Second Edition

HEMATOLOGY
Basic Principles and Practice

Second Edition

HEMATOLOGY
Basic Principles and Practice

Edited by

Ronald Hoffman, M.D.

Vice-President for Research, Systemix, Palo Alto, California;
Clinical Associate Professor, Department of Medicine,
Stanford University School of Medicine,
Stanford, California

Edward J. Benz, Jr., M.D.

Jack D. Meyers Professor and Chairman, Department of Medicine,
University of Pittsburgh School of Medicine; Attending Physician,
Department of Internal Medicine, University of Pittsburgh Medical Center,
Pittsburgh, Pennsylvania

Sanford J. Shattil, M.D.

Professor, Departments of Medicine and Pathology and Laboratory Medicine,
University of Pennsylvania School of Medicine;
Hospital of the University of Pennsylvania,
Philadelphia, Pennsylvania

Bruce Furie, M.D.

Professor, Departments of Medicine and Biochemistry,
Tufts University School of Medicine;
Chief, Hematology/Oncology Division, Department of Medicine,
New England Medical Center,
Boston, Massachusetts

Harvey J. Cohen, M.D., Ph.D.

Professor and Chairman, Department of Pediatrics,
Stanford University School of Medicine, Stanford, California;
Chief of Staff, Lucille Salter Packard Children's Hospital,
Palo Alto, California

Leslie E. Silberstein, M.D.

Professor, Departments of Medicine and Pathology and Laboratory Medicine,
University of Pennsylvania School of Medicine;
Director, Blood Bank and Transfusion Medicine Section,
Hospital of the University of Pennsylvania,
Philadelphia, Pennsylvania

Churchill Livingstone
New York, Edinburgh, London, Madrid, Melbourne, Milan, Tokyo

Library of Congress Cataloging-in-Publication Data

Hematology : basic prinicples and practice / edited by Ronald Hoffman
 . . . [et al.]. — 2nd ed.
    p. cm.
Includes bibliographical references and index.
ISBN 0–443–08914–0
1. Hematology.   I. Hoffman, Ronald, date.
[DNLM: 1. Hematologic Diseases—diagnosis. 2. Hematologic
Diseases—therapy.   WH 100 H48745 1995]
RC633.H434   1995
616.1'5—dc20
DNLM/DLC
for Library of Congress   94–27924
                                                                   CIP

Second Edition © Churchill Livingstone Inc. 1995
First Edition © Churchill Livingstone Inc. 1990

Distributed in the United Kingdom by Churchill Livingstone, Robert Stevenson House, 1–3 Baxter's Place, Leith Walk, Edinburgh EH1 3AF, and by associated companies, branches, and representatives throughout the world.

Accurate indications, adverse reactions, and dosage schedules for drugs are provided in this book, but it is possible that they may change. The reader is urged to review the package information data of the manufacturers of the medications mentioned.

The Publishers have made every effort to trace the copyright holders for borrowed material. If they have inadvertently overlooked any, they will be pleased to make the necessary arrangements at the first opportunity.

Acquisitions Editor: *Kerry Willis*
Copy Editor: *Bridgett L. Dickinson*
Production Supervisor: *Christina Hippeli*

Printed in the United States of America

First published in 1995   7 6 5 4 3 2 1

To my wife, Nan, my daughter, Judith, and my son, Michael, who have provided me with a supportive atmosphere in which to pursue this project. Their continued love has allowed me to maintain a frame of reference that has assured my happiness. To my parents, Sarah and Morris Hoffman, who made great sacrifices in order for me to pursue my education. To Esmail D. Zanjani and Ralph Zalusky, who at Mt. Sinai Hospital in New York initially kindled and promoted my interests in clinical and experimental hematology.

Ronald Hoffman, M.D.

To my wife, Peggy, for your friendship, support, and patience and for understanding why this book is important to me. To my children Tim and Jen. To my family and my mentors, whose example and caring nurtured my interest in academic hematology: Bernard G. Forget, M.D., David G. Nathan, M.D., Arthur W. Nienhuis, M.D., and Arthur B. Pardee, M.D.

Edward J. Benz, Jr., M.D.

To my wife, Gloria, my son, Jason, my parents, Arthur and Helen, my mentors, Drs. Richard A. Cooper, Neil Abramson, and James H. Jandl, and my colleagues at the University of Pennsylvania School of Medicine for their example and support.

Sanford J. Shattil, M.D.

To William J. Williams and the late Arlan J. Gottlieb for introducing me to hematology and specifically the field of blood coagulation. To Alan N. Schechter and Christian B. Anfinsen for their guidance into serious scientific research. To Robert S. Schwartz and Jane F. Desforges for their nurturance and guidance during my years at Tufts–New England Medical Center Hospital. To my family, especially, Barbara C. Furie, for their continued support.

Bruce Furie, M.D.

To my wife, Ilene, who continues to sustain me, especially during transition times; to my children, Philip and Jonathan and now Renee, who always teach me the importance and joy of being a father; and to all my family and friends who make my life so full and rewarding.

Harvey J. Cohen, M.D., Ph.D.

To my friends and family for their love and support. To Robert S. Schwartz and Eugene M. Berkman at Tufts–New England Medical Center, who continue to serve as my mentors. To Leonard Jarett for creating an environment at the University of Pennsylvania Medical Center conducive to the development of an academic transfusion medicine program and to my colleague Steven L. Spitalnik for helping me achieve that goal.

Leslie E. Silberstein, M.D.

Contributors

Camille N. Abboud, M.D.
Associate Professor of Medicine and Medical Oncology, Hematology Unit, Department of Medicine, University of Rochester School of Medicine and Dentistry, Rochester, New York

Herbert T. Abelson, M.D.
Professor and Chairman, Department of Pediatrics, University of Washington School of Medicine; Pediatrician-in-Chief, Department of Pediatrics, Children's Hospital and Medical Center, Seattle, Washington

Janis Abkowitz, M.D.
Associate Professor, Hematology Division, Department of Medicine, University of Washington School of Medicine; Director, Hematology Clinic of the University of Washington Medical Center, Seattle, Washington

Janet L. Abrahm, M.D.
Associate Professor, Hematology/Oncology Section, Department of Medicine, University of Pennsylvania School of Medicine; Acting Chief, Department of Medicine, Philadelphia Veterans Affairs Medical Center, Philadelphia, Pennsylvania

Junius G. Adams III, Ph.D.
Sickle Cell Branch, Division of Blood Diseases and Resources, National Heart, Lung, and Blood Institute, National Institutes of Health, Bethesda, Maryland

Saundra N. Aker, R.D., C.D.
Clinical Instructor, Department of Physiologic Nursing, University of Washington School of Nursing; Clinical Affiliate, Department of Nutritional Sciences, University of Washington School of Public Health; Director, Clinical Nutrition Program, Fred Hutchinson Cancer Research Center, Seattle, Washington

Jane Bradley Alavi, M.D.
Associate Professor, Department of Medicine, University of Pennsylvania School of Medicine; Attending Physician, Hematology/Oncology Division, Department of Medicine, Hospital of the University of Pennsylvania, Philadelphia, Pennsylvania

Karl E. Anderson, M.D.
Director, Human Nutrition Division, and Professor of Preventive Medicine and Community Health, Internal Medicine, and Pharmacology and Toxicology, University of Texas Medical Branch at Galveston, Galveston, Texas

Kenneth C. Anderson, M.D.
Associate Professor, Department of Medicine, Harvard Medical School; Medical Director, Blood Component Laboratory, Dana-Farber Cancer Institute, Boston, Massachusetts

Janine André-Schwartz, M.D.
Associate Professor, Department of Medicine, Tufts University School of Medicine; Hematology/Oncology Division, Department of Medicine, New England Medical Center, Boston, Massachusetts

Stylianos E. Antonarakis, M.D.
Professor, Division of Medical Genetics, Department of Medicine, University of Geneva, Geneva, Switzerland

Asok C. Antony, M.D.
Professor of Medicine, Hematology/Oncology Division, Department of Medicine, Indiana University School of Medicine, Indianapolis, Indiana

James O. Armitage, M.D.
Professor and Chairman, Department of Internal Medicine, University of Nebraska College of Medicine, Omaha, Nebraska

Robert Baehner, M.D.
Professor, Department of Pediatrics, University of Southern California School of Medicine; Staff Hematologis/Oncologist, Department of Pediatrics, University of Southern California–Los Angeles County Medical Center, Los Angeles, California

Grover C. Bagby, Jr., M.D.
Professor and Head, Hematology and Medical Oncology Division, Departments of Medicine and Medical Genetics, Oregon Health Sciences University; Director, Molecular Biology Laboratory, Department of Veterans Affairs Medical Center; Director, Oregon Cancer Center, Portland, Oregon

Dorothy Ford Bainton, M.D.
Professor, Department of Pathology, Senior Vice-Chancellor for Academic Affairs, and Attending Pathologist, Department of Pathology, University of California, San Francisco, School of Medicine, San Francisco, California

Kenneth A. Bauer, M.D.
Associate Professor, Department of Medicine, Harvard Medical School; Associate Physician, Beth Israel Hospital, Boston, Massachusetts; Chief, Hematology/Oncology Section, Brockton-West Roxbury Department of Veterans Affairs Medical Center, West Roxbury, Massachusetts

William R. Bell, M.D.
Professor of Medicine, Radiology, and Nuclear Medicine, Hematology Division, Department of Medicine, The Johns Hopkins University School of Medicine; Clinical Director, Hematology Division, and Director, Coagulation Laboratory, The Johns Hopkins Hospital, Baltimore, Maryland

Joel S. Bennett, M.D.
Professor, Department of Medicine, University of Pennsylvania School of Medicine; Member, Hematology/Oncology Division, Hospital of the University of Pennsylvania, Philadelphia, Pennsylvania

Edward J. Benz, Jr., M.D.
Jack D. Meyers Professor and Chairman, Department of Medicine, University of Pittsburgh School of Medicine; Attending Physician, Department of Internal Medicine, University of Pittsburgh Medical Center, Pittsburgh, Pennsylvania

Stacey Berg, M.D.
Pediatric Branch, National Cancer Institute, National Institutes of Health, Bethesda, Maryland

Eugene M. Berkman, M.D.
Professor, Department of Medicine, Tufts University School of Medicine; Medical Director, Hematology/Oncology Division, Department of Medicine, Transfusion Medicine Services, New England Medical Center, Boston, Massachusetts

Nancy Berliner, M.D.
Associate Professor, Hematology Section, Department of Internal Medicine and Department of Genetics, Yale University School of Medicine; Attending Physician, Departments of Internal Medicine and Hematology, Yale–New Haven Hospital, New Haven, Connecticut

Philip J. Bierman, M.D.
Associate Professor of Medicine, Oncology/Hematology Section, Department of Internal Medicine, University of Nebraska College of Medicine, Omaha, Nebraska

David H. Bing, Ph.D.
Senior Investigator and Laboratory Director, Center for Blood Research, Boston, Massachusetts

Morey A. Blinder, M.D.
Assistant Professor, Hematology and Laboratory Medicine Divisions, Departments of Medicine and Pathology, Washington University Medical School, St. Louis, Missouri

H. Scott Boswell, M.D.
Associate Professor of Medicine, Hematology/Oncology Division, Department of Medicine, Indiana University School of Medicine, Indianapolis, Indiana

Lawrence F. Brass, M.D., Ph.D.
Associate Professor, Departments of Medicine, and Pathology and Laboratory Medicine, University of Pennsylvania School of Medicine; Attending Physician, Hematology/Oncology Section, Department of Medicine, Hospital of the University of Pennsylvania, Philadelphia, Pennsylvania

Philip P. Breitfeld, M.D.
Associate Professor, Departments of Pediatrics and Biochemistry and Molecular Biology, Indiana University School of Medicine; Director, Pediatric Hematology/Oncology Division, Indiana University Medical Center, Indianapolis, Indiana

Doreen B. Brettler, M.D.
Associate Professor, Department of Medicine, University of Massachusetts Medical School; Director, New England Hemophilia Center, Medical Center of Central Massachusetts, Worcester, Massachusetts

Gary M. Brittenham, M.D.
Professor of Medicine, Hematology Division, Department of Medicine, Case Western Reserve University School of Medicine; Staff Physician, Cleveland Metropolitan General Hospital, Cleveland, Ohio

Patrick J. Buckley, M.D., Ph.D.
Professor, Department of Pathology and Laboratory Medicine, University of Wisconsin School of Medicine; Director, Hematopathology Section, and Associate Director, Laboratory Medicine Division, Department of Pathology and Laboratory Medicine, University of Wisconsin Hospital and Clinics, Madison, Wisconsin

Samuel A. Burstein, M.D.
Professor, Hematology/Oncology Section, Department of Medicine, University of Oklahoma College of Medicine, Oklahoma City, Oklahoma

James Bussel, M.D.
Associate Professor, Department of Pediatrics, Cornell University Medical College; Associate Attending, Department of Pediatrics, New York Hospital, New York, New York

Antonio C. Buzaid, M.D.
Assistant Professor, Department of Medicine, University of Texas Medical School at Houston; Internist, Department of Melanoma/Sarcoma Medical Oncology, University of Texas M.D. Anderson Cancer Center, Houston, Texas

Edwin C. Cadman, M.D.
Professor, Department of Medicine, Yale University School of Medicine; Senior Vice-President for Medical Affairs and Chief of Staff, Yale–New Haven Hospital, New Haven, Connecticut

Douglas Cines, M.D.
Associate Professor, Department of Pathology and Laboratory Medicine, University of Pennsylvania School of Medicine; Director, Hematology and Coagulation Laboratories, Hospital of the University of Pennsylvania, Philadelphia, Pennsylvania

Thomas D. Coates, M.D.
Associate Professor, Department of Pediatrics, University of Southern California School of Medicine; Head, Hematology Section, Pediatric Hematology/Oncology Division, Department of Pediatrics, Children's Hospital of Los Angeles, Los Angeles, California

Harvey J. Cohen, M.D., Ph.D.
Professor and Chairman, Department of Pediatrics, Stanford University School of Medicine, Stanford, California; Chief of Staff, Lucille Salter Packard Children's Hospital, Palo Alto, California

Désiré Collen, M.D., Ph.D.
Professor, Department of Medicine, Center for Thrombosis and Vascular Research, University of Leuven Faculty of Medicine, Leuven, Belgium

Barry S. Coller, M.D.
Murray M. Rosenberg Professor, and Chairman, Department of Medicine, Mount Sinai School of Medicine of the City University of New York, New York, New York

Steven J. Collins, M.D.
Professor, Department of Medicine, University of Washington School of Medicine; Member, Program in Molecular Medicine, Fred Hutchinson Cancer Research Center, Seattle, Washington

Isabel Cunningham, M.D.
Associate Professor, Department of Medicine, Indiana University School of Medicine, Indianapolis, Indiana

John T. Curnette, M.D., Ph.D.
Clinical Professor, Department of Pediatrics, Stanford University School of Medicine, Stanford, California; Director, Department of Immunology, Genentech, Inc., South San Francisco, California

Nicholas Dainiak, M.D.
Louis D. Lowenstein Professor of Hematology/Oncology, McGill University Faculty of Medicine; Director, Hematology/Oncology Division, Royal Victoria Hospital, Montreal, Quebec, Canada

Chi V. Dang, M.D., Ph.D.
Associate Professor, Department of Medicine, The Johns Hopkins University School of Medicine; Chief, Hematology Division, The Johns Hopkins Hospital, Baltimore, Maryland

Jane F. Desforges, M.D.
Distinguished Professor, Department of Medicine, Tufts University School of Medicine; Senior Physician, Hematology/Oncology Division, Department of Medicine, New England Medical Center, Boston, Massachusetts

Robert J. Desnick, M.D., Ph.D.
Arthur J. and Nellie Z. Cohen Professor of Pediatrics and Genetics, Chairman, Department of Human Genetics, Mount Sinai School of Medicine of the City University of New York; Attending Physician, Departments of Human Genetics and Pediatrics, The Mount Sinai Hospital, New York, New York

Kenneth Dorshkind, Ph.D.
Professor, Biomedical Sciences Division, University of California at Riverside, Riverside, California

William N. Drohan, Ph.D.
Head, Plasma Derivatives Department, Biomedical Research and Development, Jerome H. Holland Laboratory, American Red Cross, Rockville, Maryland

Thomas P. Duffy, M.D.
Professor, Hematology Section, Department of Internal Medicine, Yale University School of Medicine; Attending Physician, Yale–New Haven Hospital, New Haven, Connecticut

Walter H. Dzik, M.D.
Assistant Professor, Department of Medicine, Harvard Medical School; Director, Blood Bank and Tissue Typing Laboratory, New England Deaconess Hospital, Boston, Massachusetts

Charles S. Eby, M.D.
Assistant Professor, Departments of Pathology and Medicine, St. Louis University School of Medicine; Associate Director, Hemostasis Laboratory, St. Louis University Health Sciences Center, St. Louis, Missouri

Richard L. Edelson, M.D.
Professor and Chairman, Department of Dermatology, Yale University School of Medicine; Attending Physician, Dermatology Division, Yale–New Haven Medical Center, New Haven, Connecticut

Stephen H. Embury, M.D.
Professor, Department of Medicine, University of California, San Francisco, School of Medicine; Chief, Hematology Division of the Medical Service, San Francisco General Hospital; Director of Adult Patient Services, Northern California Comprehensive Sickle Cell Center, San Francisco, California

Pablo Engel, M.D., Ph.D.
Assistant Research Professor, Department of Immunology, Duke University School of Medicine, Durham, North Carolina

Charles T. Esmon, Ph.D.
Investigator, Research Laboratories, Howard Hughes Medical Institute; Professor, Department of Pathology, Associate Professor, Department of Biochemistry and Molecular Biology, University of Oklahoma College of Medicine; Member and Head, Cardiovascular Biology Research Program, Oklahoma Medical Research Foundation, Oklahoma City, Oklahoma

Elihu H. Estey, M.D.
Professor, Department of Medicine, University of Texas Medical School at Houston; Internist, Department of Medicine, University of Texas M.D. Anderson Cancer Center, Houston, Texas

Douglas V. Faller, M.D., Ph.D.
Professor, Departments of Medicine, Biochemistry, Pediatrics, Microbiology, and Pathology and Laboratory Medicine, Boston University School of Medicine; Director of Cancer Research Center, Boston University Medical Center Hospital, Boston City Hospital, Boston Veterans Affairs Hospital, Boston, Massachusetts

Robert J. Fallon, M.D., Ph.D.
Associate Professor, Department of Pediatrics, St. Louis University School of Medicine; Director, Pediatric Hematology/Oncology Division, Cardinal Glennon Children's Hospital, St. Louis, Missouri

Donald I. Feinstein, M.D.
Professor, Department of Medicine, University of Southern California School of Medicine; Chief of Medicine, University of Southern California/Norris Comprehensive Cancer Center and University of Southern California University Hospital; Attending Physician, Los Angeles County and University of Southern California Medical Center, Los Angeles, California

Bernard G. Forget, M.D.
Professor of Internal Medicine and Genetics, Department of Internal Medicine, Chief of Hematology Section, Yale University School of Medicine; Attending Physician, Department of Internal Medicine, Yale–New Haven Hospital, New Haven, Connecticut

Charles W. Francis, M.D.
Associate Professor, Hematology Unit, Department of Medicine, University of Rochester School of Medicine and Dentistry; Attending Physician, Department of Medicine, Strong Memorial Hospital, Rochester, New York

Glauco Frizzera, M.D.
Professor, Department of Pathology, New York University School of Medicine; Director of Hematopathology, New York University Medical Center, New York, New York

Barbara C. Furie, Ph.D.
Professor, Departments of Medicine and Biochemistry, Tufts University School of Medicine; Hematology/Oncology Division, Department of Medicine, New England Medical Center, Boston, Massachusetts

Bruce Furie, M.D.
Professor, Departments of Medicine and Biochemistry, Tufts University School of Medicine; Chief, Hematology/Oncology Division, Department of Medicine, New England Medical Center, Boston, Massachusetts

James N. George, M.D.
Professor, Hematology/Oncology Section, Department of Medicine, University of Oklahoma College of Medicine; Chief, Hematology/Oncology Section, Department of Medicine, Oklahoma Medical Center, Oklahoma City, Oklahoma

Morie A. Gertz, M.D.
Associate Professor, Department of Medicine, Mayo Medical School; Consultant, Hematology Division, Department of Internal Medicine, Mayo Clinic and Mayo Foundation, Rochester, Minnesota

Joan Cox Gill, M.D.
Associate Professor, Department of Pediatrics, Medical College of Wisconsin; Investigator, Blood Research Institute, Blood Center of Southeastern Wisconsin; Medical Director, Great Lakes Hemophilia Foundation, Milwaukee, Wisconsin

David Ginsburg, M.D.
Professor, Departments of Internal Medicine and Human Genetics, University of Michigan Medical School; Investigator, Research Laboratories, Howard Hughes Medical Institute, Ann Arbor, Michigan

Mark H. Ginsberg, M.D.
Member, Department of Vascular Biology, The Scripps Research Institute; Adjunct Professor, University of California, San Diego, School of Medicine, La Jolla, California

Bertil E. Glader, M.D., Ph.D.
Professor, Department of Pediatrics, Stanford University School of Medicine, Stanford, California; Director, Hematology/Oncology Program, Lucille Salter Packard Children's Hospital at Stanford, Stanford, California

John H. Glick, M.D.
Professor of Medicine, and Madlyn and Leonard Abramson Professor of Clinical Oncology, Hematology/Oncology Division, Department of Medicine, University of Pennsylvania School of Medicine; Director, Cancer Center, University of Pennsylvania Cancer Center, Philadelphia, Pennsylvania

John M. Goldman, D.M., F.R.C.P., F.R.C.Path
Professor of Leukaemia Biology, LRF Centre for Adult Leukaemia, Royal Postgraduate Medical School; Honorary Consultant Physician, Department of Haematology, Hammersmith Hospital, London, England

Lawrence T. Goodnough, M.D.
Associate Professor, Departments of Medicine and Pathology, Washington University School of Medicine; Director of Clinical Transfusion Services, Laboratory Medicine Division, Barnes Hospital, St. Louis, Missouri

Michael S. Gordon, M.D.
Assistant Professor of Medicine, Hematology/Oncology Division, Department of Medicine, Indiana University School of Medicine; Director, Clinical Hematology and Cytokine Program, Indiana University Medical Center, Indianapolis, Indiana

Edward C. Gordon-Smith, M.D.
University Professor of Haematology, Haematology Division, Department of Cellular and Molecular Sciences, St. George's Hospital Medical School; Consultant Physician and Haematologist, Division of Haematology, St. George's Hospital, London, England

Gregory A. Grabowski, M.D.
Professor, Departments of Pediatrics, and Molecular Genetics and Biochemistry, University of Cincinnati College of Medicine; Director, Human Genetics Division, Cincinnati Children's Hospital Research Foundation, Cincinnati, Ohio

T. Flint Gray III, M.D.
Instructor, Department of Medicine, University of North Carolina School of Medicine; Attending Physician, Department of Medicine, University of North Carolina Hospitals, Chapel Hill, North Carolina

Peter L. Greenberg, M.D.
Professor of Medicine, Hematology Division, Department of Medicine, Stanford University School of Medicine, Stanford, California

Jerome E. Groopman, M.D.
Professor of Medicine, Dina and Raphael Recanati Chair in Immunology, Department of Medicine, Harvard Medical School; Chief, Hematology/Oncology, Department of Medicine, New England Deaconess Hospital, Boston, Massachusetts

Douglas S. Harrington, M.D.
Vice-President and Medical Director, Nichols Institute, San Juan Capistrano, California

Peter W. Heald, M.D.
Associate Professor, Department of Dermatology, Yale University School of Medicine; Attending Physician, Dermatology Division, Yale–New Haven Medical Center, New Haven, Connecticut

Christopher D. Hillyer, M.D.
Assistant Professor, Department of Pathology and Laboratory Medicine, Emory University School of Medicine; Assistant Medical Director, Transfusion Medicine Services, Emory University Hospital, Atlanta, Georgia

Jack Hirsh, M.D.
Professor, Department of Medicine, McMaster University School of Medicine; Director, Hamilton Civic Hospitals Research Centre, Hamilton, Ontario, Canada

Dieter Hoelzer, M.D.
Professor of Internal Medicine, and Chief, Department of Hematology, Johann Wolfgang Goethe University, Frankfurt, Germany

Ronald Hoffman, M.D.
Vice-President for Research, Systemix, Palo Alto, California; Clinical Associate Professor, Department of Medicine, Stanford University School of Medicine, Stanford, California

James A. Hoxie, M.D.
Associate Professor of Medicine, Hematology/Oncology Division, Department of Medicine, University of Pennsylvania School of Medicine; Hematology/Oncology Division, Hospital of the University of Pennsylvania, Philadelphia, Pennsylvania

Robert Hromas, M.D.
Assistant Professor, Hematology/Oncology Division, Department of Medicine, Indiana University School of Medicine, Indianapolis, Indiana

Timothy P. Hughes, M.D., F.R.A.C.P., F.R.C.P.A.
Senior Hematologist, Hematology Department, Institute of Medical and Veterinary Science, Adelaide, South Australia, Australia

Richard A. Insel, M.D.
Professor, Departments of Pediatrics, and Microbiology and Immunology, and Chief, Pediatric Immunology, Allergy, and Rheumatology Division, University of Rochester School of Medicine and Dentistry; Director, Strong Children's Research Center, Rochester, New York

William M. Isenberg, M.D., Ph.D.
Research Pathologist, Department of Pathology, University of California, San Francisco, School of Medicine; Staff Obstetrician/Gynecologist, Department of Obstetrics, Gynecology, and Reproductive Services, University of California, San Francisco Medical Center, San Francisco, California

Petr Jarolim, M.D., Ph.D.
Assistant Professor, Department of Medicine, Tufts University School of Medicine, Boston, Massachusetts

Marshall E. Kadin, M.D.
Associate Professor, Department of Pathology, Harvard Medical School; Senior Pathologist and Director of Hematopathology, Department of Pathology, Beth Israel Hospital, Boston, Massachusetts

Hagop Kantarjian, M.D.
Professor, Department of Medicine, University of Texas Medical School at Houston; Internist, Leukemia Section, Department of Hematology, University of Texas M.D. Anderson Cancer Center, Houston, Texas

Randall J. Kaufman, Ph.D.
Professor, Department of Biological Chemistry, University of Michigan Medical School, Ann Arbor, Michigan

Michael J. Keating, M.D.
Professor of Medicine, Department of Hematology, University of Texas Medical School at Houston; Associate Vice-President for Clinical Investigations, Department of Hematology, University of Texas M.D. Anderson Cancer Center, Houston, Texas

John G. Kelton, M.D.
Professor, Departments of Medicine and Pathology, McMaster University School of Medicine; Chief, Department of Medicine, Chedoke-McMaster Hospitals, Hamilton, Ontario, Canada

Anne Kessinger, M.D.
Professor of Medicine and Chief, Oncology/Hematology Section, Department of Internal Medicine, University of Nebraska College of Medicine, Omaha, Nebraska

Harvey G. Klein, M.D.
Chief, Department of Transfusion Medicine, Warren G. Magnuson Clinical Center, National Institutes of Health, Bethesda, Maryland

Kim Kramer, M.D.
Fellow, Pediatric Hematology/Oncology Division, Memorial Sloan-Kettering Hospital, New York, New York

Sanford B. Krantz, M.D.
Professor and Director of Hematology, Department of Medicine, Vanderbilt University School of Medicine; Chief, Department of Hematology, Department of Veterans Affairs Medical Center, Nashville, Tennessee

Elissa M. Kraus, M.S.
Genetic Counselor, New England Hemophilia Center, Medical Center of Central Massachusetts, Worcester, Massachusetts

Theodore G. Krontiris, M.D., Ph.D.
Associate Professor, Department of Medicine and Program in Genetics, Tufts University School of Medicine; Physician, Hematology/Oncology Division, Department of Medicine, New England Medical Center, Boston, Massachusetts

Margot S. Kruskall, M.D.
Associate Professor, Departments of Pathology and Medicine, Harvard Medical School; Director, Laboratory Medicine Division, Beth Israel Hospital, Boston, Massachusetts

Thomas J. Kunicki, Ph.D.
Associate Member, Department of Molecular and Experimental Medicine, The Scripps Research Institute, La Jolla, California

Robert A. Kyle, M.D.
Professor, Departments of Medicine and Laboratory Medicine, Mayo Medical School; Consultant, Hematology Division, Department of Internal Medicine, Mayo Clinic and Mayo Foundation, Rochester, Minnesota

Parviz Lalezari, M.D.
Professor of Medicine and Pathology, Department of Medicine, Albert Einstein College of Medicine of Yeshiva University; Director, Immunohematology Division, Montefiore Medical Center, Bronx, New York

Stephen A. Landaw, M.D., Ph.D.
Professor, Department of Medicine, State University of New York Health Science Center at Syracuse; Associate Chief of Staff, Research and Development, Veterans Affairs Medical Center, Syracuse, New York

Richard A. Larson, M.D.
Associate Professor, Hematology/Oncology Section, Department of Medicine, University of Chicago Division of the Biological Sciences Pritzker School of Medicine; Director, Acute Leukemia Program, Hematology/Oncology Section, Department of Medicine, University of Chicago Medical Center, Chicago, Illinois

Michelle M. Le Beau, Ph.D.
Assistant Professor, Hematology/Oncology Section, Department of Medicine, University of Chicago Division of the Biological Sciences Pritzker School of Medicine, Chicago, Illinois

John P. Leddy, M.D.
Professor of Medicine and Microbiology, Department of Medicine, University of Rochester School of Medicine and Dentistry, Rochester, New York

William M. F. Lee, M.D., Ph.D.
Associate Professor, Hematology/Oncology Division, Department of Medicine, University of Pennsylvania School of Medicine, Philadelphia, Pennsylvania

Polly Lenssen, R.D., M.S., C.D.
Assistant Director, Clinical Nutrition Program, Fred Hutchinson Cancer Research Center, Seattle, Washington

Nancy Leslie, M.D.
Assistant Professor, Department of Pediatrics, University of Cincinnati College of Medicine; Head, Metabolic Disease Section, Human Genetics Division, Cincinnati Children's Hospital Research Foundation, Cincinnati, Ohio

Peter H. Levine, M.D.
Professor, Department of Medicine, University of Massachusetts Medical School; President and Chief Executive Officer, Medical Center of Central Massachusetts, Worcester, Massachusetts

Howard A. Liebman, M.D.
Associate Professor, Departments of Medicine and Pathology, University of Southern California School of Medicine, Los Angeles, California

Jane L. Liesveld, M.D.
Assistant Professor of Medicine, Hematology Unit, Department of Medicine, University of Rochester School of Medicine and Dentistry, Rochester, New York

H. Roger Lijnen, Ph.D.
Associate Professor, Department of Medicine, Center for Molecular and Vascular Biology, University of Leuven Faculty of Medicine, Leuven, Belgium

Steven A. Limentani, M.D.
Assistant Professor, Department of Medicine, Tufts University School of Medicine; Assistant Physician, Hematology/Oncology Division, Department of Medicine, Chief, Special Coagulation Laboratory, New England Medical Center, Boston, Massachusetts

Jeffrey M. Lipton, M.D.
Associate Professor, Jack and Lucy Clark Department of Pediatrics, Mount Sinai School of Medicine of the City University of New York; Chief, Pediatric Hematology/Oncology Division, Mount Sinai Medical Center, New York, New York

Johnson M. Liu, M.D.
Senior Research Investigator, Hematology Branch, National Heart, Lung, and Blood Institute, National Institutes of Health, Bethesda, Maryland

Michael W. Long, Ph.D.
Associate Professor, Department of Pediatrics, University of Michigan School of Medicine; Member, University of Michigan Comprehensive Cancer Center, University of Michigan Medical Center, Ann Arbor, Michigan

A. Thomas Look, M.D.
Professor, Department of Pediatrics, University of Tennessee, Memphis, College of Medicine; Chairman, Department of Experimental Oncology, St. Jude Children's Research Hospital, Memphis, Tennessee

Marilyn Manco-Johnson, M.D.
Associate Professor, Department of Pediatrics, University of Colorado School of Medicine, Denver, Colorado

Robert Mandle, Ph.D.
Investigator, Center for Blood Research, Boston, Massachusetts

Sridhar Mani, M.D.
Postdoctoral Fellow, Hematology/Oncology Division, Department of Internal Medicine, Yale University School of Medicine, New Haven, Connecticut

José Martinez, M.D.
Professor, and Senior Member and Associate Director for Research Education, Cardeza Foundation for Hematologic Research, Department of Medicine, Jefferson Medical College of Thomas Jefferson University, Philadelphia, Pennsylvania

Aneal S. Masih, M.D.
Professor, Department of Pathology and Laboratory Medicine, University of Florida College of Medicine, Gainesville, Florida

Ruth McCorkle, Ph.D., F.A.A.N.
American Cancer Society Professor, Adult Health and Illness Division, University of Pennsylvania School of Nursing; Associate Director, Cancer Control, University of Pennsylvania Cancer Center, Philadelphia, Pennsylvania

Rodger P. McEver, M.D.
Professor of Medicine and Biochemistry, Department of Medicine–W.K. Warren Research Institute, University of Oklahoma College of Medicine; Member, Cardiovascular Biology Program, Oklahoma Medical Research Foundation, Oklahoma City, Oklahoma

Philip B. McGlave, M.D.
Professor, Department of Medicine, University of Minnesota Medical School—Minneapolis; Director, Adult Bone Marrow Transplantation Program, University of Minnesota Hospital and Clinic of the University of Minnesota Health Sciences Center, Minneapolis, Minnesota

Jay E. Menitove, M.D.
Professor, Department of Internal Medicine, University of Cincinnati College of Medicine; Deputy Director, Medical Services, Hoxworth Blood Center, University of Cincinnati Medical Center, Cincinnati, Ohio

Steven J. Mentzer, M.D.
Assistant Professor, Department of Surgery, Harvard Medical School; Brigham and Women's Hospital, Dana-Farber Cancer Institute, Boston, Massachusetts

Dean D. Metcalfe, M.D.
Head, Allergic Diseases Section, Laboratory of Clinical Investigation, National Institute of Allergy and Infectious Diseases, National Institutes of Health, Bethesda, Maryland

Kenneth B. Miller, M.D.
Associate Professor of Medicine, Hematology/Oncology Division, Department of Medicine, Tufts University School of Medicine; Director, Leukemia Service, and Bone Marrow Transplant, New England Medical Center, Boston, Massachusetts

Wesley J. Miller, M.D.
Associate Professor, Department of Medicine, University of Minnesota Medical School; Associate Director, Adult Bone Marrow Transplantation Program, University of Minnesota Hospital and Clinic of the University of Minnesota Health Sciences Center, Minneapolis, Minnesota

Joel L. Moake, M.D.
Professor, Hematology Section, Department of Medicine, Baylor College of Medicine; Medical Hematology Section, The Methodist Hospital; Associate Director, Biomedical Engineering Laboratory, Rice University, Houston, Texas

Narla Mohandas, D.Sc.
Professor, Department of Laboratory Medicine, University of California, San Francisco, School of Medicine, San Francisco, California; Senior Staff Scientist, Lawrence Berkeley Laboratories, University of California, Berkeley, California

Robert R. Montgomery, M.D.
Clinical Professor, Departments of Pediatrics and Pathology, Medical College of Wisconsin; Vice-President and Director of Research, Blood Center of Southeastern Wisconsin, Milwaukee, Wisconsin

Jon S. Morrow, M.D., Ph.D.
Professor and Chairman, Department of Pathology, Yale University School of Medicine; Chief, Department of Pathology, Yale–New Haven Hospital, New Haven, Connecticut

Deane F. Mosher, M.D.
Professor, Department of Medicine, University of Wisconsin Medical School; Head, Hematology Section, Department of Medicine, University of Wisconsin Hospital and Clinics, Madison, Wisconsin

Sharon B. Murphy, M.D.
Professor, Department of Pediatrics, and Chair, Pediatric Oncology Group, Southwestern University School of Medicine; Chief, Hematology/Oncology Division, Children's Memorial Hospital, Chicago, Illinois

Paul M. Ness, M.D.
Associate Professor, Departments of Pathology and Medicine, The Johns Hopkins University School of Medicine; Principal Officer, The Greater Chesapeake and Potomac Blood Services, American Red Cross, Baltimore, Maryland

Peter E. Newburger, M.D.
Professor, Departments of Pediatrics and Molecular Genetics/Microbiology, University of Massachusetts Medical School; Associate Director, Cancer Center, Worcester, Massachusetts

Arthur W. Nienhuis, M.D.
Director of Hospital, and Member, Department of Hematology/Oncology, St. Jude Children's Research Hospital, Memphis, Tennessee

Rachelle Nuss, M.D.
Assistant Professor, Department of Pediatrics, University of Colorado School of Medicine; Associate Director, Mountain States Regional Hemophilia Center–Denver, Denver, Colorado

Lorrie F. Odom, M.D.
Professor, Department of Pediatrics, University of Colorado School of Medicine; Director, Clinical Oncology, Oncology/Hematology Division, Denver Children's Hospital, Denver, Colorado

Donald E. Paglia, M.D.
Professor, Department of Pathology and Laboratory Medicine, University of California, Los Angeles, UCLA School of Medicine, Los Angeles, California

Jiri Palek, M.D.
Professor, Department of Medicine, Tufts University School of Medicine; Chairman, Department of Biomedical Research, Chief, Hematology/Oncology Division, St. Elizabeth Medical Center, Boston, Massachusetts

Thalia Papayannopoulou, M.D.
Professor, Hematology Division, Department of Medicine, University of Washington School of Medicine, Seattle, Washington

Robert I. Parker, M.D.
Associate Professor, Department of Pediatrics, Vice-Chairman for Pediatric Academic Affairs, State University of New York at Stony Brook Health Sciences Center School of Medicine; Director, Department of Pediatric Hematology/Oncology, Children's Medical Center at Stony Brook, Stony Brook, New York

Robertson Parkman, M.D.
Professor, Departments of Pediatrics and Microbiology, University of Southern California School of Medicine; Head, Division of Research Immunology/Bone Marrow Transplantation, Children's Hospital of Los Angeles, Los Angeles, California

Richard T. Parmley, M.D.
Professor, Department of Pediatrics, University of Texas Medical School at San Antonio, San Antonio, Texas

Jeannie V. Pasacreta, Ph.D., R.N., C.S.
Project Director, Serious Illness Center, University of Pennsylvania School of Nursing; Psychiatric Consultation-Liason Nurse, Inpatient Oncology, Hospital of the University of Pennsylvania, Philadelphia, Pennsylvania

Dilip V. Patel, M.D.
Assistant Professor, Department of Medicine, Albert Einstein College of Medicine of Yeshiva University, Bronx, New York; Program Director, Hematology/Oncology Division, Department of Medicine, Long Island Jewish Medical Center, New Hyde Park, New York

Richard P. Phipps, Ph.D.
Associate Professor, Departments of Cancer Center, Microbiology and Immunology, and Pediatrics, University of Rochester School of Medicine and Dentistry, Rochester, New York

Lawrence D. Piro, M.D.
Director, Ida M. and Cecil H. Green Cancer Center, and Head, Hematology/Oncology Division, Scripps Clinic and Research Foundation, La Jolla, California

Philip A. Pizzo, M.D.
Professor, Department of Pediatrics, Uniformed Services University of the Health Sciences, F. Edward Hebért School of Medicine; Chief and Head, Pediatrics and Infectious Diseases Section, National Cancer Institute, National Institutes of Health, Bethesda, Maryland

Edward F. Plow, Ph.D.
Chairman, Department of Molecular Cardiology, Head of Research, Center for Thrombosis and Vascular Biology, The Cleveland Clinic Foundation, Cleveland, Ohio

David G. Poplack, M.D.
Elise C. Young Professor of Pediatric Oncology, Department of Pediatrics, Baylor College of Medicine; Head, Hematology/Oncology Section, Department of Pediatrics, Texas Children's Hospital, Houston, Texas

Carol S. Portlock, M.D.
Associate Professor of Clinical Medicine, Department of Medicine, Cornell University Medical College; Associate Attending Physician, Lymphoma Service, Memorial Sloan-Kettering Cancer Center, New York, New York

David A. Potter, M.D., Ph.D.
Assistant Professor, Department of Medicine, Tufts University School of Medicine; Assistant Physician, Hematology/Oncology Division, Department of Medicine, New England Medical Center, Boston, Massachusetts

David T. Purtilo, M.D. *
Chairman and Professor, Department of Pathology and Microbiology, University of Nebraska College of Medicine, Omaha, Nebraska

Kanti R. Rai, M.D.
Professor, Department of Medicine, Albert Einstein College of Medicine of Yeshiva University, Bronx, New York; Chief, Hematology/Oncology Division, Department of Medicine, Long Island Jewish Medical Center, New Hyde Park, New York

Elizabeth C. Reed, M.D.
Associate Professor, Oncology/Hematology Section, Department of Internal Medicine, University of Nebraska College of Medicine; Medical Director, Oncology/Hematology Special Care Units, University of Nebraska Medical Center, Omaha, Nebraska

A. Kim Ritchey, M.D.
Professor and Vice-Chairman, Department of Pediatrics, West Virginia University School of Medicine; Chief, Pediatric Hematology/Oncology Division, Department of Pediatrics, Robert C. Byrd Health Sciences Center of West Virginia University, Morgantown, West Virginia

Harold R. Roberts, M.D.
Sarah Graham Kenan Professor of Medicine, Department of Medicine, University of North Carolina at Chapel Hill School of Medicine; Attending Physician, Department of Medicine, University of North Carolina Hospitals, Chapel Hill, North Carolina

Glenn E. Rodey, M.D.
Professor, Department of Pathology and Laboratory Medicine, Emory University School of Medicine; Director, Transplantation and Immunogenetics Laboratories, Emory University Hospital, Atlanta, Georgia

Naomi Rosenberg, Ph.D.
Professor, Departments of Pathology, and Molecular Biology and Microbiology, Tufts University School of Medicine, Boston, Massachusetts

Barry E. Rosenbloom, M.D.
Clinical Professor, Department of Medicine, University of California, Los Angeles, UCLA School of Medicine; Attending Physician, Department of Medicine, Cedars–Sinai Medical Center, Los Angeles, California

David S. Rosenthal, M.D.
Associate Professor, Department of Medicine, Harvard Medical School, Boston, Massachusetts; Henry K. Oliver Professor of Hygiene, and Director, Harvard University Health Services, Cambridge, Massachusetts

Philip M. Rosoff, M.D.
Associate Professor, Departments of Medicine, Pediatrics, and Physiology, Tufts University School of Medicine; Hematology/Oncology Division, Department of Medicine, New England Medical Center, Boston, Massachusetts

Wendell F. Rosse, M.D.
Florence McAllister Professor of Medicine, Department of Medicine, Duke University School of Medicine; Hematology/Oncology Division, Department of Medicine, Duke University Medical Center, Durham, North Carolina

Kate Rothko, M.D.
Assistant Professor, Department of Pathology, The Johns Hopkins University School of Medicine, Baltimore, Maryland; Medical Director, Pathology of Laboratory Medicine Services, Veterans Affairs Medical Center, Washington, D.C.

Marc Rubin, M.D.
Director, Infectious Diseases Clinical Research Group, Glaxo Research Institute, Research Triangle Park, North Carolina

Daniel H. Ryan, M.D.
Associate Professor, Department of Pathology and Laboratory Medicine, University of Rochester School of Medicine and Dentistry; Director, Hematology Laboratory Unit, Strong Memorial Hospital, Rochester, New York

Stephen E. Sallan, M.D.
Professor, Department of Pediatrics, Harvard Medical School; Clinical Director, Department of Pediatric Oncology, Dana-Farber Cancer Institute, Boston, Massachusetts

Samuel A. Santoro, M.D., Ph.D.
Professor of Pathology and Medicine, Laboratory Medicine Division, Departments of Pathology and Medicine, Washington University School of Medicine; Director, Clinical Hematology/Hemostasis Laboratory, Barnes Hospital, St. Louis, Missouri

Alan Saven, M.D.
Associate Director for Clinical Research, Hematology/Oncology Division, Ida M. and Cecil H. Green Cancer Center, Scripps Clinic and Research Foundation, La Jolla, California

David T. Scadden, M.D.
Assistant Professor, Department of Medicine, Harvard Medical School; Director, AIDS Hematology/Oncology Research Unit, New England Deaconess Hospital, Boston, Massachusetts

David P. Schenkein, M.D.
Assistant Professor of Medicine, Hematology/Oncology Division, Department of Medicine, Tufts University School of Medicine; Director, Lymphoma Service, Hematology/Oncology Division, Department of Medicine, New England Medical Center, Boston, Massachusetts

Paul I. Schneiderman, M.D.
Associate Clinical Professor, Department of Dermatology, Columbia University College of Physicians and Surgeons, New York, New York

Stanley Schrier, M.D.
Professor of Medicine, Hematology Section, Stanford University School of Medicine, Stanford, California

Lynn M. Schuchter, M.D.
Assistant Professor of Medicine, Hematology/Oncology Division, Department of Medicine, University of Pennsylvania School of Medicine; Hematology/Oncology Division, Department of Medicine, Hospital of the University of Pennsylvania, Philadelphia, Pennsylvania

*Deceased.

Cindy L. Schwartz, M.D.
Associate Professor of Oncology and Pediatrics, Pediatric Oncology Division, Department of Pediatrics, The Johns Hopkins University School of Medicine; Associate Director for Clinical Programs, Pediatric Oncology Division, Departments of Oncology and Pediatrics, The Johns Hopkins Oncology Center, Baltimore, Maryland

Elias Schwartz, M.D.
Professor and Chair, Department of Pediatrics, University of Pennsylvania School of Medicine; Physician-in-Chief, Werner and Gertrude Henle Professor of Pediatrics, The Children's Hospital of Philadelphia, Philadelphia, Pennsylvania

Robert S. Schwartz, M.D.
Professor, Department of Medicine, Tufts University School of Medicine; Senior Physician, Hematology/Oncology Division, Department of Medicine, New England Medical Center, Boston, Massachusetts

David W. Scott, Ph.D.
Head, Department of Immunology, Jerome H. Holland Laboratory, American Red Cross, Rockville, Maryland

Gerald M. Segal, M.D.
Associate Professor, Hematology and Medical Oncology Division, Department of Medicine, Oregon Health Sciences University School of Medicine; Director, Hematopoiesis Laboratory, Oregon Health Sciences University, Portland, Oregon

Jean A. Shafer, M.A., M.T.(A.S.C.P.)
Assistant Professor, Departments of Medicine and Pathology, University of Rochester School of Medicine and Dentistry, Rochester, New York

Sanford J. Shattil, M.D.
Professor, Departments of Medicine and Pathology and Laboratory Medicine, University of Pennsylvania School of Medicine; Hospital of the University of Pennsylvania, Philadelphia, Pennsylvania

Marc A. Shuman, M.D.
Professor of Medicine, Hematology Division, Department of Medicine, Cancer Research Institute, University of California, San Francisco, School of Medicine; Chief, Hematology Division, Department of Medicine, Moffitt/Long Hospitals, University of California, San Francisco, Medical Center, San Francisco, California

Susan B. Shurin, M.D.
Professor, Department of Pediatrics, Case Western Reserve University School of Medicine; Chief, Pediatric Hematology/Oncology Division, Rainbow Babies Hospital, Cleveland, Ohio

Leslie E. Silberstein, M.D.
Professor, Departments of Medicine and Pathology and Laboratory Medicine, University of Pennsylvania School of Medicine; Director, Blood Bank and Transfusion Medicine Section, Hospital of the University of Pennsylvania, Philadelphia, Pennsylvania

Murray N. Silverstein, M.D.
Professor of Medicine, Departments of Hematology and Internal Medicine, Mayo Medical School; Consultant in Hematology, Department of Hematology, Mayo Clinic and Mayo Foundation, Rochester, Minnesota

Peter J. Sims, M.D., Ph.D.
Adjunct Professor, Department of Pharmacology, Clinical Professor, Department of Pathology, Medical College of Wisconsin; Associate Director, Blood Research Institute, The Blood Center of Southeastern Wisconsin, Milwaukee, Wisconsin

Jan J. Sixma, M.D.
Professor, Department of Hematology, University Hospital of Utrecht, The Netherlands

Sherrill J. Slichter, M.D.
Professor, Hematology Division, Department of Medicine, University of Washington School of Medicine; Director, Research and Education Division, Puget Sound Blood Center, Seattle, Washington

Melisse Sloas, M.D.
Assistant Professor, Department of Pediatrics, Uniformed Services University of the Health Sciences, F. Edward Hebért School of Medicine; Senior Clinical Investigator, Pediatric Branch, National Cancer Institute, National Institutes of Health, Bethesda, Maryland

Brian R. Smith, M.D.
Associate Professor, Departments of Laboratory Medicine, Internal Medicine, and Pediatrics, Yale University School of Medicine; Director of Research, Yale Bone Marrow Transplant Unit, Yale–New Haven Hospital, New Haven, Connecticut

Edward L. Snyder, M.D., F.A.C.P.
Professor, Department of Laboratory Medicine, Yale University School of Medicine; Director, Transfusion Service, Yale–New Haven Hospital, New Haven, Connecticut

Steven L. Spitalnik, M.D.
Associate Professor, Department of Pathology and Laboratory Medicine, University of Pennsylvania School of Medicine; Co-Director, Laboratory Medicine Division, Hospital of the University of Pennsylvania, Philadelphia, Pennsylvania

Jerry L. Spivak, M.D.
Professor of Medicine and Oncology, Hematology Division, Department of Medicine, The Johns Hopkins University School of Medicine, Baltimore, Maryland

Martin H. Steinberg, M.D.
Professor, Department of Medicine, University of Mississippi School of Medicine; Associate Chief of Staff of Research, Department of Research, Veterans Affairs Medical Center, Jackson, Mississippi

Ronald G. Strauss, M.D.
Professor, Departments of Pathology and Pediatrics, University of Iowa College of Medicine; Medical Director, DeGowin Blood Center, University of Iowa Hospitals and Clinics, Iowa City, Iowa

John L. Sullivan, M.D.
Professor, Department of Pediatrics, University of Massachusetts Medical School, Worcester, Massachusetts

Thomas F. Tedder, Ph.D.
Professor, Department of Immunology, Duke University School of Medicine, Durham, North Carolina

Marilyn J. Telen, M.D.
Associate Professor of Medicine, Hematology/Oncology Division, Department of Medicine, Duke University School of Medicine; Associate Medical Director, Transfusion Service, Duke University Medical Center, Durham, North Carolina

Douglas M. Tollefsen, M.D., Ph.D.
Professor, Hematology Division, Department of Medicine, Washington University School of Medicine, St. Louis, Missouri

Malcolm S. Trimble, M.D.
Fellow, Department of Pathology, McMaster University School of Medicine, West Hamilton, Ontario, Canada

Julie M. Vose, M.D.
Associate Professor of Medicine, Oncology/Hematology Section, Department of Internal Medicine, University of Nebraska College of Medicine, Omaha, Nebraska

Denisa D. Wagner, Ph.D.
Senior Investigator, The Center for Blood Research, Harvard Medical School, Boston, Massachusetts

Christopher E. Walsh, M.D., Ph.D.
Senior Investigator, Clinical Pathology, Hematology Service, Clinical Center, National Institutes of Health, Bethesda, Maryland

Thomas J. Walsh, M.D.
Senior Investigator, Infectious Disease Section, Pediatric Branch, National Cancer Institute, National Institutes of Health, Bethesda, Maryland

Theodore E. Warkentin, M.D., F.R.C.P.(C.), F.A.C.P.
Assistant Professor, Departments of Pathology and Medicine, McMaster University School of Medicine; Head, Transfusion Medicine and Hemostasis, Department of Laboratory Medicine, Hamilton Civic Hospitals (General Division); Research Scholar of the Heart and Stroke Foundation of Canada, Hamilton, Ontario, Canada

Irwin M. Weinstein, M.D.
Clinical Professor, Department of Medicine, University of California, Los Angeles, UCLA School of Medicine; Attending Physician, Department of Medicine, Cedars–Sinai Medical Center, Los Angeles, California

Daniel J. Weisdorf, M.D.
Professor, Department of Medicine, University of Minnesota Medical School; Associate Director, Adult Bone Marrow Transplantation Program, University of Minnesota Hospital and Clinic of the University of Minnesota Health Sciences Center, Minneapolis, Minnesota

Leon P. Weiss, M.D., Ph.D.
Professor of Cell Biology, and Chairman, Department of Animal Biology, University of Pennsylvania School of Veterinary Medicine; Professor, Hematology Division, Department of Medicine, University of Pennsylvania School of Medicine, Philadelphia, Pennsylvania

Jeffrey I. Weitz, M.D.
Professor, Department of Medicine, McMaster University School of Medicine; Director, Experimental Thrombosis and Atherosclerosis Programme, Hamilton Civic Hospitals Research Centre, Hamilton, Ontario, Canada

Gilbert C. White II, M.D.
Professor, Departments of Medicine and Pharmacology, University of North Carolina at Chapel Hill School of Medicine; Attending Physician, Department of Medicine, North Carolina Memorial Hospital, Chapel Hill, North Carolina

Therese Wiedmer, M.D.
Investigator, Blood Research Institute, The Blood Center of Southeastern Wisconsin, Milwaukee, Wisconsin

James S. Wiley, M.D.
Professorial Associate, Department of Medicine, University of Melbourne; Director, Department of Hematology, Austin Hospital, Heidelberg, Victoria, Australia

Craigenne A. Williams, B.A., R.A.C.
Research Associate, Plasma Derivatives Department, Biomedical Research and Development, Jerome H. Holland Laboratory, American Red Cross, Rockville, Maryland

David A. Williams, M.D.
Associate Professor, Departments of Pediatrics, and Medical and Molecular Genetics, Indiana University School of Medicine; Kipp Investigator of Pediatrics, Herman B. Wells Center for Pediatrics Research; Associate Investigator, Howard Hughes Medical Institute; Pediatric Hematology/Oncology Division, James Whitcomb Riley Hospital for Children, Indianapolis, Indiana

Eliot C. Williams, M.D., Ph.D.
Associate Professor, Departments of Medicine and Laboratory Medicine and Pathology, University of Wisconsin Medical School, Madison, Wisconsin

Robert M. Winslow, M.D.
Blood Component Laboratory, Dana-Farber Cancer Institute, Boston, Massachusetts

Bruce A. Woda, M.D.
Professor, Anatomic Pathologic Division, Department of Pathology, University of Massachusetts Medical School; Director, Anatomic Pathology Division, Department of Pathology, University of Massachusetts Medical Center, Worcester, Massachusetts

Sheldon M. Wolff, M.D. *
Endicott Professor and Chairman, Department of Medicine, Tufts University School of Medicine; Physician-in-Chief, New England Medical Center, Boston, Massachusetts

Neal S. Young, M.D.
Chief, Hematology Branch, National Heart, Lung, and Blood Institute, National Institutes of Health, Bethesda, Maryland

Karen A. Zaboy, M.D.
Pediatric Hematology/Oncology Division, Department of Pediatrics, St. Joseph's Children's Hospital, Tampa, Florida

Ralph Zalusky, M.D.
Professor, Department of Medicine, Albert Einstein College of Medicine of Yeshiva University, Bronx, New York; Chief, Hematology/Oncology Division, Department of Medicine, Beth Israel Medical Center, New York, New York

---

*Deceased.

Preface to the Second Edition

The first edition of *Hematology: Basic Principles and Practice* appeared in 1991. This work was intended to be a comprehensive and up-to-date textbook developed to serve a diverse group of individuals ranging from practicing general hematologists, students of the field, basic scientists involved in hematologic research, as well as practicing internists and pediatricians. During the past four years, the science and practice of hematology have continued to evolve. The rapid advancement of this field has necessitated the creation of a second edition, in order that the book remain current and useful to our readers as the field of hematology progresses.

We retained the features of the first edition that were regarded by our audience as most effective, but altered the second edition as required to further enhance the quality of the book. In response to the constructive criticisms offered in numerous positive reviews of the first edition, we have added an entirely new section titled *Immunology*. It is organized in a manner resembling the section titled *Molecular and Cellular Basis of Hematology*, which provides an overview of the basic science needed to gain insight into the field. Some chapters have been eliminated in the interest of reducing redundancy and balancing the content. The editors met twice for extended work sessions during the inception of this edition in order to organize the information to be included. These meetings led to the development of close relationships between the editors and staff which has, we believe, led to the generation of a more cohesive and comprehensive text.

The growing importance of transfusion medicine has been recognized by the appointment of Leslie E. Silberstein, M.D. to the editorial group. The second edition has 16 chapters that deal exclusively with transfusion medicine. This section provides a concise review of an increasingly significant and complex area. An understanding of transfusion medicine is required of all practicing hematologists. We hope this primer will serve as a framework by which students of hematology can gain mastery of this rapidly evolving area.

In the first edition we asked authors to contribute their personal strategies for managing difficult clinical problems in sections set apart from the main text. These boxed paragraphs were highlighted by a shaded tint so the reader could easily identify these clinical points. Such contributions now appear in an expanded form in most of the chapters dealing with clinical hematology.

The remarkably rapid progress of both experimental and clinical hematology, coupled with the accelerated entry of molecular and cellular concepts and techniques into clinical practice, has resulted in an entirely new set of terminologies relevant to the clinical hematologist. Oncogenes, chromosomal translocations, cell-surface antigens, growth factors, and specialized cellular receptors comprise but a few examples of entities that were identified only by the arcane jargon of research laboratories a few years ago, but are now important for the classification, diagnosis, and treatment of hematologic diseases. The translation of knowledge from research laboratory to the bedside has been so rapid that the names of these substances and phenomena have often remained in the shorthand of the basic research community. A formidable challenge facing the editors and publisher of this volume has been the development of a coherent approach to the terms used to identify these materials. In some cases, loose rules of usage have been developed. For example, the abbreviations used to designate human and mouse proto-oncogenes, their oncogene derivatives, and the proteins resulting from their expression are distinguished by differential use of lower case and upper case letters, italics, and so forth. However, these rules are not universally honored in either the primary research literature, or in reviews or textbooks. We have tried to conform to recommended usage in every situation in which a recommended terminology has been developed. However, we have deferred to the best judgment and preferences of the authors of individual chapters whenever they thought the conventional terminology was inappropriate for the subjects they discuss. We have attempted to alert the reader to the use of alternative terminologies, and to define potentially confusing terms.

The contributors to this edition have done an outstanding job, and the editors are indebted to them for their diligence, perseverance, and scholarly presentations.

Ronald Hoffman, M.D.

Edward J. Benz, Jr., M.D.

Sanford J. Shattil, M.D.

Bruce Furie, M.D.

Harvey J. Cohen, M.D., Ph.D.

Leslie E. Silberstein, M.D.

Preface to the First Edition

The last several decades have seen an exponential increase in new medical knowledge related to hematology. New disease entities, new diagnostic methods, and novel therapeutic modalities have been introduced into the discipline. These clinical advances have largely been based on insights into the pathophysiology of hematologic disorders and have been gained by applying the tools of cell biology, biochemistry, immunology, and molecular genetics to this discipline. Inevitably, this explosion of knowledge has also led to further subspecialization within hematology, with the appearance of experts in transfusion medicine, red cell disorders, platelet and coagulation disorders, neoplastic diseases, and immunohematology.

The practicing general hematologist, whether operating at a university or in private practice, faces the challenge of caring for patients who have a variety of hematologic disorders. It has become increasingly difficult for one individual to remain current in all aspects of this expanding discipline, yet clinical care requires intimate familiarity with the enlarging knowledge base. In addition, basic scientists without clinical training have been attracted to hematology research. To put their work in a clinical context, these scientists require a broad background in the fundamentals of hematology and comprehension of clinical presentations, diagnostics, and therapy of specific diseases. Furthermore, students of the field, including medical residents, hematology fellows, and internists with special needs for understanding hematologic diseases have a requirement for an up-to-date source of information. *Hematology: Basic Principles and Practice* is a comprehensive textbook developed to serve these diverse groups.

The structure of the book reflects the diversity of its readership. *Hematology: Basic Principles and Practice* was designed during a meeting of the Editors with Bob Hurley and Beth Barry of Churchill Livingstone in Woods Hole, Massachusetts, during the summer of 1988. As our starting point, all of the Editors stressed the importance of emphasizing the scientific underpinnings of modern hematology. Part I, *Molecular and Cellular Basis of Hematology*, is the foundation of the book and provides the overview of basic science needed to gain insight into the practice of hematology during the 1990s and into the next century. The next six parts are devoted to the major subspecialty areas, *Hematopoiesis, Red Blood Cells, White Blood Cells, Hematologic Malignancies, Hemostasis and Thrombosis*, and *Transfusion Medicine*. Each part contains an up-to-date review of the scientific fundamentals, followed by the description of specific hematologic diseases and their diagnosis and treatment. To further extend the book's clinical usefulness, Part VIII deals with *Consultative Hematology*. With nine chapters covering general medicine and surgery, we hope this section will be especially valuable to the clinician performing consultations on patients who do not have a primary hematologic disorder but whose primary disorder results in hematologic abnormalities. The book closes with a section on *Special Tests and Procedures* that are integral to the practice of hematology.

To strike a balance between the scientific and clinical, we believe the text should be academic and scholarly, yet still offer a practical approach to diagnosis and patient management. To reconcile these objectives and provide a forum for sharing clinical approaches, we asked authors to contribute their personal strategies for managing difficult problems in nonreferenced editorial sections set off from the main text. The boxed paragraphs are highlighted by a shaded tint so the reader can easily identify these clinical pearls.

We also asked the contributors to seek out and create helpful illustrations to make difficult concepts easier to understand. We have redrawn much of the art work to render primary visual material in a uniform style throughout the book, and have added color and tints to emphasize the more important points in the illustrations. We hope this makes our overall presentation more comprehensible and greatly enhances the heuristic value of these illustrations.

Ultimately, the quality of this project is closely related to the quality of the contributions received from the many participants in this multi-authored textbook. The preparation of each chapter has taken considerable effort and time, and we are grateful that the experts in the field agreed to participate in this undertaking. The contributors have done an outstanding job in writing comprehensive and timely treatises on specialized subjects, and we have responded by minimizing the delay between the preparation of each chapter and publication. We want to especially thank Les Silberstein at the University of Pennsylvania School of Medicine and Ed Snyder at the Yale University School of Medicine, who organized the section on blood banking. Their knowledge and guidance have been indispensable in editing this major section of the book.

Each of the Editors brings to the book different interests and perspectives. We all worked together as equal partners to create a shared vision of a hematology text for a new generation of scientists and clinicians. We hope that we have accomplished this lofty goal, and that this will be the initial edition of a book that will continue to serve its varied readership for many editions to come.

Ronald Hoffman, M.D.

Edward J. Benz, Jr., M.D.

Sanford J. Shattil, M.D.

Bruce Furie, M.D.

Harvey J. Cohen, M.D., Ph.D.

Acknowledgments

Churchill Livingstone has provided excellent support for this project and we thank the company for its continued confidence in our efforts. In particular, Bob Hurley, Kerry Willis, Nancy Terry, Shireen Dunwoody, and Bridgett Dickinson are acknowledged for their extraordinary contributions, which have resulted in the rapid completion of the text. The expert secretarial support provided by Nancy Blecharz and Wilda DiPietro during the preparation of this textbook is greatly acknowledged as well.

Contents

xxiii

MOLECULAR AND CELLULAR BASIS OF HEMATOLOGY

Part I

Anatomy and Physiology of the Gene

Edward J. Benz, Jr.

INTRODUCTION

Normal blood cells have limited life spans; they must be replenished in precise numbers by a continually renewing population of progenitor cells. Homeostasis of the blood requires that proliferation of these cells be efficient, yet strictly constrained. Many distinctive types of mature blood cells must arise from these progenitors by a controlled process of commitment to, and execution of, complex programs of differentiation. Thus, developing red cells must produce large quantities of hemoglobin, but not the myeloperoxidase characteristic of granulocytes, the immunoglobulins characteristic of lymphocytes, or the fibrinogen receptors characteristic of platelets. Similarly, the maintenance of normal amounts of coagulant and anticoagulant proteins in the circulation requires exquisitely regulated production, destruction, and interaction of the components. Understanding the basic biologic principles underlying cell growth, differentiation, and protein biosynthesis requires a thorough knowledge of the structure and regulated expression of genes, because the gene is now known to be the fundamental unit by which biologic information is stored, transmitted, and expressed in a regulated fashion.

Genes were originally characterized as mathematical units of inheritance. They are now known to consist of molecules of deoxyribonucleic acid (DNA). By virtue of their ability to store information in the form of nucleotide sequences, to transmit it by means of semiconservation replication to daughter cells during mitosis and meiosis, and to express it by directing the incorporation of amino acids into proteins, DNA molecules are the chemical transducers of genetic information flow. Efforts to understand the biochemical means by which this transduction is accomplished has given rise to the discipline of molecular genetics.

Our ability to study the molecular genetics of hematologic problems has been greatly advanced by the development of recombinant DNA technology, which permits one to isolate, characterize, synthesize, and manipulate individual genes controlling known proteins or biologic phenomena. A brief overview of the basic methods and terminology of recombinant DNA technology is included in this chapter.

THE GENETIC VIEW OF THE BIOSPHERE—THE CENTRAL DOGMA OF MOLECULAR BIOLOGY

The fundamental premise of the molecular biologist is that the magnificent diversity encountered in nature is ultimately governed by genes. The capacity of genes to exert this control is in turn determined by relatively simple stereochemical rules, first appreciated by Watson and Crick in the 1950s. These rules constrain the types of interactions that can occur between two molecules of DNA or ribonucleic acid (RNA).

DNA and RNA are linear polymers consisting of four types of nucleotide subunits. Proteins are linear unbranched polymers consisting of 21 types of amino acid subunits. Each amino acid is distinguished from the others by the chemical nature of its side chain, the moiety not involved in forming the peptide bond links of the chain. The properties of cells, tissues, and organisms depend largely on the aggregate structures and properties of their proteins. The central dogma of molecular biology states that genes control these properties by controlling the structures of proteins, the timing and amount of their production, and the coordination of their synthesis with that of other proteins. The intermediary transmitting the information needed to achieve these ends is a class of nucleic acid molecules called RNA. Genetic information is stored in the form of DNA nucleic acid sequences and expressed in the form of protein synthesis through the mediation of RNA. Genetic information thus flows in the direction DNA → RNA → protein. This central dogma provides, in principle, a universal approach for investigating the biologic properties and behavior of any given cell, tissue, or organism by study of the controlling genes. Methods permitting direct manipulation of DNA sequences should then be universally applicable to the study of all living entities. Indeed, the power of the molecular genetic approach lies in the universality of its utility.

One exception to the central dogma of molecular biology that is especially relevant to hematologists is the storage of genetic information in RNA molecules in certain viruses, notably the retroviruses associated with T-cell leukemia/lymphoma and the human immunodeficiency virus. When retroviruses enter the cell, the RNA genome is copied into a DNA replica by an enzyme called reverse transcriptase. This DNA representation of the viral genome is then expressed according to the rules of the central dogma. Retroviruses thus represent a variation on the theme, rather than a true exception or violation of the rules.

ANATOMY AND PHYSIOLOGY OF GENES

DNA Structure

DNA molecules are extremely long unbranched polymers of nucleotide subunits. Each nucleotide contains a sugar moiety called deoxyribose, a phosphate group attached to the 5' carbon position, and a purine or pyrimidine base attached to the 1' position (Fig. 1-1). The linkages in the chain are formed by phosphodiester bonds between the 5' position of each sugar residue and the 3' position of the adjacent residue in the chain (Fig. 1-1). The sugar phosphate links form the backbone of the polymer, from which the purine or pyrimidine bases project perpendicularly.

The haploid human genome consists of 23 long, double-stranded DNA molecules tightly complexed with histones and other nuclear proteins to form compact linear structures called chromosomes. The genome contains 3 billion nucleotides; each chromosome is thus 50–200 million bases in length. The individual genes are aligned along each chromosome. Blood cells, like most somatic cells, are diploid. Each chromosome is present in two copies, so that there are 46 chromosomes consisting of approximately 6 billion base pairs (bp) of DNA. The length of a DNA molecule is often described in terms of the length of the number of nucleotide bases it contains. Since each nucleotide contains one such base, it is equivalent to say a DNA molecule is 1,000 bases (1 kilobase [kb]) or 1,000 nucleotides in

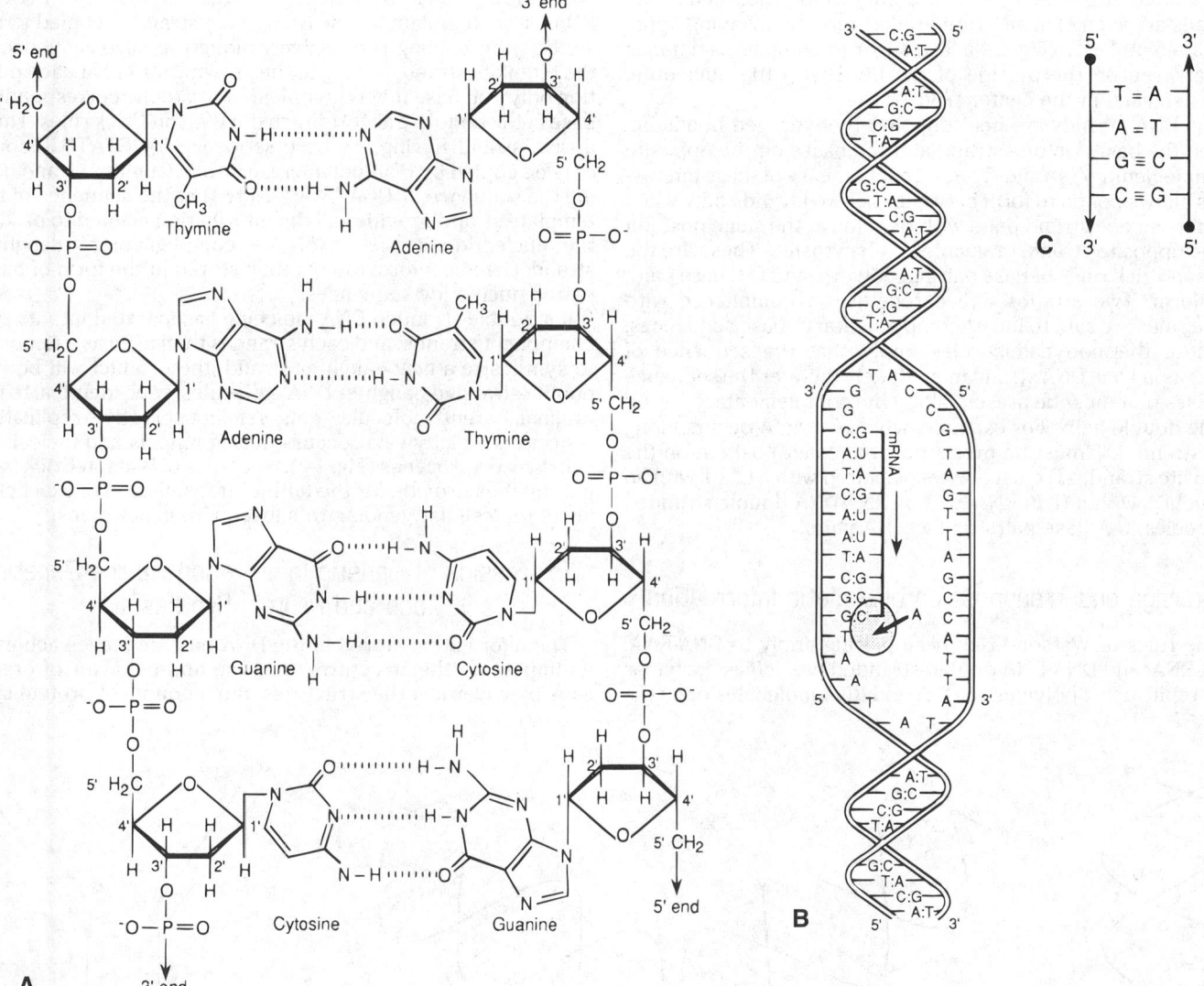

Fig. 1-1. Structure, base pairing, polarity, and template properties of DNA. **(A)** Structures of the four nitrogenous bases projecting from sugar phosphate backbones. The hydrogen bonds between them form base pairs holding complementary strands of DNA together. Note that AT and TA base pairs have only two hydrogen bonds, whereas CG and GC pairs have three. **(B)** The double helical structure of DNA results from base pairing of strands to form a double-stranded molecule with the backbones on the outside and the hydrogen-bonded bases stacked in the middle. Also shown schematically is the separation (unwinding) of a region of the helix by mRNA polymerase, which is shown utilizing one of the strands as a template for the synthesis of an mRNA precursor molecule. Note that new bases added to the growing RNA strand obey the rules of Watson-Crick base pairing (see text). Uracil (U) in RNA replaces T in DNA and, like T, forms base pairs with A. **(C)** Diagram of the antiparallel nature of the strands, based on the stereochemical 3'→5' polarity of the strands. The chemical differences between reading along the backbone in the 5' to 3' and 3' to 5' directions can be appreciated by reference to Fig. A.

length. As noted below, DNA often exists as a double-stranded structure, held together by hydrogen bonds between the bases at equivalent positions of each strand (base pairing); the length of these double-stranded molecules is described in base pairs (e.g., 1,000 bp = 1 kilobase pair [1 kbp]).

The four nucleotide bases in DNA are the purines (adenosine and guanosine) and the pyrimidines (thymine and cytosine). The basic chemical configuration of the other nucleic acid found in cells, RNA, is quite similar, except that the sugar is ribose (having a hydroxyl group attached to the 2' carbon, rather than the hydrogen found in deoxyribose) and the pyrimidine base uracil is used in place of thymine. The bases are commonly referred to by a short-hand notation: the letters A, C, T, G, and U are used to refer to adenosine, cytosine, thymine, guanosine, and uracil, respectively.

The ends of DNA and RNA strands are chemically distinct,

because of the 3'→5' phosphodiester bond linkage that ties adjacent bases together (Fig. 1-1). One end of the strand (the 3' end) will have an unlinked (free at the 3' carbon) sugar position, and the other (the 5' end) a free 5' position. There is thus a polarity to the sequence of bases in a DNA strand: the same sequence of bases read in a 3'→5' direction carries a different meaning than if read in a 5'→3' direction. Cellular enzymes can thus distinguish one end of a nucleic acid from the other; most enzymes that "read" the DNA sequence tend to do so only in one direction (3'→5' or 5'→3', but not both). Most nucleic acid-synthesizing enzymes, for instance, add new bases to the strand in a 5'→3' direction.

The ability of DNA molecules to store information resides in the *sequence* of nucleotide bases arrayed along the polymer chain. Under the physiologic conditions extant within living cells, DNA is thermodynamically most stable when two strands coil around each other to form a double-stranded helix. The strands are aligned in an "antiparallel" direction, having opposite 3'→5' polarity (Fig. 1-1). The sugar phosphate backbones are arrayed on the outside of the helix with the nucleotide bases stacked in the center (Fig. 1-1).

The DNA strands are held together by hydrogen bonds between the bases on one strand and the bases on the opposite (complementary) strand. The stereochemistry of these interactions allows bonds to form between the two strands only when adenine on one strand pairs with thymine at the same position of the opposite strand, or guanine with cytosine. These are the Watson-Crick rules of base pairing: only A-T and G-C base pairs can form. Two strands joined together in compliance with these rules are said to have "complementary" base sequences.

These thermodynamic rules imply that the sequence of bases along one DNA strand immediately dictates the sequence of bases that must be present along the complementary strand in the double helix. For example, whenever an A occurs along one strand, a T must be present at that exact position on the opposite strand; a G must always be paired with a C, a T with an A, and a C with a G. In RNA-RNA or RNA-DNA double-stranded molecules, U-A base pairs replace T-A pairs.

Storage and Transmission of Genetic Information

The rules of Watson-Crick base pairing apply to DNA-RNA, RNA-RNA, and DNA-DNA double-stranded molecules. Enzymes that replicate or polymerize DNA and RNA molecules obey the base pairing rules. By utilizing an existing strand of DNA or RNA as the template, a new (daughter) strand is copied (transcribed) by reading processively along the base sequence of the template strand, adding to the growing strand at each position only that base that is complementary to the corresponding base in the template according to the Watson-Crick rules. Thus, a DNA strand having the base sequence 5'-GCTATG-3' could only be copied by DNA polymerase into a daughter strand having the sequence, 3'-CGATAC-5'. Note that the sequence of the template strand provides all the information needed to predict the nucleotide sequence of the complementary daughter strand. Genetic information is thus stored in the form of base-paired nucleotide sequences.

If a double-stranded DNA molecule is separated into its two component strands, and each strand is then used as a template to synthesize a new daughter strand, the product will be two double-stranded daughter DNA molecules, each identical to the original parent molecule. This semiconservative replication process is exactly what occurs during mitosis and meiosis as cell division proceeds (Fig. 1-2). The rules of Watson-Crick base pairing thus provide for the faithful transmission of exact copies of the cellular genome to subsequent generations.

Expression of Genetic Information via the Genetic Code and Protein Synthesis

The information stored in the DNA base sequence achieves its impact on the structure, function, and behavior of organisms by governing the structures and amounts of protein syn-

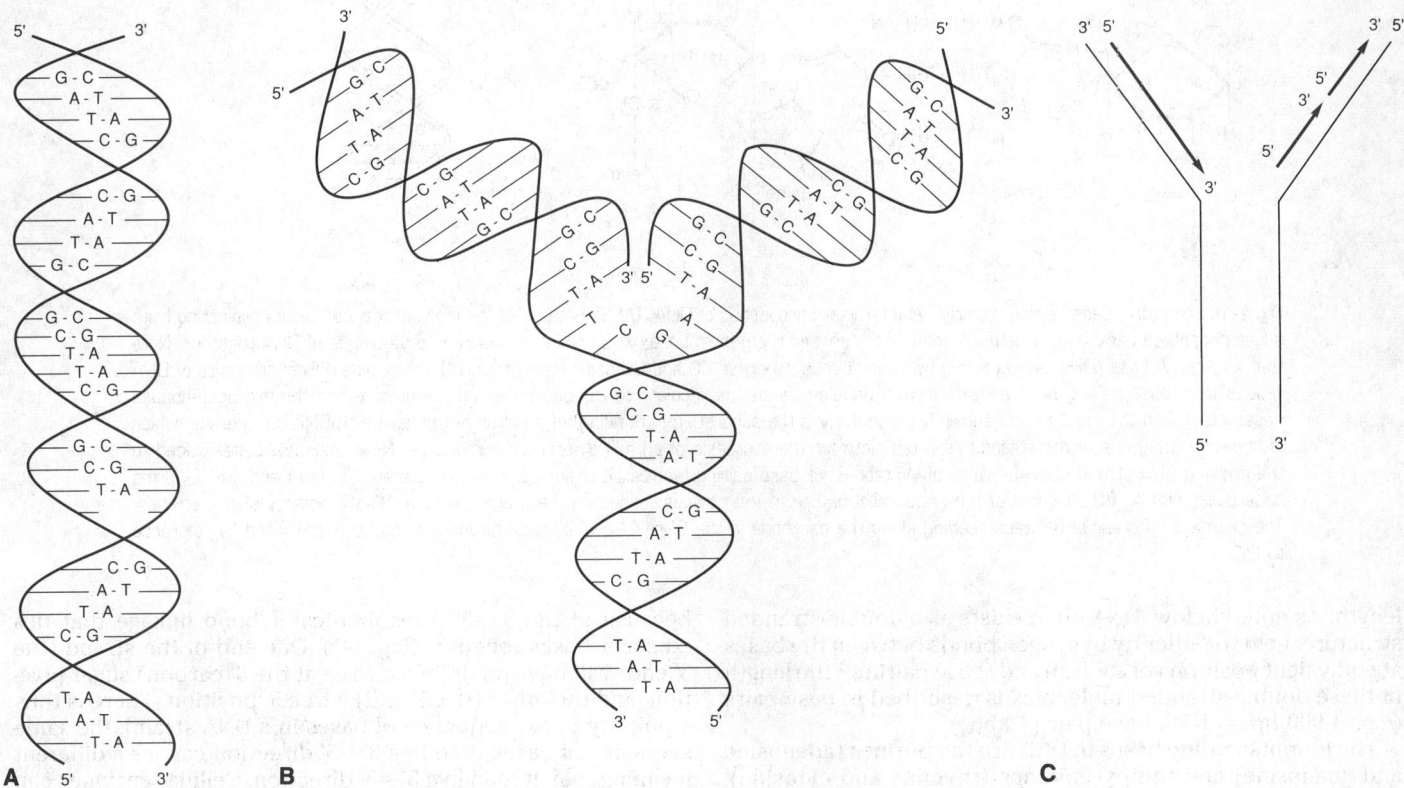

Fig. 1-2. Semiconservative replication of DNA. **(A)** The process by which the DNA molecule on the left is replicated into two daughter molecules, as occurs during cell division. Replication occurs by separation of the parent molecule into the single-stranded form at one end, reading of each of the daughter strands in the 3'→5' direction by DNA polymerase, and addition of new bases to growing daughter strands in the 5'→3' direction. **(B)** The replicated portions of the daughter molecules are identical to each other (red). Each carries one of the two strands of the parent molecule, accounting for the term *semiconservative replication*. Note the presence of the replication fork, the point at which the parent DNA is being unwound. **(C)** The antiparallel nature of the DNA strands demands that replication proceed toward the fork in one direction and away from the fork in the other (red). This means that replication is actually accomplished by reading of short stretches of DNA, followed by ligation of the short daughter strand regions to form an intact daughter strand.

thesized in the cells. The primary structure (i.e., the amino acid sequence) of each protein determines its three-dimensional conformation and therefore properties (e.g. shape, enzymatic activity, ability to interact with other molecules, stability, and so forth). In the aggregate, these proteins control cell structure and metabolism. Genes determine the structures of proteins that are synthesized, the timing of their production during development or differentiation, and the amounts produced in different cells or tissues. The process by which DNA achieves its control of cells via protein synthesis is called gene expression.

An outline of the basic pathway of gene expression in eukaryotic cells is shown in Fig. 1-3. The DNA base sequence is first copied into an RNA molecule, called premessenger RNA, by mRNA polymerase. Pre-mRNA has a base sequence complementary to the DNA coding strand. Genes in eukaryotic species consist of tandem arrays of sequences encoding mRNA (exons); these sequences alternate with sequences (introns) present in the initial mRNA transcript (pre-mRNA) but absent from the mature mRNA. The entire gene is transcribed into the large precursor, which is then further processed (spliced) in the nucleus. The introns are excised from the final mature mRNA molecule, which is then exported to the cytoplasm to be decoded (translated) into the amino acid sequence of the protein, by association with a biochemically complex group of ribonucleoprotein structures called ribosomes. Ribosomes contain two subunits; the 60S subunit contains a single large (28S) ribosomal RNA molecular complexed with multiple proteins, while the RNA component of the 40S subunit is a smaller (18S) rRNA molecule.

Ribosomes read mRNA sequence in a ticker tape fashion *three bases at a time,* inserting the appropriate amino acid encoded by each three base code words or codons into the appropriate position of the growing protein chain. This process is called mRNA translation. The glossary used by cells to know which amino acids are encoded by each DNA codon is called the genetic code (Table 1-1). Each amino acid is encoded by a sequence of three successive bases. Since there are four code letters, (A, C, G, and U), and since sequences read in the 5′→3′ direction have a different biologic meaning than sequences read in the 3′→5′ direction, there are 4^3, or 64, possible codons consisting of three bases.

There are 21 naturally occurring amino acids found in proteins. Thus, more codons are available than amino acids to be encoded. As noted in Table 1-1, a consequence of this redundancy is that some amino acids are encoded by more than one codon. For example, six distinct codons can specify incorporation of arginine into a growing amino acid chain, four codons can specify valine, two can specify glutamic acid, and only one each, methionine or tryptophan. It is important to note that in no case does a single codon encode more than one amino acid. Codons thus predict unambiguously the amino acid sequence they encode. However, one cannot easily read backward from the amino acid sequence to decipher the *exact* encoding DNA sequence. These facts are summarized by saying that the code is degenerate but not ambiguous.

Some specialized codons serve as punctuation points during translation. The methionine codon (AUG), when surrounded by a consensus sequence (the Kozak box) near the beginning (5′ end) of the mRNA, serves as the initiator codon signaling the first amino acid to be incorporated. All proteins thus begin with a methionine residue, but this is often removed later in the translational process. Three codons, UAG, UAA, and UGA serve as translation terminators, signaling the end of translation.

The adaptor molecules mediating individual decoding events during mRNA translation are small (40 bases long) RNA molecules called transfer (t)RNAs. When bound into a ribosome, each tRNA exposes a three-base segment within its sequence called the anticolon. These three bases attempt to pair with the three-base codon exposed on the mRNA. If the anticodon is complementary in sequence to the codon, a stable interaction among the mRNA, the ribosome, and the tRNA molecule will result. Within each tRNA is also a separate region that is adapted for covalent binding to an amino acid. The enzymes that catalyze the binding of each amino acid are constrained in such a way that each tRNA species can bind only to a single amino acid. For example, tRNA molecules containing the anticodon 3′-AAA-5′, which is complementary to a 5′-UUU-3′ (phenylalanine) codon in mRNA, can only be bound to or charged with phenylalanine; tRNA containing the anticodon 3′-UAG-5′ can only be charged with isoleucine, and so forth.

tRNAs and their amino acyl tRNA synthetases provide for the coupling of nucleic acid information to protein information needed to convert the genetic code to an amino acid sequence. Ribosomes provide the structural matrix on which tRNA anticodons and mRNA codons become properly exposed and aligned in an orderly, linear, and sequential fashion. As each new codon is exposed, the appropriate charged tRNA species is bound. A peptide bond is then formed between the amino acid carried by this tRNA and the C-terminal residue on the existing nascent protein chain. The growing chain is transferred to the new tRNA in the process, so that it is held in place as the next tRNA is brought in. This cycle is repeated until completion of translation. The completed polypeptide chain is then transferred to other organelles for further processing (e.g., to the endoplasmic reticulum and the Golgi apparatus) or released into cytosol for association of the newly completed chain with other subunits to form complex multimeric proteins (e.g., hemoglobin), and so forth, as discussed in Chapter 2.

Messenger RNA Metabolism

Eukaryotic and prokaryotic cells are different with respect to the way that the initial mRNA transcript is structurally related to the mature mRNA species that is ultimately translated on ribosomes. In prokaryotes, the initial transcript and the translated transcript are essentially the same. In eukaryotes, the situation is far more complex.

In eukaryotic cells, mRNA is initially synthesized in the nucleus (Figs. 1-3 and 1-4). Before the initial transcript becomes suitable for translation in the cytoplasm, several complex events, messenger RNA processing and transport, must occur: excision of the portions of the mRNA that are complementary to the introns of the gene (mRNA splicing), modification of the 5′ and 3′ ends of the mRNA to render them more stable and translatable, and transport to the cytoplasm. Moreover, the amount of any particular mRNA moiety in both prokaryotic and eukaryotic cells is governed not only by the composite rate of mRNA synthesis (transcription, processing, and transport), but also by its degradation by cytoplasmic ribonucleases (RNA degradation). Many mRNA species of special importance in hematology (e.g., mRNAs for growth factors and their receptors, proto-oncogene mRNAs, acute-phase reactants) are exquisitely regulated by control of their stability (half-life) in the cytoplasm.

Post-transcriptional mRNA metabolism is complex. Only a few relevant details are considered in this section.

mRNA Splicing

The initial transcript of eukaryotic genes contains several subregions (Fig. 1-4). Most striking is the tandem alignment of exons and introns. Precise excision of intron sequences and ligation of exons is critical for production of mature mRNA. This process is called mRNA splicing, and it occurs on complexes of small nuclear RNAs and proteins called snRNPs; the term

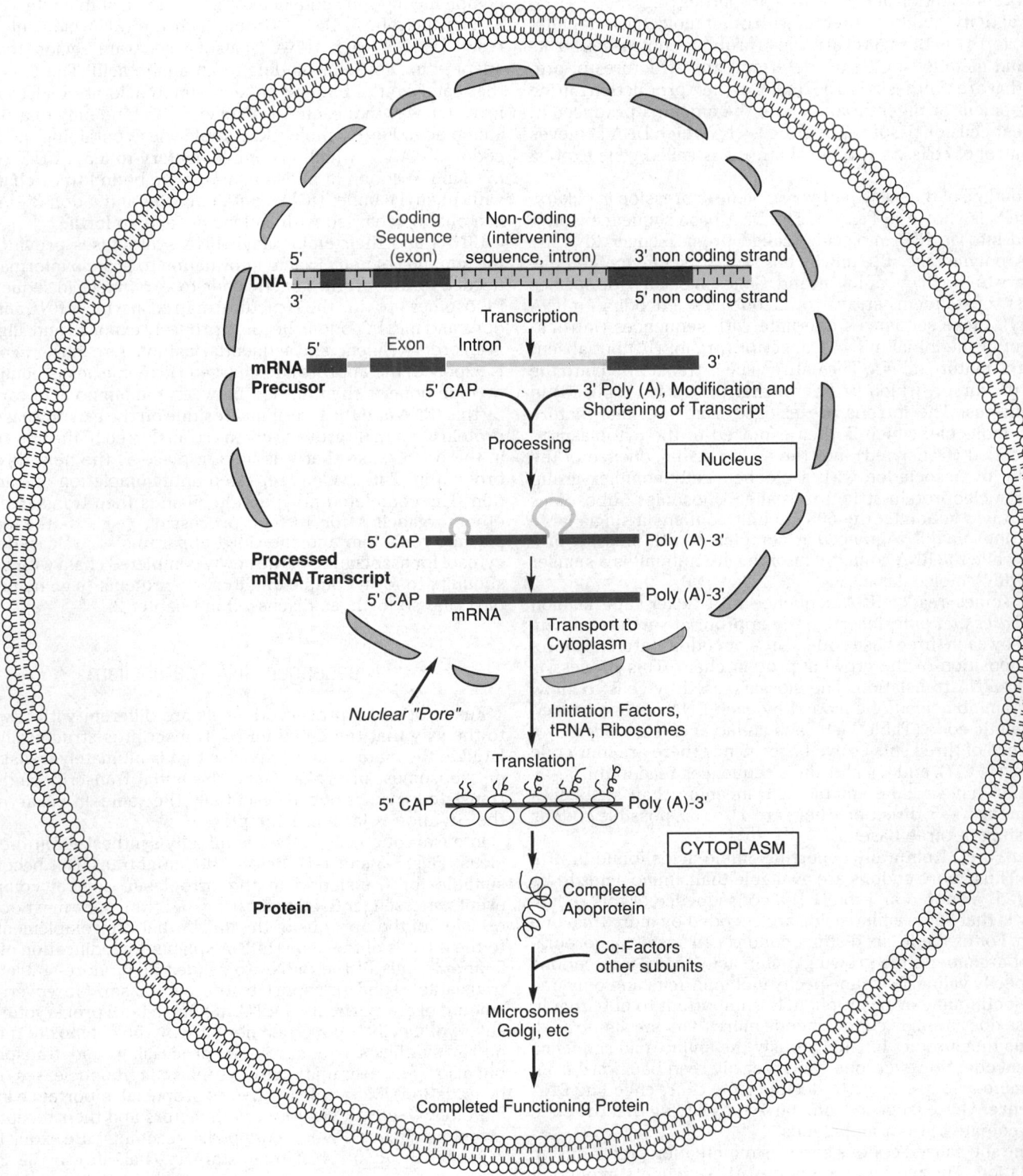

Fig. 1-3. Synthesis of mRNA and protein—pathway of gene expression. The diagram of the DNA gene shows the alternating array of exons (red) and introns (pink) typical of most eukaryotic genes. Transcription of the mRNA precursor, addition of the 5'-CAP and 3'-poly (A) tail, splicing and excision of introns, transport to the cytoplasm through the nuclear pores, translation into the amino acid sequence of the apoprotein, and post-translational processing of the protein are described in the text. Translation proceeds from the initiator methionine codon near the 5' end of the mRNA, with incorporation of the amino terminal end of the protein. As the mRNA is read in a 5'→3' direction, the nascent polypeptide is assembled in an amino→carboxyl terminal direction.

Table 1-1. The Genetic Code[a] Messenger RNA Codons for the Amino Acids

Alanine	Arginine	Asparagine	Aspartic acid	Cysteine
5'-GCU-3'	CGU	AAU	GAU	UGU
GCC	CGC	AAG	GAC	UGC
GCA	CGA			
GCG	AGA			
	AGG			

Glutamic acid	Glutamine	Glycine	Histidine	Isoleucine
GAA	CAA	GGU	CAU	AUU
GAG	CAG	GGC	CAC	AUC
		GGA		AUA
		GGG		

Leucine	Lysine	Methionine	Phenylalanine	Proline[c]
UUA	AAA	AUG[b]	UUU	CCU
UUG	AAG		UUC	CCC
CUU				CCA
CUC				CCG
CUA				
CUG				

Serine	Threonine	Tryptophan	Tyrosine	Valine
UCU	ACU	UGG	UAU	GUU
UCC	ACC		UAC	GUC
UCA	ACA			GUA
UCG	ACG			GUG
AGU				
AGC				

Chain termination codons[d]
UAA
UAG
UGA

[a] Note that most of the degeneracy in the code is in the third base positions (e.g., lysine = AA (G or C), asparagine = AA (U or G), valine = GU (N, where N is any base).

[b] AUG is also used as the chain initiation codon when surrounded by the Kozak consensus sequence.

[c] Hydroxyproline, the twenty-first amino acid, is generated by post-translational modification of proline. It is almost exclusively confined to collagen subunits.

[d] The codons that signal the end of translation, also called nonsense or terminaton codons, are described by their nicknames *amber* (UAG), *ochre* (UAA), and *opal* (UGA).

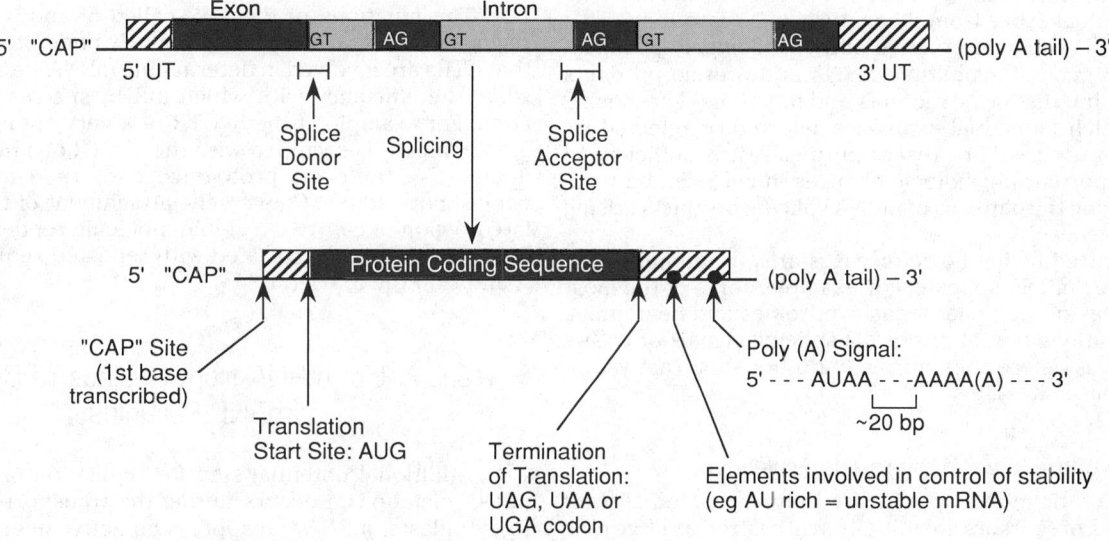

Fig. 1-4. Anatomy of the products of the structural gene (mRNA precursor and mRNA). This schematic shows the configuration of the critical anatomic elements of an mRNA precursor, which represents the primary copy of the structural portion of the gene (see text for details). The sequences GT and AG indicate, respectively, the invariant dinucleotides present in the donor and acceptor sites at which introns are spliced out of the precursor. Not shown are the less stringently conserved consensus sequences that must precede and succeed each of these sites for a short distance.

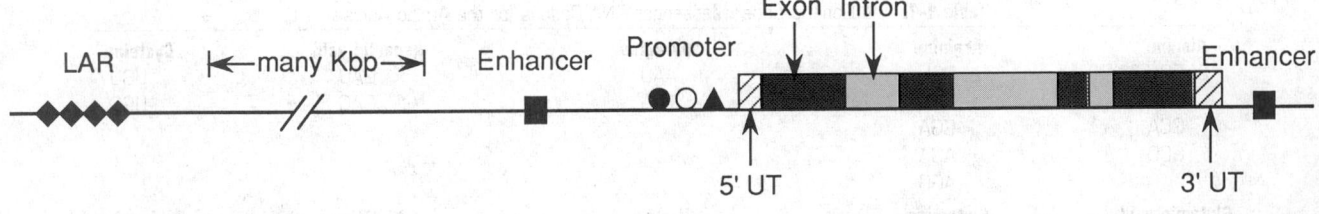

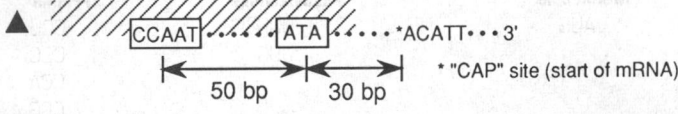

● Tissue specific elements, hormone responsive elements, etc.

○ "Octamer", conserved G-C rich regions

▲ ////// CCAAT ////// ATA //.... *ACATT...3'
|← 50 bp →|← 30 bp →| * "CAP" site (start of mRNA)

◆◆◆◆— Locus Activating Region - sequences recognized as markers of active gene clusters by tissue or differentiation specific nuclear proteins.

Fig. 1-5. Regulatory elements flanking the structural gene.

spliceosome is also used to describe the intranuclear organelle that mediates mRNA splicing reactions. The biochemical mechanism for splicing is complex. A consensus sequence, which includes the dinucleotide GT, is recognized as the donor site at the 5' end of the intron (5' end refers to the polarity of the mRNA strand coding for protein); a second consensus sequence ending in the dinucleotide AG is recognized as the acceptor site, which marks the distal end of the intron (Figs. 1-4 and 1-5). The spliceosome recognizes the donor and acceptor and forms an intermediate lariat structure that provides for both excision of the intron and proper alignment of the cut ends of the two exons for ligation in precise register.

mRNA splicing has proved to be an important mechanism for greatly increasing the versatility and diversity of expression of a single gene. For example, some genes contain an array of more exons than one actually finds in any mature mRNA species encoded by the gene. Several different mRNA protein products can arise from a single gene by selective inclusion or exclusion of individual exons from the mature mRNA products. This phenomenon is called alternative mRNA splicing. It permits a single gene to code for multiple mRNA and protein products with related, but distinct structures and functions. The mechanisms by which individual exons are selected or rejected remain totally obscure. For present purposes, it is sufficient to note that important physiologic changes in cells can be regulated by altering the patterns of mRNA splicing products arising from single genes.

Many inherited hematologic diseases arise from mutations, which derange mRNA splicing. For example, some of the most common forms of the thalassemia syndromes and hemophilia arise by mutations that alter normal splicing signals or create splicing signals where they normally do not exist (activation of cryptic splice sites).

Modification of the Ends of the mRNA Molecule

Most eukaryotic mRNA species are polyadenylated at their 3' ends. mRNA precursors are initially synthesized as large molecules that extend further downstream from the 3' end of the mature mRNA molecule. Polyadenylation results in the addition of stretches of 100–150 A residues at the 3' end. Such an addition is often called the poly-A tail, and may be a variable length. Polyadenylation facilitates rapid early cleavage of the unwanted 3' sequences from the transcript and is also important for stability or transport of the mRNA out of the nucleus.

Signals near the 3' extremity of the mature mRNA mark positions at which polyadenylation occurs. The consensus signal is AUAAA (Fig. 1-4). Mutations in the poly-A signal sequence have been shown to cause thalassemia.

At the 5' end of the mRNA, a complex oligonucleotide having unusual phosphodiester bonds is added. This structure contains the nucleotide 7-methyl-guanosine, and is called CAP (Fig. 1-4). The 5'-CAP enhances both mRNA stability and the ability of the mRNA to interact with protein translation factors and ribosomes.

5' and 3' Untranslated Sequences

The 5' and 3' extremities of mRNA extend beyond the initiator and terminator condons that mark the beginning and the end of the sequences actually translated into proteins (Figs. 1-4 and 1-5). The functions of these so-called 5' and 3' untranslated regions (5' UTR, 3' UTR) remain poorly understood. It appears that UTRs are involved in determining mRNA stability and, possibly, the efficiency with which mRNA species can be translated. For example, if the 3' UTR of a very stable mRNA (e.g., globin mRNA) is swapped with the 3' UTR of a highly unstable mRNA (e.g., the c-*myc* proto-oncogene), the c-myc mRNA becomes more stable. Conversely, attachment of the 3' untranslated region of c-*myc* to a globin molecule renders it unstable. Instability is often associated with repeated sequences rich in A and U in the 3' UT (Fig. 1-4).

Transport of mRNA from Nucleus to Cytoplasm: mRNP Particles

An additional potential step for regulation or pathology of mRNA metabolism occurs during the transport from nucleus to cytoplasm. mRNA transport is an active energy-consuming process. Moreover, at least some mRNAs appear to enter the cytoplasm in the form of complexes bound to proteins (mRNPs). mRNPs may regulate stability of the mRNAs and their access to translational apparatus. There is some evidence that certain mRNPs are present in the cytoplasm but are not translated (masked message) until proper physiologic signals are received.

GENE REGULATION

Virtually all cells of an organism receive a complete copy of the DNA genome inherited at the time of conception. The panoply of distinct cell types and tissues found in any complex organism is possible only because different portions of the genome are selectively expressed or repressed in each cell type. Each cell must "know" which genes to express, how actively to express them, and when to express them. This biologic necessity has come to be known as gene regulation or regulated gene expression. Understanding gene regulation allows an understanding of how pluripotent stem cells determine that they will express the proper sets of genes in daughter progenitor cells that differentiate along each lineage. Major hematologic disorders (such as the leukemias and lymphomas), immunodeficiency states, and myeloproliferative syndromes result from derangements in the system of gene regulation. An understanding of the ways that genes are selected for expression thus remains one of the major frontiers of biology and medicine.

Active and Inactive Configurations of Genomic DNA in Chromatin

Most of the DNA in living cells is inactivated by formation of a nucleoprotein complex called chromatin. The histone and nonhistone proteins in chromatin effectively sequester genes from enzymes needed for expression. The most tightly compacted chromatin regions are called euchromatin. Heterochromatin, less tightly packed, contains actively transcribed genes. Activation of a gene for expression (i.e., transcription) requires that it become less compacted and more accessible to the transcription apparatus. Little is known about these processes, but it is clear that both cis-acting and trans-acting factors are involved. Cis-acting elements are regulatory DNA sequences, within or flanking the genes. They are recognized by trans factors, which are nuclear DNA binding proteins needed for transcriptional regulation.

DNA sequence regions flanking genes are called cis-acting because they influence expression of nearby genes only on the same chromosome. These sequences do not usually encode mRNA or protein molecules. They alter the conformation of the gene within chromatin in such a way as to facilitate or inhibit access to the factors that facilitate transcription. These interactions may twist or kink the DNA in such a way as to increase exposure to other molecules. When exogenous nucleases are added in small amounts to nuclei, these exposed sequence regions are especially sensitive to the DNA cutting action of the nucleases. Thus, nuclease-hypersensitive sites in DNA have come to be appreciated as markers for regions in or near genes that are interacting with regulatory nuclear proteins.

Methylation is another structural feature that can be utilized to recognize differences between actively transcribed and inactive genes. Most eukaryotic DNA is heavily methylated, that is, the DNA is modified by the addition of a methyl group to the 5′ position of cytosines (5-methyl-C). In general, heavily methylated genes are inactive, while active genes are relatively hypomethylated, especially in the 5′ flanking regions containing the promoter and other regulatory elements (see below). These flanking regions frequently include DNA sequences with a high content of Gs and Cs (G-C-rich islands). Hypomethylated G-C-rich islands (detectable by methylation-sensitive restriction endonucleases) serve as markers of actively transcribed genes. For example, a search for undermethylated G-C-rich islands on chromosome 7 facilitated the search for the gene for cystic fibrosis.

Several other structural configurations of DNA and their interaction with chromatin have been implicated as important for gene regulation. These include the B or Z conformation of the DNA helix, the degree of supercoiling or torsion of DNA superstructures, acetylation, phosphorylation, or ribosylation of nuclear proteins, and so forth. However, none of these mechanisms is understood in sufficient detail to merit further discussion currently.

Enhancers, Promoters, and Silencers

Several types of cis-active DNA sequence elements have been defined according to the presumed consequences of their interaction with nuclear proteins (Fig. 1-5). *Promoters* are found just upstream (to the 5′ side) of the start of mRNA transcription (the CAP). mRNA polymerases appear to bind first to the promoter region and thereby gain access to the structural gene sequences downstream. Promoters thus serve a dual function of being binding sites for mRNA polymerase and marking for the polymerase the downstream point at which transcription should start.

Enhancers are more complicated and less well-understood DNA sequence elements. Enhancers can lie on either side of a gene, or even within the gene in introns. Enhancers appear to bind transcription factors and thereby stimulate expression of genes nearby. The domain of influence of enhancers (i.e., the number of genes to either side whose expression is stimulated) varies. Some enhancers influence only the adjacent gene; others seem to mark the boundaries of large multigene clusters (gene domains) whose coordinated expression is appropriate to a particular tissue type or a particular time. For example, the very high levels of globin gene expression in erythroid cells depend on the function of an enhancer that seems to activate the entire gene cluster and is thus called a locus-activating region. The nuclear factors interacting with enhancers are probably induced into synthesis or activation as part of the process of differentiation.

Silencer sequences serve a function that is the obverse of enhancers. When bound by the appropriate nuclear proteins, silencer sequences cause repression of gene expression. There is some evidence that the same sequence elements can act as enhancers or silencers under different conditions, presumably by being bound by different sets of proteins having opposite effects on transcription.

Transcription Factors

Assays for detecting nuclear proteins that exhibit gene-specific DNA binding are just beginning to achieve widespread utility. Considerable information is now available about these nuclear proteins and their biochemical properties, but their physiologic behavior is incompletely understood. Proteins involved in the regulation of several gene systems have been isolated and their genes cloned. Common structural features have become apparent. Most transcription factors have DNA-binding domains sharing homologous structural motifs (cytosine-rich regions called zinc fingers, leucine-rich regions called leucine zippers, etc.), but other regions appear to be unique. Many factors implicated in the regulation of growth, differentiation, and development (e.g., homeobox genes, proto-oncogenes, anti-oncogenes, etc.) appear to be DNA-binding proteins and may be involved in the steps needed for activation of a gene within chromatin. Others seem to bind to, or modify, DNA-binding proteins. These factors are discussed in more detail in Chapter 7.

Regulation of mRNA Splicing, Stability, and Translation (Post-transcriptional Regulation)

It has become increasingly apparent that *post-transcription* and *translational* mechanisms are important strategies used by cells to govern the amounts of mRNA and protein accumulating when a particular gene is expressed. The major modes of *post-transcriptional* regulation are regulated alternative mRNA splicing, control of mRNA *stability,* and control of *translational* efficiency.

By regulating the relative amounts of an mRNA precursor that are spliced along one pathway or another, a cell can regulate the relative amounts of different protein isoforms arising from a given gene (alternative mRNA splicing). Several striking examples of this type of regulation are described, including the switch in immunoglobulin types produced at different stages of lymphoid differentiation, changes in the particular isoforms of cytoskeletal proteins produced during red cell differentiation, and a switch from one isoform of the c-*myb* proto-oncogene product to another during red cell differentiation. The effect of controlling the pathway of mRNA processing utilized in a cell is to include or exclude portions of the mRNA sequence. These portions encode peptide sequences that influence the ultimate physiologic behavior of the protein, or the RNA sequences that alter stability or translationability.

The importance of the control of mRNA stability for gene regulation is being increasingly appreciated. The steady-state level of any given mRNA species ultimately depends on the balance between the rate of its production (transcription and mRNA processing) and its destruction. One means by which stability is regulated is the inherent structure of the mRNA sequence, especially the 3′ and 5′ UTRs. As already noted, these sequences appear to affect mRNA secondary structure or recognition by nucleases, or both. Different mRNAs thus have inherently longer or shorter half-lives, almost regardless of the cell type in which they are expressed. Some mRNAs tend to be highly unstable. In response to appropriate physiologic needs, they can thus be produced quickly and removed from the cell quickly when a need for them no longer exists. Globin mRNA, on the other hand, is inherently quite stable, with a half-life measured in the range of 50 hours. This is appropriate for the need of reticulocytes to continue to synthesize globin for 24–48 hours after the ability to synthetize new mRNA has been eliminated from the terminally mature erythroblasts.

mRNA stability can also be altered in response to changes in the intracellular milieu. This phenomenon usually involves nucleases capable of destroying one or more broad classes of mRNA defined on the basis of their 3′ or 5′ UTR sequences. Thus, for example, histone mRNAs are destabilized after the S phase of the cell cycle is complete. Presumably this occurs because histone synthesis is no longer needed. Induction of cell activation, mitogenesis, or terminal differentiation events often results in the induction of nucleases that destabilize specific subsets of mRNAs. Selective stablization of mRNAs probably also occurs, but specific examples are less well documented.

The amount of a given protein accumulating in a cell depends on the amount of the mRNA present, the rate at which it is translated into the protein, and the stability of the protein. Translational efficiency depends on a number of variables, including polyadenylation and presence of the 5′ CAP. The amounts and state of activation of protein factors needed for translation are also crucial. The secondary structure of the mRNA, particularly in the 5′ UTR, greatly influences the intrinsic translatability of an mRNA molecule, by constraining the access of translation factors and ribosomes to the translation initiation signal in the mRNA. Secondary structure along the coding sequence of the mRNA may also have some impact on the rate of elongation of the peptide.

Changes in capping, polyadenylation, and translation factor efficiency affect the overall rate of protein synthesis within each cell. These effects tend to be global, rather than specific to a particular gene product. However, these effects influence the relative amounts of different proteins made. mRNAs whose structures inherently lend themselves to more efficient transla-

tion will tend to compete better for rate-limiting components of the translational apparatus, whereas those mRNAs that are inherently less translatable will tend to be translated less efficiently in the face of limited access to other translational components. For example, the translation factor eIF-4 tends to be produced in higher amounts when cells encounter transforming or mitogenic events. This causes an increase in overall rates of protein synthesis, but also leads to a selective increase in the synthesis of some proteins that were underproduced prior to mitogenesis.

Translational regulation of individual mRNA species is critical for some events important to blood cell homeostasis. For example, as discussed in Chapter 38, the amount of iron entering a cell is an exquisite regulator of the rate of ferritin mRNA translation. An mRNA sequence, called the iron response element, is recognized by a specific mRNA binding protein, but only when the protein lacks iron. mRNA bound to the protein is translationally inactive. As iron accumulates in the cell, the protein becomes iron bound and loses its affinity for the mRNA, resulting in production of apoferritin molecules available to bind the iron.

Tubulin synthesis involves coordinated regulation of translation and mRNA stability. Tubulin regulates the stability of its own mRNA via a feedback loop. As tubulin concentrations rise in the cell, it interacts with its own mRNA through the intermediary of an mRNA-binding protein. This results in the formation of a mRNA-protein complex and nucleolytic cleavage of the mRNA. The mRNA is destroyed, and further tubulin production is halted.

These examples of post-transcriptional regulation emphasize that cells tend to use every step in the complex pathway of gene expression as points at which exquisite control over the amounts of a particular protein can be regulated. In other chapters, additional levels of regulation are described (e.g., regulation of the stability, activity, localization, and access to other cellular components of the proteins that are present in a cell).

Additional Structural Features of Genomic DNA

Most DNA does not code for RNA or protein molecules. The vast majority of nucleotides present in the human genome reside outside structural genes. Structural genes are separated from one another by as few as 1–5 kb, or as many as several thousand kilobases of DNA. Almost nothing is known about the reason for the erratic clustering and spacing of genes along chromosomes. It is clear that *intergenic* DNA contains a variegated landscape of structural features that provide useful tools to localize genes, identify individual human beings as unique from every other human being (DNA fingerprinting), and diagnose human diseases by linkage. A more detailed discussion of these techniques is included in Chapter 164. Only a brief introduction is provided here.

The rate of mutation in DNA under normal circumstances is approximately $1/10^6$. In other words, 1 of 1 million bases of DNA will be mutated during each round of DNA replication. If these mutations occur in bases critical to the structure or function of a protein or gene, altered function, disease, or a lethal condition will often result. Most pathologic mutations tend not to be preserved throughout many generations because of their unfavorable phenotypes. Exceptions, such as the hemoglobinopathies, occur when the heterozygous state for these mutations confers selective advantage in the face of unusual environmental conditions, such as malaria epidemics. These "adaptive" mutations drive the dynamic change in the genome with time (evolution).

The vast majority of mutations that accumulate in the DNA of *Homo sapiens* occur in either intergenic DNA, or "silent" bases of DNA, such as the degenerate third bases of codons. They do not pathologically alter the function of the gene or its products. These clinically harmless mutations are called DNA polymorphisms. DNA polymorphisms can be regarded exactly as one regards other types of polymorphisms that have been widely recognized for years (e.g., eye and hair color, blood groups, etc.). They are variations in the population that occur without apparent clinical impact. Each of us differs from other humans in the precise number and type of DNA polymorphisms that we possess.

Like other types of polymorphisms, DNA polymorphisms breed true. In other words, if an individual's DNA contains a G 1,200 bases upstream from the α-globin gene, instead of the C most commonly found in the population, that G will be transmitted to that individual's offspring. Note that if one had a means for distinguishing the G at that position from a C, one would have a linked marker for that individual's α-globin gene.

Occasionally, a DNA polymorphism will fall within a restriction endonuclease site. (Restriction enzymes cut DNA molecules into smaller pieces, but only at limited sites, defined by short base sequences recognized by each enzyme.) The change could abolish the site or create a site where one did not exist before. These polymorphisms will change the array of fragments (by creating or eliminating a fragment from the array) generated when the genome is digested by that restriction endonuclease. This permits detection by use of the appropriate restriction enzyme. This specific class of polymorphisms is thus called restriction fragment length polymorphisms (RFLPs).

RFLPs are useful because the length of a restriction endonuclease fragment on which a gene of interest resides provides a linked marker for that gene. The exploitation of this fact for diagnosis of genetic diseases and detection of specific genes is discussed in Chapter 164; Fig. 1-6 shows a simple example.

RFLPs have proved to be extraordinarily useful for the diagnosis of genetic diseases, especially when the precise mutation is not known. Recall that DNA polymorphisms breed true in the population. For example, as discussed in Chapter 105, a mutation that causes hemophilia will, when it occurs on the X chromosome, be transmitted to subsequent generations attached to the pattern (often called a framework or haplotype) of RFLPs that were present on that same X chromosome. If one knows the pattern of RFLPs in the parents, one can detect the presence of the abnormal chromosome in the offspring.

An important feature of the DNA landscape is the high degree of repeated DNA sequence. A DNA sequence is said to be repeated if it or a sequence very similar (homologous) to it occurs more than once in a genome. Some multicopy genes, such as the histone genes and the ribosomal RNA genes, are repeated DNA sequences. The vast majority of repeated DNA occurs outside genes, or within introns. Indeed, the human genome appears to consist of 30–45% repeated DNA sequences.

The function of repeated sequences remains totally unknown, but their presence has inspired useful strategies for detecting and characterizing individual genomes. For example, a pattern of short repeated DNA sequences, characterized by the presence of flanking sites recognized by the restriction endonuclease Alu-1 (called Alu-repeats) occurs 300,000 or so times in a human genome. These sequences are not present in the mouse genome. If one wishes to infect mouse cells with human DNA and then identify the human DNA sequences within the infected mouse cells, one simply probes for the presence of Alu-repeats. The Alu-repeat thus serves as a signature of human DNA.

Classes of highly repeated DNA sequences called variable number of tandem repeats (VNTRs) have proved to be useful for distinguishing genomes of each human individual. VNTRs

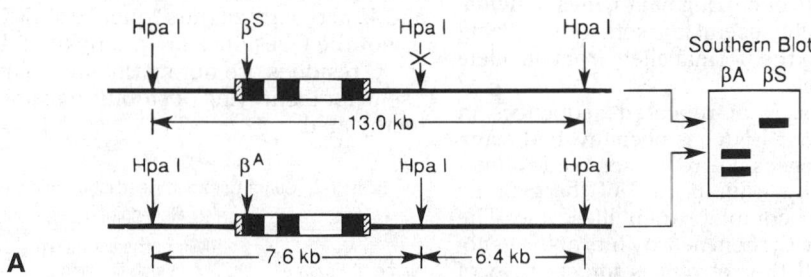

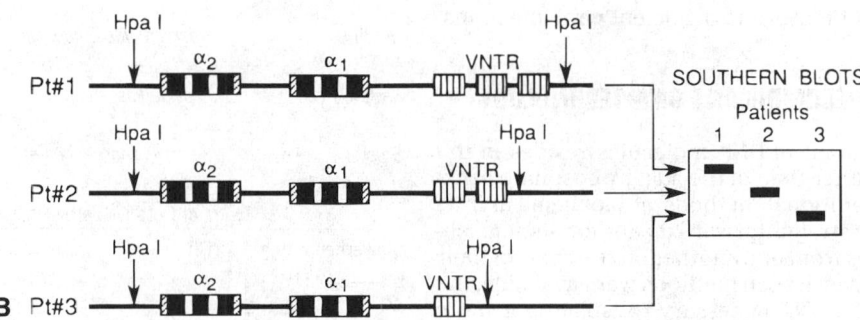

Fig. 1-6. Two useful forms of sequence variation among the genomes of normal individuals. **(A)** Presence of a DNA sequence polymorphism that falls within a restriction endonuclease site, thus altering the pattern of restriction endonuclease digests obtained from this region of DNA on Southern blot analysis. (Readers not familiar with Southern blot analysis should return to examine this figure after reading later sections of this chapter.) **(B)** A VNTR region (defined and discussed in the text). Note that individuals can vary from one to another in many ways according to how many repeated units of the VNTR are located on their genomes, whereas RFLP differences are in effect all-or-none differences, allowing for only two variables (restriction site presence or absence).

are short DNA sequences, usually less than a few hundred bases long, that tend to occur in tandem clusters (Fig. 1-6). For example, there is a VNTR near the insulin gene. In some individuals or populations it is present in only a few tandem copies, whereas in others it is present in many more. When the population as a whole is examined, there is a wide degree of variability from individual to individual as to the number of these repeats residing near the insulin gene. One can readily imagine that, if one had probes to detect a dozen or so distinct VNTR regions, each human individual would differ from virtually all other human individuals with respect to the aggregate pattern of these VNTRs. Indeed, it can be shown mathematically that the probability of any two human beings sharing exactly the same pattern of VNTRs is exceedingly small if one maps about 10–12 different VNTR elements for each person. A technique called DNA fingerprinting that is based on VNTR analysis has become widely publicized because of its forensic applications.

VNTRs can be regarded as normal sequence variations in DNA that are similar to, but far more useful than, single base change RFLP polymorphisms. Note that the odds of a single base change altering a convenient restriction endonuclease site are relatively small, so that RFLPs occurring in a useful region of the genome occur relatively infrequently. Moreover, there is only one state or variable that can be examined, that is, the presence or absence of the restriction site. By contrast, many VNTRs are scattered throughout the human genome. Most of these can be distinguished from one another quite readily by standard blotting and hybridization technology (see Ch. 164). Most importantly, the amount of variability from individual to individual at each site of a VNTR is considerably greater than for RFLPs. Rather than the mere presence or absence of a site, there is a whole array of banding patterns possible, depending on how many individual repeats are present at that site (Fig. 1-6). One can readily extend the above reasoning to appreciate that those VNTRs occurring near genes of hematologic interest can provide highly useful markers for localizing that gene, or for distinguishing the normal allele from an allele carrying a pathologic mutation.

There are many other classes of repeated sequences in human DNA. For example, human DNA has been invaded many times in its history by retroviruses. Retroviruses tend to integrate into human DNA and then "jump out" of the genome when they are reactivated, to complete their life cycle. The proviral genomes often carry with them nearby bits of the genomic DNA in which they sat. If the retrovirus infects DNA of another individual at another site, it will insert this genomic bit. Through many cycles of infection, the virus will act as a transposon, scattering its attached sequence throughout the genome. These types of sequences are called long interspersed elements. They represent footprints of ancient viral infections.

BASIC TENETS OF RECOMBINANT DNA TECHNOLOGY

The informational content of DNA molecules resides in the nucleotide sequence, rather than in the sugar phosphate backbone. Unfortunately, traditional methods of biochemical fractionation do not provide straightforward means for distinguishing nuclei acid molecules from one another on the basis of their nucleotide sequences. Even if such methods were available, the quantity of bulk genomic DNA necessary to isolate a gene of typical size (a few thousand or tens of thousands nucleotides long) from a complex genome such as the human (3 billion bp long) renders these methods impractical. In addition, genes do not exist in cells as discrete DNA molecules; rather, genes are linked together in tandem with very long stretches of intergenic DNA to form chromosomes. For example, in the human genome, each chromosome is about 100 million bp long. These facts render DNA an unworkable substance for direct physical purification of genes.

Recombinant DNA technology circumvents the biochemical problems inherent in the properties of DNA by combining enzymologic, microbiologic, and genetic approaches.

Restriction Endonucleases

Restriction endonucleases recognize short DNA base sequences and cleave DNA within or near these recognition sequences (Table 1-2). For example, EcoR1, a restriction endonuclease isolated from Escherichia coli, cuts DNA at the sequence 5'-GAATTC-3', but nowhere else. Thus, each DNA sample will be reduced reproducibly to an array of smaller sized fragments whose size ranges depend on the distribution with which 5'-GAATTC-3' is encountered in that particular genome. However, the DNA will not be degraded in any other way by the enzyme. Restriction endonucleases differ from other nucleases by the specificity and limited manner with which they degrade DNA.

Restriction enzymes are generally named after the bacteria from which they were isolated. Thus, the first restriction endonuclease activity purified from Serratia marcescens is called SmaI, the second from Haemophilus parainfluenzae, is called HpaII, and so forth. Each of the nearly 500 restriction endonucleases that have been described recognizes a unique oligonucleotide sequence and cleaves the DNA only at those points. Table 1-2 shows the names and recognition sites of some typical restriction endonucleases.

In some cases, two or more different restriction enzymes recognize exactly the same recognition sequence. Such restriction enzymes are called isoschizomers. A useful type of isoschizomer is a pair of restriction enzymes that recognize the same sequence but cut or fail to cut according to modifications of the DNA bases, notably methylation. For example, both HpaII and MspI recognize the sequence 5'-GCCG-3'. MspI cuts whether or not the C residues are methylated, but HpaII will only cut if the C residues are not methylated. These paired enzymes are useful for identifying positions in mammalian genomes that are methylated.

Table 1-2. Some Common Restriction Endonuclease Enzymes and Their Recognition Sequences

Name of Enzyme	Microorganism from Which Derived	Recognition and Cleavage Site
EcoRI	Escherichia coli	5'-GAATTC3' 3'CTTAAG5'
BamHI	Bacillus amyloliquefaciens	5'-GGATCC3' 3'CCTAGG5'
HindIII	Haemophilus influenzae	5'AAGCTT3' 3'TTCGAA5'
SauBA, Pst	Providencia stuartii	5'CTGCAG3' 3'GACGTC5'
Smal	Serratia marcescenes	5'GGGCCC3' 3'CCCGGG5'

Types of Cuts Made by Restriction Enzymes		
5' overhand: (e.g., EcoRI)		
5'------GAATTC----3' 3'------CTTAAG----5'	5'--------G3' 3'--------CTTAA-5'	5'-AATTC------3' 3'-G------5'
3' overhang: (cg PstI)		
5'------CTGCAG----3' 3'------GACGTC----5'	5'-----CTGCA3' 3'-----G5'	5'G------3' 3'-ACGTC------5'
Blunt end: (Smal)		
5'---GGGCCC---3' 3'---CCCGGG---3'	5'----GGG–3' 3'----CCC–5'	5'CCC--------3' 3'GGG--------5'

Even though their physiologic function remains unknown, restriction enzymes have proved to be extraordinarily useful in the laboratory. They reduce the sizes of DNA fragments in a controlled and reproducible manner from several hundred million base pairs long to fragment arrays ranging from a few dozen to a few tens of thousands of bases long. These ranges are far more manageable experimentally. Moreover, by digesting a DNA sample with combinations of restriction enzymes, one can construct maps or "fingerprints" of the restriction endonuclease sites in a genome. Restriction endonuclease digestion is as useful an approach for characterizing the fine structure of genomes as partial proteolytic digestion (peptide fingerprinting) has been for protein chemists.

Many restriction endonucleases cut the DNA so as to leave short single-stranded overhanging regions or "sticky ends" at the 5' or 3' end of the cutting site, while other enzymes leave blunt or flush double-stranded ends. Since many restriction endonuclease sites are palindromes (reading exactly the same on each strand, provided one reads in the same direction (e.g., 5'→3') on each strand, these overhanging ends are particularly useful. For example, if one digests DNA from two different sources (such as a bacteriophage preparation and human genomic preparation) with *Eco*RI, the "sticky ends" will be complementary by Watson-Crick base pairing and can thus be annealed at the single-stranded overhangs (Table 1-2). This is the most popular method for generating recombinant DNA molecules.

Enzymes Useful for Modifying and Synthesizing DNA

Several other nucleic acid modifying enzymes have been critical to the development of recombinant DNA technology. Notable among these are reverse transcriptase (RNA-dependent DNA polymerase) and DNA ligase. Reverse transcriptase is the enzyme packaged inside retroviruses that have an RNA genome. In order for retroviruses to reproduce themselves within their cellular hosts, their RNA genomes must be transcribed into DNA molecules (RNA→DNA) that can then be replicated (DNA→DNA) and expressed by host cell machinery (DNA→RNA).

Reverse transcriptase has a very useful property. If provided with an appropriate primer DNA sequence complementary to a small region of an mRNA molecule, it can read the mRNA strand in a 3'→5' direction and transcribe a single-stranded DNA copy (copy DNA, complementary DNA [cDNA]) of the RNA molecule. Using an oligonucleotide consisting of 12–18 dT residues (oligo dT) (recall that nearly all mRNAs in eukaryotes have a 3' poly(A) tail, complementary to the oligo dT), one can thus incubate reverse transcriptase with mRNA isolated from a cell or tissue of interest with reverse transcriptase and generate a population of single-stranded DNA molecules representing the entire array of mRNAs expressed in that cell or tissue. For example, using additional enzymes that have been characterized and purified, a DNA-dependent DNA polymerase can synthesize a complementary second strand of DNA from the single-stranded cDNA template. This creates double-stranded DNA molecules containing the sequence information originally expressed in the form of the mRNAs in the specimen. These DNA molecules can then be manipulated in the same ways that native genomic DNA molecules can, by restriction endonuclease digestion, radioactive labeling, or insertion into microbial host vectors for cloning.

DNA ligase is an enzyme that can join the ends of two DNA molecules together to form a single DNA molecule. For example, one can join double-stranded cDNA molecules with bacteriophage DNA molecules by incubating DNA from both sources together in the presence of DNA ligase. This ability to generate

artificially recombined, or recombinant, DNA molecules has given rise to the term recombinant DNA technology.

Many other important enzymes have also been useful for the development of recombinant DNA technology. These include a variety of polymerases, kinases, endonucleases, and exonucleases that are used to introduce radioactive residues into DNA molecules, to phosphorylate or dephosphorylate their termini, to synthesize new strands, to elongate the ends of DNA molecules by adding single-stranded overhanging sequences, to truncate or trim single-stranded overhangs in order to generate blunt-ended molecules, and so forth. A vast array of elegant methods have been developed to exploit these enzymes in order to synthesize, modify, and combine DNA molecules with exquisite precision, thus re-engineering DNA.

Microbial Hosts and Infectious DNA Molecules

The development of methods to fragment DNA in a controlled fashion, polymerize it, modify it, or ligate two DNA molecules from dissimilar sources represented an impressive advance. However, these tools would have been of limited value except for the discovery of certain small DNA molecules that possess remarkable biologic properties. Microbial geneticists found that many bacteria harbored DNA molecules that were not part of the single major bacterial chromosome. These novel DNA molecules are small (a few thousand to about 100 thousand bases long), have circular structures, can replicate independently in host cells, and, most remarkably, are infectious in the form of naked DNA. These DNA molecules can be thought of as elemental commensal organisms, residing in the cell and capable of infecting other host bacteria. They have come to be called extrachromosomal elements or episomes.

The most relevant episome types are plasmids and bacteriophages. Plasmids (Fig. 1-7) useful in recombinant DNA technology usually carry one or more antibiotic resistance genes, an origin of DNA replication, and a limited but useful array of restriction endonuclease sites. Many useful plasmid vectors have been engineered for customized applications. Such vectors are 3,000–10,000 bases long, carry one or two genes for antibiotic resistance, and include a short DNA sequence (polylinker) containing several tightly clustered restriction endonuclease sites. The polylinker sequence is in a noncritical region of the plasmid genome, so one can cut at a restriction site in the linker without damaging the plasmid's genes. Cells infected with these plasmids can be detected and purified by their ability to grow in media containing the relevant antibiotic.

The most useful plasmids for recombinant DNA work are those in which the plasmid or its polylinker include several restriction endonuclease sites that occur only once in the plasmic genome. A single cut in the circle will cause opening or linearization, while leaving all the biologically critical sequences intact. One can then insert a DNA molecule into the opening, reseal the loop with DNA ligase, and thereby generate a recombinant DNA molecule that retains all the useful biologic activities of the original plasmid.

Bacteriophages are viruses infective in certain species of bacteria. Their genomes are somewhat larger than plasmids (5,000–100,000 bp), and the DNA is covered during the extracellular part of the viral life span by a protein coat. However, bacterial genomes relevant to this discussion can also exist in the cell as episomes. The most useful phages for molecular genetics have been bacteriophage-λ, which can be used as a gene cloning vehicle, and the single-stranded bacteriophage M13, which is useful for DNA sequencing. Many bacteriophage genomes have been engineered to provide useful vectors.

The essential aspect of episomes important for this discussion is that they are biologically active even when they exist

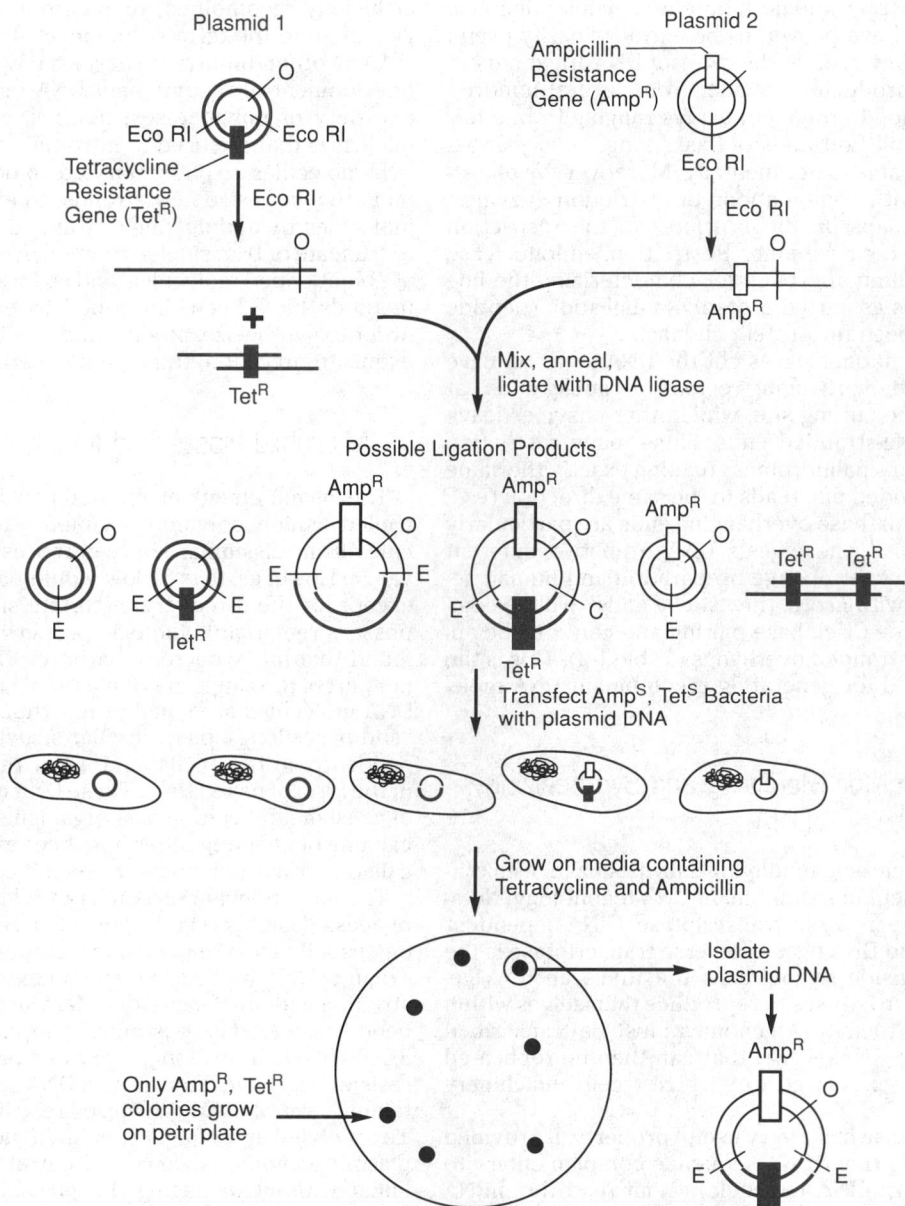

Fig. 1-7. Plasmids—structure and properties. The upper portions of the diagram outline the basic structure of bacterial plasmids in terms of two hypothetical examples (p1 and p2). The three major functional attributes of plasmids are shown at the top of the figure: origin of DNA (O), one or more phenotypic marker genes such as tetracycline resistance (Tet^R [shown in red]) or ampicillin resistance (Amp^R), and restriction endonuclease sites suitable in their location and number for a particular application, such as the *Eco* RI sites shown for p1 and p2. The remainder of the figure outlines a rudimentary recombinant DNA experiment, which results in formation of a novel new plasmid carrying the gene for tetracycline resistance in addition to the ampicillin resistance gene. Note how digestion with *Eco* RI linearizes plasmid p2 because it has only a single site, leaving the basic structure of the plasmid intact; in contrast, the two *Eco* RI sites in p1 result in fragmentation into two pieces, one of which carries the Tet^R gene. Ligation of the two digestion mixtures results in several possible ligation products, including those formed by self-ligation of the individual plasmids or plasmid fragments by means of their own "sticky ends" as well as all possible combinations formed by one fragment annealing to another. However, out of this complex mixture the desired recombinant can be clearly selected, since only it will possess both ampicillin and tetracycline resistance. Thus, one can use microbial genetics to identify and purify a DNA fragment that was created chemically or enzymatically. This illustrates the fundamental strategy of recombinant DNA technology, whereby genetic selection of biologically active macromolecules can be used to identify, isolate, purify, and amplify particular products of enzymatic reactions.

as "naked" DNA molecules. By combining the ability to attach episomal DNA to DNA from mammalian sources (via restriction enzymes and ligase) with the capacity of the episomes for infection and phenotypic alteration of host cells, one can use these molecules to introduce foreign DNA into host bacteria. Then all the useful properties of the vast array of microbial strains available become accessible for the study of genes from other

species. Individual strains of bacteria can be readily isolated as single cell clones, grown in extremely large quantities for relatively little expense, and used as factories for the production of the foreign DNA sequence contained within it, as well as any protein product encoded by the foreign DNA. Moreover, the recombinant episomal DNA can be readily isolated free of the host bacterial chromosome; this provides a simple way to retrieve large quantities of the mammalian DNA that rides as a passenger in the episomal DNA.

Advances in Nucleic Acid Chemistry

The development of automated anhydrous methods for the synthesis of DNA molecules in vitro has provided a means of synthesizing short DNA molecules without benefit of a template or DNA polymerase. For example, the polylinker sequences used to introduce restriction endonuclease sites into plasmids can be readily synthesized by automated instrumentation and ligated into a plasmid in order to alter its restriction endonuclease map. Synthetic oligonucleotides can also be radiolabeled and used as customized molecular hybridization probes, or used as primers for synthesis of DNA strands complementary to any desired region of a DNA template.

The tendency of DNA and RNA molecules to form double-stranded hybrids in physiologic solution has been exploited by nucleic acid chemists for the development of molecular hybridization assays. If DNA or RNA molecules are heated or exposed to certain denaturants, such as formamide, the hydrogen bonds holding two strands together are disrupted, and the molecule is denatured into the single-stranded form. Temperature, salt, and denaturing conditions that favor reannealing into the double-stranded form can then be restored. This reannealing process is called *molecular hybridization:* Reannealing rates under a given set of conditions of temperature, salt, and denaturant are a function of the time of incubation and the initial concentration of the annealing strands.

Denatured DNA or RNA strands will reanneal only with strands having a complementary sequence by the rules of Watson-Crick base pairing. This specificity forms the basis for the use of molecular hybridization as a means for detecting or quantifying (or both) specific DNA or RNA moieties within a complex mixture. One can incubate a specimen of denatured DNA or RNA (e.g., mRNA from human bone marrow) with a radioactively labeled, defined DNA or RNA sequence (e.g., a cloned human myeloperoxidase gene). The labeled denatured DNA probe will hybridize only to those mRNA molecules that are complementary by Watson-Crick base pairing (i.e., myeloperoxidase mRNA molecules). One can then utilize any one of several available techniques to detect the fraction of radioactively labeled DNA probe molecules that have been bound into a double-stranded form. (For example, the enzyme S_1 nuclease degrades single-stranded DNA molecules, leaving only the double-stranded hybridized molecules intact.) The result is a highly sensitive and specific assay for identifying (in our example) myeloperoxidase mRNA within the complex mix of mRNA species present in the bone marrow of mRNA. By extension of this reasoning, one can use molecular hybridization strategies to detect, quantitate, and map specific DNA or RNA sequences, provided that a complementary defined DNA probe is available.

Many hybridization assays have been devised. The range of applications, theoretical rationale, and utility of many of these assays can be appreciated by their analogy to the use of antigen/antibody reactions in immunochemistry. The DNA probe is used by the molecular geneticist in much the same way as a defined antibody probe is used by the immunologist. The principles underlying the various molecular hybridization techniques are similar to those of immunochemical assays.

Polymerase Chain Reaction

The development of the polymerase chain reaction (PCR) was a major breakthrough that has revolutionized the utility of a DNA-based strategy for diagnosis and treatment. It permits one to detect, synthesize, and isolate specific genes and to distinguish among alleles of a gene differing as little as one base. It does not require sophisticated equipment or unusual technical skills. A clinical specimen consisting of only minute amounts of tissue will suffice; in most circumstances, no special preparation of the tissue is necessary. PCR thus makes recombinant DNA techniques accessible to clinical laboratories. This single advance has produced a quantum increase in the use of direct gene analysis for diagnosis of human diseases.

PCR is based on the prerequisites for copying an existing DNA strand by DNA polymerase: an existing denatured strand of DNA to be used as the template and a primer. Primers are short oligonucleotides, 12–100 bases in length, having a base sequence complementary to the desired region of the existing DNA strand. The enzyme requires the primer in order to "know" where to begin copying. If one knows the base sequence of DNA of the gene one wishes to study, then it is a simple matter to prepare a synthetic oligonucleotide complementary to 2-base sequences flanking the region of interest (see Ch. 164). If these are the only oligonucleotides present in the reaction mixture, then the DNA polymerase can only copy daughter strands of DNA downstream from those oligonucleotides. Recall that DNA is double-stranded, that the strands are held together by the rules of Watson-Crick base pairing, and that they are aligned in antiparallel fashion. This implies that the effect of incorporation of both oligonucleotides into the reaction mix will be to synthesize two daughter strands of DNA, one originating upstream of the gene and the other originating downstream. The net effect is synthesis of only the DNA between the two primers, thus doubling only the DNA containing the region of interest. If one now heat denatures the DNA, allows hybridization of the daughter strands to the primers, and repeats the polymerization, then the region of DNA through the gene of interest is doubled again. Thus, two cycles of denaturation, annealing, and elongation result in a selective quadrupling of the gene of interest.

The cycle can be repeated 30–50 times, resulting in a selective and geometric amplification of the sequence of interest to the 2^{30}–2^{50} times. The result is a million-fold or higher selective amplification of the gene of interest, yielding microgram quantities of that DNA sequence.

The PCR reaction achieved practical utility when DNA polymerases from thermophilic bacteria were discovered, when synthetic oligonucleotides of any desired sequence could be produced efficiently, reproducibly, and cheaply by automated instrumentation, and when DNA thermocycling machines were developed. Thermophilic bacteria live in hot springs and other exceedingly warm environments. Thermophilic DNA polymerases can tolerate 100°C incubations without substantial loss of activity. Their advantage is that they retain activity in a reaction mix that is repeatedly heated to the high temperature needed to denature the DNA strands into the single-stranded form. Microprocessor-driven DNA thermocycler machines can be programmed to increase temperatures to 95°–100°C (denaturation), to cool the mix to 50°C rapidly (a good temperature for oligonucleotide annealing), and then to raise the temperature to 70°–75° (an excellent temperature for optimal activity of the thermophilic DNA polymerases). The rapidity of these changes (30–60 seconds for each phase of the cycle) allows one to include the test specimen, the thermophilic polymerase, the primers, and the chemical components (e.g., nucleotide subunits, etc.) of the reaction mix in a single tube, place it in the thermocycler, and conduct many cycles of denaturation, annealing, and polymerization in a completely automated fashion. One can thus amplify the gene of interest over 1 millionfold in a matter of a few hours. The DNA product is readily identified and isolated by routine agarose gel electrophoresis. The DNA can then be analyzed by restriction endonuclease, digestion, hybridization to specific probes, sequencing, further amplification by cloning, and so forth.

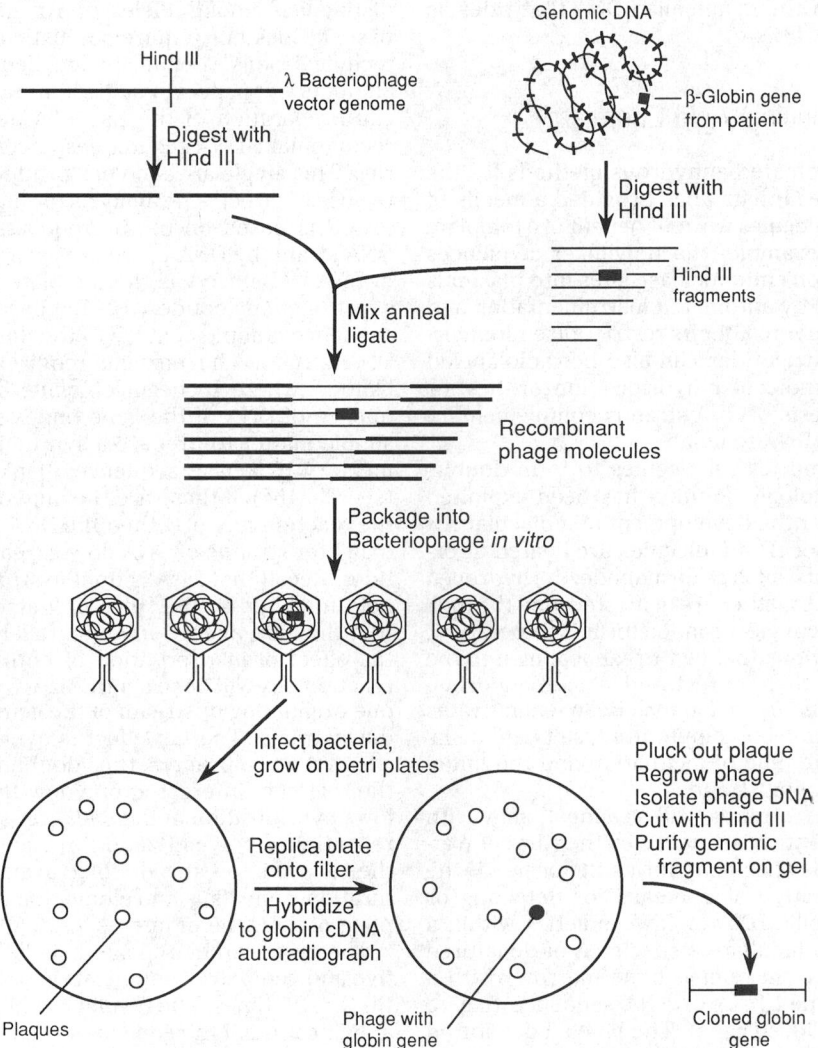

Fig. 1-8. Isolation of a genomic gene copy by molecular cloning. Illustrated here is a prototypical experiment whereby the chromosomal or genomic copy of the β-globin gene (shown in red) can be isolated by molecular cloning, using globin cDNA as a molecular hybridization probe. A suitable bacteriophage-λ cloning vector is digested with *Hind* III, which in the example cuts the phage only once, leaving two arms with "sticky ends." Genomic DNA is similarly digested. A vast array of fragments (only a few of which are shown) will result, their sizes depending on the location of the *Hind* III recognition sites. Ligation of the two digests to each other results in an array of bacteriophage DNA molecules, each containing a single fragment from the human genomic digest. The genomes are packaged into bacteriophage coats so that they become infectious viruses. These infect a culture of bacterial cells; each bacteriophage yields a plaque on a Petri plate as the result of subsequent rounds of reinfection and lysis of host cells on the plate. A replica of the plate is made by laying a filter over the plate, allowing it to absorb the colonies in situ, and hybridization of the filter to the radioactive globin cDNA probe. Only phage carrying the globin gene in the inserted genomic fragment will yield a positive autoradiography signal. This plaque is then isolated and used as starting material for isolation of the phage and the phage DNA. The globin gene can then readily be isolated by routine methods of DNA chemistry. The result is a highly purified representation of the gene and its surrounding sequences as it was configured in the original human genome.

Producing and Isolating Recombinant DNA Molecules

Most recombinant DNA methods require defined, purified DNA molecules encompassing all or part of the gene of interest. One basic algorithm for isolating genes by molecular cloning is presented (Fig. 1-8). Genomic DNA is isolated from nuclei and digested with restriction endonucleases to generate overhanging "sticky ends." (Alternatively, one can create a restricted subset of DNA sequences representing the genes expressed in a given cell by first isolating messenger RNA, converting it into cDNA by incubation with reverse transcriptase, and then converting it to double-stranded cDNA

using other enzymes.) The plasmid or bacteriophage DNA molecule to be used as a vector to carry the DNA into microbes is cut with the same restriction enzyme. The DNA molecules from the two sources thus have complementary "sticky ends." They are annealed together by means of their "sticky ends" under conditions of a slight excess of the microbial DNA vector. This procedure ensures that most of the vector molecules ligate to only one molecule from the mammalian source. The recombinant plasmids are then sealed with DNA ligase. Each recombinant molecule is thus an infectious DNA species carrying a single DNA fragment from the mammalian source as a passenger.

The plasmids are then used to infect an excess of host bacteria; the excess cell number ensures that each bacterium, on the average, acquires only a single recombinant DNA molecule. The host bacteria chosen lack some phenotypic property conferred by the infecting molecule, such as antibiotic resistance. The infected cells are then plated onto antibiotic-containing Petri plates at a density allowing detection of individual colonies or bacteriophage plaques. Each colony or phage plaque represents the progeny of a single cell or bacteriophage and is thus a clone of a single cell or phage carrying a single DNA fragment from the mammalian source. Therefore, that DNA fragment, or gene, has been physically and genetically isolated in the colony or plaque, separated from all other mammalian DNA fragments by the cloning process.

What remains is the need to identify the DNA fragment representing the specific gene one wishes to purify. One must identify within the array of plaques or colonies (called a recombinant DNA library) those cells or phages carrying the DNA sequence of interest. Numerous stratagems have been devised for screening these libraries for the presence of the occasional clone bearing the gene of interest. The approaches that are suitable depend on what information is available about the particular gene or its protein product. In some cases, one employs molecular hybridization to a DNA probe synthesized to contain a sequence encoding a known partial amino acid sequence (determined by sequencing a peptide or protein fragment of interest). In other cases, the microbial vector has the capacity to express part or all of the protein encoded by the DNA clone. The library can then be screened with antibodies raised against the protein of interest by conventional means.

Once one has identified the colony or bacteriophage plaque containing the recombinant molecule of interest, that colony or plaque can be purified free of the remainder of the library and amplified by growth in bacterial culture. In this manner, one can produce substantial quantities of recombinant DNA molecules from the cloned host cell. With respect to other DNA molecules derived from the original tissue source, the cloned gene will be pure. The purified gene can then be used as a hybridization probe, as the substrate for obtaining its DNA sequence, or as a template for controlled expression and production of its mRNA and protein products.

DNA and RNA Blotting

There are many ways that a cloned DNA sequence can be exploited to characterize the behavior of normal or pathologic genes relevant to hematology. Blotting methods deserve special mention because of their widespread use in clinical and experimental hematology. A cloned DNA fragment can be easily purified and tagged with a radioactive or nonradioactive label. The fragment provides a pure and highly specific molecular hybridization probe for the detection of complementary DNA or RNA molecules in any specimen of DNA or RNA. One set of assays that has proved particularly useful involves Southern gene blotting, named after Dr. E. Southern, who invented the method. Southern blotting allows detection of a specific gene, or region within or near a gene, in a DNA preparation (Fig. 1-9). The DNA is isolated and digested with one or more restriction endonucleases, and the resulting fragments are separated according to their molecular size by electrophoresis on agarose gels. Under conditions routinely used, the largest fragments migrate most slowly and the smallest fragments most rapidly. Unfortunately, one does not necessarily know the size of the fragment containing the gene of interest. Moreover, a human genomic DNA preparation digested with most restriction enzymes will yield many hundreds or thousands of fragments, producing a blur or streak on the gel. A final impediment to detection of the individual gene within this massive array of fragments is the unsuitability of agarose and acrylamide for molecular hybridization conditions.

Gene blotting circumvents these problems. The agarose gel is placed on top of a pad or sponge saturated in a high salt buffer. A sheet of nitrocellulose, nylon, or a similar permeable membrane is laid on top of the gel. Large numbers of dry towels are laid on top of the filter, and a weight is placed on top of

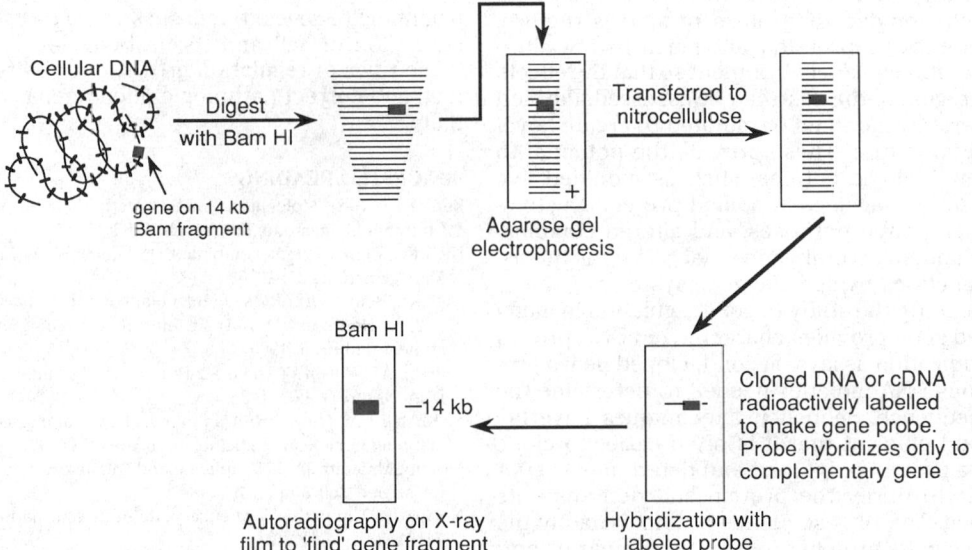

Fig. 1-9. Southern gene blotting. Detection of a genomic gene (red) that resides on a 14 kb *Eco* R1 fragment. To identify the presence of a gene in the genome and the size of the restriction fragment on which it resides, genomic DNA is digested with a restriction enzyme, and the fragments are separated by agarose gel electrophoresis. Human genomes contain from several hundred thousand to 1 million sites for any particular restriction enzyme, which results in a vast array of fragments and creates a blur or streak on the gel; one fragment cannot be distinguished from another readily. If the DNA in the gel is transferred to nitrocellulose by capillary blotting; however, it can be further analyzed by molecular hybridization to a radioactive cDNA probe for the gene. Only the band containing the gene will yield a positive autoradiography signal, as shown. If a disease state were to result in loss of the gene, alteration of its structure, or mutation (altering recognition sites for one or more restriction enzymes), the banding pattern would be changed.

the entire stack in order to ensure air- and water-tight contact among all of layers. By capillary action, fluid will be drawn from the saturated sponge or pad through the porous gel and the nitrocellulose membrane and into the dry pad of towels. The DNA will also be drawn out of the gel, but, if care is taken to denature the DNA to the single-stranded form prior to initiating the blotting, it will not pass through the semipermeable membrane. Single-stranded DNA and RNA molecules will stick noncovalently but tightly to the membrane. In this fashion the membrane becomes a replica or blot of the gel. These membranes are much more amenable to subsequent manipulation and can be used in molecular hybridization assays.

After the blotting procedure is complete, the membrane is dipped in a hybridization buffer containing the radioactively labeled probe. The probe will hybridize only to the gene of interest and render radioactive only one or a few bands containing complementary sequences. After appropriate washing and drying, the bands can be seen by autoradiography.

Digestion of a DNA preparation with several different restriction enzymes allows one to construct a restriction endonuclease map of a gene within the human genome. Southern blotting has thus become a standard way of characterizing the configuration of genes within the genome.

Northern blotting represents an analogous blotting procedure used to detect RNA. RNA cannot be digested with restriction enzymes (they cut only DNA); rather, the RNA molecules can be run intact (mRNAs are 0.5–12 kb in length), through the gel, blotted onto membranes, and probed with a DNA probe. In this fashion, one can detect the presence, absence, molecular size, number of individual species, and so forth of a particular mRNA species. Western blotting is an analogous procedure used to detect proteins with antibody probes.

SUMMARY

The elegance of recombinant DNA technology resides in the capacity it confers on investigators to examine each gene as a discrete physical entity that can be purified, reduced to its basic building blocks for decoding of its primary structure, analyzed for its patterns of expression, and perturbed by alterations in sequence or molecular environment so that the effects of changes in each region of the gene can be assessed. Purified genes can be deliberately modified or mutated to create novel genes not available in nature. These provide the potential to generate useful new biologic entities, such as modified live virus or purified peptide vaccines, modified proteins customized for specific therapeutic purposes, and altered combinations of regulatory and structural genes that allow for the assumption of new functions by specific gene systems.

Purified genes facilitate the study of gene regulation in many ways. First, a cloned gene provides characterized DNA probes for molecular hybridization assays. Second, cloned genes provide the homogenous DNA moieties needed to determine the exact nucleotide sequence. Sequencing techniques have become so reliable and efficient that it is often easier to clone the gene encoding a protein of interest and determine its DNA sequence than it is to purify the protein and determine its amino acid sequence. The DNA sequence predicts exactly the amino acid sequence of its protein product. By comparing normal sequences with the sequences of alleles cloned from patients known to be abnormal, such as the globin genes in the thalassemia or sickle cell syndromes, one can establish the normal and pathologic anatomy of genes critical to major hematologic diseases. In this manner it has been possible to iden-

tify many mutations responsible for various forms of thalassemia, hemophilia, thrombasthenia, red cell enzymopathies, porphyrias, and so forth. Similarly, single base changes have been shown to be the difference between normally functioning proto-oncogenes and their cancer-causing oncogene derivatives.

Third, cloned genes can be manipulated for studies of gene expression. Many vectors allowing efficient transfer of genes into eukaryotic cells have been perfected. Gene transfer technologies allow one to place the gene into the desired cellular environment and analyze the expression of that gene or the behavior of its products. These surrogate or reverse genetics systems allow analysis of the normal physiology of expression of a particular gene, as well as the pathophysiology of abnormal gene expression resulting from mutations.

Fourth, cloned genes enhance study of their protein products. By expressing fragments of the gene in microorganisms or eukaryotic cells, one can produce customized regions of a protein for use as an immunogen, thereby allowing preparation of a variety of useful and powerful antibody probes. Alternatively, one can prepare synthetic peptides deduced from the DNA sequence as the immunogen. Controlled production of large amounts of the protein also allows direct analysis of specific functions attributable to regions within that protein.

Finally, all of the above techniques can be extended by mutating the gene and examining the effects of those mutations on the expression of or the properties of the encoded mRNAs and proteins. By combining portions of one gene with another (chimeric genes), or abutting structural regions of one gene with regulatory sequences of another, one can investigate in previously inconceivable ways the complexities of gene regulation. These activist approaches to modifying gene structure or expression create the opportunity to generate new RNA and protein products whose applications are limited only by the collective imagination of the investigators.

The most important impact of the genetic approach to the analysis of biologic phenomena is presently the most indirect. Diligent and repeated application of the above algorithm to the study of many genes from diverse groups of organisms is beginning to reveal the basic strategies used by nature for the regulation of cell and tissue behavior. As our knowledge of these rules of regulation grows, our ability to understand, detect, and correct pathologic phenomena will increase substantially.

SUGGESTED READING

Benz EJ Jr (ed): Molecular Genetics Methods. Methods in Hematology Series. Churchill Livingstone, Edinburgh, 1989

High KA, Benz EJ Jr: Recombinant DNA technology in antenatal diagnosis. Lab Management 24:31, 1986

High KA, Benz EJ Jr: ABC's of molecular genetics: a haematologist's introduction. p. 25. In Hoffbrand AV (ed): Recent Advances in Hematology. Churchill Livingstone, Edinburgh, 1985

Jeffreys AJ, Wilson V, Thein SL: Hypervariable "minisatellite" regions in human DNA. Nature 314:67, 1985

McKusick VA: The morbid anatomy of the human genome: a review of gene mapping in clinical medicine. Medicine 66:1, 1987

Mount SM, Steitz JA: RNA splicing and the involvement of small ribonucleoproteins. Med Cell Biol 3:249, 1984

Nevins JR: The pathway of eukaryotic mRNA formation. Annu Rev Biochem 52: 441, 1983

Radin AL, Benz EJ Jr: Antenatal diagnosis of the hemoglobinopathies. Hematol Pathol 2:199, 1988

Rowley PT, Benz EJ Jr, Nienhuis AW: Molecular genetics for the hematologist. Curr Hematol Oncol 4:1, 1986

Weatherall DJ: The New Genetics and Clinical Practice. 2nd Ed. Oxford University Press, Oxford, 1985

Protein Synthesis and Intracellular Sorting

2

Philip P. Breitfeld and Robert J. Fallon

INTRODUCTION

The previous chapter discusses gene structure, transcription, RNA metabolism, and initiation of translation. This chapter focuses on distal cellular events (i.e., how cells synthesize specific proteins and then accomplish transport of the proteins to their appropriate site of function [destination]). This latter process is referred to as protein sorting, trafficking, or targeting and is critical, since the proper execution of cellular functions requires that specific proteins (e.g., enzymes, cytoskeletal proteins, DNA-binding proteins, growth factor receptors) find their way to a particular cellular location.

The importance of this process to the study of blood disorders arises from several considerations. First, several disorders exist that are primarily due to improper protein sorting. Second, orientation to the basic mechanisms of protein sorting will provide an important framework for understanding and integrating future developments in the investigation of blood disorders. Third, the understanding of the complex molecular mechanisms involved in proper protein sorting will serve as a substrate in the planned therapy of blood disorders via genetic engineering. During the discussion of the cellular mechanisms for protein sorting, examples from investigations of proteins relevant to blood diseases are stressed.

Background

Proteins are synthesized from an mRNA template through a process referred to as translation (see Ch. 1). Translation of mRNA occurs on ribosomes that are either free in the cytosol or are specifically bound to the rough endoplasmic reticulum (RER) (Fig. 2-1). The endoplasmic reticulum (ER) is a complex network of lipid membranes in which lipids and certain proteins are synthesized. The RER is that portion of the ER that contains bound ribosomes.

ER-bound ribosomes translate mRNAs coding for proteins that are secreted by the cell (e.g., von Willebrand factor [vWF] in the endothelial cell), that are expressed at the cell surface (e.g., band 3 of the red blood cell), or that span, or are contained within, the lumen of a membrane-limited organelle derived from the ER (the ER itself, the Golgi, or lysosome). Proteins synthesized on ER-bound ribosomes undergo a series of cotranslational modifications within the lumen of the ER as well as post-translational modifications within the lumen of either the ER or the Golgi. Fully modified proteins are then targeted to their destination. The protein could undergo secretion and exit from the cell or could localize in a membrane-limited organelle (ER, Golgi, lysosome) or the cell surface.

Free or cytosolic ribosomes, in contrast, translate mRNAs that code for either soluble cytosolic proteins (e.g., glycolytic enzymes, and the enzymes of the hexose monophosphate shunt, such as glucose 6-phosphate dehydrogenase), proteins that are associated with the cytosolic face of membranes (e.g., spectrin in the red blood cell), or proteins of certain organelles such as mitochondria, peroxisomes, and the nucleus. In large part, sorting of newly synthesized proteins is thought to be mediated by sorting signals contained within the proteins themselves that serve as "addresses," and thus direct proteins to the appropriate cellular destination.[1]

Relevance to Hematology

Are protein synthesis and sorting issues of importance for the study of medicine and hematology? Protein synthesis and sorting are the terminal regulators of gene expression. Therefore, any system or disease in which the regulation of gene expression is important can potentially bear on these issues. For example, it is now proposed that most of the mutations responsible for cystic fibrosis result in improper synthesis and sorting of the cystic fibrosis transmembrane conductance regulator (CFTR) protein. It has been shown that most naturally occurring mutations of the CFTR protein result in incomplete glycosylation of the protein, with subsequent degradation, most probably in the endoplasmic reticulum.[2] This leads to failure of expression of the fully glycosylated mature protein at the surface of epithelial cells. These mutations do not inhibit gene transcription or protein translation. Rather, the fully synthesized molecule fails to exit the ER—probably because the mutation led to improper folding of the molecule. Thus, the CFTR gene is functionally not expressed as a consequence of improper protein sorting.

One area of hematology in which protein synthesis and sorting has been shown to be particularly important is the fluid-phase blood clotting system. The cellular regulatory mechanisms required to generate the soluble blood protein factors responsible for proper hemostasis are vast and varied. Of particular relevance is the proper synthesis, assembly, and sorting of vWF and the vitamin K-dependent coagulation proteins (i.e., prothrombin, factor X, factor VII, factor IX, protein C, and protein S). After translation on ER-bound ribosomes, all of these proteins must travel through the appropriate cellular compartments for full chemical modification, assembly, and proteolytic processing prior to secretion of the fully functional form of the molecule. If these processes are not carried out, deficiency of the functional protein can occur. For example, certain forms of factor IX deficiency are due to point mutations in the pro sequence (see the section Chemical Modification and Post-Translational Processing) of the molecule. The molecule therefore fails to undergo γ-carboxylation, an important post-translational modification required for function, and an inactive form of factor IX is secreted.[3,4] Similarly, proteolytic cleavage of VWF precursors is thus required for proper assembly of functional multimeric complexes within Weibel-Palade bodies in endothelial cells.[5]

Defects in the synthesis and sorting of cell surface and other nonsecretory proteins have also been identified and may play a role in several disorders. Blood cells from patients with paroxysmal nocturnal hemoglobinuria (PNH) exhibit a generalized defect in expression at the plasma membrane of a family of proteins anchored to the membrane via a covalently attached glycolipid side chain.[6] This glycosylphosphatidylinositol (GPI) moiety is normally bound to the carboxyl terminus of the pro-

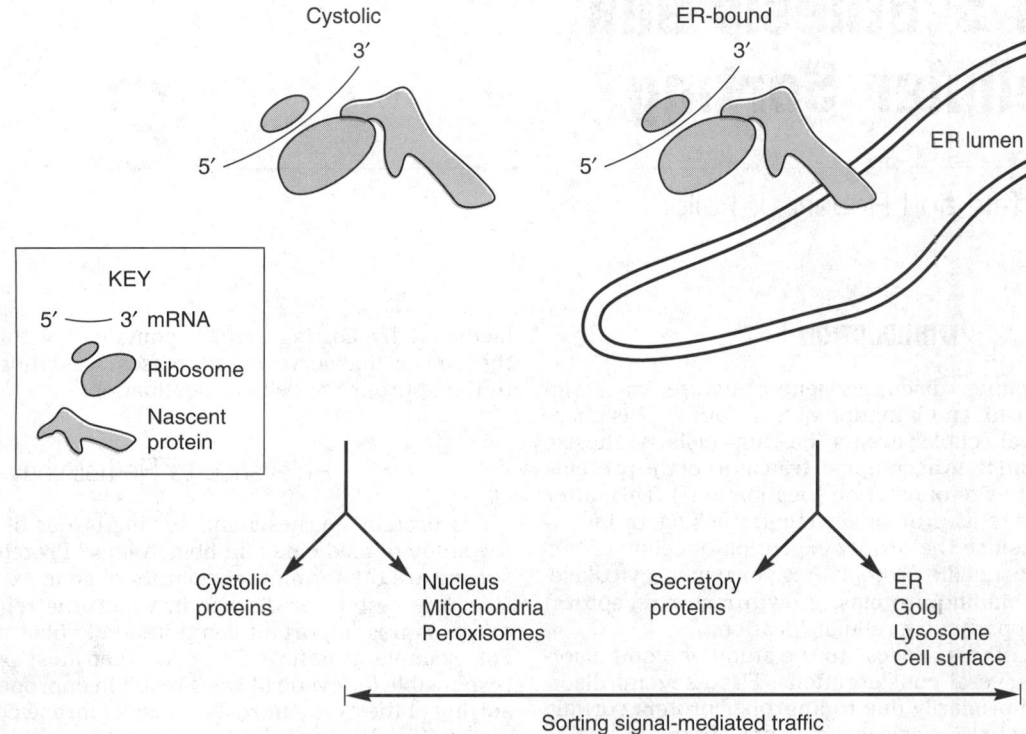

Fig. 2-1. Traffic of newly synthesized proteins. Proteins are translated from mRNA on cytosolic (free) or ER-bound ribosomes. Cytosolic ribosomes synthesize proteins that are destined for the cytosol or targeted to the nucleus, mitochondria, or peroxisomes. ER-bound ribosomes synthesize proteins that are destined for secretion or targeted to the ER, Golgi, lysosome, or cell surface. Most of this protein traffic (except for cytosolic proteins) is thought to be mediated in part by sorting signals.

tein within the ER lumen, a step that is defective in PNH.[7] The decreased expression in PNH of two GPI-linked cell surface proteins, decay-accelerating factor and membrane inhibitor of reactive lysis, is responsible for increased susceptibility to complement-mediated lysis of red blood cells.[8] Finally, the recently cloned gene *PIG-A,* which participates in the early steps of GPI anchor biosynthesis, has been demonstrated to account for these PNH defects[9] (see Ch. 25).

Nuclear-specific targeting signals have been defined.[10] They are critical for normal activity of transcription factors such as the erythroid lineage-specific factor NF-E2.[11] These targeting signals may be masked by post-translational events such as protein phosphorylation.[12]

In contrast to disorders caused by deficiencies in individual proteins, other diseases may be due to organelle dysgenesis. For example, individuals with Zellweger syndrome have severe neurologic complications and an absence of peroxisomes. Peroxisomal proteins are synthesized in these patients but do not localize to the proper organelle, suggesting that the organelle assembly/targeting apparatus is defective.[13] Defective protein targeting to granules may underlie rare phagocytic and platelet disorders. An example is Chédiak-Higashi syndrome, characterized by defective production of azurophilic granules in neutrophils and a storage pool deficiency in platelets. Selective loss of expression of two granule proteins (elastase and cathepsin G) occurs in neutrophils of patients with Chédiak-Higashi syndrome and in an animal model of this disease, beige mice.[14] Interestingly, bone marrow precursors from beige mice have a normal content of these enzymes, suggesting that protein processing or targeting to specific granules may represent the underlying defect in this disorder. These examples suggest that proper protein synthesis and intracellular transport are critical for organelle biogenesis.

SYNTHESIS AND TARGETING OF SECRETORY PROTEINS—MODEL FOR PROTEIN TRAFFIC

Secretory proteins serve as an excellent model for the cellular mechanisms involved in protein traffic. Secretory proteins are synthesized on ribosomes that are tightly bound to the ER. How does the cell determine which mRNAs should be translated on ER-bound ribosomes?

Translation/Translocation

Initially, all mRNAs undergoing translation are found associated with free, cytosolic ribosomes. However some mRNAs are more efficient than others in initiating translation. This translation efficiency is an important post-transcriptional regulator of gene expression. The translational efficiency of an individual mRNA is influenced by a number of structural features of the mRNAs themselves; for example, a favorable structure surrounding the AUG initiation codon[15] and the presence of a cap structure at the 5′ end[16] enhance translational efficiency. The presence of an out-of-frame initiation codon or stable secondary structure at the 5′ end[17] inhibits translational efficiency. A UA-rich sequence at the 3′ end of certain mRNAs coding for cytokines, growth factors, and oncoproteins (e.g., interferon, colony-stimulating factor-granulocyte/macrophage, and c-*fos*) can not only cause mRNA destabilization but also strongly inhibit translation.[18,19]

The translational control of the synthesis of the iron storage protein ferritin in response to cellular iron levels is another example of the importance of post-transcriptional control of gene expression.[20] In this system, in the presence of high levels of cellular iron, the repressor protein (iron-responsive element-binding protein) dissociates from a unique 5′ untranslated re-

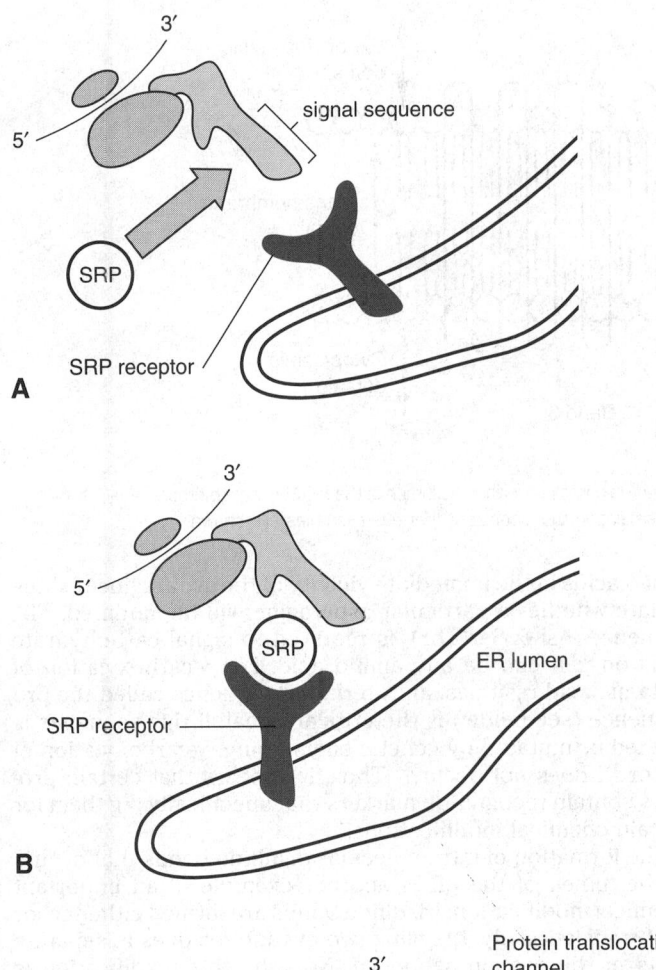

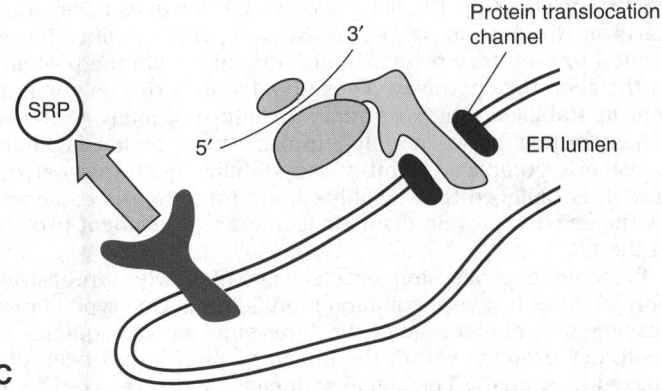

Fig. 2-2. Signal sequence targeting of ribosomes translating secretory proteins to the ER membrane. **(A)** As the N-terminal signal sequence of a secretory protein exits from the 60S subunit of the ribosome, it is specifically recognized by signal recognition particle (SRP). **(B)** SRP then binds to its receptor, thereby bringing the ribosome and attached polypeptide to the ER membrane. **(C)** SRP is released from its receptor, and the newly synthesized polypeptide chain is translocated across the membrane through a protein translocation channel into the lumen of the ER.

gion of ferritin mRNA called the iron-responsive element. This dissociation allows for increased translation of ferritin mRNA for storage of cellular iron (see Ch. 38).

Once translation has begun, the N terminus of the protein is synthesized first and gradually emerges from the 60S subunit of the ribosome (Fig. 2-2A). For almost all secretory proteins, this N terminus is composed of a 15–30-amino acid stretch that contains a highly hydrophobic core of amino acids. This N-terminal stretch of amino acids is termed the signal sequence.

It mediates a high-affinity interaction with signal recognition particle (SRP), which binds in turn to the SRP receptor at the cytoplasmic face of the ER (Fig. 2-2B & C); SRP provides the mechanism for targeting ribosomes that are translating secretory proteins to the ER.[21] In this way, secretory proteins are segregated from proteins that have other destinations such as mitochondria or the nucleus.

The importance of the signal sequence in the targeting of secreted proteins to the ER and, ultimately, the cell surface has been well demonstrated. Through genetic engineering, the signal sequence of a secretory protein has been attached to the N terminus of γ-globulin (a cytosolic protein). The resultant fusion protein is targeted to the RER and translated on ER-bound ribosomes.[22] Similarly, if the signal sequence of a secretory protein is deleted, the altered protein fails to be secreted from the cell. Thus, the signal sequence is necessary and sufficient for protein secretion. It is noteworthy that, although these signal sequences perform a single specific function, they display a great diversity at the amino acid sequence level.[23]

Once a secretory protein has been targeted to the ER membrane, translation of the mRNA continues. Interestingly, the interaction of SRP with its receptor is transient.[24] Soon after attachment of the ribosome occurs, SRP is released from its receptor and the signal sequence in a reaction dependent on guanosine triphosphate hydrolysis[25] (Fig. 2-2C). The translating ribosome remains attached to the ER. As the polypeptide chain elongates and exits from the ER-bound ribosome, the N terminus of the protein penetrates the lipid bilayer of the ER and is threaded into the lumen of the ER (Fig. 2-2C). This process of transfer of protein across the ER membrane is called translocation. The N-terminal signal sequence is then cleaved within the lumen of the RER by a specific protease called signal peptidase.[26]

What is the mechanism of protein translocation across the ER membrane? Some light has been shed on this issue recently. Translocation seems to occur through an aqueous channel in the ER membrane.[27] Two proteins in the ER membrane that bind to signal sequences were recently identified as possible structural or regulatory components of the translocation channel. They have been called signal sequence receptor-α and translocating chain-associating membrane proteins.[28,29] The organization of these proteins during channel biogenesis and the identification of new components will be a focus of intense investigation. Since model systems in yeast have yielded considerably greater complexity than these crude mammalian systems, many mammalian translocation proteins remain to be discovered.[30] Taken together, evidence is accumulating that the process of translocation is energy requiring and involves a complex series of protein-protein and protein-lipid interactions.

Proteins anchored in the membrane by a hydrophobic transmembrane domain also interact with the translocation machinery of the ER. Transmembrane or integral membrane proteins of the ER, Golgi, lysosome, and cell surface are all synthesized on ribosomes targeted to the RER. This targeting is signal sequence/SRP mediated, as has been outlined for secretory proteins. However, unlike secretory proteins, the signal sequence for several transmembrane proteins is not N terminal nor is it cleaved. For example, the transferrin receptor, which is responsible for the internalization of iron-bound transferrin, possesses a signal sequence that is not cleaved; rather, it consists of an internal stretch of amino acids.[31] The translocation process of these proteins is terminated before the entire protein is transferred across the RER membrane. A specific amino acid sequence of the protein, called the stop transfer sequence, prevents the further transfer of the growing polypeptide chain across the RER.[32] As a result, the final translation product spans the membrane. The portion of the protein in the lumen of the RER is called the extracytoplasmic domain, that portion

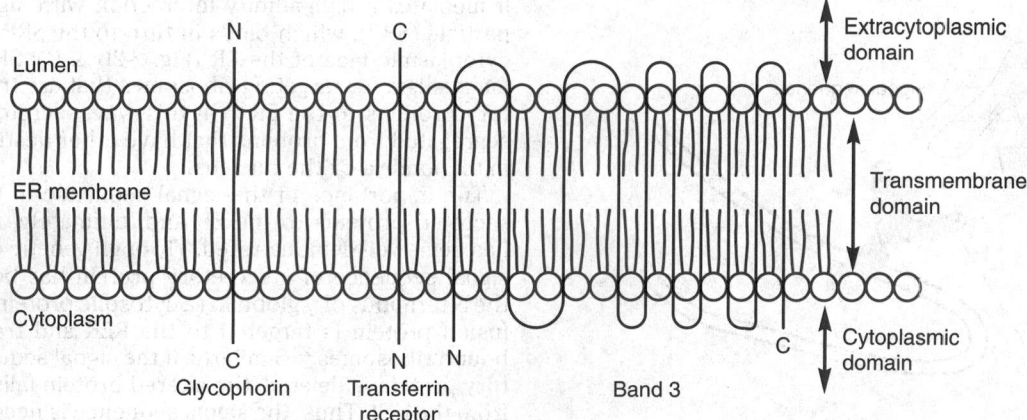

Fig. 2-3. Orientation of transmembrane proteins. The extracytoplasmic domain is contained within the lumen of the ER, the transmembrane domain is embedded within the membrane, and the cytoplasmic domain remains in the cytoplasm. Various examples are shown.

remaining embedded in the membrane is called the transmembrane domain, and the portion left in the cytoplasm is called the cytoplasmic domain (Fig. 2-3). Many transmembrane proteins are oriented with their N terminus in the lumen of the RER and their C terminus in the cytoplasm (e.g., glycophorin). Others are oriented in an opposite manner (e.g., transferrin receptor). Some proteins display a complex topology, having multiple transmembrane domains (e.g., erythrocyte band 3). Importantly, the topology of the protein in the RER is the one that the protein will display at its final destination (see Ch. 4).

Chemical Modification and Post-Translational Processing

During and after translation and translocation, a protein destined for secretion may undergo any one of a series of chemical modifications (Table 2-1). These modifications occur co- or post-translationally and fall into three major categories: chemical modifications of amino acid side chains, formation of disulfide bonds, and proteolytic processing. What purposes do these chemical modifications serve?

They are of critical importance, for example, for function of a protein such as the factor IX molecule. After translation and translocation in the ER of the liver cell the 12 N-terminal glutamic acid residues of factor IX undergo γ-carboxylation (see Ch. 100). This modification is vitamin K dependent and is essential for metal binding and for normal factor IX conformation and function. Thus, in the absence of γ-carboxylation, as occurs in vitamin K deficiency, factor IX is secreted from the liver cell in an inactive form.

The problem of specificity of chemical modification also arises. In the case of N-linked oligosaccharide addition, the amino acids in the immediate vicinity of the asparagine residue dictate whether a particular asparagine will be modified. The sequence -Asn-X-Ser(Thr)- is required to signal carbohydrate addition[33]; X can be any amino acid. For γ-carboxylation of glutamic acid residues, an N-terminal sequence called the pro sequence (see below) is the critical signal. If this sequence is deleted or mutated by genetic engineering, γ-carboxylation of factor IX does not occur.[34] Thus, it appears that certain proteins contain recognition markers that specifically tag them for certain chemical modifications.

The formation of intramolecular disulfide bonds that occurs in the lumen of the ER is another example of an important chemical modification. Disulfide bonds are formed either co- or post-translationally; they link two cystine residues in separate parts of the protein sequence. Notably, this modification is limited to secretory proteins and integral membrane proteins of the secretory pathway. These bonds are extremely important in stabilizing the secondary structure of many proteins. When formed between polypeptides, these bonds facilitate oligomeric complex assembly and stabilize quaternary structure. It is believed that disulfide bond formation is catalyzed by the enzyme protein disulfide-isomerase, a resident protein of the ER.[35]

Proteolytic processing or cleavage of newly synthesized polypeptides is a very common modification. One type of processing, that of cleavage of the N-terminal signal sequence of secretory proteins within the lumen of the ER, has been discussed previously. The signal sequence is also referred to as a pre sequence. Almost all secretory proteins contain and then have cleaved such a pre sequence. Some secretory proteins (e.g., vWF, factor IX) undergo a second cleavage event prior to secretion. The amino acid sequence so cleaved is called the pro sequence, and cleavage of this sequence yields a mature product ready for secretion (see Chs. 107 and 112). The pro sequence is N terminal and is cleaved after the molecule leaves the Golgi, but prior to secretion.[36] This cleavage event seems to require an acidic compartment and to occur in clathrin-coated secretory vesicles.[37]

An interesting example of proteolytic prepro processing occurs with the vWF molecule.[38] Prepro-vWF is translocated across the RER of endothelial cells, where its signal or pre sequence is cotranslationally cleaved, forming pro-vWF (260,000 molecular weight), which in turn forms a dimer by interchain disulfide bonding. Further assembly to multimers takes place in a late Golgi or post-Golgi compartment. Multimerization is normally accompanied by proteolytic cleavage of the pro sequence. A recently described protease of the secretory pathway, PACE/furin, is capable of mediating this cleavage

Table 2-1. Chemical Modifications of Newly Synthesized Secretory Proteins

Modification of amino acid side chains
Carbohydrate addition
N-linked (asparagine)
O-linked (serine, threonine)
Palmitylation (cystine)
Hydroxylation (proline, lysine)
γ-Carboxylation (glutamic acid)
Intra(inter)molecular disulfide bond formation (cystine-cystine)
Proteolytic processing
Signal sequence cleavage
pro sequence cleavage
Multimeric/oligomeric assembly

step.[39] Mutagenesis and deletion experiments with expressed vWF cDNA demonstrated a requirement for the pro sequence in multimer assembly. Surprisingly, this is independent of the cleavage event; the pro sequence cotransfected on a separate plasmid can substitute functionally in vWF assembly.[40] This pro sequence is unusually long (741 amino acids) and is itself secreted into plasma as the protein vWF-AgII.[41]

Another protein-processing reaction that occurs in the RER post-translationally is oligomeric assembly. Certain secretory and transmembrane proteins, such as the polymeric immunoglobulin receptor, exist as single protein units and are called monomers. Others are tightly associated with themselves and form multimers (such as vWF) or are associated with other proteins (e.g., light and heavy chains associate to form immunoglobulins). Assembly of oligomeric proteins is necessary not only for proper function but for proper sorting. How is assembly regulated in the cell? Unassembled monomers can be prevented from exiting the RER by their association with a protein called BiP, which is also called heat shock protein 78, or heavy-chain binding protein.[42,43] For example, the expression of immunoglobulin heavy chain without light chain results in its retention in the ER through its binding to BiP. Improperly assembled complexes fail to exit the RER and appear to be selectively degraded. The precise nature of the signals specifying rapid degradation in the ER are not yet defined. Retention in ER by itself is not sufficient for degradation, as ER-resident proteins escape this rapid proteolysis. Experiments with constructed chimeric proteins showed that the transmembrane domains are the major determinant of degradation.[44] These data have suggested a model for rapid ER degradation in which a signal in the hydrophobic transmembrane domain of oligomeric proteins triggers degradation. Normally masked by proper oligomeric assembly, the signal is revealed and recognized if misassembly occurs. In this way, the mis-assembled protein is targeted for degradation. The proteases and the receptors involved in this process remain to be defined. In summary, this degradation system may serve as a quality control for properly assembled multisubunit complexes.[45] Thus, proper assembly of protein oligomers is an important post-translational event that regulates the transport of proteins out of the ER to their destination.

Cellular Itinerary

After translation and translocation into the lumen of the ER, what is the pathway of a secretory protein on its way out of the cell? In general, proteins destined for secretion are transported from the lumen of the ER to the lumen of the Golgi. The Golgi is a series of membrane-limited compartments closely apposed to one another in a stack. The Golgi has been morphologically divided into cis (facing the ER), medial (in the middle), and trans (furthest from the ER but closest to the cell surface) compartments. Secretory proteins enter the cis-Golgi and mature through these compartments sequentially, exiting from the trans-Golgi. From the trans-Golgi, secretory proteins are packaged into vesicles, which then fuse with the cell surface membrane, leading to the exocytosis or secretion of the contents of the vesicle (see the section Constitutive versus Regulated Secretion).

It is now clear that the intermediate steps from one membrane limited compartment to another are achieved by vesicular transport (Fig. 2-4), that is, a membrane buds off from one compartment, forming a vesicle (the contents of which include the secretory proteins). This vesicle then meets and fuses with the next membrane compartment in the pathway, thus releasing the contents of the vesicle into the membrane-limited compartment. The vesicles act as carriers or intermediates between the ER and the cis-Golgi, between individual Golgi stacks, and between the trans-Golgi and the cell surface. Recently, it has been discovered that the vesicular transport and fusion events from ER to Golgi and between the individual Golgi stacks are biochemically similar (reviewed below).[46]

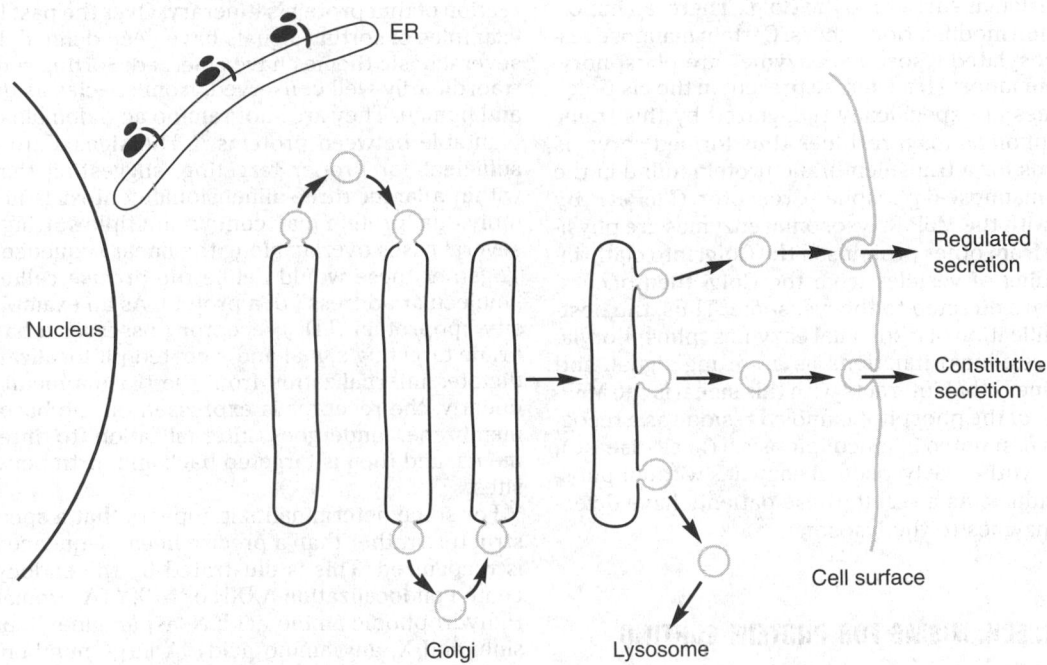

Fig. 2-4. Cellular pathways of newly synthesized secretory proteins. Soluble secretory proteins are synthesized on ER-bound ribosomes and translocated across the ER membrane into the lumen. Transfer of newly synthesized proteins from one compartment to the next involves a series of vesicular intermediates. At the trans-Golgi, three types of vesicles bud. The vesicles target their contents for regulated secretion or constitutive secretion or to the lysosome.

Constitutive Versus Regulated Secretion

Proteins can be secreted from cells in two distinct ways, regulated or constitutive (Fig. 2-4). Regulated secretion generally occurs in response to a hormone or a secretogogue. For example, tumor necrosis factor/cachectin is secreted by macrophages after stimulation by endotoxin.[47] By contrast, some proteins are secreted constitutively, in a continuous fashion (constitutive secretion) such as transferrin by the hepatocyte. On leaving the trans-Golgi, proteins are packaged in either storage (secretory) vesicles, or in transport vesicles. Secretory vesicles fuse with the cell surface on stimulation (regulated secretion), and transport vesicles continuously fuse with the cell surface (constitutive secretion). How does the cell ensure that proteins are packaged in the proper vesicle on leaving the trans-Golgi? It is now suggested that soluble proteins of the trans-Golgi selectively associate with one another in order to be targeted to secretory granules. This aggregate subsequently binds to certain secretory granule membrane proteins.[48] In addition, recent progress has been made in localizing a sorting domain contained within the cytoplasmic domain of P-selectin that targets this secretory granule membrane protein to its proper destination.[49]

Lysosomal Enzyme Sorting—A Branch of the Secretory Pathway

An important example of signal-mediated protein sorting involves the delivery of soluble lysosomal enzymes (e.g., cathepsin D) to their destination in the lysosome.[50,51] Localization in the lysosome requires these soluble proteins to be segregated from the other soluble proteins synthesized in the RER that are destined for secretion (Fig. 2-4). Following initial processing in the RER, which includes cleavage of the signal sequence and addition of N-linked oligosaccharides, lysosomal enzymes are transported by vesicular carriers to the Golgi. There, an important post-translation modification occurs. Certain mannose residues on the glycosylated lysosomal enzymes are phosphorylated by phosphomannosyl transferase present in the cis-Golgi. Lysosomal enzymes are specifically recognized by this transferase. The phosphomannosyl residues thus formed serve as high-affinity ligands for a transmembrane protein found in the Golgi called the mannose-6-phosphate receptor (M6P-R). By their interaction with the M6P-R, lysosomal enzymes are physically sorted away from other proteins in the Golgi into clathrin-coated pits. Budding of vesicles from the Golgi then occurs, and the enzymes are directed to the lysosome. Thus, the post-translational modification of lysosomal enzymes (phosphorylation of mannose residues) functions as a sorting signal, and the cellular machinery that interacts with this signal is the M6P-R. The importance of the phosphomannosyl residue as a recognition marker was first noted in mucolipidosis II (I-cell disease), in which patients synthesize lysosomal enzymes without phosphomannosyl residues. As a result, these patients have defective delivery of enzymes to the lysosome.[52]

CELLULAR MECHANISMS FOR PROTEIN SORTING

Knowledge about the elements that direct the overall flow of protein traffic (Fig. 2-4) is beginning to emerge. Protein sorting results from the complex interaction of many factors, including structural determinants on the proteins themselves, cytoskele-

Table 2-2. Cellular Mechanisms that Contribute to Protein Sorting

Acidification of cellular compartments
Sorting signals on proteins
Membrane coat proteins—clathrin, adaptins
GTP-binding proteins
Cytoskeletal elements—microtubules

tal components, lipids, and soluble factors. Table 2-2 lists several mechanisms that are thought to contribute to protein sorting.

It is known that the internal pH of successive membrane compartments in the secretory pathway becomes progressively more acidic. Proton-translocating ATPases in the vesicle membrane are responsible for generating this gradient. The acid environment modulates critical cellular functions, including receptor-ligand dissociation and the activity of lysosomal proteolytic enzymes. For example, the affinity of iron for transferrin is several orders of magnitude lower at the pH of the endosomal compartment, permitting its unloading and delivery.

Sorting Signals

How do individual proteins specify their unique intracellular destination? Sorting signals encoded in the protein's cytoplasmic domain are one essential element. The signals are short peptide domains that direct targeting of the nascent protein to ER, lysosome, nucleus, mitochondria, or peroxisome.[53,54] Similar signals mediate clustering of plasma membrane proteins at coated pits, leading to rapid endocytosis. Molecular definition of these sorting signals has been largely accomplished by site-directed mutagenesis of cloned cDNA and disruption of the targeting information. Another experimental approach has been the transfer of the signal by genetic engineering to another protein's cytoplasmic domain and redirection of that protein's itinerary. Over the past few years many examples of sorting signals have been defined. From this work several basic themes have emerged. Sorting sequences are extraordinarily well conserved, from species as diverse as yeast and human. They are short amino acid domains that are transplantable between proteins.[55] The signals are necessary and sufficient for proper targeting, suggesting that presentation within a larger three-dimensional context is not required. An individual protein may contain multiple sorting signals that in several cases overlap along the linear sequence of the protein. Together these would define the precise cellular itinerary or "molecular address" of a protein. As an example, the low-density lipoprotein (LDL) receptor possesses a basolateral membrane targeting signal and a coated pit localization signal that dictates internalization from the plasma membrane.[56] Consequently, the receptor is expressed on the basolateral plasma membrane, undergoes internalization to internal compartments, and then is targeted back and forth between these two sites.

For some determinants it appears that a specific secondary structure rather than a precise linear sequence of amino acids is recognized. This is illustrated by the endocytic signals for coated pit localization AXXH or NPXY (A, aromatic amino acid; H, hydrophobic amino acid; N, asparagine; P, proline; Y, tyrosine; and X, any amino acid). A large number of protein sequences have been identified that obey these rules. Despite their apparent diversity in primary structure, analysis with computer modeling and nuclear magnetic resonance demonstrated a secondary structural feature known as a tight β-turn that they have in common.[57,58] Amino acid substitutions that disrupt the predicted β-turn structure have been shown to interfere with efficient coated pit localization. The result is a mutant protein that is slowly endocytosed. A mutation of this type in the LDL receptor (NPVY→NPVC) has been shown to lead to defective endocytosis of LDL and to produce the phenotype of hypercholesterolemia.[59] This was one of the first molecular descriptions of a human disease caused by abnormal protein sorting.

Protein Coats

How are these peptide codes for protein sorting deciphered by the cell? The protein coats located on the cytoplasmic face of some membranes and vesicles are potential candidates. They are found in regions of the cell dedicated to protein sorting (trans-Golgi, plasma membrane) and participate in protein recognition, packaging within a nascent vesicle, and formation of the vesicle itself. Considerable progress has been made in the last several years in the description at the molecular level of protein coats. One type of protein coat contains clathrin and has been described in some biochemical detail. Clathrin is an oligomeric protein that polymerizes and thereby forms a basket-like structure. It is believed that clathrin functions in sorting and membrane traffic in large part by concentrating receptors. Thus, its contribution to sorting may be quantitative rather than absolute.[60] The inner portion of the protein coat consists of a group of polypeptides of 100 kd and 50 kd. These polypeptides have been shown to mediate the interaction of clathrin with membrane proteins (especially membrane receptors that undergo endocytosis). Thus, they have been called adaptors.[61] One set of adaptor molecules has been identified in plasma-membrane-coated pits and helps mediate the interaction of endocytosing receptors with clathrin (HA-II adaptins). Another related set of adaptor proteins is found associated with coated pits in the trans-Golgi (HA-I adaptins). These adaptors specifically interact with M6P-R, but not with other receptors.[62] Therefore, these adaptors may serve to sort M6P-R from other proteins in the Golgi. In addition, their interaction with clathrin promotes coated pit and vesicle formation from the trans-Golgi. A second family of coat proteins is involved in vesicle trafficking from ER to Golgi and between Golgi stacks. Reconstitution experiments have thus far identified seven members of a multiprotein complex, termed a coatomer, which makes up the structural unit of this coat.[63] This complex is assembled onto the membrane surface from the cytoplasm in several discrete steps.[64,65] The reaction is initiated by the binding to Golgi membranes of ADP ribosylation factor (ARF), a small GTP-binding protein of the ras protein superfamily. The stimulus for binding of ARF is exchange of GTP for GDP in its nucleotide-binding domain. ARF-GTP on the Golgi membranes then directs coatomer binding and eventually budding of the nascent coated vesicle. If ARF is unable to bind to the Golgi membrane, the entire process of anterograde transport (the ER-to-Golgi pathway) is halted, as demonstrated by studies with the drug brefeldin A, which blocks the GTP exchange reaction on ARF as well as ARF binding to membranes.[66,67] This compound thus specifically inhibits vesicle traffic from ER to the trans-Golgi network.

GTP-Binding Proteins

GTP-binding proteins (G proteins) occupy a central role in regulation of vesicle trafficking. Recent evidence shows that they participate in virtually all transport pathways known. Studies with a novel pharmacologic agent have expanded knowledge in this field. GTP-γS is a nonhydrolyzable analogue of GTP that binds and fixes G proteins in the GTP-bound or activated state. G proteins are classified on the basis of molecular structure and amino acid sequence homology into several distinct families, including heterotrimeric G proteins, dynamin-like proteins (cytoskeleton-associated G proteins), and the small G proteins structurally homologous to the proto-oncogene *ras*.[67] Members of the ras superfamily include rab, ARF, and rac and rho, which are involved in cytoskeletal organization. Members of all of these families have been implicated in vesicle trafficking. The G proteins described are not transmembrane proteins, but associate with membranes based on their tight affinity for an anchored protein, or by means of covalently bound C-terminal (isoprenyl) or N-terminal (myristate) lipid anchors. The mechanism of action of these small G proteins appears substantially similar to that described for G-protein-mediated signal transduction at the plasma membrane. They alternate between an active (GTP-bound) and an inactive (GDP-bound) state. The interconversion of these isoforms, and hence the rate of protein sorting, may be regulated by GTPase-activating proteins and nucleotide exchange proteins in a manner analogous to ras. The rab proteins illustrate many features of G-protein regulation of protein sorting. Over 30 members of this family have been described. Surprisingly, each individual rab species regulates a specific sorting pathway. For example, rab4 only regulates the endocytic pathway.[69] There is functional redundancy of rab proteins, however; more than one may act on a specific pathway. The rab proteins are themselves targeted to their appropriate site of action by means of a sorting signal expressed in the hypervariable C-terminal domain of the protein.[70] Further identification of G-protein homologues specific for protein sorting and their interaction with other components of the cellular sorting machinery will be a major focus of future investigation in this field.

How are assembled vesicles targeted to and incorporated in the correct membrane domain? The homing of vesicles involves recognition, docking, and fusion. Fusion of two lipid bilayers will not occur spontaneously. It requires ATP, cytosol, and a soluble *N*-ethylmaleimide-sensitive fusion protein (NSF).[71] In contrast to the G proteins described above, NSF has activity at multiple sites in the cell, including the ER, Golgi, and endosome. Vesicle-target membrane recognition proceeds by a receptor-ligand mechanism. The target proteins from the docking membranes that interact with NSF have recently been described. These include the soluble NSF attachment proteins and their receptors.[72] According to this model, a complementary pair of such receptors on the vesicle and target membrane is required to ensure correct recognition and docking. Amino acid sequencing revealed an extraordinary homology to proteins known to regulate secretion in the nervous system. This finding suggests that common biochemical mechanisms may underlie the processes of secretion, vesicle trafficking, and protein sorting. The critical questions of targeting of the NSF-binding proteins and their recycling within the cell remain to be answered.

Cytoskeletal Elements

Features of the cell cytoskeleton may also play a role in the efficient intracellular sorting of proteins. The cytoskeleton is a complex array of structural proteins that form discrete supramolecular structures such as microtubules, microfilaments, and intermediate filaments. The regulation of these cytoskeletal arrays plays an important role in cell development, especially erythroid development.[73] This framework may also help direct vesicles on their way from one compartment to the other. For example, microtubules form polarized units with the minus end being perinuclear and the plus end oriented toward the cell periphery. Molecular motors carry vesicles along an individual microtubule in one direction or the other.[74] If microtubules are disrupted by the drug colchicine, regulated protein secretion is inhibited, whereas constitutive secretion is not.[75] In the endocytic pathway, a protein called CLIP-170 has been described that is required for binding of coated pit-derived vesicles to microtubules.[76] This interaction is regulated by phosphorylation and may represent a additional level of specificity as vesicles make contact with the appropriate cytoskeletal component. Thus, the cytoskeleton contributes significantly to the quality of intracellular sorting of proteins. (see Chs. 4 and 32).

Interaction of Sorting Mechanisms

Several of these cellular mechanisms may act within a single compartment in the cell. For example, the Golgi, especially the trans-Golgi (sometimes called the trans-Golgi network), plays a central role in the sorting of newly synthesized proteins[77] and has been shown to segregate protein products actively into at least three unique vesicle populations: regulated secretory vesicles, vesicles with lysosomal enzymes, and vesicles with proteins possessing a GPI-linked membrane anchor destined for the apical surface of polarized cells (see the section following). The formation of each of these unique vesicle populations requires a specific and unique process. For example, lysosomal enzyme segregation occurs by interaction of the M6P-R with adaptins. Regulated products of secretion are segregated by aggregation, and apical GPI-linked proteins associate with unique lipid patches in the trans-Golgi network. Thus, the trans-Golgi network represents an excellent system in which to explore the cellular mechanisms responsible for the sorting of newly synthesized proteins.

PROTEIN SORTING IN POLARIZED CELLS

An additional level of sorting occurs in cells that demonstrate specialization of surface membrane. The most straightforward model of such specialization occurs in epithelial cells. These cells display a basolateral and apical surface membrane, separated by tight junctions. The apical surface faces the lumen, and the basolateral surface is surrounded by blood or attached to the extracellular matrix. Each surface is composed of a unique set of membrane lipids and proteins. The tight junctions serve as barriers to free diffusion of apical and basolateral membrane components. What establishes and maintains this specialization (referred to as polarity) is currently under active investigation.[78,79]

The polarity of epithelial cells was strikingly revealed with the observation that certain RNA viruses selectively bud from either the apical or basolateral surface.[80] It was then discovered that the glycoproteins of the viral membrane contain the sorting signals for polarized delivery to the proper surface.[81] Surprisingly minor changes in viral protein structure, for example insertion of a single cytoplasmic tyrosine, altered the intracellular sorting of viral hemagglutinin from apical to basolateral.[82]

Subsequent studies with model cellular proteins have addressed sorting mechanisms in polarized cells. Proteins containing a GPI-linked membrane anchor are targeted to the apical surface.[83] Recent evidence demonstrated that the lipid anchor of GPI-linked proteins associates with patches of glycosphingolipid[84] uniquely located in the trans-Golgi network and the apical membrane. Vesicles enriched in this lipid bud from the trans-Golgi network and contain GPI-linked proteins and are selectively targeted to the apical membrane.

By contrast, apical sorting signals for transmembrane proteins are presently not well understood. In some epithelia, apical sorting may result from the absence of signals specific for other destinations (i.e., default pathway).[79] The existence of a default pathway for protein sorting remains highly controversial, however.[85]

Recent studies have defined basolateral targeting signals in protein cytoplasmic domains. Examples are found in the IgG Fc receptor, the LDL receptor, and the polymeric immunoglobulin receptor.[56,86,87] These signals are relatively long (10–15 amino acids) and homologous to each other, although the precise amino acid sequence requirements have not been defined. Identification of cellular components that interact with these sorting signals is being actively pursued by several groups. As with signals for rapid endocytosis, basolateral targeting signals may possess common higher order structures.

An excellent model system illustrating the mechanisms of sorting in polarized cells is the polymeric immunoglobulin receptor (pIg-R).[88] This membrane receptor protein is responsible for the transport of polymeric immunoglobulins across various epithelia into secretions. The itinerary of the pIg-R is quite complex. After synthesis in the ER and oligosaccharide modification in the Golgi, the receptor is first specifically targeted to the basolateral surface, where it is available to bind pIg. From the basolateral surface, the receptor with bound pIg is then internalized and sorted to the apical surface. There, the extracellular portion of the receptor is cleaved to secretory component, releasing pIg. The cytoplasmic domain of this receptor protein contains at least three subdomains that specify basolateral targeting,[87] internalization,[89] and subsequent apical targeting regulated by phosphorylation.[90] Finally, intact microtubules are necessary for the fidelity of the apical targeting of the pIg-R.[91]

If apical and basolateral proteins have specific sorting signals that provide for their vectorial delivery to their destination, where in the cell do they segregate? The cellular location of this sorting apparently differs, depending on the epithelial cell type examined.[92] In some systems, for example in kidney cell lines, it appears that apical and basolaterally directed proteins travel through the same cellular compartments until the trans-Golgi. On exit from the trans-Golgi, apical proteins are sorted into vesicular carriers separate from basolateral proteins. By contrast, in hepatocytes, intrinsic apical and basolateral transmembrane proteins are transported together from the trans-Golgi to the basolateral surface. At the basolateral surface, their pathways diverge as apically directed proteins are endocytosed and travel across the cell to the apical surface through a process called transcytosis.[93] Further complexity is observed in polarized enterocytes, which utilize a combination of these pathways.[94] It is likely that new sorting mechanisms will be described as additional proteins are examined. An example is the recent demonstration of the targeting of Na^+/K^+-ATPase, which is delivered initially to both apical and basolateral surfaces. Polarity is then established by selective retention at the basolateral membrane.[95]

Polarized secretion also occurs in cells with specialized membrane domains.[96] This phenomenon has been best studied in epithelial and neurosecretory cells.[97,98] However, nonpolarized, or round, cells also demonstrate directional secretion. For example, mast cells are thought to release granules toward the region of the cell membrane at which they were stimulated.[99] These are secretory granules that release their storage contents in response to a stimulus at a particular location at the cell surface (transient polarized regulated secreton).

Lymphocytes also display aspects of transient polarity. For instance, T-helper cells reorient their microtubule-organizing centers and Golgi toward their site of interaction with antigen-presenting cells.[100] T-helper cells also constitutively secrete interleukin-4 toward the site of the cell surface occupied by T-cell receptors.[101] Finally, in response to interleukin-4, B cells become motile and polarize their surface membrane.[102] Thus, lymphocytes are able to direct the traffic of newly synthesized secretory and membrane proteins to transiently polarized regions of the cell surface.

SORTING OF CYTOSOLIC AND ORGANELLAR PROTEINS—NUCLEUS, MITOCHONDRIA, AND PEROXISOMES

Proteins translated on free, cytosolic ribosomes may be targeted to organelles not found on the secretory pathway. For instance, oncogenes that act in the nucleus must be directed through the nuclear envelope. Additionally, mitochondrial proteins such as the cytochrome oxidase involved in electron transport must be targeted to the inner mitochondrial membrane. Proteins targeted to these organelles are fully synthesized prior to their translocation into or across the appropriate membrane. Translocation is therefore post-translational, unlike translocation across the ER. It appears that specific sorting signals exist for the entry of proteins into each of these three organelles and that translocation is energy requiring. Protein import to the nucleus occurs at the nuclear pore complex, a multimeric assembly of eight structural units symmetrically arrayed around a central core.[103,104] This is a gated channel capable of admitting preformed proteins, oligomeric complexes, and particles as large as 25 nm.[105] Proteins targeted to the nucleus contain a nuclear localization sorting signal. These sequences are generally not N terminal and are not cleaved on entry. Such a sequence may consist of a single stretch of basic amino acids as defined for the viral protein simian virus 40 large T antigen or two basic regions separated by an interval of noncharged amino acids (nucleoplasmin, amphibian nuclear protein).[106] Cytoplasmic proteins that bind these nuclear localization signals and facilitate the docking and translocation process at nuclear pore complexes have been identified.[107] Ribonucleoprotein particles assembled in the cytoplasm (e.g., small nuclear RNA and protein) utilize a noncompeting pathway that depends on a trimethylguanosine cap.[108] One important principle illustrated by nuclear targeting is the reversible masking of sorting signals through mechanisms such as protein phosphorylation at a region near the sorting signal and binding to another cytoplasmic protein. In the case of the transcription factor NFkB, masking of the nuclear sorting signal is accomplished by binding of a domain of the precursor protein. Proteolytic cleavage of this fragment leads to unmasking, activation of the nuclear sorting signal, and nuclear targeting.[109]

For mitochondrial targeting, cleavable, N-terminal sorting sequences are used.[110] These sequences target proteins to the mitochondrial membranes or across both membranes into the matrix. It is clear that a membrane potential and ATP are necessary for protein translocation across mitochondrial membranes.[111] In addition, proteins of the heat-shock family (hsp70) are necessary binding factors on both faces of the membrane to maintain the transported protein in the partially unfolded state.[15,110] These proteins, which are required for translocation, are members of a family of unrelated proteins called molecular chaperones.[112] Chaperones are defined as proteins that assist in the proper folding and assembly of other polypeptides but are themselves not part of the final functional protein or protein complex. Chaperones are essential for many steps in protein synthesis and sorting, including the folding of newly synthesized proteins, oligomeric assembly, cotranslational transport across membranes such as the ER, and post-translational transport across mitochondrial membranes. In summary, the sorting of proteins destined for organelles that are not on the secretory pathway is signal mediated. In contrast to the secretory pathway, the transport of such proteins is not mediated by vesicular carriers. Finally, translocation across the organelle membrane is post-translational. A COOH-terminal signal has been identified in four peroxisomal proteins that appears to be responsible for their targeting.[112] Zellweger syndrome, a disorder associated with the absence of peroxisomes, causing profound neurologic deficits, may serve as a model system in which to identify the protein import machinery that recognizes such signals. Peroxisomal proteins appear to be present in these patients but are not in the correct membrane fraction. This finding suggests that the machinery for protein import into peroxisomes is absent or defective in Zellweger syndrome.[113]

REFERENCES

1. Blobel G: Intracellular protein topogenesis. Proc Natl Acad Sci USA 77:1496, 1980
2. Cheng SH, Gregory RJ, Marshall J et al: Defective intracellular transport and processing of CFTR is the molecular basis of most cystic fibrosis. Cell 63:827, 1990
3. Furie B, Furie BC: Molecular and cellular biology of blood coagulation. N Engl J Med 326:800, 1992
4. Bently AK, Rees DJG, Rizza C, Brownlee GG: Defective propeptide processing of blood clotting factor IX caused by mutation of arginine to glutamine at position −4. Cell 45:343, 1986
5. Wagner DD, Marder VJ: Biosynthesis of von Willebrand protein by human endothelial cells: processing steps and their intracellular localization. J Cell Biol 99:2123, 1984
6. Rosse WF: Phosphatidylinositol-linked proteins and paroxysmal nocturnal hemoglobinuria. Blood 75:1595, 1990
7. Low MG: The glycosyl-phosphatidylinositol anchor of membrane proteins. Biochim Biophys Acta 988:427, 1989
8. Wilcox LA, Ezzell JL, Bernshaw NJ, Parker CJ: Molecular basis of the enhanced susceptibility of the erythrocytes of paroxysmal nocturnal hemoglobinuria to hemolysis in acidified serum. Blood 78:820, 1991
9. Takeda J, Miyata T, Kawagoe K et al: Deficiency of the GPI anchor caused by a somatic mutation of the PIG-A gene in paroxysmal nocturnal hemoglobinuria. Cell 73:703, 1993
10. Gerace L: Molecular trafficking across the nuclear pore complex. Curr Opin Cell Biol 4:637, 1992
11. Andrews NC, Erdjument-Bromage H, Davidson MB et al: Erythroid transcription factor NF-E2 is a haematopoietic-specific basic-leucine zipper protein. Nature 362:722, 1993
12. Hunter T, Karin M: The regulation of transcription by phosphorylation. Cell 70:375, 1992
13. Shimozawa N, Tsukanoto T, Suzuki Y et al: A human gene responsible for Zellweger syndrome that affects peroxisome assembly. Science 255:1132, 1992
14. Ganz T, Metcalf JA, Gallin JI et al: Microbicidal/cytotoxic proteins of neutrophils are deficient in two disorders: Chediak-Higashi syndrome and "specific" granule deficiency. J Clin Invest 82:552, 1988
15. Beasley EM, Wachter C, Schatz G: Putting energy into mitochondrial protein import. Curr Opin Cell Biol 4:646, 1992
16. Drummond DR, Armstrong J, Colman A: The effect of capping and polyadenylation on the stability, movement and translation of synthetic messenger RNAs in Xenopus oocytes. Nucleic Acids Res 13:7375, 1985
17. Pelletier J, Sonenberg N: Insertion mutagenesis to increase secondary structure within the 5' noncoding region of a eukaryotic mRNA reduces translational efficiency. Cell 40:515, 1985
18. Kruys V, Olivier M, Shaw G et al: Translational blockade imposed by cytokine-derived UA-rich sequences. Science 245:852, 1989
19. Kruys V, Beutler B, Huez G: Translational control mediated by UA-rich sequences. Enzyme 44:193, 1990
20. Kozak M: Regulation of translation in eukaryotic systems. Annu Rev Cell Biol 8:197, 1992
21. Nunnari J, Walter P: Protein targeting to and translocation across the membrane of the endoplasmic reticulum. Curr Opin Cell Biol 4:573, 1992
22. Lingappa VR, Chaidez J, Yost CS, Hedgpath J: Determinants for protein localization: β-lactamase signal sequence directs globin across microsomal membranes. Proc Natl Acad Sci USA 81:456, 1984
23. Randall LL, Hardy SJS: Unity in function in the absence of consensus in sequence: role of leader peptides in export. Science 243:1156, 1989
24. Gilmore R, Blobel G: Transient involvement of SRP and its receptor in the microsomal membrane prior to protein translocation. Cell 35:677, 1983
25. Connolly T, Rapiejko PJ, Gilmore R: Requirement of GTP hydrolysis for dissociation of the signal recognition particle from its receptor. Science 252:1171, 1991
26. Shelness GS, Lin L, Nicchitta CV: Membrane topology and biogenesis of eukaryotic signal peptidase. J Biol Chem 268:5201, 1993

27. Simon SM, Blobel G: A protein-conducting channel in the endoplasmic reticulum. Cell 65:371, 1991

28. Krieg UC, Johnson AE, Walter P: Protein translocation across the endoplasmic reticulum membrane: identification by photo-crosslinking of a 39 kD integral membrane glycoprotein as part of a putative translocation tunnel. J Cell Biol 109:2033, 1989

29. Gorlich D, Hartmann E, Prehn S, Rapoport TA: A protein of the endoplasmic reticulum involved early in polypeptide translocation. Nature 357:47, 1992

30. Green N, Fang H, Walter P: Mutants in three novel complementation groups inhibit membrane protein insertion into and soluble protein translocation across the endoplasmic reticulum membrane of *Saccharomyces cerevisiae.* J Cell Biol 116:597, 1992

31. Schneider C, Owen MJ, Banville D, Williams JG: The primary structure of the human transferrin receptor deduced from the mRNA sequence. Nature 311:675, 1984

32. Lingappa VR: Control of protein topology at the endoplasmic reticulum. Cell Biophys 19:1, 1991

33. Lennarz W: Overview: role of intracellular membrane systems in glycosylation of proteins. Methods Enzymol 98:91, 1983

34. Jorgenson MJ, Cantor AB, Furie BC et al: Recognition site directing vitamin K-dependent γ-carboxylation resides on the propeptide of factor IX. Cell 48:185, 1987

35. Bulleid NJ, Freedman RB: Defective co-translational formation of disulphide bonds in protein disulphide-isomerase deficient microsomes. Nature 335:649, 1988

36. Orci L, Ravazzola M, Amherdt M et al: Direct identification of prohormone conversion site in insulin-secreting cells. Cell 42:671, 1985

37. Orci L, Ravazzola M, Storch MJ et al: Proteolytic maturation of insulin is a post-Golgi event which occurs in acidifying clathrin-coated secretory vesicles. Cell 49:865, 1987

38. Wagner DD: Cell biology of von Willebrand factor. Annu Rev Cell Biol 6:217, 1990

39. Wise RJ, Barr PJ, Wong PA et al: Expression of a human proprotein processing enzyme: correct cleavage of the von Willebrand factor precursor at a paired basic amino acid site. Proc Natl Acad Sci USA 87:9378, 1990

40. Wise RJ, Pittman DD, Handin RI et al: The propeptide of von Willebrand factor independently mediates the assembly of von Willebrand multimers. Cell 52:229, 1988

41. Fay PJ, Kawai Y, Wagner DD et al Propolypeptide of von Willebrand factor circulates in blood and is identical to von Willebrand antigen II. Science 232:995, 1986

42. Bole DG, Hendershott LM, Kearney JF: Post-translational association of immunoglobulin heavy chain binding protein with nascent heavy chains in nonsecreting and secreting hybridomas. J Cell Biol 102:1558, 1986

43. Mains PE, Sibley CH: The requirement of light chain for the surface deposition of the heavy chain of immunoglobulin M. J Biol Chem 258:5027, 1983

44. Bonafacino JS, Suzuki CK, Klausner RD: A peptide sequence confers retention and rapid degradation in the endoplasmic reticulum. Science 247:79, 1990

45. Hurtley SM, Helenius A: Protein oligomerization in the endoplasmic reticulum. Annu Rev Cell Biol 5:277, 1989

46. Beckers CJM, Block MR, Glick BS et al: Vesicular transport between the endoplasmic reticulum and the Golgi stack requires the NEM-sensitive fusion protein. Nature 339:397, 1989

47. Sherry B, Cerami A: Cachectin/tumor necrosis factor exerts endocrine, paracrine, and autocrine control of inflammatory responses. J Cell Biol 107:1269, 1988

48. Chanat E, Huttner W: Milieu-induced, selective aggregation of regulated secretory proteins in the trans-Golgi network. J Cell Biol 115:1505, 1991

49. Disdier M, Morrissey JH, Fugate R et al: Cytoplasmic domain of P-selectin (CD62) contains the signal for sorting into the regulated secretory pathway. Mol Cell Biol 3:309, 1992

50. Dahms NM, Lobel P, Kornfeld S: Mannose-6-phosphate receptors and lysosomal enzyme targeting. J Biol Chem 264:12115, 1989

51. Kornfeld S: Structure and function of the mannose 6-phosphate/insulinlike growth factor II receptors. Annu Rev Biochem 61:307, 1992

52. Kornfeld S: Trafficking of lysosomal enzymes in normal and diseased states. J Clin Invest 77:1, 1986

53. Hopkins CR: Selective membrane protein trafficking: vectorial flow and filter. Trends Biochem Sci 17:27, 1992

54. Walter P, Blobel G: SRP contains a 7S RNA essential for protein translocation across the endoplasmic reticulum. Nature 299:691, 1982

55. Collawn JF, Kuhn LA, Liu L-FS et al: Transplanted LDL and mannose-6-phosphate receptor internalization signals promote high-efficiency endocytosis of the transferrin receptor. EMBO J 10:3247, 1991

56. Matter K, Hunziker W, Mellman I: Basolateral sorting of LDL receptor in MDCK cells: the cytoplasmic domain contains two tyrosine-dependent targeting determinants. Cell 71:741, 1992

57. Collawn JF, Stangel M, Kuhn LA et al: Transferrin receptor internalization sequence YXRF implicates a tight turn as the structural recognition motif for endocytosis. Cell 63:1061, 1990

58. Bansal A, Gierasch LM: The NPXY internalization signal of the LDL receptor adopts a reverse-turn conformation. Cell 67:1195, 1991

59. Tolleshaug H, Hobgood KK, Brown MS, Goldstein J: The LDL receptor locus in familial hypercholesterolemia: multiple mutations disrupt transport and processing of a membrane receptor. Cell 32:941, 1983

60. Brodsky F: Living with clathrin: its molecular role in intracellular membrane traffic. Science 242:1396, 1988

61. Pearse BMF, Robinson MS: Clathrin, adaptors, and sorting. Annu Rev Cell Biol 6:151, 1990

62. Glickman JN, Conibear E, Pearse BMF: Specificity of binding of clathrin adaptors to signals on the mannose-6-phosphate/insulin-like growth factor receptor. EMBO J 8:1041, 1989

63. Waters MG, Serafini T, Rothman JE: 'Coatomer'': a cytosolic protein complex containing subunits of non-clathrin-coated Golgi transport vesicles. Nature 349:248, 1991

64. Serafini T, Orci L, Amherdt M et al: ADP-ribosylation factor is a subunit of the coat of Golgi-derived COP-coated vesicles: a novel role for a GTP-binding protein. Cell 67:239, 1991

65. Kahn RA: Fluoride is not an activator of the smaller (20–25 kDa) GTP-binding proteins. J Biol Chem 266:15595, 1991

66. Donaldson JG, Finazzi D, Klausner RD: Brefeldin A inhibits Golgi membrane-catalysed exchange of guanine nucleotide onto ARF protein. Nature 360:350, 1992

67. Helms JB, Rothman JE: Inhibition by brefeldin A of a Golgi membrane enzyme that catalyses exchange of guanine nucleotide bound to ARF. Nature 360:352, 1992

68. Bourne HR, Sanders DA, McCormick F: The GTPase superfamily: a conserved switch for diverse cell functions. Nature 348:125, 1990

69. van der Sluijs P, Hull M, Webster P et al: The small GTP-binding protein rab4 controls an early sorting event on the endocytic pathway. Cell 70:729, 1992

70. Chavrier P, Gorvel J-P, Stelzer E et al: Hypervariable C-terminal domain of rab proteins acts as a targeting signal. Nature 353:769, 1991

71. Rothman JE, Orci L: Molecular dissection of the secretory pathway. Nature 355:409, 1992

72. Sollner T, Whiteheart SW, Brunner M et al: SNAP receptors implicated in vesicle targeting and fusion. Nature 362:318, 1993

73. Palek J, Sahr KE: Mutations of the red blood cell membrane proteins: from clinical evaluation to detection of the underlying genetic defect. Blood 80:308, 1992

74. Schnapp BJ, Vale RD, Sheetz MP, Reese TS: Single microtubules from squid axoplasm support bidirectional movement of organelles. Cell 40:455, 1985

75. Rivas RJ, Moore H-PH: Spatial segregation of the regulated and constitutive secretory pathways. J Cell Biol 109:51, 1989

76. Pierre P, Scheel J, Rickard JE, Kreis TE: CLIP-170 links endocytic vesicles to microtubules. Cell 70:887, 1992

77. Griffiths G, Simons K: The trans Golgi network: sorting at the exit site of the Golgi complex. Science 234:438, 1986

78. Hopkins CR: Polarity signals. Cell 66:827, 1991

79. Mostov K, Apodaca G, Aroeti B, Okamoto C: Plasma membrane protein sorting in polarized epithelial cells. J Cell Biol 116:577, 1992

80. Rodriguez-Boulan E, Sabatini DD: Asymmetric budding of viruses in epithelial monolayers: a model system for the study of epithelial polarity. Proc Natl Acad Sci USA 75:5071, 1978

81. Rodriguez-Boulan E, Pendergast M: Polarized distribution of viral envelope proteins in the plasma membrane of infected epithelial cells. Cell 20:45, 1980

82. Brewer CB, Roth MG: A single amino acid change in the cytoplasmic domain alters the polarized delivery of influenza virus hemagglutinin. J Cell Biol 114:413, 1991

83. Lisanti MP, Sargiacomo M, Graeve L et al: Polarized apical distribution of glycosyl-phosphatidylinositol anchored proteins in a renal epithelial cell line. Proc Natl Acad Sci USA 85:9557, 1988

84. Brown DA, Rose JK: Sorting of GPI-linked proteins to glycolipid-enriched membrane subdomains during transport to the apical surface. Cell 68:533, 1992

85. Matlin KS: W(h)ither default? Sorting and polarization in epithelial cells. Curr Opin Cell Biol 4:623, 1992

86. Hunziker W, Harter C, Matter K, Mellman I: Basolateral sorting in MDCK cells requires a distinct cytoplasmic domain determinant. Cell 66:907, 1991

87. Casanova JE, Apodaca G, Mostov KE: An autonomous signal for basolateral

sorting in the cytoplasmic domain of the polymeric immunoglobulin receptor. Cell 66:65, 1991

88. Apodaca G, Bomsel M, Arden J et al: The polymeric immunoglobulin receptor: a model to study transcytosis. J Clin Invest 87:1877, 1991

89. Breitfeld PP, Casanova JE, McKinnon WC, Mostov KM: Deletions in the cytoplasmic domain of the polymeric immunoglobulin receptor differentially affect endocytotic rate and postendocytotic traffic. J Biol Chem 265:13750, 1990

90. Casanova JE, Breitfeld PP, Mostov KE: Phosphorylation of the polymeric immunoglobulin receptor required for its transcytosis. Science 248:742, 1990

91. Breitfeld PP, McKinnon WC, Mostov KM: Effect of nocodozole on vesicular traffic to the apical and basolateral surfaces of polarized Madin-Darby canine kidney cells. J Cell Biol 111:2365, 1990

92. Rodriguez-Boulan E, Salas PJI: External and internal signals for epithelial cell surface polarization. Annu Rev Physiol 51:741, 1989

93. Bartles JR, Feracci HM, Steiger B, Hubbard AL: Biogenesis of the rat hepatocyte plasma membrane in vivo: comparison of the pathways taken by apical and basolateral proteins using subcellular fractionation. J Cell Biol 105:1241, 1987

94. Matter K, Brauchbar M, Bucher K, Hauri H-P: Sorting of endogenous plasma membrane proteins occurs from two sites in cultured human intestinal epithelial cells. Cell 60:429, 1990

95. Hammerton RW, Krzemninski KA, Mays RW et al: Mechanisms for regulating cell surface distribution of Na^+/K^+-ATPase in polarized epithelial cells. Science 254:847, 1991

96. Sporn LA, Marder VJ, Wagner DD: Differing polarity of the constitutive and regulated secretory pathways for von Willebrand factor in endothelial cells. J Cell Biol 108:1283, 1989

97. Burgess TL, Kelly R: Constitutive and regulated secretion of proteins. Annu Rev Cell Biol 3:243, 1987

98. Kelly RB, Grote E: Protein targeting in the neuron. Annu Rev Neurosci 16:95, 1993

99. Lawson D, Fewtrell C, Ruff MC: Localized mast cell degranulation induced by concanavalin A-sepharose beads. J Cell Biol 79:394, 1978

100. Kupfer A, Swain SL, Janeway CA, Singer SJ: The specific direct interaction of helper T cells and antigen processing B cells. Proc Natl Acad Sci USA 83:6080, 1986

101. Poo W-J, Conrad L, Janeway CA: Receptor-directed focusing of lymphokine release by helper T cells. Nature 332:378, 1988

102. Clinchy B, Elenstro C, Moller G: The effect of T cell-derived cytokines on B cell motility in vitro. Cell Immunol 146:62, 1993

103. Silver PA: How proteins enter the nucleus. Cell 64:489, 1991

104. Gerace L: Molecular trafficking across the nuclear pore complex. Curr Opin Cell Biol 4:637, 1992

105. Hinshaw JE, Carragher BO, Milligan RA: Architecture and design of the nuclear pore complex. Cell 69:1133, 1992

106. Robbins J, Dilworth SM, Laskey RA, Dingwall C: Two interdependent basic domains in nucleoplasmin nuclear targeting sequence. Cell 64:615, 1991

107. Adam SA, Gerace L: Cytosolic proteins that specifically bind nuclear localization signals are receptors for nuclear import. Cell 66:837, 1991

108. Michaud N, Goldfarb DS: Microinjected U snRNAs are imported to oocyte nuclei via the nuclear pore complex by three distinguishable pathways. J Cell Biol 116:851, 1992

109. Henkel T, Zabel U, van Zee K et al: Intramolecular masking of the nuclear localization signal and dimerization domain in the precursor for the p50 NFkB subunit. Cell 68:1121, 1992

110. Glick B, Schatz G: Import of proteins into mitochondria. Annu Rev Genet 25:21, 1991

111. Eilers M, Schatz G: Protein unfolding and the energetics of protein translocation across biological membranes. Cell 52:481, 1988

112. Ellis RJ, van der Vies SM: Molecular chaperones. Annu Rev Biochem 60:321, 1991

113. Gould SJ, Keller G-A, Subramani S: Identification of peroxisomal targeting signals located at the carboxy terminus of four peroxisomal proteins. J Cell Biol 107:897, 1989

114. Santos MJ, Imanaka T, Shio H, Lazarow PB: Peroxisomal integral membrane proteins in control and Zellweger fibroblasts. J Biol Chem 263:10502, 1988

Protein Architecture: Relationship of Form and Function

3

Barbara C. Furie

INTRODUCTION

The previous chapters have described how the information stored in the gene is transcribed into mRNA, how the mRNA template is translated to synthesize proteins, and how newly synthesized proteins are transported to their appropriate site of function. It is the selective expression of a constellation of proteins from the genomic firmament that provides different cell types with their distinct characters. Proteins are linear polymers made up of amino acids linked together by peptide bonds. Twenty different amino acids are incorporated into these polymers when protein is synthesized from mRNA.

The features distinguishing one protein from another are determined not by the polypeptide backbone but by the different side chains of the amino acids incorporated into the protein and the sequence in which they occur. These long arrays of amino acids fold to form compact structures with a specific three-dimensional architecture. The three-dimensional structure of a protein is determined by its unique amino acid sequence. Folded proteins have the capacity to accomplish many different tasks: formation of larger structures (as in the assembly of fibrin monomers into polymers), transport of ligands (as in the binding of oxygen by hemoglobin), catalysis of chemical reactions (as in proteolytic zymogen activation during the propagation of blood coagulation), or the modulation of biologic processes (as in regulation of DNA function by DNA-binding proteins).

A mutation within the coding region of a gene can have varied consequences for synthesis of the gene product. Some mutations are silent, that is, the alteration in the gene product, usually the replacement of one single amino acid by another, has no effect on the ability of the protein to assume its normal three-dimensional structure or to perform its normal function. On the other hand, a single amino acid replacement, if it occurs at a critical position in a protein, can have profound consequences for function. The abnormal factor VIII or factor IX molecules that result in hemophilia A or B frequently arise as the result of a single point mutation (see Chs. 105 and 107). Similarly, a single point mutation at residue 6′ in the β-chain of hemoglobin, a change from glutamic acid to valine, results in sickle cell disease (see Ch. 44). Introduction of a stop codon into the translated portion of a gene, insertion or deletion of additional codons, or addition of bases leading to a shift in reading frame can all result in production of nonfunctional proteins. The altered proteins may fail to function either because a critical functional residue has been lost or because alterations in amino acid sequence prevent the protein from achieving its proper three-dimensional structure. Proteins that are improperly folded or that are drastically altered in sequence may never escape from the site of synthesis to their proper location within the cell or into the secretory pathway.

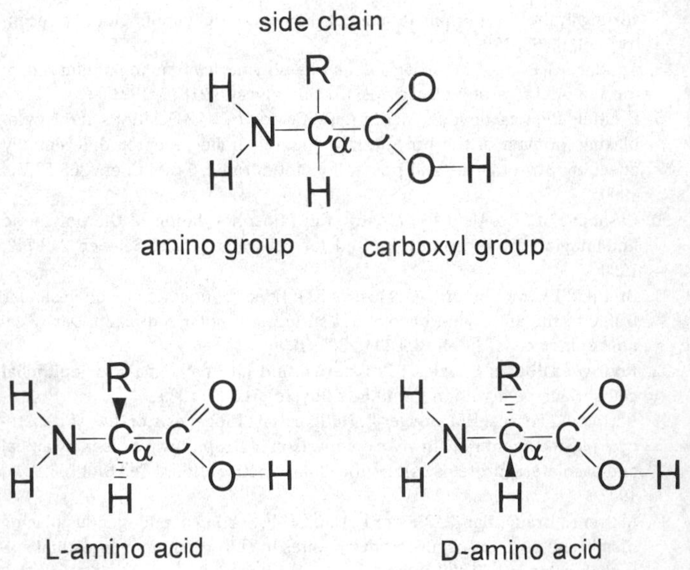

AMINO ACIDS: THE BUILDING BLOCKS OF PROTEINS

The structure of an amino acid is illustrated in Figure 3-1. The central or α-carbon atom bears four substituents: an amino group, a carboxyl group, a group of varying chemical structure

Fig. 3-1. Schematic representation of an amino acid, including an amino group, a carboxyl group, a side chain (R), and a hydrogen atom all linked to the α-carbon (C_α). Each of the substituents on the α-carbon is different, rendering the amino acid chiral. The enantiomeric forms of the amino acid, the D and L forms, are shown.

(R, usually referred to as the side chain), and a hydrogen atom. Since, with the exception of glycine, which bears two hydrogen atoms, each of the substituents carried by the α-carbon is chemically different, amino acids are chiral molecules that can exist in two different forms, the L form or the D form. These chiral forms differ from one another in the same sense as your

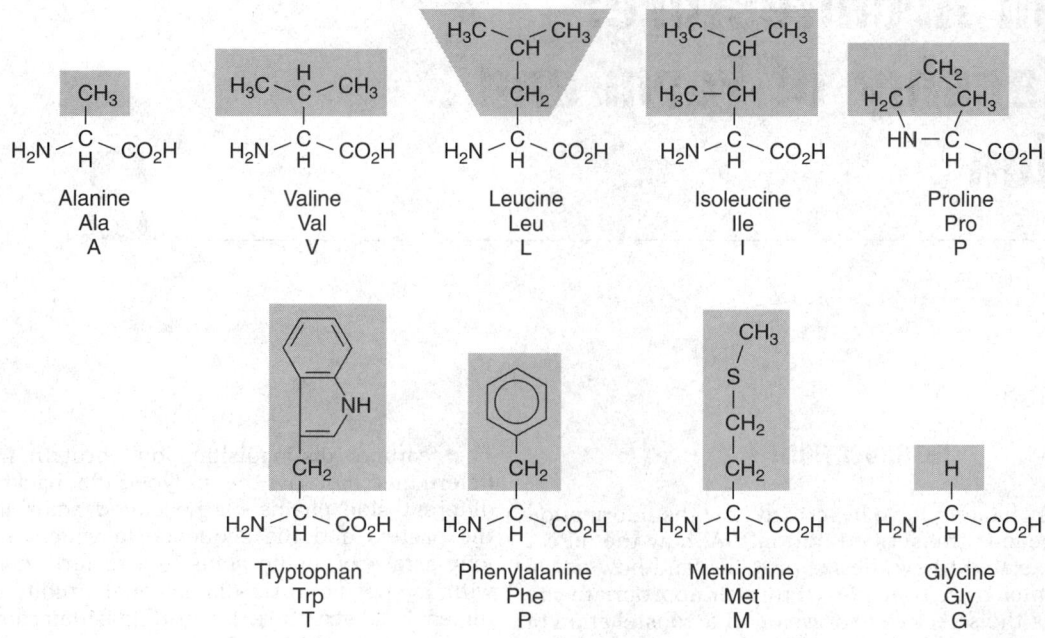

Fig. 3-2. The 20 different amino acids that are incorporated into proteins are shown with the side chain groups highlighted in pink. The amino acids are grouped according to the chemical nature of the side chains. **(A)** Hydrophobic amino acids, those that prefer a nonaqueous environment. (*Figure continues.*)

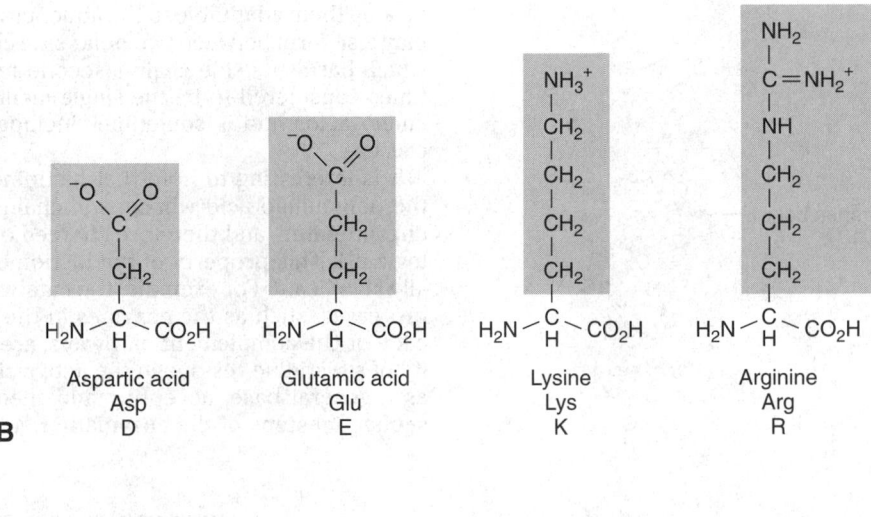

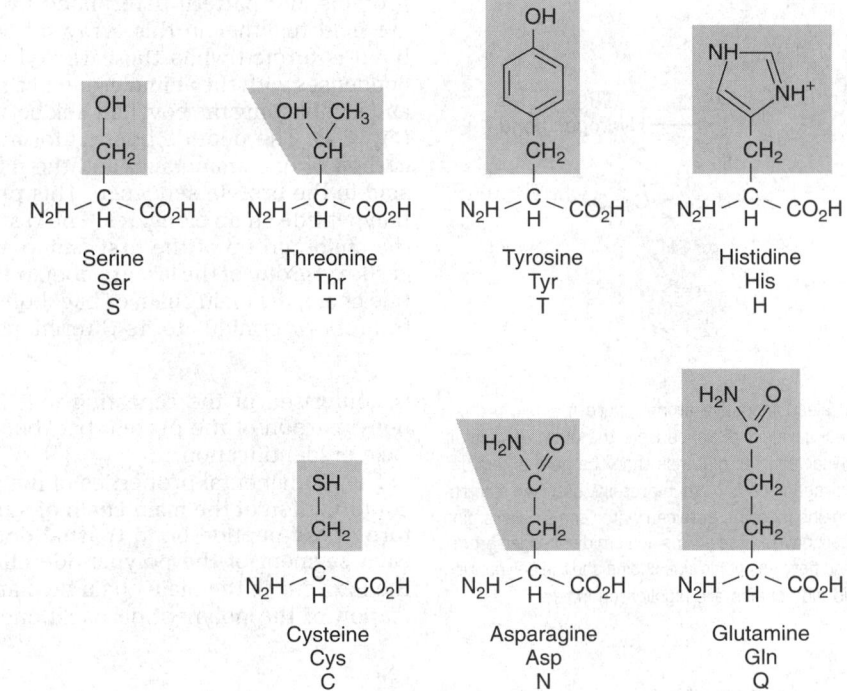

Fig. 3-2 (*Continued*). **(B)** Amino acids that bear side chains charged at physiologic pH. **(C)** Amino acids with polar side chains that can form hydrogen bonds. As described in Chapter 2, amino acids other than these 20 can appear in proteins. These additional amino acids arise by post-translational chemical modification of 1 of the 20 amino acids incorporated into a growing polypeptide chain during translation of messenger RNA. Each amino acid has a three-letter abbreviation and is also referred to by a single-letter code.

left hand differs from your right. Proteins contain only L amino acids.

The side chains of the amino acids provide each one with its distinct chemical character. The amino acids can be divided into three general classes based on the properties of their side chains, as illustrated in Figure 3-2. One group of amino acids bears side chains that are hydrophobic (i.e., they are most at home in a nonaqueous environment). Amino acids in this category include alanine, valine, leucine, isoleucine, proline,

tryptophan, phenylalanine, and methionine. A second group of amino acids, aspartic acid, glutamic acid, lysine, and arginine, contains side chains that are charged at physiologic pH and are thus at home in an aqueous environment. The side chains of the third group of amino acids, serine, threonine, tyrosine, histidine, cysteine, asparagine, and glutamine, are considered polar. The side chains of this group of amino acids may participate in hydrogen bond formation. Hydrogen bonds may be formed between these polar side chains and water molecules,

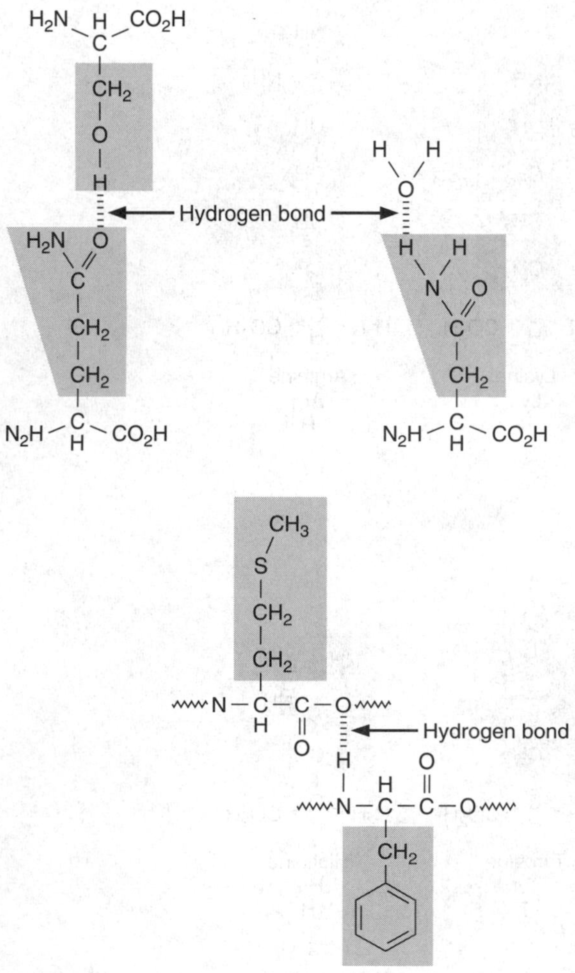

Fig. 3-3. In a hydrogen bond two electronegative atoms share a single proton. The proton is located at the normal covalent distance from the atom to which it is formally bound and at a somewhat shorter distance than the normal van der Waals contact from the other. Hydrogen bonds form in proteins between electronegative atoms in two polar side chains (shown), between water and a polar amino acid side chain (shown), between carbonyl oxygen atoms and amide nitrogen atoms of the protein backbone (shown), and between polar side chains and the polypeptide backbone (not shown). Amino acid side chains are highlighted in red.

making them adaptable to the aqueous milieu. Hydrogen bonds may also form between two polar side chains (Fig. 3-3). Glycine, which has as its side chain a second hydrogen atom, is sometimes considered to be the single member of a fourth class of amino acids and is sometimes included, as here, in the first class.

It is interesting to note that histidine is unique in that it is the only amino acid whose side chain may be protonated or unprotonated, and therefore charged or uncharged, at physiologic pH. This property of the histidine side chain is functionally significant. For example, the catalytic mechanism of serine proteases, such as the enzymes in the blood coagulation cascade or the complement pathways, are dependent on the ability of a histidine residue in the active site of the enzyme to act as a general base, accepting and then releasing a proton in sequential steps of the enzymatic reaction.

NATURE OF THE PEPTIDE BOND

The amino acid building blocks become incorporated into proteins in a pattern determined by the encoding genes and are held together in this array by peptide bonds. A peptide bond is formed when the carboxyl group of one amino acid condenses with the amino group of a second, eliminating water and establishing the covalent link between the two amino acids (Fig. 3-4). The peptide bond is formed between the carbonyl carbon of one amino acid and the nitrogen of the next amino acid in the protein sequence. This process is repeated as the polypeptide chain elongates. The result is a structure in which the amino group of the first amino acid in the chain and the carboxyl group of the last are not modified: a protein's polypeptide chain, the main chain or backbone, is described as running from its N terminus to its C terminus. The peptide backbone is comprised of the repeating unit $NH-C_\alpha-\overset{\overset{\displaystyle O}{\parallel}}{C}'-$. (The carbonyl carbon of the protein backbone is referred to as C' for ease of identification.)

The fundamental properties of the peptide bond dictate the conformation of the main chain of a protein. The chemical nature of the peptide bond (partial double-bond) requires that each segment of the polypeptide chain between one C_α and the next one in the main chain be planar (Fig. 3-5). The conformation of the polypeptide backbone is thus dictated by the

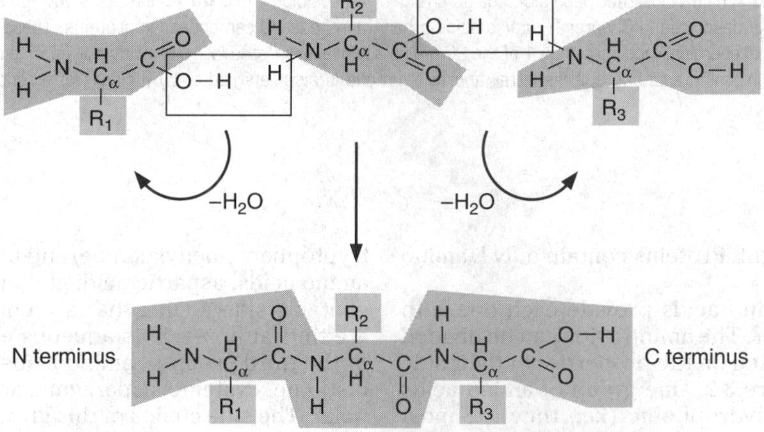

Fig. 3-4. Formation of a peptide bond occurs when the carboxyl (C) group of one amino acid condenses with the amino (N) group of the next amino acid, with concomitant loss of a water molecule.

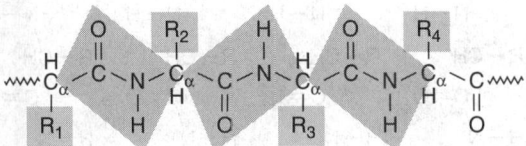

Fig. 3-5. In a peptide bond, the amide nitrogen shares its lone pair of electrons with the carbonyl oxygen, lending a considerable double-bond character to the C′—N bond. As a consequence, the main chain of a protein is planar from one C_α to the next C_α. Each planar unit has 2 degrees of freedom; it can rotate about the N—C_α bond and about the C_α—C′ bond. The peptide bonds of the polypeptide depicted are in the trans configuration; adjacent C_α carbons and the side chains they bear are on opposite sides of the planar C′—N bond. This is the preferred configuration for most amino acids, as it minimizes steric hindrance. For proline the trans configuration is not favored as much as for other amino acids, and the cis configuration occurs with significant frequency. The planar units of the polypeptide backbone are enclosed in gray boxes. The amino acid side chains are highlighted in pink.

angles between these planar segments. The angles of rotation about the N—C_α bond and the angles of rotation about the C_α—C′ bond are restricted because some angles of rotation would result in steric interference between the main chain and amino acid side chains. The only exception to these restrictions is the angles of rotation permissible for glycine residues. Since the side chain of glycine is a single hydrogen atom, a much wider range of conformations is available about the glycine C_α. Conversely, the bulky side chain of a tryptophan residue would be most restrictive of these angles of rotation.

DISULFIDE BRIDGES

In addition to the peptide bond, there is one other covalent bond between amino acid residues that frequently occurs in proteins. The sulfhydryl groups on proximal cysteine residues can be oxidized to form cystine, which contains a disulfide bond (Fig. 3-6). This reaction requires an oxidizing environment. Since the intracellular space is a reducing environment, disulfide bonds are not usually found in intracellular proteins. Disulfide bonds are frequently found in extracellular soluble and integral membrane proteins: they are formed in the lumen of the endoplasmic reticulum, the initial compartment of the

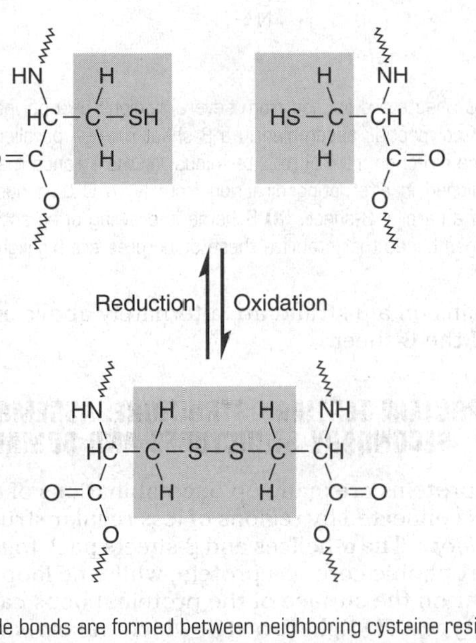

secretory pathway. Disulfide bonds may be formed from cysteines, which are members of the same polypeptide chain, in which case they are thought to stabilize an already folded polypeptide backbone. Alternatively, a disulfide bond may serve to join covalently two different polypeptide chains, for example, the heavy and light chains of immunoglobulins.

ELEMENTS OF SECONDARY STRUCTURE

The amino acid sequence of a protein is termed its primary structure. This structure is coded in the gene. When a number of consecutive amino acid residues have similar angles of rotation about N—C_α and C_α—C′, the main chain of the protein will assume a regular structure. The rotational constraints imposed on these bonds dictate that these regular structures are almost always one of two forms, α-helices and β-sheets. These structural elements of proteins are termed secondary structure.

Formation of these secondary structures resolves a dilemma posed by the folding of a polypeptide chain by permitting formation of hydrogen bonds between the NH groups and the C′=O groups of the protein main chain. The major driving force for folding of proteins in the aqueous environment is to remove nonpolar amino acid side chains from water by sequestering them in the hydrophobic core of the protein. This is akin to

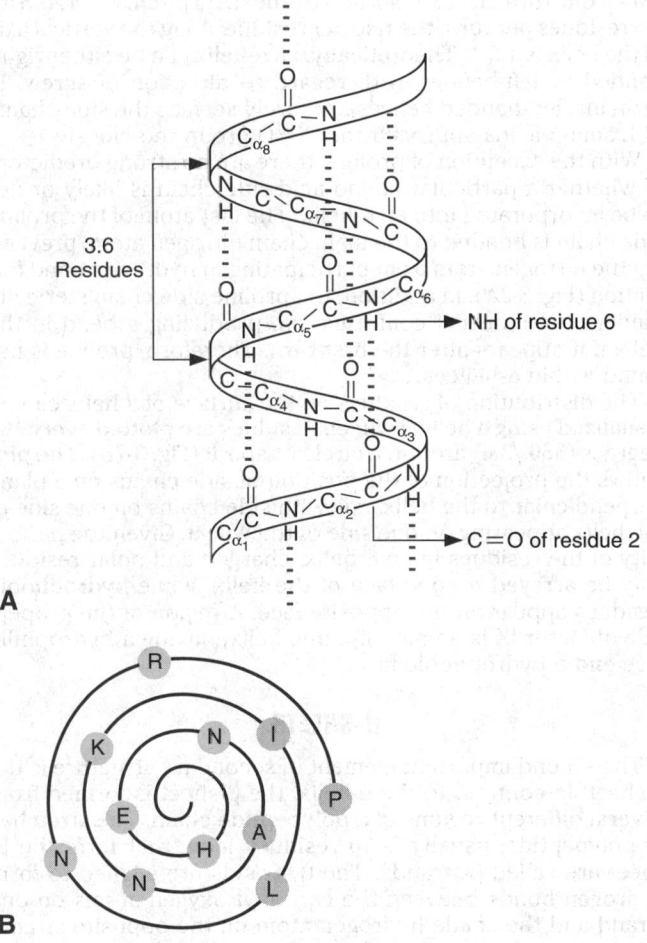

Fig. 3-7. The α-helix is formed from a continuous sequence of amino acids. **(A)** A right-handed α-helix is illustrated. The hydrogen bonds between residue n and residue n + 4, which stabilize the helix, are illustrated by the red dotted lines. **(B)** Amino acids in the propeptide of factor IX are plotted on a helical wheel. The assymetric distribution of hydrophilic amino acid side chains (red) and hydrophobic amino acid side chains (gray) about the helix is easy to visualize with this representation.

Fig. 3-6. Disulfide bonds are formed between neighboring cysteine residues in an oxidizing environment. The side chains of cysteine and cystine are highlighted in pink.

the coalescence of oil droplets when oil is dropped into water. The formation of larger globules minimizes contact of hydrophobic moieties of the oil with water. The main chain of a protein with its NH and C'═O groups is highly polar. To bring the nonpolar side chains into the hydrophobic interior of the protein the main chain must follow. The hydrophilic nature of the main chain is neutralized in regions of secondary structure by the formation of hydrogen bonds between its polar elements, as illustrated in Figure 3-3. Let us examine the nature of these secondary structures more closely.

α-HELIX

α-Helices ranging from 4 or 5 residues to 40 residues are found in compact globular proteins such as hemoglobin, while long rod-like proteins like the tail of the cytoskeletal protein myosin are made up of long helices twisted around each other to form coiled coils. The membrane-spanning regions of integral membrane proteins, for example, those of the red cell membrane protein glycophorin and the platelet α_2-adrenergic (epinephrine) receptor, are frequently α-helical regions of about 20 amino acids. An α-helix is formed from a continuous sequence of amino acid residues in a protein. One turn of an α-helix contains 3.6 amino acid residues, with hydrogen bonds forming between the carbonyl oxygen of residue n and the amide hydrogen of residue n + 4 (Fig. 3-7A). The distance between one turn of an α-helix and the next, its pitch, is 5.4 Å. With 3.6 residues per turn, the rise per residue along the vertical axis of the helix is 1.5 Å. Theoretically, an α-helix can be either right-handed or left-handed with regard to direction of screw. In proteins, left-handed helices are rarely seen as the side chains of L amino acids approach the C'═O group too closely.

With the exception of proline, there are no strong predictors of whether a particular amino acid side chain is likely or not to be incorporated into an α-helix. The last atom of the proline side chain is bonded to the main chain nitrogen atom, preventing the nitrogen atom from participating in hydrogen bond formation (Fig. 3-2A). In addition, the proline side chain sterically hinders the α-helical conformation, producing a bend in the helix if it appears after the first turn. Therefore, proline is not found within α-helices.

The distribution of residues on the surface of a helix can be visualized using a helical wheel. Residues are plotted every 100 degrees (360°/3.6) around a circle or spiral (Fig. 3-7B). The plot shows the projection of the position of side chains on a plane perpendicular to the helix axis with side chains on one side of the helix appearing on one side of the wheel. Given the periodicity of the residues in an α-helix, charged and polar residues may be arrayed on one face of the helix, while hydrophobic residues appear on the opposite face. A region of the propeptide of factor IX is an amphipathic helix, having a hydrophilic face and a hydrophobic face.

β-SHEETS

The second important element of secondary structure is the β-sheet. In contrast to the α-helix, the β-sheet is formed from several different regions of a polypeptide chain. The stretches of polypeptide, usually 5–10 residues long, that form the β-sheet are called β-strands. The β-strands are aligned to form hydrogen bonds between the carbonyl oxygen atoms on one strand and the amide hydrogen atom on the opposite strand. If in successive β-strands the amino acids are running in the same direction, N terminal to C terminal, then the β-sheet is termed parallel (Fig. 3-8A); if successive strands alternate directions, the sheet is termed antiparallel (Fig. 3-8B). Mixed β-sheets in which some of the β-strands are parallel and some antiparallel are uncommon. The hydrogen-bonding pattern is distinct in the two forms of β-sheet. In either case, however, the sheet appears pleated; alternate C_α groups appear above and below the plane of the β-sheet. Likewise, the amino acid

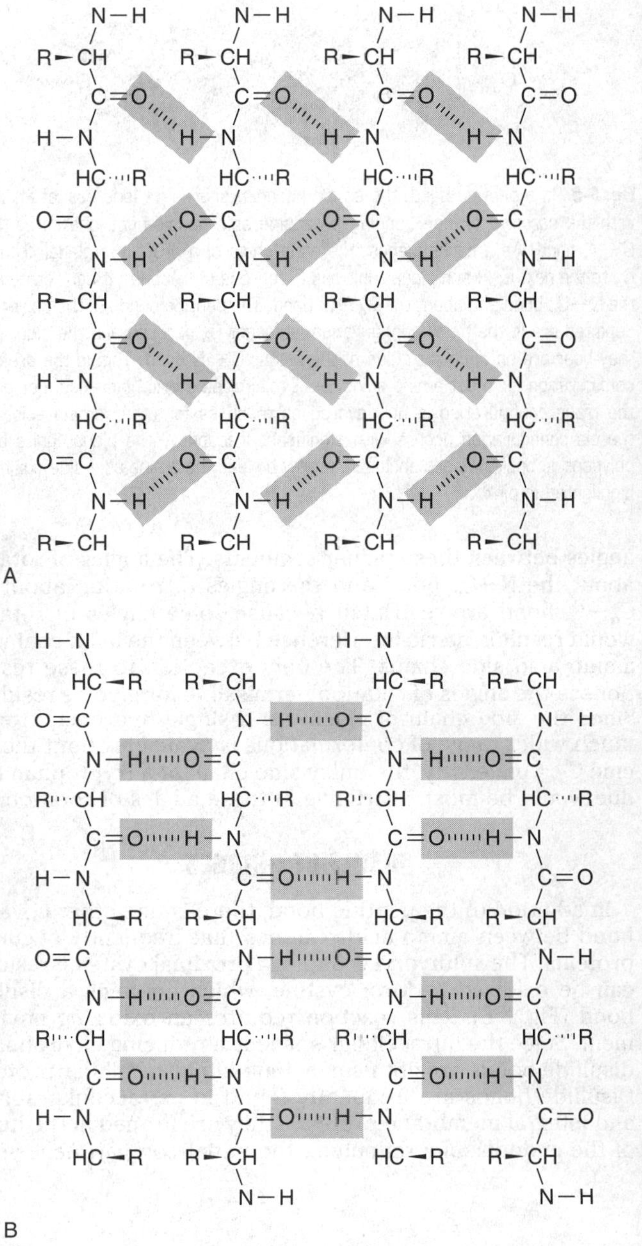

Fig. 3-8. β-Sheets are formed from several regions of a polypeptide chain. The strands of polypeptide assembled in a β-sheet may be parallel, that is, aligned in the same direction from N to C terminus, or the strands may be antiparallel, that is, aligned in alternating direction from N to C terminus. **(A)** Schematic drawing of a parallel β-sheet. **(B)** Schematic drawing of an antiparallel β-sheet. The hydrogen bonds that stabilize these structures are highlighted in red.

side chains on a β-strand are alternately above and below the plane of the β-sheet.

PROTEIN TERTIARY STRUCTURE: ASSEMBLY OF SECONDARY STRUCTURES AND DOMAINS

Most proteins are made up of combinations of α-helices and β-sheets connected by regions of less regular structure usually termed *loops*. The α-helices and β-sheets pack together to form the hydrophobic core of a protein, while the loop regions tend to appear on the surface of the protein. Loops can be of three general types: (1) tight turns, in which the carbonyl oxygen of the first residue and the amide hydrogen of the fourth residue share a hydrogen bond; (2) loops that are stabilized primarily by side chain-to-main chain hydrogen bonds; and (3) extended

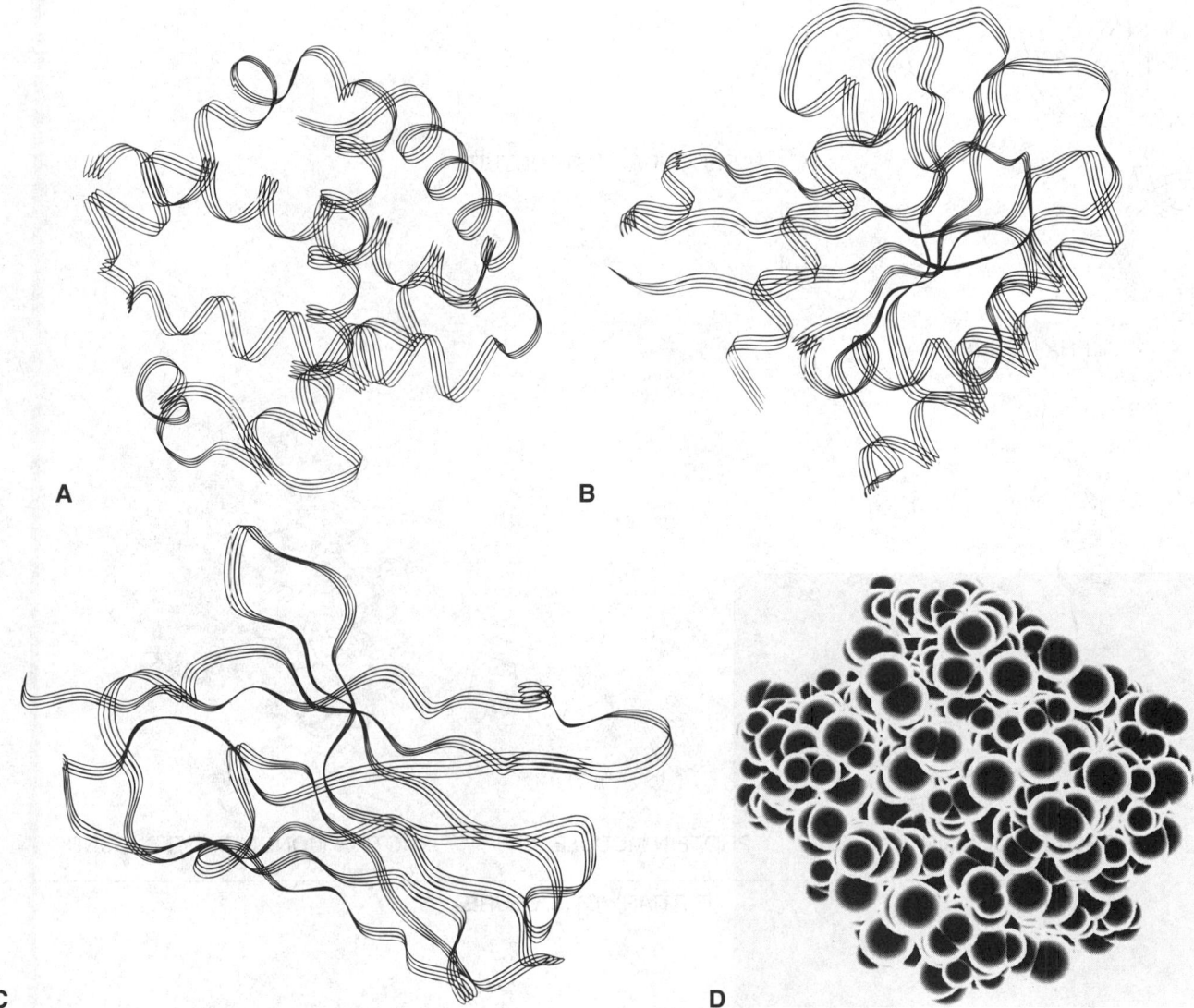

Fig. 3-9. Models illustrating the three-dimensional structures of several protein domains. **(A–C)** Ribbon diagrams, making it easy to discern the elements of secondary structure that make up a protein domain. **(A)** α-Subunit of hemoglobin composed almost entirely of α-helices. **(B)** H-*ras* oncogene protein p21 composed of both α-helices and β-sheets. **(C)** Variable domain of an immunoglobulin heavy chain composed almost entirely of β-sheets. Although the ribbon diagrams, which omit amino acid side chains and trace the protein backbone, are useful for observing the secondary structures within a protein, they give the misleading impression that there is a large amount of empty space within the molecule. This is not the case. In fact, the core of globular proteins is densely packed with atoms. **(D)** α-Subunit of hemoglobin in a space-filling model in which the atoms are represented by spheres with radii proportional to their van der Waals radii. It is clear from this representation that very little empty space is present within the protein core.

structures that do not contain hydrogen bonds. Comparison of homologous proteins among species suggests greater mutability of loop regions than of regions of regular secondary structure. The structures of the folded cores of the proteins are preserved during evolution, while insertions or deletions of several amino acids occur primarily in loop regions.

The arrangement of secondary structures within a polypeptide defines its tertiary structure. The packing of secondary structural elements into a compact folded form brings distant parts of the polypeptide chain into close proximity. Proteins may be assigned to one of four classes depending on the content and arrangement of secondary structure within the core of the protein. Proteins of the α-class are made up primarily of α-helices with connecting loop structures. Similarly, β-proteins are made up of β-sheets connected by loop regions. In αβ-proteins the two elements of secondary structure alternate, again connected by loops. A fourth class of proteins, α + β, incorporates both α-helices and β-sheets, but these elements are not arranged in an easily identifiable pattern. Most proteins studied to date are of the α-, β-, or αβ-classes. Figure 3-9 shows examples of α-, β-, and αβ-proteins.

Many proteins are made up of multiple domains. A protein domain, frequently encoded in a single exon, is a region of a polypeptide chain that can fold autonomously into a stable tertiary structure. The spatial relationship of these independent domains within a protein is part of the description of its tertiary structure. The relationship of secondary structure, protein domains, tertiary structure, and quatenary structure is illustrated in Figure 3-10.

During evolution a limited number of protein domains have been used repeatedly: related domains from different proteins share enough sequence homology to preserve the polypeptide fold but may have markedly different amino acid sequences and functions. Such domains, which appear to be associated with exon shuffling and duplication, have been termed modules. Examples of proteins whose tertiary structures are built from such conserved modules abound in plasma and as components of cells within the vasculature. A demonstration of the assembly of discrete proteins from such modules is given in Chapter 100 for the proteins involved in hemostasis and fibrinolysis. These proteins incorporate epidermal growth factor-like domains, kringle domains, and type I and type II fibronectin

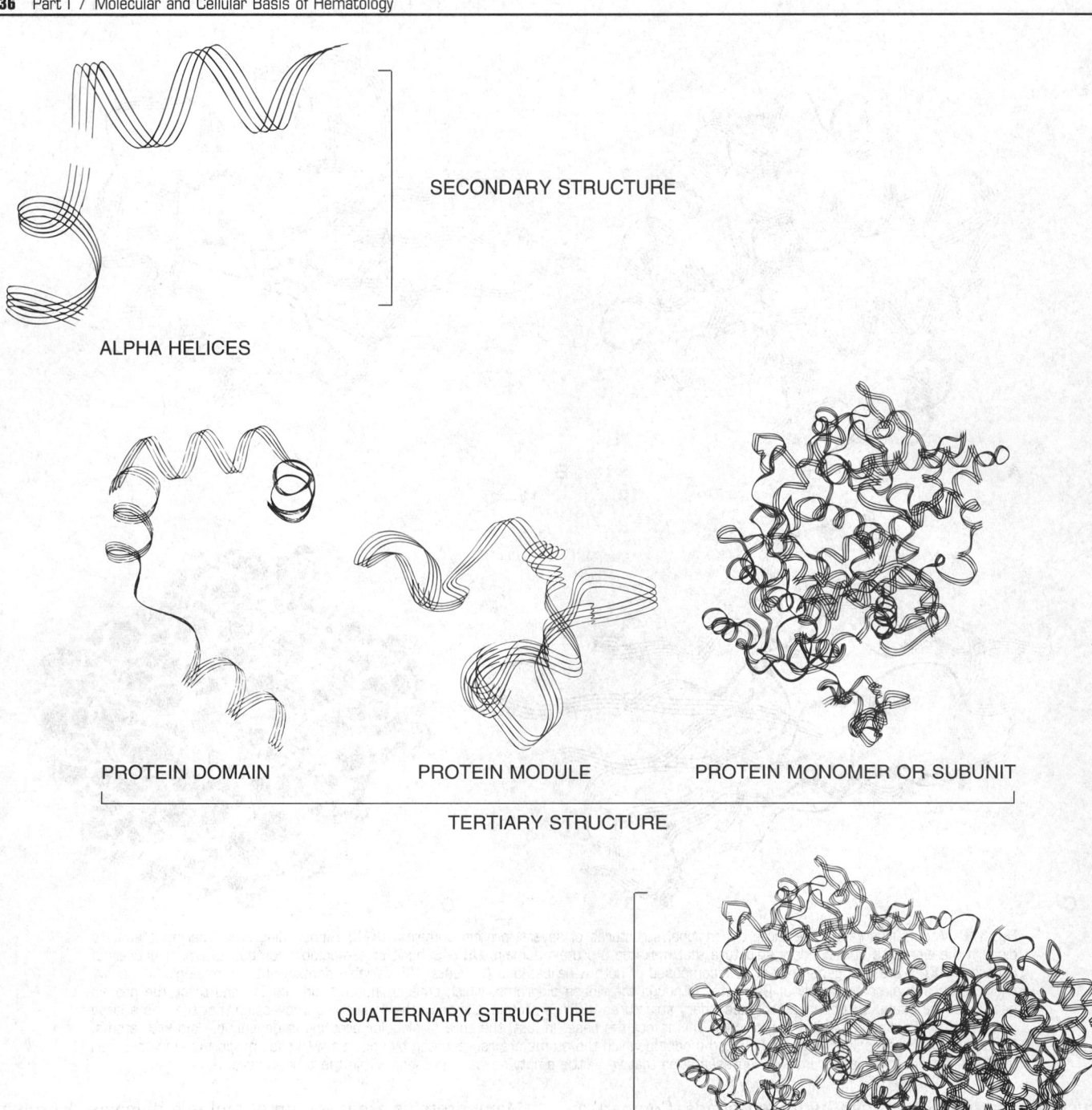

SECONDARY STRUCTURE

ALPHA HELICES

PROTEIN DOMAIN   PROTEIN MODULE   PROTEIN MONOMER OR SUBUNIT

TERTIARY STRUCTURE

QUATERNARY STRUCTURE

PROTEIN DIMER

Fig. 3-10. Structure of ovine prostaglandin H_2 synthase-1 is used to illustrate the hierarchical nature of protein folding. The organization of the secondary structures within a domain define its tertiary structure; the orientation of protein domains and protein modules within a protein subunit define its tertiary structure. When a protein is made up of more than one subunit, the spatial relationship of the subunits in the assembled protein defines the proteins quaternary structure. (The coordinates for this structure were kindly provided by Dr. Michael Garavito, Department of Biochemistry and Molecular Biology, University of Chicago; the structure is described in Picot et al.)

domains, all of which are widely distributed in mammalian proteins. The DNA-binding zinc finger domain is an example of the importance of these conserved domains to intracellular proteins as well. It is hypothesized that the modules within a given class share a stable core structure with discrete functions determined by the nonconserved amino acids expressed on the module's surface.

QUATERNARY STRUCTURE: ASSEMBLY OF POLYPEPTIDE CHAINS

For some proteins the functional unit is made up of more than one independently synthesized polypeptide chain. The orientation of the polypeptide chains to one another within the functional unit is termed the quaternary structure of a multimeric protein. A multimeric protein may be made up of identical subunits or polypeptide chains, as in glucosephosphate isomerase, a dimer of two identical polypeptide chains, or different subunits, as in hemoglobin, in which the functional protein contains two α- and two β-subunits. The interaction between the subunits of a multimeric protein may be stabilized by disulfide bonds between the polypeptide chains. The interaction of the light and heavy chains of immunoglobulin molecules and the Aα chains, Bβ chains, and γ-chains of fibrinogen are examples of such proteins. The subunits of a multimeric protein may influence one another, as in the binding of oxygen to hemoglobin, in which the occupancy of one heme group with oxygen influences the affinity of the heme groups of the remaining three subunits for oxygen. Alternatively, the subunits of the assembled multimeric protein may provide a unique function, as in the formation of the antigen-binding site of an immunoglobulin, the complementarity-determining site being formed by the variable regions of both the heavy and light chains of the immunoglobulin molecule. Finally, there are multi-subunit proteins in which each subunit has a distinct function; RNA polymerase is an example of such a protein.

SUGGESTED READINGS

Alberts B, Bray D, Lewis J et al: Molecular Biology of the Cell. 2nd Ed. Garland, New York, 1989

Baron M, Norman DG, Campbell ID: Protein modules. TIBS 16:13, 1991

Branden C, Tooze J: Introduction to Protein Structure. Garland Press, New York, 1991

Creighton TE: Proteins: Structures and Molecular Properties. 2nd Ed. WH Freeman, New York, 1993

Janin J, Chothia C: Domains in proteins: definitions, location and structural principles. Methods Enzymol 115:420, 1985

Levitt M, Chothia C: Structural patterns in globular proteins. Nature 261:552, 1976

Richardson JS: The anatomy and taxonomy of protein structure. Adv Protein Chem 34:167, 1981

Richardson JS: Describing patterns of protein tertiary structure. Methods Enzymol 115:349, 1985

Richardson JS, Richardson DC: Principles and patterns of protein conformation. p. 1. In Fasman GD (ed): Prediction of Protein Structure and the Principles of Protein Conformation. Plenum, New York, 1989

Richardson DC: The origami of proteins. p. 5. In Gierasch LM, King J (eds): Protein Folding: Deciphering the Second Half of the Genetic Code. American Association for the Advancement of Science, Washington, DC, 1990

Plasma Membrane Dynamics and Organization

4

Jon S. Morrow

INTRODUCTION

Every student of hematology must develop an understanding of the plasma membrane. So fundamental is this structure to the cellular basis of life that the concept of the membrane as a semipermeable fluid lipid bilayer is taught even in the most elementary of biology courses. However, the commonly held view of the membrane as a "soap bubble," or as only a "fluid mosaic," ignores the complexity of real cells and the rich diversity of mechanisms by which cell membranes are stabilized and organized. Of particular interest is how membranes form specialized receptor domains and achieve vectorial exchange of nutrients and information with other cells and their milieu. Perhaps as a result of this complexity and the fundamental importance of the plasma membrane, it is difficult to conceive of a disease process that at the cellular level does not involve altered membrane function, often as the primary event.

The plasma membrane consists of a complex, ordered array of lipids and protein stretched over the outer surface of the cell in the form of a lipid bilayer punctuated by penetrating or attached proteins. The membrane thus forms the interface between each cell and its environment. Biologic membranes display numerous properties that may seem paradoxical. These features issue from the general properties of the lipids and proteins that compose the plasma membrane and from specialized interactions between specific membrane proteins or lipids, or both. Three features stand out:

1. *Plasma membranes are noncovalent assemblies of billions of molecules, yet they tend to be self-assemblying, self-sealing, and stable.* A typical animal cell plasma membrane contains $>10^9$ molecules of lipid and ≤ 10 million protein molecules. All these molecules remain indefinitely associated as an extraordinarily thin (60–100 Å), continuous sheet-like membrane enveloping the cell.

2. *Plasma membranes are fluid structures, yet they are highly ordered with respect to the distribution of molecules both across the bilayer as well as within the plane of the bilayer.* Thus, the distribution of both membrane lipids and proteins is highly asymmetric. Many factors, both intrinsic and extrinsic, act to order the membrane.

3. *Plasma membranes function as a barrier, yet they readily pass ions, nutrients, and information (signals) between the cytoplasm and the extracellular environment.* They are more than simply a semipermeable membrane, since they can transport some molecules against a concentration gradient. In addition, transmembrane signaling (information transfer) often occurs without transmembrane molecular passage.

In this chapter the biochemical basis for understanding these disparate but general properties of biologic membranes is discussed, emphasizing the common principles that underlie their assembly and function. Factors that establish and maintain order within the membrane are stressed, since it is the extent of organization of the plasma membrane that distinguishes it from simple lipid bilayers. Later chapters focus on the membranes of specific cells in health and disease.[1,2]

LIPID COMPONENTS OF PLASMA MEMBRANES

Amphipathic Lipids

Lipids are organic substances that are insoluble in water but soluble in a range of organic solvents such as chloroform, alcohol, or ether. Amphipathic implies that a compound has both a hydrophobic and hydrophilic character. Therefore, an amphipathic lipid is a molecule that, although insoluble in water, does have a hydrophilic portion in its structure (the polar head group). This group would be soluble if it were not for its attached hydrophobic tail.

The simplest amphipathic lipids are the fatty acids, containing a hydrocarbon tail of variable length, linked to a carboxyl group (Fig. 4-1). When such molecules are placed in an aqueous environment, they prefer to aggregate by forming spherical micelles in which their polar head groups face the water and their hydrophobic tails face away from water. Free fatty acids are not generally found in normal plasma membranes, but are often generated during pathologic processes. Their tendency to form micelles (instead of bilayers) may induce plasma membrane instability and cell injury.

More complex amphipathic lipids are found in the plasma membranes of all eukaryotic cells. Most of these lipids fall into one of just three classes (Fig. 4-2): (1) the phospholipids, (2) the glycolipids, and (3) cholesterol. A common feature of the more complex lipids is the increased bulkiness of their hydrophobic portions, which reduces the tendency of these lipids to form spherical micelles. Rather, these lipids satisfy the need to sequester their hydrophobic tails away from water by forming planar bilayers, with their polar head groups along each surface of the bilayer and their hydrophobic tails buried in the center of the bilayer (Fig. 4-1). The basic tendency of the plasma membrane to remain as a stable self-sealing bilayer is a property bestowed by its composition of complex amphipathic lipids and by their tendency to orient with their hydrophobic portions excluded from the water environment. This tendency of hydrophobic molecules or hydrophobic regions of a molecule to be excluded from water is called the hydrophobic effect.[3] It is one of the major forces driving membrane assembly and the interaction between membrane proteins and the lipid bilayer.

Phospholipids

Two types of phospholipids commonly occur in the plasma membrane of eucaryotes: (1) phosphoglycerides, which are derived from glycerol; and (2) sphingomyelin, which is derived

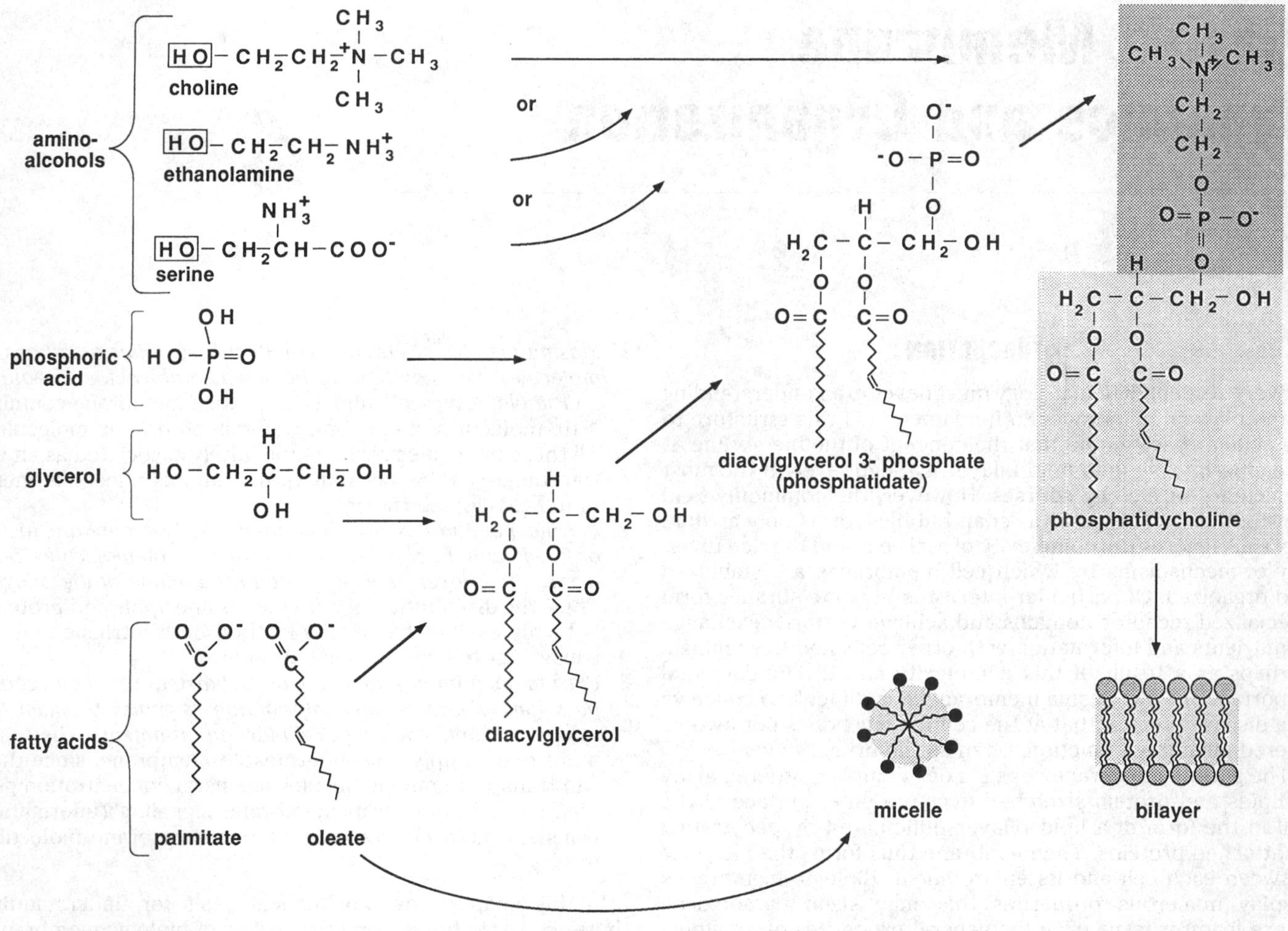

Fig. 4-1. The most basic building blocks of membranes are amphipathic lipids, such as phosphatidyl choline. This molecule is derived by the linkage of fatty acids to glycerol via an ester bond. Various amino alcohols are also linked by phosphoric acid to glycerol. Individual fatty acids will form micelles in aqueous solution. Phospholipids prefer to form planar bilayers.

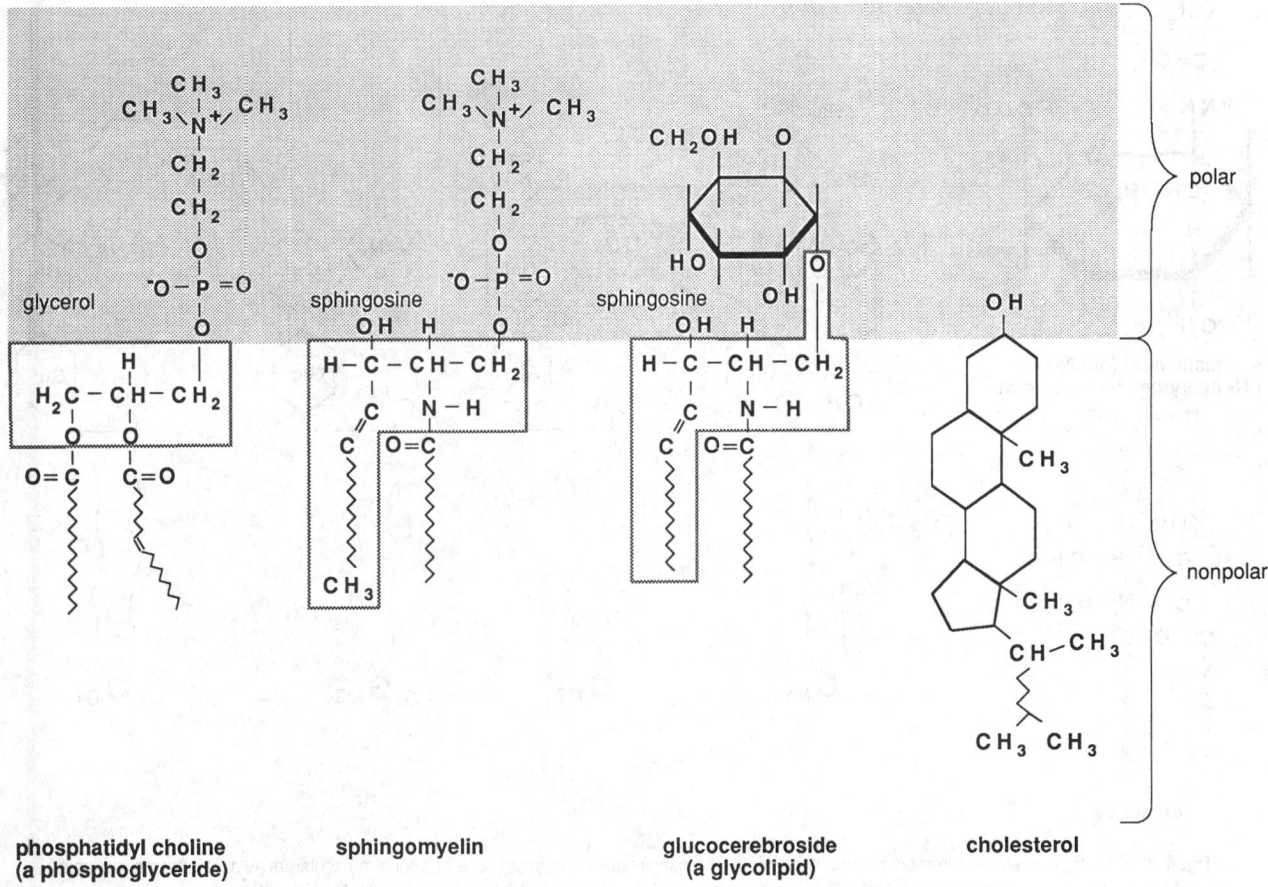

Fig. 4-2. The major types of membrane lipid are aligned to demonstrate their approximate orientation in the bilayer. Phosphatidylcholine and sphingomyelin are examples of phospholipids.

from sphingosine. These two kinds of lipids have a similar three-dimensional conformation; they function similarly in the membrane. Both also contain covalently bound fatty acid, usually with an even number of carbon atoms ranging from 14 to 24. The structure of these phospholipids is shown in Figure 4-2.

The phosphoglycerides are derived from a C_3 glycerol backbone (Fig. 4-1). Fatty acids are esterified to the C-1 and C-2 positions of the glycerol, to form diacylglycerol (DAG). The fatty acids may be either saturated or unsaturated (or both) and of variable length. The most common fatty acids in animals are saturated and include stearate (C_{18}) and palmitate (C_{16}). The introduction of a double bond(s) into the fatty acid tail (making it unsaturated) disrupts the packing of the hydrophobic tails at the center of the bilayer, and increases the overall fluidity of the membrane. Altering the degree of saturation of the phospholipids is a common mechanism by which procaryotes and plants control the fluidity of their membranes. In eucaryotes, fluidity is modulated by including variable amounts of cholesterol in the membrane, and by interactions involving the membrane proteins (see below).

A phosphoric acid molecule is esterified at the C-3 carbon of glycerol, forming diacylglycerol-3-phosphate. This compound is also known as phosphatidate and is the simplest phospholipid. It is present in only very small amounts in normal cell membranes. The more common phosphoglycerides are formed from phosphatidate by esterifying one of several alcohols to the phosphate group. The most common is choline, which after esterification forms phosphatidyl choline; other prominent phosphoglycerides include phosphatidyl ethanolamine, phosphatidyl serine, and phosphatidyl inositol (Fig. 4-1).

The other major phospholipid is sphingomyelin, which is based on the sphingosine molecule instead of glycerol (Fig. 4-2). Sphingosine is a large amino alcohol. A fatty acid is linked to the amino group through an amide bond, forming an intermediate compound called ceramide. This compound is also an intermediate in the synthesis of many glycolipids. Sphingomyelin is formed by esterifying a phosphoryl choline group to ceramide. Because C-4–C18 of sphingosine form a long hydrocarbon tail, the overall conformation of sphingomyelin in the membrane is very similar to that of phosphatidyl choline, the most common phosphoglyceride.

Glycolipids and Cholesterol

Glycolipids are lipids that contain sugar. While some of the phosphoglycerides may also contain sugar (e.g., phosphatidyl inositol), glycolipids are distinguished by the fact that phosphate esters are not involved in the linkage of the sugar to the hydrocarbon tail. Although glycolipids based on diacylglycerol are common in prokaryotes and plants, almost all glycolipids in eukaryotes are derived from ceramide (the amidated form of sphingosine). Glycolipids based on sphingosine are collectively called glycosphingolipids. In these compounds the polar head group is provided by the sugar molecules. The simplest glycosphingolipids are glucocerebroside and galactocerebroside, formed by esterifying glucose or galactose to ceramide. The more complex glycosphingolipids may contain ≤ 15 neutral sugars (the neutral glycolipids), or neutral sugars combined with one or more sialic acid residues (also called N-acetylneuraminic acid). The presence of sialic acid introduces a

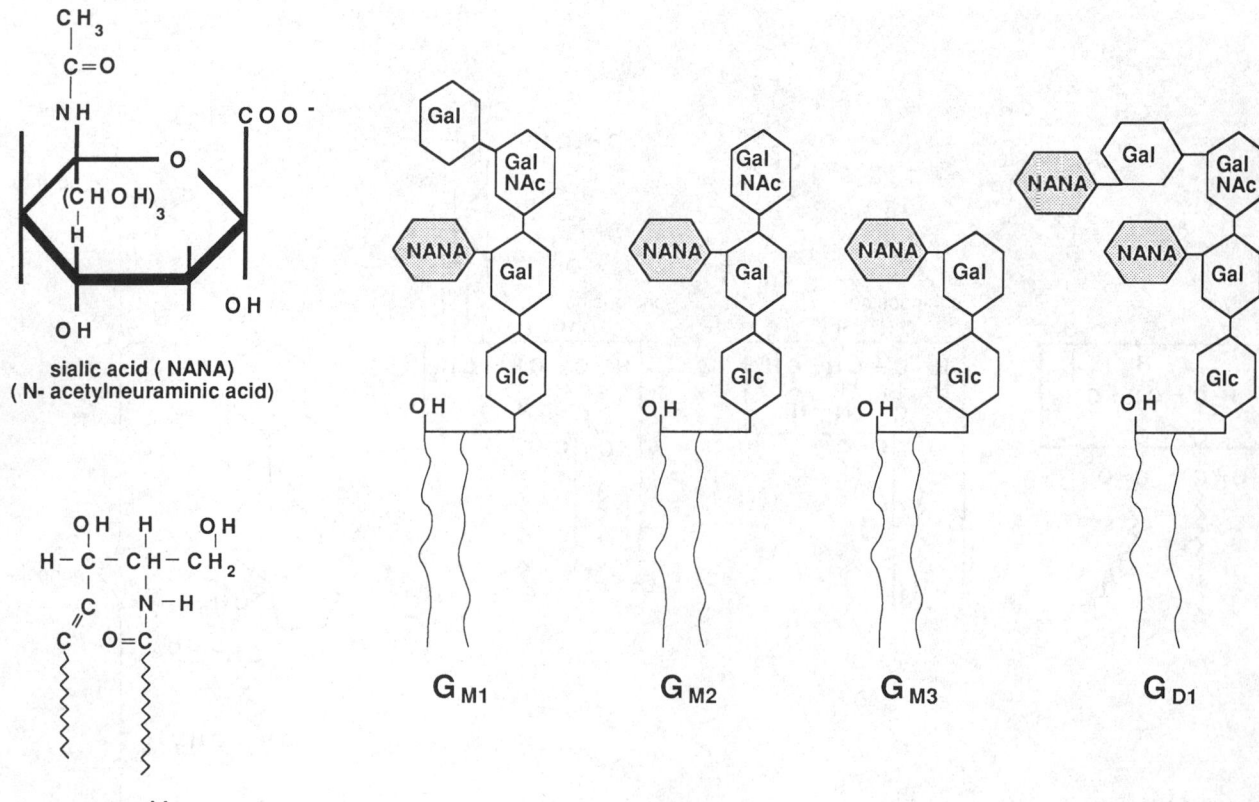

Fig. 4-3. Structure of some common glycosphingolipids. The gangliosides all contain one or more molecules of *N*-acetylneuraminic acid (NANA). Gangliosides containing one NANA group are designated G_m, (for mono); those with two NANAs, G_D (for di); those with three NANAs, G_T (for thi).

negative charge and renders the glycolipid acidic. Acidic glycolipids containing *N*-acetylneuraminic acid may be complex and as a group are called gangliosides. The structures of some of these compounds are shown in Figure 4-3.

The glycolipids are found exclusively on the extracellular face of the plasma membrane and constitute ≥5% of the total lipid of that face. Their carbohydrate structure is quite variable, even between different cells in the same organism. While their precise function is unknown, it seems likely that the cell's surface coat of carbohydrate, which is bestowed by its glycolipids (and glycoproteins and other absorbed carbohydrate, the glycocalyx), probably plays a role in intercellular recognition and the maintenance of membrane asymmetry.

Cholesterol differs from the other lipids in that it does not contain an esterified fatty acid and is entirely hydrophobic except for its hydroxyl group on C-3 (Fig. 4-2). Cholesterol is abundant in the plasma membrane of eukaryotic cells, where it may be present in amounts equimolar with all of the phospholipids combined. Its primary role appears to be in the control of membrane fluidity, since it reduces the ability of the fatty acid tails of phospholipids and glycolipids to pack in an ordered way within the bilayer. When such packing occurs, as would happen below the phase transition temperature of a lipid membrane, the bilayer becomes semisolid, and most membrane transport processes are inhibited. Sufficient amounts of cholesterol incorporated into a membrane will eliminate this phase transition. Paradoxically, although cholesterol prevents the crystallization of the fatty acid side chains below the transition temperature, its bulky sterol nucleus hinders side chain motion and fluidity near the surface of the bilayer. Thus, the net effect of cholesterol is to dampen changes in the fluidity of the membrane that might otherwise occur with changes in side chain composition or temperature.

PROTEIN COMPONENTS OF PLASMA MEMBRANE

Membrane Proteins

For most plasma membranes, about 50% of the membrane mass is composed of protein. Proteins that are associated with the membrane determine most of its tensile and functional properties. Operationally, membrane proteins have been characterized as either integral or peripheral, based on their relative ease of extraction.[4,5] Integral proteins are tightly embedded in the bilayer and are extracted only by strong detergents or organic solvents. Peripheral proteins can be removed without disruption of the lipid bilayer, usually by milder treatments such as high- or low-salt or high-pH extraction. The structural correlates of this concept of integral and peripheral proteins is shown in Figure 4-4. In general, proteins that interact strongly with the bilayer (i.e., are integral) are amphipathic molecules that span the lipid bilayer; those more easily stripped (i.e., peripheral) are associated with only one face of the bilayer, or noncovalently with integral proteins embedded in the bilayer.

Unfortunately, not all membrane-associated molecules are so easily compartmentalized. For example, many proteins may be variably associated with the membrane; may bind specific phospholipids both in vivo and in vitro; or may undergo fatty acylation by the covalent addition of myristate, palmitate, glycosylinositol phospholipids, or other fatty acids[6,7] (Table 4-1). For proteins undergoing fatty acylation, myristic acid is invariably linked via an amide bond to the amino group on an NH_2-terminal glycine; palmitate is linked by a thioester bond to internal cysteine residues; and phosphatidylinositol is joined by a complex carbohydrate-ethanolamine linkage to the COOH of the C-terminal residue. In addition, several proteins are now recognized that alternatively may be synthesized as soluble

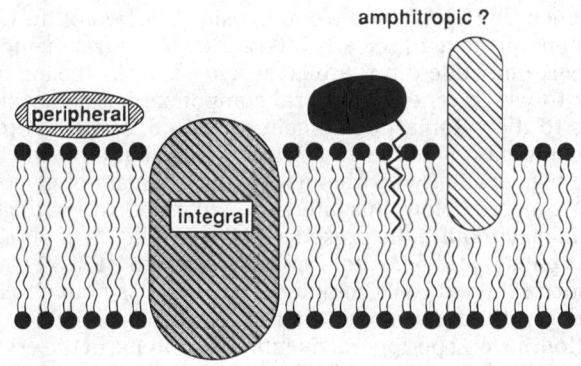

Fig. 4-4. The arrangement of membrane proteins. Some proteins interact directly with the bilayer. Others utilize indirect linkages, such as covalently bound fatty acid molecules. Proteins that reside only within the hydrophobic region of the bilayer have not been identified. Some proteins may only pass partway (dip?) into the bilayer.

precursors but that are able to insert themselves into lipid membranes coincident with a conformational rearrangement. Two proteins displaying such behavior are the C9 component of complement and perforin, the cytolytic component of natural killer and cytotoxic T lymphocytes. Both of these proteins are able to insert into membranes to form pores. Although the exact mechanism by which perforin or C9 inserts into the membrane remains unknown, it is probably similar to the mechanism deduced by x-ray diffraction studies of the pore-forming antibiotic colicin A.[8] This antibiotic is produced by *Escherichia coli* and forms voltage-sensitive channels in membranes. The key feature of this protein is a hydrophobic hairpin loop of α-helical peptide segments; once positioned over the membrane, this loop progressively inserts itself into the bilayer. Such insertion is accompanied by a conformational rearrangement and possibly a polymerization of the protein in the membrane. Yet another example of such amphiphilic behavior is exhibited by the defensins, small (3,000–4,000-MW) proteins active in the immune response that permeabilize the membranes of microorganisms and enveloped viruses.[9] Thus, under different conditions, all these proteins could be regarded as either soluble (not membrane-associated), peripheral, or integral membrane proteins. A term that has recently been applied to such proteins as a class is amphitropic.[10] The heuristic value of this classification remains to be established.

Transmembrane Proteins

Proteins that span the membrane can be roughly divided into two structural classes, based on the amount of peptide embedded in the bilayer (Fig. 4-5). Most transmembrane proteins contain large amounts of α-helix, although some with a β-structure have been identified. The first transmembrane protein to be sequenced was glycophorin A from human erythrocytes.[11] The sequence of this protein suggested the existence of three domains (Fig. 4-6): (1) a cytoplasmic 39-residue domain containing a cluster of basic residues positioned near the plasma membrane; (2) a 19-residue hydrophobic domain that forms a single α-helix spanning the bilayer; and (3) a 72-residue external domain containing 15 O-linked (to serine) and one N-linked (to asparagine) carbohydrate units. Collectively, these contain approximately 100 sugar residues and include a high content of sialic acid.

As with the glycolipids, all the carbohydrate in glycoproteins is located on the external surface of the membrane. Other integral membrane proteins also have a central hydrophobic 19–22-residue core[12] (Fig. 4-7). Almost certainly each of these

hydrophobic stretches forms a single α-helical segment spanning the bilayer. Therefore, one common structural motif found in transmembrane proteins is that of a single α-helix about 20 residues long that spans the lipid bilayer. It is worth noting that in each of these proteins, the hydrophobic core is bordered by clusters of basic and acidic residues. Presumably, these charge clusters interact with specific phospholipids asymmetrically distributed across the membrane.

A second structural pattern that has been identified in transmembrane proteins is exemplified by bacteriorhodopsin. This 25-kd protein forms organized crystalline sheets in the purple membrane of the bacterium *Halobacterium halobium*. Each molecule of bacteriorhodopsin contains a single molecule of retinal and on light stimulation transports a proton into the cytoplasm

Table 4-1. Peripheral or Soluble Proteins that Interact with Lipids

Protein	Lipid Noncovalent	Lipid Covalent
α-Actinin	DAG, FA	—
Acetylcholinesterase	—	PI
Actin	—	pal
Adducin	PC	?
Alkaline phosphatase	—	PI
Ankyrin	—	pal
Apolipoprotein A-1	—	pal
Calcineurin B	—	myr
Calpactin	PS, PI	—
cAMP kinase (catalytic unit)	—	myr
Decay-accelerating factor	—	PI
Filamin	PIP$_2$	—
5'-Nucleotidase	—	PI
Leishmania protease	—	PI
Myosin 1 (110k-CM)	PS, PIP$_2$	—
NCAM-120	—	PI
NADH-cyt b$_5$ reductase	—	myr
p15^{gag} of MM leukemia virus	—	myr
p21^{ras}	—	pal
p29$^{gag-fes}$	—	myr
p56^{lck}	—	myr
p60^{src}	—	myr
p85$^{gag-fes}$	—	myr
p120$^{gag-abl}$	—	myr
Profilin	PIP$_2$, PIP	—
Protein 4.1	PS	pal, ste, ole
Protein 4.2	—	? myr[a]
Spectrin	PS, PE	—
SV40 virus large T antigen	—	pal
T-cell activating protein	—	PI
T-cell alloantigen	—	PI
thy-1 antigen	—	PI
Trehalase	—	PI
Trypanosome VSG	—	PI
Vinculin	PI, PIP$_2$, PS	pal, myr

Abbreviations: PC, phosphatidylcholine; DAG, diacylglycerol; FA, fatty acid; PI, phosphatidylinositol; PIP, phosphatidylinositol 4-phosphate; PIP$_2$, phosphatidylinositol 4,5-bisphosphate; PS, phosphatidylserine; PE, phosphatidyl ethanolamine; pal, palmitic acid; myr, myristic acid; ste, stearic acid; ole, oleic acid; NCAM, neural cell adhesion molecule; MM, Moloney murine; SV$_{40}$, simian virus 40; VSG, variant surface glycoprotein.

[a] Korsgren, Lawler, Lambert, Speicher, and Cohen, personal communication.

(Data from references 6, 7, and 10 with modifications from references 33, 62, 63, and 64.)

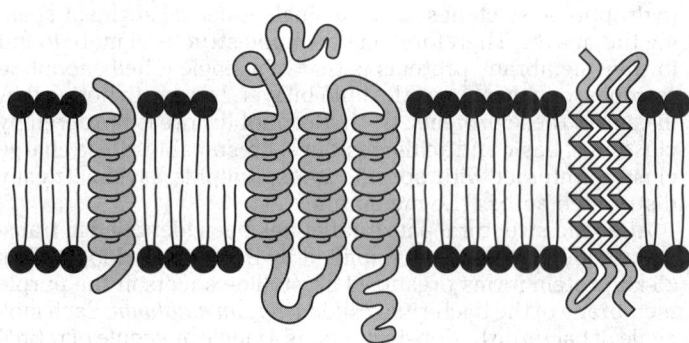

Fig. 4-5. Structural features of transmembrane proteins. Two general types of proteins are those with either a single α-helix spanning the bilayer (e.g., glycophorin) or those that are more globular with most of their mass in the bilayer. Of the latter type, either α-helical or β-pleated sheet structure may be the predominate pattern of organization. The most common pattern is α-helical, as exemplified by bacteriorhodopsin (center); porin is an example of a protein with a β-sheet.

of the bacterium. Using very low-dose electron microscopy of unstained membranes and sophisticated image reconstruction techniques, the structure of bacteriorhodopsin was determined to 7-Å resolution in 1975 by Henderson,[13] and Unwin.[14] They found that the protein was composed of seven transmembrane α-helices, each tilted slightly with respect to the plane of the membrane (Fig. 4-5). The length of each transmembrane segment was about 30 residues. Subsequently, other transmembrane proteins, such as the acetylcholine receptor[15] and the photosynthetic reaction center from a purple bacterium (*Rhodopseudomonas viridis*)[16] have also been shown to contain multiple transmembrane α-helices. Thus, it appears that transmembrane α-helices are a frequent feature of transmembrane proteins.

However, α-helices are not a universal feature of transmembrane proteins. Porin is a protein from *E. coli* outer membranes that forms voltage-dependent ion channels across the membrane. Like bacteriorhodopsin, most of its mass is embedded in the bilayer, with only very small domains that bulge into the aqueous phase. Unlike bacteriorhodopsin or glycophorin, porin contains no sizable hydrophobic domains that would be predicted to form a transbilayer α-helix on the basis of hydropathy plots.[17,18] When examined by high-angle x-ray diffraction, porin was found to consist largely of β-pleated sheet secondary structure.[19,20] In this protein, 16 strands of antiparallel β barrel span the membrane with a mean length of 10–12 residues (versus the 19–22 residues required in an α-helical configuration). These strands are oriented approximately normal (perpendicular) to the membrane and form a hydrophilic ion pore. Other transmembrane proteins that may be composed at least partly of β-barrel or pleated sheet structure include maltose binding protein of *E. coli*,[21] α-toxin of *Staphylococcus aureus*,[22] the nicotinic acetyl choline receptor,[15] defensin HNP-3,[9] and the chemotactic protein CheY from *Salmonella typhimurium*.[23]

Peripheral Membrane Proteins

Most peripheral membrane proteins are located at the cytoplasmic face of the membrane. Their nature is best understood in the mammalian erythrocyte, where they form a dense and nearly continuous protein coat that lines the inner surface of the membrane (Fig. 4-8 and Plate 4-1). Based on their extractability at pH 11, ≥10 prominent peripheral proteins have been identified in this cell by sodium dodecyl sulfate (SDS) polyacrylamide gel electrophoresis (Fig. 4-8). They are α- and β-spectrin (bands 1 and 2); ankyrin; adducin; proteins 4.1, 4.2, and 4.9; actin; tropomodulin; glyceraldehyde-3-phosphate de-

hydrogenase (G3PD); and tropomyosin.[24–26] Two of these, ankyrin and protein 4.1, clearly interact with integral membrane proteins embedded in the bilayer and serve as linking molecules to which other peripheral components attach. Ankyrin binds to the cytoplasmic domain of band 3, as well as to the α-subunit of Na/K-ATPase.[27] Protein 4.1 can bind to band 3 but has a higher affinity for the cytoplasmic domain of glycophorin.[28] As noted below, this interaction of protein 4.1 with glycophorin may require the presence of a special type of phospholipid, phosphatidylinositol 4,5-bisphosphate (PIP₂). Only a portion of the red cell's complement of G3PD is bound to band 3, along with minor amounts of other glycolytic enzymes. In addition, several peripheral membrane proteins of the erythrocyte can bind directly to the bilayer, at least under some conditions. Spectrin (and its nonerythroid analogues) is able to bind directly to a protein site on stripped plasma membranes without the participation of ankyrin,[29,30] and it may also interact directly with certain phospholipids (Table 4-1). Protein 4.1 interacts directly with phosphatidylserine[31] and may be fatty acylated[32]; adducin also interacts with phosphatidylserine[33]; and ankyrin binds to the membrane directly via a covalent linkage to palmitic acid in some species.[34]

A common structural motif has not emerged for peripheral membrane proteins. For example, spectrin (or the nonerythroid analogue of spectrin called fodrin[25]) is an approximately 500-kd heterodimeric protein that exists as an extended flexible rod about 100 nM long. Filamin is a similar sized homodimeric protein with an overall shape similar to that of spectrin. Filamin is prominent in platelets and smooth muscle. Both are peripheral membrane proteins, and both bind phospholipid, actin, and other proteins. Yet spectrin is about 70% α-helix, while filamin is largely β-sheet.[35]

A property that is frequently shared among peripheral proteins is multifunctionality or multivalency, or both. Thus, spectrin binds itself, ankyrin, protein 4.1, actin, calmodulin, adducin, and phospholipid; ankyrin binds band 3, vimentin, and spectrin; and protein 4.1 binds actin, calmodulin, spectrin, band 3, and phospholipid. Such multifunctional proteins are important since they can participate in the formation of anastamosing protein arrays at the face of the membrane and can organize constituents within the membrane. Collectively, the linked array of multifunctional proteins lining the cytoplasmic face of the plasma membrane is termed the cortical cytoskeleton or the membrane skeleton. It is an essential component of the plasma membrane, and one of the dominant structures imposing order on the membrane (Fig. 4-8 and Plate 4-1).

INTERACTIONS AND FUNCTIONS OF MEMBRANE PROTEINS AND LIPIDS

Asymetric Distribution

In the absence of other constraints, most lipids freely diffuse in the plane of the membrane, with typical diffusion coefficients of $2–4 \times 10^{-9}$ cm²/sec. The diffusional rate for unrestrained integral membrane proteins is similar, as evidenced by the diffusion rates of band 3 or glycophorin when the purified proteins are reconstituted into artificial liposomes.[36] The average distance in centimeters (δ) that a molecule will move in two dimensions is related to the diffusion coefficient (D) by:

$$\delta = (4Dt)^{1/2}$$

One therefore expects that phospholipids or proteins with unrestricted lateral mobility will diffuse from one end of a red cell to the other in <1 minute. Conversely, the transverse diffusional rate of these molecules, (i.e., the rate that they "flip-

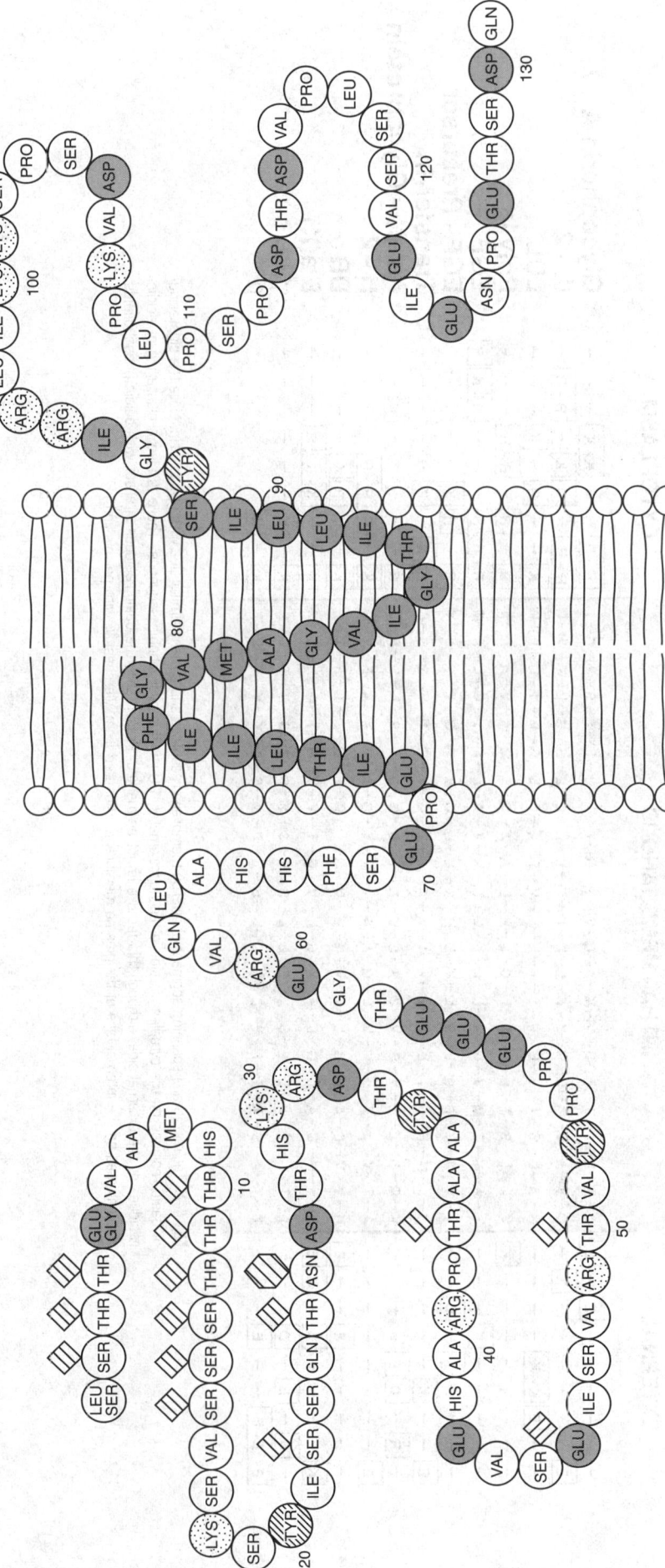

Fig. 4-6. The covalent structure of glycophorin A. Two hydrophilic domains are separated by a hydrophobic transmembrane domain (red). Note the clustering of basic residues (shaded) at the cytoplasmic face of the membrane, a property shared by other proteins that pass a single α-helix through the membrane (see Fig. 4-7). (Courtesy of Dr. V. Marchesi.)

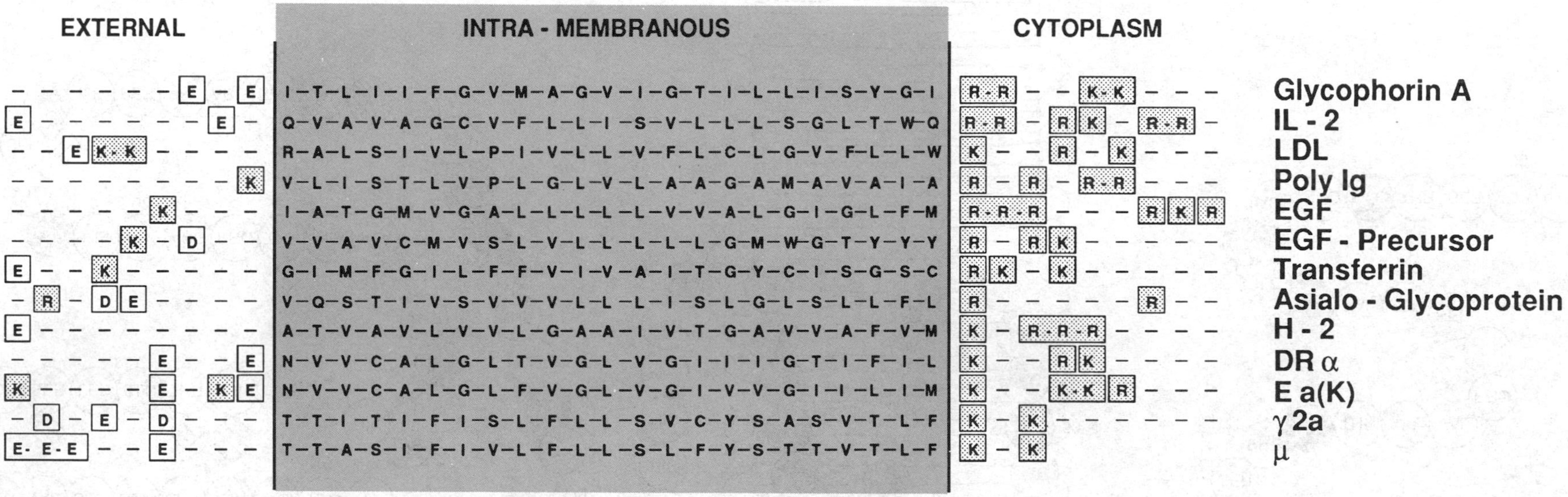

Fig. 4-7. The membrane-spanning segment of diverse membrane receptors share many similarities with glycophorin. Note the clustering of basic residues on the cytoplasmic side of an approximately 20-residue hydrophobic sequence. There is also a clustering of acidic residues on the external side, although this feature is not as marked. Presumably, the basic residues interact with acidic phospholipids concentrated on the internal face of the plasma membrane. (Adapted from Marchesi,[12] with permission.)

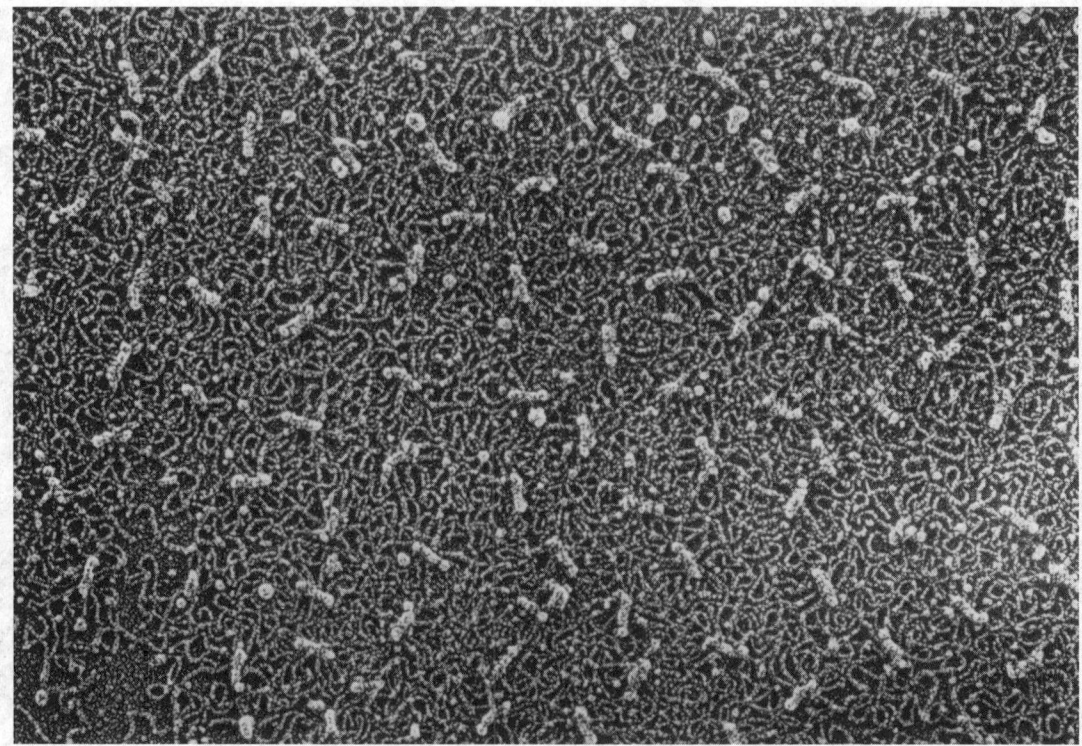

Fig. 4-8. The peripheral membrane skeleton of the mammalian erythrocyte. Erythrocyte membranes were briefly extracted with NP-40 (non-ionic detergent) and 1.5mM NaCl, quick frozen, deep etched, and then examined by electron microscopy. The view is of the cytoplasmic surface of the membrane. A dense anastamosing network of spectrin links short actin filaments. (Photograph courtesy of Dr. J. Heuser; from Coleman et al,[24] with permission.)

flop" across the bilayer) is much slower due to the unfavorable free energy change attendant on dragging a hydrophilic head group through the hydrophobic membrane. For phospholipids, a given molecule will usually require many hours before it will flip across the membrane even once,[37] and most transmembrane proteins and glycolipids probably do not flip at all. Thus, because their insertion is not random, many of the lipids and all of the proteins are asymmetrically oriented with respect to the two faces of the plasma membrane. Typically, the external surface contains all the protein, carbohydrate, and glycolipids and is rich in neutral phospholipids such as phosphatidylcholine, while the inner leaflet of the bilayer is enriched in acidic phospholipids such as phosphatidylserine and phosphatidylethanolamine. The inner half of the bilayer also contains all of the phosphatidylinositol phosphates.

Most proteins and some lipids also display restricted mobility and a nonrandom distribution in the plane of the membrane. For example, in the erythrocyte, only about 60% of band 3 and 75% of glycophorin diffuse at all, and then with a rate nearly 100 times more slowly than that of unrestricted lipids or proteins.[38] In fibroblast plasma membranes, stable, laterally segregated protein-rich domains of ≤ 1 μm across have been identified.[39] Ordered arrays involving membrane proteins such as spectrin,[40] clathrin (coated pits),[41] talin and vinculin (adhesion plaques),[42] and actin are an obvious and characteristic feature of eukaryotic cells (Fig. 4-9).

Membrane Organization

A major question in membrane biology is how the plasma membrane achieves and maintains its high level of organization. Three mechanisms that act at the membrane appear to be dominant: (1) ordering by the cytoplasmic cytoskeleton or the cortical cytoskeleton, or both; (2) ordering by specific associations between integral membrane proteins or lipids, or both, within the bilayer; and (3) ordering by extracellular ligands. In some cases, a level of organization is also established at the time of membrane assembly and is subsequently maintained by mechanisms intrinsic to the membrane. An example would be the vectoral insertion of specific membrane proteins into either the apical or basolateral domain of epithelial cells. Subsequent mixing of proteins between these two domains is prevented by the presence of the tight junctional complex that bridges the monolayer.[43] More precise levels of organization (not simply apical or basolateral) are established in the plasma membrane by factors acting on the membrane itself.

Cortical Cytoskeleton

The role of the cortical cytoskeleton in organizing the plasma membrane is now well established. Antibodies directed to spectrin lead to a reorganization of the integral membrane proteins in erythrocyte ghosts. The removal of spectrin by low-salt extraction leads to aggregation of the intramembranous particles.[44] More recent data also demonstrate that the lateral mobility of both band 3 and glycophorin are controlled by the spectrin/ankyrin/protein 4.1 assembly.[38] In other cells, various analogues of spectrin and in some cases ankyrin precisely colocalize with collections of specific receptors or transport proteins. The best characterized of these associations include Na/K-ATPase at the lateral margins of renal epithelial cells[45,46]; the voltage-dependent Na$^+$ channel at the nodes of Ranvier[47]; and the clustered acetylcholine receptors at the neuromuscular junction.[40] The most obvious way that a protein in the cortical cytoskeleton can participate in the organization of these receptor clusters is by binding strongly, either directly or indirectly, to at least two receptors at a time, thereby cross-linking the receptors and slowing their lateral diffusion.

In addition to direct cross-linking, the polyvalent properties

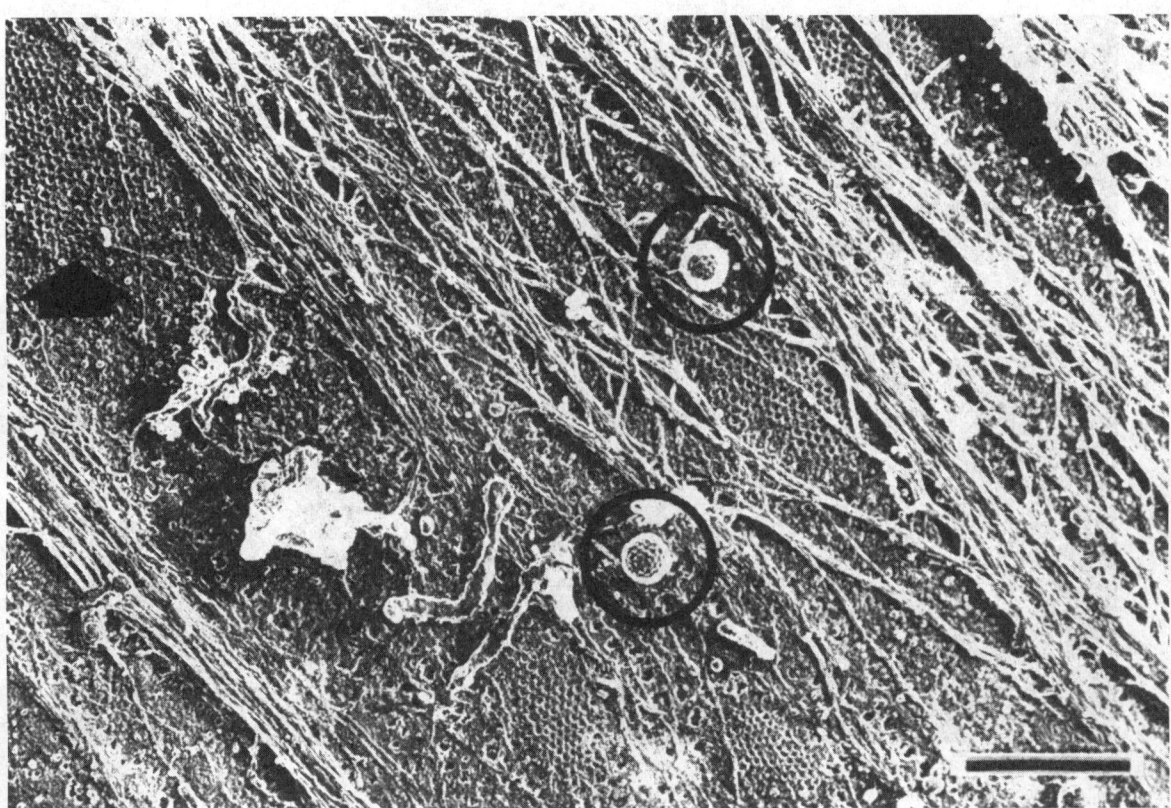

Fig. 4-9. Lateral organization at the cytoplasmic face of the plasma membrane. In this quick-freeze, deep-etch electron micrograph of the plasma membrane of a fibroblast, organized patches of clathyrin-coated membrane (arrow) and invaginating clathyrin-coated pits (circled) are evident. Organized bundles of actin also cross the membrane. Compare this with the more homogeneous membrane of the erythrocyte (Fig. 4-8). Scale bar = 0.5 μM. (From Mahaffey et al.[41] with permission.)

of large cytoskeletal proteins like spectrin (or filamin or talin) suggest that they might participate in the organization of the membrane in a more subtle way, as schematically shown in Figure 4-10. Assume for the purposes of illustration that there are two integral membrane proteins (labeled A and B) and that they can both bind to a peripheral multifunctional protein like spectrin (call it S) at different sites on S. Assume that A binds with high affinity ($K_a = 10^7/M$), while B binds with low affinity ($K_a = 10^4/M$). If the nominal concentration of S in the cell is micromolar, then only receptor A would be appreciably bound and immobilized by S. However, since the binding of S to A increases the effective concentration of S in the vicinity of the membrane, enhanced binding of B to S would be expected. Thus, the binding of S to A could induce the clustering of B in the vicinity of A. The accumulation of S at the membrane might also drive additional associations between two separate molecules of S or between S and other peripheral membrane proteins. The net effect of these interactions would be to drive the assembly of the cortical cytoskeleton about A, and to potentially recruit other integral membrane proteins that bind S, even with low affinity, into the vicinity of A. Although it is difficult to prove that such a mechanism contributes to the clustering of integral and peripheral proteins in vivo, several studies support the notion.[48–50]

Another way that polyvalent S in the above example could participate in the organization of the plasma membrane would be if clusters of B were formed in a way that created a polyvalent binding site on the membrane for S. The way that the initial clusters of B form is unimportant in this model; possible mechanisms would include direct clustering of B by intramembrane association, or by the binding of external polyvalent ligands. However, once polyvalent clusters of a membrane protein with

even low affinity for S are formed, they would collectively create a high-affinity site favorable for the binding of polyvalent S to the membrane. Thus, in this model, S would stabilize the organization of B, even though it would be difficult to measure any interaction of S with isolated B. Consequently, in the special environment of the plasma membrane, low-affinity interactions that are difficult to measure in solution may assume great significance. A mechanism very similar to this one has been postulated to play a role in at least one pathway of B-lymphocyte activation by polyvalent antigens.[51]

Protein and Lipid Associations in the Bilayer

Another way that order may arise in the membrane is via direct association between proteins embedded in the bilayer, or between such proteins and specific types of lipids. In many cases, association is required in order to form a functional assembly. For example, the active unit of Na/K-ATPase, the acetylcholine receptor, connexin (the protein of gap junctions), and several components of the complement cascade are all multimers of at least two protein subunits. Other associations seem to occur without effect on function, or between seemingly random and dissimilar proteins. The intramembranous particles seen in erythrocyte membranes by electron microscopy after freeze-cleavage probably represent such associations, since these aggregates are composed of multimers of band 3, glycophorin, and other transmembrane proteins as well. Another example of laterally organized clusters of membrane protein is seen in the purple membrane of *H. halobium*. In these membranes, bacteriorhodopsin forms such a large planar crystalline array that it was possible to determine the structure of bacteriorhodopsin by Fourier analysis.[13]

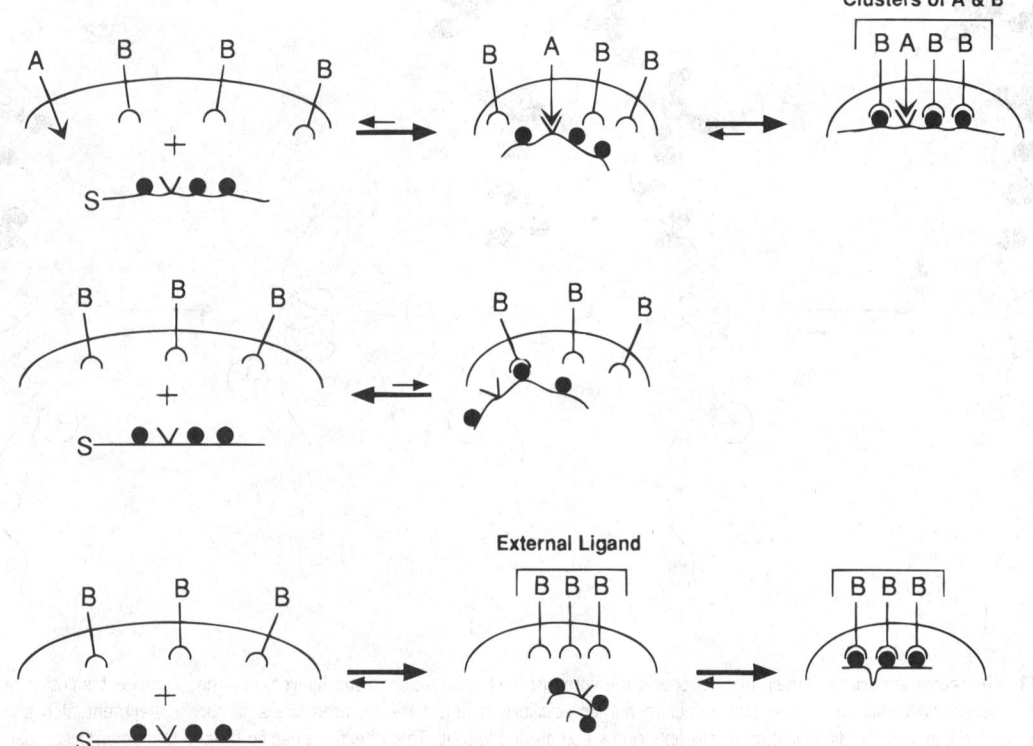

Fig. 4-10. Possible ways that a polyvalent peripheral protein might organize the membrane. **(Top)** If receptor A binds to the multifunctional protein S with high affinity, then S will be concentrated at the membrane. This promotes the binding of a high fraction of the lower affinity receptors (B) to S. The net effect is to cluster B in the vicinity of A. **(Center)** In the absence of A, the binding of S to B is so weak, that most of S remains unbound, and no clustering effect is achieved. **(Bottom)** Alternatively, B might be clustered by external forces, such as polyvalent antigen binding or by the binding of B to the substrata or other cells. In this case, the binding of S to the membrane becomes more favorable, since multiple weak interactions effectively create a strong binding site on the membrane.[48–51]

Given the extremely high concentration of protein within the bilayer of most plasma membranes, it is perhaps surprising that any integral membrane protein can remain dispersed. Indeed, as noted above, the effect of spectrin extraction on the distribution of intramembranous particles seems to suggest that in the absence of external constraints, random associations within the bilayer may dominate. However, recent experiments suggest that this assumption may not be true, at least for some integral proteins. As discussed above, many proteins share the basic structural features of glycophorin A, with a single helical transmembrane segment (Figs. 4-6 and 4-7). In detergent solution, and in the bilayer as well, glycophorin self-associates to form a dimer. The specific role of the hydrophobic core of glycophorin (rather than the hydrophilic domains external to the membrane) in mediating this association was shown by experiments with an isolated synthetic peptide that had a sequence identical to the glycophorin A transmembrane segment.[52] Incubation of glycophorin A in detergent* yielded both dimers and monomers of glycophorin. Incubation of a mixture of glycophorin A and the isolated transmembrane segment led to a reduction in the amount of glycophorin dimer present, and the formation of a complex containing a single glycophorin A and a single copy of the transmembrane peptide

(Fig. 4-11). The interaction between the transmembrane domains was specific for the synthetic peptide with the glycophorin A sequence, since similar peptides with the transmembrane sequence of glycophorin C or the interleukin-2 receptor (Fig. 4-7) did not bind to glycophorin A and did not interfere with glycophorin dimer formation. Thus, even the relatively simple α-helical transmembrane segments of proteins like glycophorin may demonstrate highly specific intra-bilayer associations. As noted below, this specificity may play a role in the regulation of activity for receptors such as the one for epidermal growth factor (EGF-R).

Specific associations between membrane lipids and between lipids and membrane proteins may also contribute to order within the membrane. As noted above, several peripheral proteins (amphitropic proteins?) may display an affinity for specific phosopholipids, such as the binding of phosphatidylserine and phosphatidylethanolamine to spectrin, or the binding of phoshatidylserine to protein 4.1. The raison d'etre of these interactions is not understood in most cases, although such binding might be one mechanism by which the lipid asymmetry of the plasma membrane is maintained. One lipid that has emerged as particularly important in cell regulation and that binds to several membrane proteins is PIP_2.[53] The structure of this phospholipid, and related compounds, is shown in Figure 4-12. PIP_2 constitutes <1% of the total cellular lipid, and it is present exclusively on the cytoplasmic face of the membrane. Under the action of phospholipase C, PIP_2 is cleaved at the C-3 position of glycerol to yield inositol triphosphate (IP_3) and DAG. IP_3 is a soluble second messenger that activates several cellular processes.[53] The affinity of membrane proteins for DAG and PIP_2 may be quite different, and thus the partitioning of these two lipids with different proteins will be a sensitive func-

---

*The detergent used in these experiments is SDS, which is usually thought to be a strongly denaturing agent. Under most conditions, this detergent will disrupt protein-protein associations. However, SDS actually promotes α-helix formation in hydrophobic peptides, and thus, while solubilizing them, may still preserve interactions that are characteristic of the interior of the membrane bilayer.

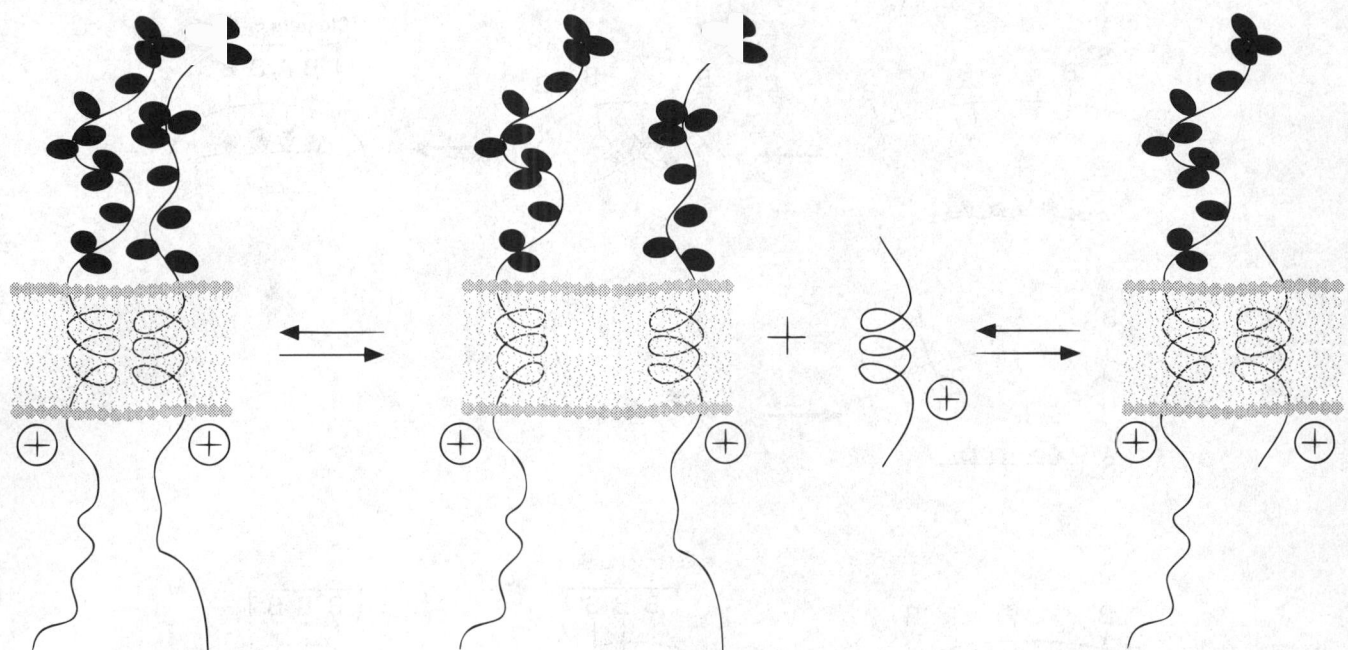

Fig. 4-11. The transmembrane domain of glycophorin mediates its self-association in the bilayer. In either detergent solution or in lipid bilayers, glycophorin exists in a reversible dimer-monomer equilibrium (left). The isolated transmembrane segment also shows this behavior, and will inhibit the dimerization of glycophorin by complexing with it. This effect is specific for the transmembrane segment of glycophorin A, since neither the transmembrane domain of glycophorin C or interleukin-2 will bind glycophorin A. (Adapted from Bormann et al,[52] with permission.)

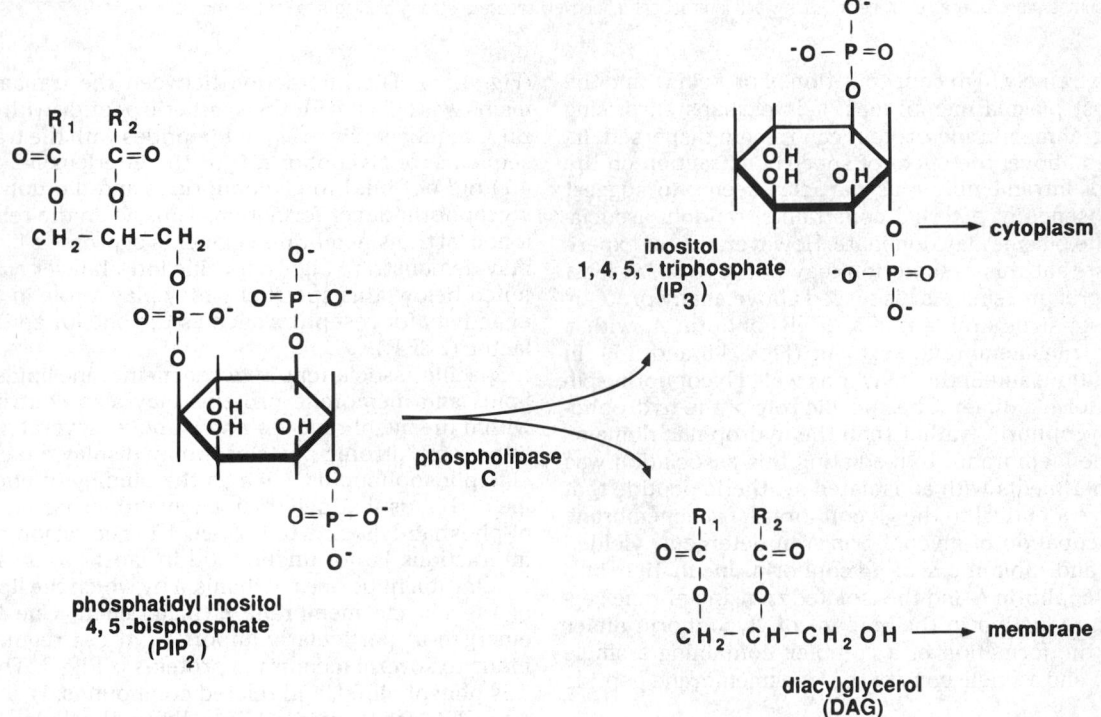

Fig. 4-12. Structure of PIP_2 and related compounds. After hydrolysis by phospholipase C, IP_3 diffuses into the cytoplasm as a second messenger, while DAG remains in the membrane, where it stimulates the activity of protein kinase C. In addition, the conversion of PIP_2 to DAG is expected to reduce the affinity of glycophorin for protein 4.1, which may lead to a rearrangement of the cortical cytoskeleton.

tion of the activity of the PIP_2/DAG cycle. These changes may have profound consequences on the plasma membrane. For example, protein kinase C (which phosphorylates many membrane and cytoskeletal proteins) requires DAG but not PIP_2 for activity, while protein 4.1 (a peripheral membrane protein) binds glycophorin/PIP_2 complexes but not glycophorin/DAG.

Finally, membrane order can be generated by the association of specific lipids alone to form lateral organized patches or domains in the plane of the membrane. Such phase separations occur readily in artificial lipid membranes. For example, a variety of laterally organized lipid phases have been demonstrated by electron spin resonance techniques and freeze cleavage microscopy in artificial liposomes.[54,55] In such experiments, the nature of the phase separation was modulated by the amount of cholesterol in the membrane. In plasma membranes treated with various lipophilic agents, similar phase separations can be induced. However, evidence for the existence of such laterally separated lipid phases in normal plasma membranes has been more difficult to generate. Electron spin resonance studies of lymphocyte membranes are consistent with the existence of such phases,[56] as are a number of other studies employing x-ray diffraction, electron microscopy, and other techniques.[56]

External Ligands

The third general way that membranes may be ordered is by the direct influence of external ligands, other cells, or the substratum. In most respects these factors are entirely analogous to the organizing interactions that occur with peripheral proteins at the cytoplasmic face; only the nature of the molecules involved has changed. One of the best examples of this sort of interaction is the ability of antibodies or polyvalent ligands to patch surface receptors in lymphocytes and other cells. Another example probably includes the ability of the extracellular matrix to guide the clustering of molecules such as the fibronectin receptor to sites of specialized cell attachment (adhesion plaques).[57] The ability of matrices containing fibronectin or type IV collagen, but not the isolated matrix molecules themselves, to alter the shape and growth characteristics of cells profoundly may also be a manifestation of receptor organization by a polyvalent ligand. (In this case, the polyvalency presumably derives from the organization of the matrix molecules in the substratum.) For example, endothelial cells grown on a type I or type III, or both, collagen substrate demonstrate rapid migration and a flattened morphology. The same cells, in exactly the same culture medium, when grown on a substrate containing fibronectin or type IV collagen, or both, will cluster their fibronectin receptors along the points of cell-substratum attachment, cease to migrate, and assume a stouter morphology. These effects cannot be mimicked by the addition of soluble peptides containing the Arg-Gly-Asp sequence, which binds to the fibronectin receptor, although such peptides can inhibit the action of fibronectin.[57]

SIGNAL TRANSDUCTION: RELIANCE ON ALTERED MEMBRANE ORDER

Many signals are propagated across the plasma membrane by the passage of effector molecules, such as steroid hormones, Ca^{2+}, Na^+ or K^+, lipophilic drugs, and so forth. Usually such events will involve specific membrane proteins that function as pores or transport molecules. Alternative pathways of signal transduction do not involve the passage of molecules across the membrane, but instead rely on changes in the orga-

nization of the membrane to transmit information. Four such signal transduction mechanisms are depicted in Figure 4-13. All involve rearrangements of either integral or peripheral membrane proteins, or of certain membrane lipids, as an essential step in the transduction process. None require the net passage of molecules across the bilayer. Two involve the generation of second messengers (cAMP and IP_3) at the cytoplasmic face of the membrane.

One of the first signal transduction pathways to be clearly elucidated was that involving the β-adrenergic receptor. Subsequently, it has been recognized that this receptor is just one of many hormone receptors coupled to their effector proteins by the intermediary of a guanyl-nucleotide-binding protein (G protein)[58,59] (Fig. 4-13A). Other receptors acting via heterotrimeric G proteins include the α_2-adrenergic receptor (a cyclase inhibitory receptor); the M_2 muscarinic receptor; and all of the rhodopsins. These receptors are all integral membrane proteins with an approximately globular structure composed of seven transmembrane α-helices (similar to bacteriorhodopsin). The nature of the G protein varies between tissues, as does the nature of the effector protein. For example, stimulation of the β-adrenergic receptor releases a G protein that subsequently activates adenylate cyclase to produce cAMP, whereas stimulation of rhodopsin (by light) energizes a different G protein (called transducin), which then activates phosphodiesterase and leads to the conversion of cGMP to 5'GMP. The product of the *ras* oncogene ($p21^{ras}$) is also a G protein of sorts, except that it appears to function as a monomer. In yeast *(Saccharomyces cerevisiae)*, this protein stimulates adenylate cyclase. Its function in mammalian cells remains uncertain. However, regardless of the variability in the specific molecules participating in different G protein receptor systems, all are activated by an allosteric rearrangement within an integral transmembrane protein, followed by a redistribution of specific peripheral membrane proteins (the G protein complex).

A similar rearrangement of peripheral proteins may also accompany activation of the PIP_2-IP_3 signal pathway. In this pathway, there is a rearrangement of membrane lipid as well, due to the hydrolysis of PIP_2 to DAG (Figs. 4-12 and 4-13B). As with the β-adrenergic receptor, recent evidence[53,58] suggests that rearrangement of a G protein is involved in the activation of phospholipase C. The activation of this enzyme has two consequences: (1) the release of IP_3 as a soluble second messenger, and (2) the conversion of PIP_2 to DAG in the membrane. DAG enhances the activity of protein kinase C and its association with the cytoplasmic face of the membrane. DAG also may cause the release of protein 4.1 from glycophorin, since the glycophorin/protein 4.1 complex is most stable in the presence of PIP_2.[28] Thus signaling via the PIP_2 pathway involves a transmembrane allosteric signal, followed by the rearrangement of phospholipid and potentially three peripheral membrane proteins: G protein, C kinase, and protein 4.1.

Another family of receptors includes those that help recognize polypeptide growth factors, and those that possess tyrosine kinase activity.[60,61] Such receptors include EGF-R, platelet-derived growth factor, and colony-stimulating factor-1 receptors. They all share a tripartite domain structure similar to that of glycophorin, with a single α-helix spanning the membrane (Fig. 4-7). On binding of ligand to their extracellular domain, tyrosine kinase activity is elicited in the cytoplasmic domain. This remarkable effect is propagated across the membrane (using a single stretch of α-helix) by the ligand-induced dimerization of the receptor in the plane of the membrane. Once two receptors are brought together, their cytoplasmic domains interact in a way that evokes their latent tyrosine kinase activity. It is uncertain whether ligand-induced allosteric changes in the external domain play a role in this process, or

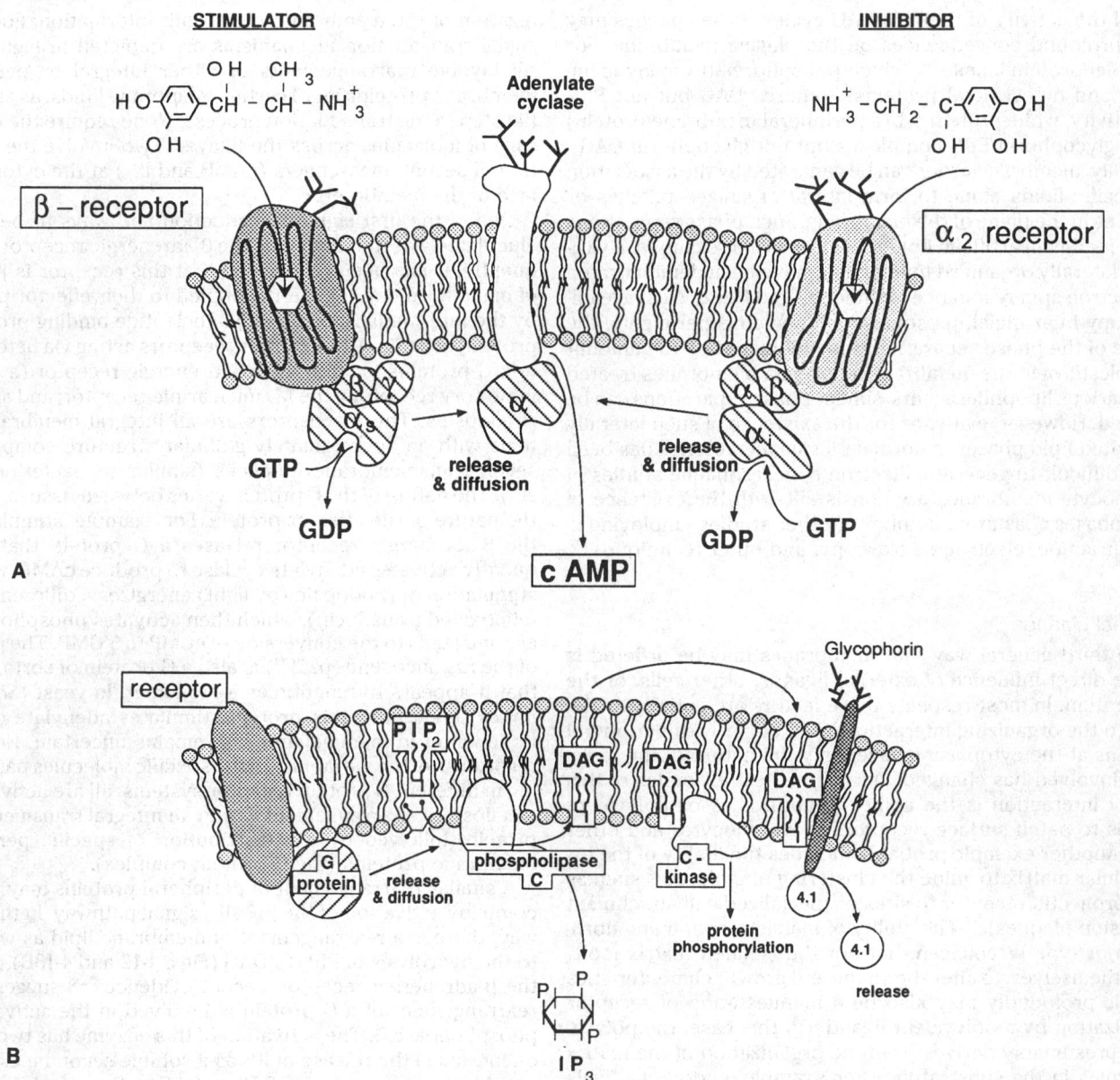

Fig. 4-13. Signal transduction pathways that require changes in membrane order. **(A)** Cascades utilizing cyclic nucleotides as second messengers rely on a redistribution of the peripheral G protein unit (a heterotrimer composed of α-, β-, and γ-subunits) from the transmembrane receptor to adenylate cyclase (or another catalytic unit, such as transducin). The same event occurs with a different G unit for inhibitory cascades. **(B)** Pathways based on the hydrolysis of PIP_2 probably require the redistribution of a G protein-like unit from the transmembrane receptor to phospholipase C. The hydrolysis of PIP_2 leads to a redistribution of these lipids in the membrane, with DAG stimulating the binding of C kinase to the membrane, and the release of protein 4.1 from the membrane. (*Figure continues.*)

whether the growth factor peptide itself may cross-link two receptors. Given the recent evidence that the transmembrane domain of glycophorin A may control its dimerization (Fig. 4-12), it is even possible that ligand-induced changes in the transmembrane domain of the growth factor receptors may activate their self-association. In any event, it appears that the actual propagation of the signal across the membrane, as measured by the activation of tyrosine kinase activity, requires only a change in the organization of the receptors in the plane of the membrane.

Although more controversial, it now seems likely that many other receptors transmit their message to the cell interior via rearrangements in the distribution of integral and peripheral membrane proteins (Fig. 4-13D). A theoretical way that cluster-

ing of receptors with weak affinity for cytoplasmic proteins might activate events in the cell was presented in Figure 4-10. A similar mechanism has been proposed for the T-cell-independent activation of B lymphocytes by polyvalent antigens.[51] The activation of B lymphocytes by such antigens appears to be a threshold phenomenon, since it was found that only certain polyvalent ligands (polyacrylamides with >20 DNP haptens/polymer unit) were capable of activating the lymphocytes. Presumably, the threshold effect arises from the need to form confluent patches of surface receptors of some minimal size, since occupancy of the same number of receptor sites by ligands of lesser valency does not activate the cells. The receptor clusters created by such activation-competent ligands were called immunons.[51] Other situations in which this type of signaling may

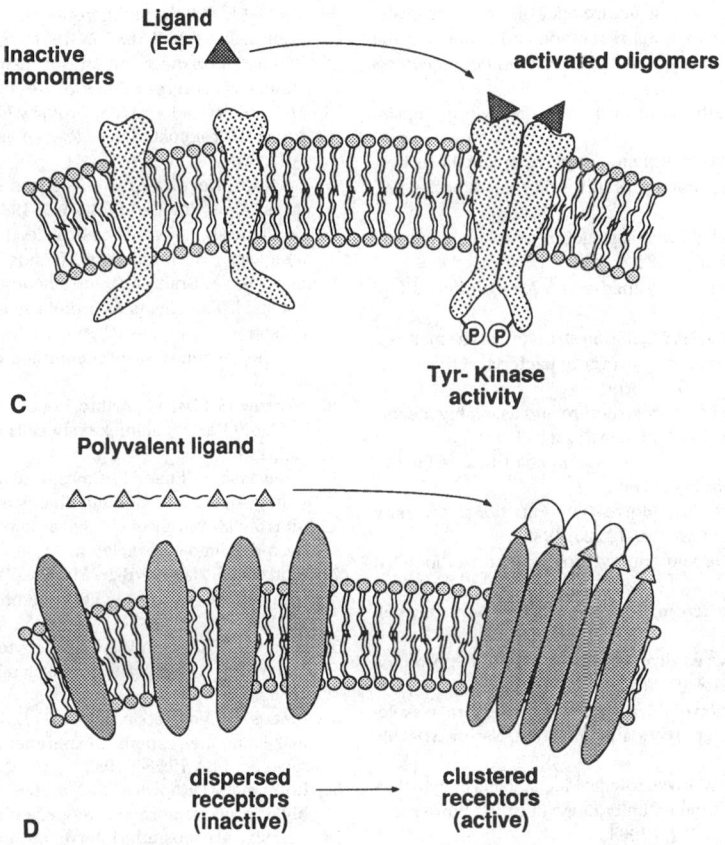

Fig. 4-13 (*Continued*). **(C)** The binding of ligands to receptors of the epidermal growth factor type (EGF-R) promotes the self-association of the receptor. Self-association appears to be a necessary and probably sufficient signal to activate the latent Tyr-kinase activity resident in the cytoplasmic domain of EGF-R. **(D)** Receptor clustering is induced by the binding of an external polyvalent ligand. In the case of B lymphocytes, if the cluster achieves a sufficient size (an immunon), cell activation will occur.[51] Note that in all of the pathways depicted here, no molecules pass across the membrane.

be important include the recognition of cell-cell and cell-substratum contact.[57]

SUMMARY

The fundamental structure of the plasma membrane is a bilayer composed of three basic types of amphipathic lipid: phospholipid, glycolipid, and cholesterol. Embedded in this lipid bilayer are integral membrane proteins and associated with either surface are peripheral membrane proteins. Some proteins are difficult to classify into these two categories because they may at times be both cytoplasmic or directly membrane associated; these have been called amphitrophic proteins. Proteins may comprise $\leq 70\%$ of the mass of a membrane. Integral membrane proteins may span the bilayer with a single α-helical segment approximately 22 residues long, or they may have most of their mass embedded in the bilayer. Proteins that are largely embedded in the bilayer usually possess α-helical secondary structure, although membrane-spanning proteins with β-sheet structure exist. Both lipids and proteins in membranes often display high degrees of lateral mobility, yet biologic membranes are distinguished by their high degree of lateral and transverse order. Thus, the external face of some membranes contain most of the neutral phospholipids and all of the glycolipids and protein-bound carbohydrates, while the internal face contains most of the acidic phospholipids. Laterally organized clusters of protein or lipid domains, or both, are also common. Alterations in the state of organization of both integral and peripheral membrane proteins is a key mechanism of signal transduction.

REFERENCES

1. Stryer L: Biochemistry. 3rd Ed. WH Freeman, New York, 1988
2. Alberts B, Bray D, Lewis J et al: Molecular Biology of the Cell. 2nd Ed. Garland, New York, 1988
3. Tanford C: The Hydrophobic Effect: Formation of Micelles and Biological Membranes. 2nd Ed. Wiley-Interscience, New York, 1980
4. Fairbanks G, Steck TL, Wallach DFH: Electrophoretic analysis of the major polypeptides of the human erythrocyte membrane. Biochemistry 10:2606, 1971
5. Reichstein E, Blostein R: Asymmetric iodination of the human erythrocyte membrane. Biochem Biophys Res Commun 54:494, 1973
6. Sefton BM, Buss JE: The covalent modification of eukaryotic proteins with lipid. J Cell Biol 104:1449, 1987
7. Cross GAM: Eukaryotic protein modification and membrane attachment via phosphatidylinositol. Cell 48:179, 1987
8. Parker MW, Postma JP, Pattus F, et al: Refined structure of the pore-forming domain of colicin A at 2.4 A resolution. J Mol Biol 224:639, 1992
9. Hill CP, Yee J, Selsted ME, Eisenberg D: Crystal structure of defensin HNP-3, an amphiphilic dimer: mechanisms of membrane permeabilization. Science 251:1481, 1991
10. Burn P: Amphitropic proteins: a new class of membrane proteins. Trends Biochem Sci 13:79, 1988
11. Tomita M, Furthmayr H, Marchesi VT: Primary structure of human erythrocyte glycophorin A. Isolation and characterization of peptides and complete amino acid sequence. Biochemistry 17:4756, 1978
12. Marchesi VT: Functional adaptations of transbilayer proteins. p. 107. In Dhindsa DS, Bahl OP (eds): Molecular and Cellular Aspects of Reproduction. Plenum, New York, 1986
13. Henderson R, Unwin PNT: Three-dimensional model of purple membrane obtained by electron microscopy. Nature 257:28, 1975
14. Unwin N, Henderson R: The structure of proteins in biological membranes. Sci Am 250:78, 1984
15. Unwin N: Nicotinic acetylcholine receptor at 9 Å resolution. J Mol Biol 229:1101, 1993

16. Deisenhofer J, Epp O, Miki N et al: X-ray structure analysis of a membrane protein complex. Electron density map at 3-Å resolution and a model of the chromophores of the photosynthetic reaction center from *Rhodopseudomonas viridis.* J Mol Biol 180:385, 1984

17. Paul C, Rosenbusch JP: Folding patterns of porin and bacteriorhodopsin. EMBO J 4:1593, 1985

18. Engleman DM, Steitz TA, Goldman A: Identifying nonpolar transbilayer helices in amino acid sequences of membrane proteins. Annu Rev Biophys Biophys Chem 15:321, 1986

19. Cowan SW, Schirmer T, Rummel G et al: Crystal structures explain functional properties of two *E. coli* porins. Nature 358:727, 1992

20. Weiss MS, Schulz GE: Structure of porin refined at 1.8 Å resolution. J Mol Biol 227:493, 1992

21. Spurlino JC, Lu GY, Quiocho FA: The 2.3-Å resolution structure of the maltose- or maltodextrin-binding protein, a primary receptor of bacterial active transport and chemotaxis. J Biol Chem 266:5202, 1991

22. Tobkes N, Wallace BA, Bayley H: Secondary structure and assembly mechanism of an oligomeric channel protein. Biochemistry 24:1915, 1985

23. Volz K, Matsumura P: Crystal structure of *Escherichia coli* CheY refined at 1.7-Å resolution. J Biol Chem 266:15511, 1991

24. Coleman T, Fishkind DJ, Mooseker MS, Morrow JS: Functional diversity among spectrin isoforms. Cell Motil Cytoskel 12:225, 1989

25. Winkelmann JC, Forget BG: Erythroid and nonerythroid spectrins. Blood 81:3173, 1993

26. Marchesi VT: The stabilizing infrastructure of cell membranes. Annu Rev Cell Biol 1:531, 1985

27. Bennett V: Ankyrins. Adaptors between diverse plasma membrane proteins and the cytoplasm. J Biol Chem 267:8703, 1992

28. Anderson RA, Marchesi VT: Regulation of the association of membrane skeletal protein 4.1 with glycophorin by a polyphosphoinositide. Nature 318:295, 1985

29. Howe CL, Sacramone LM, Mooseker MS, Morrow JS: Mechanisms of cytoskeletal regulation: modulation of membrane affinity in avian brush border and erythrocyte spectrins. J Cell Biol 101:1379, 1985

30. Steiner JP, Bennett V: Ankyrin-independent membrane protein binding sites for brain and erythrocyte spectrin. J Biol Chem 263:14417, 1988

31. Sato SB, Ohnishi S: Interaction of a peripheral protein of the erythrocyte membrane, band 4.1, with phosphatidylserine-containing liposomes and erythrocyte inside-out vesicles. Eur J Biochem 130:19, 1983

32. Keenan TW, Heid HW: Tight attachment of fatty acids to proteins associated with milk lipid globule membrane. Eur J Cell Biol 26:270, 1982

33. Wolfe M, Sayhoun A: Protein kinase C and phosphatidyl serine bind to M_r 110,000/115,000 polypeptides enriched in cytoskeletal and post-synaptic density preparations. J Biol Chem 261:13327, 1986

34. Staufenbiel M, Lazarides E: Ankyrin is fatty acid acylated in erythrocytes. Proc Natl Acad Sci USA 83:318, 1986

35. Koteliansky VE, Glukhova MA, Shirinsky VP et al: A structural study of filamin, a high-molecular-weight actin-binding protein from chicken gizzard. Eur J Biochem 121:553, 1982

36. Vaz WLC, Derzko ZI, Jacobson KA: Photobleaching measurements of the lateral diffusion of lipids and proteins in artificial phospholipid bilayer membranes. Cell Surface Rev 8:83, 1982

37. Kornberg RD, McConnell HM: Inside-outside transitions of phospholipids in vesicle membranes. Biochemistry 10:1111, 1971

38. Golan DE: Red blood cell membrane protein and lipid diffusion. p. 367. In Agre P, Parker JC (eds): Red Blood Cell Membranes, Structure, Function, Clinical Implications. Marcel Dekker, New York, 1989

39. Yechiel E, Edidin M: Micrometer-scale domains in fibroblast plasma membranes. J Cell Biol 105:755, 1987

40. Bloch R, Morrow JS: An unusual β-spectrin associated with clustered acetylcholine receptors. J Cell Biol 108:481, 1989

41. Mahaffey DT, Moore MS, Brodsky FM, Anderson RG: Coat proteins isolated from clathrin coated vesicles can assemble into coated pits. J Cell Biol 108:1615, 1989

42. Buck CA, Horwitz AF: Cell surface receptors for extracellular matrix molecules. Annu Rev Cell Biol 3:179, 1987

43. Gumbiner B, Louvard D: Localized barriers in the plasma membrane: a common way to form domains. Trends Biochem Sci 10:435, 1985

44. Elgsaeter A, Branton D: Intramembrane particle aggregation in erythrocyte ghosts. I. The effects of protein removal. J Cell Biol 63:1018, 1974

45. Nelson WJ, Veshnock PJ: Ankyrin binding to (Na⁺K)ATPase and implications for the organization of membrane domains in polarized cells. Nature 328:533, 1987

46. Morrow JS, Cianci C, Ardito T et al: Ankyrin links fodrin to alpha Na/K ATPase in Madin-Darby canine kidney cells and in renal tubule cells. J Cell Biol 108:455, 1989

47. Srinivasan Y, Elmer L, Davis J et al: Ankyrin and spectrin associate with voltage-dependent sodium channels in brain. Nature 333:177, 1988

48. Morrow JS, Marchesi VT: Self-assembly of spectrin oligomers in vitro: a basis for a dynamic cytoskeleton. J Cell Biol 88:463, 1981

49. Morrow JS, Haigh WB Jr, Marchesi VT: Spectrin oligomers: a structural feature of the erythrocyte cytoskeleton. J Supramol Struct Cell Biochem 17:275, 1981

50. Lazarides E, Nelson WJ: Erythrocyte and brain forms of spectrin in cerebellum: distinct membrane-cytoskeletal domains in neurons. Science 220:1295, 1985

51. Dintzis RZ, Vogelstein B, Dintzis HM: Specific cellular stimulation in the primary immune response: experimental test of a quantized model. Proc Natl Acad Sci USA 79:884, 1982

52. Bormann B-J, Knowles WJ, Marchesi VT: Synthetic peptides mimic the assembly of transmembrane glycoproteins. J Biol Chem 264:4033, 1989

53. Berridge MJ: Inositol triphosphate and diacylglycerol: two interacting second messengers. Annu Rev Biochem 56:159, 1987 ·

54. Wu SH, McConnell HM: Phase separations in phospholipid membranes. Biochemistry 14:847, 1975

55. Rechtenwald DJ, McConnell HM: Phase equilibria in binary mixtures of phosphatidylcholine and cholesterol. Biochemistry 20:4505, 1981

56. Karnovsky MJ, Kleinfeld AM, Hoover RL, Klausner RD: The concept of lipid domains in membranes. J Cell Biol 94:1, 1982

57. Madri JA, Pratt BM, Yannariello-Brown J: Endothelial cell-extracellular matrix interactions. p. 167. In Simionescu N, Simionescu M (eds): Endothelial Cell Biology. Plenum, New York, 1988

58. Levitzki A: Transmembrane signalling to adenylate cyclase in mammalian cells and in *Saccharomyces cerevisiae.* Trends Biochem Sci 13:298, 1988

59. Gilman AG: G proteins: transducers of receptor generated signals. Annu Rev Biochem 56:615, 1987

60. Schlessinger J: Signal transduction by allosteric receptor oligomerization. Trends Biochem Sci 13:443, 1988

61. Stahl N, Yancopoulos GD: The alphas, betas, and kinases of cytokine receptor complexes. Cell 74:587, 1993

62. Adams RJ, Pollard TD: Binding of myosin I to membrane lipids. Nature 340:565, 1989

63. Miyata H, Bowers B, Korn ED: Plasma membrane association of Acanthamoeba myosin I. J Cell Biol 109:1519, 1989

64. Skene JH, Virag I: Posttranslational membrane attachment and dynamic fatty acylation of a neuronal growth cone protein, GAP-43. J Cell Biol 108:613, 1989

Cell Adhesion

5

Rodger P. McEver

INTRODUCTION

Cell adhesion is essential for the development and maintenance of multicellular organisms. Cell-cell and cell-matrix contacts facilitate intercellular communication and define the architecture of organs. The regulated nature of cell adhesion is particularly evident in the hematopoietic system, where cells routinely make transitions between nonadherent and adherent phenotypes during differentiation and in response to stimuli in the circulation or extravascular tissues.

In the bone marrow, proliferation and differentiation of hematopoietic stem cells is controlled not only by soluble growth factors, but also by adhesion to stromal cells and matrix molecules. Weakening of these adhesive bonds is required for mature blood cells to enter the circulation. Circulating erythrocytes normally remain nonadhesive until they are finally cleared by the reticuloendothelial system. Other circulating cells often participate in regulated adhesive events during their life spans. For example, prothymocytes enter and adhere to components of the thymus, where they undergo further maturation before reentering the circulation. Lymphocytes regularly stick to the specialized high endothelial venules of lymphoid tissues, migrate into these tissues for sampling of processed antigens, and then exit via the lymphatics. During inflammation, specific classes of leukocytes roll on the endothelium, then adhere more tightly, and finally emigrate between endothelial cells into the tissues. There, neutrophils and monocytes phagocytose invading pathogens, whereas lymphocytes adhere to antigen-presenting macrophages. During hemorrhage, platelets stick to exposed subendothelial matrix components, spread, and recruit additional platelets into large aggregates that serve as an efficient surface for thrombin and fibrin generation. Leukocytes also adhere to activated platelets, a mechanism for linking hemostatic and inflammatory responses. The endothelial cells express molecules that affect the adhesiveness of platelets or leukocytes. Tight contacts between adjacent endothelial cells also limit access of blood cells to the underlying tissues.

ADHESION MOLECULES

Cells adhere through noncovalent bond formation between macromolecules on cell surfaces with macromolecules on other cell surfaces or in extracellular matrix. These interactions involve either protein-protein or protein-carbohydrate recognition. Although some adhesion molecules are expressed only by blood or endothelial cells, most are also synthesized by other cells. Many adhesion molecules can be grouped into families according to related structural and functional features.

Extracellular Matrix Proteins

The principal constituents of the extracellular matrix are adhesive proteins and proteoglycans. The major proteins are von Willebrand factor (vWF), thrombospondin, collagen, fibronectin, laminin, and vitronectin. These proteins are large, often highly extended, and consist of multiple domains with different binding functions. In some proteins such as fibronectin, alter-

native splicing can increase diversity by producing molecules with variable numbers of domains. The many binding domains allow adhesive proteins to interact with each other as well as with cell-surface receptors, resulting in multipoint contacts that stabilize matrix structure. One large adhesive protein, fibrinogen, is found predominantly in plasma but may also be deposited in exposed subendothelial matrix following vascular injury. Fibronectin, vitronectin, thrombospondin, and vWF are located predominantly in the extracellular matrix, but are also found in plasma. Several adhesive proteins are also stored in α-granules of platelets, where they are secreted following platelet activation at sites of hemorrhage.

Proteoglycans contain protein cores to which are covalently attached many glycosoaminoglycans, long linear polymers of repeating disaccharides. Most proteoglycans are in the extracellular matrix, but some are anchored on cell surfaces through a core protein that contains a membrane-spanning domain. Hyaluronan is a unique glycosoaminoglycan that forms polymers with molecular masses up to several million that are not covalently attached to a protein. Hyaluronan forms noncovalent interactions with globular domains on the protein core of proteoglycans and with a small molecule called link protein. The resultant hyaluronan-proteoglycan complexes can become very large, contributing to the structural stability of matrix. Hyaluronan can also bind to cell-surface receptors (see below).

Integrins

Integrins are a broadly distributed group of cell-surface adhesion receptors that consist of noncovalently associated α- and β-subunits (Fig. 5-1 and Table 5-1). There are ≥ 14 α- and 8 β-chains that pair in many, but not all, of the possible combinations. All blood cells have several different integrins. The three β_2 integrins, each paired with a unique α-subunit, are expressed only by leukocytes, and the $\alpha_{IIb}\beta_3$ integrin (glycoprotein [GP]IIb/IIIa) is expressed only by megakaryocytes and platelets. Multidomain adhesive proteins of the extracellular matrix are ligands for many integrins. Some integrins bind to specific domains of several different proteins, and some adhesive proteins bind to several different integrins. These interactions generally mediate cell-matrix adhesion. However, binding of fibrinogen to $\alpha_{IIb}\beta_3$ integrins on adjacent platelets serves as a molecular bridge that promotes platelet aggregation. Cell-cell contact also results from integrin recognition of cell-surface members of the immunoglobulin superfamily.

Immunoglobulin-Like Receptors

Immunoglobulin superfamily members contain a variable number of disulfide-stabilized motifs like those in antibodies that are linked to transmembrane and cytoplasmic domains (Fig. 5-1 and Table 5-2). The immunoglobulin-like motif provides a framework on which specific recognition structures for other proteins can be added. The immunoglobulin-like molecules intercellular adhesion molecule (ICAM)-1, ICAM-2, and vascular cell (VC)AM-1, expressed on endothelial cells, as well as ICAM-3, expressed on leukocytes, mediate cell-cell contact through recognition of specific integrins on leukocytes. Interac-

53

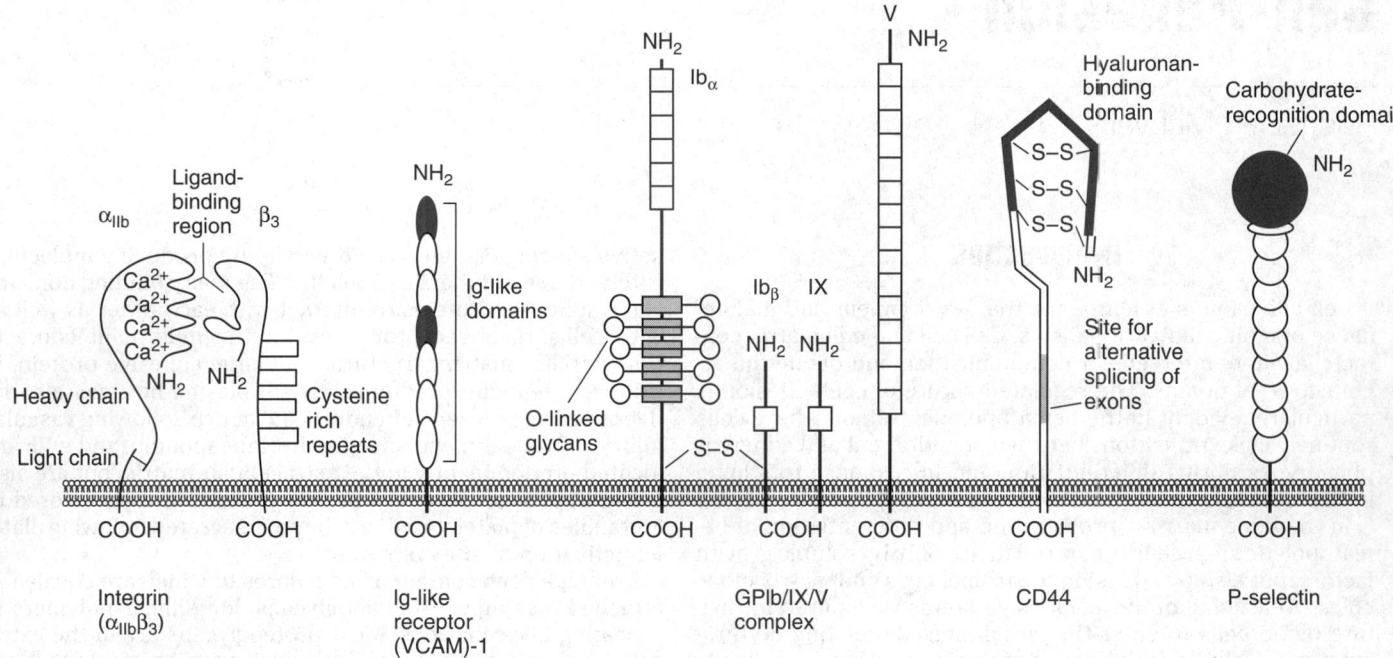

Fig. 5-1. Schematic diagrams of several types of cell-surface adhesion receptors. Integrins consist of noncovalently linked α- and β-subunits, both of which contribute to ligand binding. The platelet $\alpha_{IIb}\beta_3$ integrin is illustrated. Immunoglobulin-like receptors contain a variable number of immunoglobulin homology domains, some of which bind ligands, while others extend the ligand-binding domains from the membrane. Shown is VCAM-1, which contains seven immunoglobulin domains. The platelet GPIb/IX/V complex consists of several leucine-rich protein subunits. CD44 contains an N-terminal domain that binds to hyaluronan. Each of the selectins contains an N-terminal carbohydrate-recognition domain that binds sialylated and fucosylated oligosaccharides on specific cell-surface glycoprotein ligands. Illustrated is P-selectin, the largest of the three selectins.

tions between immunoglobulin-like molecules help to mediate adhesion between T cells and antigen-presenting cells. Thus, the immunoglobulin-like molecules CD8 and CD4 on T cells bind to the conserved membrane-proximal domains of class I and class II MHC proteins, respectively, whereas the T-cell receptor (CD3) binds to the polymorphic antigen-presenting domain. In addition, the immunoglobulin-like protein CD2 on T cells binds to the immunoglobulin-like protein leukocyte function-associated antigen-3 (LFA-3) on antigen-presenting cells. In many tissues, the immunoglobulin-like neural (N)CAM molecule mediates cell-cell contact through homotypic interactions, that is, binding of an NCAM molecule on one cell to an NCAM molecule on another cell. Similarly, the immunoglobulin-like receptor platelet and endothelial cell adhesion molecule-1 (PECAM-

Table 5-1. Integrins on Blood Cells

Integrin Designation	Other Names	Expressed by	Ligand	Function
$\alpha_1\beta_1$	VLA-1	Leukocytes, other cells	Collagens, LM	Adhesion to ECM
$\alpha_2\beta_1$	VLA-2 GPIa/IIa	Leukocytes, platelets, other cells	Collagens, LM	Adhesion to ECM
$\alpha_3\beta_1$	VLA-3	Leukocytes, other cells	Collagens, LM, FN	Adhesion to ECM
$\alpha_4\beta_1$	VLA-4	Monocytes, lymphocytes, eosinophils	VCAM-1, FN	Adhesion to cells, ECM
$\alpha_5\beta_1$	VLA-5 GPIc/IIa	Leukocytes, platelets, other cells	FN	Adhesion to ECM
$\alpha_6\beta_1$	VLA-6 GPIc/IIa	Leukocytes, platelets, other cells	LM	Adhesion to ECM
$\alpha_L\beta_2$	LFA-1 CD11a/CD18	Leukocytes	ICAM-1, -2, -3	Leukocyte aggregation and adhesion
$\alpha_M\beta_2$	MAC-1, CR3 CD11b/CD18	Neutrophils, monocytes	ICAM-1, FIB	Neutrophil aggregation and adhesion to EC
$\alpha_X\beta_2$	p150,95 CD11c/CD18	Neutrophils, monocytes	?	Adhesion to EC
$\alpha_{IIb}\beta_3$	GPIIb/IIIa	Platelets	FIB, FN, vWF, VN, TSP	Platelet adhesion and aggregation
$\alpha_V\beta_3$	VN receptor	Platelets, other cells	FIB, FN, vWF, VN, TSP, collagens	Platelet adhesion
$\alpha_4\beta_7$	LPAM-1	Lymphocytes	VCAM-1, MAdCAM-1, FN	Lymphocyte adhesion to EC and ECM

Abbreviations: CR, complement receptor; EC, endothelial cell; ECM, extracellular matrix; FIB, fibrinogen; FN, fibronectin; GP, glycoprotein; LFA-1, leukocyte function-associated antigen-1; LM, Laminin; LPAM-1, lymphocyte Peyer's patch adhesion molecule; MAdCAM-1, mucosal addressin cell adhesion molecule-1; TSP, thrombospondin; VCAM-1, vascular cell adhesion molecule-1; VN, vitronectin; vWF, von Willebrand factor.

Table 5-2. Immunoglobulin-Like Receptors

Name	Other Names	Expressed by	Ligand	Function
ICAM-1		Macrophages, EC, other cells	$\alpha_M\alpha_2$, $\alpha_L\beta_2$, FIB	T-cell responses, leukocyte adhesion to EC
ICAM-2		EC	$\alpha_L\beta_2$	Leukocyte adhesion to EC
ICAM-3		Leukocytes	$\alpha_L\beta_2$	T-cell responses, leukocyte aggregation
PECAM-1	CD31	Leukocytes, platelets, EC	PECAM-1, carbohydrate?	EC junctions, leukocyte transmigration
VCAM-1	INCAM-110	Activated EC, smooth muscle cells	$\alpha_4\beta_1$, $\alpha_4\beta_7$	Mononuclear cell adhesion to EC
MAdCAM-1		EC of Peyer's patches	$\alpha_4\beta_7$	Lymphocyte homing
CD2		T cells	LFA-3[a]	T-cell responses
CD4		T cells	Class II MHC[a]	T-cell responses
CD8		T cells	Class I MHC[a]	T-cell responses
CD3	T-cell receptor	T cells	Antigen on MHC[a]	T-cell responses

Abbreviations: ICAM-1, -2, -3, intercellular adhesion molecules; PECAM-1, platelet and endothelial cell adhesion molecule-1. For EC, FIB, LFA, MAdCAM-1, and V-CAM-1, see Table 5-1 footnote.

[a] LFA-3 and classes I and II MHC molecules are also immunoglobulin-like receptors.

1) (CD31) may promote contacts between adjacent endothelial cells through homotypic interactions, but may also augment leukocyte adhesion to platelets and endothelium by binding to unknown cell-surface ligands.

Other Adhesion Receptors that Mediate Protein-Protein Interactions

Cadherins are cytoskeletally linked membrane proteins that mediate cell-cell contact in many organs through homotypic binding to cadherins on adjacent cells (Table 5-3). Cadherins have not been described on blood cells, but are found on endothelial cells, where, like PECAM-1, they help form cell junctions.

The GPIb/IX/V complex on platelets consists of leucine-rich protein subunits (Fig. 5-1). Under conditions of high shear like those found in the arterial circulation, this complex promotes the initial platelet adhesion to injured vessels by binding avidly to vWF exposed in the subendothelium. The leucine-rich GPIbα subunit is also expressed by endothelial cells exposed to inflammatory cytokines such as tumor necrosis factor-α, but its function on the endothelium is less well understood.

CD36 is a receptor with at least two membrane-spanning domains that is expressed on many cell types. On platelets, it has been implicated as a receptor for collagen and perhaps for thrombospondin; both interactions could facilitate adhesion to subendothelial matrix at sites of hemorrhage.

Lectin Adhesion Receptors

CD44 is an unusual transmembrane glycoprotein expressed to variable degrees on many subsets of leukocytes (Fig. 5-1). It has a membrane-distal domain that is structurally related to link protein of extracellular matrix, and, like link protein, can bind to hyaluronan. The hyaluronan-binding function of CD44 may modulate a number of leukocyte responses, but its importance has been most clearly demonstrated for lymphopoiesis, in which maturation of lymphocyte precursors requires contacts with bone marrow stromal cells bearing surface hyaluronan. The membrane-proximal regions of CD44 are structurally diverse because of the insertion of variable numbers of domains through alternative splicing. These insertions may regulate the ability of CD44 to bind hyaluronan and may mediate postbinding events that affect cell signaling.

The selectins are a group of three asymmetric receptors that terminate in a membrane-distal carbohydrate-recognition domain related to those in Ca^{2+}-dependent (C-type) animal lectins such as the hepatic asialoglycoprotein receptor (Fig. 5-1). L-selectin is expressed on leukocytes, E-selectin on cytokine-activated endothelium, and P-selectin on platelets and endothelial cells exposed to secretagogues such as thrombin (Table 5-4). The selectins mediate leukocyte adhesion to platelets or endothelium through Ca^{2+}-dependent interactions of the carbohydrate-recognition domains with cell-surface carbohydrates on apposing cells. High-affinity binding appears to require specific carbohydrate structures displayed on a limited number of membrane glycoproteins. The best characterized glycoprotein ligands for selectins contain large numbers of clustered, sialylated O-linked oligosaccharides whose structures are incompletely defined.

Natural killer cells express a group of membrane proteins that are distinct from the selectins, but also have membrane-distal C-type carbohydrate-recognition domains. Although these receptors are important for interactions of natural killer cells with target cells, their carbohydrate-recognition functions have not been established.

LIGAND BINDING VERSUS CELL ADHESION

Like all macromolecular interactions, adhesion molecules bind to each other with equilibrium affinities that are defined by their on and off rates. However, the efficiency of cell adhesion is not simply a function of the solution-phase equilibrium affinities of adhesion molecules for one another. Adhesion mol-

Table 5-3. Other Adhesion Receptors

Name	Other Names	Expressed by	Ligand	Function
Cadherins		EC, many other cells	Homotypic binding	Formation of EC junctions
GPIb/IX/V		Platelets	vWF	Platelet adhesion to ECM under shear
CD36	GPIV	Platelets, many other cells	Collagens, TSP	Platelet adhesion to ECM
CD44		Leukocytes, other cells	Hyaluronan	Lymphopoiesis, lymphocyte activation?
Natural killer cell receptors		Natural killer cells	Carbohydrate? MHC molecules?	Recognition of virus-infected or other foreign cells

For abbreviations, see Table 5-1 footnotes.

Table 5-4. Selectins

Name	Other Names	Expressed by	Ligands[a]	Ligands Expressed by	Function
P-selectin	CD62P, GMP-140, PADGEM	Thrombin-activated platelets and EC, cytokine-activated EC	PSGL-1, Others?	Leukocytes	Leukocyte adhesion to activated EC and platelets
E-selectin	CD62E, ELAM-1	Cytokine-activated EC	150 kd and 280 kd glycoproteins, others?	Leukocytes	Leukocyte adhesion to activated EC
L-selectin	CD62L, LECAM-1 LAM-1	Leukocytes	GlyCAM-1, CD34, others?	EC of lymph nodes, activated EC	Leukocyte adhesion to activated EC, lymphocyte homing

Abbreviations: EC, endothelial cells; ELAM-1, endothelial leukocyte adhesion molecule-1; Gly-CAM-1, glycosylation-dependent cell adhesion molecule-1; GMP-140, granule membrane protein-140; LAM-1, leukocyte adhesion molecule-1; LECAM-1,leukocyte endothelial cell-adhesion molecule-1; PADGEM, platelet activation-dependent granule external membrane protein; PSGL-1, P-selectin glycoprotein ligand-1.

[a] The selectins bind to sialylated, fucosylated, and (in some cases) sulfated oligosaccharides on specific glycoproteins, of which only some have been identified.

ecules in cell membranes and matrix are primarily limited to two dimensions, and even low-affinity molecular interactions may allow time for additional bonds to form along the plane of cell contact, stabilizing adhesion. The efficiency of cell attachment, and the ensuing strength of adhesion, may reflect multiple factors that dictate the probability of bonds forming between adhesion molecules on cell or matrix surfaces. The requirements for cell attachment are particularly stringent in the circulation, where platelets and leukocytes must rapidly adhere to the blood vessel wall under shear conditions. Factors that affect bond formation include the number of adhesion molecules on a cell or matrix surface, the distance the binding domain of an adhesion receptor protrudes from the cell membrane, the lateral mobility of receptors, and the clustering of receptors on microvilli or other membrane domains. Cell adhesion can be further stabilized by events that occur after bond formation between adhesion molecules. For example, the cytoplasmic domains of the integrins, cadherins, CD44, L-selectin, and some immunoglobulin-like molecules interact with cytoskeletal components, allowing clustering of receptors into surface patches that strengthen adhesion and promote cell spreading or migration.

REGULATION OF ADHESION RECEPTORS

To prevent inappropriate interactions of cells with each other or with extracellular matrix, the expression and function of adhesion receptors must be tightly controlled. Three primary control mechanisms are used: (1) the rate of synthesis of the receptor, (2) the time the receptor is displayed on the cell surface, and (3) the binding affinity/avidity of the receptor for ligands (Table 5-5). All these mechanisms are used to control interactions of blood and vascular cells, examples of which are given below.

Table 5-5. Regulation of Adhesion Receptors

Mechanism	Example
Synthesis	Errythroid precursor synthesis of $\alpha_5\beta_1$
	Lymphocyte synthesis of CD44
	Cytokine-induced synthesis of E-selectin, P-selectin, ICAM-1, and VCAM-1 by endothelial cells
Surface expression	Proteolytic cleavage of L-selectin from leukocytes
	Redistribution of P-selectin from granule membranes to plasma membrane of platelets and endothelial cells
	Endocytosis of P- and E-selectin on endothelial cells
Ligand affinity	Activation-induced increased affinity of many integrins for their ligands
	Activation-induced increased affinity of CD44 for hyaluronan

For abbreviations, see Table 5-1 footnote.

Regulation of Synthesis

The synthesis of many adhesion receptors is regulated. Erythroid precursors synthesize integrins that mediate their interactions with stromal cells and with extracellular matrix in the bone marrow. As the precursors mature, synthesis ceases, resulting in loss of expression of cell-surface integrins by the time a mature erythrocyte enters the circulation. Lymphocyte precursors synthesize CD44 during differentiation in the bone marrow, stop synthesis prior to release, and resume synthesis during maturation in the thymus. On exposure to antigens, immunologically naive lymphocytes synthesize increased amounts of several adhesion receptors during their conversion to the memory phenotype; this process presumably allows these cells to become more adhesive in response to a subsequent antigenic challenge. When exposed to inflammatory cytokines such as tumor necrosis factor-α and interleukin-1, endothelial cells transiently increase synthesis of E- and P-selectin, ICAM-1, and VCAM-1, resulting in an adhesive surface for leukocytes.

Regulation of Surface Expression

The surface expression of some adhesion receptors is tightly controlled. L-selectin is present on the plasma membrane of leukocytes, where it is available to bind to inducible ligands on the endothelial cell surface. Stimulation of the leukocyte causes L-selectin to be shed into the plasma by proteolytic cleavage, a mechanism for down-regulating adhesion. P-selectin is constitutively synthesized by megakaryocytes (where it is incorporated into platelets) and by endothelial cells. Rather than being directly delivered to the plasma membrane, however, it is sorted into secretory storage granules: the α-granules of platelets and the Weibel-Palade bodies of endothelial cells. On stimulation of these cells by agonists such as thrombin or histamine, P-selectin is rapidly transported to the cell surface during fusion of granule membranes with the plasma membrane. Once on the surface of the endothelium, both E- and P-selectin are internalized and delivered to lysosomes for degradation. The cytoplasmic domain of P-selectin contains signals that direct sorting into secretory granules, internalization through coated pits of the plasma membrane, and movement from endosomes to lysosomes; the latter two signals are probably also present in the cytoplasmic domain of E-selectin. The net result of these events is to control the duration that E- and P-selectin are exposed on the endothelium, where they can mediate adhesion of leukocytes. Activation of leukocytes also mobilizes a pool of β_2 integrins from storage compartments to the plasma membrane, although some of these molecules are also constitutively expressed on the cell surface. Finally, platelet activation redistributes a portion of the GPIb/IX/V complexes from ligand-accessible positions on the plasma membrane to sequestered, invaginated membrane domains known as the surface-connected canalicular system. This process, which requires interactions of the cytoplasmic domain of GPIb/IX/V with the cytoskeleton, may serve to downregulate GPIb-mediated adhesion of platelets to immobilized vWF.

Regulation of Binding Affinity

Regulation of binding affinity is an important control mechanism for other adhesion receptors. Many integrins are constitutively present on the cell surface but interact poorly with their ligands. Cell activation by a number of agonists induces conformational changes in integrins so that they effectively recognize their ligands. An example is the $\alpha_{IIb}\beta_3$ integrin, which requires platelet stimulation to bind fibrinogen; if this binding affinity were not regulated, circulating platelets would indiscriminately aggregate in the fibrinogen-rich plasma milieu. The mechanisms for activation-induced affinity increases in integrins are still being defined. The cytoplasmic domains of integrins can have both positive and negative influences on binding affinity, and lipid mediators released by cellular activation may modulate the conformation of specific integrins. Low-affinity ligand binding may stabilize the active conformation of integrins, perhaps explaining why integrins on unactivated cells will sometimes bind to immobilized, multivalent adhesive proteins but not to the same proteins in solution. Although less well studied, the affinity of CD44 for hyaluronan is also affected by cellular activation, through mechanisms that appear to require an intact cytoplasmic domain.

CELL SIGNALING THROUGH ADHESION MOLECULES

In addition to their roles in cell-cell and cell-matrix contacts, adhesion molecules may affect cell signaling through indirect or direct mechanisms. Proteoglycans in the extracellular matrix can sequester growth factors that can be released to bind to surface receptors on nearby cells. Some chemoattractants bind to proteoglycan-like molecules on the surface of endothelial cells, where they can activate adherent leukocytes. Binding of adhesive ligands to cell-surface integrins, GPIb/IX/V, CD44, cadherins, CD36, PECAM-1, and perhaps other receptors can directly trigger intracellular events. The consequences of these signals include increases in affinity/avidity of other adhesion receptors for their ligands, shape change, secretion, proliferation, synthesis of cytokines and other molecules, and migration. In some cases, binding of a monovalent adhesive ligand to a receptor may induce a signal. More commonly, signaling requires cross-linking of several receptors through interactions with multivalent ligands in matrix or on apposing cells.

Many of the recent studies on adhesion receptor signaling have focused on integrins. Binding of the same ligand to different integrins can mediate different responses in the same cell. Furthermore, ligand binding to the same integrin expressed in different cells can result in different signals. These data suggest that very specific interactions occur between ligand-occupied integrins and intracellular components. The cytoplasmic domains of integrins are probably essential for initiating signaling. Phosphorylation of such domains, while an attractive candidate for regulation, has not been shown to have important effects on cellular responses in the integrins that have been studied. However, tyrosine kinases have been localized at the interaction zones between integrins and the cytoskeleton, and tyrosine phosphorylation of a number of proteins accompanies integrin-mediated cell signaling. The localization of tyrosine kinases near the cytoplasmic domains of integrins is analogous to the *lck*-encoded tyrosine kinase associated with the cytoplasmic domains of CD4 and CD8, which appears to function in T-cell signaling. Ligand binding to integrins also results in

generation of lipid second messengers, alkalinization of the cytoplasm, and influxes of Ca^{2+}. The latter event may be due to Ca^{2+} transport through an integrin-associated protein that has several membrane-spanning domains.

COOPERATIVE INTERACTIONS BETWEEN SIGNALING AND ADHESION MOLECULES

Signaling and adhesion molecules frequently function cooperatively in sequential cascades to enhance the specificity of cell adhesion. Three examples of how these cooperative interactions facilitate blood cell responses are illustrated.

Platelet Adhesion and Aggregation

At sites of hemorrhage in the arterial circuit, platelets rapidly adhere to the damaged vessel through interactions of GPIb/IX/V receptors with immobilized vWF exposed in the subendothelial matrix (Fig. 5-2). This interaction is actually facilitated by high shear rates, perhaps because of shear-induced conformational effects on GPIb or vWF, or both. An important feature of this initial adhesive event is that prior activation of the platelets is not required. After adhesion, however, the interaction of immobilized vWF with GPIb receptors triggers intracellular signals that lead to platelet activation. These signals may synergize with those produced by small amounts of locally produced thrombin to enhance platelet activation. Platelet activation, in turn, increases the affinity of platelet integrins for other matrix adhesive proteins such as collagen and fibronectin, which stabilize adhesion. Binding of these ligands transduces signals that propagate further activation responses such as spreading, secretion of granule contents, and recruitment of additional platelets through cell-cell contact mediated by binding of fibrinogen to activated $\alpha_{IIb}\beta_3$ integrins. This adhesion cascade allows unstimulated platelets to home to the site of vascular injury and subsequently be activated by locally generated mediators.

Neutrophil Rolling, Spreading, and Migration

Near sites of extravascular bacterial infections, neutrophils first roll, or form transient adhesive contacts, on the endothelial surface of venules through the interactions of selectins with cell-surface carbohydrate ligands (Fig. 5-3). Neutrophil rolling on the endothelium must occur under shear forces, just as platelets must adhere to subendothelial matrix under shear forces, although the shear rates in postcapillary venules are lower than those in arteries. The selectins are capable of forming rapid, yet reversible, bonds with their ligands under these conditions. Just as the initial adhesion to vWF does not require prior activation of platelets, selectin-mediated rolling does not require prior activation of neutrophils. Instead, locally generated inflammatory mediators induce expression of E- or P-selectin, and probably a ligand(s) for L-selectin, on the endothelial cell surface. The requirement for activation of endothelial cells rather than leukocytes allows the latter to adhere to vessels only at the site of microbial invasion. Once situated on the vessel wall through selectin-mediated contacts, however, the neutrophils become exposed to activators such as platelet-activating factor, a phospholipid signaling molecule, and interleukin-8, a potent chemoattractant, both of which are presented on the surface of activated endothelial cells. Neutrophil activation increases the affinity of β_2 integrins for immunoglobulin counter-receptors on the endothelial cell surface such as ICAM-1 and ICAM-2. Although these bonds will not form under shear conditions, they do form once neutrophils are transiently arrested on the endothelium by the selectins. The integrin-ICAM

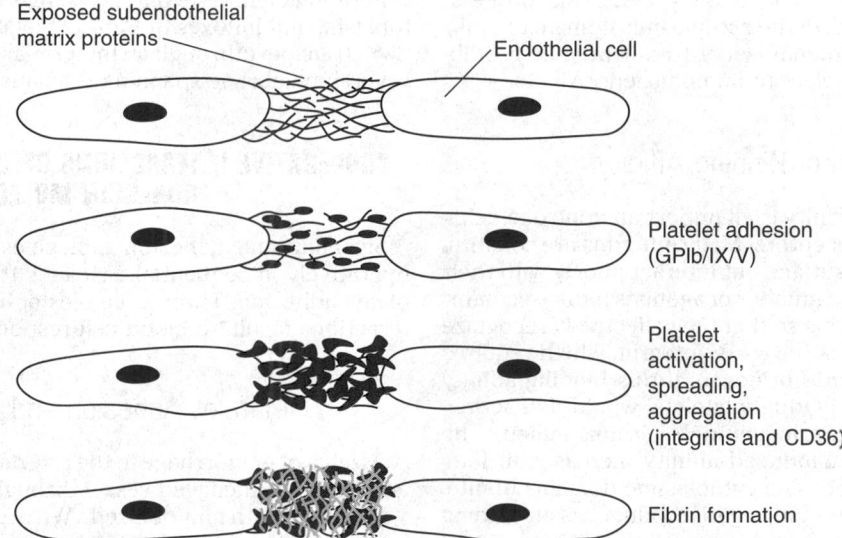

Fig. 5-2. Platelet adhesion and aggregation. In response to arterial injury under high shear forces, platelets rapidly adhere to the subendothelial matrix. The initial contacts are made between GPIb/IX/V on platelets and vWF in the matrix. These mclecular interactions help activate platelets, thereby increasing the affinity of several platelet integrins for other adhesive matrix proteins such as fibronectin, laminin, and collagen. CD36 also interacts with both collagen and thrombospondin. Fibrinogen cross-links activated platelets into aggregates by binding to $\alpha_{IIb}\beta_3$ integrins. The platelet plug then serves as an efficient surface for generation of thrombin and fibrin.

interactions strengthen adhesion, promote spreading, and ultimately favor migration, presumably because of disengagement of integrin-ICAM bonds and redistribution of integrins to the leading edge of the cell, where new bonds form. Subsequent interactions of leukocytes with PECAM-1 in interendothelial cell junctions facilitates transendothelial migration of the neu-

trophils into the underlying tissues. Both the integrin- and PECAM-1-mediated adhesive events may signal cytoskeletal redistributions that enhance migration toward chemotactic molecules released in the vicinity of the infection. Once in the tissues, integrin recognition of extracellular matrix protein ligands may trigger secretion of proteolytic enzymes and production of superoxide anions, both required for optimal bactericidal function.

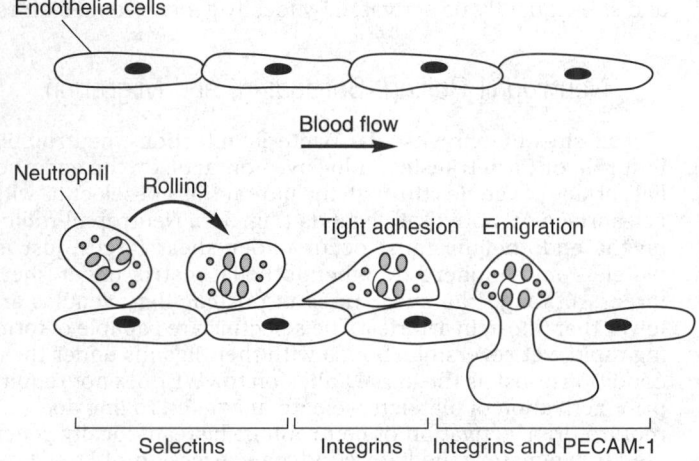

Fig. 5-3. Neutrophil rolling, spreading, and emigration. At sites of tissue injury or infection, neutrophils first roll on the endothelial cells in postcapillary venules. These transient adhesive interactions are mediated by activation-induced expression of E- or P-selectin, or a ligand for L-selectin, on the endothelial cell surface. E- and P-selectin bind to carbohydrate ligands on the neutrophil, whereas L-selectin on the neutrophil binds to a carbohydrate on the endothelial cell. These molecular bonds can form under the shear forces in the venular circulation. The rolling neutrophils are then activated by locally generated inflammatory mediators that increase the affinity of β_2 integrins for immunoglobulin-like receptors such as ICAM-1 on the endothelium. These bonds strengthen adhesion. Neutrophil migration between endothelial cells into tissues at the site of infection requires disengagement of old adhesive bonds and formation of new bonds between integrins, PECAM-1, and their respective ligands.

Adhesion of T lymphocytes to Antigen-Presenting Cells

The initial interaction of T lymphocytes with antigen-presenting cells requires that the T-cell receptor (CD3) recognize antigen presented by the polymorphic domain of MHC molecules (Fig. 5-4). Subsequent interactions include the binding of CD8

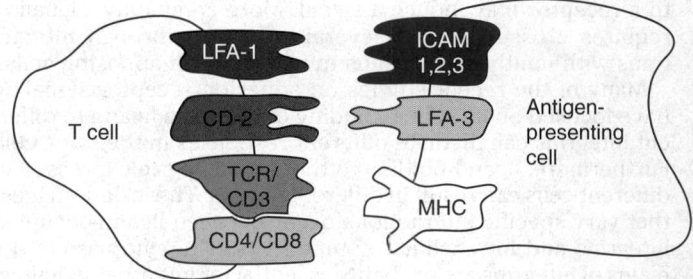

Fig. 5-4. Adhesion between T lymphocytes and antigen-presenting cells. The initial contact is mediated by the T-cell receptor (CD3), which binds with low affinity but high specificity to a specific antigen presented by an MHC molecule. Additional contacts, also of low affinity, are between CD4 (on helper cells) or CD8 (on cytotoxic cells) and MHC, and between CD2 and LFA-3. These interactions signal the T cell to increase transiently the affinity of the β_2 integrin, LFA-1, for the immunoglobulin-like molecules ICAM-1, -2, and -3 on the antigen-presenting cell. These bonds strengthen adhesion and transduce further signals to the T cell that cause proliferation and cytokine secretion. Additional signals result from binding of β_1 integrins on the T cell to adhesive proteins in the extracellular matrix.

or CD4 to MHC class I or II molecules, respectively, plus the binding of CD2 to LFA-3. These molecular contacts are all of low affinity but are highly specific, because they first require specific antigen presentation to the appropriate T cell. The combination of these binding events triggers signals that increase the affinity of LFA-1 ($\alpha_L\beta_2$), a β_2 integrin on T cells, for its ligand, ICAM-1 on antigen-presenting cells, strengthening adhesion. After ICAM-1 binds to LFA-1, the T cell is further activated, resulting in cytokine secretion and proliferation. Additional signaling is mediated through binding of other integrins on T cells to protein ligands in the extracellular matrix.

The first key principle of these three responses is that the initial adhesive event, while relatively limited, is highly specific. Thus, platelets bind only to exposed subendothelial matrix, neutrophils bind only to endothelium near the site of infection, and T cells bind only to cells presenting specific antigen. A second key principle is that subsequent activation events strengthen cell adhesion and lead to further responses such as secretion, fibrin formation, migration, proliferation, or release of cytotoxic mediators. Activation often results from cooperative signaling by soluble agonists and by binding of ligands to adhesion receptors. Co-stimulation by multiple signals can amplify, and provide specificity to, cellular responses by mechanisms not always feasible for individual mediators. Thus, adhesion and cell signaling are highly interrelated processes.

The process of reversing cell adhesion, while less well understood, is equally important for the control of cell behavior. Some molecules such as the selectins can be proteolytically cleaved or internalized. The activation-induced increases in affinity of integrins and CD44 for their ligands are generally transient, but the mechanisms for return to the inactive conformation are obscure.

ALTERED EXPRESSION OF ADHESION MOLECULES

The highly regulated nature of adhesive events by hematopoietic cells suggests that defects in, or excessive expression of, adhesion molecules could contribute to the pathogenesis of disease. A variety of clinical observations support this hypothesis.

Genetic Deficiencies in Adhesion Molecules

Genetic deficiencies in platelet adhesion receptors such as the GPIb complex (Bernard-Soulier syndrome) and the $\alpha_{IIb}\beta_3$ integrin (Glanzmann thrombasthenia) result in hemorrhagic symptoms similar to those of patients with thrombocytopenia. Genetic deficiencies in the leukocyte β_2 integrins (leukocyte adhesion deficiency-1) are associated with frequent severe bacterial infections and a failure of neutrophils to enter the infected tissues. Similar symptoms are seen in patients with a congenital defect in fucose metabolism that prevents synthesis of the carbohydrate ligands for selectins (leukocyte adhesion deficiency-2) (Table 5-6).

Dysregulated Expression of Adhesion Molecules

Inappropriate expression of adhesion molecules has been implicated in thrombotic and inflammatory disorders and in tumor metastasis. For example, erythrocytes from patients with sickle cell anemia adhere to each other and to the endothelium, contributing to vaso-occlusive crises. These adhesive events may reflect, in part, the expression of integrins not normally found on mature erythrocytes. Inappropriate adhesion and activation of platelets on exposed atherosclerotic plaques

Table 5-6. Genetic Deficiencies in Adhesion Molecules

Molecule	Disease	Laboratory Findings	Clinical Findings
$\alpha_{IIb}\beta_3$	Glanzmann thrombasthenia	Impaired platelet aggregation	Mucocutaneous bleeding
GPIb/IX/V	Bernard-Soulier Syndrome	Impaired platelet adhesion to vWF	Mucocutaneous bleeding
β_2 integrins	Leukocyte adhesion deficiency-1	Impaired adhesion of activated leukocytes to EC	Frequent infections
Selectin ligands	Leukocyte adhesion deficiency-2	Impaired fucose metabolism resulting in defective carbohydrate ligands for selectins, impaired rolling of leukocytes on venules	Frequent infections

For abbreviations, see Table 5-1 footnote.

may contribute to thrombosis. Dysregulated expression of selectins on the endothelium of ischemic blood vessels during myocardial infarction or shock may contribute to neutrophil-mediated tissue necrosis following reperfusion of the vessel. Mediators released while the neutrophils are adherent in the reperfused vessels may activate integrin function, strengthening adhesion and generating further signals that release destructive oxygen radicals and proteases within the vasculature. Finally, malignant cells appear to utilize molecules normally used for adhesion of blood cells to promote metastatic spread through interactions with platelets, endothelial cells, and extravascular matrix.

These examples underscore the importance of proper regulation of adhesion molecule expression in the physiology of blood cells. Further studies of the structure and function of these molecules may lead to effective treatments for disorders in which their expression becomes dysregulated.

SUGGESTED READINGS

Greenwalt DE, Lipsky RH, Ockenhouse CF et al: Membrane glycoprotein CD36: a review of its roles in adherence, signal transduction, and transfusion medicine. Blood 80:1105, 1992

Hynes RO: Integrins: versatility, modulation, and signaling in cell adhesion. Cell 69:11, 1992

Kjellen L, Lindahl U: Proteoglycans: structures and interactions. Annu Rev Biochem 60:443, 1991

Lasky LA: Selectins: interpreters of cell-specific carbohydrate information during inflammation. Science 258:964, 1992

Lesley J, Hyman R, Kincade PW: CD44 and its interaction with extracellular matrix. Adv Immunol 54:271, 1993

McEver RP: Leukocyte-endothelial cell interactions. Curr Opin Cell Biol 4:840, 1992

McEver RP: Selectins. Curr Opin Immunol 6:75, 1994

Roth GJ: Developing relationships: arterial platelet adhesion, glycoprotein Ib, and leucine-rich glycoproteins. Blood 77:5, 1991

Roth GJ: Platelets and blood vessels: the adhesion event. Immunol Today 13: 100, 1992

Ruggeri ZM, Ware J: von Willebrand factor. FASEB J 7:308, 1993

Ruoslahti E, Yamaguchi Y: Proteoglycans as modulators of growth factor activities. Cell 64:867, 1991

Shattil SJ, Brugge JS: Protein tyrosine phosphorylation and the adhesive functions of platelets. Curr Opin Cell Biol 3:869, 1991

Smyth SS, Joneckis CC, Parise LV: Regulation of vascular integrins. Blood 81: 2827, 1993

Springer TA: Adhesion receptors of the immune system. Nature 346:425, 1990

Takeichi M: Cadherin cell adhesion receptors as a morphogenetic regulator. Science 251:1451, 1991

Yamada KM: Adhesive recognition sequences. J Biol Chem 266:12809, 1991

Regulatory Mechanisms

Philip M. Rosoff and David A. Potter

INTRODUCTION

The maintenance of cellular homeostasis in the midst of a rapidly and continually changing extracellular environment requires the complex interaction of biochemical processes that must operate under strict regulatory control. The ability to respond to both intra- and extracellular signals in a coordinated fashion is a hallmark of a properly functioning cell. Failure to respond to stimuli, or failure to terminate a response, can lead to pathologic states in which disordered regulation of normal cellular processes achieves primacy. Eukaryotic cells have developed a number of molecular mechanisms that are used to control biochemical processes. These range from covalent modification of various rate-limiting enzymes, so as to alter their activity, to down-regulation or amplification of surface expression and function of membrane receptors leading to decreases or increases in the ability to respond to cognate stimuli. Critical to this regulation is the ability to process and integrate continually a large amount of disparate information from both local and distant sources ranging from nearby cells of similar and dissimilar tissue types to trophic hormonal signals from other organ systems within the body (Fig. 6-1).

BIOCHEMICAL MECHANISMS OF REGULATORY CONTROL

Many levels of cellular biochemical functions exist in which cells constantly regulate the activity of a number of synthetic, metabolic, and degradative processes so as to maintain homeostasis in a constantly changing environment. These include such diverse processes as controlling both transcription rates of critical genes and proteolysis rates of critical proteins. Examples of proteins whose levels fluctuate rapidly because of control of both transcription and proteolysis include the cyclins and the proto-oncogene transcription factor c-*fos*. The levels of cyclins oscillate with the period of the cell division cycle, and these proteins play a critical role in cell cycle progression. Transcription of the c-fos gene is stimulated by growth factors, and the c-fos protein acts in concert with other proteins to regulate expression of still other genes critical for cell growth. One of the best understood examples of hormone-regulated gene expression in mammals is the steroid receptor family of transcription regulators. These proteins are located intracellularly and bind with high affinity to their specific steroid hormone, be it estrogen, mineralocorticoids, glucocorticoids, or others. The complex then migrates to the nucleus, where it binds to specific regulatory sequences in steroid-responsive genes, thus stimulating transcription.

Less well understood are the genes that respond indirectly to signals generated by receptors at the cell surface. Generally speaking, transcriptional regulation of these genes is initiated in response to a cascade of signaling events that occurs on the generation of so-called second messenger molecules. Examples include genes that are expressed in response to stimulation of cells with β-adrenergic hormones or other agents that elevate cAMP. cAMP is generated by the action of adenylate cyclase on ATP at the cytosolic surface of the plasma membrane. It then activates a cAMP-dependent protein kinase that phosphorylates a number of different substrates, some of which effect transcriptional activation of genes that contain so-called cAMP-responsive elements, such as the gene for tyrosine hydroxylase.

cAMP and other second messengers may also influence more proximate regulatory events in the cell. An example of regulatory control by agents that elevate cAMP is that demonstrated by the regulation of intermediate anaerobic metabolism in hepatocytes, which is exerted at several distinct points. Both fructose-2,6-bisphosphatase and fructose 6-phosphate 2-kinase, two enzyme activities that reside on a single polypeptide chain, are phosphorylated at serine residues by the cAMP-dependent protein kinase. This covalent modification has opposite effects on each enzyme, activating the former and inhibiting the latter. The sum effect is to alter the level of fructose-2,6 bisphosphate and thereby inhibit phosphofructokinase and stimulate fructose 1,6-bisphosphatase, eventually leading to shunting of glucose-6-phosphate from the Embden-Meyerhof pathway to free glucose. cAMP-dependent protein kinase is just one of a large number of serine/threonine protein kinases.

In general, second messengers act by directly or indirectly stimulating protein kinases, which, by covalently modifying a host of substrates, effect regulatory control of enzymes, ion channels, and structural proteins. Protein kinases fall into two large families, those that modify serine or threonine residues, and those that phosphorylate tyrosine residues. The former are much more prevalent than the latter. Indeed, in resting cells, only 0.01–0.05% of the total phosphoamino acid is present as phosphotyrosine. This level rises rapidly and dramatically after stimulation with either growth factors or oncogenic transformation. Both protein-tyrosine kinases and the enzymes that remove phosphate from tyrosine residues, the tyrosine protein phosphatases, have become a central focus of research on growth regulatory mechanisms.

Just as the addition of phosphate groups can alter the activity or function of a protein, their removal can also modify activity. There are numerous substrate-specific and -nonspecific protein phosphatases, some of which also demonstrate preference for either tyrosyl- or seryl/threonyl-phosphate bonds. These enzymes cooperatively interact with the protein kinases to regulate important metabolic pathways. Thus, cellular homeostasis is achieved and maintained by a complex interplay between protein kinases and phosphatases. Changing the balance between these two apparently opposing forces can have profound consequences for the regulation of cellular activity. For example, evidence is abundant that the leukocyte common antigen, also known as CD45, which is a prototype of the receptor-like class of tyrosine protein phosphatases, participates in the generation of a mitogenic activating signal in T lymphocytes and B cells. Thus, inhibiting the function of this enzyme can block T-cell activation by antigen or mitogen. Conversely, one can also activate some cells simply by inhibiting phosphotyrosine phosphatase activity. Interestingly, these enzymes themselves are often substrates for still other kinases and phosphatases, which imposes yet another level of regulatory control. For example, CD45 may be regulated by both Ca^{2+} or Ca^{2+}-dependent kinases and protein kinase C.

Another example of regulatory control involves the compartmentalization of cellular processes. Just as it is vitally important for lysosomal proteolytic enzymes to remain safely confined in the lysosome, it is also critical that many enzymes and their substrates be localized to those parts of the cell in which

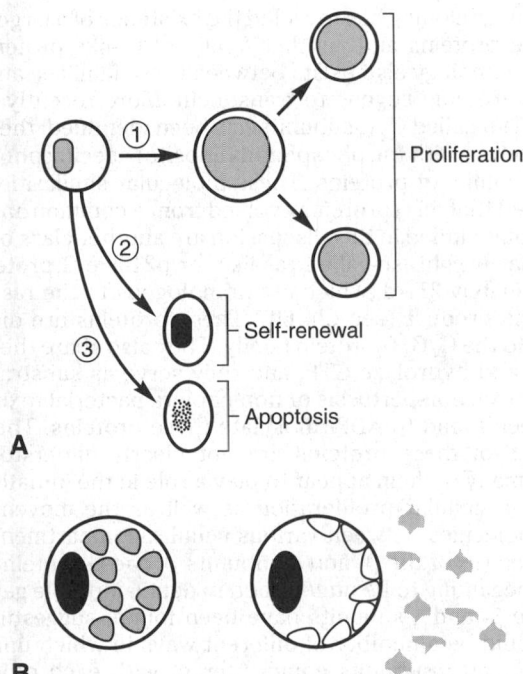

Fig. 6-1. Schematic diagram of several major types of stimulus-response reactions in nucleated quiescent cells. **(A)** In these cells (the prototypes of which are resting G_0 T lymphocytes and quiescent fibroblasts), hormone or growth factor (or antigen) stimulation results in both activation and proliferation. In the case of T cells, the initial step (induction of "competence") (1) appears to involve the secretion of lymphokines, including interleukin-2, which participates in an autocrine fashion to initiate the second step (induction of "progression") leading to DNA synthesis and cell division (see Ch. 7). This occurs only if the cell receives the appropriate signals; a "default" pathway also exists in which the cell undergoes programmed cell death or apoptosis (3) (see also Ch. 7). Finally, as best illustrated in the hematopoietic system, some types of cells demonstrate the capacity for self-renewal (2). **(B)** In these cells, typified by neutrophils and platelets that are incapable of further cell division, stimulation results in degranulation or secretion events relatively rapidly after receptor occupancy. Many of the transmembrane signaling events used by the cells to initiate proliferation and secretion are similar.

their activity is needed. Cells have also developed mechanisms by which cellular components can be rapidly moved from one cellular compartment to another, a phenomenon termed translocation. An example is the mechanism by which insulin stimulates increased glucose uptake in adipocytes. In these and many other types of cells, glucose enters the cells by a mechanism of facilitated transport via a 45-kd glucose transporter membrane protein. In the nonstimulated cell, most glucose transporters are located in cytoplasmic vesicles. Within minutes of insulin binding to its receptor, there is an apparent fusion of these vesicles with the plasma membrane, vastly increasing the density of functional transporters in the membrane, and thus increasing glucose permeability. The insulin receptor has an intrinsic protein-tyrosine kinase activity that is activated by insulin binding; this and other insulin responses in the cell are thought to involve modification of target proteins on tyrosine residues. However, only some of the protein targets that mediate these events have been identified.

Another example of regulation involving movement of components of important metabolic pathways from one cellular compartment to another involves the translocation of the Ca^{2+} and phospholipid-dependent serine/threonine protein kinase (protein kinase C [PKC]) from the cytosol to the inner leaflet of the plasma membrane on stimulation with a variety of growth factors and hormone agonists. In resting cells, most PKC can be found in the cytosol in an essentially inactive state. Within

seconds of exposure to such hormones as platelet-derived growth factor (PDGF), T-lymphocyte-specific antigens, thrombin, α_1-agonists, and others, there is a rapid shift of enzymatic activity to the membrane fraction. Indeed, many of the critical substrates for this enzyme are found within the plasma membrane; these include other enzymes as well as many of the growth factor/hormone receptors themselves, the phosphorylation of which is often associated with a loss of activity. Thus, moving an inactive, but easily activatable enzyme or rate-limiting component of a biochemical pathway from one part of the cell to another is another way in which cells can regulate transitory but critical metabolic processes.

Yet another example of the critical importance of subcellular localization for the functional activity of biomolecules involves the targeting information encoded by the post-translational addition of fatty acid moieties. There are several different types of this process, including farnesylation, isoprenylation, and fatty acylation. Examples of the former include the modifications of the *ras* proto-oncogene family of proteins, the low-molecular-weight ras-like GTP-binding proteins, and a number of α-subunits of the heterotrimeric, receptor-associated G proteins. The entire family of src-like membrane-associated tyrosine protein kinases are fatty acylated (usually by myristic acid) on their N termini in a manner determined by their amino acid sequences. Moreover, this modification is required for successful targeting of these proteins to a specific receptor located on the inner plasma membrane and thus is needed for full functioning of the proteins in vivo. Therefore, a common theme in this regulatory process is that substrate specificity is conferred not only by information encoded within the substrate recognition and binding domains of an enzyme, but also by the physical availability of the substrate to the catalyst. Thus, a mutated src or ras protein that can no longer be localized to the plasma membrane might still be enzymatically normal, but would be functionally inactive.

One final general mechanism of regulatory control that we consider concerns biochemical pathways used to turn off stimulatory processes at the plasma membrane. One can easily imagine the pathologic consequences of allowing an unregulated, constant stimulation of, for example, the cellular proliferation apparatus, or antigenic activation of lymphocytes or basophils/mast cells. In the former case, neoplastic transformation may occur, as may be the situation with cellular transformation with the *sis* oncogene, which encodes the B chain of PDGF. In the latter example, either autoimmunity or allergy may be the pathologic consequences. Cells have developed many ways to turn off a response to a stimulus. One of the better studied controls exists at the plasma membrane and involves receptor down-regulation. Binding of a hormone to its receptor often induces an aggregation of ligand-bound receptors and the consequent endocytosis or "modulation" of the complexes from the plasma membrane. In some cases, as with the epidermal growth factor (EGF) receptor and the antigen/immunoglobulin receptor on B lymphocytes, aggregation is required for receptor signaling. Once internalized, the receptors either dissociate from the hormone and return to the surface (recycle) or they become disabled or degraded (down-regulation). Therefore, even though saturating amounts of hormone may be continually present on the outside of the cell, the response can be either down-graded or attenuated by loss of receptors from the cell surface. This control may exist at several levels. For example, in the case of the EGF receptor, stimulation of PKC leads to a phosphorylation of specific serine residues on the cytoplasmic domain of the receptor. This in turn is associated with a decrease in affinity of the receptor for EGF. At the same time, aggregation of receptors in the presence of EGF leads to their endocytosis. Both processes contribute to the attenuation of the response. Covalent modification of receptors or other components of the signal-generating pathways by PKC is not an event that is limited to the EGF receptor. Indeed, it has now been described for a number of hormone receptor/second messenger systems; in many cases it is associated with the loss of membrane receptor expression or decreased ligand affinity (or both), or decreased production of second messengers such as inositol trisphosphate and diacylglycerol. Recent evidence suggests that protein tyrosine phosphatases, which appear to play a role in generating or propagating a positive signal, may also participate in attenuating a response. Presumably this is accomplished by removing phosphates from tyrosyl residues that serve activating functions, such as those on the carboxyl termini of the PDGF, EGF, and insulin receptors, for example. Heterologous expression (or overexpression) of a tyrosine protein phosphatase can lead to changes in responsiveness to growth factors or a change in apparent phenotype of v-src-transformed fibroblasts.

SIGNAL TRANSDUCTION

The ability to transduce to the cell interior the information that a specific hormone is present at the cell surface requires that the cognate receptor for this hormone rapidly generate a molecular signal capable of evoking the desired cellular response. One could imagine several ways in which this could be accomplished. However, mechanisms for signal transduction must generally satisfy the following criteria: (1) very rapid response time for cellular reactions to hormones such as glucagon or insulin; (2) the ability to amplify a response to very low concentrations of either hormone or receptor, or both; and (3) the ability to attenuate a response even in the presence of continued hormone-receptor interaction.

Eukaryotic cells have evolved at least two highly efficient mechanisms for stimulus-response coupling. One of these involve the guanine nucleotide binding proteins, or G proteins. These ubiquitous and highly conserved sets of proteins exist in macromolecular complexes of heterotrimers composed of α-, β-, and γ-subunits. Via the α-subunit, these heterotrimeric complexes interact with the cytoplasmic domains of a wide variety of receptors and couple them to second messenger generating systems. Examples of receptor systems coupled with G proteins include the β-adrenergic receptor, the vertebrate visual system, muscarinic acetylcholine receptors, and a subclass of serotonin receptors. All of these proteins have some structural similarity involving seven transmembrane α-helical regions. However, they couple to distinct G proteins that in turn produce distinct responses. Specific responses that have been shown to be mediated by physical association with specific G proteins include activation of adenylate cyclase and activation of cGMP phosphodiesterase. Other responses that may be directly mediated by G proteins include activation of polyphosphoinositide-specific phospholipase C, activation of phospholipase A_2, inhibition of adenylate cyclase, and activation of certain types of K^+ channels.

The α-subunit of the G proteins contains the binding site for both the receptor and the target protein (effector) as well as the guanine nucleotide binding site. The α-subunits can be classified as to whether they are susceptible to ADP-ribosylation by either cholera or pertussis toxins, or both. Those that fall into the former category include the G_s-like proteins, named for the prototype that couples the β-adrenergic receptor to the stimulation of adenylate cyclase, leading to an increased synthesis of cAMP. The latter includes the G_i-like α-subunits, named after the one that inhibits activity of the cyclase, leading to a fall in cellular cAMP levels. Finally, some α-subunits are ADP-ribosylated by both toxins; these are typified by transducin, the G protein that couples the visual pigment receptor rhodopsin to a cGMP phosphodiesterase. These bacterial toxins have thus played a vital role in determining the involvement of G proteins in signal transduction pathways.

Molecular cloning has revealed the existence of a large family of G_i-like proteins and another family of G_s-like proteins. Sequence homology also exists between these families, and both families are homologous to transducin. More recently, a new family of so-called G_q α-subunits has been identified: these proteins interact with the phosphatidylinositol-specific phospholipase C^β family of proteins. These molecular similarities have suggested that all G proteins evolved from a common ancestral gene. Not included in this discussion are another class of lower molecular weight, so-called ras-like, or p21-like G proteins, of approximately 21 kd, which are homologous to the ras proto-oncogene product (see Ch. 60). These proteins are distantly related to the G_i/G_s G-protein family. They also share the ability to bind and hydrolyze GTP, and they serve as substrates for other, novel, non-pertussis or non-cholera bacterial toxins that have been found to ADP-ribosylate these proteins. The exact functions of these proteins are not clearly understood, although many of them appear to play a role in the initiation and control of cellular proliferation as well as the movement of macromolecules between various cellular compartments.

The role(s) of the β- and γ-subunits of the G-protein family is only beginning to be understood in detail. Multiple genes for both the β- and γ-subunits have been found, suggesting that there could be a number of different ways in which unique β-subunits and γ-subunits could interact with each other and with unique α-subunits to couple different receptor and effector systems. Indeed, the βγ complex itself may mediate the activation of K^+ channels, possibly through effects on arachidonate metabolism, the yeast mating pheromone response, some calcium channels, and receptor-associated protein kinases. The level of complexity in this system is such that very few proteins can connect with multiple signaling pathways and endow them with a highly structured level of feedback and feedforward regulatory control.

G proteins regulate effector activation by a sequential series of conformational changes. Ligand-induced changes in receptor structure cause conformational changes in the G protein that permit GDP to be released and allow GTP to bind. The 39–43 kd α-subunits can be dissociated from the other two, but it has proved difficult to separate the β-subunit from the γ-subunit, suggesting that the βγ complex forms a natural heterodimer in vivo. The βγ complex dissociates from the G_α/GTP complex, and it is the latter (activated) complex that modulates the appropriate effector protein. The intrinsic GTPase activity of G_α results in a G_α/GDP complex. This complex reassociates with the βγ complex to bring the system back to the prestimulated condition. Whereas the ligand may bind to the receptor for 1 second, the activated G protein may exist for ≤20 seconds. A G protein may also influence a receptor's affinity for its ligand. Energy expended in maintaining the G_α/GTP complex weakens the binding of ligand to its receptor. By using nonhydrolyzable GTP analogues (e.g., GTP-γ-S), which maintain the complex in a stable, active conformation, or by using large amounts of GDP, which shifts the equilibrium to the inactive, GDP-bound state, or by observing the inhibitory effects of cholera or pertussis toxins on a biologic phenomenon, investigators have been able to determine G-protein involvement in a particular biologic or biochemical response. Thus, G-protein-complexed receptors have often been identified by the effect of GTP analogues on ligand-receptor binding. However, this simple system does not present the whole story, since isolated βγ units themselves can exert both stimulatory and inhibitory properties on receptor-activated metabolic events.

Another frequently used mechanism of hormone and growth factor signal transduction involves direct stimulation of protein-tyrosine kinase activity. Examples of receptors with intrinsic ligand-activated protein-tyrosine kinase activity include the receptors for insulin, EGF, PDGF, colony-stimulating factor-1, insulin-like growth factor-1, the fibroblast growth factor family, the *trk* nerve growth factor receptor family, and the stem cell factor receptor *kit*. These receptors consist of three distinct structural domains: (1) an extracellular domain that contains the ligand-binding site; (2) a short stretch of hydrophobic amino acids that spans the plasma membrane a single time; and (3) a cytosolic domain that has protein-tyrosine kinase activity. The extracellular and transmembrane domains of these different receptors are not homologous; however, there is significant homology in the protein-tyrosine kinase domains, suggesting that, like the G_α-subunits, these proteins all evolved from a common ancestral gene. Indeed, the level of structural complexity is such that it has been proposed that these receptors be classified into at least nine distinct families.

In these receptors, the binding of ligand activates the intrinsic receptor tyrosine kinase. In all of the receptors of this class studied to date, the receptors themselves are also substrates for phosphorylation on tyrosine residues, either by autophosphorylation or by the action of an associated kinase. The consequences of this covalent modification are not fully understood for each receptor type. However, mutations that decrease or eliminate the tyrosine kinase domains of these receptors also destroy their ability to generate intracellular signals. In many cases this requires the aggregation of receptors into complexes; it is unclear why this is necessary in order to transmit a signal successfully, but it can be clearly dissociated from aggregation necessary for internalization. For the EGF receptor, aggregation is associated with down-regulation and internalization.

Interestingly, one can derive hybrid receptors composed of the ligand-binding domain of one and the cytosolic, tyrosine kinase domain of the other, and preserve the signaling function of the latter in response to stimulation by the cognate ligand of the former. Thus, linking the insulin-binding domain of the insulin receptor to the transmembrane and kinase domains of the EGF receptor, and inserting this receptor into a suitable cellular recipient, yields a hybrid molecule that is capable of stimulating G protein-tyrosine kinase activity on stimulation with insulin. Therefore, while the intracellular domains of these receptors may exhibit exquisite substrate specificity with respect to the proteins that are targets for phosphorylation, the catalytic activity can be stimulated by any ligand that binds to the extracellular domain. These data suggest that the specificity of a hormone response is encoded by both the signal recognition and the intracellular, signal transmission domains of the receptor molecule.

Another class of receptors, which themselves do not possess intrinsic protein-tyrosine kinase activity, but that stimulate other protein-tyrosine kinases in the cell, is typified by the T-lymphocyte antigen receptor. Structurally, these receptors differ from those receptors with intrinsic kinase activity in that they lack the cytosolic tyrosine kinase domain. These receptors also differ structurally from the classic G protein-coupled systems described above. The former consist of peptides with single transmembrane-spanning domains, while the latter have at least seven membrane-spanning α-helical regions. The exact mechanism by which the cytosolic protein-tyrosine kinases are activated is unknown, but presumably involves a conformational change in the receptor following ligand binding that induces the active state in receptor-associated kinases. Phosphorylation of the T-cell antigen receptor complex on a number of its constituent chains is associated with certain types of transmembrane signaling. Indeed, the activation of tyrosine protein kinases is probably the necessary first step in transmitting a signal from the T-cell receptor to the cell. The interaction of these receptor systems with classic heterotrimeric G proteins is unclear. In the case of the T-cell receptor, for instance, the use of pertussis toxin as a probe for G-protein coupling is obscured because of the toxin's ability to stimulate second messenger generation directly via the antigen receptor. The

neutrophil chemotactic peptide receptor may be a very interesting hybrid. On binding the formylated small peptides (such as f-met-leu-phe), it signals the production of a number of second messenger compounds. All of these events are inhibited by preincubation of the cells with pertussis toxin, which inhibits the $G_{i\alpha}$ class of G proteins. This receptor also stimulates protein-tyrosine kinase activity. Thus, this receptor may represent a functional hybrid molecule. The exact mechanism of how this is accomplished remains to be elucidated. However, it is also now clear that stimulation of the T-cell receptor also activates the p21[ras] G protein as a consequence of the initiation and propagation of an activation signal from the plasma membrane.

Other events occur rapidly after hormone or growth factor binding to quiescent cells, some of which can be directly attributed to the activation of G proteins or protein-tyrosine kinase activity. Many, but not all, growth factors and hormones stimulate the appearance of both water-soluble and lipid-soluble second messengers derived from the phospholipase C-catalyzed hydrolysis of inositol-containing phospholipids. Initially thought to comprise a so-called futile cycle of phospholipid turnover, it is now known that hormone-stimulated phosphatidylinositol (PI) turnover is an integral component of growth factor- and hormone-mediated stimulus-response coupling. On receptor binding of ligand, there is a rapid stimulation of PI-specific phospholipase C activity. These enzymes comprise a large family of isoenzymes; those that are coupled to tyrosine protein kinase receptors or receptors that activate tyrosine kinases belong to the phospholipase Cγ-family, whereas those that are coupled to G protein-linked receptors belong to the β-family. Several isozymes of this family can exist in the same cell. Phospholipase Cγ is itself a substrate for tyrosine phosphorylation in response to the activation of several different receptors; this serves to activate the enzyme. This enzyme hydrolyzes a phosphorylated form of PI (PI-4,5-bisphosphate) to produce the hydrophilic inositol phosphate inositol 1,4,5-trisphosphate [$Ins(1,4,5)P_3$] and the lipophilic *sn*-1,2-diacylglycerol (DAG). $Ins(1,4,5)P_3$ is responsible for effecting the release of Ca^{2+} from the endoplasmic reticulum (ER) and perhaps also mediating its influx from outside the cell. It has a relatively short-lived half-life due to its rapid dephosphorylation to $Ins(1,4)P_2$ (by a specific phosphatase) or phosphorylation to $Ins(1,3,4,5)P_4$. The role of the tetrakisphosphate moiety is controversial. There is evidence suggesting that it may play a role in activating a Ca^{2+} re-uptake mechanism in the ER as well as stimulating Ca^{2+} entry from outside the cells.

Besides phospholipase Cγ, a number of other cytosolic proteins are common substrates for tyrosine phosphorylation by the PDGF receptor (as well as by other tyrosine kinase receptors and tyrosine protein kinases that are activated by nonkinase receptors). One that appears to be fairly ubiquitous and that is used as an example is phosphatidylinositol-3 kinase (PI-3-K). This enzyme catalyzes a reaction that may be important for growth regulation. It phosphorylates PI and other polyphosphoinositides at the D-3 position of the inositol ring to generate a series of polyphosphoinositides that are *not* in the pathway for $Ins(1,4,5)P_3$ production. Because the D-3-phosphorylated polyphosphoinositides are far less abundant than PI-4-P and PI-4,5-P_2, PI-3-K went undetected until recently. It was discovered because of its physical association in the cell with a number of protein products of proto-oncogenes of the protein-tyrosine kinase family. Although the functions of the lipid products of this enzyme are not known, the correlation of their appearance with the growth state of the cell suggests that they may contribute to the regulation of cell growth and neoplastic transformation. This enzyme has been purified to homogeneity, and the cDNAs for its subunits have been cloned. The 85-kd regulatory subunit of the heterodimeric holoenzyme contains both SH2 and SH3 domains, which presumably serve to attach the enzyme to the phosphorylated PDGF receptor, for example. PI-3-K also bears a significant structural homology to a yeast protein that appears to play a major role in protein sorting. However, it is important to mention that certain substrates are receptor-specific as well.

Much of what we know about growth factor signal transduction has come from studies of retrovirus-encoded oncogenes (see also Chs. 7 and 60). In many cases oncogenes have been shown to be mutated forms of genes that encode critical proteins in the cascade of events leading from growth factor binding to cell division. Thus, oncogenes encode mutated forms of growth factors (PDGF by v-*sis*), growth factor receptors (EGF receptor by *erb*B), cytosolic protein-tyrosine kinases (by *src*), cytosolic protein-serine/threonine kinases (by *raf*), low-molecular-weight GTP-binding proteins (by *ras*), and transcription regulatory factors (by *fos*). The mechanism by which these components of the growth factor signal transduction pathways interact to transmit signals to the nucleus is an area of intensive research.

An almost ubiquitous event after stimulation with cell growth-promoting hormones, such as PDGF or cell activation factors (like antigen for B and T lymphocytes, or chemotactic peptides for neutrophils, or thrombin for platelets), is an immediate increase in the cytosolic calcium concentration ($[Ca^{2+}]_i$). The importance of this increase in $[Ca^{2+}]_i$ has been shown by experiments in which either extracellular or intracellular Ca^{2+} (or both) were removed and stimulation with a large variety of hormone agonists was prevented. These data have been interpreted to mean that a rapid and prolonged rise in $[Ca^{2+}]_i$ is vital (although in most cases, not sufficient) for successful stimulus-response coupling.

The normal cytosolic free Ca^{2+} level is tightly regulated and held relatively constant at about 100 nM in the face of an extracellular $[Ca^{2+}]$ of 1.5–2.0 mM and a total cell $[Ca^{2+}]$ in a similar range. In the cell, the main storage sites for Ca^{2+} are the mitochondria and a specialized compartment of the ER. Maintenance of a low $[Ca^{2+}]_i$ against such large concentration gradients occurs through the activity of several ATP-driven Ca^{2+} pumps in the plasma membrane and ER and the Ca^{2+} exchange systems in mitochondria. Thus, there are several pools from which rapid increases in $[Ca^{2+}]_i$ could be derived. The rise in $[Ca^{2+}]_i$ is due to both an influx from outside the cell and an efflux from intracellular storage pools. The efflux appears to be derived from nonmitochondrial vesicles that are most probably derived from the smooth ER. $Ins(1,4,5)P_3$, produced from the hormone-stimulated hydrolysis of $PI(4,5)P_2$, binds to a receptor in the vesicles and stimulates the rapid release of Ca^{2+}. In the brain this receptor has been purified and shown to be a 220-kd protein that is widely distributed in nonplasma membrane vesicle systems. Ca^{2+} is resequestered into the calciosomes by an ATP-dependent mechanism, presumably a Ca^{2+} ATPase (to be distinguished from the pump of a similar name in the plasma membrane that has been isolated and cloned). In the past few years it has also become clear that Ca^{2+} release and re-uptake can be pulsatile in nature. The precise significance of this phenomenon is unclear, although it has been observed in several different hormone-receptor systems.

The production of $Ins(1,4,5)P_3$ and the release of Ca^{2+} from intracellular pools is relatively short lived and is usually not sufficient to permit a successful cellular response. A sustained influx of calcium from outside the cell is usually necessary to provide a complete response. The precise mechanism by which the Ca^{2+} influx occurs is obscure. In some systems, it has been noted in the absence of measurable, stimulated PI turnover, whereas in others it appears to be a prerequisite. It has recently been suggested that $Ins(1,4,5)P_3$ itself stimulates the opening of an unusual type of "ligand-gated," non-voltage-activated, low-conductance Ca^{2+} channel in the plasma membranes of human lymphocytes. The T-cell antigen receptor-driven Ca^{2+} influx is not blocked by drugs that are specific for the types of calcium channels found in electrically excitable cells such as nerve or muscle. However, the anionic cross-linking agent diisothiocyanostilbene-disulfonate is a high-affinity inhibitor of this flux. The transporter can be reconstituted in the absence of a mechanism for generating $Ins(1,4,5)P_3$. The protein component(s) of this channel has not been identified.

Both the increase in $[Ca^{2+}]_i$ and the stimulation of protein kinase C, together (or individually) stimulate the rapid transcription of a number of so-called early genes that are associated with cell activation. These include the genes for the proto-oncogenes *fos* and *myc*. The proto-oncogene product c-jun is constitutively expressed in unstimulated cells. The c-fos protein makes a complex with the c-jun protein to form a heterodimer in the nucleus that is then capable of recognizing and binding to specific DNA sequences in the 5′ upstream regulatory domains of a number of growth factor-stimulatable genes.

The heterodimer is also known as the activator protein-1 (AP-1) complex. Interestingly, the AP-1 heterodimer may also stimulate transcription of its own components; thus increased levels of *fos* and *jun* can be observed soon after growth factor activation of the cell, although the initial stimulation appears to be due to a complex of endogenous, previously synthesized protein. Thus, the cell is rapidly able to amplify and sustain a response to a short-lived signal. This complex thus falls into the family of transcriptional regulators that play a major role in controlling the inducible activation (and possibly deactivation) of nonconstitutive genes.

DAG stays within the plasma membrane and is a specific activator of the ubiquitous, membrane-associated protein PKC. This enzyme also depends on the presence of phosphatidylserine and Ca^{2+}. It is the cellular receptor for the tumor-promoting phorbol esters. These compounds activate PKC directly by a mechanism identical to that of endogenously produced DAG, possibly because of their structural homology to the DAGs. At least seven isoenzymes of PKC have been detected by molecular cloning techniques. Bacterial expression of these various proteins in pure form has also demonstrated that they have vastly different dependencies on phospholipid, divalent cations, and neutral lipids; indeed, at least one of the isoenzymes can be activated by arachidonic acid, and more recently it has been shown that another can be activated by an arachidonic acid metabolite, lipoxin A4, in nerve terminals. Another source of DAG is the phospholipase C-catalyzed hydrolysis of non-PI phospholipids. The primary phospholipid substrate is phosphatidylcholine (PC). PC may make up 25% of the total phospholipid in the cell, compared with the 2–5% for the PI-containing phospholipids. This phospholipase C is a different enzyme(s) from the one that hydrolyzes PI-phospholipids. DAG derived from PC is stimulated by a wide variety of hormones, including interleukin-1. It is unclear how the two sources of DAG interact and are regulated. What is clear is that the substrates of PKC are varied and extremely important for the transmission of a signal to the nucleus.

The rapid production of $Ins(1,4.5)P_3$ and DAG from PI-4,5-bisphosphate is triggered by receptors that couple to G proteins (e.g., muscarinic receptors), receptors with intrinsic protein-tyrosine kinase activity (e.g., PDGF and EGF receptors), receptors that indirectly activate protein-tyrosine kinases (e.g., the T-cell antigen receptor), and those that activate both G proteins and protein-tyrosine kinases (e.g., the neutrophil chemotactic peptide receptor). There are also receptors of both major families that fail to stimulate PI turnover. Thus, there appear to be multiple mechanisms for activating polyphosphoinositide-specific phospholipase C, some involving G proteins and others involving G protein-coupled tyrosine kinases.

A large number of proteins involved in transmitting a positive signal from a plasma membrane growth factor receptor (such as the PDGF, EGF, stem cell factor receptor or *kit,* and nerve

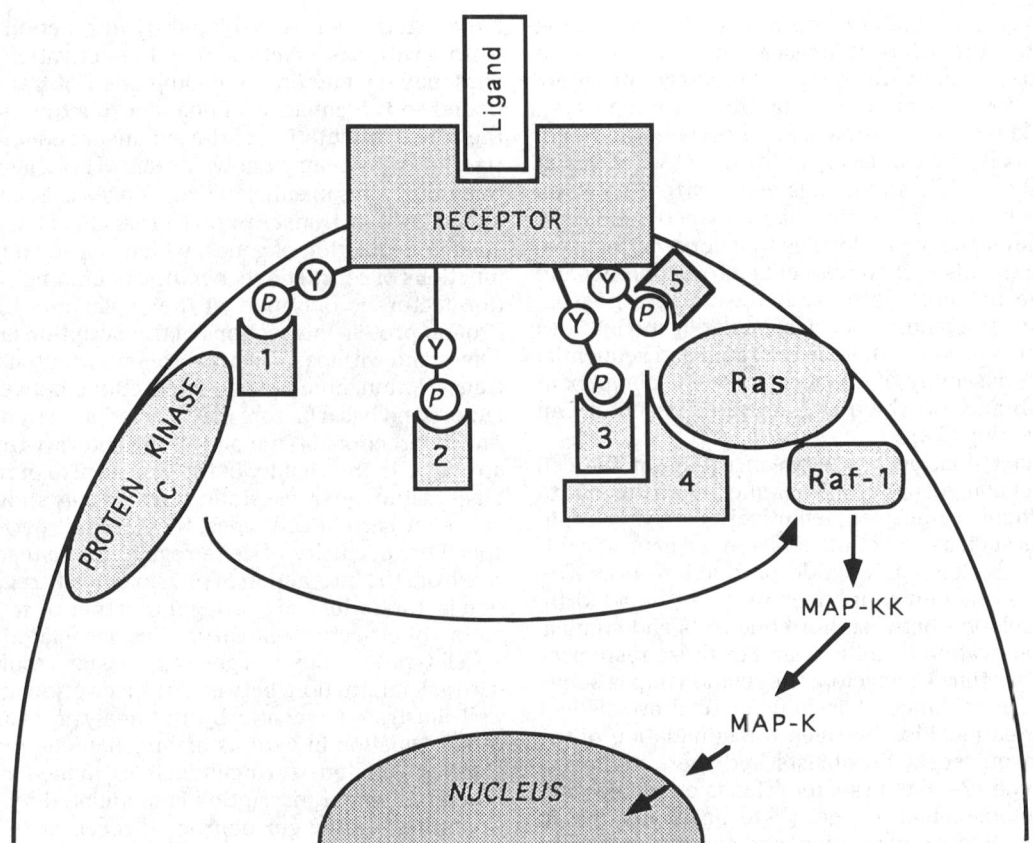

Fig. 6-2. Schematic diagram of the assembly of a signaling complex at the plasma membrane after the binding of ligand to a tyrosine kinase growth factor receptor. This event initiates a sequence of events in which the receptor, here shown as a monomer, multimerizes and its intrinsic kinase activity is activated (see text for details). This leads to phosphorylation of both the receptor and numerous other substrates. The generation of tyrosine-phosphates in the appropriate context leads to the recruitment of other components of the signaling complex, including phospholipase Cγ (1), phosphatidylinositol-3-kinase (2), Grb2 (3), Sos (4), and GAP (5). Phospholipase Cγ can now hydrolyze PI(4,5)P$_2$ to produce Ins(1,4,5)P$_3$ and diacylglycerol; the former produces an increase in cellular [Ca^{2+}], and the latter activates protein kinase C. Phosphatidylinositol-3-kinase (2) is phosphorylated on the 85-kd regulatory subunit, which can then activate its associated 100-kd catalytic subunit. Grb2 (3) attaches to the receptor by virtue of its SH2 domains and brings along the GDP-GTP exchange protein Sos (4) via its SH3 domains. ras is now capable of being activated with a negative regulator, GAP (5), which is also recruited to the complex. ras serves to activate the serine/threonine kinase raf-1 (also activated by protein kinase C), which in turn activates MAP kinase kinase (MAP-KK), which then activates MAP kinase (MAP-K), and so on.

growth factor receptors, for example) possess common structural features that have been called SH2 and SH3 domains. These domains are homologous to noncatalytic regions of the c-src proto-oncogene protein, itself a tyrosine protein kinase. SH2 domains function, at least in part, to anchor signaling molecules to proteins phosphorylated on tyrosine residues via a specific pentapeptide recognition motif. This is a very high-affinity and specific interaction and serves to assemble multiple components of a signaling complex to localized region(s) of the cell. When PDGF binds to its receptor, it immediately activates the intrinsic tyrosine protein kinase activity of the receptor, which undergoes an autophosphorylation reaction. The phosphorylated receptor is now able to bind other signaling molecules such as the SH2 domain-containing PI-3-K, phospholipase Cγ, and the GTPase-activating protein (GAP) (Fig. 6-2). In a like manner, SH3 domains have now been shown to target proteins to other sequence motifs (proline-rich regions). Indeed, there are proteins that are largely composed of SH2 and SH3 domains, such as the products of the *shc, crk,* and *nck* proto-oncogenes, and Grb2. Recent work has demonstrated that these proteins can function as molecular bridges or adapters between activated tyrosine protein kinase receptors and the p21^{ras} signaling pathway. Other proteins, such as sos (named after a mutation of a homologous protein in *Drosophila*), may also be part of this adapter complex; in particular,

this protein appears to be a GDP-GTP exchanger. SH3 domains have also been shown to direct proteins to associate with the actin cytoskeleton.

The 21-kd low-molecular-weight GTP-binding protein ras plays a critical role in transmembrane signaling in most, if not all, cells. This protein has long been known to occupy a central switch point in signal transmission, although those elements in the pathway that connect receptors to *ras* and then *ras* to downstream components have only recently been demonstrated. Under normal conditions, *ras* has a reasonable intrinsic GTPase activity, thus helping it to maintain itself in the GDP-bound (and thus inactive) state. Two other proteins play important roles in the regulation of *ras* activity, GAP, which turns *ras* off, and at least two guanine nucleotide exchange factors, which serve to keep *ras* in the GTP-bound, or "on" state. GAP can be phosphorylated on tyrosines, and in PDGF-stimulated cells it can be found complexed with the PDGF receptor. Mutations in *ras* that change it into a transforming oncogene also tend to decrease its GTPase activity and render it insensitive to the regulatory control of these other proteins. Evidence connects *ras* with several other members of the mitogenic signaling apparatus that have long been thought to play a role in connecting the tyrosine kinase and serine/threonine kinase pathways. These include raf, a proto-oncogene product that is a serine/threonine kinase phosphorylated on both serines (mostly) and tyrosines after receptor stimulation, and the mitogen-activated protein (MAP) kinases. The latter are also Ser-Thr kinases that are activated by tyrosine and serine/threonine phosphorylation, at least in part by their own kinase(s), the MAP kinase kinase. *raf* can be phosphorylated and activated by PKC. Finally, *raf* can associate with activated *ras* at the plasma membrane. These findings emphasize a common regulatory theme in that there exist nascent recognition elements in important signaling molecules that serve to join spatially and structurally distinct components into a coherent and functionally active metabolic pathway. In the case of mitogenic signaling receptors, the binding of extracellular ligand initiates a sequence of events in which there is the rapid and sequential (or simultaneous) assembly of a macromolecular complex at the plasma membrane, of which the activated receptor can serve as the nidus (Fig. 6-2).

What is the exact relationship between events at the cell membrane and cellular responses? This question turns out to be somewhat difficult to answer definitively. For very rapid cellular responses such as secretion of histamine in mast cells, degranulation in platelets, superoxide production in neutrophils, excitation-contraction coupling in muscle, and so forth, the temporal correlation between hormone or ligand stimulation and cellular activation is quite clear. For those responses that require a longer time to develop, the relationship is somewhat less clear. For instance, it is difficult to draw distinct cause-and-effect relationships between the stimulation of the PDGF receptor in quiescent fibroblasts and the initiation of DNA synthesis some 12–16 hours later. This is especially true when the known biochemical changes (PI turnover, changes in $[Ca^{2+}]_i$, stimulation of *fos* transcription, and so forth) peak and decay relatively rapidly. The observations that cellular levels of $Ins(1,3,4)P_3$ rise slowly after PDGF stimulation, and stay elevated for some time, and that the product of PI-3-K, PI-3-P, also stays elevated for prolonged periods, suggests a specific correlation. However, the discovery of the rel family of transcription regulatory proteins, and particularly the nuclear factor (NF)-κB family, has enabled us to draw a connection between membrane signaling events and consequent events in the nucleus.

REGULATION OF TRANSCRIPTION

The transcriptional regulation of mRNA-encoding genes is of primary importance in mammalian development, tissue differentiation, morphogenesis, and the response of cells to their environment. One tissue is distinct from another largely because of the specific pattern of genes expressed. The tissue- or cell-specific pattern of protein expression is determined in large measure by the corresponding pattern of transcriptional regulation. Transcription is regulated at the level of the gene (1) by basal (or general) factors—proteins that have a general role in the recruitment of RNA polymerase II (POl II); (2) by transcription factors—proteins that bind to specific cis-acting cognate DNA sequences that differ in arrangement from gene to gene; and (3) by the interaction between these two classes of factors.

Basal factors act on promoter proximal sites at or near the transcription start site (or cap site). One such site is the TATA box, located 25–35 base pairs (bp) upstream from the cap site, to which the basal factor TATA-binding protein binds as part of a complex of proteins called TFIID. Other basal factors can also contribute to the formation of a transcriptionally active Pol II complex. By contrast, transcription factors recognize cognate binding sites in cis-acting DNA sequences called enhancers, which are usually located more than 100 bp upstream of the transcription start site, but may be downstream of the gene or in intron sequences. When bound to the enhancer, transcription factors may activate or inhibit the utilization of the pro-

moter. Activation is mediated by interaction of transcription factors with basal factors. Whether activation or inhibition occurs may depend on the combination of transcription factors bound to the enhancer. Enhancer function is independent of the 5′ to 3′ orientation of the enhancer sequence and position, (i.e., both upstream or downstream of Pol II genes). By adhering to binding sites in enhancer sequences in a physiologically regulated fashion, transcription factors affect tissue- and stimulus-specific regulation of genes, which is critical for differentiated functions of cells. The recognition of binding sites by transcription factors is only part of the explanation of their function. Protein-protein interactions of transcription factors with themselves and with basal factors are important in the regulation of transcription. Some of the interactions between transcription factors and basal factors may be mediated by adaptor proteins. The interaction of transcription factors with the chromatin structure in the vicinity of the gene is also of regulatory importance. Although transcription factors may show distinct preferences for certain cell types, they are not necessarily cell-type specific. Specificity of gene regulation instead appears to derive from the interaction of physiologically regulated transcription factors, which are brought together by the specific combination of cis-acting enhancer sites associated with each gene.

Cell-type specificity of gene expression resulting from combinatorial interaction between transcription factors has been well illustrated recently by the analysis of mouse proliferin gene regulation in various mammalian cell types. Proliferin is a growth-related, serum-inducible, immediate-early protein. Proliferin gene transcription is modulated by glucocorticoids, which bind to the glucocorticoid receptor (GR), and by mitogens and phorbol esters, which induce the AP-1 transcription factor (composed of either c-fos/c-jun heterodimers or c-jun homodimers). Depending on the cell type, glucocorticoid treatment enhances, represses, or has no effect on proliferin transcription. The remarkable finding is that the direction of the cellular response depends on the combinatorial interaction of hormone-GR complex and AP-1 at a proliferin gene composite response element, which has overlapping binding sites for both factors. Glucocorticoid hormone stimulation of hormone-responsive cells results in translocation of the glucocorticoid hormone-receptor complex to the nucleus, where it can bind its cognate glucocorticoid response element. Growth factor or mitogen stimulation of the same cell results in translocation of AP-1 to the nucleus, where it can bind its cognate AP-1 site. The outcome of cellular stimulation with glucocorticoids depends on the functional ratio of c-jun to c-fos, which in turn depends on the cell type. Glucocorticoid-stimulated HeLa cells, for example, which express AP-1 predominantly as a c-jun homodimer, have increased transcription driven by the proliferin composite response element. By contrast, glucocorticoid-stimulated CV-1 cells, which express AP-1 predominantly as c-fos/ c-jun heterodimers, have decreased transcription driven by the same element. The ratio of c-fos to c-jun, determining the makeup of the AP-1 factor, is the critical variable in determining the nature of the response to glucocorticoid, not the absolute levels of these factors. This is one example of regulatory cross-talk or regulation by committee, which results in cell-type-specific gene expression.

Transcription factors generally fall into several structural families (Table 6-1). One family is composed of the helix-turn-helix proteins, of which homeobox proteins are among the best known examples. Homeobox proteins play critical roles in the development of both vertebrates and invertebrates; they have been best studied in *Drosophila*. The ubiquitous Oct1 and lymphoid-specific Oct2 factors are members of a closely related family. A second family of transcription factors is the group of zinc finger factors, which includes the steroid receptors, such as the glucocorticoid receptor. The GATA factors,

Table 6-1. Examples of Eukaryotic Transcription Factors

Class and Family	Factor	Comments
Helix-turn-helix		
Octamer	Oct1	Ubiquitous factor
	Oct2	Lymphoid-specific factor
Zn finger		
Steroid receptor	Retinoic acid receptor (RAR and RXR)	Many isoforms, critical for mammalian development
GATA family	GATA1, -2, and -3	Important in hematopoietic development
SP1	SP1	Ubiquitously found activator
Amphipathic helix		
b-ZIP family	c-fos and c-jun	Cell growth regulation
	NF-E2	Erythroid development
	C/EBP	Liver gene regulation
Helix-loop-helix (HLH)	E12 and E47	Immunoglobulin gene activation
	MyoD	Muscle differentiation
b-HLH-ZIP	c-myc mad max	Regulation of cell growth and apoptosis
rel	NF-κB, c-rel, and others	Regulation of immunoreceptors, cytokines, adhesion proteins, and acute-phase proteins

important for hematopoietic development, are also members of the zinc finger family. A third family is composed of the amphipathic helix proteins, which can engage in heterotypic dimerization leading to regulatory specificity (e.g., proliferin gene regulation). The amphipathic helix family includes the leucine zipper proteins c-fos and c-jun, which together make up the AP-1 transcription factor and are important in the response of cells to mitogenic stimuli. Other examples include NF-E2, an erythroid-specific factor involved in the regulation of globin locus control regions and C/EBP, which activates liver-specific gene expression. The amphipathic helix proteins also include the helix-loop-helix proteins (HLH) such as MyoD, important in muscle differentiation, and the myc family, which includes the proto-oncoprotein c-myc. The myc family of factors, including c-myc, max, and mad are of the bHLH-Zip variety, having a basic region that contacts DNA followed by an HLH domain and a leucine zipper that together mediate dimerization. The rel transcription factors are distinct in structure from the above families and are an example of a family of signal-transducing transcription factors. A recurring theme, demonstrated by the amphipathic helix and rel families, is the combinatorial association of subunits as homo- or heterodimers to generate regulatory diversity.

rel Family of Transcription Factors

rel family proteins, named for the v-rel oncogene, form a family of signal-transducing transcription factors with considerable functional diversity based on combinatorial homo- and heterodimerization. Functional diversity may arise in part from the ability of certain combinations of rel factors to distinguish between variants of a decameric DNA-binding site found in the enhancers of rel-regulated genes. rel factors serve as regulators of cellular responses to a myriad of stimuli, including mitogens, cytokines, bacterial and viral infection, DNA-damaging agents, oxidative stress, and ultraviolet and X-irradiation. Highly conserved in evolution and found in both vertebrate- and invertebrate-signaling systems, rel factors form critical links between

organisms and their environment. rel factors are implicated in diverse physiologic and pathophysiologic processes in humans, including cell growth, viral and translocation-mediated oncogenesis, MHC class I down-regulation in malignant cells, the progression of acquired immunodeficiency syndrome (AIDS) and other viral infections, the acute-phase response, local inflammation, and allograft rejection. The most studied member of the rel family is the pleiotropic transcription factor NF-κB.

Several lines of evidence implicate rel factors in the regulation of cell growth. The v-rel oncogene of avian reticuloendotheliosis virus induces lymphoma in birds. The lyt-10 candidate proto-oncogene identified at a B-cell non-Hodgkin lymphoma t(10;14)(q24;q32) translocation breakpoint, involving the immunoglobulin heavy chain $C\alpha_1$ switch region, is identical to a gene encoding an NF-κB factor. Furthermore, the c-rel proto-oncogene counterpart of v-rel appears to be involved in a translocation found in a human large cell lymphoma. The rel-associated bcl-3 candidate proto-oncogene was first identified at a B-cell chronic lymphocytic leukemia t(14;19)(q32;q13.1) translocation, which also involved the immunoglobulin heavy chain $C\alpha_1$ switch region. The bcl-3 protein has been shown to alter both the type and transcriptional activity of rel factors bound to κB sites.

rel factors play a role in T-cell activation. Stimulation of resting T cells by tumor necrosis factor-β (TNF-β), interleukin-1 (IL-1), IL-6, or antibodies to the CD3 and CD28 receptors appears to involve NF-κB in each case. NF-κB may also play additional roles in T-cell activation by regulating the genes encoding IL-2 and the IL-2 receptor α-chain (IL-2Rα). The rel factors are also involved in the pathogenesis of human immunodeficiency virus-1 and human T-lymphotropic virus-1 (HTLV-1), which appear to have taken advantage of the activation of rel factors in T cells for their own use. The progression of AIDS and HTLV-1 infection is thought to occur at least in part by the activation of NF-κB in infected cells.

NF-κB Model for Gene Activation

NF-κB was first described as a factor in B-lymphocyte nuclear extracts binding to the decameric immunoglobulin-κ (lg-κ) intron enhancer κB site (lg-κ κB site). The κB site is important for the function of the lg-κ intron enhancer. NF-κB is a heterodimer of two DNA-binding proteins, p50 and p65. The p50 protein was shown to be derived by proteolytic cleavage from a precursor protein, p105, located predominantly in the cytoplasm.

Two critical discoveries connecting NF-κB with signal transduction were (1) that NF-κB could be activated by a post-translational mechanism and (2) that NF-κB was present in the cytoplasm of most cell types, bound to an inhibitor of its DNA-binding activity, named inhibitor of κB (IκB). Treatment of cytoplasmic extracts with several protein kinases, including PKC, which is involved in signal transduction of mitogenic stimuli, released NF-κB DNA-binding activity from its covert complex with IκB. PKC can phosphorylate IκB in vitro, correlating with the appearance of NF-κB DNA-binding activity. A specific protease cleaves IκB, and it is suspected that proteolysis is the critical step in the inactivation of IκB.

NF-κB as a Pleiotropic Transcriptional Regulator

DNA-binding sites for rel complexes (κB sites) have been found in numerous genes falling mainly in the following categories: those encoding immunoreceptors, cytokines, acute-phase

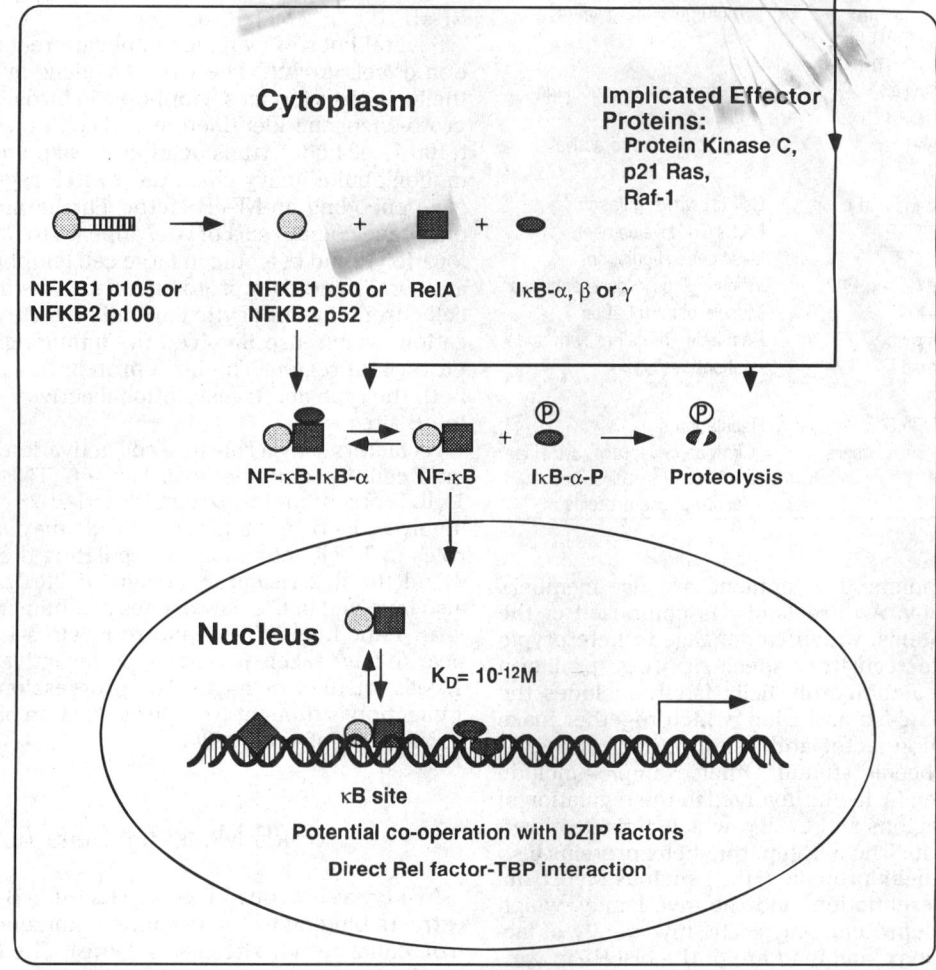

Extracellular Stimuli:

Cytokines: IL-1, TNF-α and -β
Mitogens: PMA/PHA, lectins,Ca++ ionophore
Antibodies to: CD28, TCR-α/CD3
Bacteria: LPS
Viruses: HTLV-1, HSV-1, CMV, HBV, Adenovirus
Other stimuli: Free Radicals, UV or X-irradiation

Cytoplasm

Implicated Effector Proteins:
Protein Kinase C,
p21 Ras,
Raf-1

NFKB1 p105 or   NFKB1 p50 or   RelA   IκB-α, β or γ
NFKB2 p100   NFKB2 p52

NF-κB-IκB-α   NF-κB   +   IκB-α-P   →   Proteolysis

Nucleus $K_D = 10^{-12}M$

κB site

Potential co-operation with bZIP factors

Direct Rel factor-TBP interaction

Fig. 6-3. A model for the activation of NF-κB by extracellular stimuli. The p105 and p100 proteins are post-translationally processed to generate the p50 and p52 subunits of NF-κB, respectively. Stimuli activating NF-κB include cytokines, mitogens, antibodies to membrane-signaling proteins, lipopolysaccharide (LPS), viral immediate-early proteins, free radicals, and ultraviolet or X-irradiation. Three effector proteins have been implicated in NF-κB activation: protein kinase C, ras, and raf-1. The exact roles of these effector proteins are not yet known. IκB-α is inactivated by proteolysis. Phosphorylation (indicated by a circled P) of IκB-α can also occur, and may contribute to inactivation. Once IκB is inactivated, NF-κB can then enter the nucleus and bind its cognate binding sites. The equilibrium dissociation constant (K_D) for the binding of NF-κB p50, p65 to the canonical Igκ κB site is indicated. NF-κB can interact physically and functionally with transcription factors of the bZIP family. Non-rel transcription factors binding at their different cognate sites are indicated by the diamond and by ovals.

proteins, cellular adhesion proteins, and viral proteins. The genes possessing κB sites are regulated by diverse cellular stimuli, including growth factors, cytokines mediating inflammation- and acute-phase-related signals, oxidative stress, and viral infection. The functional significance of many of the κB sites has been demonstrated by mutational analysis of those sites.

The immunoreceptor genes with κB sites include those encoding Ig-κ, T-cell receptor-β, IL-2Rα, MHC class I proteins, β2-microglobulin, and MHC class II invariant chain. Cytokine genes having κB sites include those encoding interferon-β, IL-2, IL-6, TNF-α, TNF-β (lymphotoxin), colony-stimulating factor-

granulocyte/macrophage, colony-stimulating factor-granulocyte, and proenkephalin (a cytokine precursor). Proto-oncogenes having κB sites include those encoding c-*myc* and c-ha-*ras*1. The candidate antioncogene encoding interferon regulatory factor-1 has at least three putative κB sites. The acute-phase protein genes encoding serum amyloid A precursor, angiotensinogen (also a cytokine precursor) and E-selectin have functional κB sites. Finally, the rel factors can potentially autoregulate themselves, since the c-*rel*, *NFKB1*, and *NFKB2* genes have κB sites. The complex array of NF-κB-regulated genes with related functions in cell growth, infection, inflammation, allograft, oxidation, and radiation responses suggests a coordinating role of rel factors in rapidly activating genes in the host response to environmental stresses. A model portraying the activation of this family of transcription factors is shown in Figure 6-3.

rel Factors and Cell Growth

The connection between the mammalian rel factors and cell growth became apparent when the cDNA clones for several rel factors were isolated from cDNA libraries specific for the immediate-early response of human peripheral T cells to mitogens or growth factors. These results demonstrated a connection between rel factors and the G_0-G_1 transition in the initiation of cell growth. Furthermore, it has been observed that the NF-κB DNA-binding activity is rapidly induced in growth-arrested mouse fibroblasts stimulated with serum growth factors, but not in proliferating cells. This result suggested that the induction of NF-κB is specific for the G_0-G_1 transition, during which cell growth is initiated. Recently, the connection between cell growth stimulation and NF-κB activation was strengthened by the finding that activated forms of the GTP-binding ras or the serine/threonine protein kinase raf, both involved in signal transduction, can stimulate κB site-directed transcription. raf is thought to act downstream of ras. These results delineate a possible pathway by which serum growth factors, PKC, and T-cell receptor stimulation may activate NF-κB. Despite the connection between rel factors and cell growth, the basis for the oncogenic potential of certain rel and IκB proteins remains to be determined.

SUGGESTED READINGS

Baeverle PA, Henkel T: Function and activation of NFkB in the immune system. Annu Rev Immunol 12:141, 1994

Berk A, Schmidt MC: How *do* transcription factors work? Genes Dev 4:151, 1990

Cantley LC, Auger KR, Carpenter C et al: Oncogenes and signal transduction. Cell 64:281, 1991

Cohen P: The structure and regulation of protein phosphatases. Annu Rev Biochem 58:453, 1989

Edelman AM, Blumenthal DK, Krebs EG: Protein serine/threonine kinases. Annu Rev Biochem 56:567, 1987

Fantl WJ, Johnson DE, Williams LT: Signaling by receptor tyrosine kinases. Annu Rev Biochem 62:453, 1993

Hannink M, Temin HM: Molecular mechanisms of transformation by the v-rel oncogene. Crit Rev Oncog 2:293, 1991

Herschman HR: Primary response genes induced by growth factors and tumor promoters. Annu Rev Biochem 60:281, 1991

Johnson PF, McKnight SL: Eukaryotic transcriptional regulatory proteins. Annu Rev Biochem 58:799, 1989

Lowy DR, Willumsen BM: Function and regulation of RAS. Annu Rev Biochem 62: 851, 1993

Mayer BJ, Baltimore D: Signaling through SH2 and SH3 domains. Trends Cell Biol 3:8, 1993

Miner JN, Yamamoto KR: Regulatory crosstalk at composite response elements. Trends Biochem Sci 16:423, 1991

Mitchell PJ, Tjian R: Transcriptional regulation in mammalian cells by sequence-specific DNA binding proteins. Science 245:371, 1989

Orkin SH: GATA-binding transcription factors in hematopoietic cells. Blood 80: 575, 1992

Pabo CO, Sauer RT: Transcription factors: structural families and principles of DNA recognition. Annu Rev Biochem 61:1053, 1992

Perlmutter RM, Levin SD, Appleby MW, et al: Regulation of lymphocyte function by protein phosphorylation. Annu Rev Immunol 11:451, 1993

Ptashne M, Gann AAF: Activators and targets. Nature 346:329, 1990

Walton KM, Dixon JE: Protein tyrosine phosphatases. Annu Rev Biochem 62:101, 1993

Control of Cell Growth, Differentiation, and Death

7

William M. F. Lee and Chi V. Dang

INTRODUCTION

Somatic cells undergo one of three general fates: they (1) proliferate by mitotic cell division, (2) differentiate and acquire specialized functions, or (3) die and are eliminated from the body. Proliferation ensures repletion of cells lost to terminal differentiation, cell death, or cell loss; in the case of lymphocytes, it serves the additional function of allowing amplification of the immune response to specific antigens. Differentiation provides the organism with a supply of cells to execute specific and specialized functions. Cell death as an active process, initiated by the cell itself (apoptosis), is physiologically as impor-

tant as cell proliferation and differentiation, since it allows tissue renewal and changes in cellular composition without an undesirable accumulation of cells. When the regulation of any of these three cellular processes goes awry, and their balance becomes abnormal, the consequences to the organism are usually dire and result in either functional insufficiency or neoplasia. The relevance of these events to normal tissue function and neoplasia has led to investigations of their mechanisms and regulation at a molecular level.

Cell proliferation and differentiation are frequently exclusive fates, so that a differentiating cell may lose its proliferative potential; muscle and nerves are examples of tissues composed of cells that have undergone terminal differentiation and are no longer capable of proliferation. However, these two pathways need not be mutually exclusive, so that cells may proliferate and at the same time acquire differentiated characteristics. During hematopoiesis, for example, actively proliferating cells such as erythroblasts, myeloblasts, and megakaryoblasts are already committed to particular differentiation pathways and display lineage-specific biochemical and morphologic markers of differentiation. Fully differentiated T and B lymphocytes expressing antigen-specific T-cell receptors or immunoglobulins actively proliferate when appropriately stimulated.

SIGNAL TRANSDUCTION AND CELL PROLIFERATION

Cells proliferate, differentiate, and die in response to signals from their environment. Of these, mitogenic signals and signaling mechanisms are the best understood and serve as the paradigm for how cells respond to environmental signals in general. Signaling pathways leading to differentiation and apoptosis probably use similar mechanisms but achieve a different cellular response as the end result. Cell proliferation is normally stimulated by extracellular growth factors; the process by which information about the presence of these factors at the cell surface is transmitted to the nucleus, where ultimate control of most cellular events resides, is called signal transduction. A brief overview of some of the biochemical events that constitute signal transduction is provided as an introduction to the subsequent discussion of cell cycle regulation. A detailed description of signal transduction is provided in Chapter 6.

Much of what is known about signal transduction has been learned through studies of the cellular biochemical response to platelet-derived growth factor (PDGF) and epidermal growth factor (EGF).[1,2] When these ligands bind to their cognate cell surface receptors (PDGF-R and EGF-R, respectively), the receptors dimerize and their intrinsic tyrosine kinase activity becomes activated, resulting in the transfer of phosphate groups from ATP to tyrosine residues of specific cellular proteins. Among the targets for tyrosine phosphorylation are the receptors themselves, which become autophosphorylated (Fig. 7-1). Some other types of receptors, such as the T-cell antigen receptor, do not possess intrinsic tyrosine kinase activity, and the tyrosine phosphorylation that they induce on ligand binding is mediated by associated nonreceptor tyrosine kinases that become activated.[3] The presence of phosphotyrosines in target proteins enables them to form noncovalent complexes with proteins containing SH2 (src-homology region 2) domains; the latter are peptide domains (originally defined by homology

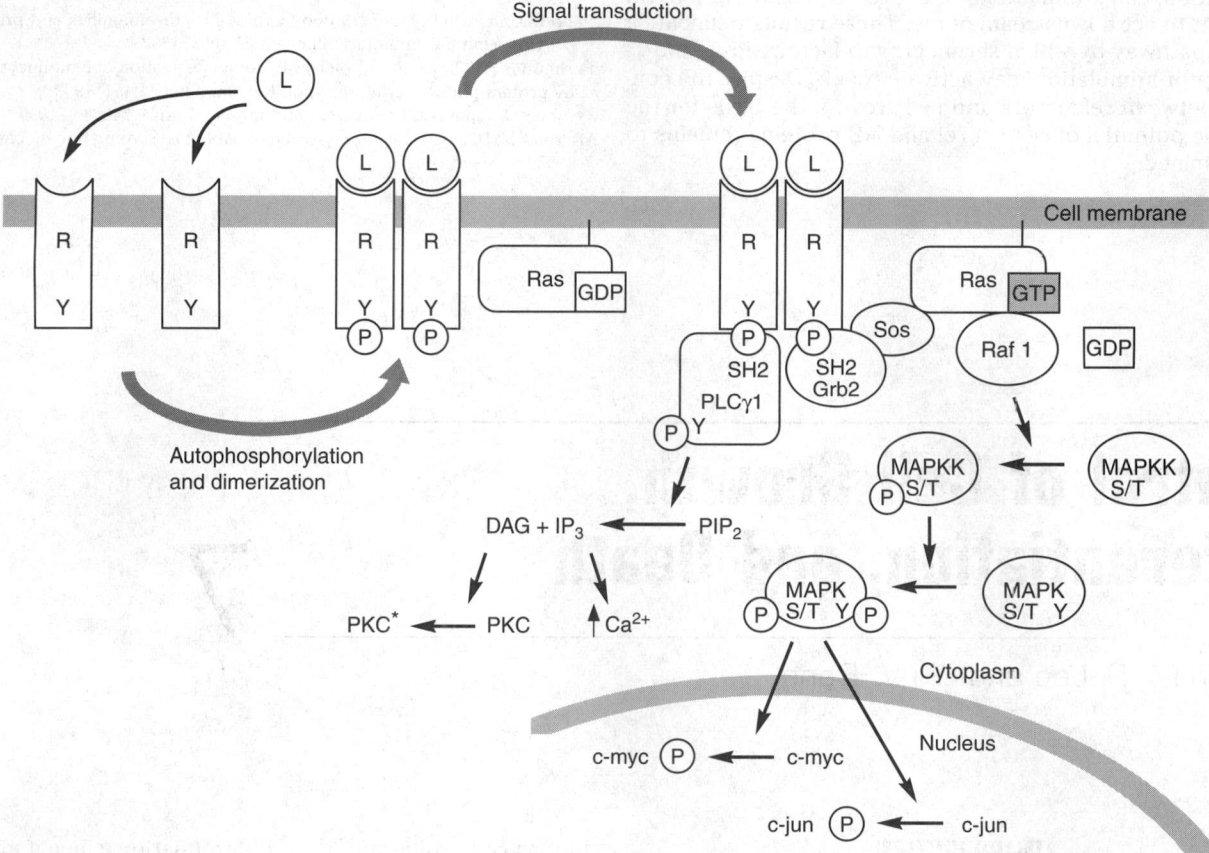

Fig. 7-1. Mitogenic signal transduction. Shown are signal transduction pathways activated by the binding of mitogenic ligands (L), such as PDGF or EGF, to their cognate receptors (R) at the cell surface. Binding results in dimerization and autophosphorylation (P) of the receptors on tyrosine residues (Y). This enables them to associate with and activate specific SH2 domain-containing downstream components of the signaling pathway. In the case of phospholipase Cγ1 (PLCγ1), association leads to tyrosine phosphorylation by the receptor kinase and an enhanced ability to hydrolyze bisphoinositol bisphosphate (PIP$_2$) to diacylglycerol (DAG) and inositol trisphosphate (IP$_3$); in turn, DAG activates protein kinase C (PKC) and IP$_3$ mobilizes Ca^{2+} from intracellular stores. In the case of Grb2-Sos, association with phosphorylated receptors stimulates its ability to facilitate ras GTP-GDP exchange; GTP-ras activates the MAP kinase (MAPK) cascade, which eventually induces serine (S)/threonine (T) phosphorylation of nuclear proteins that modulate gene transcription. Note that MAPK is activated by serine/threonine and tyrosine phosphorylation and that both result from the activity of a single dual-function kinase, MAPK kinase.

to a region in the src retroviral oncoprotein) that have affinity for phosphotyrosine-containing peptides.[4]

Autophosphorylation of EGF-R and PDGF-R enables them to interact with other proteins near or at the plasma membrane and activate proximate downstream components of the signaling pathway. Certain enzymes with SH2 domains, such as the γ1-isoform of phospholipase C, become directly associated with autophosphorylated EGF-R and PDGF-R.[5,6] This association targets these enzymes for tyrosine phosphorylation by the receptors, which, in the case of phospholipase Cγ1, results in enhancement of its enzymatic activity.[7,8] Activation of phospholipase Cγ1 catalyzes the hydrolysis of phosphatidylinositol (PIP$_2$) into diacylglycerol (DAG) and inositol(1,4,5)-trisphosphate (IP$_3$), both of which act as second messengers that launch dependent reactions inside the cell; DAG activates protein kinase C ([PKC], a kinase that phosphorylates serine/threonine residues in substrate proteins). IP$_3$ induces Ca^{2+} release from intracellular stores, which in turn activates Ca^{2+}/calmodulin-dependent serine/threonine protein kinases and other Ca^{2+}-dependent events.[9,10]

Another signaling molecule that becomes activated when receptors bind their ligand and become autophosphorylated is ras. This proto-oncoprotein is a member of the class of low-molecular-weight GTP-binding proteins that are inactive in their GDP-bound form and active in their GTP-bound form[11] (Fig. 7-1). The intrinsic GTPase activity of ras, enhanced by the presence of a GTPase-activating protein (GAP), hydrolyzes bound GTP to GDP and maintains ras in its basal, inactive state.[12] Following EGF binding by EGF-R, two cytoplasmic proteins, Grb2 and sos, that exist as heterodimers in unstimulated cells physically link EGF-R with ras in a quarternary complex through binding of phosphorylated EGF-R with the SH2 domain of Grb2 and the binding of sos to ras. Formation of this complex activates the function of sos as a guanine nucleotide exchange factor, resulting in the conversion of ras-GDP to ras-GTP and ras activation (see references within McCormick[13]). Activation of ras initiates a cascade of serine/threonine kinase activation. It may begin with the association of GTP-ras with raf-1, leading to activation of the latter's serine/threonine kinase function.[14] raf-1 phosphorylates and activates the kinase (MAPK kinase or MEK) that phosphorylates and activates MAP kinase (MAPK or mitogen-activated protein kinase.[15] Mitogen exposure thus results in activation of a host of serine/threonine kinases that phosphorylate diverse cellular proteins and modulate their activities. Among these targets are proteins that modulate gene transcription, resulting in a change in the transcriptional program of the cell. For example, activated MAP kinase can phosphorylate nuclear proteins, such as c-jun[16] and c-myc,[17] and can alter their transcriptional activities.

Ligands other than EGF and PDGF may activate signal transduction pathways differently. Neuro- and vasoactive agonists (e.g., epinephrine, bombesin, thrombin, and so forth) activate responsive cells through specific receptors that have seven membrane-spanning domains. These receptors are typically coupled to heterotrimeric G proteins that resemble ras in being regulated by GTP and GDP.[2] These receptor-coupled G proteins are linked to effector enzymes (e.g., adenylyl cyclases) that generate molecular signaling intermediates (e.g., cAMP) on ligand binding (see Ch. 98 for more details).[18] Ligands such as steroid and thyroid hormones and retinoids can access the cell interior by virtue of their lipophilic nature. Their receptors are intracellularly located, are able to bind sequence-specific DNA, and are capable of directly modulating the transcription of certain cellular genes (i.e., they are transcription factors). The effect of these receptors on the transcription of responsive genes is influenced by the binding of the cognate hormone to the receptor.[19]

Factors regulating gene transcription are final participants in the afferent signal transduction pathway and initiators of cellular responses to these signals. In general, they are se-

quence-specific DNA binding proteins that modulate the expression of the genes to which they bind. When these factors bind their cognate DNA sequence, they interact with the basal transcription machinery to initiate, enhance, or inhibit transcription. Transcription factors have peptide domains with characteristic secondary structures that are responsible for their ability to bind DNA. Many bind DNA only as dimers, and the peptide domains responsible for dimerization are essential for DNA binding. Most transcription factors use one of a limited number of peptide motifs to dimerize and bind DNA: the zinc finger motif, the basic region-leucine zipper (bZip) motif, the basic region-helix-loop-helix (bHLH) motif, a variation of this motif that adds a leucine zipper-like region (bHLHZip), or a helix-turn-helix motif.[20] The ability of transcription factors to activate or suppress the transcription of genes is usually due to a separate transcriptional activation (transactivation) domain that is frequently acidic in nature, glutamine rich, or proline rich.[21] Transcriptional gene regulation is highly complex, not only because of the multitude of transcription factors present in cells but also because of the ability of the different factors to heterodimerize. The combined pairs formed may have DNA-binding, transactivation, and regulatory properties that are different from the parental homodimers.[22] A striking example is seen in heterodimers containing the protein Id, which is an HLH protein that can dimerize with selected bHLH proteins, such as the myogenic transcription factor myoD. Id does not possess a DNA-binding basic region adjacent to its HLH dimerization domain. Id-containing heterodimers are incapable of binding DNA, making Id a negative transcriptional regulator that inhibits the function of positive factors.[23]

Transcription factors, situated at the "end" of the signal transduction pathway, are frequently the recipient of mitogenic signals delivered in the form of serine/threonine phosphorylation. Phosphorylation may directly alter their ability to bind DNA (e.g., myb[24]) or activate transcription (e.g., CREB[25] and c-myc[17]). Alternatively, phosphorylation may indirectly activate a transcription factor by inactivating its inhibitor (e.g., phosphorylation of the inhibitor IκB leads to activation of NF-κB[26]). Dephosphorylation of some residues may be coupled with phosphorylation of others to enhance the activity of certain transcription factors. Mitogen stimulation results in c-jun undergoing dephosphorylation of serine and threonine residues near its DNA-binding domain and increased phosphorylation of residues in its transactivation domain; the former enhances its ability to bind DNA,[27] while the latter enhances its transactivation function.[16] These examples demonstrate that protein phosphorylation and dephosphorylation can rapidly alter the transcriptional program of mitogen-stimulated cells independently of any new mRNA or protein synthesis. These initial post-translational changes lead to the rapid induction of transcription of genes like c-fos and c-myc. Expression of these so-called early response genes[28] occurs well before the induction of genes directly involved in DNA biosynthesis and adds to the transcriptional reprogramming that eventually enables cells to undergo DNA synthesis and later events in the cell cycle. Not surprisingly, some of the transcription factors at the end of the mitogenic signaling pathway, such as c-myc, c-fos, and c-jun, have oncogenic potential when inappropriately activated.

THE CELL CYCLE

A cell stimulated to divide may be viewed as passing through a cyclic series of states, defined by biochemical and morphologic criteria, collectively termed the cell cycle (Fig. 7-2). Passage through the cell cycle provides for an ordered and orderly sequence to the complex series of events necessary for the production of two identical progeny cells. The normal cell cycle is divided into discrete and sequential phases, S, G$_2$, M, and G$_1$.

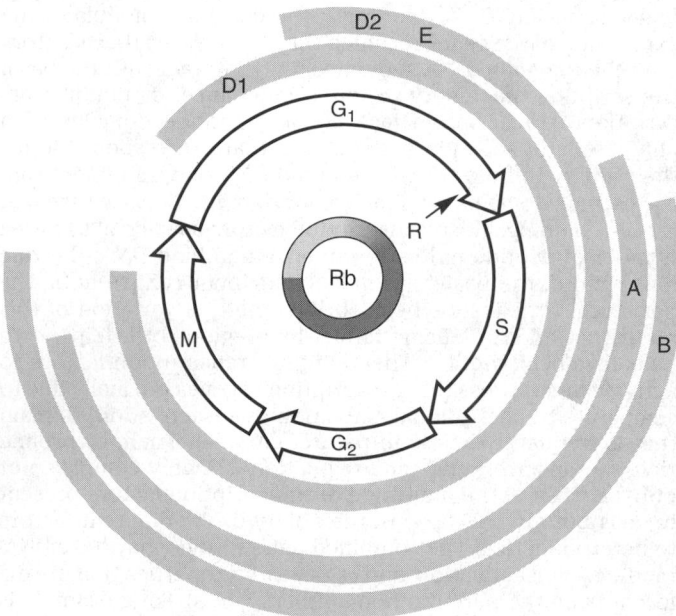

Fig. 7-2. The cell cycle. The somatic cell cycle is divided into phases of DNA replication (S), mitosis (M), and the "gaps" in between (G_1 between M and S; G_2 between S and M). G_0 is not shown for the sake of simplicity but would be a side loop exiting and entering G_1. The point in late G_1 at which cells become committed to DNA replication is called the restriction point (R). The inner circle shows the pattern of Rb phosphorylation through the cell cycle, with the density of stippling indicating the degree of RB phosphorylation. Places in the cell cycle where individual cyclins (A, B, D1, D2, E) appear are shown by the outer arcs.

S Phase

S phase is the period of wholesale DNA synthesis during which the cell replicates its genetic content[29]; a normal, diploid, somatic cell with a 2N complement of DNA at the beginning of S phase acquires a 4N complement of DNA at its end. The duration of S phase may be highly variable. It may last only a few minutes in rapidly dividing, early embryonic cells but usually lasts a few hours in most somatic cells. Early embryonic cells generally "live off" the accumulated stores of maternal RNAs and proteins present in the egg and are transcriptionally silent. Cells in later development and mature organisms must actively transcribe subsets of their genes to survive and maintain specialized functions. The "extra" time it takes for the latter to complete S phase is probably needed to coordinate DNA replication with transcription and to preserve higher order structural information influencing gene expression during DNA replication.

M Phase

M phase, or mitosis, is the period of actual nuclear and cell division during which the duplicated chromosomes are divided equally between the two daughter cells.[30] Mitosis is obvious microscopically as the period of chromosome condensation, nuclear envelope breakdown, chromosome segregation to opposite poles, reformation of nuclear envelopes (which completes nuclear division, or karyokinesis), and physical separation of the two daughter cells (which completes cell division, or cytokinesis). A cell entering the M phase has a 4N DNA content and finishes as two cells, each with an identical 2N complement of DNA.

G_1 and G_2 Phases

G_1 and G_2 phases were originally conceived of as "gaps" between the distinctive M and S phases of the cell cycle. The molecular characteristics of both "gaps" have been difficult to define but are beginning to be revealed. G_2 is the period between S and M, when cells have finished replicating their DNA, are preparing to divide, and have a 4N DNA content. For any given cell type, the duration of G_2 is generally fixed, and, except under special circumstances, is "automatic" (i.e., cells entering S almost always complete G_2 and M). Its duration can be extremely short, so that G_2 is essentially undetectable in rapidly proliferating, early embryonic cells. G_1, which occupies the period between M and S, is the most variable in duration and can be prolonged. As might be expected of the period between completion of one round of cell division and initiation of the next, its duration depends on the cell type and is regulated by environmental factors such as the availability of growth factors and essential nutrients. It is the period of cell growth. Usually, a certain increase in cell mass is required before the cell initiates the next round of cell division. As a first approximation, the amount of time a cell spends in G_1 is inversely related to its rate of proliferation. When conditions are unsuitable for proliferation, cells arrest in G_1. Those that are already in S, G_2, or M usually complete the cell cycle to which they have been committed and arrest only when they reach G_1 again. On the other hand, when rapid cell proliferation is mandated, as in embryos shortly after fertilization, there is no detectable G_1 phase and no growth. This results in the original mass of egg cytoplasm being partitioned among thousands of cells within a few hours.

G_1 has been subdivided into segments and regulatory points largely based on the study of the proliferative response of cells to sequential application of different growth factors, nutrients, and metabolic inhibitors.[31] One of the most significant of these is a point in G_1, near the G_1-S boundary, when cells become committed to entering S phase. Called the restriction point or R in cells from higher organisms, this is a point beyond which growth factor stimulation and essential amino acids are no longer needed for cells to enter S and may be analogous to the cell division commitment point in the yeast cell cycle called Start. R is obviously a particularly important point in the cell cycle from the standpoint of regulation.

G_0 Phase

Viable cells may remain for prolonged periods in a nonproliferative G_0 state.[31] Such cells have a 2N DNA content and may be difficult to distinguish from cells in prolonged G_1. The distinction, if not obvious morphologically, may be made biochemically, since cells in G_1 and G_0 exhibit differences in their protein and RNA metabolism. Terminally differentiated cells, such as neutrophilic granulocytes, have irreversibly exited the cell cycle during the process of differentiation, and are examples of cells in G_0. However, other cells reversibly enter G_0 and may be induced to return to G_1 and begin cycling with appropriate stimuli. For example, hepatocytes are usually in G_0 unless partial hepatectomy induces them to proliferate to reconstitute the functional mass of the liver. Resting, antigen-specific lymphocytes are in G_0 until antigen and cytokine stimulation induces them to proliferate.

The enforced sequence, G_1-S-G_2-M, during normal progression through the cell cycle means that a cell must duplicate its DNA before dividing and that it must divide before duplicating its DNA again. This sequence ensures euploidy, and its enforcement maintains genetic stability. The dependence of later events in the cell cycle upon completion of earlier events is ensured by control mechanisms, called checkpoints; they prevent a cell that has not successfully completed one phase of the cycle from entering the next.[32] The existence and importance of checkpoints is illustrated by yeast mutants defective in the *RAD9* gene.[33] Normally, yeasts cannot enter M until their DNA is fully replicated. Yeasts defective in the *RAD9* gene enter M even if they are prevented from completing DNA replication. They also die more rapidly, presumably because the progeny inherit incomplete or damaged genetic material. In mammalian cells, the activity of checkpoints is seen after exposure to DNA-damaging agents, such as ionizing radiation, which delay their entry into S and M by inducing temporary G_1 or G_2 arrest.[32] This delay probably allows the cells time to repair damaged DNA and prevents its replication and segregation, which would propagate the errors introduced. Caffeine antagonizes the G_2/M checkpoint mechanism, and cells that are exposed to caffeine fail to arrest in G_2 and are less viable following irradiation.[34] The tumor suppressor protein p53 participates in the G_1/S checkpoint mechanism, and cells with mutant or absent p53 function fail to arrest in G_1 following irradiation or other genotoxic insults.[35–37] Consequences of absent or aberrant p53 activity include genomic instability and, over a broader time framework, predisposition to tumors.

REGULATION OF CELL CYCLE PROGRESSION

The molecular mechanisms regulating progression of cells through the cell cycle are beginning to be defined. Currently, there is a coherent but incomplete picture of the control of cell entry into M. The control of cell entry into S is less clear. What has emerged from these studies is that serine/threonine kinases of the cell division cycle/cyclin dependent kinase (cdc/cdk) family drive cell cycle events. However, like catalytic subunits of enzyme complexes, their activities are under the stringent control of associated, noncatalytic proteins called cyclins that function as regulatory subunits. Cyclins are so named because they (cyclins A and B) were first described as proteins in marine invertebrate cells whose levels fluctuated periodically with the cell cycle.[38] Numerous cdc/cdk kinases and cyclins in the cell form various combinatorial pairs with distinct activities. Control of their activities occurs by the appearance and disappearance of the different cyclins at specific phases of the cell cycle (Figs. 7-2 and 7-3). It also occurs by post-translational modification of the subunits of the kinase/cyclin complex. Finally, these complexes associate with other cellular proteins that may modify or direct their activities.

Entry into M

The molecular mechanisms regulating cell entry into M were first revealed by studies of a conditional cell cycle mutant of *Schizosaccharomyces pombe* (fission yeasts) called *cdc2* (cell division cycle 2). Grown under nonpermissive conditions, these mutants arrest in G_1 or G_2 and do not enter S or M.[39] Cloning of the *cdc2* gene revealed that it encodes a 34-kd protein ($p34^{cdc2}$) with serine/threonine kinase activity.[40] Human cells were subsequently found to have a structurally and functionally similar protein.[41] Conservation between such phylogenetically separate organisms as yeast and human speaks to the preservation of this regulatory mechanism through evolution. An independent line of study examining the effect of microinjected cytoplasmic extracts from mature *Xenopus* frog eggs into immature frog oocytes showed that these extracts contain a material that induces oocytes to mature and undergo typical M phase changes such as nuclear membrane breakdown. After purification, the maturation-promoting factor (MPF) in these extracts was found to contain two proteins. One was identified as frog $p34^{cdc2}$,[42] and the other was identified as a B-type cyclin.[43] Cyclin B has no known enzymatic function and plays a regulatory role in the MPF complex, since $p34^{cdc2}$ exhibits kinase/MPF activity only in association with cyclin B.

Cyclin B levels gradually increase during S and G_2 (Fig. 7-2), and levels of the $p34^{cdc2}$/cyclin B complex sufficient for the G_2/M transition are reached well before the actual onset of M. Mitosis is not prematurely triggered, because the complex accumulates in an inactive form and only becomes activated just prior to the onset of M[44] (Fig. 7-3). During S and G_2, the $p34^{cdc2}$ complexed with cyclin B accumulates as a multiply phosphorylated protein. In human $p34^{cdc2}$, phosphorylation of Thr 161 stabilizes its association with cyclin B, and phosphorylation of Thr 14 and Tyr 15 suppresses its kinase activity. Thus, the $p34^{cdc2}$/cyclin B complex accumulates in an inactive form due to kinases that phosphorylate Thr 14 and Tyr 15. Phosphorylation of Tyr 15 appears to be accomplished by a human tyrosine kinase that is homologous to the product of the *S. pombe wee1* gene,[45] but the kinase responsible for Thr 14 phosphorylation is yet to be identified. Activation of $p34^{cdc2}$ prior to entry into M requires dephophorylation of both Thr 14 and Tyr 15, which can be accomplished by a single phosphatase, the product of the human homolog of the *S. pombe cdc25* gene. The timing of cell entry into M, therefore, is controlled through the activity of this phosphatase. The kinase and phosphatase that regulate $p34^{cdc2}$/cyclin B activity are themselves regulated by phosphorylation. Phosphorylation inhibits the kinase responsible for Tyr 15 phosphorylation and enhances the phosphatase function of cdc25. Once activated, $p34^{cdc2}$/cyclin B can phosphorylate cdc25 and create a self-amplifying feedback loop that generates more oocyte MPF activity from a small initial amount of active MPF and the large pre-existing stock of inactive MPF.[46] What starts this sequence of events by initially phosphorylating cdc25 is unclear, although $p34^{cdc2}$ and cdk-cyclin A have been put forth as candidates, because they are active prior to $p34^{cdc2}$/cyclin B activation and have MPF activity, and inhibition of cyclin A during S prevents entry into M.

Activated $p34^{cdc2}$/cyclin B complex can phosphorylate serine/threonine residues in many cellular proteins. Discerning its physiologic substrates is difficult, however, because of the presence of many other cyclin/kinase complexes that have similar specificities. Candidates include the lamins and vimentin, which are, respectively, nuclear and cytoplasmic proteins important for the structural organization of their compartments. These proteins undergo M-phase phosphorylation and can be shown to be in vitro kinase substrates for $p34^{cdc2}$/cyclin B. Phosphorylation of lamins is important for nuclear lamina disassembly and envelope breakdown,[47,48] and phosphorylation of vimentin may cause depolymerization of vimentin intermediate filaments.[49] If these are physiologic substrates, $p34^{cdc2}$/cyclin B kinase activity may initiate the structural reorganization that is essential for mitosis. As M-phase progresses, $p34^{cdc2}$/cyclin B is inactivated by degradation of the cyclin B component via the ubiquitin pathway.[50] Inactivation of this complex appears to be essential for cells to exit M, since a recombinant cyclin B that is resistant to proteolysis causes cells to arrest in M.[51]

Entry into S

The rate of cell proliferation in somatic cells is generally determined by events in G_1, with the "irreversible" decision to undergo DNA replication made at R, a commitment point about 2 hours before S phase begins.[31] The importance of the decisions made in G_1 and their relevance to neoplastic cell behavior have made the identification of regulatory factors involved in G_1 and the G_1-S transition a prime objective. In *S. pombe*, the

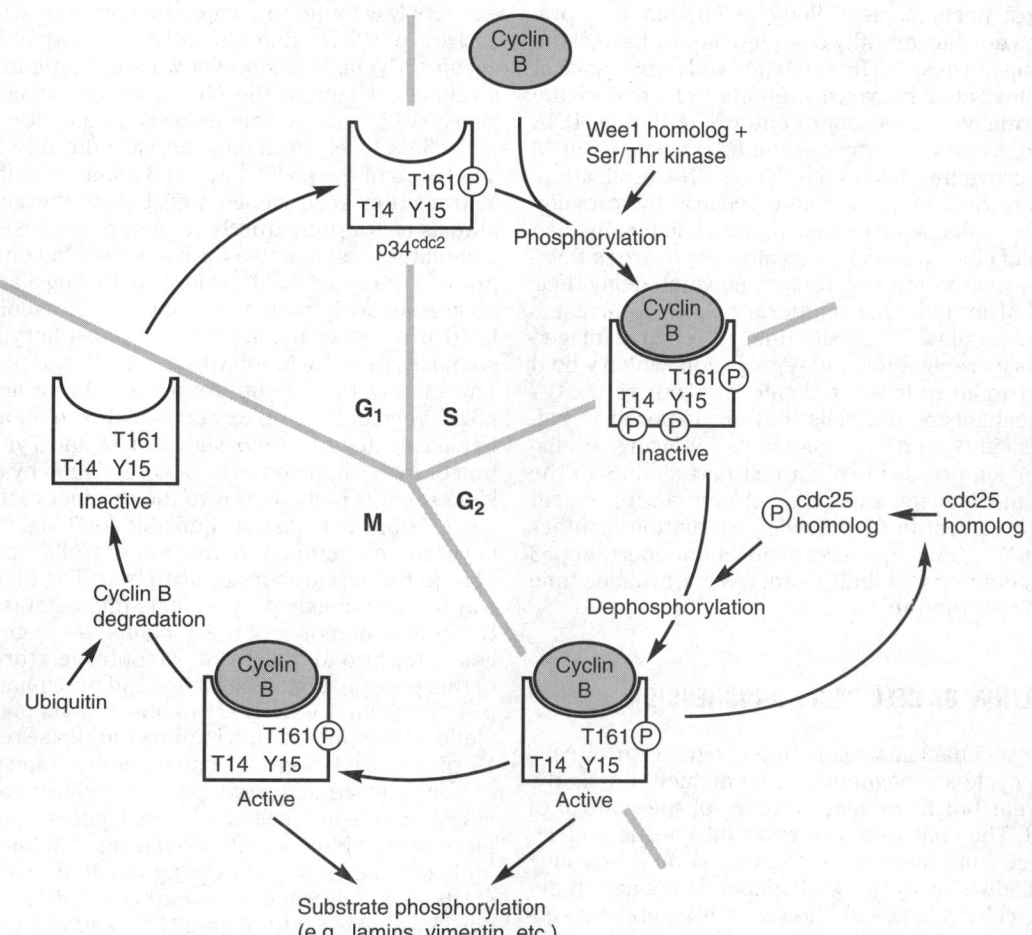

Fig. 7-3. Regulation of cell entry into M by p34^{cdc2}/cyclin B (maturation promoting factor [MPF]). p34^{cdc2} kinase activity controls cell entry into M and is regulated during the cell cycle. Association with cyclin B, which first appears during S phase is necessary for its kinase activity, and formation of the p34^{cdc2}/cyclin B complex (MPF) is stabilized by phosphorylation of Thr (T) 161. Accumulating MPF is maintained in an inactive state by phosphorylation of Thr 14 and Tyr (Y) 15, which is catalyzed by the homolog of the *S. pombe wee1* gene product and another kinase. At the G$_2$/M transition, MPF is activated by dephosphorylation of Thr 14 and Tyr 15 by the homolog of the *S. pombe cdc25* gene product. This may be a self-amplifying reaction, because activated MPF can phosphorylate and activate more cdc25. Activated MPF phosphorylates cellular substrates and brings about the biochemical changes needed for M phase. During progression through M, degradation of cyclin B generates inactive p34^{cdc2} and permits cell exit from M.

kinase produced by the *cdc2* gene is responsible for both the G$_1$-S and G$_2$-M transitions. In higher organisms, additional p34^{cdc2}-related kinases (cdks) have been identified and are candidates for involvement in G$_1$ regulation.[52,53] These cdks have been labeled cdk2, cdk3, cdk4 and cdk5, with cdk1 reserved for p34^{cdc2}. Except for p34^{cdc2}, which has a clear role in G$_2$ and M and appears unnecessary for G$_1$ and S phase events in higher organisms, their specific functions in cell cycle regulation are yet to be defined. Some, like cdk2, will certainly play important roles in G$_1$ and S phase events.[54] Their activities are probably regulated by the cyclins with which they are paired, and studies indicate that most cdks bind to a restricted number of cyclins. The permitted partnerships are likely to determine where and how in the cell cycle the individual cdks function.

The appearance of cyclins A and B during S and their disappearance during M (Fig. 7-2) preclude a role for them in G$_1$ and imply that other regulatory components are active in G$_1$ and the G$_1$-S transition. Here, as before, yeast mutants have helped to identify the proteins involved. *S. cerevisiae* (budding yeast) deficient in three G$_1$ cyclin genes *(CLN1–3)* were used to clone human genes encoding putative G$_1$ cyclins by functional complementation.[55–57] The human cyclin genes (C, D, and E) cloned by this approach cannot be assumed to encode G$_1$ cyclins on

this basis alone, because human cyclin B is also capable of rescuing the deficient yeast. D-type cyclin genes were independently identified by two other groups, one searching for an oncogene involved in parathyroid adenomas[58] and the other for genes induced during mitogenic stimulation of macrophages.[59] Currently, in addition to cyclins A and B (B1 and B2), cyclins C, D, (D1, D2, and D3) and E have been identified. Available information about cyclins D, E, and A indicate that they play important roles in G$_1$, the G$_1$-S transition, and S.

D-type cyclins appear to be important regulators of G$_1$ events, but generalizations are difficult because there are multiple family members (D1, D2, D3) with distinctive characteristics and differential expression in various cell types. In mitogen-stimulated cells, cyclin D1 expression is rapidly induced and maintained through the cell cycle; cyclin D2 expression rises later in G$_1$, peaks near the G$_1$-S boundary, and declines through S[59] (Fig. 7-2). Cyclins D1 and D3 can associate with Cdk2, -4, and -5 and other proteins, including proliferating cell nuclear antigen (PCNA), which is a cofactor necessary for DNA replication.[60] The D-type cyclins can also bind Rb, the product of the retinoblastoma susceptibility gene *(Rb)*, and the Rb-like protein, p107, via a peptide motif (Leu-X-Cys-X-Glu) that they share with Rb-binding viral oncoproteins like simian virus 40

(SV40) T antigen and adenovirus E1A. These data, combined with the observations that inhibition of cyclin D1 expression prevents cell entry into S[61] and that cyclins D1 and D2 can reverse the G_1 growth arrest induced by Rb in SaOS-2 cells,[62–64] suggest that D-type cyclins are important for G_1 progression. A regulatory rather than a "mechanical" role in G_1 is suggested by the fact that cyclin D1 is implicated as an oncoprotein in certain parathyroid adenomas, B-cell lymphomas, and various other tumors in which its gene becomes translocated or amplified.[65]

The relationship of the different D-type cyclins to Rb is potentially revealing. Rb is a "tumor suppressor" gene product whose absence or inactivation is associated with retinoblastoma and some other tumors. Rb hyperphosphorylation in late G_1 is a critical event for cell entry into S. Cyclin D2 efficiently directs Rb phosphorylation by cdk2, while cyclin D1 is less effective. This parallels their respective ability to reverse the growth-arrest phenotype induced by hypophosphorylated Rb in SaOS-2 cells. A cyclin D2 that has been mutated in its Rb-binding motif and binds Rb poorly is much less effective at inducing Rb phosphorylation and reversing the Rb-induced growth arrest,[63] while a similarly mutated cyclin D1 that binds Rb poorly is more effective at reversing Rb-induced growth arrest.[64] The contrasting behavior of these mutants indicates that the functional interaction of cyclin D1 and D2 with Rb is different. One interpretation is that cyclin D2 is an upstream regulator of Rb that binds Rb and targets it for phosphorylation and functional inactivation, leading to cell cycling; a mutant that cannot target Rb will not promote cell cycling. Cyclin D1, on the other hand, may be regulated by Rb. If Rb is an upstream regulator of cyclin D1 activity, a mutant that cannot be bound or regulated by Rb but is otherwise functional will exhibit enhanced activity.[64]

Cyclin E may play an important role in G_1 and the G_1/S transition. In mitogen-stimulated cells, it appears later in G_1, peaks near the G_1-S boundary, and declines in S, having kinetics that resemble that of cyclin D2 (Fig. 7-2). The predominant cyclin E-associated kinase in cells is cdk2 and, in cells in G_1, cyclin E is found in a quarternary complex with p107, transcription factor E2F, and cdk2.[66,67] This complex disappears as cells enter S, just as a similar complex containing cyclin A instead of E makes its appearance[68] (Fig. 7-4). Given the role that E2F is suspected to play in activating genes required for S phase (see below), the cyclin E and E2F-containing complex may activate genes important in the G_1-S transition. Cyclin E efficiently induces hyperphosphorylation of Rb and counters the G_1 growth arrest induced by hypophosphorylated Rb in SaOS-2 cells,[62] which also supports a role for cyclin E in G_1 or the G_1-S transition. Enforced overexpression of cyclin E shortens the length of G_1, decreases cell size, and reduces the serum requirement for cell entry into S. However, cell proliferation remains serum dependent, and the cells are not transformed. This could mean that cyclin E is part of a G_1 timing mechanism that coordinates cell entry into S with G_1 events and milestones.[69]

The primary role played by cyclin A may be in S phase. It first appears at the beginning of S, increases during S, and declines in G_2 and M; its rise and fall parallels but precedes that of cyclin B (Fig. 7-2). Cyclin A may associate with either $p32^{cdc2}$ or cdk2[70] and, in S phase, is found in a quarternary complex with cdk2, E2F, and p107.[68,71] Injection of anticyclin A antibodies or plasmids encoding antisense cyclin A cDNA into cells in G_1 inhibits DNA synthesis.[70,72] Furthermore, a cell-free extract made from cells in G_1 can replicate SV40 DNA only if an extract made from S-phase cells is added; the S-phase extract contains cyclin A, and addition of cyclin A is sufficient to allow the G_1 extract to start DNA replication.[73] On this basis, cyclin A has been suggested to play a major role in driving S phase events.

TRANSCRIPTIONAL REGULATION AND THE CELL CYCLE

Cells proliferate only when they express all genes necessary for cell proliferation coordinately. Proliferating cells must, therefore, orchestrate the timely expression of all these genes, beginning with their appropriately modulated transcription. Since the necessary genes are many, including those of cyclins, DNA polymerases, accessory factors for DNA replication and purine/pyrimidine biosynthesis enzymes, just to name the most obvious, the orchestration mechanism must be highly sophisticated. Investigations into the function and properties of the Rb protein have provided hints as to how this might occur. Rb is the product of the retinoblastoma susceptibility gene *Rb*, which predisposes individuals to retinoblastomas and other tumors when only one functional copy is present in the germline.[74–76] *Rb* is a tumor suppressor gene, and somatic cells of certain lineages (e.g., retinoblasts) become neoplastic when both copies are functionally inactivated. Normally, *Rb* is ubiquitously expressed, and expression is invariant through the cell cycle. This is reconciled with the antiproliferative effects of Rb by the cyclical regulation of Rb activity by phosphorylation[77] (Fig. 7-4). Rb is hypophosphorylated in early G_1. During G_1 progression and especially near the G_1-S transition, Rb acquires more phosphoserine and phosphothreonine residues and becomes hyperphosphorylated. This persists until M, at which time Rb is dephosphorylated and returned to its hypophosphorylated, early G_1 state.[78–80] The discovery that various viral oncoproteins (adenovirus E1A, SV40 large T antigen, human papillomavirus E7) that force cell cycling also bind hypophosphorylated Rb suggests that the latter is antagonistic to cell cycling and that either Rb phosphorylation or binding by these oncoproteins abrogates this effect.[81–84]

The identification of a cellular factor, E2F, that complexes with Rb suggests how hypophosphorylated Rb might modulate gene transcription and cell cycle progression.[85] E2F was originally described as a cellular factor necessary for adenovirus E2 gene transcription. Found in complex with other cellular proteins and mostly unavailable for adenoviral use, E2F can be released from these complexes and made available by the viral E1A protein. The discovery that E1A binds Rb suggested that Rb might be one of the cellular proteins sequestering E2F. It has now been shown that hypophosphorylated Rb is indeed an E2F binding protein and that either Rb phosphorylation or binding to E1A disrupts this interaction (Fig. 7-4). Thus, E2F provides a link between cyclical Rb phosphorylation and the transcription of cellular genes. Since E2F probably activates expression of genes essential for DNA synthesis, such as dihydrofolate reductase and thymidine kinase, it links the cell cycle mechanism to the production of proteins necessary for cell cycle progression. In this model, E2F is complexed to Rb in G_1 cells and is unavailable for transcriptional duties. When Rb becomes hyperphosphorylated near the G_1-S boundary, E2F is released, becomes an active transcription factor, and induces expression of genes needed for S phase. In cells in which Rb is absent or inactive because of homozygous deletion or mutation (as in retinoblastoma cells), there is an abundance of free and transcriptionally active E2F, which leads to deregulated expression of cell cycle-regulated genes and cell proliferation. In cells infected with adenovirus, a functionally equivalent effect is achieved through E1A binding of hypophosphorylated Rb. It may be a simplification to consider the Rb-E2F complex transcriptionally inert, because Rb binding to E2F may convert this transcription factor from a positive to an actively negative regulator.[86] Furthermore, Rb may associate with transcription factors other than E2F and may activate expression of certain genes, such as those encoding transforming growth factor-β (TGF-β).[87] Since TGB-β is a negative growth regulator, activa-

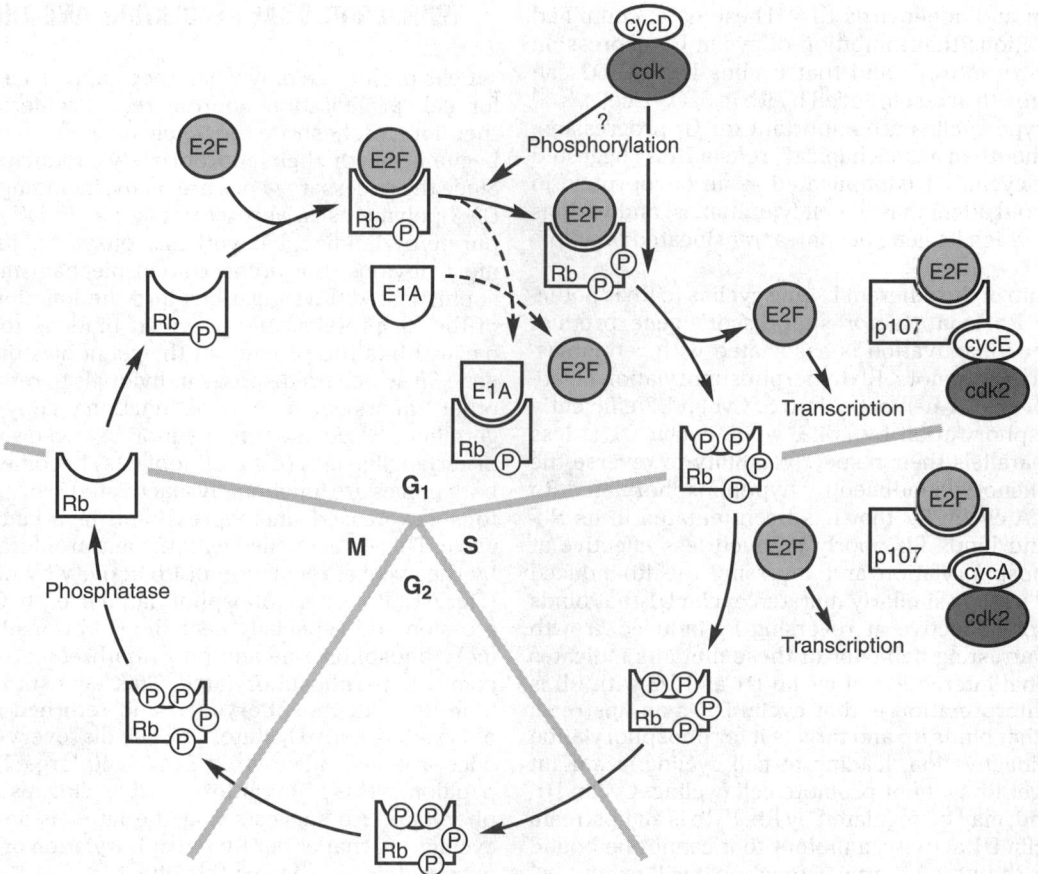

Fig. 7-4. Regulation of the retinoblastoma susceptibility gene product (Rb) through the cell cycle. Rb is regulated by serine/threonine phosphorylation (P) through the cell cycle. Non- or hypophosphorylated Rb present in early and mid-G_1 can bind transcription factor E2F and thereby alter or sequester its activity. In late G_1, Rb becomes hyperphosphorylated (perhaps due to cdk/cyclin D kinase activity), releasing E2F for transcriptional duties or formation of other complexes. Removal of phosphate groups in M restores Rb to its hypophosphorylated form. In cells transformed by adenovirus E1A, SV40 large T, or HPV E7, these oncoproteins can bind hypophosphorylated RB and displace E2F (dashed lines). The Rb-like p107 protein also binds E2F and is found in quarternary complexes with cdk2-cyclin E in G_1 or with cdk2-cyclin A in S phase.

tion of its expression is consonant with the other cellular effects of Rb.

These data are consistent with the view that Rb functions as an integral part of the cell cycling machinery that drives cells to enter S through phosphorylation-controlled interactions with factors such as E2F. Alternatively, Rb may function more as a modulator of the cycling mechanism that allows cells to stop proliferating. In this view, cyclical Rb phosphorylation-dephosphorylation permits the basic cell cycle machinery to drive proliferation, but maintenance in its dephosphorylated state is a way for differentiation and growth-inhibitory signals to induce cells to arrest in G_1 and allow initiation of differentiation pathways.[88] That Rb functions as a cell type-specific initiator of differentiation is supported by results obtained with mouse embryos that have both copies of *Rb* deleted. These embryos arise from matings of heterozygous *Rb*− mice and appear in expected numbers up to day 13 of gestation. However, they fail to develop beyond day 15 and display abnormal central nervous system development and erythropoiesis with the appearance of immature, nucleated erythrocytes.[89–91] That these embryos develop more than halfway through gestation and appear grossly normal argues against a central role in driving cell proliferation for Rb. On the other hand, the failure of nervous system and erythroid development in these embryos favors a role in enforcing terminal differentiation of these tissues for Rb. If not Rb, what is (are) the central molecular specie(s) driving the cell cycle? The answer is not known, but the

Rb-like p107 protein is a potential candidate. p107 is found in complex with E2F, cyclin E, and cdk2 in G_1 and with E2F, cyclin A, and cdk2 in S and has the properties expected of a core participant.[68] These quarternary complexes may sequester E2F activity, but since they have both the DNA binding properties of E2F and the kinase function of cdk2, they may have important additional properties, such as the ability to target kinase activity to proteins bound near E2F DNA binding sites.[85]

p53 AND CELL CYCLE CHECKPOINTS

The ability of somatic cells to respond to genotoxic insults by pausing temporarily in the G_1 or G_2 phases of the cell cycle is believed to be a protective mechanism that allows the cells time to repair damaged DNA before it becomes established in the genome by DNA replication or cell division.[32] Recently, the p53 tumor suppressor gene has been found to be important for the G_1 checkpoint activated by both chemical agents and ionizing radiation. Originally described as a 53-kd cellular protein that is overexpressed in a wide variety of transformed cells, p53 was believed to be an oncoprotein, because p53 genes cloned from nontumorigenic cell lines could immortalize and help transform primary rodent embryo cells. Subsequently, mutations were found in these p53 genes, and normal p53 was found to suppress rather than promote cell transformation.[92] The results of many studies have contributed to the current view that normal p53 is a tumor suppressor gene with a negative effect on cell proliferation, stopping cells at the G_1/ S transition, and that some mutant p53 genes exert a "dominant negative" effect and transform cells by inhibiting the activities of the normal gene.[93] That p53 is the most frequently deleted or mutated gene in human tumors and that certain kindreds prone to developing cancer (Li-Fraumeni syndrome) are heterozygous for mutated p53 in their germline[94,95] attests to its importance in malignant transformation. At a biochemical level, p53 is a sequence-specific DNA binding protein with transcriptional activation properties.[96] Mutant p53 from tumor cells lose this ability to bind DNA and fail to activate transcription.[97] p53 associates with a variety of other cellular (hsc70, $p34^{cdc2}$, casein kinase II, mdm2, and so forth) and viral (large T antigen, adenovirus E1B, and HPV E6) proteins, and these associations are presumed to alter some of p53s activities. For example, the mdm2 protein complexes with p53 and inhibits its ability to transactivate a responsive promoter.[98] (The *mdm-2* gene is amplified in a transformed murine cell line, and overexpression enhances the tumorigenic potential of cells.)

A gene that plays so prominent a role in oncogenesis might be expected to perform crucial cellular functions and be indispensible for normal development. It was a surprising finding, therefore, that mice with homozygous deletions of p53 developed normally and were abnormal only in being prone to developing spontaneous tumors.[99] How p53 prevents tumorigenesis but is not essential for normal growth and development may be explained by its role in the G_1 checkpoint mechanism. Such a role for p53 is suggested by studies of the cellular response to PALA, a drug that inhibits uridine biosynthesis, and to γ-irradiation. PALA is toxic to cells, but cellular resistance can develop through amplification of the *CAD* gene. Cells with normal p53 exposed to PALA arrest their growth in G_1, do not amplify *CAD,* and rarely develop resistance; by contrast, cells lacking normal p53 continue to proliferate when exposed to PALA and amplify *CAD.* These studies suggest that normal p53 is important for activation of the PALA-induced G_1 checkpoint and that this checkpoint inhibits the acquisition of genetic anomalies.[36,37] In normal cells, ionizing radiation induces p53 expression and delays in the G_1 and G_2 phases of the cell cycle.[35] Cells with mutant or absent p53 fail to arrest in G_1 (but do arrest in G_2) after irradiation. Transfection of a normal p53 into these cells partly restores the G_1 arrest, and overexpression of a dominant negative p53 mutant in cells with normal p53 abrogates the G_1 arrest. Thus, p53 is necessary to activate the radiation-induced G_1 checkpoint but not the G_2 checkpoint.[100] These studies indicate that p53 is an essential component of the mechanism that conditionally inhibits cell cycling in G_1 after genotoxic insults and whose activity limits the transmission of genetic changes following DNA damage. This mechanism should not operate under "normal" circumstances, and its absence might not cause developmental or growth abnormalities. However, over time, the absence of this mechanism would result in accumulation of somatic mutations that ultimately result in cell transformation. From the known properties of normal p53, it presumably affects transcription of certain cellular genes important for arresting cells at the G_1/S transition. A candidate target for p53 action is the growth arrest and DNA damage-inducible (*GADD45*) gene, which is induced by γ-radiation only if normal p53 is present and induced. A conserved sequence element in the *GADD45* gene is bound by normal but not mutant p53, and a nuclear factor that binds this element following irradiation contains p53.[100] More recently *CIP1/WAF1* was identified as a gene that produces a 21-kd protein that is a tight-binding inhibitor of cdks and cell cycle progression.[101] Its expression is induced by normal but not mutant p53 through an upstream enhancer sequence that contains a p53 consensus-binding site.[102]

CONTROL OF CELL DIFFERENTIATION

Cell proliferation stocks an organism with the necessary number of cells to allow growth and to compensate for cell loss, but differentiation is the process by which these cells become endowed with necessary specialized functions. Each year an average adult man or woman produces about 3–4 body weight equivalents (200–300 kg) of blood cells to maintain the steady-state numbers of cells in the circulation. Such a high cellular turnover suggests that the control of hematopoietic cell proliferation and differentiation must be tightly regulated. Otherwise a slight increase in proliferation rate could result in leukemia or hyperviscosity. By contrast, a tip of the balance in the opposite direction could lead to severe cytopenias.

The lineage-specific pathways of hematopoiesis have provided a paradigm for the study of cell differentiation. However, the molecular switches that determine lineage-specific cell differentiation remain incompletely understood. Nevertheless, limited insights into the molecular basis of cell differentiation have been gained through the study of various model cell culture systems. For example, conceptual paradigms on the transcriptional regulation of cell differentiation have been generated from the study of myogenesis and adipocytogenesis.

Adipogenic Differentiation Model

The tissue culture model for differentiation of 3T3-L1 fibroblastic preadipocytes into adipocytes (fat cells) exemplifies the interaction between extracellular factors and nuclear transcription factors in differentiation.[103] In this model, confluent 3T3-L1 cells are induced to differentiate by a cocktail that includes insulin and dexamethasone. The cells undergo several rounds of division, cease proliferating, and then acquire the biochemical and morphologic phenotype of differentiated adipocytes. Differentiation into adipocytes in culture is accompanied by the coordinate expression of adipocyte-specific genes. Characterization of the cis-acting regulatory elements within the promoters of adipocyte-specific genes has revealed sequences that are responsible for activating or derepressing transcription during differentiation.

Among the trans-acting factors that participate in the expression of adipocyte-specific genes, the transcription factor C/EBP has been extensively studied. C/EBP is the prototypic leucine zipper protein that binds a specific DNA sequence known as the CAAT box, which is found in promoters of adipocyte-specific genes. With induction of adipocyte differentiation, expression of C/EBPα precedes the transcription of adipocyte-specific genes.[103] Studies using antisense or enforced sense C/EBPα expression suggest that C/EBPα is necessary and sufficient for differentiation of 3T3-L1 into adipocytes. Other members of the C/EBP family of proteins are expressed at the time of differentiation induction by exogenous factors, but the levels of these C/EBPs decline after that. Although the exact roles of some C/EBPs and other transcription factors in the expression of the adipocyte phenotype remain unknown, C/EBPα appears to play a central role in the expression of adipocyte-specific genes. It is notable, however, that regulatory sequences far removed (in terms of number of DNA base pairs) from promoters of adipocyte-specific genes are required for tissue-specific expression. Thus, both proximal and far distal regulatory sequences may be required for expression of many tissue-specific genes.

The mechanisms of signal transduction from the extracellular differentiation-inducing agents to nuclear events remain to be established. This link, however, is begining to be understood through the study of promoter regions of genes that respond early to extracellular signals. For example, the promoter region of the *c/ebp* gene is found to contain an array of putative transcription factor binding sites, including those of c-myc, Krox 24, CUP, Sp1, and C/EBP itself.[104] The c-myc binding site is within a potentially repressing *cis* element within the *c/ebp* promoter. Enforced expression of c-myc in 3T3-L1 cells prevents the expression of C/EBPα and differentiation into adipocytes.[105] The c-*myc* gene expression pattern is an approximate mirror-image of the expression of *c/ebp* during adipocyte differentiation, suggesting that release from suppression by silencing cis elements may be a critical initiating event.

Myogenic Differentiation Model

The cell culture myogenesis model has also provided astounding insights into some molecular mechanisms of cell differentiation induction.[106] Early studies of myogenesis generated the idea that a single master gene may control muscle cell differentiation. Brief treatment of C3H 10T^1/$_2$ fibroblastic cells with 5-azacytidine induced the formation of many myogenic colonies and fewer numbers of chondrogenic and adipogenic colonies. Transfection experiments showed that genomic DNA from 5-azacytidine-induced myoblasts, but not DNA from parental cells, conferred the muscle phenotype to C3H 10T^1/$_2$ cells. A cDNA for the gene termed *myoD* was cloned by subtractive hybridization to identify mRNAs that were specifically expressed in myoblasts but not in parental C3H 10T^1/$_2$ cells. Transfection of *myoD* cDNA alone was sufficient for myogenic conversion of C3H 10T^1/$_2$ cells. myoD is a transcription factor that was subsequently shown to activate muscle-specific genes. As with the adipocyte differentiation model, overexpression of c-*myc* also inhibited myogenic differentiation, suggesting that signals for cell proliferation could override cues for differentiation.

myoD, a member of the HLH family of transcription factors, binds to consensus DNA sites that includes a CA–TG sequence present in most muscle-specific enhancers. myoD is also a member of a family of myogenic transcription regulators such as myogenin, myf-5, and myf6-mrf4-herculin that can confer muscle phenotype to C3H 10T^1/$_2$ cells. The myoD protein is comprised of a bHLH DNA-binding domain and an N-terminal transcriptional activation domain. myoD binds its target sites as homodimers but binds them more tightly when it is heterodimerized with ubiquitous bHLH E2A transcription factors. The association of myoD with E2A is regulated by a third factor that was sought because myoD protein is present in proliferating undifferentiated myoblasts. Indeed, the *Id* (inhibitor of differentiation) gene was cloned as a cDNA whose protein product was homologous to helix 2 of myoD. Id contains an HLH motif but lacks the DNA-binding basic region. It can form heterodimers with myoD or E2A proteins, but these dimers are unable to bind DNA. Transfection experiments have demonstrated that Id can inhibit the ability of myoD to trans-activate a muscle-specific gene and retard myogenic differentiation. The myogenic differentiation model led to the discoveries of myoD and Id which both participate in a network of protein-protein interactions that alters muscle-specific gene expression. It will become apparent in the subsequent discussions that these general paradigms hold true for myeloid maturation as well.

INTRODUCTION TO HEMATOPOIETIC DIFFERENTIATION

Hematopoiesis is a fascinating system in which pluripotent hematopoietic stem cells (PHSCs) differentiate into many highly specialized circulating blood cells.[107] The long-term repopulating PHSCs are capable of self-renewal as well as limited differentiation toward the common lymphoid stem cell or myeloid multipotent stem cell. Most PHSCs are believed to be dormant and stochastically awakened to enter the cell cycle. The common lymphoid stem cell differentiates into either mature T cells or B cells. The myeloid multipotent stem cell differentiates into a variety of circulating blood cells, including basophils, eosinophils, neutrophils, monocytes, erythrocytes, and megakaryocytes (platelets). The developmental program for each type of mature circulating cell consists of networks of cell-extracellular matrix, cell-cell, and cell-growth factor/lymphokine interactions. Some of these interactions are assuredly functional equivalents of molecular interactions revealed in the simple adipogenic or myogenic differentiation models outlined above.

It has been established experimentally that PHSCs can differentiate toward either lymphoid or common myeloid progenitor. Retroviral labeling of the genome to analyze the clonality of differentiated cells revealed that both myeloid and lymphoid cells arise from common pluripotent stem cells. The mechanisms determining the commitment of PHSCs to differentiate toward either lymphoid or myeloid progenitors remain unknown. It has been proposed that commitment to differentiate is a stochastic process based on paired daughter cell analysis. In these studies, daughter cells derived from a single parent progenitor cell frequently displayed varied combinations of cell lineages. Such observations have been construed to suggest that random activation of a group of differentiation genes might be required for single-lineage expression. This suggestion has precedence in the known random shuffling of immunoglobulin gene fragments through *V(D)J* rearrangements to generate antibody diversity. Clones of B cells are then expanded by specific antigens that select for specific antibody variable region structures arising from random *V(D)J* rearrangements. A stochastic model for hematopoietic cell differentiation has been proposed based on notions similar to those for generation of antibody diversity.

The stochastic model for commitment suggests that dormant PHSCs are recruited into the cell cycle by many lymphokines, including combinations of interleukin (IL)-1, IL-3, IL-4, IL-6, IL-11, IL-12, colony-stimulating factor-granulocyte (G-CSF), G-CSF/macrophage (M), and stem cell factor (Fig. 7-5). Although the molecular basis for synergisms between these factors remains unknown, certain functional and structural homologies among them are notable. For example, IL-6, IL-11, and leukemia inhibitory factor require cooperation with a signal-transducing protein gp130 for function.[108] Likewise, receptors for IL-3, IL-5, and GM-CSF share a common β-subunit that associates with unique factor-specific α-chains.[109] Once recruited into the cycling fraction of cells, PHSCs must survive and differentiate into a certain lineage of cells. It is hypothesized that the stochastic establishment of specific differentiation programs (perhaps by random expression of groups of differentiation genes) in PHSCs provides a population of partially committed cells that are poised to receive additional instructions. Intermediate stage-acting, lineage-nonspecific factors such as IL-3, GM-CSF, and IL-4 support the proliferation of the multipotential progenitors after they have been awakened from their dormant state.

Lineage-specific factors support the survival, proliferation, and maturation of progenitors that are committed through hypothetical stochastic expression of specific groups of differentiation genes. For example, M-CSF promotes the proliferation and differentiation of macrophage/monocytes. Erythropoietin (EPO) promotes the survival, proliferation, and differentiation of erythrocytes. IL-5 and G-CSF are thought to be specific for eosinophils and granulocytes, respectively. A late-acting lineage-specific factor for megakaryocytopoiesis remains to be identified. These late-acting lineage-specific factors could be viewed as factors that select out and promote the proliferation of subsets of committed cells whose differentiation programs have been randomly selected. The activation of groups of dif-

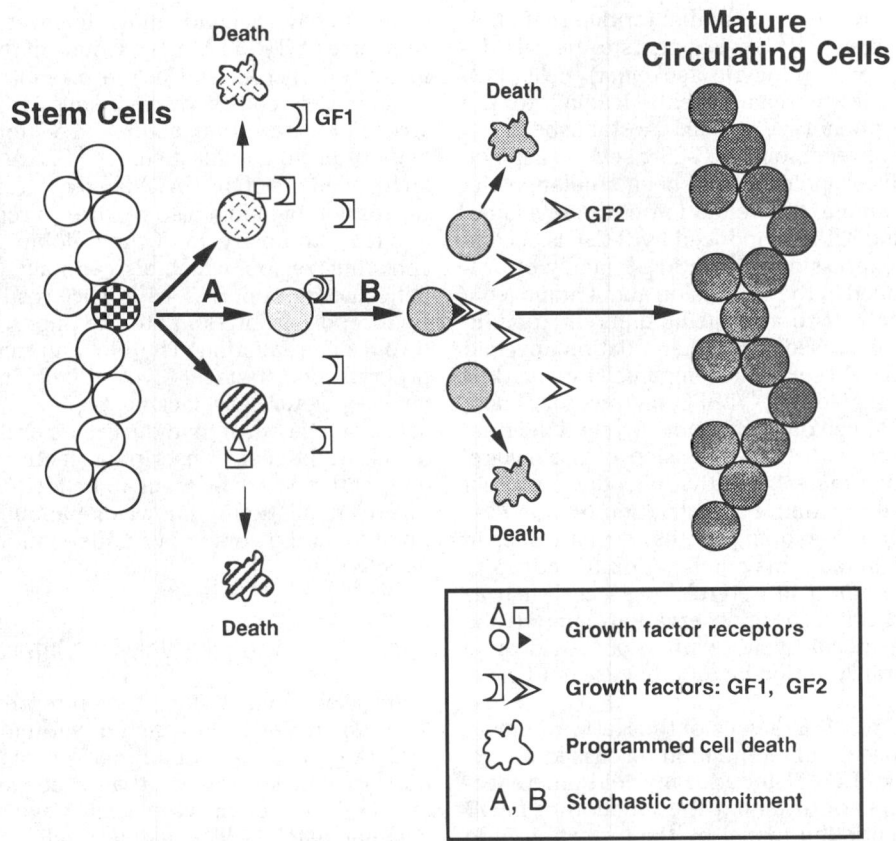

Fig. 7-5. Stochastic commitment model and selective survival in hematopoietic differentiation. Cells that are stochastically committed display specific growth factor receptor(s) and are selected for survival and proliferation by the cognate growth factor(s). Cells that bear receptors or genetic programs incompatible with the available growth factors are eliminated by programmed cell death. Sequential stochastic commitment and selective survival also contribute to differentiation of the committed cells to mature circulating cells.

ferentiation genes that are not supported by lineage-specific factors will hypothetically result in cell death (discussed at the end of this chapter).

Lymphoid Differentiation

The commitment of PHSCs to lymphohematopoietic progenitors is thought to be mediated in part by the lineage-nonspecific factors mentioned above. The mechanisms of early lymphoid development remain poorly understood. B-cell differentiation occurs in the bone marrow of adults where expression of the immunoglobulin heavy chain precedes that of the light chain. Completed immunoglobulin chains expressed on the surface lead to the surface-immunoglobulin-positive B lymphocytes that migrate to the peripheral lymphoid organs such as the spleen.[110]

Several molecular events that are critical for maturation of lymphoid cells have been identified. Study of Bruton X-linked agammaglobulinemia, which is a disorder of B-cell development, has localized the defect to a B-cell-specific cytoplasmic tyrosine kinase gene locus.[111] This tyrosine kinase, termed BPK, has classic tyrosine kinase SH2 and SH3 domains. Pre-B- or B-cell lines from X-linked agammaglobulinemia patients display reduced or absent *BPK* mRNA. Study of genetically engineered (knock-out) mice in which the recombination-mediating protein RAG1 or RAG2 (necessary for recombination events such as *V(D)J* recombination) is absent revealed that RAG1 and RAG2 are required for the normal maturation of lymphocytes.[112–114] In either case, the inability to initiate *V(D)J* recombination appears to cause maturation arrest.

Myelomonocytic Differentiation

The study of myeloid differentiation underscores our lack of understanding of early events in the commitment of PHSCs to the multipotent myeloid progenitor colony-forming unit-granulocyte/erythrocyte/monocyte/megakaryocyte (CFU-GEMM). CFUs specific for granulocytes (CFU-G) are thought to arise from a precursor common to granulocytes and monocytes (CFU-GM). The committed myeloid precursors (CFU-G) are presumably selected for and amplified by a myeloid-specific factor, G-CSF. The monocyte/macrophage lineage is selected by M-CSF (CSF-1) that stimulates growth and differentiation through the CSF-1 receptor (CSF-1R) encoded by the proto-oncogene c-*fms*.

CSF-1 exerts its effects by binding to a class of high-affinity receptor that is expressed predominantly on monocytes and macrophages.[115] The receptor CSF-1R is a member of the growth factor receptor group that displays ligand-induced tyrosine-specific protein kinase activity. Activation of CSF-1R triggers a cascade of events, many of which were described for the activation of EGF-R and PDGF-R, that convey signals from the plasma membrane to the cell nucleus. Dissection of CSF-1R by mutagenesis has led to the paradigm that a single plasma membrane receptor can give rise to separate nuclear transcription programs. Specifically, a point mutation in CSF-1R has been identified that results in the activation of the *fos* and *jun* proto-oncogenes, but not *myc,* by CSF-1.[116] This mutant receptor cannot trigger mitogenesis in transfected cultured cells unless complemented by a constitutively expressing *myc* allele. In separate studies of cell lines with the potential for differentiation into neutrophils or macrophages, the zinc finger transcription factor Egr-1 has been shown to be essential for differentiation along the macrophage lineage.[117] Egr-1 appears to restrict differentiation of HL-60 (promyelocytic leukemia) cells into macrophages. Farther downstream, events leading to the monocyte/macrophage phenotype remain unestablished.

With the availability of recombinant G-CSF, several cell culture models for granulocytopoiesis have been studied at the molecular level. For example, differentiation of the myelomonoblastic murine cell line 32D C13 induced by G-CSF is accompanied by differential expression of the C/EBP family of proteins previously mentioned in the discussion about adipogenic differentiation.[118] In contrast to adipogenic differentiation, in which C/EBPα protein increased with differentiation, myeloid differentiation of the 32D C13 cells is accompanied by a marked decrease in C/EBPα protein levels. C/EBPβ, on the other hand, is increased with 32D C13 cell differentiation. Myeloid differentiation is also associated with the expression of the *myb*-responsive myeloid-specific *mim-1* gene that encodes a protein with an as yet unknown function. Full activation of *mim-1* requires both myb and C/EBPβ binding to their cognate sites in the *mim-1* promoter.[119] In fact, this combination of activators is sufficient to activate *mim-1* in heterologous cells such as fibroblasts or erythroid cells. These observations support the hypothesis that tissue-specific gene expression could arise from combinations of transcription factors that are not tissue-specific.

Enforced expression in 32D C13 cells of the HLH protein Id, which inhibits the myogenic differentiation discussed above, has resulted in the lack of G-CSF-induced myeloid differentiation.[120] Although Id appears to inhibit the function of myoD in the myogenic differentiation model by the formation of Id heterodimers that could not bind DNA, the molecular target of Id inhibition in 32D C13 myelomonoblastic cells has not been identified. It is possible that a myeloid-specific bHLH protein might participate in myeloid differentiation. Recent studies on the myeloperoxidase gene promoter suggest that myeloid-specific expression of myeloperoxidase might in part be dictated by the cell-type-restricted transcription factor myeloid nuclear factor 1 (MyNF1).[121] MyNF1 remains to be isolated and the corresponding cDNA cloned. Identification of relevant *cis* elements and *trans*-acting factors required for myeloid-specific gene expression will provide novel avenues to connect extracellular signals from G-CSF to nuclear events that lead to the expression of the myeloid phenotype.

Erythroid Differentiation

Cells committed to differentiate stochastically into the erythroid lineage are amplified by the erythroid-specific factor EPO. EPO is thought not to determine lineage commitment, but to function as a growth factor as well as a survival factor in cell culture studies of erythroid cell lines and normal bone marrow erythroid precursors. Thus, according to the stochastic lineage commitment model, EPO serves to rescue those cells (CFU-E or burst-forming unit-erythroid) that express the EPO receptor.[122] When bound to its receptor, EPO initiates a signal transduction pathway that involves the serine/threonine protein kinase raf, PKC, and a genetic program that activates the expression of the c-*myc* proto-oncogene.[123,124] Without EPO, committed erythroid cells undergo programmed cell death with the characteristic laddering of DNA due to nuclease-mediated fragmentation.[125] In these models, hemoglobin synthesis as well as other manifestations of the erythroid phenotype follow; however, the molecular events responsible for the initiation of these events remain unknown.

Insights into the regulation of the globin gene have begun to emerge with the identification of cis and trans factors that regulate erythroid-specific genes. Erythroid-specific cis-acting

elements have been identified in several erythroid genes. The sequence (A/T)GATA(A/G) is found in the globin gene enhancer in several species and in the promoter of the EPO receptor gene.[122] This consensus sequence is recognized by a cell-restricted transcription factor GATA-1 found in megakaryocytes and erythroid and mast cells.[126] GATA-1 is one among four related members of the GATA family of transcription factors. High expression of globin also requires a regulatory region located about 20 kb upstream of the ε-globin gene termed the locus-activating region, which also contains a GATA sequence. Genetic knock-out of GATA-1 in mice results in a block in normal erythropoiesis, attesting to the importance of GATA-1 in erythroid differentiation. The block in maturation occurs at the proerythroblast stage. Myeloid cells, however, do arise from hematopoietic cells lacking GATA-1, indicating that GATA-1 acts at a later stage than the PHSCs or their immediate descendants. Additional transcription factors involved in erythroid differentiation are begining to be identified and characterized. The accumulation of knowledge about these factors will continue to fill the void in our understanding about erythroid differentiation.

Megakaryocytic Differentiation

Megakaryocytic differentiation represents an intriguing biologic phenomenon in which a cell undergoes several rounds of DNA replication without cytokinesis. The resultant mature polyploid megakaryocyte than sheds small membrane-bound, metabolically active cytoplasmic fragments, which become circulating platelets. The platelet "cell" participates in thrombosis through several signal transduction pathways including activation of the thrombin receptor and fibrinogen receptor (GPIIb/IIIa). The activated platelet lets the cellular "glue" plug up small anatomic defects in the vasculature. Although it is clinically apparent that thrombocytopenia due to peripheral destruction is accompanied by recruitment of mature megakaryocytes from precursor cells, the factors involved in this feedback loop remain to be determined. A definitive thrombopoietin remains unidentified but several lymphokines, such as IL-6, are known to stimulate megakaryocytes.

Some of the later megakaryocytic differentiation events, however, are begining to emerge from studies of megakaryotic cell lines and megakaryocyte-specific genes. Several cell lines can be induced to differentiate and express various megakaryocytic phenotypes, including the platelet-specific fibrinogen receptor GPIIb/IIIa. These cells also display repeated rounds of DNA replication that result in polyploidism. The molecular mechanisms that control polyploidism are likely to involve certain molecules that determine cell fate, the cyclins. Hypothetically, megakaryocytic differentiation is a result of alterations in cell cycle regulatory events that allow repeated DNA replication but neither mitosis nor the ensuing cytokinesis. As such, ongoing studies of cyclin gene regulation in megakaryocytic differentiation will shed more light on this fascinating phenomenon.

As the promoters of several platelet-specific genes are cloned, the mechanism of regulation of platelet-specific genes is beginning to emerge. Inspection of the promoters for platelet genes GPIb, GPIIb, and GPIIIa (Villa-Garcia M, Bray PF, personal communcation) indicates that there is a common putative DNA-binding site, termed putative meg-specific element, that may be megakaryocyte specific.[127] It is also apparent that unique combinations of many ubiquitous transcription factors are likely to dictate tissue specificity. Indeed, various DNA-binding sites have been identified in promoters of megakaryocyte-specific genes. Among these sites is the GATA sequence that was previously thought to be erythroid specific. In fact, enforced expression of GATA-1, a GATA-binding protein, in a myeloid cell line induced the megakaryocyte phenotype.[128] A clearer picture of the interplay between these GATA-1 and other transcription factors to initiate megakaryocyte-specific gene transcription is likely to be forthcoming.

PROGRAMMED CELL DEATH AND HEMATOPOIESIS

Apoptosis and Programmed Cell Death

Apoptosis is a morphologically unique process of cell death that is distinctly different from necrosis.[129] Necrosis is accidental cell death resulting from severe and sudden thermal, physical, or chemical trauma. Morphologically, there is early mitochondrial and cellular swelling with ensuing cytoskeletal disruption and ruptured plasma membrane and organelles. During necrosis, the nuclear structure remains intact. By contrast, apoptosis is a sequential process starting with condensation of the chromatin and shrinkage of cell volume. The plasma membrane becomes ruffled and blebbed. The nucleus and cytoplasm then become partitioned into membrane-bound apoptotic bodies that are shed from the dying cells. The term apoptosis was proposed by Kerr et al[130] to describe these cellular alterations and used in Greek ($\alpha\pi o\pi\tau\omega\sigma\iota\sigma$) to describe the falling off of petals from flowers or leaves from trees. Most cells in the last stages of apoptosis display a characteristic degradation of nuclear DNA into multimers of 180 bp (DNA laddering). Throughout apoptosis, the mitochondria remain morphologically normal. Apoptosis participates in many physiologic processes, including morphogenesis, death of short-lived neutrophils, elimination of self-reactive T cells, and, perhaps, death of B cells with nonproductive V(D)J gene rearrangements.

Genetic Basis of Programmed Cell Death

Although apoptosis is commonly equated with programmed cell death in vertebrate systems, a genetic program for cell death has only been established unequivocally for the death of individual cells in *Caenorhabtditis elegans* (a small worm).[131] In *C. elegans*, 131 of the organism's 1,090 somatic cells are programmed to die during development. Studies of mutant *C. elegans* have revealed ≥ 14 genes (complementation groups) that are involved in cell death. Of these, *nuc-1* is a gene that encodes an endonuclease. Mutants of *ced-3* or *ced-4*, genes that are required for cell death, have extra somatic cells. Vertebrate genes, which are structurally homologous to *ced-3* or *ced-4*, are as yet unidentified. Mutation of the locus *ced-9*, which antagonizes *ced-3* and *ced-4*, results in developmental arrest. The product of *ced-9* blocks apoptosis, and hence its loss presumably results in untimely cell death.

An understanding of the genetic regulation of programmed cell death in vertebrates is only begining to emerge. An intriguing clue to the genetics of vertebrate apoptosis came from the study of *bcl-2*, a gene that is characteristically translocated [t(14:18)] in most follicular lymphomas.[132] The protein, bcl-2, has significant sequence homology to the product of the *C. elegans ced-9* gene.[133] The expression of the bcl-2 protein is restricted to tissues characterized by apoptotic death, within which its presence is inversely correlated with apoptosis. For example, bcl-2 is found in the thymic medulla where surviving T cells are located, whereas bcl-2 is not found in cortical thymocytes destined to die.[134] The function of bcl-2 at the molecular level still eludes characterization; however the bcl-2 protein is known to exist in mitochondrial, endoplasmic reticular, as well as perinuclear membranes.[135] In transgenic mice experiments, targeted *bcl-2* expression in B cells resulted in memory cells with an extended lifetime. Targeted *bcl-2* expression in T cells

resulted in immature thymocytes that are resistant to apoptosis induced by glucocorticoids, radiation, or anti-CD3 antibody.[136] Thus, follicular lymphomas, which are characterized by a low growth fraction and deregulated expression of *bcl-2*, proliferate predominantly by a decrease in the rate of cell death.

Recently, the tumor suppressor protein p53 has been shown to participate in the regulation cell cycle G_1-S transition. It is thought to be involved in the monitoring of DNA breaks induced by various physical and chemical agents such as ionizing radiation. Through an unknown mechanism, DNA breaks are detected and p53 protein levels are subsequently increased (by post-transcriptional events), resulting in cellular arrest in G_1. Overexpression of wild-type p53 protein in tissue culture cells has been associated with an increase in the rate of apoptosis.[137] By contrast, homologous genetic knock-out of the p53 gene resulted in thymocytes that do not undergo apoptosis with exposure to ionizing radiation, but continue to die with exposure to glucocorticoid.[138] These observations suggest that several pathways leading to apoptosis in thymocytes exist and that at least one of these pathways is p53 dependent.[139]

The participation of c-myc in cell proliferation and neoplastic transformation has been established by a variety of studies.[140] A new twist on the function of the c-myc protein in cell fate, however, was unveiled when cells overexpressing myc were deprived of nutrients and growth factors through serum deprivation.[141,142] In contrast to parental fibroblastic cell lines that undergo growth arrest and withdraw into the G_0 phase with serum deprivation, the myc-overexpressing cells undergo apoptosis. The apoptotic phenotype depends on domains of the c-myc protein required for transcriptional activation and cellular transformation, suggesting that myc actively participates in apoptosis.[142] Hypothetically, the myc-overexpressing cells appear to contend with apparently conflicting signals for cell proliferation *(myc)* and for growth arrest (serum withdrawal) by executing the cell death program. While serum deprivation provides a convenient experimental maneuver, its physiologic significance is obscure unless one considers the growth of a tumor mass. In a mass that is sufficiently large, access to nutrients becomes diffusion limited toward the center of the mass as tumor size increases. Thus, cells at the center of the mass may undergo aoptosis unless additional genetic alterations are sustained. Such additional genetic alteration might be the expression of bcl-2 that can block the apoptotic effects of myc.[143,144]

Besides the nuclear and cytoplasmic effectors of apoptosis discussed above, a membrane protein termed Fas/APO-1 induces apoptosis when crosslinked by anti-Fas/APO-1 antibody.[145] The Fas protein is homologous to receptors for tumor necrosis factor and nerve growth factor. A lymphoproliferative condition is found in mice bearing the *lpr* mutation that is responsible for a defect in Fas. The signals transduced between antibody crosslinking of Fas and apoptosis will likely overlap with the roles of bcl-2, p53, or myc in programmed cell death. Another intriguing idea that stems from the discovery of fas is the possibility of therapeutically inducing cell death in neoplasia by using anti-Fas antibodies.[146]

Although the understanding of molecular mechanisms mediating or averting apoptosis is only in its infancy, several hematologic growth and differentiation systems appear to be intimately intertwined with programmed cell death. As discussed above, programmed cell death appears to be an integral component of the stochastic hematopoietic cell lineage commitment and differentiation model. Apoptosis also appears to participate in the physiology of the more mature hematopoietic cells. For example, thymocytes undergo a stringent selection process that uses apoptosis to eliminate cells that recognize self-antigen. In fact, T cells exposed to certain monoclonal anti-CD3/T-cell-receptor complex antibodies undergo activation-induced death. This process can be blocked by down-regulation of c-*myc* gene expression by antisense technology.[147] Likewise, pre-B cells that come into contact with antigen at the stage of producing IgM will abort by death. Thus, apoptosis appears to participate in the control of autoreactive T and B cells.

Eosinophils, monocytes, and neutrophils all participate in the initiation and control of inflammatory responses. Their elimination from circulation may in part be mediated by apoptosis. Isolated eosinophils undergo apoptosis after about 80 hours in culture. IL-5 appears to extend eosinophil lifetime by delaying apoptosis.[148] Mature neutrophils have also been shown to undergo apoptosis.[149] Likewise, monocytes undergo programmed cell death that can be averted by exposure to IL-1β, tumor necrosis factor-α, GM-CSF, and interferon-γ.[150]

REFERENCES

1. Cantley LC, Auger KR, Carpenter C et al: Oncogenes and signal transduction. Cell 64:281, 1991
2. Rozengurt E: Growth factors and cell proliferation. Curr Opin Cell Biol 4: 161, 1992
3. Weiss A: T cell antigen receptor signal transduction: a tale of tails and cytoplasmic protein-tyrosine kinases. Cell 73:209, 1993
4. Koch CA, Anderson D, Moran MF et al: SH2 and SH3 domains: elements that control interactions of cytoplasmic signaling proteins. Science 252:668, 1991
5. Margolis B, Rhee SG, Felder S et al: EGF induces tyrosine phosphorylation of phospholipase C-II: a potential mechanism for EGF receptor signaling. Cell 57:1101, 1989
6. Meisenhelder J, Suh P-G, Rhee SG, Hunter T: Phospholipase C-γ is a substrate for the PDGF and EGF receptor protein-tyrosine kinases in vivo and in vitro. Cell 57:1109, 1989
7. Nishibe S, Wahl MI, Hernandez-Sotomayor SMT et al: Increase of the catalytic activity of phospholipase C-γ1 by tyrosine phosphorylation. Science 250:1253, 1990
8. Kim HK, Kim JW, Zilberstein A et al: PDGF stimulation of inositol phospholipid hydrolysis requires PLC-γ1 phosphorylation on tyrosine residues 783 and 1254. Cell 65:435, 1991
9. Nishizuka Y: Turnover of inositol phospholipids and signal transduction. Science 225:1365, 1984
10. Berridge MJ, Heslop JP, Irvine RF, Brown KD: Inositol triphosphate formation and calcium mobilization in Swiss 3T3 cells in response to platelet-derived growth factor. Biochem J 222:195, 1984
11. Bourne HR, Sanders DA, McCormick F: The GTPase superfamily: conserved structure and molecular mechanism. Nature 39:117, 1991
12. McCormick F: *ras* GTPase activating protein: signal transmitter and signal terminator. Cell 56:5, 1989
13. McCormick F: How receptors turn Ras on. Nature 363:15, 1993
14. Moodie SA, Willumsen BM, Weber MJ, Wolfman A: Complexes of Ras-GTP with Raf-1 and mitogen-activated protein kinase kinase. Science 260:1658, 1993
15. Ruderman JV: MAP kinase and the activation of quiescent cells. Curr Opin Cell Biol 5:207, 1993
16. Pulverer BJ, Kyriakis JM, Avruch J et al: Phosphorylation of c-*jun* mediated by MAP kinases. Nature 353:670, 1991
17. Gupta S, Seth A, Davis RJ: Transactivation of gene expression by Myc is inhibited by mutation at the phosphorylation sites Thr-58 and Ser-62. Proc Natl Acad Sci USA 90:3216, 1993
18. Tang W-J, Gilman AG: Adenylyl cyclases. Cell 70:869, 1992
19. Evans RM: The steroid and thyroid hormone receptor superfamily. Science 240:889, 1988
20. Pabo CO, Sauer RT: Transcription factors: structural families and principles of DNA recognition. Annu Rev Biochem 61:1053, 1992
21. Ptashne M: How eukaryotic transcriptional activators work. Nature 335:683, 1988
22. Jones N: Transcriptional regulation by dimerization: two sides to an incestuous relationship. Cell 61:9, 1990
23. Benezra R, Davis RL, Lockshon D et al: The protein Id: a negative regulator of helix-loop-helix DNA binding proteins. Cell 61:49, 1990
24. Luscher B, Christenson E, Litchfield DW et al: Myb DNA binding inhibited by phosphorylation at a site deleted during oncogenic activation. Nature 344:517, 1990
25. Gonzalez GA, Montminy MR: Cyclic AMP stimulates somatostatin gene transcription by phosphorylation of CREB at serine 133. Cell 59:675, 1989
26. Ghosh S, Baltimore D: Activation *in vitro* of NF-κB by phosphorylation of its inhibitor IκB. Nature 344:678, 1990

27. Boyle WJ, Smeal T, Defize LHK et al: Activation of protein kinase C decreases phosphorylation of c-Jun at sites that negatively regulate its DNA-binding activity. Cell 64:573, 1991
28. Almendral JM, Sommer D, MacDonald-Bravo H et al: Complexity of the early genetic response to growth factors in mouse fibroblasts. Mol Cell Biol 8: 2140, 1988
29. Laskey RA, Fairman MP, Blow JJ: S phase of the cell cycle. Science 246:609, 1989
30. McIntosh JR, Koonce MP: Mitosis. Science 246:622, 1989
31. Pardee A: G$_1$ events and regulation of cell proliferation. Science 246:603, 1989
32. Hartwell LH, Weinert TA: Checkpoints: controls that ensure the order of cell cycle events. Science 246:629, 1989
33. Weinert TA, Hartwell LH: The *Rad9* gene controls the cell cycle response to DNA damage in *Saccharomyces cerevisiae*. Science 241:317, 1988
34. Rowley R: Reduction of radiation-induced G$_2$ arrest by caffeine. Radiat Res 129:224, 1992
35. Kastan MB, Onyekwere O, Sidransky D et al: Participation of p53 protein in the cellular response to DNA damage. Cancer Res 51:6304, 1991
36. Livingstone LR, White A, Sprouse J et al: Altered cell cycle arrest and gene amplification potential accompany loss of wild-type p53. Cell 70:923, 1992
37. Yin Y, Tainsky MA, Bischoff FZ et al: Wild-type p53 restores cell cycle control and inhibits gene amplification in cells with mutant p53 alleles. Cell 70:937, 1992
38. Evans T, Rosenthal ET, Youngblom J et al: Cyclin: a protein specified by maternal mRNA in sea urchin eggs that is destroyed at each cleavage division. Cell 33:389, 1983
39. Nurse P, Thuriaux P: Regulatory genes controlling mitosis in the fission yeast *Schizosaccharomyces pombe*. Genetics 96:627, 1980
40. Simanis V, Nurse P: The cell cycle control gene cdc2$^+$ of fission yeast encodes a protein kinase potentially regulated by phosphorylation. Cell 45:261, 1986
41. Lee M, Nurse P: Complementation used to clone a human homologue of the fission yeast cell cycle control gene cdc2$^+$. Nature 327:31, 1987
42. Gautier J, Norbury C, Lohka M et al: Purified maturation-promoting factor contains the product of a *Xenopus* homolog of the fission yeast cell cycle control gene cdc2$^+$. Cell 54:433, 1988
43. Gautier J, Minshull J, Lohka M et al: Cyclin is a component of maturation-promoting factor from *Xenopus*. Cell 60:487, 1990
44. Norbury C, Nurse P: Animal cell cycles and their control. Annu Rev Biochem 61:441, 1992
45. Parker LL, Piwnica-Worms H: Inactivation of the p34^{cdc2}-cyclin B complex by the human WEE1 tyrosine kinase. Science 257:1955, 1992
46. Hoffmann I, Clarke PR, Marcote MJ et al: Phosphorylation and activation of human cdc25-C by cdc2-cyclin B and its involvement in the self-amplification of MPF at mitosis. EMBO J 12:53, 1993
47. Ward GE, Kirschner MW: Identification of cell cycle-regulated phosphorylation sites on nuclear lamin C. Cell 61:561, 1990
48. Peter M, Nakagawa J, Doree M et al: In vitro disassembly of the nuclear lamina and M phase-specific phosphorylation of lamins by cdc2 kinase. Cell 61:591, 1990
49. Chou Y-H, Bischoff JR, Beach D, Goldman RD: Intermediate filament reorganization during mitosis is mediated by p34^{cdc2} phosphorylation of vimentin. Cell 62:1063, 1990
50. Glotzer M, Murray AW, Kirschner MW: Cyclin is degraded by the ubiquitin pathway. Nature 349:132, 1991
51. Murray AW, Solomon MJ, Kirschner MW: The role of cyclin synthesis and degradation in the control of maturation-promoting factor activity. Nature 339:280, 1989
52. Paris J, Guellec RL, Couturier A et al: Cloning by differential screening of a *Xenopus* cDNA coding for a protein highly homologous to cdc2. Proc Natl Acad Sci USA 88:1039, 1991
53. Meyerson M, Enders GH, Wu C-L et al: A family of human cdc2-related protein kinases. EMBO J 11:2909, 1992
54. Fang F, Newport JW: Evidence that the G1-S and G2-M transitions are controlled by different cdc2 proteins in higher eukaryotes. Cell 66:731, 1991
55. Xiong Y, Connolly T, Futcher B, Beach D: Human D-type cyclin. Cell 65:691, 1991
56. Koff A, Cross F, Fisher A et al: Human cyclin E, a new cyclin that interacts with two members of the *CDC2* gene family. Cell 66:1217, 1991
57. Lew DJ, Dulic V, Reed SI: Isolation of three novel human cyclins by rescue of G1 cyclin (Cln) function in yeast. Cell 66:1197, 1991
58. Motokura T, Bloom T, Kim HG et al: A novel cyclin encoded by a *BCL1*-linked candidate oncogene. Nature 350:512, 1991
59. Matsushime H, Roussel MF, Ashmun RA, Sherr CJ: Colony-stimulating factor 1 regulates novel cyclins during the G1 phase of the cell cycle. Cell 65:701, 1991

60. Xiong Y, Zhang H, Beach D: D type cyclins associate with multiple protein kinases and the DNA replication and repair factor PCNA. Cell 71:505, 1992

61. Baldin V, Lukas J, Marcote MJ et al: Cyclin D1 is a nuclear protein required for cell cycle progression in G1. Genes Dev 7:812, 1993

62. Hinds PW, Mittnacht S, Dulic V et al: Regulation of retinoblastoma protein functions by ectopic expression of human cyclins. Cell 70:993, 1992

63. Ewen ME, Sluss HK, Sherr CJ et al: Functional interactions of the retinoblastoma protein with mammalian D-type cyclins. Cell 73:487, 1993

64. Dowdy SF, Hinds PW, Louie K et al: Physical interaction of the retinoblastoma protein with human D cyclins. Cell 73:499, 1993

65. Motokura T, Arnold A: Cyclin D and oncogenesis. Curr Opin Genet Dev 3: 5, 1993

66. Koff A, Giordano A, Desai D et al: Formation and activation of a cyclin E-cdk2 complex during the G_1 phase of the human cell cycle. Science 257: 1689, 1992

67. Dulic V, Lees E, Reed SI: Association of human cyclin E with a periodic G_1-S phase protein kinase. Science 257:1958, 1992

68. Lees EB, Faha B, Dulic V et al: Cyclin E/cdk2 and cyclin A/cdk2 kinases associate with p107 and E2F in a temporally distinct manner. Genes Dev 6: 1874, 1992

69. Ohtsubo M, Roberts JM: Cyclin-dependent regulation of G_1 in mammalian fibroblasts. Science 259:1908, 1993

70. Pagano M, Pepperkok R, Verde F et al: Cyclin A is required at two points in the human cell cycle. EMBO J 11:961, 1992

71. Mudryj M, Devoto S, Hiebert SW et al: Cell cycle regulation of the E2F transcription factor involves an interaction with cyclin A. Cell 65:1243, 1991

72. Girard F, Strausfeld U, Fernandez A, Lamb NJC: Cyclin A is required for the onset of DNA replication in mammalian fibroblasts. Cell 67:1169, 1991

73. D'Urso G, Marraccino RL, Marshak DR, Roberts JM: Cell cycle control of DNA replication by a homologue from human cells of the p34^{cdc2} protein kinase. Science 250:786, 1990

74. Friend SH, Bernards R, Rogelj S et al: A human DNA segment with properties of the gene that predisposes to retinoblastoma and osteosarcoma. Nature 323:643, 1986

75. Lee W-H, Bookstein R, Hong F et al: Human retinoblastoma susceptibility gene: cloning, identification, and sequence. Science 235:1394, 1987

76. Fung Y-K T, Murphree AL, T'Ang A et al: Structural evidence for the authenticity of the human retinoblastoma gene. Science 236:1657, 1987

77. Goodrich DW, Wang NP, Qian Y-W et al: The retinoblastoma gene product regulates progression through the G1 phase of the cell cycle. Cell 67:293, 1991

78. DeCaprio JA, Ludlow JW, Lynch D et al: The product of the retinoblastoma susceptibility gene has properties of a cell cycle regulatory element. Cell 58:1085, 1989

79. Buchkovich KJ, Duffy LA, Harlow E: The retinoblastoma protein is phosphorylated during specific phases of the cell cycle. Cell 58:1097, 1989

80. Chen P-L, Scully P, Shew J-Y et al: Phosphorylation of the retinoblastoma gene product is modulated during the cell cycle and cellular differentiation. Cell 58:1193, 1989

81. Whyte P, Buchkovich KJ, Horowitz JM et al: Association between an oncogene and an antioncogene: the adenovirus E1A proteins bind to the retinoblastoma gene product. Nature 334:124, 1988

82. DeCaprio JA, Ludlow JW, Figge J et al: SV40 large tumor antigen forms a specific complex with the product of the retinoblastoma susceptibility gene. Cell 54:275, 1988

83. Ludlow JW, DeCaprio JA, Huang C-M et al: SV40 large T antigen binds preferentially to an underphosphorylated member of the retinoblastoma susceptibility gene product family. Cell 56:57, 1989

84. Dyson N, Howley PM, Munger K, Harlow E: The human papilloma virus-16 E7 oncoprotein is able to bind to the retinoblastoma gene product. Science 243:934, 1989

85. Nevins JR: E2F: a link between the Rb tumor suppressor protein and viral oncoproteins. Science 258:424, 1992

86. Weintraub SJ, Prater CA, Dean DC: Retinoblastoma protein switches the E2F site from positive to negative element. Nature 358:259, 1992

87. Kim S-J, Wagner S, Liu F et al: Retinoblastoma gene product activates expression of the human TGF-β2 gene through transcription factor ATF-2. Nature 358:331, 1992

88. Cooper JA, Whyte P: Rb and the cell cycle: entrance or exit? Cell 58:1009, 1989

89. Lee EY-HP, Chang C-Y, Hu N et al: Mice deficient for Rb are nonviable and show defects in neurogenesis and haematopoiesis. Nature 359:288, 1992

90. Jacks T, Fazeli A, Schmitt EM et al: Effects of an Rb mutation in the mouse. Nature 359:295, 1992

91. Clarke AR, Maandag ER, van Roon M: Requirement for a functional Rb-1 gene in murine development. Nature 359:328, 1992

92. Finlay CA, Hinds PW, Levine AJ: The p53 proto-oncogene can act as a suppressor of transformation. Cell 57:1083, 1989

93. Perry ME, Levine AJ: Tumor-suppressor p53 and the cell cycle. Curr Opin Genet Dev 3:50, 1993

94. Malkin D, Li FP, Strong LC et al: Germ line p53 mutations in a familial syndrome of breast cancer, sarcoma, and other neoplasms. Science 250:1233, 1990

95. Srivastava S, Zou Z, Pirollo K et al: Germ-line transmission of a mutated p53 gene in a cancer-prone family with Li-Fraumeni syndrome. Nature 348:747, 1990

96. Fields S, Jang SK: Presence of a potent transcription activating sequence in the p53 protein. Science 249:1046, 1990

97. Raycroft L, Wu H, Lozano G: Transcriptional activation by wild-type but not transforming mutants of the p53 anti-oncogene. Science 249:1049, 1990

98. Momand J, Zambetti GP, Olson DC et al: The mdm-2 oncogene product forms a complex with the p53 protein and inhibits p53-mediated transactivation. Cell 69:1237, 1992

99. Donehower LA, Harvey M, Slagle BL et al: Mice deficient for p53 are developmentally normal but susceptible to spontaneous tumours. Nature 356:215, 1992

100. Kastan MB, Zhan Q, El-Deiry WS et al: A mammalian cell cycle checkpoint pathway utilizing p53 and GADD45 is defective in ataxia-telangiectasia. Cell 71:587, 1992

101. Harper JW, Adami GR, Wei N et al: The p21 Cdk-interacting protein Cip1 is a potent inhibitor of G1 cyclin-dependent kinases. Cell 75:8–5, 1993

102. El-Deiry WS, Tokino T, Velculescu D et al: WAF1, a potential mediator of p53 tumor suppression. Cell 75:817, 1993

103. Vasseur-Cognet M, Lane MD: Trans-acting factors involved in adipogenic differentiation. Curr Opin Genet Dev 3:238, 1993

104. Christy RJ, Kaestner KH, Geiman DE et al: CCAAT/-break enhancer binding gene promoter: binding of nuclear factors during differentiation of 3T3-L1 preadipocytes. Proc Natl Acad Sci USA 88:2593, 1991

105. Freytag SO, Geddes TJ: Reciprocal regulation of adipogenesis by Myc and C/EPBα. Science 256:379, 1992

106. Weintraub H, Davis R, Tapscott S et al: The myoD gene family: nodal point during specification of the muscle cell lineage. Science 251:761, 1991

107. Ogawa M: Differentiation and proliferation of hematopoietic stem cells. Blood 81:2844, 1993

108. Gearing DP, Comeau MR, Friend DJ et al: The IL-6 signal transducer, gp130: an oncostatin M receptor and affinity converter for the LIF receptor. Science 255:1434, 1992

109. Nicola NA, Metcalf D: Subunit promiscuity among hemopoietic growth factor receptors. Cell 67:1, 1991

110. Rolink A, Melchers F: Molecular and cellular origins of B lymphocyte diversity. Cell 66:1081, 1991

111. Tsukada S, Saffran DC, Rawlings DJ et al: Deficient expression of a B cell cytoplasmic tyrosine kinase in human X-linked agammaglobulinemia. Cell 72:279, 1993

112. Schatz D, Baltimore D: Stable expression of immunoglobulin gene V(D)J recombinase activity by gene transfer into 3T3 fibroblasts. Cell 53:107, 1988

113. Mombaerts P, Iacomini J, Johnson RS et al: RAG-1 deficient mice have no mature B and T lymphocytes. Cell 68:869, 1992

114. Shinkai Y, Rathbun G, Lam KP et al: RAG-2 deficient mice lack mature lymphocytes owing to inability to initiate V(D)J rearrangement. Cell 68:855, 1992

115. Sherr CJ: Colony-stimulating factor-1 receptor. Blood 75:1, 1990

116. Roussel MF, Cleveland JL, Shurtleff SA et al: Myc rescue of a mutant CSF-1 receptor impaired in mitogenic signalling. Nature 353:361, 1991

117. Nguyen HQ, Liebermann BH, Liebermann DA: The zinc finger transcription factor Egr-1 is essential for and restricts differentiation along the macrophage lineage. Cell 72:197, 1993

118. Scott LM, Civin CI, Rorth P et al: A novel temporal expression pattern of three C/EBP family members in differentiating myelomonocytic cells. Blood 80:1725, 1992

119. Ness SA, Kowenz-Leutz E, Casini T et al: Myb and NF-M: combinatorial activators of myeloid genes in heterologous cell types. Genes Dev 7:749, 1993

120. Kreider BL, Benezra R, Rovera G et al: Inhibition of myeloid differentiation by the helix-loop-helix protein Id. Science 255:1700, 1992

121. Suzow J, Friedman AD: The murine myeloperoxidase promoter contains several functional elements, one of which binds a cell type-restricted transcription factor, myeloid nuclear factor 1 (MyNF1). Mol Cell Bio 13:2141, 1993

122. Youssoufian H, Longmore G, Neumann D et al: Structure, function, and activation of the erythropoietin receptor. Blood 81:2223, 1993

123. Carroll MP, Spivak JL, McMahon M et al: Erythropoietin induces Raf-1 activa-

tion and Raf-1 is required for erythropoietin mediated proliferation. J Biol Chem 266:14964, 1991

124. Spangler R, Bailey SC, Sytkowski AJ: Erythropoietin increases c-*myc* mRNA by a protein kinase C-dependent pathway. J Biol Chem 266:681, 1991

125. Koury MJ, Bondurant MC: Erythropoietin retards DNA breakdown and prevents programmed death in erythroid progenitor cells. Science 248:378, 1990

126. Orkin SH: GATA-binding transcription factors in hematopoietic cells. Blood 80:575, 1992

127. Uzan G, Prenant M, Prandini MH et al: Tissue-specific expression of the platelet GPIIb gene. J Biol Chem 266:8932, 1991

128. Visvader JE, Elefanty AG, Strasser A et al: GATA-1 but not SCL induces megakaryocytic differentiation in an early myeloid line. EMBO 11:4557, 1992

129. Raff MC: Social controls on cell survival and cell death. Nature 356:397, 1992

130. Kerr JFR, Wyllie AH, Currie AR: Apoptosis: a basic biological phenomenon with wide ranging implications in tissue kinetics. Br J Cancer 26:239, 1972

131. Ellis RE, Yuan J, Horvitz HR: Mechanisms and functions of cell death. Annu Rev Cell Biol 7:663, 1991

132. Korsmeyer SJ: Bcl-2 initiates a new category of oncogenes: regulators of cell death. Blood 80:879, 1992

133. Hengartner MO, Ellis RE, Horvitz HR: *Caenorhabditis elgans* gene, ced 9, protects cells from programmed cell death. Nature 356:494, 1992

134. Hockenbury DM, Zutter M, Hickey W et al: BCL-2 protein is topographically restricted in tissues characterised by apoptotic cell death. Proc Natl Acad Sci USA 88:6981, 1991

135. Hockenbury D, Nunez G, Milliman C et al: Bcl-2 is an inner mitochondrial membrane protein that blocks programmed cell death. Nature 348:334, 1990

136. Sentman CL, Shutter JR, Hockenbury DM et al: Bcl-2 inhibits multiple forms of apoptosis but not negative selection in thymocytes. Cell 65:879, 1991

137. Yonish-Rouach E, Resnitzky E, Loten J et al: Wild type p53 induces apoptosis

138. Lowe SW, Schmitt EM, Smith SW et al: p53 is required for radiation-induced apoptosis in mouse thymocytes. Nature 362:847, 1993

139. Clarke AR, Purdie CA, Harrison DJ et al: Thymocyte apoptosis induced by p53-dependent and independent pathways. Nature 362:849, 1993

140. Kato GJ, Dang CV: Function of the c-Myc oncoprotein. FASEB J 6:3065, 1992

141. Askew DS, Ashmun RA, Simmons BC et al: Constitutive c-myc expression in an IL-3 dependant myeloid cell line suppresses cell cycle arrest and accelerates apoptosis. Oncogene 6:1915, 1991

142. Evan GI, Wyllie AH, Gilbert CS et al: Induction of apoptosis in fibroblasts by c-myc protein. Cell 69:119, 1992

143. Fanidi A, Harrington EA, Evan GI: Cooperative interaction between c-myc and bcl-2 proto-oncogenes. Nature 359:554, 1992

144. Bissonette RP, Echeverri F, Mahboubi A et al: Apoptotic cell death induced by c-myc is inhibited by bcl-2. Nature 359:552, 1992

145. Itoh N, Yonehara S, Ishii A et al: The polypeptide encoded by the cDNA for the human cell surface antigen Fas can mediate apoptosis. Cell 66:233, 1991

146. Trauth BC, Klas C, peters AMJ et al: Monoclonal antibody mediated tumour regression by induction of apoptosis. Science 245:301, 1989

147. Shi Y, Glynn JM, Guilbert LJ et al: Role of c-myc in activation-induced apoptotic cell death in T cell hybridomas. Science 257:211, 1992

148. Stern M, Meagher L, Savill J et al: Apoptosis in human eosinophils leads to phagocytosis by macrophages and is modulated by IL-5. J Immunol 148:3543, 1992

149. Lee A, Young SK, Henson PM et al: Modulation of neutrophil programmed cell death by inflammatory mediators. FASEB J 3:1344, 1989

150. Mangan DF, Wahl SM: Differential regulation of human monocyte programmed cell death (apoptosis) by chemotactic factors and pro-inflammatory cytokines. J Immunol 147:3408, 1991

of myeloid leukemia cells that is inhibited by interleukin 6. Nature 352:345, 1991

Structure and Function of the Immune System

8

Janine André-Schwartz and Robert S. Schwartz

INTRODUCTION

Hematology and immunology have been intertwined disciplines for at least a century. The relationship began with a mutual interest in antibodies and in the diseases they cause; since the 1960s, the two fields have complemented each other in pursuit of the lymphocyte (Table 8-1). For hematologists, the molecular genetics, differentiation, and functions of lymphocytes are of special importance. These cells take a leading part in hematologic practice. They give rise to forms of malignant lymphoma, multiple myeloma, macroglobulinemia, chronic lymphocytic leukemia (CLL), and acute lymphocytic leukemia (ALL); they have a pivotal role in autoimmune thrombocytopenia and autoimmune hemolytic anemia; and they participate in other blood disorders, among which infectious mononucleosis and aplastic anemia are important examples. For hematologists, therefore, an understanding of the biology and pathology of lymphocytes is imperative.

The growth of information about lymphocytes during the past few years has been explosive. Remarkable progress has been made thanks to numerous technical advances, especially in molecular and cell biology. Powerful new techniques can elucidate the contribution of a single gene to immune function in a living animal. Transgenic mice, created by microinjection of a foreign gene into fertilized eggs, and "knockout" mice, in which the gene of interest has been functionally inactivated (gene targeting, homologous recombination), are in the vanguard of immunologic research. Gene amplification with the polymerase chain reaction (PCR) continues to provide a wealth of data on genes and molecules essential for immune function. Batteries of monoclonal antibodies with specificity for cell lineages, sets, subsets, and even activation states, combined with sophisticated fluorescence-activated cell-sorting (FACS) machines, enable high-resolution purification and analysis of live lymphocytes. Many of these new techniques have important applications in diagnosis and treatment because they can identify precisely the genotype and phenotype of malignant lymphocytes, often within a few hours.

CLASSIFICATION OF LYMPHOCYTES

About 30% of the leukocytes in the blood are lymphocytes. Of these, about 70% are T cells, 15% are B cells, and 15% are natural killer (NK) cells (Fig. 8-1). The terms T cell and B cell were proposed in 1969 by Roitt et al[1] To emphasize that the two sets of cells are distinct lineages, these investigators used T to denote thymus-dependent lymphocytes and B for bursa-dependent lymphocytes (after the bursa of Fabricius in birds). Their designations were grounded in the observations that thymectomy of newborn mice sharply reduced production of mature T cells without influencing B cells, whereas removal of the bursa of Fabricius from newly hatched chickens interrupted the development of B cells without affecting T cells.[2] The T-cell/B-cell nomenclature is convenient and universal, but in mammals no organ corresponds to the bursa of Fabricius, the sole function of which is to produce B cells. The mammalian B-cell precursor reaches maturity in the bone marrow, along with many other types of cells, all of which trace their lineage to hematopoietic stem cells[3] (Fig. 8-2).

B Cells

Structure and Function of Lymphatic Tissue

All five classes of immunoglobulin (IgM, IgG, IgA, IgD, IgE) originate from B cells; the sole function of the plasma cell, the most differentiated B cell, is to secrete these immunoglobulins into plasma or other body fluids (Fig. 8-3). Although the bone marrow contains plasma cells (≤5% of the nucleated marrow cells) the bulk of immunoglobulin synthesis and secretion occurs in specialized anatomic sites in lymph nodes, spleen, and lymphatic tissues of the gastrointestinal tract and oropharynx.[4] The gut-associated lymphoid tissue specializes in the production of IgA[5]; elsewhere, B cells produce mainly IgM and IgG antibodies.

In quiescent lymph nodes, the cortical zone contains small organized collections of B cells, T cells, and follicular dendritic cells—the primary follicles. Between these follicles lies a paracortical (marginal) zone of T cells (Plate 8-1 and Fig. 8-4). In immunologically stimulated lymph nodes, the primary follicles become sites of intense activity. Proliferating lymphocytes cause them to expand into secondary follicles. A secondary follicle consists of a germinal center and a mantle zone, the rim or cap of small lymphocytes on its perimeter. The main constituents of the germinal center are B cells in various morphologic guises, but follicular dendritic cells and small numbers of T cells are also present. When stimulated by antigen, small B cells around the lymphoid follicles proliferate, transform into primary B blasts, and enter the germinal center. There they become centroblasts (large noncleaved follicular center cells): large B cells with basophilic cytoplasm and round nuclei within which nucleoli are prominent. The germinal center also contains polymorphic B cells with clefted or angulated nuclei, the centrocytes, or cleaved follicular center cells. The functional relationship, if any, between centroblasts and centrocytes is unknown. One possibility, shown in Figure 8-5, is that centrocytes arise from centroblasts and, with continued antigenic stimulation, transform into secondary B blasts. The latter, identifiable by a distinctive antigenic marker, CD30 (Table 8-2), migrate into the mantle zone, where they differentiate into mature B cells. Tingible body macrophages, loaded with cellular debris, are numerous in active germinal centers. The medulla of the lymph node contains many T cells organized into medullary cords. Macrophages are numerous within and around these cords.

Lymphatic tissues are not static collections of lymphocytes. On the contrary, lymphocytes enter and leave these sites continuously. They crawl on uropods, blunt-ended extensions of their cytoplasm, which they point in the direction of movement

Table 8-1. Highlights in the History of Hematology and Immunology

Year	Investigators	Event
1889	H. Buchner	Discovery of complement
1890	E. von Behring and S. Kitasato	Discovery of antibodies
1900	K. Landsteiner	ABO blood group system
1904	J. Donath and K. Landsteiner	First human autoimmune disease (paroxysmal cold hemoglobinuria)
1937	P.A. Gorer and G.D. Snell	Histocompatibility complex
1938	A. Tiselius and E.A. Kabat	Antibodies are γ-globulins
1945	R.D. Owen	Red cell chimerism (immune tolerance)
1946	R.R.A. Coombs, A.E. Morant, and R.R. Race	Antiglobulin test
1948	J. Waldenström	Monoclonal gammopathies
1951	E. Lorenz and D. Uphoff	Bone marrow protects rodents against lethal irradiation
1951	W.J. Harrington and J.W. Hollingsworth	Autoantibodies are pathogenic (immune thrombocytopenia)
1954	D.W.H. Barnes and J.F. Loutit	Graft-versus-host disease
1954	J. Dausset	HLA system
1959	M. Bielschowsky, B.J. Helyer, and J.B. Howie	Autoimmune hemolytic anemia in NZB mice
1961	J.F.A.P. Miller	Function of the thymus
1961	J. Gowans	Immunologic role of the lymphocyte
1963	H.G. Kunkel and J. Oudin	Immunoglobulin idiotypes
1966	A. Mitchison	Helper T cells
1969	G. Edelman and R.R. Porter	Structure of immunoglobulins
1976	S. Tonegawa	Immunoglobulin genes
1975	G. Köhler and C. Milstein	Monoclonal antibodies

(Fig. 8-6). They enter and leave the lymph node through specialized postcapillary venules, the high endothelial venules, which display adhesion molecules and surface receptors that interact specifically with ligands on lymphocyte surfaces.[6]

In lymphatic tissues, B cells come into contact with T cells and star-shaped follicular dendritic cells. These three kinds of cells constitute a functional unit of prime importance in the immune response (Fig. 8-7). The dendritic cells ingest, digest, and present antigens to T cells and B cells[7,8]; the T cells provide signals ("help") that activate B cells and other T cells[9]; the B cells respond to those stimuli by differentiating into plasma cells. All three cell types originate from hematopoietic precursors in the bone marrow. B cells that have not yet responded to an antigen—recent emigrants from the bone marrow—belong to the pre-immune repertoire. These "naive," or "virgin," B cells display IgM on their surfaces and, when activated, secrete IgM antibodies. Under the continued influence of activated T cells these B cells switch from the production of IgM to IgG, IgA, or IgE antibodies (isotype switch). Most of the B lymphocytes in the blood are of the pre-immune type; >90% of these B lymphocytes are quiescent and display surface IgM en route from the bone marrow to lymphatic tissue.

T Cells

T cells can be readily distinguished from B cells by phenotypic (cell surface) markers (Table 8-2) or by molecular probes that detect the expression of lineage-specific genes (see below). Physical separation of the two kinds of lymphocytes by FACS or by rosetting techniques (mouse red blood cells bind to and form rosettes with human T cells; Fig. 8-8) is also possible.

T-Cell Subsets

There are two major subsets of T cells: helper T cells and cytotoxic T cells. A distinctive surface protein defines each subset: CD4 (helper T cells) and CD8 (cytotoxic T cells).[10] Of the lymphocytes in blood, about 40% are CD4$^+$ T cells and 30% are CD8$^+$ T cells. These values have a wide variation in normal subjects (Fig. 8-1). The variability in normal values is important to keep in mind when evaluating a patient suspected of having acquired immunodeficiency syndrome in which a deficiency of CD4$^+$ T cells is an important diagnostic criterion.[11] Helper T cells have a central role in the immune response. When activated by specific immunogens or nonspecific mitogens, they secrete polypeptides (cytokines or lymphokines), which par-

Table 8-2. Cell-surface markers used in FACS Analysis of Leukocytes

CD[a] Name	Function	Reactivity
CD2	E rosette (LFA-3) receptor	T cells, NK cells
CD3	CD3 complex (5 chains)	T cells
CD4	MHC class II ligand; HIV receptor	Helper T cells
CD5	CD72 ligand	T cells, B-cell subset
CD7	Fc receptor for IgM (FcµR)	Early T cells, T-cell subset, NK cells
CD8	MHC class I ligand	Cytotoxic T cells
CD10	CALLA, neutral endopeptidase	Early B cells
CD11c	β2-integrin receptor	Monocytes, NK cells, granulocytes, hairy cells
CD13	Aminopeptidase N	Granulocytes, monocytes
CD14	Phosphatidylinositol-linked membrane protein	Monocytes, granulocytes
CD16	Fcγ receptor III	NK cells, granulocytes, monocytes
CD19	B-cell receptor complex	Early and mature B cells
CD20	Ion channel?	Early B cells
CD21	C3d and EBV receptor	B cells
CD25	IL-2R β-chain (low affinity)	Activated T and B cells
CD33	?	Myeloid precursor
CD34	L-selectin ligand	Hematopoietic progenitor cells
CD38	?	Plasma cells
CD45RO	Restricted leukocyte common antigen	T-cell subset, B cells, granulocytes, monocytes
CD45RA	Restricted leukocyte common antigen	T-cell subset, B cells, granulocytes, monocytes
CD56	N-CAM adhesion molecule	NK cells

Abbreviations: EBV, Epstein-Barr virus; IL-2R, interleukin-2 receptor; HIV, human immune deficiency virus.

[a] Terminology established by an international committee to designate cellular antigens recognized by monoclonal antibodies (e.g., monoclonal antibodies termed B4, Leu12, and HD37 recognize CD19). A large number of other monoclonal antibodies recognize CD antigens in tissue sections.

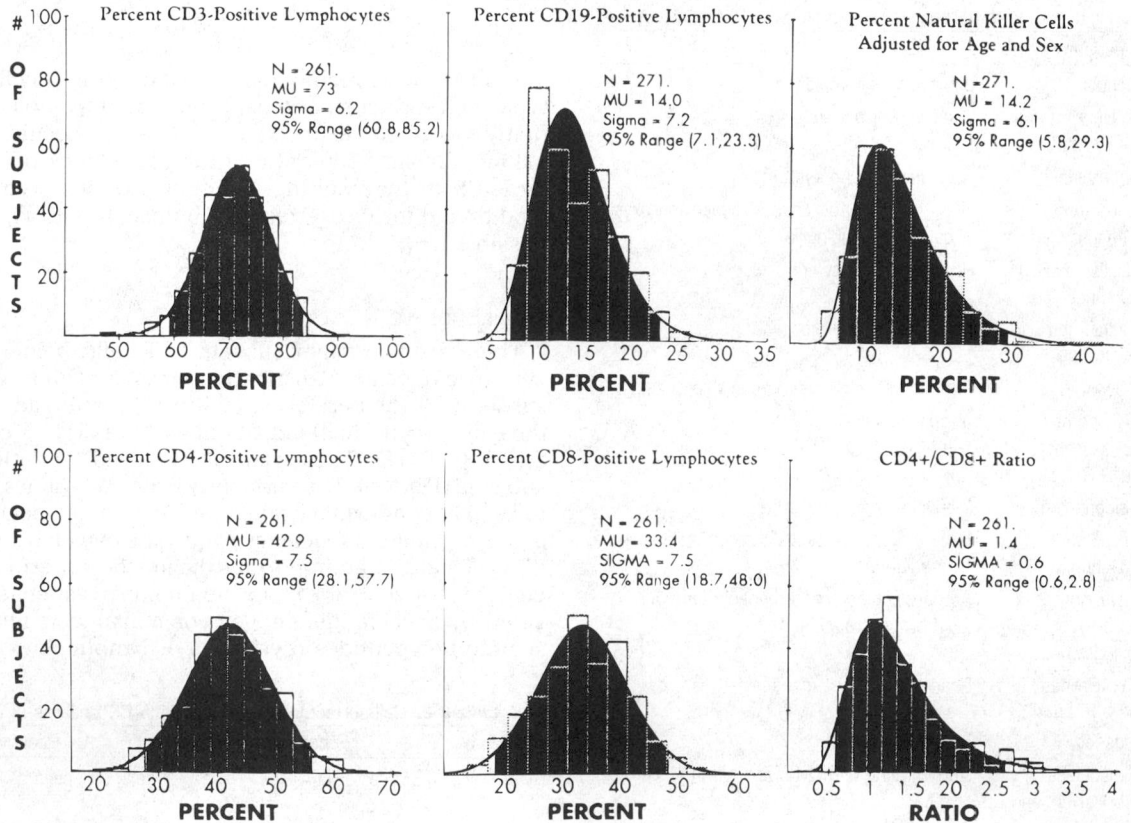

Fig. 8-1. Lymphocyte subsets in normal white adults. The values were obtained by fluorescence-activated cell-sorting (FACS) analysis of blood leukocytes with monoclonal antibodies specific for the five subsets of lymphocytes shown. (From Reichert et al.,[90] with permission.)

ticipate in the activation of B cells, cytotoxic T cells, or other $CD4^+$ T cells (Fig. 8-9). Interactions between $CD4^+$ T cells and other lymphocytes depend not only on cytokines but on intimate cell-cell contacts as well, the stability of which requires an array of adhesion molecules[9] (Fig. 8-10). Other types of adhesion molecules mediate the migration, or homing, of lymphocytes from the blood into lymphoid and other tissues.[6] Collectively, the cytokines and adhesion molecules that mediate T-B, T-T, or T-macrophage interactions are called second signals, to differentiate them from signals engendered in lymphocytes by contact with antigens.[12] The physiologic importance of second signals is discussed later in this chapter.

Subsets of Helper T Cells

Helper T cells have been subdivided into two functional types, T_{H1} and T_{H2} cells.[13] T_{H1} cells mediate delayed hypersensitivity reactions and activate macrophages. They secrete interleukin-2 (IL-2), interferon-γ, and tumor necrosis factor. T_{H2} cells "help" B cells produce antibodies. When activated, they secrete IL-4, IL-5, IL-6, and IL-10, all of which influence B-cell growth and development. T_{H1} and T_{H2} cells arise from a $CD4^+$ precursor (T_{H0}) through the action of distinct cytokines. IL-12, produced by macrophages when they become infected by certain bacteria or protozoa, shifts differentiation of the T_{H0} precursor toward T_{H1} cells, whereas IL-4 directs it into T_{H2} cells.

By contrast with helper T cells, the principal role of $CD8^+$ T cells is to induce the lysis of cells that bear a foreign antigen, such as virus-infected epithelial cells (Fig. 8-9). The functional differences between $CD4^+$ and $CD8^+$ T cells are generally clear cut, but they occasionally overlap.

Antigen Presentation

Whether they are $CD4^+$ or $CD8^+$, T cells engage their cognate antigen through receptors—antigen receptors, or, more loosely, T-cell receptors.[8] For $CD8^+$ T cells, the cognate antigen is usually a peptide of 9–12 amino acids; a longer peptide—$\leq$20 amino acids—engages the $CD4^+$ T cell. These peptides are exposed on the surface of an antigen-presenting cell (APC) (for helper T cells), or a target cell (for cytotoxic T cells).[14] They sit in a prominent groove of a cell-surface glycoprotein, for historical reasons called either the major histocompatibility complex (MHC) antigen or the human leukocyte antigen (HLA). The HLA system consists of a large and extremely polymorphic group of glycoproteins. It was discovered by serologic analysis of alloantibodies in serum from polytransfused patients and multiparous women, and it is the major barrier to the acceptance of allografts.[15] However, the physiologic role of HLA glycoproteins is to transport peptides from the cytosol to the surface of the cell; there they "present" the peptide to T cells.[7] The contact region of the T-cell receptor actually binds to a configuration made up of the peptide and a portion of the presenting HLA molecule (Fig. 8-11).

MHC molecules are of two types: class I and class II.[16] In general, class I MHC glycoproteins transport peptides derived from the enzymatic breakdown of endogenous cellular proteins, whereas class II MHC glycoproteins carry the proteolytic products of proteins that enter the cell from the exterior. These differences are not absolute, but peptides derived from viruses, which are obligatory intracellular parasites, would be presented by class I MHC glycoproteins, whereas peptides from an exogenous protein such as chicken albumin would be presented by class II HLA molecules. That the T-cell receptor recognizes peptides only in association with an MHC molecule is

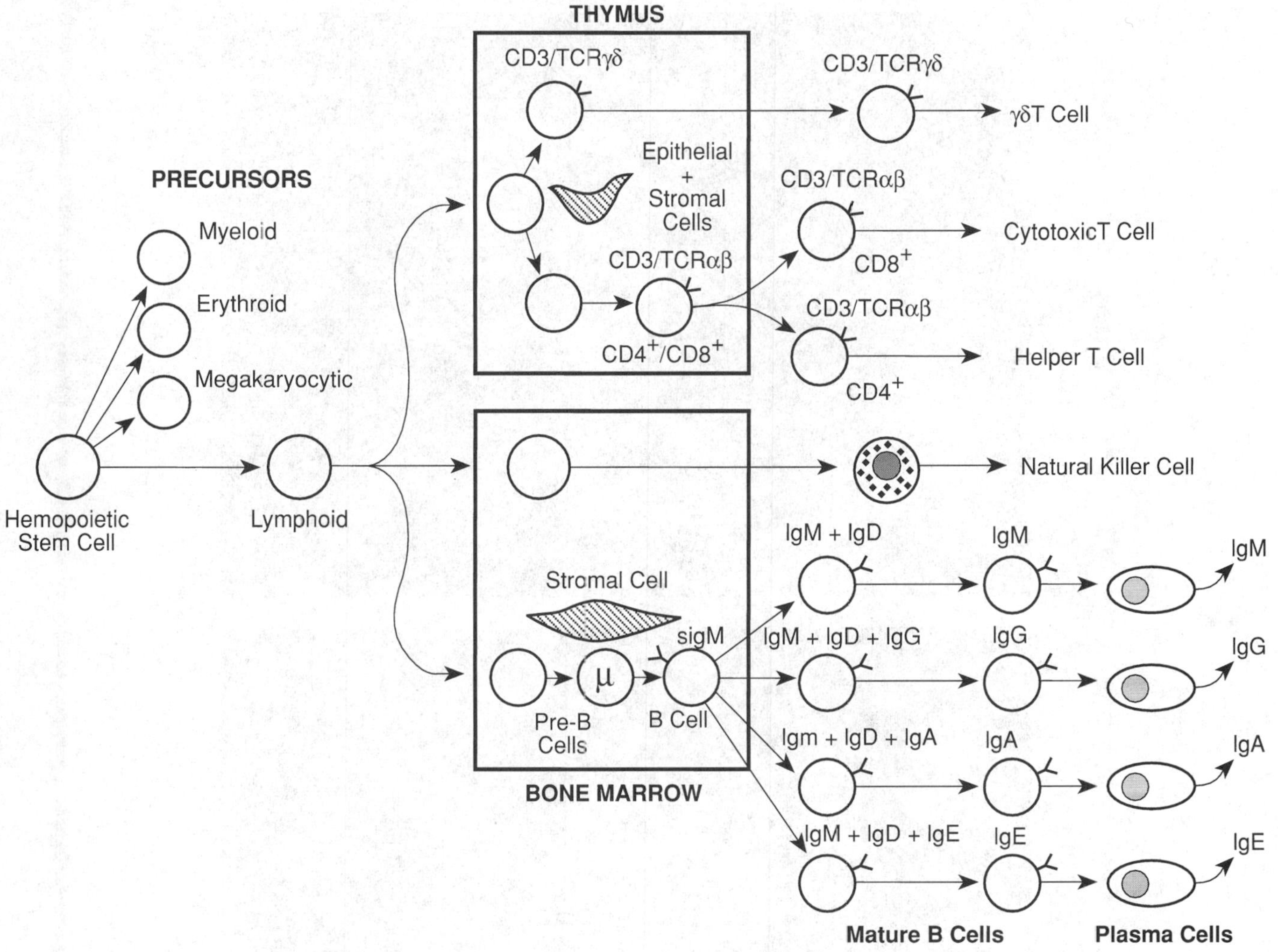

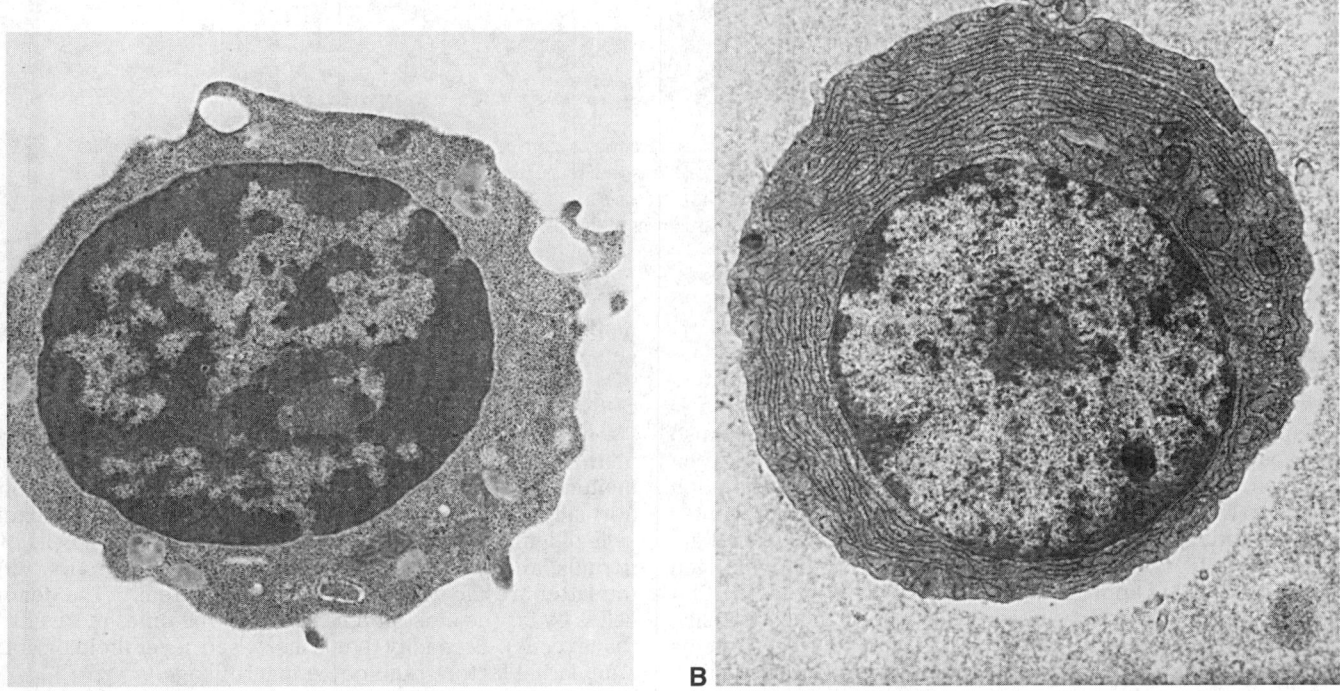

THYMUS

CD3/TCRγδ

CD3/TCRγδ → γδT Cell

PRECURSORS

Myeloid

Erythroid

Megakaryocytic

Epithelial
+
Stromal
Cells

CD3/TCRαβ

CD3/TCRαβ
CD8$^+$ → CytotoxicT Cell

CD4$^+$/CD8$^+$

CD3/TCRαβ
CD4$^+$ → Helper T Cell

Hemopoietic
Stem Cell

Lymphoid

→ Natural Killer Cell

Stromal Cell

sigM

IgM + IgD   IgM   IgM

μ

IgM + IgD + IgG   IgG   IgG

Pre-B   B Cell
Cells

Igm + IgD + IgA   IgA   IgA

BONE MARROW

IgM + IgD + IgE   IgE   IgE

Mature B Cells   Plasma Cells

Fig. 8-2. Overview of lymphocyte differentiation. All lymphocytes originate from a hematopoietic stem cell. αβ and γδ T cells arise independently. Natural killer cells share some features with T cells, but they mature in the bone marrow and do not rearrange T-cell receptor genes.

A

B

Fig. 8-3. Electron micrographs of **(A)** a quiescent B cell and **(B)** a plasma cell. The plasma cell is rich in endoplasmic reticulum, the hallmark of protein secretion. (X12,000.)

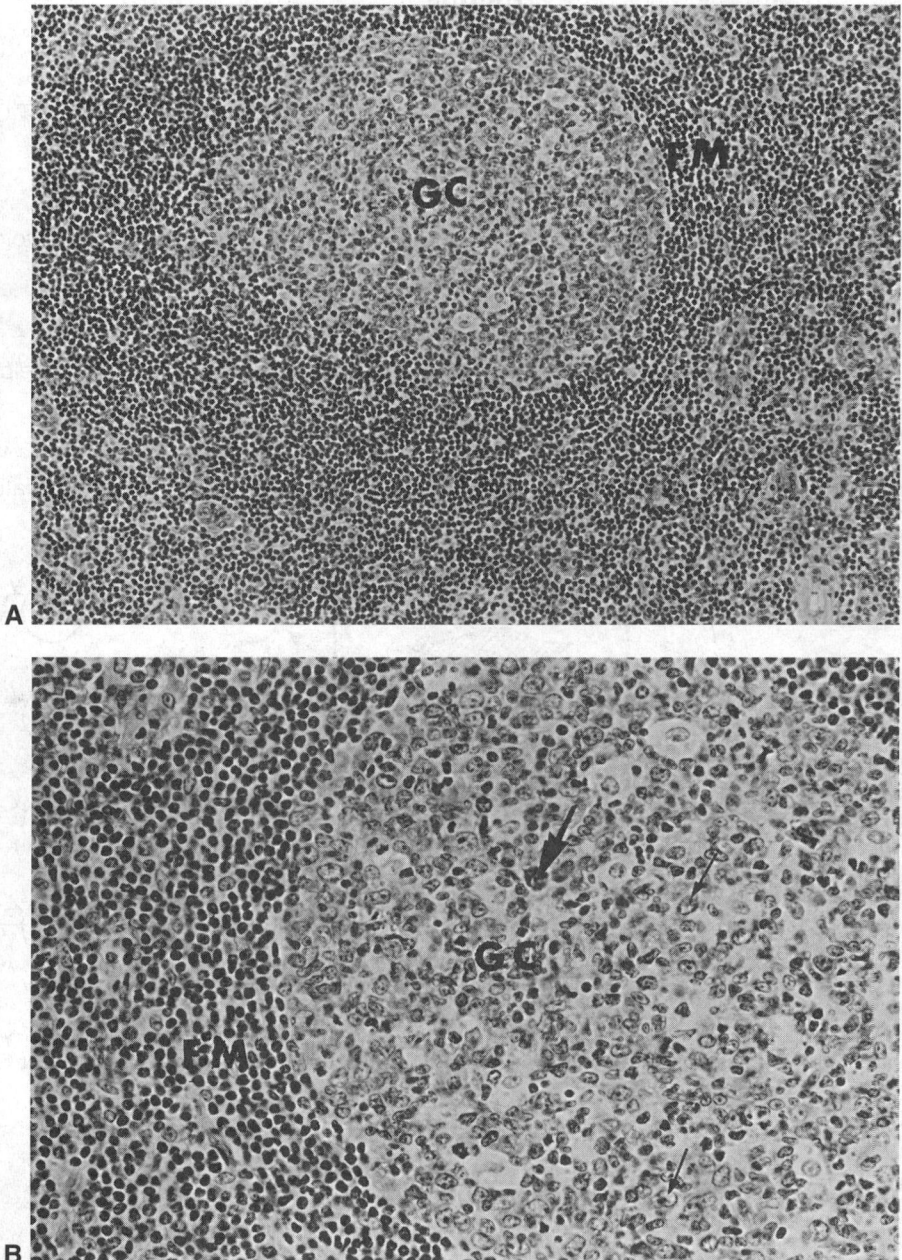

Fig. 8-4. Human lymph node. **(A)** The lymphatic follicle contains a prominent germinal center (GC) surrounded by the follicular mantle (FM). (x200.) **(B)** The germinal center is crowded with large, pale cells with round nuclei (centroblasts, thin arrows), among which a few macrophages laden with debris, the tingible bodies (thick arrow), are visible. The follicular mantle (FM) is pushed away by the expanded germinal center. (x400.) (Courtesy of Dr. Ronald Delellis, Department of Pathology, New England Medical Center.)

referred to as MHC-restriction. CD4⁺ T cells are class II restricted, whereas CD8⁺ T cells are class I restricted.[17]

The CD4 and CD8 surface molecules participate in T-cell activation; their cytoplasmic regions are physically linked to a T-cell-specific tyrosine kinase termed p56^{lck}. CD4 and CD8 also serve as adhesion molecules; they increase the bond between the T cell and the APC (or target cell).[18] This stabilizing function is important because the binding affinity of the T-cell receptor for the peptide/HLA complex in vitro is relatively low (Kd approximately 10^{-5}; by comparison, a typical antibody/antigen affinity has a Kd of approximately 10^{-9}). The ligand of the CD4 protein is an invariant region of class II MHC glycoproteins, whereas the CD8 protein binds to class I MHC glycoproteins (Fig. 8-11). Hence, class II/peptide complexes stimulate CD4⁺

helper T cells, whereas class I/peptide complexes are the targets of CD8⁺ cytotoxic T cells. These adhesive properties of CD4 and CD8 account for the MHC restriction of CD4⁺ and CD8⁺ T cells. All nucleated cells (and platelets) express class I MHC glycoproteins. This is why virus-infected epithelial cells, neurons, and erythroblasts are susceptible to destruction by immune CD8⁺ T cells. By contrast, class II MHC glycoproteins normally occur only on certain cells: macrophages, dendritic cells of lymphoid tissue and skin, B cells, epithelial cells of the thymus, and primitive hematopoietic cell precursors. All but the latter are the APCs of the immune system.[19] The dendritic cell is by far the most potent APC (50–100 times more efficient than B cells), a capacity that is increased severalfold by colony-stimulating factor-granulocyte/macrophage.

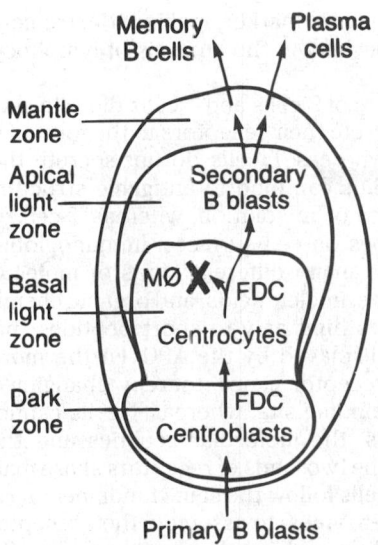

Fig. 8-5. Diagrammatic representation of a germinal center showing possible relationships between centroblasts and centrocytes. FDC, follicular dendritic cell; MØ, macrophage. (From Osmond,[91] with permission.)

Natural Killer Cells

NK cells, a peculiar subset of T cells, are cytolytic; unlike conventional CD8$^+$ cytotoxic T cells, they are not MHC restricted. NK cells do not depend on a prior immune stimulus for their lytic function (hence, their name); they are even present in mice lacking all conventional T cells and B cells, such as mice with severe combined immunodeficiency (SCID). NK cells are notable for their ability to kill virus-infected cells and tumor cells in vitro, and they probably have similar effects in vivo. Their large azurophilic cytoplasmic granules place them in the group of large granular lymphocytes (LGLs), of which there are two main types: NK cells, which lack T-cell receptors,

and a subset of CD8$^+$ T cells with surface T-cell receptors. These CD8$^+$ LGLs are atypical because their in vitro lytic effects are not MHC restricted; they are probably functional variants of conventional CD8$^+$ T cells that have been hyperactivated by IL-2. NK cells and conventional T cells share certain surface markers, such as CD7 and CD38, but CD56, an adhesion molecule, is relatively specific for NK cells.[21] NK cells are likely a distinct lineage that arises from the same precursor as conventional T cells. Benign LGL lymphoproliferative disorders, often associated with an autoimmune disease, and leukemia arising from LGLs have been described.[20]

Clinical Implications

The historic work that defined the two main types of lymphocytes has had a major impact on hematology. Classification of leukemias and lymphomas into B-cell and T-cell types is now routine. The methods of identifying cell lineage with immunohistochemical and FACS techniques—now standard practice—have substantial clinical value. For example, the morphologic diagnosis of acute leukemia can be difficult when the leukemic cells are undifferentiated blasts: are they lymphoblasts or myeloblasts? In these instances, phenotypic FACS analysis of the cells with monoclonal antibodies specific for lymphocytes, myeloid cells, and their subsets is very useful. Therapeutic decisions in acute leukemia hinge on accurate identification of the leukemic cell's lineage. The classification of lymphomas into B-cell or T-cell types also has important clinical applications. In general, B-cell lymphomas are associated with a more favorable prognosis than are T-cell lymphomas and are more likely than T-cell lymphomas to respond well to chemotherapy. The pathologic classification of lymphomas is also crucial, as knowledge of the histology and function of normal lymphatic tissue is key to understanding the terminology used by pathologists. Finally, the widespread therapeutic application of bone marrow transplantation requires familiarity with the genetics, serology, and immunology of the HLA system.

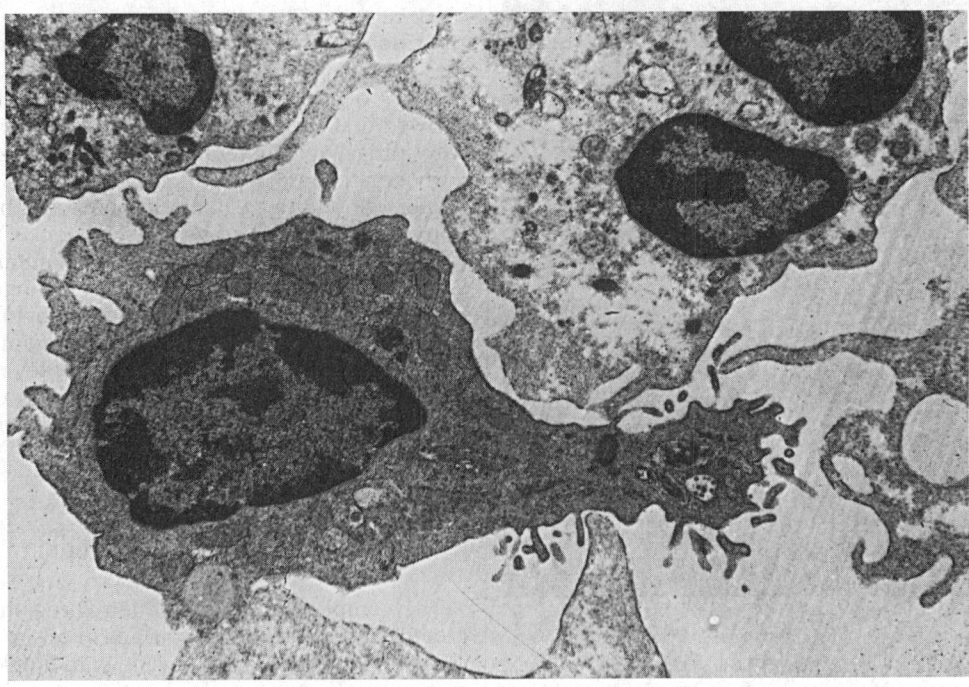

Fig. 8-6. Lymphocyte moving between two cells by means of its uropod. ($\times$ 10,000.)

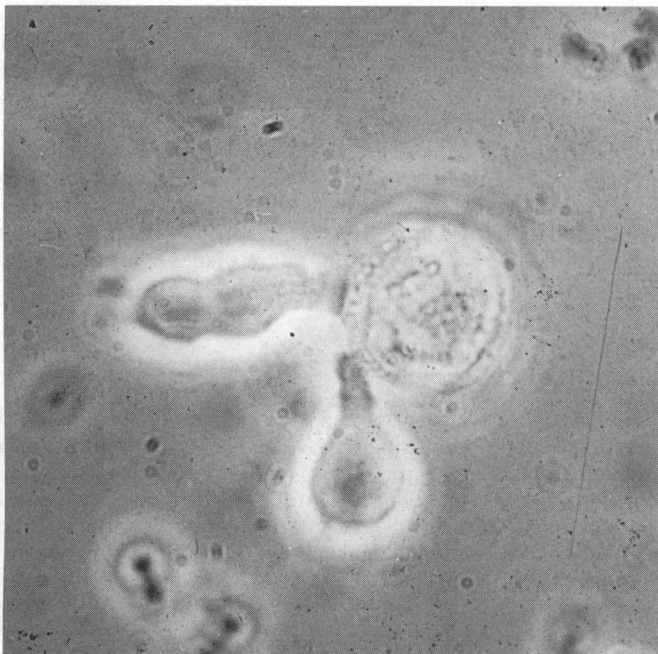

Fig. 8-7. Phase-constrast micrograph of two lymphocytes attached to a monocyte by their uropods. Note the broad adherent region of the uropod. (x 400.) (Courtesy of Dr. W. J. Mitus, Carney Hospital, Dorchester, MA.)

STRUCTURE AND MOLECULAR GENETICS OF ANTIGEN RECEPTORS

If there is one defining feature of lymphocytes, it is clonal diversity. No other cell lineage is as diverse as the lymphocyte because each clonal progenitor of a mature lymphocyte builds a structurally unique antigen receptor. The antigen receptor

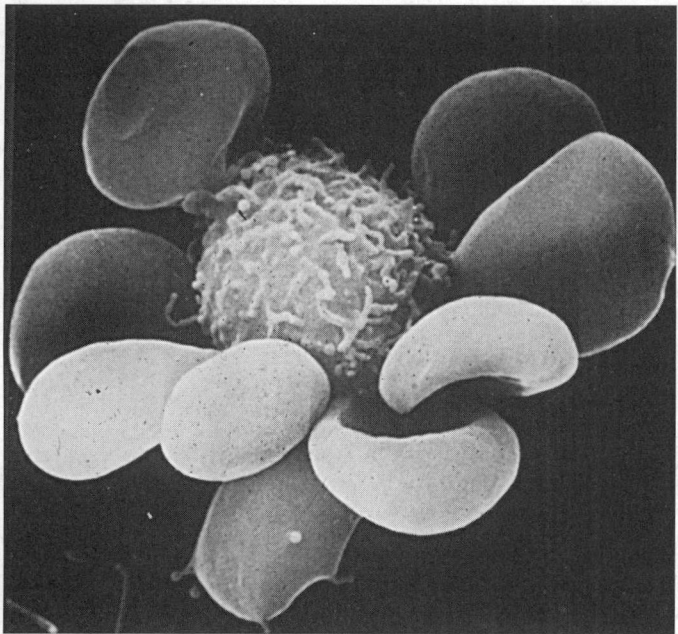

Fig. 8-8. Scanning electron micrograph of a human T cell surrounded by a rosette of mouse erythrocytes. Note the ruffled surface of the T cell. (x 5,000.) (Courtesy of Dr. Henry Wortis, Department of Pathology, Tufts University School of Medicine.)

is therefore a clonal marker, making it extremely useful in hematology, especially in the analysis of lymphocytic malignancies.

The receptors of B cells and T cells differ in several respects. B cells can secrete their receptors in the form of soluble immunoglobulins, whereas T cells do not secrete their receptors. Immunoglobulins can bind to antigenic structures (epitopes) on cell surfaces or in solution, whereas T-cell receptors bind only to epitopes on cell surfaces. Immunoglobulins can bind to epitopes on many different kinds of molecules, including proteins, sugars, nucleic acids, and organic chemicals, whereas T-cell receptors bind only to short peptides that occupy the MHC groove displayed by the APC. Furthermore, B cells can mutate their receptor genes, thereby changing the affinity of the receptor binding site, whereas T cells cannot.

Nevertheless, the molecular genetics and the phenotypic properties of the two kinds of receptors share many properties. B cells and T cells follow the same fundamental rules, and even use the same enzymes, to assemble their receptor genes. Both immunoglobulins and T-cell receptors consist of disulfide-linked polypeptides; both contain constant (C) and variable (V) regions.[22,23] Immunoglobulins have nine kinds of heavy (H) chains (IgM, four subclasses of IgG, IgA, IgD, and IgE, also called μ-, γ-, α-, δ-, and ϵ-chains) and two kinds of light (L) chains (κ and λ). Identical pairs of H and L chains (e.g., μ_2/κ_2) form the immunoglobulin molecule (Fig. 8-12). There are also two kinds of T-cell receptor pairs, $\alpha\beta$ and $\gamma\delta$.[24] Most T cells, perhaps 90%, express the $\alpha\beta$ heterodimer; γ/δ T cells occur principally in the mucosal surfaces of the intestinal tract, the vagina, and the skin. They constitute a subset of T cells that specialize in the response to certain types of bacterial antigens, among which heat shock proteins are notable.[25,26]

Variable Region

In both immunoglobulins and the T-cell receptor, the V region of each paired chain contains subregions (unfortunately, they are also called "regions") termed hypervariable regions, or complementarity determining regions (CDRs) and framework regions (FRs). This nomenclature refers to segments of the V domain that have maximal (CDR) or minimal (FR) tendencies to vary in amino acid sequence (Fig. 8-13). A statistical analysis of immunoglobulin V region amino acid sequences, showed that the CDRs contain the residues that make contact with antigens. This hypothesis was subsequently verified by x-ray crystallography, which showed that the six CDRs of the immunoglobulin V region fold on each other to form the antibody's antigen-binding surface (or pocket).[27] By contrast, the FRs comprise an infrastructure that maintains the three-dimensional shape of the V region. The arrangement in the T-cell receptor is similar.[28,29] Both in immunoglobulins and in the T-cell receptor, the third hypervariable region (CDR3) is the most diverse part of the V region. It plays a key role in antigen binding. And, because of its great structural diversity, CDR3 has important clinical applicability as a clonal marker in diagnostic hematology.

Constant Region

The complete immunoglobulin C region occurs only in secreted antibodies. It is invariant in all immunoglobulins of a particular class or subtype. The immunoglobulin C region mediates the effector functions of the antibody (e.g., complement fixation, binding to mast cells), and its compact globular shape

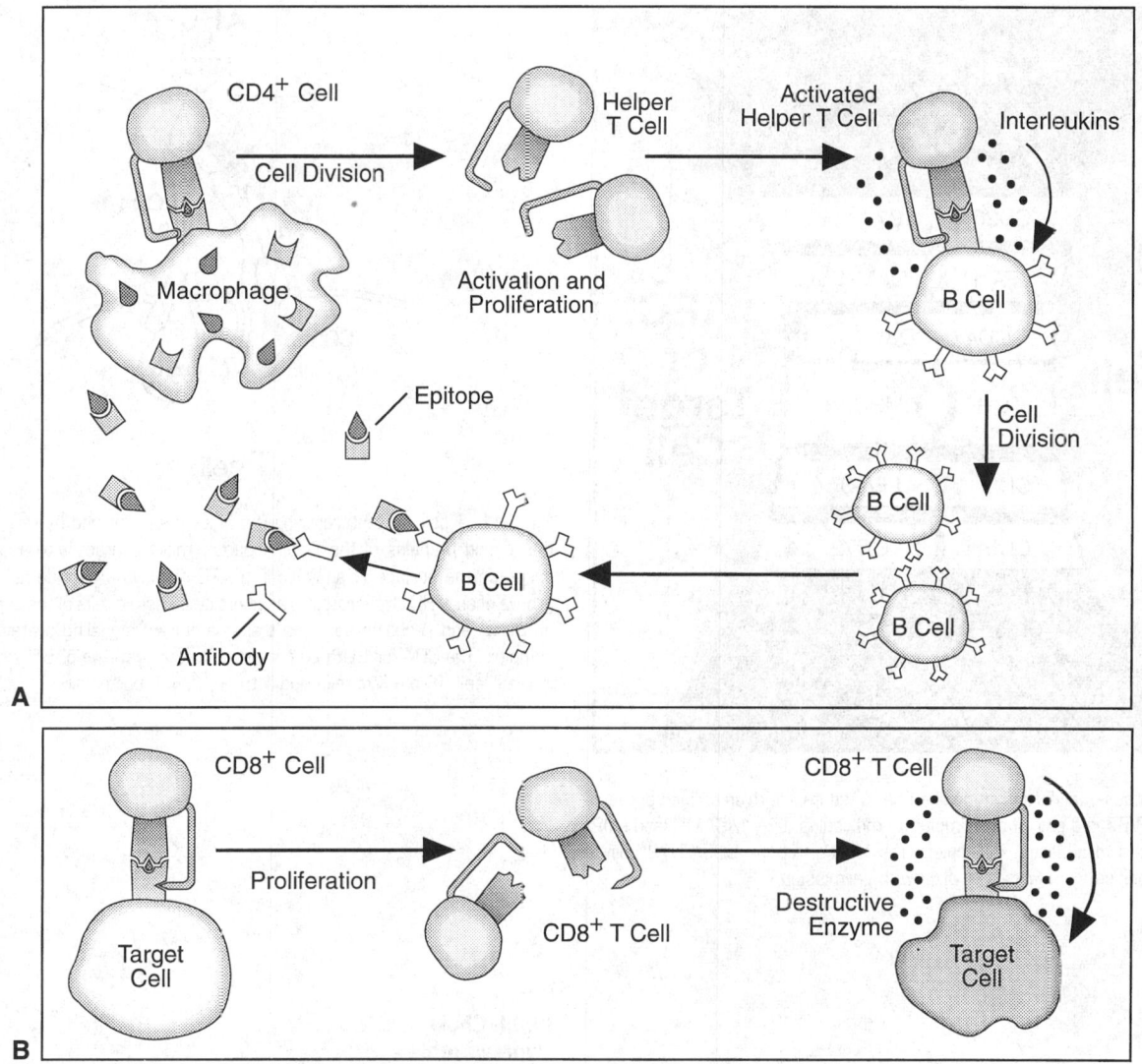

Fig. 8-9. (A) Helper and **(B)** cytotoxic T cells. Aided by co-stimulator molecules, CD4⁺ T cells become activated and proliferate when their antigen receptors bind to peptide/class II MHC complexes on APCs. The activated helper T cells bind to antigen-presenting B cells by means of adhesion molecules, the CD4 co-receptor, and their antigen-specific receptors. T-cell interleukins and intimate cell-cell contact stimulate B cells to proliferate and to differentiate into antibody-secreting plasma cells. CD8⁺ T cells (Fig. B) proliferate when their antigen receptors bind to a peptide presented by class I MHC molecules and their CD8 co-receptors bind to the invariant region of a class I MHC molecule on the surface of a target cell. Lymphokines released by activated helper T cells (e.g., IL-2) and other co-stimulatory molecules enable efficient proliferation of the CD8⁺ cells. The activated cytotoxic cell, in intimate contact with the target through adhesion molecules, releases perforins and other polypeptides from its cytolytic granules. These polypeptides induce lysis of the target cell. (Modified from von Boehmer and Kisielow,[92] with permission.)

stabilizes the molecule's folded V region. The C region of the T-cell receptor has no known effector function.

Receptor Complexes of B Cells and T Cells

The receptors of both T cells and B cells associate noncovalently with other transmembrane proteins that act as signal transducers[30,31] (Fig. 8-14). The B-cell receptor complex consists of the surface immunoglobulin molecule and four proteins termed Ig-α, Ig-β, CD19, and CD22. These four members of the complex are substrates for protein tyrosine kinases; they compensate for the limited signaling function of the very short cytoplasmic tail of the surface immunoglobulin (only three amino acids). CD22 has an additional property: it is an adhesion protein that enhances interactions between B cells and T cells. A fifth protein, CD21 (or CR2), the B-cell surface receptor for C3dg

(a breakdown product of the third component of complement), associates with CD19 on the membrane.[30] The CD19/CD21 proteins may engender activation of B cells that encounter complement-fixing antigen/antibody complexes.

The T-cell receptor also has a very short cytoplasmic tail; it too occurs in noncovalent association with other transmembrane proteins, three of which make up the CD3 complex: CD3γ, -δ, and -ε. They have highly similar structures and probably arose by gene duplication. Two other proteins, ζ and η, are also linked to the T-cell receptor; ζ can occur as a ζ–ζ disulfide-linked homodimer or as a ζ–η disulfide-linked heterodimer. These two polypeptides have very short (6–9 amino acids) extracellular domains. All these transmembrane proteins stabilize the conformation of the receptor and augment its signaling function by interacting with protein tyrosine kinases of the *src* family or other signaling pathways.[32,33]

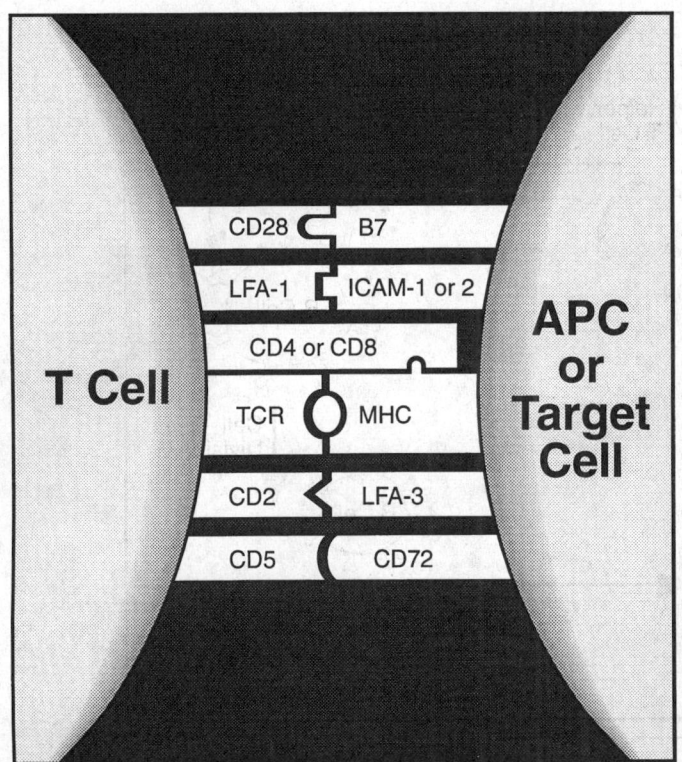

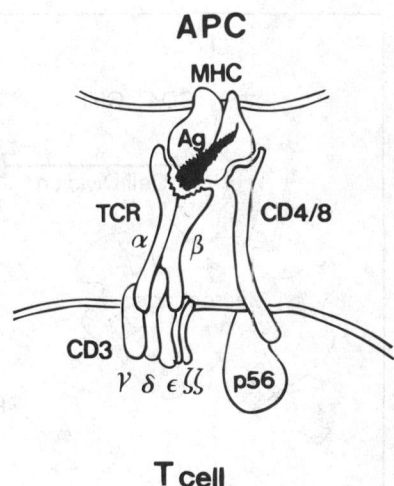

Fig. 8-11. T cell APC interaction. The binding site formed by variable regions of the α- and β-chains of the T-cell receptor make contact with a complementary shape on the surface of an APC. The APC displays a peptide held in the major groove of an MHC glycoprotein. The short cytoplasmic tails of the constant regions of the α- and β-chains abut the transmembrane signaling proteins of the CD3 complex. The CD4 (or CD8) co-receptors link up with the p56[lck] signaling protein in the T cell. (From Mustelin and Altman,[94] with permission.)

Fig. 8-10. Antigen-specific activation of a T cell by contact with an antigen-presenting cell. CD28/B7 is a pair of co-stimulatory molecules; LFA-1/ICAM-1 and CD2/LFA-3 are pairs of adhesion molecules. The function of the CD5/CD72 pair is unknown. (Modified from Fraser et al,[93] with permission.)

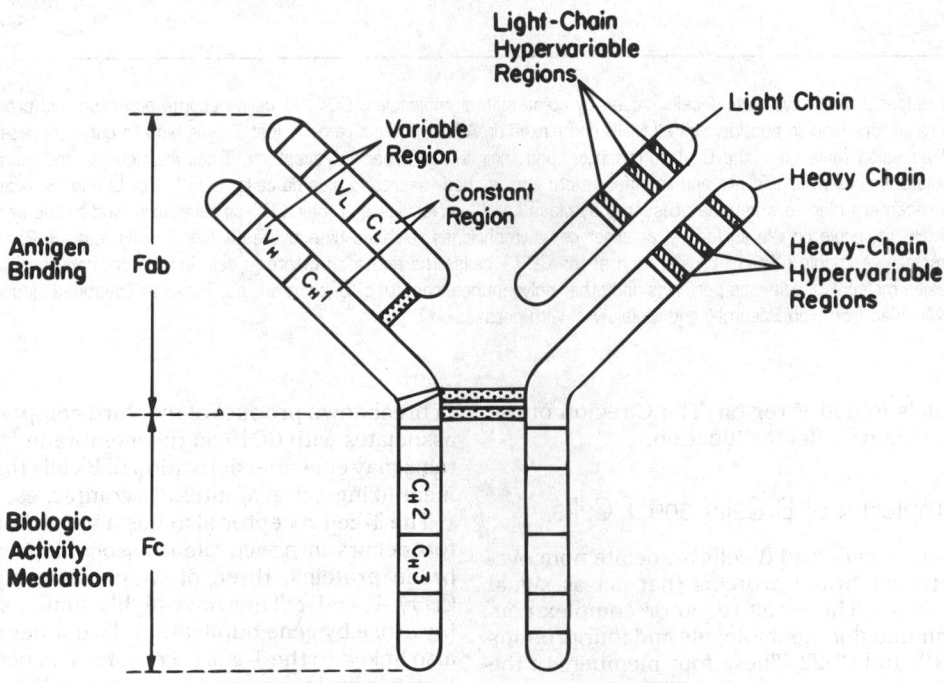

Fig. 8-12. Diagrammatic representation of an immunoglobulin molecule. Hatched bars indicate the hypervariable regions of the H and L chains. Dotted bars represent disulfide bridges. Limited proteolytic digestion splits the molecule into two regions that contain the variable (Fab) and constant (Fc) domains.

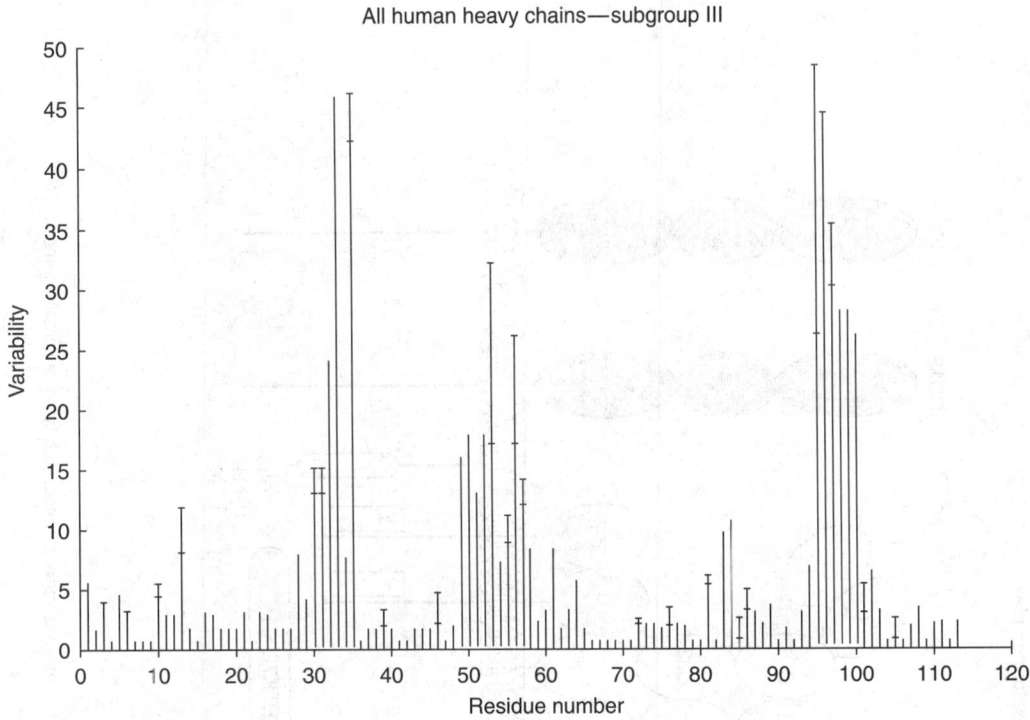

Fig. 8-13. Wu–Kabat variability plot. The three hypervariable regions stand out clearly from the relatively invariant framework regions. (From Kabat et al,[95] with permission.)

Immunoglobulin *V* Genes

The key to the clonal diversity of lymphocytes is that discrete physically separate gene segments link up to form the coding unit for a variable region polypeptide. This process is called *V* gene recombination or *V* gene rearrangement.[34,35] Before fusing, the individual *V* gene segments are in their germline configuration; after joining, they are recombined or rearranged. The molecular genetics of the immunoglobulin V region are summarized first, followed by a review of the formation of the T-cell receptor variable region. The general principles under consideration apply both to B cells and to T cells.

Light Chains

The genetic elements that encode the L chain V region are V_κ and J_κ and V_λ and J_λ (Fig. 8-15). The immunoglobulin κ-locus, on chromosome 2, contains a single C_κ gene, about 70 different V_κ genes, and 5 J_κ genes. The V_λ locus, on chromosome 22, has about 40 V_λ segments and 6 J_λ segments, each linked to a C_λ gene. The coding region for the V_κ polypeptide forms when one V_κ segment joins to one J_κ gene segment. Each V_κ segment contains its own promoter; a leader sequence important for L chain secretion; and an exon that, from 5′ → 3′, encodes FR1, CDR1, FR2, CDR2, and the NH_2-terminal part of CDR3. Recombination signals specific to *V* segments restrict joint formation to *V-J*, thereby preventing sterile *V-V* or *J-J* splicing (Fig. 8-16). The *J* segments also have a recombination signal, followed by an exon that encodes the remainder of CDR3 and FR4.

During B-cell differentiation, one V_κ segment joins to one J_κ segment by inversion or deletion of the intervening DNA, depending on the transcriptional orientation of the V_κ segment. (The orientation of most V_κ segments is 5′ → 3′, but in some cases it is 3′ → 5′.) Two proteins, RAG-1 and RAG-2, are essential for the recombination of *V* gene DNA. Their role in *V* gene recombination is unclear. These enzymes are only active in immature B cells; the mature B cell therefore has a fixed *V* gene rearrangement by the time it leaves the bone marrow.

Recombination can generate approximately 350 different V_L regions because any one of about 70 V_κ segments can juxtapose to any one of the 5 J_κ segments. The L chain repertoire acquires even more diversity by enzymatic digestion of the joining ends of V_κ and J_κ. This nibbling process can remove ≤5 basepairs (bp) from the V_κ-J_κ junctional sequence. The somatic modification of the junction by exonucleases highlights the importance of CDR3, formed by *V-J* joining, in the diversification of V_L chains. Splicing mechanisms remove the introns from the transcribed unit to yield a mature V_L-C mRNA product of approximately 1.2 kb.[36]

It is important to appreciate that recombinatorial pairing and nibbling are random events. No genetic program dictates which of the B cell's two alleles initiates recombination, which V_κ and J_κ segments join in a given B cell, or which nucleotides are removed by the exonucleases. Thus, not only does each clone construct a unique V region coding unit, but the probability of a repetition of that clone's V region sequence in another clone is extremely low.

Allelic Exclusion

The polypeptide product of a successfully assembled V_L coding region suppresses V_L gene rearrangement on the opposite allele. This process of allelic exclusion, a rule applied equally to V_L, V_H, and T-cell receptor genes, forces the B-cell clone to express only one species of L chain and a single type of H chain. In a substantial proportion of instances, the developing B cell must pause, because joining and nibbling introduced untranslatable nonsense reading frames into its V_κ-J_κ junctions. When

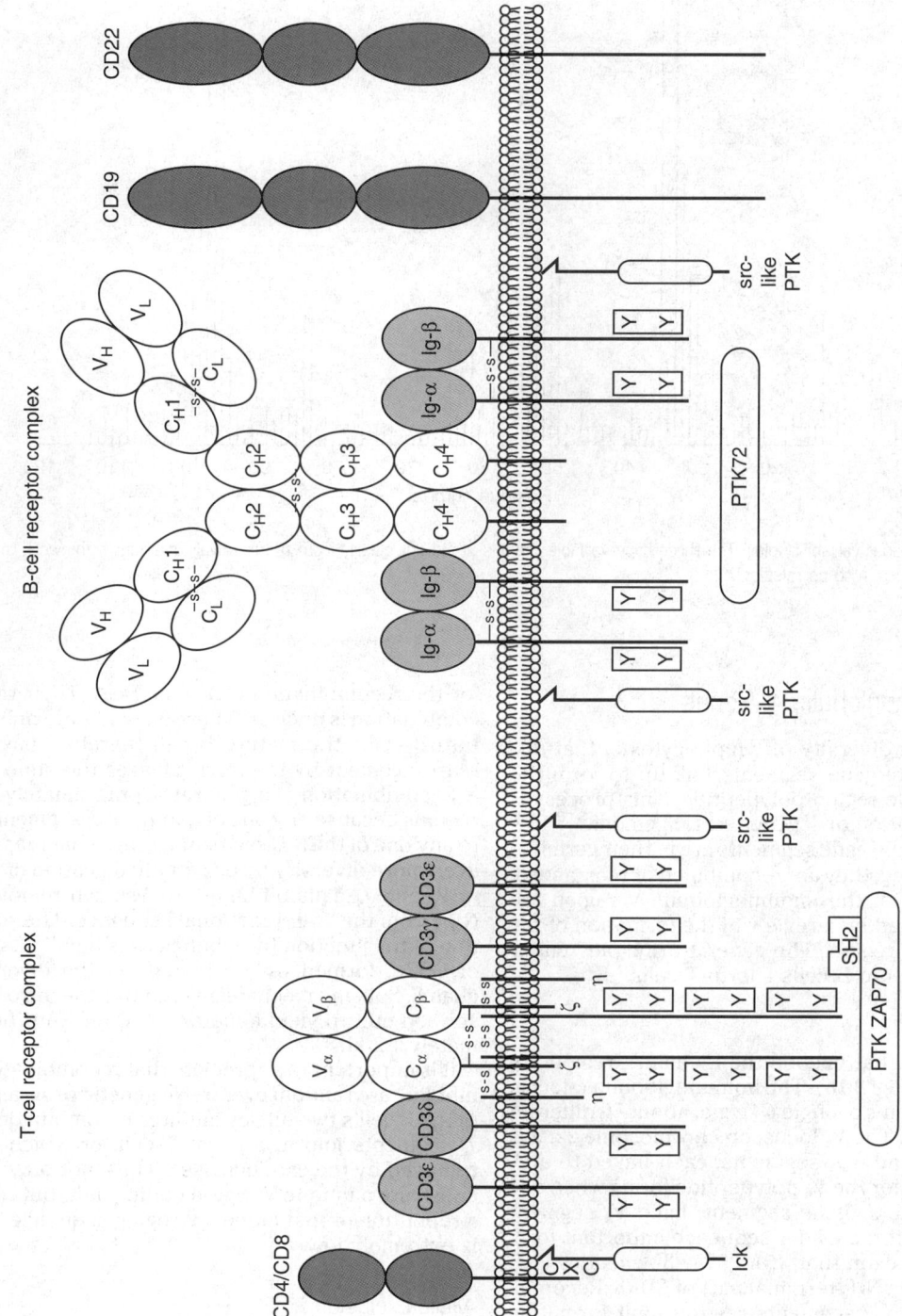

Fig. 8-14. Receptor complexes of T cells and B cells. The cytoplasmic tails of the main components of the complexes make contacts with tyrosine-containing motifs (Y Y) in cytosolic signaling components. (Modified from Borst et al,[30] with permission.)

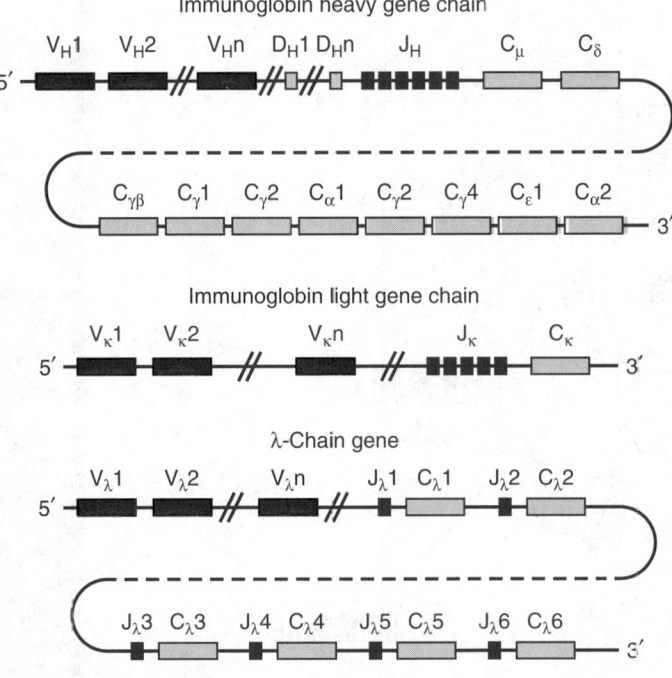

Fig. 8-15. Immunoglobulin H and L chain loci.

intervening DNA. Extensive diversity of the V_H CDR3 results from three mechanisms. One mechanism is nibbling of the terminal nucleotides of the V_H, D, and J_H segments. In contrast with V_L gene segments, ≤ 20 bp can be removed by exonucleases in the V_H-D-J_H joints. The second diversifying mechanism is the random addition, through the action of terminal deoxytransferase (TdT), of ≤ 20 nucleotides (N nucleotides, or N additions) at the D-J_H and V_H-D junctions. N nucleotides are unusual (or few) in V_L coding units because by the time the differentiating B cell begins to rearrange its L chain genes, levels of TdT are low, or production of the enzyme has stopped. An additional one or two bases that are complementary to the coding region termini (p nucleotides) can be appended to junctions that elude exonuclease nibbling. The third source of V_H diversity consists of special properties of the D segment, such as D–D fusion, which enable it to encode six different peptides.

These somatic modifications of the junctional regions give the V_H repertoire remarkable diversity. Potentially, the system can generate $>10^{14}$ CDR3s. Not all these combinations are translatable, so the number of possible functional CDR3s is less—probably 10^{12}. Since each CDR3 is clone specific, the V_H CDR3 is, in essence, a clonal B-cell marker. Its sequence can thus serve as a molecular probe for the kinds of monoclonal populations that occur in B-cell neoplasms. The pairing in the B-cell cytoplasm of independently produced H and L chains according to chemical, and not genetic, rules further increases immunoglobulin (and clonal) diversity.

Isotype Switch

Virgin B cells in the germinal center undergo remarkable changes when they interact with antigen on the fimbriated surfaces of follicular dendritic cells and with activated T cells. One important outcome of this engagement is the isotype switch, whereby the B cell converts from the synthesis of IgM to the production of IgG, IgA, or IgE.[38,39] The IgM → IgA switch is typical of B cells in lymphatic tissues of the gut; the dominant change in other lymphatic tissues is IgM → IgG. IgG antibodies, the major immunoglobulin class in normal serum (Fig. 8-18 and Table 8-3), are characteristic of antigen-stimulated B cells.

Isotype switching depends on the binding of a B-cell surface protein termed CD40 to a ligand for CD40 on activated T cells.[40] Studies of patients with X-linked immunoglobulin deficiency (HIGMX-1) have demonstrated the importance of these two proteins. The underlying defect in this immunodeficiency disease is an inability of B cells to undergo isotype switching. The serum of patients with HIGMX-1 contains normal or elevated levels of IgM, but no IgG, IgA, or IgE. Normal numbers of circulating B cells are present, none of which expresses surface IgG or IgA. Boys with the disease suffer from recurrent pyogenic infections, autoimmune diseases, and lymphomas. B cells from patients with HIGMX-1 express functionally normal CD40 molecules, and can synthesize IgG or IgE in vitro when treated with a cross-linking anti-CD40 monoclonal antibody. However, activated T cells from HIGMX-1 patients fail to express the CD40 ligand, and cannot mediate isotype switching in vitro. The molecular defect in HIGMX-1 may be due to a mutation in the CD40 ligand gene.

such defective or "abortive" rearrangements occur, the B cell tries again by rearranging the V_κ genes on the other allele. If the second attempt fails, the B-cell then rearranges its V_λ gene segments. The V_λ segments undergo rearrangement only if V_κ rearrangement miscarries. Since about 40% of B cells express V_λ L chains, V_κ rearrangements succeed only 60% of the time. B cells that fail to rearrange a functional V_λ coding unit die in the bone marrow.

Heavy Chains

Formation of the V_H coding unit is more complex than assembly of the V_L gene because there are three different kinds of V gene segments, V_H, D, and J_H, and nine different C_H segments. However, the general principles we have outlined for L chain coding units apply to H chain coding units. The IgH locus, on chromosome 14, contains, in $5' \to 3'$ order, about 100 functional V_H segments, 30 D segments, and 6 J_H segments[37] (Fig. 8-15). The numerous V_H segments fall into seven families (V_H1–V_H7); members of each family have $\geq 80\%$ sequence homology. The largest family is V_H3; V_H5, V_H6, and V_H7 contain only one or two functional segments. Members of these families occur in no particular order in the locus.* The V_H segments encode FR1, CDR1, FR2, CDR2, FR3, and the NH_2-terminal portion of CDR3. The D segment contains sequences for the middle of CDR3; J_H segments encode the remainder of the V_H polypeptide.

The B cell begins to form the H chain coding unit early in its differentiation, in almost all instances before rearranging its V_κ segments. The initial step is the joining of a D segment to a J_H segment; the resulting D-J_H combination then joins to a V_H segment (Fig. 8-17). A looping-out mechanism excises the inter-

---

*A new nomenclature designates individual V_H genes according to family and position in relation to the 3′ end of the locus (e.g., 3–23 is a V_H3 family gene that is the 23rd V_H gene from the 3′ side of IgH). This system may find wide acceptance because many V_H genes are burdened by multiple labels; in fact 3–23 has at least four other names.

Table 8-3. Immunoglobulins in Blood

Immunoglobulin	Level (mg/dl)
IgM	0.3–2.5
IgG	5.0–14
IgA	0.5–5.0
IgE	—
IgD	0.01

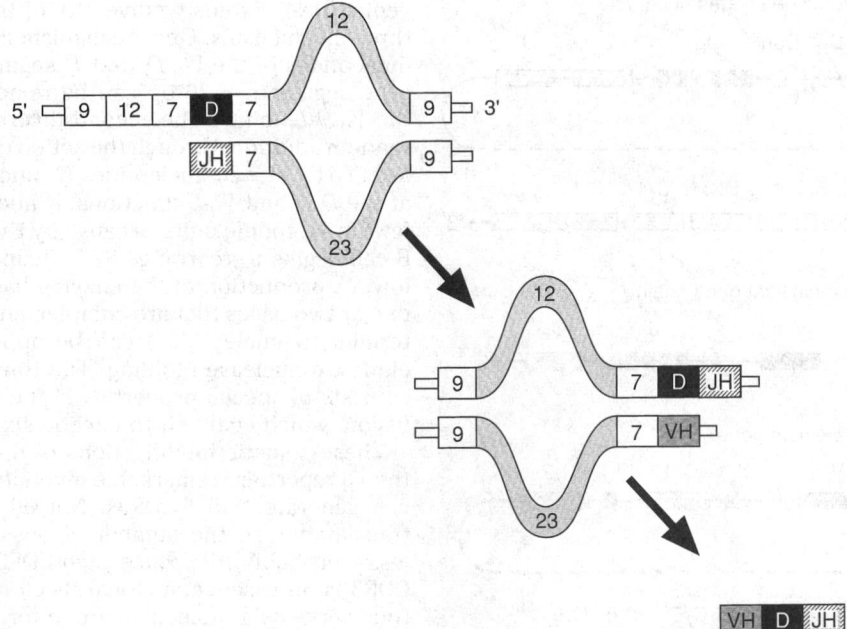

Fig. 8-16. Mechanism of joining of V region segments. Introns containing conserved heptamer (7), spacer (12), and nonamer (9) sequences flank the *D* segment. Identical heptamers and nonamers flank the J_H segment, but its spacer contains 23 instead of 12 bp. Recombination occurs only if one *V* gene segment has a 12-bp spacer, and the other a 23-bp spacer. Hybridization of the D heptamer with the J_H heptamer and of the D nonamer with the J_H nonamer causes the unmatched spacers of the D and J_H spacers to form loops. These looped introns are excised, forming a *D-J_H* joint. A similar process joins a V_H segment to the *D-J_H* pair. Although RAG-1 and RAG-2 are essential, the role of these proteins in *V* gene recombination is unknown.

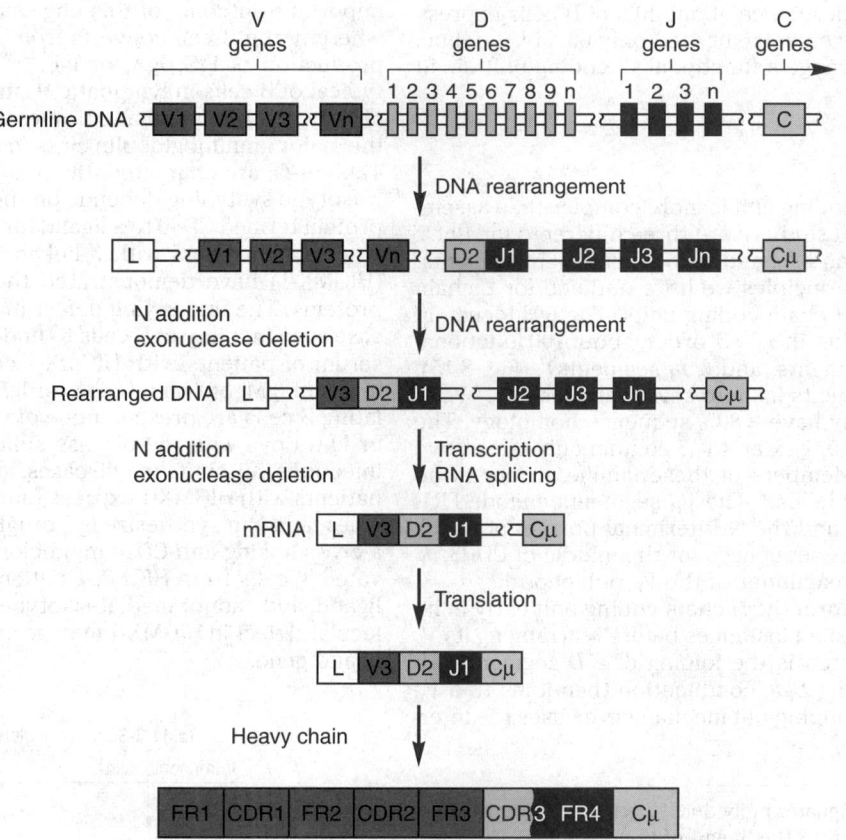

Fig. 8-17. Formation of a H chain coding region by *V* gene segment rearrangement; exonuclease deletions of terminal bases (nibbling) and N additions mediated by TdT further diversify the molecule.

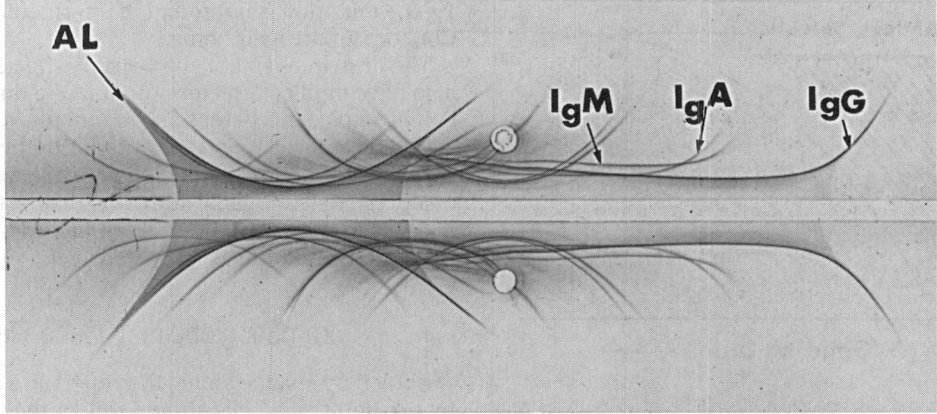

Fig. 8-18. Immunoelectrophoresis of normal serum. In this procedure, a glass microscope slide was coated with agar, normal serum was placed in the central round wells, and the serum proteins were separated electrophoretically. Next, serum from a rabbit immunized against whole human serum was added to the slot between the two samples. The rabbit antibodies and the human proteins diffused through the agar and formed precipitin bands where they met. The immunoprecipitates were stained with Coomassie blue to enhance visualization. The three main immunoglobulins (IgG, IgA, IgM) are clearly visible. The minute amounts of IgD and IgE in normal serum cannot be detected by this method. The very long precipitin arcs, especially notable in the case of IgG, are an indication of the molecular diversity of immunoglobulins.

Immunoglobulin D

IgD is an enigmatic B-cell surface molecule.[41] In adults, about 90% of surface IgM$^+$ B cells in the blood co-express IgD; in the bone marrow, only 30–40% of B cells are IgM$^+$/IgD$^+$. B cells use a distinct mechanism of isotype switching for IgD. Expression of the δ-gene, which is close to the μ-gene in the IgH locus, does not involve the usual V_H class-switch DNA rearrangement, but an alternative route of RNA processing in which a long nuclear transcript, V_H-D-J_H-C_μ-C_δ, is differentially spliced into separate V_H-D-J_H-C_μ and V_H-D-J_H-C_δ transcripts. These mRNAs are then translated into μ- and δ-chains. Therefore, the IgM and IgD surface receptors have identical V regions.[42] Activated B cells down-regulate the expression of surface IgD, but not surface IgM. Receptors for IL-6, which induces the differentiation of B cells into immunoglobulin-secreting plasma cells, are present on activated δ$^-$ B cells, but not on resting δ$^+$ resting B cells. Thus, plasma cells do not secrete IgD antibodies, and the serum level of IgD is negligible.

It is not known how the expression of two immunoglobulin isotypes with identical V regions serves the B cell. Surface IgD associates with a co-receptor molecule, IgD-α, which is structurally similar to the IgM-α co-receptor protein that associates with surface IgM. Both IgM-α and IgD-α are disulfide-linked to Ig-β. IgM-α and IgD-α might be products of recently duplicated genes, or the result of alternative splicing of the *mb-1* gene transcript (*mb-1* encodes Ig-α). All these findings suggest that surface IgD, like its IgM counterpart, has a signaling function.[43]

Clonal Selection and Immunoglobulin *V* Gene Mutation

Antigen-activated B cells undergo another process of considerable importance: clonal selection.[44,45] To understand clonal selection, let us consider how it would operate in the case of immunization with an influenza vaccine. Clonal selection depends strictly on the B lymphocyte's surface immunoglobulin—its antigen receptor. As we have seen, the pre-immune repertoire of B cells contains a vast number of structurally different receptors, each specific, through its V region, for a particular B cell clone. In the example under consideration, some B-cell clones in the germinal center would have receptors that bind to influenza virus antigens displayed by follicular dendritic cells. The cross-linking of the IgM receptors of these few cells by influenza virus epitopes transduces intracellular signals that stimulate them to proliferate. Hence, compared to

B cells whose receptors cannot bind the epitope, these activated B cells have an advantage: they have been selected by the antigen for preferential growth.

Clonal selection by antigen triggers an event that occurs only in B cells, and only in germinal center B cells: under the influence of antigen and T cells, activated B cells mutate their *V* genes.[46] The biochemistry of the mutation mechanism is poorly understood, but it has been established that somatic mutations occur only in the coding regions of *V* genes, and only in those *V* genes that have been arranged into a complete V region genetic unit. These antigen-driven mutations can alter the amino acid sequence of the V region, and thus the affinity of the B cell's receptor for the epitope. (Silent mutations, which do not change the amino acid sequence, or replacement mutations that do not affect the variable region's binding surface would not influence the receptor's affinity.) In some instances, the binding capacity of the receptor will be diminished or even abolished by the amino acid substitutions. In others, it will be increased. Mutations that improve receptor affinity protect the clone's growth advantage, whereas mutations that abolish receptor affinity annul the advantage. Somatic mutation of *V* genes thus imposes darwinian competition among B cells; clones with mutations that result in high-affinity receptors eventually dominate over their rivals. As a consequence, the antigen-specific affinity of serum antibodies against the influenza virus rises during the course of the immune response (Fig. 8-19).

By contrast with B cells, T cells are unable to mutate their *V* genes. However, since they do respond to antigenic stimulation by proliferating, they are also susceptible to clonal selection. The immunologic jargon for that process is *clonal expansion*. A T-cell population that has been stimulated by antigen has been "expanded," but the structure of its receptors has not been altered by somatic mutation.

Clinical Implications

The IgM → IgG class switch, somatic mutation of immunoglobulin *V* genes, and high antibody affinity—the hallmarks of a T-cell-dependent B-cell response—have profound biologic and clinical implications. For instance, antibodies with high affinity for a microbial antigen are much more protective than low-affinity antibodies. Moreover, immunoglobulin class switching yields IgG antibodies that can diffuse into interstitial

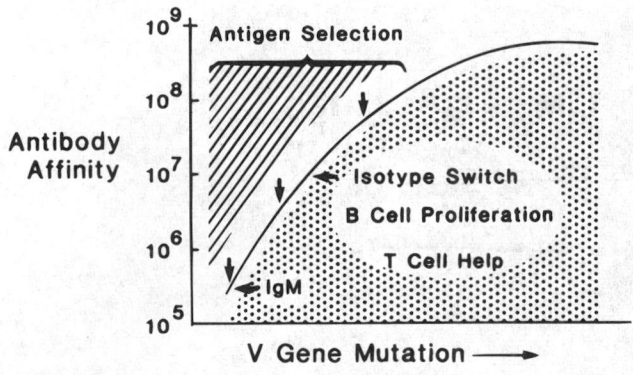

Fig. 8-19. Maturation of the antibody response. Under the influence of antigenic stimulation and T-cell help, B cells undergo the isotype switch (IgM → IgG) and their V genes mutate. There is preferential growth of B cells whose surface immunoglobulin receptors have high affinity for the immunizing antigen. The net result is an increase in affinity of serum antibodies for the immunizing antigen.

fluids; IgM antibodies, by contrast, are too large (M_r approximately 10^6) to leave the blood plasma compartment.

In almost all instances of ALL of B-cell origin, the leukemic cells rearrange their V_H genes; by contrast, V_L gene segment rearrangements occur in less than one-half. Therefore, the CDR3 sequence of the H chain is a more reliable clonal marker than that of the L chain in B-cell ALL. The absence of somatic V gene mutations in B-cell ALL reflects the origin of the disease from early B cells, whose germline V genes cannot mutate.

An abnormality in allelic exclusion, manifested by bi-allelic V_H-D-J_H recombinations, can occur in B-cell ALL. In other instances, more than two rearranged V_H genes have been found, suggesting the presence of multiple malignant clones in the same patient. Deletion of the entire J_H region has also been observed in B-cell ALL.

N addition is developmentally regulated; fetal B cells usually do not introduce N nucleotides, whereas after birth N additions are characteristic, but not universal. In a study of B-cell ALL in children <3 years of age, almost 90% of CDR3s lacked N additions. This finding is a clue that B-cell ALL in young children may arise in utero. In pre-B-cell ALL with residual recombinase and TdT activity, variants with new V_H gene segment arrangements and N additions are common. All the variants in these biclonal or oligoclonal B-cell ALL have the same abnormal karyotype; thus, they arise from a common precursor. In contrast to B-cell ALL, the malignant B cells in Burkitt lymphoma are strictly monoclonal. This difference with B-cell ALL reflects the relative maturity of the neoplastic B cell in Burkitt lymphoma; presumably, the transforming event in that disease occurs after transcription of recombinase and TdT genes has stopped.

Somatic mutations of V genes are frequent in low-grade B-cell lymphoma. This type of lymphoma arises in the germinal center, which is where B cells mutate their immunoglobulin V genes. Additional mutations can occur over time, giving rise to variants of the original lymphoma clone. The clustering of replacement mutations in the CDRs in low-grade lymphoma B cells is typical of the T-cell-dependent antigen-driven immune response in normal B cells. Multiple myeloma also seems to arise from an antigen-driven mechanism. The monoclonal immunoglobulin in myeloma is almost always IgG or IgA, an indication that the neoplastic precursor cell made an isotype switch. Moreover, somatic mutations of immunoglobulin V genes are frequent in the disease. These findings suggest that a persistent antigenic stimulus may have a role in causing, and even perpetuating, low-grade lymphoma and multiple myeloma.[47] In contrast with low-grade lymphoma and myeloma,

V gene mutation is not found in intermediate-grade lymphoma, CLL, or Burkitt lymphoma.

The principles established by investigations of normal B cells also have implications for autoimmune diseases of blood cells. For example, the detection of somatic mutations in V genes encoding anti-red blood cell autoantibodies suggests that some types of autoimmune hemolytic anemia may arise as the result of a persistent antigenic stimulus, that is, that the autoimmune process in these instances is not just the result of nonspecific B-cell activation but is antigen driven (see Ch. 33).

Immunoglobulin V Gene Repertoire

If ruled by chance alone, the repertoire of V genes expressed by pre-immune B cells should reflect the repertoire of V genes in the germline. If the germline contains 100 different functional V_H genes, each having an equal probability of undergoing a productive V_H-D-J_H rearrangement, the proportion of each V_H gene in the expressed pre-immune repertoire should be 1%. However, investigations of this question have shown a bias in the representation of particular V genes in the virgin B-cell repertoire.[48] Indeed, a large fraction of mature B cells with unmutated V_H genes use only a small group of the V_H segments available in the germline. This tendency of the primary repertoire to express certain V genes has been found in fetal, newborn, and adult B cells. Bias in the pre-immune repertoire could originate at the level of either the V gene itself or its phenotype. A gene might have an inherent tendency to rearrange because of its position in the locus; this could give it preferential accessibility to recombinases. The latter may apply to instances of CLL in which abortive rearrangement of V_κ genes were expected (i.e., where the monoclonal B cells had productively rearranged λ L chains). It was found that nonproductive rearrangements of the V_κ gene *humkv*325 occurred 10 times more frequently than expected on the basis of chance alone. At least in the malignant B cells of CLL, therefore, the rearrangement of *humkv*325 was independent of its expression as a polypeptide. This mechanism may also apply to the J_H4 segment, the only J_H segment with conventional recombinase signaling sequences. J_H4 is by far the most frequently expressed J_H segment.

It is also possible that, through its surface immunoglobulin molecule, the immature B cell undergoes a form of antigen-mediated clonal selection. This concept gains support from the demonstrations that the surface H chain and its associated B-cell receptor complex proteins have a signaling function in immature B cells. What ligand triggers these signals? Some investigators have speculated that it is a self-antigen, in line with abundant evidence that the receptors of immature T cells bind to self-peptides (see below). The proposed anti-self properties of H chains of pre-B cells can explain why a large fraction of pre-immune (unmutated V genes) IgM antibodies are low-affinity autoantibodies, the so-called natural autoantibodies present in all normal sera.

Clinical Implications

The high rearrangement frequency of certain V genes in B-cell lymphomas and leukemias may relate to the V gene bias of the normal pre-immune repertoire. For instance, normal B cells, malignant B cells in follicular lymphomas, and B cells that produce monoclonal IgM cold agglutinins frequently express the V_H4.21 segment. The repetition of the same V gene segments in both normal pre-immune B cells and their malignant counterparts suggests that the entire virgin B-cell population is at risk of neoplastic transformation. In other words, the transforming event acts randomly on the entire population.

The immunoglobulin V region polypeptide contains epitopes that can be identified by other antibodies. This serologically defined structure is termed an idiotype; the antibody used for its detection is an anti-idiotype.[49] Some anti-idiotypes detect a three-dimensional structure made up of parts of both the H and L chain V regions. In other cases, anti-idiotypes identify the product of a particular V gene segment. V gene segment-specific anti-idiotypes are especially useful in demonstrating, by immunohistochemistry or serologic analysis of secreted monoclonal antibodies, the V genes expressed by B-cell neoplasms. Treatment of B-cell lymphomas with monoclonal mouse anti-idiotypes against the immunoglobulin idiotype on the surface of the neoplastic cell has yielded promising results. However, the manufacture of mouse anti-idiotypes is tedious because they have to be tailored to each patient's needs. The recent recognition of restricted use of V genes by B-cell lymphomas suggests that lymphomas from different patients may share idiotypes. Idiotype sharing by lymphomas may permit wider applications of anti-idiotype therapy. Autoimmunization with the patient's own lymphoma cell idiotype might replace passive immunization with mouse anti-idiotypes.

T-Cell Receptor V Genes

The recombinatorial and diversity-generating mechanisms of the T cell are strikingly similar to those used by the B cell.[28,50,51] Indeed, transfected V_β T-cell receptor gene segments can undergo D-J joining in B cells, transformed by Abelson leukemia virus.[52] Parallels in the molecular genetics of T cells and B cells have important implications in clinical practice: the principles of molecular diagnosis are the same for either T-cell or B-cell neoplasms.[53] Like its H chain locus counterpart, only the V_β locus of the α/β pair contains D segments; and in the γ/δ pair, only the V_γ locus has D segments.[54] Under the influence of RAG-1 and RAG-2, discrete V gene segments recombine to form the T-cell receptor's coding unit. The principles of flexible V-D-J (or V-J) joining, exonuclease nibbling, TdT-directed N nucleotide additions, and allelic exclusion that apply to im-munoglobulin V genes also pertain to T-cell receptor V genes.[55] These molecular mechanisms give the α/β T-cell receptor repertoire enormous diversity, especially in CDR3 regions.[28] They also result in a population that consists of billions of clonally unique T cells.

T-Cell V Gene Loci

The V_β locus, on chromosome 7, contains about 70–100 V_β segments (divisible into 20 families) and two tandem $D_\beta/J_\beta/C_\beta$ complexes (Fig. 8-20). Each of the latter contains a single D_β and C_β segment; the 5' complex contains six J_β segments, whereas the 3' complex has seven J_β segments. The V_α locus is atypical because the V_δ locus lies embedded within it on band 11 of chromosome 14. Another unusual feature of the V_α locus is that it contains a very large number of J_α segments—perhaps as many as 100. There are only four V_δ, two D_δ, three J_δ, and one C_δ segments. The V_γ locus, on chromosome 7, is also uncomplicated. It has only 12 functional segments: 8 V_γ, 2 J_γ, and 2 C_γ.

Clinical Implications

T-cell receptor genes have been under intense scrutiny in ALL. Rearrangement of immunoglobulin V genes occurs in almost every case of ALL with a B-cell surface phenotype (i.e., CD19$^+$). Surprisingly, rearrangement of T-cell receptor V genes is also frequent. For unknown reasons, particular V_δ segments and V_δ-D_δ rearrangements, such as $V_\delta2$-$D_\delta3$, are common in B-cell ALL. The rearranged T-cell receptor V genes are not transcribed in most ALL cells, but weak transcription does occur in a few. All these results indicate that B-cell ALL arises in a precursor cell that has active recombinase enzymes. The rearrangement of both immunoglobulin and T-cell receptor V genes suggests that B-cell ALL arises in a cell with dual recombinatory potential, such as an uncommitted pro-lymphocyte, or that the leukemic cell has a defect in the regulation of V gene

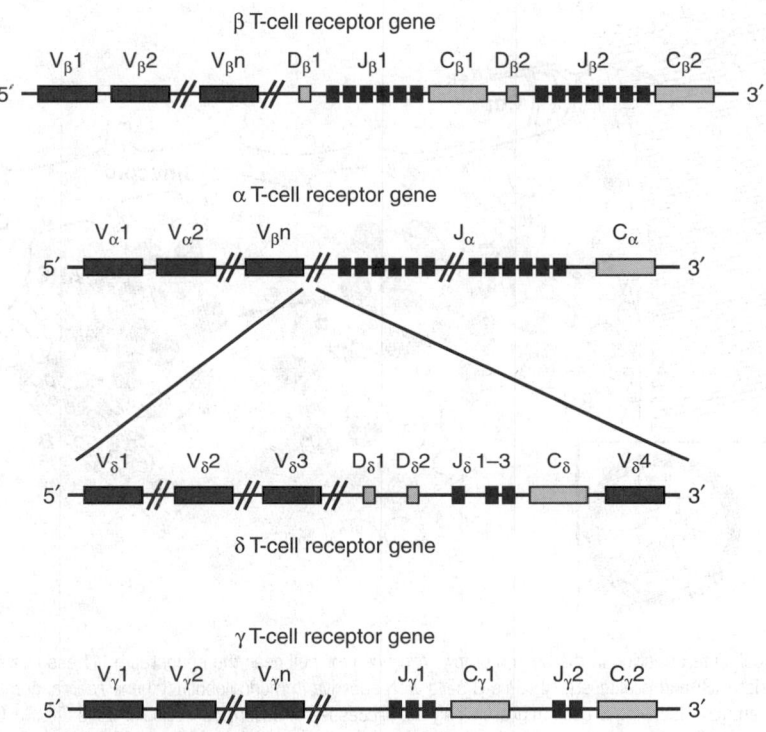

Fig. 8-20. The T-cell receptor loci. Note that the V_δ locus is embedded within the V_α locus. Both V_δ and V_γ are relatively simple loci.

recombination. The phenomenon of rearrangement of both B-cell and T-cell *V* genes in B-cell ALL (lineage promiscuity) must be distinguished from that of lineage infidelity, in which the leukemic cell has a double phenotype, expressing both lymphoid and myeloid markers.

After chemotherapy for ALL, the blood and bone marrow may appear normal, and the patient is in a remission. Nevertheless, small numbers of "invisible" leukemic cells can remain. The clonal specificity of CDR3 has been exploited to search for these residual leukemic cells (minimal residual disease). A powerful method for identifying very small numbers of leukemic cells within a population of normal blood cells entails amplification of CDR3 sequences by means of the PCR and probing the PCR product with clone-specific CDR3 oligonucleotides. This technic can detect one leukemic cell in 10^5–10^6 normal bone marrow cells; a positive result may predict an impending relapse.[56] In one report, evidence for minimal residual disease was found by the PCR method in 6 of 11 patients undergoing maintenance chemotherapy for ALL, but clonotypic DNA was undetectable in almost all patients after termination of treatment. PCR amplification and probing of V_γ and V_δ T-cell receptor genes are useful in most patients with ALL because these loci have a simple organization and they rearrange frequently in B-cell ALL.

LYMPHOCYTE DIFFERENTIATION

All lymphocytes take their origin in the bone marrow from multilineage progenitors, the immediate descendants of hematopoietic stem cells. These multipotent cells have the capacity to differentiate into precursors of granulocytes, monocytes, erythrocytes, megakaryocytes, and lymphocytes (Fig. 8-2). The program of genetic instructions that determines whether a prolymphocyte differentiates into a T cell or a B cell begins before any detectable sign of *V* gene rearrangement. Cells in that early stage of lineage commitment are either pro-T cells or pro-B cells. To develop into mature T cells or B cells, these primitive cells require microenvironmental conditions specific to the thymus or the bone marrow. Intimate contact with stromal cells and signals transduced by lineage-specific cytokines are crucial. For example, early B-cell development depends on the action of IL-7. IL-2 has an important role in T-cell maturation. Some forms of SCID, with virtual absence of T cells, have been traced to defects in the production of IL-2 or other T-cell growth factors.

Experiments in gene "knockout" mice have demonstrated conclusively that rearrangement of *V* genes is essential for the differentiation of T cells and B cells. No mature lymphocytes were found in mice homozygous for disabled *RAG*-1 or *RAG*-2 genes; moreover, T-cell maturation was completely restored in *RAG*-2-deficient mice by transgenic T-cell-receptor *V* region genes. In mice with SCID, which lack both T cells and B cells, a defective gene prevents *V-D-J* joining. Deletion of the H chain joining region, or deletion of all J_H segments by targeted mutation, have been shown to cause a severe deficiency of mature B cells. B-cell differentiation also requires a plasma membrane-bound H chain: disruption of the genetic instructions for insertion of the μ-chain into the cell membrane blocks the development of mature B cells.

It is very likely that surface μ- (B-cell) and β- (T-cell) polypeptide chains mediate the differentiation of pre-T cells and pre-B cells through transducing intracellular signals.[57] The importance of signal transduction in B-cell differentiation has been illuminated by the discovery of the molecular defect in X-linked agammaglobulinemia. This genetic disease is characterized by normal numbers of pre-B cells in the marrow, but no mature B cells. The hindrance to B-cell maturation in X-linked agammaglobulinemia is due to a mutation in pre-B cells of the *Atk* gene, a member of the *src* family of signal-transducing protein tyrosine kinases.

B-Cell Differentiation

B-cell production begins in the yolk sac, shifts to the fetal liver, and continues in the bone marrow. In the marrow, B cells develop in close proximity to stromal reticular cells (Fig. 8-21).

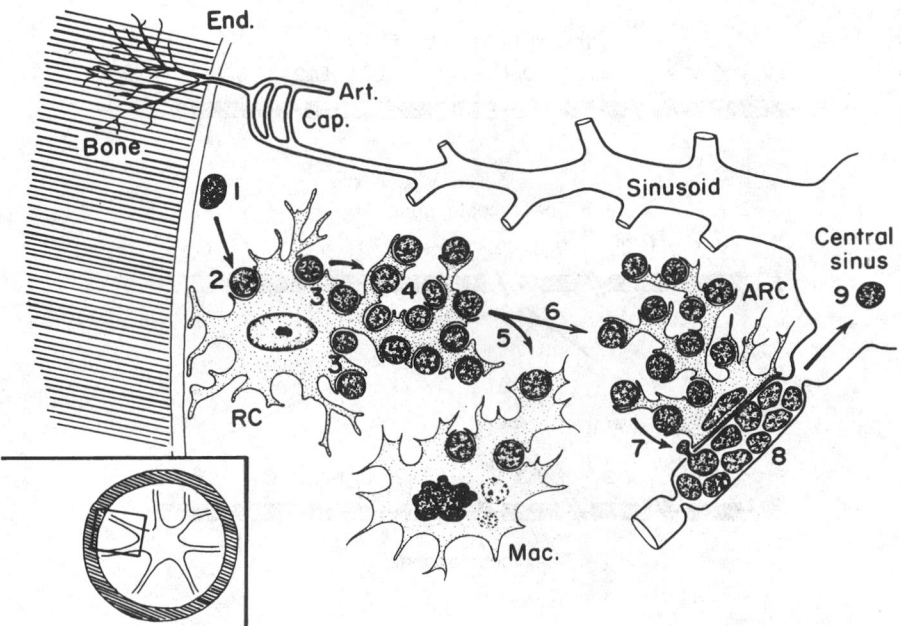

Fig. 8-21. Model of B-cell differentiation in the bone marrow. A progenitor cell near the endosteum (1) associates with stromal cells (2) and begins to differentiate (3) and proliferate (4). Pre-B cells with abortive immunoglobulin *V* gene rearrangements undergo apoptosis; macrophages ingest them (5). Surviving B cells migrate along the processes of adventitial reticular cells (7). Surface μ^+ B cells traverse a segment of a sinusoidal wall (8) and complete their differentiation in the central sinus (9). (From Jacobsen and Osmond,[96] with permission.)

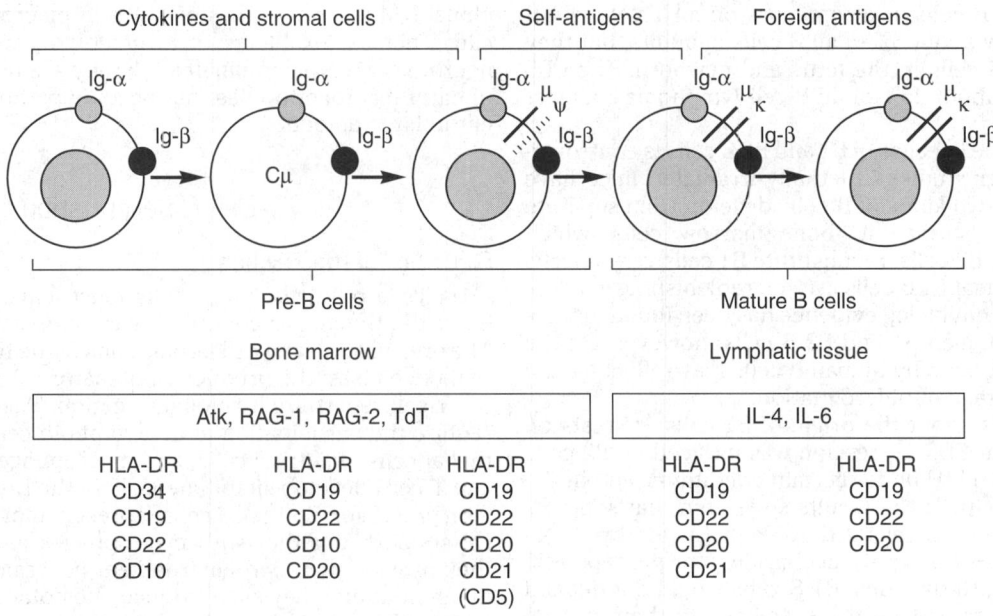

Fig. 8-22. B-cell differentiation. Ig-α and Ig-β, components of the B-cell receptor complex; Cμ, cytoplasmic IgM; Atk, the *src*-related gene that mediates a signaling function in pre-B cells; ψ, pseudo-L chain; μ, surface μ H chain; κ, surface L chain; HLA-DR, class II HLA antigen. CD antigens representative of each stage of differentiation are listed at the bottom of the diagram.

They usually occur singly or in small clusters near sinusoidal walls; lymphoid follicles are rare, except in persons >60 years of age. Paratrabecular lymphoid follicles are also unusual; their presence is highly suggestive of malignant lymphoma. The proportions of lymphoid and nonlymphoid cells in the marrow vary with age; in children, lymphoid cells constitute 20–30% of the nucleated cells, whereas in the adult marrow they represent 10–20% of the cells. An early indication of commitment to the B-cell lineage is expression of the CD19 surface protein, a member of the B-cell receptor complex. B cells express CD19 at all stages of maturation, except for terminally differentiated plasma cells; this molecule is thus a specific marker of B cells, even before they express surface immunoglobulins. Two other B-cell receptor complex proteins, Ig-α and Ig-β, appear in the cytoplasm of early B cells, perhaps at the pro-B-cell stage.[30] These very early CD19$^+$ B cells also synthesize TdT, to prepare for somatic modification of V_H-D-J_H joints by N nucleotide additions.

Pseudo-Light Chains

The major event in the differentiation of pro-B cells is the rearrangement and expression of H chain genes[58,59] (Fig. 8-22). The onset of V_H segment rearrangement defines the cell as a pre-B cell. The appearance of surface H chains (surface μ) signals allelic exclusion and triggers $V_κ$-$J_κ$ rearrangement.[60] At the surface μ$^+$-stage, the pre-B cell expresses two other genes, V_{pre-B} and λ5. They specify the ω- and ι-proteins, which make up the so-called pseudo-L chain (ψ L chain, surrogate L chain).[58,59] The function of the ψ L chain is unknown; it may transport the H chain polypeptide from the endoplasmic reticulum to the cell surface or modulate intracellular signaling by the surface H chain.[58] The ψ-chain seems essential for B-cell maturation; disruption of the λ5 gene in mice by gene targeting arrests B-cell differentiation at the pre-B-cell stage.

The surface L chain appears on the plasma membrane after the H chain. The clonal precursor has one distinctive H chain and one unique L chain on its surface. The transmembrane L chain releases the B cell from its dependence on IL-7; by that time, the ψ L chain has disappeared. The mature surface μ$^+$/κ$^+$ or μ$^+$/λ$^+$ B cell now emerges from the bone marrow, enters the blood, and within <1 hour settles into a lymphoid follicle.

B-Cell Turnover

The normal adult probably has 50×10^{10} B cells. Little is known about the life span of these cells. Most of the data have been derived from studies in mice and rats, using a variety of cell-labeling techniques, all of which have technical and interpretive drawbacks.[61–63] It is generally agreed that, in rodents, a substantial proportion of immature B cells die in the bone marrow. The underlying mechanism of the high death rate is programmed cell death, a metabolic process that degrades nuclear contents, especially DNA.[64] Programmed cell death culminates in apoptosis, a disorganization of nuclear contents that produces distinctive morphologic changes.[65,66] Macrophages in the marrow and lymphatic tissue ingest apoptotic B cells—the tingible bodies of the germinal centers. In the bone marrow, apoptosis probably accounts for the death of immature B cells that fail to express surface IgM molecules because of ineffective *V* gene rearrangements. In germinal centers of lymphatic tissues, virgin B cells undergo apoptosis unless they encounter an antigenic stimulus. In that event, transcription of the *bcl*-2 gene begins and its protein product rescues the activated B cell from apoptosis.[64] The bcl-2 protein, located on inner mitochondrial membranes, interrupts the cell's death program by an unknown mechanism. The antigen-activated bcl-2$^+$ B cell thus survives and becomes a long-lived memory cell.[64,67] Transgenic mice in which the *bcl*-2 gene was targeted for expression by a B-cell-specific promoter progressively accumulated large numbers of mature B cells and developed a lymphoproliferative disorder with huge lymph nodes filled with transgenic bcl-2$^+$ B cells. Apart from its role in normal B cells, the *bcl*-2 gene is of considerable importance in the development of certain B-cell lymphomas.[64] Bone marrow production matches the high death rate of immature and virgin B cells. The marrow in adults likely produces 10^{10} B cells daily; for comparison, it produces about 10^{11} erythrocytes daily.

CD5 (B1) B Cells

The surface antigen CD5 identifies an unconventional subpopulation of B cells,[68] variously termed CD5$^+$, Ly-1 (in the mouse), and more recently B1 B cells.[69] In the new nomenclature, conventional CD5$^-$ B cells are termed B2 B cells. CD5 is not specific for B1 B cells; it also occurs on all T cells. B1 B cells constitute only about 5% of all B cells in adults, but they account for most B cells in the fetus and newborn. The CD5 marker occurs on about 25% of all B-cell lymphomas; almost all CLLs are CD5[+].[70]

The question of the lineages of B1 and B2 B cells is controversial.[71,72] Cell-transfer studies in lethally irradiated mice have suggested that the two kinds of B cells develop from separate progenitors. CD19[-]/surface μ[-]-bone marrow cells, which readily reconstitute B2 cells, reconstitute B1 cells very poorly. By contrast, peritoneal B1 B cells are self-replenishing in adoptive recipients. No convincing evidence has been found for separate lineages for human B1 and B2 B cells, however. On the contrary, CD5 expression by human B cells may reflect a state of activation or a stage of differentiation.

A new hypothesis about the origin of B1 cells[73,74] rests on the observation that CD5 expression was induced on B2 cells by ligation of surface IgM under certain conditions, and in the absence of T-cell help. These results suggested that some B2 B cells convert into B1 B cells if they are activated by T-cell-independent antigens (e.g., polysaccharides), or perhaps self-antigens. According to this idea, B1 B cells would not depend on unique precursors, but on the specificity of their antigen receptors.

The functional significance of the CD5 transmembrane glycoprotein is unclear. The B-cell surface protein CD72 is a ligand for CD5 in both humans and mice. This arrangement is an example of the co-expression of a receptor and its ligand on the same cell; however, nothing is known about the biologic activities mediated by the interaction of CD5 with CD72. In recent studies, mice in which the CD5 gene was disabled failed to show any gross immunologic differences from normal mice.[74] In complementary studies, a CD5 transgene linked to an immunoglobulin gene promoter and enhancer was introduced into normal mice. All IgM-bearing B cells constitutively expressed high levels of CD5. Nevertheless, levels of serum IgM were no different from those in normal mice, and the transgenic CD5[+] B cells could display the typically high surface IgM/IgD ratio of B1 B cells.[74] These knockout and transgenic experiments failed to define a role for CD5 in relation to the properties of B1 B cells.

Clinical Implications

A characteristic feature of B1 B cells is the ability to produce IgM autoantibodies, among which anti-DNA antibodies and rheumatoid factor are the most frequent.[75] The B1 B-cell population is therefore thought to be the source of the natural autoantibodies present in normal serum.[76] Natural autoantibodies occur in the blood of adults, children, newborn infants, and even fetuses. They are present in low amounts, almost always bind to multiple antigens (polyreactive autoantibodies), and have low affinity for their ligands.[77] Under normal circumstances they are harmless. It is not clear whether natural autoantibody production is an exclusive property of B1 B cells; virgin B2 B cells probably have the same ability.[78]

In almost all CLLs, the monoclonal B cells are CD5[+]. The range of immunoglobulin V genes used by leukemic B cells of this disease is restricted to just a few germline segments. Those that do rearrange show no signs of somatic mutation. These two molecular features of CLL are prominent in normal CD5[+] B cells. The monoclonal IgM antibodies secreted by neoplastic B1 B cells often bind to red blood cells (cold agglutinins), glycoproteins in peripheral nerve, DNA, or IgG (rheumatoid factors). The V_H gene segment V_H4.21 encodes all monoclonal cold agglutinins that have been examined thus far, but in each instance the V_H CDR3 and the L chain are unique. In these monoclonal cold agglutinins, somatic mutations of the V_H4.21 gene are minimal or absent. Therefore, the germline V_H segment itself must encode a binding site for the red cell autoantigen. The mono-

clonal IgM autoantibodies of CLL and macroglobulinemia can cause clinical problems (e.g., hemolytic anemia, peripheral neuropathy, cryoglobulinemia)[79]; they are probably examples of natural autoantibodies that become pathogenic when present in large amounts.

T-Cell Differentiation

Structure of the Thymus

Unlike pro-B cells, pro-T cells must leave the marrow and enter the thymus to continue their differentiation program.[80] The organization and cell populations of the thymus are geared to its two tasks: the production of mature T cells, and shaping the T-cell repertoire by clonal selection. These dual functions require the participation of nonlymphoid cells, especially epithelial cells, dendritic cells, and macrophages. Dendritic cells and T cells develop simultaneously in the thymus from a common precursor. Epithelial cells represent more than a mechanical support; together with macrophages and dendritic cells, they provide the microenvironment necessary for thymocyte differentiation. They also produce chemotactic factors that facilitate the entry of pro-T cells into the highly vascularized corticomedullary junction of the thymus.[81]

The thymus contains two distinct anatomic areas, the cortex and the medulla, each having a distinct function (Fig. 8-23). Many of the thymocytes in the subcapsular cortex are large proliferating blasts. They give rise to three populations: the deep cortical small lymphocytes, the juxtamedullary and medullary medium-size thymocytes, and the mature T cells that leave the thymus to populate the periphery. The blasts in the subcapsular cortex are in close contact with epithelial cells and interdigitating dendritic cells. Some of them cluster within infoldings of the plasma membrane of large "nurse" epithelial

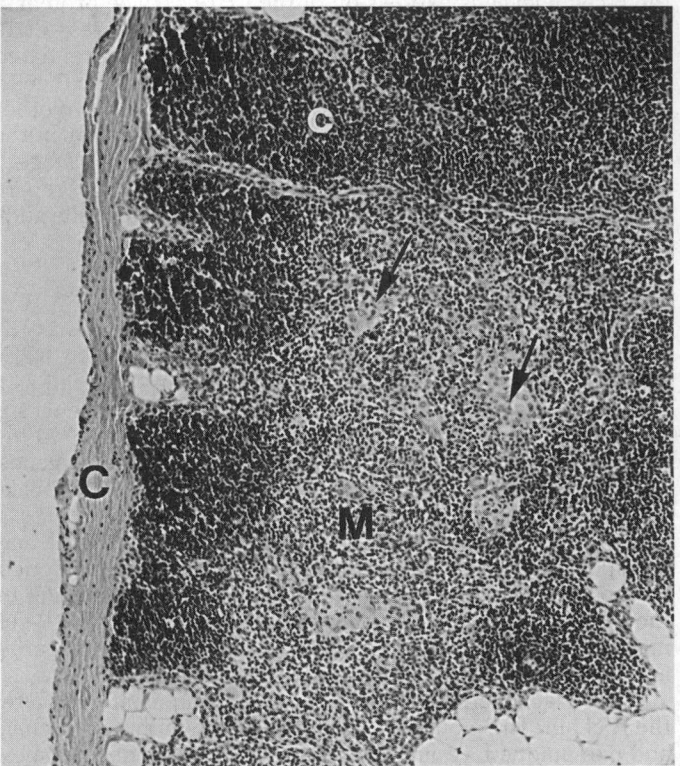

Fig. 8-23. Human thymus. Connective tissue septa divide the thymus into lobules. Each lobule has a distinct outer cortex (C) and a central medulla (M). The thymic capsule (c) is also visible. (x 250.)

cells. The deep cortex contains epithelial cells, dendritic cells, and 85% of all the thymic lymphocytes. Most of these small lymphocytes die in situ within hours or days. Indeed, <1% of all thymocytes leave the thymus. The mechanisms of the high turnover rate of thymocytes are discussed below. The deep cortical epithelial cells are in close contact with thymocytes and express high levels of class II MHC antigens.

The juxtamedullary portion of the deep cortex contains numerous medium-size mature thymocytes. Macrophages are numerous in this area. Some participate in thymocyte maturation, whereas others, engorged with cellular debris, ingest dead thymocytes. Thymocytes have another graveyard on the medul-

lary side of the cortex-medulla junction: Hassal's corpuscles, which probably originate from bone marrow-derived dendritic cells, medullary epithelial cells, and macrophages. The thymic medulla contains mature T cells, macrophages, dendritic cells, and epithelial cells. In contrast to cortical epithelial cells, those in the medulla exhibit both class I and class II MHC antigens at comparable levels.

Formation of the T-Cell Receptor Complex

Once within the thymic cortex, the pro-T cell synthesizes the δ- and ε-proteins of the CD3 T-cell receptor complex and delivers them to the cytoplasm and cell surface[51,82] (Fig. 8-24). (Note

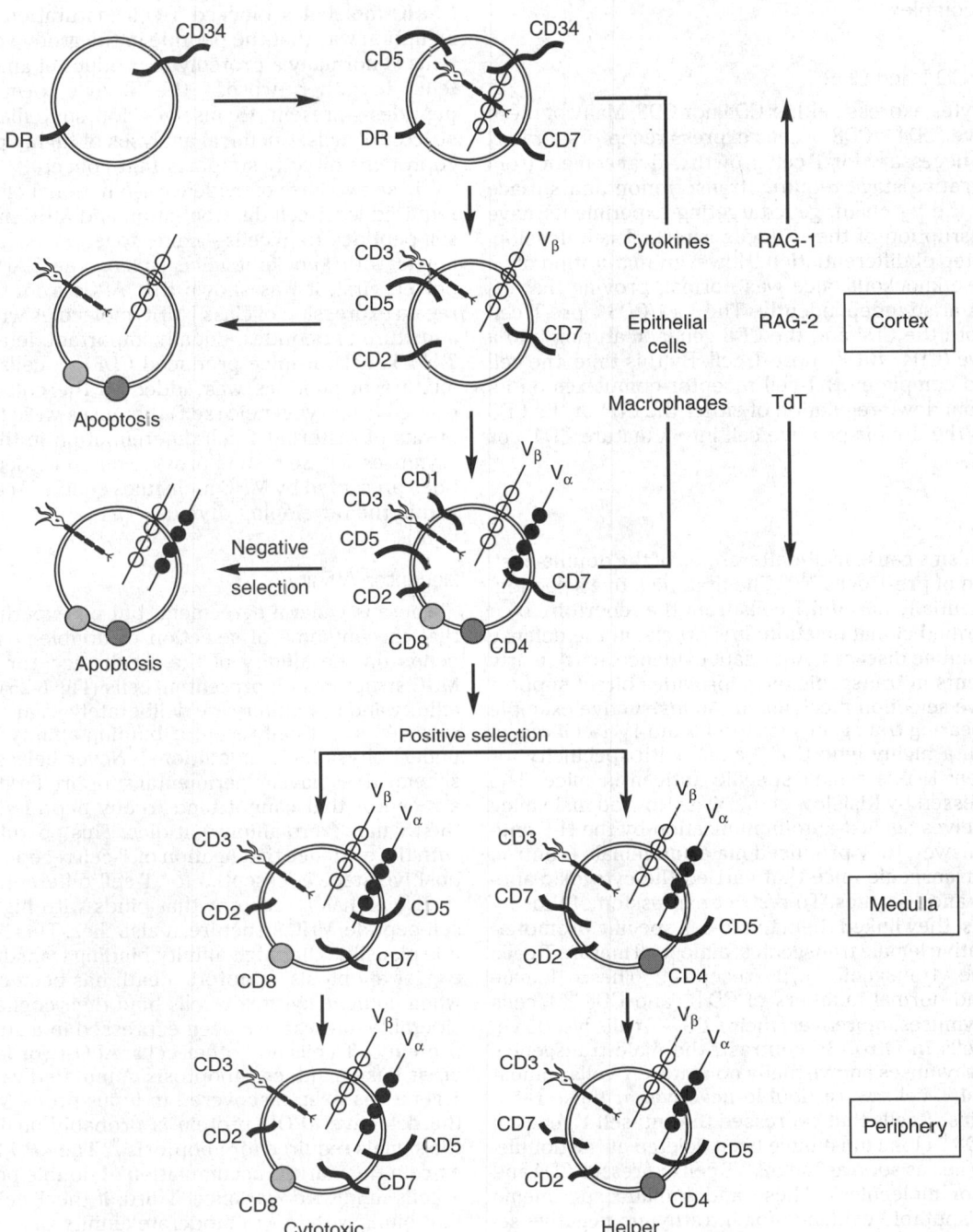

Fig. 8-24. Schematic representation of T-cell differentiation. Positive selection at the CD4+/CD8+ (double positive) stage permits further maturation of T cells into single positive CD4+ or CD8+ T cells. Down-regulation of either CD8 or CD4 by double-positive T cells may be a random process. Negative selection results in apoptotic death of the T cell. T cells that fail to rearrange V genes correctly also undergo apoptosis. CD antigens representative of each stage of T-cell differentiation are shown. DR, class II HLA antigen.

the similarity to the expression by pro-B cells of proteins of the B-cell receptor complex.) The pro-T cell, still in the cortical zone, next rearranges and transcribes its V_β gene segments. Arrival of the mature Vβ chain on the cell surface signals allelic exclusion and induces rearrangement of V_α segments. Even in the absence of the surface V_α chain, the transmembrane Vβ chain and CD3 T-cell receptor complex proteins likely have a signaling function.[32] The differentiating thymocyte has now reached the pre-T-cell stage of development. The assembly and transcription of V_α genes produces the V_α polypeptide, which permits efficient transport of V_β chains and all five accessory proteins (γ, δ, ϵ, ζ, and η). The seven polypeptides (V_α, V_β, γ, δ, ϵ, ζ, and η) then converge on the cell surface to form the T-cell receptor complex.

Expression of CD4 and CD8

Pro-thymocytes express neither CD4 nor CD8. Many of these double-negative (CD4$^-$/CD8$^-$) cells express receptors for IL-2, a lymphokine necessary for T-cell growth. Advancement from the double-negative stage requires transcription and surface expression of the V_β chain; gene-targeting experiments have shown that disruption of the V_β locus arrests T-cell development at that step of differentiation. However, maturation of $\gamma\delta$ T cells in those knockout mice was normal, proving that $\alpha\beta$ and $\gamma\delta$ T cells arise independently. The $V_\beta{}^+$/CD3$^+$ pre-T cell transcribes both the CD4 and the CD8 genes, maturing into a double-positive (CD4$^+$/CD8$^+$) pre-T cell. By this time, the cell has assembled complete $\alpha\beta$ T-cell receptor complexes on its surface. Random down-regulation of either the CD4 or the CD8 gene converts the double-positive cell into a mature CD4$^+$ or CD8$^+$ T cell.

T-Cell Selection

Two mechanisms cause major alterations of the double-positive population of pre-T cells.[83,84] The first, negative selection, eliminates potentially harmful T cells from the repertoire by a mechanism termed clonal deletion. It is crucial in the defense against autoimmune diseases. Abundant evidence, particularly from experiments in transgenic mice, provides direct support for the negative selection mechanism. An instructive example is male mice bearing transgenes for the V_α and V_β T-cell receptor genes from a highly lytic CD8$^+$ clone with specificity for the H-Y antigen. H-Y is a male-specific antigen in mice. The question addressed by Kisielow et al[85] was: How do male mice protect themselves against autoimmunization by the H-Y antigen? For the answer, they produced male and female (control, H-Y-negative) transgenic mice that carried the cytotoxic anti-H-Y clone's V_α and V_β genes. To restrict expression of those V genes to T cells, they linked them to a T-cell specific promoter. In the H-Y-negative female transgenics, almost all mature T cells expressed the transgenic α/β receptor. These female transgenics had normal numbers of CD4$^+$ and CD8$^+$ T cells and normal thymuses; moreover, their CD8$^+$ T cells lysed syngeneic male cells in vitro. By contrast, the male transgenics had shriveled thymuses and virtually no mature T cells; almost all the residual T cells were double negative. In these H-Y$^+$ male transgenics, T cells that expressed the anti-self V genes of the anti-H-Y CD8$^+$ clone must have been deleted at the double-positive stage (i.e., as soon as the $\alpha\beta^+$ T cell expresses CD4 and CD8 co-receptor molecules). These and similar experiments constitute indisputable evidence for intrathymic negative selection. Negative selection is a powerful influence on the T-cell repertoire, with almost 95% of T-cell precursors dying within the thymus because of clonal deletion or abortive V-gene rearrangements.

Positive selection is a mechanism that abrogates the death program, allowing the T cell to advance to the next stage of maturity: CD4$^+$ or CD8$^+$. It has been difficult to obtain direct experimental support for positive selection. However, recent studies have validated its importance in T-cell differentiation. These experiments were based on two premises. The first supposition was that the completion of T-cell differentiation requires ligation of the T-cell receptor by a peptide/MHC complex on the surface of an epithelial cell or macrophage in the thymic cortex. Results obtained in knockout mice, in which the peptide-transporting function of class I MHC glycoproteins was disabled by targeting the *TAP1* transporter gene, supported that idea. Disruption of *TAP1* blocked expression of class I MHC glycoproteins on cell surfaces and caused a profound deficiency of CD8$^+$ T cells. Thus, failure to express functional class I MHC molecules blocked T-cell maturation. The second assumption was that the peptide in the groove of MHC glycoproteins is normally a proteolytic product of an endogenous protein. In other words, the body's own peptides—self-peptides—present themselves for surveillance by MHC-restricted T cells. Chemical analyses of highly purified MHC glycoproteins directly supports that concept.[14]

These two lines of evidence—functional MHC molecules are required for T-cell differentiation and MHC molecules present self-peptides to T cells—came together beautifully in experiments with knockout mice lacking the TAP1 peptide transporter. First, it was shown that APCs from these mice could regain expression of class I MHC molecules when cultured with a mixture of peptides. Equally important, fetal thymuses from *TAP1* knockout mice produced CD8$^+$ T cells in vitro when a mixture of peptides was added to the culture. Peptides extracted from syngeneic (self) thymuses were the most efficient means of restoring T-cell differentiation in the TAP1-deficient thymuses. These results provide direct evidence that self-peptides presented by MHC molecules enable T-cell differentiation within the developing thymus.

Receptor Affinity

There is general agreement, but no experimental evidence, that the outcome of selection of double-positive T cells depends on the affinity of the T-cell receptor for self-peptide/MHC structures on presenting cells (Fig. 8-25). The terms high affinity and low affinity are deliberately vague because no measurements of T-cell receptor binding affinity have been made under physiologic conditions. Nevertheless, the following scheme does have experimental support. First, if the T cell has a receptor that cannot bind to any peptide/MHC complex in the thymus (zero affinity), it dies. This postulate is consistent with the evidence that ligation of T-cell receptors at the double-positive stage is essential for T-cell differentiation. Second, if the T cell has a receptor that binds with high affinity for the self-peptide/MHC structure, it also dies. This is clonal deletion. It is plausible that high-affinity binding transduces signals that trigger apoptosis; apoptotic death has been observed in vitro when immune cytotoxic cells bind their cognate peptide. Considerable interest has been expressed in a surface membrane protein of T cells and other cells, APO-1 (or fas), which, when cross-linked, induces apoptosis. A mutated variant of the *APO-1* gene has been discovered in lupus-prone MRL-*lpr/lpr* mice, the defective APO-1 protein is probably unable to transduce the signals required for apoptosis.[86] The *APO*-1 mutation could explain the marked accumulation of double-positive immature T cells in MRL-*lpr/lpr* mice. Third, if the T cell has a receptor that binds with low to moderate affinity to a self-peptide/MHC complex, it avoids cell death, probably through a bcl-2-mediated mechanism, and continues to differentiate. This postulate is consistent with the evidence in mice that mature T cells in the thymic medulla express the bcl-2 protein, whereas immature cortical thymocytes do not.

T cells thus seem to complete their differentiation only if the

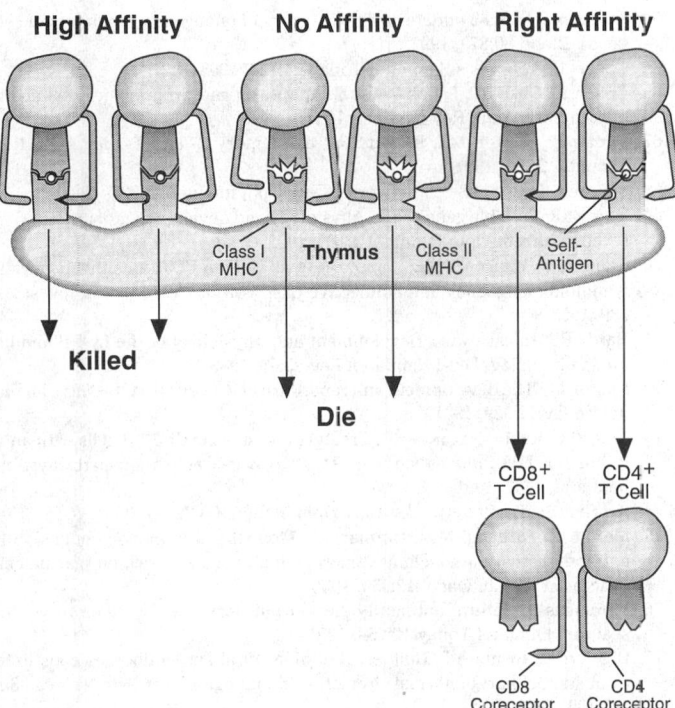

High Affinity **No Affinity** **Right Affinity**

Killed

Die

Class I MHC **Thymus** Class II MHC Self-Antigen

CD8+ T Cell   CD4+ T Cell

CD8 Coreceptor   CD4 Coreceptor

Fig. 8-25. Affinity-based model of positive and negative selection of maturing T cells within the thymus. See text for explanation. (Modified from von Boehmer and Kisielow,[92] with permission.)

binding affinity of their receptors for self-peptide/MHC complexes fall within a particular "affinity window." The T cell dies if the affinity for any of the numerous MHC/self-peptide complexes in the thymic cortex is too high or too low, but it is allowed to mature if its receptor complex transduces signals that shut off programmed cell death (positive selection). Clonal deletion reconciles the diversity-generating mechanism, which must inevitably produce potent anti-self pre-T cells, with the need to eliminate harmful (high-affinity receptors) and useless (zero-affinity receptors) T cells from the system.

Clonal Anergy

Clonal anergy is another mechanism designed to avoid auto-immunization.[87] It differs from clonal deletion in that the T cell does not die but is disabled. The anergic T cell is unable to transcribe its IL-2 gene, preventing it from proliferating in vitro in the presence of its cognate peptide/MHC complex. However, the anergic T cell can proliferate in the presence of exogenous IL-2.[88] Clonal anergy can affect both immature thymocytes and mature peripheral T cells. It occurs when T cells meet antigens in situations that fail to summon the "second signals"—cytokines and adhesion molecules—required for T-cell activation. Clonal anergy may have evolved to silence anti-self T cells that encounter a self-peptide/MHC complex in normal, uninfected, quiescent tissue.

Clinical Implications

Negative selection and clonal anergy are major natural defenses against autoimmunization. However, little information about these mechanisms in humans has been reported. It is not known whether an inherited or acquired defect in T-cell (or B-cell) selection can cause susceptibility to autoimmune diseases in humans. The second signal phenomenon may have considerable clinical relevance. For example, some patients treated for malignant diseases with high doses of IL-2 develop autoimmune disorders such as thyroiditis and hemolytic ane-

mia. A new approach to tumor therapy consists of administration of HLA-compatible tumor cell lines transfected with the IL-2 gene.[89] These cells constitutively express IL-2, and thus in principle simultaneously deliver a powerful, nonspecific T-cell-activating signal (signal 2) and a tumor antigen-specific signal (signal 1). An understanding of and manipulation of the immune system will have far-reaching implications for both the pathogenesis and treatment of many human diseases.

REFERENCES

1. Roitt IM, Greaves MF, Torrigiani G et al: The cellular basis of immunological responses: a synthesis of some current views. Lancet 2:367, 1969
2. Miller JFAP: The discovery of the immunological function of the thymus. Immunol Today 12:42, 1991
3. Lemischka JF, Raulet CH, Mulligan RC: Developmental potential and dynamic behaviour of hematopoietic stem cells. Cell 45:917, 1986
4. Nahm MH, Kroese FGM, Hoffmann JW: The evolution of immune memory and germinal centers. Immunol Today 13:438, 1992
5. Underdown BJ, Schiff JM: Immunoglobulin A: strategic defence initiative at the mucosal surface. Annu Rev Immunol 4:389, 1986
6. Picker LJ, Butcher EC: Physiological and molecular mechanisms of lymphocyte homing. Annu Rev Immunol 10:561, 1992
7. Rivett AJ: Proteasomes: multicatalytic proteinase complexes. Biochem J 291:1, 1993
8. Germain RN, Margulies DH: The biochemistry and cell biology of antigen processing and presentation. Annu Rev Immunol 11:403, 1993
9. Clark EA, Lane PJL: Regulation of human B-cell activation and adhesion. Annu Rev Immunol 9:97, 1991
10. Julius M, Maroun CR, Haughn L: Distinct roles for CD4 and CD8 as co-receptors in antigen receptor signalling. Immunol Today 14:177, 1993
11. Bowen DL, Lane HC, Fauci AA: Immunopathogenesis of the acquired immunodeficiency syndrome. Ann Intern Med 103:704, 1985
12. Schiff C, Milili M, Bossy D et al: Organization and expression of pseudo-light chain genes in human B cell ontogeny. Int Rev Immunol 8:135, 1992
13. Romagnani S: Induction of TH1 and TH2 responses—a key role for the natural immune response. Immunol Today 13:379, 1992
14. Rammensee H-G, Falk K, Rotzschke O: Peptides naturally presented by MHC class I molecules. Annu Rev Immunol 11:213, 1993
15. Dausset J: Lecture for the Nobel prize for physiology or medicine, 1980: The major histocompatibility complex in man: past, present, and future concepts. Scand J Immunol 36:145, 1992
16. Gorga JC: Structural analysis of class-II major histocompatibility complex proteins. Crit Rev Immunol 11:305, 1992
17. Zinkernagel RM, Doherty PC: MHC-restricted cytotoxic T-cells. Adv Immunol 27:51, 1979
18. Janeway CA: The T-cell receptor as a multicomponent signalling machine—CD4/CD8 coreceptors and CD45 in T-cell activation. Annu Rev Immunol 10:645, 1992
19. Steinman RM: The dendritic cell system and its role in immunogenicity. Annu Rev Immunol 9:271, 1991
20. Loughran TP: Clonal diseases of large granular lymphocytes. Blood 82:1, 1993
21. Trinchieri G: Biology of natural killer cells. Adv Immunol 47:187, 1989
22. Natvig JB, Kunkel HG: Human immunoglobulins: classes, subclasses, genetic variants, and idiotypes. Adv Immunol 16:1, 1973
23. Allison JP, Lanier LL: Structure, function, and serology of the T cell antigen receptor complex. Annu Rev Immunol 5:503, 1987
24. Marrack P, Kappler J: The T cell receptor. Science 238:1073, 1987
25. Allison JP, Havran WL: The immunobiology of T-cells with invariant γ/δ antigen receptors. Annu Rev Immunol 9:679, 1991
26. Haas W, Pereira P, Tonegawa T: γ/δ cells. Annu Rev Immunol 11:637, 1993
27. Poljak RJ: X-ray diffraction studies of immunoglobulins. Adv Immunol 21:1, 1975
28. Davis MM: T-cell receptor gene diversity and selection. Annu Rev Biochem 59:475, 1990
29. Ashwell JD, Klausner RD: Genetic and mutational analysis of the T cell antigen receptor. Annu Rev Immunol 8:139, 1990
30. Borst J, Brouns GS, Devries E et al: Antigen receptors on T-lymphocyte and B-lymphocytes: parallels in organization and function. Immunol Rev 132:49, 1993
31. Cambier JC, Bedzyk W, Campbell K et al: The B-cell antigen receptor: structure and function of primary, secondary, tertiary and quaternary components. Immunol Rev 132:85, 1993
32. Weiss A: T-cell antigen receptor signal transduction—a tale of tails and cytoplasmic protein-tyrosine kinases. Cell 73:209, 1993

33. Clevers HB, Alacron B, Willeman T et al: The T cell receptor/CD3 complex: a dynamic protein ensemble. Annu Rev Immunol 6:629, 1988

34. Gellert M: Molecular analysis of V(D)J recombination. Annu Rev Genet 26: 425, 1992

35. Yancopoulos GD, Alt FW: Regulation of the assembly and expression of variable-region genes. Annu Rev Immunol 4:339, 1986

36. Staudt LM, Lenardo MJ: Immunoglobulin gene transcription. Annu Rev Immunol 9:373, 1991

37. Walter MA, Surti U, Hofker MH et al: The physical organization of the human immunoglobulin heavy chain gene complex. EMBO J 9:3303, 1990

38. Snapper CM, Mond JJ: Towards a comprehensive view of immunoglobulin class switching. Immunol Today 14:15, 1993

39. Harriman W, Volk H, Defranoux N et al: Immunoglobulin class switch recombinations. Annu Rev Immunol 11:361, 1993

40. Noelle RJ, Ledbetter JA, Aruffo A: CD40 and its ligand, an essential ligand-receptor pair for thymus-dependent B-cell activation. Immunol Today 13: 431, 1992

41. Blattner FR, Tucker PW: The molecular biology of immunoglobulin D. Nature 307:417, 1984

42. Calame KL: Mechanisms that regulate immunoglobulin gene expression. Annu Rev Immunol 3:159, 1985

43. Cambier JC, Campbell KS: Membrane immunoglobulin and its accomplices—new lessons from an old receptor. FASEB J 6:3207, 1992

44. Wysocki L, Manser T, Gefter ML: Somatic evolution of variable region structures during an immune response. Proc Natl Acad Sci USA 83:1847, 1986

45. Manser T, Huang SY, Gefter ML: Influence of clonal selection on the expression of immunoglobulin variable region genes. Science 226:1283, 1984

46. Kocks C, Rajewsky K: Stable expression of somatic hypermutation of antibody V regions in B-cell developmental pathways. Annu Rev Immunol 7: 537, 1989

47. Schwartz RS, Beldotti L: Malignant lymphomas following allogeneic disease: transition from an immunological to a neoplastic disorder. Science 149:1511, 1965

48. Stewart AK, Huang C, Long AA et al: V_H gene representation in autoantibodies reflects the normal human B cell repertoire. Immunol Rev 128:101, 1992

49. Greenspan NS, Bona CA: Idiotypes: structure and immunogenicity. FASEB J 7:437, 1993

50. Moss PAH, Rosenberg WMC, Bell JI: The human T-cell receptor in health and disease. Annu Rev Immunol 10:71, 1992

51. Strominger JL: Developmental biology of T cell receptors. Science 244:943, 1989

52. Yancopoulos G, Blackwell TK, Heikyung S et al: Introduced T cell receptor variable region gene segments recombine in pre-B cells: evidence that B cells and T cells use a common recombinase. Cell 44:251, 1986

53. Waldmann TA, Davis MM, Bongiovanni KF et al: Rearrangements of genes for the antigen receptor on T cells as markers of lineage and clonality in human lymphoid neoplasms. N Engl J Med 313:776, 1985

54. Raulet DH: The structure, function and molecular genetics of the γ/δ T cell receptor. Annu Rev Immunol 7:175, 1989

55. Malissen M, Trucy J, Jouvin-Marche E, et al: Regulation of TCR-α and TCR-β gene allelic exclusion during T-cell development. Immunol Today 13:315, 1992

56. Potter MN: The detection of minimal residual disease in acute lymphoblastic leukemia. Blood Rev 6:68, 1992

57. Kim KM, Alber G, Weiser P et al: Signalling function of the B-cell antigen receptors. Immunol Rev 132:125, 1993

58. Burrows PD, Cooper MD: B-cell development in man. Curr Opin Immunol 5:201, 1993

59. Melchers F, Karasuyama H, Haasner D et al: The surrogate light chain in B-cell development. Immunol Today 14:60, 1993

60. Nussenzweig MC, Shaw AC, Sinn E et al: Allelic exclusion in transgenic mice that express the membrane form of immunoglobulin μ. Science 236:816, 1987

61. Freitas AA, Rocha BB: Lymphocyte lifespans—homeostasis, selection and competition. Immunol Today 14:25, 1993

62. MacLennan I, Chan E: The dynamic relationship between B-cell populations in adults. Immunol Today 14:29, 1993

63. Osmond DG: The turnover of B-cell populations. Immunol Today 14:34, 1993

64. Korsmeyer S: Bcl-2 initiates a new category of oncogenes: regulators of cell death. Blood 80:879, 1992

65. Cohen JJ: Apoptosis. Immunol Today 14:126, 1993

66. Cohen JJ, Duke RC, Fadok VA et al: Apoptosis and programmed cell death in immunity. Annu Rev Immunol 10:267, 1992

67. Vitetta ES, Berton MT, Burger C et al: Memory B- and T-cells. Annu Rev Immunol 9:193, 1991

68. Kearney JF: CD5+ B-cell networks. Curr Opin Immunol 5:223, 1993

69. Hardy RR: Variable gene usage, physiology and development of Ly+ (CD5+) B cells. Current Opin Immunol 4:181, 1992

70. Youinou P, Mackenzie LE, Lamour A et al: Human CD5– positive B-cells in lymphoid malignancy and connective tissue diseases. Eur J Clin Invest 23: 139, 1993

71. Hardy RR, Hayakawa K: Development and physiology of the Ly-1 B and its human homolog, Leu-1. Immunol Rev 93:53, 1986

72. Kantor AB: The development and repertoire of B-1 cells (CD5 B-Cells). Immunol Today 12:389, 1991

73. Ying-Zi C, Rabin E, Wortis HH: Treatment of murine CD5– B cells with anti-Ig but not LPS induces surface CD5: two B cell activation pathways. Int Immunol 3:467, 1991

74. Kearney JF: B-cell networks. Curr Opin Immunol 4:223, 1993

75. Merlini G, Farhangi M, Osserman EF: Monoclonal immunoglobulins with antibody activity in myeloma, macroglobulinemia and related plasma cell dyscrasias. Semin Oncol 13:350, 1986

76. Avrameas S: Natural autoantibodies—from horror autotoxicus to gnothi seauton. Immunol Today 12:154, 1991

77. Dighiero G, Lymberi P, Guilbert B et al: Natural autoantibodies constitute a substantial part of normal circulating immunoglobulins. Ann NY Acad Sci 475:135, 1986

78. Schwartz RS: Autoantibodies and normal antibodies: two sides of the same coin. Harvey Lect 81:53, 1987

79. Duggan DB, Schattner A: Unusual manifestations of monoclonal gammopathies. Autoimmune and idiopathic syndromes. Am J Med 81:864, 1986

80. Vanewijk W: T-cell differentiation is influenced by thymic microenvironments. Annu Rev Immunol 9:591, 1991

81. Dunon D, Imhof BA: Mechanisms of thymus homing. Blood 81:1, 1993

82. Bonati A, Zanelli P, Ferrari S et al: T-cell receptor β-chain gene rearrangement and expression during human thymic ontogenesis. Blood 79:1472, 1992

83. Sprent J, Gao EK, Webb SR: T-cell reactivity to MHC molecules: immunity versus tolerance. Science 248:1357, 1990

84. Von Boehmer H: Thymic selection: a matter of life and death. Immunol Today 13:454, 1992

85. Kisielow P, Bluthmann H, Staerz UE et al: Tolerance in T-cell-receptor transgenic mice involves deletion of nonmature CD4+ CD8+ thymocytes. Nature 333:742, 1988

86. Cohen P, Eisenberg R: The Lpr and gld genes in systemic autoimmunity—life and death in the Fas lane. Immunol Today 14:97, 1993

87. Mueller DL, Jenkins MK, Schwartz RH: Clonal expansion versus functional clonal inactivation. Annu Rev Immunol 7:45, 1989

88. Schwartz RH: A cell culture model for T lymphocyte clonal anergy. Science 248:1349, 1990

89. Hock H, Dorsch M, Kunzendorf U et al: Vaccinations with tumor cells genetically engineered to produce different cytokines: effectivity not superior to classical adjuvant. Cancer Res 15:714, 1993

90. Reichert T, DeBruyere M, Deneys V et al: Lymphocyte subset reference ranges in adult caucasians. Clin Immunol Immunopathol 60:190, 1991

91. Osmond DG: The turnover of B-cell populations. Immunol Today 14:34, 1991

92. von Boehmer H, Kisielow P: How the immune system learns about self. Sci Am 265:74, 1991

93. Fraser JD, Straus D, Weiss A: Signal transduction events leading to T-cell lymphokine gene expression. Immunol Today 14:358, 1993

94. Mustelin T, Altman A: Do CD4 and CD8 control T-cell activation via a specific tyrosine protein kinase. Immunol Today 10:89, 1989

95. Kabat EA, Wu TT, Perry HM et al: Sequences of Proteins of Immunological Interest. 5th Ed. NIH Publication no. 91-3242. US Department of Health and Human Services, Washington, DC, 1991

96. Jacobsen K, Osmond DG: Microenvironmental organization and stromal cell associations of B lymphocyte precurson cells in mouse bone marrow. Eur J Immunol 20:2395, 1990

Immunoglobulins: Structure, Function, and Uses

9

Robert Mandle and David H. Bing

INTRODUCTION

In 1845 Dr. Watson, a general practitioner, sent a urine sample obtained from a patient suffering from mollities ossium along with the following letter to Professor H. Bence Jones, an English pathologist:

Saturday, Nov. 1st, 1845

Dear Dr. Jones,—The tube contains urine of very high specific gravity. When boiled it becomes slightly opaque. On addition of nitric acid it effervesces, assumes a reddish hue, and becomes quite clear; but as it cools, assumes the consistence and appearance which you see. Heat reliquifies it. What is it?

[Signed] Dr. Watson

In 1847 Jones published the results of his analysis of the specimen. He confirmed Dr. Watson's observation and reported that the sample contained a protein substance (an "oxide albumen") distinguished from albumin by its solubility in nitric acid and lack of heat coagulability. He proceeded to demonstrate that a protein in the sample purified by alcohol precipitation retained the properties of solubility in cold water: increased solubility in boiling water, coagulation with continued boiling, and return to solution with further boiling. Acid precipitated the substance and heating solubilized the acid precipitate, but cooling led to reprecipitation. Jones[1] concluded his analysis by noting: "Each oz. of this urine contained as much nutritive matter as an oz. of blood. No supply of food could compensate for such a loss."

Over the years, the presence of such proteins, subsequently named Bence Jones proteins, became a diagnostic test for multiple myeloma because of the high association between the plasma cell disease and the urinary pattern. One hundred and ten years lapsed, however, before Jones's original insight about a possible relationship between the urinary substances and plasma proteins was confirmed by Korngold and Lipari[2] and Deutsch et al,[3] who used immunologic techniques to demonstrate the relationship of the urinary microglobulins (Bence Jones proteins) to normal and myeloma immunoglobulins.

IMMUNOGLOBULINS

Properties and Structure

The mammalian immune system responds to the almost unlimited array of antigens by producing specific antibodies, each of which will react specifically with the molecule that induced its production. During the immune response, the structure of the inducing antigen is imprinted on the immune system, as subsequent challenges with the same or structurally related molecule will cause a more rapid rise in antibody levels to much greater concentrations than were achieved following the primary antigenic challenge. Thus, the hallmarks of the immune system include induction, specific protein interaction, and memory.

Antibodies belong to the family of proteins called the immunoglobulins. The basic structure of all immunoglobulins consists of a monomer that contains four polypeptide chains: two identical heavy (H) chains and two identical light (L) chains covalently linked by disulfide bonds (Fig. 9-1). A model of the monomeric form of immunoglobulin has been prepared based on x-ray crystallographic data obtained on the IgG myeloma protein Dob (Plate 9-1). The immunoglobulin monomer consists of a Y- or T-like structure. The size of the arms, called Fab (antigen binding fragment) domain of the Y or T is $80 \times 50 \times 40$ nm and the size of the base, called Fc (fragment crystallizable) is approximately $70 \times 45 \times 40$ nm, according to models based on x-ray diffraction data.[4] The immunoglobulin molecule exhibits considerable flexibility; the angle between the Fabs has been observed in electron microscopic, low-angle x-ray scattering, transient electric birefringence, and resonance energy transfer studies to vary from 0° to 180°. All antibodies have two identical combining sites for each antigen located at the ends of the Fab domains.

The Fab and Fc represent functional domains in immunoglobulins. These were discovered by performing limited proteolytic digestion of the molecule. Both the H and L chains contribute amino acids that constitute the antigen-binding site in Fab. The Fab will combine with, but will not precipitate, multivalent antigens, in contrast to native IgG. A fragment can be prepared, called Fab$'_2$, which is devoid of Fc but still precipitates antigen. This form of immunoglobulin consists of two Fabs disulfide bonded at a part of the molecule called the hinge region. The hinge region is the part of the immunoglobulin molecule that is responsible for the molecular flexibility exhibited by all immunoglobulins. Every immunoglobulin is a glycoprotein, and the carbohydrate is always found attached to the H chain in the Fc domain. The other major function of immunoglobulin, binding to specific receptors on cells and certain effector proteins such as protein A and Clq, is associated with binding site(s) also found in Fc.

The chain structure of immunoglobulin explains neither antibody structural diversity nor antibody binding to antigen. The discovery that there are variable (V) and constant (C) regions of amino acid sequence formed the basis for understanding both phenomena. Thus, in the L chain, the 100 or so amino acids in the NH_2-terminal half of the protein (V_L) vary between antibody molecules, but in the second half (C_L) there is virtual complete correspondence in amino acids, position for position, to the COOH-terminus. H chains exhibit the same pattern and can be divided likewise into V_H and C_H. Comparison of the amino acid sequence of many V_L has shown that certain parts of the V region exhibit excess variability, while others have lesser variability. The former are called hypervariable regions or complementarity determining regions (CDRs) and the latter framework regions. H chains exhibit the same pattern in the V_H regions. Amino acid sequence analysis of the C_H region has shown there are three homologous regions—C_H1, C_H2, C_H3—in which the amino acid sequences show more similarity than could have occurred by chance. The Fab region consists of the

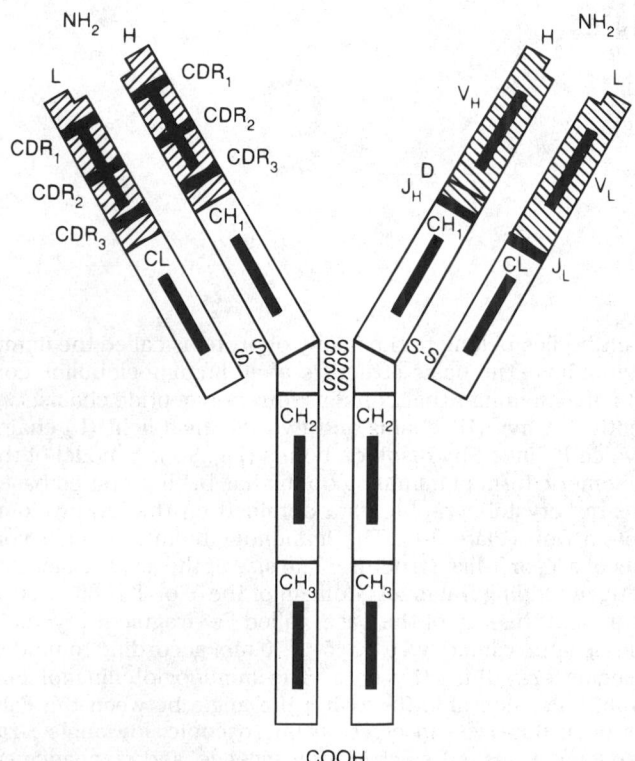

Fig. 9-1. Diagrammatic representation of the structural features of an IgG molecule. NH$_2$ indicates the NH$_2$-terminus and COOH the C terminus. The V$_H$, C$_{H_1}$, V$_L$, and C$_L$ homology domains are shown as boxes. Only the disulfide linkages that join H and L chains are shown. **(Left)** Approximate boundaries of the CDR regions in the V$_L$ and V$_H$ regions. **(Right)** Sequences encoded by V$_H$, D, J$_H$, V$_L$, and J$_L$ segments in the V$_H$ and V$_L$ regions.

intact L chain and the Fd region of the H chain, which consists of V$_H$-C$_{H_1}$ (Fig. 9-1). The combining site for antigen is a trough or a cavity composed of parts of the hypervariable regions of both the H and L chain. This small region represents only 25% of the antibody V region. The region that interacts directly with the epitope on the antigen is even smaller and is formed by the association of the CDR regions, each of which contains about 20 amino acids. Thus, the variation in a few amino acids accounts for the specificity and diversity of antibodies with respect to antigen binding.

In addition to the amino acid sequence variations at the binding site, immunoglobulins can exhibit additional physical heterogeneity. This imparts a special effector function to each immunoglobulin that is reflected in unique biologic properties additional to the antigen-binding activity. Heterologous and autologous antisera raised against immunoglobulins have been used to classify three types of physical heterogeneity. The first kind is based on the antigenic heterogeneity exhibited by immunoglobulin when it is used as an immunogen in other species. This is called class or isotypic variation. In humans five isotypes can be distinguished on the basis of unique antigenic (isotypic) determinants found on the H chain. These are designated by capital Roman letters: IgG, IgM, IgA, IgD, and IgE. The H chain of each class is designated by the small Greek letter corresponding to the Roman letter of the class. Thus the H chain for IgG is γ, for IgM is μ, for IgA is α, for IgD is δ, and for IgE is ϵ. Some of the immunoglobulin classes are composed of polymers of the basic monomer. Two antigenic varieties of the L chain (κ and λ) are found in humans. Each immunoglobulin will have two identical L chains; the κ and λ are shared by all classes. The monomeric form of any immunoglobulin is de-

scribed by its chain structure. The molecular mass of the immunoglobulins can vary from 150 kd to 1,000 kd. This variation is due to polymerization of the basic monomer form. None of the immunoglobulins, however, is a polymeric form of another class.

IgG is the most prevalent immunoglobulin, constituting 75% of the total immunoglobulins in blood. It is present in normal adults at concentrations of 600 to 1,500 mg/dl. IgG is designated $\gamma_2\kappa_2$ or $\gamma_2\lambda_2$. It is the only class of immunoglobulin that will cross the placenta.

Isotype IgM is a pentamer consisting of five monomeric units disulfide linked at the C terminus of the H chain; each monomer of IgM is 180 kd due to the presence of an additional C$_H$ domain. The complete protein has a sedimentation coefficient of 19 S, which corresponds to a molecular mass of 850–1,000 kd. IgM is designated $(\mu_2\kappa_2)_5$ or $(\mu_2\lambda_2)_5$. IgM also contains a 15-kd protein, called the J chain. In the current structural model of IgM the J chain forms a disulfide bonded clasp at the C terminus of two H chains (Fig. 9-2).

The structure of the other isotypes of immunoglobulin is summarized as follows: Isotype IgA has a variable number of monomeric units and is designated $(\alpha_2\kappa_2)_n$ or $(\alpha_2\lambda_2)_n$, where n is 2–5. Serum IgA constitutes 20% of the total serum immunoglobulin, 80% of which is monomeric. The remainder is in the form of polymers. The other form of IgA is found in external secretions such as saliva, tracheobronchial secretions, colostrum, milk, and genitourinary secretions. Secretory IgA consists of four components: a dimer of two monomeric molecules; a 70-kd secretory component that binds noncovalently to the IgA dimer; and the 15-kd J chain, believed to form a disulfide bonded clasp at the C terminus of the H chains (Fig. 9-2). Isotype IgD has a molecular mass of 180 kd. Its serum concentration is very low, approximately 3 mg/dl. IgD apparently functions as a membrane molecule, associated in mature but unstimulated B cells in association with IgM. IgE is the homocytotropic or reaginic immunoglobulin and mediates immediate hypersensitivity. It has a molecular mass of 180 kd and, like IgM, has four C$_H$ domains. The Fc portion of IgE binds strongly to a receptor on mast cells. This is how immunoglobulin exerts its particular activity. The overall properties of the immunoglobulins are summarized in Table 9-1.

In addition, subclasses of isotypes IgG, IgA, and IgM have been identified. The structural basis for this heterogeneity is antigenic variation (e.g., amino acid sequence differences) in the Fc portion of the H chain of a given class. The subclasses of IgG are the best characterized. These are called IgG1, IgG2, IgG3, and IgG4. Each has a slightly different structure, the most notable difference being the interchain disulfide bonding pattern (Fig. 9-2 and Table 9-1). IgG1 comprises 70% of the total IgG and IgG2 20%. IgG3 and IgG4 make up 8% and 2%, respectively, of the total IgG. The subclasses of IgG exhibit different catabolic rates and IgG2 crosses the placenta slightly more slowly than the other three. The other known subclasses of immunoglobulin isotypes are associated with IgM (IgM1 and IgM2) and IgA (IgA1 and IgA2). The properties and function of these subclasses are less well known.

The second type of variation is called allotypic variation, caused by genetically controlled antigenic determinants found on both the H and L chains. While every human has all immunoglobulin isotypes, an individual has only one form of each allotype on their immunoglobulin molecules. Allotypes are co-dominantly expressed, but an individual B lymphocyte secretes only one of the parental forms. This phenomenon is called allelic exclusion.

The third type of variation is due to antigenic determinants unique to each particular antibody molecule produced by an individual. These markers are called idiotypic determinants and are associated with a single species of antibody. The anti-

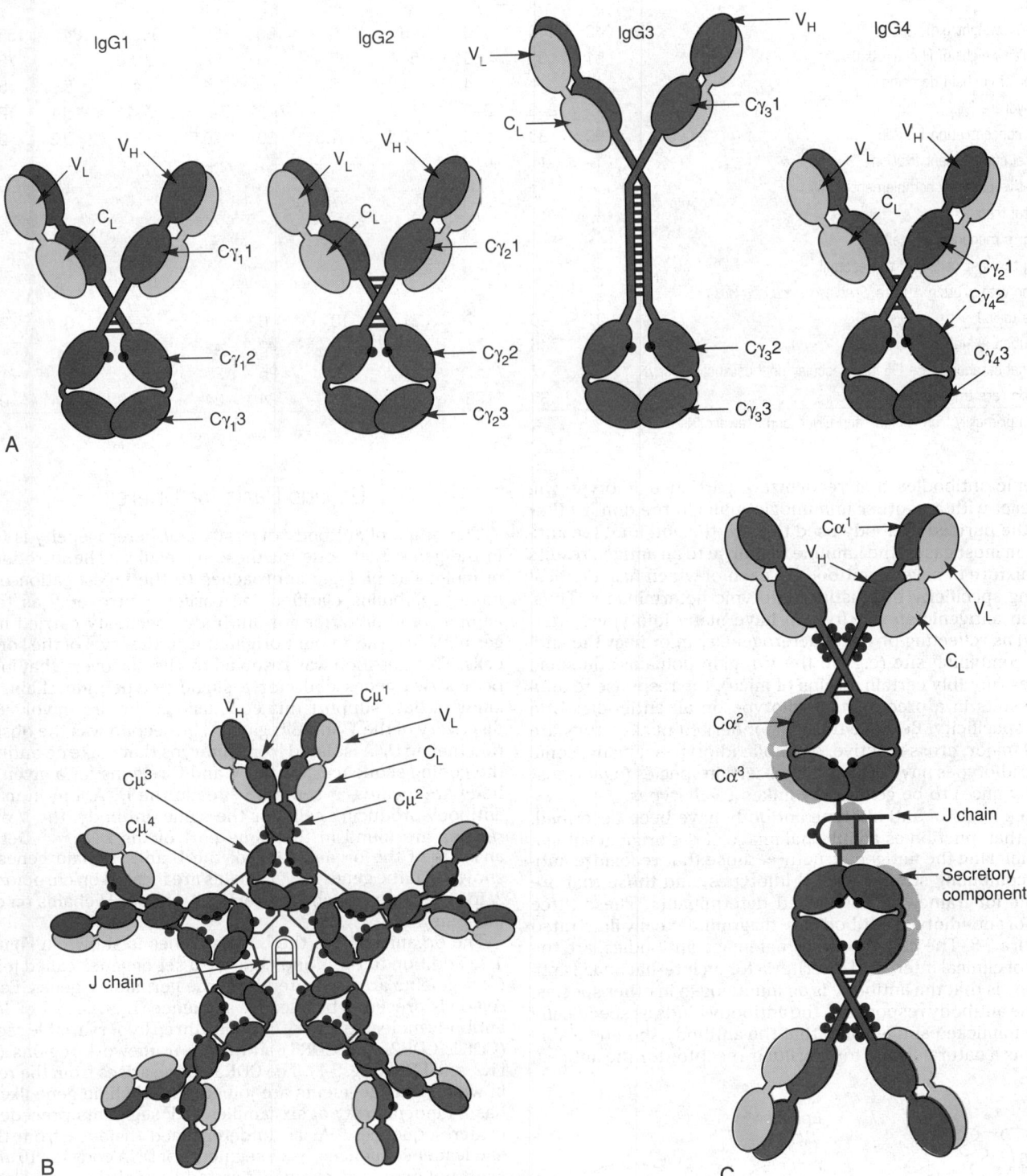

Fig. 9-2. (A) Structure of the four subclasses of human IgG. Constant region domains are indicated by Cγ_nN, where n is the subclass and N is the domain. V$_H$ (· · ·), heavy chain variable region; V$_L$ (– – –), light chain variable region. **(B)** Structure of human IgM. The J chain is shown in this model as being disulfide linked to two μ-chains. Other models have been proposed. Filled circle (●) carbohydrate. **(C)** Structure of human secretory IgA. This model shows the possible arrangement of the two IgA monomers in relationship to the secretory component and J chain. As the IgA molecule passes through the epithelial cells, the secretory components are synthesized and attached covalently to the Fc domain of the α-chains that have previously been joined to the J chain with disulfide links. Light chain, pink; heavy chain, red; disulfide bonds, black lines; carbohydrates, black circles. (From Turner,[24] with permission.)

Table 9-1. Human Immunoglobulins: Properties and Function

	IgG1	IgG2	IgG3	IgG4	IgM	IgA1	IgA2	IgA$_{6cc}$	IgD	IgE
H chain	γ1	γ2	γ3	γ4	μ	α1	α2	α1, α2	δ	ε
Molecular weight (kd)	146	146	170	146	970	160	160	385	184	188
Molecular weight of H chain (kd)	51	51	60	51	65	56	52	52–56	70	73
Number of H chain domains	4	4	4	4	5	4	4	4	5	5
Carbohydrate (%)	2–3	2–3	2–3	2–3	12	7–11	7–11	7–11	9–14	12
Serum concentration (mg/dl)	90	30	10	0.5	1.5	30	0.5	0.5	0.3	0.0005
Classical complement fixation	+ +	+	+ + +	−	+ + +	−	−	−	−	−
Alternative pathway complement activity	−	−	−	−	−	+	+	−	−	−
Placental transfer	+	+	+	+	+	−	−	−	−	−
Binding to mononuclear cells	+	−	+	−	−	−	−	−	−	−
Binding to mast cells and to basophils	−	−	−	−	−	−	−	−	−	+ + +
Reaction with protein A from *Staphylococcus aureus*	+	+	−	+	−	−	−	−	−	−
Half-life (days)	21	20	7	21	10	6	6	—	3	2
Distribution (% intravascular)	45	45	45	45	80	42	42	—	75	50
Fractional catabolic rate (% intravascular pool catabolized/day)	7	7	17	7	9	25	25	—	37	71
Synthetic rate (mg/kg/day)	33	33	33	33	3.3	24	24	—	0.4	0.002

(Data primarily from Golub[6] and Glynn and Steward.[8])

idiotypic antibodies that recognize a particular idiotype will not react with any other immunoglobulins in the donor other than the purified antibody used to raise the anti-idiotype antibody. In most cases, the immune response to an antigen results in a mixture of several antibodies, each of which has identical binding specificity but distinct idiotypic determinants. Thus, a given antigenic specificity can have many idiotypes, interpreted as reflecting physical heterogeneity in or near the antibody combining site (e.g., in the V region domains). In some species (notably certain strains of mice), the response to antigen results in a predominant idiotype on all antibodies of a given specificity. Because this is an inherited quality, they are called major, cross-reactive, or public idiotypes. Finally, some public idiotypes have been found in certain species (again most notably mice) to be genetically linked to allotypes.

Three kinds of anti-idiotype antibody have been described: those that function as an internal image of the original antigen by mimicking the antigen structure, those that recognize antibody-combining site-associated idiotypes, and those that are specific for framework-associated determinants. These three types of anti-idiotype antibody are diagrammatically illustrated in Figure 9-3. The first type, internal image antibodies, are the those of clinical interest. The criteria for an internal image antiidiotype is that the antibody is an immunogen in other species, that the antibody response to the antibody binds as specifically as the mimicked antigen, and that the antibody should be able to act as a natural ligand for a cellular receptor for the antigen.

Genetic Basis for Diversity

The origin of antibody diversity and heterogeneity is found in the genes that code for these molecules. The introduction of molecular biologic approaches to the investigation of the immunoglobulins clarified the earlier controversy as to the amount of information for antibody specificity carried in the germline and the amount originating at the level of the somatic cells. This question was resolved by the discovery that in antibodies two genes code for a single polypeptide chain. Two kinds of data support this conclusion. The first involved the discovery of the V and C regions. The second was the observation that, in DNA isolated from embryos that make no antibody, the coding sequences for the V and C regions for a given antibody are located at separate sites in the DNA, but in mature antibody-producing cells for the same antibody, the V and C regions are found in the same part of the DNA.[5,7,8] Detailed analysis of the organization of the L and H chain genes has shown that the genes for κ L chains are located on chromosome 2, for λ L chains on chromosome 22, and for H chains on chromosome 14.

The organization of the L chain genes is shown in Figure 9-4. In addition to the *V* and *C* genes, a set of genes called joining (J) segments are separated from the germline *V* genes. Each V region is preceded by a leader sequence (L$_1$, L$_2$, . . ., L$_N$). In the antibody molecule, the V$_L$ contains three hypervariable regions (CDR1, CDR2, and CDR3) and three framework regions (FR1, FR2, and FR3) (Fig. 9-1). The CDR3 region arises from the region in which gene segments are joined. The H chain gene likewise has a tandem array of six families of *V* segments preceded by leader sequences.[8] At an undetermined distance from the V and leader sequences, 5–15 segments of DNA code for 10 amino acids not found in L chains. These additional elements of variation are called the diversity (D) segments. The functional V$_H$ region is composed of a *V-D-J* segment that results from a series of rearrangements of the germline DNA (Fig. 9-5).

The rearranged *V* genes join with C regions from three families of genes, H, κ, and λ. The estimated 300 *V*κ, 2 *V*λ, and 200 *V*$_H$ genes—are not enough to account for the complete repertoire of the antibody response. It is therefore believed that antibody diversity not only originates in germline genes but is also due to somatic diversification. The possible genetic mechanisms currently under study as forming the basis for somatic diversification include somatic hypermutation and di-

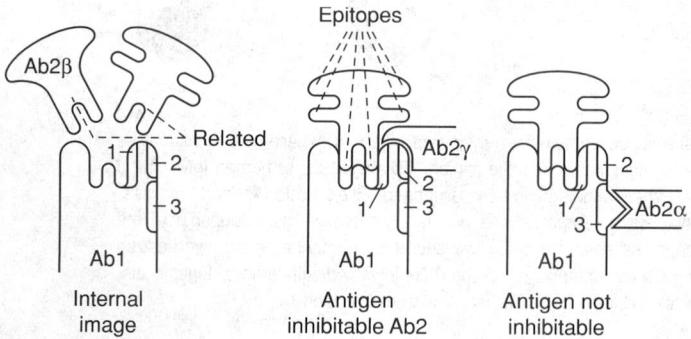

Fig. 9-3. Types of anti-idiotype antibodies. 1, paratope; 2, idiotope; 3, framework.

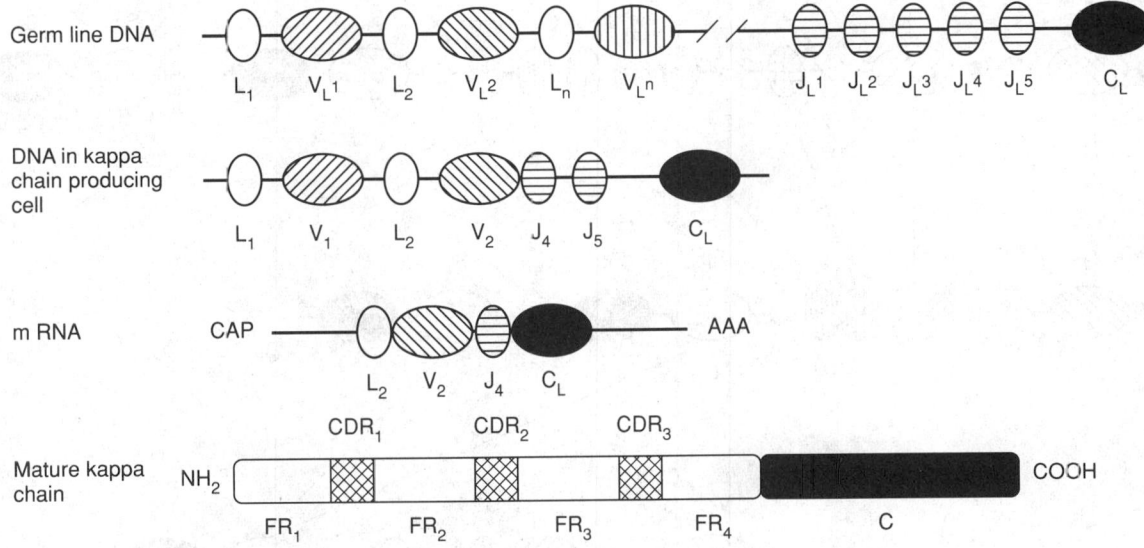

Fig. 9-4. Organization of κ-chain gene. The germline DNA is rearranged in a κ-producing cell so that one V region is brought together with one J region. The mRNA that encodes the protein has the C region adjoined to the V-J region and yields a complete κ-chain. This same motif is used in the organization of the λ-chains. L1, L2, Ln, leader sequences. CDR, hypervariable regions; FR, framework regions. (Data from Golub.[6])

versification occurring during gene rearrangement. A large number of combinations of genes can arise in this manner; calculations show that combinatorial mechanisms can result in 10^7 genes. Thus, the origin of antibody diversity and heterogeneity is believed to originate both in the germline as well as at the level of somatic cells and can be accounted for by a mechanism that joins a relatively small number of genes together in a variety of different ways.

The organization of the human C region genes is now understood. Four $C\lambda$ genes, one $C\kappa$ gene, and as many C_H genes as there are classes and subclasses have been found. The location of the C region genes is on the 3′ side of the V, D, and J regions. During the proliferation of the lymphocytes in an immune response, a class switch usually occurs. This phenomenon refers to the mechanism by which the isotype switches from μ to another class while retaining the same rearranged V region.

The switch occurs in a stretch of DNA called the S region. The DNA also has enhancer elements that are tissue specific and that function to increase the level of transcription of the DNA to mRNA[9] (Fig. 9-6).

Therapeutic Use

IgG was one of the first plasma proteins prepared in a purified state as a therapeutic agent for the treatment of clinical disorders. Along with albumin and factor VIII (antihemophilic factor), it remains the most widely used therapeutic plasma derivative. The method for purifying IgG has remained essentially unchanged from the cold ethanol method developed by Edwin J. Cohn and colleagues from 1935 to 1945. The Cohn method for purifying IgG yields a 15% protein solution that can only be

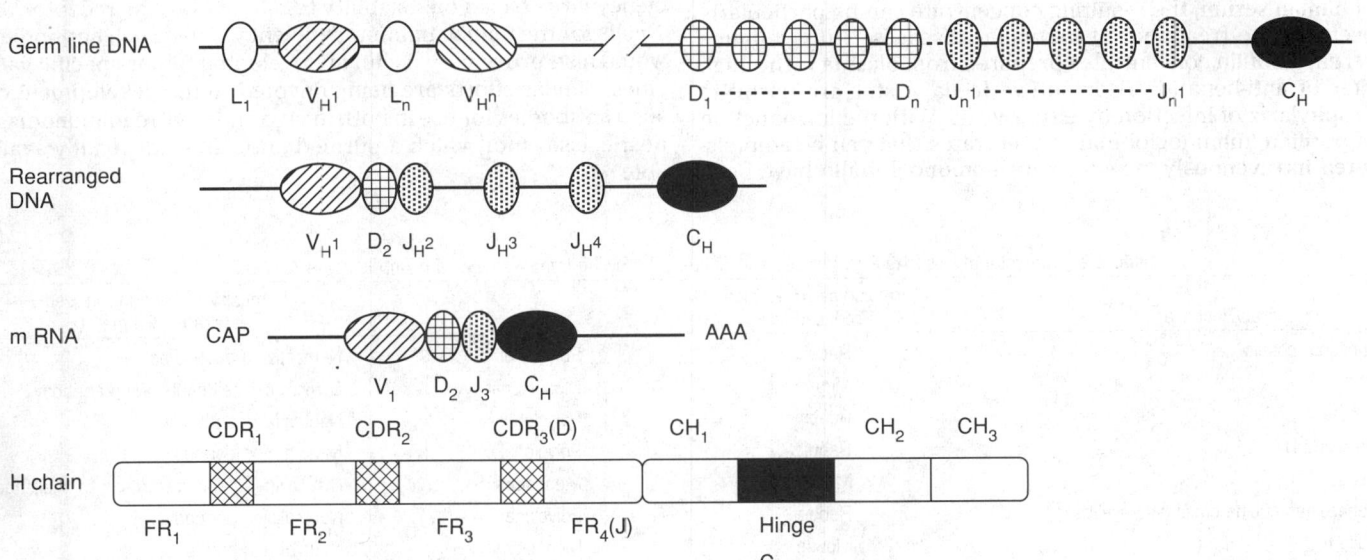

Fig. 9-5. Organization of H chain gene. The germline DNA is rearranged so that *V-D-J* joining results in a V region. In the mRNA this is joined to one of the *Cμ* genes, which encodes a complete H chain. L_1 and L_n, leader sequences. (Data from Golub.[6])

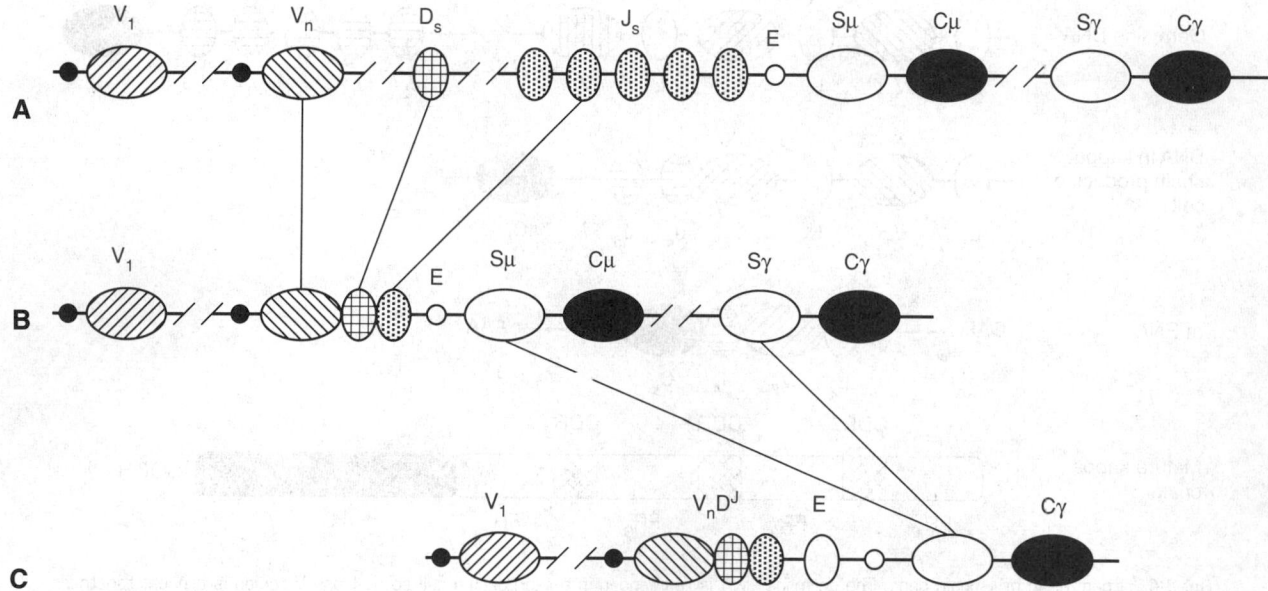

Fig. 9-6. (A) Organization of immunoglobulin H chain genes and enhancer germline DNA of μ-chain in preswitch DNA. Sμ and Sγ are areas in which switch recombination occurs. **(B)** Rearranged DNA in preswitch DNA. Note that the enhancer sequence is located between the J region and the μ-gene. **(C)** Rearranged DNA in postswitch DNA. Note that the same enhancer sequence is now between the rearranged V gene and the Cγ region. Sμ and Sγ refer to the regions in which switch recombination occurs. E, enhancer sequence. (Data from Golub.[6])

given intramuscularly. Over the past 15 years, methods have been developed for preparing IgG in a form suitable for intravenous administration. Three types of preparations are currently approved for use in the United States, all of which have additional purification steps to remove protein aggregates that lead to complications in administering the IgG concentrate intravenously. These steps include precipitation with polyethylene glycol, ion-exchange chromatography, the addition of albumin and sugars, treatment at low pH, and mild treatment with proteolytic enzymes.[10,11] The current therapeutic preparations of immunoglobulin prepared from pooled human plasma are characteristically ≥95% pure.

The principal therapeutic use of immunoglobulin developed for intramuscular injection has been for prophylaxis of disease. When such preparations are made from hyperimmune pools of human serum, the resulting concentrate can be particularly useful in the treatment of particular diseases. Thus, immune serum globulin concentrates prepared from plasma with a high titer of anti-hepatitis B or anti-varicella zoster are useful in prophylaxis of infection by either virus. With the introduction of purified immunoglobulin concentrates that can be administered intravenously, new uses for immunoglobulin have been developed. Notable are the ability to treat primary (congenital) immunodeficiency; secondary immunodeficiency associated with hematologic, traumatic, and neoplastic disease; acute and chronic idiopathic thrombocytopenia; and inflammatory illnesses such as Kawasaki disease. In addition, anti-varicella zoster immunoglobulin has been prepared in a form suitable for intravenous use for use in bone marrow transplant patients.[10,11]

A possible therapeutic and diagnostic use for internal image anti-idiotype antibodies has been suggested, particularly as prophylactic vaccines. Table 9-2 lists the viruses and bacteria to which immunity has been induced in mice with an anti-idiotype antibody.[12] Recent efforts have been devoted to the use of this method to make a vaccine against human immunodeficiency virus based on its ability to mimic CD4, the receptor on T cells for the human immunodeficiency virus. Such antibodies would also prove very useful in developing tumor-specific vaccines. Similar efforts are being devoted to the development of such antibodies for use in both in vivo and in vitro immunodiagnostic assays for which a purified antigen is not readily available.

Table 9-2. Immunity of Mice Against Viruses and Bacteria Following Immunization with Anti-Idiotype Antibodies

Virus/Bacteria	Anti-Idiotype Antibodies Produced In	Class	Immunity of Mice Immunized with α-Idiotype
Tobacco mosaic	Rabbit	Polyclonal	Neutralizing antibodies
Reo	Mouse	Monoclonal	Cytotoxic T-cell neutralizing antibody
Rabies	Rabbit	Polyclonal	Neutralizing antibody
Hepatitis B	Rabbit	Polyclonal	Neutralizing antibody
Sendai	Mouse	Monoclonal	Cytotoxic T cells; resistance to challenge
Venezuelan equine encephalomyelitis	Rabbit	Polyclonal	Neutralizing antibody
Polio II	Mouse	Monoclonal	Neutralizing antibody
Escherichia coli	Mouse	Monoclonal	Resistance to challenge
Streptococcal pneumonia	Mouse	Monoclonal	Resistance to challenge

(From Walter et al.,[12] with permission.)

POLYCLONAL AND MONOCLONAL ANTIBODIES

A fundamental concept in the immune system is the clonal nature and function of the B lymphocytes, the cell type responsible for synthesis of immunoglobulins (see Ch. 8). The constant production by the mammalian immune system of large numbers of B-lymphocyte clones that recognize different antigenic structures on different as well as single molecules leads to the production of a vast array of antibody proteins. Thus, an antiserum raised by immunization with a single cell type or a homogeneous purified antigen contains many different antibodies that have in common specific reactivity with the immunizing cell or antigen but that are also a mixture of immunoglobulins that are heterogeneous according to other criteria, such as size, charge, amino acid sequence, and binding affinity. Because such an antiserum represents a mixture of antibodies derived from many clones of B lymphocytes, all of which have produced an antibody reactive with the immunizing antigen, this is called a polyclonal antiserum; purified immunoglobulins with a single antigen specificity derived from such an antiserum are called polyclonal antibodies.

Monoclonal antibody technology, as described in 1975 by Kohler and Milstein, combines the clonal properties of B lymphocytes with the random segregation of chromosomes in hybrids formed between two cells.[13,14] This procedure produces a hybrid cell that immortalizes an individual antibody-producing B lymphocyte. Thus, each cell line derived from the hybrid produces a unique or monoclonal constant antibody molecule. These cell lines are called hybridomas. The method for obtaining a monoclonal antibody was first developed in a murine system. It is summarized as follows.

After immunization of the mouse, the B lymphocytes are harvested from the spleen or lymph nodes as a single cell suspension and fused with a mouse myeloma cell (plasmacytoma cell; see Ch. 87). The myeloma cell is immortal and has the cytoplasmic machinery with which to produce large quantities of immunoglobulin. The tumor cell used for fusion also contains an enzyme deletion that can be used to select for cells that do not have the deletion. In the murine system this is usually hypoxanthine guanine phosphoribosyltransferase (HGPRT), an enzyme required for survival of the cell in the presence of the folic acid antagonist aminopterine. Fusion of the immunized spleen cells with the myeloma cells is triggered by Sendai virus, polyethylene glycol, electric current, or directed fusion.[15,16] This mixed cell suspension is separated into small aliquots (usually by dilution into a 96-well microtiter plate holding about 200 μl/well); and each aliquot is grown in the presence of the selecting agent, hypoxanthine aminopterine thymidine. Only those hybridoma cells that have acquired the HGPRT from the immunized lymphocytes will survive. The hybrids are then cloned by limited dilution such that there is one cell per well. The growth of the newly fused hybridoma can be facilitated by the addition of interleukin-6, which can be added exogenously or provided by feeder cells. Once they have grown out, the individual clones are tested for the antibody of desired specificity, titer, and binding affinity, before being propagated in either a large-scale tissue culture system or the peritoneal cavity of a mouse as an ascites tumor. Once established, the B-cell hybridomas will exhibit autonomous growth and can be adapted to growth in synthetic media containing no serum. Since these cultures produce a single species of immunoglobulin, the antibodies can be purified by standard column chromatographic methods. However, immunoaffinity purification methods are frequently used to obtain highly purified antibody devoid of any contaminating proteins. The basic steps in the production of a monoclonal antibody from an immunized mouse are summarized in Figure 9-7.

The most widely used species for the production of monoclonal antibodies is the mouse, but hybridoma cell lines can also be obtained from rats and humans. Compared with human immunoglobulin purified from pooled plasma, human monoclonal antibodies are particularly useful as a potential therapeutic reagent for the treatment of human disease, because they have the added advantage of antigen specificity. Serious ethical considerations have been raised concerning the immunization of humans with potential toxins or tumor cells and the lack of a suitable reproducible source of antigen-activated human lymphocytes remains the major difficulty in the preparation of human monoclonal antibodies. An early approach to this problem was the use of Epstein-Barr virus to transform human B cells obtained from the peripheral circulation, allowing for an expansion of the B cells before fusion. This approach is dependent on first finding someone who is producing an antibody of the desired specificity and isotype. Another difficulty in producing human monoclonal antibodies is that a human/mouse hybridoma cell (called a heterohybridoma cell) that results from the fusion of mouse myeloma cells with human B cells tends to lose human chromosomes; this eventually leads to the loss of the ability to secrete human immunoglobulin. A mouse cell line that fuses efficiently with human B cells has been developed and used to produce stable human

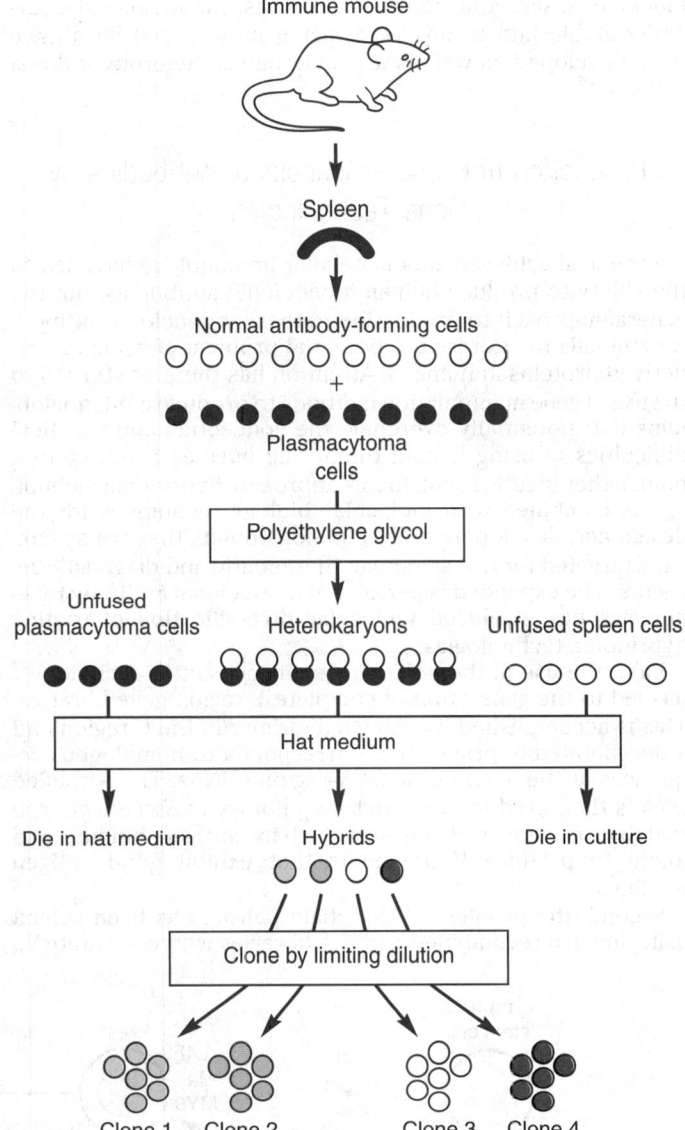

Fig. 9-7. General scheme for the production of murine monoclonal antibodies.

monoclonal secreting heterohybridomas. Simultaneously, several suitable human myeloma fusion partner cell lines have been developed as well as a human/mouse heterohybridoma cell line.[16]

Production of Human Monoclonal Antibodies by Gene Technologies

Technical achievements in cellular immunology have led to the ability to produce human monoclonal antibodies, but the general approach to production of these monoclonal antibodies still fails to address the potential problem of using tumor-derived proteins in humans. Attention has therefore turned to the use of gene manipulation methods to produce immunoglobulins that potentially overcome the conceptual and practical difficulties of using human tumor cell lines as a source of a human therapeutic agent. In this approach, hybridoma technology is combined with molecular biology techniques for the design and development of immunoglobulins that are specifically targeted for use as human therapeutic and diagnostic reagents. The expanded repertoire of monoclonal antibody technologies has produced molecular diversification of routine hybridoma technologies.

First, the use of the polymerase chain reaction technique[17] has led to the generation of complete V region gene libraries. This is accomplished by using a 3' primer in the C region and a degenerated 5" primer that corresponds to homologous sequences at the 5' end of most V-region cDNAs. The amplified DNA is then used to construct a V_H library in *Escherichia coli* that has previously been screened by antigen binding and found to produce V fragments that exhibit good antigen binding.[18]

Second, the problem of H-L chain pairing has been solved using in vitro recombined λ-phage libraries where separate V_H

and V_L fragments (inserted, respectively, on the left and right arm of the phage) are randomly combined in vitro using a unique restriction site located near the center of the phage genome. The diversity generated by this system is probably as large at that generated by the immune system ($>10^8$ antibodies). The resulting antibodies will not be the same as those generated in mammals because phage do not have mechanisms such as the use of alternative V gene fragments (V, D, or J) to form the V regions. Thus, the phage combinatorial library system is most effective when the starting animal has been immunized with the antigen of interest. It is possible, however, to obtain specific antibodies from phage libraries made from nonimmunized animals by enriching for antigen binding through panning the phage-derived immunoglobulin population on immobilized antigen.[19] Thus, the combinatorial phage library methodology represents a significant advance in monoclonal antibody technology.

Third, the problem of modifying an existing antibody to retain desired characteristics and introduce other characteristics required for the intended use forms the basis for engineering monoclonal antibody genes. The high somatic mutation rate of V regions in H and L chains during maturation of the immune response is operative in B-cell hybridomas; this has led to the development of positive screening and selective methods for the detection and enrichment of hybridoma secreted monoclonal antibodies that have altered characteristics.[20] Another approach to engineering monoclonal antibodies is based on recombinant DNA technology. Briefly, H and L chain plasmid cDNAs expressed in hybridoma cells are cloned, sequenced, and appropriately modified by replacing nucleotide sequences. These plasmids are then transfected into non-immunoglobulin secreting myeloma cells and the new cell, called a transfectoma, will secrete the engineered antibody.[21] This is the approach that has been used to humanize murine monoclonal antibodies (e.g., to convert a murine immunoglobulin to

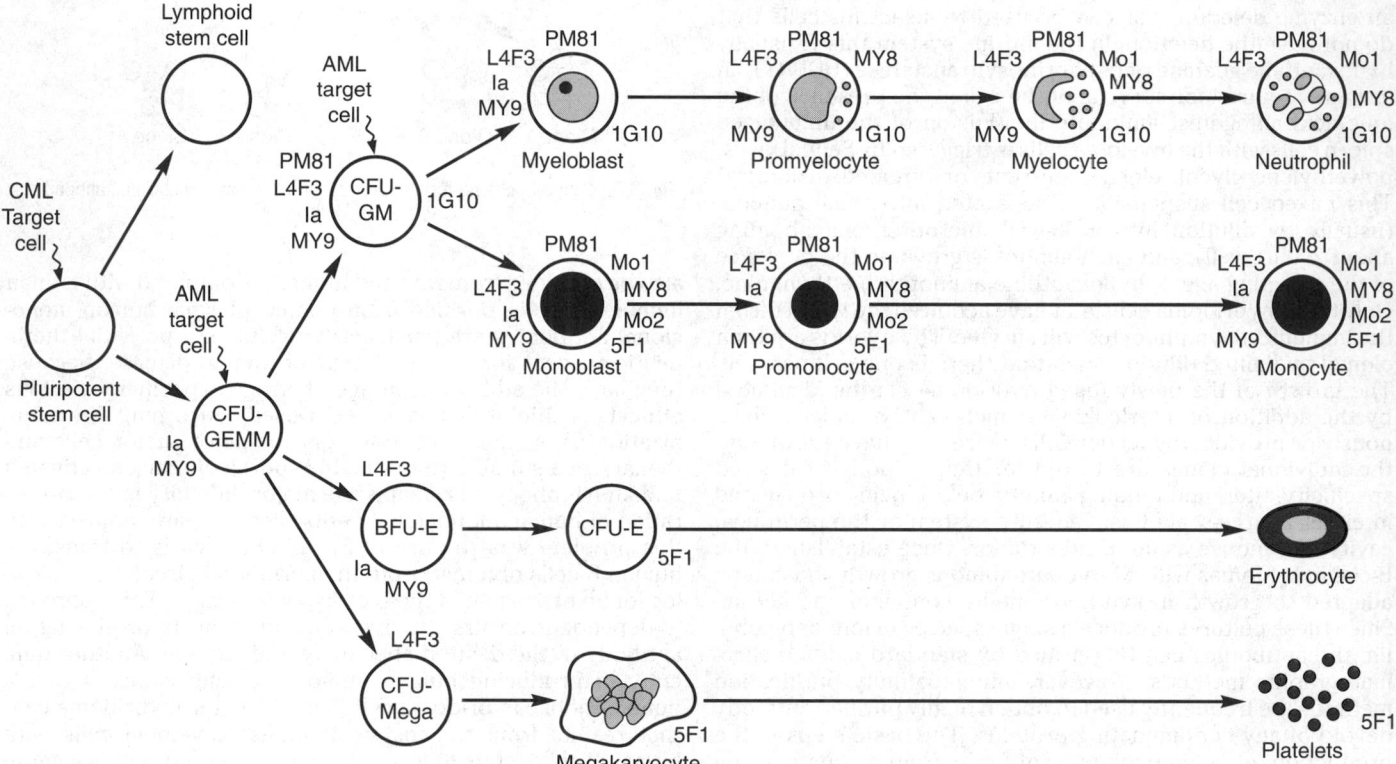

Fig. 9-8. Schematic representation of human myeloid differentiation indicating the phenotype of cell-surface markers as defined by monoclonal antibody reagents.

Table 9-3. Representative Murine Monoclonal Antibodies That Identify Human Myeloid Differentiation Antigens

	S16–114[67,68]	MYg[70,114]	82H5[83]	MY10[115,116]	L1B2[103,117]	R1B1g[67,68,77,89]	8OH.5[84]	S4-7[67,68]	AHN-7[101]	L4F3[103,117]	T5A7[103,117]	Mo1[98,114,118]	Mo5[98]	MY7[114,118,120]	1G10[98,103,117]
CFU-GEMM	+	+	+	+	+	+	+	+	+	+	+	+		+	+
CFU-GM (d 14)	+	+	+	+	+	+	+	+	+	+	+	+	+	+	+
CFU-GM (d 7)	+	+	+	+	+	+	+	+	+	+	+	+	+	+	+
Myeloblast	+	+	+	+	+	+	+	+	+	+	+	+	+	+	+
Promyelocyte	+	+	+	+	+	+	+	+	+	+	+	+	+	+	+
Myelocyte	+	+	+	+	+	+	+	+	+	+	+	+	+	+	+
Metamyelocyte	+	+	−	−	+	−	−	−	−	+	+	+	+	+	+
Neutrophil	−	−	−	+	+	−	−	−	−	+	+	+	+	+	−
Monoblast/promonocyte															
Monocyte	+	+	+	+	+	+	+	+	+	+	+	+	+	+	+
BFU-E	+	+		−	+	−	−	−	−	+	+	−	−	+	+
CFU-E	−	−		+	−	−	−	−	−	−	−	−	−	−	−
Erythroid precursor	−	−		−	−	−	−	−	−	−	−	−	−	−	−
Erythrocyte				−											
CFU-Mk	−	+		−	−	−	−	−	−	+	−	−	−	−	−
Megakaryocyte	−	−		−	−	−	−	−	−	−	−	−	−	−	−
Platelet				−											−

	PMB1[97,114]	AML-2-23[91,114,121,122]	MY-1[90,116,123]	TG-1[66,88]	PMN 6[91,122]	MY8[69,118,119]	8OH.3[84]	B13.4[77,96]	Mo2[83,114,124]	MY3/4[114,118,119]	20.3[104]	Mo4[83,124]	5F1[98,103]	SFL 23.6[126]
CFU-GEMM	−	−	−	−	−	−	−	−	−	−	−	−	−	−
CFU-GM (d 14)	+	+	+	−	−	−	−	−	−	−	−	−	−	−
CFU-GM (d 7)	+	+	+	−	−	−	−	−	−	−	−	−	−	−
Myeloblast	+	+	+	+	+	+	+	+	−	−	−	−	−	−
Promyelocyte	+	+	+	+	+	+	+	+	+	−	−	−	−	−
Myelocyte	+	+	+	+	+	+	+	+	+	+	−	−	−	−
Metamyelocyte	+	+	+	+	+	+	+	+	+	+	+	+	−	−
Neutrophil	−	+	−	+	+	+	+	+	+	+	+	+	−	−
Monoblast/promonocyte														
Monocyte	+	−	−	−	−	−	−	−	+	+	+	+	+	+
BFU-E	−	−	−	−	−	−	−	−	−	−	+	−	−	−
CFU-E	−	−	−	−	−	−	−	−	−	−	−	−	−	+
Erythroid precursor	−	−	−	−	−	−	−	−	−	−	−	−	−	−
Erythrocyte													+	−
CFU-Mk	−	−	−	−	−	−	−	−	−	−	−	−	+	−
Megakaryocyte	−	−	−	−	−	−	−	−	−	−	−	−	+	+
Platelet	−	−	−	−	−	−	−	−	−	−	−	−	−	−

Abbreviations: CFU-GEMM, GM, -E, -Mk, colony-forming unit-granulocyte/erythroid/macrophage/megakaryocyte, -granulocyte/macrophage, -erythroid, -megakaryocyte; BFU-E, burst-forming unit-erythroid.

resemble a human immunoglobulin).[22] Such engineered antibodies are designed to overcome the problem that murine monoclonal antibodies cannot be repeatedly injected into humans without the eventual development of an immune response to the foreign protein. Finally, the combination of the somatic cell method with this type of recombinant DNA method forms the basis of specific gene therapies for the treatment of inherited genetic diseases.[16]

Therapeutic Use

The potential use of monoclonal antibodies as diagnostic reagents and therapeutics is just beginning to be realized. No attempt is made here to summarize all the emerging developments. Two examples of how monoclonal antibodies have proved useful in hematology are the use of monoclonal antibodies to identify cell types that have a common myeloid cell progenitor and the understanding of human myeloid cell differentiation as demonstrated by the identification of cell-surface marker phenotypes.

At one level, monoclonal antibodies have been found that detect antigens expressed uniquely not only by T and B lymphocytes but also as more general markers of peripheral blood monocytes or neutrophils. Thus, certain reagents identify cell surface antigens common (1) to monocytes and neutrophils; (2) to monocytes, neutrophils, and large granular lymphoid cells; (3) to monocytes and platelets; or (4) to neutrophils and large granular lymphoid cells.[23]

At a second level, monoclonal antibodies have been used to correlate the presence of cell-surface antigens with pathways of normal differentiation within the myeloid lineage. These are summarized in Table 9-3, and the stage in differentiation in which the antibodies react is illustrated in Figure 9-8. Detection of the cell-surface antigens is based on either complement-dependent monoclonal antibody-mediated cell lysis (negative selection) or techniques such as fluorescence-activated cell sorting (FACS) or immune rosetting (positive selection). These methods permit the determination of antigen expression by multipotential progenitor cells (colony-forming unit [CFU]-granulocyte/erythroid/macrophage/megakaryocyte) and progenitor cells committed to the myeloid (CFU-GM), erythroid (burst-forming unit-erythroid, CFU-E), or megakaryocyte/platelet (CFU-MK) pathways of differentiation. Certain monoclonal antibodies have been used to prepare 50–100-fold enriched preparations of myeloid progenitor cells from pooled bone marrow mononuclear cells. Certain determinants have been found to be expressed uniquely by progenitor cells; other cell-surface antigens can be found on myeloid, erythroid, or platelet precursors that correspond morphologically and histochemically to distinct stages of maturation; some antigens are either lost or acquired as cells progress from myeloblasts to mature neutrophils; finally, some antigens are maintained on all recognized myeloid cells.[23]

In addition to serving as differentiation markers, many of these cell-surface antigens represent functionally significant plasma membrane proteins, glycoproteins, and glycolipids. Cell-surface antigens have been given cluster designations (CD or CDw), followed by a number. The systematic classification of monoclonal antibodies has made these reagents invaluable tools, not only for the understanding of the development of cellular aspects of hematopoiesis, but they had also found a role in the diagnosis and classification of hematologic disorders and have allowed for guidance on therapeutic decisions.

SUMMARY

The immunoglobulins modulate and mediate many physiologic functions, as well as serving as diagnostic markers of disease and monitors of changing health. Thus, the study of these molecules continues to yield new insights in fundamental biologic, biochemical, and genetic mechanisms controlling hematopoiesis and host-defense mechanisms. Now occurring is a rapid increase in new information on the immunoglobulins based on both biologic and physical/biochemical studies as illustrated by the advances in knowledge on immunoglobulin structure and function and monoclonal antibody technology.

REFERENCES

1. Jones HB: Papers on chemical pathology, lecture III. Lancet 2:88, 1847
2. Korngold L, Lipari R: Immunological studies of Bence-Jones proteins. Proc Ann Assoc Cancer Res 2:29, 1955
3. Deutsch HF, Kratovil CH, Reif AG: Immunological relation of Bence-Jones proteins to normal serum proteins. J Biol Chem 216:103, 1955
4. Getzoff ED, Tamer JA, Lerner RA et al: The chemistry and mechanism of antibody binding to protein antigens. Adv Immunol 43:1, 1988
5. Alt FW, Blackwell TK, Yancopoulos GD: Development of the primary antibody repertoire. Science 238:1079, 1987
6. Golub ES: Immunology: A Synthesis. Sinauer Associates, Sunderland, 1987
7. Blackwell TK, Alt FW: Immunoglobulin genes. In Hames BD, Glover DM (eds): Molecular immunology. IRL Press, Washington, 1988
8. Glynn LE, Steward MW (eds): Structure and Function of Antibodies John Wiley & Sons, Chichester, 1981
9. Barman JE, Mellis SJ, Pollock R et al: Control and organization of human Ig V₄ locus: definition of three new V_H families and linkage to the Ig C_H locus. EMBO J 7:727, 1988
10. Boshkov LK, Kelton JG: The use of intravenous gammaglobulin as an immune replacement and immune suppressant. Transfus Med Rev 3:82, 1989
11. Eibl MM, Wedgwood RJ: Intravenous immunoglobulin: a review. Immunodefic Rev, Suppl. 1:1, 1989
12. Walter G, Friesen HJ, Harthus HP: Anti-idiotypic antibodies: powerful tools in diagnosis and therapy. Behring Inst Mitt 82:182, 1988
13. Kohler G, Milstein C: Continuous cultures of fused cells secreting antibody of predefined specificity. Nature 256:495, 1975
14. Tyle P, Ram BR (eds): Targeted Therapeutic Systems. Marcel Dekker, New York, 1986
15. Oates KM: Therapeutic and drug delivery application of monoclonal antibodies. In Schook LB (ed): Monoclonal Antibody Production Techniques and Applications. Marcel Dekker, New York, 1987
16. Lemieux R, Bazin R: Novel approaches to the preparation and use of monoclonal antibodies. Transfus Med Rev 7:25, 1993
17. Saiki RK, Scharf S, Faloona F et al: Enzymatic amplification of beta-globin genomic sequences and restriction site analysis for diagnosis of sickle cell anemia. Science 222:721, 1985
18. Orlandi R, Gussow DH, Jones PT et al: Cloning immunoglobulin variable domains for expression by the polymerase chain reaction. Proc Natl Acad Sci USA 86:3833, 1989
19. Huse WD, Sastry L, Iverson SA et al: Generation of a large combinatorial library of the immunoglobulin repertoire in phage lambda. Science 246:1275, 1985
20. Spira G, Bargellesi A, Teillaud JL et al: The identification of monoclonal class switch variants by SIB selection and ELISA assay. J Immunol Methods 74:307, 1984
21. Morrison SL, Oi VT: Transfer and expression of immunoglobulin genes. Annu Rev Immunol 2:239, 1984
22. Bruggemann M, Winter G, Waldmann H et al: The immunogenicity of chimeric antibodies. J Exp Med 170:2153, 1989
23. Foon KA, Todd RF III: Immunologic classification of leukemia and lymphoma. Blood 68:1, 1986
24. Turner M: Molecules which recognize antigens. p. 51. In Roitt IM, Brostoff J, Mak DK (eds): Immunology. 2nd Ed. CV Mosby, St. Louis, 1989
25. Alexander MR, Alexander B, Mustion AL et al: Therapeutic use of albumin. JAMA 247:831, 1981

Lymphocyte Cell-Surface Antigens and Receptors

10

Thomas F. Tedder and Pablo Engel

INTRODUCTION

Lymphocytes are a critical cell of the immune system, since individual lymphocytes are able to recognize specific antigens. This level of specificity is achieved through the generation of a myriad of unique antigen receptors expressed on the cell surface. Many of the events that regulate the development of an immune response following antigen encounter are orchestrated through a complex series of cell-surface molecules that are expressed by different lymphocyte subpopulations at different stages of development and activation. Although a significant number of cell-surface molecules expressed by lymphocytes have been identified and their structures determined (Table 10-1), undoubtedly a large array of receptors responsible for regulating biologic processes lack molecular definition. In addition, only a portion of the molecules currently identified are known to carry out specific functions. This chapter reviews some of the known cell-surface molecules expressed by lymphocytes and indicates how these receptors are able to regulate the immune response.

CD Classification of Human Leukocyte Differentiation Antigens

The ability to produce monoclonal antibodies (mAbs) that identify single antigens has led to the discovery, functional characterization, purification, and cloning of a large number of leukocyte surface molecules (Table 10-1). At first, mAbs against leukocyte surface molecules were primarily used to identify lineage-specific markers and to define lymphocyte subpopulations. In many cases, these mAbs identified cell-surface "differentiation" antigens that were specifically expressed during different stages of leukocyte maturation. These reagents have been essential in the study of leukocyte development.

A series of International Workshops on Leukocyte Differentiation Antigens were established in 1982 to develop a nomenclature for cell-surface molecules of human white blood cells. Using a combination of flow cytometric, biochemical, and molecular analysis, individual mAbs that recognize common leukocyte surface structures have been grouped in clusters, permitting the definition of individual surface molecules by cluster designations (CDs). The subsequent determination of function and molecular structure for these antigens has greatly improved our understanding of the cellular interactions involved in the immune response. For example, many of the CDs associate with the T- and B-cell antigen receptors or serve as cell-cell interaction molecules or cytokine receptors or adhesion molecules that regulate lymphocyte activation, proliferation, and differentiation (Table 10-1). Adhesion receptors also appropriately regulate the availability and number of mature lymphocytes and regulate the generation of primary and secondary lymphoid organs that provide the microenvironments

essential for the production of immunocompetent effector cells.

Lymphocyte Development

Lymphocytes are derived from a common bone marrow stem cell that gives rise to two functionally and phenotypically distinct populations through a process described in detail in Chapter 20. Progenitor B and T lymphocytes develop in the bone marrow from a common mesenchymal stem cell that arises from the pool of stem cells that generate all hematopoietic cells. Stem cells are characterized by their cell-surface expression of CD34, a 115,000-M_r sialoglycoprotein with extensive O-linked glycosylation characteristic of cell-associated mucins.[1] Expression of CD34 is limited to a minor subset of bone marrow and fetal liver cells and to small vessel endothelium. While CD34$^+$ bone marrow cells are devoid of lineage-specific cell-surface antigens expressed by mature myeloid, T, B, and natural killer (NK) cells, both in vitro and in vivo studies have shown that most hematopoietic progenitor cells are present in the CD34$^+$ subset.[2]

B cells were the first distinguishable lymphocyte subpopulation based on their site of generation (bursa in the chicken) and expression of cell-surface immunoglobulin (sIg) (Fig. 10-1), which serves as their receptor for antigen. B lymphocytes are generated in the human fetal liver and bone marrow and are the cell lineage responsible for the production of antibodies and presenting antigen to T lymphocytes. Since antibodies generated during a immune response are soluble mediators, they are most often directed against extracellular pathogens such as bacteria, circulating viral particles, and parasites. T lymphocytes are thymus-derived cells that originate in the bone marrow but that mature in the thymus (Fig. 10-2). T lymphocytes are essential for host defense against intracellular pathogens such as viruses and are involved in regulating the function of the other lymphocytes, including B cells. In addition, T lymphocytes are responsible for the rejection of foreign tissue, and may contribute to immune surveillance against tumors. A third lineage of lymphocytes are NK cells, large granular lymphocytes closely related to T cells but that lack the T-cell receptor. NK cells provide innate antigen-nonspecific immunity against certain viruses and bacteria. They are not described in detail in this chapter.

B-LYMPHOCYTE DEVELOPMENT AND RECEPTOR EXPRESSION

B-Cell Differentiation

The maturation of human B-cell precursors into functional B cells proceeds through a highly regulated process involving the coordinated acquisition and loss of B-lineage-associated

Table 10-1. CD Antigens and Their Characterization

CD[a]	Common Name	Chromosome	M_r ($\times 10^{-3}$) (Reduced)	Structure (No. of Domains)	Pattern of Cellular Expression	Function
CD1a	T6	1q22–q23	49	Ig superfamily (1), β2 Microassociated	Thy, DC	Unknown, antigen presentation for some γδ TCR
CD1b		1q22–q23	45	Same as CD1a	Thy, DC	Same as CD1a
CD1c		1q22–q23	43	Same as CD1a	Thy, DC, B-cell subset	Same as CD1a
CD2	T11, LFA-2	1p13	50	Ig superfamily (2)	Thy, T, and NK	Sheep RBC-R, R for CD58, T-cell activation
CD2R	T11₂	1p13	50	Ig superfamily (2)	Activ. T and NK	Epitope expressed with activation
CD3γ	T3, Leu-4	11q23	25–28	Ig superfamily (1)	T	TCR complex
CD3δ	T3, Leu-4	11q23	20	Ig superfamily (1)	T	TCR complex
CD3ε	T3, Leu-4	11q23	20	Ig superfamily (1)	T	TCR complex
CD4	T4, Leu-3	12pter–p12	55	Ig superfamily (4)	T subset, low on M	Interaction molecule that binds MHC class II, signal transduction, R for HIV
CD5	T1	11q13	67	Scavenger R family (3)	Thy, T and B subset	Signal transduction
CD6	T12	11	100	Scavenger R family (3)	T, some B	Unknown
CD7		17	40	Ig superfamily (1)	Thy, T	Unknown
CD8	T8, Leu-2	α-Chain 2p12, β-chain 2	32 α-chain, 32 β-chain	Ig superfamily (1)	T subset	Interaction molecule for class I MHC, signal transduction
CD9		12p13	24	tetra-spans family	Pre-B and immature B, M, P	Signal transduction molecule, P activation
CD10	CALLA	3q21–q27	100	Metalloprotease	Immature B, lymphoid progenitors, G	Cell-surface neutral endopeptidase, enkephalinase
CD11a	LFA-1 α-chain	16p13.1–p11	180	Integrin αᴸ chain	Leukocytes	Associated with CD18, adhesion R for CD50, CD54 and CD102
CD11b	Mac-1, CR3	16p13.1–p11	165	Integrin αᴹ chain	G, M, NK	Associates with CD18, adhesion R for CD54, C3bi R
CD11c	p150,95	16p13.1–p11	150	Integrin αˣ chain	M, G, NK	Associates with CD18, adhesion R
CDw12	—	—	90–120	—	M, G, P	Not a real cluster, essentially abandoned
CD13	MY-7	15q25–q26	150	Metalloprotease	G, M	Aminopeptidase N (EC 3.4.11.2)
CD14	MY-4, Mo2	5q31	55	GPI-linked	M, G, FDC	R for LPS
CD15	Lewis X, LNF III	—	—	COH	M, G, Eo	Lewis X blood group antigen, X hapten
CD15s	sLeˣ, X hapten	—	—	Sialylated COH	M, N, T subset	Sialylated Lewis X, ligand for CD62P and CD62E
CD16	FcγRIIIA, B	1q23	50–65	Ig superfamily (2), GPI-linked and TM forms	G, M, NK subset	Low-affinity Fc-R for IgG, NK activation
CD16b	FcγRIIIB	1q23	48	Ig superfamily (2), GPI-linked	G	Low-affinity Fc-R for IgG
CDw17	LacCer	—	—	COH	G, M, P	Lactosylceramide
CD18	β₂ Integrin	21q22.3	95	Integrin β-chain	Leukocytes	Associates with CD11a, b, or c chains
CD19	B4	16p11.2	95	Ig superfamily (2)	B	Signal transduction complex with CD21 and CD81
CD20	B1	11q12–q13.1	33, 35, 37	4 TM domains	B	Ca²⁺ channel associated with cell cycle progression
CD21	CR2	1q32	145	Complement R family (15, 16)	B and FDC	C3d R, Epstein-Barr virus R, signal transduction complex with CD19

(Table continues)

Table 10-1. *(Continued)*

CD[a]	Common Name	Chromosome	M_r ($\times 10^{-3}$) (Reduced)	Structure (No. of Domains)	Pattern of Cellular Expression	Function
CD22	BL-CAM	19q13.1	130, 140	Ig superfamily (7)	B	Adhesion R for leukocytes and RBC
CD23	FcεRIIa, FcεRIIb	19p13.3	42–45	Type II molecule with C-type lectin domain	Activ. B, M, FDC	Low-affinity R for IgE, antigen focusing
CD24			42	Mucin, GPI-linked	B, G	Signal transduction
CD25	Tac, IL-2R	10p15–p14	55	Complement R family (2)	Activ. lympho-cytes, M, NK	IL-2R α-chain, complexes with CD122 to form high-affinity IL-2R
CD26	DPP IV	11pt34–p11.2	130	Endopeptidase	Activated T and B, M	Dipeptidyl peptidase IV (EC 3.4.14.5), associated with HIV infection
CD27			55, 55 homodimer	NGF-R family (2)	T, activ. B, PC	R for CD70
CD28	9.3	2q33–q34	44, 44 homodimer	Ig superfamily (1)	T subset, PC	R for CD80, signal transduction
CD29	β₁ integrin	10	135	Integrin β-chain	Leukocyte subsets, G weak	Associates with CD49 integrin α chains
CD30	Ki-1, Ber-H2	1p36	105	NGF-R family (5)	Activ. lymphocytes, Reed-Sternberg Cells	Unknown
CD31	PECAM-1		130–140	Ig superfamily (6)	M, G, P, T subset, E	May be involved in G transmigration between endothelial cells
CD32	FcγRIIA, B, and C	1q23	40	Ig superfamily (2)	M, G, P, B, E	Low-affinity FcR for aggregated IgG
CD33		19q13.3	67	Ig superfamily (2)	G, M	Unknown
CD34		1q32	105–120	Mucin	E, bone marrow progenitor cells	Marker for early hematopoietic precursor cells.
CD35	CR1	1q32	220	Complement R family (30)	B, G, M, FDC, T subset	C3bR, polymorphisms in size 190–280
CD36	GpIV		85	No homologies	M, P, E	Unknown
CD37		19	40–52	Tetra-spans family	B, (T, M)	Signal transduction?
CD38	T10, HB-7	4	45	Type II TM glycoprotein	Proliferating B and T, PC, Thy	Unknown
CD39			80	Unknown	Activated B and T	Signal transduction
CD40		20q11–q13	50	NGF-R family (4)	B, E, carcinomas	B-cell growth and inhibition of apoptosis
CD41a	GPIIb/IIIa complex	—	120, 110, 23	Integrin complex	P, megakaryocytes	P activation and aggregation, R for fibrinogen, fibronectin, von Willebrand factor, vitronectin and thrombospondin
CD41b	GPIIb	17c21.32	120, 23	Integrin α^IIb chain	P, megakaryocytes	Associates with CD61
CD42a	GP1X		17–23	Leucine-rich glycoprotein repeat (1) family	P, megakaryocytes	von Willebrand factor and thrombin R, associates with CD42b and c
CD42b	GPIB-α	17pter–p12	135–145	Leucine-rich glycoprotein repeat (7) family	P, megakaryocytes	von Willebrand factor and thrombin R, covalently associates with CD42c
CD42c	GPIB-β		22–25	Leucine-rich glycoprotein repeat (1) family	P, megakaryocytes	von Willebrand factor and thrombin R, covalently associates with CD42b
CD42d	GPV		85		P, megakaryocytes	
CD43	Sialophorin Leukosialin	16p11.2	95	Mucin	Leukocytes	Proposed adhesion R, potential role in T-cell activation
CD44	Pgp-1	11p13	80–100	Mucin, multiple isoforms	Broad, RBC	R for haluronic acid, involved in tumor metastasis
CD44R		11p13	80–100	Mucin	Broad, RBC	Restricted epitope on one CD44 isoform

(Table continues)

Table 10-1. *(Continued)*

CD[a]	Common Name	Chromosome	M_r ($\times 10^{-3}$) (Reduced)	Structure (No. of Domains)	Pattern of Cellular Expression	Function
CD45	T200	1q31–q32	220, 205, 190, 180	Protein tyrosine phosphatase family	Leukocytes	Protein tyrosine phosphatase involved in regulation of signal transduction
CD45RA	T200	1q31–q32	220, 205, 190, 180	Protein tyrosine phosphatase family	B and T subsets, M	Same as CD45, among T cells primarily on virgin or naive cells
CD45RB	B220	1q31–q32	220, 205, 220	Protein tyrosine phosphatase family	B and T subsets, G, M	Same as CD45
CD45RO	UCHL-1	1q31–q32	180	Protein tyrosine phosphatase family	B and T subsets, M	Same as CD45, among T cells primarily on memory cells
CD46	MCP	1q32	66, 56	Complement R family (4)	Leukocytes, E, Epi, F, not on RBC	Membrane cofactor protein for regulation of complement activation
CD47	GP47–52, IAP	—	47–52	COH	Broad	N-linked glycan glycoprotein
CD48	BLAST-1	1q21–q23	41	GPI-linked, Ig superfamily (2)	Broad; including T, B, NK, Eo, not on RBC	Potential ligand for CD2, signal transduction
CD49a	VLA-1		210	Integrin α-chain	Activ. T and B, M	α_1 integrin chain, associates with CD29, collagen, and laminin R
CD49b	VLA-2, gpIa	5	167	Integrin α-chain	P, activ. T, M, some B	α_2 integrin chain, associates with CD29, collagen and extracellular matrix R
CD49c	VLA-3		125	Integrin α-chain	T, some B, M	α_3 integrin chain, associates with CD29, fibronectin, and laminin R
CD49d	VLA-4	2q31–q32	150	Integrin α-chain	T, B, M	α_4 integrin chain, associates with CD29, R for CD106 and fibronectin
CD49e	VLA-5	12q11–q13	135, 25	Integrin α-chain	T, some B and M, G, P	α_5 integrin chain, associates with CD29, R for fibronectin
CD49f	VLA-6		120, 25	Integrin α-chain	P, megakaryocytes, activ. T, M	α_6 integrin chain, associates with CD29, R for extracellular matrix and laminin
CD50	ICAM-3		124	Ig superfamily	T, B, M, G	Ligand for CD11a/CD18
CD51	α^v integrin	2	120/24	Integrin α-chain	P, megakaryocytes	Associates with CD61, R for vitronectin, fibrinogen, and von Willebrand factor
CD51/CD61	GPIIb/IIIa complex	—	120, 114, 24	Integrin complex	P	Complex-dependent epitope
CD52	Campath-1		25–30	O-linked COH on GPI-linked protein	Leukocytes, but not RBC or P	Target for immunotherapy, mitogenic?
CD53	MEM-53	1p12–p13.3	32–40	Tetra-spans family	Leukocytes, PC	Signal transduction
CD54	ICAM-1	19	85	Ig superfamily (5)	Wide activ. lymphocytes, E	Ligand for CD11a/CD18 and CD11b/CD19, rhinovirus R
CD55	DAF	1q32	73	Complement R family (4), PI-linked	Broad	Decay accelerating factor, complement regulatory protein
CD56	NCAM, NKH-1	11q23–q24	220, 135	Ig superfamily (5)	NK cells	Unknown function on NK cells, proposed adhesion R
CD57	HNK-1	—	—	COH	NK (T subset)	Unknown
CD58	LFA-3	1p13	45–60	Ig superfamily (2), PI-linked or TM	Broad, RBC	Ligand for CD2
CD59	MEM-43, LY6, MIRL	11p14–p13	18–20	GPI-linked	Broad, leukocytes, E, Epi.	Membrane attack complex-inhibitor, membrane inhibitor of reactive lysis
CD60	UM4D4	—	—	COH	T subset, M, P	NeuAc-NeuAc-Gal-$^{\beta 1-4}$-(x)-Cer

(Table continues)

Table 10-1. *(Continued)*

CD[a]	Common Name	Chromosome	M_r ($\times 10^{-3}$) (Reduced)	Structure (No. of Domains)	Pattern of Cellular Expression	Function
CD61	gpIIIa	17q21.32	114	Integrin β_3-chain	P, megakaryocytes, M	Associates with CD51, vitronectin R
CD62E	ELAM-1	1q21–23	115	E-selectin	Activ. E	Adhesion R for M, G
CD62L	LAM-1	1q21–q23	74 or 95	L-selectin	Leukocyte subsets	Adhesion R for activated E and HEV
CD62P	PADGEM, GMP-140	1q21–q23	140	P-selectin	P and activ. E	Adhesion R for M, G
CD63	gp53	12q12–q13	53	Tetra-spans family	Activ. P, M (G, T, B)	Present in P lysosomes, translocated to the surface following activation
CD64	FcγRI	1q	75	Ig superfamily (3)	M, activ. G	High-affinity FcγR
CDw65	VIM-2	—		COH	G, M subset	$X^3NeuAcVII^3FucnLc10Cer$
CD66a	BGP-1		180–200	Ig superfamily (4)	G	NCA subgroup of the CEA family, biliary glycoprotein
CD66b	CD67, CGM6		95–100	Ig superfamily (3), PI-linked	G	CEA subfamily member, p100, CGM6, NCA-95
CD66c	NCA		90–95	Ig superfamily (7)	G	CEA subfamily member
CD66d	CGM1		30	Ig superfamily (7)	G	CEA subfamily member
CD66e	CEA		180–200	Ig superfamily (7)	G	Carcinoembryonic antigen, adhesion molecule
CD67	now CD66b	—	—	—	—	Now CD66b
CD68	Macrosialin		110	Mucin	M, G, B	Unknown
CD69	AIM		28, 34 homodimer	Type II glycoprotein-like CD23	Activ. B and T, M, NK	Activation inducer molecule, early activation antigen
CD70	Ki-24		55, 75, 95, 110, 170	NGF-R family	Activ. B and T	Ligand for CD27
CD71	T9	3q26.2–qter	90 homodimer	Type II glycoprotein	Proliferating cells	Transferrin R
CD72	Lyb-2	9p11.1–p24	43, 39 homodimer	CD23 like, type II molecule	B	Signal transduction
CD73	—	6q14–q21	69	GPI-linked ectoenzyme	Activ. B and T	Ecto-5′-nucleotidase, regulates nucleotide metabolism
CD74	—	5q31–q33	41	Type II glycoprotein	B, M	MHC class II invariant chain, antigen processing
CDw75		—	—	COH	Lymphocyte subpopulation	α2,6 linked sialic acid moiety
CDw76		—	—	COH	Lymphocyte subpopulation	α2,6 linked sialic acid moiety
CD77	Gb3		—	—	COH	Activated B	Globotriaocylceramide, p^k blood group, Burkitt lymphoma associated antigen
CD278	Ba	—	67?	Unknown	B, M subpopulation	Unknown
CD79α	Igα, mb-1		33	Ig superfamily (1)	B	B cell Ig-R complex
CD79β	Igβ, B29		40	Ig superfamily (1)	B	B cell Ig-R complex
CD80	B7, BB-1	3q13.3–q21	60	Ig superfamily (2)	Activ. lymphocytes and M, DC	Ligand for CD28 and CTLA-4
CD81	TAPA-1	11p11.2–p15.5	22	Tetra-spans family	B, T, NK, M, E, Epi	Component of CD19 complex
CD82	R2	11p12	50–53	Tetra-spans family	Broad, all leukocytes	Signal transduction
CD83	HB15	6p23–p21.3	43	Ig superfamily (1)	DC, weak on activated lymphocytes	Unknown
CDw84	2G7	—	Unknown	Unknown	B, T, M, P	Unknown

(Table continues)

Table 10-1. *(Continued)*

CD[a]	Common Name	Chromosome	M_r ($\times 10^{-3}$) (Reduced)	Structure (No. of Domains)	Pattern of Cellular Expression	Function
CD85	—		120	Unknown	Strong on M and PC, weak on B	Unknown
CD86	FUN-1	—	80	Unknown	Activ. B, M	Unknown
CD87	UPA-R		50–65	PI-linked glycoprotein	G, M, activ. T, E	R for urokinase plasminogen activator
CD88	C5a-R		42	7-TM domain glycoprotein	G, Eo, M	Complement component R promotes activation and chemotaxis
CD89	FcαR		55–75	Ig superfamily (2)	G, M, T and B subsets	Medium-affinity IgA-R
CDw90	Thy-1	11q22.3–q23	25–35	GPI linked Ig superfamily (1)	Subset of CD34+ stem cells	Growth of stem cells?
CD91	α₂M-R, LRP		515 α-chain, 85 β-chain	Heterodimeric TM glycoprotein	M, F, smooth muscle, hepatocytes	R for α₂-macroglobulin, plasminogen activators, chylomicron remnants, lipoprotein lipase
CDw92			70	Single chain	G, M, E, P	Unknown
CD93			110–120	Single chain	G, M, E	Unknown
CD94	KP43		43, 43	Unknown	NK	Increases with activation
CD95	APO-1, *fas*	10q24.1	42	NGF-R family (3)	Myeloid and lymphoblastoid lines	Induces apoptosis
CD96	Tactile		160	Ig superfamily	Activ. T and NK	Unknown
CD97			74, 80, 90	Unknown	Broad	Unknown
CD98	4F2, 2F3	11q12–q22	80, 40 dimer	Heavy chain is a TM glycoprotein	M (B, T, NK, G are low)	Signaling
CD99	E2, MIC2	Xp22.32-pter, Yp11.2-pter	32	TM glycoprotein	Thy, lymphocytes, RBC	Involved in T-cell rosette formation with RBC
CD99R	—	—	32	—		Restricted epitope
CD100	BB18, A8		150	Unknown	Most lymphocytes, increases with activ.	Unknown
CDw101	BB27, BA27		140 dimer	Unknown	G, M, some T cells	Unknown
CD102	ICAM-2	17q23–q25	60	Ig superfamily (2)	Lymphocytes, M, E, P	Ligand for CD11a/CD18
CD103	αᴱ integrin		150, 25	Integrin α-chain	T	Associates with β₇ to generated HML-1 antigen
CD104	β₄ integrin		220	Integrin β-chain	E, Thy	
CD105	Endoglin		95 dimer	TM with no homology	E, activ. M	Adhesion R?
CD106	VCAM-1		100, 110	Ig superfamily (6, 7)	Activ. E	Ligand for CD49d/CD29 (VLA-4) integrin
CD107a	LAMP-1		110	Mucin	P	Lysosomal vesicle protein
CD107b	LAMP-2		120	Mucin	P	Lysosomal vesicle protein
CDw108	MEM-150, MEM-121		80	GPI-linked	Activ. T and B	Unknown
CDw109	8A3, 7D1		170, 150	GPI-linked	Activ. T and P, E	Activation-dependent antigen
CD115	*c-fms*	5q33.2–q33.3	150	Ig superfamily (5)	M, committed bone marrow progenitors	CSF-1R, CSF-MR
CDw116	CSF-GMR	Xp22.32, Yp11.3	75–85	Hematopoietic cytokine R family	M, G, Eo, F, Endo	CSF-GMR
CD117	*c-kit*	4cen-q21	145	Ig superfamily (5)	Hematopoietic progenitor cells	SCFR
CDw119	IFN-γR	6q23–q24	90	TM glycoprotein	M, B, F, Epi, E	IFN-γR
CD120a	TNF-R	12p13.2	55	NGF-R family (4)	Epi, most cells	TNF-R type I
CD120b	TNF-R	1p36.3–p36.2	75	NGF-R family (4)	M, most cells	TNF-R type II

(Table continues)

Table 10-1. *(Continued)*

CD[a]	Common Name	Chromosome	M_r ($\times 10^{-3}$) (Reduced)	Structure (No. of Domains)	Pattern of Cellular Expression	Function
CDw121a	IL-1R	2q12	80	Ig superfamily (3)	Thy, T, F, E	IL-1R type I
CD121b	IL-1R	2q12–2q22	68	Ig superfamily (3)	B, M, mRNA in T cells	IL-1R type II
CD122	Il-2Rβ	22q13	75	Hematopoietic cytokine R family	Activ. T and B, NK, M	IL-2R β-chain, combines with CD25 to generate a high-affinity R
CDw124	IL-4R	16p12.1–p11.2	140	Hematopoietic cytokine R family	B, T, hematopoietic precursors, E, Epi	IL-4R
CD126	IL-6R	1	80	Ig superfamily (1), hematopoietic cytokine R family	B, PC, myelomas (low on leukocytes, E, F)	IL-6R
CDw127	IL-7R		75	Hematopoietic cytokine R family	Lymphoid precursors, pro-B, T, Thy, M	IL-7R
CDw128	IL-8R	2	58–67	7 TM domains	N, Baso, T subset, M	IL-8R
CDw130	gp130		130	Hematopoietic cytokine R family	Broad	Associates with cytokine R for signal transduction

[a] CDs that have only been partially defined are indicated with a w (for Workshop) designation.

Abbreviations: activ., activated; β2-micro, β2-microglobulin; B, B lymphocytes; Baso, basophils; CEA, carcinoembryonic antigen; COH, carbohydrate; DC, dendritic cells; E, endothelial cells; Eo, eosinophils; Epi., epithelial cells; F, fibroblasts; FDC, follicular dendritic cells; G, granulocytes and neutrophils; GPI, glycosylphosphatidylinositol; HEV, high endothelial cells of secondary lymphoid tissues; HIV, human immunodeficiency virus; Ig, immunoglobulin; IL, interleukin; LPS, lipopollysaccharide; M, monocytes; MAC, membrane attack complex; MHC, major histocompatibility complex; NCA, nonspecific cross-reacting antigen; NGF, nerve growth factor; NK, natural killer cells; P, platelets; PC, plasma cells; R, receptor; RBC, red blood cells; SCF, stem cell factor; T, T lymphocytes; TCR, T-cell antigen receptor; Thy, thymocytes; TM, transmembrane; VCAM, vascular cell adhesion molecule; VLA, very late antigen.

cell-surface molecules. Differentiation within the human B-cell lineage can generally be considered to occur in multiple stages along a linear pathway, as indicated in Figure 10-1. A series of stages have been defined based on immunoglobulin gene rearrangement and expression patterns.[3,4] Although B cells generally express additional characteristic surface structures at each stage, expression of those markers should not be considered to strictly define that maturation stage. Rather, the array of surface molecules expressed is likely to represent a continuum of independent alterations in gene expression that are influenced by maturity as well as the cells microenvironment and state of activation or antigen stimulation.

The earliest stages of B-cell development are antigen independent. The pro-B cell is defined as the earliest committed B-cell progenitor with germline immunoglobulin genes. Pro-B cells do not express cytoplasmic or sIg.[3,4] Pro-B cells do express surface MHC class II molecules, CD10, CD34, and nuclear terminal deoxynucleotidyl transferase but lack most B-lineage specific antigens, such as CD19, CD20, and CD22. CD10 expression on CD34+ stem cells is regarded as an initial event in B-cell development.[4] CD10 may also be on a subset of bone marrow pre-T cells as well as pre-B cells.[5] The next step of B-cell maturation involves rearrangement of immunoglobulin genes prior to the expression of immunoglobulin heavy or light chains and is termed the pre-pre-B cell. Although immunoglobulin genes undergo rearrangement in pre-pre-B cells, immunoglobulin heavy chain protein is not expressed.

B-cell precursors called pre-B cells are marked by rearrangement in their immunoglobulin genes and expression of cytoplasmic μ heavy chain protein[6] (Fig. 10-1). IgM (μ) heavy chains are first expressed only in the cytoplasm, since no light chains are produced at this stage. Late in pre-B cell development, μ heavy chains in combination with a pseudo (ψ) light chain complex are expressed on the surface.[7] In association with appearance of cμ, the expression of CD34 and CD10 ceases, and nu-

clear terminal deoxynucleotidyl transferase is no longer present.[4,6] Later, a pseudo-light chain complex ψLC, is produced, without light chain rearrangement, and a subset of pre-B cells express surface μ heavy chain/ψLC complexes.[6–8] Although the function of this early surface complex is unknown, it theoretically serves as a positive selection mechanism for B-cell development. At the next stage of B-cell development, immature B cells have productively rearranged their κ or λ light chain genes, synthesize κ- or λ-protein and are thereby able to express an IgM monomer (H_2-L_2) receptor on the cell surface. This receptor is the antigen-recognizing structure that gives the B cell its specificity. Although some pre-pre-B cells express CD19, CD22, CD38, and CD40 late in development, most pre-B cells express these surface antigens.[5,9] Once this process has occurred, immature B cells develop into mature B cells and sIgD is coexpressed with sIgM. At this point, B-lineage development in bone marrow is completed and B cells exit into the peripheral circulation and migrate to secondary lymphoid organs.[6,10]

As described in Chapter 20, the immunoglobulin receptor is assembled from separate gene products that generate heavy chains of multiple isotypes, μ, δ, γ1, γ2, γ3, γ4, α1, α2, and ε, and light chains that derive from two gene loci, κ and λ. Each heavy chain gene product is assembled from members of syntenic families of discrete exons that encode distinct functional immunoglobulin-like domains. Heavy chains derive from the assembly of V(ariable), D(iversity), J(oining), and C(onstant) exons, while light chains derive from V, J, and C components. This patchwork assembly of *V, D,* and *J* segments and the possibility of different heavy and light chain combinations allows for the generation of antibody molecules with tremendous diversity in specificity for antigen. Moreover, somatic mutation, in conjunction with combinatorial diversity, permits the production of millions of distinct antibody molecules, each with its own characteristic antigen-binding abilities. Since, gene

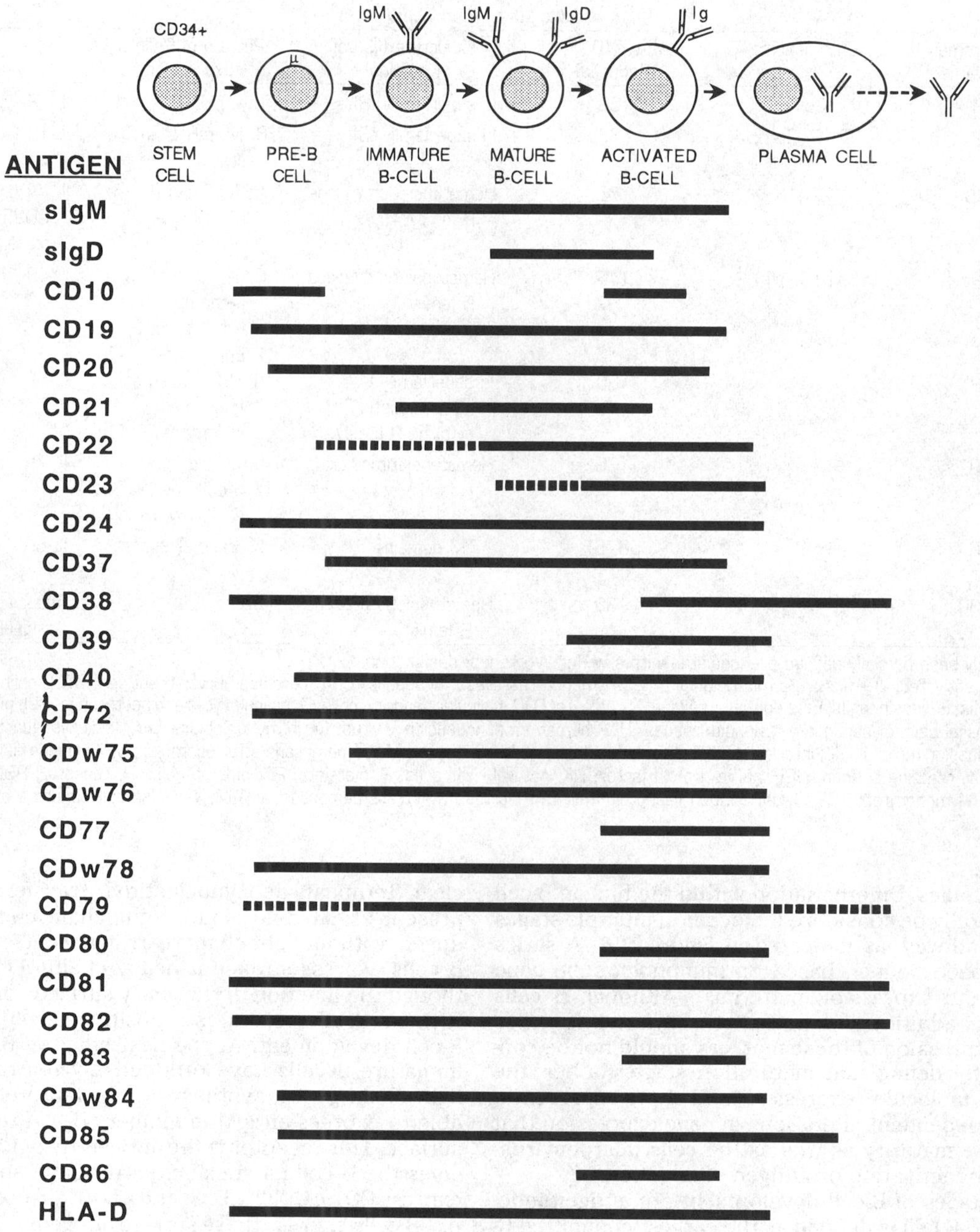

Fig. 10-1. Expression of surface molecules during B-cell development.

rearrangement is required to generate functional immunoglobulin products, successful rearrangement shuts off continued rearrangements at other loci, so that each B-cell clone produces an antibody product with a single specificity. Considering the numbers of V, D, and J gene segments and heavy chain and light chain possibilities, a multitude of different antibody specificities can be constructed. In addition, new codons can be generated at the sites of gene segment recombination. These codon modifications are generated by two mechanisms: imprecise joining of gene segments (called junctional diversity), which can act during both V_H and V_L gene assembly, and the insertion of random nucleotides at the gene segment junctions of V_H genes (called N-region diversity), which probably occurs through the action of the enzyme terminal deoxynucleotidyl transferase. Within germinal centers of secondary follicles in lymphoid tissues, additional somatic mutation of immunoglobulin genes occurs during the generation of an immune response to increase the repertoire of antigen-binding specificities.

These point mutations add more potential diversity to a maturing population of antibody producing cells.[11]

Once antibody specificity is defined by heavy chain V-D-J joining and light chain assembly, the B cell can switch from the initial production of μ heavy chains to the expression of the other heavy chain isotypes, again through gene rearrangement involving the C region exons. Through differential mRNA splicing, both secreted and membrane-anchored forms of immunoglobulin are produced. Immature B cells begin to express both sIgM and IgD, which represent the vast majority (80–90%) of circulating B cells. After an encounter with the appropriate antigen followed by T-cell help, B cells become activated and proliferate with a subsequent clonal expansion of their numbers in order to generate an effective immune response. Activated B cells gain the expression of some surface molecules like CD23, CD25, and CD38. These molecules are known as activation antigens and regulate the proliferation and further differentiation of the B lymphocytes into plasma cells. At the same

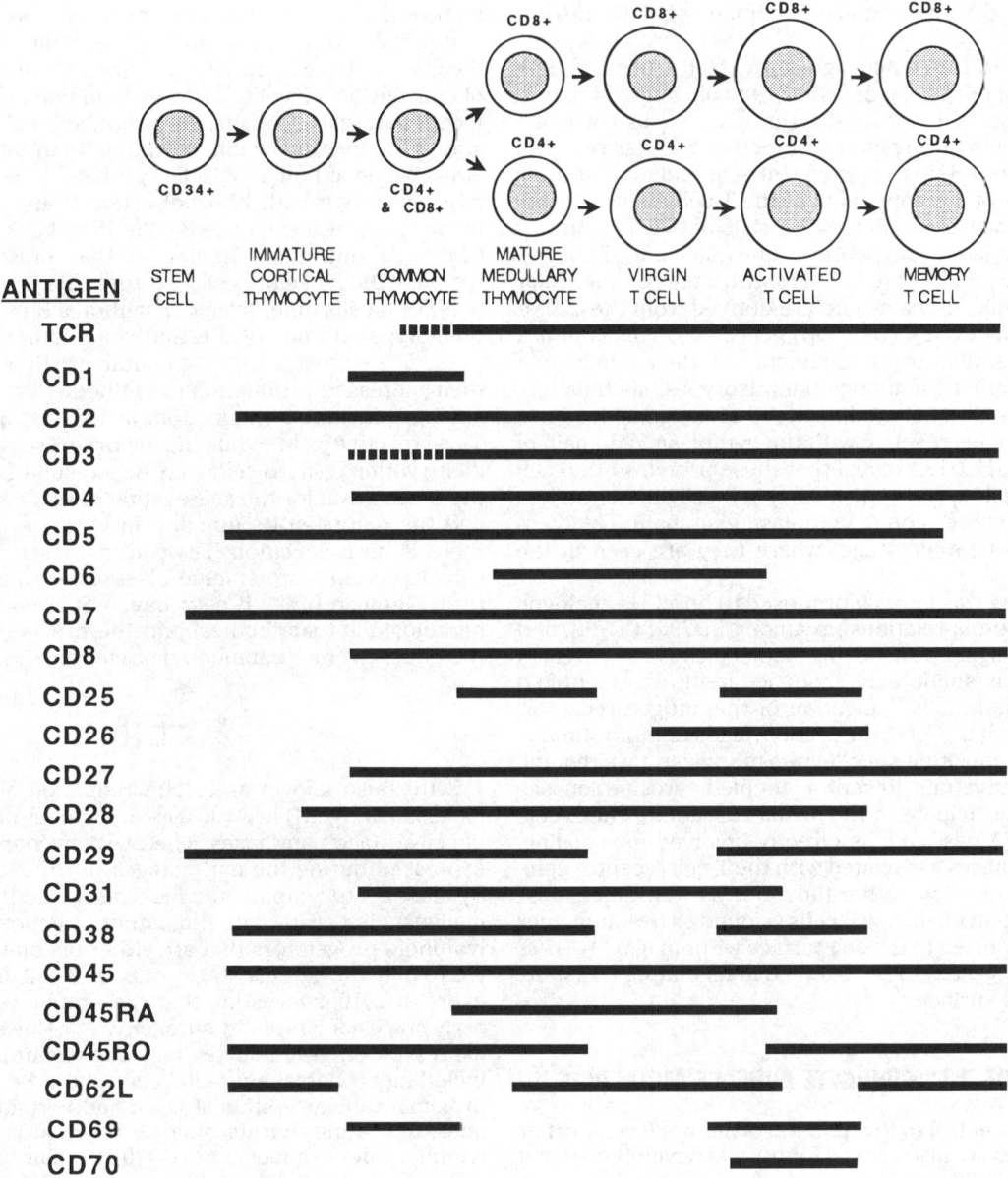

Fig. 10-2. Expression of surface molecules during T-cell development.

time that these activation antigens appear on the surface of B lymphocytes, some antigens that were previously expressed disappear from the membrane such as IgD and CD21 (Fig. 10-1). This activation process can be recapitulated in vitro using antibodies to crosslink sIg. However, cross-linking sIgM can also lead to inactivation or elimination of B cells through a mechanism whereby early B cells are tolerized to self-antigens.

Although mature B cells express both IgM and IgD on their cell surface, B cells at the border of specific stages of development can express as many as three different immunoglobulin heavy chain isotypes. However, after terminal differentiation into a plasma cell, only one antibody isoform is secreted with ≈2,000 antibody molecules produced by each plasma cell per second. Thus, the generation of a functional antigen receptor represents a complex and necessary event in the development of a functional B cell. Many cells do not undergo the appropriate gene rearrangements and are deleted from the B-cell pool through heretofore unknown mechanisms. In addition, few B cells encounter the appropriate antigen or effector T cell and therefore fail to become amplified in number and to differentiate into plasma cells. After plasma cell development, the se-

creted antibodies are then able to combine with the inducing antigen to aid in its elimination. Those antigen-specific B cells that have gone through antigen stimulation without terminal differentiation are thought to reenter the circulating pool of B cells as an amplified population of "memory" B cells. These cells are able to respond to antigen on subsequent stimulation with a hastened response.

The sIg Receptor Complex: CD79α and CD79β

The B-cell antigen receptor complex performs several highly specialized functions. Engagement of antigen by sIg triggers a signal transduction cascade that results in activation and proliferation of mature B cells, and clonal deletion of immature B cells. The receptor complex is also required for the appropriate internalization and processing of antigen, which is then externalized in association with MHC class II molecules for presentation to T cells.[12] In addition, expression of sIg may regulate B cell development by signaling the productive rearrangement of immunoglobulin genes.[6] Many of these processes may be influenced by the differential activation of signal transduction pathways.

sIg is not able to transduce signals by itself since IgM, IgD, and IgG lack a significant cytoplasmic domain, being of only 3, 3, and 28 amino acids, respectively. However, the use of gentle nonionic detergents during immunoprecipitation has revealed a set of phosphoproteins noncovalently associated with sIg analogous to the CD3 components of the T-cell antigen receptor.[13] The IgM-associated complex consists of two structurally distinct N-glycosylated polypeptides of 47,000 and 37,000 M_r, which occur as disulfide-linked dimers with single extracellular immunoglobulin-like domains and are derived from the CD79α (mb1, Igα) and the CD79β (B29, Igβ) genes.[14–16] This complex is biochemically similar to, yet distinct from, the complex that associates with other immunoglobulin isotypes, such as IgD, suggesting that additional modifications of the gene products occur.[17,18] Antibodies reactive with the cytoplasmic domain of human CD79α and CD79β reveal that these proteins are B-cell specific in expression, and appear early in B-cell differentiation, probably before expression of cytoplasmic μ-chain. They persist until the plasma cell stage, where they are seen in the cytoplasm.[19]

Although CD79α was initially proposed to be a CD3 analogue based on structure, a relationship among CD79α, CD79β, and other CD3-like signal-transducing molecules was revealed when a consensus amino acid sequence motif was identified in their cytoplasmic tails.[20] Ligation of the antigen receptor, apparently through G-protein activation, leads to rapid stimulation of a phosphoinositide-specific phosphodiesterase that initiates cellular activation. Receptor coupled tyrosine kinases also initiate or participate in the signal cascade.[21] The B-cell-specific tyrosine kinase, *blk*, is directly involved in signaling, as are tyrosine kinases associated with the T-cell receptor complex.[22,23] CD79α may have other functions as well, since most of the CD79α protein on mouse B cells is found as free monomer that can be transported to the cell surface without IgM.[24] CD79α has also been suggested to be involved in mediating transport of IgM to the cell surface.[25]

FUNCTIONS OF B-LYMPHOCYTE SURFACE MOLECULES

Although sIg is central to the function of mature B cells, other surface structures are also critical for normal development and regulation of B-cell differentiation, activation, and proliferation. Signals generated through non-immunoglobulin receptors can also modulate, either in a positive or a negative way, the signals delivered through sIg. In this way, the anatomic location, local microenvironment or milieu of localized "factors" can directly influence the outcome of a humoral response. In addition, the array of surface antigens expressed at any particular stage of differentiation on the B cell or the interacting T cell can have a directing influence as well. While many B-cell- and T-cell-restricted or associated proteins are undoubtedly involved in regulating lymphocyte development and proliferation (Table 10-1), it is likely that additional surface receptors have yet to be identified and functionally examined.

CD5

A subpopulation of human B cells express CD5, a marker found on nearly all T lymphocytes. Functional studies have suggested that CD5 B cells develop along a lineage that is distinct from conventional B cells, but this issue is highly controversial.[26] CD5$^+$ B cells appear in the human fetal peritoneal and pleural cavities at 15 weeks of gestation, however, these cells are absent from the liver before 16 weeks and are rare in the bone marrow.[27] During B-cell development, 40% of the mature B cells found in the omentum and spleen are CD5$^+$ compared with only 20% in the liver.[28] In mouse, CD5 (Ly1$^+$) B cells are also generated in a compartment distinct from that of conventional B cells.[29] However, in humans, CD5-expressing B cells may just represent a subpopulation of cells at a different stage of activation or differentiation than other B cells.[30] This is likely, since human B cells can be induced to express CD5 after treatment with phorbol esters,[31] and crosslinking sIgM on newly emerging mouse B cells stimulates the expression of CD5.[32] An intriguing finding is that most human chronic lymphocytic leukemia cells express CD5.

CD5$^+$ B cells differ from conventional B cells in their surface phenotype, tissue localization, and immunoglobulin repertoire.[30] The most intriguing characteristic of CD5$^+$ B cells is their increased production of antibodies with affinity for self-antigens, including rheumatoid factor, and anti-DNA and anti-T-cell reactivity.[33,34] While the over-representation of this specificity within CD5$^+$ B cells may be a result of antigen selection, the mechanism for the segregation of this antibody specificity and the nature of its function in vivo are unclear. Although there is an association between increased levels of CD5$^+$ B cells in certain autoimmune diseases such as rheumatoid arthritis, human CD5$^+$ B cells have not been shown to secrete pathologic autoantibodies, and the precise role they play in the etiology of autoimmune disease remains unknown.

CD10

CD10 (also known as CALLA [common acute lymphocytic leukemia antigen]) is a 100,000-M_r member of a growing family of cell-surface peptidases. The CD10 glycoprotein is primarily expressed during the early stages of pre-B-cell development, by most acute lymphocytic leukemias, and by other lymphoid malignancies with an immature phenotype.[35,36] Normal lymphoid progenitors that are either uncommitted or committed to only the earliest stages of B- or T-cell differentiation also express CD10, suggesting that the protein plays a role in the early stages of lymphoid ontogeny.[37–39] However, CD10 is also expressed on granulocytes and nonhematopoietic cell types, including bronchial epithelial cells, cultured fibroblasts, renal proximal tubular epithelial cells, and certain solid tumor cell lines, indicating that its biologic function is not restricted to lymphoid development.[40,41] CD10 is a zinc metalloproteinase neutral endopeptidase 24.11 that cleaves peptide bonds on the amino side of hydrophobic amino acids and inactivates a variety of peptide hormones.[36,42] Although the true function of CD10 on B cells remains unclear, the endopeptidase activity may serve to digest polypeptide factors present in the environment of maturing B lymphocytes, thereby altering proliferation and differentiation.

CD19

In addition to the sIg receptor complex, CD19 and CD21 are key signal transduction molecules that noncovalently associate to form multimolecular complexes on the cell surface.[43,44] CD19, a member of the immunoglobulin superfamily,[45] is associated with several proteins at the cell surface, including CD21 (CR2), a member of a family of complement receptors,[46,47] which, like CD19, is uniquely expressed by B cells and follicular dendritic cells.[48–50] Two additional members of the CD19 complex are CD81, a broadly expressed protein that is a member of a family of proteins that span the membrane four times,[51] and Leu-13, a broadly expressed protein that has not yet been structurally characterized.[52] Thus, CD19, CD21, CD81, and Leu-13 associate to generate a signal transduction complex on B lymphocytes independent of the antigen receptor complex.

CD19 is a 95,000-M_r protein whose expression is restricted to normal and neoplasic B cells.[53] CD19 is expressed from the early stages of immunoglobulin heavy chain rearrangement until plasma cell differentiation and most B-cell lineage malignancies.[54] The CD19 protein has two extracellular immunoglobulin-like domains, a membrane-spanning domain, and a highly charged approximately 240-amino acid cytoplasmic tail containing localized regions of strong net negative charge.[45,55] CD19 may be involved in growth regulation of B cells because mAb binding to CD19 inhibits the increase in free intracellular calcium concentration and the subsequent activation and proliferation that follow mitogen stimulation.[56] Transgenic mice overexpressing the human CD19 gene have been generated to dissect the in vivo role of CD19 in B-cell development and activation.[57] Expression of the human transgene product is specifically restricted to all B-lineage cells and appears early in development as occurs with human CD19. In addition, expression of human CD19 severely impairs the development of immature B cells in the bone marrow with dramatically fewer B cells found in the spleen, peripheral circulation, and peritoneal cavity. These results indicate an important role for CD19 during early B-cell development before antigen-dependent activation and suggest that CD19 may be involved in early tolerance induction of B cells.

CD20

CD20 was the first non-immunoglobulin differentiation antigen specific of human B cells to be identified by a mAb.[58] CD20 expression is found on some B-cell precursors and all mature B cells and is lost with differentiation into plasma cells.[59] CD20 is a structurally unique protein that contains three extensive hydrophobic regions of sufficient lengths to pass through the membrane four times.[60] Long C- and N-terminal ends of the molecule are located within the cytoplasm, with only a minor portion of the molecule exposed to the extracellular environment. The transmembrane and cytoplasmic regions of both mouse and human CD20 are well conserved and may allow for interactions with the multiple proteins that are co-immunoprecipitated with CD20.[61] CD20 is a dominant phosphoprotein in activated B cells with three isoforms of 33,000, 35,000, and 37,000 M_r resulting from differential phosphorylation of a single protein species at different serine and threonine residues within the cytoplasmic domain.[61,62] CD20 shares a common chromosomal location, a similar overall structure and sequence homology with the β-chain of the high-affinity IgE receptor found on mast cells,[63,64] suggesting that CD20 is a member of a new gene family.

Antibody binding to CD20 inhibits B cell entry into the S, G_2, and M stages of cell cycle after mitogen stimulation and also blocks differentiation.[65,66] CD20 is not phosphorylated in resting B cells, becomes heavily phosphorylated after mitogen stimulation, and antibody binding to CD20 generates a transmembrane signal that results in enhanced phosphorylation of the molecule.[62] The presence of four membrane-spanning domains in CD20 is reminiscent of membrane transporters or ion channels. Indeed, CD20 has been found to be a component of a homo-oligomeric complex of perhaps four CD20 molecules that forms a Ca^{2+} channel critical for normal B-cell function.[67]

CD21

CD21 is the B-cell receptor for the C3d, C3dg, and iC3b fragments of complement[68,69] and also serves as the receptor for Epstein-Barr virus.[70] CD21 is first expressed by most B cells around the time of IgD expression and is lost following activation.[49] CD21 is a 145,000 M_r protein that consists of 15 or 16 short consensus repeat units, each of 60–70 amino acids, followed by a transmembrane region and a 34-amino acid intracytoplasmic domain.[46,47] Cross-linking with CD21 mAb or C3d can deliver a costimulatory signal to B cells suboptimally activated by phorbol esters, anti-IgM antibodies, or T-cell factors.[71–73] Cross-linking of IgM with CD21 also enhances the transient increase in intracellular Ca^{2+} levels induced through IgM alone.[74,75] Capping of CD21 results in co-capping of immunoglobulin, and capping of immunoglobulin results in co-capping of CD21.[76] Thus, CD21 and immunoglobulin may not only share some similar signal transduction pathways but may also associate under appropriate conditions. These data, and the recent finding that CD21 is part of a large multimolecular complex containing CD19, CD81, and Leu-13, suggest that CD21 plays an important role in regulating the B-cell response to antigen.

CD22

CD22 is a B lineage-restricted member of the immunoglobulin-superfamily that functions as an adhesion receptor.[77,78] CD22 cDNA encodes a 140,000-M_r protein with a single N-terminal immunoglobulin V-like domain, six immunoglobulin C-type domains, a transmembrane domain, and a long cytoplasmic tail. CD22 is homologous with other adhesion receptors that are members of the immunoglobulin superfamily, CD56 and CD66. CD22 expression is restricted to normal and neoplasic B cells, with CD22 protein expressed in the cytoplasm of progenitor B and pre-B cells, but CD22 is found mainly on the surface of mature B cells.[79,80] However, most precursor-B-cell acute lymphocytic leukemias seem to express both the cytoplasmic and the membrane forms of CD22. CD22 expression increases following activation and disappears with further differentiation.[77,79] In lymphoid tissues, CD22 is expressed by follicular mantle and marginal zone B cells, but only weakly by germinal center B cells.[79] However, in situ hybridization reveals the strongest expression of CD22 mRNA within the germinal center and weaker expression within the mantle zone.[77]

CD22 may be involved in the regulation of B-cell activation, since the binding of CD22 mAb to B cells in vitro augments both the increase in intracellular free Ca^{2+} and the proliferation induced after cross-linking of sIg.[81,82] A soluble form of CD22 inhibits CD3-mediated activation of human T cells, suggesting that CD22 may be important in T cell-B cell interactions.[83]

CD23

CD23 is a low-affinity receptor for IgE (FcεRII) that may have broad effects in immunoregulation.[84] CD23 is a 45,000-M_r glycoprotein expressed on the surface of activated B cells that is a type II integral membrane protein (N_2 terminus within the cell) with a C-terminal C-type lectin domain.[85,86] Following the cloning of the FcεRII cDNA, it was quickly realized that this functionally defined structure was identical to serologically defined CD23.[87,88] Differential splicing of a single gene results in an isoform of CD23 expressed by B cells (FcεRIIa) with a second form expressed by eosinophils, monocytes, and platelets (FcεRIIb).[89] A striking feature of CD23 is that it may be cleaved into biologically active soluble fragments, some of which retain the ability to bind IgE and possess a variety of reported biologic effects. CD23 has been proposed to be involved in multiple regulatory functions, including the regulation IgE synthesis, immunoglobulin-dependent antigen focusing, B-cell growth-promoting activity and germinal center B-cell survival.[90]

CD24

CD24 is a pan-B-cell marker expressed from the pro-B-cell stage until plasma cell differentiation that is also expressed by neutrophils.[91] CD24 is a heavily glycosylated protein of 35,000–45,000 M_r,[92] attached to the plasma membrane through a glycosylphosphatidylinositol (GPI) anchor.[93] The CD24 cDNA encodes a remarkably small peptide of 31–35 amino acids with multiple sites for addition of N- and O-linked carbohydrates suggesting that the bulk of the 35,000–45,000-M_r molecule is carbohydrate.[94] Consistent with this, many of the CD24 mAb react with carbohydrate determinants present on CD24.[95] Although the function of CD24 is unknown, the high carbohydrate content of CD24 suggests a lectin-like molecule as its ligand, although such a ligand has not been identified. Several GPI-anchored cell-surface molecules, including CD24, have been found to associate with protein tyrosine kinases, key regulators of cell activation and signal transduction,[96] consistent with reported signaling through this cell surface molecule.

CD40

CD40 is a 50,000-M_r glycoprotein expressed on most B cells that delivers a potent co-stimulatory signal for cell-cycle progression.[97,98] CD40 is also expressed by epithelial and carcinoma cells.[99,100] Quiescent B cells can be directly perturbed through CD40 to enlarge, aggregate, and acquire enhanced responsiveness to mitogenic triggering.[101] B cells stimulated with anti-IgM, CD20 antibody, or phorbol esters can be stimulated to enter S phase by anti-CD40 mAb.[97,98,100] Moreover, mAb binding to CD40 can act synergistically with other growth promoting agents such as interleukin (IL)-4 to sustain B-cell proliferation.[102,103] Antibody binding to CD40 can also prevent germinal center B cells from entering apoptosis, thereby directing B cells toward plasma cell development on antigenic stimulation.[104]

CD40 is a member of the nerve growth factor receptor family.[105] The CD40 ligand is a cell-surface molecule preferentially expressed by CD4$^+$ T cells immediately after activation.[106,107] Engagement of this ligand mediates B-cell proliferation in the absence of a co-stimulus, as well as IgE production in the presence of IL-4. Thus, this receptor-ligand pair provides a rapid means of cellular communication between B and T cells when they come into intimate contact following antigen recognition.[108] Consistent with this, a defect in the CD40 ligand is the cause of X-linked hyper-IgM immunodeficiency.[109] This rare disorder is characterized by markedly decreased serum concentrations of IgA, IgE, and IgG, while concentrations of polyclonal IgMs are normal or even elevated. This clearly indicates that CD40 regulates isotype-switching of B cells.

CD72

CD72 is expressed at all stages of B-cell differentiation, except for the plasma cell stage, and is identical to the mouse Lyb-2 differentiation antigen.[110,111] CD72 is an 80,000-M_r pan-B-cell glycoprotein composed of two disulfide-linked polypeptides of 39,000 and 43,000 M_r derived from an identical protein precursor that is differentially proteolytically cleaved. CD72 is a type II integral membrane protein that, like CD23, contains a C-terminal domain homologous with C-type animal lectin domains. Functional data for human CD72 are modest, while extensive studies have been carried out on the mouse Lyb-2 molecule suggesting that Lyb-2 participates in early B-cell activation.[112] With human B cells, mAb binding to CD72 augments selective activation pathways in tonsillar B cells.[113] By itself, CD72 mAb binding provides a weak stimulus to resting B cells but provides synergistic signals when added with immobilized anti-IgM antibody.

CD80

CD80 is a cell-surface activation antigen expressed after stimulation of resting B cells by cross-linking sIg or HLA-DR antigens, by Epstein-Barr virus infection, or by exposure to IL-2 or IL-4.[114–116] CD80 identifies a subpopulation of B cells in vivo that appears to be previously activated or primed and therefore demonstrates an accelerated response to activation agents.[114] CD80 is also expressed on the surface of monocytes in response to interferon-γ activation.[117] CD80 is a 44,000–54,000-M_r glycoprotein composed of a V-type immunoglobulin-like domain, a C-type immunoglobulin-like domain, a transmembrane domain, and a short 16-amino acid cytoplasmic tail.[118]

CD80 serves as a ligand for two structurally similar molecules expressed on T lymphocytes: CD28 and CTLA-4.[119–121] Binding of CD28 by mAb or by interaction with CD80 results in enhanced production of cytokines by activated T cells due to increased mRNA stability.[116,122,123] Direct helper T-cell-induced B-cell differentiation also involves interaction between CD28 on T cells and CD80 on activated B cells.[124] CTLA-4 is expressed at a lower level on the T-cell surface than is CD28 but possesses a higher affinity for CD80.[121] Since the interaction between CD28/CTLA-4 and CD80 provides a necessary co-stimulus for the activation of T lymphocytes to respond to presented antigen, it is likely to serve as an important regulator of the cognate antigen responses, particularly in germinal centers.

The interaction between CD80 and its ligands (CD28/CTLA-4) is likely to regulate the development of an immune response, since T-cell receptor signaling in the absence of CD80 co-stimulation results in the induction of antigen-specific tolerance.[123,125,126] Recently, another ligand for the CTLA-4 T-cell receptor has been identified, termed B7-2.[127] This receptor appears 24 hours after B-cell activation and induces IL-2 secretion and T-cell proliferation.[128] This molecule also belongs to the immunoglobulin superfamily and has 26% amino acid sequence identity with CD80,[127] consistent with the observation that CD80-deficient mice still express a functional CTLA-4 ligand that can compensate for the CD80 loss.[129] This finding and the observation that B7-2 appears on the cell surface immediately following B-cell activation have suggested that there are a series of co-stimulatory steps and receptors involved in early T-cell-B cell interactions.[128,130]

HLA Class II

HLA class II antigens serve a critical role in the initiation of an immune response through their role as antigen-presenting molecules on the surface of B cells. Although the precise signal transduction role of MHC class II antigen in the biologic responses of B lymphocytes remains unknown, engagement of B-lymphocyte class II region gene products with mAb generates transmembrane signals. Thus, antibodies reactive with HLA-D can replace helper T cells in activating B lymphocytes,[131] or, conversely, can inhibit human B-cell activation, proliferation, and differentiation.[132] HLA-D-mediated signaling is associated with an increase in intracellular Ca^{2+}, activation of phospholipase C, and induction of protein phosphorylation.[133] Transmembrane signaling through murine B-cell class II molecules induces the rapid translocation of cytosolic protein kinase C to the nucleus,[134,135] and stimulation of quiescent murine B cells with IL-4 and anti-sIg antibody primes B cells to proliferate in response to class II antigen cross-linking.[136] Engagement of class II antigen also induces sustained LFA-1-dependent and

-independent B-cell adhesion. In addition, engagement of class II antigen by CD4 induces rapid homotypic adhesion of B lymphocytes.[137] Antibody ligation of other epitopes on class II antigens can also lead to heterologous desensitization of signal transduction pathways that induce homotypic adhesion in lymphocytes.[138] Thus, signal transduction through class II molecules is likely to be critical to the generation of B cell responses, in addition to the function of these surface receptors in antigen presentation.

T-LYMPHOCYTE DEVELOPMENT AND RECEPTOR EXPRESSION

T-Cell Differentiation

As with B lymphocytes, T-lymphocyte progenitor cells derive from a common CD34[+] stem cell in the bone marrow. T-cell precursors express CD45, CD34, and CD7 before and during migration to the thymus, where most T cells mature into immunocompetent effector cells.[139] The thymus can be anatomically divided into cortical and medullary regions, each containing different subsets of T lymphocytes that can be distinguished both by expression of specific cell-surface receptors (Fig. 10-2) and by function. Thymocyte subsets are primarily delineated by their expression of cell-surface CD4 and CD8. The least mature T cells are found in the cortex, where the cells express CD7 and CD2, but lack other T-cell markers, including CD3, CD4, and CD8.[140] The predominantly immature cortical thymocytes that lack CD4 and CD8 are called "double-negative" cells; these proliferating cells comprise 3–5% of the thymus. The next identifiable stage of pre-T-cell maturation in the thymus is reached when the T cells begin to rearrange their T-cell receptor genes through mechanisms similar to those used by B cells, as described in Chapter 20. Although these cells lack surface T-cell receptor expression, they are CD7[+] and cytoplasmic CD3[+].[141–143] In vitro, putative intrathymic pre-T cells give rise to T-cell receptor γδ cells, NK cells, and a small percentage of T-cell receptor αβ cells, suggesting that rearrangement of γδ genes identifies a more primitive lineage of T cell.[140–144]

Pre-T cells undergo the next discernible series of differentiation events when cell-surface CD4 and CD8 expression is initiated. These "double positive" CD4[+]/CD8[+] cells are found in the thymic cortex, where they comprise approximately 80–85% of total thymocytes. Double positive cells are rarely seen in peripheral tissues. CD4 low or negative pre-T cells express CD8 as an intermediate before becoming CD4[+]/CD8[+] cortical "common" thymocytes.[144] Common thymocytes located in the cortex are the only thymocytes that express CD1[145] (Fig. 10-2). A stage at which CD4[+] T-cell receptor-negative cells express the CD8α chain, but not the CD8β chain, has also been proposed.[146] The cortex contains the most immature and rapidly dividing thymocytes where most die in situ consistent with their rearrangement of T-cell receptor genes. T-cell receptor positive cells also express cell-surface CD3, a complex of multiple cell-surface proteins that physically associate with the T-cell receptor to provide the signal transduction machinery. T-cell receptor-bearing CD3[+] cells are found in both the cortex and the medulla of the thymus.

As immature cortical thymocytes begin to express a cell-surface T-cell receptor, the process of positive and negative thymocyte selection takes place.[147] Self-reactive thymocytes are removed from the T-cell pool by negative selection.[148] Thymocytes with T-cell receptors that are incapable of binding to self-MHC are also deleted through the process of apoptosis. Thymocytes with T-cell receptors capable of interacting with foreign antigens within the context of self-MHC antigens undergo positive selection, leading to activation and maturation.[149] The cell-receptor αβ cells that express CD4 primarily become MHC class II-restricted helper T cells, while T-cell receptor αβ cells that express CD8 become MHC class I restricted. Thymic selection processes are thought to occur sequentially.[150] Immature thymocytes that have just begun to express low levels of surface T-cell receptor first undergo positive selection, while still refractory to negative selection. However, later in T-cell development, autoreactive T cells are deleted by means of the negative selection process.[150]

Mature thymocytes that are capable of migrating from the thymus into the bloodstream are found almost exclusively in the medullary region and constitute about 10–15% of total thymocytes. When T-cell maturation is completed, the cells leave the thymus and migrate to the peripheral tissue, to become part of the recirculating pool of lymphocytes. Mature T lymphocytes can be subdivided in two groups according to the class of T-cell receptor they express. More than 90% of circulating and peripheral T cells express heterodimers of α- and β-chains, and 3–10% of T lymphocytes express the heterodimeric γδ T-cell receptor. Most of the γδ lymphocytes are CD4[−]/CD8[−], although a small number are CD4[−]/CD8[+].[151] Mature αβ T lymphocytes can be further subdivided according to expression of CD4 or CD8, where the expression of these two molecules is mutually exclusive.[145] These subsets of T lymphocytes differ not only in the way they recognize antigen, interacting with different classes of MHC molecules but also in their effector functions. CD4[+]/CD8[−] cells (about 60% of mature T cells) recognize MHC class II products and are largely involved in mediating B-cell help and inflammatory responses.[152] By contrast, CD4[−]/CD8[+] cells, which comprise about 20–30% of mature T cells, recognize MHC class I molecules and have predominantly cytotoxic functions.[153] In addition to this effector function, CD4[+] and CD8[+] lymphocytes express a large array of cell-surface receptors and are able to release a variety of soluble factors that influence the differentiation of other lymphohemotopoietic cells.

After leaving the thymus, CD4[+] T cells undergo a linear differentiation program.[154,155] Helper T cells that have recently left the thymus, have not encountered antigen, and therefore do not proliferate in a recall response to antigen exposure, express a specific 220,000-M_r isoform of CD45 known as CD45RA. These cells have been termed virgin or naive T cells.[154] When these mature T lymphocytes interact with the appropriate antigen, signals are transduced through the T-cell receptor/CD3 complex that activates the cells. In contrast to the B-cell antigen receptor that recognizes antigenic determinants in solution, T cells only recognize antigen when bound to MHC class I or class II structures on the surface of antigen-presenting cells.[156] This allows T cells to recognize cell-associated antigens such as virus particles expressed by infected cells. T cells that have previously encountered antigen and can therefore mount a recall response are CD45RA[−] and are called memory T cells.[154] Both the CD45RA[+] and CD45RA[−] subpopulations of helper T cells are able to activate B cells through direct contact and induce equivalent B-cell proliferation.[155] By contrast, only the memory subpopulation of T cells is able to induce B-cell differentiation into immunoglobulin-secreting plasma cells.[155,157] These studies suggest that memory helper T cells are induced to express surface molecules not expressed by virgin T cells. Virgin post-thymic T lymphocytes are CD44[low], CD58[low], and CD11a/18[low].[158–161] After initial antigen-induced activation of virgin T cells in the periphery, memory T cells express CD29, CD58, and the 180,000-M_r isoform of CD45 (CD45RO). Memory T cells also express high levels of a number of adhesion molecules (CD44[hi], CD58[hi], CD2[hi], CD11a/CD18[hi]) and have display expression of the fibronectin or laminin receptors (VLA-4, VLA-5, and VLA-6).[159,160,162] Activated T lymphocytes also express several surface molecules not expressed on resting cells. Some of these molecules are receptors for growth factors and nutrients, such as the α-chain of the IL-2 receptor (CD25) and the transferrin receptor (CD71).[163] Other surface molecules are involved in the regulation of T-cell proliferation, such as the CD40 ligand and the ligand for CD27 (CD70).[164] These molecules are essential for the T cell to initiate an effective immune response, since full responsiveness of a T lymphocyte requires the participation of multiple accessory molecules in addition to antigen receptor cross-linking.

T-Cell Antigen Receptor: CD3

The T-cell receptor is similar in structure to the immunoglobulin receptor of B lymphocytes (see Ch. 20). T-cell receptors are disulfide-linked heterodimers composed of either α- (45,000–60,000 M_r) and β- (40,000–50,000) chains or γ- (45,000–60,000) and δ- (40,000–60,000) chains. The T-cell receptor chains belong to the immunoglobulin superfamily and consist of an N-terminal V-like immunoglobulin domain and a C-like immunoglobulin domain, a transmembrane region, and a short cytoplasmic tail.[165] Since the T-cell receptor chains have short cytoplasmic domains, signal transduction requires associations with a set of transmembrane proteins that constitute the CD3 complex. A great diversity of α- and β-chains can be generated in the T-lymphocyte pool by the combinatorial rearrangement of different *V, D,* and *J* gene segments. However, T-cell receptor genes differ from immunoglobulin genes in that there are smaller numbers of *V* genes and larger numbers of *J*-gene segments. Junctional and N-region diversification is also generated for both α- and β-chain genes and tends to be much higher for the T-cell receptors than for the immunoglobulin molecules. By contrast, somatic mutations do not contribute to the diversification of T-cell receptor V regions.[166] The γ- and δ-genes are organized similarly and use the same strategies to generate a diversity of T-cell receptor specificity.

The CD3 signal transduction complex is composed of multiple subunits; γ (25,000 M_r), δ (20,000), and ε (20,000)[167] (Fig. 10-3). During intrathymic T-cell maturation, members of the CD3 complex are expressed in the cytoplasm but become functionally and physically linked to either the αβ or γδ T-cell receptor heterodimers once they are expressed. This event results in expression of the T-cell receptor complex on the cell surface. CD3 γ, δ, and ε are each T-cell-specific transmembrane glycoproteins that contain a single extracellular C-type immunoglobulin domain and a cytoplasmic tail. CD3 γ- and δ-chains exist as heterodimers with CD3 ε. Additional transmembrane proteins also associate with CD3; ζ (16,000 M_r) and η (22,000 M_r).[168] The T-cell receptor ζ-chain contains a 9-amino acid extracellular domain, a transmembrane region, and a 112-amino acid cytoplasmic tail. The T-cell receptor ζ-chain forms disulfide-linked homodimers or, less frequently, heterodimers with its splicing variant, the η-chain.[169] The cytoplasmic domains of CD3 γ, δ, ε, ζ, and η encode a motif found in a variety of molecules associated with signal transduction, including the proteins associated with the B-cell receptor complex components, CD79α and CD79β.[20] Like surface immunoglobulin on B cells, the T-cell receptor complex is responsible for initiating intracellular signals following receptor recognition of antigen.

FUNCTIONS OF T-LYMPHOCYTE SURFACE MOLECULES

CD1

CD1 is a transmembrane glycoprotein that shares a similar structure with MHC class I molecules; it is also associated with β2-microglobulin. However, in contrast to MHC class I molecules, CD1 does not exhibit polymorphism. Nonetheless, five CD1 genes have been cloned in humans. Comparison of nucleotide and amino acid sequences shows that members of the CD1 family are significantly less related to each other than are each of the different MHC class I isotypes.[170] Three cell-surface protein products of the CD1 family, CD1a (49,000 M_r), CD1b (45,000 M_r), and CD1c (43,000 M_r), have been identified by mAb. CD1a, CD1b, and CD1c differ from one another in tissue distribution

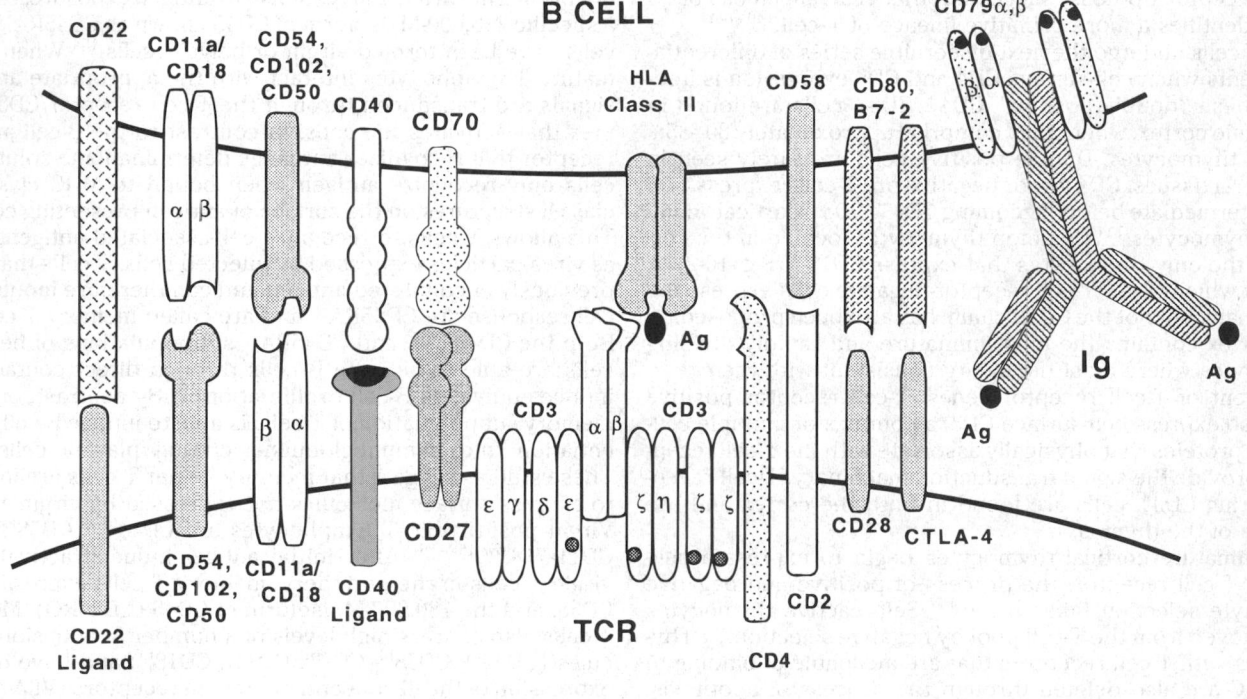

Fig. 10-3. Representative cell-surface receptors that regulate T cell-B cell interactions. TCR, T-cell receptor; Ag, antigen.

patterns and levels of expression.[171] In general, CD1 is expressed on cortical thymocytes and dendritic cells, including interdigitating cells and Langerhans cells.[172] CD1 and specially CD1c can also be found on a subset of B cells.[173] It has been proposed that CD1 functions as an antigen-presenting molecule for T-cell receptor $\gamma\delta$ cells.[174]

CD2

CD2 is a 45,000–58,000-M_r glycoprotein that contains two extracellular immunoglobulin-like domains and a large cytoplasmic domain rich in proline and basic amino acids.[175] CD2 is expressed on all T cells, including immature thymocytes and memory T cells, and is also found on a subpopulation of NK cells. The expression of a specific cell-surface epitope on CD2 (CD2R) can be induced after T-cell activation. This epitope is expressed on thymocytes and on activated mature lymphocytes but is absent from resting peripheral blood lymphocytes. Antibody binding to the CD2R epitope can induce potent T-cell proliferation analogous to that generated after cross-linking of the CD3 complex.[176] Although this activation pathway is antigen independent, CD3 has to be expressed on the cell surface for CD2 activation to occur, suggesting that they share a common signal transduction pathway.[177] Moreover, it has been shown that CD2 can physically associate with the CD3 complex. CD2 and CD3 are functionally linked, since T-cell activation via CD2 results in phosphorylation of tyrosine residues on T-cell receptor ζ-chains and serine phosphorylation of CD3 γ-chains.[178]

Human T lymphocytes were first identified by their ability to form rosettes with sheep erythrocytes; CD2 serves as the T-cell receptor for this event.[179] A CD2 ligand on sheep and human erythrocytes has been identified as the CD58 surface molecule.[180] CD2 interacts with CD58 through its N-terminal immunoglobulin-like domain. CD58 is a phospholipid-linked glycoprotein that is also a member of the immunoglobulin superfamily consisting of two immunoglobulin-like domains homologous to its receptor CD2.[181–183] CD58 is widely expressed on epithelial cells and hematopoietic cells, as well as throughout normal lymphocyte ontogeny. CD58 mediates adhesion and signal transduction to T cells and NK cells through binding to CD2 and mAb binding to CD58 inhibits sheep erythrocyte rosette formation, T-cell cytotoxicity, and NK and lymphokine-activated killer-cell killing.[183] Two other molecules, CD59 and CD48, have been proposed to be ligands for CD2; however, the physiologic relevance of the interaction of these molecules with CD2 remains to be determined.[184,185]

CD4

CD4 is a monomeric 55,000-M_r transmembrane glycoprotein that belongs to the immunoglobulin superfamily and contains four extracellular immunoglobulin-like domains. CD4 is expressed on thymocytes, on a subset of mature T lymphocytes (approximately 60%), and can also be found at very low levels on monocytes and macrophages. CD4 binding to monomorphic determinants present on MHC class II molecules serves to stabilize interactions between the T-cell receptor and antigenic peptides located on HLA molecules of antigen-presenting cells.[152,153,186] CD4 is directly involved in regulating T-cell activation and is physically associated with an intracellular lymphocyte-specific protein tyrosine kinase known as p56[lck].[187] While most CD4+ mature lymphocytes function as helper T cells, CD4 has also been found on cytotoxic T cells that are able to lyse cells bearing class II MHC molecules. CD4 also functions as a receptor for human T-cell leukemia virus-1,

whereby the viral gp120 protein binds to the N-terminal domain of the molecule.[188]

CD5

CD5 is an immunoglobulin superfamily member that is expressed on T-cell precursors, and is maintained throughout ontogeny.[189] The function of CD5 on thymocytes is unknown.

CD7

CD7 is a 40,000-M_r glycoprotein that contains a V-type immunoglobulin-like domain.[190] CD7 is expressed on early hematopoietic cells (including a subset of CD34+ bone marrow cells), as well as by immature and mature T and NK cells.[139] It was initially proposed to be a receptor for IgM, but studies with cDNA-transfected cells have not verified this hypothesis.[190]

CD8

CD8 is a heterodimer composed of α- and β-chains, although dimers of CD8α can also be found on the cell surface.[191] Both CD8α and CD8β are glycoproteins of 32,000–34,000 M_r that have one immunoglobulin-like domain separated from the transmembrane by a hinge region rich in proline, serine, and threonine residues.[191] CD8 is expressed by thymocytes and by a subpopulation (approximately 40%) of T lymphocytes.[145] CD8α has also been detected at low levels on NK cells. The immunoglobulin-like domain of CD8α binds to invariant residues in the $\alpha3$ domain of MHC class I molecules.[153] Like CD4, the cytoplasmic domain of CD8 binds to the p56[lck] tyrosine kinase.[187] Most CD8+ lymphocytes have cytotoxic capabilities. CD8 cells were also initially proposed to be suppressor T lymphocytes.[145] However, it is unclear whether suppressor cells are a separate lineage, since CD4+ T cells can also mediate suppressive effects under certain experimental circumstances. Some of the suppressor activity observed in early experiments with CD8+ cells is possibly attributable to the cytotoxic capacity of this cell lineage.

CD27

CD27 is a disulfide-linked homodimer composed of two chains of 55,000 M_r. Like CD40, CD27 is a member of the neuronal growth factor receptor family.[192] CD27 is found on a subset of mature T lymphocytes and medullary thymocytes, and the expression of CD27 is increased after T-cell activation.[193] CD27 is also expressed on some B cells, including activated B lymphocytes, B-lymphoblastoid cell lines, and plasma cells.[194] The ligand for CD27 has been identified as the CD70 activation antigen of B and T cells.[164,195] It has been proposed that the interaction of these two proteins may play a role in regulating the proliferation of T lymphocytes and the further differentiation of this cell into cytotoxic cells.

CD28

CD28 is a heavily glycosylated disulfide-linked homodimer composed of a single V-type immunoglobulin-like domain, a transmembrane region, and a cytoplasmic tail.[196] CD28 is expressed on most T lymphocytes, and its expression is augmented after T-cell activation.[119] CD28 expression has also been detected on activated B and plasma cells. CD28 binds to CD80 on activated B lymphocytes.[197] CD28 is also homologous to another ligand for CD80, known as CTLA-4.[198] The CD28-

CD80 interaction plays an important role in the interactions between B and T lymphocytes and specially in the regulation of the proliferation of T cells.

ADHESION MOLECULES

Another group of cell-surface molecules that are critical to normal lymphocyte function are the receptors that mediate cell-cell interactions and lymphocyte migration throughout the body. Many of the lineage-associated receptors previously described, such as CD2 and CD22, are adhesion molecules. However, a number of broadly expressed receptors are also critical for the adhesion of lymphocytes to the proper microenvironment and for their growth and differentiation.[199,200] For example, CD49d/CD29, CD44, CD62L, and CD11a/CD18 mediate B-cell adhesion to bone marrow stromal cells and to components of the lymph node microenvironment.

CD29/CD49

Several members of the integrin family are present on lymphocytes. One group of integrins designated very late antigens (VLA) are glycoprotein heterodimers consisting of unique CD29 α chains ($\alpha_1-\alpha_7$) noncovalently associated with a common CD49 β_1 chain that bind their ligands in a cation-dependent manner.[201,202] The β_1 integrins VLA-4 ($\alpha_4\beta_1$) and VLA-5 ($\alpha_5\beta_1$) function as extracellular matrix receptors by binding to fibronectin. VLA-4 also serves as a receptor for CD106 (vascular cell adhesion molecule-1 [VCAM-1]),[203] a member of the immunoglobulin superfamily that is widely expressed. Although VLA-5 is only expressed during early lymphocyte differentiation, VLA-4 remains on B cells even after they exit the bone marrow and enter the circulation, while it is only present on a subpopulation of circulating T cells.[204,205] The β_1 integrins generally increase in number on the cell surface after activation (Table 10-1), and lymphocyte stimulation induces a transient increase in their receptor activity providing a means of rapid adhesion/de-adhesion for cellular interactions such as cytotoxicity.[206] Differential expression of various members of the CD49 integrin family between T and B cells and the observation that the density of many members of the CD49 family are increased following T-cell activation may in part account for some of the migratory differences between activated T and B lymphocytes.[200]

CD11/CD18

Essentially all leukocytes express the CD11a/CD18 (leukocyte function-associated antigen-1 [LFA-1]) surface antigen that interacts with its ligand intercellular adhesion molecule (ICAM)-1 to facilitate cellular interactions critical for most T- and B-cell functions.[201,202] LFA-1 is a member of the leukocyte integrin family, which consists of three CD11 α-chains that form heterodimers with a common CD18 β_2-chain, CD11a/CD18 ($\alpha_L\beta_2$), CD11b/CD18 ($\alpha_M\beta_2$, Mac-1, Mo1, CR3), and CD11c/CD18 ($\alpha_x\beta_2$, p150,95). CD11b and CD11c are not expressed by most circulating lymphocytes, but CD11c is expressed on activated B cells after in vitro stimulation, on some B-cell lines, and at high levels on hairy cell leukemias.[207,208] The ligands for LFA-1 include ICAM-1 (CD54), ICAM-2 (CD102), and ICAM-3 (CD50), which are members of the immunoglobulin superfamily. ICAM-1 is expressed on activated B and T cells, monocytes, follicular dendritic cells, and cytokine-activated endothelial cells. ICAM-2 expression is largely restricted to unstimulated endothelial cells, peripheral blood T and B lymphocytes and monocytes, but not to neutrophils. Nearly all lymphocytes express low levels of ICAM-2. ICAM-3 is constitutively expressed on all leukocytes and is not expressed on endothelial cells.[209] The broad constitutive expression of ICAM-3 has led to the postulate that ICAM-3 is potentially the most important ligand for LFA-1 in initiating the immune response because expression of ICAM-1 on resting leukocytes is low, while ICAM-3 expression is high.[209]

CD44

CD44 constitutes a broadly distributed family of glycoproteins expressed on virtually all hematopoietic cells.[210] CD44 is involved in cell-cell or cell-matrix binding as a receptor for hyaluronate[211] and is functionally associated with tumor cell metastasis.[212] Lymphocyte CD44 is homologous to cartilage-link proteins and proteoglycans,[213] but different isoforms of CD44 result from differential splicing of a single complex gene.

CD62L

The ability of lymphocytes to leave the circulation and to migrate into tissues is a critical feature of the immune response involving several adhesion molecules that are sequentially involved in adhesion and transmigration of leukocytes through vascular endothelium. One molecule responsible for the initial attachment of leukocytes to endothelium is CD62L (L-selectin, LAM-1, MEL-14),[214] a 74,000-M_r glycoprotein expressed on the surface of most leukocytes.[215] Expression of CD62L is coordinately regulated during lymphocyte development with virgin, immunocompetent B and T cells uniformly expressing L-selectin.[215] However, CD62L is lost on antigen-activated lymphocytes and is differentially expressed by memory T cells.[216]

CD62L regulates lymphocyte recirculation by serving as the receptor for a constitutively expressed ligand on specialized postcapillary venules in secondary lymphoid tissues where lymphocytes leave the circulation.[217] CD62L also mediates lymphocyte, neutrophil, and monocyte attachment to endothelium at sites of inflammation where cell-surface expression of the L-selectin ligand(s) is induced only after exposure of the endothelial cells to inflammatory cytokines.[218] Similar to LFA-1, lymphocyte activation through lineage-specific stimuli induces a conformational change in CD62L that increases its affinity for ligand and thus influences lymphocyte migration.[219] Regulation of CD62L expression and function plays a major role in directing the patterns of leukocyte recirculation throughout all lymphoid tissues.[220]

B CELL-T CELL INTERACTIONS

Consistent with the critical role for the T cell in the regulation of a normal immune response, most B-cell responses are directed and regulated by T cell-B cell interactions (Fig. 10-3). Physical interactions take place between the B cell and T cell through cell-surface receptors that initiate a cascade of events that leads to the generation of an effective immune response. B cells express antigen receptors of exquisite specificity, allowing them to function as efficient antigen-presenting cells. Following internalization of the antigen by the appropriate B cell, "processed" components of the antigen are "presented" on the cell surface in association with HLA class II molecules.[221,222] This processed antigen/class II complex on the surface of B cells is recognized by T cells bearing an appropriate T-cell antigen receptor complex, with CD4 serving as an accessory interaction molecule. The interaction of CD4 on T cells and MHC class II antigen on B cells initiates conjugate formation, which is essential for T-cell activation. CD4 binding to class II also induces potent homotypic adhesion of B cells,[137] and T cell-B cell interactions are stabilized by the interaction of multiple adhesion receptors, including CD11a/CD54 and CD2/CD58. Lymphocyte activation further strengthens the adhesion between these receptors and ligands. Many adhesion molecules are capable of transmitting signals themselves, adding an additional layer of regulation to the B cell-T cell interaction.

Following initial B-cell activation through sIg, B7-2 is expressed on the cell surface, which serves as a ligand for CD28 expressed by T cells. The joint stimulation of T cells through the antigen receptor and through CD28 leads to signals that up-regulate T-cell synthesis of CTLA-4, the CD40 ligand, and IL-2 mRNA. Induction of the CD40 ligand on a subpopulation of activated T cells[106] suggests that this molecule is involved early in the activation of B cells. Binding of CD40 on B cells by the T-cell receptor for CD40 generates additional signals that further activate B cells, leading to the expression of CD80 on the B-cell surface. Delayed expression of CD80 by activated B cells suggests that it is involved during the later stages of this progression. At this time, both B7-2 and CD80 are expressed by activated B cells, and CTLA-4 and CD28 are expressed by the T cells. At some point along this pathway, both B and T cells express growth factor receptors such as IL-2 receptors, and the T cell produces IL-2 and other lymphokines necessary to initiate proliferation and terminal differentiation of the activated B cell. Thus, the specificity of the immune response is preserved through the obligate requirement for both B and T cells to interact within the context of the appropriate antigen, but a series of surface receptors regulate this process in an antigen-independent manner.

Helper T cell-B cell contact is a critical step in the induction of immunoglobulin secretion, since recombinant or T-cell-derived lymphokines cannot replace the direct contact between helper T cells and B cells in inducing optimal B-cell differentiation.[155,157] Although the receptors that mediate this phase of the interaction have not been clearly defined, a novel 30,000-M_r surface protein was recently identified that is expressed by activated CD4$^+$ cells that induce contact-dependent B-cell differentiation.[107] This protein is expressed transiently 5–6 hours after activation and antibody binding to this molecule inhibits the ability of helper T cells to direct terminal B-cell differentiation. The direct T cell-B cell interactions required for B cells to differentiate into plasma cells are also likely to involve a series of surface receptors.

SUMMARY

Current studies suggest a simplified scheme for lymphocyte activation and differentiation that is in major part regulated through a complex array of cell-surface receptors. Although not discussed in detail, a large series of receptors for soluble factors, including cytokines, lymphokines, and chemokines, are also required. Therefore, it is apparent that the function of the immune response is highly regulated through cell-cell interactions and soluble factors. It is likely that the number of receptors yet to be identified is quite large. Nonetheless, the antigen-dependent nature of the immune response is critically dependent on the specificity of the antigen receptors expressed by B and T lymphocytes that allow for the identification of a vast array of foreign determinants that initiate immune responses.

ACKNOWLEDGMENTS

This work was supported by National Institutes of Health grants AI-26872, CA54464, and CA34183. Thomas F. Tedder is a Scholar of the Leukemia Society of America.

REFERENCES

1. Civin CI, Strauss LC, Brovall C et al: Antigenic analysis of hematopoiesis: a hematopoietic progenitor cell surface antigen defined by a monoclonal antibody raised against KG-1a cells. J Immunol 133:157, 1984
2. Andrews RG, Singer JW, Bernstein ID: Human hematopoietic precursors in long-term culture: single CD34 + cells that lack detectable T cell, B cell, and myeloid cell antigens produce multiple colony-forming cells when cultured with marrow stromal cells. J Exp Med 172:355, 1990
3. Osmond DG: B cell development in the bone marrow. Semin Immunol 2:173, 1990
4. Uckun FM: Regulation of human B-cell ontogeny. Blood 76:1908, 1990
5. Loken MR, Shah VO, Dattilio KL, Civin CI: Flow cytometric analysis of human bone marrow. II. Normal B lymphocyte development. Blood 70:1316, 1987
6. Rolink A, Melchers F: Molecular and cellular origins of B lymphocyte diversity. Cell 66:1081, 1991
7. Burrows PD, Cooper MD: Regulated expression of cell surface antigens during B cell development. Semin Immunol 2:189, 1990
8. Nishimoto N, Kubagawa H, Ohno T et al: Normal pre-B cells express a receptor complex of Mu heavy chains and surrogate light chain proteins. Proc Natl Acad Sci USA 88:6284, 1991
9. LeBien TW, Elstrom RL, Moseley M et al: Analysis of immunoglobulin and T cell receptor gene rearrangements in human fetal bone marrow B lineage cells. Blood 76:1196, 1990
10. Alt FW, Blackwell TK, Yancopoulos GD: Development of the primary antibody repertoire. Science 238:1079, 1987
11. Berek C, Berger A, Apel M: Maturation of the immune response in germinal centers. Cell 67:1121, 1991
12. Lanzavecchia A: Antigen uptake and accumulation in antigen-specific B cells. Immunol Rev 99:39, 1987
13. Reth M, Hombach J, Wienands J et al: The B-cell antigen receptor complex. Immunol Today 12:196, 1991
14. Campbell KS, Hager EJ, Freidrich RJ, Cambier JC: IgM antigen receptor complex contains phosphoprotein products of B29 and mb-1 genes. Proc Natl Acad Sci USA 88:3982, 1991
15. Sakaguchi N, Kashiwamura S, Kimoto M et al: B lymphocyte lineage-restricted expression of mb-1, a gene with CD3-like structural properties. EMBO J 7:3457, 1988
16. Hermanson GG, Eisenberg D, Kincade PW, Wall R: B29: a member of the immunoglobulin gene superfamily exclusively expressed on B-lineage cells. Proc Natl Acad Sci USA 85:6890, 1988
17. Yednock TA, Stoolman LM, Rosen SD: Phosphomannosyl derivatized beads detect a receptor involved in lymphocyte homing. J Cell Biol 104:713, 1987
18. Yednock TA, Butcher EC, Stoolman LM, Rosen SD: Receptors involved in lymphocyte homing: relationship between a carbohydrate-binding receptor and the MEL-14 antigen. J Cell Biol 104:725, 1987
19. Mason DY, Cordell JL, Tse AGD et al: The IgM-associated protein mb-1 as a marker of normal and neoplastic B cells. J Immunol 147:2474, 1991
20. Reth M: Antigen receptor tail clue. Nature 338:383, 1989
21. Chin YH, Rasmussen R, Cakiroglu AG, Woodruff JJ: Lymphocyte recognition of lymph node high endothelium. VI. Evidence of distinct structures mediating binding to high endothelial cells of lymph nodes and Peyer's patches. J Immunol 133:2961, 1984
22. Dymecki SM, Niederhuber JE, Desiderio SV: Specific expression of a tyrosine kinase gene blk, in B lymphoid cells. Science 247:332, 1989
23. Hutchcroft JE, Harrison ML, Geahlen RL: Association of the 72 kDa protein-tyrosine kinase PTK72 with the B cell antigen receptor. J Biol Chem 267:8613, 1992
24. Matsuo T, Kimoto M, Sakaguchi N: Direct identification of the putative surface IgM receptor-associated molecule encoded by murine B cell-specific mb-1 gene. J Immunol 146:1584, 1991
25. Hombach J, Tsubata T, Leclercq L et al: Molecular components of the B-cell antigen receptor complex of the IgM class. Nature 343:760, 1990
26. Haughton G, Arnold LW, Whitmore AC, Clarke SH: B-1 cells are made, not born. Immunol Today 14:84, 1993
27. Bofill M, Janossy G, Janossy M et al: Human B cell development. II. Subpopulation in the human fetus. J Immunol 134:1531, 1985
28. Solvason N, Kearney JF: The human fetal omentum: a site of B cell generation. J Exp Med 175:397, 1992
29. Solvason N, Lehuen A, Kearney JF: An embryonic source of Ly1 but not conventional B cells. Int Immunol 3:543, 1991
30. Plater-Zyberk C, Maini RN, Kam K et al: A rheumatoid arthritis B cell subset expresses a phenotype similar to that in chronic lymphocytic leukemia. Arthritis Rheum 28:971, 1985
31. Freedman AS, Freeman G, Whitman J et al: Expression and regulation of CD5 on in vitro activated human B cells. Eur J Immunol 19:849, 1989
32. Cong T, Rabin E, Wortis H: Treatment of CD5$^-$ B cells with anti-Ig but not

LPS, induces suface CD5: two B cell activation pathways. Int Immunol 3: 467, 1991

33. Casali P, Burastero SE, Nakamura M et al: Human lymphocytes making rheumatoid factor and antibody to ssDNA belong to Leu-1 + B-cell subset. Science 236:77, 1987

34. Hardy RR, Hayakawa K, Shimizu M et al: Rheumatoid factor secretion from human Leu-1 B cells. Science 236:81, 1987

35. Brown G, Hogg N, Greaves M: Candidate leukemia-specific antigen in man. Nature 258:454, 1975

36. LeBien TW, McCormack RT: The common acute lymphoblastic leukemia antigen (CD10)—emancipiation from a functional enigma. Blood 73:625, 1989

37. Greaves MF, Hairi G, Newman RA et al: Selective expression of the common acute lymphoblastic leukemia (gp100) antigen on immature lymphoid cells and their malignant counterparts. Blood 61:628, 1983

38. Hokland P, Nadler LM, Griffin JM et al: Purification of common acute lymphoblastic leukemia antigen positive cells from normal human bone marrow. Blood 64:662, 1984

39. Neudorf JSM, LeBien TW, Kersey JH: Characterization of thymocytes expressing the common acute lymphoblastic leukemia antigen. Leuk Res 8: 173, 1984

40. Cossman J, Neckers LM, Leonard WJ, Greene WC: Polymorphonuclear neutrophils express the common acute lymphoblastic leukemia antigen. J Exp Med 157:1064, 1983

41. Metzgar RS, Borowitz MJ, Jones NH, Dowell BL: Distribution of common acute lymphoblastic leukemia antigen in non-hematopoietic tissues. J Exp Med 154:1249, 1981

42. LeTarte M, Vera S, Tran R et al: Common acute lymphoblastic leukemia antigen is identical to neutral endopeptidase. J Exp Med 168:1247, 1988

43. Matsumoto AK, Kopicky-Burd J, Carter RH et al: Intersection of the complement and immune systems: a signal transduction complex of the B lymphocyte containing complement receptor type 2 and CD19. J Exp Med 173:55, 1991

44. Bradbury L, Kansas GS, Levy S et al: CD19 is a component of a signal transducing complex on the surface of B cells that includes CD21, TAPA-1 and Leu-13. J Immunol 149:2841, 1992

45. Tedder TF, Isaacs CM: Isolation of cDNAs encoding the CD19 antigen of human and mouse B lymphocytes: a new member of the immunoglobulin superfamily. J Immunol 143:712, 1989

46. Weis JJ, Fearon DT, Klickstein LB et al: Identification of a partial cDNA clone for the C3d/Epstein-Barr virus receptor of human B lymphocytes: homology with the receptor for fragments C3b and C4b of the third and fourth components of complement. Proc Natl Acad Sci USA 83:5639, 1986

47. Moore MD, Cooper NR, Tack BF, Nemerow GR: Molecular cloning of the cDNA encoding the Epstein-Barr virus/C3d receptor (complement receptor type 2) of human B lymphocytes. Proc Natl Acad Sci USA 84:9194, 1987

48. Nadler LM, Stashenko P, Hardy R et al: Characterization of a human B cell-specific antigen (B2) distinct from B1. J Immunol 126:1941, 1981

49. Tedder TF, Clement LT, Cooper MD: Expression of C3d receptors during human B cell differentiation: immunofluorescence analysis with the HB-5 monoclonal antibody. J Immunol 133:678, 1984

50. Schriever F, Freedman AS, Freeman G et al: Isolated human follicular dendritic cells display a unique antigenic phenotype. J Exp Med 169:2043, 1989

51. Oren R, Takahashi S, Doss C et al: TAPA-1, the target of an antiproliferative antibody, defines a new family of transmembrane proteins. Mol Cell Biol 10:4007, 1990

52. Chen YX, Welte K, Gebhard DH, Evans RL: Induction of T cell aggregation by antibody to a 16 kd human leukocyte surface antigen. J Immunol 133: 2496, 1984

53. Nadler LM, Anderson KC, Marti G et al: B4, a human B lymphocyte-associated antigen expressed on normal, mitogen activated, and malignant B lymphocytes. J Immunol 131:244, 1983

54. Anderson KC, Bates MP, Slaughenhoupt B et al: Expression of human B cell-associated antigens on leukemias and lymphomas: a model of human B cell differentiation. Blood 63:1424, 1984

55. Zhou L-J, Ord DC, Hughes AL, Tedder TF: Structure and domain organization of the CD19 antigen of human, mouse and guinea pig B lymphocytes. Conservation of the extensive cytoplasmic domain. J Immunol 147:1424, 1991

56. Pezzutto A, Dorken B, Rabinovitch PS et al: CD19 monoclonal antibody HD37 inhibits anti-immunoglobulin-induced B cell activation and proliferation. J Immunol 138:2793, 1987

57. Zhou L-J, Smith HM, Waldschmidt TJ et al: Tissue-specific expression of the human CD19 gene in transgenic mice inhibits antigen-independent B lymphocyte development. Mol Cell Biol 1994 (in press)

58. Stashenko P, Nadler LM, Hardy R, Schlossman SF: Characterization of a human B lymphocyte-specific antigen. J Immunol 125:1678, 1980

59. Nadler LM, Korsmeyer SJ, Anderson KC et al: B cell origin of non-T cell acute lymphoblastic leukemia. A model for discrete stages of neoplastic and normal pre-B cell differentiation. J Clin Invest 74:332, 1984

60. Tedder TF, Streuli M, Schlossman SF, Saito H: Isolation and structure of a cDNA encoding the B1 (CD20) cell-surface antigen of human B lymphocytes. Proc Natl Acad Sci USA 85:208, 1988

61. Tedder TF, McIntyre G, Schlossman SF: Heterogeneity in the B1 (CD20) cell surface molecule expressed by human B lymphocytes. Mol Immunol 25: 1321, 1988

62. Tedder TF, Schlossman SF: Phosphorylation of the B1 (CD20) cell surface molecule expressed by normal and malignant human B lymphocytes. J Biol Chem 263:10009, 1988

63. Tedder TF, Disteche CM, Louie E et al: The gene that encodes the human CD20 (B1) differentiation antigen is located on chromosome 11 near the t(11;14) (q13♦2) translocation site. J Immunol 142:2555, 1989

64. Hupp K, Siwarski D, Mock BA, Kinet J-P: Gene mapping of the three subunits of the high affinity FcR for IgE to mouse chromosomes 1 and 19. J Immunol 143:3787, 1989

65. Tedder TF, Boyd AW, Freedman AS et al: The B cell surface molecule B1 is functionally linked with B cell activation and differentiation. J Immunol 135: 973, 1985

66. Tedder TF, Forsgren A, Boyd AW et al: Antibodies reactive with the B1 molecule inhibit cell cycle progression but not activation of human B lymphocytes. Eur J Immunol 16:881, 1986

67. Bubien JK, Zhou L-J, Bell PD et al: Transfection of the CD20 cell surface molecule into ectopic cell types generates a Ca++ conductance found constitutively in B lymphocytes. J Cell Biol 121:1121, 1993

68. Iida K, Nadler L, Nussenzweig V: Identification of the membrane receptor for the complement fragment C3d by means of a monoclonal antibody. J Exp Med 158:1021, 1983

69. Weiss JJ, Tedder TF, Fearon DT: Identification of a 145,000 Mr membrane protein as the C3d receptor (CR2) of human B lymphocytes. Proc Natl Acad Sci USA 81:881, 1984

70. Nemerow GR, Wolfert R, McNaughton ME, Cooper NR: Identification and characterization of the Epstein-Barr virus receptor on human B lymphocytes and its relationship to the C3d complement receptor (CR2). J Virol 55:347, 1985

71. Tedder TF, Weiss JJ, Clement LT et al: Role of receptors for complement in the induction of polyclonal B cell proliferation and differentiation. J Clin Immunol 6:65, 1986

72. Nemerow GR, McNaughton ME, Cooper NR: Binding of monoclonal antibody to the Epstein Barr virus (EBV)/CR2 receptor induces activation and differentiation of human B lymphocytes. J Immunol 135:3068, 1985

73. Bohnsack JF, Cooper NR: CR2 ligands modulate human B cell activation. J Immunol 141:2569, 1988

74. Tsokos GC, Lambris JD, Finkelman FD et al: Monovalent ligands of complement receptor 2 inhibit whereas polyvalent ligands enhance anti-Ig-induced human B cell intracytoplasmic free calcium concentration. J Immunol 144: 1640, 1990

75. Hivroz C, Fischer E, Kazatchkine MD, Grillot-Courvalin C: Differential effects of the stimulation of complement receptors CR1 (CD35) and CR2 (CD21) on cell proliferation and intracellular Ca²⁺ mobilization of chronic lymphocytic leukemia B cells. J Immunol 146:1766, 1991

76. Tanner J, Weis J, Fearon D et al: Epstein-Barr virus gp350/220 binding to the B lymphocyte C3d receptor mediates adsorption, capping and endocytosis. Cell 50:203, 1987

77. Wilson GL, Fox CH, Fauci AS, Kehrl JH: cDNA cloning of the B cell membrane protein CD22: a mediator of B-B cell interactions. J Exp Med 173:137, 1991

78. Engel P, Nojima Y, Rothstein D et al: The same epitope on CD22 of B lymphocytes mediates the adhesion of erythrocytes, T and B lymphocytes, neutrophils and monocytes. J Immunol 150:4719, 1993

79. Dorken B, Moldenhauer G, Pezzutto A et al: HD39 (B3), a B lineage-restricted antigen whose cell surface expression is limited to resting and activated human B lymphocytes. J Immunol 136:4470, 1986

80. Mason DY, Stein H, Gerdes J et al: Value of monoclonal anti-CD22 (p135) antibodies for the detection of normal and neoplastic B lymphoid cells. Blood 69:836, 1987

81. Pezzutto A, Dorken B, Moldenhauer G, Clark EA: Amplification of human B cell activation by a monoclonal antibody to the B cell-specific antigen CD22, Bp130/140. J Immunol 138:98, 1987

82. Pezzutto A, Rabinovitch PS, Dorken B et al: Role of the CD22 human B cell antigen in B cell triggering by anti-immunoglobulin. J Immunol 140:1791, 1988

83. Stamenkovic I, Sgroi D, Aruffo A et al: The B lymphocyte adhesion molecule CD22 interacts with leukocyte common antigen CD45RO on T cells and α2,6 sialyltransferase, CD75, on B cells. Cell 66:1133, 1991

84. Gordon J, Flores-Romo L, Cairns JA et al: CD23: a multi-functional receptor/lymphokine? Immunol Today 10:153, 1989
85. Kikutani H, Inui S, Sato R et al: Molecular structure of human lymphocyte receptor for immunoglobulin E. Cell 47:657, 1986
86. Ikuta K, Takami M, Kim CW et al: Human lymphocyte Fc receptor for IgE: sequence homology of its cloned cDNA with animal lectins. Proc Natl Acad Sci USA 84:819, 1987
87. Bonnefoy JY, Aubry JP, Peronne C et al: Production and characterization of a monoclonal antibody specific for human lymphocyte low affinity receptor for IgE: CD23 is a low affinity receptor for IgE. J Immunol 138:2970, 1987
88. Yukawa K, Kikutani H, Owaka H et al: A B cell-specific differentiation antigen, CD23, is a receptor for IgE (FcεR) on lymphocytes. J Immunol 138:2576, 1987
89. Yokota A, Kikutani H, Tanaka T et al: Two species of human Fc epsilon receptor II (Fc epsilon RII/CD23): tissue-specific and IL-4-specific regulation of gene expression. Cell 55:611, 1988
90. Delespesse G, Suter U, Mossalayi D et al: Expression, structure, and function of the CD23 antigen. Adv Immunol 49:149, 1991
91. Abramson CS, Kersey JH, LeBien TW: A monoclonal antibody (BA-1) reactive with cells of human B lymphocyte lineage. J Immunol 126:83, 1981
92. Pirruccello SJ, LeBien TW: The human B cell-associated antigen CD24 is a single chain sialoglycoprotein. J Immunol 136:3779, 1986
93. Fischer GF, Majdic O, Gadd S, Knapp W: Signal transduction in lymphocytic and myeloid cells via CD24, a new member of phosphoinositol-anchored membrane molecules. J Immunol 144:638, 1990
94. Kay R, Rosten PM, Humphries RK: CD24, a signal transducer modulating B cell activation responses, is a very short peptide with a glycosyl phosphatidylinositol membrane anchor. J Immunol 147:1412, 1991
95. Mehmet H, Larkin M, Tang PW et al: Monoclonal antibody BA-1 to the human B lymphocyte marker CD24 recognizes a sialic acid (N-acetylneuraminic acid) dependent epitope in multi-valent display on peptide. Clin Exp Immunol 81:489, 1990
96. Stefanova I, Horejsi V, Ansotegui IJ et al: GPI-anchored cell-surface molecules complexed to protein tyrosine kinases. Science 254:1016, 1991
97. Clark EA, Ledbetter JA: Activation of human B cells mediated through two distinct cell surface differentiation antigens, Bp35 and Bp50. Proc Natl Acad Sci USA 83:4494, 1986
98. Ledbetter JA, Shu G, Gallagher M, Clark EA: Augmentation of normal and malignant B cell proliferation by monoclonal antibody to the B cell-specific antigne Bp50 (CDw40). J Immunol 138:788, 1987
99. Paulie S, Ehlin-Henriksson B, Mellstedt H et al: A p50 surface antigen restricted to human urinary bladder carcinomas and B-lymphocytes. Cancer Immunol Immunother 20:23, 1985
100. Paulie S, Rosen A, Ehlin-Henriksson B et al: The human B lymphocyte and carcinoma antigen, CDw40, is a phosphoprotein involved in growth signal transduction. J Immunol 142:590, 1989
101. Gordon J, Millsum MJ, Guy GR, Ledbetter JA: Resting B lymphocytes can be triggered directly through the CDw40 (Bp50) antigen. J Immunol 140:1425, 1988
102. Gordon J, Millsum MJ, Guy GR, Ledbetter JA: Synergistic interaction between IL-4 and anti-Bp50 (CDw40) revealed in a novel B cell restimulation assay. Eur J Immunol 17:1535, 1987
103. Banchereau J, Rousset F: Growing human B lymphocytes in the CD40 system. Nature 353:678, 1991
104. Liu Y-J, Hoshua DE, Willimas GT et al: Mechanism of antigen-driven selection in germinal centres. Nature 342:929, 1989
105. Stamenkovic I, Clark EA, Seed B: A B-lymphocyte activation molecule related to the nerve growth factor receptor and induced by cytokines in carcinomas. EMBO J 8:1403, 1989
106. Armitage RJ, Fanslow WC, Strockbine L et al: Molecular and biological characterization of a murine ligand for CD40. Nature 357:80, 1992
107. Lederman S, Yellin MJ, Krichevsky A et al: Identification of a novel surface protein on activated CD4+ T cells that induces contact-dependent B cell differentiation. J Exp Med 175:1091, 1992
108. Lederman S, Yellin MJ, Inghirami G et al: Molecular interactions mediating T-B lymphocyte collaboration in human lymphoid follicles. Roles of T cell-B cell-activating molecule (5c8 antigen) and CD40 in contact dependent help. J Immunol 149:3817, 1992
109. Allen RC, Armitage RJ, Conley ME et al: CD40 ligand gene defects responsible for X-linked hyper-IgM syndrome. Science 259:990, 1993
110. Nakayama E, von Hoegen I, Parnes J: Sequence of the Lyb-2 B cell differentiation antigen defines a gene superfamily of receptors with inverted membrane orientation. Proc Natl Acad Sci USA 86:1352, 1989
111. von Hoegen I, Nakayama E, Parnes JR: Identification of a human protein homologous to the mouse Lyb-2 B cell differentiation antigen and sequence of the corresponding cDNA. J Immunol 144:4870, 1990
112. Yakura H, Shen F-W, Bourcet E, Boyse EA: On the function of Ly-5 in the regulation of antigen-drived B cell differentiation. Comparison and contrast with Lyb-2. J Exp Med 157:1077, 1983
113. Kamal M, Katira A, Gordon J: Stimulation of B lymphocytes via CD72 (human Lyb-2). Eur J Immunol 21:1419, 1991
114. Freedman AS, Freeman G, Horowitz JC et al: B7, a B cell-restricted antigen that identifies preactivated B cells. J Immunol 139:3260, 1987
115. Yokochi T, Holly RD, Clark EA: B lymphoblast antigen (BB-1) expressed on Epstein-Barr virus-activated B cell blasts, B lymphoblastoid cell lines, and Burkitt's lymphomas. J Immunol 128:823, 1982
116. Koulova L, Clark EA, Shu G, Dupont B: The CD28 ligand B7/BB1 provides a costimulatory signal for alloactivation of CD4+ T cells. J Exp Med 173:759, 1991
117. Freedman AS, Freeman GJ, Rhynhart K, Nadler LM: Selective induction of B7/BB-1 on interferon-γ stimulated monocytes: a potential mechanism for amplification of T cell activation through the CD28 pathway. Cell Immunol 137:429, 1991
118. Freeman GJ, Freedman AS, Segil JM et al: B7, a new member of the Ig superfamily with unique expression on activated and neoplastic B cells. J Immunol 143:2714, 1989
119. June CH, Ledbetter JA, Linsley PS, Thompson CB: Role of the CD28 receptor in T-cell activation. Immunol Today 11:211, 1990
120. Linsley PS, Clark EA, Ledbetter JA: T-cell antigen CD28 mediates adhesion with B cells by interacting with activation antigen B7/BB-1. Proc Natl Acad Sci USA 87:5031, 1990
121. Linsley PS, Brady W, Urnes M et al: CTLA-4 is a second receptor for the B cell activation antigen B7. J Exp Med 174:561, 1991
122. Linsley PS, Brady W, Grosmaire L et al: Binding of the B cell activation antigen B7 to CD28 costimulates T cell proliferation and interleukin 2 mRNA accumulation. J Exp Med 173:721, 1991
123. Gimmi CD, Freedman GJ, Gribben JG et al: B-cell surface antigen B7 provides a costimulatory signal that induces T cells to proliferate and secrete interleukin 2. Proc Natl Acad Sci USA 88:6575, 1991
124. Damle NK, Linsley PS, Ledbetter JA: Direct helper T cell-induced B cell differentiation involves interaction between T cell antigen CD28 and B cell activation antigen B7. Eur J Immunol 21:1277, 1991
125. Harding FA, McArthur JG, Gross JA et al: Cd28-mediated signaling co-stimulates murine T cells and prevents induction of anergy in T cells clones. Nature 356:607, 1992
126. Schwartz RH: Costimulation of T lymphocytes: the role of CD28, CTLA-4, and B7/BB1 in interleukin-2 production and immunotherapy. Cell 71:1065, 1992
127. Freeman GJ, Gribben JG, Boussiotis VA et al: B7-2, a novel CTLA4 counterreceptor that costimulates human T cell proliferation. Science 262:909, 1993
128. Boussiotis VA, Freeman GJ, Gribben JG et al: Activated human B lymphocytes express three CTLA4 counter-receptors which costimulate T cell activation. Proc Natl Acad Sci USA 90:11059, 1993
129. Freeman GJ, Borriello F, Hodes RJ et al: B7 deficient mice reveal an alternative functional CTLA4 counter-receptor. Science 262:907, 1993
130. Nickoloff BJ, Mitra RS, Lee K et al: Discordant expression of CD28 ligands, BB-1 and B7 on keratinocytes in vitro and psoriatic cells in vivo. Am J Pathol 142:1029, 1993
131. Palacios R, Martinez-Maza O, Guy K: Monoclonal antibodies against HLA-DR antigens replace T helper cells in activation of B lymphocytes. Proc Natl Acad Sci USA 80:3456, 1983
132. Clement LT, Tedder TF, Gartland GL: Antibodies reactive with class II antigens encoded for by the major histocompatibility complex inhibit human B cell activation. J Immunol 136:2375, 1986
133. Mooney NA, Grillot-Courvalin C, Hivroz C et al: Early biochemical events after MHC class II-mediated signaling on human B lymphocytes. J Immunol 145:2070, 1990
134. Cambier JC, Newell MK, Justement LB et al: Ia binding ligands and cAMP stimulate nuclear translocation of PKC in B lymphocytes. Nature 327:629, 1987
135. Chen ZZ, McGuire JC, Leach KL, Cambier JC: Transmembrane signaling through B cell MHC class II molecules: anti-Ia antibodies induce protein kinase C translocation to the nuclear fraction. J Immunol 138:2345, 1987
136. Cambier JC, Lehmann KR: Ia mediated signal transduction leads to proliferation of primed B lymphocytes. J Exp Med 170:877, 1989
137. Kansas GS, Cambier JC, Tedder TF: CD4 binding to MHC class II induces LFA-1-dependent and -independent homotypic adhesion of B lymphocytes. Eur J Immunol 22:147, 1992
138. Wagner N, Engel P, Vega M, Tedder TF: Ligation of MHC class I and class II molecules leads to heterologous desensitization of signal transduction pathways that regulate homotypic adhesion in human lymphocytes. J Immunol 1994 (in press)
139. Haynes BF, Denning SM, Le PT, Singer KH: Human intrathymic T cell differentiation. Semin Immunol 2:67, 1990
140. Schnittman SM, Denning SM, Greenhouse JJ et al: Evidence for susceptibility

of intrathymic T-cell precursors and their progeny carrying T-cell antigen receptor phenotypes TCRαβ+ and TCRγδ+ to human immunodeficiency virus infection: a mechanism for CD4+ (T4) lymphocyte depletion. Proc Natl Acad Sci USA 87:7727, 1990

141. de la Hera A, Marston W, Aranda C et al: Thymic stroma is required for the development of human T cell lineages in vitro. Int Immunol 1:471, 1989

142. Groh V, Fabbi M, Strominger JL: Maturation or differentiation of human thymocyte precursors in vitro. Proc Natl Acad Sci USA 87:5973, 1990

143. Denning SM, Kurtzberg J, Leslie DS, Haynes BF: Human postnatal CD4-CD8-CD3- thymic T cell precursors differentiate in vitro into T cell receptor δ-bearing cells. J Immunol 142:2988, 1989

144. Guidos GJ, Weissman IL, Adkins B: Intrathymic maturation of murine T lymphocytes from CD8+ precursors. Proc Natl Acad Sci USA 86:7542, 1989

145. Reinherz EL, Schlossman SF: The differentiation and function of human T lymphocytes. Cell 19:821, 1980

146. Hori T, Cupp J, Wrighton N et al: Identification of a novel human thymocyte subset with phenotype of CD3−CD4+CD8α+β−1. J Immunol 146:4078, 1991

147. Nikolic-Zugic J: Phenotypic and functional stages in the intrathymic development of αβ T cells. Immunol Today 12:65, 1991

148. Nossal GJV: Negative selection of lymphocytes. Cell 76:229, 1994

149. von Boehmer H: Positive selection of lymphocytes. Cell 76:219, 1994

150. Finkel TH, Kubo RT, Cambier JC: T-cell development and transmembrane signaling: changing biological responses through an unchanging receptor. Immunol Today 12:79, 1991

151. Brenner MB, Strominger JL, Krangel MS: The γδ T cell receptor. Adv Immunol 11:340, 1991

152. Doyle C, Strominger JL: Interaction between CD4 and class II MHC molecules mediates cell adhesion. Nature 330:256, 1987

153. Norment AM, Salter RD, Parham P, Englehard VH: Cell-cell adhesion mediated by CD8 and MHC class I molecules. Nature 336:79, 1988

154. Tedder TF, Clement LT, Cooper MD: Human lymphocyte differentiation antigens HB-10 and HB-11. I. Ontogeny of antigen expression. J Immunol 134:2983, 1985

155. Tedder TF, Cooper MD, Clement LT: Human lymphocyte differentiation antigens HB-10 and HB-11. II. Differential production of B cell growth and differentiation factors by distinct helper T cell subpopulations. J Immunol 134:2989, 1985

156. Schwartz R: T lymphocyte recognition of antigen in association with gene products of the major histocompatibility complex. Annu Rev Immunol 3:237, 1985

157. Sleasman JW, Morimoto C, Schlossman SF, Tedder TF: The role of functionally distinct helper T lymphocyte subpopulations in the induction of human B cell differentiation. Eur J Immunol 20:1357, 1990

158. Moy VT, Brian AA: Signaling by lymphocyte function associated antigen-1 (LFA-1) in B cells: enhanced antigen presentation after stimulation through LFA-1. J Exp Med 175:1, 1992

159. Sanders ME, Makgoba MW, Sharrow SO et al: Human memory T lymphocytes express increased levels of three cell adhesion molecules (LFA-3, CD2, and LFA-1) and three other molecules (UCHL1, CDw29, and Pgp-1) and have enhanced IFN-gamma production. J Immunol 140:1401, 1988

160. Mackay CR, Marston WL, Dudler L: Naive and memory T cells show distinct pathways of lymphocyte recirculation. J Exp Med 171:801, 1990

161. Sanders VM, Vitetta ES: B cell-associated LFA-1 and T cell-associated ICAM-1 transiently cluster in the area of contact between interacting cells. Cellular Immunol 132:45, 1991

162. Mackay CR, Kimpton WG, Brandon MR, Cahill RNP: Lymphocyte subsets show marked differences in their distribution between blood and the afferent and efferent lymph of peripheral lymph nodes. J Exp Med 167:1755, 1988

163. Weiss A, Imboden JB: Cell surface molecules and early events involved in human T lymphocyte activation. Adv Immunol 41:1, 1987

164. Bowman MR, Crimmins MAV, Yetz-Aldape J et al: The cloning of CD70 and its identification as the ligand for CD27. J Immunol 152:1756, 1994

165. Davis M: T receptor gene diversity and selection. Annu Rev Biochem 59:475, 1990

166. Ikuta K, Ogura T, Shimizu A, Honjo T: Low frequency of somatic mutation in beta-chain variable region genes of human T-cell receptors. Proc Natl Acad Sci USA 82:7701, 1985

167. Meuer SC, Fitzgerald KA, Hussey RE et al: Clonotypic structures involved in antigen-specific human T cell function. J Exp Med 157:705, 1983

168. Hendrik SM, Eidelman FJ: T lymphocyte antigen receptors. p. 383. In Paul WE (eds): Fundamental Immunology. 3rd Ed. Raven Press, New York, 1993

169. Clayton LK, DAdamio L, Howard FD et al: CD3 eta and CD3 zeta are alternatively spliced products of a common genetic locus and are transcriptionally and/or post-transcriptionally regulated during T-cell development. Proc Natl Acad Sci USA 88:5202, 1991

170. Martin LH, Calabi F, Milstein C: Isolation of CD1 genes: a family of major histocompatibility complex-related differentiation antigens. Proc Natl Acad Sci USA 83:9154, 1986

171. Amiot M, Bernard A, Raynal B et al: Heterogeneity of the first cluster of differentiation: characterization and epitopic mapping of three CD1 molecules on normal human thymus cells. J Immunol 136:1752, 1986

172. Amiot H, Dastot H, Fabbi M et al: Intermolecular complexes between three human CD1 molecules on normal thymus cells. Immunogenetics 27:187, 1988

173. Small TN, Knowles RW, Keever C et al: M241 (CD1) expression on B lymphocytes. J Immunol 138:2864, 1987

174. Poncelli S, Brenner MB, Greenstein JL et al: Recognition of differentiation 1 antigens by human CD4-8- cytolytic T lymphocytes. Nature 341:447, 1989

175. Seed B, Aruffo A: Molecular cloning of the CD2 antigen, T cell-erythrocyte receptor, by a rapid immunoselection procedure. Proc Natl Acad Sci USA 84:3365, 1987

176. Meuer SC, Hussey RE, Fabbi M et al: An alternative pathway of T-cell activation: a functional role for the 50 kd T11 sheep erythrocyte receptor protein. Cell 36:897, 1984

177. Bockenstedt LK, Goldsmith MA, Dustin M et al: The CD2 ligand LFA-3 activates T cells but depends on the expression and function of the antigen receptor. J Immunol 141:1904, 1988

178. Monostori E, Desai D, Brown MH et al: Activation of human T lymphocytes via the CD2 antigen results in tyrosine phosphorylation of T cell antigen receptor ζ-chains. J Immunol 144:1010, 1990

179. Howard FD, Ledbetter JA, Wong J et al: A human T lymphocyte differentiation marker defined by monoclonal antibodies that block E rosette formation. J Immunol 126:2117, 1981

180. Shaw S, Luce GE, Quinones R et al: Two antigen-independent adhesion pathways used by human cytotoxic T-cell clones. Nature 323:262, 1986

181. Sanchez-Madrid F, Krensky AM, Ware CF et al: Three distinct antigens associated with human T-lymphocyte-mediated cytolysis: LFA-1, LFA-2 and LFA-3. Proc Natl Acad Sci USA 79:7489, 1982

182. Seed B: An LFA-3 cDNA encodes a phospholipid-linked membrane protein homologous to its receptor CD2. Nature 329:840, 1987

183. Selvaraj P, Plunkett ML, Dustin M et al: The T lymphocyte glycoprotein CD2 binds the cell surface ligand LFA-3. Nature 326:400, 1987

184. Hahn WC, Menu E, Bothwell ALM et al: Overlapping but nonidentical binding sites on CD2 for CD58 and a second ligand CD59. Science 256:1805, 1992

185. Kato K, Koyanagi M, Okada H et al: CD48 is a counter-receptor for mouse CD2 and is involved in T cell activation. J Exp Med 176:1241, 1992

186. Bierer BE, Sleckman BP, Ratnofsky SE, Burakoff SJ: The biologic roles of CD2, CD4 and CD8 in T cell activation. Annu Rev Immunol 7:579, 1989

187. Turner JM, Brodsky MH, Irving BA et al: Interaction of the unique N-terminal region of tyrosine kinase p56 lck with cytoplasmic domains of CD4 and CD8 is mediated by cysteine motifs. Cell 66:755, 1990

188. Rosenberg ZF, Fauci AS: The immunopathogenesis of HIV infection. Adv Immunol 47:377, 1989

189. Huang H-JS, Jones NH, Strominger JL, Herzenberg LA: Molecular cloning of Ly-1, a membrane glycoprotein of mouse T lymphocytes and a subset of B cells: molecular homology to its human counterpart Leu-1/T1 (CD5). Proc Natl Acad Sci USA 84:204, 1987

190. Aruffo A and Seed B: Molecular cloning of two CD7 (T-cell leukemia antigen) cDNAs by a COS cell expression system. EMBO J 6:3313, 1987

191. Parnes JR: Molecular biology and function of CD4 and CD8. Adv Immunol 44:265, 1989

192. Camerini D, Walz G, Loenen AM et al: The T cell activation antigen CD27 is a member of the NGF/TNF receptor gene family. J Immunol 147:3165, 1991

193. de Jong R, Loenen WAM, Brower M et al: Regulation of expression of CD27: a T cell-specific member of a novel family of membrane receptors. J Immunol 146:2488, 1991

194. Maurer D, Holter W, Majdic O et al: CD27 expression by a distinct subpopulation of human B lymphocytes. Eur J Immunol 20:2679, 1990

195. Goodwin RG, Alderson MR, Smith CA et al: Molecular and biological characterization of a ligand for CD27 defines a new family of cytokines with homology to tumor necroses factor. Cell 73:447, 1993

196. Aruffo A, Seed B: Molecular cloning of a CD28 cDNA by a high-efficiency COS cell expression system. Proc Natl Acad Sci USA 84:8573, 1987

197. Turka LA, Linsley PS, Paine R et al: Signal transduction via CD4, CD8, and CD28 in mature and immature thymocytes. J Immunol 146:1428, 1991

198. Brunet J-F, Denizot F, Luciani M-F et al: A new member of the immunoglobulin superfamily, CTLA-4. Nature 328:267, 1987

199. Tedder TF, Engel P, Wagner N, Freedman AS: Adhesion receptors of B lymphocytes: expression and function on normal and malignant cells. p. 280. In Schmizu Y (ed): Lymphocyte Adhesion Molecules. RG Landes, Austin, TX, 1993

200. Springer TA: Traffic signals for lymphocyte recirculation and leukocyte emigration: the multistep paradigm. Cell 76:301, 1994

201. Hemler ME: VLA proteins in the integrin family: structure, functions, and their role on leukocytes. Annu Rev Immunol 8:365, 1990

202. Hynes RO: Integrins: versatility, modulation, and signaling in cell adhesion. Cell 69:11, 1992

203. Elices MJ, Osborn L, Takada Y et al: VCAM-1 on activated endothelium interacts with the leukocyte integrin VLA-4 at a site distinct from the VLA-4/fibronectin binding site. Cell 60:577, 1990

204. Bernardi P, Patel VP, Lodish HF: Lymphoid precursor cells adhere to two different sites on fibronectin. J Cell Biol 105:489, 1987

205. Guan J-L, Hynes RO: Lymphoid cells recognize an alternatively spliced segment of fibronectin via the integrin receptor α4β1. Cell 60:53, 1990

206. Dustin ML, Springer TA: T-cell receptor cross-linking transiently stimulates adhesiveness through LFA-1. Nature 341:619, 1989

207. Postigo AA, Corbi AL, Sanchez-Madrid F, de Landazuri MO: Regulated expression and function of CD11c/CD18 integrin on human B lymphocytes. Relation between attachment to fibrinogen and triggering of proliferation through CD11c/CD18. J Exp Med 174:1313, 1991

208. Visser L, Shaw A, Slupsky J et al: Monoclonal antibodies reactive with hairy cell leukemia. Blood 74:320, 1989

209. de Fougerolles A, Springer T: Intercellular adhesion molecule 3, a third adhesion counter-receptor for lymphocyte function-associated molecule-1 on resting lymphocytes. J Exp Med 175:185, 1992

210. Haynes BF, Telen MJ, Hale LP, Denning SM: CD44 - A molecule involved in leukocyte adherence and T-cell activation. Immunol Today 10:423, 1989

211. Miyake K, Underhill CB, Lesley J, Kincade PW: Hyaluronate can function as a cell adhesion molecule and CD44 participates in hyaluronate recognition. J Exp Med 172:69, 1990

212. Arch R, Wirth K, Hofmann M et al: Participation of normal immune responses of a metastasis-inducing splice variant of CD44. Science 257:682, 1992

213. Stamenkovic I, Amiot M, Pesando JM, Seed B: A lymphocyte molecule implicated in lymph node homing is a member of the cartilage link protein family. Cell 56:1057, 1989

214. Tedder TF, Luscinskas W, Kansas GS: Regulation of leukocyte migration by L-selectin: mechanisms, domains and ligands. Behring Inst Mitt 92:165, 1993

215. Tedder TF, Penta AC, Levine HB, Freedman AS: Expression of the human leukocyte adhesion molecule, LAM1. Identity with the TQ1 and Leu-8 differentiation antigens. J Immunol 144:532, 1990

216. Tedder TF, Matsuyama T, Rothstein DM et al: Human antigen-specific memory T cells express the homing receptor necessary for lymphocyte recirculation. Eur J Immunol 20:1351, 1990

217. Lasky LA: Selectins: interpreters of cell-specific carbohydrate information during inflammation. Science 258:964, 1992

218. Spertini O, Luscinskas FW, Gimbrone MA Jr, Tedder TF: Monocyte attachment to activated human vascular endothelium in vitro is mediated by leukocyte adhesion molecule-1 (L-selectin) under non-static conditions. J Exp Med 175:1789, 1992

219. Spertini O, Kansas GS, Munro JM et al: Regulation of leukocyte migration by activation of the leukocyte adhesion molecule-1 (LAM-1) selectin. Nature 349:691, 1991

220. Arbones ML, Ord DC, Ley K et al: Lymphocyte homing and leukocyte rolling and migration are impaired in L-selectin (CD62L) deficient mice. Immunity 1994 (in press)

221. Pierce SK, Morris JF, Grusby MJ et al: Antigen-presenting function of B lymphocytes. Immunol Rev 106:149, 1988

222. Chesnut RW, Grey HM: Antigen presentation by B cells and its significance in T-B interactions. Adv Immunol 39:51, 1986

HLA Antigen and Antibody System

11

Glenn E. Rodey

INTRODUCTION

The human leukocyte (HLA) antigen genetic system is the major histocompatibility complex (MHC) in humans. MHC gene products were initially defined in mice[1] as transplantation antigens. For several years, they were of interest primarily to transplantation immunologists. In the mid-1960s, two lines of evidence suggested that MHC genes might participate more broadly in immune responses. First, Lilly et al[2] discovered that genetic susceptibility of inbred mice to Gross virus-induced leukemia was linked to the murine MHC, H-2. This observation was the basis for a major survey of HLA and disease associations[3] that began in 1967 and has continued to the present time. Second, it was observed that certain inbred mouse strains responded poorly or not at all to selected simple antigens.[4] Genetic studies demonstrated that the capacity to respond to specific antigens was genetically determined by factors linked to the H-2 complex,[5] giving rise to the concept of immune response genes. In 1974, Zinkernagel and Dougherty[6] identified the critical role of MHC genes in immune responses by demonstrating that antigen primed T cells only recognized a foreign antigen when it was presented on cells sharing the same MHC antigens as the initial antigen-presenting cell (APC). This phenomenon became known as MHC restriction. Finally, MHC molecules were found to direct the "educational" process occurring in the thymus that ultimately determines the repertoire of expressed T-cell receptors.[7] Thus, MHC studies have merged into the mainstream of immunology. Together with the B- and T-cell receptor genes, MHC genes form a major triad of gene families responsible for the genetic control of immune responses.

This chapter provides a review of the structure and function of the HLA genetic complex, followed by a discussion of some important clinical applications of HLA testing. Analysis of HLA gene products is used in four clinical settings: (1) for selection of compatible donor and recipient pairs in organ and bone marrow transplantation, (2) for selection of HLA-compatible single donor products for thrombocytopenic patients who are refractory to random pooled platelets, (3) for analysis of genetic factors that contribute to the expression of HLA-associated diseases, and (4) for resolution of parentage disputes. This chapter limits the discussion to HLA testing in organ transplantation and blood transfusion.

HLA NOMENCLATURE

Evolution of HLA Specificity Nomenclature

Since 1962, regular International Histocompatibility Workshops have been held in which HLA investigators exchange concepts, reagents, and procedures. In 1967, an HLA nomenclature committee, formed under the auspices of the World Health Organization (WHO), recommended the following nomenclature for clearly defined specificities[8]: HL-A, followed by a numeric term, for example, HL-A2. A provision also allowed for the inclusion of probable specificities. The numerics of such specificities were preceded by a lowercase w to indicate their provisional acceptance (e.g., HL-Aw28). When formally accepted, the w is dropped from the specificity. This nomenclature replaced a number of local terminologies currently in use, such as the LA series, FOUR series, and Hu series. At that time, however, two distinct segregant series were only hinted at, so specificities of both HLA-A and -B received numbers sequentially according to their discovery. For historical reasons, HLA-A and -B alleles are still considered as a single group for sequential numbering of new specificities.

By 1975, it became clear that a new nomenclature was needed to accommodate multiple loci. By this time, three segregant series (loci) were clearly defined, as were newly recognized allelic specificities present only on B lymphocytes. The WHO committee thus adopted a revised nomenclature based on the following principles: HLA designated the MHC; a capital letter (e.g., A, B, C, D) designated the segregant series; the provisional w was retained when appropriate; and numerics for each segregant series, with the exception of the A and B series, started with the number 1.[9] Thus, the specificity HL-A2 became HLA-A2, and HL-A5 became HLA-B5.

Modifications were again made in 1984 to the nomenclature when multiple HLA-D region segregant series were found. Different D region segregant series retained the capital letter D but could be further divided into subregions by adding a second capital letter (e.g., DR, DP, DQ).[10] To prevent possible confusion between HLA-C locus alleles and complement components, a decision was made to retain the w prefix in all C locus alleles permanently.

Two additional modifications have been made since 1984. First, newly defined variant serologic specificities that detect a single gene product of known nucleotide sequence receive an extended numeric that coincides with the molecular nomenclature of the allele.[11] For example, a unique serologic specificity that detects the class I gene product HLA-A*0203 is called HLA-A203. Second, the Provisional workshop designation, w, has been dropped from all specificities except the public epitopes Bw4 and Bw6, the Dw and DP specificities defined by cellular typing techniques, and the Cw specificities.

Allelic Nomenclature

An additional nomenclature, based on nucleotide sequences, was recommended during the Tenth International Histocompatibility Workshop, in 1987.[12] Refined gene mapping and nucleotide sequence data revealed that more than one locus could code for alternate protein chains in D region molecules. Furthermore, many HLA allelic variants that are not detectable by traditional serologic techniques were discovered. This complexity necessitated the development of the following nomenclature for HLA genes: (1) HLA designates the MHC; (2) a capital letter indicates a specific region (A, B, C, D, E, F, G, H, J, . . . , n), with all genes in the D region prefixed by the letter D, followed by a second capital letter indicating the subregion of D (DM, DN, DO, DP, DQ, DR, . . . , n); (3) specific chains coding for the class II genes are next identified (e.g., A1, A2, B1, B2); and (4) specific alleles are designated by an asterisk (*) followed by a two-digit number indicating the most closely associated serologic specificity, followed by a two-digit number defining the allele. For example, the serologically defined HLA-A2 specificity actually comprises 12 distinct variant alleles. These alleles are now referred to as HLA-A*0201 through *0212. Similarly, the 12 recognized allelic variants of the serologically defined specificity, HLA-DR4, are referred to as HLA-DRB1*0401 through *0412. Occasionally, a fifth digit may appear in the nomenclature (e.g., *11041 and *11042). The fifth digit indicates two alleles that differ only by a single nucleotide that does not change the encoded amino acid.[11]

To summarize, there are now two HLA nomenclatures one is used to describe serologically or cellularly defined specificities (antigenic determinants), and a new nomenclature, formulated in 1987, is used to define alleles, based on confirmed nucleotide sequences.

STRUCTURE OF THE HLA GENETIC COMPLEX

The HLA genetic complex, located on the short arm of chromosome 6, spans a distance of approximately 4,000 kb.[13] The complex contains an estimated 70–80 genes. Thirty-one class I and II genes are officially recognized by the WHO nomenclature committee (Table 11-1). Within the MHC, defined genes are physically grouped into three regions (Fig. 11-1). The class I region encodes genes for heavy chains of the classic transplantation molecules, HLA-A, -B, -C, the nonclassic class I genes, HLA-E, -F, and -G, and several pseudogenes. The class II region encodes both α- and β-chains of HLA-DR, -DQ, -DP. At least four genes in the class II region coding proteins transport peptides into the endoplasmic reticulum for loading into class I molecules (TAP1, TAP2) or have proteosome-like sequences for molecules that potentially could partially digest endogenously derived peptides (LMP2, LMP7).[13] The class III region encodes several structurally and functionally diverse molecules (C4, 21-hydroxylase [21-OH], C2, factor B, tumor necrosis factor [TNF], heat shock protein hsp70). DRA, the most telomeric class II locus, is separated from 21-OHB by about 400 kb; The position of TNF α and β loci are approximately 200 kb centromeric to the HLA-B locus, with the β gene on the HLA-B locus side.[14]

Class I and II genes, together with variable domain genes of the B- and T-cell receptor genes, are the most polymorphic genetic systems known. More than 250 class I and II allelic gene products have been sequenced, 133 of which can be detected by serologic techniques.[11] The true number of gene products is still underestimated, as a significant number of variant alleles remain to be sequenced in nonwhite populations throughout the world.[15–18] The occurrence of the class III genes within the MHC is still puzzling. It is not clear whether this group of somewhat unrelated genes is located in this region by chance occurrence or whether these genes and the class I and II genes share a functional relationship. Because the focus of this chapter is the HLA class I and II genes and molecules, no further discussion of class III genes is presented.

Class I and II Genes

Class I and II genes, with minor exceptions, have similar structures (Fig. 11-2). These split genes contain six to eight exon-coding sequences that closely correlate with functional

Table 11-1. Names for Class I and II Genes

Name	Previous Equivalents	Molecular Characteristics
HLA-A	—	Class I α-chain
HLA-B	—	Class I α-chain
HLA-C	—	Class I α-chain
HLA-E	E, '6.2'	Associated with class I 6.2-kb *Hind*III fragment
HLA-F	F, '5.4'	Associated with class I 5.4-kb *Hind*III fragment
HLA-G	G, '6.0'	Associated with class I 6.0-kb *Hind*III fragment
HLA-H	H, AR, '12.4'	Class I pseudogene associated with 5.4-kb *Hind*III fragment
HLA-J	cda12	Class I pseudogene associated with 5.9-kb *Hind*III fragment
HLA-DRA	DRα	DR α-chain
HLA-DRB1	DRβI, DR1B	DR β1-chain determining specificities DR1, DR2, DR3, DR4, DR5, etc.
HLA-DRB2	DRβII	Pseudogene with DR β-like sequences
HLA-DRB3	DRβIII, DR3B	DR β3-chain determining DR52 and Dw24, Dw25, Dw26 specificities
HLA-DRB4	DRβIV, DR4B	DR β4-chain determining DR53
HLA-DRB5	DRβIII	DR β5-chain determining DR51
HLA-DRB6	DRBX, DRBσ	DRB pseudogene found on DR1, DR2, and DR10 haplotypes
HLA-DRB7	DRBψ1	DRB pseudogene found on DR4, DR7, and DR9 haplotypes
HLA-DRB8	DRBψ2	DRB pseudogene found on DR4, DR7, and DR9 haplotypes
HLA-DRB9	M42 β-exon	DRB pseudogene, isolated fragment
HLA-DQA1	DQα1, DQ1A	DQ α-chain as expressed
HLA-DQB1	DQβ1, DQ1B	DQ β-chain as expressed
HLA-DQA2	DXα, DQ2A	DQ α-chain-related sequence, not known to be expressed
HLA-DQB2	DXβ, DQ2B	DQ β-chain-related sequence, not known to be expressed
HLA-DQB3	DVβ, DQB3	DQ β-chain-related sequence, not known to be expressed
HLA-DOB	DOβ	DO β-chain
HLA-DMA	RING6	DM α-chain
HLA-DMB	RING7	DM β-chain
HLA-DNA	DZα, DOα	DN α-chain
HLA-DPA1	DPα1, DP1A	DP α-chain as expressed
HLA-DPB1	DPβ1, DP1B	DP β-chain as expressed
HLA-DPA2	DPα2, DP2A	DP α-chain-related pseudogene
HLA-DPB2	DPβ2, DP2B	DP β-chain-related pseudogene
TAP1	RING4, Y3, PSF1	ABC (ATP binding cassette) transporter
TAP2	RING11, Y1, PSF2	ABC (ATP binding cassette) transporter
LMP2	RING12	Proteasome-related sequence
LMP7	RING10	Proteasome-related sequence

regions of the gene product. The exons code a leader sequence, two to three extracytoplasmic domains, a transmembrane sequence, and two to three intracytoplasmic sequences.[19,20]

Only the heavy chain of the HLA class I molecule is encoded in the MHC. Genes encoding A, B, and C alleles each contain three extracytoplasmic exons coding for α_1, α_2, and α_3 domains of the heavy chain; a transmembrane, and three cytoplasmic tail exons. The associated class I light chain, β_2-microglobulin, is encoded on chromosome 15.[21] By contrast, both α- and β-protein chains of HLA class II molecules are encoded within the MHC. α-Chain genes usually contain four exons coding for a leader sequence, α_1 and α_2 domains, and a combined transmembrane-cytoplasmic tail. β-Chain genes, in addition to leader, β_1 exon, and β_2 exon, have a separate transmembrane and two distinct cytoplasmic tail exons.

Several class I and II genes, as noted in Table 11-1, are pseudogenes. Other class II genes (DQA2, DQB2, DQB3, DNA, DOB, DMA, and DMB) are potentially functional but are not known to be expressed in adults.[11] Thus, DP molecules are the product of DPA1 and DPB1 alleles, and DQ molecules are the product of DQA1 and DQB1 alleles. All DR molecules use DRA for α-chains but can use alleles coded by either DRB1 (the classic DR specificities), DRB3 (DR52 molecules), DRB4 (DR53), or DRB5 (DR51). The structures of the various HLA gene products are discussed in more detail in the section Physical Structure of HLA Gene Products.

Expression of HLA Molecules

HLA molecules are expressed constitutively on the cell membranes of many different cell types. HLA class I molecules are found on most nucleated cells.[22] They also occur on platelets, in plasma, and, to a limited extent, on reticulocytes.[23] Constitutive expression of class II, by contrast, is restricted to relatively few cells, principally B lymphocytes, tissue dendritic cells, Langerhans cells, and some endothelial cells.[24]

Expression and transcription of class I and II chains can also be up-regulated in most cells.[25] The expression of class II in certain physiologic and pathologic conditions may play a major role in the pathogenesis of the allograft rejection process and in certain types of autoimmune disease. Induction is controlled in part by regulatory sequences found in the 5′-flanking regions and intron regions contiguous with exon 1.[26,27] Different conserved sequences can be found, some that are common to all HLA genes, some that are class specific, and others that appear to confer tissue specificity. Some of the 5′ sites serve as ligands for transacting proteins or cytokines that determine the quantity of message that will ultimately be produced.[28] The major proteins that initiate the sequence of nuclear events leading to increased expression of HLA molecules in differentiated cells are the interferons, particularly interferon-γ (IFN-γ).[29–31] Class II molecules are coordinately expressed on cells exposed to interferon. However, the relative type of class II molecules induced can show variation, possibly related to variations in the interaction of transacting factors on the cis-acting regions.

Most of the human MHC has been mapped, and <1,000 kb remains to be sequenced. In addition to class I, II, and III genes of known function, there are ≥12 other potentially functional genes. Some of the novel class I molecules appear to be analogous to the murine Qa molecules. If the observed MHC-linked mating preference[32] extends to humans, some of the class I-like genes could code for pheromone-like molecules, which mediate chemosensory recognition between members of the same species.

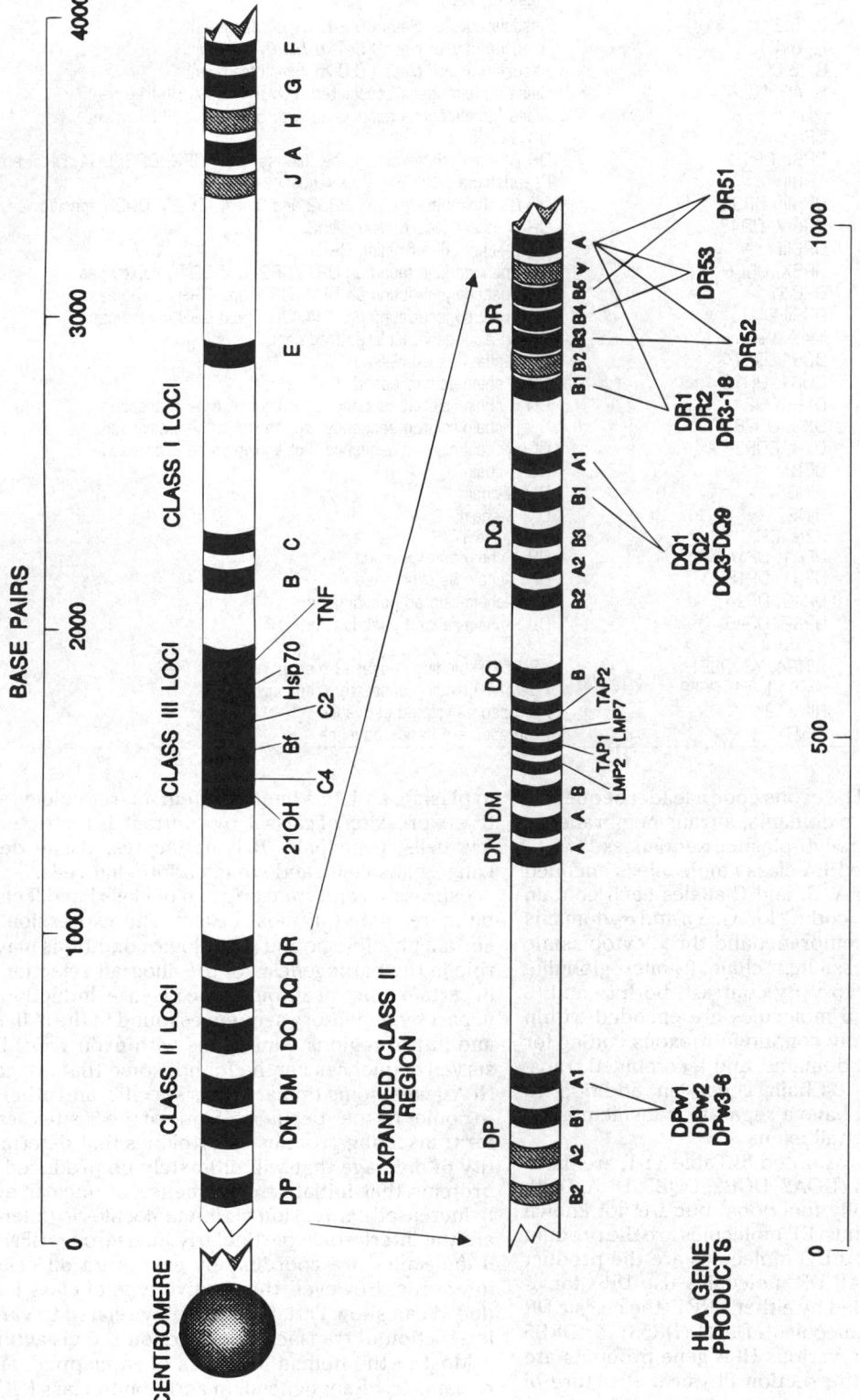

Fig. 11-1. Physical map of the HLA genetic complex, illustrating the clusters of genes according to the class of encoded gene products. Expanded view of the HLA-D region, illustrating loci used for specific HLA-D region gene products. The symbol ψ represents 6 DRB pseudogenes designated DRB6, 7, 8, and 9.

Class I

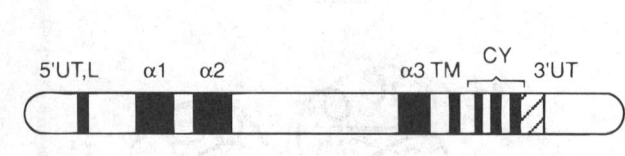

Class II

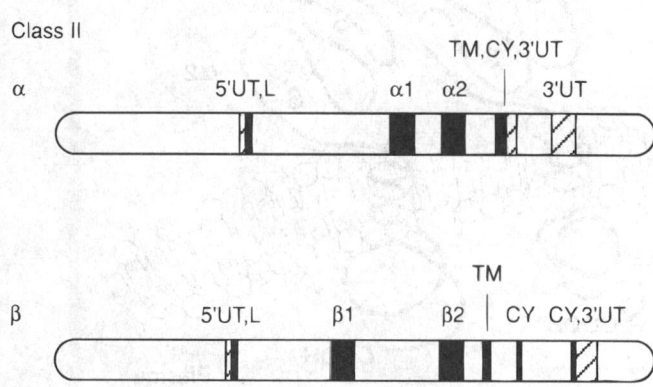

Fig. 11-2. Organization of class I and II MHC genes. 5' UT and 3' UT, untransated regions in the 5' and 3' ends of the gene; L, leader sequence; a, b, exons encoding extracellular domains; TM, transmembrane exon; CY, exons encoding the cytoplasmic tail. (From Germain,[20] with permission.)

Inheritance and Linkage Disequilibrium

Because of their close physical linkage, HLA genes are normally inherited en bloc from the parents, unless a recombination event has occurred. Thus, despite the complexity of the gene clusters, only four genotypes are normally transmitted to offspring, and the probability of genotypic HLA identity of two siblings is 25%. Recombinant HLA haplotypes (the portion of a single chromosome carrying one set of the HLA genes) are observed in about 2–3% of offspring, a frequency that would be expected on the basis of the length of the genetic complex. HLA genes are expressed co-dominantly and no null or amorphic class I or II alleles have been reported. However, specific functional HLA-DR β-loci are commonly deleted on different HLA haplotypes. The DRB1 locus, which codes for the β-chain of classic DR molecules, is found on all HLA haplotypes. Haplotypes that carry the DR1 allele do not bear the DRB3, -4, or -5 loci; DR2 haplotypes carry only DRB5; DR3, -5, and -6 haplotypes carry only DRB3; DR4, -7, and -9 haplotypes carry only DRB4; and DR8 haplotypes carry only DRB1.[13] Null alleles are common in the C4 and C2 class III genes.[33–35]

Certain combinations of genes occur in HLA haplotypes within the population far more frequently than expected on the basis of gene frequencies. This phenomenon, referred to as linkage disequilibrium, is quite common in the HLA system and has important biologic and clinical implications. In large randomly mating populations, gene frequencies rapidly achieve equilibrium within the population after one or two generations, unless some positive or negative selection pressure is acting on the gene (i.e., Hardy-Weinberg principle). When equilibrium exists, the occurrence of any two HLA genes on a particular haplotype should be an independent event governed only by the gene frequencies in the population. For example, if HLA-A1 and -B8 gene frequencies in a population are 0.16 and 0.1, respectively, the expected occurrence of an HLA haplotype bearing both A1 and B8 should be $0.16 \times 0.1 \times 100 = 1.6\%$. In certain white populations with origins in Northern Europe,

the actual occurrence of this haplotype in the population may be as high as 8%. Linkage disequilibrium effects often can be seen throughout an entire haplotype, involving class III as well as class I and II MHC-encoded genes.[33,36] The possible causes and significance of linkage disequilibrium are discussed in more detail in the section Evolution and Functions of HLA Gene Products.

PHYSICAL STRUCTURE OF HLA GENE PRODUCTS

Class I and II molecules are heterodimeric glycoproteins. Although the peptide chains are different for each class of molecules, the overall three-dimensional configurations of the molecules are probably very similar (Fig. 11-3). The protein chains of each class of molecule, the class I heavy chain, β_2-microglobulin, and the class II α- and β-chains belong to the immunoglobulin gene superfamily.[37] Each protein contains one of the immunoglobulin-like domain structures typical of this family, and these domains show sequence homologies with domains of other members of that family.

Class I Molecules

HLA class I molecules contain a heavy protein chain, of approximately 45-kd mass, that is noncovalently associated with β_2-microglobulin, a nonpolymorphic protein of 12-kd mass. The heavy chain structure correlates closely with the exonic arrangement of the gene. Beginning with the N-terminal amino acid, three extracytoplasmic domains (α_1, α_2, and α_3) are followed by a hydrophobic transmembrane stretch of amino acids, terminating in a cytoplasmic tail. β_2-Microglobulin, together with the heavy chain domain, constitutes the membrane-proximal portion of the molecule. The amino acid sequences of 40–50 class I molecules, deduced from class I nucleotide sequences,[38,39] demonstrate that amino acid sequences of the α_3 domain are highly conserved. β_2-Microglobulin appears to be nonpolymorphic. All the polymorphism detectable by serologic and cellular techniques resides in the α_1 and α_2 domains. Moreover, most of the polymorphism occurs in specific sites referred to as hypervariable regions.

Early structural models of class I molecules indicated that both the α_1 and α_2 domains contain stretches of amino acid sequences in an α-helical configuration. The significance of this observation was not appreciated until further studies conducted by Bjorkman and colleagues[40,41] elucidated the three-dimensional structure of HLA-A2 (Fig. 11-4). The α_1 and α_2 domains form a platform of eight antiparallel β-strands overlaid by the two α-helices (Fig. 11-5). This configuration forms a groove that is about 25 Å long, 10 Å wide, and 11 Å deep. This site, referred to as the peptide groove, accommodates processed peptides for presentation to T-lymphocyte receptors (see the section Evolution and Functions of the HLA Gene Products). Comparisons of the various class I amino acid sequences to HLA-A2 indicate that virtually all hypervariable sites occur within, or in close proximity to, the peptide groove.[41]

Class II Molecules

HLA class II molecules contain two noncovalently associated protein chains, an α-chain of approximately 33 kd, and a β-chain of approximately 29 kd. Each chain is a transmembrane protein that consists of a cytoplasmic tail, a hydrophobic transmembrane segment, and two membrane-distal domains (Fig. 11-3). Currently, no HLA class II molecule has been crystallized. However, simulated modeling of class II molecules, alignment of conserved amino acid sequences, and homologous segments

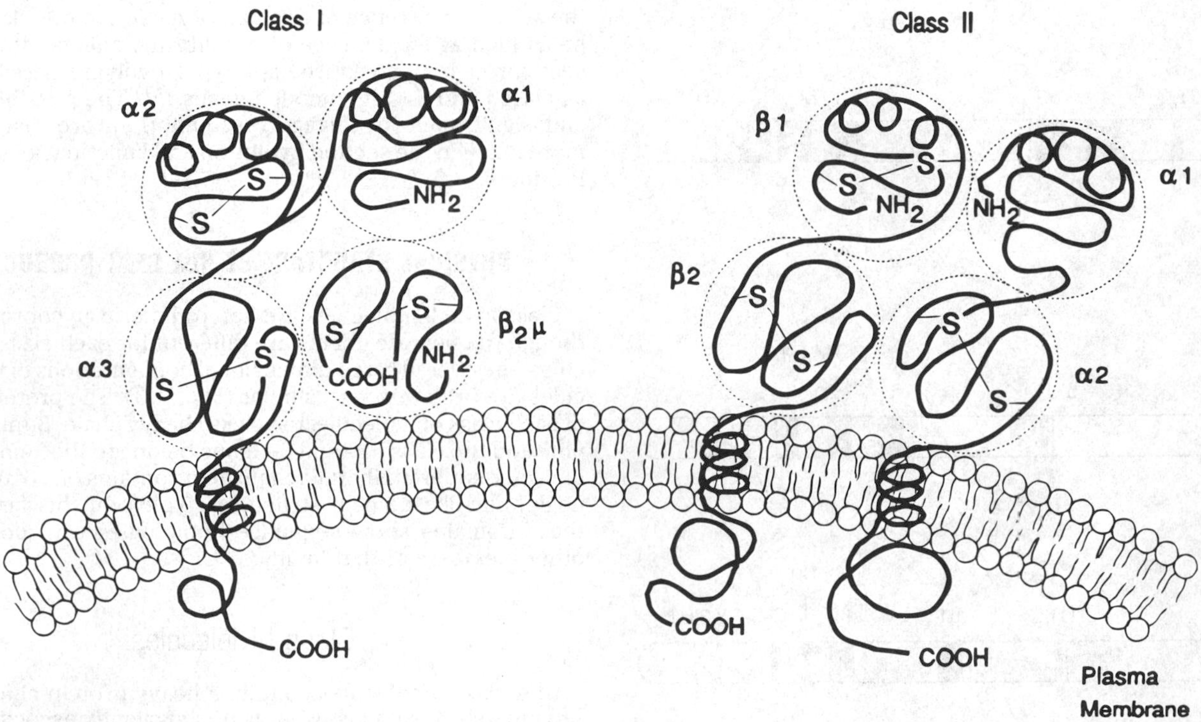

Class I   Class II

Fig. 11-3. General structure of HLA class I and II heterodimeric molecules, indicating their conformational similarities. (From Rodey and Fuller,[54] with permission.)

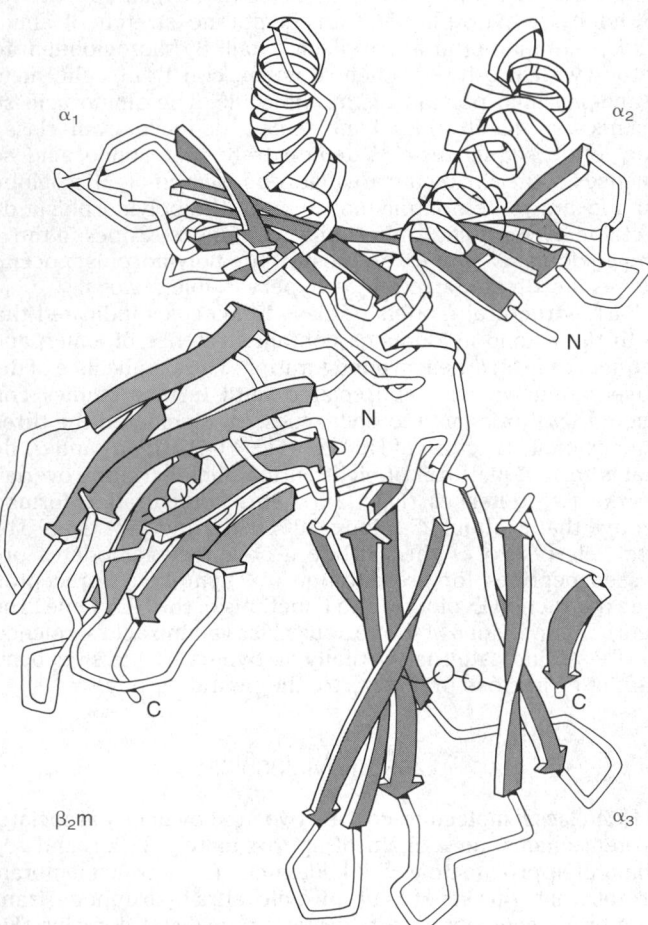

Fig. 11-4. Three-dimensional configuration of HLA-A2, modeled from x-ray crystallographic studies. (From Bjorkman et al.,[40] with permission.)

of class I and II molecules strongly indicate that a similar peptide groove exists on class II molecules.[42]

Origin of MHC-Associated Peptides

Peptides presented by MHC molecules are derived from two distinct sources. The first source is exogenously derived antigens that are taken into cells and ultimately presented on class II MHC molecules to CD4+ T lymphocytes.[43] (This is the classic

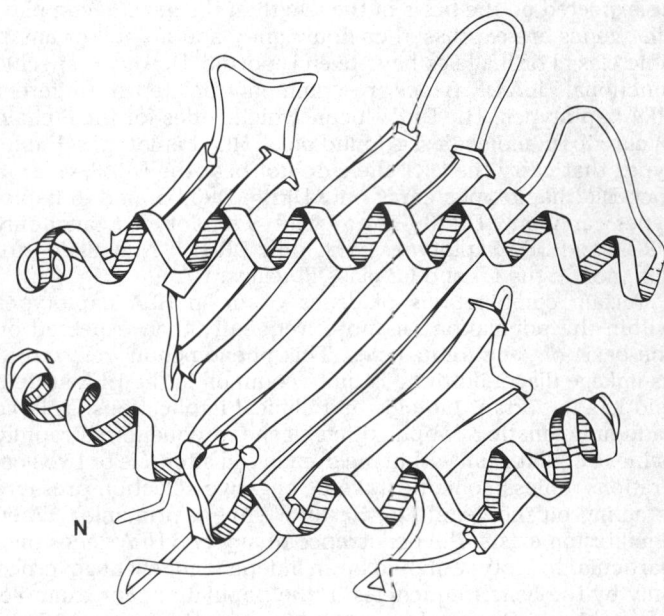

Fig. 11-5. Scheme of the peptide groove of an HLA class I molecule, formed by the α_1 and α_2 domains. The view is looking down on the vertically oriented molecule. (From Bjorkman et al.,[41] with permission.)

pathway used by APCs to capture, process, and present antigens for subsequent induction of delayed-type hypersensitivity reactions or the production of antibodies.) Another source of MHC molecules is endogenous antigens that originate in the cytosolic internal environment of the cell.[44] Endogenous peptides, which may include peptides from self-antigens, or may be derived from early viral proteins produced in a virus-infected cell, are presented primarily by class I MHC molecules and are recognized by CD8[+] cytotoxic T lymphocytes (CTL). The routes through which the peptides and the class II or I molecules pass are referred to, respectively, as the exogenous and endogenous pathways, according to the origin of the peptides.

Exogenous Pathway

With an appropriate route of administration, foreign antigen derived from the external environment is taken up by APCs via random or receptor-mediated endocytosis. The antigen undergoes limited proteolysis within membrane-bound endosomal compartments. Concurrently, MHC class II molecules are assembled in the endoplasmic reticulum. In addition to the α- and β-chains early class II molecules contain a third chain, called the invariant or γ-chain. The chain serves two important functions in the exogenous pathway: (1) it occupies the peptide binding groove and prevents most endogenously derived peptides from binding to the newly assembled class II molecules, and (2) it contains an amino acid sequence that targets the molecule to the endosomal compartments. On entry into endosomes, the invariant chain is degraded, freeing the peptide groove to bind newly formed peptides specifically derived from exogenous antigens. The peptide/MHC complex is then transported to the plasma membrane and is re-expressed on its surface.

Endogenous Pathway

Peptides presented by class I MHC molecules originate primarily from proteins found in the cytosol. Most are derived from self-proteins under normal circumstances. Endogenous peptides are also derived from viral proteins when these proteins are actively synthesized by a virus-infected cell.[45] Recent evidence indicates that peptides from phagocytosed microbial antigens can also gain access to newly synthesized class I molecules by undefined mechanisms.[46] It appears that evolution has provided the endogenous pathway and class I MHC molecules as a mechanism to survey the internal environment of the cell for antigens from replicating organs and from mutated self-proteins that would otherwise escape recognition by antibody or other extracellular immune mechanisms.

In contrast to class II molecules, whose structure is temporarily stabilized by the invariant chain before peptide binding in endosomal compartments, class I molecules must bind peptides within the endoplasmic reticulum. Otherwise, the association of the class I heavy chain with β_2-microglobulin is highly unstable.[44,47,48] Cytosolic antigens appear to be degraded into a series of short peptides through the action of proteosome-like bodies. However, the requirement for the MHC-linked proteosomal units in peptide presentation to class I molecules has recently been questioned.[49,50] The peptides, which are transported into the endoplasmic reticulum by transporter proteins, specifically bind with the assembling class I molecules to produce stable trimeric complexes. The complexes are then transported directly to the plasma membrane and re-expressed on the membrane surface.

The high degree of polymorphism found in both class I and II molecules is, as in immunoglobulin and T-cell variable domains, restricted to specific hypervariable regions of the membrane distal domains that form the peptide groove. The remaining portions of the molecules are relatively conserved, reflecting structural constraints imposed by the functions of the molecules in antigen presentation and cellular interactions.

ANTIGENIC STRUCTURE OF HLA MOLECULES

HLA molecules contain multiple alloepitopes that are capable of inducing humoral and cellular responses during alloimmunization. Serologically detected HLA alloepitopes are de-

Table 11-2. Listing of Serologically Defined HLA Specificities

A	B	C	DR	DQ
A1	B5	Cw1	DR1	DQ1
A2	B7	Cw2	DR103	DQ2
A203	B703	Cw3	DR2	DQ3
A210	B8	Cw4	DR3	DQ4
A3	B12	Cw5	DR4	DQ5(1)
A9	B13	Cw6	DR5	DQ6(1)
A10	B14	Cw7	DR6	DQ7(3)
A11	B15	Cw8	DR7	DQ8(3)
A19	B16	Cw9(w3)	DR8	DQ9(3z)
A23(9)	B17	Cw10(w3)	DR9	
A24(9)	B18		DR10	
A2403	B21		DR11(5)	
A25(10)	B22		DR12(5)	
A26(10)	B27		DR13(6)	
A28	B35		DR14(6)	
A29(19)	B37		DR1403	
A30(19)	B38(16)		DR1404	
A31(19)	B39(16)		DR15(2)	
A32(19)	B3901		DR16(2)	
A33(19)	B3902		DR17(3)	
A34(10)	B40		DR18(3)	
A36	B4005		DR51	
A43	B41		DR52	
A66(10)	B42		DR53	
A68(28)	B44(12)			
A69(28)	B45(12)			
A74(19)	B46			
	B47			
	B48			
	B49(21)			
	B50(21)			
	B51(5)			
	B5102			
	B5103			
	B52(5)			
	B53			
	B54(22)			
	B55(22)			
	B56(22)			
	B57(17)			
	B58(17)			
	B59			
	B60(40)			
	B61(40)			
	B62(15)			
	B63(15)			
	B64(14)			
	B65(14)			
	B67			
	B70			
	B71(70)			
	B72(70)			
	B73			
	B75(15)			
	B76(15)			
	B77(15)			
	B7801			
	Bw4			
	Bw6			

(Data from Bodmer et al.[11])

Table 11-3. Population Frequencies of Major Cross-reactive or Determinants Present on HLA-A and -B Gene Products

Public Epitope	Associated Private Epitopes	Approximate Epitope Frequency[a] (%)
1C	A1, 3, 9, 10, 11, 28, 29, 30, 31, 32, 33	79
2C	A2, 28, 9, 17	70
5C	B5, 15, 17, 18, 35, 53, 70	50
7C	B7, 13, 22, 27, 40, 42, 47, 48	54
8C	B8, 14, 16, 18	38
12C	B12, 21, 13, 40, 41	44
Bw4	B13, 27, 37, 38, 44, 47, 49, 51, 5102, 5103, 52, 53, 57, 58, 59, 63, 77, A24, 25, 32	79
Bw6	7, 703, 8, 18, 35, 39, 3901, 3902, 4005, 41, 42, 45, 46, 48, 50, 54, 55, 56, 60, 61, 62, 64, 65, 67, 71, 72, 73, 75, 76, 7801	87

[a] North American white populations of European origin. (Modified from Rodey and Fuller,[54] with permission.)

fined with well-characterized operationally monospecific alloantibodies and T-cell-defined epitopes with cloned T lymphocytes. Availability of HLA structure and amino acid sequence data, together with monoclonal antibodies and the technology of site-directed mutagenesis, now make precise mapping of alloepitopes on the HLA molecules technically feasible.[51] As expected, serologically definable epitopes are located principally on and adjacent to the peptide groove. The epitopes recognized by T lymphocytes are distinct from the serologically defined epitopes.[52,53] This was anticipated, since T and B lymphocytes recognize epitopes through different mechanisms (see the section Evolution and Functions of the HLA Gene Products).

Two general types of alloepitopes have been defined serologically on the basis of their distribution pattern.[54] Certain epitopes (private epitopes) occur only on a single gene product. Reagents to private epitopes have been extremely important in defining and discriminating individual HLA gene products. Additional alloepitopes are common to more than one gene product, and some of these public epitopes are fairly widely distributed among HLA molecules. Antibodies to public epitopes have been used to categorize HLA gene products into major cross-reactive groups (CREGs). The current significance of public epitopes, however, is their clinical relevance for patients awaiting transplants or requiring repetitive platelet transfusions. A single alloantibody directed against a public epitope can have devastating consequences for potential transplant recipients or for patients who require repetitive platelet transfusions (see the section HLA Testing for Transplantation and Transfusion). Table 11-2 lists the currently recognized HLA specificities.[11] Table 11-3 summarizes the major public epitopes and their approximate distribution among HLA molecules.[54]

HLA ALLOIMMUNIZATION

Alloimmunization to HLA antigens occurs through pregnancy, transfusion of blood products, or prior transplantation. HLA molecules have traditionally been considered strong immunogens because of their influence on allograft rejection and the development of graft-versus-host disease. Surprisingly, only about one-third of individuals exposed to HLA antigens develop HLA alloantibodies,[55,56] suggesting to some that these molecules may be relatively poor immunogens. Since cell-mediated immunity is a principal mechanism of graft rejection in nonimmune recipients, it is possible that HLA molecules preferentially induce T-cell-mediated responses. Such responses, however, are difficult to measure in vitro. The frequency of

precursor T lymphocytes activated in vitro to an HLA molecule is normally an order of magnitude greater than the frequency to strong antigens, such as tetanus toxoid.[57,58] Generally, there is no consistent measurable difference in precursor frequency between nonimmune and alloimmunized individuals.[59] Possible explanations for high T-cell HLA precursor frequencies are briefly discussed in the section Evolution and Functions of the HLA Gene Products.

An alternative to poor immunogenicity as an explanation for the relatively low percentage of antibody responses to alloimmunization is that the molecules are strong immunogens, but immune effector responses are modified by concurrent immune responses that down-regulate effector products such as antibodies or CTL. Increasing evidence indicates that regulatory immune responses do occur.[60,61] Suciu-Foca and others[62–64] have described the occurrence of autoanti-idiotypic-like antibodies (AB2) in the sera of many alloimmunized individuals who do not make HLA alloantibodies. AB2 appear to have specificity for cross-reactive idiotypes present on HLA-specific alloantibodies, as shown by the capacity of AB2 to inhibit binding of the HLA alloantibodies to relevant HLA targets. Reed et al.[65] report that the presence of AB2 inhibiting one or more HLA antibodies to incompatible HLA antigens on donor grafts is associated with excellent graft outcome, whereas the absence of AB2 portends early graft loss. Despite the absence of no direct evidence that these autoantibodies are important components in early activation of immune regulation, their occurrence suggests that alloimmunization with specific HLA incompatibilities will modify subsequent immune responses to these incompatibilities, either positively or negatively.

Immune regulation of effector responses may also be mediated by T lymphocytes. Helper T cells with distinctive patterns of cytokine secretion recently were identified in mice[66] and subsequently in humans.[67,68] One type, T_{H1}, which secretes predominantly interleukin-2 (IL-2), TNF-β, and IFN-γ, mediates classic delayed type hypersensitivity reactions. The second type, T_{H2}, secretes predominantly IL-4, IL-5, and IL-10, and is largely responsible for B-lymphocyte activation and differentiation into antibody-secreting cells.[69] These two helper T-cell types are mutually regulatory: IL-4 and IFN-γ each reciprocally inhibit synthesis of the other cytokine. Thus, preferential activation of one type subsequently inhibits activation of the other type. Predominant T_{H2} cytokine profiles in an allograft is associated with decreased rejection because cellular immune effector mechanisms are suppressed. Some investigators suggest that the elusive cell type responsible for suppressor T-lymphocyte function may be attributable, in part, to T_{H2} cells.

LABORATORY DETECTION OF HLA ANTIGENS AND ANTIBODIES

Historically, HLA antigens have been defined by serologic techniques, using well-characterized alloantisera. Although serology remains the keystone for clinical HLA testing, newer procedures are available that supplement serologic testing. These include cellular techniques,[15,70] one- and two-dimensional isoelectric focusing,[16,71] and DNA analysis using restriction fragment length polymorphisms and oligonucleotide probes.[72] All three supplemental procedures have defined HLA alleles that are not detectable by serologic methods. Increasingly, the use of oligonucleotide primers and probes, used in conjunction with the polymerase chain reaction or other processes that amplify the relevant gene copy,[73] is emerging as the principal adjunct procedure for class II typing. In the next few years molecular genetic typing techniques could replace serology as the primary form of HLA testing.

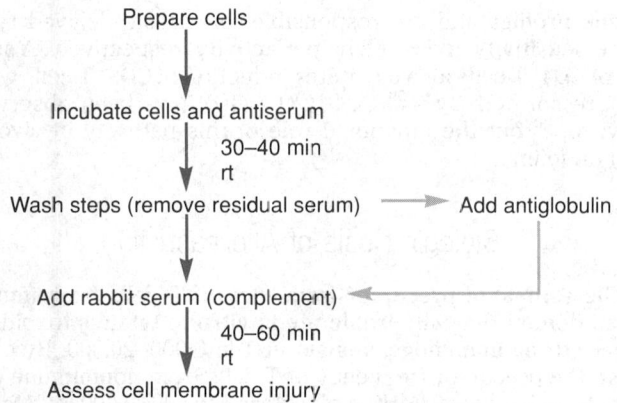

Prepare cells

↓

Incubate cells and antiserum

30–40 min
rt

↓

Wash steps (remove residual serum) ——→ Add antiglobulin

↓

Add rabbit serum (complement) ←——

40–60 min
rt

↓

Assess cell membrane injury

Fig. 11-6. Summary of the complement-dependent lymphocytotoxicity procedure, showing the optional antiglobulin augmentation step.

The most common cellular procedure used clinically is the unidirectional mixed leukocyte reaction. This procedure measures activation and proliferation of T lymphocytes from one individual primarily to HLA-D region incompatibilities on the cells of a second individual.[74] No activation or proliferation occurs in co-cultured cells from genotypic HLA-identical siblings. Variable degrees of weak or strong stimulation occur in most other combinations. Clinically, mixed leukocyte reaction is used for two purposes: (1) as a cross-match for confirming genotypic HLA identity of potential sibling donors, and (2) as a typing technique for composite typing of the D region gene products, using panels of HLA-Dw-typed cells and the unknown test cell.[15] HLA-Dw typing, used clinically to select unrelated bone marrow donors, has also been replaced by molecular genetic typing in many centers.[75]

Microlymphocytotoxicity Procedure

The standard procedure[76] for HLA testing is a complement-dependent microlymphocytotoxicity test (CDC). Because of extensive polymorphism of the HLA system, multiple antisera (or cells) must be used for thorough testing. It is not uncommon to employ 120–140 antisera to determine the HLA phenotype of an individual or 60 cells when screening patients' sera for HLA antibodies. The general procedure, summarized in Fig. 11-6, involves an initial incubation of antisera and lymphocytes, followed by the addition of rabbit serum as a source of complement. If specific binding of antibody to relevant HLA molecules has activated the complement cascade efficiently, the result is cell membrane injury, visualized microscopically by the addition of a vital dye, such as eosin Y, trypan blue, or ethidium bromide.

Class I HLA molecules are present on both T and B lymphocytes. Class II molecules, however, are normally present only on the B-cell population. To perform class II typing, relatively purified B lymphocytes must be used as targets (nylon wool adherence or antibody-specific capture to a solid phase), or B cells must be tagged so that they can be distinguished from T cells (tagged with fluorochrome-labeled B-cell-specific antibody).[77]

CDC is used for HLA typing (unknown cell tested against panels of HLA antisera), for HLA serum analysis (unknown serum tested against panels of HLA-typed cells), or for cross-matches between potential recipients and donor pairs (recipient serum tested against donor cells). A limitation of CDC in antibody detection is that not all HLA antibodies efficiently activate the complement system, and certain HLA specificities are not detected. Thus, antibody reactivity can be greatly underestimated in some patients. Failure to detect certain antibodies with CDC is referred to as the cytotoxicity negative but adsorption positive (CYNAP) phenomenon.[78] CYNAP can be largely eliminated by the addition of antiglobulin reagent.[79,80] This modified test is termed the antiglobulin-augmented microlymphocytotoxicity (AHG-CDC) test. CYNAP commonly occurs with antibodies directed against public or CREG specificities, whereas only partial specificity of the antibody is defined by CDC. An example of the CYNAP phenomenon is given in Table 11-4. The serum, directed against the 2C public epitope, shows no reactivity with the HLA-A9 (A23, A24) epitopes until tested by AHG-CDC.

Indirect immunofluorescence, using flow cytometry, is more sensitive than AHG-CDC for detection of HLA antibodies, and is gradually replacing CDC or AHG-CDC as the final cross-match procedure used for organ transplantation.[81]

Molecular Typing

HLA class II DR and DQ typing by molecular techniques is performed routinely in many clinical laboratories that support transplantation programs. Two general procedures are employed, depending on the level of resolution desired to discriminate variant alleles. One procedure, referred to as sequence-specific primer typing, uses DNA primers specific for individual or similar groups of class II alleles. The primers are used in conjunction with polymerase chain reaction to amplify the relevant genomic DNA. The amplified products for each primer pair are subjected to gel electrophoresis and are stained with ethidium bromide.[82] Amplification occurs only when the appropriate sequence is present. This technique is especially useful for typing individual patients but loses efficiency when larger numbers of patients (>50/wk) are typed. This is because of the need for larger numbers of electrophoresis units. Additional labeled probes are not necessary for routine definition of the

Table 11-4. The CYNAP Phenomenon in an Alloantibody Directed Against the 2C Public Epitope[a]

Cell Phenotype	Procedure	1:1	1:2	1:4	1:8	1:16	1:32
A1, 2, Bw53, w42	CDC	8	8	8	4	1	1
	AHG-CDC	8	8	8	8	4	1
A23, w36, Bw53, 58	CDC	1	1	1	1	1	1
	AHG-CDC	8	8	6	1	1	1
A24, w34, Bw42, 45	CDC	1	1	1	1	1	1
	AHG-CDC	8	8	8	6	4	1
A3, 28, B45 49	CDC	8	8	8	6	1	1
	AHG-CDC	8	8	8	6	4	1
A34, w36, Bw53, 42	CDC	1	1	1	1	1	1
	AHG-CDC	1	1	1	1	1	1

[a] Underlined specificities in the cell phenotypes belong to the 2C CREG. Sera were tested at doubling dilutions (1:1–1:32). AHG-CDC enhanced reactions are shown in boxed areas.

amplified DNA, and the test can be performed within 2 hours using nonradioactive techniques. Currently, the procedure is used for "low-resolution" class II typing (comparable to or slightly better than serologically defined typing), since primer pairs are not available to distinguish all known alleles.

A second common procedure, dot-blotting, uses locus-specific or group-specific primers to amplify the desired genomic DNA, followed by the application of a labeled oligonucleotide probe that binds to an allele-specific sequence. Amplified DNA is usually applied to a membrane as dots, and the labeled probes are added to each DNA dot for hybridization and subsequent visualization.[83] In reverse dot-blotting, nonlabeled probes are attached to a membrane through linking molecules and stored. Amplified labeled DNA is then added at testing. A number of sensitive nonradioactive labels are now available. This procedure is more frequently used when "high-resolution" typing is required because specific probes are available to discriminate variant alleles that cannot be distinguished by sequence-specific primers.

EVOLUTION AND FUNCTIONS OF HLA GENE PRODUCTS

MHC molecules are crucial to the general process by which an organism discriminates, at a molecular, cellular, and perhaps species member level, between self- and non-self-elements. This function is most clearly demonstrated in the immune system, which functions mainly to eliminate non-self- or altered self-products from the internal environment.

A second major function of MHC molecules is antigen presentation to T lymphocytes. After the three-dimensional structure of HLA-A2 was determined, the molecular basis of the MHC restriction became apparent. The ligand of a T-cell receptor is actually a bimolecular complex that consists of a peptide bound within the peptide groove of an MHC molecule. The configuration imparted by this combination determines the affinity of this complex for a set of T-cell receptors and subsequent activation of the T cell.[84] The estimated length of peptides that can be accommodated in the MHC peptide groove is 8–17 amino acids, depending on the class of HLA molecule.[41,85-87] The peptide groove of class II molecules, which appears to be open at both ends, can accommodate peptides 13–17 amino acids in length. Class I peptide grooves are closed at one end and will only carry peptides of 7–11 amino acids in length. Most peptides presented to T-cell receptors by MHC molecules are derived from larger protein chains through limited proteolysis within cells.[88] Although the MHC/peptide complex is essential for antigen-specific T-cell activation, it is not sufficient. APCs must provide additional signals, either cytokines or other expressed membrane receptors,[89-91] to permit T-cell activation. Finally, a variety of accessory molecules that enhance contact between APCs and T lymphocytes promote T-cell activation.[84] Two T-cell molecules, CD8 and CD4, interact directly with class I and II MHC molecules, respectively.[92,93]

Class I and II molecules have related but distinct roles in the antigen presentation process. The class I/peptide complex interacts primarily with T-cell receptors of CD8[+] T lymphocytes. This effector arm of the immune response is particularly important for endogenously derived peptides, such as early viral proteins produced by infected cells, and perhaps for early destruction of any cell that has produced aberrant self-proteins.[94] Peptide-MHC interactions occur intracellularly.[95] Thus, viral proteins produced very early during the initial replication cycle could be processed and presented before significant replication occurs.

The predominant function of class II molecules is presentation of peptides from exogenously derived proteins to CD4[+] T lymphocytes.[96,97] This heterogeneous population includes helper T-cell subsets, T_{H1} and T_{H2}[66-69] that secrete distinct cytokine profiles and are responsible for classic delayed type hypersensitivity and B-cell helper activity, respectively. A subset of CD4[+] T cells also facilitates induction of CD8[+] T cells with suppressor activity.[98,99] CD4[+] CTLs also have been observed in vitro,[100] but the functional role of this pathway in vivo is still undefined.

Biologic Basis of Alloreactivity

The estimated precursor frequency of T cells from immunized donors that will proliferate in vitro to tetanus toxoid or other strong immunogens is about 1 in 5,000–20,000. By contrast, the precursor frequency of T cells from nonimmune donors to an allogeneic MHC molecule is 1 in 500–2,000.[57-59] Similar differences are observed when CTL precursor frequencies are estimated. This large discrepancy has puzzled investigators for a number of years, particularly because exposure to allogeneic molecules does not normally occur in nature, except during pregnancy. Recognition of allogeneic MHC molecules and of self-MHC/foreign peptide complexes may not involve distinct sets of receptors, since cloned T lymphocytes that can react with both are described. This evidence suggests that MHC alloreactivity is actually a form of cross-reactivity with altered self; that is, a given allogeneic MHC molecule will have a configuration similar to that recognized by a set of T cells with reactivity of self-MHC complexed with a variety of foreign peptides.[101,102] A recently proposed alternative explanation is that, in the absence of processed foreign peptides, peptide grooves of MHC molecules are normally occupied by self-peptides. Thus, exposure to an apparently homogeneous allogeneic MHC molecule by serologic testing is at the T-cell level, exposure to MHC molecules already complexed with a large array of different peptides.[103] Consequently, a proportionally broader set of T lymphocytes are activated.

Evolutionary Basis of MHC Polymorphism

Every individual who is heterozygous for each known MHC gene product has six class I molecules (two each of HLA-A, -B, and -C gene products) and eight class II molecules (two each of DR, DP, DQ, and DRw52/w53). Within the human species, however, there are ≥300 discrete class I and II gene products. Two general theories, selectionist and neutralist, are proposed to explain the level of polymorphism.[104,105] Both theories propose that a high level of polymorphism has been established and maintained because of heterozygous advantage. However, the theories differ in proposed reason and mechanism. Selectionist theories propose that new MHC molecules are selected and maintained in the species because they confer some form of survival advantage. Neutralist theories propose that positive selection does not occur but that neutral random mutations are accumulated to favor outbreeding and heterozygosity. The conclusion that MHC heterozygosity would favor overall genetic heterogeneity is based on the observation that H-2 linked mating preference in mice promotes MHC-incompatible matings.[32]

Recent observations that positive selection appears to influence amino acid substitutions in the MHC hypervariable region favor a selectionist theory. This theory proposed that the major evolutionary pressure for developing polymorphism was a need to select large sets of alternative antigen-presenting molecules within the species to attain parity with constantly mutating environmental pathogens. The limited number of gene products carried by a single individual must be used to present all foreign peptides encountered by that individual. An MHC molecule can present many, but not all, different peptides. A single amino acid substitution in the peptide groove of an

MHC can abrogate the molecule's capacity to carry a specific peptide.[106] Therefore, the capacity of one MHC molecule to accommodate different foreign peptides is broad but not limitless. It is probable, in fact, that in a given individual some peptides cannot be effectively presented to or recognized by T cells. In inbred animals, some immune response gene phenomena are a reflection of these physiologic blind spots.

A final question concerns the mechanism through which MHC polymorphism is generated. Initially, genetic hotspots of hypermutability that favored a higher than normal mutation rate in MHC molecules were thought to exist. This mechanism would tend to produce an ever-changing set of MHC molecules of relatively recent origin. However, comparative amino acid sequence data in different animal strains indicate that most of the observed MHC polymorphism in rodents and primates actually predates speciation and has been retained for as long as 5–10 million years. Originally suggested as a major source of class I polymorphism in inbred mice,[106] gene conversion was not apparent in the highly outbred human populations. However, the study of HLA class I alleles in Amerindian populations with limited HLA gene pools indicates that gene conversion may play a prominent role in sustaining HLA heterogeneity within relatively inbred populations.[17,18]

HLA TESTING FOR TRANSPLANTATION AND TRANSFUSION

Three general procedures are used for clinical HLA testing: HLA typing to identify HLA specificities, serum analysis to detect HLA alloantibodies, and cross-match procedures to determine compatibility between specific donor/recipient pairs. Conceptually, transfusion of blood products and pregnancy are allografts. As such, they induce similar immunologic responses. The responses, however, are modified according to differences such as the physical structure of the graft, the manner in which it is introduced into the host, and the duration of time in the host. Transfused leukocytes, for example, persist for a relatively short time compared with fetal allografts or vascularized organ allografts. Immune responses also differ among solid organs. Liver allografts, which shed large amounts of HLA antigen and have a large capacity to clear preformed donor-specific antibodies, evoke different types of immunity and in turn are affected differently by immune effector responses than are other organs, such as kidney. Because of these differences, it is not possible to make categorical statements concerning HLA that apply to all transplant situations. The following sections use renal transplantation data to support most of the discussion of transplantation principles, but also provide a brief indication of instances in which the principles do not apply to other organ transplants.

Renal Transplantation

When an allogeneic organ is transplanted, incompatible alloantigens present in the tissues are recognized appropriately as foreign. This recognition initiates a complex sequence of immunologic events that lead to the production of immune effector, as well as immune regulatory, responses. In a nonimmunosuppressed recipient, effector responses usually dominate early in the course of the immune response, leading to rejection of the tissue. Although primary rejection is mediated by cellular mechanisms in the nonimmune recipient,[107] preformed donor-specific alloantibodies directed against alloantigens in the endothelium (ABH blood group antigens, HLA antigens, and possibly endothelium-specific alloantigens) can lead to the rapid loss of a vascularized graft, such as a kidney.

Three clinical strategies have been employed to increase the probability of graft acceptance: (1) use of immunosuppressive

agents to blunt immune effector mechanisms, (2) histocompatibility matching to reduce graft foreignness, and (3) pretransplant alloimmunization to initiate the early phases of specific immune tolerance to alloantigens present in the graft.[108]

Immunosuppressive agents are a keystone of transplantation. Without some form of immunosuppression, all but grafts from monozygotic twins will be rejected. The first successful combination of drugs for organ transplantation was azathioprine and prednisone.[109] This drug therapy has been replaced or supplemented with a more effective immunosuppressive drug, Cyclosporin A. A principal mode of action of Cyclosporin A as an immunosuppressive agent is the inhibition of factors that activate IL-2 and IL-2 receptor genes of T cells. IL-2 production plays a central role in the early amplification of cellular responses to the allograft.[110] Immunosuppression in transplant recipients, however, is a two-edged sword. Sufficient immunosuppression must be given to sustain engraftment while allowing the patient to respond adequately to environmental pathogens. In the absence of effective in vitro assays to quantify immunosuppression, it is difficult to define adequate immunosuppression in the organ transplant recipient. In comparison to bone marrow transplantation, in which the immune system must be ablated with lethal doses of radiation or drugs, the degree of immunosuppression used in organ transplantation appears to be quite modest, yet most grafts survive. The role of immunosuppressive drugs in organ transplantation partly may be indirect, by facilitating immunologically mediated donor-specific acquired tolerance, as well as directly suppressing immune effector responses. The success of Cyclosporin A in improving graft survival, particularly for nonrenal organ transplants, spurred an extensive search for additional immunosuppressive agents; and a number of promising drugs, such as FK506, rapamycin, mycophenolate mefotil, and brequinar, are currently undergoing preclinical and clinical testing.[111–113]

The two major transplantation antigen systems in human organ transplantation are the ABO and HLA systems. ABH substances are present in endothelial cell membranes. Naturally occurring isohemagglutinins can bind to the endothelium and cause hyperacute rejection of kidney and heart allografts. ABO matching of organs is therefore performed according to the same principles used for red cell transfusion. The second major transplantation antigen system is HLA. In humans, the most compelling evidence that HLA is the major histocompatibility complex is the superior graft survival rate of organs obtained from genotypic HLA identical siblings, as compared with any other donors.[114,115] Patients receiving these grafts have fewer rejection episodes and require lower doses of immunosuppressive drugs. Renal graft survival rates (GSRs) in this group are >90% at 2 years.

The importance of HLA-matching kidney donors derived from cadaveric sources has been difficult to establish, especially if GSRs are evaluated only during the first 2-year posttransplant period. However, statistically significant improvement in GSRs can be demonstrated in major registries that monitor renal transplant results submitted by multiple centers.[114,116,117] The half-life of a genotypic HLA-identical graft is 25 years compared with 13 years for parental one-haplotype matched grafts. By contrast, calculated half-lives for cadaveric grafts matched or mismatched for HLA-A, -B, and -DR are 17 and 8 years, respectively. This means that after 10 years, 60% of mismatched cadaveric grafts are lost.

Prior alloimmunization, through either blood transfusion, pregnancy, or prior allografts, poses an additional risk for potential recipients. The presence in a patient's serum of donor-specific HLA antibodies, especially antibodies directed against donor HLA class I antigens, is associated with a high incidence of early graft failure.[118,119] Such antibodies, detected by cross-matching procedures, preclude the use of that donor. Serum of potential recipients is regularly monitored for HLA antibodies against panels of HLA-typed cells. Antibody reactivity to the panel, expressed as percent reactive antibody, is an indication of the likelihood that a compatible donor will be found. Many alloimmunized patients' sera react against ≤80–100% of panel cells. In such patients, defining the specificity of the HLA antibodies becomes an important factor in predicting which donors will be compatible. Interestingly, the high percent reactive antibody in the highly sensitized patients is not due to multiple HLA antibodies. Rather, it is almost always due to the presence of one to two HLA antibodies with specificity to the high-frequency public or CREG epitopes (see the section HLA Alloimmunization).

Although prior alloimmunization may be detrimental to potential transplant recipients who make HLA antibodies, it paradoxically promotes graft acceptance in cross-match-negative transplants.[56,120,121] The beneficial effect of blood transfusion was found to be most striking in patients who received repetitive donor-specific blood transfusions before receiving kidneys from living-related donors.[56] Following these observations, most centers established a policy of deliberate pretransplant blood transfusion. Interestingly, the beneficial effect of blood transfusion of graft survival has not been so apparent in the cyclosporine era.[122] The apparent loss of this effect is attributed to the general use of Cyclosporin A and to improved procedures for management of early rejection episodes. Most centers now do not perform deliberate blood transfusion.

Other Organ Transplantation

Heart and liver transplantation are now established forms of therapy for end-stage organ failure. A beneficial effect of HLA matching is observed in heart and pancreas transplants.[115,123] Clearly establishing HLA effects in liver transplants has been difficult. Retransplants appear to exhibit a matching effect. Interestingly, primary nonfunction of liver grafts may occur more frequently in well-matched grafts,[124] perhaps related to recurrence of the original disease mediated by HLA-restricted effector mechanisms.

Concept of Allograft Acceptance

During the first two decades of organ transplantation, most investigations focused on mechanisms that lead to allograft rejection. An important by-product of the observed beneficial effect of blood transfusion was the raised awareness that graft acceptance might be an active immunologic process. This concept suggests that a primary role of immunosuppressive drugs in successful allograft acceptance is to facilitate the emergence of donor-specific acquired tolerance. Long-term graft survival would therefore depend on how effectively this process is achieved. Multiple mechanisms of active immune regulation have been identified in experimental transplant models. Donor-specific T-suppressor cells, adoptively transferred from an engrafted animal to a nonimmune animal, support acceptance of a similar graft in that animal.[125–127] Although the relationships between the early and late regulatory events have not been formulated, early graft acceptance may also be promoted through the induction of anti-idiotypic antibodies.[62,65] Recent studies of cytokine profiles locally secreted by graft-infiltrating cells may reflect the state of immunologic balance in the allograft. Acute rejection is associated elevations of IL-2, IFN-γ, and CTL-derived enzymes granzyme B and perforin. IL-2 and IFN-γ are secreted by the T_{H1}-type of helper T cell. By contrast, cytokine patterns characteristic of T_{H2}-type cells, IL-4 and IL-10, are observed more frequently during graft acceptance.[128,129] The T_{H1} and T_{H2} are mutually self-regulatory, and when one type predominates, the other is suppressed. Factors that favor the

induction of T_{H2} helper cells facilitate allograft survival. Finally, donor graft-derived passenger leukocytes have been observed to persist in the peripheral lymphoid tissues of some animals[130] and patients[131] with long-term allograft acceptance. Mononuclear leukocyte microchimerism has been proposed, through unknown mechanisms, to induce or sustain a state of donor-specific unresponsiveness.[132]

Thus, alloimmunization initiates two opposing immune responses that are in dynamic balance: strong effector immune responses that cause allograft rejection, and relatively weak regulatory immune responses that potentially suppress graft rejection responses that are waning or have been actively blunted through immunosuppression. The intensity of effector immune responses is less when allografts are well matched for histocompatibility antigens. When effector responses predominate, graft rejection occurs. But when regulatory mechanisms predominate, the rejection process is down-regulated and a state of graft acceptance ensues. Some of the new and promising immunosuppressive agents appear to preferentially suppress T_{H1} cells while sparing T_{H2} cells.

HLA Alloimmunization in Platelet Transfusion

HLA class I molecules, expressed on platelets, are a major cause of immunologic refractoriness in the alloimmunized thrombocytopenic patient.[133–136] Although it would be useful to provide HLA-identical platelet products to patients destined to receive repetitive platelet transfusions, extensive HLA polymorphism precludes this as a routine practice. Furthermore, additional factors contribute to the refractory state, especially in patients treated intensively with chemotherapeutic agents that damage vascular endothelium.[137] Platelet-specific antigens, such as Pl^{a1}, are uncommon causes of refractoriness, as each diallelic system contains a high-frequency allele.[138] In about one-third of transfusion events, the cause of apparent immunologic refractoriness cannot be identified. Thus, most patients receive either random pooled platelets or ABO-compatible random single-donor platelets until signs of immunologic refractoriness develop; efforts are then made to provide HLA-compatible single-donor platelet products.

The optimal clinical approach to this problem is to prevent HLA alloimmunization. Two relatively new methods that prevent or forestall the development of the refractory state show promise: leukocyte depletion of platelet products[139,140] and ultraviolet irradiation of platelet products.[141,142] Class II molecules are important during the cognitive phase of primary alloimmunization. Experimental models of alloimmunization indicate that recognition of class I alloantigens may not occur in the absence of metabolically functional class II-bearing APCs.[143] Platelets bear only class I HLA antigens. Both clinical methods remove the class II-bearing APCs (monocytes, dendritic cells) either physically (through leukocyte depletion) or functionally (through ultraviolet irradiation).

Although the number of thrombocytopenic patients alloimmunized by repetitive transfusion of blood products may be dramatically reduced with these procedures, it still can occur. Patients at risk to develop refractoriness can be alloimmunized from prior transplants, pregnancies, and transfusions in which depleted products were not used. In these cases, HLA-matched platelets may be required. The average patient needs ≥1,500–3,000 HLA-typed apheresis donors for a reasonable chance of procuring several compatible platelet products.[144,145] When compatible donors are not found, subsequent selection of donors having one or more mismatched antigens is often random. It is possible, however, to increase the likelihood of providing mismatched antigens to which the patient is not yet alloimmunized through an understanding of the types of HLA antibodies induced by alloimmunization.

Concepts of HLA Matching and Selective Mismatching

Table 11-5 summarizes a hierarchic strategy used in our laboratories for the selection of HLA-typed single-donor platelet products.[54] HLA match (also referred to as A match) requires full HLA-A and -B phenotypes in both recipient and donor and matching of all four alleles. HLA compatible means that no mismatches exist. This can occur when the donor phenotype contains "blanks" in the phenotype (fewer than four alleles identified). Incomplete phenotyping is usually due to homozygosity or to an uncommon allele for which the individual has no reagents. When it is due to homozygosity, the products are actually matched. HLA public match is also referred to as cross-reactive matching. This is an important partial matching strategy, because antibodies directed against the public epitopes are the most frequent cause of the highly alloimmunized state. Selection of donors matched for public epitopes increases the odds that the patient will not have antibodies directed against the platelet product.

Most centers that provide HLA-typed single-donor platelets already select products for refractory patients on the basis of the criteria summarized previously. When donors cannot be found in these groups, the next step is the selection of donors with one or more arbitrarily mismatched antigens. The process can be greatly improved if the specificity of HLA antibodies can be ascertained in advance. When HLA antibody specifications are known, mismatched antigens to which the patient has developed antibodies can be avoided. This strategy is referred to as selective mismatching. Because the highly HLA-sensitized state is caused by relatively few antibodies directed against high-frequency public specificities rather than many antibodies against low-frequency specificities, determination of antibody specificity is usually feasible, even in patients with reactivity against 75% of donor cells.[146,147]

Finally, selection of HLA-compatible donors by cross-matching is effective if CYNAP-insensitive procedures are used to detect antibodies. Primarily for logistical reasons, cross-matching is not the first test of donor selection in many large centers. Selection by cross-matching requires either storing cells from all donors or calling in large numbers of donors when a product is selected. However, cross-matching may be the only practical method of donor selection for some highly refractory patients in whom antibodies cannot be identified or non-HLA factors may contribute to refractoriness.

SUMMARY

HLA molecules were originally defined serologically as transplantation antigens. Clinically, the most common application of histocompatibility testing remains the selection of donors for recipients who require organ and tissue transplantation or compatible single-donor platelet products. The biologic significance of HLA molecules, however, extends far beyond their applications in transplantation, and the clinical applications of HLA in transplantation and in treatment or prevention of other diseases have not been realized. As the crucial role of HLA molecules in immunoreactivity is further defined and understood, additional therapeutic applications will undoubtedly emerge.

REFERENCES

1. Gorer PA: The detection of antigenic differences in mouse erythrocytes by employment of immune sera. Br J Exp Pathol 17:42, 1936
2. Lilly F, Boyse EA, Old LJ: Genetic basis of susceptibility to viral leukemogenesis. Lancet 2:1207, 1964
3. Amiel JL: Study of the leukocyte phenotypes in Hodgkins disease. p. 79. In Curtoni ES, Mattiuz P, Tosi RM (eds): Histocompatibility Testing 1967. Munksgaard, Copenhagen, 1967
4. Benacerraf B, Green I, Paul WE: The immune response of guinea pigs to hapten-poly-L-lysine conjugates as an example of the genetic control of the recognition of antigenicity. Cold Spring Harbor Symp Quant Biol 32:569, 1967
5. McDevitt HO, Chinitz A: Genetic control of antibody response: relationship between immune response and histocompatibility (H-2) type. Science 163:1207, 1969
6. Zinkernagel RM, Doherty PC: Restriction of in vitro T cell mediated cytotoxicity in lymphocytic choriomeningitis within a syngeneic or semiallogeneic system. Nature 248:701, 1974
7. Marrack P, Kappler J: The T-cell repertoire for antigen and MHC. Immunol Today 9:308, 1988
8. Curtoni ES, Mattiuz PL, Tosi RM: Nomenclature: HL-A. p. 449. In Curtoni ES, Mattiuz PL, Tosi RM (eds): Histocompatibility Testing 1967. Williams & Wilkins, Baltimore, 1967
9. Kissmeyer-Nielsen F: WHO-IUS Terminology Committee—nomenclature for factors of the HLA system. p. 5. In Kissmeyer-Nielsen F (ed): Histocompatibility Testing 1975. Munksgaard, Copenhagen, 1975
10. Albert ED, Baur MP, Mayr WR: Nomenclature for factors of the HLA system 1984. p. 3. In Albert ED, Baur MP, Mayr WR (eds): Histocompatibility Testing 1984. Springer-Verlag, Berlin, 1984
11. Bodmer JG, Marsh SGE, Albert ED et al: Nomenclature for factors of the HLA system, 1992. Hum Immunol 34:4, 1992
12. Dupont B: Nomenclature for factors of the HLA system, 1987. Immunogenetics 28:391, 1988
13. Trowsdale J, Campbell RD: Physical map of the human HLA region. Immunol Today 12:443, 1991
14. Spies T, Blanck G, Bresnaham M et al: A new cluster of genes within the human major histocompatibility complex. Science 243:214, 1989
15. Mickelson E, Reinsmoen N, Robbins FM et al: HLA-Dw and HLA-DP typing of the reference panel of B-lymphoblastoid cell lines. p. 38. In Dupont B (ed): Immunobiology of HLA. Vol. 1. Springer-Verlag, New York, 1989
16. Knowles RW: Assignment of HLA-class II α and β chain 2-D gel patterns for the Workshop Reference Panel of B-Lymphoblastoid Cell Lines. p. 44. In Dupont B (ed): Immunobiology of HLA. Vol. 1. Springer-Verlag, New York, 1989
17. Belich MP, Madrigal JA, Hildebrand WH et al: Unusual HLA-B alleles in two tribes of Brazilian Indians. Nature 357:327, 1992
18. Watkins DI, McAdam SN, Liu X et al: New recombinant HLA-B alleles in a tribe of South American Amerindians indicate rapid evolution of MHC class I loci. Nature 357:329, 1992
19. Malissen M, Malissen B, Jordan BR: Exon/intron organization and complete nucleotide sequence of an HLA gene. Proc Natl Acad Sci USA 79:893, 1982
20. Germain RN, Malissen B: Analysis of the expression and function of class II major histocompatibility complex-encoded molecules by DNA-mediated gene transfer. Annu Rev Immunol 4:281, 1986

Table 11-5. Search Strategy for Potential HLA-Typed Platelet Donors That Includes Analyses of Public Epitopes and Antibodies to Public Epitopes

Data needed for search
  Recipient phenotype (based on private epitopes): A1, 3, B8, 27
  Recipient phenotype (based on public epitopes): 1C, —, 7C, 8C, 4C, 6C
  (see Table 11-3)
Recipient serum analysis: anti-2C HLA antibody detected
  Prioritized donor search
    HLA match
    HLA compatible[a]
    HLA public match[b]
    Selective mismatch[c]
    Random cross-matching
  Acceptable donor phenotype(s)
    A1, 3, B8, 27 (e.g., A1, —, B3, — etc.)
    Any donor with no public epitope incompatibilities
    Any donor lacking the 2C public epitope
    Any cross-match negative donor[d]

[a] Platelet donor has "blanks" in phenotype due to either homozygosity or rare HLA alleles.
[b] Donor phenotype usually contains mismatched private epitopes, previously referred to as cross-reactive mismatching.
[c] Selection requires careful analysis of recipient serum for HLA alloantibodies.
[d] No evidence of donor-specific HLA or platelet antibodies in recipient serum.
(From Rodey and Fuller,[54] with permission.)

21. Goodfellow PW, Jones EA, van Hegringen J et al: The β-2 microglobulin gene is in chromosome 15 and not in the HL-A region. Nature 254:267, 1975

22. Daar AS, Fuggle SV, Fabre JW et al: The detailed distribution of HLA-A, B, C antigens in normal human organs. Transplantation 38:287, 1984

23. Panzer S, Mayr WR, Graninger W et al: Haemolytic transfusion reactions due to HLA antibodies. Lancet 1:474, 1987

24. Daar AS, Fuggle SV, Fabre JW et al: The detailed distribution of MHC class II antigens in normal human organs. Transplantation 38:293, 1984

25. Skoskiewicz MJ, Colvin RB, Schneeberger EE, Russell PS: Widespread and selective induction of major histocompatibility complex-determined antigens in vivo by γ-interferon. J Exp Med 162:1645, 1985

26. Kimura A, Israel A, LeBail V, Kourilsky P: Detailed analysis of the mouse H-2K^b promoter: enhancer-like sequences and their role in the regulation of class I gene expression. Cell 41:261, 1986

27. Sullivan KE, Culman AF, Nakanishi M et al: A model for the transcriptional regulation of MHC class II genes. Immunol Today 8:289, 1987

28. Amaldi I, Reith W, Berte C, Mach B: Induction of HLA class II genes by IFN-γ is transcriptional and requires a trans-acting protein. J Immunol 142:999, 1989

29. Basham TY, Merigan TC: Recombinant interferon-γ increases HLA-DR synthesis and expression. J Immunol 130:1492, 1983

30. Collins T, Korman AJ, Wake CT et al: Immune interferon activates multiple class II major histocompatibility complex genes and the associated invariant chain gene in human endothelial cells and fibroblasts. Proc Natl Acad Sci USA 81:4917, 1984

31. Paulnock-King D, Sizer KC, Freund YR et al: Coordinate induction of Ia-α B and Ii mRNA in a macrophage cell line. J Immunol 135:632, 1986

32. Boyse EA, Beauchamp GK, Yamazaki K: Critical review: the sensory perception of genotypic polymorphism of the major histocompatibility complex and other genes: some physiologic and phylogenetic implications. Hum Immunol 6:177, 1983

33. Schendel DJ, O'Neill G, Wank R: MHC-linked class III genes: analyses of C4 gene frequencies, complotypes and associations with distinct HLA haplotypes in German Caucasians. Immunogenetics 20:23, 1984

34. Cole FS, Whitehead AS, Auerbach HS et al: The molecular basis for genetic deficiency of the second component of human complement. N Engl J Med 313:11, 1985

35. Campbell RD, Law SKA, Reid KBM, Sim RB: Structure, organization, and regulation of the complement genes. Annu Rev Immunol 6:161, 1988

36. Whitehead AS, Truedsson L, Schneider PM et al: The distribution of human C4 DNA variants in relation to major histocompatibility complex alleles and extended haplotypes. Hum Immunol 21:23, 1988

37. Williams AF, Barclay AN: The immunoglobulin superfamily—domains for cell surface recognition. Annu Rev Immunol 6:381, 1988

38. Parham P, Lomen CE, Lawlor DA et al: Nature of polymorphism in HLA-A, -B, and -C molecules. Proc Natl Acad Sci USA 85:4005, 1988

39. Zemmour J, Parham P: HLA class I nucleotide sequences, 1992. Hum Immunol 34:225, 1992

40. Bjorkman PJ, Saper MA, Samraoui B et al: Structure of the HLA class I histocompatibility antigen, HLA-A2. Nature 329:506, 1987

41. Bjorkman PJ, Saper MA, Samraoui B et al: The foreign antigen binding site and T cell recognition regions of class I histocompatibility antigens. Nature 329:512, 1987

42. Brown JH, Jardetzky T, Saper MA et al: A hypothetical model of the foreign antigen binding site of class II histocompatibility molecules. Nature 332:845, 1988

43. Neefjes JJ, Ploegh HL: Intracellular transport of MHC class II molecules. Immunol Today 13:179, 1992

44. Monaco JJ: A molecular model of MHC class-I-restricted antigen processing. Immunol Today 13:173, 1992

45. Townsend A, Öhlén C, Bastin J et al: Association of class I major histocompatibility heavy and light chains induced by viral peptides. Nature 340:443, 1989

46. Pfeifer JD, Wick MJ, Roberts RL et al: Phagocytic processing of bacterial antigens for class I MHC presentation to T cells. Nature 361:359, 1993

47. Vitiello A, Potter TA, Sherman LA: The role of β$_2$-microglobulin in peptide binding by class I molecules. Science 250:1423, 1990

48. Rock KL, Rothstein LE, Gamble SR, Benacerraf B: Reassociation with β$_2$-microglobulin is necessary for K^b class I major histocompatibility complex binding of exogenous peptides. Proc Natl Acad Sci USA 87:7517, 1990

49. Arnold D, Driscoll J, Androlewicz M et al: Proteosome subunits encoded in the MHC are not generally required for the processing of peptides bound by MHC class I molecules. Nature 360:171, 1992

50. Momburg F, Ortez-Navarrete V, Neefjes J et al: Proteosome subunits encoded by the major histocompatibility complex are not essential for antigen presentation. Nature 360:174, 1992

51. Santos-Aguado J, Barbosa J, Biro PA, Strominger JL: Molecular characterizations of serologic recognition sites in the human HLA-A2 molecule. J Immunol 141:2811, 1988

52. Wraith DC, Holtkamp B, Askonas BA: Loss of serological determinants does not affect recognition of H-2K^k target cells by an influenza-specific cytotoxic T cell clone. J Immunol 13:762, 1983

53. Krangel MS, Taketani S, Pions D et al: Biochemistry of HLA structural variants with altered serological and cellular recognition determinants. J Cell Biochem, suppl. 8A:152, 1984

54. Rodey GE, Fuller TC: Public epitopes and the antigenic structure of the HLA molecules. CRC Crit Rev Immunol 7:229, 1987

55. Rodey GE, Anderson J, Kunicki J, Aster RH: Procurement and identification of HLA lymphocytotoxic antibodies in sera of non-pregnant multiparous blood donors. Transfusion 14:167, 1974

56. Salvatierra O Jr, Vincenti F, Amend W Jr et al: Four-year experience with donor-specific blood transfusions. Transplant Proc 15:924, 1983

57. van Oers MHJ, Pinkster J, Zeüylemaker WP: Quantification of antigen-reactive cells among human T lymphocytes. Eur J Immunol 8:477, 1978

58. Singal DP: Quantitative studies of alloantigen-reactive human lymphocytes in primary and secondary MLC. Hum Immunol 1:67, 1980

59. Duffy BF, Tyler JD, Anderson CB et al: The effect of donor-specific blood transfusion on in vitro alloactive precursor cell frequencies. Transplant Proc 19:753, 1987

60. Jerne NK: Towards a network theory of the immune system. Ann Immunol 125C:373, 1974

61. Nossal GJV: Cellular mechanisms of immunologic tolerance. Annu Rev Immunol 1:33, 1983

62. Suciu-Foca N, Reed E, Rohowsky C et al: Anti-idiotypic antibodies to anti-HLA receptors induced by pregnancy. Proc Natl Acad Sci USA 80:830, 1983

63. Barkley SC, Sakai RS, Ettenger RB et al: Determination of antiidiotypic antibodies to anti-HLA IgG following blood transfusions. Transplantation 44:30, 1987

64. Phelan DL, Rodey GE, Anderson CB: The development and specificity of antiidiotypic antibodies in renal transplant patients receiving single donor blood transfusions. Transplantation 48:57, 1989

65. Reed E, Hardy M, Benvenisty A et al: Effect of antiidiotypic antibodies to HLA on graft survival in renal allograft recipients. N Engl J Med 316:1450, 1987

66. Mosmann TR, Cherwinski H, Bond MW et al: Two types of murine helper T clone. I. Definition according to profiles of lymphokine activities and secreted proteins. J Immunol 136:2348, 1986

67. DelPrete GF, De Carli M, Ricci M, Romagnani S: Helper activity for immunoglobulin synthesis of T helper type 1 (Th1) and Th2 human T cell clones: the help of Th1 clones is limited by their cytolytic capacity. J Exp Med 174:809, 1991

68. Salgame P, Abrams JS, Clayberger C et al: Differing lymphokine profiles of functional subsets of human CD4 and CD8 T cell clones. Science 254:279, 1991

69. Stevens TL, Bossie A, Sanders VM et al: Subsets of antigen-specific helper T cells regulate isotype secretion by antigen-specific B cells. Nature 334:255, 1988

70. Flomenberg N: Assignment of T-cell-defined (TCD) HLA class II specificities for the Reference Panel of B-Lymphoblastoid Cell Lines. p. 46. In Dupont B (ed): Immunobiology of HLA. Vol. I. Springer-Verlag, New York, 1989

71. Yang SY: Assignment of HLA-A and HLA-B antigens for the reference panel of B-lymphoblastoid cell lines determined by one dimensional isoelectric focusing (1D-IEF) gel electrophoresis. p. 43. In Dupont B (ed): Immunobiology of HLA. Vol. I. Springer-Verlag, New York, 1989

72. Cohen D, Simons MJ, Lalouel JM, Dupont B: Nomenclature for HLA-RFLP. p. 67. In Dupont B (ed): Immunobiology of HLA. Vol. I. Springer-Verlag, New York, 1989

73. Saiki R, Gelfand D, Stoffel S et al: Primer-directed enzymatic amplification of DNA with a thermostable DNA polymerase. Science 239:487, 1988

74. Dubey DP, Yunis I, Yunis EJ: Cellular typing: mixed lymphocyte response and cell-mediated lympholysis. p. 847. In Rose NR, Friedman H, Fahey JL (eds): Manual of Clinical Laboratory Immunology. American Society of Microbiology, Washington, DC, 1986

75. Tiercy J-M, Roosneck E, Mach B, Jeannet M: Bone marrow transplantation with unrelated donors: HLA class II oligonucleotide typing as predictive of mixed lymphocyte culture reactivity. Transplant Proc 25:1243, 1993

76. Terasaki PI, McClelland JD: Microdroplet assay of human serum cytotoxins. Nature 204:998, 1964

77. van Rood JJ, Van Leeuwen A, Ploem JS: Simultaneous detection of two-cell populations by two-color fluorescence and application to the recognition of B-cell determinants. Nature 262:795, 1976

78. Yunis EJ, Ward FE, Amos DB: Observations on the CYNAP phenomenon. p.

351. In Terasaki PI (ed): Histocompatibility 1970. Munksgaard, Copenhagen, 1970

79. Fuller TC, Phelan DL, Gebel HM, Rodey GE: Antigenic specificity of antibody reactive in the antiglobulin-augmented lymphocytotoxicity test. Transplantation 34:24, 1982

80. Gebel HM, Oldfather JW, Karr RW et al: Antibodies directed against HLA-DR gene products exhibit the CYNAP phenomenon. Tissue Antigens 23:135, 1984

81. Scornik JC, Brunson ME, Howard RJ, Pfaff WW: Alloimmunization, memory, and the interpretation of crossmatch results for renal transplantation. Transplantation 54:389, 1992

82. Olerup O, Zetterquist H: HLA-DR typing by PCR amplification with sequence-specific primers (PCR-SSP) in 2 hours: an alternative to serological DR typing in clinical practice including donor-recipient matching in cadaveric transplantation. Tissue Antigens 39:225, 1992

83. Mach B, Tiercy J-M: Genotypic typing of HLA class II: from the bench to the bedside. Hum Immunol 30:278, 1991

84. Allison JP, Lanier LL: Structure, function, and serology of the T-cell antigen receptor complex. Annu Rev Immunol 5:503, 1987

85. Reddehose MJ, Rothbard JB, Koszinowski UH: A pentapeptide as minimal antigenic determinant for MHC class I-restricted T lymphocytes. Nature 337: 651, 1989

86. Margalit H, Sponge JL, Cornette JL et al: Prediction of immunodominant helper T cell antigenic sites from the primary sequence. J Immunol 138: 2213, 1987

87. Rudensky AY, Preston-Hurlburt P, Hong SC et al: Sequence of peptides bound to MHC class II molecules. Nature 353:622, 1991

88. McKean DJ, Nilson A, Infante AJ, Kazim L: Biochemical characterization of B lymphoma cell antigen processing and presentation to antigen-reactive T cells. J Immunol 131:2726, 1983

89. Hawrylowicz CM, Unanue ER: Regulation of antigen-presentation 1. IFN-γ induces antigen-presenting properties on B cells. J Immunol 141:4083, 1988

90. Lederman S, Yellin MJ, Inghirami G et al: Molecular interactions mediating T-B lymphocyte collaboration in human lymphoid follicles. Roles of T cell-B cell-activating molecules (Sc8 antigen) and CD40 in contact-dependent help. J Immunol 149:3817, 1992

91. Galvin F, Freeman GJ, Razi-Wolf Z et al: Murine B7 antigen provides a sufficient costimulatory signal for antigen-specific and MHC-restricted T cell activation. J Immunol 149:3802, 1992

92. Doyle C, Strominger JL: Interaction between CD4 and class II MHC molecules mediates cell adhesion. Nature 330:256, 1988

93. Rosenstein Y, Ratnofsky S, Burakoff SJ, Herrmann SH: Direct evidence for binding of CD8 to HLA class I antigens. J Exp Med 169:149, 1989

94. Rajan TV: Is there a role for MHC class I antigens in the elimination of somatic mutants? Immunol Today 8:171, 1987

95. Long EO: Intracellular traffic and antigen processing. Immunol Today 10: 232, 1989

96. Heber-Katz E, Hansberg D, Schwartz RH: The Ia molecule of the antigen presenting cell plays a critical role in immune response gene regulation of T cell activation. J Mol Cell Biol 1:3, 1983

97. Schwartz RH: The role of gene products of the major histocompatibility complex in T cell activation and cellular interactions. p. 379. In Paul WE (ed): Fundamental Immunology. Raven Press, New York, 1984

98. Morimoto C, Letvin NL, Boyd AW et al: The isolation and characterization of the human helper inducer T cell subset. J Immunol 134:3762, 1985

99. Damle NK, Childs AL, Doyle LV: Immunoregulatory T lymphocytes in man: soluble antigen-specific suppressor-inducer T lymphocytes are derived from the CD4+CD45R−p80+ subpopulation. J Immunol 139:1501, 1987

100. Scrivner DL, Kristoff S, Rodey GE: Human T4+ T-lymphocyte clones specific for the B fragment of tetanus toxoid. Hum Immunol 19:245, 1987

101. Finberg R, Burakoff S, Cantor H, Benacerraf B: Biological significance of alloreactivity: to cells stimulated by Sendai virus coated syngeneic cells specifically lyse allogeneic target cells. Proc Natl Acad Sci USA 75:5154, 1978

102. von Boehmer H, Hengartner H, Nabholz et al: Fine specificity of a continuously growing killer cell clone specific for the H-Y antigen. Eur J Immunol 9:592, 1979

103. Marrack P, Kappler J: T cells can distinguish between allogeneic major histocompatibility complex products on different cell types. Nature 332:840, 1988

104. Klein J: Origin of major histocompatibility complex polymorphism: the trans-species hypothesis. Hum Immunol 19:155, 1987

105. Flaherty L: Major histocompatibility complex polymorphism: a nonimmune theory for selection. Hum Immunol 21:3, 1988

106. Nathenson SG, Geliebter J, Pfaffenbach GM, Zeff RA: Murine major histocompatibility complex class-I mutants: molecular analysis and structure-function implications. Annu Rev Immunol 4:471, 1986

107. Ascher NL, Hanto DW, Simmons RL: Immunobiology of allograft rejection. p. 91. In Flye MW (ed): Principles of Organ Transplantation. WB Saunders, Philadelphia, 1989

108. Terasaki PI: The beneficial transfusion effect on kidney graft survival attributed to clonal deletion. Transplantation 37:119, 1984

109. Flye MW: Immunosuppressive therapy. p. 155. In Flye MW (ed): Principles of Organ Transplantation. WB Saunders, Philadelphia, 1989

110. Borel JF, Ryffel B: The mechanism of action of cyclosporine: a continuing puzzle. p. 24. In Schindler R (ed): Cyclosporine in Autoimmune Diseases. Springer-Verlag, New York, 1985

111. Sollinger HW, Deierhoi MH, Belger FO et al: RS-61443—a phase I clinical trial and pilot rescue study. Transplantation 53:428, 1992

112. Morris RE: Rapamycins: antifungal, antitumor, antiproliferative, and immunosuppressive macrolides. Transplant Rev 6:39, 1992

113. Cramer DV, Chapman FA, Jaffee BD et al: The effect of a new immunosuppressive drug, brequinar sodium, on heart, liver, and kidney allograft rejection in the rat. Transplantation 53:303, 1992

114. Mickey MR: HLA Matching effects. p. 303. In Terasaki PI (ed): Clinical Transplants 1987. UCLA Tissue Typing Laboratory, Los Angeles, 1987

115. Sutherland DER, Goetz FC, Najarian JS: Pancreas transplants from related donors. Transplantation 38:625, 1984

116. Opelz G: Effect of HLA matching in 10,000 cyclosporine-treated cadaveric kidney transplants. Transplant Proc 19:641, 1987

117. Sanfilippo F, Vaughn WK, LeFor WM et al: The benefits of HLA matching on renal transplantation relative to cyclosporine use and organ sharing. Transplant Proc 21:661, 1989

118. Kissmeyer-Nielsen F, Olsen S, Peterson VP, Fjeldborg O: Hyperacute rejection of kidney allografts, associated with pre-existing humoral antibodies against donor cells. Lancet 1:662, 1966

119. Patel R, Terasaki PI: Significance of the positive crossmatch in kidney transplantation. N Engl J Med 280:735, 1969

120. Opelz G, Sengar DPS, Mickey MR, Terasaki PI: Effect of blood transfusion on subsequent kidney transplants. Transplant Proc 5:253, 1973

121. Anderson CB, Sicard GA, Rodey GE, Etheredge EE: Renal allograft recipient pre-treatment with donor-specific blood and concomitant immunosuppression. Transplant Proc 16:939, 1983

122. Opelz G: Improved kidney graft survival in non-transfused recipients. Transplant Proc 19:149, 1987

123. Opelz G: Effect of HLA matching in heart transplantation. Transplant Proc 21:794, 1989

124. Markus BH, Duquesnoy RJ, Gordon RD et al: Histocompatibility and liver transplant outcome: does HLA exert a dualistic effect? Transplantation 46: 372, 1988

125. Kilshaw PJ, Brent L, Pinto M: An active suppressor mechanism preventing skin allograft rejection in mice. Transplant Proc 7:225, 1975

126. Tilney NL, Graves MJ, Strom TB: Prolongation of organ allograft survival by syngeneic lymphoid cells. J Immunol 121:1480, 1978

127. Wood ML, Monaco AP: Suppressor cells in specific unresponsiveness to skin allografts in thymectomized, ALS-treated, marrow-injected mice. Transplantation 28:387, 1980

128. Lipman ML, Stevens AC, Strom TB: Cytotoxic, pro- and anti-inflammatory cytokine gene-transcript profiles in human renal allografts. Presented at the Twelfth Annual Meeting, American Society of Transplant Physicians, Houston, 1993

129. Xu G, Wang JC, Li B et al: Human renal graft rejection: molecular characterization including quantitation of intragraft gene expressions. Presented at the Twelfth Annual Meeting, American Society of Transplant Physicians, Houston, 1993

130. Starzl TE, Demetris AJ, Murase N et al: Review article: cell migration, chimerism, and graft acceptance. Lancet 339:1579, 1992

131. Burlingham WJ, Grailer A, Oberly TD, Sollinger HW: Human renal transplant tolerance in a DST-pretreated recipient is associated with dense focal lymphocyte infiltrates and microchimerism. Presented at the Twelfth Annual meeting, American Society of Transplant Physicians, Houston, 1993

132. Starzl TE: Cell migration and chimerism—a unifying concept in transplantation—with particular reference to HLA matching and tolerance induction. Transplant Proc 25:8, 1993

133. Yankee RA, Grumet FC, Rogentine GN: Platelet transfusion therapy: the selection of compatible platelet donors for refractory patients by lymphocyte HLA typing. N Engl J Med 281:1208, 1963

134. Yankee RA, Graff KS, Dowling R, Henderson ES: Selection of unrelated compatible platelet donors by lymphocyte HLA matching. N Engl J Med 288: 760, 1973

135. Herzig RH, Herzig GP, Bull MI et al: Correction of poor platelet transfusion responses with leucocyte-poor HLA matched platelet concentrates. Blood 46:743, 1975

136. Tosato G, Applebaum FR, Deisseroth AB: HLA-matched platelet transfusion therapy of severe aplastic anemia. Blood 52:846, 1978

137. Bucher U, DeWeek A, Splengler H et al: Platelet transfusion: shortened sur-

vival of HLA-identical platelets and failure of in vitro detection of antiplatelet antibodies after multiple transfusion. Vox Sang 25:187, 1973

138. Kunicki TJ: Human platelet antigen systems. p. 15. In Smith DM Jr, Summers SH (eds): Platelets. American Association of Blood Banks, Arlington, VA, 1988

139. Eernisse JG, Brand A: Prevention of platelet refractoriness due to HLA antibodies by administration of leukocyte-poor blood components. Exp Hematol 9:77, 1981

140. Murphy MF, Metcalfe P, Thomas H et al: Use of leucocyte-poor blood components and HLA matched-platelet donors to prevent HLA alloimmunization. Br J Haematol 62:529, 1986

141. Kahn RA, Duffy BF, Rodey GE: UV-irradiation of platelet concentrates abrogates lymphocyte activation without affecting platelet function in vitro. Transfusion 25:547, 1985

142. Slichter SJ, Deeg HJ, Kennedy MS: Prevention of platelet alloimmunization

in dogs with systemic cyclosporine and by UV-irradiation or cyclosporine loading of donor platelets. Blood 69:414, 1987

143. Faustman D, Lacey PE, Davie JM, Hauptfield VE: Allograft prolongation by immunization with donor blood depleted of Ia bearing cells. Transplant Proc 15:1341, 1983

144. Mickey R: Donor pool sizes for HLA matching. Transfusion 29:285, 1989

145. Bolgiano DC, Larson EB, Slichter SJ: A model to determine required pool size for HLA-typed community donor apheresis programs. Transfusion 29: 306, 1989

146. Oldfather JW, Mora A, Phelan DL et al: The occurrence of crossreactive "public" antibodies in the sera of highly sensitized dialysis patients, abstracted. Transplant Proc 15:1212, 1982

147. Oldfather JW, Anderson CB, Phelan DL et al: Prediction of crossmatch outcome in highly sensitized patients based on the identification of serum HLA antibodies. Transplantation 43:267, 1986

Complement Biology

12

Peter J. Sims and Therese Wiedmer

INTRODUCTION

The complement system includes >20 plasma proteins that interact through two enzymatic pathways to generate products with distinct immunoregulatory, opsonic, and inflammatory activity (Table 12-1 and Fig. 12-1). In addition to these fluid-phase proteins, the complement system encompasses a variety of cell-surface proteins that have receptor function. These membrane complement receptors recognize activated fragments derived from the complement components in plasma, and through this interaction, initiate immune adherence and cell activation. Additionally, cellular receptors that bind activated components of complement can function as inhibitors, which serve to limit dissemination of the complement reaction cascades and to protect autologous cell membranes from damage by the complement system. In concert, these plasma proteins and cell membrane receptors play a central role in host defense against infection and contribute to virtually every aspect of the inflammatory response.[1-6]

Protein Structure and Function

Table 12-1 summarizes the main components of the complement system. Shared structural motifs and related function among several of these proteins permit identification of a number of distinct protein superfamilies.[6,7] Common structural elements include a serine protease domain (SPD) shared among many of the complement enzymes, including C1r, C1s, and C2 and factors B, D, and I[8]; and cysteine-rich short consensus repeats (SCRs), representing highly conserved globular domains of approximately 60 amino acids each that confer binding affinity for C3b/C4b. SCRs are found predominantly in those complement proteins and receptors that bind C3b or C4b, but are also found in several unrelated proteins,[9,10] and a cytolytic peptide motif (found in C6, C7, C8, and C9), consisting of a putative membrane-spanning domain and a cysteine-rich domain char-

acteristic of the epidermal growth factor receptor precursor.[11] This latter motif is also shared by perforin, a pore-forming cytolytic polypeptide contained in the intracellular granules of cytotoxic T cells.[12]

Shared structural and functional homology is also apparent when comparing the reaction mechanisms of the classic and alternative activation pathways (Fig. 12-1). This is most evident for the C3/C5 convertases of both pathways.[3,6,7] These enzyme complexes (C4b2a of the classic pathway and C3bBb of the alternative pathway) represent Mg^{2+}-stabilized heterodimers formed between serine proteases (C2a or Bb) and surface-bound cofactors (C4b or C3b, respectively). C2 and factor B are proenzymes containing SPD and SCR. When proteolytically activated, they each share specificity for the same substrates (i.e., C3 and C5). C3 and C4 also derive from homologous precursor polypeptides, and each contains an internal thioester bond (between a cysteinylsulfhydryl and γ-glutamylcarbonyl) that is destabilized on peptide cleavage of their α-chains.[13,14] Transacetylation through nucleophilic attack by surface amino or hydroxyl groups provides a mechanism by which the C3b and C4b domains of these components covalently attached to membrane surfaces, thereby localizing the C3/C5-convertase enzyme complexes to the target membrane of complement attack. Membrane-bound C3b also serves an important opsonic function, labeling the target for removal by the reticuloendothelial system.

Common structure and function can also be discerned among the complement regulatory proteins and cellular complement receptors (Tables 12-1 and 12-2). Cellular C1q receptors (C1qRs) appear to be closely related to cellular collagen receptors.[15,16] The cellular C3b/C4b receptors, CR1 and CR2, as well as the C3/C4 regulatory proteins, factor H, C4b-binding protein (C4b-bp), membrane cofactor protein (MCP), and decay accelerating factor (DAF), all share the SCR motif that confers ability to bind C3b and C4b. The genes for these proteins cluster as a linkage group designated regulators of complement activation (RCA).[9,10] Two other cellular C3 receptors

Table 12-1. Components and Regulatory Proteins of the Complement System

Protein	Serum Concentration (μg/ml)	Peptide Chains (N)	Structural Motifs
Components of Activation Pathways			
C1q	100	18 (6 × 3)	Collagen-type helix
C1r	50	1	Serine protease, SCR
C1s	40	1	Serine protease, SCR
C4	640	3	Internal thioester
C2	25	1	Serine protease, SCR
C3	1,200	2	Internal thioester
Factor B	200	1	Serine protease, SCR
Factor D	1	1	Serine protease, SCR
Factor I	35	1	Serine protease, SCR
Components of Membrane Attack Complex			
C5	70	2	Homologous to C3, C4
C6	65	1	Pore-forming protein, SCR
C7	55	1	Pore-forming protein, SCR
C8	55	3	Pore-forming protein
C9	60	1	Pore-forming protein
Plasma Regulatory Proteins			
C1 inhibitor	200	1	Serpin-type inhibitor
Properdin	25	4	
C4b-binding protein	250	8 (7α, 1β)	SCR
Factor H	500	1	SCR
S protein (vitronectin)	500	1	Adhesive protein (RGD sequence)
Membrane Regulatory Proteins			
DAF (CD55)		1	SCR, GPI anchor
MCP (CD46)		1	SCR
20-kd Homologous restriction factor (HRF20, CD59)		1	GPI anchor
Membrane Receptors			
CR1 (CD35)		1	SCR
CR2 (CD21)		1	SCR
CR3 (CD11b/CD18)		2	Leukocyte β_2-integrin
CR4 (CD11c/CD18)		2	Leukocyte β_2-integrin
C1q receptor		1	
C3a receptor		1	G-protein coupling
C5a receptor		1	G-protein coupling

Abbreviations: SCR, short consensus repeat; GPI, glycosylphosphatidylinositol; DAF, decay accelerating factor; MCP, membrane cofactor protein; HRF, homologous restriction factor.

(CR3 and CR4) belong to the Leu-CAM β_2-integrin family of cellular adhesion receptors that includes LFA-1.[17]

COMPLEMENT ACTIVATION PATHWAYS

Expression of the biologic activity of the complement system requires proteolytic processing of C3 and C5. Accordingly, the reaction mechanisms of this system are focused on the assembly and control of the C3/C5 convertases (Fig. 12-1). The alternative pathway C3/C5-convertase (C3bBb) is phylogenetically the older and remains the more important enzyme mechanism for C3/C5 activation. The classic activation pathway appears to reflect evolutionary adaptation to use the specificity of immune recognition provided by immunoglobulin.[6,18]

Classic Pathway

The classic pathway is initiated through the conformational activation of C1q, one of the components of the C1 enzyme complex.[19] C1 is present in plasma largely as a Ca^{2+}-dependent complex between C1q and the proenzymes C1r and C1s with the stoichiometry C1q,r$_2$,s$_2$. Ultrastructurally, C1q exhibits six globular heads joined by filamentous segments to a helical

stem-like core. This helical core is compositionally and structurally similar to collagen and can compete with collagen for binding to plasma membrane collagen receptors.[15,16] The C1r and C1s enzyme dimers bind to the collagen-like tail of C1q, whereas the binding of C1 activators generally occurs through the globular heads of C1q. Activation of C1 requires multipoint attachment of at least two globular heads of C1q to the Fc domains of immunoglobulin within immune complexes. This can be achieved by simultaneous attachment to either two closely spaced IgG molecules, or to multiple Fc parts of a single antigen-complexed molecule of IgM.[19,20] The conformational change induced in C1q on binding multiple immunoglobulin Fc is transmitted to the C1r$_2$s$_2$ subunits, resulting in proteolytic autoactivation of the C1r dimer, which then proteolytically activates C1s. Activated C1s contains the catalytic site for proteolytic activation of C4 and C2. In addition to antigen/antibody complexes and IgG aggregates, C1 activation can be initiated by C-reactive protein (CRP), certain viral and bacterial membranes, endotoxin, DNA, monosodium urate crystals, cytoskeletal proteins, and heart mitochondrial membranes.[19] Whereas immunoglobulins bind to the globular region of C1q, C1 activation by CRP occurs through the binding of this protein to the collagen-like core of C1q. Two domains on the C1q A chain have recently been identified as the CRP binding sites. These same sites have been implicated as the binding sites for DNA,

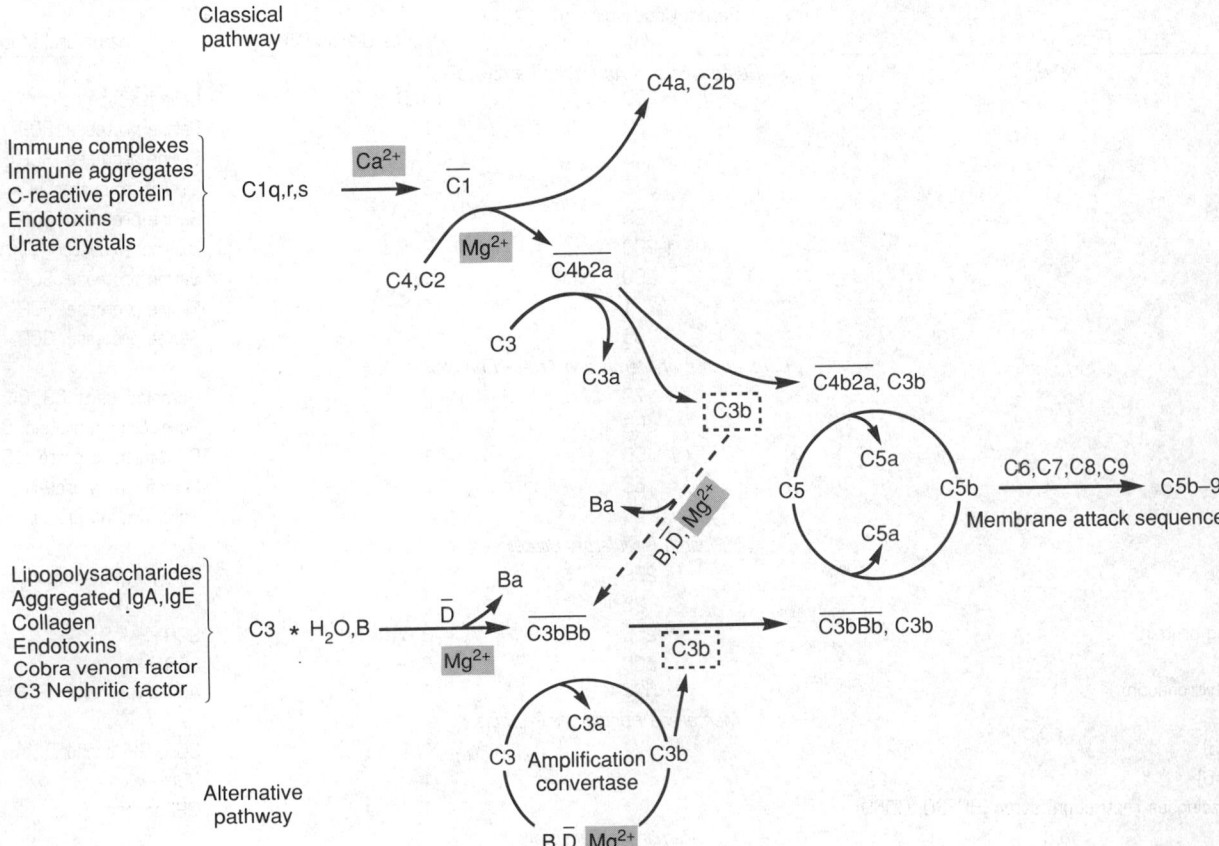

Fig. 12-1. Reaction scheme of the complement activation pathways. Components displaying enzymatic activity are denoted by a solid bar above symbol. C3*H₂O is generated from C3 by spontaneous hydrolysis of an internal thiol ester bond in the C3 α-chain (see Fig. 12-2). Dashed arrow denotes crossover between classic and alternative pathways, through which C3b generated by the classic pathway C3-convertase (C4b2a) serves as the membrane cofactor for assembly of the alternative pathway C3-convertase (C3bBb). Also note potential for self-propagation of the C3bBb enzyme complex through the cycle of the amplification convertase. See text for details. (From Sims,[201] with permission.)

which can also initiate the classic pathway by activation of C1.[21] In addition to C1, human plasma contains another enzyme complex that can initiate the reaction cascade of the classic pathway. Mannan-binding protein is a C-type lectin in plasma that binds to glycosidic residues expressed by bacteria and other pathogens, shares a similar structure to C1q and binds to C1q receptors, enhancing phagocytosis. On binding to mannose-rich surfaces, mannan-binding protein initiates proteolytic activation of C4 and C2 through an associated C1s-like serine protease.[22]

Proteolytic cleavage of the α-chain of C4 by C1s generates two fragments, C4a and C4b.[23] C4a is a vasoactive peptide of 77 amino acids, removed from the N-terminal end of the C4 α-chain.[24] In addition to liberating the C4a peptide, C1s cleavage of the α-chain of C4 exposes an intrachain thioester bond within the α-chain of the C4b domain of the molecule, which provides a short-lived and highly reactive carbonyl for covalent attachment of C4b to suitable acceptor residues (primary amines and hydroxyl groups) of the antigen/antibody complex or the target cell surface.[13,14] Polymorphism of the C4 gene is reflected in two common isotypes, C4A and C4B.[25] These isotypes differ in the reactivity of the internal thioester bond for amines versus hydroxyl groups, reflected in functional differences in hemolytic activity and in their interaction with immune complexes (see below). Once covalently bound to the cell surface or immune complex, C4b can bind C2 in a Mg²⁺-dependent complex. When complexed to C4b, C2 is proteolytically cleaved by C1s

to liberate the C2b fragment, the C2a domain of the molecule remaining attached to C4b. C2a complexed to C4b provides the catalytic site for subsequent proteolytic activation of C3 and C5.

Peptide cleavage of the α-chain of C3 by the C4b2a enzyme complex liberates the vasoactive peptide C3a, and exposes a reactive intrachain thioester bond within the α-chain of the C3b portion of the molecule[13,14,23,24,26] (Fig. 12-2). Multiple C3b is deposited on the cell surface (or within the immune complex) through reaction of this thioester bond with nearby residues containing primary amines or hydroxyl groups. Those molecules of nascent C3b that fail to react with acceptor residues undergo spontaneous hydrolysis of the internal thioester bond, thereby losing their capacity for covalent attachment to the target surface. The covalently bound C3b functions as a cofactor for subsequent activation of C5, and as cofactor for assembly of the alternative pathway C3/C5-convertase (the C3bBb complex, described below). On permissive surfaces, the recruitment of this "amplification convertase" of C3bBb provides a positive-feedback mechanism for propagating the activation of C3 and C5.

The next step in the classic pathway is the activation of C5, which is also initiated by the C4b2a enzyme complex, through proteolytic cleavage of the α-chain of C5.[27] C3b that is covalently bound to the C4b subunit of the C4b2a enzyme complex is thought to facilitate presentation of C5 to the active site in C2a, conferring enhanced specificity of the enzyme for C5.[6,28–30]

Table 12-2. Specificity and Cellular Distribution of Major Complement Receptors

Receptor	Ligand Specificity	Structural Motifs	Cellular Distribution in Humans
C1qR	C1q (collagen)		Platelets, PMNs, B lymphocytes, monocytes, fibroblasts, endothelial cells
C3aR	C3a (C4a)	G-protein coupling	Mast cells, basophils, eosinophils, PMNs, monocytes, T cells
C5aR	C5a, C5a$_{des-arg}$	G-protein coupling	PMNs, monocytes, basophils, eosinophils, mast cells
CR1 (CD35)	C3b (C4b, iC3b, C3c)	SCR	Erythrocytes, B cells, certain T cells, neutrophils, eosinophils, macrophages, follicular dendritic cells
CR2 (CD21)	C3d, C3dg, (iC3b)	SCR	B cells, T cells, follicular dendritic cells
CR3 (CD11b/CD18)	iC3b (C3d)	Leukocyte β_2-integrin	Neutrophils, eosinophils, macrophages, K and NK cells, follicular dendritic cells
CR4 CD11c/CD18, p150,95)	iC3b	Leukocyte β_2-integrin	Neutrophils, macrophages, monocytes, K and NK cells

Abbreviations: C1qR, C1q receptor; C3aR, C3a receptor; iC3b, inactivated C3b; C5aR, C5a receptor; CR1–CR4, complement receptors 1–4; NK, natural killer; PMNs, polymorphonuclear neutrophils.

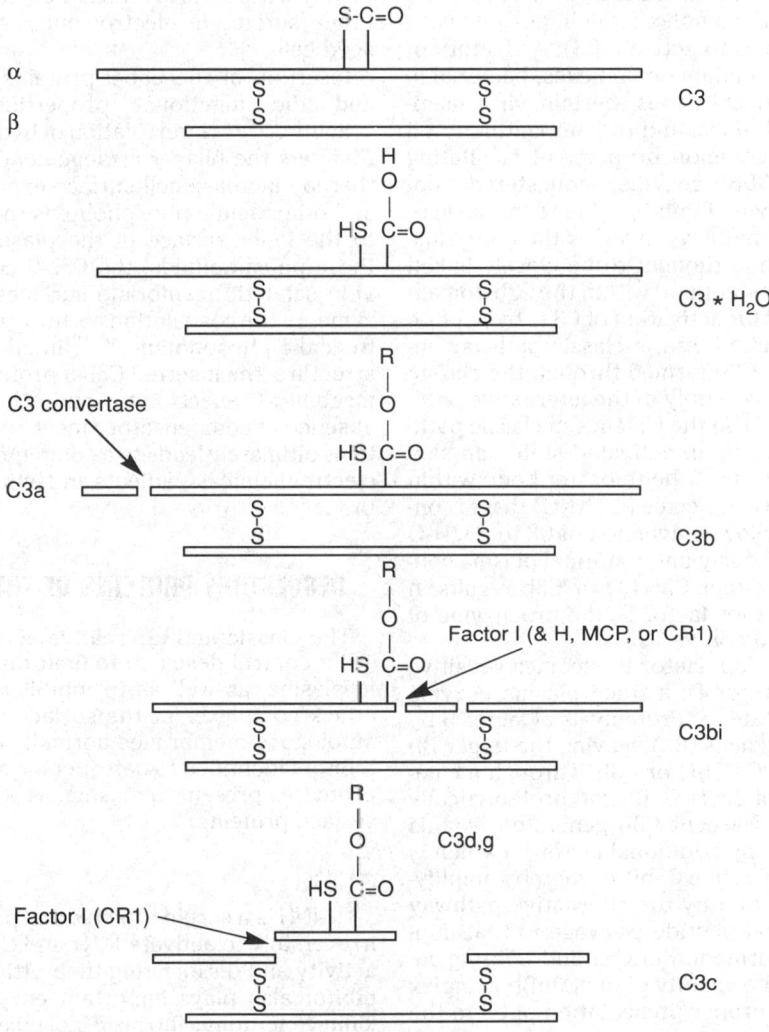

Fig. 12-2. Schematic diagram of the proteolytic processing of C3 through enzyme reactions of the complement system. Native C3 lacks biologic activity. C3*H$_2$O is a "C3b-like" molecule that is generated by spontaneous hydrolysis of the internal thiol ester bond of the C3 α-chain. C3-to-C3b conversion is mediated by either classic or alternative pathway C3-convertase through proteolytic cleavage between amino acid residues 77 and 78 of the C3 α-chain. In addition to generating C3b, this proteolysis liberates the peptide anaphylatoxin C3a. The formation of C3b exposes the carbonyl of the α-chain thiol ester, which freely reacts either with H$_2$O or with residues on the target surface to attach C3b covalently. Inactivation of C3b is initiated by the protease factor I, which cleaves a 3-kd fragment from the C3b α-chain to generate iC3b. Proteolysis by factor I requires binding of C3b either plasma component factor H or to the membrane receptors CR1 or MCP. Further proteolysis by factor I liberates the larger fragment C3c, leaving C3dg (43 kd) covalently bound to the target surface via the carbonyl of the internal thioester. Disulfide bonds linking C3 α- and β-chains are represented by dotted lines. See text for details. R, residue; S–S, disulfide bonds.

Proteolytic cleavage of C5 liberates the chemotactic peptide C5a, leaving the C5b portion of the molecule weakly attached to C3b.[27] Interaction of C5b with C6 initiates assembly of the membrane attack complex, composed of components C5b, C6, C7, C8, and C9. The resulting C5b-9 complex has the potential to insert into lipid bilayers and to initiate plasma membrane damage (see below).

Alternative Pathway

In contrast with the sequentially ordered enzyme cascade of the classic pathway, the alternative pathway entails a positive feedback interaction in which the principal activation product (C3b) serves as the cofactor of the C3-cleaving enzyme complex (C3bBb) that is responsible for its own production[6,31,32] (Fig. 12-1). This system is therefore continuously primed for explosive C3 activation, the rate of C3 activation governed by the stability of the C3bBb enzyme complex (which, analogous to the C4b2a complex, also serves to activate C5). Activators of this pathway—which include immune complexes, bacterial lipopolysaccharides and yeast cell walls, certain viral membranes and virus-infected cell lines, and the autoantibody C3 nephritic factor—share the common property of facilitating stability of the assembled C3bBb enzyme, sequestered from the regulatory control of enzyme inhibitors found in plasma.

Initiation of the alternative pathway involves the conformational activation of C3, which is thought to be closely linked to rupture of the internal thioester bond within the C3b domain of the protein.[33] One pathway for activation of C3 is by peptide cleavage to C3b (e.g., as initiated by the classic pathway enzyme C4b2a). In this manner, C3b formed through the classic pathway can directly initiate assembly of the alternative pathway enzyme complex (Fig. 12-1). In the absence of classic pathway activation, C3 conversion to an activated state can also occur by spontaneous hydrolysis of the thioester bond within the intact protein, resulting in a molecule ($C3*H_2O$) that is conformationally similar to C3b. Slow conversion of C3 to $C3*H_2O$ is believed to proceed continuously under normal plasma conditions. Conversion of C3 to either $C3*H_2O$ or C3b results in expression of a binding a site for factor B, the proenzyme of the alternative pathway C3/C5 convertase.

When bound to $C3*H_2O$ or C3b, factor B becomes sensitive to proteolytic cleavage by factor D, a trace plasma enzyme normally found in its active state.[6,34] Proteolysis of factor B by factor D liberates a 30-kd fragment (Ba), leaving the larger Bb fragment (80 kd) attached to $C3*H_2O$ or C3b. Through a catalytic site in Bb, the complex of $C3*H_2O$, Bb can proteolytically convert C3 to C3a and C3b. Nascent C3b generated by this mechanism is capable of binding additional factor B (which is then converted by factor D to active C3bBb), thereby amplifying the reaction. Activation of C5 by the alternative pathway convertase occurs by identical peptide cleavage to that initiated by C4b2a, resulting in formation of C5a and C5b. Again, C3b covalently deposited in the vicinity of the C3bBb complex is thought to be required for proper presentation of C5 to the catalytic site of the enzyme.[35]

Assembly of the Membrane Attack Complex

Membrane damage by the complement system is initiated through the interaction of C5b (generated by either the classic pathway or alternative pathway C3/C5-convertase) with plasma proteins C6, C7, C8, and C9.[1,36–39] C5 shares homology with C3 and C4, but does not contain the internal thioester bond that is found in those proteins. C6, C7, C8, and C9 share structural motifs that are also found in the cytolytic polypeptide, perforin, a membrane pore-forming protein contained in

the intracellular dense granules of cytotoxic lymphocytes. The first step in assembly of the C5b-9 complex is the formation of a complex between C5b and C6, through a short-lived interactional site that is expressed by nascent C5b.[40] Association of C6 with C5b is thought to occur while C5b remains in contact with membrane-bound C3b. On reaction of C7 with the C5b6 complex, a membrane interactional site is transiently expressed (primarily by the C7 subunit), enabling the C5b67 complex to deposit directly onto membrane surfaces.[41] Once bound to a membrane surface, the C5b67 complex expresses a stable binding site for a single molecule of C8. Association of C8 with the complex results in insertion of a portion of the molecule into the hydrophobic core of the membrane and expression of a binding site for C9.[42] The interaction of C9 with membrane-bound C5b-8, results in its elongation and insertion into the membrane interior, concomitant with a polymerization of multiple C9 into a large torus-ringed tubular structure. This tubule of polymerized C9 is readily detected projecting from the membrane surface in electron micrographs of complement-damaged cells.[43,44]

Insertion of the C5b-9 proteins affects both the structural and the functional properties of the plasma membrane.[36,38,45–47] Intercalation of hydrophobic domains of C8 and C9 alters the bilayer arrangement of membrane lipid and can thereby increase cell surface exposure of phosphatidylserine and other acidic phospholipids that are normally sequestered to the inner surface of the plasma membrane. By exposing these phospholipids, the C5b-9 complex can potentially provide catalytic membrane surfaces for assembly of those enzymes of the coagulation pathway that are stabilized by binding to acidic phospholipid.[48–50] In addition to altering membrane structure, the inserted C5b-9 proteins increase membrane permeability to electrolytes and other small molecules.[51] In the absence of compensatory mechanisms, insertion of these proteins ultimately leads to a complete collapse of transmembrane electrochemical gradients and lytic rupture of the plasma membrane.

REGULATORY PROTEINS OF THE COMPLEMENT SYSTEM

The classic and alternative activation pathways are under strict control designed to limit dissemination of the reactions in plasma, as well as to inhibit activation of the membrane attack complexes at the surface of blood cells and on other autologous membranes normally exposed to complement. Inhibitors identified to date include specific binding proteins and proteases present in plasma, as well as several important cell surface proteins.

C1-INH

C1-INH is a serpin-type (serine protease) inhibitor that binds irreversibly to activated C1r and C1s, blocking their enzymatic activity and dissociating their attachment to C1q.[52–55] This inhibitor also plays important enzyme regulatory roles in the kinin-generating, intrinsic coagulation, and fibrinolytic pathways through interaction with plasmin, kallikrein, and factors XIa and XIIa.[6,56] Inherited deficiency of C1-INH underlies the syndrome of hereditary angioedema.[55] Antibodies to C1-INH have been observed in certain lymphoproliferative disorders and can give rise to an acquired syndrome of angioedema that is analogous to hereditary angioedema seen in C1-INH-deficient patients.

Carboxypeptidase N

The biologic activity of C3a, C4a, and C5a is regulated by carboxypeptidase N, a plasma enzyme that rapidly removes the C-terminal arginine residue from each of these anaphylatoxins.[24,57] In the case of C3a, removal of this amino acid abolishes its biologic activity. By contrast, carboxypeptidase N-treated C5a (designated C5a$_{des-arg}$) retains about 5–10% of its chemotactic and neutrophil-stimulating activity (see below).[58]

C3b/C4b-Binding Proteins

The C3b/C4b-binding proteins serve to bind C3b or C4b and to regulate assembly of the C3/C5-convertases. Additionally, several of these proteins serve as physiologically important plasma membrane receptors (Tables 12-1 and 12-2). The genes for factor H, C4b-bp, DAF, MCP, CR1, and CR2 are all localized to the long arm of chromosome 1 and comprise a family of closely related genes, designated RCA.[9,10] These proteins share a common globular structure consisting of homologous cysteine-rich repeating units (or SCRs), each of approximately 60 amino acids. This characteristic structure is also found in enzymes that interact with C3 or C4, including C1s, C2, and factor B, as well as in a number of unrelated proteins.

Factor H

Factor H is a plasma protein composed of 20 SCRs that binds C3b and serves to inhibit association of either C3b or C3*H$_2$O with factor B (restricting assembly of the C3bB proenzyme).[56,59,60] Additionally, factor H promotes the dissociation of the assembled C3bBb enzyme complexes and serves as a cofactor for proteolytic degradation of C3b by factor I.[61] Limited intrachain proteolysis by factor I initially converts C3b to inactivated C3b (iC3b), which remains covalently bound to its original acceptor surface (Fig. 12-2). Subsequent degradation of the iC3b α-chain by factor I releases the large C3c fragment (150 kd), leaving C3dg (41 kd) attached to the acceptor surface through the C3d domain of the fragment.[62] Bound C3dg is normally the final C3b degradation product remaining on circulating cells in vivo.[63] By contrast to factor H (which promotes dissociation of the C3bBb), another regulatory protein found in plasma, factor P (properdin), acts to stabilize the alternative pathway enzyme complex.[64]

C4b-Binding Protein

C4b-bp is an acute-phase reactant plasma protein that binds to C4b, serving both to block its association with C2 and to accelerate dissociation of the assembled C4b2a enzyme complex.[65] C4b-bp also serves as a cofactor to facilitate proteolytic degradation of C4b by the serine protease factor I, which splits the larger C4c fragment from the molecule, leaving C4d bound to the original acceptor surface.[66] Approximately 50% of C4b-bp normally circulates in plasma as a complex with protein S, a vitamin K-dependent protein with regulatory function in the coagulation system.[67,68] C4b-bp is composed of seven α-chains, each with eight SCRs containing the binding site for C4b, and a single β-chain with three SCRs that form the binding site for protein S.[69]

Regulation at Cell Surfaces

Surfaces that promote activation of the alternative pathway are distinguished by their capacity to stabilize the C3bBb enzyme complex, away from regulatory control by factor H in plasma, whereas nonactivating surfaces facilitate factor H binding to C3b. Although the precise chemical and physical properties that distinguish complement-activating from nonactivating surfaces remain to be elucidated, it appears that the total content and chemical modification of cell-surface sialic acid residues can be a determining factor.[70,71] The inhibitory activity of factor H is increased when C3b is bound to a surface containing polyanions such as sialic acid, reflecting an increase in the apparent affinity of factor H for C3b under these conditions.[72,73] Consistent with these data, a specific polyanion binding site in factor H has been localized to the 13th SCR domain of the protein.[74] In addition to the nature of the glycosidic residues presented by the cell surface, the propensity for complement activation is governed by the expression of specific membrane proteins that exhibit avidity for C3b and C4b and that exert complement regulatory function through their interaction with these membrane-bound components of the C3/C5-convertases.[10,75–77]

Decay Accelerating Factor

DAF (CD55) is a 70-kd single-chain glycoprotein normally expressed on the surface of red cells, platelets, leukocytes, endothelium, and other cells that serves to accelerate the dissociation of the subunits of the membrane-assembled C4b2a and C3bBb enzyme complexes.[75,78,79] DAF does not function as a cofactor for the inactivation of C4b or C3b by factor I.[80] The protein is composed of four SCRs, three of which are essential for its function.[81] In addition to containing the SCR motif, DAF belongs to a class of membrane proteins (e.g., erythrocyte acetylcholinesterase, lymphocyte LFA-1, leukocyte 5′-ectonucleotidase, leukocyte Fcγ III receptors, neutrophil alkaline phosphatase, and complement regulatory protein CD59; see below) that are attached to the cell surface by glycosidic linkage to the membrane lipid phosphatidylinositol.[76,82–84]

Membrane Cofactor Protein

MCP (CD46) is a 45–70-kd glycoprotein distributed on all human leukocytes and platelets but absent on erythrocytes.[10,85] This protein contains four SCRs that function in binding C3b, C4b, and iC3b.[86] Additionally, MCP exhibits potent cofactor activity for factor I-mediated proteolysis of C3b and C4b. DAF and MCP act in concert on the membrane surface and are complementary in their activity; DAF exhibits only decay accelerating activity but no cofactor activity for factor I, while MCP serves as cofactor for factor I but does not promote decay of the C3-convertase enzymes. CR1 (CD35), the principal cellular receptor for C3b, also serves as an important cofactor for proteolysis of C3b and C4b by factor I. By contrast to MCP, CR1 also exhibits "DAF-like" function and contributes to the decay of the C3-convertases.[78,87–89]

Inhibitors of the Membrane Attack Complex

Formation of C5b on human blood cells is regulated through control of the C3/C5-convertases, exerted by DAF and other inhibitors. Furthermore, the C6 binding site that is exposed when C5 is activated to C5b is highly unstable, limiting the rate of formation of C5b6. Once formed, diffusion of the C5b67 complex to "innocent" bystander cells is limited by the very short lifetime of the membrane-interactional site exposed in this complex.[1,41] Membrane damage to autologous cells exposed to activated complement is also restricted by certain inhibitory proteins in plasma and on cell surfaces.

Vitronectin (S Protein) and Clusterin

The diffusion of functional C5b-9 complexes from the initial target of complement activation to other cells is restricted by several "scavenger" proteins in plasma that bind newly formed C5b67, preventing its dissemination to other cells. Proteins with this property include vitronectin (also referred to as S protein), as well as certain serum lipoproteins, including clusterin (SP40,40).[90–95] On binding one molecule each of C8 and C9, the vitronectin/C5b-9 complex (SC5b-9) circulates inactive in plasma until cleared, providing a serologic marker of intravascular complement activation that has proceeded to assembly of the C5b-9 complex. Vitronectin also contains the RGD (Arg-Gly-Asp) peptide sequence found in fibrinogen, fibronectin, and other integrin-binding proteins, which provides a mechanism for interaction of SC5b-9 complexes with plasma membrane integrin receptors on a variety of cells.[92,95]

CD59 (HRF20) and Other Homologous Complement Restriction Factors

In addition to the protection afforded by vitronectin and other C5b-9 scavenger proteins in plasma, human blood cells, vascular endothelial cells, and many other tissues are also protected from lytic damage by human complement due to the cell-surface expression of a protein(s) that specifically serves to inhibit intercalation of C9 into the plasma membrane.[96-103] This cell-surface inhibitor of the membrane attack complex appears to recognize specific domains contained within the human C8 α-chain and human C9 involved in the transformation of C9 from its globular conformation in plasma to a membrane-embedded homopolymer displaying cytolytic activity.[101-103] Proteins with this function have been designated homologous restriction factors because of their apparent specificity for human C8 and C9, as opposed to these same complement proteins derived from the serum of other species. The best characterized human complement homologous restriction factor, designated CD59 (HRF20) is an 18–22-kd cell-surface glycoprotein first isolated from the erythrocyte membrane.[99,100,104-106] Like DAF, CD59 is tethered to the cell surface by glycosidic linkage to membrane phosphatidylinositol.[107] Deletion of CD59 from the surface of erythrocytes and other blood cells can occur as the consequence of the glycosylphosphatidylinosital (GPI)-anchoring defect that underlies paroxysmal nocturnal hemoglobinuria (PNH), which accounts for the unusual sensitivity of the defective blood cells that arise in this disorder to lysis by the C5b-9 proteins (see Ch. 25). A 64-kd human erythrocyte membrane protein (commonly referred to as HRF or C8-binding protein) has been reported to exhibit many of the complement-inhibitory properties that are now recognized to reside in CD59.[96,108,109]

In addition to the complement-inhibitory function exhibited by CD59, recent evidence shows that this membrane protein participates in rosette formation between human erythrocytes and T lymphocytes, and also augments T-cell activation by antigen-presenting cells, activities that appear to be mediated through the capacity of CD59 to bind to CD2 on T lymphocytes.[99,110-113] In this context, it should also be noted that antibodies against CD59 (as well as several other GPI-anchored plasma membrane proteins) have been reported to elicit cell-stimulatory responses which may be related to activation of intracellular tyrosine kinases.[114,115]

CELLULAR RESPONSES MEDIATED BY COMPLEMENT RECEPTORS

Activated components of the complement system contribute to virtually every aspect of inflammatory response, including increased vascular permeability, leukocyte chemotaxis, leukocyte activation, immune adherence and phagocytosis, solubilization and clearance of immune complexes, and regulation of the lymphocytic immune response.[1-4] These proteins also play a direct role in mediating cell lysis, through both intravascular and extravascular mechanisms. In addition to their role in host defense and inflammation, evidence shows that complement proteins can also interact with components of the coagulation, fibrinolytic, and kinin systems to alter vascular hemostatic mechanisms.[6,116] In general, the biologic effects of complement

are initiated through binding of activated components to specific complement receptors distributed on the surface of various blood and vascular cells. This binding interaction can serve to remove immune complexes and other complement-coated particles from plasma, through direct adherence to circulating blood cells. In many cases, binding of a complement protein to its cell-surface receptor elicits specific cellular responses, evoked by receptor-coupled signaling across the plasma membrane. By contrast, the biologic activity of the C5b-9 complex appears to arise directly through a C5b-9-induced change in the structural and functional properties of the plasma membrane itself and does not require receptor-coupled signaling mechanisms.

C1qRs, receptors for the C1q subunit of C1, have been described for neutrophils, monocytes, endothelial cells, platelets, and certain lymphocytes.[117-120] Aggregates of C1q have also been shown to elicit oxidative bursts in neutrophils and to potentiate antibody-dependent cellular killing by peripheral blood lymphocytes through binding to C1qR. These interactions potentially contribute to the inflammatory responses elicited by C1q-containing immune complexes.

Anaphylatoxin Receptors

The N-terminal peptide fragments released from the α-chains of C3, C4, and C5 during complement activation exhibit a spectrum of biologic effects, collectively referred to as anaphylatoxin activity. These three peptides share considerable structural and functional homology.

C3a/C4a Receptor

C3a causes increased vascular permeability and stimulates the degranulation of mast cells and basophils, resulting in the release of histamine and other vasoactive compounds.[57,58] Many of the biologic effects of C3a are also shared by C4a, which appears to interact with the same cellular receptors as C3a.[58] The sensitivity of the cellular C3a response to inhibition by pertussis toxin suggests that the C3a/C4a receptor is coupled to a cellular G protein, as has now been established for the C5a receptor (below).[121]

C5a Receptor

C5a interacts with cell-surface receptors that are specific for C5a (and distinct from the C3a/C4a receptors) to stimulate degranulation of mast cells and basophils.[58,122,123] C5a also plays a major role in the recruitment and activation of human neutrophils and macrophages at sites of complement activation. C3a and C5a receptors can undergo internalization after stimulation, resulting in a desensitization of the cells to further stimulation.[121,124] The C5a receptor has recently been isolated and the protein sequence deduced from cDNA cloning. The receptor is a 42-kd polypeptide that purifies as a complex with the subunits of the GTP-binding protein, Gi.[125] The deduced amino acid sequence of the C5a receptor shows homology with the leukocyte N-formyl peptide receptor, and confirms a G protein-binding motif within the cytoplasmic domain of the polypeptide.[123] The gene for the C5a receptor is also closely linked to the formyl peptide receptor genes on chromosome 19.[126]

Through activation of it cellular receptors, C5a initiates several important inflammatory responses. First, C5a serves as a potent chemotactic agent for human neutrophil and mononuclear phagocyte migration. Stimulation by C5a has been shown to increase neutrophil adhesiveness and to initiate neutrophil aggregation. C5a also elicits oxidative metabolism and the secretory release of lysosomal enzymes from neutrophils and a variety of phagocytic cells. These proinflammatory changes in C5a-stimulated neutrophils are accompanied by increased surface expression and activity of both CR1 (CD35) and CR3 (CD11b/CD18), promoting leukocyte adhesion as well as phagocytosis of opsonized particles.[123,127] The physiologic significance of these responses is suggested by animal studies in which direct intravascular complement activation has been shown to result in transient neutropenia, leukocyte aggregation, and leukostatic vascular plugging.[128] Recent evidence also suggests that inflammatory and immunoregulatory responses to C5a may be mediated through induction of interleukin-6 (IL-6) synthesis by human monocytes.[129,130] The potent chemotactic and leukocyte-activating properties of C5a (and C5a$_{des-arg}$) suggest an important role in the vascular response to complement activation in humans. In particular, these peptides have been implicated as mediators of the neutropenia associated with hemodialysis and cardiopulmonary bypass and may give rise to the pulmonary leukostasis associated with adult respiratory distress syndrome and acute transfusion reactions.[131,132] The role of C5a in the pathogenesis of endotoxic shock syndrome is suggested by studies in primates, in which blocking antibodies against C5a have been shown to attenuate respiratory distress and enhance survival after gram-negative bacteremia.[128]

Cellular Responses Mediated by C3b Receptors

Cellular receptors that bind C3b and C4b play an important role in the inactivation of these proteins by providing cofactor function for the serum protease, factor I. By contributing to the degradation of C3b deposited onto the plasma membrane, these receptors serve to limit the accumulation of C3b on circulating blood cells and restrict dissemination of the C3/C5-convertase reaction. In addition to this function, it is now recognized that these cellular receptors for C3b (and its degradation products) play a central role in mediating cellular adherence and ultimate clearance of immune complexes and other C3b-coated particles and cells.[133–135]

The cellular distribution and ligand specificities of the various C3 receptors are summarized in Table 12-2. Although it is distributed in the plasma membrane of nearly all blood cells, the preponderance of CR1 found in the blood of humans and other primates is expressed on the surface of erythrocytes. In humans, the clearance of immune complexes from the circulation is mediated principally by an initial adsorption to red cells, which is mediated via interaction of multiple C3b and/or C4b incorporated into the immune complex with erythrocyte CR1 receptors.[135,136] After adsorption to the erythrocyte surface, proteolytic processing of C3b provides a mechanism for transfer of the bound immune complex to cells of the reticuloendothelial system: on conversion of C3b to iC3b and C3dg (by factor I), the reduced affinity of these degraded C3b fragments for CR1 promotes release of the immune complex from the erythrocyte surface (which contains only the CR1 receptor), followed by endocytic uptake of the complexes by phagocytic cells that express CR3 and CR4. Studies with radiolabeled C3b-coated immune complexes suggest that these immune complexes are stripped from the erythrocyte surface during passage through the liver and, to a lesser extent, the spleen. These data implicate hepatic Kupffer cells as the principal scavenger of C3b-containing immune complexes initially transported by red cells.[137]

In addition to serving as receptors for cellular adherence to immune complexes (and other C3-containing particles), these complement receptors are also known to provide stimulatory signals for leukocyte activation.[133,138] Binding of C3b aggregates to leukocyte membrane CR1, either alone or in concert with IgG occupancy of cell surface Fc receptors, is known to trigger an endocytic response from neutrophils and mononuclear phagocytes accompanied by enzyme secretion and a re-

spiratory burst. The capacity of iC3b-coated particles to trigger similar responses from neutrophils and monocytes suggests a similar role for CR3 and CR4. The distribution of CR1 (the C3b receptor) and CR2 (the C3dg receptor) on B lymphocytes suggests possible roles for these receptors in modulating immune responses. For example, interaction of CR1 and CR2, with their respective ligands, has been shown to promote B-lymphocyte proliferation and differentiation into memory B cells, although the physiologic significance of these responses remains to be clarified.[139] Aggregated C3-split products have also been reported to augment the response of IL-2-treated helper T lymphocytes, suggesting a co-stimulatory function.[139,140] Decreased numbers of erythrocyte CR1 receptors have been documented in patients with systemic lupus erythematosus (SLE), acquired immunodeficiency syndrome (AIDS), and lepromatous leprosy, diseases that are also associated with increased levels of circulating immune complexes, reflecting polyclonal B-cell activation. CR2 has been identified as the B-lymphocyte receptor for the Epstein-Barr virus (EBV), implicating this receptor in the pathogenesis of infectious mononucleosis and Burkitt lymphoma.[141,142] Finally, CR3 distributed on natural killer lymphocytes has been implicated in promoting adhesion and enhancing the cytotoxic response to target cells bearing surface iC3b.[143,144]

CR1

CR1 (CD35), the principal cellular receptor for C3b, is a single-chain membrane glycoprotein that is distributed on erythrocytes, neutrophils, eosinophils, monocytes, B lymphocytes, subsets of T lymphocytes, macrophages, follicular dendritic cells, and glomerular podocytes.[133,134] CR1 is not found on human platelets. Four different allotypes exist, and the cellular concentration of this receptor also exhibits genetic polymorphism.[135,145–149] The primary role of CR1 is to mediate binding of particles opsonized with C3b or iC3b to neutrophils and monocytes that express this receptor for subsequent phagocytosis. In addition to this contribution to immune adherence and clearance, CR1 contributes to the regulation of complement by acting as cofactor for the proteolytic degradation of both C3b and C4b by factor I and by accelerating decay of the C3-convertases.[78,87–89] CR1 contains 30 SCRs. The binding site for C3b has been localized to SCR 15–18, while SCR 1–4 contain the C4b binding site.[150,151]

CR2

CR2 (CD21), is a 145-kd glycoprotein found primarily on B lymphocytes, T lymphocytes, and follicular dendritic cells, but not on phagocytic cell types. This protein functions as a receptor for C3d, C3dg, and iC3b, and is the plasma membrane receptor of EBV.[134,141,152,153] CR2 contains 15 SCRs. The binding sites for both EBV and C3dg have been mapped to a common domain on CR2, which includes the first two SCRs.[142,154] CR2 on follicular dendritic cells binds C3d- or C3dg-bearing immune complexes. On B lymphocytes, stimulation through CR2 is thought to play a role in proliferation and differentiation. Recent evidence implicates CR2 in the infection of B lymphocytes by human immunodeficiency virus (HIV-1)[155,156] (see below).

CR3 and CR4

CR3 (CD11b/CD18) and CR4 (CD11c/CD18) belong to the Leu-CAM family of leukocyte adhesion molecules, which also includes LFA-1 (CD11a/CD18). They constitute the β_2-subfamily of membrane integrin receptors, two-chain glycoproteins composed of a common β-chain (CD18 antigen) and a noncovalently associated α-subunit.[17,157,158] These receptors do not contain the SCR motif that is common to CR1, CR2, and other C3b-binding proteins. Of note, "CR4" had originally designated another C3 receptor (the platelet C3dg receptor), unrelated to CD11c/CD18.[159] CR3 and CR4 are cellular receptors for iC3b, distributed on neutrophils, monocytes, and other mononuclear phagocytes, and natural killer lymphocytes. They are not found on B lymphocytes, glomerular podocytes, or erythrocytes. CR3 participates in immune adherence and phagocytosis by promoting adhesion of granulocytes and monocytes to iC3b-coated cells and particles and plays a role in lymphocyte-mediated antibody-dependent cellular toxicity.[158,160] CR4 shares these functions and has been implicated in the granulocyte-mediated lysis of erythrocytes.[160] Expression of the receptor function of these proteins requires cell activation, which entails both redistribution to the cell surface and increased affinity for their ligand, possibly through phosphorylation of cytoplasmic domains of the CD18 subunits.[161] Congenital deficiency of these receptors gives rise to the disorder leukocyte adhesion deficiency (LAD), which is associated with defective chemotaxis, reduced adhesion with impaired transmigration across endothelium, and impaired cell-mediated killing of microbial pathogens.[158,162–164]

Cellular Responses to the C5b-9 Complex

The cytolytic activity of the complement system resides in the capacity of the C5b-9 proteins to insert into phospholipid bilayers, thereby increasing membrane permeability to aqueous solute. This membrane permeability-inducing function of the C5b-9 complex can be observed for a variety of cellular and synthetic lipid membranes, suggesting that it is directly mediated through interaction of these proteins with the lipid bilayer and does not require binding to specific receptors on the surface of the target cell. The affinity of activated C5b-9 for phospholipid bilayers confers a capacity to interact with the membrane envelope of virtually every biologic cell, a feature that at least in principal enables the complement system to defend against a limitless variety of potential pathogens.

Although the cytolytic function of these proteins is consistent with their role in immunologic defense and is a prominent feature of their interaction with nonhuman cells, accumulating evidence suggests that some of the biologic manifestations of complement activation relate to the capacity of the assembled C5b-9 proteins to evoke specific cellular responses, without lytic consequence for the target cell.[36,45,47,165] It is now recognized that specific inhibitors of this protein complex are expressed on the surface of human blood cells and vascular endothelium. By limiting the extent of activation and membrane insertion of C9, the cytolytic activity of the complement system is markedly attenuated on these cell membranes. In addition to protecting these cells from lysis during intravascular complement activation, the resistance to complement-mediated cytolysis conferred by these plasma membrane inhibitors may have other biologic consequences. For example, the insertion of the C5b-9 proteins into the plasma membrane of human platelets, neutrophils, cultured vascular endothelium, and numerous other cells has been shown to elicit activation-related responses, indicating that these proteins trigger stimulatory intracellular metabolic pathways without lytic breakdown of the plasma membrane. Among the cellular changes reported to result from sublytic plasma membrane damage by C5b-9 proteins include initiation of arachidonate metabolism leading to the biosynthesis of various active prostanoids, activation of intracellular C kinases, induction of shape change, secretory exocytosis of the contents of intracellular storage granules, an oxidative burst, induction of mitogenic responses, expression of receptor sites for serum lipoproteins, vesiculation of cell-surface components from the plasma membrane, and the induction of a transbilayer migration of plasma membrane phospholipids with exposure of membrane-binding sites for coagu-

lation factors and other plasma proteins that exhibit affinity for anionic phospholipid surfaces.[166–173] The cellular changes initiated by the C5b-9 proteins generally show a dependence on the level of extracellular calcium, suggesting that the stimulatory effects observed reflect increased cytoplasmic $[Ca^{2+}]$, that arises by influx of this ion across the complement pore formed in the plasma membrane.[51]

COMPLEMENT IN DISEASE

Genetic Polymorphism and Deficiency States

Insight into the functional importance of individual complement components in humans has been provided by study of complement deficiency states. Additionally, genetic polymorphisms of many of the complement proteins have now been identified. In several cases, these have proved of serologic and immunohematologic interest and have also provided clues to specific protein structure/function relationships. cDNA and genomic clones for most of the complement proteins and receptors have been isolated and the chromosomal location of the genes identified (Table 12-3). The discussion below is limited to selected examples of complement deficiency states and allelic variants that are of particular hematologic interest. For extensive review of the structure and regulation of the complement genes and of the known complement deficiency states, the reader is referred to several excellent reviews.[174–176]

C1-INH Deficiency

Inherited deficiency of C1-INH underlies the syndrome of hereditary angioedema. The gene for this serpin protease inhibitor is localized to p11.2-q.13 of chromosome 11. Deficiency states can arise through subnormal production of functional C1-INH, or by production of dysfunctional protein.[55]

Class III Genes and C4 Polymorphism

The genes for C4, C2, and factor B form a tight cluster (with the gene for enzyme 21-hydroxylase) in the MHC on the short arm of chromosome 6, a region designated MHC class III.[177] Class III lies between the class I and II genes of the HLA system. C2 deficiency is commonly associated with SLE and is one of the most common complement deficiency states. Deficiency of factor B has not been described, which may reflect a requirement of this primary C3 activator for survival. Polymorphisms of factor B, C2, and C4 have each been described. Of greatest immunohematologic interest is the polymorphism of C4, in which two isotypes (C4A and C4B) with distinct functional and serologic properties have been characterized.[25] The functional distinction between C4A and C4B isotypes relates to the type of bond that is preferentially formed by the internal α-chain thioester group: the C4A isotype preferentially transacylates onto amino group nucleophiles, while the C4B isotype reacts with equal efficiency toward amino or hydroxyl groups. The C4B variants show greater hemolytic activity due to increased binding to the red cell surface, whereas the C4A variant binds more efficiently to C1-containing immune aggregates, which serves to inhibit immune precipitation of these complexes.[178] The haplotype C4AQ0 is linked to SLE and other autoimmune disease, which may reflect this differential processing of immune complexes. At a serologic level, the C4A and C4B isotypes give rise to the Rodgers (Rg) and Chido (Ch) immune serotypes detected in red cell cross-matching. These antisera detect the antigenic differences of the erythrocyte-bound C4d fragment that originate from the C4A and C4B isotypes; that is, C4A-coated red cells type Rg+, Ch−, while C4B-coated cells type Rg−, Ch+. For each, numerous allotypic and isotypic variants have

Table 12-3. Complement Components: Gene Location and Deficiency States

Component	Chromosomal Gene Location	Disease Associated with Deficiency
Components of Activation Pathways		
C1q	1	SLE; pyogenic infection; glomerulonephritis
C1r/C1s	12	SLE; infection; nephritis
C4	6 (MHC class III)	SLE; infection; immune complex disease
C2	6 (MHC class III)	SLE; infection; nephritis
C3	19	SLE; infection; nephritis
Factor B	6 (MHC class III)	
Factor D	X?	Neisserial infection
Factor I	4	Pyogenic infection
Components of Membrane Attack Complex		
C5	9	Neisserial infection; SLE
C6/C7	5	Neisserial infection; SLE, Sjögren
C8	α and β: 1; γ: 9	Neisserial infection
C9	5	Neisserial infection; also asymptomatic
Plasma Regulatory Proteins		
C1-INH	11	Hereditary angioedema
Properdin	X	Neisserial infection; other pyogenic infection
C4b-bp	1 (RCA gene cluster)	
Factor H	1 (RCA gene cluster)	Infection; hemolytic uremic syndrome; glomerulonephritis
Vitronectin (S protein)	17	
Membrane Regulatory Proteins		
DAF (CD55)	1 (RCA cluster)	No symptoms with isolated deficiency (Inab phenotype)[a]
MCP (CD46)	1 (RCA cluster)	
HRF-20 (CD59)	11	PNH-like symptoms with isolated deficiency[a]
Membrane Receptors		
CR1 (CD35)	1 (RCA cluster)	SLE
CR2 (CD21)	1 (RCA cluster)	
CR3 (CD11b/CD18)	16	LAD
CR4 (CD11c/CD18)	21	LAD

[a] DAF and CD59 can be deleted due to GPI-anchoring defect, which is associated with PNH.

been identified, several of which have been characterized at the molecular level, permitting precise epitope mapping.[179]

Deficiencies of Plasma Membrane Complement Receptors and Regulatory Proteins

CR1

The gene for CR1 is located within the RCA group on the long arm of chromosome 1.[180] Four different allotypes (range 160–250 kd) have been identified, and numerical expression of erythrocyte CR1 is subject to considerable polymorphic variability. Additionally, evidence has been found for acquired reduction of CR1 due to proteolysis of the receptor in vivo. In several conditions associated with immune diseases, a reduction of erythrocyte CR1 is observed, and in certain cases, this has been shown to be accompanied by increased plasma levels of the receptor, implying removal from the membrane. Decreased cell-surface CR1 may in turn alter the capacity of these cells to subsequently bind immune complexes and impair processing of C3b by factor I.

CR3/CR4

Genetic deficiency of CR3 (CD11b/CD18), CR4 (CD11c/CD18), and LFA-1 (CD11a/CD18) gives rise to the LAD syndrome.[162,163] The genes coding for the α-chains of these receptors are each located on chromosome 16, while their common β-chain (CD18) is coded by a gene on chromosome 21. LAD is caused by defective β-chain synthesis, affecting cell-surface assembly of these three heterodimeric integrin receptors. Many of the clinical manifestations of LAD, including recurrent pyogenic infections and defective wound healing, can be related to dysfunction of the adhesive and opsonic functions of CR3 and CR4.

Decay Accelerating Factor

The gene for DAF is contained within the RCA group on chromosome 1.[9] Allotypic variants of DAF give rise to the blood group antigens contained in the Cromer blood group. Genetic deficiency of DAF is associated with the Inab erythrocyte phenotype.[181] These cells lack the common antigens of the Cromer blood group (see Ch. 131). This isolated deficiency of DAF is not associated with clinical disorder, suggesting that other complement regulatory proteins are sufficient to protect these cells.[75,181,182]

CD59

The gene for CD59 has been localized to the short arm of chromosome 11. Isolated genetic deficiency of CD59 has been described in a single individual, with evidence for autosomal recessive inheritance.[183] This patient was reported to suffer episodic intravascular hemolysis with a clinical course similar to that observed in PNH. As discussed in detail in Chapter 25, PNH is an acquired stem cell disorder in which somatic mutation in a hematopoietic progenitor cell gives rise to defective biosynthesis of the GPI anchor by which DAF, CD59, and several other cell-surface proteins are normally anchored to the plasma membrane. The blood cells produced in this disorder can have several different phenotypes, depending on the extent to which individual GPI-anchored proteins are missing from the cell surface. In many cases, the affected proteins can be detected in plasma and urine. The intravascular hemolysis characteristic of this disorder appears to be most directly attributable to those cohorts of erythrocytes that are missing CD59, and therefore cannot regulate the cytolytic activity of the C5b-9 complex.

Contribution of Complement to Accelerated Destruction of Blood Cells

The complement system is known to mediate the accelerated destruction of blood cells that can arise in several hematologic disorders (see detailed discussion in Chs. 25, 47 and 125).

Autoimmune Hemolytic Anemia

Antibody-initiated activation of the complement system can result in increased deposition of C3b, C4b, and potentially C5b-9 on the red cell surface. Most commonly, the shortened survival rate of these cells reflects accelerated hepatosplenic clearance, due to endocytic uptake initiated on interaction of red cell-associated IgG and C3b (or C4b) with Fcγ- and CR1 receptors on phagocytic mononuclear cells of the reticuloendothelial system.[184,185] The rate and organ site of red cell sequestration and removal appear to depend on whether endocytic recognition is principally mediated through Fc receptor interaction with IgG or through CR1 interaction with C3b and C4b. Sequestration of IgG-coated red cells (generally associated with warm-antibody hemolytic anemia) occurs primarily in the spleen rather than liver, except when there is a very high density of cell-surface IgG.[184] The ability of noncomplement-fixing IgG antibody (e.g., anti-Rh$_0$D) to shortened red cell survival suggests that in the case of IgG antibodies against red cell antigens, splenic sequestration and clearance can be directly initiated by Fcγ-receptors on phagocytic cells.[186] Studies in complement-deficient animals and humans nevertheless suggest that complement activation does serve to accelerate the rate of clearance of these IgG-coated cells and to shift the site of clearance to the liver. It has also been suggested that in the case of noncomplement-fixing IgG antibodies, the small amounts of C3b (or C3d or C3dg) and C4b (or C4d) normally found on the red cell surface may be sufficient to initiate endocytic clearance by splenic macrophages, when presented concurrently with IgG.

In the case of IgM antibodies against erythrocyte antigens (e.g., as found in chronic cold agglutinin disease) activation of the complement system appears to be required for red cell survival to be affected.[184,185,187] When complement activation does occur, most of the affected cells (bearing IgM and C3b or iC3b) are initially sequestered in the liver. The sequestration of these cells is presumably mediated by interaction of CR1 on hepatic Kupffer cells with red cell C3b and C4b (or iC3b). A portion of the sequestered red cells are subsequently returned to the circulation and remain coated with IgM and proteolytically degraded fragments of C3b (mainly C3dg).[188] Sequestered red cells that escape endocytic clearance and return to the circulation survive normally, reflecting the general absence of receptors for IgM on phagocytic cells and the specificity of CR1 receptors for intact C3b (Table 12-2).

In addition to mediating extravascular clearance, complement activation on the red cell surface can lead to intravascular hemolysis. Nevertheless, for both IgG- and IgM-mediated immune hemolytic anemias, clinically significant intravascular hemolysis is rarely observed, even when complement-fixing antibodies are documented. Exceptions include circumstances in which massive complement activation at the erythrocyte membrane occurs due to the nature of the antibody (e.g., alloimmune hemolysis of ABO-mismatched red cells, or for the antibody of paroxysmal cold hemoglobinuria) and in PNH, where a decrease in cell-surface CD59 compromises the normal regulatory control of the terminal complement proteins (see Ch. 25).

Neutropenia and Thrombocytopenia

The potential role of C5a (and C5a$_{des-arg}$) in the neutropenia and vascular leukostasis associated with cardiopulmonary bypass procedures, hemodialysis, and bacterial sepsis has been described. Additionally, evidence for accelerated clearance of neutrophils through IgG-plus-C3b-mediated hepatosplenic sequestration has been found in patients with Felty syndrome.[189] There are also data suggesting that complement activation contributes to shortened platelet survival in cases of immune thrombocytopenia and in circumstances of alloimmune platelet transfusion. In most instances, shortened platelet survival is thought to reflect hepatosplenic sequestration and removal through the reticuloendothelial system, and not intravascular platelet lysis per se. Since deposition of the C5b-9 proteins promotes exposure of membrane binding sites for coagulation factors responsible for thrombin formation, activation of these complement proteins may underlie the increased risk of thrombosis observed in PNH, immune thrombocytopenic purpura, and other immune and inflammatory states associated with intravascular complement activation.

Acquired Immunodeficiency Syndrome

Several reports suggest that interaction of HIV-1 with components of the complement system may contribute to the pathogenesis of AIDS. Activation of the classic pathway of complement by HIV-1 has been shown to occur through both antibody-dependent and antibody-independent mechanisms, including direct binding and activation of C1 by the GP41 viral glycoprotein.[190] Complement-dependent enhancement of HIV-1 infection of numerous lymphocytic cells has also been demonstrated in vitro, with viral entry facilitated through C3dg interaction with cell-surface CR2 (CD21), either alone or in concert with the attachment of HIV-1 glycoprotein GP120 to cell-surface CD4.[155,156,191] The possibility that complement contributes to the depletion of lymphocytes expressing HIV-1-derived surface antigens has also been suggested.[192] A decrease in the surface expression of CD59 has recently been described for T lymphocytes of HIV-infected individuals, raising the possibility of increased susceptibility of these cells to lysis by complement.[193] Whether complement activation in vivo exacerbates the cellular and clinical manifestations of AIDS remains to be clarified.[194-196]

Interactions Between Complement and Coagulation Systems

Interactions among certain components of the complement, kinin, coagulation, and fibrinolytic systems are known to occur, although their physiologic significance is poorly understood.[6,197] Complement activation has been shown to affect plasma clotting, clot retraction, and clot lysis.[6,197] Complement activation can also result in platelet activation and increased expression of platelet procoagulant activity.[116] In gram-negative bacteremia, episodes of disseminated intravascular coagulation can be temporarily associated with prominent intravascular complement activation; unregulated complement activation at the platelet surface has been implicated in the recurrent deep venous thrombosis that occurs in patients with PNH.[198] Nevertheless, the precise role of the complement system in the pathogenesis of these and other coagulopathies remains to be clarified.

FUTURE DIRECTIONS

Research conducted during the past decade has yielded dramatic new insight into the structural, functional, and genetic elements that comprise the complement system, and has provided new understanding of the molecular and cellular mechanisms by which complement contributes to human health and disease. Despite widespread appreciation of the role of activated complement in a variety of immune and inflammatory disorders, the development of therapeutic agents that can directly intercede to control the complement system remains a future challenge. Recent insight into the molecular specificity of the various regulatory elements that normally control production of the biologically active products of the complement reaction cascades, combined with knowledge of the structure and function of the complement receptors that mediate the myriad of cellular responses to activated complement, enable design of inhibitors that are targeted toward individual complement proteins or selected complement receptors. In this regard, the use of soluble recombinant CR1 to ameliorate complement-mediated inflammatory responses in vivo has recently been described.[199,200] Those complement-related disorders in which a single gene defect can be identified (e.g., PNH and LAD) also hold the future prospect for targeted gene therapy.

REFERENCES

1. Müller-Eberhard HJ: Molecular organization and function of the complement system. Annu Rev Biochem 57:321, 1988
2. Gaither TA, Frank MM: Complement. p. 830. In Henry JB (ed): Clinical Diagnosis and Management by Laboratory Methods. WB Saunders, Philadelphia, 1991
3. Davies KA: Complement. Baillieres Clin Haematol 4:927, 1991
4. Boackle R: The complement system. Immunol Ser 58:135, 1993
5. Sims PJ: Plasma proteins: complement p. 1582. In Hoffman R, Benz EJ, Shattil SJ et al (eds): Hematology: Basic Principles and Practice. 1st Ed. Churchill Livingstone, New York, 1990
6. Halkier T: Mechanisms in Blood Coagulation, Fibrinolysis and the Complement System. Cambridge University Press, Cambridge, 1991
7. Bentley DR: Structural superfamilies of the complement system. Exp Clin Immunogenet 5:69, 1988
8. Neurath H: Evolution of proteolytic enzymes. Science 224:350, 1984
9. Hourcade D, Holers VM, Atkinson JP: The regulators of complement activation (RCA) gene cluster. Adv Immunol 45:381, 1989
10. Liszewski MK, Post TW, Atkinson JP: Membrane cofactor protein (MCP or CD46): newest member of the regulators of complement activation gene cluster. Annu Rev Immunol 9:431, 1991
11. Haefliger JA, Tschopp J, Vial N, Jenne DE: Complete primary structure and functional characterization of the sixth component of the human complement system. Identification of the C5b-binding domain in complement C6. J Biol Chem 264:18041, 1989
12. Podack ER: Perforin: structure, function, and regulation. Curr Top Microbiol Immunol 178:175, 1992
13. Tack BF: The beta-Cys-gamma-Glu thiolester bond in human C3, C4, and alpha$_2$-macroglobulin. Springer Semin Immunopathol 6:259, 1983
14. Tack BF, Janatova J, Thomas ML et al: The third, fourth and fifth components of human complement: isolation and biochemical properties. Methods Enzymol 80:64, 1981
15. Malhotra R, Sim RB, Reid KB: Interaction of C1q, and other proteins containing collagen-like domains, with the C1q receptor. Biochem Soc Trans 18:1145, 1990
16. Ghebrehiwet B: Functions associated with the C1q receptor. Behring Inst Mitt 84:204, 1989
17. Springer TA, Miller LJ, Anderson DC: p150, 95, the third member of the Mac-1, LFA-1 human leukocyte adhesion glycoprotein family. J Immunol 136:240, 1986
18. Farries TC, Atkinson JP: Evolution of the complement system. Immunol Today 12:295, 1991
19. Sim RB, Reid KB: C1: molecular interactions with activating systems. Immunol Today 12:307, 1991
20. Borsos T, Rapp HJ: Complement fixation on cell surfaces by 19S and 7S antibodies. Science 150:505, 1965
21. Jiang H, Robey FA, Gewurz H: Localization of sites through which C-reactive protein binds and activates complement to residues 14–26 and 76–92 of the human C1q A chain. J Exp Med 175:1373, 1992
22. Matsushita M, Fujita T: Activation of the classical complement pathway by mannose-binding protein in association with a novel C1s-like serine protease. J Exp Med 176:1497, 1992
23. Reid KBM, Porter RR: The proteolytic activation systems of complement. Annu Rev Biochem 50:433, 1981
24. Hugli TE: Biochemistry and biology of anaphylatoxins. Complement 3:111, 1986
25. Campbell RD, Dunham I, Kendall E, Sargent CA: Polymorphism of the human complement component C4. Exp Clin Immunogenet 7:69, 1990
26. Isaac L, Isenman DE: Structural requirements for thioester bond formation in human complement component C3. Reassessment of the role of thioester bond integrity on the conformation of C3. J Biol Chem 267:10062, 1992
27. DiScipio RG, Smith CA, Müller-Eberhard HJ, Hugli TE: The activation of human complement component C5 by a fluid phase C5 convertase. J Biol Chem 258:10629, 1983
28. Kim YU, Carroll MC, Isenman DE et al: Covalent binding of C3b to C4b within the classical complement pathway C5 convertase. Determination of amino acid residues involved in ester linkage formation. J Biol Chem 267:4171, 1992
29. Isenman DE, Podak ER, Cooper NR: The interaction of C5 with C3b in free solution: a sufficient condition for cleavage by a fluid phase C3/C5 convertase. J Immunol 124:326, 1980
30. Vogt W, Schmidt G, Von Buttlar B, Dieminger L: A new function of the activated third component of complement: binding to C5, an essential step for C5 activation. Immunology 34:29, 1978
31. Pangburn MK, Müller-Eberhard HJ: The alternative pathway of complement. Springer Semin Immunopathol 7:163, 1984
32. Pangburn MK: Alternative pathway of complement. Methods Enzymol 162:639, 1988
33. Pangburn MK, Schreiber RD, Müller-Eberhard HJ: Formation of the initial C3 convertase of the alternative complement pathway: acquisition of C3b-like activities by spontaneous hydrolysis of the putative thioester in native C3. J Exp Med 154:856, 1981
34. Lesavre PH, Müller-Eberhard HJ: Mechanism of action of factor D of the alternative complement pathway. J Exp Med 148:1498, 1978
35. Daha MR, Fearon DT, Austen KF: C3 requirements for formation of alternative pathway C5 convertase. J Immunol 117:630, 1976
36. Esser AF: The membrane attack pathway of complement. Year Immunol 6:229, 1989
37. Esser AF, Sodetz JM: Membrane attack complex proteins C5b-6, C7, C8, and C9 of human complement. Methods Enzymol 162:551, 1988
38. Bhakdi S, Hugo F, Tranum-Jensen J: Functions and relevance of the terminal complement sequence. Blut 60:309, 1990
39. Peitsch MC, Tschopp J: Assembly of macromolecular pores by immune defense systems. Curr Opin Cell Biol 3:710, 1991
40. Goldman JM, Ruddy S, Austen KF: Reaction mechanism of nascent C5,6,7 (reactive lysis). I. Reaction characteristics of production of EC5,6,7 and lysis by C8 and C9. J Immunol 109:353, 1972
41. Podack ER, Biesecker G, Kolb WP, Müller-Eberhard HJ: The C5b-6 complex: reaction with C7, C8, C9. J Immunol 121:484, 1978
42. Sodetz JM: Structure and function of C8 in the membrane attack sequence of complement. Curr Top Microbiol Immunol 140:19, 1989
43. Tschopp J, Müller-Eberhard HJ, Podack ER: Formation of transmembrane tubules by spontaneous polymerization of the hydrophilic complement protein C9. Nature 298:534, 1982
44. Stanley KK: The molecular mechanism of complement C9 insertion and polymerisation in biological membranes. Curr Top Microbiol Immunol 140:49, 1989
45. Hänsch GM: The complement attack phase: control of lysis and non-lethal effects of C5b-9. Immunopharmacology 24:107, 1992
46. Lachmann PJ: Biological functions of the complement system. Biochem Soc Trans 18:1143, 1990
47. Shin ML, Carney DF: Cytotoxic action and other metabolic consequences of terminal complement proteins. Prog Allergy 40:44, 1988
48. Van der Meer BW, Fugate RD, Sims PJ: Complement proteins C5b-9 induce transbilayer migration of membrane phospholipids. Biophys J 56:935, 1989
49. Wiedmer T, Esmon CT, Sims PJ: On the mechanism by which complement proteins C5b-9 increase platelet prothrombinase activity. J Biol Chem 261:14587, 1986
50. Sims PJ, Faioni EM, Wiedmer T, Shattil SJ: Complement proteins C5b-9 cause release of membrane vesicles from the platelet surface that are enriched in the membrane receptor for coagulation factor Va and express prothrombinase activity. J Biol Chem 263:18205, 1988
51. Campbell AK, Daw RA, Hallett MD, Luio JP: Direct measurement of increase in intracellular free calcium ion concentration in response to the action of complement. Biochem J 194:551, 1981

52. Davis AE: Structure and function of C1 inhibitor. Behring Inst Mitt 84:142, 1989

53. Cooper NR: The classical complement activation pathway: activation and regulation of the first component. Adv Immunol 37:151, 1985

54. Schapira M, de Agostini A, Schifferli JA, Colman RW: Biochemistry and pathophysiology of human C1 inhibitor: current issues. Complement 2:111, 1985

55. Orfan NA, Kolski GB: Angioedema and C1 inhibitor deficiency. Ann Allergy 69:167, 1992

56. Vik DP, Munoz-Canoves P, Chaplin DD, Tack BF: Factor H. Curr Top Microbiol Immunol 153:147, 1990

57. Hugli TE: Structure and function of C3a anaphylatoxin. Curr Top Microbiol Immunol 153:181, 1990

58. Meuer S, Hugli TE, Andreatta RH et al: Comparative study on biological activities of various anaphylatoxins (C4a, C3a, C5a). Inflammation 5:263, 1981

59. Weiler JM, Daha MR, Austen KF, Fearon DT: Control of the amplification convertase of complement by the plasma protein beta-1H. Proc Natl Acad Sci USA 73:3268, 1976

60. Ripoche J, Day AJ, Harris TJ, Sim RB: The complete amino acid sequence of human complement factor H. Biochem J 249:593, 1988

61. Pangburn MK, Schreiber RD, Müller-Eberhard HJ: Human complement C3b inactivator: isolation, characterization, and demonstration of an absolute requirement for the serum protein beta-1H for cleavage of C3b and C4b in solution. J Exp Med 146:257, 1977

62. Harrison RA, Lachman PJ: The physiological breakdown of the third component of complement. Mol Immunol 17:9, 1980

63. Davis AEI, Harrison RA, Lachmann PJ: Physiologic inactivation of fluid phase C3b: isolation and structural analysis of C3c, C3dg (alpha-2D) and C3g. J Immunol 132:1960, 1984

64. Medicus RG, Götze O, Müller-Eberhard HJ: Alternative pathway of complement. Recruitment of precursor properdin by the labile C3/C5 convertase and the potentiation of the pathway. J Exp Med 144:1076, 1976

65. Gigli I, Fujita T, Nussenzweig V: Modulation of the classical pathway C3 convertase by plasma proteins C4 binding protein and C3b inactivator. Proc Natl Acad Sci USA 76:6596, 1979

66. Fujita T, Tamura N: Interaction of C4-binding protein with cell bound C4b. A quantitative analysis of binding and the role of C4-binding protein in proteolysis of cell-bound C4b. J Exp Med 157:1239, 1983

67. Dahlbäck B, Stenflow J: High molecular weight complex in human plasma between vitamin K-dependent protein S and complement compnent C4b-binding protein. Proc Natl Acad Sci USA 78:2512, 1981

68. Dahlbäck B, Smith CA, Müller-Eberhard HJ: Visualization of human C4b-binding protein and its complexes with vitamin K-dependent protein S and complement protein C4b. Proc Natl Acad Sci USA 80:3461, 1983

69. Hardig Y, Rezaie A, Dahlbäck B: High affinity binding of human vitamin K-dependent protein S to a truncated recombinant beta-chain of C4b-binding protein expressed in Escherichia coli. J Biol Chem 268:3033, 1993

70. Fearon DT: Regulation by membrane sialic acid of beta-1H dependent decay-dissociation of amplification C3 convertase of the alternative complement pathway. Proc Natl Acad Sci USA 75:1971, 1978

71. Pangburn MK, Müller-Eberhard HJ: Complement C3 convertase: cell surface restriction of beta-1H control and generation of restriction on neuraminidase-treated cells. Proc Natl Acad Sci USA 75:2416, 1978

72. Meri S, Pangburn MK: Discrimination between activators and nonactivators of the alternative pathway of complement: regulation via a sialic acid/polyanion binding site on factor H. Proc Natl Acad Sci USA 87:3982, 1990

73. Pangburn MK: Reduced activity of DAF on complement enzymes bound to alternative pathway activators. Similarity with factor H. Immunology 71:598, 1990

74. Pangburn MK, Atkinson MAL, Meri S: Localization of the heparin-binding site on complement factor H. J Biol Chem 266:16847, 1991

75. Nicholson-Weller A: Decay accelerating factor (CD55). Curr Top Microbiol Immunol 178:7, 1992

76. Parker CJ: Regulation of complement by membrane proteins: an overview. Curr Top Microbiol Immunol 178:1, 1992

77. Mollnes TE, Lachmann PJ: Regulation of complement. Scand J Immunol 27:127, 1988

78. Nicholson-Weller A, Burge J, Fearon DT et al: Isolation of a human erythrocyte membrane glycoprotein with decay-accelerating activity for C3 convertases of the complement system. J Immunol 129:184, 1982

79. Pangburn MK, Schreiber RD, Müller-Eberhard HJ: Deficiency of an erythrocyte membrane protein with complement regulatory activity in paroxysmal nocturnal hemoglobinuria. Proc Natl Acad Sci USA 80:5430, 1983

80. Pangburn MK: Differences between the binding sites of the complement regulatory proteins DAF, CR1, and factor H on C3 convertase. J Immunol 2216:136, 1986

81. Coyne KE, Hall SE, Thompson S et al: Mapping of epitopes, glycosylation sites, and complement regulatory domains in human decay accelerating factor. J Immunol 149:2906, 1992

82. Davitz MA, Low MG, Nussenzweig V: Release of decay-accelerating factor (DAF) from the cell membrane by phosphatidylinositol-specific phospholipase C (PIPLC). J Exp Med 163:1150, 1986

83. Ferguson MAJ: Cell-surface anchoring of proteins via glycosyl-phosphatidylinositol structures. Annu Rev Biochem 57:285, 1988

84. Low MG: Glycosyl-phosphatidylinositol: a versatile anchor for cell surface proteins. FASEB J 3:1600, 1989

85. Liszewski MK, Atkinson JP: Membrane cofactor protein. Curr Top Microbiol Immunol 178:45, 1992

86. Adams EM, Brown MC, Nunge M et al: Contribution of the repeating domains of membrane cofactor protein (CD46) of the complement system to ligand binding and cofactor activity. J Immunol 147:3005, 1991

87. Iida K, Nussenzweig V: Functional properties of membrane-associated complement receptor CR1. J Immunol 130:1876, 1983

88. Medof ME, Iida K, Nussenzweig V: Role of the complement receptor CR1 in the processing of substrate-bound C3. Ann NY Acad Sci 421:299, 1983

89. Masaki T, Matsumoto M, Nakanishi I et al: Factor I-dependent inactivation of human complement C4b of the classical pathway by C3b/C4b receptor (CR1, CD35) and membrane cofactor protein (MCP, CD46). J Biochem 111:573, 1992

90. Podak ER, Kolb WP, Müller-Eberhard HJ: The C5b-6 complex: formation, isolation, and inhibition of its activity by lipoprotein and the S-protein of human serum. J Immunol 120:1841, 1978

91. Podak ER, Kolb WP, Müller-Eberhard HJ: The SC5b-7 complex: formation, isolation, properties, and subunit composition. J Immunol 119:2024, 1977

92. Preissner KT: Structure and biological role of vitronectin. Annu Rev Cell Biol 7:275, 1991

93. Preissner KT, Podack ER, Müller-Eberhard HJ: SC5b-7, SC5b-8 and SC5b-9 complexes of complement: ultrastructure and localization of the S-protein (vitronectin) within the macromolecules. Eur J Immunol 19:69, 1989

94. Jenne DE, Lowin B, Peitsch MC et al: Clusterin (complement lysis inhibitor) forms a high density lipoprotein complex with apolipoprotein A-I in human plasma. J Biol Chem 266:11030, 1991

95. Bhakdi S, Kaflein R, Halstensen TS et al: Complement S-protein (vitronectin) is associated with cytolytic membrane-bound C5b-9 complexes. Clin Exp Immunol 74:459, 1988

96. Zalman LS: Homologous restriction factor. Curr Top Microbiol Immunol 178:87, 1992

97. Holguin MH, Parker CJ: Membrane inhibitor of reactive lysis. Curr Top Microbiol Immunol 178:61, 1992

98. Lachmann PJ: The control of homologous lysis. Immunol Today 12:312, 1991

99. Walsh LA, Tone M, Thiru S, Waldmann H: The CD59 antigen—a multifunctional molecule. Tissue Antigens 40:213, 1992

100. Davies A, Simmons DL, Hale G et al: CD59, an LY-6-like protein expressed in human lymphoid cells, regulates the action of the complement membrane attack complex on homologous cells. J Exp Med 170:637, 1989

101. Meri S, Morgan BP, Davies A et al: Human protectin (CD59), an 18–20 kD complement lysis restricting factor, inhibits C5b-8 catalyzed insertion of C9 into lipid bilayers. Immunology 71:1, 1990

102. Ninomiya H, Sims PJ: The human complement regulatory protein CD59 binds to the alpha-chain of C8 and to the "b" domain of C9. J Biol Chem 267:13675, 1992

103. Rollins SA, Zhao J, Ninomiya H, Sims PJ: Inhibition of homologous complement by CD59 is mediated by a species-selective recognition conferred through binding to C8 within C5b-8 or C9 within C5b-9. J Immunol 146:2345, 1991

104. Holguin MH, Fredrick LR, Bernshaw NJ et al: Isolation and characterization of a membrane protein from normal human erythrocytes that inhibits reactive lysis of the erythrocytes of paroxysmal nocturnal hemoglobinuria. J Clin Invest 84:7, 1989

105. Sawada R, Ohashi K, Okano K et al: Complementary DNA sequence and deduced peptide sequence for CD59/MEM-43 antigen, the human homologue of murine lymphocyte antigen Ly-6C. Nucleic Acids Res 17:6728, 1989

106. Sugita Y, Nakano Y, Tomita M: Isolation from human erythrocytes of a new membrane protein which inhibits the formation of complement transmembrane channels. J Biochem (Tokyo) 104:633, 1988

107. Ratnoff WD, Knez JJ, Prince GM et al: Structural properties of the glycoplasmanylinositol anchor phospholipid of the complement membrane attack complex inhibitor CD59. Clin Exp Immunol 87:415, 1992

108. Zalman LS, Wood LW, Müller-Eberhard HJ: Isolation of a human erythrocyte membrane protein capable of inhibiting expression of homologous complement transmembrane channels. Proc Natl Acad Sci USA 83:6975, 1986

109. Schönermark S, Rauterberg EW, Shin ML et al: Homologous species restric-

tion in lysis of human erythrocytes: a membrane-derived protein with C8-binding capacity functions as an inhibitor. J Immunol 136:1772, 1986

110. Korty PE, Brando C, Shevach EM: CD59 functions as a signal-transducing molecule for human T cell activation. J Immunol 146:4092, 1991

111. Deckert M, Kubar J, Bernard A: CD58 and CD59 molecules exhibit potentializing effects in T cell adhesion and activation. J Immunol 148:672, 1992

112. Venneker GT, Asghar SS: CD59: a molecule involved in antigen presentation as well as downregulation of membrane attack complex. Exp Clin Immunogenet 9:33, 1992

113. Hahn WC, Menu E, Bothwell AL et al: Overlapping but nonidentical binding sites on CD2 for CD58 and a second ligand CD59. Science 256:1805, 1992

114. Cinek T, Horejsi V: The nature of large noncovalent complexes containing glycosyl-phosphatidylinositol-anchored membrane glycoproteins and protein tyrosine kinases. J Immunol 149:2262, 1992

115. Hahn WC, Burakoff SJ, Bierer BE: Signal transduction pathways involved in T cell receptor-induced regulation of CD2 avidity for CD58. J Immunol 150:2607, 1993

116. Sims PJ, Wiedmer T: The response of human platelets to activated components of the complement system. Immunol Today 12:338, 1991

117. Tenner AJ: C1q interactions with cell surface receptors. Behring Inst Mitt 84:220, 1989

118. Peerschke EI, Ghebrehiwet B: Platelet interactions with C1q in whole blood and in the presence of immune complexes or aggregated IgG. Clin Immunol Immunopathol 63:45, 1992

119. Peerschke EIB, Ghebrehiwet B: Human blood platelets possess specific binding sites for C1q. J Immunol 138:1537, 1987

120. Peerschke EI, Malhotra R, Ghebrehiwet B et al: Isolation of a human endothelial cell C1q receptor (C1qR). J Leukocyte Biol 53:179, 1993

121. Klos A, Bank S, Gietz C, Bautsch W et al: C3a receptor on dibutyryl-cAMP-differentiated U937 cells and human neutrophils: the human C3a receptor characterized by functional responses and 125I-C3a binding. Biochemistry 31:11274, 1992

122. Ember JA, Sanderson SD, Taylor SM et al: Biologic activity of synthetic analogues of C5a anaphylatoxin. J Immunol 148:3165, 1992

123. Gerard NP, Gerard C: The chemotactic receptor for human C5a anaphylatoxin. Nature 349:614, 1991

124. Chenoweth DE, Hugli TE: Demonstration of specific C5a receptor on intact human polymorphonuclear leukocytes. Proc Natl Acad Sci USA 75:3943, 1978

125. Rollins TE, Siciliano S, Kobayashi S et al: Purification of the active C5a receptor from human polymorphonuclear leukocytes as a receptor-Gi complex. Proc Natl Acad Sci USA 88:971, 1991

126. Gerard NP, Bao L, Xiao-Ping H et al: Human chemotaxis receptor genes cluster at 19q13.3–13.4. Characterization of the human C5a receptor gene. Biochemistry 32:1243, 1993

127. Monk PN, Banks P: The role of protein kinase C activation and inositol phosphate production in the regulation of cell-surface expression of Mac-1 by complement fragment C5a. Biochim Biophys Acta 1092:251, 1991

128. Stevens JH, O'Hanley P, Shapiro JM et al: Effects of anti-C5a antibodies on the adult respiratory distress syndrome in septic primates. J Clin Invest 77:1812, 1986

129. Gross V, Andus T: Human recombinant C5a enhances lipopolysaccharide-induced synthesis of interleukin-6 by human monocytes. Eur J Clin Invest 22:271, 1992

130. Morgan EL, Sanderson S, Scholz W et al: Identification and characterization of the effector region within human C5a responsible for stimulation of IL-6 synthesis. J Immunol 148:3937, 1992

131. Jacob SH, Craddock PR, Hammerschmidt DE, Moldow CF: Complement-induced granulocyte aggregation: an unsuspected mechanism of disease. N Engl J Med 302:789, 1980

132. Skubitz KM, Craddock PR: Reversal of hemodialysis granulocytopenia and pulmonary leukostasis. J Clin Invest 67:1383, 1981

133. Ross GD: Complement receptor type 1. Curr Top Microbiol Immunol 178:31, 1992

134. Fearon DT, Ahearn JM: Complement receptor type 1 (C3b/C4b receptor; CD35) and complement receptor type 2 (C3d/Epstein-Barr virus receptor; CD21). Curr Top Microbiol Immunol 153:83, 1990

135. Walport MJ, Lachmann PJ: Erythrocyte complement receptor type 1, immune complexes, and the rheumatic diseases. Arthritis Rheum 31:153, 1988

136. Medof ME, Iida K, Mold C, Nussenzweig V: Unique role of the complement receptor CR1 in the degradation of C3b associated with immune complexes. J Exp Med 156:1739, 1982

137. Cornacoff JB, Hebert LA, Smead WL et al: Primate erythrocyte-immune complex-clearing mechanism. J Clin Invest 71:236, 1983

138. Schreiber RD, Pangburn MK, Bjornson AB et al: The role of C3 fragments

139. Erdei A, Füst G, Gergely J: The role of C3 in the immune response. Immunol Today 12:332, 1991

140. Bartok I, Erdei A, Mouzaki A et al: Interaction between C3 and IL-2; inhibition of C3b binding to CR1 by IL-2. Immunol Lett 21:131, 1989

141. Molina H, Brenner C, Jacobi S et al: Analysis of Epstein-Barr virus-binding sites on complement receptor 2 (CR2/CD21) using human-mouse chimeras and peptides. At least two distinct sites are necessary for ligand-receptor interaction. J Biol Chem 266:12173, 1991

142. Carel JC, Myones BL, Frazier B, Holers VM: Structural requirements for C3d,g/Epstein-Barr virus receptor (CR2/CD21) ligand binding, internalization, and viral infection. J Biol Chem 265:12293, 1990

143. Follin P, Wymann MP, Dewald B et al: Human neutrophil migration into skin chambers is associated with production of NAP-1/IL8 and C5a. Eur J Haematol 47:71, 1991

144. Ramos OF, Patarroyo M, Yefenof E, Klein E: Requirement of leukocytic cell adhesion molecules (CD11a-c/CD18) in the enhanced NK lysis of iC3b-opsonized targets. J Immunol 142:4100, 1989

145. Dykman TR, Hatch JA, Aqua MS, Atkinson JP: Polymorphism of the C3b/C4b receptor (CR1): characterization of a fourth allele. J Immunol 134:1787, 1985

146. Morgan BP, Walport MJ: Complement deficiency and disease. Immunol Today 12:301, 1991

147. Walport MJ, Lachmann PJ: Complement deficiencies and abnormalities of the complement system in systemic lupus erythematosus and related disorders. Curr Opin Rheumatol 2:661, 1990

148. Dykman TR, Cole JL, Iida K, Atkinson JP: Structural heterogeneity of the C3b/C4b receptor (CR1) on human peripheral blood cells. J Exp Med 157:2160, 1983

149. So AK, Fielder AH, Warner CA et al: DNA polymorphism of major histocompatibility complex class II and class III genes in systemic lupus erythematosus. Tissue Antigens 35:144, 1990

150. Kalli KR, Hsu PH, Bartow TJ et al: Mapping of the C3b-binding site of CR1 and construction of a (CR1)2-F(ab')2 chimeric complement inhibitor. J Exp Med 174:1451, 1991

151. Makrides SC, Scesney SM, Ford PJ et al: Cell surface expression of the C3b/C4b receptor (CR1) protects Chinese hamster ovary cells from lysis by human complement. J Biol Chem 267:24754, 1992

152. Cooper NR, Bradt BM, Rhim JS, Nemerow GR: CR2 complement receptor. J Invest Dermatol 94:112S, 1990

153. Fischer E, Delibrias C, Kazatchkine MD: Expression of CR2 (the C3dg/EBV receptor, CD21) on normal human peripheral blood T lymphocytes. J Immunol 146:865, 1991

154. Lowell CA, Klickstein LB, Carter RH et al: Mapping of the Epstein-Barr virus and C3dg binding sites to a common domain on complement receptor type 2. J Exp Med 170:1931, 1989

155. Montefiori DC, Zhou J, Shaff DI: CD4-independent binding of HIV-1 to the B lymphocyte receptor CR2 (CD21) in the presence of complement and antibody. Clin Exp Immunol 90:383, 1992

156. Boyer V, Desgranges C, Trabaud MA et al: Complement mediates human immunodeficiency virus type 1 infection of a human T cell line in a CD4- and antibody-independent fashion. J Exp Med 173:1151, 1991

157. Sanchez-Madrid F, Nagy JA, Robbins E et al: A human leukocyte differentiation antigen family with distinct alpha-subunits and a common beta subunit: the lymphocyte function-associated antigen (LFA-1), the C3bi complement receptor (OKM1/Mac-1), and the p150,95 molecule. J Exp Med 158:1785, 1983

158. Rosen H, Law SK: The leukocyte cell surface receptor(s) for the iC3b product of complement. Curr Top Microbiol Immunol 153:99, 1990

159. Vik DP, Fearon DT: Cellular distribution of complement receptor type 4 (CR4): expression of human platelets. J Immunol 138:254, 1987

160. Kojima A, Hazeki K, Seya T: Granulocyte-dependent extracellular cytotoxicity is enhanced by complement C3bi and independent of phagocytosis. Scand J Immunol 33:707, 1991

161. Roubey RA, Ross GD, Merrill JT et al: Staurosporine inhibits neutrophil phagocytosis but not iC3b binding mediated by CR3 (CD11b/CD18). J Immunol 146:3557, 1991

162. Springer TA, Thompson WS, Miller LJ et al: Inherited deficiency of the Mac-1, LFA-1, p150, 95 glycoprotein family and its molecular basis. J Exp Med 160:1901, 1984

163. Dustin ML, Springer TA: Role of lymphocyte adhesion receptors in transient interactions and cell locomotion. Annu Rev Immunol 9:27, 1991

164. Gresham HD, Graham IL, Anderson DC, Brown EJ: Leukocyte adhesion-deficient neutrophils fail to amplify phagocytic function in response to stimula-

tion. Evidence for CD11b/CD18-dependent and -independent mechanisms of phagocytosis. J Clin Invest 88:588, 1991

165. Morgan BP: Effects of the membrane attack complex of complement on nucleated cells. Curr Top Microbiol Immunol 178:115, 1992

166. Hänsch GM: The complement attack phase: control of lysis and non-lethal effects of C5b-9. Immunopharmacology 24:107, 1992

167. Hamilton KK, Sims PJ: The terminal complement proteins C5b-9 augment binding of high density lipoprotein and its apoproteins A-I and A-II to human endothelial cells. J Clin Invest 88:1833, 1991

168. Wiedmer T, Sims PJ: Participation of protein kinases in complement C5b-9-induced shedding of platelet plasma membrane vesicles. Blood 78:2880, 1991

169. Halperin JA, Taratuska A, Nicholson-Weller A: Terminal complement complex C5b-9 stimulates mitogenesis in 3T3 cells. J Clin Invest 91:1974, 1993

170. Niculescu F, Rus H, Shin S et al: Generation of diacylglycerol and ceramide during homologous complement activation. J Immunol 150:214, 1993

171. Cybulsky AV: Release of arachidonic acid by complement C5b-9 complex in glomerular epithelial cells. Am J Physiol 261:F427, 1991

172. Chang C-P, Zhao J, Wiedmer T, Sims PJ: Contribution of platelet microparticle formation and granule secretion to the transmembrane migration of phosphatidylserine. J Biol Chem 268:7171, 1993

173. Dahlbäck B, Wiedmer T, Sims PJ: Binding of anticoagulant vitamin K-dependent protein S to platelet-derived microparticles. Biochemistry 31:12769, 1992

174. Wurzner R, Orren A, Lachmann PJ: Inherited deficiencies of the terminal components of human complement. Immunodefic Rev 3:123, 1992

175. Moulds JM, Krych M, Holers VM et al: Genetics of the complement system and rheumatic diseases. Rheum Dis Clin North Am 18:893, 1992

176. Rosen FS: Genetic defects of the complement system. Clin Immunol Immunopathol 61:S78, 1991

177. Campbell RD, Dunham I, Sargent CA: Molecular mapping of the HLA-linked complement genes and the RCA linkage group. Exp Clin Immunogenet 5:81, 1988

178. Schifferli JA, Paccaud JP: Two isotypes of human C4, C4A and C4B have different structure and function. Concours Med 6:19, 1989

179. Giles CM: C4: Rodgers and Chido typing. Concours Med 7:213, 1990

180. Ahearn JM, Fearon DT: Structure and function of the complement receptors, CR1 (CD35) and CR2 (CD21). Adv Immunol 46:183, 1989

181. Telen MJ, Green AM: The Inab phenotype: characterization of the membrane protein and complement regulatory defect. Blood 74:437, 1989

182. Holguin MH, Martin CB, Bernshaw NJ, Parker CJ: Analysis of the effects of activation of the alternative pathway of complement on erythrocytes with an isolated deficiency of decay accelerating factor. J Immunol 148:498, 1992

183. Yamashina M, Ueda E, Kinoshita T et al: Inherited complete deficiency of 20-kilodalton homologous restriction factor (CD59) as a cause of paroxysmal nocturnal hemoglobinuria. N Engl J Med 323:1184, 1990

184. Schreiber AD, Frank MM: The role of antibody and complement in the immune clearance and destruction of erythrocytes. I. In vivo effects of IgG and IgM complement-fixing sites. J Clin Invest 51:575, 1972

185. Schreiber AD, Frank MM: The role of antibody and complement in the immune clearance and destruction of erythrocytes. II. Molecular nature of IgG and IgM complement-fixing sites and effects of their interaction with serum. J Clin Invest 51:583, 1972

186. Engelfriet CP, von dem Borne AEG Jr, Fleer A et al: In vivo destruction of erythrocytes by complement-binding and non-complement-binding antibodies. p. 213. In Sanders SG, Nusbacher J, Schanfield MD (eds): Immunobiology of the Erythrocyte. Alan R Liss, New York, 1980

187. Jaffe CJ, Atkinson JP, Frank MM: The role of complement in the clearance of cold agglutinin sensitized erythrocytes in man. J Clin Invest 58:942, 1976

188. Chaplin H Jr, Coleman ME, Monroe MC: In vivo instability of red-blood-cell bound C3d and C4d. Blood 62:965, 1983

189. Rustagi PK, Currie MS, Logue GD: Activation of human complement by immunoglobulin G antigranulocyte antibody. J Clin Invest 70:1137, 1982

190. Ebenbichler CF, Thielens NM, Vornhagen R et al: Human immunodeficiency virus type 1 activates the classical pathway of complement by direct C1 binding through specific sites in the transmembrane glycoprotein gp41. J Exp Med 174:1417, 1991

191. Thieblemont N, Delibrias C, Fischer E et al: Complement enhancement of HIV infection is mediated by complement receptors. Immunopharmacology 25:87, 1993

192. Daniel V, Süsal C, Prodeus AP et al: CD4+ lymphocyte depletion in HIV-infected patients is associated with gp120-immunoglobulin-complement attachment to CD4+ cells. Vox Sang 64:31, 1993

193. Weiss L, Okada N, Haeffner-Cavaillon N et al: Decreased expression of the membrane inhibitor of complement-mediated cytolysis CD59 on T-lymphocytes of HIV-infected patients. AIDS 6:379, 1992

194. Füst G, Ujhelyi E, Hidvegi T et al: The complement system in HIV disease. Immunol Invest 20:231, 1991

195. Senaldi G, Peakman M, McManus T et al: Activation of the complement system in human immunodeficiency virus infection: relevance of the classical pathway to pathogenesis and disease severity. J Infect Dis 162:1227, 1990

196. Montefiori DC, Lefkowitz LB Jr, Keller RE et al: Absence of a clinical correlation for complement-mediated, infection-enhancing antibodies in plasma or sera from HIV-1-infected individuals. Multicenter AIDS Cohort Study Group. AIDS 5:513, 1991

197. Blajchman MA, Ozge-Anwar AH: The role of the complement system in hemostasis. Prog Hematol 14:149, 1986

198. Rosse WF: Paroxysmal nocturnal hemoglobinuria. Curr Top Microbiol Immunol 178:163, 1992

199. Hill J, Lindsay TF, Ortiz F et al: Soluble complement receptor type 1 ameliorates the local and remote organ injury after intestinal ischemia-reperfusion in the rat. J Immunol 149:1723, 1992

200. Homeister JW, Satoh PS, Kilgore KS, Lucchesi BR: Soluble complement receptor type 1 prevents human complement-mediated damage of the rabbit isolated heart. J Immunol 150:1055, 1993

201. Sims PJ: Interaction of human platelets with the complement system. p. 354. In Kunicki TJ, George JN (eds): Platelet Immunology. JB Lippincott, Philadelphia, 1989

Cellular Aspects of Immunity and Their Control

13

David W. Scott and Richard P. Phipps

OVERVIEW OF THE DICHOTOMY OF THE IMMUNE SYSTEM

Immune System as Part of the Circulatory System

Approximately one-third of all blood leukocytes are the B and T lymphocytes. An important concept is that to maximize the chances for encountering a foreign invader (e.g., bacteria, virus), these cells must have a defined migration pathway throughout the body.[1] This is particularly important, as only a small subset of lymphocytes can recognize and respond to a given antigen. These recirculating lymphocytes must also be capable of surveillance of most of the body tissues, since the invading microorganism can enter the host through a variety of sites (e.g., skin, mucosal surfaces).

Lymph Nodes

A unique set of peripheral lymphoid organs has developed to facilitate lymphocyte circulation and antigen encounter. The lymph nodes are situated along the lymphatic channels in most tissues of the body. Invading microorganisms that enter through any body portal usually locate in these channels, which direct the lymph to flow into a lymph node (Fig. 13-1). Lymph nodes have three cardinal features: (1) provide a mechanism to trap or filter invading microorganisms, (2) act as a portal of entry for recirculating lymphocytes, and (3) serve as a specialized microenvironment for the generation of effector lymphocytes. The lymph node capsule is penetrated by a series of valved lymphatic channels to allow the lymph fluid to percolate throughout the node. Macrophages line the subcapsular sinuses, where they encounter and destroy microorganisms and subsequently release the degraded components. These degraded products may then be picked up and presented by lymphoid dendritic cells or B lymphocytes (see later in this chapter for details). Deeper within the node, lie the more organized B- and T-lymphocyte regions. The outer aspect of the node, the cortex, includes the B-cell-rich follicles, which also contain the antigen-retaining follicular dendritic cells.[2,3] Deeper within the lymph node is the paracortex, which includes the postcapillary venules, surrounded by dense aggregates of T lymphocytes interspersed with lymphoid dendritic cells.[4] The inner medullary region contains large numbers of macrophages, as well as some lymphocytes, dendritic cells, and plasma cells. The lymph fluid exits via the efferent lymphatics, where it can "drain" into the next node.

The postcapillary venules in the paracortical region are structures important for lymphocyte entry from blood into the lymph node. These venules are especially important, since they contain special endothelial cells that permit the binding and transendothelial cell migration of blood lymphocytes (especially T lymphocytes).[5] Once inside the node, the lymphocytes may be retained or may exit through the efferent lymphatics, progressing to the next lymph node and eventually entering the thoracic duct to be returned to the circulating blood through the pulmonary vein. The other mode of lymphocyte entry into the node is through the afferent lymphatic drainage that penetrates the node capsule. Here, B and T lymphocytes can travel through the node, ultimately exiting through the efferent lymphatic channels.

The concept behind the organized structures of the lymph node and the ability of lymphocytes to enter the lymph nodes through the lymphatics or the postcapillary venules is to permit the lymphocytes to "sample" a variety of tissues. If foreign antigens are present and "processed," this permits high-affinity interactions between antigen-presenting cells (APCs), such as macrophages, lymphoid dendritic cells, and B lymphocytes, as well as the receptive T lymphocytes. These interactions result in sequestration of appropriate antigen-specific B and T lymphocytes followed by their activation and clonal expansion (see the section Recirculation and the Immune Response). On antigenic stimulation the B-cell areas (follicles) enlarge and form the so-called germinal centers, which contain nests of proliferating B lymphocytes as well as a few T cells (Fig. 13-1A). The T-dependent paracortical zones also swell with T cells. This results in nodule enlargement, due in part to the increased number of responding lymphocytes. In addition to the clonal expansion that occurs, some B and T lymphocytes differentiate into effector cells, such as plasma cells, T-helper cells, and cytotoxic T cells, which are ultimately released into the circulation.

Spleen

Events similar to those described above also occur in the spleen, a more complex organ that serves to filter the blood. The blood is dumped into the spleen via the splenic artery and its arterioles. As occurs in the lymph nodes, splenic lymphocytes are organized into discrete regions. Aggregates of primarily T lymphocytes surround the central arterioles and form the periarteriolar lymphoid sheath with the attached B-cell-rich lymphoid follicles. These dense aggregates of lymphocytes comprise the white pulp of the spleen. The arterioles terminate in vascular sinusoids containing large numbers of resident macrophages and dendritic cells, as well as blood erythrocytes (the red pulp). Here blood-borne microorganisms can be trapped and killed by phagocytic cells (macrophages). The blood is then returned by the sinusoids. These sinusoids form venules that collect the splenic vein, returning the blood to the portal circulation.

Thus, the spleen and lymph node provide a nurturing microenvironment that facilitates the complete interaction of APCs and T cells. These structures permit dissemination of the end-stage effector B and T lymphocytes and their products (antibodies and lymphokines) through the lymph node lymphatics or, in the case of the spleen, through the venous system.

Humoral Versus Cell-Mediated Immunity

Antigen-specific immune responses have classically been divided into two broad categories: humoral immunity and cell-mediated immunity. This classification is based on the ability to transfer components of specific immunity to a naive (i.e., unimmunized) recipient. For example, humoral immunity can

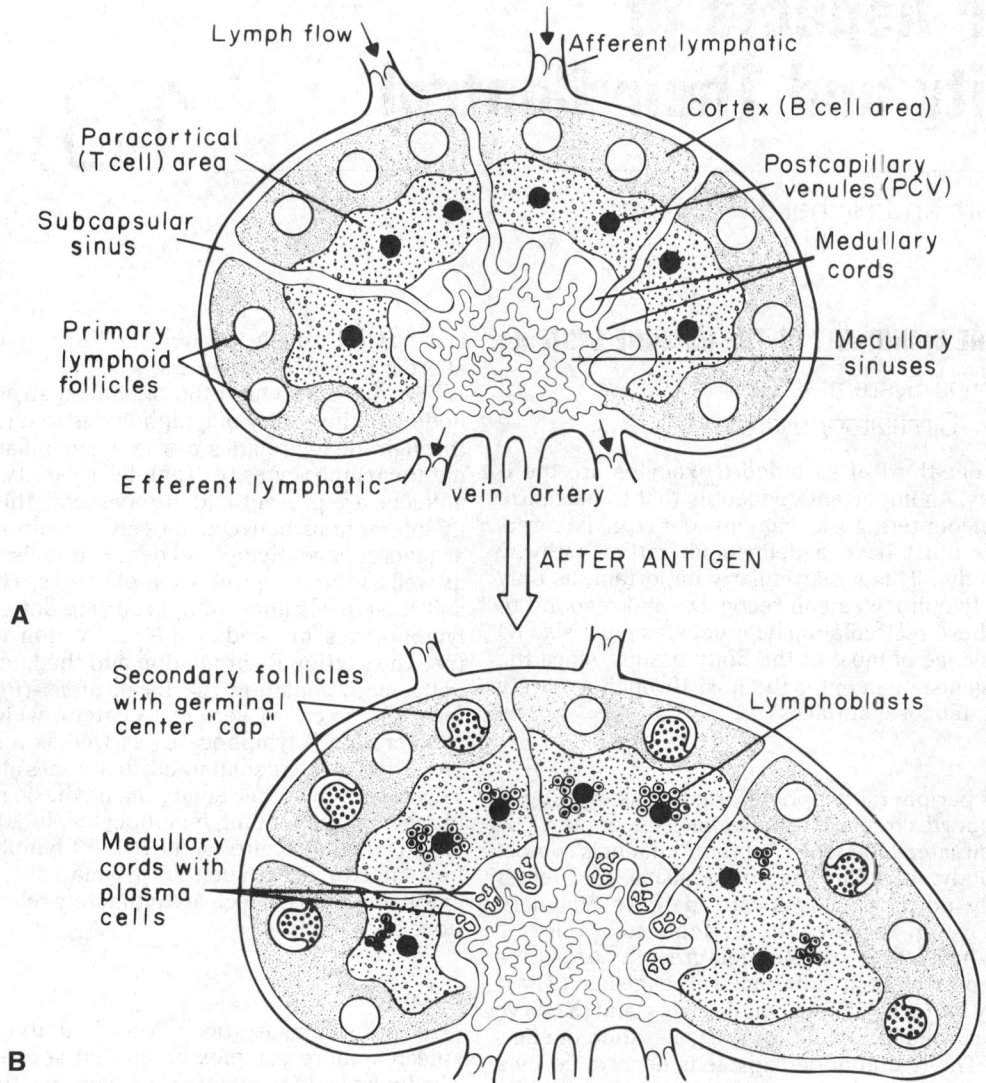

Fig. 13-1. Diagrammatic representation of the human lymph node. **(A)** Quiescent (non-antigen-stimulated) lymph node. Lymphocytes migrate through the node through the postcapillary venules or via entry through the afferent lymphatics. They exit the node by way of the efferent lymphatics, where they may travel to the next node in the chain. **(B)** Morphologic changes that occur in an antigen-stimulated lymph node. The B-cell-dependent follicular regions in the cortex transform into secondary follicles containing germinal centers—areas of lymphocyte proliferation. In the T-cell-dependent paracortical regions, many lymphoblasts are observed. Plasma cells can be found accumulating in the medullary cord region. These events serve to expand the pool of effective T and B lymphocytes and to increase the size of the node.

be transferred by the injection of blood whose cellular components have been removed. This would include the transfer of serum or plasma. Humoral immunity consists primarily of the antibody molecules (immunoglobulins) made by B lymphocytes. These proteins are responsible for the specific recognition and elimination of invading microorganisms. By contrast, cell-mediated immunity is defined by the transference to naive patients of antigen-specific components mediated by cellular elements of the blood. Antigen-specific lymphocytes (i.e., T lymphocytes) are responsible for cell-mediated immunity.

Humoral immunity can be demonstrated in many ways. Practical examples include the delivery of antibodies (or cell-free fluids containing antibodies) to provide protection against certain microorganisms or their toxins. The antibodies may function because of a number of attributes: (1) neutralization of bacterial toxins (e.g., cholera toxin, diphtheria toxin), preventing their uptake by sensitive cells or by inducing a conformational change in the toxin; (2) possession of a directly lytic effect through their ability to activate the components of the

complement system; (3) prevention of the attachment of bacteria or viruses to tissue structures or cellular receptors; and (4) behavior similar to that of opsonins, that is, facilitating the uptake of, and killing by, phagocytic cells. Thus, humoral immunity is primarily effective against those microorganisms and toxins that operate at the extracellular level, and mediated by B lymphocytes.

Specific cell-mediated-immunity can be demonstrated by the transference of cells, using a variety of in vitro or in vivo systems. The key cells that mediate cell-mediated immunity are the T lymphocytes. These cells provide antigen-specific immunity against microorganisms that invade or divide within the host cells (e.g., *M. tuberculosis,* viruses). Thus, cell-mediated immunity is a crucial element in host defense against intracellular microorganisms. T lymphocytes promote intracellular destruction of microbes by inducing direct or indirect T-cell-mediated lysis of infected cells. Cell-mediated immunity is also responsible for the destruction of both transplanted tissue (e.g., lung, kidney, skin) and malignant cells.

CELLULAR BASIS OF IMMUNE RESPONSIVENESS

T- and B-Cell Development: Introduction

In human fetal development, precursors of T and B lymphocytes originate in the yolk sac and migrate to the fetal liver; later they are found in the bone marrow. These stem cells give rise to the first B cells as early as 8 weeks' gestation. Identified by their large size, scant cytoplasm, and staining for μ heavy (H) chains, these so-called pre-B cells possess rearranged H chains (for details of this process, see Ch. 20) but lack light (L) chains and are therefore unable to express a complete IgM receptor on their surface. Synthesis of L chains is followed by the expression of the IgM monomer (H_2/L_2) receptor on the surface of the B cells. This receptor is the antigen-recognizing structure that gives the B lymphocyte its specificity.

By 12 weeks' gestation, most pre-B-cell formation occurs in the bone marrow. At 8–20 weeks, the numbers of IgM^+ B cells rise rapidly and begin to appear in the spleen. Cells expressing both IgM and IgD receptors can be observed by 14 weeks' gestation but are still in the minority in the liver and marrow throughout gestation. IgM^+/IgD^+ (double-positive) B cells begin to predominate in the spleen and circulating blood, resulting in cord blood that contains mostly double-positive B cells. By birth, human B cells not only express IgM and IgD but are also positive for HLA-D region (class II MHC) molecules and bear receptors for the Fc portion of IgG molecules. Class II antigen expression is critical for cellular interactions with T cells (see below), whereas the latter receptor results in regulatory signals that develop from IgG/antigen complexes as part of the immune response.

By definition, T cells are derived from a thymic maturation pathway. Unlike B cells, whose differentiation occurs at many sites, T cells develop predominantly in the thymus. The earliest thymic primordium develops by invagination of the third and fourth pharyngeal pouches, beginning at 4–5 weeks' gestation. Studies in other species indicate that T-cell precursors, which like B-cell precursors are derived from pluripotential hematopoietic stem cells, soon begin to arrive through the blood from the yolk sac and then from the liver to colonize the epithelial thymic rudiment. Migration of T-cell precursors into the thymus continues postnatally, but their source shifts from fetal liver to the bone marrow. These immigrant cells continue to differentiate in situ into mature immunocompetent T cells, which eventually leave the thymus to populate peripheral lymphoid tissues, such as the spleen and lymph nodes.[6]

The thymus can be divided anatomically into cortical (immature) and medullary (more mature) regions, each containing different sets of T lymphocytes that can be distinguished functionally and by the expression of a variety of specific cell-surface molecules. The role of the thymus in the T-cell development is discussed in detail in Chapter 20.

Clonal Selection and Programmed Development of the Repertoire

The human infant is relatively mature immunologically, at birth. Although human neonates are able to respond to a multitude of antigens, they are unresponsive to a variety of antigens. Several reasons for this initial lack of responsiveness have been suggested: (1) maternal antibodies of the IgG class cross the placenta and not only provide protective passive immunity but also prevent the neonatal response; (2) some antigens, such as the capsular polysaccharide of *Haemophilus influenzae*, are unable to trigger the human infant's immune system, at least in their native polysaccharide form[7]; and (3) B cells of the appropriate specificities have not yet productively rearranged their IgM receptors. When exposed to antigen, in the absence

of cells with surface receptors for that antigen, no response can ensue.

Evidence for the last category of unresponsiveness abounds in the literature. Silverstein and co-workers[8] demonstrated nearly 30 years ago that fetal sheep could respond to a simple bacterial virus before midgestation yet could not make antibody to *Salmonella typhosa* until after birth. In examining precursor frequencies to different haptens in mice, Klinman[9] found responsiveness to certain epitopes to precede precursor detection to other haptens consistently. Indeed, a programmed pattern of repertoire development could be mapped and predicted for a given mouse strain. While such an acquisition has not been delineated for T-cell responsiveness in humans (although it has been seen in sheep), it is assumed to be generalizable.

What is the basis for this repertoire acquisition? Recent data suggest that the rearrangements necessary to make a complete immunoglobulin H (and L) chain may occur in a predetermined order, with the initial rearrangements involving V_H gene segments most proximal to the constant region.[10,11] Details of this process are discussed in Chapter 20.

The net result is that B cells (and T cells) each express surface receptors determined by these rearrangements. Importantly, each B or T cell expresses only one receptor specificity. That is, of 1,000 randomly chosen cells, specificity for 1,000 different antigens would be found, each cell specific for only one of these. Antigen is therefore the ultimate *selector* of a responding T or B lymphocyte. This process, known as clonal selection, results in the recruitment of specific lymphocytes out of the circulation to become part of the immune response (Fig. 13-2).

Recirculation and the Immune Response

One of the hallmarks of the immune system and its specific T or B lymphocytes is its ability to be rapidly recruited to respond to a wide variety of antigens entering the body through portals or breaks in its physical barriers. Since the immune system possesses a wide array of lymphocytes, how do these dispersed lymphocytes respond so rapidly? The answer is based on a fundamental property of lymphocytes not possessed by all other white (or red) blood cells: the ability to recirculate (Fig. 13-3). More than 35 years ago, Sir James Gowans[12] inserted an indwelling cannula into the thoracic duct of an adult rat and was impressed by the numbers of cells that flowed out. Curious as to their destination and origin, he labeled these cells and reinjected them into the venous system. Surprisingly, the vast majority of these thoracic duct lymphocytes began to appear in the outgoing lymph within hours, traversing from the blood back to the lymph. Indeed, lymphocytes traffic around the body in <1 hour and traverse lymph nodes through either afferent lymphatics or the postcapillary venules. Once inside a lymph node, they percolate through the cortex and leave through the efferent lymphatics—unless they encounter an antigen.

If a lymphocyte encounters its specific antigen as it migrates through a lymph node, it is recruited out of the circulation, and into the immune response.[13] That is, circulation through the node is delayed once antigen is encountered and an immune response is initiated. This response includes the interaction of specific T and B cells with antigen, generally presented on the surface of cells such as dendritic cells or macrophages (APCs); the interaction of T cells with B cells, and the ultimate production of the mediators characteristic of an immune response (specific antibody to that antigen, specific T cells and/or cytokines).

The process by which specific lymphocytes are recruited out of the circulation into the immune response is called clonal selection. The changes that occur in a lymph node, draining where a specific antigen has entered the body, are discussed below. Shortly after these initial stages of lymphocyte recruit-

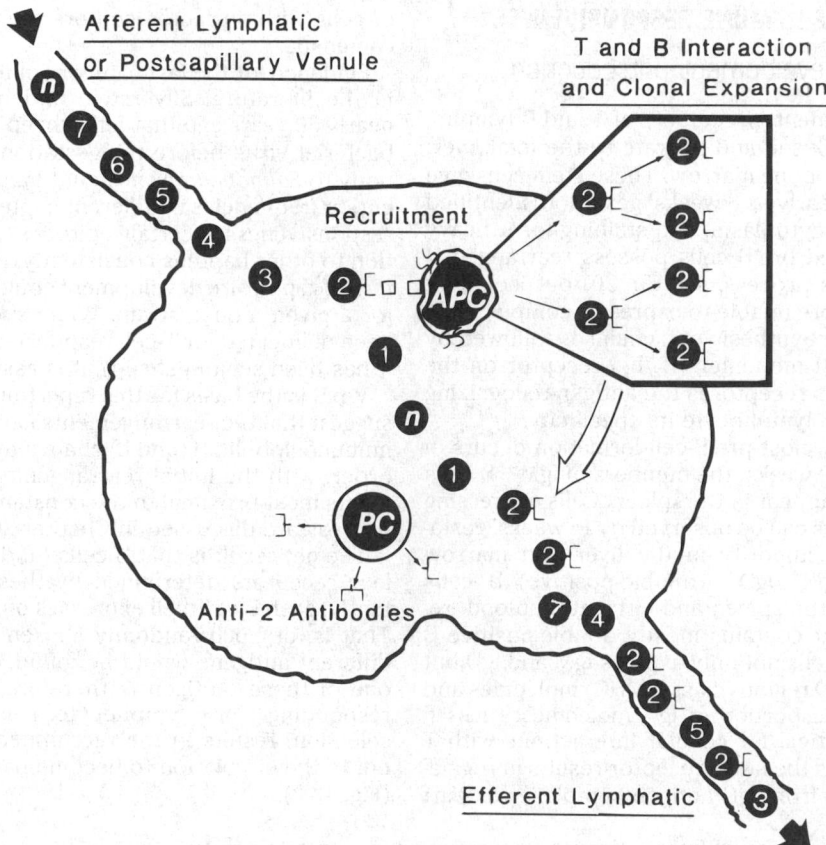

Fig. 13-2. Scheme of a lymph node draining a site of antigen exposure and demonstrating the clonality of the immune system. Recirculating lymphocytes (1–n) enter the lymph node either by the afferent lymphatics or by the blood through the postcapillary venule. They percolate through and exit by the efferent lymphatics if no antigen to which they have an affinity is trapped therein. Here, antigen 2 has been filtered and presented on an antigen-presenting cell (APC). Lymphocyte 2 can bind to this antigen by virtue of its receptors (IgM, for example, on B cells) and is then recruited from the circulating pool. It has been demonstrated that the efferent lymph from such a node is depleted of reactivity to antigen 2 within 1 day after antigen 2 is delivered to the node. However, reactivity to all other antigens (1 and 3–n) is still present in the efferent lymph. Cellular interactions then occur and lymphocyte 2 clonally expands to make more effective cells (such as plasma cell [PC] secreting anti-2 antibody), which then join the circulating pool and exit by days 5–7 after antigenic stimulation.

ment, clonal selection, expansion, and differentiation, antigen-specific T and B cells re-enter the circulating pool of lymphocytes and disseminate throughout the body as effector cells. The entire process occurs over a period of days with the initial recruitment leading to a temporary enlargement of the draining lymph nodes (Fig. 13-1B), due to proliferation of specific cells, and to nonspecific vascular effects, secondary to the release of molecules such as prostaglandins on the activation of T cells and macrophages. Once they begin the activation process, both T cells and B cells may express new differentiation markers that both promote their interaction, as well as prevent their emigration out of the active lymph node. These surface markers are involved both in the attachment of lymphoid cells to each other, and to the vascular endothelium.

Morphology of Lymphoid Tissue Changes in Immunity

Antigen processed by APCs, such as macrophages, dendritic cells, and B cells, serves to recruit and stimulate specific T lymphocytes, which, in turn, stimulate B cells to make specific antibody. Within 24–48 hours, the lymphoid cells in the lymph node deep cortex begin a process known as blast transformation, in which their cytoplasm can be stained intensively with pyronin, a dye that interacts with RNA. In the deep cortex, the T-cell-dependent area, a significant number of lymphoblastoid cells and dividing cells are seen over the next few days (Fig. 13-1B). Division continues asymmetrically to yield clones of progeny, as well as differentiated T cells producing cytokines, and B cells that are the precursors of antibody-screening cells. Some daughter cells persist as so-called memory cells. By 3–5 days after an intense antigenic stimulation in the draining lymph node, activated T cells and B cells migrate to form secondary follicles and germinal centers characteristic of an active immune response. Subsequently, antibody-secreting plasma cells are seen in the medullary cords. These changes persist for varying degrees of time, depending on the intensity of the antigenic stimulus, as well as the route of injection. The lymph nodes diminishes in size back to a normal range, often within approximately 2 weeks, but will often persist in the appearance of secondary follicles and germinal centers for months. Characteristically, the lymphoid tissue of normal persons exposed to a variety of environmental stimuli will contain many germinal

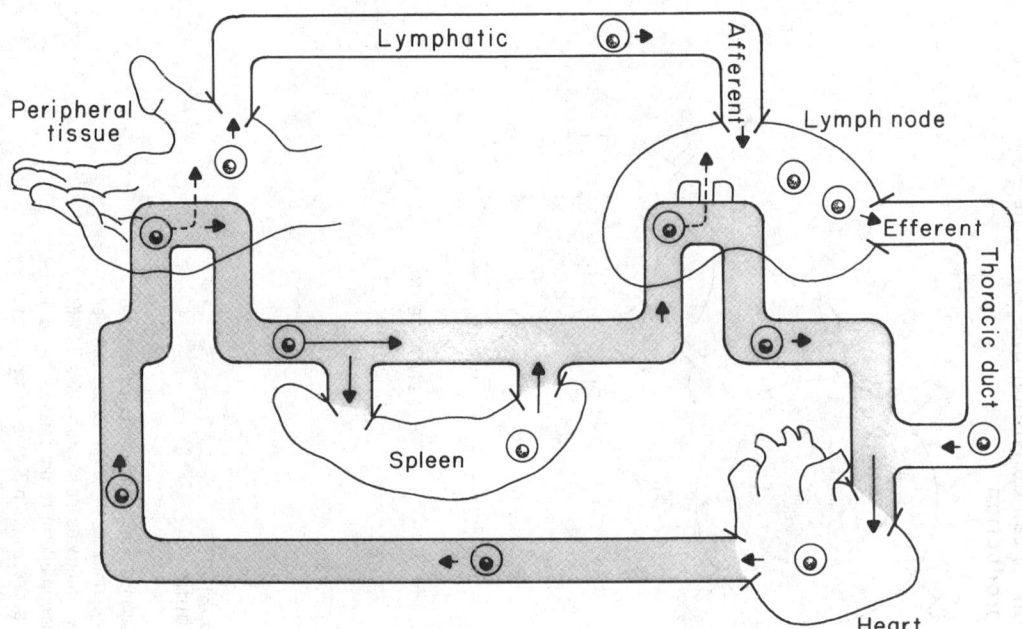

Fig. 13-3. Lymphocyte recirculation pathway throughout the body. B and T lymphocytes can migrate throughout the body via the blood or the lymphatics. Lymphocytes in the blood enter tissues and lymph nodes by passing through the specialized high-walled endothelium (see also Fig. 13-1). They may then exit the tissues via the efferent lymphatics. The efferent lymphatics eventually drain into the thoracic duct, where the lymphocytes are returned to the circulation. In the spleen, the T and B lymphocytes enter the white pulp via the splenic arterioles and eventually migrate to the red pulp sinusoids, where they exit via the splenic vein.

centers, a sign indicative of previous antigen exposure. Only in patients with immunodeficiencies do lymph nodes lack secondary follicles.[14]

Antigen Presentation and T- and B-Cell Collaboration

In order for humoral and cell-mediated immunity to develop, the B and T lymphocytes (particularly T-helper lymphocytes) must be activated by antigen. This occurs in a complex process of antigen presentation and T- and B-cell collaboration.[15,16] One of the fundamental differences between B and T lymphocytes is in their ability to recognize antigens. B lymphocytes with their surface immunoglobulins can bind or recognize native (undenatured) protein antigens. By contrast, the T lymphocyte and its surface receptor, the T-cell receptor (TCR), typically recognizes denatured or "processed" antigens in association with MHC antigens (the CD4$^+$ T-helper cells use class II MHC and the CD8$^+$ T cytotoxic cells use class I MHC).[17]

One of the key aspects for T cells to recognize and respond to foreign protein antigens is that they must encounter the antigen on the surface of another cell type. The critical process of antigen presentation occurs when APCs express the foreign antigen in association with class II MHC on their surface.[15] For many years, macrophages were thought to be the dominant cell type capable of presenting antigen and activating T cells. However, it is now known that many other cell types, including lymphoid dendritic cells, Langerhans cells in the skin, B lymphocytes, and even fibroblasts, can participate in this process.[16]

This complex process of antigen presentation may be explored using the paradigm of bacterial infection. Bacteria finding their way into one of the lymphatic channels, would first be encountered by macrophages that line the entry way to the node. Here, they may be phagocytosed and killed by powerful intracellular digestive enzymes. Some of the degraded bacterial proteins bind with high affinity to the intracellular class II MHC

molecules (e.g., HLA-DR, DP, DQ). The complexes of class II MHC and peptide are then transported to the surface of the macrophage. Migrating T lymphocytes recognize this peptide/MHC complex and, in conjunction with other co-stimulatory activities, the T cell will enlarge, begin to synthesize lymphokines, and divide.

Another mechanism exists for other potential APCs to participate in this process. Several other cells in lymph node and spleen can also activate T-helper cells. Specialized lymphoid dendritic cells that inhabit the T-cell-dependent zones of spleen and lymph node express very high levels of class II MHC; in rodents and humans, they are exceptionally potent in their ability to activate T cells.[4] However, the lymphoid dendritic cells are not phagocytic and would be unable to kill and dismantle intact bacteria. However, the processed or degraded bacterial proteins (peptides) that are released from macrophages would flow through the node through the lymph, where they could be accessible to the lymphoid dendritic cells, allowing these cells to bind to and activate recirculating T-helper cells.

An alternative pathway of antigen presentation of increasing importance involves B lymphocytes, which also possess the elements needed to activate T-helper cells.[15,18] Although they are not phagocytic, the B lymphocytes do possess an outstanding antigen capture system (i.e., surface immunoglobulin), express class II MHC, and can process simple proteins into a form recognized by helper T cells (Fig. 13-4). During the process of B-cell presentation of antigen to T cells, these cells form conjugates; the activation of the T cells further activates the B cell, stimulating it to express even higher levels of class II MHC antigen. This increased B-lymphocyte activation makes these cells even better at stimulating T cells. The activated T lymphocytes produce a variety of lymphokines critical for this mutual stimulation (i.e., T- and B-cell collaboration). The lymphokines (see below) are necessary for B-cell proliferation, isotype switching, and differentiation into the powerful antibody secreting plasma cells.[19] Overall, this process of antigen capture, presentation, clonal selection, conjugate formation, and lymphokine production results in B- and T-cell clonal expan-

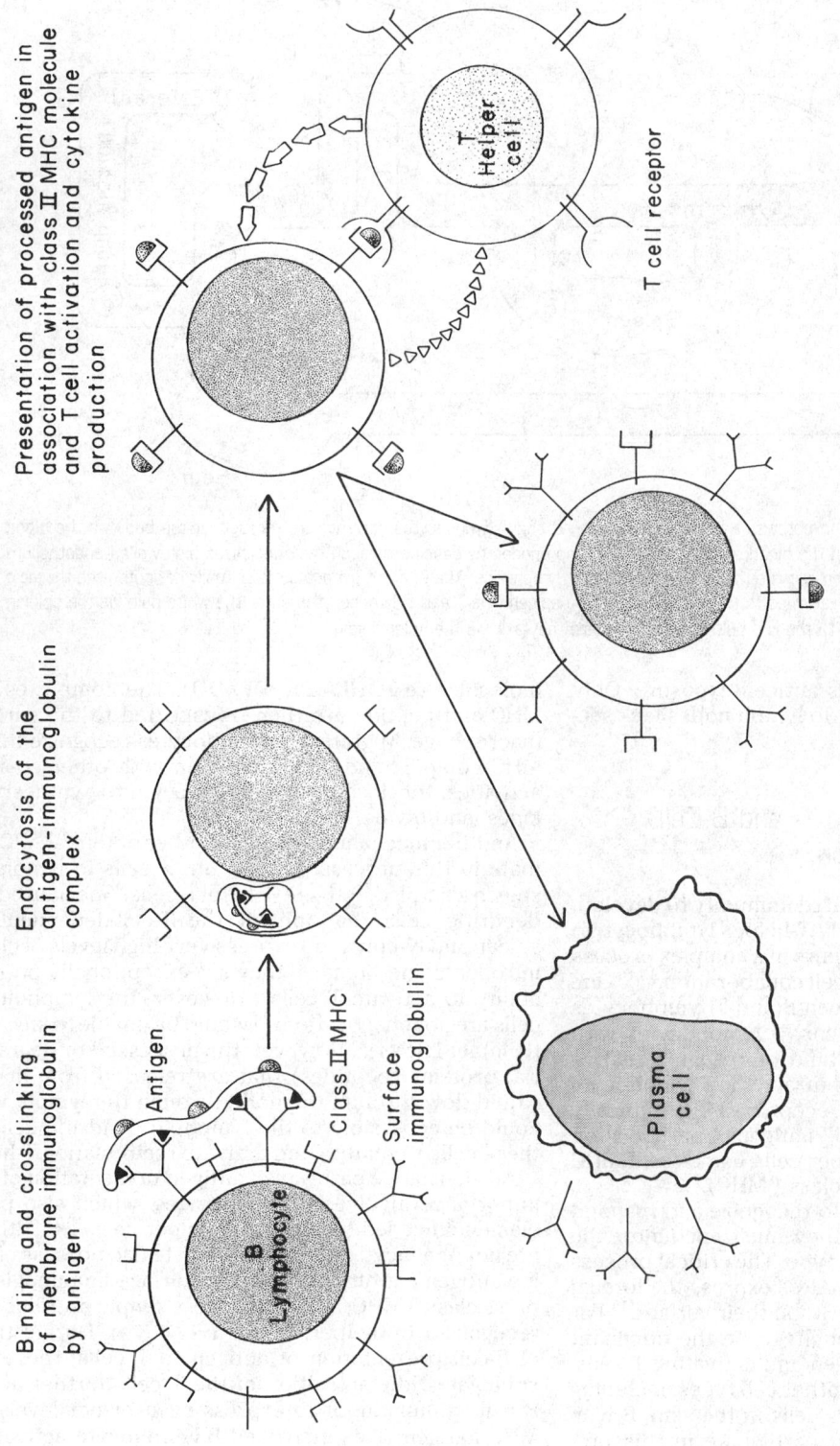

Binding and crosslinking of membrane immunoglobulin by antigen

Endocytosis of the antigen-immunoglobulin complex

Presentation of processed antigen in association with class II MHC molecule and T cell activation and cytokine production

Antigen

Class II MHC

Surface immunoglobulin

B Lymphocyte

Helper cell

T cell receptor

Plasma cell

B lymphocyte re-expression of surface immunoglobulin

Fig. 13-4. antigen capture, processing, and presentation by B lymphocytes. the B-lymphocyte surface immunoglobulin binds exposed determinants on an intact protein antigen, triggering the antigen/immunoglobulin complex to be internalized. the endocytosed complex is degraded into small peptides. this degradation process exposes these peptide determinants, which now associate with class II MHC molecules. In a matter of hours, the peptide/MHC complex is expressed on the B-cell surface, now in a form recognizable by helper T cells. The antigen presentation and conjugation process of B and T cells result in their mutual activation, with T cells enlarging and synthesizing cytokines that help B cells differentiate into antibody secreting plasma cells. Some B cells do not differentiate into plasma cells but re-express surface immunoglobulin and may survive as B-memory cells.

sion and differentiation to effector cells. This would include B-cell differentiation to antibody-secreting plasma cells and T-cell proliferation and differentiation into a lymphocyte that provides the lymphokines needed for B-cell proliferation and differentiation.

CELL-MEDIATED IMMUNITY

T-Cell Subpopulations and Cytokine Production

The T-cell maturation process in the thymus has been partially delineated using two CD markers[20,21]: CD4 and CD8. One subset that fails to express both CD4 and CD8 uses the $\gamma\delta$ TCR gene products in association with the CD3 complex and appears in the periphery in the epidermis and intestinal epithelium and in lung.[22,23] The function of the $CD3^+$, $CD4^-$, $CD8^-$ $\gamma\delta$ T cells is unclear, but some evidence suggests that they are important in initiating immune responses to microbial antigens at epithelial cell interfaces. In contrast to the $CD4^-/CD8^- \gamma\delta$ T cells, the mature thymocytes in the thymic medulla display either CD4 or CD8, in conjunction with the TCR $\alpha\beta$-gene products and CD3.[17] These cells serve to seed the peripheral circulating pool with mature T lymphocytes.

One major subset of peripheral mature T cells is composed of approximately 20–30% $CD4^-/CD8^+$ cells. This subset of cells is restricted to recognizing processed protein antigens associated with class I MHC (e.g., HLA, A, B, C region gene products). Functionally, they are characterized as cytolytic (or cytotoxic) T cells and, in some cases, as the so-called T-suppressor cells. These CD8 expressing cytolytic T lymphocytes are critical effectors in killing host cells that contain intracellular microorganisms, particularly viruses. These intracellular organisms are not accessible to the humoral elements of the immune response. Once generated (in concert with lymphokines produced by T-helper cells), the cytolytic T cells recognize non-self- peptides in association with class I MHC antigens. After the $CD8^+$ T cells encounter the peptide/class I MHC complex, there is a brief conjugation with the target cell, followed by $CD8^+$ T-cell activation and killing of the target cell. Some viruses are cytopathic, while others are noncytopathic. This presents a problem, as the cytolytic T cells are very effective at killing host cells that may not be virally damaged and are of no real threat to the host. For example, in humans much of the damage of viral hepatitis is not caused by the virus, but by the extensive liver damage caused by cytolytic T cells.

Finally, the $CD8^+$ T cells are also critically important effector cells for attacking transplanted tissue (in concert with $CD4^+$ T cells), as well as for some types of malignant cells. Unfortunately, relatively little is known about the peptides recognized on class I MHC expressing tumor cells which stimulate cytotoxic T cells. Moreover, the potential for $CD8^+$ secretion of lymphokines is only beginning to be uncovered.[24]

The other major fraction of peripheral T lymphocytes display only CD4 and are typically characterized as "helper" T cells. Earlier in this chapter, the ability of B cells to present antigen to $CD4^+$ T cells was discussed. One of the reasons the $CD4^+$ T cells are called "helper" cells is that they produce the crucial lymphokines[19,25] necessary for B lymphocytes to become activated, proliferate, and differentiate into plasma cells (Fig. 13-4). In addition to their key role in antibody production, $CD4^+$ T cells are needed to mediate delayed-type hypersensitivity (DTH) reactions. An example is the skin testing procedure, which uses purified protein derivative of old tuberculin broth to test for prior exposure to tubercle bacilli. Examination of the cellular infiltrate reveals predominantly a mononuclear cell (macrophages/lymphocytes) infiltrate. Analysis of the surface antigens on the lymphocytes demonstrates that the dominant effector cells are $CD4^+/CD8^-$. These DTH reactions are

Table 13-1. Cytokine Synthesis Patterns of $CD4^+$ T Lymphocytes

	IL-2	IFN-γ	LT	IL-4	IL-5	IL-10	IL-3	CSF-GM
T_{H0}	+	+	+	+	+	+	+	+
T_{H1}	+	+	+	–	–	–	+	+
T_{H2}	–	–	–	+	+	+	+	+

Abbreviations: LT, lymphotoxin; IFN, interferon; IL, interleukin; CSF-GM, colony-stimulating factor-granulocyte/macrophage.

critically dependent on the lymphokines secreted by $CD4^+$ cells (see below and the section Delayed-Type Hypersensitivity and Cytotoxic T-Cell Responses).

The immune system has distinct elements that tend to specialize in one aspect of immunity or another, including humoral versus cell-mediated immunity and $CD8^+$ cytolytic versus $CD4^+$ helper T lymphocytes. A very exciting concept has recently emerged. Careful analysis of mouse and human $CD4^+$ T lymphocyte clones showed that these clones could generally be divided into two major subsets, clarifying the division of labor between $CD4^+$ T cells that act to help B cells make antibody, yet must also function to stimulate cell-mediated immunity and DTH reactions. Mouse, and more recently human, $CD4^+$ T cells, have been further divided into subsets called T_{H1} and T_{H2} cells.[19,25,26] Table 13-1 presents cytokine profiles of these cells. The important points are that the T_{H1} cells that synthesize interleukin-2 (IL-2) and interferon-γ (IFN-γ) specialize in cell-mediated immune responses (e.g., DTH), while the T_{H2} subset produces IL-4, IL-5, and IL-10 and assists in B-cell production of antibody (particularly IgM, IgG, and IgE) for humoral responses. Another subset of T cells called T_{H0} may be precursors to T_{H1} and T_{H2} and synthesize a variety of cytokines (Table 13-1). The preferential development of one T-cell subset over another could dictate the outcome of an immune response. For example, different mouse strains infected with *Leishmania major* induce either a T_{H1} or T_{H2} response.[27] Strains that make a T_{H1} response eliminate the organism and survive. Those that make a predominant T_{H2} response die. In humans, a predominant T_{H1} response leads to a tuberculoid form of leprosy, in which the organisms are contained and the clinical course generally benign, whereas a T_{H2} response leads to the devastating progressive lepromatous form.[28] In allergic patients, many investigators find a predominance of T_{H2} cells that secrete IL-4, the cytokine needed for B-cell production of IgE antibody.[26,29] It is becoming clear that dominance of one type of T-helper cell can lead to either a predominant humoral response (T_{H2}) or toward the cell-mediated, DTH response (T_{H1}). This may result in future therapy whereby the immune response is guided by using the proper cytokines or cytokine inhibitors to generate the type of T-cell response desired.

Delayed-Type Hypersensitivity and Cytotoxic T-Cell Responses

Typically immediate (humoral) and DTH reactions differ in terms of the time course of their expression, mediators, and cellular infiltrates. For example, most immediate reactions are transferable by serum and peak within minutes to hours. By contrast, DTH reactions develop over a period of 24–48 hours and, as discussed above, can only be transferred to naive individuals by immune effector T cells. The period required for the development of a full-fledged DTH is a function of the requirement of a massive cellular infiltrate of mononuclear cells to migrate to the scene, be activated, and begin to destroy and eliminate the invading organism. The tuberculin skin test is a classic (noninfectious) example of such a reaction in which the dermis provides a window to observe what occurs in an infected milieu in the body. A more extensive example is seen in tuberculous and lepromatous reactions in the lung and extremities, respectively.

Mechanistically, the DTH response is initiated by CD4$^+$ T cells, which actively recruit the inflammatory cells from rapidly dividing bone marrow precursors. Adoptive transfer experiments performed several decades ago demonstrated that the numbers of lymphocytes required for a DTH response was only a fraction (1–5%) of the final cellular infiltrate. In addition, using the migration inhibition assay, in vitro analyses could be carried out with only 1% sensitized T cells plus 99% normal macrophages. In vivo, this reaction is attributable to the recognition by specific T cells of defined antigenic peptides presented on the surface of an APC, these T cells begin to secrete a series of cytokines (see below). As demonstrated by adoptive transfer of labeled lymphocytes and bone marrow cells, most of the cells that migrate to the site arrive by the bloodstream from these short-lived myeloid precursors in the bone marrow.

The T cells responsible for initiating this reaction remain at the site of antigenic invasion and synthesize a number cytokines important for recruiting, activating, and retaining macrophages at that location.[25] One cytokine is a monocyte/macrophage chemotactic factor that stimulates monocyte/macrophage migration to the tissue site.[30] Once, there IFN-γ, a powerful cytokine produced by T$_{H1}$ cells, helps blunt the T$_{H2}$ response and serves as an important activator of macrophages.[25] Macrophage activation involves enlargement, expression of class II MHC antigens (so they will act as better APCs), and an increase in their ability to kill microbes due to stimulation of the respiratory burst and enhanced synthesis of proteolytic enzymes. Finally, CD4$^+$ T cells synthesize migration inhibition factor(s), which tends to immobilize macrophages and retain them where they are needed. Therefore, the DTH reaction is a paradigm of the elimination of invading organisms by the immune system. It demonstrates a combination of specific recognition of antigen by T cells on APCs, recruitment of effector mononuclear cells from the bloodstream via cytokines, their activation, and subsequent intracellular destruction of the invader.

Another form of DTH response is that provoked by contact sensitization (e.g., dinitrochlorobenzene, nickel, poison ivy). Typically, the cellular infiltrate and kinetics are identical to a tuberculin reaction, although some evidence shows that the initiating effector cells include CD8$^+$ cells. Since the nature of the cytokines produced by CD8$^+$ cells is less well defined, the mechanism of infiltration and inflammation in contact reactions may be somewhat different.

The removal of an invading organism is carried out in DTH through an indirect pathway. Another form of cell-mediated immunity involves the direct destruction of an infected target cell. Thus, when a virus invades a particular host cell and begins to replicate, some viable proteins are brought to the surface, and are presented in a groove of the HLA class I molecules. These viral peptides thus are displayed as flags on any infected cell. Cytotoxic T cells destroy cells bearing these flags.

The process of cytotoxic T-cell destruction initially involves recognition by the TCR, followed by rapid signal transduction and activation of these cells, and finally the effector activity causes the infected host cells to literally explode. While the detailed mechanism of cytotoxicity has been studied for decades, it is not entirely clear whether there is a single pathway of destruction. However, a set of proteins called the perforins are released as granules by cytotoxic cells and appear to enter the target cells to mediate their destruction.[31] In addition, other actions of the cytotoxic cell, which may require host metabolic activity, lead to the dissolution of the nuclear membrane and ultimately to apoptosis.

REGULATION OF IMMUNE RESPONSIVENESS

B-Cell and T-Cell Tolerance as a Lifelong Process

One of the salient features of the immune system is that it is able to discriminate between self and foreign epitopes. The process by which this occurs is learned and occurs both during early development of the immune system, and throughout life. This property, termed immunologic tolerance or unresponsiveness, leads to either the elimination or the silencing of specific self-antigen-reactive clones by several possible mechanisms. These processes include (1) clonal deletion, (2) clonal anergy, and (3) active suppression of anti-self-reactivity. While evidence for each of these mechanisms has been obtained, the dominance of one or another pathway may depend on the nature of the antigen, its distribution and concentration, and the time at which it is expressed during human development.

Historically, that individuals do not respond to their own self-proteins was recognized as early as 1900. However, an experimental basis for the lack of anti-self-reactivity was not provided until the observations of Owen,[32] who noted that nonidentical (dizygotic) cattle twins possessed and tolerated blood cells from their fraternal sibling. Interestingly, these animals shared a blood supply in utero. Moreover, the twins could exchange and maintain skin grafts. These observations led to the suggestion that exposure of an individual's (immature) immune system during development led to the induction of tolerance to those antigens. This was formally tested in the elegant experiments conducted by Medawar and colleagues,[33] who demonstrated that perinatal injection of allogeneic lymphoid cells into mice caused subsequent acceptance of those skin grafts as if they were self, while still allowing different foreign skin grafts to be rejected. Thus, immunologic tolerance was specific and was due to an early exposure to antigen. This has led to the concept that one of the parameters for tolerance induction is the interaction of immature, developing T (and B) cells, incapable of mounting a full-blown immune response against that antigenic epitope. This notion is essentially correct, although it does not exclude the development of tolerance in more mature cells by other mechanisms. The assumption is that such potentially autoreactive cells are actually eliminated (deleted) during this process early in life. Hence, one would not expect to see any significant number of anti-self-binding B or T cells in the circulation, an observation that is generally supported, despite observations of low-affinity reactivity to self.

Tolerance is both dose dependent and of finite duration. If one were to induce tolerance experimentally in a neonatal animal, it would persist into adult life. but tolerance would eventually wane, unless the antigen were capable of establishing a persistent chimeric state, such as the lymphoid cells in the Medawar's experiments. In fact, once the number of antigenic moieties diminishes below a specific threshold level, tolerance begins to wane as new cells that develop are not exposed to these antigens during development. Hence, maintenance of tolerance is a lifelong process requiring periodic antigen exposure as new clones arise.

Tolerance or unresponsiveness is a property of both T and B cells. Over 20 years ago, Weigle and colleagues[34] demonstrated that both types of lymphocytes were rendered unresponsive in vivo, and that tolerance persisted for a longer period in T cells than in B cells (Fig. 13-5). Presumably the longer persistence of tolerance in the T-cell repertoire reflects the length of time needed for T-cell development and the long-lived nature of these lymphocytes; while B cells generally turn over more rapidly. T-cell tolerance typically requires lower doses of antigen than B-cell tolerance. The molecular basis for this phenomenon is not understood, although it may reflect a difference in the chemistry of the epitopes normally recognized by B cells

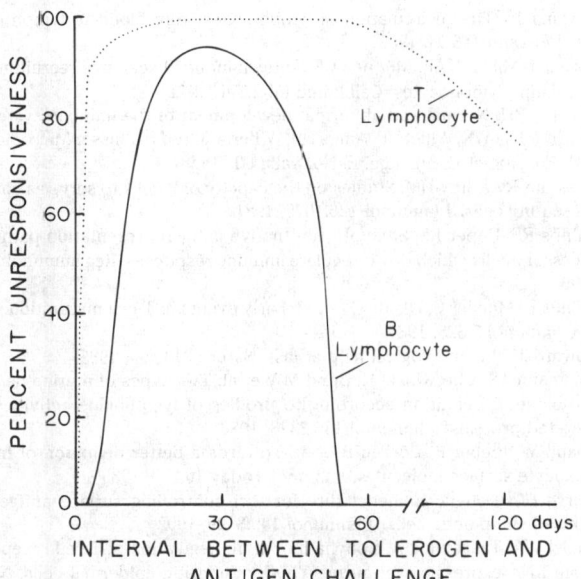

Fig. 13-5. Kinetics of T- and B-lymphocyte tolerance induction. On exposure to a protein tolerogen (e.g., the intravenous administration of a high dose of a monomeric protein), T cells and shortly thereafter B cells become refractory to that same protein presented in an immunogenic form. In some instances, the B and T cells may be clonally deleted, and in others they remain viable but are rendered anergic (unable to be triggered by antigen). Eventually, both B- and T-cell compartments recover from the tolerance protocol. The B cells recover faster, perhaps because of their more rapid turnover in vivo.

(conformational) versus T cells (denatured proteins), and the nature of antigen presentation to both cells.

While deletion has been assumed to be a major mechanism of unresponsiveness, definitive proof of this process was difficult since the disappearance of rare antigen-reactive cells would be nearly impossible to detect. The recent development of transgenic mouse systems has helped address this issue. When transgenic mice are made that contain a rearranged TCR or IgM receptor, endogenous rearrangements are generally suppressed, and virtually all the T or B cells, respectively, express the rearranged TCR or immunoglobulin gene. Thus, exposure of these animals to the antigen recognized by their rearranged receptor can lead to unresponsiveness during development. Therefore, TCR transgenic mice exposed to antigen, by breeding with an animal that expresses that epitope, may show a loss of specific T cells; similarly, immunoglobulin transgenic mice reactive to a given peptide show disappearance of B cells when exposed to that peptide or bred to other transgenic mice expressing that peptide.[35]

Anergy has also been demonstrated in such model systems. That is, in some transgenic mice, exposure to the putatively tolerated epitope leads to functional inactivation, but not a disappearance of reactive lymphocytes. Hence, one can observe B cells that can bind the tolerated antigen in vitro, yet cannot be simulated to produce antibodies. This form of functional anergy has also been demonstrated for T-cell clones exposed to certain antigens on inappropriate APCs in vitro. Thus, both deletion and anergy can be seen as mechanisms for tolerance. It is not clear which mechanism predominates, although the nature of the antigen clearly plays a role; that is, membrane-bound antigens tend to cause anergy. In addition, expression of IgD on B cells can provide a resistance to deletion and lead to anergy.[36]

Suppression is defined as a state of unresponsiveness that is maintained by cells capable of preventing other reactive cells from responding. Although numerous examples for suppression of immune responses, both specific and non-specific, have

been described, there is no formal demonstration that this is due to a new type of so-called suppressor cell. Rather, down-regulation of immune responsiveness seems to be a property of T cells in general and of their cytokines in particular. Thus, cytokines such as IFN-γ, tumor necrosis factor, or IL-10 may modulate immune responsiveness or be directly cytotoxic for other cells in the immune system.

As stated earlier, tolerance is a property that is considered to be induced during early development of the immune system. Numerous systems have evolved in which unresponsiveness also can be elicited in adult life. This occurs by virtue of exposure of T cells to peptides on nonprofessional APCs such as keratinocytes.[16] Moreover, ultracentrifuged immunoglobulin carriers (consisting of monomeric protein) have been used to induce tolerance in experimental systems.[37] Nonetheless, tolerance induced either as in the neonatal period or in the adult is still of finite duration. Therefore, it is necessary to continue to expose the developing immune system to antigen to prevent the inappropriate development of autoreactivity. Since potentially autoreactive rearrangement may occur randomly, the maintenance of tolerance must be ensured by an exposure mechanism and a window of opportunity to induce tolerance even later in life. The best example of a naturally occurring loss of self-tolerance is the response of adults to human fetal hemoglobin. That is, with time and the disappearance of fetal hemoglobin, new cells can develop that are not tolerant to this protein. Therefore, if challenged with fetal hemoglobin, adults make antibodies.

Antibody Feedback and Idiotype Regulation

The immune system is regulated by its own products. That is, cytokines produced in the immune system may down-regulate the responses of other subpopulations of cells and antibody can feedback to regulate its own formation. An example of this is seen in the treatment of erythroblastosis fetalis or hemolytic disease of the newborn. Mothers who are RhD⁻ and who bear an RhD⁺ child are exposed to an antigen to which they are not tolerant at parturition. These mothers have the potential to form anti-RhD antibodies that can cause this devastating disease during their second pregnancy and with an RhD⁺ child. Treatment of this disease uses an anti-RhD antibody administered at the time of delivery of the first child. This treatment is virtually 100% successful at preventing the formation of anti-RhD antibodies and subsequent disease. The most obvious mechanism to explain how this works is the removal of antigen. Evidence for this clearly exists. A second mechanism involves the formation of immune complexes that can feed back and inhibit antigen-reactive B cells.[37]

Antibody regulates its own formation in vivo as the immune system matures, and there is a competition for available antigen leading to antibody-producing clones of increasing affinity. By eliminating antigen, the immune system is in fact depleting itself of the stimulus for continued immune responsiveness, while at the same time selecting for higher-affinity responses to develop at a later time.

Immunoglobulins also bear antigenic determinants that are believed to be recognized by the immune system and used to regulate responsiveness. The particular epitopes expressed in immunoglobulin V regions, for example, are called idiotypes and theoretically can be recognized to elicit an anti-idiotypic response. Presumably, humans are not tolerant to these epitopes because the immune system is not exposed to high enough quantities of idiotype early in life. Once an immune response occurs, the amount of a given idiotype will increase and immune complexes form that can be immunogenic for the idiotype. The initiation of an anti-idiotype response can then be imagined as a controlling factor to down-regulate idiotype formation. Therefore, anti-idiotype might directly inactivate antibody (idiotype) producing cells by interaction with the surface receptors to give a negative signal or merely block antigen recognition.

SUMMARY

The immune system is organized to provide a multifaceted response that is appropriate for a given organism. The nature of the invader will partially control the kind of response elicited. Moreover, the cytokines produced by immune effector cells influence the extent of the response and modulate other forms of responsiveness. By design, the immune system is structured to make molecules (antibodies and cytokines) that rapidly respond to particular invasions from outside, while tolerating self, and preventing ineffective responses.

ACKNOWLEDGMENTS

We thank Sandy Lynah for her expert secretarial help with this manuscript and Melinda Borrello for critically reading the manuscript. This work was supported by grants Al29691 and CA55644 (DWS) and by CA42739, CA55305, and CA11198 (RP).

REFERENCES

1. Gowans JL, McGregor DD: The immunological activities of lymphocytes. Prog Allergy 9:1, 1966
2. Tew JG, Kosco MH, Burton GF, Szakal AK: Follicular dendritic cells as accessor cells. Immunol Rev 117:185, 1990
3. Tew JG, Phipps RP, Mandel TE: Role of follicular antigen-binding dendritic reticular cells in the regulation of humoral antibody responses. Immunol Rev 53:175, 1980
4. Steinman RM, Nussenzweig MC: Dendritic cells: features and functions. Immunol Rev 53:53, 1980
5. Pickes LJ, Butcher EC: Physiological and molecular mechanisms of lymphocyte homing. Annu Rev Immunol 10:561, 1992
6. Scolley RG, Butcher EC, Weissman IL: Thymus cell migration: quantitative aspects of cellular traffic from the thymus to the periphery in mice. Eur J Immunol 10:210, 1980
7. Kayhty H, Pehtola H, Karanko V, Makela PH: The protective level of serum antibodies to the capsular polysaccharide of Haemophilus influenzae type b. J Infect Dis 76:52, 1983
8. Silverstein AM, Uhr JW, Kramer K, Lukes RJ: The fetal responses to antigenic stimulus. II. Antibody production by the fetal lamb. J Exp Med 117:799, 1963
9. Klinman NR: The acquisition of B-cell competence and diversity. Am J Pathol 85:695, 1976
10. Alt FW, Blackwell TK, Yankopoulos GD: Development of the primary antibody repertoire. Science 238:1079, 1987
11. Perlmutter RM, Kearney JF, Chang SP, Hood LE: Developmentally controlled expression of immunoglobulin genes. Science 227:1597, 1985
12. Gowans JL: The recirculation of lymphocytes from blood to lymph in the rat. J Physiol 146:54, 1959
13. Sprent J, Miller JFAP, Mitchell GF: Antigen-induced selective recruitment of circulating lymphocytes. Cell Immunol 2:171, 1971
14. Buckley RH: Normal and abnormal development of the immune system. p. 226. In Joklik WK, Willet HP, Amos DB, Wilfert CM (eds): Zinsser Microbiology. 19th Ed. Appleton & Lange, E. Norwalk, CT, 1988
15. Chestnut RW, Grey HM: Studies on the capcity of B cells to serve as antigen-presenting cells. J Immunol 126:1075, 1981
16. Phipps RP, Roper RL, Stein SH: Alternative antigen presentation pathways: accessory cells which down-regulate immune responses. Reg Immunol 2:326, 1989
17. Adkins B, Mueller C, Okada CY et al: Early events in T-cell maturation. Annu Rev Immunol 5:325, 1987
18. Howard JC: Immunological help at last. Nature 314:494, 1985
19. Mosmann TR, Cherwinski H, Bond MW et al: Two types of murine helper T cell clone. I. Definition according to profiles of lymphokine activities and secreted proteins. J Immunol 136:2348, 1986
20. Knapp W, Rieber P, Dörken B et al: Towards a better definition of human leukocyte surface molecules. Immunol Today 10:253, 1989
21. Morse HC: Genetic nomenclature for loci controlling surface antigens of mouse hemopoietic cells. J Immunol 149:3129, 1992
22. Kuziel WA, Takashima A, Bonyhadi M et al: Regulation of T-cell receptor γ-chain RNA expression in murine Thy-1$^+$ dendritic epidermal cells. Nature 328:263, 1987
23. Goodman T, LeFrancois L: Expression of the gamma/delta T-cell receptor on intestinal CD8$^+$ intraepithelial lymphocytes. Nature 333:855, 1988
24. Fong TA, Mosmann TR: Alloreactive murine CD8$^+$ T cell clones secrete the TH1 pattern of cytokines. J Immunol 144:1744, 1990
25. Street NE, Mosmann TR: Functional diversity of T lymphocytes due to secretion of different cytokine patterns. FASEB J 5:171, 1991
26. Kapsenberg ML, Wieenga EA, Bos JD, Jensen HM: Functional subsets of allergen reactive human CD4$^+$ T cells. Immunol Today 12:392, 1991
27. Heinzel FP, Sadick MD, Mutha SS, Locksley RM: Production of IFNγ, IL-2, IL-4 and IL-10 by CD4 lymphocytes in vivo during healing and progressive murine leishmaniasis. Proc Natl Acad Sci USA 88:7011, 1991
28. Yamamura M, Uyemura K, Deans RJ et al: Defining protective responses to pathogens: cytokine profiles in leprosy legions. Science 254:277, 1991
29. Robinson DS, Hamid Q, Ying S et al: Evidence for a predominant "TH2 type" bronchoalveolar lavage T-lymphocyte population in atopic asthma. N Engl J Med 326:298, 1992
30. Muramori K, Mitsuyama M, Handa T et al: A dissociated induction of MCF-producing and MAF-producing T cells specific for Listeria monocytogenes in the in vitro primary culture system. Immunology 72:373, 1991
31. Podack ER, Hengartner H, Lichtenheld MG: A central role in perforin in cytolysis? Annu Rev Immunol 9:129, 1991
32. Owen RD: Immunogenetic consequences of vascular anastomoses between bovine twins. Science 102:400, 1945
33. Billingham RE, Brent L, Medawar PB: Quantitative studies on tissue transplantation immunity. III. Activity acquired tolerance. Philos Trans R Soc Lond Biol 239:257, 1956
34. Chiller J, Habicht G, Weigle WO: Kinetic differences in unresponsiveness of thymus and bone marrow cells. Science 171:813, 1971
35. Nossal JGV: Cellular and molecular mechanisms of B lymphocyte tolerance. Adv Immunol 52:283, 1992.
36. Scott DW: Analysis of B cell tolerance in vitro. Adv Immunol 54:393, 1993
37. Fedyk ER, Borrello MA, Brown DM, Phipps RP: Regulation of B cell tolerance and triggering by immune complexes. Chem Immunol 58:67, 1994

BIOLOGY OF STEM CELLS AND DISORDERS OF HEMATOPOIESIS

Part III

Stem Cell Model of Hematopoiesis

14

David A. Williams

INTRODUCTION

Healthy individuals require adequate production of enormous numbers of differentiated blood cells daily. Mature blood cells are derived from undifferentiated stem and progenitor cells in a complex series of maturational and divisional steps not yet completely understood. The complexity of this system is enormous, since as many as 10^{10} erythrocytes and 10^8-10^9 white blood cells are produced each hour each day during the lifetime of the individual. Additional complexities include the need for rapid responses to acute stress (blood loss or infection) and the need to maintain a pool of undifferentiated cells from which mature cells are derived. Finally, mature blood cells must function in anatomic locations widely separated from the bone marrow, where most cells arise. Abnormalities of this process are manifested by sometimes life-threatening diseases such as aplastic anemia, cytopenias, leukemias, and other myeloproliferative disorders.

Understanding the complex relationships involved in blood cell production has been possible due to continued basic science research by experimental hematologists, radiobiologists, and immunologists. Careful staining and microscopic observation of bone marrow cells by pathologists and hematopathologists have led to a clear understanding of the maturational steps involved in precursor cell differentiation. In 1961 Till and McCullough[1] developed an in vivo colony assay that identified a murine pluripotent and self-renewing stem cell, the colony-forming unit-spleen (CFU-S); this assay allowed initial characterization of a transplantable primitive bone marrow cell. Pluznik and Sachs[2] and Bradley and Metcalf[3] later described in vitro colony assays for hematopoietic progenitor cells, which led to new understanding of the role of growth-stimulatory proteins in hematopoietic cell survival and differentiation. The molecular cloning of a number of growth factors, including several now in clinical use, is in part due to these early accomplishments. The influence of the bone marrow environment on hematopoiesis was initially suggested by Wolf and Trentin.[4] Again, progress in our understanding of the role of environmental signals in hematopoiesis was brought about by the description by Dexter et al[5] of an in vitro culture system that mimicked the medullary environment and allowed continued production of myeloid hematopoietic cells for months in culture flasks.

HEMATOPOIETIC CELL HIERARCHY

The experimental systems described above, as well as many other experimental approaches and observations, have led to some general hematopoietic concepts. Blood cell formation occurs as a result of a series of maturational cell divisions. The hematopoietic system, which gives rise to all circulating blood cells, can be envisioned as a series of overlapping functional compartments (Fig. 14-1). The stem cell compartment is made up of rare primitive cells that are multipotential (maintain the capacity to give rise to all lineages of blood cells) and have a high self-renewal capacity (give rise to "identical" daughter stem cells).[6] A characteristic of the stem cell compartment is that most stem cells are mitotically quiescent.

A process termed commitment describes the transition from pluripotent, self-renewing cells in the stem cell compartment to the progenitor cell compartment. The process is incompletely understood, but is characterized by restriction in the stem cell differentiative and proliferative capacity. Progenitor cell compartments are comprised mainly of cells with the capacity to differentiate along one lineage (unipotential progenitors), with lower frequencies of bipotential and multipotential primitive cells. Therefore, commitment involves the acquisition of some specific growth factor receptors and loss of others. Progenitor cells are generally defined functionally, that is, by the capacity of the cells to form colonies in in vitro assays; they demonstrate little self-renewal capacity. Mitotically active cells are far more frequent in progenitor compartments compared with stem cell compartments.

Most cells in the bone marrow make up the precursor compartment. These cells exhibit easily recognized nuclear and cytoplasmic morphologic characteristics that can be used to classify the lineage of commitment of the precursor cell. For example, a myeloblast has distinguishing morphologic characteristics that allow classification into the lineage of cells destined to become granulocytes. Little self-renewal capacity exists in this compartment, but because of the large number of precursor cells and the high mitotic activity of these less primitive cells, considerable amplification in absolute cell numbers occurs within these compartments. Therefore, early cells have the capacity to give rise to large numbers of progeny cells on a clonal basis during the transition from stem cell to differentiated and functional cell.

PURIFICATION AND FUNCTIONAL CHARACTERISTICS OF HEMATOPOIETIC STEM AND PROGENITOR CELLS

Stem cells have been defined functionally by the ability to reconstitute both lymphoid and myeloid hematopoiesis when transplanted into a recipient. Initial studies used radioprotection as an assay for this rare cell,[7] while Till and McCulloch[1] developed the first quantitative assay for stem cells based on reinfusion of cells into an irradiated recipient (Fig. 14-2). Detailed understanding of the biology of the hematopoietic stem cell has been hindered by the low frequency of this cell in the bone marrow nucleated cell population, the lack of reagents to distinguish the stem cell from other immature cell types, and the lack of practical and quantitative assays for human hematopoietic stem cells. Recent advances have been made in all of these problematic areas. Hematopoietic stem cells have been reported to be purified to a high degree using density gradient centrifugation, labeling with antibodies, lectins, or dyes, and separation on fluorescence-activated cell sorters. Additional separation methods include immunomagnetic bead selection or the use of immunopanning.[8] Immunologic characteristics of murine hematopoietic cells include lack of antigens present on more lineage-restricted progenitors (termed Lin⁻), expression of the antigens Sca-1 (Ly6),[9] Qa-m7,[10] and Thy-1.[9] In addition, several investigators have used the intensity of mitochondrial staining with rhodamine 123, which is related

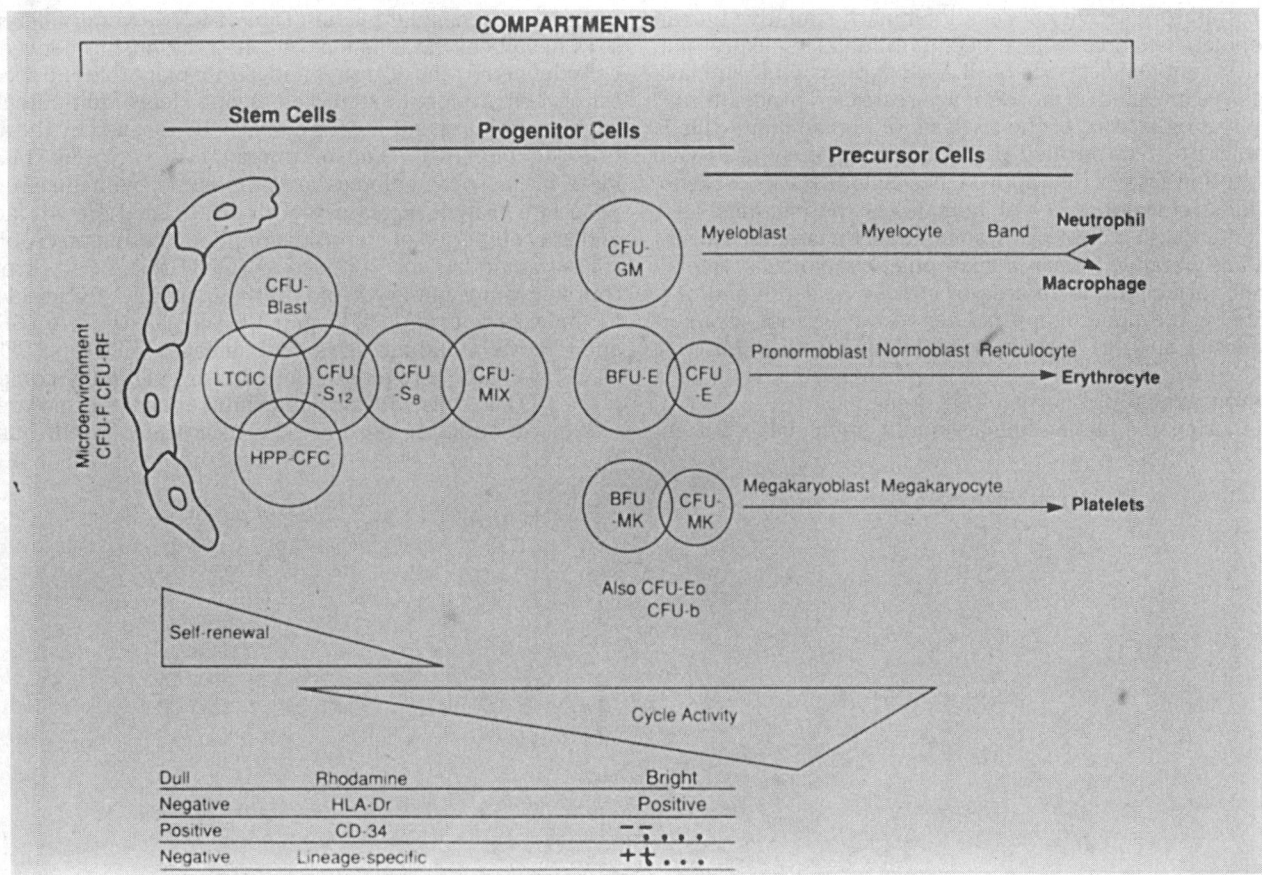

Figure 14-1. Schematic view of hematopoietic compartments. Primitive stem cells reside in close association with cells making up the hematopoietic microenvironment. Several in vitro and in vivo assays are represented by the Venn diagram, since the relationship of these cells and the reconstituting hematopoietic stem cell is unclear. Cells in the progenitor compartments are defined by in vitro colony assays. Precursor cells are morphologically recognizable cells in the bone marrow environment. See text for full details.

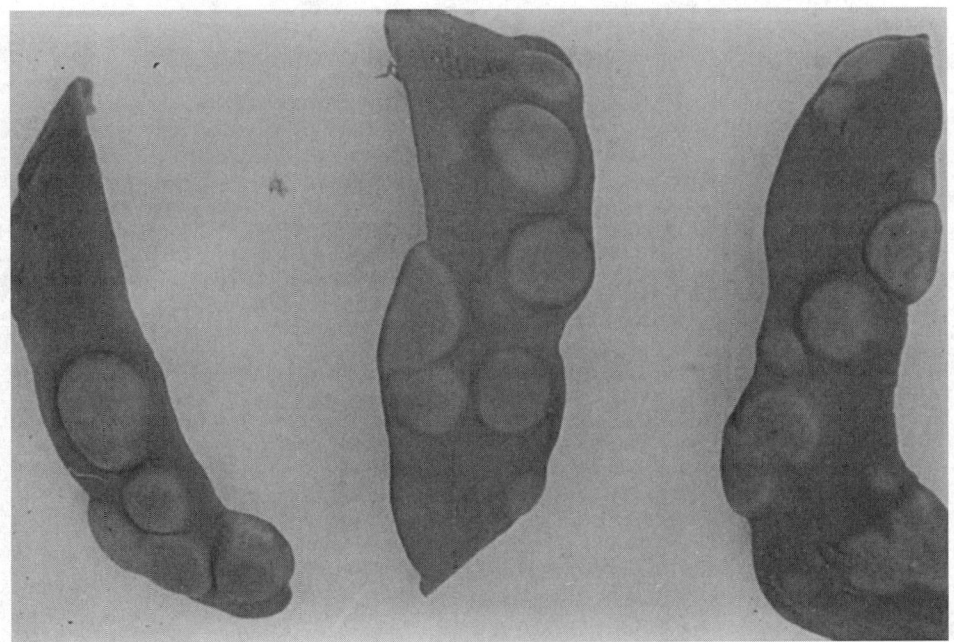

Figure 14-2. CFU-S assay. Hematopoietic colonies arising from the CFU-S stem/progenitor cell 14 days after injection of murine bone marrow into lethally irradiated mice.

to the respiratory activity of cells.[11] Similarly, putative human hematopoietic stem cells have been purified using expression of the CD34 antigen,[12,13] lack of HLA-DR expression,[14] and lack of antigens expressed on more lineage-restricted progenitors.[15] A complicating feature of the analysis of human stem cells is the inability to test purified populations routinely in in vivo reconstitution assays. New approaches include the use of xenografts for "reconstitution" of human cell populations after transplantation.[16,17] Table 14-1 summarizes characteristics of murine and putative human hematopoietic stem cells. Human stem cell purification is an area of intense research and may provide new therapeutic approaches to the treatment of certain diseases, such as chronic myeloloid leukemia (CML), for which the goal of current work is to purify normal stem cells from cytogenetically abnormal CML stem cells.

Both murine and human hematopoietic stem cells can form colonies in semisolid media (Table 14-2). Several different assays have been established, but the relationship between the cells defined by these assays and a transplantable and reconstituting hematopoietic stem cell is not clear. Multipotent and unipotential progenitor cells can also be assayed by the ability to form colonies in semisolid medium in vitro (Fig. 14-3 and Plate 14-1). These colonies are stimulated by inclusion of appropriate growth regulatory proteins, termed growth factors, and are comprised of maturing granulocytes and macrophages (CFU-granulocyte/macrophage [CFU-GM]), erythrocytes (burst-forming unit-erythroid [BFU-E], and CFU-erythroid [CFU-E], megakaryocytes, (BFU- and CFU-megakaryocyte [BFU-Mk and CFU-Mk]), and mixtures of all lineages (CFU-mix [CFU-Mix or CFU-GEMM]). Progenitor colonies are generally composed of 50–100,000 cells, most which exhibit a relatively mature phenotype. In addition, murine[5] and to a lesser extent human[18]

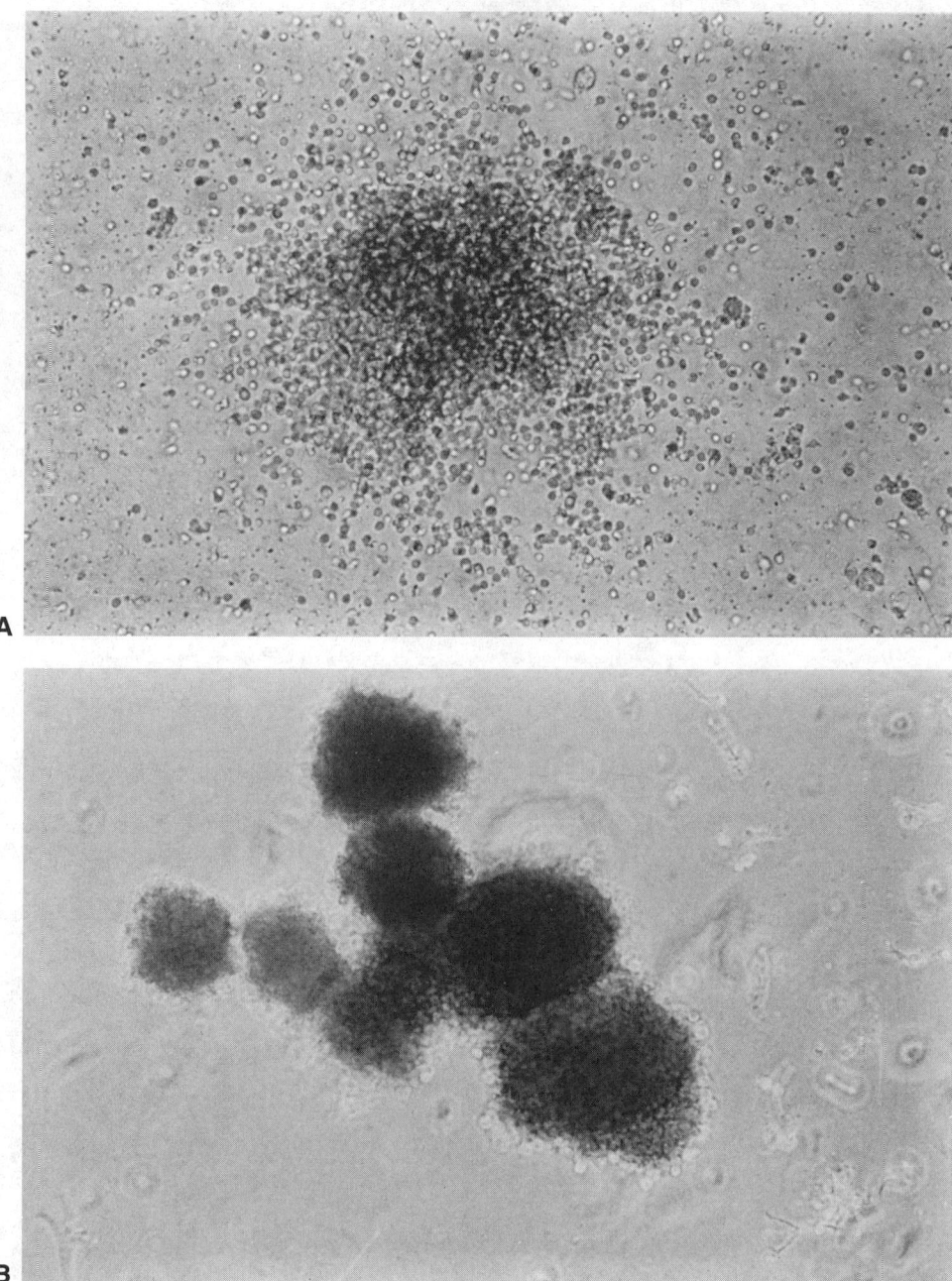

Figure 14-3. Progenitor assay. Colonies arising in vitro in semisolid medium after plating of human bone marrow cells. **(A)** Colony-forming unit-granulocyte/macrophage (CFU-GM). **(B)** Burst-forming unit-erythroid (BFU-E). (*Figure continues.*)

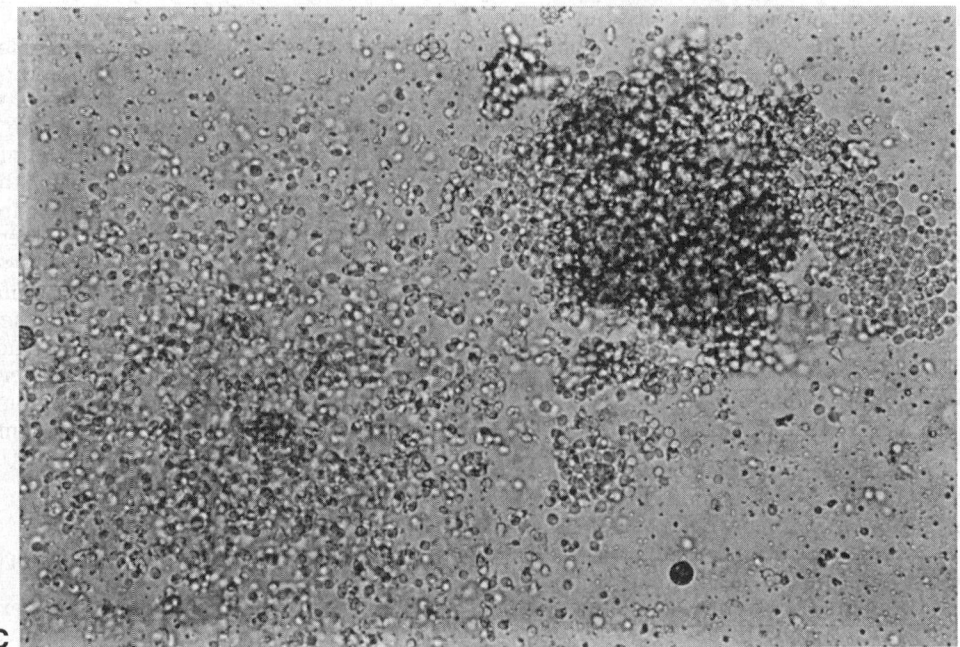

Figure 14-3 *(Continued).* **(C)** Colony-forming unit-megakaryocyte (CFU-Mk), upper right and CFU-GM, lower right. (See also Plate 14-1.)

hematopoietic stem and progenitor cells can be cultured for prolonged periods in vitro in a culture system, termed long-term marrow or Dexter cultures, which allows direct contact between these hematopoietic cells and supporting cells derived from the medullary cavity.

Commitment

The factors that regulate hematopoietic cell proliferation and differentiation, including commitment, remain unknown. Theories of stem cell behavior include the stochastic model,[19] which considers stem cell renewal versus differentiation to be based on probability, and the hematopoietic inductive environment theory,[4] which links commitment to local environmental signals. In either case, the survival and differentiation of hematopoietic stem cells can be influenced by an ever-increasing number of glycoproteins, termed cytokines, which stimulate both cell division and survival.[20] Recent evidence suggests that the provision of appropriate cytokines in vitro can induce the expansion of primitive progenitor cells without the loss of reconstitution capacity.[21] Growth factors that appear to be important in the survival of stem cells and expansion of progenitor cells in vitro include steel factor (also called stem cell factor, kit ligand, and mast cell growth factor), interleukin-1 (IL-1), IL-6 and possibly IL-11, colony-stimulating factor-granulocyte (CSF-G),[22] and leukemia inhibitory factor (LIF).[23]

Table 14-1. Phenotypic Characterization of Murine and Human Hematopoietic Stem Cells

Mouse	Human
Ly6A (Sca-1)+	CD34+
Lin−	HLA-DR−
thy 1+	c-kit+
c-kit+	CD15−, CD77−
Rhodamine^dull	thy 1+
5-FU resistant	Rhodamine^dull
	5-FU resistant
	4-HC resistant

(From Williams,[22] with permission.)

Based on in vitro data, Ogawa[24] has proposed that these factors may function by triggering cell cycle-dormant primitive cells into proliferation. Some of these factors (CSF-G, IL-3, and steel factor) may be required for the survival of primitive hematopoietic cells in G_0. Interestingly, IL-6, IL-11, and LIF appear to interact with distinct receptors, but may share common signal-transduction pathways, while IL-6 and CSF-G share some structural homology.

At the molecular level, little is known about the process of commitment. Although it is clear that differentiation is accompanied by increased expression of certain lineage-specific genes, the regulation of gene expression during hematopoietic cell differentiation is due to largely unknown transcriptional regulatory proteins. These regulatory proteins bind to DNA sequences that either up- or down-regulate the expression of a nearby gene.[25] The best studied transcription regulators in hematopoietic cell differentiation are the GATA-1 and NF-E2 proteins. Both of these proteins appear to be critical for expression of many erythroid-specific genes. DNA sequences that lie within the regulatory regions of erythroid-specific genes are recognized by these proteins. GATA-1-binding protein recognizes a specific DNA sequence [T/A(GATA)A/G] (hence the name GATA) that is present near the promoter, enhancer, or locus control region (LCR) of erythroid genes.[26] Protein binding to the cognate DNA stretch via domains resembling "zinc fingers" transactivates the neighboring promoter.[25] GATA-1 motifs appear to be required for full promoter activity of a wide variety of erythroid-specific genes, including α- and β-globin, erythropoietin-receptor gene, porphobilinogen deaminase, pyruvate kinase, and glycophorin.[26] Genetic disruption of the murine GATA-1-binding protein gene is incompatible with development of erythrocytes either in vitro or in vivo.[27] Other members of the GATA family, especially GATA-2, may play an important role in hematopoietic cell differentiation. Both GATA-1 and

Table 14-2. Assays for Primitive Human Hematopoietic Cells

High proliferative potential-colony forming cell[76]
Colony-forming cell blast[77]
Long-term culture-initiating cell[78]

GATA-2 are expressed not only in erythroid cells, but also in megakaryocytes and mast cell lineages.[28,29] Several promoters of lineage-specific genes in these lineages have been demonstrated to contain GATA-1 sites.

NF-E2 binds to an activator protein-1-like site upstream of several erythroid-specific promoters and in the LCR of both β- and α-globin. NF-E2 has the same tissue expression profile as GATA-1. However, NF-E2 affects transcriptional activation as a heterodimer with a ubiquitous protein, p18.[30] Thus NF-E2 and GATA-1 proteins function together and largely control the tissue-specific expression of a great number of genes expressed only in red blood cells.

C-*kit* Proto-oncogene and Its Ligand

Two mouse mutants have contributed significantly to our understanding of the hematopoietic stem cell biology. The murine mutants of bone marrow failure syndromes, *dominant white spotting (W)* and *steel (Sl)* have now been fully characterized at the molecular level. Because of the key role of these mutations in our understanding of the basic biology of hematopoietic stem cells, a summary of the phenotypic abnormalities and molecular biology is included here.

Phenotypically the *Sl* and the better characterized *W* mutants are black-eyed white mice with reduced fertility and macrocytic anemia[31] (Fig. 14-4). All hematopoietic lineages are affected.[31-33] The hematopoietic abnormalities associated with the *W* mutation can be corrected by bone marrow transplantation, while the abnormalities of *Sl* mutants are manifested in supporting cells, such as stromal cells in the bone marrow environment. In recent years, the molecular basis of both mutations have been delineated. The *W* mutations affect the c-*kit* proto-oncogene, a growth factor receptor and member of the tyrosine kinase receptor family, which includes the receptor for CSF-1.[34,35] This receptor is expressed on primitive hematopoietic stem and progenitor cells. Specific c-*kit* mutations and the severity of the phenotypic abnormalities have been corre-

lated with functional impairment of the c-*kit*-associated tyrosine kinase activity.[36] Piebald syndrome in humans appears to be associated with genetic mutations of the c-*kit* receptor[37] (Fig. 14-5).

The molecular and biochemical nature of *Sl* mutations has also been identified.[38-40] The gene identified in these studies encodes a protein that is the ligand for the c-*kit* receptor mutated in *W* mice.[41-43] The gene maps to chromosome 10 in mice and is deleted in alleles associated with embryonic lethal phenotypes.[42-44] The cloned *Sl* cDNA predicts a membrane-associated and glycosylated protein with structural homology to CSF-1. Recombinant growth factor expressed from the cloned cDNA, which has been called stem cell factor, kit ligand, mast cell growth factor, and steel factor, corrects the bone marrow manifestations of the mutation when administered to mice.[42] The protein has pleiotropic effects on hematopoietic stem and progenitor cells in vitro and is currently being tested in early human trials in vivo.[45]

Hematopoietic Microenvironment

Hematopoiesis occurs within a complex environment in the medullary cavity of adults and the fetal liver[46] and yolk sac[47,48] of the developing fetus.[49] Many cells making up this hematopoietic microenvironment (HM) are not derived from hematopoietic stem cells, while hematopoietic cells develop in nests termed "cobblestone areas"[50] (Fig. 14-6). Adventitial reticular cells reside on the adluminal surface of venous endothelial cells, which branch through the medullary cavity.[51] These cells appear to provide a reticular network that supports developing blood cells. In addition, both adventitial reticular cells and adipocytic cells play an active role in hematopoiesis by producing both soluble and membrane-associated growth factors.[52] These cells also respond to hematopoietic stress by changing volume; impaired hematopoiesis is associated with increased accumulation of fat inclusions in both cell types, and accelerated hematopoiesis is associated with loss of fat vacuoles and

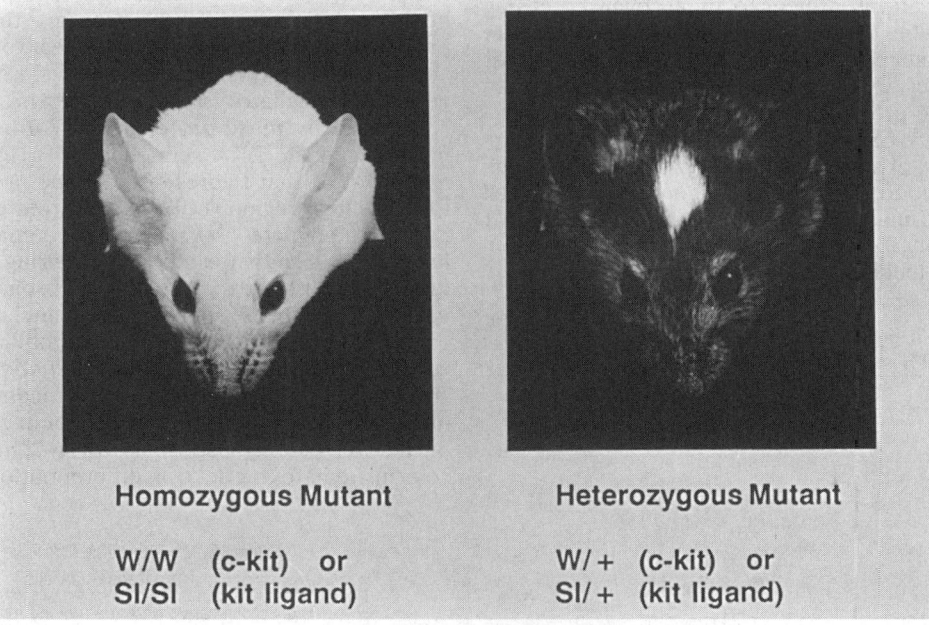

Homozygous Mutant

W/W (c-kit) or
Sl/Sl (kit ligand)

Heterozygous Mutant

W/+ (c-kit) or
Sl/+ (kit ligand)

Figure 14-4. *Sl* and *W* mouse mutants. Photograph of homozygote (left) and heterozygote (right) mice showing characteristic coat color abnormalities characteristics of *Sl* and *W* mouse mutations. (Photographs courtesy of Dr. Roger Fleischman.)

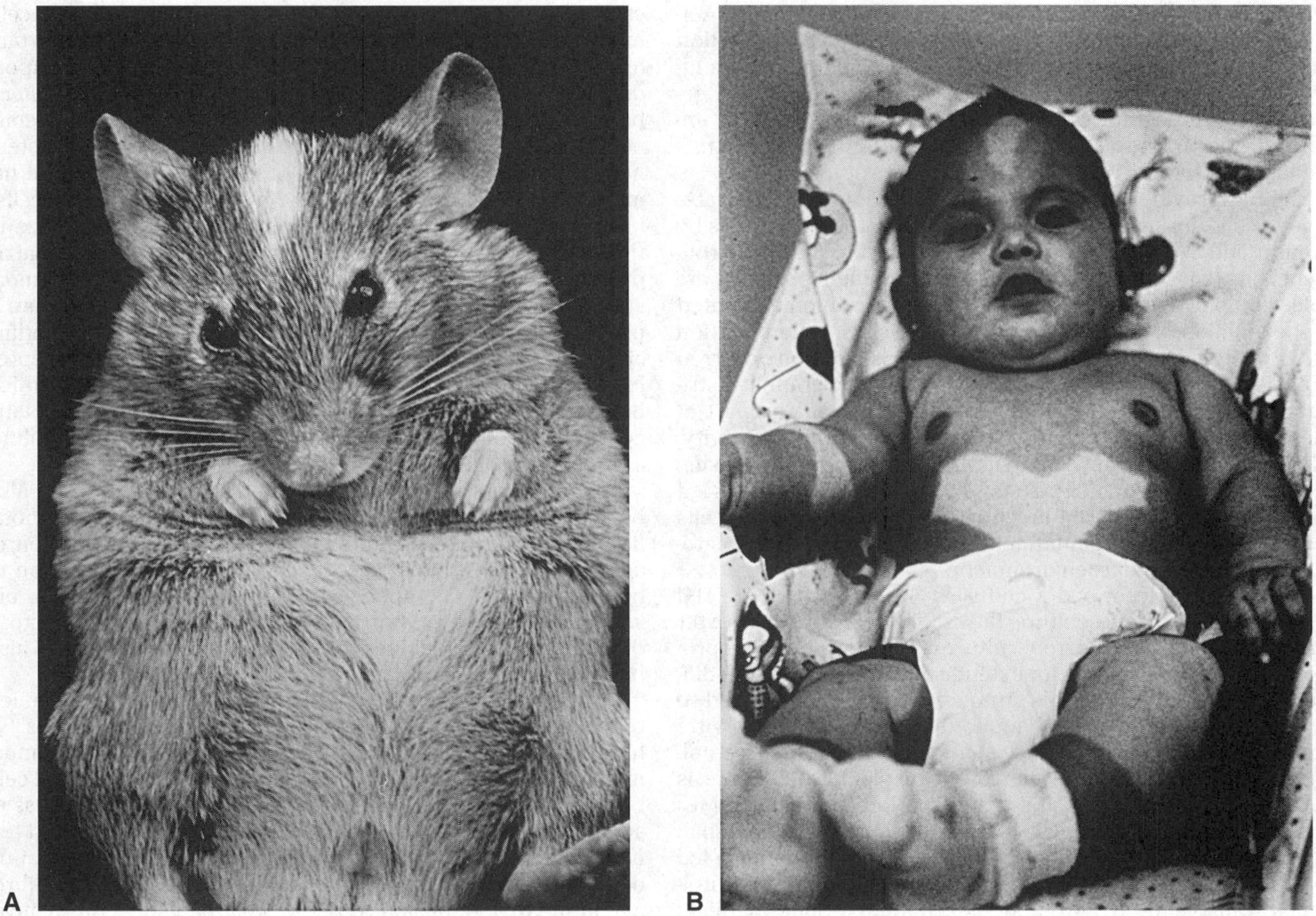

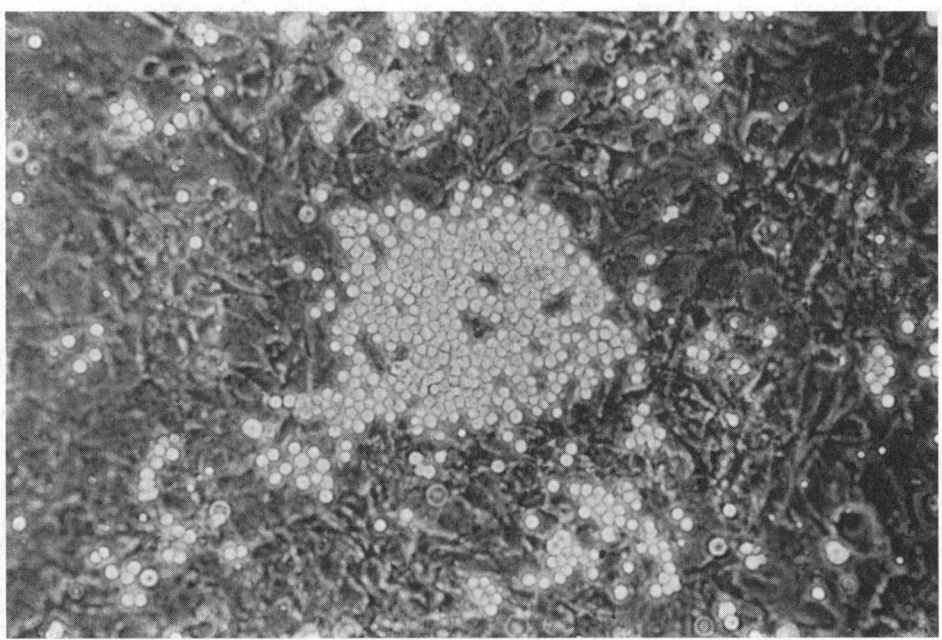

Figure 14-5. Comparison of **(A)** mouse *W* heterozygote and **(B)** infant with piebald syndrome. (From Fleischman et al.,[37] with permission.)

Figure 14-6. Hematopoietic nest arising in long-term marrow (Dexter et al.[5]) culture. Round refractile cells in the middle represent area of active hematopoiesis within the stromal hematopoietic microenvironment of the adherent layer.

the provision of increased space for hematopoietic cells.[53] Adipocytes may play an additional role in blood cell production as a reservoir for lipids needed in cell metabolism during proliferation. Macrophages and osteoclasts, cells derived from hematopoietic precursor cells and osteoblasts, may also play important roles in the HM. The organization of the HM in situ is detailed in Chapter 15.

The HM provides more than structural support for hematopoietic cells during proliferation and differentiation. Studies by Trentin and Wolf[4] show the effects of specific microenvironments on stem cell differentiation. Femoral shafts placed in the spleen pulp of mice give rise to hematopoietic colonies located at the junction of the spleen and femur tissues. Differentiation of cells derived from a single stem cell at this junction occurred in a lineage-specific manner according to the geographic distribution of the colony. Myeloid cells developed in the part of the stem cell-derived colony arising in the medullary cavity, while erythroid cells developed in the part of the colony arising in the splenic environment. These and similar observations led to the theory that the HM in which stem and progenitor cells reside influences the commitment process, termed the hematopoietic inductive microenvironment.

Dexter et al.[5] described a culture system in which the HM is replicated in tissue culture flasks. These cultures (Dexter cultures or long-term marrow cultures) allow survival and proliferation of primitive cells for extended periods in vitro. Modifications of the cultures allow support of lineages restricted to myeloid, erythroid,[54,55] or lymphoid (termed Whitlock-Witte cultures)[56] cells. Cells produced in such cultures can be collected and used for bone marrow transplantation. There is some evidence that CML and acute myeloid leukemia (AML) stem or progenitor cells survive less well in such cultures than phenotypically normal cells.[57,58] These observations have led to the use of long-term marrow cultures for experimental autologous transplants in CML and AML patients. Some patients treated with these protocols have re-established normal hematopoiesis, although it remains unclear whether long-term sustained remissions can be obtained using this approach.

The HM provides support for hematopoietic stem cell proliferation and differentiation both in vivo and in vitro. At least two hematopoietic growth factors have been shown to be important in vivo in the normal function of the HM. Mice deficient in steel factor (homozygous *Sl/Sl* mice [see above]) and LIF (LIF-deficient mice generated by gene targeting)[23] have hematopoietic deficiencies as a result of the lack of presentation by the HM of each protein. *Sl/Sl*[d] mice (from a viable mutant allele of *Sl*) have deficient CFU-S stem cells and low peripheral blood counts.[42,59] LIF-deficient mice have normal peripheral blood counts but are deficient in CFU-S and committed progenitor cells. The bone marrow of both animals is capable of reconstituting normal hematopoiesis when transferred by bone marrow transplantation into a normal HM.

Several theories concerning the physiologic roles of HM in the regulation of hematopoiesis have been proposed and are under investigation (Table 14-3). The HM provides adhesive interactions important for co-localization of stem and progenitor cells and growth regulatory proteins within the medullary cavity. Long[60] has suggested the categories of cell/cell, cell/matrix, and cell/growth factor for these interactions. Important matrix adhesive molecules include fibronectin, thrombospondin, glycosaminoglycans, and proteoglycans. Integral membrane proteins important in these interactions include haemonectin and vascular cell adhesion molecule-1. Pluripotent hematopoietic stem cells (CFU-S$_{12}$, reconstituting murine hematopoietic stem cells, and CD34$^+$ human bone marrow cells) have been demonstrated to adhere to the CS-1 sequence in the alternatively spliced IIICS region of the extracellular matrix protein fibronectin.[61,62] Other investigators have demonstrated adhesion of primitive hematopoietic cells to the matrix protein thrombospondin and the high-affinity heparin binding site in the C-terminal sequence of fibronectin.[63,64] The receptor for the fibronectin CS-1 sequence is the integrin VLA-4, which has been shown to be expressed on primitive hematopoietic cells. The thrombospondin receptor is expressed on multilineage human progenitor cells.

Adhesion of primitive cells to the HM via lectins has also been demonstrated. Aizawa and Tavossoli,[65] using sugar-modified bovine serum albumin, have demonstrated inhibition of adhesion of CFU-S to stromal cells in vitro and inhibition of homing in vivo. The specificity of this interaction is via unknown core proteins, but appears to be related to galactose or mannose sugar residues (or both). CD44 expression has also been detected on early hematopoietic progenitor cells.[66]

Both myeloid and erythroid differentiation are accompanied by changes in adhesive interactions. Patel and colleagues[67,68] have demonstrated that erythroid differentiation is accompanied by increased adhesion to the RGDS-containing central cell-binding domain of fibronectin via the VLA-5 receptor. Loss of adhesion to RGDS is temporally related to enucleation and terminal differentiation, and increased efficiency of enucleation of some erythroid cell lines has been demonstrated on fibronectin in vitro. Adhesion to the protein haemonectin by myeloid progenitor and precursor cells has been demonstrated.[69] Loss of adhesion to this protein has been postulated to be involved in maturing granulocyte egress from the marrow.

The HM may also provide binding sites for hematopoietic growth factors. Proteoglycans and glycosaminoglycans are produced by several cells in the HM.[70] Both CSF-GM and IL-3 have been shown to bind noncovalently to glycosaminoglycans in the extracellular matrix of bone marrow.[71,72] Co-localization of hematopoietic cells with locally high concentrations of growth factors bound in this fashion may be one way in which local area networks are established throughout the medullary cavity.[73] Multiple other adhesive interactions have been studied and are important in lymphocyte homing and leukocyte trafficking in the periphery.[74] These interactions utilize receptors in the immunoglobulin superfamily, integrins, selectin/LEC-CAM, and CD44. Many hematopoietic cell/stromal cell adhesive interactions have been described with receptor/ligand pairs of unknown identity.[75]

PRECURSOR CELL DIFFERENTIATION

Most cells present in the bone marrow of a healthy individual are recognizable precursor cells of the myeloid or erythroid lineage. The ratio of myeloid/erythroid precursors (M/E) is normally 3:1, with approximately 10% of nucleated cells recognizable as lymphocytes, plasma cells, macrophages and rare morphologically indistinct blasts, progenitor cells, and stem cells. Megakaryocytes are present at a frequency of 4–5/1,000 nucleated bone marrow cells. Alterations in the M/E can be determined by staining bone marrow aspirates and are often useful in the evaluation of peripheral cytopenias. However, absolute cellularity is difficult to determine by examination of aspirate samples and is best determined by bone marrow biopsy. A

Table 14-3. Possible Roles of the Hematopoietic Microenvironment in Hematopoiesis

Direct communication via tight cell-to-cell contact

Stabilization of growth factors via binding to extracellular matrix molecules or membrane proteins

Production of both positive and negative regulators of hematopoiesis

Co-localization of growth factors and hematopoietic cells in a local area network, allowing receptor modulation by small quantities of cytokines

(From Williams,[22] with permission.)

relative lymphocytosis and variation in the M/E ratio are normal developmental differences seen in the bone marrow of infants and young children and make the interpretation of these bone marrow samples more difficult.

As seen on standard Wright-Giemsa staining at the light microscope level, the normal differentiation of erythrocytes occurs in well-defined stages. The first identifiable and also largest precursor of the erythroid lineage is the erythroblast (Plate 14-2). The cell diameter is 14–19 μm, and the nucleus is large, oval and homogeneously staining (violet) with indistinct nucleoli. The cytoplasm is darkly basophilic, with lighter staining areas (hyaloplasm) usually near the nucleus that reflect the position of the Golgi apparatus and lipid-containing mitochondria. Maturation to the basophilic normoblast is accompanied by reduction in cell size and pronounced changes in the nuclear chromatin structure (Plate 14-3). The basophilic normoblast is 12–17 μm in diameter, with basophilic cytoplasm, and the nuclear chromatin shows a coarsening and prominent clumping leading to descriptions of a spoked wheel or cartwheel appearance. Nucleoli are generally not seen. The polychromatic normoblast is nearly the same size as the basophilic normoblast (Plate 14-4). The accumulation of hemoglobin is now seen by the presence of less basophilic and muddy gray-colored cytoplasm. The nucleus shows further condensation and is nearly black. The last nucleated red cell precursor is the orthochromatic normoblast (Plate 14-3). The cell now approaches the diameter of a reticulocyte (8–12 μm), and the eosinophilic staining cytoplasm contains nearly a full amount of hemoglobin. The nucleus is now fully condensed and pyknotic.

Extrusion of the nucleus results in the reticulocyte, a cell slightly larger than a fully mature erythrocyte. The reticulocyte is characterized by the presence of a fine granular or reticular network of ribosomal RNA observed with supravital stains such as cresyl violet or methylene blue. Such cells are present at low frequency in the peripheral blood of normal individuals but are increased in response to stress on the erythroid lineage, such as hemolysis or blood loss. Stress reticulocytes are prematurely released into the peripheral blood, where further maturation is completed. Characteristics of stress reticulocytes include a larger cell diameter and more basophilic cytoplasm than reticulocytes.

Additional morphologic indications of stress erythropoiesis include polychromatophilia (violet tinting seen with Wright-Giemsa staining) and basophilia (blue or black stippling diffusely distributed throughout the cell). These staining characteristics are the result of RNA remnants that stain in the cytoplasm of the erythrocyte. The premature destruction of erythroid precursors in the medullary cavity, termed ineffective erythropoiesis, is accompanied by elevation of serum lactate dehydrogenase, decreased levels of serum haptoglobin, slight elevation of the reticulocyte count (1.5–4%), and the occasional appearance of nucleated red blood cells in the peripheral blood. The destruction of erythrocyte precursors in the medullary cavity normally occurs in <10% of developing erythrocytes. Increased destruction of erythrocyte precursors, termed ineffective erythropoiesis, accompanies hemoglobinopathies, iron deficiency anemia, megaloblastic anemias, and other rarer congenital anemias, such as congenital dyserythropoietic anemias.

The final stage of erythroid maturation is the erythrocyte. The cell is a biconcave, relatively flat, non-nucleated disk 7–8 μm in diameter. Normal erythrocyte survival is 100–120 days in humans.

Leukocytes that circulate in the peripheral blood are divided into those of the myeloid, monocyte/macrophage, and lymphocytic lineages. The differentiation and function of the lymphocyte lineage is discussed elsewhere (see Ch. 19). In myeloid and monocyte lineages, four distinct granule populations are seen that distinguish these cells morphologically during differentiation. Azurophilic granules are present in cells of both lineages, stain pink with Romanowsky dyes, and contain myeloperoxidase, acid phosphatase, basic cationic protein, and other hydrolases. Eosinophilic granules are a conspicuous reddish orange, and basophilic granules are intensely blue. Specific neutrophilic granules do not stain intensely with standard Wright-Giemsa stains.

The earliest identifiable cell of the myeloid lineage is the myeloblast (Fig. 14-7). The cell is approximately 12–14 μm in diameter, with a round or oval nucleus and basophilic cytoplasm that lacks granules. Nuclear chromatin is fine, and one to five nucleoli are easily visible. The nucleus often stains reddish. Promyelocytes are the largest and most frequent of the primi-

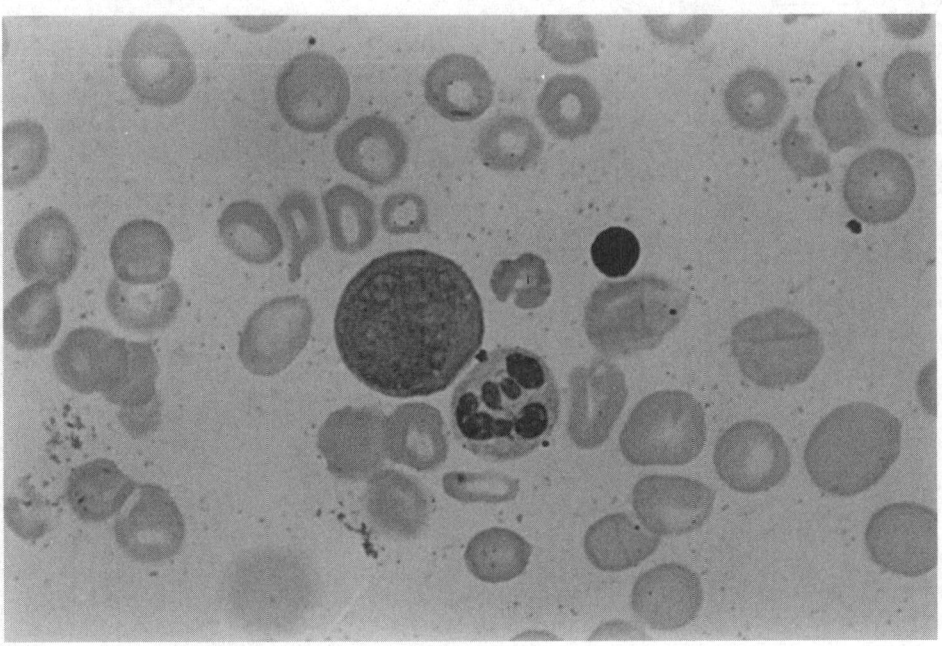

Figure 14-7. Myeloblast transition to promyelocyte. Neutrophil below.

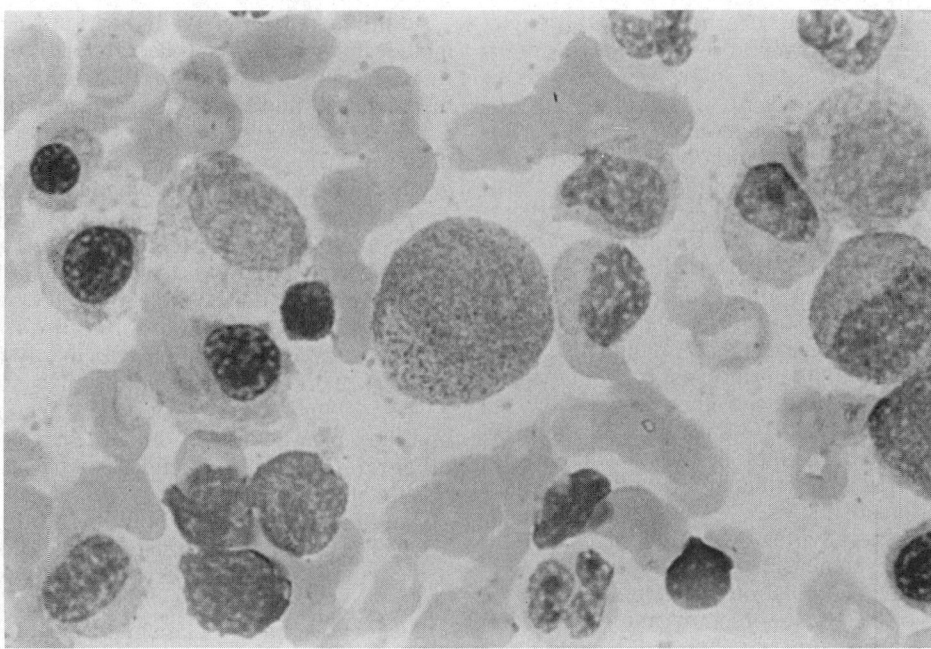

Figure 14-8. Promyelocyte in the middle. Eosinophilic myelocyte on the left.

tive myeloid precursor (Fig. 14-8). Promyelocytes are variable in nuclear shape, with less prominent nucleoli, and chromatin of medium density that is coarser than that of the myeloblast. The cytoplasm is deeply basophilic and contains variable numbers of peroxidase-positive granules. These granules can overlie the nucleus and can vary in color from deep red to blue; they distinguish the promyelocyte from the myeloblast.

Myelocytes are characterized by round-to-oval nuclei with characteristic nuclear indentations, indistinct nucleoli, and unevenly stained, coarse chromatin structure (Fig. 14-9). The cytoplasm stains pale gray-brown or pink-brown, with numerous specific granules covering the nucleus and throughout the cytoplasm except in a clear area near the nuclear indentation (centrosphere), which represents the Golgi apparatus. The my-

elocyte is also characterized by the first appearance of specific granules and is the last cell capable of cell division during myeloid differentiation. The metamyelocyte exhibits a characteristic bean-shaped nucleus, the band neutrophil a horseshoe- or S-shaped nuclear structure without recognizable nuclear constrictions, and the segmented neutrophil is characterized by the typical nuclear segmentations for which it is named, which divide the nucleus into two to five lobes (Fig. 14-9). These myeloid forms exhibit cytoplasmic characteristics similar to the myelocyte without the centrosphere and with progressive reduction in the overall cell size. An additional nuclear lobule, termed a drumstick, is seen in 10–12% of neutrophils of females.

Maturation of the eosinophil and basophil follows the same

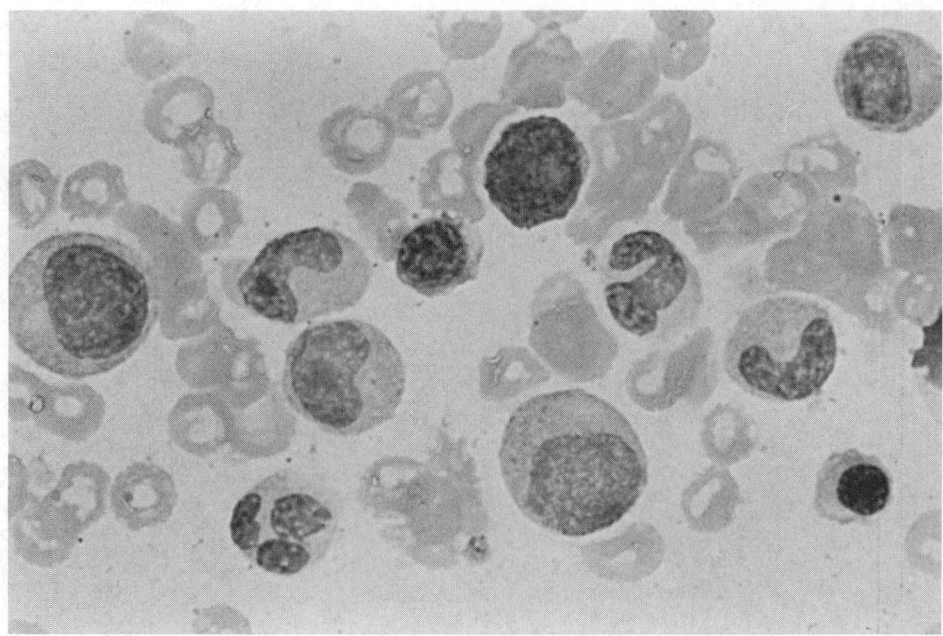

Figure 14-9. Myeloid maturation. Myelocytes, metamyelocytes, band, and segmented neutrophils.

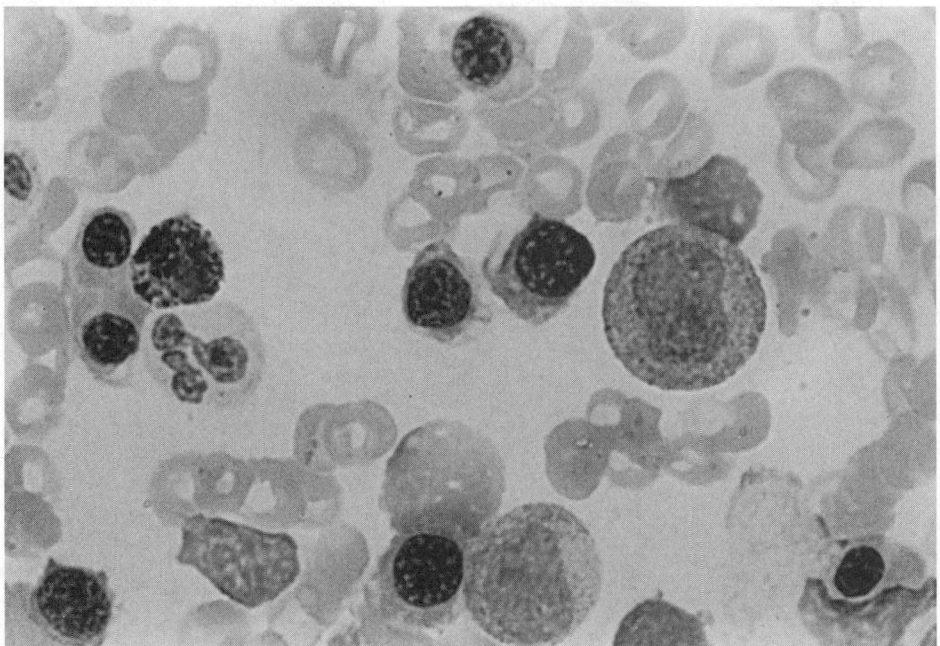

Figure 14-10. Eosinophilic myelocyte (left) and basophil (right).

morphologic steps as the neutrophil until the appearance of specific granules (Fig. 14-10). The eosinophil exhibits a bilobed nucleus, and the basophilic cytoplasm is filled with prominent orange-red granules (Fig. 14-11). Basophils exhibit less segmentation of the nucleus and cytoplasm that is sparsely filled with deeply staining blue-to-purple metachromatic granules (Fig. 14-10). The granules often obscure the nucleus and cytoplasm, which stains pink to reddish pink and frequently exhibits vacuoles. Frequencies in the peripheral blood of normal individuals are 0–4% and 0–0.5%, respectively, for eosinophils and basophils.

The earliest cell of the monocyte/macrophage lineage is difficult to distinguish from the myeloblast. The cell is 12–18 µm in diameter, with a round or oval nucleus that is frequently

convoluted. The chromatin is fine, and nucleoli are sometimes present. The cytoplasm is basophilic, with a grayish cast and, although devoid of granules, may contain vacuoles. Blunt pseudopodia are sometimes present. The naphthol-AS-acetate esterase reaction is positive and is inhibited by fluoride. The promonocyte is a large cell with an indented nucleus exhibiting fine chromatin and a single nucleolus (Fig. 14-12). The cytoplasm stains light blue with azurophilic granules and a small centrosphere. The monocyte is the largest cell present in the peripheral blood and measures 13–20 µm in diameter (Fig. 14-13). The nucleus is large, lobulated, or bean-shaped, with coarse nuclear chromatin; it lacks nucleoli and is often eccentric in location. The cytoplasm stains a characteristic smoke-blue with azurophilic granules. The chromatin structure of the

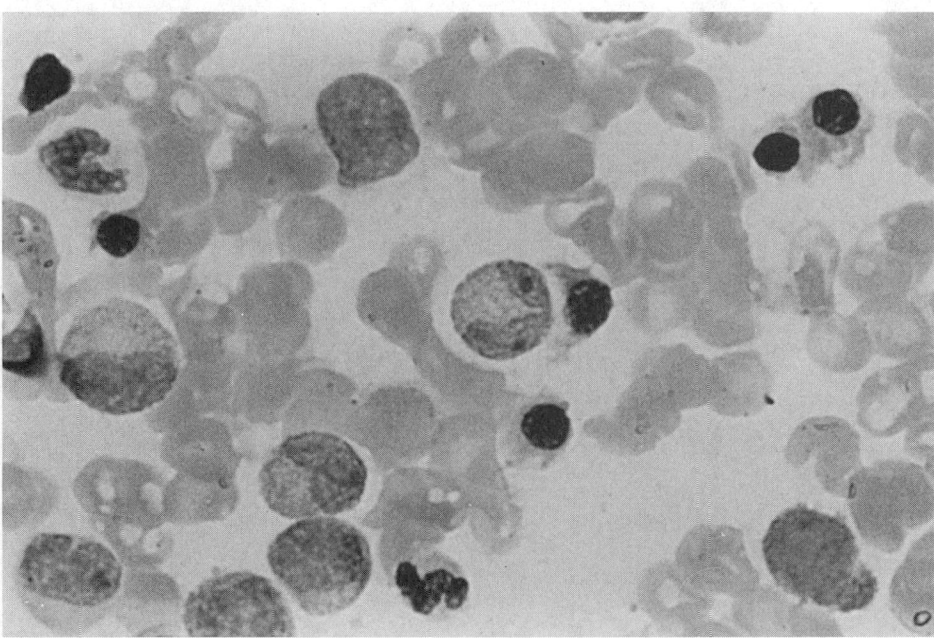

Figure 14-11. Mature, bilobed eosinophils (middle and right).

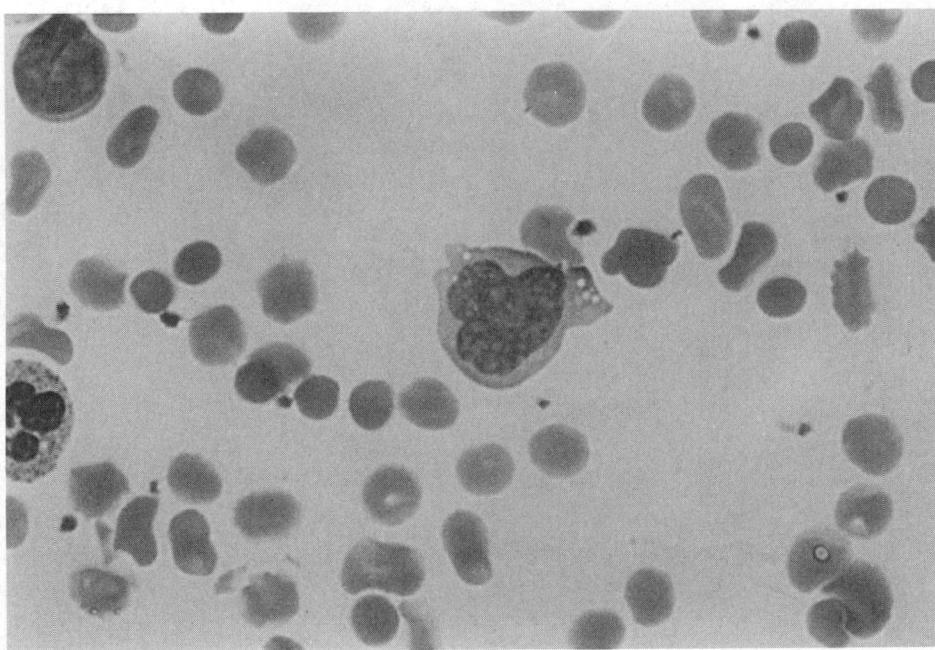

Figure 14-12. Promonocyte in peripheral blood.

monocyte is less clumped and the cytoplasm grayer than the lymphocyte, characteristics that (along with nuclear convolutions) help to distinguish these cells from moderate-size lymphocytes in the peripheral blood. Other helpful distinguishing characteristics are blunt pseudopodia. Monocytes usually make up ≤5–10% of the peripheral leukocytes. Egress of monocytes from the blood into tissues is associated with increased cell size and larger, more lightly staining nucleus. These cells, termed macrophages or histiocytes, are phagocytic and mobile, and intracellular debris is often present.

Morphologic differentiation of platelet-forming cells is distinctly different from either erythroid or leukocyte cell lineages. Distinct morphologic maturational steps and divisions

do not take place; these processes are instead replaced by the process of polyploidization. In the process, successive nuclear divisions without concomitant cytoplasmic divisions lead to megakaryocytes with 1–32 nuclei representing diploid to 64N nuclear content. The first identifiable cell in this lineage is the megakaryoblast, a distinctly large cell with a high nuclear/cytoplasmic ratio. The nucleus shows variable chromatin coarseness and may contain nucleoli. The nuclear shape varies, but the nucleus frequently displays convolutions or deep furrows. The cytoplasm stains basophilic, does not contain granules, and may exhibit fraying at the cytoplasmic membrane. Some megakaryoblasts may contain multiple nuclei. The promegakaryocyte exhibits a lobulated nuclear structure without nu-

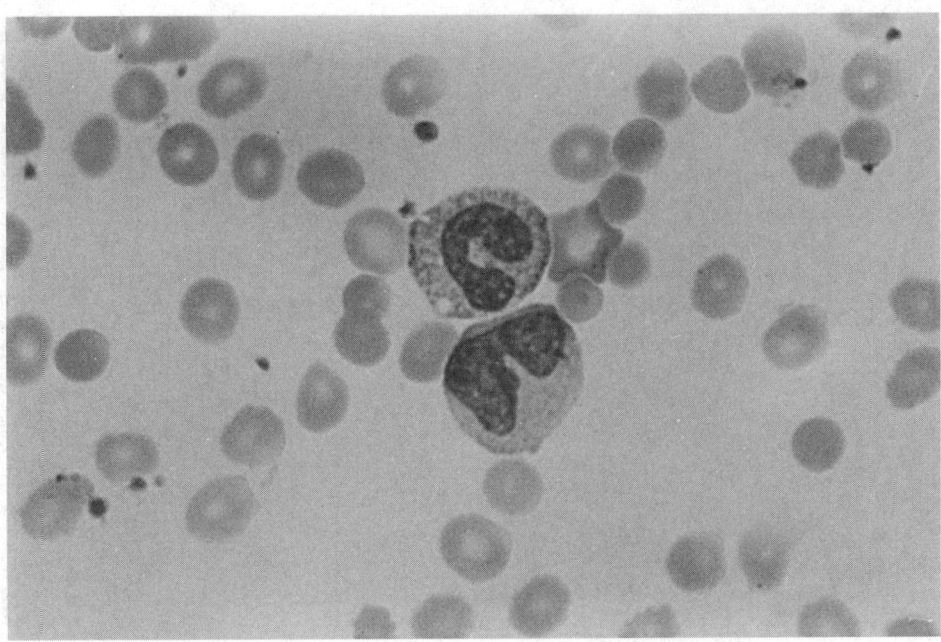

Figure 14-13. Monocyte with band neutrophil (below).

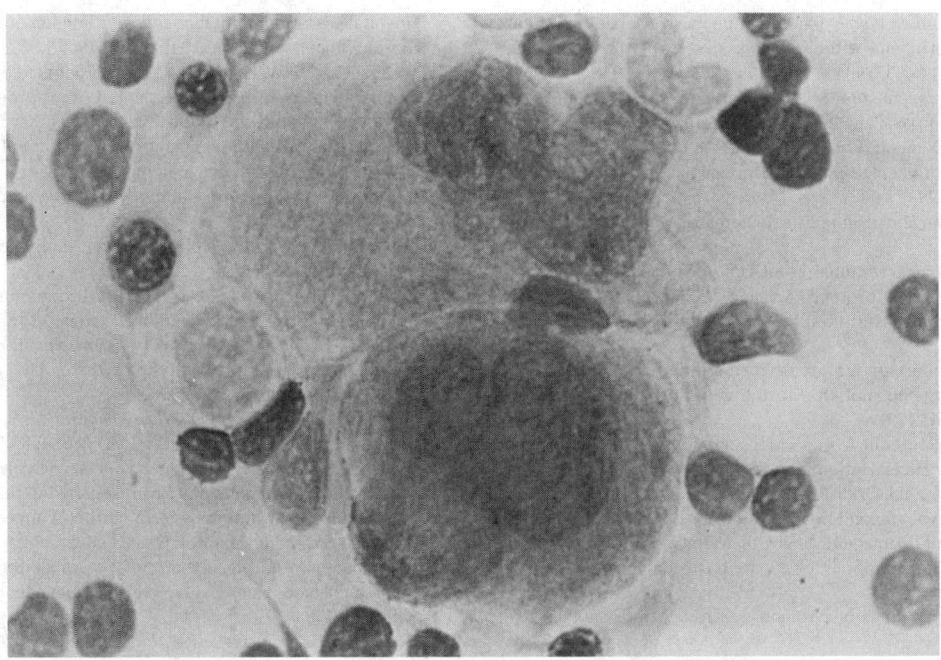

Figure 14-14. Megakaryocytes.

cleoli and with a coarse chromatin structure. The cytoplasm is basophilic, with azurophilic granules adjacent to the nucleus, and formed platelets are seen on the cytoplasmic cell surface.

Occasionally the presence of other cells apparently within the cytoplasm (emperipolesis) of the promegakaryocyte is noted, although the mechanism leading to this occurrence is unknown. Mature megakaryocytes are the largest hematopoietic cell in the bone marrow (Fig. 14-14). The nucleus is lobulated and exhibits coarse and clumped chromatin. Nuclear number varies from eight diploid nuclei (65% of marrow megakaryocytes) to four nuclei (10% of marrow megakaryocytes). The cytoplasm is basophilic, with numerous azurophilic granules. Platelets can be seen at the periphery of the cytoplasm and are attached to the cell membrane. Megakaryocytes constitute 0.1–0.5% of cells in the medullary cavity of normal individuals.

SUMMARY

The formation of blood cells represents a complex interaction between stem cells, cells making up the HM, and growth regulatory proteins, which are presented in soluble and localized forms. These interactions give rise to an enormous number and diversity of cells that function in widely separated parts of the body to transport oxygen, defend against infectious agents, and provide a stimulus for clotting. Abnormalities that affect this process can lead to life-threatening illness such as aplastic anemia and myeloproliferative diseases. In addition to contributing to our understanding of the basic pathophysiology of these diseases, research in hematopoiesis is providing new therapeutic tools, such as growth factors, which are being used in treatment of both congenital and induced hypoplastic conditions of the bone marrow.

ACKNOWLEDGMENT

Special thanks to Atillio Orazi, MD, Department of Pathology, Indiana University School of Medicine, Indiana University Medical Center, Indianapolis, Indiana.

REFERENCES

1. Till JE, McCulloch EA: A direct measurement of the radiation sensitivity of normal mouse bone marrow cells. Radiat Res 14:213, 1961
2. Pluznik DH, Sachs L: The cloning of normal "mast" cells in tissues cultures. J Cell Comp Physiol 66:319, 1965
3. Bradley TR, Metcalf D: The growth of mouse bone marrow cells in vitro. Aust J Exp Biol Med Sci 44:287, 1966
4. Wolf NS, Trentin JJ: Hemopoietic colony studies: V. Effect of hemopoietic organ stroma on differentiation of pluripotent stem cells. J Exp Med 127:205, 1968
5. Dexter TM, Allen TD, Lajtha LG: Conditions controlling the proliferation of haemopoietic stem cells in vitro. J Cell Physiol 91:335, 1976
6. Botnick LE, Hannon EC, Hellman S: Nature of the hematopoietic stem cell compartment and its proliferative potential. Blood Cells 5:195, 1979
7. Jacobson LO, Simmons EL, Marks EK et al: Further studies on recovery from radiation injury. J Lab Clin Med 37:683, 1951
8. Visser JWM, VanBekkum DW: Purification of pluripotent hemopoietic stem cells: past and present. Exp Hematol 18:248, 1990
9. Spangrude GJ, Heimfeld S, Weissman IL: Purification and characterization of mouse hematopoietic stem cells. Science 241:58, 1988
10. Bertoncello I, Bartelmez SH, Bradley TR et al: Isolation and analysis of primitive hemopoietic progenitor cells on the basis of differential expression of Qa-m7 antigen. J Immunol 136:3219, 1986
11. Visser JWM, deVries P: Isolation of spleen-colony forming cells (CFU-S) using wheat germ agglutinin and rhodamine 123 labeling. Blood Cells 14:369, 1988
12. Civin CI, Strauss LC, Brovall C et al: Antigenic analysis of hematopoiesis. III. A hematopoietic progenitor cell surface antigen defined by a monoclonal antibody raised against KG-1a cells. J Immunol 133:157, 1984
13. Berenson RJ, Andrews RG, Bensinger WI et al: Antigen CD 34+ marrow cells engraft lethally irradiated baboons. J Clin Invest 81:951, 1988
14. Srour EF, Brandt JE, Briddell RA et al: Human CD34+ HLA-DR bone marrow cells contain progenitor cells capable of self-renewal, multilineage differentiation, and long-term in vitro hematopoiesis. Blood Cells 17:287, 1991
15. Williams DA: In search of the self-renewing hematopoietic stem cell. Blood Cells 17:296, 1991
16. Kamel-Reid S, Dick JE: Engraftment of immune-deficient mice with human hematopoietic stem cells. Science 242:1706, 1988
17. Zanjani ED, Pallavicini MG, Ascensao JL et al: Engraftment and long-term expression of human fetal hematopoietic stem cells in sheep following transplantation in utero. J Clin Invest 89:1178, 1992
18. Gartner S, Kaplan HS: Long-term culture of human bone marrow cells. Proc Natl Acad Sci USA 77:4756, 1980
19. Siminovitch L, Till JE, McCulloch EA: The distribution of colony-forming cells among spleen colonies. J Cell Comp Physiol 62:327, 1963
20. Clark SC, Kamen R: The human hematopoietic colony-stimulating factors. Science 236:1229, 1987
21. Muench MO, Firpo MT, Moore MAS: Bone marrow transplantation with in-

terleukin-1 plus kit-ligand *ex vivo* expanded bone marrow accelerates hematopoietic reconstitution in mice without the loss of stem cell lineage proliferative potential. Blood 81:3463, 1993

22. Williams DA: *Ex vivo* expansion of hematopoietic stem and progenitor cells—robbing Peter to pay Paul? Blood 81:3169, 1993

23. Escary JL, Perreau J, Dumenil D et al: Leukaemia inhibitory factor is necessary for maintenance of haematopoietic stem cells and thymocyte stimulation. Nature 363:361, 1993

24. Ogawa M: Differentiation and proliferation of hematopoietic stem cells. Blood 81:2844, 1993

25. Mitchell PJ, Tjian R: Transcriptional regulation in mammalian cells by sequence-specific DNA binding proteins. Science 245:371, 1989

26. Orkin SH: GATA-binding transcription factors in hematopoietic cells. Blood 80:3:575, 1992

27. Perry L, Simon MC, Robertson E et al: Erythroid differentiation in chimeric mice blocked by a targeted mutation in the gene for transcription factor GATA-1. Nature 349:257, 1991

28. Pomeo PH, Prandini MH, Joulin V et al: Megakaryocytic and erythropoietic lineages share specific transcription factors. Nature 334:447, 1990

29. Martin DIK, Zon LI, Mutter IS, Orkin SH: Expression of an erythroid transcription factor in megakaryocytic and mast cell lineages. Nature 344:444, 1990

30. Andrews NC, Erdjument-Bromage H, Davidson MB et al: Erythroid transcription factor NF-E2 is a haematopoietic-specific basic-leucine zipper protein. Nature 362:722, 1993

31. Russell ES: Hereditary anemias of the mouse: a review for geneticists. Adv Genet 20:357, 1979

32. Ruscetti FW, Boggs DR, Torok BJ, Boggs SS: Reduced blood and marrow neutrophils and granulocytic colony-forming cells in S1/S1/^{d} mice (39405). Proc Soc Exp Biol Med 152:398, 1976

33. Ebbe S, Phalen E, Stohlman F Jr: Abnormalities of megakaryocytes in S1/S1^d mice. Blood 42:865, 1973

34. Chabot B, Stephenson DA, Chapman VM et al: The proto-oncogenic *c-kit* encoding a transmembrane tyrosine kinase receptor maps to the mouse W locus. Nature 335:88, 1988

35. Geissler EN, Ryan MA, Housman DE: The dominant-white spotting (W) locus of the mouse encodes the c-kit proto-oncogene. Cell 55:185, 1988

36. Reith AD, Rottapel R, Giddens E et al: *W* mutant mice with mild or severe developmental defects contain distinct point mutations in the kinase domain of the *c-kit* receptor. Genes Dev 4:390, 1990

37. Fleischman RA, Saltman DL, Stastny V, Zneimer S: Deletion of the c-kit protooncogene in the human developmental defect piebald trait. Proc Natl Acad Sci USA 88:10885, 1991

38. Martin FH, Suggs SV, Langley KE et al: Primary structure and functional expression of rat and human stem cell factor DNAs. Cell 63:203, 1990

39. Anderson DM, Lyman SD, Baird A et al: Molecular cloning of mast cell growth factor a hematopoietin that is active in both membrane bound and soluble forms. Cell 63:235, 1990

40. Nocka K, Buck J, Levi E, Besmer P: Candidate ligand for the *c-kit* transmembrane kinase receptor: KL, a fibroblast derived growth factor stimulates mast cells and erythroid progenitors. EMBO J 9:3287, 1990

41. Williams DE, Eisenman J, Baird A et al: Identification of a ligand for the *c-kit* proto-oncogene. Cell 63:167, 1990

42. Zsebo KM, Williams DA, Geissler EN et al: Stem cell factor (SFC) is encoded at the S1 locus of the mouse and is the ligand for the c-kit tyrosine kinase receptor. Cell 63:213, 1990

43. Huang E, Nocka K, Beier DR et al: The hematopoietic growth factor KL is encoded at the S1 locus and is the ligand of the *c-kit* receptor, the gene product of the *W* locus. Cell 63:225, 1990

44. Copeland NG, Gilbert DJ, Cho BC et al: Mast cell growth factor maps near the steel locus on mouse chromosome 10 and is deleted in a number of steel alleles. Cell 63:175, 1990

45. Lyman SD, Williams DE: Biological activities and potential therapeutic uses of steel factor: a new growth factor active on multiple hematopoietic lineages. Am J Pediatr Hematol Oncol 14:1, 1992

46. Weissman I, Papaioannou V, Gardner R: Fetal hematopoietic origins of the adult hematolymphoid system. p. 371. In: Clarkson B, Marks PA, Till JE (eds): Differentiation of Normal and Neoplastic Hematopoietic Cells. Cold Spring Harbor Laboratory Press, Cold Spring Harbor, 1978

47. Moore MAS, Metcalf D: Ontogeny of the haemopoietic system: yolk sac origin of *in vivo* and *in vitro* colony forming cells in the developing mouse embryo. Br J Haematol 18:279, 1970

48. Tyan ML: Studies on the ontogeny of the mouse immune system. I. Cell bound immunity. J Immunol 100:535, 1968

49. Trentin JJ, Curry JC, Wolf N, Cheng V: Factors controlling stem cell differentiation and proliferation: the hematopoietic inductive microenvironment (HIM). p. 713. In: The Proliferation and Spread of Neoplastic Cells. M.D. Anderson Hospital 21st Annual Symposium on Fundamental Cancer Research, Baltimore, Williams & Wilkins, Baltimore, 1967

50. Weilbaecher K, Weissman I, Blume K, Heimfeld S: Culture of phenotypically defined hematopoietic stem cells and other progenitors at limiting dilution on Dexter monolayers. Blood 78:945, 1991

51. Weiss L: The hematopoietic microenvironment of the bone marrow: an ultrastructural study of the stroma in rats. Anat Rec 186:161, 1976

52. Gimble JM: The function of adipocytes in the bone marrow stroma. New Biol 2:304, 1990

53. Tavassoli M: Marrow adipose cells and hemopoiesis: an interpretative review. Exp Hematol 12:139, 1984

54. Eliason JF, Testa NG, Dexter TM: Erythropoietin-stimulated erythropoiesis in long term bone marrow culture. Nature 281:382, 1979

55. Corey CA, DeSilva A, Williams DA: Erythropoiesis in murine long term marrow cultures following transfer of the erythropoietic cDNA into marrow stromal cells. Exp Hematol 18:201, 1990

56. Whitlock CA, Robertson D, Witte ON: Murine B cell lymphopoiesis in long term cultures. J Immunol Methods 67:353, 1984

57. Chang J, Coutino L, Morgenster G et al: Reconstitution of haematopoietic system with autologous marrow taken during relapse of acute myeloblastic leukemia and grown in long-term culture. Lancet 2:294, 1986

58. Coulombel L, Kalousek DK, Eaves CJ et al: Long term marrow culture reveals chromosomally normal hematopoietic progenitor cells in patients with Philadelphia chromosome positive chronic myelogenous leukemia. N Engl J Med 308:1493, 1983

59. Bodine DM, Orlic D, Birkett NC et al: Stem cell factor increases CFU-S number *in vitro* in synergy with interleukin-6, and *in vivo* as a single factor. Blood 79:913, 1992

60. Long MW: Blood cell cytoadhesion molecules. Exp Hematol 20:288, 1992

61. Williams DA, Rios M, Stephens C, Patel V: Fibronectin and VLA-4 in haematopoietic stem cell-microenvironment interactions. Nature 352:438, 1991

62. Verfaillie CM, McCarthy JB, McGlave PB: Differentiation of primitive human multipotent hematopoietic progenitors is accompanied by alterations in their interaction with fibronectin. J Exp Med 174:693, 1991

63. Long MW, Dixit Vishva M: Thrombospondin functions as a cytoadhesion molecular for human hematopoietic progenitor cells. Blood 75:2311, 1990

64. Verfaillie C, McCarthy J, McGlave P: Differentiation of primitive human lin-34+DR-hematopoietic progenitors is accompanied by transition of adhesion from the heparin-binding domain to the cell-binding domain of fibronectin (FN), abstracted. Blood 76:10, 1992

65. Aizawa S, Tavassoli M: Molecular basis of the recognition of intravenously transplanted hemopoietic cells by bone marrow. Proc Natl Acad Sci USA 85:3180, 1988

66. Lewinsohn DM, Nagler A, Ginzton N et al: Hematopoietic progenitor cell expression of the H-CAM (CD44) homing-associated adhesion molecule. Blood 75:589, 1990

67. Patel VP, Lodish HF: Loss of adhesion of murine erythroleukemia cells to fibronectin during erythroid differentiation. Science 224:996, 1984

68. Patel VP, Ciechanover A, Platt O, Lodish HF: Mammalian reticulocytes lose adhesion to fibronectin during maturation to erythrocytes. Proc Natl Acad Sci USA 82:440, 1985

69. Campbell AD, Long MW, Wicha MS: Haemonectin, a bone marrow adhesion protein specific for cells of granulocytic lineage. Nature 329:744, 1987

70. Gordon MY, Greaves MF: Physiological mechanisms of stem cell regulation in bone marrow transplantation and haemopoiesis. Bone Marrow Transplant 4:335, 1989

71. Gordon MY, Riley GP, Watt SM, Greaves MF: Compartmentalization of a haematopoietic growth factor. Nature 326:403, 1987

72. Roberts R, Gallagher J, Spooncer E et al: Heparan sulphate bound growth factors: a mechanism for stromal cell mediated haemopoiesis. Nature 332:376, 1988

73. Toksoz D, Zsebo KM, Smith KA et al: Support of human hematopoiesis in long-term bone marrow cultures by murine stromal cells selectively expressing the membrane-bound and secreted forms of the human homolog of the steel gene products, stem cell factor. Proc Natl Acad Sci USA 89:7350, 1992

74. Khwaja KYA: Leucocyte cellular adhesion molecules. Blood Rev 4:211, 1990

75. Clark BR, Gallagher JT, Dexter TM: Cell adhesion in the stromal regulation of haemopoiesis. Baillieres Clin Hematol 5:619, 1992

76. Bertoncello I, Bradley TR, Hodgson GS: The concentration and resolution of primitive hemopoietic cells from normal mouse bone marrow by negative selection using monoclonal antibodies and dynabead monodisperse magnetic microspheres. Exp Hematol 17:171, 1989

77. Hara H, Ogawa M: Murine hemopoietic colonies in culture containing normoblasts, macrophages, and megakaryocytes. Am J Hematol 4:23, 1978

78. Sutherland HJ, Eaves CJ, Eaves AC et al: Characterization and partial purification of human marrow cells capable of initiating long-term hematopoiesis *in vitro*. Blood 74:1563, 1989

Functional Organization of Hematopoietic Tissues

15

Leon P. Weiss

BASIC ORGANIZATION

The principal hematopoietic tissues that produce the blood cells in adult humans and participate in immune reactions and other functions of blood cells are bone marrow, thymus, lymph nodes and mucosa-associated lymphatic tissue (MALT), spleen, the immunologically competent pool of recirculating lymphocytes (RLP), and the blood itself.[1-6] The marrow contains the great majority of hematopoietic stem cells and provides the diverse microenvironments that induce their differentiation into each of the blood cell types.[5,7-9] The thymus receives T-cell progenitors from bone marrow and permits or surveils their differentiation into mature T cells.[5,10-12] The spleen supports late phases of differentiation in at least several blood cell types, which immediately precede the definitive circulatory phase of the cells.[5,13] Bone marrow and the thymus produce blood cells (including lymphocytes and their accessory cells) and are termed primary or central hematopoietic or immune tissues.[5] Spleen, lymph nodes, and MALT engage in immune reactions and are designated peripheral or secondary hematopoietic or immune tissues. The RLP accounts for 2–3% of the lymphocytes of the body and consists of immunologically competent long-lived T and B cells that circulate and recirculate through blood, lymph, and lymphatic tissue.[1,14-18] Lymphocytes of RLP engage in immune reactions after being presented with the appropriate antigen in the appropriate way.[2,3] Stem cells, progenitor cells, and other hematopoietic cells regularly travel in the blood among hematopoietic tissues and from hematopoietic tissues to target tissues. The presence of these undifferentiated cells in the circulating blood makes blood a hematopoietic tissue, blurring the distinction between blood cell and hematopoietic cell.

Erythrocytes differentiate from progenitor cells, ultimately from stem cells in marrow.[5,9,19] Differentiation normally proceeds in marrow until reticulocytes are produced. Reticulocytes in marrow constitute a reserve equal in number to the level of circulating reticulocytes. Released in marrow, reticulocytes circulate to the spleen, where they are briefly conditioned before joining the general circulation. In rats, at least, eosinophils also differentiate rather fully in marrow, and then circulate to the spleen for a few days of "tuning up" before release to the general circulation. Neutrophilic differentiation may also be supported by a marrow/spleen partnership. Data are not yet available for the basophil. Putative platelets outlined in the megakaryocytes by specialized endoplasmic reticulum (demarcation membranes) are shed from the cytoplasm of megakaryocytes. As demarcation membranes fuse, platelets are released from megakaryocytes.

Full maturation of T cells means joining the RLP.[2,14-18] T cells differentiate from marrow stem cells and then travel to the thymus, where they undergo the greatest part of their differentiation.[4,12,20-22] They become mature T cells, but are "unsophisticated." They must travel to the spleen, which has a library of antigens with which the body must deal. If thymus-released T cells interact with one of these antigens, they are stabilized and become both mature and "sophisticated." Only then do they join the RLP and begin a potentially long life as a migra-

tory, immunologically competent T cell. B cells in birds display a parallel pattern of differentiation, starting in bone marrow, traveling from there to the bursa of Fabricius, a lymphoepithelial organ organized as a diverticulum of the cloaca, a "cloacal thymus" as it were, for most of their maturation. They then move to the spleen, where they, like T cells, become both mature and "sophisticated" before joining RLP. Mammals lack a bursa; the bone marrow likely assumes bursal functions.

Monocytes are produced in marrow from promonocytes and may well be released directly to the general circulation. They differentiate readily into macrophages, which are classified as stromal cells.[1,3,23] Additional blood cell/stromal cell types have been recognized among mononuclear blood cells.

Veiled cells are produced in marrow and released to blood.[5] By light microscopy, they resemble monocytes, but their nucleus is often more irregular in contour, and they possess long, veil-like cytoplasmic processes. They may possess distinctive Birbeck granules. Veiled cells circulate to stratified squamous epithela, leave the vasculature, and penetrate the epithelium. They were recognized in gold-toned skin preparations in 1894 by a medical student, Paul Langerhans, and for this reason were eponymically termed Langerhans cells. Their significance was not appreciated for many years—effete macrophages and damaged epithelial cells were considered as possibilities. In fact, Langerhans cells trap and hold onto their surface antigens, which penetrate the skin. When replete with antigens, Langerhans cells leave the epithelium and home to regional lymph nodes or the spleen. There, as interdigitating cells (IDCs), they cluster T cells, present antigen to them, and, perhaps, control the migration of T cells within lymphatic tissues. While it has not yet been demonstrated, it may well be that IDC after completing the processes of antigen presentation and intralymphatic tissue migration, re-enter the circulation as veiled cells. The follicular dendritic cell (FDC), whose life cycle is not well known, is the counterpart of the IDC, dedicated to B cells.

Barrier cells were identified in my laboratory as fibroblastic, contractile, hematopoietic stromal cells that fuse with one another to form complex branched, extensive syncytial membranes deployed in a variety of barrier formations. Barrier cell syncytia in the spleen, marrow, and thymus may envelop hematopoietic colonies, protecting them against parasitization and confining hematopoietic regulatory factors at high concentration. They may surround collections of immunocompetent lymphocytes, protecting them from epiphenomenal antigen after the initiation of an immune response. They may form channels regulating blood flow. They produce interleukins and, probably, other hematopoietic inflammatory factors. In the spleen, where these barriers have been closely studied, they constitute a dynamic component of the filtration beds.[24-27] Barrier cells may be as far-flung as macrophages, present not only in hematopoietic tissues, but in virtually any tissue of the body. They appear to originate in marrow and, like monocytes and other leukocytes, use the circulation to reach appropriate target tissues.

The two major types of lymphocytes, as indicated above, are T cells and B cells. A third type is the null cell, defined as lymphocytes that are neither T nor B cells. Null cells are variegated. They include natural killer cells, hematopoietic stem cells, and progenitor cells. T cells, B cells, and null cells circulate and are recognized as lymphocytes in standard Romanovsky-stained smears. Only by the delineation of selective or specific cell markers using immunologic as well as other methods can these cells be separated into specific cell types.

As one considers blood cell development one realizes that blood and connective tissues, including the hematopoietic and immunologic tissues, are interactive and that stem cells and the more restricted progenitor cells, as well as connective tissue cells, are mobile and niche-seeking cells. The hematopoietic stroma makes major contributions in the construction of such niches or hematopoietic microenvironments.

HEMATOPOIETIC STROMA

The hematopoietic stroma mechanically supports the differentiating hematopoietic cells, the blood cells, and the vasculature.[5,7,9,19,21,23,24-36] This is best illustrated by reticular cells, which are large, branched, probably contractile cells that envelop reticular fibers (selectively stained by silver and intimately associated with collagen, which they appear to produce). Reticular cells (reinforced to varying degrees by reticular fibers) associate with one another to form meshworks that hold hematopoietic and blood cells, the makeup and proportions of which vary from tissue to tissue and within a tissue. Reticular meshworks in lymph nodes are disproportionately rich in lymphocytes, for example, while those in splenic red pulp are often crowded with erythrocytes, macrophages, and platelets. Because these reticular meshworks may receive lymph (as in lymph nodes) or blood (as in spleen) and differentially clear and support the cells of the lymph or blood, I have recognized them as filtration beds, but the more subtle roles played by the stroma in regulating hematopoiesis are being increasingly appreciated. Marrow adipocytes, for example, possess the mechanical function of controlling hematopoietic volume in the relatively fixed, large, dispersed spaces encased in bone, dedicated to marrow.[5] However, adipocytes also possess metabolic and inductive functions. They solubilize testosterone, which drives erythropoiesis, and aromatize it to estrogen, which maintains bone. They, and the reticular cells of which they are a variant, appear to induce granulopoiesis. The salient function of macrophages is phagocytosis. Macrophages are thereby important in the clean-up of ineffective erythropoiesis and in the removal of the nuclear pole, produced when a normoblast becomes a reticulocyte. However, macrophages are important in regulating hematopoiesis not only by phagocytosis, but by the secretion of colony-stimulating factors, monokines, interleukins, leukotrienes, prostaglandins, and other factors, all of which may be loosely grouped as growth or signaling factors. Macrophages regulate the immune response by phagocytizing antigen and lymphocytes capable of autoimmune actions, by making antigen immunogenic, by presenting antigen, and, again, by secreting factors. Macrophages also illustrate the difficulty in delineating stromal cells from hematopoietic and blood cells. Regarded as stromal cells, macrophages originate from monocytes. They are mobile cells, moreover, capable of homing to, or migrating from, serous cavities, where they collect in great number, via blood and lymphatic vessels. IDCs and Langerhans cells also originate from a circulating precursor, the veiled cell. Barrier cells also possess a circulating progenitor. Many of the inductive and regulatory capacities associated with the stroma, moreover, are shared by blood cells. T cells secrete interleukin-2 and regulate B-cell differentiation. B cells present antigen. There are clearly dynamic, interactive relationships between the connective and hematopoietic tissues and between stroma and blood cells. In this perspective, we turn to the structure and function of bone marrow.

BONE MARROW

The yolk sac, gut wall, liver, spleen, and thymus precede the development of bone marrow.[5-9,23,30-39] At around 5 months in human gestation ossification begins and marrow quickly follows and acts pre-emptively, gathering in circulating hematopoietic stem cells and concentrating them in the layer of bone lining cells or endosteum[30] (Fig. 15-1). This seminal layer contains osteoblasts and osteoclasts and their progenitor cells, pointed toward bone, and hematopoietic stem cells and progenitor cells of the blood cells and stromal cells, pointed toward the bone marrow. If the marrow in murine femur is mechanically forced out, >90% of the stem cells remain and can be scraped from the marrow surface of the bone. The layer of bone-lining cells may well be the true capsule of bone marrow.

Not only does bone contain hematopoietic stem cells, its marrow provides a number of domains or, as LaPushin and Trentin[31] termed them, hematopoietic inductive microenvironments. These environments support the inductive forces that cause the multipotent hematopoietic stem cell to differentiate into one or more blood cell lines. Thus, there may be erythropoietic inductive microenvironments, eosinophilopoietic inductive microenvironments, and so forth.[5,31] Marrow, spleen, and thymus possess distinguishing microenvironments. Those of marrow produce leukocytes preponderantly, three or four to every erythrocyte. Those in mouse spleen produce two erythrocytes for every leukocyte. The thymus specializes in T-cell production. Since reticular cells and barrier cells physically form locules or enclosures in bone marrow, spleen, thymus, and lymph nodes, as do epithelial cells in thymus, and since macrophages are omnipresent, these dendritic stromal cells have been put forth, as yet uncertainly, as candidates for the creation of hematopoietic microenvironments.

Bone marrow is organized into vascular and hematopoietic compartments[7-9,19,31,37] (Fig. 15-2). The vascular compartment is dominated by large, thin-walled veins—vascular sinuses—that drain from the periphery of the marrow toward the center, where, in long bones, they are received by one or more central veins. This venous system carries blood back toward the heart and receives blood cells delivered transmurally from the hematopoietic compartments.[38,39] Most of the blood cells received by the veins of marrow are not carried directly into the general circulation. Instead they travel to other hematopoietic tissues for further maturation, conditioning, and testing before joining the general circulation.

The wall of the vascular sinus is simple but highly specialized[5] (Fig. 15-2), consisting of an endothelium and adventitia separated by a poorly developed basement membrane. Its endothelium consists of large sheet-like cells that bulge into the lumen in their nuclear zone, but over much of their cytoplasmic expanse they are quite thin, often 0.2 μm, just at or below the level of resolution of the light microscope. Endothelial cells display moderately specialized intercellular adherent membranous junctions. The endothelium permits transmural passage of cells from the hematopoietic compartment into the vascular lumen. Such passage occurs not through interendothelial junctions but through endothelial cytoplasm near interendothelial junctions and away from the cell center. It is likely that this passage, initiated by endocytosis at the basal endothelial surface, is receptor mediated. The receptors, moreover, likely include differentiation markers on the blood cell surface, since, under normal conditions, only blood cells that are rather mature leave the hematopoietic compartment and cross into the venous vasculature.

The second cellular layer comprising the wall of the venous sinuses of the marrow consists of adventitial reticular cells, large branched or dendritic stromal cells that lie on the outside, or adventitial, surface of the endothelium. These cells, as reticular cells in the spleen and other locations, branch out

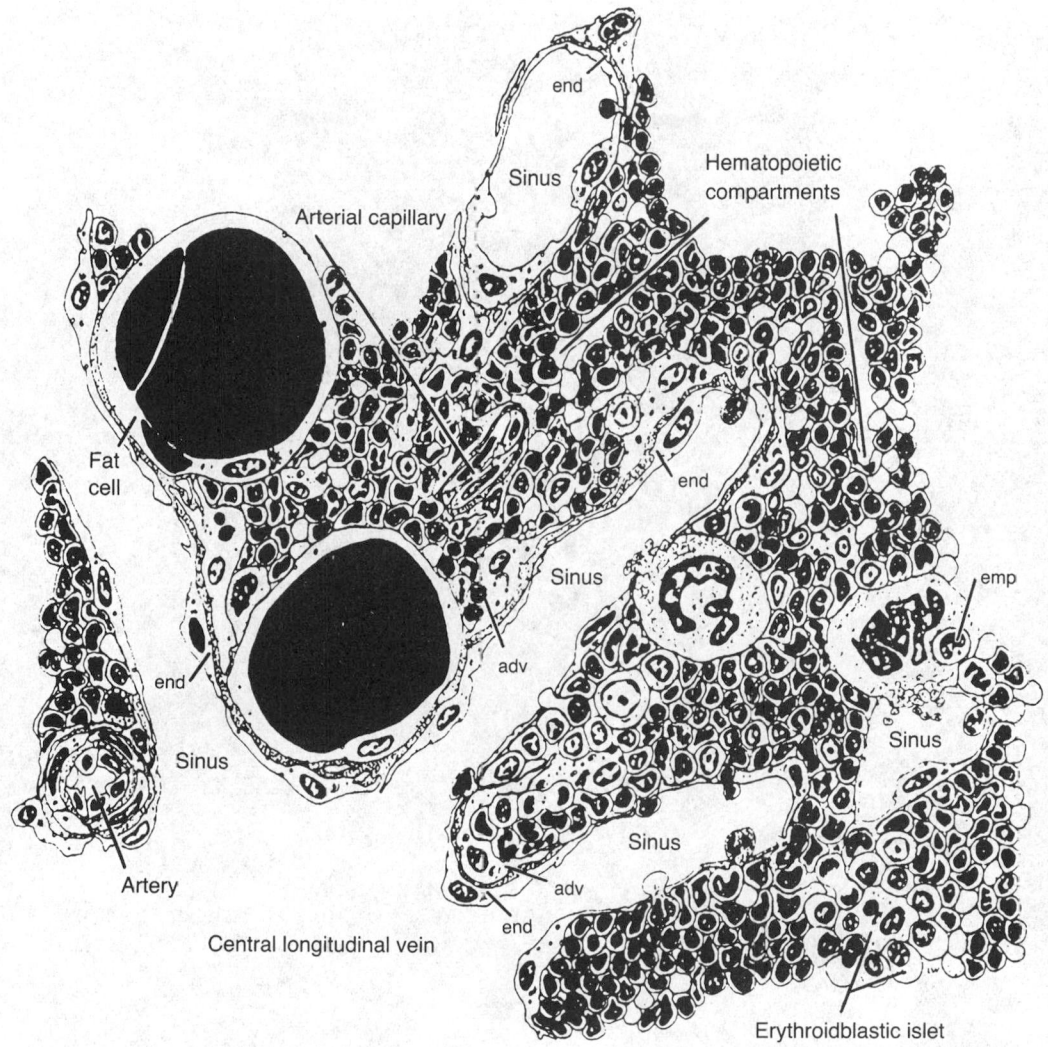

Fig. 15-1. Bone marrow, schematic view of cross section near the central longitudinal vein. Several sinuses drain into the central longitudinal vein, in cross section. A portion of the nutrient artery is present, as is an arterial capillary. Hematopoietic cells lie between the sinuses, in the hematopoietic compartment. Where hematopoiesis is relatively quiet, the wall of the sinus and of the central longitudinal vein is trilaminar, consisting of endothelium (end), a basement membrane, and adventitial cell (adv). The adventitial cell may become voluminous, encroaching on the hematopoietic space and thereby displacing hematopoietic cells. The increased volume of the adventitial cell may be due to a gelatinous change wherein its cytoplasm becomes rarefied, presumably because of hydration. If this change is widespread, the marrow may become grossly white and gelatinous. A second and more common basis for the large bulk of adventitial cells is fatty change, wherein they become adipocytes. Contrariwise, when hematopoiesis is active the hematopoietic compartment is large and packed with myelocytes, erythroblasts, megakaryocytes, promonocytes, and lymphocytes. The sinus wall becomes thin, reduced to an endothelial layer alone as the adventitial cells are displaced or lifted from the wall by infiltrating hematopoietic cells. Apertures appear in the endothelium, moreover, as maturing hematopoietic cells cross the sinus wall and enter the sinus lumen. Megakaryocytes (meg) characteristically lie against the outside of the sinus wall. Occasionally the cytoplasm of megakaryocytes is entered by other cell types, which remain visible and later leave the megakaryocyte. The phenomenon is known as emperilopoiesis (emp). Erythroblasts tend to be present in clusters near the sinus wall. They often occur as erythroblastic islets, ensembles of erythroblasts and macrophages. Granulocytes usually develop near the center of the hematopoietic space and move toward the sinus wall as postmitotic relatively mature cells. Lymphocytes occur throughout the marrow, as do macrophages. (From Weiss,[5] with permission.)

from the adventitial surface of the sinuses and, by their branches, form a perivascular scaffolding in the hematopoietic compartment that holds the developing blood cells. The amount of the adventitial surface of endothelium covered by adventitial reticular cells in active, hematopoietic marrow is about 40% in mice, much less in dogs and not yet measured in humans. The reticular cells providing adventitial cover are dynamic: when there is increased transmural passage associated with increased blood cell delivery, the adventitial reticular cells move away, reducing their cover and thereby exposing more of the outside surface of the endothelium to the cells in passage.

Adventitial reticular cells therefore regulate cell passage across the venous sinuses, covering or uncovering the endothelium as needed. Adventitial reticular cells play another major regulatory role. They may become fatty and, when they do so, constitute the adipocytes of bone marrow (Fig. 15-1). Adipocytes control the volume of the hematopoietic compartment available for hematopoietic cells, since the bone marrow, encased as it is by bone, does not readily change its volume by flux in bone. The modulation of adventitial reticular cells to and from adipocytes occurs rather readily in the hematopoietic marrow of the axial skeleton (where, as Tavossoli[7] showed, the adipocyte fat is unsaturated), but not as readily in the yellow

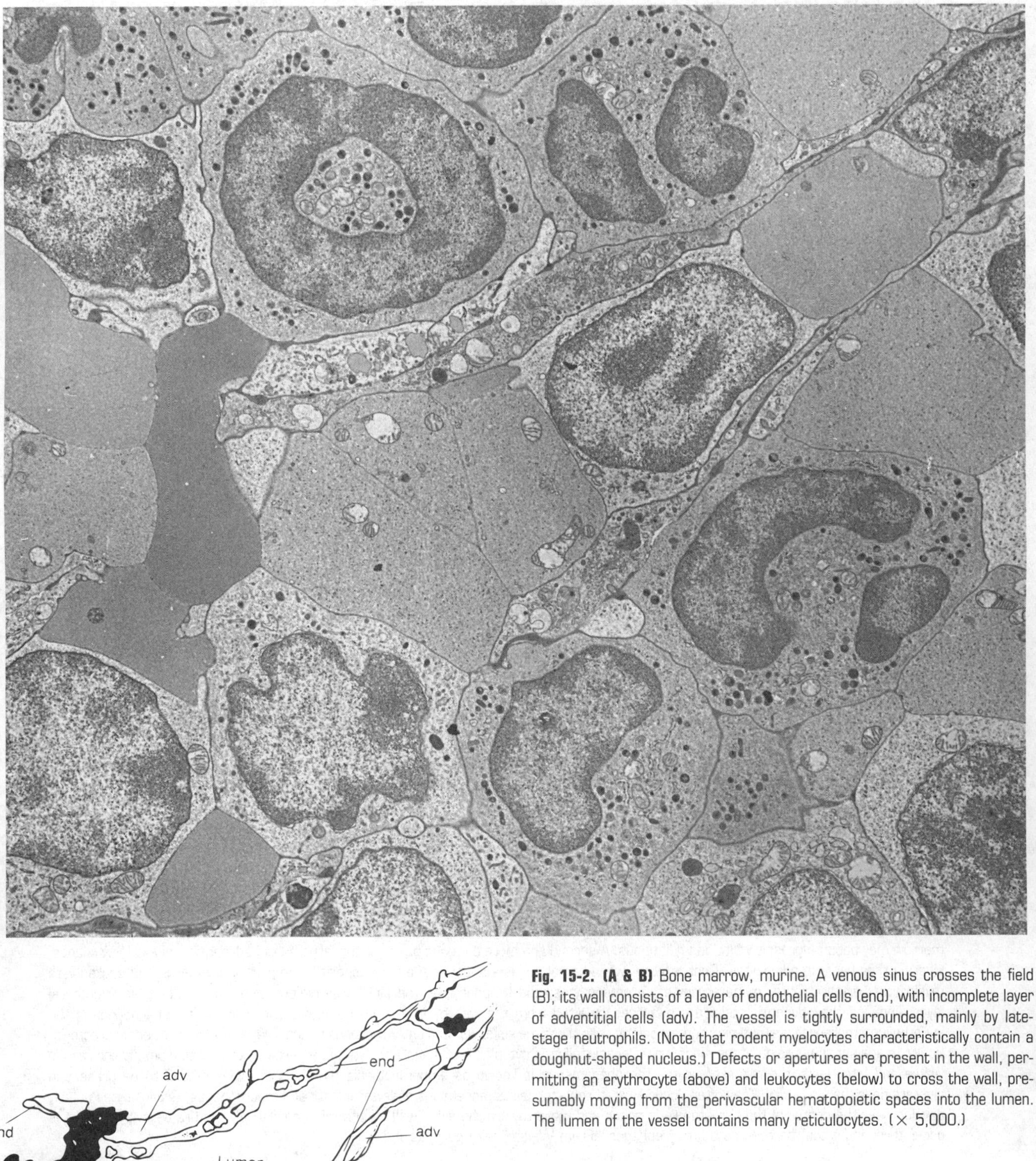

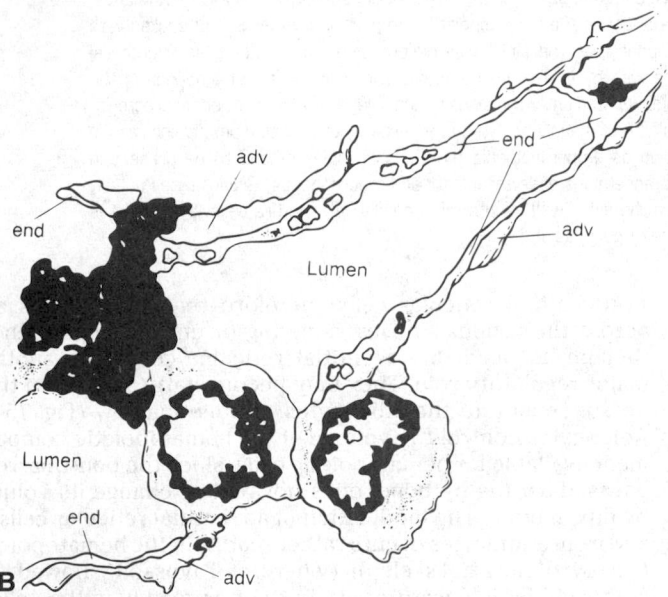

Fig. 15-2. (A & B) Bone marrow, murine. A venous sinus crosses the field (B); its wall consists of a layer of endothelial cells (end), with incomplete layer of adventitial cells (adv). The vessel is tightly surrounded, mainly by late-stage neutrophils. (Note that rodent myelocytes characteristically contain a doughnut-shaped nucleus.) Defects or apertures are present in the wall, permitting an erythrocyte (above) and leukocytes (below) to cross the wall, presumably moving from the perivascular hematopoietic spaces into the lumen. The lumen of the vessel contains many reticulocytes. (× 5,000.)

marrow of the peripheral skeleton (where the fat is saturated and less easily mobilized). Indeed, yellow bone marrow contains a sufficient number of adipocytes grossly to impart the yellow color. Red bone marrow is taken to be hematopoietic, the color due to the erythropoietic component of hematopoiesis. However, a hypoplastic marrow may sometimes be red, not because of hemoglobin-containing hematopoietic cells, but because of engorgement of the venous vasculature with erythrocytes. Marrow adventitial reticular cells are also capable of gelatinous transformation. Here the adventitial cells become voluminous, not with fat, but, in all likelihood, by increased hydration, imparting a white, gelatinous character to the marrow. This gelatinous change may be a transient intermediary stage between red hematopoietic and yellow hypoplastic marrow. It may also be long-lasting, associated with starvation or certain marrow toxins.

The hematopoietic compartment of marrow occupies the perivascular spaces and contains hematopoietic colonies, arterial vasculature, and accessory cells. Only rarely are hematopoietic colonies as discrete and spherical as those observed in tissue culture or in stem cell-seeded marrow beginning to recover from irradiation. Erythroid colonies often do approach this conformation; they have been termed erythroblastic islets (Fig. 15-1). Colonies of the other cell lineages tend to be confluent, overlapping, and mixed, extending in irregular sheet-like formations. The colonies consist of differentiating blood cells tightly packed together and regularly include both macrophages and barrier cells. Erythroblastic islets occur right against the adventitial surface of vascular sinuses. The more differentiated cells (i.e., reticulocytes and normoblasts) lie against the vascular wall, while the earlier forms (i.e., the basophilic erythroblasts) are most distant from the venous vasculature. Those normoblasts that lie against the wall, moreover, are polarized into nuclear and cytoplasmic poles. The cytoplasmic pole is pressed into the adventitial surface of the endothelium (the adventitial reticular cell has typically retracted from the vascular wall), and the nuclear pole, consisting of the dense nucleus and surrounding rim of cytoplasm, faces toward the hematopoietic compartment. The arrangement clearly puts those erythroid cells that are more differentiated, and therefore more prepared for delivery to the circulation, in a favored position for delivery. A macrophage typically occupies a central position in the colony, its many slender cytoplasmic branches threading among the differentiating erythroid cells so that virtually every differentiating cell is partially enveloped by macrophage cytoplasm. The macrophage so situated is prepared for the phagocytosis of broken-off nuclear poles, a necessary occurrence as erythroblasts become reticulocytes, and for the phagocytosis of any imperfectly produced erythroid cell, representing ineffective erythropoiesis. The macrophages are also well situated for the efficient delivery of the regulatory factors they produce. Syncytial sheets of barrier cells may also compartmentalize the colony and partially encapsulate it.

Megakaryocytes, like erythroblastic islets, lie against the outside surface of venous sinuses (Fig. 15-2). They originate from small lymphocyte-like cells, which, in rodents, are marked by the presence of the enzyme acetylcholinesterase. These small acetylcholinesterase cells or "sache" cells move to the outside surface of the vascular sinus and, in that hematopoietic microenvironment, continue their differentiation, which involves the final endomitotic divisions resulting in polyploidy (they can go to 64N). Set against an aperture in the wall of a vascular sinus, these large, polyploid cells may deliver platelets efficiently into the vascular sinus through the aperture, while "stoppering" it so that the vessel remains competent. Full development of megakaryocytes and platelet production and release may require emigration of megakaryocytes, from marrow to other tissues, such as the lung.[40] A mature polyploid megakaryocyte may be fairly regarded as an hematopoietic colony; from this

perspective, it is not surprising that it is usually enveloped by barrier cells. Indeed, during the early stages of differentiation, reticular cells or barrier cells typically reach from their pericytic location in the wall of a venous sinus to a megakaryocyte progenitor some distance from the sinus and may well play a role in bringing the progenitor to the characteristic mural megakaryocyte position.

Granulocytes typically develop in the perivascular space away from the vascular wall. When they become mature enough to move, usually as metamyelocytes, they move to the sinus wall. Just preceding their transmural passage and release from the hematopoietic compartment into the circulation, they develop microvilli, which probe the adventitial cell cover of the vascular sinus, inducing it to move away, baring the endothelial cell. The microvilli then press on the outside surface of the endothelium, setting in motion the special transcytotic process that results in the leukocyte crossing the endothelium, deeply constricted in a transient mural aperture, and gaining the lumen.[39] During periods of hematopoietic stress, granulocyte colonies, as well as all other kinds of hematopoietic colonies, may display a meshwork of barrier cells that support and protect the hematopoietic cells (Fig. 15-3). Even fully hematopoietic bone marrow has scattered adipocytes, consisting of adventitial reticular cells that have accumulated fat droplets that have enlarged and coalesced.

THYMUS

The thymus is a central immunologic organ that receives T-cell progenitors from the bone marrow, supports their differentiation to mature T cells, and exports them to other, so-called peripheral lymphatic tissues.[1,5,10,11,20–22,32–34,41–45] The process of T-cell maturation is complicated by the large-scale death of differentiating T cells. Fewer than 10% survive to mature T cells. Rather on release from the thymus, they home to the spleen, where some are stabilized (perhaps those capable of responding to antigen in the spleen's library of antigens with which the body is experienced) then are released to the recirculating pool of long-lived immunologically competent lymphocytes (RLP).

The thymus is a lymphoepithelial organ, an epithelial-rich medullary core surrounded by a lymphocyte-rich cortex[1,5,11,33] (Fig. 15-4). The prepubertal thymus is fully developed, organized into side-by-side lobules, each consisting of a thick cortical cap on a medullary prolongation extending from the central medullary core. The cortex may well look like a solid blanket of lymphocytes; indeed, it contains more than 95% of the lymphocytes of the thymus, but it is also rich in less visible epithelial cells that form a network or reticulum supporting the lymphocytes. These epithelial cells, pushed apart by infiltrating T cells, remain attached to one another by desmosomes and thereby assume a reticular dendritic conformation. Accordingly, they are termed epithelial-reticular cells. Circulating T-cell progenitors homing to the thymus leave the vasculature and enter the thymic parenchyma high in the cortex, just under the capsule. They form a poorly defined layer of relatively large lymphocytes there, showing active proliferation, marked preferentially in autoradiographs after a pulse of tritiated thymidine. They then move deeper into the cortex toward the corticomedullary junction. The migration of T-cell progenitors is associated with their differentiation; they acquire successively more mature differentiation markers, until they become mature T cells. During this intrathymic migration and maturation, differentiating T cells are in intimate association with stromal cells, including epithelial-reticular cells[10,43,46] reticular cells, barrier cells, and macrophages. These stromal cells regulate differentiation in at least three ways: (1) secretion of thymosin and other factors that enhance or diminish T-cell differentiation, proliferation, and migration; (2) formation of sacs or en-

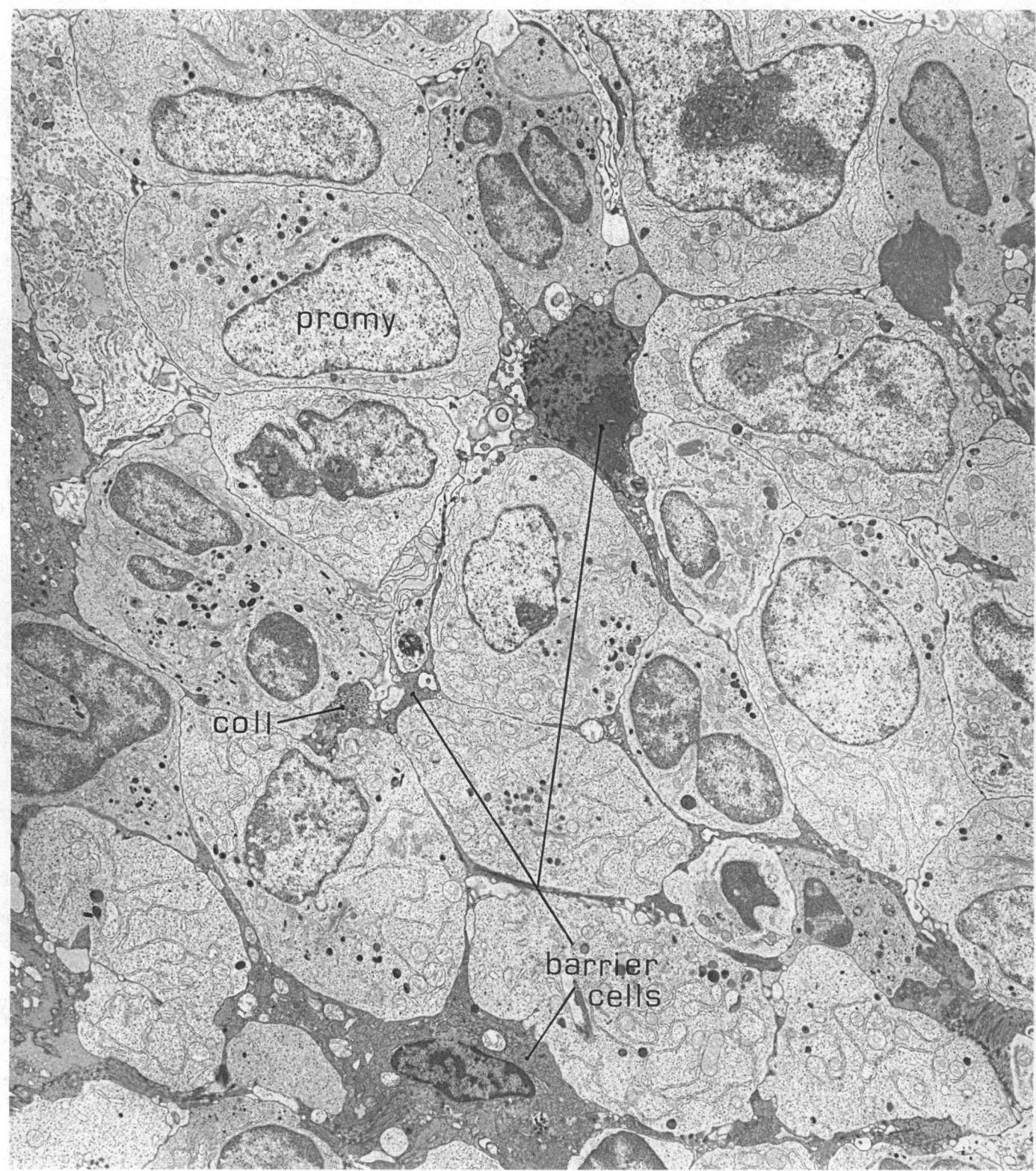

Fig. 15-3. Bone marrow, murine. This field consists of a portion of a large granulocyte colony, particularly rich in promyelocytes (promy) and myelocytes. The dark branched cells lying within the colony are barrier cells, in some places associated with collagen (coll). They form a syncytial meshwork closely holding the granulocytes. (× 3,000.)

closures, very much like brood sacs, that isolate and protect the differentiating T cells and hold regulatory factors in high concentration; and (3) surveillance of T-cell maturation by means of cell surface MHC antigens, which give physical and practical expression to the idea of self. As T cells differentiate, their MHC antigens emerge, and stromal cells, notably epithelial cells, wrap cell processes about differentiating T cells and establish cell-surface/cell-surface contact. These epithelial cells determine through their own MHC cell-surface antigens whether the "self" that the differentiating T cells will assume, as expressed through their developing cell surface MHC anti-gens, is congenial or hostile to the tissues of the body. If hostile, and therefore threatening autoimmune reaction, the development and even survival of those T lymphocytes are suppressed. In part, as a consequence of such epithelial cell surveillance, a large proportion of differentiating T cells quickly die. Only about 5% survive to be released from the thymus as mature, immunologically competent, but naive, T cells. They are released into the blood and lymphatic vasculature at the corticomedullary junction or within the medulla. They go to the spleen for final conditioning and culling before their release to the general circulation and long life in RLP.

Cortical epithelial cells assume conformations in addition to

that of epithelial-reticular cells[5,11,33,41] (Fig. 15-4). As flat cells, joined by desmosomes, they form a rim or border about the thymic lobule and ensheath intrathymic blood vessels. The thymic cortex is thereby effectively isolated from many outside influences, only the selective entrance of certain cells (e.g., the T-cell progenitors released from bone marrow) is permitted, and particulates and macromolecules as antigen are excluded. A blood-thymic barrier, effected largely by the epithelial cells ensheathing blood vessels, contributes to this thymic isolation. Epithelial cells, moreover, are present in some variety (e.g., dark and light epithelial cells). Their distinctive functions have not yet been sorted out. Nurse cells, large dendritic cells, specialized in containing groups of developing T cells, occur in

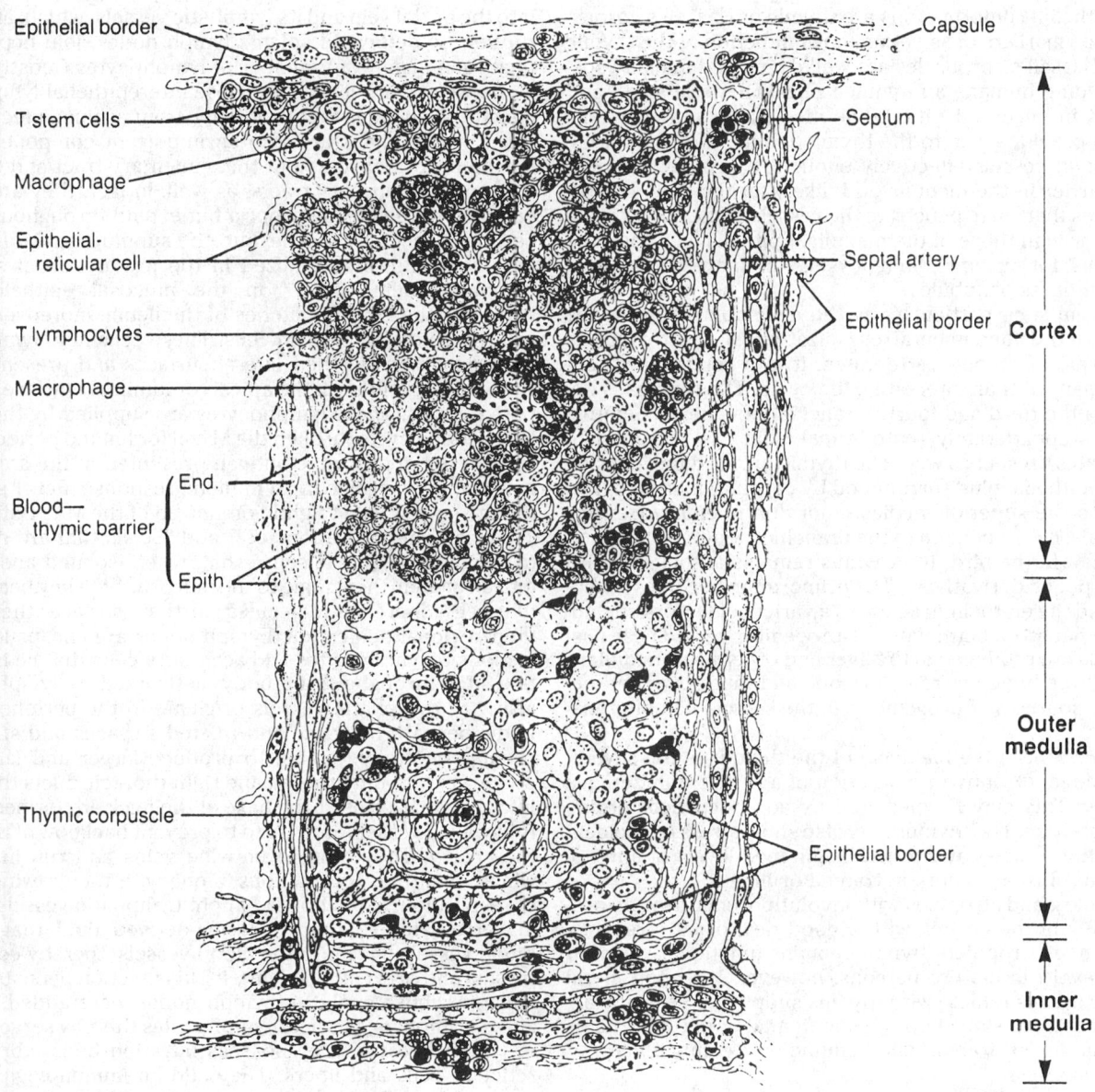

Fig. 15-4. Schema of portion of thymus lobule. The cortex is heavily infiltrated with lymphocytes. As a result, the epithelial cells become stellate and remain attached to one another by desmosomes. These epithelial cells are termed epithelial-reticular cells because they form a meshwork or reticulum. The medulla is closer to a pure epithelium, although it too is commonly infiltrated by lymphocytes. A thymic corpuscle, consisting of concentrically arranged epithelial cells, is shown. A border of somewhat flattened epithelial cells is joined by desmosomes, and tight junctions surround the cortex and outer medulla, serving to shield the lobule from outside influences. This epithelial layer surrounds blood vessels that penetrate the cortex and outer medulla of the thymus, providing a thymic-blood barrier. A capsule and septae made up mainly of collagenous connective tissue, and containing granulocytes and lymphocytes, lies outside the epithelial border, forming the outermost cover of the thymus. (From Weiss,[5] with permission.)

the cortex. Other stromal cells are present, including reticular cells, with associated collagen fibers, and barrier cells.[5,11] Interdigitating cells are present in the medulla.[5,11,33]

The medulla of the thymus, like the cortex, is lymphoepithelial, but only about 5% of thymic lymphocytes are held there. Medullary lymphocytes, in contrast to those of the cortex, are rather differentiated. They are, as is characteristic of mature T cells, resistant to cortisone, which induces widespread cell death in the immature T-cell cortical populations. The dominant cell types of the medulla are epithelial cells that, not pressed apart by large, proliferating populations of interepithelial lymphocytes, as occurs in the cortex, tend to be polyhedral as opposed to the reticular shape of the cortex. In places, medullary epithelial cells take on a circumferential, lamellated, conformation that is often irregular and, when large in size, tends to show central necrosis, calcification, and cyst formation. These epithelial conformations are thymic or Hassall's corpuscles, unique markers of as yet unknown function of the thymic medulla. Hassall's corpuscles are well developed in many species, including humans and guinea pigs. They are small and infrequent in mice and rats. While medullary epithelial cells appear to provide a rim to the thymic lobule, they do not ensheath blood vessels effectively enough to provide a blood-thymic barrier in the medulla and, likely, in the deep cortex. Particulates that fail to penetrate the vessels of the cortex readily enter through those of the medulla. Epithelial cells assume other forms, for example, lining cysts, which are remnants of embryonal ducts or tubules.

Aside from such particulars as the development of thymic corpuscles, the fundamental organization of the thymus is rather invariant among vertebrates. It is a remarkably conserved organ, with an interesting life cycle. The thymus is derived from the third and fourth branchial pouches. Its epithelium is preponderately entodermal, but an ectodermal component is present as well. The thymic primordium, consisting of an epithelial plug surrounded by capsular mesenchyme, moves into the superior mediastinum during embryogenesis of mammals; its connection to the branchial pouch withers and disappears. (In the bird, the thymus remains associated with branchial pouch derivatives.) The primordium becomes vascularized, and the epithelium secretes a variety of factors, including those that attract circulating T-progenitor cells. These nascent T cells are produced in the liver and other extramedullary sites, until the bone marrow develops and takes over and becomes the source of T progenitors in the second half of prenatal life.

A major event in the life cycle of the thymus is the severe, rather sudden, atrophy or involution of age that it undergoes at puberty. This may be mediated by adrenocorticosteroids and testosterone. The thymus may also show stress or accidental involution caused by sudden heightened levels of adrenocortical steroids, as occurs in trauma or illness.

The whole gland atrophies with involution, occurring disproportionately in the cortex, with a good deal of fatty replacement. Even an atrophied thymus remains functional, albeit at reduced levels. In mature persons, however, with peripheral lymphatic tissues replete with thymus-supplied T cells, the activity of the thymus need not be maintained at prepubertal or young-adult levels, to maintain immunologic competence.

LYMPH NODES AND MUCOSA-ASSOCIATED LYMPHATIC TISSUE

Lymphocytes and many of their accessory cells are migratory, capable of forming immunologically responsive aggregations virtually anywhere in the body; in pathologic states, they may do so. There are, nonetheless, certain sites or microenvironments that regularly support formal, well-organized, immunologically distinctive and powerful collections of lymphocytes and supporting cells.[1,3,5] Collectively, these sites are termed peripheral lymphatic tissues because they tend to be the sites where immunologic reactions occur, rather than the central lymphatic tissues (i.e., bone marrow and thymus), where the immunologically competent and accessory cells are generated. (In fact, the bone marrow and the septae of the thymus can engage in immunologic reactions, showing that this useful dichotomy is not rigorous.)

A major concentration of peripheral lymphatic tissue is in the gut mucosa, reaching to the submucosa, perhaps because the gut is a major site at which antigen is encountered. The spleen originates as a specialized portion of the lamina propria near the stomach and migrates from the gut to its nearby independent location. However, its vasculature keeps it tied into the gastrointestinal tract, particularly its veins, which drain into the portal vein and its lymphatic vessels, which, after interruption by dedicated splenic lymph nodes, join hepatic lymphatics. A significant number of lymphocytes (mostly T cells) lie between epithelial cells. These interepithelial lymphocytes constitute an important protective front against infectious disease. Lymphocytes are also an important component of the lamina propria throughout the alimentary tract and of the respiratory and urinary tracts, as well. In fact, they are seldom confined to the lamina propria but extend throughout the mucosa and spill into and beyond the submucosa. MALT is rich in B cells and is specialized in the production of secretory immunoglobulin (IgA).[47] In the mucosal epithelium surmounting the Peyer's patches of the ileum, moreover, lie specialized epithelial cells, M cells. These cells hold lymphocytes in invaginations in their lateral surfaces and present antigen to them, brought from the apical (or lumimal) surface by transport vesicles. These lymphocytes are supplied by the Peyer's patches and cycle through the M cell for limited periods. If they receive the appropriate antigen presented in the appropriate manner, they engage in an immune response. Peyer's patches are the largest, most tightly organized of the MALT structures. They contain populations of B and T cells that are dedicated to the mucosa, in the sense that, when isolated and injected into an animal, they home to the mucosa.[14,15] They bear distinctive cell adherence molecules on their surface, the basis of their regional dedication. Lymph nodes are encapsulated collections of lymphocytes and accessory cells that lie in distinctive sites throughout the body, networked by lymphatic vessels.[48–50] Lymphatic vessels originate in the periphery of the body, beneath mucosae and related surfaces and structures, running centrally, joining to produce larger and larger lymphatic vessels, until the left and right thoracic ducts that empty into the great veins at the base of the neck are formed.[5] These thin-walled vessels are valved to prevent backflow of the lymph they carry. They tend to entwine veins and run in muscles whose remitting contractions, along with the drawing actions of respiration, propel their lymph. Lymphatic vessels evolved in vertebrates to return plasma-derived fluid that escapes blood vessels back into the blood vessels, thereby conserving plasma and preventing edema.[51] This function persists in mammals, in whose evolution lymph nodes were added, inserted across lymphatic vessels. Lymph nodes thereby serve as filters of lymph because they possess filtration beds fabricated of reticular cells and fibers. They add an immunologic role because they collect lymphocytes of the RLP in their filtration beds. Lymph nodes thus serve as immunologically competent depots specialized in responding to antigen introduced regionally and brought to them by the regional lymphatic vessels. Lymph nodes contrast with the spleen, which receives blood-borne antigen. Indeed, lymph nodes and spleen display specializations in lymphocyte populations, hence, in function. The spleen and Peyer's patches specialize in humoral immunity and are B-cell rich. The peripheral lymph nodes and the skin, in-

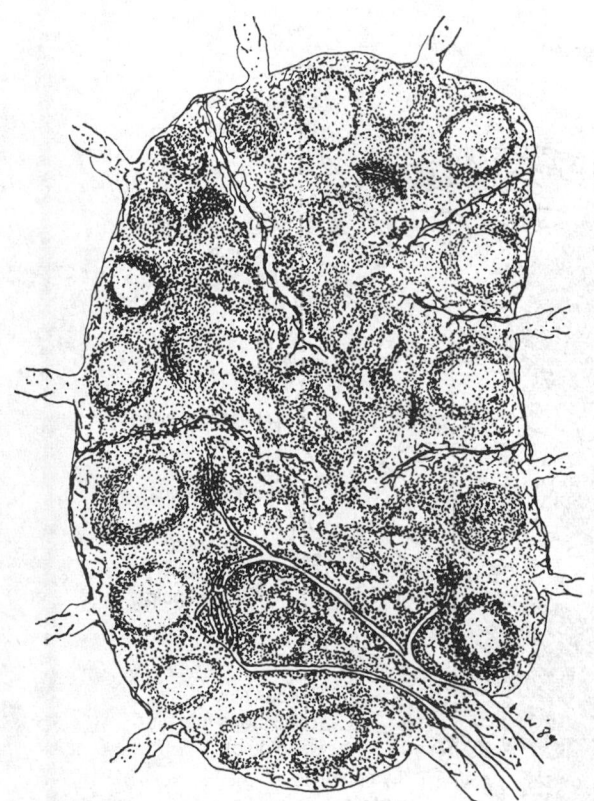

Fig. 15-5. Schema of lymph node. Afferent lymphatic vessels, some showing valves, pierce the capsule along its convexity. Efferent lymphatic vessels leave the node at the hilus. The nodular cortex consists of spherical lymphatic nodules, some of which contain germinal centers. The diffuse cortex lies between the nodules and deep to them. The diffuse cortex is separated into internodular cortex and deep or tertiary cortex. Within the center of the node lie the linear medullary cords, rich in lymphocytes and plasma cells, converging on the hilus. A subcapsular sinus, into which the afferent lymphatic vessels empty, lies beneath the full expanse of capsule. Radial sinuses run from the subcapsular sinus toward the hilus. They run along trabeculae, and, in the medulla, between medullary cords. Arteries enter the node at the hilus and branch richly, penetrating the node. Postcapillary venules lie in the diffuse cortex. Veins leave the node at the hilus.

volved in delayed hypersensitivity and other manifestations of cellular immunity, are, accordingly, rather rich in T cells. Further specializations derive from skewed distributions of T-cell subtypes in mucosal and nonmucosal lymphatic tissues. As one charts the distribution of T and B cells and their subtypes, it becomes evident that the lymphatic system is mosaic, richly, minutely, and subtly specialized.

Lymph nodes are small encapsulated structures (Fig. 15-5) that receive lymph via afferent lymphatic vessels, which pierce the capsule, and from which lymph drains via efferent lymphatic vessels.[52,53] The inside of the node consists of specialized meshworks, or filtration beds, fabricated of reticular cells and their associated reticular fibers. These filtration beds receive T and B cells of the RLP and their accessory cells, sorting them out into T- and B-cell zones.[16,17] About the periphery of a lymph node is a broad dense band of lymphocytes. Nodules of lymphocytes, termed lymphatic nodules, lie within this band, toward its outside margin. Lymphocytes in the band are preponderantly T cells, while those in nodules are mostly B cells. As a result of the placement of the lymphatic nodules, the T-cell domain is divided into two zones: a deeper paracortex and a more superficial internodular cortex. Lymphatic nodules, internodular cortex, and paracortex make up the cortex of the lymph node. Within the cortex lymphocytes are the dominant cell type, so much so that it may appear, on first view, that

they are the exclusive cell type. However, they are supported by meshworks of reticular cells and fibers, augmented by barrier cells when functional demands increase. These fibroblastic stromal cells provide filtration beds, as in splenic white pulp, which selectively filter out B and T cells of the RLP. Furthermore, macrophages and other antigen-presenting cells and accessory cells are present, again as in splenic white pulp. The center, or medulla, of the lymph node, deep to the cortex, is organized as medullary cords of reticular cells enmeshing lymphocytes, plasma cells, macrophages, and granulocytes. Medullary cords are separated by medullary sinuses. These intranodal lymphatic vessels converge on the hilus and exit.[49,50]

Lymphatic vessels run through the node.[1,5,18] Afferent lymphatics pierce the capsule and empty into a large subcapsular sinus. Radial vessels run from the subcapsular sinus through the cortex, often along trabeculae, and enter the medulla, where, as medullary sinuses, they run between the medullary cords and out the lymph node at its hilus, via efferent lymphatics. Afferent lymphatic vessels bring antigen into a lymph node; if that node is central, receiving lymph from a peripheral node, the afferent lymphatics also bring lymphocytes of the RLP from the peripheral node. Lymph nodes possess a good blood supply, arteries entering and veins leaving through the hilus. Distinctive postcapillary venules are concentrated in the paracortex. Often termed high endothelial venules because their endothelium can be cuboidal instead of squamous, they represent the major pathway by which recirculating lymphocytes enter the node.[5,14,15] On the basis of specific surface receptors, T and B cells recognize and adhere to the high endothelium and then pass through it into the node, the B cells moving peripherally into lymphatic nodules and the T cells into the paracortex and the internodular cortex.[14,16,17] There, facing one another and served by IDC, which present antigen to T cells, and FDC, which present antigen to B cells, an immune response may be initiated. In sustained primary responses or in secondary responses, germinal centers, sites specialized in the generation of lymphocytes and accessory cells, develop within lymphatic nodules. If the T and B cells fail to engage in an immune response, they leave the node via lymphatic vessels within a matter of hours, rejoining the RLP.

SPLEEN

By means of its unique circulation, the spleen filters lymphocytes, monocyte/macrophages, granulocytes, and platelets from the blood and positions them to protect efficiently against blood-borne infection.[5,24,25,36,54–61] The unique splenic circulation lacks endothelial continuity between the ending of its arteries and the beginning of its veins (Fig. 15-6). Instead, diverse filtration beds, which confer on the spleen its extraordinary capacity to clear the blood of circulating cells and particles, are interposed between arteries and veins. The basic filtration beds are made up of large branched fibroblastic stromal cells, reticular cells. Reticular cells are considered stable or "fixed."[5,23,24] They are associated with reticular fibers, which are ensheathed by their branches. Reticular cell filtration beds are augmented by other stromal cell types, including macrophages, interdigitating cells, and follicular dendritic cells. In addition, newly recognized stromal cells, termed barrier cells, are present with heightened splenic activity. Barrier cells are fibroblastic and probably contractile. They are related to reticular cells but are rapidly responsive and mobile, and fuse to form syncytial sheets deployed as diverse barriers.[23–26] These cells are insinuated into the basic reticulum and, by their flexibility and responsiveness, adapt to deal with heightened levels of splenic activities, such as blood filtration and hematopoiesis.

Two types of filtration beds, the periarterial lymphatic

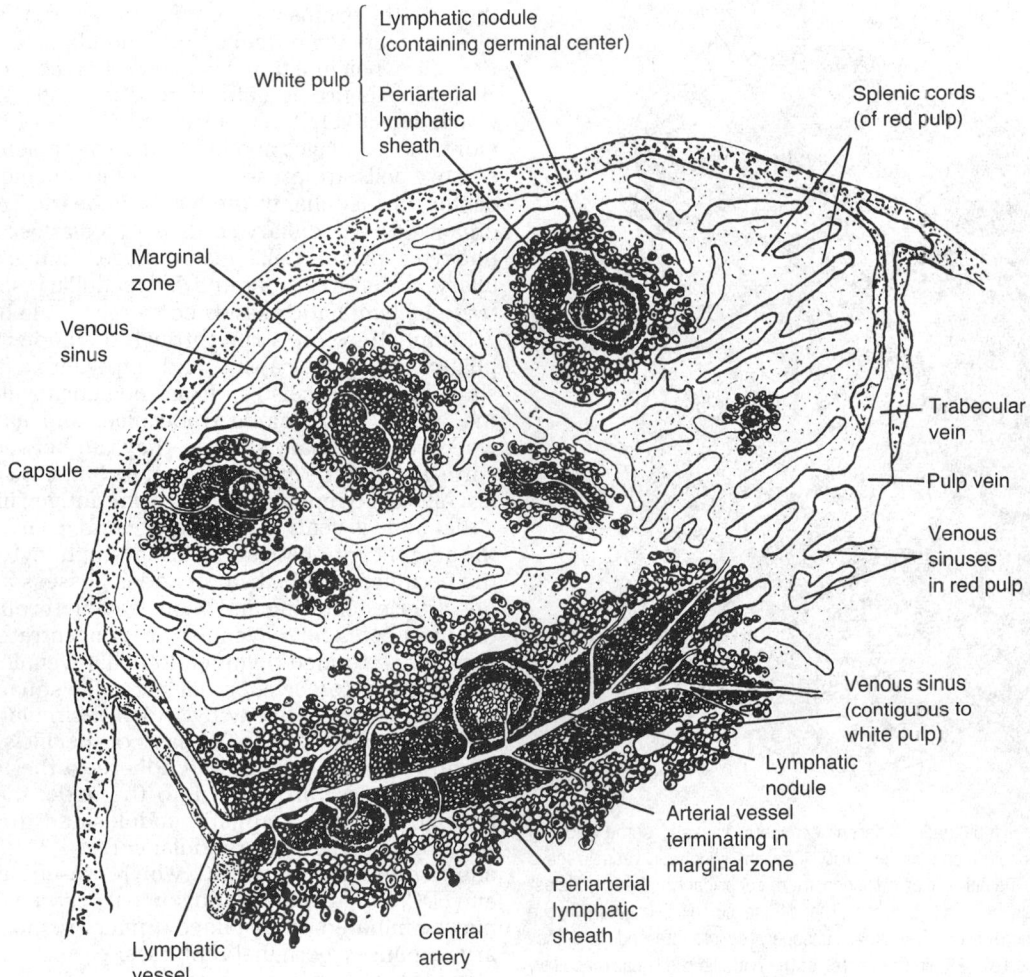

Fig. 15-6. Schematic view of the organization of the human spleen. The white pulp has two components: periarterial lymphatic sheath (T-cell zone) and lymphatic nodules (B-cell zones). The latter may be a solid nodule of small cells or be made up of a germinal center (representing a high-level antibody-producing center) and a surrounding mantle zone of small cells. The WP is surrounded by an MZ. The remainder of the tissue depicted is RP, whose salient structures are splenic (or venous) sinuses separated by splenic cords. The pattern of blood flow is as follows. A trabecular artery enters the WP and becomes the central artery. The central artery runs in the central axis of the periarterial lymphatic sheath and gives rise to many branches. Many end within the WP, supplying the periarterial lymphatic sheath, the germinal center, and mantle zone of the secondary nodule. Most terminate at the periphery of the WP, emptying in or near the MZ. A number of arterial vessels emerge from the WP, pass into the MZ, reach the RP, and curve back to empty into the MZ. Other arterial branches, as well as the main stem of the central artery, run into RP. Almost all terminate in the filtration beds of the cords. Here, too, variation exists. Some arterial vessels terminate adjacent to a venous sinus, whereas others terminate away from a sinus. Arterial vessels may terminate as capillaries or as somewhat larger vessels. Some arterial vessels may be surrounded by macrophage sheaths shortly before termination. Venous sinuses drain into pulp veins, which in turn drain into trabecular veins. Thus, the vasculature of the spleen is "anatomically open" with filtration beds interposed between fine arterial and venous vessels. Efferent lymphatic vessels lie about the proximal portion of the central artery and run out of the spleen through the trabeculae carrying out T and B cells of the WP that had not engaged antigen, to rejoin the RLP. (From Weiss and Tavassoli,[61] with permission.)

sheath, which selectively clears T cells (with their accessory cells and antigen) from the blood, and the lymphatic nodules, which clear B cells (with their accessory cells and antigen) from the blood, make up the white pulp (WP) (Figs. 15-6 and 15-7), the immunologically competent portion of the spleen.[5,24,25,58–60] The WP is bounded by specialized reticular cells that cover its surface, assuming a circumferential configuration. WP is supplied by slender branching arterioles that run through WP, running to its periphery, terminating at its very edge by flaring out and merging with the circumferential reticulum. These terminating arterial vessels release their blood into the filtration beds within and outside WP. The red pulp (RP), consisting of filtration beds that clear erythrocytes, monocyte/macrophages, platelets, granulocytes, and lymphocytes from the blood, forms the periphery of splenic nodules, enclosing

the WP, and extending centrally as broad bands between lobules of WP.

The marginal zone (MZ) consists of fine-meshed filtration beds that lie between WP and RP. These filtration beds tightly surround the WP, receiving blood from many arterial vessels that course and end in the MZ. On its periphery, the MZ merges into RP. The MZ thus serves as a major portal, a vestibule, to the spleen. Many blood cells are processed in the MZ; damaged erythrocytes are detained and phagocytized or modified; monocytes are held and permitted to differentiate into macrophages; platelets are stored; granulocytes are detained or destroyed; and microbes are cleared and destroyed. Veins penetrate the MZ and drain blood from the spleen.

The RP (Figs. 15-6 and 15-8) is the most peripheral component of the spleen.[5,24,25,55,56,58–60] It has three major elements:

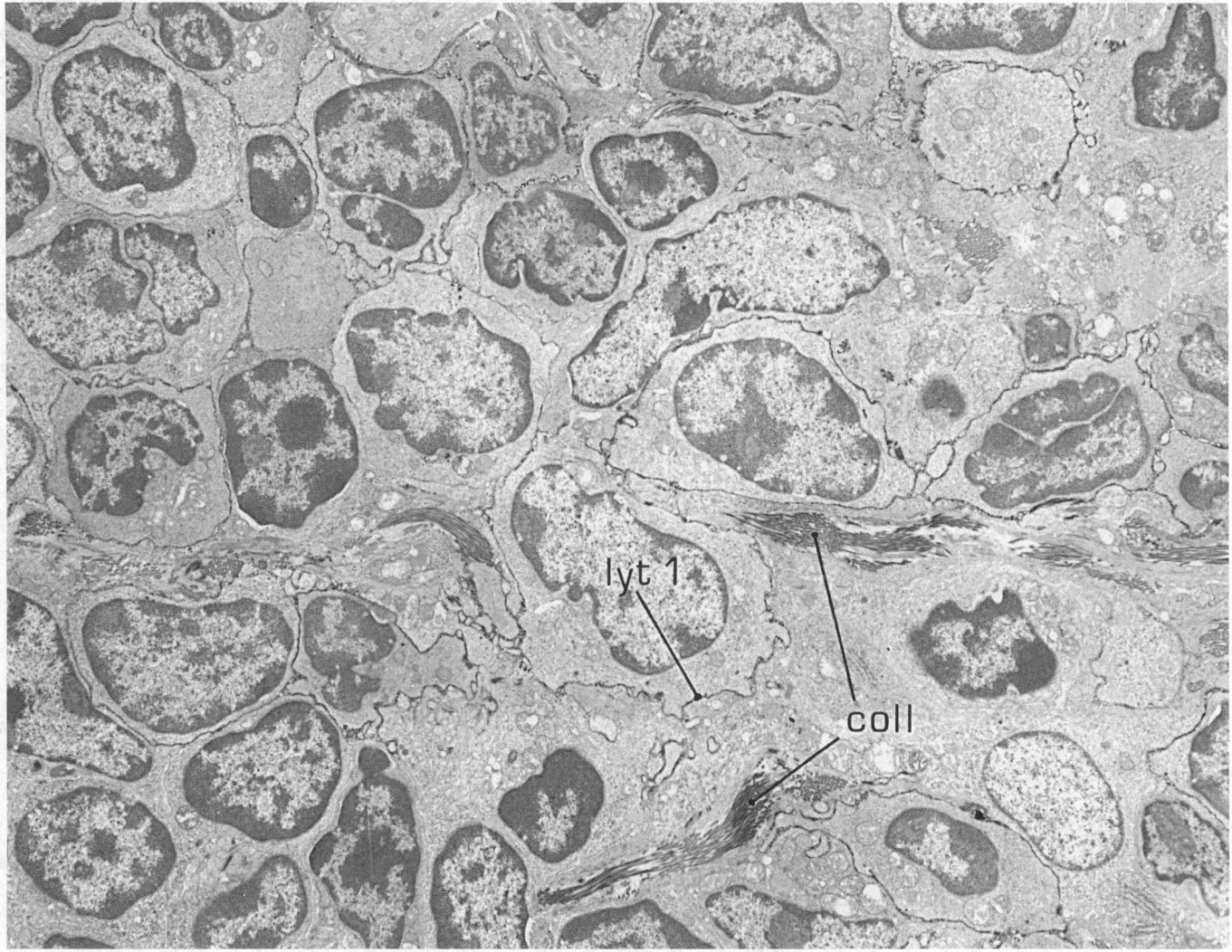

Fig. 15-7. Murine spleen, white pulp. The field consists preponderantly of packed small lymphocytes lying among processes of reticular cells associated with collagen (coll). An immunocytochemical reaction has stained the surface of the LyT 1 T cells. (× 3,000)

arterial vessels that branch from arteries of WP and terminate as fine vessels; a large system of pulp veins that drain the spleen, flowing into trabecular veins and then out of the spleen as splenic veins; and filtration beds interposed between arterial terminals and veins. The clearance patterns of RP are not unlike those of the MZ. Imperfect erythrocytes are modified or destroyed. Erythroid progenitors (burst-forming unit-erythroid and colony-forming unit-erythroid) and frank, effective erythropoiesis are regularly present in rodents, but not in humans. Most of the body's large platelet reserve is held in the filtration beds of the RP, where granulocytes are stored and plasmacytopoiesis may occur. Those lymphocytes that do not follow the immunologically selective route through WP flow through the RP, where they may be detained and differentiate into immunologically reactive forms or rapidly exit the spleen to continue as part of the RLP.

The extraordinary capacity of the spleen to clear the blood has been demonstrated both experimentally and clinically. Other major splenic functions (e.g., homing, cell sorting, progenitor cell differentiation or hematopoiesis, immunologic reactivity, and phagocytosis) depend on the primary function of blood clearance. Splenic functions depend on the selective clearance of a given cell type in a splenic filtration bed and

then on the capacity of the bed to support that cell type in function or differentiation. Thus, monocytes are cleared from the blood and held in the filtration beds of the MZ, RP, and WP, where they undergo differentiation into macrophages. Filtration beds are thereby bolstered by macrophages, which add phagocytosis and other attributes to mechanical filtration. Lymphocytes are cleared from the blood in the RP and MZ, home to the WP, where they are separated into T- and B-cell zones, set up to meet antigen and accessory cells, and respond immunologically or rejoin the RLP. Their arrangements are similar to those in the cortex of lymph nodes. Further examples can be provided by each of the other blood cell types.

While the filtration beds consist of a meshwork or reticulum of reticular cells and reticular fibers interposed between arteries and veins, such a structure, by itself, would not appear to account for the behavior of the normal or stressed spleen. How does >90% of the blood normally circulate through the spleen at a rate as fast as blow flow through vascularly conventional tissues? Why do most lymphocytes rapidly pass through the RP and out of the spleen uncleared, while a few, a highly significant few to be sure, enter the WP in immunologically significant passage?[24–27] Only a small proportion of red cells, rendered imperfect by almost any means, are cleared from the circula-

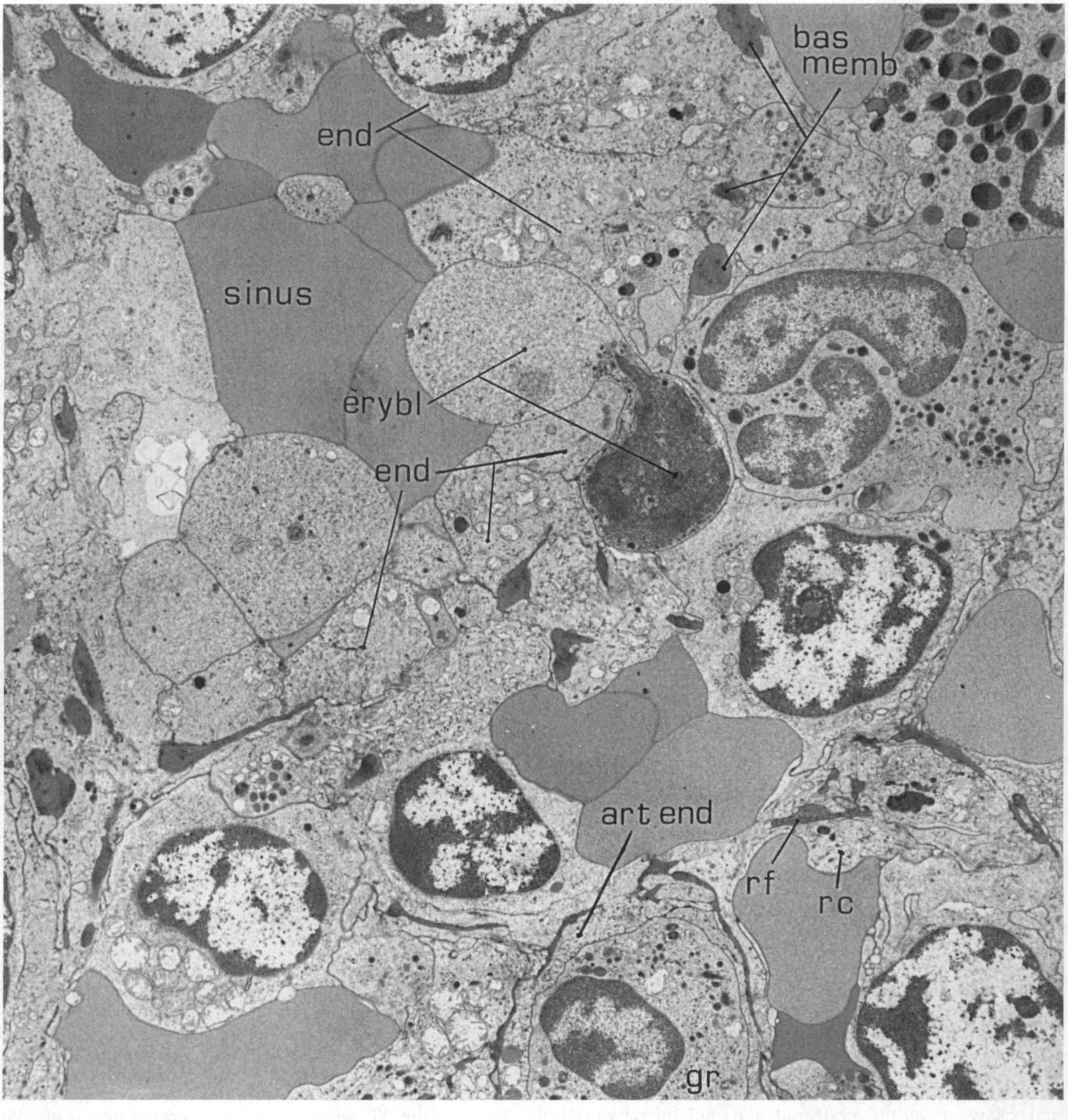

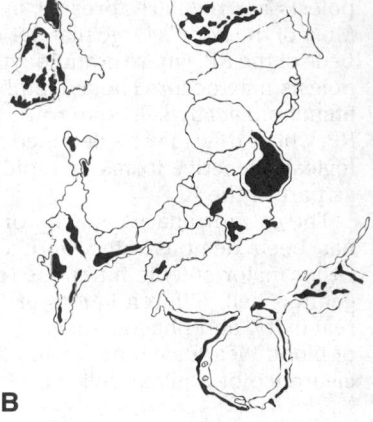

A

Fig. 15-8. Human spleen, red pulp in β-thalassemia. The upper portion of the field contains a venous sinus (sinus) cut in cross section. Its rod-shaped endothelium (end) is thereby cut in cross section, and the fenestrated subendo-thelium basement membrane (bas mem) is present in short segments. An erythroblast (erybl) is crossing the endothelium, probably passing from the perisinusoidal filtration bed into the lumen. Its nuclear portion still lies in the cord; being less flexible than the cytoplasm, it probably has difficulty in squeezing through the narrow interendo-thelial slit. It is here that relatively rigid structures, such as malarial parasites and Heinz bodies, are pitted from erythrocytes. The surrounding cord contains erythocytes, mononuclear cells, and strands of the reticular cells (rc) and fibers (rf), which create the filtration beds of RP. An arterial capillary distended by a neutrophil lies in the cord. Its endothelium is labeled (art end). Discontinuities in its basement membrane suggest that it is a terminating vessel, emptying its blood into the cord. From the cord, the normal path of flow is through the interendothelial slits of the venous sinus into its lumen and then on into pulp and trabecular veins and into the splenic veins and out. (× 4,000.) (Tissue obtained through the courtesy of Drs. Roy Gay, Presbyterian Hospital of Philadelphia, and Elias Schwartz, Children's Hospital of Philadelphia.)

B

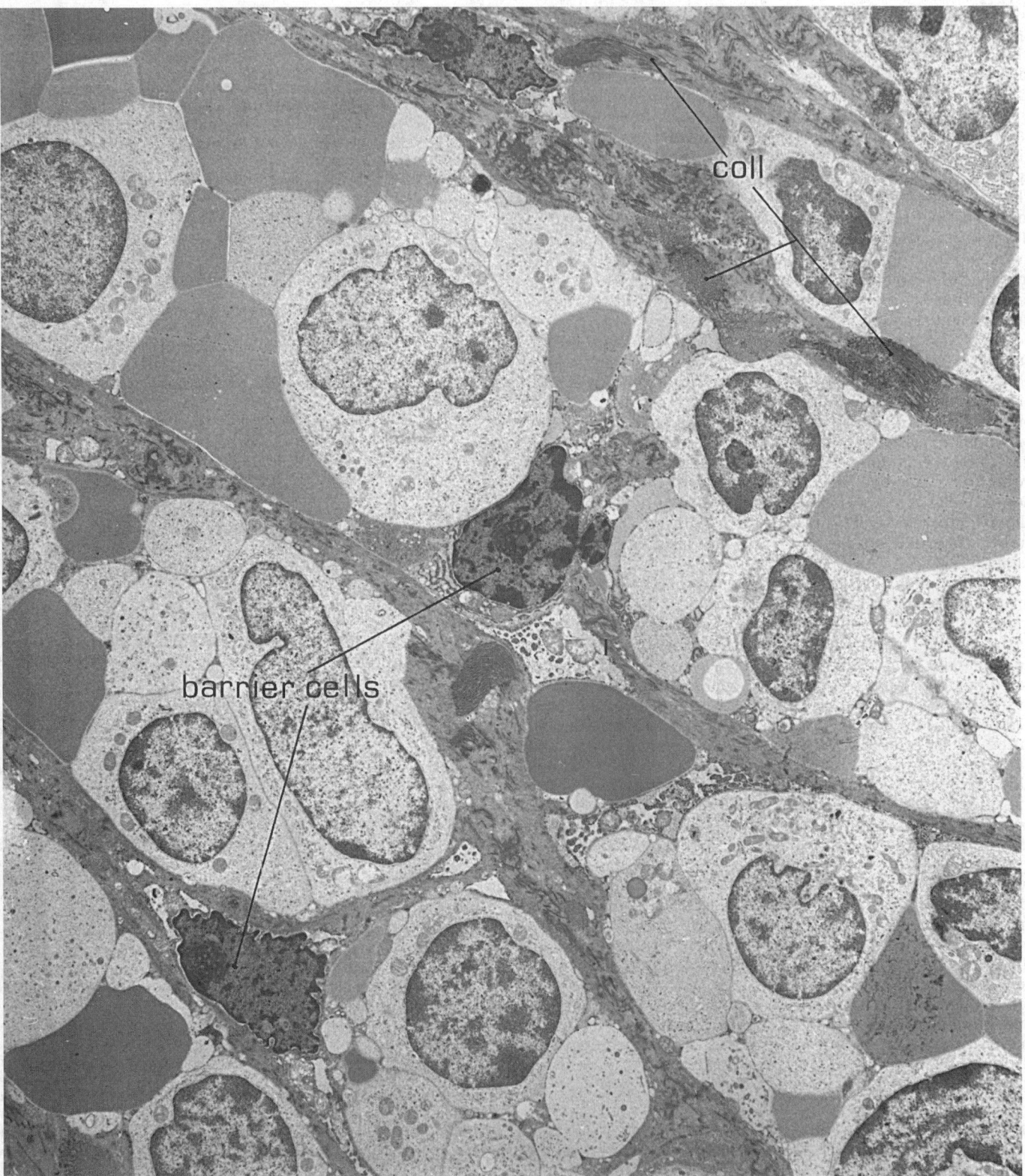

Fig. 15-9. Human spleen, sickle cell disease, red pulp. Barrier cells form a syncytial meshwork that penetrates the red pulp, augmenting the normal reticular cell meshwork. The barrier cells are characteristically electron-dense and envelope collagen fibers (coll), which they probably produce. As sickle cell disease progresses, increasing numbers of barrier cells enter the spleen, and more and more collagen is laid down. The end-stage fibrotic spleen of sickle cell disease thus appears to be caused by the increasing number and activity of barrier cells called out in this disease, not, as would be intuitively supposed, by cumulative microinfarctions that occur when irreversibly sickled cells obstruct blood flow. Similar processes occur in the thalassemias, but are not as marked. (× 3,000.) (Tissue obtained through the courtesy of Drs. Roy Gay, Presbyterian Hospital, and Elias Schwartz, Children's Hospital of Philadelphia.)

tion in a single passage through the spleen. It takes many passages to approach complete clearance. Because the whole blood volume circulates through the spleen in about 4 minutes, clearance of any given circulating cell type can be accomplished within hours, masking that, for all its specialization, the normal spleen, handling normal loads, is modest, indeed, rather inefficient, in clearing the blood. However, this inefficient clearance most likely serves the body well. The normal spleen has a "quiet" appearance, with limited requirements to clear the blood: enough lymphocytes and accessory cells to maintain the RLP, small numbers of macrophages to handle the measured turnover in erythrocytes, and enough granulocytes and macrophages to clear the occasional surges of bacteremia stemming from as everyday an event as chewing. The normal spleen can quickly recruit the cellular resources it needs when stressed and can enlarge easily.

The behavior of the enlarged spleen may be dangerous and erratic. In sickle cell disease in children, it may veer unpredictably to the acute sequestration syndrome, a lethal hypersplenism, to functional asplenia, in which the clearance capacity of the spleen is so diminished that debilitating and even lethal infectious diseases occur. It should be understood, however, that there are circumstances in which such exaggerated polar swings of splenic behavior are constructive. The acute resolution of malaria, the so-called crisis, is due to hypersplenism, albeit quite selectively directed to parasitized erythrocytes, and the precrisis spleen, preparing for crisis, is functionally asplenic.[26]

Recent studies have identified a lineage of barrier cells: distinctive fibroblasts, closely related to reticular cells, which may well provide a structural basis for understanding the behavior of the stressed spleen.[23-26] Barrier cells probably originate in bone marrow and circulate into the spleen as branched, activated mononuclear cells, which, on reaching the perivascular tissues, fuse with one another to form extensive, complex, highly branched syncytial sheets. These sheets are adapted in the spleen to form a variety of enclosures, envelopes, and barriers. Barrier cells may ensheath blood vessels, forming blood-spleen barriers, restricting blood flow into and out of the spleen. They form channels, which may shunt blood away from the filtration beds. Barrier cells may seal off zones of WP after an antigenic stimulus, rendering them inaccessible to further immunologic stimulus. They may enclose hematopoietic colonies, isolating them, concentrating hematopoietic regulatory factors, and, as is the case with erythropoietic colonies in malaria, protecting the developing blood cells from parasitization. Barrier cells are normally present in small numbers; in stressed and enlarged spleens, they are present in large numbers and may be the cellular basis of splenic fibrosis in sickle cell disease (Fig. 15-9). Barrier cells form a flexible, dynamic, rapidly mobilized system that, augmenting the relatively stable, static reticular meshwork, provides the morphologic substrate by which many of the diverse actions of the stressed spleen may be understood.

REFERENCES

1. Friedman H, Escobar MR, Reichard SM: The Reticuloendothelial System: A Comprehensive Treatise. Vols. 1–10. Plenum, New York, 1979–1988
2. Golub ES: Immunology. Sinauer, Sunderland, MA, 1987
3. Klauss GGB (ed): Microenvironments in the Lymphoid System: Advances in Experimental Medicine and Biology. Vol. 186. Plenum, New York, 1985
4. Scollay R, Bartlett P, Shortman K: T cell development in the adult murine thymus: changes in the expression of the surface antigens Ly 2L3T4 and B2A2 during development from early precursor cells to emigrants. Immunol Rev 82:79, 1984
5. Weiss L: Bone marrow; spleen; thymus; lymphatic vessels and lymph nodes. In Weiss L (ed): Cell and Tissue Biology: A Textbook of Histology. 6th Ed. Urban & Scharzenburg, Baltimore, 1988
6. Gilmour JR: Normal hematopoiesis in intrauterine and neonatal life. J Pathol 52:25, 1941
7. Tavassoli M: Marrow adipose cells—histochemical identification of labile and stable components. Arch Pathol Lab Med 100:16, 1976
8. Weiss, L, Chen LT: The organization of hematopoietic cords and vascular sinuses in bone marrow. Blood Cells 1:617, 1975
9. Weiss L: The hematopoietic microenvironment of the bone marrow: an ultrastructural study of the stroma in rats. Anat Rec 186:161, 1976
10. Ezine S, Weissman IL, Rouse RV: Thymus clonogenic bone marrow cells. p. 223. In Klauss GGB (ed): Microenvironments in the Lymphoid System. Plenum, New York, 1985
11. Kendall MD: The Thymus Gland. Academic Press, London, 1981
12. Scollay R: Intrathymic events in the differentiation of T lymphocytes: a continuing enigma. Immunol Today 4:282, 1983
13. Groom AC, Song SH: Effects of norepinephrine on washout of red cells from the spleen. Am J Physiol 22:255, 1971
14. Butcher EC: The regulation of lymphocytic traffic. Curr Top Microbiol Immunol 128:85, 1986
15. De Sousa MAB: Lymphocyte Circulation. Experimental and Clinical Aspects. John Wiley & Sons, New York, 1981
16. Gowans JL: The recirculation of lymphocyte from blood to lymph in the rat. J Physiol (Lond) 146:54, 1959
17. Gowans JL, Knight EJ: The route of recirculation of lymphocytes in the rat. Proc R Soc Lond [Biol] 159:257, 1964
18. Butcher EC, Weissman IL: Lymphoid tissues and organs. p. 109. In Paul W (ed): Fundamental Immunology. Raven Press, New York, 1986
19. McCuskey RS, Meinke HA: Studies of the hematopoietic microenvironment. III. Differences in the splenic microvascular system and stroma between S1/S1† and W/Wᵒ mice. Am J Anat 137:187, 1973
20. Scollay R, Andrews P, Boyd R, Shortman K: The role of the thymic cortex and medulla in T cell differentiation. Immunol Today 6:229, 1985
21. Shortman K, Scollay R, Andrews P, Boyd R: Development of T lymphocytes within the thymus and within thymic nurse cells. Curr Top Microbiol Immunol 126:5, 1986
22. Smith K: Inside the thymus: Workshop Basel Institute for Immunology. Immunol Today 5:83, 1984
23. Weiss L, Geduldig U: Barrier cells: Stromal regulation of hematopoiesis and blood cell release in normal and stressed murine bone marrow. Blood 78:975, 1991
24. Weiss L: Barrier cells in the spleen. Immunol Today 12:24, 1991
25. Weiss L: Mechanisms of splenic clearance of the blood. p. 23. In Bowdler AJ (ed): The Spleen: Structure, Functions, and Clinical Significance. Chapman & Hall, London, 1989
26. Weiss L, Geduldig U, Weidanz WP: Mechanisms of splenic control of malaria: reticular cell activation and the development of blood-spleen barrier. Am J Anat 170:447, 1984
27. Weiss L, Sakai H: The hematopoietic stroma. Am J Anat 170:447, 1984
28. Halpern PN, Benecerraf B, Delafresnaye JF (eds): Physiology of the Reticuloendothelial System, A Symposium. The Council for International Organizations for Medical Sciences. UNESCO and WHO, Paris. Blackwell, Oxford, 1957
29. Parker FG, Barnes EN, Kaye GI: The pericryptal fibroblast sheath. Gastroenterology 67:607, 1974
30. Deldar A, Lewis H, Weiss L: Bone lining cells and hematopoiesis: an electron microscopic study of canine bone marrow. Anat Rec 213:187, 1985
31. LaPushin RW, Trentin JJ: Identification of distinctive stromal elements in erythroid and neutrophil granuloid spleen colonies: light and electron microscopic study. Exp Hematol 5:505, 1977
32. Jenkinson EJ: Stromal cell populations in the developing thymus of normal and nude mice microenvironments in the lymphoid system. p. 245. In Klauss GGB (ed): Microenvironments in the Lymphoid System. Plenum, New York, 1985
33. Ritter MA, Crispe: In: The Thymus. IRL Press at Oxford University Press, Oxford, 1992
34. Wekerle H, Ketelson UP, Ernst M: Thymic nurse cells. Lymphoepithelial cell complexes in murine thymuses: morphological and serological characterization. J Exp Med 151:925, 1980
35. Jaffee RH: The reticulo-endothelial system. p. 973. In Downey H (ed): The Handbook of Hematology. Hoeber, New York, 1988
36. Knisely MH: Spleen studies. I. Microscopic observations of the circulatory system of living unstimulated mammalian spleen. Anat Rec 65:23, 1936
37. Bloom W, Bartelmez GW: Hematopoiesis in young human embryos. Am J Anat 67:21, 1940
38. Braanemark PI: Vital microscopy of bone marrow in rabbit. Scand J Clin Lab Invest, suppl. 38. 11:1, 1959
39. Campbell F: Ultrastructural studies of transmural migration of blood cells in the bone marrow of rats, mice and guinea pigs. Am J Anat 135:521, 1972
40. Levine RF et al: Circulating megakaryocytes: turnover of megakaryocyte cytoplasm in the lungs is equal to the platelet production rate. Blood (in press)

41. Bearman RM, Levine GD, Bensch KG: The ultrastructure of the normal human thymus. Anat Rec 190:755, 1978

42. Harris JE, Barnes DWH, Evans CP: Cellular traffic of the thymus: experiments with chromosome markers. II. Evidence from parabiosis for an afferent stream of cells. Nature 201:886, 1964

43. Moore MAS, Owens JJT: Experimental studies in the development of the thymus. J Exp Med 126:715, 1967

44. Parrott DMV, De Sousa MAB, East J: Thymus-dependent areas in the lymphoid areas of neonatally thymectomized mice. J Exp Med 123:191, 1966

45. Weissman IL: Thymus cell migration. J Exp Med 126:291, 1967

46. Goldstein AD (ed): Thymic Hormones and Lymphokines. Plenum, New York, 1984

47. Crabb ED, Kelsall MA: Organization of the mucosa and lymphatic structures of the rabbit appendix. J Morphol 67:351, 1940

48. Anderson AO, Anderson ND: Studies on the structure and permeability of the microvasculature in normal rat lymph nodes. Am J Pathol 80:387, 1975

49. Belisle C, Sainte-Marie G: Tridimensional study of the deep cortex of the rat lymph node. III. Morphology of the deep cortex units. Anat Rec 199:213, 1981

50. Belisle C, Sainte-Marie G: The narrowing of high endothelial venules of the rat lymph node. Anat Rec 211:284, 1985

51. Crandall LA, Barker SB, Graham DG: A study of the lymph flow from a patient with thoracic duct fistula. Gastroenterology 1:1040, 1943

52. Drinker CK, Field ME, Ward HK: The filtering capacity of lymph nodes. J Exp Med 59:393, 1934

53. Drinker CK, Wislocki GB, Field ME: The structure of the sinuses in the lymph nodes. Anat Rec 56:261, 1933

54. Fujita T, Kashimura M, Adachi K: Scanning electron microsopy and terminal circulation. Experientia 40:167, 1985

55. Schmidt EE, MacDonald IC, Groom AC: Circulatory pathways in the sinusal spleen of the dog, studied by scanning electron microscopy of microcorrosion casts. J Morphol 178:111, 1983

56. Schmidt EE, MacDonald IC, Groom AC: Microcirculatory pathways in normal human spleen demonstrated by scanning electron microscopy of corrosion casts. Am J Anat 181:253, 1988

57. Tablin F, Weiss L: Equine spleen: an electron microscopic analysis. Am J Anat 166:393, 1983

58. Tischendorf F: On the evolution of the spleen. Experientia 41:243, 1985

59. Weiss L, Powell R, Schiffman FJ: Terminating arterial vessels in red pulp of the spleen. Experientia 41:233, 1985

60. van Ewijk W, Nieuwenhius P: Compartments, domains and migration pathways of lymphoid cells in the splenic pulp. Experientia 41:199, 1985

61. Weiss L, Tavassoli M: Anatomical hazards to the passage of erythrocytes through the spleen. Semin Hematol 7:732, 1970

Growth Factors and the Control of Hematopoiesis

16

Grover C. Bagby, Jr. and Gerald M. Segal

INTRODUCTION

Mammalian tissues have an astonishing capacity to respond to environmental stimuli. The hematopoietic system, responsible for efficient oxygen delivery, hemostasis, and all phases of the inflammatory response, is a paradigm of such adaptable control. The responsiveness of each lineage of the hematopoietic system results from coordinate increases in the production and functional activity of appropriate hematopoietic cell types, without expansion of irrelevant ones. A mountaineer at high altitude, for instance, will develop a specific expansion of the erythroid bone marrow and subsequent erythrocytosis, but the bone marrow will not increase production of neutrophils, monocytes, eosinophils, mast cells, T lymphocytes, or B lymphocytes. This particular response results from a hypoxia-induced[1-5] increase in circulating levels of erythropoietin (EPO), a glycoprotein hormone that specifically stimulates the proliferation and differentiation of cells of the erythroid lineage.[6-9] EPO is but 1 of ≥19 well-characterized hematopoietic growth factors that regulate the production and activity of blood cells. Although there are undoubtedly many as yet undiscovered hematopoietic growth factors, one fundamental feature of hematopoietic regulation is incontrovertible—the nature of all lineage-specific hematopoietic reflexes depends in large part on the levels of proteins in hematopoietic tissues that stimulate or inhibit the production of mature blood cells.

Fully characterized recombinant hematopoietic growth factors and the genes encoding their receptors have recently become available, enabling hundreds of laboratories to test exactly how a given change in the environment incites expression of the right genes at the right time. In vitro experiments in many laboratories using genomic and cDNA clones, in vitro transcripts, and recombinant proteins have uncovered new levels of complexity and provided new explanations of how biologic organisms work. Results of therapeutic trials in which recombinant hematopoietic growth factors and interleukins (ILs) were administered to experimental animals[10-23] and humans[10,24-33] document hematopoietic responses predicted by scientists using in vitro techniques. In vivo work has therefore legitimized the use of in vitro clonal assays as windows through which biologically relevant in vivo hematopoietic events can be observed. What has emerged from research on hematopoietic growth factors and ILs is a clear picture of an extraordinarily complex and highly efficient intercellular molecular communication system.

Although much has been learned in the past decade, research on hematopoietic growth factors and related cytokines is still in its infancy. Each new year brings with it new factors and new bioactivities for old ones. To attempt to memorize the growth factors and ILs in chronologic order (e.g., IL-1 through IL-13) would be a task for Sisyphus. Consequently, without a cohesive a set of rules, it would be virtually impossible to remember the complex details of all the growth factors with hematopoietic activity of one kind or another: not only will new factors be described, but with each new month new activities will be found for old factors. Fortunately, in the past few years

Table 16-1. General Rules of Hematopoietic Growth Factor and Interleukin Biology

1. Hematopoietic growth factors and ILs have multiple biologic activities.
2. Those growth factors and ILs that induce proliferation of hematopoietic precursor cells often have the capacity to enhance the functional activity of the terminally differentiated progeny of these precursor cells.
3. Factors exerting an effect on hematopoiesis can do so directly or indirectly.
4. ILs and growth factors commonly act synergistically with other cytokines.
5. Hematopoietic regulatory cytokines are organized in a highly complex interdependent network with some concrete elements of hierarchic structure.
6. The cytokine network exhibits many signal amplification circuits.
7. The genes encoding hematopoietic growth factors and ILs share important structural and functional attributes.
8. Receptors for hematopoietic growth factors share many structural and functional attributes.
9. Structural abnormalities of hematopoietic growth factors or their receptors may result in abnormalities of hematopoiesis.

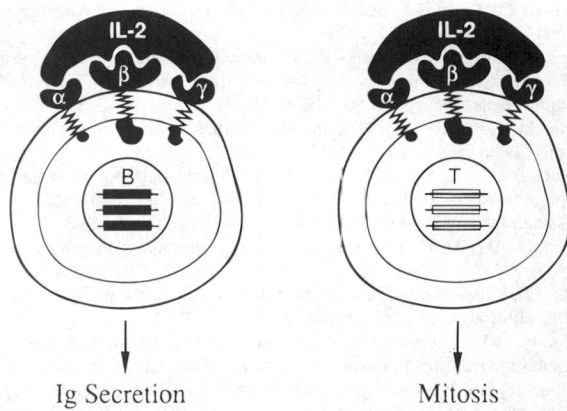

Ig Secretion   Mitosis

Fig. 16-1. Although B and T lymphocytes share the same IL-2 receptor, the repertoires of IL-2-induced gene expression are different. The B cell can be induced to secrete immunoglobulin, but productive immunoglobulin gene rearrangement and immunoglobulin secretion is forbidden in T cells.

it has become clear that certain biologic themes are steadily recapitulated in the science of hematopoietic control. Nine of these themes are presented as general rules in Table 16-1. Although virtually all of the hematopoietic growth factors and interleukins can be used as examples of each rule, only one or two selected examples are used here, and most of the factors known to stimulate hematopoiesis are presented in the context of these nine rules.

RULE 1. HEMATOPOIETIC GROWTH FACTORS AND INTERLEUKINS HAVE MULTIPLE BIOLOGIC ACTIVITIES

IL-2

IL-2, formerly known as T-cell growth factor, is encoded by a gene located on the long arm of chromosome 4.[34] The 23-kd gene product is produced by T lymphocytes induced by mitogens, antigens, certain antibodies, phorbol esters, and lectins.[34-43] The IL-2 receptor (IL-2R), a heterotrimer of 55 (α)-, 75 (β)-, and 64 (γ)-kd subunits,[44] is expressed by T cells,[42,45,46] B cells,[47-49] and natural killer (NK) cells.[50,51] The biologic activities of IL-2 include induction of growth and activation of T lymphocytes,[42,45,46] B lymphocytes,[47-49] and NK cells[50,51] both in vitro and in vivo. Recent intense interest in IL-2 and IL-2-stimulated lymphocytes as effectors of clinical tumor cytotoxicity[52-55] have provided unambiguous evidence of in vivo immunomodulatory activity of IL-2 in humans.

Although there are a number of plausible explanations for the heterogeneous activities of IL-2, most of the variations seen in the induced biologic responses are not determined by differences in receptor structure (in B cells, for example, the IL-2R is the same heterotrimer as that present on the surface of T lymphocytes).[42,45,46,56,57] Responses induced by IL-2 vary among lineages of cells bearing the receptor because permissible gene programs in those cells are different; some of them are also lineage-specific. In the example shown in Fig. 16-1, IL-2 binds to its receptor on both B lymphocytes and T lymphocytes, but the induced B-cell repertoire involves expression of immunoglobulin genes, an effect that is forbidden in T lymphocytes. Three IL-2R affinities have been defined. Low-affinity receptors contain IL-2Rα, intermediate-affinity receptors contain the γ- and β-chains, and the high-affinity receptors contain all three chains.[58,59] Nonetheless, no evidence suggests that differential expression of intermediate- or high-affinity receptors accounts for lineage-specific responses. Additional mechanisms of biologic heterogeneity may include cell type- or cell stage-specific differences in stimulus-response coupling mechanisms

in the cellular targets of the specific protein. The heterogeneous biologic activities of each of the hematopoietic growth factors and ILs are reviewed in Table 16-2.

IL-2
Also known as: T-cell growth factor
Chromosome: 4q
Gene product: 23 kd
Produced by: T lymphocytes
Induced by: mitogens, antigens, some antibodies, phorbol esters, lectins, and IL-1
Receptor: α/β/γ heterotrimer on T lymphocytes, B lymphocytes, and NK cells
Bioactivity: see Table 16-2

LIF/HILDA

The murine cDNA encoding leukemia inhibitory factor (LIF)[60] (also known as human interleukin for DA cells [HILDA]), a protein first identified by its capacity to induce differentiation and inhibit self-renewal simultaneously in certain murine leukemic cells,[60-62] was used as a hybridization probe to identify the human homologue[63] located on chromosome 22q12.[64] LIF is expressed by marrow stromal cells,[65,66] monocytes,[67] and blastocysts,[66,68] and expression is augmented by IL-1 and transforming growth factor-β (TGF-β). The human gene encodes a glycoprotein with 78% amino acid sequence identity with murine LIF, which, like the murine factor, induces differentiation of murine M1 leukemic cells.[63] Although it has no inhibitory activity on its own against the leukemic cell lines HL60 and U937, LIF, when combined with colony-stimulating factor-granulocyte/macrophage (CSF-GM) or CSF-G, reduces in vitro clonal proliferative capacity of these cell lines[69] and induces differentiation.[70] LIF enhances the efficiency of retroviral mediated gene transfer in hematopoietic cells,[71] expands megakaryocyte mass in mice,[72] and exerts additional in vitro activities. For example, when added to cultures of totipotential embryonic stem cells, LIF suppresses the natural tendency of these cells to commit to differentiation.[73,74] Whether LIF will function to inhibit commitment in other types of cells remains to be proven. It may prove to play an essential role in regulating the self-replication of not only hematopoietic stem cells, but other progenitors as well. The LIF receptor (LIF-R) is a heterodimer consisting of an α-chain and a second chain, gp130, which is shared with the IL-6 receptor α-chain.[75] The LIF-R/gp130 heterodimer is also a receptor for oncostatin M.[75]

Table 16-2. Heterogeneous Biologic Activities of the Hematopoietic Growth Factors and Interleukins

Factor	Bioactivities	Factor	Bioactivities

Direct-acting lineage-specific factors

EPO
Stimulates clonal growth of CFU-E and a subset of BFU-E[269,324,611–613]

Induces release of reticulocytes from marrow

Induces globin synthesis in erythroid precursor cells

Stimulates murine megakaryocyte colony growth and terminal maturation in vitro[255,256,258] but has no apparent thrombopoietic activity in vivo

CSF-G
Stimulates growth of progenitor cells committed to the neutrophil lineage[27,170,208–211]

Stimulates neutrophil maturation of certain leukemic cells[327,614,615]

Activates phagocytic function of mature neutrophils[191,196,212]

Stimulates quiescent pluripotent hematopoietic progenitor cells to enter G_1-S phase[343,394]

CSF-M
Induces monocyte/macrophage growth and differentiation[170,209,210,213–216,274,395,616,617]

Activates macrophage phagocytic function[218,219]

Activates macrophage secretory function[217,278]

IL-7
Induces clonal growth of pre-B cells[280–282]

Stimulates growth of pre-T cells[282]

Stimulates growth of chronic lymphocytic leukemia, acute leukemia,[283] and Sézary cells[284]

Enhances IL-3 and CSF-GM production by activated T cells[285]

Induces expression of IL-6, IL-1, TNF-α, and IL-8 in peripheral blood monocytes[286,287]

IL-12
Induces the differentiation of naive T-helper cells into T_{H1} cells[145]

Augments functional activity of NK cells[136,152,618]

Acts synergistically with TNF-α to stimulate IFN-γ production by NK cells[156]

Induces lymphokine-activated killer activity in NK cells[154,155]

Direct-acting factors that induce proliferation of multipotential progenitors and stem cells

IL-3
Stimulates multilineage colony growth[171,215,294,325,391,619,620]

Stimulates growth of primitive hematopoietic cell lines with multilineage potential[327,328]

Stimulates BFU-E proliferation in vitro[165,294,324]

Stimulates proliferation of murine CFU-S[11]

Induces B-lymphocyte differentiation[336]

Co-stimulates T-cell proliferation with IL-2[334]

Induces macrophages to express CSF-M[330] (this may explain reports that IL-3 induces clonal growth of pulmonary alveolar macrophages[342])

Stimulates growth of myeloid leukemic cells in vitro[327,328,571,574,575,621–623]

CSF-GM
Stimulates multilineage hematopoietic progenitor cell growth[166,168,170–172,209,210,624]

Stimulates BFU-E growth[11,164,165,169,174,310]

Stimulates granulocyte, macrophage, and eosinophil colony growth[164,165,168,171,184,205,625]

Stimulates functional activity of eosinophils, neutrophils, monocytes, and macrophages[13,181,184,187,190,194,197,199–201,204,205,626,627]

Induces IL-1 gene expression in neutrophils[189,198] and peripheral blood mononuclear leukocytes[399]

Co-stimulates T-cell proliferation with IL-2[334]

Induces[628] or co-induces TNF-α gene expression with IFN-γ in monocytes[539]

Stimulates proliferation of myeloid leukemic cells[183,577,623,629–632]

Stimulates growth of certain nonhematopoietic cancer cells in vitro[633,634]

Induces migration and proliferation of vascular endothelial cells in vitro[177]

Indirect-acting factors whose function in hematopoiesis includes regulating expression of direct-acting factors by auxiliary cells

IL-1
Induces expression of CSF-GM, CSF-G, IL-6, and IL-1 in fibroblasts, endothelial cells, keratinocytes, and thymic epithelial cells[302–304,307–312,315,354,355,369,375,496,499,501]

Induces proliferation of preactivated T cells[334,560,592]

Induces acute-phase protein synthesis[635–639]

Induces fever and sleep in vivo[638,639]

Stimulates release of corticotropin[640–645]

Promotes transendothelial passage of neutrophils[646]

Synergizes with IL-3 in stimulating proliferation in primitive hematopoietic progenitor cells in vitro[326]

Stimulates prostaglandin E production in fibroblasts, monocytes, and neutrophils[493,647–650]

Modulates EGF receptor expression[651]

TNF-α
Induces expression of CSF-GM, CSF-G, IL-6, and IL-1 in fibroblasts and endothelial cells[16,306,310,311,367,494,495,510,652]

Enhances mitogen-induced CSF-GM expression in T cells[316]

Induces release of CSF-GM and CSF-M in vivo[16]

Inhibits virus replication synergistically with interferons[653]

Stimulates prostaglandin E production in fibroblasts and neutrophils[647,648]

Enhances parasite and tumor cell cytotoxicity of eosinophils[654] and macrophages[202,655,656]

Inhibits proliferation of hematopoietic progenitor cells,[505,506,509] lymphocytes,[657] and certain leukemia cell lines in vitro[658]

Mediates the hemodynamic and toxic effects of endotoxin[659–666]

Induces expression of IL-6 in fibroblasts[367]

Induces expression of adhesion molecules in myeloid cells[667]

Activates phagocytic function of neutrophils[647,668–671]

Induces expression of monocyte-derived neutrophil chemotactic factor[81]

Increases production of plasminogen-activator inhibitor in vascular endothelial cells[672,673]

Suppresses transcription of the thrombomodulin gene in endothelial cells[674]

Modulates endothelial growth factor receptor expression[651]

Promotes transendothelial passage of neutrophils[646]

Induces expression of NF-κB trans-activating protein in lymphoid cells[675,676]

IL-2
Induces proliferation and activation of T lymphocytes[42,45,46,50]

Induces proliferation and activation of B lymphocytes[47–49]

Induces proliferation and activation of NK cells[50,51]

Induces expression of IL-1 in monocytes and macrophages[398]

Co-induces (with IL-1) expression of IFN-γ in T cells[589]

IL-10
Inhibits monocyte/macrophage-dependent synthesis of $T_{H}1$-derived cytokines (IL-2, IFN-γ, lymphotoxin) in humans and mice[401,404]

Inhibits monocyte/macrophage-dependent synthesis of "$T_{H}2$-type" (IL-3, IL-4, IL-5) and NK-derived cytokines (IFN-γ and TNF-α) in humans[156,349,405,406]

Inhibits monocyte/macrophage-dependent T-cell proliferation[407,408]

Inhibits proliferation of and IL-2 production by purified T-cells[409]

Acts as co-stimulator of B-cell proliferation[410]

Represses constitutive and IFN-γ-induced MHC class II antigen expression on mononuclear phagocytes[407,408]

Inhibits the production of IL-1, TNF-α, IL-6, IL-8, CSF-G, CSF-GM, and IL-10 by mononuclear phagocytes[347,411]

Inhibits the production of reactive oxygen species and nitric oxide by mononuclear phagocytes[412,413]

(Table continues)

Table 16-2. *(Continued)*

Factor	Bioactivities	Factor	Bioactivities
Direct-acting factors that directly (either alone or synergistically) stimulate growth, differentiation, or functional activation of multiple cell types		IL-9	Stimulates the clonal growth of BFU-E in combination with EPO[110,111]
IL-4	Induces proliferation of activated B cells[422,432,433]		Stimulates the clonal growth of fetal CFU-Mix and CFU-GM[111]
	Inhibits IL-2-stimulated proliferation of B cells[441,442]		Augments IL-3-induced growth of murine bone marrow-derived mast cells[112]
	Co-induces immunoglobulin secretion and isotype switching[47,230,233,437–440,677]		Stimulates the proliferation of preactivated peripheral blood mononuclear cell-derived T-cell lines[113]
	Induces proliferation of T cells[426–428,591,678,679]	IL-11	Stimulates proliferation of murine plasmacytoma and hybridoma cell lines[115,118]
	Induces proliferation of fibroblasts[435]		Stimulates CD4$^+$ T-cell-dependent proliferation of antigen-specific plaque-forming B cells[115,120,121]
	Co-induces (with PMA) IL-2 receptor expression in T cells[427]		Shortens the duration of G_0 of primitive hematopoietic progenitor cells[122,123]
	Induces the differentiation of naive T-helper cells into T$_{H2}$ cells[148,149]		Acts synergistically with IL-3 or Steel factor to stimulate the clonal growth of erythroid (BFU-E and CFU-E) and primitive megakaryocytic (BFU-Mk) progenitors[124–126]
	Inhibits induction and function of lymphokine-activated killer cells[680]		Increases the ploidy of cultured megakaryocytes[127]
	Inhibits IL-1 release[681]		Increases peripheral platelet and neutrophil counts[128,129]
	Induces expression of CSF-M and CSF-G genes in monocytes[400]		Increases the numbers and cycling activity of committed progenitor cells[128,129]
	Induces expression of an inhibitor of hematopoiesis by mixed murine marrow stromal cells[444]		Hastens hematopoietic recovery following cytotoxic chemotherapy, ionizing radiation, and bone marrow transplantation[129,130]
	Enhances murine BFU-E and CFU-E growth (with EPO)[682]		Acts as an autocrine growth factor for certain megakaryoblastic cell lines[131]
	Enhances CFU-GM growth (with CSF-G and CSF-GM)[682]		Stimulates hepatic acute-phase reactant production[132]
IL-5	Activates cytotoxic T cells[228,229]		Suppresses adipogenesis in preadipocytes[117]
	Induces or co-induces immunoglobulin secretion[47,49,225,231,232,234]	Steel factor	Promotes the proliferation and differentiation of pre-CFCs[455,477,478]
	Stimulates eosinophil production[220,236,237,239,241] and activation[239,240]		Acts synergistically with IL-3, CSF-GM, and EPO to support clonal growth of CFU-GEMM, BFU-E, and CFU-Mk[124,479–481]
IL-6	Is synergistic with IL-3 in promoting CFU-GEMM colony growth[325,378,388,391,392]		Enhances hematopoietic colony growth in cultures of marrow cells from patients with congenital marrow failure states[482–484]
	Is synergistic with CSF-M in promoting macrophage colony growth[395] and with CSF-GM in promoting granulocyte colony growth[380]		Stimulates the proliferation and differentiation of mast cell precursors[460,485]
	Is synergistic with IL-4 in inducing T-cell proliferation,[379] immunoglobulin secretion,[230] and hematopoietic colony formation[378]		Chemotactic for mast cells[486]
	Is synergistic with IL-2[356,390] and IL-1[387] in inducing T-cell proliferation		Independently stimulates mast cell degranulation and enhances IgE-dependent mediator release from mast cells[487,488]
	Co-induces differentiation of B cells[230,360,361,396]		Stimulates expansion of committed progenitor cell compartment in vivo[489]
	Induces terminal differentiation of myeloid leukemic cell lines[373,683,684]		Stimulates mast cell hyperplasia in vivo[490]
	Induces neuronal differentiation in certain pheochromocytoma cell lines[685]		Supports melanocyte development and migration[445,491]
	Co-induces cytotoxic T cells in vitro[389]		Supports gametogenesis[445,472]
	Stimulates plasmacytoma growth[358,371,576,686,687]		
	Induces acute-phase responses in vivo[17,358,637,688–690]		
	Induces acute-phase protein synthesis in hepatocytes[690,691]		
	Stimulates megakaryocytopoiesis in vitro and in vivo[381–385]		
IL-8	Stimulates neutrophil chemotaxis,[87,88] exocytosis,[90,91] respiratory burst,[89,92] shape change,[89] adhesion molecule expression,[692,693] and complement receptor type 1 expression[693,694]		
	Stimulates T-lymphocyte chemotaxis[95]		
	Stimulates basophil chemotaxis,[96] histamine release,[695,696] and leukotriene release[696]		
	Stimulates endothelial cell chemotaxis and proliferation[97]		
	Stimulates angiogenesis[97]		

LIF

Also known as: human interleukin for DA cells (HILDA)

Chromosome: 22q

Gene product: 58 kd

Produced by: peripheral blood mononuclear leukocytes and Krebs II ascites tumor cells

Induced by: IL-1, TGF-β

Receptor: A heterodimer consisting of gp130 and LIF-Rα subunits

Bioactivity: see Table 16-2

IL-8

Despite its name, IL-8 is more properly considered a chemoattractant than a growth factor. IL-8 is a member of the so-called intercrine family of 8–10-kd basic polypeptide cytokines involved in various proinflammatory and tissue reparative activities.[76,77] The intercrine family is composed of two subfamilies of cytokines encoded by closely linked genes on chromosomes 4 and 17. IL-8 is a member of the subfamily on chromosome 4, which also includes platelet factor 4, β-thromboglobulin, GROα, GROβ, GROγ, ENA-78, interferon-γ (IFN-γ) inducible protein (IP10), and neutrophil-activating peptide-2 (NAP-2).[78] After its secretion, extracellular N-terminal processing of the mature IL-8 polypeptide yields several active species 69–79 amino acids in length, with the predominant species consisting of 72 amino acids.[79,80] IL-8 is produced by mononuclear phagocytes, endothelial cells, fibroblasts, and other connective tissue cells, and by neutrophils themselves in response to IL-1, tumor necrosis factor (TNF), and a variety of other inflammatory stimuli and proinflammatory cytokines.[81–84] Neutrophils express two closely related G protein-coupled IL-8 receptor molecules, which each possess seven membrane-spanning domains and share significant sequence homology with receptors for the neutrophil chemoattractants f-Met-Leu-Phe and C5a.[85,86]

IL-8 is a potent neutrophil agonist, inducing neutrophil chemotaxis,[87,88] shape change,[89] exocytosis of storage granule proteins,[90,91] and the respiratory burst.[89,92] NAP-2, the GRO proteins, and ENA-78 also bind IL-8 receptors and induce similar neutrophil responses.[86,93,94] IL-8 is also chemotactic for T lymphocytes,[95] basophils,[96] and endothelial cells[97] and is a potent angiogenic agent.[97] In addition to playing a crucial role in host defense by promoting neutrophil activation and directed migration to sites of infection, IL-8 is also an important mediator of the destructive inflammatory processes that characterize such disease states as rheumatoid arthritis and psoriasis.[98–100]

IL-8

Also known as: neutrophil attractant/activation peptide-1

Chromosome: 4q12-21

Gene product: 8 kd

Produced by: mononuclear phagocytes, fibroblasts, endothelial cells, neutrophils, keratinocytes, synovial cells, chondrocytes

Induced by: IL-1, TNF, lipopolysaccharide (LPS), IL-3, CSF-GM, immune complexes, phorbol esters

Receptor: Two G protein-coupled receptors (350 and 355 amino acids in length)

Bioactivity: see Table 16-2

IL-9

The cytokine now known as IL-9[101,102] was originally identified as a 40-kd growth factor (P40) for certain murine T-cell clones.[103,104] The human protein was identified as a factor produced by a human T-cell leukemia virus (HTLV) I-transformed T-cell line that stimulates the proliferation of MO7E human megakaryoblastic leukemia cells.[105] Sequence comparison of the respective cDNAs demonstrated that P40 was the murine homologue of the human protein, both of which were subsequently designated IL-9.[104,105] The human IL-9 gene resides on the portion of the long arm of chromosome 5 that also contains the genes that encode CSF-GM, IL-3, IL-4, IL-5, CSF-M and its receptor (c-fms), and a number of other cytokines and growth factor receptors[106,107] (see Rule 7 below). IL-9 is produced by activated T lymphocytes, primarily CD4+ lymphocytes.[104,108] The IL-9 receptor is a member of the hematopoietic growth factor superfamily and is expressed in membrane-bound and soluble forms.[109]

In combination with EPO, IL-9 supports burst-forming unit-erythroid (BFU-E)-derived colony growth from both unfractionated and highly progenitor-enriched marrow cells.[110,111] In contrast to its effects on adult progenitors, which appear confined to the erythroid lineage, IL-9 supports the clonal growth of fetal erythroid, multipotential, and granulocyte macrophage progenitors.[111] Despite its stimulatory effects on MO7E cells, IL-9 lacks megakaryocytopoietic activity. IL-9 acts synergistically with IL-3 in promoting murine mast cell growth.[112] Although

originally identified as a murine T-cell growth factor, it has been difficult to demonstrate comparable activity in the human system. Recently, however, IL-9 has been shown to stimulate the proliferation of human peripheral blood-derived T-cell lines and clones that had been preactivated with phytohemagglutinin (PHA), IL-2, and irradiated allogeneic feeder cells.[113]

IL-9 is also produced by certain lymphoid cell lines and neoplasms, including HTLV-I- and -II-transformed T lymphocytes,[105] Hodgkin disease cells (particularly Reed-Sternberg cells),[114] and large cell anaplastic lymphoma cells.[114] It has been proposed that IL-9 may be acting as an autocrine growth factor in such cases.

IL-9

Also known as: T-cell growth factor P40, mast cell-enhancing activity

Chromosome: 5q31.2-31.3

Gene product: 20–30 kd

Produced by: T lymphocytes

Induced by: PHA, PMA, calcium ionophore A23187, anti-CD3, IL-1, IL-2, HTLV-I or -II

Receptor: 522-amino acid member of hematopoietic growth factor receptor superfamily

Bioactivity: see Table 16-2

IL-11

The IL-11 cDNA was isolated from a bone marrow stromal cell line PU-34 by an expression cloning strategy based on the capacity of the encoded protein to stimulate the proliferation of a murine plasmacytoma cell line.[115] The human IL-11 gene has been mapped to the long arm of chromosome 19.[116] IL-11 is produced by fibroblasts and bone marrow stromal cells, and its production is markedly increased by IL-1.[115,117,118]

IL-11 is a pleiotropic cytokine with growth stimulatory effects, which overlap those of IL-6, on multiple classes of lymphoid and myeloid cells.[118,119] IL-11 is mitogenic for a number of murine plasmacytoma and hybridoma cell lines.[115,118] IL-11 enhances CD4+ T-cell-dependent proliferation of antigen-specific plaque-forming B cells.[115,120,121] IL-11 shortens the duration of G_0 of primitive hematopoietic progenitor cells as measured in the blast cell colony assay of Ogawa's group.[122,123] It acts synergistically with IL-3 or Steel factor to support the clonal growth of erythroid (BFU-E and colony-forming unit-erythroid [CFU-E]) and primitive megakaryocytic (BFU-Mk) progenitor cells.[124–126] In combination with IL-3, IL-11 induces an upward shift in the ploidy values of cultured megakaryocytes.[127] In vivo, IL-11 administration stimulates megakaryocytopoiesis, increases peripheral platelet and neutrophil counts, and increases the numbers and cycling activity of all classes of committed hematopoietic progenitor cells.[128,129] IL-11 hastens hematopoietic recovery following treatment with cytotoxic agents or ionizing radiation and accelerates hematopoietic reconstitution following bone marrow transplantation.[129,130] These results underscore the potential therapeutic value of this cytokine in the management of thrombocytopenia and chemotherapy- or radiation-induced myelosuppression. Recent studies suggest that IL-11 may act as an autocrine growth factor for certain megakaryoblastic cell lines.[131] Outside the hematopoietic system, IL-11 stimulates hepatic production of acute-phase reactant proteins[132] and suppresses adipogenesis and heparin-releasable lipoprotein lipase activity in murine preadipocytes.[117]

The similarity in the biologic activities of IL-11 and IL-6 suggests the possibility of a common receptor or overlapping signal transduction pathways for these two cytokines. Recent studies by Yin et al.[133,134] demonstrate that IL-6 and IL-11 bind to distinct receptor molecules. However, these studies implicate gp130, the common signal-transducing protein utilized by

IL-6, LIF, oncostatin M, and ciliary neurotrophic factor[75,135] in IL-11 signal transduction pathways.[134]

IL-11

Also known as: adipogenesis inhibitory factor

Chromosome: 19q13.3–13.4

Gene product: 24 kd

Produced by: fibroblasts, bone marrow stromal cells

Induced by: IL-1, PMA, calcium ionophore A23187

Receptor: 151-kd ligand-binding subunit possibly linked to the gp130 signal-transducing protein

Bioactivity: see Table 16-2

IL-12

The novel cytokine IL-12 is a 75-kd heterodimer composed of disulfide-linked 35- and 40-kd (p35 and p40, respectively) subunits.[136–138] Isolation of their respective cDNAs demonstrated that p35 and p40 are encoded by distinct genes and that expression of both genes is necessary for production of the biologically active molecule.[139,140] p35 bears minor sequence homology with IL-6 and CSF-G, while p40 demonstrates homology with the soluble IL-6 receptor, leading to the suggestion that IL-12 represents a cytokine-soluble receptor complex.[141,142] IL-12 expression was originally demonstrated in Epstein-Barr virus (EBV)-transformed B-cell lines.[136,138,140] Subsequently, mononuclear phagocytes were shown to be an important source of IL-12. A variety of pathogens or their products (LPS, *Staphylococcus aureus*, *Mycobacterium tuberculosis*, *Toxoplasma gondii*, *Listeria monocytogenes*, *Leishmania major*) induce IL-12 production by mononuclear phagocytes.[143–145] A high-affinity IL-12 receptor has been identified and partially characterized on T lymphocytes and NK cells.[146,147]

Recent studies have demonstrated the vital role of IL-12 in cell-mediated immunity. IL-12 induces the differentiation of naive murine CD4+ T-helper cells into T_{H1} cells,[145] a process analogous to IL-4-induced differentiation of naive T-helper cells into T_{H2} cells.[148,149] IL-12-mediated generation of antigen-specific IFN-γ-producing T_{H1} cells is an essential component of the host response to infection by obligate intracellular pathogens, leading to reduction in the microbial burden in several experimental mouse models.[144,145,150,151]

As suggested by its original name (NK cell stimulatory factor), IL-12 has profound effects on NK cells. Exposure to IL-12 augments the functional activity of NK cells and induces lymphokine-activated killer activity in NK cells.[136,152–155] IL-12 also acts synergistically with TNF-α to induce IFN-γ production by NK cells.[156]

IL-12

Also known as: NK cell stimulatory factor, cytotoxic lymphocyte maturation factor

Chromosome: not reported

Gene product: 75-kd heterodimer of 35- and 40-kd subunits

Produced by: mononuclear phagocytes, EBV-transformed B-cell lines

Induced by: LPS, various pathogens

Receptor: single class of high-affinity receptors approximately 110 kd in size

Bioactivity: see Table 16-2

RULE 2. FACTORS THAT STIMULATE GROWTH OF PROGENITORS OFTEN ACTIVATE FUNCTION OF THE TERMINALLY DIFFERENTIATED DAUGHTER CELLS OF THE SAME PROGENITOR

CSF-GM

CSF-GM, a glycoprotein of 14–35 kd[157–159] (the wide range of molecular weight reflects variable degrees of glycosylation) encoded by a gene located on the long arm of chromosome

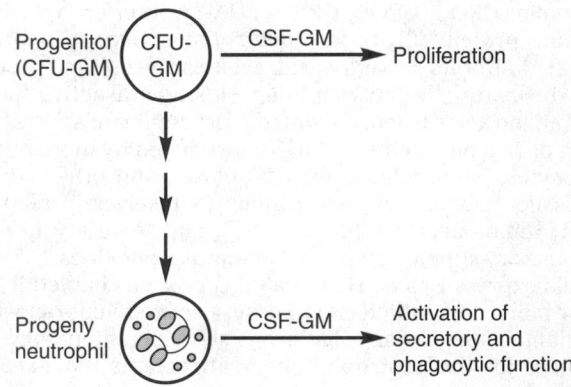

Fig. 16-2. CSF-GM induces proliferation of progenitor cells (CFU-GM) and also stimulates mature progeny of CFU-GM, the neutrophil, activating phagocytic and secretory function.

5,[160–162] stimulates clonal growth of multipotential CFUs (CFU-granulocyte / erythrocyte / macrophage / megakaryocyte [GEMM]), BFU-E, CFU-Mk, granulocyte/macrophage progenitor cells (CFU-GM), and eosinophil colony-forming cells (CFU-Eo),[163–178] although some evidence suggests that the effect of CSF-GM on neutrophil colony growth is indirect[179,180] (e.g., CSF-GM induces auxiliary cells to release neutrophil-specific growth factors[179]). However, CSF-GM also activates the functional activity of most phagocytes, including neutrophils[173,181–200] (Fig. 16-2), macrophages,[201–204] and eosinophils,[184,187,205] cells that can no longer proliferate. In neutrophils and eosinophils, cells that in all likelihood bear the same CSF-GM receptor as their progenitors,[183,206] the stimulatory effect of CSF-GM is on phagocytic function (permitted), not replication (forbidden in a terminally differentiated cell).

CSF-GM

Chromosome: 5q

Gene product: 18–28 kd

Produced by: mast cells, T lymphocytes, endothelial cells, fibroblasts, and thymic epithelial cells

Induced by: TNF-α, IL-1, LPS, phorbol esters, calcium ionophore A23187

Receptor: heterodimer composed of CSF-GM-specific α-subunit and a β-subunit shared with high-affinity IL-3 and IL-5 receptors

Bioactivity: see Table 16-2

CSF-G and CSF-M

CSF-G, an 18-kd protein encoded by a gene on the long arm of chromosome 17,[207] stimulates proliferation of granulocyte progenitor cells[170,208–211] and activates neutrophil function.[191,196,212] CSF-M, encoded by a gene on the long arm of chromosome 5, which gives rise to two glycoprotein species (70–90 kd and 40–50 kd) as a result of alternative splicing of the pre-mRNA transcript,[161,213] stimulates monocyte/macrophage proliferation[170,209,210,213–216] and activation of secretory[217] and phagocytic[218,219] function of monocytes and macrophages.

CSF-G

Chromosome: 17q

Gene product: 18 kd

Produced by: monocytes, macrophages, endothelial cells, fibroblasts

Induced by: IL-1 (α and β), TNF-α, endotoxin

Receptor: 813 and 840 amino acid polypeptides

Bioactivity: see Table 16-2

CSF-M

Also known as: CSF-1

Chromosome: 5q

Gene product: 40–90 kd

Produced by: monocytes, macrophages, fibroblasts, epithelial cells, vascular endothelial cells, osteoblasts

Induced by: IL-3, IL-4, TNF-α

Receptor: a cell-surface receptor tyrosine kinase, encoded by c-fms, a cellular proto-oncogene located on human chromosome 5q

Bioactivity: see Table 16-2

IL-5

IL-5,[162,220–223] the gene for which is also located on the long arm of chromosome 5,[162,222] serves as a final example of the notion that growth factors stimulate both proliferation of progenitors and function of the progeny. IL-5 was known as T-cell-replacing factor and eosinophil differentiation factor.[220,221,223] IL-5 is produced by T lymphocytes induced by antigen, mitogens, and phorbol esters.[220,221,223–225] The high-affinity IL-5 receptor is dimer composed of an IL-5 specific ligand-binding α-chain and a β-chain also common to the CSF-GM and IL-3 receptors[226,227] (see Rule 8 below). IL-5 activates cytotoxic T-cells[228] and induces immunoglobulin secretion.[47,49,229–234] IL-5 also induces eosinophil production in vitro[220,221,223,235–238] and, as predicted by rule 2, activates the functional activity of eosinophils.[239–241]

IL-5

Also known as: T-cell-replacing factor, eosinophil differentiation factor

Chromosome: 5q

Gene product: 50–60 kd

Produced by: T lymphocytes

Induced by: antigen, mitogen, phorbol esters

Receptor: heterodimer composed of IL-5-specific α-subunit and β-subunit shared with the high-affinity CSF-GM and IL-3 receptors

Bioactivity: see Table 16-2

The consistency of this particular rule has a number of implications, including the obvious one that the expression of growth factor receptors does not disappear when the cell has differentiated to a nonreplicative form.[183,206,212,242,243]

RULE 3. HEMATOPOIETIC GROWTH FACTORS CAN ACT DIRECTLY OR INDIRECTLY, OR BOTH

Direct-Acting Lineage-Specific Factors

Certain of the growth factors alter the activity of hematopoietic cells by binding to receptors on the surface of those same cells. Other factors that induce growth of hematopoietic cells do so indirectly, by binding to receptors in the membranes of auxiliary cells and through the receptor, inducing the expression of hematopoietic growth factor genes (the products of which act directly). Of these direct-acting factors (Table 16-2), some exert largely lineage-specific effects. In molecular terms, there are at least two potential explanations for lineage specificity of hematopoietic growth factors. First, as a variation on the theme presented in Fig. 16-1, cells of multiple lineages might express the receptor, but the repertoire of intracytoplasmic or nuclear events may permit only the cells of one lineage to respond. Second, cells of only one lineage may express the gene for a particular growth factor receptor. The importance of the latter mechanism[178] is nicely exemplified by the observa-

tions of Roussel and co-workers,[244] who noted that the receptor for the monocyte/macrophage lineage-specific CSF-M is enforced, by transfection of its gene, in fibroblasts (which ordinarily neither express the receptor nor respond to CSF-M). As a result of such "promiscuous" receptor expression, the fibroblasts become capable of proliferating in response to CSF-M.

Erythropoietin

EPO, an 18-kd protein[245] (34–39 kd when fully glycosylated[246]) encoded by a gene[245–247] stationed on the long arm of chromosome 7,[248] is expressed largely by cells in the liver in embryonic life,[249,250] cells of the kidney,[251] and, to a lesser extent, liver[249] in adult life, and by certain hepatoma cell lines.[1] The production of EPO is induced by reductions of tissue oxygenation,[3,252,253] a mechanism that may involve the initial activation, by hypoxia,[1,5] of heme proteins that stimulate EPO gene expression.[5] EPO stimulates growth and differentiation[246] of erythroid progenitor cells and stimulates proliferation and RNA synthesis in more well-differentiated erythroid precursors as well.[252–254] While EPO has been reported to stimulate various levels of megakaryocytopoiesis in vitro and platelet production in experimental animals[255–258] and although high-affinity EPO receptors have been reported in rodent megakaryocytes,[259] the physiologic relevance of these observations is unclear. First, this is not an effect seen in serum-free cultures[258] or in cultures of cells enriched for progenitors[9] (and relatively free, therefore, of accessory cells). Moreover, others have failed to observe an effect of EPO on megakaryocyte colony growth in human bone marrow cell cultures.[9,260] Certainly, in clinical trials, recombinant human EPO has shown no consistent effects on platelet counts.[261–263]

EPO was the first hematopoietic growth factor to be identified experimentally,[3,4,251,264] and the use of the recombinant protein has been shown to be effective in the management of anemia associated with renal failure.[261–263] It is widely anticipated that expression of EPO receptors will be demonstrated to be a unique attribute of cells committed to erythropoiesis. This prophecy may be self-fulfilling, however, because to date most studies on EPO binding have been performed using murine[265–268] and human[265,269–271] erythroid cells. Indeed, some investigators have suggested that high-affinity EPO-binding sites may exist in IL-3-responsive cell lines that lack erythroid characteristics (but may have erythroid potential) and in megakaryocytes.[259] The cloning of the murine[272] and human[273] EPO receptor genes will help to answer the question of EPO's lineage specificity.

EPO

Chromosome: 7q

Gene product: 34–39 kd

Produced by: kidney in adult, liver during development, hepatoma lines

Induced by: hypoxia

Receptor: 508-amino acid peptide

Bioactivity: see Table 16-2

Other Direct-Acting Lineage-Specific Factors

Growth factors other than EPO also interact directly with progenitor and precursor cells largely committed to one lineage. CSF-G stimulates differentiation of granulopoietic progenitor cells along the neutrophil pathway and only along that pathway.[208] CSF-G also activates the functional activity of neutrophils in vitro and in vivo.[191,196]

CSF-M (Table 16-2) induces replication of monocytes and

macrophages[39,170,172,209,210,215,216,274] and activates the functional capacity of those cells as well[209,217–219,275–278] (rule 2). Although IL-5 has lymphoid bioactivity,[47,49,228,231–234,241,279] its effect on phagocyte production seems to be rather specific for the eosinophil lineage.[220,221,239–241] IL-7 demonstrates relative specificity for lymphoid cells, inducing the clonal growth of normal pre-B cells,[280–282] pre-T cells,[282] and various types of neoplastic lymphoid cells[283,284] and enhancing IL-3 and GM-CSF production by activated T-cells.[285] However, IL-7 was recently shown to induce IL-6, IL-1, TNF-α, and IL-8 production by peripheral blood monocytes.[286,287]

IL-7

Also known as: pre-B cell CSF

Chromosome: 8q12–13

Gene product: 17 kd

Produced by: marrow stromal cells, spleen, and thymus tissue

Induced by: unknown

Receptor: 439-amino acid polypeptide

Bioactivity: see Table 2

Thrombopoietin

The gene encoding thrombopoietin (TPO) has not yet been cloned, and in that sense it is unique among the proteins discussed in this chapter. As was the case with EPO, TPO was first identified as a factor in serum or plasma from thrombocytopenic animals that stimulates thrombopoiesis in a dose-dependent fashion. Plasma from normal animals has less activity, and plasma from thrombocytotic animals has no activity.[288,289] These observations demonstrate the existence of a humoral regulator of platelet production. TPO has been partially purified from the serum of thrombocytopenic animals, and it is a glycoprotein apparently distinct from EPO.[290,291] A 15-kd glycoprotein sharing biologic and immunochemical properties with TPO has been reported to be purified from human embryonic kidney cell-conditioned medium.[291,292] TPO and the kidney cell-derived protein induce not only thrombopoiesis in vivo, but also maturation of megakaryocyte precursor cells in vitro.[293]

Direct-Acting, Multilineage Growth Factors

Two growths factors, IL-3[171,172,294–296] and CSF-GM,[157,166,168,171] have obvious direct effects on multilineage progenitor cells (Table 16-2) and are thus capable of stimulating hematopoietic precursors before they have become fully committed to one lineage or another.

IL-3

IL-3 was known as multi-CSF and multipotential colony growth factor-1.[170,178,209] The human IL-3 gene encodes a 14–28-kd protein and resides on the long arm of chromosome 5 only 9 kb upstream of the gene for CSF-GM, another multipotential colony growth stimulator. To date, only T lymphocytes (induced by mitogens, phorbol esters, and certain antigens)[297] mast cells,[298] and certain cell types in mouse brain tissue[299] have been found to express the IL-3 gene. It is interesting that, although the coding regions of the CSF-GM and IL-3 genes are only separated by 9 kb of intervening DNA, the genes are very differently regulated. CSF-GM is produced by stromal cells[35,174,300–312] and IL-3 is not.[174,310,311] Although T lymphocytes can be induced to produce both IL-3[297,313,314] and CSF-GM,[43,313–316] evidence is clear-cut that each is regulated independently of the other.[35] The high-affinity IL-3 receptor is a heterodimer composed of an IL-3-specific ligand-binding α-subunit and a β-subunit shared in common with the IL-5 and CSF-GM receptors.[226,227] The receptor seems to transduce signals coupled to the cellular response via activation of protein kinase C[317–320] and tyrosine kinases[321] and involves guanyl regulatory nucleotide protein activation.[322,323]

The biologic activity of IL-3, outlined in Table 16-2, like many of the hematopoietic growth factors, is the result of direct effects on progenitors and other more indirect effects. The direct growth-stimulatory effects of IL-3 seem to be largely limited to very primitive committed progenitors like the BFU-E[165,294,324] and hematopoietic progenitor cells with multilineage potential,[165,170,178,209,210,294,295,325–329] including the CFU-spleen (S).[11] The direct proliferation effect of IL-3 and its recently described ability to induce expression of other hematopoietic factors by mature hematopoietic cells[202,330] have complicated efforts to clarify the roles of this factor in hematopoiesis. For example, although it is clear that IL-3 induces formation of multilineage colonies in cultured human bone marrow cells,[165,294,325,331] the full biologic potential of the cytokine is only apparent when it is combined with other factors.[15,215,324,326,332,333] Consequently, reports that IL-3 stimulates proliferation or function of certain mature hematopoietic cells[171,240,334–337] may be a result of its ability to induce expression of other factors that actually do the real work. One particularly intriguing problem in this regard is the apparent ability of IL-3 to stimulate the full developmental potential of basophils and mast cells in vitro,[337,338] a phenomenon that seems to be inconsistent in cultures of human marrow cells[339] but invariable in long-term cultures of rodent tissue marrow cells.[328,340] In fact, administration of IL-3 to nude mice induces marked intestinal and splenic mastocytosis.[341] Nonetheless, the presence of accessory cells (including IL-3-responsive macrophages[202,330,342]) in such settings is universal, as is, therefore, the potential for a number of indirect effects.

Perhaps in part because they are also capable of stimulating proliferation of cells that have made early commitments to a lineage (e.g., the BFU-E[165,294,324]), multilineage growth factors almost always enhance the overall proliferative response of bone marrow cells exposed to lineage-specific factors as well. Both IL-3 and CSF-GM, for example, will enhance the effect of EPO on clonal erythropoiesis in vitro,[11,165,294,324] and, although IL-3 does not induce granulocyte or monocyte colony growth, it does increase self-replication of progenitors in granulocyte and macrophage colonies.[215,332,343,344] Taking these considerations into account, it is very likely that, as hematopoietic cells differentiate, they lose the capacity to proliferate in response to IL-3.[178,327,329]

IL-3

Also known as: multi-CSF, mast cell growth factor-1

Chromosome: 5q

Gene product: 14–28 kd

Produced by: T lymphocytes, mast cells

Induced by: mitogens, phorbol esters, calcium ionophore A23187, IgE receptor activation (mast cells)

Receptor: heterodimer of IL-3-specific α-subunit and β-subunit shared in common with IL-5 and CSF-GM receptors

Bioactivity: see Table 16-2

Indirect-Acting Hematopoietic Factors

Some proteins that regulate hematopoiesis in vivo and in vitro do so indirectly[304,310–312,345,346] (Table 16-2), that is, in some cases they incite bystander cells, also known as accessory or auxiliary cells, to release direct-acting factors.[347–349]

IL-1

IL-1 was formerly known as endogenous pyrogen, lymphocyte-activating factor, and by many other names. IL-1 exists in two molecular forms (IL-1α and IL-1β) that are encoded by two

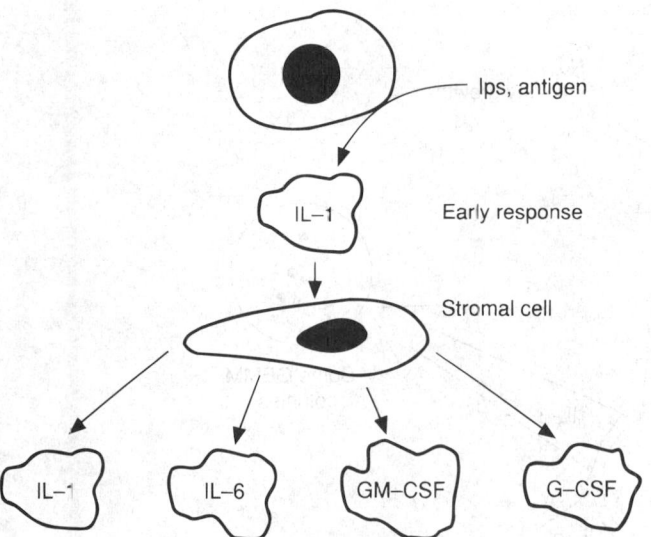

Fig. 16-3. IL-1 is an indirect-acting hematopoietic factor that recruits other cells (including T cells, macrophages, fibroblasts, vascular endothelial cells, keratinocytes, and thymic epithelial cells) to produce hematopoietic growth factors. These induced factors can be direct-acting factors (CSF-G), indirect-acting factors (IL-1 and IL-6), or both direct- and indirect-acting (CSF-GM).

genes on chromosome 2. Each of these genes encodes 31-kd precursor molecules that are cleaved to 17-kd peptides. IL-1, originally thought to be produced only by monocytes and macrophages, is produced by almost all cells. Gene expression is induced by endotoxin, IL-1, CSF-GM, TNF-α, and IL-2. There are two high-affinity IL-1 receptors, the 80-kd type I receptor and the 68-kd type II receptor, which show differential patterns of tissue expression. Both are members of the immunoglobulin superfamily and share 28% amino acid homology in their extracellular ligand-binding domains.[350–352] The bioactivity of IL-1 is tremendously broad, and there is good evidence that it regulates expression of most genes encoding mediators of inflammation.

IL-1 has no colony-stimulating activity itself. However, when administered in vivo, it universally induces neutrophilic leukocytosis, which results from the induction of CSF-G and CSF-GM expression by other cells, including fibroblasts,[305,308,309,311,353,354] endothelial cells,[174,301,303,304,307,310–312] thymic epithelial cells,[355] and T lymphocytes.

The broad activity of IL-1 derives in large part from its ability to induce the expression of other IL and CSF genes, which themselves function as subordinate effector molecules in the inflammatory process. The temporal pattern of IL-1 gene expression in the inflammatory response and its hierarchic dominance over a variety of other cytokines is shown graphically in Fig. 16-3, in which an activated macrophage produces IL-1 and thereby induces stromal cells (e.g., fibroblasts and endothelial cells) to express IL-1, IL-6, CSF-GM, and CSF-G.

IL-1α and -β

Also known as: endogenous pyrogen, leukocyte-activating factor, leukocyte-adhesion molecule, other names

Chromosome: 2q

Gene product: 31-kd precursor, mature 17-kd cleavage product

Produced by: most cells

Induced by: endotoxin, IL-1, CSF-GM, TNF-α, IL-2

Receptors: 68- and 80-kd members of immunoglobulin superfamily

Bioactivity: see Table 16-2

IL-6

IL-6 was formerly known as IFN-β_2, 26-kd protein, B-cell stimulatory factor-2, and hybridoma growth factor.[356–361] The gene resides on the short arm of chromosome 7[362,363] and encodes a 21–26-kd protein.[357,359,364,365] The expression of the gene is seen in heterogeneous cell types, including fibroblasts,[359,366,367] endothelial cells,[365,368–370] monocyte/macrophages,[359,366,371–373] and T lymphocytes[374] and is induced by IL-1,[312,367,369,375–377] TNF-α,[367] mitogens,[374] and endotoxin.[370] The IL-6 receptor consists of a 468-amino acid (90 of which are in an immunoglobulin superfamily domain) ligand-binding subunit coupled to the gp130 signal-transducing protein.[75,135] The biologic activity of IL-6 is exceedingly broad (Table 16-2). It functions synergistically with IL-3 in promoting CFU-GEMM and BFU-E proliferation,[378] with IL-4 and CSF-G promoting in GM colony formation,[378] with IL-4 in inducing T-cell proliferation,[379] and with IL-2 in inducing immunoglobulin secretion[47]; it also increases the self-replicative potential of cells in CSF-M- and CSF-GM-stimulated colonies.[312,378,380] IL-6 is a potent thrombopoietic factor both in vitro and in vivo. It acts synergistically with IL-3 and CSF-GM in supporting CFU-Mk-derived colony growth, it promotes megakaryocytic maturation, and it increases peripheral platelet counts.[381–385] IL-6 may be a humoral mediator of the reactive thrombocytosis that accompanies chronic inflammatory states.

Recombinant human IL-6 has no clearly demonstrable direct effect on the proliferation of any human hematopoietic cell (although it stimulates murine granulocyte/macrophage colony formation[380,386]), yet IL-6 acts synergistically with many direct-acting hematopoietic growth factors.[325,376,378–380,387–396] In concert with IL-3, for example, IL-6 induces proliferation of primitive hematopoietic progenitors[325,388,391,392] (Fig. 16-4). Thus, recent in vivo studies in rats demonstrating that recombinant human IL-6 stimulates replication of CFU-S, may reflect the ability of IL-6 to act in concert with other constitutively produced factors.

As outlined above, some ILs and growth factors act directly, while some act, almost exclusively, indirectly. Other factors, however, are capable of acting in both ways, that is, some of the peptides with hematopoietic activity directly stimulate growth or proliferation, or both, of one cell type while in other cells the same proteins induce expression of other growth factor genes and thus act indirectly as well. IL-2, for example, induces T-cell proliferation and B-cell differentiation and also induces the expression of TNF-α and IL-1 by mononuclear leukocytes.[397,398] Additional factors that exert both direct and indirect effects include CSF-GM (stimulates growth of progenitors and induces IL-1 expression[198,399]), IL-3 (stimulates progenitor cell growth and induces CSF-M gene expression[330]), and IL-4 (directly stimulates isotype switching in B lymphocytes and induces expression of CSF-M and -G in monocytes[400]). Attributing to any protein, therefore, a discrete set of biologic activities may be very difficult if that protein stimulates event X directly and event Y indirectly. It becomes most confusing when a direct-acting factor also induces a second factor that has broad hematopoietic activity (e.g., IL-1).

IL-6

Also known as: IFN-β_2, 26-kd protein, B-cell stimulatory factor-2, hybridoma growth factor

Chromosome: 7p

Gene product: 21–26 kd

Produced by: macrophages, endothelial cells, fibroblasts, T lymphocytes

Induced by: IL-1, mitogens, endotoxin

Receptor: 468-amino acid (90 of which are in an immunoglobulin superfamily domain) ligand-binding protein coupled to gp130

Bioactivity: see Table 16-2

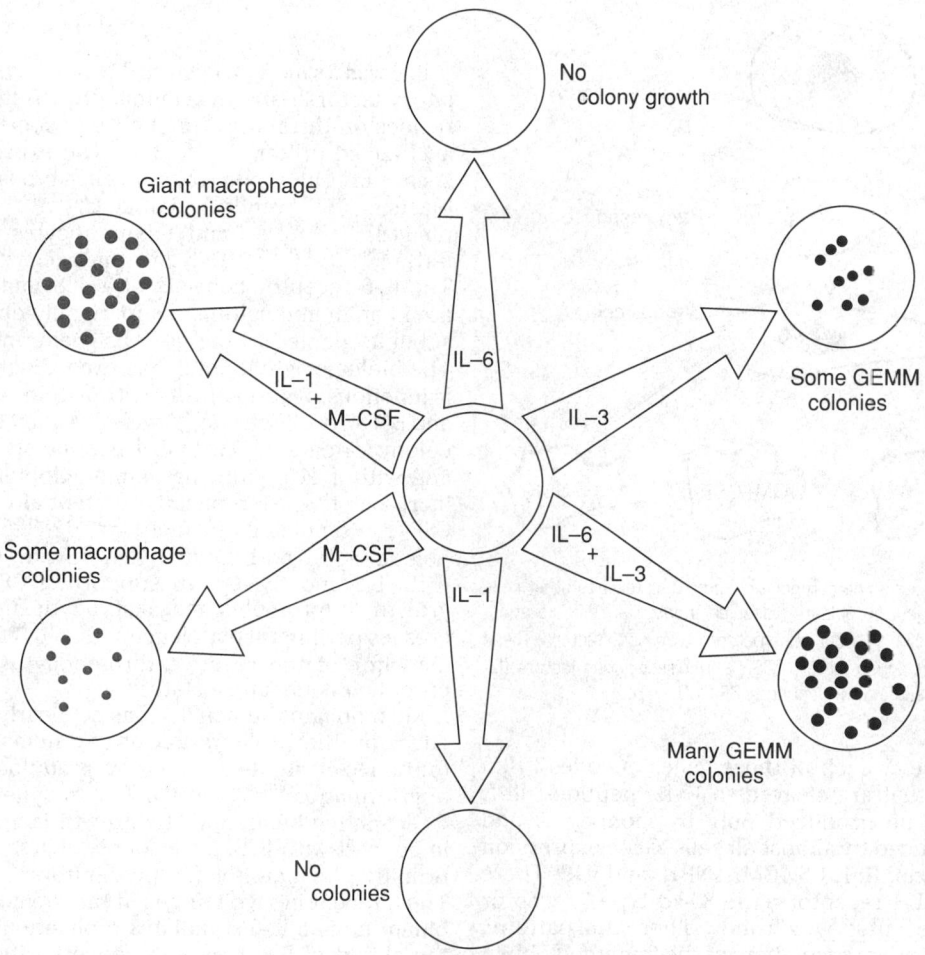

Fig. 16-4. Two examples of synergy. IL-3 and IL-6 are synergistic. Recombinant human IL-6 is, by itself, incapable of inducing hematopoietic colony formation. IL-3 does induce multilineage colony growth (also known as GEMM colonies). The combination of IL-6 and IL-3 induces not only a greater number of GEMM colonies but the colonies are bigger (i.e., the daughters of the progenitor that gave rise to the colony undergo more replicative events per unit time). IL-1 and CSF-M are also synergistic. As is the case with IL-6, IL-1 treatment of bone marrow cells has no colony-stimulating effect whatever, but, when combined with CSF-M, a lineage-specific factor that induces clonal monocyte and macrophage growth, IL-1 enhances the number and size of CSF-M-induced colonies.[420,421]

IL-10

One of the indirect regulators of hematopoiesis, IL-10, is largely an inhibitory factor.[349] IL-10 was originally identified as a cytokine elaborated by murine T_H2 clones that inhibits the production of cytokines such as IFN-γ by T_H1 clones.[401] The cDNA for human IL-10 was isolated by virtue of its sequence homology with the murine cDNA.[402] Subsequently, IL-10 expression was demonstrated in all classes of CD4$^+$ T cells, CD8$^+$ T cells, mononuclear phagocytes, and activated B cells.[349] Human IL-10 is an 18-kd protein[402] expressed as a noncovalent homodimer[349] and is encoded by a gene on chromosome 1.[403]

IL-10 was formerly termed cytokine synthesis inhibitory factor (CSIF) because of its capacity to inhibit the production of cytokines by T lymphocytes.[401] Whereas the murine protein seems to inhibit specifically the production of cytokines (IL-2, IFN-γ, and lymphotoxin) by T_H1 cells,[401,404] human IL-10 inhibits, in addition, the production of "T_H2-type" cytokines (IL-3, IL-4, and IL-5)[349] and NK-cell-derived cytokines (IFN-γ and TNF-α).[156,405,406] This effect is largely indirect, reflecting IL-10-induced inhibition of mononuclear phagocyte antigen-presenting cell function (due in part to down-regulation of MHC class II antigen expression).[407,408] In systems in which cells other than mononuclear phagocytes, such as B cells, present antigen, IL-

10 is devoid of CSIF activity. IL-10 inhibits mononuclear phagocyte-dependent T-cell proliferation[407,408] but can also directly inhibit the proliferation of highly purified T cells (due primarily to suppression of IL-2 production).[409] Human IL-10 can act as a co-stimulator (e.g., with IL-4) of human B-lymphocyte proliferation.[410] IL-10 is a potent inhibitor of mononuclear phagocyte function, suppressing MHC class II antigen expression,[407] monokine (IL-1α, IL-1β, TNF-α, IL-6, IL-8, CSF-G, CSF-GM, and IL-10 itself)[347,411] synthesis, and production of reactive oxygen species and nitric oxide.[412,413]

As a result of its inhibitory effects on "T_H1-type" immune functions, IL-10 appears to play an important role, at least in murine models, in the maintenance and progression of infections by obligate intracellular pathogens that infect macrophages (e.g., listeria, *Schistosoma mansoni*, and mycobacteria).[414-416] In such infections, T_H1-derived cytokines and efficient macrophage function may be crucial in reducing the microbial burden.[417]

It is of considerable interest that the EBV genome contains an open reading frame encoding a protein, termed BCRF1 or viral IL-10 (vIL-10), that has 84% amino acid sequence homology with human IL-10 and that displays many of the activities of IL-10.[402,405] vIL-10, which is expressed in the late phase of the EBV lytic cycle,[418] may contribute to the B-cell proliferative responses and immune defects characteristic of EBV infection. In addition, B-cell lines derived from patients with the acquired immunodeficiency syndrome and Burkitt lymphoma elaborate large quantities of IL-10 (not vIL-10),[419] which may play a role in promoting neoplastic B-cell proliferation.

IL-10

Also known as: Cytokine synthesis inhibitory factor

Chromosome: 1

Gene product: 18 kd

Produced by: T cells, activated B cells and B-cell lymphomas, mononuclear phagocytes, keratinocytes

Induced by: LPS, anti-CD3, PMA

Receptor: not characterized

Bioactivity: see Table 16-2

RULE 4. INTERLEUKINS AND GROWTH FACTORS COMMONLY ACT SYNERGISTICALLY WITH OTHER CYTOKINES

This rule, some examples of which (IL-1 and IL-6) have been mentioned above, is illustrated here by three examples. The first two are the synergies that occur with IL-3 and IL-6 and with IL-1 and CSF-M. Experiments demonstrating synergy between IL-6 and IL-3[392] and between IL-1 and CSF-M[420,421] are summarized in Fig. 16-4. The third example is the complex synergistic activities of IL-2, IL-4, and IL-5 in immunoglobulin isotype switching, depicted in Fig. 16-5. In addition, Steel factor (SF), a cytokine with broad synergistic activity, will be discussed in connection with this rule.

IL-4

IL-4 was formerly known as B-cell stimulatory factor-1, B-cell differentiation factor-γ, T-cell growth factor-2, and mast cell growth factor-2.[422–428] The IL-4 gene resides on the long arm of chromosome 5[162,362,429] and encodes an 18-kd protein[424,430] produced by T lymphocytes induced by phorbol esters, lectins, and certain antigens.[431] IL-4 induces proliferation of activated

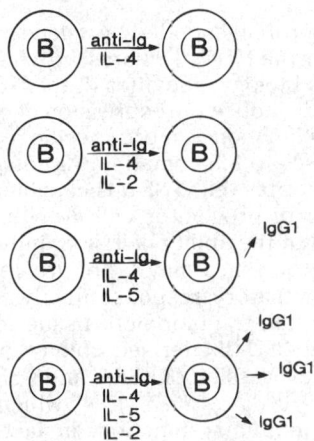

Fig. 16-5. IL-2, IL-4, and IL-5 are synergistic in isotype switching. Experiments performed by Purkerson et al.[47] are summarized here. Although IL-4 was found to be capable of inducing isotype switching in endotoxin-stimulated B cells (not shown), it did not induce switching in B cells activated by anti-immunoglobulin. Combinations of IL-4 and IL-2 were inactive, and the combination of IL-4 and IL-5 was minimally active. However, when recombinant IL-4, IL-5, and IL-2 were combined, maximal production and release of IgG1 occurred.

B cells,[422,432–434] T cells,[379,423,427,428] mast cells,[423] and fibroblasts.[435] It induces expression of its own receptor in B cells and T cells,[279,436] isotype switching to IgG and IgE in activated B cells,[230,233,437–440] and expression of IL-2R in T cells exposed to phorbol esters[427]; it suppresses IL-2-induced B-cell proliferation[441,442] and IL-2-induced IgM secretion.[443] IL-4 induces expression of CSF-M and CSF-G genes in human monocytes,[400] as well as expression of TNF-α and an inhibitor of hematopoiesis (they may be the same factor) in mixed murine marrow stromal cells.[444]

IL-4

Also known as: B-cell stimulatory factor-1, B-cell differentiation factor-γ, T-cell growth factor-2, mast cell growth factor-2

Chromosome: 5q

Gene product: 18 kd

Produced by: T lymphocytes (both CD4⁺ and CD8⁺)

Induced by: phorbol esters, calcium ionophore A23187

Receptor: two domains with homology to the receptors for IL-2, IL-3, IL-6, and EPO

Bioactivity: see Table 16-2

Figure 16-5 demonstrates results of recent experiments performed by Purkerson et al.[47] demonstrating synergy between IL-4, IL-2, and IL-5. Other examples of synergy in hematopoiesis are outlined in Table 16-3.

Steel Factor

Identification of SF and its receptor, the c-*kit* gene product, came after years of study of mice carrying mutations in the dominant white spotting (*W*) or Steel (*Sl*) loci.[445,446] These animals display defects of varying severity in hematopoiesis (macrocytic anemia and reduced numbers of stem cells and tissue mast cells), skin pigmentation, and fertility. Reciprocal marrow transplantation studies with *W*, *Sl*, and normal mice clearly demonstrated that the hematopoietic defect in *W* mice resides in progenitor cells while the defect in *Sl* animals was in the hematopoietic microenvironment.[447–450] Subsequently, *W* mutations were localized to the c-*kit* gene, which encodes a transmembrane protein of the tyrosine kinase class of growth factor receptors.[451,452] In the hematopoietic system, the c-kit protein, encoded by a gene on the long arm of human chromosome 4,[453,454] is expressed on "pre-colony-forming cell (CFC)" progenitor cells,[455,456] CFCs,[457–459] and mast cells and their precursors.[460] The *Sl* locus, which is deleted or defective in Steel mice, was shown to encode the ligand of the c-*kit* gene product.[461–465] Heterozygous defects in the human c-*kit* gene have been associated with several cases of the piebald trait, a dominantly inherited depigmenting state reminiscent of the murine *W* trait.[466,467] No inherited SF defects analogous to the murine *Sl* trait have yet been identified in humans.

SF is a highly glycosylated protein encoded by a gene on the long arm of human chromosome 12.[468] Alternative splicing gives rise to two mRNA species, one containing exon 6 (exon 6⁺) and a second in which exon 6 has been spliced out (exon 6⁻).[469,470] The ratio of exon 6⁺ to exon 6⁻ transcripts is approximately 3:1.[471] SF expression has been demonstrated in fibroblasts, bone marrow stromal (fibroblast-like) cells, vascular endothelial cells, and Sertoli cells, as well as in various embryonic tissues.[471–473] No inductive cytokines for SF expression have yet been convincingly documented,[471] although we have found that TGF-β represses SF expression.[474] SF is elaborated in both membrane-bound and soluble forms, the latter resulting from protease cleavage of the exon 6⁺ transcript-encoded protein at an exon 6-encoded consensus cleavage site.[470,475,476]

Table 16-3. Interleukins, Interferons, and Hematopoietic Growth Factors: Examples of Synergy

1. IL-2, IL-4, and IL-5 in stimulating immunoglobulin isotype switching in B lymphocytes[47]
2. IL-1 and TNF-α in stimulating prostaglandin production by fibroblasts[648]
3. TNF-α and IFN-γ in suppressing hematopoiesis in vitro[505]
4. IL-1 and IL-2 in inducing IFN production in T lymphocytes[697]
5. IL-3 and CSF-M in stimulating proliferation of murine progenitor cells in clonal assays[215]
6. IL-1 and TNF-α in inducing differentiation of murine myeloid leukemic cells[568]
7. IL-4 and IL-2 in inducing T-lymphocyte proliferation[426]
8. IL-3 and CSF-G in inducing proliferation of multipotential progenitor cells[343]
9. IL-6 and IL-1 in activating T lymphocytes[387]
10. IL-3 and both CSF-G and CSF-GM in stimulating granulocyte and granulocyte/macrophage colony growth[332]
11. IL-4 and IL-6 in induction of T-lymphocyte proliferation[379]
12. IFN-γ and TNF-α in induction of CSF-G and CSF-GM release from T lymphocytes[316]
13. IL-3 and IL-2 in stimulation of T-cell proliferation[334]
14. CSF-GM and IFN-γ in induction of TNF-α gene expression by monocytes[539]
15. IL-3 and EPO in stimulation of BFU-E growth in vitro[324]
16. CSF-G and IL-3 in induction of megakaryocyte colony growth[333]
17. IL-1 and TNF-α in induction of IL-1 gene expression in vascular endothelial cells[652]
18. CSF-M and IL-6 in stimulating macrophage colony growth of human marrow cells[395]
19. CSF-GM and IL-6 in promoting granulocyte differentiation[380]
20. IL-1, IL-3, and CSF-M in supporting clonal growth of macrophages[420] and primitive myeloid progenitor cells[326]
21. IL-6, IL-3, EPO, and IL-4 in supporting erythroid and megakaryocytic colony growth[378]
22. IL-9 augments EPO-induced BFU-E growth,[698] IL-4 induced immunoglobulin production by B lymphocytes,[699,700] and IL-3-induced growth of murine mast cells[112]
23. IL-11 acts synergistically with IL-3 and Steel factor to stimulate clonal growth of erythroid (BFU-E and CFU-E) and megakaryocytic (BFU-Mk) progenitor cells[115,126]
24. IL-12 synergizes with TNF-α to stimulate IFN-γ production by NK cells[156]
25. Steel factor acts synergistically with IL-3, CSF-GM, and EPO to support optimal clonal growth of hematopoietic progenitor cells of all lineages[21,701,702] and also synergistically functions with IL-6 to augment CFU-S growth[703] and with IL-9 to stimulate proliferation of the human leukemic cell line MO7E[704]

The membrane-bound and soluble forms of SF display equivalent bioactivity in clonogenic assays in vitro.[469] However, the particular relevance of the membrane-bound form to normal hematopoiesis, gametogenesis, and pigmentation is clearly illustrated by mice homozygous for the Sl^d allele in which a genomic deletion gives rise to a soluble protein lacking the anchoring transmembrane and cytoplasmic domains.[470,476] Although the soluble protein retains full biologic activity in vitro, these animal are anemic, sterile, and nonpigmented.[470,476]

SF promotes the proliferation and differentiation of the most primitive hematopoietic progenitor cells ("pre-CFCs") into committed progenitor cells (CFU-GEMM, BFU-E, CFU-GM, and CFU-Mk).[455,477,478] Whether SF promotes self-renewal of pre-CFCs is controversial. While SF has no independent colony-stimulating activity, it acts synergistically with IL-3, CSF-GM, and EPO to promote CFU-GEMM-, BFU-E, and CFU-Mk-derived colony growth.[124,479–481] SF improves the deficient in vitro colony growth of bone marrow cells from patients with Diamond-Blackfan anemia or Fanconi anemia,[482–484] suggesting a poten-

tial therapeutic use of SF in these congenital marrow failure states (note that neither SF nor c-*kit* are defective in these conditions). SF promotes the survival, proliferation, and differentiation of mast cell precursors.[460,485] In addition, SF is chemotactic for mast cells[486] and enhances the release of mast cell mediators such as histamine.[487,488] SF administration in vivo induces a marked expansion in the compartment of committed hematopoietic progenitor cells and striking mast cell hyperplasia.[489,490] Outside the hematopoietic system, appropriate developmentally regulated SF expression is necessary for normal melanocyte development and migration and gametogenesis.[445,469,491]

Steel Factor

Also known as: Stem cell factor, kit ligand, mast cell growth factor

Chromosome: 12q22-24

Gene product: approximately 40 kd

Produced by: fibroblasts, endothelial cells, bone marrow stromal cells, Sertoli cells, hepatocytes, various embryonic tissues

Induced by: expression is constitutive

Receptor: c-kit protein

Bioactivity: see Table 16-2

RULE 5. HEMATOPOIETIC REGULATORY CYTOKINES ARE ORGANIZED IN A HIGHLY COMPLEX INTERDEPENDENT NETWORK BUT RETAIN SOME CONCRETE ELEMENTS OF HIERARCHIC STRUCTURE

New students of hematopoiesis are often dismayed at the complexity of the growth factor network with all its synergies and feedback loops. One rule that seems to place the networks into some understandable framework is that most cytokine responses are hierarchic.[312] The central roles of IL-1 and TNF-α in hematopoietic regulation serve as particularly obvious examples.[304,311,312] Both IL-1 (Fig. 16-3) and TNF-α genes are expressed early in the inflammatory response. These two gene products induce the expression of a wide variety of subordinate IL and growth factor genes.[16,174,301–309,311,312,315,345,355,369,375,492–501]

TNF-α

TNF-α, a 17-kd protein encoded by a gene stationed on chromosome 6[502] near the MHC,[503] shares with IL-1 a large number of heterogeneous biologic activities (Table 16-2) and, like IL-1, functions largely to induce the expression of other subordinate genes that in turn function as more specific regulators of hematopoietic responses to inflammation. Although a good deal of evidence demonstrates that TNF-α is capable of functioning as a direct inhibitor of progenitor cell growth,[504–509] some evidence suggests that the ability of TNF to induce expression of other growth factor genes may be of greater importance, at least in the inflammatory response involving lymphopoiesis and granulopoiesis. In granulopoietic tissue, for example, while TNF-α can inhibit CFU-GM-derived colony growth,[505,506,509] it also induces the expression of CSF-G and CSF-GM genes in accessory cells,[16,306,310,311,316,354,494,495,510] which likely functions to override the inhibitory function. In fact, that EPO gene expression is not induced by TNF-α may account for the vulnerability of erythropoiesis in chronic inflammatory diseases wherein many patients are anemic. Indeed, Roodman and colleagues[507] have proposed that the anemia of chronic disease results from TNF-α production. When factors like TNF-α have confusing double-edged biologic functions, we are obliged to assess the function of the molecule in vivo to assign weight to one or the other in vitro response. This has been done recently, and it is clear that the stimulatory effect of TNF-α dominates

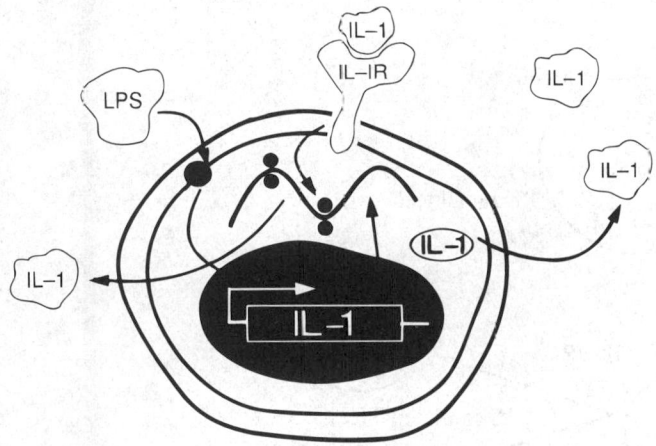

Fig. 16-6. Autocrine signal amplification of IL-1 gene expression. A macrophage exposed to endotoxin (lps), transcribes the IL-1 gene (shown in the nucleus of the cell). The wavy line attached to the dots represents IL-1 mRNA attached to ribosomes. The half-life of IL-1 mRNA is quite short.[609,610] However, certain molecular events, reviewed in detail later, transpire to stabilize IL-1 mRNA. Specifically, IL-1 is translated, is secreted by the cell, and binds to IL-1 receptors (IL-1R) on the same cell. Signals induced by IL-1 binding to the receptor result in the stabilization of its own mRNA.

in granulopoiesis[16,511] but inhibitory effects dominate erythropoiesis.[507,512] Other examples of the double-edged bioactivity of TNF-α exist, some of which have been evaluated by in vivo studies. For example, while the growth of cultured vascular endothelial cells in vitro is inhibited by TNF, TNF administered in vivo is angiogenic.[513,514]

TNF-α

Also known as: cachectin

Chromosome: 6p

Gene product: 17 kd

Produced by: macrophages, B lymphocytes, NK cells

Induced by: endotoxin, CSF-GM, IL-3, poly(I):poly(C), phorbol esters, calcium ionophore A23187

Receptor: 55 kd protein homologous to nerve growth factor receptor

Bioactivity: see Table 16-2

RULE 6. CYTOKINE NETWORK EXHIBITS MANY SIGNAL AMPLIFICATION CIRCUITS

Certain gene products that appear early in the inflammatory response, such as IL-1, enhance the expression of their own genes,[312,496,499,501,515–517] and TNF-α induces IL-1 gene expression.[16,518–520] More trying complexities exist. IL-1 gene expression is induced by proteins that IL-1 itself induces.[189,198,312] Thus, such signal amplification mechanisms can be autocrine, paracrine, or both. Examples of these two mechanisms are reviewed in Figs. 16-6 and 16-7.

RULE 7. GENES ENCODING HEMATOPOIETIC GROWTH FACTORS AND INTERLEUKINS SHARE IMPORTANT STRUCTURAL AND FUNCTIONAL ATTRIBUTES

Two issues are considered here: (1) the evidence for evolutionary relatedness among cytokines, and (2) the function of cis-acting elements in the 3′ untranslated region of many hematopoietic growth factors and ILs.

Importance of Chromosome 5

Many of the cytokine genes are located on the long arm of chromosome 5 (Fig. 16-8). Recent studies using pulsed transverse field electrophoresis have suggested that IL-4, IL-5, IL-3, and CSF-GM are located within 500 kb of each other.[162] IL-3 is only 9 kb upstream of CSF-GM.[160] Other cytokine genes and genes involved in the regulation of cell growth or differentiation (or both) located on chromosome 5 include CSF-M,[161,521,522] c-*fms*[161,522] (a cellular proto-oncogene that encodes the CSF-M receptor[523–526]), IL-9,[106,107] IFN regulatory factor-1,[527] endothelial cell growth factor,[528] the B chain of platelet-derived growth factor receptor,[529] the β2-adrenergic receptor,[529] and the monocyte differentiation antigen CD14.[530] The proximity of these genes is of significant evolutionary interest as well as of potential clinical interest in patients with the hematopoietic disorder known as the 5q minus syndrome in which many of these genes are deleted from one of the chromosomes 5 in hematopoietic cells.[222,521,522,527]

mRNA Instability and the 3′ AU-Rich Motifs of ILs and CSFs

There are also important functional similarities of genetic structure among the ILs, one example of which will be addressed here. Most of the genes encoding ILs and hematopoietic growth factors have, in their 3′ untranslated regions, motifs that contain reiterated ATTTA pentamers[531,532] (Fig. 16-9). Therefore, these domains in IL gene transcripts read AUUUA. Shaw and Kamen[531] have demonstrated that motifs containing these AU-rich clusters can destabilize certain otherwise stable heterologous mRNAs to which they are attached. Thus, as shown in Fig. 16-9, in which CSF-GM is actively transcribed, the 3′ untranslated region containing the AU-rich motif somehow targets the mRNA for rapid degradation by ribonucleases. After stimulation of the cell by IL-1, the pace of CSF-GM mRNA decay is slowed. We have recently found that the accumulation of CSF-GM mRNA in endothelial cells or fibroblasts results not from transcriptional activation by IL-1, but from stabilization of mRNA[533] (Fig. 16-10) and that this is also true for other IL-1 induced genes, including IL-6, CSF-G, and IL-1 (unpublished data).

Given these observations, we can explain a number of rules for IL-1, including its breadth of activity (although it has not yet been proved, the mRNA stabilization effect of IL-1 may occur with any constitutively transcribed mRNA bearing the destabilizer motif), its autocrine amplification loop (IL-1 gene transcripts also have the AU-rich 3′ element[531]), and its ability to synergize with other factors. We review the latter issue, synergy, in more detail.

Molecular Models of Synergy

When in vitro assays of biologic activity are used, the targets of ILs may be the cell whose function is being observed (in Fig. 16-11, it is a progenitor cell that forms colonies). However, the target of the IL might be another cell that can be induced to make additional factors that directly affect the progenitors. Such cells are known to cell biologists as auxiliary or accessory cells. To make it even more complicated, over time in any assay system, cells that are progeny of the progenitors (i.e., daughter cells within the colonies) can become capable of producing factors themselves. A monocyte or promonocyte that appeared early in a macrophage colony would be capable of being induced to produce CSF-G,[217,330,400,534,535] CSF-M,[330,400,535] IL-1,[501,536,537] TNF-α,[202,397,538–541] or IL-6.[359,371–374] Keeping the importance of the auxiliary cell in mind, two theoretical molec-

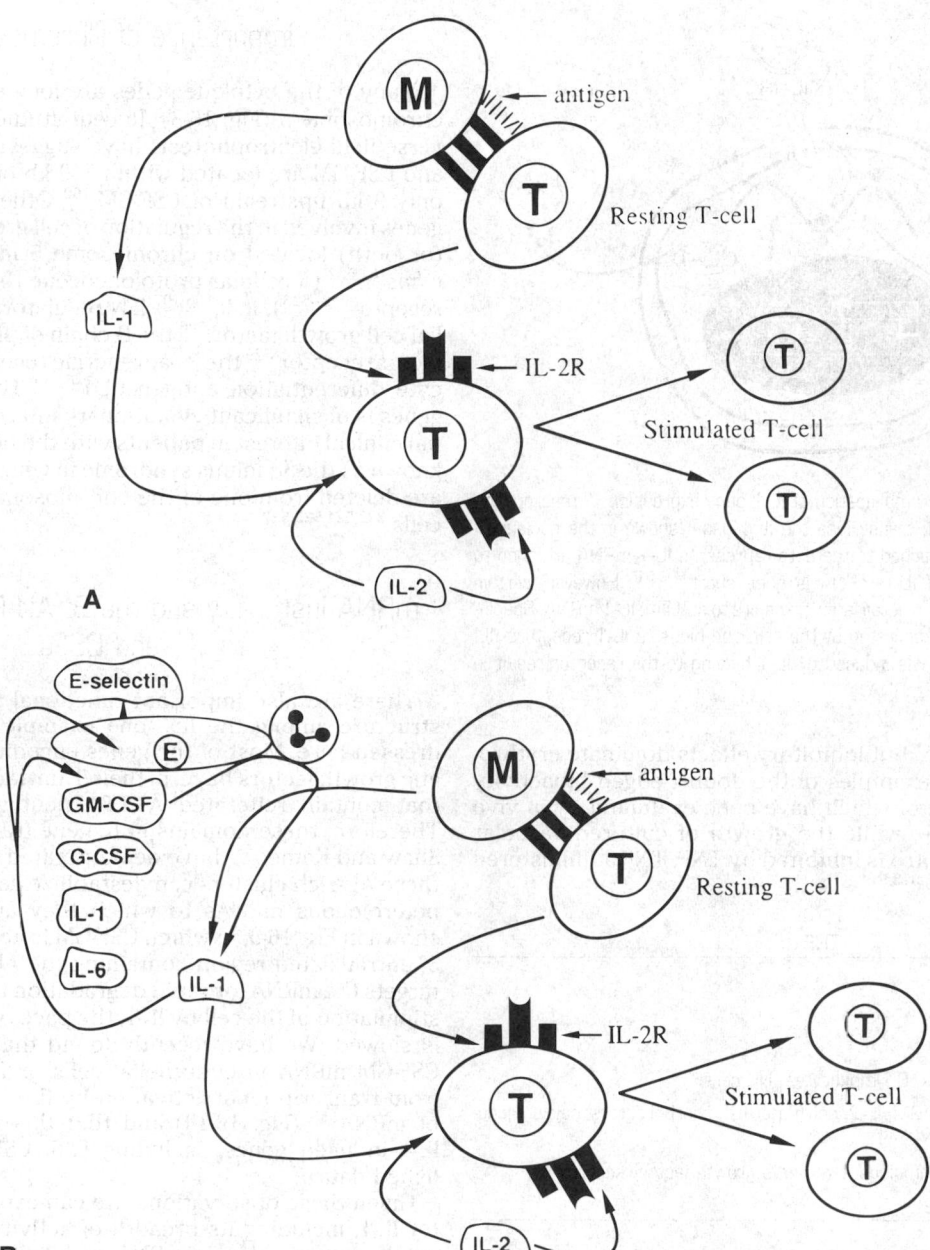

Fig. 16-7. Paracrine signal Amplification. **(A)** A T cell (T) exposed to antigen processed by a macrophage (M) expresses IL-2 receptor (IL-2R) and secretes IL-2, a process that is enhanced by the IL-1 produced by the antigen-stimulated macrophage. As a result, T cells will proliferate. In any tissue or lymph node, the amplification process is far more complex. For example, IL-2 can amplify the expression of IL-1 (not shown). **(B)** Macrophages and T cells do not interact in a vacuum. There are always stromal cells nearby (to which the interacting T cells and macrophages might even be directly attached) that contribute to additional complexities. For example, the IL-1 released by the same macrophage will induce expression of CSF-GM, CSF-G, IL-6, and more IL-1 in endothelial cells. E-selectin, an adhesion molecule for neutrophils induced by IL-1, will cause the attachment of neutrophils, which will doubtless come under the influence of CSF-GM, which induces expression of IL-1 mRNA in neutrophils.

ular models of synergy are worthy of consideration (Fig. 16-12 and 16-13). In these examples, we use IL-1 and three hypothetical ILs, IL-X, IL-Y, and IL-Z in a culture system that includes a few auxiliary cells of one kind or another.

In the first example (Fig. 16-12), a colony growth assay is being performed with exogenous IL-Z as a colony growth stimulator. In this system, IL-1 has no direct colony-stimulating effect, yet it synergizes with IL-Z. IL-1 essentially functions to induce the expression by auxiliary cells of an additional direct-acting factor, IL-X.

In the second theoretical example of synergy (Fig. 16-13), neither IL-1 nor IL-Z have any direct colony-stimulating effects on their own, but together they can induce colony growth. The effectors of the colony growth response are the direct-acting colony stimulating factors IL-Y and IL-X, both of which are effectively induced by IL-1 and IL-Z.

Can synergy be more complex than this? Of course. Consider that this bioassay system is one that excludes multiple tissues and organs that might otherwise participate fruitfully in the network. Imagine what additional complexities unfold when pu-

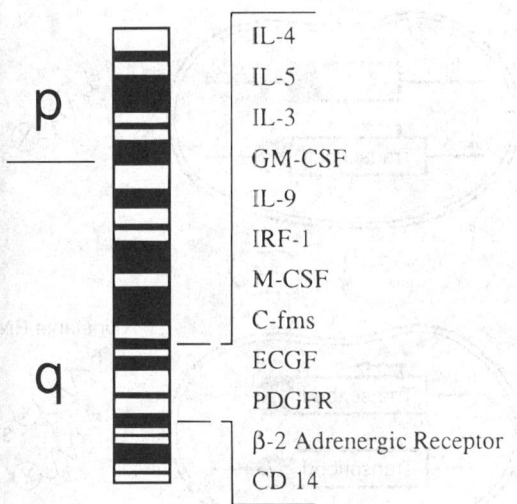

Fig. 16-8. A number of hematopoietic growth factors and ILs are found on the long arm of chromosome 5 in humans, including IL-4, IL-5, IL-3, and CSF-GM.[160,162] Other cytokine genes and genes involved in the regulation of cell growth and differentiation located on chromosome 5 include CSF-M,[161,521,522] c-fms[161,522], which encodes the CSF-M receptor,[523–526] IL-9,[106,107] endothelial cell growth factor,[528] the B chain of platelet-derived growth factor receptor[529] the β_2-adrenergic receptor,[529] and the monocyte differentiation antigen CD14[530] In the 5q— syndrome, some of these genes are deleted from one of the chromosomes 5 in hematopoietic cells.[221,521,522]

rified recombinant ILs or hematopoietic growth factors are injected intravenously, when any cell in any organ may function as an auxiliary cell. One reason for emphasizing these molecular models of synergy is largely to underscore the single most important pitfall encountered in dealing with new scientific reports on the biologic activity of any hematopoietic growth factor or IL: when a new factor stimulates any hematopoietic event (e.g., stimulation of mast cell colony growth), the cells whose behavior demonstrates the event (e.g., mast cell progenitors) may not even possess receptors for the new factor at all. Instead, the factor may only nudge the first in a long line of molecular dominoes, the last of which is a production of a protein that binds to a receptor on the indicator cell (the mast cell progenitor).

RULE 8. RECEPTORS FOR HEMATOPOIETIC GROWTH FACTORS SHARE MANY STRUCTURAL AND FUNCTIONAL ATTRIBUTES

There are two hematopoietic growth factor receptor superfamilies, one in which the cytoplasmic domains of each receptor possess tyrosine kinase activity, and the other, substantially larger, superfamily whose members do not have cytoplasmic tyrosine kinase domains.

Receptors with Cytoplasmic Tyrosine Kinase Domains

Amino acid sequence analysis has provided a framework for the categorization of three subclasses of a tyrosine kinase receptor family. Subclass 1 includes the *neu/HER-2* proto-oncogene and epidermal growth factor, subclass 2 includes the insulin and IGF-1 receptors, and subclass 3 includes the receptors for CSF-M, SF, and platelet-derived growth factor. Because subclass 3 includes receptors for some hematopoietic growth factors, it will be discussed further here.

C-*kit* and c-*fms* are genes that encode two related hematopoi-

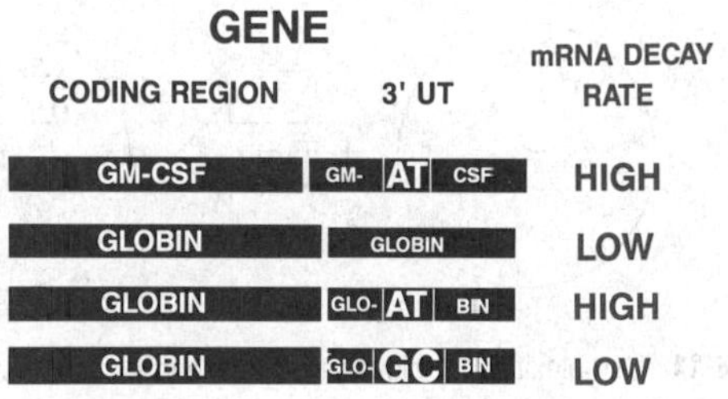

Fig. 16-9. The AU-rich motif in the 3′ untranslated region of the CSF-GM transcript is a destabilizing element for heterologous mRNA. Shown is the location of the coding region of this destabilizing element in the CSF-GM gene and the homologous sequences present in other genes whose products display hematopoietic activity. Shaw and Kamen[531] synthesized a double-stranded copy of the CSF-GM 3′ element (AU) and placed it into the 3′ untranslated region of the rabbit β-globin gene. They noted that when the globin transcript possessed this motif, its ordinarily long half-life was shortened. When a mutant element (GC) of equal size containing no reiterated ATTTA sequences was inserted in place of the AT-rich region, the half-life of the globin transcript was normal.

etic growth factor receptors, the ligands for which are SF and CSF-M, respectively. Along with PDGF (A and B) receptors, they constitute a subclass of receptor tyrosine kinases with similar topologies.[542] All receptors with tyrosine kinase activity possess large glycosylated extracellular domains, a single transmembrane-spanning region, and a cytoplasmic domain that contains one or more tyrosine kinase catalytic sites (Fig. 16-14).

Hematopoietic Growth Factor Receptor Superfamily

The characterization of receptors for many of the growth factors has permitted the identification of a group that includes receptors for LIF, IL-1, IL-2, IL-3, IL-4, IL-5, IL-6, IL-7, IL-9, CSF-GM, CSF-G, EPO, prolactin, growth hormone, ciliary and c-*mpl*.[543,544] As shown in Figure 16-14, a number of repetitive structural and functional themes occur in this unique integral membrane protein superfamily, including (1) four cysteine residues in the extracellular domain; (2) the sequence W-S-X-W-S in the ligand-binding extracellular domain; (3) a capacity for enhanced binding or signal transduction, or both, when expressed as a heterodimer or homodimer; (4) lack of a known catalytic domain in the cytoplasmic portion of the molecule, and (5) the presence of fibronectin type III domains[545] in the

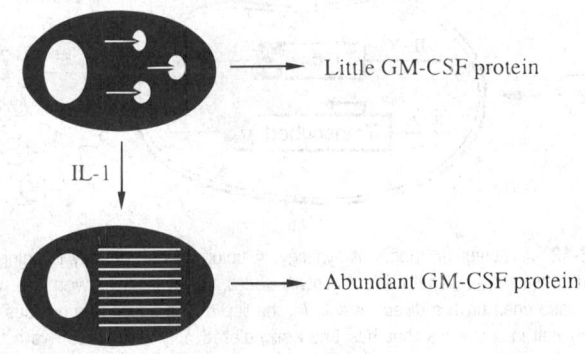

Fig. 16-10. The CSF-GM gene, containing the AU-rich 3′ element, is transcribed, giving rise to a transcript that becomes, quite rapidly, the target of ribonucleases, shown here as Pac Men. The half-life of such transcripts in cells exposed to IL-1 is markedly prolonged (from 1 hour in control cells to >24 hours in IL-1-stimulated cells). Therefore, IL-1 functions to induce the expression of CSF-GM by somehow inhibiting ribonucleolytic decay of the transcripts.

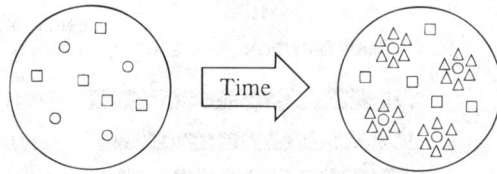

Fig. 16-11. Complexities of bioassays in hematopoiesis. Cells from blood, bone marrow, lymph nodes, thymus, or other hematopoietic sites are cultured in vitro and exposed to a variety of factors that induce some of the cells present to do something measurable. In the example shown here, the assay is designed to measure hematopoietic colony development over time. Each colony is formed by a single progenitor cell (circles). If a factor is added to this system and stimulates colony growth, it might act directly on the progenitor cell itself. However, because other cells that can be induced to produce direct-acting factors (squares) are present in the culture system, one cannot presume that the factor tested is a direct-acting factor. To make it still more complicated, over time in any assay system, cells (triangles) that are progeny of the progenitors (that is, daughter cells within the colonies) can become capable of producing factors themselves.

extracellular regions. Apart from these shared homologous domains, there is not much sequence homology among these receptors, and the sizes of their cytoplasmic domains (Fig. 16-14) are immensely variable. Nonetheless, these homologies are likely of substantial functional importance and also give clues to the evolution of this family. For example, fibronectin type III domains are shared with several cell-adhesion molecules, suggesting that cytokine receptors evolved from ancestors whose products functioned largely to facilitate cellular adhesion to both substrates and other cells.

Another interesting feature of some of these receptor molecules is their capacity to share peptide subunits with other receptors. For example, IL-5, CSF-GM, and IL-3 have unique low-

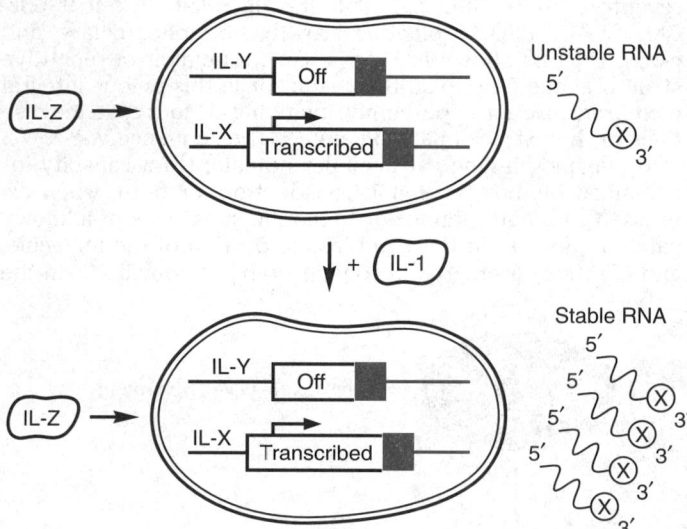

Fig. 16-12. A molecular model of synergy. A colony growth assay is being performed in which IL-1 has no direct growth effect, yet synergizes with IL-Z, which in this case does have a direct effect. At the top of the figure is a nucleus of an auxiliary cell in a culture that has been stimulated only with IL-Z. Two cytokine genes, IL-X and IL-Y, are present in this cell. Both IL-X and IL-Y genes encode proteins that stimulate colony growth. Both have mRNA instability elements. Only IL-X is transcribed in the steady state, but because of the decay element, in the absence of IL-1, the IL-X mRNA is unstable and produces no protein. After IL-1 is added to the culture, however, IL-X mRNA is stabilized, IL-X is produced, and it induces a greater colony growth response than is seen with IL-Z alone. Thus, IL-X and IL-Z are additively stimulatory, and IL-1 and IL-Z are synergistic.

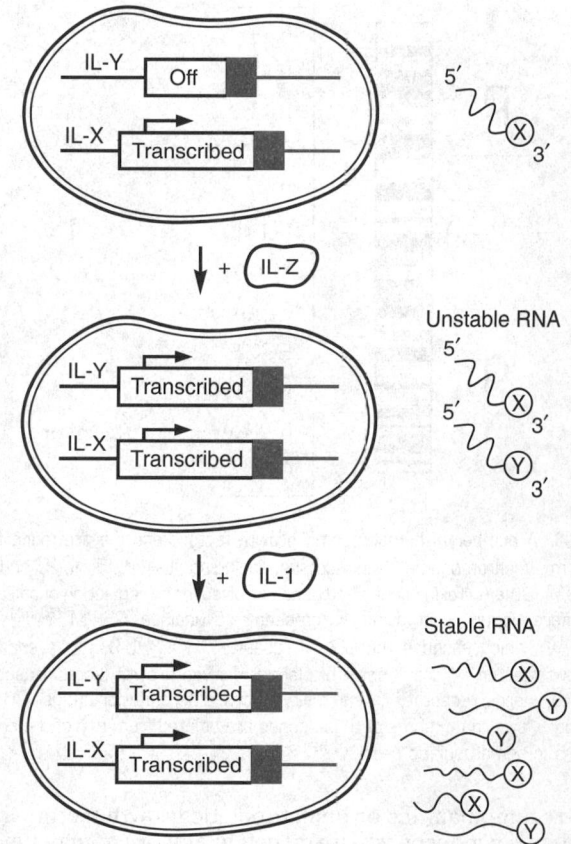

Fig. 16-13. A second molecular model of synergy. In this case, neither IL-1 nor IL-Z have any direct colony-stimulating effects on their own, but together they can induce colony growth. The effectors of the colony growth response are actually the gene products IL-Y and IL-X, which themselves are direct-acting colony-stimulating factors. In the cell at the top, only IL-X is transcribed, but, as before, IL-X mRNA is degraded and makes no protein. The addition of IL-Z to the culture stimulates the transcription of IL-Y. However, because IL-Y also has a destabilizer motif (shown again in red) at the 3′ end of the gene, it too gives rise to unstable and untranslated message. However, on addition of IL-1, both transcripts are stabilized and expressed, giving rise to IL-X and IL-Y proteins, which directly induce colony growth.

affinity (α-chain) receptors, but they share the same β-chain,[226,227] and association of the two chains results in the formation of a specific high-affinity subunit capable of effective signal transduction (Fig. 16-15). The role of each chain in signal transduction is now being carefully examined. For example, distinct regions within the cytoplasmic domain of the CSF-GM receptor β-chain have been identified recently.[546] A membrane proximal region is necessary for the chain to activate c-*myc* gene expression, while a more distal region, between residues 626 and 763, is required for activation of *ras, raf*-1, and MAP kinase and induction of c-*fos* and c-*jun*.[546] Shared subunits have also been identified for high-affinity complexes that serve as receptors for LIF, IL-6, ciliary neurotrophic factor, and oncostatin M[75,135] (Fig. 16-16). In this case, gp130 functions as a signal-transducing component of the IL-6Rα/gp130 and CNTF-Rα/LIF-Rα/gp130 complexes. The details of the stimulus-response coupling pathways are not yet known, but it has been reported that gp130 is phosphorylated at tyrosine residues on stimulation of cells with the ligand.[547]

In many instances, soluble forms of the receptor can be found, sometimes resulting from translation of differentially spliced mRNA. Soluble forms have been described for IL-4, IL-5, IL-7, CSF-G, SF, EPO, and CSF-GM receptors.[548–552] Although the biologic significance of this phenomenon is not yet fully

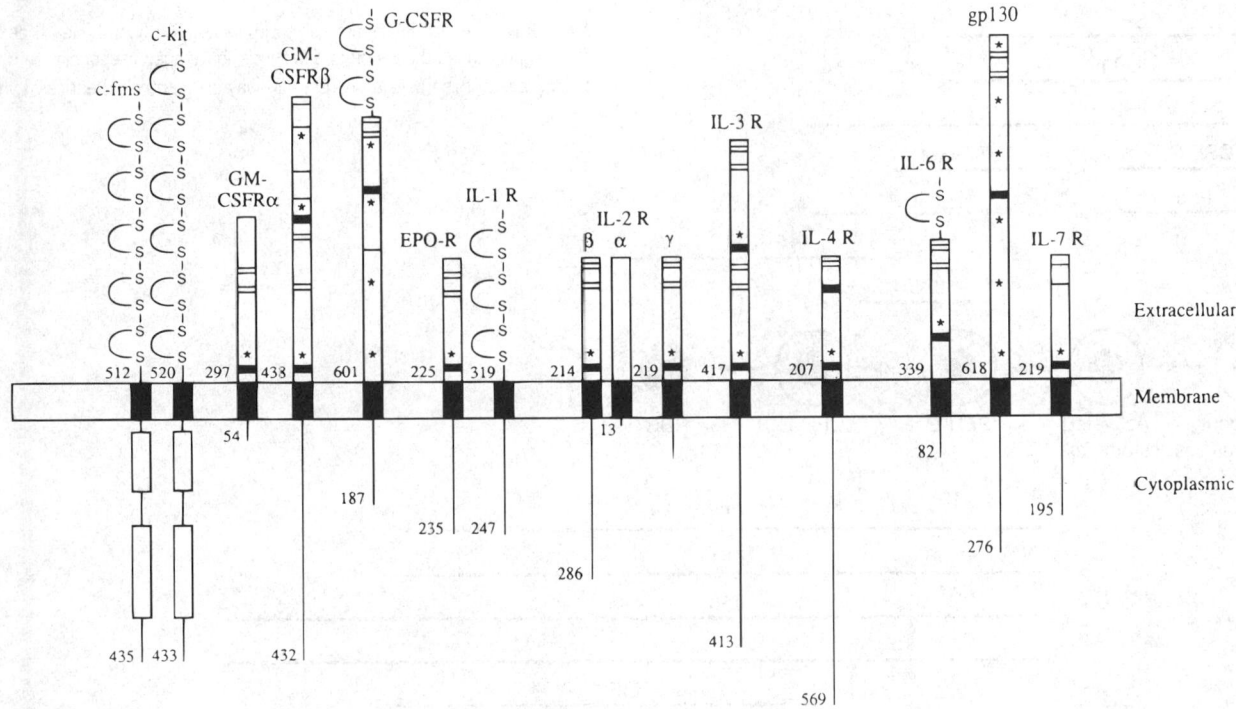

Fig. 16-14. Structures for a variety of hematopoietic growth factor receptors. c-fms and c-kit are integral membrane proteins with tyrosine kinase domains. Tyrosine kinase domains are indicated as cytoplasmic boxes. The other growth factor receptors shown are members of the hematopoietic growth factor superfamily. The extracellular domains include the immunoglobulin-like regions shown as loops (c-fms, c-kit, IL-1R, and IL-6R). The superfamily members have conserved cysteines in the extracellular domains (parallel lines). The dark box above the membrane region of the receptors represents the WSXWS motif. Locations of the fibronectin type III motifs are indicated by stars. Only two of the many known heterodimeric subunits are illustrated: the CSF-GM receptor β-subunit (a subunit it shares with IL-3R and IL-5R) is paired with CSF-GM-Rα and the gp130 subunit paired with IL-6Rα.

understood, the soluble forms may act as competitive binding proteins for the ligand and, as is clearly the case for the soluble IL-4 receptor,[552] serve as natural in vivo antagonists for specific cytokines.

Another shared feature of hematopoietic growth factor receptors is that they transduce signals that prevent programmed cell death (apoptosis). Apoptosis is characterized by chromatin condensation at the edge of the nuclear envelope, followed by convolution, and then fragmentation of the nucleus in terminally differentiated cells or in undifferentiated cells after mild injury, factor deprivation, or exposure to mitotic inhibitors.[553] DNA fragmentation occurs internucleosomally and can be monitored by agarose gel electrophoresis.[553] The capacity of hematopoietic growth factors to inhibit apoptosis

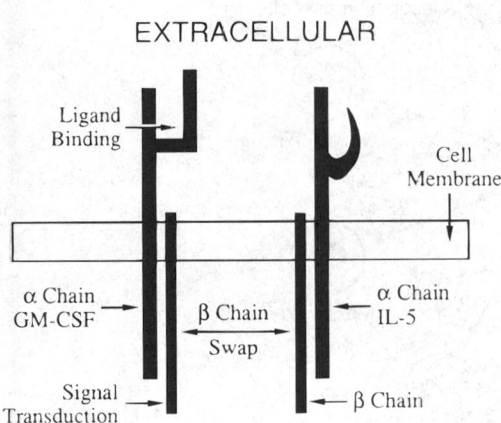

Fig. 16-15. The high-affinity receptors for IL-3, IL-5, and CSF-GM each consist of unique α-chains and a shared β-chain. Competition for a limited number of β-chains, shown here as a "swap" between the α-chain of the IL-5 receptor and the α-chain of the CSF-GM receptor, accounts for the capacity of one ligand to reduce high-affinity binding of the other two ligands.

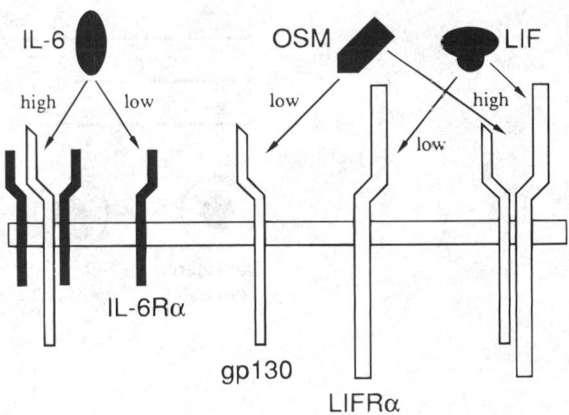

Fig. 16-16. As is the case with the IL-3, IL-5, and CSF-GM, receptors, the high-affinity receptors for IL-6, oncostatin M (OSM), and leukemia inhibitory factor (LIF) are also heterodimers. Specifically, when IL-6Rα pairs with the signal-transducing gp130 protein, it is converted from a low-affinity monomeric receptor to a high-affinity heterodimeric receptor. The LIF receptor α-chain (LIF-Rα) functions as a low-affinity receptor for LIF. When gp130 and LIF-Rα dimerize, they function together as high-affinity receptors for both OSM and LIF.

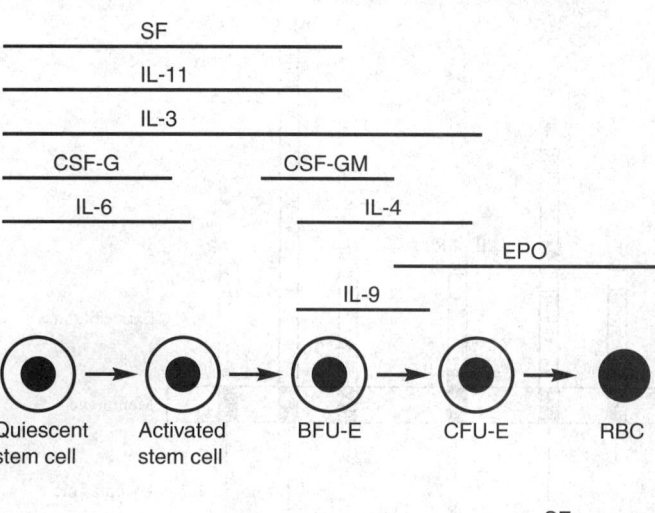

Fig. 16-17. Factors influencing erythropoiesis. The lines beneath each growth factor encompass the range of differentiation stages responsive to that factor. Late stages of the developmental pathway are controlled entirely by EPO.

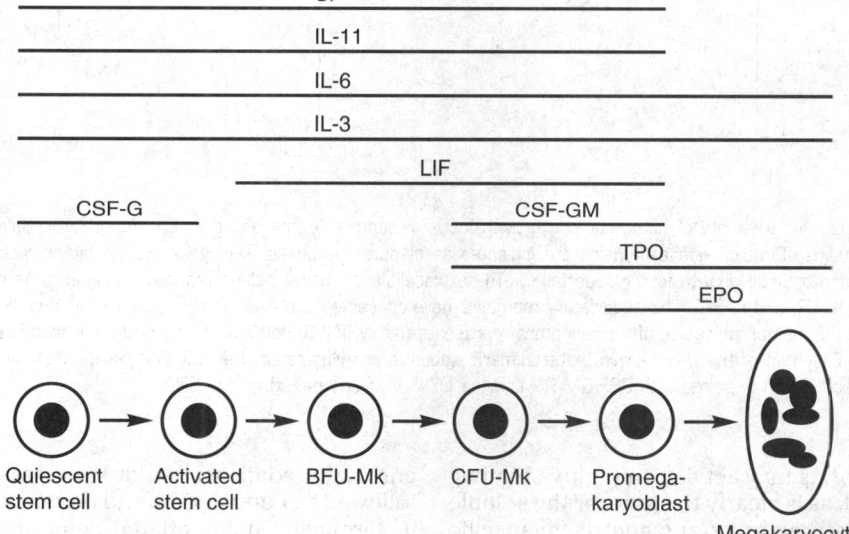

Fig. 16-18. Factors influencing megakaryocyte development. The lines beneath each growth factor encompass the range of differentiation stages responsive to that factor.

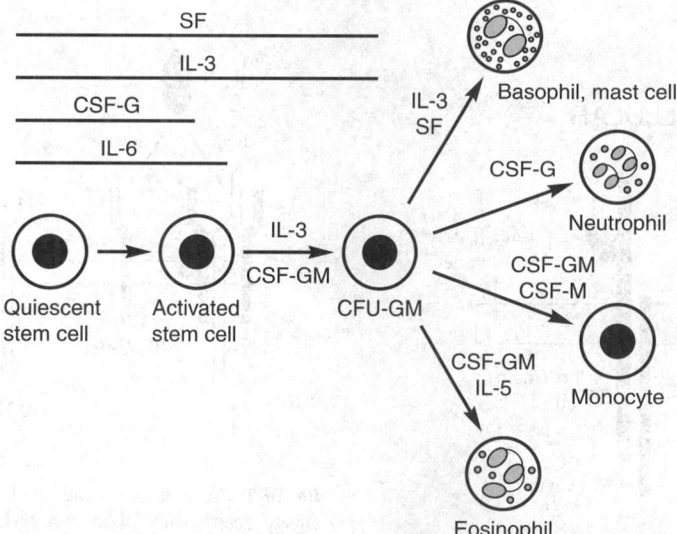

Fig. 16-19. Factors influencing granulopoiesis. The lines beneath each growth factor encompass the range of differentiation stages responsive to that factor. Those factors shown here to control the production of terminally differentiated cells are those that, on the strength of existing data, seem to be sufficient to induce production of cells in that lineage, (i.e., the factor listed requires no help from accessory cells).

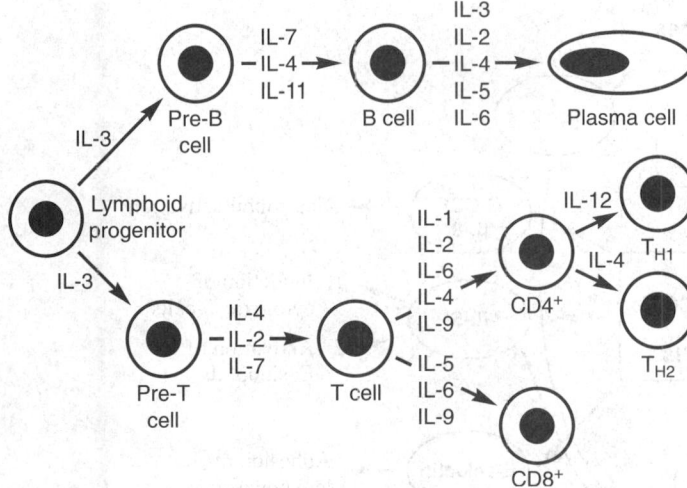

Fig. 16-20. Factors influencing lymphopoiesis. Some of the factors involved in regulating growth and differentiation of lymphoid cells are sufficient to induce growth or differentiation, or both. However, most of the factors act synergistically and some (e.g., IL-6 in B-cell differentiation) cannot induce the change without "help" from other factors (e.g., IL-2).

has been most clearly documented in factor-dependent cell lines[554–556] and in terminally differentiated phagocytes, including neutrophils (CSF-GM prolongs survival) and eosinophils (IL-5 prolongs survival).[557,558] That the results of studies on these cell types were reflective of activities of growth factor receptors in human progenitor cells was clearly demonstrated by Krantz's group, who found that EPO greatly reduced the amount of DNA fragmentation in CFU-E. They also reported that SF and insulin-like growth factor type 1 also inhibited apoptosis to some degree in this same cell population, clarifying a role

for these factors in erythropoiesis. SF can suppress programmed cell death in primordial germ cells as well.[559]

RULE 9. STRUCTURAL ABNORMALITIES OF HEMATOPOIETIC GROWTH FACTORS OR THEIR RECEPTORS MAY RESULT IN ABNORMALITIES OF HEMATOPOIESIS

Certain elements of the hierarchic network of hematopoietic growth factors and ILs can fail. When cells produce their own growth factor, they are said to exhibit autocrine growth. While there exist some autocrine functions in normal cells,[496,499,501,516,560] they rarely affect cell growth directly. For the most part, cells that produce their own growth factors are transformed or neoplastic. An increasing number of neoplastic cells or cell lines, either of the wild type or molecularly engineered, have been found to depend on autocrine growth factors, including IL-1,[496,560–569] IL-2,[36,570] IL-3,[571–575] IL-4,[428] IL-6,[574,576] IL-11,[131] CSF-GM,[573,574,577–580] CSF-M,[581,582] and EPO.[8]

Hematopoietic growth factor receptors also participate in autostimulatory growth. For example, an elegant series of studies on the structure and function of the CSF-M receptor by Sherr and co-workers indicates that (1) the CSF-M receptor is the cellular proto-oncogene c-*fms*[523] located on chromosome 5 in humans[161,521]; and (2) when portions of the c-*fms* gene are transduced by a retrovirus (in which the c-*fms* homolog is known as v-*fms*), critical regulatory regions are excluded.[525,526,583] Thus, after infection by this virus, cells exhibit constitutive proliferative activity, not by autocrine release of a growth factor, but by autoactivation of the receptor for a growth factor.[525,526,584] These observations are in line with other work on receptors for other growth factors, including epidermal growth factor[585,586] and EPO.[587,588]

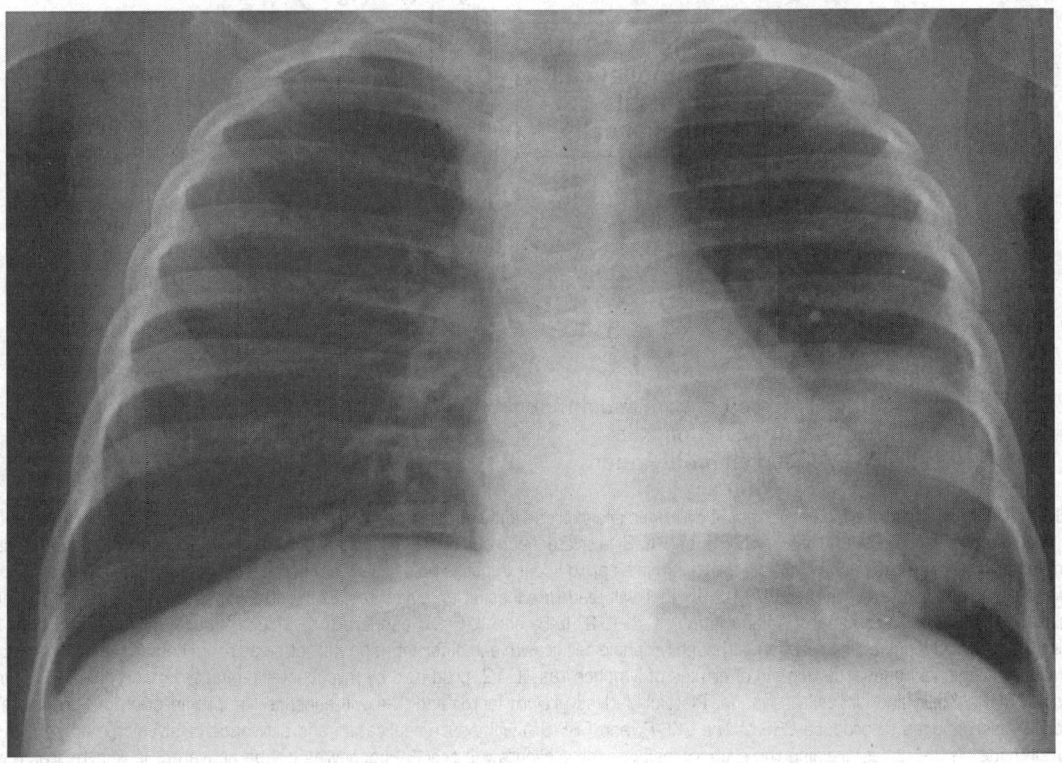

Fig. 16-21. Chest radiograph of a 2-year-old child with fever, failure to thrive, diarrhea, and leukocytosis, all of which were found to have resulted from primary pulmonary tuberculosis. Note the infiltrate in the left lung field, and both hilar and paratracheal adenopathy. Some of the important molecular events in the lung, lymph node, and bone marrow of this child are reviewed in Fig. 16-22.

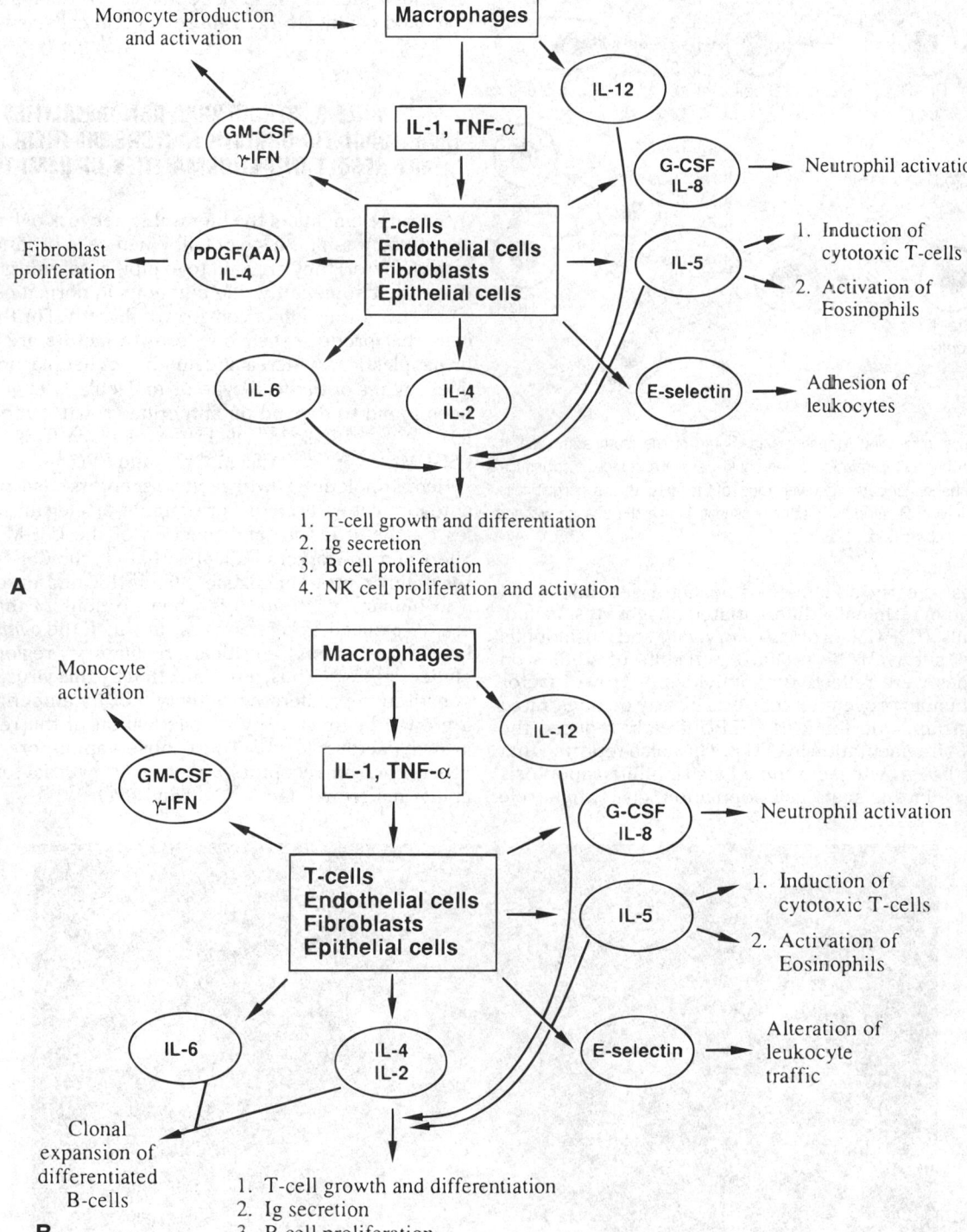

Fig. 16-22. (A) The lung. In the lung, a variety of cytokines are expressed by auxiliary cells, many produced by armed alveolar macrophages under the influence of IL-1 and TNF-α. CSF-G and IL-8 activate neutrophils. IL-5 induces cytotoxic T cells and may, under certain circumstances, activate eosinophils, although this is more apt to occur in parasitic or allergic disorders of the lung. Induction of E-selectin and intercellular adhesion molecule-1 (ICAM-1) by IL-1 will lead to adhesion of leukocytes to endothelium and likely enhance the egress of circulating cells into the region of inflammation. IL-4, IL-2, IL-6, and IL-5 will cooperate to induce T-cell expansion and both B-cell proliferation and immunoglobulin secretion, although lymphoid cell growth and differentiation will not be as prominent in the lung parenchyma as it will be in regional nodes, the domain of armies of lymphocytes. IL-12, produced by mycobacteria-infected macrophages, will induce production of T_H1 cells and NK cell activation. Platelet-derived growth factor and IL-4 will enhance the proliferation of fibroblasts, IL-4 will induce macrophages to produce CSF-M and CSF-G, and CSF-GM will induce replication and activation of alveolar macrophages. **(B)** The lymph node. In the nodes draining the primary lesion, similar events will occur. Phagocytes will be activated, leukocyte traffic will be altered by adhesion molecules, macrophages will be produced and activated, and processed antigen will be delivered to masses of competent lymphoid cells, which abound in this particular microenvironmental niche. The lymphoid cells will be armed and, through the release of IFN-γ, will rearm macrophages. An enormous measure of T-cell expansion and clonal expansion of differentiated B cells will follow. (*Figure continues.*)

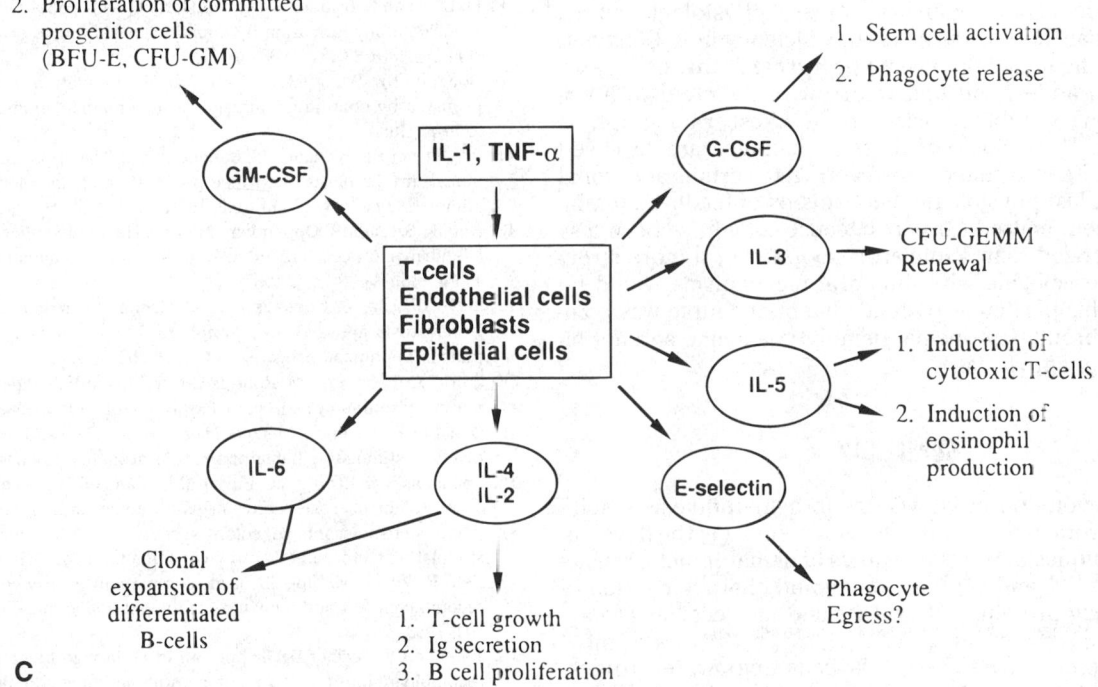

Fig. 16-22 (*Continued*). **(C)** The bone marrow. The marrow will also respond to the cytokine signals of TNF-α and IL-1. CSF-G induces stem cell activation, neutrophil production, and phagocyte release. IL-3 will induce renewal of CFU-GEMM. IL-5 will induce eosinophil production as well as cytotoxic T cells. Egress of phagocytes from the marrow may be effected by adhesion molecule expression. Although the intensity of lymphopoiesis is greater in the lymph node, some may occur in the marrow. Thus, IL-4, IL-1, and IL-6 will induce the production and differentiation of B cells, IL-4 will induce CSF-G and CSF-M gene expression in mononuclear phagocytes, and, finally, CSF-GM will activate phagocytes and induce proliferation of progenitors committed to granulopoiesis.

Regulation of Hematopoiesis

Humoral Factors Directly Involved in Production of Discrete Lineages

Erythropoiesis

As shown in Figure 16-17, the factors involved in effective production of red cells include IL-3, IL-9, IL-11, and CSF-GM, which induce proliferation of primitive erythroid progenitors. None of these factors, however, will induce erythroid proliferation in the absence of the lineage-specific factor EPO, which is the only humoral factor known to stimulate the growth of more committed erythroid progenitor cells and their progeny.

Megakaryocytopoiesis

CSF-GM and IL-3 can stimulate proliferation of megakaryocyte progenitors. IL-3, IL-6, IL-11, LIF, SF, and EPO have been reported to support terminal maturation of megakaryocytes as well. However, although TPO has not yet been fully characterized, it is probably the factor that, like EPO in the erythroid lineage, acts on more committed progenitors and megakaryocytes to augment megakaryocytopoiesis and platelet production in response to thrombocytopenia (Fig. 16-18).

Granulopoiesis

As shown in Fig. 16-19, the production of granulocytes involves a variety of different factors. Both CSF-GM and IL-3 induce proliferation of primitive progenitor cells. CSF-GM can, in fact, induce macrophage and eosinophil colony growth, although there is some disagreement on whether it can induce neutrophil differentiation in the absence of CSF-G.[179] It is

known, for example, that CSF-GM can induce IL-1 gene expression,[189,198] which in turn can induce expression of CSF-G[302,307,309–312] by a variety of cell types. No one has yet studied the possibility that the impact of CSF-GM on eosinophil colony growth might be an indirect effect by means of induction of IL-5 gene expression in auxiliary cells.

Eosinophil growth depends on CSF-GM and IL-5, the latter being the more cell-type-specific of the two, at least in granulopoiesis (Fig. 16-19). Incubation of human bone marrow cells in suspension culture with IL-5 induces production of a greater fraction of eosinophils.[235,237,238]

The production of basophils and mast cells is induced by IL-3 and SF, which seem to be sufficient in vitro to stimulate production and viability of this cell type (Fig. 16-19), although the relationship between these factors and IL-4 (which some investigators find can also induce mast cell production in vitro[423]) has not been clarified.

Lymphopoiesis

The growth and development of lymphoid cells occurs in multiple anatomic locations where different factors may influence these processes. Many of the hematopoietic growth factors and ILs have been shown to play a role in the growth and development of T lymphocytes[34,36,45,282,334,356,374,389,390,426–428, 560,570,589–592] and B lymphocytes.[47,49,221,230,233,280,281,336,360,361,432, 433,437,439,440,593–598] These factors are reviewed in Fig. 16-20.

Coordination of the Inflammatory Response

Even when selected lineages are conceptually or experimentally isolated, as in Figs. 16-17 through 16-20, complexities are apparent. In real life, the lineages act at the same time and interact with each other to accomplish complicated tasks. Accordingly, the complexities of the inflammatory response are enormous. Although the known cytokines are only now beginning to fill in some of the gaps of a colossal physiologic puzzle, we can see that there is tremendous efficiency in it. Consider, for example, the molecular events occurring in the lung, mediastinal lymph nodes, and bone marrow of the child with primary pulmonary tuberculosis whose chest radiograph is shown in Fig. 16-21. Some of these phenomena are reviewed in Fig. 16-22. Keep in mind, however, that certain additional complexities, like physiologic mechanisms of feedback inhibition, have been omitted (in part because they have been less well characterized than stimulatory loops). For a more strenuous exercise, imagine what humoral mechanisms would be operative if this particular patient's hospital course was complicated by thrombocytopenia, hemolytic anemia, and antibiotic-induced anaphylaxis.

SUMMARY

The brisk evolution of knowledge in hematopoiesis results in large part from two scientific developments: (1) the development of techniques permitting studies of hematopoietic regulation in vitro,[599,600] and (2) the cloning and characterization of genes encoding proteins with direct and indirect hematopoietic activities.[157,159,220,221,223,245,246,424,430,502,601-608] As a result of these developments, we know that cells empowered to produce these factors do so in response to early inductive stimuli and that these inductive signals are quite predictable. Some are even simple; hypoxia induces EPO gene expression, but inflammatory stimuli do not. Clearly, most responses to environmental stresses are more complex, including those induced by microbial assault. These are met by a multipronged inflammatory response by hematopoietic cells under the influence of a complex network of hematopoietic growth factors and interleukins. Despite its complexity, cause-and-effect relationships (e.g., factor X induces expression of factor Y) are clearly testable using molecular methods. As a result, the network model is orderly and hierarchic. In it, an initial environmental signal induces the expression of a limited number of primary genes, the products of which function largely to "recruit" the expression of a larger number of subordinate genes, which subsequently both amplify the original signal and induce lineage-specific responses. Taking into account the degree to which certain cytokines like IL-1 have been conserved throughout evolution, this hematopoietic control network is a molecular paradigm of biologic efficiency with profound implications for clinicians, developmental biologists, cell biologists, and molecular biologists alike.

REFERENCES

1. Goldberg MA, Glass GA, Cunningham JM, Bunn HF: The regulated expression of erythropoietin by two human hepatoma cell lines. Proc Natl Acad Sci USA 84:7972, 1987
2. Eckardt K-U, Boutellier U, Kurtz A et al: Rate of erythropoietin formation in humans in response to acute hypobaric hypoxia. J Appl Physiol 66:1785, 1989
3. Stohlman F Jr, Rath CE, Rose JC: Evidence for a humoral regulation of erythropoiesis: studies on a patient with polycythemia secondary to regional hypoxia. Blood 9:721, 1954
4. Erslev AJ: Humoral regulation of red cell production. Blood 8:349, 1953
5. Goldberg MA, Dunning SP, Bunn HF: Regulation of the erythropoietin gene: evidence that the oxygen sensor is a heme protein. Science 242:1412, 1988
6. Nijhof W, Wierenga PK, Sahr K et al: Induction of globin mRNA transcription by erythropoietin in differentiating erythroid precursor cells. Exp Hematol 15:779, 1987
7. Shouval D, Anton M, Galun E, Sherwood JB: Erythropoietin-induced polycythemia in athymic mice following transplantation of a human renal carcinoma cell line. Cancer Res 48:3430, 1988
8. Semenza GL, Traystman MD, Gearhart JD, Antonarakis SE: Polycythemia in transgenic mice expressing the human erythropoietin gene. Proc Natl Acad Sci USA 86:2301, 1989
9. Lu L, Bruno E, Briddell RA et al: Effects of hematopoietic growth factors on in vitro colony formation by human megakaryocyte progenitor cells. Behring Inst Mitt 83:181, 1988
10. Donahue RE, Wang EA, Stone DK et al: Stimulation of haematopoiesis in primates by continuous infusion of recombinant human GM-CSF. Nature 321:872, 1986
11. Broxmeyer HE, Williams DE, Hangoc G et al: The opposing actions in vivo on murine myelopoiesis of purified preparations of lactoferrin and the colony stimulating factors. Blood Cells 13:31, 1987
12. Neta R, Sztein MB, Oppenheim JJ et al: The in vivo effects of interleukin 1. I. Bone marrow cells are induced to cycle after administration of interleukin 1. J Immunol 139:1861, 1987
13. Mayer P, Lam C, Obenaus H et al: Recombinant human GM-CSF induces leukocytosis and activates peripheral blood polymorphonuclear neutrophils in nonhuman primates. Blood 70:206, 1987
14. Stork LC, Peterson VM, Rundus CH, Robinson WA: Interleukin-1 enhances murine granulopoiesis in vivo. Exp Hematol 16:163, 1988
15. Donahue RE, Seehra J, Metzger M et al: Human IL-3 and GM-CSF act synergistically in stimulating hematopoiesis in primates. Science 241:1820, 1988
16. Kaushansky K, Broudy VC, Harlan JM, Adamson JW: Tumor necrosis factor-α and tumor necrosis factor-β (lymphotoxin) stimulate the production of granulocyte-macrophage colony-stimulating factor, macrophage colony-stimulating factor, and IL-1 in vivo. J Immunol 141:3410, 1988
17. Neta R, Vogel SN, Sipe JD et al: Comparison of in vivo effects of human recombinant IL 1 and human recombinant IL 6 in mice. Lymphokine Res 7: 403, 1988
18. Johnson CS, Keckler DJ, Topper MI et al: In vivo hematopoietic effects of recombinant interleukin-1α in mice: stimulation of granulocytic, monocytic, megakaryocytic, and early erythroid progenitors, suppression of late-stage erythropoiesis, and reversal of erythroid suppression with erythropoietin. Blood 73:678, 1989
19. Suzuki C, Okano A, Takatsuki F et al: Continuous perfusion with interleukin 6 (IL-6) enhances production of hematopoietic stem cells (CFU-S). Biochem Biophys Res Commun 159:933, 1989
20. Lord BI, Molineux G, Pojda Z et al: Myeloid cell kinetics in mice treated with recombinant interleukin-3, granulocyte colony-stimulating factor (CSF), or granulocyte-macrophage CSF in vivo. Blood 77:2154, 1991
21. Molineux G, Migdalska A, Szmitkowski M et al: The effects of hematopoiesis of recombinant stem cell factor (ligand for c-kit) administered in vivo to mice either alone or in combination with granulocyte colony-stimulating factor. Blood 78:961, 1991
22. Uchida T, Yamagiwa A: Kinetics of rG-CSF-induced neutrophilia in mice. Exp Hematol 20:152, 1992
23. Schwartz GN, Patchen ML, Neta R, MacVittie TJ: Radioprotection of mice with interleukin-1: relationship to the number of erythroid and granulocyte-macrophage colony-forming cells. Radiat Res 121:220, 1990
24. Morstyn G, Campbell LM, Keech J et al: Effect of granulocyte colony stimulating factor on neutropenia induced by cytotoxic chemotherapy. Lancet 1: 667, 1988
25. Brandt SJ, Peters WP, Atwater SK et al: Effect of recombinant human granulocyte-macrophage colony-stimulating factor on hematopoietic reconstitution after high-dose chemotherapy and autologous bone marrow transplantation. N Engl J Med 318:869, 1988
26. Gabrilove JL, Jakubowski A, Scher H et al: Effect of granulocyte colony-stimulating factor on neutropenia and associated morbidity due to chemotherapy for transitional-cell carcinoma of the urothelium. N Engl J Med 318: 1414, 1988
27. Kodo H, Tajika K, Takahashi S et al: Acceleration of neutrophilic granulocyte recovery after bone-marrow transplantation by administration of recombinant human granulocyte colony-stimulating factor. Lancet 2:38, 1988
28. Vadhan-Raj S, Buescher S, Broxmeyer HE et al: Stimulation of myelopoiesis in patients with aplastic anaemia by recombinant human granulocyte-macrophage colony-stimulating factor. N Engl J Med 319:1628, 1988
29. Duhrsen U, Villeval J-L, Boyd J et al: Effects of recombinant human granulocyte colony-stimulating factor on hematopoietic progenitor cells in cancer patients. Blood 72:2074, 1988
30. Yamasaki Y, Izumi Y, Sawada H, Fujita K: Probable in vivo induction of differentiation by recombinant human granulocyte colony stimulating factor (rhG-CSF) in acute promyelocytic leukaemia (APL). Br J Haematol 78: 579, 1991
31. Armitage JO: The use of granulocyte-macrophage colony-stimulating factor in bone marrow transplantation. Semin Hematol, suppl. 29. 3:14, 1992

32. Freund MRF, Luft S, Schöber C et al: Differential effect of GM-CSF and G-CSF in cyclic neutropenia. Lancet 336:313, 1990

33. Ganser A, Lindemann A, Seipelt G et al: Effects of recombinant human interleukin-3 in patients with normal hematopoiesis and in patients with bone marrow failure. Blood 76:666, 1990

34. Seigel LJ, Harper ME, Wong-Staal F et al: Gene for T-cell growth factor: location on human chromosome 4q and feline chromosome B1. Science 223:175, 1984

35. Bickel M, Tsuda H, Amstad P et al: Differential regulation of colony-stimulating factors and interleukin 2 production by cyclosporin A. Proc Natl Acad Sci USA 84:3274, 1987

36. Arima N, Daitoku Y, Ohgaki S et al: Autocrine growth of interleukin 2-producing leukemic cells in a patient with adult T cell leukemia. Blood 68:779, 1986

37. Gromo G, Geller RL, Inverardi L, Bach FH: Signal requirements in the stepwise functional maturation of cytotoxic T-lymphocytes. Nature 327:424, 1987

38. Ayanlar-Batuman O, Shevitz J, Traub UC et al: Lymphocyte interleukin 2 production and responsiveness are altered in patients with primary myelodysplastic syndrome. Blood 70:494, 1987

39. Schrader JW, Ziltener HJ, Leslie KB: Structural homologies among the hemopoietins. Proc Natl Acad Sci USA 83:2458, 1986

40. Kronke M, Leonard WJ, Depper JM et al: Cyclosporin A inhibits T-cell growth factor gene expression at the level of mRNA transcription. Proc Natl Acad Sci USA 81:5214, 1984

41. Efrat S, Kaempfer R: Control of biologically active interleukin 2 messenger RNA formation in induced human lymphocytes. Proc Natl Acad Sci USA 81:2601, 1984

42. Smith KA: Interleukin-2: inception, impact, and implications. Science 240:1169, 1988

43. Lindsten T, June CH, Ledbetter JA et al: Regulation of lymphokine messenger RNA stability by a surface-mediated T-cell activation pathway. Science 244:339, 1989

44. Taniguchi T, Minami Y: The IL-2/IL-2 receptor system: a current overview. Cell 73:5, 1993

45. Crabtree GR: Contingent genetic regulatory events in T lymphocyte activation. Science 243:355, 1989

46. Farrar WL, Cleveland JL, Beckner SK et al: Biochemical and molecular events associated with interleukin 2 regulation of lymphocyte proliferation. Immunol Rev 92:49, 1986

47. Purkerson JM, Newberg M, Wise G et al: Interleukin 5 and interleukin 2 cooperate with interleukin 4 to induce IgG1 secretion from anti-Ig-treated B cells. J Exp Med 168:1175, 1988

48. Fotedar R, Diener E: The role of recombinant IL-2 and IL-1 in murine B cell differentiation. Lymphokine Res 7:393, 1988

49. Matsui K, Nakanishi K, Cohen DI et al: B cell response pathways regulated by IL-5 and IL-2. Secretory μH chain-mRNA and J chain mRNA expression are separately controlled events. J Immunol 142:2918, 1989

50. Ben Aribia MH, Leroy E, Lantz O et al: rIL-2-induced proliferation of human circulating NK cells and T lymphocytes: synergistic effects of IL-1 and IL-2. J Immunol 139:443, 1987

51. Anegon I, Cuturi MC, Trinchieri G, Perussia B: Interaction of Fc receptor (CD16) ligands induces transcription of interleukin 2 receptor (CD25) and lymphokine genes and expression of their products in human natural killer cells. J Exp Med 167:452, 1988

52. Foon KA: Biological response modifiers: the new immunotherapy. Cancer Res 49:1621, 1989

53. Oliver RT: The clinical potential of interleukin-2. Br J Cancer 58:405, 1988

54. Hadden JW: Recent advances in the preclinical and clinical immunopharmacology of interleukin-2: emphasis on IL-2 as an immunorestorative agent. Cancer Detect Prev 12:537, 1988

55. Ciolli V, Gabriele L, Sestili P et al: Combined interleukin 1/interleukin 2 therapy of mice injected with highly metastatic Friend leukemia cells: host antitumor mechanisms and marked effects on established metastases. J Exp Med 173:313, 1991

56. Smith KA: The interleukin 2 receptor. Adv Immunol 42:165, 1989

57. Greene WC: The human interleukin-2 receptor: a molecular and biochemical analysis of structure and function. Clin Res 35:439, 1989

58. Voss SD, Seondel PM, Robb RJ: Characterization of the interleukin 2 receptors (IL-2R) expressed on human natural killer cells activated in vivo by IL-2: association of the p64 IL-2R τ chain with the IL-2Rβ chain in functional intermediate-affinity IL-2R. J Exp Med 176:531, 1992

59. Noguchi M, Yi H, Rosenblatt HM et al: Interleukin-2 receptor gamma chain mutation results in X-linked severe combined immunodeficiency in humans. Cell 73:147, 1993

60. Gough NM, Hilton DJ, Gearing DP et al: Biochemical characterization of murine leukaemia inhibitory factor produced by Krebs ascites and by yeast cells. Blood Cells 14:431, 1988

61. Metcalf D, Hilton DJ, Nicola NA: Clonal analysis of the actions of the murine leukemia inhibitory factor on leukemic and normal murine hemopoietic cells. Leukemia 2:216, 1988

62. Hilton DJ, Nicola NA, Metcalf D: Purification of a murine leukemia inhibitory factor from Krebs ascites cells. Anal Biochem 173:359, 1988

63. Gough NM, Gearing DP, King JA et al: Molecular cloning and expression of the human homologue of the murine gene encoding myeloid leukemia-inhibitory factor. Proc Natl Acad Sci USA 85:2623, 1988

64. Sutherland GR, Baker E, Hyland VJ et al: The gene for human leukemia inhibitory factor (LIF) maps to 22q12. Leukemia 3:9, 1989

65. Wetzler M, Talpaz M, Lowe DG et al: Constitutive expression of leukemia inhibitory factor RNA by human bone marrow stromal cells and modulation by IL-1, TNF-α, and TGF-β. Exp Hematol 19:347, 1991

66. Derigs HG, Boswell HS: LIF mRNA expression is transcriptionally regulated in murine bone marrow stromal cells. Leukemia 7:630, 1993

67. Grolleau D, Soulillou J-P, Anegon I: Control of HILDA/LIF gene expression in activated human monocytes. Ann NY Acad Sci 628:19, 1991

68. Murray R, Lee F, Chiu C-P: The genes for leukemia inhibitory factor and interleukin-6 are expressed in mouse blastocysts prior to the onset of hemopoiesis. Mol Cell Biol 10:4953, 1990

69. Maekawa T, Metcalf D: Clonal suppression of HL60 and U937 cells by recombinant human leukemia inhibitory factor in combination with GM-CSF or G-CSF. Leukemia 3:270, 1989

70. Brach MA, Riedel D, Mertelsmann RH, Herrmann F: Synergistic effect of recombinant human leukemia inhibitory factor (LIF) and 1-β-D arabinofuranosylcytosine (Ara-C) on proto-oncogene expression and induction of differentiation in human U 937 cells. Leukemia 4:646, 1990

71. Fletcher FA, Moore KA, Williams DE et al: Effects of leukemia inhibitory factor (LIF) on gene transfer efficiency into murine hematolymphoid progenitors. Adv Exp Med Biol 292:131, 1991

72. Metcalf D, Nicola NA, Gearing DP: Effects of injected leukemia inhibitory factor on hematopoietic and other tissues in mice. Blood 76:50, 1990

73. Williams DA, Lemischka IR, Nathan DG, Mulligan RC: Introduction of new genetic material into pluripotent haematopoietic stem cells of the mouse. Nature 310:476, 1984

74. Smith AG, Heath JK, Donaldson DD et al: Inhibition of pluripotential embryonic stem cell differentiation by purified polypeptides. Nature 336:688, 1988

75. Gearing DP, Comeau MR, Friend DJ et al: The IL-6 signal transducer, gp130: an oncostatin M receptor and affinity converter for the LIF receptor. Science 255:1434, 1992

76. Oppenheim JJ, Zachariae COC, Mukaida N, Matsushima K: Properties of the novel proinflammatory supergene "intercrine" cytokine family. Annu Rev Immunol 9:617, 1991

77. Baggiolini M, Clark-Lewis I: Interleukin-8, a chemotactic and inflammatory cytokine. FEBS Lett 307:97, 1992

78. Modi WS, Dean M, Seuanez HN et al: Monocyte-derived neutrophil chemotactic factor (MDNCF/IL-8) resides in a gene cluster along with several other members of the platelet factor 4 gene superfamily. Hum Genet 84:185, 1990

79. Yoshimura T, Robinson EA, Appella E et al: Three forms of monocyte-derived neutrophil chemotactic factor (MDNCF) distinguished by different lengths of the amino-terminal sequence. Mol Immunol 84:87, 1989

80. Schroder J-M, Sticherling M, Hennicke HH et al: IL-1 alpha or tumor necrosis factor alpha stimulate release of three NAP-1/IL-8-related neutrophil chemotactic proteins in human dermal fibroblasts. J Immunol 144:2223, 1990

81. Matsushima K, Morishita K, Yoshimura T et al: Molecular cloning of a human monocyte-derived neutrophil chemotactic factor (MDNCF) and the induction of MDNCF mRNA by interleukin 1 and tumor necrosis factor. J Exp Med 167:1883, 1988

82. Larsen CG, Anderson AO, Oppenheim JJ, Matsushima K: Production of interleukin-8 by human dermal fibroblasts and keratinocytes in response to interleukin-1 or tumour necrosis factor. Immunology 68:31, 1989

83. Sica A, Matsushima K, Van Damme J et al: IL-1 transcriptionally activates the neutrophil chemotactic factor/IL-8 gene in endothelial cells. Immunology 69:548, 1990

84. Strieter RM, Phan SH, Showell HJ et al: Monokine-induced neutrophil chemotactic factor gene expression in human fibroblasts. J Biol Chem 264:10621, 1989

85. Holmes WE, Lee J, Kuang W-J et al: Structure and functional expression of a human interleukin-8 receptor. Science 253:1278, 1991

86. Murphy PM, Tiffany HL: Cloning of complementary DNA encoding functional human interleukin-8 receptor. Science 253:1280, 1991

87. Yoshimura TK, Matsushima K, Tanaka S et al: Purification of a human monocyte-derived neutrophil chemotactic factor that shares sequence homology with other host defense cytokines. Proc Natl Acad Sci USA 84:9233, 1987

88. Baggiolini M, Walz A, Kunkel SL: Neutrophil-activating peptide-1/interleukin-8, a novel cytokine that activates neutrophils. J Clin Invest 84:1045, 1989

89. Thelen M, Peveri P, Kernen P et al: Mechanism of neutrophil activation by NAF, a novel monocyte-derived peptide agonist. FASEB J 2:2702, 1988

90. Peveri P, Walz A, Dewald B, Baggiolini M: A novel neutrophil activating factor produced by human mononuclear phagocytes. J Exp Med 167:1547, 1988

91. Djeu JY, Matsushima K, Oppenheim JJ et al: Functional activation of human neutrophils by recombinant monocyte-derived neutrophil chemotactic factor/IL-8. J Immunol 144:2205, 1990

92. Schroder J-M, Mrowietz U, Morita E, Christophers E: Purification and partial biochemical characterization of a human monocyte-derived neutrophil-activating peptide that lacks interleukin 1 activity. J Immunol 139:3474, 1987

93. Moser B, Schumacher C, von Tscharner V et al: Neutrophil-activating peptide 2 and GRO/melanoma growth-stimulatory activity interact with neutrophil-activating peptide-1/interleukin-8 receptors on human neutrophils. J Biol Chem 266:10666, 1991

94. Walz A, Burgener R, Car B et al: Structure and neutrophil-activating properties of a novel inflammatory peptide (ENA-78) with homology to interleukin 8. J Exp Med 174:1355, 1991

95. Larsen CG, Anderson AO, Appella E et al: Neutrophil activating peptide (NAP-1) is also chemotactic for T lymphocytes. Science 243:1464, 1989

96. Leonard EJ, Skeel A, Yoshimura T et al: Leukocyte specificity and binding of human neutrophil attractant/activating protein 1. J Immunol 144:1323, 1990

97. Koch AE, Polverini PJ, Kunkel SL et al: Interleukin-8 as a macrophage-derived mediator of angiogenesis. Science 258:1798, 1992

98. Seitz M, Dewald B, Gerber N, Baggiolini M: Enhanced production of neutrophil-activating peptide-1/interleukin-8 in rheumatoid arthritis. J Clin Invest 87:463, 1991

99. Peichl P, Ceska M, Broell H et al: Human neutrophil activating peptide/interleukin-8 acts as an autoantigen in rheumatoid arthritis. Ann Rheum Dis 51:19, 1992

100. Schroder J-M, Christophers E: Identification of C5a-des-arg and an anionic neutrophil-activating peptide (ANAP) in psoriatic scales. J Invest Dermatol 87:53, 1986

101. Yang Y-C: Human interleukin-9: a new cytokine in hematopoiesis. Leuk Lymphoma 8:441, 1992

102. Renaud J-C, Houssiau F, Druez C et al: Interleukin-9. Int Rev Exp Pathol 34:99, 1993

103. Uyttenhove C, Simpson RJ, Van Snick J: Functional and structural characterization of P40, a mouse glycoprotein with T-cell growth factor activity. Proc Natl Acad Sci USA 85:6934, 1988

104. Van Snick J, Goethals A, Renauld J-C et al: Cloning and characterization of a cDNA for a new mouse T cell growth factor (P40). J Exp Med 169:363, 1989

105. Yang Y-C, Ricciardi S, Ciarletta A et al: Expression cloning of a cDNA encoding a novel human hematopoietic growth factor: human homologue of murine T-cell growth factor P40. Blood 74:1880, 1989

106. Mock BA, Krall M, Kozak CA et al: *IL9* maps to mouse chromosome 13 and human chromosome 5. Immunogenetics 31:265, 1990

107. Kelleher K, Bean K, Clark SC et al: Human interleukin-9: genomic sequence, chromosomal location, and sequences essential for its expression in human T-cell leukemia virus (HTLV)-I-transformed human T cells. Blood 77:1436, 1991

108. Renauld J-C, Goethals A, Houssiau F et al: Human P40/IL-9: expression in activated CD4⁺ T cells, genomic organization, and comparison with the mouse gene. J Immunol 144:4235, 1990

109. Renauld J-C, Druez C, Kermouni A et al: Expression cloning of the murine and human interleukin 9 receptor cDNAs. Proc Natl Acad Sci USA 89:5690, 1992

110. Donahue RE, Yang Y-C, Clark SC: Human P40 T-cell growth factor (interleukin-9) supports erythroid colony formation. Blood 75:2271, 1990

111. Holbrook ST, Ohls RK, Schibler KR et al: Effect of interleukin-9 on clonogenic maturation and cell-cycle status of fetal and adult hematopoietic progenitors. Blood 77:2129, 1991

112. Hultner L, Druez C, Moeller J et al: Mast cell growth-enhancing activity (MEA) is structurally related and functionally identical to the novel mouse T cell growth factor P40/TCGFIII (interleukin 9). Eur J Immunol 20:1413, 1990

113. Houssiau FA, Renauld J-C, Stevens M et al: Human T cell lines and clones respond to IL-9. J Immunol 150:2634, 1993

114. Merz H, Houssiau FA, Orscheschek K et al: Interleukin-9 expression in human malignant lymphomas: unique association with Hodgkin's disease and large cell anaplastic lymphoma. Blood 78:1311, 1991

115. Paul SR, Bennett F, Calvetti JA et al: Molecular cloning of a cDNA encoding interleukin 11, a stromal cell-derived lymphopoietic and hematopoietic cytokine. Proc Natl Acad Sci USA 87:7512, 1990

116. McKinley D, Wu Q, Yang-Feng T, Yang Y-C: Genomic sequence and chromosomal location of human interleukin-11 gene (IL11). Genomics 13:814, 1992

117. Kawashima L, Ohsumi L, Mita-Honjo K et al: Molecular cloning of cDNA encoding adipogenesis inhibitory factor and identity with interleukin-11. FEBS Lett 283:199, 1991

118. Suzow J, Friedman AD: The murine myeloperoxidase promoter contains several functional elements, one of which binds a cell type-restricted transcription factor, myeloid nuclear factor 1 (MyNF1). Mol Cell Biol 13:2141, 1993

119. Paul SR, Schendel P: The cloning and biological characterization of recombinant human interleukin 11. Int J Cell Cloning 10:135, 1992

120. Yin T, Schendel P, Yang Y-C: Enhancement of in vitro and in vivo antigen-specific antibody responses by interleukin 11. J Exp Med 175:211, 1992

121. Anderson KC, Morimoto C, Paul SR et al: Interleukin-11 promotes accessory cell-dependent B-cell differentiation in humans. Blood 80:2797, 1992

122. Musashi M, Yang Y-C, Paul SR et al: Direct and synergistic effects of interleukin 11 on murine hemopoiesis in culture. Proc Natl Acad Sci USA 88:765, 1992

123. Musashi M, Clark SC, Sudo T et al: Synergistic interactions between interleukin-11 and interleukin-4 in support of proliferation of primitive hematopoietic progenitors of mice. Blood 78:1448, 1991

124. Tsuji K, Lyman SD, Sudo T et al: Enhancement of murine hematopoiesis by synergistic interactions between Steel factor (ligand for c-kit), interleukin-11, and other early acting factors in culture. Blood 79:2855, 1992

125. Quesniaux VFJ, Clark SC, Turner K, Fagg B: Interleukin-11 stimulates multiple phases of erythropoiesis in vitro. Blood 80:1218, 1992

126. Bruno E, Briddell RA, Cooper RJ, Hoffman R: Effects of recombinant interleukin 11 on human megakaryocyte progenitor cells. Exp Hematol 19:378, 1991

127. Teramura M, Kobayashi S, Hoshino S et al: Interleukin-11 enhances human megakaryocytopoiesis in vitro. Blood 79:327, 1992

128. Neben TY, Loebelenz J, Hayes L et al: Recombinant human interleukin-11 stimulates megakaryocytopoiesis and increases peripheral platelets in normal and splenectomized mice. Blood 81:901, 1993

129. Hangoc G, Yin T, Cooper S et al: In vivo effects of recombinant interleukin-11 on myelopoiesis in mice. Blood 81:965, 1993

130. Du XX, Neben T, Goldman S, Williams DA: Effects of recombinant human interleukin-11 on hematopoietic reconstitution in transplant mice: acceleration of recovery of peripheral blood neutrophils and platelets. Blood 81:27, 1993

131. Kobayashi S, Teramura M, Sugawara I et al: Interleukin-11 acts as an autocrine growth factor for human megakaryoblastic cell lines. Blood 81:889, 1993

132. Bauman H, Schendel P: Interleukin-11 regulates the hepatic expression of the same plasma protein genes as interleukin-6. J Biol Chem 266:20424, 1993

133. Yin T, Miyazawa K, Yang Y-C: Characterization of interleukin-11 receptor and protein tyrosine phosphorylation induced by interleukin-11 in mouse 3T3-L1 cells. J Biol Chem 267:8347, 1992

134. Yin T, Taga T, Tsang ML-S et al: Interleukin (IL)-6 signal transducer, GP130, is involved in IL-11 mediated signal transduction, abstracted. Blood, suppl. 1. 80:151a, 1992

135. Ip NY, Nye SH, Boulton TG et al: CNTF and LIF act on neuronal cells via shared signaling pathways that involve the IL-6 signal transducing receptor component gp130. Cell 69:1121, 1992

136. Kobayashi M, Fitz L, Ryan M et al: Identification and purification of natural killer cell stimulatory factor (NKSF), a cytokine with multiple biologic effects on human lymphocytes. J Exp Med 170:827, 1989

137. Podlaski FJ, Nanduri VB, Hulmes JD et al: Molecular characterization of interleukin 12. Arch Biochem Biophys 294:230, 1992

138. Stern AS, Podlaski FJ, Hulmes JD et al: Purification to homogeneity and partial characterization of cytotoxic lymphocyte maturation factor from human B-lymphoblastoid cells. Proc Natl Acad Sci USA 87:6808, 1990

139. Wolf SF, Temple PA, Kobayashi M et al: Cloning of cDNA for natural killer cell stimulatory factor, a heterodimeric cytokine with multiple biologic effects on T and natural killer cells. J Immunol 146:3074, 1991

140. Gubler U, Chua AO, Schoenhaut DS et al: Coexpression of two distinct genes is required to generate secreted bioactive cytotoxic lymphocyte maturation factor. Proc Natl Acad Sci USA 88:4143, 1991

141. Gearing DP, Cosman D: Homology of the p40 subunit of natural killer cell stimulatory factor (NKSF) with the extracellular domain of the interleukin-6 receptor. Cell 66:9, 1991

142. Merberg DM, Wolf SF, Clark SC: Sequence similarity between NKSF and the IL-6/G-CSF family. Immunol Today 13:77, 1992

143. D'Andrea A, Regaraju M, Caliante N et al: Production of natural killer cell stimulatory factor (IL-12) by peripheral blood mononuclear cells. J Exp Med 176:1387, 1992

144. Gazzinelli RT, Hieny S, Wynn TA et al: Interleukin 12 is required for the T-

lymphocyte-independent induction of interferon gamma by an intracellular parasite and induces resistance in T-cell-deficient hosts (see comments). Proc Natl Acad Sci USA 90:6115, 1993

145. Hsieh C-S, Macatonia SE, Tripp CS et al: Development of T_H1 CD4+ T cells through IL-12 produced by *Listeria*-induced macrophages. Science 260:547, 1993

146. Chizzonite R, Truitt T, Desai BB et al: IL-12 receptor. I. Characterization of the receptor on phytohemagglutinin-activated human lymphoblasts. J Immunol 148:3117, 1992

147. Desai BB, Quinn PM, Wolitzky AG et al: IL-12 receptor. II. Distribution and regulation of receptor expression. J Immunol 148:3125, 1992

148. Swain S, Weinberg A, English M, Huston G: IL-4 directs the development of Th2-like helper effectors. J Immunol 145:3796, 1990

149. LeGros G, Ben-Sasson S, Seder R et al: Generation of interleukin 4 (IL-4)-producing cells in vivo and in vitro: IL-1 and IL-4 are required for in vitro generation of IL-4-producing cells. J Exp Med 172:921, 1990

150. Scott P: IL-12: Initiation cytokine for cell-mediated immunity. Science 260:496, 1993

151. Locksley RM: Interleukin 12 in host defense against microbial pathogens. Proc Natl Acad Sci USA 90:5879, 1993

152. Chan SH, Perussia B, Gupta JW et al: Induction of interferon gamma production by natural killer cell stimulatory factor: characterization of the responder cells and synergy with other inducers. J Exp Med 173:869, 1991

153. Naume B, Gately M, Espevik T: A comparative study of IL-12 (cytotoxic lymphocyte maturation factor)-, IL-2-, and IL-7-induced effects on immunomagnetically purified CD56+ NK cells. J Immunol 148:2429, 1992

154. Robertson MJ, Soiffer RJ, Wolf SF et al: Response of human natural killer (NK) cells to NK cell stimulatory factor (NKSF): cytolytic activity and proliferation of NK cells are differentially regulated by NKSF. J Exp Med 175:779, 1992

155. Chehimi J, Starr SE, Frank I et al: Natural killer (NK) cell stimulatory factor increases the cytotoxic activity of NK cells from both healthy donors and human immunodeficiency virus-infected patients. J Exp Med 175:789, 1992

156. Tripp CS, Wolf SF, Unanue ER: Interleukin 12 and tumor necrosis factor alpha are costimulators of interferon gamma production by natural killer cells in severe combined immunodeficiency mice with listeriosis, and interleukin 10 is a physiologic antagonist. Proc Natl Acad Sci USA 90:3725, 1993

157. Wong GG, Witek JAS, Temple PA et al: Human GM-CSF: molecular cloning of the complementary DNA and purification of the natural and recombinant proteins. Science 228:810, 1985

158. Kaushansky K, Shoemaker SG, Alfaro S, Brown C: Hematopoietic activity of granulocyte/macrophage colony-stimulating factor is dependent upon two distinct regions of the molecule: functional analysis based upon the activities of interspecies hybrid growth factors. Proc Natl Acad Sci USA 86:1213, 1989

159. Cantrell MA, Anderson D, Cerretti DP et al: Cloning, sequence, and expression of a human granulocyute/macrophage colony-stimulating factor. Proc Natl Acad Sci USA 82:6250, 1985

160. Yang Y-C, Kovacic S, Kriz R et al: The human genes for GM-CSF and IL 3 are closely linked in tandem on chromosome 5. Blood 71:958, 1988

161. Le Beau MM, Pettenati MJ, Lemons RS et al: Assignment of the GM-CSF, CSF-1, and FMS genes to human chromosome 5 provides evidence for linkage of a family of genes regulating hematopoiesis and for their involvement in the deletion (5q) in myeloid disorders. Cold Spring Harbor Symp Quant Biol LI:899, 1986

162. Van Leeuwen BH, Martinson ME, Webb GC, Young IG: Molecular organization of the cytokine gene cluster, involving the human IL-3, IL-4, IL-5, and GM-CSF genes, on human chromosome 5. Blood 73:1142, 1989

163. Vadhan-Raj S, Keating M, LeMaistre A et al: Effects of recombinant human granulocyte-macrophage colony-stimulating factor in patients with myelodysplastic syndromes. N Engl J Med 317:1545, 1987

164. Socinski MA, Cannistra SA, Elias A et al: Granulocyte-macrophage colony stimulating factor expands the circulting haemopoietic progenitor cell compartment in man. Lancet 1:1194, 1988

165. Migliaccio G, Migliaccio AR, Adamson JW: In vitro differentiation of human granulocyte/macrophage and erythroid progenitors: comparative analysis of the influence of recombinant human erythropoietin, G-CSF, GM-CSF, and IL-3 in serum-supplemented and serum-deprived cultures. Blood 72:248, 1988

166. Kaushansky K, O'Hara PJ, Berkner K et al: Genomic cloning, characterization, and multilineage growth-promoting activity of human granulocyte-macrophage colony-stimulating factor. Proc Natl Acad Sci USA 83:3101, 1986

167. Cantrel MA, Anderson D, Cerretti DP et al: Cloning, sequence, and expression of a human granulocyte-macrophage colony-stimulating factor. Proc Natl Acad Sci USA 82:6250, 1985

168. Tomonaga M, Golde DW, Gasson JC: Biosynthetic (recombinant) human granulocyte-macrophage colony-stimulating factor: effect on normal bone marrow and leukemic cell lines. Blood 67:31, 1986

169. Sieff CA, Emerson SG, Donahue RE et al: Recombinant granulocyte-macrophage colony-stimulating factor: a multilineage hemopoietin. Science 230:1171, 1985

170. Clark SC, Kamen R: The human hematopoietic colony-stimulating factors. Science 236:1229, 1987

171. Koike K, Ogawa M, Ihle HN et al: Recombinant murine granulocyte-macrophage (GM) colony-stimulating factor supports formation of GM and multipotential blast cell colonies in culture: comparison with the effects of interleukin-3. J Cell Physiol 131:458, 1987

172. Strife A, Lambek C, Wisniewski D et al: Activities of four purified growth factors on highly enriched human hematopoietic progenitor cells. Blood 69:1508, 1987

173. Fleischmann J, Golde DW, Weisbart RH, Gasson JC: Granulocyte-macrophage colony stimulatory factor enhances phagocytosis of bacteria by human neutrophils. Blood 68:708, 1986

174. Segal GM, McCall E, Bagby GC: The erythroid burst promoting activity produced by interleukin-1 stimulated endothelial cells is granulocyte macrophage colony stimulating factor. Blood 72:1364, 1988

175. Morstyn G, Burgess AW: Hemopoietic growth factors: a review. Cancer Res 48:5624, 1988

176. Sonoda Y, Yang Y-C, Wong GG et al: Erythroid burst-promoting activity of purified recombinant human GM-CSF and interleukin-3: studies with anti-GM-CSF and anti-IL-3 sera and studies in serum-free cultures. Blood 72:1381, 1988

177. Bussolino F, Wang JM, Defilippi P et al: Granulocyte- and granulocyte-macrophage-colony stimulating factors induce human endothelial cells to migrate and proliferate. Nature 337:471, 1989

178. Metcalf D: The molecular control of cell division, differentiation commitment and maturation in haemopoietic cells. Nature 339:27, 1989

179. Ferrero D, Tarella C, Badoni R et al: Granulocyte-macrophage colony-stimulating factor requires interaction with accessory cells or granulocyte-colony stimulating factor for full stimulation of human myeloid progenitors. Blood 73:402, 1989

180. Bot FJ, Van Eijk L, Schipper P, Löwenberg B: Human granulocyte-macrophage colony-stimulating factor (GM-CSF) stimulates immature marrow precursors but no CFU-GM, CFU-G, or CFU-M. Exp Hematol 17:292, 1989

181. Gasson JC, Weissbart RH, Kaufman SE et al: Purified human granulocyte-macrophage colony-stimulating factor: direct action on neutrophils. Science 226:1339, 1984

182. Weisbart RH, Golde DW, Clark SC et al: Human granulocyte-macrophage colony-stimulating factor is a neutrophil activator. Nature 314:361, 1985

183. Gasson JC, Kaufman SE, Weisbart RH et al: High affinity binding of granulocyte-macrophage colony-stimulating factor to normal and leukemic human myeloid cells. Proc Natl Acad Sci USA 83:669, 1986

184. Lopez AF, Williamson DJ, Gamble JR et al: Recombinant human granulocyte-macrophage colony-stimulating factor stimulates in vitro mature human neutrophil and eosinophil function, surface receptor expression, and survival. J Clin Invest 78:1220, 1986

185. Arnaout MA, Wang EA, Clark SC, Sieff CA: Human recombinant granulocyte-macrophage colony-stimulating factor increases cell-to-cell adhesion and surface expression of adhesion-promoting surface glycoproteins on mature granulocytes. J Clin Invest 78:597, 1986

186. Weisbart RH, Golde DW, Gasson JC: Biosynthetic human GM-CSF modulates the number and affinity of neutrophil f-met-leu-phe receptors. J Immunol 137:3584, 1986

187. Vadas MA, Nicola NA, Metcalf D: Activation of antibody-dependent cell-mediated cytotoxicity of human neutrophils and eosinophils by separate colony-stimulating factors. J Immunol 130:795, 1983

188. Weisbart RH, Kwan L, Golde DW, Gasson JC: Human GM-CSF primes neutrophils for enhanced oxidative metabolism in response to major chemoattractants. Blood 69:18, 1987

189. Lindemann A, Riedel D, Oster W et al: Granulocyte/macrophage colony-stimulating factor induces interleukin 1 production by human polymorphonuclear neutrophils. J Immunol 140:837, 1988

190. Baldwin GC, Gasson JC, Quan SG et al: GM-CSF enhances neutrophil function in AIDS patients. Blood 70:130, 1987

191. Weisbart RH, Kacena A, Schuh A, Golde DW: GM-CSF induces human neutrophil IgA-mediated phagocytosis by an IgA Fc receptor activation mechanism. Nature 332:647, 1988

192. Sayers TJ, Wiltrout TA, Bull CA et al: Effect of cytokines on polymorphonuclear neutrophil infiltration in the mouse: prostaglandin- and leukotriene-independent induction of infiltration by IL-1 and tumor necrosis factor. J Immunol 141:1670, 1988

193. Socinski MA, Cannistra SA, Sullivan R et al: Granulocyte-macrophage colony-stimulating factor induces the expression of the CD11b surface adhesion molecule on human granulocytes in vivo. Blood 72:691, 1988

194. Atkinson YH, Lopez AF, Marasco WA et al: Recombinant human granulocyte-macrophage colony-stimulating factor (rH GM-CSF) regulates f Met-Leu-Phe receptors on human neutrophils. Immunology 64:519, 1988

195. Buescher ES, McIlheran SM, Vadhan-Raj S: Effects of in vivo administration of recombinant human granulocyte-macrophage colony-stimulating factor on human neutrophil chemotaxis and oxygen metabolism. J Infect Dis 158:1140, 1988

196. Nathan CF: Respiratory burst in adherent human neutrophils: Triggering by colony-stimulating factors CSF-GM and CSF-G. Blood 73:301, 1989

197. Kaplan SS, Basford RE, Wing EJ, Shadduck RK: The effect of recombinant human granulocyte macrophage colony-stimulating factor on neutrophil activation in patients with refractory carcinoma. Blood 73:636, 1989

198. Lindemann A, Riedel D, Oster W et al: Granulocyte-macrophage colony-stimulating factor induces cytokine secretion by human polymorphonuclear leukocytes. J Clin Invest 83:1308, 1989

199. Sullivan R, Fredette JP, Socinski M et al: Enhancement of superoxide anion release by granulocytes harvested from patients receiving granulocyte-macrophage colony-stimulating factor. Br J Haematol 71:475, 1989

200. Sullivan R, Griffith JD, Simons ER et al: Effects of recombinant human granulocyte and macrophage colony-stimulating fctors on signal transduction pathways in human granulocytes. J Immunol 139:3422, 1987

201. Kleinerman ES, Knowles RD, Lachman LB, Gutterman JU: Effect of recombinant granulocyte/macrophage colony-stimulating factor on human monocyte activity in vitro and following intravenous administration. Cancer Res 48:2604, 1988

202. Cannistra SA, Vellenga E, Groshek P et al: Human granulocyte-monocyte colony-stimulating factor and interleukin 3 stimulate monocyte cytotoxicity through a tumor necrosis factor-dependent mechanism. Blood 71:672, 1988

203. Wing EJ, Magee DM, Whiteside TL et al: Recombinant human granulocyte/macrophage colony-stimulating factor enhances monocyte cytotoxicity and secretion of tumor necrosis factor α and interferon in cancer patients. Blood 73:643, 1989

204. Morrissey PJ, Grabstein KH, Reed SG, Conlon PJ: Granulocyte/macrophage colony stimulating factor. A potent activation signal for mature macrophages and monocytes. Int Arch Allergy Appl Immunol 88:40, 1989

205. Owen WF, Rothenberg ME, Silberstein DS et al: Regulation of human eosinophil viability, density and function by granulocyte/macrophage colony-stimulating factor in the presence of 3T3 fibroblasts. J Exp Med 166:129, 1987

206. Park LS, Friend D, Gillis S, Urdal DL: Characterization of the cell surface receptor for granulocyte-macrophage colony-stimulating factor. J Biol Chem 261:4177, 1986

207. Simmers RN, Webber LM, Shannon MF et al: Localization of the G-CSF gene on chromosome 17 proximal to the breakpoint in the t(15;17) in acute promyelocytic leukemia. Blood 70:330, 1987

208. Ohara A, Suca T, Saito M et al: Effect of recombinant human granulocyte colony-stimulating factor on hemopoietic cells in serum-free culture. Exp Hematol 15:695, 1987

209. Sieff CA: Hematopoietic growth factors. J Clin Invest 79:1549, 1987

210. Metcalf D: The molecular biology and functions of the granulocyte-macrophage colony-stimulating factors. Blood 67:257, 1986

211. Suda T, Suda J, Kajigaya S et al: Effects of recombinant murine granulocyte colony-stimulating factor on granulocyte-macrophage and blast colony formation. Exp Hematol 15:958, 1987

212. Uzumaki H, Okabe T, Sasaki N et al: Characterization of receptor for granulocyte colony-stimulating factor on human circulating neutrophils. Biochem Biophys Res Commun 156:1026, 1988

213. Ralph P, Warren MK, Nakoinz I et al: Biological properties and molecular biology of the human macrophage growth factor, CSF-1. Immunobiology 172:194, 1986

214. Kawasaki ES, Ladner MB, Wang AM et al: Molecular cloning of a complementary DNA encoding macrophage-specific colony stimulating factor (CSF-1). Science 230:291, 1985

215. Williams DE, Hangoc G, Cooper S et al: The effects of purified recombinant murine interleukin-3 and/or purified natural murine CSF-1 in vivo on the proliferation of murine high and low-proliferative potential colony forming cells: demonstration of in vivo synergism. Blood 70:401, 1987

216. Broxmeyer HE, Williams DE, Cooper S et al: Recombinant human granulocyte-colony stimulating factor and recombinant human macrophage-colony stimulating factor synergize in vivo to enhance proliferation of granulocyte-macrophage, erythroid, and multipotential progenitor cells in mice. J Cell Biochem 38:127, 1988

217. Warren MK, Ralph P: Macrophage growth factor CSF-1 stimulates human monocyte production of interferon, tumor necrosis factor, and colony-stimulating activity. J Immunol 137:2281, 1986

218. Mufson RA, Aghajanian J, Wong G et al: Macrophage colony-stimulating factor enhances monocyte and macrophage antibody-dependent cell-mediated cytotoxicity. Cell Immunol 119:182, 1989

219. Cheers C, Hill M, Haigh AM, Stanley ER: Stimulation of macrophage phagocytic but not bactericidal activity by colony-stimulating factor 1. Infect Immun 57:1512, 1989

220. Campbell HD, Tucker WQJ, Hort Y et al: Molecular cloning, nucleotide sequence, and expression of the gene encoding human eosinophil differentiation factor (interleukin 5). Proc Natl Acad Sci USA 84:6629, 1987

221. Yokota T, Coffman RL, Hagiwara H et al: Isolation and characterization of lymphokine cDNA clones encoding mouse and human IgA-enhancing factor and eosinophil colony-stimulating factor activities: relationship to interleukin 5. Proc Natl Acad Sci USA 84:7388, 1987

222. Sutherland GR, Baker E, Callen DF et al: Interleukin-5 is at 5q31 and is deleted in the 5q- syndrome. Blood 71:1150, 1988

223. Campbell HD, Sanderson CJ, Wang Y et al: Isolation, structure and expression of cDNA and genomic clones for murine eosinophil differentiation factor. Comparison with other eosinophilopoietic lymphokines and identity with interleukin-5. Eur J Biochem 174:345, 1988

224. Swain SL, McKenzie DT, Weinberg AD, Hancock W: Characterization of T helper 1 and 2 cell subsets in normal mice. Helper T cells responsible for IL-4 and IL-5 production are present as precursors that require priming before they develop into lymphokine-secreting cells. J Immunol 141:3445, 1988

225. Jabara HH, Ackerman SJ, Vercelli D et al: Induction of interleukin-4-dependent IgE synthesis and interleukin-5-dependent eosinophil differentiation by supernatants of a human helper T-cell clone. J Clin Immunol 8:437, 1988

226. Tavernier J, Devos R, Cornelis S et al: A human high affinity interleukin-5 receptor (IL5R) is composed of an IL-5-specific α chain and a β chain shared with the receptor for GM-CSF. Cell 66:1175, 1991

227. Kitamura T, Sato N, Arai K, Miyajima A: Expression cloning of the human IL-3 receptor cDNA reveals a shared β subunit for the human IL-3 and GM-CSF receptors. Cell 66:1165, 1991

228. Takatsu K, Kikuchi Y, Takahashi T et al: Interleukin 5, a T-cell-derived B-cell differentiation factor also induces cytotoxic T lymphocytes. Proc Natl Acad Sci USA 84:4234, 1987

229. Yokota T, Arai N, De Vries J et al: Molecular biology of interleukin 4 and interleukin 5 genes and biology of their products that stimulate B cells, T cells and hemopoietic cells. Immunol Rev 102:137, 1988

230. Vercelli D, Geha RS: Regulation of IgE synthesis in humans. J Clin Immunol 9:75, 1989

231. Pène J, Rousset F, Brière F et al: Interleukin 5 enhances interleukin 4-induced IgE production by normal human B cells. The role of soluble CD23 antigen. Eur J Immunol 18:929, 1988

232. Matsumoto R, Matsumoto M, Mita S et al: Interleukin-5 induces maturation but not class switching of surface IgA-positive B cells into IgA-secreting cells. Immunology 66:32, 1989

233. Pène J, Chrétien I, Rousset F et al: Modulation of IL-4-induced human IgE production in vitro by IFN-gamma and IL-5: the role of soluble CD23 (s-CD23). J Cell Biochem 39:253, 1989

234. Alderson MR, Pike BL, Harada N et al: Recombinant T-cell replacing factor (interleukin 5) acts with antigen to promote the growth and differentiation of single hapten-specific B lymphocytes. J Immunol 139:2656, 1987

235. Clutterbuck EJ, Sanderson CJ: Human eosinophil hematopoiesis studied in vitro by means of murine eosinophil differentiation factor (IL5): production of functionally active eosinophils from normal human bone marrow. Blood 71:646, 1988

236. Sonoda Y, Arai N, Ogawa M: Humoral regulation of eosinophilopoiesis in vitro: analysis of the targets of interleukin-3, granulocyte/macrophage colony-stimulating factor (GM-CSF), and interleukin-5 Charleston. Leukemia 3:14, 1989

237. Yamaguchi Y, Suda T, Suda J et al: Purified interleukin 5 supports the terminal differentiation and proliferation of murine eosinophilic precursors. J Exp Med 167:43, 1988

238. Warren DJ, Moore MA: Synergism among interleukin 1, interleukin 3, and interleukin 5 in the production of eosinophils from primitive hemopoietic stem cells. J Immunol 140:94, 1988

239. Yamaguchi Y, Hayashi Y, Sugama Y et al: Highly purified murine interleukin 5 (IL-5) stimulates eosinophil function and prolongs in vitro survival. IL-5 as an eosinophil chemotactic factor. J Exp Med 167:1737, 1988

240. Rothenberg ME, Pomerantz JL, Owen WF et al: Characterization of a human eosinophil proteoglycan, and augmentation of its biosynthesis and size by interleukin 3, interleukin 5, and granulocyte/macrophage colony stimulating factor. J Biol Chem 263:13901, 1988

241. Sanderson CJ, Campbell HD, Young IG: Molecular and cellular biology of eosinophil differentiation factor (interleukin-5) and its effects on human and mouse B cells. Immunol Rev 102:29, 1988

242. Park LS, Friend D, Price V et al: Heterogeneity in human interleukin-3 receptors. A subclass that binds human granulocyte/macrophage colony stimulating factor. J Biol Chem 264:5420, 1989

243. Hedzat C, Baldwin GC, Golde DW et al: Biological activities of human G-CSF and characterization of the human G-CSF receptor. Blood 70:165, 1987

244. Roussel MF, Dull TJ, Rettenmier CW et al: Transforming potential of the c-fms proto-oncogene (CSF-1 receptor). Nature 325:549, 1987

245. Lin F-K, Suggs S, Lin C-H et al: Cloning and expression of the human erythropoietin gene. Proc Natl Acad Sci USA 82:7580, 1985

246. Browne JK, Cohen AM, Egrie JC et al: Erythropoietin: gene cloning, protein structure and biological properties. Cold Spring Harbor Symp Quant Biol 51:693, 1986

247. Jacobs K, Shoemaker C, Rurensdorf R et al: Isolation and characterization of genomic and cDNA clones of human erythropoietin. Nature 313:806, 1985

248. Powell JS, Berkner KL, Lebo RV, Adamson JW: Human erythropoietin gene: high level expression in stably transfected mammalian cells and chromosome localization. Proc Natl Acad Sci USA 83:6465, 1986

249. Fried W: The liver as a source of extrarenal erythropoietin. Blood 40:671, 1972

250. Zanjani ED, Ascensao JL, McGlave PB et al: Studies on the liver to kidney switch of erythropoietin production. J Clin Invest 67:1183, 1981

251. Jacobson LO, Goldwasser E, Fried W, Pizak L: Studies on erythropoiesis. VII. The role of the kidney in the production of erythropoietin. Trans Assoc Am Physicians 70:305, 1957

252. Kubanek B, Ferrari L, Tyler WS et al: Regulation of erythropoiesis. XXIII. Dissociation between stem cell and erythroid response to hypoxia. Blood 32:586, 1968

253. Stohlman F Jr: Some aspects of erythrokinetics. Semin Hematol 4:304, 1967

254. Stohlman F Jr, Ebbe S, Morse B et al: Regulation of erythropoiesis. XX. Kinetics of red cell production. Ann NY Acad Sci 149:156, 1968

255. McDonald TP, Cottrell MB, Clift RE et al: High doses of recombinant erythropoietin stimulate platelet production in mice. Exp Hematol 15:719, 1987

256. Ishibashi T, Koziol JA, Burstein SA: Human recombinant erythropoietin promotes differentiation of murine megakaryocytes in vitro. J Clin Invest 79:286, 1987

257. Dessypris EN, Gleaton JH, Armstrong OL: Effect of human recombinant erythropoietin on human marrow megakaryocyte colony formation in vitro. Br J Haematol 65:265, 1987

258. Clark DA, Dessypris EN: Effects of recombinant erythropoietin on murine megakaryocytic colony formation in vitro. J Lab Clin Med 108:423, 1986

259. Fraser JC, Tan AS, Lin FK, Berridge MV: Expression of specific high-affinity binding sites for erythropoietin on rat and mouse megakaryocytes. Exp Hematol 17:10, 1989

260. Bruno E, Miller ME, Hoffman R: Interacting cytokines regulate in vitro human megakaryocytopoiesis. Blood 73:671, 1989

261. Eschbach JW, Egrie JC, Downing MR et al: Correction of the anemia of end-stage renal disease with recombinant human erythropoietin. Results of a combined phase I and II clinical trial. N Engl J Med 316:73, 1987

262. Lim VS, DeGowin RL, Zavala D et al: Recombinant human erythropoietin treatment in pre-dialysis patients: a double-blind placebo-controlled trial. Ann Intern Med 110:108, 1989

263. Winearls CG, Oliver DO, Pippard MJ et al: Effect of human erythropoietin derived from recombinant DNA on the anaemia of patients maintained by chronic haemodialysis. Lancet 2:1175, 1986

264. Reissmann KR: Studies on the mechanism of erythropoietic stimulation in parabiotic rats during hypoxia. Blood 5:372, 1950

265. Broudy VC, Lin N, Egrie J et al: Identification of the receptor for erythropoietin on human and murine erythroleukemia cells and modulation by phorbol ester and dimethyl sulfoxide Seattle 98195. Proc Natl Acad Sci USA 85:6513, 1988

266. Tojo A, Fukamachi H, Saito T et al: Induction of the receptor for erythropoietin in murine erythroleukemia cells after dimethyl sulfoxide treatment, University of Tokyo, Japan. Cancer Res 48:1818, 1988

267. Tojo A, Fukamachi H, Kasuga M et al: Identification of erythropoietin receptors on fetal liver erythroid cells. Biochem Biophys Res Commun 148:443, 1988

268. Sawyer ST, Krantz SB, Luna J: Identification of the receptor for erythropoietin by cross-linking to Friend virus-infected erythroid cells. Proc Natl Acad Sci USA 84:3690, 1987

269. Sawada K, Krantz SB, Kans JS et al: Purification of human erythroid colony-forming units and demonstration of specific binding of erythropoietin J Clin Invest 80:357, 1987

270. Hitomi K, Fujita K, Sasaki R et al: Erythropoietin receptor of a human leukemic cell line with erythroid characteristics. Biochem Biophys Res Commun 154:902, 1988

271. Fraser JK, Lin FK, Berridge MV: Expression of high affinity receptors for erythropoietin on human bone marrow cells and on the human erythroleukemic cell line, HEL Medicine, New Zealand. Exp Hematol 16:836, 1988

272. D'Andrea AD, Lodish HFM, Wong GG: Expression cloning of the murine erythropoietin receptor. Cell 57:277, 1989

273. Winkelmann JC, Penny LA, Deaven LL et al: The gene for the human erythropoietin receptor: analysis of the coding sequence and assignment to chromosome 19p. Blood 76:24, 1990

274. Hamilton JA, Vairo G, Nicola NA et al: Activation and proliferation signals in murine macrophages: synergistic interactions between the hematopoietic growth factors and with phorbol ester for DNA synthesis. Blood 71:1574, 1988

275. Lu L, Walker D, Graham CD et al: Enhancement of release from MHC class II antigen-positive monocytes of hematopoietic colony stimulating factors CSF-1 and G-CSF by recombinant human tumor necrosis factor-alpha: synergism with recombinant human interferon-gamma. Blood 72:34, 1988

276. Sampson-Johannes A, Carlino JA: Enhancement of human monocyte tumoricidal activity by recombinant M-CSF. J Immunol 141:3680, 1988

277. Vairo G, Hamilton JA: Activation and proliferation signals in murine macrophages: stimulation of Na$^+$, K$^+$-ATPase activity by hemopoietic growth factors and other agents. J Cell Physiol 134:13, 1988

278. Broxmeyer HE, Juliano L, Waheed A, Shadduck RK: Release from mouse macrophages of acidic isoferritins that suppress hematopoietic progenitor cells is induced by purified L cell colony stimulating factor and suppressed by human lactoferrin. J Immunol 135:3224, 1985

279. Paul WE: Pleiotropy and redundancy: T cell-derived lymphokines in the immune response. Cell 57:521, 1989

280. Namen AE, Lupton S, Hjerrild K et al: Stimulation of B-cell progenitors by cloned murine interleukin-7. Nature 333:571, 1988

281. Goodwin RG, Lupton S, Schmierer A et al: Human interleukin 7: molecular cloning and growth factor activity on human and murine B-lineage cells. Proc Natl Acad Sci USA 86:302, 1989

282. Takeda S, Gillis S, Palacios R: *In vitro* effects of recombinant interleukin 7 on growth and differentiation of bone marrow pro-B- and pro-T-lymphocyte clones and fetal thymocyte clones. Proc Natl Acad Sci USA 86:1634, 1989

283. Digel W, Schmid M, Heil G et al: Human interleukin-7 induces proliferation of neoplastic cells from chronic lymphocytic leukemia and acute leukemias. Blood 78:753, 1991

284. Dalloul A, Laroche L, Bagot M et al: Interleukin-7 is a growth factor for Sézary lymphoma cells. J Clin Invest 90:1054, 1992

285. Dokter WHA, Sierdsema SJ, Esselink MT IL-7 enhances the expression of IL-3 and granulocyte-macrophage-CSF mRNA in activated human T cells by post-transcriptional mechanisms. J Immunol 150:2584, 1993

286. Alderson MR, Tough TW, Ziegler SF, Grabstein KH: Interleukin 7 induces cytokine secretion and tumoricidal activity by human peripheral blood monocytes. J Exp Med 173:923, 1991

287. Standiford TJ, Strieter RM, Allen RM et al: IL-7 up-regulates the expression of IL-8 from resting and stimulated human blood monocytes. J Immunol 149:2035, 1992

288. Levin J, Evatt BL: Humoral control of thrombopoiesis. Blood Cells 5:105, 1979

289. McDonald TP: Assays for thrombopoietin. Scand J Haematol 18:5, 1977

290. Evatt BL, Spivak JL, Levin J: Relationships between thrombopoiesis and erythropoiesis: with studies of the effects of preparations of thrombopoietin and erythropoietin. Blood 48:547, 1976

291. Tayrien G, Rosenberg RD: Purification and properties of a megakaryocyte stimulatory factor present both in the serum-free conditioned medium of human embryonic kidney cells and in thrombocytopenic plasma. J Biol Chem 262:3262, 1987

292. McDonald TP, Andrews RB, Clift R, Cottrell M: Characterization of a thrombocytopoietic-stimulating factor from kidney cell culture medium. Exp Hematol 9:288, 1981

293. Long MW, Williams N, McDonald TP: Immature megakaryocytes in the mouse: in vitro relationship to megakaryocyte progenitor cells and mature megakaryocytes. J Cell Physiol 112:339, 1982

294. Sieff CA, Niemeyer CM, Nathan DG et al: Stimulation of human hematopoietic colony formation by recombinant gibbon multi-colony-stimulating factor or interleukin 3. J Clin Invest 80:818, 1987

295. Lopez AF, To LB, Yang YC et al: Stimulation of proliferation, differentiation, and function of human cells by primate interleukin 3. Proc Natl Acad Sci USA 84:2761, 1987

296. Bot FJ, Dorssers L, Wagemaker G, Lowenberg B: Stimulating spectrum of human recombinant multi-CSF (IL-3) on human marrow precursors: importance of accessory cells. Blood 71:1609, 1988

297. Niemeyer CM, Sieff CA, Mathey-Prevot B et al: Expression of human interleukin-3 (multi-CSF) is restricted to human lymphocytes and T-cell tumor lines. Blood 73:945, 1989

298. Wodnar-Filipowicz A, Heusser CH, Moroni C: Production of the haemopoietic growth factors GM-CSF and interleukin-3 by mast cells in response to IgE receptor-mediated activation. Nature 339:150, 1989

299. Farrar WL, Vinovour M, Hill JM: In situ hybridization histochemistry localization of interleukin-3 mRNA in mouse brain. Blood 73:137, 1989

300. Rennick D, Yang G, Gemmell L, Lee F: Control of hemopoiesis by a bone marrow stromal cell clone: lipopolysaccharide- and interleukin-1-inducible production of colony-stimulating factors. Blood 69:682, 1987

301. Bagby GC, Dinarello CA, Wallace P et al: Interleukin-1 stimulates granulocyte macrophage colony stimulating activity release by vascular endothelial cells. J Clin Invest 78:1316, 1986

302. Broudy VC, Kaushansky K, Harlan JM, Adamson JW: Interleukin-1 stimulates human endothelial cells to produce granulocyte macrophage colony-stimulating factor and granulocyte colony-stimulating factor. J Immunol 139:464, 1987

303. Sieff CA, Tsai S, Faller DV: Interleukin 1 induces cultured human endothelial cell production of granulocyte-macrophage colony-stimulating factor. J Clin Invest 79:48, 1987

304. Bagby GC: Production of multilineage growth factors by hematopoietic stromal cells: an intercellular regulatory network involving mononuclear phagocytes and interleukin-1. Blood Cells 13:147, 1987

305. Zucali JR, Broxmeyer HE, Dinarello CA et al: Regulation of early human hematopoietic (BFU-E and CFU-GEMM) progenitor cells in vitro by interleukin 1-induced fibroblast conditioned medium. Blood 69:33, 1987

306. Munker R, Gasson J, Ogawa M, Koeffler HP: Recombinant human TNF induces production of granulocyte macrophage colony-stimulating factor. Nature 323:79, 1986

307. Zsebo KM, Yuschenkoff V, Schulter S et al: Vascular endothelial cells and granulopoiesis: interleukin-1 stimulates release of G-CSF and GM-CSF. Blood 71:99, 1988

308. Lee M, Segal GM, Bagby GC: Interleukin-1 induces human bone marrow-derived fibroblasts to produce multilineage hematopoietic growth factors. Exp Hematol 15:983, 1987

309. Kaushansky K, Lin N, Adamson JW: Interleukin 1 stimulates fibroblasts to synthesize granulocyte-macrophage and granulocyte colony-stimulating factors. J Clin Invest 81:92, 1988

310. Segal GM, Bagby GC: Vascular endothelial cells and hematopoietic regulation. Int J Cell Cloning 6:306, 1988

311. Sieff CA, Niemeyer CM, Mentzer SJ, Faller DV: Interleukin-1, tumor necrosis factor, and the production of colony-stimulating factors by cultured mesenchymal cells. Blood 72:1316, 1988

312. Bagby GC: Interleukin 1 and hematopoiesis. Blood Rev 3:152, 1989

313. Davignon J-L, Kimoto M, Kindler V et al: Selective production of interleukin 3 (IL3) and granulocyte-macrophage colony-stimulating factor (GM-CSF) in vitro by murine L3T4+ T cells: lack of spontaneous IL3 and GM-CSF production by Ly-2−/L3T4− lpr subset. Eur J Immunol 18:1367, 1988

314. Kelso A, Gough NM: Coexpression of granulocyte-macrophage colony-stimulating factor, gamma interferon, and interleukins 3 and 4 is random in murine alloreactive T-lymphocyte clones. Proc Natl Acad Sci USA 85:9189, 1988

315. Herrmann F, Oster W, Meuer SC et al: Interleukin 1 stimulates T lymphocytes to produce granulocyte-monocyte colony-stimulating factor. J Clin Invest 81:1415, 1988

316. Lu L, Srour EF, Warren DJ et al: Enhancement of release of granulocyte- and granulocyte-macrophage colony-stimulating factors from phytohemagglutinin-stimulated sorted subsets of human T lymphocytes by recombinant human tumor necrosis factor-α: synergism with recombinant human IFN-gamma. J Immunol 141:201, 1988

317. Evans SW, Rennick D, Farrar WL: Multilineage hematopoietic growth factor interleukin 3 and direct activators of protein kinase C stimulate phosphorylation of common substrates. Blood 68:906, 1986

318. Whetton AD, Monk PN, Consalvey SD et al: Interleukin 3 stimulates proliferation via protein kinase C activation without increasing inositol lipid turnover. Proc Natl Acad Sci USA 85:3284, 1988

319. Ferris DK, Willet-Brown J, Martensen T, Farrar WL: Interleukin 3 stimulation of tyrosine kinase activity in FDC-P1 cells. Biochem Biophys Res Commun 154:991, 1988

320. Whetton AD, Vallance SJ, Monk PN et al: Interleukin-3-stimulated haemopoietic stem cell proliferation. Evidence for activation of protein kinase C and Na+/H+ exchange without inositol lipid hydrolysis. Biochem J 256:585, 1988

321. Morla AO, Schreurs J, Miyajima A, Wang JYJ: Hematopoietic growth factors

322. activate the tyrosine phosphorylation of distinct sets of proteins in interleukin-3-dependent murine cell lines. Mol Cell Biol 8:2214, 1988

322. Kelvin DJ, Shreeve M, McAuley C et al: Interleukin 3-stimulated proliferation is sensitive to pertussis toxin: evidence for a guanyl nucleotide regulatory protein-mediated signal transduction mechanism. J Cell Physiol 138:273, 1989

323. He Y, Hewlett E, Temeles D, Quesenberry P: Inhibition of interleukin 3 and colony-stimulating factor 1-stimulated marrow cell proliferation by pertussis toxin. Blood 71:1187, 1988

324. Migliaccio G, Migliaccio AR, Visser JWM: Synergism between erythropoietin and interleukin-3 in the induction of hematopoietic stem cell proliferation and erythroid burst colony formation. Blood 72:944, 1988

325. Ikebuchi K, Wong GC, Clark SC et al: Interleukin 6 enhancement of interleukin 3-dependent proliferation of multipotential hemopoietic progenitors. Proc Natl Acad Sci USA 84:9035, 1987

326. Bartelmez SH, Bradley TR, Bertoncello I et al: Interleukin 1 plus interleukin 3 plus colony-stimulating factor 1 are essential for clonal proliferation of primitive myeloid bone marrow cells. Exp Hematol 17:240, 1989

327. Valtieri M, Tweardy DJ, Caracciolo D et al: Cytokine-dependent granulocytic differentiation: regulation of proliferative and differentiative responses in a murine progenitor cell line. J Immunol 138:3829, 1987

328. Conscience JF, Verrier B, Martin G: Interleukin-3-dependent expression of the c-myc and c-fos proto-oncogenes in hemopoietic cell lines. EMBO J 5:317, 1986

329. Lopez AF, Dyson PG, To LB et al: Recombinant human interleukin-3 stimulation of hematopoiesis in humans: loss of responsiveness with differentiation in the neutrophilic myeloid series. Blood 72:1797, 1988

330. Vellenga E, Rambaldi A, Ernst TJ et al: Independent regulation of M-CSF and G-CSF gene expression in human monocytes. Blood 71:1529, 1988

331. Yang Y-C, Ciarietta AB, Temple PA et al: Human IL-3 (multi-CSF): identification by expression cloning of a novel hematopoietic growth factor related to murine IL-3. Cell 47:3, 1986

332. Paquette RL, Zhou J-Y, Yang Y-C et al: Recombinant Gibbon interleukin-3 acts synergistically with recombinant human G-CSF and GM-CSF in vitro. Blood 71:1596, 1988

333. McNiece IK, McGrath HE, Quesenberry PJ: Granulocyte colony-stimulating factor augments in vitro megakaryocyte colony formation by interleukin-3. Exp Hematol 16:807, 1988

334. Santoli D, Clark SC, Kreider BL et al: Amplification of IL-2-driven T cell proliferation by recombinant human IL-3 and granulocyte-macrophage colony-stimulating factor. J Immunol 141:519, 1988

335. Rothenberg ME, Owen WF, Silberstein DS et al: Human eosinophils have prolonged survival, enhanced functional properties, and become hypodense when exposed to human interleukin 3. J Clin Invest 81:1986, 1988

336. Tadmori W, Feingersh D, Clark SC, Choi YS: Human recombinant IL-3 stimulates B cell differentiation. J Immunol 142:1950, 1989

337. Valent P, Schmidt G, Besemer J et al: Interleukin-3 is a differentiation factor for human basophils. Blood 73:1763, 1989

338. Kirshenbaum AS, Goff JP, Dreskin SC et al: IL-3-dependent growth of basophil-like cells and mastlike cells from human bone marrow. J Immunol 142:2424, 1989

339. Ishizaka T, Saito H, Hatake K et al: Preferential differentiation of inflammatory cells by recombinant human interleukins. Int Arch Allergy Appl Immunol 88:46, 1989

340. Haig DM, Mcmenamin C, Redmond J et al: Rat IL-3 stimulates the growth of rat mucosal mast cells in culture. Immunology 65:205, 1988

341. Abe T, Ochiai H, Minamishima Y, Nawa Y: Induction of intestinal mastocytosis in nude mice by repeated injection of interleukin-3. Int Arch Allergy Appl Immunol 86:356, 1988

342. Chen BD-M, Mueller M, Olencki T: Interleukin-3 (IL-3) stimulates the clonal growth of pulmonary alveolar macrophage of the mouse: role of IL-3 in the regulation of macrophage production outside the bone marrow. Blood 72:685, 1988

343. Ikebuchi K, Clark SC, Ihle JN et al: Granulocyte colony-stimulating factor enhances interleukin 3-dependent proliferation of multipotential hemopoietic progenitors. Proc Natl Acad Sci USA 85:3445, 1988

344. Sieff CA, Ekern SC, Nathan DG, Anderson JW: Combinations of recombinant colony-stimulating factors are required for optimal hematopoietic differentiation in serum-deprived culture. Blood 73:688, 1989

345. Bagby GC, Wilkinson B, McCall E, Lee M: Abnormalities of the hematopoietic regulatory network. p. 255. In Tavassoli M, Zanjani ED, Ascensao JL et al (eds): Advances in Experimental Medicine and Biology. Plenum, NY, 1988

346. Bagby GC, Rigas VD, Bennett RM et al: Interaction of lactoferrin, monocytes, and T-lymphocyte subsets in the regulation of steady-state granulopoiesis in vitro. J Clin Invest 68:56, 1981

347. De Waal Malefyt R, Abrams J, Bennett B et al: Interleukin 10 (IL-10) inhibits

cytokine synthesis by human monocytes: an autoregulatory role of IL-10 produced by monocytes. J Exp Med 174:1209, 1991

348. Ralph P, Nakoinz I, Sampson-Johannes et al: IL-10, T lymphocyte inhibitor of human blood cell production of IL-1 and tumor necrosis factor. J Immunol 148:808, 1991

349. Moore KW, O'Garra A, Malefyt RdeW et al: Interleukin-10. Annu Rev Immunol 11:165, 1993

350. Bomsztyk K, Sims JE, Stanton TH et al: Evidence for different interleukin 1 receptors in murine B- and T-cell lines. Proc Natl Acad Sci USA 86:8034, 1989

351. Sims JE, March CJ, Cosman D et al: cDNA expression cloning of the IL-1 receptor, a member of the immunoglobulin superfamily. Science 241:585, 1988

352. McMahan CJ, Slack JL, Mosley B et al: A novel IL-1 receptor, cloned from B cells by mammalian expression, is expressed in many cell types. EMBO J 10:2821, 1991

353. Fibbe WE, Van Damme J, Billiau A et al: Human fibroblasts produce granulo-cyte-CSF, macrophage-CSF, and granulocyte-macrophage-CSF following stimulation by interleukin-1 and poly(rI)·poly(rC). Blood 72:860, 1988

354. Seelentag W, Mermod J-J, Vassalli P: Interleukin 1 and tumor necrosis factor-α additively increase the levels of granulocyte-macrophage and granulocyte colony-stimulating factor (CSF) mRNA in human fibroblasts. Eur J Immunol 19:209, 1989

355. Ridgway D, Borzy MS, Bagby GC: Granulocyte macrophage colony stimulating activity production by cultured human thymic non-lymphoid cells is regulated by endogenous interleukin-1. Blood 72:1230, 1988

356. Garman RD, Jacobs KA, Clark SC, Raulet DH: B-cell-stimulatory factor 2 (β₂ interferon) functions as a second signal for interleukin 2 production by mature murine T cells. Proc Natl Acad Sci USA 84:7629, 1987

357. Tosato G, Seamon KB, Goldman ND et al: Monocyte-derived human B-cell growth factor identified as interferon-β2 (BSF-2, IL-6). Science 239:502, 1988

358. Vink A, Coulie PG, Wauters P et al: B cell growth and differentiation activity of interleukin-HP1 and related murine plasmacytoma growth factors. Synergy with interleukin 1. Eur J Immunol 18:607, 1988

359. May LT, Ghrayeb J, Santhanam U et al: Synthesis and secretion of multiple forms of β₂-interferon/B-cell differentiation factor 2/hepatocyte-stimulating factor by human fibroblasts and monocytes. J Biol Chem 263:7760, 1988

360. Muraguchi A, Hirano T, Tang B et al: The essential role of B cell stimulatory factor 2 (BSF-2/IL-6) for the terminal differentiation of B cells. J Exp Med 167:332, 1988

361. Takatsuki F, Okano A, Suzuki C et al: Human recombinant IL-6/B cell stimula-tory factor 2 augments murine antigen-specific antibody responses in vitro and in vivo. J Immunol 141:3072, 1988

362. Sutherland GR, Baker E, Callen DF et al: Interleukin 4 is at 5q31 and interleu-kin 6 is at 7p15. Hum Genet 79:335, 1988

363. Ferguson-Smith AC, Chen YF, Newman MS et al: Regional localization of the interferon-beta 2/B-cell stimulatory factor 2/hepatocyte stimulating factor gene to human chromosome 7p15-p21. Genomics 2:203, 1988

364. Yamasaki K, Taga T, Hirata Y et al: Cloning and expression of the human interleukin-6 (BSF-2/IFNβ 2) receptor. Science 241:825, 1988

365. May LT, Torcia G, Cozzolino F et al: Interleukin-6 gene expression in human endothelial cells: RNA start sites, multiple IL-6 proteins and inhibition of proliferation. Biochem Biophys Res Commun 159:991, 1989

366. Van Damme J, Schaafsma MR, Fibbe WE et al: Simultaneous production of interleukin 6, interferon-β and colony-stimulating activity by fibroblasts after viral and bacterial infection. Eur J Immunol 19:163, 1989

367. Walther Z, May LT, Sehgal PB: Transcriptional regulation of the interferon-β2/B cell differentiation factor BSF-2/hepatocyte-stimulating factor gene in human fibroblasts by other cytokines. J Immunol 140:974, 1988

368. Norioka K, Hara M, Harigai M et al: Production of B cell stimulatory factor-2/interleukin-6 activity by human endothelial cells. Biochem Biophys Res Commun 153:1045, 1988

369. Sironi M, Breviario F, Proserpio P et al: IL-1 stimulates IL-6 production in endothelial cells. J Immunol 142:549, 1989

370. Jirik FR, Podor TJ, Hirano T et al: Bacterial lipopolysaccharide and inflamma-tory mediators augment IL-6 secretion by human endothelial cells. J Immu-nol 142:144, 1989

371. Aarden LA, DeGroot ER, Schaap OL, Lansdorp PM: Production of hybridoma growth factor by human monocytes. Eur J Immunol 17:1411, 1987

372. Bauer J, Ganter U, Geiger T et al: Regulation of interleukin-6 expression in cultured human blood monocytes and monocyte-derived macrophages. Blood 72:1134, 1988

373. Miyaura C, He Jin C, Yamaguchi Y et al: Production of interleukin 6 and its relation to the macrophage differentiation of mouse myeloid leukemia cells (M1) treated with differentiation-inducing factor and 1α, 25-dihydroxyvita-min D₃. Biochem Biophys Res Commun 158:660, 1989

374. Horii Y, Muraguchi A, Suematsu S et al: Regulation of BSF-2/IL-6 production by human mononuclear cells: macrophage-dependent synthesis of BSF-2/IL-6 by T cells. J Immunol 141:1529, 1988

375. Van Damme J, Cayphas S, Opdenakker G et al: Interleukin 1 and poly (rI)·poly (rC) induce production of a hybridoma growth factor by human fibroblasts. Eur J Immunol 17:1, 1987

376. Helle M, Brakenhoff JPJ, de Groot ER, Aarden LA: Interleukin 6 is involved in interleukin 1-induced activities. Eur J Immunol 18:957, 1988

377. Bendtzen K: Interleukin 1, interleukin 6 and tumor necrosis factor in infec-tion, inflammation and immunity. Immunol Lett 19:183, 1988

378. Rennick D, Jackson J, Yang G et al: Interleukin-6 interacts with interleukin-4 and other hematopoietic growth factors to selectively enhance the growth of megakaryocytic, erythroid, myeloid, and multipotential progenitor cells. Blood 73:1828, 1989

379. Hodgkin PD, Bond MW, O'Garra A et al: Identification of IL-6 as a T cell-derived factor that enhances the proliferative response of thymocytes to IL-4 and phorbol myristate acetate. J Immunol 141:151, 1988

380. Caracciolo D, Clark SC, Rovera G: Human interleukin-6 supports granulo-cytic differentiation of hematopoietic progenitor cells and acts synergisti-cally with GM-CSF. Blood 73:666, 1989

381. Stahl CP, Zucker-Franklin D, Evatt BL, Winton EF: Effects of human interleu-kin-6 on megakaryocyte development and thrombocytopoiesis in primates. Blood 78:1467, 1991

382. Ishibashi T, Shikama Y, Kimura H et al: Thrombopoietic effects of interleu-kin-6 in long-term administration in mice. Exp Hematol 21:640, 1993

383. Ishibashi T, Kimura H, Uchida T et al: Human interleukin 6 is a direct pro-moter of maturation of megakaryocytes in vitro. Proc Natl Acad Sci USA 86:5953, 1989

384. Ishibashi T, Kimura H, Shikama Y et al: Interleukin-6 is a potent thrombo-poietic factor in vivo in mice. Blood 74:1241, 1989

385. Quesenberry PJ, McGrath HE, Williams ME et al: Multifactor stimulation of megakaryocytopoiesis: effects of interleukin 6. Exp Hematol 19:35, 1991

386. Wong GG, Witek-Giannotti JS, Temple PA et al: Stimulation of murine hemo-poietic colony formation by human IL-6. J Immunol 140:3040, 1988

387. Houssiau FA, Coulie PG, Olive D, Van Snick J: Synergistic activation of human T cells by interleukin 1 and interleukin 6. Eur J Immunol 18:653, 1988

388. Leary AG, Ikebuchi K, Hirai Y et al: Synergism between interleukin-6 and interleukin-3 in supporting proliferation of human hematopoietic stem cells: comparison with interleukin-1α. Blood 71:1759, 1988

389. Okada M, Kitahara M, Kishimoto S et al: IL-6/BSF-2 functions as a killer helper factor in the in vitro induction of cytotoxic T cells. J Immunol 141:1543, 1988

390. Tosato G, Pike SE: Interferon-β₂/interleukin 6 is a co-stimulant for human T lymphocytes. J Immunol 141:1556, 1988

391. Koike K, Nakahata T, Takagi M et al: Synergism of BSF-2/interleukin 6 and interleukin 3 on development of multipotential hemopoietic progenitors in serum-free culture. J Exp Med 168:879, 1988

392. Ogawa M, Clark SC: Synergistic interaction between interleukin-6 and in-terleukin-3 in support of stem cell proliferation in culture. Blood Cells 14:329, 1988

393. Suda T, Yamaguchi Y, Suda J et al: Effect of interleukin 6 (IL-6) on the differ-entiation and proliferation of murine and human hemopoietic progenitors. Exp Hematol 16:891, 1988

394. Ikebuchi K, Ihle JN, Hirai Y et al: Synergistic factors for stem cell prolifera-tion: further studies of the target stem cells and the mechanism of stimula-tion by interleukin-1, interleukin-6, and granulocyte colony-stimulating fac-tor. Blood 72:2007, 1988

395. Bot FJ, Van Eijk L, Broeders L et al: Interleukin-6 synergizes with M-CSF in the formation of macrophage colonies from purified human marrow progenitor cells. Blood 73:435, 1989

396. Emilie D, Crevon M-C, Auffredou MT, Galanaud P: Glucocorticosteroid-de-pendent synergy between interleukin 1 and interleukin 6 for human B lym-phocyte differentiation. Eur J Immunol 18:2043, 1988

397. Strieter RM, Remick DG, Lynch JP III et al: Interleukin-2-induced tumor necro-sis factor-alpha (TNF-α) gene expression in human alveolar macrophages and blood monocytes. Am Rev Respir Dis 139:335, 1989

398. Numerof RP, Aronson FR, Mier JW: IL-2 stimulates the production of IL-1α and IL-1β by human peripheral blood mononuclear cells. J Immunol 141:4250, 1988

399. Sisson SD, Dinarello CA: Production of interleukin-1α, interleukin-1β and tumor necrosis factor by human mononuclear cells stimulated with granulo-cyte-macrophage colony-stimulating factor. Blood 72:1368, 1988

400. Wieser M, Bonifer R, Oster W et al: Interleukin-4 induces secretion of CSF for granulocytes and CSF for macrophages by peripheral blood monocytes. Blood 73:1105, 1989

401. Fiorentino DF, Bond MW, Mosmann TR: Two types of mouse helper T cells.

IV. Th2 clones secrete a factor that inhibits cytokine production by Th1 clones. J Exp Med 170:2081, 1989

402. Vieira P, de Waal-Malefyt R, Dang M-N et al: Isolation and expression of human cytokine synthesis inhibitory factor cDNA clones: homology to Epstein-Barr virus open reading frame BCRFI. Proc Natl Acad Sci USA 88:1172, 1991

403. Kim JM, Brannan CI, Copeland NG et al: Structure of the mouse IL-10 gene and chromosomal localization of the mouse and human genes. J Immunol 148:3618, 1992

404. Fiorentino DF, Zlotnik A, Vieira P et al: IL-10 acts on the antigen-presenting cell to inhibit cytokine production by Th1 cells. J Immunol 146:3444, 1991

405. Hsu D-H, De Waal Malefyt R et al: Expression of interleukin-10 activity by Epstein-Barr virus protein BCRF1. Science 250:830, 1990

406. Hsu D-H, Moore KW, Spits H: Differential effects of interleukin-4 and -10 on interleukin-2-induced interferon-gamma synthesis and lymphokine-activated killer activity. Int Immunol 4:563, 1992

407. de Waal-Malefyt R, Haanen J, Spits H et al: IL-10 and viral IL-10 strongly reduce antigen-specific human T cell proliferation by diminishing the antigen-presenting capacity of monocytes via down-regulation of class II MHC expression. J Exp Med 174:915, 1991

408. Ding L, Shevach EM: IL-10 inhibits mitogen-induced T cell proliferation by selectively inhibiting macrophage costimulatory function. J Immunol 148:3133, 1992

409. Taga K, Mostowski H, Tosato G: Human interleukin-10 can directly inhibit T-cell growth. Blood 81:2964, 1993

410. Rousset F, Garcia E, DeFrance T et al: Interleukin 10 is a potent growth and differentiation factor for activated human B lymphocytes. Proc Natl Acad Sci USA 89:1890, 1992

411. Fiorentino DF, Zlotnik A, Mosmann TR et al: IL-10 inhibits cytokine production by activated macrophages. J Immunol 147:3815, 1991

412. Bogdan C, Vodovotz Y, Nathan C: Macrophage deactivation by interleukin 10. J Exp Med 174:1549, 1991

413. Gazzinelli RT, Oswald IP, James SL, Sher A: IL-10 inhibits parasite killing and nitric oxide production by IFN-gamma-activated macrophages. J Immunol 148:1792, 1992

414. Heinzel FP, Sadick MD, Mutha SS, Locksley RM: Production of interferon gamma, interleukin 2, interleukin 4, and interleukin 10 by CD4-positive lymphocytes in vivo during healing and progressive murine leishmaniasis. Proc Natl Acad Sci USA 88:7011, 1993

415. Silva JS, Morrissey PJ, Grabstein KH et al: Interleukin 10 and interferon gamma regulation of experimental *Trypanosoma cruzi* infection. J Exp Med 175:169, 1992

416. Sher A, Fiorentino DF, Caspar P et al: Production of IL-10 by CD4+ lymphocytes correlates with down-regulation of Th1 cytokine synthesis in helminth infection. J Immunol 147:2713, 1991

417. Sher A, Coffman RL: Regulation of immunity to parasites by T cells and T cell-derived cytokines. Annu Rev Immunol 10:385, 1992

418. Hudson GS, Bankier AT, Satchwell SC, Barrell BG: The short unique region of the B95-8 Epstein-Barr virus genome. Virology 147:81, 1985

419. Benjamin D, Knobloch TJ, Dayton MA: Human B-cell interleukin-10: B-cell lines derived from patients with acquired immunodeficiency syndrome and Burkitt's lymphoma constitutively secrete large quantities of interleukin-10. Blood 80:1289, 1992

420. Zhou YQ, Stanley ER, Clark SC et al: Interleukin-3 and interleukin-1 alpha allow earlier bone marrow progenitors to respond to human colony-stimulating factor 1. Hôpital Paul Brousse, Villejuif, France. Blood 72:1870, 1988

421. Stanley ER, Bartocci A, Patinkin D et al: Regulation of very primitive, multipotent, hemopoietic cells by hemopoietin-1. Cell 45:667, 1986

422. Peschel C, Green I, Ohara J, Paul WE: Role of B cell stimulatory factor 1/interleukin 4 in clonal proliferation of B cells. J Immunol 139:3338, 1987

423. Mosmann TR, Bond MW, Coffman RL et al: T-cell and mast cell lines respond to B-cell stimulatory factor 1. Proc Natl Acad Sci USA 83:5654, 1986

424. Yokota T, Otsuka T, Mosmann T et al: Isolation and characterization of a human interleukin cDNA clone homologous to mouse B-cell stimulatory factor 1 that expresses B-cell and T-cell-stimulating activities. Proc Natl Acad Sci USA 83:1, 1986

425. Kanakura Y, Kuriu A, Waki N et al: Changes in number and types of mast cell colony-forming cells in the peritoneal cavity of mice after injection of distilled water: evidence that mast cells suppress differentiation of bone marrow-derived precursors. Blood 71:573, 1988

426. Carding SR, Bottomly K: IL-4 (B cell stimulatory factor 1) exhibits thymocyte growth factor activity in the presence of IL-2. J Immunol 140:1519, 1988

427. Brown M, Hu-Li J, Paul WE: IL-4/B cell stimulatory factor 1 stimulates T cell growth by an IL-2-independent mechanism. J Immunol 141:504, 1988

428. Fernandez-Botran R, Sanders VM, Oliver KG et al: Interleukin 4 mediates autocrine growth of helper T cells after antigenic stimulation. Proc Natl Acad Sci USA 83:9689, 1986

429. Le Beau MM, Lemons RS, Espinosa R III et al: Interleukin-4 and interleukin-5 map to human chromosome 5 in a region encoding growth factors and receptors and are deleted in myeloid leukemias with a del(5q). Blood 73:647, 1989

430. Arai N, Nomura D, Villaret D et al: Complete nucleotide sequence of the chromosomal gene for human IL-4 and its expression. J Immunol 142:274, 1989

431. Lewis DB, Prickett KS, Larsen A et al: Restricted production of interleukin 4 by activated human T cells. Proc Natl Acad Sci USA 85:9743, 1988

432. Hofman FM, Brock M, Taylor CR, Lyons B: IL-4 regulates differentiation and proliferation of human precursor B cells. J Immunol 141:1185, 1988

433. Jankovic DL, Abehsira-Amar O, Korner M et al: IL-4, but not IL-5, can act synergistically with B cell activating factor (BCAF) to induce proliferation of resting B cells. Cell Immunol 117:165, 1988

434. Sanderson CJ, O'Garra A, Warren DJ, Klaus GGB: Eosinophil differentiation factor also has B-cell growth factor activity. Proc Natl Acad Sci USA 83:437, 1986

435. Monroe JG, Haldar S, Prystowsky MB, Lammie P: Lymphokine regulation of inflammatory processes: interleukin-4 stimulates fibroblast proliferation. Clin Immunol Immunopathol 49:292, 1988

436. Ohara J, Paul WE: Up-regulation of interleukin 4/B-cell stimulatory factor 1 receptor expression. Proc Natl Acad Sci USA 85:8221, 1989

437. Del Prete G, Maggi E, Parronchi P et al: IL-4 is an essential factor for the IgE synthesis induced in vitro by human T cell clones and their supernatants. J Immunol 140:4193, 1988

438. Snapper CM, Paul WE: B cell stimulatory factor-1 (interleukin 4) prepares resting murine B cells to secrete IgG1 upon subsequent stimulation with bacterial lipopolysaccharide. J Exp Med 139:10–17, 1987

439. Bergstedt-Lindqvist S, Moon H-B, Persson U et al: Interleukin 4 instructs uncommitted B lymphocytes to switch to IgG$_1$ and IgE. Eur J Immunol 18:1073, 1988

440. DeFrance T, Vanbervliet B, Pène J, Banchereau J: Human recombinant IL-4 induces activated B lymphocytes to produce IgG and IgM. J Immunol 141:2000, 1988

441. DeFrance T, Vanbervliet B, Aubry J-P, Banchereau J: Interleukin 4 inhibits the proliferation but not the differentiation of activated human B cells in response to interleukin 2. J Exp Med 168:1321, 1988

442. Jelinek DF, Lipsky PE: Inhibitory influence of IL-4 on human B cell responsiveness. J Immunol 141:164, 1988

443. Tigges MA, Casey LS, Koshland ME: Mechanism of interleukin-2 signaling: mediation of different outcomes by a single receptor and transduction pathway. Science 243:781, 1989

444. Peschel C, Green I, Paul WE: Interleukin-4 induces a substance in bone marrow stromal cells that reversibly inhibits factor-dependent and factor-independent cell proliferation. Blood 73:1130, 1989

445. Williams DE, deVries P, Namen AE et al: The Steel factor. Dev Biol 151:368, 1992

446. Ratajczak MZ, Luger SM, Gewirtz AM: The c-kit proto-oncogene in normal and malignant human hematopoiesis. Int J Cell Cloning 10:205, 1992

447. McCulloch EA, Siminovitch L, Till JE et al: The cellular basis of the genetically determined hemopoietic defect in anemic mice of genotype Sl/Sld. Blood 26:399, 1964

448. Russell ES, Bernstein SE: Proof of whole-cell implant in therapy of W-series anemia. Arch Biochem Biophys 125:594, 1968

449. Bernstein SE: Tissue transplantation as an analytic and therapeutic tool in hereditary anemias. Am J Surg 119:448, 1970

450. Russell ES: Hereditary anemias of the mouse: a review for geneticists. Adv Genet 20:357, 1979

451. Chabot B, Stephenson DA, Chapman VM et al: The proto-oncogene c-kit encoding a transmembrane tyrosine kinase receptor maps to the mouse W locus. Nature 335:88, 1988

452. Geissler EN, Ryan MA, Housman DE: The dominant-White spotting (W) locus of the mouse encodes the c-kit proto-oncogene. Cell 55:185, 1988

453. Yarden Y, Kuang W-J, Yang-Feng T et al: Human proto-oncogene c-kit: a new cell surface receptor tyrosine kinase for an unidentified ligand. EMBO J 6:3341, 1987

454. Hsieh CL, Navankasattusas S, Escobedo JA et al: Chromosomal localization of the gene for AA-type platelet-derived growth factor receptor (PDGFRA) in humans and mice. Cytogenet Cell Genet 56:160, 1991

455. Brandt J, Briddell RA, Srour EF et al: Role of c-kit ligand in the expansion of human hematopoietic progenitor cells. Blood 79:634, 1992

456. Weiss M, Yetz-Aldape J, Crosier PS et al: Committed hematopoietic progenitors of human bone marrow are restricted to the CD38+34+ fraction

whereas c-kit expression is greatest in CD38−34+ cells, abstracted. Blood, suppl. 1. 78:161a, 1991

457. Papayannopoulou T, Brice M, Broudy VC, Zsebo KM: Isolation of c-kit receptor-expressing cells from bone marrow, peripheral blood, and fetal liver: functional properties and composite antigenic profile. Blood 78:1403, 1991

458. Broudy VC, Lin N, Zsebo KM et al: Isolation and characterization of a monoclonal antibody that recognizes the human c-kit receptor. Blood 79:338, 1992

459. Ogawa M, Matsuzaki Y, Nishikawa S et al: Expression and function of c-*kit* in hemopoietic progenitor cells. J Exp Med 174:63, 1991

460. Galli SJ, Tsai M, Wershil BK: The c-kit receptor, stem cell factor, and mast cells. What each is teaching us about the others. Am J Pathol 142:965, 1993

461. Williams DE, Eisenman J, Baird A et al: Identification of a ligand for the c-*kit* proto-oncogene. Cell 63:167, 1990

462. Copeland NG, Gilbert DJ, Cho BC et al: Mast cell growth factor maps near the steel locus on mouse chromosome 10 and is deleted in a number of steel alleles. Cell 63:175, 1990

463. Flanagan JG, Leder P: The *kit* ligand: a cell surface molecule altered in steel mutant fibroblasts. Cell 63:185, 1990

464. Zsebo KM, Williams DA, Geissler EN et al: Stem cell factor is encoded at the *Sl* locus of the mouse and is the ligand for the c-*kit* tyrosine kinase receptor. Cell 63:213, 1990

465. Huang E, Nocka K, Beier DR et al: The hematopoietic growth factor KL is encoded by the *Sl* locus and is the ligand of the c-*kit* receptor, the gene product of the *W* locus. Cell 63:225, 1990

466. Giebel LB, Spritz RA: Mutation of the *KIT* (mast/stem cell growth factor receptor) protooncogene in human piebaldism. Proc Natl Acad Sci USA 88:8696, 1991

467. Fleischman RA, Saltman DL, Stastny V, Zneimer S: Deletion of the c-*kit* protooncogene in the human developmental defect piebald trait. Proc Natl Acad Sci USA 88:10885, 1991

468. Anderson DM, Williams DE, Tushinski R et al: Alternate splicing of the mRNAs encoding human mast cell growth factor and localization of the gene to chromosome 12q22–q24. Cell Growth Differ 2:373, 1991

469. Anderson DM, Lyman SD, Baird A et al: Molecular cloning of mast cell growth factor, a hematopoietin that is active in both membrane bound and soluble forms. Cell 63:235, 1990

470. Flanagan JG, Chan DC, Leder P: Transmembrane form of the *kit* ligand growth factor is determined by alternative splicing and is missing in the *Sl*^d mutant. Cell 64:1025, 1991

471. Heinrich MC, Dooley DC, Freed AC et al: Constitutive expression of steel factor gene by human stromal cells. Blood 82:771, 1993

472. Rossi P, Albanesi C, Grimaldi P, Geremia R: Expression of the mRNA for the ligand of c-kit in mouse Sertoli cells. Biochem Biophys Res Comm 176:910, 1991

473. Keshet E, Lyman SD, Williams DE et al: Embryonic RNA expression patterns of the c-*kit* receptor and its cognate ligand suggest multiple functional roles in mouse development. EMBO J 10:2425, 1991

474. Heinrich MC, Dooley DC, Freed AC et al: TGF-beta-1 represses Steel factor (SF) gene expression in long term human bone marrow culture (LTBMC) adherent cells, abstracted. Blood, suppl. 1. 80:95a, 1992

475. Lu HS, Clogston CL, Wypych J et al: Amino acid and post-translational modification of stem cell factor isolated from Buffalo rat liver conditioned medium. J Biol Chem 266:8102, 1991

476. Huang EJ, Nocka KH, Buck J, Besmer P: Differential expression and processing of two cell associated forms of the Kit-ligand: KL-1 and KL-2. Mol Biol Cell 3:349, 1992

477. Bernstein ID, Andrews RG, Zsebo KM: Recombinant human stem cell factor enhances the formation of colonies of CD34+ and CD34+lin− cells, and the generation of colony-forming cell progeny from CD34+lin− cells cultured with interleukin-3, granulocyte colony-stimulating factor, or granulocyte-macrophage colony-stimulating factor. Blood 77:2316, 1991

478. Lansdorp PM, Dragowska W: Long-term erythropoiesis from constant numbers of CD34+ cells in serum-free cultures initiated with highly purified progenitor cells from human bone marrow. J Exp Med 175:1501, 1992

479. McNiece IK, Langley KE, Zsebo KM: Recombinant human stem cell factor synergises with GM-CSF, G-CSF, IL-3 and Epo to stimulate human progenitor cells of the myeloid and erythroid lineages. Exp Hematol 19:226, 1991

480. Broxmeyer HE, Cooper S, Lu L et al: Effect of murine mast cell growth factor (c-kit proto-oncogene ligand) on colony formation by human marrow hematopoietic progenitor cells. Blood 77:2142, 1991

481. Briddell RA, Bruno E, Cooper RJ et al: Effect of c-*kit* ligand on in vitro human megakaryocytopoiesis. Blood 78:2854, 1991

482. Olivieri NF, Grunberger T, BenDavid Y et al: Diamond-Blackfan anemia: heterogeneous response of hematopoietic progenitor cells in vitro to the protein product of the Steel locus. Blood 78:2211, 1991

483. Abkowitz JL, Sabo KM, Nakamoto B et al: Diamond-Blackfan anemia: in vitro response of erythroid progenitors to the ligand for c-*kit*. Blood 78:2198, 1991

484. Bagnara GP, Strippoli P, Bonsi L et al: Effect of stem cell factor on colony growth from acquired and constitutional (Fanconi) aplastic anemia. Blood 80:382, 1992

485. Tsai M, Takeishi T, Thompson H et al: Induction of mast cell proliferation, maturation and heparin synthesis by rat c-kit ligand, stem cell factor. Proc Natl Acad Sci USA 88:6382, 1991

486. Meininger CJ, Yano H, Rottapel R et al: The c-*kit* receptor ligand functions as a mast cell chemoattractant. Blood 79:958, 1992

487. Columbo M, Horowitz EM, Botana LM et al: The human recombinant c-kit receptor ligand, rhSCF, induces mediator release from human cutaneous mast cells and enhances IgE dependent mediator release from both skin mast cells and peripheral blood basophils. J Immunol 149:599, 1992

488. Lynch DH, Jacobs C, DuPont D et al: Pharmacokinetic parameters of recombinant murine mast cell growth factor (rMGF). Lymphokine Cytokine Res 11:233, 1992

489. Andrews RG, Knitter GH, Bartelmez SH et al: Recombinant human stem cell factor, a c-*kit* ligand, stimulates hematopoiesis in primates. Blood 78:1975, 1991

490. Tsai M, Shih L, Newlands GFJ et al: The rat c-kit ligand, stem cell factor, induces the development of connective tissue-type and mucosal mast cells in vivo. Analysis by anatomical distribution, histochemistry and protease phenotype. J Exp Med 174:125, 1991

491. Murphy M, Reid K, Williams DE et al: Steel factor is required for maintenance, but not differentiation, of melanocyte precursors in the neural crest. Dev Biol 153:396, 1992

492. Fibbe WE, Van Damme J, Billiau A et al: Interleukin 1 (22K factor) induces release of granulocyte-macrophage colony-stimulating activity from human mononuclear phagocytes. Blood 68:1316, 1986

493. Zucali JR, Dinarello CA, Oblon DJ et al: Interleukin-1 stimulates fibroblasts to produce granulocyte-macrophage colony stimulating activity and prostaglandin E2. J Clin Invest 77:1857, 1986

494. Koeffler HP, Gasson J, Ranyard J et al: Recombinant human TNF alpha stimulates production of granulocyte colony-stimulating factor. Blood 70:55, 1987

495. Broudy VC, Kaushansky K, Segal GM et al: Tumor necrosis factor type α stimulates human endothelial cells to produce granulocyte-macrophage colony-stimulating factor. Proc Natl Acad Sci USA 83:7467, 1986

496. Warner SJC, Auger KR, Libby P: Interleukin 1 induces interleukin 1. II. Recombinant human interleukin 1 induces interleukin 1 production by adult human vascular endothelial cells. J Immunol 139:1911, 1987

497. Lee MA, Segal GM, Bagby GC: The hematopoietic microenvironment in the elderly: defects in IL-1 induced CSF expression. Exp Hematol 17:952, 1989

498. Fibbe WE, Goselink HM, van Eeden G et al: Proliferation of myeloid progenitor cells in human long-term bone marrow cultures is stimulated by interleukin-1 beta. Blood 72:1242, 1988

499. Mauviel A, Temime N, Charron D et al: Interleukin-1 α and β induce interleukin-1 β gene expression in human dermal fibroblasts. Biochem Biophys Res Commun 156:1209, 1988

500. Raines EW, Dower SK, Ross R: Interleukin-1 mitogenic activity for fibroblasts and smooth muscle cells is due to PDGF-AA. Science 243:393, 1989

501. Dalton BJ, Connor JR, Johnson WJ: Interleukin-1 induces interleukin-1α and interleukin-1β gene expression in synovial fibroblasts and peripheral blood monocytes. Arthritis Rheum 32:279, 1989

502. Goeddel DV, Aggarwal BB, Gray PW et al: Tumor necrosis factors: gene structure and biological activities. p. 597. In: Molecular Biology of Homo Sapiens. Cold Spring Harbor Laboratory Press, Cold Spring Harbor, 1986

503. Spies T, Blanck G, Bresnahan M et al: A new cluster of genes within the human major histocompatibility complex. Science 243:214, 1989

504. Migliaccio AR, Migliaccio G: Human embryonic hemopoiesis: control mechanisms underlying progenitor differentiation in vitro. Dev Biol 125:127, 1988

505. Broxmeyer HE, Williams DE, Lu L et al: The suppressive influences of human tumor necrosis factors on bone marrow hematopoietic progenitor cells from normal donors and patients with leukemia: synergism of tumor necrosis factor and interferon-gamma. J Immunol 136:4487, 1986

506. Pelus LM, Ottmann OG, Nocka KH: Synergistic inhibition of human marrow granulocyte-macrophage progenitor cells by prostaglandin E and recombinant interferon-α, -β, and -τ and an effect mediated by tumor necrosis factor. J Immunol 140:479, 1988

507. Roodman GD: Mechanisms of erythroid suppression in the anemia of chronic disease. Blood Cells 13:171, 1987

508. Roodman GD, Bird A, Hutzler D, Montgomery W: Tumor necrosis factor-alpha and hematopoietic progenitors: effects of tumor necrosis factor on the growth of erythroid progenitors CFU-E and BFU-E and the hematopoietic cell lines K562, HL60, and HEL cells. Exp Hematol 15:928, 1987

509. Cannistra SA, Groshek P, Griffin JD: Monocytes enhance gamma-interferon-

induced inhibition of myeloid progenitor cell growth through secretion of tumor necrosis factor. Exp Hematol 16:865, 1988

510. Koeffler HP, Gasson J, Tobler A: Transcriptional and posttranscriptional modulation of myeloid colony-stimulating factor expression by tumor necrosis factor and other agents. Mol Cell Biol 8:3432, 1988

511. Vogel SN, Douches SD, Kaufman EN, Neta R: Induction of colony stimulating factor in vivo by recombinant interleukin 1 alpha and recombinant tumor necrosis factor alpha 1. J Immunol 138:2143, 1987

512. Moldawer LL, Marano MA, Wei H et al: Cachectin/tumor necrosis factor-α alters red blood cell kinetics and induces anemia in vivo. FASEB J 3:1637, 1989

513. Frater-Schroder M, Risau W Hallmann R et al: Tumor necrosis factor type alpha, a potent inhibitor of endothelial cell growth in vitro, is angiogenic in vivo. Proc Natl Acad Sci USA 84:5277, 1987

514. Leibovich SJ, Polverini PJ, Shepard HM et al: Macrophage-induced angiogenesis is mediated by tumour necrosis factor-α. Nature 329:630, 1987

515. Niitsu Y, Watanabe N, Neda H et al: Induction of synthesis of tumor necrosis factor in human and murine cell lines by exogenous recombinant human tumor necrosis factor. Cancer Res 48:5407, 1988

516. Ghezzi P, Dinarello CA: IL-1 induces IL-1. III. Specific inhibition of IL-1 production by IFN-gamma[1]. J Immunol 140:4238, 1988

517. Manson JC, Symons JA, Di Giovine FS et al: Autoregulation of interleukin 1 production. Eur J Immunol 19:261, 1989

518. Nawroth PP, Bank I, Handley D et al: Tumor necrosis factor/cachectin interacts with endothelial cell receptors to induce release of interleukin 1. J Exp Med 163:1363, 1986

519. Le JM, Weinstein D, Gubler U, Vilcek J: Induction of membrane-associated interleukin 1 by tumor necrosis factor in human fibroblasts. J Immunol 138:2137, 1987

520. Kurt-Jones EA, Fiers W, Pober JS: Membrane interleukin 1 induction on human endothelial cells and dermal fibroblasts. J Immunol 139:2317, 1987

521. Pettenati MJ, Le Beau MM, Lemons RS et al: Assignment of CSF-1 to 5q33.1: evidence for clustering of genes regulating hematopoiesis and for their involvement in the deletion of the long arm of chromosome 5 in myeloid disorders. Proc Natl Acad Sci USA 84:2970, 1987

522. Le Beau MM, Westbrook CA, Diaz MO et al: Evidence for the involvement of GM-CSF and FMS in the deletion (5q) in myeloid disorders. Science 231:984, 1986

523. Sacca R, Stanley ER, Sherr CJ, Rettenmier CW: Specific binding of the mononuclear phagocyte colony-stimulating factor CSF-1 to the product of the v-fms oncogene. Proc Natl Acad Sci USA 83:3331, 1986

524. Rettenmier CW, Sacca R, Furman WL et al: Expression of the human c-fms proto-oncogene product (colony-stimulating factor-1 receptor) on peripheral blood mononuclear cells and choriocarcinoma cell lines. J Clin Invest 77:1740, 1986

525. Roussel MF, Downing JR, Ashmun RA et al: Colony-stimulating factor 1-mediated regulation of a chimeric c-fms/v-fms receptor containing the v-fms-encoded tyrosine kinase domain. Proc Natl Acad Sci USA 85:5903, 1988

526. Sherr CJ, Roussel MF, Rettenmier CW: Colony-stimulating factor-1 receptor (c-fms). J Cell Biochem 38:179, 1988

527. Willman CL, Sever CE, Pallavicini MG et al: Deletion of IRF-1, mapping to chromosome 5q31.1, in human leukemia and preleukemic myelodysplasia. Science 259:968, 1993

528. Jaye M, Howk R, Burgess W et al: Human endothelial cell growth factor: cloning, nucleotide sequence, and chromosome localization. Science 233:541, 1986

529. Kobilka BK, Dixon RA, Frielle T et al: cDNA for the human beta 2-adrenergic receptor: a protein with multiple membrane-spanning domains and encoded by a gene whose chromosomal location is shared with that of the receptor for platelet-derived growth factor. Proc Natl Acad Sci USA 84:46, 1987

530. Goyert SM, Ferrero En, Rettig WJ et al: The CD14 monocyte differentiation antigen maps to a region encoding growth factors and receptors. Science 239:497, 1988

531. Shaw G, Kamen R: A conserved AU sequence from the 3′ untranslated region of GM-CSF mRNA mediates selective mRNA degradation. Cell 46:659, 1986

532. Caput D, Beutler B, Hartog K et al: Identification of a common nucleotide sequence in the 3′ untranslated region of mRNA molecules specifying inflammatory mediators. Proc Natl Acad Sci USA 83:1670, 1986

533. Bagby GC, Shaw G, Segal GM: Human vascular endothelial cells, granulopoiesis, and the inflammatory response. J Invest Dermatol 93:48S, 1989

534. Nioche S, Tazi A, Lecossier D, Hance AJ: Production of granulocyte colony-stimulating factor (G-CSF) by human cells: T lymphocyte-dependent and T lymphocyte-independent release of G-CSF by blood monocytes. Eur J Immunol 18:1021, 1988

535. Ernst TJ, Ritchie AR, Demetri GD, Griffin JD: Regulation of granulocyte- and monocyte-colony stimulating factor mRNA levels in human blood mono-

cytes is mediated primarily at a post-transcriptional level. J Biol Chem 264:5700, 1989

536. Haq AU: Failure of hydrocortisone to suppress the interferon-gamma-induced augmentation of interleukin 1 secretion of aged human monocytes. Immunobiology 177:245, 1988

537. Turner M, Chantry D, Feldman M: Post-transcriptional control of IL-1 gene expression in the acute monocytic leukemia line THP-1. Biochem Biophys Res Commun 156:830, 1988

538. Sariban E, Imamura K, Luebbers R, Kufe D: Transcriptional and posttranscriptional regulation of tumor necrosis factor gene expression in human monocytes. J Clin Invest 81:1506, 1988

539. Hart PH, Whitty GA, Piccoli DS, Hamilton JA: Synergistic activation of human monocytes by granulocyte-macrophage colony-stimulating factor and IFN-gamma. Increased TNF-α but not IL-1 activity. J Immunol 141:1516, 1988

540. Martinet Y, Yamauchi K, Crystal RG: Differential expression of the tumor necrosis factor/cachectin gene by blood and lung mononuclear phagocytes. Am Rev Respir Dis 138:659, 1988

541. Goldfeld AE, Maniatis T: Coordinate viral induction of tumor necrosis factor α and interferon β in human B cells and monocytes. Proc Natl Acad Sci USA 86:1490, 1989

542. Ullrich A, Schlessinger J: Signal transduction by receptors with tyrosine kinase activity. Cell 61:203, 1990

543. Nicola NA, Metcalf D: Subunit promiscuity among hemopoietic growth factor receptors. Cell 67:1, 1991

544. Bazan JF: Structural design and molecular evolution of a cytokine receptor superfamily. Proc Natl Acad Sci USA 87:6934, 1990

545. Patthy L: Homology of a domain of the growth hormone/prolactin receptor family with type III modules of fibronectin, letter. Cell 61:13, 1990

546. Sato N, Sakamaki K, Terada N et al: Signal transduction by the high-affinity GM-CSF receptor: two distinct cytoplasmic regions of the common β subunit responsible for different signaling. EMBO J 12:4181, 1993

547. Taga T, Hibi M, Murakami M et al: Interleukin-6 receptor and signals. Chem Immunol 51:181, 1992

548. Kuramochi S, Ikawa Y, Todokoro K: Characterization of murine erythropoietin receptor genes. J Mol Biol 216:567, 1990

549. Goodwin RG, Friend D, Ziegler SF et al: Cloning of the human and murine interleukin-7 receptors: demonstration of a soluble form and homology to a new receptor superfamily. Cell 60:941, 1990

550. Honda M, Yamamoto S, Cheng M et al: Human soluble IL-6 receptor: its detection and enhanced release by HIV infection. J Immunol 148:2175, 1992

551. Fukunaga R, Seto Y, Mizushima S, Nagata S: Three different mRNAs encoding human granulocyte colony-stimulating factor receptor. Proc Natl Acad Sci USA 87:8702, 1990

552. Fanslow WC, Clifford KN, Park LS et al: Regulation of alloreactivity in vivo by IL-4 and the soluble IL-4 receptor. J Immunol 147:535, 1991

553. Kerr JFR, Harmon BV: Definition and incidence of apoptosis: an historical perspective. p. 5. In Tomei LD, Cope FO (eds): Apoptosis: The Molecular Basis of Cell Death. Cold Spring Harbor Laboratory Press, Cold Spring Harbor, 1993

554. Baffy G, Miyashita T, Williamson JR, Reed JC: Apoptosis induced by withdrawal of interleukin-3 (IL-3) from an IL-3-dependent hematopoietic cell line is associated with repartitioning of intracellular calcium and is blocked by enforced Bcl-2 oncoprotein production. J Biol Chem 268:6511, 1993

555. Magnelli L, Cinelli M, Turchetti A, Chiarugi VP: Apoptosis induction in 32D cells by IL-3 withdrawal is preceded by a drop in the intracellular calcium level. Biochem Biophys Res Commun 194:1394, 1993

556. Collins MK, Marvel J, Malde P, Lopez-Rivas A: Interleukin 3 protects murine bone marrow cells from apoptosis induced by DNA damaging agents. J Exp Med 176:1043, 1992

557. Yamaguchi Y, Suda T, Ohta S et al: Analysis of the survival of mature human eosinophils: interleukin-5 prevents apoptosis in mature human eosinophils. Blood 78:2542, 1991

558. Brach MA, deVos S, Gruss HJ, Herrmann F: Prolongation of survival of human polymorphonuclear neutrophils by granulocyte-macrophage colony-stimulating factor is caused by inhibition of programmed cell death. Blood 80:2920, 1992

559. Pesce M, Farrace MG, Piacentini M et al: Stem cell factor and leukemia inhibitory factor promote primordial germ cell survival by suppressing programmed cell death (apoptosis). Development 118:1089, 1993

560. Tartakovsky B, Finnegan A, Muegge K et al: IL-1 is an autocrine growth factor for T cell clones. J Immunol 141:3863, 1988

561. Scala G, Morrone G, Tamburrini M et al: Autocrine growth function of human interleukin 1 molecules on ROHA-9, an EBV-transformed human B cell line. J Immunol 138:2527, 1987

562. Busson P, Braham K, Ganem G et al: Epstein-Barr virus-containing epithelial

cells from nasopharyngeal carcinoma produce interleukin 1 alpha. Proc Natl Acad Sci USA 84:6262, 1987

563. Bagby GC, Dinarello CA, Neerhout RC et al: Interleukin-1 dependent para-crine granulopoiesis in chronic granulocytic leukemia of the juvenile type. J Clin Invest 82:1430, 1988

564. Furukawa Y, Ohta M, Miura Y, Saito M: Interleukin-1 derived from human monocytic leukemia cell line JOSK-I acts as an autocrine growth factor. Biochem Biophys Res Commun 147:39, 1987

565. Furukawa Y, Ohta M, Kasahara T et al: Constitutive production of interleukin 1 by human monocytic leukemia cell line JOSK-I and the production mecha-nism. Cancer Res 47:2589, 1987

566. Furukawa Y, Ohta M, Miura Y, Saito M: Interleukin-1 producing ability of leukaemia cells and its relationship to morphological diagnosis. Br J Haema-tol 65:11, 1987

567. Ohta M, Furukawa Y, Ide C et al: Establishment and characterization of four human monocytoid leukemia cell lines (JOSK-I, -S, -M and -K) with capabili-ties of monocyte-macrophage lineage differentiation and constitutive pro-duction of interleukin 1. Cancer Res 46:3067, 1986

568. Onozaki K, Urawa H, Tamatani T et al: Synergistic interactions of interleukin 1, interferon-β, and tumor necrosis factor in terminally differentiating a mouse myeloid leukemic cell line (M1). J Immunol 140:112, 1988

569. Cozzolino F, Rubartelli A, Aldinucci D et al: Interleukin 1 as an autocrine growth factor for acute myeloid leukemia cells. Proc Natl Acad Sci USA 86: 2369, 1989

570. Duprez V, Lenoir G, Dautry-Varsat A: Autocrine growth stimulation of a human T-cell lymphoma line by interleukin 2. Proc Natl Acad Sci USA 82: 6932, 1985

571. Schrader JW, Leslie KB, Ziltener HJ, Schrader S: Autostimulatory mecha-nisms in myeloid leukemogenesis. J Cell Biochem 34:39, 1987

572. Zipori D, Lee F: Introduction of interleukin-3 gene into stromal cells from the bone marrow alters hemopoietic differentiation but does not modify stem cell renewal. Blood 71:586, 1988

573. Stocking C, Löliger C, Kawai M et al: Identification of genes involved in growth autonomy of hematopoietic cells by analysis of factor-independent mutants. Cell 53:869, 1988

574. Humphries RK, Abraham S, Krystal G et al: Activation of multiple hemopoi-etic growth factor genes in Abelson virus-transformed myeloid cells. Exp Hematol 16:774, 1988

575. Hapel AJ, Vande Woude G, Campbell HD et al: Generation of an autocrine leukaemia using a retroviral expression vector carrying the interleukin-3 gene. Lymphokine Res 5:249, 1986

576. Kawano M, Hirano T, Matsuda T et al: Autocrine generation and requirement of BSF-2/IL-6 for human multiple myelomas. Nature 332:83, 1988

577. Young DC, Griffin JD: Autocrine secretion of GM-CSF in acute myeloblastic leukemia. Blood 68:1178, 1986

578. Lang RA, Metcalf D, Gough NM et al: Expression of a hemopoietic growth factor cDNA in a factor-dependent cell line results in autonomous growth and tumorigenicity. Cell 43:531, 1985

579. Cheng GYM, Kelleher CA, Miyauchi J et al: Structure and expression of genes of GM-CSF and G-CSF in blast cells from patients with acute myeloblastic leukemia. Blood 71:204, 1988

580. Schuler GD, Cole MD: GM-CSF and oncogene mRNA stabilities are indepen-dently regulated in trans in a mouse monocytic tumor. Cell 55:1115, 1988

581. Rambaldi A, Wakamiya N, Vellenga E et al: Expression of the macrophage colony-stimulating factor and c-fms genes in human acute myeloblastic leu-kemia cells. J Clin Invest 81:1030, 1988

582. Rettenmier CW, Roussel MF, Ashmun RA et al: Synthesis of membrane-bound colony stimulating factor 1 (CSF-1) and downmodulation of CSF-1 receptors in NIH 3T3 cells transformed by cotransfection of the human CSF-1 and c-fms (CSF-1 receptor) genes. Mol Cell Biol 7:2378, 1987

583. Browning PJ, Bunn HF, Cline A et al: Replacement of COOH-terminal trunca-tion of v-fms with c-fms sequences markedly reduces transformation poten-tial. Proc Natl Acad Sci USA 83:7800, 1986

584. Wheeler EF, Askew D, May S et al: The v-fms oncogene induces factor-inde-pendent growth and transformation of the interleukin-3-dependent myeloid cell line FDC-P1. Mol Cell Biol 7:1673, 1987

585. Schlessinger J: Regulation of cell growth and transformation by the epider-mal growth factor receptor. Adv Exp Med Biol 234:65, 1988

586. Yarden Y, Ullrich A: Growth factor receptor tyrosine kinases. Annu Rev Biochem 57:443, 1988

587. Yoshimura A, Longmore G, Lodish HF: Point mutation in the exoplasmic domain of the erythropoietin receptor resulting in hormone-independent activation and tumorigenicity. Nature 348:647, 1990

588. Longmore GD, Lodish HF: An activating mutation in the murine erythropoie-tin receptor induces erythroleukemia in mice: a cytokine receptor superfam-ily oncogene. Cell 67:1089, 1991

589. Wilson AB, Harris JM, Coombs RRA: Interleukin-2-induced production of interferon-gamma by resting human T cells and large granular lymphocytes: requirement for accessory cell factors, including interleukin-1. Cell Immunol 113:130, 1988

590. Nabel GJ, Gorka C, Baltimore D: T-cell-specific expression of interleukin 2: evidence for a negative regulatory site. Proc Natl Acad Sci USA 85:2934, 1988

591. Heeg K, Gillis S, Wagner H: IL-4 bypasses the immune suppressive effect of cyclosporin A during the in vitro induction of murine cytotoxic T lympho-cytes. J Immunol 141:2330, 1988

592. Lichtman AH, Chin J, Schmidt JA, Abbas AK: Role of interleukin 1 in the activation of T lymphocytes. Proc Natl Acad Sci USA 85:9699, 1988

593. DeFranco AL: Molecular aspects of B-lymphocyte activation. Annu Rev Cell Biol 3:143, 1987

594. Hirohata S, Jelinek DF, Lipsky PE: T cell-dependent activation of B cell prolif-eration and differentiation by immobilized monoclonal antibodies to CD3. J Immunol 140:3736, 1988

595. Shirakawa F, Chedid M, Suttles J et al: Interleukin 1 and cyclic AMP induce kappa immunoglobulin light-chain expression via activation of an NF-kap-paB-like DNA-binding protein. Mol Cell Biol 9:959, 1989

596. Freedman AS, Freeman G, Whitman J et al: Pre-exposure of human B cells to recombinant IL-1 enhances subsequent proliferation. J Immunol 141:3398, 1988

597. King AG, Wierda D, Landreth KS: Bone marrow stromal cell regulation of B-lymphopoiesis. I. The role of macrophages, IL-1, and IL-4 in pre-B cell maturation. J Immunol 141:2016, 1988

598. Pene J, Chretien I, Rousset F et al: Modulation of IL-4-induced human IgE production in vitro by IFN-γ and IL-5: the role of soluble CD23 (s-CD23). J Cell Biochem 39:253, 1989

599. Bradley TR, Metcalf D: The growth of mouse bone marrow cells in vitro. Aust J Exp Biol Med Sci 44:287, 1966

600. Pluznik DH, Sachs L: The induction of clones of normal "mast" cells in tissue culture. J Cell Comp Physiol 66:319, 1965

601. Otsuka T, Miyajima A, Brown N et al: Isolation and characterization of an expressible cDNA encoding human IL-3: induction of IL-3 mRNA in human T cell clones. J Immunol 140:2288, 1988

602. Bensi G, Raugei G, Palla E et al: Human interleukin-1 beta gene. Gene 52:95, 1987

603. Brakenhoff JPJ, de Groot ER, Evers RF et al: Molecular cloning and expres-sion of hybridoma growth factor in Escherichia coli. J Immunol 139:4116, 1987

604. Clark BD, Collins KL, Gandy MS et al: Genomic sequence for human proin-terleukin 1 beta: possible evolution from a reverse transcribed prointerleu-kin 1 alpha gene. Nucleic Acids Res 14:7897, 1986

605. Tanabe O, Akira S, Kamiya T et al: Genomic structure of the murine IL-6 gene: high degree conservation of potential regulatory sequences between mouse and human. J Immunol 141:3875, 1988

606. Lomedico PT, Gubler U, Hellmann CP et al: Cloning and expression of murine interleukin-1 cDNA in Escherichia coli. Nature 312:458, 1984

607. March CJ, Mosley B, Larsen A et al: Cloning, sequence and expression of two distinct human interleukin-1 complementary DNAs. Nature 315:641, 1985

608. Gearing DP, King JA, Gough NM: Complete sequence of murine myeloid leukaemia inhibitory factor (LIF). Nucleic Acids Res 16:9857, 1988

609. Lee SW, Tsou A-P, Chan H et al: Glucocorticoids selectively inhibit the tran-scription of the interleukin 1β gene and decrease the stability of interleukin 1β mRNA. Proc Natl Acad Sci USA 85:1204, 1988

610. Fenton MJ, Vermeulen MW, Clark BD et al: Human pro-IL-1β gene expression in monocytic cells is regulated by two distinct pathways. J Immunol 140: 2267, 1988

611. Axelrad AA, McLeod DL, Suzuki S, Shreeve MM: Regulation of the population size of erythropoietic progenitor cells. p. 155. In Clarkson AB, Marks PA, Till JE (eds): Differentiation of Normal and Neoplastic Hematopoietic Cells, Cold Spring Harbor Laboratory Press, Cold Spring Harbor, 1978

612. Eaves CJ, Eaves AC: Erythropoietin (Ep) dose-response curves for three classes of erythroid progenitors in normal human marrow and in patients with polycythemia vera. Blood 52:1196, 1978

613. Iscove NN: The role of erythropoietin in regulation of population size and cell cycling of early and late erythroid precursors in mouse bone marrow. Cell Tissue Kinet 10:323, 1977

614. Tsuda H, Neckers LM, Pluznik DH: Enhanced c-fos expression in differen-tiated monomyelocytic cells is associated with differentiation and not with the position of the differentiated cells in the cell cycle. Exp Hematol 15:700, 1987

615. Nicola NA, Metcalf D: Binding of the differentiation-inducer, granulocyte-colony-stimulating factor to responsive but not unresponsive leukemic cell lines. Proc Natl Acad Sci USA 81:3765, 1984

616. Akagawa KS, Kamoshita K, Tokunaga T: Effects of granulocyte-macrophage colony-stimulating factor and colony-stimulating factor-1 on the proliferation and differentiation of murine alveolar macrophages. J Immunol 141: 3383, 1988

617. Becker S, Warren MK, Haskill S: Colony-stimulating factor-induced monocyte survival and differentiation into macrophages in serum-free cultures. J Immunol 139:3703, 1987

618. McCall E, Bagby GC: Monocyte-derived recruiting activity. Kinetics of production and effects of endotoxin. Blood 65:689, 1985

619. Merchav S, Nagler A, Sahar E, Tatarsky I: Production of human pluripotent progenitor cell colony stimulating activity (CFU-GEMM CSA) in patients with myelodysplastic syndromes. Leuk Res 3:273, 1987

620. Dorssers L, Burger H, Bot F et al: Characterization of a human multilineage-colony-stimulating factor cDNA clone identified by a conserved noncoding sequence in mouse interleukin-3. Gene 55:115, 1987

621. Miyauchi J, Kelleher CA, Yang Y-C et al: The effects of three recombinant growth factors, IL-3, GM-CSF, and G-CSF on the blast cells of acute myeloblastic leukemia maintained in short-term suspension culture. Blood 70:657, 1987

622. Delwel R, Dorssers L, Touw I et al: Human recombinant multilineage colony stimulating factor (interleukin-3): stimulator of acute myelocytic leukemia progenitor cells in vitro. Blood 70:333, 1987

623. Löwenberg B, Salem M, Delwel R: Effects of recombinant multi-CSF, GM-CSF, G-CSF and M-CSF on the proliferation and maturation of human AML in vitro. Blood Cells 14:539, 1988

624. Williams DE, Straneva JE, Cooper S et al: Interactions between purified murine colony-stimulating factors (natural CSF-1, recombinant GM-CSF, and recombinant IL-3) on the in vitro proliferation of purified murine granulocyte-macrophage progenitor cells. Exp Hematol 15:1007, 1987

625. Champlin RE, Nimer SD, Ireland P et al: Treatment of refractory aplastic anemia with recombinant human granulocyte-macrophage-colony-stimulating factor. Blood 73:694, 1989

626. Baldwin GC, Gasson JC, Quan SG et al: Granulocyte-macrophage colony-stimulating factor enhances neutrophil function in acquired immunodeficiency syndrome patients. Proc Natl Acad Sci USA 85:2763, 1988

627. Naccache PH, Faucher N, Borgeat P et al: Granulocyte-macrophage colony-stimulating factor modulates the excitation-response coupling sequence in human neutrophils. J Immunol 140:3541, 1988

628. Cannistra SA, Rambaldi A, Spriggs DR et al: Human granulocyte-macrophage colony-stimulating factor induces expression of the tumor necrosis factor gene by the U937 cell line and by normal human monocytes. J Clin Invest 79:1720, 1987

629. Vellenga E, Delwel HR, Touw IP, Lowenberg B: Patterns of acute myeloid leukemia colony growth in response to recombinant granulocyte-macrophage colony-stimulating factor (rGM-CSF). Exp Hematol 15:652, 1987

630. Vellenga E, Young DC, Wagner K et al: The effects of GM-CSF and G-CSF in promoting growth of clonogenic cells in acute myeloblastic leukemia. Blood 69:1771, 1987

631. Hoang T, Nara N, Wong G et al: Effects of recombinant GM-CSF on the blast cells of acute myeloblastic leukemia. Blood 68:313, 1986

632. Schwartz EL, Maher AM: Enhanced mitogenic responsiveness to granulocyte-macrophage colony-stimulating factor in HL-60 promyelocytic leukemia cells upon induction of differentiation. Cancer Res 48:2683, 1988

633. Dedhar S, Gaboury L, Galloway P, Eaves C: Human granulocyte-macrophage colony-stimulating factor is a growth factor active on a variety of cell types of nonhemopoietic origin. Proc Natl Acad Sci USA 85:9253, 1988

634. Berdel WE, Danhauser-Riedl S, Steinhauser G, Winton EF: Various human hematopoietic growth factors (interleukin-3, GM-CSF, G-CSF) stimulate clonal growth of nonhematopoietic tumor cells. Blood 73:80, 1989

635. Mortensen RF, Shapiro J, Lin B-F et al: Interaction of recombinant IL-1 and recombinant tumor necrosis factor in the induction of mouse acute phase proteins. J Immunol 140:2260, 1988

636. Arcone R, Gualandi G, Ciliberto G: Identification of sequences responsible for acute-phase induction of human C-reactive protein. Nucleic Acids Res 16:3195, 1988

637. Nishimoto N, Yoshizaki K, Tagoh H et al: Elevation of serum interleukin 6 prior to acute phase proteins on the inflammation by surgical operation. Clin Immunol Immunopathol 50:399, 1989

638. Dinarello CA: Biology of interleukin 1. FASEB J 2:108, 1988

639. Dinarello CA, Savage N: Interleukin-1 and its receptor. CRC Crit Rev Immunol 9:1, 1989

640. Lumpkin MD: The regulation of ACTH secretion by IL-1. Science 238:452, 1987

641. Berkenbosch F, van Oers J, del Rey A et al: Corticotropin-releasing factor-producing neurons in the rat activated by interleukin-1. Science 238:524, 1987

642. Sapolsky R, Rivier C, Yamamoto G et al: Interleukin-1 stimulates the secretion of hypothalamic corticotropin-releasing factor. Science 238:522, 1987

643. Bernton EW, Beach JE, Holaday JW et al: Release of multiple hormones by a direct action of interleukin-1 on pituitary cells. Science 238:519, 1987

644. Uehara A, Gottschall PE, Dahl RR, Arimura A: Interleukin-1 stimulates ACTH release by an indirect action which requires endogenous corticotropin releasing factor. Endocrinology 121:1580, 1987

645. Besedovsky H, del Rey A, Sorkin E, Dinarello CA: Immunoregulatory feedback between interleukin-1 and glucocorticoid hormones. Science 233:652, 1986

646. Moser R, Schleiffenbaum B, Groscurth P, Fehr J: Interleukin 1 and tumor necrosis factor stimulate human vascular endothelial cells to promote transendothelial neutrophil passage. J Clin Invest 83:444, 1989

647. Conti P, Reale M, Fiore S et al: Recombinant interleukin 1 and tumor necrosis factor acting in synergy to release thromboxane, 6-KETO-PGF$_{1\alpha}$ and PGE$_2$ by human neutrophils. Scand J Rheumatol, suppl. 75. 17:318, 1988

648. Elias JA, Gustilo K, Baeder W, Freundlich B: Synergistic stimulation of fibroblast prostaglandin production by recombinant interleukin 1 and tumor necrosis factor. J Immunol 138:3812, 1987

649. Friteau L, Francesconi E, Lando D et al: Opposite effect of interferon-gamma on PGE$_2$ release from interleukin-1-stimulated human monocytes or fibroblasts. Biochem Biophys Res Commun 157:1197, 1988

650. Korn JH, Downie E, Roth GJ, Ho S-Y: Synergy of interleukin 1 (IL-1) with arachidonic acid and A23187 in stimulating PGE synthesis in human fibroblasts: IL-1 stimulates fibroblast cyclooxygenase. Clin Immunol Immunopathol 50:196, 1989

651. Bird TA, Saklatvala J: IL-1 and TNF transmodulate epidermal growth factor receptors by a protein kinase C-independent mechanism. J Immunol 142: 126, 1989

652. Howells GL, Chantry D, Feldmann M: Interleukin 1 (IL-1) and tumour necrosis factor synergise in the induction of IL-1 synthesis by human vascular endothelial cells. Immunol Lett 19:169, 1988

653. Wong GH, Goeddel DV: Tumour necrosis factors alpha and beta inhibit virus replication and synergize with interferons. Nature 323:819, 1986

654. Silbertein DS, David JR: Tumor necrosis factor enhances eosinophil toxicity to Schistosoma mansoni larvae. Proc Natl Acad Sci USA 83:1055, 1986

655. Inmaculada E, Mannel D, Ruppel A et al: Interferon gamma and lymphotoxin or tumor necrosis factor act synergistically to induce macrophage killing of tumor cells and schistosomula of Schistosoma mansoni. J Exp Med 166: 589, 1987

656. Chen L, Suzuki Y, Wheelock EF: Interferon-γ synergizes with tumor necrosis factor and with interleukin 1 and requires the presence of both monokines to induce antitumor cytotoxic activity in macrophages. J Immunol 139:4096, 1987

657. Kashiwa H, Wright SC, Bonavida B: Regulation of B cell maturation and differentiation. I. Suppression of pokeweed mitogen-induced B cell differentiation by tumor necrosis factor (TNF). J Immunol 138:1383, 1987

658. Trinchieri G, Rosen M, Perussia B: Retinoic acid cooperates with tumor necrosis factor and immune interferon in inducing differentiation and growth inhibition of the human promyelocytic leukemic cell line HL-60. Blood 69:1218, 1987

659. Tracey KJ, Fong Y, Hesse DG et al: Anti-cachectin/TNF monoclonal antibodies prevent septic shock during lethal bacteraemia. Nature 330:662, 1987

660. Bauss F, Droge W, Mannel DN: Tumor necrosis factor mediates endotoxic effects in mice. Infect Immun 55:1622, 1987

661. Michie HR, Manogue KR, Spriggs DR et al: Detection of circulating tumor necrosis factor after endotoxin administration. N Engl J Med 318:1481, 1988

662. Weinberg JR, Wright DJM, Guz A: Interleukin-1 and tumour necrosis factor cause hypotension in the conscious rabbit. Clin Sci 75:251, 1988

663. Beutler B, Cerami A: Tumor necrosis, cachexia, shock, and inflammation: a common mediator. Annu Rev Biochem 57:505, 1988

664. Mathison JC, Wolfson E, Ulevitch RJ: Participation of tumor necrosis factor in the mediation of gram negative bacterial lipopolysaccharide-induced injury in rabbits. J Clin Invest 81:1925, 1988

665. Hesse DG, Tracey KJ, Fong Y et al: Cytokine appearance in human endotoxemia and primate bacteremia. Surg Gynecol Obstet 166:147, 1988

666. Ulich TR, Guo K, Del Castillo J: Endotoxin-induced cytokine gene expression in vivo: I. Expression of tumor necrosis factor mRNA in visceral organs under physiologic conditions and during endotoxemia. Am J Pathol 134:11, 1989

667. Simmons D, Makgoba MW, Seed B: ICAM, an adhesion ligand of LFA-1, is homologous to the neural cell adhesion molecule NCAM. Nature 331:624, 1988

668. Shlaby MR, Palladino MA, Hirabayashi SE et al: Receptor binding and activation of polymorphonuclear neutrophils by tumor necrosis factor-alpha. J Leuk Biol 41:196, 1987

669. Tsujimoto M, Yokota S, Vilcek J, Weissmann G: Tumor necrosis factor provokes superoxide anion generation from neutrophils. Biochem Biophys Res Commun 137:1094, 1986

670. Perussia B, Kobayashi M, Rossi ME et al: Immune interferon enhances functional properties of human granulocytes: role of Fc receptors and effect of lymphotoxin, tumor necrosis factor, and granulocyte-macrophage colony-stimulating factor. J Immunol 138:765, 1987

671. Klebanoff SJ, Vadas MA, Harlan JM et al: Stimulation of neutrophils by tumor necrosis factor. J Immunol 136:4220, 1986

672. Van Hinsbergh VWM, Kooistra T, Van den Berg EA et al: Tumor necrosis factor increases the production of plasminogen activator inhibitor in human endothelial cells in vitro and in rats in vivo. Blood 72:1467, 1988

673. Medina R, Socher SH, Han JH, Friedman PA: Interleukin-1, endotoxin or tumor necrosis factor/cachectin enhance the level of plasminogen activator inhibitor messenger RNA in bovine aortic endothelial cells. Thromb Res 54: 41, 1989

674. Conway EM, Rosenberg RD: Tumor necrosis factor suppresses transcription of the thrombomodulin gene in endothelial cells. Mol Cell Biol 8:5588, 1988

675. Lowenthal JW, Ballard DW, Böhnlein E, Greene WC: Tumor necrosis factor α induces proteins that bind specifically to kappaB-like enhancer elements and regulate interleukin 2 receptor α-chain gene expression in primary human T lymphocytes. Proc Natl Acad Sci USA 86:2331, 1989

676. Osborn L, Kunkel S, Nabel GJ: Tumor necrosis factor α and interleukin 1 stimulate the human immunodeficiency virus enhancer by activation of the nuclear factor kappaB. Proc Natl Acad Sci USA 86:2336, 1989

677. Vercelli D, Jabara HH, Arai K-I, Geha RS: Induction of human IgE synthesis requires interleukin 4 and T/B cell interactions involving the T cell receptor/CD3 complex and MHC class II antigens. J Exp Med 169:1295, 1989

678. Widmer MB, Grabstein KH: Regulation of cytolytic T-lymphocyte generation by B-cell stimulatory factor. Nature 326:795, 1987

679. Ho SN, Abraham RT, Nison A et al: Interleukin 1-mediated activation of interleukin 4 (IL-4)-producing T lymphocytes. Proliferation by IL-4 dependent and IL-4 independent mechanisms. J Immunol 139:1532, 1987

680. Gallagher G, Wilcox F, Al-Azzawi F: Interleukin-3 and interleukin-4 each strongly inhibit the induction and function of human LAK cells. Clin Exp Immunol 74:166, 1988

681. Hurme M, Palkama T, Sihvola M: Interleukin-4 inhibits interleukin-1 synthesis by a posttranscriptional mechanism. Biochem Biophys Res Commun 157:861, 1988

682. Peschel C, Paul WE, Ohara J, Green I: Effects of B cell stimulatory factor-1/interleukin 4 on hematopoietic progenitor cells. Blood 70:254, 1987

683. Miyaura C, Onozaki K, Akiyama Y et al: Recombinant human interleukin 6 (B-cell stimulatory factor 2) is a potent inducer of differentiation of mouse myeloid leukemia cells (M1). FEBS Lett 234:17, 1988

684. Shabo Y, Lotem J, Rubinstein M et al: The myeloid blood cell differentiation-inducing protein MGI-2A is interleukin-6. Blood 72:2070, 1988

685. Satoh T, Nakamura S, Taga T et al: Induction of neuronal differentiation in PC12 cells by B-cell stimulatory factor 2/interleukin 6. Mol Cell Biol 8:3546, 1988

686. Klein B, Zhang X-G, Jourdan M et al: Paracrine rather than autocrine regulation of myeloma-cell growth and differentiation by interleukin-6. Blood 73: 517, 1989

687. Chiu C-P, Moulds C, Coffman RL et al: Multiple biological activities are expressed by a mouse interleukin 6 cDNA clone isolated from bone marrow stromal cells. Proc Natl Acad Sci USA 85:7099, 1988

688. Ramadori G, Van Damme J, Rieder H, Meyer zum Büschenfelde K-H: Interleukin 6, the third mediator of acute-phase reaction, modulates hepatic protein synthesis in human and mouse. Comparison with interleukin 1 β and tumor necrosis factor-α. Eur J Immunol 18:1259, 1988

689. Koj A, Gordon AH, Gauldie J: An alternative regulatory pathway of the acute phase response: the role of fibroblast-derived interferon-β₂. Experientia 44: 9, 1988

690. Morrone G, Ciliberto G, Oliviero S et al: Recombinant interleukin 6 regulates the transcriptional activation of a set of human acute phase genes. J Biol Chem 263:12554, 1988

691. Ganapathi MK, May LT, Schultz D et al: Role of interleukin-6 in regulating synthesis of C-reactive protein and serum amyloid A in human hepatoma cell lines. Biochem Biophys Res Commun 157:271, 1988

692. Carveth HJ, Bohnsack JF, McIntyre TM et al: Neutrophil activating factor (NAF) induces polymorphonuclear leukocyte adherence to endothelial cells and to subendothelial matrix proteins. Biochem Biophys Res Comm 162: 387, 1989

693. Detmers PA, Li SK, Olsen-Egbert E et al: Neutrophil activating protein 1/interleukin 8 stimulates the binding activity of the leukocyte adhesion receptor CD11b/CD18 on human neutrophils. J Exp Med 171:1155, 1990

694. Paccaud J-P, Schifferli JA, Baggiolini M: NAP-1/IL 8 induces up-regulation of CR1 receptors in human neutrophil leukocytes. Biochem Biophys Res Commun 166:187, 1990

695. White MV, Yoshimura T, Hook W et al: Neutrophil attractant/activation protein 1 (NAP-1) causes human basophil histamine release. Immunol Lett 22: 151, 1989

696. Dahinden CA, Kurimoto Y, DeWeck AL et al: The neutrophil-activating peptide NAF/NAP-1 induces histamine and leukotriene release by interleukin 3-primed basophils. J Exp Med 170:1787, 1989

697. Le J, Lin J-X, Henriksen-DeStefano D, Vilcek J: Bacterial lipopolysaccharide-induced interferon-gamma production: roles of interleukin 1 and interleukin 2. J Immunol 136:4525, 1986

698. Birner A, Hueltner L, Mergenthaler HG et al: Recombinant murine interleukin 9 enhances the erythropoietin-dependent colony formation of human BFU-E. Exp Hematol 20:541, 1992

699. Dugas B, Renauld JC, Pène J et al: Interleukin-9 potentiates the interleukin-4-induced immunoglobulin (IgG, IgM and IgE) production by normal human B lymphocytes. Eur J Immunol 23:1687, 1993

700. Petit-Frere C, Dugas B, Braquet P, Mencia-Huerta JM: Interleukin-9 potentiates the interleukin-4-induced IgE and IgG1 release from murine B lymphocytes. Immunology 79:146, 1993

701. Ulich TR, Del Castillo J, Yi ES et al: Hematologic effects of stem cell factor in vivo and in vitro in rodents. Blood 78:645, 1991

702. Migliaccio G, Migliaccio AR, Druzin ML et al: Effects of recombinant human stem cell factor (SCF) on the growth of human progenitor cells in vitro. J Cell Physiol 148:503, 1991

703. Bodine DM, Orlic D, Birkett NC et al: Stem cell factor increases colony-forming unit-spleen number in vitro in synergy with interleukin-6, and in vivo in Sl/Sl^d mice as a single factor. Blood 79:913, 1992

704. Miyazawa K, Hendrie PC, Kim Y-J et al: Recombinant human interleukin-9 induces protein tyrosine phosphorylation and synergizes with steel factor to stimulate proliferation of the human factor-dependent cell line, M07e. Blood 80:1685, 1992

Biology of Erythropoiesis, Erythroid Differentiation, and Maturation

17

Thalia Papayannopoulou and Janis Abkowitz

INTRODUCTION

The production of erythroid cells is a dynamic and exquisitely regulated process. The mature red cell is only the final phase of a complex but orderly series of genetic events that are initiated at the time a multipotent stem cell becomes committed to express the erythroid program. Expression of the erythroid program occurs several divisions later in a greatly amplified population of erythroid cells, which have a characteristic morphology, maturation sequence, and function. These maturing cells are the erythroid precursor cells and reticulocytes. As these terminally differentiated cells have a finite life span, they are constantly replenished by influx from earlier compartments of a spectrum of cells that are irreversibly committed to express the erythroid phenotype. These erythroid progenitor cells consist of burst-forming unit-erythroid (BFU-E) and colony-forming unit-erythroid (CFU-E). Erythroid progenitors and precursors proliferate and mature at specific anatomic sites (e.g., bone marrow cavities), in which they are in intimate contact with other cells (stromal cells and hematopoietic accessory cells) comprising their microenvironment. Within this microenvironment, erythroid development is influenced by cytokines, which are either elaborated by microenvironmental cells or produced elsewhere and then entrapped in their extracellular matrix.

An understanding of the properties of cells within the various erythroid compartments and their complex interactions with the microenvironment is essential for understanding the pathophysiology of erythropoiesis. Aberrations either in the intrinsic generation and/or amplification of functional erythroid cells or in the regulatory influences of microenvironmental cells or cytokines form the basis for the various disorders, including aplasias, dysplasias, and neoplasias, of the erythroid tissue.

ERYTHROID PROGENITOR CELL COMPARTMENT

The erythroid progenitor cell compartment, occurring functionally between the multipotent stem cell and the morphologically recognizable erythroid precursor cells, contains a spectrum of cells with a parent-to-progeny relationship, all irreversibly committed to erythroid differentiation. Basic understanding of how erythroid commitment is achieved at the biochemical or molecular level is lacking. Evidence from in vitro cultures of single multipotent progenitor cells allowed to differentiate in competent environments, as well as evidence obtained by studying the phenotype of leukemic cells, suggests that commitment to a specific hematopoietic lineage is accomplished not by acquisition of new genetic information but rather by restriction (probably on a stochastic basis) to specific programs from a wider repertoire available to pluripotent progenitor cells.[1,2] Although the irreversible commitment to express the erythroid phenotype is a feature common to all progenitor cells within this compartment, their properties progressively diverge as they become separated by several divisions.

Little direct information is available about the properties of erythroid progenitor cells, as these are both sparse (Table 17-1) and difficult to isolate in sufficient numbers for study. Their existence and characteristics have been inferred from their ability to generate hemoglobinized progeny in vitro in clonal erythroid cultures (Fig. 17-1). Through this approach two classes of progenitors have been identified.[3] The first, more primitive, class consists of the BFU-E, named for their ability to give rise to multiclustered colonies (erythroid bursts) of hemoglobin-containing cells. BFU-E represent the earliest progenitors committed exclusively to erythroid differentiation and a quiescent reserve, since only 10–20% are in cycle at any given time. However, once stimulated to proliferate in the presence of appropriate cytokines, they demonstrate a significant proliferative capacity in vitro, giving rise to colonies of ≥30,000–40,000 cells, which are fully hemoglobinized after 2–4 weeks, with a peak incidence at 14–16 days. They also have a limited self-renewal capacity, since at least a subset of BFU-E is capable of generating bursts when replated in secondary cultures. In contrast to this class of progenitor cells, a second, more differentiated class of progenitors consists of the CFU-E. Most (60–80%) of these progenitors are already in cycle and thus proliferate immediately after initiation of culture to form erythroid colonies within 7 days. Since CFU-E are more differentiated than BFU-E, they require fewer divisions to generate colonies of hemoglobinized cells, and the colonies are small (8–65 cells).

Although the two classes of committed erythroid progenitors, BFU-E and CFU-E, appear distinct from each other, in reality progenitor cells constitute a continuum, with graded changes in their properties. Only progenitor cells at both ends of the differentiation spectrum have distinct properties. Perhaps the earliest cell with the potential to generate hemoglobinized progeny is an oligopotent progenitor, which is capable of giving rise to mature cells of at least one other lineage (granulocytic, macrophage, or megakaryocytic) in addition to the erythroid. This progenitor, a multilineage CFU called CFU-granulocyte/erythrocyte/macrophage/megakaryocyte (GEMM), and the most primitive BFU-E have physical and functional properties that are shared by both pluripotent stem cells and progenitor cells committed to nonerythroid lineages. These properties include high proliferative potential, low rate of cycling, response to several cytokines, and presence of specific surface antigens or surface receptors (Tables 17-1 and 17-2). By contrast, the latest CFU-E have many similarities to erythroid precursor cells and little in common with primitive BFU-E. Their proliferative potential is limited, they cannot self-renew, they lack the cell surface antigens common to all early progenitors, and they are exquisitely sensitive to erythropoietin (EPO) (Tables 17-1 and 17-2).

Although clonal erythroid cultures are indispensable for the study of erythroid progenitors, they do not faithfully reproduce the in vivo kinetics of red cell differentiation/maturation, and many maturing cells have a megaloblastic appearance and lyse before they reach the end stage of red cell development. In vivo, erythropoiesis probably occurs faster than would be pre-

Table 17-1. Erythroid Progenitors: General Properties

	CFU-GEMM	BFU-E	CFU-E
Self-renewal	+ +	+	0
Differentiation potential	Multipotent	Committed to erythropoiesis	Committed to erythropoiesis
Cycling status % suicide with ^{3}H Thymidine	15–20	30–40	60–80
Cell density (g/ml)	<1.077	<1.077	<1.077
Incidence/10^5 cells	2–5	40–120	200–600
Circulate in blood	+	+	0
Growth factor response			
CSF-G, IL-6, IL-1	+[a]	0	0
KL	+	+	+
CSF-GM, IL-3	+	+	+
Erythropoietin	+	+	+ +
Insulin, insulin-like growth factor, activin	0	0	+
TGF-β1	−	−	+ +

[a] These effects include synergistic action.

Table 17-2. Erythroid Progenitors: Surface Antigen/Receptors

Receptor/Antigen	CFU-GEMM	BFU-E	CFU-E
CD34	+ +	+ +	−
CD33	+	+	0
c-kit	+ +	+ +	±
HLA-DR (-DP, -DQ)	+ +	+ +	±
EPO receptor	+	+	+ +
Tumor necrosis factor receptor	+	+	+ +
Ep-1[119]	±	+	+ +
23.6[120a]	0	0	+
CD36	0	0	+
Glycophorin A	0	0, ±	+
ABH, il[b]	0	+	+
Adhesion molecules			
ICAM-1	+ +	+ +	+
HCAM	+	+	
VLA-4	+ +	+ +	+ +
VLA-5	+	+	+ +

[a] 23.6 (SFL 23.6) is a monoclonal antibody reactive with CFU-E, erythroblasts, and erythrocytes.
[b] ABH and il are blood group antigens.

dicted from culture data. For example, studies in dogs with cyclic hematopoiesis, a genetic stem cell defect leading to pulses of hematopoiesis, provide evidence that BFU-E mature to CFU-E over 2–3 days in vivo (Fig. 17-2), although this process may require 5–6 days in canine marrow cultures.[4] Erythroid progenitors can be cultured under serum-depleted conditions,[5] as well as in serum-containing media. Although the effects of recombinant growth factors can be studied in serum-depleted cultures without the complicating influences of multiple or unknown factors present in serum, no physiologic advantage for these conditions can be advocated. However, conditions that imitate the lower oxygen pressures found in bone marrow in vivo do favorably influence erythroid development in culture and may be advantageous.[6]

In vivo

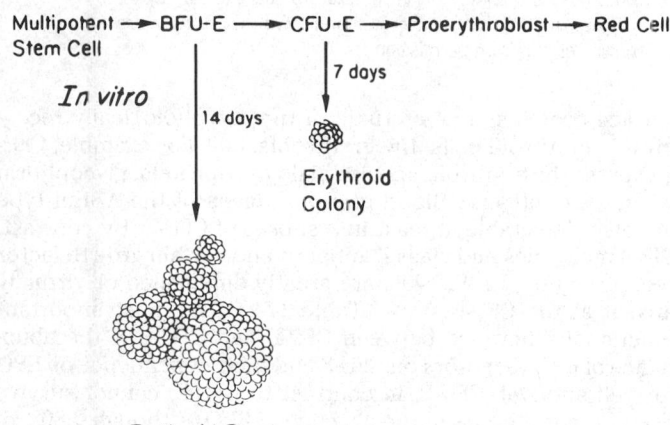

Multipotent → BFU-E → CFU-E → Proerythroblast → Red Cell
Stem Cell

In vitro

7 days

14 days

Erythroid Colony

Erythroid Burst

Fig. 17-1. Erythroid differentiation. BFU-E and CFU-E occur infrequently in the marrow (approximately 0.3% of mononuclear cells) and cannot be distinguished by morphologic or cytochemical techniques. Their existence is inferred by their ability to differentiate in culture. If marrow is placed in semisolid medium (e.g., methylcellulose) to decrease cell motility, with appropriate nutrients and growth factors (e.g., transferrin, insulin, EPO, and IL-3), CFU-E (after approximately 7 days) differentiate into small clusters of hemoglobinized or red cells termed erythroid colonies. Most BFU-E present in the inoculum differentiate to form multiclustered colonies of hemoglobinized cells, erythroid bursts, by days 14–16. Each erythroid colony or burst derives from one CFU-E or BFU-E, respectively.

As BFU-E are generated from the multipotent or oligopotent progenitors within the marrow, they are dependent for their survival and proliferation on the presence of cytokines, elaborated by either stromal cells or immunoregulatory accessory cells within the microenvironment. The most potent of these cytokines is interleukin 3 (IL-3), produced mainly by a subset of T cells.[7] Also, the recently identified kit ligand (KL) has been assigned a dominant role in early erythropoiesis.[8] IL-3 and KL affect the proliferation of all stages of BFU-E. By contrast, other cytokines with proliferative effects on BFU-E, such as colony-stimulating factor-granulocyte/macrophage (CSF-GM) or with ill-defined burst-promoting activities, are capable of stimulating only a subset of IL-3-responsive BFU-E. The defined cytokines (IL-3, CSF-GM, KL) exert their effects through interaction with specific receptors present on the BFU-E surface. The presence of such receptors has also been documented in the leukemic counterparts of normal BFU-E and in leukemic cell lines.[9] BFU-E cannot survive in the absence of cytokines for more than a few days in culture, and if they are deprived of cytokines for >6 days, >80% of them are lost.[10] In addition to positive regulators (IL-3, CSF-GM, or KL), substances with negative influences on BFU-E proliferation have been identified. These include tumor necrosis factor-α, transforming growth factor β, and interferon-γ.[10,12] The latter two factors seem to prevent BFU-E from entering the synthetic (S) phase of the cell cycle. Circulating progenitors along with repopulating stem cells can be mobilized to significant numbers post chemotherapy and/or cytokine treatments. Because of this, their use for transplantation purposes is expanding.

BFU-E and immediate progeny (but not CFU-E) are motile cells and are found in significant numbers in peripheral blood. As with BFU-E, the ability of stem cells and progenitor cells to circulate is physiologically important for the redistribution of marrow cells when there is local damage to the microenvironment and for the reconstitution of hematopoiesis after transplantation. The spectrum of BFU-E in circulation is probably narrower (consisting mostly of early, quiescent BFU-E) than that of BFU-E in the bone marrow, but otherwise their properties are similar to those of marrow BFU-E.

Surface antigens of BFU-E have been explored through the use of monoclonal antibodies.[13,14] The antibodies tested thus far include two broad categories, antibodies raised against leukemic cells or cell lines and antibodies raised against normal, terminally differentiated red cells. Enrichment in BFU-E (or CFU-E) following labeling with these antibodies or their loss after complement-dependent lysis have been considered indic-

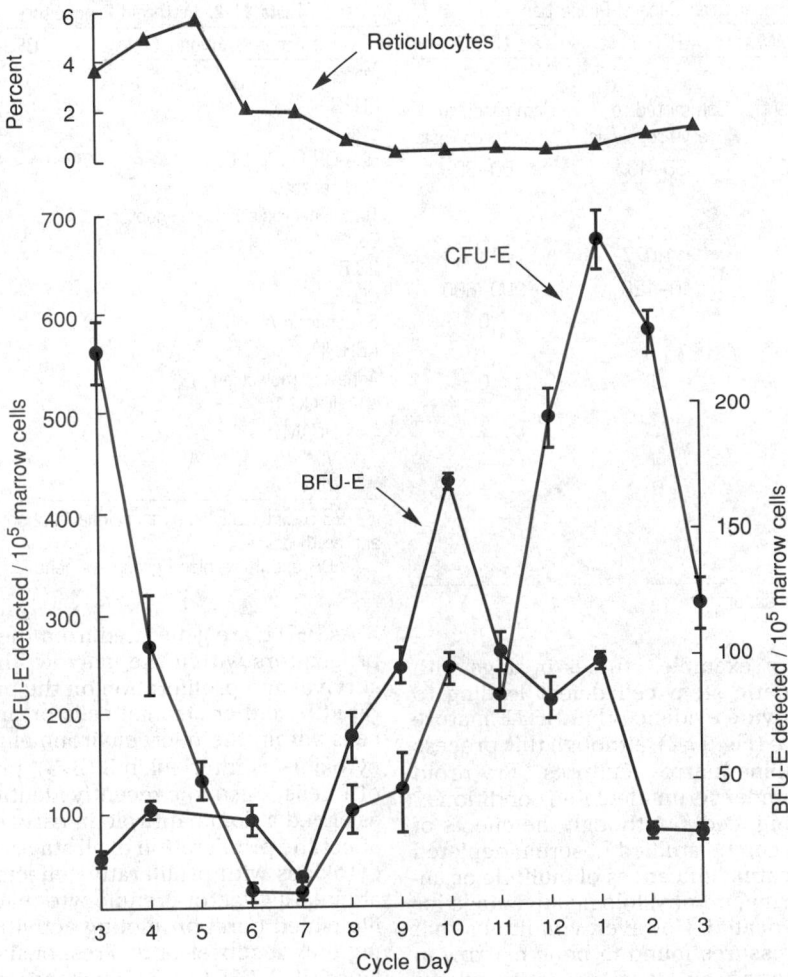

Fig. 17-2. Studies in a gray collie dog with cyclic hematopoiesis, an inherited disorder of hematopoietic stem cells in which granulocytes, monocytes, platelets, and reticulocyte counts fluctuate (or "cycle") at 12-day intervals. It is thought that multipotent stem cells intermittently contribute to hematopoiesis, thus giving rise to pulses of differentiating cells. As shown here, the peak frequency of BFU-E (cycle day 10) occurs 3 days before the peak of CFU-E (cycle day 1), which in turn precedes the peak in the reticulocyte count (cycle day 4). These data confirm that BFU-E are the precursors of CFU-E in vivo and suggest that erythroid differentiation in vivo may occur more quickly than would be predicted from maturation time in culture. (From Abkowitz et al.,[4] with permission.)

ative of the presence of test antigens on the BFU-E surface. Reactivities of BFU-E with several antibodies directed against defined surface antigens are listed in Table 17-2. Like other hematopoietic progenitors, BFU-E display HLA class I and class II antigens on their surface, but class II antigens, especially the products of DR locus, are, in contrast to class I, variably expressed among BFU-E. This may relate to variations in their cycling status, as myeloid progenitors in S phase have been shown to have relatively higher expression of class II antigens.[15] The presence of class II antigens (DR and, to a lesser extent, DP and DQ) most likely allows BFU-E to recognize and interact with the immunoregulatory cells (e.g., T cells, monocytes), which also express class II determinants.[16] In addition to HLA antigens, several other antigenic structures have been found on cells within the BFU-E compartment (Table 17-2). The best representative of these is the CD34 molecule (identified through monoclonal antibody MY10, 12.3, or HPCA1), which has been successfully exploited for the isolation of BFU-E and other progenitors. Its function in hematopoiesis, however, remains unknown. Furthermore, through the use of antibodies or conjugated ligands it was determined that BFU-E present in enriched progenitor preparations display KL, CSF-GM, IL-3, or IL-6 receptors.

As BFU-E mature to the CFU-E stage, they begin to express

surface proteins characteristic of the morphologically recognizable erythroid cells, the erythroblasts.[14] For example, CFU-E express the erythroid-specific sialoglycoprotein, glycophorin A, and Rh antigens. Blood group antigens of the ABH,iI type are also detectable at least in a subset of CFU-E. By contrast, CD34 molecules and class II antigens and certain growth factor receptors (i.e., IL-3R, c-kit) are greatly diminished or virtually absent at the CFU-E stage (Table 17-2). The most important functional difference between BFU-E and CFU-E is the abundance of EPO receptors on CFU-E and their dependence on EPO for cell survival. CFU-E, in contrast to BFU-E, cannot survive even for a few hours in the absence of EPO. Although >80% of CFU-E have detectable EPO receptors,[17] only a small proportion of BFU-E have receptors[18,19] and can terminally differentiate in culture in the presence of EPO alone.[20] Direct binding studies show that the number of EPO receptors peaks at the CFU-E/proerythroblast level and progressively declines when cells mature further[18] (Table 17-2), reflecting the decline in the influence of EPO. In addition to the presence of EPO receptors, erythroid progenitors are distinguished from other marrow progenitors by the presence of abundant transferrin receptors.[19,21,22] The latter play a unique role in iron transport and in hemoglobin synthesis. Peak levels of transferrin receptors are seen on CFU-E and erythroid precursors, and lower levels are present on reticulocytes.[14,21]

ERYTHROID PRECURSOR CELL COMPARTMENT

The erythroid precursor cell compartment, also termed the erythron includes cells that, in contrast to the erythroid progenitor cells (BFU-E and CFU-E), are defined by morphologic criteria. The earliest recognizable erythroid cell is the proerythroblast, which after four to five mitotic divisions and serial morphologic changes gives rise to mature erythroid cells. Its progeny includes basophilic erythroblasts, which are the earliest daughter cells, followed by polychromatophilic and finally orthochromatic erythroblasts. Their morphologic characteristics reflect the accumulation of erythroid-specific proteins (i.e., hemoglobin) and the decline in nuclear activity (Fig. 17-3). After the last mitotic division, the inactive, dense nucleus of the orthochromatic erythroblast moves to one side of the cell and is extruded encased by a thin cytoplasmic layer. Expelled nuclei are ingested by marrow macrophages, and the resulting enucleated cell is a reticulocyte. Although all mammals have enucleated cells in their circulation, the evolutionary advantage of enucleation is not readily apparent. It may allow for more red cell deformability when traveling through the small vasculature or it may minimize the cardiac work load.

It is unlikely that maturation from the proerythroblast to the reticulocyte always adheres to a rigid sequence in which each division is associated with the production of two more differentiated and morphologically distinct daughter cells (i.e., with a basophilic erythroblast giving rise to two polychromatophilic ones). Rather, significant flexibility may be allowed, both in the number and rate of divisions and in the rate of enucleation. Such deviations from the normal, orderly maturation sequence may be dictated by the level of EPO. Thus, when there is an acute demand for red cell production (because of blood loss or hemolysis), the kinetics of formation of new reticulocytes are significantly more rapid. Resulting red cells may be larger (i.e., with increased mean corpuscular volume). This has led to the concept of "skipped" divisions.[23]

The alterations in cell morphology as erythroid precursor cells mature (Fig. 17-3) are determined by complex biochemical changes, which accommodate the accumulation of erythroid-specific proteins and the progressive decline in proliferation. As compared with erythroid progenitor cells, erythroid precursor cells have been more accessible to study, and considerable information is available about their maturation-related biochemical changes.

The shape and deformability of the red cell is determined by its membrane proteins. Most membrane cytoskeletal proteins (spectrin, glycophorin, band 3, band 4.1, and ankyrin) accumulate after the CFU-E stage (i.e., within the precursor cell compartment). Specifically, expression of membrane glycoproteins such as band 3 and band 4.1 is greatly enhanced at the later stages of erythroid maturation.[24,25] Likewise, the quantity of polylactosaminoglycan, a specific carbohydrate chain that carries blood group ABH and ii antigenic determinants, is much higher in mature erythrocytes than in erythroblasts.[26] Whereas a linear, virtually unbranched polylactosamine structure is present in fetal and newborn erythroid cells (reflected by i antigenic reactivity), a branched polylactosaminyl structure is present in adult erythroblasts (reflected by I antigenic reactivity), and branching increases further as maturation progresses.[26] Glycophorins, especially glycophorin A, are expressed fully at the CFU-E or proerythroblast level just before the expression of globin, and there are few changes during maturation.[14] By contrast, the membrane glycoproteins p105 and p95 decline during the later stages of maturation,[26] and yet other membrane glycoproteins, such as vimentin (an intermediate filament protein) are totally lost.[24] The loss of vimentin expression at the late erythroblastic stages most likely facilitates enucleation.

In addition to quantitative changes during maturation, there are gradual switches in subunit composition of some cytoskeletal proteins. For example, exclusively erythroid subunits of α- and β-spectrin are displayed only in end-stage cells.[25] Likewise, multiple transcripts of ankyrin or protein 4.1 have been identified and the ratios of these transcripts found to change during maturation.[27] It is likely that the initial expression of many of these membrane components begins at the progenitor cell level. In these cells, however, final assembly may be discouraged because of the higher turnover of these proteins, which minimizes mutual interactions, or because of asynchrony in their synthesis. Prevention of cytoskeletal assembly at these early stages may secure more membrane fluidity and cell motility needed during this proliferative phase of differentiation. Since molecular probes for many of the red cell cytoskeletal components have been developed, detailed information about the transcription and processing of these proteins should soon be available.

Gene activity during erythroid maturation is dominated by the expression of globin. Although globin represents <0.1% of protein at the proerythroblast level, it reaches 95% of all protein at the level of reticulocytes.[28] Its expression has been extensively studied, and it is one of the better understood proteins of red cells in molecular terms. Major steps in its transcription and processing are now known in considerable detail and are summarized elsewhere in this volume. The globin type synthesized by the adult precursors is hemoglobin (Hb) A $(\alpha_2\beta_2)$. In addition, two other minor globin components, Hb A$_2$ $(\alpha_2\delta_2)$ and Hb F $(\alpha_2\gamma_2)$, are present. Of significant biologic interest are the low amounts of Hb F that continue to be synthesized throughout life.

This small amount of Hb F, which is present in all normal individuals, has the following characteristics[29]: (1) It is confined to a small fraction of red cells, called F cells, which are detected by sensitive immunofluorescence assays or acid elution techniques and usually constitute 2–5% of all red cells. Within each F cell, Hb F (or γ-globin) constitutes 14–25% of total globin. (2) The number of F cells is genetically determined, and gene(s) linked or nonlinked to the β-locus are responsible for F-cell formation. (3) F cells do not display other features of "fetalness," since their membrane components and enzymes are characteristically adult. (4) Synthesis of Hb F peaks earlier than that of Hb A so that the proportion of fetal hemoglobin is higher in immature cells compared with mature, fully hemoglobinized cells. (5) F cells and cells that contain only Hb A are not derived from distinct stem cell populations but from a common adult stem cell. Whether this cell will form F or non-F (i.e., A) cells is determined at the BFU-E and throughout the CFU-E level. In vitro the great majority of BFU-E have the potential to express Hb F, whereas in vivo only a very small proportion of red cells contain Hb F; this potential appears to be gradually lost during normal cell differentiation and maturation in vivo. This concept links the potential for Hb F expression to the pathway of erythroid differentiation and thus may have implications for interpreting the reactivation of Hb F that occurs in adults under diverse circumstances (e.g., after chemotherapy or with acute bleeding).[29] Many of these circumstances seem to influence Hb F levels by directly or indirectly modifying the kinetics of the normal differentiation/maturation process.[30,31]

The synthesis of globin appears to be coordinated with the synthesis of heme throughout erythroid maturation, so that functional hemoglobin tetramers are formed rapidly and spontaneously after the release of newly synthesized globins from polysomes. Information about the accumulation of heme and its synthetic intermediaries has been provided thus far by

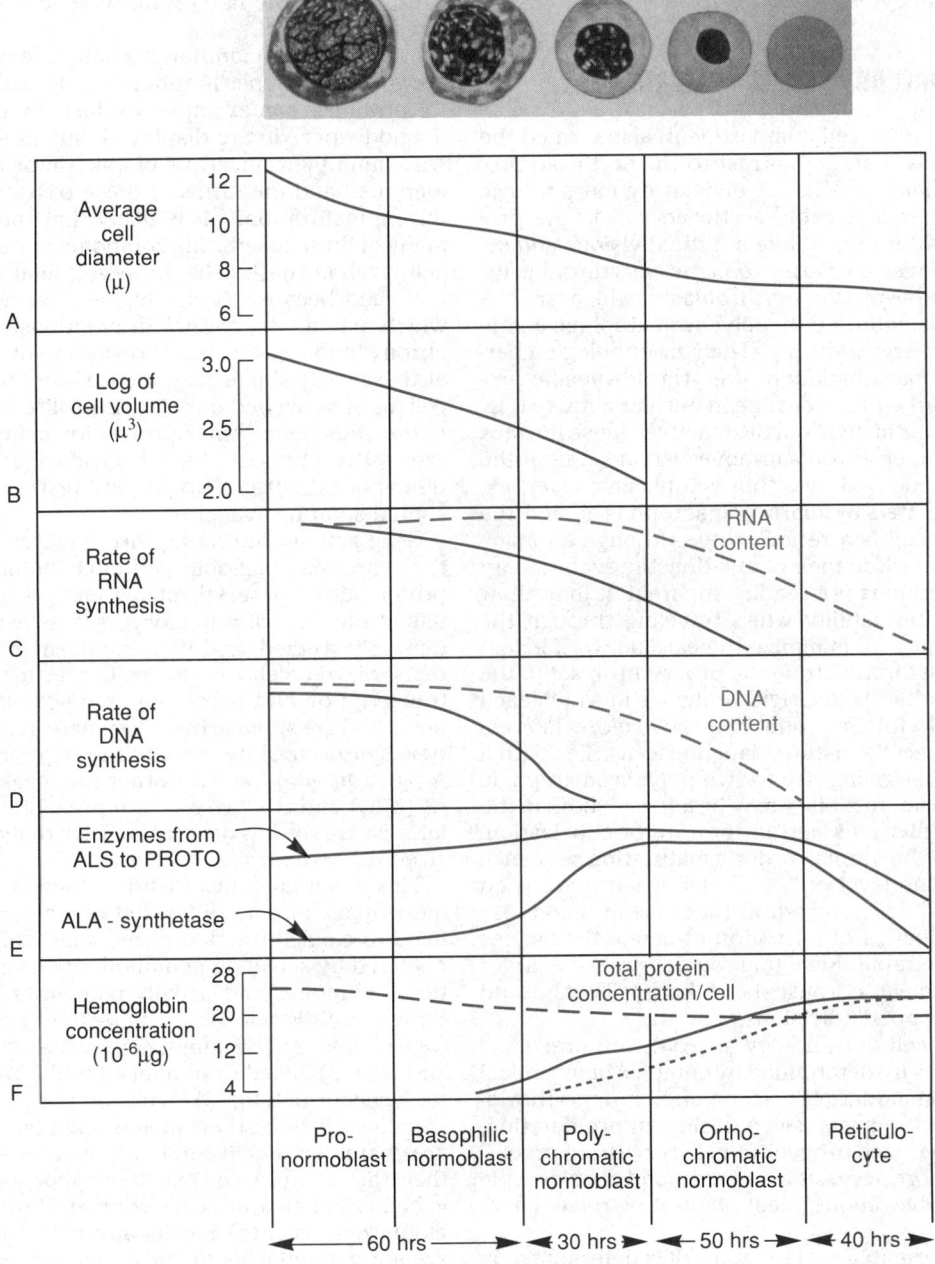

Fig. 17-3. Erythroid maturation sequence. As proliferation parameters (i.e., rates of DNA and RNA synthesis) and cell size decrease, accumulation of erythroid-specific proteins (i.e., heme and globin) increases, and the cells adapt their characteristic morphology. (Adapted from Granick and Levere,[122] with permission.)

crude biochemical approaches (Fig. 17-3). However, as the genes for several enzymes in the heme synthetic pathway have now been cloned (i.e., genes for δ-aminolevulinic acid synthetase, porphobilinogen deaminase, and heme synthetase), future studies will shed more light on their transcriptional regulation and processing as erythroid maturation progresses. In this context it is intriguing that the erythroid DNA-binding factor NF-E2, which presumably regulates high hemoglobin output, is also linked to iron trafficking.[32]

Crucial to the functional response of erythroid precursors is the expression of EPO receptors and of transferrin receptors. EPO receptors decrease progressively (from about 1,000 to <300 receptors/percell) as proerythroblasts mature, and they

are undetectable at the reticulocyte level.[17,33] Through these receptors, EPO exerts its proliferative influence on proerythroblasts and basophilic erythroblasts, but maturation beyond these stages can proceed in the absence of EPO.

Transferrin receptors are found in characteristic abundance in erythroid cells (300–800,000/cell).[34] This is a reflection not only of the proliferative needs of erythroid cells but also of their extreme requirements for iron for hemoglobin synthesis. It is for this reason that transferrin receptors persist in maturing, nondividing erythroblasts and in reticulocytes. Transferrin receptors belong to a large group of receptors that internalize their ligand through the general pathway of receptor-mediated endocytosis. This cycle allows for reutilization both of the ligand (transferrin) to be resaturated with iron and of the receptor to enter an additional route of endocytosis.[35] Transferrin receptor density decreases with maturation, and after the reticulocyte stage, receptors appear to be shed as small lipid vesicles.[36] There is an inverse relationship between receptor density and the availability of iron. Deprivation of iron results in receptor induction, and excess iron results in receptor suppression.[35] However, the mechanisms that regulate the number of transferrin receptors throughout the maturation of precursors (even within progenitors) are largely unknown. Evidence has been recently presented that erythroid cells differ from nonerythroid cells not only by requiring a higher number and higher occupancy of transferrin receptors but by displaying immunologically distinct receptor isoforms.[22] Whether the antigenically distinct form of transferrin receptor in erythroid cells is of physiologic significance to the unique role of erythroid cells in iron metabolism remains to be seen. However, monoclonal antibodies recognizing distinct receptor isoforms are useful in the isolation of erythroid cells from bone marrow.[22,37]

ERYTHROPOIETIN AND THE ERYTHROID DIFFERENTIATION/MATURATION PROCESS

EPO, a 35-kd glycoprotein,[38] is an obligatory growth factor for erythroid development. It is produced in the kidney, presumably by peritubular cells.[39] A heme-containing protein senses oxygen need and then triggers the synthesis of EPO and its release into the bloodstream.[40] Through the interaction of EPO with receptor-bearing cells within the bone marrow, physiologic oxygen demands are translated into increased red cell production. Thus, EPO is a true hormone, manufactured at one anatomic site and transported through the bloodstream to the site of activity.

According to the prevailing model of hematopoiesis, progenitor cells committed to erythroid differentiation (i.e., BFU-E) are generated in a stochastic fashion from pluripotent stem cells.[1] Neither EPO nor other lineage-restricted regulators play any role in determining lineage commitment. According to this model, EPO influences erythroid differentiation by rescuing cells that express the EPO receptor and amplifying them further. Whether EPO receptors are present on all BFU-E (although only detectable on a subset of BFU-E) is not clear.[18] Thus, it is not known whether the presence of the EPO receptor in BFU-E is synchronous with the initial commitment event or follows it. In addition to the permissive role that the stochastic theory ascribes to EPO, experiments in vivo, in anemic states, or after pharmacologic doses of EPO, suggest that high levels of EPO, may hasten the transition from BFU-E to hemoglobin-synthesizing cells either by decreasing the number of divisions required for this transition[23] or by decreasing the resting periods between cell divisions.[41] Autoradiographic studies in purified BFU-E populations indicate that EPO receptors increase as BFU-E mature to CFU-E, with the highest level observed at the CFU-E/proerythroblast boundary.[18] As the transition from BFU-E to CFU-E occurs under the influence of EPO, it may suggest ligand (EPO)-induced receptor up-regulation. Whether the magnitude of such up-regulation is EPO dose dependent and whether it can modulate the rate of entry of these cells into the maturing compartment is unclear.

Although a direct inductive role for EPO in BFU-E differentiation remains to be established, CFU-E proliferate and are triggered to terminal maturation when exposed to EPO. Thus, in these cells EPO seems to stimulate all the biochemical processes characterizing erythroid cells (i.e., heme synthesis, globin synthesis, and synthesis of cytoskeletal proteins). However, the precise role of EPO in these processes has not been determined. Whether EPO only increases the number of cells

engaged in these biochemical functions or directly influences the intracellular mechanism of transcription of erythroid-specific proteins is unclear. Indeed, experiments in vitro showing complete maturation of BFU-E in the absence of EPO suggest that other factors or combination of factors can influence red cell maturation (such as insulin, insulin-like growth factors, activin).[42-44] It is possible that the biochemical and morphologic changes are predictable consequences of erythroid cell proliferation if these cells are allowed to survive and complete a certain number of divisions. In all previous studies temporal correlations between exposure to EPO and initiation of biochemical changes—before cell division occurs—have been compromised by the cell's prior in vivo exposure to EPO. Experiments on appropriate target cells (i.e., BFU-E) in the absence of prior internalization of EPO and with the use of newer molecular approaches are required for firm conclusions.

Whatever the precise mode of EPO action, it directly affects the number of CFU-E and the maturation of their progeny. This control is achieved by influencing CFU-E survival and not their cycling status.[43] CFU-E are irrevocably lost after one cycle of DNA synthesis if EPO is not present.[44a]

With the availability of radiolabeled recombinant EPO and of purified or enriched populations of progenitors and precursors, information about the characteristics of EPO receptors in erythroid cells is continuously emerging. Direct binding studies have shown that as CFU-E and proerythroblasts mature to reticulocytes, there is a progressive decrease in the number of EPO receptors.[18,19,33] Pure reticulocyte populations show no detectable binding to EPO. The maturation-associated decline in the number of EPO receptors parallels the declining influence of EPO on erythroid cells during the terminal phase of maturation. Whether the receptor complex consists of more than one subunit or of more than one protein species, or both, is currently under investigation. In addition, recent studies show that the EPO receptor in early progenitors differs qualitatively compared with late progenitors.[45] In early progenitors, a truncated form of EPO receptor, arising by alternative splicing, is displayed. This type of receptor has greatly reduced function compared with the full-length EPO receptor mRNA present in later progeny (CFU-E). As a result, the cellular responses elicited by EPO (survival, proliferation, differentiation) may depend on the stage of differentiation of erythroid cells and may be qualitatively different in the two populations of cells.

The intracellular events that follow the binding of EPO to its receptor are not fully understood. In addition to early effects on RNA synthesis, DNA synthesis, cell division, iron uptake, and hemoglobin synthesis, several other cellular processes are stimulated.[43] These include acetylation and methylation of nuclear proteins, incorporation of glucosamine, transmembrane calcium fluxes, and production of cyclic nucleotides. Elevated cAMP levels were observed in EPO-stimulated cells by some investigators but not by others. Effects of EPO on cGMP seem to be secondary to EPO-induced cell cycle changes. Undoubtedly several of these effects are secondary to the EPO-induced activation of an initial, yet to be defined, signal transduction pathway. Studies on the signaling pathway of EPO receptor following binding to its ligand have suggested that tyrosine-phosphorylation is involved, based on changes in the phosphorylation state of specific proteins and of the EPO receptor itself.[46] Specifically, EPO induces the tyrosine-phosphorylation of JAK-2 kinase and a correlation between tyrosine-phosphorylation and EPO-induced mitogenesis has been found.[47] Recent molecular studies of the EPO receptor have provided additional insights. EPO mutations in the extracellular domain of the EPO receptor have been found to lead to EPO-independent proliferation of cells in vitro.[46a] Mutations, however, in the cytoplasmic region lead to EPO hypersensitivity in vitro.[49] It is intriguing that a similar mutation in humans giving rise to a truncated protein was thought to be responsible for autosomal dominant familiar erythrocytosis.[50] EPO-receptor expression is not entirely restricted to erythroid cells. Megakaryocytes, lymphocytes, and endothelial cells, as well as placental cells in mice and rats, have been reported to express EPO receptor. Their function, however, in these cells is unclear.

TRANSCRIPTIONAL FACTORS IN ERYTHROPOIESIS

It is widely believed that lineage-specific transcriptional factors are responsible for regulating the expression of erythroid genes during both development and the erythroid differentiation process. Experiments with somatic cell fusions and with transgenic mice have provided compelling evidence for this belief.[49–51] Recent studies using terminally differentiated cells, leukemic cells of different lineages and, more importantly, studies in mice with gene disruption have identified trans-acting elements and proto-oncogenes that are essential for erythroid development. Most notable among these factors are the GATA family of transcriptional factors (GATA-1, GATA-2, GATA-3) and NF-E2, a factor important for the function of the locus control region that regulates globin gene expression.[52] The GATA protein family of factors interacts with the WGATAR DNA motif frequently found in erythroid genes. Both GATA-1 and GATA-2 are expressed early in multipotential progenitors; however, their expression ratios change as the cells differentiate, suggesting that the ratio of these two factors may be important at specific stages of erythroid differentiation.[53,54] In mice with gene-targeted deletions, both GATA-1 and GATA-2 have been found to be indispensable for normal red cell development, although other lineages appear to mature properly. As GATA-1 and GATA-2 are present in nonerythroid cells (i.e., megakaryocytes, mast cells, eosinophils, or cell lines with different phenotypic features) the precise role of these factors in erythroid cells compared to other cells is not clear. Thus, how the erythroid specificity is being achieved or what governs the initial activation of GATA-1 in multipotential progenitors, or its upregulation in erythroid cells, remain to be elucidated. Some in vitro experiments suggest that certain oncogenes (i.e., c-erb A, c-ets) may be involved in the initial activation of GATA factors in early progenitors. Consistent with this view is that c-myb[55] or Rb gene[56] ablation in mice was accompanied by failure to establish erythropoiesis. Furthermore, since there is no selective activation of GATA proteins in erythroid cells, it is possible that the presence of other factors or that sequences surrounding the GATA-binding sites in erythroid cells are important determinants of the GATA function.[57] Thus, the association of GATA-1 with other, more promiscuous, DNA-binding proteins (i.e., A-1 or AP-1) may be important for achieving transactivation of erythroid genes. It is also likely that GATA-1 may be involved in the displacement of specific or nonspecific repressors and the establishment of stable initiation complexes within erythroid cells.

Thus, the emerging picture in erythropoiesis is that certain genes (i.e., c-myb, GATA-2) have to be active in early, proliferating progenitors, and are responsible for their expansion, whereas others are necessary to direct high levels of expression of erythroid-specific genes (i.e., GATA-1, SCL,[58] NF-E2[59]. Failure to activate both types of genes can lead to death at respective stages or erythroid cell development. According to this scheme, what is unique in erythroid cells, at early or later stages of differentiation, is the combination of factors expressed rather than any one particular factor. As research in this area has already gained a significant momentum, the order of regulatory events in erythroid differentiation and the hierarchy in expression of specific transcriptional factors during this process should be delineated in the near future.

HEMATOPOIETIC MICROENVIRONMENT

In invertebrates such as worms and sessile marine creatures, erythropoiesis takes place adjacent to peritoneal and endothelial cells. In premammalian species the spleen is the primary site of erythropoiesis, and with evolutionary advancement this gradually shifts to the liver and the sinusoidal cavities of bones.[3] These observations suggest that sufficient oxygen, a stagnated flow of blood to avoid dispersion of factors produced locally, and extensive and redundant surfaces for cell-cell interactions may be essential. Similar sites support erythropoiesis during human development. During phylogeny and ontogeny the liver and spleen are primarily erythropoietic organs, while granulocytic cells are dominant in bone marrow.[3] Studies in mice indicate that BFU-E and CFU-E are not randomly distributed within bone cavities.[3] Thus, elements of the local anatomy or a specific hematopoietic microenvironment may influence the regulation of erythropoiesis.

Such an influence is exemplified in the Steel mouse model, in which there is a genetic defect of KL production.[8,60] Although S1/S1 mice die in utero with anemia, mice with an allelic variant of the Steel mutation (S1/S1^d) are viable but severely anemic. When marrow cells from S1/S1^d animals are transplanted into irradiated normal recipients, they can reconstitute normal hematopoiesis, demonstrating that S1/S1^d progenitor cells function appropriately. However, anemia persists after transplantation of normal marrow cells into S1/S1^d recipients, which suggests that the defect is host derived and resides in structural, not easily transplantable microenvironmental cells.[61] Subsequent studies have shown that murine, and human, marrow stromal cells produce KL.[8] Human transplantation studies have demonstrated that certain microenvironmental cells (e.g., macrophages, monocytes, T cells) are of hematopoietic cell origin and thus derive from donor cells, while fibroblasts, endothelial cells, adipocytes, and smooth muscle cells, which constitute the structural components of the microenvironment, are of host origin.[62,63] In addition to the cellular components, an integral part of the hematopoietic microenvironment is the extracellular matrix, a protein-carbohydrate scaffolding, which is laid down by microenvironmental cells and fills the spaces between them.[64] Although microenvironmental influence is defined through in vivo studies of mice, dissection of the cellular components of the microenvironment, definition of the cytokines elaborated, and elaboration of the nature of cell-cell interactions require an in vitro model. Long-term marrow cultures provide an experimental method that allows such studies.[65] Under these conditions murine hematopoiesis may be maintained for several months. A stromal (adherent) layer consisting of fibroblasts, adipocytes, and macrophages is a crucial component of this culture system. Islands of differentiating hematopoietic cells appear adjacent to stromal cells. As hematopoiesis occurs in "niches" rather than diffusely throughout the culture, interactions of several cell types are required for optimal differentiation. In human long-term bone marrow cultures, early erythroid progenitors (BFU-E) usually persist for a few (2–10) weeks and are more prevalent among adherent cells than in the nonadherent cell pool.[66] Adherent BFU-E are generally quiescent (not actively cycling). Because of the lack of EPO, CFU-E and subsequent red cell maturation are not seen in murine or human cultures; however, when EPO is added, terminal erythroid maturation proceeds.[65] It is also possible that other factors absent in stromal layers, or whose production is suppressed by the corticosteroids added to these cultures, are important.

Studies of the interactions of stromal cells with hematopoietic progenitors suggest a complex regulation mediated through several mechanisms.[16] Marrow-derived stromal cells, as well as endothelial cells and fibroblasts, elaborate cytokines such as CSF-GM, CSF-G, IL-1, IL-6, KL, activin-A, or basic fibroblast growth factor, which influence, alone and in combination, the growth of all marrow progenitors.[66,67] In addition to these positive regulators, these cells are capable of elaborating factors such as transforming growth factor-β, interferon-γ, and tumor necrosis factor, which exert a negative influence on proliferation and may help to maintain a dormant state in progenitors. Since some of these negative regulators may inhibit differentiation along certain lineages but not others, there is an intriguing possibility that lineage-specific regulation within the microenvironment may be achieved through negative rather than positive factors.[11] Because of the close proximity of stromal and progenitor cells, the latter are exposed to high concentrations of these growth factors. Thus, such interactions, as well as direct stromal cell-progenitor cell contact, may influence the balance between self-renewal and differentiation.[65-68]

The extracellular matrix that surrounds the stromal cells also influences erythropoiesis. This matrix contains proteoglycans, glycoproteins with glycosaminoglycan side chains (such as chondroitan sulfate), and heparan sulfate.[64] The glycosaminoglycan moieties have been shown to bind cytokines such as IL-3, CSF-GM, and EPO and may help to concentrate these factors within the microenvironment.[68,69] In addition to grounding the growth factor components, the extracellular matrix itself may directly influence lineage-specific development. Fibronectin, a glycoprotein produced by fibroblasts, is universally present in long-term marrow cultures and sections of bone marrow. Erythroid progenitors, specifically late BFU-E and CFU-E (but not CFU-GM), attach to fibronectin via its RGD (Arg-Gly-Asp) cell recognition domain.[70] By contrast, hemonectin, a second extracellular matrix glycoprotein first described in 1987, is associated with granulocytic adherence.[71] More recent data suggest that fibronectin also stimulates erythroid (but not granulocytic) maturation.[70] Fibronectin may therefore be important for the "homing" of circulating early BFU-E to appropriate sites in the marrow or for the retention of erythroid precursor cells to complete their maturation, or for both processes.[72] With terminal erythroid maturation, however, the surface expression of these adhesion molecules decreases, and fibronectin receptors, for example, are no longer present in reticulocytes, which are freely released into the circulation.[70] Other adhesion molecules in the extracellular matrix or on the surface of fibroblasts or endothelial cells have been defined that bind ligands on progenitor cells.[62,73-75] Although these interactions help to direct the geography and physiology of erythropoiesis within the marrow space, their physiologic relevance has not been demonstrated in vivo.

Besides stromal cells, accessory cells of hematopoietic origin (monocytes, macrophages, and lymphocytes) are active participants in the microenvironment.[76] Each can elaborate cytokines that directly or indirectly affect erythroid differentiation. T cells may have a unique role in IL-3 production. Negative regulators such as interferon-γ or lymphotoxin are all products of activated lymphocytes or natural killer (NK) cells. Other cytokines (IL-1 and IL-6) produced by accessory cells may mediate growth factor production by stromal cells and vice versa. T lymphocytes or NK cells may also influence erythropoiesis through cell-cell contacts. These influences may require HLA-DR (HLA class II) recognition of target (progenitor) cells by T cells (CD4+ or CD8+).[16] Interactions of T cells with macrophages leading to amplification of cytokine production may also be HLA class II-restricted. In addition, intercellular adhesion molecule, ICAM-1, present in BFU-E and CFU-GM, is the ligand for LFA-1, a receptor on the surface of macrophages, T cells, and NK cells.[77] These products of the integrin gene family are also involved in the cell-matrix and cell-cell interactions. A special relationship between marrow macrophages and erythroid cells had been recognized long before the nature of cytokines elaborated by macrophages was established. In sections of normal marrow, islands of maturing erythroblasts surround a central macrophage.[78] These macrophages, termed nurse cells, have

cytoplasmic processes in direct contact with developing red cells and have more mature cells at the periphery within erythroblastic islands.[78] The exact role of the nurse cells is not known. As tissue macrophages express mRNA for EPO, local as well as systemic (renal) production of EPO may contribute to the regulation of erythropoiesis.[79] In long-term marrow cultures, areas of erythropoiesis also contain central macrophages.

Interactions of erythroid cells, accessory cells, and stromal cells are complex. The microenvironment does not serve as a passive surface for adherence of progenitor and precursor cells but rather exerts a crucial and interactive role in the differentiation and maturation of red cells.

ONTOGENY OF ERYTHROPOIESIS

During human development different anatomic areas for production of erythroid cells are recruited sequentially, with a temporal succession that allows overlapping (Fig. 17-4). In addition, there are parallel changes in the morphology and functional properties of the erythroid cells themselves.

As in all mammals, erythropoiesis in humans is initiated outside the embryo and arises from the mesoderm in the blood islands of the yolk sac.[80] During this phase of embryonic erythropoiesis, aggregates of immature erythroid cells go through maturation synchronously as a single cohort. Before their maturation is completed, they begin to circulate, and by the fifth gestational week they are found in the vascular spaces of the rudimentary liver (Fig. 17-5). At about the same time, foci of immature erythroid cells emerge within the fetal liver as the fetal, or hepatic phase of erythropoiesis commences.[81] The stem cells from which the fetal phase of erythropoiesis is established are thought to have migrated to the liver from the yolk sac rather than to have been generated de novo in the fetal liver.[82] From the seventh week onward the liver is progressively filled with erythroid precursors and becomes the dominant site of erythroid cell production until about the 30th gestational week. Although some red cell production can be found in the thymus, the spleen, or occasionally in the lymph nodes, these other sites are never dominant. From the sixth month onward the cavities of long bones are invaded by vascular sprouts and become competent to support red cell development. At birth all bone cavities are actively engaged in erythroid production, and the hepatic (fetal) phase of erythropoiesis comes to an end, as the final (adult) phase of erythropoiesis unfolds exclusively within the bone marrow.

In addition to the anatomic shifts in the sites of erythropoiesis, there are associated shifts in the phenotypic characteristics of erythroid cells. Embryonic erythroid cells (derived from the yolk sac) are large (about 200 μm), retain their nuclei at terminal stages of maturation, and have a megaloblastic appearance (Fig. 17-5). Fetal erythroid cells (produced in the fetal liver and later in fetal bone marrow spaces) are smaller than embryonic cells (about 125 μm) but have a macrocytic appearance when compared with adult, normocytic red cells (about 80 μm). Like adult cells, however, they eject their nuclei during maturation.

Apart from variations in size and morphology, embryonic and fetal erythroid cells differ from each other and from their adult counterparts in several other characteristics, including hormonal requirements, proliferative potential, and cellular composition. For example, whereas fetal erythropoiesis is under the control of EPO,[83] the nature of EPO's influence on embryonic erythropoiesis has not been established.[84,85] EPO levels increase between the 9th and the 32nd week of gestation, and fetuses respond to hypoxia or anemia with increased EPO as early as 24 weeks. Fetal erythroid progenitors when studied in vitro appear more sensitive to EPO than do adult progenitors; by contrast, their in vitro response to lymphokines (e.g., IL-3 or CSF-GM) is minimal compared with that of adult ery-

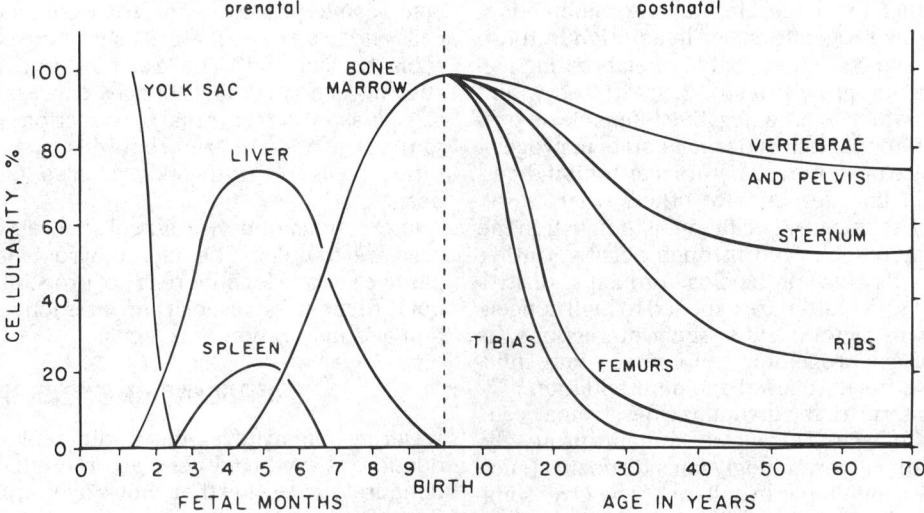

Fig. 17-4. Sites of hematopoiesis during fetal development and after birth. Only erythroid cells, and possibly lymphocytes, are generated by the yolk sac and early embryo. Significant megakaryopoiesis and granulopoiesis develop at 4–5 months. After birth, hematopoiesis occurs in the sinusoidal cavities of the tibias, femurs, and axial skeleton. (Adapted from Erslev and Gabuzda,[123] with permission.)

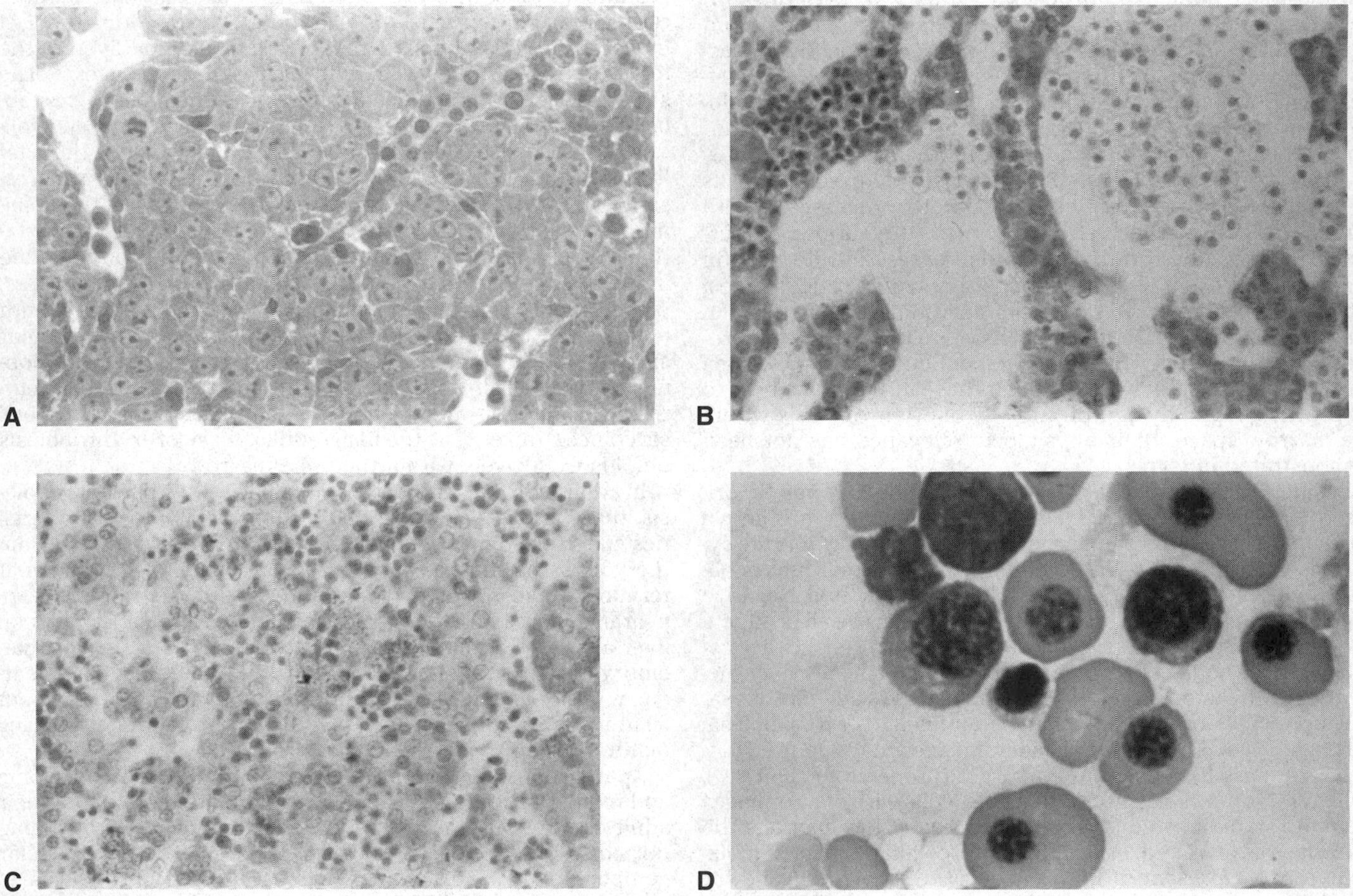

Fig. 17-5. (A) Section of an 8-mm embryo depicting a portion of hepatic parenchymal cells with embryonic erythroblasts present within primitive sinusoidal cavities. **(B)** At 6–8 weeks, discrete aggregates of definitive erythroblasts appear within the liver parenchyma, whereas mature embryonic erythroblasts persist in well-developed sinusoids (PAS stain). **(C)** Later on definitive erythroblasts are spread throughout the liver (100-day fetus) (PAS stain). **(D)** Cytologic spread from disaggregated fetal liver cells of a 55-day embryo. The characteristic morphology of embryonic erythroblasts and immature (basophilic) definitive erythroblasts is shown.

throid progenitors.[86,87] It is noteworthy that in the early stages of fetal liver erythropoiesis, only erythroid differentiation/maturation is promoted.[88] Although progenitors committed to other lineages are abundant in the fetal liver, very few mature cells from other lineages (granulocytes, megakaryocytes, or monocytes) are seen. In addition to their heightened sensitivity to EPO, fetal erythroid progenitors and precursors are characterized by high proliferative potential and shorter doubling times than adult cells when cultured in vitro.[87,88] Furthermore, the enzymatic activity of several enzymes in the glycolytic pathway is greater in fetal than in adult red cells.[89] By contrast, carbonic anhydrase levels are very low during intrauterine and early neonatal life.[90] Distinct isozyme patterns for several enzymes (phosphoglycerate kinase, acetylcholinesterase, etc.) also distinguish fetal from adult red cells.[91,92]

The surface antigenic profiles of erythroid cells are distinct at each ontogenic stage. For example, HLA class I and class II antigens are not detected in embryonic erythroid progenitor cells but reach adult levels about the ninth week of gestation.[93] Furthermore, fetal BFU-E and CFU-E express similar levels of HLA class II antigens, whereas adult CFU-E are largely devoid of these antigens.[93,94] Fetal red cells display on their surface a straight, unbranched polylactosaminyl chain (i antigen), whereas this structure, which bears ABH blood group determinants, is highly branched in adult cells (I antigen).[26]

The most widely studied changes during red cell ontogeny are the shifts or "switches" in globin types. Embryonic erythroblasts are characterized by their avid accumulation of iron, which is stored as ferritin[95] (0.3–1% of total protein) and by the synthesis of the unique hemoglobins Gower I ($\zeta_2\epsilon_2$), Gower II ($\alpha_2\epsilon_2$), and Hb Portland ($\zeta_2\gamma_2$). The ζ- and ϵ-globin chains are embryonic α-like and β-like chains, respectively.[29] These three embryonic types of hemoglobin are most likely synthesized in succession, as the concentration of Gower I is highest in smaller embryos. Thus, a switch from ζ- to α- and ϵ- to γ-globin gene production is initiated during the embryonic phase of erythropoiesis but is not complete until fetal erythropoiesis is well established. During the transition from yolk sac to fetal liver erythropoiesis (6–9 weeks), erythroid precursors within the fetal liver co-express embryonic (ζ- or ϵ-) and fetal (α-, γ-) globin both in vivo and in vitro.[96,97] The predominant type of hemoglobin synthesized during fetal liver erythropoiesis is Hb F ($\alpha_2\gamma_2$), with a high proportion of Gγ (Gγ Aγ = 7:3). Adult hemoglobin A ($\alpha_2\beta_2$), detectable at the earliest stages of fetal liver erythropoiesis, is also synthesized as a minor component throughout this period, but Hb A_2 ($\alpha_2\delta_2$), a minor hemoglobin in the adult, is undetectable in these early stages. From about the 30th gestational week onwards, β-globin synthesis steadily increases, so that by term 50–55% of hemoglobin synthesized is Hb A. By 4–5 weeks of postnatal age, 75% of the hemoglobin is Hb A, the proportion increasing to 95% by 4 months as the fetal-to-adult hemoglobin switch is completed. Hb F levels in circulating red cells are in a plateau for the first 2–3 weeks (owing to the decline in total erythropoiesis that follows birth), but Hb F gradually declines, so that normal levels (<1%) are achieved by 200 days after birth.[98]

Several in vitro and in vivo approaches have been used to study the basis of globin switching through development. Beyond its biologic interest, rigorous research in this area was propelled by the possibility of manipulating globin switching to ameliorate the clinical symptoms of disorders of the β-globin locus (e.g., sickle cell anemia, thalassemia). Transplantation experiments and ablative endocrine maneuvers in the sheep model have failed to provide convincing support for effects of environmental or humoral factors on the switching process, although some modulation of the rate of switching was seen in these models.[99,100] The most important determinant of fetal to adult hemoglobin switching seems to be postconceptual age, with the sharpest period for transition between 30 and 52 weeks.[101] The fetal-to-adult switch appears to be unaffected by the time at which birth occurs or by changes in the kinetics of erythropoiesis induced by perinatal hemolysis.[101] A delay in switching is usually observed in cases of general developmental retardation and in patients with certain chromosomal abnormalities (e.g., trisomy 13). Integration of the data available from in vitro and in vivo approaches indicates that control of switching is intrinsic to erythroid cells, which provides support for the concept of a "developmental clock."[100] Stage-specific transcriptional forces with negative or positive influences (or both) on specific globin genes may provide the molecular basis for differential transcriptional activity during development. This view is favored by experiments in transgenic mice[102] and in heterokaryons (produced by fusion of human with mouse cells),[103] as well as by the isolation of stage-specific transcriptional factors in other erythroid systems (e.g., avian).[104] Furthermore, as β-like and α-like globin genes are activated sequentially in the order of their location in chromosome 11 or chromosome 16, respectively, it is possible that polarity of the transcriptional activity and promoter competition for developmental stage-specific transcriptional factors contribute to this regulation.[105]

In summary, throughout human development waves of hematopoiesis are initiated sequentially in newly recruited sites. The only organ that gives rise to its own stem cells is the yolk sac, and an uncommitted progeny from these cells colonizes subsequent hematopoietic organs, initiating fetal and later adult erythropoiesis. Although the early embryonic phase of erythropoiesis may be autonomous, fetal and adult erythropoiesis are under the control of EPO and distinct environmental influences. The erythroid populations that follow each other in ontogeny have distinct phenotypes and intrinsic programs, which are dependent on gestational time and not on the sites at which they mature. The sequential activation of globin genes in the order of their location in chromosome 11 (β-like globin) or 16 (α-like globin) is likely mediated through interactions between stage-specific transcriptional factors and cis-regulatory sequences within the globin loci.

CELLULAR DYNAMICS IN ERYTHROPOIESIS

The primary function of the end product of erythropoiesis, the mature red cell, is to transport oxygen efficiently through the circulation to the tissues. To achieve this goal the adult marrow must release approximately 3×10^9 new red cells, or reticulocytes/kg/day.[106] This number of reticulocytes represents 1/100th of the total red cell mass and is derived from an estimated 5×10^9 erythroid precursor/kg.[106] In addition to maintaining homeostasis (i.e., a stable hematocrit) the erythron must be able to respond quickly and appropriately to increased oxygen demands, either acute (e.g., following red cell loss) or chronic (e.g., with hypoxia from pulmonary disease or a right-to-left cardiac shunt). It is now well established that EPO is responsible both for maintaining normal erythropoiesis and for increasing red cell production in response to oxygen needs. The overall marrow response, however, is a complex one and requires not only the participation of erythroid cells responsive to EPO but also a structurally intact microenvironment and an optimal iron supply within the marrow.

EPO stimulation elicits two types of measurable responses, changes in proliferative activity and changes in maturation rates. The first detectable response to increased serum EPO is amplification of CFU-E and erythroid precursors, cells that are extremely sensitive to EPO. Since virtually all these cells are already in cycle, increases in their numbers cannot be achieved by increasing their fraction in cycle. Either additional divisions are involved or new cells are recruited to the CFU-E pool (from a fraction of CFU-E less sensitive to EPO or from a pre-CFU-E pool). Additional divisions of CFU-E or precursor cells would increase their transit time within the marrow and potentially delay the delivery of new red cells to the periphery.

Since a shortened maturation time has been observed instead and the proliferative potentials of CFU-E and proerythroblasts are finite, high levels of amplification cannot be achieved through this mechanism. Therefore, such needs are met by influx into the CFU-E and precursor pools of newly differentiating cells from earlier progenitor compartments.

Such a surge of newly produced cells has been observed in all previous experiments.[41,107,108] A rapid influx of fresh cells was particularly notable in polycythemic mice that were experimentally depleted of CFU-E and erythroid precursors at the time the stimulus was applied.[23,41] Because of the rapidity of response (e.g., within 24 hours in the polycythemic animals), it appeared that the orderly progression from BFU-E to CFU-E to proerythroblast had been compressed. Such acceleration of differentiation is possible through shortened intermitotic intervals, fewer mitotic divisions, or differentiation without divisions. This short circuiting in differentiation requires high serum levels of EPO and adequate numbers of BFU-E (e.g., either a previously hypertransfused, polycythemic animal stimulated by EPO or marrow suddenly recovering from acquired pure erythroid aplasia). Once CFU-E and precursors are expanded through this mechanism, most persisting erythropoietic demands can be met through this pool without excess input from pre-CFU-E pools. Thus, acute demands for erythropoiesis are met by influx from pre-CFU-E pools through an accelerated differentiation and maturation sequence. By contrast, chronic demands (i.e., demands in chronic hemolytic anemia) are mainly satisfied through a greatly amplified late erythroid pool and with a minimum distortion in the differentiation sequence.[29,109] That the kinetics of erythroid differentiation/maturation are different in acute versus chronic marrow regeneration is supported by differing qualitative changes in the newly formed red cells. An increase in i antigen and Hb F expression as well as an increase in cells with higher mean corpuscular volumes is seen with an acute response, whereas these are minimal or less pronounced with chronic responses.[29,110] When anemia persists, erythroid production can undergo an ≤10-fold increase above baseline.[109] This is possible not only because of maximally expanded erythropoietic pools but also because the sites of active erythropoiesis extend to include those that support red cell differentiation during fetal life. Thus, although the marrow space in axial bones (vertebrae, pelvis, ribs, sternum, clavicles) is sufficient for normal erythropoiesis, the femur, humerus, spleen and/or liver, and (rarely) thymus may support red cell production. Expanded erythropoiesis in children with congenital hemolytic anemia (e.g., thalassemia major) may lead to skeletal deformities, hepatosplenomegaly, or erythropoiesis in the soft tissues adjacent to bone.

Quantitative assessments of changes in erythroid progenitor cell pools in response to EPO stimulation can be made through cultures of bone marrow cells. Despite sampling errors, erythroid cultures can provide rough estimates of relative progenitor abundance within an aspirated marrow specimen and have shown consistent increases in the frequency of CFU-E in proportion to the level of EPO stimulation.[111,112] Conversely, with increases in the hematocrit or in polycythemic animals, a decrease in CFU-E frequency has been observed.[113,114] In contrast to CFU-E, the incidence of BFU-E was found to fluctuate less with either acute or chronic expansion of erythropoiesis, probably because a few BFU-E can generate progeny of several thousand cells. Furthermore, BFU-E can increase their fraction in cycle and thus increase the number of differentiated progeny without a significant change in their total numbers. Most BFU-E detectable in marrow or blood erythroid cultures probably represent a reservoir of progenitors not normally participating in day-to-day erythropoiesis. The parameters needed to maintain a healthy or appropriate BFU-E pool in hemopoiesis are not defined. As hemopoietic expansion is curtailed in mice with Steel mutations and anemia develops in mice treated with anti-

c-kit Ab antibody,[115] one may suggest that adequate levels of normal KL may be crucial for early constitutive erythropoietic expansion.[116]

The rate of red cell production also can be accurately evaluated through ferrokinetics (i.e., the study of iron incorporation into developing red cells) (see Ch. 34). In addition, a marrow scan, typically with ^{99m}Tc, can document the extent of active erythropoiesis. These approaches, however, are seldom necessary in clinical practice, since estimates of erythropoiesis can be obtained from the reticulocyte index.[109] First, the observed percentage of reticulocytes is normalized for the hematocrit to calculate the total marrow output of reticulocytes. This number is termed the absolute reticulocyte count. However, since under conditions of acute need, younger reticulocytes are prematurely released into the circulation, the total number of reticulocytes overestimates the true level of red cell production as measured by iron kinetics.[109] Therefore, a second correction is made to account for the maturation of early circulating reticulocytes, or "shift" cells (polychromatophilic red cells) when present in the blood smear. The resulting reticulocyte index gives excellent estimates of effective red cell production.

Although the presence or density (or both) of EPO receptors on developing erythroid cells determines the responses to EPO, other properties (e.g., surface antigens on BFU-E versus CFU-E versus end-stage red cells) may provide the basis for selective suppression of CFU-E versus BFU-E or selective immune destruction of red cells versus erythroblasts. For example, suppression of CFU-E or erythroblasts can occur in acquired pure red cell aplasia[117] or B19 parvovirus infection,[118] respectively, whereas BFU-E in both these conditions remain largely unperturbed. Thus, the boundary from BFU-E to CFU-E and erythroblast may be biologically important for the pathophysiology of these disease states. Furthermore, in acquired hemolytic anemia selective destruction at a given stage of maturation (of red cells only or of both erythroblasts and red cells) can be observed depending on the type of antibody produced and the density of its antigen on maturing erythroid cells. Qualitative aberrations in the response of erythroid progenitors to cytokines or EPO may underlie the abnormalities of congenital erythroid aplasia (Diamond-Blackfan syndrome).[119] Analogous qualitative or functional defects can be observed in neoplastic erythropoiesis, as erythroid progenitors from patients with polycythemia vera and other myeloproliferative syndromes have altered sensitivities to EPO.[120]

Therefore, detailed knowledge of the structural and functional properties of erythroid cells throughout their differentiation may provide significant insights into the pathogenesis of hematopoietic disorders affecting the red cell lineage.

REFERENCES

1. Ogawa M, Porter PN, Nakahata T: Renewal and commitment to differentiation of hemopoietic stem cells (an interpretive review). Blood 61:823, 1983
2. Fairbairn LJ, Cowling GJ, Reipert BM, Dexter TM: Suppression of apoptosis allows differentiation and development of a multipotent hemopoietic cell line in the absence of added growth factor. Cell 74:823, 1993
3. Testa NG: Structure and regulation of the erythroid system at the level of progenitor cells. CRC Crit Rev Oncol Hematol 9:17, 1989
4. Abkowitz JL, Holly RD, Hammond WP IV: Cyclic hematopoiesis in dogs: studies of erythroid burst-forming cells confirm an early stem cell defect. Exp Hematol 16:941, 1988
5. Iscove NN, Guilbert LJK, Weyman C: Complete replacement of serum in primary cultures of erythropoietin-dependent red cell precursors (CFU-E) by albumin, transferrin, iron, unsaturated fatty acid, lecithin and cholesterol. Exp Cell Res 126:121, 1980
6. Rich IN, Kubanek B: The effect of reduced oxygen tension on colony formation of erythropoietic cells in vitro. Br J Haematol 52:579, 1982
7. Clark SC, Kamen R: The human hematopoietic colony-stimulating factors. Science 236:1229, 1987
8. Bernstein A, Forrester L, Reith AD et al: The murine W/c-kit and Steel loci and the control of hematopoiesis. Semin Hematol 28:138, 1991
9. Park LS, Waldron PE, Friend D et al: Interleukin-3, GM-CSF, and G-CSF recep-

tor expression on cell lines and primary leukemia cells: receptor heterogeneity and relationship to growth factor responsiveness. Blood 74:56, 1989

10. Leary AG, Ogawa M: Blast cell colony assay for umbilical cord blood and adult bone marrow progenitors. Blood 69:953, 1987

11. Keller JR, Mantel C, Sing GK et al: Transforming growth factor β1 selectively regulates early murine hematopoietic progenitors and inhibits the growth of IL-3 dependent myeloid leukemia cell lines. J Exp Med 168:737, 1988

12. Broxmeyer HE, Williams DE: The production of myeloid blood cells and their regulation during health and disease. CRC Crit Rev Oncol Hematol 8: 173, 1988

13. Civin CI, Loken MR: Cell surface antigens on human marrow cells: dissection of hematopoietic development using monoclonal antibodies and multiparameter flow cytometry. Int J Cell Cloning 5:267, 1987

14. Sieff CA: Membrane antigen expression during hemopoietic differentiation. CRC Crit Rev Oncol Hematol 5:1, 1986

15. Broxmeyer HE: Relationship of cell-cycle expression of Ia-like antigenic determinants on normal and leukemia human granulocyte-macrophage progenitor cells to regulation in vitro by acidic isoferritins. J Clin Invest 69: 632, 1982

16. Torok-Storb B: Cellular interactions. Blood 72:373, 1988

17. Sawada K, Krantz SB, Sawyer ST, Civin CI: Quantitation of specific binding of erythropoietin to human erythroid colony-forming cells. J Cell Physiol 137:337, 1988

18. Sawada K, Krantz SB, Dai CH et al: Purification of human blood burst-forming units-erythroid and demonstration of the evolution of erythropoietin receptors, abstracted. Exp Hematol 17:513, 1989

19. Broudy VC, Lin N, Brice M et al: Erythropoietin receptors (EpoR) on normal human erythroid precursor cells, abstracted. Blood 74:266, 1989

20. Migliaccio G, Migliaccio AR, Adamson JW: In vitro differentiation of human granulocyte/macrophage and erythroid progenitors: comparative analysis of the influence of recombinant human erythropoietin, G-CSF, GM-CSF, and IL-3 in serum-supplemented and serum-deprived cultures. Blood 72:248, 1988

21. Sawyer ST, Krantz SB: Transferrin receptor number, synthesis and endocytosis during erythropoietin-induced maturation of Friend virus-infected erythroid cells. J Biol Chem 261:9187, 1986

22. Cotner T, Das Gupta A, Papayannopoulou T, Stamatoyannopoulos G: Characterization of a novel form of transferrin receptor preferentially expressed on normal erythroid progenitors and precursors. Blood 73:214, 1989

23. Stohlman F Jr, Ebbe S, Morse B et al: Regulation of erythropoiesis. XX. Kinetics of red cell production. Ann NY Acad Sci 149:156, 1968

24. Lazarides E: From genes to structural morphogenesis: the genesis and epigenesis of a red blood cell. Cell 51:345, 1987

25. Woods CM, Lazarides E: The erythroid membrane skeleton: expression and assembly during erythropoiesis. Annu Rev Med 39:107, 1988

26. Hakomori SI: Blood group ABH and Ii antigen of human erythrocytes: chemistry, polymorphism and their developmental change. Semin Hematol 18: 39, 1981

27. Chasis JA, Coulombel L, Conboy JG, Mohandas N: Protein 4.1 isoforms are differentially expressed during erythroid maturation, abstracted. Blood 74: 104a, 1989

28. Nienhuis AW, Benz EJ: Regulation of hemoglobin synthesis during the development of the red cell. N Engl J Med 297:1318, 1371, 1430, 1977

29. Stamatoyannopoulos G, Nienhuis AW: Hemoglobin switching. p. 66. In Stamatoyannopoulos G, Nienhuis AW, Leder P, Majerus P (eds): Molecular Basis of Blood Diseases. WB Saunders, Philadelphia, 1987

30. Papayannopoulou T, Vichinsky E, Stamatoyannopoulos G: Foetal Hb production during acute erythroid expansion. I. Observations in patients with transient erythroblastopenia and post-phlebotomy. Br J Haematol 44:535, 1980

31. Blau CA, Constantoulakis P, Al-Khatti A et al: Fetal hemoglobin in acute and chronic states of erythroid expansion. Blood 81:227, 1993

32. Peters LL, Andrews NC, Eicher EM et al: Mouse microcytic anaemia caused by a defect in the gene encoding the globin enhancer-binding protein NF-E2. Nature 362:768, 1993

33. Sawada K, Krantz SB, Kans JS et al: Purification of human erythroid colony-forming units and demonstration of specific binding of erythropoietin. J Clin Invest 80:357, 1987

34. Iacopetta BJ, Morgan EH, Yeoh GCT: Transferrin receptors and iron uptake during erythroid cell development. Biochim Biophys Acta 687:204, 1982

35. Seligman PA, Klausner RD, Huebers HA: Molecular mechanisms of iron metabolism. p. 219. In Stamatoyannopoulos G, Nienhuis AW, Leder P, Majerus P (eds): Molecular Basis of Blood Diseases. WB Saunders, Philadelphia, 1987

36. Huebers HA, Finch CA: The physiology of transferrin and transferrin receptors. Physiol Rev 67:520, 1987

37. Yokochi T, Brice M, Radinovitch PS et al: Monoclonal antibodies detecting

antigenic determinants with restricted expression on erythroid cells: from the erythroid committed progenitor level to the mature erythroblast. Blood 63:1376, 1984

38. D'Andrea AD, Lodish HF, Wong, GG: Expression cloning of the murine erythropoietin receptor. Cell 57:277, 1989

39. Koury ST, Bondurant MC, Koury MJ: Localization of erythropoietin synthesizing cells in murine kidneys by in situ hybridization. Blood 71:524, 1988

40. Goldberg MA, Dunning SP, Bunn HF: Regulation of the erythropoietin gene: evidence that the oxygen sensor is a heme protein. Science 242:1412, 1988

41. Papayannopoulou T, Finch CA: On the in vivo action of erythropoietin: a quantitative analysis. J Clin Invest 51:1179, 1979

42. Takeshita K, Benz EJ: Analysis of gene expression during hematopoiesis: present and future applications. CRC Crit Rev Oncol Hematol 4:67, 1985

43. Spivak JL: The mechanisms of action of erythropoietin. Int J Cell Cloning 4:139, 1986

44. Correa PN, Axelrad AA: Production of erythropoietin bursts by progenitor cells from adult human periphral blood in an improved serum-free medium: role of insulin-like growth factor 1. Blood 78:2823, 1992

44a. Koury MJ, Bondurant MC: Erythropoietin retards DNA breakdown and prevents programmed death in erythroid progenitor cells. Science 248:378, 1990

45. Nakamura Y, Komatsu N, Nakauchi H: A truncated erythropoietin receptor that fails to prevent programmed cell death of erythroid cells. Science 257: 1138, 1992

46. Witthuhn BA, Quelle FW, Silvennoinen O et al: JAK2 associates with the erythropoietin receptor and is tyrosine phosphorylated and activated following stimulation with erythropoietin. Cell 74:227, 1993

46a. Longmore, GD, Lodish HF: An activating mutation in the murine erythropoietin receptor induces erythroleukemia in mice: a cytokine receptor superfamily oncogene. Cell 67:1089, 1991

47. D'Andrea AD, Yoshimura A, Youssoufian H, et al: The cytoplasmic region of the erythropoietin receptor contains nonoverlapping positive and negative growth-regulatory domains. Mol Cell Biol 11:1980, 1991

48. de La Chappelle A, Träskelin A-L, Juvonen E: Truncated erythropoietin receptor causes dominantly inherited benign human erythrocytosis. Proc Natl Acad Sci USA 90:4496, 1993

49. Baron MH, Maniatis R: Rapid reprogramming of globin gene expression in transient heterokaryons. Cell 46:591, 1986

50. Papayannopoulou T, Enver T, Takegawa S et al: Activation of developmentally mutated human globin genes by cell fusion. Science 242:1056, 1988

51. Grosveld F, Blom van Assendelft G, Greaves DR, Kollias G: Position-independent, high level expression of the human β-globin gene in transgenic mice. Cell 51:975, 1987

52. Orkin SH: GATA-binding transcription factors in hematopoietic cells. Blood 80:575, 1992

53. Sposi NM, Zon LI, Care A et al: Cell cycle-dependent initiation and lineage-dependent abrogation of GATA-1 expression in pure differentiating hemopoietic progenitors. Proc Natl Acad Sci USA 89:6353, 1992

54. Leonard M, Brice M, Engel JD, Papayannopoulou T: Dynamics of GATA transcription factor expression during erythroid differentiation. Blood 82:1071, 1993

55. Mucenski ML, McLain K, Kier AB et al: A functional c-myb gene is required for normal murine fetal hepatic hematopoiesis. Cell 65:677, 1991

56. Jacks T, Fazeli A, Schmitt EM et al: Effects of an Rb mutation in the mouse. Nature 359:295, 1992

57. Walters M, Martin DK: Functional erythroid promoters created by interaction of the transcription factor GATA-1 with CACCC and AP-1/NFE-2 elements. Proc Natl Acad Sci USA, 89:10,444 1992

58. Green AR, Begley CG: SCL and related hemopoietic helix-loop-helix transcription factors. Int J Cell Cloning 10:269, 1992

59. Andrews NC, Erdjument-Bromage H, Davidson MB et al: Erythroid transcription factor NF-E2 is a haematopoietic-specific basic-leucine zipper protein. Nature 362:722, 1993

60. McCulloch EA, Siminovitch L, Till JE et al: The cellular basis of the genetically determined hemopoietic defect in anemic mice of genotype S1/S1^d. Blood 26:399, 1965

61. Anklesaria P, Fitzgerald TJ, Kase K et al: Improved hematopoiesis in anemic S1/S1^d mice by splenectomy and therapeutic transplantation of a hematopoietic microenvironment. Blood 74:1144, 1989

62. Simmons PJ, Prezepiorka D, Thomas ED, Torok-Storb B: Host origin of bone marrow stromal cells following allogenic bone marrow transplantation. Nature 328:429, 1987

63. Gordon MY: The origin of stromal cells in patients treated by bone marrow transplantation. Bone Marrow Transplant 3:247, 1988

64. Gordon MY: Extracellular matrix of the marrow microenvironment. Br J Hematol 70:1, 1988

65. Dexter TM, Testa NG, Allen TD et al: Molecular and cell biological aspects of erythropoiesis in long-term bone marrow cultures. Blood 58:699, 1981

66. Cashman JD, Eaves AC, Raines EW et al: Mechanisms that regulate the cell cycle status of very primitive hematopoietic cells in long-term human marrow cultures. I. Stimulatory role of a variety of mesenchymal cell activators and inhibitory role of TGF-β. Blood 75:96, 1990

67. Shao L, Frigon NL, Sehy DW et al: Regulation of production of activin A in human marrow stromal cells and monocytes. Exp Hematol 20:1235, 1992

68. Dexter MT, Spooncer E, Schofield R et al: Hemopoietic stem cells and the problem of self-renewal. Blood Cells 10:315, 1984

69. Roberts R, Gallagher J, Spooncer E et al: Heparan sulphate bound growth factors: a mechanism for stromal cell mediated haemopoiesis. Nature 332: 376, 1988

70. Vuillet-Gaugler MH, Breton-Gorius J, Vainchenker W et al: Loss of attachment to fibronectin with terminal human erythroid differentiation. Blood 75:865, 1990

71. Campbell AD, Long MW, Wicha MS: Haemonectin, a bone marrow adhesion protein specific for cells of granulocyte lineage. Nature 329:744, 1987

72. Weinstein R, Riordan MA, Wenc K et al: Dual role of fibronectin in hematopoietic differentiation. Blood 73:111, 1989

73. Papayannopoulou T, Brice M: Integrin expression profiles during erythroid differentiation. Blood 79:1686, 1992

74. Long MC, Briddell R, Walter AW et al: Human hemopoietic stem cell adherence to cytokines and matrix molecules. J Clin Invest 90:251, 1992

75. Teixido J, Hemler ME, Greenberger JS, Anklesaria P: Role of β₁ and β₂ integrins in the adhesion of human CD34^{hi} stem cells to bone marrow stroma. J Clin Invest 90:358, 1992

76. Trinchieri G, Murphy M, Perussia B: Regulation of hematopoiesis by T lymphocytes and natural killer cells. CRC Crit Rev Oncol Hematol 7:219, 1987

77. Arkin S, Naprstek B, Guarini L et al: Expression of ICAM-1 on hematopoietic progenitors, abstracted. Blood 74:148a, 1989

78. Lichtman MA: The ultrastructure of hemopoietic environment of the marrow: a review. Exp Hematol 9:391, 1981

79. Rich IN: Haemopoietic regulation and the role of the macrophage in erythropoietic gene expression. Adv Exp Med Biol 241:55, 1988

80. Le Douarin NM: Cell migrations in embryos. Cell 38:353, 1984

81. Hoyes AD, Riches DJ, Martin BGH: The fine structure of haemopoiesis in the human fetal liver. J Anat 115:99, 1973

82. Moore, MAS, Metcalf D: Ontogeny of the haemopoietic system: yolk sac origin of in vivo and in vitro colony forming cells in the developing mouse embryo. Br J Haematol 18:279, 1970

83. Zanjani ED, Poster J, Brulington H et al: Liver as the primary site of erythropoietin formation in the fetus. Lab Clin Med 89:640, 1977

84. Wong PMC, Chung SW, Reicheld SW, Chui DHK: Hemoglobin switching during murine embryonic development: evidence for two populations of embryonic erythropoietic progenitor cells. Blood 67:716, 1986

85. Labastie MC, Thiery JP, Le Douarin NM: Mouse yolk sac and intraembryonic tissues produce factors able to elicit differentiation of erythroid burst-forming units and colony-forming units, respectively. Proc Natl Acad Sci USA 81: 1453, 1984

86. Valtieri M, Gabbianelli M, Pelosi E et al: Erythropoietin alone induces erythroid burst formation by human embryonic but not adult BFU-E in unicellular serum-free culture. Blood 74:460, 1989

87. Migliaccio AR, Migliaccio G: Human embryonic hemopoiesis: control mechanisms underlying progenitor differentiation in vitro. Dev Biol 125:127, 1988

88. Migliaccio G, Migliaccio AR, Petti S et al: Human embryonic hemopoiesis: kinetics of progenitors and precursors underlying the yolk sac → liver transition. J Clin Invest 78:51, 1986

89. Kahn A, Boyer C, Cottreau D et al: Immunologic study of the age-related loss of activity of six enzymes in the red cells from newborn infants and adults—evidence for a fetal type of erythrocyte phosphofructokinase. Pediatr Res 11:271, 1977

90. Weatherall DJ, McIntyre PA: Developmental and acquired variations in erythrocyte carbonic anhydrase isozymes. Br J Haematol 13:106, 1967

91. Chen S-H, Anderson JE, Giblett ER, Stamatoyannopoulos G: Isozyme patterns in erythrocytes from human fetuses. Am J Hematol 2:23, 1977

92. Garre C, Ravazzolo R, Ajmar F, Bruzzone G: Electrophoretic difference between fetal and adult acetylcholinesterase of human red cell membranes. Cell Differ Dev 9:165, 1980

93. Gabbianelli M, Boccoli G, Petti S et al: Expression and in-vitro modulation of HLA antigens in ontogenic development of human hemopoietic system. Ann NY Acad Sci 511:138, 1987

94. Robinson J, Sieff C, Delia D et al: Expression of cell-surface HLA-DR, HLA-ABC and glycophorin during erythroid differentiation. Nature 289:68, 1981

95. Theil EC: The abundance of ferritin in yolk-sac derived red blood cells of the embryonic mouse. Br J Haematol 33:437, 1976

96. Stamatoyannopoulos G, Constantoulakis P, Brice M et al: Coexpression of embryonic, fetal and adult globins in erythroid cells of human embryos: relevance to the cell-lineage models of globin switching. Dev Biol 123:191, 1987

97. Peschle C, Migliaccio AR, Migliaccio G et al: Embryonic fetal Hb switch in humans: studies on erythroid bursts generated by embryonic progenitors from yolk sac and liver. Proc Natl Acad Sci USA 81:2416, 1984

98. Young NS, Nienhuis AW: Hemoglobin switching in sheep and man. p. 103. In Silber R, LaBue J, Gordon AS (eds): The Year in Hematology. Plenum, New York, 1978

99. Wintour EM, Smith MB, Bell RJ et al: The role of fetal adrenal hormones in the switch from fetal to adult globin synthesis in the sheep. J Endocrinol 104:165, 1985

100. Wood WG, Bunch C, Kelly S et al: Control of haemoglobin switching by a developmental clock? Nature 313:320, 1985

101. Wood WG, Howes S, Bunch C: Developmental clocks and hemoglobin switching. p. 521. In Stamatoyannopoulos G, Nienhuis AW (eds): Developmental Control of Globin Gene Expression. Alan R Liss, New York, 1987

102. Costantini F, Radice G, Magram J et al: Developmental regulation of human globin genes in transgenic mice. Cold Spring Harb Symp Quant Biol L 50: 361, 1985

103. Baron MH, Maniatis T: Rapid reprogramming of globin gene expression in transient heterokaryons. Cell 46:591, 1986

104. Choi RB, Engel JD: Developmental regulation of β-globin gene switching. Cell 55:17, 1988

105. Enver T, Raich N, Ebens AJ et al: Development regulation of human fetal-to-adult globin gene switching in transgenic mice. Nature 344:309, 1990

106. Donohue DM, Reiff RH, Hanson ML et al: Quantitative measurement of the erythrocytic and granulocytic cells of the marrow and blood. J Clin Invest 37:1571, 1958

107. Alpen EL, Cranmore D: Observations on the regulation of erythropoiesis and on cellular dynamics by Fe^{59} autoradiography. p. 240. In Stohlman F Jr (ed): The Kinetics of Cellular Proliferation. Grune & Stratton, Orlando, FL, 1959

108. Deubelbeiss KA, Dancey JT, Harker LA et al: Marrow erythroid and neutrophil cellularity in the dog. J Clin Invest 55:825, 1975

109. Hillman RS, Finch CA: Erythropoiesis: normal and abnormal. Semin Hematol 4:327, 1967

110. Papayannopoulou T, Chen P, Maniatis A, Stamatoyannopoulos G: Simultaneous assessment of i-antigenic expression and fetal hemoglobin in single red cells by immunofluorescence. Blood 55:221, 1980

111. Ogawa M, Grush OC, O'Dell RF et al: Circulating erythropoietic precursors assessed in culture: characterization in normal men and patients with hemoglobinopathies. Blood 50:1081, 1977

112. Umemura T, Papayannopoulou T, Stamatoyannopoulos G: The mechanism of expansion of late erythroid progenitors during erythroid regeneration: target cells and effects of erythropoietin and interleukin-3. Blood 73:1993, 1989

113. Iscove NN: The role of erythropoietin in regulation of population size and cell cycling of early and late erythroid precursors in mouse bone marrow. Cell Tissue Kinet 10:373, 1977

114. Peschle C, Magli MC, Cillo C et al: Regulatory mechanisms of erythroid stem cell kinetics. p. 86. In Murphy MJ Jr (ed): In Vitro Aspects of Erythropoiesis. Springer-Verlag, New York, 1978

115. Ogawa M, Matsuzaki Y, Nishikawa S et al: Expression and function of c-kit in hemopoietic progenitor cells. J Exp Med 174:63, 1991

116. Papayannopoulou T, Brice M, Blau T: Kit ligand in synergy with interleukin-3 amplifies the erythropoietin-independent, globin-synthesizing progeny of normal human burst-forming units-erythroid in suspension cultures: physiologic implications. Blood 81:299, 1993

117. Krantz SB, Zaentz SD: Pure red cell aplasia. p. 153. In Silver R, Golden AS, Bueg LE (eds): Year in Hematology. Plenum, New York, 1977

118. Young NS, Mortimer PP, Moore JG, Humphries RD: Characterization of a virus that causes transient aplastic crisis. J Clin Invest 73:224, 1984

119. Lipton JM, Kudisch M, Gross R, Nathan DG: Defective erythroid progenitor differentiation system in congenital hypoplastic (Diamond-Blackfan) anemia. Blood 67:962, 1986

120. Mladenovic J, Adamson JW: Characteristics of circulating erythroid colony-forming cells in normal and polycythemic man. Br J Haematol 51:337, 1982

121. Das Gupta A, Samoszuk M, Papayannopoulou T, Stamatoannopoulos G: SFL 23.6: a monoclonal antibody reactive with CFU-E, erythroblasts, and erythrocytes. Blood 66:522, 1985

122. Granick S, Levere RD: Heme synthesis in erythroid cells. p. 1. In Moore CV, Brown EB (eds): Progress in Hematology. Vol. 4. Grune & Stratton, Orlando, FL, 1964

123. Erslev AJ, Gabuzda TG: Pathophysiology of Blood. 2nd Ed. WB Saunders, Philadelphia, 1979

Granulopoiesis and Monocytopoiesis

18

Camille N. Abboud and Jane L. Liesveld

INTRODUCTION

This chapter details the process of granulopoiesis (production of neutrophils, eosinophils, and basophils) and monocytopoiesis (production of monocytes and tissue-fixed macrophages). The need for rapid adjustment in production rates in response to acute stress (infection, inflammation) as well as the enormous number of short-lived mature cells that are produced each day have necessitated the development of a very intricate cytokine network and a series of progenitor compartments to meet those requirements.[1,2] The hematopoietic growth factor combinations required for the proliferation, survival, and maturation of these cells are analyzed, and the functional similarities in signaling of colony-stimulating factor receptors (CSF-R) and interleukin receptors (IL-Rs) are highlighted. Mechanisms of lineage commitment to the granulocyte versus monocyte differentiation pathways are delineated, and the interactions of cytokines with mature cellular elements as well as other accessory cells demonstrated, as are the paracrine and autocrine feedback loops that regulate this complex process.

Understanding the properties and regulatory cytokine networks affecting each progenitor compartment within the marrow microenvironment will facilitate an understanding of the pathophysiology of disorders of granulopoiesis and monocytopoiesis. These may include aberrant cell proliferation and impaired differentiation in leukemic disorders, excessive precursor production in the setting of inflammation, infection, or allergic diseases, and impaired cellular production or excessive precursor destruction (or both) due to apoptosis in myelodysplastic diseases or congenital neutropenia.

STEM CELL AND PROGENITOR HIERARCHY

Growth factors important for myelopoiesis exert their effects at the level of the stem cell or the progenitor cell, or both. Stem cells are defined by their capacity for long-term self-renewal and by their ability to differentiate along multiple lineage pathways.[2,3] Progenitor cells, on the other hand, retain proliferative potential but are committed to the production of cells from a limited array of lineages.[2-4] Progenitor cells are often defined as colony-forming cells (CFCs) because of their ability to generate clonal colonies in vitro; such colonies can be erythroid, granulocyte, eosinophil, macrophage, megakaryocyte, mast cell, or T or B lymphocyte.[5-8] In humans, stem cells are defined by surrogate assays such as the high proliferative potential CFC (CFC-HPP),[9] the so-called CFC-blast,[10] or the long-term culture initiating cell assay (LTC-IC).[11] For obvious reasons, no in vivo definition of such a population is feasible in humans, but studies using fetal sheep transplantation have allowed the long-term detection of transplanted stem cell progeny, thereby providing the means to study early events in hematopoiesis.[12-14]

Multipotential cells are largely unresponsive to single growth factors, but they often respond synergistically to combinations of growth factors.[3] For example, the combination of colony-stimulating factor-macrophage (CSF-M) and IL-1 stimulates the proliferation of CFC-HPP,[15,16] whereas the combination of IL-3, IL-6, and CSF-granulocyte (G) is one of many cytokine combinations to have activity in CFC-blast.[17,18] Although cytokines influence the growth of these cells, they do not alter the proportion of stem cells that self-renew or differentiate along a given hematopoietic lineage. This has led to the postulation of a stochastic model for hematopoiesis in which a cell randomly becomes committed to differentiate along any given myeloid lineage pathway.[3]

Progenitor Characterization

Early hematopoietic progenitors are CD34$^+$/CD33$^-$ and are negative for lineage-specific markers.[19] When CD34$^+$ cells are isolated from bone marrow or blood, most have CD13 and HLA-DR surface antigens. Only a minor subset co-express CD33.[20] CD33 is an antigen expressed by clonogenic leukemia cells and also by normal myeloid progenitor cells.[21] After 7 days in culture in the presence of CSF-GM and IL-3, CD33 expression is found in 50% of these cells. Concurrently, CD34 is lost, and CD13 and HLA-DR expression also diminishes. By 14 days of culture, most cells are CD33$^+$.[22] Patients receiving marrow grafts purged with anti-CD33 have been found to require a significantly longer time to achieve polymorphonuclear neutrophils (PMNs) >500/mm^3, underscoring the importance of these committed granulocytic progenitors during the early phase of hematopoietic reconstitution after bone marrow transplantation.[23] Moreover, such marrow grafts depleted of CD33 cells result in durable engraftment after myeloablative treatment, implying that CD33 is absent or expressed in very low amounts on primitive pluripotent hematopoietic stem cells.[23]

The pluripotent stem cell has been defined by long-term in vivo repopulating assays; it belongs to the CD34-antigen-positive cell compartment,[15,24] displays the multidrug resistance gene (mdr-1)[25] also measured by the efflux of the fluorescent mitochondrial dye rhodamine 123,[26] has low levels of the Thy-1 antigen,[27,28] and displays no lineage commitment markers (CD38$^-$, CD33$^-$).[29-31] Other surrogate in vitro assays, developed in lieu of reconstitution assays, have also established the presence of a whole continuum of myeloid progenitors of decreasing proliferative potential and multilineage commitment.[2] These assays include the long-term marrow initiating cells (LTC-IC),[11,32] the CFC-HPP-1 and -2,[9,33] the CFU-blast,[10,34] and the mixed progenitor assays (colony-forming unit-granulocyte/erythroid/macrophage/megakaryocyte [CFU-GEMM]).[35] Subsets of committed granulocyte and macrophage progenitors can be enumerated in vitro after 7–14 days in culture, using semisolid colony assays and specific histochemical staining techniques,[36] allowing identification of CFU-granulocyte/macrophage (CFU-GM), granulocyte (CFU-G), macrophage (CFU-M), eosinophil (CFU-Eo), and basophil (CFU-Baso).[5-7] Figure 18-1 illustrates examples of CFC-HPP, CFU-GM, and CFU-M colonies assayed in semisolid media.

The advent of sophisticated flow cytometric cell separation techniques, coupled with improved progenitor and long-term reconstitution assays, has established that the earliest CD34$^+$

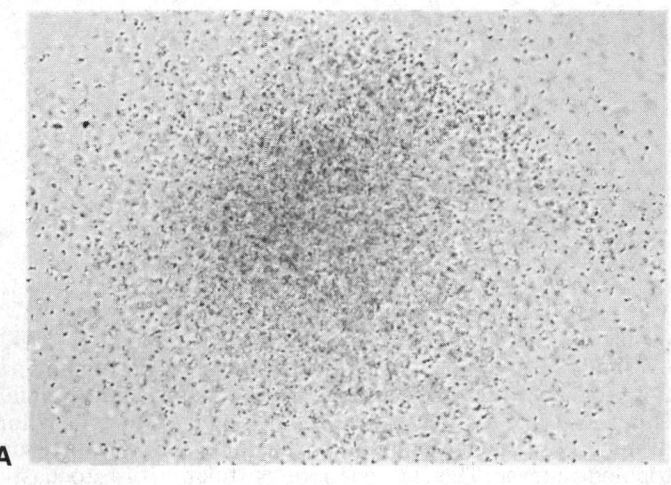

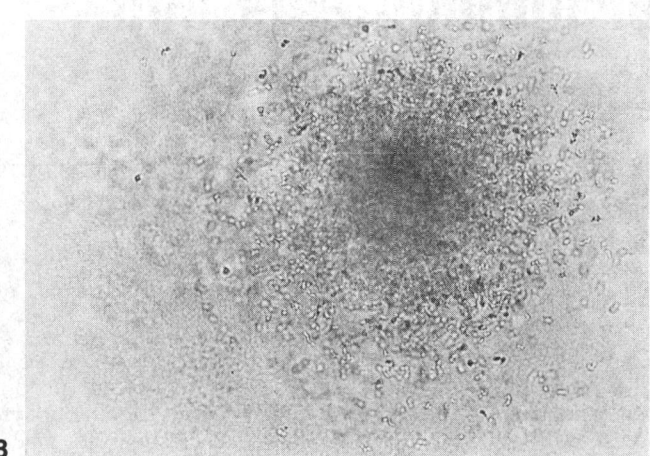

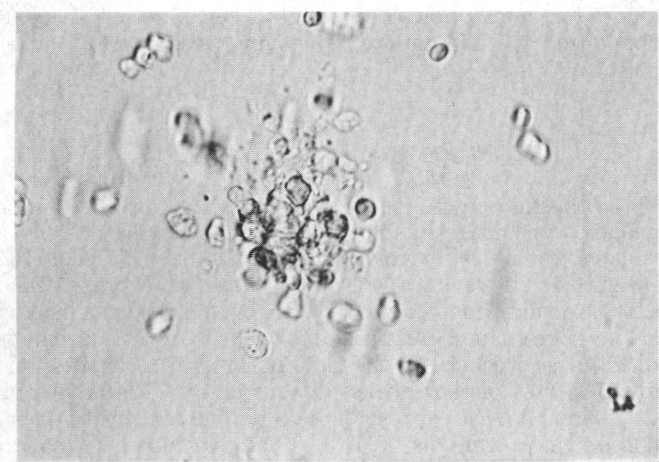

Fig. 18-1. **(A)** Large, diffuse CFC-HPP. (× 8) at day 25 of culture. **(B)** CFU-GM at day 14 of culture. (× 100.) **(C)** Smaller CFU-M at day 14 of culture. (× 160.)

stem cell compartment appears not to express CD45RA, as well as antigens associated with lineage commitment (CD33⁻, CD38⁻), but is CD45RO positive.[37–39] CD34⁺ progenitors begin to loose myeloid potential and become lymphoid progenitors after acquiring CD10 and CD19 (B-cell lineage) or CD7 and CD45RA⁺ (T-cell lineage).[40,41] The CD34⁺, CD10⁻, CD19⁻ populations contain mostly LTC-ICs and myeloid progenitors, while the CD34⁺, CD10⁺, CD19⁻ population gives rise to macrophage colonies and are CD33⁺.[40] This overlap in B-cell/macrophage lineage development is underscored by the plasticity of hemopoietic cells and is also validated by the identification of bipotential B-cell macrophage progenitors in fetal liver,[42] and by the observed lineage switching between early B cells to macrophages associated with expression of the proto-oncogene c-*fms,* which is the CSF-1 receptor.[43,44] The earliest bipotential myeloid progenitor, CFU-GM, has been characterized as CD34⁺, CD33⁺, CD13⁺, CD45RA⁺ and myeloperoxidase positive.[45] Figure 18-2 recapitulates the salient phenotypic changes that human progenitors undergo as they differentiate into specialized lymphoid and myeloid precursors.

GROWTH FACTOR REGULATION

Synergistic Growth Factors

Hematopoietins exert their effects in concert on primitive stem cells (synergistic early-acting factors) and continue to influence progenitor expansion (intermediate-acting factors); later, one or two factors influence progenitor maturation along specific lineages (late-acting factors).[46,47] These growth factors

were initially defined by colony assays, hence the name colony-stimulating factors; they include CSF-G, CSF-GM, and CSF-M.[5,48–50] Other myeloid-active cytokines include the ILs such as IL-3, (multi-CSF, a multilineage growth factor),[51] IL-4 (B-cell stimulatory factor I, a basophil/mast cell growth factor),[52] IL-5 (B-cell stimulatory factor II, eosinophil differentiation factor, an eosinophil growth factor),[53] and the kit-ligand stem cell factor (SCF/KL, a mast cell growth factor).[54,55]

While the initial process of stem cell lineage commitment is stochastic (random), stem cells are likely to display multiple cytokine receptors, thereby explaining the synergistic overlapping properties of hematopoietic growth factors.[3,47] These early-acting factors are shown in Figure 18-3 and include CSF-G (produced by stromal cells, fibroblasts, endothelial cells, and monocyte/macrophages),[48,56] IL-1 (produced by many cell types, including stromal cells, fibroblasts, endothelial cells, keratinocytes, epithelial cells, monocyte/macrophages, and B cells),[2,57] IL-6 (produced by T and B cells, stromal cells, fibroblasts, endothelial cells, keratinocytes, and mast cells),[58] IL-11 (produced by stromal cells),[59] IL-12 (produced by B cells and macrophages),[60] leukemia inhibitory factor (LIF) (present in serum and produced by stromal cells, fibroblasts, T cells, astrocytes, and monocytes/macrophages),[61] basic fibroblast growth factor (bFGF) (present in serum, megakaryocytes, platelets, immature granulocytes, and stromal cells and within an extracellular matrix reservoir),[62–64] and lastly, two tyrosine kinase receptor ligands, SCF/KL (produced by stromal cells, and synthesized in a soluble as well as membrane-bound form)[54,55] and the FLK-2/FLT3 ligand (stromal cells).[65,66]

The cytokines mentioned above participate at various levels in the steady-state regulation of granulopoiesis and monocyto-

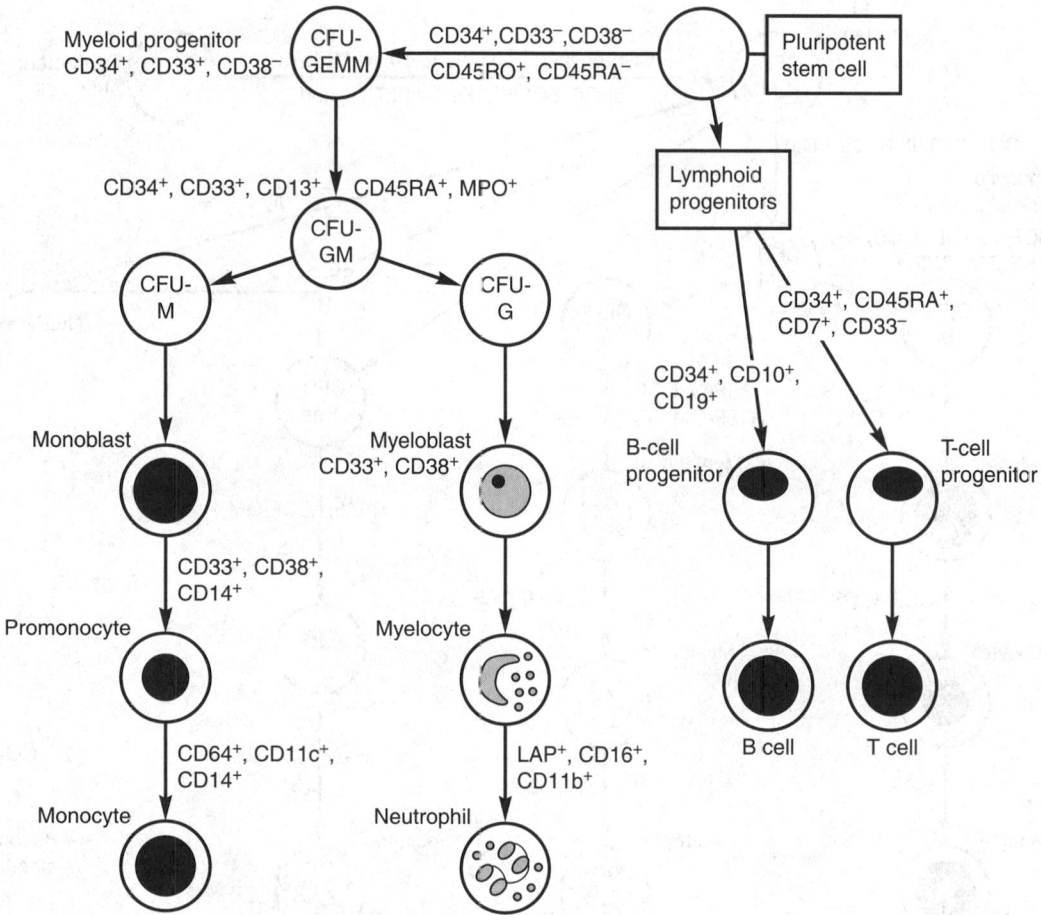

Fig. 18-2. This schematic lineage diagram illustrates some of the significant surface antigen features of both progenitor CFCs and those of the morphologically distinguishable precursors of monocytes and neutrophils. The pluripotent stem cell, which can give rise to both lymphoid and myelocytic progenitors, expresses CD34 and CD45RO but not CD45RA. At the myeloid progenitor level, CD34 persists, but CD33 and CD13 expression eventually emerges, as does RNA and protein production of myeloperoxidase (MPO). Monocytic precursors develop CD14 expression. The characteristics of the various CD antigens are more extensively defined in the text. CD64 = FcRI; CD16 = FcRIII; LAP, leukocyte alkaline phosphatase.

poiesis by promoting the survival of noncycling early progenitors and by shortening the G_0 period of early progenitors and triggering the proliferation and maturation of committed progenitors.[3,67] These synergistic interactions have been deduced from in vitro early progenitor assays (LTC-IC, CFC-HPP, CFU-blast) as well as intermediate-to-late progenitor assays (CFU-GEMM and CFU-GM)[32,68–80] (Fig. 18-3). Such interactions occur in vivo when more than one compartment of progenitors is stimulated.

Lineage-Specific Growth Factors

Cytokine receptor expression becomes more restricted as progenitors differentiate along separate granulocyte or monocyte pathways. Thus, at later stages of lineage commitment they express fewer cytokine receptors, and granulocytic maturation and differentiation is then governed by fewer growth factors, such as CSF-GM and -G for neutrophil production, CSF-1 and CSF-GM for monocyte precursor growth, IL-5 for eosinophil growth and maturation, and SCF, nerve growth factor, and IL-3 for basophil and mast cell growth[3,81] (Fig. 18-3). Also shown in Figure 18-3 are a superfamily of immune cytokines termed chemokines that regulate leukocyte trafficking and tissue distribution.[82] Neutrophil migration is mediated by the chemokines IL-8, neutrophil-activating peptide-2 (NAP-2), and Gro-α

(Gro = growth related). Monocytes are recruited by monocyte chemotactic protein(s) (MCP-1, -2, -3), interferon-inducible protein (IP-10), and macrophage inflammatory protein (MIP-1α), whereas RANTES (a T-cell-derived chemokine) affects monocytes, eosinophils, and basophils alike.[82,83]

CSF-G leads to only weak in vitro colony growth by itself, but when it is combined with SCF or CSF-GM in vitro, larger colonies are stimulated.[47,75] Similarly, CSF-G does not display its maximal range of in vivo activity when administered to W/W mice defective in their c-kit signaling,[47,84] while appreciable circulating levels of SCF in normal subjects[85] amplify its effects in vivo, thus explaining its potent activity on neutrophil production and progenitor expansion.[86] This in vivo synergism also occurs on administration of SCF and CSF-G either alone or together, leading to early and committed progenitor expansion and mobilization.[87–89] Indeed, while commitment decisions of pluripotent cells have been shown to evolve from random asymmetric cell divisions not affected by external growth factors, it is evident that cytokine receptors with overlapping specificities and at times opposing effects govern in large part lineage-specific maturation of intermediate and late progenitors by promoting the proliferation and survival of precursors expressing the appropriate growth factor receptors.[3,90] These include the granulocyte CSF receptor (CSF-GR) on neutrophils, the macrophage CSF receptor (CSF-MR, CSF-1R) on monocytes/macrophages),[91,92] the IL-5 receptor (IL-5R) on eosinophils and baso-

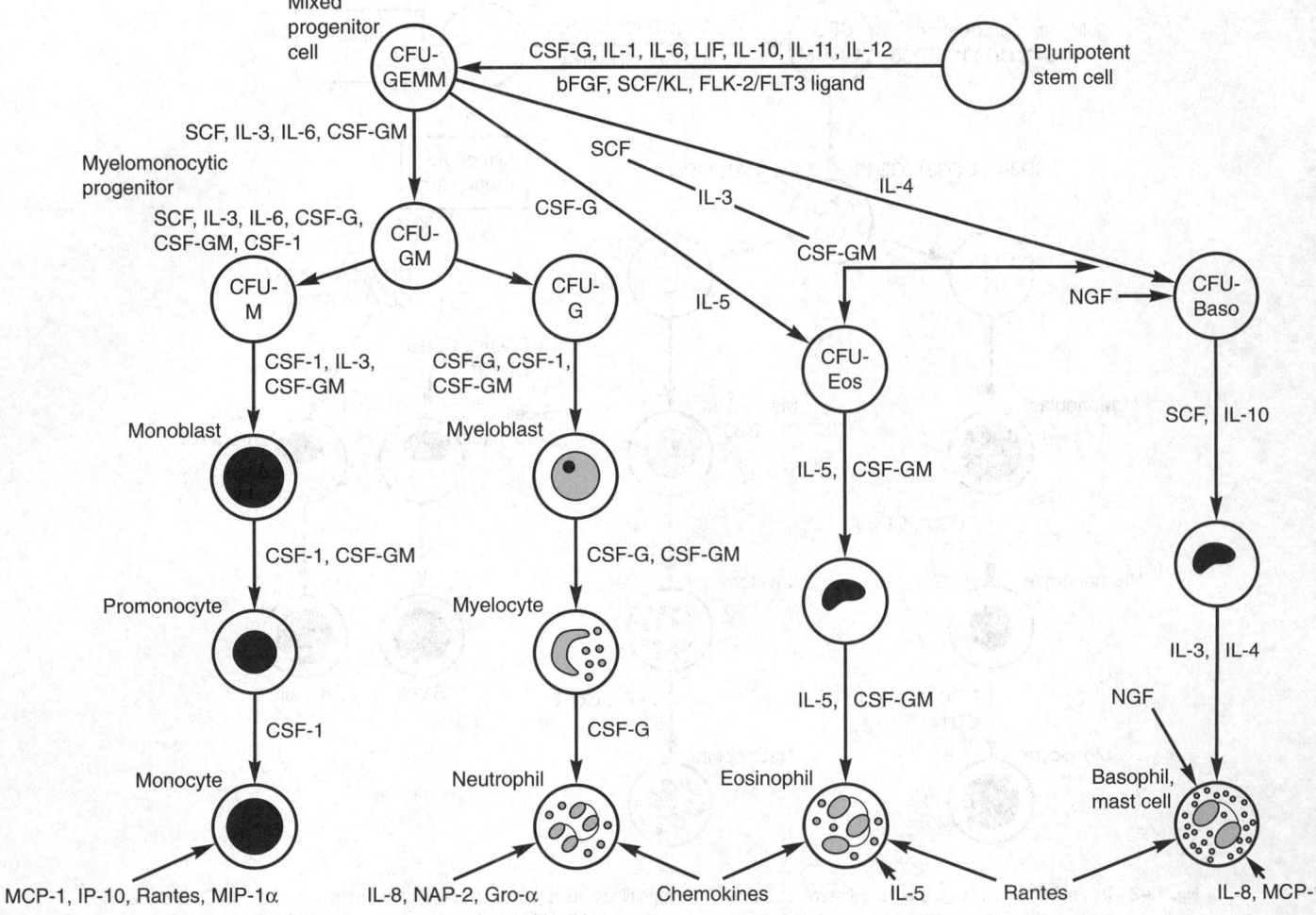

Fig. 18-3. Various cytokines and chemokines that act at different levels of granulopoiesis and monocytopoiesis. Multiple cytokines regulate progenitor cells or mature effector cells at each stage of maturation/differentiation from the primitive pluripotent stem cell to nondividing terminally differentiated precursors (monocytes, neutrophils, eosinophils, and basophil/mast cells). The cytokines and chemokines also have varying degrees of specificity; some, such as CSF-1 and IL-5, act predominantly on the monocytic and eosinophilic pathways, respectively, while others, such as CSF-GM, act on multiple granulocytic/monocytic (erythroid not shown) cell types.

phils,[93,94] and the c-kit (SCF) receptor (SCF-R) on mast cells[55] (Fig. 18-3). The in vivo lineage specificity of these factors is demonstrated in a canine model of neutropenia. Administration of CSF-G to dogs leads to the generation of neutralizing antibodies to their endogenous CSF-G and consequently neutropenia.[95] Transgenic mice expressing IL-5 display hypereosinophilia,[96] while IL-5-blocking antibody administration inhibits helminth-induced eosinophilia in mice.[97] In the op/op mouse osteopetrosis model, the op locus is the CSF-1 gene on murine chromosome 3. These mice do not produce CSF-1 because of a stop codon mutation within the CSF-1 gene; they also have a deficiency in their monocyte/macrophage compartment and suffer from osteopetrosis due to the absence of osteoclasts, which mediate bone resorption.[98,99] CSF-1 is essential for osteoclast proliferation and differentiation,[100] but in addition, CSF-GM promotes these monocyte-derived precursors to differentiate into multinucleated osteoclasts.[101] These op/op mice improve over time,[102] suggesting that other factors, such as IL-6, tumor necrosis factor-α (TNF-α), or CSF-GM, can stimulate macrophage progenitors in lieu of CSF-1.[103–106] Lastly, animal models such as the W/W have a defective c-kit receptor and mast cell deficiency,[107] whereas an activating mutation in c-kit, the SCF-R, has been identified in a mast cell leukemia,[108] underscoring the importance of SCF in terminal mast cell differentiation. As knock-out mice are produced, we may soon ascertain the function of CSF-GM and CSF-G in macrophage and neu-

trophil production with greater certainty.[47] Indeed, the first report of a CSF-GM knock-out murine model has shown normal hematopoiesis, but the mice have developed alveolar proteinosis, suggesting a role for this cytokine in normal lung physiology.[108a]

GROWTH FACTOR RECEPTOR STRUCTURE AND FUNCTION

Receptor Structure

The hematopoietic growth factors that regulate granulopoiesis and monocytopoiesis are a diverse group of glycoproteins whose actions are mediated through lineage-restricted specific cytokine receptors.[109] Cytokine receptors can be placed in four subgroups based on their structural characteristics, as shown in Table 18-1.[110–120] We restrict ourselves here to the two cytokine families that encompass most of the growth factors. The hemopoietin type I cytokine receptor family includes IL-2R, -3R, -4R, -5R, -6R, -7R, -9R, -11R, and -12R, erythropoietin (EPO), CSF-GMR and CSF-GR, the common signaling β-subunit KH97 for human CSF-R and the gp130 subunit for IL-6R, LIF receptor (LIF-R), ciliary neurotrophic factor receptor (CNTF-R), and oncostatin M receptor (OSM-R)[110–118]; all of these factors share a structural similarity to the growth hormone prolactin receptor family. The immunoglobulin superfamily includes the receptors for hemopoietic active growth

Table 18-1. Cytokine Receptor Subgroups

Type I cytokine receptors—hematopoietin receptor family
- IL-2Rβ, -γ
- IL-3Rα
- IL-4Rα
- IL-5Rα
- IL-6Rα
- IL-7Rα
- IL-9Rα
- IL-12Rα
- EPO-R
- CSF-GMRα
- AIC2A (IL-3 murine receptor)
- AIC2B (murine) or KH97 (human) (common β-chain for IL-3, -5/CSF-GM)
- CSF-GR
- Myeloproliferative leukemia virus
- LIF-R
- OSM-R
- CNTF-Rα
- gp130 (common signal transducer)
- Growth hormone (GH-R)
- Prolactin (PRL-R)

Immunoglobulin superfamily receptors
- IL-1R
- FGF-R
- SCF/KL-R
- CSF-R
- PDGF-R

Type II cytokine receptors
- Interferon receptors
- (IFN-Rα, IFN-Rβ, IFN-Rγ)

TNF-like receptors
- CD40 (gp39)
- CD27
- CD30
- OX40
- 4-1BB
- Fas
- Low-affinity nerve growth factor receptor

factors, such as IL-1R, and the tyrosine kinase-containing receptors: CSF-1R, SCF/KL-R, FGF-R, and platelet-derived growth factor (PDGF-R).[110]

High-affinity receptor interactions require homodimeric ligand receptor interactions such as those for CSF-G,[121] CSF-1,[122,123] SCF/KL,[124] and EPO,[125] or heterodimeric receptor ligand interactions via multichain receptors like PDGF-R[126] as well as receptors with a common signal transducer such as the IL-3/IL-5/CSF-GM common β-chain,[111,115] or the gp130 receptor subunit shared by IL-6R,[116,117] LIF-R,[111,127] OSM-R,[128] CNTF-R,[111,129] and IL-11R.[130] In addition, shared signaling receptor subunits like the IL-2Rγ subunit common to IL-2, IL-4,[131] IL-7,[132] and perhaps IL-13[133] may account for the functional redundancy of these factors in hematopoiesis and immune regulation.

Most cytokines have pleiotropic activities and exhibit multiple functions on multiple cell types, and several CSFs may exert the same function when interacting with a given cell type.[47,112] Growth factor receptors exist in high- and low-affinity forms on many hematopoietic and nonhematopoietic cells.[110,115,134-139] High-affinity CSF-GMRs are expressed in low numbers on progenitors (50–100/cell) and increase as neutrophil and monocyte precursors undergo terminal maturation.[110,140] All CSF interactions with high-affinity receptors at 37°C are associated with internalization and subsequent degradation of internalized CSF.[122,136,141] This can in effect serve as a negative feedback mechanism.[142,143] Low-affinity receptors have a high rate

of ligand dissociation; as such, they may serve as a reserve pool that can be used by new high-affinity receptors as they become available.[144]

Another common growth factor receptor theme is receptor trans-modulation.[145,146] Such modulation of receptor number can occur through a variety of mechanisms.[147-151] First, several ligands that do not directly interact at the CSF-binding domains of receptors can down-modulate CSF-Rs. With the CSF-1R, such modulators include lipopolysaccharide (LPS), phorbolesters 12-0-tetradecanoyl-phorbol-13-acetate (TPA), and TNF-α; for CSF-GR, they include LPS, TPA, and the chemotactic peptide f-met-leu-phe (FMLP); and for CSF-GMR, they include TPA, FMLP, and TNF-α. Second, the loss of high-affinity binding sites through internalization is a mode of receptor down-regulation. Third, CSFs can trans-modulate other CSF-Rs. This means that the binding of one CSF to its own receptor at 37°C results in a loss of high-affinity binding sites for another CSF. In the mouse, IL-3R can transmodulate CSF-MR, -GR, and -GMR; CSF-GMRs can modulate CSF-MR and -GR; CSF-GRs can transmodulate CSF-MRs; and CSF-MRs can transmodulate CSF-GMRs. In mice, the multipotential CSFs (IL-3/CSF-GM) seem able to down-modulate lineage-specific CSF-Rs (CSF-G/GM), but not vice versa.[110] In humans, the trans-modulation between IL-3, CSF-GM, and IL-5 is reciprocal.[144,148]

Unlike the IL-2R β-subunit, the CSF-GM/IL-5/IL-3 common β-subunit does not bind ligand but rather alters the affinity of the ligand for α-subunits. This finding might help to explain receptor trans-modulation: if β-subunits are limiting, then binding of ligand (IL-3) to its α-subunit will deplete β-subunits since the α/β high-affinity receptor complex will be internalized.[144] The possession of common receptor subunits may help to explain some overlapping activities of these growth factors, but it does not fully explain the unique spectrum of activities of each growth factor or their pleiotropic actions in a given cell type. The β-subunits are responsible for CSF-GM/IL-3/IL-5 signal transduction in responsive cells.[115,144,152]

Indeed, cross-regulation of cytokine receptors by other factors is a constant theme in hematopoiesis and has been demonstrated with several early- and late-acting cytokines such as SCF, IL-1, IL-6, IL-3, CSF-GM, TNF-α, and transforming growth factor-β (TGF-β).[81,153-160] This complex regulation serves as an additional checkpoint to regulate specific precursor survival and maturation after the initial commitment process.[3,81,91] All hemopoietin family receptors have common structural features: two fibronectin type III modules, four conserved cysteines residues in the N-terminal module, and a unique sequence Trp-Ser-X-Trp-Ser (WSXWS) in the C-terminal module.[111,115] These structural features ensure appropriate receptor dimerization and ligand receptor three-dimensional interactions.[161] Lastly, these receptors have no intrinsic kinase activity of their own, hence they require activation (phosphorylation of β-chains) and the additional docking action of intracellular serine threonine/tyrosine kinase(s)/signaling complexes to transduce a mitogenic signal effectively.[115]

Receptor-Mediated Signaling

In contrast to type I cytokine receptors of the hematopoietin family, tyrosine kinase-containing receptors like CSF-1R (c-fms),[162,163] PDGF-R,[164,165] FLK-2/FLT3,[66,166] and c-kit[54] mediate signaling directly after ligand/receptor dimerization and interchain phosphorylation by interacting with multiple signaling molecules with adapter domains for src-homology regions (SH2/SH3).[165]

Cytokine receptor-mediated signal transduction results in cell activation, priming, proliferation, and/or maturation, depending on the particular target cell being analyzed.[3,135,158,163] A complex cascade of events following CSF-GM/IL-3 high-affinity receptor engagement has been uncovered and includes (1) G-binding protein(s) translocation,[167-172] (2) phosphatidylinositol pathway activation,[173,174] (3) phospholipase A_2 and D activation,[175–177] (4) p21ras activation,[178,179] (5) *raf* kinase phosphorylation,[180] (6) protein kinase C (PKC) activation[181] and Na^+/H^+ antiporter activation,[182] and (7) mitogen-associated activated protein (MAP) kinase phosphorylation.[183–185] Similar events also occur with CSF-1R-*(fms)*-mediated signaling, leading to Na^+ antiporter activation,[162,186] *raf* kinase phosphorylation and activation,[162,187] cell proliferation[163] and cyclin D1 expression,[188] and activation events such as enhanced phagocytosis,[189] chemotaxis,[190,191] chemokine gene expression,[192] and integrin expression[193] of c-*fms*-positive target cells. The convergence of these various CSF-R-mediated signaling pathways, involving PKC or MAP kinase (MAPK), on the nucleus results in the transcriptional regulation of new genes, such as *EGR-1*, c-*jun*, and *AP1*, in both proliferating and terminally differentiated myeloid cells.[115,194–198] with enhanced expression of AP-1, nuclear factor (NF)-AT, and NF-κB after induction of MAPK in T cells.[199]

Most hematopoietin receptors, such as CSF-GR and CSF-GMR, are devoid of tyrosine kinase activity and require additional molecules to mediate their mitogenic activity.[111,115] For example, for CSF-GMR, neither subunit is a tyrosine kinase and neither has domains similar to those found in G-protein-associated receptors. The finding of common substrates phosphorylated on tyrosine residues after activation of several cytokine receptors, as well as the necessity of tyrosine kinase activity to activate p21*ras,* suggested that these receptors were undergoing phosphorylation after ligand interaction by associating with intracytoplasmic signaling complexes with adapter proteins containing 2 SH2 in a variety of cells.[115,178] Furthermore, insights into the physiology of proteins with SH2 domains revealed their capacity to act as transducers of several tyrosine kinase signaling pathways.[200] The seminal discovery has been the isolation of an SH2 domain containing transforming protein with a unique sequence (SHC).[201,202] The SHC cDNA encodes overlapping proteins of 46.8 and 51.7 kd, while antibodies recognize three components, (46, 52, and 66 kd). SHC proteins are rapidly phosphorylated by *src* kinases and form a complex with the 23-kd polypeptide of the adapter molecule Grb2 with an SH3 domain and its partner binding protein sos (a guanine nucleotide exchange factor).[203,204] This activated complex mediates *ras* activation after receptor/ligand interactions, as shown for the epidermal growth factor (EGF)/erbB-2 receptor[205–208] and for the insulin/insulin receptor substrate-1 (IRS-1).[209–211] The demonstrated role of the SH2/SH3 domains of Grb2 in coupling EGF signaling to the ras activator sos provided the final link for growth factor-mediated p21*ras* activation.[212] Soon thereafter came the discovery of the JAK tyrosine kinase family and the realization that either JAK1 or JAK2 can serve as receptor-associated tyrosine kinases to transduce multiple growth factor/receptor proliferative signals,[213] as illustrated by the signaling mediated through growth hormone,[213] interferon-α (via JAK1) and interferon-γ (both JAK1 or JAK2).[214–216]

This tyrosine kinase pathway linked to receptor subunits and Grb2/sos adapters offered the necessary explanation for the frequently seen p21*ras* activation, which leads to the MAPK kinase extracellular signal-regulated kinase activation[217] seen with CSF-GM,[115,184,185] SCF, and IL-3.[115,178,179] As shown in Figure 18-4, hemopoietins such as IL-6, IL-3/CSF-GM/IL-5 and the immunoglobulin-like receptor for IL-1 use distinct but somewhat overlapping intracytoplasmic signaling pathways, eventually leading to new gene (c-*myc*, cyclin D2, c-*jun,* c-*fos*) transcription.[115] Multiple cytokines, with the exception of IL-4, stimulated the phosphorylation of a p97-kd protein (JAK2) and p42 MAPK.[218–221] CSF-GM and IL-3 phosphorylated the same sets of proteins, including raf kinase and MAPK, in a factor-dependent cell line (MO7), while SCF, in addition, phosphorylated phospholipase Cγ on tyrosine,[220] like the kinase-containing receptors such as PDGF-R, CSF-1R, and FLK-2/FLT3.[163–166] Distinct cytoplasmic regions of the common β-subunit mediating the signaling for the IL-3/IL-5/CSF-GM ligands have been mapped by reconstitution experiments using a factor-dependent hematopoietic cell line of 3T3 fibroblasts.[222–229] The importance of both α- and β-chains for CSF-GM signal transduction is illustrated in Figure 18-4,[225,227] as is polypeptide signaling to the nucleus via JAK kinase.[230]

Mounting evidence is also implicating the IL-6 signal transducer gp130 protein in JAK2 kinase activation.[231] In the event that this activation leads to tyrosine phosphorylation of an interferon-stimulated factor (ISGF), this may provide a direct transcriptional signal to the nucleus without activating the *ras-raf*-MEK-MAPK cascade, which is reminiscent of the JAK1/2-mediated tyrosine phosphorylation of several cytoplasmic *STAT* (signal transducers and activators of transcription) proteins[231,232] (Fig. 18-4). These transduction pathways have also been confirmed by the demonstration of JAK2 kinase association with several type I cytokine receptor/ligand complexes, such as IL-3,[233,234] EPO,[235,236] and CSF-GM,[237,238] which have also been found to be associated with SHC and sos, leading to p21*ras* activation.[233–238] Similarly, SCF[239] and the p210bcr/*abl* kinase[240] recapitulate the same events, leading to receptor subunit phosphorylation[239] and activation of the SHC signaling component of the p21*ras* pathway via tyrosine phosphorylation, underscoring the importance of this cascade and its common utilization by several cytokine-receptor interactions.[201,240–242]

Receptor reconstitution experiments showing a divergence in cellular signaling events between hematopoietic cells and nonhematopoietic cells such as 3T3 fibroblasts, as well as subtle differences between SCF and IL-3 and CSF-GM action on the same target cells, require additional explanation.[220,224,241] The discovery of the tyrosine phosphorylation of many endogenous cytoplasmic transcription factors with SH2/SH3 domains by JAK1 or JAK2 kinases[243,244] at last provided a *ras*-independent growth factor signaling pathway.[245] The detailed analysis of signaling complexes has shown a p80-kd component in cells stimulated by IL-3, CSF-GM, or IL-5, while interferon-γ-treated cells activated several transcription factors containing the p91-kd component of ISGF-3.[244] Thus, the cellular specificity of signaling may be provided by individual receptor subunits (such as α-chains of CSF-R) that activate unique cytoplasmic transcription factors.[243] In addition, the CSF-GMR α-subunit participates in glucose transport without requiring tyrosine phosphorylation, thus providing a link to the increased survival of precursors induced by CSF-GM.[245a]

Another issue in cytokine receptors is the pleiotropic nonreceptor tyrosine kinases (such as src kinases) and transforming proto-oncogenes (such as *abl, myb, vav*) that have been identified in hematopoietic cells.[246,247] While the exact function(s) of these molecules is far from being totally understood, gene knock-out experiments have started to shed some light on the role of these molecules in hematopoiesis.[246,247] For instance, *Pim*-1 is induced by IL-3/CSF-GM-treated cells,[115] and its expression parallels the growth of cytokine-exposed cells.[248] The tyrosine kinase c-fps/fes has been implicated in CSF-GMR and EPO-R signaling,[249–251] the *src* kinase lyn, normally associated with the high-affinity Fc receptor I, is regulated by IL-3 in myeloid cells,[252] and the syk kinase participates in CSF-GM/IL-5-induced eosinophil differentiation.[253] These potential regulatory kinase complexes are also illustrated in Figure 18-4.

CSF-GR, which is also devoid of kinase activity, by itself forms a three-component complex with *lyn* and *syk* protein kinases.[254] The study of patients with severe congenital neutropenia offers insights into the role of this receptor, as patients display normal CSF-GR on their neutrophils,[255] but their CFU-GM growth in response to CSF-G alone is poor, while a combination of SCF and CSF-G reveals normal growth patterns.[256] Indeed, molecular characterization of CSF-GR showed distinct cytoplasmic regions involved in the induction of proliferation or differ-

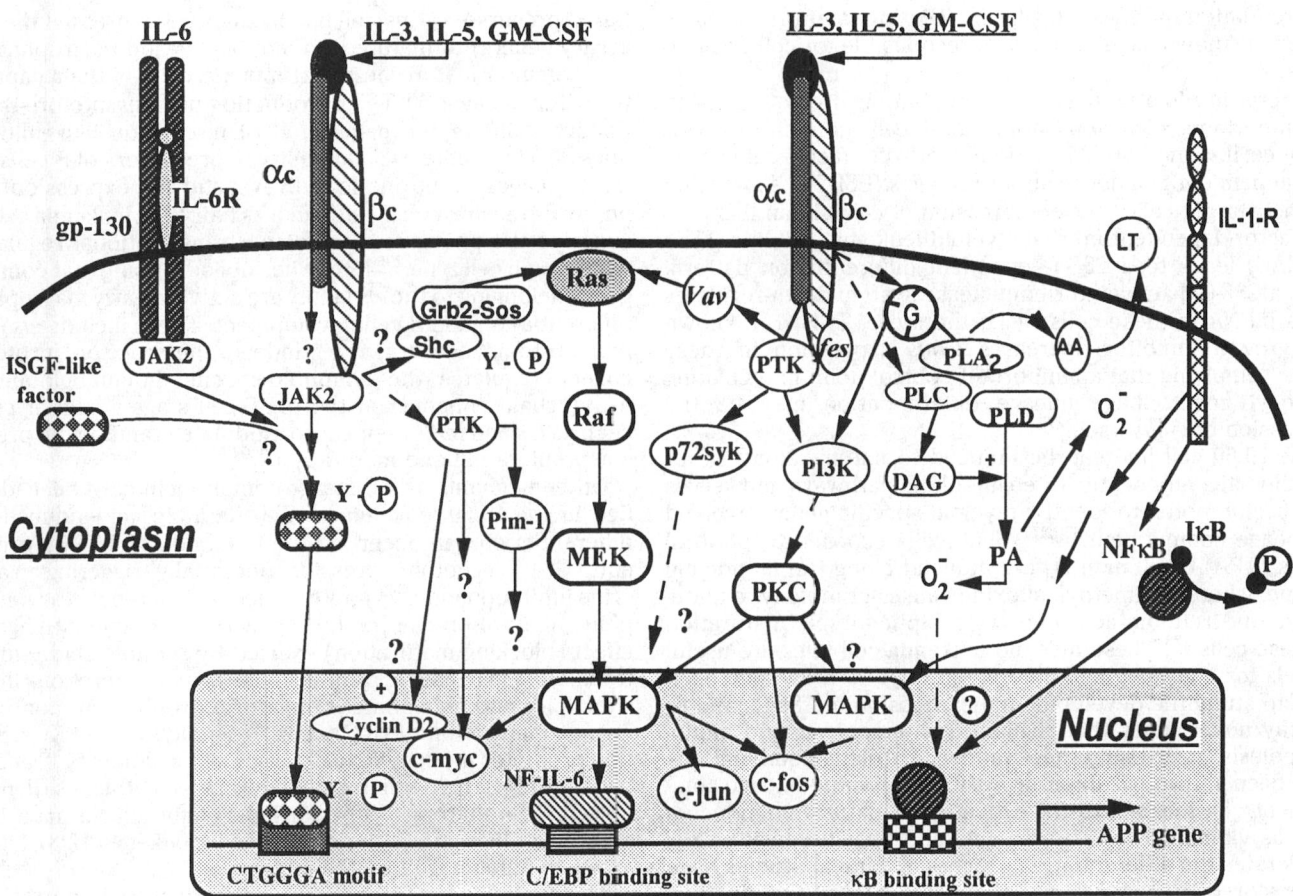

Fig. 18-4. Multiple signaling pathways involved in granulopoiesis including the IL-6R/gp130 receptor and the IL-3Rα, IL-5Rα, and CSF-GMRα receptors, which possess a common β-subunit (βc). Also shown is the ability of IL-1 to act synergistically with these other growth factors. Complex intracytoplasmic cross-talk between mediators of these pathways occurs, and many aspects remain to be elucidated (denoted by ?). The β-chain of the IL-3/CSF-GM/IL-5 receptor family has no intrinsic protein tyrosine kinase (PTK)-activating capacity and can associate with the JAK2 tyrosine kinase. The common β-chain and gp130 interact with JAK2, resulting in receptor phosphorylation. The α-chain of these receptors confers specificity for the individual cytokine signals, as shown by receptor reconstitution studies. Grb2-sos, growth factor receptor-binding protein and mammalian son of sevenless; PL, phospholipase; SHC, *src* homology; DAG, diacylglycerol; NF, nuclear factor; MAP, mitogen-activated protein; ERK, extracellular signal-regulated kinase; MEK, MAP kinase/ERK-activating kinase; ISGF, interferon-stimulated gene factor; APP, acute-phase protein; AA, arachidonic acid; LT, leukotriene.

entiation,[257] and transfection analysis showed cross-phosphorylation of IL-3R by CSF-G stimulation of cells expressing both receptors, indicating potential functional redundancy of cytokine receptor signaling[258] (Fig. 18-4). Moreover, the identification of a truncated CSF-G receptor in a case of severe congenital neutropenia[259] offers an example of the important role of receptor-associated signaling complexes leading to p21ras and MAPK activation in mediating cell proliferation.[260] Finally, the importance of PKC in CSF-G-mediated neutrophil survival underscores the potential for this activation pathway in the cytokine receptor signaling process diagrammed in Figure 18-4.[261]

Along with the characterization of protein kinases came the realization that in these dynamic phosphorylation/dephosphorylation processes, distinct protein tyrosine phosphatases were an integral part of turning off or in some instances turning on a given signaling cascade.[262] In the case of hematopoiesis, the CD45-associated phosphatase has been shown to modulate IL-3-, CSF-GM-, and SCF-mediated progenitor growth,[263] whereas CSF-1 phosphorylates[264] and SCF associates with a tyrosine phosphatase.[265] Similarly, a cell-associated phosphatase has been shown to associate with the IL-3 receptor β-chain and to mediate the down-regulation of IL-3-induced tyrosine phosphorylation and cell proliferation,[266] and an IL-3-induced serine/threonine phosphatase may regulate c-*jun* expression in monocytes.[267]

Lastly, the regulation of myeloid proliferation and differentiation may also include small intracellular messenger molecules such as nitric oxide, which has been implicated in the modulation of the cell differentiation and c-*myc* and c-*fos* gene expression in the HL60 human myeloid leukemia cell line, also adding more complexity to the cytokine transduction pathways regulating myeloid cell proliferation or differentiation, or both.[268]

Lineage Commitment

The mechanism(s) of lineage commitment toward granulopoiesis and monocytopoiesis and the roles of cytokines, cytokine receptors, and specific myeloid genetic programs are still incompletely understood.[269,270] In vitro studies of murine embryonic stem cells and embryoid bodies reveal a temporal coordinated expression of growth factor receptor genes during cell maturation.[271] Certain genes are expressed constitutively during development of these cells, such as c-*kit* and the α-subunits of the growth factor receptor genes, while the common β-subunit of the IL-3/IL-5/CSF-GM receptors, as well as SCF, are induced early. By contrast, c-*fms*, CSF-GR, and CD34 are induced later, at an intermediate stage of development, reflecting the initiation of myeloid commitment.[271] The extent to which growth factors and cytokine receptor expression determine the differentiation pathway taken by GM progenitors remains largely unknown, as do the genes responsible for cell commitment.

Several in vitro models of differentiation provide clues to the importance of various stimuli to lineage commitment. For instance, IL-3 and CSF-GM act dominantly in a factor concentration-dependent manner to suppress c-fms (CSF-1R) expression on their target cell.[272] Overexpression of c-fms in an IL-3/CSF-GM factor-dependent murine myeloid leukemia cell line (FDC-P1/MAC) leads to a CSF-1-dependent differentiation pattern. Also, a CSF-GM-activated ribonuclease system down-regulates c-fms mRNA in these cells.[273] Furthermore, TGF-β1, a known cell growth inhibitor, increases c-fms expression in these cells,[274] implying that an important control point in regulating monocyte/macrophage lineage differentiation may be the expression of c-fms itself.[275]

The HL60 cell line can be induced to mature along either granulocytic, monocytic, or eosinophilic pathways and serves as a useful model to identify myeloid-specific genes involved in lineage commitment.[276,277] HL60 cells exposed to phorbol esters (TPA) or vitamin D_3 are induced along the monocytic lineage, whereas dimethylsulfoxide causes granulocytic maturation, and retinoic acid induces a biphenotypic maturation of these cells.[278] These myeloid leukemia cell lines are useful models for analyzing cell differentiation, and they have been used to study the developmental expression of CSF-Rs and to identify novel genes that regulate granulopoiesis and monocytopoiesis.[135,279] Using these models, cytokine combinations have been shown to inhibit growth and promote lineage commitment,[280] while sequential exposure to maturation inducers such as vitamin D_3 or retinoic acid and lineage-specific CSFs accelerates the differentiation process.[281] Similar studies have underscored the central role of specific genes in modulating myeloid commitment, such as the c-myc,[282,283] c-myb,[284] SCL,[285] and EGR-1 genes.[194,286] Furthermore, they have demonstrated the importance of c-myc expression on cell proliferation[283] and the need to down-regulate its function prior to the induction of terminal differentiation.[287,288]

CSF-GM concentration determines myeloid versus monocytic commitment by controlling c-fms expression.[103] At low concentrations of CSF-GM, macrophage colony formation is favored due to relatively high expression of c-fms, whereas at higher CSF-GM concentrations, mixed colony formation (GM) is preferred due to the lower levels of c-fms expression.[103,272] Similarly, EGR-1, a DNA-binding zinc-finger transcription factor, is an early response gene up-regulated by macrophage inducers (TPA and CSFs)[163,194]; it functions by restricting myeloblast differentiation to the macrophage lineage.[286] The essential role of CSF-1R in monocyte/macrophage lineage commitment is also illustrated by a c-fms-dependent HL60 cell differentiation model[289] in which monocytic differentiation and retinoblastoma (Rb) gene expression depend on the presence of active CSF-1R on the cell surface.[289]

Similar cross-regulation of CSF-Rs occurs in the 32DC13(G) IL-3-dependent murine cell line, which can be primed by CSF-G to express CSF-GMRs and thereby differentiate into monocytes and granulocytes.[290] Such findings are in keeping with the observed synergistic effects between CSF-GM and CSF-G on highly purified progenitor cells.[291] Moreover, as with c-fms and monocytic maturation, expression of CSF-GR promotes granulocytic differentiation in the WEHI-3B D⁺ cell line,[292] while the up-regulation of CSF-GR mRNA appears to be an early commitment event in normal myeloid differentiation that is often dysfunctional in leukemic cells.[293] Thus, the cellular milieu in which CSF-R expression is modulated plays an important part in overall lineage commitment. This fact is underscored by a multipotential stem cell line that requires stromal induction to mature and does not alter its maturation program following premature expression of CSF-1R,[294] implying that (unlike more differen-

tiated precursors) this cell line has not yet expressed the necessary gene(s) to mature into monocytes and macrophages.

A common feature of hematopoietic cells is their capacity to switch lineages.[270] The introduction of v-fms into pre-B lymphocytes allows the generation of monocytic leukemic cell lines.[295] The bipotential capability of precursors of B cells and macrophages in murine fetal liver[42] and the expression of c-fms by B-transformed B cells such as hairy cell leukemia cells[191] suggests the presence of common transcriptional regulators within each cell type.[296] Hence it is not surprising that common genes belonging to the ets family are active in early macrophage differentiation and B-cell development. These include ets2 and pu.1 proto-oncogene(s).[297,298] Indeed, the pu.1/spi-1 proto-oncogene regulates the lymphoid-specific immunoglobulin μ heavy chain enhancer at the pre-B-cell stage.[299] Other genes such as fes and MZF-1 appear to modulate granulocytic precursor proliferation and maturation.[300,301]

Other mechanisms for lineage commitment have been identified in the HL60 leukemia model. Retinoic acid-induced cell differentiation can occur via the induction of TGF-β1 protein and TGF-β1 receptor expression, potentially triggering an autocrine inhibition loop.[302] Another mechanism regulating neutrophilic maturation can be the easing of the dominant negative effect (blocking maturation) exerted by retinoic acid α-fusion transcripts in leukemic promyelocytes.[295,303] Alterations in inositol lipids and phosphates regulate neutrophilic or monocytic lineage maturation of HL60 cells.[304] Finally, while PKC activation promotes monocytic maturation of myeloblasts[305] and enhances CFU-GM growth in conjunction with cytokines (IL-6 and CSF-G),[306] inhibitors of myosin light chain kinase have been shown to differentiate the monoblastic leukemia U937 line,[307] an effect antagonized by CSF-GM.

The central role of transcriptional regulators in normal and leukemic cells has been increasingly appreciated as sites of chromosomal translocations have been characterized.[295] Undoubtedly, complex regulatory signaling pathways involving receptor and nonreceptor kinases and phosphatases must affect specific genetic programs responsible for the lineage commitment process.

CELLULAR PRODUCTION

Granulocytes are derived from a common myeloid stem cell and comprise neutrophils, eosinophils, and basophil/mast cells. Neutrophils (PMNs) and monocytes/macrophages constitute two important elements of the host defense system: (1) mucosal immunity (basophil/mast cells), and (2) responses to allergens and parasitic infections (eosinophils, basophils, mast cells). In this role, they must have the capacity to migrate, phagocytize, and produce inflammation-inducing substances in order to achieve antimicrobial destruction or to contribute to inflammatory reactions. In addition to combating microorganisms, tissue macrophages constitute the "resident" reticuloendothelial system of many organs such as liver, spleen, and bone marrow.[308] In these sites, they may also serve to eliminate debris and senescent cells, to aid in antigen presentation and processing, and in some cases, to effect antitumor cytotoxicity. Since these effector cells are constantly utilized, the need to maintain appropriate cell numbers in an equilibrium state as well as to have the capacity for increased production in times of stress requires a finely controlled regulation of both neutrophil and monocyte production.

Neutrophil and Monocyte Production

Briefly, in the adult, the marrow is the source of both neutrophils and monocytes, which circulate until they exit the vascular spaces for the tissues. In the marrow, the CFU-GM is the earliest cell type that can be identified in culture as having commitment to differentiate along the myeloid pathway. This cell type is distinguished by its ability to form clonal cell groups (colonies) when grown in vitro in semisolid media such as agar or methylcellulose in the presence of CSFs (Fig. 18-1). CFU-GM, which numbers about 50–100/10⁶ nucleated cells in a normal human marrow specimen, is a bipotential progenitor and can respond to CSF-GM differentially based on growth factor concentration. As discussed previously, at high concentrations of CSF-GM, the granulocytic pathway is favored, whereas at low concentrations, monocytic/macrophagic differentiation occurs preferentially (Fig. 18-3). CSF-1 appears to control its own expression on maturing progenitor cells, providing another feedback regulatory pathway to limit unchecked monocyte production,[309] while anti-inflammatory agents such as cyclosporine and dexamethasone regulate CSF-1 and c-*fms* expression at a post-transcriptional level.[310]

Progenitor cells cannot be recognized morphologically in marrow, but rather have the appearance of nondescript mononuclear cells (lymphoid appearance). The myeloblast is the first morphologically identifiable precursor. Myeloblasts, promyelocytes, and myelocytes are mitotic, but metamyelocytes, band neutrophils, and mature PMNs constitute what is known as the postmitotic compartment (Fig. 18-2). Azurophilic granules appear at the promyelocyte stage, but the specific granules containing such substances as lactoferrin and cytochrome b do not appear until the myelocyte stage. The adult human harbors an estimated 7.7×10^9 PMNs/kg. In addition to neutrophils found in the vascular space and tissues, there is a large marginated pool and a large marrow reserve, allowing for rapid recruitment of effector cells in times of need. Neutrophils spend approximately 6–7 days in the marrow. On egress, they spend only a short time in the circulation (half-life 6.7 hours). The released PMN is differentiated and can no longer divide. Neutrophils live in tissues for only a few days.

Monocytic cells, of which the promonocyte is the earliest recognizable stage, spend less time in the bone marrow than do PMNs, so they are released into the circulation with the ability to mature further. No marrow reserve exists. Monocytes spend 1–3 days in transit through the marrow and 8–72 hours in the blood. On entry into tissues, further maturation and possible proliferation can occur. Monocytes can survive in tissues for long periods, reportedly >80 days. The tissue-fixed macrophages derived from monocytes include alveolar macrophages, which can proliferate when exposed to IL-3 with CSF-1,[311] the Kupffer cells in the liver and splenic macrophages,[308] and oligodendrocytes/glial cells, which elaborate cytokines and express CSF-GMRs.[312,313]

Additional specialized cells include dendritic cells, which appear to be derived from CD34⁺ progenitors,[314,315] since colonies with a dendritic appearance grew in the same colonies as macrophages, suggesting a common origin. The dendritic cells were HLA-DR⁺ and CD4⁺, but they lacked nonspecific esterase and other macrophage surface markers. They were HLA-DQ⁺ and were able to stimulate allogeneic mixed lymphocyte cultures. In the presence of TNF-α and CSF-GM, these cells proliferate and acquire the characteristic morphologic appearance of dendritic cells.[316] Furthermore, dendritic cells in the lungs as well as pleural and peritoneal macrophages are subject to local control by CSF-GM,[317] a process also seen in transgenic mice expressing CSF-GM.[318]

To maintain steady-state hematopoiesis, it is estimated that 8.7×10^8 PMNs/kg and 5.7×10^6 monocytes/kg must be produced every day. The cytokine factors that influence the proliferation and maturation of these cells must thus be finely tuned to be able to accommodate ever-changing and sometimes urgent demands for increased production. CFU-M generally need two factors, CSF-GM plus CSF-1 or IL-6 plus CSF-1 to express full colony-forming potential.[291] CSF-GM synergizes with CSF-G

in the formation of granulocytic colonies (CFU-G) with respect to number and size of the colonies. Also, CSF-GM synergizes with CSF-1 (CSF-M) to increase the number and size of macrophage colonies (CFU-M).[47,291] A significant proportion of CFU-M growth requires the presence of IL-6, indicating that an intricate regulatory cytokine network probably influences marrow promonocyte production.[319,320] Additional studies have also identified a monocyte-specific inducer elaborated by activated macrophages undergoing phagocytosis or at sites of inflammation.[321] This cytokine, termed factor-increasing monocytopoiesis, differs from IL-1 and CSF-1 and regulates marrow monocyte production in a specific long-range manner.[322] Its relationship to the newly identified monocyte-active chemokines such as MCP-1, -2, and -3 remains to be determined.[82,83]

Another example of complex cell-cell interactions and cytokine networks is illustrated by the in vitro actions of IL-4 on myelopoiesis. This cytokine inhibits TNF-α, IL-1α and -β, IL-6, and IL-8 expression at the transcriptional level in monocytes,[323–325] while it increases CSF-1 output in fibroblasts.[326] Lastly, IL-4 has been shown to release stromal inhibitory factors that may further complicate cellular production.[327] In vitro, IL-4 stimulates neutrophilic colony growth in CD34⁺/DR²⁺ progenitors, while it specifically inhibits IL-3 and CSF-GM-driven macrophage colony growth in vitro.[328,329] On the other hand, in the presence of IL-3 produced by activated T cells or natural killer cells, IL-4 facilitates the growth of basophils.[7] The net effects of these complex interactions following IL-4 administration in vivo are not clear and will require extensive clinical testing. IL-10 is another cytokine with anti-inflammatory properties able to promote basophil growth[330] while also inhibiting monocytic cytokines (IL-1α, -β, IL-6, IL-8, TNF-α, CSF-GM, and CSF-G) synthesis at the transcriptional level.[331]

The cytopenias frequently associated with infections and other bone marrow disorders reflect a complex regulatory network of soluble factors such as positive regulatory cytokines, inhibitory cytokines (TGF-β, TNF-α)[160,332] and chemokines (MIP-1α, IP-10, MCP-1),[82,333–337] soluble cytokine receptors,[111,338] and short-range regulatory signals mediated by leukotrienes,[339,340] prostaglandins,[341] and cytomatrix-bound factors regulating the interactions of stromal cell and progenitors.[342–345] Furthermore, macrophages developing within the marrow may differ in their function and phenotype.[346,347] These complex cytokine/cell-cell interactions are illustrated in Figure 18-5, which recapitulates intramedullary regulatory events occurring during active immune stimulation or chronic infections.[2,348] Mature mononuclear cells including granulocytes, monocytes, and T lymphocytes release cytokines when exposed to activating agents such as bacterial antigens or inflammatory stimuli, as shown in Figure 18-5 and Table 18-2, emphasizing the potential for localized regulation of progenitor output by mature precursors.[349–351]

Eosinophil Production

The eosinophil is a type of granulocyte characterized by distinct granules that become apparent at the early myelocyte stage of development.[94] Eosinophils are derived from CD34⁺ committed progenitors, and they proliferate and mature within the marrow. As illustrated in Figure 18-3, eosinophil production requires early-acting factors such as SCF, IL-3, and CSF-G,[352–354] as well as late-acting lineage-specific factors such as IL-5,[354] and CSF-GM.[355] Eosinophilic colonies in culture have been identified by luxol fast blue or peroxidase staining.[5,94] Their distinctive morphology and enzymatic granule content account for their staining properties and are described in greater detail in Chapter 51. The normal concentration of eosinophils in the blood is $<0.7 \times 10^9$ cells/L. Many diseases are associated with eosinophilia, including parasitic infestation with tissue-inva-

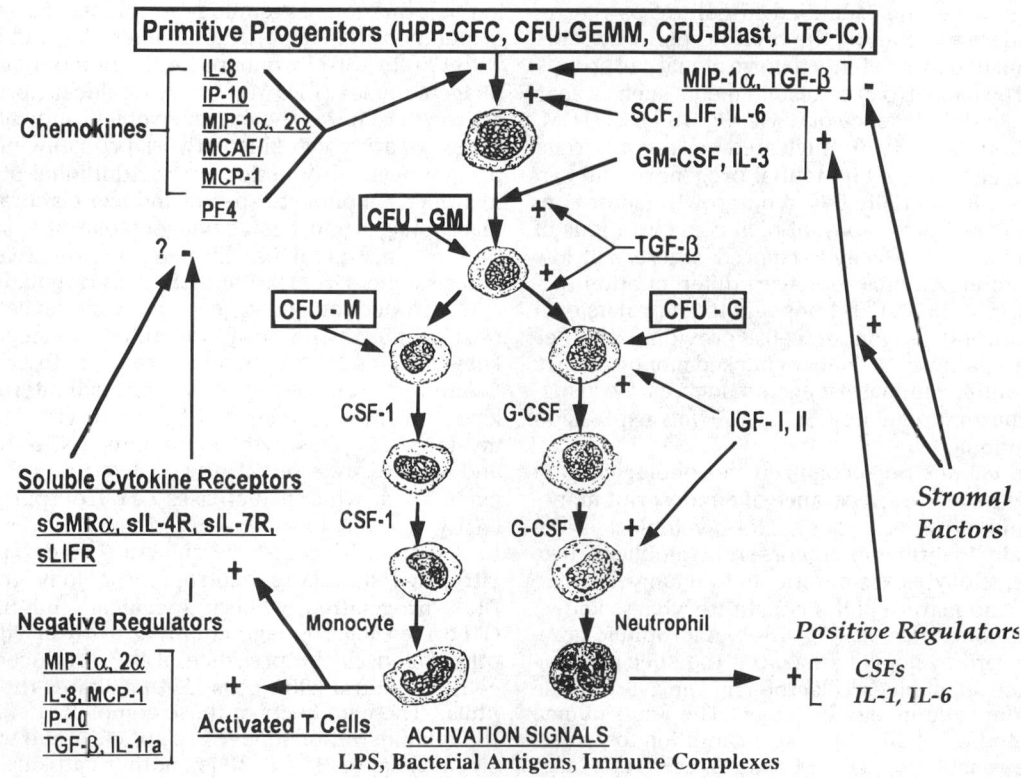

Fig. 18-5. Positive and negative regulators of monocytopoiesis and granulocytopoiesis (neutrophil component). Mediators of both a positive and negative nature are active at all levels of development. Also, certain cytokines at different concentrations and in different isoforms (e.g., TGF-β) can act in either an inhibitory or stimulatory fashion at various levels of maturation. MIP, macrophage inflammatory protein; PF4, platelet factor-4; IP-10, interferon-inducible protein 10; MCAF, monocyte chemotactic activating factor; ra, receptor antagonist; IGF, insulin-like growth factor; sIL-R, soluble interleukin receptor.

sive organisms, allergic states (bronchial asthma, allergic rhinitis, pulmonary aspergillosis), vasculitides, various collagen vascular diseases, and paraneoplastic conditions.[356,357]

The sequential action of eosinophil-active cytokines and their cellular derivation are shown in detail in Figure 18-6. Several growth factors have been found to act on early eosinophil progenitors, sometimes in a synergistic fashion. These include factors such as CSF-G and kit ligand (SCF) that are not specific for this lineage.[352,355] IL-3 is capable of inducing colonies from CD34+/CD33− cells, whereas IL-5 by itself does not have this capability.[355] When CD34+/CD33− cells are grown in IL-3 followed by IL-5, CFU-Eo emerge. CD34−/CD33+ cells will form CFU-Eo if first exposed to CSF-G or to IL-3 and then replated in IL-5.[355] IL-3, CSF-GM, and IL-5 have additional activity at intermediate stages of eosinophilopoiesis, and they are also active on mature eosinophils.[94,358]

In vivo experiments in mice and humans infected with filarial parasites have shown IL-5 to be the principal regulator of eosinophil production.[97,359,360] IL-2 administration leads to eosinophilia, which can be blocked by a monoclonal antibody to IL-5.[361] This in vivo IL-2 administration is associated with increased IL-5 RNA expression in the spleens of treated mice.[361] Transgenic mice expressing IL-5 develop eosinophilia and autoantibody production.[96] Moreover, IL-5 has also been found to be elevated in patients with hypereosinophilia[362] and has been identified along with CSF-GM and IL-3 in the eosinophilia associated with T-cell lymphoma.[363]

T cells and eosinophils are implicated in the pathogenesis of many disease states such as asthma.[94,356,357] The role of human types 1 and 2 T-helper-derived cytokines in eosinophilic states is highlighted in Figure 18-6.[364,365] The activation of IL-5-producing T cells in atopic states may lead to eosinophilia; additional

factors, some of which have not been cloned yet, are also operational in these conditions.[366] Also, in the hypereosinophilic syndrome, there is evidence in some patients for clonal proliferation of type 2 helper T cells.[367,368] A case has been reported of a patient with hypereosinophilia who had T-cell clones that produced IL-4 and IL-5 and demonstrated clonal rearrangements of the β-chain of the T-cell receptor.[368] Moreover, the importance of cell-cell intercrine stimulation is illustrated by the finding that CSF-GM-induced LTB4 secretion can lead to increased IL-5 elaboration by T cells, thereby amplifying eosinophilic precursor maturation at the sites of antigenic stimulation.[369] Lastly, eosinophils in the circulation and at the sites of allergic inflammation express IL-5 and CSF-GM[370,371] and in addition elaborate a potent angiogenic factor, TGF-α, as indicated by Table 18-2.[372]

Basophil Production

The basophil is a granulocyte subtype derived from marrow precursors; it functions in allergic disease, whereas tissue mast cells do not circulate in the blood but complete their maturation in tissues, where they provide mucosal immunity as well as a source of cytokines and a variety of agents on activation by allergens.[373] Mast cells are derived from CD34+, c-*kit*-positive progenitors, and not from monocytes, as previously thought.[374] The production of basophils as well as tissue-fixed mast cells is regulated by a complex array of cytokines elaborated by T-cell subsets, macrophages, and stromal cells/fibroblasts (Fig. 18-6). Basophilopoiesis is regulated by overlapping cytokines such as SCF, IL-3,[373,375,376] and IL-5,[7,94,377] which are active in eosinophilopoiesis, but it also relies on IL-4[7,378] and IL-10,[330]

Table 18-2. Cytokines Released by Activated Mature Precursors

Cytokine	Neutrophil	Monocyte/ Macrophage	Eosinophil	Mast Cell
IL-1α/IL-1β	+ + +	+ + +	+ + +	+ + +
IL-1 receptor antagonist	+ + +	+ + +	– – –	– – –
CSF-G	– – –	+ + +	– – –	– – –
CSF-GM	+ + +	+ + +	+ + +	+ + +
CSF-M	+ + +	+ + +	– – –	– – –
IL-3	– – –	– – –	+ + +	+ + –
IL-4	– – –	+ + +	– – –	+ + –
IL-5	– – –	– – –	– – –	+ + –
IL-6	+ + +	+ + +	+ + +	+ + –
OSM	– – –	+ + +	– – –	– – –
LIF	– – –	+ + +	– – –	– – –
IL-8	+ + +	+ + +	– – –	+ + –
Gro-α/MGSA	+ + +	+ + +	– – –	– – –
IL-10	– – –	+ + +	– – –	– – –
IL-12	– – –	+ + +	– – –	– – –
MCP-1/MCAF	– – –	+ + +	– – –	– – –
IP-10	– – –	+ + +	– – –	– – –
MIP-1α/MIP-1β	– – –	+ + +	– – –	+ + –
TNF-α	+ + +	+ + +	– – –	+ + –
IFN-α	+ + +	+ + +	– – –	– – –
TGF-β	– – –	+ + +	+ + +	– – –
TGF-α	– – –	+ + +	+ + +	– – –
Nerve growth factor	– – –	+ + +	– – –	– – –

Abbreviations: MGSA, melanoma growth-stimulatory activity; MCAF, monocyte chemotactic and activating factor.

cytokines with anti-inflammatory roles that do not affect eosinophil production.[7]

Also, at later stages of development, mast cells are differentially influenced by IL-3 and SCF (kit ligand), whereas basophils are regulated by IL-10, IL-3, and IL-4.[373,375] A rat model with an abnormal *W* locus has been developed that has no mast cells but has normal numbers of basophils,[379] implying that additional regulators such as nerve growth factor and IL-10 can substitute for SCF in mast cell development (Fig. 18-6). SCF (c-kit ligand) also induces mast cell proliferation, maturation, and heparin synthesis.[380] SCF also allows the emergence of mast cells from marrow mononuclear cells in long-term culture.[376] Nerve growth factor promotes murine mast cell colony formation[381] and has been found to be synergistic with CSF-GM in normal and leukemic basophilic cell differentiation[377,382] (Figs. 18-3 and 18-6).

CELLULAR DYNAMICS

Cytokine Expression by Mature Cells

Macrophages synthesize and release CSF-GM and CSF-G and display a large spectrum of heterogeneity.[347,349] Very little CSF is produced by resting macrophages, but stimulation with substances such as endotoxin can increase CSF-GM or -G production, while bone marrow-derived macrophages can elaborate SCF in small amounts.[346] Since tissue macrophages are separated from proliferating granulopoietic cells in the marrow, it is uncertain whether CSFs produced by these resident macrophages have any proliferative effects on the marrow progenitor compartment; they may serve only to activate granulocytes/macrophages locally. Monocytes also produce IL-1 and -6 as well as TNF-α[383] (Table 18-2). Disruption of the microtubule network of human monocytes induces expression of IL-1 but not that of IL-6 or of TNF-α. The IL-1 production is mediated by the stimulation of protein kinase A.[384]

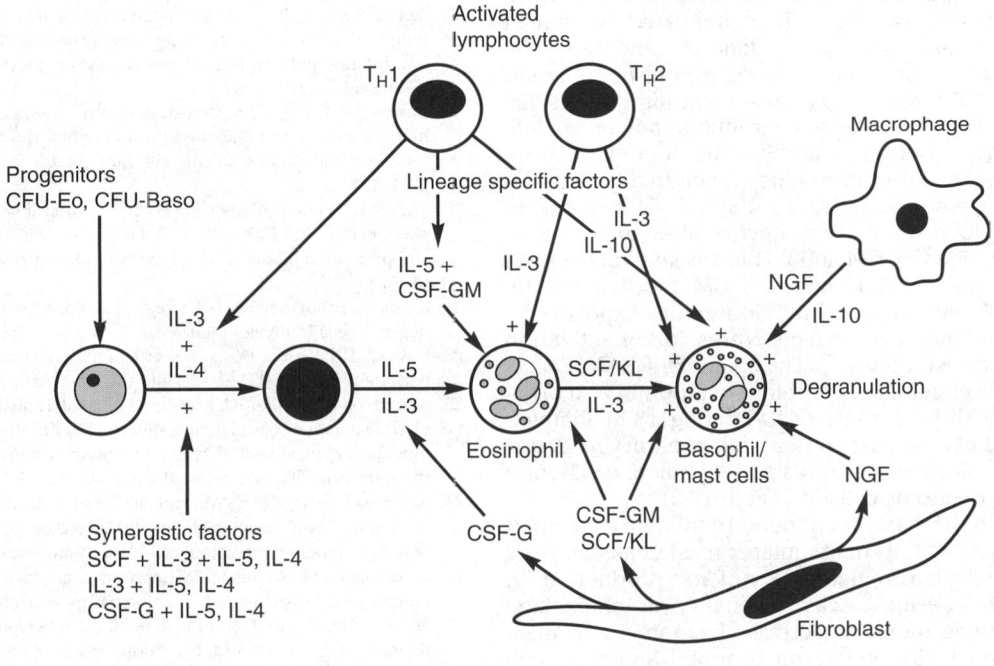

Fig. 18-6. Regulatory cytokines and accessory cells that modulate eosinophilopoiesis and basophilopoiesis. Factors produced by T-lymphocyte subsets, macrophages, and fibroblasts control the development of these cell types. These cytokines act individually or synergistically within each maturation pathway to promote cell proliferation or inhibit apoptosis. Several cytokines can activate mature precursors and thereby prime them for degranulation, migration, and enhanced effector function.

Neutrophils as well as eosinophils express IL-6 mRNA and secrete IL-6 protein.[372] This expression is rapidly down-regulated after cells are removed from the blood. Neutrophils can thus modulate T- and B-lymphocyte functions, granulocyte self-priming, and endothelial interactions through secretion of IL-6. CSF-GM has also been found to induce c-*fos, egr*-1, IL-1, CSF-G, CSF-M, and TNF-α genes in neutrophils, again suggesting that neutrophils can play a role in regulating the inflammatory response.[135,385–388] One can assume that there are active autocrine loops in both mature neutrophils and monocytes.[389,390] As with other granulocytic effector cells, eosinophils and mast cells also express cytokines upon activation (Table 18-2).

Cytokine Modulation of Mature Effector Cell Function

Growth factors are released at sites of inflammation and can exert both priming and direct effects on mature monocytes and neutrophils. These influences can effectively arm effectors for improved response to other physiologic substances that are also active at sites of inflammation and infection such as chemotactic factors, ILs, and leukotrienes. CSF-GM, as an example, can decrease random migration of macrophages and neutrophils, increase surface expression of Mo1, and increase leukocyte aggregation.[391,392] These represent only a few of the many effects of CSF-GM on mature neutrophils, which generally include accentuating host defense mechanisms such as adhesion, chemotaxis, phagocytosis, superoxide production, antibody-dependent cell-mediated cytotoxicity, and synthesis and release of inflammatory mediators and cytokines. Many of these effects have clinical significance, such as the profound drop in neutrophil counts after intravenous boluses of CSF-GM and CSF-G, possibly due to sequestration of these activated cells in lungs.[392]

Numerous cytokines also have effects on the mature eosinophil. IL-5 can prevent apoptosis in mature human eosinophils.[358] CSF-GM, IL-5, and IL-3 can activate eosinophils, manifested in many ways. The FcRγ II is activated in human eosinophils in response to these cytokines,[393] and each one has a priming effect on the eosinophil respiratory burst[394] and on responses to FMLP and to platelet-activating growth factor.[395] IL-5, CSF-GM, and IL-3 cause degranulation in an eosinophilic HL60 subline,[396] but CSF-G and IL-1 did not demonstrate this activity. Also, these three cytokines result in different patterns of activation; when IL-1, IL-3, IL-5, and CSF-GM are compared, anti-staphylococcal activity occurs after exposure to CSF-GM and IL-3, while CSF-GM and IL-1 increase phagocytosis of *Candida* organisms.[397] Moreover, CSF-GM and IL-3 amplify leukotriene C4 production after Ca^{2+} ionophore exposure.[397] Cytokines also modulate cell-surface expression of activation antigens on mature eosinophils.[398] The chemokine RANTES has been shown to be a chemoattractant for eosinophils,[399] a property not shared by MCP-1 MIP-1α, or IL-8[400] (Fig. 18-3). Platelet-activating factor is also another potent inflammatory mediator that can activate mature eosinophils and stimulate eosinophil production from precursor cells[401] (Table 18-2).

CSF-GM, IL-3, and IL-5 have been found to influence basophil functional activity.[7,373,402] IL-10 stimulates mast cells and their progenitors[330] and also regulates cytokine production in mouse marrow-derived mast cells.[403] Finally, the chemokine MIP-1α has also been found to activate basophils and mast cells.[404] In addition to its effects on basophil and mast cell development, SCF (c-kit ligand) potentiates release of mediators from mast cells[405] and activates their adhesion to fibronectin.[406] Both cyclosporine and FK506 have been found to inhibit cytokine production from mast cells[407,408] and basophils.[409] Table 18-2 illustrates the panel of cytokines released by basophil/mast cells on activation.

REFERENCES

1. Brennan JK, Lichtman MA, DiPersio JF, Abboud CN: Chemical mediators of granulopoiesis: a review. Exp Hematol 8:441, 1980
2. Moore MAS: Clinical implications of positive and negative hematopoietic stem cell regulators. Blood 78:1, 1991
3. Ogawa M: Differentiation and proliferation of hematopoietic stem cells. Blood 81:2844, 1993
4. Watt SM, Visser JWM: Recent advances in the growth and isolation of primitive human haemopoietic progenitor cells. Cell Prolif 25:263, 1992
5. Metcalf D: The Hemopoietic Colony Stimulating Factors. Elsevier. Amsterdam, 1984
6. Slovick FT, Abboud CN, Brennan JK, Lichtman MA: Modulation of in vitro eosinophil progenitors by hydrocortisone: role of accessory cells and interleukins. Blood 66:1072, 1985
7. Denburg JA: Basophil and mast cell lineages in vitro and in vivo. Blood 79:846, 1992
8. Fauser AA, Messner HA: Granuloerythropoietic colonies in human peripheral blood and cord blood. Blood 52:1243, 1978
9. McNiece IK, Bertoncello I, Kriegler AB, Quesenberry PJ: Colony-forming cells with high proliferative potential (HPP-CFC). Int J Cell Cloning 8:146, 1990
10. Leary AG, Ogawa M: Blast cell colony assay for umbilical cord blood and adult marrow progenitors. Blood 69:953, 1987
11. Udomsakdi C, Lansdorp PM, Hogge DE et al: Characterization of primitive hematopoietic cells in normal peripheral blood. Blood 80:2513, 1992
12. Zanjani ED, Pallavicini MG, Ascensao JL et al: Engraftment and long-term expression of human fetal hemopoietic stem cells in sheep following transplantation in utero. J Clin Invest 89:1178, 1992
13. Srour EF, Zanjani ED, Brandt JE et al: Sustained human hematopoiesis in a sheep transplanted in utero during early gestation with fractionated adult human bone marrow cells. Blood 79:1404, 1992
14. Srour EF, Zanjani ED, Cornetta K et al: Persistence of human multilineage, self-renewing lymphohematopoietic stem cells in chimeric sheep. Blood 82:3333, 1993
15. Mochizuki DY, Eisenman JA, Conlon PJ et al: Interleukin-1 regulates hematopoietic activity, a role previously ascribed to hemopoietin-1. Proc Natl Acad Sci USA 84:5267, 1987
16. McNiece IK, Kriegler AB, Quesenberry PJ: Studies on myeloid synergistic factor from 5637: comparison with interleukin-1 alpha. Blood 73:919, 1989
17. Ikebuchi K, Clark SC, Ihle JN et al: Granulocyte colony-stimulating factor enhances interleukin-3-dependent proliferation of multipotential hemopoietic progenitors. Proc Natl Acad Sci USA 85:3445, 1988
18. Ikebuchi K, Ihle JN, Hirai Y et al: Synergistic factors for stem cell proliferation: further studies of the target stem cells and the mechanism of stimulation by interleukin-1, interleukin-6 and granulocyte colony-stimulating factor. Blood 72:2007, 1988
19. Andrews RG, Singer JW, Bernstein ID: Precursors of colony forming cells in humans can be distinguished from colony forming cells by expression of the CD33 and CD34 antigens and light scatter properties. J Exp Med 169:1721, 1989
20. Pierelli L, Teofili L, Menichella G et al: Further investigations on the expression of HLA-DR, CD33 and CD13 surface antigens in purified bone marrow and peripheral blood CD34+ haematopoietic progenitor cells. Br J Haematol 84:24, 1993
21. Kabral A, Bradstock KF, Grimsley P, Favaloro EJ: Immunophenotype of clonogenic cells in myeloid leukemia. Leuk Res 12:51, 1988
22. Haylock DN, To LB, Dowse TL et al: Ex vivo expansion and maturation of peripheral blood CD34+ cells into the myeloid lineage. Blood 80:1405, 1992
23. Robertson MJ, Soiffer RJ, Freedman AS et al: Human bone marrow depleted of CD33-positive cells mediates delayed but durable reconstitution of hematopoiesis: clinical trial of MY9 monoclonal antibody-purged autografts for the treatment of acute myeloid leukemia. Blood 79:2229, 1992
24. Andrews RG, Bryand EM, Bartelmez SH et al: CD34+ marrow cells, devoid of T and B lymphocytes, reconstitute stable lymphopoiesis and myelopoiesis in lethally irradiated allogeneic baboons. Blood 80:1693, 1992
25. Chaudhary PM, Roninson IB: Expression and activity of P-glycoprotein, a multidrug efflux pump, in human hematopoietic stem cells. Cell 66:85, 1991
26. Srour EF, Leemhuis T, Brandt JE et al: Simultaneous use of rhodamine 123, phycoerythrin, Texas red, and allophycocyanin for isolation of human hematopoietic progenitor cells. Cytometry 12:179, 1991
27. Baum CM, Weissman IL, Tsukamoto AS et al: Isolation of a candidate human hematopoietic stem-cell population. Proc Natl Acad Sci USA 89:2804, 1992
28. Terstappen LWMM, Huang S, Safford M et al: Sequential generations of hemopoietic colonies derived from single nonlineage-committed CD34+ CD38- progenitor cells. Blood 77:1218, 1991
29. Srour EF, Brandt JE, Briddell RA et al: Human CD34+ HLA-DR- bone mar-

row cells contain progenitor cells capable of self-renewal multilineage, differentiation, and long-term in vitro hematopoiesis. Blood Cells 17:287, 1991

30. Terstappen LWMM, Buescher S, Nguyen M, Reading C: Differentiation and maturation of growth factor expanded human hematopoietic progenitors assessed by multidimensional flow cytometry. Leukemia 6:1001, 1992
31. Mayani H, Dragowska W, Lansdorp PM: Characterization of functionally distinct subpopulations of CD34+ cord blood cells in serum-free long-term cultures supplemented with hemopoietic cytokines. Blood 82:2664, 1993
32. Sutherland HJ, Hogge DE, Eaves CJ: Growth factor regulation of the maintenance and differentiation of human long-term culture-initiating cells (LTC-IC). Leukemia, suppl. 2. 7:S122, 1993
33. Yoder MC, Du XX, Williams DA: High proliferative potential colony-forming cell heterogeneity identified using counterflow centrifugal elutriation. Blood 2:385, 1993
34. Suda T, Suda J, Ogawa M: Proliferative kinetics and differentiation of murine blast cell colonies in culture: evidence for variable G0 periods and constant doubling rates of early pluripotent hemopoietic progenitors. J Cell Physiol 117:308, 1989
35. Carow CE, Hangoc G, Broxmeyer H: Human multipotential progenitor cells (CFU-GEMM) have extensive replating capacity for secondary CFU-GEMM: an effect enhanced by cord plasma. Blood 81:942, 1993
36. Slovick FT, Abboud CN, Brennan JK, Lichtman MA: Survival of granulocytic progenitors in the adherent and non-adherent compartments of human long-term marrow cultures. Exp Hematol 12:327, 1984
37. Lansdorp PM, Sutherland HJ, Eaves CJ: Selective expression of CD45 isoforms on functional subpopulations of CD34+ hemopoietic cells from human bone marrow. J Exp Med 172:363, 1991
38. Fritsch G, Buchinger P, Printz D et al: Rapid discrimination of early CD34+ myeloid progenitors using CD45-RA analysis. Blood 81:2301, 1993
39. Kinniburgh D, Russell NH: Comparative study of CD34-positive cells and subpopulations in human umbilical cord blood and bone marrow. Bone Marrow Transplant 12:489, 1993
40. Pontvert-Delucq S, Breton-Gorius J, Schmitt C et al: Characterization and functional analysis of adult human bone marrow cell subsets in relation to B-lymphoid development. Blood 82:417, 1993
41. Schmitt C, Ktorza S, Sarun S et al: CD34-expressing human thymocyte precursors proliferate in response to interleukin-7 but have lost myeloid differentiation potential. Blood 82:3675, 1993
42. Cumano A, Paige CJ, Iscove NN, Brady G: Bipotential precursors of B cells and macrophages in murine fetal liver. Nature 356:612, 1992
43. Borzillo GV, Ashmun RA, Sherr CJ: Macrophage lineage switching of murine early pre-B lymphoid cells expressing transduced fms genes. Mol Cell Biol 10:2703, 1990
44. Martin M, Strasser A, Baumgarth N et al: A novel cellular model (SPGM 1) of switching between the pre-B cell and myelomonocytic lineages. J Immunol 150:4395, 1993
45. Strobl H, Takimoto M, Majdic O et al: Myeloperoxidase expression in CD34+ normal human hematopoietic cells. Blood 82:2069, 1993
46. Demetri GD: Hematopoietic growth factors: current knowledge, future prospects. Curr Probl Cancer 16:179, 1992
47. Metcalf D: Hematopoietic regulators: redundancy or subtlety? Blood 82:3515, 1993
48. Demetri GD, Griffin JD: Granulocyte colony-stimulating factor and its receptor. Blood 78:2791, 1991
49. Clark SC, Kamen R: The human hematopoietic colony-stimulating factors. Science 236:1229, 1987
50. Sherr CJ, Stanley ER: Colony stimulating factor 1. p. 667. In Sporn MB, Roberts AB (eds): Peptide Growth Factors and their Receptors. Springer-Verlag, New York, 1990
51. Yang YC, Clark SC: Interleukin-3: molecular biology and biologic activities. Hematol Oncol Clin North Am 3:441, 1989
52. Mosmann TR, Zlotnick A: Multiple functions of interleukin 4 and its role in immune regulation. p. 129. In Habenicht A (ed): Growth Factors, Differentiation Factors, and Cytokines. Springer-Verlag, Berlin, 1990
53. Takatsu K: Interleukin-5. Curr Opin Immunol 4:299, 1992
54. Zsebo KM, Williams DA, Geissler EN et al: Stem cell factor is encoded at the Sl locus of the mouse and is the ligand for the c-kit tyrosine kinase receptor. Cell 63:213, 1990
55. Williams DE, Lyman SD: Biology of the Steel factor. Curr Opin Hematol 5, 1993
56. Hollingshead LM, Goa KL: Recombinant granulocyte colony-stimulating factor (rG-CSF): a review of its pharmacological properties and prospective role in neutropenic conditions. Drugs 42:300, 1991
57. Schindler R, Dinarello CA: Interleukin 1. p. 85. In Habenicht A (ed): Growth Factors, Differentiation Factors, and Cytokines. Springer-Verlag, Berlin, 1990

58. Van Snick Nordan RP: Interleukin 6. p. 163. In Habenicht A (ed): Growth Factors, Differentiation Factors, and Cytokines. Springer-Verlag, Berlin, 1990
59. Paul SR, Bennett F, Calvetti JA et al: Molecular cloning of a cDNA encoding interleukin-11, a stromal cell-derived lymphopoietic and hematopoietic cytokine. Proc Natl Acad Sci USA 87:7512, 1990
60. Ploemacher RE, van Soest PL, Boudewijn A, Neben S: Interleukin-12 enhances interleukin-3 dependent multilineage hematopoietic colony formation stimulated by interleukin-11 or steel factor. Leukemia 7:1374, 1993
61. Metcalf D: The leukemia inhibitory factor (LIF). Int J Cell Cloning 9:95, 1991
62. Schweigerer L: Basic fibroblast growth factor: properties and clinical implications. p. 42. In Habenicht A (ed): Growth Factors, Differentiation Factors, and Cytokines. Springer-Verlag, Berlin, 1990
63. Gabbianelli M, Sargiacomo M, Pelosi E et al: "Pure" human hemopoietic progenitors: permissive action of basic fibroblast growth factor. Science 249:1562, 1990
64. Brunner G, Nguyen H, Gabrilove J et al: Basic fibroblast growth factor expression in human bone marrow and peripheral blood. Blood 81:631, 1993
65. Lyman SD, James L, Vanden Bos T et al: Molecular cloning of a ligand for the flt3/flk-2 tyrosine kinase receptor: a proliferative factor for primitive hematopoietic cells. Cell 75:1157, 1993
66. Small D, Levenstein M, Kim E et al: The human homolog of Flk-2/Flt-3 is selectively expressed in CD34+ human bone marrow cells and is involved in the proliferation of early progenitor/stem cells. Proc Natl Acad Sci USA 91:459, 1994
67. Katayama N, Clark SC, Ogawa M: Growth factor requirement for survival in cell-cycle dormancy of primitive murine lymphohematopoietic progenitors. Blood 81:610, 1993
68. Bartelmez SH, Bradley TR, Bertoncello I et al: Interleukin 1 plus interleukin 3 plus colony-stimulating factor 1 are essential for clonal proliferation of primitive myeloid bone marrow cells. Exp Hematol 17:240, 1989
68a. Musashi M, Yang YC, Paul SR et al: Direct and synergistic effects of interleukin 11 on murine hemopoiesis in culture. Proc Natl Acad Sci USA 88:765, 1991
69. Tsuji K, Zsebo KM, Ogawa M: Enhancement of murine blast cell colony formation in culture by recombinant rat stem cell factor, ligand for c-kit. Blood 78:1223, 1991
70. Musashi M, Clark SC, Sudo T et al: Synergistic interactions between interleukin-11 and interleukin-4 in support of proliferation of primitive hematopoietic progenitors of mice. Blood 78:1448, 1991
71. Tsuji K, Lyman SD, Sudo T et al: Enhancement of murine hematopoiesis by synergistic interactions between steel factor (ligand for c-kit), interleukin-11, and other early acting factors in culture. Blood 79:2855, 1992
72. Leary AG, Zeng HQ, Clark SC, Ogawa M: Growth factor requirements for survival in G0 and entry into the cell cycle of primitive human hemopoietic progenitors. Proc Natl Acad Sci USA 89:4013, 1992
73. Gabrilove JL, White K, Rahman Z, Wilson EL: Stem cell factor and basic fibroblast growth factor are synergistic in augmenting committed myeloid progenitor growth. Blood 83:907, 1994
74. Lowry PA, Zsebo KM, Deacon DH et al: Effects of rrSCF on multiple cytokine responsive HPP-CFC generated from SCA+ Lin− murine hematopoietic progenitors. Exp Hematol 19:994, 1991
75. Broxmeyer HE, Cooper S, Lu L et al: Effect of murine mast cell growth factor (c-kit proto-oncogene ligand) on colony formation by human marrow hematopoietic progenitor cells. Blood 77:2142, 1991
76. Metcalf D: The cellular basis for enhancement interactions between stem cell factor and the colony stimulating factors. Stem Cells, suppl. 2. 11:1, 1993
77. Tsujino Y, Wada H, Misawa M et al: Effects of mast cell growth factor, interleukin-3, and interleukin-6 on human primitive hematopoietic progenitors from bone marrow and cord blood. Exp Hematol 21:1379, 1993
78. Lemoli RM, Fogli M, Fortuna A et al: Interleukin-11 stimulates the proliferation of human hematopoietic CD34+ and CD34+CD33−DR− cells and synergizes with stem cell factor, interleukin-3, and granulocyte-macrophage colony-stimulating factor. Exp Hematol 21:1668, 1993
79. Jacobsen SE, Veiby OP, Smeland EB: Cytotoxic lymphocyte maturation factor (interleukin 12) is a synergistic growth factor for hematopoietic stem cells. J Exp Med 178:413, 1993
80. Hirayama F, Katayama N, Neben S et al: Synergistic interaction between interleukin-12 and Steel factor in support of proliferation of murine lymphohematopoietic progenitors in culture. Blood 83:92, 1994
81. Peschle C, Testa U, Valtieri M et al: Stringently purified human hematopoietic progenitors/stem cells: analysis of cellular/molecular mechanisms underlying early hematopoiesis. Stem Cells 11:356, 1993
82. Kelvin DJ, Michiel DF, Johnston JA et al: Chemokines and serpentines: the molecular biology of chemokine receptors. J Leukoc Biol 54:604, 1993

83. Schall TJ: The chemokines. The Cytokine Handbook. 2nd Ed. Academic Press, New York, (in press)

84. Cynshi O, Satoh K, Shimonaka Y et al: Reduced response to granulocyte colony-stimulating factor in W/Wv and Sl/Sld mice. Leukemia 5:75, 1991

85. Langley KE, Bennett LG, Wypych J et al: Soluble stem cell factor in human serum. Blood 81:656, 1993

86. Bodine DM, Seidel NE, Zsebo KM, Orlic D: In vivo administration of stem cell factor to mice increases the absolute number of pluripotent hematopoietic stem cells. Blood 82:445, 1993

87. Tong J, Gordon MS, Srour EF et al: In vivo administration of recombinant methionyl human stem cell factor expands the number of human marrow hematopoietic stem cells. Blood 82:784, 1993

88. Teshima T, Harada M, Takamatsu Y et al: Granulocyte colony-stimulating factor (G-CSF)-induced mobilization of circulating haemopoietic stem cells. Br J Haematol 84:570, 1993

89. Briddell RA, Hartley CA, Smith KA, McNiece IK: Recombinant rat stem cell factor synergizes with recombinant human granulocyte colony-stimulating factor in vivo in mice to mobilize peripheral blood progenitor cells that have enhanced repopulating potential. Blood 82:1720, 1993

90. Mayani H, Dragowska W, Lansdorp PM: Lineage commitment in human hematopoiesis involves asymmetric cell division of multipotent progenitors and does not appear to be influenced by cytokines. J Cell Physiol 157:579, 1993

91. Metcalf D: Lineage commitment of hemopoietic progenitor cells in developing blast cell colonies: influence of colony-stimulating factors. Proc Natl Acad Sci USA 88:11310, 1991

92. Metcalf D, Nicola NA: The clonal proliferation of normal mouse hematopoietic cells: enhancement and suppression by colony-stimulating factor combinations. Blood 79:2861, 1992

93. Sonoda Y, Arai N, Ogawa M: Humoral regulation of eosinophilopoiesis in vitro: analysis of the targets of interleukin-3, granulocyte/macrophage colony-stimulating factor (GM-CSF), and interleukin-5. Leukemia 3:14, 1989

94. Sanderson CJ: Interleukin-5, eosinophils and disease. Blood 79:3101, 1992

95. Hammond WP, Csiba E, Canin A et al: Chronic neutropenia. A new canine model induced by human granulocyte colony-stimulating factor. J Clin Invest 87:704, 1991

96. Tominaga A, Takaki S, Koyama M et al: Transgenic mice expressing a B cell growth and differentiation factor gene (IL-5) develop eosinophilia and autoantibody production. J Exp Med 173:429, 1991

97. Coffman RL, Seymour BWP, Hudak S et al: Antibody to interleukin-5 inhibits helminth-induced eosinophilia in mice. Science 245:308, 1989

98. Yoshida H, Hayashi S-I, Kunisada T et al: The murine mutation osteopetrosis is in the coding region of the macrophage colony stimulating factor gene. Nature 345:442, 1990

99. Wiktor-Jedrzejczak W, Ratajczak MZ, Patsznik A et al: CSF-1 deficiency in the op/op mouse has differential effects on macrophage populations and differentiation stages. Exp Hematol 20:1004, 1992

100. Tanaka S, Takahashi N, Udagawa N et al: Macrophage colony-stimulating factor is indispensable for both proliferation and differentiation of osteoclast progenitors. J Clin Invest 91:257, 1993

101. Liggett W Jr, Shevde N, Anklesaria P et al: Effects of macrophage colony stimulating factor and granulocyte-macrophage colony-stimulating factor on osteoclastic differentiation of hematopoietic progenitor cells. Stem Cells 11:398, 1993

102. Begg SK, Radley JM, Pollard JW et al: Delayed hematopoietic development in osteopetrotic (op/op) mice. J Exp Med 177:237, 1993

103. Caracciolo D, Shirsat N, Wong GG et al: Recombinant human macrophage colony-stimulating factor (M-CSF) requires subliminal concentrations of granulocyte/macrophage (GM)-CSF for optimal stimulation of human macrophage colony formation in vitro. J Exp Med 166:1851, 1987

104. Mak N-K, Fung M-C, Leung K-N, Hapel AJ: Monocytic differentiation of a myelomonocytic leukemic cell (WEHI 3B JCS) is induced by alpha-tumor necrosis factor (TNF-α). Cell Immunol 150:1, 1993

105. Cheung DL, Hamilton JA: Regulation of human monocyte DNA synthesis by colony-stimulating factors, cytokines, and adenosine monophosphate. Blood 79:1972, 1992

106. Jansen JH, Kluin-Nelemans JC, Van Damme J et al: Interleukin 6 is a permissive factor for monocytic colony formation by human hematopoietic progenitor cells. J Exp Med 175:1151, 1992

107. Tei H, Kasugai T, Tsujimura T et al: Characterization of cultured mast cells derived from Ws/Ws mast cell-deficient rats with a small deletion at tyrosine kinase domain of c-kit. Blood 83:916, 1994

108. Furitsu T, Tsujimura T, Tono T et al: Identification of mutations in the coding sequence of the proto-oncogene c-kit in a human mast cell leukemia cell line causing ligand-independent activation of c-kit product. J Clin Invest 92:1736, 1993

108a. Dranoff G, Crawford AD, Sadelain M et al: Involvement of granulocyte-macrophage colony-stimulating factor in pulmonary homeostasis. Science 264:713, 1994

109. Kaushansky K, Karplus PA: Review: hematopoietic growth factors: understanding functional diversity in structural terms. Blood 82:3229, 1993

110. Nicola NA: Hematopoietic growth factors and their receptors. p. 51. In Donnall Thomas (ed): Application of Basic Science to Hematopoiesis and Treatment of Disease. Raven Press, New York, 1993

111. Cosman D: The hematopoietin receptor superfamily. Cytokine 5:95, 1993

112. Paul WE, Seder RA: Lymphocyte responses and cytokines. Cell 76:241, 1994

113. Bazan JF: Structural design and molecular evolution of a cytokine receptor superfamily. Proc Natl Acad Sci USA 87:6934, 1990

114. Youssoufian H, Longmore G, Neuman D et al: Structure, function, and activation of the erythropoietin receptor. Blood 81:2223, 1993

115. Miyajima A, Mui AL-F, Ogorochi T, Sakamaki K: Receptors for granulocyte-macrophage colony-stimulating factor, interleukin-3, and interleukin-5. Blood 82:1960, 1993

116. Hibi M, Murakami M, Saito M et al: Molecular cloning and expression of an IL-6 signal transducer, gp-130. Cell 63:1149, 1990

117. Taga T, Kishimoto T: Role of a two-chain IL-6 receptor system in immune and hematopoietic cell regulation. Crit Rev Immunol 11:265, 1992

118. Gearing DP, Ziegler SF: The hematopoietic growth factor receptor family. Curr Opin Hematol 19, 1993

119. Mallett S, Barclay AN: A new superfamily of cell surface proteins related to the nerve growth factor receptor. Immunol Today 12:220, 1991

120. Barbacid M: Nerve growth factor: a tale of two receptors. Oncogene 8:2033, 1993

121. Fukunaga R, Ishizaka Ikeda E, Nagata S: Growth and differentiation signals mediated by different regions in the cytoplasmic domain of granulocyte colony-stimulating factor receptor. Cell 74:1079, 1993

122. Li W, Stanley ER: Role of dimerization and modification of the CSF-1 receptor in its activation and internalization during the CSF-1 response. EMBO J 10:277, 1991

123. Pandit J, Bohm A, Jancarik J et al: Three-dimensional structure of dimeric human recombinant macrophage colony-stimulating factor. Science 258:1358, 1992

124. Blechman JM, Lev S, Givol D, Yarden Y: Structure-function analyses of the kit receptor for the Steel factor. Stem Cells, suppl. 2. 11:12, 1993

125. Watowich SS, Yoshimura A, Longmore GD et al: Homodimerization and constitutive activation of the erythropoietin receptor. Proc Natl Acad Sci USA 89:2140, 1992

126. Herren B, Rooney B, Weyer KA et al: Dimerization of extracellular domains of platelet-derived growth factor receptors: a revised model of receptor-ligand interactions. J Biol Chem 268:15088, 1993

127. Owczarek CM, Layton MJ, Metcalf D et al: Inter-species chimeras of leukaemia inhibitory factor define a major human receptor binding determinant. EMBO J 12:3487, 1993

128. Gearing DP, Comeau MR, Friend DJ et al: The IL-6 signal transducer, gp130: an oncostatin M receptor and affinity converter for the LIF receptor. Science 255:1434, 1992

129. Davis S, Aldrich TH, Valenzuela DM et al: LIFRβ and gp130 as heterodimerizing signal transducers of the tripartite CNTF receptor. Science 259, 1736, 1993

130. Yin T, Taga T, Tsang ML-S et al: Involvement of interleukin-6 signal transducer gp130 in interleukin-11-mediated signal transduction. J Immunol 151:2555, 1993

131. Kondo K, Takeshita T, Ishi N et al: Sharing of the interleukin-2 (IL-2) receptor γ chain between receptors for IL-2 and IL-4. Science 262:1874, 1993

132. Noguchi M, Nakamura Y, Russel SM et al: Interleukin-2 receptor γ chain: a functional component of the interleukin-7 receptor. Science 262:1877, 1993

133. Zurawski G, de Vries JE: Interleukin 13, an interleukin 4-like cytokine that acts on monocytes and B cells, but not on T cells. Immunol Today 15:19, 1994

134. Jacobsen FW, Veiby OP, Skjonsberg C, Jacobsen SE: Novel role of interleukin 7 in myelopoiesis: stimulation of primitive murine hematopoietic progenitor cells. J Exp Med 178:1777, 1993

135. Rapoport AP, Abboud CN, DiPersio JF: Granulocyte-macrophage colony-stimulating factor (GM-CSF) and granulocyte colony-stimulating factor (G-CSF): receptor biology, signal transduction, and neutrophil activation. Blood Rev 6:43, 1992

136. Cannistra SA, Groshek P, Garlick R et al: Regulation of surface expression of the granulocyte/macrophage colony-stimulating factor receptor in normal human myeloid cells. Proc Natl Acad Sci USA 87:93, 1990

137. Baldwin GC, Gasson JC, Kaufman SE et al: Nonhematopoietic tumor cells express functional GM-CSF receptors. Blood 73:1033, 1989

138. Avalos BR, Gasson JC, Hedvat C et al: Human granulocyte colony-stimulating factor: biologic activities and receptor characterization on hematopoietic cells and small cell lung cancer cell lines. Blood 75:851, 1990

139. Hampson J, McLaughlin PJ, Johnson PM: Low-affinity receptors for tumour necrosis factor-alpha, interferon-gamma and granulocyte-macrophage colony-stimulating factor are expressed on human placental syncytiotrophoblast. Immunology 79:485, 1993

140. Elliott MJ, Vadas MA, Eglinton JM et al: Recombinant human interleukin-3 and granulocyte-macrophage colony-stimulating factor show common biological effects and binding characteristics on human monocytes. Blood 74:2349, 1989

141. DiPersio JF, Hedvat C, Ford CF et al: Characterization of the soluble human granulocyte-macrophage colony-stimulating factor receptor complex. J Biol Chem 266:279, 1991

142. Layton JE, Hockman H, Sheridan WP, Morstyn G: Evidence for a novel *in vivo* control mechanism of granulopoiesis: mature cell-related control of regulatory factor. Blood 74:1303, 1989

143. Roth P, Stanley ER: The biology of CSF-1 and its receptor. Curr Top Microbiol Immunol 181:141, 1992

144. Lopez AF, Elliott MJ, Woodcock J, Vadas MA: GM-CSF, IL-3 and IL-5: cross-competition on human haemopoietic cells. Immunol Today 13:495, 1992

145. Walker F, Nicola NA, Metcalf D, Burgess AW: Hierarchical down modulation of hemopoietic growth factor receptors. Cell 43:269, 1985

146. Nicola NA, Metcalf D: Subunit promiscuity among hemopoietic growth factor receptors. Cell 67:1, 1991

147. Lopez AF, Lyons AB, Eglinton JM et al: Specific binding of human interleukin-3 and granulocyte-macrophage colony-stimulating factor to human basophils. J Allergy Clin Immunol 85:99, 1990

148. Lopez AF, Eglinton JM, Lyons AB et al: Human interleukin-3 inhibits the binding of granulocyte-macrophage colony-stimulating factor and interleukin-5 to basophils and strongly enhances their functional activity. J Cell Physiol 145:69, 1990

149. Onetto-Pothier N, Aumont N, Haman A et al: IL-3 inhibits the binding of GM-CSF to AML blasts, but the two cytokines act synergistically in supporting blast proliferation. Leukemia 4:329, 1990

150. Lopez AF, Vadas MA, Woodcock JM et al: Interleukin-5, interleukin-3, and granulocyte-macrophage colony-stimulating factor cross-compete for binding to cell surface receptors on human eosinophils. J Biol Chem 266:24741, 1991

151. Tavernier J, Devos R, Cornelius S et al: A human high affinity interleukin-5 receptor (IL-5R) is composed of an IL-5-specific alpha-chain and a beta chain shared with the receptor for GM-CSF. Cell 66:1175, 1991

152. Kitamura T, Miyajima A: Functional reconstitution of the human interleukin-3 receptor. Blood 80:84, 1992

153. Sato N, Caux C, Kitamura T et al: Expression and factor-dependent modulation of the interleukin-3 receptor subunits on human hematopoietic cells. Blood 82:752, 1993

154. Kitamura T, Takaku F, Miyajima A: IL-1 upregulates the expression of cytokine receptors on a factor-dependent human hemopoietic cell line TF-1. Int Immunol 3:571, 1991

155. Shieh J-H, Gordon M, Jakubowski A et al: Interleukin-1 modulation of cytokine receptors on human neutrophils: in vitro and in vivo studies. Blood 81:1745, 1993

156. Elbaz O, Budel LM, Hoogerbrugge H et al: Tumor necrosis factor regulates the expression of granulocyte-macrophage colony-stimulating factor and interleukin-3 receptors on human acute myeloid leukemia cells. Blood 5:989, 1991

157. Brailly H, Pebusque MJ, Tabilio A, Mannoni P: TNF alpha acts in synergy with GM-CSF to induce proliferation of acute myeloid leukemia cells by upregulating the GM-CSF receptor and GM-CSF gene expression. Leukemia 7:1557, 1993

158. Löwenberg B, Touw IP: Hematopoietic growth factors and their receptors in acute leukemia. Blood 81:281, 1993

159. Jacobsen SE, Ruscetti FW, Dubois CM et al: Transforming growth factor-beta trans-modulates the expression of colony stimulating factor receptors on murine hematopoietic progenitor cell lines. Blood 77:1706, 1991

160. Keller JR, Jacobsen SEW, Dubois CM et al: Transforming growth factor-β: a bidirectional regulator of hematopoietic cell growth. Int J Cell Cloning 10:2, 1992

161. Miura O, Ihle JN: Dimer- and oligomerization of the erythropoietin receptor by disulfide bond formation and significance of the region near the WSXWS motif in intracellular transport. Arch Biochem Biophys 306:200, 1993

162. Lee AW-M: Signal transduction by the colony-stimulating factor-1 receptor: comparison to other receptor tyrosine kinases. Curr Top Cell Regul 32:73, 1992

163. Roussell MF, Sherr CJ: Signal transduction by the macrophage colony-stimulating factor receptor. Curr Opin Hematol 1:11, 1993

164. Coughlin SR, Escobedo JA, Williams LT: Role of phosphatidylinositol kinase in PDGF receptor signal transduction. Science 243:1191, 1989

165. Schlesinger J: Signal transduction by receptors with protein kinase activity.

166. Dosil M, Wang S, Lemischka IR: Mitogenic signalling and substrate specificity of the Flk2/Flt3 receptor tyrosine kinase in fibroblasts and interleukin 3-dependent hematopoietic cells. Mol Cell Biol 13:6572, 1993

167. McColl SR, Kreis C, DiPersio JF et al: Involvement of guanine nucleotide binding proteins in neutrophil activation and priming by GM-CSF. Blood 73:588, 1989

168. DiPersio JF, Naccache PH, Borgeat P et al: Characterization of the priming effects of human granulocyte-macrophage colony-stimulating factor on human neutrophil leukotriene synthesis. Prostaglandins 36:673, 1988

169. McColl SR, Beauseigle D, Gilbert C, Naccache PH: Priming of the human neutrophil respiratory burst by granulocyte-macrophage colony-stimulating factor and tumor necrosis factor-alpha involves regulation at a post-cell surface receptor level. Enhancement of the effect of agents which directly activate G proteins. J Immunol 145:3047, 1990

170. Townsend PV, Crouch MF, Mak NK, Hapel AJ: Localization of the GTP-binding protein Gi alpha in myelomonocytic progenitor cells is regulated by proliferation (GM-CSF, IL-3) and differentiation (TNF) signals. Growth Factors 9:21, 1993

171. Durstin M, McColl SR, Gomez-Cambronero J et al: Up-regulation of the amount of Gi alpha 2 associated with the plasma membrane in human neutrophils stimulated by granulocyte-macrophage colony-stimulating factor. Biochem J 292:183, 1993

172. Al Aoukaty A, Giaid A, Sinoff C et al: Priming effects of granulocyte-macrophage colony-stimulating factor are coupled to cholera toxin-sensitive guanine nucleotide binding protein in human T lymphocytes. Blood 83:1299, 1994

173. MacPhee CH: Granulocyte/macrophage colony-stimulating factor affects myoinositol metabolism in a novel manner. Implications for its priming action on human neutrophils. Biochem J 286:535, 1992

174. Nishimura M, Kaku K, Azuno Y et al: Stimulation of phosphoinositol turnover and protein kinase C activation by granulocyte-macrophage colony-stimulating factor in HL-60 cells. Blood 80:1045, 1992

175. Wirthmueller U, de Weck AL, Dahinden CA: Studies on the mechanism of platelet-activating factor production in GM-CSF primed neutrophils: involvement of protein synthesis and phospholipase A2 activation. Biochem Biophys Res Commun 170:556, 1990

176. Bourgoin S, Plante E, Gaudry M et al: Involvement of a phospholipase D in the mechanism of action of granulocyte-macrophage colony-stimulating factor (GM-CSF): priming of human neutrophils in vitro with GM-CSF is associated with accumulation of phosphatidic acid and diradylglycerol. J Exp Med 172:767, 1990

177. Bourgoin S, Poubelle PE, Liao NW et al: Granulocyte-macrophage colony-stimulating factor primes phospholipase D activity in human neutrophils in vitro: role of calcium, G-proteins and tyrosine kinases. Cell Signal 4:487, 1992

178. Duronio V, Welham MJ, Abraham S et al: p21ras activation via hemopoietin receptors and c-kit requires tyrosine kinase activity but not tyrosine phosphorylation of p21ras GTPase-activating protein. Proc Natl Acad Sci USA 89:1587, 1992

179. Satoh T, Uehara Y, Kaziro Y: Inhibition of interleukin 3 and granulocyte-macrophage colony-stimulating factor stimulated increase of active ras.GTP by herbimycin A, a specific inhibitor of tyrosine kinases. J Biol Chem 267:2537, 1992

180. Carroll MP, Clark-Lewis I, Rapp UR, May WS: Interleukin-3 and granulocyte-macrophage colony-stimulating factor mediate rapid phosphorylation and activation of cytosolic c-raf. J Biol Chem 265:19812, 1990

181. Baxter GT, Miller DL, Kuo RC et al: PKC epsilon is involved in granulocyte-macrophage colony-stimulating factor signal transduction: evidence from microphysiometry and antisense oligonucleotide experiments. Biochemistry 31:10950, 1992

182. Ghigo D, Brizzi MF, Avanzi GC et al: Evidence for a role of the Na+/H+ exchanger in the colony-stimulating-factor-induced ornithine decarboxylase activity and proliferation of the human cell line M-07e. J Cell Physiol 145:147, 1990

183. Rajotte D, Haddad P, Haman A et al: Role of protein kinase C and the Na+/H+ antiporter in suppression of apoptosis by granulocyte-macrophage colony-stimulating factor and interleukin-3. J Biol Chem 267:9980, 1992

184. Raines MA, Golde DW, Daeipour M, Nel AE: Granulocyte-macrophage colony-stimulating factor activates microtubule-associated protein 2 kinase in neutrophils via a tyrosine kinase-dependent pathway. Blood 79:3350, 1992

185. Gomez-Cambronero J, Colasanto JM, Huang CK, Shaafi RI: Direct stimulation by tyrosine phosphorylation of microtubule-associated protein (MAP) kinase activity by granulocyte-macrophage colony-stimulating factor in human neutrophils. Biochem J 291:211, 1993

p. 39. In Donnall Thomas (ed): Application of Basic Science to Hematopoiesis and Treatment of Disease. Raven Press, New York, 1993

186. Imamura K, Kufe D: Colony-stimulating factor 1-induced Na+ influx into human monocytes involves activation of a pertussis toxin-sensitive GTP-binding protein. J Biol Chem 263:14093, 1988

187. Baccarini M, Sabatini DM, App H et al: Colony stimulating factor-1 (CSF-1) stimulates temperature dependent phosphorylation and activation of the RAF-1 proto-oncogene product. EMBO J 9:3649, 1990

188. Matsushime H, Roussel MF, Ashmun RA, Sherr CJ: Colony-stimulating factor 1 regulates novel cyclins during the G1 phase of the cell cycle. Cell 65:701, 1991

189. Nemunaitis J: Macrophage function activating cytokines: potential clinical application. Crit Rev Oncol Hematol 14:153, 1993

190. Pierce JH, DiMarco E, Cox GW et al: Macrophage-colony-stimulating factor (CSF-1) induces proliferation, chemotaxis, and reversible monocytic differentiation in myeloid progenitor cells transfected with the human *c-fms*/CSF-1 receptor cDNA. Proc Natl Acad Sci USA 87:5613, 1990

191. Burthem BJ, Baker PK, Hunt JA, Cawley JC: The function of *c-fms* in hairy-cell leukemia: macrophage colony-stimulating factor stimulates hairy-cell movement. Blood 83:1381, 1994

192. Wickham LL, Hagan JP, Hsieh H-J et al: Human monocyte colony-stimulating factor stimulates the gene expression of monocyte chemotactic protein-1 and increases the adhesion of monocytes to endothelial monolayers. J Clin Invest 92:1745, 1993

193. De Nichilo MO, Burns GF: Granulocyte-macrophage and macrophage colony-stimulating factors differentially regulate αv integrin expression on cultured human macrophages. Proc Natl Acad Sci USA 90:2517, 1993

194. Varnum BC, Lim RW, Kujubu DA et al: Granulocyte-macrophage colony-stimulating factors and tetradecanoyl phorbol acetate induce a distinct, restricted subset of primary response TIS genes in both proliferating and terminally differentiated myeloid cells. Mol Cell Biol 9:3580, 1989

195. Liu JW, Lacy J, Sukhatme VP, Coleman DL: Granulocyte-macrophage colony-stimulating factor induces transcriptional activation of Egr-1 in murine peritoneal macrophages. J Biol Chem 266:5929, 1991

196. Adunyah SE, Unlap TM, Wagner F, Kraft AS: Regulation of c-jun expression and AP-1 enhancer activity by granulocyte-macrophage colony-stimulating factor. J Biol Chem 266:5670, 1991

197. Beaulieu AD, Paquin R, Rathanaswami P, McColl SR: Nuclear signaling in human neutrophils. Stimulation of RNA synthesis is a response to a limited number of proinflammatory agonists. J Biol Chem 267:426, 1992

198. Mufson RA, Szabo J, Eckert D: Human IL-3 induction of c-jun in normal monocytes is independent of tyrosine kinase and involves protein kinase C. J Immunol 148:1129, 1992

199. Park JH, Levitt L: Overexpression of mitogen-activated protein kinase (ERK1) enhances T-cell cytokine gene expression: role of AP1, NF-AT, and NF-KB. Blood 82:2470, 1993

200. Margolis B: Proteins with src homology 2 domains: transducers in the tyrosine kinase signaling pathway. Cell Growth Differ 3:73, 1992

201. Pelicci G, Lanfrancone L, Grignani F et al: A novel transforming protein (SHC) with an SH2 domain is implicated in mitogenic signal transduction. Cell 70:93, 1992

202. Birge RB, Hanafusa H: Closing in on SH2 specificity. Science 262:1522, 1993

203. McCormick F: How receptors turn Ras on. Nature 363:15, 1993

204. Egan SE, Giddings BW, Brooks MW et al: Association of Sos Ras exchange protein with Grb2 is implicated in tyrosine kinase signal transduction and transformation. Nature 363:45, 1993

205. Segatto O, Pelicci G, Giuli S et al: Shc products are substrates of erbB-2 kinase. Oncogene 8:2105, 1993

206. Ruff-Jamison S, McGlade J, Pawson T et al: Epidermal growth factor stimulates the tyrosine phosphorylation of SHC in the mouse. J Biol Chem 268:7610, 1993

207. de Vries-Smits AMM, Burgering BMT, Leevers SJ et al: Involvement of p21ras in activation of extracellular signal-regulated kinase 2. Nature 357:602, 1992

208. Buday L, Downward J: Epidermal growth factor regulates p21ras through the formation of a complex of receptor, Grb2 adapter protein, and Sos nucleotide exchange factor. Cell 73:611, 1993

209. Skolnik EY, Lee CH, Batzer A et al: The SH2/SH3 domain-containing protein GRB2 interacts with tyrosine-phosphorylated IRS1 and Shc: implications for insulin control of ras signaling. EMBO J 12:1929, 1993

210. Skolnik EY, Batzer A, Li N et al: The function of GRB2 in linking the insulin receptor to Ras signaling pathways. Science 260:1953, 1993

211. Pronk GJ, McGlade J, Pelicci G et al: Insulin-induced phosphorylation of the 46- and 52-kDa Shc proteins. J Biol Chem 268:5748, 1993

212. Rozakis-Adcock M, Fernley R, Wade J et al: The SH2 and SH3 domains of mammalian Grb2 couple the EGF receptor to the Ras activator mSos1. Nature 363:83, 1993

213. Argetsinger LS, Campbell GS, Yang X et al: Identification of JAK2 as a growth hormone receptor-associated tyrosine kinase. Cell 74:237, 1993

214. Silvennoinen O, Ihle JN, Schlessinger J, Levey DE: Interferon-induced nuclear signalling by Jak protein tyrosine kinase. Nature 366:583, 1993

215. Watling D, Guschin D, Muller M et al: Complementation by the protein tyrosine kinase JAK2 of a mutant cell line defective in the interferon-gamma signal transduction pathway. Nature 366:166, 1993

216. Silvennoinen O, Ihle JN, Schlessinger J, Levy DE: Interferon-induced nuclear signalling by Jak protein tyrosine kinases. Nature 366:583, 1993

217. Hall A: Ras-related proteins. Curr Opin Cell Biol 5:265, 1993

218. Kanakura Y, Druker B, Cannistra SA et al: Signal transduction of the human granulocyte-macrophage colony-stimulating factor and interleukin-3 receptors involves tyrosine phosphorylation of a common set of cytoplasmic proteins. Blood 76:706, 1990

219. Sakamaki K, Miyajima I, Kitamura T, Miyajima A: Critical cytoplasmic domains of the common beta subunit of the human GM-CSF, IL-3 and IL-5 receptors for growth signal transduction and tyrosine phosphorylation. EMBO J 11:3541, 1992

220. Hallek M, Druker B, Lepisto EM et al: Granulocyte-macrophage colony-stimulating factor and steel factor induce phosphorylation of both unique and overlapping signal transduction intermediates in a human factor-dependent hematopoietic cell line. J Cell Physiol 153:176, 1992

221. Linnekin D, Evans G, Michiel D, Farrar WL: Characterization of a 97-kDa phosphotyrosylprotein regulated by multiple cytokines. J Biol Chem 267:23993, 1992

222. Sato N, Sakamaki K, Terada N et al: Signal transduction by the high-affinity GM-CSF receptor: two distinct cytoplasmic regions of the common beta subunit responsible for different signaling. EMBO J 12:4181, 1993

223. Takaki S, Murata Y, Kitamura T et al: Reconstitution of the functional receptors for murine and human interleukin 5. J Exp Med 177:1523, 1993

224. Eder M, Griffin JD, Ernst TJ: The human granulocyte-macrophage colony-stimulating factor receptor is capable of initiating signal transduction in NIH3T3 cells. EMBO J 12:1647, 1993

225. Weiss M, Yokoyama C, Shikama Y et al: Human granulocyte-macrophage colony-stimulating factor receptor signal transduction requires the proximal cytoplasmic domains of the alpha and beta subunits. Blood 82:3298, 1993

226. Watanabe S, Mui AL, Muto A et al: Reconstituted human granulocyte-macrophage colony-stimulating factor receptor transduces growth-promoting signals in mouse NIH 3T3 cells: comparison with signalling in BA/F3 pro-B cells. Mol Cell Biol 13:1440, 1993

227. Polotskaya A, Zhao Y, Lilly ML, Kraft AS: A critical role for the cytoplasmic domain of the granulocyte-macrophage colony-stimulating factor alpha receptor in mediating cell growth. Cell Growth Differ 4:523, 1993

228. Areces LB, Jucker M, San Miguel JA et al: Ligand-dependent transformation by the receptor for human granulocyte/macrophage colony-stimulating factor and tyrosine phosphorylation of the receptor beta subunit. Proc Natl Acad Sci USA 90:3963, 1993

229. Kastelein RA, Shanafelt AB: GM-CSF receptor: interactions and activation. Oncogene 8:231, 1993

230. Shuai K, Ziemiecki A, Wilks AF et al: Polypeptide signalling to the nucleus through tyrosine phosphorylation of Jak and Stat proteins. Nature 366:580, 1993

231. Narazaki M, Witthuhn BA, Ihle JN et al: Activation of JAK2 kinase mediated by the IL-6 signal transducer, gp130. Proc Natl Acad Sci USA 91:2285, 1994

232. Kishimoto T, Taga T, Akira S: Cytokine signal transduction. Cell 76:253, 1994

233. Silvennoinen O, Witthuhn BA, Quelle FW et al: Structure of the murine Jak2 protein-tyrosine kinase and its role in interleukin 3 signal transduction. Proc Natl Acad Sci USA 90:8429, 1993

234. Cutler RL, Liu L, Damen JE, Krystal G: Multiple cytokines induce the tyrosine phosphorylation of Shc and its association with Grb2 in hemopoietic cells. J Biol Chem 268:21463, 1993

235. Witthuhn BA, Quelle FW, Silvennoinen O et al: JAK2 associates with the erythropoietin receptor and is tyrosine phosphorylated and activated following stimulation with erythropoietin. Cell 74:227, 1993

236. Damen JE, Liu L, Cutler RL, Krystal G: Erythropoietin stimulates the tyrosine phosphorylation of Shc and its association with Grb2 and a 145-Kd tyrosine phosphorylated protein. Blood 82:2296, 1993

237. Eder R, Inhorn M, Sattler T et al: Binding of GM-CSF induces association of the α and β receptor subunits at the cell surface and tyrosine phosphorylation of the β subunit and JAK-2. Blood, suppl. 1. 82:438a, 1993

238. Schrader JW, Welham MJ, Duronio V, Bowtell D: Shc and mSos-1 are involved in activation of p21ras by hemopoietin. Blood, suppl. 1. 82:438a, 1993

239. Liu L, Cutler RL, Mui ALF, Krystal G: Steel factor stimulates the serine/threonine phosphorylation of the interleukin-3 receptor. Blood, suppl. 1. 82:439a, 1993

240. Matulonis U, Salgia R, Okuda K et al: Interleukin-3 and p210 BCR/*ABL* activate

both unique and overlapping pathways of signal transduction in a factor-dependent myeloid cell line. Exp Hematol 21:1460, 1993

241. Matsuguchi T, Salgia R, Hallek M et al: Shc phosphorylation in myeloid cells is regulated by GM-CSF, IL-3, Steel factor and is constitutively increased by p210bcr/abl. Blood, suppl. 1. 82:438a, 1993

242. Tauchi T, Boswell HS, Leibowitz D, Broxmeyer HE: Coupling between p210bcr-abl and Shc and Grb2 adaptor proteins in hematopoietic cells permits growth factor receptor-independent link to ras activation pathway. J Exp Med 179:167, 1994

243. Montminy M: Trying on a new pair of SH2s. Science 261:1694, 1993

244. Larner AC, David M, Feldman GM et al: Tyrosine phosphorylation of DNA binding proteins by multiple cytokines. Science 261:1730, 1993

245. Sivennoinen O, Schindler C, Schlessinger J, Levy DE: Ras-independent growth factor signaling by transcription factor tyrosine phosphorylation. Science 261:1736, 1993

245a. Ding DX-H, Rivas CI, Heaney ML et al: The α subunit of the human granulocyte-macrophage colony-stimulating factor receptor signals for glucose transport via a phosphorylation-independent pathway. Proc Natl Acad Sci USA 91:2537, 1994

246. Varmus HE, Lowell CA: Cancer genes and hematopoiesis. Blood 83:5, 1994

247. Bolen JB: Nonreceptor tyrosine kinases. Oncogene 8:2025, 1993

248. Lilly M, Le T, Holland P, Hendrickson SL: Sustained expression of the pim-1 kinase is specifically induced in myeloid cells by cytokines whose receptors are structurally related. Oncogene 7:727, 1992

249. Hanazono Y, Chiba S, Sasaki K et al: c-fps/fes protein-tyrosine kinase is implicated in a signaling pathway triggered by granulocyte-macrophage colony-stimulating factor and interleukin-3. EMBO J 12:1641, 1993

250. Hanazono Y, Chiba S, Sasaki K et al: Erythropoietin induces tyrosine phosphorylation and kinase activity of the c-fps/fes proto-oncogene product in human erythropoietin-responsive cells. Blood 81:12:3193, 1993

251. Quelle FW, Quelle DE, Wojchowski DM: Interleukin-3, granulocyte-macrophage colony-stimulating factor, and transfected erythropoietin receptors mediate tyrosine phosphorylation of a common cytosolic protein (pp100) in FDC-ER cells. J Biol Chem 267:17055, 1992

252. Torigoe T, O'Connor R, Santoli D, Reed JC: Interleukin-3 regulates the activity of the lyn protein kinase in myeloid-committed leukemic cell lines. Blood 80:617, 1992

253. Baumann MA, Corey SJ, Tolbert M et al: Signal transduction through cytokine receptors during eosinophilic differentiation: definition of signals mediating differentiation vs proliferation. Blood, suppl. 1. 82:107a, 1993

254. Corey S, Burkhardt A, Bolen J et al: G-CSF receptor signaling involves formation of a three component complex with lyn and syk protein tyrosine kinases. Blood, suppl. 1. 82:439a, 1993

255. Kyas U, Pietsch T, Welte K: Expression of receptors for granulocyte colony-stimulating factor on neutrophils from patients with severe congenital neutropenia and cyclic neutropenia. Blood 79:114, 1992

256. Hestdal K, Welte K, Lie SO et al: Severe congenital neutropenia: abnormal growth and differentiation of myeloid progenitors to granulocyte colony-stimulating factor (G-CSF) but normal response to G-CSF plus stem cell factor. Blood 82:2991, 1993

257. Dong F, van Buitenen C, Pouwels K et al: Distinct cytoplasmic regions of the human granulocyte colony-stimulating factor receptor involved in induction of proliferation and maturation. Mol Cell Biol 13:7774, 1993

258. Pan CX, Fukunaga R, Yonehara S, Nagata S: Unidirectional cross-phosphorylation between the granulocyte colony-stimulating factor and interleukin 3 receptors. J Biol Chem 268:25818, 1993

259. Dong F, Hoefsloot LH, Schelen AM et al: Identification of a nonsense mutation in the granulocyte-colony-stimulating factor receptor in severe congenital neutropenia. Proc Natl Acad Sci USA 91:4480, 1994

260. Bashey A, Healy L, Marshall CJ: Proliferative but not nonproliferative responses to granulocyte colony-stimulating factor are associated with rapid activation of the p21ras/MAP kinase signalling pathway. Blood 83:949, 1994

261. Adachi S, Kubota M, Matsubara K et al: Role of protein kinase C in neutrophil survival enhanced by granulocyte colony-stimulating factor. Exp Hematol 21:1709, 1993

262. Fischer EH, Charbonneau H, Cool DE, Tonks NK: Tyrosine phosphatases and their possible interplay with tyrosine kinases. Ciba Found Symp 164:132, 1992

263. Broxmeyer HE, Lu L, Hangoc G et al: CD45 cell surface antigens are linked to stimulation of early human myeloid progenitor cells by interleukin-3 (IL-3), granulocyte/macrophage colony-stimulating factor (GM-CSF), a GM/IL-3 fusion protein, and mast cell growth factor (a c-kit ligand). J Exp Med 174:447, 1991

264. Yeung YG, Berg KL, Pixley FJ et al: Protein tyrosine phosphatase-1C is rapidly phosphorylated in tyrosine in macrophages in response to colony stimulating factor-1. J Biol Chem 267:23447, 1992

265. Yi T, Ihle JN: Association of hematopoietic cell phosphatase with c-kit after stimulation with c-kit ligand. Mol Cell Biol 13:3350, 1993

266. Yi T, Mui AL, Krystal G, Ihle JN: Hematopoietic cell phosphatase associates with the interleukin-3 (IL-3) receptor beta chain and down-regulates IL-3-induced tyrosine phosphorylation and mitogenesis. Mol Cell Biol 13:7577, 1993

267. Rao P, Mufson RA: Interleukin-3 inhibits cycloheximide induction of C-jun mRNA in human monocytes: possible role for a serine/threonine phosphatase. J Cell Physiol 156:560, 1993

268. Magrinat G, Mason SN, Shami PJ, Weinberg JB: Nitric oxide modulation of human leukemia cell differentiation and gene expression. Blood 80:1880, 1992

269. Whetton AD, Dexter TM: Influence of growth factors and substrates on differentiation and haemopoietic stem cells. Curr Opin Cell Biol 5:1044, 1993

270. Liebermann DA, Hoffman-Liebermann B: Genetic programs of myeloid cell differentiation. Curr Opin Hematol 1:24, 1994

271. McClanahan T, Dalrymple S, Barkett M, Lee F: Hematopoietic growth factor receptor genes as markers of lineage commitment during in vitro development of hematopoietic cells. Blood 81:2903, 1993

272. Gliniak BC, Rohrschneider LF: Expression of the M-CSF receptor is controlled posttranscriptionally by the dominant actions of GM-CSF or multi-CSF. Cell 63:1073, 1990

273. Gliniak BC, Park LS, Rohrschneider LR: A GM-CSF activated ribonuclease system trans-regulates MCSF receptor expression in the murine FDC-P1/MAC myeloid cell line. Mol Biol Cell 3:535, 1992

274. Chen AR, Rohrschneider LR: Mechanism of differential inhibition of factor-dependent cell proliferation by transforming growth factor-β1: selective uncoupling of fms from myc. Blood 81:2539, 1993

275. McArthur GA, Rohrschneider LR, Johnson GR: Induced expression of c-fms in normal hematopoietic cells shows evidence for both conservation and lineage restriction of signal transduction in response to macrophage colony-stimulating factor. Blood 83:972, 1994

276. Leglise MC, Dent GA, Ayscue LH, Ross DW: Leukemic cell maturation: phenotypic variability and oncogene expression in HL60 cells: a review. Blood Cells 3:319, 1988

277. Meier RW, Chen T, Mathews S et al: The differentiation pathway of HL-60 cells is a model system for studying the specific regulation of some myeloid genes. Cell Growth Differ 3:663, 1992

278. Hsu HC, Yang K, Kharbanda S et al: All-trans retinoic acid induces monocyte growth factor receptor (c-fms) gene expression in HL-60 leukemia cells. Leukemia 7:458, 1993

279. Hromas R, Collins SJ, Hickstein D et al: A retinoic-acid responsive human zinc finger gene, MZF-1, preferentially expressed in myeloid cells. J Biol Chem 266:14183, 1991

280. Maekawa T, Metcalf D: Clonal suppression of HL-60 and U937 cells by recombinant leukemia inhibitory factor in combination with GM-CSF or G-CSF. Leukemia 3:270, 1989

281. Valtieri M, Boccoli G, Testa U et al: Two-step differentiation of AML-193 leukemic line: terminal maturation is induced by positive interaction of retinoic acid with granulocyte colony-stimulating factor (CSF) and vitamin D3 with monocyte CSF. Blood 77:1804, 1991

282. Holt JT, Redner RL, Nienhuis AW: An oligomer complementary to c-myc mRNA inhibits proliferation of HL-60 promyelocytic cells and induces differentiation. Mol Cell Biol 8:3683, 1988

283. Schwartz EL, Chamberlain H, Brechbuhl AB: Regulation of c-myc expression by granulocyte-macrophage colony-stimulating factor in human leukemia cells. Blood 77:2716, 1991

284. Ferrari S, Donelli A, Manfredini R et al: Differential effects of c-myb and c-fes antisense oligodeoxynucleotides on granulocytic differentiation of human myeloid leukemia HL-60 cells. Cell Growth Differ 1:543, 1990

285. Tanigawa T, Elwood N, Metcalf D et al: The SCL gene product is regulated by and differentially regulates cytokine responses during myeloid leukemic cell differentiation. Proc Natl Acad Sci USA 90:7864, 1993

286. Nguyen HQ, Hoffman-Liebermann B, Liebermann D: The zinc finger transcription factor Egr-1 is essential for and restricts differentiation along the macrophage lineage. Cell 72:197, 1993

287. Weinberg B, Mason SN, Wortham TS: Inhibition of tumor necrosis factor-α (TNF-α) and interleukin-1β (IL-1β) messenger RNA (mRNA) expression in HL-60 leukemia cells by pentoxifylline and dexamethasone: dissociation of acivicin-induced TNF-α and IL-1β mRNA expression from acivicin-induced monocytoid differentiation. Blood 79:3337, 1992

288. Selvakumaran M, Liebermann D, Hoffman-Liebermann B: Myeloblastic leukemia cells conditionally blocked by myc-estrogen receptor chimeric transgenes for terminal differentiation coupled to growth arrest and apoptosis. Blood 81:2257, 1993

289. Yen A, Forbes ME, Varvayanis S et al: C-fms dependent HL-60 cell differentiation and regulation of RB gene expression. J Cell Physiol 157:379, 1993

290. Kreider BL, Phillips PD, Prystowsky MB et al: Induction of the granulocyte-macrophage colony-stimulating factor (CSF) receptor by granulocyte CSF increases the differentiative options of a murine hematopoietic progenitor cell. Mol Cell Biol 10:4846, 1990

291. Bot FJ, van Eijk L, Schipper P et al: Synergistic effects between GM-CSF and G-CSF or M-CSF on highly enriched human marrow progenitor cells. Leukemia 4:325, 1990

292. Li J, Koay DC, Xiao H, Sartorelli AC: Regulation of the differentiation of WEHI-3B D+ leukemia cells by granulocyte colony-stimulating factor receptor. J Biol Chem 120:1481, 1993

293. Steinman RA, Tweardy DJ: Granulocyte colony-stimulating factor receptor mRNA upregulation is an immediate early marker of myeloid differentiation and exhibits dysfunctional regulation in leukemic cells. Blood 83:119, 1994

294. Kinashi T, Lee KH, Ogawa M et al: Premature expression of macrophage colony-stimulating factor receptor on a multipotential stem cell line does not alter differentiation lineages controlled by stromal cells used for coculture. J Exp Med 173:1267, 1993

295. Heard JM, Roussel MF, Rettenmier CW, Sherr CJ: Multilineage hematopoietic disorders induced by transplantation of bone marrow cells expressing the v-fms oncogene. Cell 51:663, 1987

296. Hromas R, Zon L, Friedman AD: Hematopoietic transcription regulators and the origins of leukemia. Crit Rev Oncol Hematol 12:167, 1992

297. Boulukos KE, Pognomec P, Sariban E et al: Rapid and transient expression of Ets2 in mature macrophages following stimulation with cMGF, LPS, and PKC activators. Genes Dev 4:401, 1990

298. Hromas R, Orazi A, Neiman RS et al: Hematopoietic lineage- and stage-restricted expression of the ets oncogene family member pu.1. Blood 82:2998, 1993

299. Nelsen B, Tian G, Erman B et al: Regulation of lymphoid-specific immunoglobulin μ heavy chain gene enhancer by ets-domain proteins. Science 261:82, 1993

300. Manfredini R, Grande A, Tagliafico E et al: Inhibition of c-fes expression by an antisense oligomer causes apoptosis of HL60 cells induced to granulocytic differentiation. J Exp Med 178:381, 1993

301. Bavisotto L, Kaushansky K, Lin N, Hromas R: Antisense oligonucleotides from the stage-specific myeloid zinc finger gene MZF-1 inhibit granuloiesis in vitro. J Exp Med 174:1097, 1991

302. Falk LA, De Benedetti F, Lohrey N et al: Induction of transforming growth factor-β1 (TGF-β1) receptor expression and TGF-β1 protein production in retinoic acid-treated HL-60 cells: possible TGF-β1-mediated autocrine inhibition. Blood 77:1248, 1991

303. Tsai S, Collins SJ: A dominant negative retinoic acid receptor blocks neutrophil differentiation at the promyelocyte stage. Proc Natl Acad Sci USA 90:7153, 1993

304. French PJ, Bunce CM, Stephens LR et al: Changes in the levels of inositol lipids and phosphates during the differentiation of HL-60 promyelocytic cells towards neutrophils or monocytes. Proc R Soc Lond [Biol] 245:193, 1991

305. Bunce CM, Patton WN, Pound JD et al: Phorbol myristate acetate treatment of normal myeloid blast cells promotes monopoiesis and inhibits granulopoiesis. Leuk Res 14:1007, 1990

306. Heyworth CM, Dexter TM, Nicholls SE, Whetton AD: Protein kinase C activators can interact synergistically with granulocyte colony-stimulating factor or interleukin-6 to stimulate colony formation from enriched granulocyte-macrophage colony-forming cells. Blood 81:894, 1993

307. Makishima M, Honma Y, Hozumi M et al: Differentiation of human monoblastic leukemia U937 cells induced by inhibitors of myosin light chain kinase and prevention of differentiation by granulocyte-macrophage colony-stimulating factor. Biochim Biophys Acta 1176:245, 1993

308. van Furth R: Development and distribution of mononuclear phagocytes. p. 325. In Gallin JI, Goldstein IM, Snyderman R (eds): Inflammation: Basic Principles and Clinical Correlates. 2nd Ed. Raven Press, New York, 1992

309. Panterne B, Zhou YQ, Hatzfeld J et al: CSF-1 control of C-FMS expression in normal human bone marrow progenitors. J Cell Physiol 155:282, 1993

310. Chambers SK, Gilmore Hebert M, Wang Y et al: Posttranscriptional regulation of colony-stimulating factor-1 (CSF-1) and CSF-1 receptor gene expression during inhibition of phorbol-ester-induced monocytic differentiation by dexamethasone and cyclosporin A: potential involvement of a destabilizing protein. Exp Hematol 21:1328, 1993

311. Chen BD-M, Mueller M, Olencki T: Interleukin-3 (IL-3) stimulates the clonal growth of pulmonary alveolar macrophage of the mouse: role of IL-3 in the regulation of macrophage production outside the bone marrow. Blood 72:685, 1988

312. Raivich G, Gehrmann J, Moreno-Floros M, Kreutzberg GW: Microglia: growth factor and mitogen receptors. Clin Neuropathol 12:293, 1993

313. Baldwin GC, Benveniste EN, Chung G-Y et al: Identification and characterization of a high-affinity granulocyte-macrophage colony-stimulating factor receptor on primary rat oligodendrocytes. Blood 82:3279, 1993

314. Inaba K, Inaba M, Deguchi M et al: Granulocytes, macrophages and dendritic cells arise from a common major histocompatibility complex class II-nega-

tive progenitor in mouse bone marrow. Proc Natl Acad Sci USA 90:3038, 1993

315. Reid CD, Stackpoole A, Tikerpae J: TNF and GM-CSF dependent growth of an early progenitor of dendritic Langerhans cells in human bone marrow. Adv Exp Med Biol 329:257, 1993

316. Santiago-Schwarz F, Divaris N, Kay C, Carsons SE: Mechanisms of tumor necrosis factor-granulocyte-macrophage colony-stimulating factor-induced dendritic cell development. Blood 82:3019, 1993

317. Tazi A, Bouchonnet F, Grandsaigne M et al: Evidence that granulocyte-macrophage colony-stimulating factor regulates the distribution and differentiated state of dendritic cells/Langerhans cells in human lung and lung cancers. J Clin Invest 91:566, 1993

318. Elliott MJ, Strasser A, Metcalf D: Selective up-regulation of macrophage function in granulocyte-macrophage colony-stimulating factor transgenic mice. J Immunol 147:2957, 1991

319. Jansen JH, Kluin Nelemans JC, Van Damme J et al: Interleukin 6 is a permissive factor for monocytic colony formation by human hematopoietic progenitor cells. J Exp Med 175:1151, 1992

320. Kerst JM, Slaper-Cortenbach IC, van der Schoot CE et al: Interleukin-6 is a survival factor for committed myeloid progenitor cells. Exp Hematol 21:1550, 1993

321. Sluiter W, Husing-Hesselink E, Elzenga-Claasen I et al: Macrophages as origin of factor increasing monocytopoiesis. J Exp Med 166:909, 1987

322. Annema A, Sluiter W, van Furth R: Effect of interleukin 1, macrophage colony-stimulating factor, and factor increasing monocytopoiesis on the production of leukocytes in mice. Exp Hematol 20:69, 1992

323. Essner R, Rhoades K, McBride WH et al: IL-4 down-regulates IL-1 and TNF gene expression in human monocytes. J Immunol 142:3857, 1989

324. te Velde AA, Huijbens RJF, Heije K et al: Interleukin 4 (IL-4) inhibits secretion of IL-1β, tumor necrosis factor α, and IL-6 by human monocytes. Blood 76:1392, 1990

325. Standiford TJ, Strieter RM, Chensue SW et al: IL-4 inhibits the expression of IL-8 from stimulated human monocytes. J Immunol 145:1435, 1990

326. Henschler R, Mantovani L, Oster W et al: Interleukin-4 regulates mRNA accumulation of macrophage-colony stimulating factor by fibroblasts: synergism with interleukin-1β. Br J Haematol 76:7, 1990

327. Peschel C, Green I, Paul WE: Interleukin-4 induces a substance in bone marrow stromal cells that reversibly inhibits factor-dependent and factor-independent cell proliferation. Blood 73:1130, 1989

328. Snoeck HW, Lardon F, van Bockstaele DR, Peetermans ME: Effects of interleukin-4 on myelopoiesis: localization of the action of IL-4 in the CD34+HLA-DR++ subset and distinction between direct and indirect effects of IL-4. Exp Hematol 21:635, 1993

329. Snoeck HW, Lardon F, van Brockstaele DR, Peetermans ME: Effects of interleukin-4 (IL-4) on myelopoiesis: studies on highly purified CD34+ hematopoietic progenitor cells. Leukemia 7:625, 1993

330. Thompson-Snipes L-A, Dhar V, Bond MW et al: Interleukin-10: a novel stimulatory factor for mast cells and their progenitors. J Exp Med 173:507, 1991

331. de Waal Malefyt R, Abrams J, Bennett B et al: Interleukin 10 (IL-10) inhibits cytokine synthesis by human monocytes: an autoregulatory role for IL-10 produced by monocytes. J Exp Med 174:1209, 1991

332. Kreisberg R, Detrick MS, Moore RN: Opposing effects of tumor necrosis factor alpha and leukemia inhibitory factor in lipopolysaccharide-stimulated myelopoiesis. Infect Immun 61:418, 1993

333. Broxmeyer HE, Sherry B, Lu L et al: Enhancing and suppressing effects of recombinant murine macrophage inflammatory proteins on colony formation in vitro by bone marrow myeloid progenitor cells. Blood 76:1110, 1990

334. Lu L, Xiao M, Grigsby S et al: Comparative effects of suppressive cytokines on isolated single CD34+++ stem/progenitor cells from human bone marrow and umbilical cord blood plated with and without serum. Exp Hematol 21:1442, 1993

335. Cooper S, Mantel C, Broxmeyer HE: Myelosuppressive effects in vivo with very low dosages of monomeric recombinant murine macrophage inflammatory protein-1α. Exp Hematol 22:186, 1994

336. Van Damme J, Proost P, Lenaerts J-P, Opdenakker G: Structural and functional identification of two human, tumor-derived monocyte chemotactic proteins (MCP-2 and MCP-3) belonging to the chemokine family. J Exp Med 176:59, 1992

337. Broxmeyer HE, Cooper S, Lu L et al: Synergistic suppressive interactions and enhanced specific activity of human chemokines on human myeloid progenitor cell proliferation. Exp Hematol 21:1031, 1993

338. Heaney ML, Golde DW: Soluble hormone receptors. Blood 82:1945, 1993

339. McDonald PP, Pouliot M, Borgeat P, McColl SR: Induction by chemokines of lipid mediator synthesis in granulocyte-macrophage colony-stimulating factor-treated human neutrophils. J Immunol 151:6399, 1993

340. Pasquale D, Chikkappa G: Lipoxygenase products regulate proliferation of granulocyte-macrophage progenitors. Exp Hematol 21:1361, 1993

341. Lee M-T, Kaushansky K, Ralph P, Ladner MB: Differential expression of M-CSF, G-CSF, and GM-CSF by human monocytes. J Leukoc Biol 47:275, 1990

342. Gordon MY, Ford AM, Greaves MF: Interactions of hematopoietic progenitor cells with extracellular matrix. p. 152. In Long MW, Wicha MS (eds): The Hematopoietic Microenvironment. The Johns Hopkins University Press, Baltimore, 1993

343. Moore SC, Theus SA, Barnett JB, Soderberg LSF: Bone marrow natural suppressor cells inhibit the growth of myeloid progenitor cells and the synthesis of colony-stimulating factors. Exp Hematol 20:1178, 1992

344. Lowry PA, Deacon D, Whitefield P et al: Stem cell factor induction of in vitro murine hematopoietic colony formation by "subliminal" cytokine combinations: the role of "anchor factors." Blood 80:663, 1992

345. Verfaillie CM: Soluble factor(s) produced by human bone marrow stroma increase cytokine-induced proliferation and maturation of primitive hematopoietic progenitors while preventing their terminal differentiation. Blood 82:2045, 1993

346. Temeles DS, McGrath HE, Kittler ELW et al: Cytokine expression from bone marrow derived macrophages. Exp Hematol 21:388, 1993

347. Wijffels JFAM, de Rover Z, Kraal G, Beelen RHJ: Macrophage phenotype regulation by colony-stimulating factors at bone marrow levelf. J Leukoc Biol 53:249, 1993

348. Schwartz GN, Hudgins WR, Perdue JF: Glycosylated insulin-like growth factor II promoted expansion of granulocyte-macrophage colony-forming cells in serum-deprived liquid cultures of human peripheral blood cells. Exp Hematol 21:1447, 1993

349. Adams DO, Hamilton TA: Macrophages as destructive cells in host defense. p. 637. In Gallin JI, Goldstein IM, Snyderman R (eds): Inflammation: Basic Principles and Clinical Correlates. 2nd Ed. Raven Press, New York, 1992

350. Cicco NA, Lindemann A, Content J et al: Inducible production of interleukin-6 by human polymorphonuclear neutrophils: role of granulocyte-macrophage colony-stimulating factor and tumor necrosis factor-alpha. Blood 75:2049, 1990

351. Kita H, Ohnishi T, Okubo Y et al: Granulocyte/macrophage colony-stimulating factor and interleukin-3 release from human peripheral blood eosinophils and neutrophils. J Exp Med 174:745, 1991

352. Kobayashi H: Effect of c-kit ligand (stem cell factor) in combination with interleukin-5, granulocyte-macrophage colony-stimulating factor, and interleukin-3, on eosinophil lineage. Int J Hematol 58:21, 1993

353. Paul CC, Tolbert M, Mahrer S et al: Cooperative effects of interleukin-3 (IL-3), IL-5, and granulocyte-macrophage colony-stimulating factor: a new myeloid cell line inducible to eosinophils. Blood 81:1193, 1993

354. Clutterbuck EJ, Hirst EMA, Sanderson CJ: Human interleukin-5 (IL-5) regulates the production of eosinophils in human bone marrow cultures: comparison and interaction with IL-1, IL-3, IL-6 and GM-CSF. Blood 73:1504, 1989

355. Ema H, Suda T, Nagayoshi K et al: Target cells for granulocyte colony-stimulating factor, interleukin-3, and interleukin-5 in differentiation pathways of neutrophils and eosinophils. Blood 76:1956, 1990

356. Corrigan CJ, Kay AB: T cells and eosinophils in the pathogenesis of asthma. Immunol Today 13:501, 1992

357. Liesveld JL, Abboud CN: State of the art: the hypereosinophilic syndromes. Blood Rev 5:29, 1991

358. Yamaguchi Y, Suda T, Ohta S et al: Analysis of the survival of mature eosinophils: interleukin-5 prevents apoptosis in mature human eosinophils. Blood 78:2542, 1991

359. Sher A, Coffman RL, Hieny S et al: Interleukin 5 is required for the blood and tissue eosinophilia but not granuloma formation induced by infection with Schistosoma mansoni. Proc Natl Acad Sci USA 87:61, 1991

360. Limaye AP, Abrams JS, Silver JE et al: Regulation of parasite-induced eosinophilia: selectively increased interleukin-5 production in helminth-infected patients. J Exp Med 172:399, 1990

361. Yamaguchi Y, Suda T, Shiozaki H et al: Role of IL-5 in IL-2-induced eosinophilia. In vivo and in vitro expression of IL-5 mRNA by IL-2. J Immunol 145:873, 1990

362. Enokihara H, Kajitani H, Nagashima S et al: Interleukin-5 activity in sera from patients with eosinophilia. Br J Haematol 75:458, 1990

363. Fermand J-P, Mitjavila M-T, Le Couedic J-P et al: Role of granulocyte-macrophage colony-stimulating factor, interleukin-3 and interleukin-5 in the eosinophilia associated with T cell lymphoma. Br J Haematol 83:359, 1993

364. Kay AB: Origin of type 2 helper T cells. N Engl J Med 330:567, 1994

365. Wierenga EA, Backx B, Snoek M et al: Relative contribution of human types 1 and 2 T-helper cell-derived eosinophilotrophic cytokines to development of eosinophilia. Blood 82:1471, 1993

366. Ohshima Y, Morita M, Hirashima M et al: Characterization of an eosinophilic leukemia cell differentiation factor (ELDF) produced by a human T cell leukemia cell line, HIL-3. Exp Hematol 21:749, 1993

367. Schrezenmeier H, Thomé SD, Tewald F et al: Interleukin-5 is the predominant eosinophilopoietin produced by cloned T lymphocytes in hypereosinophilic syndrome. Exp Hematol 21:358, 1993

368. Cogan E, Schandene L, Crusiaux A et al: Clonal proliferation of type 2 helper T cells in a man with the hypereosinophilic syndrome. N Engl J Med 330:535, 1994

369. Yamaoka KA, Kolb JP: Leukotriene B4 induces interleukin 5 generation from human T lymphocytes. Eur J Immunol 23:2392, 1993

370. Broide DH, Paine MM, Firestein GS: Eosinophils express interleukin-5 and granulocyte macrophage-colony-stimulating factor mRNA at sites of allergic inflammation in asthmatics. J Clin Invest 90:1414, 1992

371. Melani C, Mattia GF, Silvani A et al: Interleukin-6 expression in human neutrophil and eosinophil peripheral blood granulocytes. Blood 81:2744, 1993

372. Walz TM, Nishikawa BK, Malm C, Wasteson: Production of transforming growth factor alpha by normal blood eosinophils. Leukemia 7:1531, 1993

373. Galli SJ, Hammel I: Mast cell and basophil development. Curr Opin Hematol 1:33, 1994

374. Agis H, Willheim M, Sperr WR et al: Monocytes do not make mast cells when cultured in the presence of SCF. Characterization of the circulating mast cell progenitor as a c-kit +, CD34 +, Ly −, CD14 −, CD17 − colony-forming cell. J Immunol 151:4221, 1993

375. Tsai M, Takeishi T, Thompson H et al: Induction of mast cell proliferation, maturation, and heparin synthesis by rat c-kit ligand, stem cell factor. Proc Natl Acad Sci USA 88:6382, 1991

376. Valent P, Spanblochl E, Sperr WR et al: Induction of differentiation of human mast cells from bone marrow and peripheral blood mononuclear cells by recombinant human stem cell factor/kit-ligand in long-term culture. Blood 80:2237, 1992

377. Denburg JA, Silver JE, Abrams JS: Interleukin-5 is a human basophilopoietin: induction of histamine content and basophilic differentiation of HL-60 cells and of peripheral blood basophil-eosinophil progenitors. Blood 77:1462, 1991

378. Coleman JW, Holliday MR, Kimber I et al: Regulation of mouse mast cell secretory function by stem cell factor, IL-3 or IL-4. J Immunol 150:556, 1993

379. Tei H, Kasugai T, Tsujimura T et al: Characterization of cultured mast cells derived from Ws/Ws mast cell-deficient rats with a small deletion at tyrosine kinase domain of c-kit. Blood 83:916, 1994

380. Rottem M, Goff JP, Albert JP, Metcalfe DD: The effects of stem cell factor on the ultrastructure of Fc epsilon RI + cells developing in IL-3-dependent murine bone marrow-derived cell cultures. J Immunol 151:4950, 1993

381. Kannan Y, Matsuda H, Ushio H et al: Murine granulocyte-macrophage and mast cell colony formation promoted by nerve growth factor. Int Arch Allergy Immunol 102:362, 1993

382. Tsuda T, Wong D, Dolovich J et al: Synergistic effects of nerve growth factor and granulocyte-macrophage colony-stimulating factor on human basophilic cell differentiation. Blood 77:971, 1991

383. Greene WC: The interleukins. p. 233. In Gallin JI, Goldstein IM, Snyderman R (eds): Inflammation: Basic Principles and Clinical Correlates. 2nd Ed. Raven Press, New York, 1992

384. Manie S, Schmid-Alliana A, Kubar J et al: Disruption of microtubule network in human monocytes induces expression of interleukin-1 but not that of interleukin-6 nor tumor necrosis factor-α. Involvement of protein kinase A stimulation. J Biol Chem 268:13675, 1993

385. Colotta F, Wang JM, Polentarutti N, Mantovani A: Expression of c-fos protooncogene in normal peripheral blood granulocytes. J Exp Med 165:1224, 1987

386. Lindemann A, Reidel D, Oster W et al: Granulocyte/macrophage colony-stimulating factor induces interleukin 1 production by human polymorphonuclear neutrophils. J Immunol 140:837, 1988

387. Lindemann A, Riedel D, Oster W et al: GM-CSF induces cytokine secretion by polymorphonuclear neutrophils. J Clin Invest 83:1308, 1989

388. Cicco NA, Lindemann A, Content J et al: Inducible production of interleukin-6 by human polymorphonuclear neutrophils: role of granulocyte-macrophage colony-stimulating factor and tumor necrosis factor-alpha. Blood 75:2049, 1990

389. Lloyd AR, Oppenheim JJ: Poly's lament: the neglected role of the polymorphonuclear neutrophil in the afferent limb of the immune response. Immunol Today 13:169, 1992

390. Baggiolini M, Dewald B: Cytokine regulation of mononuclear phagocyte activation. Curr Opin Hematol 1:133, 1993

391. Gasson JC: Molecular physiology of granulocyte-macrophage colony-stimulating factor. Blood 77:1131, 1991

392. DiPersio JF, Abboud CN: Activation of neutrophils by granulocyte-macrophage colony-stimulating factor. Immunol Ser 57:457, 1992

393. Koenderman L, Hermans SWG, Capel PJA, van de Winkel JGJ: Granulocyte-macrophage colony-stimulating factor induces sequential activation and deactivation of binding via a low-affinity IgG Fc receptor, FcγRII, on human eosinophils. Blood 81:2413, 1993

394. van der Bruggen T, Kok PTM, Raaijmakers JAM et al: Cytokine priming of the respiratory burst in human eosinophils is Ca^{2+} independent and accompanied by induction of tyrosine kinase activity. J Leukoc Biol 53:347, 1993

395. Tomioka K, MacGlashan DW Jr, Lichtenstein LM et al: GM-CSF regulates human eosinophil responses to F-Met peptide and platelet activating factor. J Immunol 151:4989, 1993

396. Fabian I, Lass M, Kletter Y, Golde DW: Differentiation and functional activity of human eosinophilic cells from an eosinophil HL-60 subline: response to recombinant hematopoietic growth factors. Blood 80:788, 1992

397. Fabian I, Kletter Y, Mor S et al: Activation of human eosinophil and neutrophil functions by haematopoietic growth factors: comparisons of IL-1, IL-3, IL-5 and GM-CSF. Br J Haematol 80:137, 1992

398. Hartnell A, Robinson DS, Kay AB, Wardlaw AJ: CD69 is expressed by human eosinophils activated in vivo in asthma and in vitro by cytokines. Immunology 80:281, 1993

399. Kameyoshi Y, Dörschner A, Mallet AI et al: Cytokine RANTES released by thrombin-stimulated platelets is a potent attractant for human eosinophils. J Exp Med 176:587, 1992

400. Meurer R, Van Riper G, Feeney W et al: Formation of eosinophilic and monocytic intradermal inflammatory sites in the dog by injection of human RANTES but not human monocyte chemoattractant protein 1, human macrophage inflammatory protein 1 alpha, or human interleukin 8. J Exp Med 178:1913, 1993

401. Saito H, Koshio T, Yanagihara Y et al: Platelet-activating-factor-induced augmentation of production of eosinophil-lineage cells in hematopoietic precursor cells obtained from human umbilical cord blood. Int Arch Allergy Immunol 102:375, 1993

402. Meade R, Neddermann KM, Greenfield RS et al: Granulocyte-macrophage colony-stimulating factor plays a role in the functional activity of mast cells. J Leukoc Biol 54:523, 1993

403. Hultner L, Huls C, Kremer J-P et al: IL-1 and IL-10 are major regulators of cytokine production in mouse bone marrow-derived mast cells. Exp Hematol 21:1077, 1993

404. Alam R, Forsythe PA, Stafford S et al: Macrophage inflammatory protein-1 alpha activates basophils and mast cells. J Exp Med 176:781, 1992

405. Bischoff SC, Dahinden CA: c-kit ligand: a unique potentiator of mediator release by human lung mast cells. J Exp Med 175:237, 1992

406. Dastych J, Metcalfe DD: Stem cell factor induces mast cell adhesion to fibronectin. J Immunol 152:213, 1994

407. Hatfield SM, Roehm NW: Cyclosporine and FK506 inhibition of murine mast cell cytokine production. J Pharmacol Exp Ther 260:680, 1992

408. Hatfield SM, Mynderse JS, Roehm NW: Rapamycin and FK506 differentially inhibit mast cell cytokine production and cytokine-induced proliferation and act as reciprocal antagonists. J Pharmacol Exp Ther 261:970, 1992

409. Casolaro V, Spadaro G, Patella V, Marone G: In vivo characterization of the anti-inflammatory effect of cyclosporin A on human basophils. J Immunol 151:5563, 1993

Thrombocytopoiesis

19

Michael W. Long and Ronald Hoffman

INTRODUCTION

The clinical consequences of alterations in platelet levels are well known, ranging from severe thromboembolic episodes occurring in some patients with thrombocytosis to hemorrhage resulting from thrombocytopenia. With the exception of instances of increase peripheral destruction (e.g., trauma, infection), most quantitative and qualitative disorders of platelet function result from intrinsic errors that occur within the megakaryocyte. As platelets lack a nucleus and, for the most part, a rough endoplasmic reticulum, they have limited ability to alter their biochemical composition or structure. Consequently, an understanding of the biochemical and molecular mechanisms underlying thrombocytopoiesis rests on understanding the development of the platelet within its precursor cell, the megakaryocyte. Until recently, however, megakaryocyte differentiation has been difficult to study because the low frequency and fragility of these cells makes them difficult to purify in sufficient numbers for biochemical and molecular studies. Recent scientific advances, together with new developments in cytokine therapy and bone marrow transplantation, suggest that therapeutic tools to alter platelet production will soon be available.

Megakaryocyte development is a complex process in which a wide variety of regulatory signals work in concert to direct a highly specific response to thrombopoietic demand. The cells of the megakaryocyte lineage are the primitive, actively proliferating progenitors cells as well as the mature postmitotic megakaryocytes undergoing maturational development (Fig. 19-1). The complex nature of this developmental hierarchy is underscored by the wide variety of hematopoietic growth factors that stimulate these cells (i.e., the various colony-stimulating factors and interleukins). Developing megakaryocytes also interact with surrounding extracellular molecules, which further modulate the developmental process. Each of these key elements (i.e., cells, growth factors, and extracellular molecules) thus defines a highly organized and localized regulatory system known as the megakaryocytic microenvironment. It is this system that coordinately regulates megakaryocyte development and the daily production of approximately 2×10^{11} platelets.[1]

Although the precise makeup of the megakaryocyte microenvironment is unknown, many of its important elements have been defined. The cellular components are the parenchymal cells (i.e., cells committed to megakaryocyte lineage) and the neighboring stromal cells (e.g., fibroblasts, endothelial cells, and macrophages). These stromal cells produce both membrane-associated and soluble cytokines (growth factors), as well as extracellular molecules important to megakaryocyte function. To date, approximately 19 hematopoietic growth factors have been identified and molecularly cloned (interleukins [IL] 1–13), colony-stimulating factor-granulocyte, -granulocyte/macrophage, and -macrophage (CSF-G, -GM, -M), leukemia in-

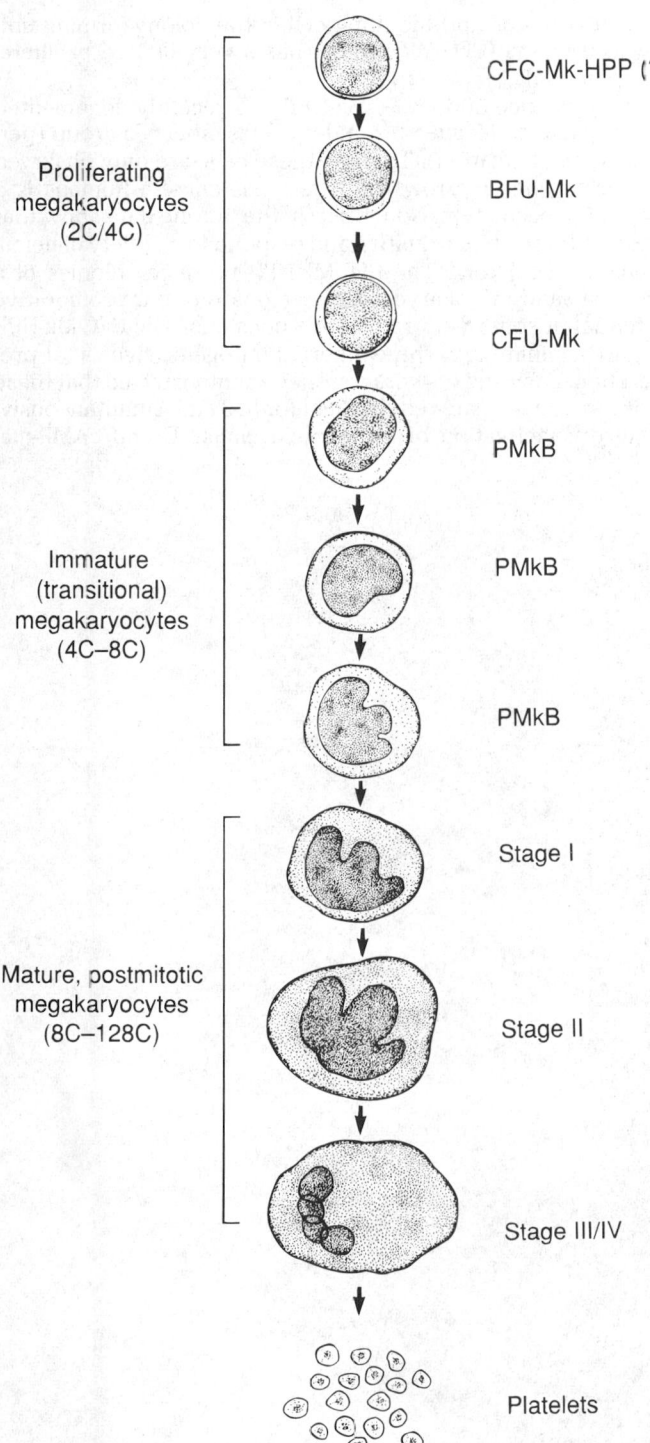

Proliferating
megakaryocytes
(2C/4C)

CFC-Mk-HPP (?)

BFU-Mk

CFU-Mk

Immature
(transitional)
megakaryocytes
(4C–8C)

PMkB

PMkB

PMkB

Mature, postmitotic
megakaryocytes
(8C–128C)

Stage I

Stage II

Stage III/IV

Platelets

Fig. 19-1. Cellular hierarchy of megakaryocyte development. Megakaryocytes can be conceptually divided into three stages: the proliferating progenitor cells, which have the typical 2C/4C DNA content; the immature megakaryocytes, which have an intermediate DNA content and are transitional between the progenitor cells and the more mature cells; and the mature postmitotic cells, which have an 8C to 128C DNA content (see text). CFC-Mk-HPP, colony-forming cell-megakaryocyte-high-proliferative-potential; BFU-Mk, burst-forming unit-megakaryocyte; CFU-Mk, colony-forming unit-megakaryocyte; PMkB, promegakaryoblast.

hibitory factor [LIF], c-kit ligand, and erythropoietin). A variety of other regulatory factors, such as the interferons, tumor necrosis factor, and transforming growth factor-β (TGF-β) are capable of inhibiting and/or stimulating hematopoiesis. Among these 20 or so growth factors, at least four interleukins (IL-3,

IL-6, IL-9, and IL-11) as well as c-kit ligand (also known as stem cell factor, or mast cell growth factor), CSF-GM, and possibly erythropoietin, stimulate both in vivo and in vitro megakaryocyte development.[2] The final component of megakaryocytic microenvironment is the extracellular matrix (ECM). Once referred to as basement membrane, ECM is no longer thought to be an inert structural scaffold for various organs. Rather, it is a dynamic, complex cellular substrate, whose components stimulate cells to proliferate, differentiate, or migrate.[3–7] Recent studies demonstrate that, like other lineages, megakaryocytes have unique developmental requirements modulated by interactions with specific ECM molecules.[8–12]

Interestingly, megakaryocytopoiesis occurs within a number of locations throughout the body. Clearly, the primary site of megakaryocyte development (and hence platelet production) is the bone marrow. However, it is known that megakaryocyte precursors and some mature megakaryocytes circulate,[13–15] which suggests that capillary beds might filter (trap) such cells. If the surrounding microenvironment is appropriate, megakaryocytes may develop in this extramedullary tissue. This is true for both the spleen and lungs, each of which contains megakaryocytes and produces platelets.[16–18] Their contribution to total thrombocytopoiesis, however, is on the order of only 7–15%.[1,18]

An understanding of the disorders of platelet production clearly requires insights into the complex regulatory events that occur during normal megakaryocytopoiesis. Moreover, a rational approach to therapeutic interventions that might alter the clinical course of megakaryocyte disorders must take into consideration the precise nature of the developmental control mechanism(s) affected. This chapter focuses on the current concepts of megakaryocyte/platelet development, examining the various types of megakaryocytic cells, their responses to cytokines and other extracellular influences, and recent observations on the biochemical and molecular control lineage-specific gene expression.

BIOLOGY OF MEGAKARYOCYTES

Megakaryocyte Progenitor Cells

The cellular hierarchy of megakaryocytopoiesis is best understood if megakaryocyte development is artificially divided into three stages: progenitor cells, immature megakaryocytes (promegakaryoblasts [PMkB]), and mature megakaryocytes (Fig. 19-1). Megakaryocyte progenitor cells are responsible for the expansion of the megakaryocyte numbers and proliferate in response to a number of mitotic growth factors. The PMkB are transitional in nature, bridging the progenitor cells with the more mature postmitotic cells. Mature megakaryocytes no longer proliferate but have the unique ability to continue and/or increase DNA synthesis, without undergoing mitosis, during maturation (see below). Mature megakaryocytes are markedly larger than other marrow cells and, thus, have a dramatically increased cell volume. As a result, an individual megakaryocyte produces on the order of 2,000–3,000 platelets.[19]

Most of our knowledge concerning the nature of hematopoietic progenitor cells comes from the ability to assay these cells in vitro. The most primitive hematopoietic progenitor cells are multi- or pluripotential, giving rise to cells of different lineages. These, in turn, give rise to committed progenitor cells, defined as proliferating cells capable of generating progeny of a given lineage(s). The development of either progenitor type in vitro thus results in a clonal expansion of cells, leading to the formation of a "colony" in semisolid media. Originally, the entity generating a colony was called a colony-forming unit (CFU), to reflect the concept that it was unclear whether a colony was derived from a single cell; this is now definitively proven.

In vitro studies demonstrate that megakaryocyte progenitor cells, like other lineages, progressively lose proliferative potential as they develop. The proliferating cells of this lineage are themselves heterogeneous and are of at least three distinct cell populations, each marked by varying degrees of proliferative potential. Reports from animal studies suggest that the earliest detectable cell in this lineage, the colony-forming cell-mega-karyocyte-high-proliferative-potential (CFC-Mk-HPP), is the most primitive progenitor cell of this lineage. Unlike most other progenitor cells, this cell proliferates in vitro to the extent that its colonies are macroscopically visible. The burst-forming unit-megakaryocyte (BFU-Mk) is more mature than the CFC-Mk-HPP, but retains a high degree of proliferative potential developing "bursts" of individual colony-forming cells (Fig. 19-2).

The most mature proliferating cell is the colony-forming unit megakaryocyte (CFU-Mk), which has a very limited proliferative potential.

The existence of the CFC-Mk-HPP was recently documented by Long and colleagues[20,21] and by Quesenberry's group (personal communication). To date, these cells are only observed in murine bone marrow, and their existence in humans is a matter of speculation. Nonetheless, the murine data show that these cells are quite primitive and respond to a variety of hematopoietic regulators. The CFC-Mk-HPP produce colonies of a few thousand megakaryocytes, demonstrating a proliferative potential of some 8–10 replicative divisions. The CFC-Mk-HPP require a minimum of three different mitogenic signals for proliferation. Long and co-workers[20] have demonstrated that these cells have an obligate requirement for IL-3 and, simultaneously, require co-activation of the protein kinase C and cAMP-me-

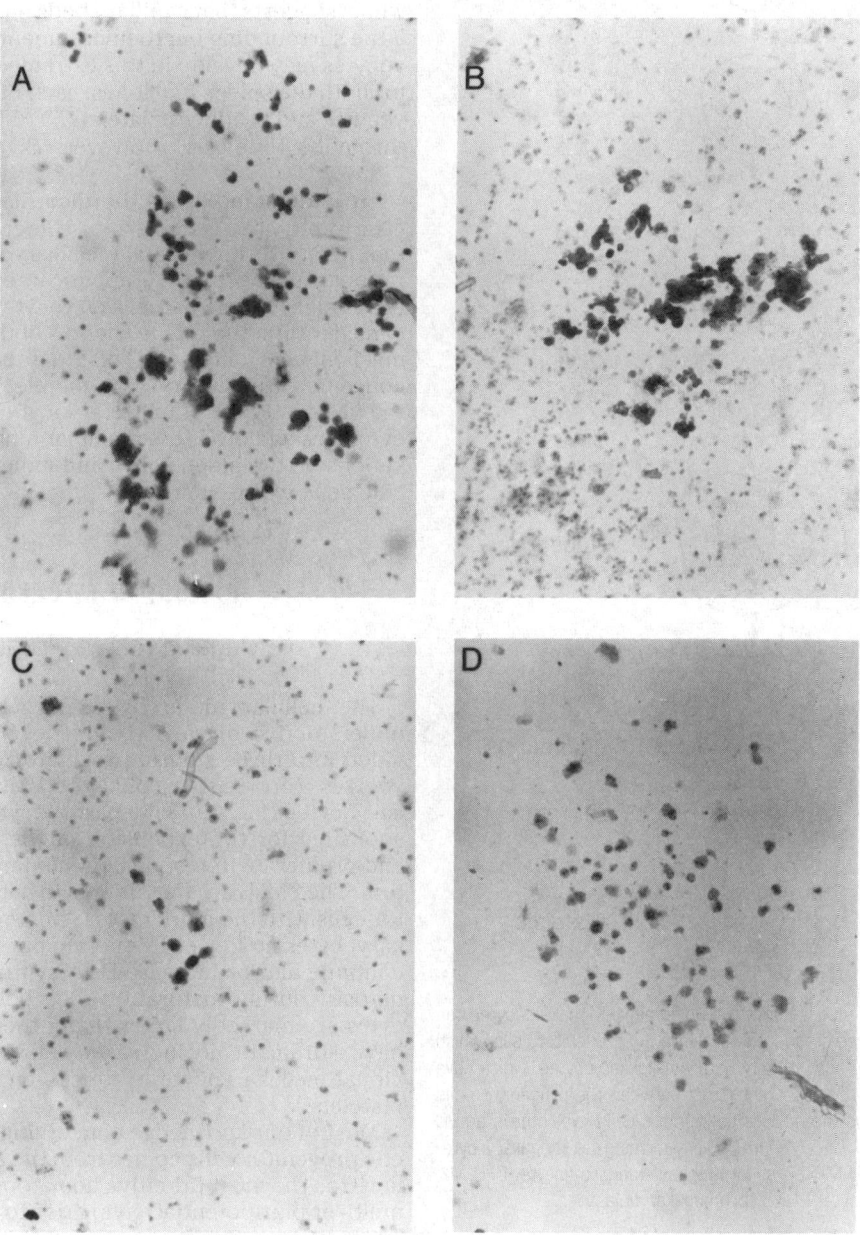

Fig. 19-2. Megakaryocyte progenitor cells. **(A & B)** The cellular hierarchy of the megakaryocyte lineage is believed to begin with a primitive, highly proliferative burst-forming cell, BFU-Mk, which divides, migrates, and differentiates to generate multicentric clusters of megakaryocytes. **(C & D)** Each BFU-Mk gives rise to several nonmotile, less proliferative CFU-Mk, each of which generates a small cluster of megakaryocytes in culture. (From Long et al.,[22] with permission.)

diated signal transduction pathways. The results from Quesenberry et al. confirmed and extended these observations, demonstrating that three to five recombinant hematopoietic growth factors are required to sustain the proliferation of these early megakaryocyte progenitor cells. Interestingly, colonies observed in these latter studies contained cells of multiple hematopoietic lineages, with large numbers of megakaryocytes present. The relationship between these two colony phenotypes as well as the existence of the CFC-Mk-HPP in humans remains to be determined.

The BFU-Mk has a high proliferative potential, generating 100–500 megakaryocytes per cell, representing a proliferative capacity of some five to seven replicative events.[22] These cells are believed to be the progeny of the CFC-Mk-HPP and to be the immediate ancestors of the CFU-Mk.[21] The BFU-Mk colonies morphologically resemble the burst-forming cell-erythroid in that the BFU-Mk colonies consist of multiple foci of megakaryocyte development, each of which is attributed to the presence of a single CFU-Mk (Fig. 19-2). The human BFU-Mk have in vitro characteristics similar to those of the murine cells and, additionally, are resistant to treatment in vitro with 5-fluorouracil.[23,24] Proliferation of these cells in chemically defined media (i.e., serum-free cultures) has permitted precise determination of their growth factor responsiveness. The BFU-Mk requires two categories of growth factors for in vitro development. They have an obligate requirement for mitogenic growth factors such as IL-3 or CSF-GM. In addition, optimal development of BFU-Mk requires the presence of a synergistic co-regulator that augments hematopoietic growth factor-driven proliferation and differentiation (see the section Cytokines).[20] In humans, these cells respond to IL-3, CSF-GM, and CSF-Mk as proliferative stimuli.[24] In addition, c-kit ligand, IL-11, as well as IL-1α synergize with IL-3 to augment BFU-Mk development.[24–28] A number of other putative megakaryocyte co-regulators (i.e., IL-6, erythropoietin, CSF-G, IL-4) fail to synergize with IL-3, CSF-GM, or CSF-Mk in stimulating BFU-Mk.[24]

The most differentiated of the megakaryocyte progenitor cells is the CFU-Mk. This was the first megakaryocyte progenitor cell to be assayed in vitro. Both CFU-Mk and its progenitors have relatively fastidious requirements for in vitro growth. As a result, the first murine in vitro CFU-Mk colony assay was developed 9 years[29–31] after the first in vitro hematopoietic progenitor cell assay (the granulocyte progenitor cell),[32] and the first human megakaryocyte colony assay was not reported until 5 years later.[33,34] The CFU-Mk have a restricted proliferative potential, generating only 4–32 megakaryocytes (i.e., two to five divisions).[35] This progenitor cell responds to a variety of single growth factors (e.g., IL-3, CSF-GM) and also interacts with co-regulators such as c-kit ligand and crudely purified sources of thrombopoietin-like activities.[25,28,36,37] Interestingly, the CFU-Mk are not the first cells in the lineage to respond to thrombocytopenia. In fact, increases in CFU-Mk numbers occur as a late response to decreased platelet numbers.[38,39] This finding suggests that megakaryocyte progenitor cells somehow sense megakaryocyte (and not platelet) mass, thus increasing in number to supply an increased need for megakaryocytes. This type of regulatory network was first suggested by Ebbe and Phalen,[40] who demonstrated that decreased megakaryocyte numbers resulted in a correcting stimulus that was independent of platelet level.

A number of reports suggest that other types of multi- or pluripotential cells express megakaryocytic potential (e.g., the colony-forming unit-granulocyte/erythrocyte/megakaryocyte/macrophage [CFU-GEMM]). Notably, a developmental relationship seems to exist between the erythroid and megakaryocyte lineage. Early work by Nicola and Johnson[41] documented the progressive loss of lineage potential by pluripotential progenitor cells resulting in a bipotential erythroid/megakaryocytic progenitor cell. This concept was strengthened by observa-

tions made by Papayannopoulou et al.[42,43] and by Long et al.[44] showing that cell lines derived from patients with erythroleukemia either express some megakaryocyte phenotypic markers or can be induced to undergo megakaryocyte commitment and differentiation, or both. Other investigators have documented the existence of transplantable megakaryocyte progenitors (CFC-Mk)[45] and that megakaryocyte colonies can be composed of megakaryocytes at various stages of development.[46]

Immature Megakaryocytes (Promegakaryoblasts)

PMkB are transitional cells intermediate between the proliferating progenitor cells and the postmitotic mature megakaryocytes.[47,48] These immature cells are not readily observed morphologically in vitro, or in bone marrow specimens, but can be identified by their expression of megakaryocyte/platelet-specific markers, such as platelet peroxidase, platelet glycoprotein IIb/IIIa, and von Willebrand factor (vWF).[49,50] PMkB are quite restricted (or lacking) in their proliferative potential. They therefore are the developmental stage at which megakaryocytes cease to proliferate but rather continue to acquire an increased DNA content. As such, they are endomitotic (a mechanism of acquiring polyploid nuclei) and contain an intermediate (6C–8C), DNA content (MWL, personal communication). The PMkB respond to a variety of hematopoietic growth factors (IL-3, c-kit ligand, IL-6) in vitro, maturing into single large megakaryocytes.[51–53] Observations of the early phases of CFU-Mk colony formation demonstrate that progenitor cells pass through a PMkB stage during development, confirming the parent:progeny relationship between PMkB and megakaryocytes.[54] Studies in animals document the responsiveness of these cells in vivo. PMkB are highly sensitive to thrombopoietic demand and are the first cells to increase in number after the induction of thrombocytopenia or to decrease following conditions of thrombocytosis.[55,56] Subsequently, increases and reductions (respectively) are seen in megakaryocyte numbers, again confirming the kinetic and developmental relationship between the PMkB and their more differentiated progeny. PMkB are also a heterogeneous group of cells, and during development increase in nuclear and cytoplasmic complexity.[52,54,57–59] Three distinct subpopulations of these cells exist, differing in their physicochemical characteristics, morphology, antigen expression, and enzymatic content.[49,52,57,60]

Mature Megakaryocytes

Morphologically recognizable megakaryocytes exist in four maturational stages as defined by their morphology (Fig. 19-3). The megakaryoblast (stage I) is characterized by a high nucleus cytoplasm ratio and scanty basophilic cytoplasm, reflecting the large amounts of protein syntheses occurring in these cells. The promegakaryocyte (stage II) is the cell in which both the cytoplasmic volume and number of platelet-specific granules increase. The granular or "platelet-shedding" megakaryocyte (stages III and IV) is the most mature of the megakaryocytes, and is supposedly the platelet-shedding cell. It should be understood that these morphologic classifications also represent a maturation progression and are, themselves, heterogeneous with respect to many other developmental characteristics, such as antigenic expression, enzymatic content, and DNA content.

Platelets

The final event of megakaryocyte development is the release of platelets into the circulation. Interestingly, the platelets were the first element of this lineage to be identified and among the

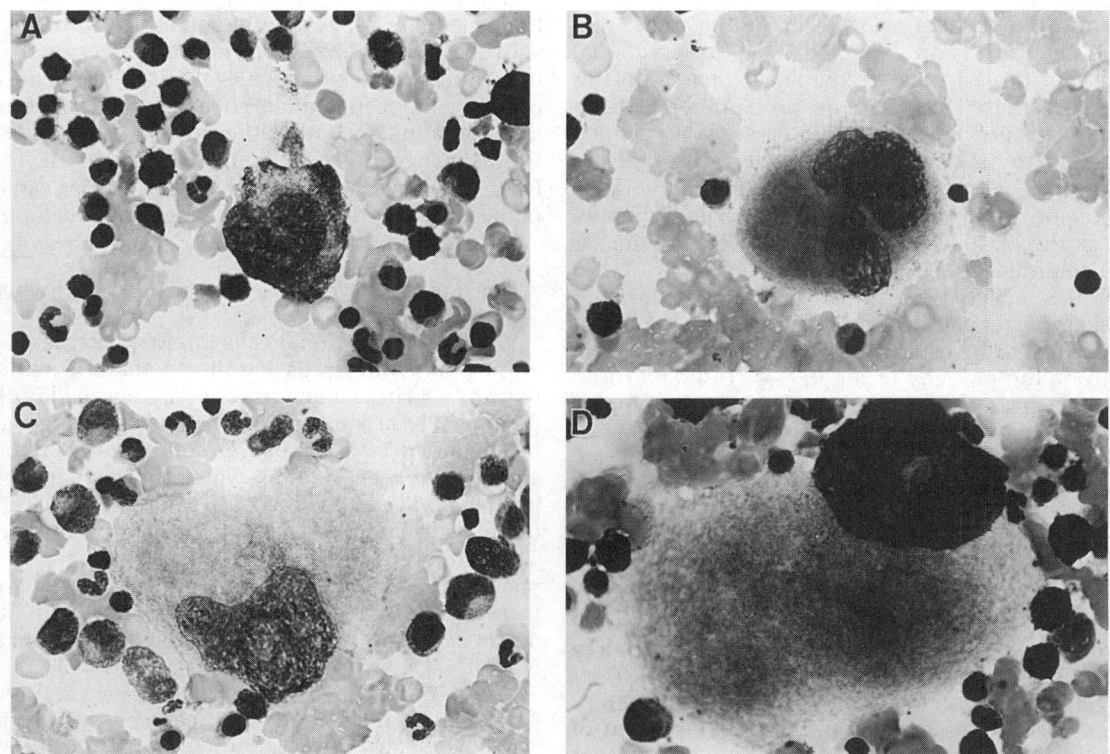

Fig. 19-3. Mature human megakaryocytes. **(A)** Megakaryoblast. **(B)** Promegakaryocyte (stage II). **(C)** Granular megakaryocyte (stage III). **(D)** Granular megakaryocyte (stage IV). (Figure courtesy of Dr. Maryann Weller.)

first of the blood cells observed. During the late 1800s, both William Oster, in 1874, and Georges Hayem, in 1878, described and illustrated blood platelets.[61] In 1882, Julius Bizzorzero coined the term platelet *(Blutplättchen)* and noted their shape change with activation, and their involvement with homeostasis.[61] However, it was not until 1906 that Homer Wright linked platelets with the megakaryocyte[62,63] and not until the 1950s that this hypothesis was proven.[19,64] Given that the existence of platelets has been recognized for more than a century, it is surprising that the mechanisms by which platelets are produced and released remain poorly understood. During maturation, proliferation and invagination of the megakaryocyte plasma membrane occur, resulting in the development of a tubular network known as the demarcation membrane system. The demarcation membrane system is thought to divide the megakaryocyte cytoplasm into platelet fields (Fig. 19-4), although its precise role in the formation of individual platelets remains obscure and, thus, controversial. Finally, megakaryocytes seem to extend pseudopods into the sinusoidal lumins from which platelets are shed into the circulation.[65] Unfortunately, the lack of adequate in vitro assays of platelet production has precluded (to date) examination of the biochemical and molecular control of this process.

REGULATION OF MEGAKARYOCYTE DEVELOPMENT

Physiologic control over the megakaryocyte lineage is relevant in three areas: expansion of megakaryocyte numbers (proliferation), regulation of megakaryocyte maturation, and control of platelet shedding. Many investigators have detailed the role of cytokines in the first two areas. Moreover, increasing evidence suggests the importance of the extracellular matrix components to megakaryocyte or platelet production or both. The actual process of both platelet formation and shedding is poorly understood. Given the lack of definitive data, the regulation of platelet production, per se, is not discussed here. Instead, this section examines megakaryocyte antigenic expression and the regulation of megakaryocytes by cytokines and the ECM.

Markers of Megakaryocyte Development

Megakaryocytes and their precursors express antigenic determinants that are developmentally regulated. The expression of these cell-surface structures allows for both the isolation and purification of subpopulations of marrow cells, which are enriched for the various megakaryocyte progenitor cells. One of the antigens on megakaryocytes and their precursors is CD34, a panhematopoietic cell antigen first identified by Civin and co-workers.[66–68] This antigen is expressed on all hematopoietic progenitor cells and allows their separation from other bone marrow cells by a variety of immunologic procedures. Subsequent examination of CD34+ subsets for other developmental markers has yielded the beginnings of an immunophenotypic analysis of the megakaryocytic lineage.

As expected, cells of the megakaryocyte lineage from the BFU-Mk to the mature cells express CD34, although its expression is reduced in mature cells. Subsequent characterization of CD34+ cells, based on the expression of the human major histocompatibility class II complex, HLA-DR yields further segregation of progenitor cell phenotypes. In general, expression of the HLA-DR antigen characterizes a more mature subset of hematopoietic progenitor cells (i.e., CD34+ DR− cells are more primitive than CD34+ DR+ cells).[8,69] Among megakaryocyte progenitors, this distinction separates the BFU-Mk (which are CD34+ DR−) from the more mature CFU-Mk (CD34+ DR+).[70] Importantly, CD34+ DR− cells can sustain long-term megakaryocytopoiesis in growth factor-driven cultures for 10–12 weeks,

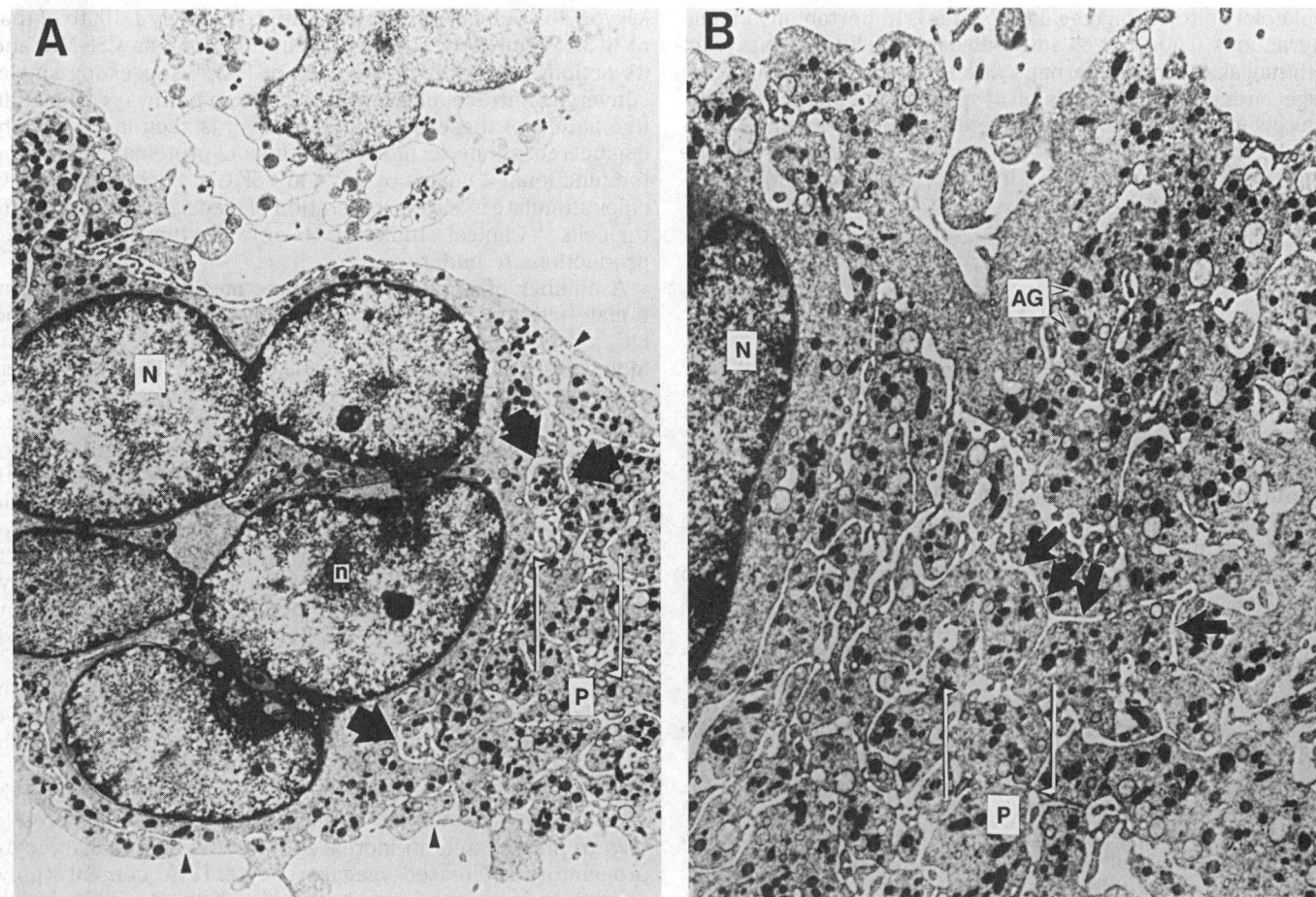

Fig. 19-4. Megakaryocyte Demarcation System (DMS). The DMS is thought to evolve from an invagination and proliferation of the plasma membrane and is involved in platelet formation. **(A & B)** Transmission electron micrographs of two separate stage III/IV human megakaryocytes. P, a platelet field within the megakaryocyte cytoplasm (the distance between the vertical bars is approximately 2 μm); N, nucleus; n, nucleolus; AG, α-granules; arrows, the DMS; arrowheads, opening of the DMS to the extracellular environment. (Figure courtesy of Dr. Maryann Weller.)

demonstrating the marked proliferative potential of these cells.[70] Megakaryocyte CD34$^+$ DR$^-$ burst-forming progenitor cells also express the c-kit receptor (the receptor that interacts with stem cell factor).[71] It should be realized, however, that the progression of cells through a differentiation sequence results in a spectrum of phenotypes (immunologic, morphologic, or otherwise) and that cells do not exist as "compartments." While most of a given cell type may express (or lack) a given antigen, this does not mean that antigenic expression is phenotypically exclusive.

Platelet glycoprotein IIb/IIIa (CD41) is another important marker of the megakaryocyte lineage. This antigenic structure results from the interaction of two gene products (glycoproteins IIb and IIIa) on the surface of cells and is expressed on cells of this lineage from the progenitor cells through the platelets.[49,50,72] Co-expression studies demonstrate that CD41$^+$ cells represent approximately 2% of the CD34$^+$ cells subpopulation (i.e., 0.06% of total nucleated bone marrow cells). This number is consistent with the frequency of the assayable megakaryocyte progenitor cells in human bone marrow.

Studies of human PMkB by Vainchenker and co-workers[60] show that these cells also express CD34. Three antigenically distinct subpopulations of human PMkB can be identified based on the co-expression of CD34 and platelet glycoprotein IIIa (i.e., CD34$^+$ IIIa$^-$, CD34$^+$ IIIa$^+$, and CD34$^-$ IIIa$^+$). These cells are thus transitional in antigenic expression, being the point

at which megakaryocytes alter expression CD34 and begin to express platelet glycoprotein IIIa. Based on proliferative capacity and granular content, the CD34$^-$ IIIa$^+$ are the most mature, having a high granular content and a low proliferative potential. The CD34$^+$ IIIa$^+$ cells are intermediate, and the CD34$^+$ IIIa$^-$ the most primitive, having a higher proliferative capacity and giving rise to more polyploid progeny. Nonetheless, the overall proliferative capacity of the PMkB remains low, since only 10% of these double-positive cells are capable of forming megakaryocyte colonies.[60] These studies show that CD34 is still expressed on the (polyploid) transitional PMkB and suggest that CD34 expression occurs in those cells capable of some degree of DNA synthesis (mitosis or endomitosis). Also, platelet glycoprotein IIIa is present on both PMkB and those megakaryocyte progenitor cells that exhibit a low proliferative capacity.

Immunophenotypic analysis demonstrates that despite limited (if any) expression of CD34 by mature megakaryocytes, they do express multiple markers associated with the platelet lineage (i.e., platelet factor 4 [PF4], platelet glycoprotein IIb/IIIa, vWF, thrombospondin, and thrombomodulin) but are heterogeneous for the degree of expression of these antigens. The functional significance of such antigenic heterogeneity among the various subpopulations of mature megakaryocytes remains unresolved. Although the exact function of platelet antigen heterogeneity on megakaryocytes is unknown, it may be clinically relevant. For example, Stahl et al.[73] have shown that expression of platelet epitopes on megakaryocytes is important in immune interactions. Thus, not all antibodies to platelet antigens react with megakaryocytes, perhaps due to lack of exposure of the target antigen. Also, expression of specific (but undefined) antigens occurs in megakaryocyte progenitor cells.[74] Such antigens may be the targets of antibodies that lead to certain autoimmune disorders, such as acquired amegakaryocytic thrombocytopenias.[75]

Cytokines

The ability to assay megakaryocyte progenitor cells in vitro goes hand in hand with the ability to identify growth factors important to megakaryocyte development. In 1969, an elegant study by Harker and Finch[1] demonstrated that, in vivo, thrombocytopoiesis is regulated by alterations in both megakaryocyte number and megakaryocyte volume (mass). During the late 1970s and early 1980s, investigators struggling with crude sources of megakaryocyte growth factors (conditioned medium from various tissues or cell lines) discovered the in vitro correlates of the Harker-Finch hypothesis: that distinct factors (bioactivites) seem to regulate the proliferative and maturational events occurring during in vitro megakaryocyte development.[37,52,76–79] The purification of these activities proved difficult, but the rapid identification and cloning of numerous human recombinant hematopoietic growth factors during the mid- to late 1980s and early 1990s markedly improved our understanding of the cytokine control of megakaryopoiesis.

A number of cytokines affect megakaryocyte proliferation in vitro, raising the questions of growth factor redundancy and combinatorial control. Given the importance of hematopoiesis, it is not surprising that each of the lineages is controlled by redundant mechanisms. The concept of combinatorial control is illustrated by studies in which multiple cytokines provide a better (in vitro) stimulus than do single growth factors. Studies in which purified progenitor cells are cultured in defined serum-free media demonstrate that as many as two to seven recombinant hematopoietic growth factors have additive proliferative effects on megakaryocyte progenitor cell proliferation.[36,37,80]

Among the many possible cytokine combinations, the most physiologically relevant class of interactions are growth factor combinations that are synergistic (i.e., pharmacologically nonadditive). This type of control is biologically important, as synergistic responses strongly suggest that differing intracellular signal transduction pathways are co-activated, leading to dramatic and rapid increases in proliferation. This has been clearly demonstrated in other developmental systems and for murine as well as human megakaryocytopoiesis.[20,37,81,82] Furthermore, the identification of such synergistic control mechanisms in vitro point to possibly more effective forms of therapeutic intervention in platelet disorders.

Of the hematopoietic growth factors that affect megakaryocytes proliferation, IL-3 (a 17–30 kd glycoprotein) is the most potent.[23,24,83] It stimulates each of the three classes of megakaryocyte progenitor cells, the immature cells, as well as the mature megakaryocytes. However, the physiologic role of IL-3 is unknown. Exogenous IL-3 stimulates in vivo expansion of megakaryocyte progenitor cells, but by itself IL-3 has little (significant) effect on platelet production.[84] Moreover, IL-3 is only produced by antigen-activated T lymphocytes, suggesting a minimal role in maintaining basal hematopoiesis or platelet production.

Another pleiotropic cytokine affecting megakaryocyte development is CSF-GM, a glycoprotein of approximately 23 kd. CSF-GM stimulates development of BFU-Mk and CFU-Mk. However, parallel cell culture experiments demonstrate that its mega-

karyocyte-stimulatory activity is approximately 1/100th of that of IL-3.[83] Nonetheless, this protein functions as CSF-Mk, and its actions are additive to those of IL-3,[36] suggesting single, converging intracellular mitotic signalling pathways. The additive nature of these two cytokines also is seen in genetically engineered chimeric molecules (fusion proteins) containing the functional domains of IL-3 and CSF-GM. Such hybrid molecules stimulate in vitro proliferation of megakaryocyte progenitor cells.[71] Clinical studies of its role in stimulating platelet production are under way.

A number of growth factors have megakaryocyte maturational activities (e.g., IL-6, IL-3, IL-1α, IL-11, CSF-G, and LIF).[24–27,85–90] While none of these purified and/or recombinant molecules is megakaryocyte lineage specific, some are synergistic co-regulators. Such auxiliary growth factors were first defined in vitro as cytokines that lack the solutary ability to simulate megakaryocyte proliferation, but do function as co-regulators to augment megakaryocyte size, DNA content, antigen expression and other factors.[24,37,91] Of the hematopoietic growth factors identified, only a few fall into this category: c-kit ligand (stem cell factor), IL-1α, IL-6, and IL-11.[24,26,89,92] Each of these growth factors is capable of augmenting the megakaryocytic activity of other growth factors, such as IL-3, albeit at differing developmental levels. For example, IL-1, c-kit ligand, and IL-11 each interact with IL-3 at the level of BFU-Mk,[24] whereas IL-6 and c-kit ligand each synergize with IL-3 to modulate CFU-Mk development.[92] IL-11 has multiple effects on in vivo and in vitro megakaryocytopoiesis.[27,28] It not only affects IL-3-dependent megakaryocyte colony formation but also has a potent effect on megakaryocyte maturation. Neben et al.[93] showed that recombinant human IL-11 when administered in vivo to mice results in increased numbers of megakaryocyte progenitors, increased megakaryocyte DNA content (polyploidy), and increased peripheral platelet counts. Phase I trials of this growth factor in humans are ongoing. Finally, a number of animal and preclinical trials have shown that some of these cytokines (e.g., IL-3, IL-6, IL-1, IL-11, LIF) have platelet stimulatory affects in vivo.[87,93–98]

Recently, megakaryocytes and platelets were shown to express basic fibroblast growth factor (bFGF), a potent modulator of hematopoiesis.[99,100] bFGF stimulates adherent stromal cells in human long-term bone marrow cultures, thereby promoting hematopoietic cell development.[101,102] bFGF is deposited in a complex with heparan sulfate proteoglycans within the ECM and is also found on the cell surface of stromal cells.[101,102] Bikfalvi et al.[99] reported the presence of bFGF receptor mRNA in human leukemic cell lines that express megakaryocyte properties, in normal megakaryocytes, and in platelets. bFGF also appears to affect human megakaryocytopoiesis by directly promoting progenitor cell proliferation, as well as stimulating marrow accessory cells to release an unknown megakaryocyte growth factor(s).[103] Thus, bFGF is probably a component of megakaryocyte microenvironment that may play an important role in the control of human megakaryocytopoiesis.

The most notable of the megakaryocyte maturational promoters is IL-6. This cytokine stimulates megakaryocyte maturation, and its actions are (partially) additive to those of IL-3.[80,87,88] Although in vivo IL-6 stimulates platelet production (and speeds recovery from thrombocytopenia in animals), its actions may be via the secondary activation of accessory (stromal) cells.[92,95] From a clinical perspective, however, the mechanism of therapeutic manipulation of platelet levels is immaterial, and the possible two- to four-fold increase in platelets resulting from IL-6 therapy[94–98] may be therapeutically useful. The efficacy of IL-6 remains to be seen, as its other functions (it is an inflammatory cytokine) suggest that side effects may limit its clinical value.

It should be understood that IL-6 is not thrombopoietin

(TPO). While TPO is addressed in more detail below, its lack of relationship to IL-6 has been demonstrated in a number of studies. Recently, a carefully controlled study by Hill et al.[104] indicated that IL-6 levels are essentially unchanged after the induction of acute, severe thrombocytopenia in animals. Underscoring this experimental observation, three prospective studies of patients with platelet disorders demonstrated that IL-6 is elevated only in patients with reactive, but not primary, thrombocytosis.[105–107] Studies conducted by Straneva et al.[106] and Hollen et al.[107] also show that 80–90% of the patients with increased IL-6 had definitive ongoing inflammatory processes. Furthermore, no observations were made of a reciprocal correlation relationship between IL-6 levels and platelet count.[104,105,107] Taken as a whole, these data demonstrate that IL-6 is unlikely to be thrombopoietin. Increased levels of IL-6 may account, however, for the secondary thrombocytosis seen in some patients with inflammation.

TPO is a (putative) lineage-specific regulator of platelet production. Classically defined as an *activity* in the plasma of thrombocytopenic animals or humans, when transferred to a secondary recipient, it stimulates platelet production (as monitored by radiolabeled amino acid incorporation).[108–110] To date, TPO has not been purified to homogeneity, nor has the gene for this protein been cloned. A number of studies with partially purified TPO or TPO-like activities demonstrate that, in vitro, this activity mimics most of the known in vivo responses of megakaryocyte to thrombopoietic demand. These changes include increased megakaryocyte size, DNA content, cytoplasmic content, morphologic maturation status, and antigen or enzyme expression.[37,82,111–113] A number of other regulators are also proposed as lineage-specific modulators of megakaryocytopoiesis (e.g., megakaryocyte stimulatory factor, thrombopoietic stimulator factor, megakaryocyte maturation promoting activity).[114–116] The lack of purification or molecular cloning of a TPO protein/gene is notable, given the numerous academic and commercial laboratories attempting this task. The absence of definitive information on the existence or molecular structure of a TPO gene, coupled with the pleiotropic and overlapping nature of most hematopoietic growth factors, suggests that the *activity* known as TPO may actually be a group of interacting cytokines.

An alternative, and perhaps more likely, explanation for the lack of isolation of TPO is that it is the ligand for a rare and, thus, poorly understood, member of a receptor family (i.e., an orphan receptor). Recently, Vignon and colleagues[116a,b] cloned the human and murine homologues of the v-*mpl* oncogene that is transduced by the myeloproliferative leukemia virus. The c-*mpl* gene encodes a protein with strong homologies to the highly conserved hematopoietin receptor superfamily, and is expressed in low levels in cells of hematopoietic origin.[116b] As it pertains to thrombocytopoiesis, Mothia et al.[116c] used reverse-transcriptase-based PCR studies to demonstrate c-*mpl* expression in CD34+ cells, megakaryocytes, and platelets. As well, they showed that antisense c-*mpl* oligonucleotides specifically inhibited in vitro megakaryocyte colony formation. These data clearly show a role for this receptor in megakaryocytopoiesis, and further suggest that the as yet unidentified mpl ligand may be the elusive TPO.

Finally, a number of cytokines can inhibit megakaryocytopoiesis. Platelets release specific and general inhibitors of megakaryocytopoiesis, such as TGF-β,[117–119] PF4,[120,121] and a low-molecular weight protein known as platelet-released glycoprotein, all of which inhibit megakaryocyte development. However, the physiologic role for platelet-derived inhibitors is unclear. Theoretically, one would hypothesize that increased platelet destruction would stimulate (rather than inhibit) platelet production, raising the paradoxical situation of increasing

inhibitors with increased platelet destruction. Other inhibitors, such as the interferons, also inhibit megakaryocyte development.[123,124] Again, the mechanism of action is unknown.

Extracellular Influences and Cell Interactions

The cellular concentration of bone marrow is roughly 10^9 cells/ml. This suggests that blood cells develop within the context of their interactions with neighboring cells and extracellular molecules. Within the past decade, a number of investigations demonstrated that stromal cells and ECM are dynamic and inductive (or permissive) components of all developing cells systems.[4,5,125] With respect to hematopoiesis, numerous studies have shown that hematopoietic progenitor cells interact with growth factors, accessory cells such as T cells, stromal cells, and ECM components.[126,127] This developmental network is further complicated by observations that stromal cells express membrane-associated growth factors[128,129] and that ECM both binds hematopoietic growth factors and presents these cytokines in a biologically functional manner.[130,131]

Both cell-cell and cell-ECM communications among development megakaryocytes are poorly understood. Structurally, mature (platelet-shedding) megakaryocytes are located on the abluminal surface of the bone marrow sinusoid. It is postulated that megakaryocytes extend pseudopods through or between sinusoidal endothelial cells, thus allowing sheer forces to fragment platelets into the circulation.[65] Both the location and putative mechanism of platelet shedding imply that megakaryocyte-ECM or megakaryocyte-(endothelial) cell interactions are important to thrombocytopoiesis. Isolated megakaryocytes adhere to (bovine corneal endothelial) cell-derived ECM and proplatelet-like structures are induced under these conditions.[10,12] In addition, megakaryocytes adhere to collagen and secrete both a collagenase and a gelatinase,[9,12] suggesting a possible mechanism for pseudopod infiltration of the surrounding ECM.

Studies of megakaryocyte progenitor cells show that cell-ECM relationships are important to megakaryocyte proliferation. Approximately 30% of CFU-Mk cells in bone marrow adhere to the ECM proteins fibronectin or thrombospondin.[132] Interestingly, 60–80% of primitive CD34+ HLD-DR− BFC-Mk attach to thrombospondin, whereas they fail to bind to fibronectin.[8] Therefore, primitive megakaryocyte progenitor cells show both altered expression of cytoadhesion molecule attachment and altered responsiveness to complex matrix-cytokine regulatory signals.

MOLECULAR AND BIOCHEMICAL CONTROL OF MEGAKARYOCYTE COMMITMENT AND DIFFERENTIATION

Transcriptional Control of Megakaryocyte Gene Expression

One of the fundamental goals of molecular hematology is the identification of specific genes, or sets of genes, that direct the activation of lineage-specific differentiation events. A related and equally important aim is to identify the specific nuclear proteins (transcription factors) involved in the (trans-) activation of such master control genes. The activation of lineage-specific gene expression during the commitment of multi- or pluripotential progenitor cells requires a great deal of transcriptional specificity, which is complicated by the observation that DNA-binding transcription factors recognize short (6–8 basepair [bp]) DNA sequences.[133] For example, cis-acting DNA regulatory sequences recognized by factors involved in transcription include TATA, which binds transcription factor IID; CCAAT, found in many gene promotor regions; and GATA, a regulatory element observed in genes of hematopoietic, endothelial, and neural cells.[133]

To date, the nature of lineage master control genes remains obscure. Nonetheless, a number of cis-regulatory elements have been identified, and their regulatory motifs are found in the control regions of specific genes. Of these, the GATA motif is an important control element for erythroid and, perhaps, megakaryocyte development.[133] The GATA sequence was first observed in the promotor region of chicken globin genes,[134] and later in the enhancer region of the human β-globin gene.[135] In fact, all currently identified erythroid genes contain GATA sequences within their control regions.[133] In addition, the core regions of the locus control region of the human β- and α-globin gene clusters contain GATA sequences.[133] A family of nuclear DNA-binding proteins interacts with GATA sequences. GATA-1 (also known as NF-E1, GF-1, eryf-1) was the first such protein identified and is an abundant nuclear protein in erythroid cells and megakaryocytes.[136,137] GATA-2 and GATA-3 were subsequently identified by molecular cloning techniques.[133,138] GATA-1 is a 413-amino acid 50-kd polypeptide containing two highly conserved zinc finger regions both of which are necessary and sufficient for DNA binding. In hematopoietic tissue, expression of GATA-1 is observed in the erythroid, megakaryocyte, and mast cell lineages.[136] GATA-2 is present in megakaryocytes and mast cells,[133] and GATA-3 expression is restricted to T cells, being found in the enhancer region of the T-cell receptor α-gene.[139] Interestingly, GATA-1 expression is detectable in CD34+ CD38+ bone marrow cells, but not in the more primitive CD34+ CD38− cells, suggesting a role for GATA-1 in the function of more differentiated progenitor cells.[140]

GATA-binding proteins are observed in various tissues or cell lines, but the mere presence of a transcriptional factor does not define its role in lineage-specific gene expression or hematopoietic differentiation.[133] The function of such transcription factors is best examined in transgenic animals in which the gene of interest is rendered inoperative. This has been achieved for GATA-1 by Pevny et al.,[141] who disrupted the GATA-1 gene in embryonic stem cells by homologous recombination. The resultant "knock-out" cells were analyzed both in vitro and in vivo. In vitro differentiation of GATA-1-deficient embryonic stem cells failed to generate erythroid cells. Confirming its role in erythropoiesis, the inoperative transgene also failed to contribute to hematopoiesis in transgenic animals. GATA-1-deficient mice either died in utero or had severe anemia. Importantly, these animals sustained white blood cell production and generated clonogenic myeloid progenitor cells,[141] indicating that GATA-1 had a predominant role in erythroid differentiation. However, because platelet counts were not reported as being altered, the function of GATA-1 in megakaryocyte development is not obvious.

While the role of GATA-1 (or GATA-2) in megakaryocytopoiesis remains to be resolved, a number of megakaryocyte/platelet specific genes (thrombomodulin, PF4, platelet glycoprotein IIb, platelet glycoprotein IX) have GATA sequences in their promotor regions,[142–144] as do megakaryocytes and megakaryocyte cell lines.[133] A recent study indicated that transfection and 50-fold over expression of GATA-1 in a murine myeloid cell line restored some of its (previously) lost megakaryocyte potential.[145] Cells expressing high levels of GATA-1 (again) acquired some, but not all, of the appropriate megakaryocyte characteristics. For example, consistent with the presence of GATA sequences in its promotor, PF4 levels were increased, as was the level of acetylcholinesterase (a marker for megakaryocytes in certain rodents and cats). Likewise, a limited number (20–40%) of GATA-transfected cells increase their cell size and volume. In most of these cells, the volume increase was modest, but a small number (3–8%) became both large and polyploid. However, the degree of polyploidy appeared to be limited to 8C.[145] These studies suggest that GATA-1 is important to certain aspects of megakaryocyte differentiation, but its presence (even in 50-fold excess) is insufficient to drive full megakaryocyte differentiation. Perhaps GATA-1 itself is down stream of specific lineage commitment genes. Alternatively, other cis-regulating sequences may confer specificity control. For example, platelet glycoprotein IIb is specifically expressed in cells of the megakaryocyte lineage.[146] It contains both GATA and the *ets* sequences in its 5′-untranslated region; mutations in both regions markedly decrease promotor activity without altering tissue expression, suggesting that tissue specificity is controlled elsewhere.[147] Corroborating this possibility, two other control regions in the 5′-untranslated region of IIb gene interact with proteins present only in megakaryocytes, and deletion of these domains significantly decrease IIb promotor activity.[146] Thus, other proteins are involved in transcriptional control of megakaryocyte-specific genes, and multiple transcription factors may be required for full differentiation.

Megakaryocyte Cell Cycle Control and Endomitosis

Unlike other cells, megakaryocytes continue to synthesis DNA during differentiation. During this process, megakaryocytes become polyploid,[148–150] having a DNA content of 8C–128C, where 2C is the DNA content of a somatic cell. Megakaryocytes are not multinucleate cells but contain this increased DNA content within a single, albeit highly lobulated, nucleus.[151,152] Using tritiated thymidine incorporation, Ebbe and Stohlman[153] and Feinendegen et al.[154] demonstrated that mature (stage II and III) megakaryocytes do not take up this label, demonstrating that they are not undergoing DNA synthesis.[153,154] Stage I megakaryocytes are the only recognizable cells capable of synthesizing DNA, but only 20–40% of these cells do so. With a prolonged exposure to tritiated thymidine, 100% of the megakaryocytes become labeled, indicating that DNA synthesis takes place primarily in the immediate precursor of the megakaryoblast (i.e., the PMkB). The cell cycle of megakaryocytes, is therefore different from other cells, in that the normal 2C → 4C → 2C cell cycle progression is abolished. However, this release from normal cell-cycle control does not imply that megakaryocyte DNA synthesis is dysregulated. The acquisition of a polyploid nucleus is tightly or globallly controlled, as megakaryocytes show progressive doublings of their DNA content, and no intermediate ploidy classes (e.g., 3C, 6C) are seen.

Two observations indicate that formation of a polyploid nucleus requires alterations in the megakaryocyte cell cycle: (1) the immediate precursors of the stage I megakaryocytes (i.e., the promegakaryoblasts) actively synthesize DNA, for a prolonged period[153,154]; and (2) megakaryoblasts do not undergo the usual processes of mitosis, as few if any cells reach metaphase and none progress into anaphase or telophase. As important as these historical observations are, they are based on either morphologic evidence or the analysis of a limited number of megakaryocytes. Indeed, the term generally applied to this type of polyploidization—endomitosis—is a morphologic classification. The definition of endomitosis refers to the replication of nuclear elements within an intact nuclear envelop without subsequent chromosomal movement or cytokinesis.[155] This term is best used to describe megakaryocyte polyploidization.[151] Frequently, the term endoreduplication is erroneously applied to megakaryocytes. Endoreduplication is the mechanism that results in polytenic (diplo- and quatro- chromosome number) cells in insects and is a chromosome duplication cycle not associated with endomitotic-like changes.[155]

Given that the polyploid nature of megakaryocytes is unique among mammalian bone marrow cells, the question arises as to the biologic significance of this altered DNA content. A related question is whether polyploidization occurs as a prerequisite to, or a consequence of, the increase megakaryocyte in cell volume that occurs within these cells. It is known that megakaryocyte DNA content is related to megakaryocyte cell size and thus to the eventual numbers of platelets produced.[151,156] A number of studies have documented the stimulatory actions of partially purified thrombopoietin or other cytokines or megakaryocyte DNA content both in vivo and in vitro.[35,113,157,158] For example, acute thrombocytopenia results in an increased DNA content prior to increased platelet production.[151] Likewise, increases in cytoplasmic volume and cytoplasmic maturation occur predominantly, if not completely, in stage II and III megakaryocytes,[151,156] which do not appear to synthesize DNA. Therefore, whatever its functional significance, polyploidization precedes the increase in megakaryocyte cell volume. This association of increased DNA content and increased cell volume implies that the large DNA content in megakaryocytes is in some unknown manner relevant to the process of platelet formation. For example, increased DNA content may be associated with increased mRNA expression which, in turn, drives the marked degree of biosynthesis required for platelet formation. While this remains to be proven, it is clear that megakaryocytes synthesize increased amounts of DNA prior to increases in cytoplasmic volume and cytoplasmic maturation.

It is now recognized that two classes, or families, of proteins control cell cycle in mammalian cells. These are the cell division kinases (also known as cyclin-dependent kinases, [CDK]), and the cyclins, so named for their cyclical synthesis and degradation. Together, these two classes of proteins form a protein-kinase complex in which the catalytic unit is a CDK, and the regulatory unit is a cyclin. These proteins are highly conserved[159,160] and are important at two points of the cell cycle: the regulation of G_1/S transit,[161,162] and mitosis.[163] The role of these kinase complexes in cell-cycle control is complex. Currently, there are five members of the cyclin gene family,[164,165] as well as at least seven distinct CDK genes.[166] The role of the kinase known as cdc2, and its cognate cyclin (B) is best understood. Together these proteins form a mitosis-initiating cdc2 kinase complex, also known as maturation (or mitosis) promoting factor. The cdc2/cyclin B kinase complex regulates the initiation of mitosis at the G_2/M transition as well as subsequent events, such as spindle fiber formation and cytokinesis.[164] Regarding the regulation of the early phases of the cell cycle, other cyclins (e.g., cyclin A) appear to complex not only with cdc2 but other cell cycle kinases (e.g., cdk2) to regulate both G_1/S transition and subsequent S-phase events.[164,167,168]

The role of CDK and cyclin proteins in megakaryocyte endomitosis is unknown. Currently, a number of laboratories are examining these proteins, but definitive studies have not been published. Nonetheless, a general hypothesis can be put forward concerning the biochemical control of endomitosis. Not surprisingly, megakaryocytes show demonstrable alterations at the two control (or restriction) points evident in all cycling cells. They have a prolonged S-phase period and synthesize increased amounts of DNA (i.e., they are altered in G_1 or S phase); they also undergo an abrogation of mitosis (M phase). Interestingly, in normal cells, the cdc2/cyclin B complex kinase activity peaks in early metaphase.[169] This is just the point at which megakaryocytes fail to progress through mitosis. Moreover, recent observations demonstrate that stabilizing mutations of the cyclin B gene (e.g., the loss of its N-terminal domain) results in persistence of this protein, and its sustained presence leads to mitotic arrest.[170–172] Preliminary biochemi-

cal studies in a human megakaryocyte cell line show that induction of endomitotosis is associated with elevated and sustained levels of cyclin B (MWL, personal communication). Therefore, one aspect of megakaryocyte endomitosis may be the generation of a uninucleate cell as a result of biochemical modulation of the mitosis-promoting cdc2/cyclin B kinase complex. Clearly, the overall regulation of endomitosis is much more complicated. For example, it is not clear whether the changes in cyclin B abundance are either necessary or sufficient to induce endomitosis, nor have the multiple events regulating the increased DNA content of megakaryocytes been examined.

SUMMARY

Our increased understanding of the cellular and molecular basis of megakaryocytopoiesis has had an immediate impact on clinical medicine. Numerous megakaryocyte dyscrasias result in abnormal platelet production, such as amegakaryocytic thrombocytopenia, thrombocytopenia with absent radii, and essential thrombocythemia. While the molecular and biochemical basis of these disorders remains unknown, a number of preliminary studies have documented alterations in the frequency of megakaryocyte colony-forming cells in these conditions.[173–176] Amegakaryocytic thrombocytopenia is associated with increased levels of circulating regulatory factors,[75,77] and myeloproliferative disorders have been described in which patients have increased megakaryocytes and thrombocytosis presumably due to altered cellular defects.[1] The myelofibrosis that characterizes agnogenic myeloid metaplasia is perhaps due to mitogenic factors released from abnormal megakaryocytes that stimulate fibroblast proliferation and ECM deposition.[177] Interestingly, neoplastic disorders of the megakaryocyte lineage are rare, and those observed are variants of acute or chronic myelocytic leukemia in which blast cells express some megakaryocyte antigenic determinants.[178] Neoplastic proliferation of mature megakaryocytes has not been observed, perhaps because of the endomitotic nature of these cells.

Effective control of platelet production requires examination of both normal and abnormal megakaryocyte development at the biomolecular level. This requires that the interacting ECM-cytokine complexes that regulate platelet production be defined. Similarly, the megakaryocytic signal transduction pathways activated by these thrombopoietic signals must be understood. Ultimately, the understanding of megakaryocyte development requires the identification of those genes that regulate megakaryocyte commitment and differentiation. These requirements not withstanding, current clinical trails of single hematopoietic growth factors (e.g., c-kit ligand), as well as hematopoietic growth factor combinations (e.g., IL-3 plus IL-6, or IL-11),[93,96–98,124] will likely result in the development of an effective strategy for the therapeutic manipulation of thrombocytopoiesis.

REFERENCES

1. Harker LA, Finch CA: Thrombokinetics in man. J Clin Invest 48:963, 1969
2. Gordon M, Hoffman R: Growth factors affecting human thrombocytopoiesis: potential agents for the treatment of thrombocytopenia. Blood 80:302, 1992
3. Wicha MS, Lowrie G, Kohn E et al: Extracellular matrix promotes mammary epithelial growth and differentiation in vitro. Proc Natl Acad Sci USA 79:3213, 1982
4. Gospodarowicz D, Ill C: Extracellular matrix and control of proliferation of vascular endothelial cells. J Clin Invest 65:1351, 1980
5. Gospodarowicz D, Delagado D, Vlodavsky I: Permissive effect of the extracellular matrix on cell proliferation in vitro. Proc Natl Acad Sci USA 77:4094, 1980

6. Zuckerman KS, Wicha MS: Extracellular matrix production by the adherent cells of long-term murine bone marrow cultures. Blood 61:540, 1983

7. Campbell A, Wicha MS, Long MW: Extracellular matrix promotes the growth and differentiation of murine hematopoietic cells in vitro. J Clin Invest 75:2085, 1985

8. Long MW, Briddell R, Walter AW et al: Human hematopoietic stem cell adherence to cytokines and matrix molecules. J Clin Invest 90:251, 1992

9. Leven RM, Yee T: Collagenase production by guinea pig megakaryocytes in vitro. Exp Hematol 18:743, 1990

10. Eldor A, Fuks Z, Levine RF, Vlodavsky I: Measurement of platelet and megakaryocyte interaction with the subendothelial extracellular matrix. Methods Enzymol 169:76, 1989

11. Kelm RJ Jr, Hair GA, Mann KG, Grant BW: Characterization of human osteoblast and megakaryocyte-derived osteonectin (SPARC). Blood 80:3112, 1992

12. Tablin F, Castro M, Leven RM: Blood platelet formation in vitro. The role of the cytoskeleton in megakaryocyte fragmentation. J Cell Sci 97:59, 1990

13. Hansen M, Pedersen NT: Circulating megakaryocytes in patients with pulmonary inflammation and in patients subjected to cholecystectomy. Scand J Haematol 23:211, 1979

14. Berridge MV, Fraser JK, Carter JM, Lin F-K: Effects of recombinant human erythropoietin on megakaryocytes and on platelet production in the rat. Blood 72:970, 1988

15. Zauli G, Vitale L, Brunelli MA, Bagnara GP: Prevalence of the primitive megakaryocyte progenitors (BFU-meg) in adult human peripheral blood. Exp Hematol 20:850, 1992

16. Ihzumi T, Hattori A, Sanada M, Muto M: Megakaryocyte and platelet formation: a scanning electron microscope study in mouse spleen. Arch Histol Jpn 40:305, 1977

17. Grouls V, Helpap B: Megakaryocytopoiesis in the spleen of growing rats. Am J Anat 157:429, 1980

18. Kaufman KM, Ario R, Pollack S et al: Origin of pulmonary megakaryocytes. Blood 25:767, 1965

19. Thiery JP, Bessis M: Mécanisme de la plaquettogénèse. Etude in vitro par la microcinématographie. Rev Hematol 11:162, 1956

20. Long MW, Heffner CH, Gragowski LL: Cholera toxin and phorbol diesters synergistically modulate murine hematopoietic progenitor cell proliferation. Exp Hematol 16:195, 1988

21. Long MW: Signal transduction events in in vitro megakaryocytopoiesis. Blood Cells 15:205, 1989

22. Long MW, Gragowski LL, Heffner CH, Boxer LA: Phorbol diesters stimulate the development of an early murine progenitor cell. The burst-forming unit-megakaryocyte. J Clin Invest 67:431, 1985

23. Briddell RA, Brandt JE, Straneva JE et al: Characterization of the human burst-forming unit-megakaryocyte. Blood 74:145, 1989

24. Briddell RA, Hoffman R: Cytokine regulation of the human burst-forming unit-megakaryocyte. Blood 76:516, 1990

25. Briddell RA, Bruno E, Cooper RJ et al: Effect of c-kit ligand on in vitro human megakaryocytopoiesis. Blood 78:2854, 1991

26. Bruno E, Briddell RA, Cooper RJ, Hoffman R: Effects of recombinant interleukin 11 on human megakaryocyte progenitor cells. Exp Hematol 19:378, 1991

27. Teramura M, Kabayashi S, Hoshiro S et al: Interleuken-11 enhances human megakaryocytoporens in vitro. Blood 32:791, 1992

28. Avraham H, Scadden DT, Chi S et al: Interaction of human bone marrow fibroblasts with megakaryocytes role of c-kit ligand. Blood 80:1679, 1992

29. Nakeff A, Dicke KA, van Noord MJ: Megakaryocytes in agar cultures of mouse bone marrow. Semin Haemat 8:4, 1975

30. Metcalf D, MacDonald HR, Odartchenko N, Sordat B: Growth of mouse megakaryocyte colonies in vitro. Proc Natl Acad Sci USA 72:1744, 1975

31. McLeod DL, Shreeve MM, Axelrad AA: Induction of megakaryocyte colonies with platelet formation in vitro. Nature 261:492, 1976

32. Bradley TR, Metcalf D: The growth of mouse bone marrow cells in vitro. Aust J Exp Biol Med Sci 44:287, 1966

33. Fauser AA, Messner HA: Identification of megakaryocytes, macrophages, and eosinophils in colonies of human bone marrow containing neutrophilic granulocytes and erythroblasts. Blood 53:1023, 1979

34. Vainchenker W, Bougeut J, Guichard J, Breton-Gorius J: Megakaryocyte colony formation from human bone marrow precursors. Blood 54:940, 1979

35. Williams N, Jackson H: Kinetic analysis of megakaryocyte numbers and ploidy levels in developing colonies from mouse bone marrow cells. Cell Tissue Kinet 15:483, 1982

36. Bruno E, Miller ME, Hoffman R: Interacting cytokines regulate in vitro human megakaryocytopoiesis. Blood 73:671, 1989

37. Long MW, Hutchinson RJ, Gragowski LL et al: Synergistic regulation of human megakaryocyte development. J Clin Invest 82:1779, 1988

38. Burstein SA, Adamson JW, Erb SK, Harker LA: Megakaryocytopoiesis in the mouse: response to varying platelet demand. J Cell Physiol 109:333, 1981

39. Levin J, Levin FC, Metcalf D: The effects of acute thrombocytopenia an megakaryocyte-CFC and granulocyte-macrophage-CFC in mice: studies on bone marrow and spleen. Blood 56:274, 1980

40. Ebbe S, Phalen E: Does autoregulation of megakaryocytopoiesis occur? Blood Cells 5:123, 1979

41. Nicola NA, Johnson GR: The production of committee hemopoietic colony-forming cells from multipotential precursor cells in vitro. Blood 60:1019, 1982

42. Papayannopoulou T, Nakamoto B, Kurachi S et al: Surface antigenic profile and globin phenotype of two new human erythroleukemia cell lines: characterization and interpretation. Blood 72:1029, 1988

43. Papayannopoulou T, Raines E, Collins S et al: Constitutive and inducable secretion of platelet-derived growth factor analogs by human leukemic cell lines coexpressing erythroid and megakaryocytic markers. J Clin Invest 79:859, 1987

44. Long MW, Heffner CH, Williams JL et al: Regulation of megakaryocyte potential in human erythroleukemia cells. J Clin Invest 85:1072, 1990

45. Thean LE, Hodgson GS, Bertoncello I, Radley JM: Characterization of megakaryocyte spleen colony-forming units by response to 5-fluorouracil and by unit gravity sedimentation. Blood 62:896, 1983

46. Stenberg PE, Levin J: Ultrastructural analysis of murine megakaryocyte maturation in vitro: comparison of big-cell and heterogeneous megakaryocyte colonies. Blood 70:1509, 1987

47. Long MW, Williams N: Differences in the regulation of megakaryocytopoiesis in the murine bone marrow and spleen. Leuk Res 6:721, 1982

48. Pizzolo G, Chilosi M, Perona G: The use of anti beta-thromboglobulin serum for the diagnosis of megakaryoblastic leukaemia. Haematologica 67:804, 1982

49. Rabellino EM, Levene RB, Leung LLK, Nachman RL: Human megakaryocytes. II. Expression of platelet proteins in early marrow megakaryocytes. J Exp Med 154:88, 1981

50. Rabellino EM, Nachman RL, Williams N et al: Human megakaryocytes. I. Characterization of the membrane and cytoplasmic components of isolated marrow megakaryocytes. J Exp Med 149:1273, 1979

51. Vainchenker W, Guichard J, Deschamps JF et al: Megakaryocyte cultures in the chronic phase and in the blast crisis of chronic myeloid leukaemia: studies on the differentiation of the megakaryocyte progenitors and on the maturation of megakaryocytes in vitro. Br J Haematol 51:131, 1982

52. Long MW, Williams N, Ebbe S: Immature megakaryocytes in the mouse: physical characteristics, cell cycle status, and in vitro responsiveness to thrombopoietic stimulatory factor. Blood 59:569, 1982

53. Hegyi E, Navarro S, Debili N et al: Regulation of human megakaryocytopoiesis: analysis of proliferation, ploidy and maturation in liquid cultures. Int J Cell Cloning 8:236, 1990

54. Long MW, Williams N, McDonald TP: Immature megakaryocytes in the mouse: in vitro relationship to megakaryocyte progenitor cells and mature megakaryocytes. J Cell Physiol 112:339, 1982

55. Long MW, Henry RL: Thrombocytosis-induced suppression of small acetylcholinesterase positive cells in bone marrow of rats. Blood 54:1339, 1979

56. Jackson CW: Cholinesterase as a possible marker for early cells of the megakaryocytic series. Blood 42:413, 1973

57. Long MW, Williams N: Immature megakaryocytes in the mouse: morphology and quantitation acetylcholinesterase staining. Blood 58:1032, 1981

58. Vainchenker W, Guichard J, Breton-Gorius J: Growth of human megakaryocyte colonies in culture from fetal, neonatal, and adult peripheral blood cells: ultrastructural analysis. Blood Cells 5:25, 1979

59. Breton-Gorius J, Vainchenker W, Nurden A et al: Defective alpha-granule production in megakaryocytes from gray platelet syndrome. Ultrastructural studies of bone marrow cells and megakaryocytes growing in culture from blood precursors. Am J Pathol 102:10, 1981

60. Debili N, Issaad C, Masse JM et al: Expression of CD34 and platelet glycoproteins during human megakaryocytic differentiation. Blood 80:3022, 1992

61. Spaet TH: Platelets: The blood dust. p. 549. In Wintrobe MM (ed): Blood Pure and Eloquent. McGraw-Hill, New York, 1980

62. Wright JH: The origin and nature of the blood plates. Boston Med Surg J 23:643, 1906

63. Wright JH: The histogenesis of blood platelets. J Morphol 21:263, 1906

64. Zajicek J: Studies on the histogenesis of blood platelets. Acta Haemaol 12:238, 1954

65. Zucker-Franklin D, Petursson SR: Thrombocytopoiesis: analysis by membrane tracer and freeze-fracture studies on fresh human and cultured mouse megakaryocytes. J Cell Biol 99:390, 1984

66. Civin CI, Strauss LC, Brovall C et al: Antigenic analysis of hematopoiesis. III. A hematopoietic progenitor cell surface antigen defined by a monoclonal antibody raised against KG-1a cells. J Immunol 133:157, 1984

67. Civin CI, Banquerigo ML, Strauss LC, Loken MR: Antigenic analysis of hema-

topoiesis. VI. Flow cytometric characterization of My-10-positive progenitor cells in normal human bone marrow. Exp Hematol 15:10, 1987

68. Strauss LC, Rowley SD, La Russa VF et al: Antigenic analysis of hematopoiesis. V. Characterization of My-10 antigen expression by normal lymphohematopoietic progenitor cells. Exp Hematol 14:878, 1986

69. Brandt J, Srour EF, van Vesien K et al: Cytokine-dependent long term culture of highly enriched precursors of hematopoietic progenitor cells from human marrow. J Clin Invest 86:932, 1990

70. Briddell RA, Brandt JE, Leemhuis TB, Hoffman R: Role of cytokines in sustaining long-term human megakaryocytopoiesis in vitro. Blood 79:332, 1992

71. Bruno E, Briddell RA, Cooper RJ et al: Recombinant GM-CSF/IL-3 fusion protein: its effect on in vitro human megakaryocytopoiesis. Exp Hematol 20: 494, 1992

72. Levene RB, Lamaziere JMD, Broxmeyer HE et al: Human megakaryocytes. V. Changes in the phenotypic profile of differentiating megakaryocytes. J Exp Med 161:457, 1985

73. Stahl CP, Zucker-Franklin D, McDonald TP: Incomplete antigenic cross-reactivity between platelets and megakaryocytes: relevance to ITP. Blood 67: 421, 1986

74. Jackson H, Rabellino EM, Williams N: A level of differentiation of megakaryocyte progenitors and subsequent modulation of megakaryocyte antigens on developing colony cells. Leukemia 4:490, 1990

75. Hoffman R, Bruno E, Elwell J et al: Acquired amegakaryocytic thrombocytopenic purpura: a syndrome of diverse etiologies. Blood 60:1173, 1982

76. Williams N, Jackson H: Regulation of the proliferation of murine megakaryocyte progenitor cells by cell cycle. Blood 52:163, 1978

77. Hoffman R, Yang HH, Bruno E, Straneva JE: Purification and partial characterization of a megakaryocyte colony-stimulating factor from human plasma. J Clin Invest 75:1174, 1985

78. Straneva JE, Briddell RA, Hui SL, Hoffman R: Serum from patients with various thrombopoietic disorders alters terminal cytoplasmic maturation of human megakaryocytes in vitro. Eur J Haematol 42:293, 1989

79. Gewirtz AM, Bruno E, Elwell J, Hoffman R: In vitro studies of megakaryocytopoiesis in thrombocytotic disorders of man. Blood 61:384, 1983

80. Quesenberry PJ, McGrath HE, Williams ME et al: Multifactor stimulation of megakaryocytopoiesis: effects of interleukin 6. Exp Hematol 19:35, 1991

81. Yoshimasa T, Sibley DR, Bouvier M et al: Cross-talk between cellular signalling pathways suggested by phorbol-ester-induced adenylate cyclase phosphorylation. Nature 327:67, 1987

82. Roth BJ, Sledge GW Jr, Straneva JE et al: Analysis of phorbol ester stimulated human megakaryocyte development. Blood 72:202, 1988

83. Emerson SG, Yang YC, Clark SC, Long MW: Human recombinant granulocyte-macrophage colony stimulating factor and intelleukin 3 have overlapping but distinct activities. J Clin Invest 82:1282, 1988

84. Lindemann A, Ganser A, Herrmann F et al: Biologic effects of recombinant human interleukin-3 in vivo. J Clin Oncol 9:2120, 1991

85. Ishibashi T, Burstein SA: Interleukin 3 promotes the differentiation of isolated single megakaryocytes. Blood 67:1512, 1986

86. Segal GM, Stueve T, Adamson JW: Analysis of murine megakaryocyte colony size and ploidy: effects of interleukin-3. J Cell Physiol 137:537, 1988

87. Stahl CP, Zucker-Franklin D, Evatt BL, Winton EF: Effects of human interleukin-6 on megakaryocyte development and thrombocytopoiesis in primates. Blood 78:1467, 1991

88. Kimura H, Ishibashi T, Uchida T et al: Interleukin 6 is a differentiation factor for human megakaryocytes in vitro. Eur J Immunol 20:1927, 1990

89. Teramura M, Kobayashi S, Hoshino S et al: Interleukin-11 enhances human megakaryocytopoiesis in vitro. Blood 79:327, 1992

90. McNiece IK, McGrath HE, Quesenberry PJ: Granulocyte colony-stimulating factor augments in vitro megakaryocyte colony formation by interleukin-3. Exp Hematol 16:807, 1988

91. Debili N, Hegyi E, Navarro S et al: In vitro effects of hematopoietic growth factors on the proliferation, endoreplication, and maturation of human megakaryocytes. Blood 77:226, 1991

92. Bruno E, Hoffman R: Effect of interleukin 6 on in vitro human megakaryocytopoiesis: its interaction with other cytokines. Exp Hematol 17:1038, 1989

93. Neben TY, Loebelenz J, Hayes L et al: Recombinant human interleukin-11 stimulates megakaryocytopoiesis and increases peripheral platelets in normal and splenectomized mice. Blood 81:901, 1993

94. Geissler K, Valent P, Bettelheim P et al: In vivo synergism of recombinant human interleukin-3 and recombinant human interleukin-6 on thrombopoiesis in primates. Blood 79:1155, 1992

95. Herodin F, Mestries JC, Janodet D et al: Recombinant glycosylated human interleukin-6 accelerates peripheral blood platelet count recovery in radiation-induced bone marrow depression in baboons. Blood 80:688, 1992

96. Weber J, Yang JC, Topalian SL et al: Phase I trial by subcutaneous interleukin 6 in patients with advanced malignancies. J Clin Oncol 11:499, 1993

97. Demetri GD, Samuels B, Gordon M et al: Recombinant human interleukin-6 (IL-6) increases circulating platelet counts and C-reactive protein levels in vitro: initial results as a phase I trial in sarcoma patients with normal hemopoiesis. Blood, suppl 1. 80:88a, 1992

98. Gordon MS, Neumantis J, Hoffman R et al: Phase I trial of subcutaneous (SC) recombinant human interleukin-6 (IL-6) in patients with myelodysplasia (MDS) and thrombocytopenia. Blood, suppl 1. 80:249a, 1992

99. Bikfalvi A, Han C, Fuhrmann G: Interaction of fibroblast growth factor (FGF) with megakaryocytopoiesis and demonstration of FGF receptor expression in megakaryocytes and megakaryocyte-like cells. Blood 80:1905, 1992

100. Brunner G, Nguyen H, Gabrilove JR et al: Basic fibroblast growth factor expression in human bone marrow and peripheral blood cells. Blood 81: 63, 1993

101. Oliver LJ, Rifkin DB, Gabrilove J et al: Long-term culture of human bone marrow stromal cells in the presence of basic fibroblast growth factor. Growth Factors 3:231, 1990

102. Wilson EL, Rifkin DB, Velley F et al: Basic fibroblast growth factor stimulates myelopoiesis in very long term human bone marrow cultures. Blood 77:954, 1991

103. Bruno E, Wilson EL, Cooper RJ et al: Basic fibroblast growth factor promotes the proliferation of human megakaryocyte progenitor cells. Blood 81:1091, 1993

104. Hill RJ, Warren MK, Levin J, Gauldie J: Evidence that interleukin-6 does not play a role in the stimulation of platelet production after induction of acute thrombocytopenia. Blood 80:346, 1992

105. Hollen CW, Henthorn J, Koziol JA, Burstein SA: Serum interleukin-6 levels in patients with thrombocytosis. Leuk Lymphoma 8 235, 1992

106. Straneva JE, van Besien KW, Derigs G, Hoffman R: Is interleukin 6 the physiological regulator of thrombopoiesis? Exp Hematol 20:47, 1992

107. Hollen CW, Henthorn J, Koziol JA, Burstein SA: Elevated serum interleukin-6 levels in patients with reactive thrombocytosis. Br J Haematol 79:286, 1991

108. Spector B: In vivo transfer of a thrombopoietic factor (26874). Proc Soc 108: 146, 1961

109. Odell TT Jr, McDonald TP, Detwilder TC: Stimulation of platelet production by serum of platelet-depleted rats. Proc Soc Exp Biol Med 108:428, 1961

110. Schulman I, Abildgaard CF, Cornet JA et al: Studies on thrombopoiesis. II. Assay of human plasma thrombocytopoietic activity. J Pediatr 66:604, 1965

111. Straneva JE, Goheen MP, Hui SL et al: Terminal cytoplasmic maturation of human megakaryocytes in vitro. Exp Hematol 14:919, 1986

112. Hill RJ, Levin J, Levin FC: Correlation of in vitro and in vivo biological activities during the partial purification of thrombopoietin. Exp Hematol 20:354, 1992

113. Hill RJ, Leven RM, Levin FC, Levin J: The effect of partially purified thrombopoietin on guinea pig megakaryocyte ploidy in vitro. Exp Hematol 17:903, 1989

114. Tayrien G, Rosenberg RD: Purification and properties of a megakaryocyte stimulatory factor present both in the serum-free conditioned medium of human embryonic kidney cells and in thrombocytopenic plasma. J Biol Chem 262:3262, 1987

115. McDonald TP, Nolan C: Partial purification of a thrombocytopoietic-stimulating factor from kidney cell culture medium. Biochem Med 21:146, 1979

116. Grant BW, Nichols WL, Solberg LA et al: Quantitation of human in vitro megakaryocytopoiesis by radioimmunoassay. Blood 69:1334, 1987

116a. Vigon I, Florindo C, Fichelson S et al: Characterization of the murine Mpl proto-oncogene, a member of the hematopoietic cytokine receptor family: molecular cloning, chromosomal location and evidence for a function in cell growth. Oncogene 8:2607, 1993

116b. Vigon I, Momon JP, Cocault L et al: Molecular cloning and characterization of MPL, the human homolog of the v-mpl oncogene: identification of a member of the hematopoietic growth factor receptor superfamily. Proc Natl Acad Sci USA 89:5640, 1992

116c. Mothia N, Louache F, Vainchenker W, Wendling F: Oligodeoxynucleotides antisense to the proto-oncogene c-mpl specifically inhibit in vitro megakaryocytopoiesis. Blood 82:1395, 1993

117. Ishibashi T, Miller SL, Burstein SA: Type beta transforming growth factor is a potent inhibitor of murine megakaryocytopoiesis in vitro. Blood 69: 1737, 1987

118. Kuter DJ, Gminski DM, Rosenberg RB: Transforming growth factor-B inhibits megakaryocyte growth and endomitosis. Blood 79:619, 1992

119. Fava RA, Casey TT, Wilcox J et al: Synthesis of transforming growth factor-B1 by megakaryocytes and its localization to megakaryocytes and platelet alpha granules. Blood 76:1946, 1990

120. Gewirtz AM, Calabretta B, Rucinski B et al: Inhibition of human megakaryocytopoiesis in vitro by platelet factor 4 (PF4) and a synthetic COOH-terminal PF4 peptide. J Clin Invest 83:1477, 1989

121. Han C, Senselbe L, Abgrall JF, Briere J: Platelet factor 4 inhibits human megakaryocytopoiesis in vitro. Blood 75:1234, 1990

122. Dessypris EN, Gleanton JH, Sawyer ST, Armstron OL: Suppression of maturation of megakaryocyte colony forming units in vitro by a platelet glycoprotein. J Cell Physiol 130:361, 1987

123. Griffin CG, Grant BW: Effects of recombinant interferons on human megakaryocyte growth. Exp Hematol 18:1013, 1990

124. Tong J, Gordon MS, Srour EF et al: Effects of the in vivo administration of recombinant methionyl human stem cell factor on human hematopoietic stem cells. Proc Am Assoc Cancer Res 34:1289, 1993

125. Majack RA, Cook SC, Bornstein P: Control of smooth muscle cell growth by components of the extracellular matrix: autocrine role for thrombospondin. Proc Natl Acad Sci USA 83:9050, 1986

126. Springer TA: Adhesion receptors of the immune system. Nature 346:425, 1990

127. Long MW: Blood cell cytoadhesion molecules. Exp Hematol 20:288, 1992

128. Yamazaki K, Roberts RA, Spooncer E et al: Cellular interactions between 3T3 cells and interleukin-3-dependent multipotent haemopoietic cells: a model system for stromal-cell-mediated haemopoiesis. J Cell Physiol 139:301, 1989

129. Anderson DM, Lyman SD, Baird A et al: Molecular cloning of mast cell growth factor, a hematopoietin that is active in both membrane bound and soluble forms. Cell 63:235, 1990

130. Gordon MY, Riley GP, Watt SM, Greaves MF: Compartmentalization of a haematopoietic growth factor (GM-CSF) by glycosaminoglycans in the bone marrow microenvironment. Nature 326:403, 1987

131. Roberts R, Gallagher J, Spooncer E et al: Heparan sulphate bound growth factors: a mechanism for stromal cell mediated haemopoiesis. Nature 332:376, 1988

132. Long MW, Dixit VM: Thrombospondin functions as a cytoadhesion molecule for human hematopoietic progenitor cells. Blood 75:2311, 1990

133. Orkin SH: GATA-binding transcription factors in hematopoietic cells. Blood 80:575, 1992

134. Evans T, Reitman M, Felsenfeld G: An erythrocyte-specific DNA-binding factor recognizes a regulatory sequence common to all chicken globin genes. Proc Natl Acad Sci USA 85:5976, 1988

135. Wall L, deBoer E, Grosveld F: The human beta-globin gene 3′ enhancer contains multiple binding sites for an erythroid-specific protein. Genes Dev 2:1089, 1988

136. Martin DI, Zon LI, Mutter G, Orkin SH: Expression of an erythroid transcription factor in megakaryocytic and mast cell lineages. Nature 344:444, 1990

137. Romeo PH, Prandini MH, Joulin V et al: Megakaryocytic and erythrocytic lineages share specific transcription factors. Nature 344:447, 1990

138. Yamamoto M, Ko LJ, Leonard MW et al: Activity and tissue-specific expression of the transcription factor NF-E1 multigene family. Genes Dev 4:1650, 1990

139. Ho IC, Vorhees P, Marin N et al: Human GATA-3: a lineage-restricted transcription factor that regulates the expression of the T cell receptor alpha gene. EMBO J 10:1187, 1991

140. Mouthon MA, Bernard O, Mitjavila MT et al: Expression of tal-1 and GATA-binding proteins during human hematopoiesis. Blood 81:647, 1993

141. Pevny L, Simon MC, Robertson E et al: Erythroid differentiation in chimaeric mice blocked by a targeted mutation in the gene for transcription factor GATA-1. Nature 349:257, 1991

142. Prandini MH, Uzan G, Martin F et al: Characterization of a specific erythro-megakaryocytic enhancer within the glycoprotein IIb promoter. J Biol Chem 267:10370, 1992

143. Hickey MJ, Roth GJ: Characterization of the gene encoding human platelet glycoprotein IX. J Biol Chem 268:3438, 1993

144. Ravid K, Doi T, Beeler DL et al: Transcriptional regulation of the rat platelet factor 4 gene: interaction between an enhancer/silencer domain and the GATA site. Mol Cell Biol 11:6116, 1991

145. Visvader JE, Elefanty AG, Strasser A, Adams JM: GATA-1 but not SCL induces megakaryocytic differentiation in an early myeloid line. EMBO J 11:4557, 1992

146. Uzan G, Prenant M, Prandini MH et al: Tissue-specific expression of the platelet GPIIb gene. J Biol Chem 266:8932, 1991

147. Lemarchandel V, Ghysdael J, Mignotte V et al: GATA and ets cis-acting sequences mediate megakaryocyte-specific epxression. Mol Cell Biol 13:668, 1993

148. Odell TT, Jackson CW, Friday TJ: Megakaryocytopoiesis in rats with special reference to polyploidy. Blood 35:775, 1970

149. Odell TT Jr, Jackson CW: Polyploidy and maturation of rat megakaryocytes. Blood 32:102, 1968

150. Odell TT Jr, Jackson CW, Gosslee DG: Maturation of rat megakaryocytes studied by microspectrophotometric measurement of DNA. Proc Soc Exp Biol Med 119:1194, 1965

151. Ebbe S: Biology of megakaryocytes. Prog Hemost Thromb 3:211, 1976

152. De Leval M, Paulus JM: Megakaryocytes: uninucleate plurinucleate cells? p. 190. In Paulus JM (ed): Platelet Kinetics. North-Holland, Amsterdam, 1971

153. Ebbe S, Stohlman F Jr: Megakaryocytopoiesis in the rat. Blood 26:20, 1965

154. Feinendegen LE, Odartchenko N, Cottier H, Bond VP: Kinetics of megakaryocyte proliferation. Proc Soc Exp Biol Med 111:177, 1962

155. Therman E, Sarto GE, Stubblefield PA: Endomitosis: a reappraisal. Hum Genet 63:13, 1983

156. Ebbe S, Stohlman F Jr, Overcash J et al: Megakaryocyte size in thrombocytopenic and normal rats. Blood 32:383, 1968

157. Ebbe S, Yee T, Carpenter D, Phalen E: Megakaryocytes increase in size within ploidy groups in response to the stimulus of thrombocytopenia. Exp Hematol 16:55, 1988

158. Kuter D, Rosenberg RD: Regulation of megakaryocyte ploidy in vivo in the rat. Blood 75:74, 1990

159. Riabowol K, Draetta G, Brixuela L et al: The cdc2 kinase is a nuclear protein that is essential for mitosis in mammalian cells. Cell 57:393, 1989

160. Pines J, Hunter T: Isolation of a human cyclin cDNA: Evidence for cyclin mRNA and protein regulation in the cell cycle and for interaction with p34-CDC2. Cell 58:833, 1989

161. Lee M, Nurse P: Cell cycle control genes in fission yeast and mammalian cells. Trends Biochem Sci 4:287, 1988

162. Nurse P, Bisset Y: Gene requires for G1 committment to the cell cycle and in G2 for control of mitosis in fission yeast. Nature 292:558, 1981

163. Arion D, Meijer L, Brizuela L, Beach D: CDC2 is a component of the M phase-specific histon H1 kinase: evidence for identity with MPF. Cell 55:317, 1988

164. Hunter T, Pines J: Cyclins and cancer. Cell 66:1071, 1991

165. Matsushime H, Roussel M, Ashmun R, Sherr C: Colony-stimulating factor 1 regulates novel cyclins during the G1 phase of the cell cycle. Cell 65:701, 1991

166. Meyerson M, Enders GH, Wu C-L et al: A family of human cdc2-related protein kinases. EMBO J 11:2909, 1992

167. Girard F, Strausfeld U, Fernandez A, Lamb NJ: Cyclin A is required for the onset of DNA replication in mammalian fibroblasts. Cell 67:1169, 1991

168. Mudryl M, Devoto SH, Hiebert SW et al: Cell cycle regulation of the E2F transcription factor involves an interaction with cyclin A. Cell 65:1243, 1991

169. Draetta G, Beach D: Activation of cdc2 protein kinase during mitosis in human cells: cell-cycle-dependent phosphorylation and subunit rearrangement. Cell 54:17, 1988

170. Luca FC, Shibuya EK, Dohrmann CE, Ruderman JV: Both cyclin A delta 60 and B delta 97 are stable and arrest cells in M-phase, but only cyclin B delta 97 turns on cyclin destruction. EMBO J 10:4311, 1991

171. Gallant P, Nigg EA: Cyclin B2 undergoes cell cycle-dependent nuclear translocation and, when expressed as a non-destructible mutant, causes mitotic arrest in HeLa cells. J Cell Biol 117:213, 1992

172. Glotzer M, Murray AW, Kirschner MW: Cyclin is degraded by the ubiquitin pathway. Nature 349:132, 1991

173. Kimura H, Ishibashi T, Sato T et al Megakaryocytic colony formation (CFU-Meg) in essential thrombocythemia: quantitative and qualitative abnormalities of bone marrow CFU-Meg. Am J Hematol 24:23, 1987

174. Greenberg SM, Chandrasekhar C: Hematopoietic factor-induced synthesis of von Willebrand factor by the Dami human megakaryoblastic cell line and by normal human megakaryocytes. Exp Hematol 19:53, 1991

175. Geissler D, Zwierzina H, Pechlaner C et al: Abnormal megakaryopoiesis in patients with myelodysplastic syndromes: analysis of cellular and humoral defects. Br J Haematol 73:29, 1989

176. Homas AC, Cohen JL, Mazur EM: Defective megakaryocytopoiesis in the syndrome of thrombocytopenia with absent radii. Br J Haematol 70:205, 1988

177. Castro-Malaspina H, Rabellino EM, Yen A et al: Human megakaryocyte stimulation of proliferation of bone marrow fibroblasts. Blood 57:781, 1981

178. Matolcsy A, Kalman E, Pajor L et al: Morphologic and flow cytometric analysis of circulating megakaryoblasts in chronic myeloid leukaemia. Leuk Res 15:887, 1991

Lymphopoiesis

20

Kenneth Dorshkind

INTRODUCTION

In 1956 Glick and colleagues[1] reported that bursectomy of chickens shortly after birth resulted in a severe agammaglobulinemia. Five years later a classic study by J.F.A.P. Miller[2] concluded that selected immunocompetent cells are generated in the thymus. Taken together, these observations were among the first to establish that the immune system is comprised of B cells responsible for humoral immunity and T lymphocytes, which mediate cellular immunity. Since these first reports, the use of cell culture and molecular biologic approaches to investigate immune system development has made it possible to define precursor-progeny relationships as well as regulatory mechanisms operative during lymphopoiesis.

These studies, which have provided a basis for understanding disorders of lymphocyte development that result in neoplasia and immunodeficiency diseases, have established that the bone marrow and thymus are the sites of primary B- and T-cell development, respectively, in adult mammals. However, during embryogenesis lymphopoiesis occurs transiently in many different embryonic tissues. Accordingly, the present chapter begins with a brief review of fetal blood cell development before addressing the specifics of marrow and thymic lymphopoiesis.

EMBRYONIC HEMATOPOIESIS

One of the first sites of blood cell development in the embryo is the yolk sac[3,4](Fig. 20-1). Whether yolk sac hematopoiesis originates from resident stem cells or, as suggested by avian studies, from an intraembryonic immigrant[5] is unresolved. Although erythropoiesis is a predominant feature of yolk sac hematopoiesis, murine studies have demonstrated that precursors with lymphoid developmental potential are present at that site.[6,7] Following its seeding by yolk sac-derived[4,8] hematopoietic precursors at 5–6 weeks of gestation, the liver assumes a major role in fetal blood cell production. Studies in mice have demonstrated that B- and T-cell precursors are present in that organ and that it is a site of B lymphopoiesis.[9,10] By the time liver hematopoiesis has subsided during the third trimester of pregnancy, the spleen and bone marrow have become sites of blood cell production.

Splenic hematopoiesis initiates by week 5 of development, and that organ remains hematopoietic until late fetal life. In the adult it functions as a secondary lymphoid tissue that houses mature T and B cells.[8,11] Hematopoiesis in the bone marrow is evident by 3 months of development, and after birth that tissue becomes the primary site of myeloid and B-lymphocyte development. Most T-cell production, however, takes place in the thymus. At 7–8 weeks of development the thymic rudiment is seeded by blood-borne precursors[11–13] and in the adult traffic of marrow-derived precursors to that organ is thought to be responsible for maintenance of T lymphopoiesis.[14,15]

In addition to the above organs, other embryonic tissues, including the omentum, placenta, and blood have been reported to contain B-cell progenitors.[16–18]

HEMATOPOIETIC HIERARCHY

Figure 20-2 shows a scheme of adult hematopoiesis in the marrow with emphasis on the development of lymphoid lineage cells. At the head of the human hematopoietic hierarchy is a CD34-expressing pluripotent hematopoietic stem cell that can self-renew as well as differentiate into all blood cell populations.[19–23] Its progeny include a restricted, multipotential precursor that has the capacity to generate erythroid and myeloid cells but not B or T lymphocytes.[19,20] The existence of a comparable stage of lymphoid development restricted to the B- and T-cell lineages has been proposed,[24] but such a population has not been isolated. Therefore, the possibility remains that progenitors committed to the B- and T-cell developmental pathways are direct descendants of the pluripotent stem cell.

B-LYMPHOCYTE DEVELOPMENT

B-lymphocyte development in the adult occurs in two distinct phases. The first is antigen independent and culminates in the production of surface immunoglobulin expressing B lymphocytes. The second is antigen dependent and takes place in secondary lymphoid tissues such as the spleen and lymph nodes in response to cellular and soluble signals provided by T cells, macrophages, and other accessory cell populations. Antigen-independent, or primary, B-cell production occurs in the bone marrow of adult mammals and is the focus of the present review.[25,26]

As shown in Figure 20-3, it is possible to distinguish intermediates in the B-cell developmental pathway using antibodies that recognize immunoglobulin and nonimmunoglobulin cell surface and cytoplasmic determinants.[26] In the mouse, cells committed to B-cell differentiation but that have their immunoglobulin genes in the germline configuration are referred to as pro-B cells. As these cells mature they express the CD45RA cell-surface antigen, a tyrosine phosphatase whose function in B-cell development is unknown.[7,26,27] Subsequently, μ heavy chain protein appears in the cytoplasm of a population now designated as a pre-B cell[28,29] and is largely retained there by an immunoglobulin-binding protein known as BiP.[30] Once light chain protein is expressed in the cell, the immunoglobulin molecule is assembled and appears on the surface of cells now defined as B lymphocytes. Light chain proteins in the mouse are predominantly of the κ-isotype. Additional cell-surface determinants (including cytokine receptors) that appear during development are shown in Figure 20-3 and Table 20-1.

Models of human B-cell development are based on analysis of leukemic B-cell precursors and investigation of B-cell reconstitution following bone marrow transplantation, as well as on flow cytometric study of normal bone marrow aspirates. Figure 20-3 shows that the most immature human B-cell precursors express CD34 and CD19, an antigen present on all B-lineage cells. At the progenitor cell stage, CD34 expression is lost and cell surface CD10 is acquired. Subsequently, pre-B cells, defined by the presence of cytoplasmic μ-protein, express CD20.

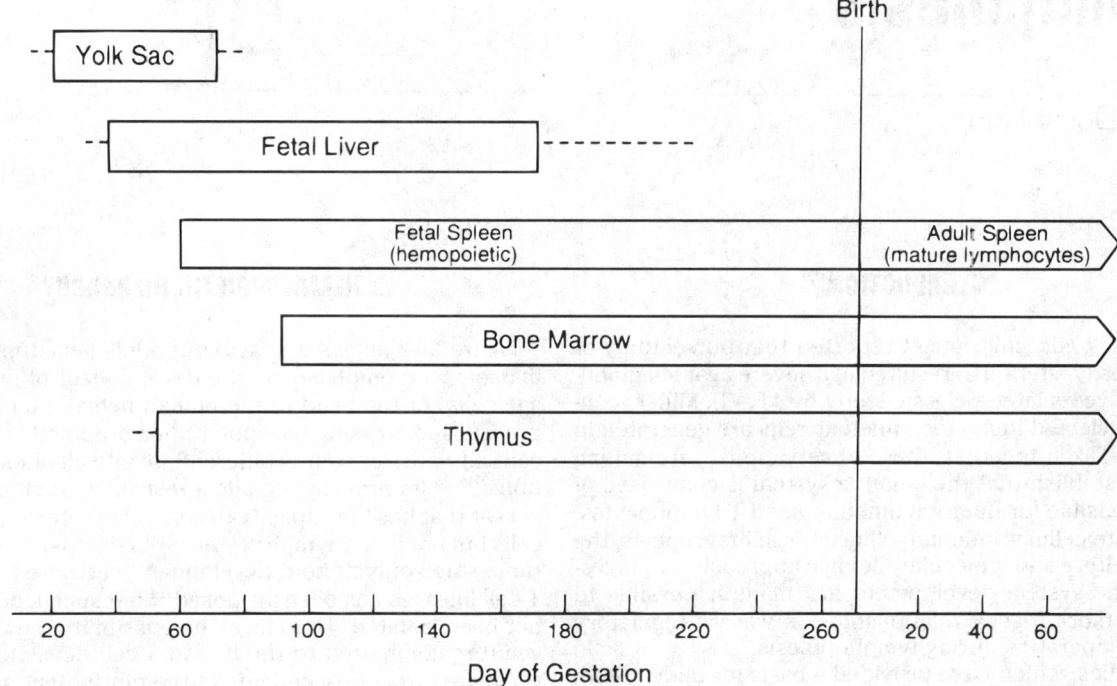

Fig. 20-1. Onset of hematopoiesis/lymphopoiesis in different tissues at various times of human gestation.

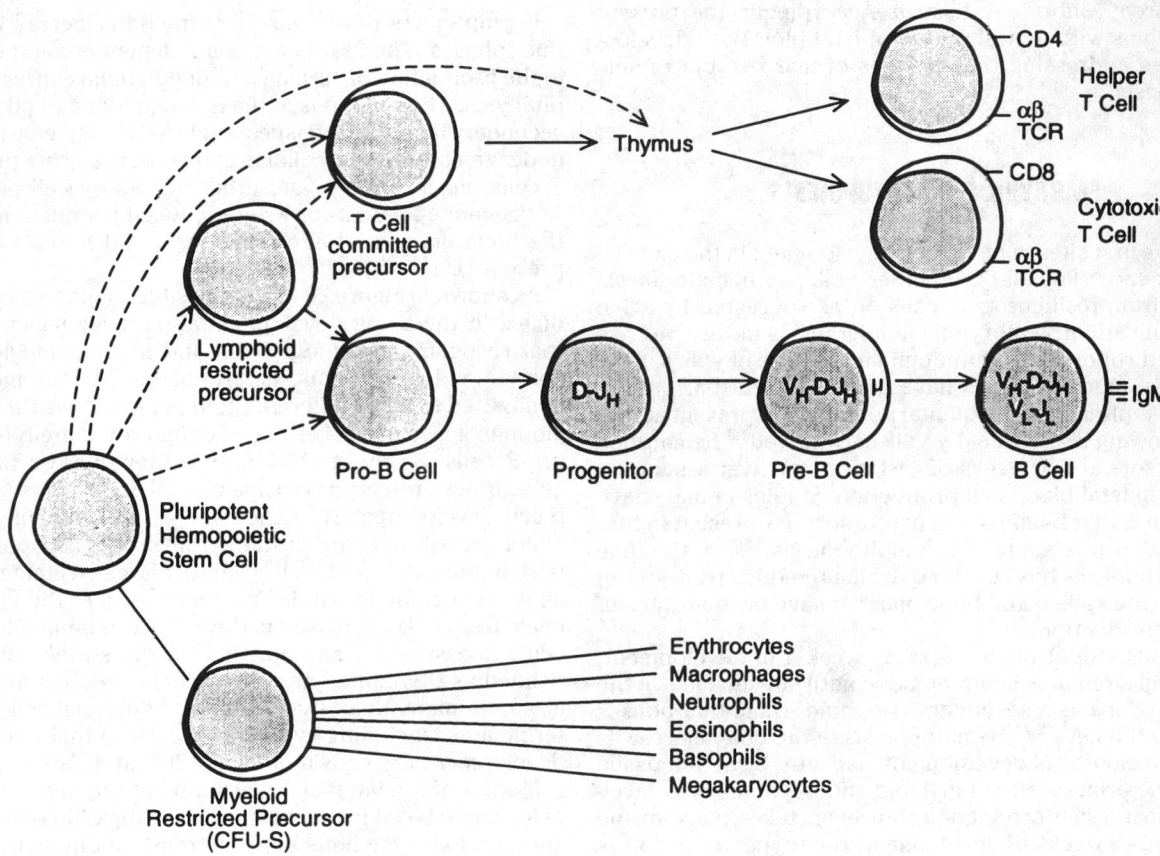

Fig. 20-2. Adult hematopoietic system. Dashed lines indicate that lineage relationships have not been established. Although natural killer cells are derived from the pluripotent stem cell, their absence from the diagram indicates that the lineage from which they originate in unknown. (A detailed discussion of lymphocyte development from stem cells during embryonic and adult life can be found in the article by Ikuta et al.[90])

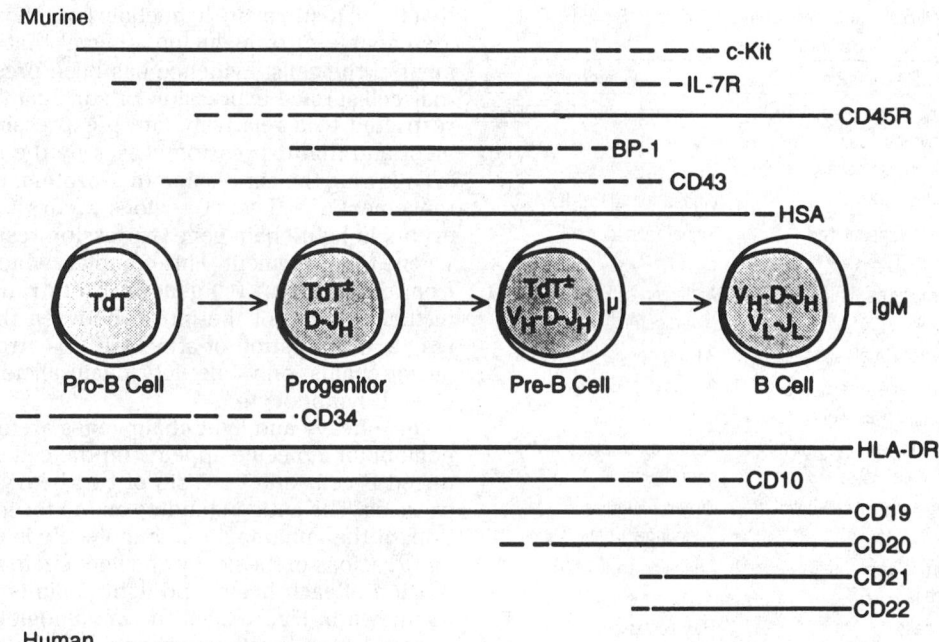

Fig. 20-3. Stages of murine and human B-cell development as defined by the expression of various cell surface and cytoplasmic determinants. (For more detailed information on stages of human and murine B-cell development, consult references 32–34 and 78.) The terms used to indicate particular stages of development have not been standardized.

During the pre-B to B cell transition, the loss of CD10 and acquisition of CD21, CD22, and surface IgM occurs[31–34] (Table 20-1).

B lymphopoiesis is characterized by a considerable degree of cell proliferation, which is most evident at the progenitor cell stage.[28,29] By the time cells have matured to small pre-B cells that express cytoplasmic μ-protein, cell division ceases. Kinetic studies on murine marrow cell turnover have demonstrated that in addition to the tremendous expansion of progenitor cells, there is considerable loss of B-lineage cells at the pre-B cell stage. Deleted cells may include those that have undergone defective immunoglobulin gene rearrangements or that express autoreactive heavy chain genes. The cells that progress to the surface IgM stage of development leave the bone marrow and migrate to the spleen, where they undergo further maturation. These cells survive for a few days unless they become stimulated by antigen.[28,29]

B1 (CD5) B Cells

It has been hypothesized that three distinct B-cell lineages, distinguished by phenotypic and functional properties, exist. B1a cells, which express CD5, and B1b cells, which do not express CD5, are further characterized by high levels of surface IgM and low levels of membrane IgD. These populations are largely confined to the peritoneal and pleural cavities in the adult and predominantly secrete IgA and IgM antibodies, which are thought to provide defense against environmental flora. These populations are distinguished from conventional, or B2, B cells, which predominate in secondary lymphoid organs such as the spleen and lymph node.[35,36]

While the existence of B cells with these different phenotypic and functional properties is accepted, debate is considerable regarding the origin of such cells. Some investigators propose that B1 cells constitute a distinct B-cell subpopulation derived from a fetal stem cell present in the omentum and liver during embryonic development. The hypothesis further proposes that stem cells present in adult bone marrow can no longer generate B1 cells and are committed to the production of conventional B2 cells. Others believe that B1 cells are conventional B cells whose characteristics result from selective pressures following stimulation with thymus-independent antigen.[37] Resolution of this issue has important implications for understanding potential differences between fetal and adult stem cell populations.[35] The propensity of cells with a B1 phenotype to secrete autoantibodies and generate lymphomas makes their understanding of clinical relevance.[38]

Immunoglobulin Genes and Their Expression

Immunoglobulin is the unique marker of B-lineage cells, and its expression depends on an ordered series of gene rearrangements at the heavy and light chain loci.[39,40] The heavy chain locus (Fig. 20-4) includes variable (V), diversity (D), and joining (J) segments and is the first to rearrange during B-cell development. Initial events in heavy chain gene rearrangement juxtapose one of several D-region segments to a J_H segment. Subsequently, a V_H gene rearranges to the D/J_H complex. During rearrangement of heavy chain genes, nucleotides not encoded in the germline can be added to D-J_H and V_H-DJ$_H$ junctions by the enzyme terminal deoxynucleotidyl transferase (TdT).[41] As shown in Figure 20-3, TdT is expressed in cells undergoing immunoglobulin gene rearrangements.

The heavy chain constant (C_H) region remains separated from the rearranged VDJ complex by an intron, and this entire sequence is transcribed. Subsequent RNA processing leads to deletion of the intron between the VDJ complex and the most proximal C-region gene; following translation, the μ heavy chain protein is expressed in the cytoplasm of pre-B cells. Even though each B-cell precursor has two sets of immunoglobulin heavy chain genes, only one allele is expressed in any given cell. The production of μ-protein, as a result of successful rearrangement and transcription of one allele, inhibits further heavy chain rearrangements in the cell. The mechanism by which this process, known as allelic exclusion, occurs is undefined.[42]

Table 20-1. Selected Cell-Surface Determinants Involved in B- and T-Cell Development

Determinant	Distribution	Function
CD1	Cortical and medullary thymocytes, dendritic cells	Proposed ligand for TCRγδ
CD2	T cells	Ligand for CD58 (LFA-3)
CD3 complex	T cells (associated with TCR)	Signal transduction
CD4	Thymocytes, helper T cells	Adhesion to class II MHC antigens
CD5	T cells; B cell subset	? Lymphocyte activation
CD7	Thymocytes, fetal liver T-cell precursors	?
CD8	Thymocytes, cytotoxic T cells	Adhesion to class I MHC antigens
CD10 (CALLA)	Progenitor/pre-B cells	Enzyme neutral endopeptidase
CD11a (LFA-1α) CD18 (LFA-1β)	Thymocytes and T cells	Adhesion to ICAM-I
CD16	NK cells, granulocytes, macrophage	FCγ receptor
CD19	B lineage	?
CD20	B cells	?
CD21	B cells	Epstein-Barr virus receptor
CD22	B cells	?
CD29	Broad	β-chain of VLA integrins
CD34	?Pluripotent stem cells; immature hematopoietic precursors	?
CD43	Many leukocytes; murine B-cell progenitors	?
CD44 (Pgp-1)	Most leukocytes	Receptor for matrix molecules, including hyaluronate
CD45	Family of leukocyte common antigens (T200); different molecular weight forms distinguish distinct lineages	Tyrosine phosphatase
CD54 (ICAM-1)	Broad	Ligand for LFA-1
CD56	NK cells	Adhesion
CD58	Broad	CD2 ligand
CD72	B cells	CD5 ligand

Abbreviations: ICAM-I, intercellular adhesion molecule-1; LFA, leukocyte function-associated antigen; NK, natural killer; TCR, T-cell receptor.

Traditionally, μ-protein was believed to be expressed on the surface of B-lineage cells only in association with κ or λ light chain proteins. However, recent work on two proteins encoded by the V_{pre-B} and λ5 genes has challenged this view.[43-46] As shown in Figure 20-5, the V_{pre-B} and λ5 proteins associate with one another to form a light chain-like structure known as the surrogate light chain, which can form immunoglobulin-like complexes with the μ heavy chain protein. The genes encoding V_{pre-B} and λ5 proteins are located on human chromosome 22 along with the λ light chain genes. It has been hypothesized

that these μ-surrogate light chain complexes on the cell surface are capable of transducing a signal that affects the development of the cells. Evidence has been presented in the human that cell-surface expression of surrogate light chain genes is restricted to a relatively late μ-expressing stage of development and that expression ceases by the B-cell stage.[46]

Following the expression of μ-protein, light chain gene rearrangement of V, J, and C regions occurs[47] (Fig. 20-6). The initial events in light chain gene expression result in the joining of a V gene to a J segment. This complex, which remains separated from the constant (C) gene by an intron, is transcribed, and further splicing of the intron between the J and C segments results in formation of a mature V-J-C transcript. As with the heavy chains, only one light chain allele is expressed in any given B lymphocyte.

Once heavy and light chain genes are expressed, the immunoglobulin molecule appears on the cell surface of newly produced B cells and consists of two heavy and two light chain proteins. The antigen-binding amino terminus, or variable portion, of the immunoglobulin molecule is encoded by the V, D, and J regions of the heavy and light chain genes. The remaining portion of each heavy and light chain is relatively invariable. As shown in Figure 20-5, the immunoglobulin molecule is anchored in the B-cell membrane, but the cytoplasmic carboxy tail of the heavy chain consists of only three amino acids, suggesting that the immunoglobulin molecule itself can not generate an intracellular signal. Recently, two transmembrane proteins (Ig-α and Ig-β), noncovalently associated with the heavy chain molecule, have been described.[48] Their rapid tyrosine phosphorylation after cross-linking of membrane IgM, and their association with distinct cytoplamic effectors involved in cell signaling, indicate that these molecules are involved in signal transduction.[49] Knowledge of signaling in B cells is a rapidly evolving topic, and recent evidence indicates that defects in these pathways can result in severe B-cell developmental disorders. For example, deficient expression of a specific tyrosine kinase during B-cell development has been implicated in X-linked agammaglobulinemia.[50,51]

Regulation of Immunoglobulin Gene Expression

The rearrangement and subsequent expression of immunoglobulin genes is a highly ordered process regulated at both the recombinatorial and transcriptional levels.[52,53] As noted above, the recombinatorial machinery deletes intronic sequences and forms coding joints between V, D, and J region-coding genes. Enzymes responsible for these events function in part via the recognition of specific DNA sequences located 3' of each V-region exon, 5' of each J segment, and 5' and 3' of each D-region segments. Figure 20-4 shows the association of these recognition sequences with one D-region and one J-region exon. Each recognition signal consists of conserved heptamer and nonamer sequences, separated by nonconserved DNA segments of 12 or 23 base pairs (bp). During immunoglobulin gene recombination, these recognition sequences form loops of DNA, which in turn bring the coding exons in apposition to one another. These loops are subsequently deleted and degraded.[53] Two genes, referred to as RAG-1 and RAG-2, which play a role in stimulating immunoglobulin gene recombination, have recently been identified and are expressed in developing B cells. It is unknown whether RAG-1 and RAG-2 encode recombinases that directly stimulate immunoglobulin gene recombination or regulatory proteins that control the expression of those factors.[54] Further elements that function in immunoglobulin gene rearrangements are yet to be defined, but it is likely they include enzymes that act as exonucleases and ligases.

The transcription of productively rearranged heavy and light

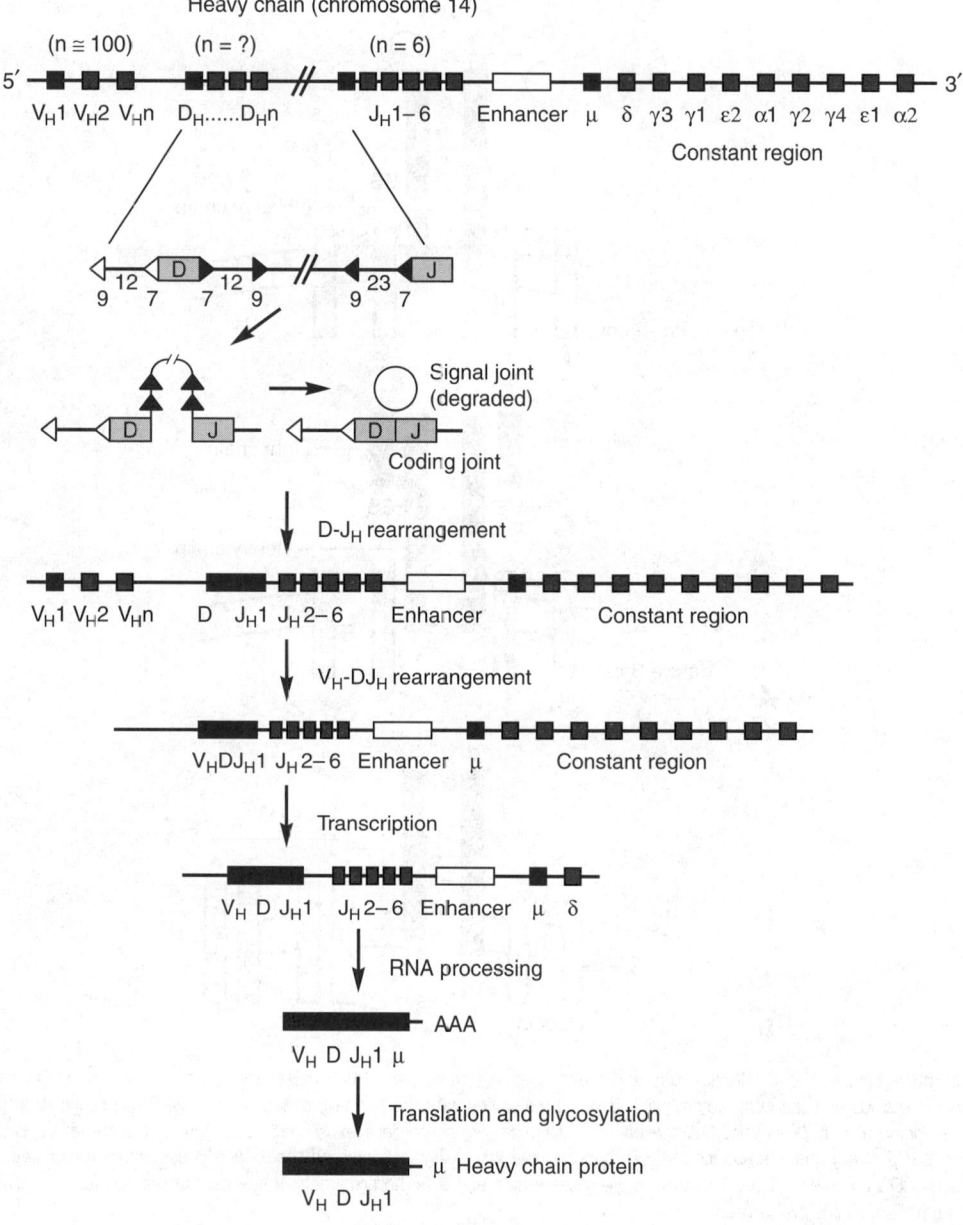

Fig. 20-4. The human heavy chain gene. Immunoglobulin diversity is generated in part by the formation of the heavy chain molecule from one V_H, one D, and one J_H segment. $D\text{-}J_H$ rearrangements occur first, followed by rearrangement of a V_H gene to the rearranged DJ_H complex. Following transcription and RNA processing, a mature heavy chain transcript is generated. Synthesis of μ heavy chain protein is shown. It is unknown whether the primary transcript contains all C regions. The figure also shows the conserved heptamer (7) and nonamer (9) sequences that flank the D and J_H genes and their role in rearrangement. These are separated from each other by nonconserved regions of 12 or 23 bp. While these signal sequences are associated with each V, D, and J segment, for simplicity they are shown for only one of the D and one of the J_H genes. (For additional details consult the articles by Alt et al.[39] and Tonegawa.[40])

chain genes is controlled by promoter sequences located 5' of the heavy and light chain V-region genes and one or more heavy and light chain enhancer regions. The latter include regions located in the μ- and κ-intron, respectively. Activation of promoter and enhancer regions is regulated in part by the binding of multiple transcription factors to specific segments of DNA located in those regions. Many of these DNA-binding proteins have been identified and the genes that encode them cloned.[52,55] The ability of these trans-activating proteins to initiate transcription is regulated by their interactions with one another and by binding to negative regulatory proteins that inhibit their activity.[56,57]

Immunoglobulin Repertoire

The use of multiple heavy and light chain V, D, and J segments, the loss and gain of nucleotides at coding joints during rearrangement, and somatic mutations in V-region genes result in formation of a murine B-cell repertoire of $\geq 10^8$ possible antigen-binding specificities.[58,59] However, the complete immunoglobulin repertoire is not present at birth. Instead, the repertoire develops in an ordered manner resulting from an apparently programmed pattern of V-gene segment utilization during development in which the most 3' V-region genes are initially expressed.[60]

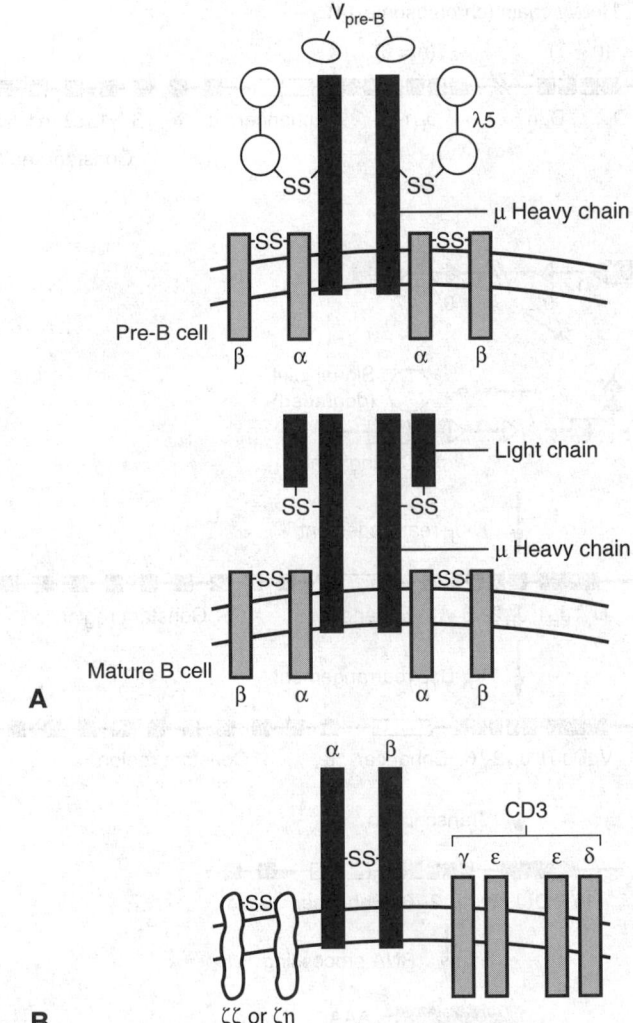

Fig. 20-5. Immunoglobulin, the T-cell receptor, and their accessory molecules. **(A)** Pre-B-cell stage of development and association of the covalently linked λ5 and the noncovalently linked V_{pre-B} molecules with the μ heavy chain. By the pre-B-cell stage, the Ig-α and Ig-β chains are associated with μ-protein, but the earliest stage at which they are expressed is unclear. By the mature B-cell stage of development, the μ heavy chain is associated with conventional κ or λ light chains and the α- and β-accessory molecules. **(B)** αβ TCR and associated CD3 complex. CD3 consists of a γε heterodimer and a δε heterodimer. These complexes are further associated with either a ζζ homodimer or a ζη heterodimer.

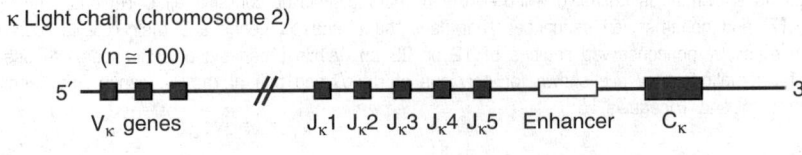

Fig. 20-6. Organization of the human κ and λ light chain genes. The mechanisms of light chain gene rearrangements are analogous to those for heavy chain. λ-Chain enhancers are not shown but have been mapped 3′ of $C_\lambda 1$ and $C_\lambda 4$. Rearrangements occur first at the κ-locus. Rearrangements of the λ-locus occur only if both κ-genes are unable to code a functional protein. Not all the six $J_\lambda C_\lambda$ clusters are shown. Approximately 60% of human B cells express κ light chains.

One important requirement during development of the B-cell repertoire is that lymphocytes expressing membrane immunoglobulin with self-reactive determinants be eliminated. Experimental evidence using transgenic mouse systems suggests that self-reactive cells can be physically eliminated or functionally inactivated. In the former case, cells might be killed by other cells or undergo programmed death on receptor engagement. In the latter case, self-reactive B cells may persist and enter an anergic state characterized by defects in the ability to proliferate and differentiate into immunoglobulin-secreting cells.[61,62] The mechanisms that underlie these processes remain to be defined.

Cells and Cytokines that Regulate B-Cell Development

Morphologic analyses of the bone marrow have demonstrated that hematopoiesis occurs in association with a fixed population of stromal cells present in the intersinusoidal spaces of the medullary cavity.[63,64] The development of methods for the long-term, stromal cell-dependent culture of bone marrow made it possible to isolate stromal cell populations and demonstrate that they regulate B lymphopoiesis via direct cell-cell interactions and through secretion of soluble mediators.[65,66]

Several in vitro studies have demonstrated that developing B lymphocytes express the VLA-4 integrin that interacts with a stromal cell ligand identified as vascular cell adhesion molecule-1 (VCAM-1).[67–69] CD44 on developing B-lineage cells has also been implicated in mediating stromal cell-lymphocyte interactions via binding to stromal cell-derived hyaluronate.[70] The physiologic result of such contacts is not clear, but stromal cells could be stimulated to secrete factors that potentiate B-cell differentiation on binding immature lymphoid cells. In some cases, cytokines themselves serve as cell-surface receptors for developing B-lineage cells. Kit-ligand is a stromal cell-derived factor[71–73] that can be presented by the stromal cell in a membrane-bound form.[74] Its receptor, c-*kit*, is a tyrosine kinase widely distributed on hematopoietic cells.[75] Finally, the surrogate light chain complexes described above have been hypothesized to mediate binding of B-lineage cells to the stroma.[43]

Studies with stromal cell lines have revealed that they are a major source of cytokines that regulate the proliferation and differentiation of hematopoietic cells (Table 20-2). One important stromal cell-derived cytokine, interleukin-7 (IL-7), functions in stimulating proliferation of developing B-lineage cells.[76] A hallmark of B lymphopoiesis is its high rate of cell production,[28,29] and molecules such as IL-7 appear to play a key role in this expansion. The precise stage of development at which cells first become sensitive to IL-7 is unclear, but progenitors that have undergone D-J_H rearrangements are IL-7 responsive.[77,78] The proliferation-stimulating effects of IL-7 can be augmented by additional cytokines such as kit-ligand.[79] While the latter factor alone has no apparent effects on B-cell growth or differentiation, it interacts with IL-7 to potentiate the proliferation of B-cell progenitors. Table 20-2 lists additional stromal cell-derived cytokines involved in B-cell development. For example, insulin-like growth factor-1 has been shown to play a role in the maturation of murine pro-B cells to cμ-expressing pre-B cells,[80] and an IL-4-like molecule appears to function during the maturation of murine pre-B cells to B lymphocytes.[81]

Although the above discussion has focused on positive regulation of B-cell development, some agents may inhibit growth or differentiation, or both, of B-lineage cells. For example, transforming growth factor-β (TGF-B) has been shown to inhibit IL-

Table 20-2. Selected Cytokines and Their Effects on B- and T-Cell Development[a]

Cytokine	Source	B Cells	T Cells
IL-1	Macrophages, TE cells	?Direct effects: stimulates IL-4 production in murine stroma	Thymocyte proliferation
IL-2	T cells, thymocytes	—	Proliferation of DN thymocytes and T cells
IL-3	T cells	?Differentiation of immature precursors	Proliferation of DN thymocytes if IL-1 and CSF-GM present
IL-4	T cells; BM stroma (murine)	Expression of immunoglobulin light chains (murine)	Proliferation of DN thymocytes
IL-6	BM stroma, TE cells	Plasma cell development	Proliferation of DN thymocytes if IL-1 and mitogen present
IL-7	BM stroma (murine)	Progenitor/pre-B cell proliferation	CD3⁻, DN thymocyte proliferation
IGF-1	BM stroma	Development of pre-B cells (murine) from pro-B cells; enhances IL-7 proliferative responses (murine)	
kit-ligand	BM stroma	Enhances IL-7 proliferative responses (murine)	?Enhances IL-7 proliferative responses (murine)
TGF-β	BM stroma (murine)	Inhibits IL-7 effects (murine)	Inhibits thymocyte proliferation (murine)

Abbreviations: CSF-GM, colony-stimulating factor-granulocyte/macrophage; IGF, insulin-like growth factor; IL, interleukin; TGF, transforming growth factor; DN, double negative; TE, thymic epithelial; BM, bone marrow.

[a] Cytokine biology is a rapidly evolving field, and current references must be consulted for new or better defined effects of the above factors as well as identification of additional soluble mediators with lymphopoietic effects. The above summary is compiled from both human and murine studies. Effects are from human studies unless so indicated.

7-induced proliferation.[82] In other cases, abnormal concentrations of factors, such as various colony-stimulating factors, may result in increased myeloid cell production at the expense of B lymphopoiesis.[83] Finally, cytokines that are stimulatory at some stages may be inhibitory at other points in the developmental hierarchy. In this regard, IL-4 is believed to inhibit the pro-B to pre-B transition even though, as noted above, it stimulates the formation of B cells from pre-B cells.[84]

T-LYMPHOCYTE DEVELOPMENT

At week 4 of human embryonic development, the thymic rudiment forms from ectoderm of the third pharyngeal cleft and endoderm of the third pharyngeal pouch[85–87] and is colonized by hematopoietic precursors at 7–8 weeks of gestation. After birth the thymus retains its role as the site of T lymphopoiesis. As discussed in detail below, T-cell development is dependent on a complex process in which immature T-cell precursors present in the cortical areas of the thymus mature into functional T-cell subpopulations.

A feature of thymocyte development is the high rate of cell production, and an unanswered question is whether thymopoiesis is maintained by an intrathymic pool of precursors or is dependent on continual input by a bone marrow-derived precursor. One recent study of parabiotic mice presents evidence that the thymus is continually replenished by blood-borne precursors.[15] Even in that case, however, the number of cells that migrate from marrow to thymus appears to be extremely low. A second unresolved issue is the developmental status of the immigrant cells. Pluripotent hematopoietic stem cells have the ability to generate T lymphocytes and could continually migrate to the thymus. However, the possibility remains that precursors that populate the thymus are already committed to T-cell development (Fig. 20-2).

Extrathymic T-cell maturation has been described.[88] However, since thymic agenesis in the human results in depressed cell-mediated immunity with recurrent infections,[89] it is clear that an intact thymus is critical for the optimal development of T lymphocytes. Therefore, the focus of the remaining discussion is on the thymus and intrathymic T-cell development.

Intrathymic T-Cell Development

Distinct stages of thymocyte development can be delineated based on expression of various cell surface and cytoplasmic molecules, cytokine receptors, and the rearrangement status of T-cell receptor (TCR) genes. The TCR is a heterodimeric complex formed by association of α- and β- and γ- and δ-subunits. Each of these subunits is encoded by a separate gene. Analogous to B-cell development, murine studies have made significant contributions to the understanding of T-cell development, and the events in that species overlap considerably with those in the human. For example, in both species CD4$^-$/CD8$^-$ precursor cells differentiate into CD4$^+$ helper and CD8$^+$ cytotoxic T cells. While parallels between human and murine intrathymic development are discussed below, further details regarding the latter species can be found in recent reviews.[90–92]

Figure 20-7 presents a schema of human intrathymic T-cell development and shows that the most immature precursor cells in that organ express CD7. Some of these early T-cell precursors are also CD44$^+$ (Pgp-1$^+$). CD44 functions as a receptor for hyaluronate and could play a role in homing of T-cell precursors to the thymus. These immature precursors then generate CD2$^+$/CD7$^+$ progeny in which cytoplasmic CD3 is present. Subsequently, CD4 and CD8 are expressed. By this time the α- and β-genes are rearranging, and the TCRαβ/CD3 receptor complex is expressed on the cell surface. As these CD4$^+$/CD8$^+$ TCR-expressing double-positive cells pass from the thymic cortex to the medulla, they mature into single positive CD4$^+$ helper T-cells or CD8$^+$ cytotoxic T cells. Cells that mature to the single positive stage of development comprise <5% of thymocytes. CD4$^+$ T cells mediate a helper or regulatory function and recognize antigen in the context of class II MHC molecules. CD8$^+$ T cells function as cytotoxic cells and recognize antigen in association with class I MHC molecules. Single positive T cells leave the thymus and populate secondary lymphoid tissues such as the spleen and lymph node.[93–97]

Figure 20-7 further shows that some T-cell populations can be characterized by their expression of the TCRγδ gene. γδ-T cells, which express CD3 but not CD4 or CD8 molecules,[98–100] are the first TCR-bearing cells to appear during development. Although the issue is not resolved, recent work suggests that αβ- and γδ-T cells are distinct lineages that separate prior to

initiation of TCR gene rearrangement.[101,102] In this regard, it has been hypothesized that γδ-T cells and B1 cells are analogous populations that develop in parallel.[35]

γδ-T cells are found in various tissues, including the spleen, the epidermis, and the mucosal epithelium of the uterus, vagina, and tongue. A number of γδ-cell lines that exhibit cytolytic activity and cytokine secretory activity have been described, suggesting that this cell population may have an immune surveillance role in the above tissues.[100,103]

T-Cell Receptor Genes

Mature T cells express a T-cell receptor comprised of a heterodimeric αβ- or γδ-complex.[97–109] Analogous to the immunoglobulin heavy and light chain molecules, the genes that encode the TCR proteins undergo a process of somatic rearrangement that bring coding segments in apposition to one another and delete intervening sequences. Figure 20-8 shows a map of the TCR genes that points out several important structural features. First, each TCR gene includes V,J,C, and, in the case of the TCR β- and δ-chains, D regions. Second, the TCRδ-chain genes are located within the α-gene in the intron between V_α and J_α. A consequence of this is that productive α-rearrangements result in a deletion of the entire δ-locus.

γδ-Genes

γ- and δ-gene rearrangements appear to take place simultaneously. During γ-gene rearrangements, V-region genes rearrange to one of the five J-region segments. During δ-gene rearrangements, joining of a V-region gene to a DJ complex can occur. In addition, direct V- to J-segment rearrangements have also been observed.[103] There are relatively few γ and δ V gene segments compared with the number at the α- and β-loci. Nevertheless, since considerable junctional diversity can occur during assembly of γ- and δ-chains, the potential to generate an extensive repertoire exists.[98,110–112]

Murine γδ cells that appear first during development are unusual in that their TCRs display limited diversity. These cells home to the epidermis and mucosal epithelium of the uterus, vagina, and tongue. Subsets that display considerable TCRγδ diversity appear subsequently and traffic to the blood and peripheral lymphoid organs.[101,103,112]

αβ-Genes

The initial rearrangement events during the expression of the TCRαβ occur at the β-locus.[37,104–109] D_β to J_β rearrangements occur first, followed by rearrangement of a V_β gene to the rearranged DJ_β complex. This rearranged complex is then transcribed, and the mature transcript is formed by deletion of intronic sequences present between the VDJ complex and the C_β gene. Rearrangements at the α-locus involve the joining of V_α and J_α regions. The rearranged gene is then transcribed and, as with the β-chain, post-transcriptional processing deletes intronic sequences between the J and C regions. Diversity of the TCRαβ complex is achieved partly because multiple V, D, and J gene segments can be used to assemble the rearranged TCR gene. In addition, the enzyme TdT can randonly add nucleotides at VD, DJ, and VJ junctions. The total potential TCRαβ repertoire has been estimated to include 10^{16} binding specificities.[100]

It is believed that signal transduction through the molecules that form the heterodimeric TCR does not occur, because of the short intracytoplasmic carboxy tails of these molecules.

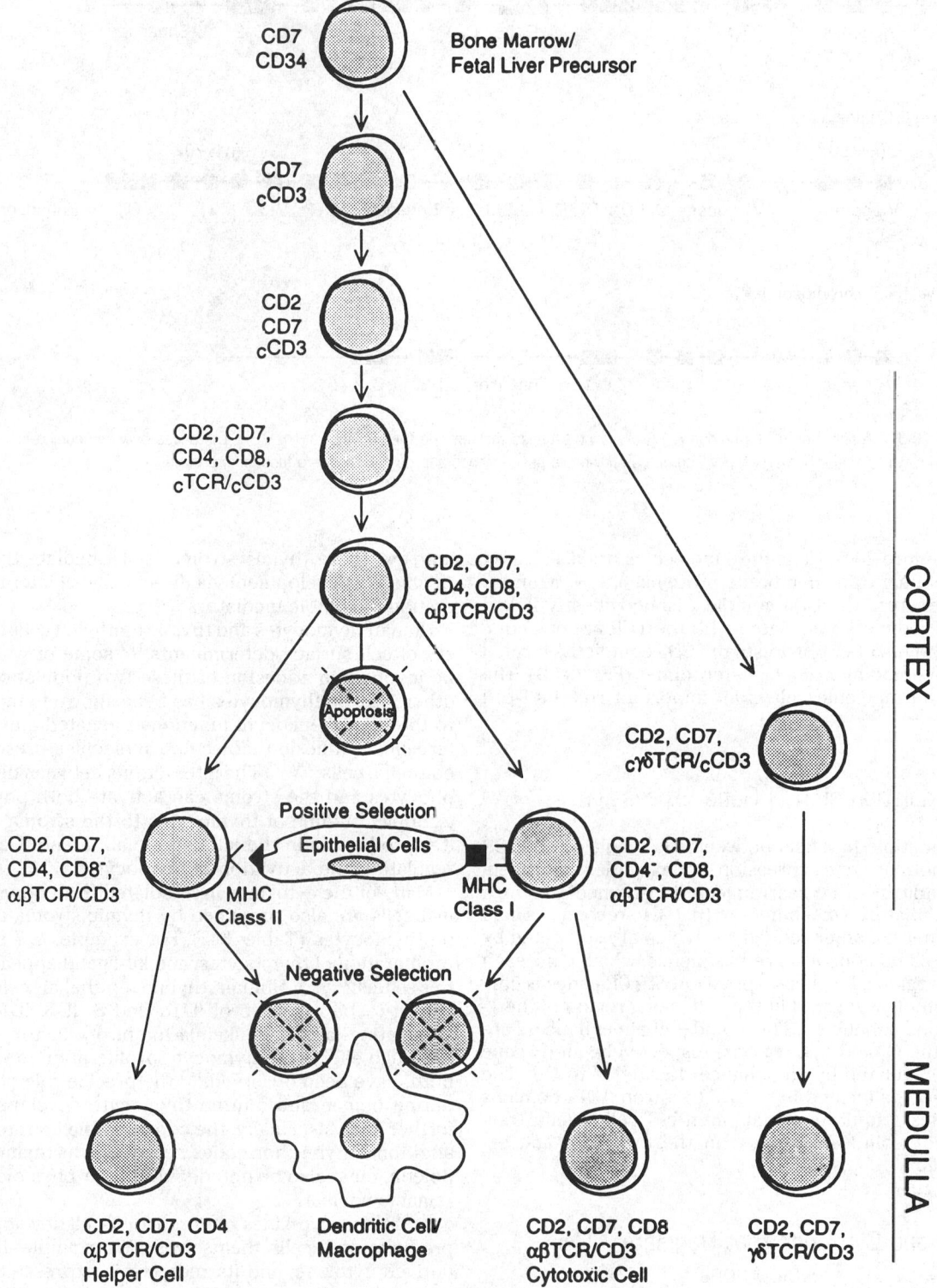

Fig. 20-7. Model of T-cell development in the thymus; stages of human thymocyte development as delineated by the expression of various CD molecules. (For a more detailed delineation of cellular stages based on expression of additional cell surface and cytoplasmic determinants see the article by Haynes et al.[96]) The figure also demonstrates that positive selection is mediated by thymic epithelial cells in the cortex and that dendritic cells/macrophages in the medulla are involved in negative selection. Cells not selected may be deleted or undergo apoptosis (i.e., programmed cell death). (The article by von Boehmer[135] should be consulted for a concise, up-to-date discussion of current issues in thymic selection.) $_c$CD3, cytoplasmic CD3; $_c\gamma\delta$, cytoplasmic $\gamma\delta$ chains; $_c$TCR, cytoplasmic $\alpha\beta$ TCR chains.

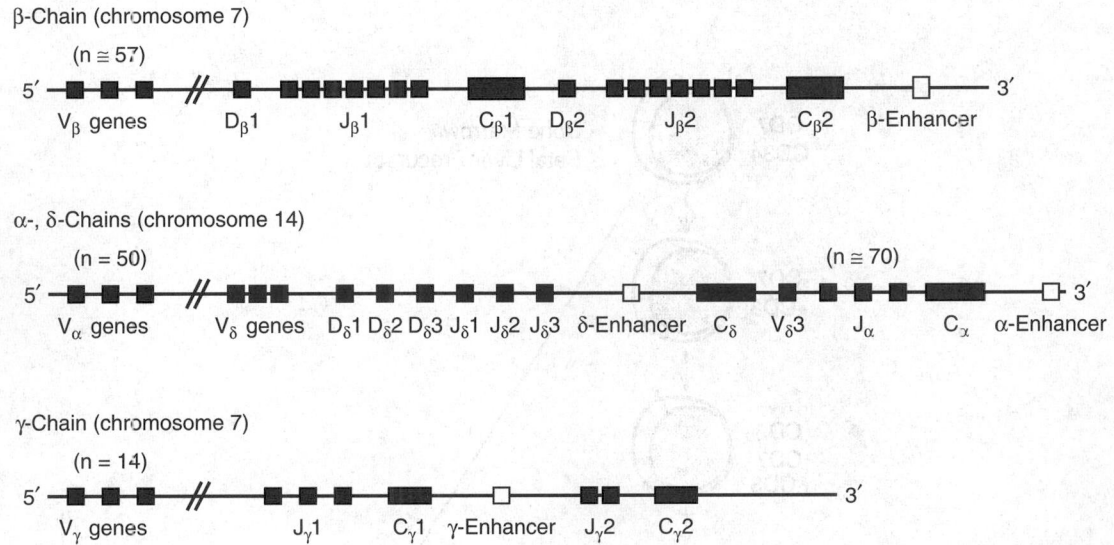

Fig. 20-8. Organization of the human α-, β-, γ-, and δ-genes that encode the subunits of the TCR. Distances between coding loci are not drawn to scale. Some of the V segments shown are pseudogenes and do not encode a functional protein.

As shown in Figure 20-5, γδ- and αβ-molecules are associated with five additional transmembrane proteins, δ, ε, γ, η, and ζ, which together form the CD3 complex. Noncovalently linked δε and γε heterodimers associated with the TCR are one component of CD3. The other portion of the CD3 complex is formed by either a ζζ-homodimer or a ζη-heterodimer (Fig. 20-5B). The CD3 complex of molecules plays an important role in T-cell signaling.[113–115]

Regulation of TCR Gene Expression

There are multiple parallels between the regulation of TCR and immunoglobulin gene expression. For example, experimental evidence indicates that rearrangements are mediated by a similar recombinatorial machinery[116] that also recognizes conserved heptamer-nonamer sequences, which are separated by either a 12- or 23-bp nonconserved sequence, which flank each of the coding regions. Further, expression of TCR genes is controlled by promoters located in the 5′ flanking region of the V-region genes and enhancers. The α- and β-chain enhancers are located 3′ of the C_α and $C_\beta 2$ regions, respectively, and γ-gene expression is regulated by an enhancer located 3′ to $C_\gamma 1$. The δ-chain enhancer is located in the $J_\delta 3$-C_δ intron. DNA domains to which various ubiquitous and apparently T-cell-specific transcription factors bind are located in the promoter and enhancer regions.[117]

Cells and Cytokines that Regulate T-Cell Development

The thymus gland is organized into distinct cortical and medullary regions. This architectural feature is a consequence of lower thymocyte numbers and differences in stromal cell composition in the latter region. Stromal cells form a three-dimensional network within the thymus that provides a supporting framework for thymocyte development. Many of these cells are derived from the epithelium of the third pharyngeal pouch. In addition, dendritic cells and macrophages believed to be of bone marrow origin are present in the medulla. As in the bone marrow, these thymic stromal cells mediate their effects on thymocyte development via direct cell-cell interactions and secretion of soluble mediators.[96,118]

Human thymocytes and thymic epithelial cells express a variety of cell surface determinants,[119] some of which appear to be involved in adhesion of these two populations to one another. CD2 on thymocytes has been shown to mediate binding to the CD58 (leukocyte function-associated antigen-3) and intercellular adhesion molecule-1 molecules present on thymic epithelial cells.[120,121] The interactions between developing lymphocytes and the stroma can activate both populations. For example, binding of thymocytes to the stroma can stimulate IL-1 production in the latter population and IL-2 receptor upregulation and activation of thymocytes.[122]

Many of the cytokines first isolated from bone marrow stromal cells are also produced by thymic stroma and are active on thymocytes (Table 20-2). For example, IL-7 stimulates the proliferation of thymocytes, and kit-ligand appears to augment this effect.[123,124] Human thymic epithelial cells have been shown to be a source of IL-1α and β, IL-3, IL-6, IL-8 colony-stimulating factors, leukemia inhibitory factor, and TGF-α.[119] Although effects on thymocyte proliferation or maturation, or both, have been observed,[125] the precise role of these factors during human and murine thymocyte development requires further analysis. Finally, the considerable literature describing additional thymic hormones, referred to as thymosin or thymopoietin, must also be noted,[126] but their physiologic relevance remains unclear.

Additional cytokines required for T-cell development may be products of T cells themselves. For example, Il-2 is a T-cell-derived cytokine, and its receptor is expressed on immature thymocytes. Thymocytes have also been reported to produce interferon-γ, TNF-α, IL-3, and, based on the detection of its transcripts, IL-4.[119,125]

Positive and Negative Selection in the Thymus

A major event during thymic development is the amplification of thymocyte populations expressing TCRs that recognize non-self foreign antigens and the deletion of populations reactive with self-determinants.[127] These latter cells may constitute the major population in the thymus, since only about 5% or less of cells in the thymus ever mature and leave that organ. Both processes are thought to occur during thymocyte development and are known as positive and negative selection, respectively. Much of what is known about these processes is derived from studies of transgenic mice.

The key point in understanding positive selection is to appreciate that the TCR recognizes foreign antigen in association with self-MHC antigens. In the case of CD4+ helper populations, this occurs in the context of MHC class II molecules, while CD8+ cytotoxic T cells recognize foreign antigen in association with MHC class I molecules. During development, TCR-expressing thymocytes that recognize self-MHC class I and II determinants present on thymic epithelial cells appear to be rescued from programmed cell death. Accordingly, the latter stromal cells are considered to be a critical population involved in thymic education[128–130] (Fig. 20-7). An unresolved issue is the stage of development at which positive selection occurs. Instructive models argue that this occurs at the CD4+/CD8+ stage. Those double-positive cells expressing receptors that recognize MHC class II molecules down-regulate CD8 and further develop into CD4+ helper cells. Similarly, double-positive cells that express MHC class I receptors down-regulate CD4 expresion and develop into a CD8+ cytotoxic T cell. A tenet of selective or stochastic models is that double-positive cells randomly differentiate into CD4 or CD8 single-positive cells regardless of TCR specificity. Subsequently, rescue from programmed cell death occurs if the TCR receptor complex on the cell then engages the appropriate class I or class II MHC molecules on stromal cells.[131,132]

During the process of negative selection, T cells that express TCRs reactive against self-proteins are deleted. Negative selection seems to occur in the thymic medulla mediated by bone marrow-derived stromal elements. Dendritic cells or macrophages, or both, in the medulla are thought to present self-antigens, and thymocytes that recognize those complexes undergo clonal anergy or deletion[133] (Fig. 20-7). However, it remains unclear whether all potential self-antigens are encountered by thymocytes during intrathymic development or if self-antigens in the periphery also play a role.

NATURAL KILLER CELLS

Natural killer (NK) cells are defined by their ability to lyse selected cellular targets spontaneously that are virally infected or tumorigenic. Human NK cells express CD16 and CD56 but not TCR or CD3. NK cells are also known as large granular lymphocytes, because of the presence of large cytoplasmic granules. While NK cells are of hematopoietic origin, little is known about the lineage from which they develop.[134]

REFERENCES

1. Glick B, Chang TS, Jaap RG: Experimental modification of the growth of the bursa of fabricius. Poultry Sci 35:224, 1956
2. Miller JFAP: Immunological function of the thymus. Lancet 2:748, 1961
3. Moore MAS, Metcalf D: Ontogeny of the haemopoietic system: yolk sac origin of in vivo and in vitro colony forming cells in the developing mouse embryo. Br J Hematol 18:279, 1970
4. Metcalf D, Moore MAS: Haemopoietic Cells. North Holland Publishing, Amsterdam, 1971
5. Dieterlen-Lievre F: On the origin of hemopoietic stem cells in the avian embryo: an experimental approach. J Embryol Exp Morphol 33:607, 1975
6. Paige CJ, Kincade PW, Moore MAS, Lee G: The fate of fetal and adult B-cell

7. Kincade PW: Formation of B lymphocytes in fetal and adult life. Adv Immunol 31:177, 1981
8. Moore KL: The Developing Human, Clinically Oriented Embryology. WB Saunders, Philadelphia, 1982
9. Tyan ML, Herzenberg LA: Studies on the ontogeny of the mouse immune system. II. Immunoglobulin producing cells. J Immunol 101:446, 1968
10. Owen JJT, Cooper MD, Raff MC: In vitro generation of B lymphocytes in mouse foetal liver, a mammalian 'bursa equivalent'. Nature 249:361, 1974
11. Klein J: Immunology: The Science of Self-Nonself Discrimination. John Wiley & Sons, New York, 1982
12. Moore MAS, Owen JJT: Experimental studies on the development of the thymus. J Exp Med 126:715, 1967
13. Ritter MA: Embryonic mouse thymic development: stem cell entry and differentiation. Immunology 34:69, 1978
14. Scollay R, Smith J, Stauffer V: Dynamics of early T cells: prothymocyte migration and proliferation in the adult mouse thymus. Immunol Rev 91:129, 1986
15. Donskoy E, Goldschneider I: Thymocytopoiesis is maintained by blood-borne precursors throughout postnatal life. J Immunol 148:1604, 1992
16. Solvason N, Kearney JF: The human fetal omentum: a site of B cell generation. J Exp Med 175:397, 1992
17. Melchers F: Mouse embryonic B lymphocyte development in the placenta. Nature 277:219, 1979
18. Melchers F, Abramczuk J: Murine embryonic blood between day 10 and 13 of gestation as a source of immature precursor B cells. Eur J Immunol 10:763, 1980
19. Keller G, Paige C, Gilboa E, Wagner EF: Expression of a foreign gene in myeloid and lymphoid cells derived from multipotent hemopoietic precursors. Nature 318:149, 1985
20. Dick JE, Magli MC, Huszar D et al: Introduction of a selectable gene into primitive stem cells capable of long-term reconstitution of the hematopoietic system of W/W mice. Cell 42:71, 1985
21. Jordan CT, Lemischka IR: Clonal and systemic analysis of long-term hematopoiesis in the mouse. Genes Dev 4: 220, 1990
22. Fialkow PJ, Jacobson RJ, Papayannopoulou T: Chronic myelocytic leukemia: clonal origin in a stem cell common to the granulocyte, erythrocyte, platelet, and monocyte/macrophage. Am J Med 63:125, 1977
23. Andrews RG, Singer JW, Bernstein ID: Human hematopoietic precursors in long-term culture: single CD34+ cells that lack detectable T cell, B cell, and myeloid cell antigens produce multiple colony-forming cells when cultured with marrow stromal cells. J Exp Med 172:355, 1990
24. Fulop GM, Phillips RA: Use of SCID mice to identify and quantitate lymphoid-restricted stem cells in long-term bone marrow cultures. Blood 74:1537, 1989
25. Brahim F, Osmond DG: Migration of bone marrow lymphocytes demonstrated by selective bone marrow labeling with thymidine-³H. Anat Rec 168:139, 1970
26. Kincade PW: Experimental models for understanding B lymphocyte formation. Adv Immunol 41:181, 1987
27. Tonks NK, Charbonneau H, Diltz CD et al: Demonstration that the leukocyte common antigen CD45 is a protein tyrosine phosphatase. Biochemistry 27:8696, 1988
28. Landreth KS, Rosse C, Clagett J: Myelogenous production and maturation of B lymphocytes in the mouse. J Immunol 127:2027, 1981
29. Park YH, Osmund DG: Phenotype and proliferation of early B lymphocyte precursor cells in mouse bone marrow. J Exp Med 165:444, 1987
30. Haas IG, Wabl M: Immunoglobulin heavy chain binding protein. Nature 306:387, 1983
31. Ryan DH, van Dongen JJM: Detection of residual disease in acute leukemia using immunological markers. p. 173. In Bennett JM, Foon KA (eds): Immunologic Approaches to the Classification and Management of Lymphomas and Leukemias. Kluwer Publishers, Norwell, MA, 1988
32. Ukun FM, Haissig S, Ledbetter JA et al: Developmental hierarchy during early human B-cell ontogeny after autologous bone marrow transplantation using autografts depleted of CD19+ B-cell precursors by anti-CD19 pan-B cell immunotoxin containing pokeweed antiviral protein. Blood 79:3369, 1992
33. Loken MR, Shah VO, Dattilio KL, Civin CI: Flow cytometric analysis of human bone marrow. II. Normal B lymphocyte development. Blood 70:1316, 1987
34. Clark EA, Ledbetter JA: Structure, function and genetics of human B cell associated surface molecules. Adv Cancer Res 52:81, 1989
35. Kantor AB, Herzenberg LA: Origin of murine B cell lineages. Annu Rev Immunol 11:501, 1993
36. Stall AM, Adams S, Herzenberg LA, Kantor AB: Characteristics and development of the murine B-1b (Ly-1 B sister) cell populations. Ann NY Acad Sci 651:33, 1992

progenitors grafted into immunodeficient CBA/N mice. J Exp Med 150:548, 1979

37. Haughton G, Arnold LW, Whitmore AC, Clarke SH: B-1 cells are made, not born. Immunol Today 14:84, 1993

38. Hayakawa K, Hardy RR: Normal, autoimmune, and malignant CD5⁺ B cells: the Ly-1 lineage? Annu Rev Immunol 6:197, 1988

39. Alt F, Blackwell T, Yancopolous G: Development of the primary antibody repertoire. Science 238:1079, 1987

40. Tonegawa S: Somatic generation of antibody diversity. Nature 302:575, 1983

41. Desiderio SV, Yancopoulos GD, Paskind M et al: Insertion of N region into heavy-chain genes is correlated with expression of terminal deoxytransferase in B cells. Nature 311:752, 1984

42. Storb U: Transgenic mice with immunoglobulin genes. Annu Rev Immunol 5:151, 1987

43. Melchers F, Karasuyama H, Haasner D et al: The surrogate light chain in B-cell development. Immunol Today 14:60, 1993

44. Pillai S, Baltimore D: The omega and iota surrogate immunoglobulin light chains. Curr Top Microbiol Immunol 137:136, 1988

45. Tsubata T, Reth M: The products of the pre-B cell-specific genes (λ5 and V$_{pre-B}$) and the immunoglobulin μ heavy chain form a complex that is transported onto the cell surface. J Exp Med 172:973, 1990

46. Lassoued K, Nunez L, Billips L: Expression of surrogate light chain receptors is restricted to a late stage in pre-B cell differentiation. Cell 73:73, 1993

47. Reth M, Petrac E, Wiese P et al: Activation of V$_k$ gene rearrangement in pre-B cells follows the expression of membrane-bound immunoglobulin heavy chain. EMBO J 6:3299, 1987

48. Reth M: Antigen receptors on B lymphocytes. Annu Rev Immunol 10:97, 1992

49. Clark MR, Campbell KS, Kazlauskas A et al: The B cell antigen receptor complex: association of Ig-α and Ig-β with distinct cytoplasmic effectors. Science 258:123, 1992

50. Vetrie D, Vorechovsky, Sideras P et al: The gene involved in X-linked agammaglobulinanemia is a member of the src family of protein-tyrosine kinases. Nature 361:226, 1993

51. Tsukada S, Saffran DC, Rawlings DJ et al: Deficient expression of a B cell cytoplasmic tyrosine kinase in human X-linked agammaglobulinemia. Cell 72:279, 1993

52. Staudt LM, Lenardo MJ: Immunoglobulin gene transcription. Annu Rev Immunol 9:373, 1991

53. Schatz DG, Oettinger MA, Schlissel MS: V(D)J recombination: molecular biology and regulation. Annu Rev Immunol 10:359, 1992

54. Oettinger MA, Schatz DG, Gorka C, Baltimore D: Rag-1 and Rag-2, adjacent genes that synergistically activate V(D)J recombination. Science 248:1517, 1990

55. Libermann TA, Baltimore D. Transcriptional regulation of immunoglobulin gene expression. p. 399. In Cohen P, Foulkes JG (eds): The Hormonal Control of Gene Transcription. Elsevier Science Publishing, Amsterdam, 1991

56. Baeuerle AP, Baltimore D: IκB: a specific inhibitor of the NK-κB transcription factor. Science 242:540, 1988

57. Wilson KB, Kiledjian M, Shen CP: Repression of immunoglobulin enhancers by the helix-loop-helix protein Id: implications for B-lymphoid development. Mol Cell Biol 11:6185, 1985

58. Rajewsky K, Forster I, Cumano A: Evolutionary and somatic selection of the antibody repertoire on the mouse. Science 283: 1088, 1987

59. Leder P: The genetics of antibody diversity. Sci Am 246:72, 1982

60. Malynn BA, Yancopoulos GD, Barth JE et al: Biased expression of the J$_H$-proximal V$_H$ genes occurs in the newly generated repertoire of neonatal and adult mice. J Exp Med 171:843, 1990

61. Goodnow CC: Transgenic mice and analysis of B-cell tolerance. Annu Rev Immunol 10:489, 1992

62. Nemazee D, Russel D, Arnold B et al: Clonal deletion of autospecific B lymphocytes. Immunol Rev 122:117, 1991

63. Weiss L: The structure of bone marrow. Functional interrelationships of vascular and hematopoietic compartments in experimental hemolytic anemia: an electron microscopic study. J Morphol 117:467, 1965

64. Lichtman MA, Packman CH, Constine LS: Molecular and cellular traffic across the marrow sinuses. p. 87. In Tavassoli M (ed): Handbook of the Hemopoietic Microenvironment. Humana Press, Clifton, NJ, 1989

65. Dorshkind K: Regulation of hemopoiesis by bone marrow stromal cells and their products. Annu Rev Immunol 8:111, 1990

66. Kincade PW, Lee G, Pietrangeli CE et al: Cells and molecules that regulate B lymphopoiesis in bone marrow. Annu Rev Immunol 7:111, 1989

67. Miyake K, Weissman IL, Greenberger JS, Kincade PW: Evidence for a role of the integrin VLA-4 in lymphohemopoiesis. J Exp Med 173:599, 1991

68. Kina T, Majumdar AS, Heimfeld S et al: Indentification of a 107-kD glycoprotein that mediated adhesion between stromal cells and hematolymphoid cells. J Exp Med 173:373, 1991

69. Ryan DH, Nuccie BL, Abboud CN, Winslow JM: Vascular cell adhesion molecule-1 and the integrin VLA-4 meiate adhesion of human B cell precursors to cultured bone marrow cells. J Clin Invest 88:995, 1991

70. Miyake K, Underhill CB, Lesley J, Kincade PW: Hyaluronate can function as a cell adhesion molecule and CD44 participates in hyaluronate recognition. J Exp Med 172:69, 1990

71. Williams DE, Eisenman J, Baird A et al: Identification of a ligand for the c-kit proto-oncogene. Cell 63:167, 1990

72. Zsebo KM, Wypych J, McNiece IK et al: Identification, purification, and biological characterization of hematopoietic stem cell factor from buffalo rat liver-conditioned medium. Cell 63:195, 1990

73. Huang E, Nocka K, Beier DR et al: The hematopoietic growth factor KL is encoded at the Sl locus and is the ligand of the c-kit receptor, the gene product of the W locus. Cell 63:225, 1990

74. Flanagan JG, Leder P: The kit ligand: a cell surface molecule altered in steel mutant fibroblasts. Cell 63:185, 1990

75. Chabot B, Stephenson DA, Chapman VM et al: The proto-oncogene c-kit encoding a transmembrane tyrosine kinase receptor maps to the mouse W locus. Nature 335:88, 1988

76. Namen AE, Lupton S, Hjerrild K, Wagnall, et al: Stimulation of B-cell progenitors by cloned murine interleukin-7. Nature 333:571, 1988

77. Rolink A, Kudo A, Karasuyama H et al: Long-term proliferating early pre-B cell lines and clones with the potential to develop to surface Ig positive, mitogen reactive B cells in vitro and in vivo. EMBO J 10:327, 1991

78. Hardy RR, Carmack CE, Shinton SA et al: Resolution and characterization of pro-B and pre-pro B cell stages in normal mouse bone marrow. J Exp Med 173:1213, 1991

79. McNeice IK, Langley KE, Zsebo KM: The role of recombinant stem cell factor in early B cell development. J Immunol 146:3785, 1991

80. Landreth KS, Narayanan R, Dorshkind K: Insulin-like growth factor-I regulates pro-B cell differentiation. Blood 80:1207, 1992

81. King AG, Wierda D, Landreth KS: Bone marrow stromal cell regulation of B-lymphopoiesis. I. The role of macrophages, IL-1, and IL-4 in pre-B cell maturation. J Immunol 141:2016, 1988

82. Lee G, Namen AE, Gillis et al: Normal B cell precursors responsive to recombinant murine IL-7 and inhibition of IL-7 activity by transforming growth factor-α. J Immunol 142:3875, 1989

83. Dorshkind K: In vivo administration of recombinant granulocyte-macrophage colony-stimulating factor results in a reversible inhibition of primary B lymphopoiesis. J Immunol 146:4204, 1991

84. Peschel C, Green I, Paul WE: Preferential proliferation of immature B lineage cells in long-term stroma cell dependent cultures with IL-4. J Immunol 142: 1558, 1989

85. Weller GL: Development of the thyroid, parathyroid, and thymus gland in man. Contrib Embryol Carnegie Inst 24:95, 1993

86. Lobach DF, Haynes BF: Ontogeny of the human thymus during fetal development. J Clin Immunol 7:81, 1987

87. Haynes BF, Scearce RM, Lobach DM, Hensley LL: Phenotypic characterization and ontogeny of mesodermal-derived and endocrine epithelial components of the human thymic microenvironment. J Exp Med 150:1149, 1984

88. Rocha B, Vassalli P, Guy-Grand D: The extrathymic T-cell development pathway. Immunol Today 13:449, 1992

89. DiGeorge AM: Congenital absence of the thymus and its immunologic consequences: concurrence with congenital hypoparathyroidism. Birth Defects 4:116, 1968

90. Ikuta K, Uchida NH, Friedman J, Weissman IL: Lymphocyte development from stem cells. Annu Rev Immunol 10:759, 1992

91. Rothenberg EV: The development of functionally responsive T cells. Adv Immunol 51:85, 1992

92. Mathieson BJ, Fowlkes BJ: Cell surface antigen expression on thymocytes: development and phenotypic differentiation of intrathymic subsets. Immunol Rev 82:141, 1984

93. Lobach DF, Hensley IL, Ho W, Haynes BF: Human T cell antigen expression during the early stages of fetal thymic maturation. J Immunol 135:1752, 1985

94. Campana D, Janossy G, Coustane-Smith E et al: The expression of T cell receptor-associated proteins during T cell ontogeny in man. J Immunol 142:57, 1989

95. Haynes BF, Telen MJ, Hale LP, Denning SM: CD44—a molecule involved in leukocyte cellular adherence and T cell activation. Immunol Today 10:423, 1989

96. Haynes BF, Denning SM, Le PT, Singer KH: Human intrathymic T cell differentiation. Semin Immunol 2:67, 1990

97. Moss PAH, Rosenberg WMC, Bell JI: The human T cell receptor in health and disease. Annu Rev Immunol 10:71, 1992

98. Allison JP, Havran WL: The immunobiology of T cells with invariant $\gamma\delta$ antigen receptors. Annu Rev Immunol 9:679, 1991

99. Pardoll DM, Fowlkes BJ, Bluestone JA et al: Differential expression of two distinct T-cell receptors during thymocyte development. Nature 326:79, 1987

100. Abbas AK, Lichtman, AH, Pober JS: Cellular and Molecular Immunology. WB Saunders, Philadelphia, 1991

101. Itohara S, Mombaerts P, Lafaille J et al: T cell receptor delta gene mutant mice: independent generation of $\alpha\beta$ T cells and programmed rearrangements of gamma delta TCR genes. Cell 72:337, 1993

102. Winoto A, Baltimore D: Separate lineages of T cells expressing the $\alpha\beta$ and $\gamma\delta$ receptors. Nature 338:430, 1989

103. Raulet DH: The structure, function, and molecular genetics of the $\gamma\delta$ T cell receptor. Annu Rev Immunol 7:175, 1989

104. Raulet DH, Garman RD, Saito HY, Tonegawa S: Developmental regulation of T-cell receptor gene expression. Nature 314:103, 1985

105. Kronenberg M, Siu G, Hood LE, Shastri N: The molecular genetics of the T-cell antigen receptor and T-cell antigen recognition. Annu Rev Immunol 4:529, 1986

106. Davis MM: T cell receptor gene diversity and selection. Annu Rev Biochem 59:475, 1990

107. Wilson RK, Lai E, Concannon P et al: Structure, organization and polymorphism of murine and human T-cell receptor α and β chain gene families. Immunol Rev 101:149, 1988

108. Yanagi Y, Yoshikai Y, Leggeth K et al: A human T cell specific cDNA clone encodes a protein having extensive homology to immunoglobulin chains. Nature 308:145, 1984

109. Hedrick SM, Cohen DI, Nielsen EA, Davis MM: Isolation of cDNA clones encoding T cells specific membrane associated proteins. Nature 308:149, 1984

110. Lafaille JJ, DeCloux A, Bonneville M et al: Junctional sequences of T cell receptor $\gamma\delta$ genes: implications for $\gamma\delta$ T cell lineages and for a novel intermediate of V-(D)-J joining. Cell 59:859, 1989

111. Elliott JF, Rock EP, Patten et al: The adult T-cell receptor δ chain is diverse and distinct from that of fetal thymocytes. Nature 331:627, 1988

112. Haas W, Pereira P, Tonegawa S: Gamma/delta cells. Annu Rev Immunol 11:637, 1993

113. Clevers HC, Alarcon B, Wileman TE, Terhorst C: The T cell receptor/CD3 complex: a dynamic protein ensemble. Annu Rev Immunol 6:629, 1988

114. Bauer A, McConkey DJ, Howard FD et al: Differential signal transduction via T-cell receptor $CD3\zeta_2$, $CD3\zeta\eta$ and $CD3\eta_2$ isoforms. Proc Natl Acad Sci USA 88:3842, 1991

115. Ashwell JD, Klausner RD: Genetic and mutational analysis of the T-cell antigen receptor. Annu Rev Immunol 8:139, 1990

116. Yancopoulos G, Blackwell T, Suh H et al: Introduced T cell receptor variable gene segments on pre-B cell: evidence that B and T cells use a common recombinase. Cell 44:251, 1986

117. Leiden JM: Transcriptional regulation of T cell receptor genes. Annu Rev Immunol 11:539, 1993

118. van Ewijk W: T-cell differentiation is influenced by thymic microenvironments. Annu Rev Immunol 9:591, 1991

119. Le PT, Singer KH: Human thymic epithelial cells: adhesion molecules and cytokine production. Clin Lab Res 23:56, 1993

120. Vollger LW, Tuck DT, Springer TA et al: Thymocyte binding to human thymic epithelial cells is inhibited by monoclonal antibodies to CD2 and LFA-3 antigens. J Immunol 138:358, 1987

121. Notoyama S, Nakayama, Shiohara T, Yata J: Only dull CD3+ thymocytes bind to thymic epithelial cells. The binding is elicited by both CD2/LFA/3 and LFA-1/ICAM-1 interaction. Eur J Immunol 19:1631, 1989

122. Denning SM, Kurtzberg J, Le PT et al: Human thymic epithelial cells directly induce activation of autologous immature thymocytes. Proc Natl Acad Sci USA 85:3125, 1988

123. Watson JD, Morrissey PJ, Namen AE et al: Effect of IL-7 on the growth of fetal thymocytes in culture. J Immunol 143:1215, 1989

124. Conlon PJ, Morrissey PJ, Nordan RP et al: Murine thymocytes proliferate in direct response to interleukin-7. Blood 74:1368, 1989

125. Carding SR, Hayday AC, Bottomly K: Cytokines in T-cell development. Immunol Today 12:239, 1991

126. Goldstein AL: Thymic Hormone and Lymphokines, Basic Chemistry and Clinical Applications. Plenum, New York, 1984

127. Blackman M, Kappler J, Marrack P: The role of the T cell receptor in positive and negative selection of developing T cells. Science 248:1335, 1990

128. Fink PJ, Bevan MJ: H-2 antigens of the thymus detemine lymphocyte specificity. J Exp Med 148:766, 1978

129. von Boehmer H: Developmental biology of T cells in T cell-receptor transgenic mice. Annu Rev Immunol 8:531, 1990

130. Fowlkes BJ, Pardoll DM: Molecular and cellular events of T cell development. Adv Imunol 44:207, 1989

131. Chan SH, Cosgrove D, Waltzinger C et al: Another view of the selective model of thymocyte selection. Cell 73:225, 1993

132. Davis CB, Killeen N, Crooks MEC: Evidence for a stochastic mechanism in the differentiation of mature subsets of T lymphocytes. Cell 73:237, 1993

133. Kappler JW, Roehm N, Marrack P: T cell tolerance by clonal elimination in the thymus. Cell 49:273, 1987

134. Trinchieri G: Biology of natural killer cells. Adv Immunol 47:187, 1989

135. von Boehmer H: Thymic selection: a matter of life and death. Immunol Today 13:454, 1992

Pathogenesis and Pathophysiology of Aplastic Anemia

21

Neal S. Young

INTRODUCTION

An empty bone marrow, the pathognomonic morphologic picture of aplastic anemia, has multiple causes, yet the mechanisms by which marrow failure occurs are relatively limited.

Our understanding of certain forms of bone marrow failure has increased greatly in recent years. Advances in cell biology, virology, toxicology, and immunology have brought better realization of the complex interactions involved in the pathobiology of this disorder. We review here the pathophysiology of aplastic anemia and related marrow failure states. My recent

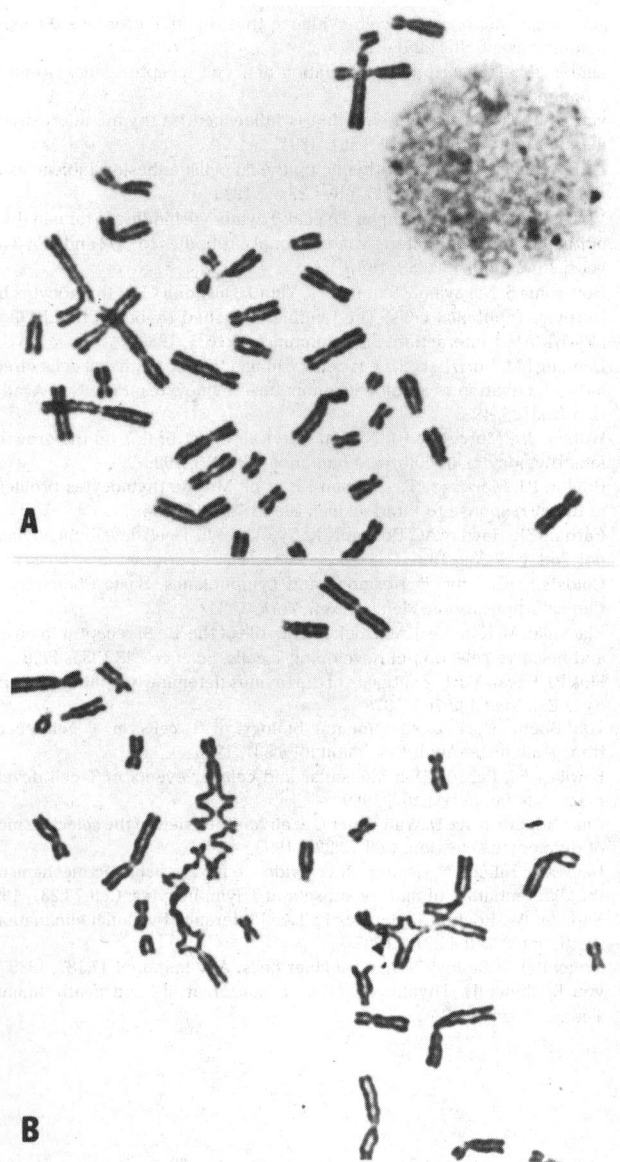

Fig. 21-1. Chromosomal appearance in Fanconi's anemia. Chromosomes present on metaphase spreads of cultured peripheral blood lymphocytes are shown in the **(A)** absence and **(B)** presence of a bifunctional cross-linking agent. Note that the abnormalities typical of this disease—chromosomal breaks, gaps, rearrangements, chromatid interchanges, and endoreduplication—are apparent after chemical treatment. (Courtesy of Dr. A. Auerbach.)

monograph on this subject can be consulted for a more detailed description and a full bibliography.[1]

Erhlich[2] described the pathology of the first case of aplastic anemia. As regards the etiology, bone marrow failure was historically regarded as secondary to physical, chemical, or infectious insults or nutritional deficiencies. Marrow failure is now thought to arise from either intrinsic stem cell defects or from damage after an extrinsic insult. Two observations can be used to illustrate this paradigm. In Fanconi's anemia, the inheritable defect is detected in vitro with the addition of chemicals (Fig. 21-1). Patients often present with pancytopenia after chemical exposure. In this genetic disease, stem cell susceptibility at the level of DNA repair underlies the development bone marrow failure.

The most remarkable feature of the epidemiology of aplastic anemia is an apparently large and as yet unexplained geographic variation in its incidence.[3–5] Aplastic anemia is more common in the Orient than in the West; hundreds of cases may be seen annually at a single hospital in the Orient, making it nearly as frequent an admitting diagnosis as acute myeloid leukemia. The impression of a high prevalence in the Orient has been apparently confirmed by comparison of incidence in population surveys[6–8] (Table 21-1), autopsy series, and age-adjusted mortality statistics. This geographic variation is probably mainly environmental rather than genetic, since Japanese in Hawaii suffer from aplastic anemia at the same rate as whites.[7] Individual susceptibility must play a permissive role, however.

CLINICAL ASSOCIATIONS AND PATHOGENESIS

Genetic Factors

Causes and clinical associations of the inherited and acquired forms of aplastic anemia are listed in Table 21-2. Diagnostic cytogenetic testing has revealed that about 30% of patients with Fanconi's anemia lack the "typical" physical stigmata, and probably 10% present at ages beyond childhood.[1,9] The diagnosis is determined by cytogenetic analysis of peripheral blood cells of children or patients who are middle-aged. The peculiar features of penetrance in Fanconi's anemia, especially the wide variation in phenotypic expression (even within kindreds), the long delay in the appearance of pancytopenia in some individuals, and the apparent link between drug or chemical exposure and clinical manifestations, suggest that genetic factors probably predispose rather than predetermine the development of aplasia. Other as yet undefined genetic variabilities in DNA repair enzymes (and also in drug-metabolizing enzymes or the immune response) may underlie susceptibility to inciting drugs and viruses. Perhaps the reportedly abnormal susceptibility of lymphocytes to bleomycin,[10] a DNA strand breaker, and to ultraviolet light[11] in adult acquired aplastic anemia reflects a Fanconi-like defect in some cases.

Fanconi's anemia is characterized by pancytopenia and congenital defects in the cutaneous, musculoskeletal, and urogenital systems.[1,12,13] Like other rare hereditary diseases associated with aplastic anemia, such as dyskeratosis congenita and Shwachman-Diamond syndrome, Fanconi's anemia patients may not develop bone marrow failure until adulthood. In the case of Fanconi's anemia, the striking cytogenetic abnormality (Fig. 21-1) suggests a general mechanism of bone marrow failure, which in these patients is inherited but in other individuals may be acquired. Cells of patients with Fanconi's anemia proliferate slowly and resist cell division, accumulating in the G_2 phase of the cell cycle.[14,15] All cells share the same genetic defect, but the proliferative failure of hematopoiesis is the most common manifestation; the same defect presumably explains the propensity for malignant transformation of nonhematopoietic tissues as well as in the bone marrow of these patients. Most patients will die of marrow failure. Pancytopenia may be precipitated or exacerbated by chemical exposure or viral infection, consistent with the abnormal sensitivity of Fanconi's anemia cells to in vitro exposure to a wide range of physical and chemical agents that damage DNA.

Attempts to define the genetic lesion biochemically in Fanconi's anemia have yielded equivocal results. At least four complementation groups have been defined by somatic cell hybridization studies, and it is clear that distinct lesions in different genes on separate chromosomes can result in the characteristic cytogenetic and clinical phenotypes.[16] Basic defects in excision of damaged DNA and DNA ligase and topoisomerase activity have been advocated as the underlying pathologic lesions.[17] Chromosomal abnormalities are worsened by high oxygen tension[18] or the addition of oxidants,[19] while addition of superoxide dismutase or antioxidants[19,20] to cultures of Fanconi's anemia cells has been found to decrease the number of chromosomal breaks and increase cell survival. Cells obtained

Table 21-1. Epidemiology of Aplastic Anemia[a]

Study	Dates	Method, Database	Size $\times 10^6$	No.	Incidence/10^6
U.S. Army[78]	1942–1945	Retrospective, marrow tissue	—	57	0.4–1.8 6.6–28.4[b]
California[77]	1960	Retrospective, death certificates	15.7	81	5.2
California[76]	1963–1964	Death certificates	2.4	93	7.8
Uppsala, Sweden[218]	1964–1968	Retrospective, discharge diagnosis	1.28	13	
Uppsala[322]	1973–1977	Retrospective, medical records	1.3	90	14
Israel[721]	1961–1965	Retrospective, hospital/clinic records	17.5	93	7.8
Japan[185]	1970–1973	Prospective, nationwide hospital survey	—	471	13.9
Japan[722]	1970–1973	Prospective, industry survey	11.3	166	14.7
Baltimore[723]	1970–1978	Retrospective, medical records and death certificates	2.1	118	6.1
Northern Region, UK[724]	1971–1978	Hospital records	3.25	174	6.8
United Kingdom[725]	1985	Prospective survey of hematologists	21	49	2.3
Denmark[726]	1967–1982	Retrospective registry (children only)	1.13	39	2.2
Europe[727]	1980–1984	Population-based case control survey	22.3	168	2.2
Buenos Aires[728]	1966–1977	Retrospective, medical records	0.45	35	6
France[729]	1984–1987	Prospective, medical records	81.5	250	1.4
China[730]	1986–1988	Case collection	17.3	387	7.4
Bangkok[5]	1989	Population-based case control survey	8.8	32	3.7

[a] Studies are listed in order of their date of publication. Size, population size; No., total number of cases.
[b] Pacific theater.

from these patients generate superoxide ions at a high rate[21] and have low levels of superoxide dismutase,[22] the enzyme that scavenges free radicals. Treatment of a few patients with the bovine enzyme has temporarily improved their cytogenetic scores and blood counts.[23]

Table 21-2. A Classification of Aplastic Anemia

Acquired Aplastic Anemia	Inherited Aplastic Anemia
Secondary aplastic anemia	Fanconi's anemia
Radiation	Dyskeratosis congenita
Drugs and chemicals	Shwachman-Diamond syndrome
Regular effects	
Cytotoxic agents	Reticular dysgenesis
Benzene	Amegakaryocytic thrombocytopenia
Idiosyncratic reactions	
Chloramphenicol	Familial aplastic anemias
Nonsteroidal anti-inflammatory drugs	Preleukemia (monosomy 7, etc.)
Antiepileptics	
Gold	Nonhematologic syndromes (Down, Dubovitz, Seckel)
Other drugs and chemicals	
Viruses	
Epstein-Barr virus (infectious mononucleosis)	
Hepatitis (non-A, non-B, non-C hepatitis)	
Parvovirus (transient aplastic crisis, pure red cell aplasia)	
Human immunodeficiency virus (AIDS)	
Immune diseases	
Eosinophilic fasciitis	
Hypoimmunoglobulinemia	
Thymoma and thymic carcinoma	
Graft-versus-host disease in immunodeficiency	
Paroxysmal nocturnal hemoglobinuria	
Pregnancy	
Idiopathic aplastic anemia	

The proliferative defect in Fanconi's anemia cells has been corrected by DNA transfection.[24,25] Recently the gene mutated in Fanconi's anemia type C has been cloned and localized to chromosome 9,[26] and several distinct mutations have been described in individual patients.[27–29] While the function of this novel gene and its relationship to the biochemical defects described above are still unknown, its identification offers the possibility of gene therapy for correcting this abnormality in some patients.

Familial forms of aplastic anemia other than Fanconi's are rare. Occasionally relatives of patients with acquired aplastic anemia will have the same condition.[30] Leukemia has also been noted with a higher frequency in relatives of aplastic anemia patients;[31] some of these cases probably represent Fanconi's anemia presenting late in life. Similar considerations apply to reports of siblings with acquired aplastic anemia. Aplastic anemia and leukemia have occurred in a few families with C-group monosomy, but the course in certain cases suggests that they may represent hypocellular preleukemic syndromes.[32,33] In other families, aplasia has been associated with neurologic defects and complex chromosomal abnormalities.[34,35] In general, however, cytogenetic abnormalities are infrequent in acquired aplastic anemia; in one large series chromosomal abnormalities were found in only 4% of 183 cases.[36]

One form of genetic susceptibility is dramatically exemplified by the high frequency of aplastic anemia in boys with the X-linked lymphoproliferative syndrome, which is characterized by an abnormal immune response to Epstein-Barr virus (EBV) infection.[37] Acquired aplasia has occurred in siblings exposed to drugs[38] or viruses.[39] Increased representation of some class I (HLA-A2)[40] and class II (HLA-DR2, HLA-DR4, HLA-DPw3)[41,42] antigens among patients with acquired aplastic anemia has been reported.

Ionizing Radiation

Acute Exposure

Marrow aplasia is a major acute toxicity of radiation.[43–47] It is worth noting, however, that following the atomic bomb explosions over Hiroshima and Nagasaki, radiation accounted directly for only about 15% of the total casualties (burn and blast injuries predominating[48]) and that even in restricted episodes such as the Chernobyl reactor accident, most fatalities were the result of skin burns and damage to the gastrointestinal and pulmonary systems[49]; collateral local injuries, especially burns, also greatly complicate the management of pancytopenia.

Precisely how radiant energy damages cells is uncertain.[50,51] Radiant energy generates ions, peroxides, and free radicals. Radiation doses are defined in terms of ionization in tissue: 1 Gy equals absorbed energy equivalent to 1 J/kg of mass. Macromolecules such as DNA are damaged directly by large amounts of radiant energy, which can rupture covalent bonds, or indirectly, by interaction with highly charged and reactive small molecules resulting from ionization of free radicals formed in solution. That a round of replication is required for radiation damage to become manifest (except for lymphocytes) and that mitotically active tissue (such as bone marrow) is exquisitely radiosensitive strongly implicate DNA as the primary site of radiation damage. In atomic bomb explosions, γ-radiation has been the major effector of tissue damage, while α-, β-, γ-, and neutron emissions all figure to variable degrees in civilian accidents. Bone marrow cells are probably most affected by high-energy γ-rays, which penetrate the viscera, and only secondarily by ingested or absorbed α- and β-particles (low-energy β-particles burn but do not penetrate beyond the skin).

Cytotoxicity and bone marrow hypoplasia occur with radiation doses >1.5–2 Gy to the total body. Lethal exposure in animals begins at about 4 Gy, and whole-body exposures of 8 Gy are normally incompatible with survival[44] (Fig. 21-2). Experience with humans is more limited, fortunately, and determination of a median lethal dose (LD$_{50}$) depends on the quality of medical care applied. For the Hiroshima atomic bomb explosion, which effectively destroyed the medical support system, the LD$_{50}$ was estimated at 2.2–3.0 Gy.[52] However, the LD$_{50}$ has been estimated at about 4.5 from assessment of the outcome of radiation accidents and from the high-dose irradiation of patients with Ewing sarcoma, who were relatively few in number and all of whom had received more comprehensive medical support.[52–54] Animal studies used to extend the limited human data cannot be simply extrapolated to humans, first because interspecies differences in radiation sensitivity are large and second because of the substantial differences between controlled and accidental exposures. Physical structures and the body itself can create complicated patterns of shielding, and exposure is much more heterogeneous in accidental than in experimental irradiation.

It is at intermediate radiation doses around the LD$_{50}$ that bone marrow toxicity limits survival. Mitosis is much more sensitive to radiation than are the viability functions of a cell, and the dose-related occurrence of pancytopenia 2–4 weeks following a single large exposure is due to injury to the actively replicating pool of marrow progenitor and precursor cells. An exception is the lymphocyte, which is uniquely sensitive to radiation and is directly lysed by relatively low doses independent of its proliferative status. The ability to recover hematopoietic function following even massive single irradiation exposures is considerable, reflecting the resistance of the quiescent stem cell to damage and the enormous marrow-repopulating potential of even a greatly reduced stem cell pool. Autopsies of atomic bomb victims in Japan showed acellular bone marrows in persons dying within the first 2 weeks of the explosion, but regenerating marrow was frequently found in those who survived for 6 weeks.[55] Serial monitoring of blood counts provides a good measure of radiation dose. For atomic bomb victims exposure correlated with the degree of pancytopenia.[56] Lymphocytes are particularly sensitive to radiation, undergoing rapid changes in number and morphology. The rate of fall

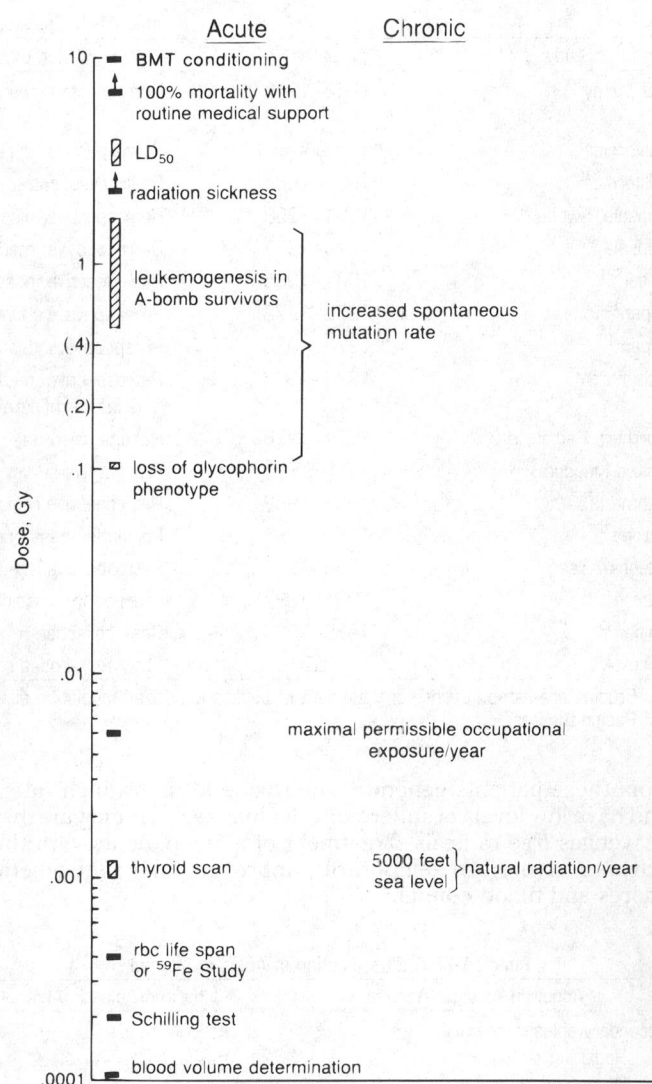

Fig. 21-2. Scale of biologic effects in humans of whole-body radiation doses. One gray (Gy) is a measure of absorbed dose equivalent to 1 J/kg unit mass (1 Gy = 100 rads). Radiation represents radiant energy. When absorbed into biologic tissue, radiant energy causes electron release and molecular ionization, which in turn results in further energy release. Radiant energy can directly break chemical bonds and indirectly damage macromolecules through generation of high-energy free-radical forms. The relationship between increased mutation rate and radiation dose is very approximate (hatched bars). Measurement of phenotype of an autosomal recessive gene such as glycophorin[731] would be expected to be a more sensitive indicator than frank malignant transformation, which is almost certainly a two-step process.

in lymphocyte numbers is a dose-related function of exposure to about 3 Gy of total body irradiation[43,56]; at higher doses, the fall in granulocytes and the severity of thrombocytopenia and reticulocytopenia can be used to estimate dose.[45–57]

Aplastic anemia, in contrast to acute leukemia, is not a late consequence of atomic bomb exposure or fallout.[58–60] Both single large doses and chronic radiation exposure result in prolonged depression of progenitor cell number and the self-renewing capacity of the stem cell compartment as a whole,[61] but the stem cells that survive radiation damage behave normally.[62] As is the case following other insults to the bone marrow, normal blood counts and normal marrow morphology can be maintained from a limited stem cell pool. Experiments using irradiation of single limbs in animals have suggested that the degree of injury to stromal cells, which are much less sensitive to irradiation (and may tolerate >40 Gy), ultimately may determine recovery in a localized region of marrow. "Second" waves of aplasia in irradiated limbs are presumably due to stromal failure. Late aplasia may not occur in whole-body exposures because the high doses that would ablate the stroma invariably produce more acute and fatal cutaneous, gastrointestinal, and neurologic damage.

Chronic Exposure

Repeated exposures to low doses of radiation are less damaging to stromal cells, which may tolerate 40–50 Gy of fractionated irradiation with some repair.[44] Continuous low-dose γ-irradiation produces aplasia in about 50% of exposed dogs after a total dose of 20 Gy.[61] Repeated low doses of radiation can damage human bone marrow and have been associated with aplastic anemia. Some dial painters in the luminous watch industry died of aplastic anemia,[63] and mesothorium that was injected rather than ingested (in the form of the contrast material thorotrast) produced iatrogenic aplasia, as well as acute leukemia and myelofibrosis, often decades after the injection, owing to the relentless destruction of marrow cells by the slowly disintegrating isotope.[64] Excessive numbers of deaths from aplastic anemia (and acute leukemia) have occurred after therapeutic irradiation of the spine for ankylosing spondylitis.[65] Excessive deaths from aplastic anemia and to a lesser degree from acute leukemia and multiple myeloma occurred among American radiologists who died between 1948 and 1961, presumably the victims of chronic exposure to γ-ray scatter.[66] While the distinction between aplastic anemia and myelodysplasia in some of the older reports is not reliable, it seems probable that chronic radiation exposure can cause accumulated stem cell injury, depletion of stem cells through continued recruitment from a quiescent reserve, or stromal injury.

Drugs and Chemicals

Drug or chemical exposure is the most frequently cited specific etiology for aplastic anemia in both clinical series of patients and epidemiologic surveys[67–72] (Tables 21-3 and 21-4 and Figs. 21-3 and 21-4). The agents cited vary with place and over time: benzene and chloramphenicol have been replaced by hydantoin and phenylbutazone with changing patterns of industrial exposure and choice of medications. While drugs and chemicals are commonly cited as causes of bone marrow failure, clear clinical associations have been established in very few instances, and relative risk has usually been overestimated. The literature on idiosyncratic reactions—cases reports and collections of cases—should be approached with skepticism. The data are often of poor quality, underlying mechanisms are seldom offered, and detection bias is an especially important problem. Patients with aplastic anemia are undoubtedly more closely questioned about potentially toxic exposures than individuals with other diseases. Interpretation of single cases is often confounded because many drugs are used in combination. The onset of marrow failure is notoriously difficult to date accurately and therefore to place temporally in relation to drug use; the delay in marrow disease following benzene use may be years or decades, and conversely there are trivial case reports of drug use virtually coincident with the onset of marrow failure. Association does not establish causality: some drugs may be preferentially employed in a patient population with an inherently high risk of marrow failure. It is remarkable that, in contrast to patients with idiopathic disease, aplastic anemia patients who have a history of drug or toxin exposure have identical demographic and clinical characteristics, a similar prognosis, and equivalent responses to therapy. In more formal studies (a European cooperative survey[73] and a small case-control study[74]), neither drug use nor chemical exposure figured significantly in a case-control study of aplastic anemia. Drug use has been calculated to account for only about 25% of the total cases of aplastic anemia.[75]

While the associations of some agents and marrow failure are convincing, being based on cumulative case reports and in some cases epidemiologic surveys, the estimated risk of aplastic anemia remains extremely small relative to the use of the drug. Quantitation of the probability of aplastic anemia with drug use has until recently been based on retrospective studies, in which cases are collected, drug use ascertained,

Table 21-3. Drug and Chemical Associations with Aplastic Anemia[a]

	Clinical Series									
	1950–1959		1960–1969		1970–1979		1980–1989		Far East 1970–1979	
Agent	No.	(%)	No.	(%)	No.	(%)	No.	(%)	No.	(%)
Chloramphenicol	227	(30)	90	(27)	194	(17)	28	(3)	626	(19)
Phenylbutazone	1	(<1)	30	(9)	67	(6)	22	(3)	81	(2)
Sulfonamides	27	(4)	3	(1)	13	(1)	5	(1)	42	(1)
Anticonvulsants	15	(2)	8	(2)	16	(2)	4	(<1)	35	(1)
Gold	0	(0)	3	(1)	12	(1)	12	(2)	11	(<1)
Benzene, solvents	24	(6)	14	(4)	37	(3)	21	(3)	95	(3)
Insecticides	9	(1)	29	(9)	15	(1)	11	(1)	122	(4)
Other drugs	118	(16)	26	(8)	169	(13)	60	(7)	451	(12)
Total drug cases	427	(57)	203	(60)	523	(45)	163	(20)	1,469	(43)
Total cases	756	(100)	339	(100)	1,292	(100)	811	(100)	3,391	(100)

	Epidemiologic Surveys			
Country	Dates	Design	No.	Drug Cases (%)
Israel	1961–1965	Nationwide, retrospective hospital survey	93	45[721]
Sweden	1964–1968	Provincial retrospective survey	80	28[218]
Japan	1970–1973	Nationwide survey	1,594	17[6]
England	1971–1978	Provincial retrospective survey	174	36[724]

[a] Data are derived from published collected series of adult patients in the United States, Europe, and Far East; dates indicate publication period.
(Data from Alter et al.,[732] with additional material from Heimpel and Heit[72] and for Far Eastern data, Abe and Komiya[733] (Japan), Whang[734] (Korea), and personal communication from S. Issaragrasil [Sirriraj Hospital, Thailand].)

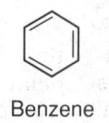

Benzene

Explosive

Trinitrotoluene

Pentachlorophenol

Wood preservative

insecticides

Chlordane

Lindane

Parathion

DDT

Antisyphilitic

Arsphenamine

Arsenamide

Antihelminthic

Antirheumatic

CH_2COONa
|
AuSCHCOONa

Gold sodium thiomalate

Fig. 21-3. Structure of some chemicals associated with aplastic anemia.

and calculations made on the basis of the amount of drug produced and an average dose; each of these procedures is prone to error. This method has been used to estimate the risk of aplastic anemia from a course of chloramphenicol at 1 in 20,000 to 1 in 60,000 on the assumptions of an average therapeutic course of 4 g.[76,77] On the basis of these figures, a course of chloramphenicol was estimated to increase the risk of aplastic anemia 13-fold. For quinacrine the risk has been estimated at 1 in 40,000 (a 10-fold increase over the control population)[78] and for phenylbutazone at 1 in 100,000 (a 5-fold increase).[79] In view of the nature of the data and the lack of rigor in the analysis, these numbers are probably not significantly different from each other and may not even be accurate within an order of magnitude. Furthermore, risk estimates based on more stringent case-control studies have often reduced the risk estimates substantially.

The distinction between regular and idiosyncratic reactions is useful but not absolute. Many drugs associated with idiosyncratic development of aplastic anemia are linked much more commonly with other forms of marrow suppression, for example, phenylbutazone and gold with neutropenia and chloramphenicol with reticulocytopenia. A low incidence of aplastic anemia may be a function of the doses commonly employed in clinical practice; at very high doses chloramphenicol, phenytoin, chlorpromazine, thiouracil, and methicillin all have been reported to produce reversible marrow depression in human subjects, and large doses of phenylbutazone have been reported to produce aplastic anemia in horses. Presumably, many other agents could be shown to affect marrow function at very high doses, were such doses attainable without toxicity to other organ systems. Some dose relationship probably exists even for idiosyncratic occurrences; there seems little likelihood that exquisitely small doses of drugs (e.g., a whiff of insecticide, an eyedrop of chloramphenicol) play a role in the development of aplastic anemia.[71] Dose-related and idiosyncratic marrow depression have only rarely been reported in the same person,[80] but it is reasonable to assume that at least one mechanism responsible for rare drug reactions is a meta-

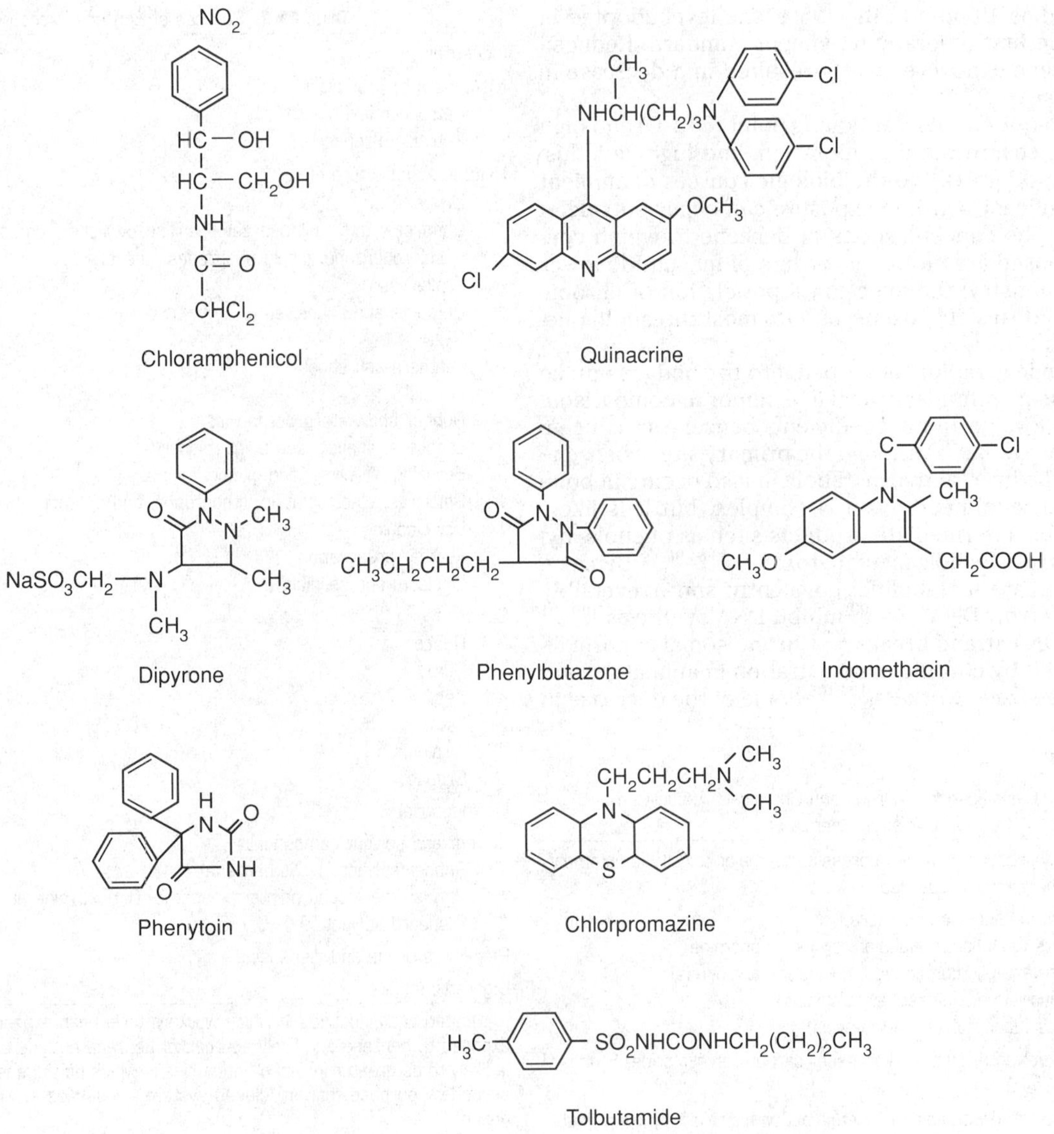

Fig. 21-4. Structure of some drugs associated with aplastic anemia.

bolic pathway that reproduces in the unusual individual the condition of excess drug administration. Similarly, the probability of developing aplastic anemia following a course of drug may be a quantitative reflection of the gene frequency for metabolic enzymes or histocompatibility types in the human population.

Cytotoxic Chemotherapy

Aplastic anemia is regularly produced by a chemically diverse group of drugs, the chemotherapeutic agents employed in the treatment of cancer.[81] Acute myelosuppression resulting from their use is dose dependent and predictable. In most cases they have relatively well-defined effects on fundamental cell processes, usually DNA replication but in some cases also RNA transcription, protein synthesis, or the mechanics of mitosis. While it is true that virtually all chemotherapeutic drugs exert dose-dependent myelotoxicity, higher doses are not well correlated with late or irreversible damage to stem cells. Some agents, such as busulfan, at doses that cause relatively limited immediate reductions in colony-forming unit-spleen (CFU-S) number and self-renewal capacity, can cause profound delayed depression of bone marrow and reduced marrow regenerative capacity. By contrast, 5-fluorouracil and cyclophosphamide appear to spare the regenerating cell population, and long-term administration of cyclophosphamide in animals does not reduce CFU-S number or repopulating ability. Late effects of chemotherapeutic agents are well documented in animal models of bone marrow failure, such as the latent aplastic anemia of the busulfan-treated mouse. The marrow of patients who have been subjected to chemotherapy is similarly damaged. Nevertheless, late frank marrow failure in humans as a result of cytotoxic chemotherapy is rare.[82]

Benzene

Benzene has been most convincingly linked to aplastic anemia by clinical and epidemiologic studies and by animal and in vitro data.[70,83] Enormous quantities of benzene are produced, employed in industry, released into the atmosphere, and found in the household.[69,84,85] The highest exposures are experienced by workers in the large number of industries that use benzene (Table 21-5); the number of American workers exposed has been estimated at 2 million.[84] The limit of benzene exposure was established as 10 ppm in the 1950s, the level adopted in the 1970s in the first federal government standard. Reduced industrial benzene exposure clearly resulted in a decrease in hematologic disease.[86-88]

Benzene is ubiquitous. Its low boiling point (80.1°C) and high vapor pressure ensure rapid evaporation, and fugitive industrial emissions add greatly to the biologic sources of ambient benzene.[84] Significant benzene exposure can occur outside of industry.[84,89,90] The concentrations of benzene to which consumers are exposed are, however, orders of magnitude lower than those in industry; the effect on a population of chronic exposure to low doses of benzene, as with most threshold phenomena, is unknown.[91]

Inhaled benzene is rapidly absorbed into the body[92]; uptake through mucous membranes and skin is minor in comparison. Because of its low partition coefficient, benzene is concentrated in the marrow fat[93]; although the primary site of benzene metabolism is the liver, active metabolism also occurs in bone marrow.[94,95] Benzene metabolism is complex, but it is likely that water-soluble intermediate products such as phenols, hydroquinones, and catechols mediate toxicity.[83,84,96-98] Benzene and its intermediate metabolites covalently and irreversibly bind to bone marrow DNA,[94,99,100] inhibit DNA synthesis,[100,101] and introduce DNA strand breaks.[102] Chromosomal abnormalities are produced by chronic administration in animals[103] and are present in benzene workers.[104,105] Some of the decrease in

Table 21-4. Classification of Drugs and Chemicals Associated with Aplastic Anemia

Agents that regularly produce marrow depression as major toxicity in commonly employed doses or normal exposures

Cytotoxic drugs used in cancer chemotherapy

Alkylating agents (busulfan, melphalan, cyclophosphamide)

Antimetabolites (antifolic compounds, nucleotide analogues)

Antimitotics (vincristine, vinblastine, colchicine)

Some antibiotics (daunorubicin, Adriamycin)

Benzene (and other solvents, such as kerosene, carbon tetrachloride, Stoddard solvent, chlorophenols)

Agents probably associated with aplastic anemia but with a relatively low probability relative to their use

Chloramphenicol

Insecticides

Antiprotozoals (quinacrine and chloroquine)

Nonsteroidal anti-inflammatory drugs (indomethacin, ibuprofen, sulindac, and others)

Anticonvulsants (hydantoins, carbamazapine, phenacemide)

Heavy metals (gold, arsenicals, bismuth, mercury)

Sulfonamides (antibiotics, antithyroid [methimazole, methylthiouracil], antidiabetes drugs [tolbutamide, chlorpropamide], carbonic anhydrase inhibitors [methazolamide])

D-penicillamine

Estrogens

Agents very rarely associated with aplastic anemia

Antibiotics (streptomycin, tetracycline, methicillin, mebendazole, griseofulvin, flucytosine)

Antihistamines (chlorpheniramine, cimetidine)

Sedatives and tranquilizers (chlorpromazine, prochlorperazine, piperacetazine, chlordiazepoxide, meprobamate, methyprylon)

Allopurinol (may potentiate marrow suppression by cytotoxic drugs)

Quinidine

Lithium carbonate

Guanidine

Potassium perchlorate

Thiocyanate

Carbimazole

(Based on review of primary references: 67, 68, 70, 72, 735–737.)

Table 21-5. Sources of Benzene Exposure[a]

Industrial[a]

Made as a by-product in

Petrochemical plants

Petroleum refineries

Used in manufacture of

Drugs

Chemicals (e.g., nitrobenzene, aniline, styrene, cumene, maleic anhydride, chlorobenzene, dichlorobenzenes, phenol)

Explosives

Cements and adhesives

Dyes

Leathers and shoes

Enamel

Rubber and waterproof fabrics

Lacquers, shellac, and paint thinners

Bronzing, silvering, and gilding liquids

Batteries, electroplating, lithography, and photography

Dry cleaning

Feather preparation

Linoleum and celluloid

Solvent for

Rubber

Gum

Resins

Fats

Alkaloids

Grease

Nonindustrial

Solvent and solvent component

Rubber solvent (1.5% benzene)

Varnish maker and painters' naphtha (0.1%), mineral spirits

Stoddard solvent (0.1–0.7%)

Gasoline storage and dispensing

Cigarette smoke

[a] Listed are industries in which workers have been exposed or continue to be exposed to benzene and likely sources of benzene outside of industry. Exposure is likely to be greater in "open" industries in which benzene is employed for some secondary purpose than in "closed system" industries in which benzene is produced.

cell proliferation that has frequently been measured in vitro and in animals could result from any number of indirect effects on cell function, such as irreversible protein binding, as well as from direct action on DNA.[106,107]

Administration of benzene to animals produces bone marrow depression.[69,84] However, there are practical difficulties in reproducing the route and duration of typical industrial exposure. The metabolism of benzene varies among animal species[108,109] and tissues.[95,108] In general, benzene administration to animals decreases marrow cell proliferation. Acutely, the more mature, mitotically active marrow precursor cells are preferentially damaged compared with more primitive progenitors, but marked depression of CFU-erythroid (CFU-E), CFU-granulocyte macrophage (CFU-GM), burst-forming unit-erythroid (BFU-E), and CFU-S can be measured within days.[110-114] Intermittent exposure is more damaging to stem cell number than continuous exposure.[113,115] The stroma is also damaged by benzene, and marrow from chronically exposed mice does not support in vitro long-term hematopoiesis.[116-118] In benzene-treated mice, CFU-S-derived colonies fail to implant,[113] and physically extirpated marrow will not regenerate.[119] Benzene adversely affects macrophage support of hematopoiesis in vitro.[120] Benzene has other diverse effects on the immune system, depleting lymphocyte numbers and suppressing lymphocyte function.[121,122] In vitro, low concentrations of benzene are mildly stimulatory of myeloid colony number, while benzene metabolites are strongly inhibitory, results perhaps consistent with the leukocytosis and marrow hypercellularity seen in the early stages of human and animal benzene poisoning.[123]

The range of hematologic disease attributable to benzene is quite broad, from relatively common alterations in blood counts to aplastic anemia or hematologic malignancy.[124-128] The risk of aplastic anemia is 3-4% in workers exposed to benzene concentrations >300 ppm. One-half of the people exposed to 100 ppm show some blood count depression. The prevalence of some form of marrow suppression in heavily exposed workers can still be astonishingly high: >10% of workers surveyed in China in the 1950s developed leukopenia; with improved hygiene the figure was lowered to 0.5%, a proportion that still represented >2,000 cases in 500,000 workers.[129] The incidence of aplastic anemia in one group of Chinese shoemakers was estimated to be increased sixfold over that in the general population (there was a 2% prevalence of aplastic anemia in a single factory).[129] In 217 apparently healthy Turkish shoe factory workers, 25% had some combination of leukopenia, thrombocytopenia, and/or pancytopenia.[130] Leukopenia,[128] thrombocytopenia,[130] and anemia,[126] and lymphocytopenia have all been cited as the most frequent hematologic consequences of benzene. Other manifestations include macrocytosis, acquired Pelger-Huët anomaly, eosinophilia, basophilia, elevated fetal hemoglobin, and, more rarely, polycythemia, leukocytosis, thrombocytosis, and splenomegaly.[127,128,131,132] The marrow of healthy workers is usually normocellular but may show moderate hypo- or hypercellularity.[128] The predictive value of abnormal blood counts is uncertain: the borderline values of workers exposed to benzene followed in one large clinic returned to normal, despite continued exposure to benzene,[127] and one-half of 44 patients with pancytopenia in another series completely recovered.[133] Chronic benzene exposure also clearly increases the risk of developing acute myeloid leukemia[134] and a variety of lymphohematopoietic malignancies.[135,136] Both aplastic anemia and acute leukemia in benzene workers can manifest decades after exposure, but, as with the after effects of irradiation, malignancy may be the more frequent late consequence. Cumulative benzene exposure best correlates with the risk of acute leukemia and probably is an important variable for marrow failure also.

Other Aromatic Hydrocarbons

The common perception that other compounds resembling benzene in structure or containing a benzene ring might also cause marrow suppression is not well supported. Neither the closely related alkylbenzenes[137] nor pure toluene and xylenes[138,139] are marrow toxins. The total number of bone marrow failure cases reported following aromatic hydrocarbon exposure is small, considering the very large populations exposed to this heterogeneous group of chemicals. In the case of insecticides, for example, surveys of aplastic anemia patients found only 2-6%[68,73,140] of cases associated with insecticide exposure, and the significance of a handful of case reports in the context of vast use is dubious.[141] Perhaps their visibly lethal effect on insects has created a prejudice; it is worth recalling that insecticides were associated with far fewer cases of pancytopenia reported to the American Medical Association Drug Registry than were tetracyclines and penicillins.[142]

Case reports greatly outnumber series of patients. Twenty-four aplastic anemia cases reported for the British explosives industry in two world wars were attributed to trinitrotoluene.[143] Dinitrophenol used to effect weight reduction,[144] pen-

tachlorophenol used as a wood preservative,[145] and substituted aromatic hydrocarbons employed in the wood pulp industry[146] have also been associated with a few cases of aplasia. Only 14 cases of aplasia related to hair dyes could be collected in 1985 despite their abundant use.[147] Heavy insecticide exposure was implicated in 16 of 20 cases of aplastic anemia. Insecticides were implicated in the high incidence of the disease in Mexico[148] and were blamed for aplasia in children in California,[149] among heavily exposed professional users in Germany,[150] and in agricultural workers in Brazil.[151] In 1967, however, only 44 cases could be collected from the literature.[150] The most frequently cited insecticides in these case reports and summaries are chlordane,[152,153] lindane,[150,154-156] or these products in combination with DDT.[156-160]

The results of systematic epidemiologic surveys of users of aromatic hydrocarbons are mixed. British Columbia farmers had a statistically significant increase in mortality, with most of the increase occurring within a single 10-year period.[161] In a special study the U.S. Census Bureau coded the usual occupation and industry from 1975 death certificates for four rare diseases, including aplastic anemia; job exposure matrices, which allowed cross-classification of employment with agents found in industries, were then used to measure chemical exposure as a variable for disease.[162] Significant numbers of aplastic anemia cases were found in employees in printing and publishing, lumber and wood products manufacturing, agriculture, and construction, but neither pesticide nor wood preservative exposures were significantly associated with the development of aplastic anemia. Neutropenia was correlated with insecticide exposure among Canadian apple pickers and exposed residents.[163] However, most other surveys of pesticide makers or heavy users[164-167] and farmers[168-171] have failed to show an increased mortality rate due to aplastic anemia, even though these workers have detectable blood levels of pesticide.[172]

Some organophosphate insecticides depress rodent blood counts and inhibit hematopoietic colony formation in vitro.[173,174]

Chloramphenicol

The first published case of aplastic anemia associated with chloramphenicol was reported in 1950, followed by such an explosion of case reports that the Food and Drug Administration collected several hundred cases within a few years.[175,176] A still more remarkable feature of chloramphenicol was that, in contrast to most other agents associated with marrow suppression, its most common hematologic toxicity was pancytopenia, frequently fatal. Most patients died, and a few of the survivors developed acute leukemia.[177,178] (Leukemia also occurred independently of aplastic anemia.[179]) From 1949 to 1952 47% of 296 cases of aplastic anemia collected were associated with prior chloramphenicol use[176]; from 1952 to 1954, following much adverse publicity, 15% of 607 patients were found to have had prior exposure.[175] However, chloramphenicol use rebounded, and the drug continued to be the one most frequently associated with aplastic anemia for several decades. In clinical series, chloramphenicol use was associated with 20-30% of total cases and one-half of drug-associated cases; in epidemiologic surveys in California in the early 1960s, chloramphenicol was associated with the great majority of drug-related cases of aplastic anemia.[76,77] With narrowing indications for the use of chloramphenicol, aplastic anemia associated with its use has almost disappeared. In nearly 200 patients with acquired aplastic anemia studied at the National Institutes of Health from 1978 to 1989, we have obtained only a single history of (distant) chloramphenicol exposure. The International Agranulocytosis and Aplastic Anemia Study failed to find chloramphenicol use in any of 135 patients with aplastic anemia (in 1980–1986 in Europe and Israel).[180] While medical use of the drug has substantially diminished, it has not disappeared, especially in surgical services[181] and eye clinics,[182] and it has occasionally been detected in the muscle tissue of animals brought to slaughter.[183]

During the period of unrestrained use, chloramphenicol was considered the most common cause of aplastic anemia in the United States. While its introduction into the American market was perceived as having increased the total number of cases of bone marrow failure,[140,184] this assumption was only weakly supported by epidemiologic data.[77] Nor was the fall in chloramphenicol use in Japan[185] and Sweden[186] associated with a decrease in the incidence of aplastic anemia, and where chloramphenicol continues to be popular, associated aplastic anemia is either infrequent[187,188] or may even have declined since its introduction (Colombia[189]). Perhaps chloramphenicol affects a subpopulation prone to drug effects on the bone marrow, and only the rapid introduction and popularity of the antibiotic led to its recognition as a dramatic destructive agent. Genetic susceptibility is supported by the appearance of aplasia in family members treated with chloramphenicol.[190,191]

The dose relationship of chloramphenicol to aplastic anemia has never been satisfactorily resolved. The earliest publications stressed excessive dosage, often given in repeated or intermittent courses, and included a high proportion of children, who may not metabolize the drug efficiently; in a later collection of nearly 600 cases, however, most patients had received less than a 10-g dose.[192] In most patients the duration between exposure and onset of symptoms has been brief, around 2 months, and the culpability of chloramphenicol administered years prior to the appearance of aplastic anemia seems low. A dose relationship is also suggested by the occurrence of anemia, leukopenia, or pancytopenia with the therapeutic,[193] accidental,[194] or experimental[195,196] administration of extremely large amounts of chloramphenicol, usually >40 g; these blood changes are reversible but have been fatal in some cases.[80] Hematologic toxicity has been associated with high blood levels[196] and delayed clearance of chloramphenicol, due either to failure of the liver to conjugate the drug or to poor renal excretion.[197] The bioavailability of chloramphenicol is higher following administration of the palmitate (the form of chloramphenicol in oral suspensions given to children) than in the free base formulation of pills and is lowest after injection of the succinate salt parenterally[198] (although the rarity of cases following intravenous dosing may simply be a function of the relative infrequency of parenteral use[199]).

At the usual therapeutic doses, a stereotypical pattern of reversible alterations in erythropoiesis occurs in virtually every patient treated with chloramphenicol.[200] Suppression of erythropoiesis is probably secondary to drug inhibition of mitochondrial protein synthesis, especially of enzymes important in heme synthesis (e.g., ferrochelatase, which catalyzes the insertion of iron into protoporphyrin[201]); other enzymes that are inhibited include cytochrome oxidase, cytochrome b, and an ATPase.[202] The typical vacuolization of erythroblasts after chloramphenicol exposure represents mitochondria with condensed and fragmented matrices.[203] Increased iron utilization and reticulocytopenia may occur earlier in patients than in normal volunteers because of their increased erythropoietic activity.[204] Suppression of erythropoiesis has never been correlated with the later occurrence of aplastic anemia.[205]

Chloramphenicol can inhibit in vitro hematopoietic colony formation,[206–210] but usually at doses greater than those achieved in patients; inhibition of marrow stromal cell proliferation[211] and production of growth factors[212] has also been reported. Chloramphenicol also suppresses some lymphocyte

functions,[213] and karyotype abnormalities have been described in a few cases of chloramphenicol-associated aplasia.[213] Marrow cells from affected patients are resistant to chloramphenicol toxicity, perhaps because they have survived a drug insult.[214]

Nonsteroidal Anti-Inflammatory Drugs

Nonsteroidal anti-inflammatory drugs been most frequently employed in the treatment of rheumatologic syndromes; other therapies (gold and penicillamine) have also been associated with aplastic anemia. Neutropenia is far more common than pancytopenia as a hematologic toxicity associated with phenylbutazone.[215,216]

The prevalence of association with aplastic anemia may be lower for phenylbutazone than for chloramphenicol. In England, mortality figures of 1–6 per 100,000 treated patients were calculated[79]; other estimates have ranged from 1 in 100,000 to 1 in 1 million treatment courses, the uncertainty as usual being due to the number of treatment courses.[217,218] Other nonsteroidal anti-inflammatory drugs, including aspirin, have occasionally been associated with aplastic anemia.[219] The large case-control investigation conducted by the International Agranulocytosis and Aplastic Anemia Study not only confirmed the association of aplastic anemia with phenylbutazone but identified even higher risks following the use of other nonsteroidal anti-inflammatory drugs (equivalent to excess risks of 10.1 per million for indomethacin, 6.8 per million for diclofenac, and 6.6 per million for the butazones).[220] There was some suggestion of increased risk for drugs taken regularly over a prolonged period. Many of the early cases of butazone-associated aplasia had been treated with very high doses.[216] As with chloramphenicol, hematologic toxicity has been associated with decreased clearance rates.[221] In vitro hematopoietic colony formation in marrow cells obtained from patients with drug-associated neutropenia was shown to be abnormally sensitive to phenylbutazone,[222] but these studies suffer from the common defect of poor controls.

Neuroleptic Drugs

A variety of anticonvulsants have been associated with aplastic anemia, especially the hydantoins and carbamazapine, as well as antidepressants and tranquilizers. Many of these compounds are also associated with neutropenia and agranulocytosis. Carbamazapine (Tegretol), a tricyclic compound structurally related to imipramine, is of particular interest. Laboratory studies of carbamazapine implicated sensitivity of a patient's cells to a toxic metabolic intermediate of the drug.[223] Carbamazapine in the schizophrenic population was associated with frequently fatal aplastic anemia in about 6 case reports during the 1960s.[224] More demanding regimens for monitoring patients' blood counts were recommended by the manufacturer and then disseminated in the *Physicians' Desk Reference* beginning in 1969 and in standard pharmacology textbooks. The cost of hematologic monitoring was estimated to far exceed that of the drug itself.[225] Monitoring regimens were recommended despite the <24 total cases reported by 1982,[226] doubt about the validity of many cases in the literature,[227] multiple large series of patients without hematologic toxicity,[225,228] and an estimated aplastic anemia case rate of about 1 in 200,000 treated patients.[225,229] Routine monitoring is costly and inconvenient and often leads to diagnostic confusion with modest leucopenia, which commonly occurs. Even advocates of hematologic monitoring acknowledge that all cases will not be prevented by the procedure and that the management of modestly depressed granulocyte and platelet numbers is uncertain.[230] Many authorities no longer recommend routine hematologic monitoring[228,231-233] or suggest monitoring with considerable latitude for clinical judgment and common sense.[233,234]

Gold and Other Heavy Metals

Gold salts have been associated with an extraordinarily high frequency of fatal adverse reactions, estimated at 1.6 per 10,000 prescriptions. Dose-dependent neutropenia is common, but several dozen cases of aplastic anemia have also been reported.[235,236] Gold has been demonstrated in the bone marrow by electron microscopy.[237] Bone marrow failure has also been associated in the past with the use of inorganic and organic (hydrocarbon) arsenic compounds, and with mercury and bismuth compounds. Chelation therapy does not reverse gold aplasia, but patients have been successfully treated with bone marrow transplantation[238] and immunosuppression.[239-241] High concentrations of gold salts inhibit hematopoietic colony formation in vitro,[242] and there is some evidence for a dose relationship.[243]

Drug Metabolism and Toxic Reactive Intermediate Compounds

Many drugs and chemicals, especially if they have limited water solubility, must be enzymatically degraded before conjugation and excretion. Degradative pathways for xenobiotics, such as most drugs and chemicals, are complex, specific, redundant, and interrelated (Fig. 21-5). Polar groups are added to some aromatic hydrocarbons by phase I enzymes, part of the cytochrome P-450 mitochondrial system; these metabolites become the substrates for phase II enzyme systems, which add glucuronide, sulfate, acetate, or glycine moieties to increase water solubility and permit excretion. Other xenobiotics are directly metabolized by addition of methyl or acetyl groups. Intermediate compounds, especially arene oxides, are often very electrophilic and therefore highly reactive with macromolecules, especially DNA.[244]

Toxic intermediate molecules are difficult to study because they may be produced in relatively small concentrations by a minor metabolic pathway, and they are intrinsically unstable. Metabolic pathways in other species, especially rodents, are often quite different from those in humans. The rarity of idiosyncratic responses requires large numbers of animals or normal humans to detect a metabolic defect. The four detoxifying enzyme systems described below have been chosen because they are directly applicable to bone marrow failure and also demonstrate genetic variability.

Aryl Hydrocarbon Hydroxylase

Aromatic hydrocarbons are metabolized by the P-450 enzyme system, a microsomal catalytic group of monooxygenases that are inducible by specific substrates.[245] Metabolism to reactive intermediates by the cytochrome P-450 monooxygenases appears to be required for mutagenesis, carcinogenesis, and toxicity of many aromatic compounds. The *Ah* locus in the mouse regulates the induction of numerous drug-metabolizing enzymes, of which aryl hydrocarbon hydroxylase is most easily measured. Aryl hydrocarbon hydroxylase can be induced by polycyclic aromatic hydrocarbons in wild mice that bear the *Ah^b* locus, which encodes a cytosolic receptor for the aromatic hydrocarbon. Unresponsive *Ah^d* animals develop aplastic anemia when they ingest benzo[a]pyrene, while responsive animals with a functioning *Ah* gene are resistant. Animals can be protected against marrow failure by phenobarbital, which induces drug-conjugating enzyme activities,[246] and α-napthoflavone, which inhibits P-450 metabolism. In vitro, *Ah^b/Ah^b* myeloid cells are paradoxically more sensitive than *Ah^d/Ah^d* cells to benzo[a]pyrene, probably because they themselves generate toxic metabolites more efficiently. In intact *Ah^b/Ah^b* animals, the marrow is protected by first-pass detoxification of metabolites in the intestine and liver, while large concentrations of unaltered hydrocarbon reach the marrow of *Ah^d/Ah^d* animals.

Most of the chemicals and drugs implicated in human aplastic anemia are probably metabolized by similar P-450 enzyme systems. Genetic variation in chemical metabolism and detoxification in the liver and gut and generation of toxic intermediates in the bone marrow would be predicted to correlate with susceptibility of hematopoietic tissue to chemical damage. Fibroblasts of patients with aplastic anemia form benzo[a]pyrene-DNA adducts more readily than normal subjects, but the levels of these adducts are within the normal range.[247]

Epoxide Hydrolases

One mechanism of detoxification of arene oxides is conversion of epoxides to phenols, a function of a large and poorly defined system of epoxide hydroxylases. These enzymes are substrate specific, and their activity varies widely among individuals and ethnic groups. Epoxide hydroxylase activity has been measured indirectly by generating reactive intermediates in vitro from a test compound by use of rat hepatic microsomes and then testing these intermediates for cytotoxicity against lymphocytes; the patient's cells serve as a source of the detoxifying enzyme and as a marker for the effect of the toxic intermediates. This system has identified individuals susceptible to phenytoin hepatotoxicity and birth defects. In a patient who had recovered from phenytoin-associated aplastic anemia, there was dose-dependent killing of the patient's lymphocytes, no toxicity for normal donors' cells, and intermediate killing of cells from the patient's mother.[223] The patient's cells were unaffected by the drug alone or by the metabolites generated from closely related compounds.

S-Methylation

Methylation is an important step in the metabolism of many drugs, chemicals, and neurotransmitters.[248] Thiopurine methyltransferase catalyzes the S-methylation of 6-mercaptopurine, 6-thioguanine, and azathioprine. The activity of this enzyme can be measured in erythrocytes, and population and family studies have shown a pattern of inheritance of a single genetic locus, with estimated gene frequencies of 94% for high enzyme activity (TPMT^H) and 6% for low (TPMT^L). Most individuals have high (89%) or intermediate (11%) levels of activity, but those homozygous for TPMT^L, who represent only 0.03% of the population, have undetectable enzyme, and it is these individuals who, on treatment with azathioprine or 6-mercaptopurine accumulate intracellular 6-thioguanine, a purine analogue that can be incorporated into DNA. 6-Thioguanine levels were elevated in the red blood cells of patients with thiopurine-induced myelosuppression.[249,250] Enzyme levels were undetectable in two of three patients with hematologic complications of azathioprine and intermediate in the third.[251]

N-Acetylation

N-acetyltransferase activity is inherited as an autosomal recessive trait.[252] Acetylation rates vary greatly among the races; fast acetylation is far more frequent among Orientals than among whites. Acetylation phenotypes have been associated with isoniazid failure in tuberculosis (fast), drug-induced lupus

Model

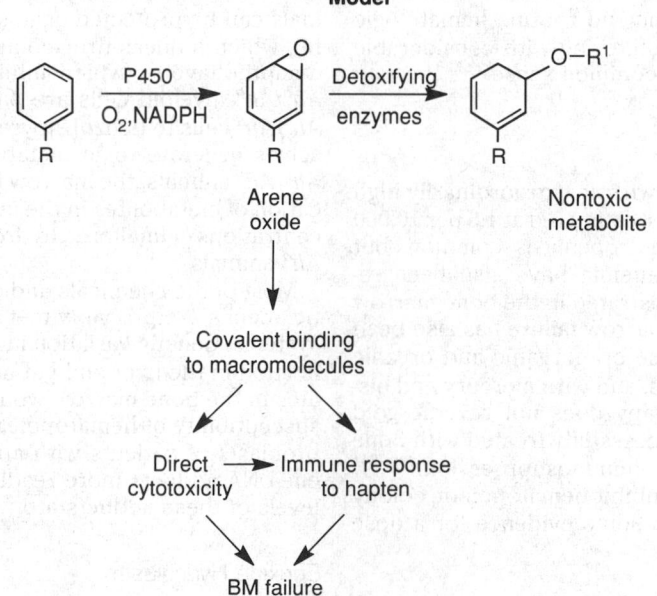

Arene oxide → Covalent binding to macromolecules

Direct cytotoxicity ← → Immune response to hapten

BM failure

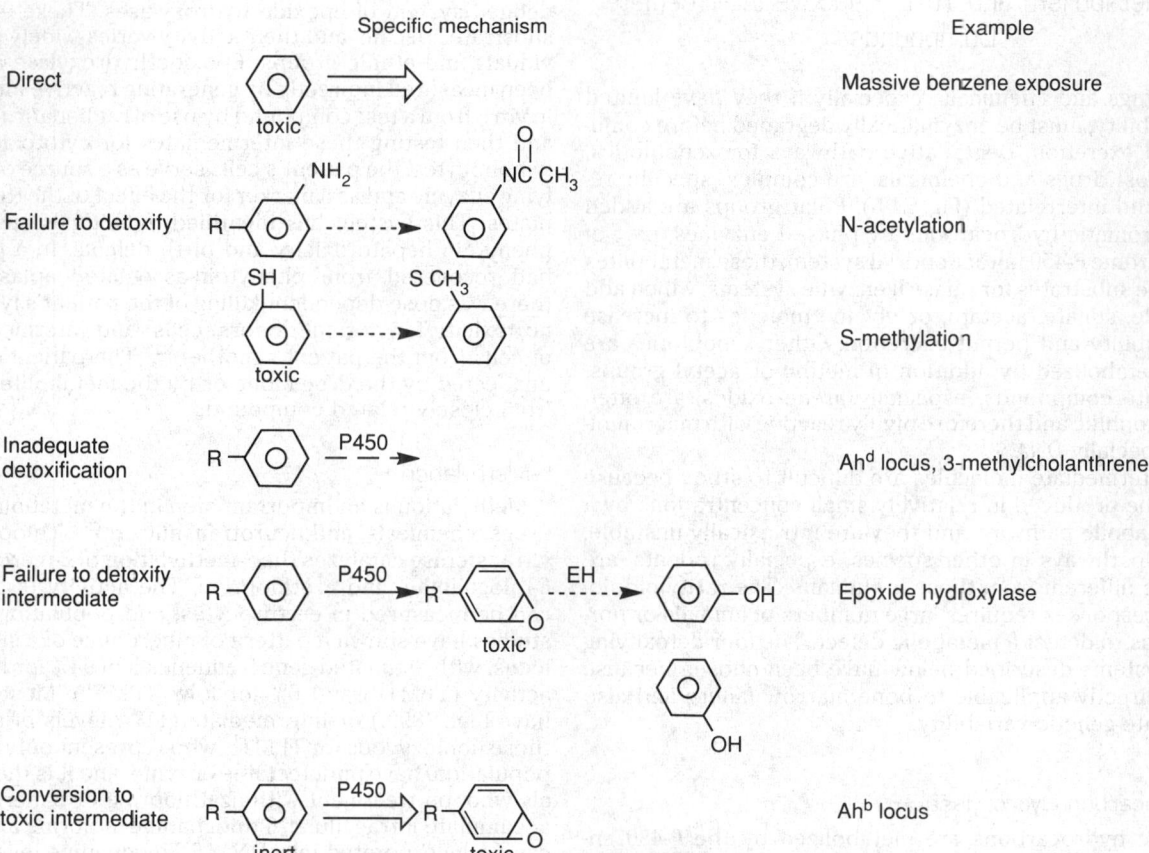

Fig. 21-5. A general model for the generation of toxic intermediate metabolites and some specific mechanisms, with examples of chemical- or drug-mediated toxicity.

erythematosus, leprosy, and bladder cancer (slow). The association of sulfonamide toxicity with the slow acetylation phenotype is strong.[253] Under these circumstances sulfonamide drugs may be shunted away from the acetylation detoxification pathway to a cytochrome P-450 pathway, with generation of a toxic intermediate such as a hydroxylamine. N-acetylation is also a major metabolic pathway of procainamide, which can

be further processed to a toxic hydroxylamine intermediate. Slow acetylation may protect against drug-induced lupus.[254]

Chloramphenicol Metabolism

No biochemical explanation for chloramphenicol-associated aplastic anemia is satisfactory; the precise toxic intermediates involved, mechanisms of cellular damage, and basis of rare individual susceptibility are unknown. Thiamphenicol, in which the *p*-nitro group is replaced by a methylsulfonyl group, was originally thought to be a nontoxic relative of chloramphenicol, but it has been associated with at least six cases of irreversible aplastic anemia,[255] a frequency of serious marrow failure that may be only proportional to its use. Both chloramphenicol and thiamphenicol cause dose-related reversible suppression of erythropoiesis in patients, and both similarly inhibit hematopoietic colony formation.[214] However, these drugs are relatively nontoxic against mammalian cells. Although the cellular uptake and metabolism of chloramphenicol and thiamphenicol differ, neither is concentrated in the bone marrow. Yunis and colleagues[257] have shown that nitrosochloramphenicol (in which the *p*-nitro group has been reduced to the nitroso form) can efficiently degrade isolated[256] and cellular DNA. However, the nitroso derivative is not made in the bone marrow and has a very brief half-life. Dehydrochloramphenicol, another toxic metabolite, is produced by gut bacteria[258]; individual susceptibility is hypothesized to be due to differences in intestinal bacteria, clearance of toxic metabolites, or hematopoietic cell sensitivity. Others have proposed that chloramphenicol toxicity is due to covalent binding to cellular proteins of reactive oxidative metabolites, to an oxalic acid derivative produced by P-450 cytochrome-mediated oxidative dehalogenation, or to an inability to produce a chloramphenicol free radical and hydroxylamine intermediate, all capable of acylating proteins.[259,260]

Viruses

Temporary depression of blood counts is frequently observed during common viral infections.[261] Virus species of many different families are capable of infecting human bone marrow cells and inducing damage either by direct cytotoxicity or by invoking a pathophysiologic host immune response (Table 21-6). Evidence exists for several mechanisms of virus-hematopoietic cell interactions that probably apply to human disease (Fig. 21-6).

Parvovirus

B19 parvovirus infection is more closely related clinically to pure red cell aplasia than to aplastic anemia, but of all the viruses its interaction with hematopoietic cells and the immune system is best understood[262] (Fig. 21-7). The Parvoviridae, which are small, single-stranded DNA viruses, are common animal pathogens. Feline panleukopenia virus was the first virus experimentally demonstrated to cause disease in animals; this virus infects cat hematopoietic and lymphocytic cells and causes fatal neutropenia.[263] The first parvovirus shown to cause human disease was only discovered in 1975. Acute infection with B19 parvovirus (named from the blood bank code for the donor from whom the virus was isolated) causes childhood exanthem fifth disease (erythema infectiosum) (Fig. 21-8).[264,265] Children with fifth disease are usually not very ill, but the characteristic rash (the "slapped cheek" facial erythema and a lacy, reticular, evanescent maculopapular eruption over the trunk and proximal extremities), combined with extreme contagion, is diagnostic for individuals and in epidemics. Adults with fifth disease more commonly suffer joint pains or frank arthritis than a rash, and symptoms that mimic rheumatoid arthritis can occasionally persist for months and even years.[266,267]

Transient Aplastic Crisis

In persons with an underlying hemolytic disorder, acute parvovirus infection causes transient aplastic crisis, which is an abrupt cessation of erythropoiesis characterized by reticulocytopenia, absence of marrow erythroid precursors, and precipitous worsening of anemia (Fig. 21-8). The aregenerative quality of the anemic crisis was first recognized in patients with hereditary spherocytosis and other forms of hemolysis.[268,269] Owren[269] introduced the term aplastic crisis and stressed the relationship of anemic crisis to preceding infection and the temporary nature of red cell failure. Transient aplastic crisis occurs in patients with sickle cell disease, erythrocyte membrane defects, enzymopathies, and thalassemias, under circumstances of erythroid stress (such as hemorrhage and iron deficiency), and following bone marrow transplantation. In retrospect, parvovirus infection was almost certainly responsible for cases of transient erythropoietic failure that were blamed on kwashiorkor, folate deficiency, some drugs (especially immunosuppressive agents), and a variety of bacterial infections. It is not accidental that many of the reported cases of aplastic crisis occurred in hospitalized patients, as the virus is easily transmitted nosocomially to patients[270] (as well as to hospital personnel[271] and in blood products[272]).

The patient with an aplastic crisis may be profoundly ill due to the severity of the anemia; symptoms can include not only dyspnea and fatigue but extreme lassitude, confusion, and congestive heart failure. An aplastic crisis may be the first evidence of an underlying compensated hemolytic disorder.[273,274] The crisis is readily treated by blood transfusion but can be fatal. Transient aplastic crisis,[275–277] as well as experimental parvovirus infection in humans,[278] is often associated with variable degrees of neutropenia and thrombocytopenia; rarely, bone marrow necrosis may be present.[279] Transient pancytope-

Table 21-6. Viruses that Infect Bone Marrow Cells[a]

Virus Family	Animal Model	In Vitro Target	Human Disease
Parvovirus	Feline panleukopenia virus (FePV)	FePV: hematopoietic progenitors, lymphocyte	Transient aplastic crisis
			Pure red cell aplasia
		B19:CFU-E, BFU-E	Nonimmune hydrops fetalis
Herpesvirus	Murine cytomegalovirus	CMV: fibroblast, hematopoietic progenitors(?)	Post-bone marrow transplant
		EBV: lymphocyte, macrophage, BFU-E(?)	Infectious mononucleosis-AA
Flavivirus	Bovine viral diarrhea	Dengue fever: macrophage, hematopoietic progenitors	Hematodepressive diseases
			Hepatitis C-AA(?)
Retrovirus	Feline leukemia virus (FeLV)	FeLV: BFU-E	Acquired immunodeficiency syndrome
	Friend Leukemia virus (FLV)	FLV: CFU-E	
		HIV: macrophage, megakaryocyte	

Abbreviations: CFU-E, colony-forming unit erythroid; BFU-E, burst-forming unit erythroid; HIV, human immunodeficiency virus; EBV, Epstein-Barr virus.
[a] For references, see text and also individual reviews in Young.[738]

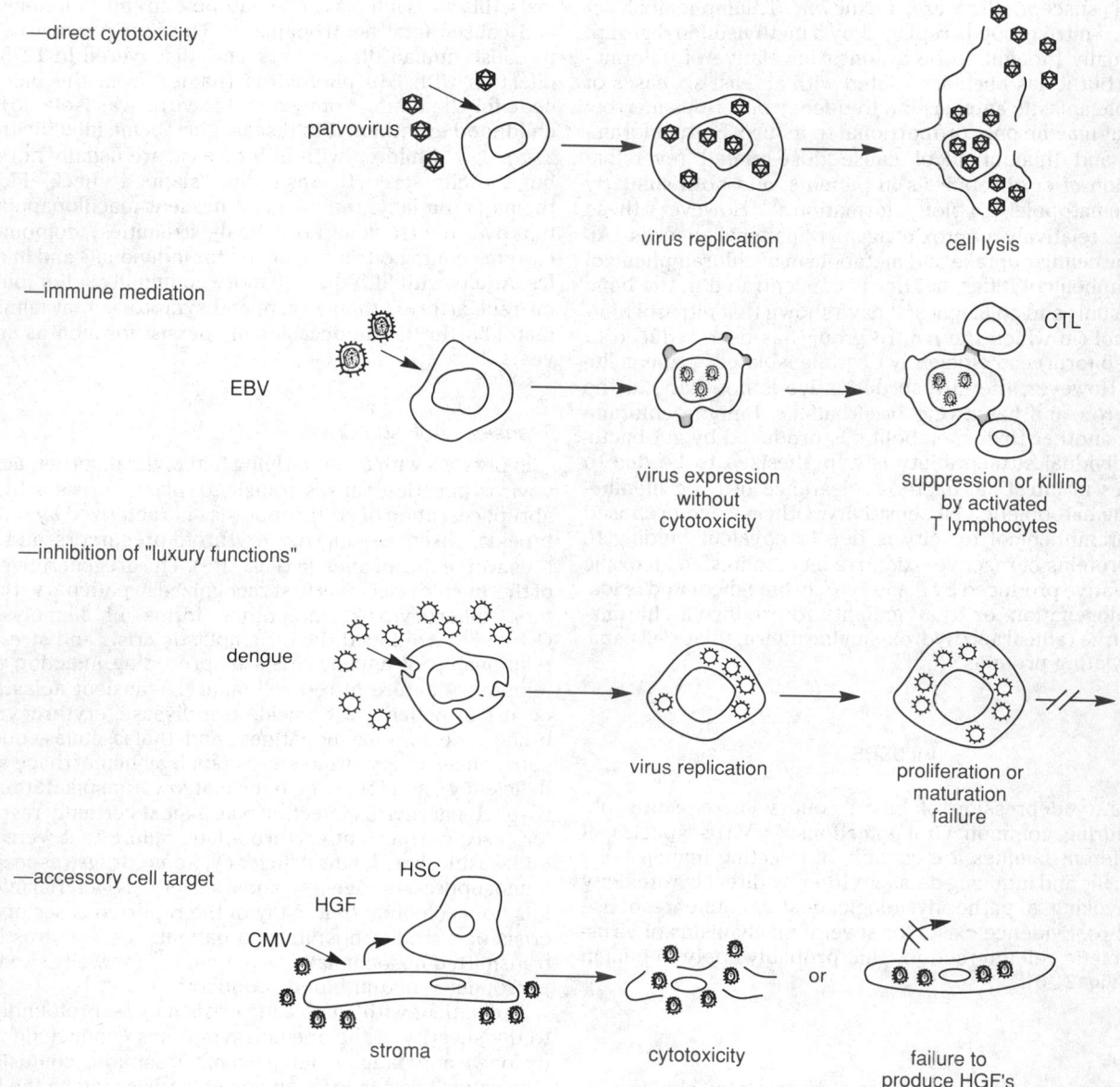

Fig. 21-6. Mechanisms of virus-mediated bone marrow failure; the four models are not mutually exclusive. In parvovirus infection, direct cytotoxicity for a progenitor cell dominates. For Epstein-Barr virus (and perhaps also other herpesviruses such as cytomegalovirus), viral infection of hematopoietic cells is postulated to be noncytotoxic, but the immune response to viral antigens targets the stem cell for suppression or destruction by cytotoxic lymphocytes. Flavivirus infection is also noncytotoxic, but in addition to provoking a cellular immune response, the virus infection itself alters the growth properties of the host hematopoietic cell. Cytomegalovirus probably infects stromal fibroblasts and disturbs hematopoiesis by altering the function of supporting accessory cells.

nia[280,281] and a case of typical severe aplastic anemia[282] have been reported to follow acute parvovirus infection.

Community-acquired aplastic crisis is almost always due to parvovirus infection.[273,283,284] B19 parvovirus should be the presumptive diagnosis in transient aplastic crisis and should be sought in any patient with anemia due to an abrupt cessation of erythropoiesis. Patients with transient aplastic crisis are often viremic at presentation, with concentrations of viral genomes as high as 10^{14}/ml as determined by DNA dot blot hybridization of serum.[285,286] Immunoglobulin M antibody appears during the first week of convalescence and is a specific indicator of recent infection.[287] IgG antibody to parvovirus is present in about 50% of the adult population. Both IgG and IgM antibodies to parvovirus can be measured,[287,288] but these tests have not been generally available because of the limited

amounts of antigen recoverable from infected sera; expression of recombinant empty capsids in baculovirus systems should remedy the antigen shortage[289] and also provide a vaccine reagent.[290] Immunoglobulin assays are not useful in cases of persistent infection.

Hydrops Fetalis Due to B19 Parvovirus

In utero infection is a cause of nonimmune hydrops fetalis, in which death occurs as a result of severe anemia.[291] Hydropic infants born of mothers infected with parvovirus show leukoerythroblastosis, iron deposition in the liver, and viral cytopathic alterations of erythroblasts in the liver. Virus has been demonstrated in liver cells.[292,293] The risk of a fatal fetal outcome is probably greatest when infection occurs during the first two

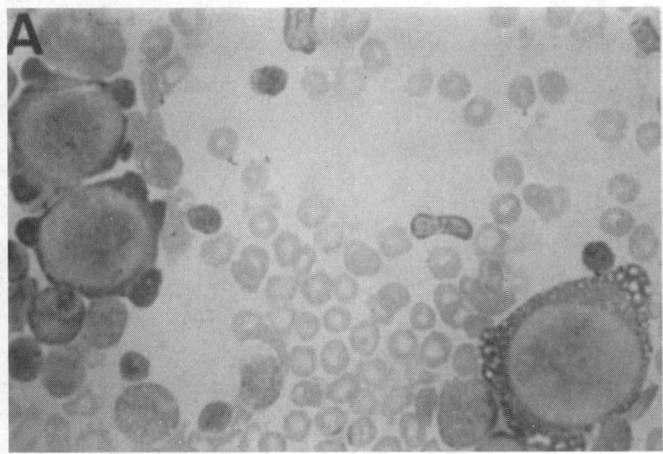

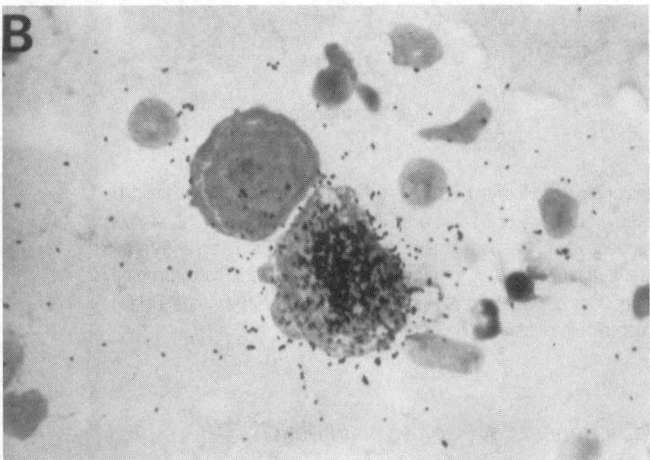

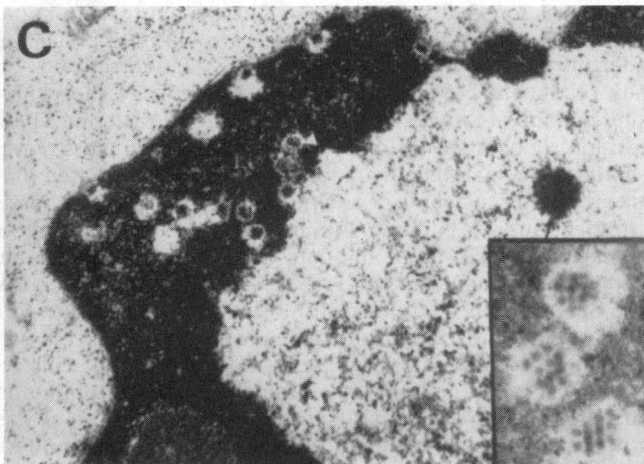

Fig. 21-7. B19 parvovirus infection of bone marrow cells. **(A)** Giant pronormoblasts in the bone marrow of a patient with chronic anemia due to persistent infection. **(B)** Viral protein detected by immunoperoxidase staining with a specific anti-B19 parvovirus capsid antibody in the bone marrow cells of a patient with acquired immunodeficiency syndrome (AIDS) and persistent parvovirus infection. **(C)** Electron micrograph of a human late erythroid progenitor infected in vitro with B19 parvovirus. Inset shows viral particles in the marginated chromatin of the cell's nucleus.

trimesters. The probability of stillbirth remains unknown, but is almost certainly low: of 170 reported cases of seroconversion during pregnancy, only a small minority have resulted in stillborn deliveries; in some normal newborns, the umbilical cord blood tested positive for IgM antibody to parvovirus.[291] An increased risk of spontaneous abortion during the first trimester is being investigated in several large epidemiologic surveys[294,295]; a preliminary estimate is that about 5% of infected women aborted. Congenital anomalies have not been associated with intrauterine parvovirus infection, either prospectively or in retrospective analysis of banked fetal tissue, although viral infection of myocardial cells was shown by in situ hybridization at autopsy of one hydropic infant.[296]

While the overall risk of a poor outcome to pregnancy is probably low, the concern of the potentially exposed pregnant mother is valid. Parvovirus infection is extremely contagious. Pregnant women are commonly exposed to fifth disease through other children in the household, at schools and day care centers, and (among nursing and medical personnel) by caring for persistently infected patients. About one-half of the pregnant population has acquired protective immunity, as determined by assay for IgG antibody to parvovirus. Evidence of seroconversion should be sought in IgG-negative women. Hydrops can be detected by ultrasound, and treatment of a suspected hydropic infant with intrauterine red blood cell transfusion has been reported.[297] The usefulness of this type of intervention and of administration of commercial immunoglobulin preparations containing antiparvovirus antibodies requires investigation.

Parvovirus infection of the fetus need not be fatal but may persist after birth.[298] We have studied three infants born with chronic anemia in whom there was a history of both maternal exposure to parvovirus during pregnancy and hydrops either in utero or at birth. Congenital infection is characterized by the low-level viral infection: virus could be detected in the bone marrow by gene amplification but did not circulate. Presumably infection early in ontogeny allows more efficient suppression of red cell production than infection of a mature marrow. One patient died, and at autopsy virus was found in other tissues, including thymus, brain, heart, liver, and spleen, suggesting the possibility of congenital malformation of other organ systems as a result of in utero B19 parvovirus infection. Exposure of the fetal immune system to virus early in pregnancy would also be predicted to result in tolerance to the capsid proteins and absence of an antibody response despite continued virus production.

Persistent Parvovirus Infection

Patients with persistent B19 parvovirus infection have pure red cell aplasia. Persistence is possible because patients fail to mount a neutralizing antibody response to the virus; as a result they lack the immune complex-mediated symptoms of fifth disease, fever, rash, and polyarthralgia/polyarthritis. Persistent parvovirus infection and pure red cell aplasia have been documented in three patient populations: those with congenital immunodeficiency (Nezelof syndrome),[299] children with lymphocytic leukemia in remission on chemotherapy,[300] and patients with the acquired immunodeficiency syndrome (AIDS).[301] However, defective antibody production also occurs in other diseases associated with pure red cell aplasia, such as chronic lymphocytic leukemia and malignancies treated with cytotoxic drugs; some of these cases may also represent occult viral infection.

Clinically, the anemia is severe and the patients depend on erythrocyte transfusions. There may be associated neutropenia. The bone marrow contains giant pronormoblasts, the

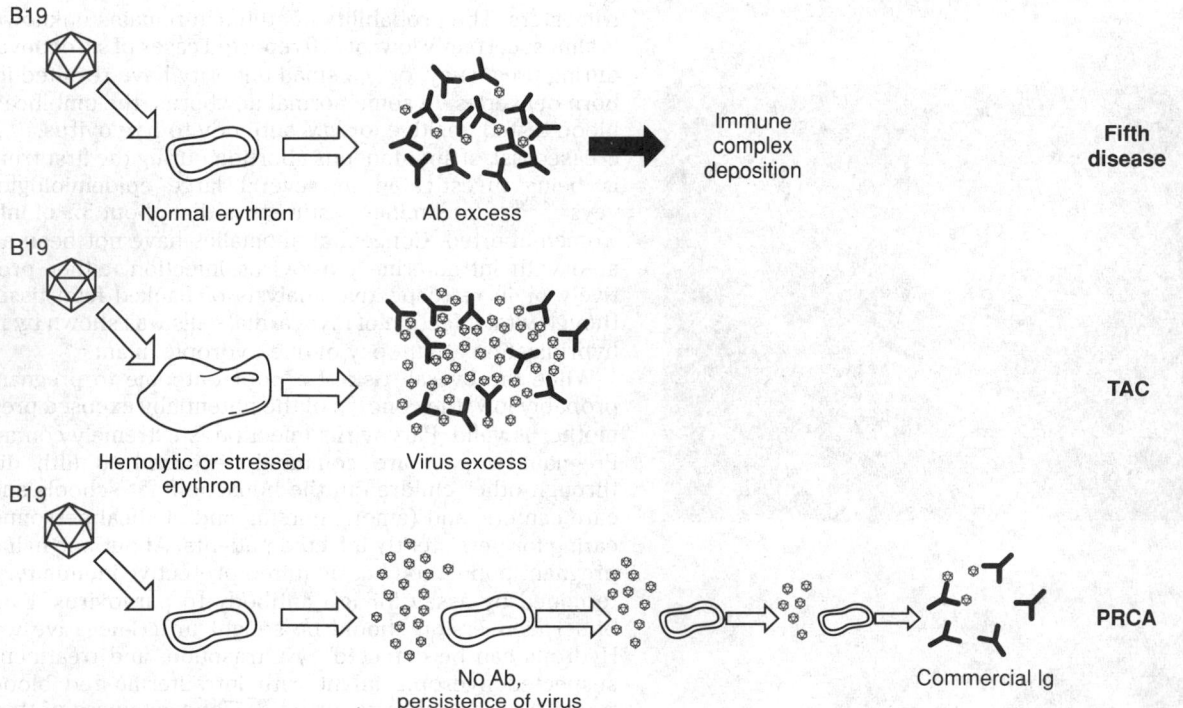

Fig. 21-8. Models of parvovirus-induced disease. Fifth disease and transient aplastic crisis (TAC) are acute infections and should be contrasted with each other and with persistent infection resulting in chronic pure red cell aplasia (PRCA). The relatively small amount of virus produced by normal bone marrow is neutralized by a vigorous antibody (Ab) response, and the relative antibody excess favors immune complex formation and deposition in skin and joints. In TAC, virus is neutralized but immune complex disease is rare, probably because of a relatively larger amount of virus than antibody. Persistent infection results in gradual shrinkage of the erythron and smaller amounts of viral production. Virus infection can be interrupted by administered immunoglobulin.

cytopathic sign of parvovirus infection, but these are usually infrequent and may not be present at all. The anemia may be intermittent, with periods of relapse associated with viremia and remission periods characterized by spontaneous disappearance of the virus from the circulation, possibly due to depletion of the erythroid target cell population. The diagnosis is established by detection of B19 parvovirus genome in the serum, blood, or bone marrow cells by DNA dot blot hybridization, although polymerase chain reaction amplification of viral DNA may be necessary in rare cases.[302,303] Antibodies to parvovirus, as determined in capture immunoassays or enzyme-linked immunosorbent assay, are not present in most patients, but a pattern of antibody response suggestive of early infection (IgM antibody and IgG antibody directed to the major capsid protein) may be found in patients with congenital immunodeficiency.[304] A poor reaction on immunoblot testing is a consistent finding and correlates with poor neutralizing activity for the virus in erythroid colony assays.[304] It should be stressed that persistent parvovirus infection may be the dominant manifestation of some inherited immunodeficiency states.

Effective therapy consists of infusion of commercial immunoglobulin preparations, which are a good source of neutralizing antibodies because most of the adult population has been exposed to the virus. An optimal treatment regimen has not been established. One patient with congenital immunodeficiency was cured by a 10-day course followed by intermittent injections until virus had disappeared from his serum.[299] Patients with AIDS respond to a 5- to 10-day course but may relapse some months later; they can respond to a second course.[301] Patients with AIDS have had high virus serum concentrations, and they should be considered highly infectious. Measurement of serum virus is helpful in predicting relapse and may assist in determining optimal treatment regimens.

Pathogenesis of Parvovirus Infection

The pattern of disease that follows parvovirus infection is the result of balance among virus, marrow target cell, and the immune response (Fig. 21-8). Bone marrow depression in parvovirus infection occurs during the early viremic phase and under normal conditions is terminated by a neutralizing antibody response. The immune response produces the clinical manifestations of fifth disease (the childhood rash illness and the adult rheumatic syndrome); these occur during the period of antibody formation and are immune complex-mediated (fifth disease symptoms can be precipitated by treatment of persistent infection with immunoglobulin). In patients with hyperactive erythropoiesis, large amounts of virus are produced, and the immune response may be weak, resulting in greater quantities of antigen in relation to antibody and little immune complex formation; rash and joint pains are rare in patients with transient aplastic crisis.[275] In persistent infection in children and adults as well as in in utero infection, failure to mount a neutralizing antibody response allows parvovirus to persist and cause chronic anemia.[302] In acute infection, the period of viremia is brief, usually 1–3 days, and virus titers are extremely high (10^{11}–10^{14} genome copies/ml). In persistent infection, virus can be demonstrated in serum samples obtained months apart; the viral titer is often lower (10^{6}), although AIDS patients may have serum concentrations equal to those seen in acute infection.

B19 parvovirus is extraordinarily trophic for human erythroid progenitor cells. Viral replication occurs only in erythroid marrow cells,[305] and replicative double-stranded DNA forms can be detected in the marrow of infected patients.[276,300,306] The virus has been propagated only in the erythroid cells of human bone marrow,[307] blood,[308] and fetal liver[309] (and in semipermissive leukemic cell lines adapted to growth in erythropoietin[310,311]). Erythroid colony formation, but not CFU-GM, is strongly inhibited by virus.[312] Parvovirus is directly cytotoxic and induces characteristic light[307,313] and electron[314] microscopic morphologic changes in erythroid precursors (Fig. 21-8). Tropism for erythroid cells is largely determined by cell entry, as the cellular receptor for the virus is a red cell antigen, globoside, or P antigen.[315] Rare individuals of p erythrocyte phenotype are resistant to parvovirus infection.[316] The virus cytopathic effect manifests as giant pronormoblasts.[269,307] Virus toxicity is the result of expression of the single nonstructural protein of the virus,[317] and limited expression of this gene may explain inhibition of myelopoiesis and megakaryocytopoiesis in patients in the absence of virus replication in these cells.[318]

Hepatitis

Aplastic anemia may follow an episode of acute hepatitis.[319–321] The association of hepatitis and aplastic anemia is not rare, and the literature to 1972 reported almost 200 cases.[320] As an identifiable clinical event, a prior episode of hepatitis is recognized in 2–5% of aplastic anemia patients in the Western series[322] and about twice this proportion in the Far East.[4] About one-fourth of children with aplastic anemia in Taiwan have a history of recent acute hepatitis.[323] A previous episode of hepatitis was a significant risk factor in a case control study of aplastic anemia.[74] In a far higher proportion of cases, antecedent hepatitis may be subclinical, as about 50% of patients may have abnormally elevated hepatic transaminases on presentation.[320] While hepatitis is frequently associated with mild blood count depression, aplasia is a rare sequela, estimated at <0.07% of total pediatric hepatitis cases[324] and at <2% of hepatitis C.[325–327] Aplastic anemia developed in an astonishing 28% (9 of 32) of patients after liver transplant for hepatic failure following hepatitis C.[328]

Hepatitis-associated aplastic anemia has several peculiar features. Bone marrow depression usually occurs just when the patient is recovering from acute liver inflammation, as judged by serum transaminase elevation, generally about 2 months after the episode of hepatitis. A large proportion of patients are young males. Hepatitis confers a particularly poor prognosis: in Hagler et al.'s[320] collection of 174 cases, >90% of patients had died within 1 year of diagnosis, and the average survival was only 11 weeks from the onset of pancytopenia. Aplastic anemia has occurred in some family members affected with hepatitis[329]; a genetic predisposition is suggested by the prevalence of the HLA-B8 antigen (which is also associated with autoimmune hepatitis).[330] Hematopoietic depression during the course of hepatitis is common. The leukopenia, atypical lymphocytosis, erythroid macrocytosis, and thrombocytopenia are less severe than the hematologic changes of aplastic anemia. Transient pancytopenia,[331] pure red cell aplasia,[332,333] and hypoplastic acute lymphocytic leukemia[334] have also been reported in association with hepatitis.

Hepatitis-associated aplastic anemia has been considered an indication for early bone marrow transplantation, because of the severity of the pancytopenia.[335] Many such patients have been successfully transplanted.[335–337] However, hepatitis increases the risk of veno-occlusive disease of the liver, a frequently fatal post-transplant complication.[338] Patients with hepatitis-associated aplasia have also responded to antilymphocyte globulins,[339–341] high-dose methylprednisolone,[342,343] cyclosporine,[344] and androgens.[319] Some may even recover spontaneously.[331]

Altered liver function has been invoked to explain the findings of decreased hematopoietic stimulatory activity in the sera of patients with hepatitis-associated aplasia[345] and cases in which chloramphenicol use was followed by jaundice and aplasia.[346] Hepatitis-associated aplastic anemia has been associated with diminished immune responsiveness, including decreased T-cell number and function and lower serum immunoglobulins as compared with patients who had idiopathic disease.[347,348] Other investigators have reported heightened immune responsiveness, with increased numbers of circulating activated suppressor lymphocytes, in children with hepatitis-associated aplasia.[349,350]

In one series of 16 patients, hepatitis A and B could be confidently excluded in 13 and was doubtful as a preceding illness in the remaining 3[321]; subsequently additional serologically well-defined cases have been reported.[325–328,351] Hepatitis C has until recently been a diagnosis of exclusion, but in 1989 the hepatitis C virus was molecularly cloned. By serologic testing for antibody to a nonstructural protein of the virus, hepatitis C virus infection has been associated with virtually all transfusion-acquired hepatitis C and with about 50% of cases of community-acquired hepatitis C. Because hepatitis C virus is small, enveloped, and contains positive-stranded RNA,[352] it has been classified as a flavivirus-like virus.

Flaviviruses are the etiologic agents of the arbovirus hemorrhagic fevers, dengue fever (Thai hematodepressive disease),[353,354] Russian spring-summer fever,[355] South American hemorrhagic fever,[356] Omsk fever, and many other disorders.[357] These are acute infectious hematodepressive syndromes. In dengue fever, the neutrophil and platelet counts fall, often to very low levels, during the early, viremic phase of illness, while immune events, probably secondary to cytokine release and reflected by atypical lymphocytosis, predominate during the second (often fatal shock) phase of the disease. The bone marrow in dengue fever is hypocellular, with an abnormal megakaryocyte appearance.[353,354] Experimental inoculation of flaviviruses into human volunteers has produced pancytopenia and marrow aplasia.[358] Flaviviruses propagate efficiently in human bone marrow cultures and hematopoietic cell lines.[359] While not directly cytotoxic to marrow cells,[359] dengue fever infection in vitro induces lymphocyte activation (both cytotoxic and helper phenotypes) and release of cytokines such as interferon-γ (IFN-γ) that suppress hematopoiesis.[360] Children with dengue fever also have high circulating levels of IFN-γ interleukin-2 (IL-2), and the soluble forms of the receptor for IL-2, CD4, and CD8; those with the shock syndrome have particularly high concentrations of soluble CD8.[361]

However, hepatitis C virus does not appear to be an etiologic agent in the pathogenesis of aplastic anemia. Occasional case reports signal absence of antibody to hepatitis C as well as antibodies to hepatitis A and B.[362] A serologic study of hepatitis C virus antibody in patients with aplastic anemia found no difference in the titer of antihepatitis virus antibody in patients with hepatitis-associated marrow failure compared with those who had marrow failure from other causes, although the rate of seropositivity was high in all groups (10–22%).[363] Using the polymerase chain reaction to amplify viral RNA, an extremely sensitive and specific assay for hepatitis C virus, we have examined large numbers of sera from different patient populations. Hepatitis C viremia is common among Thai patients presenting with aplastic anemia, but the incidence is not different from the 5% found in a control population.[364] In American, European, and Japanese patients with clinically defined posthepatitis aplastic anemia, neither virus nor antibody was present in sera collected before transfusions in any cases; no virus was found in bone marrow from these patients or in hepatic tissue from patients who had undergone liver transplantation for fulminant hepatitis and developed aplastic anemia afterward.[365] In an analysis of several hundred serum samples drawn from patients with aplastic anemia, from patients with other hematologic disease requiring multiple transfusions, and from patients undergoing cardiac surgery, the rate of hepatitis C viremia correlated strongly only with the number of transfusions administered, and acquisition of virus did not adversely correlate with blood counts.[365] These results indicate that a non-A, non-B, and non-C agent produces posthepatitis aplastic anemia. An indirect, immune-mediated pathophysiology rather than direct viral toxicity is suggested by the following points: recovery of hepatitis/aplasia patients with marrow transplantation; the requirement for immunosuppression prior to syngeneic transplantation; the effectiveness of immunotherapy alone in other cases; and a suggestion of HLA linkage.[366]

Occasional case reports of aplasia following hepatitis B,[367,368] hepatitis A,[369,370] and hepatitis C[371] have not been supported by epidemiologic evidence.[363,364,372] All are common pathogens, and perhaps some of the patients were coinfected with another hepatitis agent. Hematopoietic colony formation in vitro can be (modestly) inhibited by hepatitis B,[373,374] hepatitis A,[375,376] and perhaps hepatitis C.[377] Hepatitis B surface antigen has been detected in the nuclei of immature myeloid cells[378] and hepatitis B DNA in circulating white blood cells.[379] Hepatitis C has been found in macrophages.[379] Murine hepatitis virus, a coronavirus, also causes pancytopenia and bone marrow necrosis associated with acute liver inflammation.[380,381]

Epstein-Barr Virus

Herpesviruses are large, genetically complex DNA viruses; two herpesviruses have been associated clinically and experimentally with bone marrow failure. Acute infection with EBV causes infectious mononucleosis, which can rarely be complicated by aplastic anemia. Only nine cases of pancytopenia immediately following infectious mononucleosis could be collected in 1981, and bone marrow hypocellularity was not documented in all; some patients recovered spontaneously, others recovered with corticosteroid therapy, and some died.[382] EBV may be involved in marrow failure more frequently than would be inferred from the history alone.[383,384] EBV has been demonstrated by immunologic and molecular techniques in bone marrow cells of six patients with aplastic anemia; all of them had serologic evidence of recent infection or reactivation, but only two had a previous history of typical infectious mononucleosis.[383]

Cytotoxic T cells are activated during infectious mononucleosis.[385] Lymphocyte suppression of hematopoiesis was demonstrated in one patient with postmononucleosis aplastic anemia who responded to antithymocyte globulin therapy.[386] An aberrant genetically determined immune response to the virus is also suggested by the frequent mortality from bone marrow failure in boys with the X-linked lymphoproliferative syndrome, a familial syndrome characterized by various combinations of hypogammaglobulinemia, chronic or fatal acute infectious mononucleosis, B-cell lymphomas, and aplastic anemia.[37] Hematopoietic cells might be targets of EBV infection. Although the B lymphocyte is the most obvious target, EBV has also been detected in T lymphocytes in some patients with lymphoma[387] and in nasopharyngeal epithelial cells.[388,389] The virus was present in monocyte/macrophage cell lines established from children with a variety of clinical defects in hematopoiesis.[390]

Cytomegalovirus

Like EBV, cytomegalovirus infection is common and usually benign in its effects. Even in immunosuppressed patients, cytomegalovirus infection resulting either from reactivation or from new exposure is not associated with a characteristic clinical syndrome. Graft failure after marrow transplantation has been linked to cytomegalovirus infection in humans[391] and in mice.[392] Anemia, neutropenia, thrombocytopenia, or pancytopenia frequently occur in patients with hematologic malignancies who are infected with cytomegalovirus.[393]

Cytomegalovirus promiscuously infects fibroblasts of many tissues, and its infection of bone marrow stromal cells is the probable mechanism of marrow failure.[394,395] In mice, at least, CFU-GM can be rescued from cytomegalovirus-inoculated adherent cell layers, indicating that the infected stroma was the sole site of defective myelopoiesis.[396] Cytomegalovirus suppression of myelopoiesis in human long-term bone marrow culture resulted from infection of stromal cells, and CSF-G transcription by these cells appeared to be specifically inhibited.[397] As regards infectivity of human hematopoietic progenitor cells by cytomegalovirus, the data are conflicting. Some investigators have been unable to inhibit colony formation with laboratory strains of cytomegalovirus.[397] In one study, colony formation (especially of progenitors responsive to CSF-G) was diminished by infection with a laboratory strain (Towne) and wild-type cytomegalovirus. Cytomegalovirus was detected in some progeny cells by immunofluorescence and in situ hybridization.[398] Some clinical isolates of cytomegalovirus inhibited colony formation (both CFU-GM and BFU-E derived), but there has not been a good correlation between these in vitro effects and the presence of neutropenia in the patient donor.[397,399] In our studies, both laboratory strains and clinical isolates inhibited myeloid and erythroid colony formation; expression of early and late antigens as well as immediate early proteins indicated that infection was productive and not simply abortive.[400] Furthermore, both CD34+ cells and monocytes could be productively infected, and their surviving progeny expressed viral proteins.

As in EBV infection, cytomegalovirus infection is associated with reversal of the helper/suppressor lymphocyte ratio, but in contrast to EBV, T-cell function is diminished.[401] The constitutive production of IFN-γ and tumor necrosis factor by lymphocytes, seen in recipients after human marrow transplantation, is greatly enhanced by in vitro incubation of blood mononuclear cells with cytomegalovirus-infected autologous marrow fibroblasts.[402]

Human Herpesvirus 6

Herpesvirus 6 is responsible for the childhood rash illness called exanthema subitum.[403] Human herpesvirus 6 was isolated from marrow mononuclear cells in immunosuppressed patients after bone marrow transplantation.[404] In vitro, the virus suppresses hematopoietic colony formation, as well as marrow stromal cell proliferation.[405]

Human Immunodeficiency Virus

Hematologic changes are common in patients with AIDS. The effects of human immunodeficiency virus and other retroviruses on hemtopoiesis are discussed in Chapter 155.

Other Viruses

As an organ of actively proliferating cells accessible to the circulation, the bone marrow undoubtedly provides an attractive milieu for many types of viruses. Infection of human megakaryocytes has been inferred in congenital and acquired rubella,[406–408] measles,[409] and mumps,[410] as well as following live attenuated measles vaccination[411] and in experimental varicella.[412] Viral effects on hematopoiesis have been observed in animals infected with cytomegalovirus,[389] Newcastle disease virus,[413] encephalomyocarditis virus,[414] and coxsackie B virus.[415]

Paroxysmal Nocturnal Hemoglobinuria

Aplastic anemia and paroxysmal nocturnal hemoglobinuria (PNH) are closely related syndromes.[416–419] Because PNH has a defined genetic basis (see Ch. 25), this relationship is potentially of great importance in understanding the pathophysiology of marrow failure. During the course of PNH, pancytopenia is common; about one-third of patients will die of bone marrow failure. Red cell lysis in the presence of activated complement is the defining laboratory feature of PNH, and many patients with pancytopenia and marrow hypocellularity will have either a positive sucrose hemolysis test or a positive acidified serum hemolysis test on presentation or during the course of otherwise typical aplastic anemia.[420-422] Overlap with aplastic anemia is particularly striking among younger patients with PNH, who much less frequently present with hemoglobinuria (15% of children versus 50% of adults) and more commonly have moderate-to-severe marrow failure (58% compared with about one-half this number in adults), commonly leading to an initial diagnosis of aplastic anemia.[423] PNH, aplastic anemia, and acute myeloid leukemia have all occurred in a single patient.[424] When leukemia replaced hemolysis as the dominant clinical manifestation,[425] the blast cells have been shown to be derived from the abnormal complement-sensitive clone.[426,427]

PNH and aplastic anemia share several pathophysiologic and epidemiologic features. Hematopoietic progenitor number is severely decreased in patients with cytopenias and PNH, even when the marrow is cellular.[428,429] Studies of fractionated erythrocytes[430] and progenitor cell cultures[431] have suggested that complement-sensitive cells are relatively frequent in aplastic anemia. Flow cytometric analysis for the PNH phenotype, characterized by the absence of specific proteins from the cell surface, is more sensitive than the Ham test, detecting affected granulocytes and monocytes in the absence of erythrocyte defects[432] and phenotypically absent proteins despite negative Ham tests.[433] In contrast to patients with PNH, who display predominantly hemolytic or thrombotic features, aplastic patients show a smaller subpopulation of abnormal cells (10–20% compared with 30–100%).[433] Aplastic patients with positive Ham tests can respond to immunosuppressive therapies such as antithymocyte globulin and cyclosporine.[434] PNH, like aplastic anemia, is also relatively common in the Far East. In Thailand[435] and India[436] the disease is more commonly associated with aplastic anemia and less commonly with thrombotic episodes, similar to the pattern in younger American patients.[423]

The concept of PNH as a clonal disorder was based on the initial observation of a single glucose-6-phosphate dehydrogenase isoenzyme in the affected erythrocytes of two female patients heterozygous at this locus.[437] Using DNA analysis of females heterozygous for markers susceptible to digestion with restriction enzymes that recognize methylation sites, virtually all such cases of PNH have been shown to be of clonal origin.[438] Both normal and sensitive erythrocytes circulate, and identification of distinct populations of complement-sensitive and normal progenitors has been reported by some[439,440] but not others.[441,442] Expression of the surface membrane molecules that regulate complement degradation changes with hematopoietic differentiation.[443]

The biochemical basis of PNH lies in the defective attachment of a class of membrane proteins that are joined to the cell surface by a glycolipid anchor (see Ch. 25). In PNH, the glycosylphosphatidylinositol anchor is not synthesized, and the affected proteins remain in the cytoplasm.[444] Although multiple enzymatic steps are involved in the production of the anchor, surprisingly, only a single defect has been found in all patients so far examined; this defect affects synthesis of the first intermediate, N-acetylgucosaminyl-phosphotidylinositol.[445] A gene called PIG-A, required for this early step in anchor synthesis, has been cloned and sequenced.[446]

For the PNH clone to dominate hematopoiesis, PIG-A cells must have a selective advantage over normal cells. However, such an advantage has not been shown by in vitro studies.[428,429] No growth factor or growth factor receptor has been shown to be phosphoinositol linked to the cell surface. Some cytoadhesion molecules, and proteoheparin sulfate share this linkage, and their disruption might affect the hematopoietic stem cell's proximity to local high concentrations of growth factors in the marrow microenvironment. At least three immune system proteins are also affected by the PNH defect: the type III Fc$_\gamma$ receptor, monocyte antigen CD14 (of unknown function), and lymphocyte function-associated antigen 3, which is the ligand for the T-cell glycoprotein CD2; a second phosphoinositol-linked protein, CD59, the membrane inhibitor of lysis that also blocks complement lysis of erythrocytes, represents a second ligand for CD2 on T cells.[447] There is little evidence that PNH cells have growth advantages over normal cells under physiologic conditions; for example, syngeneic bone marrow transplants have succeeded without prior ablation of the recipient's marrow,[448] but absence of a recognition site for cytotoxic lymphocytes would provide a growth advantage in a hematopoietic system under immune system attack (see below). Hypotheses accounting for the emergence of clonal disease in aplastic anemia are treated more fully elsewhere.[449]

Immunologic Abnormalities

Eosinophilic Fasciitis

Aplastic anemia commonly occurs during the course of eosinophilic fasciitis.[450,451] Of the first 100 cases reported in the literature, nearly 10% of patients with eosinophilic fasciitis had bone marrow failure. Eosinophilic fasciitis is a severe, scleroderma-like disease characterized clinically by a peculiar fibrosis of subcutaneous and fascial tissue, localized areas of skin induration, peripheral blood eosinophilia, hypergammaglobulinemia, and an elevated erythrocyte sedimentation rate. While the rheumatologic symptoms of fasciitis respond to corticosteroids, the associated aplastic anemia has a very poor prognosis,[450] although some cases have responded to immunosuppression.[452]

Runt Disease

Iatrogenic fatal aplastic anemia has occurred following the transfusion of competent lymphocytes into immunodeficient hosts.[453] Such hosts include thymic dysplasia patients treated with bone marrow infusion[454] or blood transfusion[455]; children with progressive vaccinia infection who received leukocyte transfusions[456] neonate who received intrauterine transfusion of red blood cells[457]; and neonates who underwent exchange transfusion for hemolytic disease of the newborn.[458] Runt disease in some animal species (chicken, rat, and rabbit) may also be accompanied by aplasia, resulting in histiocytic, phagocytic cell infiltrates.

Graft-versus-host disease occurs following solid organ transplants, particularly when the spleen is included in the pedicle of a pancreas transplant[459] or after liver transplants.[460] In these instances, graft-versus-host disease is due to the inclusion of sufficient numbers of donor lymphocytes in the transplanted organ. As with transfusion-associated graft-versus-host disease, aplastic anemia occurs in these cases. Marrow aplasia has also occurred after infusion of donor lymphocytes into post-transplant patients who have relapsed with chronic myeloid leukemia.[461,462]

Hypoimmunoglobulinemia

Aplastic anemia occasionally occurs in individuals with hypogammaglobulinemia[463,464] or in association with thymoma, thymic hyperplasia,[465] or thymic carcinoma.[466] In one case, suppressor T cells, already implicated in B-cell inhibition, were shown to suppress erythroid colony formation.[467]

Aside from the specific and possibly pathophysiologic immunologic abnormalities described below, immune system function is not severely impaired in most cases of aplastic anemia. Patients with aplastic anemia generally have normal immunoglobulin levels and normal antibody titers to common viral antigens.[464,468–470] About one-half of patients are anergic, but in vitro lymphocyte proliferation is normal.[468] Monocytopenia and lymphocytopenia are responsible for reported specific abnormalities, such as deficient differentiation of B cells on lectin stimulation[464] or lymphocyte proliferation that requires monocyte help.[470] Aplastic patients do not behave clinically as if they were immunodeficient, and their apparent susceptibility to viral and protozoan organisms is solely related to immunosuppressive therapy.

Pregnancy

Pregnancy is common in the age groups most susceptible to marrow failure, and in many cases its association is probably only coincidental. A causal relationship is suggested by the temporal relationship between the onset of pancytopenia and pregnancy and remissions with delivery[471–473] or abortion.[474,475] Occasional patients have developed aplastic anemia during pregnancy and remitted after each delivery.[476] The paucity of cases is apparent from periodic literature reviews: in 1958 only 16 cases were collected[477]; in 1976 there were 27 cases[478]; and in 1975 there were 43 cases, of which only 30 were actually diagnosed during the pregnancy.[479] Several larger series have been reported from the Orient.[480,481] Bone marrow hypoplasia may be relatively common during pregnancy, since it was detected in 8 of 101 anemic pregnant women without overt iron deficiency.[482]

Estrogens might be related to the aplasia of pregnancy. Estrus-associated aplastic anemia occurs in ferrets,[483] and administration of large doses of estrogens can produce blood count depression in ferrets[484] and dogs.[485–488] Estrogens can blunt the erythrokinetic response to erythropoietin in rats.[489] Estrogen administration decreases the number of CFU-S in the spleen and bone marrow of mice.[490]

PATHOPHYSIOLOGY

Hematopoietic Stem Cells

Certainly the most consistent laboratory finding in aplastic anemia is very low numbers of blood and bone marrow hematopoietic progenitor cells.[491–502] Some preservation of progenitor cells and precursors has been associated with an improved prognosis.[494,498,501] Depressed progenitor cell numbers persist in patients long after successful treatment by bone marrow transplantation,[503] immunosuppression,[497,504] or anabolic steroids.[505] Long-term culture-initiating cells, an in vitro surrogate for repopulating cells, are reduced in number when compared with normal: in aplastics, they are found at a frequency of 1:8,260–1:30,898 compared with the normal frequency of 1:341–1:6,200. In enriched progenitor fractions, the frequency in aplastic patients was 1:4,269 on average compared with the normal 1:229.[506] An absence of the most primitive stem cells is reasonably inferred from these culture data and seemingly confirmed by the dramatic efficacy of stem cell replacement in the form of bone marrow transplantation. However, the success of immunosuppressive therapies in aplastic anemia has made a simple thesis untenable: that quantitative aplastic anemia is due to a deficiency of the most primitive stem cells. The relative maintenance of lymphocyte function and number and other stem cell-derived compartments in aplastic anemia also places the point of injury distal to the most primitive repopulating cell.

The W/W^v mouse is an animal model of stem cell-based bone marrow failure; these heterozygotes have a macrocytic anemia that is curable by transplantation, but their own cells form microscopic rather than macroscopic spleen colonies in normal host animals.[507–509] The anemia (which is out of proportion to depression of other blood counts) and the CFU-S assay itself reflect mainly an erythropoietic lesion.[510] The phenotype is the result of mutations at the c-*kit* locus; the c-*kit* gene is primarily expressed in erythroid cells and encodes a cell-surface protein with tyrosine kinase activity, probably a receptor for a hematopoietin (see Ch. 14). The W/W^v mouse is a possible model for human hereditary bone marrow failure disorders such as pure red cell aplasia and congenital neutropenia. It has less relevance to acquired aplastic anemia because a somatic mutation in a stem cell would probably not result in predominance of a cell clone with a growth disadvantage.

The stem cell compartment is not homogeneous but is organized along a hierarchy of cells according to generational age[511,512] (Fig. 21-9). If a mouse is treated with a cell cycle-active drug such as hydroxyurea[513,514] or 5-fluorouracil,[515] the remaining hematopoietic stem cells have increased capacities to proliferate, differentiate, and self-renew. Similar results can be seen in long-term bone marrow cultures, in which the initial phase of establishing the culture leaves a population in the adherent cell layer that has a high proliferative capacity.[516] The hierarchical model predicts that as stem cells age by undergoing repeated cell divisions, they increase their probability of entering another division and of being recruited in an orderly but random fashion to leave the stem cell compartment and differentiate.

The number of true stem cells is limited. In the mouse, their frequency has been estimated as 1 or $2/10^5$ bone marrow cells, which corresponds to a total of 400–1,000 stem cells/animal.[517,518] If the ratio is similar for humans, the total stem cell number in a 70-kg person would be about 9.8×10^6 to 2.6×10^7. A very small proportion of primitive stem cells is likely to be in the mitotic phase of the cell cycle at any time; by inference from the distribution of glucose-6-phosphate dehydrogenase phenotype in heterozygous individuals, 10–24 cells have been estimated to be actively maintaining hematopoiesis.[519] Repopulating cells and CFU-S can be physically separated.[520] Primitive repopulating cells are only about one-tenth as frequent as CFU-S while 5–50 CFU-S are needed to reconstitute the bone marrow of an irradiated mouse,[521,522] clonal analysis has shown that a single pluripotent stem cell will repopulate.[523,524] However, normal hematopoiesis is maintained from these small numbers of cell for the life span of the animal, and there is very little evidence for aging of hematopoiesis—indeed, elderly mice are as good bone marrow donors as young ones.[525] The same stem cells when serially transplanted can maintain normal blood counts in animals through several life spans.[525]

Given its enormous capacity and highly regulated structure, it is paradoxical that the stem cell compartment suffers drastic loss in number and especially in self-renewal capacity in a wide variety of experimental situations. Late CFU-S numbers decline in colony-forming ability following serial transplantation.[526] The same loss of self-renewal capacity occurs when repopulation is the end point,[527] in the shielded limb of an irradiated animal,[528] after a single bone marrow transplantation,[528] or in parabiotic W/W^v animals.[529] Similar permanent loss of self-renewal capacity can be observed at the initiation of a long-term bone marrow culture[530] and after irradiation of in vitro cultures.[62] The limited numbers of stem cells that repopulate after marrow damage has been illustrated in cats; in animals that are heterozygous for glucose-6-phosphate dehydrogenase, clonal evolution of hematopoiesis can be monitored after chemotherapy.[531] Deregulation of hematopoiesis appears to result not only in reduction in the size of the stem cell compartment but also in alteration of its most important functional properties.

The busulfan-treated mouse is an animal model of aplastic anemia due to direct injury to stem cell DNA. In contrast to the effect of hydroxyurea in "improving" the number and qualities of the hematopoietic stem cell compartment, treatment

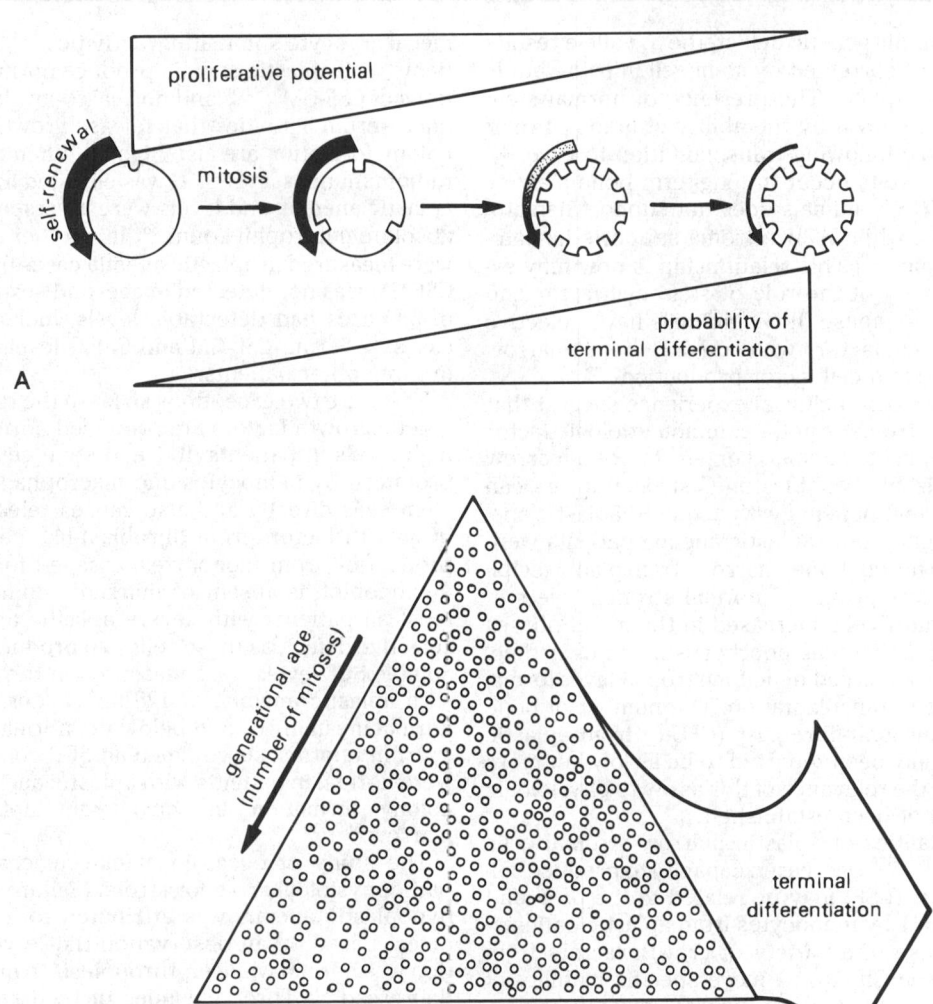

Fig. 21-9. Stem cell "aging" and a model of stem cell hierarchical organization by generational age. **(A)** Functional changes in an individual cell followed through several mitotic cycles. With each cell cycle, the cell's proliferative potential for expansion or self-renewal decreases, and its likelihood of entering a pathway of terminal differentiation increases. Proliferation, self-renewal, and differentiation are regulated by a combination of internal cell mechanisms (genetic) and environmental influences (cell-cell interactions, growth factors, hormones). For example, increasing cell-surface receptors would be one way to increase the probability of a response to a specific proliferative or differentiative stimulus, such as a constant concentration of hematopoietic growth factor molecules in the environment. **(B)** Each mitosis also increases the number of cells. Here, the organization of the entire compartment is diagrammed. The stochastic or random nature of regulatory events can be envisioned from this model. As cell number increases owing to mitosis, the number of cells available to a signaling event is much higher among the mitotically older members of the population. Amplification in cell number also occurs during terminal differentiation. All the members of this compartment are stem cells, as they are capable of both self-renewal and differentiation along multilineage pathways; cells at the top of the pyramid would be further characterized as pluripotent repopulating cells, those in the middle as CFU-S, and those near the bottom as cells capable of forming multipotent colonies in semisolid medium (CFU-GEMM, some BFU-E).

with busulfan produces latent bone marrow failure[532–534]; similar bone marrow damage can be produced by other alkylating agents[535] and frequent small doses of γ-irradiation.[536] At an appropriate dose, busulfan-treated mice maintain normal or near normal blood counts and bone marrow cellularity and near normal or only moderately reduced progenitor cell and stem cell numbers for 1 year, until the CFU-S number falls and the animals develop frank aplasia. Estimates that hematopoiesis failed when the CFU-S number fell to 10%, based on the effects of busulfan or split-dose irradiation, can now be reinterpreted as a disappearance of the last repopulating cell.[536] A self-renewal deficit in busulfan-treated animals can be demonstrated in vitro.[535,537] A marrow transplant largely reverses busulfan-induced marrow failure.[531,538,539]

Hematopoietic Stroma and Growth Factors

The hypothesis that bone marrow failure could be the result of a lesion of "soil" rather than "seed" was based on several experimental observations: regeneration in isolated limbs after irradiation[540]; defects of the sinusoidal vasculature in animals rejecting allogeneic bone marrow grafts; and intrinsic differences in the ability of red and yellow, or predominantly fatty, marrow to support hematopoiesis after transplantation to extramedullary sites.[541] Abnormal adipocyte proliferation has even been proposed as the primary lesion in aplastic anemia,[542] but direct evidence for a microenvironmental defect in aplastic anemia patients has not been found.[543,544]

Bone marrow failure due to a stromal defect occurs in the

Sl/Sl^d mouse.[507,508] In this genetic defect, the Sl^d allele results in an anemia that is not corrected by stem cell infusion but is curable by spleen transplant. The presence of normal stem cells in Sl/Sl^d mice is shown by the ability of grafts of their spleen or bone marrow following transplantation to cure W/W^v animals. Parallel results occur in long-term bone marrow cultures: stroma of Sl/Sl^d animals does not support hematopoiesis by W/W^v cells, while W/W^v stroma supports hematopoiesis from Sl/Sl^d mice.[545] This relationship is now fully explained by the discovery of the role of stem cell factor and its receptor, c-kit, in the mouse. W/W^v animals have defective receptors for stem cell factor, while Sl/Sl^d bone marrow stroma is deficient in stem cell factor production.

However, most in vitro and clinical experience suggest that an abnormal marrow stroma is not a common etiologic factor in the pathology of aplastic anemia. Long-term bone marrow cultures with recognizable "cobblestone" stromal layers can be established from most patients with acquired aplastic anemia.[546–550] In one recent study, aplastic anemia patients were compared with recovering bone marrow transplant recipients.[551] Aplastic patients produced normal stromal layers in vitro, myeloid progenitor cells increased in the initial phases of culture, but their number was poorly sustained over time. By contrast, there was a marked deficit in stromal layer formation after bone marrow transplantation. The number of bone marrow colony-forming unit-fibroblast (CFU-F) from aplastic marrow has occasionally been reported to be as low but more usually normal[552–554]; the relevance of this assay to physiologic stroma function has not been established.

Functional abnormalities of aplastic marrow stromal cells have been described.[553–556] Decreased capacity to produce colony-stimulating factors (CSF) may be related to the profound inability to generate IL-1 by monocytes from aplastic patients. IL-1 induces the release of a variety of growth factors from fibroblast-like cells (see Ch. 16). A more specific inability of aplastic anemia cells in long-term culture to increase colony-stimulating activities (mainly CSF-G) in response to IL-1 was noted in about one-half of patients studied.[557] Nonetheless, when directly measured by immunoassays, the release of growth factors—CSF-G, CSF-GM, and IL-6—by marrow stromal cells was normal in 29 aplastic anemia patients. These cells also responded normally to IL-1 stimulation in vitro, and growth factor production was not affected by antithymocyte globulin therapy.[558] When examined by reverse polymerase chain reaction, IL-6 and CSF-GM mRNA were abundant in long-term bone marrow cultures of marrow cells from patients with acquired aplastic anemia.[559] In a "cross-over" experiment with bone marrow from seven recovered aplastic anemia patients, the patients' cells behaved normally when used to establish the adherent layer of long-term bone marrow culture for normal CD34$^+$ progenitors; by contrast, the reduced number of CD34$^+$ cells from the aplastic patients grew poorly on normal stroma.[550] Similar data have been obtained with a blast colony assay of isolated CD34$^+$ cells grown on stroma.[560] Some investigators have reported the production of hematopoietic inhibitory activity by adherent cells isolated from aplastic bone marrow[561] or peripheral blood.[562,563]

The factors that stimulate hematopoiesis are almost always abundant in patients with aplastic anemia. The urine of these patients has been a favored source of erythropoietin for purification, and high levels of this hormone circulate.[564] Indeed, for the same hemoglobin level, serum erythropoein values are higher in children with aplastic anemia when compared with children who have iron-deficiency anemia.[565] Production of burst-promoting activity by aplastic anemia patients' mononuclear cells in vitro is high,[566–568] and high activity levels have been measured in patients' sera.[569,570] Similarly, CSF-GM activities usually,[571,572] if not always,[573] have been elevated, as have

megakaryocyte-stimulating activities.[574–578] T cells from patients with aplastic anemia produce normal-to-high concentrations of CSF-GM[579,580] and normal-to-low levels of IL-3.[580] Undefined serum activities that release growth factors or enhance colony formation are also high.[581] When directly measured by radioimmunoassay, CSF-G was elevated in 9 of 11 patients with aplastic anemia, and levels were inversely correlated with the absolute neutrophil count.[582] In another series, CSF-GM levels were measured in aplastic anemia cases on presentation: while CSF-GM was not detected in age- and sex-matched controls, 25 of 33 cases had detectable levels, including 17 of 19 severe cases.[583] Serum CSF-GM and CSF-G levels have been elevated in three other patients.[584]

There are two exceptions so far to the rule that most hematopoietic growth factors are produced normally or at normal-to-high levels in patients: IL-1 and stem cell factor (SCF). IL-1 is produced by monocytes and macrophages; the factor affects stem cells directly and also causes release of a wide variety of growth factors from fibroblast-like cells (see Ch. 16). IL-1 production from monocytes, assayed for biologic activity or immunoblot, is absent or markedly diminished in vitro in almost all patients with severe aplastic anemia[585,586]; this is a selective defect, as these cells can produce IL-6 and CSF-GM.[586] Soluble SCF levels were measured in the serum of 32 patients with aplastic anemia; of 128 specimens, SCF was below the normal mean in 107 and below the normal range in 26.[587] However, in another survey median SCF concentrations in blood were normal in patients with aplastic anemia.[588] SCF increased colony formation in vitro from aplastic anemia bone marrow.[589,590]

The study of occassional clinical cases has suggested a pathophysiologic role for stromal failure. A case of congenital hypoplastic anemia was attributed to a microenvironmental defect based on an observation that erythroid colony formation was normal while erythropoiesis in marrow fragments was depressed.[591] Three episodes of recurrent graft failure after syngeneic marrow transplantation were credited to stromal failure in an aplastic patient who lacked in vitro evidence of host-mediated hematopoietic suppression.[592] In total, however, there is little evidence for a stromal cell defect in most cases of acquired aplastic anemia, and, when observed, deficient growth factor production may be secondary rather than primary in the pathology of this disease.

Immunosuppression of Hematopoiesis

Clinical observations have provided a powerful impetus to the development of an immune theory of aplastic anemia. Mathé et al[593] first suggested an immune mechanism when they observed improvement in autologous bone marrow function after failed, mismatched bone marrow transplantation; their patients had been conditioned with antilymphocyte sera; other cases of endogenous recovery were reported following cyclophosphamide conditioning.[594–596] Immunosuppressive drug regimens, using antilymphocyte globulins and cyclosporine, have a high rate of success, $\geq 50\%$ hematopoietic recovery (see Ch. 22). As further evidence, about one-half of bone marrow transplants between syngeneic twins fail unless the host receives cytotoxic conditioning treatment,[597] and marrow graft failure can occur even with adequate preparation.[598]

Lymphocytes

Mixing and Depletion Experiments

T cells were first implicated in the etiology of aplastic anemia by in vitro studies of a patient's bone marrow. Hematopoietic colony formation only occurred after physical separation of myeloid cells from lymphocytes; colony formation was improved by addition of antilymphocyte serum; and the patient's bone marrow cells inhibited normal bone marrow colony formation.[599,600] In several larger series cellular inhibition of hematopoiesis was detected in most[601,602] or many[603-606] cases, but in other studies only a small minority or no patients showed evidence of inhibitory activity.[607-610] In some cases suppressor cell activity disappeared with successful therapy[611]; in others it was present in patients who had improved hematologically.[602,612]

Major criticisms of such studies were made based on the argument that prior transfusion affected the patient's lymphocyte function measured in vitro. Small numbers of blood transfusions in dogs sensitized recipients' lymphocytes so that they either failed to stimulate or actively depressed colony formation in co-culture experiments.[613] Co-culture inhibition was observed with much higher frequency when cells from patients who had received transfusions were used and in co-culture with histoincompatible marrow; in only 3 of 16 patients who had not received transfusions were HLA-compatible hematopoietic progenitors inhibited.[614,615] In a parallel study, removal of T cells from patient bone marrow was proposed as a means of distinguishing the transfusion effect: BFU-E-derived colony formation was increased by this maneuver in 8 of 32 patients (and no correlation between this test and co-culture inhibition was found).[616] Although other studies either had used patients with diverse hematologic diseases who had received massive transfusions as controls or were based on the T-cell depletion assay, enthusiasm for the hypothesis of immune mediation was tempered.

Analysis of Cell Surface Phenotype and Cytokine Expression

Bacigalupo et al[617] generated suppressor cells from normal bone marrow by in vitro lectin stimulation. The bone marrow cells of aplastic patients were spontaneously inhibitory, and their blood lymphocytes required only mild activation. In addition, the inhibitory activity was found in the supernatants of cultured cells. Inhibitory activity was generated by a specific subset of radiation-sensitive lymphocytes bearing receptors for IgG (T_G^+ or Tγ cells, the subpopulation that functionally suppresses immunoglobulin production by B lymphocytes), which were present in all of seven aplastic anemia patients tested but not in normal bone marrow.[505,617] The soluble inhibitor produced by stimulated normal lymphocytes was identified as IFN-γ.[618] The interferons are known to be potent inhibitors of hematopoietic colony formation.[619-625] Experimental data support the notion that IFN-γ acts both directly on progenitors[625] and through accessory immune system cells.[626] Coexpression of lymphokines by activated T lymphocytes is common, and lymphotoxins and the interferons act synergistically to suppress hematopoiesis.[504,627-630]

Heightened lymphokine production has been associated in vitro with acquisition of activation markers on stimulated lymphocytes, with IL-2 receptor (IL-2R) appearing early and HLA-DR late.[631] Inhibitory activity for hematopoiesis was localized to Fcγ receptor-bearing cells,[632] to CD8$^+$,[633-635] or nonhelper cells,[636] but only rarely to helper inducer lymphocytes CD4$^+$ or to both populations.[637,638] Triggering of the CD3 antigen receptor complex with antibody also leads to IL-2R acquisition, dependence of proliferation on IL-2, and IFN-γ mediation, at least in part, of BFU-E inhibition.[638,639]

Distinctive immune system changes have been observed in many cases of aplastic anemia. The evidence of increased activity of some components of the immune system in patients is analogous to the changes produced experimentally by stimulation of normal lymphocytes. For example, IFN-γ was overproduced by mononuclear cells from aplastic anemia patients

both following lectin stimulation or spontaneously,[640] and IL-2 production in vitro was also excessive.[641] IFN-gg activity was present in sera, and addition of antibodies to IFN-γ enhanced in vitro aplastic marrow progenitor growth.[640] Recent studies have examined cytokine gene expression in unmanipulated bone marrow using gene amplification techniques. By this method, mRNA for IFN-γ has been detected in most patients with acquired aplastic anemia, but not in normal subjects, in patients with other forms of marrow failure, or in heavily transfused control patients.[642,643] Quantitative measurements of specific mRNA also showed that tumor necrosis factor-β or lymphotoxin, while present in normal marrow, was much overexpressed in severe aplastic anemia.[644]

Cytotoxic lymphocytes also appear to be pathophysiologic in aplastic anemia. Many patients displayed inverted helper-inducer/suppressor-cytotoxic lymphocyte ratios in blood[645,646] and predominantly suppressor lymphocytes in bone marrow.[645,647,648] In addition, a distinctive population of activated cytotoxic lymphocytes was identified by the presence of CD8, HLA-DR, and IL-2R on the cell surface.[648] This population mediated suppression of hematopoiesis in vitro through lymphokine production.[649] Lymphocyte activation and lymphokine release do not relate to patients' transfusion status.[649,650] Recent studies have suggested that activated cytotoxic lymphocytes may be more easily detected in marrow samples than in peripheral blood.[651] The expanded T-cell population in aplastic anemia appears to be polyclonal[652] (Kurtzman and Young, unpublished data).

The biologic importance of immunologic dysfunction has been further supported by the observed reduction in activated lymphocytes following successful immunosuppressive therapy.[653] CD8$^+$ T-cell, IFN-γ-mediated immune suppression in nine patients disappeared after antithymocyte globulin treatment; the presence of this cell population correlated with the probability of improvement using immunosuppression.[654] Interferon gene expression also fell following successful treatment but was present in relapsed cases;[641] one study has suggested that the finding of interferon mRNA in aplastic marrow predicted responsiveness to immunosuppressive therapy.[642] In another setting—experimental immunotherapy of cancer—IL-2 administration has been associated with lymphocyte activation in vivo, release of IFN-γ and tumor necrosis factor, and hematopoietic suppression.[655-657]

The most likely explanation for the immune system abnormalities in aplastic anemia is that activated cytotoxic lymphocytes function as pathophysiologic mediators of marrow suppression. These cells might suppress hematopoiesis directly or through the release of inhibitory cytokines. Other, more subtle effects may also be important. One important role of IFN-γ is to increase cell surface expression of HLA-DR on target cells,[658] thus enhancing their recognition by lymphocytes; IFN-γ also induces the production of other inhibitory molecules such as tumor necrosis factor.[659] However, the relationships between cells of the immune and hematopoietic systems are complex. Some hematopoietic growth factors (IL-3, CSF-GM) are produced by stimulated lymphocytes, including cells of the cytotoxic/suppressor phenotype[660] (although in vitro the kinetics are different from the kinetics of production of inhibitory molecules.[632] IL-2 can enhance T-cell release of colony-stimulating[661] and burst-promoting activities,[662] and inhibitory molecules like interferon and tumor necrosis factor can promote production of colony-stimulating activities.[663,664] Under some conditions even IFN-γ may have positive effects on hematopoiesis.[665]

Findings of lymphocyte activation and lymphokine overproduction in aplastic anemia have been broadly if not uniformly

Table 21-7. Summary of Studies of Immune Pathophysiology in Aplastic Anemia

Phenomenon	Positive Studies	Negative Studies
Activated T cells	CD8+, DR+, IL-2R+ in 10/12[659] Tac+ pre-BMT[739] T8+ mediate suppression[663]	DR+ in 4/21[351] nl mean[623,664,740]
High IFN-γ production	Spontaneous and stimulated[652,664,741] Stimulated only[663]	Normal 7/7[742]
Serum IFN-γ	Bioassay[652] RIA[564]	RIA[664,741]
High IL-2 production	12/17[653] 18/34[583]	
CD4+/CD8+ ≤ 1	15/28[654] 8/31[655] 12/22[743] 10/21[350] Low mean[739] 11/18[744]	3/18[349] 3/18[657] 6/27[740] nl mean[663] 2/19[623] 2/7[742]
Clinical correlation	Decreased IL-2R+ T cells with recovery[662] CD4+/CD8+ with recovery[743] Falling IL-2R+ cells with ATG[745] CD8+ number, activation with BMT[739] IFN-γ production with ATG[663]	IFN-γ production with ATG[746] CD4+/CD8+ with ATG[744] CD4+/CD8+ with therapy[740]

Abbreviations: RIA, radioimmunoassay; ATG antithymocyte globulin; IL-2R, interleukin-2; BMT, bone marrow transplantation.

confirmed (Table 21-7). As described above, study of the marrow, the site of disease, while more technically challenging, may also be more rewarding for detection of abnormal cells and their products. Other markers of immune system activation may also be present in aplastic anemia. Most patients also have elevated serum-soluble levels of CD8[666] and the soluble form of IL-2R (Maron, Young, and Nelson, unpublished data). In lymphocyte cytotoxicity studies that used autologous or HLA-identical target cells, about 30% of patients showed autoreactivity,[667,668] and 50% showed alloreactivity, apparently independently of transfusion history.[668] Atypical lymphocytes, a morphologic sign of lymphocyte activation, are also commonly present in aplastic anemia patients.

Natural Killer Cells

Natural killer (NK) cells,[669] like cytotoxic lymphocytes, also express CD8 antigen on the cell surface[670] and they can produce IFN-γ, IL-2, and colony-stimulating activities.[671,672] That NK cell activity can be generated from cloned murine cytotoxic T cells[673] implies a close ontogenic relationship between the two cell types. Like cytotoxic/suppressor lymphocytes, NK cells can suppress hematopoiesis. Human NK cells inhibit myeloid[674–677] and erythroid[676–678] colony formation. Analysis of individual human NK cell clones has suggested that some cells may preferentially affect erythroid or myeloid progenitor cells.[677] Murine NK cells have been reported to inhibit either differentiating marrow cells[679,680] or more primitive CFV-S cells.[681,683] Usually NK cell action requires intimate cell contact between effector and target, but soluble inhibitors, including IFN-γ, can function as effectors and in addition can increase NK activity and target cell recognition.[675,677,683] In some cases NK cell inhibition of hematopoiesis may behave as if it were HLA-DR restricted,[676] a property of cytotoxic T cells. A pathologic rather than physiologic function for NK cells in bone marrow is suggested by normal hematopoiesis in the presence of these cells.[684]

NK cells are pathogenic in at least one disease, Tγ-lymphoproliferative disease, a large granular lymphocytosis of which neutropenia and other single-cell cytopenias are common manifestations.[682,685] Some patients with idiopathic or cyclic neutropenia may also show increased circulating[686] or bone marrow[687] large granular lymphocytes. Both direct cytotoxicity and IFN-γ-mediated[688] suppression of hematopoiesis may be pathogenic. NK cells have also been implicated in graft rejection following bone marrow transplantation.[689,690] NK cell activity may play a dominant role in hematopoietic suppression mediated by IL-2-stimulated lymphocytes (lymphokine-activated cells).[691]

However, there is little evidence for a role of NK cells in aplastic anemia. Multiple studies of aplastic anemia patients have shown low NK cell activity and low numbers of phenotypically defined NK cells in blood and bone marrow[692–695]; both return toward normal with hematopoietic recovery.[692,695] NK cell activity has been implicated in the normal host immune defense against viral infection, and an interesting question is whether a NK cell deficiency state might predispose to chronic viral infections that suppress the bone marrow.

Stimuli for T-Cell Activation

Cytotoxic lymphocytes are a major component of the primary response to viral infection. In some series of aplastic anemia patients, immunologic abnormalities have clustered in a subset of patients whose marrow failure is associated with a virus, usually hepatitis (e.g., low helper-inducer/suppressor-cytotoxic lymphocyte ratios and elevated numbers of activated suppressor-cytotoxic cells).[350,351] Cell lines with the activated suppressor-cytotoxic cell phenotype have been isolated from the blood of a patient with hepatitis-associated aplastic anemia[696] and from a patient with EBV-associated aplastic anemia (Baranski and Young, unpublished data); these cell lines produced IFN-γ and suppressed hematopoiesis in vitro.

Activation of cytotoxic lymphocytes is a feature of the immune response to viruses,[697] some of which have been implicated in marrow failure, such as the flaviviruses[698] and herpesviruses.[699] In aplasia, the lymphocyte response itself may be more destructive than the original viral infection. Murine lymphocytic choriomeningitis virus is the paradigm of cytotoxic lymphocyte- and lymphokine-mediated pathology.[700] Detailed studies of this model and others have shown that the amount of virus may be small yet provoke a cytopathic immune response. Cytotoxic lymphocytes may be targeted to cells by nonstructural viral proteins synthesized in latently infected cells or by viral peptides passively attached to the MHC antigens on the cell surface; exposure to a virus may provoke attack on normal cells by molecular mimicry.[701–703] Viruses differ in the pattern of host response they provoke, with great variation in experimental infection in the relative importance of CD8+, CD4+, NK, and antibody responses. Finally, the presence and magnitude of the host immune response are genetically regulated.[704] In humans, permissivity for persistent parvovirus infection appears as a restricted immunodeficiency syndrome and susceptibility to the malignant and destructive complications of EBV, an X-linked trait. Similar considerations apply to the immune response to other antigens, especially drugs or chemicals presented to the immune system as haptens. Genetic differences among viruses and among people offer ample explanation for the variability in the consequences of bone marrow infection.

Antibodies

Immunoglobulin-mediated inhibition of hematopoiesis is less important in the pathology of aplastic anemia than in the single-cell cytopenias, especially pure red blood cell aplasia and agranulocytosis (see Ch. 52). In most cases of aplastic anemia, the clinical significance and specificity of serum inhibitors are uncertain. In a study published in 1978, sera from seven of eight aplastic anemia patients was reported to inhibit myeloid progenitor cells[707] serum inhibitory activity has been reported in a substantial minority of patients in subsequent series.[495,706–708] However, serum inhibitory activity in most cases is associated with transfusions, often directed against HLA antigens and frequently not reactive with the patient's own cells.[706,707] Serum inhibitors may be present in multiparous women, in patients with other hematologic diseases who have received multiple transfusions, and in occasional normal individuals.[496,708–710]

Well-characterized antibody inhibitors have been described in rare cases of rather atypical bone marrow failure and occasional patients with drug-associated aplastic anemia. In the first category are individual patients with unusual patterns of disease; these include episodic panleukopenia[711] and aplasia with normal in vitro colony formation[712] and, more frequently, aplastic anemia associated with systemic lupus erythematosus.[713–716] (Systemic lupus is also associated with antibody immune-mediated neutropenia, thrombocytopenia, and autoimmune hemolytic anemia.) Some of these patients have recovered with the aid of plasmapheresis or immunosuppressive drug therapy.

Antibody inhibitors have been defined by their ability to inhibit hematopoietic colony formation in vitro. A convincing demonstration of antibody-mediated disease requires isolation and identification of an immunoglobulin fraction, determination of complement dependence, and some clinical correlation between the presence of the inhibitor and the course of the disease. Antibody activity is usually complement dependent,[707,713,715,716] but it may be independent of complement.[713] In some cases both humoral and cellular inhibition of in vitro hematopoiesis have been detected in the same patient.[712,714] Antibodies to progenitor cells also have been demonstrated in drug-associated bone marrow failure, but much more rarely in pancytopenia as compared with drug-associated agranulocyto-

sis and pure red cell aplasia. In one patient with aplastic anemia following quinidine, acute-phase serum plus drug (but not either serum alone or convalescent phase serum plus drug) inhibited normal bone marrow colony formation.[717] For drug-associated antibody formation in general, progenitor cells often appear to act as "innocent bystanders" that bind antibody-drug complexes.[718] For metamizole and diclofenac agranulocytosis, putative drug metabolites present in urine, rather than the parent compounds, were antigenic[718]; detection of antibodies to metabolites greatly complicates detection of a specific antibody response. Autoantibodies have also been found in the sera of some patients with drug-associated agranulocytosis,[718,719] but whether they are pathogenic or represent an immune response to a damaged cell membrane or lysed cell constituent is unknown.

MODEL(S) OF BONE MARROW FAILURE

The mechanisms of bone marrow failure are complex but perhaps not infinitely so. Hematopoiesis may be blocked because of defects in stroma or growth factor production in some inherited bone marrow failure states, and antibodies are important in some monocytopenias, but these are not major pathogenic mechanisms in most cases of acquired aplastic anemia.

Stem cell damage or loss almost certainly underlies adult aplasia. Two different pathways of bone marrow injury, based on the paradigms of animals treated with busulfan or hydroxyurea, are diagrammed in Figure 21-10. Common to both pathways is the crucial position of the most primitive hematopoietic stem cells. These cells are mitotically quiescent. Quiescence serves to prevent stem cell compartment depletion in the course of normal hematopoietic demands. Quiescence also protects stem cells from a variety of environmental toxins and viruses, which would be expected to be most injurious to metabolically active cells.

In pathway I, damage to the hematopoietic compartment is random, striking all cells with an equal probability. This path-

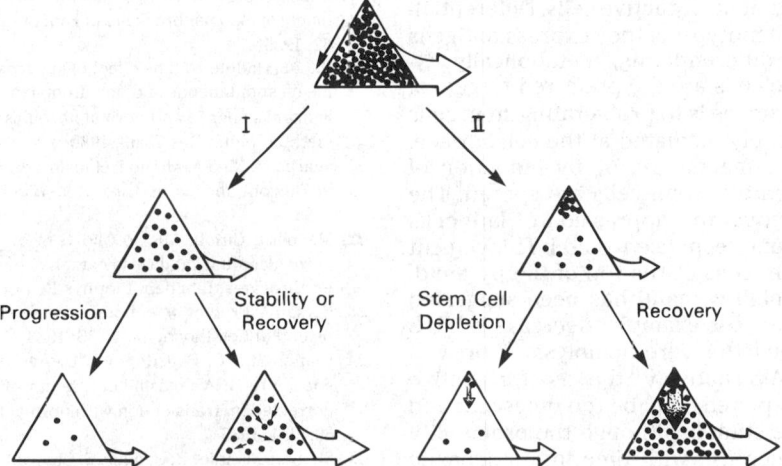

Fig. 21-10. Simplified diagram showing two mechanisms of stem cell compartment damage. Stem cells are depicted in outline according to the scheme of Figure 21-10. Type I damage is directed at the DNA; examples of agents include irradiation, radiomimetic agents such as busulfan, and some drugs (perhaps chloramphenicol); Fanconi's anemia would represent genetic susceptibility to type I damage due to inability to repair DNA damage. Type II damage would occur at the level of the cell membrane, the metabolic machinery of the cell, or by induction of apoptosis and would include most drugs, viruses, and immune-mediated marrow failure. Some exogenous agents may act to injure a late cell's metabolic machinery and also to introduce genetic damage (benzene may be an example); genetic susceptibility as in Fanconi's anemia implies an external precipitating event. Very primitive stem cells would feed recovery when loss has occurred to actively cycling cells (right), while later stem cells would be needed to repair random damage (left). At some point in either scheme, qualitative alterations in the compartment can become an absolute, quantitative loss of stem cells. Nonetheless, hematopoietic recovery should be easier with type II damage, in which the repopulating cells are preserved.

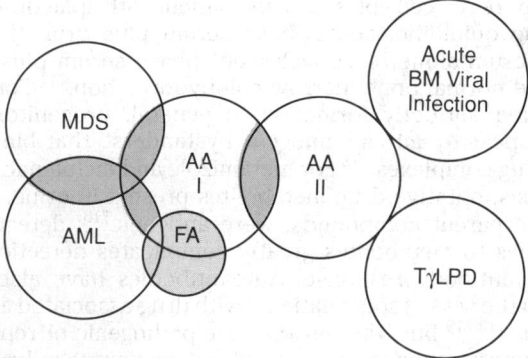

Fig. 21-11. Venn diagram that relates types I and II aplastic anemia to related hematologic diseases. Real overlap exists between type I aplastic anemia and myelodysplastic and leukemic syndromes because of the commonality of DNA damage to these diseases. That only some ordinary viral infections result in aplasia is probably a function of the immune response. Monoclonal (if not malignant) proliferation of similar cytotoxic lymphocytes such as those detected in some cases of type II aplastic anemia results in Tγ-lymphoproliferative disease.

way is the likely mechanism of direct injury to cellular DNA; examples of exogenous agents include irradiation, alkylating drugs, reactive benzene metabolites, and perhaps also chloramphenicol. While the likelihood of injury would be the same for all cells, the effect would be selective for more primitive cells because primitive cells require many mitoses to mature, while late cells have accomplished most of their mitotic life and need only a few divisions to reach terminal maturation. Recovery would occur throughout the compartment, but a permanent severe defect in stem cell number and self-renewal capacity would ensue, as a result of busulfan or radiation treatment. The introduction of DNA defects is probably rare aside from iatrogenic or experimental drug and x-ray exposure. The genetic defects that cause Fanconi's anemia, in which repair of DNA is inadequate, would be the commonest examples of bone marrow failure by pathway I. By contrast, most environmental damage to the stem cell compartment is probably directed at mitotically and metabolically active cells. Differentiating cells acquire a distinct phenotype as they express antigens absent on immature cells; differentiating, metabolically dynamic, and mitotically active cells are the preferred targets of most viruses. In pathway II damage is to proliferating stem cells and progenitors and is probably mediated at the cell surface, through the cell's metabolic machinery, or by induction of apoptosis, but the most primitive stem cells are spared. The response to continuous removal or suppression of late cells by viral infection or an immune response would be movement from the most primitive stem cells at the top of the pyramid. Depletion of stem cells by high demand has been suggested by some experimental results, for example, decreased CFU-S self-renewal following prolonged severe hemolysis[530] or with growth factor therapy.[720] Alternatively, the most primitive stem cells, even when not depleted, may be too quiescent and too unresponsive to positive stimuli, although the probability of such a response might increase with time in a stochastic model.

The high recovery rate from aplastic anemia following immunosuppressive therapy would imply that most patients suffer from type II damage to the stem cell compartment. Type II aplastic anemia would be related mechanistically to hematopoietic depression in many viral infections, which is usually transient and moderate when terminated by an appropriate immune response, and to the Tγ-lymphoproliferative diseases, in which monoclonal (but not necessarily frankly malignant) proliferation of cytotoxic lymphocytes can result in bone marrow depression (Fig. 21-11).

REFERENCES

1. Young NS, Alter BF: Aplastic Anemia, Acquired and Inherited. WB Saunders, Philadelphia, 1994
2. Ehrlich P: Ueber einen Fall von Anämie mit Bemerkungen über regenerative Veränderungen des Knochenmarks. Charite Ann 13:300, 1888
3. Young NS, Issaragrisil S, Ch'en WC, Takaku F: Aplastic anemia in the Orient. Br J Haematol 62:1, 1986
4. Gordon-Smith EC, Issargrisil S: Epidemiology of aplastic anaemia. Baillieres Clin Haematol 5:475, 1992
5. Issargrisil S, Sriratanasatavorn C, Piankijagum A et al: The incidence of aplastic anemia in Bangkok. Blood 77:2166, 1991
6. Aoki K: Epidemiology. p. 1. In Hibino S, Takaku F (eds): Aplastic Anemia. Igaku-Shoin, Tokyo, 1979
7. Yin D, Wu Y, Lin Z et al: Epidemiological and etiological studies on aplastic anemia in the Mudanjiang area. Chin J Hematol 1:33, 1980
8. Whang KS: Aplastic anemia in Korea: a clinical study of 309 cases. p. 225. In Hibino S, Takaku F, Shahidi NT (eds): Aplastic Anemia. University Park Press, Baltimore, 1978
9. Auerbach AD, Rogatko A, Traute M, Schroeder-Kurth TM: International Fanconi anemia registry: relation of clinical symptoms to diepoxybutane sensitivity. Blood 73:391, 1989
10. Turner DR, Morley AA, Seshadri RS: Lymphocyte DNA in aplastic anaemia. Br J Haematol 48:207, 1981
11. Kovacs E, Nissen C, Speck B, Signer E: Repair of UV-induced DNA damage in aplastic anaemia: changes after treatment with antilymphocyte globulin (ALG). Eur J Haematol 40:430, 1988
12. Gordon-Smith EC, Rutherford TR: Fanconi anaemia—constitutional, familial aplastic anaemia. Baillieres Clin Haematol 2:139, 1989
13. Shahidi NT: Fanconi's anemia, dyskeratosis congenita, and WT syndrome. Am J Med Genet, suppl. 3:263, 1987
14. Kaiser TN, Lojewski A, Dougherty C et al: Flow cytometric characterization of the response of Fanconi's anemia cells to mitomycin C treatment. Cytometry 2:291, 1989
15. Kubbies M, Schindler D, Hoehn H et al: Endogenous blockage and delay of the chromosome cycle despite normal recruitment and growth phase expain poor proliferation and frequent endomitosis in Fanconi anemia cells. Am J Hum Genet 37:1022, 1985
16. Strathdee CA, Duncan AMV, Buchwald M: Evidence for at least four Fanconi anaemia genes including FACC on chromosome 9. Nature Genet 1:196, 1992
17. Timme TL, Moses RE: Diseases with DNA damage-processing defects. Am J Med Sci 295:40, 1988
18. Joenje H, Arwert F, Eriksson AW et al: Oxygen-dependence of chromosomal aberrations in Fanconi's anaemia. Nature 290:142, 1981
19. Dallapiccola B, Porfirio B, Mokini V et al: Effect of oxidants and antioxidants on chromosomal breakage in Fanconi anemia lymphocytes. Hum Genet 69:62, 1985
20. Raj AS, Heddle JA: The effect of superoxide dismutase, catalase and L-cysteine on spontaneous and on mitomycin C induced chromosomal breakage in Fanconi's anemia and normal fibroblasts as measured by the micronucleus method. Mutat Res 78:59, 1980
21. Scarpa M, Rigo A, Momo F et al: Increased rate of superoxide ion generation in Fanconi anemia erythrocytes. Biochem Biophys Res Commun 130:127, 1985
22. Mavelli I, Ciriolo MR, Rotilio G et al: Superoxide dismutase, glutathione peroxidase and catalase in oxidative hemolysis. A study of Fanconi's anemia erythrocytes. Biochem Biophys Res Commun 106:286, 1982
23. Petkau A: Protection of bone marrow progenitor cells by superoxide dismutase. Mol Cell Biochem 84:133, 1988
24. Diatloff-Zito C, Papadopoulo D, Averbek D, Moustacchi E: Abnormal response to DNA crosslinking agents of Fanconi anemia fibroblasts can be corrected by transfection with normal human DNA. Proc Natl Acad Sci USA 83:7034, 1986
25. Shaham M, Adler B, Ganguly S, Chaganti RSK: Transfection of normal human and Chinese hamster DNA corrects diepoxybutane-induced chromosomal hypersensitivity of Fanconi anemia fibroblasts. Proc Natl Acad Sci USA 84:5853, 1987
26. Strathdee CA, Gavish H, Shannon WR, Buchwald M: Cloning of cDNAs for Fanconi's anaemia by functional complementation. Nature 356:763, 1992
27. Strathdee CA, Buchwald M: Molecular and cellular biology of Fanconi anemia. Am J Pediatr Hematol Oncol 14:177, 1992
28. Gavish H, dos Santos CC, Buchwald M: A Leu554-to-Pro substitution completely abolishes the functional complementing activity of the Fanconi anemia (FACC) protein. Hum Mol Genet 2:123, 1993
29. Whitney MA, Saito H, Jakobs PM et al: A common mutation in the FACC gene causes Fanconi anaemia in Ashkenazi Jews. Nature Genet 4:202, 1993

30. Sleifer DT, Mulder NH, Nieweg HO et al: Acquired pancytopenia in relatives of patients with aplastic anaemia. J Intern Med 207:397, 1980
31. Garriga S, Crosby WH: The incidence of leukemia in families of patients with hypoplasia of the marrow. Blood 14:1008, 1959
32. Li FP, Potter NU, Buchanan GR et al: A family with acute leukemia, hypoplastic anemia and cerebellar ataxia. Am J Med 65:933, 1978
33. Chitambar CR, Robinson WA, Glode LM: Familial leukemia and aplastic anemia associated with monosomy 7. Am J Med 75:756, 1983
34. Nagata M, Hara T, Sakamoto K, Ueda K: Aplastic anemia associated with ataxia and chromosome translocation (1;20). Acta Haematol 84:198, 1990
35. Alter CL, Levine PH, Bennett J et al: Dominantly transmitted hematologic dysfunction clinically similar to Fanconi's anemia. Am J Hematol 32:241, 1989
36. Appelbaum FR, Barrall J, Storb R et al: Clonal cytogenetic abnormalities in patients with otherwise typical aplastic anemia. Exp Hematol 15:1134, 1987
37. Purtilo DT, Sakamoto K, Barnabei V et al: Epstein-Barr virus-induced diseases in boys with the X-linked lymphoproliferative syndrome (XLP). Update on studies of the registry. Am J Med 73:49, 1982
38. Dameshek W: Chloramphenicol aplastic anemia in identical twins—a clue to pathogenesis. N Engl J Med 281:42, 1969
39. McLaren GD, Doukas MA, Muir WA: Methyprylon-induced bone marrow suppression in siblings. JAMA 240:1744, 1978
40. Dausset J, Gluckman E, Lemarchand F et al: Excès d'HLA-A2 et d'homozygotes HLA-A2 parmi les malades atteints d'aplasie médullaire et maladie de Fanconi. Nouv Rev Franc Hematol 18:315, 1977
41. Chapuis B, Von Fliedner VE, Jeannet M et al: Increased frequency of DR2 in patients with aplastic anaemia and increased DR sharing in their parents. Br J Haematol 63:51, 1986
42. Odum N, Platz P, Morling N et al: Increased frequency of HLA-DPw3 in severe aplastic anemia (AA). Tissue Antigens 29:184, 1987
43. Cronkite EP: Hematology, diagnosis and therapy of radiation injury. US Armed Forces Med J 56:661, 1951
44. Knospe WH: Long-term bone marrow damage after irradiation. p. 93. In Testa NG, Gale RP (ed): Hematopoiesis. Long-Term Effects of Chemotherapy and Radiation. Marcel Dekker, New York, 1988
45. Champlin R: Bone marrow aplasia due to radiation accidents: pathophysiology, assessment and treatment. Baillieres Clin Haematol 2:69, 1989
46. Wald N, Thoma GE, Broun G Jr: Hematological manifestations of radiation exposure in man. Prog Hematol 3:1, 1962
47. Andrews GA: The medical management of accidental total-body irradiation. p. 297. In Hübner KF, Fry SA (eds): The Medical Basis for Radiation Accident Preparedness. Elsevier/North Holland, New York, 1980
48. Bruegge CFV: Radiation injury following an A-bomb explosion. Ann Intern Med 36:1444, 1952
49. Gale RP: Immediate medical consequences of nuclear accidents. Lessons from Chernobyl. JAMA 258:625, 1987
50. Pollard EC: The biological action of ionizing radiation. Am Sci 57:206, 1969
51. Puck TT: The action of radiation on mammalian cells. Am Naturalist 94:95, 1960
52. Baverstock KF, Ash PJND: A review of radiation accidents involving whole body exposure and the relevance to LD50/60 for man. Br J Radiol 56:837, 1983
53. Adams GE: Lethality from acute and protracted radiation exposure in man. Int J Radiat Biol 46:209, 1984
54. Mole RH: The LD50 for uniform low LET irradiation of man. Br J Radiol 57:355, 1984
55. Liebow AA, Warren S, DeCoursey E: Pathology of atomic bomb casualties. Am J Pathol 25:853, 1949
56. LeRoy GV: Hematology of atomic bomb casualties. Arch Intern Med 86:691, 1950
57. Fliedner TM: The bone marrow syndrome: signs, symptoms, time course of hematological and pathological findings, dose-response functions; replacement therapy. p. 14. In Bond VP, Cronkite EP (eds): Workshop on Short-Term Health Effects of Reactor Accidents: Chernobyl, August 8–9, 1986. Brookhaven National Laboratory, Upton, NY, 1986
58. Kirshbaum JD, Marsuo T, Sato K et al: A study of aplastic anemia in an autopsy series with special reference to atomic bomb survivors in Hiroshima and Nagasaki. Blood 38:17, 1971
59. Lange RD, Wright SW, Tomonaga M et al: Refractory anemia occurring in survivors of the atomic bombing in Nagasaki, Japan. Blood 10:312, 1955
60. Conrad RA, Cronkite EP, Bond VP et al: Fallout radiation: effects on Marshallese people. p. 308. In Behrens CF, King ER, Carpender JWJ (eds): Atomic Medicine. 5th Ed. Williams & Wilkins, Baltimore, 1969
61. Fliedner TM, Nothdurft W, Calvo W: The development of radiation late effects to the bone marrow after single and chronic exposure. Int J Radiat Biol 49:35, 1986
62. Reincke U, Hannon EC, Hellman S: Residual radiation injury exhibited in long-term bone marrow cultures. J Cell Physiol 112:345, 1982
63. Martland HS: Occupational poisoning in manufacture of luminous watch dials. JAMA 92:466, 1929
64. Kamiyama R, Ishikawa Y, Hatakeyama S et al: Clinicopathologic study of hematological disorders after thorotrast administration in Japan. Blut 56:153, 1988
65. Court-Brown WM, Doll R: Leukemia and aplastic anaemia in patients irradiated for ankylosing spondylitis. (British) Medical Research Council Special Report Series, No. 295. H.M. Stationery Office, London, 1957
66. Lewis EB: Leukemia, multiple myeloma, and aplastic anemia in American radiologists. Science 142:1492, 1963
67. Bithell TC, Wintrobe MM: Drug-induced aplastic anemia. Semin Hematol 4:194, 1967
68. Williams DM, Lynch RE, Cartwright GE: Drug-induced aplastic anemia. Semin Hematol 10:195, 1973
69. Le Gall E, Guerin MN, Le Prise PV et al: The role of pharmacologic and industrial agents in the etiology of aplastic anemia. p. 13. In Najean Y (ed): Medullary Aplasia. Masson Publishing, New York, 1980
70. Young N: Drugs and chemicals as agents of bone marrow failure. p. 131. In Testa N, Gale RC (eds): Hematopoiesis. Long-Term Effects of Chemotherapy and Radiation. Marcel Dekker, New York, 1988
71. Gordon-Smith EC: Aplastic anaemia—aetiology and clinical features. Bailleres Clin Haematol 2:18, 1989
72. Heimpel H, Heit W: Drug-induced aplastic anaemia: clinical aspects. Clin Haematol 9:641, 1980
73. Aksoy M, Erdem S, Dincol G et al: Aplastic anemia due to chemicals and drugs: a study of 108 patients. Sex Transm Dis 11:347, 1984
74. Linet MS, Markowitz JA, Sensenbrenner LL et al: A case-control study of aplastic anemia. Leuk Res 13:3, 1989
75. Kaufman DW, Kelly JP, Levy M, Shapiro S: The Drug Etiology of Agranulocytosis and Aplastic Anemia. Oxford University Press, New York, 1991
76. Wallerstein RO, Condit PK, Kasper CK et al: Statewide study of chloramphenicol therapy and fatal aplastic anemia. JAMA 208:2045, 1969
77. Smick KM, Condit PK, Proctor RL, Sutcher V: Fatal aplastic anemia: an epidemiological study of its relationship to the drug chloramphenicol. J Chronic Dis 17:899, 1964
78. Custer RP: Aplastic anemia in soldiers treated with atabrine. Am J Med Sci 212:211, 1946
79. Inman WHW: Study of fatal bone marrow depression with special reference to phenylbutazone and oxyphenbutazone. BMJ 1:1500, 1977
80. Daum RS, Cohen DL, Smith AL: Fatal aplastic anemia following apparent "dose-related" chloramphenicol toxicity. J Pediatr 94:403, 1979
81. Testa NG, Hendry JH, Molineux G: Long-term bone marrow damage after cytotoxic treatment: stem cells and microenvironment. p. 75. In Testa NG, Gale RP (eds): Hematopoiesis. 8th Ed. Marcel Dekker, New York, 1988
82. Bowcock SJ, Galton DAG, Goldman JG: Marrow aplasia developing 3 years after treatment with busulphan for chronic myeloid leukemia. Eur J Haematol 42:496, 1989
83. Snyder R, Kocsis JJ: Current concepts of chronic benzene toxicity. CRC Crit Rev Toxicol 3:265, 1975
84. Fishbein L: An overview of environmental and toxicological aspects of aromatic hydrocarbons. I. Benzene. Sci Total Environ 40:189, 1984
85. Brief RS, Lynch J, Bernath T, Scala RA: Benzene in the workplace. Am Ind Hyg Assoc J 41:616, 1980
86. Hamilton A: Benzene (benzol) poisoning. Arch Pathol Lab Med 11:434, 1931
87. Rejsek K, Rejsková M: Long term observation of chronic benzene poisoning. J Intern Med 152:71, 1955
88. Vigliani EC, Forni A: Benzene and leukemia. Environ Res 11:122, 1976
89. Wester RC, Maibach HI, Gruenke LD, Craig JC: Benzene levels in ambient air and breath of smokers and nonsmokers in urban and pristine environments. J Toxicol Environ Health 18:567, 1986
90. Brandi L, Nilsson PG, Mitelman F: Non-industrial exposure to benzene as leukaemogenic risk factor. Lancet 2:1074, 1977
91. Cronkite EP: Benzene hematotoxicity and leukemogenesis. Blood Cells 12:129, 1986
92. Srbová J, Teisinger J, Skramovsky S: Absorption and elimination of inhaled benzene in man. Arch Ind Hyg Occup Med 2:1, 1950
93. Sato A, Nakajima T, Fujiwara Y, Hirosawa K: Pharmacokinetics of benzene and toluene. Int Arch Occup Environ Health 33:169, 1974
94. Irons RD, Dent JG, Baker TS, Rickert DE: Benzene is metabolized and covalently bound in bone marrow in situ. Chem Biol Interact 30:241, 1980
95. Andrews LS, Sasame HA, Gillette JR: ^{3}H-benzene metabolism in rabbit bone marrow. Life Sci 25:567, 1979
96. Kalf GF, Post GB, Snyder R: Solvent toxicology: recent advances in the toxi-

cology of benzene, the glycol ethers, and carbon tetrachloride. Annu Rev Pharmacol Toxicol 27:399, 1987

97. Sawahata T, Rickert DE, Greenlee WF: Metabolism of benzene and its metabolites in bone marrow. p. 141. In Irons RD (ed): Toxicology of the Blood and Bone Marrow. Raven Press, New York, 1985

98. Greenlee WF, Sun JD, Bus JS: A proposed mechanism of benzene toxicity: formation of reactive intermediates from polyphenol metabolites. Toxicol Appl Pharmacol 59:187, 1981

99. Lutz WK, Schlatter CH: Mechanism of the carcinogenic action of benzene: irreversible binding to rat liver DNA. Chem Biol Interact 18:241, 1977

100. Lee EW, Garner CD, Johnson JT: A proposed role played by benzene itself in the induction of acute cytopenia: inhibition of DNA synthesis. Res Commun Chem Pathol Pharmacol 60:27, 1988

101. Kissling M, Speck B: Further studies on experimental benzene induced aplastic anemia. Blut 25:97, 1972

102. Pellack-Walker P, Blumer JL: DNA damage in L5178YS cells following exposure to benzene metabolites. Mol Pharmacol 30:42, 1986

103. Rithidech K, Au WW, Ramanujam VMS et al: Induction of chromosome aberrations in lymphocytes of mice after subchronic exposure to benzene. Mutat Res 188:135, 1987

104. Tough IM, Brown WMC: Chromosome aberrations and exposure to ambient benzene. Lancet I:684, 1965

105. Jablonická A, Vargová M, Karelová J: Cytogenetic analysis of peripheral blood lymphocytes in workers exposed to benzene. J Hyg Epidemiol Microbiol Immunol 31:127, 1987

106. Snyder R, Lee EW, Kocsis JJ: Binding of labeled benzene metabolites to mouse liver and bone marrow. Res Commun Chem Pathol Pharmacol 20: 191, 1978

107. Tunek A, Platt KL, Bentley P, Oesch F: Microsomal metabolism of benzene to species irreversibly binding to microsomal protein and effects of modifications of this metabolism. Mol Pharmacol 14:920, 1978

108. Harper C, Drew RT, Fouts JR: Species differences in benzene hydroxylation to phenol by pulmonary and hepatic microsomes. Drug Metab Dispos 3: 381, 1975

109. Sabourin PJ, Bechtold WE, Birnbaum LS et al: Differences in metabolism and disposition of inhaled [3H]benzene by F344/N rats and B6C3F1 mice. Toxicol Appl Pharmacol 94:128, 1988

110. Moeschlin S, Speck B: Experimental studies on the mechanism of action of benzene on the bone marrow (radioautographic studies using H-thymidine). Acta Haematol 38:104, 1967

111. Uyeki EM, Ashkar AE, Shoeman DW, Bisel TU: Acute toxicity of benzene inhalation to hemopoietic precursor cells. Toxicol Appl Pharmacol 40:49, 1977

112. Hilderbrand RL, Murphy MJ: The effects of benzene inhalation on murine hematopoietic precursor cells (CFU-e, BFU-e and CFU-gm). Int J Cell Cloning 1:240, 1983

113. Gill DP, Jenkins VK, Kempen RR, Ellis S: The importance of pluripotential stem cells in benzene toxicity. Toxicology 16:163, 1980

114. Seidel HJ, Barthel E, Zinser D: The hematopoietic stem cell compartments in mice during and after long-term inhalation of three doses of benzene. Exp Hematol 17:300, 1989

115. Green JD, Snyder CA, LoBue J et al: Acute and chronic dose/response effects of inhaled benzene on multipotential hematopoietic stem (CFU-S) and granulocyte/macrophage progenitor. Toxicol Appl Pharmacol 58:492, 1981

116. Garnett HM, Cronkite EP, Drew RT: Effect of in vivo exposure to benzene on the characteristics of bone marrow adherent cells. Leuk Res 7:803, 1983

117. Gaido K, Wierda D: In vitro effects of benzene metabolites on mouse bone marrow stromal cells. Toxicol Appl Pharmacol 76:45, 1984

118. Chertkov JL, Lutton JD, Jiang S et al: Hematopoietic effects of benzene inhalation assessed by murine long-term bone marrow culture. J Lab Clin Med 119:412, 1992

119. Steinberg B: Bone marrow regeneration in experimental benzene intoxication. Blood 4:550, 1949

120. Thomas DJ, Reasor MJ, Wierda D: Macrophage regulation of myelopoiesis is altered by exposure to the benzene metabolite hydroquinone. Toxicol Appl Pharmacol 97:440, 1989

121. Aoyama K: Effects of benzene inhalation on lymphocyte subpopulations and immune response in mice. Toxicol Appl Pharmacol 85:92, 1986

122. Hsieh GC, Sharma RP, Parker RDR: Subclinical effects of groundwater contaminants. I: Alteration of humoral and cellular immunity by benzene in CD-1 mice. Arch Environ Contam Toxicol 17:151, 1988

123. Bostrom B, Smith K, Ramsay N: Low concentrations of benzene stimulate CFU/GM. Blood 66:119, 1985

124. Hunter FT: Chronic exposure to benzene (benzol). II. The clinical effects. J Ind Hyg Toxicol 21:331, 1939

125. Erf LA, Rhoads CP: The hematological effects of benzene (benzol) poisoning. J Ind Hyg Toxicol 21:421, 1939

126. Goldwater LJ: Disturbances in the blood following exposure to benzol. J Lab Clin Med 26:957, 1941

127. Oldfeldt CO: Benzene poisoning; clinical considerations. J Intern Med 119: 380, 1944

128. Aksoy M, Koray D, Akgun T et al: Haematological effects of chronic benzene poisoning in 217 workers. Br J Med 28:296, 1971

129. Yin S-N, Li Q, Liu Y et al: Occupational exposure to benzene in China. Br J Ind Med 44:192, 1987

130. Savilhati M: Mehr als 100 Vergiftungsfälle durch Benzol in einer Schuhfabrik. Arch Gewerbepathol Gewerbehyg 15:147, 1956

131. Moszczynski P, Lisiewicz J: Hematological indices of peripheral blood in workers occupationally exposed to benzene, tolvene and xylene. Zentralbl Bakteriol Mikrobiol Hyg[B] 178:329, 1983

132. Aksoy M, Dincol K, Erdem S et al: Details of blood changes in 32 patients with pancytopenia associated with long-term exposure to benzene. Br J Ind Med 29:56, 1972

133. Aksoy M, Erdem S: Follow-up study on the mortality and the development of leukemia in 44 pancytopenic patients with chronic exposure to benzene. Blood 52:285, 1978

134. Jacobs A: Benzene and leukemia. Br J Haematol 72:119, 1989

135. Arp EW, Wolf PH, Checkoway H: Lymphocytic leukemia and exposures to benzene and other solvents in the rubber industry. J Occup Med 25:598, 1983

136. Decoufle P, Blattner WA, Blair A: Mortality among chemical workers exposed to benzene and other agents. Environ Res 30:16, 1983

137. Gerarde HW: Toxicological studies on hydrocarbons. II. A comparative study of the effect of benzene and certain mono-n-alkylbenzenes on hemopoiesis and bone marrow metabolism in rats. AMA Arch Ind Health 13:468, 1956

138. Wolf MA, Rowe VK, McCollister DD et al: Toxicological studies of certain alkylated benzenes and benzene. AMA Arch Ind Health 14:387, 1956

139. Jenkins LJ Jr, Jones RA, Siegel J: Long-term inhalation screening studies of benzene, toluene, o-xylene, and cumene on experimental animals. Toxicol Appl Pharmacol 16:818, 1970

140. Scott JL, Cartwright GE, Wintrobe MM: Acquired aplastic anemia: an analysis of thirty-nine cases and review of the pertinent literature. Medicine 38: 119, 1958

141. Mastromatteo E: Hematological disorders following exposure to insecticides. Can Med Assoc J 90:1166, 1964

142. Erslev AJ, Wintrobe MM: Detection and prevention of drug-induced blood dyscrasias. JAMA 181:114, 1962

143. Crawford MAD: Aplastic anaemia due to trinitrotoluene intoxication. BMJ 2:430, 1954

144. Imerman SW, Imerman CP: Dinitrophenol poisoning with thrombocytopenia, granulopenia, anemia and purpura complicated by lung abscess. JAMA 106:1085, 1936

145. Roberts HJ: Aplastic anemia due to pentachlorophenol and tetrachlorophenol. South Med J 56:632, 1963

146. Carlson GW: Aplastic anemia following exposure to products of the sulfite pulp industry. Ann Intern Med 24:277, 1946

147. Hopkins JE, Manoharan A: Severe aplastic anaemia following the use of hair dye: report of two cases and review of literature. Postgrad Med J 61:1003, 1985

148. Sánchez-Medal L, Castanedo JP, Garcia-Rojas F: Insecticides and aplastic anemia. N Engl J Med 269:1365, 1963

149. Reeves JD, Driggers DA, Kiley VA: Household insecticide associated aplastic anaemia and acute leukaemia in children. Lancet 2:300, 1981

150. Stieglitz R, Stobbe H, Schüttmann W: Knochenmarkschäden nach beruflicher Einwirkung des Insektizids gamma-Hexachlorcyclohexan (Lindan). Acta Haematol 38:337, 1967

151. Lorand IC, Souza CA, Costa FF: Haematological toxicity associated with agricultural chemicals in Brazil, letter. Lancet 1:404, 1984

152. Infante PF, Epstein SS, Newton WA: Blood dyscrasias and childhood tumors and exposure to chlordane and heptachlor. Scand J Work Environ Health 4:137, 1978

153. Epstein SS, Ozonoff D: Leukemias and blood dyscrasias following exposure to chlordane and heptachlor. Teratogen Carcinogen Mutagen 7:527, 1987

154. Loge JP: Aplastic anemia following exposure to benzene hexachloride (Lindane). JAMA 193:104, 1965

155. West I: Lindane and hematologic reactions. Arch Environ Health 15:97, 1967

156. Woodliff HJ, Connor PM, Scopa J: Aplastic anaemia associated with insecticides. Med J Aust 1:628, 1966

157. Jenkyn LR, Budd RC, Fein SH, Cornell CJ: Insecticide/herbicide exposure, aplastic anaemia, and pseudotumor cerebri. Lancet 2:368, 1979

158. Stormont RT: Pharmacologic and toxicologic aspects of DDT (chlorophenothane U.S.P.). JAMA 135:728, 1951
159. Friberg L, Martensson J: Case of panmyelopthisis after exposure to chlorphenothane and benzene hydrochloride. AMA Arch Ind Hyg 8:166, 1953
160. Clinico-pathologic conference: Exposure to insecticides, bone marrow failure, gastrointestinal bleeding, and uncontrollable infections. Am J Med 19:274, 1955
161. Gallagher RP, Threlfall WJ, Jeffries E et al: Cancer and aplastic anemia in British Columbia farmers. J Natl Cancer Inst 72:1311, 1984
162. Spirtas R, Hoar SK, Kaminski R, Rosenberg H: Aplastic anemia mortality and occupational exposures. p. 53. In: Proceedings of the 1985 Public Health Conference on Records and Statistics. Publication No. PHS 86-1214. U S. Department of Health and Human Services, Washington, DC, 1986
163. Davignon LF, St-Pierre J, Charest G, Tourangeau FJ: A study of the chronic effects of insecticides in man. Can Med Assoc J 92:597, 1965
164. Blair A, Grauman DJ, Lubin JH, Fraumeni JF: Lung cancer and other causes of death among licensed pesticide applicators. J Natl Cancer Inst 71:31, 1983
165. Frinci F, Spurbeck GH: A study of workers exposed to the insecticides chlordan, aldrin, dieldrin. Arch Ind Hyg Occup Med 3:64, 1951
166. Ditraglia D, Brown DP, Namekata T, Iverson N: Mortality study of workers employed at organochlorine pesticide manufacturing plants. Scand J Work Environ Health 7:140, 1981
167. Samuels AJ, Milby TH: Human exposure to lindane. Clinical, hematological and biochemical effects. J Occup Med 13:147, 1971
168. Wang HH, Grufferman S: Aplastic anemia and occupational pesticide exposure: a case-control study. J Occup Med 23:364, 1981
169. Burmeister LF, Everett GD, Van Lier SF, Isacson P: Selected cancer mortality and farm practices in Iowa. Am J Epidemiol 118:72, 1983
170. Blair A, Thomas TL: Leukemia among Nebraska farmers: a death certificate study. Am J Epidemiol 110:264, 1979
171. Linos A, Kyle RA, O'Fallon WM, Kurland LT: A case-control study of occupational exposures and leukaemia. Int J Epidemiol 9:131, 1980
172. Milby TH, Samuels AJ, Ottoboni F: Human exposure to lindane: blood lindane levels as a function of exposure. J Occup Med 10:584, 1968
173. Gallicchio VS, Casale GP, Bartholomew PM, Watts TD: Altered colony-forming activities of bone marrow hematopoietic stem cells in mice following short-term in vivo exposure to parathion. Int J Cell Cloning 5:231, 1987
174. Gallicchio VS, Casale GP, Watts T: Inhibition of human bone marrow-derived stem cell colony formation (CFU-E, BFU-E, and CFU-GM) following in vitro exposure to organophosphates. Exp Hematol 15:1099, 1987
175. Lewis CN, Putnam LE, Hendricks FD et al: Chloramphenicol (chloromycetin) in relation to blood dyscrasias with observations on other drugs. A special study. Antibiot Chemother 2:601, 1952
176. Welch H, Lewis CN, Kerlan I: Blood dyscrasias. A nationwide survey. Antibiot Chemother 4:607, 1954
177. Hellriegel KP, Gross R: Follow-up studies in chloramphenicol-induced aplastic anaemia. Postgrad Med J 50:136, 1974
178. Brauer MJ, Dameshek W: Hypoplastic anemia and myeloblastic leukemia following chloramphenicol therapy. N Engl J Med 277:1003, 1967
179. Xiao OS, Yu TG, Linet MS et al: Chloramphenicol use and childhood leukaemia in Shanghai. Lancet 2:934, 1987
180. Kelly JP, Kaufman DW: Anti-infective drug use in relation to the risk of agranulocytosis and aplastic anemia. Arch Intern Med 149:1036, 1989
181. Fink TJ, Gump DW: Chloramphenicol: an inpatient study of use and abuse. J Infect Dis 138:690, 1978
182. Besamuca FW, Bastiaensen LA: Blood dyscrasias and topically applied chloramphenicol in ophthamology. Doc Ophthalmol 64:87, 1986
183. Settepani JA: The hazard of using chloramphenicol in food animals. J Am Vet Med Assoc 184:930, 1984
184. Wolff JA: Anemias caused by infections and toxins, idiopathic aplastic anemia and anemia caused by renal disease. Pediatr Clin North Am 469, 1957
185. Aoki K, Ohtani M, Shimizu H: Epidemiological approach to the etiology of aplastic anemia. p. 155. In Hibino S, Takaku F, Shahidi NT (eds): Aplastic Anemia. University Park Press, Baltimore, 1978
186. Böttiger LE: Epidemiology and aetiology of aplastic anemia. Hematol Blood Transfusion 24:27, 1979
187. Kumana CR, Li KY, Chau PY: Worldwide variation in chloramphenicol utilization: should it cause concern? J Clin Pharmacol 28:1071, 1988
188. Weiner H: Less drug reactions in Jews?, letter. N Engl J Med 281:740, 1969
189. Ghitis J: Chloramphenicol in South America, letter. N Engl J Med 282:813, 1970
190. Nagao T, Mauer AM: Concordance for drug induced aplastic anemia in identical twins. N Engl J Med 281:7, 1969
191. Yunis AA: Chloramphenicol-induced bone marrow suppression. Semin Hematol 10:225, 1973
192. Polak BCP, Wesseling H, Schut D et al: Blood dyscrasias attributed to chloramphenicol. J Intern Med 192:409, 1972
193. Volini IF, Greenspan I, Ehrlich L et al: Hemopoietic changes during administration of chloramphenicol (chloromycetin). JAMA 142:1333, 1950
194. Ozer FL, Truax WE, Levin WC: Erythroid hypoplasia associated with chloramphenicol therapy. Blood 16:997, 1960
195. Krakoff IH, Karnofsky DA, Burchenal JH: Effects of large doses of chloramphenicol on human subjects. N Engl J Med 253:7, 1950
196. Scott JL, Finegold SM, Belkin GA, Lawrence JS: A controlled double-blind study of the hematologic toxicity of chloramphenicol. N Engl J Med 272:1137, 1965
197. Suhrland LG, Weisberger AS: Delayed clearance of chloramphenicol from serum in patients with hematologic toxicity. Blood 34:466, 1969
198. Kramer WG, Rensimer ER, Ericsson CD, Pickering LK: Comparative bioavailability of intravenous and oral chloramphenicol in adults. J Clin Pharmacol 24:181, 1984
199. Alavi JB: Aplastic anemia associated with intravenous chloramphenicol. Am J Hematol 15:375, 1983
200. Gussoff BD, Lee SL: Chloramphenicol-induced hematopoietic depression: a controlled comparison with tetracycline. Am J Med Sci 251:8, 1966
201. Abou-Khalil S, Salem Z, Yunis AA: Mitochondrial metabolism in normal, myeloid, and erythroid hyperplastic rabbit bone marrow: effect of chloramphenicol. Am J Hematol 8:71, 1980
202. Smith AL, Weber A: Pharmacology of chloramphenicol. Pediatr Clin North Am 30:209, 1983
203. Rosenbach LM, Caviles AP, Mitus WJ: Chloramphenicol toxicity: reversible vacuolization of erythroid cells. N Engl J Med 263:724, 1960
204. Rubin D, Weisberger AS, Botti RE, Storaasli JP: Changes in iron metabolism in early chloramphenicol toxicity. J Clin Invest 37:1286, 1958
205. Oski FA: Hematologic consequences of chloramphenicol therapy. J Pediatr 94:515, 1979
206. Ratzan RJ, Moore MAS, Yunis AA: Effect of chloramphenicol and thiamphenicol on the in vitro colony-forming cell. Blood 43:363, 1974
207. Bostrom B, Smith K, Ramsay NKC: Stimulation of human committed bone marrow stem cells (CFU-GM) by chloramphenicol. Exp Hematol 14:156, 1986
208. Sawada H, Tezuka H, Kamamoto T et al: Effects of chloramphenicol on hemopoietic cells and their microenvironment in vitro. Acta Haematol 48:1323, 1985
209. Hara H, Kohsaki M, Noguchi K, Nagai K: Effect of chloramphenicol on colony formation from erythrocytic precursors. Am J Hematol 5:123, 1978
210. Firkin FC, Sumner MA, Bradley TR: The influence of chloramphenicol on the bone marrow haemopoietic stem cell compartment. Exp Hematol 2:264, 1974
211. Nara N, Bessho M, Hirashima K, Momoi H: Effects of chloramphenicol on hematopoietic inductive microenvironment. Exp Hematol 10:20, 1982
212. Couderc J, Perrodon Y, Ventura M et al: Specification of the immune response: its suppression induced by chloramphenicol in vitro. Biosci Rep 3:19, 1983
213. Rowley JD, Blaisdell RK: Abnormal marrow karyotype in chloramphenicol associated aplastic anemia, abstracted. Clin Res 15:287, 1967
214. Howell A, Andrews TM, Watts RWE: Bone marrow cells resistant to chloramphenicol in chloramphenicol-induced aplastic anaemia. Lancet 1:65, 1975
215. Venning GR: Identification of adverse reactions to new drugs. II. How were 18 important adverse reactions discovered and with what delays? Br Med J 286:365, 1983
216. McCarthy DD, Chalmers TM: Hematological complications of phenylbutazone therapy: review of the literature and report of two cases. Can Med Assoc J 90:1061, 1964
217. Chaplin S: Bone marrow depression due to mianserin, phenylbutazone, oxyphenbutazone, and chloramphenicol. Part I. Adverse Drug React Acute Poisoning Rev 5:97, 1986
218. Bottiger LE, Westerholm B: Aplastic anaemia: I. Incidence and aetiology. J Intern Med 192:315, 1972
219. Wijnja L, Snijder JAM, Nieweg HO: Acetylsalicylic acid as a cause of pancytopenia from bone-marrow damage. Lancet 2:768, 1966
220. The International Aplastic Anemia and Agranulocytosis Study: Risks of agranulocytosis and aplastic anemia: a first report of their relation to drug use with special reference to analgesics. JAMA 256:1749, 1986
221. Cunningham JL, Leyland MJ, Delamore IW, Price Evans DA: Acetanilide oxidation in phenylbutazone-associated hypoplastic anaemia. BMJ 3:313, 1974
222. Smith CS, Chinn S, Watts RWE: The sensitivity of human bone marrow granulocyte/monocyte precursor cells to phenylbutazone, oxyphenbutazone and gamma-hydroxyphenylbutazone in vitro, with observations on the bone marrow colony formation in phenylbutazone-induced granulocytopoenia. Biochem Pharmacol 26:847, 1977
223. Gerson WT, Fine DG, Spielberg SP, Sensenbrenner LL: Anticonvulsant-in-

duced aplastic anemia: increased susceptibility to toxic drug metabolites in vitro. Blood 61:889, 1983

224. Livingston S, Pauli LL, Pruce I: No proven relationship of carbamazapine therapy to blood dyscrasias, letter. Neurology 28:101, 1978

225. Hart RG, Easton JD: Carbamazepine and hematological monitoring. Ann Neurol 11:309, 1982

226. Joffe RT, Post RM, Roy-Byrne PP, Uhde TW: Hematological effects of carbamazepine in patients with affective illness. Am J Psychiatry 142:1196, 1985

227. Pisciotta AV: Hematologic toxicity of carbamazepine. p. 355. In Penry JK, Daly DD (eds): Advances in Neurology. Raven Press, New York, 1975

228. Camfield C, Camfield P, Smith E, Tibbies JAR: Asymptomatic children with epilepsey: little benefit from screening for anticonvulsant-induced liver, blood, or renal damage. Neurology 36:838, 1986

229. Pellock JM: Carbamazepine side effects in children and adults. Epilepsia, suppl. 3. 28:S64, 1987

230. Wyllie E, Wyllie R: Routine laboratory monitoring for serious adverse effects of antiepileptic medications: the controversy. Epilepsia, suppl. 5. 32:S74, 1991

231. Camfield P, Camfield C, Dooley J et al: Routine screening of blood and urine for severe reactions to anticonvulsant drugs in asymptomatic patients is of doubtful value. Can Med Assoc J 140:1303, 1989

232. McEvoy GK (ed): AHFS Drug Information 1990. American Society of Hospital Pharmacists, Bethesda, MD, 1990

233. Sobotka JL, Alexander B, Cook BL: A review of carbamazepine's hematologic reaction and monitoring recommendations. DICP Ann Pharm 24:1214, 1990

234. Israel M, Beaudry P: Carbamazepine in psychiatry: a review. Can J Psychiatry 33:577, 1988

235. MacCarty DJ, Brill JM, Harrop DH: Aplastic anemia secondary to gold-salt therapy. Report of fatal case and a review of literature. JAMA 179:655, 1962

236. Shearer CA, Parker WA: Chrysotherapy-induced aplastic anemia: a case report. Am J Hosp Pharm 35:1095, 1978

237. Cheson BD, Clegg DO, Moatamed F: Ultrastructural evidence for persistent gold in the bone marrow of a patient with aplastic anemia. Arthritis Rheum 29:128, 1986

238. Baldwin JL, Storb R, Thomas ED, Mannik M: Bone marrow transplantation in patients with gold-induced marrow aplasia. Arthritis Rheum 20:1043, 1977

239. Mant MJ, Russell AS, Percy JS et al: Immunosuppression as initial treatment for gold induced aplastic anemia. J Rheumatol 14:1026, 1987

240. Alvaro-Gracia JM, Castañeda-Sanz S, Arranz R et al: Antithymocyte globulin in the treatment of gold induced severe aplastic anemia. J Rheumatol 15:43, 1988

241. Doney K, Storb R, Buckner CD, Thomas ED: Treatment of gold-induced aplastic anaemia with immunosuppressive therapy. Br J Haematol 68:469, 1988

242. Howell A, Gumpel JM, Watts RWE: Depression of bone marrow colony formation in gold-induced neutropenia. BMJ 1:432, 1975

243. Kay AGL: Myelotoxicity of gold. BMJ 1:1266, 1976

244. Jerina DM, Daly JW: Arene oxides: a new aspect of drug metabolism. Science 185:573, 1974

245. Nebert DW, Gonzalez FJ: P450 genes: structure, evolution and regulation. Annu Rev Biochem 56:945, 1987

246. Gill DP, Kempen RR, Nash JB, Ellis S: Modifications of benzene myelotoxicity and metabolism by phenobarbitol, SKF-525A and 3-methylcholanthrene. Life Sci 25:1633, 1979

247. Meyer A, Nowak D, Hossfeld D, Rudiger HW: Increased formation of DNA adducts in cultured fibroblasts of patients with aplastic anemia after in vitro incubation with benzo(a)pyrene. Int Arch Occup Environ Health 62:525, 1990

248. Weinshilboum R: Pharmacogenetics of methyl conjugation and thiopurine drug toxicity. Prog Clin Biol Res 135:167, 1983

249. Lennard L, Rees CA, Lilleyman JS, Maddocks JL: Childhood leukaemia: a relationship between intracellular 6-mercaptopurine metabolites and neutropenia. Br J Clin Pharmacol 16:359, 1983

250. Lennard L, Murphy MF, Maddocks JL: Severe megaloblastic anaemia associated with abnormal azathioprine metabolism. Br J Clin Pharmacol 17:171, 1984

251. Lennard L, VanLoon JA, Lilleyman JS, Weinshilboum RM: Thiopurine pharmacogenetics in leukemia: correlation of erythrocyte thiopurine methyltransferase activity and 6-thioguanine nucleotide concentrations. Clin Pharmacol Ther 41:18, 1987

252. Price DA: Acetylation. p. 209. In Kalow W, Goedde HW, Agarwal DP (eds): Ethnic Differences in Reactions to Drugs and Xenobiotics. Alan R Liss, New York, 1986

253. Shear NH, Spielberg SP, Grant DM et al: Differences in metabolism of sulfonamides predisposing to idiosyncratic toxicity. Ann Intern Med 105:179, 1986

254. Uetrecht JP, Sweetman BJ, Woosley RL, Oates JA: Metabolism of procainam-

ide to a hydroxylamine by rat and human hepatic microsomes. Drug Metab Dispos 12:77, 1984

255. Ferrari V: Salient features of thiamphenicol: review of clinical pharmacokinetics and toxicity. Sex Transm Dis 11:336, 1984

256. Murray TR, Downey KM, Yunis AA: Chloramphenicol-mediated DNA damage and its possible role in the inhibitory effects of chloramphenicol on DNA synthesis. J Lab Clin Med 102:926, 1983

257. Yunis AA, Arimura GK, Isildar M: DNA damage induced by chloramphenicol and its nitroso derivative: damage in intact cells. Am J Hematol 24:77, 1987

258. Jimenez JJ, Arimura GK, Abou-Khalil et al: Chloramphenicol-induced bone marrow injury: possible role of bacterial metabolites of chloramphenicol. Blood 70:1180, 1987

259. Krishna G, Aykac I, Siegel D: Recent studies on the mechanisms of chloramphenicol activation responsible for aplastic anemia. p. 5. In Najean Y (ed): Safety Problems Related to Chloramphenicol and Thiamphenicol Therapy. Raven Press, New York, 1981

260. Pohl LR, Reddy GB, Krishna G: A new pathway of metabolism of chloramphenicol which influences the interpretation of its irreversible binding to protein in vivo. Biochem Pharmacol 28:2433, 1979

261. Baranski B, Young N: Hematologic manifestations of viral illness. Hematol Oncol Clin North Am 1:167, 1987

262. Young N: Hematologic and hematopoietic consequences of B19 parvovirus infection. Semin Hematol 25:159, 1988

263. Kurtzman G: Feline panleucopenia virus. p. 119. In Young NS (ed): Viruses and Bone Marrow. Marcel Dekker, New York, 1993

264. Balfour HH Jr: Erythema infectiosum (fifth disease): clinical review and description of 91 cases seen in an epidemic. Clin Pediatr 8:721, 1969

265. Chorba TL, Coccia P, Holman RC et al: Role of parvovirus B19 in aplastic crisis and erythema infectiosum (fifth disease). J Infect Dis 154:383, 1986

266. White DG, Woolf AD, Mortimer PP et al: Human parvovirus arthropathy. Lancet 1:419, 1985

267. Reid DM, Reid TMS, Rennie JAN et al: Human parvovirus-associated arthritis: a clinical and laboratory description. Lancet 1:422, 1985

268. Gasser C: Aplasia of erythropoiesis. Pediatr Clin North Am 4:445, 1957

269. Owren PA: Congenital hemolytic jaundice: the pathogenesis of the "hemolytic crisis." Blood 3:231, 1948

270. Evans JPM, Rossiter MA, Kumaran TO et al: Human parvovirus aplasia: case due to cross infection in a ward, letter. BMJ 288:681, 1984

271. Bell LM, Naides SJ, Stoffman P et al: Human parvovirus B19 infection among hospital staff members after contact with infected patients. N Engl J Med 321:485, 1989

272. Mortimer PP, Luban NLC, Kelleher JF, Cohen BJ: Transmission of serum parvovirus-like virus by clotting-factor concentrates. Lancet 2:482, 1983

273. Lefrère J, Courouc A, Bertrand Y et al: Human parvovirus and aplastic crisis in chronic hemolytic anemias: a study of 24 observations. Am J Hematol 23:271, 1986

274. McLellan NJ, Rutter N: Hereditary spherocytosis in sisters unmasked by parvovirus infection. Postgrad Med J 63:49, 1987

275. Nunoue T, Koike T, Koike R et al: Infection with human parvovirus (B19), aplasia of the bone marrow and a rash in hereditary spherocytosis. J Infect 14:67, 1987

276. Kurtzman G, Gascon P, Caras M et al: B19 parvovirus replicates in circulating cells of acutely infected patients. Blood 71:1448, 1988

277. Doran HM, Teall AJ: Neutropenia accompanying erythroid aplasia in human parvovirus infection, letter. Br J Haematol 69:287, 1988

278. Anderson MJ, Higgins PG, Davis LR et al: Experimental parvoviral infection in humans. J Infect Dis 152:257, 1985

279. Conrad ME, Studdard H, Anderson LJ: Case report: aplastic crisis in sickle cell disorders: bone marrow necrosis and human parvovirus infection. Am J Med Sci 295:212, 1988

280. Saunders PWG, Reid MM, Cohen BJ: Human parvovirus induced cytopenias: a report of five cases, letter. Br J Haematol 63:407, 1986

281. Hanada T, Koike K, Takeya T et al: Human parvovirus B19-induced transient pancytopenia in a child with hereditary spherocytosis. Br J Haematol 70:113, 1988

282. Hamon MD, Newland AC, Anderson MJ: Severe aplastic anaemia after parvovirus infection in the absence of underlying haemolytic anaemia, letter. J Clin Pathol 41:1242, 1988

283. Serjeant GR, Topley JM, Mason K et al: Outbreak of aplastic crises in sickle cell anaemia associated with parvovirus-like agent. Lancet 2:595, 1981

284. Saarinen UM, Chorba TL, Tattersall P et al: Human parvovirus B19-induced epidemic acute red cell aplasia in patients with hereditary hemolytic anemia. Blood 67:1411, 1986

285. Anderson MJ, Jones SE, Minson AC: Diagnosis of human parvovirus infection by dot-blot hybridization using cloned viral DNA. J Med Virol 15:163, 1985

286. Clewley JP: Detection of human parvovirus using a molecularly cloned probe. J Med Virol 15:173, 1985

287. Cohen BJ, Mortimer PP, Pereira MS: Diagnostic assays with monoclonal antibodies for the human serum parvovirus-like virus (SPLV). J Hyg (Camb) 91:113, 1983

288. Erdman DD, Usher MJ, Tsou C et al: Human parvovirus B19 specific IgG, IgA, and IgM antibodies and DNA in serum specimens from persons with erythema infectiosum. J Med Virol 35:110, 1991

289. Kajigaya S, Fujii H, Field AM et al: Self-assembled B19 parvovirus capsids, produced in a baculovirus system, are antigenically and immunogenically similar to native virions. Proc Natl Acad Sci USA 88:4646, 1991

290. Bansal GP, Hatfield J, Dunn FE et al: Candidate recombinant vaccine for human B19 parvovirus. J Infect Dis 167:1034, 1993

291. Anderson LJ, Hurwitz ES: Human parvovirus B19 and pregnancy. Clin Perinatol 15:273, 1988

292. Anand A, Gray ES, Brown T et al: Human parvovirus infection in pregnancy and hydrops fetalis. N Engl J Med 316:183, 1987

293. Cotmore SF, McKie VC, Anderson LJ et al: Identification of the major structural and nonstructural proteins encoded by human parvovirus B19 and mapping of their genes by procaryotic expression of isolated genomic fragments. J Virol 60:548, 1989

294. Rodis JF, Quinn DL, Gary GW Jr, Anderson LJ: Management and outcomes of pregnancies complicated by human B19 parvovirus infection: a prospective study. Am J Obstet Gynecol 163 (4 Pt. 1):1168, 1990

295. Public Health Laboratory Service Working Party on Fifth Disease: Prospective study of human parvovirus (B19) infection in pregnancy. Br Med J 300: 1166, 1990

296. Porter HJ, Quantrill AM, Fleming KA: B19 parvovirus infection of myocardial cells, letter. Lancet 1:535, 1988

297. Schwarz TF, Roggendorf M, Hottentrager B et al: Human parvovirus B19 infection in pregnancy, letter. Lancet 2:566, 1988

298. Brown KE, Green SW, Antunez de Mayolo J et al: Congenital anemia following transplacental B19 parvovirus infection. Lancet 343:895, 1994

299. Kurtzman G, Frickhofen N, Kimball J et al: Pure red-cell aplasia of 10 years' duration due to persistent parvovirus B19 infection and its cure with immunoglobulin therapy. N Engl J Med 321:519, 1989

300. Kurtzman G, Cohen B, Myers P et al: Persistent B19 parvovirus infection as a cause of severe anemia in children with acute lymphocytic leukemia in remission. Lancet 2:1159, 1988

301. Frickhofen N, Abkowitz J, Safford M et al: Persistent B19 parvovirus infection in patients infected with human immunodeficiency virus 1: a treatable cause of anemias in AIDS. Ann Intern Med 113:926, 1990

302. Frickhofen N, Young NS: Persistent parvovirus B19 infections in humans. Microb Pathog 7:1989

303. Frickhofen N, Young NS: A rapid method of sample preparation for detection of DNA viruses in human serum by polymerase chain reaction. J Virol Methods 45:65, 1991

304. Kurtzman G, Cohen B, Field AM et al: The immune response to B19 parvovirus infection and an antibody defect in persistent viral infection. J Clin Invest 84:1114, 1989

305. Ozawa K, Kurtzman G, Young NS: Replication of the B19 parvovirus in human bone marrow cultures. Science 233:883, 1986

306. Kurtzman G, Ozawa K, Hanson GR et al: Chronic bone marrow failure due to persistent B19 parvovirus infection. N Engl J Med 317:287, 1987

307. Ozawa K, Kurtzman G, Young N: Productive infection by B19 parvovirus of human erythroid bone marrow cells in vitro. Blood 70:384, 1987

308. Schwarz TF, Serke S, Hottentrager B et al: Replication of parvovirus B19 in hematopoietic progenitor cells generated in vitro from normal human peripheral blood. J Gen Virol 66:1273, 1992

309. Yaegashi N, Shiraishi H, Takeshita T et al: Propagation of human parvovirus B19 in primary culture of erythroid lineage cells derived from fetal liver. J Virol 63:2422, 1989

310. Shimomura S, Komatsu N, Frickhofen N et al: First continuous propagation of B19 parvovirus in a cell line. Blood 79:18, 1992

311. Munshi NC, Zhou S, Woody MJ et al: Successful replication of parvovirus B19 in the human megakaryocytic cell line MB-02. J Virol 67:562, 1993

312. Mortimer PP, Humphries RK, Moore JG et al: A human parvovirus-like virus inhibits hematopoietic colony formation in vitro. Nature 302:426, 1983

313. Morey AL, Fleming KA: Immunophenotyping of fetal haemopoietic cells permissive for human parvovirus B19 replication in vitro. Br J Haematol 82: 302, 1992

314. Young NS, Harrison M, Moore JG et al: Direct demonstration of the human parvovirus in erythroid progenitor cells infected in vitro. J Clin Invest 74: 2024, 1984

315. Brown KE, Anderson S, Young S: Erythrocyte P antigen: cellular receptor for B19 parvovirus. Science 262:114, 1993

316. Brown KE, Hibbs J, Gallinella G et al: Resistance to parvovirus B19 infection due to lack of virus receptor (erythrocyte P antigen). N Engl J Med 330: 1192, 1994

317. Ozawa K, Ayub J, Kajigaya S et al: The gene encoding the nonstructural protein of B19 (human) parvovirus may be lethal in transfected cells. J Virol 62:2884, 1962

318. Srivastava A, Bruno E, Briddell R et al: Parvovirus B19-induced perturbation of human megakaryocytopoiesis in vitro. Blood 76:1997, 1990

319. Ajlouni K, Doeblin TD: The syndrome of hepatitis and aplastic anaemia. Br J Haematol 27:345, 1974

320. Hagler L, Pastore RA, Bergin JJ, Wrensch MR: Aplastic anemia following viral hepatitis: report of two fatal cases and literature review. Medicine 54: 139, 1975

321. Zeldis JB, Dienstag JL, Gale RP: Aplastic anemia and non-A, non-B hepatitis. Am J Med 74:64, 1983

322. Böttiger LE. Westerholm B: Aplastic anemia. III. Aplastic anaemia and infectious hepatitis. J Intern Med 192:323, 1972

323. Liang D-C, Lin K-H, Lin D-T et al: Post-hepatitic aplastic anaemia in children in Taiwan, a hepatitis prevalent area. Br J Haematol 74:487, 1990

324. Pikis A, Kavaliotis J, Manios S: Incidence of aplastic anemia in viral hepatitis in children. Scand J Infect Dis 20:109, 1988

325. Cargnel A, Vigano P, Davoli C et al: Sporadic acute non-A non-B hepatitis complicated by aplastic anemia. Am J Gastroenterol 78:245, 1983

326. Sandberg T, Lindquist O, Norkrans G: Fatal aplastic anaemia associated with non-A, non-B hepatitis. Scand J Infect Dis 16:403, 1984

327. Perrillo RP, Pohl DA, Roodman ST, Tsai CC: Acute non-A, non-B hepatitis with serum sickness-like syndrome and aplastic anemia. JAMA 245:494, 1981

328. Tzakis AG, Arditi M, Whitington PF et al: Aplastic anemia complicating orthotopic liver transplantation for non-A, non-B hepatitis. N Engl J Med 319: 393, 1988

329. Boga M, Szemere PA: Infectious hepatitis and aplastic anaemia in two sisters, letter. Lancet 2:703, 1971

330. Albert E, Thomas ED, Nisperos B, Storb R: HLA antigens and haplotypes in 200 patients with aplastic anemia. Transplantation 22:528, 1976

331. Dhingra K, Michels SD, Winton EF, Gordon DS: Transient bone marrow aplasia associated with non-A, non-B hepatitis. Am J Hematol 29:168, 1988

332. Sears DA, George JN, Gold MS: Transient red blood cell aplasia in association with viral hepatitis. Occurrence four years apart in siblings. Arch Intern Med 135:1585, 1975

333. Wilson HA, McLaren GD, Dworken HJ, Tebbi K: Transient pure red-cell aplasia: cell-mediated suppression of erythropoiesis associated with hepatitis. Ann Intern Med 92:196, 1980

334. Ireland R, Gillett D, Mieli-Vergani G, Mufti G: Pre-ALL and non-A, non-B hepatitis infection. Leuk Res 12:795, 1988

335. Camitta BM, Nathan DG, Forman EN et al: Posthepatic severe aplastic anemia—an indication for early bone marrow transplantation. Blood 43:473, 1974

336. Kojima S, Matsuyama K, Kodera Y: Bone marrow transplantation for hepatitis-associated aplastic anemia. Acta Haematol 79:7, 1988

337. Witherspoon RP, Storb R, Shulman H et al: Marrow transplantation in hepatitis-associated aplastic anemia. Am J Hematol 17:269, 1984

338. McDonald GB, Sharma P, Matthews DE et al: Venocclusive disease of the liver after bone marrow transplantation: diagnosis, incidence, and predisposing factors. Hepatology 4:116, 1984

339. Strafuss AC, Linares M, Jarque I et al: Recovery from aplastic anemia after non A non B post transfusion hepatitis, letter. Ann Intern Med 109:513, 1988

340. Shannon K, Koehne W, Heyman MB, Koerper MA: Relapsing post-hepatitis aplastic anemia. Immunosuppressive therapy. Clin Pediatr 29:25, 1990

341. Shimokawa T, Suzue T: Successful treatment of a case with hepatitis-associated severe aplastic by anti-lymphocyte globulin (ALG). Jpn J Clin Hematol 31:1836, 1990

342. Ozsoylu S, Coskun T, Minassazi S: High dose intravenous glucocorticoid in the treatment of childhood acquired aplastic anaemia. Scand J Haematol 33:309, 1984

343. Tohda S, Suzuki T, Nagata K et al: Successful treatment of a patient with posthepatitic severe aplastic anemia with bolus methylprednisolone. Jpn J Med 29:191, 1990

344. Pant A, Kale P, Harjai K et al: Non-A non-B hepatitis induced aplastic anemia. J Postgrad Med 38:85, 1992

345. Karp JE, Schacter LP, Burke PJ: Humoral factors in aplastic anemia: relationship of liver dysfunction to lack of serum stimulation of bone marrow growth in vitro. Blood 51:397, 1978

346. Hodgkinson R: Blood dyscrasias associated with chloramphenicol. Lancet 1:285, 1954

347. Foon KA, Mitsuyasu RT, Schroff RW et al: Immunologic defects in young

male patients with hepatitis-associated aplastic anemia. Ann Intern Med 100:657, 1984

348. Strauss RG, Bove KE, Lake A, Kisker CT: Acquired immunodeficiency in hepatitis-associated aplastic anemia. J Pediatr 86:910, 1975

349. Wang WC, Herrod HG, Presbury GJ: Lymphocyte subsets in children with aplastic anemia. Am J Med Sci 291:304, 1986

350. Kojima S, Matsuyama K, Kodera Y, Okada J: Circulating activated suppressor T lymphocytes in hepatitis-associated aplastic anaemia. Br J Haematol 71:147, 1989

351. Bannister P, Miloszewski K, Barnard D, Losowsky MS: Fatal marrow aplasia associated with non-A, non-B hepatitis. Br Med J 286:1314, 1983

352. Choo QL, Kuo G, Weiner AJ et al: Isolation of cDNA clone derived from a blood-borne non-A, non-B viral hepatitis genome. Science 244:359, 1989

353. Bierman HR, Nelson ER: Hematodepressive disease of Thailand. Ann Intern Med 62:867, 1965

354. Halstead SB: Dengue: hematologic aspects. Semin Hematol 19:116, 1982

355. Casals J, Hoogstraal H, Johnson KM et al: A current appraisal of hemorrhagic fevers in the U.S.S.R. Am J Trop Med Hyg 15:751, 1966

356. Johnson KM, Halstead SB, Cohen SM: Hemorrhagic fevers of Southeast Asia and South America: a comparative appraisal. Prog Med Virol 9:106, 1967

357. Young NS: Hypothesis: flaviviruses are agents of bone marrow failure. JAMA 263:3065, 1990

358. Tigertt WD, Crosby WH, Berge TO et al: The virus of Venezuelan equine encephalomyelitis as an antineoplastic agent in man. Cancer 15:628, 1962

359. Nakao S, Lai C-J, Young NS: Dengue virus, a flavivirus, propagates in human bone marrow progenitors and hematopoietic cell lines. Blood 74:1235, 1989

360. Kurane I, Innis BL, Nisalak A et al: Human T cell responses to dengue virus antigens. Proliferative responses and interferon gamma production. J Clin Invest 83:506, 1989

361. Kurane I, Innis BL, Nimmannitya S et al: Activation of T lymphocytes in dengue virus infections. High levels of soluble interleukin 2 receptor, soluble CD4, soluble CD8, interleukin 2, and interferon gamma in sera of children with dengue. J Clin Invest 88:1473, 1991

362. Lorenz T, Heinemann V, Jehn U: Panzytopenie nach non-A-non-B-Hepatitis. Internist (Berl) 33:559, 1992

363. Pol S, Driss F, Devergie A et al: Is hepatitis C virus involved in hepatitis-associated aplastic anemia? Ann Intern Med 113:435, 1990

364. Hibbs J, Issaragrisil S, Young NS: High prevalence of hepatitis C viremia among aplastic anemia case patients and controls in Thailand. Am J Trop Med Hyg 46:564, 1992

365. Hibbs J, Rosenfeld S, Feinstone SM et al: Hepatitis/aplasia syndrome: non A, non B, non C? JAMA 267:2051, 1992

366. Royal Marsden Hospital Bone Marrow Transplant Team: Failure of syngeneic bone marrow graft without preconditioning in post-hepatitis marrow aplasia. Lancet 2:742, 1977

367. Nakamura S, Sato T, Maeda T, Sato Y: Viral hepatitis B and aplastic anemia. Tohoku J Exp Med 116:101, 1975

368. Casciato DA, Klein CA, Kaplowitz N, Scott JL: Aplastic anemia associated with type B viral hepatitis. Arch Intern Med 138:1557, 1978

369. Aoyagi K, Ohhara N, Okamura S: Aplastic anemia associated with type A viral hepatitis—possible role of T lymphocytes. Jpn J Med 26:348, 1987

370. Doménech P, Palomeque A, Martinez-Gutiérrez A et al: Severe aplastic anemia following hepatitis A. Acta Haematol 76:227, 1986

371. Gruber A, Grillner L, Norder H et al: Severe aplastic anemia associated with seronegative community-acquired hepatitis C virus infection. Ann Haematol 66:157, 1993

372. Lin CK, Gau JP: Aplastic anaemia is not aetiologically associated with hepatitis-B in Taiwan, letter. Eur J Haematol 42:505, 1989

373. Zeldis JB, Mugishima H, Steinberg HN et al: In vitro hepatitis B infection of human bone marrow cells. J Clin Invest 78:411, 1986

374. Zeldis JB, Farraye FA, Steinberg HN: In vitro hepatitis B virus suppression of erythropoiesis is dependent on the multiplicity of infection and is reversible with anti-HBs antibodies. Hepatology 8:755, 1988

375. Busch FW, deVos S, Flehmig B et al: Inhibition of in vitro hematopoiesis by hepatitis A virus. Exp Hematol 15:978, 1987

376. Busch FW, Kunst A, Flehmig B et al: Myelopoiesis in vitro is suppressed by hepatitis A virus. Ann Hematol 64:A132, 1992

377. Zeldis JB, Boender PJ, Hellings JA, Steinberg H: Inhibition of human hemopoiesis by non-A, non-B hepatitis. J Med Virol 27:34, 1989

378. Lie-Injo LE, Balasagaram M, Lopez CG, Herrera AR: Hepatitis B virus DNA in liver and white blood cells of patients with hepatoma. DNA 2:301, 1983

379. Shimizu YK, Iwamoto A, Purcell RH, Yoshikura H: Evidence for in vitro replication of hepatitis C virus genome in a human T-cell line. Proc Natl Acad Sci USA 89:5477, 1992

380. Piazza M, Piccinino F, Matano F: Haematological changes in viral (MHV-3) murine hepatitis. Nature 205:1034, 1965

381. Hunstein W, Perings E, Eggeling B, Uhl N: Panmyelophthise und Virushepatitis. Experimentelle Untersuchungen mit dem Mäusehepatitis-Virus MHV3. Acta Haematol 42:336, 1969

382. Lazarus KH, Baehner RL: Aplastic anemia complicating infectious mononucleosis: a case report and review of the literature. Pediatrics 67:907, 1981

383. Baranski B, Armstrong G, Truman JT et al: Epstein-Barr virus in the bone marrow of patients with aplastic anemia. Ann Intern Med 109:695, 1988

384. Ahronheim GA, Auger F, Ghibu F et al: Primary infection by Epstein-Barr virus presenting as aplastic anemia, letter. N Engl J Med 309:313, 1983

385. Tosato G, Magrath I, Koski I et al: Activation of suppressor T cells during Epstein-Barr-virus-induced infectious mononucleosis. N Engl J Med 301:1133, 1979

386. Shadduck RK, Winkelstein A, Zeigler Z et al: Aplastic anemia following infectious mononucleosis: possible immune etiology. Exp Hematol 7:264, 1979

387. Jones JF, Shurin S, Abramowsky C et al: T-cell lymphomas containing Epstein-Barr viral DNA in patients with chronic Epstein-Barr virus infections. N Engl J Med 318:733, 1988

388. Sixbey JW, Vesterinen EH, Nedrud JG et al: Replication of Epstein-Barr virus in human epithelial cells infected in vitro. Nature 306:480, 1983

389. Sixbey JW, Nedrud JG, Raab-Traub N et al: Epstein-Barr virus replication in oropharyngeal epithelial cells. N Engl J Med 310:1225, 1983

390. Revoltella RP, Vigneti E, Fruscalzo A et al: Epstein-Barr virus DNA sequences in precursor monocyte-macrophage cell lines established from the bone marrow of children with maturation defects of haematopoiesis. J Gen Virol 70:1203, 1989

391. Verdonck LF, de Gast GC, Van Heugten HG et al: Cytomegalovirus infection causes delayed platelet recovery after bone marrow transplantation. Blood 78:844, 1991

392. Mutter W, Reddehase MJ, Busch FW et al: Failure in generating hemopoietic cells is the primary cause of death from cytomegalovirus disease in the immunocompromised host. J Exp Med 167:1645, 1988

393. Bussel A, Danon F, Ferchal F, Pérol Y: Cytomegalovirus infection in malignant blood diseases. Clinical and laboratory data in 29 patients. Nouv Rev Fr Hematol 20:67, 1978

394. Apperley JF, Dowding C, Hibbin J et al: The effect of cytomegalovirus on hemopoiesis: in vitro evidence for selective infection of marrow stromal cells. Exp Hematol 17:38, 1989

395. Reddehase MJ, Dreher-Stumpp L, Angele P et al: Hematopoietic stem cell deficiency resulting from cytomegalovirus infection of bone marrow stroma. Ann Hematol 64:A125, 1992

396. Busch FW, Mutter W, Koszinowski UH, Reddehase MJ: Rescue of myeloid lineage-committed preprogenitor cells from cytomegalovirus-infected bone marrow stroma. J Virol 65:981, 1991

397. Simmons P, Kaushansky K, Torok-Storb B: Mechanisms of cytomegalovirus-mediated myelosuppression: perturbation of stromal cell function versus direct infection of myeloid cells. Proc Natl Acad Sci USA 87:1386, 1990

398. Sing GK, Ruscetti FW: Preferential suppression of myelopoiesis in normal human bone marrow cells after in vitro challenge with human cytomegalovirus. Blood 75:1965, 1990

399. Rakusan TA, Juneja HS, Fleischmann WR Jr: Inhibition of hemopoietic colony formation by human cytomegalovirus in vitro. J Infect Dis 159:127, 1989

400. Maciejewski JP, Bruening E, Young NS, St Jeor SC: Infection of hematopoietic progenitor cells by human cytomegalovirus. Blood 80:170, 1992

401. Carney WP, Rubin RH, Hoffman RA et al: Analysis of T lymphocyte subsets in cytomegalovirus mononucleosis. J Immunol 126:2114, 1981

402. Duncombe AS, Meager A, Grant Prentice H et al: Gamma interferon and tumor necrosis factor production after bone marrow transplantation is augmented by exposure to marrow fibroblasts infected with cytomegalovirus. Blood 76:1046, 1990

403. Yamanishi K: Human herpesvirus 6. Microbiol Immunol 36:551, 1992

404. Yoshikawa T, Nakashima T, Asano Y et al: Endonuclease analyses of DNA of human herpesvirus-6 isolated from blood before and after bone marrow transplantation. J Med Virol 374:228, 1992

405. Knox KK, Carrigan DR: In vitro suppression of bone marrow progenitor cell differentiation by human herpesvirus 6 infection. J Infect Dis 165:925, 1992

406. Zinkham WH, Medearis DN, Osborne JE: Blood and bone-marrow findings in congenital rubella. J Pediatr 71:512, 1967

407. Rausen AR, Richter P, Tallal L, Cooper LZ: Hematologic effects of intrauterine rubella. JAMA 199:75, 1967

408. Bayer WL, Sherman FE, Michaels RH et al: Purpura in congenital and acquired rubella. N Engl J Med 273:1362, 1965

409. Gresser I, Chany C: Isolation of measles virus from the washed leucocytic fraction of blood. Proc Soc Exp Biol Med 113:695, 1963

410. Graham DY, Brown CH III, Benrey J, Butel JS: Thrombocytopenia: a complication of mumps. JAMA 227:1162, 1974

411. Oski FA, Naiman JL: Effect of live measles vaccine on the platelet count. N Engl J Med 275:352, 1966

412. Espinoza C, Kuhn C: Viral infection in megakaryocytes in varicella with purpura. Am J Clin Pathol 61:203, 1974

413. Jerushalmy Z, Kaminski E, Kohn A, DeVries A: Interaction of Newcastle disease virus with megakaryocytes in cell cultures of guinea pig bone marrow. Proc Soc Exp Biol Med 114:687, 1963

414. Modai Y, Oren R, de Vries A, Kohn A: Thrombocytopenia in guinea pigs infected by encephalomyocarditis virus (EMC). Thromb Haemost 18:686, 1967

415. Fikrig SM, Berkovich S: Virus induced aplastic crisis in mice. Blood 33:582, 1969

416. Lewis SM, Dacie JV: The aplastic anaemia-paroxysmal nocturnal haemoglobinuria syndrome. Br J Haematol 13:236, 1967

417. Conrad ME, Barton JC: The aplastic anemia-paroxysmal nocturnal hemoglobinuria syndrome. Am J Hematol 7:61, 1979

418. Rotoli B, Luzzatto L: Paroxysmal nocturnal hemoglobinuria. Semin Hematol 26:201, 1989

419. Rosse WF: Dr. Ham's test revisited. Blood 78:547, 1991

420. Quagliana JM, Cartwright GE, Wintrobe MM: Paroxysmal nocturnal hemoglobinuria following drug-induced aplastic anemias. Ann Intern Med 61:1045, 1964

421. Aksoy M: Different types of malignancies due to occupational exposure to benzene: a review of recent observations in Turkey. Environ Res 23:181, 1980

422. Vogel SJ, Reinhard EH: Paroxysmal nocturnal hemoglobinuria associated with infectious mononucleosis. Blood 54:351, 1979

423. Ware RE, Hall SE, Rosse WF: Paroxysmal nocturnal hemoglobinuria with onset in childhood and adolescence. N Engl J Med 325:991, 1991

424. Wasi P, Kruetrachue M, Na-Nakorn S: Aplastic anemia-paroxysmal nocturnal hemoglobinuria syndrome-acute leukemia in the same patient. The first record of such occurrence. J Med Assoc Thailand 53:656, 1970

425. Hirsch VJ, Neubach PA, Parker DM et al: Paroxysmal nocturnal hemoglobinuria. Termination in acute myelomonocytic leukemia and reappearance after leukemic remission. Arch Intern Med 141:525, 1981

426. Devine DV, Gluck WL, Rosse WF, Weinberg JB: Acute myeloblastic leukemia in paroxysmal nocturnal hemoglobinuria. Evidence of evolution from the abnormal paroxysmal nocturnal hemoglobinuria clone. J Clin Invest 79:314, 1987

427. Shichishima T, Terasawa T, Hashimoto C et al: Discordant and heterogeneous expression of GPI-anchored membrane proteins on leukemic cells in a patient with paroxysmal noctural hemoglobinuria. Blood 81:1855, 1993

428. Moore JG, Humphries RK, Frank MM, Young N: Characterization of the hematopoietic defect in paroxysmal nocturnal hemoglobinuria. Exp Hematol 14:222, 1986

429. Rotoli B, Robledo R, Luzzatto L: Decreased number of circulating BFU-Es in paroxysmal nocturnal hemoglobinuria. Blood 60:157, 1982

430. Ben-Bassat I, Brok-Simoni F, Ramot B: Complement-sensitive red cells in aplastic anemia. Blood 46:357, 1975

431. Nissen C, Gratwohl A, Speck B et al: Acquired aplastic anaemia: a PNH-like disease? Br J Haematol 64:355, 1986

432. Schubert J, Alvarado M, Uciechowski P et al: Diagnosis of paroxysmal nocturnal haemoglobinuria using immunophenotyping of peripheral blood cells. Br J Haematol 79:487, 1991

433. Van der Schoot CE, Huizinga TWJ, Van't Veer-Korthof ET et al: Deficiency of glycosyl-phosphatidylinositol-linked membrane glycoproteins of leukocytes in paroxysmal nocturnal hemoglobinuria, description of a new diagnostic cytofluorometric assay. Blood 76:1853, 1990

434. Kusminsky GD, Barazzutti L, Korin JD et al: Complete response to antilymphocyte globulin in a case of aplastic anemia-paroxysmal noctural hemoglobinuria syndrome, letter. Am J Hematol 29:123, 1988

435. Kruatrachue M, Wasi P, Na-Nakorn S: Paroxysmal nocturnal haemoglobinuria in Thailand with special reference to an association with aplastic anaemia. Br J Haematol 39:267, 1978

436. Koduri PR, Gowrishankar S: Paroxysmal nocturnal haemoglobinuria in Indians. Acta Haematol 88:126, 1992

437. Oni SB, Osunkoya BO, Luzzatto L: Paroxysmal noctural hemoglobinuria: evidence for monoclonal origin of abnormal red cells. Blood 36:145, 1970

438. Josten KM, Tooze JA, Borthwick-Clarke C et al: Acquired aplastic anemia and paroxysmal nocturnal hemoglobinuria: studies on clonality. Blood 78:3162, 1991

439. Dessypris EN, Clark DA, McKee LC Jr, Krantz SB: Increased sensitivity to complement of erythroid and myeloid progenitors in paroxysmal nocturnal hemoglobinuria. N Engl J Med 309:690, 1983

440. Rotoli B, Robledo R, Scarpato N, Luzzatto L: Two populations of erythroid cell progenitors in paroxysmal nocturnal hemoglobinuria. Blood 64:847, 1984

441. Moore JG, Frank MM, Muller-Eberhard HJ, Young NS: Decay accelerating factor is present on PNH hematopoietic progenitors and lost during in vitro erythropoiesis. J Exp Med 162:1182, 1985

442. Shichishima T, Terasawa T, Uchida T, Kariyone S: Complement sensitivity of erythroblasts and erythropoietic precursors in paroxysmal nocturnal haemoglobinuria (PNH). Br J Haematol 72:578, 1989

443. Terstappen LWMM, Nguyen M, Lazarus HM, Medof ME: Expression of the DAF (CD55) and CD59 antigens during normal hematopoietic cell differentiation. J Leuk Biol 52:652, 1992

444. Rotoli B, Bessler M, Alfinito F, del Vecchio L: Membrane proteins in paroxysmal nocturnal hemoglobinuria. Blood Rev 7:75, 1993

445. Hirose S, Ravi L, Prince GM et al: Synthesis of mannosylglucosaminylinositol phospholipids in normal but not paroxysmal nocturnal hemoglobinuria cells. Proc Natl Acad Sci USA 89:6025, 1992

446. Miyata T, Takeda J, Lida Y et al: The cloning of PIG-A, a component in the early step of GPI-anchor biosynthesis. Science 259:1318, 1993

447. Hahn WC, Menu E, Bothwell ALM et al: Overlapping but nonidentical binding sites on CD2 for CD58 and a second ligand CD59. Science 256:1805, 1993

448. Fefer A, Freeman H, Storb R et al: Paroxysmal noctural hemoglobinuria and marrow failure treated by infusion of marrow from an identical twin. Ann Intern Med 84:692, 1976

449. Young NS: The problem of clonality in aplastic anemia. Dr. Dameshek's riddle, restated. Blood 79:1385, 1992

450. Hoffman R, Young N, Ershler WB et al: Diffuse fasciitis and aplastic anemia: a report of four cases revealing an unusual association between rheumatologic and hematologic disorders. Medicine 61:373, 1982

451. Moore TL, Zuckner J: Eosinophilic fasciitis. Semin Arthritis Rheum 9:228, 1980

452. Debusscher L, Bitar N, De Maubeuge J et al: Esoinophilic fasciitis and severe aplastic anemia: favorable response to either antithymocyte globulin or cyclosporine A in blood and skin disorders. Transplant Proc 10:310, 1988

453. Anderson KC, Weinstein HJ: Transfusion-associated graft versus-host disease. N Engl J Med 323:315, 1990

454. Miller ME: Thymic dysplasia ("Swiss agammaglobulinemia"). I. Graft versus host reaction following bone-marrow transfusion. J Pediatr 70:730, 1967

455. Hathaway WE, Fulginiti VA, Pierce CW et al: Graft-vs-host reaction following a single blood transfusion. JAMA 201:1015, 1967

456. Hathaway WE, Githens JH, Blackburn WR et al: Aplastic anemia histiocytosis and erythrodermia in immunologically deficient children. Probable human runt disease. N Engl J Med 273:953, 1965

457. Naiman JL, Punnett HH, Lischner HW et al: Possible graft-versus-host reaction after intrauterine transfusion for Rh erythroblastosis fetalis. N Engl J Med 281:697, 1969

458. Parkman R, Mosier D, Umansky I et al: Graft-versus-host disease after intrauterine and exchange transfusions for hemolytic disease of the newborn. N Engl J Med 290:359, 1974

459. Deierhoi MH, Sollinger HW, Bozdech MJ, Belzer FO: Lethal graft-versus-host disease in a recipient of a pancreas-spleen transplant. Transplantation 41:544, 1986

460. Burdick JF, Vogelsang GB, Smith WJ et al: Severe graft-versus-host disease in a liver-transplant recipient. N Engl J Med 318:689, 1988

461. Drobyski WR, Keever CA, Roth MS et al: Salvage immunotherapy using donor leukocyte infusions as treatment for relapsed chronic myelogenous leukemia after allogeneic bone marrow transplantation: efficacy and toxicity of a defined T-cell dose. Blood 82:2310, 1993

462. Leber B, Walker IR, Rodriguez A et al: Reinduction of remission of chronic myeloid leukemia by donor leukocyte transfusion following relapse after bone marrow transplantation: recovery complicated by initial pancytopenia and late dermatomyositis. Bone Marrow Transplant 12:405, 1993

463. Mir MA, Geary CG, Delamore IW: Hypoimmunoglobulinaemia and aplastic anaemia. Scand J Haematol 19:225, 1977

464. Uchiyama T, Nagai K, Yamagishi M et al: Pokeweed mitogen-induced B cell differentiation in idiopathic aplastic anemia associated with hypogammaglobulinemia. Blood 52:77, 1978

465. Josse JW, Zacks SI: Thymoma and pancytopenia. N Engl J Med 259:113, 1958

466. Thomas CV, Manivel JC: Thymic carcinoma and aplastic anemia: report of a previously undocumented association. Am J Hematol 25:333, 1987

467. Littman BH, Cooke CL, Hoffman R: Hypogammaglobulinemia followed by aplastic anemia with suppressor lymphocytes: a case report. Clin Immunol Immunopathol 10:344, 1978

468. Elfenbien GJ, Kallman CH, Tutschka PJ et al: The immune system in 40 aplastic anemia patients receiving conventional therapy. Blood 53:652, 1989

469. Falcao RP, Voltarelli JC, Bottura C: Some immunological studies in aplastic anaemia. J Clin Lab Immunol 10:25, 1983

470. Sabbe LJM, Haak HL, Te Velde J et al: Immunological investigations in aplastic anemia patients. Acta Haematol 71:178, 1984

471. Goldstein IM, Coller BS: Aplastic anemia in pregnancy: recovery after normal spontaneous delivery, letter. Ann Intern Med 82:537, 1975

472. Maizels G: Aplastic anaemia of pregnancy with recovery. South Afr Med J 25:973, 1951

473. Collins DJ, Rosenthal DS, Goldstein DP, Moloney F: Aplastic anemia in pregnancy. Obstet Gynecol 39:884, 1972

474. Evans IL: Aplastic anaemia in pregnancy remitting after abortion, letter. BMJ 3:166, 1968

475. Crisp AJ: Remission of pregnancy hypoplastic anaemia and "malignant" pre-eclampsia after delivery: a case report and discussion. Br J Clin Pract 34:304, 1900

476. Fleming AF: Hypoplastic anaemia in pregnancy. Br J Obstet Gynaecol 75: 138, 1968

477. Rovinsky JJ: Primary refractory anemia complicating pregnancy and delivery. Obstet Gynecol Surv 14:149, 1959

478. Knispel JW, Lynch VA, Viele BD: Aplastic anemia in pregnancy: a case report, review of the literature, and a re-evaluation of management. Obstet Gynecol Surv 31:523, 1976

479. Suda T, Omine M, Tsuchiya J, Maekawa T: Prognostic aspects of aplastic anemia in pregnancy. Experience in six cases and review of literature. Blut 36:285, 1978

480. Issaragrisil S, Vanachivanavin V, Piankijagum A, Kruatrachue M: Aplastic anemia with pregnancy. J Med Assoc Thai 65:111, 1982

481. Hsu MC, Ho HN, Lee TY et al: Aplastic anemia and pregnancy. J Formosan Med Assoc 83:1128, 1984

482. Holly RG: Hypoplastic anemia in pregnancy. Obstet Gynecol 1:535, 1953

483. Kociba GJ, Caputo CA: Aplastic anemia associated with estrus in pet ferrets. J Am Vet Med Assoc 178:1293, 1981

484. Bernard SL, Leathers CW, Brobst DF, Gorham JR: Estrogen-induced bone marrow depression in ferrets. Am J Vet Res 44:657, 1983

485. Tyslowitz R, Dingemanse E: Effect of large doses of estrogens on the blood picture of dogs. Endocrinology 29:817, 1941

486. Crafts RC: The effects of estrogens on the bone marrow of adult female dogs. Blood 3:276, 1948

487. Van Kruiningen HJ, Friedland TB: Responsive estrogen-induced aplastic anemia in a dog. Clin Reprod Fertil 191:91, 1987

488. Castrodale D, Bierbaum O, Helwig EB, MacBryde CM: Comparative studies of the effects of estradiol and stilbestrol upon the blood, liver, and bone marrow. Endocrinology 29:363, 1941

489. Dukes PP, Goldwasser E: Inhibition of erythropoiesis by estrogens. Endocrinology 69:21, 1961

490. Fried W, Tichler T, Dennenberg I et al: Effects of estrogens on hematopoietic stem cells and on hematopoiesis of mice. J Lab Clin Med 83:807, 1974

491. Kurnick JE, Robinson WA, Dickey CA: In vitro granulocytic colony-forming potential of bone marrow from patients with granulocytopenia and aplastic anemia. Proc Soc Exp Biol Med 137:917, 1971

492. Ragab AH, Gilkerson E, Crist WM, Phelan E: Granulopoiesis in childhood aplastic anemia. J Pediatr 88:790, 1976

493. Kern P, Heimpel H, Heit W, Kubanek B: Granulocytic progenitor cells in aplastic anemia. Br J Haematol 35:613, 1977

494. Haak HL, Goselink HM, Veenhof W et al: Acquired aplastic anemia in adults. IV. Histological and CFU studies in transplanted and non-transplanted patients. Scand J Haematol 19:159, 1977

495. Barrett AJ, Faille A, Balitrand N et al: Bone marrow culture in aplastic anaemia. J Clin Pathol 32:660, 1979

496. Rickard KA, Brown RD, Wilkinson T, Kronenberg H: The colony forming cell in the myeloproliferative disorders and aplastic anaemia. Scand J Haematol 22:121, 1979

497. Yoshida K, Miura I, Takahashi T et al: Quantitative and qualitative analysis of stem cells of patients with aplastic anemia. Scand J Haematol 30:317, 1983

498. Hinterberger W, Geissler K, Fischer M et al: Aplastic anemia: assessment of myeloid progenitor cells in the bone marrow and blood provides prognostic information. Acta Haematol 73:1, 1985

499. Hansi W, Rich I, Heimpel H et al: Erythroid colony forming cells in aplastic anaemia. Br J Haematol 37:483, 1977

500. Moriyama Y, Sato M, Kinoshita Y: Studies on hematopoietic stem cells: XI. Lack of erythroid burst-forming units (BFU-E) in patients with aplastic anemia. Am J Hematol 6:11, 1979

501. Umemura T, Takeichi N, Kaneko S et al: Significance of abnormally high endogenous CFU-E numbers in aplastic anemia. Acta Haematol Jpn 49:837, 1985

502. Hara H, Kai S, Fushimi M et al: Pluripotent hemopoietic precursors in vitro (CFU$_{mix}$) in aplastic anemia. Exp Hematol 8:1165, 1980

503. Li S, Champlin R, Fitchen JH, Gale RP: Abnormalities of myeloid progenitor cells after "successful" bone marrow transplantation. J Clin Invest 75:234, 1985

504. Bacigalupo A, 'Podesta M, Mingari MC et al: Immune suppression of hematopoiesis in aplastic anemia: activity of T-gamma lymphocytes. J Immunol 125:1449, 1981

505. Heit W, Heimpel H, Kubanek B: Granulocytic and erythroid progenitor cells in recovering aplastic anemia. p. 97. In Heimpel H, Gordon-Smith EC, Heit W, Kubanek B (eds): Aplastic Anemia—Pathophysiology and Approaches to Therapy. Springer-Verlag, Berlin, 1979

506. Schrezenmeier H, Gerok M, Heimpel H, Raghavachar A: Assessment of frequency of hematopoietic stem cells in aplastic anemia by limiting dilution type long term marrow culture, abstracted. Exp Hematol 20:806, 1992

507. Harrison DE: Use of genetic anaemias in mice as tools for haematological research. Clin Haematol 8:239, 1979

508. Russell ES: Hereditary anemias of the mouse: a review for geneticists. Adv Genet 200:357, 1979

509. Lewis JP, O'Grady LF, Bernstein SE et al: Growth and differentiation of transplanted W/Wv marrow. Blood 30:601, 1967

510. Geissler EN, Ryan MA, Housman DE: The dominant-white spotting (W) locus of the mouse encodes the c-kit proto-oncogene. Cell 55:185, 1988

511. Spangrude G: Enrichment of murine haemopoietic stem cells: diverging roads. Immunol Today 10:344, 1989

512. Ogawa M, Porter PN, Nakahata T: Renewal and commitment to differentiation of hemopoietic stem cells (an interpretive review). Blood 61:823, 1983

513. Sinclair WK: Hydroxyurea: differential lethal effects on cultured mammalian cells during the cell cycle. Science 150:1729, 1965

514. Rosendaal M, Hodgson GS, Bradley TR: Haemopoietic stem cells are organised for use on the basis of their generation-age. Nature 264:68, 1976

515. Hodgson GS, Bradley TR: Properties of haematopoietic stem cells surviving 5-fluorouracil treatment: evidence for a pre-CFU-S cell? Nature 281:381, 1979

516. Mauch PM, Greenberger JS, Botnick LE et al: Evidence for structured variation in self-renewal capacity in long-term bone marrow cultures. Proc Natl Acad Sci USA 77:2927, 1980

517. Harrison DE, Astle CM, Lerner C: Number and continuous proliferative pattern of transplanted primitive immunohematopoietic stem cells. Proc Natl Acad Sci USA 85:822, 1988

518. Spangrude GJ, Smith L, Uchida N et al: Mouse hematopoietic stem cells. Blood 78:1395, 1991

519. Fialkow P: Primordial cell pool size and lineage relationships of five human cell types. Ann Hum Genet 37:39, 1973

520. Spooncer E, Lord BI, Dexter TM: Defective ability to self-renew in vitro of highly purified primitive haematopoietic cells. Nature 316:62, 1985

521. Boggs DR, Boggs SS, Saxe DF et al: Hematopoietic stem cells with high proliferative potential. Assay of their concentration in marrow by the frequency and duration of cure of W/Wv mice. J Clin Invest 70:242, 1982

522. Wiktor-Jedrejczak W, Sharkis SJ, Ahmed A et al: Engraftment of bone marrow transplants in W anemic mice measured by electronic determination of the red blood cell size profile. Exp Hematol 7:416, 1979

523. Nakano T, Waki N, Asai H, Kitamura Y: Long-term monoclonal reconstitution of erythropoiesis in genetically anemic W/Wv mice by injection of 5-fluorouracil-treated bone marrow cells of Pgk-1b/Pgk-1a mice. Blood 70:1758, 1987

524. Mintz B, Anthony K, Litwin S: Monoclonal derivation of mouse myeloid and lymphoid lineages from totipotent hematopoietic stem cells experimentally engrafted in fetal hosts. Proc Natl Acad Sci USA 81:7835, 1984

525. Harrison DE: Normal production of erythrocytes by mouse marrow continuous for 73 months. Proc Natl Acad Sci USA 70:3184, 1973

526. Siminovitch L, Till JE, McCulloch EA: Decline in colony-forming ability of marrow cells subjected to serial transplantation into irradiated mice. Cell Comp Physiol 64:23, 1964

527. Ross EAM, Anderson N, Micklem HS: Serial depletion and regeneration of the murine hematopoietic system. Implications for hematopoietic organization and the study of cellular aging. J Exp Med 155:432, 1982

528. Mauch P, Hellman S: Loss of hematopoietic stem cell self-renewal after bone marrow transplantation. Blood 74:872, 1989

529. Harrison DE, Astle CM: Loss of stem cell repopulating ability upon transplantation. Effects of donor age, cell number, and transplantation procedure. J Exp Med 156:1767, 1982

530. MacMillan JR, Wolf NS: Depletion of reserve in the hemopoietic system. II. Decline in CFU-S self-renewal capacity following prolonged cell cycling. Stem Cells 2:45, 1982

531. Abkowitz JL, Ott RM, Holly RD, Adamson JW: Clonal evolution following chemotherapy-induced stem cell depletion in cats heterozygous for glucose-6-phosphate dehydrogenase. Blood 71:1687, 1988

532. Morley A, Trainor K, Blake J: A primary stem cell lesion in experimental chronic hypoplastic marrow failure. Blood 45:681, 1975

533. Morley A, Blake J: An animal model of chronic aplastic marrow failure. I. Late marrow failure after busulfan. Blood 44:49, 1974

534. Fitchen JH, Cline MJ: The effect of granulopoietic stress in mice with "latent" bone marrow failure. Exp Hematol 8:788, 1980

535. Botnick LE, Hannon EC, Hellman S: Limited proliferation of stem cells surviving alkylating agents. Nature 262:68, 1976

536. Chervenick PA, Boggs DR: Patterns of proliferation and differentiation of hematopoietic stem cells after compartment depletion. Blood 37:568, 1971

537. Fitchen JH, Deregnaucourt J, Cline MJ: An in vitro model of hematopoietic injury in chronic hypoplastic anemia. Cell Tissue Kinet 14:85, 1981

538. McManus PM, Weiss L: Busulfan-induced chronic bone marrow failure: changes in cortical bone, marrow stromal cells, and adherent cell colonies. Blood 64:1036, 1984

539. Fried W, Kedo A, Barone J: Effects of cyclophosphamide and of busulfan on spleen colony-forming units and on hematopoietic stroma. Cancer Res 37:1205, 1977

540. Knospe WH, Crosby WH: Aplastic anaemia: a disorder of the bone-marrow sinusoidal microcirculation rather than stem-cell failure? Lancet 1:20, 1971

541. Tavassoli M, Maniatis A, Crosby WH: Induction of sustained hemopoiesis in fatty marrow. Blood 43:33, 1974

542. Islam A: Do bone marrow fat cells or their precursors have a pathogenic role in idiopathic aplastic anaemia? Med Hypotheses 25:209, 1988

543. Malik F, Gordon MY, Goldman JM, Gordon-Smith EC: Comparisons of the composition of fat cells obtained from the marrow of normal individuals or of subjects with aplastic anemia and from bone marrow cultures. Exp Hematol 12:191, 1984

544. Samsom JP, Hulstaert CE, Molenaar I, Nieweg HO: Fine structure of the bone marrow sinusoidal wall in idiopathic and drug-induced panmyelopathy. Acta Haematol 48:218, 1972

545. Dexter TM, Moore MAS: In vitro duplication and 'cure' of haemopoietic defects in genetically anaemic mice. Nature 269:412, 1977

546. Yoshida K, Takatsu H, Miura I et al: Long-term liquid culture of marrow CFU-C from normal subjects and patients with aplastic anemia. Acta Haematol Jpn 49:829, 1986

547. Juneja HS, Gardner FH, Minguell JJ, Helmer RE III: Abnormal marrow fibroblasts in aplastic anemia. Exp Hematol 12:221, 1984

548. Hotta T, Kato T, Maeda H et al: Functional changes in marrow stromal cells in aplastic anaemia. Acta Haematol 74:65, 1985

549. Juneja HS, Lee S, Gardner FH: Human long-term bone marrow cultures in aplastic anemia. Int J Cell Cloning 7:129, 1989

550. Marsh JCW, Chang J, Testa NG et al: In vitro assessment of marrow 'stem cell' and stromal cell function in aplastic anaemia. Br J Haematol 78:258, 1991

551. Bacigalupo A, Figari O, Tong J et al: Long-term marrow culture in patients with aplastic anemia compared with marrow transplant recipients and normal controls. Exp Hematol 20:425, 1992

552. Wiktor-Jedrzejczak W, Siekierzynski M, Szczylik C et al: Aplastic anaemia with marrow defective in formation of fibroblastoid cell colonies in vitro. Scand J Haematol 28:82, 1982

553. Juneja HS, Gardner FH: Functionally abnormal marrow stromal cells in aplastic anemia. Exp Hematol 13:194, 1985

554. Hirata J, Umemura T, Kaneko S et al: Difference of bone marrow adipocyte colony-forming capacity between aplastic anemia and iron deficiency anemia. Leuk Res 12:179, 1988

555. Gordon MY, Gordon-Smith EC: Bone marrow fibroblast function in relation to granulopoiesis in aplastic anemia. Br J Haematol 53:483, 1983

556. Nissen C, Moser Y, dalle Carbonare V et al: Complete recovery of marrow function after treatment with anti-lymphocyte globulin is associated with high, whereas early failure and development of paroxysmal nocturnal haemoglobinuria are associated with low endogenous G-CSA-release. Br J Haematol 72:573, 1989

557. Migliaccio AR, Migliaccio G, Adamson JW, Torok-Storb B: Production of granulocyte colony-stimulating factor and granulocyte/macrophage-colony-stimulating factor after interleukin-1 stimulation of marrow stromal cell cultures from normal or aplastic anemia donors. J Cell Physiol 152:199, 1992

558. Kojima S, Matsuyama T, Kodera Y: Hematopoietic growth factors released by marrow stromal cells from patients with aplastic anemia. Blood 79:2256, 1992

559. Stark R, Andre C, Thierry D, Cherel M, Galibert F, Gluckman E: The expression of cytokine and cytokine receptor genes in long-term bone marrow culture in congenital and acquired bone marrow hypoplasias. Br J Haematol 83:560, 1993

560. Novitzky N, Jacobs P: Marrow stem cell and stroma cell function in aplastic anaemia, letter. Br J Haematol 79:531, 1991

561. Merchav S, Tatarsky I, Sharon R: Aplastic anemia associated with in vitro inhibition of erythropoiesis by bone marrow-adherent cells. Eur J Haematol 41:429, 1988

562. Suda T, Mizoguchi H, Miura Y et al: Suppression of in vitro granulocyte-macrophage colony formation by the peripheral mononuclear phagocytic cells of patients with idiopathic aplastic anaemia. Br J Haematol 47:433, 1981

563. Hanada T, Abe T: The effect of peripheral blood adherent cells from patients with aplastic anemia on in vitro hematopoiesis. Exp Hematol 11:298, 1983

564. Alexanian R: Erythropoietin excretion in bone marrow failure and hemolytic anemia. J Lab Clin Med 82:438, 1973

565. Bray GL, Taylor B, O'Donnell R: Comparison of the erythropoietin response in children with aplastic anemia, transient erythroblastopenia, and iron deficiency. J Pediatr 120:528, 1992

566. Takeichi N, Umemura T, Nishimura J et al: Regulation of erythropoietin and burst-promoting activity production in patients with aplastic anemia and iron deficiency anemia. Acta Haematol 80:145, 1988

567. Okamoto T, Kanamaru A, Hara H, Nagai K: Burst-promoting activity (BPA) without erythropoietin (Ep) activity in sera of aplastic anemia patients fractionated by chromatofocusing column. Exp Hematol 10:844, 1982

568. Fukamachi H, Urabe A, Saito T et al: Burst-promoting activity in anemia and polycythemia. Int J Cell Cloning 4:74, 1986

569. Hara H, Okamoto T, Ohe Y, Kanamaru A: Mixed colony inducing activity in sera from patients with acquired aplastic anemia. Acta Haematol 46:35, 1983

570. Yen YP, Zabala P, Doney K et al: Hematopoietic growth factors in human serum. Erythroid burst-promoting activity in normal subjects and in patients with severe aplastic anemia. J Lab Clin Med 106:384, 1985

571. Entringer MA, Robinson WA, Dreging CJ: Colony stimulating activity in normal human serum tested against human bone marrow. Exp Hematol 8:1232, 1980

572. Nissen C, Moser Y, Weis J et al: The release of interleukin-2 (IL-2) and colony stimulating activity (CSA) in aplastic anemia patients: opposite behaviour with improvement of bone marrow function. Blut 52:221, 1986

573. Weatherly TL, Fleisher TA, Strong DM: Reduced granulocyte-macrophage colony-stimulating activity by mitogen-stimulated lymphocytes from patients with aplastic anemia. Br J Haematol 43:335, 1979

574. Enomoto K, Kawakita M, Kishimoto S et al: Thrombopoiesis and megakaryocyte colony stimulating factor in the urine of patients with aplastic anemia. Br J Haematol 45:551, 1980

575. Adams JA, Barrett AJ: Haematopoietic stimulators in the serum of patients with severe aplastic anaemia. Br J Haematol 52:327, 1982

576. Miyake T, Kawakita M, Enomoto K et al: Partial purification and biological properties of thrombopoietin extracted from the urine of aplastic anemia patients. Stem Cells 2:129, 1982

577. Hoffman R, Mazur E, Bruno E et al: Assay of an activity in the serum of patients with disorders of thrombopoiesis that stimulates formation of megakaryocytic colonies. N Engl J Med 305:533, 1981

578. Ogata K, Kuriya S, Dan K, Nomura T: Partial purification of human urinary megakaryocyte colony-stimulating factor. Exp Cell Biol 57:19, 1989

579. Nimer SD, Golde DW, Kwan K et al: In vitro production of granulocyte-macrophage colony stimulating factor in aplastic anemia: possible mechanisms of action of antithymocyte globulin. Blood 78:163, 1991

580. Kawano Y, Takaue Y, Hirao A et al: Production of interleukin 3 and granulocyte-macrophage colony-stimulating factor from stimulated blood mononuclear cells in patients with aplastic anemia. Exp Hematol 20:1125, 1992

581. Nissen C, Moser Y, Weis J, Speck B: Stimulatory serum factors in aplastic anaemia. I. Serum 'releaser' activity for haemopoietic growth factors, a regulator? Br J Haematol 61:491, 1985

582. Watari K, Asano S, Shirafuji N et al: Serum granulocyte colony-stimulating factor levels in healthy volunteers and patients with various disorders as estimated by enzyme immunoassay. Blood 73:117, 1989

583. Schrezenmeier H, Raghavachar A, Heimpel H: Granulocyte-macrophage colony-stimulating factor in the sera of patients with aplastic anemia. Clin Invest 71:102, 1993

584. Omori F, Okamura S, Shimoda K et al: Levels of human serum granulocyte colony-stimulating factor and granulocyte-macrophage colony-stimulating factor under pathological conditions. Biotherapy 4:147, 1992

585. Nakao S, Matsushima K, Young N: Deficient interleukin 1 production by aplastic anemia monocytes. Br J Haematol 71:431, 1989

586. Childs B, Tomelden C, Chasseing NA et al: Stimulated monocytes from severe aplastic anemia patients are deficient in production of IL-1-beta, variably deficient in production of IL-6, but not deficient in GM-CSF production, abstracted. Blood, suppl. 1. 78:367a, 1991

587. Wodnar-Filipowicz A, Yancik S, Moser Y et al: Levels of soluble stem cell factor in serum of patients with aplastic anemia. Blood 81:3259, 1993

588. Holmberg LA, Yancik S, Zsebo K, Torok-Storb B: Circulating levels of kit ligand (KL) in serum of patients with aplastic anemia, myelodysplasia or

following allogeneic bone marrow transplantation, abstracted. Exp Hematol 20:775, 1992

589. Wodnar-Filpowicz A, Tichelli A, Zsebo KM et al: Stem cell factor stimulates the in vitro growth of bone marrow cells from aplastic anemia patients. Blood 79:3196, 1992

590. Bacigalupo A, Bagnara GP, Ramenghi U et al: In vitro effect of stem cell factor on colony growth from acquired and constitutional (Fanconi) severe aplastic anemia, abstracted. Exp Hematol 805, 1992

591. Ershuin WB, Ross J, Finlay JL, Shahidi NT: Bone-marrow microenvironment defect in congenital hypoplastic anemia. N Engl J Med 302:1321, 1980

592. Marsh JCW, Harhalakis N, Dowding C et al: Recurrent graft failure following syngeneic bone marrow transplantation for aplastic anemia. Bone Marrow Transplant 4:581, 1989

593. Mathé G, Amiel JL, Schwarzenberg L et al: Bone marrow graft in man after conditioning by antilymphocytic serum. BMJ 2:131, 1970

594. Thomas ED, Storb R, Giblett ER et al: Recovery from aplastic anemia following attempted marrow transplantation. Exp Hematol 4:97, 1976

595. Bussel A, Dumont J, Schenmetzler C et al: Long-term complete autologous reconstitution following cyclophosphamide and allogeneic marrow infusion in a case of severe aplastic anemia. Nouv Rev Fr Hematol 27:15, 1985

596. Territo MC: Autologous bone marrow repopulation following high dose cyclophosphamide and allogeneic marrow transplantation in aplastic anemia. Br J Haematol 36:305, 1977

597. Champlin RE, Feig SA, Sparkes RS, Gale RP: Bone marrow transplantation from identical twins in the treatment of aplastic anaemia: implication for the pathogenesis of the disease. Br J Haematol 56:455, 1984

598. Appelbaum FR, Cheever MA, Fefer A et al: Recurrence of aplastic anemia following cyclophosphamide and syngeneic bone marrow transplantation: evidence for two mechanisms of graft failure. Blood 65:553, 1985

599. Kagan WA, Ascensao JA, Pahwa RN et al: Aplastic anemia: presence in human bone marrow of cells that suppress myelopoiesis. Proc Natl Acad Sci USA 73:2890, 1976

600. Ascensao J, Kagan W, Moore M et al: Aplastic anaemia: evidence for an immunological mechanism. Lancet 1:669, 1976

601. Hoffman RA, Zanjani ED, Lutton JD et al: Suppression of erythroid-colony formation by lymphocytes from patients with aplastic anemia. N Engl J Med 296:10, 1977

602. Nissen C, Cornu P, Gratwohl A, Speck B: Peripheral blood cells from patients with aplastic anaemia in partial remission suppress growth of their own bone marrow precursors in culture. Br J Haematol 45:233, 1980

603. Shionoya S, Motoyoshi K, Saito M et al: Immunosuppressive therapy in aplastic anemia based on in vitro culture studies. Acta Haematol Jpn 49: 1282, 1986

604. Bacigalupo A, 'Podesta M, van Lint MT et al: Severe aplastic anaemia: correlation of in vitro tests with clinical response to immunosuppression in 20 patients. Br J Haematol 47:423, 1981

605. Takaku F, Suda T, Mizoguchi H et al: Effect of peripheral blood mononuclear cells from aplastic anemia patients on the granulocyte-macrophage and erythroid colony formation in samples from normal human bone marrow in vitro—a cooperative work. Blood 55:937, 1980

606. Da WM: In vitro studies on the pathogenesis of aplastic anemia in Chinese patients. Exp Hematol 16:336, 1988

607. Abdou NI, Verdirame JD, Amare M, Abdou NL: Heterogeneity of pathogenetic mechanisms in aplastic anemia. Ann Intern Med 95:43, 1981

608. Morris TCM, Vincent PC, Young GAR et al: CFU-C inhibitors in aplastic anaemia. Blut 48:61, 1984

609. Nagasawa T, Abe T, Hanada T: Inhibitory effects of T cells on in vitro granulopoiesis, erythropoiesis, and immunoglobulin production in patients with aplastic anemia. Scand J Haematol 28:389, 1982

610. Sullivan R, Quesenberry PJ, Parkman R et al: Aplastic anemia: lack of inhibitory effect of bone marrow lymphocytes on in vitro granulopoiesis. Blood 56:625, 1980

611. Hanada T, Aoki Y, Ninomiya H, Abe T: T cell-mediated inhibition of haematopoiesis in aplastic anemia: serial assay of inhibitory activities of T cells to autologous CFU-E during immunosuppressive therapy. Br J Haematol 63: 69, 1986

612. Bacigalupo A, 'Podesta M, Raffo MR et al: Lack of in vitro colony (CFU$_C$) formation and myelosuppressive activity in patients with severe aplastic anemia after autologous hematologic reconstitution. Exp Hematol 8:795, 1980

613. Torok-Storb BJ, Storb R, Graham TC et al: Erythropoiesis in vitro: effect of normal versus "transfusion-sensitized" mononuclear cells. Blood 52:706, 1978

614. Singer JW, Brown JE, James MC et al: Effect of peripheral blood lymphocytes from patients with aplastic anemia on granulocytic colony growth from HLA-matched and mismatched marrows: effect of transfusion sensitization. Blood 52:37, 1978

615. Singer JW, Doney KC, Thomas ED: Coculture studies of 16 untransfused patients with aplastic anemia. Blood 54:180, 1979

616. Torok-Storb BJ, Sieff C, Storb R et al: In vitro tests for distinguishing possible immune-mediated aplastic anemia from transfusion-induced sensitization. Blood 55:211, 1980

617. Bacigalupo A, 'Podesta M, Frassoni F et al: Generation of CFU-C suppressor T cells in vitro. V. A multistep process. Br J Haematol 52:421, 1982

618. Zoumbos NC, Djeu JY, Young NS: Interferon is the inhibitor of hematopoiesis generated by stimulated lymphocytes in vitro. J Immunol 133:769, 1984

619. Rigby WFC, Ball ED, Guyre PM, Fanger MW: The effects of recombinant-DNA-derived interferons on the growth of myeloid progenitor cells. Blood 65:858, 1985

620. Mamus SW, Beck-Schroeder S, Zanjani ED: Suppression of normal human erythropoiesis by gamma interferon in vitro. Role of monocytes and T lymphocytes. J Clin Invest 75:1496, 1985

621. Broxmeyer HE, Cooper S, Rubin BY, Taylor MW: The synergistic influence of human interferon-gamma and interferon-α on suppression of hematopoietic progenitor cells is additive with the enhanced sensitivity of these cells to inhibition by interferons at low oxygen tension in vitro. J Immunol 135:2502, 1985

622. Ganser A, Carlo-Stella C, Greher J et al: Effect of recombinant interferons alpha and gamma on human bone marrow-derived megakaryocytic progenitor cells. Blood 70:1173, 1987

623. Koren S, Klimpel GR, Fleischmann WR Jr: Treatment of mice with macrophage colony stimulating factor (CSF-1) prevents the in vivo myelosuppression induced by murine alpha, beta, and gamma interferons. J Biol Response Mod 5:481, 1986

624. Talpaz M, Spitzer G, Hittelman W et al: Changes in granulocyte-monocyte colony-forming cells among leukocyte-interferon-treated chronic myelogenous leukemia patients. Exp Hematol 14:668, 1986

625. Raefsky E, Platanias L, Zoumbos N, Young NS: Studies of interferon as a regulator of hematopoietic proliferation. J Immunol 135:2507, 1985

626. Conta BS, Powell MB, Ruddle NH: Production of lymphotoxin, IFN-gamma and IFN-α, β by murine T cell lines and clones. J Immunol 130:2231, 1983

627. Murphy M, Loudon R, Kobayashi M, Trinchieri G: Gamma-interferon and lymphotoxin released by activated T cells synergize to inhibit granulocyte/monocyte colony formation. J Exp Med 164:263, 1986

628. Williams TW, Bellanti JA: In vitro synergism between interferons and human lymphotoxin: enhancement of lymphotoxin-induced target cell killing. J Immunol 130:518, 1983

629. Lee SH, Aggarwal BB, Rinderknecht E et al: The synergistic anti-proliferative effect of gamma-interferon and human lymphotoxin. J Immunol 133:1083, 1984

630. Broxmeyer HE, Williams DE, Lu L et al: The suppressive influences of human tumor necrosis factors on bone marrow hematopoietic progenitor cells from normal donors and patients with leukemia: synergism of tumor necrosis factor and interferon-gamma. J Immunol 136:4487, 1986

631. Weiss A: T lymphocyte activation. p. 467. In Paul WE (ed.) Fundamental Immunology. Raven Press, New York, 1993

632. Spitzer G, Verma DS, Abramowitz S, Tomasovic B: Cells with Fc gamma receptors from normal donors suppress granulocytic macrophage colony formation. Blood 60:758, 1982

633. Broxmeyer HE, Lu L, Bognacki J: Transferrin, derived from an OKT8-positive subpopulation of T lymphocytes, suppresses the production of granulocyte-macrophage colony-stimulatory factors from mitogen-activated T lymphocytes. Blood 62:37, 1983

634. Nakao S, Harada M, Kondo K et al: Effect of activated lymphocytes on the regulation of hematopoiesis: suppression of in vitro granulopoiesis by OKT8$^+$ Ia$^+$ T cells induced by alloantigen stimulation. J Immunol 132:160, 1984

635. Verma DS, Johnston DA, McCredie KB: Evidence for the separate human T-lymphocyte subpopulations that collaborate with autologous monocyte/macrophages in the elaboration of colony-stimulating activity and those that suppress this collaboration. Blood 62:1088, 1983

636. Torok-Storb B, Martin PJ, Hansen JA: Regulation of in vitro erythropoiesis by normal T cells: evidence for two T-cell subsets with opposing function. Blood 58:171, 1981

637. Harada M, Nakao S, Kondo K et al: Effect of activated lymphocytes on the regulation of hematopoiesis: enhancement and suppression of in vitro BFU-E growth by T cells stimulated by autologous non-T cells. Blood 67:1143, 1986

638. Burdach ST, Shatsky M, Wagenhorst B, Levitt L: The T-cell CD2 determinant mediates inhibition of erythropoiesis by the lymphokine cascade. Blood 72: 770, 1988

639. Burdach SEG, Levitt LJ: Receptor-specific inhibition of bone marrow erythropoiesis by recombinant DNA-derived interleukin-2. Blood 69:1368, 1987

640. Zoumbos N, Gascon P, Djeu J, Young NS: Interferon is a mediator of hematopoietic suppression in aplastic anemia in vitro and possibly in vivo. Proc Natl Acad Sci USA 82:188, 1985

641. Gascon P, Zoumbos N, Djeu J et al: Lymphokine abnormalities in aplastic anemia. Implications for the mechanism of action of ATG. Blood 65:407, 1985

642. Nisticò A, Young NS: Gamma-interferon gene expression in the bone marrow of patients with aplastic anemia. Ann Intern Med 120:463, 1994

643. Nakao S, Yamaguchi M, Shiobara S, et al: Interferon gamma gene expression in unstimulated bone marrow mononuclear cells predicts a response to cyclosporine therapy in aplastic anemia. Blood 79:2532, 1992

644. Katevas P, Maciejewski JP, Rosenfeld S et al: Expression of tumor necrosis factor-6 mRNA in bone marrow of patients with aplastic anemia. Blood, suppl. 1 82:90a, 1993

645. Zoumbos NC, Ferris WO, Hsu S-M et al: Analysis of lymphocyte subsets in patients with aplastic anemia. Br J Haematol 58:95, 1984

646. Ruiz-Argüelles GJ, Katzmann JA, Greipp PR et al: Lymphocyte subsets in patients with aplastic anemia. Am J Hematol 16:267, 1984

647. Janossy G, Tidman N, Selby WS et al: Human T lymphocytes of inducer and suppressor type occupy different microenvironments. Nature 288:81, 1980

648. Falcao RP, Voltarelli JC, Bottura C: T-lymphocyte subpopulations in the peripheral blood and bone marrow of patients with aplastic anemia. Blut 50:103, 1985

649. Zoumbos N, Gascon P, Trost S et al: Circulating activated suppressor T lymphocytes in aplastic anemia. N Engl J Med 312:257, 1985

650. Hinterberger W, Adolf G, Aichinger G et al: Further evidence for lymphokine overproduction in severe aplastic anemia. Blood 72:266, 1988

651. Maciejewski JP, Hibbs JR, Anderson S et al: Bone marrow and peripheral blood lymphocyte phenotyping in patients with bone marrow failure. Br J Haematol (in press)

652. Mehta AB, Chiu E, Harhalakis N et al: A T-cell lymphoma of suppressor phenotype arising in a patient with severe aplastic anaemia, letter. Br J Haematol 1989:287, 1972

653. Platanias L, Gascon P, Bielory L et al: Lymphocyte subsets and lymphokines following anti-thymocyte globulin therapy in patients with aplastic anemia. Br J Haematol 66:433, 1987

654. Laver J, Castro-Malaspina H, Kernan NA et al: In vitro interferon-gamma production by cultured T-cells in severe aplastic anaemia: correlation with granulomonopoietic inhibition in patients who respond to anti-thymocyte globulin. Br J Haematol 69:545, 1988

655. Ettinghausen SB, Moore JG, Platanias L et al: Hematologic toxicity of lymphokine activated killer (LAK) cells and recombinant interleukin 2 in cancer patients. Blood 69:1654, 1987

656. Heslop HE, Gottlieb DJ, Bianchi ACM et al: In vivo induction of gamma interferon and tumor necrosis factor by interleukin-2 infusion following intensive chemotherapy or autologous marrow transplantation. Blood 74:1374, 1989

657. Tritarelli E, Rocca E, Testa U et al: Adoptive immunotherapy with high-dose interleukin-2: kinetics of circulating progenitors correlate with interleukin-6, granulocyte colony-stimulating factor level. Blood 77:741, 1991

658. Basham TY, Merigan TC: Recombinant interferon-gamma increases HLA-DR synthesis and expression. J Immunol 130:1492, 1983

659. Collart MA, Belin D, Vassalli J-D et al: Gamma interferon enhances macrophage transcription of the tumor necrosis enhances macrophage transcription of the tumor necrosis factor/cachectin, interleukin 1, and urokinase genes, which are controlled by short-lived repressors. J Exp Med 164:2113, 1986

660. Wisniewski D, Strife A, Wachter M, Clarkson B: Regulation of human peripheral blood erythroid burst-forming unit growth by T lymphocytes and T lymphocyte subpopulations defined by OKT_4 and OKT_8 monoclonal antibodies. Blood 65:456, 1985

661. Estrov Z, Roifman C, Mills G et al: The regulatory role of interleukin 2-responsive T lymphocytes on human marrow granulopoiesis. Blood 69:1161, 1987

662. Skettino S, Phillips J, Lanier L et al: Selective generation of erythroid burst-promoting activity by recombinant interleukin 2-stimulated human T lymphocytes and natural killer cells. Blood 71:907, 1988

663. Piacibello W, Lu L, Williams D et al: Human gamma interferon enhances release from phytohemagglutinin-stimulated $T4^+$ lymphocytes of activities that stimulate colony formation by granulocyte-macrophage, erythroid, and multipotential progenitor cells. Blood 68:1339, 1986

664. Koeffler HP, Gasson J, Ranyard J et al: Recombinant human TNFα stimulates production of granulocyte colony-stimulating factor. Blood 70:55, 1987

665. Caux C, Moreau I, Saeland S, Banchereau J: Interferon-gamma enhances factor-dependent myeloid proliferation of human CD34+ hematopoietic progenitor cells. Blood 79:2628, 1992

666. Raghavachar A, Frickhofen N, Taniguchi Y et al: Soluble interleukin-2 receptors and CD8 like molecules in the sera of patients with aplastic anemia, abstracted. Blut 57:240, 1988

667. Warren RP, Storb R, Thomas ED et al: Autoimmune and alloimmune phenomena in patients with aplastic anemia: cytotoxicity against autologous lymphocytes and lymphocytes from HLA identical siblings. Blood 56:683, 1980

668. Carpenter N, Fontannaz J, Jeannet M et al: Characteristics and clinical relevance of autolymphocytotoxins in patients with aplastic anemia. Transplantation 42:159, 1986

669. Trinchieri G: Biology of natural killer cells. Adv Immunol 47:187, 1989

670. Perussia B, Fanning V, Trinchieri G: A human NK and K cell subset shares with cytotoxic T cells expression of the antigen recognized by antibody OKT8. J Immunol 131:223, 1983

671. Kasahara T, Djeu JY, Dougherty SF, Oppenheim JJ: Capacity of human large granular lymphocytes (LGL) to produce multiple lymphokines: interleukin 2, interferon, and colony stimulating factor. J Immunol 131:2379, 1983

672. Pistoia V, Ghio R, Nocera A et al: Large granular lymphocytes have a promoting activity on human peripheral blood erythroid burst-forming units. Blood 65:464, 1985

673. Brooks CG: Reversible induction of natural killer cell activity in cloned murine cytotoxic T lymphocytes, letter. Nature 305:155, 1983

674. Hansson M, Beran M, Andersson B, Kiessling R: Inhibition of in vitro granulopoiesis by autologous allogeneic human NK cells. J Immunol 129:126, 1982

675. Degliantoni G, Perussia B, Mangoni L, Trinchieri G: Inhibition of bone marrow colony formation by human natural killer cells and by natural killer cell-derived colony-inhibiting activity. J Exp Med 161:1152, 1985

676. Vinci G, Vernant JP, Nakazawa M et al: In vitro inhibition of normal human hematopoiesis by marrow $CD3^+$, $CD8^+$, $HLA-DR^+$, HNK_1^+ lymphocytes. Blood 72:1616, 1988

677. Herrmann F, Schmidt RE, Ritz J, Griffin JD: In vitro regulation of human hematopoiesis by natural killer cells: analysis at a clonal level. Blood 69:246, 1987

678. Mangan KF, Hartnett ME, Matis SA et al: Natural killer cells suppress human erythroid stem cell proliferation in vitro. Blood 63:260, 1984

679. O'Brien T, Kendra J, Stephens H et al: Recognition and regulation of progenitor marrow elements by NK cells in the mouse. Immunology 49:717, 1983

680. Holmberg LA, Miller BA, Ault KA: The effect of natural killer cells on the development of syngeneic hematopoietic progenitors. J Immunol 133:2933, 1984

681. Barlozzari T, Herberman RB, Reynolds CW: Inhibition of pluripotent hematopoietic stem cells of bone marrow by large granular lymphocytes. Proc Natl Acad Sci USA 84:7691, 1987

682. Reynolds CW, Foon KA: T_{gamma}-lymphoproliferative disease and related disorders in humans and experimental animals: a review of the clinical, cellular, and functional characteristics. Blood 64:1146, 1984

683. Gibson FM, Malkovska V, Myint AA et al: Mechanism of suppression of normal hemopoietic activity by lymphokine-activated killer cells and their products. Exp Hematol 19:659, 1991

684. Niemeyer CM, Sieff CA, Smith BR et al: Hematopoiesis in vitro coexists with natural killer lymphocytes. Blood 74:2376, 1989

685. Loughran TP: Clonal disease of large granular lymphocytes. Blood 82:1, 1993

686. Loughran TP Jr, Clark EA, Price TH, Hammond WP: Adult-onset cyclic neutropenia is associated with increased large granular lymphocytes. Blood 68:1082, 1986

687. Picker LJ, Furst A, Robinson SH, Kadin ME: Immunoarchitecture of the bone marrow in neutropenia: increased HNK-1+ cells define a subset of neutropenic patients. Am J Hematol 25:29, 1987

688. Hooks JJ, Haynes BF, Detrick-Hooks B et al: Gamma (immune) interferon production by leukocytes from a patient with a T_G cell proliferative disease. Blood 59:198, 1982

689. Murphy WJ, Reynolds CW, Tiberghien P, Longo DL: Natural killer cells and bone marrow transplantation. JNCI 85:1475, 1993

690. Yu YY, Kumar V, Bennett M: Murine natural killer cells and marrow graft rejection. Annu Rev Immunol 10:189, 1992

691. Takahashi M, Oshimi K, Saito H, Mizoguchi H: Inhibition of human granulocyte-macrophage colony formation by interleukin 2-treated lymphocytes. Exp Hematol 16:226, 1988

692. Gascon P, Zoumbos N, Young NS: An analysis of natural killer cells in aplastic anemia. Blood 67:1349, 1986

693. Porwit A, Hast R, Stenke L et al: Decreased blood natural killer cell activity and immunoglobulin synthesis in vitro in aplastic anemia. J Intern Med 224:391, 1988

694. Yoda Y, Kawakami Z, Abe T: Decreased frequency of bone marrow NK progenitors in aplastic anemia. Br J Haematol 71:545, 1989

695. Myint AA, Malkovska V, Morgan S et al: Antilymphocyte globulin therapy enhances impaired function to natural killer cells and lymphokine activated killer cells in aplastic anemia. Br J Haematol 75:578, 1990

696. Herrmann F, Griffin JD, Meuer SG, Zum Buschenfelde K-HM: Establishment of an interleukin 2-dependent T cell line derived from a patient with severe

aplastic anemia, which inhibits in vitro hematopoiesis. J Immunol 136:1629, 1986

697. Long EO, Jacobson S: Pathways of viral antigen processing and presentation to CTL: defined by the mode of virus entry? Immunol Today 10:45, 1989

698. Kurane I, Meager A, Ennis FA: Dengue virus-specific human T cell clones. Serotype crossreactive proliferation, interferon gamma production, and cytotoxic activity. J Exp Med 170:763, 1989

699. Lotz M, Tsoukas CD, Fong S et al: Release of lymphokines after Epstein Barr virus infection in vitro. I. Sources of and kinetics of production of interferons and interleukins in normal humans. J Immunol 136:3636, 1986

700. Ahmed R, Oldstone MBA: Mechanisms and biological implications of virus-induced polyclonal B-cell activation. p. 231. In Notkins AL, Oldstone MBA (eds): Concepts in Viral Pathogenesis. Springer-Verlag, New York, 1984

701. Kurtz CIB, Fujinami RS: Immune response to viral infections. p. 31. In Young NS (ed): Viruses and the Bone Marrow. Marcel Dekker, New York, 1993

702. Welsh RM, McFarland HI: Mechanisms of viral pathogenesis. p. 3. In Young NS (ed): Viruses and the Bone Marrow. Marcel Dekker, New York, 1993

703. Hibbs JR, Young NS: Host response to viruses. In Young NS (ed): Viruses and Hematology. London, Ballière Tindall (in press)

704. Brinton MA, Nathanson N: Genetic determinants of virus susceptibility: epidemiologic implication in murine models. Epidemiol Rev 3:115, 1981

705. Gordon MY: Circulating inhibitors of granulopoiesis in patients with aplastic anaemia. Br J Haematol 39:491, 1978

706. Fitchen JH, Cline MJ: Serum inhibitors of myelopoiesis. Br J Haematol 44: 7, 1980

707. Takahashi M: Complement-dependent hematopoietic inhibitors in the sera of patients with aplastic anemia and paroxysmal nocturnal hemoglobinuria. Int J Cell Cloning 5:242, 1987

708. Chudomel V, Rerábková E. Cinátl J et al: Progenitor white cells and serum inhibitors in patients with bone marrow aplasia. Folia Haematol (Leipz) 106: 358, 1979

709. Chan SH, Metcalf D: Inhibition of bone marrow colony formation by normal and leukemic human serum. Nature 227:845, 1980

710. Vincent PC, Sutherland R, Morris TCM, Chapman GV: Inhibitor of in-vitro granulopoiesis in plasma of patients with renal failure. Lancet 2:864, 1978

711. Cline MJ, Opelz G, Saxon A et al: Autoimmune panleukopenia. N Engl J Med 295:1489, 1976

712. Freedman MH, Gelfand EW, Saunders EF: Acquired aplastic anemia: antibody-mediated hematopoietic failure. Am J Hematol 6:135, 1979

713. Fitchen JH, Cline MJ, Saxon A, Golde DW: Serum inhibitors of hematopoiesis in a patient with aplastic anemia and systemic lupus erythematosus. Am J Med 66:537, 1979

714. Dainiak N, Hardin J, Floyd V et al: Humoral suppression of erythropoiesis in systemic lupus erythematosus (SLE) and rheumatoid arthritis. Am J Med 69:537, 1980

715. Brooks BJ Jr, Broxmeyer HE, Bryan CF, Leech SH: Serum inhibitor in systemic lupus erythematosus associated with aplastic anemia. Arch Intern Med 144:1474, 1984

716. Bailey FA, Lilly M, Bertoli LF, Ball GV: An antibody that inhibits in vitro bone marrow proliferation in a patient with systemic lupus erythematosus and aplastic anemia. Arthritis Rheum 32:901, 1989

717. Kelton HG, Huang AT, Mold N et al: The use of in vitro technics to study drug-induced pancytopenia. N Engl J Med 301:621, 1979

718. Salama A, Schütz B, Kiefel V et al: Immune-mediated agranulocytosis related to drugs and their metabolites: mode of sensitization and heterogeneity of antibodies. Br J Haematol 72:127, 1989

719. Taetle R, Lane TA, Mendelsohn J: Drug-induced agranulocytosis: in vitro evidence for immune suppression of granulopoiesis and a cross-reacting lymphocyte antibody. Blood 54:501, 1979

720. Hornung RL, Longo DL: Hematopoietic stem cell depletion by restorative growth factor regimens during repeated high-dose cyclophosphamide therapy. Blood 80:77, 1992

721. Modan B, Segal S, Shani M, Sheba C: Aplastic anemia in Israel: evaluation of the etiological role of chloramphenicol on a community-wide basis. Am J Med Sci 270:441, 1975

722. Shima S, Kato Y: Incidence of aplastic anemia among workers in major indus-

tries in Japan and suspected causal factors. p. 53. In Aoki K, Hosoda Y, Yanagawa H et al: (eds): Epidemiology of Intractable Diseases in Japan. Department of Preventive Medicine, Nagoya University School of Medicine, Nagoya, 1986

723. Szklo M, Sensenbrenner L, Markowitz J et al: Incidence of aplastic anemia in metropolitan Baltimore: a population-based study. Blood 66:115, 1985

724. Davies SM, Walker DJ: Aplastic anaemia in the Northern Region 1971–1978 and follow-up of long-term survivors. Clin Lab Haematol 8:307, 1986

725. Cartwright RA, McKinney PA, Williams L et al: Aplastic anaemic incidence in parts of the United Kingdom in 1985. Leuk Res 12:459, 1988

726. Clausen N: A population study of severe aplastic anemia in children: incidence, etiology and course. Acta Paediatr Scand 75:58, 1986

727. The International Agranulocytosis and Aplastic Anemia Study: Risks of agranulocytosis and aplastic anemia: a first report of their relation to drug use with special reference to analgesics. JAMA 256:1749, 1986

728. Aggio MC, Alvarez RV, Bartomioli MA, Maguitman O: Incidence and etiology of aplastic anemia in a defined population of Argentina (1966–1977). Medicina 48:231, 1988

729. Mary JY, Baumelou E, Guiguet M: Epidemiology of aplastic anemia in France: a prospective multicenter study. Blood 75:1646, 1990

730. Chongli Y, Xiaobo Z: Incidence survey of aplastic anemia in China. Chin Med Sci J 6:203, 1991

731. Langlois RG, Bigbee WL, Kyoizumi S et al: Evidence for increased somatic cell mutations at the glycophorin A locus in atomic bomb survivors. Science 236:445, 1987

732. Alter BP, Potter NU, Li FP: Classification and aetiology of the aplastic anaemias. Clin Haematol 7:431, 1978

733. Abe T, Komiya M: Some clinical aspects of aplastic anemia. p. 197. In Hibino S, Takaku F, Shahidi NT (eds): Aplastic Anemia. University Park Press, Baltimore, 1978

734. Whang KS: Aplastic anemia in Korea: a clinical study of 309 cases. p. 225. In Hibino S, Takaku F, Shahidi NT (eds): Aplastic Anemia. University Park Press, Baltimore, 1978

735. Wintrobe MM, Lee GR, Bogg DR et al: Pancytopenia, aplastic anemia, and pure red cell aplasia. p. 698. In Wintrobe MM, Lee GR, Boggs DR et al (eds): Clinical Hematology. 8th Ed. Lea & Febiger, Philadelphia, 1981

736. Erslev AJ: Aplastic anemia: p. 151. In Williams WJ, Beutler E, Erslev AJ, Lichtman MA (eds): Hematology. 3rd Ed. McGraw-Hill, New York, 1983

737. Vincent PC: Drug-induced aplastic anemia and agranulocytosis. Incidence and mechanisms. Drugs 31:52, 1986

738. Young NS (ed): Viruses and Bone Marrow. Marcel Dekker, New York, 1993

739. Mangan KF, Mullaney MT, Rosenfeld CS, Shadduck RK: In vitro evidence for disappearance of erythroid progenitor T suppressor cells following allogenic bone marrow transplantation for severe aplastic anemia. Blood 71:144, 1988

740. De Planque MM, Brand A, Kluin-Nelemans HC et al: Haematopoietic and immunologic abnormalities in severe aplastic anaemia patients treated with anti-thymocyte globulin. Br J Haematol 71:421, 1989

741. Torok-Storb B, Johnson G, Bowden R, Storb R: Gamma-interferon in aplastic anemia: inability to detect significant levels in sera or demonstrate hematopoietic suppressing activity. Blood 69:629, 1987

742. Hanada T, Yamamura H, Ehara T et al: Inhibitory activity of T cells on hematopoiesis and gamma-IFN production by T cells from peripheral blood in patients with aplastic anemia. Acta Haematol Jpn 51:571, 1988

743. Kuriyama K, Tomonaga M, Jinnai I et al: Reduced helper (OKT4+):suppressor (OKT8+) T ratios in aplastic anaemia: relation to immunosuppressive therapy. Br J Haematol 57:329, 1984

744. Lumm LG, Seigneuret MC, Doney KC, Storb R: In vitro immunoglobulin production, proliferation, and cell markers before and after antithymocyte globulin therapy in patients with aplastic anemia. AM J Hematol 26:1, 1987

745. López-Karpovitch X, Zarzosa ME, Cárdenas MR, Piedras J: Changes in peripheral blood mononuclear cell subpopulations during antithymocyte globulin therapy for severe aplastic anemia. Acta Haematol 81:176, 1989

746. Kunicka JE, Platsoucas CD: Defective helper function of purified T4 cells and excessive suppressor activity of purified T8 cells in patients with B-cell chronic lymphocytic leukemia: T4 suppressor effector cells are present in certain patients. Blood 71:1551, 1988

Acquired Aplastic Anemia

22

Edward C. Gordon-Smith

INTRODUCTION

Acquired aplastic anemia is characterized by the development of peripheral blood pancytopenia and a hypocellular bone marrow in which normal hematopoietic tissue is replaced to a greater or lesser extent by fatty marrow. Examination of the peripheral blood reveals a decrease in all granulocytic cells, neutrophils, eosinophils, and basophils, as well as monocytes, platelets, and reticulocytes, with a variable reduction in the lymphocyte count. Malignant or markedly dysplastic cells are not seen. In the bone marrow all hematopoietic cell lines are reduced, malignant cells are not present, and macrophages, lymphocytes, mast cells, and fibroblasts may be prominent, but the striking characteristic is the expansion of fatty marrow, which replaces the hematopoietic marrow without an increase in reticulin. Such appearances may be produced in a number of ways (Table 22-1).

This chapter is concerned with idiosyncratic acquired aplastic anemia. The diagnosis of the disease is mainly one of exclusion, made by eliminating the other causes of marrow hypocellularity listed in Table 22-1. Typically, the condition arises in a previously healthy person who has no evidence of malignant disease and who has not been exposed to cytotoxic drugs or irradiation.

Aplastic anemia was first described in 1888 by Paul Ehrlich,[1] who considered it a variant of pernicious anemia. Chauffard[2] first used the phrase "anémie pernicieuse aplastique," but, as this name implies, still considered it a variant of pernicious anemia. That drugs might be involved in the etiology of aplastic anemia was recognized early in the twentieth century, but proper clinical and epidemiologic studies only became possible when examination of the bone marrow, particularly by trephine biopsy, became a routine procedure. Much of the early literature is bedeviled by the inclusion of patients with pancytopenia under the title of aplastic anemia regardless of whether they had a hypocellular or proliferative bone marrow. The introduction of bone marrow transplantation for the treatment of aplastic anemia in 1969 by Thomas and colleagues led to the search for acceptable criteria for the diagnosis of acquired aplastic anemia and for criteria by which its severity might be judged.

INCIDENCE AND EPIDEMIOLOGY

The true incidence of acquired aplastic anemia is uncertain. An early attempt at defining the incidence in a known population at risk in Sweden put the incidence at 13 in 1 million/yr, which was an overestimate, since patients with pancytopenia due to other causes were included.[3] More recent surveys in Western Europe[4,5] and the United States[6] suggest that the incidence is on the order of 3–6 in 1 million population/yr. There is a suggestion of a biphasic age distribution, with a peak in the early twenties and a rising incidence again after the age of 65.[6] It is tempting to suppose that this may reflect differences in etiology, with viruses perhaps being a more common cause in the younger age group and exposure to drugs in the older. However, data are not firm enough to draw any definite conclusions. People of all ages may be affected.

The incidence in the Far East, particularly China and south-

east Asia, is higher than that in Western Europe and the United States, probably by three or four times.[7,8] This does not appear to reflect a genetic or racial predisposition, since people from these countries who settle in the West have the same incidence as the indigenous population. More likely the higher incidence is related to the greater prevalence of virus infections, particularly hepatitis, to the more widespread use of potentially toxic antibiotics, and perhaps to the wide use of industrial and agricultural chemicals without adequate protection.

In any idiosyncratic disease (i.e., a disease that afflicts a very small minority of people exposed to the same etiologic agents), genetic factors may play a role. In aplastic anemia the evidence for a genetic predisposition is weak, although cases of blood dyscrasias in twins have been reported, including one case of chloramphenicol-induced aplasia.[9] However, the nature of the blood dyscrasia in these families is not typical of idiosyncratic acquired aplastic anemia. Other possible genetic predispositions that have been studied are association with particular HLA types[10–13] and differences in drug metabolism.[14] Occasional clusters of aplastic anemia cases have been described in certain localities, but as with all cases of clustering of rare diseases, interpretation is difficult without adequate knowledge of pathogenesis.[15,16]

BIOLOGY AND ETIOLOGY

The presence of peripheral blood pancytopenia, together with a hypocellular marrow, would suggest that aplastic anemia is the consequence of failure of hematopoietic stem cells to proliferate and differentiate. Such a failure might result from intrinsic damage to hematopoietic stem cells, a failure of the bone marrow stroma to support hematopoiesis, or the presence of inhibitors of hematopoiesis in the environment of the bone marrow.[17] The question of the pathogenesis of aplastic anemia is addressed in greater detail in Chapter 21.

It is possible that several mechanisms operate at the same time to prevent the proliferation of hematopoietic cells and that in any individual different mechanisms may be more or less important. Evidence that there is damage to hematopoietic stem cells comes from the observation that committed progenitor cells, defined in short-term bone marrow culture systems, are markedly reduced in aplastic anemia[18] and the observation that about one-half the patients given bone marrow infusions from identical twins recover without additional immunosuppression or chemotherapy.[19] Abnormalities of bone marrow stroma have been observed by the use of short-term culture systems from patients with aplastic anemia[20]; however, in long-term bone marrow cultures the stroma appears to be normal and capable of supporting hematopoiesis from normal individuals. Stem cells from patients with aplastic anemia, however, proliferate poorly in long-term culture on normal stroma.[21,22] On the other hand, aplastic anemia patients who have an identical twin but who do not respond to simple infusion of syngeneic bone marrow may recover following treatment with cyclophosphamide or other cytotoxic therapy and further infusion of bone marrow.[19,23–25] The assumption is that such conditioning is immunosuppressive and that immune mechanisms play a part, at least, in the pathobiology of aplastic anemia.

Following allogeneic bone marrow transplantation, the stro-

Table 22-1. Classification of Aplastic Anemia

Pathogenesis	Etiology	Characteristics
Inevitable	Cytotoxic drugs Irradiation	Dose-dependent Predictable Onset and recovery dependent on the dose and nature of the etiologic agent
Idiosyncratic	Drugs Viruses Idiopathic	Rare: unpredictable in onset; prolonged course
Inherited	Fanconi anemia Dyskeratosis congenita Others	Inherited disorders with delayed but progressive aplasia
Immune	Infectious mononucleosis Associated with autoimmune disease	Rare; usually self-limited; circulating inhibitors of hematopoiesis may be detected
Industrial	Benzene	Dose-dependent, proliferative pancytopenia with rare aplasia
Malignant	Acute lymphocytic leukemia Acute myeloid leukemia Myelodysplastic aplastic aplasia	Mainly but not exclusively in children; spontaneous or steroid-induced remission followed by later appearance of leukemia

mal cells, with the exception of macrophages, remain of recipient origin,[26] which suggests that no major stromal defect is present in aplastic anemia patients. Erythropoietin levels are elevated in these patients,[27] and other hematopoietic growth factors are probably also increased.[28,29] It has been suggested that inhibitors of hematopoiesis (e.g., interferon[30]) are increased in aplastic anemia (although this has not been confirmed[31]) and that other growth factors (e.g., interleukin-1 [IL-1] derived from monocytes) are reduced.[32] It seems most likely that intrinsic damage to hematopoietic stem cells indeed occurs but that this damage either is reversible or does not affect all hematopoietic stem cells.

Autologous recovery from aplastic anemia is slow and is characterized by hematopoietic proliferative abnormalities.[33,34] Thrombocytopenia may persist for months or even years after the granulocyte count and hemoglobin return to normal. Even when the granulocyte count does return to normal, it is possible to demonstrate relative deficiencies of committed precursor cells (colony-forming unit-granulocyte/macrophage [CFU-GM]) persisting for many years.[34] Erythropoiesis may remain macrocytic for several years after recovery. These abnormalities in hematopoiesis during recovery are probably the basis for the incidence of relapse and the development of later clonal disorders in patients who achieve remission.[35,36]

The etiology of aplastic anemia is discussed in detail in Chapter 21.

CLINICAL MANIFESTATIONS

The manifestations of acquired aplastic anemia are basically due to deficiency of the cellular products of hematopoiesis. Symptoms and signs at presentation are related directly to the effects of the peripheral blood pancytopenia; there are no specific clinical features, the spleen and liver are not enlarged, and there is no lymphadenopathy or bone pain. The platelet count is depressed early in the course of the disease in most cases, and increased bruising, gum bleeding, buccal hemorrhage, and visual disturbance due to retinal hemorrhages may be presenting features. The hemoglobin falls relatively gradually so that patients adapt to the anemia quite well, but fatigue and apparent shortness of breath on exercise may also be presenting features. The neutrophil and monocyte counts may fall to very low levels, but severe infection is a less common presentation than bleeding or fatigue, at least in Western countries. As with other neutropenic patients, ulcers on the tongue or in the mouth may occur, as may infections of the skin or air sinuses. Severe infection as the presenting feature of aplastic anemia, with high fever and malaise, particularly in a young person, should raise the possibility of an underlying acute leukemia.[37] Presentation with infection and a severely depressed neutrophil count carries a poor prognosis.[38]

In most aplastic anemia patients the hemoglobin, white blood cell count, and platelet count are all low at presentation, but in occasional patients aplasia may develop after a prolonged period during which only one cell line has been deficient. The best documentation of these uncommon presentations is found in those patients who have amegakaryocytic thrombocytopenia that subsequently progresses to aplastic anemia.[39] Occasionally patients may have isolated neutropenia for months or years, with subsequent failure of all hematopoietic lineages, and even more rarely a refractory anemia may progress to true aplastic anemia (personal observation).

Aplastic anemia during pregnancy is an uncommon but well-documented event.[40,41] The rarity of the anemia and the commonness of pregnancy make it difficult to be certain that there is a causal relationship. Apart from cases that present during pregnancy, patients may relapse at this time.[41] Remission of the aplastic anemia follows delivery or termination of pregnancy in about one-third of patients.[41] These clinical observations make a direct association between pregnancy and aplastic anemia highly likely, but the mechanism remains unknown. One may speculate that the immunologic changes that occur during pregnancy, hormonal changes, and even the stress of pregnancy on a subclinically damaged marrow may each play a part, but no good data exist to support any of these hypotheses. Whatever the mechanism, patients who have previously suffered from aplastic anemia, whether or not their peripheral blood counts show complete remission, should be cautioned about the risks of pregnancy. Management of the disease during pregnancy will depend on the stage at which the pancytopenia develops and the degree of difficulty in supporting the mother's blood count throughout gestation.[42] It is essential to monitor the growth and development of the fetus with great care in those cases in which the pregnancy is allowed to continue with blood product support. The baby should be delivered electively with maximum support available, in most instances by cesarean section. The blood count of the baby is not affected by the aplastic anemia of the mother.

LABORATORY EVALUATIONS

The diagnosis of acquired aplastic anemia depends entirely on the laboratory evaluations, which are designed to demonstrate the diagnosis and to exclude other disorders that may present in a similar way. A second purpose of the evaluation is to determine the severity of the disease at any particular time.

Peripheral Blood

The peripheral blood count shows pancytopenia, although occasionally the lymphocyte count is preserved to such an extent that the total leukocyte count is within the normal range.

The differential count shows a decrease in neutrophils, monocytes, and eosinophils, with a variable decrease in lymphocytes. The morphology of the cells shows nonspecific variations from normal. The red blood cells show some degree of anisocytosis, and the mean cell volume may be increased. A degree of macrocytosis indicates some residual underlying erythropoiesis and is perhaps associated with a better prognosis.[43] Neutrophils, although reduced in number, are normal in morphology apart from a tendency to increased granulation (the so-called toxic granulation of neutropenia). In the early stages of aplastic anemia, circulating myelocytes may be seen, and their occasional presence does not exclude the diagnosis. Platelets are reduced in number and tend to be small. Careful examination of the peripheral blood is required to exclude the presence of blasts or evidence of dysplastic myelopoiesis. The morphology of the lymphocyte is generally normal, but sometimes there are reactive changes in the population, which can lead to confusion in the differential diagnosis from malignant disorders associated with marrow hypocellularity.

Bone Marrow Examination

Both bone marrow aspirate and trephine marrow biopsy are required for the diagnosis and evaluation of a patient with aplastic anemia. Aspiration of aplastic bone marrow is usually easy, and fragments are readily obtained. The fragments are typically hypocellular, with prominent fat spaces within the fine stromal structure. The cell trails have reduced cellularity, with a variable amount of residual hematopoietic cells present. Erythroid precursors commonly show quite marked degrees of dyserythropoiesis, but the granulocyte precursors that remain are usually normal. Megakaryocytes characteristically are reduced or absent; if seen, they are normal in appearance and do not possess the micromegakaryocytic features associated with the myelodysplastic syndrome. Macrophages may be particularly prominent and may show evidence of accumulation of iron and even phagocytosis of cellular debris.

The failure of hematopoiesis in aplastic anemia may not be total, and patches of active hematopoiesis may remain.[44,45] The bone marrow aspirate may not, under these circumstances, show any of the features already described but may be cellular or even hypercellular in patients with severe pancytopenia due to aplasia. Even in these hypercellular aspirates megakaryocytes are reduced. It may be necessary to repeat the bone marrow aspirate from a different site in order to document hypocellularity. Imaging techniques such as radioisotope scanning with [52]Fe or magnetic resonance imaging may also be used to delineate cellular and fatty areas of marrow.

A bone marrow trephine biopsy is essential to assess the overall cellularity of the bone marrow and to exclude proliferative dysplasias. Typically, the normal hematopoietic marrow is replaced by fat spaces, with lymphocytes, plasma cells, and macrophages remaining in the normal distribution. Islands of apparently normal hematopoietic tissue may be seen, although it is rare to have an adequate trephine biopsy that does not show some evidence of marrow failure in part of the specimen. Reticulin is not increased. The pattern of nonhematopoietic cells was formerly thought to relate to response to immunosuppressive therapy, particularly if follicles of lymphoid cells were seen,[46] but later studies have not confirmed these predictions.[47] Examples of a bone marrow aspirate and a trephine biopsy from aplastic anemia patients are shown in Figure 22-1.

Additional Hematologic Tests

The acidified serum lysis test (Ham test) and sucrose-lysis test should be carried out on all patients at presentation. A positive Ham test indicates the possibility of paroxysmal nocturnal hemoglobinuria (PNH) as a major component in the pancytopenia. A small population of PNH cells may be detected for 10–20% of patients with aplastic anemia during the course of the disease, although most commonly during partial remission.[48] A positive Ham test together with the presence of hemosiderin in the urine would shift the diagnosis from aplastic anemia to PNH. Serum vitamin B_{12} and folate levels, together with red cell folate levels, should also be measured to exclude the rare possibility that vitamin deficiency has produced a hypoplastic state. PNH clones may also be detected using fluorescence-labeled antibodies directed against phosphatidylinositol glycan-anchored proteins, which are deficient in PNH cells.

Biochemical Investigations

No specific biochemical abnormalities are associated with aplastic anemia. Liver function tests are helpful in detecting those patients who have an antecedent hepatitis. Abnormal liver function tests or renal function may modify subsequent treatment.

Immunologic Investigations

It is helpful to genotype the blood group antigens, if possible at presentation, before the patient has been transfused. HLA typing should also be carried out as soon as the diagnosis becomes apparent, not least because there may be difficulties in establishing the HLA types in severely leucopenic patients.

Viral Studies

The presence or absence of antibodies to cytomegalovirus (CMV) in the serum should be determined at presentation. Patients who have no evidence of previous CMV infection should receive CMV-negative blood products until the possibility of bone marrow transplantation has been excluded. Evidence of recent infection with hepatitis A, B, and C should be established. It may be of interest to screen for a recent parvovirus infection.[49]

Radiologic Investigations

A chest radiograph is useful at presentation to exclude a potential infection and for comparison with subsequent films if a chest infection does develop. Sinus infections may be a problem during the course of aplastic anemia, and radiologic evaluation at presentation may be helpful for later comparisons. In younger patients radiographs of the forearms and hands may be helpful. The features of Fanconi anemia may be obvious from clinical examination but not always, and changes in radiologic appearances, particularly of the thumbs (Fig. 22-2), may strengthen the suspicion that the patient has congenital aplastic anemia. Another congenital syndrome is the association of radioulnar fusion with an inherited late-onset aplastic anemia.[50] Typical appearances of the fusion are shown in Figure 22-3. Ultrasound examination of the abdomen may be helpful in children and younger adults. Anatomically displaced or abnormal kidneys raise the possibility of Fanconi anemia, while a bulky spleen, particularly in a child, raises the possibility of a malignant hematopoietic disorder as a cause of the pancytopenia.

Cytogenetic Investigations

Cytogenetic investigations are important to exclude Fanconi anemia[51] and preleukemic myelodysplastic syndromes.[52] The definitive test for Fanconi anemia, increased chromosome fra-

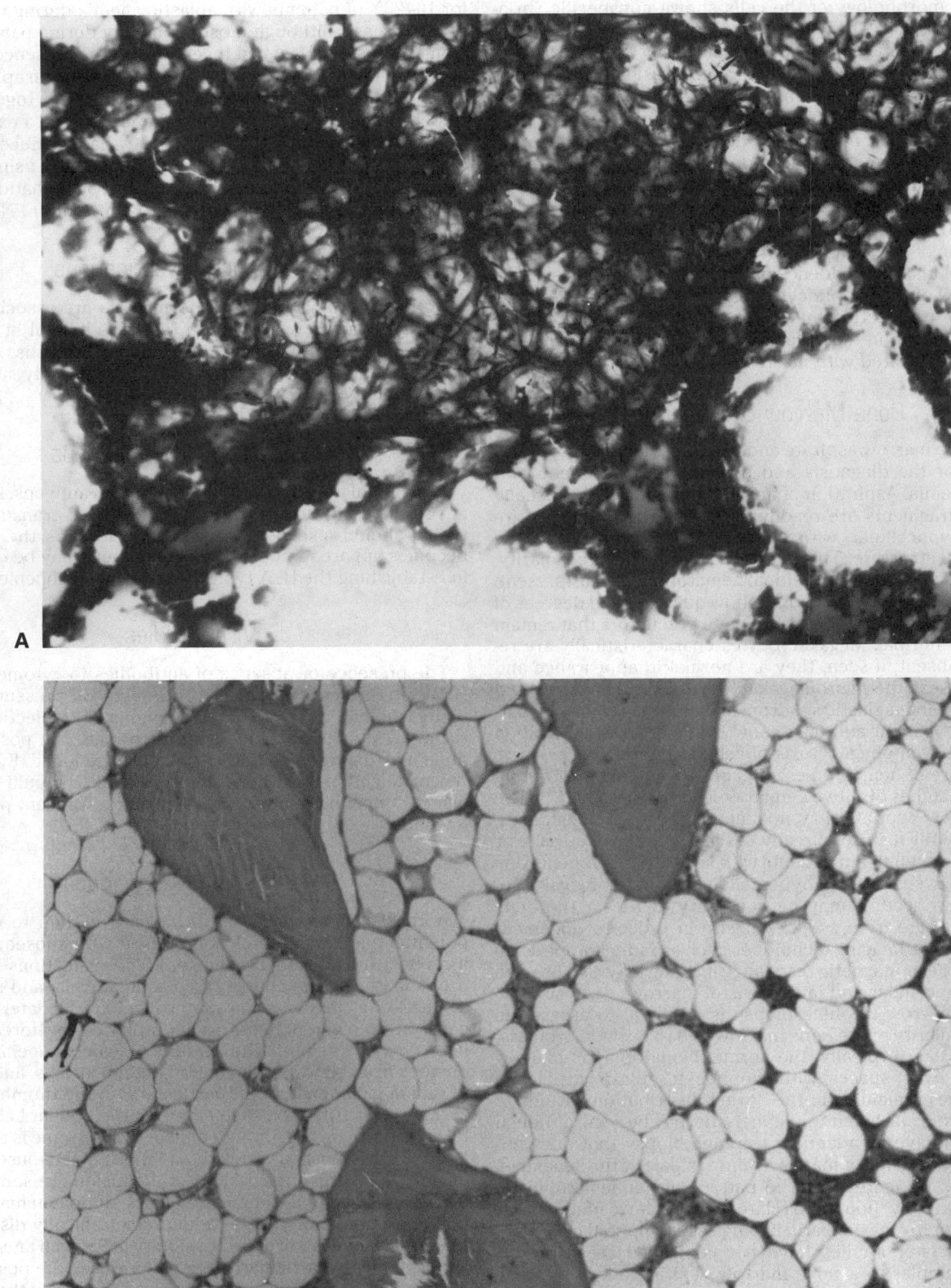

Fig. 22-1. (A) A fragment of tissue obtained by bone marrow aspiration in aplastic anemia showing typical lacy appearance of the hypocellular fragment. (× 80.) **(B)** Bone marrow trephine biopsy from a patient with aplastic anemia showing replacement of normal hematopoietic tissue by fat cells. (× 40.)

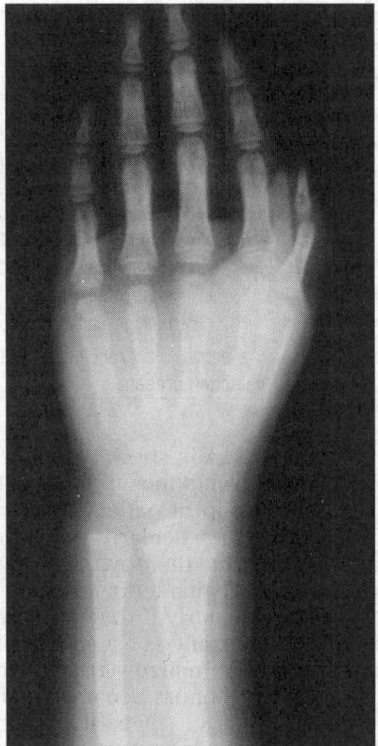

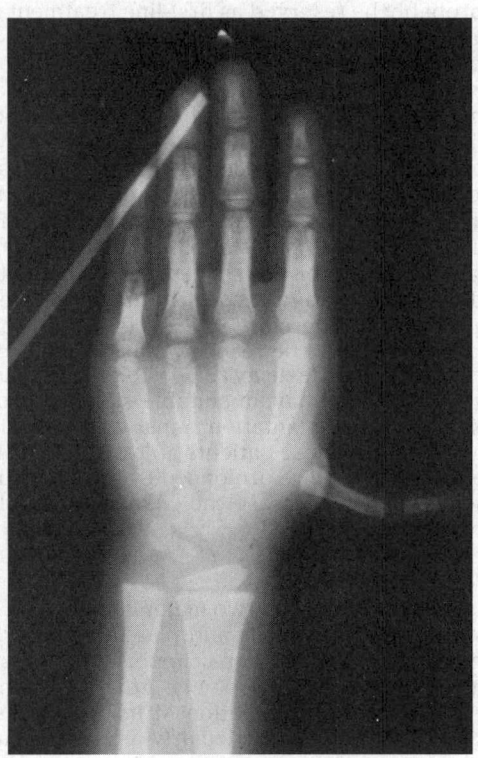

Fig. 22-2. Radiographs of the **(A)** left wrist and hand and **(B)** right wrist and hand of a child with Fanconi anemia. Note the abnormalities of the thumbs and that in this patient these abnormalities are not symmetric.

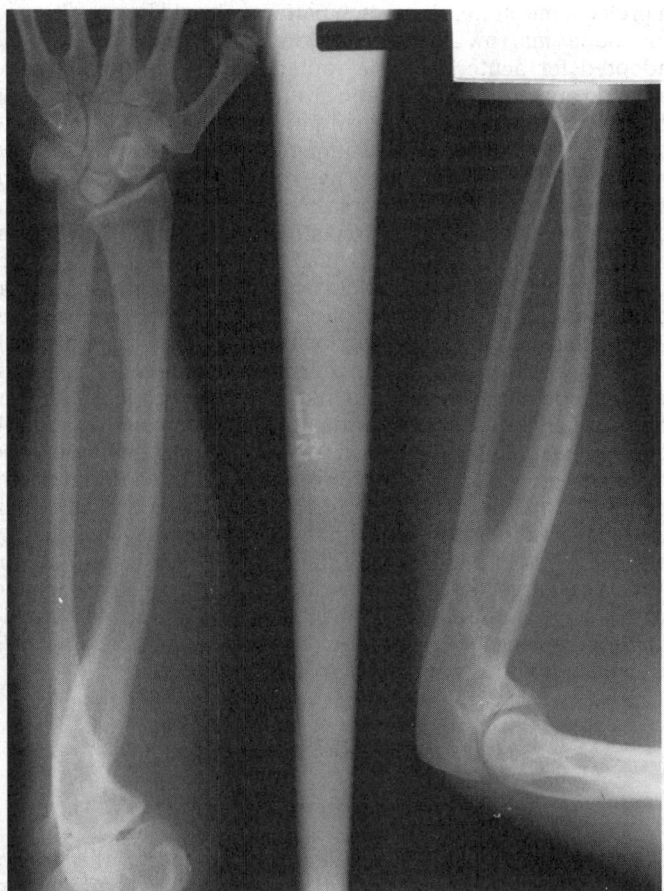

Fig. 22-3. Radiograph of the radius and ulna from a patient with late-onset bone marrow failure associated with proximal fusion of the radius and ulna. (Courtesy of Dr. I. Dokal, Royal Postgraduate Medical School, London.)

gility in the presence and absence of stress from DNA cross-linking agents,[53] is carried out on peripheral blood lymphocytes. A search for a chromosomal rearrangement, which may demonstrate the presence of a preleukemic state, is carried out on hematopoietic cells obtained from the bone marrow.

DIFFERENTIAL DIAGNOSIS

The differential diagnosis of acquired aplastic anemia includes inherited aplastic anemia (Fanconi anemia), hypoplastic leukemia, and hypoplastic myelodysplastic syndrome. Fanconi anemia should be excluded in all children and young adults presenting with aplastic anemia, even when no somatic features to suggest the disease are present. Peripheral blood lymphocytes should be examined for the presence of nonspecific chromosomal breaks and the sensitivity of chromosomes to diepoxybutane or mytomycin C. In aplastic anemia the chromosome stability is normal. Acute leukemia presenting as aplastic anemia may be indistinguishable from the nonmalignant condition in the early stages, but careful examination of the peripheral blood and bone marrow aspirate and trephine biopsy may raise the suspicion of a leukemia. Such a presentation is more common in childhood, particularly with acute lymphocytic leukemia.[37] An apparent spontaneous or steroid-induced remission frequently occurs within 3–6 weeks of presentation.[54] Hypocellular acute leukemia frequently presents following an obvious infection or febrile episode; the platelet count is frequently better preserved than in acquired aplastic anemia, and the spleen may be enlarged, which is not a characteristic of acquired aplastic anemia.[37] Hypoplastic myelodysplastic syndrome is difficult to distinguish from acquired aplastic anemia, and there seems to be considerable overlap in that dyshematopoietic changes, particularly in the erythroid series, are common in aplastic anemia.[55–57] It is mainly important to distinguish between these two disorders when there is a cytogenetic abnormality in hematopoietic bone marrow,[52] which suggests a preleukemic state, since such patients should be conditioned for bone marrow transplantation by using the regimens adopted for acute leukemia rather than those for acquired aplastic anemia.[58] Cytogenetic studies on hematopoietic bone marrow should therefore be attempted, even though the small number of cells that can be induced into metaphase may be insufficient to produce conclusive results. The above disorders are characterized by a hypoplastic marrow and pancytopenia and are frequently difficult to distinguish from acquired aplastic anemia. Other conditions also may be confused with acquired aplastic anemia, particularly when there is a peripheral blood pancytopenia with few circulating abnormal cells associated with a marrow aspiration, resulting in a dry tap. Hairy cell leukemia appears to be one of the most common misdiagnoses, often producing a bloody marrow tap. Hairy cell leukemia can occasionally be associated with a trephine biopsy that superficially appears hypocellular but in which normal hematopoietic tissue is replaced by amorphous eosinophilic material partly composed of the cytoplasm of the hairy cells and in which there is an increase in reticulin. Confusion in diagnosis nearly always arises in patients with hairy cell leukemia who do not have an enlarged spleen. Anorexia nervosa may be associated with pancytopenia and a hypocellular marrow, but eosinophilic material replaces the hematopoietic marrow, and the diagnosis is usually obvious on clinical grounds.

MANAGEMENT

General Considerations

Management may be considered in two parts, the first of which, replacement therapy with blood products and support for the patient, is provided while the second phase of definitive treatment is being instituted. The two main therapeutic options are immunosuppressive therapy and bone marrow transplantation. Which of these options offers the best hope of recovery depends on a number of factors, including the age of the patient, the severity of the disease, and the availability of a suitable donor. Treatment strategy needs to be determined early in the disease, particularly the decision about whether the patient should proceed to bone marrow transplantation. It is urgent to confirm early that the condition is uncomplicated acquired aplastic anemia and not one of the several disorders that may superficially resemble aplastic anemia, as well as to assess marrow damage. The main importance of the correct diagnosis and assessment of disease severity lies in the decision of whether to proceed with bone marrow transplantation, since acquired aplastic anemia requires conditioning that differs from that for the other disorders, and immunosuppressive therapy is less effective in severe or very severe disorders. While it is important to decide the etiology of the disease in individual patients so that they may avoid contact with the supposed agent, the outcome of treatment depends not on etiology but only on disease severity.[59]

Acquired aplastic anemia may remit spontaneously. There have been several attempts to define which patients are most likely to recover and which are likely to die early in the course of the disease.[44,59–62] The most widely used classification is that of Camitta and colleagues,[63] who divided patients into those with severe aplastic anemia (SAA) and those with nonsevere aplastic anemia (NSAA) on the basis of peripheral blood counts and bone marrow appearance and showed that patients with SAA had a <20% chance of surviving for 1 year if managed only with support with or without androgens.[63] These observations were made before the introduction of immunosuppressive therapy with antilymphocyte globulin (ALG),[64,65] which has improved the prognosis for patients with SAA, although their long-term (5-year) survival rate is still only about

Table 22-2. Grading of Severity of Aplastic Anemia

Designation	Criteria

Severe aplastic anemia[59]	Peripheral blood: two of three values
	  Granulocytes $<0.5 \times 10^9$/L
	  Platelets $<20 \times 10^9$/L
	  Reticulocytes <1% (corrected for hematocrit)
	Bone marrow trephine
	  Markedly hypocellular, <25% cellularity
	  Moderately hypocellular, 25–50% normal cellularity with <30% of remaining cells hematopoietic

Very severe aplastic anemia[62]	As above, but granulocytes $<0.2 \times 10^9$/L Infection present

30–40%.[44] The definition of SAA is shown in Table 22-2. More recent analysis of response to immunosuppressive therapy has suggested that there is a group of patients with very severe aplastic anemia who have a particularly poor chance of responding to immunosuppressive therapy.[66] These are patients within the SAA group who have markedly reduced granulocyte counts ($<0.2 \times 10^9$/L), particularly if they are infected at the time of assessment. The importance of such classification will become more evident as bone marrow transplantation from matched unrelated volunteer donors becomes more practical. The prognosis is related to age, since HLA-matched sibling transplants are less effective than immunosuppression in patients >50 years old, and at present nonsibling transplants would probably be reserved as first-line treatment for patients <25 years of age.[66]

The possibility of bone marrow transplantation means that certain other investigations need to be carried out at presentation. The presence or absence of anti-CMV antibodies should be established at once, and if these are absent, CMV-negative blood products should be used until such time as a decision on bone marrow transplantation is reached.[67] The HLA type of the patient should be determined as soon as possible and the availability of HLA-matched siblings ascertained. Bone marrow transplantation has a higher success rate in patients who have not had transfusions and those who have received <10 U of blood products.[68] Therefore the decision on bone marrow transplantation should be reached quickly and the procedure carried out with as little delay as possible. These measures will identify patients who have a suitable sibling donor who may be referred for transplantation; most patients will not have such an option. For these patients aplastic anemia is a chronic disorder that will require prolonged transfusion support, with therapy designed to increase the chances of autologous marrow recovery.

Supportive Measures

Supportive care falls into two major categories, replacement therapy with red blood cells and platelets and prevention or treatment of infection. Of equal importance is psychological support for the patient and family. Aplastic anemia is a rare disease, so a careful explanation of its nature and potential seriousness is required, particularly as the patient feels well for much of the time and may resent the restrictions that the pancytopenia puts on normal activity. The chronic nature and slow response to therapy, but also the ultimate possibility of recovery, should be stressed early in the disease. The morale of the patient, family, and staff may sag when recovery has not occurred at 6 months or even 1 year, but the temptation to give up must be resisted.

Red Cell Transfusion

Red cell transfusions should be given as required. Although keeping the patient anemic, thereby promoting erythropoietic drive, offers no benefit in terms of recovery, red cell transfusions should be used sparingly, particularly in the early stages of aplastic anemia while decisions about bone marrow transplantation are being made. Red cell transfusions should also be kept to a minimum to decrease the risk of transmission of hepatitis C, which may halt or reverse recovery. CMV-negative blood should be used for CMV-negative recipients, particularly those who will receive transplants.[69] Sensitization to HLA antigens can be avoided by giving white cell-depleted blood, which may be obtained by transfusing through white cell-depleting filters, which decrease the white cell count by two or more orders of magnitude.[70-74]

Transfusion of red cells may lead to minor subclinical reactions, perhaps involving the complement system, which in turn will lead to a lowering of the platelet count. In the severely thrombocytopenic patient (platelet count $<20 \times 10^9/L$), it is advisable to give platelets at the end of the red cell transfusion to reduce the risk of cerebral hemorrhage. Despite the chronic nature of the disorder, iron overload from recurrent red cell transfusions is rarely a problem in patients with aplastic anemia, since it may take ≥ 2 years to accumulate sufficient iron to produce clinical damage. Desferrioxamine may be given with the transfusions but is unnecessary as a continuing subcutaneous treatment, particularly in view of the risk of hemorrhage or local infection from such injections.

Platelet Transfusion

Platelet transfusions are an essential part of management. There is debate as to whether they should be given only in response to bleeding or whether they should be used prophylactically.[75,76] In practice this becomes more of a theoretical argument than a practical decision. When platelets are given in response to bleeding manifestations, it soon becomes apparent whether the patient is going to require regular platelet transfusions. There is no way of telling in an individual patient whether a fatal hemorrhage is likely to occur. Fatal hemorrhage, usually cerebral, is more common in patients who have $<10 \times 10^9/L$ platelets, extensive retinal hemorrhages, buccal hemorrhage, or rapidly spreading purpura, but may also be the first major bleed in patients who have none of these conditions. The advantage of prophylactic administration of platelets two or three times a week is partly logistic and partly due to the opportunity to assess the patient at regular intervals. Platelet transfusions, however, lead to sensitization of the patient, with subsequent failure of random donor platelets to produce an increment in the platelet count.[75,76] Sensitization is mainly due to HLA antigens, but in some cases specific platelet antigen can cause development of antibodies. About 40% of patients will become sensitized if given random donor platelets, but sensitization may be reduced if white cell-depleted platelets are given.[71] Filters for platelet transfusion are available, which will reduce the white cell contamination by ≥ 3 orders of magnitude. Use of such filters would seem advisable in order to avoid sensitization and also to prevent possible transmission of CMV.[77-79] If white cell-depleted platelets are used, they should be given from the beginning of treatment and used throughout; of course, white cell-depleted red cell transfusions should also be used. Once sensitization to HLA antigens has occurred, HLA-matched platelets should be used.[75]

Infection Prevention

The risk of systemic or local infection is determined by the patient's granulocyte and monocyte counts.[80,81] Patients with granulocyte counts $>0.5 \times 10^9/L$ have a low risk and patients with counts $<0.2 \times 10^9/L$ have a high risk of infection, whereas those with intermediate counts have a moderate risk; the risk level should be determined on an individual basis, as some patients have repeated infections and some have none.[82] Pa-

tients with a high risk of infection need to be managed in a sterile or clean environment when in the hospital and should receive nonabsorbable antifungal and antibacterial agents, food of low bacterial content, scrupulous mouth care, and regular bacteriologic surveillance.[83-85] A suitable regimen in the hospital consists of chlorhexadine mouth washes, amphotericin lozenges, amphotericin or nystatin suspension to prevent *Candida* overgrowth in the esophagus, and nystatin tablets to prevent overgrowth in the gastrointestinal tract. Nonabsorbable antibiotics designed to remove potential aerobic pathogens may be given at the same time.[83,84] Such precautions are advisable for all patients while they are receiving immunosuppressive therapy.

Less obvious is the advice one should give to outpatients. Mouth care is particularly important, as local infection may promote gingival bleeding, and continuation of antiseptic mouth washes and amphotericin lozenges is advisable if the patient will comply. Patients with very low granulocyte counts should be encouraged to continue with nonabsorbable antibiotics and freshly cooked food, avoiding salads, fruits, and other foods that may be contaminated with bacteria or fungal pathogens.

Difficulties may also arise over how to deal with pet animals. While transmission of some infections is theoretically possible, such events seem to be exceedingly rare, and it is not necessary to ban pets completely. Sensible advice is to avoid intimate contact with such animals. Children with a granulocyte count $<0.2 \times 10^9/L$ should be kept away from school, but family flora are unlikely to be a major problem. Patients with less severe disease may be encouraged to lead a more normal life but should be warned about the dangers related to trauma and thrombocytopenia.

Therapy for Infection

As with all severely neutropenic patients, fever suggesting infection in acquired aplastic anemia patients requires treatment urgently before results of bacteriologic investigations are available.[86] Gram-positive infections, particularly with *Staphylococcus epidermidis,* are more common than gram-negative infections in patients who have indwelling central venous catheters,[87] but it is the gram-negative infections that kill the patient rapidly. Most "blind" antibiotic regimen are thus designed to cover gram-negative infection while awaiting the result of microbiologic cultures.[85,88,89] The most commonly employed regimens include a synergistic combination of antibiotics such as an aminoglycoside and a β-lactam penicillin. If the fever fails to resolve in 48 hours, gram-positive antibiotic coverage may be introduced, even in the absence of microbiologic confirmation. Difficulty arises over how long to continue antibiotic therapy once the fever or documented infection has cleared. In patients with severe neutropenia it is unlikely that infection will be eradicated even with bactericidal antibiotics. Such patients may eventually require prolonged intravenous antibiotic therapy. Initially, however, it is reasonable to stop antibiotics after 5 fever-free days.

If the fever persists or returns with failure to respond to antibiotic administration, antifungal agents may be needed, although the use of such agents, particularly amphotericin, is problematic. *Candida* spp. and *Aspergillus* are the two major fungal pathogens. Each may be difficult to detect with microbiologic methods, although *Candida* may be suspected if it is cultured from three or more superficial sites. Fungal infections are more common in the neutropenic patient who has received prolonged antibiotic therapy, but this is by no means universal, and such infections may occur early in the disease. Systemic candidiasis may lead to abscess formation in the liver, which gives a characteristic pattern on ultrasound examination.[90]

Documented fungal infection is unlikely to be eradicated

until such time as the granulocyte and monocyte counts return to normal.

Granulocyte Transfusion

Early enthusiasm for granulocyte transfusions in the febrile neutropenic patient has diminished considerably, and the benefit of such transfusions is debated.[91,92] There is no clear role for prophylactic granulocyte transfusion.[93] There may be a role for granulocyte transfusions in the management of localized infective lesions, but the prolonged nature of the neutropenia in aplastic anemia makes any benefits marginal.

Colony-Stimulating Factor-Granulocyte and -Granulocyte/ Macrophage

Since the introduction of recombinant human colony-stimulating factor-granulocyte (CSF-G)[94] and colony-stimulating factor-granulocyte/macrophage (CSF-GM),[95,96] much interest has arisen in the potential of these growth factors to stimulate granulocyte and macrophage production and activation in patients with neutropenia, including those with aplastic anemia.[97,98] In aplastic anemia, CSF-GM given either intravenously or subcutaneously will increase the granulocyte and monocyte counts in those patients who have some granulopoietic reserve, as demonstrated by the presence of circulating neutrophils $>0.4 \times 10^9/L$.[99] Neutrophils, eosinophils, and monocytes all increase, and the bone marrow becomes cellular with an increase in granulopoiesis, but CFU-GM does not increase. The increase in granulocyte count persists for as long as CSF-GM is given, and the count then returns to the baseline. Antibodies have been described that developed against recombinant human CSF-GM prepared from *Escherichia coli,* a preparation that leads to nonglycosylated growth factor.[100] Patients who have severe impairment of hematopoiesis with circulating granulocytes $<0.2 \times 10^9/L$ show no or modest changes in granulocyte levels following treatment with CSF-GM.[99] CSF-GM not only increases the production of granulocytes but also activates circulating and tissue granulocytes and macrophages[101] and inhibits their spontaneous migration.[102] It is not yet clear whether the increase in circulating granulocytes achieved with CSF-GM is of benefit in the management of infections in neutropenic patients, although early indications suggest that it may be. CSF-G given intravenously also raised the granulocyte count in a proportion of children with aplastic anemia, and increasing the dose produced a response in some of the nonresponders to a lower dose.[103] Another hematopoietic growth factor, IL-3, has also been tried in aplastic anemia. Treatment with IL-3 increased leukocyte counts in most patients, but few patients responded with increases in platelet and reticulocyte counts.[104]

Medical Management

In the absence of detailed knowledge of the pathogenesis of acquired aplastic anemia, treatment remains somewhat empirical and, apart from bone marrow transplantation, rests on the premises that immunosuppressive therapy may allow the bone marrow to recover function and that immunosuppression may be coupled to attempts to stimulate residual hematopoiesis. The two most widely used treatments have been anabolic steroids and derivatives to stimulate hematopoiesis and ALG or antithymocyte globulin (ATG) for immunosuppression. Cyclosporine has now been added to the list of effective immunosuppressive agents.

Antilymphocyte Globulin

ALG was first introduced in 1970 as treatment for acquired aplastic anemia by Mathé and colleagues[105] in Paris. They used a preparation of crude serum from a horse that had been immunized with peripheral blood lymphocytes from humans. The results of this therapeutic trial were inconclusive. However, Speck[106] from Basel pursued the use of ALG, using rabbits with benzene-induced aplastic anemia as an experimental model. He demonstrated that ALG in combination with anabolic steroids and infusion of haploidentical bone marrow would lead to a recovery in a significant proportion of rabbits. Further clinical trials in 1977, using a preparation of ALG from a horse immunized with human thoracic duct lymphocytes or lymphocytes from the thymus removed at operation, or both, led to recovery from aplastic anemia in a significant proportion of patients, even those with SAA.[65] These early uncontrolled clinical trials also suggested that it was unnecessary to give haploidentical marrow and that the role of anabolic steroids was unclear. The suggestion that ALG was effective in aplastic anemia was eventually confirmed by controlled clinical trials in the United States.[107] Although there was much variation in the reported results of ALG treatment, with survival figures ranging from 35% to 76%,[108,109] the randomized studies confirmed that ALG was more effective than supportive care alone in the treatment of SAA and that ALG, haploidentical bone marrow, and androgens given together were more effective than androgens alone.[110]

Information derived from the European Bone Marrow Transplant Group (EBMTG) registry and a variety of published reports on the use of ALG defines more clearly which patients are likely to benefit from its use. Disease severity is clearly related to response[43]—patients with SAA have about a 35% recovery rate, whereas those with less severe disease have about 65% long-term survival. A subgroup with a particularly poor prognosis is comprised of patients with very severe aplastic anemia, who have $<0.2 \times 10^9/L$ neutrophils, particularly in conjunction with infection at presentation.[38] Age also influences the outcome with ALG.[111] Patients with similar disease severity do as well, if not better, with immunosuppressive therapy, at least in terms of survival, as with bone marrow transplantation if they are >25 years old,[38,109] with the exception of the very severe aplastic anemia group. Children <6 years old respond poorly to treatment with ALG,[38,43,109] and this difference probably extends up to the age of 16, although the age effect is not statistically significant for those >6 years old.[111]

ALG is a biologic product prepared by a number of commercial laboratories and some university- or transfusion-based departments. The immunogen may consist of thoracic duct lymphocytes, lymphocytes extracted from the thymus removed during cardiothoracic surgery, or lymphoblastoid cell lines. Antibodies are raised either in horses or rabbits, and the resulting immunoglobulins are purified and absorbed with a variety of human tissues, including red blood cells and human placenta. When thoracic duct- or thymus-derived lymphocytes are used as the immunogen, the product may be called ATG, but there seems little evidence for a distinction between ALG and ATG. The product may be standardized by a variety of tests, including cytotoxicity assay and preservation of skin grafts in monkeys, but the tests do not correlate well in the same sample and may show wide variation between batches. It is not clear whether differences in results with ALG represent differences in effectiveness of particular batches or in the different way in which ALG is prepared commercially.[112,113] No trial has been conducted that demonstrates ALG to be more effective than horse immunoglobulin alone. The mode of action of ALG is also unclear[114]: while it is presumed to be immunosuppressive and leads to a decrease in lymphocyte count,[115,116] it also has possible immunostimulatory effects, particularly in relationship to the production of lymphokines,[117] and may also act on the surface receptors of hematopoietic progenitor cells, directly stimulating these cells[118,119] or making them more responsive to hematopoietic growth factors.[120]

The dose of ALG varies according to the method of preparation; the manufacturers often recommend a dosage based on the number of vials to be used rather than a weight-for-weight dose. ALG is diluted in 0.9% normal saline and is infused through a central venous catheter to avoid sclerosis of peripheral veins. The duration of infusion varies somewhat, but if the drug is given slowly over 18 hours, most of the severe reactions are avoided. A test dose of 10 mg diluted in 100 ml of saline and given intravenously should be used before starting treatment to exclude the possibility of anaphylactic reactions to animal proteins. Subcutaneous testing is not helpful, because a potent ALG will almost always provoke a skin reaction if given in this way. In Europe ALG is given mainly for 5 days. Other schedules have varied from 8 to 28 days, but there is no indication that a more prolonged course influences the outcome.

Adverse effects of ALG may be immediate or delayed.[114] All preparations cause lymphopenia, and some preparations have produced a neutropenia, although this is a relatively rare occurrence. Some antiplatelet activity is present in most preparations, and platelets should be given daily after the infusion of ALG. Fevers and rigors may occur, usually during the first or second day of administration, together with a variety of rashes, including urticaria. These effects are usually reversed by concomitant administration of hydrocortisone and antihistamines. More serious side effects include hypertension and fluid retention, which in susceptible individuals may lead to seizures. Hypotension has also been reported. Serum sickness is a late manifestation of treatment, occurring 7–13 days after beginning ALG; it is caused by circulating immune complexes involving the horse or rabbit protein and antibodies. Fever, joint pains, and rashes are the most common manifestations.[121] In experimental serum sickness, glomerulonephritis and proteinuria may occur, but this is rare in the therapeutic situation. Serum sickness occurs in about 75% of patients given ALG unless corticosteroids are given prophylactically. The dose of methylprednisone used to suppress serum sickness should be kept as low as possible, certainly <2 mg/kg/day, to reduce or avoid the risk of avascular necrosis of the hip.[122] Analysis of patients who developed serum sickness compared with those who did not failed to show any correlation with recovery.[121,123] Throughout the course of treatment patients are at greater risk of infection, owing to the immunosuppression caused by both the ALG and the corticosteroids required to manage the side effects. Patients should be in isolation throughout the therapy.

Response to ALG therapy is slow, and evidence of recovery in those patients who respond occurs 6–12 weeks after treatment. Later responses may be seen, but it is difficult to know whether these are related to the ALG. There are no definitive tests to show which patients will recover, but an early sign of improvement is an increase in the mean cell volume of the red cells.[43] For patients who do not respond to the first course of ALG, a second course using an alternative animal source may be tried after 4 months; response to the second course is achieved in about one-third of patients.[124]

High-Dose Methylprednisolone

High-dose methylprednisolone given intravenously by bolus injection has been tried as an alternative form of immunosuppressive treatment for aplastic anemia.[125] The dose used was 20 mg/kg/day initially, with a sliding scale over a period of 1 month. In the relatively small trials using this form of therapy, response rates seem to be comparable with those achieved using ALG.[126] Toxicity is considerable, however; infections during the administrative program are most troublesome, but diabetes and hypertension are also difficult to manage. A trial of ALG combined with high-dose methylprednisolone failed to show any clear-cut benefit.[127] More conventional doses of prednisolone are not effective in the treatment of SAA.[128]

Cyclosporine

In the late 1980s interest centered on cyclosporine as an alternative immunosuppressive agent to ALG for the management of patients with aplastic anemia.[129] Individual case reports have described patients who responded well to cyclosporine after failing one or more courses of treatment with ALG.[130,131] A more systematic, nonrandomized study suggested that cyclosporine might produce a response in about one-third of patients who had failed ALG therapy, but few patients responded in the first 3 months of therapy, and in the remaining patients recovery followed only on the introduction of corticosteroids or stopping the immunosuppressive therapy.[132] A randomized study of ALG versus cyclosporine as first-line treatment suggested that cyclosporine is as effective as ALG.[133,134] In a second European trial ALG was given with or without cyclosporine, and again results were obtained suggesting that addition of cyclosporine to the ALG regime may increase the chance of response.[135] The dose of cyclosporine used is generally 5 mg/kg PO given twice a day, with adjustment of the dose according to cyclosporine levels in the blood and to toxicity as monitored by creatinine levels and liver function tests. Prolonged cyclosporine administration may produce renal impairment and a syndrome resembling thrombotic thrombocytopenic purpura, but long-term toxicity is minimal if doses of 5 mg/kg/day are used and creatinine levels carefully monitored.[136] Most patients who respond to cyclosporine have a durable response, but some relapse when the drug is withdrawn and a second response following reinstitution of the drug is usual. It is advisable to withdraw cyclosporine gradually once a response has been obtained.

Anabolic (Androgenic) Steroids

Androgens were introduced in 1959 as a treatment for aplastic anemia.[137] It was already known that androgens would raise the hemoglobin levels in women with carcinoma of the breast and that they had some effect on hemoglobin levels in patients with myelofibrosis.[138] Analysis of the early results of androgen therapy in aplastic anemia proved difficult because patients with Fanconi anemia as well as acquired aplastic anemia were treated, and most patients with Fanconi anemia will respond to androgen therapy, at least in the short term.[137,139] Patients with NSAA frequently show some improvement in hemoglobin levels and also in granulocyte and platelet levels in response to high doses of androgens, but the severe side effects of prolonged use make this a difficult form of therapy to manage. The role of androgens in SAA is unclear. A randomized study suggested that in severe disease anabolic steroids were of no benefit,[140] whereas retrospective analysis of patients reported to the EBMTG registry suggested that there was a definite benefit and improved recovery when androgens were given, particularly in children.[141] Further randomized studies may help to resolve these discrepancies.

Androgenic steroids are usually used in the form of anabolic steroids, which have been modified from the basic testosterone molecule to diminish virilizing effects and to allow absorption from the gastrointestinal tract. Most of the orally absorbed anabolic steroids have a methyl substitution at the 17-α position, which allows absorption but also causes hepatotoxicity.

Splenectomy

Before the introduction of immunosuppressive therapy and bone marrow transplantation for the treatment of aplastic anemia, splenectomy was recommended in some cases, particularly those in which blood transfusion support was difficult.[128] Splenectomy may still play a role in patients managed with immunosuppressive therapy when it is difficult to obtain a rise in the platelet count even with HLA-matched platelets.[142]

Prognosis Following Immunosuppressive Therapy

Recovery of bone marrow function following treatment with ALG and other forms of immunosuppressive therapy is generally slow, and a totally normal peripheral blood count is obtained in only a proportion of patients who have become free from transfusion requirements. Even when the blood count returns to normal, it is possible to demonstrate abnormalities of bone marrow function by in vitro culture techniques.[143] Of the patients who survive, some 10–15% will develop further hematologic abnormalities manifested by either relapse of the aplastic anemia, the development of PNH, or the appearance of leukemic clones.[143,144] It is not entirely clear whether there is ever a true plateau of survival following immunosuppression or whether there is an increased risk of conversion to a more malignant condition in all patients with aplastic anemia so treated.[145]

Role of Hematopoietic Growth Factor Therapy

The introduction of recombinant human hematopoietic growth factors such as CSF-GM, CSF-G, and IL-3 has added a new dimension to the management of patients with pancytopenia produced by chemotherapy or radiotherapy. Whether they will have a major role in the management of idiosyncratic aplastic anemia remains to be seen. CSF-GM can raise the granulocyte and monocyte count in patients with aplastic anemia who have some residual bone marrow function,[146,147] but such temporary improvement in the leukocyte count does not occur in patients with severe marrow failure.[99] IL-3 has been used as a single agent in a small number of patients with aplastic anemia without any clear-cut improvement in the blood count. Nevertheless, it may well be that growth factors will have an important role to play in the management of patients with aplastic anemia, perhaps as an adjunct to other measures to prevent bleeding and infection rather than as curative agents.

Bone Marrow Transplantation

Mention has already been made of bone marrow transplantation from identical twins in aplastic anemia, a proportion of such patients having been cured by infusion of normal syngeneic marrow.[24] Treatment of the disorder by allogeneic bone marrow transplantation from HLA-matched siblings was introduced in 1969 in Seattle by Thomas and Storb[148] and Storb and colleagues.[149] Their early experience suggested that immunosuppression with cyclophosphamide alone was superior to cyclophosphamide plus total body irradiation in this disease. The standard conditioning measurement for patients with aplastic anemia has subsequently become cyclophosphamide (50 mg/kg/day) for 4 days. Initially, there was a high rate of graft failure or graft rejection, possibly associated with the use of methotrexate for prophylaxis of graft-versus-host disease.[150,151] The importance of an adequate cell dose from the donor was recognized, as was the influence of blood transfusions on the outcome of transplantation.[152] Patients who receive 3.0×10^8 cells/kg body weight are less likely to reject the transplant than those who receive a smaller dose, and patients who have not received blood have less transplant-related morbidity than those who received multiple transfusions.[152] The introduction of cyclosporine to prevent graft rejection has improved survival of patients who received transplants from HLA-matched sibling donors,[153] and there may be an advantage in using a short course of methotrexate together with prolonged cyclosporine in these patients.[154] Late graft failure may occur after stopping treatment with cyclosporine, and it is advisable to continue with the postgraft immunosuppression for ≥1 year.[155] Although graft failure rates have fallen, rejection is still a problem. Second transplants may rescue ≤30% of such patients,[156] and rejection may be averted by giving CSF-GM.[156]

The superiority of bone marrow transplantation over supportive care with or without androgen was confirmed in an early multicenter trial.[63] Comparison of matched sibling transplants with immunosuppressive therapy using ALG has not been made in a formal randomized study, but data from the EBMTG registry suggest that younger patients with severe disease who have a matched sibling should receive transplants, and the sensitizing influence of blood transfusion suggests that transplantation should be carried out as a matter of urgency.[157] Attempts to prevent graft-versus-host disease by T-cell depletion without increasing immunosuppression have proved disappointing in aplastic anemia, in which the incidence of graft rejection reaches unacceptable levels in the T-cell-depleted grafts unless additional immunosuppression is used.[158] For HLA-matched sibling transplants, the most widely used regimen currently in use is cyclophosphamide (50 mg/kg/day) for 4 days and cyclosporine started on day −1 at 5 mg/kg/day for 2 days, thereafter adjusted according to blood levels and toxicity and continuing with an oral preparation for 12 months postgraft. Methotrexate 10 mg/m^2 on days 1, 3, and 5 is also recommended by some centers.[154] In a patient highly sensitized by multiple blood transfusions it may be desirable to provide additional immunosuppression with ALG. The use of monoclonal antibodies directed against the host's immune system is under investigation, and results are promising. Addition of either total lymphoid irradiation or modified thoracoabdominal irradiation decreases the incidence of graft failure but does not improve overall survival.[159,160] The difficulties are more acute when unrelated or mismatched donors are used.

Phenotypically unrelated volunteer donors or partially matched family donors offer an obvious alternative to matched sibling donors for those patients with very severe aplastic anemia who are unlikely to respond to ALG or for those patients who fail one or more courses of immunosuppression. Earlier results using phenotypically matched volunteer donors showed that such a course was feasible, at least in patients who had not been grossly sensitized by multiple transfusions.[161] Subsequent experience has suggested that a more cautious or selective approach is necessary. It would appear that fully phenotypically matched unrelated donors produce results almost as successful as those achieved with the genotypically matched sibling transplants once comparable analyses have been made and that mismatch at a single HLA locus, whether class I or class II, is acceptable. Greater degrees of mismatch are associated with unacceptable transplant-related mortality. As registries of volunteer donors expand and the speed with which a suitable donor can be identified increases, this form of therapy will almost certainly become more widespread and more successful for patients unlikely to respond to immunosuppressive therapy. The post-transplant problems encountered by patients with aplastic anemia are less than those found in leukemic patients, in whom irradiation is routinely used. One advantage of transplants for aplastic anemia, at least for those cases in which irradiation is not used, is that these patients develop normally and are normally fertile following the transplant.

SUMMARY

The treatment of aplastic anemia depends on the severity of the disease, the age of the patient, and the availability of an HLA-matched donor. Patients <50 years old with severe bone marrow failure who have an HLA-matched sibling donor, particularly if they have not received blood transfusions, are best treated by bone marrow transplantation. For most other patients a trial of immunosuppressive therapy is appropriate, but for children <10 years old with severe disease who do not have a sibling donor, an urgent hunt for an HLA-matched volunteer donor should be instigated and transplantation carried out early if a suitable donor is identified.

REFERENCES

1. Ehrlich P: Über einen Fall von Anämie mit Bemerkungen über regenerative Veränderungen des Knochenmarks. Charité Ann 13:300, 1888
2. Chauffard M: Un cas d'anémie pernicieuse aplastique. Bull Mem Soc Med Hop Paris 21:313, 1904
3. Böttiger LE, Westerholm B: Aplastic anaemia: I. Incidence and aetiology. J Intern Med 192:315, 1972
4. International Agranulocytosis and Aplastic Anemia Study: Incidence of aplastic anemia: the relevance of diagnostic criteria. Blood 70:1718, 1987
5. Mary JY, Baumelou E, Guiguet M, the French Cooperative Group for Epidemiological Study of Aplastic Anaemia: Epidemiology of aplastic anemia in France: a prospective multicentre study. Blood 75:1646, 1990
6. Szklo M, Sensenbrenner L, Markowitz J et al: Incidence of aplastic anemia in metropolitan Baltimore: a population based study. Blood 66:115, 1985
7. Young NS, Issaragrasil S, Chieh CW, Takaku F: Annotation: aplastic anaemia in the Orient. Br J Haematol 62:1, 1986
8. Gordon-Smith EC, Issaragrisil S: Epidemiology of aplastic anaemia. Clin Haematol 5:475, 1992
9. Nagao T, Mauer AM: Concordance for drug induced aplastic anemia in identical twins. N Engl J Med 281:7, 1969
10. Albert E, Thomas ED, Nisperos B et al: HLA antigens and haplo-types in 200 patients with aplastic anemia. Transplantation 22:528, 1976
11. Werner-Favre C, Jeannet M: HLA compatibility in couples with children suffering from acute leukemia or aplastic anemia. Tissue Antigens 13:307, 1979
12. D'Amaro J, Van Rood JJ, Rimm AA, Bortin MM: HLA associations in Italian and non-Italian caucasoid aplastic anaemia patients. Tissue Antigens 21:184, 1983
13. Chapuis B, Von Fliedner E, Jeannet M et al: Increased frequency of DR-2 in patients with aplastic anaemia and increased sharing in their parents. Br J Haematol 63:51, 1986
14. Suhrland LG, Weisberger AS: Delayed clearance of chloramphenicol from serum in patients with hematologic toxicity. Blood 34:466, 1969
15. Linet MS, Tielsch JM, Markowitz JA et al: An apparent cluster of aplastic anemia in a small population of teenagers. Arch Intern Med 145:635, 1985
16. Morgan GJ, Palmer SR, Onions D et al: A cluster of three cases of aplastic anaemia in children. Clin Lab Haematol 10:29, 1988
17. Camitta BM, Storb R, Thomas ED: Aplastic anemia (first of two parts); pathogenesis, diagnosis, treatment, and prognosis. N Engl J Med 306:645, 1982
18. Singer JW, Brown JE: In vitro marrow culture techniques in aplastic anaemia and related disorders. Clin Haematol 7:487, 1978
19. Thomas ED, Storb R: Acquired aplastic anemia: progress and perplexity. Blood 64:325, 1984
20. Reynolds M, McCann SR: Human marrow stromal cells in short term semisolid bone marrow culture in aplastic anemia. Scand J Haematol 34:101, 1985
21. Marsh JCW, Chang J, Testa NG et al: In vitro assessment of marrow "stem cell" and stromal cell function in aplastic anaemia. Br J Haematol 79:258, 1991
22. Gibson FM, Scopes J, Laurie A, Gordon-Smith EC: Contribution of the marrow stroma to the pathogenesis of aplastic anaemia. Exp Hematol 18:628, 1990
23. Pillow RP, Epstein RB, Buckner CD et al: Treatment of bone marrow failure by isogeneic marrow infusion. N Engl J Med 275:94, 1966
24. Applebaum FR, Fefer A, Cheever MA et al: Treatment of aplastic anemia by bone marrow transplantation in identical twins. Blood 55:1033, 1980
25. Lu D-P: Syngeneic bone marrow transplantation for treatment for aplastic anemia: report of a case and review of the literature. Exp Hematol 9:257, 1981
26. Simmons PJ, Przepiorka D, Thomas ED, Torok-Storb B: Host origin of marrow stromal cells following allogeneic bone marrow transplantation. Nature 328:429, 1987
27. Alexanian R: Erythropoietin excretion in bone marrow failure and hemolytic anemia. J Lab Clin Med 82:438, 1973
28. Nissen C, Moser Y, Weiss J et al: Stimulatory serum factors in aplastic anaemia. I. Serum "releasor" activity for haemopoietic growth factors, a regulator? Br J Haematol 61:491, 1985
29. Yen YP, Zabala P, Doney K et al: Hematopoietic growth factors in human serum: erythroid burst-promoting activity in normal subjects and in patients with severe aplastic anemia. J Lab Clin Med 106:384, 1985
30. Zoumbos NC, Gascon P, Djeu JY et al; Circulating activated suppressor T lymphocytes in aplastic anemia. N Engl J Med 312:257, 1985
31. Torok-Storb B, Johnson G, Bowden R et al: Gamma-interferon in aplastic anemia: inability to detect significant levels in sera or demonstrate hematopoietic suppressing activity. Blood 69:629, 1987
32. Nakao S, Matsushima K, Young NS: Deficient interleukin-I by aplastic anaemia monocytes. Br J Haematol 71:431, 1989
33. Haak H, Goselink HM, Veenhof W et al: Acquired aplastic anaemia in adults. Part IV. Histological and CFU studies in transplanted and non-transplanted patients. Scand J Haematol 19:159, 1977
34. Heit W, Heimpel H, Kubanek B: Granulocytic and erythroid progenitor cells in recovering aplastic anemia. p. 97. In Heimpel H, Gordon-Smith EC, Heit W, Kubanek B (eds): Aplastic Anemia, Pathophysiology and Approaches to Therapy. Springer-Verlag, Berlin, 1979
35. Tichelli A, Gratwohl A, Würsch A et al: Late haematological complications in severe aplastic anaemia. Br J Haematol 69:413, 1988
36. De Planque MM, Kluin-Nelemans JC, Van Krieken JHJM et al: Evolution of acquired severe aplastic anaemia to myelodysplasia and subsequent leukaemia in adults. Br J Haematol 70:55, 1988
37. Breatnach F, Chessels JM, Greaves MF: The aplastic presentation of childhood leukaemia: a feature of common ALL. Br J Haematol 49:387, 1981
38. Bacigalupo A, Hows J, Gluckman E et al: Bone marrow transplantation (BMT) versus immunosuppression for the treatment of severe aplastic anaemia (SAA): a report of the EBMT SAA working party. Br J Haematol 70:177, 1988
39. Stoll DB, Blum S, Pasquale B, Murphy S: Thrombocytopenia with decreased megakaryocytes. Evaluation and prognosis. Ann Intern Med 94:170, 1981
40. Atchison RGM, Marsh JCW, Hows JM et al: Pregnancy associated aplastic anaemia: a report of 5 cases and review of current management. Br J Haematol 73:541, 1989
41. Fleming AF: Hypoplastic anaemia in pregnancy. Br Med J 3:166, 1973
42. Doney K, Storb R, Buckner CD et al: Marrow transplantation for treatment of pregnancy associated aplastic anemia. Exp Hematol 13:1080, 1985
43. Marsh JCW, Hows JM, Bryett KA et al: Survival after antilymphocyte globulin for aplastic anemia depends on disease severity. Blood 70:1046, 1987
44. Lewis SM: Course and prognosis in aplastic anaemia. Br Med J I:1027, 1965
45. Kansu E, Erslev AJ: Aplastic anaemia with "hot pockets." Scand J Haematol 17:326, 1976
46. Te Velde J, Haak HL: Aplastic anaemia. Histological investigation of methacrylate embedded bone marrow biopsy specimens: correlation with survival after conventional treatment in 15 adult patients. Br J Haematol 35:61, 1977
47. Sale GE, Rajantie J, Doney K et al: Does histologic grading of inflammation in bone marrow predict the response of aplastic anaemia patients to antithymocyte globulin? Br J Haematol 67:261, 1987
48. Lewis SM, Dacie JV: The aplastic anaemia paroxysmal nocturnal haemoglobinuria syndrome. Br J Haematol 13:236, 1967
49. Kurtzman N, Young N: Viruses and bone marrow failure. Clin Haematol 2:51, 1989
50. Dokal I, Ganly P, Ribeiro L et al: Late onset bone marrow failure associated with proximal fusion of radius and ulna: a new syndrome. Br J Haematol 71:277, 1989
51. Cervenka J, Arthur D, Yasis C: Mitomycin C test for diagnostic differentiation of idiopathic aplastic anaemia and Fanconi anaemia. Pediatrics 67:119, 1981
52. Appelbaum FR, Barrall J, Storb R et al: Clonal cytogenetic abnormalities in patients with otherwise typical aplastic anemia. Exp Hematol 15:1134, 1987
53. Auerbach AD, Adler B, Chaganti RFK: Pre-natal and post-natal diagnosis and carrier detection of Fanconi anemia by a cytogenetic method. Pediatrics 67:128, 1981
54. Melhorn DK, Gross S, Newman AJ: Acute childhood leukemia presenting as aplastic anemia: the response to corticosteroids. J Pediatr 77:647, 1970
55. Dameshek W: Riddle—what do aplastic anemia, paroxysmal nocturnal haemoglobinuria and hypoplastic leukemia have in common? Blood 30:251, 1967
56. Editorial: Aplasia leukemia syndrome. Lancet 1:1425, 1989
57. Fohlmeister I, Fischer R, Modder B et al: Aplastic anaemia and the hypocellular myelodysplasias: histomorphological diagnosis and prognostic features. J Clin Pathol 39:1218, 1985
58. Appelbaum FR, Storb R, Ramberg RE et al: Treatment of preleukemic syndromes with marrow transplantation. Blood 69:92, 1987
59. Fraunfelder FT, Bagby GC Jr: Ocular chloramphenicol and aplastic anemia. N Engl J Med 308:1536, 1983
60. Lynch RE, Williams DM, Reading JC, Cartwright GE: The prognosis in aplastic anemia. Blood 45:517, 1975
61. Najean Y, Pecking A: Prognostic factors in acquired aplastic anemia. A study of 352 cases. Am J Med 67:564, 1979

62. Camitta BM, Rappaport JM, Parkman R, Nathan DG: Selection of patients for bone marrow transplantation in severe anemia. Blood 45:355, 1975

63. Camitta BM, Thomas ED, Nathan DG et al: Severe aplastic anemia: a prospective study of the effect of early marrow transplantation on acute mortality. Blood 48:63, 1976

64. Mathé G, Amiel JL, Schwarzenberg L et al: Bone marrow graft in man after conditioning by antilymphocyte serum. Br Med J 2:131, 1970

65. Speck B, Gluckman E, Haak HL, Van Rood JJ: Treatment of aplastic anaemia by antilymphocyte globulin with and without allogeneic bone marrow infusions. Lancet 2:1145, 1977

66. Bacigalupo A, Van Lint MT, Congui M et al: Treatment of SAA in Europe 1970–1985: a report of the SAA working party. Bone Marrow Transplant, suppl. 1. 1:19, 1986

67. Meyers JD, Fourney N, Thomas ED: Risk factors for cytomegalovirus infection after human marrow transplantation. J Infect Dis 153:478, 1986

68. Storb R, Thomas ED, Buckner CD et al: Marrow transplantation in 30 "untransfused" patients with severe aplastic anemia. Ann Intern Med 92:30, 1980

69. Saral R, Burns WH, Prentice HG: Herpes virus infections: clinical manifestations and therapeutic stratagems in immunocompromised patients. Clin Haematol 13:645, 1984

70. Eernisse JG, Brand A: Prevention of platelet refractoriness due to HLA antibodies by administration of leucocyte-poor blood components. Exp Hematol 9:77, 1981

71. Brand A, Claas FHJ, Voogt PJ et al: Allo-immunisation after leucocyte-depleted multiple random donor platelet transfusions. Vox Sang 54:160, 1988

72. Vakkila J, Myllylä G: Amount and type of leucocytes in "leucocyte-free" red cell and platelet concentrates. Vox Sang 53:76, 1987

73. Menitove JE: Platelet transfusion for allo-immunised patients. Clin Oncol 2: 587, 1983

74. Snyder EL: Clinical use of white cell-poor blood components. Transfusion 29:568, 1989

75. Klingemann HG, Self S, Benaji M et al: Refractoriness to random platelet transfusions in patients with aplastic anemia: a multivariant analysis from 264 cases. Br J Haematol 66:115, 1987

76. Dutcher JP, Schiffer CA, Aisner J, Wiernik PH: Alloimmunisation following platelet transfusion: the absence of a dose-response relationship. Blood 57: 395, 1981

77. Luban NLC, Williams AE, MacDonald NG et al: Low incidence of acquired cytomegalovirus in neonates transfused with washed red blood cells. Am J Dis Child 141:416, 1987

78. Gilbert GL, Hayes K, Hudson IL, James J: Prevention of transfusion-acquired cytomegalovirus infection in infants by blood filtration to remove leucocytes. Lancet 1:1228, 1989

79. Murphy MF, Grint PCA, Hardiman AE et al: Use of leucocyte-poor blood components to prevent primary cytomegalovirus (CMV) infection in patients with acute leukaemia. Br J Haematol 70:253, 1988

80. Bodey GP, Bolivar R, Fainstein V: Infectious complications in leukaemic patients. Semin Hematol 19:193, 1982

81. Keidan AJ, Tsatalas C, Cohen J et al: Infective complications of aplastic anaemia. Br J Haematol 63:503, 1986

82. Bodey GP, Buckley BA, Sathe YS, Freireich EJ: Quantitative relationships between circulating leucocytes and infection in patients with acute leukemia. Ann Intern Med 64:328, 1966

83. Hann IM, Prentice HG: Infection prophylaxis in the patient with bone marrow failure. Clin Haematol 13:523, 1984

84. Van Saene HKF, Stoutenbeek CP: Selective decontamination. J Antimicrob Chemother 20:462, 1987

85. Gaya H: Rational basis for the choice of regimens for empirical therapy of sepsis in granulocytopenic patients. Clin Haematol 13:573, 1984

86. Young LS: Nosocomial infections in the immunocompromised adult. Am J Med 70:398, 1981

87. Young LS: Antimicrobial prophylaxis against infection in neutropenic patients. J Infect Dis 147:611, 1983

88. Joshi JH, Schimpff SC: Therapy of infection in granulocytopenic patients with cancer. Clin Oncol 2:611, 1983

89. Love LJ, Schimpff SC, Schiffer CA, Wiernik PH: Improved prognosis for granulocytopenic patients with gram-negative bacteraemia. Am J Med 68:643, 1980

90. Maxwell AJ, Mamtora H: Fungal liver abscesses in acute leukemia. Clin Radiol 39:197, 1988

91. Buckner CD, Clift RA: Prophylaxis and treatment of infection of the immunocompromised host by granulocyte transfusions. Clin Haematol 13:557, 1984

92. Christensen RD, Anstall H, Rothstein G: Neutrophil transfusion in septic neutropenic neonates. Transfusion 22:151, 1982

93. Navari IM, Buckner CD, Clift RA et al: Prophylaxis of infection in patients with aplastic anemia receiving allogeneic marrow transplants. Am J Med 76:564, 1984

94. Nagata S, Tsuchiya M, Asano S et al: Molecular cloning and expression of cDNA for human granulocyte colony-stimulating factor. Nature 319:415, 1986

95. Gough NM, Gough J, Metcalf D et al: Molecular cloning of cDNA encoding a murine haematopoietic growth regulator, granulocyte-macrophage colony stimulating factor. Nature 309:763, 1984

96. Wong GG, Witek JS, Temple PA et al: Human GM-CSF: molecular cloning of the complementary DNA and purification of natural and recombinant proteins. Science 228:810, 1985

97. Vadhan-Raj S, Buescher S, LeMaistre A et al: Stimulation of haematopoiesis in patients with bone marrow failure and in patients with malignancy by recombinant human granulocyte-macrophage colony stimulating factor. Blood 72:134, 1988

98. Champlin RE, Niemer SD, Ireland P et al: Treatment of refractory aplastic anemia with recombinant human granulocyte-macrophage colony stimulating factor. Blood 73:694, 1989

99. Nissen C, Tichelli A, Gratwohl A et al: Failure of recombinant human granulocyte-macrophage colony-stimulating factor therapy in aplastic anemia patients with very severe neutropenia. Blood 72:2045, 1988

100. Gribben JG, Devereux S, Thomas NSB et al: Development of antibodies to unprotected glycosylation sites on recombinant human GM-CSF. Lancet 1: 434, 1990

101. Weisbart RM, Golde DW, Clark SC et al: Human granulocyte-macrophage colony-stimulating factor is a neutrophil activator. Nature 314:361, 1985

102. Wang JM, Colella S, Allavena P, Mantovani A: Chemotactic activity of human recombinant granulocyte-macrophage colony-stimulating factor. Immunology 60:439, 1987

103. Kojima S, Fukuda M, Miyajima Y, Matsuyama T, Honbe K: Treatment of aplastic anemia in children with recombinant human granulocyte colony-stimulating factor. Blood 77:937, 1991

104. Ganser A, Lindemann A, Seipelt G et al: Effect of recombinant human interleukin-3 in aplastic anemia. Blood 76:1287, 1990

105. Mathé G, Amiel JL, Schwarzenberg L et al: Bone marrow grafts in man after conditioning by antilymphocyte serum. Br Med J 2:131, 1980

106. Speck B: Toxische Knochenmarkinsuffizienz. Hamatol Bluttransfus 16:235, 1975

107. Champlin R, Ho W, Gale RP: Antithymocyte globulin treatment in patients with aplastic anemia. N Engl J Med 308:113, 1983

108. Speck B, Gratwohl A, Nissen C et al: Treatment of severe aplastic anaemia with antilymphocyte globulin or bone marrow transplantation. Br Med J 282:860, 1981

109. Doney KC, Weiden PL, Buckner CD et al: Treatment of severe aplastic anemia using antilymphocyte globulin with or without an infusion of HLA haploidentical marrow. Exp Hematol 9:829, 1981

110. Doney K, Kopecky K, Storb R et al: Long term comparison of immunosuppressive therapy with antithymocyte globulin to bone marrow transplantation in aplastic anemia. p. 104. In Shahidi NT (ed): Aplastic Anemia and Other Bone Marrow Failure Syndromes. Springer-Verlag, New York, 1990

111. Werner EJ, Stout RD, Valdez LP, Herres RE: Immunosuppressive therapy versus bone marrow transplantation for children with aplastic anemia. Pediatrics 83:61, 1989

112. Smith AG, O'Reilly RJ, Hansen JA, Martin PJ: Specific antibody-blocking activities in antilymphocyte globulin as correlates with efficacy for the treatment of aplastic anemia. Blood 66:721, 1985

113. Gratwohl A, Wursch A, Speck B et al: Absence of lot to lot variation of antilymphocyte globulin in the treatment of severe aplastic anaemia. Bone Marrow Transplant, suppl. 1. 1:23, 1986

114. Marsh JCW, Gordon-Smith EC: The role of antilymphocyte globulin in the treatment of chronic acquired bone marrow failure. Blood Rev 2:141, 1988

115. Platanias L, Gascon P, Bielory L et al: Lymphocyte phenotype and lymphokines following antithymocyte globulin therapy in patients with aplastic anaemia. Br J Haematol 66:437, 1987

116. Greco B, Bielory L, Stephany D et al: Antithymocyte globulin reacts with many normal human cell types. Blood 62:1047, 1983

117. Gascon P, Zoumbos NC, Scala G et al: Lymphokine abnormalities in aplastic anemia: implications for the mechanism of action of antithymocyte globulin. Blood 65:407, 1985

118. Faille EA, Barrett AJ, Balitrand N et al: The effect of ATG on granulocyte precursors in aplastic anaemia. Br J Haematol 42:371, 1979

119. Netzel B, Rodt H, Hoffman-Fezer G et al: The effect of crude and differently absorbed anti-human T cell globulin on granulocytic and erythropoietic colony formation. Exp Haematol 6:410, 1978

120. Hunter RF, Mold NG, Mitchell RB, Huang AT: Differentiation of normal marrow and HL60 cells induced by antithymocyte globulin. Proc Natl Acad Sci USA 82:4823, 1985

121. Lawley TJ, Bielory L, Gascon P et al: A prospective clinical and immunological analysis of patients with serum sickness. N Engl J Med 311:1407, 1984

122. Marsh JCW, Zomas A, Hows JM et al: Avascular necrosis after treatment of aplastic anaemia with antilymphocyte globulin and high-dose methylprednisolone. Br J Haematol 84;731, 1993

123. Bielory L, Gascon P, Lawley PJ et al: Serum sickness and haemopoietic recovery with antithymocyte globulin in bone marrow failure patients. Br J Haematol 63:729, 1986

124. Marsh JCW, Hows JM, Bryat KA, Gordon-Smith EC: Antilymphocyte globulin therapy for aplastic anemia. Report of UK study group on 164 patients. Blood, suppl. 1. 70:139A, 1987

125. Bacigalupo A, Giordano D, Van Lint MT et al: Bolus methyl prednisolone in severe aplastic anemia. N Engl J Med 300:501, 1979

126. Bacigalupo A, Podesta M, Van Lint MT et al: Severe aplastic anaemia. Correlation of in vitro tests with clinical response to immunosuppression in 20 patients. Br J Haematol 47:423, 1981

127. Gluckman E, Devergie A, Poros A, Degaoulet P: Results of immunosuppression in 170 cases of severe aplastic anaemia: report of the European group of bone marrow transplant. Br J Haematol 51:541, 1982

128. Scott JL, Cartwright GE, Wintrobe MM: Acquired aplastic anemia: an analysis of 39 cases and review of the pertinent literature. Medicine 38:119, 1959

129. Shahidi NT, Wang W, Shurin S et al: Treatment of acquired aplastic anemia with cyclosporine and androgens. p. 155. In Shahidi NT (ed): Aplastic Anemia and Other Bone Marrow Failure Syndromes. Springer-Verlag, New York, 1990

130. Stryckmans PA, Dumont JP, Velu TH, Debusscher L: Cyclosporine in refractory severe aplastic anemia. N Engl J Med 310:655, 1984

131. Finlay JL, Toretsky J, Hoffman R et al: Cyclosporin A (CyA) in refractory aplastic anemia (AA). Blood 64:326, 1984

132. Leonard F, Raefsky E, Nienhuis AW et al: Cyclosporin A therapy of aplastic anemia and pure red cell aplasia. Blood, suppl. 1. 70:403, 1987

133. Gluckman E, Esperou H, Devergie A: Comparison of cyclosporin A (CyA) and horse antithymocyte globulin (HATG) for treatment of severe aplastic anaemia (SAA): a multicentre prospective randomised study. Blood, suppl. 1. 72:78a, 1988

134. Gluckman E, Esperou-Bourdeau H, Baruchel A et al: Multicentre randomized study comparing cyclosporin-A alone and antithymocyte globulin with prednisone for treatment of severe aplastic anemia. Blood 79:2540, 1992

135. Frickhofen N, Kaltwasser JP, Schrezenmeier H et al: Treatment of aplastic anemia with antilymphocyte globulin and methylprednisolone with or without cyclosporine. N Engl J Med 324:1297, 1991

136. Assan R, Timsit J, Fentren G et al: The kidney in cyclosporin A-treated diabetic patients: a long-term clinicopathological study. Clin Nephrol 41:41, 1994

137. Shahidi NT, Diamond LK: Testosterone-induced remission in aplastic anemia. Am J Dis Child 98:293, 1959

138. Gardener SH, Nathan DG: Androgens and erythropoiesis. N Engl J Med 274:420, 1966

139. Li FP, Alter BP, Nathan DG: The mortality of acquired aplastic anemia in children. Blood 40:153, 1972

140. Champlin RE, Ho WG, Feig SA et al: Do androgens enhance the response to antithymocyte globulin in patients with aplastic anemia? A prospective randomised trial. Blood 66:184, 1985

141. Locasciulli A, Porta F, Vossen JM, Bacigalupo A: Treatment of acquired severe aplastic anaemia (SAA) in children: an analysis of the EBMT-SAA working party. Bone Marrow Transplant, suppl. 2. 4:90, 1989

142. Tichelli A, Speck B: Indikationen zur Splenektomie bei hämatologischen Erkränkungen. Aktuel Probl Chir Orthop 30:19, 26, 1985

143. De Planque MM, Brand A, Kluin-Nelemans HC et al: Haematopoietic and immunological abnormalities in severe aplastic anaemia patients treated with anti-thymocyte globulin. Br J Haematol 71:421, 1989

144. Tichelli A, Gratwohl A, Würsch A et al: Late haematological complications in severe aplastic anaemia. Br J Haematol 69:413, 1988

145. Moore MAS, Castro-Malaspina H: Immunosuppression in aplastic anemia—postponing the inevitable? N Engl J Med 324:1358, 1991

146. Vadhan-Raj S, Buescher S, Broxmeymer HE et al: Stimulation of myelopoiesis in patients with aplastic anemia by recombinant human granulocyte-macrophage colony-stimulating factor. N Engl J Med 319:1628, 1988

147. Antin JH, Smith BR, Holmes W, Rosenthal DS: Phase 1/2 study of recombinant human granulocyte macrophage colony stimulating factor in aplastic anemia and myelodysplastic syndromes. Blood 72:705, 1988

148. Thomas ED, Storb R: Technique for human marrow grafting. Blood 36:507, 1970

149. Storb R, Thomas ED, Buckner CD et al: Allogeneic marrow grafting for treatment of aplastic anemia. Blood 43:157, 1974

150. Storb R, Prentice RL, Thomas ED: Marrow transplantation for aplastic anemia: factors associated with rejection. N Engl J Med 296:61, 1977

151. Storb R, Prentice RL, Thomas ED et al: Factors associated with graft rejection after HLA identical marrow transplantation. Br J Haematol 55:563, 1983

152. Storb R, Thomas ED, Buckner CD et al: Marrow transplantation in 30 "untransfused" patients with severe aplastic anemia. Ann Intern Med 92:30, 1980

153. Hows JM, Palmer S, Gordon-Smith EC: The use of cyclosporin A in allogeneic bone marrow transplantation for severe aplastic anemia. Transplantation 33:382, 1982

154. Storb R, Deague HJ, Fairwell V et al: Marrow transplantation for severe aplastic anemia: methotrexate alone compared with a combination of methotrexate and cyclosporin for prevention of acute graft versus host disease. Blood 68:119, 1986

155. Hows JM, Yin JL, Chipping PM et al: Post graft immunosuppression with cyclosporine in allogeneic bone marrow transplantation for severe aplastic anemia. Transplant Proc suppl. 1. 4:2634, 1983

156. McCann SR, Bacigalupo A, Gluckman E et al: Graft rejection and second bone marrow transplants for acquired aplastic anaemia: a report from the aplastic anaemia working party of the European Bone Marrow Transplant Group. Transplantation 13:233, 1994

157. Bacigalupo A, Gordon-Smith EC, Van Lint MT et al: Bone marrow transplantation (BMT) vs immunosuppression (IS) in the management of severe aplastic anemia. Bone Marrow Transplant, suppl. 1. 2:99, 1987

158. Bacigalupo A, Hows J, Gordon-Smith EC et al: Bone marrow transplantation for severe aplastic anemia from donors other than HLA identical siblings: a report of the BMT working party. Bone Marrow Transplant 3:531, 1988

159. Ramsay NKC, Kim TH, McGlave P et al: Total lymphoid irradiation and cyclophosphamide conditioning prior to bone marrow transplantation for patients with severe aplastic anemia. Blood 62:622, 1983

160. Gluckman E, Devergie A, Dutreux A et al: Total body irradiation in bone marrow transplantation. Hôpital St Louis results. Pathol Biol (Paris) 27:349, 1979

161. Gordon-Smith EC, Fairhead SM, Chipping PM et al: Bone marrow transplantation for severe aplastic anaemia using histocompatible unrelated volunteer donors. Br Med J 2:835, 1982

Acquired Pure Red Cell Aplasia

23

Sanford B. Krantz

INTRODUCTION

Pure red cell aplasia (PRCA) was first described by Kaznelson.[1] This disorder is characterized by severe anemia, a reticulocyte count of <1%, and a marrow containing <0.5% mature erythroblasts.[1-8] The blood leukocyte and platelet counts remain normal, and the bone marrow is normocellular.[4,6] Congenital forms of PRCA have been called chronic (congenital) hypoplastic anemia, Diamond-Blackfan anemia, or erythrogenesis imperfecta. Acquired PRCA in children is generally referred to as transient erythroblastopenia of childhood.[9] In adults, acquired PRCA is known as isolated aplastic anemia, aplastic crisis, erythroblastopenia, erythrophthisis, chronic erythrocytic hypoplasia, red cell aplastic anemia, and red cell agenesis. In this chapter, PRCA refers to red cell aplasia in adults, while congenital hypoplastic anemia and transient erythroblastopenia of childhood (TEC) refer to the congenital and acquired forms of this syndrome in children.

ETIOLOGY AND PATHOGENESIS

A classification of PRCA is presented in Table 23-1. Congenital hypoplastic anemia occurs within the first 18 months of life. It differs from acquired PRCA in that it is characterized by residual erythropoiesis, a 25% incidence of congenital abnormalities, and a remarkable therapeutic response to small doses of corticosteroids.[10,11]

Acquired primary PRCA occurs in children and adults and has frequently been shown to be associated with immunoglobulins or T cells that inhibit marrow erythropoiesis. When such a mechanism of disease cannot be identified, the cases are termed idiopathic, but frequently such patients respond to immunosuppressive treatment in a similar fashion to those in whom an immunologic mechanism has been determined. PRCA was thought of as a rare condition, as only 56 cases had been reported by 1967.[4] While the precise incidence is unknown, within a period of 5 years our group learned of 80 new cases, indicating that the incidence of PRCA may be slightly greater than previously appreciated. Males and females are equally affected, and no evidence has appeared for any racial predisposition.[3,6,7,12]

Primary PRCA must be distinguished from secondary forms of PRCA. Of particular interest is the association of PRCA with thymomas, reported in as many as 50% of PRCA cases in the literature.[2,4] This figure is probably an exaggeration of the strength of the association of these two disorders. In a more recent series, of 37 consecutive patients with PRCA, 1 individual had a coexistent thymoma, while a second had a thymoma resected before the onset of PRCA.[13] The incidence of PRCA in patients with thymomas has ranged from 1% to 15%.[8]

A variety of hematologic malignancies have been associated with PRCA (Table 23-1). PRCA is most frequently reported in patients with chronic lymphocytic leukemia (CLL). PRCA is found in 6% of CLL patients, of which two-thirds are B-cell, and one-third are T-cell CLL.[8,14-18] PRCA has been reported in patients with Hodgkin disease and non-Hodgkin lymphoma.[2,16,]

[20-28] In most of these cases, the PRCA has remitted with treatment of the lymphoma. PRCA has also been associated with acute lymphocytic leukemia.[29-31]

Chronic myeloid leukemia[12,33-35] and myelofibrosis with myeloid metaplasia have been reported with PRCA.[8,12,33-37] While the PRCA may precede the development of a myeloproliferative disease, it generally occurs during the course of the latter and may respond to immunosuppressive treatment.[34]

Several nonhematologic neoplasms have been reported to occur with PRCA (Table 23-1). However, an etiologic relationship between many of these neoplasms and PRCA has not been established. In only one case did treatment of the malignancy lead to a remission of the PRCA.[38]

In contrast to acquired chronic PRCA, which may occur as a primary or secondary disease, an acute and self-limited form of PRCA can arise during the course of a number of infectious processes (Table 23-1). A similar marrow erythroblastopenia has been reported after exposure to several drugs and chemicals[4,12,27,70-86] (Table 23-2). When the infection resolves, or the drug or chemical is removed, normal erythropoiesis is generally re-established. PRCA has also been reported to occur following exposure to herbicides or insecticides.[68-70] Chronic hemolytic anemias are occasionally complicated by an acute, self-limited form of PRCA that has been called "aplastic" crisis.[8,49, 62-68,87-91] This event generally occurs in children, lasts 5-10 days, and is often associated with a parvovirus infection.[58-68] Chronic autoimmune hemolytic anemia has also been reported with PRCA[8,92,93]; several cases of PRCA with systemic lupus erythematosus and chronic rheumatoid arthritis have also been published.[8,91,95,96] PRCA occurring during pregnancy has been noted in which the PRCA remitted following the delivery of a normal child.[97-99] In another case, PRCA occurred with megakaryocytic aplasia in a pregnant woman. After delivery of a normal baby, hematologic improvement was observed over a period of 1.5 years.[8] One mother with PRCA had three pregnancies in which PRCA and hydrops fetalis developed in each of the infants. Only the third fetus, which had received intrauterine red cell transfusions, survived. This infant's PRCA remitted after 3 months, and it is possible that the PRCA could have been due to a placentally transferred antibody to erythroid progenitor cells.[100]

PRCA also occurs in patients with renal failure[101] and in those with severe nutritional deficiency, such as marasmus and kwashiorkor.[102] Riboflavin deficiency has been implicated as a possible cause of anemia; some PRCA patients have responded to riboflavin administration.[79,102] In addition, severe megaloblastic anemia due to vitamin B_{12} or folic acid deficiency may lead to erythroid hypoplasia.[103] Because of these findings and the high incidence of pernicious anemia associated with PRCA, serum vitamin B_{12} and folic acid levels should be obtained in all patients with PRCA.[104-106]

BIOLOGIC AND MOLECULAR ASPECTS

Immunoglobulin Inhibitors

While marrow erythroblasts are clearly absent in PRCA, erythroid progenitor cells are often present. The marrow cells from 52% of these patients respond in vitro by increasing hemo-

Table 23-1. Classification of PRCA

I. Congenital
   Congenital hypoplastic anemia (Diamond-Blackfan syndrome)
II. Acquired
   A. Primary
      1. Autoimmune
         a. Immunoglobulin inhibitors
            i. Directed to marrow erythroid cells
            ii. Directed to erythropoietin
         b. T-cell inhibition of marrow erythroid cells
      2. Idiopathic
   B. Secondary
      1. Thyoma[2,4,8,13]
      2. Hematologic malignancies
         a. Chronic lymphocytic leukemia (CLL)
            i. B-cell type[8,14-16]
            ii. T-cell type[8,17-19]
         b. Malignant lymphomas
            i. Hodgkin disease[20-23]
            ii. Non-Hodgkin lymphomas[16,24-28]
         c. Acute lymphocytic leukemia[29-31]
         d. Multiple myeloma[32]
         e. Chronic myeloid leukemia[12,33-35]
         f. Myelofibrosis with myeloid metaplasia[8,35-37]
      3. Nonhematologic solid tumors
         a. Adenocarcinoma of stomach[38]
         b. Carcinoma of breast[39,40]
         c. Adenocarcinoma of bile duct[41]
         d. Carcinoma of lung[42-44]
         e. Carcinoma of thyroid[45]
         f. Adenocarcinoma (unknown primary)[46]
         g. Carcinoma of skin[44]
         h. Kaposi sarcoma[4,47,48]
      4. Infections
         a. Human immunodeficiency virus[49] and T-cell leukemia virus[50]
         b. Atypical pneumonia
         c. Mumps
         d. Viral hepatitis[51,52]
         e. Meningococcemia
         f. Staphylococcemia
         g. Infectious mononucleosis[53-56]
         h. Cytomegalovirus[57]
         i. B19 parvovirus[58-68]
         j. Leishmaniasis[69]
      5. Drugs and chemicals[4,12,27,70-86] (see Table 23-2)
      6. Hemolytic anemias[8,54,62-68,87-93]
      7. Systemic lupus erythematosus[8,91,94] and rheumatoid arthritis[8,95,96]
      8. Pregnancy[97-100]
      9. Severe renal failure[101]
      10. Severe nutritional deficiencies[79,102,103]

(Modified from Krantz and Zaentz,[6] with permission.)

Table 23-2. Drugs and Chemicals Associated with the Onset of PRCA

Allopurinol	Halothane
α-Methyldopa	Isoniazid
Aminopyrine	Maloprim (dapsone and pyrimethamine)
Anagyrine	Mepacrine
Arsphenamine	Methazolamide
Azathioprine	Penicillin
Benzene hexachloride	d-Penicillamine
Bromsulphalein	Pentachlorophenol
Calomel	Phenobarbital
Carbamazepine	Phenylbutazone
Cephalothin	Procainamide
Chenopodium	Salicylazosulfapyridine
Chloramphenicol	Santonin
Chlorpropamide	Sodium dipropylacetate
Co-trimoxazole	Sodium valproate
Diphenylhydantoin	Sulfasalazine
Estrogens	Sulfathiazol
Fenbufen	Sulindac
Fenoprofen	Thiamphenicol
Gold	Tolbutamide

(Data from Dessypris.[3])

tor is detectable in 40% of PRCA patients, and PRCA is the first human disease in which immune injury to the bone marrow has been demonstrated.

Erythropoietin, erythroid progenitor cells, or erythroblasts could each serve as potential targets for IgG inhibitors of erythropoiesis. Detection of large amounts of erythropoietin in the plasma of PRCA patients[70,112] has indicated that the inhibitor in PRCA is most likely directed to the marrow cells. Several investigators have administered PRCA plasma or sera to mice and found a marked impairment in erythropoiesis that was not observed with normal plasma, plasma from patients with other hematologic conditions, or plasma from the same PRCA patients in remission.[8,24,42,113-115] Normal rat bone marrow, which contains erythroblasts, absorbed the inhibitor, while the bone marrow cells from hypertransfused rats with a paucity of erythroblasts failed to absorb the inhibitor, again identifying erythroid marrow elements as a target for the inhibitor.[115]

The PRCA inhibitor appears to be directed against the erythroblasts in some cases and against the erythropoietin-responsive progenitor cells in others. When a patient's remission erythroblasts were radiolabeled with ^{59}Fe, and then incubated with the patient's pretreatment plasma and post-treatment remission plasma in the presence of complement, the pretreatment plasma produced a 50–100% increase in the release of radioactive hemoglobin, an index of cytotoxic damage to the erythroblasts.[34,112] The same findings occurred with the patient's pretreatment IgG, indicating that some PRCA patients have antibody that specifically damages their own erythroblasts. No similar cytotoxic effect was detected when blood lymphocytes or red cells served as the IgG target.[112] Light or electron microscopy also was used to identify IgG on the membranes of PRCA erythroblasts.[116,117] Since PRCA plasma frequently contains alloantibody to normal erythroblasts, acquired as a consequence of multiple transfusions, such assays must be performed with the patient's own cells to be certain an autoimmune phenomenon is occurring.

PRCA sera have also been shown to contain IgG that inhibits the development of the patient's own erythroid progenitor cells, the colony-forming unit-erythroid (CFU-E) as well as the burst-forming unit-erythroid (BFU-E). This has been observed both in adults with acquired primary and secondary PRCA[34,94,118,119] and in children with TEC.[110-120] The IgG was shown to act directly at the level of the CFU-E and BFU-E by removal of the IgG from these cells after short incubation periods.[110,119] A study was performed with a group of 12 children with TEC.[110] An IgG inhibitor of autologous erythroid colony development was found in 3 patients. In addition, 5 children who were not

globin synthesis by two- to ninefold.[70,71,107,108] When PRCA marrow cells are assayed in semisolid media, 60% have normal numbers of assayable erythroid progenitor cells, while 56% of children with TEC have a similar cloning efficiency pattern.[109,110] In the adults, increased erythropoietic proliferative capacity in vitro correlates with the therapeutic response to immunosuppressive therapy.[35,111]

The presence of erythroid progenitor cells that proliferate normally in vitro, but that will not produce red cells in vivo, is a remarkable feature of PRCA and TEC. The most likely reason for the exuberant erythropoiesis in vitro is the presence of an inhibitor in vivo that blocks effective erythropoiesis. It has been shown in these patients that incubation of marrow cells with patient plasma, or IgG, results in a marked inhibition of heme synthesis, but plasma, or plasma IgG, obtained after remission of the disease, is not inhibitory.[70,112] Such an inhibi-

previously transfused had an IgG that inhibited normal marrow CFU-E and BFU-E development but that did not inhibit the development of granulocyte/macrophage colonies. None of the IgG fractions neutralized erythropoietin, and erythroblast cytotoxicity was not demonstrable. Three of the IgG inhibitors were complement dependent, while one was inhibitory without the presence of complement. Among nine adult patients with acquired PRCA who were studied at one institution from 1980 to 1984, an IgG inhibitor to autologous CFU-E or BFU-E was found in six.[8] A similar IgG inhibitor, which inhibits granulocyte/macrophage progenitor cells in vitro, has been found in a patient with pure white blood cell aplasia,[121] while in megakaryocyte aplasia an IgG inhibitor of megakaryocyte progenitor cells has been identified.[122,123] Patients with combined PRCA and agranulocytosis, including one with an IgG inhibitor of erythropoiesis and granulopoiesis, have also been reported.[124]

Two unusual PRCA patients have been reported in whom erythropoietin levels were low.[125,126] Both patients appeared to have an IgG inhibitor directed against erythropoietin. In one case, the addition of goat antihuman γ-globulin to the patient's serum led to the removal of the serum erythropoietin along with the patient's IgG.[126] When the serum was boiled to denature the IgG, the detectable activity of the hormone was greatly increased.[126] Administration of the patient's IgG to mice led to severe anemia without the presence of increased erythropoietin levels, while other PRCA IgG preparations appeared to act on the marrow cells and produced anemia with increased erythropoietin levels. The precise incidence with which antibody to erythropoietin leads to PRCA is unknown, but it is thought to be far less common than in cases due to antibody to marrow erythroid cells.

T-Cell Inhibition of Marrow Erythroid Cells

A 6% incidence of PRCA in patients with CLL has been noted.[6,8,14,17,18,81,127,128] Serum inhibitors of erythropoiesis in these patients have not been found.[17,81,127] Initial investigations of a patient with T-cell CLL showed that blood lymphocytes inhibited normal marrow CFU-E growth and that treatment of the patient's marrow with antithymocyte globulin plus complement produced increased numbers of erythroid colonies in vitro.[17] Nagasawa et al.[18] studied a patient with T-cell CLL, PRCA, and hypogammaglobulinemia, in whom the T lymphocytes had membrane receptors for the Fc portion of the IgG molecule (Tγ). The Tγ lymphocytes were frozen and stored; they were shown to have a great inhibitory effect on CFU-E development by the patient's own post-treatment, remission bone marrow cells. No effect of media conditioned by these lymphocytes on erythropoiesis was observed, suggesting that direct cellular contact is required for this inhibition to occur. Since blood transfusions can induce sensitization of lymphocytes, and activated lymphocytes can inhibit erythropoiesis in vitro, these experiments were necessary to eliminate the possibility that these results were an epiphenomenon of alloimmunization.[129,130] No effect of Tγ cells was observed on myeloid colony formation. A similar inhibition of erythropoiesis in vitro by large granular lymphocytes has been demonstrated in two other patients with PRCA.[50,131] In an additional case of T-cell CLL, the suppressive effect of T cells was shown to be genetically restricted.[19]

PRCA occurs more commonly in association with B-cell CLL. In these cases, an increased percentage of marrow Tγ cells that inhibit CFU-E development has also been found. After removal of these Tγ cells, a large increase in CFU-E growth in vitro was observed.[127,132] Granulocyte/macrophage colony growth was not suppressed by these cells. In patients with B-cell CLL who did not have PRCA, an increased number of Tγ cells was present in the blood, but not in the marrow, suggesting that the PRCA may be attributable to enhanced migration of these cells into the marrow or to enhanced proliferation within the marrow. Thus, PRCA may occur only when a critical mass of Tγ cells are present in the marrow and may not necessarily be related to the number of these cells in the peripheral blood. While it seems clear that T cells may produce PRCA in T- and B-cell CLL, and possibly in certain viral illnesses,[52,55] this relationship is not clear in acquired primary PRCA.[8] In some cases, the increased number of T cells may be an epiphenomenon rather than of pathogenetic significance.[133]

Thymoma and PRCA

Attempts to induce anemia in animals by administering extracts of thymic tumors have been unsuccessful.[39] Some studies have indicated that the presence of a serum IgG inhibitor of erythroid development accounts for the PRCA, but these studies were performed with mice or allogeneic human marrow cells. The results might therefore merely be the result of alloimmunization, and their significance is unknown.[21,47,113–115,134] In another report, a patient with PRCA and a thymoma was found to have a bone marrow infiltrate with 30% activated T-suppressor cells similar to T cells in the pleural fluid invaded by the thymoma.[135] The patient's serum did not suppress marrow erythropoiesis in vitro, but removal of the marrow T cells increased marrow erythroid colony growth significantly; this process was reversed by reconstitution with the T cells. Immunosuppressive treatment that reduced the marrow lymphocytes by 75% led to remission of the disease. Altogether, studies on the pathogenesis of PRCA with thymoma are quite sparse, but the latter case indicates that suppression of erythropoiesis by T lymphocytes may occur in some of these patients.

Viral Infection and PRCA

Infection with the B19 parvovirus, which has been associated with fifth disease (erythema infectiosum), has also been associated with acute transient erythroblastopenia in patients with hemolytic anemia[58,60,64,65] and chronic PRCA.[66,67] Serum containing this DNA virus inhibits normal marrow CFU-E development in vitro; this inhibition can be prevented by antibody to the virus.[59,61] Little effect of the virus was found on granulocyte/macrophage colony formation. This virus has been identified in proliferating CFU-E and appears to be directly toxic for these cells.[59] A similar infection might occur in persons without hemolytic anemia and may produce a transient PRCA, yet go unrecognized, because of the normal red cell survival in these patients. In patients with immunodeficiency, from a variety of causes, PRCA may occur due to B19 parvovirus and this often responds to high-dose immunoglobulin therapy.[67,136–140] Of 56 patients with PRCA, 14% were chronically infected with the virus, identified by polymerase chain reaction amplification of B19 DNA from the patients' sera, and 6% had elevated anti-B19 serum IgM levels.[141] PRCA has also been reported in patients with viral hepatitis and Epstein-Barr virus; in one of these cases, an increase in T-suppressor cells in the marrow was associated with marked inhibition of autologous marrow CFU-E by the patient's bone marrow T cells, but not blood T cells.[52,55]

Autoimmune Hemolytic Anemia and PRCA

PRCA occurs in association with autoimmune hemolytic anemia. Several investigators postulated that the red cell antibodies might affect erythroid progenitor cells and produce the

PRCA.[89] In two cases of PRCA and autoimmune hemolytic anemia, an IgG eluate from the patient's red cells inhibited normal marrow and the patient's autologous marrow CFU-E development in vitro.[8,91] The latter effect appeared to be dependent on complement. In two other cases, antibody to red cell ee or E antigens appeared to be distinct from a serum IgG inhibitor of marrow CFU-E and BFU-E.[92,93]

Systemic Lupus Erythematosus or Rheumatoid Arthritis and PRCA

Cavalcant et al[94] demonstrated a serum IgG inhibitor to autologous marrow BFU-E in a patient with systemic lupus erythematosus. Dessypris et al.[95] demonstrated a similar inhibition of autologous CFU-E and BFU-E by the serum IgG of a patient with PRCA and rheumatoid arthritis. These two very carefully studied cases suggest that an antibody to a patient's erythroid progenitor cells can lead to PRCA in systemic lupus erythematosus or rheumatoid arthritis.

Drugs and PRCA

Drug-induced PRCA was clearly demonstrated in a patient receiving diphenylhydantoin. This patient achieved remission of the disease following cessation of the drug; with rechallenge, the PRCA was reinduced. The mechanism for this effect was thought to be a direct toxic effect on DNA synthesis by marrow erythroid cells.[142] In another case of diphenylhydantoin-associated PRCA, Dessypris et al.[73] showed that the patient's IgG markedly inhibited normal marrow CFU-E and BFU-E only in the presence of diphenylhydantoin. Diphenylhydantoin had no effect on the marrow cells in the presence of normal IgG or IgG prepared from the patient's serum after remission of PRCA. Autologous erythroid progenitor cells were inhibited in the same way, while no inhibitory effect on granulocyte/macrophage colony development, marrow erythroblasts, or erythropoietin was detected. The precise mechanism of inhibition remains unknown. A similar study of patients with isoniazid-associated PRCA and procainamide-associated PRCA failed to demonstrate a similar effect.[77] These discrepancies could be due to the presence of multiple pathogenetic mechanisms leading to drug-associated PRCA.

Figure 23-1 summarizes data indicating that erythropoietin-responsive cells, erythroblasts, or erythropoietin are the targets of immunoglobulin inhibitors in acquired primary PRCA. The most frequent target appears to be the erythroid progenitor cells. In CLL, T-cell inhibition of the erythroid progenitor cells is also well documented but is less clearly operational in cases of primary PRCA. The acute pure red cell aplastic crisis that occurs in patients with hemolytic anemia is most often due to direct toxicity of the parvovirus to the CFU-E.

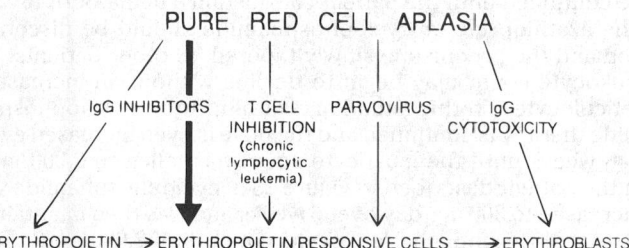

Fig. 23-1. Different mechanisms by which erythropoiesis may be inhibited in PRCA. (Modified from Krantz and Dessypris,[7] with permission.)

CLINICAL MANIFESTATIONS

Patients with PRCA feel weak and tired. The degree of this weakness is proportional to the degree of the anemia. Since red cells normally survive 120 days in the circulation, a complete cessation of erythropoiesis leads to a decline of the red cell count of approximately 1%/day. With such a slowly progressive anemia, sufficient time is available for adjustment of the patient's blood volume. PRCA patients are often ambulatory at hematocrits of 15–20%. TEC often is preceded by symptoms of a viral illness. The physical examination is generally unremarkable, except for pallor. No organomegaly related to the PRCA or TEC is present. In primary acquired PRCA, additional physical findings are more likely to be related to other conditions, while in secondary PRCA they may reflect the primary condition that is predisposing to the PRCA. Those patients who have received multiple transfusions for PRCA may eventually exhibit signs of hepatitis or hemosiderosis, or both.

LABORATORY EVALUATION

The red cells in acquired PRCA are generally normochromic and normocytic, but early in the disease, a macrocytosis may be present. Polychromatophilic red cells are usually absent. The reticulocyte count is <1.0%, and most often no reticulocytes are observed.[4] The white blood cell and platelet counts are normal, but an occasional patient may have a mild leukopenia or thrombocytopenia and, occasionally, a mild lymphocytosis or eosinophilia is evident.[4] Patients should be screened for B19 parvovirus by serum anti-B19 IgM and B19 DNA identification.[141]

The bone marrow is characterized by an almost complete absence of erythroblasts.[2] In some cases, however, small numbers of proerythroblasts (3–4%) are present, with a smaller number of mature erythroblasts, showing a "maturation arrest."[9,71,89,108] On rare occasions, PRCA may either recur or begin with a period of ineffective erythropoiesis and erythroblast phagocytosis.[143,144] In a previously diagnosed patient, this may be taken as an indication of recurrence of PRCA, but in a new patient the correct diagnosis may not be apparent until the PRCA appears. Unlike aplastic anemia, PRCA is associated with normal marrow cellularity. Granulopoiesis and megakarocytopoiesis are normal. Increased numbers of small aggregated or diffusely scattered lymphocytes may be present.[4,47] Adequate marrow particle sections or a bone marrow biopsy must be obtained to ascertain the ratio of cells to fat spaces. Plate 23-1A shows a marrow particle section from such a patient and indicates normal cellularity. Both the marrow particle section and particle smear (Plate 23-1B) show that most of the cells are of the granulocytic lineage with additional small lymphocytes, but no erythroblasts are present. After treatment, a large number of erythroblasts appear (Plate 23-1C). On rare occasions, an increased marrow cellularity due to a granulocytic or lymphocytic hyperplasia may be observed.[4,47,108] Stainable iron in the marrow is generally increased because of a lack of iron utilization, as well as iron deposition following red cell transfusions. Cytogenetic studies in acquired PRCA are most often normal. Of 37 consecutive patients with PRCA, only 1, in whom acute myelomonocytic leukemia subsequently developed, had an abnormal karyotype (47,XY, +G).[5,8] Ferrokinetic studies show prolonged clearance of ^{59}Fe and extremely low red cell ^{59}Fe incorporation.[47,145] After remission, ferrokinetics generally return to normal, but an occasional patient may have evidence of ineffective erythropoiesis, and some may have evidence of an expanded marrow distribution.[145] ^{111}In, which binds selectively to transferrin, can also be used to scan the marrow for erythropoietic activity; this shows minimal uptake in PRCA but normal uptake during remission.[146] No specific radiographic findings are present other than those relating to the presence of a thymoma. A computed tomography scan of the mediastinum should be performed in all cases, because of a high incidence of thymomas. Uptake of selenomethionine ^{75}Se or gallium citrate ^{67}Ga has also been used to detect this tumor.[147,148]

Chronic acquired PRCA has been associated with a large number of abnormalities of the immune system.[8,149] These include thymomas,[2,4] paraproteins,[71] hypogammaglobulinemia,[3,149] pyroproteins,[71] hypocomplementemia,[150] anergy,[6] presence of antinuclear antibodies,[70,134,151] reduced phytohemagglutinin-induced lymphocyte-mediated cytotoxicity,[152] angioimmunoblastic lymphadenopathy,[153,154] and autoimmune hemolytic anemia.[3,89,92] When PRCA occurs in conjunction with chronic active hepatitis,[51,52] myasthenia gravis,[149,155,156] systemic lupus erythematosus,[8,91,94] acquired immunodeficiency syndrome,[49,67] multiple endocrine glandular insufficiency,[157] hypothyroidism,[118,158,159] or pernicious anemia,[104–106] the immunologic abnormalities characteristic of those diseases may be seen as well.

THERAPY

Initially, all drugs being given to patients with PRCA should be discontinued, and any infection should be treated. Drug- or infection-induced PRCA generally remits within 1–3 weeks of removal of the inciting agent. If B19 parvovirus is identified, the PRCA often responds to the administration of anti-parvovirus

DIFFERENTIAL DIAGNOSIS

Because of its unique bone marrow morphology, PRCA is usually readily identifiable. PRCA is generally easily distinguished from aplastic anemia, which is characterized by reduced marrow cellularity and is accompanied by leukopenia and thrombocytopenia. Examination of a bone marrow aspirate permits rapid differentiation of PRCA from megaloblastic anemia or myelodysplastic disorders with marked ineffective erythropoiesis. However, PRCA may be confused with cases of myelodysplasia with erythroid hypoplasia. In these cases, the bone marrow has more erythroblasts (2–5%) than generally observed with other forms of PRCA, and evidence for a maturation arrest is lacking. Ringed sideroblasts may be present, cytogenetic abnormalities are frequent, and the number of blasts may be increased. In addition, patients with myelodysplasia may have reduced neutrophil alkaline phosphatase or myeloperoxidase activity and neutrophils with Pelger-Huët nuclei. The megakaryocytes may have immature single large nuclei. Platelets of a patient with a myelodysplastic disorder may function abnormally and produce a prolonged bleeding time.

In children, TEC must be distinguished from congenital hypoplastic anemia. The latter generally occurs during the first 18 months of life and may be associated with other congenital abnormalities. Red cells in congenital hypoplastic anemia often have an increased erythrocyte mean corpuscular volume and increased levels of hemoglobin F, i antigen, and glycolytic enzymes. These changes appear to reflect increased erythropoiesis with fetal characteristics, compared with the complete lack of erythropoiesis seen in TEC. Patients with the latter also often have a preceding history of a viral illness.

antibodies in pooled serum IgG.[66,67,136,137,140] Any malignancy should be treated. A thymoma should be resected before further treatment of the PRCA is considered. Removal of a thymoma has resulted in a remission of PRCA within 4–8 weeks in 29% of cases and has improved the response rate to corticosteroids in others.[2,4] Many patients did not respond to further treatment unless the thymoma was first resected, although some have mounted a response.[4] If the thymoma cannot be resected, radiotherapy should be used, and this may produce a remission.[24,160] Removal of a normal thymus gland has not proved of value.[8] If treatment of a thymoma does not provide a remission, the patient should be treated similarly to other patients with primary PRCA.

With increasing evidence for an autoimmune pathogenesis of PRCA, therapy now consists mainly of the use of immunosuppressive agents. In a recent study, no remissions resulted from folic acid or vitamin B_{12} therapy; of 22 patients treated with androgenic steroids, only 1 patient had a temporary response.[13]

Since cytotoxic immunosuppressive drugs increase the incidence of acute leukemia and skin and gastrointestinal carcinomas and also lead to the development of infertility, corticosteroids should be the initial therapy of choice in PRCA, particularly among younger patients.[161–164] Administration of prednisone (60 mg/day) has resulted in a 37% remission rate.[13] These remissions have always occurred within 4 weeks. After the hematocrit rose to 35%, the corticosteroids were slowly tapered and discontinued. A high incidence of recurrence of the PRCA was noted and, although further remissions could be induced in some patients, others became refractory to corticosteroids. Nevertheless, because of the short period of treatment, the limited number of complications, the reduced expense, and the ambulatory nature of this treatment, corticosteroids continue to be the initial form of treatment for chronic acquired primary PRCA.

If corticosteroid administration fails to produce remission, several alternate modes of therapy are available. Steroids should be rapidly reduced to a dose of 30 mg/day, and treatment with either azathioprine, cyclophosphamide, or antithymocyte globulin (ATG) should be initiated. One of the former two drugs should be administered at a dose of 50–100 mg/day and gradually increased to doses of 2.2 mg/kg over 2–3 weeks.[13,59,70–72,112,165–169] Blood counts should be obtained each week to detect leukopenia or thrombocytopenia. If no toxicity is apparent, these drugs should be continued for an additional 4–8 weeks, with blood counts performed every 1–2 weeks. When normal erythropoiesis is re-established, or when the leukocyte count falls to <2,000/mm³, or the platelet count drops below 80,000/mm³, the cytotoxic drug should be discontinued. If this has not occurred, the dose of azathioprine or cyclophosphamide can be increased by 50-mg increments every 3–4 weeks until either normal erythropoiesis commences or toxicity necessitates interruption of therapy.

In some patients, the first sign of a response is an increase in reticulocytes with a disappearance of transfusion requirement and subsequent rise in hematocrit (Fig. 23-2). The drugs should be continued until the patient can sustain a hematocrit of 35%. The azathioprine or cyclophosphamide should be discontinued and the prednisone slowly tapered. In other patients, the leukocyte count may begin to decline without an increase in reticulocytes. In this situation, azathioprine or cyclophosphamide therapy is continued and the dose is even increased every 4–8 weeks until the leukocyte count has fallen to 2,000/mm³. In the patient described in Figure 23-3, cyclophosphamide was increased to 300 mg/day over 6 weeks and was then maintained at that dose until the leukocyte count was 2,000/mm³. Only then did the first reticulocytes appear in the blood. The cyclophosphamide was then decreased, and the patient's erythropoiesis increased. In other patients, if no response is evident,

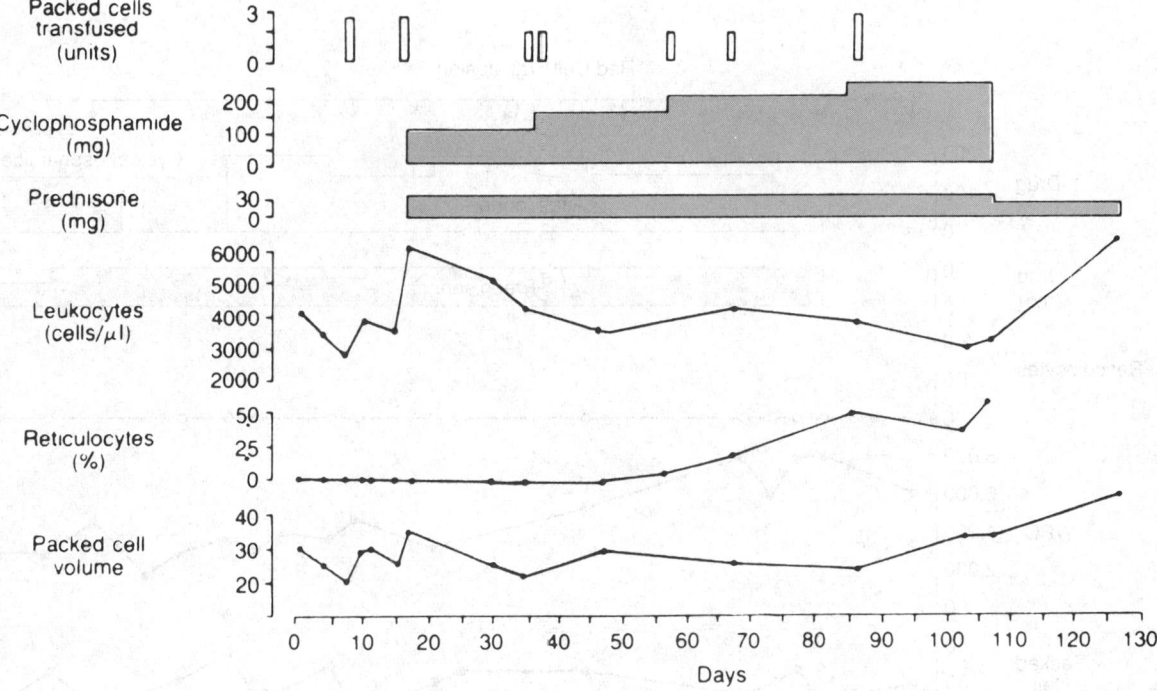

Fig. 23-2. Gradual response of a 43-year-old man with PRCA to cyclophosphamide and prednisone. Patient needed frequent red cell transfusions during the first 40 days of treatment to maintain his packed red cell volume, but reticulocytes gradually increased to 5%, and the patient then maintained a normal packed red cell volume without further transfusions. Both drugs were subsequently discontinued. (Modified from Hartmann and Krantz,[167] with permission.)

and the white blood cells continue to decline below 2,000/mm³, azathioprine or cyclophosphamide should be discontinued and prednisone therapy maintained. Once the marrow recovers within 3–5 weeks, increased reticulocytes may appear. In this event, when the hematocrit reaches 35%, prednisone

therapy should be slowly tapered and discontinued. In a series of 37 PRCA patients, 56% had a remission with this form of therapy, even though many had previously failed treatment with prednisone alone.[13] Crossover from one cytotoxic agent to the other also has been reported to produce a remission in

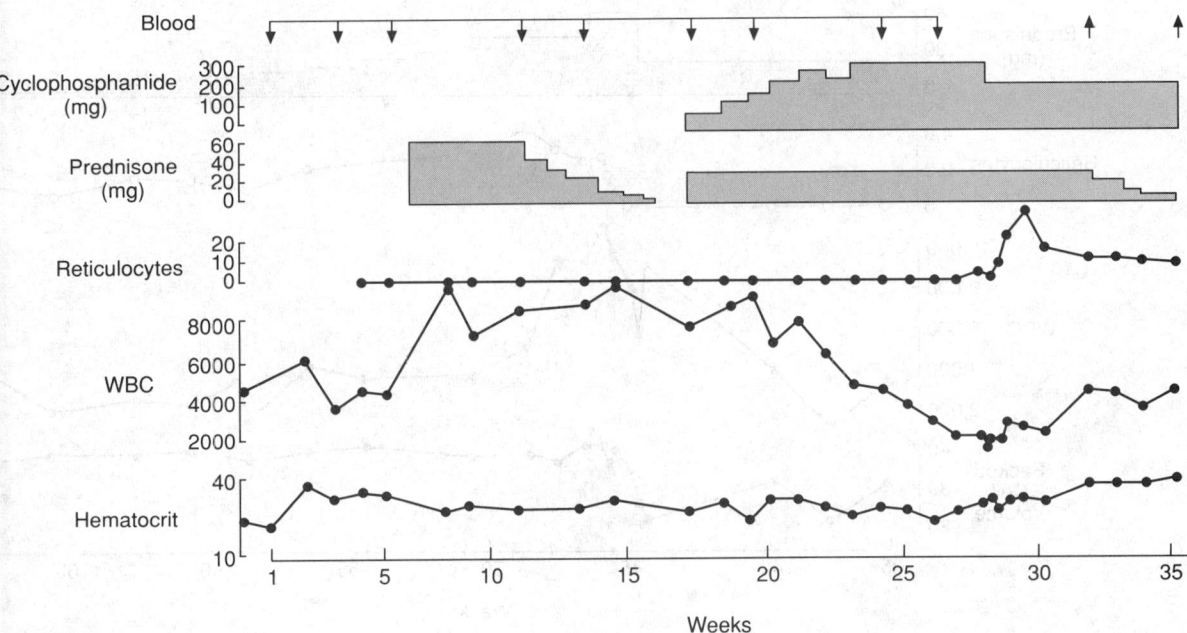

Fig. 23-3. Response of PRCA to cyclophosphamide and prednisone simultaneous to the appearance of marrow toxicity. This 38-year-old man had little response to prednisone alone. Cyclophosphamide was added and gradually increased until the leukocyte count was 2,000 cells/mm³; at this point, reticulocytes first appeared. The cyclophosphamide dose was reduced; the patient was then able to sustain his hematocrit while being phlebotomized for the removal of iron. (Modified from Krantz,[169] with permission.)

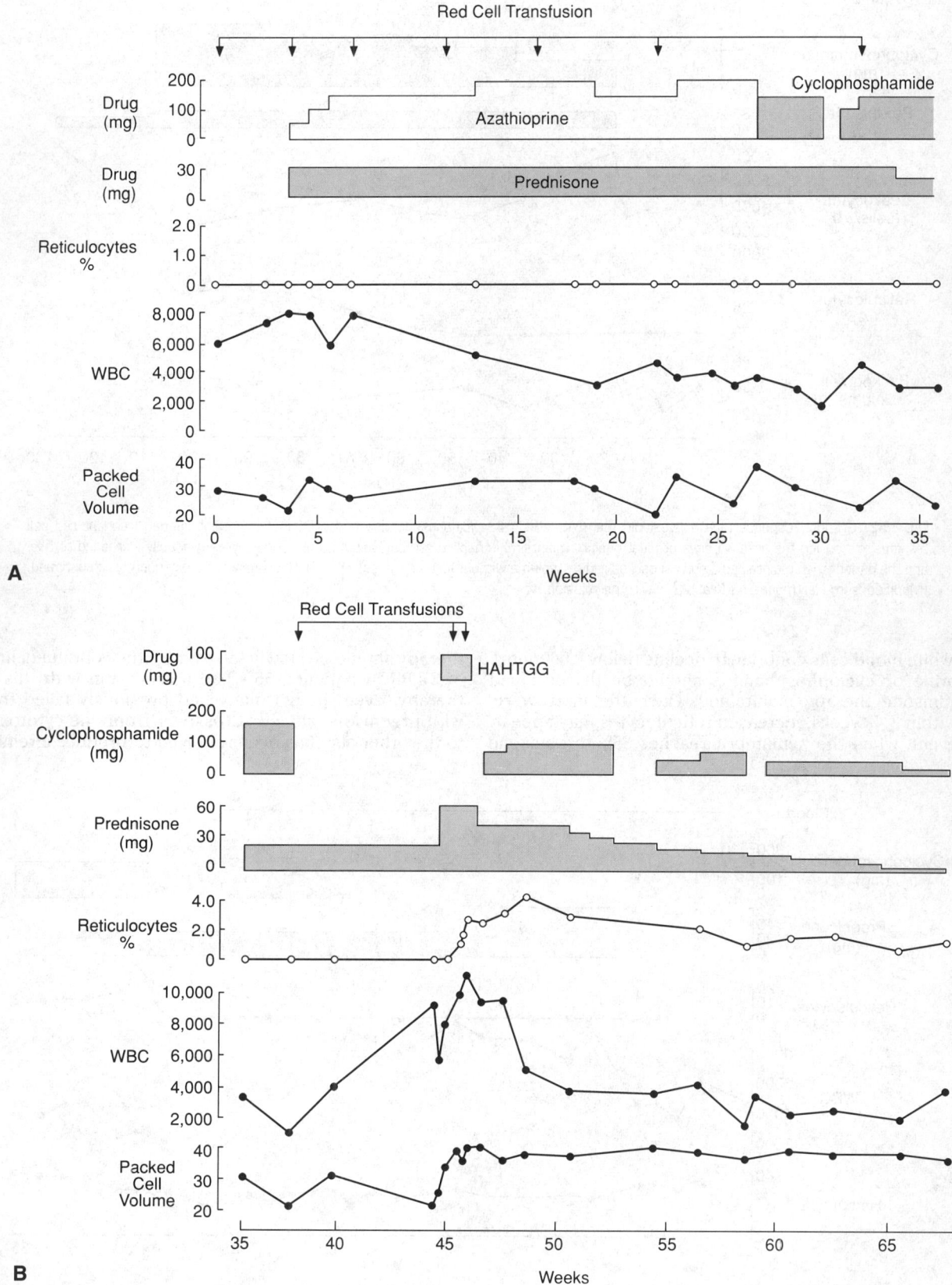

Fig. 23-4. Fifty-year-old woman with PRCA. **(A)** After failure to respond to azathioprine or cyclophosphamide, and prednisone, **(B)** response to horse antihuman thymocyte γ-globulin (HAHTGG) (20 mg/kg/day IV) for 8 days is shown. (Modified from Krantz,[171] with permission.)

three of five patients who failed initial therapy with the other drug.[168]

An alternate mode of therapy is the administration of ATG.[35,47,81,150,170–172] Figure 23-4 demonstrates the response of a patient to horse antihuman thymocyte γ-globulin (HAHTGG) (Atgam; Upjohn, Kalamazoo, MI). This patient failed to respond to azathioprine, cyclophosphamide, or corticosteroid therapy (Fig. 23-4A) but had a dramatic response to 8 days of HAHTGG infused at 20 mg/kg/day according to the schedule recommended by Champlin et al[178] (Fig. 23-4B). This patient has remained in remission for 5 years. In a recent series of nine PRCA patients treated with HAHTGG, six responded to therapy, with five obtaining normal hematocrits and one a hematocrit of 32%.[172] Four of the responders suffered from primary PRCA, while one had PRCA secondary to B-cell CLL, and another had PRCA secondary to infectious mononucleosis. Fever and serum sickness were the most common complications of this therapy and were seen in seven of nine patients. Three of the patients remained in a complete remission, whereas two relapsed. In another report, one patient with T-cell CLL had a transient response to ATG.[174] These patients can receive a second course of HAHTGG or an antithymocyte serum or globulin produced by another species and often will have a complete remission after such a second course.[171,175] Since ATG has no known leukemogenic or teratogenic effects, it may be especially useful for treating PRCA in young patients who may still wish to have children.

In patients refractory to the above therapies, cyclosporine may be tried. This agent has been primarily used for prevention of graft-versus-host disease following organ transplantation but has also been used for the treatment of autoimmune diseases.[176–178] Patients with primary PRCA, as well as PRCA secondary to CLL, have responded to cyclosporine when administered at 8–12 mg/kg/day PO in divided doses.[8,179–185] Prednisone (30 mg/day PO) should be added to this regimen to obtain a synergistic depression of the immune system.[176] Although reports of its use in PRCA are scarce, recent studies have indicated that 3 of 4,[8] 5 of 6,[184] 6 of 9,[185] and 6 of 8[186] patients responded very rapidly, consistent with individual case reports that generally show a response within the first 8–12 weeks.[8,179–184] The advantage of this drug is its rapid effect and its ability to be administered in an ambulatory setting. The disadvantage of cyclosporine lies in the severe renal toxicity that can result if the patients are not followed carefully. Weekly serum creatinine, bilirubin, transaminase, and alkaline phosphatase levels should also be obtained; at the first sign of organ toxicity, the dose of cyclosporine should be adjusted downward. When remission is produced, the drug dose should be gradually tapered. In some patients, it can be withdrawn completely, while in other cases, small maintenance doses may be necessary to maintain remission and, in the event of a relapse, second remissions can be induced with retreatment.[8,183,184]

Other forms of therapy available for primary acquired PRCA are administration of danazol[187] the use of plasmapheresis[119,188–192] and lymphocytopheresis,[189,192] and administration of high-dose intravenous γ-globulin.[8,16,66,67,193–195] As only small numbers of individual case reports citing results with these treatments are available, a precise incidence of remission and duration of remission is not known. Finally, splenectomy has been reported to have a 17% response rate[8]; most of these patients have had durable, long-standing remissions.[13] In addition, some patients, previously refractory to treatment, have responded to immunosuppressive drugs only after splenectomy.[6,13,196] Altogether, many modes of immunosuppressive therapy are now available for PRCA and these should be tried in succession, as it is not possible to predict which might be most effective in an individual patient.

Although spontaneous remissions have been reported in

APPROACH TO THERAPY FOR ACQUIRED PRCA

Once it is clear that the acquired PRCA is not due to an infection, drugs, or neoplasm, it is then most likely secondary to an autoimmune process. Many immunosuppressive therapies are now available and I start with the safest, easiest to use, and least expense choices. If the PRCA does not remit, I subsequently escalate the therapy to combinations of drugs that have enhanced immunosuppressive capacity, but also, unfortunately, increased complications and expense. Thus, prednisone (60 mg/day) is my preferred initial therapy, but if it does not work within 4 weeks I reduce the dose to 30 mg/day and add other immunosuppressive drugs. The reason for reducing the dose is that with the addition of other immunosuppressive agents I have encountered a very high incidence of infections.

After 4 weeks of high-dose prednisone either azathioprine, cyclophosphamide, antithymocyte globulin (ATG), or cyclosporine should be initiated with prednisone (30 mg/day). Overall, each of these drugs has an approximate 55–75% remission rate and the choice should be made based on the characteristics of each individual case and on local physician expertise and experience. Cyclophosphamide is probably more immunosuppressive than azathioprine, but also has more toxicity. Cyclosporine is more expensive and its use has to be accompanied by costly weekly serum chemistries to minimize serious renal toxicity. ATG is very effective and has few long-term complications, but the patient needs to be hospitalized during its administration because of the possibility of an anaphylactic reaction to the foreign protein. Nevertheless, the major point is that each of these therapies is effective, and when used in succession, one can expect a remission rate of ≥80%. Since patients can be completely resistant to some forms of therapy and very sensitive to others, it is necessary to be very persistent and thorough in treating PRCA.

10–15% of PRCA patients, these usually occur at the onset of the disease but have occurred ≤14 years after diagnosis.[13]

PROGNOSIS

Of patients with PRCA, 80% will have either a spontaneous remission (14%) or remission induced by immunosuppressive treatment (66%).[8,13,35,81] More than one-half of patients in complete remission will relapse, but with additional treatment a second remission can be induced in 80% of these patients.[13] By retreating several times or continuing maintenance immunosuppression in those patients with a tendency to relapse, 70% of relapsing patients, including those with spontaneous remissions, or slightly more than one-half (54%) of patients with drug-induced remissions, can be maintained transfusion-free for years thereafter.[13] Because additional effective modes of immunosuppression have become available since these reports, it is likely that current remission rates are now higher. The median survival of patients with primary acquired PRCA in a recent series was 14 years.[13] Nevertheless, immunosuppressive therapy must be administered carefully, since one-third of these patients acquired serious infections as a consequence of therapy.[13] Rarely, patients with PRCA have had a progression of their disease to aplastic anemia, and some have developed leukopenia or thrombocytopenia.[3,4] Acute myeloid

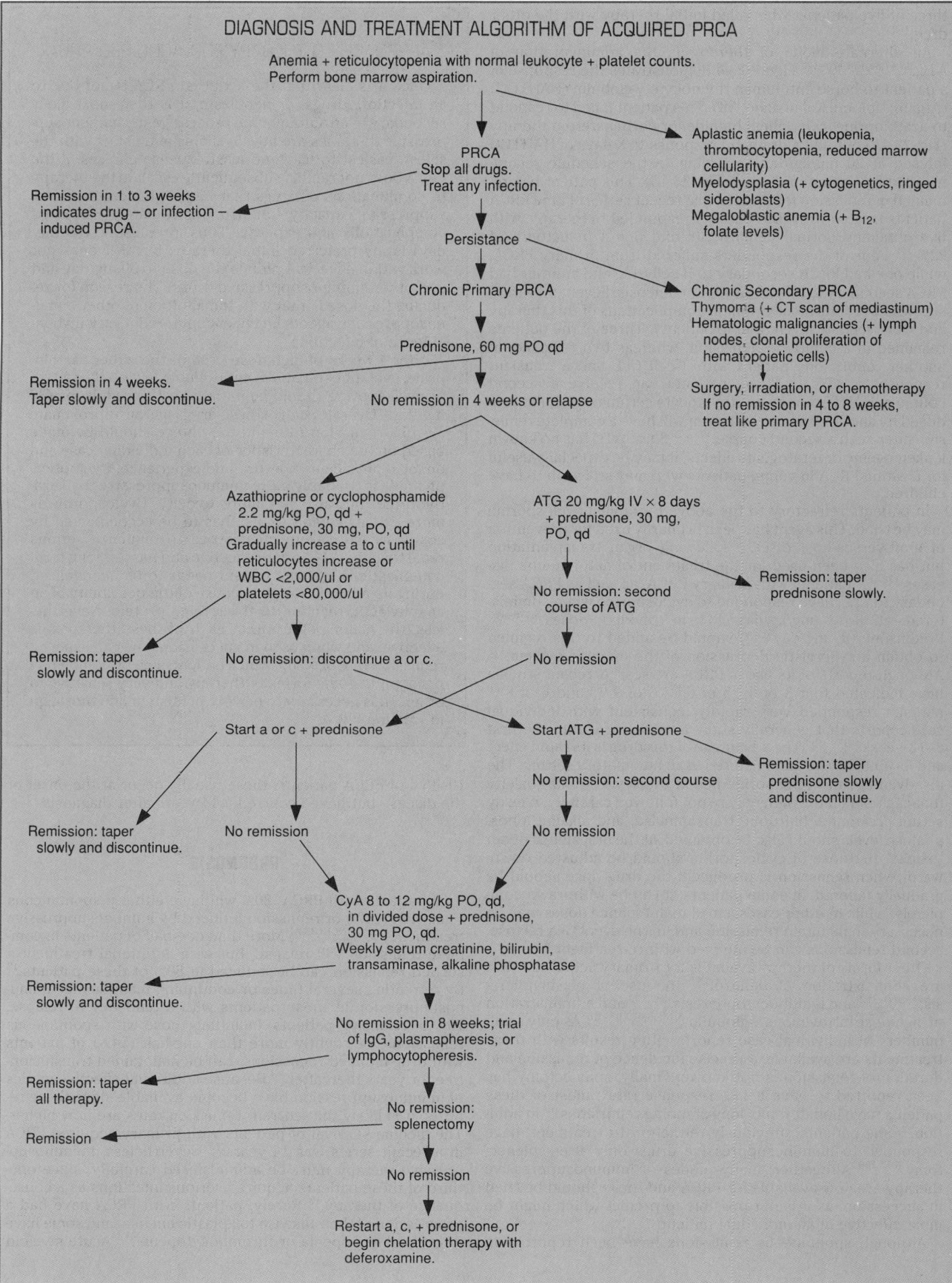

DIAGNOSIS AND TREATMENT ALGORITHM OF ACQUIRED PRCA

Anemia + reticulocytopenia with normal leukocyte + platelet counts.
Perform bone marrow aspiration.

Aplastic anemia (leukopenia,
thrombocytopenia, reduced marrow
cellularity)
Myelodysplasia (+ cytogenetics, ringed
sideroblasts)
Megaloblastic anemia (+ B_{12},
folate levels)

PRCA
Stop all drugs.
Treat any infection.

Remission in 1 to 3 weeks
indicates drug – or infection –
induced PRCA.

Persistance

Chronic Primary PRCA

Chronic Secondary PRCA
Thymoma (+ CT scan of mediastinum)
Hematologic malignancies (+ lymph
nodes, clonal proliferation of
hematopoietic cells)

Surgery, irradiation, or chemotherapy
If no remission in 4 to 8 weeks,
treat like primary PRCA.

Prednisone, 60 mg PO qd

Remission in 4 weeks.
Taper slowly and discontinue.

No remission in 4 weeks or relapse

Azathioprine or cyclophosphamide
2.2 mg/kg PO, qd +
prednisone, 30 mg, PO, qd
Gradually increase a to c until
reticulocytes increase or
WBC <2,000/ul or
platelets <80,000/ul

ATG 20 mg/kg IV × 8 days
+ prednisone, 30 mg,
PO, qd

Remission: taper
prednisone slowly.

No remission: second
course of ATG

Remission: taper
slowly and discontinue.

No remission: discontinue a or c.

No remission

Start a or c + prednisone

Start ATG + prednisone

Remission: taper
prednisone slowly
and discontinue.

Remission: taper
slowly and discontinue.

No remission

No remission: second course

No remission

CyA 8 to 12 mg/kg PO, qd,
in divided dose + prednisone,
30 mg PO, qd.
Weekly serum creatinine, bilirubin,
transaminase, alkaline phosphatase

Remission: taper
slowly and discontinue.

No remission in 8 weeks; trial
of IgG, plasmapheresis, or
lymphocytopheresis.

Remission: taper
all therapy.

No remission:
splenectomy

Remission

No remission

Restart a, c, + prednisone, or
begin chelation therapy with
deferoxamine.

leukemia has developed in 4% of patients with PRCA.[8] Patients refractory to all modes of therapy, who continue to have PRCA, suffer the consequences of frequent red cell transfusions: hepatitis, hemosiderosis, transfusion reactions, and recurrent infections. Iron chelation therapy should be started before organ dysfunction ensues, by infusing deferoxamine mesylate subcutaneously, using a portable pump.[197]

REFERENCES

1. Kaznelson P: Zur Entstehung der Blutplattchen. Verh Dtsch Ges Inn Med 34:557, 1922
2. Jacobs EM, Hutter RV, Pool JL, Ley AB: Benign thymoma and selective erythroid aplasia of the bone marrow. Cancer 12:47, 1959
3. DiGiacomo J, Furst SW, Nixon DD: Primary acquired red cell aplasia in the adult. Mt Sinai J Med 33:382, 1966
4. Hirst E, Robertson TI: The syndrome of thymoma and erythroblastopenic anemia: a review of 56 cases including 3 case reports. Medicine 46:225, 1967
5. Dessypris EN, Fogo A, Russell M et al: Studies on pure red cell aplasia. X. Association with acute leukemia and significance of bone marrow karyotype abnormalities. Blood 56:421, 1980
6. Krantz SB, Zaentz SD: Pure red cell aplasia. p. 153. In Gordon AS, Silber R, LoBue J (eds): The Year in Hematology. Plenum, New York, 1977
7. Krantz SB, Dessypris EN: Pure red cell aplasia. p. 229. In Golde DW, Takaku F (eds): Hematopoietic Stem Cells. Marcel Dekker, New York, 1985
8. Dessypris EN: Pure Red Cell Aplasia. Johns Hopkins University Press, Baltimore, 1988
9. Wranne L: Transient erythroblastopenia in infancy and childhood. Scand J Haematol 7:76, 1970
10. Diamond LK, Wang WC, Alter BP: Congenital hypoplastic anemia. Adv Pediatr 22:349, 1976
11. Wang WC, Mentzer WC: Differentiation of transient erythroblastopenia of childhood from congenital hypoplastic anemia. J Pediatr 88:784, 1976
12. Schmid JR, Kiely JM, Pease GL, Hargraves MM: Acquired pure red cell agenesis: report of 16 cases and review of the literature. Acta Haematol 30:255, 1963
13. Clark DA, Dessypris EN, Krantz SB: Studies on pure red cell aplasia. XI. Results of immunosuppressive treatment of 37 patients. Blood 63:227, 1984
14. Chikkappa G, Zarrali MH, Tsan MF: Pure red cell aplasia in patients with chronic lymphocytic leukemia. Medicine 65:339, 1986
15. Mangan KF, Chikkappa G, Farley PC: T-gamma (Tγ) cells suppress growth of erythroid colony forming units in vitro in the pure red cell aplasia of B-cell chronic lymphocytic leukemia. J Clin Invest 70:1148, 1982
16. Clauvel JP, Vainchenker W, Herrera A et al: Treatment of pure red cell aplasia by high-dose intravenous immunoglobulins. Br J Haematol 55:380, 1983
17. Hoffman R, Kopel S, Hsu SD et al: T cell chronic lymphocytic leukemia: presence in bone marrow and peripheral blood of cells that suppress erythropoiesis in vitro. Blood 52:255, 1978
18. Nagasawa T, Abe T, Nakagawa T: Pure red cell aplasia and hypogammaglobulinemia associated with Tγ-cell chronic lymphocytic leukemia. Blood 57:1025, 1981
19. Lipton JM, Nadler LM, Canellos GP et al: Evidence for genetic restriction in the suppression of erythropoiesis by a unique subset of T-lymphocytes in man. J Clin Invest 72:694, 1983
20. Bove JR: Combined erythroid hypoplasia and symptomatic hemolytic anemia. N Engl J Med 255:135, 1956
21. Field EO, Caughi MN, Blackett NM, Smithers DW: Marrow suppressing factors in the blood in pure red cell aplasia, thymoma and Hodgkin's disease. Br J Haematol 15:101, 1968
22. Guerra L, Najman A, Homberg JC et al: Auto-anticorps multiples au cours d'une maladie de Hodgkin: interpretation d'une erythroblastopenie. Nouv Rev Fr Hematol 9:601, 1969
23. Morgan E, Pang KM, Goldwasser E: Hodgkin's disease and red cell aplasia. Am J Hematol 5:71, 1978
24. Jepson JH, Vas M: Decreased in vivo and in vitro erythropoiesis induced by plasma of ten patients with thymoma, lymphosarcoma or idiopathic erythroblastopenia. Cancer Res 34:1325, 1974
25. Hunt FA, Lander CM: Successful use of combination chemotherapy in pure red cell aplasia associated with malignant lymphoma of histiocytic type. Aust NZ J Med 5:469, 1975
26. Prasad AS, Tranchida L, Palutke M, Ponlik DM: Red cell hypoplasia and monoclonal gammopathy in a patient with lymphoproliferative disorder. Am J Med Sci 271:355, 1976
27. Lee CH, Firkin FC, Grace CS, Rozenberg MC: Pure red cell aplasia: a report

of three cases with studies on circulating toxic factors against erythroid precursors. Aust NZ J Med 8:75, 1978
28. Carloss HW, Saab GA, Tavassoli M: Pure red cell aplasia and lymphoma. JAMA 242:67, 1979
29. deAlarcon PA, Miller ML, Stuart MJ: Erythroid hypoplasia: an unusual presentation of childhood acute lymphoblastic leukemia. Am J Dis Child 132:763, 1978
30. Imamura N, Kuramoto A, Morimoto T, Ihara A: Pure red cell aplasia associated with acute lymphoblastic leukemia of pre-T cell origin. Med J Aust 144:724, 1986
31. Sallan SE, Buchanan GR: Selective erythroid aplasia during therapy for acute lymphoblastic leukemia. Pediatrics 59:895, 1977
32. Gilbert EF, Harley JB, Anido V et al: Thymoma, plasma cell myeloma, red cell aplasia and malabsorption syndrome. Am J Med 44:820, 1968
33. Kitahara M: Pure RBC aplasia associated with chronic granulocytic leukemia. JAMA 240:376, 1978
34. Dessypris EN, McKee LC, Metzantonakis C et al: Red cell aplasia and chronic granulocytic leukemia. Br J Haematol 48:217, 1981
35. Lacombe C, Casadevall N, Muller O, Varet B: Erythroid progenitors in adult chronic pure red cell aplasia: relationship of in vitro erythroid colonies to therapeutic response. Blood 64:71, 1984
36. Bentley SA, Murray KH, Lewis SM, Roberts PD: Erythroid hypoplasia in myelofibrosis: a feature associated with blastic transformation. Br J Haematol 36:41, 1977
37. Barosi G, Baraldi A, Cazzola M et al: Red cell aplasia in myelofibrosis with myeloid metaplasia: a distinct functional and clinical entity. Cancer 52:1290, 1983
38. Gajwani B, Zinner EN: Pure red cell aplasia associated with adenocarcinoma of stomach. NY State J Med 76:2177, 1976
39. Clarkson BC, Prockop DJ: A regenerative anemia associated with benign thymoma. N Engl J Med 259:253, 1958
40. Slater LM, Schlutz MJ, Armentrout SA: Remission of pure red cell aplasia associated with non thymic malignancy. Cancer 44:1879, 1979
41. Lee CH, Clark AR, Thorpe ME et al: Bile duct adenocarcinoma with Leser-Trelat sign and pure red blood cell aplasia. Cancer 46:1657, 1980
42. Entwistle CC, Fentem PH, Jacobs A: Red cell aplasia with carcinoma of the bronchus. Br Med J 2:1504, 1964
43. Brafield AJ, Verbov J: A case of thrombocythemia with red cell aplasia. Postgrad Med J 42:525, 1966
44. Guthrie TH, Thornton RM: Pure red cell aplasia obscured by a diagnosis of carcinoma. South Med J 76:532, 1983
45. Iannuci A, Perini A, Pizzolo G: Acquired pure red cell aplasia associated with thyroid carcinoma: a case report. Acta Haematol 69:62, 1983
46. Mitchell ABS, Pinn G, Pegrum GD: Pure red cell aplasia and carcinoma. Blood 37:594, 1971
47. Marmont A, Peschle C, Sanguinetti M, Condorelli M: Pure red cell aplasia: response of three patients to cyclophosphamide and/or antilymphocyte globulin (ALG) and demonstration of two types of serum IgG inhibitors to erythropoiesis. Blood 45:247, 1975
48. Shimm DS, Logue GL, Rohlfing MB, Gaede JT: Primary amyloidosis, pure red cell aplasia and Kaposi's sarcoma in a single patient. Cancer 44:1501, 1979
49. Berner YN, Berrebi A, Green L et al: Erythroblastopenia in acquired immunodeficiency syndrome (AIDS). Acta Haematol 70:273, 1983
50. Levitt LJ, Reyes GR, Moonka DK et al: Human T cell leukemia virus-1 associated T-suppressor cell inhibition of erythropoiesis in a patient with pure red cell aplasia and chronic Tγ-lymphoproliferative disease. J Clin Invest 81:538, 1988
51. Sears DA, George JN, Gold MS: Transient red blood cell aplasia in association with viral hepatitis. Arch Intern Med 135:1585, 1974
52. Wilson HA, McLaren GD, Dworken HJ, Tebbi K: Transient pure red cell aplasia: cell-mediated suppression of erythropoiesis associated with hepatitis. Ann Intern Med 92:196, 1980
53. Purtilo DT, Zelkowitz L, Harada S et al: Delayed onset of infectious mononucleosis associated with acquired agammaglobulinemia and red cell aplasia. Ann Intern Med 101:180, 1984
54. Chernoff AI, Josephson AM: Acute erythroblastopenia in sickle cell anemia and infectious mononucleosis. Am J Dis Child 82:310, 1951
55. Socinski MA, Ershler WB, Tosato G, Blaese RM: Pure red blood cell aplasia associated with chronic Epstein-Barr virus infection: evidence for T-cell-mediated suppression of erythroid colony-forming units. J Lab Clin Med 104:995, 1984
56. Bruyn GA, Schelfhout LJ: Transient syndrome of inappropriate antidiuretic hormone secretion in a patient with infectious mononucleosis and pure red cell aplasia. Neth J Med 29:167, 1986

57. Sao H, Yoshikawa H, Akao Y et al: An adult case of acute erythroblastopenia. Rinsho Ketsueki 23:1453, 1982

58. Anderson MJ, Davis LR, Hodgson J et al: Occurrence of infection with a parvovirus-like agent in children with sickle cell anemia during a two-year period. J Clin Pathol 35:744, 1982

59. Young NS, Harrison M, Mortimer PP et al: Direct demonstration of the human parvovirus in erythroid progenitor cells infected in vitro. J Clin Invest 74:2024, 1984

60. Young NS, Mortimer PP: Viruses and bone marrow failure. Blood 63:729, 1984

61. Young NS, Mortimer PP, Moore JG, Humphries RK: Characterization of a virus that causes transient aplastic crisis. J Clin Invest 73:224, 1984

62. Duncan JR, Potter CB, Cappelini MD et al: Aplastic crisis due to parvovirus infection in pyruvate kinase deficiency. Lancet 2:14, 1983

63. Kelleher JF, Luban NL, Mortimer PP, Kamimura T: Human serum "Parvovirus": a specific cause of aplastic crisis in chidlren with hereditary spherocytosis. J Pediatr 102:720, 1983

64. Pattison JR, Jones SE, Hodgson J et al: Parvovirus infections and hypoplastic crisis in sickle cell anaemia. Lancet 1:664, 1981

65. Serjeant GR, Mason K, Topley JM et al: Outbreak of aplastic crises in sickle cell anemia associated with parvovirus-like agent. Lancet 2:595, 1981

66. Kurtzman G, Frickhofen N, Kimball J et al: Pure red-cell aplasia of 10 years' duration due to persistent parvovirus B19 infection and its care with immunoglobulin therapy. N Engl J Med 321:519, 1989

67. Frickhofen N, Abkowitz JL, Safford M et al: Persistent B19 parvovirus infection in patients infected with human immunodeficiency virus-1: a treatable cause of anemia in AIDS. Ann Intern Med 113:926, 1990

68. Rao KRP, Patel AR, Anderson MJ et al: Infection with parvovirus-like virus and aplastic crisis in chronic hemolytic anemia. Ann Intern Med 98:930, 1983

69. Solano C, Gomez-Reino F, Fernandez-Ranada JM: Pure red cell aplasia in Kala Azar. Acta Haematol 72:205, 1984

70. Krantz SB, Kao V: Studies on red cell aplasia. I. Demonstration of a plasma inhibitor to heme synthesis and an antibody to erythroblast nuclei. Proc Natl Acid Sci USA 58:493, 1967

71. Krantz SB, Kao V: Studies on red cell aplasia. II. Report of a second patient with an antibody to erythroblast nuclei and a remission after immunosuppressive therapy. Blood 34:1, 1969

72. Zaentz SD, Krantz SB, Brown EB: Studies on pure red cell aplasia. VIII. Maintenance therapy with immunosuppressive drugs. Br J Haematol 32:47, 1976

73. Dessypris EN, Redline S, Harris JW, Krantz SB: Diphenylhydantoin-induced pure red cell aplasia. Blood 65:789, 1985

74. Geary CG: Drug-related red cell aplasia. Br Med J 1:51, 1978

75. Reid G, Patterson AC: Pure red-cell aplasia after gold treatment. Br Med J 2:1457, 1977

76. Jurgenson JC, Abraham JP, Hardy WW: Erythroid aplasia after halothane hepatitis: report of a case. Am J Dig Dis 15:577, 1970

77. Hoffman R, McPhedram P, Benz EJ, Duffy TP: Isoniazid-induced pure red cell aplasia. Am J Med Sci 286:2, 1983

78. Lewis CR, Manoharan A: Pure red cell hypoplasia secondary to isonazid. Postgrad Med J 63:309, 1987

79. Foy H, Kondi A: A case of true red cell aplastic anemia successfully treated with riboflavin. J Pathol 65:559, 1953

80. Agudelo CA, Wise CM, Lyles MF: Pure red cell aplasia in procainamide induced systemic lupus erythmatosus. Report and review of the literature. J Rheumatol 15:1431, 1988

81. Peschle C, Marmont A, Perugini S et al: Physiopathology and therapy of adult pure red cell aplasia: a cooperative study. p. 285. In Hibino S (ed): Aplastic Anemia. University Park Press, Baltimore, 1978

82. MacDougall-Lorna G: Pure red cell aplasia associated with sodium valproate therapy. JAMA 247:53, 1982

83. Dunn AM, Kerr GD: Pure red cell aplasia associated with sulphasalazine. Lancet 2:1288, 1981

84. Antilla PM, Välimäki M, Pentikäinen PJ: Pure-red-cell aplasia associated with sulphasalazine but not 5-aminosalicylic acid. Lancet 2:1006, 1985

85. Strauss AM: Erythrocyte aplasia following sulfathiazole. Am J Clin Pathol 13:249, 1943

86. Sanz MA, Martinez JA, Gomis F, Garcia-Borras JJ: Sulindac-induced bone marrow toxicity. Lancet 2:802, 1980

87. Bouroncle BA: Familial crises in hereditary spherocytosis. J Am Med Wom Assoc 19:1045, 1969

88. Pavlic GJ, Bouroncle BA: Megaloblastic crisis in paroxysmal nocturnal hemoglobinuria. N Engl J Med 273:789, 1965

89. Eisenmann G, Dameshek W: Splenectomy for pure red cell hypoplastic aregenerative anemia associated with autoimmune hemolytic disease: report of a case. N Engl J Med 251:1044, 1954

90. Pirofsky B: The idiopathic autoimmune hemolytic anemias. p. 73. In Autoimmunization and the Autoimmune Hemolytic Anemias. Williams & Wilkins, Baltimore, 1969

91. Meyer RJ, Hoffman R, Zanjani ED: Autoimmune hemolytic anemia and periodic pure red cell aplasia in systemic lupus erythematosus. Am J Med 65:342, 1978

92. Mangan KF, Besa EC, Shadduck RK et al: Demonstration of two distinct antibodies in autoimmune hemolytic anemia with reticulocytopenia and red cell aplasia. Exp Hematol 12:788, 1984

93. Taniguchi S, Shibuya T, Morioka E et al: Demonstration of three distinct immunological disorders on erythropoiesis in a patient with pure red cell aplasia and autoimmune haemolytic anaemia associated with thymoma. Br J Haematol 68:473, 1988

94. Cavalcant J, Shadduck RK, Winkelstein A et al: Red cell hypoplasia and increased bone marrow reticulin in systemic lupus erythematosus: reversal with corticosteroid therapy. Am J Hematol 5:253, 1978

95. Dessypris EN, Baer MR, Sergent JS, Krantz SB: Rheumatoid arthritis and pure red cell aplasia. Ann Intern Med 100:202, 1984

96. Rodrigues JF, Harth M, Barr RM: Pure red cell aplasia in rheumatoid arthritis. J Rheumatol 15:1159, 1988

97. Aggio MC, Zunini C: Reversible pure red cell aplasia in pregnancy. N Engl J Med 297:221, 1977

98. Miyoshi I, Hikita T, Koi B, Kimura I: Reversible pure red cell aplasia in pregnancy. N Engl J Med 299:777, 1978

99. Lehman G, Alcoff J: Reversible pure red cell hypoplasia in pregnancy. JAMA 247:1170, 1982

100. Oie BK, Hertel J, Seip M, Friis-Hansen B: Hydrops foetalis in three infants of a mother with acquired chronic pure red cell aplasia: transitory red cell aplasia in one of the infants. Scand J Haematol 33:466, 1984

101. Pasternack A, Wahlberg P: Bone marrow in acute renal failure. Acta Med Scand 181:505, 1967

102. Foy H, Kondi A, MacDougall L: Pure red cell aplasia in marasmus and kwashiorkor treated with riboflavin. Br Med J 1:937, 1961

103. Chanarin I: Investigation and management of megaloblastic anemia. Clin Haematol 5:747, 1976

104. Hotchkiss DJ Jr: Pure red cell aplasia following pernicious anemia. p. 133. In Proceedings of the Eighth International Congress of Haematology. JF Lehmans, Munich, 1970

105. Zucker S, Likhite VV, Weintraub LR, Crosby WH: Remission in pure red cell aplasia following immunosuppressive therapy. Arch Intern Med 134:317, 1974

106. Robins-Browne RM, Green R, Katz J, Becker D: Thymoma, pure red cell aplasia, pernicious anemia and candidiasis: a defect in immunohomeostasis. Br J Haematol 36:5, 1977

107. Krantz SB: Studies on red cell aplasia. IV. Treatment with immunosuppressive drugs. p. 312. In Gordon AS, Condorelli M, Peschle C (eds): Regulation of Erythropoiesis. Il Ponte, Rome, 1972

108. Zaentz SD, Krantz SB, Sears DA: Studies on pure red cell aplasia. VII. Presence of proerythroblasts and response to splenectomy: a case report. Blood 46:261, 1975

109. Katz JL, Hoffman R, Ritchey AK, Dainiak N: The proliferative capacity of pure red cell aplasia bone marrow cells. Yale J Biol Med 54:89, 1981

110. Dessypris EN, Krantz SB, Roloff JS, Lukens JN: Mode of action of the IgG inhibitor of erythropoiesis in transient erythroblastopenia of childhood. Blood 59:114, 1982

111. Krantz SB: Pure red cell aplasia. N Engl J Med 291:345, 1974

112. Krantz SB, Moore WH, Zaentz SD: Studies on red cell aplasia. V. Presence of erythroblast cytotoxicity in γG-globulin fraction of plasma. J Clin Invest 52:324, 1973

113. Jepson JH, Lowenstein L: Inhibition of erythropoiesis by a factor present in the plasma of patients with erythroblastopenia. Blood 27:425, 1966

114. al-Mondhiry H, Zanjani ED, Spivack M et al: Pure red cell aplasia and thymoma: loss of serum inhibitor of erythropoiesis following thymectomy. Blood 38:576, 1971

115. Zalusky R, Zanjani ED, Gidari AS, Ross J: Site of action of a serum inhibitor of erythropoiesis. J Lab Clin Med 81:867, 1973

116. Bjorkholm M, Holm G, Mellstedt H et al: Membrane bound IgG on erythroblasts in pure red cell aplasia following thymectomy: case report. Scand J Haematol 17:341, 1976

117. Romano E, Layrisse M, Romano M et al: Electron microscopic demonstration of IgG antibodies directed to erythroblasts in primary acquired pure red cell aplasia. Clin Immunol Immunopathol 17:330, 1980

118. Browman GP, Freedman MH, Blajchman MA, McBride JA: A complement independent erythropoietic inhibitor acting on the progenitor cell in refractory anemia. Am J Med 61:572, 1976

119. Messner HA, Fauser AA, Curtis JE, Dotten D: Control of antibody-mediated pure red cell aplasia by plasmapheresis. N Engl J Med 304:1334, 1981

120. Koenig HM, Lightsey AL, Nelson DP, Diamond LK: Immune suppression of erythropoiesis in transient erythroblastopenia of childhood. Blood 54:742, 1979

121. Levitt LJ, Ries CA, Greenberg PL: Pure white-cell aplasia: antibody mediated autoimmune inhibition of granulopoiesis. N Engl J Med 308:1141, 1983

122. Hoffman R, Bruno E, Elwell J et al: Acquired amegakaryocytic thrombocytopenic purpura: a syndrome of diverse etiologies. Blood 60:1173, 1982

123. Hoffman R, Zaknoen S, Yang HH et al: An antibody cytotoxic to megakaryocyte progenitor cells in a patient with immune thrombocytopenic purpura. N Engl J Med 312:1170, 1985

124. Hanada T, Ehara T, Nakahara S: Simultaneous transient erythroblastopenia and agranulocytosis: IgG-mediated inhibition of erythrogranulopoiesis. Eur J Haematol 38:200, 1987

125. Jepson JH, Lowenstein L: Panhypoplasia of the bone marrow. I. Demonstration of a plasma factor with anti-erythropoietin-like activity. Can Med Assoc J 99:99, 1968

126. Peschle C, Marmont AM, Marone G et al: Pure red cell aplasia: studies on an IgG serum inhibitor neutralizing erythropoietin. Br J Haematol 30:411, 1975

127. Mangan KF, Chikkappa G, Scharfman WB, Desforges JF: Evidence for reduced erythroid burst promoting function of T lymphocytes in the pure red cell aplasia of chronic lymphocytic leukemia. Exp Hematol 9:489, 1981

128. Linch DC, Cawley JC, MacDonald SM et al: Acquired pure red cell aplasia associated with an increase of T-cells bearing receptors for the Fc of IgG. Acta Haematol 65:270, 1981

129. Torok-Storb BJ, Siell G, Storb R et al: In vitro tests for distinguishing possible immune-mediated aplastic anemia from transfusion-induced sensitization. Blood 55:211, 1980

130. Bacigalupo A, Podesta M, Mingari MC et al: Generation of CFU-C/suppressor T cells in vitro; an experimental model for immune-mediated marrow failure. Blood 57:491, 1981

131. Abkowitz JL, Kadin ME, Powell JS, Adamson JW: Pure red cell aplasia: lymphocyte inhibition of erythropoiesis. Br J Haematol 63:59, 1986

132. Mangan KF, D'Alessandro L: Hypoplastic anemia in B-cell chronic lymphocytic leukemia: evolution of T-cell mediated suppression of erythropoiesis in early stage and late stage disease. Blood 66:533, 1985

133. De La Concha EG, Oldham G, Webster ADB et al: Quantitative measurements of T- and B-cell function in "variable" primary hypogammaglobulinemia: evidence for a consistent B-cell defect. Clin Exp Immunol 27:208, 1977

134. Barnes RD: Refractory anemia with thymoma. Lancet 2:1464, 1966

135. Mangan KF, Volkin R, Winkelstein A: Autoreactive erythroid progenitor-T suppressor cells in the pure red cell aplasia associated with thymoma and panhypogammaglobulinemia. Am J Hematol 23:167, 1986

136. Kurtzman GJ, Ozawa K, Cohen B et al: Chronic bone marrow failure due to persistent B19 parvovirus infection. N Engl J Med 317:287, 1987

137. Kurtzman GJ, Meyers P, Cohen B et al: Persistent B19 parvovirus infection as a cause of severe chronic anaemia in children with acute lymphocytic leukaemia. Lancet 2:1159, 1988

138. Van Horn DK, Mortimer PP, Young N, Hanson GR: Human parvovirus-associated red cell aplasia in the absence of underlying hemolytic anemia. Am J Pediatr Hematol Oncol 8:235, 1986

139. Weiland HT, Salimans MMM, Fibbe WE et al: Prolonged parvovirus B19 infection with severe anaemia in a bone marrow transplant recipient, letter. Br J Haematol 71:300, 1989

140. Griffin TC, Squires JE, Timmons CF, Buchanen GR: Chronic human parvovirus B19-induced erythroid hypoplasia as the indirect manifestation of human immunodeficiency virus infection. J Pediatr 118:899, 1991

141. Frickhofen N, Cohen B, Young NS et al: Parvovirus B19 as a cause of acquired chronic pure red cell aplasia (PRCA), abstracted. Blood, suppl. 1. 78:366a, 1991

142. Yunis AA, Arimura GK, Lutcher CL et al: Biochemical lesion in dilantin-induced erythroid aplasia. Blood 30:587, 1967

143. Beard MJE, Krantz SB, Johnson SAN et al: Pure red cell aplasia. Q J Med 187:339, 1978

144. Keefer MJ, Solanki DL: Dyserythropoiesis and erythroblast-phagocytosis preceding pure red cell aplasia. Am J Hematol 27:132, 1988

145. Wibulyachainunt S, Price P, Brill AB, Krantz SB: Studies on red cell aplasia. IX. Ferrokinetics during remission of the disease. Am J Hematol 4:233, 1978

146. Bunn HF, McNeil BJ, Rosenthal DS, Krantz SB: Bone marrow imaging in pure red cell aplasia. Arch Intern Med 136:1169, 1976

147. Min KW, Waddell C, Pircher FJ et al: Selective uptake of ^{75}Se-selenomethionine by thymoma with pure red cell aplasia. Cancer 41:1323, 1978

148. Higasi T, Nakayama Y, Murata A et al: Clinical evaluation of ^{67}Ga citrate scanning. J Nucl Med 13:196, 1972

149. Rogers BH, Manligod JR, Blazek WV: Thymoma associated with pancytopenia and hypogammaglobulinemia: report of a case and review of the literature. Am J Med 44:154, 1968

150. Krantz SB: Studies on red cell aplasia. III. Treatment with horse antihuman thymocyte gamma globulin. Blood 39:347, 1972

151. Holborow EJ, Asherson GL, Johnson GD et al: Anti-nuclear factor and other antibodies in blood and liver disease. Br Med J 1:656, 1963

152. Frøland SS, Wisloff F, Stavem P: Abnormal lymphocyte populations in pure red cell aplasia. Scand J Haematol 17:241, 1976

153. Mannoji M, Shimoda M, Koresawa S et al: A case of angioimmunoblastic lymphadenopathy with dysproteinemia associated with autoimmune hemolytic anemia and pure red cell aplasia with special references to its pathogenesis. Rinsho Ketsueki 22:1751, 1981

154. al-Hilali MA, Joyner MV: Pure red cell aplasia secondary to angioimmunoblastic lymphadenopathy. J R Soc Med 76:894, 1983

155. MacKechnie HLN, Squires AH, Platts M, Pruzanski W: Thymoma, myasthenia gravis, erythroblastopenic anemia, and systemic lupus erythematosus in one patient. Can Med Assoc J 109:733, 1973

156. DeSevilla E, Forrest JV, Zirmuska FR, Sagel SS: Metastatic thymoma with myasthenia gravis and pure red cell aplasia. Cancer 36:1154, 1975

157. Myers TJ, Bower FB, Hild DH: Pure red cell aplasia and the syndrome of multiple endocrine gland insufficiency. Am J Med Sci 280:29, 1980

158. Gill PJ, Amare M, Larsen WE: Pure red cell aplasia: three cases responding to immunosuppression. Am J Med Sci 273:213, 1977

159. Francis DA: Pure red cell aplasia: association with systemic lupus erythematosus and primary autoimmune hypothyroidism. Br Med J 284:85, 1982

160. Penn CR, Hope-Stone HF: The role of radiotherapy in management of malignant thymoma. Br J Surg 59:533, 1972

161. Greene MH, Boice JD Jr, Greer BE: Acute nonlymphocytic leukemia after therapy with alkylating agents for ovarian cancer. A study of five randomized clinical trials. N Engl J Med 307:1416, 1982

162. Berk PD, Goldberg JD, Donovan PD et al: Therapeutic recommendations in polycythemia vera based on polycythemia vera study group protocols. Semin Hematol 23:132, 1986

163. Fairley FK, Barrie JU, Johnson W: Sterility and testicular atrophy related to cyclophosphamide therapy. Lancet 1:568, 1972

164. Uldall PR, Kerr DNS, Tacchi D: Sterility and cyclophosphamide therapy. Lancet 1:693, 1972

165. Bottiger LE, Rausing A: Pure red cell anemia: immunosuppressive treatment. Ann Intern Med 76:593, 1972

166. Vilan J, Rhyner K, Ganzoni A: Immunosuppressive treatment of pure red cell aplasia. Lancet 2:51, 1971

167. Hartmann RC, Krantz SB: Paroxysmal nocturnal hemoglobinuria and pure red cell aplasia. Two rare anemias with immunologic implications. Postgrad Med 55:141, 1974

168. Firkin FC, Maher D: Cytotoxic immunosuppressive drug treatment strategy in pure red cell aplasia. Eur J Haematol 41:212, 1988

169. Krantz SB: Implications of studies on pure red cell aplasia (PRCA) for the study of aplastic anemia. p. 305. In Japan Medical Research Foundation (eds): Aplastic Anemia. University of Tokyo Press, Tokyo, 1978

170. Hagberg H, Nilsson P, Nissell J: Treatment of pure red cell anemia with antilymphocyte globulin: report of two cases. Scand J Haematol 24:360, 1980

171. Krantz SB: Special feature: new therapies for aplastic anemia. Am J Med Sci 29:371, 1986

172. Abkowitz JL, Powell JS, Nakamura JM et al: Pure red cell aplasia: response to therapy with anti-thymocyte globulin. Am J Hematol 23:363, 1986

173. Champlin R, Ho R, Gale AP: Antithymocyte globulin treatment in patients with aplastic anemia. N Engl J Med 308:113, 1983

174. Hocking W, Champlin R, Mitsuyasu R: Transient response of pure red cell aplasia to anti-thymocyte globulin in a patient with T-cell chronic lymphocyte leukemia. Am J Hematol 24:284, 1987

175. Means RT, Krantz SB, Dessypris EN et al: Re-treatment of aplastic anemia with antithymocyte globulin or antilymphocyte serum. Am J Med 84:678, 1988

176. Cohen DJ, Loertscher R, Rubin MF et al: Cyclosporin: a new immunosuppressive agent for organ transplantation. Ann Intern Med 101:667, 1984

177. Boitard C, Feutren G, Castano L: Effect of cyclosporin A treatment on the production of antibody in insulin-dependent (type I) diabetic patients. J Clin Invest 80:1607, 1987

178. Castano L, Boitard C, Bougneres P-F: Cyclosporin A suppresses insulin autoantibodies and heterologous insulin antibodies in type I diabetic children. Diabetes 37:1049, 1988

179. Tötterman TH, Nisell J, Killander A et al: Successful treatment of pure red cell aplasia with cyclosporin. Lancet 2:693, 1984

180. Debusscher L, Parideaus R, Stryckmans P: Cyclosporine for pure red cell aplasia. Blood 65:249, 1985

pure red cell aplasia. Haematologica 72:537, 1987

183. Chikkappa G, Pasquale D, Phillips PG et al: Cyclosporin-A for the treatment of pure red cell aplasia in a patient with chronic lymphocytic leukemia. Am J Hematol 26:179, 1987

184. Tötterman TH, Bengtsson M: Treatment of pure red cell aplasia with cyclosporin: suppression of activated T suppressor/cytotoxic and NK-like cells in marrow and blood correlates with haematological response. Eur J Haematol 41:204, 1988

185. Means RT Jr, Dessypris EN, Krantz SB: Treatment of refractory pure red cell aplasia with cyclosporine A: disappearance of IgG inhibitor associated with clinical response. Br J Haematol 78:114, 1991

186. Raghavachar A: Pure red cell aplasia: review of treatment and proposal for a treatment strategy. Blut 61:47, 1990

187. Lippman SM, Durie BGM, Garewal HS et al: Efficacy of danazol in pure red cell aplasia. Am J Hematol 23:373, 1986

188. Marinone G, Mombelloni P, Marini G et al: Bone marrow erythroblastic recovery after plasmapheresis in acquired pure red cell anemia: case report. Hematologica 66:796, 1981

189. Young NS, Klein HG, Griffith P, Nienhuis AW: A trial of immunotherapy in aplastic anemia and pure red cell aplasia. J Clin Apheresis 1:95, 1983

190. Khelif A, Van HV, Tremis JP et al: Remission of acquired pure red cell aplasia

following plasma exchanges. Scand J Haematol 34:13, 1985

191. Freund LG, Hippe E, Strandgaard S et al: Complete remission in pure red cell aplasia after plasmapheresis. Scand J Haematol 35:315, 1985

192. Berlin G, Lieden G: Long-term remission of pure red cell aplasia after plasma exchange and lymphocytapheresis. Scand J Haematol 36:121, 1986

193. Etzioni A, Atias D, Pollack S et al: Complete recovery of pure red cell aplasia by intramuscular gammaglobulin therapy in a child with hypoparathyroidism. Am J Hematol 22:409, 1986

194. Katakkar SB: Pure red cell aplasia: response to intravenous immunoglobulin, a blocking antibody. Arch Intern Med 146:2288, 1986

195. McGuire WA, Yang HH, Bruno E et al: Treatment of antibody-mediated pure red cell aplasia with high-dose intravenous gammaglobulin therapy. N Engl J Med 317:1004, 1987

196. Safdar SH, Krantz SB, Brown EB: Successful immunosuppressive treatment of erythroid aplasia appearing after thymectomy. Br J Haematol 19:435, 1970

197. Propper RD, Cooper B, Rufo RR et al: Continuous subcutaneous administration of deferoxamine in patients with iron overload. N Engl J Med 297:418, 1977

Congenital Pure Red Cell Aplasia

24

Jeffrey M. Lipton

INTRODUCTION

Congenital pure red cell aplasia, or Diamond-Blackfan anemia (DBA), is a rare aregenerative anemia of childhood characterized by decreased or absent bone marrow erythroid precursor cells, reticulocytopenia, a normal or only slightly decreased granulocyte count, and a normal or increased platelet count. It is frequently associated with a variety of somatic malformations and, rarely, with mental retardation. Most patients respond to corticosteroids with an improvement in, or complete remission of, their anemia.[1,2] Since the first description of this syndrome >55 years ago,[3] a number of theories have been proposed regarding its etiology. The myriad explanations include humoral[4] or cellular[5,6] suppression of erythropoiesis, a microenvironmental defect,[7] accessory cell failure,[8] and an intrinsic progenitor defect.[9–12] These data suggest that at various stages of differentiation the pathway from the multipotent hematopoietic progenitor cell to the proerythroblast and beyond is defective.[9–12] With this model in mind, the following discussion concentrates on the development of rational diagnostic criteria and treatment strategy based on an understanding of pathophysiology rather than an exhaustive compilation of the clinical syndrome of DBA, a task that has already been expertly accomplished.[13]

CELLULAR BIOLOGY AND ETIOLOGY

Normal erythropoiesis is dependent on the interaction among erythroid progenitors, accessory cells, and the bone marrow stroma.[14] The erythropoietic failure in DBA may poten-

tially arise from an absence of, or abnormality in, any one of these elements. Studies performed over the past two decades have suggested multiple etiologies for this condition. Some investigators describe a marrow microenvironmental defect[7] or implicate accessory cell dysfunction.[8] Others support the notion that the red cell failure in DBA is due to the presence of cytotoxic or autoreactive T cells[5,6] or humoral inhibitors of erythropoiesis.[4] These findings have not been substantiated in most patients.[9,10,15–17] Thus, the pathophysiology of DBA remains controversial and may reflect multiple etiologies. Most recent studies, however, point to an intrinsic progenitor defect.[9–12,17–20] Freedman et al.[10] first suggested that some patients have decreased numbers of colony-forming unit-erythroid (CFU-E). In addition, studies by Nathan et al.,[9] using chronically affected (either multiply transfused or steroid-dependent) patients, suggested a block in maturation between the earliest committed multipotent hematopoietic progenitor cell and the immature burst-forming unit-erythroid (BFU-E). In addition, these investigators found that DBA progenitor cells were relatively insensitive to erythropoietin (EPO). Chan et al.[18,19] provided additional data to support the concept of progenitor hyporesponsiveness to EPO and suggested that this abnormality could be corrected in part by the addition of glucocorticoids in vitro. Such work provided a potential means of establishing a relationship between clinical response to corticosteroids and in vitro progenitor cell behavior. In a study by Lipton et al.[11] of nine predominantly young DBA patients, minimally transfused and off corticosteroids for ≥5 months, assayable marrow, CFU-E, and BFU-E were normal or only moderately decreased in number. In fact, in five of the nine patients, normal in vitro progenitor cell responsiveness to crude EPO preparations and adequate erythroid colony numbers were observed, demonstrating no detectable quantitative in vitro abnormality. However, the colonies themselves appeared less cellular than normal, suggesting the presence of a defect in all patients and providing the stimulus for further study, using recombinant rather than crude preparations of EPO. Indeed, in another study, in vitro insensitivity to recombinant EPO of BFU-E and CFU-E obtained from a steroid-responsive patient was documented.[12] Apparently, growth factors present in crude preparations of EPO had prevented the detection of such an abnormality in the earlier study. In addition, a relationship between an in vitro response to recombinant EPO and clinical steroid responsiveness was also established, confirming the observation of Chan et al.[19] In these studies, some patients expressed normal (or near-normal) numbers of BFU-E-derived colonies but had decreased CFU-E cloning efficiency, while other patients demonstrated normal numbers of both progenitor cells. These data support the impression that DBA is a heterogeneous disorder in which erythropoiesis may be blocked at different stages along the erythroid differentiation pathway.

It is impossible to determine whether these in vitro abnormalities are the result of an intrinsic progenitor cell defect or dysfunctional accessory cells when studies are performed on unfractionated marrow mononuclear cells containing progenitors as well as accessory cells. Indeed, it is even possible that cytokines supplied to the culture system by stimulation of endogenous accessory cells could overcome a cellular or humoral inhibitor. Tsai et al.[12] used physical and immunologic techniques to fractionate marrow into progenitor and accessory cell populations, permitting the study of progenitor cell behavior in the absence of accessory cells. In this study, enriched populations of erythroid progenitor cells from a spontaneously remitting DBA patient required increased concentrations of burst-promoting activity, a crude cell supernatant containing multiple cytokine activities (at a suboptimal concentration of recombinant EPO), to achieve optimal erythroid colony formation compared with normal controls. In vitro progenitor cell differentiation from a steroid-refractory patient was more severely defective, with decreased erythroid colony formation even in the presence of high levels of recombinant EPO and burst-promoting activity. On the basis of these data, the erythroid failure in DBA appears to be the consequence of an intrinsic defect in the erythroid progenitor cell, which involves the inability of these cells to respond normally to inducers of erythroid proliferation and differentiation. Such defects could involve the expression or function of receptors for hematopoietic growth factors and are likely heterogeneous in nature. In addition, the defect in DBA may not be confined to the erythroid compartment, as suggested by evidence of subtle T-lymphocyte dysfunction[8] as well as the presence of a mildly decreased leukocyte count and hypogammaglobulinemia in some DBA patients.

Thus, the consensus is that in most patients an intrinsic abnormality in the erythroid progenitor cell is present. The nature of this intrinsic defect was recently explored by Perdahl et al.,[20] who observed accelerated programmed cell death (apoptosis) in DBA erythroid progenitors and precursors compared with normal controls when EPO was withheld in vitro. Whether this is the primary defect or the consequence of abnormal EPO or cytokine responsiveness remains to be explored.

A number of studies indicate that recombinant cytokines may increase the in vitro clonogenicity of DBA progenitors from unfractionated cell preparations. Halperin et al.[21] reported that the size and number of marrow BFU-E was improved when interleukin-3 (IL-3) was added to DBA marrow mononuclear cell cultures in the presence of EPO. Several groups have examined the effect of the c-kit ligand or stem cell factor (SCF) on in vitro erythroid progenitor colony expression from patients with DBA. Bagnara et al.[22] observed a lack of response of enriched CD34+ progenitors to EPO, IL-3, colony-stimulating factor-granulocyte/macrophage (CSF-GM), and erythroid potentiating activity in cultures from 10 DBA patients. SCF in combination with IL-3 and EPO dramatically stimulated BFU-E colony expression in three patients. Abkowitz et al.[23] showed a response of unfractionated marrow BFU-E from four patients to SCF and EPO alone or in combination with IL-3, CSF-GM, or conditioned media. Differences in the dose response to SCF corroborate the concept of disease heterogeneity. Olivieri et al.[24] observed normal, intermediate, and no response to SCF, again confirming the heterogenous nature of the syndrome. Alter et al.[25] found that 15 of 16 DBA marrow cultures had increased erythropoiesis in the presence of SCF plus erythropoietin compared with EPO alone; 10 of the 16 cultures had normal numbers of BFU-E-derived colonies with the combination. These and other studies indicate that in many instances abnormalities of erythropoiesis in DBA can be corrected in vitro by a variety of cytokines. This, however does not confirm the presence of a defect in any one of these cytokine receptors.

The W/W^v and Sl/Sl^d mice with macrocytic anemias and mutations in the c-kit proto-oncogene and kit ligand gene, respectively, have been suggested as potential models for DBA. However, recent molecular studies have failed to identify mutations in either the kit or SCF gene in DBA.[24,26–28] Furthermore, human kit mutations do not have a DBA phenotype,[29] and these proposed murine models lack the corticosteroid effect seen in DBA.[30] The observation that superphysiologic amounts of a growth factor may stimulate in vitro hematopoiesis even when that growth factor or its receptor is not defective suggests that EPO, IL-3, and SCF may be clinically useful in DBA. In one human trial, IL-3 was clinically effective in 4 of 18 DBA patients.[31] In another study, two of six patients had sustained responses to IL-3.[32] These results are in contrast to another recent study in which none of the 10 patients studied responded.[33] However, significant side effects associated with IL-3 may preclude further clinical trials.[31] Sufficient clinical trials of EPO therapy have not been performed in DBA patients,[34] although preliminary results are not encouraging. There may still be a role for recombinant growth factors, such as EPO, IL-3, and SCF as single agents or in combination in the therapy of DBA. Such trials are suggested by in vitro and preliminary in vivo studies if nontoxic dosing schedules can be developed. Although new cytokines are being studied, it is particularly discouraging that there appears to be a lack of correlation between clinical in vivo and in vitro responsiveness to growth factors.[31]

GENETICS

DBA most frequently presents at <1 year of age.[1] Indeed, in one reported case, the initial manifestation appears to have been hydrops fetalis (although parvovirus was not ruled out).[35] Thus, DBA is considered a congenital disorder. The sex ratio is 1:1, and, although most cases appear to be sporadic, Alter[36] estimates that more than one family member is affected in approximately 10% of cases. In these families, same and opposite sex siblings,[37–40] including identical twins[41] and maternal or paternal half-siblings, have been affected.[42–45] Parental transmission has also occurred.[1,44,46–52]

The most striking instances of autosomal dominant inheritance are a case report of DBA in a male infant who had an affected mother and maternal grandfather[50] and another report in which seven members of one kindred were affected over three generations.[51] In support of an autosomal recessive mode, parental consanguinity has been observed.[53,54] Thus, evidence is ample for both autosomal recessive and dominant modes of inheritance. It is also possible that families with only affected males could be explained by X-linked inheritance rather than an autosomal recessive mode. Most cases, however, seem to be sporadic, implying new mutations or that the syndrome is acquired. The incidence of genetically determined cases is probably underestimated because of the inability to characterize the carrier state, as well as the apparent variable penetrance of the autosomal dominant cases, in which an elevated fetal hemoglobin (Hb F), mean corpuscular volume (MCV), or erythrocyte ADA activity may be the only abnormality in a parent of a child with typical DBA.[40,43–45] Therefore, pending the availability of a molecular diagnosis, families of affected individuals should be evaluated to determine Hb F levels, MCV, and erythrocyte ADA activity. A number of cases currently believed to be sporadic or autosomal-recessive in nature will no doubt be recategorized as carrier state determination improves.

The vast majority of DBA patients have a normal karyotype, but two cases with abnormalities of chromosome 1 have been reported.[55,56] These findings have not been corroborated in other patients using more modern banding techniques. The chromosomal breaks and rearrangement characteristic of Fanconi anemia have not been found in the peripheral blood cells of DBA patients.[36]

CLINICAL MANIFESTATIONS

Approximately 400 reported cases of DBA have been reviewed by Alter.[13] DBA usually presents in infancy. Severe anemia was recognized at birth in 10% of patients, with 25% by 1 month of age, 80% by 6 months and 90% within the first year of life.[13] Rarely, the disease may present in older children[36] and adults.[57] The incidence in males equals that in females. Most cases are seen in whites, but the disorder has been reported in virtually all ethnic groups.[13] An unusually high proportion of mothers of patients have a prior history of fetal loss, through either miscarriages or still births.[13] Other perinatal problems include premature, low-birthweight, and small-for-gestational-age babies.[13] Drug and toxin exposures appear to be nonspecific.[13]

The first description of red cell failure in infants was noted by Josephs[58] in 1936 and by Diamond and Blackfan[3] in 1938. The variety of descriptive names for what is now preferably called congenital pure red cell aplasia or DBA, which includes congenital pure red cell hypoplastic anemia, congenital red cell aregenerative anemia, erythrogenesis imperfecta, chronic erythroblastopenia, primary red cell aplasia, and Josephs-Diamond-Blackfan anemia,[1,36] reflects the historic lack of a precise clinical definition as well as uncertainty regarding the pathophysiology of the disorder. The diagnostic criteria for DBA, which derive from the careful clinical analyses performed by Diamond and colleagues[1] and by Alter,[13,36] have recently been more precisely defined. These criteria are summarized in Table 24-1.

Table 24-1. Diagnostic Criteria for Diamond-Blackfan Anemia

Normochromic, normocytic or (frequently) macrocytic anemia, developing in early childhood[a]

Normal or moderately increased platelet count[b]

Normal or slightly decreased leukocyte count

Normocellular bone marrow characterized by a paucity of erythroid precursors[c] with normal myeloid and megakaryocyte precursors

[a] Anemia is present at birth in 10% of patients, and in 90% by 1 year of age. Only occasionally is anemia diagnosed at >4 years of age.

[b] Less frequently, mild thrombocytopenia is present.

[c] Rarely, the numbers of erythroid precursors with a maturational arrest are normal or increased.

(Data from Diamond et al.[1] and Alter.[13,36])

Table 24-2. Physical Abnormalities in Patients with Diamond-Blackfan Anemia[a]

Feature	Patients (N)	%
Low birthweight	30	11
Short stature, no steroids	15	6
Head and face	35	13
"Cathie" facies[b]	15	
Other facies	8	
Small head	10	
Large head	2	
Jaw and mouth	15	6
Small jaw alone	2	
Small jaw plus cleft palate (Pierre-Robin syndrome)	5	
Cleft palate alone	4	
Cleft palate and lip	2	
Cleft lip alone	1	
Macroglossia	1	
Flat nasal bridge	5	2
Abnormal ears	7	3
Abnormal eyes	33	12
Hypertelorism	10	
Epicanthal folds	7	
Ptosis	2	
Strabismus	6	
Blue sclerae	2	
Congenital cataracts	3	
Microphthalmia	2	
Glaucoma	1	
Neck	16	
Short	3	
Webbed	13	
Thumb	24	9
Triphalangeal	12	
Duplicated or bifid	7	
Subluxed	2	
Hypoplastic	3	
Renal	9	3
Dysplastic	1	
Absent	1	
Horseshoe	3	
Duplicated ureters	3	
Caliectasis	1	
Congenital heart disease	10	4
Ventricular septal defect	3	
Atrial septal defect	1	
Coarctation of aorta	1	
Other	5	
Mental retardation	10	4
Hypogonadism	5	2
Asplenia	1	0.4
At least one anomaly	70[a]	26

[a] Total number is >70 because many patients had multiple anomalies. Total number of cases reported with physical examinations = 270. Most references are included in Diamond et al.[1] and in Alter.[13,36]

[b] "Tow-colored hair, snub nose, wide set eyes, thick upper lip, and an intelligent expression"[104]

(From Alter,[13] with permission.)

It is of interest that approximately 30% of DBA patients have at least one associated physical anomaly. The constellation of physical findings in cases of DBA with typical hematologic manifestations outlined in Table 24-2 includes a high percentage of anomalies of the head, face, eyes, and thumbs, as well as renal and cardiac abnormalities. Thus, efforts to define discrete syndromes on the basis of any particular physical findings[37,39] seem unwarranted. The relationships of abnormal thumbs to hematopoietic failure in DBA as well as Fanconi anemia,[59,60] and radial abnormalities in patients with thrombocytopenia-absent radius (TAR) syndrome, are particularly fascinating.[60,61] However, despite the detailed cataloguing of these anomalies, their relationship to the pathogenesis of DBA as well as to the other syndromes remains obscure. It has been suggested that DBA may be the result of a contiguous gene syndrome.[62] Alternatively, it is possible that in DBA a mutation in a growth factor receptor occurs, leading to an abnormal receptor-ligand interaction or a signal transduction abnormality resulting in a defect in differentiation that is critical to morphogenesis as well as erythropoiesis.

LABORATORY EVALUATION

DBA is characterized by severe anemia with hemoglobins in typical patients ranging from 2.8 to 8.5 g/dl[11] (Table 24-1). Reticulocytopenia, is marked and frequently the count is zero. Occasionally abnormalities are present in the other cell lines. Neutropenia may be mild,[1,13,36] although significant neutropenia has been observed.[63] Thrombocytopenia occurs as well,[57] but thrombocytosis of 400,000–700,000/mm^3 is more common.[1,13,36,64] Platelet dysfunction is not evident.[64] Although originally described as a normochromic, normocytic anemia, macrocytosis was noted at diagnosis in approximately 30% of cases reviewed by Alter.[36] The percentage of patients with macrocytosis increases with the age of the patients as the disease becomes chronic and the normal red cell MCV decreases. Indeed, the persistence of fetal-like red cells, with macrocytosis, i antigen, increased Hb F, and red cell glycolytic and hexose monophosphate (HMP) shunt enzyme activities characteristic of fetal cells, is a consistent finding. The Hb F is typical of fetal cells,[36,65] with an elevated glycine/alanine ratio at position 136 of the γ-chain (Gly/Al^{136}). Of note is that the fetal-like characteristics are not concordant; cells with high Hb F are not necessarily those with the i antigen. Although red cells contain significant Hb F, as determined by hemoglobin electrophoresis, the distribution is uneven, as evaluated by the Kleihauer-Betke method. Alter[36] points out that red cells contain both fetal and adult hemoglobin and that the "re-expression of fetal erythropoiesis is thus incomplete, and not clonal." Although glycolytic and HMP shunt enzymes have a fetal pattern, erythrocyte ADA, a purine salvage pathway enzyme, is increased in activity in DBA patients but not in fetal or cord blood erythrocytes.[66] Compared with control blood with normal erythrocyte ADA activity obtained from normal patients, cord blood, and blood from patients with hemolytic anemia, Fanconi anemia, and those with steroid-dependent nephrosis as well as virtually all patients with transient erythroblastopenia of childhood (TEC), nearly 90% of blood from patients with typical DBA shows elevated erythrocyte ADA activity.[66–68] In some DBA patients with normal ADA activity, there is markedly elevated orotidine decarboxylase activity.[67,69] Although abnormalities in purine or pyrimidine biosynthesis are a consistent finding in most DBA patients, this observation has not yet been helpful in understanding the pathophysiology of DBA. Red cells of some patients with acute leukemia, adult-type chronic myeloid leukemia, myeloproliferative disorder with Down syndrome, dyskeratosis with pancytopenia, and megaloblastic anemia were also found to have increased ADA activity.[68] This finding suggests an association of elevated ADA activity with abnormal progenitor function, supporting the concept that DBA is the consequence of an intrinsic progenitor defect. Also of interest is the observation that W/W^v and Sl/Sl^d mice with genetically determined red cell failure have elevated erythrocyte nucleoside deaminase levels.[70] Further advances in this area must await a detailed understanding of the biochemistry of hematopoiesis. However, from a practical prospective ADA activity

determinations provide a reasonably useful means for distinguishing DBA from TEC.

Vitamin B$_{12}$, folate, serum iron, and transferrin saturation are elevated or normal in patients with DBA.[1,13] Sufficient data are lacking, but EPO levels seem to reflect the degree of anemia, although they remain elevated even in steroid-responsive patients.[1,13] Approximately one-third of patients evaluated by Alter[36] had hypogammaglobulinemia[71] consistent with the finding of in vitro immunologic abnormalities in some DBA patients.[8]

Although abnormal urinary metabolites have been reported in some patients, findings are not consistent.[36] The standard urinalysis is normal. Other sporadic abnormalities found in these patients may ultimately be of interest, but they are not diagnostic, nor do they currently shed light on the pathophysiology of the disorder.

Examination of the bone marrow biopsy and aspirate usually reveals normal cellularity with a paucity of erythroid precursors. Myeloid and megakaryocyte lineages appear normal. Myeloid/erythroid ratios at diagnosis are usually around 10:1 and with time may become as high as 100:1.[1] This progression of erythroid failure (with time) seems to parallel the more severe abnormalities detected when using in vitro progenitor cell assays to study older chronically affected patients compared with those newly diagnosed.[11,12] The heterogeneity of the disorder is reflected in the marrow. In one series of nine patients, all had marked erythroid hypoplasia: four had virtually no erythroid precursors, two had erythroid maturation up to the polychromatophilic or orthochromatic normoblast stage, and three had a maturation arrest at the proerythroblast stage with 2–7% of the total nucleated cells being proerythroblasts.[11] In Alter's review,[36] 28 of 29 patients had erythroid hypoplasia. One had erythroid hyperplasia with a maturation arrest. Several of Alter's patients had normal numbers of proerythroblasts but no differentiation beyond that stage. In a series of patients from Bernard et al.[72] 90% had erythroid hypoplasia, 5% had normal erythroid precursors, and 5% had erythroid hyperplasia. Although all patients have a profound reticulocytopenia, the erythroid developmental arrest in DBA has been demonstrated by progenitor assays, or morphologically, to occur at all stages of maturation from the multipotent myeloid progenitor to the late normoblast. These observations also suggest that the defect may become more profound with age, the erythroid arrest seeming to occur at an earlier stage of differentiation as patients get older. However, serial studies of a significant group of patients have not been performed.

Imaging studies are useful to help delineate congenital abnormalities that may be present in patient with DBA. Skeletal surveys are not usually warranted, but selected radiographs may define suspected bony anomalies. Abdominal and cardiac ultrasonography may detect or diagnose suspected and perhaps significant renal or cardiac anomalies.

Prenatal diagnosis may be possible for DBA. Erythrocyte ADA activity could be increased in a fetus with DBA, and DBA fetal blood BFU-E might be decreased in number or cellularity, but these phenomena have not been examined. As only a few DBA cases appear to be familial, the opportunities for prenatal testing are quite limited.

DIFFERENTIAL DIAGNOSIS

DBA must be distinguished from the normochromic normocytic (or macrocytic) anemias that are present from birth through the first year of life. These anemias are pathophysiologically distinct from pure red cell aplasia seen in adults, which is frequently associated with an underlying disorder. For example, the association of pure red cell aplasia with thymoma, as described in adults, has not been described in infancy, although it has been observed in a 5-year-old girl.[73] A careful history, physical examination, and examination of the peripheral blood smear can usually rule out hemorrhage, myelosuppression due to infection, renal failure, infiltrative disease, severe protein malnutrition, or drug-related red cell failure, as well as the aplastic crisis of a chronic hemolytic anemia (e.g., sickle cell anemia or hereditary spherocytosis). Other less frequent forms of pure red cell failure such as antibody- or T-lymphocyte-mediated acquired autoimmune pure red cell aplasia, as well as hepatitis, Epstein-Barr or human T-cell leukemia-1 virus-associated, and drug-induced aplasia have been recently reviewed by Freedman[74] and should be considered in the differential diagnosis. Since folate deficiency as a cause of the hypoplastic crises associated with chronic hemolytic anemia is prevented by prophylactic administration of the vitamin, acquired hypoplastic anemia in these patients is now most frequently a consequence of human parvovirus (HPV) infection. Evidence of HPV infection has been found in patients with a variety of sickle cell syndromes,[75,76] hereditary spherocytosis,[76,77] pyruvate kinase deficiency,[78] and thalassemia[76] following an aplastic crisis. Red cell aplasia in otherwise normal neonates resulting in fetal hydrops, in a patient undergoing treatment for acute lymphocytic leukemia,[79] and in other immunosuppressed patients[74] has also been described, apparently due to HPV infection. Chronic red cell aplasia due to HPV infection in an otherwise normal individual has been reported as well.[80] This patient was cured after 10 years of transfusion-dependent anemia by the use of intravenous immunoglobulin. Thus HPV infection should be ruled out in all instances of red cell failure in children. The etiology of the red cell failure resulting from HPV infection is suggested by in vitro studies in which erythroid differentiation is inhibited by the presence of this small DNA virus in erythroid precursors derived from proliferating progenitors grown in the presence of HPV-containing serum.[81]

A bone marrow examination, revealing red cell aplasia or severe hypoplasia with no abnormalities in the myeloid or megakaryocyte lineages, as well as no evidence of infiltrative disease, congenital dyserythropoietic anemia, or the giant proerythroblasts often observed in HPV infection in an infant or young child, suggests either DBA or TEC. Table 24-3 outlines the important features that distinguish TEC from BDA. TEC is characterized by a temporary suppression of erythropoiesis that frequently follows a viral infection. Anemia is moderate to severe with reticulocytopenia. The disease is not familial, although the simultaneous occurrence in family members has been reported,[74] and there are no associated anomalies. The age of onset is usually a bit older than that for DBA. One key point in differentiating between DBA and TEC is the presence of fetal characteristics in the erythrocytes of many patients with DBA. These characteristics include an elevated MCV (>90 μm^3), elevated levels of Hb F and i antigen, and a fetal erythrocyte glycolytic and HMP shunt enzyme pattern.[36,82] These fetal characteristics are probably the consequence of "stress erythropoiesis" associated with chronic DBA. The presence of "fetal-like" cells is much less reliable in differentiating DBA from TEC in very young infants, in whom red cells normally possess fetal characteristics. Thus, as more children with TEC under 1 year of age are being described, the differential diagnosis is becoming more difficult. Even in older children, only 30% of DBA patients will have fetal-like erythrocytes at diagnosis. In addition, the erythroid recovery from TEC is also characterized by "stress erythropoiesis," giving rise to erythrocytes with fetal characteristics."[83] To add to this difficulty, Glader and co-workers[84] described a 16-year-old girl who presented with transfusion-dependent pure red cell aplasia that remitted after 7 months with no residual erythrocyte abnormalities. Making a prompt diagnosis is important because patients with transient erythroblastopenia of childhood usually recover spontaneously, hence appearing to respond rapidly when steroids are

Table 24-3. Diamond-Blackfan Anemia Versus Transient Erythroblastopenia of Childhood

	Diamond-Blackfan Anemia	Transient Erythroblastopenia of Childhood
Pure red cell aplasia	Present	Present
Age at onset	10% at birth; 90% by 1 year	0–4 years
Mode of inheritance	Autosomal dominant and recessive	Not inherited
Associated anomalies	≥1 in 30% of patients	Absent
Fetal hemoglobin	Elevated	Normal
i Antigen	Present	Absent
MCV	Elevated (30%) at diagnosis	Normal
Fetal pattern of red cell glycolytic and HMP shunt enzymes	Present	Absent
ADA activity	Elevated in the vast majority of patients	Normal
Response to corticosteroid therapy	Frequent (~70%)	Spontaneous recovery without therapy
Prognosis	Long periods of control; potential iron overload for those dependent on red cell transfusion requiring Desferal chelation; in long-term survivors, development of leukemia	Excellent for total recovery without sequelae

mistakenly instituted. A diagnosis of TEC in these instances may only be made retrospectively after completion of a long course of corticosteroids. Studies by Glader and co-workers[66–68] demonstrated that elevated red cell ADA activity can be used to distinguish DBA from TEC. Unfortunately, many patients are transfused before a complete initial evaluation, making an accurate erythrocyte ADA activity determination impossible. Although in vitro progenitor assays have shed important light on the pathophysiology of DBA and TEC, we do not advocate their use as a diagnostic test. Freedman[74] defined TEC in a recent review as "(1) gradual onset of pallor in previously healthy children one to four years of age (85%) with older and younger exceptions; (2) normochromic-normocytic anaemia with varying reticuloytopenia unless recovery has already ensued; (3) marrow erythroid hypoplasia (60% of cases) or aplasia (10% of cases), or a recovery picture (30% of cases); spontaneous recovery usually within four to eight weeks without recurrence, with rare exceptions." Based on the differences listed in Table 24-3, a high index of suspicion of transient erythroblastopenia of childhood should prompt avoidance of steroids, minimal red cell transfusions, and alleviation of parental concern.

THERAPY

If the diagnosis of DBA versus TEC is in doubt and the patient is symptomatic from anemia, the patient should only be modestly transfused to a hemoglobin level of 7–8 g, so that erythropoiesis will not be suppressed, delaying recovery in those patients who have TEC. In 1951, corticosteroid treatment in the

THERAPY FOR DIAMOND-BLACKFAN ANEMIA

Most patients with DBA respond to corticosteroids with improvement in, or resolution of, their anemia. If, however, the diagnosis of DBA versus TEC is in doubt and the patient has symptomatic anemia, our approach is to transfuse the patient modestly to a hemoglobin level of 7–8 g/dl. Thus, erythropoiesis will not be suppressed, delaying recovery in those patients who do have TEC. Most patients with TEC will improve within 1 month or so from diagnosis, usually after receiving only one transfusion. When TEC is suspected and recovery is not prompt, we generally withhold corticosteroid therapy in favor of additional transfusions before instituting prednisone.

In patients with DBA, we use prednisone (2 mg/kg/day PO) in three to four divided doses. On this regimen, a reticulocyte response usually occurs within 1–2 weeks of starting prednisone. If no response occurs within 2 weeks, the dose can be increased to 3 or even 4 mg/kg/day. Responses are variable. Approximately 20–30% of patients never respond to corticosteroids. Some patients respond rapidly and can be tapered off prednisone, remaining in remission for extended periods; others respond but require continued therapy with erythropoiesis, ceasing rapidly if steroids are discontinued. Care should be taken during steroid tapers, as overzealous tapering leading to erythroid failure requires reinstitution of prednisone at the original dose. The ability in responders to achieve our goal of an effective every-other-day dose schedule is also variable, but most can be tapered to such a regimen. Over time, some patients may even be tapered off steroids completely, while others may require increasing doses, eventually becoming refractory to treatment. If no response occurs within 1 month, prednisone is discontinued in favor of transfusion and chelation regimens following established guidelines. Nonresponders receive periodic (approximately yearly) prednisone trials, since they may respond at a later date.

In steroid nonresponders, high-dose corticosteroid pulses may evoke an erythroid response. We do not advocate this approach, since the potential side effects and the need for repeat pulses limit efficacy. Likewise, trials of cyclosporine in DBA have not been particularly encouraging. In some patients who fail to respond to prednisone, there may be a response when oxymetholone (2.0–5 mg/kg/day) is added. However, we prefer transfusion and chelation over the use of androgens in infants and young children.

For patients in whom a response occurs, the hemoglobin is followed until a level of 8–10 g/dl is achieved. The steroid dose is then tapered until the patient is on the smallest possible alternate-day dose. A Monday-Wednesday-Friday dose schedule is usually effective and easier to comply with than a strict every-other-day regimen. The dosage on a Monday-Wednesday-Friday schedule may range from a few milligrams (even in adolescents) to as much as 40–50 mg. Another dose schedule uses 1 week of daily prednisone during a 3-week to monthly cycle. Although this regimen may reduce side effects such as growth retardation, some patients may not maintain their hemoglobin level; thus, we prefer the Monday-Wednesday-Friday schedule. For patients who are steroid refractory or in whom the dose cannot be tapered to an alternate-day regimen and thus require high daily doses that cause toxicity, chronic transfusion is instituted. Occasionally, patients have significant steroid-related side effects, such as osteonecrosis, even on a small every-other-day dose; these patients may also require the discontinuation of corticosteroids in favor of chronic transfusion therapy.

As preparative regimens and infection control have improved and graft-versus-host disease has become more amenable to treatment and prevention, thereby reducing morbidity and mortality, bone marrow transplantation (BMT) has been used in a handful of DBA patients with good results. Because of the substantial short-term risks associated with BMT, the decision regarding BMT versus transfusion and chelation in those patients unable to achieve an every-other-day steroid schedule must be individualized in those patients with HLA-matched sibling donors. Modern chelation regimens seem very effective in reducing the consequences of iron overload in chronically transfused patients, but the long-term results of these programs are unknown. This uncertainty, the rate of leukemia and myelodysplasia, and the other risks of transfusion (i.e., sensitization and infection) make the decision regarding BMT (when a suitable donor exists) versus chelation therapy for DBA patients who are steroid refractory or steroid nontolerant one that must be individualized and constantly re-evaluated. Indeed, the leukemia, myelodysplasia risk, and possibility of late-occurring steroid failure or side effects suggest that BMT be considered even in those DBA patients responding to low alternate-day steroid doses.

---

form of corticotropin was first found to be effective in DBA.[85,86] Currently, all patients are initially given prednisone (2 mg/kg/day PO) in three to four divided doses. A reticulocyte response usually occurs within 1–2 weeks. If no response occurs within 2 weeks, the dose can then be increased to 3 or even 4 mg/kg/day. Approximately 20% of patients never respond to corticosteroids. Some patients respond rapidly and can be tapered off prednisone, remaining in remission for extended periods of time; others respond but require continued therapy, with erythropoiesis ceasing rapidly if steroids are discontinued. The frequency with which responders achieve an effective every-other-day dose schedule is variable. Some patients may be tapered off steroids even after many years, while others may require increasing doses of steroids and eventually become refractory to treatment. Approximately 50% of patients will respond to a tolerable every-other-day dose. Although high-dose corticosteroid pulses may evoke an erythroid response in some patients,[87,88] the potential side effects and the need for repeat pulses limit its efficacy. Likewise, trials of Cyclosporin A in DBA have not been particularly encouraging.[89] Some patients who fail to respond to prednisone may respond to oxymetholone (2–5 mg/kg/day).[1,40] However, most clinicians do not advocate the use of androgens in infants and young children. If no response occurs within approximately 1 month, prednisone is discontinued in favor of supportive care, with transfusion and iron chelation regimens being instituted. Such patients should receive periodic prednisone trials, since they may respond at a later date.

For patients in whom there is a response to therapy, the hemoglobin is followed until an adequate level of 8–10 g/dl is achieved. The steroid dose is then tapered until the patient is on the smallest possible alternate day dose. A Monday-Wednesday-Friday dose schedule is usually effective and easier to comply with than a strict every-other-day regimen. The dosage in a Monday-Wednesday-Friday schedule may range from a few milligrams, even in adolescents, to ≤40–50 mg. In another approach, daily prednisone is administered for 1 week out of a 3–4-week cycle.[90] This regimen may reduce side effects such as growth retardation, but some patients may not maintain their hemoglobin levels. Arbitrary discontinuation of therapy should be discouraged since re-establishing erythropoiesis, after an effective every-other-day course of prednisone is discontinued, requires reinstitution of the original daily dose. For patients who are steroid refractory or who cannot be maintained on an alternate-day regimen and who thus require high daily doses that cause toxicity, chronic transfusion is instituted. Occasional patients have significant steroid-related side effects, such as osteonecrosis, even on a small every-other-day dose, and may also require the discontinuation of corticosteroids in favor of chronic transfusion therapy.

As preparative regimens and infection control have improved and graft-versus-host disease has become more amenable to treatment and prevention, thereby reducing morbidity and mortality, bone marrow transplantation has been used in a handful of DBA patients with reasonably good results.[91–95] Because of the substantial short-term risks associated with bone marrow transplantation (BMT), the decision regarding BMT versus transfusion and chelation therapy must be individualized in those patients unable to be maintained on an every-other-day steroid schedule and who have an HLA-matched sibling donor. New oral chelators may soon be available, and modern chelation regimens seem to be highly effective in reducing the consequences of iron overload in chronically transfused patients, but the long-term results of these programs are unknown. This uncertainty, the risk of leukemia and myelodysplasia in DBA, the possibility of spontaneous remission, and the other risks of transfusion (i.e., sensitization and infection) make the decision regarding BMT (when a suitable donor exists) versus transfusion and chelation therapy for DBA patients who are steroid refractory or steroid nontolerant one that must be constantly re-evaluated. Indeed, the leukemia, the myelodysplasia risk, and the possibility of late-occurring steroid failure or side effects suggest that BMT be considered even in those DBA patients responding to low alternate-day steroid doses.

PROGNOSIS

The outcome for the approximately 50% of patients who respond to tolerable every-other-day corticosteroids is generally quite good, although a few may eventually experience significant steroid-related side effects requiring temporary or permanent discontinuation of therapy. Short stature, however, is thought to be a consequence of the underlying disorder, at least in part.

As a result of advances in therapy, the published projected median survival rate of 31 years[13] is not particularly helpful for determining the prognosis of patients diagnosed today. Deaths due to infection in splenectomized patients with DBA are now dramatically reduced through the use of pneumococcal and *Haemophilus influenzae* vaccines, prophylactic penicillin, and careful follow-up and management. In addition, splenectomy is only performed for problems due to hypersplenism and an increased transfusion requirement, not as specific therapy for DBA. Modern chelation schemes seem to be able to postpone dramatically, if not eliminate, clinically significant transfusion-related hemosiderosis. However, the morbidity and mortality from transfusion-acquired infection is difficult to access, and

despite better selection and screening of donors, problems for these chronically transfused patients may continue. Leukemia has been reported in eight patients,[96–100] and three other patients have developed myelodysplastic syndromes[101] at ages 13, 21, and 22; two subsequently developed leukemia, and one died from complications of myelodysplasia. As Glader[102] points out, it will take more time to determine whether "acute leukemia [is] a real complication of Diamond-Blackfan anemia," and although the number of cases is small and is over-represented with regard to the total number of DBA cases reported (proportionally more leukemic cases than nonleukemic cases are reported), these data indicate that the incidence of leukemia and myelodysplastic syndromes in DBA is increased. Thus, the use of cytokines, which are currently only available for experimental clinical trials, and the role of BMT must be assessed in the context of the risk of leukemia and myelodysplasia. Due to the small number of histocompatible related donors, too few DBA patients are currently undergoing BMT to determine the impact of this modality on prognosis.

FUTURE DIRECTIONS

Advances in cellular and molecular biology have begun to increase our understanding of the pathophysiology of DBA. The recent observation that DBA is characterized by the accelerated apoptosis of erythroid progenitors and precursor[20] suggests new lines of inquiry. The application of basic research in hematopoiesis to the problem of DBA has given rise to a number of clinical trials. More trials are forthcoming, but unfortunately these trials[31–34] have thus far met with only limited success.

With a reasonable degree of confidence that most instances of DBA are the consequence of an intrinsic progenitor defect, efforts are being made to determine the molecular defect. Recently, a kindred containing seven affected family members, all with short stature (but no dysmorphic features), elevated MCV, Hb F, and erythrocyte ADA activity, has been described.[51] Abnormalities in the EPO and insulin-like growth factor-1 receptor are being investigated in this family.[51] Although this is a preliminary approach, basic research will certainly reveal more candidate genes, and the improved survival in DBA patients will no doubt result in larger kindreds for study. The recently established Diamond-Blackfan Anemia Registry has enrolled 190 patients.[103] Detailed epidemiologic and treatment outcome data obtained through the registry will be of great value in defining the etiology and pathogenesis of this disorder.

For a handful of investigators, the study of DBA is the sine qua non of pediatric hematology. Careful clinical investigation has defined the syndrome, and the study of the cellular biology of the disorder has borrowed from, and contributed to, an understanding of the mechanism of hematopoietic progenitor cell differentiation. That the anemia of DBA seems to result from hyporesponsiveness to inducers of erythroid differentiation should allow a return to the bedside with therapeutic modalities derived directly from laboratory investigations.

REFERENCES

1. Diamond LK, Wang WC, Alter BP: Congenital hypoplastic anemia. Adv Pediatr 22:349, 1976
2. Lipton JM, Nathan DG: Aplastic and hypoplastic anemia. Pediatr Clin North Am 27:217, 1980
3. Diamond LK, Blackfan KD: Hypoplastic anemia. Am J Dis Child 56:464, 1938
4. Ortega JA, Shore NA, Dukes PP, Hammond D: Congenital hypoplastic anemia: inhibition of erythropoiesis by sera from patients with congenital hypoplastic anemia. Blood 45:83, 1975
5. Hoffman R, Zanjani ED, Vila J et al: Diamond-Blackfan syndrome: lymphocyte mediated suppression of erythropoiesis. Science 193:899, 1976
6. Sawada K, Koyonagawa Y, Sakamura S et al: Diamond-Blackfan syndrome:

a possible role of cellular factors for erythropoietic suppression. Scand J Haematol 35:158, 1985

7. Ershler WB, Ross J, Finlay JL, Shahidi NT: Bone marrow microenvironmental defect in congenital hypoplastic anemia. N Engl J Med 302:1321, 1980
8. Finlay JL, Shahidi NT, Horowitz S et al: Lymphocyte dysfunction in congenital hypoplastic anemia. J Clin Invest 70:619, 1982
9. Nathan DG, Clarke BJ, Hillman DG et al: Erythroid precursors in congenital hypoplastic (Diamond-Blackfan) anemia. J Clin Invest 61:489, 1978
10. Freedman MH, Amato D, Saunders EF: Erythroid colony growth in congenital hypoplastic anemia. J Clin Invest 57:673, 1976
11. Lipton JM, Kudisch M, Gross R, Nathan DG: Defective erythroid progenitor differentiation system in congenital hypoplastic (Diamond-Blackfan) anemia. Blood 67:962, 1986
12. Tsai PH, Arkin S, Lipton JM: An intrinsic progenitor defect in Diamond-Blackfan anemia. Br J Haematol 73:112, 1989
13. Alter BP: The bone marrow failure syndromes. p. 216. In Nathan DG, Oski FA (eds): Hematology of Infancy and Childhood. 4th Ed. WB Saunders, Philadelphia, 1993
14. Lipton JM, Nathan DG: Cell-cell interactions in the regulation of erythropoiesis. Br J Haematol 53:361, 1983
15. Geller G, Krivit N, Zalusky R: Lack of erythropoietic inhibitory effect from patients with congenital pure red cell aplasia. J Pediatr 86:198, 1975
16. Freedman MH, Saunders EF: Diamond-Blackfan syndrome: evidence against cell mediated erythropoietic suppression. Blood 51:1125, 1978
17. Nathan DG, Hillman DG, Chess L et al: Normal erythropoietic helper T-cells in congenital hypoplastic anemia. N Engl J Med 298:1049, 1978
18. Chan HSL, Saunders EF, Freedman MH: Diamond-Blackfan syndrome. I. Erythropoiesis in prednisone responsive and resistant disease. Pediatr Res 16:474, 1982
19. Chan HSL, Saunders EF, Freedman MH: Diamond-Blackfan syndrome. II. In vitro corticosteroid effect on erythropoiesis. Pediatr Res 16:477, 1982
20. Perdahl EB, Naprstek BL, Wallace WC, Lipton JM: Erythroid failure in Diamond-Blackfan anemia is characterized by apoptosis. Blood 83:645, 1994
21. Halperin DS, Estrov Z, Feedman MH: Diamond-Blackfan anemia: promotion of marrow erythropoiesis in vitro by recombinant interleukin-3. Blood 73:1168, 1989
22. Bagnara GP, Zauli G, Rosito P et al: In vitro growth and regulation of bone marrow enriched CD34+ hematopoietic progenitors in Diamond-Blackfan anemia. Blood 78:2203, 1991
23. Abkowitz JL, Sabo KM, Nakamoto B et al: Diamond-Blackfan anemia: in vitro response of erythroid progenitors to the ligand for c-kit. Blood 78:2198, 1991
24. Olivieri NF, Grunberger T, Ben-David Y et al: Diamond-Blackfan anemia: heterogenous response of hematopoietic progenitor cells in vitro to the protein product of the Steel locus. Blood 78:2211, 1991
25. Alter BP, Knobloch ME, He L et al: Effect of stem cell factor and other hematopoietic growth factors on in vitro erythropoiesis in patients with bone marrow failure syndromes. Blood 80:3000, 1992
26. Drachtman RA, Geissler EN, Alter BP: TaqI RFLP at the c-kit oncogene locus (KIT). Nucleic Acids Res 19:6975, 1991
27. Abkowitz JL, Broudy VC, Bennett LG et al: Absence of abnormalities of c-kit or its ligand in two patients with Diamond-Blackfan anemia. Blood 79:25, 1992
28. Dractman RA, Geissler EN, Alter BP: The molecular defect in Diamond-Blackfan anemia. Blood 79:2177, 1992
29. Giebel LB, Spritz RA: Mutation of the KIT (mast/stem cell growth factor receptor) protooncogene in human piebaldism. Proc Natl Acad Sci USA 88:8696, 1991
30. Alter BP, Gaston T, Lipton JM: Lack of effect of corticosteroids in W/W^v and Sl/Sl^d mice: these mice are not a model for Diamond-Blackfan anemia. Eur J Haemaol 50:275, 1993
31. Gillio AP, Faulkner LB, Alter BP et al: Treatment of Diamond-Blackfan anemia with recombinant human interleukin-3. Blood 52:744, 1993
32. Dunbar CE, Smith DA, Kimball J et al: Treatment of Diamond-Blackfan anemia with haematopoietic growth factors, granulocyte-macrophage colony stimulating factor and interleukin 3: sustained remissions following IL-3. Br J Haematol 79:316, 1991
33. Olivieri NF, Berriman AM, Davis S et al: Response to the hematopoietic growth factor IL-3 in patients with Diamond-Blackfan anemia. Blood 78:153A, 1991
34. Niemeyer CM, Baumgarten E, Holldack J et al: Treatment trial with recombinant human erythropoietin in children with congenital hypoplastic anemia. Contrib Nephrol 88:276, 1991
35. Scimeca PG, Weinblatt ME, Slepowitz G et al: Diamond-Blackfan syndrome: an unusual cause of hydrops fetalis. Am J Pediatr Hematol Oncol 10:241, 1988

36. Alter BP: Childhood red cell aplasia. Am J Pediatr Hematol Oncol 2:121, 1980
37. Aase JM, Smith DW: Congenital anemia and triphalangeal thumbs: a new syndrome. J Pediatr 74:471, 1969
38. Gordon RR, Varadi S: Congenital hypoplastic anaemia (pure red-cell anaemia) with periodic erythroblastopenia. Lancet 1:296, 1962
39. Sensenbrenner LA: Congenital hypoplastic anemia of Blackfan and Diamond in sibs. p. 166. In Bergsma D (ed): The Clinical Delineation of Birth Defects. Part XIV: Blood. Williams & Wilkins, Baltimore, 1972
40. Starling KA, Fernbach DJ: Hypoplastic anemia. J Pediatr 82:735, 1973
41. Waterkotte GW, McElfresh AE: Congenital pure red cell hypoplasia in identical twins. Pediatrics 54:646, 1974
42. Förare SA: Pure red-cell anemia in step siblings. Acta Paediatr 52:159, 1963
43. Altman AC, Gross S: Severe congenital hypoplastic anemia transmission from a healthy female to opposite sex step-siblings. Am J Pediatr Hematol Oncol 5:99, 1983
44. Mott MG, Apley J, Raper AB: Congenital (erythroid) hypoplastic anaemia: modified expression in males. Arch Dis Child 44:757, 1969
45. Hunter RE, Hakami N: The occurrence of congenital hypoplastic anemia in half brothers. J Pediatr 81:346, 1972
46. Hamilton PJ, Dawson AA, Galloway WH: Congenital erythroid hypoplastic anaemia in mother and daugher. Arch Dis Child 49:71, 1974
47. Michelson AD: Inheritance of Diamond-Blackfan anaemia. Med J Aust 2:409, 1982
48. Lawton JWM, Aldrich JE, Turner TL: Congenital erythroid hypoplastic anemia: autosomal dominant transmission. Scand J Haematol 13:276, 1974
49. McFarland G, Say B, Carpenter NJ et al: A condition resembling congenital hypoblastic anemia occurring in a mother and son. Clin Pediatr 12:755, 1982
50. Gray PH: Pure red-cell aplasia: occurrence in three generations. Med J Aust 1:519, 1982
51. Viskochil DH, Casey JC, Glader BE et al: Congenital hypoplastic (Diamond-Blackfan) anemia in seven members of one hundred. Am J Med Gen 35:251, 1990
52. Hurst JA, Baraitser M, Wonke B: Autosomal dominant transmission of congenital erythroid hypoplastic anemia with radial abnormalities. Am J Med Gen 40:482, 1991
53. Diamond LK, Allen DM, Magill FB: Congenital (erythroid) hypoplastic anemia. Am J Dis Child 102:403, 1961
54. Tada K, Kudo T, Nakagawa I et al: Anémie congénitale hypoplastique. Arch Fr Pediatr 15:183, 1958
55. Tartaglia AP, Propp S, Amarose AP et al: Chromosome abnormality and hypocalcemia in congenital erythroid hypoplasia (Blackfan-Diamond syndrome). Am J Med 41:990, 1966
56. Heyn R, Kurczynski E, Schmickel R: The association of Blackfan-Diamond syndrome, physical abnormalities, and an abnormality of chromosome 1. J Pediatr 85:531, 1974
57. Balban EP, Buchanan GR, Graham M, Frenkel DP: Diamond-Blackfan syndrome in adult patients. Am J Med 78:533, 1985
58. Josephs HW: Anemia of infancy and early childhood. Medicine 15:307, 1936
59. Alter BP: Thumbs and anemia. Pediatrics 62:613, 1978
60. Alter BP: Arm anomalies and bone marrow failure may go hand in hand. J Hand Surg 17A:566, 1992
61. Hedberg VA, Lipton JM: Thrombocytopenia with absent radii: a review of 100 cases. Am J Pediatr Hematol Oncol 10:51, 1988
62. Schmickel RD: Contiguous gene syndromes: a component of recognizable syndromes. J Pediatr 109:231, 1986
63. Schofield KP, Evans DK: Diamond-Blackfan syndrome and neutropenia. J Clin Pathol 44:742, 1991
64. Buchanan GR, Alter BP, Holtkamp CA, Walsh EG: Platelet number and function in Diamond-Blackfan anemia. Pediatrics 68:238, 1981
65. Schroeder WA, Huisman THJ, Brown AK et al: Postnatal changes in the chemical heterogeneity of human fetal hemoglobin. Pediatr Res 9:493, 1971
66. Blader BE, Backer K, Diamond LK: Elevated erythrocyte adenosine deaminase activity in congenital hypoplastic anemia. N Engl J Med 309:1486, 1983
67. Glader BE, Backer K: Comparative activity of erythrocyte adenosine deaminase and orotidine decarboxylase in Diamond-Blackfan anemia. Am J Hematol 23:135, 1986
68. Glader BE, Backer K: Elevated red cell adenosine deaminase activity: a marker of disordered erythropoiesis in Diamond-Blackfan anaemia and other haematologic diseases. Br J Haematol 68:165, 1988
69. Zielke HR, Ozand PT, Luddy RE et al: Elevation of pyrimidine enzyme activities in the RBC of patients with congenital hypoplastic anemia and their parents. Br J Haematol 42:381, 1979
70. Harrison DE, Malathi VG, Silber R: Elevated erythrocyte nucleoside deaminase levels in genetically anemic W/W^v and Sl/Sl^d mice. Blood Cells 1:605, 1975

71. Brookfield EG, Singh P: Congenital hypoplastic anemia associated with hypogammaglobulinemia. J Pediatr 85:529, 1974

72. Bernard J, Seligmann M, Chassigneux J, Dresch C: Anaémie de Blackfan-Diamond. Nouv Rev Fr Hematol 2:721, 1962

73. Talerman A, Amigo A: Thymoma associated with regenerative and aplastic anemia in a five year-old child. Cancer 21:1212, 1968

74. Freedman MH: Pure red cell aplasia in childhood and adolescence: pathogenesis and approaches to diagnosis. Br J Haematol 84:246, 1993

75. Pattison JR, Jones SE, Hodgson J et al: Parvovirus infection and hypoplastic crisis in sickle cell anaemia. Lancet 1:664, 1981

76. Rao KRP, Patel AR, Anderson MD et al: Infection with parvovirus-like virus and aplastic crisis in chronic hemolytic anemia. Ann Intern Med 98:930, 1983

77. Kelleher JF, Luban NLC, Mortimer PP, Kamimura T: Human serum "parvovirus": a specific cause of aplastic crisis in children with hereditary spherocytosis. J Pediatr 102:720, 1983

78. Ducan J, Potter CG, Cappellini MD et al: Aplastic crisis due to parvovirus infection in pyruvate kinase deficiency. Lancet 2:14, 1983

79. Van Horn DK, Mortimer PP, Young N, Hanson GR: Human parvovirus-associated red cell aplasia in the absence of underlying hemolytic anemia. Am J Pediatr Hematol Oncol 8:235, 1986

80. Kurtzman G, Frickhofen N, Kimball J et al: Pure red-cell aplasia of 10 years' duration due to persistent parvovirus B19 infection and its cure with immunoglobulin therapy. N Engl J Med 321:519, 1989

81. Young N, Harrison M, Moore JG et al: Direct demonstration of the human parvovirus in erythroid progenitor cells infected in vitro. J Clin Invest 74:2024, 1984

82. Wang WC, Mentzer WC: Differentiation of transient erythroblastopenia of childhood from congenital hypoplastic anemia. J Pediatr 88:784, 1976

83. Link MP, Alter BP: Fetal-like erythropoiesis during recovery from transient erythroblastopenia of childhood (TEC). Pediatr Res 15:1036, 1981

84. Zwerdling T, Finlay J, Glader BE: Transient erythroblastopenia of adolescence. Clin Pediatr 25:563, 1986

85. Hill JM, Hunter RB: ACTH therapy in refractory anemias. p. 181. In Mote JR (ed): Proceedings of the Second Clinical ACTH Conference. Vol. II. Blakiston, New York, 1951

86. Gasser C: Aplastische Anamie (chronische Erythroblastophthise) und Cortison. Schweiz Med Wochenschr 81:1241, 1951

87. Ozsoylu S: High-dose intravenous corticosteroid for a patient with Diamond-Blackfan syndrome refractory to classical prednisone treatment. Acta Haematol 71:207, 1984

88. Ozsoylu S: High-dose intravenous corticosteroid treatment for patients with Diamond-Blackfan syndrome resistent on refractory to conventional treatment. Am J Pediatr Hematol Oncol 10:217, 1988

89. Leonard EM, Raefsky E, Griffith P et al: Cyclosporine therapy of aplastic anaemia, congenital and acquired red cell aplasia. Br J Haematol 72:278, 1989

90. Sjölin S, Wranne L: Treatment of congenital hypoplastic anaemia with prednisone. Scand J Haematol 7:63, 1970

91. August CS, King E, Githens JH et al: Establishment of erythropoiesis following bone marrow transplantation in a patient with congenital hypoplastic anemia (Diamond-Blackfan syndrome). Blood 48:491, 1976

92. Iriondo A, Garijo J, Baro J et al: Complete recovery of hemopoiesis following bone marrow transplant in a patient with unresponsive congenital hypoplastic anemia (Blackfan-Diamond syndrome). Blood 64:348, 1984

93. Lenarsky C, Weinberg K, Guinan E et al: Bone marrow transplantation for constitutional pure red cell aplasia. Blood 71:226, 1988

94. Greinix HT, Storb R, Sanders JE et al: Long term survival and cure after marrow transplantation for congenital hypoplastic (Diamond-Blackfan syndrome). Br J Haemetol 84:515, 1993

95. Gluckman E, Esperou H, Deverqie A et al: Pediatric bone marrow transplantation for leukemia and aplastic anemia. Report of 222 cases transplanted in a single center. Nouv Rev Fr Hematol 31:111, 1989

96. D'Oelsnitz M, Vincet L, DeSwarte M et al: À propos d'un cas de leucémie aigüe lymphoblastique survenue guérison d'une maladie de Blackfan-Diamond, abstracted. Arch Fr Pediatr 32:532, 1975

97. Krishnan EU, Wegner K, Garg SK: Congenital hypoplastic anemia terminating in acute promyelocytic leukemia. Pediatrics 61:898, 1978

98. Wasser JS, Yolken R, Miller DR, Diamond L: Congenital hypoplastic anemia (Diamond-Blackfan syndrome) terminating in acute myelogenous leukemia. Blood 51:991, 1978

99. Basso G, Cocito MG, Rebuffi L et al: Congenital hypoplastic anaemia developed in acute megakarioblastic leukemia: a case report. Helv Paediat Acta 36:267, 1981

100. Mori PG, Haupt R, Fugazza G et al: Pentasomy 21 in leukemia complicating Diamond-Blackfan anemia. Cancer Genet Cytogenet 63:70, 1992

101. Glader BE, Flam MS, Dahl GV et al: Hematologic malignancies in Diamond Blackfan anemia. Pediatr Res 27:142A, 1990

102. Glader BE: Diagnosis and management of red cell aplasia in children. Hematol Oncol Clin North Am 1:431, 1987

103. Vlachos A, Alter B, Buchanan G et al: The Diamond Blackfan Anemia Registry (DBAR): preliminary data. Blood 80:88A, 1993

104. Cathie IAB: Erythrogenesis imperfecta. Arch Dis Child 25:313, 1950

Paroxysmal Nocturnal Hemoglobinuria

25

Wendell F. Rosse

INTRODUCTION

Paroxysmal nocturnal hemoglobinuria (PNH) is a clonal disorder of the hematopoietic stem cell that results in the production of blood cells with characteristic defects.[1] The defect that was first detected was the unusual susceptibility of erythrocytes to the hemolytic action of complement[2]; this characteristic was first definitively demonstrated by Ham and his associates in 1938[2] and has been used as the principle means by which the laboratory diagnosis of this disorder is made.

The first descriptions of PNH emphasized the hemoglobinuria, which characteristically occurred at night and often in paroxysms, at times initiated by infections.[3,4] The recognition that hemosiderinuria was "perpetual" suggested that more hemolysis occurred than was demonstrated by the dark urine.[5] With the advent of diagnostic tests, it became apparent that the disease was much more complex than first realized. In addition to hemolytic anemia, patients often had venous thromboses in unusual places such as the sagittal sinus, the hepatic veins, and the dermal veins.[6] Many patients had granulocytopenia or thrombocytopenia, or both, in addition to the hemolytic anemia.[7] Although most patients had erythroid hyperplasia of the marrow, a sizable proportion had relative or absolute hypoplasia. Finally, a small proportion of patients developed acute myeloid leukemia.[8,9]

These nonerythrocytic manifestations led to the hypothesis that the other blood elements were also abnormal and tests showed abnormalities similar to those found in cells of other hematopoietic lineages.[10] This finding suggested that the disorder originated at the level of the hematopoietic stem cell.[11] The finding that most patients had a normal as well as an abnormal population of erythrocytes and that the abnormal cells appeared to be clonal gave rise to the hypothesis that the disorder was the result of a clonal proliferation of an abnormal hematopoietic stem cell.[12]

More recently, the nature of the abnormality has been described. It has been found that the abnormal cells in PNH lack a number of membrane proteins that have in common fixation to the plasma membrane by a complex glycolipid anchor.[13] In the abnormal cells in PNH, this anchor cannot be synthesized because of a defect early in the biosynthetic pathway[14-17]; since the anchor cannot be made, the proteins cannot be affixed to the membrane. Most if not all PNH manifestations can or will probably be traced to the lack of these proteins on the abnormal cells.

PATHOBIOLOGY

In PNH, normal and abnormal erythrocytes, granulocytes, monocytes, and platelets are present in the peripheral blood at the same time, suggesting that the abnormal cells arose as a clone within the marrow. The clonal origin of the abnormal population was supported by the finding in women heterozygous for variants of the enzyme glucose-6-phosphate dehydrogenase that the abnormal PNH erythrocytes were all of one isozyme[18]; since the gene for this enzyme is located on the X chromosome, the assumption is that the abnormal cells are derived from a single precursor that possessed that isozyme after meiotic suppression of the other X chromosome.

More recent studies have confirmed this hypothesis. Using probes for detecting polymorphisms in genes located on the X chromosome, a monoclonal pattern was found in the marrow cells in five of five PNH patients, strongly indicating that the abnormal cells had arisen from a single precursor.[19]

Defect in Glycosylphosphatidylinositol Anchor

The nature of the defect in the abnormal cells in PNH was difficult to understand, as evidence of missing membrane proteins accumulated. The observation by Low and colleagues[20,21] that acetylcholinesterase (one of the proteins missing on the abnormal cells[22]) could be removed from the membrane by an enzyme, phosphatidylinositol-specific phospholipase C, without injury to its enzymatic activity, suggested that this protein was attached to the membrane in the same way as the variable surface glycoproteins of trypanosomes (i.e., by a glycosylphosphatidylinositol [GPI] anchor rather than by a transmembrane sequence of hydrophobic amino acids).[21,22] When decay accelerating factor (DAF) was also found to be attached by this anchor, a defect in this anchoring mechanism was proposed as the fundamental defect in PNH.[23]

The structure of the GPI anchor has remained fundamentally unchanged from the simplest life forms (e.g., trypanosomes) to mammals, including humans[24,25] (Fig. 25-1). It consists of a molecule of phosphatidylinositol to which are attached four sugars (a molecule of N-glucosamine and three molecules of mannose); the last mannose is attached to the carboxyl end of the protein through phosphoethanolamine. Phosphoethanolamine molecules may be attached to each of the other two mannose residues but do not attach to the protein. A palmitoyl moiety is added to the inositol but may later be removed. The N-glucosamine is derived from N-acetylglucosamine that is added and then deacetylated.[26] The source of the mannose residues is dolichyl phosphoryl mannose, which is synthesized from GDP-mannose and dolichol phosphate (a long-chain polymer of isoprene) by a specific enzyme.[27] The source of the phosphoethanolamines is not entirely clear, but they are probably derived from phosphatidylethanolamine.

Once the synthesis of the anchor is complete, it is attached to the protein in the cisterna of the endoplasmic reticulum by transamidation of the amino group of the terminal phosphoethanolamine to the carboxyl group in the protein.[28] Once the protein has been attached to the anchor, it then proceeds through the Golgi apparatus and on to the membrane surface.

Evidence for a Biosynthetic Defect

The absence of all GPI-linked proteins on the abnormal cells in PNH is due to a defect in the biosynthesis of the GPI anchor at a step prior to the addition of N-acetylglucosamine to the phosphatidylinositol moiety. This was shown in two ways: (1) the abnormal cells synthesize little or no biosynthetic intermediates containing N-glucosamine or mannose,[14,16] and (2) when the abnormal cells were fused with mouse cell lines defective in the synthesis of the anchor, those fused with cells of the class A phenotype did not complement (i.e., exhibit GPI-linked proteins on the surface), whereas those fused with lines of the other phenotypes did complement.[15,16,29] This means that the PNH cells were defective at the same step as the class A murine cells. Although the protein (?enzyme) mediating this step has not been identified, the gene responsible for it has been identified and is called the *pig-a* gene.[17,30] Abnormal PNH cells are able to express GPI-linked proteins when this gene is transfected into them. In the cells of several patients, the mRNA for this protein has been found to be abnormal in different respects (absence, reduced amount, truncation, etc.), suggesting that different abnormalities in the gene occur in different patients (Ware RE, Howard T, unpublished data).[30a-30c] It is likely that some of these abnormalities result in reduced production of the gene product and limited quantities of the final product, the complete anchor. This limitation may account for the cells of intermediate abnormality that have reduced amounts of GPI-linked proteins.

The *pig-a* gene is located on the X chromosome[17] at Xp.22 (at the end of the short arm) near the gene for the glycine receptor[31]; this means that a disabling acquired abnormality cannot be complemented by an allelic chromosome. Thus, it appears likely that the abnormalities in PNH result from a single "hit" to this gene in the hematopoietic stem cell and that the clinical manifestations result from the lack of proteins dependent on the GPI anchor for their surface expression.

Effects of the Deficiency of the Membrane Proteins

To date, about 15 proteins have been found to be lacking on the abnormal cells of patients with PNH (Table 25-1); not surprisingly, the deficiency, whether partial or complete, of so many proteins has profound effects on the function of the abnormal cells. These proteins can be divided into several

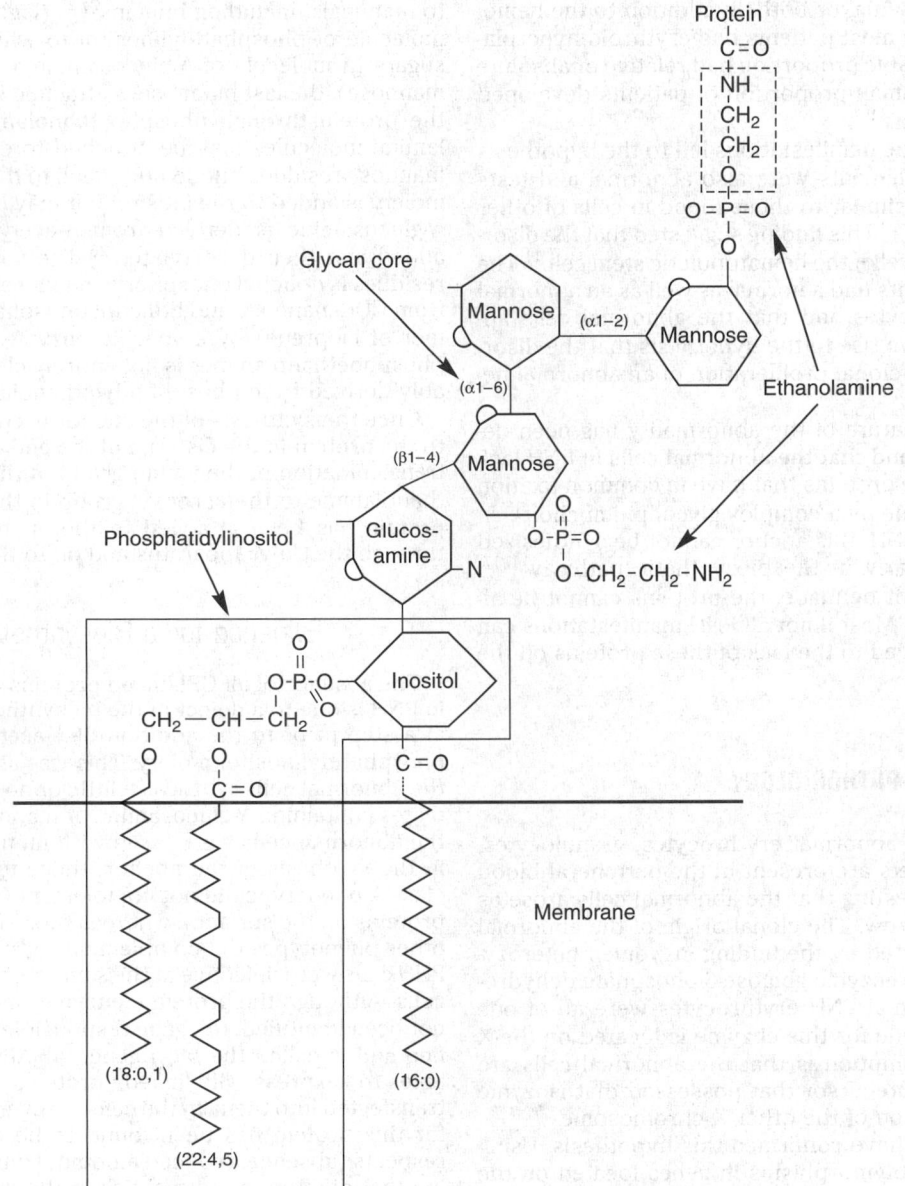

Fig. 25-1. Structure of the glycosylphosphatidylinositol (GPI) anchor. Phosphatidylinositol (with unusual fatty acids and an extra fatty acid attachment to the inositol) is inserted into the lipid core of the membrane. The glycan core consists of four sugars: one molecule of *N*-glucosamine and three molecules of mannose. Ethanolamine is attached to these sugars; the one on the terminal mannose is attached by an amide bond to the carboxyl terminus of the protein.

functional groups, and one of the aims of modern research in PNH is to explain the complex clinical syndrome in terms of the lack of these proteins.

Complement Defense Proteins

The manifestation that has been used to define PNH is the unusual sensitivity of the red cells to the hemolytic action of complement. This is due to reduced control of the activation of complement on the cell surface because of the lack of two (perhaps three) membrane proteins.

Complement consists of a group of proteins that circulate in the plasma in an inactive form; these proteins are sequentially activated on cellular sites to mediate some of the cellular destruction of the immune system[42-44] (Fig. 25-2). Inactivation mechanisms are in place to be certain that the reactions are controlled. Several fluid-phase proteins inhibit the enzymatic activity of some of the complexes[45]; other proteins cleave the

cell-bound components, thus inactivating them. Membrane proteins on the cell surface are more important for the protection of homologous cells against the attack by activated complement. Such proteins include DAF (CD55),[32] membrane inhibitor of reactive lysis (MIRL, CD59, protectin,[33] and perhaps C8-binding protein (homologous restriction factor).[34,35]

Decay Accelerating Factor

DAF, a glycoprotein of 68,000 molecular weight, increases the rate at which the convertase complexes (the enzyme complexes responsible for the activation of C3 and C5 [C4b2a of the classic pathway and C3bBb of the alternative pathway]) are dissociated or decayed. In disrupting the convertase complexes, it reduces the amount of C3 that is cleaved and thus reduces, ultimately, the number of membrane attack complexes that are formed.

The deficiency of CD55 on the abnormal PNH cells results in

Table 25-1. Membrane Proteins Missing from the Blood Cells in PNH

Complement defense proteins
    Decay accelerating factor (DAF, CD55)[32]
    Membrane inhibitor of reactive lysis (MIRL, CD59, protectin)[33]
    C8-binding protein[34] (homologous restriction factor)[35]

Immunologic proteins
    Fc$_\gamma$ receptor IIIa[36]
    Lymphocyte function-associated antigen-3 (LFA-3, CD58)[37]
    Endotoxin-binding protein receptor (CD14)[38]

Enzymes
    Acetylcholinesterase[22]
    Leukocyte alkaline phosphatase[39]

Receptors
    Urokinase (plasminogen activator) receptor[40]
    Folate receptor[a]

Granulocyte proteins of unknown function
    CD24[41]
    Two others[41]

[a] Rothenberg S, personal communication.

a greater activity of the convertases; hence, much more C3 is deposited on the membrane when either the classic or alternative pathway is activated.[46] The deficiency of this activity was thought at first to account for the greater sensitivity of PNH cells to complement, but in fact its deficiency plays a relatively minor role in that phenomenon.

The platelets in PNH also lack DAF but compensate by the release of factor H from internal granules[47]; factor H is a fluid-phase regulatory molecule with the same molecular action as DAF. This release is stimulated by activation of complement on the platelet surface and results in the local down-regulation of the convertase complexes.

Membrane Inhibitor of Reactive Lysis

MIRL (CD59), a glycoprotein of 19,000 molecular weight, is more important than DAF in the cellular regulation of complement action. It is related in structure to toxic proteins of the elapid snakes (bungarotoxin, erabutoxin)[48] and prevents the interaction between C8 and C9 in the final steps of complement activation.[49] Complement penetrates the lipid bilayer by the insertion of polymeric C9 into it; fluid-phase C9 is rendered amphipathic by interaction with C8 of the C5b/8 complex that is situated at the membrane surface.[44]

The absence of CD59 on PNH red cells is primarily responsible for their increased susceptibility to complement lysis.[50] Inhibition of its activity on normal erythrocytes renders them as susceptible to complement lysis as the most abnormal (PNH III) cells. Insertion of CD59 into the deficient PNH cells increases their resistance to complement lysis almost to normal. It is this increased susceptibility to lysis by complement that is responsible for the hemolysis of PNH cells in vivo.

The absence of CD59 on the abnormal platelets of PNH does not result in their lysis in vivo but may play a role in a serious complication of PNH, venous thrombosis. The response of the normal and PNH platelet to the insertion of the polymeric C9 into the membrane is to gather the offending complexes and remove them by exovesiculation[51] (Fig. 25-3). The vesicles that are so generated cannot maintain the acidic phospholipids on the internal leaflet and hence externalized phosphotidylserine serves as a site for prothrombinase complexes. These complexes generate thrombin. Since the formation of polymeric C9 complexes is not regulated on the PNH platelet, many more are inserted into the membrane, resulting in many more vesicles, which generate more thrombin.

The abnormal platelets in PNH appear to be specifically sensitive to the aggregating activity of thrombin. Much smaller amounts of thrombin cause aggregation of these platelets than are needed to aggregate normal platelets. The combination of these two reactions—increased production of thrombin and increased sensitivity to it—undoubtedly accounts for the markedly increased incidence of thrombosis in these patients.

Fc$_\gamma$ Receptor IIIa (CD16a)

The FC receptors on phagocytic cells bind to immunoglobulin, which is attached to antigens of the target cell. Several types exist, but only one is linked to the membrane by the GPI anchor FC$_\gamma$ receptor IIIa, it is the primary IgG receptor present on granulocytes. Its absence on PNH granulocytes[36] may contribute to the suggested propensity of these patients to infections, especially blood-borne ones (septicemia, bacterial endocarditis, etc).

Other Proteins Missing from PNH Cells

A number of other proteins are known to be missing from the blood cells in PNH (Table 25-1). Some are enzymes that have no known function in the biology of the cells. Some are related to immunologic function; their absence may play a role

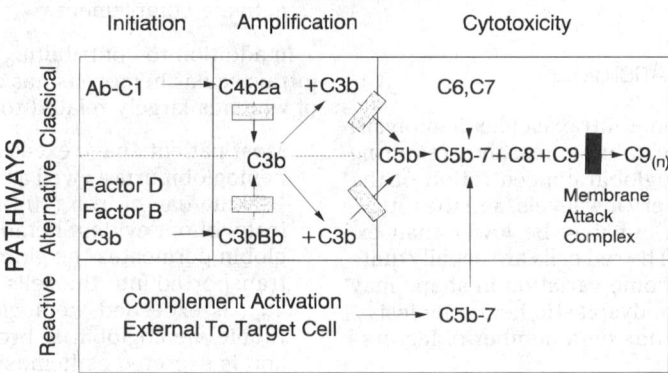

Fig. 25-2. The activation complexes of complement and their down-regulation by membrane proteins. Activation can take place by three pathways: the classic pathway involving antibody, the alternative pathway involving surface-bound C3b, and the reactive pathway involving the elements of the terminal complex C5b-7, which has been activated elsewhere (not on the target surface). Initiation complexes localize the reaction, amplification complexes amplify the effect by bimolecular enzymes (convertases), and cytotoxicity complexes insert protein into the lipid of the membrane to breach it. Decay accelerating factor inhibits the amplification complexes; membrane inhibitor of reactive lysis inhibits the formation of the membrane attack complex.

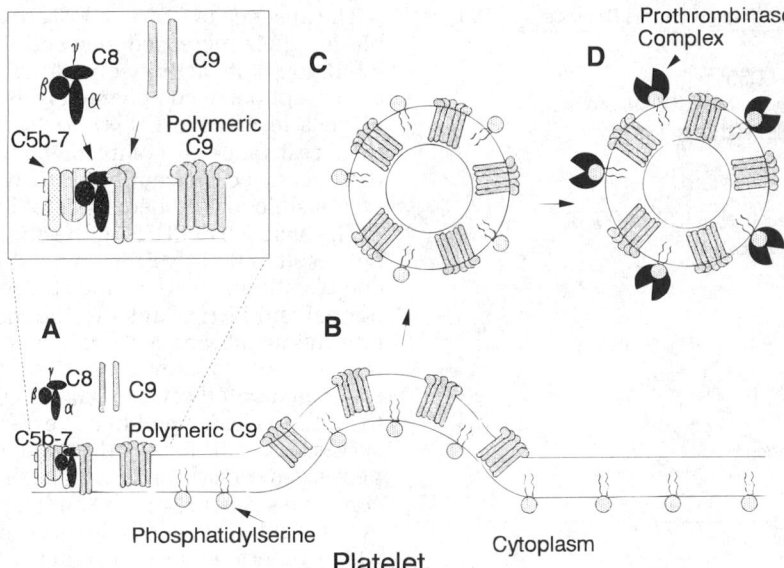

Fig. 25-3. Effect of polymeric C9 on the platelet membrane. **(A and Inset)** When the membrane attack complex is assembled on the membrane, aggregates of polymeric C9 result. **(B)** These polymeric C9 complexes are gathered into a region of the membrane and are removed by vesiculation. **(C)** The vesicles that result are not able to maintain phosphatidylserine on the internal leaflet of the bilayer. **(D)** The phosphatidylserine molecules become binding sites for the components of the prothrombinase complex, which is able to activate prothrombin.

in the pathogenesis of the syndrome, but the data for this hypothesis are not available. The lack of the folate receptor (?) and urokinase receptor (40) may alter the way in which those molecules are metabolized, but associated pathophysiology has not been identified. Future research will no doubt identify more missing proteins and will explain all the manifestations of the disease on the basis of the missing proteins (if the current algorithm is correct).

CLINICAL MANIFESTATIONS

Because of the variety of missing proteins on the hematopoietic cells, PNH is a highly protean syndrome with different manifestations in different patients. In addition, because it is clonal and the size of the abnormal clone is different in different patients, the severity of a given manifestation varies greatly from patient to patient. For these reasons, PNH must be considered in a number of hematologic clinical settings.

Hemolytic Anemia

All patients with PNH have some intravascular hemolysis, which can range from barely detectable to massive, requiring repeated transfusions. The hemoglobin concentration of the blood may range from normal to very low levels, and the reticulocyte count is usually elevated but may be lower than expected for the degree of anemia.[7] The red cells are usually quite normal in appearance, although some variation in shape may occur in some patients with more dysplastic hematopoiesis. The amount of hemolysis depends on a number of factors:

1. *The size of the abnormal clone:* the proportion of complement-sensitive red cells in the circulation can vary from 1% to >90%. Since these are the cells at risk for hemolysis,[52] the amount of hemolysis will be greater according to the number of abnormal cells, all other things being equal.
2. *The abnormality of the red cells:* the red cells may vary greatly in their abnormality because of differences in the content of

the complement defense proteins on the surface. The most abnormal (the so-called PNH III) cells completely lack these proteins and thus are very readily lysed in the circulation by minimal activation of complement. Cells of intermediate sensitivity (PNH II cells) display limited expression of the proteins on the surface and are not as readily lysed by complement activated *in vivo*.[53]

3. *The degree of complement activation:* the abnormal cells in PNH can be lysed by complement even when it is activated on other cells or in the plasma. Thus, situations in which complement is activated (infections, transfusion reactions, etc.) result in increased lysis of these red cells. The characteristic nocturnal hemolysis maybe due to the activation of complement by the absorption of endotoxin (a potent activator of the alternative pathway) from the gut, resulting in C5b/7 complexes that initiate attack through the reactive pathway (Fig. 25-2); normal cells are protected against this attack, whereas the defective PNH cells are not. Paroxysms of hemolysis often occur in conjunction with infections that activate complement.

In addition to contributing to the anemia of the patient, the intravascular hemolysis has several other effects, the severity of which is largely related to the degree of hemolysis:

1. Most patients have excessive iron loss both because of the hemoglobinuria as well as the "perpetual" hemosiderinuria; ≥20 mg/day of iron (10 times the normal amount) may be lost without evident hemoglobinuria.[54] In the kidney, hemoglobin permeates the glomerulus as a dimer and is actively transported into the cells of the proximal tubule; when the T_{max} is exceeded, hemoglobinuria results. In the proximal tubule, hemoglobin is broken down, but the iron remains and is excreted as hemosiderin.
2. In acute and massive hemolytic episodes, the kidneys may undergo acute tubular necrosis because of the large amount of hemoglobin being passed; this occurs most readily if the patient is also dehydrated and can be prevented by adequate hydration.[55]
3. In patients with long-lasting hemoglobinuria, defects in kidney function may occur. These may be as mild as renal Fan-

AN APPROACH TO PNH

Diagnosis

The diagnosis of PNH is ultimately made by the laboratory tests demonstrating complement sensitivity of the red cells or deficiency of the GPI-linked proteins. Diagnostic tests should be obtained in patients with (1) hemolytic anemia, with or without hemoglobinuria, with normal-appearing red cells, and without other hemolytic diagnosis; (2) signs of marrow dysfunction including aplastic anemia, granulocytopenia, or thrombocytopenia not otherwise explained, or myelodysplastic disease (if the test is initially negative, it should be repeated at intervals as it may become positive); (3) unexplained thromboses, particularly venous thromboses in unusual places; and (4) recurrent bouts of abdominal pain, or neurologic symptoms and headaches.

Treatment

The appropriate treatment depends on the symptoms. All patients should receive iron supplements unless they are receiving transfusions.

Anemia

The anemic patient with signs of hemolysis should be tried with prednisone at a dose of 20–40 mg every other day; if this is successful, it may be tapered, but not below a dose of about 20 mg every other day. If it is not helpful (the hemoglobin does not rise after 1 month or so), it should be discontinued unless the patient is having thrombotic complications. Some patients respond to androgens; danazol (400 mg/day) is best tolerated. Again, if no response is seen within 2 months, it should be discontinued. Transfusions should be given as needed.

Thrombosis

Patients with acute thrombosis should be given thrombolytic agents (streptokinase, urokinase, or tissue plasminogen activator) as rapidly as possible; studies are under way to determine whether these are useful on a more chronic basis for patients with insidious thrombosis, particularly of the liver. Full-dose heparin therapy should be instituted for ≥7–10 days, followed by appropriate treatment with Coumadin. Patients with documented thrombosis should be maintained on Coumadin for long periods. Antiplatelet agents (aspirin, ibuprofen, etc.) may be useful but their action is unproved.

Deficient Hematopoiesis

If the patient has an identical twin, syngeneic transplantation should be done. If the patient has a histocompatibility antigen-compatible sibling, transplantation should be considered if any complications due to the PNH are present; this is particularly true for children. Transplantation with the marrow of an antigen-compatible unrelated donor should be reserved only for patients with major complications.

Patients with marrow hypofunction (manifested by low reticulocyte count, thrombocytopenia, and/or granulocytopenia) may be candidates for antithymocyte globulin. The usual dose is 15 mg/kg/day for 10 days or 45 mg/kg/day for 4 days; this must be given with high doses of prednisone and usually results in worsening of the platelet count during and shortly after administration. The use of cyclosporine is also being explored.

General Comments

PNH is a chronic disease, and most patients are quickly tired of having it. Careful follow-up and good patient education are important parts of their care. The hope can be held out that patients who do not have serious complications may eventually be rid of their disease and that gene therapy may be possible.

coni syndrome (excretion of other molecules normally reabsorbed by the proximal tubule). Rarely, mild renal tubular acidosis of the proximal tubular type may be seen.[56,57] In a few patients, renal failure may intervene after many years of hemoglobinuria.

Relative and Absolute Bone Marrow Failure

In all patients with PNH, an element of diminished hematopoiesis is present. In its most severe form, it is manifest as aplastic anemia with the virtual absence of bone marrow precursors; in these cases, relatively few red cells are being made, so little hemolysis is evident. In many patients, the bone marrow is actively producing cells, particularly erythrocyte precursors, and in fact may be hyperplastic and yet an hematopoietic defect can be demonstrated.

At least two-thirds of all PNH patients have thrombocytopenia or granulocytopenia during the course of the illness.[58] Since the survival of platelets[59] and granulocytes[60] in the circulation in PNH is normal, these diminished numbers are due to deficient or ineffective production of these cells. These cytopenias may be important aspects of the patient's clinical syndrome.

The hematopoietic defect can be detected in most if not all patients on culturing the bone marrow. Even when the bone marrow is hyperplastic, many fewer hematopoietic colonies result when PNH progeniter cells are assayed in vitro than when normal marrow progenitor cells are assayed.[61–63] It is this characteristic that places the syndrome in the class of myelodysplastic rather than myeloproliferative syndromes.

The reason for the relative or absolute hematopoietic defect is not clear. It may have to do with missing GPI-anchored proteins on the abnormal stem cells themselves or on the lymphocytes and monocytes that may control hematopoiesis. The presence of the defect is all the more perplexing since the abnormal stem cell must have some proliferative advantage over the normal clones of cells to be able to dominate the marrow in most patients.

The effects of the diminution in hematopoiesis can be dramatic. It magnifies the effects of the hemolysis, since the response to anemia is inadequate. The granulocytopenia and thrombocytopenia may be so severe as to result in infections and bleeding. Bone marrow aplasia may intervene, with fatal results.

Thrombosis

Venous thrombosis, one of the most feared complications of PNH, was described in earlier reports and recognized as part of the syndrome by Crosby[6] in 1952. About 20% of patients with PNH experience thrombotic episodes, while others may have symptoms related to such events that are difficult to document. These thromboses commonly occur at several specific sites, as described below.

Hepatic Veins (Budd-Chiari Syndrome)

The hepatic veins are one of the most common sites of venous thrombosis in PNH.[64] The onset may be acute and dramatic, causing severe right upper quadrant pain, jaundice, hepatomegaly, and ascites[65]; this often occurs during a hemolytic crisis, suggesting that the activation of complement is responsible for both. In other instances, the onset is more gradual and insidious.[66] In either case, serum levels of enzymes indicative of hepatic injury (SGPT, [AST]) are elevated; this must not be confused with the marked elevation of lactate dehydrogenase and significant elevation of SGOT, which are indicative of hemolysis of the red cells. The serum alkaline phosphatase level may also be elevated. The most direct diagnostic test is the demonstration of the clots in the hepatic veins by computed tomography scan, magnetic resonance imaging (MRI), or ultrasound, particularly with Doppler flow measurements.[67] Sometimes the clots may not be demonstrable, but characteristic abnormalities in flow may indicate clots in the smaller vessels. Contrast injection into the hepatic veins may demonstrate the clots but should be done with caution. Imaging of the liver with colloid ^{99m}Tc may show a relative enhancement of the caudal lobe, which is spared the effects of hepatic vein thrombosis because the veins that drain this part of the liver go directly to the inferior vena cava and are not involved.[68] The thrombosis in the hepatic veins may extend to the inferior vena cava in extreme cases.[69]

The process, once initiated, tends to persist, with periodic exacerbations and remissions. Although patients may live for some years with chronic Budd-Chiari syndrome, it is usually ultimately fatal.

Cerebral Veins

The cerebral veins and sinuses are also prone to thrombosis, particularly the sagittal sinus and the veins covering the parietal lobes.[6,70–72] This results in severe headache, focal and nonfocal neurologic symptoms (depending on the location of the thrombosis), and, if sufficiently severe, coma and death. The spinal fluid is often xanthochromic or bloody. Careful examination of the flow of the cerebral veins with MRI or Doppler flow ultrasound may be needed to demonstrate the presence of the veins. Although less common than hepatic vein thrombosis, cerebral venous thrombosis also tends to be chronic and does not portend a good prognosis.

Abdominal Veins

The large and small veins of the abdomen may be thrombosed, resulting in a variety of syndromes. The most common is severe abdominal pain, often recurrent, usually lasting 3–5 days, with or without signs of inertial intestinal obstruction. The symptoms tend to occur in the same part of the abdomen with each attack. The thromboses are difficult to demonstrate radiologically. In some patients, the problem is so severe that

intestinal infarction requiring resection occurs. In other patients with recurrent pain, evidence of scarring and thrombosis may be found at operation; removal of the area may relieve the symptoms.[73]

The larger veins of the abdomen may be thrombosed, resulting in symptoms related to their site. Splenic venous thrombosis may result in splenomegaly and even splenic rupture. Portal venous thrombosis may result in ascites, esophageal varices, and other indications of rerouted circulation. Thrombosis of the veins of the stomach and duodenum may result in lesions that are detectable with gastroduodenal endoscopy.

Dermal Veins

Thrombosis of the veins of the skin may occur in two clinical patterns.[74,75] Areas of thrombosis may appear as painful, swollen, discolored lesions, usually measuring 5–10 cm over various parts of the body. These usually resolve but on occasion may ulcerate. These are recurrent dermal thromboses but do not necessarily occur at the same site. Alternatively, patients may have localized lesions resembling purpura fulminans, with purple discoloration of larger areas of skin, demarcation, and often necrosis. If sufficiently extensive, death may result.

Other Sites

Thromboses may occur at other sites. Thrombosis of the veins of the lower extremity occurs with greater frequency than is common in the population, but death by pulmonary embolism is rare. Thrombosis of the epididymal veins leads to a syndrome much like acute orchitis. Arterial thrombosis is rare.

Other Symptoms and Complications

Patients with PNH may have other symptoms that are probably related to their disease but for which there is no current explanation.

1. Many patients complain of dysphagia during episodes of intravascular hemolysis; this appears to be due to the generation in the esophagus of very strong peristaltic waves. When the hemolysis is nocturnal, the dysphagia is present in the morning but disappears by noon.
2. Many men with PNH note impotence during the periods of hemoglobinuria. In some cases, this impotence lasts beyond the hemoglobinuric period and becomes more permanent. Studies have not revealed an anatomic or physiologic defect to account for this symptom.
3. Many patients note a feeling of fatigue that may be disabling during periods of hemoglobinuria. This is not related to hemoglobin level, as it disappears when the hemoglobinuria stops.
4. Rarely, patients may have severe low back pain. Blood chemistries at the time suggest that there may be muscle destruction, and this symptom has been ascribed to small and undetectable thromboses in the muscles.

DIAGNOSIS

Since the observations of Ham and Dingle,[2] the abnormal sensitivity of the red cells to the hemolytic action of complement has been the basis of the diagnostic tests for PNH. In the original Ham test, complement is activated by acidification of the serum to a pH of 6.2; PNH cells will lyse in such serum, whereas normal cells will not.[2] The test is specific (there is no other cause for a positive test other than the very different syndrome hereditary erythroblastic multinuclearity with positive acidified serum test (HEMPAS, congenital dyserythropoie-

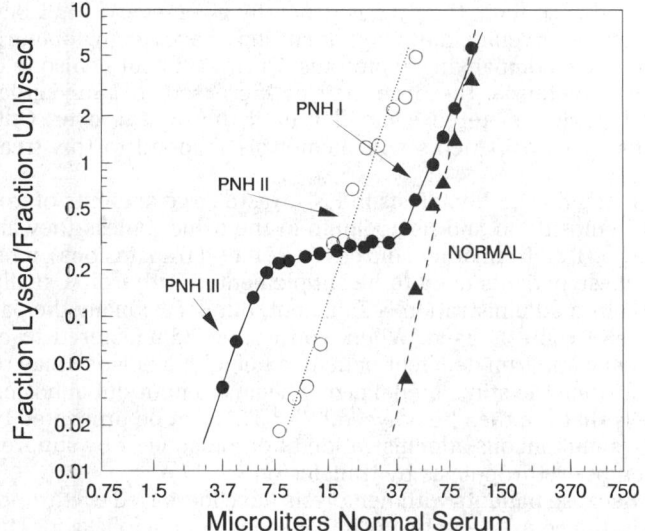

Fig. 25-4. Demonstration of the sensitivity of PNH red cells to the lytic action of complement by the complement lysis sensitivity (CLS) test. Red cells, sensitized with a potent antibody, are treated with graded amounts of normal human serum (abscissa). This is plotted against a function of the amount of lysis that results (fraction lysed divided by fraction unlysed). The resultant curve is straight for normal cells (closed triangles), indicating a single population of cells that are resistant to complement lysis. In one patient (closed circles), two populations are seen: one much like normal (PNH I), and the other requiring markedly less complement for lysis (PNH III). In a second patient (open circles), a single population of intermediate sensitivity was found.

tic anemia type II).[76] The sensitivity of this test is dependent on the concentration of Mg^{2+} in serum. The test becomes more sensitive if the Mg^{2+} concentration is raised to 0.005 M[77]; even then, the test may not detect small populations of abnormal cells and cells of intermediate sensitivity. Furthermore, the test seems to be technically difficult since many false-positive and false-negative reactions occur during routine laboratory practice.

Complement is also activated when the serum is mixed with a medium of low ionic strength; sucrose is the solute usually used to replace the salt solution in maintaining isomotic conditions, and the test is often called the sugar water test.[78,79] This test is quite sensitive and usually does not fail to lyse the abnormal PNH cells; however, it is less specific since cells in other conditions (autoimmune hemolytic anemia, leukemia, etc.) may be lysed.

Many tests have been proposed in which complement is activated by antibody to red cell antigens. The most revealing of these is the complement lysis sensitivity test in which limiting amounts of complement are activated by either a cold agglutinin or a strong rabbit anti-human red cell antibody.[12] By careful titration, both the proportion of abnormal cells and their abnormality can be demonstrated (Fig. 25-4).

Markedly abnormal (PNH III) cells can be demonstrated in the blood of about 75% of patients; these cells require only $\frac{1}{15}$ to $\frac{1}{25}$ the amount of complement for lysis as normal cells. Cells of intermediate sensitivity (PNH II cells) can be readily demonstrated in about 20–25% of patients.[53,80] In some patients, these seem to constitute a separate population of cells; in others, the sensitivity is widely dispersed (Fig. 25-4).

Tests Based on Detection of GPI-Linked Proteins

Since the finding that the abnormal cells lack the GPI-linked proteins, the demonstration that these proteins are deficient on the blood cells has been used as a diagnostic test for PNH.

In general, monoclonal antibodies to CD59 or CD55 (DAF) are used with flow cytometric analysis.[81,82] These tests have the advantage that they can be readily performed on granulocytes and platelets; the proportion of abnormal cells in these populations is greater than that of red cells, since the abnormal granulocytes and platelets have a normal survival time in the circulation.

In patients whose cells are partially deficient, some proteins are more deficient than others; in general, CD59 is the most deficient and (on granulocytes) CD16 (the FC_γ receptor IIIa) is the least deficient.[83]

The results of the examination of CD55 and CD59 on lymphocytes obtained from PNH patients are less clear. In some patients, a population of abnormal cells could be detected in all three lymphocyte cell lineages (T cell, B cell, and natural killer cells)[84,85] (often in surprisingly small numbers), whereas in others, they could not.[86] Small numbers of normal lymphocytes lack expression of these proteins, further complicating the use of lymphocytes in diagnostic studies.[85]

Even with these caveats, the use of monoclonal antibodies is likely to prove to be the optimal way of ascertaining the diagnosis of PNH.

Differential Diagnosis

Hemoglobinuria is a relatively unusual symptom in clinical medicine and is easily confused with two other symptoms: myoglobinuria and hematuria. Myoglobinuria can be identified by examination of the serum (which is without red pigment), differential solubility of the two pigments (hemoglobin is more easily precipitated by ammonium sulfate), or reaction with specific antibodies against myoglobin and hemoglobin. In hematuria, red cells are present in the freshly collected urine and the supernatant does not contain heme-reactive pigments after centrifugation.

Several other hemolytic diseases may cause hemoglobinuria. Severe autoimmune hemolytic anemia, particularly paroxysmal cold hemoglobinuria, may result in enough intravascular lysis to produce hemoglobinuria. Severe traumatic hemolytic anemia from prosthetic cardiac devices or from microangiopathic causes may also lead to hemoglobinuria; schistocytes are always evident on examination of the peripheral blood film. Rarely, toxic hemolytic anemia (as occurs during clostridial infection, copper poisoning, oxidant ingestion in a patient deficient in glucose-6-phosphate dehydrogenase, etc.) may result in hemoglobinuria.

The other more common and more subtle symptoms of PNH are more readily missed and may only be identified as part of the clinical constellation of PNH by doing the diagnostic tests for PNH. The abdominal pain that patients with PNH experience can be confused with ileitis. Budd-Chiari syndrome can be confused with cirrhosis or other parenchymal liver disease; the elevation of the liver enzymes (SGOT and lactate dehydrogenase) usually seen in PNH may add to the confusion. The effects of sagittal venous thrombosis (headaches, edema of the optic nerve, etc.) may resemble pseudotumor cerebri or other cerebral vascular events.

Most commonly, PNH is confused with other hematologic syndromes, particularly other stem cell disorders. The relationship to aplastic anemia has been described. In recent surveys,[87–89] an average of 6.8% (range 4.1% to 20.8%) of untransplanted patients with aplastic anemia evolve to PNH. Most of these patients have clinical symptoms attributable to PNH, but some have only cells with the defects characteristic of PNH. The occurrence of PNH in other stem cell disorders is far more rare but far too common to be due to chance alone. Erythroleukemia, chronic myeloid leukemia, and myelofibrosis are the most common accompanying diseases,[90] but patients with refractory anemia with excess blasts,[91] megakaryocytic myelosis,[90] and polycythemia vera (personal observation) have been associated with cells expressing the PNH defect. Rotoli and Luzzatto[90] have determined that 11 of 113 patients with myelodysplastic syndrome had a positive Ham test, suggesting the presence of the PNH defect in 1–12% of the cells. In one series, PNH developed before the development of an identifiable myelodysplastic syndrome (5 of 47 patients) and after the development of agnogenic myeloid metaplasia (4 patients).[93] The incidence of the defect in this population might be even higher if granulocytes and platelets were examined for the deficiency of GPI-linked cells.

COURSE AND PROGNOSIS

The clinical outcome in PNH is extremely variable. Estimates of mean life span from the time of diagnosis have been about 8–10 years,[93] but many patients have the disease for longer periods. The most common causes of death are the consequences of thrombosis (particularly of the hepatic veins) or of the effects of hypoproliferation of the bone marrow (infections, bleeding).

The population of abnormal cells may decrease with time in patients surviving for prolonged periods (15–20 years).[93] Rarely, the abnormal cells may disappear completely; more commonly, a small population remains, but the patient is asymptomatic. In unusual patients, the abnormal population may disappear before that time.

Progression to Acute Leukemia

In about 3–5% of patients with PNH, the illness progresses to acute leukemia.[8,9] This is usually of myeloid origin but occasionally the leukemic cells are positive for terminal deoxynucleotidyl transferase, suggesting a lymphocytic origin.[95] The onset is typically about 5 years after the onset of symptoms related to PNH. As the leukemic cells appear, the abnormal red cells disappear but will reappear if (in the rare case) the leukemia is successful treated.[96] The leukemic cells have the PNH phenotype of deficient GPI-linked proteins[97,98] and may show cytogenetic changes suggestive of subclonal evolution.[99]

THERAPY

Treatment in PNH depends on the symptoms of the patient. In general several modalities are available:

1. Correction of the anemia by
   a. Interruption of complement activation
   b. Replacement of missing nutrients
   c. Transfusion
2. Treatment and prevention of thrombosis
3. Modification of the bone marrow by transplantation or stimulation

Each of these modalities of therapy may be applied as needed and as circumstances permit.

Correction of the Anemia

Since the hemolytic component of the disorder is ultimately due to the activation of complement, measures that prevent this event lead to amelioration of the hemolysis. At present, the only agents that do so are glucocorticoids; the dose required is relatively large (0.3–0.5 mg/kg/day). The action of the steroids is very rapid; administration of a sufficient dose at 6 PM will present a nocturnal hemolytic episode. Because the dose required is so high, the drug is generally given every other day; on the intervening day, the patient may have hemoglobinuria and its accompanying symptoms. During an acute episode of hemoglobinuria, the dose may be increased to 1 mg/kg/day and be administered every day until the bout is over. Only about 60% of patients with hemolysis respond to this treatment.

Patients with hemolysis in PNH waste large amounts of iron as hemosiderin and hemoglobin in the urine. Unless they are getting iron from other sources (e.g., blood transfusions), most of these patients need to be supplemented with iron. Usually, oral iron administration is sufficient, but occasionally the parenteral route is used. When iron is first administered to an anemic and iron-deficient patient, a hemolytic episode may result when the stimulated marrow begins to pour out abnormal cells that are then hemolysed.[100,101] This can be prevented by the simultaneous administration of prednisone or by suppression of erythropoiesis by transfusion.

Because patients with hemolysis have increased erythropoiesis, they may theoretically become deficient in folic acid. This deficiency seems to be rare; it may be that the intravascular hemolysis releases red cell folate into the serum, where it again becomes available for metabolism.

Some patients require transfusion to maintain an adequate oxygen-carrying capacity, which may result in the lysis of a small number of the patients' own cells and resulting hemoglobinuria. Such lysis is probably rarer than commonly thought and may be due to minor sensitization either to red cells or to other blood elements.[101,102] When it occurs, it is confused with a hemolytic transfusion reaction due to incompatibility. The reaction can be prevented by washing the donor cells prior to transfusion.

Therapy for and Prevention of Thrombosis

When acute thrombosis occurs, it should be treated as an emergency. Thrombolytic agents (streptokinase, urokinase, or tissue plasminogen activator) should be administered at once unless otherwise contraindicated.[104,105] The results may be dramatic; the enlarged, swollen liver may reduce in size over a period of a few minutes to a few hours. Although thrombolytic agents are less effective if not used quickly after the clot has formed, they may be of some use even days later and should be tried.

Once it is safe, the patient suffering acute thrombosis should be given heparin in the usual fashion (a bolus of 5,000 U followed by an infusion of 25,000 U/day followed by careful monitoring of appropriate parameters of anticoagulation.) Although hemolytic reactions after heparin administration have been reported,[6,106] they are rare. As the acute episode passes, the patient should be anticoagulated with warfarin derivatives and should be maintained on anticoagulation therapy for ≥6 months.

These measures for preventing and treating thrombosis are inadequate. Most patients with Budd-Chiari syndrome never get rid of the problem entirely. With the development of better antithrombin agents (e.g., recombinant hirudin) and better ways of controlling the activation of platelets by thrombin, more successful ways of dealing with this complication may be found.

Modification of Hematopoiesis

Until recently, alteration of hematopoietic function was difficult and ineffective. Androgens and modified cogeners may, in some patients, stimulate erythropoiesis.[107] More recently, recombinant cytokines have been used, particularly erythropoietin and colony-stimulating factor-granulocyte; however, these are usually only moderately effective and are difficult to administer.

Antithymocyte Globulin

Based on the assumption that T lymphocytes modify hematopoiesis and may play a role in its diminution, patients with aplastic anemia were given equine antiserum to human thoracic duct lymphocytes (antithymocyte globulin); remission of the aplastic anemia was seen in abut 60%, although the reason for this response is not entirely clear.[108,109] On the basis of the similarities of PNH and aplastic anemia, antithymocyte globulin was given to patients with evidence of deficient hematopoiesis.[110] About 70% of these patients had correction of their cytopenia; reversal of thrombocytopenia was the most common. In most cases, the increase in the proportion of complement-sensitive cells was not great, and the amount of hemolysis did not usually increase.

Allogeneic Bone Marrow Transplantation

PNH can be cured by replacement of the abnormal cells of the bone marrow with normal bone marrow.[111,112] In the past, such replacement has been limited to patients with bone marrow failure who have histocompatible sibling donors, either (optimally) identical twins or HLA-A, -B, and -D matched siblings. As bone marrow transplantation has become safer, patients with other complications of PNH have undergone bone marrow transplantation, particularly children, in whom transplantation is safer and in whom the prognosis of the disease is known to be relatively poor.[113]

Syngeneic transplantation is easier to perform than allogeneic. In at least one instance, the syngeneic marrow (from an identical twin) was infused without prior conditioning (treatment of the patient with immunosuppressive and marrow-ablative drugs), disappearance of the abnormal PNH cells resulted[114]; in other instances, this has not been the case. In a recent personal case, a patient with severe Budd-Chiari syndrome was successfully given a syngeneic transplant, following which the liver disease improved.

Allogeneic marrow transplantation still carries a considerable risk of complications, including graft-versus-host disease, intercurrent infections, and failure of engraftment. However, when faced with the poor prognosis of the complicated patient, the benefits are worth the risks in many cases. To date, few patients have been given allogeneic transplants from unrelated donors; although some of these are successful, the complications are even greater than those of allogeneic transplantation from a sibling.

Gene Therapy

With the identification of the gene that is abnormal in PNH, treatment by reinsertion of the gene becomes possible. Experiments are currently under way to ascertain the appropriate conditions.

REFERENCES

1. Rosse WF: Paroxysmal nocturnal hemoglobinuria. p. 593. In: Clinical Immunohematology: Basic Concepts and Clinical Applications. Blackwell Scientific Publications, Oxford, 1990
2. Ham TH, Dingle JH: Studies on destruction of red blood cells. II. Chronic hemolytic anemia with paroxysmal nocturnal hemoglobinuria: certain immunological aspects of the hemolytic mechanism with special reference to serum complement. J Clin Invest 18:657, 1938
3. Gull WW: A case of intermittent haematinuria, with remarks. Guys Hosp Rep 12:381, 1866
4. Strubing P: Paroxysmale haemoglobinurie. Dtsch Med Wochenschr 8:1, 1882
5. Marchiafava E: Anemia emolitica con emosiderinuria perpetua. Policlin Sez Med 35:109, 1928
6. Crosby WH: PNH. Relation of the clinical manifestations to underlying pathogenic mechanisms. Blood 8:769, 1953
7. Dacie JV, Lewis SM: Paroxysmal nocturnal hemoglobinuria: variation in clinical severity and association with bone-marrow hypoplasia. Br J Haematol 7:442, 1961
8. Holden D, Lichtman H: Paroxysmal nocturnal hemoglobinuria with acute leukemia. Blood 33:283, 1969

9. Jenkins DE Jr, Hartmann RC: Paroxysmal nocturnal hemoglobinuria terminating in acute myeloblastic leukemia. Blood 33:274, 1969
10. Aster RH, Enright SE: A platelet and granulocyte membrane defect in paraoxysmal nocturnal hemoglobinuria: usefulness for the detection of platelet antibodies. J Clin Invest 48:1199, 1969
11. Hartmann RC, Arnold AB: Paroxysmal nocturnal hemoglobinuria as a clonal disorder. Annu Rev Med 28:187, 1977
12. Rosse WF, Dacie JV: Immune lysis of normal human and paroxysmal nocturnal hemoglobinuria red blood cells. I. The sensitivity of PNH red cells to lysis by complement and specific antibody. J Clin Invest 45:736, 1966
13. Rosse WF: Phosphatidylinositol-linked proteins and paroxysmal nocturnal hemoglobinuria. Blood 75:1595, 1990
14. Hirose S, Rav L, Prince GM et al: Synthesis of mannosylglucosaminylinositol phospholipids in normal but not paroxysmal nocturnal hemoglobinuria cells. Proc Natl Acad Sci USA 89:6025, 1992
15. Armstrong C, Schubert J, Ueda E et al: Affected paroxysmal nocturnal hemoglobinuria T lymphocytes harbor a common defect in assembly of N-acetyl-D-glucosamine inositol phospholipid corresponding to that in class A Thy-1-murine lymphoma mutants. J Biol Chem 267:25347, 1992
16. Takahashi M, Takeda J, Hirose S et al: Deficient biosynthesis of N-acetylglucosaminyl phosphatidylinositol, the first intermediate of glycosyl phosphatidylinositol anchor biosynthesis in cell lines established from patients with paroxysmal nocturnal hemoglobinuria. J Exp Med 177:517, 1993
17. Takeda J, Miyata T, Kawagoe K et al: Deficiency of the GPI anchor caused by a somatic mutation of the PIG-A gene in paroxysmal nocturnal hemoglobinuria. Cell 73:703, 1993
18. Oni SB, Osukoya BO, Luzzato L: Paroxysmal nocturnal hemoglobinuria: evidence for monoclonal origin of abnormal red cells. Blood 36:145, 1970
19. Josten KM, Tooze JA, Borthwick-Clarke C et al: Acquired aplastic anemia and paroxysmal nocturnal hemoglobinuria: studies on clonality. Blood 78:3162, 1991
20. Low MG, Finean JB: Release of alkaline phosphatase from membranes by a phosphatidylinositol-specific phospholipase C. Biochem J 167:281, 1977
21. Ferguson MAH, Low MG, Cross GAM: Glycosyl-sn-1,2-dimyristylphosphatidylinositol is covalently linked to Trypanosoma brucei variant surface glycoprotein. J Biol Chem 260:14547, 1985
22. Auditore JV, Hartmann RC, Flexner JM, Balchum OJ: The erythrocyte acetylcholinesterase enzyme in paroxysmal nocturnal hemoglobinuria. Arch Pathol 69:53, 1960
23. Davitz MA, Low MG, Nussenzweig V: Release of decay-accelerating factor (DAF) from the cell membrane by phosphatidylinositol specific phospholipase C (PIPLC). J Exp Med 163:1150, 1986
24. Ferguson MA, Homans SW, Dwek RA, Rademacher TW: Glycosyl-phosphatidylinositol moiety that anchors Trypanosoma brucei variant surface glycoprotein to the membrane. Science 239:753, 1988
25. Roberts WL, Santikarn S, Reinhold VN, Rosenberry TL. Structural characterization of the glycoinositol phospholipid membrane anchor of human erythrocyte acetylcholinesterase by fast atom bombardment mass spectrometry. J Biol Chem 263:18776, 1988
26. Doering TL, Masterson WJ, Englund PT, Hart GW: Biosynthesis of the glycosyl phosphatidylinositol membrane anchor of the trypanosome variant surface glycoprotein. Origin of the non-acetylated glucosamine. J Biol Chem 264:11168, 1989
27. DeGasperi R, Thomas LJ, Sugiyama E et al: Correction of a defect in mammalian GPI anchor biosynthesis by a transfected yeast gene. Science 250:988, 1990
28. Berger J, Howard AD, Brink L et al: COOH-terminal requirements for the correct processing of a phosphatidylinositol-glycan anchored protein. J Biol Chem 263:10016, 1988
29. Norris J, Hall S, Ware RE et al: Glycosyl-phosphatidylinositol anchor synthesis in paroxysmal noctural hemoglobinuria: partial or complete defect in an early step. Blood 83:816, 1994
30. Miyata T, Takeda J, Iida Y et al: The cloning of PIG-A, a component in the early step of GPI-anchor biosynthesis. Science 259:1318, 1993
30a. Bessler M, Mason PJ, Hillmen P et al: Paroxysmal nocturnal hemoglobinuria (PNH) is caused by somatic mutations in the PIG-A gene. EMBO J 13:110, 1994
30b. Miyata T, Yamada N, Iida Y et al: Abnormalities of PIG-A transcripts in granulocytes from patients with paroxysmal nocturnal hemoglobinuria. N Engl J Med 330:249, 1994
30c. Ware RE, Rosse WF, Howard TA: Mutations within the PIG-a gene in patients with paroxysmal nocturnal hemoglobinuria. Blood 83:2418, 1994
31. Ware RE, Howard TA, Kamitani T et al: Chromosomal assignment of genes involved in glycosylphosphatidylinositol anchor biosynthesis: implications for the pathogenesis of paroxysmal nocturnal hemoglobinuria. Blood 1994 (in press)
32. Nicholson-Weller A, March JP, Rosenfeld SI, Austen KF: Affected erythrocytes of patients with paroxysmal nocturnal hemoglobinuria are deficient

in the complement regulatory protein, decay accelerating factor. Proc Natl Acad Sci USA 80:5430, 1983

33. Holguin MH, Wilcox LA, Bernshaw NJ et al: Relationship between the membrane inhibitor of reactive lysis and the erythrocyte phenotypes of paroxysmal nocturnal hemoglobinuria. J Clin Invest 84:1387, 1989

34. Hansch GM, Schonermark S, Roelcke D: Paroxysmal nocturnal hemoglobinuria type III. Lack of an erythrocyte membrane protein restricting the lysis of C5b-9. J Clin Invest 80:7, 1987

35. Zalman LS, Wood LM, Frank MM, Muller-Eberhard HJ: Deficiency of the homologous restriction factor in paroxysmal nocturnal hemoglobinuria. J Exp Med 165:572, 1987

36. Selvaraj P, Rosse WF, Silber R, Springer TA: The major Fc receptor in blood has a phosphotidylinositol anchor and is deficient in paroxysmal nocturnal hemoglobinuria. Nature 333:565, 1988

37. Selvaraj P, Dustin ML, Silber R et al: Deficiency of lymphocyte function-associated antigens 3 (LFA-3) in paroxysmal nocturnal hemoglobinuria. Functional correlates and evidence for a phosphatidylinositol membrane anchor. J Exp Med 166:1011, 1987

38. Simmons DL, Tan S, Tenen DG et al: Monocyte antigen CD14 is a phospholipid anchored membrane protein. Blood 73:284, 1989

39. Beck WS, Valentine WN: Biochemical studies on leucocytes. II. Phosphatase activity in chronic lymphatic leukemia, acute leukemia, and miscellaneous hematologic conditions. J Lab Clin Med 38:245, 1951

40. Ploug M, Plesner T, Ronne E et al: The receptor for urokinase-type plasminogen activator is deficient on peripheral blood leukocytes in patients with paroxysmal nocturnal hemoglobinuria. Blood 79:1447, 1992

41. van der Schoot CE, Huizinga TWJ, Gadd S et al: Identification of three novel PI-linked proteins on granulocytes. p. 887. In Knapp W, Dorken B, Gilks WR et al (eds): Leucocyte Typing IV: White Cell Differentiation Antigens. Oxford, 1989

42. Davies KA: Complement. Baillieres Clin Haematol 4:927, 1991

43. Muller-Eberhard HJ: The membrane attack complex. Springer Semin Immunopathol 7:93, 1984

44. Pangburn MK, Muller-Eberhard HJ: The alternative pathway of complement. Springer Semin Immunopathol 7:163, 1984

45. Ross GD, Newman SL, Lambris JD et al: Generation of three different fragments of bound C3 with purified factor I or serum. II. Localization of binding sites in the C3 fragments for factors B and H, complement receptors and bovine conglutinin. J Exp Med 158:334, 1983

46. Parker CJ, Baker PJ, Rosse WF: Increased enzymatic activity in the alternative pathway convertase when bound to the erythrocytes of paroxysmal nocturnal hemoglobinuria. J Clin Invest 69:337, 1982

47. Devine DV, Rosse, WF: Regulation of the activity of platelet-bound alternative pathway C3 convertase by intracellular factor H. Proc Natl Acad Sci USA 84:5673, 1987

48. Petranka J, Norris J, Hall S et al: The structure of CD59: disulfide requirements and relationship to snake venom toxins. (in preparation)

49. Rollins SA, Zhao J, Ninomiya H, Sims PJ: Inhibition of homologous complement by CD59 is mediated by a species-selective recognition conferred through binding to C8 within C5b-8 or C9 within C5b-9. J Immunol 146:2345, 1991

50. Holguin MH, Wilcox LA, Bernshaw NJ et al: Relationship between the membrane inhibitor of reactive lysis and the erythrocyte phenotypes of paroxysmal nocturnal hemoglobinuria. J Clin Invest 84:1387, 1989

51. Sims PJ, Faioni EM, Wiedmer T, Shattil SJ: Complement proteins C5b-9 cause release of membrane vesicles from the platelet surface that are enriched in the membrane receptor for coagulation factor Va and express prothrombinase activity. J Biol Chem 263:18205, 1988

52. Rosse WF: The life-span of complement-sensitive and -insensitive red cells in paroxysmal nocturnal hemoglobinuria. Blood 37:556, 1971

53. Rosse WF, Hoffman S, Campbell M et al: The erythrocytes in paroxysmal nocturnal hemoglobinuria of intermediate sensitivity to complement lysis. Br J Haematol 79:99, 1991

54. Sears DA, Anderson PR, Foy AL et al: Urinary iron excretion and renal metabolism of hemoglobin in hemolytic diseases. Blood 28:708, 1966

55. Jackson GH, Noble RS, Maung ZT et al: Severe haemolysis and renal failure in a patient with paroxysmal nocturnal haemoglobinuria. J Clin Pathol 45: 176, 1992

56. Riley AL, Ryan IM, Roth DA: Renal proximal tubular acidosis and paroxysmal nocturnal hemoglobinuria. Am J Med 62:125, 1977

57. Clark DA, Butler SA, Braren V et al: The kidneys in paroxysmal nocturnal hemoglobinuria. Blood 57:83, 1981

58. Dacie JV: Paroxysmal nocturnal haemoglobinuria. Proc R Soc Med 56:587, 1963

59. Devine DV, Siegel RS, Rosse WF: Interactions of the platelets in paroxysmal nocturnal hemoglobinuria with complement. J Clin Invest 79:131, 1987

60. Brubaker L, Essig LJ, Mengel CE: Neutrophil life span in paroxysmal nocturnal hemoglobinuria. Blood 50:657, 1977

61. Sultan C, Marquet M, Joffrey Y: Étude des leucemies myeloides chroniques par culture de moelle "in vitro." Nouv Rev Fr Hematol 15:161, 1975

62. Tumen J, Kline LB, Fay J et al: Complement sensitivity of paroxysmal nocturnal hemoglobinuria bone marrow cells. Blood 55:1040, 1980

63. Moore JG, Humphries RK, Frank MM, Young N: Characterization of the hematopoietic defect in paroxysmal nocturnal hemoglobinuria. Exp Hematol 14: 222, 1986

64. Peytremann R, Rhodes RS, Hartmann RC: Thrombosis in paroxysmal nocturnal hemoglobinuria (PNH) with particular reference to progressive, diffuse hepatic venous thrombosis. Seri Haematol 5:115, 1972

65. Hartmann RC, Luther AB, Jenkins DE Jr et al: Fulminant hepatic venous thrombosis (Budd-Chiari syndrome) in paroxysmal nocturnal hemoglobinuria: definition of a medical emergency. Johns Hopkins Med J 146:247, 1980

66. Valla D, Dhumeaux D, Babany G et al: Hepatic vein thrombosis in paroxysmal nocturnal hemoglobinuria. A spectrum from asymptomatic occlusion of hepatic venules to fatal Budd-Chiari syndrome. Gastroenterology 93:569, 1987

67. Birgens HS, Hancke S, Rosenklint A, Hansen NE: Ultrasonic demonstration of clinical and subclinical hepatic venous thrombosis in paroxysmal nocturnal haemoglobinuria. Br J Haematol 64:737, 1986

68. Staab EV, Hartmann RC, Parrott JA: Liver imaging in the diagnosis of hepatic venous thrombosis in paroxysmal nocturnal hemoglobinuria. Radiology 117:341, 1975

69. Ishiguchi T, Fukatsu H, Itoh S et al: Budd-Chiari syndrome with long segmental inferior vena cava obstruction: treatment with thrombolysis, angioplasty, and intravascular stents. J Vasc Interv Radiol 3:421, 1992

70. Johnson RV, Kaplan SR, Blailock ZR: Cerebral venous thrombosis in paroxysmal nocturnal hemoglobinuria. Marchiafava-Micheli syndrome. Neurology 20:681, 1970

71. Donhowe SP, Lazaro RP: Dural sinus thrombosis in paroxysmal nocturnal hemoglobinuria. Clin Neurol Neurosurg 86:149, 1984

72. al-Hakim M, Katirji B, Osorio I, Weisman R: Cerebral venous thrombosis in paroxysmal nocturnal hemoglobinuria: report of two cases. Neurology 43: 742, 1993

73. Blum SF, Gardner FH: Intestinal infarction in paroxysmal nocturnal hemoglobinuria. N Engl J Med 274:1137, 1966

74. Hansen NE, Killmann SA: Paroxysmal nocturnal haemoglobinuria. A clinical study. Acta Med Scand 184:525, 1968

75. Rietschel RL, Lewis CW, Simmons RA, Phyliky RL: Skin lesions in paroxysmal nocturnal hemoglobinuria. Arch Dermatol 114:560, 1978

76. Crookston JH, Crookston MC, Burnie KL et al: Hereditary erythroblastic multinuclearity associated with a positive acidified-serum test: a type of congenital dyserythropoietic anaemia. Br J Haematol 17:11, 1969

77. May JE, Frank MM, Rosse WF: Alternate complement-pathway-mediated lysis induced by magnesium. N Engl J Med 298:705, 1973

78. Hartmann RC: Diagnostic specificity of the sucrose hemolysis test for paroxysmal nocturnal hemoglobinuria. Blood 35:462, 1970

79. Hartmann RC, Jenkins DE Jr: The "sugar water" test for paroxysmal nocturnal hemoglobinuria. N Engl J Med 275:155, 1966

80. Rosse WF, Adams JP, Thorpe AM: The population of cells in paroxysmal nocturnal hemoglobinuria of intermediate sensitivity to complement lysis—significance and mechanism of increased immune lysis. Br J Haematol 28:181, 1974

81. Schubert J, Alvarado M, Uciechowski P et al: Diagnosis of paroxysmal nocturnal haemoglobinuria using immunophenotyping of peripheral blood cells. Br J Haematol 79:487, 1991

82. van der Schoot CE, Huizinga TW, van't Veer Korthof ET et al: Deficiency of glycosyl-phosphatidylinositol-linked membrane glycoproteins of leukocytes in paroxysmal nocturnal hemoglobinuria, description of a new diagnostic cytofluorometric assay. Blood 76:1853, 1990

83. Edberg JC, Salmon JE, Whitlow M, Kimberly RP: Preferential expression of human Fc(γ) RIIIPMN (CD16) in paroxysmal nocturnal hemoglobinuria. Discordant expression of glycosyl phosphatidylinositol-linked proteins. J Clin Invest 87:58, 1991

84. Schubert J, Uciechowski P, Delany P et al: The PIG-anchoring defect in NK lymphocytes of PNH patients. Blood 76:1181, 1990

85. Nagakura S, Nakakuma H, Horikawa K et al: Expression of decay-accelerating factor and CD59 in lymphocyte subsets in healthy individuals and paroxysmal nocturnal hemoglobinuria patients. Am J Hematol 43:14, 1993

86. Hillmen P, Bessler M, Crawford DH, Luzzatto L: Production and characterization of lymphoblastoid cell lines with the paroxysmal nocturnal hemoglobinuria phenotype. Blood 81:193, 1993

87. Najean Y, Haguenauer O: Long-term (5 to 20 years) evolution of nongrafted aplastic anemias. The Cooperative Group for the Study of Aplastic and Refractory Anemias. Blood 76:2222, 1990

87. Najean Y, Haguenauer O: Long-term (5 to 20 years) evolution of nongrafted aplastic anemias. The Cooperative Group for the Study of Aplastic and Refractory Anemias. Blood 76:2222, 1990

88. de Planque MM, Bacigalupo A, Wursch A et al: Long-term follow-up of severe aplastic anaemia patients treated with antithymocyte globulin. Severe Aplastic Anaemia Working Party of the European Cooperative Group for Bone Marrow Transplantation (EBMT). Br J Haematol 73:121, 1989

89. Nissen C, Moser Y, dalle-Carbonare V et al: Complete recover of marrow function after treatment with anti-lymphocyte globulin is associated with high, whereas early failure and development of paroxysmal nocturnal haemoglobinuria are associated with low endogenous G-CSA-release. Br J Haematol 72:573, 1989

90. Rotoli B, Luzzatto L: Paroxysmal nocturnal hemoglobinuria. Semin Hematol 26:201, 1989

91. Aymard JP, Buisine J, Gregoire MJ et al: Refractory anaemia with excess of blasts as a terminal evolution of paroxysmal nocturnal haemoglobinuria. A case report with chromosomal analysis. Acta Haematol 74:181, 1985

92. Graham DL, Gastineau DA: Paroxysmal nocturnal hemoglobinuria as a marker for clonal myelopathy. Am J Med 93:671, 1992

93. Sirchia G, Lewis SM: Paroxysmal nocturnal haemoglobinuria. Clin Haematol 4:199, 1975

94. Charache S: Prolonged survival in paroxysmal nocturnal hemoglobinuria. Blood 33:877, 1969

95. Katahira J, Masako A, Oshimi K et al: Paroxysmal nocturnal hemoglobinuria terminating in TdT-positive acute leukemia. Am J Hematol 14:79, 1983

96. Hirsch VJ, Neubach PA, Parker DM et al: Paroxysmal nocturnal hemoglobinuria. Termination in acute myelomonocytic leukemia and reappearance after leukemic remission. Arch Intern Med 141:525, 1981

97. Devine DV, Gluck WL, Rosse WF, Weinberg JB: Acute myeloblastic leukemia in paroxysmal nocturnal hemoglobinuria: evidence of evolution for the abnormal PNH clone. J Clin Invest 79:314, 1987

98. Shichishima T, Terasawa T, Hashimoto C et al: Discordant and heterogeneous expression of GPI-anchored membrane proteins on leukemic cells in a patient with paroxysmal nocturnal hemoglobinuria. Blood 81:1855, 1993

99. Teyssier JR, Pigeon F, Behar C et al: Chromosomal subclonal evolution in paroxysmal nocturnal hemoglobinuria evolving into acute megakaryoblastic leukemia. Cancer Genet Cytogenet 25:259, 1989

100. Mengel CE, Kann HE Jr, O'Malley BW: Increased hemolysis after intramuscular iron administration in patients with paroxysmal nocturnal hemoglobinuria. Blood 26:74, 1965

101. Rosse WF, Gutterman LA: The effect of iron therapy in paroxysmal nocturnal hemoglobinuria. Blood 36:559, 1970

102. Brecher ME, Taswell HF: Paroxysmal nocturnal hemoglobinuria and the transfusion of washed cells. A myth revisited. Transfusion 29:681, 1989

103. Rosse WF: Transfusion in paroxysmal nocturnal hemoglobinuria. To wash or not to wash, editorial. Transfusion 29:663, 1989

104. Sholar PW, Bell WR: Thrombolytic therapy for inferior vena cava thrombosis in paroxysmal nocturnal hemoglobinuria. Ann Intern Med 103:539, 1985

105. Kwan T, Hansard P: Recombinant tissue-plasminogen activator for acute Budd-Chiari syndrome secondary to paroxysmal nocturnal hemoglobinuria. NY State J Med 92:88, 1992

106. Fritzche W, Martin H: Properdin und Hamolyse. Zur Hemmung der Hamolyse der Erythrocyten von Kranken mit paroxymaler nachtlicher Hamoglobiurie durch Heparin. Klin Wochenschr 35:1166, 1957

107. Hartmann RC, Jenkins DE Jr, McKee LC, Heyssel RM: Paroxysmal nocturnal hemoglobinuria: clinical and laboratory studies relating to iron metabolism and therapy with androgen and iron. Medicine 45:331, 1966

108. Jeannet M, Speck B, Rubinstein A et al: Reconstitution in severe aplastic anaemia after ALG pretreatment and HL-A semi-incompatible bone marrow cell transfusion. Acta Haematol 55:129, 1976

109. Young N, Griffith P, Brittain E et al: A multicenter trial of antithymocyte globulin in aplastic anemia and related diseases. Blood 72:1861, 1988

110. Herbert ME, Huang AT, Panella T et al: The treatment of hematocytopenia in paroxysmal nocturnal hemoglobinuria with antithymocyte globulin. (submitted)

111. Antin JH, Ginsburg D, Smith BR et al: Bone marrow transplantation for paroxysmal nocturnal hemoglobinuria: eradication of the PNH clone and documentation of complete lymphohematopoietic engraftment. Blood 66:1247, 1985

112. Kawahara K, Witherspoon RP, Storb R: Marrow transplantation for paroxysmal nocturnal hemoglobinuria. Am J Hematol 39:283, 1992

113. Ware RE, Hall SE, Rosse WF: Paroxysmal nocturnal hemoglobinuria with onset in childhood and adolescence. N Engl J Med 325:991, 1991

Congenital Dyserythropoietic Anemias

26

Bertil E. Glader

INTRODUCTION

Congenital dyserythropoietic anemias (CDAs) comprise a heterogeneous group of genetic disorders characterized by ineffective erythropoiesis and dyserythropoiesis. Ineffective erythropoiesis is a kinetic term indicating increased marrow erythroid activity, intramedullary red cell destruction, and decreased release of red blood cells (RBCs) into the circulation. Dyserythropoiesis is a descriptive term indicating the presence of morphologically abnormal erythroblasts with multinuclearity, karyorrhexis, or megaloblastic changes.

The first case of familial anemia with ineffective erythropoiesis and abnormal erythroblast nuclear maturation was reported by Wolff and von Hofe,[1] almost 40 years ago. Subsequently, other cases of hereditary anemia with atypical hemolysis and abnormal erythroblast morphology were described; collectively, these have come to be known as the congenital dyserythropoietic anemias.[2-4] In 1968, Heimpel and Wendt[2] classified these disorders into three groups (CDA types I, II, and III), based on differences in RBC morphology and marrow erythroblast abnormalities. Crookston et al.[5] further observed that serologic differences occur between the different types of CDA. The CDAs are still considered relatively rare disorders, and only a few hundred cases have been described. A working classification is depicted in Table 26-1. It should be noted, however, that many cases do not fit this classification and there is much clinical and laboratory overlap among the three types. A more precise classification awaits a specific biochemical and molecular definition of this disorder.

Table 26-1. Types of Congenital Dyserythropoietic Anemias

	Type I	Type II (HEMPAS)	Type III
Genetics	Recessive	Recessive	Dominant
Anemia	Mild–moderate	Moderate–severe	Mild
RBC size	Macrocytic	Normocytic	Macrocytic
Marrow erythroblasts			
Light microscopy	Megaloblastic	Binucleated	Gigantoblasts (≤12 nuclei)
	Binucleated	Multinucleated	
	Interchromatin bridges		
Electron microscopy	Widened nuclear pore space	Increased endoplasmic reticulum resembling a "double" cytoplasmic membrane	Nonspecific
	Cytoplasmic invagination into chromatin, giving appearance of a "spongy" nucleus		
Acid lysis test	Negative	Positive	Negative
Sugar water test	Negative	Negative	Negative
Source of reaction			
Anti-i antigen	Slight	Strong	Slight
Anti-I antigen	Slight	Strong	Slight

ETIOLOGY AND PATHOGENESIS

The CDAs are considered genetic disorders, since often more than one family member is affected. The specific patterns of inheritance vary among the different types of CDA (Table 26-1). To date, there are no known abnormalities of chromosome structure, and no specific DNA gene has been identified. Most of what is known about these disorders is based on studies of erythrocytes from patients with type II CDA, the most common form. At the stem cell level, in vitro culture of erythroid progenitors from patients with type II CDA produces colony-forming unit-erythroid and burst-forming unit-erythroid with erythroblast multinuclearity.[6] Chemical abnormalities that have been identified in CDA erythrocytes include unbalanced globin chain synthesis,[7,8] abnormal lipid composition,[9] and altered red cell membrane protein patterns following two-dimensional electrophoresis.[10] The latter abnormality is considered a major defect in CDA type II erythrocytes and is presumably due to impaired glycosylation of membrane proteins. Normal RBC membrane protein bands 3 and 4.5 contain significant amounts of lactosaminoglycans, but in type II CDA erythrocytes these membrane proteins are glyosylated to a much lesser extent.[11–14] In addition, decreased protein glycosylation in type II CDA erythrocytes is associated with a secondary accumulation of glycolipids.[15] One explanation for these phenomena is that in some type II CDA patients the RBCs are deficient in N-acetylglucosaminyltransferase II (GnTII), an enzyme responsible for glycosylation of membrane proteins by lactosaminoglycans.[16] However, in other HEMPAS cases, GnTII activity is normal while activity of another enzyme (α-mannosidase II [α-MII]) involved in protein glycosylation is reduced.[17,18] Furthermore, multinucleated erythroblasts are formed in vitro when normal bone marrow is cultured in the presence of an inhibitor of α-MII.[18] On the basis of these observations, it is likely that the primary defects in CDA type II erythrocytes are due to impaired production of enzymes responsible for glycosylation of membrane proteins. This impaired membrane glycoprotein synthesis and secondary glycolipid accumulation may thus be responsible for the abnormal erythroid features seen in these disorders.

CLINICAL MANIFESTATIONS

There is a wide variation in age of onset of clinical problems related to CDA. Most patients are diagnosed in late childhood or adolescence; however, a few CDA cases have now been reported in newborn infants presenting with hydrops fetalis.[19–21]

Clinical manifestations may include intermittent jaundice and dark urine due to increased hemoglobin catabolism, or signs and symptoms of anemia may be present. Rarely, hyperbilirubinemia without anemia may be the initial presentation of CDA patients.[22] The degree of splenomegaly and hepatomegaly is quite variable. Cholelithiasis may be present as a consequence of chronic hyperbilirubinemia. In some patients, evidence of hemosiderosis (i.e., skin hyperpigmentation, diabetes mellitus, hypogonadism, or delay of secondary sexual characteristics) is often present. It is noteworthy that hemosiderosis occurs in both transfused and nontransfused CDA patients. In the latter, iron overload is a direct consequence of ineffective erythropoiesis and increased gastrointestinal absorption of iron.[23] As a corollary, mild CDA should be considered in the differential diagnosis of older patients with unexplained iron overload.[24]

LABORATORY EVALUATION

A variable degree of anemia is usually present; there is also evidence of accelerated RBC destruction (i.e., hyperbilirubinemia, elevated serum lactate dehydrogenase activity). Moreover, this evidence of hemolytic anemia generally reflects ineffective erythropoiesis in that marrow erythroid activity is increased, while the reticulocyte count is less than expected for the magnitude of anemia. Ineffective erythropoiesis is further documented by isotopic studies with ^{59}Fe, which reveal accelerated isotope clearance from the plasma, while effective utilization of iron (i.e., ^{59}Fe incorporation into circulating RBCs) is markedly reduced. The serum iron concentration is usually normal to elevated, and the percentage of iron saturation is elevated.

Although ineffective erythropoiesis characterizes the CDA, it is of interest that survival of those erythrocytes that exit the marrow is normal to only slightly reduced. Several RBC glycolytic enzymatic abnormalities have been observed in CDA erythrocytes, but these are nonspecific changes similar to those seen in the dyserythropoiesis associated with other acquired disorders.[25] None of these RBC enzyme alterations is diagnostic of CDA. The specific erythrocyte morphologic and size abnormalities vary with the type of CDA. In all cases, the bone marrow reveals marked erythroid hyperplasia, and there are dyserythropoietic changes that vary according to the type of CDA. Myeloid precursors and megakaryocytes appear normal under light microscopy. Gaucher-like histiocytes are occasionally seen in type II CDA, presumably as a consequence of ineffective erythropoiesis and cellular processing by marrow macrophages.[26,27]

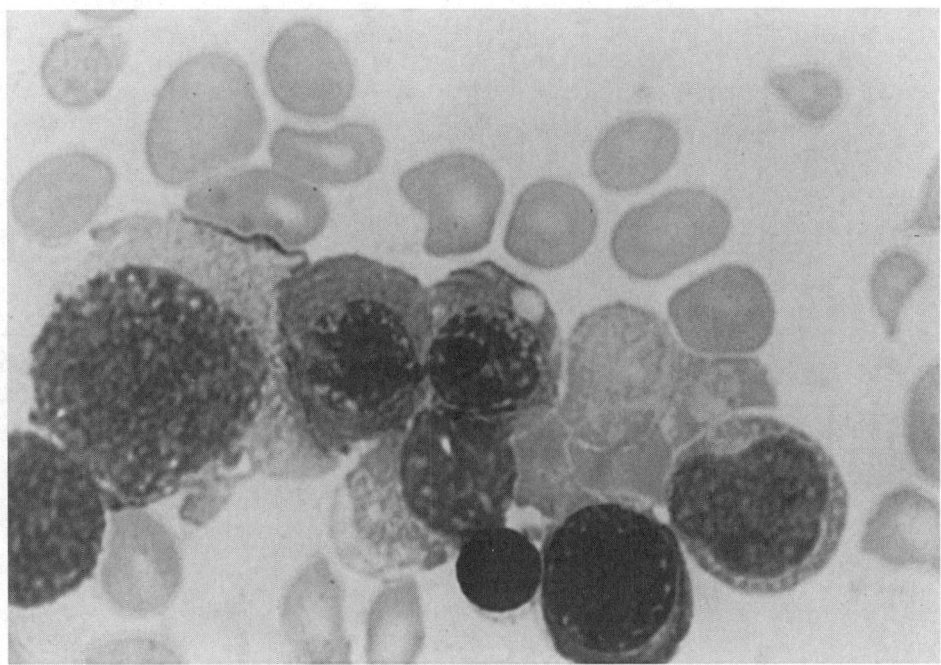

Fig. 26-1. Bone marrow from patient with type I CDA. Erythroblasts are connected by internuclear chromatin bridges connecting two cells. (Provided by Jean Shafer, MD, Rochester, NY.)

DIFFERENTIAL DIAGNOSIS

Dyserythropoiesis with erythroblast multinuclearity occurs in association with several other hematologic disorders, but these conditions are rarely confused with CDA. The dyserythropoiesis seen with megaloblastic anemias is readily distinguished by the presence of neutrophil hypersegmentation, abnormalities in red cell folic acid content, or reduced serum levels of vitamin B_{12}. The β-thalassemic syndromes, which also can have a similar RBC morphologic appearance, are distinguished by the presence of marked microcytosis with abnormal levels of either hemoglobin A_2 or fetal hemoglobin, or both. The acquired and congenital sideroblastic anemias, which can also have dyserythropoietic features, are identified by the presence of ringed sideroblasts in the bone marrow. Finally, the myelodysplastic syndromes are another major cause of dyserythropoiesis, distinguished by concomitant morphologic abnormalities in myeloid maturation and megakaryopoiesis.

SPECIFIC FEATURES OF MAJOR TYPES OF CONGENITAL DYSERYTHROPOIETIC ANEMIA

Type I

Type I CDA is a rare cause of anemia that accounts for a minority of all cases (Table 26-1). Family studies suggest that this disorder has an autosomal recessive inheritance pattern.[28] In several families more than one sibling is affected, and the disorder has been seen in fraternal and identical twins. The onset of anemia, jaundice, or other symptoms may be noted at any age. Affected patients often manifest some degree of icterus and splenomegaly. The degree of anemia is usually mild to moderate (hemoglobin in the range of 8 to 12 g/dl), and RBCs are macrocytic. Peripheral RBC morphology is characterized by anisocytosis and poikilocytosis, and occasionally Cabot rings are seen. White blood cells and platelets are normal. Examination of the bone marrow reveals erythroid hyperplasia with some megaloblastic erythropoiesis, and a small number of erythroblasts (1–5% of all RBCs present) manifest dyserythropoietic features. The unique morphologic abnormality seen in type I CDA is the presence of interchromatin bridges between nuclei of two separate erythroblasts, a reflection of impaired cellular division (Fig. 26-1). This internuclear bridging of erythroblasts seen with light microscopy is also a common feature seen in most patients with myelodysplastic syndromes.[29,30] Electron microscopy reveals additional abnormalities that include widening of the nuclear membrane pore space

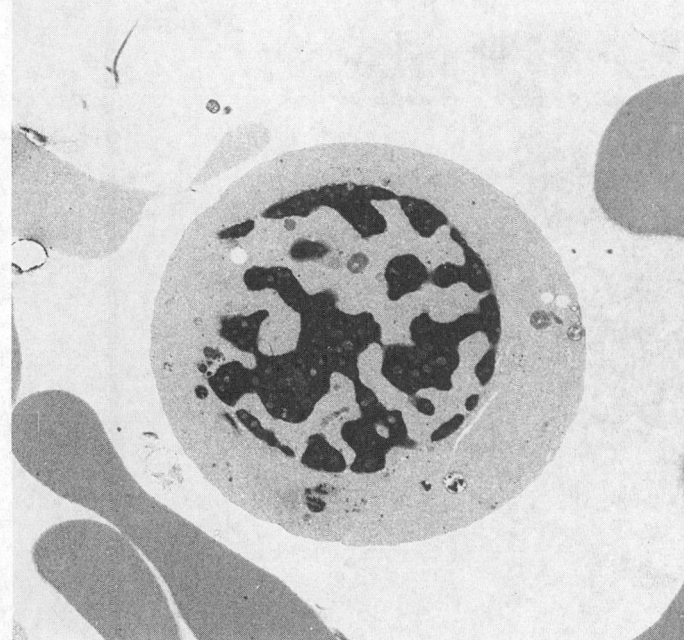

Fig. 26-2. Bone marrow-electron microscopy of CDA type I. Note the "spongy" appearance of nucleus due to uneven chromatin with cytoplasmic invagination into the nucleus. (Provided by Raoul Fresco, MD, Loyola University, Maywood, IL.)

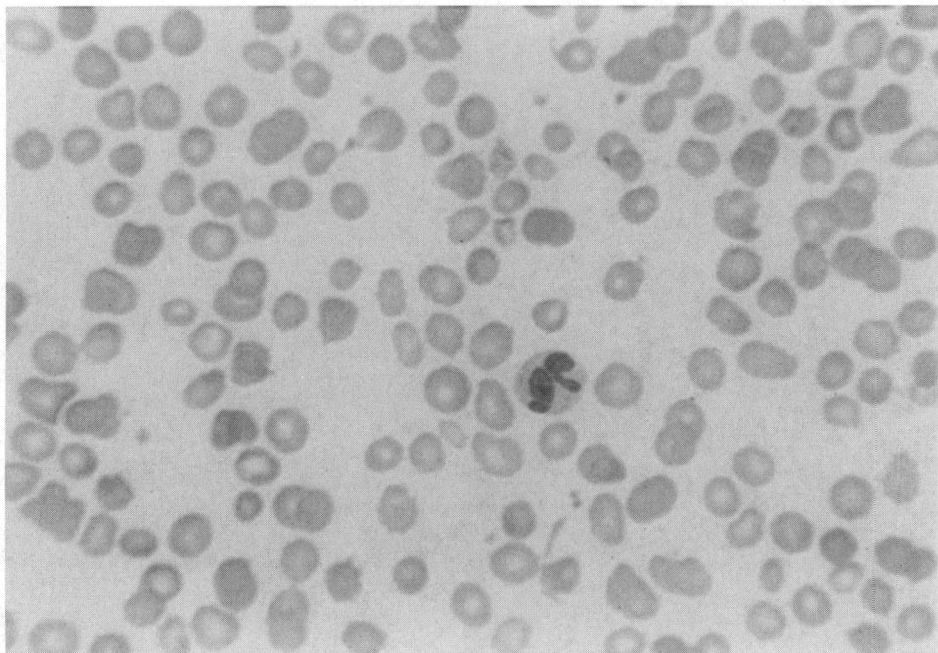

Fig. 26-3. Peripheral blood smear from patient with CDA type II. Note the marked variation in size and shape.

with cytoplasmic invagination into the nucleus, separation of nuclear chromatin, and chromatin condensation, all of which give the general appearance of a spongy nucleus[28,31,32] (Fig. 26-2). On rare occasions, these electron microscopic abnormalities have been used to diagnose type I CDA in the absence of internuclear bridging seen with light microscopy.[33] In contrast to type II CDA, there are no unique serologic features. Splenomegaly is common, although splenectomy has not been helpful. Gallstones have been a problem in some patients. The most important long-term complication may be hemosiderosis due to ineffective erythropoiesis and its associated increase in in-

testinal absorption of iron. The role of iron chelation therapy in this disorder remains to be determined.

Type II

Type II is the most common congenital dyserythropoietic anemia variant, accounting for almost two-thirds of affected patients.[2,4,34] More than 150 cases of this autosomal recessive disorder have been reported. Some of the clinical and laboratory features in type II CDA are similar to those seen in type

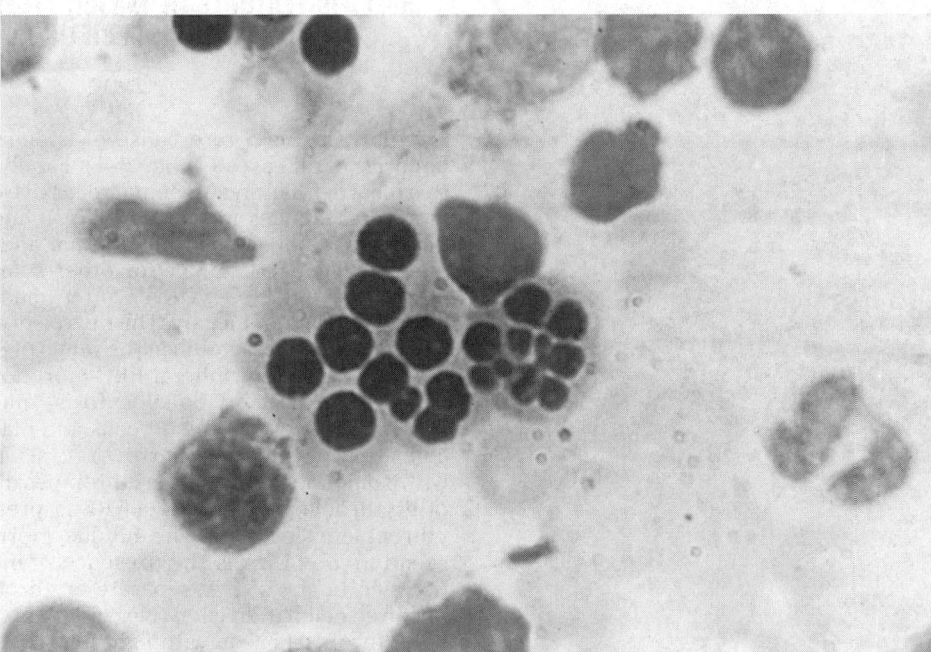

Fig. 26-4. Bone marrow aspirate from a patient with HEMPAS (type II CDA) showing erythroid hyperplasia and multinucleated erythroblasts. (Provided by Jean Shafer, MD, Rochester, NY.)

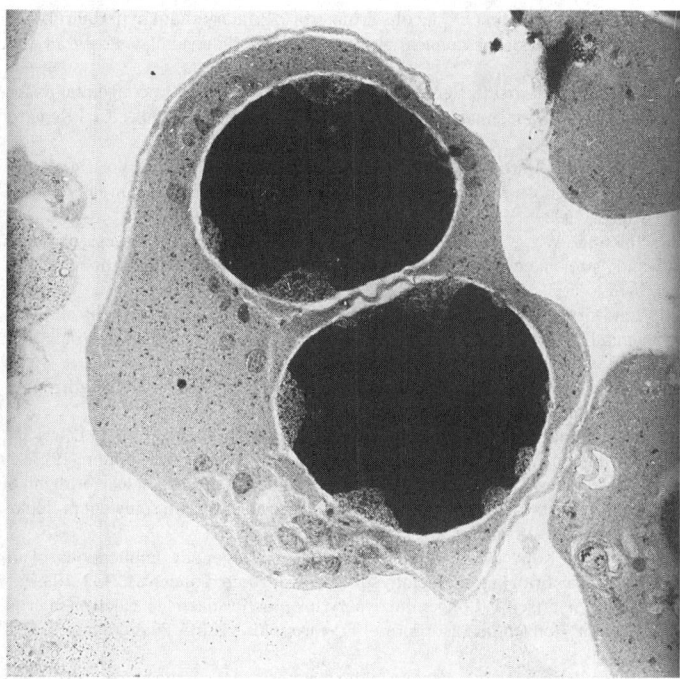

Fig. 26-5. Electron micrograph of bone marrow erythroblast from patients with HEMPAS (type II CDA). Note the appearance of a double cell membrane reflecting an excess of endoplasmic reticulum. (Provided by Raoul Fresco, MD, Loyola University, Maywood, IL.)

I, but there are differences. One major difference is that the magnitude of anemia is usually more severe, and patients with type II CDA often require RBC transfusions. The RBC are usually normocytic, and the peripheral blood reveals anisocytosis and poikilocytosis (Fig. 26-3). A second major difference is that the bone marrow in type II CDA reveals more abnormal erythroblasts (≤30%), with binuclearity, multinuclearity, and abnormal lobulation (Fig. 26-4). These nuclear abnormalities are seen only in the late erythroblasts, not in basophilic erythroblasts. Electron microscopy of late erythroblasts also reveals an excess of endoplasmic reticulum parallel to the cell membrane, giving the appearance of a double cell membrane[31,35] (Fig. 26-5). A third major difference, which is also a pathognomonic finding, is that type II CDA red cells are lysed by acidified (pH 6.8) sera obtained from approximately 30% of normal persons, but there is no lysis when RBCs are incubated with the patient's own acidified serum. In type II CDA, the combination of erythroblast multinuclearity and the sensitivity of circulating RBCs to lysis by acidified normal serum accounts for the acronym HEMPAS (*h*ereditary *e*rythroblastic *m*ultinuclearity with a *p*ositive *a*cidified *s*erum test).[5] This lysis is due to a naturally occurring IgM antibody that binds complement, and this antibody can be removed by preincubating normal sera with HEMPAS erythrocytes. However, the specific HEMPAS antigen recognized by this antibody is not known. In contrast to HEMPAS, the erythrocytes of patients with paroxysmal nocturnal hemoglobinuria (PNH) undergo lysis when the acidified serum is from the PNH patient or from normal donors. Another difference is that PNH erythrocytes undergo lysis in isotonic sucrose, whereas HEMPAS red cells do not lyse in sucrose solution.

HEMPAS red cells show increased reactive strength of the i antigen (which usually is a marker of fetal erythropoiesis) and are strongly agglutinated by both anti-i and anti-I sera.[36] In certain conditions, such as Diamond-Blackfan anemia and sickle cell anemia, both I and i antigens may be present, but these are expressed on different erythrocytes, reflecting that a frac-

tion of RBCs is a product of fetal-like erythropoiesis. In CDA type II, however, all RBCs manifest both I and i antigenicity. In view of the latter, it is noteworthy that the RBC surface antigenicity of I and i are both determined by the presence of *N*-acetylactosamines associated with membrane proteins and membrane lipids (i.e., ceramides).[18]

Patients with HEMPAS and severe anemia usually require blood transfusions. Splenectomy is occasionally helpful, as demonstrated by a decreased need for transfusions. Iron overload occurs as a consequence of RBC transfusions and ineffective erythropoiesis. In select patients, iron chelation therapy should be considered.

Type III

The first case of CDA, reported by Wolff and von Hofe[1] in 1951, was that of a woman and her three children who had mild anemia with bone marrow containing multinucleated erythroblasts. This initial case is now recognized as type III CDA; there are approximately 30 known patients.[37] These patients have macrocytosis and a mild-to-moderate degree of anemia. In contrast to the other CDAs, type III is inherited as an autosomal dominant defect. Bone marrow examination reveals erythroid hyperplasia with many multinucleated erythroblasts (i.e., gigantoblasts), containing ≤12 nuclei; these may be similar to some of the large multinucleated cells seen in type II CDA (Fig. 26-4). Type III CDA erythrocytes resemble HEMPAS red cells in that they are strongly agglutinated by anti-i and anti-I sera. In contrast to HEMPAS RBCs, however, type III CDA erythrocytes are not lysed by any acidified sera. Sodium dodecyl sulfate (SDS) polyacrylamide gel electrophoresis of the RBC membranes from two patients has suggested that minor alterations in the degree of band 3 *N*-glycosylation may be present, a defect similar to that observed in HEMPAS erythrocytes.[38]

Variants

Many reported patients with CDAs do not fit the conventional classification of type I, II, or III CDA.[39,40] In some instances this may reflect a completely different type of defect. For example, a recent patient has been described with dysplastic erythroblastic nuclei and intracellular inclusions, thought to reflect excessive synthesis or impaired degradation of intracytoplasmic membranes.[20] In most cases, variants of CDA differ from type II CDA in that they have similar erythroblast morphologic abnormalities, but lack one or more of the other features of type II CDA. For example, the absence of the double cell membrane may be seen on electron microscopy, or the inheritance pattern may be autosomal dominant instead of recessive. In the most common variants, patients differ from type II CDA in that they have a negative reaction in the acid lysis test; some investigators consider this a type IV CDA.[41,42] However, the type IV concept is not universally agreed on, and there are too few cases to define these variants more specifically. Moreover, since only 30% of normal sera contain an antibody that reacts with HEMPAS red cells, it is necessary to test with many normal sera before concluding definitively that a patient with CDA does not have a positive acid lysis test. (In order to rule out HEMPAS with a *P* value <0.005, it has been determined that the patient's RBCs need to be tested against 30 normal sera.)

REFERENCES

1. Wolff JA, von Hofe FH: Familial erythroid multinuclearity. Blood 6:1274, 1951
2. Heimpel H, Wendt F: Congenital dyserythropoietic anemia with karyorrhexis and multinuclearity of erythroblasts. Helv Med Acta 34:103, 1968
3. Verwilghen R, Verhaegen H, Waumans P, Beert J: Ineffective erythropoiesis

with morphologically abnormal erythroblasts and unconjugated hyperbilirubinaemia. Br J Haematol 17:27, 1969

4. Lewis SM, Verwilghen RL (eds): Dyserythropoiesis. Academic Press, San Diego, 1977

5. Crookston JH, Crookston MC, Burnie KL, Francombe WH: Hereditary erthroblastic multinuclearity associated with a positive acidified serum test: a type of congenital dyserythropoietic anaemia. Br J Haematol 17:11, 1969

6. Roodman GD, Clare CN, Mills G: Congenital dyserythropoietic anaemia type II (CDA-II): chromosomal banding studies and adherent cell effects on erythroid colony (CFU-E) and burst (BFU-E) formation. Br J Haematol 50:499, 1982

7. Hruby MA, Mason RG, Honig GR: Unbalanced globin chain synthesis in congenital dyserythropoietic anemia. Blood 42:843, 1973

8. Wickramasinghe SN, Goudsmit R: Precipitation of beta-globin chains within the erythropoietic cells of a patient with congenital dyserythropoietic anaemia, type III. Br J Haematol 65:250, 1987

9. Joseph KC, Gockerman JP, Alving CR: Abnormal lipid composition of the red cell membrane in congenital dyserythropoietic anemia type II (HEMPAS). J Lab Clin Med 85:34, 1975

10. Anselstetter V, Horstmann H-J, Heimpel H: Congenital dyserythropoietic anaemia, types I and II; aberrant pattern of erythrocyte membrane proteins in CDA II, as revealed by two-dimensional polyacrylamide gel electrophoresis. Br J Haematol 35:209, 1977

11. Scartezzini P, Forni GL, Baldi J et al: Decreased glycosylation of band 3 and band 4.5 glycoproteins of erythrocyte membrane in congenital dyserythropoietic anaemia type II. Br J Haematol 51:569, 1982

12. Baines AJ, Banga JPS, Gratzer WB et al: Red cell membrane protein anomalies in congenital dyserythropoietic anaemia, type II (HEMPAS). Br J Haematol 50:563, 1982

13. Mawby WJ, Tanner MJA, Anstee DJ, Clamp JR: Incomplete glycosylation of erythrocyte membrane proteins in congenital dyserythropoietic anaemia type II (CDA II). Br J Haematol 55:357, 1983

14. Fukuda MN, Papayannopoulou T, Gordon-Smith EC et al: Defect in glycosylation of erythrocyte membrane proteins in congenital dyserythropoietic anaemia type II (HEMPAS). Br J Haematol 56:55, 1984

15. Zdebska E, Anselstetter V. Pacuska T et al: Glycolipids and glycopeptides of red cell membranes in congenital dyserythropoietic anaemia type II (CDA II). Br J Haematol 66:385, 1987

16. Yukuda MN, Dell A, Scartezzini P: Primary defect of congenital dyserythropoietic anemia type II. J Biol Chem 262:7195, 1987

17. Fukuda MN, Masri KA, Dell A et al: Incomplete synthesis of N-glycans in congenital dyserythropoietic anemia type II caused by a defect in the gene encoding α-mannosidase II. Proc Natl Acad Sci USA 87:7443, 1990

18. Fukuda MN: Congenital dyserythropoietic anaemia type II (HEMPAS) and its molecular basis. Baillieres Clin Haematol 6:493, 1993

19. Carter C, Darbyshire PJ: A congenial dyserythropoietic anaemia variant presenting as hydrops foetalis. Br J Haematol 72:289, 1989

20. Wickramasinghe SN, Illum N, Wimberley PD: Congenital dyserythropoietic anaemia with novel intra-erythroblastic and intra-erythrocytic inclusions. Br J Haematol 79:322, 1991

21. Williams G, Lorimer S, Merry CC et al: A variant congenital dyserythropoietic anaemia presenting as a fatal hydrops foetalis. Br J Haematol 76:438, 1990

22. Brid AR, Knottenbelt EK, Jacobs P, Maigrot J: Primary shunt hyperbilirubinaemia: a variant of the congenital dyserythropoietic anaemias. Postgrad Med J 67:396, 1991

23. Cazzola M, Barosi G, Bergamaschi G et al: Iron loading in congenital dyserythropoietic anaemias and congenital sideroblastic anaemias. Br J Hematol 54:649, 1983

24. Greiner TC, Burns CP, Dick FR et al: Congenital dyserythropoietic anemia type II diagnosed in a 69-year-old patient with iron overload. Am J Clin Pathol 98:522, 1992

25. Valentine WN, Konrad PN, Paglia DE: Dyserythropoiesis, refractory anemia and "preleukemia": metabolic features of the erythrocytes. Blood 41:857, 1973

26. Van Dorpe A, Broeckaert-Van Orshoven A et al: Gaucher-like cells and congenital dyserythropoietic anaemia, type II (HEMPAS). Br J Haematol 25:165, 1973

27. Enquist RW, Gockerman JP, Jenis EH et al: Type II congenital dyserythropoietic anemia. Ann Intern Med 77:371, 1972

28. Heimpel H: Congenital dyserythropoietic anaemia, type I. p. 55. In Lewis SM, Verwilghen RL (eds): Dyserythropoiesis. Academic Press, London, 1977

29. Bethlenfalvay NC, Phaure TAJ, Phyliky RL, Bowman RP: Nuclear bridging of erythroblasts in acquired dyserythropoiesis: an early and transient preleukemic marker. Am J Hematol 21:315, 1986

30. Head DR, Kopecky K, Bennett JM et al: Pathogenetic implications of internuclear bridging in myelodysplastic syndrome. Cancer 64:2199, 1989

31. Lewis SM, Frisch B: Congenital dyserythropoietic anaemias: electron microscopy. In: Congenital Disorders of Erythropoiesis. CIBA Found Symp 37:171, 1976

32. Fresco R: Electron microscopy in the diagnosis of the bone marrow disorders of the erythroid series. Semin Hematol 18:279, 1981

33. Facon T, Zandecki M, Caulier MT et al: Usefulness of electron microscopy in the diagnosis of congenital dyserythropoietic anemia type I: report of a case. Am J Hematol 37:277, 1991

34. Punt K, Borst-Eilers E, Nijessen JG: Congenital dyserythropoietic anaemia, type II (HEMPAS). p. 71. In Lewis SM, Verwilghen RL (eds): Dyserythropoiesis. Academic Press, London, 1977

35. Hug G, Wong KY, Lampkin BC: Congenital dyserythropoietic anaemia type II. Lab Invest 26:11, 1972

36. Lewis SM, Grammaticos P, Dacie JV: Lysis by anti-I in dyserythropoietic anaemias: role of increased uptake of antibody. Br J Haematol 18:465, 1970

37. Goudsmit R: Congenital dyserythropoietic anaemia, type III. p. 83. In Lewis SM, Verwilghen RL (eds): Dyserythropoiesis. Academic Press, London, 1977

38. Wickramasinghe SN, Wahlin A, Anstee D et al: Observations on two members of the Swedish family with congenital dyserythropoietic anaemia, type III. Eur J Haematol 50:213, 1993

39. David G, Van Dorpe A: Aberrant congenital dyserythropoietic anaemias. p. 93. In Lewis SM, Verwilghen RL (eds): Dyserythropoiesis. Academic Press, London, 1977

40. Boogaerts MA, Verwilghen RL: Variants of congenital dyserythropoietic anaemia: an update. Haematologia 15:211, 1982

41. McBride JA, Wilson WEC, Baillien J: Congenital dyserythropoietic anaemia, type IV. Blood 38:837, 1971

42. Benjamin JT, Rosse WF, Dalldorf FG, McMillan CW: Congenital dyserythropoietic anemia–type IV. J Pediatr 87:210, 1975

Transplantation Biology

27

Robertson Parkman

INTRODUCTION

The biology of bone marrow transplantation is determined by the three different cell types transplanted from the donor: mature T lymphocytes, lymphoid stem cells, and hematopoietic stem cells. The biology of the different cell types defines the clinical and biologic events that occur following transplantation.

T LYMPHOCYTES

Unlike bone marrow transplantation in animals, in which lymphoid and hematopoietic stem cells can be transplanted relatively devoid of mature T lymphocytes, human bone marrow obtained for transplantation is contaminated by a significant percentage (10–20%) of peripheral blood T lymphocytes. The presence of the T lymphocytes in the human bone marrow has important clinical consequences, particularly the probability of hematopoietic stem cell rejection and the development of graft-versus-host disease (GVHD).

Immunosuppression

The preparative regimens used for allogeneic bone marrow transplantation contain agents to eradicate the recipient's immune system.[1] Pretransplant immunosuppression is necessary, since the mass of the recipient's lymphoid system exceeds that of the infused donor lymphoid cells. Without immunosuppression, the recipient immune system would reject the infused donor cells. Following immunosuppression of the recipient, the magnitude of the donor and of the recipient immune systems is relatively equivalent. If the residual recipient immune system becomes the dominant immune system, the infused donor lymphoid and hematopoietic stem cells are rejected. If the infused donor T lymphocytes and lymphoid stem cells become the predominant immune system, donor lymphoid and hematopoietic engraftment will occur, and GVHD may develop. The factors that influence the likelihood of graft rejection/engraftment and GVHD are shown in Tables 27-1 and 27-2. Factors that may contribute to an increased incidence of graft rejection include presensitization of the recipient immune system by blood transfusions, a reduced number of donor bone marrow cells, and T-lymphocyte depletion of the donor bone marrow.[2-4] The factors that may contribute to an increased incidence of GVHD are ineffective GVHD prophylaxis; an increased dose of donor immunocompetent cells, particularly if patients are transfused with donor peripheral blood leukocytes following transplantation; an increased frequency of donor T lymphocytes with specificity for recipient histocompatibility antigens; increased donor/recipient age; and increased donor/recipient histoincompatibility.[5-10]

The balance between the donor and immunosuppressed recipient immune systems is a narrow one; minor increases in recipient immunoreactivity can result in a significant increase in graft rejection. Rejection rates as high as 50% were initially (1970–1975) seen in aplastic anemia patients because most patients were multiply transfused.[2] The decreased incidence of hematopoietic stem cell rejection now seen in patients with aplastic anemia is attributable to three factors: (1) transplantation before significant transfusions are given, (2) use of blood products from which leukocytes (particularly monocytes and dendritic cells) have been removed, and (3) use of multiagent immunosuppression regimens (antithymocyte globulin and procarbazine in addition to cyclophosphamide) or the addition of total lymphoid/total nodal irradiation.[11-15] When a combination of techniques (i.e., early transplantation and multiagent immunosuppression) is used, the recipient's immune system is less likely to reject the donor-derived cells.

The use of one or two HLA antigen-mismatched family or matched unrelated donors is associated with an increased incidence of graft rejection.[16] The presence in the recipient of anti-HLA antibodies to unique donor antigens results in a high rate of nonengraftment that cannot be overcome by increased immunosuppression or irradiation. In addition to antibody-mediated rejection, residual recipient cytotoxic T lymphocytes with specificity for donor antigens have been identified in recipients who have rejected transplanted bone marrow.[17,18] Thus, both cellular and humoral recipient antidonor immunity can produce bone marrow graft rejection or nonengraftment.

T-Lymphocyte Depletion

On the basis of animal studies in which the elimination of mature donor T lymphocytes has prevented GVHD, many transplant centers have undertaken the use of T-lymphocyte-depleted bone marrow.[19,20] T-lymphocyte depletion can be achieved either by the lysis of mature donor T lymphocytes with monoclonal antibodies to T-lymphocyte differentiation antigens and complement or by their physical removal.[21,22] Both techniques have been successful in achieving a significant reduction in the incidence of GVHD in histocompatible, haploidentical, and matched unrelated bone marrow transplantation. However, the effective removal of donor T lymphocytes has resulted in an increased incidence of graft rejection, presumably because the removal of mature donor T lymphocytes results in predominance of the recipient's immune system.[4] The use and appropriate role of T-lymphocyte-depleted transplants in histocompatible donor-recipient pairs remain to be clarified because of the increased incidence of graft rejection in recipients of such grafts.

The successful use of T-lymphocyte-depleted transplants can be seen in the adult recipients of matched unrelated bone marrow, with T-lymphocyte depletion resulting in a significant reduction of acute GVHD from 64% to 26%, although the incidence of chronic GVHD did not decrease.[16] Since T-lymphocyte depletion can tip the balance between the donor and recipient immune systems in favor of the recipient, if standard doses of immunosuppression are used, the use of T-lymphocyte-depleted bone marrow requires the use of increased immunosuppression, usually total body irradiation exceeding 13.5 Gy.

Haploidentical T-lymphocyte-depleted transplantation has been successful, particularly in the treatment of patients with severe combined immunodeficiency (SCID), with a survival rate of 70–90%, depending on the clinical condition of the patients at transplantation.[23] The successful engraftment of donor lymphoid stem cells in the recipients of haploidentical T-lymphocyte-depleted bone marrow is dependent on whether functional natural killer (NK) cells are present in the recipient. Suc-

Table 27-1. Factors that Influence the Likelihood of Hematopoietic Engraftment

Increase	Decrease
↑ Bone marrow cell dose	↓ Bone marrow cell dose
Donor leukocyte transfusions	T-lymphocyte depletion
No prior red cell transfusions	Prior transfusions
Multiagent immunosuppression	Cyclophosphamide alone
Donor/recipient histocompatibility	Donor/recipient histoincompatibility

cessful lymphoid engraftment in patients without NK function can be achieved without the use of agents (busulfan/irradiation) that eliminate hematopoietic stem cells, while potential recipients with normal NK function must receive such therapy in order to eliminate their NK cells. NK cells appear capable of mediating the rejection of lymphoid and hematopoietic stem cells and may be the human analog of hybrid resistance seen in murine models.[24]

Graft-Versus-Host Disease

If successful donor engraftment occurs and the donor-derived immune system predominates, patients are at risk of GVHD, which is still the principal post-transplant problem in both histocompatible and histoincompatible bone marrow transplantation. Studies both in humans and in animal models indicate that acute GVHD is caused by the attack by donor-derived leukocytes, primarily T lymphocytes, against recipient cells.[25] Initially, acute GVHD was thought to be primarily due to the cytotoxic destruction of recipient cells by donor cytotoxic cells, either T lymphocytes or NK cells. Recent evidence has indicated a role for cytokine-mediated damage in the pathogenesis of GVHD.[26–28]

Animal experiments, primarily in rodents, demonstrate that the effector mechanisms involved in acute GVHD can be divided into those that are operative in GVHD due to major histocompatibility antigenic differences and those due to minor histocompatibility antigen differences within the context of major histocompatibility identity.[29–31] The primary cellular effector mechanisms in acute GVHD due to major histocompatibility differences are CD4+ T lymphocytes with specificity for the class II histocompatibility differences and CD8+ T lymphocytes with specificity for the class I histocompatibility differences. Mouse strain combinations that differ at only the class I or II histocompatibility antigens demonstrate the specificity of the effector mechanisms. Acute GVHD in histocompatible transplantation is caused by minor histocompatibility antigen differences; the cellular effector mechanisms involved in minor antigen GVHD are more complex. Both CD4+ and CD8+ T lymphocytes are involved in the pathogenesis of minor antigen GVHD.[21] The CD8+ T lymphocytes may be cytotoxic T lymphocytes with specificity for the recipient-restricted minor histocompatibility antigens, while the CD4+ T lymphocytes supply the cytokines necessary for the in vivo proliferation and differentiation of CD8+ T lymphocytes. In addition, the CD4+ and CD8+ T lymphocytes, which are capable of producing cytokines (interferon-γ [IFN-γ], tumor necrosis factors [TNF-α and TNF-β]) may be directly involved in the pathogenesis of acute GVHD.

Table 27-2. Factors that Increase Acute and Chronic GVHD

Acute GVHD	Chronic GVHD
Female → male if donor is alloimmunized	Acute GVHD > grade 2
No GVHD prophylaxis	↑ Donor/recipient age
↑ Donor/recipient age	Donor buffy coat transfusion
Prior recipient infections with herpes virus	Female → male, if donor is alloimmunized
↑ Frequency of donor anti-recipient cytotoxic T-lymphocyte precursor	
Positive skin explant assay	

Research in human GVHD has focused on the identification of donor-recipient pairs at increased risk of acute GVHD. Based on the assumption that cytotoxic T lymphocytes are the principal effector mechanism, the frequency of cytotoxic T-lymphocyte precursors (pCTL) has been shown to predict the likelihood of acute GVHD.[12] Recipients of bone marrow from donors with a low frequency of antirecipient pCTL do not develop acute GVHD, while the recipients of bone marrow from donors with a high frequency of pCTL are likely to develop the acute disease. A skin explant model has provided additional insight. Donor leukocytes are stimulated with recipient cells in a sensitization phase and are then incubated with recipient skin biopsies, which are histologically assessed for the presence of acute GVHD.[11] The assay has been successful in predicting acute GVHD; the sensitivity of the sensitization phase is increased by the addition of interleukin-2 (IL-2) and of the effector phase by IFN-γ. Thus, in acute GVHD, T lymphocytes with specificity for recipient-restricted histocompatibility antigens can be generated and their presence determined prior to transplantation.

A decreased incidence of acute GVHD has been observed in recipients transplanted in laminar flow isolation or in gnotobiotic mice, suggesting an influence of environmental factors on acute GVHD.[32,33] The donor-derived T lymphocytes with specificity for recipient antigens that develop following transplantation are either cytotoxic T lymphocytes or produce cytokines such as IFN-γ that can activate macrophages/monocytes that then can produce TNF-α or IL-1α following stimulation with endotoxin, bacteria, and so forth.[34] Antibodies to TNF-α and antagonists to the IL-1α receptor can reduce the mortality and histopathologic changes of acute GVHD in mice.[26,27]

Initially, chronic GVHD was thought to be a chronic form of the acute disease.[35] Whereas acute GVHD is characterized by the cytotoxic destruction of the skin, gastrointestinal tract, and liver, chronic GVHD is characterized primarily by increased collagen deposition and fibrosis and has many similarities to human autoimmune diseases, particularly scleroderma.[36] Analysis of the T lymphocytes found in patients and animals with chronic GVHD has shown them to be primarily autoreactive T lymphocytes (i.e., T lymphocytes with specificity for histocompatibility antigens shared by donor and recipient cells).[37,38] Humans with chronic GVHD have been shown to have an increased frequency of autoreactive T lymphocytes; autoreactive T lymphocytes are the only clonogenic T lymphocytes found in mice with chronic GVHD due to minor histocompatibility antigen differences. Cellular analyses are consistent with the clinical observations that chronic GVHD has greater similarity to autoimmune diseases than it does to acute GVHD.

Several factors may contribute to the presence of autoreactive T lymphocytes in chronic GVHD: (1) the decreased elimination of autoreactive T lymphocytes during thymic differentiation following transplantation and (2) the decreased production of autoregulatory cells following transplantation.[38,39] Current dogma states that autoreactive T lymphocytes (i.e., T lymphocytes capable of reacting with autoantigens) are eliminated during thymic differentiation at the double-positive (CD4+, CD8+) stage following interaction with thymic dendritic cells.[40,41] The elimination of autoreactive T lymphocytes requires the expression of both CD4 by the T lymphocytes and the appropriate autoantigens by the dendritic cells. The antigen specificity of the autoreactive T lymphocytes found in animals and humans with chronic GVHD is for class II histocompatibility antigens. Decreased numbers of thymic dendritic cells are found following irradiation, acute GVHD, or administration of cyclosporine.[42,43] The decreased number of dendritic cells can result in the decreased elimination of autoreactive T lymphocytes.[44] Furthermore, the administration of cyclosporine may result in the decreased production of autoregulatory cells, which normally regulate the autoreactive T lymphocytes. The dysregulated reactivity of autoreactive T lymphocytes can result in cytokine production. IL-4 is produced by autoreactive T lymphocytes and may explain many of the immunologic abnormalities seen during chronic GVHD, including the increased incidence of autoantibody production.[45] Multiple cytokines in addition to IL-4 can be detected in the serum of recipients with chronic GVHD, including IFN-γ, IL-1α, TNF-α, and TNF-β, all of which are capable of stimulating fibroblast proliferation and collagen production. The increased collagen deposition seen in chronic GVHD is most likely a consequence of the cytokines produced by the autoreactive cells and not of cytotoxic damage.

The control of chronic GVHD is currently centered on immunosuppression, as is the case with other human autoimmune diseases.[46] The ultimate control of chronic GVHD will involve the re-establishment of the normal regulation of the post-transplant immune system.[47] Such regulation could consist of (1) reducing the number of the autoreactive T lymphocytes present during the early post-transplant period, (2) stimulating the repopulation of the thymus with donor-derived dendritic cells, or (3) stimulating the production of the autoregulatory cells necessary for the regulation of the autoreactive T lymphocytes.

LYMPHOID STEM CELLS

The engraftment of donor lymphoid stem cells is followed by a recapitulation of normal immunologic ontogeny.[48] The recapitulation of immunologic ontogeny is the most important biologic feature of the immune system following transplantation. There is little evidence for the clinically significant persistence of antigen-specific donor T lymphocytes following transplantation. Since pretransplant chemoradiotherapy eradicates pre-existing recipient T- and B-lymphocyte immunity, including recipient immunity to infectious agents such as chickenpox and measles, pre-existing recipient immunity is absent following transplantation. Thus, patients need to be reimmunized with the standard childhood immunizations following transplantation. Investigators have demonstrated that the immunization of allogeneic donors during the immediate pretransplant period, followed by the repeat immunization of recipients following transplantation, can result in the post-transplant production of specific antibody.[49] The use of such experimental protocols can demonstrate the transfer of some donor immunity. However, at the clinical level, the carryover of protective donor immunity cannot be routinely demonstrated. The recipients of unpurged autologous bone marrow may have detectable antibody levels following transplantation, suggesting that the drugs (methotrexate, cyclosporine) used to treat or prevent GVHD in allogeneic recipients may eliminate the mature donor-derived antigen-specific T and B lymphocytes.

In mammals, normal immunologic ontogeny is characterized by the sequential appearance of phenotypic T lymphocytes, followed by immunologic function. Phytohemagglutinin-responsive T lymphocytes can be detected by 10–12 weeks' gestation, and T lymphocytes capable of responding to allogeneic lymphocytes (mixed lymphocyte culture) can be detected by 12–16 weeks.[50] The production of specific antibody to viral pathogens can be detected by 20 weeks' gestation.[51]

Normal postnatal thymocytes are characterized by the expression of the CD1 on the majority of thymocytes (60%) and by the co-expression of CD4 and CD8 on most CD3-expressing thymocytes.[52] Analysis of peripheral blood T lymphocytes from 24-week fetuses has shown an increased frequency of CD1 T lymphocytes, as well as circulating CD4+/CD8+, CD3-expressing T lymphocytes. Thus, fetal ontogeny is characterized by the presence in the peripheral circulation of T lymphocytes normally found only in the thymus in postnatal life.

A recapitulation of normal immunologic ontogeny occurs following transplantation. Thymocyte-like T lymphocytes are found in the peripheral blood of transplant recipients early following bone marrow transplantation. Both CD1-expressing, as well as CD4+/CD8+, T lymphocytes can be detected.[48] During post-transplant immunologic reconstitution, phenotypic T lymphocytes are first identified, followed by the capacity to respond to mitogenic stimulation and later by the capacity to respond to allogeneic lymphocytes. During the early post-transplant period, immunization with antigens such as tetanus toxoid may result in the production of no antigen-specific T lymphocytes. Antigen-specific T lymphocytes are usually first identified 2–6 months following transplantation. Factors that influence the appearance of antigen-specific T lymphocytes include recipient age (thymic function), the presence of GVHD, and the need for ongoing GVHD prophylaxis or therapy.

Following transplantation, the recipient's immune response should be monitored, first for the appearance of phenotypic T lymphocytes and then for functional T lymphocytes. In vitro T-lymphocyte proliferation requires both the production of IL-2 and the expression of the IL-2 receptor (IL-2R) by T lymphocytes.[53] Most T lymphocytes following mitogenic stimulation are capable of expressing IL-2Rs, while only those T lymphocytes that have a T-cell receptor for a specific antigen express IL-2R following antigen-specific stimulation. Although most T lymphocytes can express IL-2R, fewer than 10% of T lymphocytes are capable of producing IL-2 after mitogenic stimulation.[54] Thus, while most normal T lymphocytes are capable of IL-2R expression, only a few are capable of IL-2 production. Following transplantation, IL-2R-expressing T lymphocytes appear earlier in ontogeny than do IL-2-producing T lymphocytes[55] (Fig. 27-1). Thus, when the proliferative response of

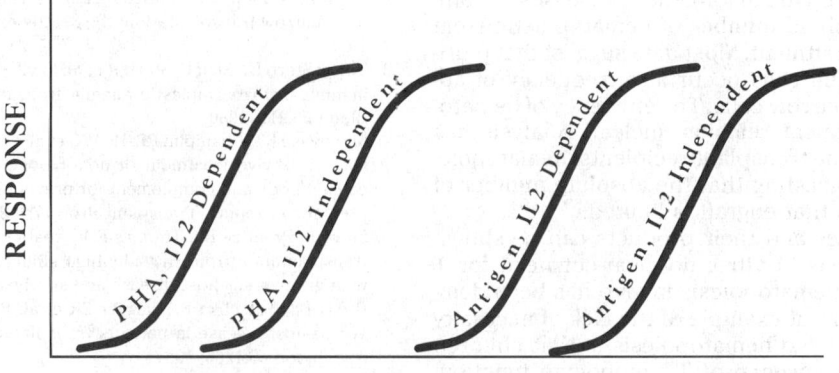

Fig. 27-1. Restoration of defective in vitro T-lymphocyte proliferation following bone marrow transplantation.

patients' T lymphocytes is determined without the addition of exogenous IL-2, a lack of proliferation can be detected following either mitogen or antigen stimulation. The addition of exogenous IL-2 can normalize the responses, demonstrating the presence of mitogen- or antigen-specific T lymphocytes but an absence of the IL-2 producing subpopulation.

Protection against encapsulated respiratory pathogens requires the immune system to produce antibodies to carbohydrate antigens. In normal immunologic development, the capacity of the immune system to respond to carbohydrate antigens is not fully developed until 18–24 months of life.[56] The same delay in the capacity of the immune system to produce anticarbohydrate antibodies occurs following transplantation. The deficiency in the production of anticarbohydrate antibodies is even more prolonged in the case of patients with chronic GVHD, presumably because of further delays in immunologic ontogeny and as a consequence of the immunosuppressant drugs they receive. The delay in the capacity to produce anticarbohydrate antibodies is the biologic basis for the increased frequency of bacterial infections seen in patients with chronic GVHD.[57] The prophylactic administration of trimethoprim/sulfamethoxazole and intravenous immunoglobulin has reduced the frequency and severity of bacterial infections in patients with chronic GVHD.

An additional immunologic problem seen in patients receiving T-lymphocyte-depleted haploidentical transplants is a lack of T- and B-lymphocyte cooperation.[23] Recipients of T-lymphocyte-depleted haploidentical transplants can have T lymphocytes of donor origin, while the B lymphocytes and hematopoietic cells may be of recipient origin, depending on their pretransplant conditioning. In spite of relatively normal T-lymphocyte function and the presence of B lymphocytes, a lack of specific antibody production can occur, necessitating long-term immunoglobulin administration. It is unclear whether the lack of T- and B-lymphocyte cooperation in such patients is due to defects in thymic processing, a lack of antigen presentation, or intrinsic defects in the recipient-derived B lymphocytes.

HEMATOPOIETIC STEM CELLS

For most recipients, the successful engraftment of donor hematopoietic stem cells is an absolute requirement for successful transplantation. The only exception to the rule is in the transplantation of children with SCID, whose abnormalities are restricted to the lymphoid stem cells and, therefore, in whom complete hematopoietic engraftment is not required.[58] Otherwise, almost all transplant recipients either are devoid of hematopoietic stem cells (aplastic anemia) or are cytoablated to eliminate their hematopoietic stem cells before transplantation (irradiation for leukemia, busulfan for genetic diseases). In animal experiments, a threshold number of hematopoietic stem cells are required for engraftment. Most data suggest that pluripotent hematopoietic stem cells occur at a frequency of approximately $1:10^5$ bone marrow cells. The efficiency of hematopoietic stem cell engraftment remains unclear. Analysis has demonstrated that, in some transplant recipients, hematopoiesis is clonal in origin, suggesting that the absolute number of hematopoietic stem cells that engraft is limited.[59]

Although T lymphocytes and their products can be shown to stimulate hematopoiesis in vitro, no clear-cut need for T lymphocytes to support hematopoiesis in vivo has been demonstrated. The most clear-cut example of the lack of necessity for T lymphocytes for in vivo hematopoiesis is that children with SCID, who have an absence of T-lymphocyte function, have normal hematopoiesis. Indeed, in some patients who receive T-lymphocyte-depleted transplants, post-transplant hematopoiesis is established more rapidly than in recipients of untreated bone marrow. The more rapid establishment of donor hematopoiesis may be partly attributable to the lack of post-transplant immunosuppression used in recipients of T-lymphocyte-depleted bone marrow.

Nevertheless, growth factors are required for successful hematopoietic engraftment and growth. In most cases, the growth factors are produced by the bone marrow stroma cells.[60,61] The prolonged chemotherapy given before transplantation may result in bone marrow stroma cells having a reduced capacity to support normal hematopoietic differentiation and proliferation.[62] Most evidence indicates that the bone marrow stroma cells continue to be of recipient origin following transplantation.[63] It is possible that the newly engrafted donor hematopoietic stem cells might not proliferate and differentiate maximally, due to defects in the recipient's stromal cells. Under such conditions, it might be expected that the administration of exogenous growth factors would result in a more rapid normalization of hematopoiesis. The administration of colony-stimulating factor-granulocyte or colony-stimulating factor-granulocyte/macrophage following autologous transplantation has resulted in the earlier recovery of granulocyte counts.[64,65] Growth factors have not been routinely given following allogeneic bone marrow transplantation because of concerns related to whether their administration might increase the incidence or severity of GVHD. Growth factors have been used in allogeneic recipients in whom engraftment is delayed or who are infected without significant increases in GVHD or leukemic relapse.[66] The administration of recombinant growth factors to these patients has resulted in myelopoiesis but no significant erythropoiesis or platelet production. In patients who respond to growth factors, the peripheral blood count drops following the discontinuation of growth factor administration. Theoretical arguments can be made that the administration of hematopoietic growth factors that stimulate differentiation is counterproductive, as it may reduce the capacity of the hematopoietic stems cells to undergo self-renewal.

SUMMARY

The biologic events that occur following bone marrow transplantation are determined by the presence of the mature T lymphocytes, lymphoid stem cells, and hematopoietic stem cells infused at transplantation. A greater understanding of the interrelationships between the different cell types may result in improved transplantation results.

REFERENCES

1. Thomas ED, Storb R, Clift RA et al: Bone marrow transplantation. N Engl J Med 292:832, 1975
2. Storb R, Weiden PL, Prentice R et al: Aplastic anemia (AA) treated by allogeneic marrow transplantation: the Seattle experience. Transplant Proc 9:181, 1977
3. Torok-Storb BJ, Sieff C, Storb R et al: In vitro tests for distinguishing possible immune-mediated aplastic anemia from transfusion-induced sensitization. Blood 55:211, 1980
4. Mitsuyasu RT, Champlin RE, Ho WG et al: Prospective randomized controlled trial of ex vivo treatment of donor bone marrow with monoclonal anti-T cell antibody and complement for prevention of graft-versus-host disease: a preliminary report. Transplant Proc 17:482, 1985
5. Storb R, Prentice RL, Thomas ED: Treatment of aplastic anemia by marrow transplantation from HLA-identical siblings. Prognostic factors associated with graft-versus-host disease and survival. J Clin Invest 59:625, 1977
6. Bross DS, Tutschka PJ, Farmer ER et al: Predictive factors for acute graft-versus-host disease in patients transplanted with HLA-identical bone marrow. Blood 63:1265, 1984
7. Beatty PG, Clift RA, Mickelson EM et al: Marrow transplantation from related donors other than HLA-identical siblings. N Engl J Med 313:765, 1985
8. Gingrich R, Howe C, Goeken N et al: Successful bone marrow transplantation with partially matched unrelated donors. Transplant Proc 17:450, 1985

9. Bortin MM: Risk factors for acute graft-versus-host disease. Exp Hematol 13: 406, 1985

10. Storb R, Doney KC, Thomas ED et al: Marrow transplantation with or without donor buffy coat cells for 65 transfused aplastic anemia ptients. Blood 59: 236, 1982

11. Vogelsang GB, Hess AD, Berkman AW et al: An in vitro predictive test for graft versus host disease in patients with genotypic HLA-identical bone marrow transplants. N Engl J Med 313:645, 1985

12. Irschick EU, Hladik F, Niederwieser D et al: Studies on the mechanism of tolerance of graft-versus-host disease in allogeneic bone marrow recipients at the level of cytotoxic T-cell precursor frequencies. Blood 79:1622, 1992

13. Parkman R, Rappeport J, Camitta B et al: Successful use of multiagent immunosuppresion in the bone marrow transplantation of sensitized patients. Blood 52:1163, 1978

14. Ramsay NKC, Kim T, Nesbit ME et al: Total lymphoid irradiation and cyclophosphamide as preparation for bone marrow transplantation in severe aplastic anemia. Blood 55:344, 1980

15. Storb R, Thomas ED, Buckner CD et al: Marrow transplantation in thirty "untransfused" patients with severe aplastic anemia. Ann Intern Med 92:30, 1980

16. Kernan NA, Bartsch G, Ash RC et al: Analysis of 462 transplantations from unrelated donors facilitated by the National Marrow Donor Program. N Engl J Med 328:593, 1993

17. Kernan NA, Flomenberg N, Dupont B, O'Reilly RJ: Graft rejection in recipients of T-cell-depleted HLA-nonidentical marrow transplants for leukemia: identification of host-derived antidonor allocytotoxic T lymphocytes. Transplantation 43:842, 1987

18. Fleischhauer K, Kernan NA, O'Reilly RJ et al: Bone marrow-allograft rejection by T lymphocytes recognizing a single amino acid difference in HLA-B44. N Engl J Med 323:1818, 1990

19. Korngold R, Sprent J: Lethal graft-versus-host disease after bone marrow transplantation across minor histocompatibility barriers in mice. Prevention by removing mature T cells from marrow. J Exp Med 148:1687, 1978

20. Hamilton BL, Parkman R: Acute and chronic graft-versus-host disease produced by minor histocompatibility antigens in mice. Transplantation 36:150, 1983

21. Reisner Y, Kapoor N, Kirkpatrick D et al: Transplantation for acute leukaemia with HLA-A and B nonidentical parental marrow cells fractionated with soybean agglutinin and sheep red blood cells. Lancet 1:327, 1981

22. Reinherz EL, Geha R, Rappeport JM et al: Reconstitution after transplantation with T lymphocyte depleted HLA haplotype-mismatched bone marrow for severe combined immunodeficiency. Proc Natl Acad Sci USA 79:6047, 1982

23. O'Reilly RJ, Keever CA, Small TN, Brochstein J: The use of HLA-non-identical, T-cell depleted marrow transplants for correction of severe combined immunodeficiency disease. Immunodef Rev 1:273, 1989

24. Cudkowicz G, Bennett M: Peculiar immunobiology of bone marrow allografts. II. Rejection of parental grafts by resistant F_1 hybrid mice. J Exp Med 134:1513, 1971

25. Billingham RE: The biology of graft versus host reactions. Harvey Lect 62: 21, 1967

26. Piquet P, Grau GE, Allet B, Vasili P: Tumor necrosis factor/cachectin is an effector of skin and gut lesions of the acute phase of graft-versus-host disease. J Exp Med 166:1280, 1987

27. McCarthy PL, Abhyankar S, Neben S et al: Inhibition of interleukin-1 by an interleukin-1 receptor antagonist prevents graft-versus-host disease. Blood 798:1915, 1991

28. Symington FW, Sullivan KM, Pepe M, Chen AB, Deliganis A: Serum tumor necrosis factor alpha associated with acute graft-versus-host disease in humans. Transplantation 50:518, 1990

29. Sprent J, Schaefer M, Lo D, Korngold R: Properties of purified T cell subsets. II. In vivo responses to class I vs. class II H-2 differences. J Exp Med 163:998, 1986

30. Korngold R, Sprent J: Negative selection of T cells causing lethal graft-versus-host disease across minor histocompatibility barriers: role of the H-2 complex. J Exp Med 151:1114, 1980

31. Korngold R, Sprent J: Variable capacity of L3T4+ T cells to cause lethal graft-versus-host disease across minor histocompatibility barriers in mice. J Exp Med 165:1552, 1987

32. Storb R, Prentice RL, Buckner CD et al: Graft-versus-host disease and survival in patients with aplastic anemia treated by marrow grafts from HLA-identical siblings. Beneficial effect of a protective environment. N Engl J Med 308:302, 1983

33. Beelen DW, Haralambie E, Brandt H et al: Evidence that sustained growth suppression of intestinal anaerobic bacteria reduces the risk of acute graft-versus-host disease after sibling marrow transplantation. Blood 80:2668, 1992

34. Nestel FP, Price KS, Seemayer TA, Lapp WS: Macrophage priming and lipo-

polysaccharide-triggered release of tumor necrosis factor α during graft-versus-host disease. J Exp Med 175:405, 1992

35. Sullivan KM, Shulman HM et al: The spectrum of chronic graft-versus-host disease in man. p. 69. In Gale RP, Fox CF (eds): Biology of Bone Marrow Transplantation. Academic Press, San Diego, 1980

36. Slavin RE, Woodruff JM: The pathology of bone marrow transplantation. Pathol Annu 9:291, 1974

37. Parkman R: Clonal analysis of murine graft-vs-host disease. I. Phenotypic and functional analysis of T lymphocyte clones. J Immunol 136:3543, 1986

38. Rosenkrantz K, Dupont B, Williams D, Flomenberg N: Autocytotoxic and autosuppressor T-cell lines generated from autologous lymphocyte cultures. Hum Immunol 19:189, 1987

39. Rosenkrantz K, Keever C, Kirsch J et al: In vitro correlates of graft-host tolerance after HLA-matched and mismatched marrow transplants: suggestions from limiting dilution analysis. Transplant Proc, suppl 7. 19:98, 1987

40. Kappler JW, Staerz U, White J, Marrack PC: Self-tolerance eliminates T cell specific for M1s-modified products of the major histocompatibility complex. Nature 332:35, 1988

41. Kisielow P, Bluthmann H, Staerz UD et al: Tolerance in T-cell-receptor transgenic mice involves deletion of nonmature CD4+8+ thymocytes. Nature 333:742, 1988

42. Beschorner WE, Di Gennaro KA, Hess AD, Santos GW: Cyclosporine and the thymus: influence of irradiation and age on thymic immunopathology and recovery. Cell Immunol 110:350, 1987

43. Shinozawa T, Beschorner WE, Hess AD: The thymus and prolonged administration of cyclosporine: irreversible immunopathologic changes associated with autologous pseudo-graft-versus-host disease. Transplantation 50:106, 1990

44. Urdahl KB, Pardoll DM, Jenkins MK: Self-reactive T cells are present in the peripheral lymphoid tissues of cyclosporine A-treated mice. Int Immunol 4: 1341, 1992

45. Sakaguchi S, Sakaguchi N: Thymus and autoimmunity. Transplantation of the thymus from cyclosporin A-treated mice causes organ-specific autoimmune disease in athymic nude mice. J Exp Med 167:1479, 1988

46. Sullivan KM, Shulman HM, Storb R et al: Chronic graft-versus-host disease in 52 patients: adverse natural course and successful treatment with combination immunosuppression. Blood 57:267, 1981

47. Rosenkrantz K, Dupont B, Flomenberg N: Generation and regulation of autocytotoxicity in mixed lymphocyte cultures: evidence for active suppression of autocytotoxic cells. Proc Natl Acad Sci USA 82:4508, 1985

48. Rappeport JM, Dunn MJ, Parkman R: Immature T lymphocytes in the peripheral blood of bone marrow transplant recipients. Transplantation 36:674, 1983

49. Wimperis JZ, Prentice HG, Karayiannis P et al: Transfer of a functioning humoral immune system in transplantation of T-lymphocyte-depleted bone marrow. Lancet 1:339, 1986

50. August CS, Berkel AI, Driscoll S, Merler E: Onset of lymphocyte function in the developing human fetus. Pediatr Res 5:539, 1971

51. Furth R, van Schuit HR, Hijmans W: The immunological development of the human fetus. J Exp Med 122:1173, 1965

52. Reinherz EL, Kung PC, Goldstein G et al: Discrete stages of human intrathymic differentiation: analysis of normal thymocytes and leukemic lymphoblasts of T-cell lineage. Proc Natl Acad Sci USA 77:1588, 1980

53. Green WC, Leonard WJ: The human interleukin-2 receptor. Annu Rev Immunol 4:69, 1986

54. Granelli-Piperno A: In situ hybridization for interleukin-2 and interleukin-2 receptor mRNA in T cells activated in the presence or absence of cyclosporin A. J Exp Med 168:1649, 1988

55. Lenarsky C, Weinberg K, Petersen J, Parkman R: Interleukin 2 (IL-2) restoration of defective in vitro lymphocyte proliferation following bone marrow transplantation (BMT), abstracted (841). Pediatr Res 21:313A, 1987

56. Smith RT, Eitzman DV, Catlin ME et al: The development of the immune response: characterization of the response of the human infant and adult to immunization with salmonella vaccines. Pediatrics 33:163, 1964

57. Atkinson K, Storb R, Prentice RL et al: Analysis of late infections in 89 long-term survivors of bone marrow transplantation. Blood 53:720, 1979

58. Parkman R, Gelfand EW, Rosen FS et al: Severe combined immunodeficiency and adenosine deaminase deficiency. N Engl J Med 292:714, 1975

59. Turhan AG, Humphries RK, Phillips GL et al: Clonal hematopoiesis demonstrated by X-linked DNA polymorphisms after allogeneic bone marrow transplantation. N Engl J Med 320:1655, 1989

60. Clark SC, Kamen R: The human hematopoietic colony-stimulating factors. Science 236:1229, 1987

61. Ogawa M: Differentiation and proliferation of hematopoietic stem cells. Blood 81:2844, 1993

62. Cairo MS, Suen Y, Sender L et al: Circulating granulocyte colony-stimulating factor (G-CSF) levels after allogeneic and autologous bone marrow transplantation: endogenous G-CSF production correlates with myeloid engraftment. Blood 79:1869, 1992

63. Simmons PJ, Przepiorka D, Thomas ED, Torok-Storb B: Host origin of marrow stromal cells following allogeneic bone marrow transplantation. Nature 328: 429, 1987

64. Brandt SJ, Peters WP, Atwater SK et al: Effect of recombinant human granulocyte-macrophage colony-stimulating factor on hematopoietic reconstitution after high-dose chemotherapy and autologous bone marrow transplantation. N Engl J Med 14:869, 1988

65. Nemunaitis J, Singer JW, Buckner CD et al: Use of recombinant human granulocyte-macrophage colony-stimulating factor in autologous marrow transplantation for lymphoid malignancies. Blood 72:834, 1988

66. Nemunaitis J, Anasetti C, Storb R et al: Phase II trial of recombinant human granulocyte-macrophage colony-stimulating factor in patients undergoing allogeneic bone marrow transplantation for unrelated donors. Blood 79:2572, 1992

Autologous Bone Marrow Transplantation

28

Elizabeth C. Reed and Anne Kessinger

INTRODUCTION

Small increments in the dose of radiation or an anticancer drug may increase the number of cancer cells killed by several logs for some malignancies. The maximum dose of a drug is determined by toxicity to normal tissues, and for cancer therapy the dose is often limited by toxicity to the bone marrow. Autologous hematopoietic stem cell rescue allows the treatment of tumors with doses of chemotherapy and radiation that exceed bone marrow tolerance; stem cell rescue re-establishes hematopoiesis after treatment by an infusion of previously stored hematopoietic stem cells. The use of the patient's own stem cells avoids the complications of graft rejection or graft-versus-host disease (GVHD) that can occur after allogeneic marrow transplant. The disadvantages are that autologous bone marrow may be contaminated with tumor cells, and the immunologic control of tumor seen after some allogeneic marrow transplants, referred to as graft versus leukemia, is not achieved with autologous rescue.[1]

The advantages of autologous transplant were recognized by many early investigators who developed techniques for bone marrow transplant. In the late 1950s investigators used high doses of radiation and in some cases nitrogen mustard for the treatment of solid tumors and then infused bone marrow that had been stored before therapy.[2,3] The results of the treatment were difficult to interpret because of mortality and the inability to determine whether hematopoiesis was re-established by residual marrow cells or the infused marrow. The appearance of more effective cytoreductive agents rekindled interest in autologous transplant, and the technique is increasingly considered for salvage therapy in patients with hematologic malignancies and selected solid tumors.[4]

COLLECTION OF THE AUTOGRAFT PRODUCT

Guidelines for collecting autologous marrow were initially adapted from the already established criteria based on the allogeneic marrow collection experience. The minimum dose of marrow cells needed to achieve autologous engraftment has been studied in preclinical models,[5] but a similar study in humans is unthinkable. As clinical experience grew, the definition of a suitable bone marrow autograft product evolved. A collection that contains 2.5×10^8 mononuclear cells/kg patient weight is considered adequate,[6] although marrow autografts with lower numbers of cells have successfully served as grafts. The progenitor cell content of these marrow collections approximates $2-3 \times 10^4$ colony-forming unit-granulocyte/macrophage (CFU-GM)/kg patient weight.[7] Since progenitor cell culture assays have not been standardized, this number may vary from one center to another. Recently, the ability to enumerate the number of CD34 cells in a graft using flow cytometric methods has become available. This approach could potentially provide a more timely estimate of progenitor cell content.[8] Although one report has suggested that 1×10^6 CD34$^+$ marrow cells/kg body weight, selected with a biotin-avidin immunoadherence technique, is sufficient for sustained engraftment,[9] no consensus regarding the number of CD34$^+$ marrow cells required has been reached. Some centers assay an aliquot of the cryopreserved marrow for CFU-GM, to ensure that the cells composing the graft have survived the cryopreservation process.[7]

While $750-1,000$ cm^3 of harvested marrow typically provides a product suitable for autografting,[10] a total of 40 L of peripheral blood processed for about 3 hours at a time over 3-6 days with an apheresis apparatus will usually supply a sufficient number of peripheral progenitors for a successful autologous transplant.[11] Peripheral blood progenitor cells can be collected during a period of unperturbed marrow function, and the presence of $6.5-8 \times 10^8$ mononuclear cells/kg patient weight in the final product has served as a reliable predictor of a harvest that will provide engraftment.[12] Currently, however, collections during steady-state marrow function are not commonly performed. Peripheral stem cell collections are much more likely to be done while marrow function is being manipulated in a deliberate attempt to expand the number of circulating progenitors. This expansion is called mobilization and is accomplished by administering either myelosuppressive chemotherapy or growth factor(s), or both.[13-15] The definition of an adequate mobilized peripheral progenitor cell autograft product is more dependent on the number of progenitors (CFU-GM) in the collection than the number of mononuclear cells. Presumably, a certain number of mononuclear cells will continue to predict engraftment in this circumstance, but mobilized progenitor cells and possibly stem cells are expected to provide not only sustained but also rapid engraftment. This is thought to result from the presence of a larger number of late progenitors in the graft than nonmobilized peripheral stem cells or bone marrow can provide. The number of CFU-GM necessary to predict rapid engraftment has not been determined and, in fact, varies from one institution to another. The reasons for this disparity are likely to include the lack of a standardized culture assay for CFU-GM, the variety of mobilization methods currently employed, and the different characteristics of the patient population treated. The number of CFU-GM believed to indicate an adequately mobilized transplant product has varied from 15 to 50×10^4 CFU-GM/kg patient weight.[16,17] The CD34$^+$ cell content of a peripheral progenitor cell product has been suggested as a surrogate for the CFU-GM content to define an adequate collection for transplant.[18] The major advantage to this approach is that the CD34 assay requires only a few hours, while the CFU-GM assay requires 2 weeks to complete. Therefore, a satisfactory collection could be identified immediately. Using the CFU-GM assay, if an insufficient number of progenitors were collected for a transplant, the mobilization effect in the patient would be gone when the deficiency was detected. Investigators are working to design CD34 assays that can be standardized and that predict for rapid engraftment. Initial reports have suggested that 8×10^6 CD34$^+$ peripheral blood mononuclear cells/kg body weight will support both rapid and sustained engraftment.[19]

PURGING

In those patients who experience relapse of their malignancies after a complete response to high-dose therapy and autologous bone marrow transplant, either complete eradication of disease was not achieved with the therapy, or else malignant cells capable of re-establishing disease were infused with the hematopoietic cell transplant. A continued concern with hematopoietic progenitor cell collections from patients with malignancies is that they might contain occult malignant cells. Use of cell culture tumor cell assays, as well as molecular and monoclonal antibody techniques, has demonstrated that some patients with lymphoma, neuroblastoma, and breast cancer have occult tumor cells in their histopathologically normal bone marrows and peripheral blood.[20-22] However, the clinical significance of these malignant cells (i.e., their clonogenic potential) when reinfused in an autograft product is not certain. Some reports suggest that successful manipulation of the autograft product to eliminate occult tumor cells leads to a better patient outcome,[23,24] although prospective randomized trials are not available.

Autograft products have been purged (manipulated to remove tumor cells) with several techniques. Either the suspected tumor cells are destroyed or isolated (negative selection), or the normal progenitors and stem cells are separated from the terminally differentiated cells and tumor cells (positive selection). A number of negative selection techniques have been employed, including treatment of the harvested marrow with cytotoxic chemotherapy designed to kill malignant cells without damaging the more primitive hematopoietic progenitors and stem cells.[25] Complement-dependent cytotoxicity generated by adding tumor-directed monoclonal antibodies and complement to marrow harvests has been used for purging,[26] as has dye-sensitized photoirradiation.[27] Malignant cells have been separated from marrow by adding tumor cell-directed

monoclonal antibody-coated magnetic beads to the marrow. After the beads attach to the targeted tumor cells, the harvest is passed through a magnetic field, which extracts tumor cells attached to magnetic beads from the harvest.[28] Selecting out only the CD34$^+$ cells from a marrow harvest, and thereby possibly excluding tumor cells from the transplant product, has also been used as a purging technique.[19,29,30] The absolute efficiency of these and various other purging methods has not been precisely determined, but it is not likely to be 100%. However, the minimum number of tumor cells that can be reinfused without re-establishing disease is also unknown, and the role that purging currently plays or may play in the future continues to be a subject for speculation. Currently, many centers do not purge marrow harvests at all, while others purge only those harvests from patients with specific malignancies that tend to involve the bone marrow.

CRYOPRESERVATION

Without the ability to store hematopoietic stem cells in a functional condition for a prolonged period, autologous bone marrow transplantation would have little clinical application. Most high-dose regimens require several days, even 1 week, to be completed, and the graft must be collected before the marrow-ablative therapy begins. The cells can be stored in a viable state for years if they are cryopreserved. The most common method of cryopreservation involves the addition of dimethyl sulfoxide (DMSO), 10% by volume, to the cell suspension prior to freezing to help prevent formation of lethal intracellular ice crystals. In addition, the cells are frozen at a controlled rate to retard cellular dehydration and still provide intracellular freezing. After cryopreservation, the cells are stored in a liquid nitrogen freezer to prevent growth of extracellular ice.[31] More recently, an alternate method has been described that uses 5% DMSO and 6% hydroxyethyl starch as cryoprotectants, and does not require controlled-rate freezing. Cells cryopreserved in this manner can be stored at $-80°C$, providing a less expensive alternative method of cryopreservation.[7]

AUTOGRAFT INFUSION

At the time of the transplant, the cryopreserved cells are removed from the freezer and taken to the bedside of the patient. For a bone marrow transplant, the entire graft product is usually included in a single bag, while a peripheral progenitor cell transplant product may occupy three to eight or more freezing bags, depending on the number of apheresis procedures performed. One bag is placed in a 40°C water bath and thawed in a matter of seconds. The cells are then administered intravenously. The next bag (if any) is not thawed until all the cells in the first bag are infused. A few centers thaw and wash the cells in the laboratory prior to infusion. Washing permits the removal of DMSO, which may cause side effects when infused; the disadvantage is that some progenitor cells are lost with the wash.[32] A bone marrow transplant requires approximately 30 minutes to complete, while most peripheral progenitor cell transplants are completed within 4 hours.

Infusion of unwashed marrow and unwashed peripheral blood progenitor cells can be associated with a number of side effects, usually attributed to the DMSO or the cell fragments, or both, that result when red cells and granulocytes lyse during the freeze-thaw process.[33] Some combination of drugs (including mannitol, hydrocortisone, diphenhydramine, and/or meperidine hydrochloride) is commonly administered prior to peripheral blood progenitor cell infusions to diminish the side effects. Reported side effects include flushing, dyspnea, nausea, abdominal cramping, hypertension, and bradycardia. Peripheral progenitor cell transplants are more likely to be associated with more side effects than are bone marrow transplants.[34] The side effects are generally short-lived and begin to abate as soon as the infusion is complete.

PREPARATIVE REGIMENS

The autologous preparative regimen must be effective against the tumor with tolerable extrahematopoietic side effects, whereas the preparative regimen for allogeneic marrow transplant must also be sufficiently immunosuppressive to allow engraftment. Since autologous regimens do not include continued immunosuppression for GVHD, more aggressive therapy can be used in autologous patients. Nonetheless, treatment regimens used for allogeneic bone marrow transplant have been adopted for the autologous setting, particularly the combinations of cyclophosphamide and total body irradiation and cyclophosphamide and busulfan. Preparative regimens have also been developed by escalating the dose of single agents, combining non-cross-resistant agents or selecting agents that demonstrate nonoverlapping toxicities, thereby allowing maximum dosing of each drug in a multiagent regimen.

Cyclophosphamide and total body irradiation are used extensively for allogeneic and autologous marrow transplants of patients with hematopoietic malignancies. The radiation is usually fractionated to reduce toxicity. Radiation doses exceeding 12 Gy decrease relapse rates, but disease-free survival is unchanged due to an increase in early toxic deaths.[35] Regimens substituting busulfan for total body irradiation are comparable in efficacy to radiation-containing regimens in the treatment of leukemia.[36,37] Other agents such as cytosine arabinoside, melphalan, and etoposide are substituted for or added to total body irradiation.[38-40] No studies are available that show any one preparative regimen to be superior for the treatment of leukemia.

Alkylating agents such as cyclophosphamide, ifosphamide, busulfan, melphalan, thiotepa, and carmustine are used extensively in high-dose therapy because they show a steep dose-response curve for most hematologic malignancies and some solid tumors such as breast cancer. Alkylating agents also have the advantage of non-cross-resistance so that tumors refractory to one alkylating agent are often still sensitive to other alkylating agents.[41] An analysis of high-dose treatment for metastatic breast cancer suggests that therapy with more than one alkylating agent is superior to treatment with a single alkylating drug and that the addition of total body irradiation does not improve tumor response.[42] High-dose chemotherapy regimens

for breast cancer are usually combinations of two or more alkylating agents.

The action of etoposide, a topoisomerase II inhibitor, may be synergistic with alkylating drugs.[43] Alkylating agents are combined with etoposide alone or with cytosine arabinoside or total body irradiation for the high-dose treatment of hematologic malignancies.[44-47] Although several high-dose regimens exist, no single regimen is clearly superior. Disease relapse continues to be the major cause of death after high-dose therapy, and although overall survival is better through improved supportive care, the ability to eradicate tumors has not improved. Several strategies for better tumor reduction are being explored. Aside from the continued search for more active chemotherapy agents, novel ways to deliver radiation through targeting tumors with polyclonal or monoclonal antibodies are being developed.[48,49] Tandem or double transplants have also been used as a means of intensifying treatment.[50] Sequencing treatment or pretreating with agents that can overcome mechanisms of drug resistance in tumors are other areas of research. Immunotherapy following transplant to improve tumor surveillance or simulate the graft-versus-tumor effect observed after allogeneic marrow transplant is also being used.[51]

INDICATIONS

Lymphomas were among the first malignancies that were cured with chemotherapy or radiation. Today, the initial use of chemotherapy or radiotherapy, or both, cures about 70% of patients with Hodgkin disease and about 50% of patients with intermediate or high-grade non-Hodgkin lymphoma. Conversely, 30–50% of patients with lymphoma relapse or are primarily refractory to treatment. These patients can have a complete remission after salvage therapy, but it is unlikely they will have a lengthy disease-free survival. A dose-response relationship between dose of the chemotherapeutic agent and tumor cell kill appears to exist for Hodgkin disease and some non-Hodgkin lymphomas, making high-dose therapy a logical approach to the treatment of refractory or relapsed disease. Results of high-dose therapy for treatment of relapsed or refractory lymphoma are presented in Table 28-1.

Hodgkin Disease

CBV (cyclophosphamide, carmustine [BCNU], etoposide [VP-16]) have been widely used for high-dose therapy of relapsed or refractory Hodgkin disease. A group of 128 patients

Table 28-1. Autologous Bone Marrow Transplant for Lymphoma

Type of Lymphoma	Ref.	Patients (N)	Regimen	Early Death (%)	DFS (Follow-up) (%)
Hodgkin	52	128	CVB	9	25 at 77 mo (median)
	53	54	CVB[a]	21	56 at 15 mo (median)
	54	155	BEAM	10	50 actuarial at 5 yr
	56	26	Cy TBI	23	26 at 3.8 yr (median)
Non-Hodgkin	69	100	Multiple regimens, some with TBI	21	19 actuarial at 3 yr
	68	50	Multiple regimens, no TBI	18	14 at 19–78 mo[b]
	67	46	Multiple regimens, some TBI	7	54 at 8–104 mo[b]
	70	101	Multiple regimens, most with TBI	21	11 actuarial at 5 yr
	71	68	Cy TBI	21	16 at 4–10 yr[b]
			Cy TBI		
	72	70	BCNU + CY + ara-C	13	23 at 1–6.5 yr[b]
	73	78	CBV	8	54 actuarial at 3 yr

Abbreviations: BCNU + Cy + ara-C, carmustine, cyclophosphamide, and cytosine arabinoside; BEAM, cyclophosphamide, etoposide, cytosine arabinoside, and melphalan; CVB, cyclophosphamide, etoposide, and carmustine; Cy TBI, cyclophosphamide and total body irradiation; DFS, disease-free survival.
[a] Augmented dose of CVB.
[b] Continuous complete remission.

transplanted at the University of Nebraska Medical Center and the M.D. Anderson Cancer Center has been followed for a median of 77 months.[52] The overall survival and failure-free survival at 4 years was estimated at 45% and 25%, respectively. The treatment was well tolerated, with an incidence of early toxic death of about 9%. Escalated doses of CBV have been used and resulted in an improved complete response rate.[53] However, 21% of the patients died of toxicity, resulting in an overall survival that was comparable to the lower dose CBV.

Other high-dose chemotherapy regimens have included melphalan. A cohort of 155 patients treated with BEAM (carmustine [BCNU], etoposide, cytosine arabinoside, melphalan) showed an estimated 5-year overall survival of 55% and progression-free survival of 50%.[54] Although the early fatal toxicity in the patients treated with BEAM was only 10%, excessive lung toxicity after treatment with melphalan, etoposide, and carmustine has also been reported.[55]

Many Hodgkin disease patients are treated with extensive radiotherapy, precluding the use of total body irradiation for high-dose therapy. However, Hodgkin disease is typically radiosensitive, and radiation may have a role in the salvage of relapsed or refractory patients. Phillips et al.[56] treated 26 patients who had progressive Hodgkin disease with cyclophosphamide, total body irradiation, and, in selected patients, involved field irradiation. Of 26 patients, 18 responded completely, and 27% of patients remained progression-free for a median of 3.8 years. Idiopathic interstitial pneumonitis caused death in 3 patients, each of whom had received mediastinal irradiation. Accelerated hyperfractionated total-lymphoid irradiation with high-dose therapy in relapsed or refractory patients achieved an actuarial disease-free survival of 50% at 6.5 years.[57] A phase I trial of ^{90}Y-labeled antiferritin and CBV in poor prognosis Hodgkin disease resulted in an estimated 21% progression-free survival at 1 year; the early mortality was comparable to the early mortality seen in poor prognosis patients treated with chemotherapy alone. Further trials are needed to evaluate the role of conventional radiotherapy and antibody-directed radiotherapy in high-dose therapy of Hodgkin disease.[58]

It is important to identify characteristics that accurately predict the benefit of high-dose therapy for a given patient. Factors that predict a poor outcome for various high-dose regimens include a poor pretransplant performance status, failure of two or more therapies, bulky tumor mass, and a long duration of disease.[56,59] Patients with good prognostic factors (i.e., a good performance status and failure of at most one treatment) who are treated with CBV have an estimated 4-year failure-free survival of 53% compared with a failure-free survival of 25% for unselected patients.[52] Reducing tumor bulk before high-dose chemotherapy may improve outcome. The use of dexamethasone, cisplatin, and cytarabine and in some cases local radiation reduces tumor size in 43% of relapsed Hodgkin patients before proceeding to high-dose treatment.[60]

The proper time to use high-dose therapy has become a key question. Conventional-dose salvage therapy following the first chemotherapy failure is unlikely to achieve long-term disease-free survival, particularly if the first remission lasted <1 year.[61] Since less heavily pretreated patients are more likely to benefit from high-dose therapy, optimal management may be high-dose therapy at second remission or first relapse with minimal disease.[62] Alternatively, a historical analysis of patients treated with conventional or high-dose salvage therapy concludes that failure-free outcome is dependent on predictive factors such as initial stage, B symptoms at relapse, and length of the initial disease-free interval rather than the type or doses of salvage therapy.[63]

Allogeneic bone marrow transplants have also been used for rescue following high-dose salvage therapy for Hodgkin disease. Allogeneic rescue provides a tumor-free rescue product and possibly a graft-versus-lymphoma effect.[64] These advantages are offset by the morbidity and mortality associated with GVHD and the lack of donors for many patients. Jones et al.[65] treated Hodgkin disease patients who had matched donors with allogeneic transplants, while patients without donors received autologous bone marrow purged with 4-hydroperoxy-cyclophosphamide (4-HC). The overall actuarial probability of event-free survival at 3 years for the entire group was 30%. Event-free survival is influenced by factors predicting for refractory disease but not by an autologous versus an allogeneic graft. Appelbaum et al.[66] compared disease-free survival in 100 patients with Hodgkin and non-Hodgkin lymphoma and found no difference among patients receiving allogeneic, syngeneic, or autologous transplants.

Non-Hodgkin Lymphoma

Patients with relapsed or refractory non-Hodgkin lymphoma are even more unlikely than patients with Hodgkin disease to achieve a long-term disease-free survival with conventional salvage chemotherapy. Again, the steep dose-response curves for some drugs for non-Hodgkin lymphoma encouraged the use of high-dose therapy and autologous marrow or peripheral blood rescue for salvage therapy. Few conclusions can be drawn from comparison of the single-arm high-dose treatment trials in this group of patients. Early trials treated only those patients that were refractory to other forms of treatment and often grouped Hodgkin disease and non-Hodgkin lymphomas together, while later trials have treated more selected patients. It is apparent that high-dose therapy can achieve long-term remission in patients that otherwise would not be "cured." The long-term remission rates on average are 20–25%, but patients with favorable prognostic factors may have long-term remission rates in the 50–60% range.[64,67–73]

As in Hodgkin disease, performance status and sensitivity to chemotherapy are important prognosticators for outcome following high-dose therapy. The superior outcome of patients with disease that is still responsive to conventional salvage chemotherapy has been reported by several groups.[64,67–73] Conversely, Philip et al.[69] reported no disease-free survival after high-dose therapy in patients with primary refractory non-Hodgkin lymphoma. Most centers treat the relapsed non-Hodgkin patient with conventional chemotherapy in an effort to test chemotherapy sensitivity and reduce the tumor size before undertaking high-dose therapy. Autologous bone marrow transplant in the first partial or complete remission when the tumor is still likely to be chemotherapy-sensitive may be a better curative strategy. Patients with poor prognostic features are treated with autologous transplant after partial induction with initial chemotherapy.[74] The overall and progression-free survival in these patients appears to be better than what would have been expected with conventional chemotherapy, but a randomized prospective trial is needed to confirm the advantage of early autologous transplant as initial therapy for patients with a poor prognosis. Poor prognostic groups that may be considered for autologous transplant in first remission are adults with stage IV lymphoblastic lymphoma and bone marrow involvement, central nervous system disease, or presentation with a high lactate dehydrogenase and adults with small non-cleaved cell lymphomas and central nervous system involvement.[75]

The general condition of the patient is the other factor that has consistently predicted outcome.[70,71,76] A pretransplant Karnofsky score of <70 predicts a poor outcome. Older age does not consistently have a negative predictive value, but the older patients that have been reported to have received an autologous bone marrow transplant may have been highly selected.[68,70–72]

Prior radiation and the presence of bulky disease, extranodal disease, and/or disease in the marrow were prognostic variables in some studies, while others did not find a similar correlation with outcome.[67,68,71,72,76,77] Tumor phenotype does not appear to predict outcome after high-dose treatment, but there is disagreement regarding the impact of tumor histology.[76] Some centers have shown a better outcome in patients with intermediate-grade lymphomas as opposed to high-grade lymphomas, while others found no difference.[67,71,72,77] Low-grade lymphomas present an interesting dilemma. This disease is not curable with conventional therapy, but patients may experience long disease-free periods or have very slow progression of disease.[78] Patients are generally older, and the bone marrow is often involved. Studies treating low-grade lymphoma with high-dose therapy and autologous transplant are small and have a short follow-up relative to the natural history of the disease.[79–81] Nonetheless, some patients have remained disease-free after high-dose therapy, an outcome that is not expected after conventional therapy. Larger numbers and longer follow-up are needed to determine whether high-dose therapy is curing some patients with low-grade lymphoma or whether relapse has just been delayed.

Although the presence of tumor in the marrow is not always predictive of a poor outcome, purging continues to be an issue in autologous marrow transplant. Several centers have failed to demonstrate an advantage to purging.[60,70,72] An interesting exception is a study by Gribben et al.[24] using antibody and complement to purge bone marrow with lymphoma cells detected by polymerase chain reaction. Patients with lymphoma cells identified in the bone marrow by the same detection methods after purging were significantly more likely to relapse. This finding suggests that relapse may indeed be due to tumor cells infused with the rescue product rather than residual tumor. Other studies may not show the effects of tumor in the marrow because the methods for tumor detection are insensitive.

Allogeneic bone marrow and peripheral blood stem cells are two alternative rescue products for high-dose therapy. Patients treated with allogeneic transplant for non-Hodgkin lymphoma and registered by the Europen Bone Marrow Transplant Group were retrospectively compared with autologous patients who had matched prognostic characteristics.[75] No differences were evident, for any histologic category, in progression-free survival between the two groups. The similar outcome coupled with the greater long-term morbidity associated with allogeneic bone marrow transplants is persuasive to many physicians, leading them to reserve allogeneic transplant for those patients who fail autologous transplant or in whom autologous transplant is not feasible. Peripheral blood progenitor cell grafts are used to hasten engraftment, but perhaps more interestingly, they are also used when bone marrow is of poor quality or is involved with tumor. The University of Nebraska Medical Center has used peripheral blood progenitor cells as the rescue product for patients with non-Hodgkin lymphoma and initial or persistent marrow involvement. A comparison of this group with patients who never had tumor found in the bone marrow and who received autologous bone marrow showed better overall and disease-free survival for the group receiving the peripheral progenitor cell graft.[82] A randomized study comparing outcome after these two autologous rescue products is being planned.

Leukemia

The use of autologous bone marrow transplant for the treatment of leukemia differs somewhat between the United States and Europe.[4] The most frequent indication for autologous transplant in the United States has been for the treatment of lymphoma and solid tumors, while in Europe it is most commonly used for the treatment of leukemia.[83] The role of autologous transplant in the treatment of leukemia has been debated for some time. Two issues at the center of the debate are, first, the benefit of high-dose therapy and autologous rescue over conventional chemotherapy alone and second, the need for purging of autologous bone marrow. Again, firm conclusions are difficult to make because most of the trials have been single-arm studies and the numbers of patients treated have been small. In earlier trials the time from remission induction to transplant was not always reported, and the selective and censoring effects of time could have biased historical comparisons of high-dose therapy and conventional therapy. Analysis of leukemia studies is aided by the more uniform use of cyclophosphamide and total body irradiation or cyclophosphamide and busulfan as the preparative regimens. Purging is most often done with derivatives of cyclophosphamide such as 4-HC or mafosfamide.[37,84] Immunologic purging, employing monoclonal antibodies and complement or magnetic beads or immunotoxins is also used.[85–87] Positive selection for early progenitor cells such as those staining for CD34 is a more recent approach to the problem of providing a tumor-free rescue product.[88]

Acute Myeloid Leukemia

High-dose therapy with autologous rescue performed for patients in the first complete remission of acute myeloid leukemia (AML) results in about a 50% disease-free survival at a median of 2 years. A randomized trial comparing autologous bone marrow transplant with conventional therapy, treated patients <50 years of age with standard induction followed by one standard course of therapy for consolidation.[89] Patients with an HLA-matched donor were treated with an allogeneic bone marrow transplant, while the remaining patients were randomized between tandem treatment with high-dose melphalan and rescue with unpurged marrow versus treatment with etoposide, high doses of arabinoside, and amsacrine given as four 1-month cycles. The relapse rates of 18%, 50%, and 83% in the allogeneic group, autologous group, and conventional chemotherapy group, respectively, were significantly different for the three groups. A further study with intensified conventional chemotherapy also showed inferior diease-free survival in the conventional treatment group compared with high-dose therapy.[90] Amadori et al.[91] randomized children with AML in first remission between autologous transplant and sequential postremission chemotherapy if the patient did not have an HLA-matched donor. They reported a superior disease-free survival in the allogeneic group, but saw no difference between the autologous and sequential chemotherapy groups.

No randomized studies have compared outcome after purged versus unpurged autologous bone marrow transplantation for AML. Gorin[92] retrospectively analyzed patients with AML treated for a median of 5 months after entering a complete remission with high-dose therapy and rescue with unpurged marrow or marrow purged with mafosphamide. He reported that the relapse rate of 35% in the purged group was superior to the 47% relapse rate in patients rescued with unpurged marrow. The greatest difference was seen in the group of patients who received a transplant within the first 6 months of achieving a complete remission.

The results of autologous bone marrow transplant in patients with advanced AML are inferior to the results of transplant in first complete remission. However, the long-term survivors of advanced leukemia are few with conventional therapy, so autologous transplant is still a consideration. Yeager et al.[37] collected bone marrow in second or third remission and treated it with 4-HC, using it for rescue after cyclophosphamide and total body irradiation or cyclophosphamide and busulfan. Forty-three percent of patients remained disease-free a median of 400 days after transplant. Others have reported that after a median of 24 months following autologous transplant, about 15–25% of patients remained disease-free.[37,85,93]

Acute Lymphocytic Leukemia

Seventy percent of children with acute lymphocytic leukemia (ALL) treated with conventional chemotherapy remain disease-free.[94] Unfortunately, adults have a poorer prognosis, and conventional chemotherapy is unlikely to result in a long-term disease-free survival for any patient who relapses.[95] Many centers use purged and unpurged autologous marrow transplant for patients in remission after at least one relapse and report disease-free survival of about 10–40%, with varying lengths of follow-up.[96] The European Cooperative Group for Bone Marrow Transplantation reported that better outcome occurs in children and adults who received fractionated rather than single-dose radiation and purged marrow.[97] The group at the Dana Farber Cancer Center reported that the duration of the initial remission was an important predictor of outcome, with no event-free survival of patients who had an initial remission of <24 months.[98] Horowitz et al.[99] treated patients in first complete remission of ALL and found no advantage of allogeneic bone marrow transplant over conventional therapy. Therefore, a role for autologous transplant in first remission ALL seems unlikely unless a particularly poor-risk subgroup can be defined. The only controlled trial comparing allogeneic bone marrow transplant with autologous rescue reported that relapse occurred in 37% of patients who received an allogeneic bone marrow transplant and developed GVHD, while allogeneic patients without GVHD and autologous patients had similar rates of relapse of 75% and 79% respectively.[100] This study suggests that for ALL, strategies to improve the outcome after autologous therapy may be better aimed at modulation of the immune system rather than earlier timing of high-dose therapy.

Chronic Myeloid Leukemia

Allogeneic bone marrow transplant, particularly when done in the early chronic phase, offers the best chance for prolonged disease-free survival for patients with chronic myeloid leukemia (CML).[101,102] The patient's age, physical condition, or lack of a donor may preclude an allogeneic transplant, and autologous transplant can be considered. Most patients treated with autologous transplant in the chronic phase will have a partial or complete remission, measured by the establishment of Philadelphia chromosome-negative hematopoiesis.[103] However, <5% of patients remain leukemia free after 3 years. Autologous transplant can convert 80% of CML patients in transformation back to the chronic phase, but the duration of remission is typically less than 1 year.[104] The absence of GVHD after an allogeneic bone marrow transplant is highly predictive for relapse.[105] Inducing a graft-versus-leukemia effect after autologous transplant could improve outcome. Another encouraging approach is the in vitro culture of early, Philadelphia chromosome-negative, progenitor cells for restoration of hematopoiesis after high-dose therapy.[106]

Multiple Myeloma

Conventional chemotherapy for multiple myeloma achieves few complete responses, and the median survival is less than 3 years.[107] There is a steep dose-response curve to melphalan; for single-agent high-dose therapy, melphalan appears to be more efficacious than thiotepa or cyclophosphamide.[108] Combining melphalan with total body irradiation and autologous rescue achieves a better complete response rate than conventional chemotherapy, and the median relapse-free survival is extended to 12 months. Post-transplant therapy with interferon-α may further extend the period of remission.[108] For autologous transplant to have a significant effect in myeloma, which typically affects older patients, the therapy must be easily tolerated. The use of peripheral progenitor cell grafts and growth factors has reduced the toxicity of high-dose therapy so that it is a feasible treatment modality for the newly diagnosed multiple myeloma patient.

Solid Tumors

High-dose therapy for nonhematologic malignancy is most often applied to the solid tumors, such as testicular cancer, ovarian cancer, small cell lung cancer, selected sarcomas, neuroblastomas, and breast cancer, which have a good response rate to conventional chemotherapy. The most frequent use of high-dose chemotherapy in solid tumors has been in the setting of recurrent or refractory disease, although the use of high-dose therapy in the adjuvant setting for high-risk breast cancer is being studied. Fewer patients with nonhematologic tumors have been treated with high-dose therapy, and the exact role of this treatment modality has not been established for many solid tumors. The encouraging results of high-dose therapy for refractory germ cell tumors and neuroblastoma certainly warrant further investigation.

Breast Cancer

The great interest in high-dose therapy for breast cancer is partly because the disease is very common and because no curative conventional therapy for the treatment of advanced breast cancer currently exists. High-dose therapy, most often a combination of two or more alkylating agents, was first used for the treatment of metastatic disease. Most studies report complete response rates higher than those reported for conventional chemotherapy. There are no long-term disease-free periods in women with refractory disease. Antman[42] has summarized the results of several centers treating patients with metastatic disease responding to high-dose therapy and reports an overall continuous complete response rate of 28% with a follow-up of 24–44 months from the start of induction therapy. High-dose therapy is also used in patients with high-risk stage II disease, defined as multiple positive nodes, and stage III disease. The disease-free interval of patients with ≥10 positive nodes treated with induction therapy followed by high-dose therapy is significantly longer than that of historical controls treated with conventional therapy alone.[109] Randomized trials are currently under way to compare high-dose therapy with conventional treatment in patients with ≥10 positive lymph nodes.

SUMMARY

High-dose therapy is used increasingly for hematologic and solid tumors. Although the usefulness of this approach has been established for tumors such as lymphomas, many pertinent issues need to be addressed. Defining the optimal timing of high-dose therapy will most likely improve the overall results. New drugs or better sequencing of drugs, modulation of the immune system, and manipulation of the autologous rescue product should also improve the usefulness of high-dose therapy.

REFERENCES

1. Weiden PL, Flournoy N, Thomas ED et al: Antileukemia effect of graft versus host disease in human recipients of allogeneic marrow grafts. N Engl J Med 300:1068, 1979
2. Clifford P, Clift RA, Duff JK: Nitrogen-mustard therapy combined with autologous marrow infusion. Lancet 1:687, 1961
3. Kurnick NB: Autologous and isologous bone marrow storage and infusion in the treatment of myelosuppression. Transfusion 2:178, 1962

4. Advisory Committee of the International Autologous Bone Marrow Transplant Registry (ABMTR): Autologous bone marrow transplants: different indications in Europe and North America. Lancet 2:317, 1989

5. Calvo W, Fliedner TM, Herbst E et al: Regeneration of blood forming organs after autologous leukocyte transfusion in lethally irradiated dogs. II. Distribution and cellularity of the marrow in irradiated and transfused animals. Blood 47:593, 1975

6. Keating A: Autologous bone marrow transplantation. p. 162. In Armitage JO, Antman KH (eds): High-dose Cancer Therapy. Williams & Wilkins, Baltimore, 1992

7. Stiff PJ, Koester AR, Weidner MK et al: Autologous bone marrow transplantation using unfractionated cells cryopreserved in dimethylsulfoxide and hydroxyethyl starch without controlled-rate freezing. Blood 70:974, 1987

8. Serke S, Sauberlich S, Abe Y, Huhn D: Analysis of CD34-positive hemopoietic progenitor cells from normal human adult peripheral blood: flow-cytometrical studies and in-vitro colony (CFU-GM, BFU-E) assays. Ann Hematol 62:45, 1991

9. Berenson RJ, Bensinger WI, Hill RS et al: Engraftment after infusion of CD34+ marrow cells in patients with breast cancer or neuroblastoma. Blood 77:1717, 1991

10. Kessinger A, Armitage JO: Harvesting marrow for autologous transplantation from patients with malignancies. Bone Marrow Transplant 2:15, 1987

11. Kessinger A, Armitage JO, Landmark JD et al: Autologous peripheral hematopoietic stem cell transplantation restores hematopoietic function following marrow ablative therapy. Blood 71:723, 1988

12. Kessinger A, Vose JM, Bierman PJ, Armitage JO: High-dose therapy and autologous peripheral stem cell transplantation for patients with bone marrow metastases and relapsed lymphoma: an alternative to bone marrow purging. Exp Hematol 19:1013, 1991

13. Elias AS, Ayash L, Anderson KC et al: Mobilization of peripheral blood progenitor cells by chemotherapy and granulocyte-macrophage colony-stimulating factor for hematologic support after high-dose intensification for breast cancer. Blood 79:3036, 1992

14. Socinski MA, Cannistra AS, Elias A et al: Granulocyte-macrophage colony stimulating factor expands the circulating hematopoietic progenitor cell compartment in humans. Lancet 1:1194, 1988

15. To LB, Shepperd KM, Haylock DN et al: Single high dose of cyclophosphamide enables the collection of high numbers of hemopoietic stem cells from the peripheral blood. Exp Hematol 18:442, 1990

16. Reiffers J, Leverger G, Castaigne S et al: Autologous blood stem cell transplantation in patients with haematological malignancies. Bone Marrow Transplant, suppl. 4:167, 1988

17. To LB, Haylock DN, Thorp D et al: The optimization of collection of peripheral blood stem cells for autotransplantation in acute myeloid leukaemia. Bone Marrow Transplant 4:41, 1989

18. Siena S, Bregni M, Brando B et al: Flow cytometry for clinical estimation of circulating hematopoietic progenitors for autologous transplantation in cancer patients. Blood 77:400, 1991

19. Giani AM, Siena S, Bregni M et al: Granulocyte-macrophage colony stimulating factor to harvest circulating haemopoietic stem cells for autotransplantation. Lancet 2:580, 1989

20. Horning SJ, Galili N, Cleary M, Sklar J: Detection of non-Hodgkin's lymphoma in the peripheral blood by analysis of antigen receptor gene rearrangements: results of a prospective study. Blood 75:1139, 1990

21. Moss TJ, Sanders DG, Lasky LC, Bostrom B: Contamination of peripheral blood stem cell harvests by circulating neuroblastoma cells. Blood 76:1879, 1990

22. Sharp JG, Joshi SS, Armitage JO et al: Significance of detection of occult non-Hodgkin's lymphoma in histologically uninvolved bone marrow by a culture technique. Blood 79:1074, 1992

23. Gorin NC, Aegerter P, Auvert B: Autologous bone marrow transplantation for acute leukemia in remission: an analysis of 1322 cases. Haematol Blood Transfusion 33:666, 1990

24. Gribben JG, Freedman AS, Neuberg D et al: Immunologic purging of marrow assessed by PCR before autologous bone marrow transplantation for B-cell lymphoma. N Engl J Med 325:1525, 1991

25. Kaiser H, Stuart RK, Brookmeyer R et al: Autologous bone marrow transplantation in acute leukemia: a phase I study of in vitro treatment of marrow with 4-hydroperoxycyclophosphamide to purge tumor cells. Blood 65:1504, 1985

26. Ritz J, Bast RC Jr, Clavell LA et al: Autologous bone marrow transplantation in calla-positive acute lymphoblastic leukaemia after in vitro treatment with J5 monoclonal antibody and complement. Lancet 2:60, 1982

27. Sieber F: Marrow purging by merocyanine 540-mediated photolysis. Bone Marrow Transplant 2:29, 1987

28. Kemshead JT, Heath L, Gibson FM et al: Magnetic microspheres for the depletion of neuroblastoma cells from bone marrow: experiences, improvements and observations. Br J Cancer 54:771, 1986

29. Hardwick A, Law P, Mansour V et al: Development of a large-scale immunomagnetic separation system for harvesting CD34-positive cells from bone marrow. p. 583. In Worthington-White DA, Gee A, Gross S (eds): Advances in Bone Marrow Purging and Processing. Wiley-Liss, New York, 1992

30. Okarma T, Lebkowski J, Schain L et al: The AIS collector: a new technology for stem cell purification. p. 487. In Worthington-White DA, Gee A, Gross S (eds): Advances in Bone Marrow Purging and Processing. Wiley-Liss, New York, 1992

31. Law P, Meryman H: Cryopreservation of human bone marrow grafts. p. 331. In Gee A (ed): Bone Marrow Processing and Purging, A Practical Guide. CRC Press, Boca Raton, FL, 1991

32. Beaujean F, Hartman O, Kuentz M et al: A simple, efficient washing procedure for cryopreserved human hematopoietic stem cells prior to reinfusion. Bone Marrow Transplant 8:291, 1991

33. Davis JM, Rowley SD, Hayden G et al: Clinical toxicity of cryopreserved bone marrow graft infusion. Blood 76:781 1990

34. Kessinger A, Schmit-Pokorny K, Smith D, Armitage J: Cryopreservation and infusion of autologous peripheral blood stem cells. Bone Marrow Transplant, suppl. 1:25, 1990

35. Clift RA, Buckner CD, Appelbaum FR et al: Allogeneic marrow transplantation in patients with acute myeloid leukemia in first remission: a randomized trial of two irradiation regimens. Blood 76:1867, 1990

36. Santos GW, Tutschka PJ, Brookmeyer R et al: Marrow transplantation for acute nonlymphocytic leukemia after treatment with busulfan and cyclophosphamide. N Engl J Med 309:1347, 1983

37. Yeager AM, Kaizer H, Santow GX et al: Autologous bone marrow transplantation in patients with acute nonlymphocytic leukemia, using ex vivo marrow treatment with 4-hydroperoxcyclophosphamide. N Engl J Med 315:141, 1986

38. Blume KG, Forman SJ, O'Donnell MR et al: Total body irradiation and high dose etoposide: a new preparatory regimen for bone marrow transplantation in patients with advanced hematologic malignancies. Blood 69:1015, 1987

39. Geller RB, Myers S, Devine S et al: Phase I study of busulfan, cyclophosphamide, and timed sequential escalating doses of cytarabine followed by bone marrow transplantation. Bone Marrow Transplant 9:41, 1992

40. Phillips GL, Shepherd JD, Barnett MJ et al: Busulfan, cyclophosphamide, and melphalan conditioning for autologous bone marrow transplantation in hematologic malignancy. J Clin Oncol 9:1880, 1991

41. Schabel FM, Trader MW, Laster WR et al: Patterns of resistance and therapeutic synergism among alkylating agents. Antibiot Chemother 23:200, 1987

42. Antman KH: Dose-intensive therapy in breast cancer. p. 706. In Armitage JO, Antman KH (eds): High-Dose Cancer Therapy. Williams & Wilkins, Baltimore, 1992

43. Zwelling LA: Topoisomerase II as target of antileukemia drugs. a review of controversial areas. Hematol Pathol 3:101, 1989

44. Jagannath S, Dicke KA, Armitage JO et al: High-dose cyclophosphamide, carmustine, and etoposide and autologous bone marrow transplantation for relapsed Hodgkin's disease. Ann Intern Med 104:163, 1986

45. Linker CA, Ries CA, Damon LE et al: Autologous bone marrow transplantation for acute myeloid leukemia using busulfan plus etoposide as a preparative regimen. Blood 81:311, 1992

46. Chao NJ, Stein AS, Long GD et al: Busulfan/etoposide-initial experience with a new preparatory regimen for autologous bone marrow transplantation in patients with acute nonlymphoblastic leukemia. Blood 81:319, 1992

47. Broun ER, Tricot G, Akard L et al: Treatment of refractory lymphoma with high dose cytarabine, cyclophosphamide and either TBI or VP-16 followed by autologous bone marrow transplantation. Bone Marrow Transplant 5:431, 1990

48. Appelbaum FR: Radiolabeled monoclonal antibodies in the treatment of non-Hodgkin's lymphoma. Hematol Oncol Clin North Am 5:1013, 1991

49. Vriesendorp HM, Herpst JM, Germack MA et al: Phase I–II studies of yttrium-labeled antiferritin treatment for end-stage Hodgkin's disease, including Radiation Therapy Oncology Group 87-01. J Clin Oncol 9:918, 1991

50. Spitzer G, Huan S, Dunphy F et al: Double high-dose therapy in human solid tumors: an emphasis on breast cancer. p. 437. In Champlin RE, Gale RP (eds): New Strategies in Bone Marrow Transplantation. Alan R Liss, New York, 1990

51. Klingemann HG, Phillips GL: Immunotherapy after bone marrow transplantation. Bone Marrow Transplant 8:73, 1991

52. Bierman PJ, Bagin RG, Jagannath S: High dose chemotherapy followed by autologous hematopoietic rescue in Hodgkin's disease: long term follow-up in 128 patients. Ann Oncol 4:767, 1993

53. Reece D, Barnett M, Connors J et al: Intensive chemotherapy with cyclo-

phosphamide, BCNU, and etoposide followed by autologous bone marrow transplantation for relapsed Hodgkin's disease. J Clin Oncol 9:1871, 1991

54. Chopra R, McMillan AK, Linch DC et al: The place of high dose BEAM therapy and autologous bone marrow transplantation in poor-risk Hodgkin's disease. A single-center eight-year study of 155 patients. Blood 5:1137, 1993

55. Zulian GB, Selby P, Milan S et al: High dose melphalan, BCNU and etoposide with autologous bone marrow transplantation for Hodgkin's disease. Br J Cancer 59:631 1989

56. Phillips GL, Wolff SN, Herzig RH et al: Treatment of progressive Hodgkin's disease with intensive chemoradiotherapy and autologous bone marrow transplantation. Blood 73:2086, 1989

57. Yahalom J, Gulati SC, Toia M et al: Accelerated hyperfractionated total-lymphoid irradiation, high-dose chemotherapy, and autologous bone marrow transplantation for refractory and relapsing patients with Hodgkin's disease. J Clin Oncol 11:1062, 1993

58. Bierman PJ, Vose JM, Leichner PK et al: Yttrium 90-labeled antiferritin followed by high-dose chemotherapy and autologous bone marrow transplantation for poor-prognosis Hodgkin's disease. J Clin Oncol 11:698, 1993

59. Jagannath S, Armitage JO, Dicke KA et al: Prognostic factors for response and survival after high-dose cyclophosphamide, carmustine and etoposide with autologous bone marrow transplantation for relapsed Hodgkin's disease. J Clin Oncol 7:179, 1989

60. Brandwein JM, Callum SB, Sutcliffe JG et al: Evaluation of cytoreductive therapy prior to high dose treatment with autologous bone marrow transplantation in relapsed and refractory Hodgkin's disease. Bone Marrow Transplant 5:99, 1990

61. Longo DL, Duffey PL, Young RC et al: Conventional-dose salvage combination chemotherapy in patients relapsing with Hodgkin's disease after combination chemotherapy: the low probability for cure. J Clin Oncol 10:210, 1992

62. Desch E, Lasala MR, Smith TJ, Hillner BE: The optimal timing of autologous bone marrow transplantation in Hodgkin's disease patients after a chemotherapy relapse. J Clin Oncol 10:200, 1992

63. Lohri A, Barnett M, Randall N et al: Outcome of treatment of first relapse of Hodgkin's disease after primary chemotherapy: identification of risk factors from the British Columbia experience 1970 to 1988. Blood 77:2292, 1991

64. Jones RJ, Ambinder RF, Piantadosi S et al: Evidence of a graft-versus-lymphoma effect associated with allogeneic bone marrow transplanation. Blood 3:649, 1991

65. Jones RJ, Piantadosi S, Mann RB et al: High-dose cytotoxic therapy and bone marrow transplantation for relapsed Hodgkin's disease. J Clin Oncol 8:527, 1990

66. Appelbaum FR, Sullivan KM, Buckner CD et al: Treatment of malignant lymphoma in 100 patients with chemotherapy, total body irradiation, and marrow transplantation. J Clin Oncol 5:1340, 1987

67. Colombat P, Gorin NC, Lemonnier MP et al: The role of autologous bone marrow transplantation in 46 adult patients with non-Hodgkin's lymphomas. J Clin Oncol 8:630, 1990

68. Gribben JG, Goldstone AH, Linch DC et al: Effectiveness of high-dose combination chemotherapy and autologous bone marrow transplantation for patients with non-Hodgkin's lymphomas who are still responsive to conventional-dose therapy. J Clin Oncol 7:1621, 1989

69. Philip T, Armitage JO, Spitzer G et al: High-dose therapy and autologous bone marrow transplantation after failure of conventional chemotherapy in adults with intermediate-grade or high-grade non-Hodgkin's lymphoma. N Engl J Med 316:1493, 1987

70. Petersen FB, Appelbaum FR, Hill R et al: Autologous marrow transplantation for malignant lymphoma: a report of 101 cases from Seattle. J Clin Oncol 8:638, 1990

71. Phillips G, Fay JW, Herzig RH et al: The treatment of progressive non-Hodgkin's lymphoma with intensive chemoradiotherapy and autologous marrow transplantation. Blood 75:831, 1990

72. Weisdorf DJ, Haake R, Miller WJ et al: Autologous bone marrow transplantation for progressive non-Hodgkin's lymphoma: clinical impact of immunophenotype and in vitro purging. Bone Marrow Transplant 8:135, 1991

73. Wheeler C, Strawderman M, Ayash L et al: Prognostic factors for treatment outcome in autotransplantation of intermediate-grade and high-grade non-Hodgkin lymphoma with cyclophosphamide, carmustine and etoposide. J Clin Oncol 11:1085, 1993

74. Philip T, Hartmann O, Biron P et al: High-dose therapy and autologous bone marrow transplantation in partial remission after first-line induction therapy for diffuse non-Hodgkin's lymphoma. J Clin Oncol 6:1118, 1988

75. Goldstone AH, McMillan K, Chopra R: High-dose therapy for the treatment of non-Hodgkin's lymphoma. p. 668. In Armitage JO, Antman KH (eds): High-Dose Cancer Therapy. Williams & Wilkins, Baltimore, 1992

76. Vose JM, Peterson C, Bierman PJ et al: Comparison of high-dose therapy and autologous bone marrow transplantation for T-cell and B-cell non-Hodgkin's lymphomas. Blood 76:424, 1990

77. Goldstone AH, Singer CRJ, Gribben JG, Jarrett M: Fifth report of EBMTG experience of ABMT in malignant lymphoma. Bone Marrow Transplant, suppl. 1:3, 1988

78. Bastion Y, Berger F, Bryon PA et al: Follicular lymphomas: assessment of prognostic factors in 127 patients followed for 10 years. Ann Oncol 2:123, 1991

79. Freedman AS, Jerome R, Neuberg D et al: Autologous bone marrow transplantation in 69 patients with a history of low-grade B-cell non-Hodgkin's lymphoma. Blood 77:2524, 1991

80. Fouillard L, Gorin NC, Laporte J et al: Feasibility of autologous bone marrow transplantation for early consolidation of follicular non-Hodgkin's lymphoma. Eur J Haematol 46:279, 1991

81. Rohatiner AZS, Price CGA, Arnott S et al: Myeloblative therapy with autologous bone marrow transplantation as consolidation of remission in patients with follicular lymphoma. Ann Oncol, suppl 2:147, 1991

82. Vose JM, Anderson JR, Kessinger A et al: High-dose chemotherapy and autologous hematopoietic stem cell transplantation for aggressive non-Hodgkin's lymphoma. J Clin Oncol, 1993 (in press)

83. Bortin MM, Horowitz MM, Rimm A: Increasing utilization of allogeneic bone marrow transplantation. Ann Intern Med 116:505, 1992

84. Rizzoli V, Mangoni L, Carella M et al: Autologous bone marrow transplantation for acute leukemia: optimal timing and mafosfamide treatment. p. 13. In Dickey KA, Spitzer G, Jagannath S, Evinger-Hodges MJ (eds): Autologous Bone Marrow Transplantation Proceedings of the Fourth International Symposium. The University of Texas M.D. Anderson Cancer Center, Houston, 1989

85. Ball ED, Mills LE, Cornwell GC III et al: Autologous bone marrow transplantation for acute myelogenous leukemia using monoclonal antibody-purged bone marrow. Blood 75:1119, 1990

86. Thorpe PE, Matson DW, Brown AN et al: A selective killing of malignant cells in a leukemic rat bone marrow using an antibody-ricin conjugate. Nature 297:594, 1982

87. Trickett AE, Ford DJ, Lam-Po-Tang, Vowels MR: Comparison of magnetic particles for immunomagnetic bone marrow purging using an acute lymphoblastic leukemia model. Transplant Proc 22:2177, 1990

88. Berenson RJ, Andrews RG, Bensinger WI et al: Antigen CD34 positive marrow cells engraft lethally irradiated baboons. J Clin Invest 81:951, 1988

89. Reiffers J, Gaspard MH, Maraninchi D et al: Comparison of allogeneic or autologous bone marrow transplantation and chemotherapy in patients with acute myeloid leukaemia in first remission: a prospective controlled trial. Br J Haematol 72:57, 1989

90. Reiffers J, Maraninchi D, Rigal-Hoguet F et al: Does more intensive treatment cure more patients with acute myeloid leukemia? In Gale RP (ed): Keystone Symposia Workshop: Curing Leukemia. Semin Hematol, suppl. 4. 3:90, 1991

91. Amadori S, Testi AM, Arico M et al: Prospective comparative study of bone marrow transplantation and postremission chemotherapy for childhood acute myelogenous leukemia. J Clin Oncol 11:1046, 1993

92. Gorin NC: High-dose therapy for acute myelocytic leukemia. p. 569. In Armitage JO, Antman KH (eds): High-Dose Cancer Therapy. Williams & Wilkins, Baltimore, 1992

93. Meloni G, De Fabritis P, Petti MC et al: BAVC regimen and autologous bone marrow transplantation in patients with acute myelogenous leukemia in second remission. Blood 75:2282, 1990

94. Clavell LA, Gelber RD, Cohen HJ et al: Four-agent induction and intensive asparaginase therapy for treatment of childhood acute lymphoblastic leukemia. N Engl J Med 315:657, 1986

95. Buchanan GR: Diagnosis and management of relapse in acute lymphoblastic leukemia. Hematol Oncol Clin North Am, suppl. 54:971, 1990

96. Ramsey N, LeBien T, Weisdorf D et al: Autologous BMT for patients with acute lymphoblastic leukemia. p. 57. In Gale RP (ed): Bone Marrow Transplantation: Current Controversies. Alan R Liss, New York 1989

97. Gorin NC, Aegerter P, Auvert B et al: Autologous bone marrow transplantation for acute myelocytic leukemia in first remission: a European survey of the role of marrow purging. Blood 74:1606, 1990

98. Billett AL: High-dose therapy in acute lymphoblastic leukemia. p. 607. In Armitage JO, Antman KH (eds): High-Dose Cancer Therapy. Williams & Wilkins, Baltimore, 1992

99. Horowitz MM, Messerer D, Hoelzer D et al: Chemotherapy compared with bone marrow transplantation for adults with acute lymphoblastic leukemia in first remission. Ann Intern Med 115:13 1991

100. Kersey JH, Weisdorf D, Nesbit ME et al: Comparison of autologous and allogeneic bone marrow transplantation for treatment of high-risk refractory acute lymphoblastic leukemia. N Engl J Med 317:461, 1987

101. Thomas ED, Cliff RA, Fefer A et al: Marrow transplantation for the treatment of chronic myelogenous leukemia. Ann Intern Med 104:155, 1986
102. McGlave P, Arthur D, Haoke R et al: Therapy of chronic myelogenous leukemia with allogeneic bone marrow transplantation. J Clin Oncol 5:1033, 1987
103. Butturini A, Keating A, Goldman JM, Gale RP: Autotransplants in chronic myelogenous leukemia: strategies and results. Lancet 1:1255, 1990
104. Reiffers J, Bernard P, David B, Broustet A: Autografting for chronic myelogenous leukemia in transformation. Am J Hematol 18:105, 1985
105. Horowitz MM, Gale RP, Sondel PM et al: Graft-versus-leukemia reactions after bone marrow transplantations. Blood 75:555, 1990
106. Barnett MJ, Eaves CJ, Phillips GL et al: Successful autografting in chronic

myeloid leukemia after maintenance of marrow in culture, Bone Marrow Transplant 4:345, 1989
107. Kyle RA: Long-term survival in multiple myeloma. N Engl J Med 308:314, 1983
108. Jagannath S, Vesole D, Barlogie B: High-dose therapy, autologous stem cells and hematopoietic growth factors for the management of multiple myeloma. p. 638. In Armitage JO, Antman KH (eds): High-Dose Cancer Therapy. Williams & Wilkins, Baltimore, 1992
109. Peters WP, Ross M, Vredenburgh JJ et al: High-dose chemotherapy and autologous bone marrow support as consolidation after standard-dose adjuvant therapy for high-risk primary breast cancer. J Clin Oncol 11:1132, 1993

Allogeneic Bone Marrow Transplantation

29

Isabel Cunningham

INTRODUCTION

Allogeneic bone marrow transplantation (BMT) is a therapy of established curative potential that is useful in the treatment of hematologic malignancies, aplastic anemia, a variety of congenital anemias, immunodeficiency disorders, and metabolic storage diseases. It involves the infusion of healthy donor hematopoietic cells into a patient who has in most cases undergone preparative therapy. The purpose of this preparative therapy is to eradicate malignancy, when necessary, as well as the host immune system's ability to reject the transplanted marrow. The success of a marrow transplant requires that (1) the patient's malignancy be sensitive to, and potentially curable by, chemotherapy or radiotherapy, or both; (2) in a nonmalignant disease, the restoration of normal hematopoiesis will improve the quality and length of the patient's life; (3) the patient be of an age and medical condition to tolerate the treatment and the subsequent period of immunosuppression; (4) a suitable donor be available; (5) extensive supportive care and the means to prevent and treat infectious complications be available. The risks of marrow transplants include graft failure, toxicity due to the preparative regimen, graft-versus-host disease (GVHD), infectious complications, and relapse of the underlying disease. The first reported marrow transplant from a sibling donor was performed in 1968, and since then there has been a steady increase in the number of transplants done annually (currently >5,000) and in the number of institutions where they are performed (>340).[1] Advances in clinical transplantation have led to a decrease in transplant-related mortality, which has made it possible to broaden the accessibility of BMT to include older patients and those without matched sibling donors. Traditionally, marrow donors have been identical twins (syngeneic BMT) or siblings who share identical haplotypes at the HLA locus present on chromosome 6 (allogeneic BMT). With syngeneic grafts there is little immunologic reaction following transplantation in the form of graft rejection or GVHD; following allogeneic grafts, the most significant problem is GVHD, which is a major factor in transplant mortality. GVHD

is presumed to be a consequence of minor alloantigens that differ between donor and host and that are not identified in routine donor testing. Because the incidence and severity of GVHD increases with patient age, most transplants have been performed in patients <40 years. As only 30–40% of patients have identically matched family donors, attempts have been made to use nonidentical family donors and unrelated volunteer donors. Unrelated donor programs are growing rapidly in numbers, size, and ethnic diversity.[2] Protocols are being created to decrease the risk of graft failure and GVHD, problems that increase with the degree of genetic incompatibility of donor and host.[3] With techniques such as T-cell depletion of donor marrow, which have decreased the incidence and severity of GVHD, it is becoming feasible to increase the age of patients who are candidates for BMT.[4]

The basic structure of a transplant protocol involves treatment of the patient with immunosuppressive therapy, alone or in combination with myeloablative therapy, followed by infusion of the marrow graft. The most commonly used preparative protocols include cyclophosphamide (Cy) given in sequence with total body irradiation (TBI) or busulfan (Bu). TBI may be given in single, fractionated, or hyperfractionated dosing schedules.[5] Following allogeneic BMT, treatment is begun to prevent or decrease the severity of GVHD once engraftment occurs, except after syngeneic BMT or in some protocols using T-cell depletion of grafts in which GVHD is not anticipated. The agents most commonly used for GVHD prophylaxis are methotrexate (MTX) and Cyclosporin A (CsA) given alone or in combination, for ≥6 months.[6] Recovery of hematopoiesis is evident about 2–3 weeks after infusion of allogeneic grafts, but immunologic recovery requires months to years.

SPECIFIC INDICATIONS

Severe Aplastic Anemia

Acquired severe aplastic anemia (defined as anemia with <1% reticulocytes, neutropenia <200–500/mm^3, and thrombocytopenia <20 × 10^3/mm^3) may result from damage to marrow stem cells and/or the marrow microenvironment caused by chemicals, drugs, viruses, or immunologic processes.[7] BMT is now successful in restoring normal hematopoiesis and in curing the disease in most patients transplanted with matched sibling donor marrow. Published studies have shown a progressive increase in the percentage of patients who are cured with BMT, from 50% to 90%. The median patient age in most of these studies is 16–22 years.[8–14]

Early experience with syngeneic transplantation demonstrated an inherent risk of graft failure associated with BMT in patients with severe aplastic anemia. Although some patients were durably engrafted without the use of immunosuppressive conditioning, most such grafts failed, and immunosuppressive therapy followed by a second graft was required.[8,14] When Cy (50 mg/kg for 4 days) was first used as conditioning for patients with HLA-matched sibling donors (with MTX for GVHD prophylaxis), graft failure occurred in 38% of patients.[8] Among patients who had not been previously transfused, and were thus not sensitized to donor antigens, rejection was observed in only 10%, and a survival rate of ≥82% was reported.[15] The risk of rejection has been found to increase with the number of transfusions patients have received prior to BMT.[16] For transfused patients, the risk of rejection has decreased to ≤9% with the implementation of protocols in which either the cell dose of the graft has been increased by adding buffy coat cells to the harvested marrow cells, or additional immunosuppressive therapy has been added to CY. Various protocols have added antithymocyte globulin (ATG) with or without procarbazine,[11,17] TBI,[13,18] total lymphoid irradiation,[9] or total abdominal irradiation in order to provide greater degrees of immunosuppression.[10] With these protocols, increases in GVHD and transplant-related mortality have, however, been observed, particularly when radiation-containing regimens are used.[16,18] A decrease in the incidence of graft failure has been observed since the introduction in 1980 of CsA for GVHD prophylaxis. Early graft failure has since been reported in <9% of previously transfused patients.[8,13,16,18] Failure to sustain initial engraftment has been reported in 14–23% of patients at the time the dose of CsA is being tapered, at 3 months following BMT. It has been suggested that continuing CsA for 1 year may decrease the incidence of late graft failure.[8,12,13] In a review of patients with severe aplastic anemia treated with BMT who had experienced graft failure, Champlin et al.[16] reported that second transplants after the administration of additional immunosuppression were successful in 33% of those patients who had shown transient engraftment after the first BMT, but in none of 19 patients with no evidence of engraftment.

Acute GVHD is a significant problem in BMT for aplastic anemia and is the main factor contributing to transplant mortality. Grade II–IV acute GVHD occurs in 21–54% of patients, and chronic GVHD in 26–56% of those who survive 100 days.[8,9,18] Both complications occur more commonly and with greater severity in adults. McGlave et al.[9] noted a difference in the frequency of GVHD between groups of adults and children treated with an identical BMT protocol for aplastic anemia. Acute and chronic GVHD were observed in 54% and 56% of adults and 24% and 12% of children, respectively. The most commonly used regimen for GVHD prophylaxis is CsA/MTX, which has been associated with an incidence of acute GVHD of 15–35%.[6,14,18] A low incidence of acute GVHD (12%) was noted in a study in which ATG was given along with Cy before sibling graft in 33 patients, with CsA/MTX prophylaxis. Disease-free survival was reported to be 90% in this study.[17]

No significant impact has been made on decreasing the incidence of chronic GVHD, except with the use of T-cell depletion of donor marrow. GVHD has been reduced or eliminated, depending on the method of depletion utilized.[19] T-cell depletion of the graft would ideally make BMT safer for older patients. There has been reluctance, however, to use T-cell depletion in

this setting because of the potential for graft failure following BMT for aplastic anemia, as well as with T-cell depletion techniques, and the poor results observed when T-cell depleted grafts were initially used for BMT in aplastic anemia patients.[12,16] However, in one study, eight previously transfused adult patients were treated with hyperfractionated TBI followed by Cy and matched sibling grafts depleted of T-cells.[20] One graft was rejected, and acute or chronic GVHD did not occur. Six of eight patients were alive and disease-free at 3–51 (median 10) months following BMT.[21]

For patients without matched sibling donors, partially or phenotypically matched family or unrelated donors have been utilized in small series of young patients with severe aplastic anemia. The Seattle group reported that 8 of 9 patients treated with Cy alone and given phenotypically identical grafts survived for 0.5–14 years.[8] This regimen was less successful when grafts mismatched at one HLA locus or at two loci were utilized (2 of 7 and 0 of 11 patients survived, respectively). By adding TBI to increase immunosuppression, three of six patients with one-locus, and two of five patients with two-locus disparate grafts were alive 1–6 years post-BMT.[8] Camitta et al.[22] treated 12 children, (median age 6 years), with a regimen of arabinosyl-cytosine (ara-C), Cy, steroids, TBI (1,400 cGy), and nonidentical grafts depleted of T cells. Two transplants of marrow matched at only one haplotype resulted in graft failure, while the other 10, with one- or two-antigen disparate grafts, were fully engrafted. Transplant-related mortality was 42%, and 7 patients (54%) were alive 1–5 years post-BMT. Limited experience using matched unrelated donors, in mostly young patients, produced 20–36% disease-free survival.[8,23–25] Moderate-to-severe acute GVHD occurred in 64–86% of these cases and was associated with a high mortality.[24,25] Hows et al.[24] noted the influence of age on survival in unrelated transplants for severe aplastic anemia: 64% of patients <15 years old survived compared with 17% of patients >15 years.

Allogeneic BMT in severe aplastic anemia has been compared with immunosuppressive therapy alone using ATG or antilymphocyte globulin (ALG) and androgens, in two nonrandomized studies. Overall survival was comparable at 62–69% for BMT groups and 59–65% for patients treated with immunosuppressive therapy.[26,27] However, for patients <15 years old, the response rate was significantly better for patients treated with BMT than ATG (82% versus 43%).[26] Most centers recommend that the young patient with a matched donor undergo BMT soon after diagnosis, prior to the initiation of transfusion if possible.[15,26,27] For the patient >40 years of age, disease-free survival with immunosuppressive therapy may be comparable to that with BMT.[28]

Malignancy has been reported, particularly squamous cell cancers and hematologic cancers, after both immunosuppressive therapy and BMT for severe aplastic anemia. The Seattle group[8] reported an incidence of malignancy of 3.8% of 330 patients; the onset was 8 years after BMT. In a French study of 147 BMT patients with aplastic anemia, tumors developed in 4 male patients at a median of 7 years after BMT.[29] In the review by Speck[27] of 122 patients treated with ALG and androgens, without BMT, 23 patients were reported to have developed myelodysplasia or paroxysmal nocturnal hemoglobinuria (PNH) between 1.5 and 8 years following treatment. As both myelodysplastic syndrome (MDS) and PNH may present with marrow hypoplasia, it is possible that these clonal stem cell malignancies may have been present but were not detected prior to immunosuppressive treatment.[27]

Paroxysmal Nocturnal Hemoglobinuria

Severe aplastic anemia may occur in approximately 25% of cases of PNH.[7] Both the aplastic and nonaplastic forms of PNH are curable with BMT. As PNH is a clonal disorder of pluripotent stem cells, myeloablation may be required to eradicate the disease, in addition to immunosuppression.[7,30] Protocols employing preparative regimens that include Cy alone, Bu and Cy, and procarbazine/rabbit ATG/Cy with HLA-matched grafts have resulted in full donor chimerism and survival for ≥19 years after BMT in >85% of cases of PNH given transplants.[30-32]

Acute Lymphocytic Leukemia

First Remission

Intensive chemotherapy protocols result in long-term disease-free survival in most children with acute lymphocytic leukemia (ALL) and approximately 35% of adult patients.[33] BMT in first remission is, therefore, an option for those patients unlikely to be cured by chemotherapy alone. The largest BMT experience in ALL primarily involves children in second remission, or children and adults with poor prognostic factors who have attained first remission. Patients in this high-risk group include those with high white blood cell (WBC) counts at diagnosis (20,000–100,000/mm^3), extramedullary disease, cytogenetic abnormalities, including translocations of chromosomes 4;11, 8;14, and 9;22, and the inability to attain complete remission within 1 month of starting chemotherapy.[33-36] Matched sibling transplants of 56 children in this high-risk group resulted in 56% disease-free survival.[37] The most common causes of failure in this series were relapse (27%) and transplant-related death (18%). In another study of 32 children with poor prognostic features who were treated with allogeneic BMT, there were 4 transplant-related deaths and 3 relapses within 7 months of BMT. Disease-free survival in this series was 84%, with a median follow-up of 30 months.[38]

Results of the treatment of >500 adults with ALL who were transplanted in first remission have been reported.[34-37,39-43] The median age of these patients is 22–24 years. The most common preparative regimen utilized was Cy/TBI. Experience with the Bu/Cy regimen is limited, but results appear to be comparable.[44,45] In published series, leukemia-free survival has varied from 21% to 72%. Significant GVHD has occurred in 28–48% of these patients, and 20–50% of patients have died of transplant-related toxicity. Transplant-related mortality is significantly less in those patients who do not develop GVHD, and in patients transplanted with T-cell-depleted marrow grafts.[41,46] The reported relapse rates in ALL have varied from 0% to 50%, probably reflecting the heterogeneity of patients referred for BMT in first complete remission (CR). The use of MTX as part of GVHD prophylaxis resulted in a fivefold decrease in relapse rate, possibly due to its antileukemic effect in ALL.[39] A decreased relapse rate has been noted in those patients who develop GVHD, suggesting that there is a graft-versus-leukemia effect associated with GVHD in ALL.[41,44,47,48] Low relapse rates (0–18%) have been reported when TBI is given with hyperfractionated dosing (125 cGy × 11–12) prior to Cy or etoposide. Disease-free survival has been reported to be 72–91%.[34,35] Factors correlated with high relapse rates following BMT have been increased age, elevated WBC count at diagnosis,[34,35,37] history of extramedullary, particularly central nervous system, disease,[44,47,49] and longer intervals between diagnosis and CR and between CR and BMT.[50] Fewer than 25% of transplants for ALL in first CR have been performed using in vitro T-cell depletion as a means of preventing GVHD. Relapse rates have been reported to be 15–35% in patients in these trials.[42,46,51-53]

Experience with BMT in two forms of high-risk ALL have been reported separately. Philadelphia (Ph) chromosome-positive ALL occurs in approximately 5% of pediatric cases of ALL and in ≥20% of patients >25 years of age.[54] Although most patients with Ph+ ALL achieve CR with chemotherapy, cure of the disease by chemotherapy is rare.[54,55] Allogeneic BMT for patients with Ph+ ALL in first remission has resulted in long disease-free survival in 38–75% of patients.[55,56] Burkitt lymphoma, or the L3 type of ALL, is characterized by an 8;14 translocation and poor long-term survival. In one study, nine adults with bone marrow and central nervous system involvement were treated successfully with chemotherapy and cranial irradiation and then given allogeneic transplants. Seven of nine were reported to be disease-free at a median of 43 months.[57]

No randomized studies are available to determine whether it is preferable to treat adult patients in first CR with BMT or with chemotherapy consolidation. Attempts have been made to analyze comparable groups of patients retrospectively in order to obtain this information. Recently the results of 234 cases, treated with various BMT protocols, were compared with 484 patients concurrently treated with protocols utilizing continued chemotherapy.[58] The relapse rate was higher with continued chemotherapy than with BMT (59% versus 32%), but treatment-related mortality was much higher in the BMT group (39% versus 4%). Overall 5-year disease-free survival was similar at 38% and 44%, respectively.[53] The French Group of Adult ALL[59] analyzed 256 adults who had received uniform remission induction regimens prior to consolidation with allogeneic or autologous marrow transplants or continuation of chemotherapy. A significant survival advantage was noted for those who underwent allogeneic BMT compared with those who were treated with either continued chemotherapy or autologous BMT.[59]

Second Remission

Published reports of BMT for ALL in second remission (where most patients are <24 years old) have shown that lengthy disease-free survival is possible in 40–64% of patients when TBI-based protocols are used.[36,60-63] Mortality is significant (23–39%) in these studies. Relapse rates vary from 6% to 32%. In an attempt to decrease the rate of relapse, several groups replaced the Cy in the preparative regimen with high-dose ara-C. In 18 children treated with this regimen the relapse rate was only 6%, but 33% of patients died, and disease-free survival occurred in 61%.[62] A retrospective multicenter survey of 213 patients treated with this protocol noted 42% disease-free survival at 3 years, with higher relapse and mortality rates occurring in older patients.[63] In the TAM study,[64] using TBI, high-dose ara-C, and melphalan prior to BMT in 57 children, 5-year survival was 54%, with 22% of patients relapsing and a 26% mortality rate. Encouraging results have been reported in patients with the use of hyperfractionated or fractionated TBI followed by etoposide or Cy, with >50% of patients reported to be in CR >2 years post-transplant.[65-68]

The German Cooperative Study[69] attempted to identify which children with ALL in second remission should receive BMT rather than continued chemotherapy. Patients were treated with uniform protocols from the time of diagnosis; after relapse, 51 patients underwent allogeneic BMT in second remission and 280 continued chemotherapy. Disease-free survival in the BMT group was comparable, whether relapse had occurred earlier (56%) or later (47%) than 18 months after first CR was attained. Patients who had relapsed within 18 months did poorly with continued chemotherapy (5% long disease-free survival), but for those who relapsed later, chemotherapy produced disease-free survival similar to BMT.[68] This study suggests that allogeneic BMT should be recommended for pediatric patients who relapse within 18 months of attaining CR or within 6 months of discontinuing chemotherapy. If there is no potential related donor, matched unrelated or autologous BMT can be considered.[68] For adults with ALL in second remission, no data suggest that any subset of patients treated with chemotherapy can attain disease-free survival comparable to that achieved with BMT. BMT is, therefore, recommended for an age-eligible adult patient in second CR who has a matched sibling donor.[64] For patients without sibling donors, the option of searching for an unrelated donor can be considered, with the knowledge that the average time required to identify a donor has been 5.5 months for the National Marrow Donor Registry.[25] The published experience with unrelated transplants for ALL in remission is limited. Primarily young patients have received such grafts. In a study including 30 patients, with a median age of 13 years, disease-free survival was 45% at 2 years.[25]

Advanced or Refractory Disease

Reports of patients transplanted in third remission of ALL are limited. Reports exist of disease-free survival of 25–42% in a small number of patients and relapse rates of 25–48%.[36,60] When transplants have been done for patients with refractory disease and Cy/TBI regimens, relapse has occurred in 50–60%, with disease-free survival being achieved in 0–25% of cases.[36,37,43,47,60] Some refractory patients may obtain prolonged survival when other drugs are added to the preparative regimen, but this approach may be associated with significant additional toxicity and mortality.[67,68,70–73] For this reason, the use of BMT earlier in the disease is advisable.

BMT using haploidentical family, or matched unrelated, donors has been performed in young patients with advanced ALL. Trigg et al.[74] reported that 10 of 18 children (56%) with ALL in second or third CR who received such grafts depleted of T cells were disease-free at a median of 8.5 months.

Results from the National Marrow Donor Program on the use of unrelated donor transplants in 53 patients with advanced acute leukemia revealed a disease-free survival of 19%. The risk of relapse was noted to be lowest in patients <18 years at the time of transplant.[25]

Acute Myeloid Leukemia

Most allogeneic transplants for acute myeloid leukemia (AML) are performed in patients during the first remission. In 1979, Thomas et al.[75] reported disease-free survival in 63% of patients after a regimen that included Cy, single-dose TBI (920 cGy), and allogeneic BMT. There was a marked difference in survival between patients <25 and >25 years of age (90% versus 14%); almost all deaths were due to interstitial pneumonia and GVHD.[75] With follow-up of >11 years, disease-free survival in this group is 47%.[76] Since this report, 5-year disease-free survival has been reported in 45–69% of adult and pediatric patients with AML treated with BMT in first CR.[60,76–80] Relapse rates have varied from 0% to 35%, and relapses rarely occur after 2 years.[60,79,80] The means of delivering TBI have been varied in attempts to maximize leukemia cell kill and to decrease relapse rates. A randomized study by the Seattle group[81] noted that increasing the total dose of TBI, given in 6 or 7 fractions, from 1,200 to 1,575 cGy resulted in a decrease in relapse rate from 35% to 12%, but also led to a concomitant increase in mortality associated with the higher radiation dose. Most of the deaths occurred in the setting of GVHD. Results of studies in which TBI was given in a single dose (500–750 cGy) at a rapid rate (26–58 cGy/min) show a comparable relapse rate.[43,80] Two groups reported the use of hyperfractionated TBI (1,320 cGy in 11 fractions) given prior to Cy or etoposide with 66–68% disease-free survival at 2–5 years, and no relapses.[60,78]

The first results of a radiation-free preparative regimen were published by Santos et al.[82] in 1983, using oral Bu (16 mg/kg) and Cy (200 mg/kg) followed by Cy-based GVHD prophylaxis. There was a 66% incidence of significant GVHD, and 39% of the patients died. Disease-free survival was 44% at 2 years.[82] When this regimen was subsequently used with CsA for 6 months for GVHD prophylaxis, a decrease in mortality was observed, and

a 3-year disease-free survival of 64% was noted.[83] The relapse rate with this regimen has been reported to be 14% by two groups.[45,83] Reduction of Cy to 120 mg/kg has resulted in rates of relapse (14–24%) and disease-free survival (63–69%) comparable to those attained with the higher (200 mg/kg) Cy dose.[84,85] The French cooperative group[86] performed a prospective, randomized study of 101 adults to compare the Bu/Cy (120 mg/kg) regimen and Cy/TBI. The GVHD prophylaxis regimen was CsA/MTX. The relapse rate was found to be higher in the Bu/Cy group (34% versus 14% with Cy/TBI), and transplant-related mortality was also higher with Bu/Cy (29% versus 8%). Disease-free survival was 72% with the radiation protocol and 47% with the Bu/Cy.[86] These and other authors noted that both relapse rate and mortality were higher in Bu/Cy-treated patients if BMT is undertaken within 4 months of diagnosis.[85,86] A similar study in children found little difference between the regimens, with mortality <7%, a relapse rate of 15%, and disease-free survival of 78–85%.[87]

AML with monocytic differentiation (FAB M4-5) and elevated WBC count at diagnosis are associated with a high relapse rate following BMT.[80,85,88–90] The occurrence of acute and chronic GVHD following BMT for AML has been correlated in some studies with a decrease in relapse rate.[41] This observation and the increased relapse risk noted following syngeneic transplants for AML suggest that a graft-versus-leukemia effect may be associated with GVHD. This potential benefit of GVHD is, however, offset by an increase in mortality in patients who develop GVHD.[41]

The problems of GVHD and mortality due to infectious complications are significant following BMT for AML. Prophylactic treatment for GVHD in most studies has involved MTX or CsA, or both, with or without steroids or ATG. The combination of CsA/MTX was found to decrease the incidence and severity of acute GVHD in AML transplants, but it has had no impact on the incidence of chronic GVHD, which has been reported in 26–38% of patients.[86,91] Methods of in vitro T-cell depletion of marrow grafts used as a means of GVHD prophylaxis have included monoclonal antibodies and complement,[46,51,52,92] counterflow centrifugal elutriation,[53,93,94] and soybean lectin agglutination/sheep red blood cell (E)-rosetting.[20,95,96] Depending on the method used, acute GVHD has been reduced to 5–28% of cases and the incidence of chronic GVHD to 0–25%. Failure of engraftment has been reported in 3–23% of patients receiving T-cell-depleted grafts.[46,52,53,92,95] In individual reports using various T-cell-depletion techniques, relapse rates vary from 5% to 30%.[46,51–53,92,94,95] A review of 159 BMT patients with AML in first remission given grafts depleted of T cells by various methods suggested that the relapse rate in these patients was increased compared with that of unmanipulated grafts (30% versus 17%). Relapse was found to occur more often in grafts depleted by monoclonal antibodies against T and natural killer cells than by methods such as elutriation and soybean lectin agglutination with E-rosetting.[42] The use of T-cell depletion by soybean lectin agglutination followed by sheep red blood cell rosetting resulted in the virtual elimination of acute and chronic GVHD in matched sibling BMT for AML.[95] However, failure of engraftment was seen in 16% in one report. In this study, disease-free survival was 45% after a median follow-up of 5 years. Relapse rate was 15%, and there were no relapses after 8 months.[95] In a subsequent study utilizing this method of T-cell depletion, with the addition of thiotepa and ATG to increase leukemia kill and immunosuppression,[96,97] there were no graft rejections encountered among 11 patients, and no early treatment-related mortality.[98] In this and other trials using T-cell-depleted BMT in AML in first remission, the loss of GVHD did not apparently result in a loss of graft-versus-leukemia effect, suggesting that in this disease these effects are not related.[52,92,94,95] Significant advantages exist for T-cell-depleted BMT in AML in early remission, particularly in adults.

Several studies have shown that allogeneic BMT for AML in first CR is superior to continuation of chemotherapy or autologous BMT. These studies were not randomized, as age-eligible patients with donors were offered allogeneic BMT and the other patients received either additional chemotherapy or autologous transplants. In two multicenter studies of children with AML, 5–6-year disease-free survival was 43–51% for the group receiving allogeneic BMT and 21–31% for the group treated with autologous BMT or continued chemotherapy.[99,100] Similar results were observed in studies of adult patients.[101] In five studies with >1 year of follow-up, median disease-free survival was better for transplanted patients (36–66% versus 16–35%) than for those who continued chemotherapy. In each of these studies the relapse rate is higher among the chemotherapy-treated patients (60–85%), while treatment-related mortality has been much higher in patients who were transplanted. These studies are limited in numbers and are heterogeneous with regard to patient age, medical condition, and risk factors. It will take further study with the accrual of larger numbers of patients to assess whether all age-eligible AML patients with good prognostic factors should undergo BMT in first remission.

Later Remissions

Published reports of BMT for advanced leukemia (AML in first relapse, second or later remissions, or refractory disease) include a heterogeneous group of patients treated with different regimens. These limitations make any firm conclusion about the utility of this form of therapy difficult. Disease-free survival after BMT in advanced leukemia treated with the Cy/TBI and Bu/Cy protocols is reported at 24–35%, principally because of relapse rates of 20–60%. The highest risk of relapse is seen among patients transplanted with frank leukemia.[42,83,85,94,102] Promising results have been reported in a small number of studies that used hyperfractionated TBI in the preparative regimen for the treatment of advanced leukemia. When given prior to Cy for patients in second CR, disease-free survival was reported at 64–75% in adults and children.[60,77] When the Cy was replaced by etoposide at 25–70 mg/kg in patients in later remissions or relapse, 10 of 25 patients in two studies were reported to be alive at a median of 28 months.[66,68]

For the newly diagnosed patient with AML <50 years of age, the presence of good or poor prognostic factors that might influence survival with chemotherapy alone should be determined. One should perform HLA typing of the patient and siblings to determine whether there is a potential marrow donor available. The physician should contact a transplant center while the patient is receiving induction therapy in order to discuss treatment options following the achievement of CR. The best results with BMT are attained in patients in early remission, and early referral may decrease the risks of mortality and relapse, which are highest when BMT is performed late in the course of leukemia.

Myelofibrosis

Acute megakaryoblastic leukemia (FAB M7) and acute or chronic myelofibrosis are characterized by marrow fibrosis and poor response to chemotherapy. Although occurring rarely in children, acute megakaryoblastic leukemia was successfully treated with BMT in 5 of 13 published cases reviewed by deOliveira et al.[103] In adults, marrow fibrosis may occur in chronic myeloid leukemia (CML) or acute myelofibrosis.[104] BMT in these patients may be complicated by graft failure or slow engraftment, and transfusion requirements may be large, particularly in patients in whom splenectomy has not been performed.[104,105] In the Seattle experience with 47 patients transplanted with fibrosis on marrow biopsy, graft failure occurred in 33% of those transplated with severe fibrosis. Reversal of fibrosis occurred in >80% of patients. Relapse occurred in 50% of those with severe fibrosis, but in only 1 of 24 with mild fibrosis. Overall disease-free survival was 20% at 2–3 years after BMT.[104] One report documented the gradual clearing of evidence of primary myelofibrosis over 30 months in a patient given a T-cell-depleted graft who had prompt engraftment and was well at 39 months.[106] In contemplating BMT for a patient with significant marrow fibrosis, the high rates of graft failure and relapse should be considered, as well as the potential benefit of pretransplant splenectomy on engraftment.[104,105]

Myelodysplasia

MDS usually occurs in patients >50 years of age. In MDS, lengthy remissions are rare, and, following transformation into acute leukemia, the rate of CR with chemotherapy is lower than for de novo acute leukemia.[107] The published experience of BMT in MDS includes approximately 300 patients, with median ages of 23–36 years and a median time from diagnosis to BMT of 3 months.[108–115] Comparable numbers of patients have been transplanted who had refractory anemia (RA), refractory anemia with excess blasts (RAEB), refractory anemia with excess blasts in transition (RAEB-T), and secondary AML (sAML). Overall disease-free survival has varied from 27% to 78% and has been correlated in several reports with patient age. For patients >30–35 years, disease-free survival was 9–40% compared with 58–83% for younger patients.[108,109,111,113] Failure was most often due to high transplant-related mortality (30–45%), usually in the setting of GVHD, which occurred in 37–53% of the patients. Relapse rates varied from 0% to 50%, depending on the presence of marrow blasts at the time of transplant.[108,110] Relapse is rare in patients transplanted with stable RA,[108,109,111,112] but relapse has occurred in 25–36% of patients with RAEB and in 20–50% of patients with RAEB-T.[109,110,112,113] Patients with sAML, following another malignancy or MDS, had the lowest disease-free survivals (17–27%).[111,112,115] DeWitte et al.[112] noted significantly better disease-free survival for patients in CR rather than partial remission at the time of transplant (63% versus 20%). However, controversy remains about whether remission induction should be attempted in sAML in view of the high treatment-related mortality in this group.[111,112,115,116] Experience using unrelated donor BMT for MDS patients is limited.[25] More than 50% of the patients died by day 100, and disease-free survival was only 18% at 2 years.[25] As the toxicity and relapse rates may be significant in MDS, it has been suggested that patients <40 years with an HLA-compatible donor undergo BMT early, and that patients >40 years be evaluated for BMT on an individual basis.[108] Better regimens to decrease the risk of relapse without increasing toxicity need to be developed for the treatment of these disorders.

Chronic Lymphocytic Leukemia

Chronic lymphocytic leukemia (CLL) is the most common form of leukemia. Only 10% of patients with CLL are <50 years old, and the median survival in this group may be ≤12 years. However, patients with poor prognostic features survive <3 years.[117,118] These features include advanced stage of disease, rapid lymphocyte doubling time, a diffuse bone marrow infiltration pattern, and abnormal cytogenetics.[117,118] Experience with allogeneic BMT for CLL is limited. Michallet et al.[119] reported on 17 patients with CLL who underwent allogeneic transplants. Complete clinical remission was attained in 15 patients (88%). Acute GVHD occurred in 100% of patients, and 63% developed chronic GVHD. Transplant-related mortality was 35%. Two patients relapsed at 7 and 54 months post-BMT. Nine patients (53%) continued in remission at a median of 25 months. Molecular techniques to detect minimal residual disease confirmed the CR status in two patients studied 19 and 48 months post-BMT. Survival after BMT correlated with the stage of CLL at the time of BMT, with only one of eight patients transplanted in Rai stage IV surviving, compared with eight of nine with stage III or less.[119]

Few data exist on the use of T-cell-depleted grafts to decrease the risk of GVHD in BMT for CLL. In a study of eight patients with poor prognostic factors, a minimal disease state was achieved before conditioning was begun. All patients received T-cell-depleted grafts, and all engrafted and achieved clinical remission. Five of six patients in remission evaluated within 6 months of BMT had evidence of residual CLL cells by phenotype and molecular analysis. However, after 6 months, no CLL cells were detected by phenotypic analysis in six patients, and five showed no molecular evidence of the malignant clone.[118] Because of the long median survival that characterizes this disease, longer follow-up will be required to know how many such patients may be cured. It is unlikely that allogeneic BMT will be a practical treatment for most patients, in view of the age of patients with CLL and the toxicity of transplant. Currently BMT is a reasonable option for selected young patients with matched donors who have poor prognostic factors and who experience good response to chemotherapy.

Chronic Myeloid Leukemia

CML is characterized by a chronic phase lasting a median of 3–4 years before transformation to the blastic phase, which is invariably fatal. No regimen can reliably induce cytogenetic remission during the chronic phase, and treatment (most commonly hydroxyurea or interferon-α) is generally used to control elevated blood counts and splenic enlargement. Once CML has accelerated or transformed, it is usually poorly responsive to therapy. Therefore, marrow transplantation has the highest potential for curing CML when performed during the chronic phase. In contrast to patients with acute leukemia, chronic-phase CML patients generally will not have had intensive chemotherapy or transfusions prior to beginning conditioning for transplant and will not be in remission. The median age of patients transplanted for CML is 32–39 years, ≥10 years older than the average age of acute leukemia BMT candidates. As in acute leukemia, CML patients <30 years have been found to have a better survival than older patients after BMT, but patients in this younger age group represent a minority of patients with CML.[120-125]

The traditional Cy/TBI conditioning regimens used during the treatment in the chronic phase have resulted in disease-free survival of 46–68% at 3–5 years.[123-128] Bu/Cy regimens have resulted in comparable survival figures,[129,130] but there are reports suggesting greater hepatic toxicity with Bu/Cy.[45,84,131] The limiting problem with all CML BMT regimens has been the 25–45% mortality encountered during the first year.[121-127,129] Most deaths are a consequence of GVHD, with the main cause of death being interstitial pneumonia. The risk of interstitial pneumonia in CML patients has been correlated with a history of treatment with Bu to control the disease during the chronic phase[122,131] and also with the type of TBI administered in the preparative regimen.[126,132] Among 281 CML patients who underwent allogeneic BMT, interstitial pneumonia was noted in 37% of patients who received single-dose TBI compared with 17% in those who received fractionated TBI.[126,132] The incidence of interstitial pneumonia has varied from 12% to 36% in trials using Bu/Cy conditioning.[129,131] Moderate-to-severe acute GVHD occurs in 33–79% of patients with CML,

with an increase in severity associated with increased patient age.[122,123] As in acute leukemia, MTX/CsA for GVHD prophylaxis has led to a decrease in the incidence of acute GVHD to about 33%.[45,91,129] The occurrence of acute GVHD has a negative effect on survival. Two studies demonstrated that 74–75% of patients with minimal (stage 0–1) acute GVHD survived compared with 20–35% for those with stages II–IV.[122,124] No drug regimen has changed the incidence of chronic GVHD in CML patients. Chronic GVHD occurs in 24–67% of patients who survive 100 days after BMT.[91,123-126,129] Although a graft-versus-leukemia effect associated with chronic GVHD has been suggested in some CML studies, it is in these patients that infectious mortality is highest.[41,125] Following BMT using unrelated donors, the incidence and severity of GVHD are significantly increased, with a consequent increase in morbidity.[133] Among 115 patients with chronic-phase CML who underwent BMT from unrelated donors, significant acute GVHD occurred in 82%, chronic GVHD occurred in 52%, and 60% of patients died within 1 year of BMT. A 16% incidence of graft failure also occurred. Overall 2-year disease-free survival was reported to be 37%. Disease-free survival was 43% for patients <30 years old and 27% for older patients.[133]

Because of the advanced age of most CML patients and the incidence and mortality of GVHD following BMT with unmanipulated grafts, the potential benefits of in vitro T-cell depletion have been thought to be considerable in CML. Monoclonal antibodies including Campath-I, anti-CD6, and anti-CD8,[46,127,133-135] or physical methods such as counterflow centrifugal elutriation[53,93] and soybean lectin agglutination with sheep red blood cell E-rosetting[20,136] have been utilized to deplete grafts of T cells. These methods remove different amounts of T cells (1–3 logs) and have reduced the incidence of GVHD to varying degrees.[19] Acute GVHD (>grade II) has been reported in 5–20% of patients receiving such grafts, and chronic GVHD has been observed in 0–35% of such patients.[125,135,137] The soybean lectin/E-rosetting method results in the greatest degree of depletion of T cells (2.5–3.0 logs), so that 99.8% of T cells may be removed, and patients do not require post-transplant immunosuppression to prevent GVHD.[138] With this method, acute GVHD rarely occurs, and chronic GVHD has not been reported.[19] Following less extensive T-cell depletion, CsA is given after the transplant for ≥6 months. Early regimen-related mortality has decreased in some studies, so that 1-year survival has increased to 75–85%.[53,123,136,137] T-cell depletion may be particularly useful in matched unrelated transplants for CML in which GVHD is the limiting factor to greater success. A significant decrease in severe acute and extensive chronic GVHD has been noted among those patients given T-cell-depleted grafts, with a trend toward better disease-free survival.[25,133] A problem associated with T-cell depletion in matched sibling grafts is an increased incidence of graft failure. Graft failure has been reported in 5–30% of patients receiving T-cell-depleted grafts.[42,46,123,135,139] Residual host lymphocytes have been noted in patients who experience graft failure.[3,139] Various means of increasing immunosuppression before BMT have been tried to eliminate these host immunocompetent cells, including the addition of ATG to the conditioning regimen, or increasing the total dose of TBI. A decrease in graft failure has been seen following the implementation of these approaches.[42,139,140]

Hematologic relapse of CML after Cy/TBI and infusion of an unmanipulated graft has been reported to occur in 0–24% of patients.[121-127,141,142] The more recently published studies have reported the higher relapse rates. This disturbing trend could reflect the change over 20 years in the administration of TBI from single-dose to fractionated dosing. Currently, most groups use fractionated (e.g., 200 cGy × 6) or hyperfractionated TBI (125 cGy × 11–12). Low relapse rates were noted in trials in which single-dose radiation was used[43,126,132,141-143] and when higher total fractionated doses were given.[128] Although routine pretransplant splenectomy has not been found to affect relapse rate after BMT, several of the studies that used single-dose TBI and reported no relapses included splenectomy.[141–143] In a review of 405 patients with CML undergoing allogeneic BMT, 27% had undergone splenectomy, and in this group the relapse rate was 6%.[125] Hematologic relapse following use of the Bu/Cy preparative regimen has been reported to be <3%, with a median follow-up over 2 years.[129] In reports of T-cell-depleted transplants, in which preparation is routinely with Cy and TBI, an increased relapse rate has been observed in most studies (40–86%).[53,94,125,127,136] However, in a study using selective T-cell depletion with anti-CD8 antibodies, no relapses were reported after a median follow-up of 2 years.[135] Several factors have been associated with an increased risk of relapse following T-cell depletion of grafts, including fractionation of TBI, lower total doses of radiation, and use of monoclonal antibody methods for T-cell depletion rather than physical methods.[42]

That the relapse rate is not increased with the use of similar T-cell depletion protocols for AML patients in CR may reflect the higher tumor burden in CML patients prior to BMT.[41,46] A possible explanation for the increased relapse rate is that the removal of T cells results in a loss of a T-cell-mediated graft-versus-leukemia effect which is crucial in CML. This could explain the observation of the persistence of Ph+ cells in the first marrow analysis after BMT in 8 of 28 CML patients who received T-cell-depleted grafts, compared with 2 of 20 patients given unmanipulated transplants.[144] Most marrows after T-cell-depleted BMT manifest mixed hematologic chimerism (the presence of both donor and host cells). In addition, patients with T-cell-depleted grafts who have the longest time to engraftment have an increased risk of relapse. These findings suggest that there is competition between donor and host cells for marrow space.[46] Hale et al.[46] and others have suggested that increasing immunosuppressive conditioning and decreasing engraftment time would provide a growth advantage to donor stem cells to offset the loss of graft-versus-leukemia effect, which is a consequence of the removal of T cells. For this reason, splenectomy could be potentially useful in decreasing the relapse rate. Patients transplanted following splenectomy achieve marrow engraftment 5–9 days earlier than nonsplenectomized patients.[145,146] Splenic radiation does not produce a similar shortening of engraftment time.[137,147] It was demonstrated in mice that the incidence of complete donor chimerism after T-cell-depleted BMT could be significantly increased by the addition of dimethylbusulfan to TBI/Cy conditioning.[97] When this agent was used in patients prior to 1979 with Cy and single-dose TBI, hepatic and pulmonary toxicity were significant.[148] However, in twins with CML in chronic phase treated with this agent, a lower relapse rate and longer time to relapse was observed in comparison with patients treated with Cy and single-dose TBI.[121] As this alkylating agent is no longer available, thiotepa has been utilized and was found to have similar effects in mice.[97] This observation led to clinical trials in which thiotepa was added to Cy/TBI; complete chimerism was attained in most patients, and a decrease in the number of early relapses was noted.[140]

Clinical relapse is usually preceded by the reappearance of Ph+ cells in the marrow of CML patients following BMT. Cytogenetic relapse may herald clinical hematologic relapse within weeks to months, or it may represent a transient occurrence followed by the return of normal donor chromosomes.[121,127,136,144] The more sensitive polymerase chain reaction (PCR) technique, which can detect bcr/abl mRNA transcript in 1 in 10[6] cells, has been used to detect minimal residual disease in CML patients at various intervals after BMT. Evidence of bcr/abl rearrangement has been reported in 20–83% of patients ≤7 years after BMT in patients who are otherwise judged to be in clinical remission.[127,134,149–151] The use of PCR to detect minimal residual disease requires expertise to minimize the incidence of false-positive results. Inadequate information is available to be sure of the value of a positive PCR test in predicting CML relapse. Several authors suggest that there is a higher risk of hematologic relapse in cases in which bcr/abl is evident on every follow-up marrow or in samples studied more than 1 year post-transplant.[127,134,149,150,152]

For patients who relapse after BMT, several immunomodulatory approaches have been studied to try to promote the growth of donor cells to achieve a graft-versus-leukemia effect. In one report, CsA prophylaxis was discontinued at the time Ph+ cells were first detected (clinical relapse had not occurred). Marrows examined after CsA was stopped demonstrated a return to 100% Ph-negative metaphases in 2–7 months.[153] Interferon-α has been utilized in patients in both cytogenetic and hematologic relapse following BMT and has been successful in returning 11–33% of patients to complete cytogenetic remission, in a median of 3 months, with absence of the bcr/abl rearrangement noted in some cases.[154,155] It is postulated that interferon promotes a graft-versus-leukemia effect by increasing the expression of major histocompatibility antigens or by increasing natural killer cell number.[154,155] Interferon therapy, however, may be associated with significant toxicity.[154,155] Another approach to treat relapsed CML post-BMT has been to infuse donor blood leukocytes alone, or with interferon, into patients in cytogenetic or hematologic relapse. Following such infusions, cytogenetic and molecular remission has resulted in a small number of cases.[156,157–159] In one study, evidence of the Ph chromosome disappeared in five of six patients at 1–3 months, and four became negative for bcr/abl by PCR.[159] All these approaches carry the risk of inducing severe GVHD and irreversible marrow aplasia. Longer follow-up is needed to know if the remissions attained with these methods are durable, and if these methods are best instituted when relapse is detected cytogenetically or molecularly, before clinical relapse. Second transplants performed at a median of 2–3 years after the first have been successful in >40% of relapsed CML patients, with the duration of disease-free survival in some patients now exceeding that after the first BMT.[127,160] Bu/Cy has been utilized as a conditioning regimen when the patient had previously had TBI. The risk of transplant-related mortality may be as high as 69%, particularly if the second transplant is performed within 6 months of the first.[161] It has been suggested that a less intensive conditioning regimen (e.g., Bu without Cy) might be effective, particularly when there is evidence of persisting donor engraftment in the relapsed patient.[127,160]

Advanced and Juvenile Chronic Myeloid Leukemia

BMT performed during the accelerated or blastic phases of CML results in higher mortality and higher relapse rates. Following BMT for patients in the accelerated phase, 17–29% disease-free survival has been reported, and relapse rates have varied from 25% to 65% in protocols using Cy/TBI conditioning.[42,43,122,124,126] This wide range of relapse rates may result from different definitions of what constitutes an accelerated phase, as well as the inclusion of cases in some studies that other investigators might have considered to be in chronic or blastic phases. BMT for patients in blastic phase results in disease-free survival of 15–23%, with ≤80% of patients relapsing.[42,121,122,126] Better results have been reported in patients receiving different preparative regimens (Bu/Cy with or without ara-C), with disease-free survival of 41–54% and 0–12% relapse rate for patients transplanted in accelerated phase, and 27–63% disease-free survival with 12–27% relapse rates for patients transplanted in blastic phase.[129,162,163] Unrelated donor transplants for patients with advanced phase CML results in disease-free survival of 22–27% and a 50% mortality by 6 months. There were no survivors after unrelated BMT in 14 patients transplanted during blastic phase.[133] For patients with blastic CML who are treated with chemotherapy and attain second chronic phase and then undergo matched-sibling BMT, 45–58% disease-free survival has been reported.[122,126] This patient group is small, since achieving a second chronic phase and remaining in a suitable condition to undergo BMT after transformation is relatively uncommon. Rarely, intensive chemotherapy of blastic CML results in CR, as in acute leukemia. Two such patients, who attained complete marrow and cytogenetic remission following idarubicin and high-dose Ara-C therapy and then underwent T-cell-depleted transplants, continue in CR over 5 years[164] (personal observations).

Juvenile CML is a Ph-negative myeloproliferative disorder that occurs in young children and is characterized by splenomegaly, leukocytosis, and increased levels of fetal hemoglobin. The median survival is <2 years.[165] Allogeneic BMT has produced 43–50% disease-free survival in a small number of children. Preparative regimens have included Cy/TBI and Bu/Cy with and without TBI or splenic irradiation and additional chemotherapy.[165-167]

Allogeneic BMT is currently the best treatment option for CML patients <50 years of age with matched sibling donors. The best results are achieved when transplant is performed in the chronic phase, because the regimen-related toxicity and relapse rates in advanced disease are much higher. The decision of how soon after diagnosis to undergo transplant is a difficult one, particularly in view of the sometimes lengthy survival achieved with minimal therapy and the significant morbidity and mortality associated with transplant. Some authors have suggested that transplants performed within 1 year of diagnosis are associated with better survival due to less regimen-related mortality, but there is no evidence that the risk of relapse is less when transplant is performed earlier in the chronic phase.[121-123,125] The decisions whether to utilize TBI- or Bu-based conditioning regimens, and whether the marrow should be depleted of T cells, are also difficult, and definitive conclusions about these options will require greater numbers of controlled studies and longer follow-up time. If no matched sibling donor is available, a search for an unrelated donor can be begun through a transplant center with access to national and international donor registries. The potential patient should understand the time and cost involved in such a search, the difficulties involved in finding donors with certain haplotypes, and the risks of such transplants, evident in the experience published to date.[2,133]

Lymphoma

Most transplants performed for Hodgkin disease and non-Hodgkin lymphoma (NHL) have been autologous, using the patient's own marrow or peripheral blood stem cells. Less than 15% of published transplants of lymphoma patients have been allogeneic, and at least 85% of these have been in patients with NHL.[168] Allogeneic BMT offers the potential advantages of a lower relapse rate (with no risk of infusing residual lymphoma cells) and a potential graft-versus-lymphoma effect.[168] Use of allogeneic BMT has been limited by patient age and donor availability and by transplant-related toxicity.[168] Because of the 50–70% chance of prolonged disease-free survival for Hodgkin disease and intermediate and high-grade NHL achieved with current chemotherapy regimens, allogeneic transplants are not routinely performed during first remission of these disorders.[168,169] Exceptions are patients in first remission of Burkitt lymphoma or lymphoblastic lymphoma, because of their high risk of relapse with continued chemotherapy.[57,170,171] In a small study of adults who received allogeneic transplants for Burkitt lymphoma, seven of nine were disease-free after a median fol-

low-up of 4 years.[57] Milpied et al.[170] reported on 25 patients with lymphoblastic lymphoma in first remission transplanted in four centers. Most had prognostic features known to be associated with poor long-term results using chemotherapy (marrow, central nervous system, or mediastinal involvement, high serum lactate dehydrogenase, older age). In comparing the results of allogeneic BMT with mafosfamide- or antibody-purged autologous BMT, disease-free survival at 4 years was found to be similar, at 67–70%, with relapse occurring in 26% of patients.[170] Among patients with lymphoblastic lymphoma, similar disease-free survival has been noted following autologous and allogeneic BMT (44% and 57%, respectively); however, the relapse rate was 48% with autologous BMT and 24% with allogeneic transplants.[171]

Most other published series of allogeneic BMT for lymphoma have involved the treatment of patients with NHL or Hodgkin disease transplanted after relapse or with refractory disease. The results and limitations of BMT have been comparable in NHL and Hodgkin disease. Status of disease at transplant is thought to be the most significant prognostic feature in BMT for lymphoma.[172-175] Patients given either allogeneic or autologous transplants when their diseases are in "sensitive relapse," that is, after being found to respond to chemotherapy after relapse, have comparable disease-free survivals, ranging from 37% to 56% at 2–4 years.[171,173,174] In studies in which comparable protocols are used, relapse rates after allogeneic BMT have been lower (18–23%) than after autologous transplants (38–46%). In both types of transplant, relapse occurs most commonly at sites of previous disease.[171-173] The apparent advantage of grafting allogeneic marrow is offset by an increase in regimen-related mortality following allogeneic (28–52%) transplant compared with autololgous BMT (14–24%).[171,173,174] Mortality has been noted to be higher in patients with poor pulmonary function, a history of prior chest irradiation, and unresponsiveness to several chemotherapy regimens.[172,173] For patients transplanted with refractory or resistant disease, BMT results have been poor, with relapse occurring in 90–100% of patients and rare survivors beyond 8–14 months after BMT.[171,173] Most conditioning regimens have been TBI based, although limited experience using Bu/Cy in previously irradiated patients has shown comparable survival data.[173,174] Additional agents, such as etoposide or ara-C, have been added to the preparative regimen to increase the efficacy of the conditioning protocol.[175,176] In one study of 17 patients with refractory lymphoma, high-dose ara-C and high-dose methylprednisone, with or without local radiation, were added to Cy/TBI prior to T-cell-depleted transplants using the T10B9 (anti-CD3) antibody, and disease-free survival was reported to be 55% at a median >2 years.[176]

For the patient with Hodgkin disease or NHL who has relapsed after initial therapy and remains sensitive to chemotherapy, allogeneic BMT may have an advantage over autologous transplant, particularly if the bone marrow has been previously involved. There is some evidence of a graft-versus-lymphoma effect occurring in patients with Hodgkin's disease and lymphoblastic lymphoma who develop GVHD.[171,174] This possible advantage of allogeneic BMT in decreasing the rate of relapse must be weighed against the potentially higher mortality associated with GVHD. Patients with lymphoma resistant to therapy have a minimal chance of attaining successful long-term outcome with the use of current treatment protocols.

Experience with allogeneic BMT for low-grade lymphoma is very limited. In making the decision about BMT for such patients, the mortality rate associated with BMT should be weighed against the potentially lengthy prognosis seen in this form of lymphoma. It is recommended that patients with low-grade lymphoma be entered on protocols so that the results of such transplants may help define the indications for BMT in this disease.

Multiple Myeloma

Multiple myeloma, a disease with a median age of onset of 65 years, is generally sensitive to chemotherapy, but complete remissions are rarely obtained. The overall median survival is approximately 3 years.[177,178] There has been great interest in using BMT as curative therapy for this disease. Most trials in myeloma patients have been performed using high-dose chemotherapy and autologous marrow and/or peripheral blood cell rescue. It is estimated that only 7% of myeloma patients are age-eligible for allogeneic BMT.[179] About 200 cases of allogeneic transplants have been reported in the literature, mostly by cooperative groups such as the European Bone Marrow Transplant Group.[178,180] The median patient age in these reports has been between 40 and 45 years, most of the patients have had advanced or poorly responsive disease, and only a minority of cases have been in CR at the time of BMT. Conditioning regimens include TBI and Cy, Bu/Cy, and multiagent protocols.[178,180,181] After the conditioning regimen, there are major (>50%) decreases in tumor burden in most patients, but CR has been attained in only 20–60% of patients.[178,180–182] Bone lesions rarely improve following BMT,[178,180,182] and only 15–20% of patients with significant bone lesions were observed to respond following BMT.[177] Attaining CR is the most important determinant of survival; 62–72% of patients who attain CR after BMT survive for ≥3 years post-transplant, but only 10–39% of patients who do not attain CR survive for >3 years.[178,180] CR after BMT is more likely to occur in patients who have responsive disease, who undergo transplant after the first chemotherapy regimen, and who have earlier stage disease at the time of BMT.[178,180] Survival is likewise longest in these patients. The reported mortality associated with allogeneic BMT has ranged from 31% to 67% and most of the deaths have occurred within 100 days of BMT.[178,180,181] Regimens in which more chemotherapy is added to TBI with the hope of decreasing relapse rates have resulted in increased toxicity.[180] Some investigators believe that remissions may be more durable following allogeneic rather than autologous transplants, suggesting that there may be a graft-versus-myeloma effect. Significant GVHD has, however, been correlated with poor survival.[177,178] To decrease the risk of GVHD, some groups have explored the use of T-cell-depleted grafts. In a study of 13 myeloma patients with <10% plasma cells before conditioning (with Cy or melphalan and TBI), using T-cell-depleted grafts, Anderson et al.[183] noted significantly lower mortality (one case), and 30% of the patients were disease-free between 1 and 2 years post-transplant. In a case report a 13-year-old with multiple extramedullary plamacytomas and an IgA-κ paraprotein was given a matched sibling T-cell-depleted graft and subsequent intermittent donor T-cell infusions. She was reported to be in clinical remission, with no paraprotein 4 years after BMT.[184]

No evidence of cure for multiple myeloma by BMT exists as yet. In fact, it is unclear whether overall survival is prolonged in patients receiving this type of therapy.[177] After transplant, even if residual disease is not evident, most patients continue to have monoclonal gammopathy.[178] The disappearance of this protein 2 years after BMT has, however, been reported.[185] Even for patients in remission, as judged by marrow and paraprotein analysis, molecular evidence of minimal residual disease has been found.[186] Larger studies and more follow-up time will be required to know which type of stem cell rescue is most useful after high-dose therapy in multiple myeloma. In view of the high mortality associated with allogeneic BMT, no overall survival advantage has yet been shown for allogeneic versus autologous marrow or peripheral blood cell transplants in this disease.[177]

Congenital Diseases

Severe Combined Immunodeficiency

The diseases encompassed by the term severe combined immunodeficiency (SCID) are characterized by defects in the differentiation of lymphoid cells, resulting in profound immunodeficiency. They may be inherited in a sex-linked or autosomal recessive manner. Typically, the diagnosis of SCID is made within 3 months of birth, and the infant dies of infection in the first year unless BMT is performed.[187,188] It is possible to engraft healthy marrow without cytoreductive preparation for those variants of SCID restricted to abnormal lymphoid development. In such cases, 50–80% survival has been reported in series of genotypically and phenotypically matched allogeneic transplants.[189–191] The survival of patients transplanted more recently has been estimated at ≤90%, due to earlier diagnosis, more rapid treatment, and improved treatment of infection.[189,190,192] After transplant, T-cell function returns to normal in most patients within months, but B-cell engraftment may be significantly delayed or may not occur at all.[193] Most treatment regimens contain no GVHD prophylaxis, as severe acute GVHD occurs in ≤20% of patients with SCID, and chronic GVHD is rare.[188,191,194] In the ADA-deficient form of SCID and in the other forms that affect hematopoietic as well as lymphoid stem cells, immunosuppression is necessary for engraftment to occur.[189,191,194,195]

It has been estimated that <10% of eligible patients with these disorders have HLA-matched sibling donors.[196,197] Haploidentical, usually parental, grafts have been explored as potential sources of normal marrow. Prior to 1977, partially compatible transplants resulted in rejection in ≥30% of cases, and >90% of such patients died of infection or severe GVHD.[187] Since 1981, T-cell depletion of grafts has been used.[20,189,190,194,198,199] Preparative regimens vary; most of these transplants have been performed without immunosuppression, but Bu, TBI, and other agents have also been used.[194,198,199] Overall, the use of T-cell-depleted grafts has produced long disease-free survival in ≤60% of cases, results comparable to those achieved with matched-sibling transplants. Graft failure has occurred in ≤39% of patients on these protocols. Haploidentical BMT is particularly difficult in ADA-deficient SCID patients, in whom the incidence of graft failure has been observed to be ≤65% with T-cell-depleted grafts.[189,191]

Attempts to decrease the incidence of graft failure following mismatched BMT have led to the addition of immunosuppression to the Bu/Cy conditioning regimen. The European Cooperative Group[200] studied the effect of administering antibody to the lymphocyte function-associated antigen-1 adhesion molecule (LFA-1 [CD11a] antibody), before and after the infusion of T-cell-depleted parental marrow. Graft failure occurred in 2 of 11 patients, and disease-free survival was 64%. Grade II or III acute GVHD occurred in only four patients.[200] Limited experience has been reported using unrelated donor transplants in SCID. Filipovich et al.,[196] using a preparative regimen of Bu/Cy/ATG with phenotypically matched or one-antigen mismatched unrelated, unmanipulated marrow, reported that six of eight patients were doing well 18–47 months post-BMT.

B-cell lymphoproliferative disorders associated with Epstein-Barr virus are a recognized complication of immunodeficiency diseases. These disorders have also been observed within a few months of bone marrow transplant for SCID, rarely in the setting of matched sibling grafts, but with increased frequency in mismatched transplants.[201] The reported incidence varies from 6% to 32% of cases, and these lymphoproliferative disorders are associated with a high mortality.[189,195,197,200]

Wiskott-Aldrich Syndrome

Wiskott-Aldrich syndrome (WAS) is a sex-linked disorder characterized by immunodeficiency and thrombocytopenia. Most patients will die before age 20, unless BMT is performed.[188,202] WAS is associated with both defective lymphocyte glycoprotein (CD43) and defective platelet glycoprotein la/Ib.[194] The successful engraftment of both lymphoid and hematopoietic elements following BMT for the treatment of WAS requires that additional agents (TBI with or without procarbazine, or Bu) be given in addition to Cy as part of the preparative regimen.[203] Bu followed by Cy has been widely used to avoid the potential long-term complications associated with TBI in young patients. Depending on patient age and need for myeloablation, lower Bu doses (2 mg/kg/day × 4) may not be adequate, and higher Bu doses (4 mg/kg/day × 4) may be required.[194,203] In >50 reported cases of HLA-matched BMT, 60–90% of patients are long-term survivors.[188,191,202] However, transplantation using haploidentical donors, even with T-cell depletion, has led to poor results in WAS, with only 16–23% of cases surviving.[190,194,202] The problems of graft failure and posttransplant lymphomas have been particularly significant.[200,202] Promising results have been achieved when additional treatment is added to the conditioning regimen. In one study using myeloablative therapy (Cy and ara-C with TBI or Bu) and haploidentical marrow depleted of T cells, three of four patients survived for 10–30 months.[204] Two patients with WAS received one-antigen mismatched unmanipulated grafts and are reported to be well at 20 and 33 months post-BMT. Although allogeneic BMT is regarded as the treatment of choice for WAS with matched sibling donors, the use of nonidentical donors and HLA-compatible unrelated donors remains experimental.

Disorders of Myeloid Function

For patients with diseases of granulocyte function who have recurrent and often life-threatening bacterial infections, BMT may be curative. Such diseases include infantile (Kostmann) agranulocytosis, Chédiak-Higashi syndrome, familial erythrophagocytic lymphohistiocytosis, leukocyte adhesion deficiency, chronic granulomatous disease, and Langerhans cell histiocytosis.[188,190,191,193,195,205–208] Experience with allogeneic BMT is limited to a number of case studies, so the overall incidence of success of BMT in these diseases cannot be determined. As with WAS, both immunosuppression and myeloablation are required for successful engraftment to occur. Higher doses of Bu (16 mg/kg) or TBI, often with additional agents, have been used as conditioning regimens.[191,206,207] There are reports of successful transplants using nonidentical family and unrelated donors in a limited number of patients.[200,205–207] Graft failure, mortality due to infection, and Epstein-Barr virus lymphoma have been major complications of such efforts. With T-cell depletion in mismatched patients, survival of approximately 30% has been reported in two small studies.[192,205]

Not all patients with these diseases are candidates for BMT. Many of them may not experience sufficient morbidity due to repeated infections to warrant the risks of BMT.[194] In some diseases there are alternate therapies, such as growth factors for the treatment of infantile agranulocytosis and interferon-γ for the treatment of chronic granulomatous disease, which may decrease or eliminate the need for BMT.[194] For the individual patient with one of the other diseases of granulocyte function, age, severity of infectious complications, and the availability of a suitable donor should be taken into account when considering BMT.[194]

Erythroid Disorders

Thalassemia Major

The largest experience using BMT as treatment for thalassemia major has been that of Lucarelli et al.[209,210] In 350 matched thalassemic patients transplanted between 1983 and 1990, using a regimen of Bu (14 mg/kg) and Cy (200 mg/kg), a 73% event-free survival was reported at ≤8 years post-BMT.[209] Graft failure occurred in 12% of these heavily transfused patients. Acute GVHD occurred in 25% of patients and chronic GVHD in 5%. Overall, the mortality rate was 19%, and most deaths occurred within 100 days of BMT in patients who developed GVHD.[209] Factors found to predict poor survival were hepatomegaly, portal fibrosis on liver biopsy prior to transplant, and a need for iron chelation therapy to prevent the complication of hemosiderosis. The likelihood of thalassemic patients having these high-risk factors increases with patient age.[210] Disease-free survival was reported to be 49% in patients with all three factors and 94% for patients with none.[210] Beginning in 1989, the dose of Cy was reduced to 120 mg/kg, and ALG was added to this regimen.[210] In 34 patients with all three bad prognostic factors, overall survival improved to 91%, but graft failure with autologous recovery and reappearance of the thalassemia occurred in 37%.[210] An increased incidence of mixed chimerism 2 months after BMT was noted using this protocol compared with the former protocol (57% versus 21%), and mixed chimerism at 2 months was associated with a 17–30% incidence of graft failure during the first year.[211] In 17 patients transplanted from haploidentical donors using the same conditioning regimen, a similar rejection rate was noted (35%). Forty-one percent of these patients died; only 4 (24%) were disease-free at 2–9 years.[210]

BMT for thalassemia major remains a matter of controversy.[212] Although HLA-matched transplants can cure the disease in most patients, early transplant-related mortality is considerable. According to Lucarelli et al.,[209] the recommended time for BMT is within the first 5 years of life. Alternative therapy, which is currently chronic transfusion therapy and iron chelation treatment, has significantly improved the survival of patients with thalassemia, so that 94% are alive 15 years after diagnosis in a large Italian study.[209] Transfusion therapy is associated with significantly less immediate mortality, but such patients require chronic, costly, therapy, which has its own infectious risks. Such therapy may not be available to all patients, particularly those in developing countries.[212] The potential exists for oral iron-chelation agents and for gene therapy for the treatment of these patients in the future. Until such treatments become widely available, and until transplant mortality is lessened, the decision about treatment of an affected child with a potential donor may be based on the availability of the different modes of therapy and the likelihood of patient compliance and careful follow-up.[212]

Sickle Cell Anemia

Sickle cell anemia is an inherited disorder of hemoglobin synthesis characterized by hemolytic anemia and vaso-occlusive crises related to the sickle shape of red blood cells. Complications include strokes, painful or aplastic crises, infections, and the need for chronic transfusions. BMT has been utilized in an attempt to cure the disease in a limited number of patients. The largest experience with matched sibling BMT has been reported in a Belgian and French cooperative study of 42 patients ranging in age from 1 to 23 years.[213] Acute GVHD was reported in 31% and chronic in 14%, but there was only one infectious death. At 36 months median follow-up, >90% were free of disease.[213] Return of splenic function was documented by the absence of Howell-Jolly bodies in the peripheral blood smear and normal technetium spleen scans in some patients.[214] Graft failure was noted in 12%, associated with the use of mismatched grafts and with patients who were heavily transfused.[213] The problems of patient selection and the relative costs of BMT versus long-term transfusion and chelation therapy in this disease are addressed in two reviews.[214,215]

Fanconi Anemia

Fanconi anemia is an autosomal recessive disorder characterized by congenital malformations, chromosomal instability, progressive bone marrow failure, and an increased incidence of malignancy. The mean age at which bone marrow failure is diagnosed is between 5 and 10 years.[216,217] Early experience with BMT using the dose of Cy widely used for severe aplastic anemia of other etiologies (50 mg/kg × 4) demonstrated a high early mortality related to unusually severe Cy side effects and grade IV GVHD, with reports of disease-free survival varying from 20% to 65%.[218,219] Gluckman[218] pioneered a regimen using Cy at 5 mg/kg × 4 followed by TAI (500 Gy). She reported that 72% of 39 patients survived.[218,220] Similar results have been reported using TBI (600 cGy), with 80% engraftment and 60% survival.[221] In an analysis of 89 matched sibling transplants, graft failure occurred in <10%, acute GVHD in 50–55%, and chronic GVHD in 51% of patients. No difference in graft failure or GVHD was seen when comparing protocols of Cy alone, or with TAI or TBI.[216] Harris and Kumar[222] used a regimen of Cy, TAI, ATG, steroids, and CsA and reported 100% survival in 12 children, with no acute GVHD.[222] Transplants performed after transition of Fanconi anemia to myelodysplasia or leukemia have had poor results, with only one survivor of eight cases reported in two studies.[219,221]

Mismatched related and matched unrelated donor transplants for Fanconi anemia have been reported, with very high mortality associated with GVHD and graft failure. Rare reports of long-term survival have been published.[220,221]

A newer source of hematopoietic stem cells, placental blood from the umbilical cord of an unaffected HLA-matched sibling, was first used successfully to engraft a 5-year-old patient in 1988.[223] Peripheral signs of engraftment became apparent on day 22, and marrow cellularity gradually increased until it was normal at 4 months. A limited number of such transplants have been performed.[224,225]

BMT has also been used successfully as a treatment for other constitutional anemias including dyskeratosis congenita, Schwachman-Diamond syndrome, and Diamond-Blackfan syndrome.[218,226–228]

Osteopetrosis

Osteopetrosis is an autosomal recessive disorder in which deficient osteoclast activity is manifest by inadequate bone resorption, resulting in overgrowth of bones and compression of cranial nerve foramina and marrow spaces; aplasia and death occur in childhood.[188] Transplantation of healthy marrow restores normal osteoclast activity such that marrow space is re-created over a period of 4–6 months. The early experience with HLA-matched grafts demonstrated that both myeloablation and immunosuppression are necessary for durable engraftment to occur and that transplantation during the first year of life provided the best chance of avoiding severe post-transplant hypercalcemia and permanent neurologic damage.[188,229] In most cases HLA-matched marrow will engraft with full or partial resolution of bone and marrow abnormalities, but neurosensory deficits may persist.[191] Early BMT is therefore advocated. Following mismatched transplants, graft failure has been reported to occur in 29–37% of cases.[192,230] Of 25 children who received such high-risk transplants, 12 survived a median of 12 months after mismatched BMT.[192,230]

Enzyme-Deficiency Diseases

Many diseases that result from the congenital deficiency of particular enzymes and that lead to tissue damage related to the buildup of unmetabolized substrate are treatable by alloge-

neic BMT. This therapy has been called "installing a donor enzyme factory for life."[231] In general, engraftment of a normal marrow results in normalization of enzyme levels and elimination of stored substrate with improvement in disease symptoms. In these diseases, there is patient variability in enzyme level, mode of presentation, and degree of irreversible damage to vital organs. Such factors may prevent patients from being candidates for BMT. More than 150 allogeneic transplants have been reported in patients with these diseases, usually after Bu/Cy conditioning.[232,233] The successes and limitations of transplant are addressed in several reviews.[232,233–236]

In Gaucher disease, signs and symptoms result from glucocerebroside accumulation in reticuloendothelial cells; tissues involved may include the spleen, liver, bones, lungs, heart, and central nervous system. After successful BMT, normal enzyme levels may be appreciated within 1 month of BMT,[194] and clearing of Gaucher cells from marrow, liver, and spleen occurs progressively over 1–3 years.[231,234] In two reports, which document this improvement, eight of nine patients treated with Bu/Cy or Cy/TBI survived for 1–5 years post-BMT.[231,234]

In diseases such as the mucopolysaccharidoses (Hunter, Hurler, Hurler-Scheie, and Sanfilippo syndromes) and the leukodystrophies, in which the principal manifestations are in the central nervous system, improvements in intellectual function and development post-BMT have been variable, even when visceral signs have diminished. This may be related to the slow entry of enzyme into the central nervous system and the extent of central nervous system damage at the time of BMT.[232] In cases of metachromatic leukodystrophy, globoid cell leukodystrophy, and X-linked adrenoleukodystrophy, there have been reports of stabilization of neurologic dysfunction clinically[235,236] and at least one case of gradual normalization of cerebral abnormalities by magnetic resonance imaging over months to years in a patient with adrenoleukodystrophy.[237] In many cases deterioration of the central nervous system and intellectual function has continued despite normal leukocyte enzyme levels.[233]

Whether patients with severe neurologic dysfunction should be subjected to BMT is controversial, and the ethical considerations are important in patient selection.[233] A consortium of North American transplant physicians has suggested restricting BMT to patients <3 years old and to those identified before severe and rapidly progressive neurologic disability occurs.[233]

FUTURE DIRECTIONS

Allogeneic BMT has become an important tool for the treatment of a variety of hematologic malignancies, marrow failure states, and inherited disorders. A major barrier to allogeneic BMT remains the limited access to immunologically compatible donors. Unrelated marrow donor banks have been established to overcome these limitations. Transplants from unrelated or related mismatched donors have met with only limited success. Such transplants frequently present an unacceptable risk to the patient. Development of new, innovative strategies will be required to overcome these immunologic barriers if allogeneic BMT is to make an impact on these diseases for larger numbers of patients.

REFERENCES

1. Bortin MM, Horowitz MM, Rimm AA: Increasing utilization of allogeneic bone marrow transplantation. Results of the 1988–1990 survey. Ann Intern Med 116:505, 1992
2. Champlin R, Coppo P, Howe C: National Marrow Donor Program: progress and challenges. Bone Marrow Transplant, suppl. 1. 2:41, 1993
3. Anasetti C, Amos D, Beatty PG et al: Effect of HLA compatibility on engraftment of bone marrow transplants in patients with leukemia or lymphoma. N Engl J Med 320:197, 1989

4. Bortin MM, Horowitz MM, Gale RP et al: Changing trends in allogeneic bone marrow transplantation for leukemia in the 1980s. JAMA 268:607, 1992
5. Cosset JM, Girinsky T, Malaise E et al: Clinical basis for TBI fractionation. Radiother Oncol, suppl. 1. 60, 1990
6. Nash RA, Pepe MS, Storb R et al: Acute graft-versus-host disease: analysis of risk factors after allogeneic marrow transplantation and prophylaxis with cyclosporine and methotrexate. Blood 80:1838, 1992
7. Shahidi NT: Acquired aplastic anemia: classification and etiologic considerations. p. 25. In Shahidi N (ed): Aplastic Anemia and Other Bone Marrow Failure Syndromes. Springer-Verlag, New York, 1990
8. Storb R, Longton G, Anasetti C et al: Changing trends in marrow transplantation for aplastic anemia. Bone Marrow Transplant, suppl. 1. 10:45, 1992
9. McGlave PB, Haake R, Miller W et al: Therapy of severe aplastic anemia in young adults and children with allogeneic bone marrow transplantation. Blood 70:1325, 1987
10. Gluckman E, Socie G, Devergie A et al: Bone marrow transplantation in 107 patients with severe aplastic anemia using cyclophosphamide and thoraco-abdominal irradiation for conditioning: long-term follow-up. Blood 78:2451, 1991
11. Smith BR, Guinan EC, Parkman R et al: Efficacy of a cyclophosphamide-procarbazine-antithymocyte serum regimen for prevention of graft-rejection following bone marrow transplantation for transfused patients with aplastic anemia. Transplantation 39:671, 1985
12. Hows JM, Marsh JCW, Yin JL et al: Bone marrow transplantation for severe aplastic anaemia using cyclosporin: long-term follow-up. Bone Marrow Transplant 4:11, 1989
13. May WS, Sensenbrenner LL, Burns WH et al: BMT for severe aplastic anemia using cyclosporine. Bone Marrow Transplant 11:459, 1993
14. Champlin RE, Ho WG, Nimer SD et al: Bone marrow transplantation for severe aplastic anemia. Transplantation 49:720, 1990
15. Anasetti C, Doney KC, Storb R et al: Marrow transplantation for severe aplastic anemia: long-term outcome in fifty untransfused patients. Ann Intern Med 104:461, 1986
16. Champlin RE, Horowitz MM, van Bekkum DW et al: Graft failure following bone marrow transplantation for severe aplastic anemia: risk factors and treatment results. Blood 73:606, 1989
17. Storb R, Etzioni R, Anasetti C et al: Cyclophosphamide combined with antithymocyte globulin in preparation for allogeneic marrow transplants in patients with aplastic anemia. Blood, suppl. 1. 80:170a, 1992
18. Gluckman E, Horowitz MM, Champlin RE et al: Bone marrow transplantation for severe aplastic anemia: influence of conditioning and graft-versus-host disease prophylaxis regimens on outcome. Blood 79:269, 1992
19. O'Reilly RJ, Kernan NA, Cunningham I et al: T-cell depleted marrow transplants for the treatment of leukemia, p. 477. In: Bone Marrow Transplant: Current Controversies. Alan R Liss, New York, 1989
20. Reisner Y, Kapoor N, Kirkpatrick D et al: Transplantation for acute leukemia with HLA-A and B nonidentical parental marrow cells fractionated with soybean agglutinin and sheep red blood cells. Lancet 1:327, 1981
21. Castro-Malaspina H, Childs B, Cunningham I et al: T-cell depleted BMT for severe aplastic anemia in adults. Blood, suppl. 1. 74:282a, 1989
22. Camitta B, Ash R, Menitove J et al: Bone marrow transplantation for children with severe aplastic anemia: use of donors other than HLA-identical siblings. Blood 74:1852, 1989
23. Gajewski JL, Ho WG, Feig SA et al: Bone marrow transplantation using unrelated donors for patients with advanced leukemia or bone marrow failure. Transplantation 50:244, 1990
24. Hows J, Szydlo R, Anasetti C et al: Unrelated donor marrow transplants for severe acquired aplastic anemia. Bone Marrow Transplant, suppl. 1. 10:102, 1992
25. Kernan NA, Bartsch G, Ash RC et al: Analysis of 462 transplantations from unrelated donors facilitated by the National Marrow Donor Program. N Engl J Med 328:593, 1993
26. Doney K, Kopecky K, Storb R et al: Long-term comparison of immunosuppressive therapy with antithymocyte globulin to bone marrow transplantation in aplastic anemia, p. 104. In Shahidi N (ed): Aplastic Anemia and Other Bone Marrow Failure Syndromes. Springer-Verlag, New York, 1990
27. Speck B: Allogeneic bone marrow transplantation for severe aplastic anemia. Semin Hematol 28:319, 1991
28. Champlin R: Treatment of aplastic anemia: bone marrow transplantation, immunomodulatory therapy, and hematopoietic growth factors. p. 121. In Shahidi N (ed): Aplastic Anemia and Other Bone Marrow Failure Syndromes. Springer-Verlag, New York, 1990
29. Socie G, Henry-Amar M, Cosset JM et al: Increased incidence of solid malignant tumors after bone marrow transplantation for severe aplastic anemia. Blood 78:277, 1991
30. Kolb HJ, Holler E, Bender-Gotze C et al: Myeloablative conditioning for marrow transplantation in myelodysplastic syndromes and paroxysmal nocturnal haemoglobinuria. Bone Marrow Transplant 4:29, 1989
31. Kawahara K, Witherspoon RP, Storb R: Marrow transplantation for paroxysmal nocturnal hemoglobinuria. Am J Hematol 39:283, 1992
32. Antin JH, Ginsburg D, Smith BR et al: Bone marrow transplantation for paroxysmal nocturnal hemoglobinuria: eradication of the PNH clone and documentation of complete lymphohematopoietic engraftment. Blood 66:1247, 1985
33. Hoelzer DF: Therapy of the newly diagnosed adult with acute lymphoblastic leukemia. Hematol Oncol Clin North Am 7:139, 1993
34. Blume KG, Forman SJ, Snyder DS et al: Allogeneic bone marrow transplantation for acute lymphoblastic leukemia during first complete remission. Transplantation 43:389, 1987
35. Chao NJ, Forman SJ, Schmidt GM et al: Allogeneic bone marrow transplantation for high-risk acute lymphoblastic leukemia during first complete remission. Blood 78:1923, 1991
36. Wingard JR, Piantadosi S, Santos GW et al: Allogeneic bone marrow transplantation for patients with high-risk acute lymphoblastic leukemia. J Clin Oncol 8:820, 1990
37. Barrett AJ, Horowitz MM, Gale RP et al: Marrow transplantation for acute lymphoblastic leukemia: factors affecting relapse and survival. Blood 74:862, 1989
38. Bordigoni P, Vernant JP, Souillet G et al: Allogeneic bone marrow transplantation for children with acute lymphoblastic leukemia in first remission: a cooperative study of the Groupe d'Etude de la Greffe de Moelle Osseuse. J Clin Oncol 7:747, 1989
39. Blaise D, Gaspard MH, Stoppa AM et al: Allogeneic or autologous bone marrow transplantation for acute lymphoblastic leukemia in first complete remission. Bone Marrow Transplant 5:7, 1990
40. Vernant JP, Marit G, Maraninchi D et al: Allogeneic bone marrow transplantation in adults with acute lymphoblastic leukemia in first complete remission. J Clin Oncol 6:227, 1988
41. Horowitz MM, Gale RP, Sondel PM et al: Graft-versus-leukemia reactions after bone marrow transplantation. Blood 75:555, 1990
42. Marmont AM, Horowitz MM, Gale RP et al: T-cell depletion of HLA-identical transplants in leukemia. Blood 78:2120, 1991
43. Fyles GM, Messner HA, Lockwood G et al: Long-term results of bone marrow transplantation for patients with AML, ALL and CML prepared with single dose total body irradiation of 500 cGy delivered with a high dose rate. Bone Marrow Transplant 8:453, 1991
44. Copelan EA, Biggs JC, Avalos BR et al: Radiation-free preparation for allogeneic bone marrow transplantation in adults with acute lymphoblastic leukemia. J Clin Oncol 10:237, 1992
45. von Buelzingsloewen A, Belanger R, Perreault C et al: Acute graft-versus-host disease prophylaxis with methotrexate and cyclosporine after busulfan and cyclophosphamide in patients with hematologic malignancies. Blood 81:849, 1993
46. Hale G, Cobbold S, Waldmann H: T cell depletion with Campath-1 in allogeneic bone marrow transplantation. Transplantation 45:753, 1988
47. Doney K, Fisher LD, Appelbaum FR et al: Treatment of adult acute lymphoblastic leukemia with allogeneic bone marrow transplantation. Multivariate analysis of factors affecting acute graft-versus-host disease, relapse, and relapse-free survival. Bone Marrow Transplant 7:453, 1991
48. Weisdorf DJ, Nesbit ME, Ramsay NKC et al: Allogeneic bone marrow transplantation for acute lymphoblastic leukemia in remission: prolonged survival associated with acute graft-versus-host disease. J Clin Oncol 5:1348, 1987
49. Thompson CB, Sanders JE, Flournoy N et al: The risks of central nervous system relapse and leukoencephalopathy in patients receiving marrow transplants for acute leukemia. Blood 67:195, 1986
50. Niederwieser D, Granena A, Hermans J et al: Slow response to induction chemotherapy is an indicator of poor survival after bone marrow transplantation for acute lymphoblastic leukemia. Bone Marrow Transplant 9:439, 1992
51. Maraninchi D, Gluckman E, Blaise D et al: Impact of T-cell depletion on outcome of allogeneic bone-marrow transplantation for standard-risk leukaemias. Lancet 2:175, 1987
52. Prentice HG, Brenner MK, Gottlieb D: T cell depleted bone marrow transplantation in acute myeloblastic leukaemia: the way ahead. Bone Marrow Transplant, suppl. 1. 4:225, 1989
53. Schattenberg A, De Witte T, Preijers F et al: Allogeneic bone marrow transplantation for leukemia with marrow grafts depleted of lymphocytes by counterflow centrifugation. Blood 75:1356, 1990
54. Lestingi TM, Hooberman AL: Philadelphia chromosome-positive acute lymphoblastic leukemia. Hematol Oncol Clin North Am 7:161, 1993
55. Barrett AJ, Horowitz MM, Ash RC et al: Bone marrow transplantation for

Philadelphia chromosome-positive acute lymphoblastic leukemia. Blood 79: 3067, 1992

56. Forman SJ, O'Donnell MR, Nademanee AP et al: Bone marrow transplantation for patients with Philadelphia chromosome-positive acute lymphoblastic leukemia. Blood 70:587, 1987

57. Troussard X, Leblond V, Kuentz M et al: Allogeneic bone marrow transplantation in adults with Burkitt's lymphoma or acute lymphoblastic leukemia in first complete remission. J Clin Oncol 8:809, 1990

58. Horowitz MM, Messerer D, Hoelzer D et al: Chemotherapy compared with bone marrow transplantation for adults with acute lymphoblastic leukemia in first remission. Ann Intern Med 115:13, 1991

59. Sebban C, Lepage E, Vernant JP et al: Allogeneic bone marrow transplantation is the best post-remission therapy for high risk adult acute lymphoblastic leukemia: a study from the French Group of Adult ALL. Proc Am Soc Clin Oncol 11:259, 1992

60. Brochstein JA, Kernan NA, Groshen S et al: Allogeneic bone marrow transplantation after hyperfractionated total-body irradiation and cyclophosphamide in children with acute leukemia. N Engl J Med 317:1618, 1987

61. Sanders JE, Thomas ED, Buckner CD et al: Marrow transplantation for children with acute lymphoblastic leukemia in second remission. Blood 70:324, 1987

62. Coccia PF, Strandjord SE, Warkentin PI et al: High-dose cytosine arabinoside and fractionated total-body irradiation: an improved preparative regimen for bone marrow transplantation of children with acute lymphoblastic leukemia in remission. Blood 71:888, 1988

63. Weyman C, Graham-Pole J, Emerson S et al: Use of high dose cytosine arabinoside and fractionated total body irradiation as conditioning for allogeneic marrow transplantation in patients with acute lymphoblastic leukemia: a multicenter survey. Bone Marrow Transplant 11:43, 1993

64. Hervé P, Cahn JY, Flesch M et al: Successful graft-versus-host disease prevention without graft failure in 32 HLA-identical allogeneic bone marrow transplantations with marrow depleted of T cells by monoclonal antibodies and complement. Blood 69:388, 1987

65. Dinsmore R, Kirkpatrick D, Flomenberg N et al: Allogeneic bone marrow transplantation for patients with acute lymphoblastic leukemia. Blood 62: 381, 1983

66. Blume KG, Forman SJ, O'Donnell MR et al: Total body irradiation and high-dose etoposide: a new preparatory regimen for bone marrow transplantation in patients with advanced hematologic malignancies. Blood 69:1015, 1987

67. Blume KG, Kopecky KJ, Henslee-Downey JP et al: A prospective randomized comparison of total body irradiation-etoposide versus busulfan-cyclophosphamide as preparatory regimens for bone marrow transplantation in patients with leukemia who were not in first remission: a Southwest Oncology Group study. Blood 81:2187, 1993

68. Schmitz N, Gassmann W, Rister M et al: Fractionated total body irradiation and high-dose VP 16-213 followed by allogeneic bone marrow transplantation in advanced leukemias. Blood 72:1567, 1988

69. Dopfer R, Henze G, Bender-Gotze C et al: Allogeneic bone marrow transplantation for childhood acute lymphoblastic leukemia in second remission after intensive primary and relapse therapy according to the BFM-and CoALL-protocols: results of the German cooperative study. Blood 78:2780, 1991

70. Biggs JC, Horowitz MM, Gale RP et al: Bone marrow transplants may cure patients with acute leukemia never achieving remission with chemotherapy. Blood 80:1090, 1992

71. Cahn JY, Bordigoni P, Souillet G et al: The TAM regimen prior to allogeneic and autologous bone marrow transplantation for high-risk acute lymphoblastic leukemias: a cooperative study of 62 patients. Bone Marrow Transplant 7:1, 1991

72. Yau JC, LeMaistre CF, Andersson BS et al: Allogeneic bone marrow transplantation for hematological malignancies following etoposide, cyclophosphamide, and fractionated total body irradiation. Am J Hematol 41:40, 1992

73. Arcese W, Meloni G, Giona F et al: Idarubicin plus ARA-C followed by allogeneic or autologous bone marrow transplantation in advanced acute lymphoblastic leukemia. Bone Marrow Transplant, suppl. 2. 7:38, 1991

74. Trigg ME, Gingrich R, Goeken N et al: Low rejection rate when using unrelated or haploidentical donors for children with leukemia undergoing marrow transplantation. Bone Marrow Transplant 4:431, 1989

75. Thomas ED, Buckner CD, Clift RA et al: Marrow transplantation for acute nonlymphoblastic leukemia in first remission. N Engl J Med 301:597, 1979

76. Clift R, Buckner CD, Bianco J et al: Marrow transplantation in patients with acute myeloid leukemia. Leukemia, suppl. 2. 6:104, 1992

77. Dinsmore R, Kirkpatrick D, Flomenberg N et al: Allogeneic bone marrow transplantation for patients with acute nonlymphocytic leukemia. Blood 63: 649, 1984

78. Chao NJ, Amylon MD, Long GD et al: Bone marrow transplantation for hema-

tologic malignancies: the Stanford experience. p. 157. In Terasaki P (ed): Clinical Transplants 1990. UCLA Tissue Typing Laboratory, Los Angeles, 1990

79. Forman SJ, Spruce WE, Farbstein MJ et al: Bone marrow ablation followed by allogeneic marrow grafting during first complete remission of acute non-lymphocytic leukemia. Blood 61:439, 1983

80. McGlave PB, Haake RJ, Bostrom BC et al: Bone marrow transplantation for acute nonlymphocytic leukemia in first remission. Blood 72:1512, 1988

81. Clift RA, Buckner CD, Appelbaum FR et al: Allogeneic marrow transplantation in patients with acute myeloid leukemia in first remission: a randomized trial of two irradiation regimens. Blood 76:1867, 1990

82. Santos GW, Tutschka PJ, Brookmeyer R et al: Marrow transplantation for acute nonlymphocytic leukemia after treatment with busulfan and cyclophosphamide. N Engl J Med 309:1347, 1983

83. Geller RB, Saral R, Piantadosi S et al: Allogeneic bone marrow transplantation after high-dose busulfan and cyclophosphamide in patients with acute nonlymphocytic leukemia. Blood 73:2209, 1989

84. Nevill TJ, Barnett MJ, Klingemann HG et al: Regimen-related toxicity of a busulfan-cyclophosphamide conditioning regimen in 70 patients undergoing allogeneic bone marrow transplantation. J Clin Oncol 9:1224, 1991

85. Copelan EA, Biggs JC, Thompson JM et al: Treatment for acute myelocytic leukemia with allogeneic bone marrow transplantation following preparation with BuCy2. Blood 78:838, 1991

86. Blaise D, Maraninchi D, Archimbaud E et al: Allogeneic bone marrow transplantation for acute myeloid leukemia in first remission: a randomized trial of a busulfan-cytoxan versus cytoxan-total body irradiation as preparative regimen: a report from the Groupe d'Etudes de la Greffe de Moelle Osseuse. Blood 79:2578, 1992

87. Michel G, Gluckman E, Blaise D et al: Improvement in outcome for children receiving allogeneic bone marrow transplantation in first remission of acute myeloid leukemia: a report from the Groupe d'Etude des Greffes de Moelle Osseuse. J Clin Oncol 10:1865, 1992

88. Maraninchi D, Vernant JP, Gluckman E et al: Greffes de moelle allogéniques dans les leucémies aigues myeloides. Presse Med 15:2093, 1986

89. Bostrom B, Brunning RD, McGlave P et al: Bone marrow transplantation for acute nonlymphocytic leukemia in first remission: analysis of prognostic factors. Blood 65:1191, 1985

90. Zwaan R, Hermans J, Barrett AJ, Speck B: Bone marrow transplantation for acute nonlymphoblastic leukaemia: a survey of the European Group for Bone Marrow Transplantation. Br J Haematol 56:645, 1984

91. Storb R, Deeg HJ, Pepe M et al: Methotrexate and cyclosporine versus cyclosporine alone for prophylaxis of graft-versus-host disease in patients given HLA-identical marrow grafts for leukemia: long-term follow-up of a controlled trial. Blood 73:1729, 1989

92. Champlin R, Ho W, Gajewski J et al: Selective depletion of CD8+ T lymphocytes for prevention of graft-versus-host disease after allogeneic bone marrow transplantation. Blood 76:418, 1990

93. Wagner JE, Donnenberg AD, Noga SJ et al: Lymphocyte depletion of donor bone marrow by counterflow centrifugal elutriation: results of a phase I clinical trial. Blood 72:1168, 1988

94. Wagner J, Vogelsang G, Santos G: Graft-vs-leukemia: the effect of acute and chronic graft-vs-host disease and marrow T-cell depletion at a single institution. Blood, suppl. 1. 76:571a, 1990

95. Young JW, Papadopoulos EB, Cunningham I et al: T-cell-depleted allogeneic bone marrow transplantation in adults with acute nonlymphocytic leukemia in first remission. Blood 79:3380, 1992

96. Aversa F, Terenzi A, Carotti A et al: T-cell depletion in allogeneic bone marrow transplantation for acute leukaemias. Bone Marrow Transplant, suppl. 4. 4:69, 1989

97. Terenzi A, Lubin I, Lapidot T: Enhancement of T cell-depleted bone marrow allografts in mice by thiotepa. Transplantation 50:717, 1990

98. Papadopoulos E, Carabasi M, Young J et al: Results of T-cell depleted allogeneic BMT after TBI, thiotepa and cyclophosphamide in patients with leukemia. Blood, suppl. 1. 80:170a, 1992

99. Amadori S, Testi AM, Arico M et al: Prospective comparative study of bone marrow transplantation and postremission chemotherapy for childhood acute myelogenous leukemia. J Clin Oncol 11:1046, 1993

100. Dahl GV, Kalwinsky DK, J. Mirro J et al: Allogeneic bone marrow transplantation in a program of intensive sequential chemotherapy for children and young adults with acute nonlymphocytic leukemia in first remission. J Clin Oncol 8:295, 1990

101. Christiansen NP: Allogeneic bone marrow transplantation for the treatment of adult acute leukemias. Hematol Oncol Clin North Am 7:177, 1993

102. Clift RA, Buckner CD, Appelbaum FR et al: Allogeneic marrow transplanta-

tion during untreated first relapse of acute myeloid leukemia. J Clin Oncol 10:1723, 1992

103. deOliveira JS, Sale GE, Bryant EM et al: Acute megakaryoblastic leukemia in children: treatment with bone marrow transplantation. Bone Marrow Transplant 10:399, 1992

104. Rajantie J, Sale GE, Deeg HJ et al: Adverse effect of severe marrow fibrosis on hematologic recovery after chemoradiotherapy and allogeneic bone marrow transplantation. Blood 67:1693, 1986

105. Schmitz N, Suttorp M, Schlegelberger B et al: The role of the spleen after bone marrow transplantation for primary myelofibrosis. Br J Haematol 81: 616, 1992

106. Dokal I, Jones L, Deenmamode M et al: Allogeneic bone marrow transplantation for primary myelofibrosis. Br J Haematol 71:158, 1989

107. Loffler H, Schmitz N, Gassmann W: Intensive chemotherapy and bone marrow transplantation for myelodysplastic syndromes. Hematol Oncol Clin North Am 6:619, 1992

108. Anderson JE, Appelbaum FR, Fisher LD et al: Allogeneic bone marrow transplantation for 93 patients with myelodysplastic syndrome. Blood 82:677, 1993

109. Appelbaum FR, Barrall J, Storb R et al: Bone marrow transplantation for patients with myelodysplasia: pretreatment variables and outcome. Ann Intern Med 112:590, 1990

110. O'Donnell MR, Nademanee AP, Snyder DS et al: Bone marrow transplantation for myelodysplastic and myeloproliferative syndromes. J Clin Oncol 5: 1822, 1987

111. Longmore G, Guinan EC, Weinstein HJ et al: Bone marrow transplantation for myelodysplasia and secondary acute nonlymphoblastic leukemia. J Clin Oncol 8:1707, 1990

112. DeWitte T, Zwaan F, Hermans J et al: Allogeneic bone marrow transplantation for secondary leukaemia and myelodysplastic syndrome: a survey by the Leukaemia Working Party of the European Bone Marrow Transplantation Group. Br J Haematol 74:151, 1990

113. Nevill TJ, Shepherd JD, Reece DE et al: Treatment of myelodysplastic syndrome with busulfan-cyclophosphamide conditioning followed by allogeneic BMT. Bone Marrow Transplant 10:445, 1992

114. Ratanatharathorn V, Karanes C, Uberti J et al: Busulfan-based regimens and allogeneic bone marrow transplantation in patients with myelodysplastic syndromes. Blood 81:2194, 1993

115. Sutton L, Leblond V, LeMaignan C et al: Bone marrow transplantation for myelodysplastic syndrome and secondary leukemia: outcome of 86 patients. Bone Marrow Transplant, suppl. 2. 7:39, 1991

116. Bandini G, Rosti G, Calori E et al: Allogeneic bone marrow transplantation for secondary leukaemia and myelodysplastic syndrome. Br J Haematol 75: 442, 1990

117. Montserrat E, Gale RP, Rozman C: Bone marrow transplants for chronic lymphocytic leukaemia. Leukemia 6:619, 1992

118. Rabinowe SN, Soiffer RJ, Gribben JG et al: Autologous and allogeneic bone marrow transplantation for poor prognosis patients with B-cell chronic lymphocytic leukaemia. Blood 82:1366, 1993

119. Michallet M, Corront B, Hollard D et al: Allogeneic bone marrow transplantation in chronic lymphocytic leukemia: 17 cases. Report from the EBMTG. Bone Marrow Transplant 7:275, 1991

120. Delage R, Ritz J, Anderson KC: The evolving role of bone marrow transplantation in the treatment of chronic myelogenous leukemia. Hematol Oncol Clin North Am 4:369, 1990

121. Fefer A, Thomas ED: Bone marrow transplantation for the treatment of chronic myelogenous leukemia. Important Adv Oncol 143, 1990

122. Thomas ED, Clift RA, Fefer A et al: Marrow transplantation for the treatment of chronic myelogenous leukemia. Ann Intern Med 104:155, 1986

123. Wagner JE, Zahurak M, Piantadosi S et al: Bone marrow transplantation of chronic myelogenous leukemia in chronic phase: evaluation of risks and benefits. J Clin Oncol 10:779, 1992

124. McGlave P, Arthur D, Haake R et al: Therapy of chronic myelogenous leukemia with allogeneic bone marrow transplantation. J Clin Oncol 5:1033, 1987

125. Goldman JM, Gale RP, Horowitz MM et al: Bone marrow transplantation for chronic myelogenous leukemia in chronic phase: increased risk of relapse associated with T-cell depletion. Ann Intern Med 108:806, 1988

126. Devergie A, Reiffers J, Vernant JP et al: Long-term follow-up after bone marrow transplantation for chronic myelogenous leukemia: factors associated with relapse. Bone Marrow Transplant 5:379, 1990

127. Marks DI, Hughes TP, Szydlo R et al: HLA-identical sibling donor bone marrow transplantation for chronic myeloid leukaemia in first chronic phase: influence of GVHD prophylaxis on outcome. Br J Haematol 81:383, 1992

128. Clift RA, Buckner CD, Appelbaum FR et al: Allogeneic marrow transplantation in patients with chronic myeloid leukemia in the chronic phase: a randomized trial of two irradiation regimens. Blood 77:1660, 1991

129. Biggs JC, Szer J, Crilley P et al: Treatment of chronic myeloid leukemia with allogeneic bone marrow transplantation after preparation with BuCy2. Blood 80:1352, 1992

130. Buckner CD, Clift RA, Appelbaum FR et al: A randomized study comparing two transplant regimens for CML in chronic phase. Blood, suppl. 1. 80:72a, 1992

131. Morgan M, Dodds A, Atkinson K et al: The toxicity of busulphan and cyclophosphamide as the preparative regimen for bone marrow transplantation. Br J Haematol 77:529, 1991

132. Socie G, Devergie A, Girinsky T et al: Influence of the fractionation of total body irradiation on complications and relapse rate for chronic myelogenous leukemia. Int J Radiat Oncol Biol Phys 20:397, 1991

133. McGlave P, Bartsch G, Anasetti C et al: Unrelated donor marrow transplantation therapy for chronic myelogenous leukemia: initial experience of the National Marrow Donor Program. Blood 81:543, 1993

134. Delage R, Soiffer RJ, Dear K et al: Clinical significance of bcr-abl gene rearrangement detected by polymerase chain reaction after allogeneic bone marrow transplantation in chronic myelogenous leukemia. Blood 78:2759, 1991

135. Champlin R, Giralt S, Przepiorka D et al: Selective depletion of CD8-positive T-lymphocytes for allogeneic bone marrow transplantation: engraftment, graft-versus-host disease and graft-versus leukemia. Prog Clin Biol Res 377: 385, 1992

136. Offit K, Burns JP, Cunningham I et al: Cytogenetic analysis of chimerism and leukemia relapse in chronic myelogenous leukemia patients after T cell-depleted bone marrow transplantation. Blood 75:1346, 1990

137. Apperley JF, Jones J, Hale G et al: Bone marrow transplantation for patients with chronic myeloid leukaemia: T-cell depletion with Campath-1 reduces the risk of graft-versus-host disease but may increase the risk of leukaemic relapse. Bone Marrow Transplant 1:53, 1986

138. Frame JN, Collins NH, Cartagena T et al: T cell depletion of human bone marrow. Transplantation 47:984, 1989

139. Kernan NA, Bordignon C, Heller G et al: Graft failure after T-cell-depleted human leukocyte antigen identical marrow transplants for leukemia: I. Analysis of risk factors and results of secondary transplants. Blood 74:2227, 1989

140. Aversa F, Pelicci PG, Terenzi A et al: Results of T-depleted BMT in chronic myelogenous leukaemia after a conditioning regimen that included thiotepa. Bone Marrow Transplant, suppl. 2. 7:24, 1991

141. Lehn P, Devergie A, Benbunan M et al: Bone marrow transplantation for chronic granulocytic leukemia. J Natl Cancer Inst 76:1301, 1986

142. Messner HA, Curtis JE, Minden MM: The combined use of cytosine arabinoside, cyclophosphamide, and total body irradiation as preparative regimen for bone marrow transplantation in patients with AML and CML. Sem Oncol, suppl. 3. 12:187, 1985

143. Speck B, Gratwohl A, Osterwalder B et al: Bone marrow transplantation for chronic myeloid leukemia. Semin Hematol 21:48, 1984

144. Arthur CK, Apperley JF, Guo AP et al: Cytogenetic events after bone marrow transplantation for chronic myeloid leukemia in chronic phase. Blood 71: 1179, 1988

145. Baughan ASJ, Worsley AM, McCarthy DM et al: Haematological reconstitution and severity of graft-versus-host disease after bone marrow transplantation for chronic granulocytic leukaemia: the influence of previous splenectomy. Br J Haematol 56:445, 1984

146. Banaji M, Bearman SI, Buckner CD et al: The effects of splenectomy on engraftment and platelet transfusion requirements in patients with chronic myelogenous leukemia undergoing marrow transplantation. Am J Hematol 22:275, 1986

147. Gratwohl A, Hermans J, von Biezen A et al: No advantage for patients who receive splenic irradiation before bone marrow transplantation for chronic myeloid leukaemia: results of a prospective randomized study. Bone Marrow Transplant 10:147, 1992

148. Kanfer EJ, Buckner CD, Fefer A et al: Allogeneic and syngeneic marrow transplantation following high dose dimethylbusulfan, cyclophosphamide and total body irradiation. Bone Marrow Transplant 1:339, 1987

149. Roth MS, Antin JH, Ash R et al: Prognostic significance of Philadelphia chromosome-positive cells detected by the polymerase chain reaction after allogeneic bone marrow transplant for chronic myelogenous leukemia. Blood 79:276, 1992

150. Hughes TP, Morgan GJ, Martiat P et al: Detection of residual leukemia after bone marrow transplant for chronic myeloid leukemia: role of polymerase chain reaction in predicting relapse. Blood 77:874, 1991

151. Guerrasio A, Saglio G, Rosso C et al: Minimal residual disease status in transplanted chronic myelogenous leukemia patients: low incidence of polymerase chain reaction positive cases among 48 long disease-free subjects

who received unmanipulated allogeneic bone marrow transplants. Leukemia 6:507, 1992

152. Cross NCP, Feng L, Martiat P et al: The use of PCR to detect MRD after BMT for CML: associations with GVHD and relapse. Blood, suppl. 1. 80:300a, 1992

153. Frassoni F, Sessarego M, Bacigalupo A et al: Competition between recipient and donor cells after bone marrow transplantation for chronic myeloid leukaemia. Br J Haematol 69:471, 1988

154. Arcese W, Mauro FR, Alimena G et al: Interferon therapy for Ph1 positive CML patients relapsing after T cell-depleted allogeneic bone marrow transplantation. Bone Marrow Transplant 5:309, 1990

155. Higano CS, Raskind WH, Singer JW: Use of alpha interferon for the treatment of relapse of chronic myelogenous leukemia in chronic phase after allogeneic bone marrow transplantation. Blood 80:1437, 1992

156. Kolb HJ, Mittermuller J, Clemm C et al: Donor leukocyte transfusions for treatment of recurrent chronic myelogenous leukemia in marrow transplant patients. Blood 76:2462, 1990

157. Cullis JO, Jiang YZ, Schwarer AP et al: Donor leukocyte infusions for chronic myeloid leukemia in relapse after allogeneic bone marrow transplantation. Blood 79:1379, 1992

158. Frassoni F, Fagioli F, Sessarego M et al: The effect of donor leukocyte infusion in patients with leukemia following allogeneic bone marrow transplantation. Exp Hem 20:712, 1992

159. Bar BMAM, Schattenberg A, Mensink EJBM et al: Donor leukocyte infusions for chronic myeloid leukemia relapsed after allogeneic bone marrow transplantation. J Clin Oncol 11:513, 1993

160. Wagner JE, Vogelsang GB, Zehnbauer BA et al: Relapse of leukemia after bone marrow transplantation: effect of second myeloablative therapy. Bone Marrow Transplant 9:205, 1992

161. Atkinson K: Who should get a second marrow transplant? Bone Marrow Transplant, suppl. 1. 10:82, 1992

162. Copelan EA, Grever MR, Kapoor N et al: Marrow transplantation following busulfan and cyclophosphamide for chronic myelogenous leukemia in accelerated or blastic phase. Br J Haematol 71:487, 1989

163. Devine S, McKeithan T, LeBeau M et al: Allogeneic bone marrow transplantation utilizing a busulfan-containing preparative regimen as effective treatment for advanced chronic myelogenous leukemia. Blood, suppl. 1. 78:502a, 1991

164. Berman E, Raymond V, Gee T et al: Idarubicin in acute leukemia: results of studies at Memorial Sloan-Kettering Cancer Center. Sem Oncol, suppl. 2. 16:30, 1989

165. Sanders JE, Buckner CD, Thomas ED et al: Allogeneic marrow transplantation for children with juvenile chronic myelogenous leukemia. Blood 71:1144, 1988

166. Rassam SMB, Katz F, Chessells JM et al: Successful allogeneic bone marrow transplantation in juvenile CML: conditioning or graft-versus-leukaemia effect? Bone Marrow Transplant 11:247, 1993

167. Bunin NJ, Casper JT, Lawton C et al: Allogeneic marrow transplantation using T cell depletion for patients with juvenile chronic myelogenous leukemia without HLA-identical siblings. Bone Marrow Transplant 9:119, 1992

168. Armitage JO: Bone marrow transplantation in the treatment of patients with lymphoma. Blood 73:1749, 1989

169. Phillips GL, Herzig RH, Lazarus HM et al: High-dose chemotherapy, fractionated total-body irradiation, and allogeneic marrow transplantation for malignant lymphoma. J Clin Oncol 4:480, 1986

170. Milpied N, Ifrah N, Kuentz M et al: Bone marrow transplantation for adult poor prognosis lymphoblastic lymphoma in first complete remission. Br J Haematol 73:82, 1989

171. Chopra R, Goldstone AH, Pearce R et al: Autologous versus allogeneic bone marrow transplantation for non-Hodgkin's lymphoma: a case-controlled analysis of the European Bone Marrow Transplant Group registry data. J Clin Onc 10:1690, 1992

172. Appelbaum FR, Sullivan KM, Buckner CD et al: Treatment of malignant lymphoma in 100 patients with chemotherapy, total body irradiation, and marrow transplantation. J Clin Oncol 5:1340, 1987

173. Jones RJ, Piantadosi S, Mann RB et al: High-dose cytotoxic therapy and bone marrow transplantation for relapsed Hodgkin's disease. J Clin Oncol 8:527, 1990

174. Jones RJ, Ambinder RF, Piantadosi S et al: Evidence of graft-versus-lymphoma effect associated with allogeneic bone marrow transplantation. Blood 77:649, 1991

175. Shepherd JD, Barnett MJ, Connors JM et al: Allogeneic bone marrow transplantation for poor prognosis non-Hodgkin's lymphoma. Blood, suppl. 80:67a, 1992

176. Lundberg JH, Hansen RM, Chitambar CR et al: Allogeneic bone marrow transplantation for relapsed and refractory lymphoma using genotypically HLA-identical and alternative donors. J Clin Oncol 9:1848, 1991

177. Barlogie B, Gahrton G: Bone marrow transplantation in multiple myeloma. Bone Marrow Transplant 7:71, 1991

178. Gahrton G, Tura S, Ljungman P et al: Allogeneic bone marrow transplantation in multiple myeloma. N Engl J Med 325:1267, 1991

179. Barlogie B: Toward a cure for multiple myeloma? N Engl J Med 325:1304, 1991

180. Tura S, Cavo M: Allogeneic bone marrow transplantation in multiple myeloma. Hematol Oncol Clin North Am 6:425, 1992

181. Bensinger WI, Buckner CD, Clift RA et al: Phase I study of busulfan and cyclophosphamide in preparation for allogeneic marrow transplant for patients with multiple myeloma. J Clin Oncol 10:1492, 1992

182. Reece DE, Shepherd JD, Nantel SH et al: Intensive therapy and allogeneic bone marrow transplantation for multiple myeloma patients: the Vancouver experience. Blood, suppl. 1. 80:362a, 1992

183. Anderson KC, Soiffer R, Freedman A et al: Bone marrow transplantation for multiple myeloma. Blood, suppl. 1. 80:362a, 1992

184. Or R, Mehta J, Naparstek E et al: Successful T-cell-depleted allogeneic bone marrow transplantation in a child with recurrent multiple extramedullary plasmacytomas. Bone Marrow Transplant 10:381, 1992

185. Angelucci E, Baronciani D, Lucarelli G et al: Long-term complete remission after allogeneic bone marrow transplantation in multiple myeloma. Bone Marrow Transplant 8:307, 1991

186. Deane M, Samson D: Detection of minimal residual myeloma after bone marrow transplantation. Br J Haematol 79:134, 1991

187. Kenny AB, Hitzig WH: Bone marrow transplantation for severe combined immunodeficiency disease. Eur J Pediatr 131:155, 1979

188. O'Reilly RJ, Brochstein J, Dinsmore R et al: Marrow transplantation for congenital disorders. Semin Hematol 21:188, 1984

189. O'Reilly RJ, Keever CA, Small TN et al: The use of HLA-non-identical T-cell-depleted marrow transplants for correction of severe combined immunodeficiency disease. Immunodefic Rev 1:273, 1989

190. Buckley RH: Advances in the correction of immunodeficiency by bone marrow transplantation. Pediatr Ann 16:412, 1987

191. Fischer A, Griscelli C, Friedrich W et al: Bone-marrow transplantation for immunodeficiencies and osteopetrosis: European survey, 1968–1985. Lancet 2:1080, 1986

192. Fischer A: Bone marrow transplantation for immunodeficiencies and osteopetrosis. Bone Marrow Transplant, suppl. 2. 7:101, 1991

193. Dror Y, Gallagher R, Wara DW et al: Immune reconstitution in severe combined immunodeficiency disease after lectin-treated, T-cell-depleted haplocompatible bone marrow transplantation. Blood 81:2021, 1993

194. Lenarsky C, Parkman R: Bone marrow transplantation for the treatment of immune deficiency states. Bone Marrow Transplant 6:361, 1990

195. Parkman R: The application of bone marrow transplantation to the treatment of genetic diseases. Science 232:1373, 1986

196. Filipovich AH, Shapiro RS, Ramsay NKC et al: Unrelated donor bone marrow transplantation for correction of lethal congenital immunodeficiencies. Blood 80:270, 1992

197. Filipovich AH: Bone marrow transplantation from unrelated donors for congenital immunodeficiencies. Bone Marrow Transplant, suppl. 1. 11:78, 1993

198. Moen RC, Horowitz SD, Sondel PM et al: Immunologic reconstitution after haploidentical bone marrow transplantation for immune deficiency disorders: treatment of bone marrow cells with monoclonal antibody CT-2 and complement. Blood 70:664, 1987

199. Reinherz EL, Geha R, Rappeport JM et al: Reconstitution after transplantation with T-lymphocyte-depleted HLA haplotype-mismatched bone marrow for severe combined immunodeficiency. Proc Natl Acad Sci USA 79:6047, 1982

200. Fischer A, Friedrich W, Fasth A et al: Reduction of graft failure by a monoclonal antibody (Anti-LFA-1 CD11a) after HLA nonidentical bone marrow transplantation in children with immunodeficiencies, osteopetrosis, and Fanconi's anemia: a European Group for Immunodeficiency/European Group for Bone Marrow Transplantation Report. Blood 77:249, 1991

201. Shapiro RS, McClain K, Frizzera G et al: Epstein-Barr virus associated B cell lymphoproliferative disorders following bone marrow transplantation. Blood 71:1234, 1988

202. Brochstein JA, Gillio AP, Ruggiero M et al: Marrow transplantation from human leukocyte antigen-identical or haploidentical donors for correction of Wiskott-Aldrich syndrome. J Pediatr 119:907, 1991

203. Parkman R, Rappeport JM, Hellman S et al: Busulfan and total body irradiation as antihematopoietic stem cell agents in the preparation of patients with congenital bone marrow disorders for allogeneic bone marrow transplantation. Blood 64:852, 1984

204. Rumelhart SL, Trigg ME, Horowitz SD et al: Monoclonal antibody T-cell-depleted HLA-haploidentical bone marrow transplantation for Wiskott-Aldrich syndrome. Blood 75:1031, 1990

205. Filipovich AH, Jyonouchi H, Loechelt B et al: Non-sibling bone marrow transplantation for congenital disorders associated with lethal hemophagocytic lymphohistiocytoses. Blood, suppl. 80.:333a, 1992

206. Hobbs JR, Monteil M, McCluskey DR et al: Chronic granulomatous disease 100% corrected by displacement bone marrow transplantation from a volunteer unrelated donor. Eur J Pediatr 151:806, 1992

207. LeDeist F, Blanche S, Keable H et al: Successful HLA nonidentical bone marrow transplantation in three patients with the leukocyte adhesion deficiency. Blood 74:512, 1989

208. Stoll M, Freund M, Schmid H et al: Allogeneic bone marrow transplantation for Langerhans' cell histiocytosis. Cancer 66:284, 1990

209. Lucarelli G, Galimberti M, Polchi P et al: Bone marrow transplantation in thalassemia. Hematol Oncol Clin North Am 5:549, 1991

210. Lucarelli G: For debate: bone marrow transplantation for severe thalassaemia: "the view from Pesaro." Br J Haematol 78:300, 1991

211. Nesci S, Manna M, Andreani M et al: Mixed chimerism in thalassemic patients after bone marrow transplantation. Bone Marrow Transplant 10:143, 1992

212. Weatherall DJ: For debate: bone marrow transplantation for severe thalassaemia: "to be or not to be." Br J Haematol 78:301, 1991

213. Vermylen C, Cornu G, Ferster A et al: Bone marrow transplantation in sickle cell anemia: the Belgian and French experience. Blood, suppl. 1. 80:344a, 1992

214. Ferster A, DeValck C, Azzi N et al: Bone marrow transplantation for severe sickle cell anaemia. Br J Haematol 80:102, 1992

215. Kirkpatrick DV, Barrios NJ, Humbert JH: Bone marrow transplantation for sickle cell anemia. Semin Hematol 28:240, 1991

216. Gluckman E, Auerbach A, Ash RC et al: Allogeneic bone marrow transplants for Fanconi anemia. A preliminary report from the International Bone Marrow Transplant Registry. Bone Marrow Transplant, suppl. 1. 10:53, 1992

217. Alter BP: Constitutional aplastic anemia. p. 38. In Shahidi N (ed): Aplastic Anemia and Other Bone Marrow Failure Syndromes. Springer-Verlag, New York, 1990

218. Gluckman E: Bone marrow transplantation for Fanconi anemia. p. 134. In Shahidi N (ed): Aplastic Anemia and Other Bone Marrow Failure Syndromes. Springer-Verlag, New York, 1990

219. Flowers MED, Doney KC, Storb R et al: Marrow transplantation for Fanconi anemia with or without leukemic transformation: an update of the Seattle experience. Bone Marrow Transplant 9:167, 1992

220. Gluckman E: Bone marrow transplantation for Fanconi anemia. P. 714. In: Workshop on Molecular, Cellular, and Clinical Aspects of Fanconi Anemia. Exp Hematol 21:703, 1993

221. Hows JM, Chapple M, Marsh JCW et al: Bone marrow transplantation for

Fanconi's anaemia: the Hammersmith experience 1977–89. Bone Marrow Transplant 4:629, 1989

222. Harris RE, Kumar M: Bone marrow transplantation for Fanconi anemia in the United States. p. 714. In: Workshop on Molecular, Cellular, and Clinical Aspects of Fanconi Anemia. Exp Hematol 21:703, 1993

223. Gluckman E, Broxmeyer HE, Auerbach AD et al: Hematopoietic reconstitution in a patient with Fanconi's anemia by means of umbilical-cord blood from an HLA-identical sibling. N Engl J Med 321:1174, 1989

224. Broxmeyer HE, Hangoc G, Cooper S: Clinical and biological aspects of human umbilical cord blood as a source of transplantable hematopoietic stem and progenitor cells. Bone Marrow Transplant, suppl. 7. 9:7, 1992

225. Rubinstein P, Rosenfield RE, Adamson JW et al: Stored placental blood for unrelated bone marrow reconstitution. Blood 81:1679, 1993

226. Alter BP: Congenital hypoplastic anemia. p. 166. In Shahidi N (ed): Aplastic Anemia and Other Bone Marrow Failure Syndromes. Springer-Verlag, New York, 1990

227. Barrios N, Kirkpatrick D, Regueira O et al: Bone marrow transplant in Schwachman Diamond syndrome. Br J Haematol 2:337, 1990

228. Lenarsky C, Weinberg K, Guinan E et al: Bone marrow transplantation for constitutional pure red cell aplasia. Blood 71:226, 1988

229. Coccia PF, Krivit W, Cervenka J et al: Successful bone-marrow transplantation for infantile malignant osteopetrosis. N Engl J Med 302:701, 1980

230. Fasth A, Porras O, Baltorano A et al: Campath-1M antibodies for T-cell depletion of haploidentical marrow transplanted to children with malignant osteopetrosis. Prog Clin Biol Res 377:385, 1992

231. Hobbs JR, Jones KH, Shaw PJ et al: Beneficial effect of pre-transplant splenectomy on displacement bone marrow transplantation for Gaucher's syndrome. Lancet 1:1111, 1987

232. Krivit W, Shapiro EG: Bone marrow transplantation for storage diseases. p. 203. In Desnick RJ (ed): Treatment of Genetic Diseases. Churchill Livingstone, New York, 1991

233. Krivit W, Shapiro E, Hoogerbrugge PM et al: State of the art review. Bone marrow transplantation treatment for storage diseases. Bone Marrow Transplant, suppl. 1. 10:87, 1992

234. Ringden O, Groth CG, Erickson A et al: Long-term follow-up of the first successful bone marrow transplantation in Gaucher disease. Transplantation 46:66, 1988

235. Krivit W, Shapiro E, Kennedy W et al: Treatment of late infantile metachromatic leukodystrophy by bone marrow transplantation. N Engl J Med 322:28, 1990

236. Parkman R: Bone marrow transplantation for genetic diseases. Pediatr Ann 20:677, 1991

237. Aubourg P, Blanche S, Jambaque I et al: Reversal of early neurologic and neuroradiologic manifestations of X-linked adrenoleukodystrophy by bone marrow transplantation. N Engl J Med 322:1860, 1990

Complications of Bone Marrow Transplantation

30

Daniel J. Weisdorf, Wesley J. Miller, and Philip B. McGlave

INTRODUCTION

The high-dose chemotherapy and radiotherapy used in bone marrow transplantation (BMT) have intrinsic clinical toxicities that are consequences directly of the treatments and secondarily of the prolonged immunodeficiency and extended recovery process following their administration. Recognition of clinical risk factors for particular complications allows risk-specific

supportive care regimens to be designed that can reduce the overall morbidity and mortality accompanying transplantation (Table 30-1)

EARLY TRANSPLANT-ASSOCIATED COMPLICATIONS

High-dose chemotherapy and radiation regimens are used prior to transplantation for both antineoplastic and immuno-

Table 30-1. Major Noninfectious Complications of BMT

Time After BMT	Complication	Incidence (%)
Early (0–30 days)	Regimen-related toxicity	60–75
	Mucositis	
	Cyclophosphamide/radiation myocarditis or pericarditis	Rare
	Cystitis	10
	Veno-occlusive disease	5–40
	Pneumonitis	10–20
	Infections	75
	Graft failure	2–10
	Adverse drug reactions from polypharmacy	Common
Intermediate (1–3)	Acute GVHD	20–50; more frequent with nonsibling donors
Late (beyond 3 months)	Chronic GVHD	20–40
	Hypothyroidism	30–50
	Growth disturbances	Common in prepubertal children
	Sterility/hypogonadism	Common
	Cataracts	25–40
	Avascular necrosis of bone	5–15
	Malignant relapse	Variable
	Second malignancy	2–10, but total incidence is uncertain

suppressive effects. However, these treatments may also damage host tissues, resulting in significant clinical morbidity.[1] These toxicities may include oropharyngeal mucositis,[2] hepatic veno-occlusive disease (VOD), interstitial pneumonitis (IP), and hemorrhagic cystitis.[3] Each of these toxicities may simulate infections or be compounded by concurrent infections. In addition, because epithelial tissue repair may be delayed by ongoing neutropenia and local microinvasive infection, delay in hematopoietic engraftment can exaggerate and prolong these toxicities.

GRAFT FAILURE

Failure to establish hematologic engraftment (primary graft failure) and loss of an established graft (late graft failure) are serious complications of both autologous and allogeneic marrow transplantation. Delayed or poor graft function can exaggerate and prolong the risks of infection and can substantially increase peritransplant mortality. Failure to engraft can occur if insufficient stem cells are infused. Approximately 2×10^4 colony-forming cells/kg recipient weight are needed to establish autologous engraftment. This is accomplished by infusing approximately 1×10^8 bone marrow mononuclear cells/kg. Most investigators recommend infusion of a minimum of 2×10^8 cells/kg to ensure establishment of an allogeneic graft. Stem cells may be damaged by cryopreservation or by ex vivo purging, and additional cells are required if intensive purging, especially with alkylators such as 4-hydroperoxycyclophosphamide, is used.

Recipient myelofibrosis or splenomegaly may also interfere with engraftment. Splenomegaly may delay hematologic recovery,[4] presumably because both progenitors and mature blood cells are sequestered in the spleen. Prior splenectomy is associated with a shorter interval to engraftment.[5] The presence of moderate or severe myelofibrosis also delays engraftment, perhaps because of faulty homing of stem cells in the marrow microenvironment.[6,7]

Post-transplant therapy may also jeopardize engraftment. Graft failure or poor graft function with continuing pancytopenia has been associated with use of methotrexate, antithymocyte globulin (ATG), acyclovir, ganciclovir, trimethoprim/sulfamethoxazole (TMP/sulfa), and 5-fluocytosine, as well as histamine blockers. Post-transplant complications such as cytomegalovirus (CMV), mycobacterial or fungal infection, acute and chronic graft-versus-host disease (GVHD), or, rarely, Epstein-Barr virus- associated lymphoma may also compromise successful engraftment.

Allogeneic marrow transplantation, especially using unrelated or mismatched donors, poses unique problems with engraftment. Transplants between siblings matched at HLA-A, -B, and -DR loci are rarely (1–5%) associated with graft failure; however, the probability of graft failure in the related donor transplant setting increases to 10–20% with greater degrees of HLA incompatibility.[8–12] The problem is frequent (5–15%) in the unrelated donor setting, in which graft failure may occur even after transplantation from donors serologically matched at the HLA-A, -B, and -DR loci.[13,14] In some cases, failure of unrelated donor marrow to engraft may result from reactivity against important histocompatibility determinants not recognized by current serologic HLA-typing methods.[15] Early failure of an allogeneic graft may be accompanied by emergence of cytotoxic T lymphocytes of host origin,[16] presumably representing immune-mediated graft rejection.

T-lymphocyte depletion of donor marrow performed as GVHD prophylaxis can also adversely affect engraftment, even from matched sibling donors.[8,12,17–19] Ex vivo marrow manipulation may deplete stem cells. Alternatively, T-cell derived soluble factors that support engraftment may not be available after T-lymphocyte depletion.[20] Correction of this deficiency by preservation of specific T-cell subsets in the graft is under study.

The availability of recombinant human growth factors such as colony-stimulating factor-granulocyte (CSF-G) and CSF-granulocyte/macrophage (GM), which stimulate myelopoiesis, has revolutionized the treatment of graft failure.[21] Of patients experiencing poor graft function, 50–60% will have a myelopoietic response within 14–21 days after initiation of growth factor therapy, although patients receiving purged autografts may be less likely to respond. Clinical trials testing the relative merits of different growth factors, growth factor combinations, and dose schedules are under way. These studies may resolve the possibilities that growth factors may stimulate either residual host cells (augmenting mixed chimerism) or residual myeloid leukemia cells (increasing the risks of relapse). Currently available growth factors increase peripheral blood leukocytes but have no major effect on platelet recovery.[22] Limited experience suggests the possible value of erythropoietin in reducing red cell transfusion needs.[23]

A second stem cell infusion may be useful if graft failure occurs.[24] In the case of a failed autograft, infusion of previously harvested and frozen marrow or peripheral blood cells will frequently re-establish a graft. Procurement and storage of "back-up" stem cells should be considered in the case of autograft protocols in which a high rate of graft failure is anticipated. In the case of marrow failure after related donor transplant, a second infusion of donor marrow (sometimes after reconditioning with reduced doses of cytotoxic agents or after further immunosuppression with ATG, corticosteroids, or cyclosporine) may allow successful engraftment.

The incidence of graft failure after unrelated donor transplant is high and poses special problems.[8,13,25] Unrelated donors may not be available for a second donation or may not have recovered sufficiently from the first harvest to undergo marrow extraction. Even if the unrelated donor is willing to undergo a second harvest, delays of >4 weeks from the time of request may occur. For these reasons, it is prudent to store autologous marrow stem cells from patients undergoing unrelated donor transplantation.

HOST DEFENSE DEFECTS

Multiple immunologic deficiencies are induced by marrow transplantation (Table 30-2). Mucocutaneous barriers to invasion of colonizing pathogens are disrupted. Early neutropenia and hypogammaglobulinemia further compromise the ability to eliminate these organisms.[26] Severe cellular immune dysfunction, including T-cell lymphopenia and anergy persist for some months after engraftment and are usually prolonged in patients with ongoing GVHD. Interestingly, natural killer cell activity regenerates much earlier, often by 4–8 weeks post-transplant.[27,28]

In the early post-transplant period, nearly all patients develop fever, although infectious pathogens are identified in only 50% of patients. Fevers may also be due to tissue inflammation (oropharyngeal or enteric mucositis), transfusions, amphotericin, or other drug fever. During initial neutropenia, the most common infections identified are due to aerobic bacteria (frequently coagulase-negative staphylococci, viridans streptococci, and enteric gram-negative bacilli). Colonizing yeasts also invade because of neutropenia and disruption of normal host flora, thus leading to systemic mycotic infections in 10–15% of patients.[29,30]

Prophylactic strategies may include suppressive antibiotics such as vancomycin, quinolones, TMP/sulfa. In some centers, a pathogen-free environment with laminar flow isolation, gut sterilization, special diets, and broad-spectrum prophylactic antibiotics are used to reduce risks of infection. However, these intensive isolation measures are both cumbersome and expensive and have not proved helpful in preventing early post-transplant mortality. Newer antifungal agents, including fluconazole, have been strikingly effective in preventing systemic candidiasis, although resistant species (Candida krusei or Torulopsis glabrata) have emerged as secondary pathogens and may require additional attention.[31]

Treatment of fever in the neutropenic transplant recipient requires strategies similar to those that have been effective in leukemia patients.[32] Broad-spectrum antibacterial coverage should be initiated early. Patients with persistent unexplained fever, particularly those colonized with yeasts, should receive empiric amphotericin. Repeated vigorous investigation to identify sources of infection, even for fever recurring after initial defervescence, is essential. In many centers, third-generation cephalosporins and aminoglycosides have been effective in treating the most common gram-negative enteric bacilli (Escherichia coli, Klebsiella spp., Enterobacter spp., and Pseudomonas spp.). However, resistant gram-negative pathogens, including Citrobacter spp., Acinetobacter, and Xanthomonas spp., have emerged in recent years as secondary pathogens in the antibiotic-exposed neutropenic population. Institutional antibiotic sensitivity profiles must guide empiric and therapeutic antibiotic choices and should, of course, be individualized based on specific pathogenic isolates and their sensitivities.

Infection with invasive fungal organisms remains a significant hazard despite the use of protected environments, high-efficiency particular air filters and reverse isolation.[33] Up to 10% of transplant recipients may develop invasive fungal infections, usually with Aspergillus spp. but Fusarium, Alternaria, and other less common isolates have been reported. Therefore, aggressive and repeated evaluation for mycotic infection, particularly in the persistently febrile neutropenic host, is essential, along with early initiation of amphotericin. Liposomal amphotericin preparations, itraconazole, or growth factors designed to accelerate neutrophil recovery or activate inflammatory phagocytes (CSF-GM, CSF-G, CSF-M) have all been proposed as newer therapies for fungal infection, but their specific role and value is as yet unclear.

All categories of infection are seen more frequently in allogeneic transplant recipients, in whom immune reconstitution (even after resolution of neutropenia) is delayed. Chronic GVHD (see the section Graft-versus-Host Disease) is accompanied by persistent hypogammaglobulinemia, cellular immune dysfunction, and a continuing risk of infection with bacterial, fungal, and viral pathogens.[34] Late infections may include varicella-zoster virus[35,36] (usually dermatomal shingles that may disseminate); encapsulated bacterial infections (pneumococcus or Haemophilus influenzae), suggesting an immunologic defect similar to that seen with hypo- or asplenia; and Pneumocystis carinii pneumonia (PCP).[37–39] These all are common in the late (3–12 months) post-transplant period and require additional prophylaxis or prompt therapy, or both, especially in allograft recipients with chronic GVHD.

VENO-OCCLUSIVE DISEASE

VOD is a serious liver disorder complicating ≤50% of marrow transplants.[40] Signs of VOD usually occur within 1 month of marrow infusion but may be recognized much sooner, even during administration of the preparative regimen.[41] Clinical evidence of VOD includes hyperbilirubinemia, hepatomegaly, ascites, and weight gain.[42,43] VOD is an hepatotoxic lesion involving obstruction of small, intrahepatic venules and damage to the surrounding centrilobular hepatocytes and sinusoids.[44] Concentric fibrosis with obliteration of the hepatic venules, fibrosis of the centrilobular zone, and atrophy of adjacent hepatocytes may occur.[44] Deposition of fibronectin and factor VIII/von Willebrand factor at the site of the damaged endothelium may be associated with activation of the coagulation system and subsequent postsinusoidal obstruction.[42,45,46] Such changes are often associated with depressed plasma protein-C levels[47] and may be associated with other evidence of procoagulant activity, including depressed factor VIII and antithrombin III levels as well as elevated fibrinogen levels.[44,48,49] Tumor necrosis factor-α levels are elevated in VOD[50,51] and may be causally related to endothelial damage.

VOD can result in encephalopathy or renal, pulmonary, or multiorgan failure.[43,44,52] The mortality of VOD is highly variable in different series, perhaps due to differing stringency of diagnostic criteria,[43,44,53] but severe VOD is often fatal within several weeks of onset.[43,52]

Table 30-2. Host Defense Defects After BMT

Time After BMT	Immune Defects	Major Infections

Early (0–30 days)	Mucosal and skin injury
	Neutropenia
		Aerobic bacteria
		  Gram-positive, especially
		    coagulase-negative
		    staphylococci, viridans
		    streptococci
		  Gram-negative bacilli
		Fungi
		  Candida spp.
		  Molds
		  (Aspergillus spp.)
		Viruses
		  Herpes simplex virus

Intermediate (1–3 months)	T-cell dysfunction
	Hypogammaglobulinemia
	Acute GVHD
		Fungi, molds, Candida spp.
		P. carinii
		Viruses
		  Cytomegalovirus
		Encapsulated bacteria,
		  pneumococci, H. influenzae

Late (3–12 months)	Slow T-cell reconstitution Chronic GVHD	P. carinii Varicella-zoster virus Encapsulated bacteria Cytomegalovirus

AN APPROACH TO TRANSPLANT-RELATED INFECTIOUS COMPLICATIONS

A typical comprehensive regimen for BMT patients has all patients nursed in single, high-efficiency particulate air-filtered, positive-air-pressure, sealed rooms with strict hand washing as the primary protective isolation measure. All patients should receive TMP/sulfa and fluconazole daily, and parenteral vancomycin may be used soon after marrow infusion. Fevers occurring during the initial conditioning and neutropenic period are first treated with a semisynthetic penicillin plus an aminoglycoside or with ceftazidime for patients receiving cyclosporine. After 72 hours of unexplained fever, patients should be treated with empiric amphotericin (0.5 mg/kg/day or 0.3 mg/kg/day in patients receiving cyclosporine), but amphotericin should be initiated earlier and in higher doses in those patients colonized with yeasts or with lesions suspicious for invasive mycotic infection (sinusitis or nodular pulmonary lesions).

Herpes simplex virus-seropositive patients require acyclovir to prevent viral reactivation. CMV-seronegative patients receive seronegative or leukocyte-depleted (by filtration) blood products, and CMV-seropositive patients should receive antiviral suppression with ganciclovir and perhaps with intravenous immunoglobulin.

Antiinfection prophylaxis later in the course includes oral fluconazole or mycostatin until day 100 for all patients and ongoing anticandidal therapy for patients being treated for continuing GVHD. All patients receive pneumocystis prophylaxis for 1 year post-BMT (TMP/sulfa double strength bid 2 days/wk or aerosolized pentamidine 300 mg once monthly).

Patients with ongoing GVHD receive continuing candida and pneumocystis prophylaxis until 1 month after discontinuation of all immunosuppression and in addition receive daily penicillin or erythromycin for protection against pneumococcal bacteremia.

Establishing a definite diagnosis is difficult. Most investigators require two of three clinical criteria, including jaundice, hepatomegaly, or ascites occurring within 2 weeks of marrow infusion.[40,42,43,53] However, other causes of hyperbilirubinemia and weight gain early after transplant (e.g., drugs [especially cyclosporine, TMP/sulfa, methotrexate, or estrogens], capillary leak, and salt and colloid overloading) complicate the differential diagnosis. Percutaneous or transabdominal needle biopsy of the liver is extremely hazardous in thrombocytopenic marrow transplant recipients and should be avoided.[54] Transvenous biopsies may provide sufficient histologic material for diagnosis and may allow determination of hepatic wedge pressure product (>10 mm is associated with VOD)[55] but may be associated with hemorrhagic complications as well.[55–57] Ultrasound Doppler flow studies demonstrating reversal of portal flow or a higher portal vein resistive index have been suggested as noninvasive means of confirming the diagnosis, but their validity has not been established.[58–60]

Risk factors associated with development of VOD include a history of pretransplant hepatitis, intensive preparative regimens, increased radiation dose and dose rate, and increased busulfan dose.[1,40,41,43,52,61–65] VOD may also be more frequent following mismatched related or unrelated donor transplants.[40,41]

Effective methods for prevention and treatment of VOD have not been defined. Promising approaches include preventive therapy with low-dose heparin,[66–68] prostaglandin E,[69] or pentoxifylline (a TNF-α blocking agent).[70] Recombinant tissue plasminogen activator has been used successfully to treat established VOD,[71,72] as has administration of urokinase,[73] although both agents are associated with increased risk of hemorrhage.

INTERSTITIAL PNEUMONITIS

IP is a common and frequently fatal complication, affecting ≤35% of allogeneic marrow recipients,[74,75] although recent advances in supportive care may substantially reduce this risk.[26] It is characterized by diffuse, nonbacterial interstitial inflammation. Risk factors reported in association with IP include (1) prolonged methotrexate therapy for GVHD prophylaxis, (2) age >21, (3) severe GVHD, (4) >6 months from the diagnosis of hematologic disease until transplant, (5) <100% Karnofsky pre-BMT performance score, and (6) radiation dose rate >4 cGy/min.[75] Remarkably, when none of these factors was present, the reported risk of IP was 8%, and that risk rose to 94% when all six were present. It has been hypothesized that unrelated donor transplantation is more immunosuppressive and is thus associated with more severe opportunistic infections and greater risk of IP, but this has not been rigorously investigated.

The course of IP is often catastrophic, presenting acutely with rapidly progressive tachypnea, dyspnea, hypoxemia, and hemodynamic compromise. Therefore, therapeutic intervention must frequently occur before the return of definitive diagnostic tests, and must be initiated based on the assessment of clinical risk factors, associated clinical clues, and clinical setting (especially the type of transplant and the time of onset).

Infectious Causes

Cytomegalovirus Infection

Risk Factors

IP due to CMV is the most common cause of IP (50% of all cases).[76] Prevention of CMV pneumonia as well as other manifestations (enteritis, hepatitis, retinitis) depends on an understanding of risk factors and institution of specific preventive measures.

Seropositive Recipients. The most powerful risk factor predisposing to CMV infection is seropositivity of the recipient.[77,78] Clinical observations strongly suggest that reactivation of latent CMV is the most important mechanism resulting in CMV disease, although the virologic and molecular confirmation of this suspicion has been difficult. The approach to CMV prevention in the seropositive patient must include chemo- or immunoprophylaxis, or both. An additional role for preventing exogenous exposure (through choosing seronegative bone marrow or blood donors) has not been proved. Chemoprophylaxis has been very useful in preventing CMV pneumonia among seropositive recipients. The use of acyclovir was associated with a decrease in CMV pneumonia incidence from 40% to 19% among seropositive recipients,[79] while ganciclovir given prophylactically,[80,81] or when administered at the time of viremia[82] or recovery of virus by bronchoalveolar lavage (BAL)[83] from asymptomatic patients has reduced the incidence of CMV pneumonia to <5%. Ganciclovir induced significant neutropenia in these trials and sometimes secondary sepsis as well. Intravenous immunoglobulin may also be useful in reducing CMV infections, perhaps through its effect in reducing risks of GVHD.[26,74]

Seronegative Recipients. It is clear that nearly all CMV infections in seronegative recipients are the result of exogenous exposure (primary CMV infection), either from a seropositive bone marrow donor or from cellular blood products from seropositive donors. Noncellular blood products do not transmit CMV.[84] Delivery of only CMV-seronegative blood products to seronegative recipients reduces the risk of CMV infection to <5% and nearly eliminates the risk of CMV pneumonia.[85,86] Unfortunately, the demand for "CMV-safe" blood is greater than the supply of seronegative blood donors at most centers. Excellent clinical and laboratory data point to leukocytes as the carriers of infectious CMV in blood products, and preliminary studies suggest that removal of white blood cells from transfused unscreened products by sedimentation or filtration will be an effective alternative in prevention of primary CMV infections.[87–89] The frequent use of intravenous immunoglobulin for CMV prevention[90] has largely been supplanted by delivery of "CMV-safe" blood products to seronegative patients.

Autologous Recipients. A second powerful risk factor for CMV pneumonia is allogeneic (as compared to autologous) BMT.[91] Enright et al.[91] reported CMV pneumonia complicating the course in 12% of >400 allogeneic recipients, but only 3% of 229 autologous recipients. However, CMV pneumonia was as severe in autologous as in allogeneic recipients, with a high case-fatality rate. Other studies have also defined a similar incidence of CMV pneumonia among autologous recipients[92] or have shown delayed engraftment among autologous recipients developing CMV infection.[93] Thus, prevention of CMV infection through use of noninfective blood products (for seronegative recipients) or chemoprophylaxis (for seropositive recipients) is still indicated. Viremia or recovery of virus from BAL fluid should be likewise be treated aggressively.

Viremia. Post-BMT CMV viremia is a strong predictor of CMV pneumonia[94] and should probably be treated regardless of the patient's previous risk group. CMV pneumonia follows 60% of asymptomatic viremias within 14 days (median). Treatment of viremia with ganciclovir can reduce the incidence of CMV pneumonia to 5%.[82]

Diagnosis of CMV Pneumonia

CMV pneumonia usually presents as an interstitial pneumonitis associated with fever and hypoxia. While lung biopsy showing CMV inclusions is the gold standard for diagnosis of CMV pneumonia, shell vial culture of BAL fluid is positive in most cases of CMV pneumonia[95] and is a less risky approach to diagnosis. Shell vial culture of CMV from BAL is not, however, specific to CMV pneumonia and is frequently positive in asymptomatic seropositive individuals who are shedding CMV in oral or respiratory secretions without pneumonia.[96–98] Despite this lack of specificity, even in asymptomatic individuals, finding CMV in BAL is a strong predictor for development of CMV pneumonia and should be treated. The practical approach is to use the combination of a compatible clinical syndrome plus either BAL direct staining or shell vial cultures to diagnose CMV pneumonia. If BAL is undertaken for other indications and CMV is found coincidentally, it should be treated to prevent development of clinical CMV pneumonia.

Therapy for CMV Pneumonia

CMV pneumonia should be diagnosed and treated as promptly as possible. If patients are already respirator dependent at the time of institution of therapy, therapy is nearly always ineffective, and mortality is nearly 100%.[91] The combined use of ganciclovir and immunoglobulin has been the most successful treatment for CMV pneumonia, with resolution in 50–75% of patients (non-respirator dependent).[91,99–101] Prolonged therapy (≤2 months) with the combination is indicated, since shorter treatment regimens have been associated with recurrence of CMV pneumonia.[92]

APPROACH TO PREVENTION OF AND THERAPY FOR CMV

Prevention

1. *Seronegative recipient with seronegative donor (allogeneic and autologous):* Transfuse only seronegative blood products. Leukocyte depletion by filtration may be a reasonable alternative.
2. *Seronegative recipient with seropositive donor (allogeneic):* Deliver only CMV-safe blood products (seronegative or leukocyte-depleted), but administer chemoimmunoprophylaxis as well as prevent reactivation of endogenous virus.
3. *Seropositive recipients:* Prophylaxis with acyclovir appears to be useful. Use of immunoglobulin may be beneficial (especially by modulation of GVHD). Seronegative blood products have no proven role. Ganciclovir is highly effective when given prophylactically, but is toxic to the bone marrow. Patients who must interrupt the course of ganciclovir because of leukopenia are at risk of developing CMV pneumonia. Ganciclovir is currently the best prophylaxis in high-risk patients but probably is not indicated for autologous recipients.

Therapy

1. *Asymptomatic infections (all types of transplant):* Ganciclovir treatment of asymptomatic CMV infection detected by either BAL or blood culture is recommended to prevent development of CMV pneumonia. Intensive treatment followed by a maintenance phase of 5 days/wk therapy is necessary. Asymptomatic viruria suggests a need for close follow-up and for serial blood viral cultures, but does not usually require therapy.
2. *CMV pneumonia:* Ganciclovir in combination with immunoglobulin is the recommended regimen. This should be instituted as promptly as possible. Once the disease has progressed to cause respiratory failure and ventilator dependence, therapeutic success is rare.

No Therapy

The following situations are important negatives in which ganciclovir is not indicated for empiric therapy of interstitial pneumonitis; in these circumstances CMV pneumonia is unlikely to be present.

1. Seronegative recipients with seronegative bone marrow and blood donors.
2. Any patient in whom BAL is negative by direct staining and shell vial culture. However, BAL CMV studies do have a small (<5%) false-negative rate so CMV IP cannot be absolutely excluded.

Fungal Infections

Pulmonary fungal infections may be associated with an interstitial pattern, alveolar infiltrates, or nodules on chest radiograph.[33,102] Aspergillus pneumonia has been very difficult to treat, partly due to the difficulty in making the diagnosis antemortem.[33] Aspergillus infections may occur early post-BMT (during the neutropenic phase) or later, especially complicating the immunosuppression associated with acute or chronic GVHD.[33,103,104] Allogeneic BMT (versus autologous), prolonged neutropenia, and GVHD all predispose to aspergillus infections.[104,105] Exposure to construction sites has also been associated with aspergillus infections.[106] Measures to prevent aspergillus include prophylactic low-dose amphotericin, inhaled amphotericin, early empiric use of amphotericin, and close attention to air filtration in patient care areas, although the relative effectiveness of these approaches has not yet been defined.

Nasal and bronchial washings for aspergillus may be inadequately sensitive,[107,108] and lung biopsy may be required to obtain a definitive diagnosis. The pattern of the infiltrate may be helpful diagnostically and can sometimes be better defined by computed tomography scan of the chest.[109] Persistent high-grade fever that does not improve on antibacterials is often assumed to be due to fungal infection.

Although it is unquestionably the treatment of choice for fungal infections, the use of high-dose amphotericin may be limited by renal dysfunction. Novel approaches to treatment of fungal pneumonia are currently under investigation, including liposomal amphotericin, itraconazole, and CSF-M.

Pneumocystis Carinii Pneumonia

P. carinii causes IP, typically bilateral, with a "butterfly" pattern on radiograph.[37] While the 5–15% risk of PCP has largely been eliminated by the use of TMP/sulfa given for 2 consecutive days/wk,[110] TMP/sulfa is not tolerated by all patients due to allergy or to bone marrow depression by the drug. Recently the use of inhaled pentamidine (300 mg every 4 weeks) or dapsone has offered effective alternatives.[38,111] TMP/sulfa therapy virtually eliminates PCP from the differential diagnosis, but only if patient compliance with the prophylaxis is certain. Inhaled pentamidine or dapsone, although partially effective, do not totally eliminate the risk of PCP. PCP can be diagnosed by cytologic evaluation of silver-stained preparations (BAL) cells or sputum. It is effectively treated by high-dose TMP/sulfa or parenteral pentamidine. Supplemental steroid therapy has improved therapeutic results in acquired immunodeficiency syndrome patients[112] and may be helpful after BMT as well. Prophylaxis against PCP should be continued during the period of immunosuppression (6–12 months after BMT) and for the duration of any therapy for chronic GVHD. PCP has been recognized as late as 1–3 years after BMT, especially following relapse of a malignancy that is not rapidly fatal (e.g., chronic myeloid leukemia or low-grade lymphoma).[37] Ongoing prophylaxis for such patients should be considered.

Respiratory Syncytial Virus

Respiratory syncytial virus (RSV) is a potentially fatal cause of IP[113] that is seasonal, occurring most frequently in the fall and winter months. RSV should be suspected if the patient has had nasal congestion and if RSV has been frequently recognized either in the community or in the hospital. Diagnosis may be made by rapid antigen testing on nasal washings or BAL specimens. Due to the possibility of horizontal transmission, patients with RSV should be isolated. Treatment is with inhaled aerosolized ribavirin (usually 6 g/day) for 3–7 days.[113,114] A similar but nonseasonal syndrome due to parainfluenza virus has been described.[115] No rapid antigen test for parainfluenza is available, and its response to ribavirin therapy is uncertain.

Noninfectious Causes

Idiopathic Interstitial Pneumonitis

Idiopathic IP (IIP) is a diagnosis of exclusion based on typical findings and ruling out infectious causes. Its timing is somewhat earlier than other causes of IP,[74,76,116] typically occurring within the first 2–7 weeks post-BMT. Interestingly, the recognized clinical risk factors for IIP have been similar to those for IP and include (1) extensive pretransplant chemotherapy, (2) high-dose cyclophosphamide, (3) total body irradiation (TBI; increased by higher total dose and dose rate), (4) blood transfusions, (5) administration of methotrexate, and (6) GVHD.[117]

The observation that IIP is as frequent among syngeneic as among allogeneic recipients[118] suggests that immunosuppression is less of a risk factor for IIP than it is for infectious IP. Clinical observations support a toxic cause of IIP,[117] and radiation-induced lung damage appears to be the major contributor.[119] These clinical observations are supported by animal studies suggesting that irradiation is the major contributor to post-BMT lung damage,[120] while cyclophosphamide makes only a minor contribution.[121] In addition, in controlled trials, higher-dose TBI has increased the incidence of IIP.[65] Effective therapy has not been established, although high-dose corticosteroid therapy is often administered.

Diffuse Alveolar Hemorrhage

Diffuse alveolar hemorrhage (DAH) has been recently recognized, primarily in autologous bone marrow recipients.[122,123] It is likely that some allogeneic BMT recipients develop a similar complication, which, because of its early timing, has been included with the diagnosis of IIP. Diagnostic criteria include (1) diffuse consolidation on chest radiograph, (2) hypoxia requiring oxygen supplementation, and (3) progressively bloody BAL on aliquots from more than one lung segment.[122] Although alveolar hemorrhage is the critical diagnostic criterion, the most typical radiologic findings at presentation are bilateral interstitial infiltrates, with alveolar infiltrates developing later in the course.[124] DAH presents early (within the first 2 weeks post-BMT) with dyspnea, hypoxia, and cough, but usually not overt hemoptysis. This syndrome is very serious, with a reported mortality of 77–100%. Treatment includes correction of any coagulopathy and aggressive ventilatory support. Limited, although uncontrolled, experience suggests that high-dose corticosteroids may be effective therapy for this syndrome.[125]

It seems likely that DAH is a subcategory of IIP and is due to lung injury from chemotherapy and irradiation. Two observations suggest that neutrophils may contribute to its pathogenesis by causing inflammatory damage to injured lung cells. First, the appearance of DAH often occurs at the time of neutrophil recovery. Second, when BAL was undertaken prior to autologous BMT for 123 patients (of whom 14 eventually developed DAH), the presence of >20% polymorphonuclear leukocytes or >0% eosinophils prior to BMT both predicted development of DAH (43% if both were present, 4% if neither).[126]

GRAFT-VERSUS-HOST DISEASE

Acute GVHD develops in the first 1–3 months after allogeneic transplantation and can involve the skin, the liver, or the gastrointestinal tract. It manifests in the skin as a maculopapular dermatitis, which when severe can lead to large bullae or can even resemble toxic epidermal necrolysis. GVHD can produce cholestatic hepatitis with marked elevation of serum bilirubin and alkaline phosphatase, but usually only mild transaminase alterations. Hepatocellular function (protein synthesis, coagulation factor production) is not impaired. In the intestine, upper gastrointestinal tract GVHD can produce nausea, vomiting, and anorexia,[127] while small bowel and colon GVHD produce large-volume secretory diarrhea.[128] Histologically, acute GVHD manifests as single cell degeneration and necrosis in the "stem cell" compartment of the skin epidermis or the intestinal or biliary epithelium. This yields basal epidermal cell vacuolization with

APPROACH TO INTERSTITIAL PNEUMONITIS

The presentation of IP following BMT should be looked on as an urgent medical situation; empiric, broad-spectrum therapy must be initiated. The choice of therapy is influenced by the following:

1. *Timing:* Within the first 3 weeks following BMT, IP is more likely to be idiopathic (including diffuse alveolar hemorrhage) or fungal than caused by CMV. Beyond 6 weeks, idiopathic pneumonitis is unusual, and the etiology is more likely infectious. PCP is rare beyond 1 year after BMT. RSV infections are seasonal (fall and winter), and community outbreaks may be prevalent.

2. *CMV serology and prophylaxis:* If a seronegative recipient has received seronegative marrow and noninfective (seronegative or leukocyte-depleted) blood, CMV pneumonia is unusual. Seropositive recipients are at higher risk, although with ganciclovir prophylaxis the risk is markedly reduced. Other prophylactic regimens for CMV such as acyclovir $\pm$ intravenous IgG have still been associated with significant risk of serious CMV infection in the seropositive recipient.

3. *Prolonged neutropenia:* This factor is associated with infectious etiologies, particularly with fungal pneumonias.

4. *Type of BMT:* DAH (early post-BMT) has been reported more frequently in autologous recipients. CMV pneumonia is unusual (2–3%) in autologous recipients, although it still has a high case-fatality rate. All infectious causes are more common following allogeneic BMT. More intensive conditioning regimens (e.g., higher dose TBI, BCNU) are associated with more frequent pneumonitis.

5. *Compliance and prophylaxis:* A thorough assessment of what the patient has actually been receiving (e.g., TMP/sulfa, penicillin, CMV prophylaxis, transfusions outside at the BMT center, etc.) is critical to assess risk.

6. *Chest radiograph:* The pattern and distribution of the infiltrate may narrow the differential diagnosis. Cardiac enlargement or pleural effusions may suggest pulmonary edema. A chest computed tomography scan may be useful, especially if nodularity or cavitary lesions (possibly fungal) are suspected.

7. *Epidemiology:* What are the etiologies of other recent cases of IP? This may be most helpful with infections that are horizontally transmitted (RSV) or have common environmental risk factors (aspergillus associated with construction).

8. *Bronchoalveolar lavage:* BAL can be extremely useful for establishing a specific diagnosis or excluding others. CMV rarely causes pneumonia without positive BAL findings (either direct staining of CMV-associated antigens in BAL cells or shell vial culture). BAL also usually detects RSV and pneumocystis and can identify alveolar bleeding. It is less sensitive for fungal pneumonias.

9. *Lung biopsy:* Although this is the gold standard for definitive diagnosis of most of the possible causes of IP, it can often be avoided through use of the clinical data listed above. It may be necessary for diagnosis of fungal pneumonias, pulmonary changes associated with chronic GVHD (lymphocytic bronchitis or bronchiolitis obliterans), or IIP.

10. *Ventilator therapy:* Progressive respiratory failure after BMT is rarely (<5%) reversible, especially in adults. While aggressive diagnostic and therapeutic measures are essential, some centers offer patients (and their families) the option of foregoing mechanical ventilatory support if survival is not expected. Preliminary discussion of this possible complication in pretransplant patient counseling may facilitate decision making if respiratory failure does occur.

---

dyskeratosis, exocytosis, and when more advanced, dermal/epidermal clefting with bullae formation. These changes are accompanied by a modest lymphoid infiltrate, typically of CD8+ T lymphocytes. Similarly, the basal cells of the intestinal glands or the colonic crypts show single epithelial cell degeneration, satellite (lymphocyte) cell necrosis, and sometimes crypt abscesses progressing to mucosal sloughing. In hepatic portal tracts, single cells of bile ducts are affected first, with eventual disruption or disappearance, or both, of the bile ducts.

Current understanding of the pathogenesis of GVHD suggests that alloreactive donor T lymphocytes recognize histocompatibility antigens on host cells and initiate secondary inflammatory injury leading to the clinical symptoms of GVHD.[128] The antigenic targets of GVHD are not well defined. Developing even after MHC-identical sibling donor allografts,[129,130] the frequency of GVHD suggests that minor histocompatibility antigens may be involved. In addition, antigens expressed after tissue damage from chemoradiotherapy conditioning or by environmental pathogens can serve as immune targets for GVHD. GVHD is more frequent and more severe in recipients of partially matched or histoincompatible transplants,[13,131] suggesting that MHC-encoded molecules may be the prime antigenic targets initiating the alloreactive T-cell response. However, autologous recognition of host tissue antigens may also occur

(autologous GVHD) because of poor immune regulation, which can be exaggerated by cyclosporine therapy.[132] This initiating T-cell response leads to a modest lymphoid infiltrate of primarily cytotoxic (CD8+) T cells within the injured tissue targets. However, recent evidence strongly suggests that secondary cytokine release (possibly including tumor necrosis factor and interleukin-1) may amplify and exaggerate the clinical severity of GVHD.[133–135]

Acute GVHD develops more commonly in older patients, in those with previously alloimmunized donors (usually parous females), or in recipients of marrow from other than a histocompatible related donor. Even with current immunoprophylaxis, 25–50% of patients receiving HLA-identical sibling donor marrow[129,130] and 70–90% of patients receiving unrelated donor marrow develop GVHD.[9,13,14] The diagnosis is established by the clinical symptomatology (diffuse maculopapular skin rash, cholestasis, or watery diarrhea) but frequently requires histologic confirmation to distinguish it from other frequent toxicities in the early post-transplant period (e.g., hypersensitivity drug rash, drug-induced cholestasis, or infectious enteritis). Severe GVHD (clinical grade III–IV) is associated with poor survival because of the ongoing morbidity and the debility of chronic illness, because of progression to chronic GVHD, and, most importantly, because of secondary opportunistic infection with bacterial, viral, and fungal pathogens.[136,137] GVHD of lesser severity (grade I–II) is less often life-threatening, may be accompanied by the graft-versus leukemia effect, and may offer protection against malignant relapse.

Prophylaxis

The most effective techniques for GVHD prevention have involved depletion of donor T lymphocytes from the donor marrow inoculum, most often coupling immunologic recognition (monoclonal anti-T-cell antibodies) with depletion techniques (immunomagnetic beads, complement cytotoxicity, or toxin immunoconjugates). Although vigorous T-lymphocyte depletion prevents acute GVHD, it also increases the risk of graft failure and neoplastic relapse after transplantation (due to the absence of the graft-versus-leukemia effect).[138–140]

Pharmacologic immunosuppression administered in the first several months after transplantation can prevent or blunt the initiating T-cell recognition and proliferative response that triggers GVHD and can allow the development of immune tolerance and complete lymphohematopoietic chimerism. Methotrexate, corticosteroids, ATG, and, most importantly, cyclosporine have been used for prophylaxis of GVHD and have successfully reduced both the frequency and severity of clinical GVHD.[131,141–143] The balance of complications has made it impossible to demonstrate a clear survival advantage for the use of either T-depletion or pharmacologic GVHD prophylaxis. It is clear, however, that some form of GVHD prophylaxis is needed following allogeneic BMT.

Therapy for Acute GVHD

Therapy for acute GVHD requires both immunosuppression (to blunt the T-cell-induced inflammatory tissue injury) and appropriate supportive care. Therapy should be intensified in order to achieve a complete or partial response to GVHD therapy because effective treatment of acute GVHD can both protect against chronic GVHD and improve survival. Limited area (<50%) skin GVHD can be treated with topical cortiosteroids alone. Corticosteroids (prednisone 1–2 mg/kg/day) ATG, and cyclosporine (for those not receiving it as prophylaxis) have been the mainstays of immunosuppressive therapy for GVHD.[136,137,144] Steroids produce a complete or partial response in approximately 40% of patients, while salvage therapy with ATG can control GVHD in 25–40% of the remainder. GVHD of lesser severity and involving only single organs responds to immunosuppressive therapy in 50–60% of patients, while only 25–30% of patients with multiorgan GVHD, especially involving the liver, respond to therapy.[136,137,145] GVHD after unrelated donor BMT may also be relatively more resistant to therapy.[146]

Newer immunosuppressive agents, including monoclonal antibodies or immunotoxins directed against T cells or inflammatory cytokines, may be used to limit the severity of GVHD.[133,134] However, in addition to effective immunosuppression, successful management of acute GVHD involves attention to supportive care in order to reduce the morbidity and opportunistic infections that accompany GVHD. Adequate nutritional support and fluid replacement for severe diarrhea are required. Avoidance of unnecessary medications can simplify the therapeutic regimen and lessen the chances of adverse drug interactions or hypersensitivity skin rashes, or both. Most importantly, infection prophylaxis directed against fungi, encapsulated bacteria, CMV, and PCP are essential elements of GVHD treatment.

Therapy for Chronic GVHD

A related syndrome, which occurs later after allotransplantation, is called chronic GVHD.[147,148] This syndrome developed in 30–40% of allograft recipients[149] and usually manifests between 50 and 200 days after transplantation. It occurs most frequently in patients with preceding acute GVHD, but may also occur in 10% of sibling allograft recipients de novo, without any preceding acute GVHD. The manifestations of chronic GVHD resemble autoimmune disease, somewhat similar to scleroderma. An inflammatory dermatitis may progress to severe dermal and periarticular fibrosis with loss of skin appendages (hair and sweat glands) as well as significant skin tightness and loss of joint flexibility. Additional manifestations may include dry eyes and dry mouth, which can resemble Sjögren syndrome clinically and histologically; enteritis with anorexia, early satiety, malabsorption, weight loss, and wasting; or severe cholestatic jaundice. Bronchiolitis obliterans occurs in ≤10% of patients with chronic GVHD.[150]

The pathogenesis of chronic GVHD may differ from acute GVHD. Autoimmune manifestations (the clinical similarity to scleroderma) and autoantibody formation (antinuclear antibodies, anti-RBC antibodies, rheumatoid factor, lupus-like anticoagulants) are frequent. In addition, the major complications of chronic GVHD include secondary infection due to hypogammaglobulinemia, severely impaired cellular immune responses (skin test anergy and hypoproliferative T-cell mitogen responses), and splenic dysfunction. This chronic inflammatory syndrome may also be accompanied by stable lymphohematopoietic engraftment, but poor myeloid function with leukopenia, anemia, and often an immune complex or autoimmune consumptive thrombocytopenia may be present.

The treatment of chronic GVHD, even more than acute GVHD, demands particular attention to prophylaxis and aggressive therapy for secondary opportunistic infection in addition to specific immunosuppressive treatment. Consequently, antibacterial, antifungal, and antiviral prophylaxis need to be administered as well as intravenous immunoglobulin support for patients manifesting persistent hypogammaglobulinemia. After the onset of chronic GVHD, 25–40% of patients die within 2 years, often of secondary infections.

Like acute GVHD the specific immunosuppressive therapy of chronic GVHD is most often corticosteroids.[151,152] However, the ongoing and long-lasting nature of the syndrome demands that reduced doses and, if possible, alternate-day steroid therapy be employed to minimize the chronic complications of corticosteroid treatment, including osteoporosis, avascular necrosis of bone,[153] cataracts, muscle wasting, hyperglycemia, and cutaneous atrophy. In addition to corticosteroids, azathioprine, cyclosporine, and newer agents, including thalidomide, have been employed to blunt the T-cell-mediated proliferative responses that sustain the autoimmune syndrome.[154] Most successful strategies for chronic GVHD, however, incorporate reduced-dose immunosuppressive treatment, aggressive antimicrobial prophylaxis, and long-term therapy for 6–9 months beyond any active GVHD symptoms followed by slow withdrawal of therapy. Much longer therapy may be required for some patients, and early withdrawal of therapy has been frequently accompanied by flares of chronic GVHD.

LATE COMPLICATIONS

Beyond the initial post-transplant period, subsequent complications result from cumulative organ injury induced by the pretransplant conditioning, from residual ill effects of any acute complications, and from ongoing immunodeficiency leading to late infections.[155] TBI, alkylating agents, and corticosteroids all contribute to the formation of cataracts, which

AN APPROACH TO GRAFT-VERSUS-HOST DISEASE

1. *Donor selection:* Lower risks of GVHD follow BMT from a genotypically identical sibling donor versus a closely matched related or an unrelated donor. Given equivalent donor-recipient histocompatibility, GVHD risks will be lower with younger donors; those who are not previously alloimmunized (by prior pregnancy or transfusion); and gender pairings other than female donor/male recipient. If the recipient is CMV seronegative, a seronegative donor will also be a better choice.

2. *GVHD prophylaxis:* Nearly complete T-lymphocyte depletion (to $<10^5$ T cells/kg recipient weight) offers the best protection against acute GVHD although outcome is compromised by greater risks of graft failure and leukemia relapse. Short-course methotrexate (15 mg/m^2 IV on day +1 and 10 mg/m^2 IV on day +3, +6, +11) plus cyclosporine (6 mg/kg IV from day −1 to day +50, then taper); or cyclosporine/steroids; or methotrexate/cyclosporine/steroids have been the most effective chemoprophylaxis regimens.[142,143]

3. *GVHD diagnosis:* Early recognition of GVHD symptoms are important in successful management. Skin biopsy to distinguish a GVHD rash from a drug eruption is advised. Nausea, vomiting, or diarrhea suggest gastrointestinal GVHD, and endoscopy is necessary to distinguish gut GVHD from infectious or peptic upper gastrointestinal symptoms or from infectious, toxic, or osmotic diarrhea.

4. *Acute GVHD treatment:* Corticosteroids (usually methylprednisolone 1–2 mg/kg/day) for several weeks and a slow tapering schedule are the usual initial therapy.[136,137,144,145]

5. *Chronic GVHD treatment:* Initial therapy with modest-dose prednisone (0.5–1 mg/kg/day) and cyclosporine followed by 9–12 months of maintenance therapy with alternate-day prednisone + cyclosporine has been widely used. Chronic GVHD induction therapy with high-dose methylprednisolone (15 mg/kg IV weekly × 6–8 weeks) can be added to this regimen. Azathioprine (1 mg/kg/day) can be used but may enhance the risks of infection without better symptom control. Adequate nutrition, vitamin and mineral supplementation, and liberal fluid intake are also important.

6. *Infection prevention during GVHD treatment:* Prophylaxis against fungi (*Candida* spp.: fluconazole 100 mg/day PO or mycostatin); encapsulated bacteria (penicillin VK 250 mg bid or erythromycin 250 mg bid if allergic); *P. carinii* (TMP/sulfa DS bid 2–3 days/wk or pentamidine 300 mg by aerosol once monthly); and CMV (dependent on serostatus) is essential during immunosuppressive therapy of GVHD (acute or chronic). Consider intravenous IgG replacement if hypogammaglobulinemia persists. Prompt and aggressive treatment of all infections is important.

replacement. Permanent sterility is expected in nearly all men and in most women undergoing transplantation,[159] although transplantation without TBI may be fertility sparing in nearly one-third of men and women. Prepubertal children may retain fertility, although secondary sexual development may be delayed.

Growth retardation is frequently seen in children receiving TBI,[160] as 40–50% of children have markedly depressed growth rates for 2 years following BMT. This may be complicated by nutritional deficiency and chronic illness, and especially by chronic GVHD. Regimens without TBI have been proposed as less likely to cause the late growth and development complications in children,[161] but definitive evidence of lesser toxicity is not available. Neurologic complications, including toxic encephalopathy, peripheral neuropathy and seizures, may result from damage due to previous high-dose therapy and radiation, neurotropic viral infections (e.g., herpes group viruses) or from cyclosporine. Destructive or inflammatory arthropathy may develop. Radiation, steroid therapy, and GVHD may produce avascular necrosis of bone[153] or periarticular contractures, which limit mobility.

Finally, pretransplant chemoradiotherapy conditioning may be carcinogenic. Secondary neoplasia may develop after BMT, especially if extensive antineoplastic therapy was administered before transplantation.[162] A sixfold higher risk of cancer for BMT recipients has been reported—mostly nonHodgkin lymphoma, but recently secondary myelodysplastic syndromes and leukemia have been seen as well.[163]

BMT survivors eventually return to full and complete functional status. Several quality of life studies have shown that by 1 year after transplantation more than three-fourths of patients are back to work, and nearly 90% of autologous BMT recipients report an above-average to excellent quality of life.[164] Allograft recipients recover more slowly, especially those >30 years of age and those with chronic GVHD, in whom ongoing physical and psychological problems delay their return to good health.[165,166]

REFERENCES

1. Bearman SI, Appelbaum FR, Buckner CD et al: Regimen-related toxicity in patients undergoing bone marrow transplantation. J Clin Oncol 6:1562, 1988
2. Weisdorf DJ, Bostrom B, Raether D et al: Oropharyngeal mucositis complicating bone marrow transplantation: prognostic factors and the effect of chlorhexidine mouth rinse. Bone Marrow Transplant 4:89, 1989
3. Sencer SF, Haake RJ, Weisdorf DJ: Hemorrhagic cystitis following bone marrow transplantation: risk factors and complications. Transplantation 56:875, 1993
4. Banaji M, Bearman SI, Buckner CD et al: The effects of splenectomy on engraftment and platelet transfusion requirements in patients with chronic myelogenous leukemia undergoing marrow tranplantation. Am J Hematol 22:275, 1986
5. Baughan ASJ, Worsley AM, McCarthy DM et al: Haematological reconstitution and severity of graft-versus-host disease after bone marrow transplantation for chronic granulocytic leukaemia: the influence of previous splenectomy. Br J Haematol 56:445, 1984
6. McGlave PB, Brunning RD, Hurd DD et al: Reversal of severe myelofibrosis and osteosclerosis following allogeneic bone marrow transplantation for chronic myelogenous leukemia. Br J Hematol 52:189, 1982
7. Rajantie J, Sale GE, Deeg HJ et al: Adverse effect of severe marrow fibrosis on hematological recovery after chemoradiotherapy and allogeneic bone marrow transplantation. Blood 67:1693, 1986
8. Ash RC, Casper JT, Chitambar CR et al: Successful allogeneic transplantation of T-cell-depleted bone marrow from closely HLA-matched unrelated donor. N Engl J Med 322:485, 1990
9. Beatty PG, Hansen JA, Longton GM et al: Marrow transplantation from HLA-matched unrelated donors for treatment of hematologic malignancies. Transplantation 51:443, 1991
10. Beatty PG, Clift RA, Mickelson EM et al: Marrow transplantation from related donors other than HLA-identical siblings. N Engl J Med 313:765, 1985
11. Anasetti C, Amos D, Beatty PG et al: Effect of HLA compatibility on en-

develop in over one-third of patients by 5 years post-transplantation and often require surgical therapy.[156] Hypothyroidism (in 30–50% of patients) and hypogonadism (60–90%) are also common.[157–159] Therefore, appropriate follow-up care should include monitoring of thyroid and gonadal function with particular attention to menopausal symptomatology and sexual dysfunction, which may be ameliorated by appropriate hormone

graftment of bone marrow transplants in patients with leukemia or lymphoma. N Engl J Med 320:197, 1989

12. Ash RC, Horowitz MM, Gale RP et al: Bone marrow transplantation from related donors other than HLA-identical siblings: effect of T cell depletion. Bone Marrow Transplant 7:443, 1991

13. Kernan NA, Bartsch G, Ash RC et al: Retrospective analysis of 462 unrelated marrow transplants facilitated by the National Marrow Donor Program. N Engl J Med 328:593, 1993

14. McGlave P, Bartsch G, Anasetti C et al: Unrelated donor bone marrow transplantation therapy for chronic myelogenous leukemia: initial experience of the National Marrow Donor Program. Blood 81:543, 1993

15. Fleishhauer K, Kernan NA, O'Reilly RJ et al: Bone marrow-allograft rejection by T-lymphocytes recognizing a single amino acid difference in HLA-B44. N Engl J Med 323:1818, 1990

16. Bordignon C, Keever CA, Small TN et al: Graft failure after T-cell-depleted human leukocyte antigen identical marrow transplants for leukemia: II. In vitro analysis of host effector mechanisms. Blood 74:2237, 1989

17. O'Reilly RJ, Collins NH, Kernan NA et al: Transplantation of marrow-depleted T cells by soybean lectin agglutination of E-rosette depletion: major histocompatibility complex-related graft resistance in leukemic transplant recipients. Transplant Proc 17:455, 1985

18. Trigg ME, Billing R, Sondel PM et al: Clinical trial depleting T lymphocytes from donor marrow for matched and mismatched allogeneic bone marrow transplants. Cancer Treat Rep 69:377, 1985

19. Bunjes D, Wiesneth M, Hertenstein B et al: Graft failure after T cell-depleted bone marrow transplantation: clinical and immunological characteristics and response to immunosuppressive therapy. Bone Marrow Transplant 6:309, 1990

20. Martin PJ: The role of donor lymphoid cells in allogeneic marrow engraftment. Bone Marrow Transplant 6:283, 1990

21. Neumanitis J, Singer JW, Buckner CD et al: Use of recombinant human granulocyte-macrophage colony-stimulating factor in graft failure after bone marrow transplantation. Blood 76:245, 1990

22. DeWitte T, Gratwohl A, Van Der Lely N et al: Recombinant human granulocyte-macrophage colony-stimulating factor accelerates neutrophil and monocyte recovery after allogeneic T-cell-depleted bone marrow transplantation. Blood 79:1359, 1992

23. Vannucchi AM, Bosi A, Grossi A et al: Stimulation of erythroid engraftment by recombinant human erythropoietin in ABO-compatible, HLA-identical, allogenic bone marrow transplant patients. Leukemia 6:215, 1992

24. Davies SM, Weisdorf DJ, Haake RJ et al: Second infusion of bone marrow for treatment of graft failure after allogeneic bone marrow transplantation. Bone Marrow Transplant 1994 (in press)

25. Davies SM, Ramsay NKC, Haake RJ et al: A comparison of engraftment in recipients of matched sibling or unrelated donor marrow allografts. Bone Marrow Transplant 13:51, 1994

26. Sullivan KM, Kopecky KJ, Jocom J et al: Immunomodulatory and antimicrobial efficacy of intravenous immunoglobulin in bone marrow transplantation. N Engl J Med 323:705, 1990

27. Wingard JR: Advances in the management of infectious complications after bone marrow transplantation. Bone Marrow Transplant 6:371, 1990

28. Lum LG: Recapitulation of immune ontogeny: a vital component for the success of bone marrow transplantation. p. 27. In Champlin R (ed): Bone Marrow Transplantation. Kluwer Academic Publishers, The Netherlands, 1990

29. Verfaillie C, Weisdorf D, Haake R et al: Candida infections in bone marrow transplant recipients. Bone Marrow Transplant 8:177, 1991

30. Goodrich JM, Reed EC, Mori M et al: Clinical features and analysis of risk factors for invasive candidal infection after marrow transplantation. J Infect Dis 164:731, 1991

31. Goodman JL, Winston DJ, Greenfield RA et al: A controlled trial of fluconazole to prevent fungal infections in patients undergoing bone marrow transplantation. N Engl J Med 236:845, 1992

32. Pizzo PA: Management of fever in patients with cancer and treatment-induced neutropenia. N Engl J Med 328:1323, 1993

33. Morrison VA, Haake RJ, Weisdorf DJ: The spectrum of non-*Candida* fungal infections following bone marrow transplantation. Medicine 72:78, 1993

34. Zaia J: Viral infections with bone marrow transplantation. Hematol Oncol Clin North Am 4:603, 1990

35. Locksley RM, Flournoy N, Sullivan KM et al: Infection with varicella-zoster after marrow transplantation. J Infect Dis 152:1172, 1985

36. Han CS, Miller W, Haake R et al: Varicella zoster infection after bone marrow transplantation: incidence, risk factors and complications. Bone Marrow Transplant 13:277, 1994

37. Tuan I-Z, Dennison D, Weisdorf D: *Pneumocystis carinii* pneumonitis following bone marrow transplantation. Bone Marrow Transplant 10:267, 1992

38. Girard P-M, Landman R, Gaudebout C et al: Dapsone-pyrimethamine compared with aerosolized pentamidine as primary prophylaxis against *Pneumocystis carinii* pneumonia and toxoplasmosis in HIV infection. N Engl J Med 328:1514, 1993

39. Hughes W, Leoung G, Kramer F et al: Comparison of atovaquone (566C80) with trimethoprim–sulfamethoxazole to treat *Pneumocystis carinii* pneumonia in patients with AIDS. N Engl J Med 328:1521, 1993

40. McDonald GB, Hinds MS, Fisher LD et al: Veno-occlusive disease of the liver and multiorgan failure after bone marrow transplantation: a cohort study of 355 patients. Ann Intern Med 118:255, 1993

41. McDonald GB, Hinds M, Fisher L et al: Liver toxicity following cytoreductive therapy for marrow transplantation: risk factors, incidence, and outcome. Hepatology 14:162A, 1991

42. Shulman HM, McDonald GB, Matthews D et al: An analysis of hepatic venocclusive disease and centrilobular hepatic degeneration following bone marrow transplantation. Gastroenterology 79:1178, 1980

43. Jones RJ, Lee KSK, Beschorner WE et al: Venocclusive disease of the liver following bone marrow transplantation. Transplantation 44:778, 1987

44. Shulman HM, Hinterberger W: Hepatic veno-occlusive disease—liver toxicity syndrome after bone marrow transplantation. Bone Marrow Transplant 10:197, 1992

45. McDonald GB, Shulman HM, Wolford JL: Liver disease after human marrow transplantation. Semin Liver Dis 7:210, 1987

46. Shulman HM, Gown AM, Nugent DJ: Hepatic veno-occlusive disease after bone marrow transplantation. Immunohistochemical identification of the material within occluded central venules. Am J Pathol 127:549, 1987

47. Faioni EM, Bearman SI, Krachmalnicoff A et al: Procoagulant imbalance due to low levels of protein C in patients with veno-occlusive disease (VOD) of the liver after marrow transplantation. Blood 78:193a, 1991

48. Harper PL, Jarvis J, Jennings I et al: Changes in the natural anticoagulants following bone marrow transplantation. Bone Marrow Transplant 5:39, 1990

49. Scrobohaci ML, Drouet L, Monem-Mansi A et al: Liver veno-occlusive disease after bone marrow transplantation: changes in coagulation parameters and endothelial markers. Thromb Res 63:509, 1991

50. Tanaka J, Imamura M, Kasai M et al: Rapid analysis of tumor necrosis factor-alpha mRNA expression during venoocclusive disease of the liver after allogeneic bone marrow transplantation. Transplantation 55:430, 1993

51. Holler E, Kolb HJ, Moller A et al: Increased serum levels of tumor necrosis factor-α precede major complications of bone marrow transplantation. Blood 75:1011, 1990

52. McDonald GB, Sharma P, Matthews DE et al: The clinical course of 53 patients with venocclusive disease of the liver after marrow transplantation. Transplantation 39:603, 1985

53. Blostein MD, Paltiel OB, Thibault A et al: A comparison of clinical criteria for the diagnosis of veno-occlusive disease of the liver after bone marrow transplantation. Bone Marrow Transplant 10:439, 1992

54. Sharma P, McDonald GB, Banaji M: The risk of bleeding after percutaneous liver biopsy: relation to platelet count. J Clin Gastroenterol 4:451, 1982

55. Shulman HM, McDonald GB: Utility of transvenous liver biopsy and hepatic venous pressure measurements in Seattle marrow transplant recipients, abstracted (569). Exp Hematol 18:699, 1990

56. Carreras E, Granena A, Navasa M et al: Transjugular liver biopsy in BMT. Bone Marrow Transplant 11:21, 1993

57. Keefe EB: Transjugular liver biopsy. p. 167. In Hoofnagle JH, Goodman Z (eds): Liver Biopsy Interpretation for the 1990s. Clinicopathologic Correlations in Liver Disease. American Association for the Study of Liver Diseases. Thorofare, NJ, 1991

58. Hommeyer SC, Teefey SA, Jacobson AF et al: Venocclusive disease of the liver: prospective study of US evaluation. Radiology 184:683, 1992

59. Herbetko J, Grigg AP, Buckley AR et al: Venocclusive liver disease after bone marrow transplantation: findings at duplex sonograph. AJR 158:1001, 1992

60. Brown BP, Abu-Yousef M, Farner R et al: Doppler sonography: a noninvasive method for evaluation of hepatic venocclusive disease. AJR 154:721, 1990

61. Ganem G, Saint-Marc Girardin M-F, Kuentz M et al: Veno-occlusive disease of the liver after allogeneic bone marrow transplantation in man. Int J Radiat Oncology Biol Phys 14:879, 1988

62. Carreras E, Granena A, Rozman C: Hepatic veno-occlusive disease after bone marrow transplant. Blood Rev 7:43, 1993

63. Nevill TJ, Barnett MJ, Klingemann H-G et al: Regimen-related toxicity of a busulfan-cyclophosphamide conditioning regimen in 70 patients undergoing allogeneic bone marrow transplantation. J Clin Oncol 9:1224, 1991

64. Rollins BJ: Hepatic veno-occlusive disease. Am J Med 81:297

65. Clift RA, Buckner CD, Appelbaum FR et al: Allogeneic marrow transplantation in patients with acute myeloid leukemia in first remission: a randomized trial of two irradiation regimens. Blood 76:1867, 1990

66. Attal M, Huguet F, Rubie H et al: Prevention of hepatic veno-occlusive dis-

ease after bone marrow transplantation by continuous infusion of low-dose heparin: a prospective randomized trial. Blood 80:2834, 1992

67. Bearman SI, Hinds MS, Wolford JL et al: A pilot study of continuous infusion heparin for the prevention of hepatic veno-occlusive disease after bone marrow transplantation. Bone Marrow Transplant 5:407, 1990

68. Marsa-Vila L, Gorin NC, Laporte JP et al: Prophylactic heparin does not prevent liver veno-occlusive disease following autologous bone marrow transplantation. Eur J Haematol 47:346, 1991

69. Gluckman E, Jolivet I, Scrobohaci ML et al: Role of PGE1 to prevent veno-occlusive disease of the liver after bone marrow transplantation. Nouv Rev Fr Hematol 32:1, 1990

70. Bianco JA, Appelbaum FR, Neumanitis J et al: Phase I–II trial of pentoxifylline for the prevention of transplant related toxicities following allogeneic bone marrow transplantation. Blood 78:1205, 1991

71. Bearman SI, Shuhart MC, Hinds MS et al: Recombinant human tissue plasminogen activator for the treatment of established severe venocclusive disease of the liver after bone marrow transplantation. Blood 80:2458, 1992

72. Baglin TP, Harper P, Marcus RE: Veno-occlusive disease of the liver complicating ABMT successfully treated with recombinant tissue plasminogen activator (rt-PA). Bone Marrow Transplant 5:439, 1990

73. Fogteloo AJ, Smid WM, Kok T et al: Successful treatment of veno-occlusive disease of the liver with urokinase in a patient with non-Hodgkin's lymphoma. Leukemia 7:760, 1993

74. Sullivan K, Meyers J, Flournoy N et al: Early and late interstitial pneumonia following human bone marrow transplantation. Int J Cell Cloning 4:107, 1986

75. Weiner RS, Bortin MM, Gale RP et al: Interstitial pneumonitis after bone marrow transplantation. Assessment of risk factors. Ann Intern Med 104:168, 1986

76. Inoue T, Masaoka T, Shibata H: Difference in onset between cytomegalovirus and idiopathic interstitial pneumonitis following allogeneic bone marrow transplantation for leukemia. Strahlenther Onkol 166:322, 1990

77. Meyers JD, Flournoy N, Thomas ED: Risk factors for cytomegalovirus infection after human marrow transplantation. J Infect Dis 153:478, 1986

78. Miller W, Flynn P, McCullough J et al: Cytomegalovirus infection after bone marrow transplantation: an association with acute graft-v-host disease. Blood 67:1162, 1986

79. Meyers JD, Reed EC, Shepp DH et al: Acyclovir for prevention of cytomegalovirus infection and disease after allogeneic bone marrow transplantation. N Engl J Med 318:70, 1988

80. Goodrich J, Bowden RA, Fisher L et al: Ganciclovir prophylaxis to prevent cytomegalovirus disease after allogeneic marrow transplant. Ann Intern Med 118:173, 1993

81. Winston DJ, Ho WG, Bartoni K et al: Ganciclovir prophylaxis of cytomegalovirus infection and disease in allogeneic bone marrow transplant recipients. Ann Intern Med 118:179, 1993

82. Goodrich JM, Mori M, Gleaves CA et al: Early treatment with ganciclovir to prevent cytomegalovirus disease after allogeneic bone marrow transplantation. N Engl J Med 325:1601, 1991

83. Schmidt GM, Horak DA, Niland JC et al: A randomized, controlled trial of prophylactic ganciclovir for cytomegalovirus pulmonary infection in recipients of allogeneic bone marrow transplants. N Engl J Med 324:1005, 1991

84. Bowden R, Sayers M: The risk of transmitting cytomegalovirus infection by fresh frozen plasma. Transfusion 30:762, 1990

85. Miller WJ, McCullough J, Balfour HH Jr et al: Prevention of CMV infection following bone marrow transplantation: a randomized trial of blood product screening. Bone Marrow Transplant 7:227, 1991

86. Bowden RA, Sayers M, McIver J et al: Comparative trial of intravenous cytomegalovirus globulin and seronegative blood products for the prevention of primary cytomegalovirus infection following marrow transplant. N Engl J Med 314:1006, 1986

87. Bowden RA, Slichter SJ, Sayers MH et al: Use of leukocyte-depleted platelets and cytomegalovirus-seronegative red blood cells for prevention of primary cytomegalovirus infection after marrow transplant. Blood 78:246, 1991

88. Gilbert GL, Hayes K, Hudson IL et al: Prevention of transfusion-acquired cytomegalovirus infection in infants by blood filtration to remove leucocytes. Lancet 1:1228, 1989

89. de Graan-Hentzen YCE, Gratama JW, Mudde GC et al: Prevention of primary cytomegalovirus infection in patients with hematologic malignancies by intensive white cell depletion of blood products. Transfusion. 29:757, 1989

90. Winston DJ, Ho WG, Cheng-Hsien L et al: Intravenous immune globulin for prevention of cytomegalovirus infection and interstitial pneumonia after bone marrow transplantation. Ann Intern Med 106:12, 1987

91. Enright H, Haake R, Weisdorf D et al: Cytomegalovirus pneumonia after bone marrow transplantation. Risk factors and response to therapy. Transplantation 55:1339, 1993

92. Reusser P, Fisher LD, Buckner CD et al: Cytomegalovirus infection after autologous bone marrow transplantation: occurrence of cytomegalovirus disease and effect on engraftment. Blood 75:1888, 1990

93. Wingard JR, Yen-Hung Chen D, Burns WH et al: Cytomegalovirus infection after autologous bone marrow transplantation with comparison to infection after allogeneic bone marrow transplantation. Blood 71:1432, 1988

94. Meyers JD, Ljungman P, Fisher LD: Cytomegalovirus excretion as a predictor of cytomegalovirus disease after marrow transplantation: importance of cytomegalovirus viremia. J Infect Dis 162:373, 1990

95. Crawford SW, Bowden RA, Hackman RC et al: Rapid detection of cytomegalovirus pulmonary infection by bronchoalveolar lavage and centrifugation culture. Ann Intern Med 108:180, 1988

96. Erice A, Hertz MI, Snyder LS et al: Evaluation of centrifugation cultures of bronchalveolar lavage fluid for the diagnosis of cytomegalovirus pneumonitis. Diagn Microbiol Infect Dis 10:205, 1988

97. Ruutu P, Ruutu T, Volin L et al: Cytomegalovirus is frequently isolated in bronchoalveolar lavage fluid of bone marrow transplant recipients without pneumonia. Ann Intern Med 112:913, 1990

98. Saltzman RL, Quirk MF, Jordan MC: Cytomegalovirus (CMV) DNA in bronchoalveolar lavage fluid from patients with and without CMV pneumonitis. Program and Proceedings of the Twenty-seventh Interscience Conference on Antimicrobial Agents and Chemotherapy, abstract (795). American Society for Microbiology. Sept 17–20, 1989, Houston, TX

99. Emanuel D, Cunningham I, Jules-Elysee K et al: Cytomegalovirus after bone marrow transplantation successfully treated with the combination of ganciclovir and high-dose intravenous immune globulin. Ann Intern Med 109:777, 1988

100. Reed EC, Bowden RA, Dandliker PS et al: Treatment of cytomegalovirus pneumonia with ganciclovir and intravenous cytomegalovirus immunoglobulin in patients with bone marrow transplants. Ann Intern Med 109:783, 1988

101. Schmidt GM, Kovacs A, Zaia JA et al: Ganciclovir/immunoglobulin combination therapy for the treatment of human cytomegalovirus-associated interstitial pneumonia in bone marrow allograft recipients. Transplantation 46:905, 1988

102. Allan BT, Patton D, Ramsay NKC et al: Pulmonary fungal infections after bone marrow transplantation. Pediatr Radiol 18:118, 1988

103. Wingard JR, Beals SU, Santos GW et al: Aspergillus infections in bone marrow transplant recipients. Bone Marrow Transplant 2:175, 1987

104. Morrison VA, Haake RJ, Weisdorf DJ: Non-candida fungal infections after bone marrow transplantation: risk factors and outcome. Am J Med 1994 (in press)

105. Pannuti C, Gingrich R, Pfaller MA et al: Nosocomial pneumonia in patients having bone marrow transplant. Attributable mortality and risk factors. Cancer 69:2653, 1992

106. Rhame FS, Streifel AJ, Kersey JH, McGlave PB: Extrinsic risk factors for pneumonia in the patient at high risk of infection. Am J Med, suppl. 51. 76:42, 1984

107. Treger TR, Visscher DW, Bartlett MS et al: Diagnosis of pulmonary infection caused by Aspergillus: usefulness of respiratory cultures. J Infect Dis 152:572, 1985

108. Pannuti CS, Gingrich RD, Pfaller MA et al: Nosocomial pneumonia in adult patients undergoing bone marrow transplantation: a 9-year study. J Clin Oncol 9:77, 1991

109. Mori M, Galvin JR, Barloon TJ et al: Fungal pulmonary infections after bone marrow transplantation: evaluation with radiography and CT. Radiology 178:721, 1991

110. Hughes WT, Rivera GK, Schell MJ et al: Successful intermittent chemoprophylaxis for Pneumocystis carinii pneumonitis. N Engl J Med 316:1627, 1987

111. Link H, Vohringer HF, Wingen F et al: Pentamidine aerosol for prophylaxis of Pneumocystis carinii pneumonia after BMT. Bone Marrow Transplant 11:403, 1993

112. Bozzette SA, Sattler FR, Chiu J et al: A controlled trial of early adjunctive treatment with corticosteroids for Pneumocystis carinii pneumonia in the acquired immunodeficiency syndrome. N Engl J Med 323:1451, 1990

113. Hertz MI, Englund JA, Snover D et al: Respiratory syncytial virus-induced acute lung injury in adult patients with bone marrow transplants: a clinical approach and review of the literature. Medicine 68:269, 1989

114. Win N, Mitchell D, Pugh S et al: Successful therapy with ribavirin of late onset respiratory syncytial virus pneumonitis complicating allogeneic bone transplantation. Clin Lab Haematol 14:29, 1992

115. Wendt CH, Weisdorf DJ, Jordan CM et al: Parainfluenza virus respiratory infection after bone marrow transplantation. N Engl J Med 326:921, 1992

116. Meyers JD, Flournoy N, Thomas ED: Nonbacterial pneumonia after allogeneic marrow transplantation: a review of ten years' experience. Rev Infect Dis 4:1119, 1982

117. Cardozo BL, Hagenbeek A: Interstitial pneumonitis following bone marrow transplantation: pathogenesis and therapeutic considerations. Eur J Cancer Clin Oncol 21:43, 1985

118. Appelbaum FR, Meyers JD, Fefer A et al: Nonbacterial nonfungal pneumonia following marrow transplantation in 100 identical twins. Transplantation 33:265, 1982

119. Weshler Z, Breuer R, Or R et al: Interstitial pneumonitis after total body irradiation: effect of partial lung shielding. Br J Haematol 74:61, 1990

120. Cardozo BL, Zoetelief H, van Bekkum DW et al: Lung damage following bone marrow transplantation: I. The contribution of irradiation. Int J Radiat Oncol Biol Phys 11:907, 1985

121. Varekamp Ae, de Vries AJ, Zurcher C et al: Lung damage following bone marrow transplantation: II. The contribution of cyclophosphamide. Int J Radiat Oncol Biol Phys 13:1515, 1987

122. Robbins RA, Linder J, Stahl MG et al: Diffuse alveolar hemorrhage in autologous bone marrow transplant recipients. Am J Med 87:511, 1989

123. Jules-Elysee K, Stover DE, Yahalom J et al: Pulmonary complications in lymphoma patients treated with high-dose therapy and autologous bone marrow transplantation. Am Rev Respir Dis 146:485, 1992

124. Witte RJ, Gurney JW, Robbins RA et al: Diffuse pulmonary alveolar hemorrhage after bone marrow transplantation: radiographic findings in 29 patients. AJR 157:461, 1991

125. Chao NJ, Duncan SR, Long GD et al: Corticosteroid therapy for diffuse alveolar hemorrhage in autologous bone marrow transplant recipients. Ann Intern Med 114:145, 1991

126. Sisson JH, Thompson AB, Anderson JR et al: Airway inflammation predicts diffuse alveolar hemorrhage during bone marrow transplantation in patients with Hodgkins Disease. Am Rev Respir Dis 146:439, 1992

127. Weisdorf D, Snover D, Haake R et al: Acute upper gastrointestinal graft versus host disease: clinical significance and response to immunosuppressive therapy. Blood 76:624, 1990

128. Vogelsang GB, Hess AD, Santos GW: Acute graft-versus-host disease: clinical characteristics in the cyclosporine era. Medicine 67:163, 1988

129. Weisdorf D, Haake R, Blazar B et al: Risk factors for acute graft-versus-host disease in histocompatible donor bone marrow transplantation. Transplantation 51:1197, 1991

130. Gale RP, Bortin MM, Van Bekkum DW et al: Risk factors for acute graft-versus-host disease. Br J Haematol 67:397, 1987

131. Nash RA, Pepe MS, Storb R et al: Acute graft-versus-host disease: analysis of risk factors after allogeneic marrow transplantation and prophylaxis with cyclosporine and methotrexate. Blood 80:1838, 1992

132. Kennedy MJ, Vogelsang GB, Beveridge RA et al: Phase I trial of intravenous cyclosporine A to induce GVHD in women undergoing autologous BMT for breast cancer. J Clin Oncol 11:478, 1993

133. Flesch PHM, Tiberghien P, Wijdenes J et al: Phase I–II trial of a monoclonal antitumor necrosis factor α antibody for the treatment of refractory severe acute graft-versus-host disease. Blood 79:3362, 1992

134. McCarthy PL, Abhyankar S, Neben S et al: Inhibition of interleukin-1 by an interleukin-1 receptor antagonist prevents graft-vs-host disease. Blood 78:1915, 1991

135. Roy J, Platt JL, Weisdorf DJ: Immunopathology of upper gastrointestinal acute graft-versus-host disease: lymphoid cells and endothelial adhesion molecules. Transplantation 55:572, 1993

136. Weisdorf D, Haake R, Blazar B et al: Treatment of moderate/severe acute graft versus host disease after allogeneic bone marrow transplantation: an analysis of clinical risk features and outcome. Blood 75:1024, 1990

137. Martin PJ, Schock G, Fisher L et al: A retrospective analysis of therapy for acute graft-versus-host disease: initial treatment. Blood 76:1464, 1990

138. Young JW, Papadopoulos EB, Cunningham I et al: T-cell-depleted allogeneic bone marrow transplantation in adults with acute nonlymphocytic leukemia in first remission. Blood 79:3380, 1992

139. Vallera DA, Blazar BR: T cell depletion for graft-versus-host disease prophylaxis: a perspective on engraftment in mice and humans. Transplantation 47:751, 1989

140. Poynton CH: T cell depletion in bone marrow transplantation. Bone Marrow Transplant 3:165, 1988

141. Ramsay NKC, Kersey JH, Robison LL et al: A randomized study of the prevention of acute graft-versus-host disease. N Engl J Med 306:392, 1982

142. Storb R, Deeg HJ, Pepe M et al: Methotrexate and cyclosporine versus cyclosporine alone for prophylaxis of graft-versus-host disease in patients given HLA-identical marrow grafts for leukemia: long-term follow-up of a controlled trial. Blood 73:1729, 1989

143. Chao NJ, Schmidt GM, Niland JC et al: Cyclosporine, methotrexate, and prednisone compared with cyclosporine and prednisone for prophylaxis of acute graft-versus-host disease. N Engl J Med 329:1225, 1993

144. Deeg HJ, Henslee-Downey PJ: Management of acute graft-versus-host disease. Bone Marrow Transplant 6:1, 1990

145. Hings IM, Filipovich AH, Miller WJ et al: Prednisone therapy for acute graft-versus-host disease: short- versus long-term treatment. Transplantation 56:577, 1993

146. Roy J, McGlave PB, Filipovich A et al: Acute graft-versus-host disease following unrelated donor marrow transplantation: failure of conventional therapy. Bone Marrow Transplant 10:77, 1992

147. Atkinson K: Chronic graft-versus-host disease. Bone Marrow Transplant 5:69, 1990

148. Wingard JR, Piantadosi S, Vogelsang GB et al: Predictors of death from chronic graft-versus-host disease after bone marrow transplantation. Blood 74:1428, 1989

149. Ochs LA, Miller WJ, Filipovich et al: Predictive factors for chronic graft-versus-host disease after histocompatible sibling donor bone marrow transplantation. Bone Marrow Transplant 13:455, 1994

150. Holland HK, Wingard JR, Beschorner WE et al: Bronchiolitis obliterans in bone marrow transplantation and its relationship to chronic graft-versus-host disease and low serum IgG. Blood 72:621, 1988

151. Loughran TP Jr, Sullivan KM: Early detection and monitoring of chronic graft-versus-host disease. p. 631. In Burakoff SJ, Deeg HJ, Ferrara J, Atkinson K (eds): Graft-versus-Host Disease: Immunology, Pathophysiology, and Treatment. Marcel Dekker, New York, 1990

152. Sullivan KM, Witherspoon RP, Storb R et al: Alternating-day cyclosporine and prednisone for treatment of high-risk chronic graft-v-host disease. Blood 72:555, 1988

153. Enright H, Haake R, Weisdorf D: Avascular necrosis of bone: a common serious complication of allogeneic bone marrows transplantation. Am J Med 89:733, 1990

154. Vogelsang GB, Farmer ER, Hess AD et al: Thalidomide for the treatment of chronic graft-versus-host disease. N Engl J Med 326:1055, 1992

155. Deeg HJ: Delayed complications and long-term effects after bone marrow transplantation. Hematol Oncol Clin North Am 4:641, 1990

156. Deeg HJ, Flournoy N, Sullivan KM et al: Cataracts after total body irradiation and marrow transplantation: a sparing effect of dose fractionation. Int J Radiat Oncol Biol Phys 10:957, 1984

157. Serafino L, Arcese W, Papa G et al: Thyroid and pituitary function following allogeneic bone marrow transplantation. Arch Intern Med 148:1066, 1988

158. Katsanis E, Shapiro RS, Robison LL et al: Thyroid dysfunction following bone marrow transplantation: long-term follow-up of 80 pediatric patients. Bone Marrow Transplant 5:335, 1990

159. Sanders JE: Impact of marrow transplantation on subsequent fertility. p. 579. In Bern M, Frigoletto F (eds): Hematologic Disorders in Maternal-Fetal Medicine. Wiley-Liss, New York, 1990

160. Sanders JE, Seattle Marrow Transplant Team: The impact of marrow transplant preparative regimens on subsequent growth and development. Semin Hematol 28:244, 1991

161. Wingard JR, Plotnick LP, Freemer CS et al: Growth in children after bone marrow transplantation: busulfan plus cyclophosphamide versus cyclophosphamide plus total body irradiation. Blood 79:1068, 1992

162. Witherspoon RP, Fisher LD, Schoch G et al: Secondary cancers after bone marrow transplantation for leukemia or aplastic anemia. N Engl J Med 321:784, 1989

163. Miller JS, Arthur DC, Litz CE et al: Myelodysplastic syndrome after autologous bone marrow transplantation: an additional late complication of curative cancer therapy. Blood 83:1, 1994

164. Chao NJ, Tierney DK, Bloom JR et al: Dynamic assessment of quality of life after autologous bone marrow transplantation. Blood 80:825, 1992

165. Andrykowski MA, Henslee PJ, Farrall MG: Physical and psychosocial functioning of adult survivors of allogeneic bone marrow transplantation. Bone Marrow Transplant 4:75, 1989

166. Wingard JR, Curbow B, Baker F et al: Health, functional status, and employment of adult survivors of bone marrow transplantation. Ann Intern Med 114:113, 1991

Gene Therapy for Hematologic Disorders

31

Johnson M. Liu, Christopher E. Walsh, and Arthur W. Nienhuis

INTRODUCTION

Advances in recombinant DNA technology over the past several decades have offered the promise that inherited disorders may be treated by gene replacement. Acquired disorders such as the acquired immunodeficiency syndrome (AIDS) and cancer may also become amenable to modulation via the introduction of selected genes that block viral replication or neoplasia. While the concept of human gene therapy is simple, progress in its application to clinical disorders has been slow. The most direct model for gene therapy is the introduction of a correctly functioning gene into the appropriate target cell of an affected individual. The newly inserted gene is transcribed and translated into a protein that alters the phenotype of the target cell. For hematologic disorders, the cells in which gene expression is required may be lymphocytes, monocytes, neutrophils, or other mature blood elements. In the ideal case, gene transfer could be targeted to the pluripotent hematopoietic stem cell (HSC). Introduction of the genetic material into the HSC would ensure the continuous production of genetically modified blood elements over the lifetime of the patient. Theoretically, any genetic disease affecting one of the stem cell-derived lineages could be treated by gene insertion into a repopulating cell, provided that regulated, cell-specific gene expression could be maintained. Alternatively, long-lived mature blood elements such as lymphocytes could be targeted for gene transfer. Gene therapy has also been proposed as a strategy to treat neoplastic diseases. Genetic alteration of cancer cells might suppress or change their phenotype. Alternatively, gene transfer strategies might be used to enhance the immune response to tumor-specific antigens.

GENE DELIVERY

Transduction, the process of stable transfer of foreign genetic material to the host chromosome, must be safe and efficient. Most methods of gene delivery use viral vectors to capitalize on the inherent efficiency with which viruses transfer and express genetic material in host cells. Typically, viruses bind specific cellular receptors and enter host cells by endocytosis. Subsequently, the viral genome is transported to the nucleus; viral genes direct the production of viral proteins and enzymes. Viral infection leads to the production of progeny virions, lysis of the host cell in some cases, and release of virion particles. Alternatively, a latent viral infection may occur, with the viral genome maintained either integrated in the cellular genome or in an extrachromosomal state. Murine retroviruses, adeno-associated virus (AAV), adenoviruses, herpesviruses, and vaccinia viruses are currently being developed for use in humans. At the present time, only retroviruses and AAV have been shown to transduce murine or human hematopoietic progenitors (see below). Each of these vectors establishes a latent infection in cells wherein a recombinant genome is integrated into a host cell chromosome.

Retroviral Vectors

Retroviruses are single-stranded RNA viruses that enter cells by specific receptors.[1] Following transport to the cell nucleus, the viral RNA is converted into a double-stranded DNA molecule by an enzyme known as reverse transcriptase. The viral DNA is integrated into the host chromosome as a provirus and serves as a template for encoding viral-specific proteins and enzymes.

The retroviral vectors currently used for gene transfer are derived from the murine leukemia virus family. Figure 31-1 depicts the integrated proviral form of the Moloney murine leukemia virus. The genome is flanked by long terminal repeat (LTR) elements that contain the transcriptional control elements (promoter), polyadenylation and termination signals, and sequences required for replication and integration.[2,3] The viral coding sequence encodes for structural proteins (gag), reverse transcriptase (pol), other viral enzymes, and envelope proteins (env). A packaging signal (ψ), located at the 5' end of the coding sequence, facilitates the incorporation of viral RNA into the capsid. Efficient packaging also requires a portion of the gag sequence. Retroviruses capable of infecting murine cells are termed ecotropic; target cells must express a specific receptor that binds the viral envelope glycoprotein (GP)70.[4,5] Retroviruses capable of infecting human cells are termed amphotropic; the cellular receptor for these retroviruses has recently been cloned.[6]

The ability to use retroviruses as vectors has been greatly enhanced by the development of packaging cell lines engineered to produce recombinant retroviruses (Fig. 31-2). The cell lines contain the coding sequences for the viral structural proteins. Bacterial plasmids are constructed that link the foreign gene to be transferred to the elements necessary for viral RNA encapsidation, replication, and integration.[7,8] Transfection of the packaging cell line with the recombinant plasmid results in the production of recombinant virus. To prevent the production of replication competent virus, the helper genome within the packaging line and the viral genome within the plasmid are designed to minimize overlapping sequence, thus making homologous recombination and the production of replication competent virus unlikely. Viral supernatants from producer cell clones are assayed for virion production. Typically, producer clones that generate 10^6–10^7 vector particles/ml can be obtained.

Retroviral transduction requires that target cells be actively replicating; quiescent cells are refractory to proviral integration.[9,10] Virus binding and internalization are independent of cell cycling, but reverse transcriptase and integrase are active only in dividing cells. This requirement for target cell replication is a major limitation of retroviral gene transfer into HSCs.

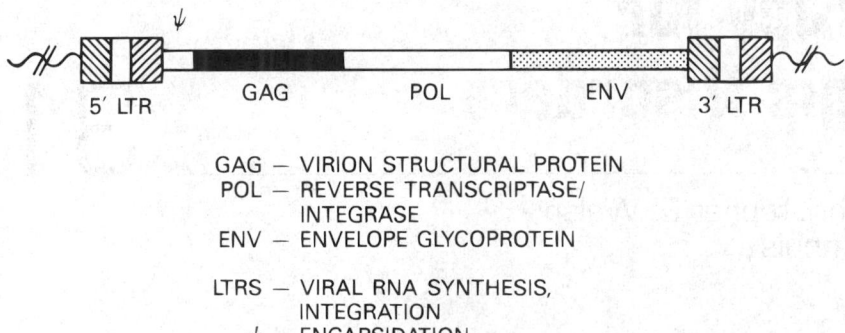

GAG — VIRION STRUCTURAL PROTEIN
POL — REVERSE TRANSCRIPTASE/
INTEGRASE
ENV — ENVELOPE GLYCOPROTEIN

LTRS — VIRAL RNA SYNTHESIS,
INTEGRATION
ψ — ENCAPSIDATION

Fig. 31-1. Integrated proviral form of the Moloney murine leukemia virus depicting structural features. GAG, virion structural protein; POL, reverse transcriptase/integrase; ENV, envelope glycoprotein; LTR, viral RNA synthesis, integration; ψ, encapsidation.

The safety of retroviral vectors has been studied in several animal models. Notably, lethally irradiated rhesus monkeys developed thymic lymphomas following bone marrow transplantation with progenitors transduced by recombinant retroviruses contaminated with replication-competent virus.[11] Multiple copies of replication-competent proviral genome were detected in the tumor cell material, implicating viral insertional mutagenesis as a mechanism of carcinogenesis. These experiments underscore the absolute necessity of eliminating replication-competent virus from packaging cell systems. To prevent the production of replication-competent virus by recombination between vector and helper genomes, areas of homology between the two have been eliminated, mutations have been introduced into residual viral coding sequences in the vector genome, and the structural genes required for helper function have been separated into two transcriptional units. Newer packaging lines have virtually eliminated detectable production of replication-competent virus. Nevertheless, vector preparations intended for human gene therapy should be routinely monitored for replication-competent virus using standardized assays.

Adeno-Associated Virus Vectors

AAV is a single-stranded DNA parvovirus that requires helper virus (adenovirus or herpesvirus) co-infection for replication and subsequent viral propagation. In the absence of helper virus, AAV can persist in host cell genomic DNA as an integrated provirus similar to a retrovirus vector.[7,12] Viral integration has no known deleterious effect on cell growth or morphology. AAV has a broad host range. Virtually every mammalian cell line can be productively or latently infected. Despite its wide host range, no disease has been associated with wild-type AAV infection in human or animal populations. Unlike other viral vectors, wild-type AAV is unusual because the viral genome integrates at a specific site on human chromosome 19.[13]

Recombinant AAV (rAAV) generation is hampered currently by the lack of packaging cell lines analogous to those used in retroviral production. Instead, rAAV generation relies upon co-transfection of the recombinant plasmid with a helper plasmid containing the AAV capsid genes (Fig. 31-3). The recombinant plasmid is configured with the transcriptional unit (gene of interest driven by a promoter) flanked by the AAV inverted

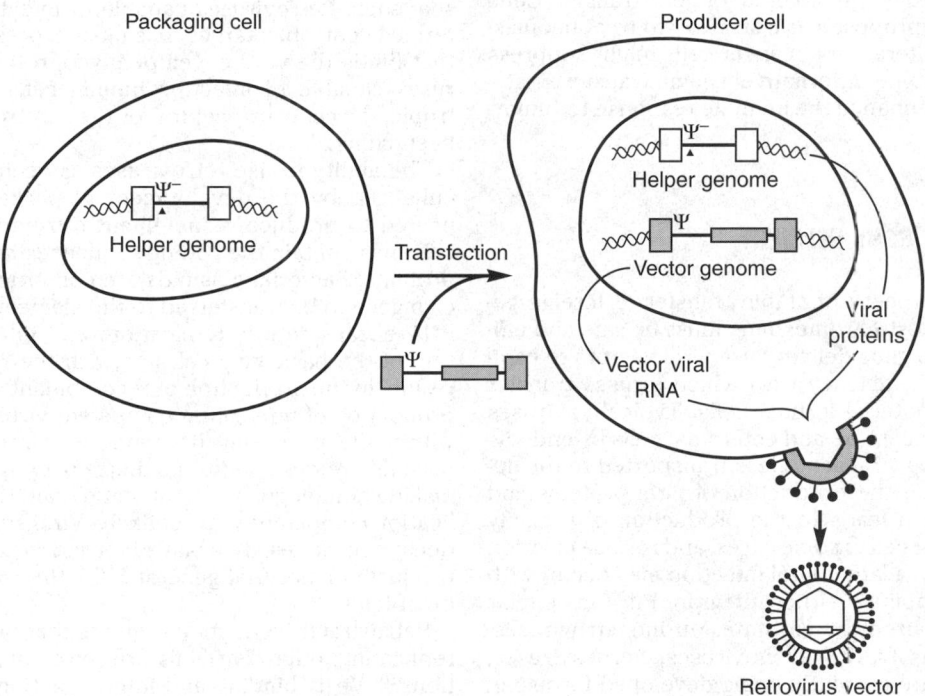

Fig. 31-2. Generation of a producer cell line following transfection of a packaging cell line with a recombinant retroviral vector genome. The ψ element refers to the encapsidation signal, which is provided by the transfected vector genome (see text for details).

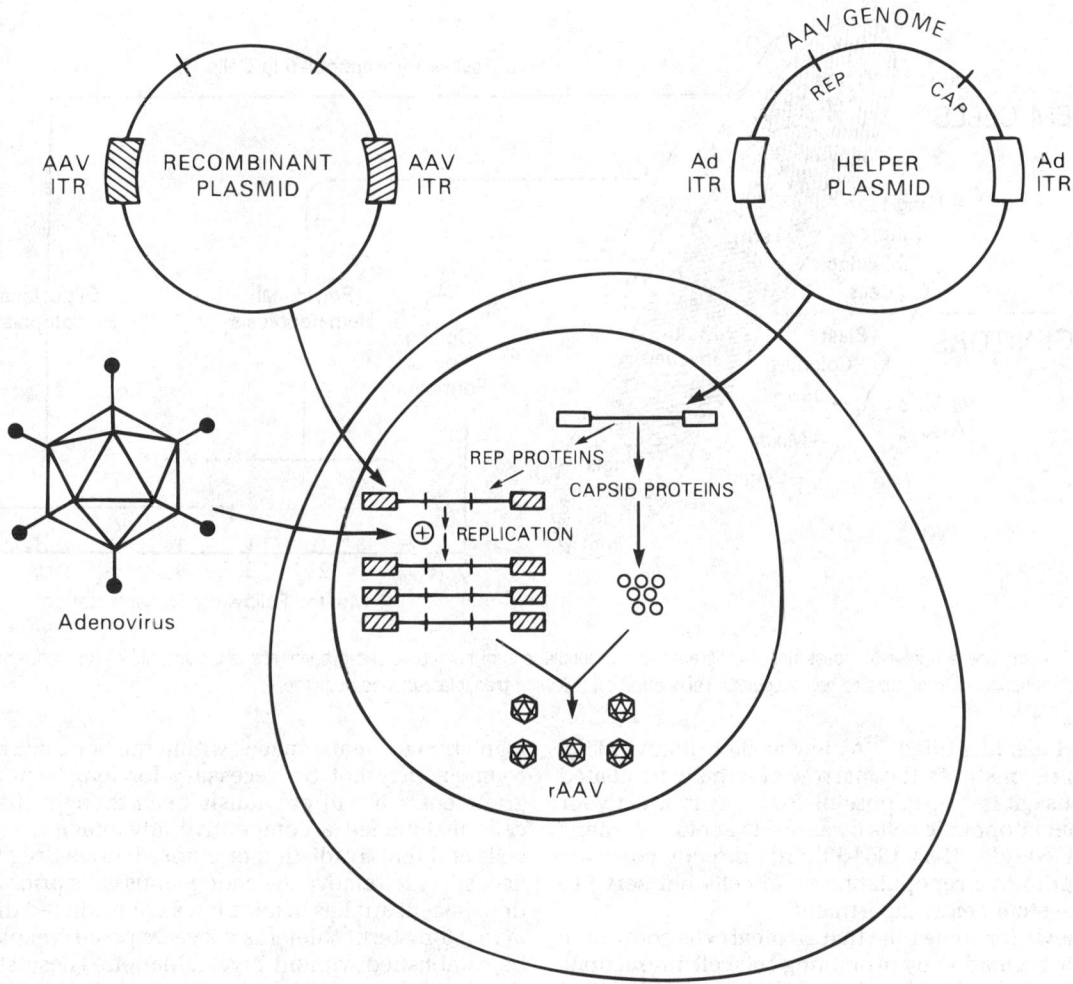

Fig. 31-3. Generation of rAAV by co-transfection of recombinant and helper genomes and co-infection with adenovirus.

terminal repeats (ITRs). The AAV ITRs contain the necessary signals for integration, packaging, and replication. Concomitant infection of the transfected cell line with adenovirus provides the necessary replication function for the production of AAV virions. The titer of rAAV generated in this way is low (10^4–10^6 infectious particles/ml) but is free of wild-type AAV. Contaminating adenovirus can be removed by gradient centrifugation or inactivated by heating (since AAV is heat resistant).

Work in our laboratory has explored the potential of rAAV vectors to transfer genes to hematopoietic progenitors. Apparent efficiencies of 60–70% have been achieved with a vector containing the β-galactosidase gene, used because its enzymatic product is readily detectable cytochemically.

Nonviral Methods of Gene Transfer

Nonviral methods of gene transfer have also been developed.[14] Originally, these methods relied on adsorption and entry of DNA into cells by physical means such as calcium phosphate co-precipitation, liposomal encapsulation, or direct microinjection of DNA into target cells. Complexes between the expression plasmid and liposomes have been used to transfer DNA to various cell types. One problem has been toxicity from the lipid moiety of these complexes. A recent report has described in vivo expression from a reporter gene in various mouse tissues following a single intravenous injection of plasmid/liposome complex.[15] Interest has also centered on gene transfer mediated by specific receptors. Whether these methods will be reliable and as efficient as viral gene transfer

is unclear at present. Transduction of repopulating hematopoietic progenitor cells using these methods has not yet been achieved.

HEMATOPOIETIC STEM CELLS

HSCs are essential for production of the formed elements of the blood. Stem cells are defined by their ability to repopulate the bone marrow after experimental marrow ablation and transplantation. These cells are rare, with an estimated frequency of 1/10,000–1/100,000 mononuclear bone marrow cells. The earliest studies of stem cell biology relied on functional and indirect assays (Fig. 31-4) such as the spleen colony assay, clonal suspension culture assays, and reconstitution of a lethally irradiated or genetically deficient animal (usually mouse).[16,17] It is thought that most primitive stem cells are quiescent, with only 1–5% of cells actively cycling and contributing to hematopoiesis. These cells appear to reenter the cell cycle randomly. In animal models, individual stem cells may vary in their contribution to hematopoiesis over time, giving rise to a pattern of "clonal succession."[18]

More recently, HSCs and progenitor cells have been characterized on the basis of unique cell surface antigens. In particular, both primitive and committed cells express the CD34 molecule on their cell surfaces.[19–21] Subsets of CD34$^+$ cells have recently been identified based on the pattern of antigen expression. Cells having the phenotype CD34$^+$, CD33$^-$, CD38$^-$, HLA-DR$^-$, and Thy1$^+$ are thought to include the repopulating stem cells.[22–24] Cell surface antigens that mark primitive murine

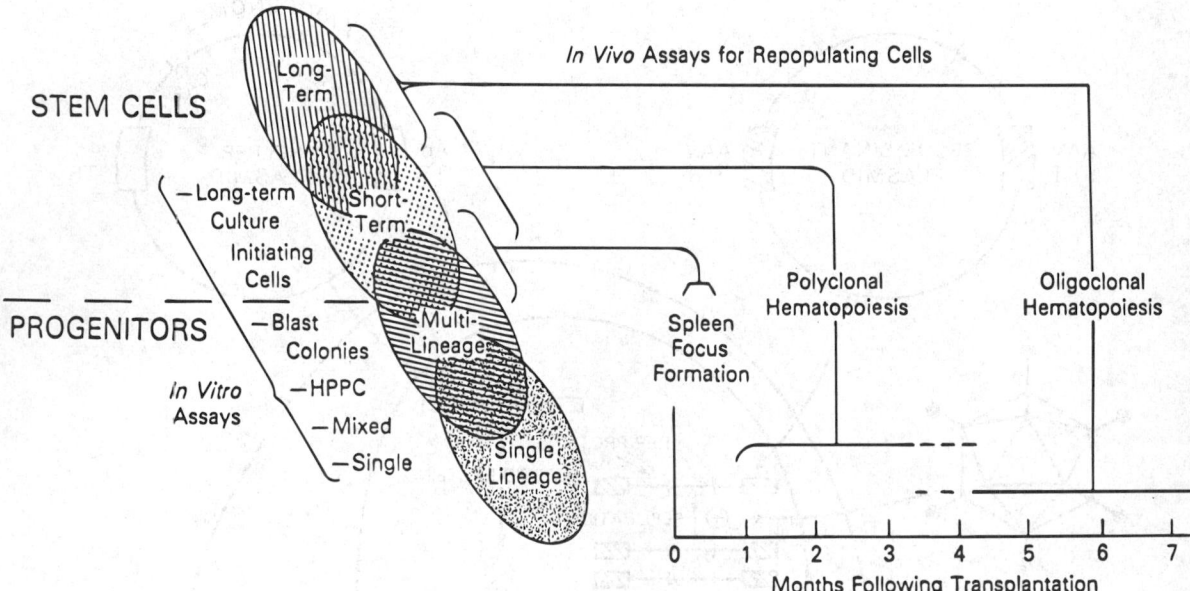

Fig. 31-4. In vitro and in vivo assays used to detect various populations of hematopoietic progenitors and stem cells. The contribution of each subpopulation of cells to hematopoietic reconstitution following transplantation is depicted.

HSCs have also been identified.[25] As few as 50 primitive HSCs are sufficient to reconstitute the marrow of lethally irradiated mice. In the mouse, it has been possible to assay indirectly for very primitive hematopoietic cells by assessing colony-forming unit-spleen (CFU-S) (Fig. 31-4). CFU-S do not directly correlate with the most primitive repopulating stem cells but serve to approximate the stem cell compartment.

It has been known for some time that stromal cells contribute to hematopoietic regulation by promoting cell-cell interactions and secreting cytokines. Multiple factors have been identified and cloned by recombinant DNA techniques. In vitro, these factors may have stimulatory or inhibitory effects on the growth and differentiation of hematopoietic progenitors; they may influence the entry of cells into cycle.[26] Stromal cells can express cell-surface adhesion molecules that promote clustering of progenitors; local cytokine concentrations may be higher within these defined microenvironments.

Hematopoietic stem cells also circulate in the peripheral blood,[27–29] with an estimated frequency ≥100-fold less than in bone marrow. To increase this frequency, growth factors produced by recombinant DNA methods, such as colony-stimulating factor-granulocyte, can be used to mobilize stem cells from the marrow to the peripheral blood. Peripheral blood hematopoietic progenitors and stem cells can then be collected by leukapheresis and used for gene transduction. The extent of engraftment following transplantation with purified populations of peripheral blood progenitors and stem cells is being actively investigated.

Gene Transfer Into HSCs

Progress toward the introduction of genetic material into HSCs has been slow and hampered by a lack of information regarding stem cell biology. In mice, it is thought that pretreatment with agents that induce stem cell cycling (such as 5-fluorouracil or cytokines like interleukin-6 and stem cell factor) improves gene transduction of HSCs.[30] Based on these types of studies, nearly 80–100% of primitive murine hematopoietic cells (such as CFU-S) can be transduced. The optimal conditions for gene transfer into transplanted hematopoietic cells are still under study. Recently, it has been suggested that mye-

loablation to "make space" within the bone marrow microenvironment may not be necessary for long-term transplant engraftment.[31] It had previously been thought that endogenous cells maintained a competitive advantage over transplanted cells and that irradiation or cytoreductive drug treatment was necessary to remove the endogenous cells prior to transplantation. Recent studies in mice have contradicted this assumption in that long-term chimeras ≤2 years post-transplantation could be established without myeloablation. These studies suggest that gene therapy might be accomplished by transplantation of cells into unprepared hosts.

In contrast to the situation with mice, it has proved difficult to transfer genes efficiently into the repopulating HSCs of large outbred animals.[32] Canine, feline, and nonhuman primate (cynomolgus and rhesus monkey) bone marrow progenitors have been successfully transduced with amphotropic retroviruses and reinfused in transplantation models. Unfortunately, the proportion of cells in the myeloid and lymphoid lineages containing the transferred gene after transplantation of transduced stem cells has been disappointingly low, approximately 1%.

PROGENITOR MARKING STUDIES

Genetic marking of hematopoietic progenitor cells obtained for autologous bone marrow transplantation is currently being assessed. Autologous bone marrow progenitors marked by the bacterial neomycin phosphotransferase gene were reinfused into children with acute myeloid leukemia.[33] Sensitive polymerase chain reaction methods were used to monitor the efficiency of gene transduction following hematopoietic reconstitution. Of 18 patients enrolled in this marking protocol, 2 patients who relapsed had gene-marked cells in the leukemic blasts. This information can establish the origin (multilineage or lineage restricted) of the cell involved in relapsing acute myeloid leukemia. Furthermore, these studies have demonstrated the feasibility of gene transfer into primitive hematopoietic cells.

SITE-SPECIFIC VASCULAR GENE TRANSFER

For certain hematologic disorders, direct application of foreign gene expression to vascular sites may be desirable. Particularly relevant for this discussion are disorders of thrombosis and hemostasis, which may be treated by gene therapy. The ability to achieve local increases in gene expression at vascular or endothelial sites serves several purposes. First, local delivery of genes involved in thrombosis or hemostasis by vectors may be preferable to systemic administration of the gene product, thereby obviating systemic side effects. Second, surgical interventions mediated by catheters might be combined with vascular gene transfer in a simple manner, avoiding complex transplantation procedures. Third, local vascular wall defects might be directly targeted. Gene transfer has been achieved directly into vasculature by two different means. First, cultured endothelial cells have been transduced and reimplanted along vascular walls.[34] Second, direct in vivo gene transfer into cells lining the vessel wall has been reported using both viral vectors and physical methods of gene transfer.[35] Limitations of these approaches include difficulty in culturing primary human endothelial cells and low efficiency of gene transfer. Recently, replication-deficient adenovirus vectors have been used to transfer foreign genes to cells lining the blood vessel wall.[36,37]

GENE TRANSFER IN HEMATOLOGIC DISORDERS

The treatment of various hematologic disorders by gene therapy is under active investigation by laboratories around the world. Gene transfer into hematopoietic pluripotent stem cells is envisioned as a potential treatment for both inherited and acquired disorders (Table 31-1). The procedure might involve gene transduction of the recipient's bone marrow or peripheral blood hematopoietic progenitors ex vivo, perhaps in the setting of autologous bone marrow transplantation (Fig. 31-5). As mentioned above, gene therapy of non-myeloablated, unprepared hosts may be possible in certain hematologic applications.

Single Gene Defects

Adenosine Deaminase Deficiency

ADA deficiency is the current paradigm for gene replacement therapy.[38] This rare, inherited, life-threatening illness of children manifests clinically as a severely immunocompromised state. Accumulated purine metabolic intermediates that result from ADA deficiency cause profound lymphocyte dysfunction and destruction. Current therapy includes allogeneic bone mar-

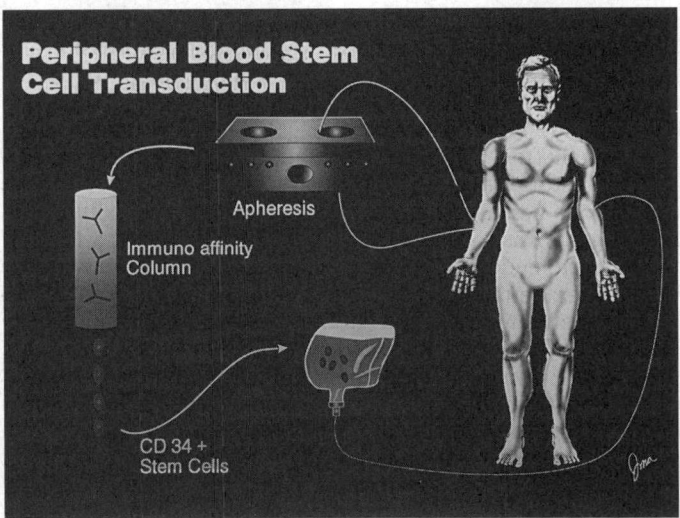

Fig. 31-5. Schema for the transduction and reinfusion of peripheral blood progenitors and stem cells collected by apheresis.

row transplantation for patients with unaffected sibling donors[39] and infusional enzyme replacement.[40] Patients without a suitable donor or receiving no benefit from enzyme replacement are potential candidates for gene therapy.

A recombinant retroviral vector was constructed with the cDNA for the ADA gene linked to a selectable marker, the bacterial neomycin phosphotransferase gene. In vitro experiments demonstrated that this vector could correct the defective phenotype of lymphocytes derived from ADA patients.[41] Transplantation of ADA-deficient human T lymphocytes transduced with the retroviral vector restored lymphocyte function in a murine severe combined immunodeficiency model.

The clinical protocol for ADA deficiency has utilized genetically modified peripheral blood T lymphocytes. Lymphocytes were expanded ex vivo by exposure to interleukin-2 and anti-T-cell receptor antibodies, infected with recombinant virus, and reinfused into the patients (who were maintained on enzyme replacement). Cells were repeatedly incubated with viral supernatant, and a transduction frequency of 5–10% was achieved. T-cell number and function, and ADA serum levels rose in the two patients tested. Whether the improvement in lymphocyte function was due to the effect of ADA gene transduction rather than ex vivo expansion is not entirely clear. Subsequent reinfection of peripheral lymphocytes by the retroviral vectors has been required to maintain adequate T-cell levels, presumably due to the normal turnover of the lymphocytes.

Recently, work has focused on ADA gene transduction of lymphohematopoietic stem cells; if successful, reinfusion of these stem cells might obviate the need for repeated correction of lymphocytes. Transduction of murine hematopoietic progenitors and transplantation following marrow ablation demonstrated ≤80% transfer efficiency in CFU-S and pluripotent stem cells. Long-term expression was demonstrated in all hematopoietic lineages.[42,43] Transduction of repopulating stem cells from larger animals has proved to be more difficult (see above), with stem cell transduction efficiencies of 1–2%.[44] Nevertheless, these preclinical data have formed the basis for trials of stem cell transduction in several ADA patients.

Hemoglobinopathies

Gene therapy for severely affected patients with sickle cell anemia and β-thalassemia has recently been reviewed.[45] High-level regulated globin gene expression is required for such therapy to be effective. Expression of a normal β-globin gene

Table 31-1. Disorders Amenable to Gene Therapy

Inherited
    Immunodeficiencies
        Lymphocytes
            ADA deficiency
            Purine nucleoside phosphorylase deficiency
            X-linked severe combined immunodeficiency
        Neutrophils
            Chronic granulomatous disease
            Leukocyte adhesion deficiency
    Anemias
        Erythrocytes
            Hemoglobinopathies
    Lysosomal storage disorders
        Monocyte/macrophages
            Gaucher disease
            Mucopolysaccharidoses
    Clotting disorders
        Hemophilias
Acquired
    Acquired immunodeficiency syndrome
    Cancer

would be useful in correcting the defect of homozygous β-thalassemia. Alternatively, increased γ-globin gene expression and fetal hemoglobin (α_2, γ_2) production would ameliorate the severity of sickle cell disease and β-thalassemia.

One of the major obstacles for globin gene transfer is the requirement for high-level, regulated gene expression. Retroviral vectors have been used to transfer the β-globin gene into murine hematopoietic progenitor cells.[46,47] The human β-globin gene was expressed in most animals but at a level of 1–2% of the endogenous murine β-globin gene, too low to be of any therapeutic value. Discovery of regulatory control elements upstream from the globin gene cluster, collectively termed the locus control region (LCR), offered new hope that gene correction of hemoglobinopathies might be feasible.[48] Linking powerful enhancer elements from the LCR to the globin genes substantially increases globin gene expression in transgenic mouse models and transfected erythroid cell lines. Unfortunately, retroviral vectors containing LCR-globin cassettes suffered from low titer and proviral rearrangement. Recently, retroviral vectors utilizing truncated LCR elements linked to a human β-globin gene have yielded nearly equivalent levels of gene expression as the endogenous globin genes in both cultured cell lines and murine hematopoietic cells.[49]

One approach that we have taken to overcome some of the problems with globin gene transfer is to use rAAV vectors. We found that rAAV vectors containing LCR elements linked to a γ-globin gene were capable of expressing the γ-globin gene at levels nearly equivalent to those of the native gene in a cultured human erythroid cell line.[50] Expression of a globin gene linked to elements from the LCR has recently been documented in erythroblasts derived from transduced hematopoietic progenitors. In summary, while more work is needed to improve the transduction frequency and expression of globin genes, there is reason to believe that gene therapy of hemoglobinopathies may become feasible in the near future.

Gaucher Disease

Gaucher disease is one of several lysosomal storage disorders in which gene therapy may be therapeutic. Deficient glucocerebrosidase leads to lipid accumulation in mononuclear phagocytes. Phenotypic correction of patients' fibroblasts and lymphocytes has been demonstrated following retrovirus-mediated transfer of the glucocerebrosidase gene.[51] Transduction of murine hematopoietic stem cells has been achieved, with long-term expression in macrophages of transplanted mice.[52,53] Glucocerebrosidase expression in human hematopoietic progenitors has also been described and is the basis of a recently approved clinical protocol utilizing retroviral vectors.[54]

Chronic Granulomatous Disease

Deficiencies of both membrane-associated and cytosolic components have been described in the phagocytic NADPH oxidase (phox) system.[55] Although several of the *phox* genes had been cloned and characterized, only recently has gene transduction been achieved in vitro. Lymphoblastoid cell lines derived from patients initially served as targets for testing retroviral gene correction. A retroviral vector expressing the cDNA for the cytosolic p47[phox] supported increased superoxide generation in cultured cells.[56] Recent studies have demonstrated that a p91[phox]-expressing retrovirus can generate superoxide in both lymphoblast cells and peripheral blood CD34[+] hematopoietic progenitors. Since heterozygous women with only 10% of cells having normal enzymatic activity are clinically normal with respect to white cell function, correction of only a small percentage of cells in affected patients should result in clinical benefit.

Clotting Disorders

Hemophilias A and B are deficiencies of factors VIII and IX, respectively. Severely affected individuals (in whom factor levels are <5% of normal) can suffer from life-threatening bleeding complications. Such patients usually benefit from factor replacement therapy. In these disorders, a low level of factor gene expression in corrected target cells might be sufficient since patients making as little as 2–5% of normal levels of clotting factor tend to be less susceptible to serious bleeding complications. Work has focused on transduced keratinocytes, myoblasts, and fibroblasts, any of which might secrete the deficient factor into the circulation. At Fudan University in China, two hemophilia B patients received transplanted autologous fibroblasts that had been transduced with a retroviral vector carrying the factor IX gene.[57] Many questions remain, however, as to whether transplanted gene-corrected cells will express factor genes over long periods. Furthermore, the conditions favoring successful transplantation of gene-corrected cells are unknown.

Recently, sustained gene transfer of factor IX was reported in factor-deficient hemophilia B dogs.[58] The factor IX gene-retroviral vector was delivered directly to the liver by portal vein injection. Because retroviral vectors only insert genetic material into cellular DNA of dividing cells, partial hepatectomy was performed on the dogs to stimulate liver cell regeneration and division. Of four dogs undergoing this procedure, one animal died from liver damage suffered during surgery, and three dogs showed evidence of factor IX production. Unfortunately, the level of clotting factor production was only 0.1% of normal, too low to be of clinical value.

Acquired Disorders

Acquired Immunodeficiency Syndrome

Gene therapy for AIDS is conceptually based on the premise that introduction of anti-human immunodeficiency virus (HIV) genes might serve as "intracellular immunization" against HIV. Presumably, lymphohematopoietic cells would be the targets for gene therapy. Current strategies can be divided into (1) elimination of HIV-infected cells, (2) interference with HIV replication or gene expression by intracellular means, and (3) protection against HIV infection by extracellular means.

Elimination of Infected Cells

A "suicide gene," which can be selectively activated by HIV control elements, can be introduced into HIV-infected cells.[59] As an example, a potent inhibitor of protein synthesis such as the diphtheria toxin can be engineered so that toxin expression is controlled by the promoter element within the HIV LTR. The HIV LTR contains a sequence known as the TAT-activating region (TAR), which is responsive to up-regulation by the HIV TAT protein. Presumably, toxin production would be selectively "switched on" in HIV-infected cells that produced TAT, thus sparing non-HIV-infected cells. Plans have been made to test this general approach to kill infected cells in vivo. Because the exact mechanism involved in HIV-induced immunosuppression is unknown, it is currently unclear whether accelerated destruction of cells harboring the HIV virus would benefit an infected patient.

Interference with Replication

By "intracellular immunization," lymphoid cells can be genetically altered so that they become resistant to HIV replication or infection.[60] Several ingenious ideas have been proposed based on the life cycle of HIV. For example, small molecules containing TAR sequences, when overexpressed, may act as "decoys" for the HIV TAT protein, perhaps preventing binding to the authentic regulatory region of the HIV genome.[61] Alternatively, expression of antisense sequences complementary to various portions of the HIV genome might inhibit HIV protein translation.[62] One new idea is to introduce directly into the target cell an antibody that might interfere with some aspect of HIV infection. Recently, specially engineered antibodies against the HIV GP120 envelope protein were introduced into cultured HIV-permissive cells.[63] HIV particles released from these antibody-producing HIV-transfected cells proved to be less infectious than wild-type HIV.

There is little doubt that "intracellular immunization" can be achieved in cultured lymphoid cell lines, but formidable problems must be overcome before this approach becomes therapeutically useful. Most of the in vitro experiments have been done with HIV laboratory isolates that may not behave like wild-type HIV. The ability to block HIV replication might be critically dependent on the stage of HIV infection. As outlined above, gene delivery into the desired target, either hematopoietic stem cells or peripheral blood T lymphocytes, is currently inefficient. More effective means of gene delivery are needed. Furthermore, the fundamental concept that an HIV-resistant T-cell population will be of clinical benefit to the patient remains to be established.

Inhibition of HIV Infection

Extracellular protection against HIV infection is one strategy suggested by the tropism of HIV. CD4, a transmembrane molecule, acts as a receptor for HIV entry into T cells. The external domain of CD4 is soluble and capable of interacting with the major HIV envelope protein, GP120. Soluble CD4 inhibits HIV infection of susceptible CD4-expressing cells. Attempts to use soluble CD4 as a pharmacologic agent have been limited by the very high concentrations required for inhibition. An alternative strategy envisions the genetic engineering of cells to produce soluble CD4. Cell lines transduced with a retroviral vector capable of synthesizing soluble CD4, when co-cultured with HIV-susceptible cells, elaborated sufficient CD4 to decrease virus production when subsequently challenged with HIV.[64]

Cancer

Gene therapy of neoplastic disorders can be divided into several broad categories: toxin or prodrug delivery, immunomodulation and immunotherapy, and inhibition of the tumor phenotype.

Toxin Delivery

The introduction of conditionally toxic genes into tumor cells is one promising approach. Typically, the foreign gene encodes an enzyme that activates a prodrug via selective gene expression in the tumor cell. Ingenious examples have included introduction of prodrug enzymes such as the herpesvirus thymidine kinase (HSV-tk). This enzyme phosphorylates gancyclovir to toxic metabolites. Subsequent administration of gancyclovir would be expected to destroy tumor cells expressing HSV-tk. This strategy has recently been applied to experimental treatment for brain tumors.[65]

Immunomodulation and Immunotherapy

The first protocols for cancer gene therapy have focused on the use of tumor-specific lymphocytes as vehicles for gene delivery. Tumor-infiltrating lymphocytes (TILs) target tumors such as malignant melanoma and renal cell carcinoma. In the first approved gene therapy protocol, TIL cells marked by a retroviral vector bearing the bacterial neomycin phosphotransferase gene were reintroduced into patients parenterally.[66]

Despite a low transduction frequency, genetically tagged cells were recovered at tumor sites without apparent toxicity to the patients. These studies have now progressed to enhancing TIL cytotoxicity to tumor cells by the insertion of potent cytokines such as tumor necrosis factor, interferon-γ, and various interleukin molecules.

Another example of immunomodulation via gene therapy is specific stimulation of an antitumor immune response by alteration of the antigenic state of the tumor cell. Deficient expression of MHC antigens on tumor cells may allow such clones to escape immune surveillance. A novel strategy has been proposed in which a specific antitumor immune response is provoked by introducing histocompatibility genes directly into tumor cells: this strategy formed the basis for a gene therapy trial for malignant melanoma. In a preclinical murine model, gene transfer of an allogeneic MHC class I gene into melanoma cells was found to induce a cytotoxic T-cell response that resulted in partial regression of the tumor.[67] The human trial involving patients with melanoma is also the first application of a nonviral vector in human gene therapy: the HLA-B7 gene was encapsulated in liposomes and injected directly into melanoma tissue of patients. Five patients have been treated thus far without serious toxicities.

Suppression of the Tumor Phenotype

Unraveling the genetic mechanisms responsible for oncogenesis has been the focus of intense investigation. Molecular approaches to suppress the tumor phenotype might include specific inactivation of oncogene expression or replacement of a tumor suppressor gene. For these applications to be successful, gene transduction of tumor cells would need to be very efficient since residual tumor cells would presumably continue to grow. Although protocols have been proposed to test transfer of antisense molecules to oncogenes, it remains unclear whether neoplasia can be effectively treated using these strategies.

SUMMARY

In many respects, gene therapy has been a logical extension of the application of molecular biology to medicine. The first genetic disease elucidated at the molecular level was sickle cell anemia. Since then, our understanding of inherited and acquired blood disorders has continued to become more sophisticated. While gene therapy of the hemoglobinopathies has been more difficult to achieve than anticipated, it seems likely that at least certain genetic hematologic disorders, such as ADA deficiency, will soon become amenable to effective gene replacement therapy. To some extent, scientific progress in this field will depend on a better understanding of human hematopoiesis as well as the development of simple and reliable vectors for gene transfer. Whether or not complex disorders such as neoplasia can be effectively treated by gene transfer is unclear at present, but it seems reasonable to expect that novel and important research will continue to result from the interface between this applied science and hematology.

REFERENCES

1. Varmus H: Form and function of retroviral proviruses. Science 216:812, 1982
2. Shoemaker C, Goff S, Gilboa E et al: Structure of the cloned circular Moloney murine leukemia virus DNA molecule containing an inverted segment: implications for retroviral integration. Proc Natl Acad Sci USA 77:3932, 1980
3. Leis J, Baltimore D, Bishop JM et al: Standardized and simplified nomenclature for proteins common to all retroviruses. J Virol 62:1808, 1988
4. Hunter E, Swanstrom R: Retrovirus envelope glycoproteins. Curr Top Microbiol Immunol 171:95, 1991
5. Wang H, Kavanaugh MP, North RA, Kabat D: Cell surface receptor for eco-

tropic murine retroviruses is a basic amino-acid transporter. Nature 352:729, 1991

6. Miller DG, Edwards RH, Miller AD: Cloning of the cellular receptor for amphotropic murine retroviruses reveals homology to that for gibbon ape leukemia virus. Proc Natl Acad Sci USA 91:78, 1994

7. Nienhuis AW, Walsh CE, Liu J: Viruses as therapeutic gene transfer vectors. p. 353. In Young NS (ed): Viruses and Bone Marrow. Marcel Dekker, New York, 1993

8. Miller AD: Retroviral vectors. Curr Top Microbiol Immunol 171:95, 1991

9. Harel J, Rassert E, Jolicoeur P: Cell cycle dependence of synthesis of unintegrated viral DNA in mouse cells newly infected with murine leukemia virus. Virology 110:202, 1981

10. Miller DG, Adam MA, Miller AD: Gene transfer by retrovirus vectors occurs only in cells that are actively replicating at the time of infection. Mol Cell Biol 10:4239, 1990

11. Donahue RE, Kessler SW, Bodine D et al: Helper virus induced T-cell lymphoma in non-human primates after retroviral mediated gene transfer. J Exp Med 176:1125, 1992

12. Muzyczka N: Use of AAV as a general transduction vector for mammalian cells. Curr Top Microbiol Immunol 158:97, 1992

13. Samulski RJ: Adeno-associated virus: integration at a specific chromosomal locus. Curr Opin Genet Dev 3:74, 1993

14. Mulligan RC: The basic science of gene therapy. Science 260:926, 1993

15. Zhu N, Liggitt D, Liu Y, Debs R: Systemic gene expression after intravenous DNA delivery into adult mice. Science 261:209, 1993

16. Becker AJ, McCulloch EA, Siminovitch L, Till JE: The effect of differing demands for blood cell production on DNA synthesis by hematopoietic colony forming cells of mice. Blood 26:296, 1965

17. Hodgson GS, Bradley TR: Properties of haematopoietic stem cells surviving 5-fluorouracil treatment: evidence for a pre-CFU-S cell? Nature 281:381, 1979

18. Snodgrass R, Keller G: Clonal fluctuations within the haemopoietic system of mice reconstituted with retrovirus-infected stem cells. EMBO J 6:3955, 1987

19. Andrews RG, Singer JW, Bernstein ID: Precursors of colony-forming cells in humans can be distinguished from colony-forming cells by expression of the CD33 and CD34 antigens and light scatter properties. J Exp Med 169:1721, 1989

20. Andrews RG, Singer JW, Bernstein ID: Human hematopoietic precursors in long-term culture: single CD34+ cells that lack detectable T cell, B cell, and myeloid cell antigens produce multiple colony-forming cells when cultured with marrow stromal cells. J Exp Med 172:355, 1990

21. Berenson RJ, Andrews RG, Bensinger WI et al: Antigen CD34+ marrow cells engraft lethally irradiated baboons. J Clin Invest 81:951, 1988

22. Lansdorp PM, Schmitt C, Sutherland HJ et al: Hematopoietic stem cell characterization. Prog Clin Biol Res 377:475, 1992

23. Craig W, Kay R, Cutler RL, Lansdorp PM: Expression of Thy-1 on human hematopoietic progenitor cells. J Exp Med 177:1331, 1993

24. Lansdorp PM, Dragowska W, Mayani H: Ontogeny-related changes in proliferative potential of human hematopoietic cells. J Exp Med 178:787, 1993

25. Spangrude GJ, Heimfeld S, Weissman IL: Purification and characterization of mouse hematopoietic stem cells. Science 241:58, 1988

26. Leary AG, Zeng HQ, Clark SC, Ogawa M: Growth factor requirements for survival in G_0 and entry into the cell cycle of primitive hematopoietic progenitors. Proc Natl Acad Sci USA 89:4013, 1992

27. Goodman JW, Hodgson GS: Evidence for stem cells in the peripheral blood of mice. Blood 19:702, 1962

28. Bender JG, Unverzagt KL, Walker DE et al: Identification and comparison of CD34-positive cells and their subpopulations from normal peripheral blood and bone marrow using multicolor flow cytometry. Blood 77:2591, 1991

29. Eaves CJ: Peripheral blood stem cells reach new heights. Blood 82:1957, 1993

30. Bodine DM, Karlsson S, Nienhuis AW: Combination of interleukins 3 and 6 preserves stem cell function in culture and enhances retrovirus-mediated gene transfer into hematopoietic stem cells. Proc Natl Acad Sci USA 86:8897, 1989

31. Stewart FM, Crittenden RB, Lowry PA et al: Long-term engraftment of normal and post-5-fluorouracil murine marrow into normal nonmyeloablated mice. Blood 81:2566, 1993

32. Karlsson S: Treatment of genetic defects in hematopoietic cell function by gene transfer. Blood 78:2481, 1991

33. Brenner MK, Rill DR, Moen RC et al: Gene marking to trace the origin of relapse after autologous bone marrow transplantation. Lancet 341:85, 1993

34. Nabel EG, Plautz G, Boyce FM et al: Recombinant gene expression in vivo within endothelial cells of the arterial wall. Science 244:1342, 1989

35. Nabel EG, Plautz G, Nabel GJ: Site-specific gene expression in vivo by direct gene transfer into the arterial wall. Science 249:1285, 1990

36. Lee SW, Trapnell BC, Rade JJ et al: In vivo adenoviral vector-mediated gene transfer into balloon-injured rat carotid arteries. Circ Res 73:797, 1993

37. Lemarchand P, Jones M, Yamada I, Crystal RG: In vivo gene transfer and expression in normal uninjured blood vessels using replication-deficient recombinant adenovirus vectors. Circ Res 72:1132, 1993

38. Blaese RM: Development of gene therapy for immunodeficiency: adenosine deaminase deficiency. Pediatr Res, suppl. 1. 33:s49, 1993

39. Wijnaendts L, Le Deist F, Griscelli C, Fischer A: Development of immunologic functions after bone marrow transplantation in 33 patients with severe combined immunodeficiency. Blood 74:2212, 1989

40. Hershfield MS, Buckley RH, Greenberg ML et al: Treatment of adenosine deaminase deficiency with polyethylene glycol-modified adenosine deaminase. N Engl J Med 316:589, 1987

41. Kantoff PW, Kohn DB, Mitsuya H et al: Correction of adenosine deaminase deficiency in cultured human T and B cells by retrovirus-mediated gene transfer. Proc Natl Acad Sci USA 83:6563, 1986

42. Lim B, Apperley JF, Orkin ST, Williams DA: Long-term expression of human adenosine deaminase in mice transplanted with retrovirus-infected hematopoietic stem cells. Proc Natl Acad Sci USA 86:8892, 1989

43. Wilson JM, Danos O, Grossman M et al: Expression of human adenosine deaminase in mice reconstituted with retrovirus-transduced hematopoietic stem cells. Proc Natl Acad Sci USA 87:439, 1990

44. Bodine D, Moritz T, Donahue RE et al: Long term expression of a murine adenosine deaminase (ADA) gene in rhesus hematopoietic cells of multiple lineages following retroviral mediated gene transfer into CD 34+ bone marrow cells. Blood 82:1975, 1993

45. Walsh CE, Liu J, Miller JL et al: Gene therapy for human hemoglobinopathies. Proc Soc Exp Med Biol 204:289, 1993

46. Bender MA, Miller AD, Gelinas RE: Expression of the human β-globin gene after retroviral transfer into murine erythroleukemia cells and human BFU-E cells. Mol Cell Biol 8:1725, 1988

47. Dzierzak EA, Papayannopoulou T, Mulligan RC: Lineage-specific expression of a human β-globin gene in murine bone marrow transplant recipients reconstituted with retrovirus-transduced stem cells. Nature 331:35, 1988

48. Grosveld F, van Assendelft B, Greaves DR, Kollias G: Position-independent, high level expression of the human β-globin gene in transgenic mice. Cell 51: 975, 1987

49. Plavec I, Papayannopoulou T, Maury C, Meyer F: A human β-globin gene fused to the human β-globin locus control region is exposed at high levels in erythroid cells of mice engrafted with retrovirus transduced hematopoietic stem cells. Blood 81:1384, 1993

50. Walsh CE, Liu JM, Young NS et al: Regulated high level expression of a human γ-globin gene introduced into erythroid cells by an adeno-associated virus vector. Proc Natl Acad Sci USA 89:7257, 1992

51. Sorge J, Kuhl W, West C, Beutler E: Complete correction of the enzymatic defect of type 1 Gaucher disease fibroblasts by retroviral gene transfer. Proc Natl Acad Sci USA 84:906, 1987

52. Nolta JA, Sender LS, Barranger JA, Kohn DB: Expression of human glucocerebrosidase in murine long-term bone marrow culture after retroviral vector-mediated transfer. Blood 75:787, 1990

53. Correll PH, Fink JK, Brady RO et al: Production of human glucocerebrosidase in mice after retroviral gene transfer into multipotential hematopoietic progenitor cells. Proc Natl Acad Sci USA 86:8912, 1989

54. Xu LC, Dave HPG, Correll PH et al: High efficiency transfer of the glucocerebrosidase gene into human CD34+ hematopoietic progenitors using a clinically acceptable protocol. Blood, suppl. 1. 80:179a, 1992

55. Curnutte JT: Molecular basis of the autosomal recessive forms of chronic granulomatous disease. Immunodefic Rev 3:149, 1992

56. Cobbs CS, Malech HL, Leto T et al: Retroviral expression of recombinant p47phox protein by Epstein-Barr virus-transformed B lymphocytes from a patient with autosomal chronic granulomatous disease. Blood 79:1829, 1992

57. Tolstoshev P: Gene therapy, concepts, current trials and future directions. Annu Rev Pharmacol Toxicol 32:573, 1993

58. Kay MA, Rothenberg S, Landen CN et al: In vivo gene therapy of hemophilia B: sustained partial correction in factor IX-deficient dogs. Science 262:117, 1993

59. Venkatesh LK, Arens MQ, Subramanian T, Chinnadurai G: Selective induction of toxicity to human cells expressing human immunodeficiency virus type 1 Tat by a conditionally cytotoxic vector. Proc Natl Acad Sci USA 87:8746, 1990

60. Baltimore D: Gene therapy: intracellular immunization. Nature 335:395, 1988

61. Sullenger BA, Gallardo HF, Ungers GE, Gilboa E: Overexpression of TAR sequences renders cells resistant to human immunodeficiency virus replication. Cell 63:601, 1990

62. Chatterjee S, Johnson PR, Wong KK Jr: Dual-target inhibition of HIV-1 in vitro by means of an adeno-associated virus vector. Science 247:1485, 1992

63. Marasco W, Haseltine WA, Chen SY: Design, intracellular expression, and

activity of a human anti-human immunodeficiency virus type 1 gp120 single-chain antibody. Proc Natl Acad Sci USA 90:7889, 1993

64. Morgan RA, Looney DJ, Muenchau DD et al: Retroviral vectors expressing soluble CD4: a potential gene therapy for AIDS. AIDS Res Hum Retroviruses 6:183, 1990

65. Oldfield EH, Ram Z, Culver KW et al: Gene therapy for the treatment of brain tumors using intra-tumoral transduction with the thymidine kinase gene and intravenous ganciclovir. Hum Gene Ther 4:39, 1993

66. Rosenberg SA, Aebersold P, Cornetta K et al: Gene transfer into humans—immunotherapy of patients with advanced melanoma. using tumor infiltrating lymphocytes modified by retroviral gene transduction. N Engl J Med 326: 370, 1990

67. Plautz GE, Yang ZY, Wu B et al: Immunotherapy of malignancy by in vivo gene transfer into tumors. Proc Natl Acad Sci USA 90:4645, 1993

Appendix 31-1

Glossary of Terms

Amphotropic: Term used to describe a retrovirus capable of infecting nonmurine (human) as well as murine cells.

Antisense: Nucleic acid (RNA or DNA) complementary in sequence to the mRNA transcript of a target gene. Antisense molecules are thought to inhibit translation of the target mRNA.

Ecotropic: Term used to describe a retrovirus capable of infecting murine cells.

Gene marking: The introduction of foreign viral sequences into the chromosomal DNA of a patient's bone marrow to mark or track cells.

Insertional mutagenesis: Occurs when the retroviral genomes insert into the human genome at or near a gene and cause that nearby gene to behave in a deranged manner that disrupts normal control of cell growth or differentiation.

Integration: Process whereby exogenous genetic material becomes incorporated into the host cell genome. Usually refers to the latent or proviral state of certain viruses in infected cells.

Intracellular immunization: Genetic alteration of a cell to induce resistance to viral (e.g., HIV) replication or infection.

Locus control region: Control elements that flank the human β-globin gene cluster and modulate globin gene expression.

Long terminal repeat: Terminal sequences of a retrovirus that usually contain the transcriptional control elements (promoters), polyadenylation signals, and sequences involved in replication and integration.

Promoter: Control element responsible for transcription of a gene.

Provirus: Integrated form of a transducing virus, such as a retrovirus.

Selectable marker: To optimize and enrich for transduced cells, genes encoding for bacterial antibiotic resistance proteins (such as neomycin or hygromycin) are incorporated into the vector. Following transduction, incubation with the antibiotic selects for transduced cells resistant to the antibiotic.

Transduction: The stable transfer of genetic material into a cell, usually implying integration of DNA into the nuclear genome.

Transfection: The uptake of foreign genetic material into a cell. Transfection is usually accomplished by physical means such as co-precipitation of the DNA with insoluble calcium phosphate. Transfected DNA can either exist in the cell as an episomal (extrachromosomal) element or be integrated within the nuclear genome. The efficiency of DNA transfer into cells depends on the particular method used.

Vector: Vehicle for gene transfer

RED BLOOD CELLS

Part IV

The Red Cell Membrane

32

Narla Mohandas

INTRODUCTION

The human red cell leaves the bone marrow in the form of the reticulocyte; thereafter, the mature erythrocyte spends its circulatory lifetime of approximately 120 days performing its function of oxygen delivery. To provide this function optimally, it must possess a remarkable ability to undergo cellular deformation. The diameter of the human red cell ($8\ \mu m$) far exceeds that of the capillaries ($2-3\ \mu m$) through which it must pass in the process of delivering oxygen to the tissues. The ability of normal red blood cells to undergo marked deformation during passage through capillaries was originally documented by Leeuwenhoek in 1675, who noted that the globules underwent deformation into an ellipsoidal shape during passage through the microvasculature, but resumed their original shape when they returned to large vessels. After observing a smear of his own blood, Leeuwenhoek noticed, with remarkable prescience, that when he was greatly "disordered," globules of his blood appeared hard and rigid but grew softer and more pliable as his health returned to normal. Since these insightful original observations, a substantial body of evidence has been gathered that suggests that the ability of the red cell to undergo extensive passive deformation is essential, not only for its function but also for its survival.[1-5]

The capacity of the red blood cell to negotiate narrow splenic channels and capillaries (Fig. 32-1) while withstanding continuous circulatory stresses is programmed into its geometry, the viscosity of the intracellular milieu, and the material properties of the membrane.[6] The biochemical composition and anatomic organization of various components of the red cell membrane determine these various cellular characteristics. The red cell is unique among eukaryotic cells in that its principal physical structure is its membrane, which encloses a concentrated hemoglobin solution. In contrast with other cells, the red blood cell has no cytoplasmic structures or organelles and does not have a nucleus. Thus, all the structural elements of the red cell are in one way or other linked to the cell membrane. This chapter summarizes the mechanisms by which different membrane components and their interactions with one another contribute to these unique features.

MEMBRANE STRUCTURAL ORGANIZATION

The red cell membrane is composed of a lipid bilayer to which is anchored a filamentous network of proteins lining the cytoplasmic surface of the membrane. This network, also referred to as the membrane skeleton, is important for maintaining red cell shape and regulating membrane properties of deformability and mechanical stability.[6] The red cell membrane has been well characterized biochemically. The structural organization of the various lipid and protein components has been well delineated.[7-13] About 52% of the membrane mass is protein, 40% is lipid and 8% is carbohydrate. The major lipid components are unesterified cholesterol and phospholipids, present in nearly equimolar quantities. Free fatty acid and glycolipids are present in small amounts.[7] The phospholipid of the membrane has the following composition: phosphatidylcholine (PC) 30%, sphingomyelin (SM) 25%, phosphatidylethanolamine (PE) 28%, and phosphatidylserine (PS) 14%. Phospho-

lipids such as phosphatidic acid, phosphatidylinositol-4-phosphate, and phosphatidylinositol-4,5-diphosphate comprise about 2–3% of the total. These phospholipids are asymmetrically distributed in the membrane: >75% of the choline-containing uncharged phospholipids PC and SM lies in the outer monolayer of lipid bilayer, while 80% of PE and all PS, the charged phospholipids, reside in the inner monolayer.[8]

The maintenance of asymmetric phospholipid distribution in the normal red cell membrane appears to be the result of (1) a slow and symmetric rate of passive diffusion of choline-containing phospholipids (PC and SM) across the two lipid monolayers (half-times on the order of hours), and (2) active transport of the aminophospholipids (PS and PE) by an ATP-dependent aminophospholipid translocase or "flipase" from the outer to the inner monolayer.[9] In contrast to phospholipids, cholesterol diffuses across the membrane on a physiologic time scale (a half-time of seconds or less).[14] The mature red cell is unable to synthesize lipids de novo, but a number of lipid renewal pathways produce considerable turnover of the various phospholipids with no net change in lipid composition. In addition, the cholesterol content of the membrane is regulated by the exchange that takes place between plasma cholesterol and membrane cholesterol.

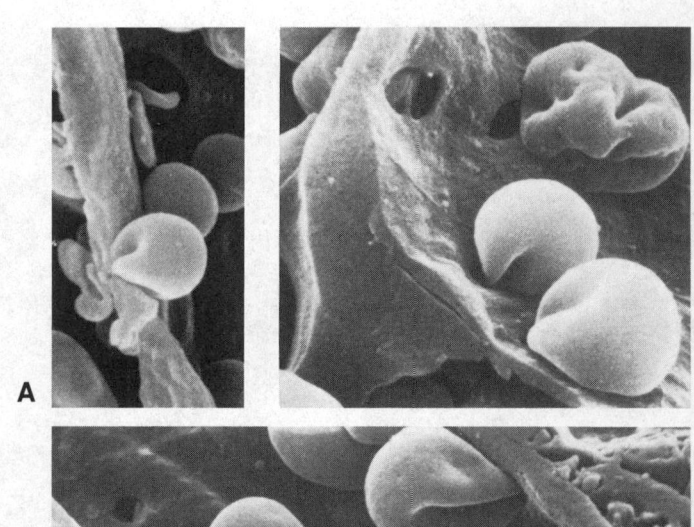

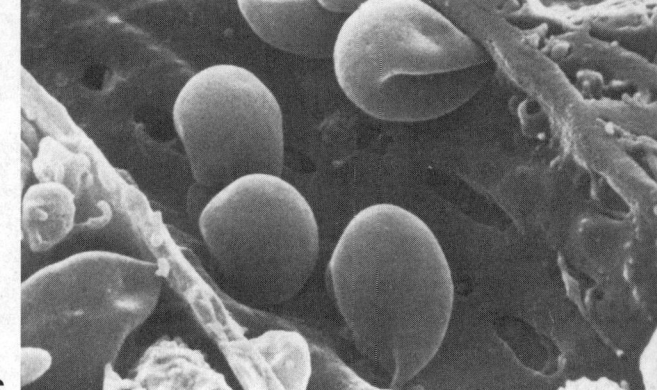

Fig. 32-1. (A–C) Scanning electron micrographs of red blood cells passing through splenic endothelial slits. Note the remarkable deformation exhibited by the red cells during their transit through these structures. The cell with lobular and irregular surface in Fig. B is a reticulocyte in transit.

The function of the phospholipid bilayer is to provide physical continuity to the membrane. This membrane continuity, in turn, is responsible for solute impermeability. The lipid bilayer also serves as the matrix in which transmembrane proteins reside. The fluidity of this matrix is regulated by lipid composition.

Analysis of proteins of the red cell membrane by sodium dodecyl sulfate/polyacrylamide gel electrophoresis (SDS/PAGE) in one dimension indicates the presence of about a dozen distinct species, most of which have been well characterized. By contrast, two-dimensional separation employing isoelectric focusing and SDS/PAGE shows the membrane to be composed of >100 different proteins, many of which are yet to be characterized. The proteins of the membrane are divided into two general groups: integral and peripheral proteins. The integral proteins are tightly bound to the membrane through hydrophobic interactions with the lipids in the bilayer. Band 3 and glycophorins belong to this class; these proteins span the membrane and have distinct structural and functional domains, both within the bilayer and on either side of the membrane. The peripheral proteins are located on the cytoplasmic surface of the lipid bilayer and can be readily released from the membrane by manipulation of ionic strength of the milieu or other protein perturbants. The peripheral proteins, which include spectrin, actin, and protein 4.1, constitute the membrane skeleton (Fig. 32-2).

The most abundant and best-studied integral proteins of the red cell membrane are band 3 and a family of sialoglycoproteins called glycophorins.

Band 3, the anion exchanger, is the major integral protein, constituting about 25% of total membrane protein. Recent cloning studies have demonstrated that this protein is the product of a gene residing on chromosome 17 that encodes a 911-amino acid protein ($101,791$ M_r).[15] Each red cell contains approximately 1×10^6 copies of band 3. This protein is composed of three dissimilar and functionally distinct domains. The hydrophilic cytoplasmic domain (residues 1–403) interacts with a variety of peripheral membrane and cytoplasmic proteins, including ankyrin, protein 4.1, protein 4.2, hemoglobin, and a variety of glycolytic enzymes. The hydrophobic transmembrane domain (residues 404–882) contains multiple membrane spanning domains and forms the anion transporter. The acidic C-terminal domain (residues 883–911) has no known function. Band 3 contains a single N-glycosidically linked oligosaccharide that possesses the blood group antigen activities I and i. The two clearly established functions of band 3 in the membrane are (1) anion transport, resulting in one-for-one exchange

of HCO_3^- or Cl^- across the membrane; and (2) physical linkage of the lipid bilayer to the underlying membrane skeleton, primarily through its interaction with ankyrin and secondarily through binding to protein 4.1 or protein 4.2.

Four sialic acid-rich glycoproteins (glycophorins A, B, C, and D) comprise a class of integral proteins termed glycophorins, constituting approximately 2% of the total red cell membrane proteins.[16–18] Glycophorins A, B, and C are distinctly different polypeptides containing 131, 72, and 128 residues, respectively. Recent cloning and sequencing studies have shown that these proteins are the product of distinct genes. The genes coding for glycophorins A and B reside on chromosome 4' and glycophorin C is encoded on chromosome 2. Glycophorins consist of three domains: a cytoplasmic domain, containing a cluster of basic residues positioned near the plasma membrane; a hydrophobic domain, which forms a single α-helix spanning the bilayer; and an extracellular domain, which is heavily glycosylated. The glycophorin A molecule carries the MN blood group specificity, glycophorin B the Ss specificity, and glycophorin C the Gerbich blood group specificity. The presence of carbohydrates imparts a strong net negative charge to the cell surface; this is functionally important in reducing the interaction of red cells with one another as well as of red cells with other cells, including vascular endothelium. Glycophorin C appears to interact with protein 4.1; through this association it may regulate the membrane content of protein 4.1.

A number of other integral proteins are present in the red cell membrane. These carry blood group-specific determinants, such as Rh, Duffy, and Kell. These proteins are beginning to be characterized. It is likely that some of these integral proteins possess transmembrane transport functions.

The filamentous network of peripheral proteins is anchored to the bilayer by interaction with several integral proteins. The network, generally referred to as the membrane skeleton, is composed of three principal components: spectrin, actin, and protein 4.1 (Fig. 32-2). Spectrin is a flexible, rod-like molecule present in red cells at approximately 200,000 copies per cell. It is composed of two nonidentical subunits of 260,000 daltons (spectrin, α-subunit) and 246,000 daltons (spectrin β-subunit) intertwined side to side, forming a heterodimer with a contour length of approximately 100 nm. The gene that codes for α-spectrin resides on chromosome 1 and that for β-spectrin on chromosome 14. Each polypeptide is organized into a number of independently folded domains, each containing 106 residues. The subunits are linked by flexible joining regions like beads on a string.

Spectrin heterodimers associate head to head to form $(\alpha\beta)_2$-

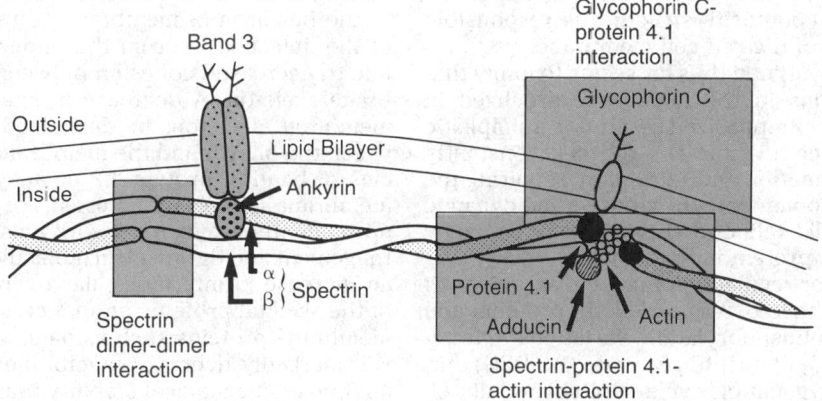

Fig. 32-2. Schematic diagram of the red cell membrane organization based on our current understanding of various protein associations. The key protein interactions identified to be important in regulating red cell membrane mechanical stability include spectrin dimer-dimer interaction, spectrin-actin-protein 4.1 interaction, band 3-ankyrin-spectrin interaction, and glycophorin C-protein 4.1 interaction. Adducin, a membrane skeleton-associated calmodulin-binding protein, also promotes spectrin-actin interaction.

tetramers, which have a contour length of approximately 200 nm. Tetrameric species of spectrin appear to predominate in the membrane skeleton. Oligomers larger than the tetramers are also observed; they appear to be formed by spectrin dimers joined by head-to-head linkages into a central ring.[19] The tail ends of spectrin tetramers are associated with short oligomers of actin composed of 12 monomers. Red cell actin is unusual in being organized into short, highly uniform filaments of approximately 35 nm in length. The strict control of actin filament length may be modulated by the proteins tropomyosin and tropomodulin.[20] On average, six spectrin ends complex with each actin oligomer, creating an irregular network with an approximately hexagonal lattice.

Each spectrin-actin junction is stabilized by the formation of a ternary complex with protein 4.1. The gene coding for protein 4.1 has been sequenced and localized to chromosome 1. The protein is composed of 622 amino acids; approximately 200,000 copies of this molecule are present in each red cell. Spectrin-actin interactions that are independently weak are greatly stabilized by protein 4.1.[13] This stabilization occurs through direct interaction of protein 4.1 with spectrin at sites on the molecule close to the region in which spectrin interacts with actin oligomers. Adducin is yet another skeletal protein that stabilizes the interaction of spectrin with actin. However, in contrast to protein 4.1, adducin is much less abundant in the red cell, with only 30,000 molecules present in each cell. An interesting feature of adducin is that it is a target for the calcium-dependent regulating protein, calmodulin; as such, its ability to promote spectrin-actin interactions is regulated by intracellular calcium concentrations.

The red cell membrane skeleton can be envisioned as an irregular network in which the basic unit is composed of a hexagonal lattice with six spectrin molecules. The structural model for organization of the membrane skeleton has been confirmed by high resolution electron micrographs of isolated membranes.[21] These micrographs show a highly repeated and remarkably regular organization of the spectrin/actin/protein 4.1 complexes in which each complex is linked to adjacent complexes by multiple spectrin tetramers.

The physical linkage of membrane skeleton to the lipid bilayer is accomplished primarily by ankyrin (band 2.1), which simultaneously interacts with spectrin in the skeleton and band 3 localized in the bilayer.[13] The gene coding for ankyrin has been sequenced and localized to chromosome 8. Ankyrin is 1,879 amino acids long. It contains distinct binding sites for both β-spectrin and band 3 and is present in the red cell at 100,000 copies per cell. The ankyrin-binding site on β-spectrin is located approximately 20 nm from the C-terminus. Through this linkage, the lipid bilayer is mechanically coupled to the membrane skeleton; this composite structure is responsible for the unique properties of the red cell membrane.

Much of the discussion outlined thus far seems to imply that protein-protein associations in the membrane are fixed in space and time. It should be emphasized that this is a simplistic view. During its time in circulation, the red cell constantly undergoes cycles of deformation and relaxation, requiring the membrane skeleton to accommodate to extensive and dynamic changes in cell shape. In all likelihood, this is accomplished by dynamic regulation of the protein interactions.

Potential mechanisms for regulation of protein associations within the skeleton and those between skeletal proteins and integral proteins include phosphorylation, variations in intracellular magnesium and 2,3-diphosphoglycerate (2,3-DPG) during the oxygenation/deoxygenation cycle, and calmodulin effects due to elevated intracellular calcium.[13] Only limited information is available regarding these regulatory pathways, but most available evidence suggests that phosphorylation tends to lower the affinity of protein-protein interactions. For example, phosphorylation of protein 4.1 results in a fivefold decrease in its affinity for spectrin and in its ability to promote spectrin-actin association. Similarly, increased levels of intracellular 2,3-DPG and elevated cytoplasmic concentrations of calcium, in association with calmodulin, appear to destabilize spectrin-actin-protein 4.1 and spectrin-actin-adducin interactions, respectively. Thus, the red cell membrane is a dynamic structure in which multiple protein-protein associations are subjected to regulation. The most important function of these protein assemblies is to provide the cell with a flexible yet mechanically resilient and stable, membrane.

MEMBRANE MECHANICS AND SKELETAL PROTEINS

During its 120-day life span, the erythrocyte must undergo extensive passive deformation and resist fragmentation. These two essential qualities require a highly deformable yet remarkably stable membrane. The property of membrane deformability determines the extent of membrane deformation that can be induced by a defined level of applied force. The more deformable the membrane, the less applied force necessary to allow the cell to pass through the capillaries. By contrast, membrane stability is defined as the maximum extent of deformation that a membrane can undergo, beyond which it cannot completely recover its initial shape, that is, the point at which it fails. Normal membrane stability allows red cells to circulate without fragmenting, while decreased stability leads to cell fragmentation under normal circulating stresses.

A model designed to conceptualize how these membrane properties are regulated by the membrane components is presented in Figure 32-3.[6,22] This model takes into account the known structure, associations, and stoichiometry of the skeletal proteins. In the nondeformed state, spectrin molecules exist in a folded confirmation. Reversible deformation of the red cell membrane occurs with a change in geometric shape, but at constant surface area. During reversible deformation, a rearrangement of the skeletal network occurs in which some spectrin molecules become uncoiled and extended, while others are more compressed and folded. With increased deformation, the membrane becomes increasingly extended; some of the spectrin molecules attain their maximal linear extension. This point is the limit of reversible deformability. A continued application of force would necessitate an increase in surface area and the breaking of junctional complexes. When the red cells are exposed to fluid forces great enough to require an increase in surface area, the membrane fails. This failure will occur at the weakest of the lateral protein-protein associations (spectrin-spectrin junction or spectrin-actin-protein 4.1 junction), leading to membrane fragmentation.

Another form of membrane failure involves the separation of the lipid bilayer from the underlying membrane skeleton, due to decreased cohesion between the bilayer and the membrane skeleton. A decrease in spectrin density beneath the membrane skeleton, or decreased numbers of linkages between the bilayer and the membrane skeleton, due to deficiencies of band 3, protein 4.2 or ankyrin, leads to this form of membrane failure. By contrast, for the membrane to deform normally, the skeletal network must be able to undergo rearrangement and the spectrin molecules to fold and unfold. Thus, an increase in intermolecular or intramolecular associations of the skeletal proteins or an increased association of integral membrane proteins such as band 3 with the skeletal network will markedly decrease membrane deformability.[6,22] Deformability and mechanical stability than measurements on pathologic red cells with different mutant forms of membrane proteins, as well as on biochemically perturbed normal red cells, strongly support this model and point unequivocally to a crucial role for membrane proteins and their associations in regulating these two membrane properties.[6,22]

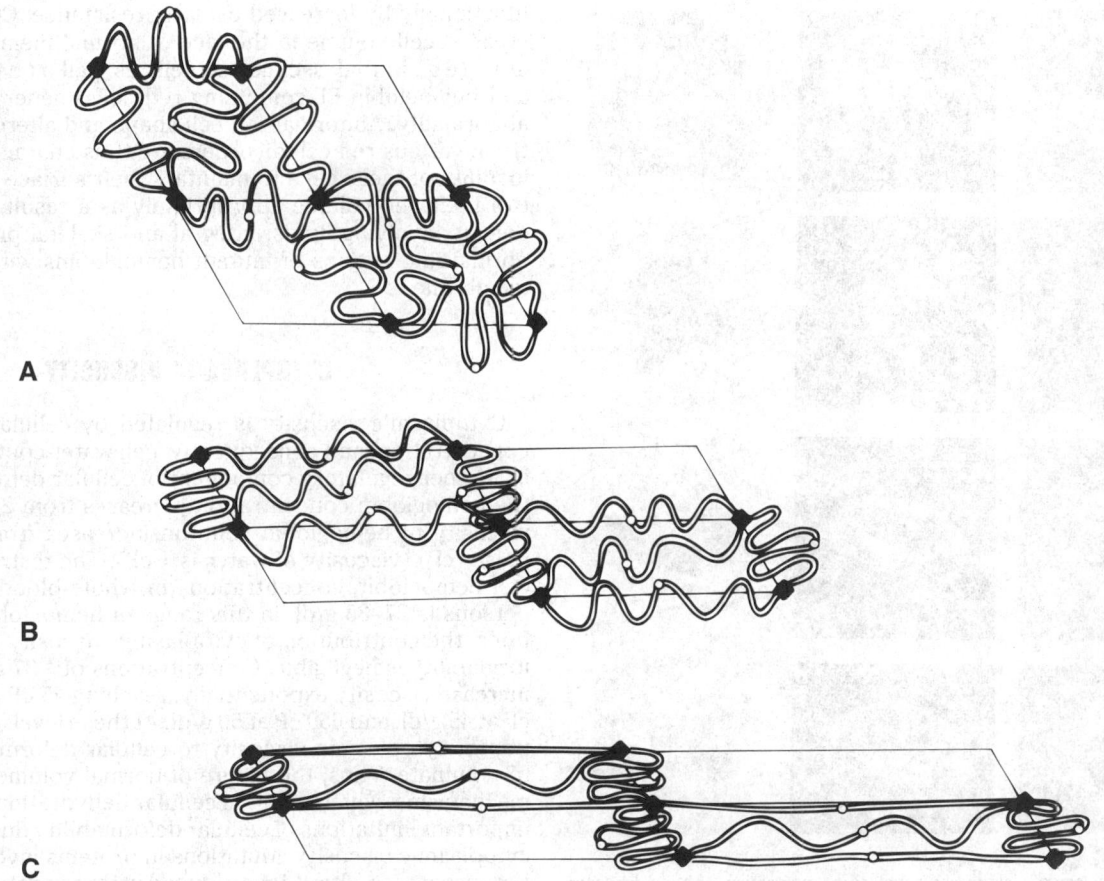

Fig. 32-3. Conceptual depiction of rearrangements in membrane skeleton during reversible deformation of red cells. Reversible deformation occurs with a change in geometric shape, but at a constant surface area. **(A)** Organization of membrane skeleton in the nondeformed membrane. **(B & C)** With increased deformation, the membrane becomes increasingly extended. **(C)** Further extention beyond this membrane would result in an increase in surface area and the breaking of lateral junction points. This is the stage at which membrane fragmentation occurs. ◆, protein 4.1-actin-spectrin junction; ○, spectrin-spectrin junction; linear coils are spectrin dimer.

ROLE OF MEMBRANE IN DETERMINING SHAPE AND DEFORMABILITY OF THE RED CELL

Cellular deformability is the term generally used to characterize the ability of the red cell to undergo deformation during flow. This property is influenced by three distinct cellular components: cell shape or cell geometry, which determines the ratio of cell surface area to cell volume; cytoplasmic viscosity, which is regulated by intracellular hemoglobin concentration; and membrane deformability.[6] Membrane deformability, in and of itself, is regulated by multiple membrane properties, which include elastic shear modulus, bending modulus, and yield stress. Either directly or indirectly, membrane components and their organization play an important role in regulating each factor that influences cellular deformability.

CELL SHAPE

The biconcave disc shape of the normal red cell creates an advantageous surface area/volume relationship, allowing the red cell to undergo marked deformation while maintaining a constant surface area. The normal human adult red cell has a volume of 90 μm^3 and a surface area of 140 μm^2. If the red cell were a sphere of identical volume, it would have a surface area of only 98 μm^2. Therefore, the discoid shape provides half again as much surface area as would a sphere of equivalent volume, and it is this excess surface area of approximately 40 μm^2 that allows the red cell to undergo extensive deformation.

Most deformations occurring in vivo, and in vitro, involve no increase in surface area. The normal red cell can undergo large linear extensions of ≤230% of its original dimension, but an increase of even 3–4% in surface area results in cell lysis. Because the acquisition and maintenance of a favorable surface area/volume relationship is crucial to red cell function, it is useful to understand how the cell acquires a discoid shape during its development from a nucleated erythroid precursor cell.

The immediate precursor of the mature discocytic red cell is the non-nucleated reticulocyte, produced when the normoblast extrudes its nucleus (Fig. 32-4). In contrast to red cells, these immature reticulocytes are multilobular and motile, contain mitochondria and ribosomes, and synthesize hemoglobin and certain membrane components, including protein 4.1 and glycophorin C. Reticulocytes exhibit much less cellular deformability and mechanical stability than is displayed by mature red cells. Both deformability and mechanical stability improve during maturation.[23] In 2–3 days, motile reticulocytes evolve further in the bone marrow, first to become deep cup-shaped nonmotile cells that still contain ribosomes, and finally to mature fully hemoglobinized discocytic red blood cells lacking organelles.

Major reorganizations of membrane phospholipids, skeletal proteins, and integral proteins, accompany the acquisition of discoid shape and enhanced deformability. These include loss of membrane lipids, loss of integral proteins such as transferrin receptors, insulin receptors, and fibronectin receptors, and a major reorganization of the skeletal protein network.

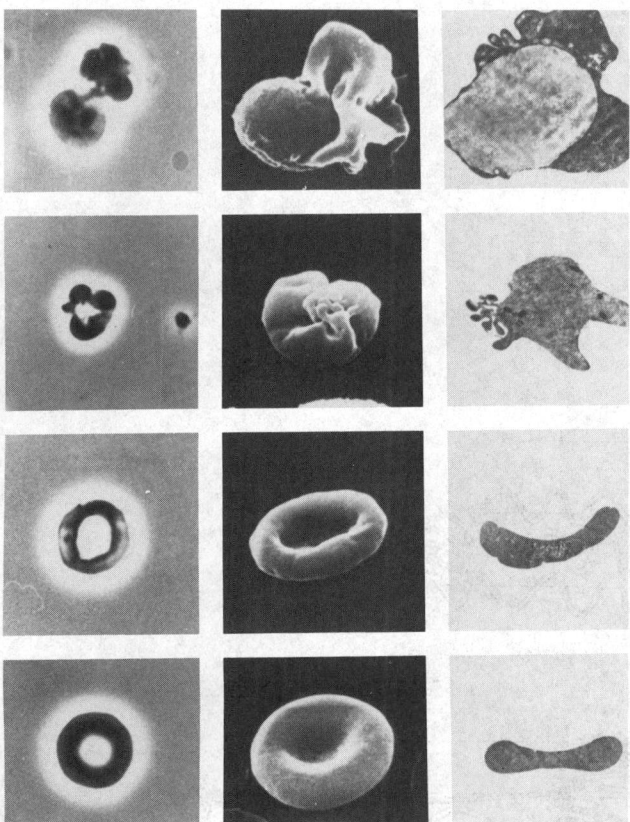

Fig. 32-4. Morphology of cells during reticulocyte maturation. Left-hand column, phase-contrast microscopy; middle column, scanning electron microscopy; right-hand column, transmission electron microscopy. The nuclear extrusion process is illustrated in the top row. The least mature reticulocytes, which are motile and multilobular, are shown in the second horizontal panel. The more mature reticulocytes, which are cup shaped and nonmotile, are depicted in the third horizontal panel. Mature red cells are illustrated in the bottom panel.

Having acquired the discoid shape with its favorable geometric parameters during reticulocyte maturation, the red cell must maintain this favorable surface area/volume relationship during its circulating life span. Either membrane loss, leading to reduction in surface area, or an increase in cell water content, leading to an increase in cell volume, will create a more spherical shape with less redundant surface area. This loss of surface area redundancy leads to decreased cellular deformability, compromised red cell function, and reduced survival.

Skeletal protein defects involving either spectrin or protein 4.1 lead to a mechanically unstable membrane, resulting in cell fragmentation and generation of cells with reduced surface area in congenital hemolytic anemias, such as hereditary spherocytosis and hereditary elliptocytosis (see Ch. 46).[24-25] Similarly, partial phagocytosis of the red cell by macrophages leads to reduced surface area and generation of spherocytes in certain immune hemolytic anemias. By contrast, in some forms of hereditary stomatocytosis, increased cell volume results from a membrane defect and results in deranged volume regulation, generating red cells with reduced redundant surface area. Increased osmotic fragility is a characteristic feature of all these red cell populations with less than normal surface redundancy.

A different type of red cell abnormality is manifested in patients with liver disease. In this instance, elevated membrane cholesterol content causes increased cell surface area; in the face of normal cell volume, this results in higher than normal redundant surface area. This excess surface area, in turn, is manifested morphologically by the presence of target cells and

functionally by increased osmotic resistance. Conversely, decreased cell volume in the face of normal membrane surface area, (e.g., in thalassemic red cells as well as hemoglobin CC- and hemoglobin EE-containing red cells) generates the same abnormality. Abnormal red cell shape and altered cell geometry in various red cell disorders are thus characterized by the inability of these cells to maintain their surface area and control their cell volume appropriately as a result of membrane defects involving lipids, integral and skeletal proteins, or abnormal interactions of mutant hemoglobins with the red cell membrane.

CYTOPLASMIC VISCOSITY

Cytoplasmic viscosity is regulated by cellular hemoglobin concentration, and consequently, cell water content. Viscosity is another regulatory component of cellular deformability.[6] As the hemoglobin concentration increases from 27–35 g/dl, the viscosity of hemoglobin solution increases from 5–15 centipoise (cP) (viscosity of water is 1 cP). The distribution of red cell hemoglobin concentrations in whole blood from normal persons is 27–35 g/dl. In this range of hemoglobin concentrations, the contribution of cytoplasmic viscosity to cellular deformability is negligible. Concentrations of ≥37 g/dl, however, increase viscosity exponentially, reaching 45 cP at 40 g/dl, 170 cP at 45 g/dl, and 650 cP at 50 g/dl. At these levels, the contribution of cytoplasmic viscosity to cellular deformability begins to dominate. Thus, the failure of normal volume homeostasis mechanisms, which result in cellular dehydration, can result in important limitations of cellular deformability due to increased cytoplasmic viscosity. Mutations in proteins involved in transport processes, alterations induced in these proteins as a result of membrane oxidation, or other changes due to mutant hemoglobin interacting with the membrane can lead to marked cellular dehydration. Reduced cellular deformability of hereditary xerocytosis, sickle red cells, and hemoglobin CC red cells is primarily due to increased cytoplasmic viscosity as a consequence of cellular dehydration.[4] The lipid components and the integral proteins of the red cell membrane play a crucial role in volume homeostasis of the red cell in order to maintain the cell hemoglobin concentration at levels that do not unduly influence the ability of the cell to deform.

MEMBRANE MATERIAL PROPERTIES

The mechanical behavior of the red cell membrane is complex. Its responses depend on the duration and magnitude of applied stresses.[6,26,27] At small values of applied force for short duration, the red cell membrane behaves as a viscoelastic solid; that is, it is capable of undergoing large elastic extensions and completely recovers its initial shape. A reversible unfolding and refolding of spectrin networks is crucial for the elastic behavior of the membrane.

By contrast, when small forces are applied over a long period, or when large forces are applied for a short period, the membrane yields and is unable to recover its initial shape. Under these circumstances, the membrane exhibits permanent "plastic" deformation due to the inability of the skeletal network to recover its prestressed configuration. While normal red cells completely recover their shape following repeated cycles of deformation in the circulation, pathologic red cells with weakened junctions between skeletal proteins fail to recover their initial shape and undergo plastic deformation. This explains in part the generation of elliptocytic shapes in congenital hemolytic anemias with defective spectrin oligomerization and decreased spectrin-actin-protein 4.1 association. The generation of irreversibly sickled cells in sickle cell anemia is also the result of plastic deformation of the membrane due to skeletal protein reorganization during repeated cycles of sickling and unsickling in the circulation.

In addition to contributing significantly to the regulation of the elastic behavior of the membrane, the membrane skeleton has a crucial role in regulating membrane mechanical stability. The junctional complexes in the skeletal network are the key regulators of mechanical stability. Decreased membrane mechanical stability is a hallmark of hereditary elliptocytosis due to either weakened spectrin-spectrin association as a result of mutations in either α- or β-spectrin or a weakened spectrin-actin-protein 4.1 junction due to mutations in protein 4.1.[6,22] A decrease in the number of linkages between the bilayer and the membrane skeleton also results in membrane surface area loss such as that seen in hereditary spherocytosis. By contrast, an increased number of linkages between the bilayer and the membrane skeleton results in decreased membrane deformability.[6] Although substantial changes in lipid composition of the membrane have little effect on membrane mechanical properties, small changes in individual protein components can profoundly alter membrane behavior. The integral proteins in association with the skeletal protein network determine the complex mechanical behavior of the red cell membrane.

The complex and regulated assembly of lipids and proteins in membrane lends the unique shape and deformability characteristics to the red cell, enabling it to survive its tortuous and at times turbulent journey through the vasculature. Derangement in the structural organization as a result of changes in any of the individual components of the membrane, either lipid or protein moieties, leads to altered cell shape or deformability characteristics, or both, the hallmarks of many red cell disorders.

REFERENCES

1. Weed RI: The importance of erythrocyte deformability. Am J Med 49:147, 1970
2. LaCelle PL, Weed RI: The contribution of normal and pathologic erythrocytes to blood rheology. Prog Hematol 7:1, 1971
3. Weiss L, Tavassoli M: Anatomic hazards to the passage of erythrocytes through the spleen. Semin Hematol 7:372, 1970
4. Mohandas N, Phillips WM, Bessis M: Red blood cell deformability and hemolytic anemias. Semin Hematol 16:95, 1979
5. Chien S: Red cell deformability and its relevance to blood flow. Annu Rev Physiol 49:177, 1987
6. Mohandas N, Chasis JA: Red cell deformability, membrane material properties and shape: regulation by transmembrane, skeletal and cytosolic proteins and lipids. Semin Hematol 30:171, 1993
7. Ways P, Hanahan DJ: Characterization and quantitation of red cell lipids in normal man. J Lipid Res 5:318, 1964
8. Verkleij AJ, Zwaal RFA, Roelofsen B et al: The asymmetric distribution of phospholipids in the human red cell membrane. A combined study using phospholipases and freeze-etch electron microscopy. Biochim Biophys Acta 323:178, 1973
9. Devaux PF: Static and dynamic lipid asymmetry in cell membranes. Biochemistry 30:1163, 1991
10. Fairbanks G, Steck TL, Wallach DFH: Electrophoretic analysis of the major polypeptides of the human erythrocyte membrane. Biochemistry 10:2606, 1971
11. Steck TL: The organization of proteins in the human red cell membrane. J Cell Biol 62:1, 1974
12. Marchesi VT: The stabilizing infrastructure of cell membranes. Annu Rev Cell Biol 1:531, 1985
13. Bennett V: The spectrin-actin junction of erythrocyte membrane skeleton. Biochim Biophys Acta 988:107, 1989
14. Lange Y, Dolde J, Steck TL: The rate of transmembrane movement of cholesterol in the human erythrocyte. J Biol Chem 256:5321, 1981
15. Lux SE, John KM, Kopito RR, Lodish HF: Cloning and characterization of band 3, the human erythrocyte and anion-exchange protein (AE1). Proc Natl Acad Sci USA 86:9089, 1989
16. Anstee DJ: The blood group MNSs active-sialoglycoproteins. Semin Hematol 18:13, 1981
17. Furthmayr H: Structural comparison of glycoprotein and immunochemical analysis of genetic variants. Nature 271:519, 1978
18. Chasis JA, Mohandas N: Red cell glycophorins. Blood 80:1869, 1992
19. Morrow JS, Marchesi VT: Self-assembly of spectrin oligomers in vitro: a basis for a dynamic cytoskeleton. J Cell Biol 88:463, 1981
20. Gilligan DM, Bennett V: The junctional complex of the membrane skeleton. Semin Hematol 30:74, 1993
21. Liu SC, Derick LH, Palek J: Visualization of the hexagonal lattice in the erythrocyte membrane skeleton. J Cell Biol 104:527, 1987
22. Chasis JA, Mohandas N: Erythrocyte membrane deformability and stability: two distinct membrane properties that are independently regulated by skeletal protein associations. J Cell Biol 103:343, 1986
23. Chasis JA, Prenant M, Leung A, Mohandas N: Membrane assembly and remodeling during reticulocyte maturation. Blood 74:1112, 1989
24. Palek J: Hereditary elliptocytosis, spherocytosis and related disorders: consequences of a deficiency or a mutation of membrane skeletal proteins. Blood Rev 1:147, 1987
25. Davies KA, Lux SE: Hereditary disorders of the red cell membrane skeleton. Trends Genet 5:222, 1989
26. Evans EA, La Celle PL: Intrinsic material properties of erythrocyte membrane indicated by mechanical analysis of deformation. Blood 45:29, 1975
27. Hochmuth RM, Waugh RE: Erythrocyte membrane elasticity and viscosity. Annu Rev Physiol 49:209, 1987

Biochemistry of the Red Cell

33

Donald E. Paglia

INTRODUCTION

The final stage of mammalian erythroid maturation produces anucleate globules composed of plasma membranes enveloping a viscous solution of concentrated hemoglobin. As such, the mature erythrocyte represents a highly specialized, yet remarkably simplified, cell—particularly as compared to nucleated cells containing complex cytoplasmic organelles, with their diverse and redundant metabolic capacities.

In the few days required for reticulocytes to mature, they

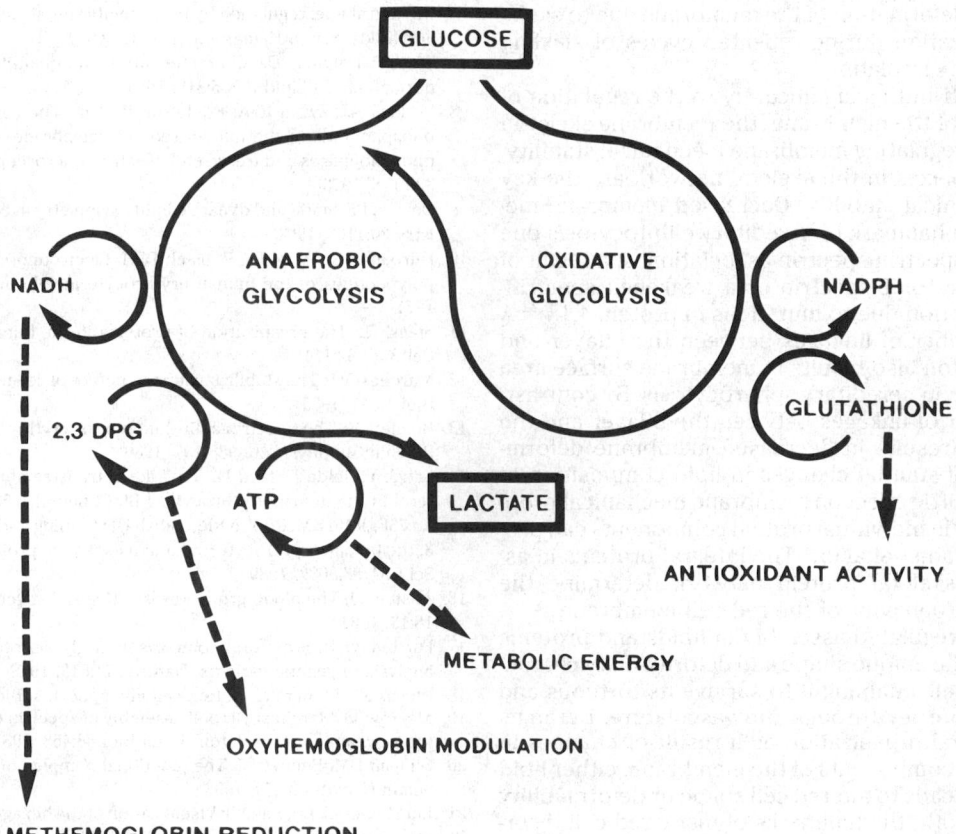

Fig. 33-1. Energy metabolism of the erythrocyte. Generation of high-energy phosphates and reducing compounds is accomplished principally by glucose catabolism. (Modified from Paglia and Valentine,[22] with permission.)

lose their last vestiges of ribosomal and mitochondrial function, having already dispatched their nuclei by pitting and karyolytic digestion. The resultant mature erythrocytes are therefore incapable of protein or lipid synthesis, oxidative phosphorylation, tricarboxylic acid cycling or most of the activities and capacities exhibited by nucleated cells.

The erythrocyte's raison d'être—gas transport and exchange—is accomplished entirely without alteration in energy states. Certain cellular functions, however, do require generation and expenditure of energy if the cell is to survive and function effectively for its full anticipated life span of 4 months. Among these energy-requiring processes are those that (1) initiate and maintain glycolysis, (2) synthesize glutathione and other essential compounds, such as phosphoribosylpyrophosphate, (3) mediate nucleotide salvage reactions, (4) maintain hemoglobin iron in its functional ferrous form, (5) protect hemoglobin and structural and enzymatic proteins from oxidative denaturation, (6) maintain appropriate cation concentrations despite electrochemical gradients, and (7) participate in phosphorylations and other reactions involving cytoskeletal components necessary for maintaining membrane phospholipids and plasticity.

These energy requirements are fulfilled almost entirely by the catabolism of glucose with storage of the generated energy as high-energy phosphate, particularly ATP, or as reducing compounds in the form of reduced glutathione (GSH) and pyridine cofactors nicotinamide adenine dinucleotide (NADH) and nicotinamide adenine dinucleotide phosphate (NADPH). Figure 33-1 summarizes this process of energy metabolism diagrammatically.

Plasma glucose provides an abundant carbon source that is assimilated by erythrocytes through a facilitated transport system. Generally, about 90% of the glucose taken into the erythrocyte is consistently catabolized through the anaerobic Embden-Meyerhof pathway, providing the cell's principal means of ATP generation. Small, and quite variable, amounts of glucose may be diverted through the hexose monophosphate shunt, also known as the pentose phosphate pathway. Glucose degradation via this oxidative shunt provides the erythrocyte with a pool of reducing energy with which to combat ambient oxidative effects on hemoglobin and other essential cellular proteins. When necessary, glucose shunting through this pathway can increase by an order of magnitude or more.

ANAEROBIC GLYCOLYSIS

Figure 33-2 shows in greater detail the biochemical pathways available to mature erythrocytes to accommodate their energy needs. Glucose catabolism is initiated by its phosphorylation to glucose-6-phosphate (G6P), a reaction catalyzed by hexokinase. This enzyme has the lowest activity of all the glycolytic enzymes in mature erythrocytes, and its catalytic rate is highly sensitive to pH, to intracellular concentrations of its product G6P, and to other metabolites, such as inorganic phosphate (P_i), 2,3-diphosphoglycerate (2,3-DPG), and disulfide compounds. By virtue of these enzyme characteristics, the phosphorylation of glucose becomes an important rate-limiting step in glycolysis.

Isomerization of G6P to fructose-6-phosphate (F6P) provides the substrate for a second major rate-limiting reaction, phosphorylation at the C-1 position, catalyzed by phosphofructokinase. Like hexokinase, this enzyme requires magnesium, is optimally active at alkaline pH, and is sensitive to stimulation by inorganic phosphate. The product of this reaction, fructose-1,6-diphosphate ($F1,6P_2$), is produced at the expense of 2 mol

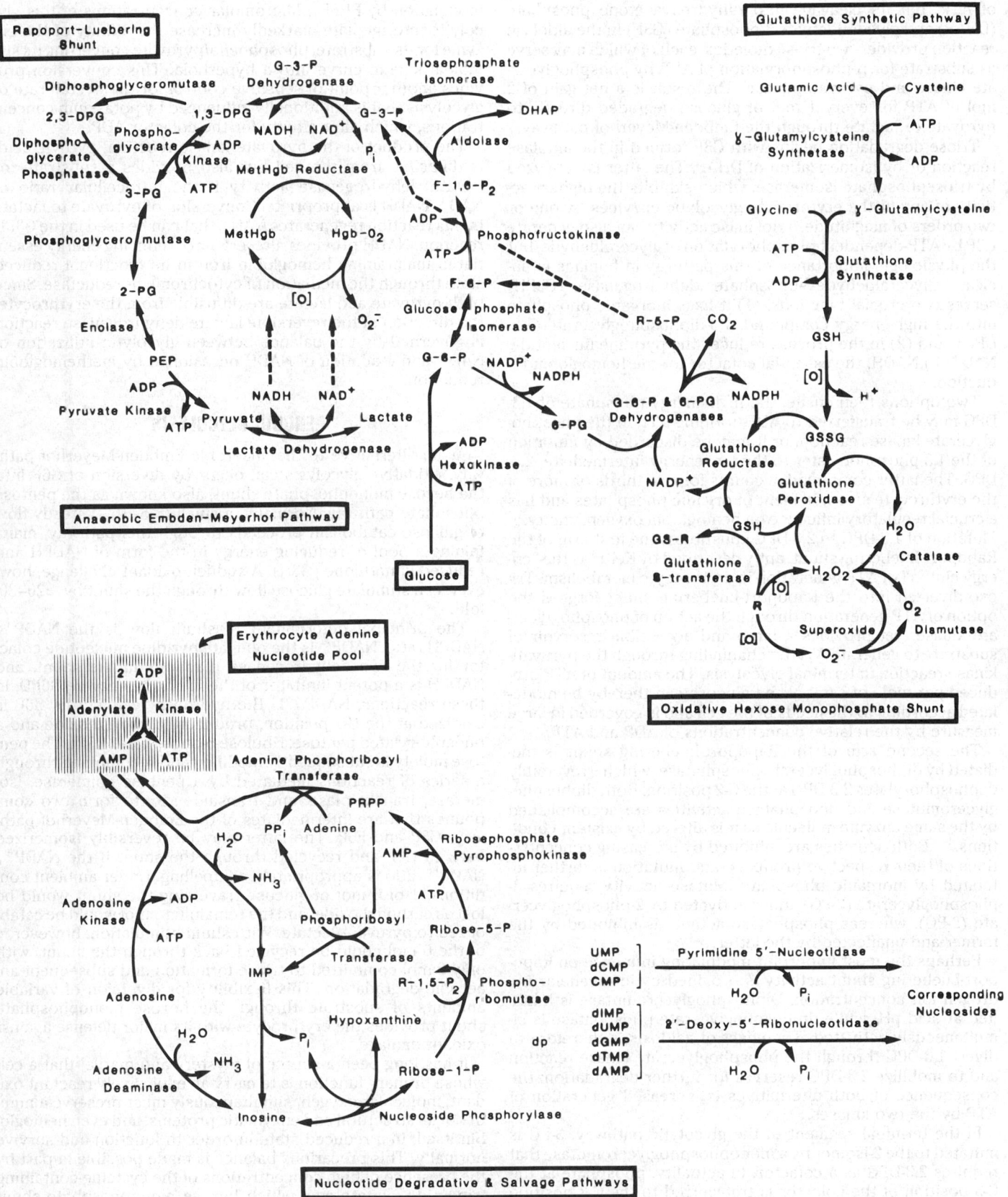

Fig. 33-2. Biochemical pathways of metabolism in the erythrocyte. Glucose is degraded to lactate anaerobically via the Embden-Meyerhof pathway or oxidatively by diversion of glucose-6-phosphate (G6P) into the hexose monophosphate shunt (pentose phosphate pathway) on the right. Pentose phosphates (R5P) generated by this pathway or by nucleoside degradation can be transformed into intermediates of anaerobic glycolysis for further catabolism. NADH serves as physiologic cofactor for methemoglobin reductase activity. NADPH is the obligate cofactor for maintenance of adequate reduced glutathione (GSH) to combat ambient oxidative stresses. The Rapoport-Luebering shunt shelters an abundant intracellular store of 2,3-DPG, which can be catabolized to regenerate ATP in response to altered ADP/ATP ratios.

of ATP, but its cleavage into dihydroxyacetone phosphate (DHAP) and glyceraldehyde-3-phosphate (G3P) in the aldolase reaction provides two triose moieties, each of which may serve as substrate for rephosphorylation of ADP by phosphoglycerate kinase and pyruvate kinase. The result is a net gain of 2 mol of ATP for every 1 mol of glucose degraded directly to pyruvate or lactate through the Embden-Meyerhof pathway.

Triose degradation begins with G3P formed in the aldolase reaction or by isomerization of DHAP. The latter is catalyzed by triosephosphate isomerase, which exhibits the highest activity of any of the erythrocyte glycolytic enzymes by one or two orders of magnitude. Triokinase activity can also generate G3P by ATP-dependent phosphorylation of glyceraldehyde, but the physiologic importance of this pathway in humans is unclear. Glyceraldehyde-3-phosphate dehydrogenase (G3PH) serves two crucial functions: (1) it fixes inorganic phosphate into the high-energy compound, 1,3-diphosphoglycerate (1,3-DPG); and (2) in the process reduces the pyridine nucleotide, NAD^+, to NADH, the essential cofactor for methemoglobin reduction.

Two options then ensue: the high-energy phosphate of 1,3-DPG may be transferred to ADP, forming ATP in the phosphoglycerate kinase reaction, or it may be discarded by mutation of the 1,3-phosphodiester to the low-energy intermediate, 2,3-DPG. The latter compound accounts for two-thirds or more of the erythrocyte's complement of organic phosphates and has a crucial regulatory influence on hemoglobin oxygen affinity.[1,2] Mutation of 1,3-DPG to 2,3-DPG constitutes the first arm of the Rapoport-Luebering shunt, aptly described by Keitt[3] as the "energy clutch" of ATP generation in erythrocyte metabolism. Triose diverted into the Rapoport-Luebering shunt forgoes the option of ATP generation through the action of phosphoglycerate kinase, yet provides a large and accessible reservoir of substrate to generate ATP by channeling through the pyruvate kinase reaction in terminal glycolysis. The amount of ATP produced per mole of catabolized glucose can thereby be modulated according to the needs of the cell and is governed in large measure by the relative concentrations of ADP and ATP.

The second arm of the Rapoport-Luebering shunt is mediated by diphosphoglycerate phosphatase, which irreversibly dephosphorylates 2,3-DPG at the C-2 position. Both diphosphoglyceromutase and phosphatase activities are accomplished by the same enzyme molecule as it is altered by existent conditions.[4-6] Both activities are inhibited by increasing concentrations of their respective products, and mutation is further inhibited by inorganic phosphate. Mutase activity requires 3-phosphoglycerate (3-PG) and is activated by 2-phosphoglycerate (2-PG), whereas phosphatase activity is inhibited by the former and unaffected by the latter.

Perhaps the most important modulating influence on Rapoport-Luebering shunt activity is provided by intracellular hydrogen ion concentration. Diphosphoglyceromutase is inhibited at acid pH, while diphosphoglycerate phosphatase is simultaneously activated. The effect of acidosis is therefore to divert 1,3-DPG through the phosphoglycerate kinase reaction and to mobilize 2,3-DPG reserves for further degradation; the consequence of both alternatives is increased generation of ATP by the two kinases.

In the terminal segment of the glycolytic pathway, 3-PG is mutated to the 2-isomer by a monophosphoglyceromutase that requires 2,3-DPG as a cofactor. In actuality, phosphate at the C-3 position of the cofactor is transferred to the C-2 position of 3-PG, transforming the original substrate into 2,3-DPG and allowing the triose of the original cofactor to continue down the pathway of terminal glycolysis. Enolization of 2-PG by phosphopyruvate hydratase produces phospho*enol*pyruvate, the substrate for pyruvate kinase in the last ATP-generating step in glycolysis.

Erythrocyte pyruvate kinase is highly sensitive to allosteric modulation by $F1,6P_2$. Micromolar concentrations of this glycolytic intermediate markedly increase the affinity of the enzyme for its substrate, phospho*enol*pyruvate converting its sigmoidal kinetic curve into a hyperbola. This conversion provides another point of sensitive control for the overall rate of glycolysis that is additionally influenced by potassium concentrations, which alter affinity for the cofactor ADP.

The product of the pyruvate kinase reaction, pyruvic acid, is diffusible from the cell but also provides a substrate for lactate dehydrogenase activity if the intracellular ratio of NAD^+/NADH is appropriate. Conversion of pyruvate to lactate in this reaction regenerates NAD^+ that can be used in the G3PD reaction. NADH provides a reservoir of reducing energy essential in maintaining hemoglobin iron in its functional reduced state through the mediation of cytochrome b_5 reductase. Since both pyruvate and lactate are diffusible from the erythrocyte, the direction of the reversible lactate dehydrogenase reaction is governed by the balance between glycolytic utilization of NAD^+ and oxidation of NADH occasioned by methemoglobin reduction.

AEROBIC GLYCOLYSIS

As an alternative to the anaerobic Embden-Meyerhof pathway, oxidative glycolysis can occur by diversion of G6P into the hexose monophosphate shunt, also known as the pentose phosphate pathway. Normally, a small ($\leq 5-10\%$) steady flow of glucose catabolism proceeds through this pathway, maintaining a pool of reducing energy in the form of NADPH and reduced glutathione (GSH). A sudden oxidant challenge, however, can stimulate glucose flow through the shunt by $\geq 20-30$-fold.

The principal determinant of shunt flow is the $NADP^+$/NADPH ratio. $NADP^+$ is the obligate pyridine nucleotide cofactor for the two dehydrogenase reactions in the shunt, and NADPH is a potent inhibitor of the initiating enzyme G6PD. In these reactions, $NADP^+$ is the hydrogen recipient as G6P is oxidized at the C-1 position, producing carbon dioxide and a phosphorylated pentose, ribulose-5-phosphate (R5P). The pentose moiety is subsequently modified and recombined through a series of reactions mediated by a pentose epimerase, isomerase, transketolase, and transaldolase, to form two compounds that are intermediates of the Embden-Meyerhof pathway, G3P and F6P. The latter may be reversibly isomerized back to G6P and recycled through the shunt if the $NADP^+$/NADPH ratio is appropriately compelling. Under ambient conditions, 1 of 6 mol of glucose traversing the shunt would be lost as carbon dioxide, and the remaining 5 mol would be catabolized to pyruvate/lactate. With shunt stimulation, however, 4 of the 6 mol could be recycled back through the shunt, with only 2 mol committed to triose formation and subsequent anaerobic degradation. This flexibility for diversion of variable amounts of substrate through the hexose monophosphate shunt provides the erythrocyte with its major defense against oxidant damage.

It has long been a source of mystery and marvel that a cell whose primary function is to carry an explosively reactant oxidant, molecular oxygen, simultaneously must preserve a number of its structural and enzymatic proteins, and even hemoglobin itself, in a reduced state in order to function and survive normally. This precarious balance is made possible in part by the presence of high concentrations of the cysteine-containing tripeptide, glutathione, which hexose monophosphate shunt activity serves to maintain in the reduced state (i.e., GSH). Because of its low oxidation potential, this compound readily serves as a sacrificial reductant, protecting other, less reactive, sulfhydryl groups of cellular proteins from oxidant damage. Glutathione has a relatively rapid turnover rate in erythrocytes and must constantly be resynthesized from its constituent amino acids as shown in Figure 33-2.

Hydrogen peroxide is one such potent oxidant, posing a serious threat because it is constantly generated in small amounts physiologically and in large amounts by pathologic conditions, as well as by certain drugs such as primaquine. Hydrogen peroxide can be detoxified directly by catalase, an iron porphyrin enzyme that is by far the most highly active enzyme in human red cells. Each catalase dimer is tightly bound to 4 molecules of NADPH, which are necessary for its full enzymatic activity and stability.[7] In addition, the selenium metalloenzyme, glutathione peroxidase, catalyzes the conversion of hydrogen peroxide to water by coupling it to the oxidative condensation of 2 molecules of GSH. The latter (GSSG) can be reduced back to functional tripeptides through disulfide cleavage mediated by the flavin enzyme, glutathione reductase, with NADPH serving as the physiologic hydrogen donor. Oxidants may also induce formation of mixed disulfides between glutathione and other sulfhydryl-containing proteins, including hemoglobin; many of these may also be reduced again through mediation of glutathione reductase. With the catalytic assistance of glutathione S-transferase, GSH also forms conjugates with a number of degradation products of nutrients and xenobiotics (R), either neutralizing their toxic qualities or converting them to forms more readily metabolized and excreted, or both.

Potentially even more damaging than hydrogen peroxide, superoxide anions and other highly reactive oxygen species and free radicals can also be generated physiologically, as in the auto-oxidation of hemoglobin to methemoglobin, or more rapidly under a variety of pathologic conditions. The metalloenzyme, superoxide dismutase, serves to neutralize this process by catalyzing conversion of superoxide anions to molecular oxygen and hydrogen peroxide, which in turn can be degraded by catalatic or peroxidative action.

NUCLEOTIDE METABOLISM

Only trace amounts of non-adenine nucleotides are normally found in mature circulating erythrocytes. Since these cells cannot synthesize nucleotides de novo, they have evolved mechanisms that effectively preserve the complement provided them as they emerge from the reticulocyte stage. Some of the known reactions pertinent to erythrocytes are summarized in Figure 32-2.

The adenine nucleotide pool in erythrocytes consists mostly of ATP (85–90%), with lesser amounts of the diphosphate ADP (10–12%), and monophosphate, AMP (1–3%), maintained in rapid equilibrium by an active adenylate kinase. Glycolysis serves to generate appropriate amounts of ATP, but this action is limited to the amounts of ADP available for phosphotransfer by kinase activity. The third component, AMP, although present in the smallest concentration, is in a particularly vulnerable position. If it is either deaminated to inosine monophosphate or dephosphorylated to diffusible adenosine, the purine moiety is effectively lost to the cell, unless some salvage mechanism intervenes.

Two potential salvage pathways are shown in Figure 33-2. Adenine phosphoribosyl transferase in erythrocytes is sufficient in activity to convert adenine to AMP, but this substrate does not seem to be readily available in plasma. Subjects with complete deficiency of the enzyme show no demonstrable alteration in erythrocyte function, longevity, or nucleotide concentrations.[8]

The evidence in support of a physiologic role for adenosine kinase in nucleotide salvage is compelling. This pathway accounts for the accumulation of high concentrations of deoxyadenine nucleotides in red cells from some subjects with marked deficiency of adenosine deaminase found in severe combined immunodeficiency disease.[9–11] Conversely, patients with hyperactive adenosine kinase show depletion of their

erythrocyte nucleotides.[12–15] Since the kinase and the deaminase compete for the same substrate, these observations indicate that nucleotide salvage through adenosine kinase is normally important to maintain the adenine nucleotide pool at constant concentrations.

With the exception of pyrimidine nucleotidase, none of the other reactions depicted in the nucleotide cycle represented in Figure 33-2 seems to have physiologic significance with regard to erythrocytes. Deficiencies and hyperactivity states exist for a number of these, including nucleoside phosphorylase, hypoxanthine-guanine phosphoribosyltransferase, and ribosephosphate pyrophosphokinase. All are apparently devoid of deleterious effects on red cell function or longevity.[16]

Pyrimidine nucleotidase is physiologically important during reticulocyte maturation. Its substrate specificity allows it to dephosphorylate only the pyrimidine products of RNA degradation. In this way, they are converted to diffusible nucleosides and cleared from the cell without simultaneously affecting AMP and the adenine nucleotide pool.[17–19] Red cells also contain a separate deoxyribonucleotidase that may have a corresponding function in DNA catabolism during the maturation of erythroid precursors.[20,21]

A number of other enzymes are detectable within erythrocytes, with no apparent physiologic functions. Some may represent vestigial remnants of metabolic pathways, such as the Krebs cycle, that were previously active in erythroid precursors but that no longer contribute to cellular metabolism.

REFERENCES

1. Benesch RE, Benesch R, Yu CI: The oxygenation of hemoglobin in the presence of 2,3-diphosphoglycerate: effect of temperature, pH, ionic strength and hemoglobin concentration. Biochemistry 8:2567, 1969
2. Caldwell PRB, Nagel RL, Jaffé ER: The effect of oxygen, carbon dioxide, pH, and cyanate on the binding of 2,3-diphosphoglycerate to human hemoglobin. Biochem Biophys Res Commun 44:1504, 1971
3. Keitt AS: Pyruvate kinase deficiency and related disorders of red cell glycolysis. Am J Med 41:762, 1966
4. Rosa R, Gaillardon J, Rosa J: Diphosphoglycerate mutase and 2,3-diphosphoglycerate phosphatase activities of red cells: comparative electrophoretic study. Biochem Biophys Res Commun 51:536, 1973
5. Rosa R, Audit I, Rosa J: Evidence for three enzymatic activities in one electrophoretic band of 3-phosphoglycerate mutase from red cells. Biochemie 57:1059, 1975
6. Sasaki R, Ikura K, Sugimoto E, Chiba H: Purification of biphosphoglycerate phosphatase and phosphoglyceromutase from human erythrocytes. Eur J Biochem 50:581, 1975
7. Kirkman HN, Galiano S, Gaetani GF: The function of catalase-bound NADPH. J Biol Chem 262:660, 1987
8. Van Acker KJ, Simmonds HA, Potter C, Cameron JS: Complete deficiency of adenine phosphoribosyltransferase. Report of a family. N Engl J Med 297:127, 1977
9. Agarwal RP, Crabtree GW, Parks RE Jr et al: Purine nucleoside metabolism in the erythrocytes of patients with adenosine deaminase deficiency and severe combined immunodeficiency. J Clin Invest 57:1025, 1976
10. Schmalstieg FC, Goldman AS, Mills GC et al: Nucleotide metabolism in adenosine deaminase deficiency. Pediatr Res 10:393, 1976
11. Coleman MS, Donofrio J, Hutton JJ et al: Identification and quantitation of adenine deoxynucleotides in erythrocytes of a patient with adenosine deaminase deficiency and severe combined immunodeficiency. J Biol Chem 253:1619, 1978
12. Valentine WM, Paglia DE, Tartaglia AP, Gilsanz F: Hereditary hemolytic anemia with increased red cell adenosine deaminase (45- to 70-fold) and decreased adenosine triphosphate. Science 195:783, 1977
13. Paglia DE, Valentine WN, Tartaglia AP et al: Control of red blood cell adenine nucleotide metabolism. Studies of adenosine deaminase. p. 319. In Brewer GJ (ed): The Red Cell. Alan R Liss, New York, 1978
14. Perignon JL, Hamet M, Buc HA et al: Biochemical study of a case of hemolytic anemia with increased (85-fold) red cell adenosine deaminase. Clin Chim Acta 124:205, 1982
15. Miwa S, Fujii H, Matsumoto N et al: A case of red-cell adenosine deaminase overproduction associated with hereditary hemolytic anemia found in Japan. Am J Hematol 5:107, 1978
16. Paglia DE, Valentine WN: Haemolytic anaemia associated with disorders of

the purine and pyrimidine salvage pathways. Baillieres Clin Haematol 10:81, 1981

17. Valentine WN, Fink K, Paglia DE et al: Hereditary hemolytic anemia with human erythrocyte pyrimidine 5′-nucleotidase deficiency. J Clin Invest 54: 866, 1974

18. Paglia DE, Valentine WN: Characteristics of a pyrimidine-specific 5′-nucleotidase in human erythrocytes. J Biol Chem 250:7973, 1975

19. Paglia DE, Valentine WM: Hereditary and acquired defects in the pyrimidine nucleotidase of human erythrocytes. Curr Top Hematol 3:75, 1980

20. Paglia DE, Valentine WN, Brockway RA: Identification of thymidine nucleotidase and deoxyribonucleotidase activities among normal isozymes of 5′-nucleotidase in human erythrocytes. Proc Natl Acad Sci USA 81:588, 1984

21. Paglia DE, Valentine WN, Brockway RA, Nakatani M: Substrate specificity and pH sensitivity of deoxyribonucleotidase and pyrimidine nucleotidase activities in human hemolysates. Exp Hematol 15:1041, 1987

22. Paglia DE, Valentine WN: Genetically induced enzyme anomalies: insights into normal cellular processes. Ann NY Acad Sci 459:344, 1985

Homeostasis, Survival, and Red Cell Kinetics: Measurement and Imaging of Red Cell Production

34

Stephen A. Landaw

INTRODUCTION

The red blood cell (RBC) has long been a favorite object of kinetic studies. This cell is enucleated and without mitochondria in mammals. It lives out its finite life span unable to renew any of its critical enzymes and structural proteins, although it is able to repair some oxidative damage to its component parts. A typical RBC living 120 days in a human has been estimated to have made a total trip of some 300 miles.[1] This corresponds to about 170,000 recirculations through the heart,[2] with an attendant number of deformations in the capillary beds and osmotic shrinking and swelling cycles in the pulmonary and renal circulation.[3] The final events that cause the aging RBC in the normal individual to be "unfit to continue to circulate" have not been clearly delineated, although this signal most likely originates in the cell membrane.

In clinical and experimental situations, the number of RBCs in the circulation is related to an interplay between the loss of blood, if any, from the body, the rate of RBC production, and the rate of RBC destruction. In any one patient multiple alterations may occur in one or more of these three basic processes. Thus, patients with congenital spherocytosis may develop gastrointestinal bleeding, patients with thalassemia may have a temporarily decreased rate of production of RBCs due to an intercurrent infection, and previously normal patients may spontaneously develop an antibody to their own RBCs, resulting in sudden hemolysis. It is the task of this chapter to discuss those studies that may be performed in an effort to quantify these three basic processes, with emphasis on the latter two.

Alterations in plasma volume may also cause problems in interpretation. For example, the three most useful clinical tests for assessing RBC mass, namely, hemoglobin concentration, hematocrit, and RBC count, are all ratios, with their numerators an RBC property and their denominators the volume of circulating blood containing both RBCs and plasma. This issue is most evident in the example of a patient with sickle cell disease and a rising hematocrit. This is hardly ever a good sign; rather than indicating increased RBC production or reduced RBC destruction (or both), it usually indicates serious dehydration with attendant decreases in circulating plasma volume. Similarly, in a patient with steadily decreasing RBC values, it may be that the worsening "anemia" is due to an expansion of the plasma volume (as in the hydremia of pregnancy) rather than to a decrease in RBC mass.

MEASUREMENT OF RED BLOOD CELL SURVIVAL

The RBC has a number of convenient properties that permit studies of its kinetics. The most prominent is our virtually unlimited and continuous access to large numbers of cells through venipuncture, something one cannot say, for example, about the crypt cells in the small intestine. Other properties useful in performing RBC survival studies are listed in Table 34-1.

Random Label Method

In the random label method, RBCs are removed from the circulation, labeled with an appropriate tracer in vitro, and reintroduced into the circulation. Blood samples are taken at regular intervals and assayed for the concentration of the tracer. Provided that certain basic assumptions hold, the rate of loss of the tracer from serial blood samples will accurately reflect the rate of loss of RBCs from the circulation. This is the rationale behind the use of any label for determining RBC

RBC TURNOVER: CLINICAL MEANING

For normal humans, RBC turnover is approximately 0.8%/day. This number sets a natural limit on the rate of loss of certain RBC properties during treatment. For example, the amounts of hemoglobin, free erythrocyte protoporphyrin, and folate do not appear to change as the RBC ages. Thus, as in these three examples, if there is instantaneous onset of RBC aplasia, effective chelation therapy for lead poisoning, or complete dietary insufficiency of folate, it is expected that the concentrations of these RBC constituents could fall no faster than the RBC turnover rate.

As an example, consider the effect of 10 days' worth of erythroid aplasia on two subjects, one with normal RBC survival and the other with a mean overall RBC survival of 20 days. In the first case, RBC loss continues at the rate of 0.8%/day, or 8%/10 days. Since input of new RBCs has been stopped, the RBC mass will drop by 8%, which would mean, for the concentration of hemoglobin, a drop from 15 g/dl to 13.8, which is not expected to be clinically evident.

For the subject with shortened RBC survival and a RBC turnover of 100/20, or 5%/day, one-half of the RBC mass will have been lost at the end of 10 days of aplasia, which is quite likely to have serious clinical consequences. This kinetic approach explains the well-known observation that short episodes of RBC aplasia (the so-called aplastic crisis) go virtually unnoticed in normal subjects and may be quite disastrous in subjects with congenital hemolytic anemias such as thalassemia, congenital spherocytosis, or sickle cell disease.[42]

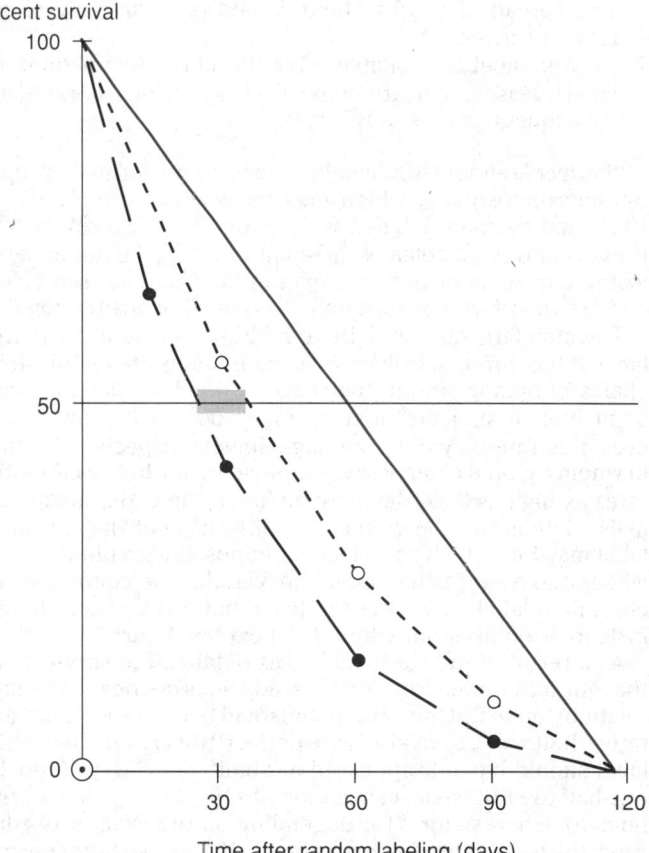

Fig. 34-1. ^{51}Cr-labeled RBCs—disappearance from circulation. The percentage of survival of a random label experiment is illustrated here for rates of label elution of zero (red line), 1%/day (open circles), and 2%/day (closed circles). Note that survival is linear for the first case and "exponential" for the latter two cases. In all three cases, the last of the labeled RBCs leave the circulation at the same time (120 days), the "extinction time." The pink area represents the accepted range for the ^{51}Cr half-time in normal humans.

survival; the general method is called a random labeling procedure, since the RBC sample to be labeled is a random selection of circulating RBCs of all ages. Virtually all RBC survival studies performed for clinical reasons are of this type.

In a steady-state situation, as many RBCs are dying per day as are being delivered into the circulation, which is another way of saying that the rates of RBC production and destruction are equal. Since RBC survival is known to be approximately 120 days[4,5,14] this means that 1/120, or 0.833%, of the circulating RBC mass is replaced each day. Thus, in 1 week 0.83 × 7 RBCs, or 5.8%, will have been lost and replaced, and in 60 days 0.83 × 60 RBCs, or 50%, will have been replaced. In

Table 34-1. Labels Available for Performance of RBC Survival Studies

Erythrocyte Component	Labels Available	Isotopes	Selected References
Surface antigens			
Ashby random label	—	—	4
Cholinesterase[a]			
Random label	DFP	[3]H, ^{14}C, [32]P	5, 6
Cohort label	DFP	[32]P	7
Globin chains			
Random label	Chromate	[51]Cr	4, 8
Random label	Cyanate	[14]C	9, 10
Cohort label	Selenomethionine	[75]Se	11
Heme			
Cohort label	Glycine	[14]C, [15]N	6, 7, 12, 13
Cohort label	Iron	[55]Fe, [59]Fe	14–16

Abbreviation: DFP, diisopropyl fluorophosphate.
[a] Also binds to other uncharacterized intracellular material.

a normal subject, RBCs withdrawn randomly from the circulation, labeled, and reinfused should disappear at this rate.

Mathematically, we have stated that

$$A(t) = A_0[1 - (1/T)t]$$

where $A(t)$ is the activity of the RBC mass at time (t), A_0 is the initial activity of the RBC mass at $t = 0$, and T is the time of senescent death of RBCs, here 120 days.

The RBC survival parameter T is called the *mean potential RBC life span,* which is the time at which the average RBC dies or leaves the circulation due to senescent processes. Plotting the above equation yields a straight line, with an extrapolated value of A_0 at $t = 0$ and a value of zero at $t = T$. The slope of this line $(1/T)$ is the fractional RBC turnover rate, 0.83%/day (Fig. 34-1, red line).

It will be useful to list the various assumptions underlying this approach. The method will be valid only under the following circumstances:

1. No change in circulating RBC mass occurs during this time.
2. No loss of RBCs from the body occurs during this period (blood sampling and blood loss are negligible).
3. The label is "perfect": it labels RBCs of all ages equally and does not dissociate from the red cell.
4. Correction is made for any radioactive decay (important for ^{51}Cr, but unimportant for ^{14}C or [3]H[tritium].
5. All RBCs die of senescence at age T days, there is no gaus-

sian spread of deaths about T, and cells die only of age-related causes.

6. No free label is available after the initial incubation, and label released on death of the cell is not reincorporated into subsequent groups of RBCs.

"Perfect" random RBC labels do exist in the form of diisopropyl fluorophosphate, which may be labeled with ^{14}C, ^{3}H, or ^{32}P,[5,6] and cyanate (labeled with ^{3}H or ^{14}C.[9,10] However, since these cannot be labeled with γ-emitters, they do not allow for isotopic imaging or in vivo organ uptake studies (see below) and are therefore not routinely used in clinical situations.

The standard random label for RBCs, ^{51}Cr, is not a perfect label. It has a rate of leakage from its binding site on the globin chains of hemoglobin in the range of 0.7–1.3%/day in normal adult human subjects[8] and average about 0.9%/day.[4,8] However, this rate may differ among subjects, especially in those in whom a globin chain variant is present, in which case elution rates as high as 2.3%/day may be found.[6] In experimental animals such as the sheep, the rate of leakage of the chromium label may be so high as to make it impossible to obtain worthwhile studies with this label.[17] A variable percentage of the chromium label may enter the RBCs but not be fixed therein; instead, it diffuses out within the next few hours.[8]

As a result of the elutional losses of label, the survival time that one may obtain from such a study does not bear any simple relationship to RBC survival but instead becomes a semiquantitative index of survival. For a perfect tracer, one-half of the label should have disappeared at about 55–60 days (equal to one-half the RBC senescence time of 110–120 days in a normal human), whereas for ^{51}Cr, depending on the exact procedure used, the usual range for loss of one-half the label (after correcting for radioactive decay) is within the range of 25–35 days[8,18] (Fig. 34-1).

An exact RBC survival parameter can be obtained from chromium studies, namely the *extinction time,* defined as the time at which the last labeled RBC leaves the circulation; it reflects the time taken for the very youngest circulating RBC labeled at the beginning of the study to leave the circulation (i.e., to die). This value is, to a good first approximation, the average time of senescent (age-dependent) death of RBCs in that patient (i.e., the value of T) and may be compared directly with the normal value of 110–120 days (Fig. 34-1).

Senescent, or age-dependent, RBC destruction is not the only mode of RBC death encountered in clinical or experimental situations. The other RBC destruction mode is independent of RBC age and is termed random destruction or random hemolysis. The rate of random hemolysis (k) is low in normal humans,[4] about ≤0.04–0.50%/day while it is within the range of zero (dog[19]) to 1.5%/day in various experimental animals.[13,16,19]

Random label RBC survival curves, which show both these processes, have the form

$$A(t) = A_0[1 - (t/T)]e^{-kt}$$

As might be expected from the exponential component, results of such survival studies do not yield straight lines when graphed on rectangular coordinate paper, although the first portion of such curves tends to be linear when the data are plotted on semilogarithmic paper.[18]

Role in Predicting Benefit of Splenectomy

An animal model of splenomegaly and resulting splenic RBC sequestration may be helpful in understanding these processes. If a rat is given multiple intraperitoneal injections of the nonmetabolizable material methylcellulose, a progressive splenomegaly is produced, and the rat develops an increased

reticulocyte count, consistent with a clinical picture of compensated hemolysis and hypersplenism.[20,21] RBC survival studies show that T, the time of senescent death of RBCs, is virtually unchanged, whereas k, the rate of random hemolysis, is increased almost sixfold.[21] Following splenectomy, the reticulocyte percentage returns to normal, as does the rate of random hemolysis. This combination of normal senescence time and increased rate of random hemolysis is what one expects to see in a patient with clinical hemolysis in whom a splenic trapping mechanism is postulated as the inciting cause. Such may be the case in Coombs-positive hemolytic anemia due to a warm-acting antibody or in congestive splenomegaly with hypersplenism. We might therefore conclude that the survival parameter k represents an estimate of the chance, per unit time, that the RBC will pass through a critical portion of the splenic circulation[22] and be destroyed. Clinically, this would be useful because hemolysis would be expected to abate after splenectomy.

The γ-emitting properties of ^{51}Cr are helpful in this context because it is possible to measure in vivo the count rates over the spleen and liver during the RBC survival study. These counts can be compared with those obtained over the heart to display the activity within the circulation. Progressively increasing counting rates over the spleen as compared with the heart or liver indicate the presence of splenic trapping and tend to predict reversal of the overall RBC destruction following splenectomy. A number of different methods for quantitating such splenic trapping have been presented. Each varies according to patient and probe placement, correction for activity in the circulating blood (or precordial count rate, which is taken to be its in vivo equivalent), and whether activity in the spleen is given as a splenic value alone or as the spleen/liver ratio[23–26] (Table 34-2).

The *sequestration index* proposed by Jandl et al[23] corrects for potential confusion resulting from the expanded amount of blood found in a grossly enlarged spleen by performing in vivo counting within a few minutes after reinjection of the labeled RBC and again when one-half the RBC activity has been lost.[23] In the studies reported by Jandl et al,[23] the sequestration index

Table 34-2. Representative Data in a ^{51}Cr Red Cell Sequestration Study

Organ Counted	In Vivo Organ Counting Rate[a] (cpm)			
	Day 0	Day 1	Day 8	Day 14
Heart (precordium) observed	1,000	850	670	370
Liver observed	670	670	640	530
Liver expected[b]	—	570	449	248
Liver excess counts[c]	—	100	191	282
Spleen observed	970	1,265	2,130	2,020
Spleen expected[b]	—	825	650	359
Spleen excess counts[c]	—	440	1,480	1,661
Spleen/liver observed	1.45	1.89	3.33	3.81
Spleen/liver "normalized"[d]	1.00	1.30	2.30	2.63

[a] These data illustrate the various methods available to determine organ sequestration, as noted in text. The study is continued until the precordium count rate has fallen to slightly less than one-half the initial value. This occurs in this example between days 8 and 14. The sequestration index[23] can also be calculated from these data; values are 76 for the liver (normal 23–35) and 449 for the spleen (normal 38–48). Using all methodologies, results suggest splenic sequestration and the likelihood that splenectomy would be beneficial (see text).

[b] Expected counts are those expected if the count rate over that organ is falling at the same rate as that over the precordium (signifying blood pool activity).

[c] Excess counts are simply the observed counts minus the expected counts.

[d] The spleen/liver ratio can be plotted directly or can be normalized to the ratio present on the day the study is started (day 0). In this case each subsequent spleen/liver ratio is divided by 1.45, the ratio present on day 0.

(Data from International Committee for Standardization in Hematology.[18])

averaged 27 for liver and 43 for spleen in normal subjects. In subjects with congenital or acquired hemolytic anemia, values for the liver index were in the normal range (30–60), whereas those for the spleen were as high as 120–180. Goldberg et al[24] suggested that a rising spleen/liver ratio during the course of a ^{51}Cr study is a more favorable indication for splenectomy than a falling one. They found this ratio to be 0.6–1.3 in normal subjects at the time of loss of 50% of circulating activity. When this ratio exceeded 2.1 in patients with pancytopenia or 2.3 in patients without leukopenia and thrombopenia, this was considered an indication for splenectomy. The *excess count rate* method (Table 34-2) corrects spleen and liver counts for the falling activity in the circulating blood[26] or under the precordial probe.[25] However, Ahuja et al[25] noted that 17 of their 18 patients improved postsplenectomy, even though there was no close correlation between the magnitude of the accumulation of splenic activity, as measured by excess counts, and the degree of response.

The International Committee for Standardization in Hematology has recommended either the excess count rate method or the spleen/liver method for prediction of benefit after splenectomy.[18] However, no method permits setting strict guidelines that will reliably predict who will or will not respond to splenectomy. There have been many instances of patients responding to splenectomy whose chromium studies did not show progressive splenic uptake; these may be examples of technical difficulties such as suboptimal placement of the splenic probe,[26] but they might just as easily be because removing the spleen also removes a major source of antibody production (in autoimmune hemolytic anemia) or due to a normalization of the expanded plasma volume often seen in patients with enlarged spleens.[25]

RBC Survival

Cohort Studies

Cohort RBC survival studies are currently performed almost exclusively in investigational situations owing to their time-consuming nature. They are performed by administering a labeled RBC precursor to the subject, and following the appearance of the label in and its subsequent disappearance from the circulating RBCs (Table 34-1). Thus, glycine, a precursor of hemoglobin heme, may be used with a nonradioactive ^{15}N label[12] or with a radioactive ^{14}C or ^{3}H label.[6,7] Similarly, radioactive iron may be given as part of an iron kinetics study or may be given solely for RBC survival studies.[14,15,16] Other amino acid precursors, such as selenomethionine, may also be used.[11] The single most important issue other than steady state is the requirement that the label not be reincorporated to any great extent into a new cohort of RBCs once released from an RBC that has just died. This problem exists for all cohort labels but is most severe for iron, about 95% of which is reincorporated

into subsequent cohorts.[27] This can be partially overcome by periodically injecting nonradioactive iron to compete with the labeled iron.[14] This maneuver can reduce reincorporation to <20% and allows the resulting curves to be analyzed.[14,16,19]

Cohort studies may also be performed by sampling the degradative products that result from catabolism of RBC hemoglobin heme. Under the action of the enzymes heme oxygenase and biliverdin reductase, 1 mol of heme is catabolized to 1 mol of bilirubin and 1 mol of carbon monoxide,[30–32] these products eventually being excreted into the stool[33] and breath,[13,34,35] respectively. If ^{14}C-labeled glycine (glycine-2-^{14}C) is administered, both products will contain the label and can be quantitated.[32] With ^{15}N-labeled glycine, only bilirubin and the fecal bile pigments will be tagged. These latter techniques have the advantage of being noninvasive, since only collection of excreta or expired air is needed. This may be especially important in very small subjects, such as the human newborn, in which case repeated blood sampling or the use of radioactive isotopes may not be practical.[36,37]

Significance

Having performed either a random or cohort label study, one has obtained RBC survival parameters that will require interpretation (Table 34-3). Thus, for a ^{51}Cr random label experiment with determination of extinction time and organ uptake studies, one will have determined the time of senescent death (the extinction time T). If T is normal and the rate of label elution is normal, there would be every reason to expect a survival half-time within the normal range (25–35 days) (Fig. 34-1). If T is normal, the half-time is short, and there is no reason to expect an increase rate of label elution, one is justified in concluding that there must be increased random hemolysis (an increase in the parameter k) and will know from the organ studies whether splenic processes predominate. Since the random label studies are generally not taken to the extinction time, one only knows from a reduced ^{51}Cr half-time that RBC survival is shortened without knowing whether this is due to an acceleration of senescence or to an increase in the rate of random hemolysis, or both. However, one should always be aware that this might be due to an increase in the rate of label elution alone.

By contrast, cohort studies give the time of senescent death (T) and the rate of random hemolysis k directly, as well as a parameter indicating the size of the labeled cohort, which in the case of glycine studies is related in a semiquantitative manner to the erythropoietic rate.[21] While most clinical situations resulting in decreased survival do so by increasing the rate of random hemolysis, in a few circumstances senescence is accelerated, as during the newborn period[36,37] and during the rapid production of new RBCs (stress erythropoiesis).[38–40] In general, RBC survival is never markedly longer than normal, but minor prolongation of the phase of senescent RBC death has been seen in the postsplenectomy state (10%), in hibernat-

Table 34-3. Changes in Erythrocyte Survival Parameters According to Destructive Process[a]

Erythrocyte Destruction Processes	Condition(s) under Which These Processes Are		
	Reduced or Slowed	Normal	Increased or Accelerated
Random hemolysis	Not described	Low to absent in humans Present in most experimental animals	Hypersplenism Defective RBCs (spherocytes)[b] Some "stress" RBCs
Senescence	Poikilotherms at low temperature Hibernating mammals Hypothyroidism Postsplenectomy	Mice: 40–50 days Rats: 60–70 days Dogs: 100–110 days Humans: 110–120 days	Some "stress" RBCs Newborn and fetal animals and humans Genetic differences

[a] For particulars see text and review references 13, 19, 28, 29, 40, 41.
[b] Hemolysis of abnormal cells.

ing animals, and in animals post-thyroidectomy or posthypophysectomy (12–15%).[41]

IRON KINETICS

Huff et al[43,44] published a model of iron kinetics in the early 1950s, according to which iron disappears from a single plasma pool to appear in circulating RBCs (Fig. 34-2). In this model, radioactive iron is incubated with plasma and reinjected into the patient and plasma samples are obtained two to four times per hour for the next few hours. Blood is obtained 2 weeks later to determine the percentage of radioactive iron incorporated into RBCs. Since the radioactive iron is plasma protein bound, it is also possible to determine plasma volume accurately in this method.

The plasma iron pool is determined from the plasma iron concentration and the size of the plasma volume, and the rate of iron loss from the plasma is the product of the plasma iron pool and the single exponential rate constant describing the rate of decrease of the plasma iron radioactivity with time after injection. This value for plasma iron turnover (PIT), stated in terms of milligrams of iron leaving the plasma per kilogram per day, serves to define iron utilization in the patient. If the circulating RBC mass is also known, RBC survival can be estimated by dividing circulating RBC hemoglobin iron (in milligrams of iron) by the iron turnover (in milligrams per day). This calculation overestimates erythroid iron incorporation and underestimates RBC survival in normal humans. Thus, the Huff model was modified to take into account that <100% of the iron leaving the plasma appears in circulating RBCs. If plasma iron turnover is modified by multiplying its value in milligrams per day by the fraction of tracer iron incorporated into circulating RBCs at 2 weeks, the erythroid iron turnover (EIT) is obtained, which when used for estimating RBC survival, yields values close to those obtained from other measures of RBC survival.

An example from the original paper by Huff et al[43] illustrates the method. A hypothetical patient weighs 77.1 kg and has a measured plasma volume of 36.4 ml/kg (2,800 ml of plasma) and an RBC mass of 30.5 ml/kg (2,350 ml of RBCs). Since 1 ml of packed RBCs contain approximately 1 mg of iron, the circulating RBC mass contains 2.35 g of iron. Plasma iron concentration is 130 µg/100 ml plasma (1.3 mg/L), and the total plasma iron pool is 2.74 mg. For this hypothetical patient an iron disappearance study is performed, and the resulting iron disappearance half-time ($T_{1/2}$) is noted to be 101 minutes, or 1.69 hours. This yields a fractional turnover rate constant k:

$$k = \ln 2/T_{1/2} = 0.693/1.69$$
$$= 0.41/hr \ (41\%/hr)$$

The patient's PIT equals the plasma iron pool multiplied by this single exponential fractional turnover rate, or

$$PIT = \text{plasma iron pool (mg)} \times (k \ hr) \times 24 \ (hr/day)$$
$$= 2.74 \times 0.41 \times 24$$
$$= 27 \ mg/day$$

Since the total amount of iron in circulating RBCs is 2.35 g (2,350 mg) and the amount of iron leaving the plasma per day is 27 mg/day (if one assumes that all the iron leaving plasma is destined for circulating RBC hemoglobin heme), the fractional turnover rate of circulating RBC hemoglobin iron is

$$\text{Fractional RBC hemoglobin heme iron turnover} = 27/2,350$$
$$= 0.0115/day$$

RBC survival in this patient is therefore the reciprocal of this value:

$$\text{Estimated RBC survival} = 1/0.0115$$
$$= 87 \ days$$

This is clearly an underestimate of RBC survival (expected value within the range of 110–120 days), and our assumption that all the iron leaving plasma is destined for incorporation into circulating RBCs must be incorrect. In fact, Huff et al[43] found incorporation to average about 74% at 2 weeks. If one assumes that the EIT can be estimated by multiplying the PIT by the fractional iron incorporation at 2 weeks, then

$$EIT = PIT \times RBC \text{ incorporation}$$
$$\text{(2 weeks)}$$
$$= 27 \ (mg/day) \times 0.74$$
$$= 20 \ mg/day$$

$$\text{Fractional RBC hemoglobin heme turnover} = EIT/RBC \text{ iron content}$$
$$= 20/2,350$$
$$= 0.0085$$
$$\text{Estimated RBC survival} = 1/0.0085$$
$$= 118 \ days$$

Although the patient is fictitious, these are the actual average values obtained for the normal subjects described by Huff et

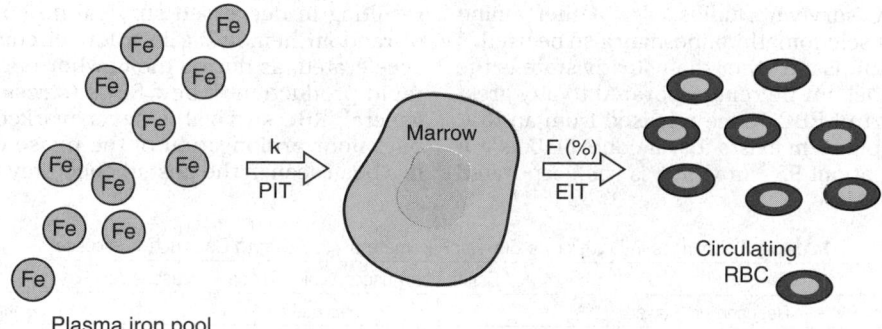

Plasma iron pool

Fig. 34-2. Huff model of iron kinetics. This simple one-compartment model assumes that all iron leaves the plasma ultimately destined for incorporation into the marrow and thence into the circulating RBCs. A certain fraction of this plasma iron pool leaves for the marrow per unit time, here given as the rate constant k. Of the iron leaving the plasma for marrow, <100% is finally incorporated into circulating RBCs here given by the fraction F.

In our hypothetical case, the plasma iron pool contained 2.74 mg iron (see text), and the fractional turnover k was 0.41/hr (41%/hr). Plasma iron turnover (PIT) is therefore (2.74) × (0.41) = 1.12 mg/hr, or 27 mg/day. Of the injected iron, only 74% was incorporated into circulating RBCs at 14 days (F = 0.74). The erythroid iron turnover (EIT) according to this model is therefore EIT = (27) × (0.74) = 20 mg/day. (Adapted from Huff et al,[43] with permission.)

Table 34-4. Selected Red Cell and Red Cell Kinetic Parameters in Normal Humans

Parameter		Value and Units		Reference
RBC mass	Males:	28.7 ± 3.8	ml/kg	86
	Females:	25.3 ± 2.6		86
Plasma volume	Males:	36.9 ± 4.2		86
	Females:	41.9 ± 4.4		86
^{51}Cr disappearance half-time	Range:	28–35	days	8
	Males:	30.1 ± 4.0		86
	Females:	29.4 ± 2.1		86
Rate of ^{51}Cr label elution	Range:	0.68–1.31	%/day	8
Plasma iron disappearance half-time		85 ± 5	min	45
	Range:	87–112		43
Incorporation of ^{59}Fe into erythrocytes	Range:	79–89	% at 14 days	51
		74 (mean)		43
		82 ± 1		45
Plasma iron turnover	Mean	0.35	mg/kg/day	43
		0.75 ± 0.02	mg/dl whole blood/day	45
	Mean:	32.5	mg/day	27
		121 ± 17	μM/L WB/day	53
Erythroid iron turnover	Mean:	20	mg/day	43
		21.4	mg/day	27
		0.56	mg/dl WB/day	52
		86 ± 10	μmol/L WB/day	53

al.[43] and the calculated value for RBC survival agrees well with that expected from cohort studies.

Cook et al[45] have taken a slightly different approach to iron kinetics by normalizing PIT to circulating estimated blood volume. Thus, in their six normal subjects PIT was 0.75 + 0.02 mg/dl whole blood per day. These investigators estimated EIT by subtracting a fixed percentage of PIT in order to correct for that portion of iron going to nonerythroid tissues. Their resulting EIT value of 0.60 ± 0.20 mg/dl blood per day[45] is said to be a quantitative measurement of the nucleated RBC precursors in the marrow and their hemoglobin-synthesizing capacity.

It is instructive at this point to understand what these kinetics say clinically about the movements of iron. First, only a very small pool of iron (about 2–3 mg) feeds the very large pool of RBC hemoglobin heme iron (>2,000 mg), which requires the plasma iron pool to turn over about 10 times per day to supply the needed iron. Instantaneous increases or decreases in erythropoietic rate (such as might occur in a patient with pernicious anemia started on treatment or in a patient with acute onset of pure RBC aplasia) would be expected to have profound immediate changes on the plasma iron pool, resulting, respectively, in a dramatic decrease or increase in plasma iron concentration. Similarly, onset of acute hemolysis of only 1% of the total circulating RBC mass in a 24-hour period, corresponding to a rate of random hemolysis k of 0.01/day, would lead to the acute addition of about 24 mg of iron to plasma, an amount equal to 1 day's worth of marrow iron needs.

Such dramatic changes have, in fact, been noted for serum iron in healthy normal subjects, changes of 20% in a 10-minute period and 200% in a 10-day period being not uncommon.[46] Lynch and Moede[47] demonstrated a significant correlation between serum iron, indirect bilirubin, and carbon monoxide excretion rates in normal human subjects, as well as increases in heme catabolism during the premenstrual half of the menstrual cycle. Given such an exquisitely sensitive character for the plasma iron pool, it is wise to be extremely suspicious of any single estimation of serum iron as being fully representative of that pool.

PIT or EIT values obtained according to either of these models can be used to determine increased or decreased erythropoiesis by comparing the obtained values with normal ranges (Table 34-4). Since it is important to minimize exposure

to radioactivity whenever possible, Lowman and Krivit[48] showed the feasibility of employing the nonradioactive ^{58}Fe isotope for the plasma iron disappearance portion of an iron kinetics study, with subsequent assay by neutron activation analysis.

Various investigators have employed more complex models containing five or more discrete pools. The interested reader is invited to seek out the original articles for a more complete discussion of this complex subject.[27,45,49–53]

In Vivo Organ Counting of Iron

The ability to place radioactivity-sensing probes over various organs becomes a powerful part of an iron kinetics study.[27,44] Probes may be placed over the liver, spleen, sacrum (marrow), and precordium to determine dynamic changes in radioactive iron patterns. All probes, wherever placed, are normalized to the maximum count rate obtained immediately after injection of the plasma protein-bound radioactive iron. This initializes the counts for each probe to the blood volume space sensed by the probe; this initial count is given the value of 1.0 for that probe.

For the sacral (marrow) probe in normal subjects, the count rate increases progressively during the first 24–48 hours postinjection as the tracer iron is transported to the erythropoietic elements in the marrow. This is followed by a release of accumulated activity over the next week, as labeled RBCs leave the marrow to enter into the circulation, resulting in a return of the count to the initial value of 1.0. This is the pattern characteristic of effective erythropoiesis (Fig. 34-3A). In the case of ineffective erythropoiesis, in which RBC precursors are destroyed at some critical time in their development within the marrow, the pattern seen is rapid uptake, followed by incomplete return of the counts back to the 1.0 baseline. The failure of the counting rate over the marrow to return to baseline is due to two effects: (1) iron contained in the destroyed RBC precursors is taken up by marrow macrophages, thus remaining in the marrow; and (2) any iron recycled back into plasma from the destroyed RBC precursors is immediately taken up again by the marrow for incorporation into subsequent cohorts of developing RBC. In the case of erythroid hypoplasia or

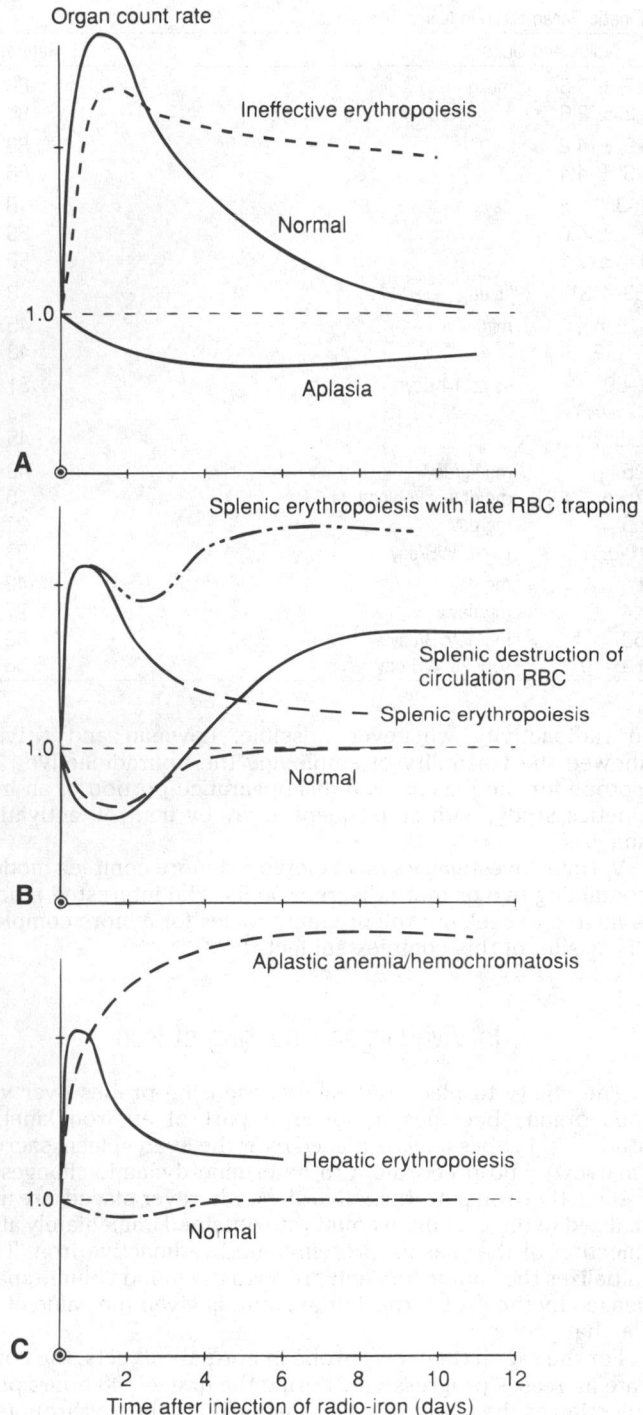

Fig. 34-3. Various patterns seen in iron kinetic studies using in vivo organ imaging. Results with **(A)** bone marrow probes, **(B)** splenic probes, and **(C)** liver probes. Results for all probes are "normalized" to initial count rates in order to correct for the blood volume space "seen" by each probe. See text for descriptions. (Adapted from Pollycove,[27] with permission.)

aplasia, little or no uptake of iron is displayed by the marrow under the probe, resulting in a blunted or flat profile, respectively.

The liver, while it takes up a variable percentage of the injected iron, places this iron in stores that turn over slowly, with little or no release over the first 2 weeks. The spleen does not take up iron initially in the normal subject, and a slight decrease in count rate is seen over that organ as iron leaves the plasma for liver and marrow. After 1–2 weeks, when the radioactive iron returns to the circulation as labeled RBCs, the count rate over the spleen returns to 1.0 (Fig. 34-3B).

In the case of hepatic or splenic erythropoiesis, as in myeloid metaplasia, a pattern of immediate uptake and release may be seen over these organs, similar to that seen for the marrow probe. In the case of the spleen, however, the initial rapid uptake may be followed by a pattern of incomplete release, because of either ineffective erythropoiesis or subsequent splenic trapping of RBCs after they have entered the circulation, or both. In hemolysis, the counting rates show secondary rises over the liver or spleen, usually beginning a few days after injection of tracer iron, corresponding to the lag time between isotope injection and the first appearance of labeled RBCs in the circulation (Fig. 34-3B).

IN VIVO IMAGING OF ERYTHROPOIESIS

The use of probes placed over liver, spleen, and marrow facilitates numerical or graphic analysis of uptake and release, but pictorial displays are not as easily obtained. ^{59}Fe is not easily imaged by conventional scanners. Owing to its high-energy emissions, heavily shielded collimators are required, which are not generally available.[54–56] However, when available, such scanners can pictorially display patterns of radioactive iron uptake and release for entire organs and for the entire skeleton rather than the patterns for a single area that are available with the probes.[54] ^{52}Fe, the positron-emitting isotope of iron, has energies suitable for imaging, but access to a cyclotron is needed for its production, and its short half-life of 8 hours makes it suitable only for imaging the initial (uptake) portion of an iron kinetics study.[57–59]

In an effort to make up for these shortcomings, attempts have been made to use carrier-free ^{111}In as a longer half-life analogue of iron, since ^{111}In is bound to transferrin and may be delivered to RBC precursors. However, the kinetics of iron and indium are not identical, and care should be taken when clinical conclusions are made based on ^{111}In uptake.[60–62]

Whether the marrow is imaged with ^{59}Fe or ^{52}Fe, such studies may give important information that cannot otherwise be easily obtained. Thus, one may see patchy areas of poor marrow uptake signifying tumor encroachment, areas of absent marrow uptake due to aplasia or damage from prior irradiation, expansion of marrow, and/or loss of central marrow as in myelofibrosis.[54,57,58]

PROBE SITES

Probes may be placed over other organs as well as the liver, spleen, and marrow to determine the fate of labeled RBCs. Thus, probes placed over the kidneys in paroxysmal nocturnal hemoglobinuria will show the progressive renal accumulation of labeled hemoglobin from hemolyzed RBCs, while a probe placed over the lung in Goodpasture syndrome will show accumulated activity due to hemorrhage of labeled RBCs into that organ.[27] Probe placement may show active erythropoiesis in abnormal areas, such as the knees and ankles in myelofibrosis. Similarly, there may be a prolonged period of erythroid hypofunction postirradiation. Thus, the use of a sacral probe as a representative sampling of an active marrow site might be inappropriate in a patient who had undergone radiation therapy in that area within the previous 2 years. In such cases alternative sites such as the iliac crest or upper portion of the femur might be chosen.

THE TRANSFERRIN RECEPTOR: IRON KINETICS IN A TEST TUBE?

The transferrin receptor (TfR) is a transmembrane glycoprotein expressed on the surface of erythroid cells[68] that binds diferric transferrin, and transfers it into the cytoplasm for heme synthesis. When the receptor is recycled back to the membrane, some of it is lost into the circulation, where it can be measured by radioimmunoassay.[69-71] Serum TfR levels were found to be increased in subjects with increased erythropoiesis and decreased in hypoplastic states.[69,70] Beguin et al.[71] showed a direct and statistically significant correlation between TfR and plasma iron turnover in experimental animals and Huebers et al.[70] showed that TfR was directly correlated with erythron transferrin uptake in humans. It appears that, within the limitations of the methodology,[72] measurement of serum TfR in humans may have wide clinical applicability for quantitation of erythropoiesis in humans. Thus, measurement of serum TfR may replace iron kinetics to the same extent that measurement of serum ferritin has replaced bone marrow aspiration/biopsy for quantitation of iron stores.

Magnetic Resonance Imaging of the Bone Marrow

Recently, magnetic resonance imaging (MRI) has shown great promise for becoming the technique of choice for imaging bone marrow. Signals arising from T_1-weighted MRI scans of bone are strongly influenced by marrow cellularity and arise mainly from the fat and water content of marrow, since cortical and trabecular bone and marrow cells themselves yield little or no MRI signal.[63] Thus, areas of bone containing fatty marrow yield a strong (bright) signal on T_1-weighted images, normocellular (approximately 50% fat) marrow an intermediate signal, and hypercellular marrow a minimal signal.[63,64] This technique has shown great utility in evaluating patchy areas of aplastic marrow (as often seen in idiopathic aplasia or following radiotherapy), marrow infarction, recovery of marrow cellularity after radiotherapy or chemotherapy, infiltration with malignancy, and other instances.[63-67]

WHOLE BODY COUNTING OF IRON

After iron has been given to the subject either by mouth or by injection, it is possible to quantitate the amount of iron in the body through whole body counting. The patient is isolated in a small room, usually lined by pre-World War II battleship steel, because of its low contamination with the γ-emitter ^{60}Co. A single large crystal or multiple small crystals are then used, with suitable geometry, to count the whole body activity. These systems can typically count iron body burdens accurately with doses as low as 1 μCi of ^{59}Fe. For determination of iron absorption, the isotope can be given orally with or without accompanying food, nonradioactive iron, or putative inhibitors of iron absorption.[73,74] A count is made immediately after the patient receives the dose of iron to establish the amount given, and subsequent counts are made over the following weeks to determine the percentage of the total dose retained in the body (i.e., the fractional amount absorbed). For determination of blood loss, especially the episodic or low-grade type (which may escape the clinician's attention or the detection limits of commercially available occult blood-testing devices), the iron can be given intravenously, which ensures that most of it will be incor-

ORAL IRON TOLERANCE TEST

Multiple kinetic approaches to the issue of iron absorption have been taken that use combinations of whole body counting, iron kinetics, and isotope imaging.[27,54,75] Using multiple isotopes of iron in a patient with gastric retention, Fawwaz et al.[75] were able to show absence of iron absorption when the orally ingested iron bolus was still in the stomach and maximum absorption when it had reached the proximal jejunum.

Ekenved[76] showed that iron absorption as determined by whole body counting could also be studied by serially determining plasma iron concentrations 30 minutes to 6 hours after ingestion of iron salts. In effect, the oral iron bolus, usually in the form of a single tablet of $FeSO_4$ serves as its own tracer, since a single 325-mg tablet of $FeSO_4$ contains about 64 mg of elemental iron, as compared with about 2-3 mg of iron in the entire plasma iron pool. Increases of iron of 21-23 μmol/L of plasma were noted at about 2-4 hours after ingestion of 100 mg of elemental iron in normal subjects, which is equivalent to a rise in plasma iron of 120 μg/dl of plasma. Peak plasma levels were higher than normal in iron-deficient patients, and blunted curves were noted when poorly absorbed preparations were ingested. Given the high correlation between this oral iron tolerance test and isotopic studies of iron absorption, this simple nonradioactive test retains a kinetic approach and has much to recommend it as an important clinical tool.

porated into circulating RBCs. Serial counts may then be made over a prolonged period to determine the rate of iron loss, if any, from the body. It has been estimated that the normal adult loses $\leq$2 mg/day of iron out of a total RBC iron pool of about 2.5 g.[27] This should result in a rate of about 0.1 %/day. Indeed, Price[73] noted losses of about this magnitude (0.136 $\pm$ 0.039%/day) in normal subjects at 20-100 days after isotope administration. Losses in excess of this rate are prima facie evidence of excessive loss of iron from the body. Although blood loss should always be the primary suspect, losses from the skin in extensive exfoliative dermatitis, lactation, and urinary tract losses of iron in chronic hemoglobinuric states (paroxysmal nocturnal hemoglobinuria, prosthetic valve hemolysis) are other possible causes of excessive losses.

BILE PIGMENT AND CARBON MONOXIDE KINETICS

Just as iron kinetics is a valuable tool for the study of erythropoiesis (because most iron leaving the plasma is destined for RBC production), production of bile pigment and of carbon monoxide is also important, since production of these substances represents mainly but not exclusively turnover of RBC hemoglobin heme. It was the very early glycine studies using ^{15}N and mass spectroscopy that revealed that a small percentage of isotope was excreted into the bile or feces (or both) within the first few days after glycine ingestion or injection, before any appreciable amount of the isotope was found to be incorporated into circulating RBCs.[33,77] The origin of this "early-appearing" bile pigment was at first obscure and was attributed to anabolic pathways that produced bilirubin without an intermediate heme molecule. This could be directly tested, since catabolic processes produce both carbon monoxide and bile pigment,[30] while anabolic processes would be expected to produce only bile pigment. The presence of an "early labeled" peak for both carbon monoxide and bile pigment made anabolic processes less likely[34,35] and suggested that this fraction was derived from the catabolism of hemes that undergo rapid turnover.

Evidence in support of this explanation was provided by Robinson et al,[78] who studied bilirubin production in the isolated saline-perfused rat liver. The amount of labeled bilirubin in the bile of these preparations and the timing of its appearance were similar to those in the early labeled peak for bilirubin in the intact rat, which firmly established this organ as a major contributor to overall heme catabolism/bilirubin production.

It has now been estimated that in both normal humans and rats this early-appearing material represents about 25% of total heme catabolism.[21,79] The consensus opinion from these studies is that there are three major contributors to heme catabolism. The first results from destruction of aged circulating RBCs and represents the "late peak" production of carbon monoxide or bile pigment, or both. The second is a fraction that appears early and represents the portion of erythropoietic heme formation that is ineffective or that does not result in heme incorporation into circulating RBCs.[21,80] Such heme could be that contained in the scarf or cytoplasm extruded with the normoblast nucleus. Bessis et al[81] estimated that this represents about 3–10% of total normoblast cytoplasm; this value corresponds well with the 8–9% estimated from kinetic studies in both animals and humans.[21,79] The third component of total heme catabolism is turnover of nonhemoglobin heme, such as the hepatic cytochromes, which appear mainly during the early peak phase and represent about 15–18% of total heme catabolism.

As mentioned above, bilirubin, bile pigment, or carbon monoxide production rates, turnover rates, and isotopic appearance curves can be obtained in animals and humans and have added significantly to our understanding of RBC survival, ineffective erythropoiesis, hepatic heme turnover, and the like. Given the multiple pools involved, bilirubin kinetics models can be as complex as those given for iron.[79,82,83]

Since each of the disciplines outlined in this chapter corresponds to a different mix of metabolic pools, they have been mutually reinforcing. For example, Berk et al[84] measured simultaneous bilirubin turnover and survival of RBCs labeled with tritiated diisopropyl fluorophosphate. They found excellent correlation between the values for mean RBC life span calculated by each method.[84] The two techniques showed extremely close agreement for mean life spans of <60 days; above that, RBC life span values derived from the bilirubin turnover technique (which assumed that 15% of total bilirubin turnover arose from nonhemoglobin heme catabolism) were consistently shorter than those obtained from the random label technique. This suggested that nonerythropoietic processes in normal subjects are responsible for >15% of total heme turnover, which has been substantiated in subsequent papers from that group.[79] Indeed, since hepatic heme turnover and RBC turn-

Table 34-5. Erythropoietic Heme Turnover (Effective)

Methodology	Original Units	µmol/day	Reference
Carbon monoxide production	6.1 µl/kg/hr	340–410 (derived value)	34
Bilirubin turnover	2.7 mg/kg/day	323	79
Iron turnover	21.4 mg/day	383	27
DFP RBC survival	116 days	366	5
Cohort RBC survival	127 days	334	12

Abbreviation: DFP, diisopropyl fluorophosphate.

over are governed by different stimuli, it is not intuitively evident that they should have any fixed relationship except in normal subjects, and even then influences from the menstrual cycle, certain drugs, and other conditions may make that conclusion suspect.[47]

Once a value for the fractionation of heme turnover arising from erythropoietic and nonerythropoietic sources is established (see above), it is possible to determine RBC survival not only from bilirubin turnover[79] but also from studies of endogenous carbon monoxide production. This technique does not require isotopes and is carried out either by determining excretion rates for carbon monoxide in subjects breathing carbon monoxide-free air[85] or by measuring the build-up of carbon monoxide-hemoglobin levels in the blood of subjects in a rebreathing apparatus.[31,34] Such studies have indicated that the production rate of carbon monoxide in normal adults averages about 19–23 µmol/hr, or 450–545 µmol/day.[31,34] In view of the prior estimate of 25% of total heme catabolism not arising from effective erythropoiesis, this would amount to 340–410 µmol/day of carbon monoxide arising from circulating RBCs. It would be expected that this value should agree closely with the EIT estimated from iron kinetics studies, with the erythropoietic component of bilirubin turnover, and also with RBC heme turnover as measured by cohort or random RBC survival methods. That this is the case is shown in Table 34-5. For all values in the table, a body weight of 70 kg and a hemoglobin mass of 10.3 g/kg and molecular weight for hemoglobin of 68,000 are assumed and each publication cited is from a different laboratory.

CONCLUSIONS

Red blood cell kinetics had its heyday in the 1950s and 1960s, when these techniques were used to establish the pathophysiology of many hematologic disorders. Once established, these did not need to be repeated, for example, whenever a clinician saw a new patient with pernicious anemia or congenital spherocytosis. The hematologist now has other well-characterized clinical and laboratory methods for determining the presence or absence of bleeding, for estimating erythropoietic rate and RBC destruction, and so forth, which may not involve the use of isotopes or other kinetic studies. However, one should always remember that our understanding of the tests employed, the pathophysiology, and the diseases themselves ultimately depends on our ability to understand the kinetic aspects of the system(s) under study, as well as the assumptions made. If we keep these in mind, we will better understand our test results, the diseases we treat, and our patients.

BILIRUBIN KINETICS AND BILIRUBIN TURNOVER

An interesting clinical observation can be made from the kinetic approaches to bilirubin turnover. This occurs because one can define the range of values for uptake of preformed bilirubin by the normal liver, as well as the range of values for heme turnover seen in most clinical situations. Given maximal possible steady-state bilirubin production rates and normal hepatic bilirubin kinetics, the plasma indirect bilirubin should not exceed 4.0 mg/dl; values in excess of this mean that there is a component of hepatic dysfunction.[83]

REFERENCES

1. Lux SE: Spectrin-actin membrane skeleton of normal and abnormal red blood cells. Semin Hematol 16:21, 1979
2. Allison AC: Turnovers of erythrocytes and plasma proteins in mammals. Nature 188:37, 1960

3. Li CKN, Li EKH: Mechanical fatigue as a possible determinant of *in vivo* longevity of red blood cells. Trans Biomed Eng 30:226, 1983

4. Eadie GS, Brown IW, Curtis WG: The potential life span and ultimate survival of fresh red blood cells in normal healthy recipients as studied by simultaneous Cr^{51} tagging and differential hemolysis. J Clin Invest 34:629, 1955

5. Cohen JA, Warringa MGPJ: The fate of P^{32} labelled diisopropyl fluorophosphonate in the human body and its use as a labelling agent in the study of the turnover of blood plasma and red cells. J Clin Invest 33:459, 1954

6. Cline MJ, Berlin NI: The red cell chromium elution rate in patients with some hematologic diseases. Blood 21:63, 1963

7. Cline MJ, Berlin NI: Red blood cell life span using DFP^{32} as a cohort label. Blood 19:715, 1962

8. Mollison PL: Further observations on the normal survival curve of ^{51}Cr-labeled red cells. Clin Sci 21:21, 1961

9. Landaw SA: The use of ^{14}C-cyanate for red blood cell survival studies. Proc Soc Exp Biol Med 142:712, 1973

10. Eschbach JW, Korn D, Finch CA: ^{14}C-cyanate as a tag for red cell survival in normal and uremic man. J Lab Clin Med 89:823, 1977

11. Smedsrod B, Aminoff D: Use of ^{75}Se-labeled methionine to study the sequestration of senescent red blood cells. Am J Hematol 18:31, 1985

12. Shemin D, Rittenberg D: The life span of the human red blood cell. J Biol Chem 166:627, 1946

13. Landaw SA, Winchell HS: Endogenous production of ^{14}CO: a method for calculation of RBC lifespan in vivo. Blood 36:642, 1970

14. Burwell EL, Brickley BA, Finch CA: Erythrocyte life span in small animals. Comparison of two methods employing radioiron. Am J Physiol 172:718, 1953

15. Shapiro SI, Landaw SA, Winchell HS, Williams MC: Independence of mechanical fragility and red blood cell age in the rat. Proc Soc Exp Biol Med 131:1206, 1969

16. Belcher EH, Harriss EB: Studies of red cell life span in the rat. J Physiol (Lond) 146:217, 1959

17. Giles RC, Berman A, Hildebrandt PK, McCaffrey RP: The use of ^{51}Cr for sheep red blood cell survival studies. Proc Soc Exp Biol Med 148:795, 1975

18. International Committee for Standardization in Hematology: Recommended method for radioisotope red-cell survival studies. Br J Haematol 45:659, 1980

19. Eadie GS, Brown IW: Red blood cell survival studies. Blood 8:1110, 1953

20. Palmer JG, Eichwald EJ, Cartwright GE, Wintrobe MM: Experimental production of splenomegaly, anemia and leukopenia in albino rats. Blood 8:72, 1953

21. Landaw SA: Kinetic aspects of endogenous carbon monoxide production. II. The erythroid component of the early labeled peak. p. 134. In Berk PD, Berlin NI (eds): Proceedings of Fogarty International Symposium on Chemistry and Physiology of Bile Pigments. Publication # NIH 77-110. Department of Health and Human Services, Washington, DC, 1977

22. Song SH, Groom AC: Storage of blood cells in spleen in the cat. Am J Physiol 220:779, 1971

23. Jandl JH, Greenberg MS, Yonemoto RH, Castle WB: Clinical determination of the sites of red cell sequestration in hemolytic anemias. J Clin Invest 35:842, 1956

24. Goldberg A, Hutchison HE, MacDonald E: Radiochromium in the selection of patients with haemolytic anaemia for splenectomy. Lancet 1:109, 1966

25. Ahuja S, Lewis SM, Szur L: Value of surface counting in predicting response to splenectomy in haemolytic anaemia. J Clin Pathol 25:467, 1972

26. Najean Y, Cacchione R, Dresch C, Rain JD: Methods of evaluating the sequestration site of red cells labelled with ^{51}Cr: a review of 96 cases. Br J Haematol 29:495, 1975

27. Pollycove M: Iron metabolism and kinetics. Semin Hematol 3:235, 1966

28. Berlin NI, Waldmann TA, Weissman SM: Life span of red blood cell. Physiol Rev 39:577, 1959

29. Berlin NI, Hewitt C, Lotz C: Hippuric acid synthesis in man after the administration of [α-^{14}C]glycine. Biochem J 58:498, 1954

30. Tenhunen RS, Marver HS, Schmid R: Microsomal heme oxygenase. Characterization of the enzyme. J Biol Chem 44:638, 1969

31. Berk PD, Rodkey FL, Blaschke TF et al: Comparison of plasma bilirubin turnover and carbon monoxide production in man. J Lab Clin Med 83:29, 1974

32. Landaw SA, Callahan EW, Schmid R: Catabolism of heme in vivo: comparison of the simultaneous production of bilirubin and carbon monoxide. J Clin Invest 49:914, 1970

33. London IM, West R, Shemin D, Rittenberg D: On origin of bile pigment in normal man, abstracted. J Biol Chem 184:351, 1950

34. Coburn RF, Blakemore WS, Forster RE: Endogenous carbon monoxide production in man. J Clin Invest 42:1172, 1963

35. White P, Coburn RF, Williams WJ et al: Carbon monoxide production associated with ineffective erythropoiesis. J Clin Invest 46:1986, 1967

36. Landaw SA, Guancial RL: Shortened survival of fetal erythrocytes in the rat. Pediatr Res 11:1155, 1977

37. Vest M, Strebel L, Hauenstein D: The extent of "shunt bilirubin" and erythrocyte survival in the newborn infant measured by the administration of (^{15}N)glycine. Biochem J 95:11c, 1965

38. Sorbie J, Valberg LS: Splenic sequestration of stress erythrocytes in the rabbit. Am J Physiol 218:647, 1970

39. Berlin NI, Lotz C: Life span of the red blood cell of the rat following acute hemorrhage. Proc Soc Exp Biol Med 78:788, 1951

40. Landaw SA: Biological aspects of senescence in red cells. p. 303. In Elias MF, Eleftheriou BE, Elias PK (eds): Special Review of Experimental Aging Research. Progress in Biology. EAR, Bar Harbor, ME, 1976

41. Landaw SA: Factors that accelerate or retard red blood cell senescence. Blood Cells 14:47, 1988

42. Owren PA: Congenital hemolytic jaundice: the pathogenesis of the "hemolytic crisis." Blood 3:231, 1948

43. Huff RL, Hennessy TG, Austin RE et al: Plasma and red cell iron turnover in normal subjects and in patients having various hematopoietic disorders. J Clin Invest 29:1041, 1950

44. Huff RL, Elmlinger PJ, Carcia JF et al: Ferrokinetics in normal persons and in patients having various erythropoietic disorders. J Clin Invest 30:1512, 1951

45. Cook JD, Marsaglia G, Eschbach JW et al: Ferrokinetics: a biological model for plasma iron exchange in man. J Clin Invest 49:197, 1970

46. Cavill I: Diagnostic methods. Baillieres Clin Haematol 11:259, 1982

47. Lynch SR, Moede AL: Variation in the rate of endogenous carbon monoxide production in normal human beings. J Lab Clin Med 79:85, 1972

48. Lowman JT, Krivit W: New in vivo tracer method with the use of nonradioactive isotopes and activation analysis. J Lab Clin Med 61:1042, 1963

49. Wasserman LR, Sharney L, Gevirtz NR: Studies of iron kinetics: I. Interpretation of ferrokinetic data in man. Mt Sinai J Med 32:262, 1965

50. Pollycove M, Mortimer R: The quantitative determination of iron kinetics and hemoglobin synthesis in human subjects. J Clin Invest 40:753, 1961

51. Ricketts C, Jacobs A, Cavill I: Ferrokinetics and erythropoiesis in man: the measurement of effective erythropoiesis, ineffective erythropoiesis and red cell lifespan using ^{59}Fe. Br J Haematol 31:65, 1975

52. Finch CA, Deubelbeiss K, Cook JD et al: Ferrokinetics in man. Medicine 49:17, 1970

53. Barosi G, Cazzola M, Morandi S et al: Estimation of ferrokinetic parameters by a mathematical model in patients with primary acquired sideroblastic anaemia. Br J Haematol 39:409, 1978

54. Ronai P, Winchell HS, Anger HO, Lawrence JH: Whole-body scanning of ^{59}Fe for evaluating body distribution of erythropoietic marrow, splenic sequestration of red cells and hepatic disposition of iron. J Nucl Med 10:469, 1969

55. Chaudhuri TK, Ehrhardt JC, DeGowin RL, Christie JH: ^{59}Fe whole-body scanning. J Nucl Med 15:667, 1974

56. Van Zyl WH, Lotter MG, Kok JC et al: Bone marrow imaging with ^{59}Fe. S Afr Med J 51:13, 1977

57. Van Dyke DC, Anger HO, Yano Y: Progress in determining bone marrow distribution in vivo. p. 65. In Lawrence JH (ed): Progress in Atomic Medicine. Grune & Stratton, Orlando, FL, 1968

58. Van Dyke DC, Anger HO: Patterns of marrow hypertrophy and atrophy in man. J Nucl Med 6:109, 1965

59. Knospe WH, Rayudu VMS, Cardello M et al: Bone marrow scanning with $^{52}iron$ (^{52}Fe). Regeneration and extension of marrow after ablative doses of radiotherapy. Cancer 37:1432, 1976

60. McNeil BJ, Holman L, Button LN, Rosenthal DS: Use of indium chloride scintigraphy in patients with myelofibrosis. J Nucl Med 15:647, 1974

61. McNeil BJ, Rappeport JM, Nathan DG: Indium chloride scintigraphy: an index of severity in patients with aplastic anaemia. Br J Haematol 34:599, 1976

62. Rojer RA, Mulder NH, Nieweg HO et al: Analysis of extramedullary erythropoiesis in the spleen by a semiquantitative method using indium-111. Acta Med Scand 203:481, 1978

63. Steiner RM, Mitchell DG, Rao VA et al: Magnetic resonance imaging of diffuse bone marrow disease. Radiol Clin North Am 31:383, 1993

64. Kaplan KR, Mitchell DG, Steiner RM et al: Polycythemia vera and myelofibrosis: correlation of MRI, clinical, and laboratory findings. Radiology 183:329, 1992

65. Porter BA, Shields AL, Olson DO: MRI of bone marrow disorders. Radiol Clin North Am 24:269, 1986

66. Rosen BR, Fleming DM, Kushner DC et al: Hematologic bone marrow disorders: quantitative chemical shift MRI. Radiology 169:799, 1988

67. Mankod VN, Williams JP, Harpen MD et al: Magnetic resonance imaging of bone marrow in sickle cell disease: clinical, hematologic, and pathologic correlations. Blood 75:274, 1990

68. Liebman A, Aisen P: Transferrin receptor of the rabbit reticulocyte. Biochemistry 16:1268, 1977

69. Kohgo Y, Niitsu Y, Kondo H et al: Serum transferrin receptor as a new index of erythropoiesis. Blood 70:1955, 1987

70. Huebers HA, Beguin Y, Pootrakul P et al: Intact transferrin receptors in human plasma and their relation to erythropoiesis. Blood 75:102, 1990

71. Beguin Y, Huebers HA, Josephson B, Finch CA: Transferrin receptors in rat plasma. Proc Natl Acad Sci USA 85:637, 1988

72. Beguin Y, Clemons GK, Pootrakul P, Fillet G: Quantitative assessment of erythropoiesis and functional classification of anemia based on measurements of serum transferrin receptor and erythropoietin. Blood 81:1067, 1993

73. Price DC: Iron turnover in man. p. 537. In Kniseley RM, Tauxe WN, Anderson EB (eds): Dynamic Clinical Studies with Radioisotopes. U.S. Atomic Energy Commission, Oak Ridge, Tennessee, 1964

74. DeAlarcon PA, Donovan ME, Forbes GB et al: Iron absorption in the thalassemia syndromes and its inhibition by tea. N Engl J Med 300:5, 1979

75. Fawwaz RA, Winchell HS, Pollycove M et al: Kinetics of oral iron absorption using iron-52, iron-55, and iron-59. J Nucl Med 7:349, 1966

76. Ekenvad G: Iron absorption studies. Scand J Haematol, suppl. 28:31, 1976

77. Gray CH, Neuberger A, Sneath PHA: Studies in congenital porphyria. II. Incorporation of 15 N in the stercobilin in the normal and in the porphyric. Biochem J 47:87, 1950

78. Robinson SH, Owen CA, Flock EV, Schmid R: Bilirubin formation in the liver from nonhemoglobin sources. Experiments with isolated, perfused liver. Blood 26:823, 1965

79. Berk PD, Blaschke TF, Scharschmidt BF et al: A new approach to quantitation of the various sources of bilirubin in man. J Lab Clin Med 87:767, 1976

80. Robinson SH: Formation of bilirubin from erythroid and nonerythroid sources. Semin Hematol 9:43, 1972

81. Bessis M, Berton-Gorius J, Thiery JP: Rôle possible de l'hémoglobine accompagnant le noyau des érythroblastes dans l'origine de la stercobiline eliminée précocement. C R Acad Sci III 252:2300, 1961

82. Shames DM, Kirshenbaum G, Schmid R: Kinetics of hepatic and extrahepatic bilirubin production in man: a new compartmental model. p. 216. In Berk PD, Berlin NI (eds): Chemistry and Physiology of Bile Pigments. Publication NIH #77-1100. Department of Health and Human Services, Washington, DC, 1977

83. Berlin NI, Berk PD: Quantitative aspects of bilirubin metabolism for hematologists. Blood 57:983, 1981

84. Berk PD, Bloomer JR, Howe RB et al: Bilirubin production as a measure of red cell life span. J Lab Clin Med 79:364, 1972

85. Sjöstrand T: Endogenous formation of carbon monoxide in man under normal and pathological conditions. Scand J Clin Lab Invest 1:201, 1949

86. Berk PD, Howe RB, Bloomer JR, Berlin NI: Studies of bilirubin kinetics in normal adults. J Clin Invest 48:2176, 1969

Hemoglobin Synthesis, Structure, and Function

35

Martin H. Steinberg and Edward J. Benz, Jr.

INTRODUCTION AND HISTORICAL ASPECTS

Hemoglobins are the major oxygen transport properties of the body. Hoppe-Seyler first used the term hemoglobin to describe the pigment in erythrocytes that had the property of reversibly binding oxygen. During this same period it was determined that hemoglobin consists of heme and globin and that iron is a constituent of heme. The early twentieth century saw the elucidation of the structure of heme, ascertainment of the molecular weight of hemoglobin, and description of the hemoglobin/oxygen dissociation curve. The three-dimensional structure of hemoglobin was described by Perutz. The primary amino acid sequence of globin chains was determined by a number of investigators, including Braunitzer, Konigsberg, Schroeder, and Ingram.*

Hemoglobins bear strong structural and functional similarities to related proteins that are present in many organisms. The root nodules of leguminous plants contain a closely related molecule, leghemoglobin, which has the property of binding oxygen. True hemoglobins are present in some invertebrates, while other invertebrates have oxygen-carrying proteins distinct from hemoglobin that may serve other than respiratory

functions. Invertebrate oxygen-carrying proteins may exist as large polymers in body fluids or may be encapsulated within cells. Most vertebrate hemoglobins are intracellular. The enveloping erythrocytes may be nucleated (e.g., avian) or anuclear (e.g., mammalian) depending on whether erythropoiesis is intra- or extravascular. Within erythrocytes, the function of hemoglobin is invariably influenced by organic phosphates and protons.

While there are major differences in the primary structure of various vertebrate hemoglobins, all are heterotetramers consisting of two pairs of unlike globin polypeptides (α_2 non-α_2). Cloning, sequencing, and chromosomal localization of globin genes have provided glimpses into the evolutionary history of globin. Vertebrate α- and β-globin genes are probably derived from a single ancestral gene. By the process of duplication, this gene gave rise to the progenitors of present-day globins. Study of the phylogeny of globin genes has taught us much about evolution in general. Genes may proliferate by duplication, be lost during recombination events, be inactivated by mutations, and "jump" by different means to different locales within the genome.

The study of hemoglobin has been in the vanguard of science since antiquity from the earliest studies applying microscopy, through the elegant dissection of the structure and function of hemoglobin and the physiology of the erythrocyte, to the present-day determination and manipulation of the DNA sequences that encode and control globin genes. Hemoglobin research has been a major contributor to the advance of biology and the translation of these advances into improved diagnosis and therapy. Familiarity with the basic aspects of hemo-

---

* No attempt is made in this introductory survey to provide citations to the vast literature that has accumulated about the hemoglobins. Rather, we have provided a list of readings at the end of the chapter. Each of these excellent works provides access to the original literature. The reader should also consult Chapters 17, 35, 43, 44, 161 for other aspects of hemoglobin relevant to human disease

globin structure, function, synthesis, and ontogeny is critical in understanding important hematologic diseases such as β-thalassemia and sickle cell anemia. The basic features of human hemoglobins and their encoding genes are discussed in the following sections.

HEMOGLOBIN STRUCTURE

The hemoglobin tetramer consists of two pairs of unlike globin polypeptide chains: one pair of α-like chains, and one pair of non-α chains. Each chain enfolds a single heme group. Each heme group, in turn, consists of a single molecule of protoporphyrin IX coordinately bound to a single ferrous (Fe^{2+}) ion (see Ch. 38). If the iron moiety is oxidized to the ferric (Fe^{3+}) state, the protein is called methemoglobin. The normal human hemoglobins most relevant to the material in this textbook are Hb A($\alpha_2\beta_2$), the major adult hemoglobin; Hb F(α_2,γ_2), the major fetal hemoglobin; and Hb A_2 (α_2,δ_2), a minor hemoglobin in adults (Table 35-1).

The behavior of hemoglobin is determined by its primary structure, the covalent linking of amino acids to form the amino acid sequence of the polypeptide globin. The higher-order structures of hemoglobin are dependent on this sequence. The α-globin chains contain 141 residues, while the β-like chains are 146 amino acids long. These globins show considerable homology, especially among the non-α-chains. While the α-globin chains result from a very remote gene duplication, the non-α-globin chains are the result of more recent gene duplications and thus are more akin to each other than they are to the α-like globin genes. Gene conversion events also ensure the similarity of duplicated genes. Despite their overall similarity, individual human globin chains, and the hemoglobins they form, differ sufficiently to be readily separable by techniques (e.g., electrophoresis, isoelectric focusing) suitable for routine diagnostic use. This permits rapid screening of patients for the presence of abnormal hemoglobins (see Ch. 161).

Elements of the secondary structure of globin are shown in Figure 35-1. About 75% of the globin polypeptide chain forms an α-helix. The eight helical segments, A–H, are separated by short stretches from which the α-helix is absent. These nonhelical segments permit folding of the polypeptide on itself and are often dictated by the presence of prolyl residues, which are generally unable to participate in the formation of α-helices. Although the helical segments of the α- and non-α-globin chains do not precisely correspond, it is possible to define amino acid residues in all globin peptides by their helical and nonhelical residue number, as indicated in Figure 35-1. This permits greater appreciation of the homology among globins. Some of the amino acids of globin are invariant, or conserved, in the sense that they are preserved during phylogeny. These residues occur at portions of the molecule that are critical for its stability and function. Examples include heme-binding residues, hydrophobic amino acids of the interior of the molecule, and certain subunit contacts at the α_1-β_2 interface. The introduction of prolyl residues into α-helical segments by mutation leads to interruption of the α-helix and instability of the resulting hemoglobin molecule.

Table 35-1. Structural Features of the Human Hemoglobins

Name	Globin Chain Composition	Comment
Hb A	$\alpha_2\ \beta_2$	Major (95–98% of total) adult hemoglobin
Hb A_2	$\alpha_2\ \delta_2$	Minor (1.5–3.5%) adult hemoglobin
Hb F	$\alpha_2\ \gamma_2$	Major fetal hemoglobin; 0.5–1% in adult
Hb Gower-1	$\zeta_2\ \epsilon_2$	Embryonic hemoglobin
Hb Gower-2	$\alpha_2\ \epsilon_2$	Embryonic hemoglobin
Hb Portland	$\zeta_2\ \gamma_2$	Embryonic hemoglobin

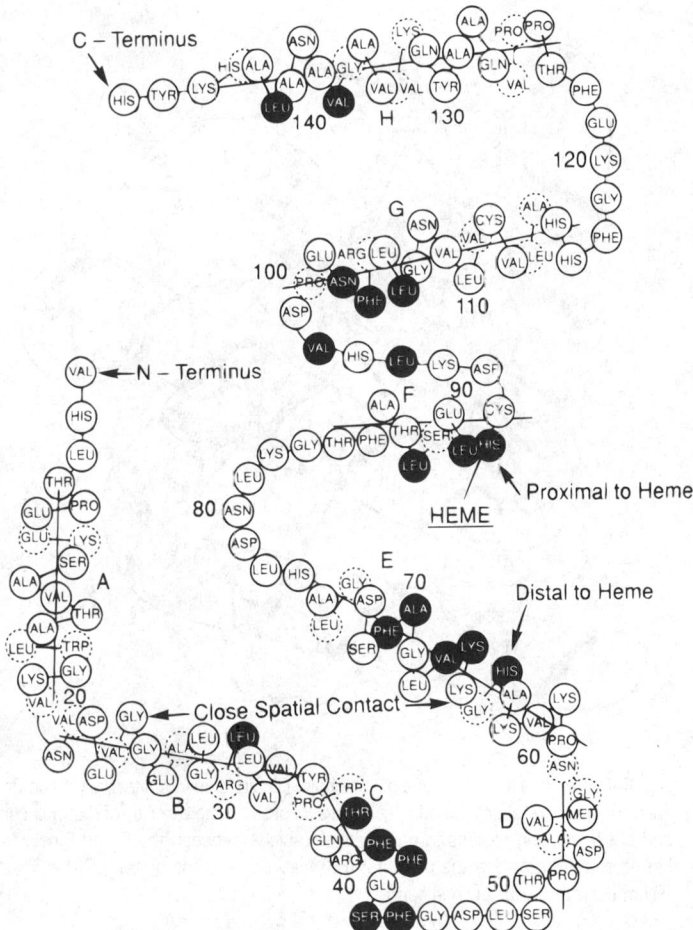

Fig. 35-1. β-Globin chain, showing helical and nonhelical segments. Helical segments are labeled A–H, while nonhelical segments are designated NA for those residues between the N terminus and the A helix, CD for residues between the C and D helices, and so forth. (From Huisman and Schroeder,[9] with permission.)

The poorly understood laws that govern the folding of proteins are responsible for the tertiary structure of globin (Fig. 35-2). This folding pattern places polar residues exteriorly and provides a hydrophobic niche for the heme ring between the E and F helices. Numerous noncovalent bonds are formed between the heme and surrounding amino acid residues of globin. An iron atom at the center of the porphyrin ring forms an important bond with the F8, or proximal histidine, and through the linked oxygen, with the E7, or distal histidine residue. Oxygenation and deoxygenation of hemoglobin occur at the heme iron.

Two α-globin chains and two non-α-globin chains fit together specifically to form a hemoglobin tetramer with a molecular weight of about 64,000, with the quaternary structure shown in Figure 35-3. The motion of individual globin chains, as well as the movement of globin chains relative to each other during oxygenation and deoxygenation, gives hemoglobin its unique value as a respiratory protein. Each heme group can bind a single oxygen molecule; thus, each hemoglobin tetramer can reversibly bind and transport ≤4 molecules of oxygen. Oxygen-laden hemoglobin is called oxyhemoglobin; hemoglobin containing no bound oxygen is deoxyhemoglobin.

HEMOGLOBIN FUNCTION

Evolution has honed the hemoglobin tetramer into a molecule ideally suited to its tasks. Owing to the exigencies of molecular evolution, we can find in the genome of all animals, includ-

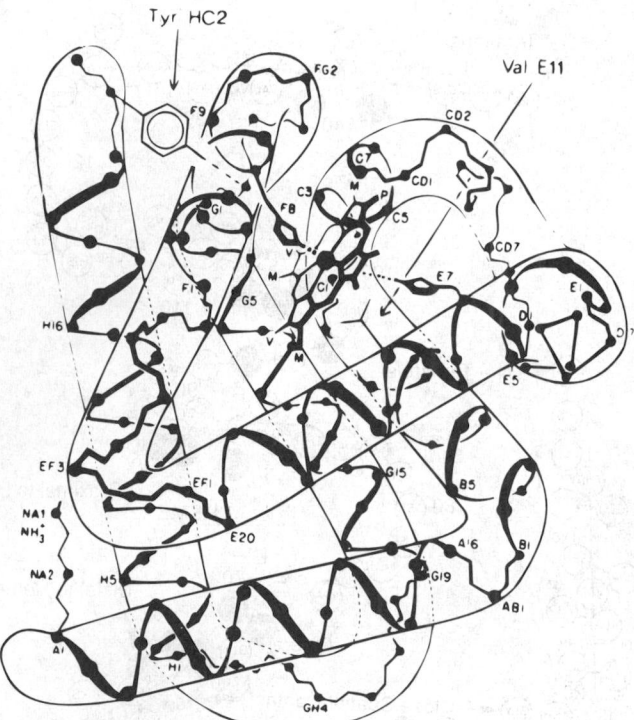

Fig. 35-2. Tertiary structure of a globin chain. Globin folds into a tertiary structure such that polar or charged amino acids are located on the exterior of the molecule and the heme ring resides in a hydrophobic niche between the E and F helices. Linked to the heme are the proximal (F8) histidine and the distal (E7) histidine. (From Perutz,[10] with permission.)

ing humans, attempts of nature to propagate a variety of different globin genes; each codes for a variant of the same basic molecular design. Crystallographic studies have defined the oxygenated and deoxygenated structures of hemoglobin at Ångstrom unit resolution and have provided an exquisitely detailed picture of how the globin chains and individual amino acid residues respond to the loading and unloading of oxygen. Thus, we know more about the function of hemoglobin than about that of virtually any other protein. Our knowledge of this mechanism provides a beautiful and intellectually satisfying culmination to decades of study by many investigators.

The oxygen dissociation curve of hemoglobin (Fig. 35-4), describes the percentage of saturation of hemoglobin with oxygen at different oxygen tensions. The sigmoidal shape of this curve is a result of interaction among the subunits of hemoglobin. Communication within the tetramer is called *heme-heme* interaction or cooperativity. This implies that the four heme groups do not undergo simultaneous oxygenation or deoxygenation, but rather that the state of each individual heme unit with regard to the presence or absence of bound oxygen influences the binding of oxygen to other heme groups. Myoglobin, a heme-containing protein with virtually the same tertiary structure as globin, exists in muscle as a monomer. The oxygen equilibrium curve of myoglobin is a rectangular hyperbola; in physiologic terms, it rapidly becomes fully saturated at low oxygen tensions and remains saturated as the oxygen tension plateaus. The difference between the oxygen equilibrium curves of myoglobin and hemoglobin lies in the tetrameric nature of the hemoglobin molecule and the cooperativity permitted by the association of similar but nonidentical subunits. Myoglobin, as compared with hemoglobin, has a very low P_{50} (the oxygen partial pressure at which the molecule is half-saturated with oxygen). It therefore has an extremely high oxygen affinity. It can acquire oxygen readily but would not be useful

for delivering oxygen to tissues, because it cannot release oxygen at physiologic oxygen tensions. The oxygen in myoglobin is passed on to the mitochondria, where oxidative metabolism occurs.

The shape of the oxygen dissociation curve of hemoglobin is sigmoidal. The totally deoxygenated hemoglobin tetramer is slow to acquire the first oxygen molecule by binding to a heme group but, as oxygenation proceeds, the reaction of the remaining hemes with oxygen accelerates. Perutz has drawn an analogy in which the "appetite" of heme for oxygen grows with the "eating," and conversely, loss of oxygen from heme lowers the oxygen affinity of the remaining heme groups. This phenomenon is sometimes summarized by saying that oxygen binding begets more oxygen binding, while oxygen release begets more oxygen release.

The Hill coefficient n, which can be calculated from plots of oxygen equilibrium curves, is a description of heme-heme interaction or cooperativity that explains in part the oxygen-binding properties of hemoglobin and myoglobin. The Hill coefficient for myoglobin is 1, indicating no cooperativity; n is about 3 for the normal hemoglobin molecule.

Transition from the deoxy (T [tense]) to the oxy (R [relaxed]) form of hemoglobin is accompanied by rotation of the $\alpha\beta$ dimers along the α_1-β_2 contact region (Fig. 35-5). The T structure is stabilized by salt bridges, which are broken as the molecule switches into the R structure. Some abnormal hemoglobins with an intrinsically high oxygen affinity, or low P_{50}, occur as a result of an amino acid substitution that leads to loss of bonds that stabilize the tetramer in the T conformation. Hydrogen ions, chloride ions, and carbon dioxide all decrease the affinity of hemoglobin for oxygen by strengthening the salt bridges that lock the molecule into its T conformation.

The corollary of the lowering of hemoglobin oxygen affinity by protons (lower pH) is the combination of hemoglobin with protons on deoxygenation. This is known as the Bohr effect and is responsible for carbon dioxide transport in blood, another critical function of the hemoglobin molecule. Deoxyhemoglobin binds the hydrogen ion liberated by the reaction of carbon dioxide with water, thus increasing the concentration of bicarbonate. Within the lungs, this hydrogen ion is released as hemoglobin binds oxygen; therefore, carbon dioxide leaves solution and is excreted from the body via the lungs. Deoxyhemoglobin can also directly bind carbon dioxide; however, this process involves the minority of carbon dioxide exchanged by the red blood cells.

The oxygen affinity of hemoglobin within the erythrocyte does not depend solely on the intrinsic properties of the tetramer. The position of the hemoglobin/oxygen dissociation curve and, therefore, the P_{50}, can be influenced by a number of heterotopic modifiers, including temperature, pH, and small organic phosphate molecules in the cell. The effects of these modifiers on P_{50} are shown in Figure 35-4.

Hemoglobin is the prototype of an allosteric protein; its structure and function are influenced by other molecules. The major intracellular modulator of hemoglobin/oxygen affinity in human erythrocytes is 2,3-bis(phosphoglyceric acid) (2,3-BPG), an intermediate product of glycolysis present within the erythrocyte at concentrations equimolar to hemoglobin. 2,3-BPG is also often called 2,3-diphosphoglyceric acid (2,3-DPG). The synthesis of 2,3-BPG is enzymatically regulated. Its levels may change depending on the conditions extant. 2,3-BPG is able to bind stereospecifically within the central cavity of the hemoglobin tetramer. In the absence of 2,3-BPG, hemoglobin has a very high oxygen affinity but, as 2,3-BPG is added to a hemoglobin solution, the oxygen affinity progressively decreases. BPG is a polyanion that binds strongly to the deoxygenated form of hemoglobin but poorly to its oxygenated or other liganded forms. Specific amino acids are involved in the binding of 2,3-BPG; these β-chain residues include the N-terminal va-

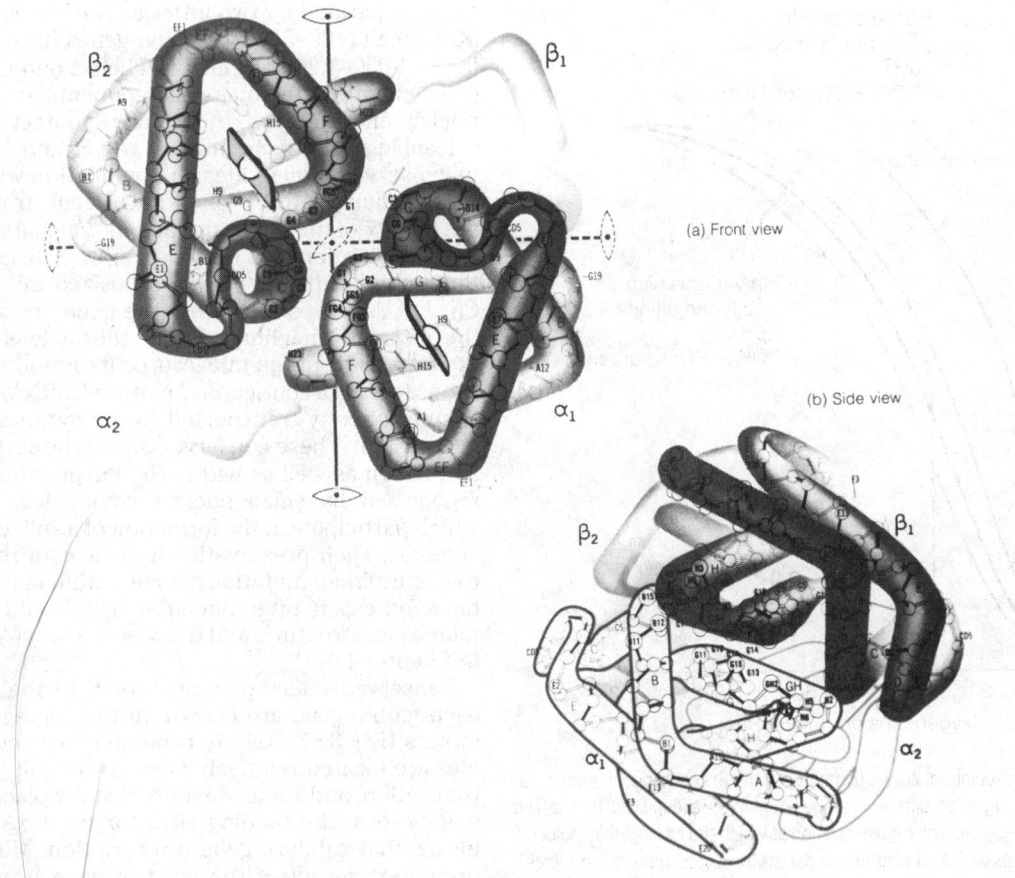

Fig. 35-3. Quaternary structure of hemoglobin. Contacts between subunits are shown as circled amino acids. **(A)** Front view, α_1-β_2 contacts. **(B)** Side view, α_1-β_1 contacts. (From Dickerson and Geis,[6] with permission.)

lines, the H21 histidine (position 143), and the EF6 lysine (position 82). In oxyhemoglobin the H helices of the β-chains are insufficiently spread to permit firm binding of 2,3-BPG; this, along with other conformational changes, favors the binding of this anion to the deoxygenated, rather than the oxygenated, form of hemoglobin. The binding of 2,3-BPG stabilizes the T structure of the deoxygenated form at the expense of the R structure of the oxyhemoglobin tetramer.

Red cells containing high levels of fetal hemoglobin (Hb F) exhibit high oxygen affinity because Hb F binds 2,3-BPG poorly. Physiologically this ensures that the hemoglobin of the fetus is oxygenated at the expense of the maternal Hb A. The high oxygen affinity of Hb F (i.e., its low affinity for 2,3-DPG) is accounted for by a single change in its primary structure, the presence of a serine residue at helical position H21 in place of the histidine found in the β-globin chain. This weakens the binding of 2,3-BPG and leads to stabilization of the molecule in its R state. Mutations of the α- or β-globin chains that affect 2,3-BPG binding have been identified; these mutant hemoglobins exhibit altered oxygen affinity.

A physiologically important property of hemoglobin is its high degree of solubility. This depends, to a first approximation, on the abundance of hydrophilic (charged) amino acids exposed to the aqueous milieu of the red cell cytoplasm by the folding of the polypeptide around the hydrophobic interior in which the heme-binding cleft resides. The integrity of the tetramer, which requires the proper configuration of amino acid residues at the points of α/non-α-chain contact, is also important, since free globin chains are far less soluble.

The solubility of hemoglobin is critical because precipitated hemoglobin, globin, and their catabolic by-products are deleterious to erythrocytes. These materials either oxidize delicate cellular components or adhere to membrane cytoskeletal proteins, or both, leading ultimately to altered membrane surfaces, increased viscosity, and deranged shapes that result in recognition and premature destruction (hemolysis) of the affected red cells by macrophages of the reticuloendothelial system. Mutations that alter hemoglobin stability (the "unstable hemoglobins") are thus often characterized by varying degrees of hemolytic anemia, that can be exacerbated by exposure to oxidative agents (see Chs. 44, 47, and 48).

The primary amino acid structure of α- and non-α-globin chains dictates the inevitable quaternary structure in which resides the ability of hemoglobin to serve as a soluble respiratory protein. Cooperativity ensures rapid binding of oxygen in the lungs and unloading in tissues. Similarly, carbon dioxide is transported from tissues to lungs. The function of hemoglobin may be influenced by mutation, as well as by heterotopic effectors such as protons and 2,3-BPG. The molecule itself changes shape as it provides oxygen for metabolism; it is a lung in miniature, breathing as it allows the body to respire.

GLOBIN GENE CLUSTERS

The amounts and types of human hemoglobin produced at any given age are determined primarily by the selective expression of the individual genes encoding each globin chain. The globin genes of humans are located in two clusters (Fig. 35-6): α-like genes in about 30 kb of DNA on the short arm of chromosome 16 between band P13.2 and the telomere, and β-like genes in about 70 kb of DNA on the terminal portion of the short arm of chromosome 11 (P15) (Fig. 35-6). Each gene shares certain basic organizational features. Each contains three

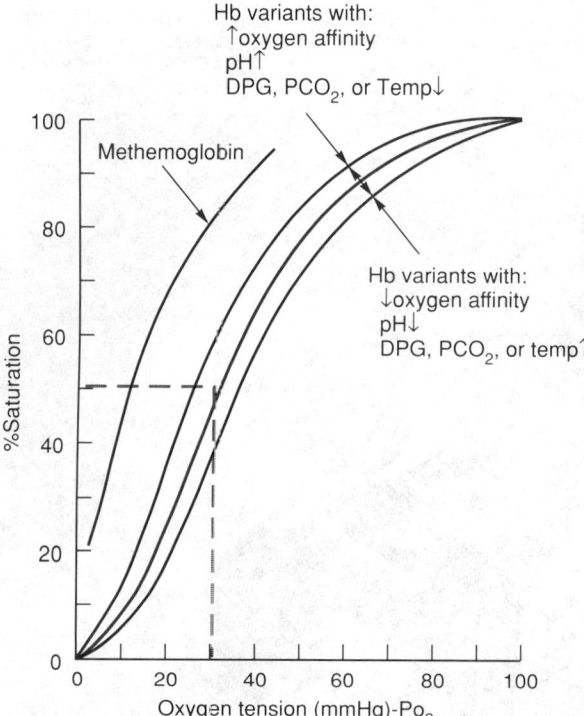

Fig. 35-4. Oxygen dissociation curve of hemoglobin. Percentage of saturation of hemoglobin with oxygen at different oxygen tensions is depicted by the red sigmoidal curve. The P_{50} (i.e., the oxygen tension at which the hemoglobin molecule is half saturated) is about 27 mmHg in normal erythrocytes (pink dotted lines). Heterotopic modifiers of hemoglobin function can shift the curve leftward by increasing or rightward by decreasing its oxygen affinity. (From Benz,[1] with permission.)

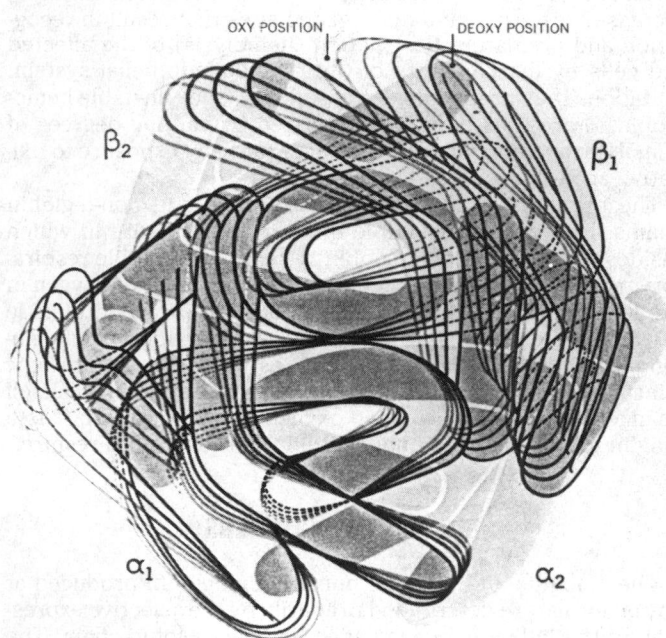

Fig. 35-5. Subunit motion in the hemoglobin tetramer, showing relative motion of hemoglobin subunits on oxygenation and deoxygenation. $\alpha_1\beta_1$ Dimer (black) is moving relative to the $\alpha_2\beta_2$ dimer (shaded). The oxyhemoglobin tetramer (R state) is more compact than the deoxyhemoglobin configuration (T state). (From Dickerson and Geis,[6] with permission.)

exons separated by two introns. The introns of the α-gene are both small (100–300 bp); non-α-genes have one small and one large (1,000–1,200-bp) intron. The second exon of each globin gene encodes the major components of the heme-binding pocket, and the third, the α/non-α contact points.

Flanking each gene at both the 5′ and 3′ ends are groups of conserved nucleotides; in conjunction with protein factors, these influence the promotion of gene transcription, ensure the fidelity of the transcript and its translatability, specify sites for the initiation and termination of translation, and improve the stability of the newly synthesized mRNA (Fig. 35-7) (see Ch. 1). Also encoded within the gene are signals that permit the enzymatic machinery within the nucleus to excise precisely the introns from the mRNA precursor and splice together the exons to form a contiguous "mature" mRNA. The spliced mRNA is subsequently transported to the cytoplasm and translated into protein. These conserved signals lie at the junction of exon and intron as well as within the introns themselves. They are recognized by small nuclear ribonuclear protein particles, which participate in the formation of a spliceosome, or splicing complex. Their preservation is critical for the splicing process to occur. When mutations occur within splice signal sites, globin synthesis is often impaired. The 5′ end of the mRNA contains a cap structure, and the 3′ end, a poly(A) tail, as described in Chapter 1.

Conserved nucleotide clusters 5′ to the coding portion of each globin gene are known, in the aggregate, to act as promoters (Fig. 35-7). Globin promoters are modular. Some modules are located relatively close to the initiation site of mRNA translation, and some are more distally placed. Promoters ultimately form the binding sites for the RNA polymerase complexes that catalyze gene transcription. Mutations within the promoter can affect the level of gene transcription and the amount of globin made. Surrounding and within each gene are other sequence elements that play important roles in its transcriptional regulation (Fig. 35-6). These clusters, termed enhancers, and silencers (see Ch. 1) may lie within introns or 5′ and 3′ to the coding sequences; in some instances, they are quite remote from the gene. The higher-order structure of DNA in chromatin may permit close approximation of these remote enhancers to the gene during transcription. Enhancers play important roles in the tissue-specific regulation of globin gene expression. The best defined of the regulatory sequences near any gene, including globin genes, are shown in Figure 35-7. DNA elements controlling globin genes are described in more detail later.

The α-like and β-like globin genes are ordered in the 5′ to 3′ direction in the same sequence expressed during embryonic, fetal, and adult development (Figs. 35-7 and 35-8). The functional significance of this arrangement is unclear. However, recent evidence suggests that the ordering of the ϵ-, α-, and β-genes is an important factor influencing the ability of each locus to interact with distant control elements at different developmental stages.

The α-like and β-like gene clusters are likely the results of an ancient duplication of a primordial globin gene, which existed early in the history of vertebrates, approximately 500 million years ago. Each gene cluster probably developed from duplication of ancestral genes and subsequent divergence through eons of evolution. Within the α-like gene cluster, the ζ-globin gene is expressed only very early in embryogenesis and partakes in the formation of embryonic hemoglobins. The α-globin genes are duplicated, a characteristic of most globin genes, and their encoded amino acid sequences are identical; therefore, only a single α-globin polypeptide results. Minor differences within the second intervening sequence and the 3′-flanking regions of the α-globin gene permit identification of transcripts from each gene. The 5′, or α_2-gene is expressed more efficiently than the 3′, or α_1-gene, so that abnormalities of this gene are more apt to be clinically apparent. Both clusters

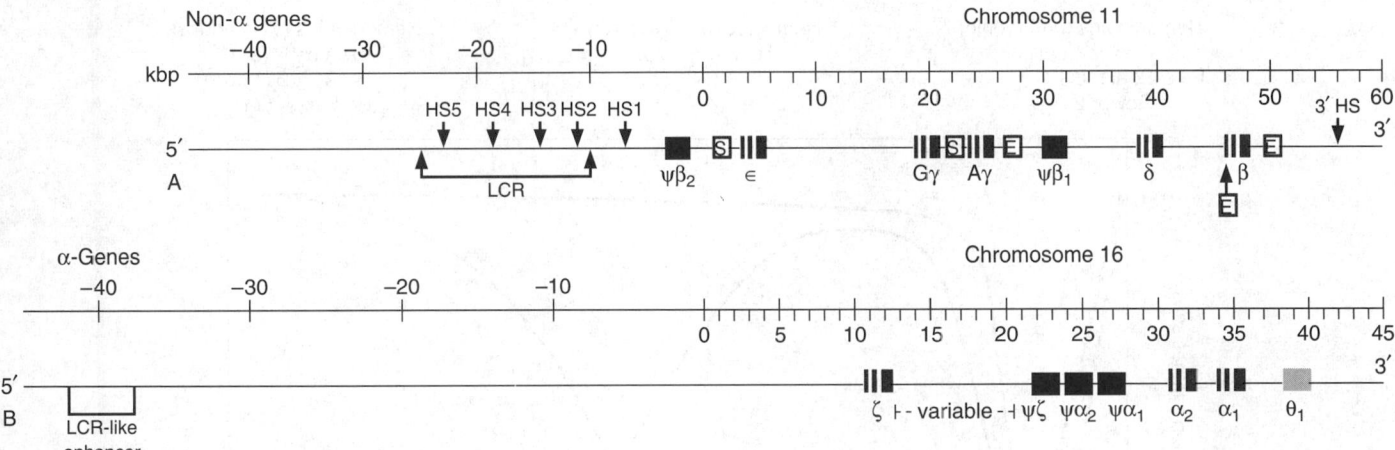

Fig. 35-6. Maps of the β-like and α-like globin gene clusters located on **(A)** chromosome 11 and **(B)** chromosome 16. Within each gene cluster are pseudogenes, which are remnants of previously expressed globin genes that have become inactivated as a result of mutation. Active genes are shown in red boxes filled with clear introns; inactive or pseudogenes are shown in solid boxes, and the θ-globin gene is shown as a pink box. While this gene is transcribed, it is not clear whether it is represented in a cellular protein. The distance between the functional ζ- and pseudo-ζ-globin gene is variable, owing to the presence of repeated elements. The distant upstream LCR control elements (see text) are shown, as are representative enhancer E and silencer S elements. There is at least one intragenic enhancer (in a β-globin gene intron). This is shown by the arrow attached to an enhancer E. HS refers to DNA hypersensitive sites (see Ch. 1) *that mark the subcomponents of the LCR and a downstream enhancer E.*

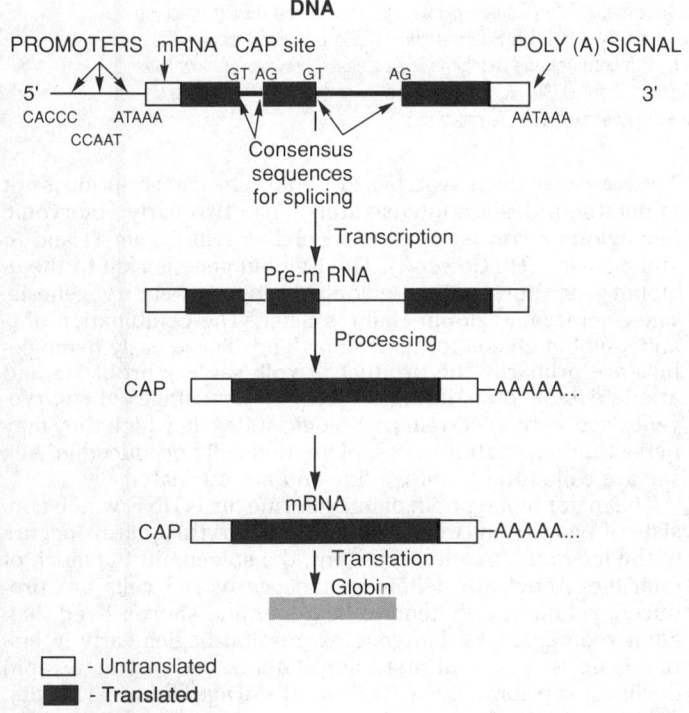

Fig. 35-7. Pathway of globin biosynthesis. Transcription of the globin gene results in a large pre-mRNA molecule containing intervening sequences. During intranuclear processing of this molecule, the intervening sequences are excised and the coding sequences ligated to form a contiguous stretch of RNA, which codes for the globin protein. The message is further processed by the addition of a CAP and a poly(A)tail. The mature message is transported from the nucleus to cytoplasm, where it is translated on polyribosomes by the addition of activated amino acids to a growing polypeptide chain. Globin acquires heme, α/non-α dimers are formed, and the hemoglobin tetramer is assembled. (From Steinberg,[13] with permission.)

contain genes that are actively transcribed, as well as pseudogenes whose defective structures prohibit expression at any time.

The gene 3′ to the α$_1$-gene is the θ-gene, a somewhat mysterious element of the α-gene cluster. While θ-gene transcripts are found in fetal tissue and adult erythroid marrow, it is unclear whether this gene's translation product is able to partake in the formation of a functional tetramer. To date no θ-globin protein has been found, and deletion of the θ-globin gene does not appear to have any implications for the developing fetus.

The β-like-globin gene cluster consists of the embryonic ε-gene, transcribed only during the first 6–11 weeks of life, the duplicated γ-globin genes that code for the dominant non-α-globin of fetal life, and the δ- and β-globin genes that code for the hemoglobins of the adult. The coding sequences of the two γ-globin genes are identical, except at codon 136, where the 5′, or (Gγ) gene, codes for glutamic acid and the 3′, or Aγ gene, an alanine residue. These genes are unequally expressed during fetal development. A switch in their relative rates of expression leads to a similar disparity between the amounts of Gγ and Aγ chains in adults. While the Gγ/Aγ switch is interesting from the standpoint of the control of gene expression, it is of little clinical importance. Hb F in both the fetus and the adult consists of a mixture of Gγ and Aγ chains; the functional qualities of these hemoglobins are identical.

The δ- and β-globin genes are probably the result of a duplication event that occurred >40 million years ago. The β-globin gene has become the predominant gene, coding for most of non-α chains of the adult. The δ-globin gene has undergone mutation in several critical areas, so its expression is greatly curtailed. Its product, minor adult hemoglobin (Hb A$_2$), has become functionally insignificant by virtue of its very low level in the erythrocyte. It is likely that the δ-globin gene is a "pseudogene in evolution." In time its expression may be totally abolished as it acquires an inactivating mutation. The pseudogenes dispersed within both globin gene clusters provide interesting glimpses into the evolutionary history of globin genes. Pseudogenes are inactive remnants of previously expressed genes. As a result of relaxed selection, their mutation rate is higher than that of surrounding active genes.

The expression of the human globin genes is highly regu-

Hemoglobins (embryonic)	Hemoglobins (% at birth)	Hemoglobins (% in adults)
Gower 1 $\zeta_2\epsilon_2$	Hb F $\alpha_2\gamma_2$ (75)	Hb A $\alpha_2\beta_2$ (97)
Portland 1 $\zeta_2\gamma_2$	Hb A $\alpha_2\beta_2$ (25)	Hb A$_2$ $\alpha_2\delta_2$ (2.5)
Gower 2 $\alpha_2\epsilon_2$		Hb F $\alpha_2\gamma_2$ (<1)

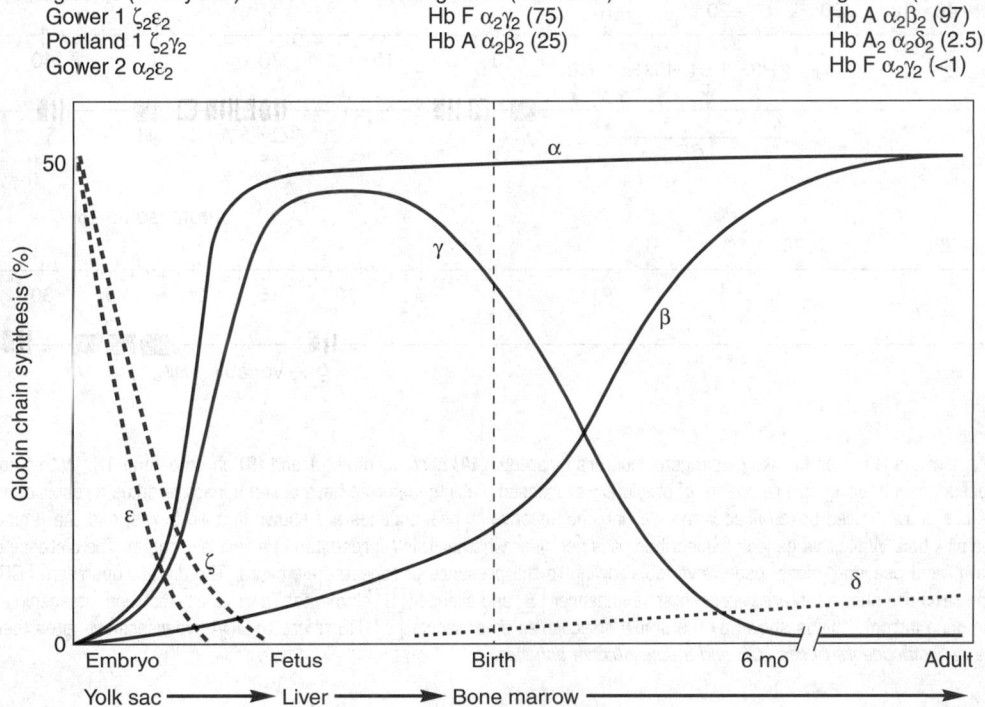

Fig. 35-8. Hemoglobin switching during embryonic, fetal, and adult development. The ζ- and ϵ-genes are transcribed during embryonic development and are soon replaced by the fetal γ- and adult α-globin gene. At birth, Hb F forms about 75% and Hb A about 25% of the total. Transcription of the γ-gene begins to fall prior to birth, and by 6 months of age this gene is expressed only at very low levels. Expression of the δ-globin gene begins near birth. In adults, Hb A makes up about 97%, Hb A$_2$ about 2.5%, and Hb F <1% of the total. Hemoglobins predominating during adult life are shown in black. (From Steinberg,[13] with permission.)

lated. The mechanisms thought to control expression are described in a later section. Globin is synthesized in only one tissue, erythroid cells, and only during a narrowly defined stage of erythroid progenitor cell differentiation—the 5–7 days that commence with the proerythroblast stage and end when the anucleate reticulocyte loses the last traces of its RNA. Within the confines of these strict tissue-specific and differentiation stage-specific boundaries, the globin genes are extraordinarily active. By the late normoblast and reticulocyte stages, 90–95% of all protein synthesis in these cells is globin synthesis. This devotion of metabolic resources to synthesis of a single set of proteins represents one of the most striking examples of specialized gene expression known in nature.

Individual globin genes are expressed at different levels in developing erythroblasts of the human embryo, fetus, and "adult" (i.e., 37–38 weeks' gestation and beyond). Different subsets of α- and non-α-genes are expressed and silenced at each developmental stage. Moreover, the overall balance of non-α-globin, α-globin, and heme production is maintained throughout each of these complex switching events. The mechanisms ensuring the proper tissue-, differentiation stage-, and ontologic stage-specific expression are complex and incompletely defined. Much recent information about relevant DNA control elements and transcription factors is emerging. These are discussed later. First, however, the ontogeny of hemoglobin should be reviewed as necessary background.

ONTOGENY OF HEMOGLOBIN

The hemoglobin composition of the erythrocyte varies depending on when in gestation or postnatal development it is measured (Table 35-1). These changes, known as hemoglobin switches, result from sequential activation and inactivation of genes within the α- and non-α-globin gene clusters (Fig. 35-8).

The control of these switches in globin gene transcription is not understood, despite intense study. The two early embryonic hemoglobins consist of ζ- and ϵ-chains (Hb Gower-1) and α- and ϵ-chains (Hb Gower-2). The ζ-globin gene is akin to the α-globin genes but is expressed only during early embryogenesis. The ϵ-embryonic globin chain is β-like. The combination of ζ- and γ-globin chains forms Hb Portland. These early hemoglobins are primarily the product of yolk sac erythroblasts and are detectable only during the very earliest stages of embryogenesis, except in certain pathologic states, in which they may persist until gestation is complete. Red cells produced in yolk sac are called the primitive line and are nucleated.

The major hemoglobin of intrauterine life is Hb F, which consists of two α- and two γ-globin chains. Erythropoiesis occurs in the liver and, to a lesser extent, the spleen, during much of fetal life. Anucleate definitive lineages of red cells are produced. Fetal red cells tend to be larger and shorter lived than adult red cells. γ-Globin gene expression begins early in embryogenesis, peaks during midgestation, and begins a rapid decline just prior to birth. By 6 months of age in normal infants, only a remnant of prior γ-globin gene expression remains, and the level of fetal hemoglobin in the blood is <1% of the total. Under normal circumstances, this shutdown of γ-globin gene activity is not reversed throughout life.

α-Globin gene expression starts early in the first trimester, peaks by about 10–12 weeks' gestation, and is sustained for life. β-Globin gene expression commences early in gestation, rises slowly, and reaches its zenith within a few weeks of birth. The combination of α- with β-globin chains forms hemoglobin A (Hb A), the predominant hemoglobin (95–97%) after birth. Also present in adult cells is Hb A$_2$. The δ-globin gene, which directs synthesis of the non-α-chain of Hb A$_2$, is very inefficiently expressed. Thus, only low levels of Hb A$_2$ (1.5–3.5%) are present. Defects in the δ-globin gene are of no clinical consequence. In adult blood, fetal hemoglobin is not evenly distributed among erythrocytes but is present in only a very small number of red cells, termed F cells. F cells retain some fetal characteristics and seem to arise from different subsets of primitive stem cells. Their number appears to be genetically determined in normal kindreds.

An important consequence of these hemoglobin switching phenomena is that pathologic states (hemoglobinopathies) arising from defects of a particular globin gene will have different effects at different developmental stages. Mutations of the α-, ζ-, ε-, and γ-genes will be phenotypically apparent in embryonic and fetal life. The more severe defects will cause early miscarriage or late fetal loss and therefore may go undetected as globin gene defects, particularly if embryo survival is compromised. By contrast, β-globin gene mutations will produce their phenotypic impact only after the Hb F→Hb A switch. Because of the prolonged circulating survival times of red cells, actual replacement of Hb F-containing cells by Hb A-containing cells takes 4–10 months after birth. β-Globin hemoglobinopathies are therefore compatible with normal fetal survival. Symptoms appear only during the middle to late months of the first year of life, or even later in mild forms of the diseases.

A corollary of the preceding considerations is that prevention or reversal of the Hb F→Hb A switch should provide effective therapy for β-chain hemoglobinopathies. Two of these conditions, sickle cell anemia and β-thalassemia, are prominent clinical problems in hematology. Strategies designed to manipulate switching are discussed in Chapters 42 and 43.

HEMOGLOBIN BIOSYNTHESIS AND ITS REGULATION

Throughout development, α- and non-α-globin genes and heme exhibit coordinated expression (Fig. 35-7). Nearly equal amounts of each of the moieties that ultimately constitute the hemoglobin tetramer are made. Excess unpaired globin chains resulting from minor imbalances of α- and non-α-globin gene expression and mutant globins are removed from the cell by ATP-dependent proteases, maintaining a balance between α- and non-α-chain synthesis. Balanced chain synthesis and coordination of globin chain production with synthesis of heme are important because hemoglobin tetramers are highly soluble, while the components of hemoglobin (i.e., unpaired chains, protoporphrin, and iron) are not. Precipitation of any of these is deleterious to cell survival. Erythroblast proteases are not efficient enough to eliminate the substantial excesses of unpaired chains that accumulate when an α- or non-α-gene is selectively impaired by severe thalassemia mutations. The mechanisms regulating heme production, and some of the interactions between heme and globin synthesis, are discussed in Chapters 38 and 39.

The proper production of the individual globin chains within erythroid tissues at the appropriate stages of differentiation and development is regulated predominantly at the level of transcription. The onset of phenotypic maturation at the proerythroblast stage is marked by the onset of globin mRNA biosynthesis in dramatically increasing quantities. α- and non-α-globin gene expression begin at essentially the same time, although some studies suggest a slightly earlier onset of α-globin gene expression. Transcription persists at a high level throughout most of the remainder of erythropoiesis, declines as the nucleus condenses, and is eventually lost in late erythroblasts. Even as the absolute rates of globin gene transcription begin to fall; however, the relative percentage of total transcriptional activity devoted to globin gene expression continues to rise; this reflects the silencing of transcription of nearly every other gene in the erythroblast.

The transcriptional activation of the globin genes is the major event that must be understood in order to define and manipulate the regulation of hemoglobin biosynthesis and hemoglobin switching. However, post-transcriptional mechanisms contribute to the final distribution of globin and nonglobin mRNAs, and the to balance of α- and non-α-globins within the erythroblasts. When compared with many other mRNAs, such as cytokine mRNAs, globin mRNAs are extraordinarily stable. Their half-lives have been estimated at 30–50 hours. Most other mRNAs have turnover rates, or half-lives, measured within the range of a few minutes, to 5–6 hours. Thus, the rise in the percentage of total mRNA that is globin mRNA is greatly accentuated because the newly transcribed globin mRNAs accumulate and remain quite stable in the cell, while nonglobin mRNAs, which are no longer being produced, are also disappearing at a faster rate. Consequently, the mRNA content of the reticulocytes consists of 90–95% globin mRNA.

The transcription rates of the α- and non-α-globin genes are not precisely equal. (This phenomenon has been studied in detail only in adult reticulocytes expressing the α- and β-globin genes.) A slight, but reproducibly detectable, excess of α-globin mRNA is present in erythroblasts. However, β-globin mRNA is translated somewhat more efficiently than α-globin mRNA. These counterbalancing forces result in nearly equal synthesis of α- and β-globin polypeptide chains. In fact, there is a very slight excess of α-globin production, resulting in a small pool of free α-chains. Newly synthesized β-chains are thus rapidly and completely incorporated into functional hemoglobin tetramers. Hemoglobin tetramers are remarkably stable throughout the life span of the circulating red cell. Only small amounts suffer oxidative or proteolytic damage. Hemoglobin molecules are thus exposed to changes in the milieu of the bloodstream for prolonged periods. They often become nonenzymatically modified by such processes as glycosylation, acetylation, and sulfation. One of these modifications, glycosylation, occurs more extensively during periods of hyperglycemia and leads to elevated levels of the glycosylated form of Hb A, Hb A_{1c}. This phenomenon is the basis of a useful test for control of the blood sugar in diabetics. Other post-translational modifications are of little clinical consequence.

Transcriptional Regulation of Globin-Gene Expression

Two decades of intensive study are beginning to uncover the molecular mechanisms regulating the individual globin genes. The major molecular elements mediating regulation are proteinaceous transcription factors, and short, specialized regions of DNA sequence that are recognized by some of these factors. The interaction causes these DNA elements to act as promoters, enhancers, or silencers of gene activity. Nuclear proteins that interact with the globin gene clusters include DNA-binding proteins and proteins that interact with the DNA-binding proteins by means of specific protein-protein interactions, such as leucine zipper domains (see Ch. 7 for background information about the basic features and properties of transcription factors and proteins with which they interact). Control of the α- and non-α-globin genes is further complicated by the fact that each gene cluster functions as a larger unit, or DNA domain. The "open" or "closed" state of these domains, with respect to access to transcriptional activating machinery, appears to be under the influence of an enhancer sequence, the locus control region (LCR). Each is located several tens of kilobases upstream of the ε-gene on chromosome 11 and the ζ-gene on chromosome 16.

LCRs are modular DNA sequence elements. For example, several DNase I-hypersensitive sites (see Ch. 1) can be detected within the β-globin cluster LCR locus in chromatin from erythroid, but not nonerythroid, cells (Fig. 35-8). Minichromosome constructs, in which globin genes are attached directly to the

LCR in the absence of most intervening DNA sequences, will be expressed at rates approaching those of endogenous globin genes in cultured erythroid cells and transgenic mice. Some nonglobin genes will also be expressed at very high levels in erythroid cells when attached to these LCR sequences. Thus, to a first approximation, the LCR regions can be regarded as master switches that promote access of other regulatory factors to individual globin promoters and enhancers within the clusters. The LCRs contain binding sites for the major erythroid transcription factors, GATA-1, and NFE-2, as well as the sites for generic factors found more widely distributed in many cell types.

The LCR is unquestionably essential for the quantitatively high rates of globin gene expression during erythroid differentiation. The role of the LCR in dictating tissue specificity, that is, shutdown of globin gene expression in other tissues, or the sequential activation and silencing of genes during hemoglobin switching, is less clear. Studies suggest that tissue specificity and qualitatively proper switching of γ- and β-globin gene expression in transgenic mice could be obtained with DNA constructs lacking the LCR. However, these genes were invariably expressed only 0.5–5% as actively as the endogenous globin genes of the host cell. The degree and fidelity of tissue-specific expression also appeared to be dependent on several factors, such as the site of transgene integration.

The interrelationships among the LCR, and individual promoters, enhancers, and silencers during erythroid differentiation and hemoglobin switching remain incompletely understood. However, most investigators agree that both tissue and developmental specificity and highly active and efficient expression of individual globin genes require interaction between the LCR and the individual promoter/enhancer elements flanking the globin gene selected for expression. A variety of looping and tracking models have been put forward as hypotheses to explain how a distant DNA sequence element and its bound transcription factors can interact with sequences located close to the transcription start site of a globin gene. No model has explained all the experimental findings or biologic phenomena.

Despite uncertainty as to the precise molecular mechanisms involved, most investigators agree that opening of the globin gene cluster by the LCR is an essential prerequisite for expression of any globin genes; this change in chromatin configuration is presumably mediated by the interaction of the LCR with specific transcription factors. The essential role of promoters and enhancers located near the globin genes is suggested by the discovery of mutations in these regions that affect hemoglobin switching or that cause thalassemia-like syndromes. Moreover, competition for the stimulating activity of the LCR can be appreciated by manipulation of the number of copies of globin genes attached to the LCR, the order in which they appear, or the orientation in which they are transcribed. These manipulations alter both the relative amounts of globin mRNA produced from each locus and the stages of development at which individual genes are expressed. Evidence for the existence of LCR-globin gene interactions is thus clear, even though the nature of the interaction remains obscure.

The shutdown of the embryonic genes late in the first trimester and, possibly, the decline of γ-gene expression during the perinatal period may also require the participation of active silencing mechanisms. The predominance of β-globin gene expression over γ-gene expression in adult life is thus not merely the result of preferential stimulation of β-gene expression. Active repression of the γ-genes may also be relevant; these mechanisms, if they exist, may have to be reversed if one hopes to manipulate hemoglobin switching therapeutically.

The nuclei of erythroid cells contain numerous proteins that have been identified as transcription factors. Many of these are found in a wide variety of tissues. At least two factors, GATA-1 and NFE-2, are much more restricted in their range of expression and have been implicated as particularly important for globin gene expression.

GATA-1 is named on the basis of the DNA sequence motif (T/A) GATA(A/G), the GATA motif that it recognizes and binds. It is a zinc finger class DNA-binding protein (see Ch. 7). GATA-1 has been shown to activate promoters containing the cognate DNA sequence motif, even when placed in nonerythroid cells. NFE-2 recognizes the DNA sequence motif (T/C) GCT GA (C/G) TCA (T/C). It is a member of the B-zip class of transcriptional activators. Both GATA-1 and NFE-2 were originally identified and cloned on the basis of their interaction with their cognate sequences in the globin genes. Initially, each was thought to be present only in erythroid cells. However, further work has demonstrated that each protein has a wider range of tissue expression. For example, GATA-1 is also present in other hematopoietic cell lineages, whereas NFE-2 consists of two subunits: one that is widely expressed, and one that is expressed in several hematopoeitic lineages and the intestine.

Clearly, neither GATA-1 or NFE-2 alone can be the sole determinants of tissue specificity of the globin genes; otherwise, globin gene expression should occur at some level in other tissues in which these proteins are present. However, there is no doubt that each of these proteins is indispensable for both globin gene expression and erythropoiesis. Gene knockout studies have shown that absence of either protein results in greatly impaired erythropoiesis.

GATA-1 and NFE-2 probably interact with each other, either directly or by means of binding to intermediary proteins, to activate the expression of globin genes and other genes necessary for erythroid maturation. Several other proteins have been identified as binding to various control elements in the globin gene cluster. Some of these appear to be stage-specific selector elements that bind predominantly to the γ- or β-globin gene enhancers and promoters. Others are generic transcription factors. Regulation at these sites is probably hierarchical, depending on the appropriate combination of DNA-binding proteins, the types of proteins that interact with them, and the activation state of the bound proteins through such processes as ribosylation and phosphorylation. It is also possible that the same sequence element may interact with different combinational sets of proteins, with a different resulting effect on transcriptional activity, depending on the stage of differentiation and/ or embryonic/fetal/adult development. Thus, it is curious that the consenses binding site for NFE-2 contains within it the sequence motif that is recognized by individual members of the *jun* and *fos* families of transcription factors (AP-1).

The precise molecular machinery necessary for regulation of transcription of individual globin genes is beginning to be defined. It is important to realize, however, that these molecular mechanics are susceptible to cellular, microenvironmental, and humoral influences affecting the proliferation and differentiation state of primitive erythroid stem cells in yolk sac, fetal liver, or bone marrow. Overwhelming evidence supports the hypothesis that the potential for expression of γ- and/or β-genes is determined in primitive erythroid stem cells (i.e., burst-forming unit-erythroid), long before actual expression of the globin genes is initiated at a later stage of differentiation. The relative percentage of maturing erythroblasts that will ultimately express Hb F or Hb A, or both, can be altered by factors, such as cytotoxic drugs or bone marrow stress, that alter the relative percentages of Hb F-potent or Hb A-potent stem cells undergoing cell-cycle events, differentiation, and so forth. Drugs currently in use in an effort to manipulate Hb F switching seem to work primarily through these cellular mechanisms (see Ch. 17).

Post-transcriptional, Translational, and Post-translational Mechanisms

Processed globin mRNA is exported from the nucleus to the cytoplasm by a mechanism that is not yet clearly defined. mRNA translation occurs in the cytoplasm (Fig. 35-7). The triplet codons of mRNA are recognized by the anticodons of specific tRNAs, that bring activated amino acid residues to the nascent polypeptide chains. The process of translation, in which an mRNA template directs the synthesis of protein, is typically divided into three phases: initiation, elongation, and termination (see Ch. 1). Each phase is regulated by a variety of protein factors.

The globin mRNA molecule becomes associated with four to six ribosomes, forming the polyribosome. At least 11 eukaryotic translation initiation factors interact with the polyribosome. These mediate stabilization of a preinitiation complex, binding of the initiator methionine tRNA to ribosomal subunits, binding of mRNA to the preinitiation complex, stabilization of mRNA binding, recognition of the cap site at the 5′ end of mRNA, and release of initiation factors from the preinitiation complex. Several elongation and termination factors have also been defined. Initiation, or early steps in the elongation process, are rate limiting.

The first post-translational step in tetramer formation is the combination of α- and non-α-chains to form dimers, an event that appears to depend on the relative charge of each globin subunit (Fig. 35-1). The dimers then spontaneously form tetrameric hemoglobin. Because of charge differences among non-α-globin chains, there is a hierarchy of affinity of these chains for α-chains. The combination of α- and β-chains is most favored, followed by a combination of α- with γ- and δ-globin chains. Certain mutant hemoglobins that have either gained or lost a charge may alter this hierarchical arrangement. This may influence the proportion of variant hemoglobin present, especially when the patient also inherits an α-thalassemia syndrome, in which the synthesis of α-globin chains is reduced. The supply of available α-chains is then limited and non-α-chains compete with one another to form tetramers with the limiting α-chain pool.

Globin chain biosynthesis and heme synthesis are mutually important. Heme plays a role in the regulation of the initiation complex. A deficiency of heme (e.g., in iron deficiency) is associated with the accumulation of a repressor of translation initiation, a protein kinase capable of phosphorylating one of the initiation factors. β-mRNA appears to be initiated more efficiently than α-mRNA. A deficit of heme selectively retards the synthesis of α-globin, conferring on the associated anemia some of the features of mild α-thalassemia. This phenomenon occurs because heme deficiency depresses the availability of initiating factors for which the less efficient α-mRNA must compete with the more efficient β-mRNA.

Hemoglobinopathies—Nosology

Inherited abnormalities of the hemoglobin molecules that cause morbidity are called hemoglobinopathies and thalassemias. Many of these conditions produce disease, (e.g., sickle cell anemia, thalassemia, methemoglobinemia) that are especially important to hematologists. A few acquired conditions lead to modification of hemoglobin (e.g., carbon monoxide exposure, producing carboxyhemoglobinemia) that produce clinial abnormalities. These situations are summarized by the term acquired hemoglobinopathies.

Most of the enormous number (nearly 1,000) of mutations of the globin gene that have been described produce no, or only trivial, clinical effect. The remainder can be classified ac-

Table 35-2. Classification of Hemoglobinopathies and Thalassemias

Structural hemoglobinopathies—mutations altering the amino acid sequence of a globin chain and altering physical or chemical properties of the hemoglobin tetramer in such a way that function is deranged.
   Abnormal hemoglobin polymerization—sickle hemoglobin (Hb S); hemolysis, vaso-occlusion
   Abnormal hemoglobin crystallization (e.g., Hb C)
   High oxygen affinity—polycythemia (Hb Zurich)
   Low oxygen affinity—cyanosis (Hb Kansas)
   Hemoglobins that oxidize or precipitate too readily—unstable hemoglobins (Hb Köln)
   M hemoglobins—methemoglobinemia, cyanosis (e.g., Hb Milwaukee)
Thalassemia—defective production of globin chains with hypochromia, anemia, hemolysis, altered erythropoiesis
   α-Thalassemia
   β-Thalassemia
   δβ-Thalassemias, γδβ-thalassemias, αβ-thalassemias
"Thalassemic" hemoglobinopathies—mutations altering both synthesis and structure or function of the hemoglobin gene products (e.g., Hb E, Hb Terre Haute, Hb Lepore, Hb Constant Spring)
Hereditary persistence of fetal hemoglobin—persistence of high levels of Hb F into adult life
   Pancellular—high HbF levels in all red cells
      Nondeletion forms
      Deletion forms
      Hb Kenya
   Heterocellular—inherited increases in the percentage of F cells
   Acquired hemoglobinopathies
      Methemoglobinemia due to toxic exposures
      Sulfhemoglobinemia due to toxic exposures
      Carboxyhemoglobinemia due to toxic exposures
      Hb H in erythroleukemias
      Acquired elevations in F cells and Hb F
         Erythroid stress (e.g., recovery from bone marrow suppression)
         Bone marrow dysplasias
         Exposure to agents altering stem cells or gene expression (e.g., hydroxyurea, butyric acid)

cording to the hematologic and clinical phenotypes that cause: reduced solubility with hemolytic anemia (unstable hemoglobins, polymerizing hemoglobins such as sickle hemoglobin), hemoglobins with altered oxygen affinity, methemoglobins, and the thalassemias involving abnormal synthesis of one or more globin chains with anemia, hemolysis, and alterations of erythropoiesis; some mutations, such as that responsible for Hb E, can alter both the structure and synthesis of the molecule. The classification of hemoglobinopathies and thalassemias is summarized in Table 35-2. Individual conditions are discussed in the chapters already cross-referenced in earlier sections of this chapter.

SUGGESTED READINGS

1. Benz EJ Jr: Synthesis, structure, and function of hemoglobin. p. 236. In Kelly WN, DeVita VT (eds): Textbook of Internal Medicine. Vol. 1. JB Lippincott, Philadelphia, 1989
2. Benz EJ Jr, Forget BG: The biosynthesis of hemoglobin. Semin Hematol 11: 463, 1974
3. Bollekins JA, Forget BG: γδ Thalassemia and hereditary persistence of fetal hemoglobin. Hematol Oncol Clin North Am 5:399, 1991
4. Bunn HF: Sickle hemoglobin and other hemoglobin mutants. p. 207. In Stamatoyannopoulos G, Nienhuis AW, Majerus PW, Varmus H (eds): The Molecular Basis of Blood Disease. WB Saunders, Philadelphia, 1993
5. Bunn HF, Forget BG: Hemoglobins: Molecular, Genetic and Clinical Aspects. WB Saunders, Philadelphia, 1986
6. Dickerson RE, Geis I: Hemoglobin: Structure, Function, and Evolution Pathology. Benjamin-Cummings, Menlo Park, CA, 1983
7. Embury SH, Hebbel RP, Mohandas N, Steinberg MH: Vasoocclusion. p. 311. In Embury SH, Hebbel RP, Mohandas N, Steinberg MH (eds): Sickle Cell Disease: Basic Principles and Clinical Practice. Raven, New York, 1994

8. Honig GR, Adams JG III: Human Hemoglobin Genetics. Springer-Verlag, New York, 1985
9. Huisman THJ, Schroeder WA: New Aspects of the Structure, Function, and Synthesis of Hemoglobin. CRC Press, Boca Raton, FL, 1971
10. Perutz MF: Molecular anatomy, physiology, and pathology of hemoglobin. p. 127. In Stammatoyannopoulos G, Nienhuis AW, Leder P, Majerus PW (eds): The Molecular Basis of Blood Diseases. WB Saunders, Philadelphia, 1987
11. Stamatoyannopoulos G, Nienhuis AW: Hemoglobin switching. p. 107. In Sta-

maloyannopoulos G, Nienhuis AW, Majerus PW, Varmus H (eds): The Molecular Basis of Blood Diseases. WB Saunders, Philadelphia, 1993
12. Stamatoyannopoulos G, Nienhuis AW: The Regulation of Hemoglobin Switching. Johns Hopkins University Press, Baltimore, 1991
13. Steinberg MH: Hemoglobinopathies and thalassemias. p. 852. In: Internal Medicine. 4th Ed. Mosby-Year Book, St. Louis, MO, 1994
14. Weatherall DJ, Clegg JB: The Thalassaemia Syndromes. 3rd Ed. Blackwell Scientific, Oxford, 1981, p. 876

Approach to the Adult and Child with Anemia

36

Nancy Berliner, Thomas P. Duffy, and Herbert T. Abelson

ANEMIA IN THE ADULT

Cycle of Erythropoiesis

Anemia represents a reduction in the body's red cell mass, a quantity that, under normal conditions, is maintained within prescribed limits through the regulatory feedback stimulus of the humoral factor erythropoietin.[1,2] A sensing device responsive to tissue oxygen content within the kidney determines the degree of erythropoietin release from renal peritubular cells.[3,4] In response to this humoral control mechanism, a population of erythropoietin-responsive marrow cells, derived from the pluripotent stem cell population, undergoes increased proliferation and acceleration of maturation. These red blood cells (RBCs) circulate in the peripheral blood for approximately 90–120 days, necessitating replacement of the approximately 1% of the body's red cells lost each day to senescence. The spleen is the major site for removal of aged RBCs: splenic macrophages may recognize an acquired RBC "senescence" antigen, which facilitates trapping of these cells within the microvasculature of the spleen.[5,6]

Mechanisms of Anemia

The erythropoietic feedback loop ensures that the hemoglobin mass for oxygen delivery matches the body's needs and that production equals destruction of red cells under stable conditions. Anemia, a deficiency in the RBC mass and the hemoglobin content of blood, occurs whenever any malfunction in this cycle upsets normal coupling of production with destruction. This pathologic condition may have its origins in a primary hematologic disorder within the marrow and/or an accelerated loss or destruction of RBCs in the periphery. Moreover, a myriad of systemic disorders may perturb the cycle of erythropoiesis and secondarily result in anemia. The hematopoietic microenvironment exists in the macroenvironment of the body; anemia, like the sedimentation rate, is thus often a "sickness index" of the body. It is this consideration that constitutes the diagnostic challenge in the workup of the anemic state; anemia is a sign of an underlying pathology whose recognition requires an approach to the whole patient for delineation of the mechanism and cause(s) of the red cell deficit.

Normal Hematologic Values

Identification of the anemic state requires knowledge of the normal hematologic values established by sampling large populations of men and women (Table 36-1). These levels show a gender difference because androgen enhances both renal erythropoietin secretion and enlistment of precursor cells into an erythropoietin-responsive state. Geographic differences also exist for these standards because ambient oxygen tensions affect hemoglobin oxygen saturation; the lower oxygen tensions at high altitudes are associated with increased RBC hemoglobin levels.

Three measurements that were previously performed manually, the hemoglobin level (in grams per deciliter), RBC number $\times 10^{12}$L, and hematocrit (in percent) are now generated by electronic counters. Both the RBC number and the mean corpuscular volume (MCV) are directly measured from a gated window pool, and the hemoglobin concentration is determined by chromatographic quantitation of the hemoglobin present in a defined volume of RBCs. These values are used to calculate the hematocrit, the mean corpuscular hemoglobin (MCH), and the mean mean corpuscular hemoglobin concentration (MCHC). The Coulter counter can also generate a red cell sizing index (the RDW), permitting recognition of different-size populations of red cells. In addition to this quantitative characterization of RBCs, the Coulter counter measures the white blood cell (WBC) and platelet counts, permitting a rapid and important assessment of the involvement of cell lines other than red cells. Such multilineage involvement implies that the anemia is part of a stem cell disorder common to all three cell lines or involves exaggerated peripheral destruction of these cells as seen in hypersplenic states.

Table 36-1. Criteria of Anemia in Adult Men and Women

	Women	Men
RBC × 10^{12}/L	<4.0	<4.5
Hemoglobin (g/dl)	<12	<14
Hematocrit (%)	<37	<40

Hyporegenerative Versus Hyperregenerative Anemias

The feedback control system of erythropoiesis provides the basis for an important means of characterizing the cause(s) of anemia. Each day approximately 0.8% of the RBC pool needs to be replaced by young erythrocytes released from the marrow. Reticulocytes are larger than mature RBCs, and they still contain portions of polyribosomal RNA material; supravital stains of peripheral blood detect these reticulated cells, and their number permits an assessment of the marrow's response to peripheral anemia. When the cause of anemia is blood loss or hemolytic destruction in the periphery, erythropoietin overdrive of the marrow leads to reticulocytosis (>1.5–2.0%) to compensate for the peripheral RBC deficit. An absence of an appropriate reticulocytosis in the setting of anemia indicates that a lesion that interferes with RBC production is responsible. The reticulocyte count provides an easy means of implicating either the marrow or the periphery as the primary source of anemia. This differentiation dictates further investigative workup by narrowing the focus to the marrow in reticulocytopenic states but to peripheral blood loss or hemolytic abnormalities, or both, when reticulocytosis is present.

Reticulocyte count is usually expressed as a percentage of RBCs examined in an individual patient. This number must be corrected for the presence of anemia because the initial count, being a percentage, is spuriously elevated when it is related to a reduced anemic RBC pool. This correction is generated according to the formula in Table 36-2. An additional correction in this index is necessary because reticulocytes released under heavy erythropoietin stimulation remain in the peripheral blood for twice the usual 1-day survival time of "nonstress" reticulocytes. An alternative to this somewhat cumbersome corrected reticulocyte index is expression of the reticulocyte count in absolute numbers. The original reticulocyte percentage is multiplied by the RBC number to yield an absolute reticulocyte count; any value >100 × 10^9/L is considered evidence for an erythroid marrow compartment that is responding appropriately to a hematologic lesion outside the marrow.

Red Blood Cell Size as a Classification of Anemia

The Coulter counter generates a value for the MCV of the red cells, which provides an important means of categorizing the types and causes of anemia. The normal MCV is 80–95 fl; values above and below this range define macrocytic and microcytic anemias, respectively. The latter have their origins in any lesion that results in deficient hemoglobin synthesis. This includes iron-deficiency anemia and the anemia of chronic disease, which are, respectively, the overall most common anemia and the most common anemia encountered in hospitalized patients. Inherited defects in globin synthesis, in thalassemia, as well as abnormalities in heme synthesis, as in the sideroblastic anemias, may also result in a hemoglobin-deficient hypochromic microcytic anemia.

Severely macrocytic anemias (MCV >115 fl) almost always

Table 36-2. Reticulocyte Count

Corrected reticulocyte count = % reticulocytes × $\dfrac{\text{patient hematocrit}}{45}$

Absolute reticulocyte count = % reticulocytes × RBC count/mm³

Absolute reticulocyte count >100,000/mm³ = hemolytic anemia

have their cause in folate or vitamin B_{12} deficiency, since both vitamins play an essential role in DNA metabolism. Less striking macrocytosis is usually caused by liver disease or alcoholism; hypothyroidism also may be associated with macrocytic indices. Inherited abnormalities in purine/pyrimidine metabolism are rare causes of macrocytic anemias. The development of a refractory macrocytic anemia, especially in the elderly, should raise consideration of a myelodysplastic or leukemic syndrome.

Two causes of pseudomacrocytosis should not be overlooked: (1) since reticulocytes are polychromatophilic macrocytes, macrocytosis increases with increasing reticulocytosis; and (2) agglutination of RBCs in the presence of cold agglutinins or cryoglobulins may lead to false elevation of the MCV because aggregates may be counted as large RBCs. Reversal of a high MCV by heating the specimen is proof that the latter phenomenon is involved.

The normocytic anemias comprise variously caused hemolytic anemias (in the absence of striking reticulocytosis, which can elevate the MCV), aplastic anemias (although some are macrocytic), and the early stages of almost all anemias (the residual normal population counterbalancing the population of abnormal cells). It is important to realize that the MCV is an average value representing the arithmetic mean volume of red cells. Combined abnormalities or deficiencies can result in a normal MCV when iron deficiency (decreased MCV) is accompanied by folate deficiency (increased MCV) or pernicious anemia supervenes on thal-assemia. Failure to appreciate that the MCV represents an average RBC size creates the potential for overlooking the real cause(s) of the anemia. The RDW now permits recognition of this phenomenon because it demonstrates graphically the heterogeneity of RBC populations.

The MCH and MCHC values do not provide very much additional information for the categorization of anemias. Both values are low in iron-deficient hematopoiesis, but the reduction in MCV is the most commonly used marker of this state and occurs earlier than the reduction in hemoglobin concentration. However, one disease, hereditary spherocytosis, is characterized by an elevation of the MCHC because it is associated with a varying population of dense microspherocytes. The data generated from the Coulter counter can also be used as an internal control on the hemoglobin and hematocrit parameters. The hematocrit is usually three times the measured hemoglobin value; a departure from this ratio occurs when intravascular hemolysis releases large amounts of hemoglobin beyond that contained in intact RBCs. Clostridial sepsis may advertise itself in this fashion. Agglutination of RBCs due to cold-reactive antibodies may falsely decrease the RBC value without altering the hemoglobin content of the specimen.

Examination of the Peripheral Blood Smear

Examination of the peripheral blood smear is a diagnostic maneuver of overriding importance—it is at least equal in importance and complementary to the machine-generated hematologic data. It confirms the RBC size categorization of the Coulter counter and permits recognition of the many variations in RBC size and shape that are frequently signposts of the causes of hemolytic anemias. Since nucleated RBCs are counted as WBCs by the Coulter counter, the smear must be examined to recognize and correct for this contribution to pseudoleukocytosis. Such erythroblastic findings are helpful clues to the diagnosis of myelophthisis or marrow infiltrative disorders.[7] Examination of the WBCs may reveal hypersegmentation of polymorphonuclear cells as the earliest manifestation of a megaloblastic process[8] (Fig. 36-1); this may be the critical marker

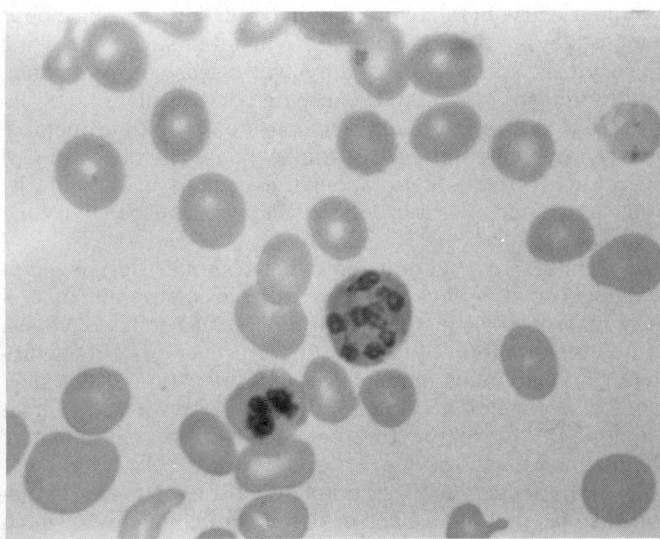

Fig. 36-1. Hypersegmentation of polymorphonuclear cell and macrocytosis as peripheral blood evidence for an underlying megaloblastic process.

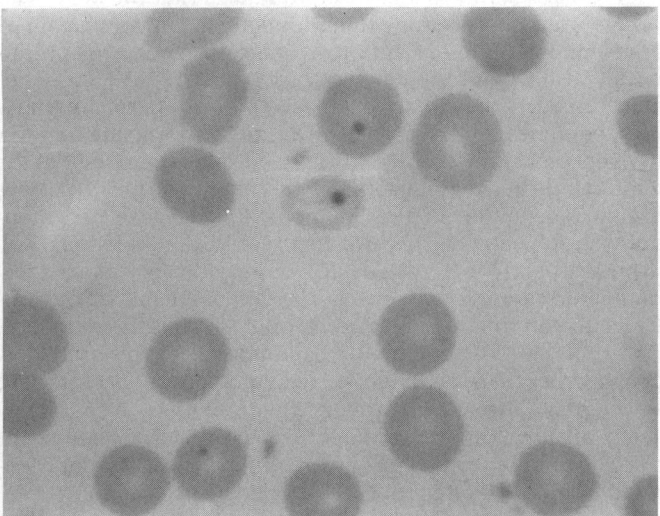

Fig. 36-2. Howell-Jolly bodies in RBCs of asplenic patient.

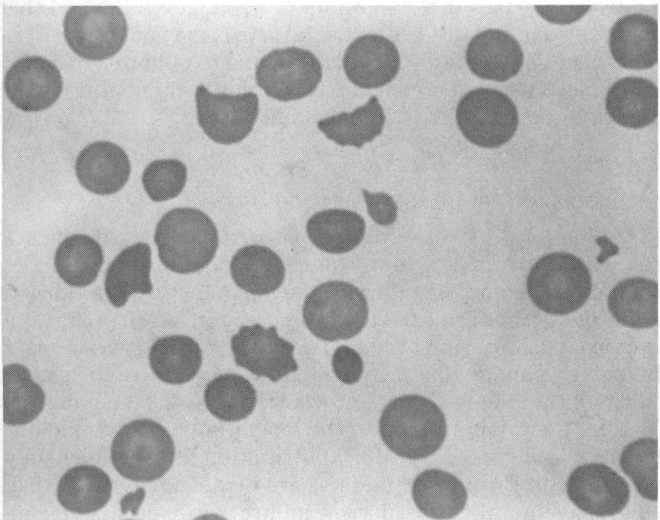

Fig. 36-3. Helmet cells, microspherocytes, and RBC fragments in microangiopathic hemolytic anemia.

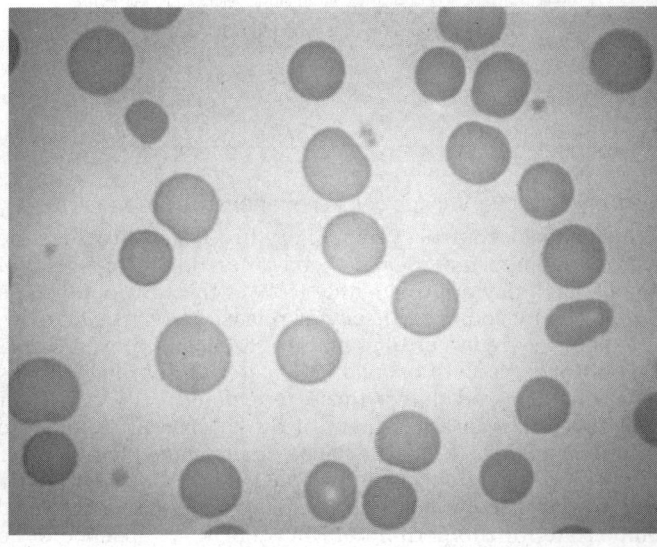

Fig. 36-4. Spherocytes and polychromatophilia in hereditary spherocytosis.

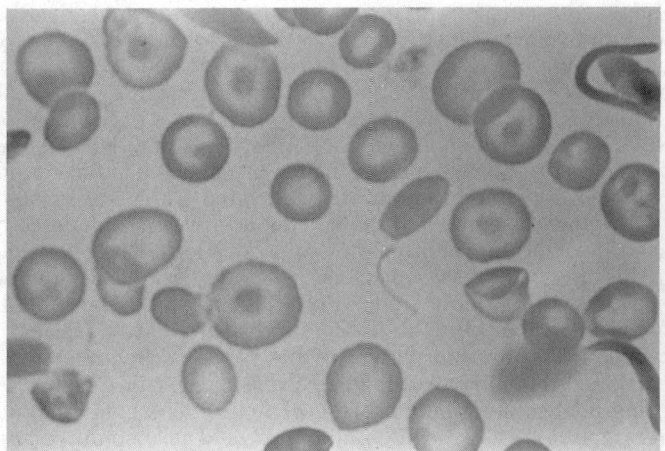

Fig. 36-5. Sickle cells in sickle cell disease.

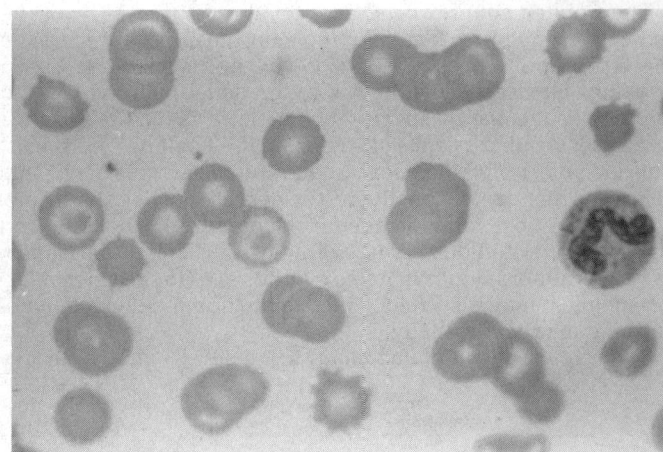

Fig. 36-6. Target cells, acanthocytes, and macrocytes in liver disease.

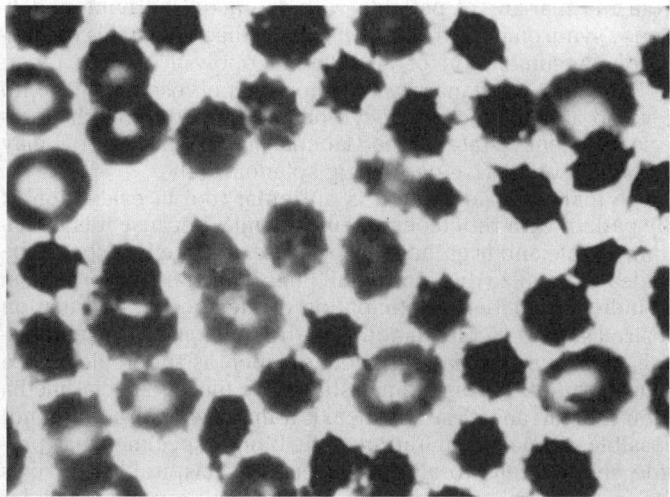

Fig. 36-7. Marked acanthocytosis in advanced liver disease.

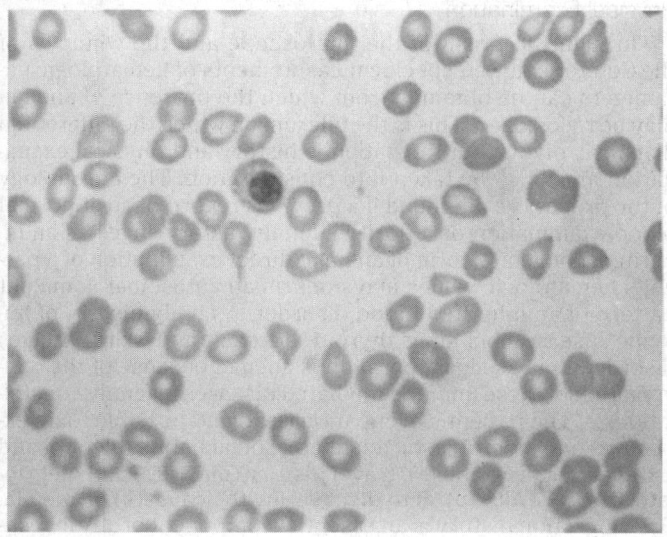

Fig. 36-8. Teardrop and nucleated RBCs in myelophthisic anemia.

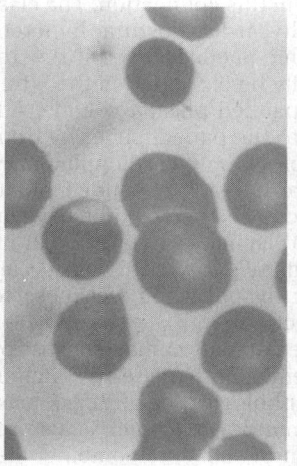 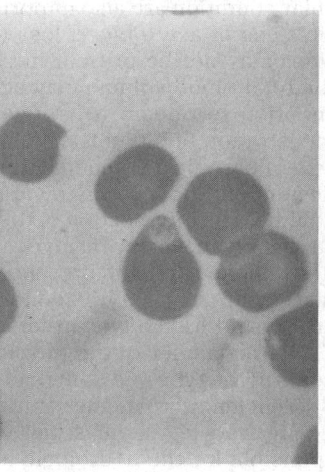

Fig. 36-9. Blister RBCs in drug-related hemolytic anemia.

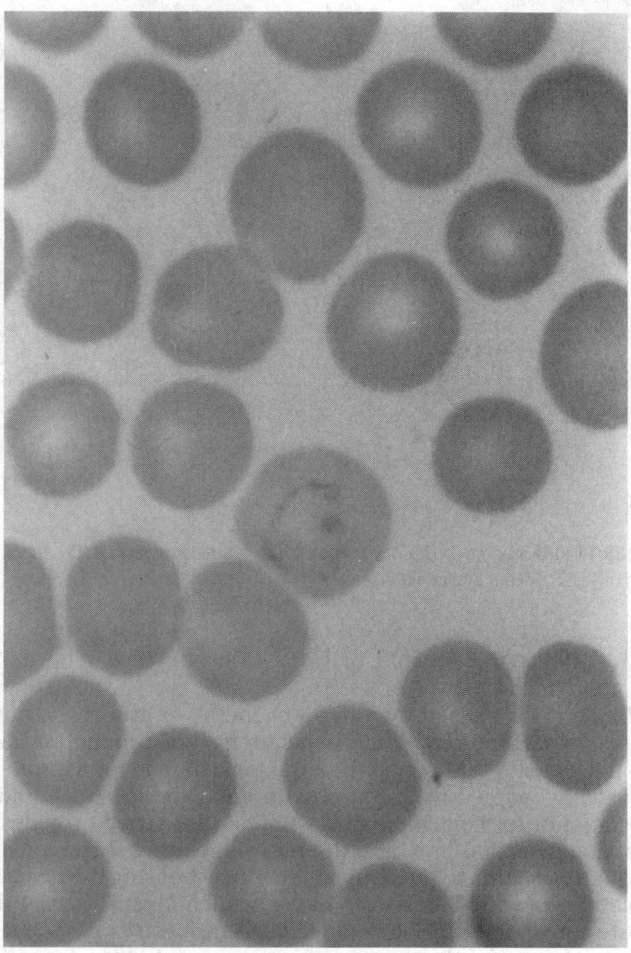

Fig. 36-10. Intraerythrocytic parasites in malaria.

in pregnancy or in alcoholics, in whom a normal MCV may occur because of a mixed iron-folate deficiency. Target cells, Howell-Jolly bodies, and nucleated RBCs may be clues to functional or anatomic asplenia (Fig. 36-2).

The red cell shape is frequently the most helpful aid in the differential diagnosis of hemolytic disorders. Diagnostic findings include RBC fragmentation as a result of traumatic hemolysis on artificial cardiac valves (Fig. 36-3); spherocytes as a marker of hereditary spherocytosis (Fig. 36-4); the oakleaf and sickle cells of sickle cell disease (Fig. 36-5); the target cell of thalassemia and hemoglobin C and liver disease (Fig. 36-6); the spur cell of liver failure (Fig. 36-7); the teardrop form of myelophthisic processes (Fig. 36-8); and the blister forms of glucose-6-phosphate dehydrogenase (G6PD) deficiency (Fig. 36-9). In addition, detection of intraerythrocytic parasites may demonstrate that a fever is caused by malaria (Fig. 36-10). The marked elevation in serum proteins in myelomatous states may result in a "protein" backdrop to RBCs stacked in rouleau formation (Fig. 36-11A); aggregation of RBCs into crowded masses (as opposed to their stacking into rouleaux) should suggest cold agglutinin disease (Fig. 36-11B).

None of the quantitative values generated by the Coulter machine substitute substitutes for the plethora of information derived from a careful, informed examination of the peripheral smear. It is the omission of this simple and inexpensive undertaking that deprives the clinician of what is often the critical clue to the etiology of anemia, and even the etiology of nonhematologic disease.

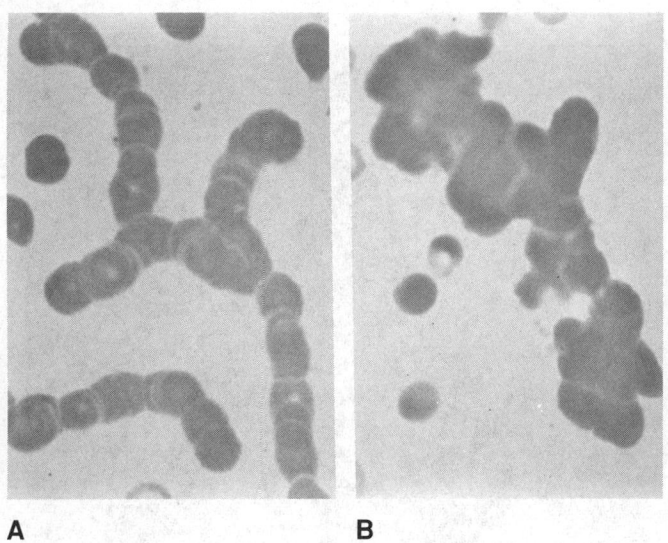

A　　　　　　　　**B**

Fig. 36-11. **(A)** Stacking of RBCs with rouleaux formation in myeloma. **(B)** Aggregation of RBCs in cold agglutinin disease.

Examination of the Bone Marrow

If anemia is caused by a hyporegenerative process, a bone marrow examination permits evaluation of the production fault responsible for reticulocytopenic anemia. A marrow aspiration is usually coupled with a marrow biopsy; the former permits observation of cellular detail, whereas the latter provides a histologic section in which the marrow contents are not disturbed in relation to the bony architecture housing the hematopoietic elements. The site of such examinations is usually the posterior or anterior iliac spine; marked obesity may prevent successful use of these sites and is commonly the reason for attempting sternal marrow aspiration. Sternal aspirates have been complicated by perforation, which entails the dire consequence of cardiac tamponade. The iliac spines are the sites of choice, although previous radiotherapy to the pelvis or overlying skin infection may necessitate shift of the examination to the sternal area. Biopsy of the sternum is not recommended.

The marrow is the final arbiter in the diagnosis of iron-deficiency anemia, since iron-deficient erythropoiesis does not result in anemia until all iron has been mobilized from the marrow. In microcytic anemias due to all other causes detectable iron stores are present in the marrow; the ringed sideroblast can only be recognized on marrow study as another sign of a hypochromic anemia. A marrow aspirate will reveal the megaloblastic origin of some macrocytic anemias and concomitantly provide an assessment of iron stores. A biopsy of the marrow permits recognition of general aplasia or hypoplasia, pure RBC aplasia, or hematologic malignancy (leukemia, lymphoma, or myeloma) as a cause of anemia. Infiltrative diseases of the marrow, sometimes heralded by a leukoerythroblastic picture (teardrop RBCs, nucleated RBCs, early WBC precursors, and/ or platelet-shape abnormalities) in the peripheral blood, may be the initial presentation of malignancy. Small cell carcinoma of the lung and breast, and prostate cancers frequently involve the marrow, creating so-called myelophthisic anemia. Myelofibrosis, a heavy deposition of collagen fibers within the marrow, can be demonstrated with special silver stains of the biopsy specimen; this abnormality is a component of myeloid metaplasia (myelofibrosis and extramedullary hematopoiesis) but may accompany such disparate states as hairy cell leukemia or mastocytosis.

The marrow may contain granulomas in tuberculosis or histoplasmosis[9;] culture of *Mycobacterium avium intracellulare*

from the marrow of patients with the acquired immunodeficiency syndrome is a frequent means of diagnosing this complication. Accumulation of an acid-mucopolysaccharide ("ceroid") occurs in the marrows of anorexia nervosa patients who develop anemia and other cytopenias secondary to their caloric deficiency state.[10] The Gaucher cell in the marrow may explain an otherwise perplexing splenomegaly.[11]

The marrow examination is an initial tool in evaluation of the patient with reticulocytopenic anemia. Because it is an uncomfortable and frightening procedure, every effort should be made to minimize the number of times it must be performed on an individual patient. Anticipation of the specific information desired should dictate handling of the specimen. Culture materials should be on hand if infection such as tuberculosis is a consideration; chromosomal studies requiring special media should be arranged in advance. If a marrow aspiration is not possible, a touch preparation of the biopsy specimen may provide enough cells to allow a diagnosis. Inaspirable marrows are frequent in myeolofibrotic states; the very hypercellular marrows of leukemia or megaloblastic anemias may also resist aspiration.

Integration of the Laboratory Data with the History and Physical Examination

Through the prism of the microscope and the windows of the Coulter counter, specific measurements of hematologic parameters can be obtained from which the presence of anemia may be recognized. This is the fulcrum on which the differential diagnosis pivots, but the patient's history and physical examination must also be taken into consideration. The chronology of the process is simplified if a previous record of an abnormal blood examination or a positive family history suggests an inherited, congenital form of anemia; direct examination of a parent's hematologic values may confirm an autosomal dominant pattern of an inherited blood disorder. A family history of immune disease, including thyroid, adrenal, and skin (vitiligo) disorders, may suggest pernicious anemia because of the congregation of these immune-mediated diseases in family constellations.[12] The patient's occupation (lead and possible toxin exposures and sideroblastic anemias), social habits (alcohol and intravenous drug abuse), travel history (malaria), and diet (folate, iron) are all central to discovering the cause(s) of anemia. Drug ingestion history is an essential component of any investigation of anemia; some perplexing anemias have only been explained after the contents of the medicine cabinet were individually reviewed.

The rate at which the anemia develops usually determines the symptoms experienced by the patient. Age and cardiovascular condition are also important in this connection. The classic signs of acute blood loss (tachycardia, postural hypotension) may not be present in chronic anemias, even if severe; the total blood volume may actually be increased in the latter situation secondary to an overexpanded plasma volume. Administration of blood transfusion to the patient suffering from severe chronic anemia may then precipitate cardiopulmonary decompensation by aggravating an already expanded blood volume. The intersection of the decreased hemoglobin oxygen-carrying capacity with myocardial ischemia can result in elderly anemic patients presenting initially to a cardiologist. Cardiac symptoms may extend from dyspnea and weakness to angina and frank myocardial infarction.

The remainder of the physical examination may suggest or confirm the type and source of anemia. Both folate and vitamin B_{12} deficiency create the same morphologic type of megaloblastic, macrocytic anemias, but vitamin B_{12} deficiency is also responsible for the neurologic lesion of subacute combined degeneration, with loss of vibratory and position sensation in the lower extremities. Telangiectasis on the buccal mucosa may be the external evidence of the internal bleeding telangiectatic lesions in Osler-Weber-Rendu disease; this hereditary hemorrhagic disease usually presents as a chronic iron deficiency anemia. Jaundice may be the clue to hemolysis. A caput medusae vascular pattern over the abdominal wall indicates portal hypertension with splenomegaly, resulting in a hypersplenic, pancytopenic state. Leg ulcers may accompany hemolytic anemias, especially sickle cell disease. The entire body merits examination to help uncover the etiology of anemia.

Since the hematologic system acts as a "sickness index" of the body's condition, hematologic abnormalities are frequently the clue to the presence of systemic disorders. The anemia of chronic disorders is an involvement of erythropoiesis in the host response to a broad range of bodily insults.[13] Infection, inflammation, and malignancy are all accompanied by this form of anemia.[14]

The problem in diagnosing these disorders may be complicated because fever, a common accompaniment of infection, inflammation, or malignancy, may also be caused by the primary hematologic process. Both hemolytic and megaloblastic anemias can have significant fever as a component of their presentation. Additional confusion arises because classic manifestations of infection, such as Roth spots, may be due to severe anemia without any contribution of endocarditis.

Malignancies are also frequently accompanied by anemia even in the absence of direct marrow involvement by the tumor. Anemia may advertise the silent presence of a hypernephroma or pancreatic neoplasm.[15] Both acute and chronic renal disease have a direct effect on erythropoiesis, which is not surprising in light of the kidney's function as the source of erythropoietin.[16] The appearance of anemia in the diabetic may be the key indication that renal deterioration secondary to diabetic nephropathy has occurred. Anemia becomes an almost universal cause of morbidity as renal failure advances.

Endocrine disease also involves anemia as a frequent complication since most of the body's hormones have direct effects on erythrocyte production. Hypothyroidism is associated with an anemia that represents a down-tuning of the erythroid mass to parallel the lowered metabolic demands of the body. Parathyroid, adrenal, and pituitary disorders may all be contributors to an anemic state.[17,18]

Mild anemias that accompany primary nonhematologic disorders may be the "minor detail" that leads to the major diagnosis. Examination of the blood may provide a computer readout of the body, but this information must be integrated into the patient's history and physical examination. It is this that constitutes the challenge in the approach to the patient with anemia—the breadth of the diagnostic possibilities that needs recognition and understanding.

Approach to Anemia with Decreased Red Cell Production

Patients with anemia and a low reticulocyte count have inadequate red blood cell production. As noted earlier, evaluation of the etiology of such anemias may be guided by the MCV of the circulating red cells.[19,20] None of the distinctions made below in characterizing microcytic, normocytic, and macrocytic anemias is absolute; nevertheless, the MCV can provide a useful guide to the analysis and laboratory investigation of the anemic patient.

Evaluation of Microcytic Anemia

Microcytic anemias generally result from inadequate hemoglobin synthesis. The failure of hemoglobin production may be caused by hereditary defects in globin synthesis, as in thalassemia; by defects in heme synthesis, as in sideroblastic ane-

---

APPROACH TO ANEMIA WITH LOW MCV AND LOW RETICULOCYTES

Differential diagnosis
  Iron deficiency
  Sideroblastic anemia
  Thalassemia trait
  Anemia of chronic disease
Laboratory evaluation
  Iron, iron-binding capacity, and ferritin
  Examination of peripheral blood smear for evidence of target cells, stippling, etc.
  Hemoglobin electrophoresis for evidence of thalassemia
  Bone marrow aspirate for definition of iron stores, presence of ring sideroblasts

---

mias; or by inadequate iron incorporation into the heme moiety because of either iron deficiency or failure of iron mobilization, as seen in the anemia of chronic disease.

The laboratory evaluation of microcytic anemia should include determination of iron indices, namely serum iron, iron-binding capacity, and ferritin; examination of the peripheral blood smear for evidence for thalassemia trait or coarse basophilic stippling suggestive of sideroblastic anemia; and hemoglobin electrophoresis to assist in defining a potential thalassemia trait. Definitive diagnosis frequently requires bone marrow aspiration to assess both iron stores and the effectiveness of iron incorporation into developing red cell precursors.

Iron deficiency is by far the most common cause of anemia in general and of microcytic anemia in particular. In iron deficiency, the total serum iron should be low, and saturation of the serum iron-binding capacity should be <10%.[21] In patients who are iron deficient but who have recently ingested iron supplements, however, these measurements are unreliable. By contrast, serum ferritin, which is a reflection of total body iron stores, is essentially always low in iron deficiency regardless of iron therapy.[22] It must also be remembered that early iron deficiency is generally a normocytic anemia. Consequently, evaluation of iron indices is indicated in virtually all anemic patients. Since iron deficiency is essentially always a sign of chronic blood loss, confirmation of the diagnosis in adult males and postmenopausal women obligates the physician to a full evaluation of the gastrointestinal tract to rule out a malignant bleeding source.

In sideroblastic anemia and in thalassemia trait, iron is usually normal to high, iron-binding capacity is normal, and ferritin is normal to high.[23] Although associated with profound microcytosis, thalassemia intermedia and thalassemia major do not present a diagnostic problem in this setting, as they are both associated with a slightly elevated reticulocyte (2–7%) count and characteristic physical stigmata of massive bone marrow expansion. Sideroblastic anemia is confirmed by the presence of ringed sideroblasts in a bone marrow aspirate. Confirmation of β-thalassemia trait is by hemoglobin electrophoresis. α-Thalassemia trait, in which two of the α-globin alleles are deleted, causes microcytosis, but minimal anemia, if any. If the diagnosis is suspected, it should be evaluated on peripheral blood smear because the hemoglobin electrophoresis in α thalassemia is normal. Definitive confirmation can only be obtained with DNA analysis of the α-globin gene loci.[24]

The most troublesome diagnostic difficulty involving analysis of microcytic anemia lies in the identification of the anemia of chronic disease. Although usually presenting as a normocytic anemia, this disorder must always be considered in the

---

APPROACH TO ANEMIA WITH ELEVATED MCV AND LOW RETICULOCYTES

Differential diagnosis
- Megaloblastic anemia
    - Vitamin B_{12} deficiency
    - Folate deficiency
    - Myelodysplastic syndrome
    - Drug-induced anemia
- Nonmegaloblastic anemia
    - Liver disease
    - Hypothyroidism
    - Reticulocytosis
- Laboratory evaluation
    - Serum vitamin B_{12}, RBC folate
    - Examination of peripheral smear for hypersegmented neutrophils, giant platelets
    - Thyroid function tests, liver function tests
    - Bone marrow aspirate for evaluation for myelodysplastic features

---

differential diagnosis of microcytic anemia.[25,26] No definitive test will confirm a diagnosis of anemia of chronic disease; patients with this anemia classically have low serum iron, low iron-binding capacity, and elevated serum ferritin. In general, the saturation of the iron-binding capacity is >10%. Confirmation of the diagnosis is primarily one of exclusion and should include a bone marrow aspirate showing confirmed adequate iron stores with poor iron incorporation into siderocytes.

Evaluation of Macrocytic Anemia

The macrocytic anemias can be divided into two major groups, the megaloblastic anemias and the nonmegaloblastic macrocytic anemias. The distinction between the two can be made on examination of the peripheral blood smear. Megaloblastic anemias affect all hematopoietic cell lines, and the peripheral smear shows evidence of hypersegmented neutrophils and large platelets.[27,28] In addition, these cell lines often are also depressed in megaloblastic anemia, and patients may in fact present with pancytopenia. By contrast, the nonmegaloblastic macrocytic anemias, other than those due to reticulocytosis, usually reflect membrane cholesterol defects related to constitutional abnormalities such as liver disease or hypothyroidism; consequently, the WBCs and platelets are morphologically normal.

Additional laboratory evaluations include determination of RBC folate and serum vitamin B_{12} levels in patients with megaloblastic anemia and thyroid and liver function tests in patients with isolated macrocytosis.

The main diagnostic challenge in evaluating patients with macrocytic anemia is identification of myelodysplastic syndromes. Although these syndromes are classically associated with megaloblastic changes, evidence of megaloblastic abnormalities in the peripheral blood of patients with myelodysplasia is frequently subtle or absent.[29,30] Patients in whom megaloblastic anemia occurs despite normal serum folate and vitamin B_{12} levels should undergo bone marrow aspiration and biopsy in order to evaluate the presence of a myelodysplastic syndrome. Moreover, patients with unexplained macrocytic anemia should also undergo bone marrow examination. Marrow evaluation should include cytogenetics.

Further studies in patients with megaloblastic anemia related to vitamin B_{12} deficiency should include a Schilling test to evaluate the diagnosis of pernicious anemia. If that diagnosis

is confirmed, patients should be investigated for evidence of other endocrine abnormalities, notably thyroid or adrenal insufficiency.

Evaluation of Normocytic Anemia

The evaluation of normocytic anemias is complicated by the consideration that many of the anemias classically associated with microcytosis or macrocytosis may, in fact, present with a normal MCV, especially in the early stages. Iron deficiency, acquired sideroblastic anemia, myelodysplasia, and the anemia of chronic disease all present frequently as normocytic anemias. In addition, mixed anemias (e.g., anemia in a patient who is both folate and iron deficient) may often result in a normal MCV determination. Examination of the peripheral blood smear in the latter group of patients will reveal a mixed population of RBCs, which may help resolve the dilemma. The guide to differential diagnosis of normocytic anemia outlined below is consequently not an exhaustive list. Early stages or mixtures of microcytic and macrocytic anemias must be considered as well.

Initial evaluation of the patient with a normocytic anemia should include iron studies because of the frequency with which iron deficiency can present as a normocytic anemia, as noted above. The main focus of the evaluation beyond this step is an attempt to establish the presence or absence of a primary bone marrow failure syndrome. Diagnosis of aplastic anemia, red cell aplasia, or myelophthisis ultimately rests on examination of the bone marrow aspirate and biopsy specimen (to assess marrow cellularity, red cell production, and the presence of abnormal cells within the marrow); however, an inappropriately low reticulocyte count is usually a major initial clue. Examination of the peripheral smear may give clues to the presence of myelophthisis, which is associated with teardrop cells and other morphologic red cell abnormalities.

Secondary causes of bone marrow failure are sometimes readily recognizable. Most common among these is the anemia associated with uremia. A frequent dilemma in diagnosing uremia as the cause of anemia is the poor correlation between the level of the serum creatinine and the degree of anemia seen in

---

APPROACH TO ANEMIA WITH NORMAL MCV AND LOW RETICULOCYTES

Differential diagnosis
- Primary bone marrow failure
    - Aplastic anemia
    - Constitutional red cell aplasia (Diamond-Blackfan)
    - Acquired red cell aplasia
    - Myelophthisis
- Secondary bone marrow failure
    - Uremia
    - Endocrinology
    - Human immunodeficiency virus infection
    - Anemia of chronic disease
- Laboratory evaluation
    - Iron, iron-binding capacity, and ferritin
    - Examination of peripheral blood smear for evidence of myelophthisis: teardrops, helmet cells, etc.
    - Serum creatinine, thyroid function tests, liver function tests, cortisol levels if appropriate
    - Erythropoietin level
    - Bone marrow aspirate and biopsy to assess iron stores, red cell production, marrow cellularity

---

the patient. This probably reflects the lack of a direct correlation between the loss of erythropoietin production and loss of glomerular function in the failing kidney.[31,32] It is now possible to assess the impact of renal dysfunction on RBC production, owing to the availability of assays of erythropoietin levels. Patients with anemia secondary to renal failure have low erythropoietin levels; virtually all other anemic patients have normal or elevated levels.

As noted earlier, many endocrine disorders, including hypothyroidism, hypoadrenalism, and hypopituitarism, are associated with mild anemia.[33] Although hypothyroidism may cause macrocytic anemia, it is more commonly associated with a normocytic anemia.[34] Hyperthyroidism is also associated with anemia. Serum tests of endocrine function should be obtained as appropriate to the clinical picture of the patient.

The anemia in patients with human immunodeficiency virus infection is multifactorial and is discussed in detail in Chapter 155. Bone marrow examination most commonly shows features compatible with the anemia of chronic disease. Other findings include plasmacytosis, lymphoid aggregates, and evidence for granulomatous disease in the marrow.[35]

Approach to Anemia with Increased Red Blood Cell Turnover

Patients with anemia and an elevated reticulocyte count usually have adequate marrow function. They have increased red cell turnover due to acute blood loss, RBC sequestration, or hemolysis. If the reticulocyte response is adequate, bone marrow examination is usually not necessary in these patients because the disease process is extrinsic to the marrow. Initial evaluation should also establish whether there is evidence of acute bleeding or an enlarged spleen. The remainder of the evaluation is directed at determining the etiology of the hemolytic diathesis.

Patients who have spherocytes in the peripheral blood should be studied for the presence of warm antibody-mediated immune hemolysis by a direct and an indirect Coombs test.[36] Patients with negative Coombs test should be tested for the presence of cold agglutinins and for other, rarer immune hemolytic disorders such as paroxysmal cold hemoglobinuria.[37,38]

Evaluation of nonimmune hemolytic disorders is guided by the peripheral blood smear findings and the clinical history. Microangiopathic changes on the peripheral blood smear should be viewed in the clinical context in which they occur. The presence of low-grade anemia in a patient with a prosthetic heart valve is probably due to a mechanical hemolysis, which may be chronic and insignificant, but an acute increase in hemolysis from a prosthetic valve should lead to evaluation for perivalvular leak or other valvular dysfunction.[39] Other causes of microangiopathic changes, specifically disseminated intravascular coagulation (DIC) and thrombotic thrombocytopenic purpura (TTP) usually present as acute medical emergencies.[40,41] In both settings, the platelet count is usually decreased. The distinction can be made by clinical evaluation for evidence of a basis for DIC and by the presence of other markers of TTP, such as fever, neurologic dysfunction, or renal insufficiency. The diagnosis of DIC can be supported by elevations in the prothrombin time (PT) and partial thromboplastin time (PTT), which are most often normal in TTP. Low-grade chronic DIC, as can be seen in association with malignancy, may require more extensive evaluation of fibrinogen and fibrin degradation products.[42]

The peripheral smear will also provide ample evidence for most hereditary hemolytic anemias. Sickle cell anemia and thalassemia are usually readily diagnosable on peripheral blood smear, and appropriate follow-up with hemoglobin electrophoresis will confirm the diagnosis. Hereditary membrane defects

---

APPROACH TO ANEMIA WITH ELEVATED RETICULOCYTE COUNT

Differential diagnosis
  Acute blood loss
  Splenic sequestration
  Hemolysis
    Immune hemolytic anemia
    Mechanical hemolysis
      Valve hemolysis
      Microangiopathic hemolytic anemia (DIC, TTP)
    Hereditary hemolytic anemia
      Hemoglobinopathies
      Enzyme defects: G6PD deficiency, pyruvate kinase deficiency, etc.
      Membrane defects: spherocytosis
      Unstable hemoglobins
    Acquired membrane defects: PNH, spur cell anemia
    Infection-related hemolysis: *Clostridia* infection, malaria, babesiosis
Laboratory evaluation
  Examination of the peripheral blood smear for evidence of spherocytes, microangiopathic changes, features of hemoglobinopathies, bite cells
  Urinary hemosiderin
  Direct and indirect Coombs test
  Cold agglutinin titer
  Appropriate further tests as indicated by preliminary evaluation: hemoglobin electrophoresis, G6PD screen, Heinz-body preparation, isopropanol stability test, P_{50}, sucrose lysis test, bacterial cultures, examination of smear for malaria, babesiosis, bartonellosis

---

that give rise to spherocytosis or elliptocytosis are also diagnosed by examination of the peripheral smear.

Enzyme defects of the red blood cell, most commonly G6PD deficiency, may present quite late in life, usually in the setting of an acute oxidant stress.[43] Evidence of disorder on the periph-

---

EVALUATION OF HEMOLYTIC ANEMIA

The evaluation of hemolytic anemia can be guided by the findings on the peripheral blood smear. The smear may allow the crucial distinction to be made between immune and nonimmune hemolysis; this determination will then guide further evaluation. Spherocytes and microspherocytes are classic markers of immune hemolytic anemia; fragmented RBCs are markers of intravascular, nonimmune hemolytic anemia. Since extravascular hemolysis within the spleen does not result in hemoglobinemia, hemoglobinuria, or hemosiderinuria, detection of any of these implies an intravascular hemolytic process. Acute severe intravascular hemolysis may cause detectable hemoglobinemia, which can be seen on visual inspection of the patient's plasma. Hemoglobinuria may be detected with recent intravascular hemolysis. Chronic intravascular hemolysis can be detected by assays for urinary hemosiderin.

Table 36-3. Red Blood Cell Values at Various Ages: Mean and Lower Limit of Normal (− 2 SD)

Age	Hemoglobin (g/dl)		Hematocrit (%)		Red Cell Count (10¹²/L)		MCV (fl)		MCH (pg)		MCHC (g/dl)	
	Mean	− 2 SD	Mean	− 2 SD	Mean	− 2 SD	Mean	− 2 SD	Mean	− 2 SD	Mean	− 2 SD
Birth (cord blood)	16.5	13.5	51	42	4.7	3.9	108	98	34	31	33	30
1–3 days (capillary)	18.5	14.5	56	45	5.3	4.0	108	95	34	31	33	29
1 wk	17.5	13.5	54	42		3.9	107	88	34	28	33	28
2 wk	16.5	12.5	51	39	4.9	3.6	105	86	34	28	33	28
1 mo	14.0	10.0	43	31	4.2	3.0	104	85	34	28	33	29
2 mo	11.5	9.0	35	28	3.8	2.7	96	77	30	26	33	29
3–6 mo	11.5	9.5	35	29	3.8	3.1	91	74	30	25	33	30
0.5–2 yr	12.0	11.0	36	33	4.5	3.7	78	70	27	23	33	30
2–6 yr	12.5	11.5	37	34	4.6	3.9	81	75	27	24	34	31
6–12 yr	13.5	11.5	40	35	4.6	4.0	86	77	29	25	34	31
12–18 yr												
Female	14.0	12.0	41	36	4.6	4.1	90	78	30	25	34	31
Male	14.5	13.0	43	37	4.9	4.5	88	78	30	25	34	31
18–49 yr												
Female	14.0	12.0	41	36	4.6	4.0	90	80	30	26	34	31
Male	15.5	13.5	47	41	5.2	4.5	90	80	30	26	34	31

(Adapted from Dallman and Siimes,[53] with permission, as appeared in Oski FA: Pallor. p. 62. In Kaye R, Oski FA, Barness LA (eds): Core Textbook of Pediatrics, 3rd Ed. JB Lippincott, Philadelphia, 1989.)

eral blood smear is detectable as bite cells, which reflect splenic conditioning of red cells containing precipitated hemoglobin.[44] Patients in whom this diagnosis is suspected should have a Heinz-body smear to look for precipitated hemoglobin in circulating red cells and should have an assay of G6PD levels. However, in the setting of an acute hemolytic episode, the circulating young red cells will have higher levels of G6PD, and most or all of the older cells with a very low G6PD level will have been cleared. Consequently, both the Heinz-body smear and the G6PD assay may be negative. In this case the G6PD level should be reassayed when the patient has recovered from the acute hemolytic episode.

Heinz-body anemia is also seen in patients with unstable hemoglobins.[45,46] Diagnosis can sometimes be made by hemoglobin electrophoresis, although many unstable hemoglobins are electrophoretically normal. Some show decreased stability in isopropyl alcohol and others show an altered oxygen dissociation curve.

Other rare causes of nonimmune hemolysis include paroxysmal nocturnal hemoglobinuria (PNH), which results in an acquired membrane defect in the red cell, thereby predisposing the cell to complement-mediated lysis.[47] Patients with PNH may be diagnosed by acid hemolysis and sucrose lysis tests. The leukocyte alkaline phosphatase score in patients with PNH is also low. Another acquired membrane defect, which can be readily diagnosed on the peripheral blood smear, is spur cell anemia, which is seen in patients with advanced cirrhosis. The smear reveals striking acanthocytosis; hemolysis results from splenic destruction of the abnormal red cells.[48]

Toxic hemolysis can result from parasitic and bacterial infections. Malaria, babesiosis, and bartonellosis cause hemolysis by direct parasitization of RBCs.[49–51] Appropriate diagnosis can be made on smears of the peripheral blood; in malaria and babesiosis, thick smears are frequently necessary to visualize the parasites. Dramatic overwhelming hemolysis may be seen in patients with clostridial sepsis. The course of these patients is usually one of fulminant hemolytic anemia, shock, and death before the bacterial diagnosis can be made.[52]

ANEMIA IN THE CHILD

The classification of anemia (Greek "without blood") can be based on physiologic, morphologic, or etiologic factors. The prospective approach to any individual patient, however, re-

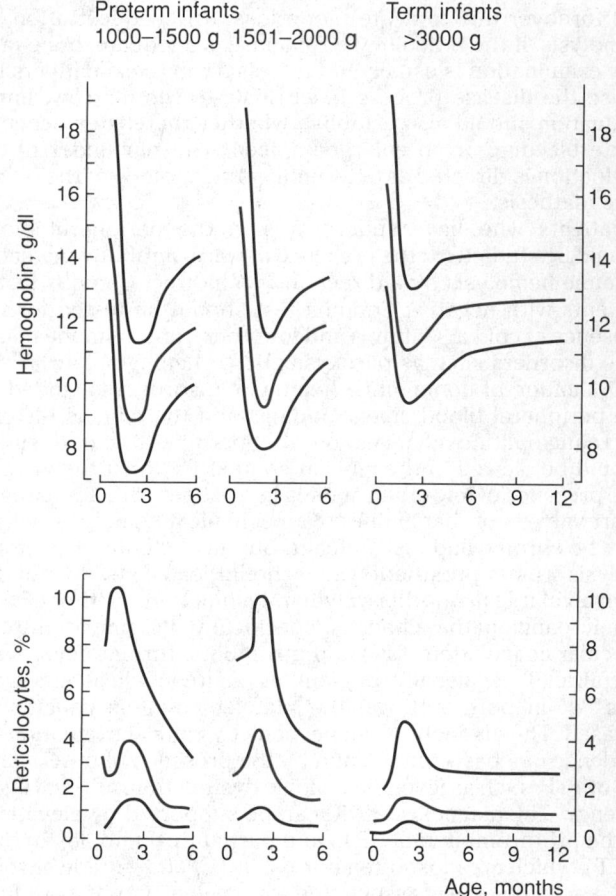

Fig. 36-12. Hemoglobin concentration and reticulocyte count in preterm and term infants. Median values (red line) and 95% confidence limits are indicated for each of three birthweight categories. (Hemoglobin values from Lundström et al.[55] and Saarinen and Siimes,[56] reticulocyte values from unpublished data on the same infants from whom hemoglobin values were derived.) (From Dallman,[57] with permission.)

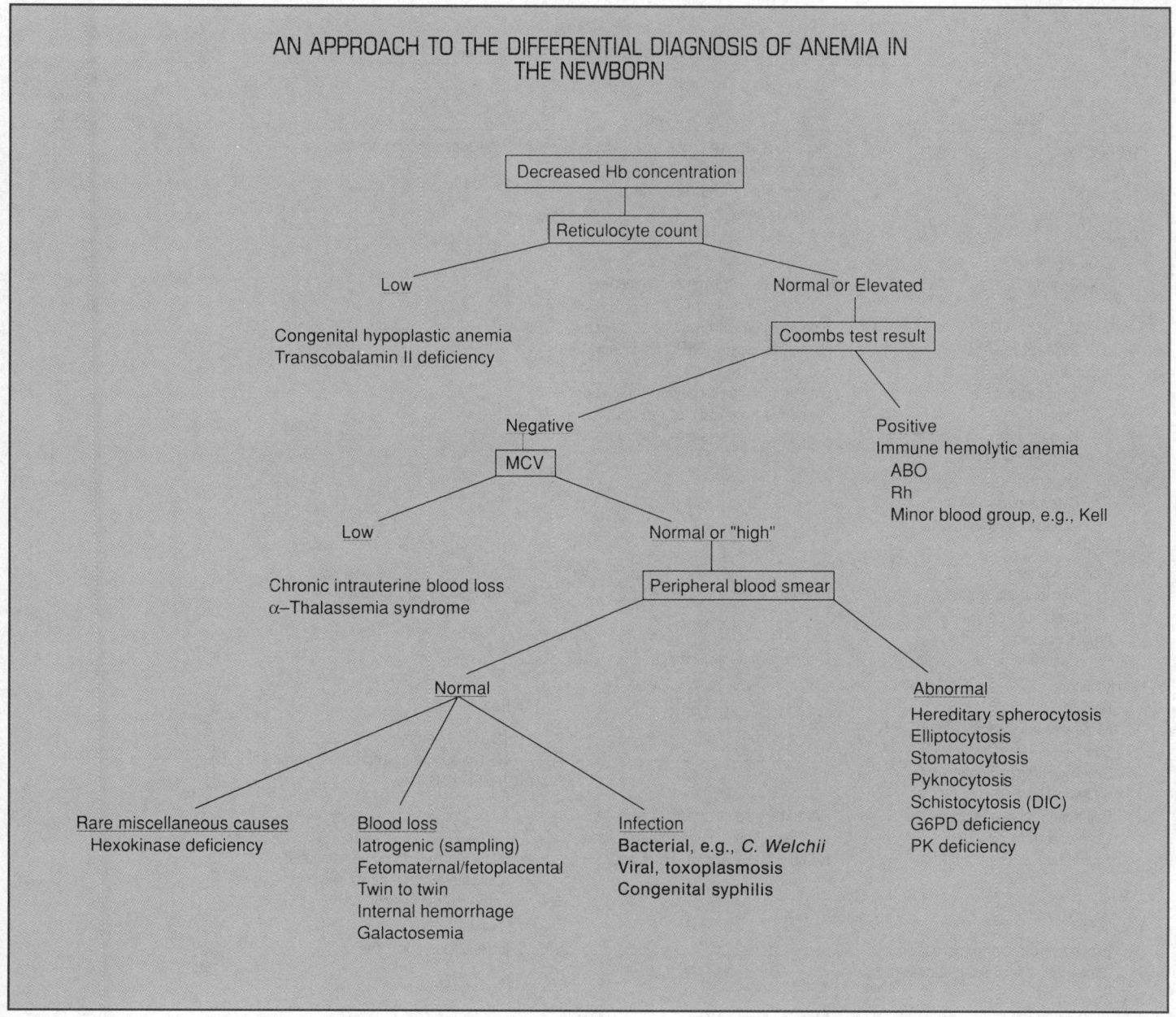

AN APPROACH TO THE DIFFERENTIAL DIAGNOSIS OF ANEMIA IN THE NEWBORN

quires integration of history, physical findings, blood count, red cell indices, reticulocyte count, RBC morphology, specific tests (e.g., Coombs), hemoglobin electrophoresis, and finally search for or determination of the underlying disease or process. This section emphasizes only the special aspects of evaluating anemia in children.

The most straightforward approach to the diagnosis of anemia in both children and adults considers several broad categories: (1) decreased production of RBCs or blood loss; (2) size of RBCs: normal (normocytic), too large (macrocytic), or too small (microcytic); (3) knowledge of the relative frequency of the causes of anemia at various ages; and (4) appreciation that the diagnosis of anemia depends on "normal" values related to the patient's age, sex (Table 36-3),[53] cardiopulmonary status, and residence. Children from 6 months to 12 years of age appear anemic compared with adults, but children have higher concentration of 2,3-diphosphoglycerate and ATP in their RBCs with a corresponding shift to right of the oxygen disassociation curve. Increased tissue oxygenation compensates for the lower hemoglobin concentrations. The "anemia" is thus a physiologically appropriate adaptation of the red cell mass to the increased efficiency of oxygen delivery.

The approach to a child with anemia differs from that for an adult in several ways, because of factors related to (1) age differences in what are accepted as normal values for hemoglobin/hematocrit (Hb/Hct) (Table 36-3)[53]; (2) much lower incidence of neoplastic disease in childhood as either a direct or an indirect cause of anemia (<7,000 of the 1,000,000* new cases of cancer each year in the United States occur in individuals <15 years of age); (3) iron deficiency, which is almost always secondary to nutritional factors in children and requires less intensive follow-up evaluation; (4) relative rarity of alcoholism and its related liver disease, as an underlying problem; (5) anemia associated with thyroid disease, which is much less common in childhood; (6) rarity of cardiovascular disease other than congenital heart disease so that valve replacement, malignant hypertension, and use of certain drugs are not usually factors; and (7) frequent difficulty of obtaining adequate specimens for evaluation in the newborn and neonatal period (especially for hemolytic processes, e.g., pyknocytosis). Clinically

---

* Excludes basal cell carcinoma of the skin and carcinoma in situ of the cervix.

Table 36-4. Historical Factors that May Be of Importance in the Diagnosis of Anemia

Factors	Newborn–1 mo	1 mo–1 yr	Older Infants, Children, and Adolescents
Prematurity	Blood loss due to procedures, vitamin E deficiency, "anemia of prematurity" may respond to erythropoietin	Predisposes to iron deficiency	
Maternal			
Drug ingestion			
Dilantin	Bleeding due to hypothrombinemia, treated with vitamin K		
Warfarin			
Diuretics	Bleeding due to thrombocytopenia		
Sulfa, etc.	Hemolysis due to G6PD deficiency		
Infections			
Toxoplasmosis	Bleeding due to thrombocytopenia or anemia secondary to red cell aplasia, hemolysis, or inflammation		
Syphilis			
Herpes			
Rubella			
Hepatitis			
Cytomegalovirus			
Group B streptococcus			
Mechanical			
Placenta previa			
Abruptio placentae	Blood loss	Predisposes to iron deficiency	
Precipitous delivery			
Amniocentesis			
Cesarean section	Fetomaternal hemorrhage		
Family history			
Black		Hemoglobins S, C	
Mediterranean origin		β-Thalassemia	
Southeast Asian origin		α-Thalassemia syndromes, hemoglobin E	
Greeks, Turkish, Sephardic Jews, Sardinians		G6PD deficiency	
Gallstones, cholestectomy, splenectomy, jaundice	Hereditary spherocytosis, elliptocytosis, and stomatocytosis		
Isoimmunization, either Rh or ABO	Hemolytic disease of the newborn	Sequelae to mild or undiagnosed problem in the newborn, predisposes to iron deficiency	
Travel			
Exposure to malaria, parasites, or other unusual infections		Intracellular parasites	
Sex			
X-linked (males)	Most enzymopathies		
Jaundice	Appearance at <24 hr of age suggests severe isoimmunization or intrauterine infection	Persistent jaundice suggests hemolytic process	
Diet	Iron-deficiency anemia related to diet is rare in the first 6 mo		
		Document milk intake, sources of iron, modifiers of iron absorption, vitamin B$_{12}$ (macrobiotic diets), goat's milk-folic acid deficiency (drug interactions, i.e., dilantin), and pica (lead, ice, clay).	
Drugs			
Sulfa, etc.		Hemolytic anemia, particularly with G6PD deficiency	
Chloramphenicol and others			Aplastic anemia
Dilantin			Megaloblastic anemia
Hydralazine			Coombs test positive reaction but rarely produces anemia
Socioeconomic		Pica: lead	
		Prevalence of intoxication of iron deficiency is inversely related to status	

(Table continues)

Table 36-4. *(Continued)*

Factors	Newborn–1 mo	1 mo–1 yr	Older Infants, Children, and Adolescents
Systemic illnesses			
Cardiac disease: prosthetic values or intracardiac patches		"Waring blender" syndrome and hemolysis	
Endocarditis			
			Anemia of chronic disease
Gastrointestinal			
Celiac disease, regional enteritis, ileal resection, chronic atrophic gastritis			Iron and vitamin B_{12} deficiency
Ulcerative colitis and Osler-Weber-Rendu disease			Iron deficiency
Cystic fibrosis		Vitamin K and E deficiency and anemia responsive to protein enrichment	
Liver disease			
Active processes		Shortened red blood cell survival and increased Heinz-body formation	
Renal disease			
Uremia		Shortened red blood cell survival	
		Decreased Red blood cell production	
Bloody diarrhea		Microangiopathic process (e.g., hemolytic uremic syndrome or thrombotic thrombocytopenic purpura)	
Dialysis			Folate deficiency
Hypothyroidism		Normochromic normocytic anemia with occasional irregularly contracted cells	
Collagen vascular diseases		Anemia of chronic disease with or without iron deficiency	
Infectious diseases			
Mild infections (e.g., otitis media, pharyngitis, gastroenteritis)		Transient mild decrease in hemoglobin/hematocrit (beware of evaluating mild anemias in children with intercurrent infections/inflammation)	
Sepsis (bacterial, viral, *Mycoplasma*)		Hemolytic anemias	

significant anemia in childhood is more often associated with a primary hematologic abnormality (e.g., hypoplastic or hemolytic anemia), whereas in adulthood, anemia is more often a secondary manifestation of underlying illness. It is often emphasized that anemia is a symptom, not a disease; this is equally true in children, but one finds the primary cause in the hematopoietic system more frequently in children.

Anemia of clinical importance is relatively uncommon in pediatrics. When it does occur, the patient's age is often a helpful guide in identifying the underlying process. In the newborn, anemia is most often associated with blood loss or hemolysis. During neonatal and early infancy periods one must consider pure red cell aplasia and blood loss becomes a less important cause. Physiologic anemia also develops during this time and is accentuated in preterm infants[54–57] (Fig. 36-12). From 6 months of age through 2 years, nutritional anemias and those associated with acute inflammation predominate, after which bone marrow infiltration (e.g., acute lymphocytic leukemia) becomes an important factor. Nutritional deficiency, in particular, iron deficiency, becomes a major consideration again during adolescence.

Children who are anemic do not often present "in extremis," thus, there is ample opportunity to review history (Table 36-4) and physical findings before ordering laboratory tests. In addition, patients who are anemic (in this section, a value of the hematocrit or hemoglobin 2 SD below normal for age is taken as the definition of anemia) may be functionally normal with respect to oxygen delivery in the microcirculation because of a compensatory shift to the right of the oxygen disassociation curve.

The history can often help focus on a diagnosis, but physical examination is more often nonspecific. In children, signs of anemia include pallor (often misleading), sallow hue, color of mucous membranes, jaundice, tachycardia, palpitation, wide pulse pressure, fatigue, dyspnea, poor feeding, and weight gain or other evidence of cardiac decompensation or decreased oxygen transport. Bruising, petechial and overt bleeding, splenomegaly, other abdominal organomegaly, and lymphadenopathy may point to an underlying process responsible for the anemia. In children it is important to be alert to the specific dysmorphic features of Diamond-Blackfan and Fanconi anemias, vascular and skin changes of sickle cell anemia and sickle C disease, and the facies of β-thalassemia major, since these congenital defects usually become symptomatic early in life.

History is particularly important when deciding which patients should undergo further evaluation when deviations of Hb/Hct from the normal range are small. Mild infections are common and recurrent during childhood, especially during the first several years. These mild infections can result in a transient decrease in Hb/Hct of sufficient magnitude to suggest the presence of iron-deficiency anemia, long considered the most likely cause of mild anemia in childhood.[58–60] In fact, iron-deficiency anemia has recently become much less common in low-

FEATURES OF THE PERIPHERAL BLOOD SMEAR OF DIAGNOSTIC IMPORTANCE FOR ANEMIA INTERPRETATION

Red Blood Cell Morphology	Interpretation
Normochromic normocytic	Acute inflammation
Hypochromic microcytic	Iron deficiency, thalassemias, lead poisoning, vitamin B_6 deficiency, sideroblastic processes, chronic inflammation
Macrocytic	Normal newborn, "shift" cells (reticulocytes), folate or vitamin B_{12} deficiency (macro-ovalocytes)
Target cells	Thalassemias, hemoglobins C, E, and S, liver disease, abetalipoproteinemia, postsplenectomy
Basophilic stippling	Hemolytic anemias, iron deficiency, thalassemias, lead poisoning
Heinz bodies	Normal newborn, hexose-monophosphate shunt abnormalities (e.g., G6PD deficiency, unstable hemoglobins, postsplenectomy)
Howell-Jolly bodies	Splenic hypofunction or absence, megaloblastic anemia
Teardrop cells	Bone marrow infiltration (leukoerythroblastosis)
Sperocytes	ABO incompatibility, G6PD deficiency or other hemolytic anemias, hereditary spherocytosis, hypophosphatemia
Schistocytes	Thalassemia, microangiopathic process (DIC)
Nucleated RBCs	Normal for first several days; hemolytic anemia, acute blood loss, or metaplasia
Polychromasia	"Shift" cells

If the hematocrit level is determined after capillary tube centrifugation, plasma trapping may lead to slightly higher values than those obtained by automated electronic methods. This difference can be accentuated by extreme anisocytosis, as in sickle cell disease, severe iron deficiency, and thalassemia.

In practice, one is usually confronted with a hemoglobin and/or hematocrit value that falls below the accepted range of normal. If these values are obtained in a laboratory with electronic cell counting, then red cell indices, RBC count, WBC count, and often platelet count are included. The smear may or may not be noted. The physician is then faced with the decision of whether to order further investigations (e.g., the free erythrocyte protoporphyrin is a simple rapid alternative approach to detecting iron deficiency), or (if the history is consistent and there has been no infection within the previous month) undertaking a therapeutic trial of iron (3 mg/kg/day of ferrous sulfate or its equivalent for 1 month) and rechecking the hemoglobin at that time. An increase in hemoglobin of at least 1 g% after treatment indicates that iron deficiency was the correct diagnosis. If the patient is unresponsive or the response is incomplete, compliance must be reviewed (color of stools and amount of ferrous sulfate remaining in the bottle), RBC indices obtained, and the smear reviewed. This latter approach is justified because iron deficiency is such a frequent cause of anemia in children.

Microcytosis out of proportion to the reduction in hemoglobin concentration suggests thalassemia trait, which can be confirmed by hemoglobin electrophoresis. The hemoglobin electrophoresis should be deferred until iron stores are deemed adequate, since hemoglobin A_2 production may be affected. In a patient with microcytic red cells, normal hemoglobin A_2 value, and adequate iron homeostasis, α-thalassemia trait is inferred. This inference is strengthened by a brilliant cresyl blue preparation that is positive for Heinz bodies. Depending on location and time of year, lead poisoning is an important

income families as well as middle-class families.[61,62] In the latter, a 3% prevalence of iron-deficiency anemia was found in healthy children in Minneapolis.[62] The very low prevalence is almost identical to the 2.4% of normal individuals whose Hb/Hct falls to <2 SD in a normal distribution. This makes screening, further evaluation, and subsequent treatment uncertain on the basis of Hb/Hct alone. The decision concerning further evaluation in the setting of mild anemia should include the historical factors listed in Table 36-4, socioeconomic status, and temporal relationship to mild infections. This will facilitate the differentiation of iron deficiency, thalassemia trait, and acute inflammation, the most common causes of anemia in childhood.

The basic laboratory evaluation for anemia, including accurate interpretation of the blood smear, often confirms the underlying process or suggests what further tests need to be done.

Collection and processing of specimens are considered routine but may introduce confounding variables, especially in very young children and in those who are quite ill. Finger sticks or heel sticks often produce Hb/Hct values greater than simultaneous venous samples, as a result of stasis in the finger or heel. The extremity must therefore be warmed before obtaining the specimen. An erroneously low Hb/Hct value can also be obtained by using excessive pressure or "milking" the extremity, thereby diluting the sample. Perfusion problems related to hydration status, cardiac disease, or infection must also be considered.

Table 36-5. Differentiation of Diamond-Blackfan Anemia from Transient Erythroblastopenia of Childhood

	Diamond-Blackfan	Transient Erythroblastopenia
Frequency	Rare	Common (? increasing)
Age of diagnosis	<1 yr (90% <6 mo)	0.5–4 yr
Etiology	Probably genetic	Acquired
Antecedent history	None	Viral illness
Physical abnormalities	Present (25%)	Absent
Course	Prolonged transfusion or steroid dependence	Spontaneous recovery in weeks to months
Laboratory		
MCV	Macrocytic	Normocytic
Hemoglobin F	Increased	Normal[a]
i Antigen	Present	Absent[a]
Fetal pattern of RBC glycolytic and HMP shunt enzymes	Present	Absent[a]
Elevated RBC ADA activity	Usually present	Usually absent

[a] During recovery phase of transient erythroblastopenia, fetal RBC features may be detected.

(Data from Glader[63] and Lanzkowsky.[64])

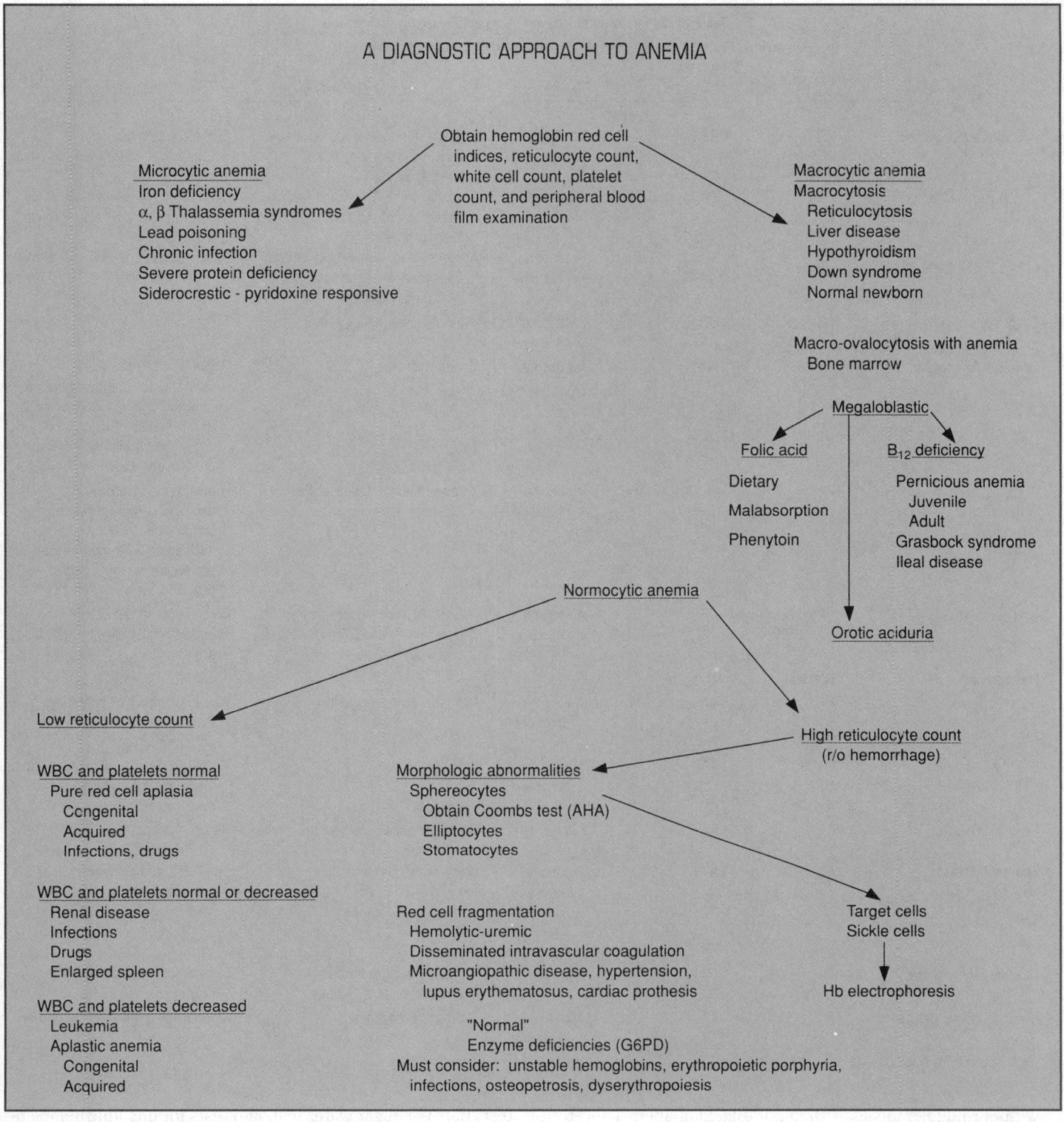

A DIAGNOSTIC APPROACH TO ANEMIA

Obtain hemoglobin red cell indices, reticulocyte count, white cell count, platelet count, and peripheral blood film examination

Microcytic anemia
Iron deficiency
α, β Thalassemia syndromes
Lead poisoning
Chronic infection
Severe protein deficiency
Siderocrestic - pyridoxine responsive

Macrocytic anemia
Macrocytosis
    Reticulocytosis
    Liver disease
    Hypothyroidism
    Down syndrome
    Normal newborn

Macro-ovalocytosis with anemia
    Bone marrow

Megaloblastic

Folic acid
Dietary
Malabsorption
Phenytoin

B_{12} deficiency
Pernicious anemia
    Juvenile
    Adult
Grasbock syndrome
Ileal disease

Orotic aciduria

Normocytic anemia

Low reticulocyte count

High reticulocyte count
(r/o hemorrhage)

WBC and platelets normal
Pure red cell aplasia
    Congenital
    Acquired
    Infections, drugs

WBC and platelets normal or decreased
Renal disease
Infections
Drugs
Enlarged spleen

WBC and platelets decreased
Leukemia
Aplastic anemia
    Congenital
    Acquired

Morphologic abnormalities
    Sphereocytes
        Obtain Coombs test (AHA)
    Elliptocytes
    Stomatocytes

Red cell fragmentation
    Hemolytic-uremic
    Disseminated intravascular coagulation
    Microangiopathic disease, hypertension,
        lupus erythematosus, cardiac prothesis

    "Normal"
    Enzyme deficiencies (G6PD)
Must consider: unstable hemoglobins, erythropoietic porphyria,
    infections, osteopetrosis, dyserythropoiesis

Target cells
Sickle cells

Hb electrophoresis

consideration, not so much for the correction of anemia but for the prevention of neurologic sequelae. History of pica and presence of basophilic stippling and elevated free erythrocyte protoporphyrin would suggest lead intoxication.

Careful examination of the peripheral smear often indicates abnormalities that point to a specific diagnosis or underlying abnormalities. Perhaps the most difficult group of patients are those with hemolytic anemias and red cell aplasia. In these circumstances as well as in hemoglobinopathies, critical information can often be obtained by examining the hemograms and peripheral blood smears from the parents. For these pa-

tients, the reticulocyte count, corrected as the reticulocyte index,† is an important guide to further evaluation.

The three major causes of pure red cell aplasia in children are Diamond-Blackfan anemia, transient erythroblastopenia of childhood (TEC), and acquired hypoplastic anemia associated

_____

† Correct for both degree of anemia and presence of polychromatophilic or "shift" cells, the reticulocyte index is calculated as follows: Reticulocyte index = (reticulocyte count × Hct/age-appropriate Hct) × ½.

Table 36-6. Features of Common Congenital Hemolytic Anemias

| Diagnosis | Hemoglobin Electrophoresis Pattern | | Pattern of Inheritance | Predominant Ethnic Group | Morphology |
	Cord Blood	Adult			
Sickle cell diseases					
Sickle cell anemia	FS	SS	Autosomal recessive	Africans, black Americans, Arabs, East Indians, Hispanics, Mediterraneans	Sickle cells, target cells, elliptocytes, nucleated red blood cells, reticulocytosis
S-β-thalassemia	FSA	SA (A_2 >3.5%)	Autsomal recessive	Africans, black Americans, Arabs, East Indians, Hispanics, Mediterraneans	Microcytes, occasional nucleated RBCs, reticulocytosis, variable sickle cells
SC	FSC	SC	Autosomal recessive	Africans, black Americans, Arabs, East Indians, Hispanics, Mediterraneans	Target cells, rare sickle cells, mild reticulocytosis
CC disease	FC	CC	Autosomal recessive	West Africans, black Americans	Target cells
Unstable hemoglobin	FA	AA	Autosomal recessive	Varies with type	Occasional schistocytes, spherocytes, and basophilic stippling and polychromatophilia (Heinz bodies after brilliant cresyl blue stain accentuated post splenectomy)
β-Thalassemia major and intermedia	FF	FF (A_2 >3.5%)	Autosomal recessive	Mediterraneans, Chinese, East Asians, East Indians	Hypochromic macrocytes, microcytes, basophilic stippling, target cells, ovalocytes, nucleated RBCs, and marked poikilocytosis, anisocytosis, and reticulocytosis
Hb H disease	FA and Barts >15%	AH	Autosomal recessive	Asians, Filipinos, Indonesians, occasionally Mediterraneans, rarely Africans	Microcytes, target cells (Heinz bodies after brilliant cresyl blue stain)
Hydrops fetalis	Barts	Nonviable			
Spherocytosis	FA	AA	Autosomal dominant	Northern European whites	Variable number of spherocytes (usually >10%), polychromatophilia
Elliptocytosis	FA	AA	Autosomal dominant	Various	Increased number of elliptocytes (may present in infancy as pyknocytosis)
Pyropoikilocytosis	FA	AA	Autosomal recessive	Black and occasionally white Americans	Bizarre poikilocytes
Stomatocytosis	FA	AA	Autosomal recessive and dominant forms	Unknown	10–50% stomatocytes, reticulocytosis
Glucose-6-phosphate	FA	AA	X-linked	Africans, black Americans, Mediterranneans, Asians	Spherocytes, nucleated RBCs, polychromatophilia
Pyruvate kinase deficiency	FA	AA	Autosomal recessive	Northern Europeans	Macrocytosis, polychromatophilia

(Adapted from Addiego et al.,[65] with permission.)

with chronic hemolysis.[63] Diamond-Blackfan anemia and transient erythroblastopenia are differentiated by features listed in Table 36-5).[63,64] Aplastic crises associated with chronic hemolytic anemias are characterized by the underlying process, the precipitous decrease in reticulocytes and hemoglobin concentration, and the frequent association of human parvovirus B19 (see Ch. 43).

The hemolytic anemias are a complex group of disorders associated with an elevated reticulocyte index (Table 36-6).[65] The correct diagnosis for an individual patient may be apparent after the history, physical examination, and routine blood studies. Frequently, however, additional tests, including hemoglobin electrophoresis, haptoglobin determination, red cell osmotic fragility, specific assays of RBC enzymes, acid hemolysis

test (Ham) or sugar water test, and tests for unstable hemoglobin, must be performed as outlined in other chapters.

Examination of bone marrow is important in the diagnosis of relatively few causes of anemia in childhood. These include megaloblastic, sideroblastic, aplastic, and dyserythropoietic anemias; acute leukemia; neuroblastoma; and lipid storage diseases.

Anemia is always an important finding that should prompt the physician to consider what underlying process may be responsible. In children, the most common causes of mild anemia, iron deficiency, acute inflammation, and thalassemia trait can be recognized and appropriately treated after a thorough medical history, physical examination, and performance of routine laboratory tests. Acquired acute anemias often produce diagnostic and treatment difficulties that demand the critical application of specialized laboratory tests and clinical expertise for appropriate management.

REFERENCES

1. Erslev A: Humoral regulation of red cell production. Blood 8:349, 1953
2. Adamson JW: The erythropoietin/hematocrit relationship in normal and polycythemic man: implications of marrow regulation. Blood 32:597, 1968
3. Jacobson L, Goldwasser E, Fried W et al: Role of the kidney in erythropoiesis. Nature 179:633, 1957
4. Lacombe C, Da Silva J, Brumeval P et al: Peritubular cells are the site of erythropoietin synthesis in the murine hypoxic kidney. J Clin Invest 81:620, 1988
5. Kay MB: Mechanism of removal of senescent cells by human macrophages in situ. Proc Natl Acad Sci USA 72:3521, 1975
6. Rosse W: The spleen as a filter. N Engl J Med 317:704, 1987
7. Weick J, Hagedorn A, Linman J: Leukoerythroblastosis—diagnostic and prognostic significance. Mayo Clin Proc 49:110, 1974
8. Herbert V: Experimental nutritional folate deficiency in man. Trans Assoc Am Physicians 75:307, 1962
9. Bodem C, Hamory B, Taylor H et al: Granulomatous bone marrow disease. Medicine 62:372, 1983
10. Mant MJ, Faraghen BS: The haematology of anorexia nervosa. Br J Haematol 23:737, 1972
11. Kitchens C: Clinical observations of human bone marrow macrophages. Medicine 56:503, 1977
12. Conley C, Misiti J, Laster A: Genetic factors predisposing to chronic lymphocytic leukemia and to autoimmune disease. Medicine 59:323, 1980
13. Zucker S, Friedman S, Lysck RM: Bone marrow erythropoiesis in the anemia of infection, inflammation and malignancy. J Clin Invest 53:1132, 1974
14. Cartwright GE: The anemia of chronic disorders. Semin Hematol 3:351, 1966
15. Doll D, Weiss R: Neoplasia and the erythron. J Clin Oncol 3:429, 1985
16. Eschbach J, Adamson J: Anemia of end-stage renal disease. Kidney Int 28:1, 1985
17. Boxer M, Ellman L, Geller R et al: Anemia in primary hyperparathyroidism. Arch Intern Med 137:588, 1977
18. Nagy E, Berczi I: Pituitary dependence of bone marrow function. Br J Haematol 71:457, 1989
19. Bessman JD, Gilmer PR, Gardner FH: Improved classification of anemias by MCV and RDW. Am J Clin Pathol 80:322, 1983
20. Witte DL, Kraemer DF, Johnson GF et al: Prediction of bone marrow iron findings from tests performed on peripheral blood. Am J Clin Pathol 85:202, 1986
21. Beutler E: Clinical evaluation of iron stores. N Engl J Med 256:692, 1957
22. Lipschitz DA, Cook JD, Finch CA: A clinical evaluation of serum ferritin as an index of iron stores. N Engl J Med 290:1213, 1974
23. Johnson CS, Tegos C, Beutler E: Thalassemia minor: routine erythrocyte measurements and differentiation from iron deficiency. Am J Clin Pathol 80:31, 1983
24. Beutler E: The common anemias. JAMA 259:2433, 1988
25. Douglas SW, Adamson JW: The anemia of chronic disorders: studies of marrow regulation and iron metabolism. Blood 45:55, 1975
26. Lee GR: The anemia of chronic disease. Semin Hematol 20:61, 1983
27. Beck WS: The metabolic basis of megaloblastic erythropoiesis. Medicine 43:715, 1964
28. Lindenbaum J, Nath BJ: Megaloblastic anemia and neutrophil hypersegmentation. Br J Haematol 44:511, 1980
29. Bennett JM, Catovsky D, Daniel MT et al: Proposals for the classification of myelodysplastic syndromes. Br J Haematol 51:189, 1982
30. Greenberg PL: The smoldering myeloid leukemic states: clinical and biologic features. Blood 61:1035, 1983
31. Fried W: Erythropoietin and the kidney. Nephron 15:327, 1975
32. Adamson JW, Eschbach J, Finch CA: The kidney and erythropoiesis. Am J Med 44:725, 1968
33. Tudhope GR, Wilson GM: Anaemia in hypothyroidism. Q J Med 29:513, 1960
34. Daughaday WH, Williams RH, Daland GA: The effect of endocrinopathies on the blood. Blood 3:1342, 1948
35. Castella A, Croxson TS, Mildvan D et al: The bone marrow in AIDS. Am J Clin Pathol 84:425, 1985
36. Bell CA, Zwicker J, Sacks HJ: Autoimmune hemolytic anemia: routine serologic evaluation in a general hospital population. Am J Clin Pathol 60:903, 1973
37. Pisciotta AV: Cold hemagglutination in acute and chronic hemolytic syndromes. Blood 10:295, 1955
38. Levine P, Celano MJ, Falkowski F: The specificity of the antibody in paroxysmal cold hemoglobinuria (PCH). Transfusion 3:278, 1963
39. Marsh GW, Lewis SM: Cardiac haemolytic anaemia. Semin Hematol 6:133, 1969
40. Brain MC, Dacie JV, Hourihane DO'B: Microangiopathic haemolytic anaemia: the possible role of vascular lesions in pathogenesis. Br J Haematol 8:358, 1962
41. Amorosi EL, Ultmann JE: Thrombotic thrombocytopenic purpura: report of 16 cases and review of the literature. Medicine 45:139, 1966
42. Antman KH, Skarin AT, Mayer RJ et al: Microangiopathic hemolytic anemia and cancer: a review. Medicine 58:377, 1979
43. Beutler E: The hemolytic effect of primaquine and related compounds: a review. Blood 14:103, 1959
44. Greenberg MS: Heinz body hemolytic anemia: bite cells—a clue to diagnosis. Arch Intern Med 136:153, 1976
45. Schmid R, Brecher G, Clemens T: Familial hemolytic anemia with erythrocyte inclusion bodies and a defect in pigment metabolism. Blood 14:991, 1959
46. Grimes AJ, Meisler A: Possible cause of Heinz bodies in congenital Heinz-body anemia. Nature 194:190, 1962
47. Rosse WF, Dacie JV: Immune lysis of normal human and paroxysmal nocturnal hemoglobinuria (PNH) red blood cells. I. The sensitivity of PNH red cells to lysis by complement and specific antibody. J Clin Invest 45:736, 1966
48. Smith JA, Lonergan ET, Sterling K: Spur-cell anemia. N Engl J Med 271:396, 1966
49. Conrad ME: Pathophysiology of malaria: hematologic observations in human and animal studies. Ann Intern Med 70:134, 1969
50. Ruebush TK, Cassaday PB, Marsh HJ et al: Human babesiosis on Nantucket Island: clinical features. Ann Intern Med 86:6, 1977
51. Reynafarje C, Ramos J: The hemolytic anemia of human bartonellosis. Blood 17:562, 1961
52. Dean HM, Decker CL, Baker LD: Temporary survival in clostridial hemolysis with absence of circulating red cells. N Engl J Med 277:700, 1967
53. Dallman PR, Siimes MA: Percentile curves for hemoglobin and red cell volume in infancy and childhood. J Pediatr 94:26, 1979
54. Stockman JA III: Anemia of Prematurity. Pediatr Clin North Am 33:111, 1986
55. Lundström U, Siimes MA, Dallman PR: At what age does iron supplementation become necessary in low-birth-weight infants? J Pediatr 91:878, 1977
56. Saarinen UM, Siimes MA: Developmental changes in red blood cell counts and indices of infants after exclusion of iron deficiency by laboratory criteria and continuous iron supplementation. J Pediatr 92:412, 1978
57. Dallman PR: Blood and blood-forming tissues. p. 1011. In Rudolph AM (ed): Pediatrics. 18th Ed. Appleton & Lange, E. Norwalk, CT, 1987
58. Reeves JD, Yip R, Kiley V, Dallman PR: Iron deficiency in infants: the influence of antecedent infection. J Pediatr 105:874, 1984
59. Dallman PR, Yip R: Changing characteristics of childhood anemia. J Pediatr 114:161, 1989
60. Beutler E: The common anemias. JAMA 259:2433, 1988
61. Yip R, Binkin NJ, Fleshood L, Trowbridge FL: Declining prevalence of anemia among low-income children in the United States. JAMA 258:1619, 1987
62. Yip R, Walsh KM, Goldfard MG, Binkin NJ: Declining childhood anemia prevalence in middle-class setting: a pediatric success story? Pediatrics 80:330, 1987
63. Glader BE: Diagnosis and management of red cell aplasia in children. Hematol Oncol Clin North Am 1:431, 1987
64. Lanzkowsky P: Pediatric Hematology-Oncology. McGraw-Hill, New York, 1980, p. 41
65. Addiego JE, Hurst D, Lubin BH: Congenital hemolytic anemia. Pediatr Rev 6:201, 1985

Erythrocytosis

37

Jerry L. Spivak

INTRODUCTION

Under normal circumstances, the red cell mass is maintained within narrow limits and is relatively constant in a given person, although it can vary between individuals of the same age and sex by 10%. In the presence of adequate nutrients, the red cell mass is in a dynamic equilibrium in which the red cells lost from the circulation each day through senescence are replaced by newly formed ones. Red cell production is regulated by erythropoietin (EPO), a glycoprotein hormone produced primarily in the kidneys in adults. EPO is a highly conserved protein, which bears no homology with any other protein.[1] Its gene is located on the long arm of chromosome 7 in humans,[2] and it encodes a protein that is identical, except that one more amino acid (Arg 166) is present,[3] to human urine EPO, the only native form of EPO purified to date.[4] In keeping with the constancy of the red cell mass in a given individual, the circulating level of EPO also remains constant unless hypoxia, anemia, or sudden blood loss intervenes. Indeed, EPO appears to be such an important regulatory or trophic factor that it is never absent from the plasma, even in the anephric state or when erythrocytosis is extreme. This chapter examines the mechanisms leading to erythrocytosis and the role of EPO in this process.

PHYSIOLOGY

Oxygen Transport

The principal function of the blood is to deliver oxygen from the lungs to the tissues. The primacy of oxygen transport in the body's economy can be easily inferred from the fact that basal metabolic processes consume oxygen at a rate of 4 ml/kg/min, while oxygen stores amount to only 20 ml/kg. Overall, oxygen transport is a complex process involving a variety of components, including ventilatory rate and volume, pulmonary diffusing capacity, cardiac output, red cell mass, hemoglobin/oxygen affinity, regional blood flow, and tissue capillary density, as well as ambient oxygen tension. The constancy of the red cell mass indicates that acute or transient changes in tissue oxygen demands or in ambient oxygen tension are met primarily by alterations in minute ventilation, cardiac output, distribution of blood flow, and hemoglobin oxygen affinity.[5-7] A sustained hypoxic stimulus, however, engenders changes in the red cell mass, in plasma volume, and eventually, in vascularity at the capillary level.[7,8] Erythrocytosis therefore suggests the presence of either sustained tissue hypoxia, autonomous EPO production, or (in the absence of an appropriate or inappropriate increase in EPO production) autonomous red cell proliferation.

Red Cell Production and Regulation

An understanding of EPO physiology is central to understanding the pathophysiology of erythrocytosis. Under normal circumstances, EPO is produced constitutively by peritubular interstitial cells in the inner cortex of the kidney.[9-11] The identity of these cells is unknown, but it appears that they are the site not only of EPO production but also of the oxygen sensor

that stimulates EPO production.[12] The oxygen sensor appears to be a heme protein that controls the accumulation of EPO mRNA in an unknown fashion.[13]

EPO production by individual renal peritubular interstitial cells appears to be an all-or-none phenomenon, since anemia or hypoxia recruits additional cells to produce EPO, rather than increasing hormone production in the cells that produce it constitutively.[11] As a corollary, the kidney has no performed stores of EPO, and changes in circulating EPO are a direct consequence of changes in the production of the hormone.[14] With correction of anemia or hypoxia, EPO production ceases except in those cells that were producing it constitutively. Since no evidence has been found to suggest that hypoxia or anemia alters the plasma clearance of EPO, it appears that its concentration in the circulation is regulated at the level of gene expression. Indeed, studies in hypoxic rodents show a close correlation between renal EPO and plasma EPO concentrations, with the latter lagging behind the former.[15]

EPO is also constitutively produced in the liver in both hepatocytes and interstitial cells. In contrast to the situation in the kidneys, however, EPO production in hepatocytes is not all or none but can be regulated in each cell.[16] The degree of hypoxia required to up-regulate liver EPO production is, however, greater than that required to induce renal EPO production. Thus, with mild hypoxia, the liver contributes little to the plasma EPO concentration; with more severe hypoxia, because of its bulk, the liver becomes a substantial source of EPO.[17]

Although small but significant changes in serum immunoreactive EPO can be detected with hypoxia[18] or changes in the hematocrit if serial measurements are obtained,[19] unequivocal elevations of serum EPO outside the normal range (4–26 mU/ml) do not occur until the hemoglobin level falls to <10.5 g%.[20] Thus, random EPO determinations are not a useful means for establishing the adequacy of EPO production in situations of slight anemia. Whether a similar threshold exists for hypoxia is unclear because no simple means is available for analyzing oxygen delivery at the tissue level. Careful studies in patients with cyanotic congenital heart disease suggest that such a threshold does not exist.[18]

The changes in the level of EPO in the circulation in response to hypoxia are instructive with regard to the body's mechanisms in compensating for this state. Exposure to hypobaric hypoxia results in a detectable increase in circulating EPO within a few hours.[21] The elevation in the EPO level is not usually sustained, however, even though the hypobaric hypoxia persists,[15,21-24] and the level usually falls to within the normal range, unless the hypoxia is extreme.[24] However, because the normal range for plasma EPO is wide (4–26 mU/ml), an increase of 10–20 mU/ml, while still within the normal range, constitutes a doubling of the plasma concentration and would be expected to elevate basal red cell production.

This unusual behavior can be explained as follows. Hypoxia generates acute changes in minute ventilation, heart rate, tissue blood flow, and hemoglobin/oxygen affinity. Hyperventilation improves alveolar oxygen delivery, increases arterial oxygen tension (PaO_2) and arterial oxygen saturation (SaO_2), and maintains the diffusion gradient between the blood and the tissues. An additional effect of hyperventilation is reduction in carbon dioxide tension, resulting in respiratory alkalosis. The change in arterial pH stimulates the synthesis in erythrocytes of the organic phosphate 2,3-diphosphoglycerate (2,3-DPG). This important compound, which is present in red cells in amounts equimolar with hemoglobin,[25] binds to hemoglobin and reduces its oxygen affinity. Although alkalosis increases hemoglobin/oxygen affinity—that is, reduces the P_{50} of the hemoglobin (the partial pressure of oxygen at which hemoglobin is half-saturated with oxygen)—the increase in red cell 2,3-DPG not only counteracts the increase in hemoglobin/oxygen affinity but actually reduces it (increases P_{50}) and enhances oxygen unloading at the tissue level. The net effect is improved oxygen delivery to tissues.

If the adaptive mechanisms described effectively correct hypoxia and improve tissue oxygen delivery, the stimulus for EPO production will be removed, and plasma EPO will diminish to the extent that the hypoxia is corrected. If, however, hypoxia is extreme, 2,3-DPG production alone cannot compensate for the respiratory alkalosis; hemoglobin/oxygen affinity will remain increased and elevated EPO production will persist. Hypoxia does not, however, have to be continuous, or even extreme, to stimulate EPO production. Thus, intermittent hypobaric hypoxia can produce erythrocytosis in rodents,[26] while supine hypoventilation or sleep apnea has the same effect in humans.[27-29]

It is worth emphasizing that in addition to the EPO-mediated elevation of the red cell mass, hypoxia is also associated with a diminution in plasma volume. This abnormality appears to be independent of the cause of hypoxia since it occurs not only at high altitudes[8] but also in cyanotic congenital heart disease[30] and in cigarette smokers.[31] Whether the reduction in plasma volume is part of a physiologic adaptation to tissue hypoxia is unclear. When it is extreme (as described below), it can have a deleterious effect.

An interesting but unexplained effect of erythrocytosis is suppression of EPO production independent of tissue oxygenation.[32] The observed reduction in plasma volume associated with hypoxic erythrocytosis probably serves as a means of facilitating this effect, thereby preventing an overexuberant response to hypoxia, since simple elevation of plasma viscosity inhibits EPO production.[33] This explains in part the observation that EPO levels are often within the normal range in patients with secondary erythrocytosis and compensated hypoxia.

CLINICAL MANIFESTATIONS

The signs and symptoms associated with erythrocytosis are nonspecific. Unless the cause of hypoxia is evident or unless erythrocytosis is extreme, there may be no unequivocal evidence of its presence. Indeed, William Osler, who provided one of the early and important descriptions of polycythemia rubra vera, also cautioned that even anemic patients could appear plethoric (anemia rubra). Thus, a high hematocrit, hemoglobin, or erythrocyte count, rather than a characteristic symptom or physical finding, may be the first clue to an elevation of the red cell mass. Since alterations in the plasma volume can influence these measurements, they cannot be relied on as indicators of the absolute red cell mass. Even when the plasma volume is not diminished, the hematocrit and the red cell mass are not directly correlated. Therefore, consideration of the causes of a high hematocrit must include a number of possibilities that could artifactually raise the hematocrit, hemoglobin, or erythrocyte values (see the section Serum Erythropoietin).

When considering these diagnostic possibilities, it is important not to overlook clues provided by the peripheral blood smear and the red cell indices. For example, in true plethora a properly prepared blood smear obtained from the fingertip will reveal red cell crowding out of proportion to what is expected from the apparent hematocrit value. Furthermore, an

---

CAUSES OF A HIGH HEMATOCRIT

Relative or spurious erythrocytosis
   Hemoconcentration secondary to dehydration (diarrhea, diaphoresis, diuretics, deprivation of water, emesis, ethanol), hypertension, preeclampsia, pheochromocytoma, carbon monoxide intoxication
Absolute erythrocytosis: hypoxia
   Carbon monoxide intoxication
   High oxygen-affinity hemoglobin
   High altitude
   Pumonary disease
   Supine hypoventilation syndrome
   Sleep apnea syndrome
   Right to left cardiac shunts
   Neurologic defects (respiratory center dysfunction)
Renal disease
   Cysts, hydronephrosis
   Renal artery stenosis
   Focal glomerulonephritis
   Renal transplantation
Tumors
   Hypernephroma
   Hepatoma
   Cerebellar hemangioblastoma
   Uterine fibromyoma
   Adrenal tumors
   Meningioma
   Pheochromocytoma
Antrogen therapy
Bartter syndrome
Familial erythrocytosis (with normal hemoglobin function)
Polycythemia vera

---

elevated red cell count in association with microcytosis should suggest the presence of autonomous or EPO-driven erythrocytosis, since this situation otherwise only occurs with thalassemia minor, a disorder not associated with a high hematocrit or hemoglobin level.[34] The presence of leukocytosis, thrombocytosis, or splenomegaly should also suggest the presence of polycythemia vera, but these abnormalities are not always present early in the course of that illness.

LABORATORY EVALUATION

Red Cell Mass Determination

The first obligation of the physician when confronted with a reproducibly high hematocrit or hemoglobin level is to determine whether the red cell mass shows an absolute increase. This can only be done accurately by direct measurement, using the technique of isotope dilution. With this technique, an aliquot of the patient's red cells is labeled with a radioactive tracer and reinfused. The red cell mass can then be calculated from the degree of dilution of the isotopically labeled red cells. It is important to remember in this regard that, in erythrocytosis (particularly in patients with splenomegaly), equilibration of the injected labeled red cells with the total blood pool may be delayed relative to the situation when the blood volume is normal. Therefore, serial blood samples should be taken over a period of approximately 90 minutes to ensure that equilibration is complete.

A direct measurement of the red mass effectively separates those patients with a reduced plasma volume from those with absolute erythrocytosis. Once the presence of erythrocytosis has been established, the cause must be sought. Depending on the severity of the plethora, one may be required to initiate treatment, even while the diagnostic evaluation is proceeding.

Serum Erythropoietin

Many factors can cause erythrocytosis. Defining the precise cause may not be possible either initially or even after prolonged evaluation; nonetheless, some guidelines can be suggested. Since erythropoiesis is regulated by EPO, a serum EPO level can provide an indication of whether the erythrocytosis is hormonally mediated or autonomous. Although prior assays for EPO in the serum were insensitive and not widely available, the production of recombinant EPO has led to development of a specific, sensitive, accurate, reproducible and commercially available radioimmunoassay.[35]

In patients with erythrocytosis due to uncompensated hypoxia, serum immunoreactive EPO is elevated; in those with compensated hypoxia, the serum immunoreactive EPO level is usually within the range of normal,[18,36,37] and in patients with polycythemia vera, serum immunoreactive EPO is either normal or low.[20,38] The number of patients with autonomous EPO production studied with a sensitive and specific EPO assay is too small to date to permit firm conclusions, but EPO levels in these patients can be either high or normal and may even fluctuate, suggesting that serial measurements may be necessary to detect an abnormality.[38] This would also be important in those patients with the supine hypoventilation syndrome or sleep apnea in whom serum EPO may be only intermittently elevated.[27] Thus, while an elevated serum EPO level suggests that erythrocytosis is a secondary phemonenon and a low EPO level supports the possibility of autonomous erythropoiesis, a normal serum EPO level excludes neither hypoxia nor autonomous EPO production as the cause of erythrocytosis.

Blood Gas Measurements

An elevated EPO level indicates that erythrocytosis is hormonally driven but does not establish the cause of this mechanism. A normal level does not exclude hypoxia as a cause of erythrocytosis. Therefore, a concomitant assessment of PaO_2 and SaO_2 is required in the evaluation of all patients with erythrocytosis because hypoxia is a correctable cause of this disorder. Patients with polycythemia vera will invariably have a normal PaO_2 and an SaO_2 of 90% unless there is coexisting pulmonary disease.[39] However, it is important to be aware that the PaO_2 is a relatively insensitive indicator of hypoxia. This is because heme-heme interactions during oxygen binding render hemoglobin fully saturated over a wide PaO_2 range. It is only when the PaO_2 falls to <67 mmHg that one encounters an appreciable increase in red cell mass.[40]

SaO_2 is, however, a more sensitive indicator of potential tissue hypoxia, since it is directly related to red cell mass.[40] In this regard, it is important to remember that in the presence of an elevated red cell mass, the serum EPO level may be normal even if the SaO_2 is low, owing to the compensatory increase in tissue oxygenation produced by the erythrocytosis.

There are also two situations causing hypoxic erythrocytosis in which the SaO_2 can be misleading: high oxygen affinity (low P_{50}) hemoglobins and carbon monoxide intoxication. In the former condition, the SaO_2 will be normal, but tissue hypoxia will exist; at ambient tissue oxygen tensions, high oxygen-affinity hemoglobins will not release their oxygen.

One must also be aware of the complexities of interpreting SaO_2 values in carbon monoxide poisoning. If an indirect method for determining SaO_2 is employed (e.g., calculating it from the measured PaO_2 and a standard oxygen dissociation curve), a normal value will be obtained when, SaO_2 is in fact low owing to the binding by hemoglobin of carbon monoxide.[41] Thus, for detection of a high oxygen-affinity hemoglobin, determination of its oxygen affinity (P_{50}) is mandatory. Detection of carbon monoxide intoxication requires both a direct determination of SaO_2 by oximetry and quantitation of the percentage of carboxyhemoglobin.

ETIOLOGIES

Hypoxic Erythrocytosis

Hypobaric Hypoxia

The prototypical model for hypoxic erythrocytosis is high-altitude hypoxia. Exposure to high altitudes leads acutely to the predictable changes in minute ventilation, heart rate, blood flow, and hemoglobin/oxygen affinity described earlier. Serum EPO is elevated initially but eventually falls to within the normal range if the hypoxia is not extreme. This decline, however, does not prevent an increase in red cell mass, which will be sustained. This effect occurs both because EPO can potentiate its own effects and because expansion of the erythroid progenitor cell pool is exponential—only picomolar quantities of the hormone are required to sustain the red cell mass under normal circumstances. Since early erythroid progenitor cells, at least in vitro, require 10^3 times as much EPO as do late erythroid progenitor cells,[42] the early unsustained increase in serum EPO probably serves to facilitate recruitment of additional erythroid progenitor cells to expand the progenitor cell pool, while smaller quantities of the hormone can maintain this pool once it is expanded.

Concomitant with the changes cited above is a reduction in plasma volume.[8] While initially this could be the consequence of fluid loss associated with hyperventilation and the low humidity of high altitude, similar changes are also seen at sea level in patients with hypoxic erythrocytosis due to cyanotic congenital heart disease,[30] in those with chronic carbon monoxide intoxication,[31] and in those with end-stage renal disease who are receiving recombinant human EPO.[43] Thus, a decrease in plasma volume appears to be a component of the compensatory EPO-induced erythrocytosis associated with hypoxia. Other noteworthy compensatory changes associated with high-altitude hypoxia are developmental and require sustained altitude exposure; they include an increase in lung volume and capillary density and a blunted ventilatory response to hypoxia.[7,44,45] Since the latter also occurs in patients with cyanotic congenital heart disease,[44] it is not peculiar to hypobaric hypoxia.

Chronic mountain sickness is an extreme response to hypobaric hypoxia in which the elevation of the red cell mass fails to compensate adequately for hypoxia.[46] In this situation, the erythrocytosis far exceeds that expected for the degree of hypobaric hypoxia, and there is symptomatic hyperviscosity. Chronic mountain sickness appears to be the consequence of an additional acquired ventilatory defect superimposed on the adaptive blunted ventilatory response that occurs during chronic exposure to high altitude.[45]

Chronic Pulmonary Disease

Hypoxia occurring with chronic lung disease represents a more complicated clinical situation than hypobaric hypoxia, since the erythrocytosis expected for the measured degree of hypoxia is not always present. This, however, appears to be more a matter of patient selection than an indication of a new paradigm.[40,47] For example, in some patients an increase in plasma volume due to fluid retention masks the increase in red cell mass.[48] In other patients clinical measurements of tissue oxygenation may not accurately reflect the actual level of tissue oxygenation, while in still others, inflammation, infection, or renal disease may impair erythropoiesis, thus blunting the marrow's response to EPO. Finally, as observed in certain patients with high-affinity hemoglobins, there may be tolerance to a particular level of tissue hypoxia.[49] In general, however, patients with impaired pulmonary function demonstrate the expected correlation between SaO_2 and red cell mass and may even have a "steeper" response than that of healthy persons.[40] Their ability to produce EPO is also more vigorous and the threshold for this is reduced.[50]

The sleep apnea syndrome and supine hypoventilation due to premature airway closure are two special situations in which hypoxia can develop without overt evidence of pulmonary disease.[27–29] In each instance, hypoxia is intermittent. A random blood gas or EPO measurement may thus fail to reveal the underlying cause of the erythrocytosis.

Chronic Carbon Monoxide Intoxication

Chronic carbon monoxide intoxication, usually as the consequence of cigarette use, is probably the commonest cause of erythrocytosis encountered clinically. It is responsible for the syndrome commonly referred to as stress erythrocytosis,[51] benign polycythemia,[52] or spurious erythrocytosis.[53] Carbon monoxide is the perfect respiratory poison. Odorless and colorless, carbon monoxide has an affinity for hemoglobin 210 times as great as that of oxygen. This is attributable not to a greater rate of association of carbon monoxide with hemoglobin as compared with oxygen but rather to its slower rate of dissociation from hemoglobin. Not only does the binding of carbon monoxide with hemoglobin reduce the quantity of oxygen that can be bound, it also shifts the oxyhemoglobin dissociation curve to the left, thereby reducing the ability of hemoglobin to unload oxygen to the tissues.[54] Furthermore, carboxyhemoglobin has a reduced affinity for 2,3-DPG. At a high carbon monoxide concentration, red cell 2,3-DPG production is suppressed.[55] Thus, carbon monoxide not only causes tissue hypoxia but also subverts the mechanisms designed to compensate for the hypoxia.

An additional, but often unrecognized, effect of carbon monoxide intoxication is diminution of plasma volume.[31] When combined with an elevation of the red cell mass, this creates a situation in which erythrocytosis occurs with a normal total blood volume, with the attentant problem of hyperviscosity. The variable extent to which elevation of the red cell mass and depression of the plasma volume can occur in patients with carbon monoxide intoxication has led to the description of syndromes of spurious erythrocytosis due to a "high normal red cell mass" or a "low normal plasma volume,"[53] but these syndromes probably only represent part of the continuum of carbon monoxide toxicity.

Although the term *benign polycythemia* has been used to describe erythrocytosis-associated carbon monoxide intoxication, the syndrome is anything but benign. Several series have demonstrated a substantial incidence of thromboembolic events, and in one study a mortality rate six times as great as expected for unaffected individuals of the same age was observed.[56]

Cyanotic Congenital Heart Disease

Congenital heart disease with anatomic right-to-left shunting is a predictable cause of erythrocytosis.[57] Such patients are similar to those with hypobaric hypoxia with respect to having a blunted ventilatory response and a low plasma volume, but in addition, they may have a coagulopathy with a low fibrinogen and a low platelet count.[57–59] When the erythrocytosis compensates for arterial oxygen desaturation, the serum EPO level will be normal.[18] However, phlebotomy will result in a marked increase in serum erythropoietin owing to the reversal of the compensatory erythrocytosis. In a manner similar to that encountered in hypobaric hypoxia, patients with cyanotic congenital heart disease can develop a syndrome resembling chronic mountain sickness. This phenomenon results from hypoxia that cannot be compensated for by erythrocytosis.[60]

High Oxygen-Affinity Hemoglobins

High oxygen-affinity hemoglobins that are unable to unload oxygen to the tissues at an acceptable tissue oxygen tension are an uncommon but interesting cause of hypoxic erythrocytosis. The first high-affinity hemoglobin, hemoglobin Chesapeake, was identified in 1966 in an 81-year-old man who was being evaluated for angina pectoris.[61] As of 1989, >40 such mutant hemoglobins have been described. These mutants may be stable or unstable; a few are not associated with erythrocytosis.[62]

Hemoglobin normally exists in an equilibrium between its oxygenated (relaxed or R) state and its deoxygenated (tense or T) state (see Ch. 161). The transition between these states involves changes in molecular conformation and intramolecular bonding. In the deoxy or T state, hemoglobin has a high affinity for 2,3-DPG and hydrogen ions, while in the oxygenated or R state, these affinities are reduced. In general, high oxygen-affinity hemoglobins arise from amino acid substitutions that prevent the obligatory conformational changes in the molecule during oxygenation and deoxygenation, particularly those that (1) involve the α_1-β_2 interface of the globin chains within the hemoglobin tetramer and stabilize it in the oxygenated state; (2) involve the C-terminal end of the β-globin chain and prevent the formation of ionic bonds; or (3) impair 2,3-DPG binding.[62]

Clinically, erythrocytosis is the major abnormality associated with a high oxygen-affinity hemoglobin, and its extent is proportional to the P_{50} of the mutant hemoglobin.[63] Interestingly, occasional patients have a low plasma volume. Affected individuals are heterozygotes, with the mutant hemoglobin accounting for approximately 40% of their total hemoglobin. The inheritance pattern is therefore dominant. A family history can be revealing, if positive. A negative history does not rule out the diagnosis, however, because of the high frequency of spontaneous mutations. Because of the nature or position of the amino acid substitution, not all high oxygen-affinity hemoglobins can be detected by routine electrophoretic techniques. An electrophoretic abnormality would not, however, establish that the hemoglobin had a high oxygen affinity. A P_{50} determination is the only reliable means of establishing this. Of course, carboxyhemoglobin or a low red cell 2,3-DPG can cause a low P_{50}. In evaluating the possibility of a high oxygen-affinity hemoglobin, a study of other family members is also important.

Inappropriate Erythropoietin Secretion

Erythrocytosis Due to Renal Disease

Since the kidneys are the major site of EPO production in adults, renal disease may cause erythrocytosis as well as anemia. Although it has been suggested that a high hematocrit associated with hypertension may be a clue to the presence of renal artery stenosis,[64] it must be remembered that hypertension per se is associated with a reduction in plasma volume.[65] Experimentally, renal artery stenosis does cause an increase in serum EPO, but this is usually modest and not of the magnitude associated with anemia.[66] It has been suggested that this effect reflects a decline in renal oxygen consumption as renal blood flow falls. Whatever the mechanism, while examples of renal artery stenosis associated with erythrocytosis have been described, they are not common.[67,68]

Renal cysts have been implicated as a cause of inappropriate EPO production, but the most striking example of this has been in patients with autosomal dominant polycystic disease and renal failure, in whom anemia is unexpectedly mild while EPO levels are elevated.[70] Acquired cystic disease has also been described in patients undergoing chronic renal dialysis and presenting with a similar clinical picture.[71] More frequently, however, renal cysts develop in these patients without any amelioration of anemia or erythrocytosis.[72] In other patients, the erythocytosis identified with renal cysts was actually due to polycythemia vera.[73]

Patients with focal glomerulonephritis, with or without the nephrotic syndrome, constitute another group in whom renal disease is associated with erythrocytosis.[74,75] Indeed, this association has been described with sufficient frequency to suggest that renal function should be examined in patients with unexplained erythrocytosis. In general, the erythrocytosis is a temporary event during the course of the renal disease.

Erythrocytosis can also be a complication of renal transplantation.[76–78] The mechanism for this is unclear, but it does not appear to involve rejection and has been seen with cadaver kidneys as well as with kidneys from living donors.[79] It has been postulated that the erythrocytosis in this situation does not arise from the transplanted kidney but rather from the patient's own kidneys.[80,81] In some instances, the erythrocytosis may actually be spurious and due to overzealous use of diuretics.[82] A rare cause of erythrocytosis associated with renal disease is Bartter syndrome.[83,84]

Tumor-Associated Erythrocytosis

Erythrocytosis associated with a tumor is a rare paraneoplastic syndrome, which has excited the imagination of physicians far beyond its clinical frequency. Unfortunately, few studies of this phenomenon have used a sensitive and specific assay for EPO. Renal tumors, both benign and malignant, have been associated with erythrocytosis and the production of EPO mRNA by renal carcinoma cells has recently been demonstrated.[86] It is of interest that erythrocytosis associated with renal, hepatic, or cerebellar tumors is more common in men.[85] It is also of interest that three of the tumors associated with erythrocytosis—hypernephroma, cerebellar hemangioma, and pheochromocytoma—are part of the constellation of von Hippel-Lindau disease, which suggests a common underlying genetic mechanism.[89] It is also noteworthy that, in patients with hepatomas, an expanded plasma volume can obscure the presence of erythrocytosis.[85] Although one might, on the basis of studies of EPO excretion,[98] expect EPO levels to be inappropriately high in patients with tumor-associated erythrocytosis, this issue has not yet been resolved.

Familial Erythrocytosis

Familial erythrocytosis is an uncommon condition for which the identified syndromes and causes are listed above. Depending on the syndrome, inheritance may be dominant or recessive.[99–107] Few such families, however, have been studied with a sensitive and specific assay for EPO. When carefully studied, EPO levels were either normal or elevated and not always influenced by phlebotomy. Erythroid progenitor cell sensitivity to EPO was either normal or increased. In several families, no evidence for abnormalities of EPO receptor gene expression or binding affinity was observed.[107] In one family, however, erythrocytosis was genetically linked to the EPO receptor gene, suggesting that a receptor mutation was responsible for the erythrocytosis, since plasma EPO levels in this family were normal or low.[108] Most recently, DNA sequence analysis has revealed truncation of this receptor with loss of the last 70 amino acids of the C-terminal domain only in affected siblings.[108a] Since, experimentally, removal of the C-terminal domain of the EPO receptor increases its sensitivity to EPO,[108b] it is likely that the observed genetic mutation has had the same effect in this kindred. In one patient with erythrocytosis and a low erythrocyte 2,3-DPG level, a deficiency of diphosphoglycerate mutase was found.[106] Some patients with familial erythrocytosis, however, had an elevated red cell 2,3-DPG level, suggesting an unrecognized cause for hypoxia, while in others the cause may have been unidentified renal disease or cigarette smoking. Whatever the mechanism, erythrocytosis has been observed to have adverse effects in a number of these patients,

---

BEST ESTABLISHED ASSOCIATIONS BETWEEN TUMORS AND INAPPROPRIATE ERYTHROPOIETIN PRODUCTION

Hypernephroma[85–88]	More common in men. Erythrocyte sedimentation rate is often elevated. Associated with von Hippel-Lindau disease.
Wilms tumor[85] Renal adenoma[85] Undifferentiated renal carcinoma[85]	
Hepatoma[85,90,91]	More common in men. Increase in plasma volume may obscure the elevated red cell mass.
Liver hamartoma[85]	
Cerebellar hemangioblastoma[85,92,93]	More common in men. Metastases can be confused with those of a hypernephroma. Associated with von Hippel-Lindau disease.
Uterine fibromyoma[94,95]	Tumor extracts (only from very large tumors) contain erythropoietic activity.
Pheochromocytoma[85]	Rare. Spurious elevation of the hematocrit can occur owing to decreased plasma volume. Associated with von Hippel-Lindau disease.
Adrenal adenoma or hemangioblastoma[89] Paraganglioma[96] Meningioma[97]	Associated with van Hippel-Lindau disease.

FAMILIAL ERYTHROCYTOSIS

High oxygen-affinity hemogloblin
Diphosphoglycerate mutase deficiency
    With increased erythropoietin production
    With normal erythropoietin production
    Polycythemia vera

and phlebotomy therapy should be employed to maintain the red cell mass at a safe level.[99,100] It should also be remembered that polycythemia vera is occasionally familial.

Polycythemia Vera Rubra

Polycythemia vera is a form of myeloproliferative syndrome in which the granulocyte, monocyte, and platelet counts as well as the red cell count, are usually elevated (see Ch. 72). This disorder appears to represent occupancy of the marrow by the progeny of a neoplastic clone of stem cells, which proliferates with inappropriate exuberance for any given level of external stimulus. Since polycythemia vera is discussed in detail in Chapter 72, it is not considered further here, except to note that elevation of the counts in all three major cell lineages (red blood cells, white blood cells, and platelets) and the presence of splenomegaly should lead one to suspect this diagnosis strongly as a cause of erythrocytosis.

EVALUATION AND MANAGEMENT

The two goals in dealing with a patient with erythrocytosis are identification of a correctable cause and reduction of the red cell mass. With respect to the medical history, prior blood counts are important in documenting the onset and duration of the erythrocytosis. The blood counts of family members may be useful in establishing an inherited basis for it. In general, with the exception of pruritus, the symptoms associated with polycythemia vera are not different from those associated with secondary erythrocytosis. The occupational, environmental, and social history of the patient may also yield important clues, especially with regard to pulmonary disease and carbon monoxide intoxication. The drug history should not be overlooked, since androgenic steroids, which may be administered for therapeutic, cosmetic, or competitive purposes or mistakenly to improve libido, can cause erythrocytosis.[109-111] The physical examination may suggest a cardiac or pulmonary cause and, with respect to the latter, sleep apnea syndrome must not be ignored. Splenomegaly should suggest the presence of a myeloproliferative disorder, but its absence does not exclude this possibility.

Laboratory evaluation should be dictated by common sense. Leukocytosis and thrombocytosis suggest polycythemia vera but, once again, their absence does not exclude this disorder. A urinalysis is mandatory, and a serum EPO measurement should always be obtained, but only by an assay using recombinant-derived reagents.[35] If it is normal, a repeat assay may be worthwhile if an EPO-producing lesion is suspected.[38] If supine erythrocytosis is suspected, a blood sample for assay should be obtained under the appropriate circumstances. A direct measurement of SaO_2 should be obtained, as should a carboxyhemoglobin level. Since the half-life of carboxyhemoglobin is approximately 7 hours, the measurement may be normal if exposure has been interrupted before the patient seeks medical attention.

If the evaluation to this point has not been revealing, renal evaluation with respect to kidney size, presence of anatomic abnormalities, and blood flow is indicated. In the absence of neurologic signs or symptoms, an abdominal computed tomography scan should complete the evaluation for paraneoplastic erythrocytosis. Since high oxygen-affinity hemoglobins may not migrate abnormally on electrophoresis, and even an electrophophoretic abnormality does not by itself establish an oxygen-binding abnormality, a P_{50} determination should be obtained if the history is suggestive and no other cause of erythrocytosis is evident.

In the absence of a clinical assay for establishing clonality with respect to erythrocytosis, even after all the tests mentioned above have been performed, the diagnosis may not be forthcoming. This problem should not influence the management protocol; treatment of unexplained erythrocytosis is no different from that of polycythemia vera. In each instance, the problem is an expanded red cell mass, which in the case of secondary erythrocytosis may be coupled with a reduction in plasma volume. The net result of these abnormalities is an increase in peripheral vascular resistance, a reduction in cardiac output, and a decline in systemic oxygen transport.[112] Cerebral blood flow is invariably reduced with any form of erythrocytosis,[113-115] and this may result in impaired glucose delivery to the brain.[116] Therefore, there is no such thing as "benign" erythrocytosis, as thromboembolic complications have been recorded with every form of the disorder and no symptoms may have been exhibited beforehand. It is therefore recommended that all patients with erythrocytosis without a correctable cause undergo phlebotomy.

In patients with pulmonary disease, cyanotic congenital heart disease, or a high oxygen-affinity hemoglobin, the extent of phlebotomy can be dictated by the patient's symptomatic response or by the serum EPO level as a measure of tissue hypoxia. In these disorders, even limited phlebotomy has proved symptomatically beneficial.[117-121] In cyanotic congenital heart disease, proteinuria may be reduced[122] and the coagulopathy improved.[58] In patients with a low plasma volume, phlebotomy is not deleterious and actually stimulates an increase in the plasma volume. If possible, phlebotomy should be continued until the hematocrit is <45%, since anything less vigorous may be associated with a persistent reduction in cerebral blood flow.[114] Contrary to published commentary, it is always possible to control the red cell mass by phlebotomy if venous access is adequate, because sustained phlebotomy induces iron deficiency with certainty. Phlebotomy does not, despite anecdotal beliefs, cause hyperviscosity by producing rigid microcytotic red cells. In adults, induced iron deficiency never causes clinically significant hyperviscosity due to the rigidity of iron-poor red cells.[123] This is because it is impossible to increase the red cell mass sufficiently to cause hyperviscosity in true iron deficiency. Furthermore, it has been well demonstrated that chronic iron deficiency in adults in the absence of anemia does not impair functional aerobic performance.[124]

In summary, erythrocytosis presents a diagnostic challenge to the physician, and in some cases no conclusive answer concerning its mechanism will be immediately evident. The clinical evaluation should follow a logical progression, and even in the absence of a firm diagnosis, therapeutic phlebotomy can and should be employed. Chemotherapeutic agents are never indicated for reduction of the red cell mass.[125] Since this is true in polycythemia vera as well as in secondary erythrocytosis, lack of a definite diagnosis will not adversely affect prognosis as long as the red cell mass is adequately controlled.

REFERENCES

1. Shoemaker CB, Mitsock LD: Murine erythropoietin gene: cloning, expression, and gene homology. Mol Cell Biol 6:849, 1986
2. Law ML, Cai G-Y, Lin F-K et al: Chromosomal assignment of the human erythropoietin gene and its DNA polymorphism. Proc Natl Acad Sci USA 83: 6920, 1986
3. Recny MA, Scoble HA, Kim Y: Structural characterization of natural human urinary and recombinant DNA-derived erythropoietin. J Biol Chem 262: 17156, 1987
4. Miyake T, Kung CK-H, Goldwasser E: Purification of human erythropoietin. J Biol Chem 252:5558, 1977
5. Torrance JD, Lenfant C, Cruz J et al: Oxygen transport mechanisms in residents at high altitude. Respir Physiol 11:1, 1970
6. Heistad DD, Abboud FM: Circulatory adjustments to hypoxia. Circulation 61:463, 1980
7. Frisancho AR: Functional adaptation to high altitude hypoxia. Science 187: 313, 1975
8. Sanchez C, Merino C, Figallo M: Simultaneous measurement of plasma volume and cell mass in polycythemia of high altitude. J Appl Physiol 28:775, 1970
9. Koury ST, Bondurant MC, Koury MJ: Localization of erythropoietin synthesizing cells in murine kidneys by in situ hybridization. Blood 71:524, 1988

10. Lacomb C, DaSilva L, Bruneval P et al: Peritubular cells are the site of erythropoietin synthesis in the murine hypoxic kidney. J Clin Invest 81:620, 1988

11. Koury ST, Koury MJ, Bondurant MC et al: Quantitation of erythropoietin-producing cells in kidneys of mice by in situ hybridization: correlation with hematocrit, renal erythropoietin mRNA, and serum erythropoietin concentration. Blood 74:645, 1989

12. Schuster SJ, Badiavas EV, Costa-Giomi P et al: Stimulation of erythropoietin transcription during hypoxia and cobalt exposure. Blood 73:13, 1989

13. Goldberg MA, Dunning SP, Bunn HF: Regulation of the erythropoietin gene: evidence that the oxygen sensor is a heme protein. Science 242:1412, 1988

14. Schooley JC, Mahlmann LJ: Evidence for the de novo synthesis of erythropoietin in hypoxic rats. Blood 40:662, 1972

15. Jelkmann W: Temporal pattern of erythropoietin titers in kidney tissue during hypoxic hypoxia. Pflugers Arch 393:88, 1982

16. Koury ST, Bondurant MC, Doury MJ et al: Localization of cells producing erythropoietin in murine liver by in situ hybridization. Blood 77:2497, 1991

17. Tan CC, Eckardt K-U, Firth JD et al: Feedback modulation of renal and hepatic erythropoietin mRNA in response to graded anemia and hypoxia. Am J Physiol 263:F474, 1992

18. Haga P, Cotes PM, Till JA et al: Serum immunoreactive erythropoietin in children with cyanotic and acyanotic congenital heart disease. Blood 70:822, 1987

19. Kickler TS, Spivak JL: Effect of repeated whole blood donations on serum immunoreactive erythropoietin levels in autologous donors. JAMA 260:65, 1988

20. Spivak JL, Hogans BB: Clinical evaluation of a radioimmunoassay for serum erythropoietin using reagents derived from recombinant erythropoietin, abstracted. Blood 70:143a, 1987

21. Caro J, Erslev AJ: Biologic and immunologic erythropoietin in extracts from hypoxic whole rat kidneys and in their glomerular and tubular fractions. J Lab Clin Med 103:922, 1984

22. Abbrecht PH, Littell JK: Plasma erythropoietin in men and mice during acclimatization to different altitudes. J Appl Physiol 32:54, 1972

23. Fried W, Johnson C, Heller P: Observations on regulation of erythropoiesis during prolonged periods of hypoxia. Blood 36:607, 1970

24. Milledge JS, Cotes PM: Serum erythropoietin in humans at high altitude and its relation to plasma renin. J Appl Physiol 59:360, 1985

25. Benesch R, Benesch RE: Intracellular organic phosphates as regulators of oxygen release by haemoglobin. Nature 221:618, 1969

26. Seferynska I, Brookins J, Rice JC et al: Erythropoietin production in exhypoxic polycythemic mice. Am J Physiol 256:C925, 1989

27. Ward HP, Bigelow DB, Petty TL: Postural hypoxemia and erythrocytosis. Am J Med 45:880, 1968

28. Zwillich CW, Sutton FD, Pierson DJ et al: Decreased hypoxic ventilatory drive in the obesity-hypoventilation syndrome. Am J Med 59:343, 1975

29. Moore-Gillon JC, Treacher DF, Gaminara EJ et al: Intermittent hypoxia in patients with unexplained polycythaemia. Br Med J 293:588, 1986

30. Verel D: Blood volume changes in cyanotic congenital heart disease and polycythemia rubra vera. Circulation 23:749, 1961

31. Smith JR, Landau S: Smokers' polycythemia. N Engl J Med 298:6, 1978

32. Kilbridge TM, Fried W, Heller P: The mechanism by which plethora suppresses erythropoiesis. Blood 33:104, 1969

33. Singh A, Eckardt KU, Zimmermann A et al: Increased plasma viscosity as a reason for inappropriate erythropoietin formation. J Clin Invest 91:251, 1992

34. Bessman JD: Microcytic polycythemia. Frequency of nonthalassemic causes. JAMA 238:2391, 1977

35. Egrie JC, Cotes PM, Lane J et al: Development of radioimmunoassays for human erythropoietin using recombinant erythropoietin as tracer and immunogen. J Immunol Methods 99:235, 1987

36. Tyndall MR, Teitel DF, Lutin WA et al: Serum erythropoietin levels in patients with congenital heart disease. J Pediatr 110:538, 1987

37. Gidding SS, Stockman JA: Erythropoietin in cyanotic heart disease. Am Heart J 116:128, 1988

38. Cotes PM, Dore CJ, Liu Yin JA et al: Determination of serum immunoreactive erythropoietin in the investigation of erythrocytosis. N Engl J Med 315:283, 1986

39. Murray JF: Arterial studies in primary and secondary polycythemic disorders. Am Rev Respir Dis 92:435, 1965

40. Weil JV, Jamieson G, Brown DW et al: The red cell mass-arterial oxygen relationship in normal man. J Clin Invest 47:1627, 1968

41. Moore-Gillon J, Pearson TC: Smoking, drinking and polycythaemia. Br Med J 292:1617, 1986

42. Gregory CJ: Erythropoietin sensitivity as a differentiation marker in the hemopoietic system: studies of three erythropoietic colony responses in culture. J Cell Physiol 89:289, 1976

43. Lim DS, DeGowin RL, Zavola D et al: Recombinant human erythropoietin treatment in predialysis patients: a double-blind placebo controlled trial. Ann Intern Med 110:108, 1989

44. Kryger M: Breathing at high altitude: lessons learned and application to hypoxemia at sea level. Adv Cardiol 27:11, 1980

45. Kryger M, McCullough R, Doekel R et al: Excessive polycythemia of high altitude: role of ventilatory drive and lung disease. Am Rev Respir Dis 118:659, 1978

46. Monge CC, Whittembury J: Chronic mountain sickness. Johns Hopkins Med J 139:87, 1976

47. Stradling JR, Lane DJ: Development of secondary polycythaemia in chronic airways obstruction. Thorax 36:321, 1981

48. Vanier T, Dulfano MJ, Wu C et al: Emphysema, hypoxia and the polycythemic response. N Engl J Med 269:169, 1963

49. Charache S, Achuff S, Winslow R et al: Variability of the homeostatic response to altered P_{50}. Blood 52:1156, 1978

50. Wedzicha JA, Cotes PM, Empey DW et al: Serum immunoreactive erythropoietin in hypoxic lung disease with and without polycythaemia. Clin Sci 69:413, 1985

51. Lawrence JH, Berlin NI: Relative polycythemia—the polycythemia of stress. Yale J Biol Med 24:498, 1952

52. Russell RP, Conley CL: Benign polycythemia: Gaisböck's syndrome. Arch Intern Med 114:734, 1964

53. Weinreb NJ, Shih C-F: Spurious polycythemia. Semin Hematol 12:397, 1975

54. Hlastala MP, McKenna HP, Franada RL et al: Influence of carbon monoxide on hemoglobin-oxygen binding. J Appl Physiol 41:893, 1976

55. Astrup P: Intraerythrocytic 2,3-diphosphoglycerate and carbon monoxide exposure. Ann NY Acad Sci 174:252, 1970

56. Burge PS, Johnson WS, Prankerd TAJ: Morbidity and mortality in pseudopolycythaemia. Lancet 1:1266, 1975

57. Perloff JK, Rosove MH, Child JS et al: Adults with cyanotic congenital heart disease: hematologic management. Ann Intern Med 109:406, 1988

58. Jackson DP: Hemorrhagic diathesis in patients with cyanotic congenital heart disease: preoperative management. Ann NY Acad Sci 115:235, 1964

59. Colon-Otero G, Gilchrist GS, Holcomb GR et al: Preoperative evaluation of hemostasis in patients with congenital heart disease. Mayo Clin Proc 62:379, 1987

60. Rosove MH, Hocking WG, Canobbio MM et al: Chronic hypoxaemia and decompensated erythrocytosis in cyanotic congenital heart disease. Lancet 2:313, 1986

61. Charache S, Weatherall DJ, Clegg JB: Polycythemia associated with a hemoglobinopathy. J Clin Invest 45:813, 1966

62. Bunn HF, Forget BG: Hemoglobin: Molecular, Genetic and Clinical Aspects. WB Saunders, Philadelphia, 1986

63. Adamson JW: Familial polycythemia. Semin Hematol 12:383, 1975

64. Tarazi RC, Frohlich ED, Dustan HP et al: Hypertension and high hematocrit. Another clue to renal arterial disease. Am J Cardiol 18:855, 1955

65. Tarazi RC, Dustan HP, Frohlich ED et al: Plasma volume and chronic hypertension. Arch Intern Med 125:835, 1970

66. Pagel H, Jelkmann W, Weiss C: A comparison of the effects of renal artery constriction and anemia on the production of erythropoietin. Pflugers Arch 413:62, 1988

67. Maezawa M, Takaku F, Muto Y et al: A case of intrarenal artery stenosis associated with erythrocytosis. Scand J Haematol 21:278, 1978

68. Bacon BR, Rothman SA, Ricanati ES et al: Renal artery stenosis with erythrocytosis artery renal transplantation. Arch Intern Med 140:1206, 1980

69. Rosse WF, Waldmann TA, Cohen P: Renal cysts, erythropoietin and polycythemia. Am J Med 34:76, 1963

70. Eckardt K-U, Mollmann M, Neumann R et al: Erythropoietin in polycystic kidneys. J Clin Invest 84:1160, 1989

71. Shalhoub RJ, Rajan U, Goldwasser E et al: Erythrocytosis in patients on long-term hemodialysis. Ann Intern Med 97:686, 1982

72. Hughson MD, Hennigar GR, McManus JFA: Atypical cysts, acquired renal cystic disease, and renal cell tumors in end stage dialysis kidneys. Lab Invest 42:475, 1980

73. Koplan JP, Sprayregan S, Ossias AL et al: Erythropoietin-producing renal cyst and polycythemia vera. Am J Med 54:819, 1973

74. Basu TK, Stein RM: Erythrocytosis associated with chronic renal disease. Arch Intern Med 133:442, 1974

75. Sonneborn R, Perez G, Epstein M et al: Erythrocytosis associated with the nephrotic syndrome. Arch Intern Med 137:1068, 1977

76. Wickre CG, Norman DJ, Bennison A et al: Postrenal transplant erythrocytosis: a review of 53 patients. Kidney Int 23:731, 1983

77. Besarab A, Caro J, Jarrell BE et al: Dynamics of erythropoiesis following renal transplantation. Kidney Int 32:526, 1987

78. Sun CH, Ward JH, Paul WL et al: Serum erythropoietin levels after renal transplantation. N Engl J Med 321:151, 1989

79. Wu KK, Gibson TP, Freeman RM et al: Erythrocytosis after renal transplantation. Arch Intern Med 132:898, 1973

80. Dagher FJ, Ramos E, Erslev AJ et al: Are the native kidneys responsible for erythrocytosis in renal allorecipients? Transplantation 28:496, 1979

81. Dagher FJ, Ramos E, Erslev A et al: Erythrocytosis after renal allotransplantation: treatment by removal of the native kidneys. South Med J 73:940, 1980

82. Pollak R, Maddux MS, Cohan J et al: Erythrocythemia following renal transplantation: influence of diuretic therapy. Clin Nephrol 29:119, 1988

83. Erkelens DW, Statius van Eps LW: Bartter's syndrome and erythrocytosis. Am J Med 55:711, 1973

84. Montagnac R, Manceaux JC, Boffa G et al: Syndrome de Bartter et erythrocytose. Sem Hop Paris 61:1513, 1985

85. Thorling EB: Paraneoplastic erythrocytosis and inappropriate erythropoietin production. Scand J Haematol 17:13, 1972

86. Da-Silva JL, Lacombe C, Bruneval P et al: Tumor cells are the site of erythropoietin synthesis in human renal cancers associated with polycythemia. Blood 75:577, 1990

87. Nielsen OJ, Jespersen FF, Hilden M: Erythropoietin-induced secondary polycythemia in a patient with a renal cell carcinoma. APMIS 96:688, 1988

88. Downing V, Levine S: Erythrocytosis and renal cell carcinoma with pulmonary metastases: case report with 18-year follow up and brief discussion of literature. Cancer 35:1701, 1975

89. Burns C, Levine PH, Reichman H et al: Case report: adrenal hemangioblastoma in von Hippel-Lindau disease as a cause of secondary erythrocytosis. Am J Med Sci 292:119, 1987

90. Kew MC, Fisher JW: Serum erythropoietin concentrations in patients with hepatocellular carcinoma. Cancer 58:2485, 1986

91. Raphael B, Cooperberg AA, Niloff P: The triad of hemochromatosis, hepatoma and erythrocytosis. Cancer 43:690, 1979

92. Trimble M, Caro J, Talalla A et al: Secondary erythrocytosis due to a cerebellar hemangioblastoma: demonstration of erythropoietin mRNA in the tumor. Blood 78:599, 1991

93. Jankovic GM, Ristic MS, Pavlovic-Kentera V: Cerebellar hemangioblastoma with erythropoietin in cerebrospinal fluid. Scand J Haematol 36:511, 1986

94. Ossias AL, Zanjani ED, Zalusky R et al: Case report: studies on the mechanism of erythrocytosis associated with a uterine fibromyoma. Br J Haematol 25:179, 1973

95. Naets JP, Wittek M, Delwiche F et al: Polycythaemia and erythropoietin producing uterine fibromyoma. Scand J Haematol 19:75, 1977

96. Imai T, Funahashi H, Sato Y et al: Multiple functioning paraganglioma associated with polycythemia. J Surg Oncol 39:279, 1988

97. Bruneval P, Sassy C, Mayeux P et al: Erythropoietin synthesis by tumor cells in a case of meningioma associated with erythrocytosis. Blood 81:1593, 1993

98. Adamson JW: The erythropoietin/hematocrit relationship in normal and polycythemic man: implications of marrow regulation. Blood 32:597, 1968

99. Adamson JW, Stamatoyannopoulos G, Kontras S et al: Recessive familial erythrocytosis: aspects of marrow regulation in two families. Blood 41:641, 1973

100. Yonemitsu H, Yamaguchi K, Shigeta H et al: Two cases of familial erythrocytosis with increased erythropoietin activity in plasma and urine. Blood 42:793, 1973

101. Greenberg BR, Golde DW: Erythropoiesis in familial erythrocytosis. N Engl J Med 296:1080, 1977

102. Howarth C, Chanarin I, Janowski-Wieczorek A et al: Familial erythrocytosis. Scand J Haematol 23:217, 1979

103. Dainiak N, Hoffman R, Lebowitz AI et al: Erythropoietin-dependent primary pure erythrocytosis. Blood 53:1076, 1979

104. Ly B, Meberg A, Kannelonning K et al: Dominant familial erythrocytosis with low plasma erythropoietin activity. Studies on four cases. Scand J Haematol 30:11, 1983

105. Mankad VN, Moore B, McRoyan D et al: Erythrocytosis associated with spontaneous erythroid colony formation and idiopathic hypererythropoietinemia. J Pediatr 111:743, 1987

106. Rosa R, Prehu M-O, Beuzard Y et al: The first case of a complete deficiency of diphosphoglycerate mutase in human erythrocytes. J Clin Invest 62:907, 1978

107. Emanuel PD, Eaves CJ, Broudy VC et al: Familial and congenital polycythemia in three unrelated families. Blood 79:3019, 1992

108. de la Chapelle A, Sistonen P, Lehvaslaiho H et al: Familial erythrocytosis genetically linked to erythropoietin receptor gene. Lancet 341:82, 1993

108a. de la Chapelle A, Traskelin A-L, Juvonen E et al: Truncated erythropoietin receptor causes dominantly inherited benign human erythrocytosis. Proc Natl Acad Sci USA 90:4495, 1993

108b. Yoshimura A, Longmore G, Lodish HF: Point mutation in the exoplasmic domain of the erythropoietin receptor resulting in hormone-independent activation and tumorigenicity. Nature 348:647, 1990

109. Alexanian R, Vaughn WK, Ruchelman MW: Erythropoietin excretion in man following androgens. J Lab Clin Med 70:777, 1967

110. Kennedy BJ, Gilbersten AS: Increased erythropoiesis induced by androgenic-hormone therapy. N Engl Med 256:719, 1957

111. Barton IK, Mansell MA: Erythrocytosis induced by danazol in an anephric patient. Br Med J 294:615, 1987

112. Murray JF, Gold P, Johnson BL, Jr: The circulatory effects of hematocrit variations in normovolemic and hypervolemic dogs. J Clin Invest 42:1150, 1963

113. Thomas DJ, Marshall J, Russell RWR et al: Effect of haematocrit on cerebral blood-flow in man. Lancet 2:941, 1977

114. Thomas DJ, Marshall J, Russell R et al: Cerebral blood-flow in polycythaemia. Lancet 2:161, 1977

115. Humphrey PRD, Marshall J, Russell RWR et al: Cerebral blood-flow and viscosity in relative polycythaemia. Lancet 2:873, 1979

116. Rosenkrantz TS, Philipps AF, Skrzypczak PS et al: Cerebral metabolism in the newborn lamb with polycythemia. Pediatr Res 23:329, 1988

117. Dayton LM, McCullough RE, Scheinhorn DJ et al: Symptomatic and pulmonary response to acute phlebotomy in secondary polycythemia. Chest 68: 785, 790, 1975

118. York EL, Jones RL, Menon D et al: Effects of secondary polycythemia on cerebral blood flow in chronic obstructive pulmonary disease. Am Rev Respir Dis 121:813, 1980

119. Wallis PJW, Skehan JD, Newland AC et al: Effects of erythrapheresis on pulmonary haemodynamics and oxygen transport in patients with secondary polycythaemia and cor pulmonale. Clin Sci 70:91, 1986

120. Rosenthal A, Nathan DG, Marty AT et al: Acute hemodynamic effects of red cell volume reduction in polycythemia of cyanotic congenital heart disease. Circulation 42:297, 1970

121. Oldershaw PJ, Sutton MG: Haemodynamic effects of haematocrit reduction in patients with polycythaemia secondary to cyanotic congenital heart disease. Br Heart J 44:584, 1980

122. De Jong PE, Weening JJ, Donker AJM et al: The effect of phlebotomy on renal function and proteinuria in a patient with congenital cyanotic heart disease. Nephron 33:225, 1983

123. Birgegard G, Carlsson M, Sandhagen B et al: Does iron deficiency in treated polycythemia vera affect whole blood viscosity? J Intern Med 216:165, 1984

124. Rector WG Jr, Fortuin NJ, Conley CL: Non-hematologic effects of chronic iron deficiency: a study of patients with polycythemia vera treated solely with venesections. Medicine 61:382, 1982

125. Bagley GC, Richert-Boe K, Koler RD: 32P and acute leukemia: development of leukemia in a patient with memoglobin Yakima. Blood 52:350, 1978

Disorders of Iron Metabolism: Iron Deficiency and Overload

38

Gary M. Brittenham

INTRODUCTION

Iron is an essential nutrient required by every human cell. A transition metal (atomic number 26, atomic weight 55.85), it can serve as a carrier for oxygen and electrons and as a catalyst for oxygenation, hydroxylation, and other critical metabolic processes, in part because of its ability to reversibly and readily cycle between the ferrous (Fe^{2+}) and ferric (Fe^{3+}) oxidation states. Iron is quantitatively the most important biocatalytic element in human enzymology, with vital roles in oxidative metabolism, in cellular growth and proliferation, and in oxygen transport and storage.

Iron functions, travels, and is stored as a component of a variety of iron compounds, not as a free cation. The very reactivity that is metabolically useful in iron porphyrin complexes and metalloenzymes makes the iron in inorganic compounds or ionized forms potentially hazardous. Ionic iron can participate in a number of reactions to produce free radical species. These in turn damage cellular constituents. Thus, either a decrease or an increase in body iron may be clinically significant. If too little iron is available (iron deficiency), limitations on the synthesis of physiologically active iron-containing compounds may have deleterious consequences. If too much iron accumulates (iron overload) and exceeds the body's capacity for safe transport and storage, iron toxicity may produce widespread organ damage and death.

IRON METABOLISM

Biologic and Molecular Aspects

Proteins of Iron Transport, Storage, and Regulation

Within the body, the supply and storage of iron are mediated by three principal proteins—transferrin, transferrin receptor, and ferritin. Their expression is, in turn, regulated by a fourth protein—the iron-responsive element-binding protein (IRE-BP). Transferrin, a transport protein, carries iron in the plasma and extracellular fluid to supply tissue needs. Transferrin receptor, a glycoprotein on cell membranes, binds the transferrin/iron complex and is internalized in a vesicle where the iron is released intracellularly; the transferrin/transferrin receptor assemblage then returns to the cell membrane, where apotransferrin is liberated into the plasma. Ferritin, an iron storage protein, sequesters iron in a presumably nontoxic form while holding it ready for prompt mobilization in time of need. The IRE-BP (also known as iron-regulatory factor (IRF), ferritin-repressor protein (FRP), and p90) is an mRNA-binding protein that coordinates the intracellular expression of transferrin receptor, ferritin, and other proteins important for iron metabolism. Each of the principal proteins has been isolated, purified, and characterized. The chromosomal locations of the corresponding genes have been identified and their sequences determined. The available information is summarized in Table 38-1, and the structures of the proteins are shown diagrammatically in Figure 38-1.

Transferrin

Transferrin mediates iron exchange between body tissues.[1,2] A single gene for apotransferrin has been identified and located[3] at q21-qter on chromosome 3, near the gene for the transferrin receptor.[4] Structural analysis suggests that the transferrin gene originated as the result of an unequal crossover between two primordial transferrin genes.[5] Apotransferrin is a single-chain glycoprotein (M_r 79,570; 6% glucosidic) with 678 amino acid residues and is composed of two homologous N-terminal and C-terminal lobes[6] (Fig. 38-1A). Each lobe can independently bind a single ferric ion, so the molecule can exist as apotransferrin or monoferric or diferric transferrin. The lobes are in the shape of prolate ellipsoids, and each is further divided into two dissimilar domains. Each iron-binding site is located within the interdomain cleft, where the iron is bound by two tyrosines, a histidine, and an aspartic acid residue.[6,7] An anion (bicarbonate or carbonate) is bound with each ferric ion, serving as a bridging ligand between the iron and protein.[1]

Transferrin binds ferric iron with high affinity; under physiologic conditions the effective stability constant[1,8] is about 10^{20} M^{-1}. Binding of two atoms of ferric iron by transferrin results in conformational changes making the molecule more compact, more soluble, and more resistant to oxidative or tryptic denaturation. The two iron-binding domains are similar but differ in their detailed spectroscopic, thermodynamic, kinetic, and chemical properties.[9] The functional importance of these differences remains uncertain. In fresh sera from healthy individuals, the N-terminal monoferric species (Fe_NTf) is more common than the C-terminal form (Fe_CTf)[9–12] but so little is known about the manner in which transferrin acquires iron from macrophages and enterocytes that the significance of this difference remains uncertain.

Most apotransferrin is produced by hepatocytes.[1,13] Other potential sites of synthesis have been identified, including lactating mammary gland, testis, central nervous system, lymphocytes, and macrophages; none seems to be a quantitatively important source of plasma transferrin in vivo. The total amount of apotransferrin in humans is about 240 mg/kg, equally divided between the plasma and extravascular fluids.[2] Apotransferrin is a true carrier. It is not lost in delivering iron, so its turnover is unrelated to the plasma iron turnover; its half-life is about 8 days.[14]

Transferrin Receptor

The transferrin receptor not only provides transferrin-bound iron access into the cell but also plays a critical role in the release of iron from transferrin within the cell. A single gene for the transferrin receptor has been identified. It is located

Table 38-1. Proteins of Iron Transport and Storage

	Transferrin	Transferrin Receptor	Ferritin	IRE-BP
Chromosomal location of gene(s)	3q21-qter	3q26.2-qter	H subunit: 11; L subunit: 19	9
Structure	Single-chain glycoprotein with two iron-binding sites	Transmembrane glycoprotein dimer with two transferrin-binding sites	Spherical protein of 24 subunits; binds ≤4,500 iron atoms	A four-domain [4Fe-4S] cluster protein
Function	Iron transport in plasma and extracellular fluid	Receptor-mediated endocytosis of ferric transferrin; is recycled	Iron storage	Coordinate translational regulation of critical proteins of iron metabolism

on the distal portion of the long arm of chromosome 3 in the region q26.2-qter.[4,15,16] The transferrin receptor is a transmembrane glycoprotein dimer composed of two identical subunits (each with M_r 94,000) linked by a disulfide bond (Fig. 38-1B). The transferrin receptor is amphipathic, with a small hydro-

philic cytoplasmic tail (62 amino acid units, M_r about 5,000), a large hydrophilic extracellular domain (648 amino acids, M_r about 140,000), and a central hydrophobic region anchoring the receptor into the membrane (28 amino acids).[17]

The transferrin receptor can bind two molecules of trans-

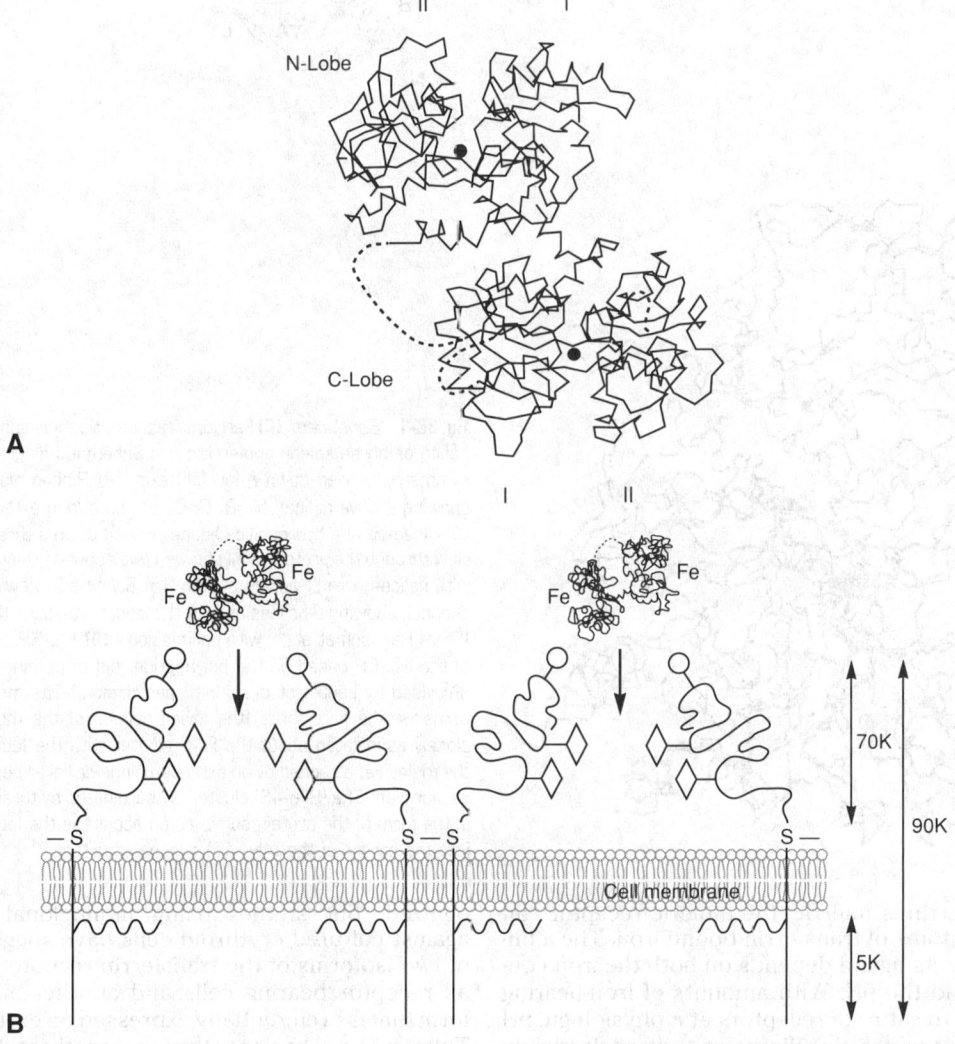

Fig. 38-1. Structures of proteins of iron transport, uptake, storage, and regulation. **(A)** Apotransferrin. Schematic representation of the polypeptide chain shows that it is folded into two lobes, each in the shape of a prolate ellipsoid and containing a single iron-binding site, represented by a dot. Each lobe is in turn composed of two dissimilar domains, labeled I and II. The N- and C-terminal lobes are indicated. (From Bailey et al.,[6] with permission.) **(B)** Transferrin receptor. Schematic representation of the transferrin receptor on the cell surface shows it as a transmembrane glycoprotein dimer composed of two identical subunits linked by a disulfide bond. The transferrin receptor is amphipathic with a small hydrophilic cytoplasmic tail, a large hydrophilic extracellular domain, and a central hydrophobic region anchoring the receptor into the membrane. The receptor can bind two molecules of transferrin. (From Huebers and Finch,[2] with permission as modified from Newman et al.,[414] with permission.) *(Figure continues.)*

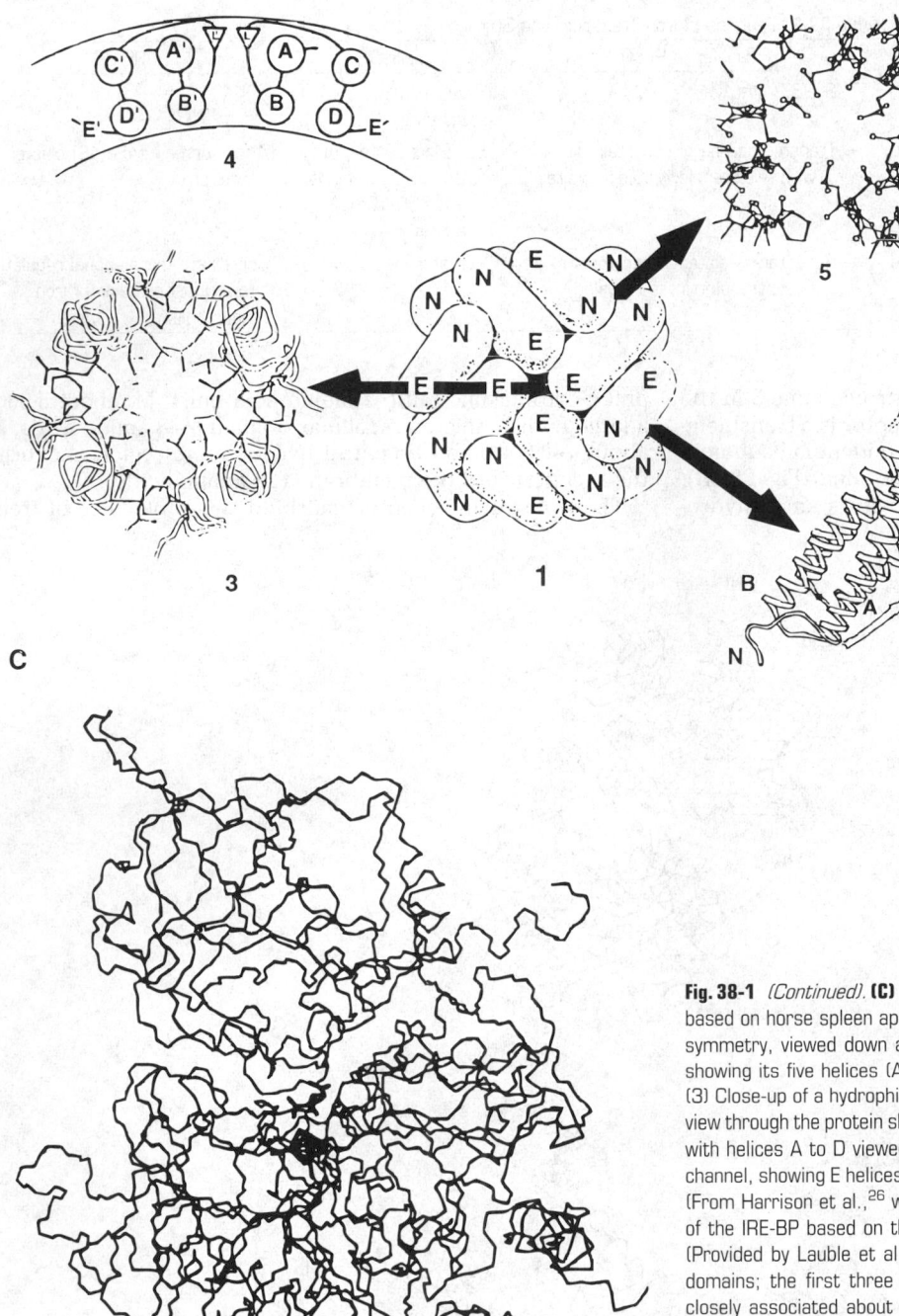

Fig. 38-1 *(Continued).* **(C)** Ferritin. A schematic representation of ferritin structure based on horse spleen apoferritin. (1) Schematic diagram of 24 subunits in 432 symmetry, viewed down a fourfold axis. (2) Ribbon diagram of a single subunit showing its five helices (A, B, C, D, E) and a long extended interhelical loop (L). (3) Close-up of a hydrophilic channel viewed down a threefold axis. (4) Schematic view through the protein shell showing two subunits related by a twofold symmetry with helices A to D viewed end-on. (5) Schematic view of a fourfold hydrophobic channel, showing E helices and the 12 leucine residues that surround the channel. (From Harrison et al.,[26] with permission.) **(D)** IRE-BP. Schematic representation of the IRE-BP based on the polypeptide fold of porcine mitochondrial aconitase. (Provided by Lauble et al.,[53] with permission.) The molecule is folded into four domains; the first three (the lower portion of the molecule in the figure) are closely associated about the Fe-S cluster with the fourth (the upper portion of the molecule) attached by an extended hinge or linker peptide, creating a intermolecular cleft. The [3Fe-4S] cluster is coordinated by three cysteine residues, while in the form of the protein active as an aconitase the fourth iron atom is inserted into the corner of the [4Fe-4S] cubane structure.[51,88]

ferrin; if each transferrin is diferric, the dimeric receptor can carry a total of four atoms of transferrin-bound iron. The affinity of the receptor for its ligand depends on both the iron content of transferrin and the pH. With amounts of iron-bearing transferrin sufficient to saturate receptors at a physiologic pH of 7.4, the receptor has very little affinity for apotransferrin, an intermediate affinity for monoferric transferrin, and the highest affinity for diferric transferrin, estimated at $2-7 \times 10^{-9}$ M.[18] Under such physiologic conditions, the affinity of the transferrin receptor for diferric transferrin is about 4.2 times that for monoferric transferrin.[19] At a pH of about 5, the affinity of the transferrin receptor for apotransferrin increases to that for diferric transferrin.[20,21]

Only a single gene for the transferrin receptor has been rec-

ognized, but studies using monoclonal antibodies raised against cultured erythroid cells have suggested the existence of two isoforms of the transferrin receptor: one expressed on all receptor bearing cells and another antigenically distinct form that is preferentially expressed on erythroid precursors.[22] The structural basis for this apparently erythroid-specific form of the transferrin receptor has not been determined. Functional differences, if any, between the two forms of the receptor have not been characterized.

Transferrin receptors appear to be expressed on virtually all nucleated cells. They are present in large numbers in erythroid precursors, placenta, and liver. The number of transferrin receptors on the cell surface seems to reflect cellular iron requirements and is a prime determinant of cellular iron supply.

In nondividing cells, the receptor number is constant. Numbers increase markedly in proliferating cells. The number of receptors seems to reflect cellular iron requirements; in the rat, the estimated number of transferrin receptors was found to be about 300,000 per cell in the early normoblast, about 800,000 per cell in the intermediate normoblast, and about 100,000 per cell in the reticulocyte.[23] The half-time for disappearance of transferrin receptors from the cell has been reported to range from <24 hours to 2–3 days.[24,25]

Ferritin

Ferritin, the major iron storage protein, is composed of 24 subunits of at least two types: L (or light: M_r 19,700; more acidic with pI 4.5–5.0) and H (or heavy: M_r 21,100; more basic with pI 5.0–5.7).[26] Genes for both the H and L chains belong to multigene families with members on several chromosomes, but most are pseudogenes, lacking introns or carrying mutations that render the gene inactive.[27] A functional H gene and a functional L gene have been mapped to chromosomes 11 and 19, respectively,[28–30] but the details of the organization and expression of the ferritin genes are still being examined.[31]

Apoferritin (M_r 440,000) consists of a spherical protein shell about 1 nm in thickness and 12 nm in diameter, which is composed of mixtures of oblong H and L subunits (Fig. 38-1C) whose proportions depend on the tissue and iron status of the cell. Tissues functioning as major iron storage depots, such as liver and spleen, have a preponderance of the L subunit, while tissues that do not normally act as iron storage sites, such as heart, have higher proportions of H subunits.

Within a specific tissue, greater amounts of storage iron are associated with a greater predominance of L subunits. These patterns have suggested that ferritins enriched in L subunits may have a long-term iron storage function, while ferritins with a predominance of H subunits may be more active in iron metabolism.[31] Recent studies using site-directed mutagenesis have found that the ferritin H subunit contains a ferrioxidase site lacking from the L subunit. Using recombinant human homopolymers, those composed solely of H subunits have been found to take up iron at a rate several times that of homopolymers composed only of L subunits.[32,33] These variations in the proportions of H and L subunits[34] and other factors such as the extent of glycosylation give rise to tissue isoferritins with different isoelectric points.

Within the apoferritin shell, the component subunits are arranged so that a total of eight hydrophilic channels are formed near the N-terminal ends of the subunits along the four threefold axes of symmetry, while an additional six hydrophobic channels lie along the three fourfold axes of symmetry.[26] These apparently provide routes for movement of iron and small molecules in and out of the interior of the sphere. Each ferritin molecule can reversibly store ≤4,500 iron atoms within the shell in an inorganic polynuclear core of ferric hydroxyphosphate. Typically only about half that amount is present. Ferritin is found in virtually all cells. It provides an accessible reserve of iron for synthesis of functional iron-containing compounds and a means of sequestering iron in a soluble, apparently nontoxic form. Ferritin is especially abundant in cells with specialized roles in the synthesis of iron-containing compounds (erythroid precursors) and in iron metabolism and storage (macrophages, hepatocytes).

The half-life of hepatic ferritin is about 60 hours.[35] Catabolism may result in digestion of the protein shell with reutilization of the iron core, or in conversion to hemosiderin, an amorphous water-insoluble storage compound with a higher iron content and slower turnover than ferritin.[36,37] Ascorbic acid seems to retard ferritin degradation by reducing lysosomal autophagy of the protein.[38,39] Intracellular ferritin is synthesized by the smooth endoplasmic reticulum in amounts required to replace catabolized products and to store any additional iron entering the cell. Small amounts of ferritin are also secreted into the plasma. Normally, the amount of plasma ferritin synthesized and secreted seems to be proportional to the amount of cellular ferritin produced in the internal iron storage pathway. The plasma ferritin concentration is thus related to the magnitude of body iron stores.[26,40–45]

Iron-Responsive Element Binding Protein

The pivotal protein that allows iron to self-regulate its intracellular availability is the IRE-BP.[46] The IRE-BP is a trans-acting cytoplasmic RNA binding protein that regulates the expression of mRNAs containing a cis-acting regulatory structure termed the IRE.[47–49] The IRE consists of a conserved 28-nucleotide sequence in a hairpin-shaped stem loop with bulge conformation that serves as the binding site for the IRE-BP (Fig. 38-2).

The IRE-BP has been found in all tissues examined but with tissue-specific variations in the amounts present; the quantities of IRE-BP seem to be highest in those tissues (e.g., liver and spleen) that have the highest concentrations of non-heme iron.

Studies of amino acid composition, molecular weight, isoelectric point, and sequences of random peptides have shown that the physicochemical and structural characteristics of the IRE-BP are identical to those of cytosolic aconitase.[50] Aconitase (citrate [isocitrate] hydrolase) is an iron-sulfur protein that catalyzes the stereo-specific interconversion of citrate to isocitrate within the Krebs cycle. It exists in both a mitochondrial and cytoplasmic form. The cytoplasmic form, the product of a gene on chromosome 9, can function both enzymatically as an aconitase and as the RNA-binding IRE-BP.[51] The mitochondrial form, encoded by a gene on chromosome 22, is enzymatically functional but lacks IRE-BP activity. The 18 active site residues of mitochondrial aconitase and of the IRE-BP are identical.[52] The catalytically active site of aconitase contains a cubane [4Fe-4S] cluster with three of the iron atoms bound to cysteines in the protein skeleton and the fourth ligated to inorganic sulfur within the cluster.[53]

The available evidence now suggests that the IRE-BP can be reversibly converted from an enzymatically active aconitase (with low RNA-binding affinity) to a high-affinity RNA-binding form (with no aconitase activity) by alterations in the Fe-S cluster in response to changes in intracellular iron availability,[51] without changes in IRE-BP synthesis or degradation.[54] The Fe-S cluster functions as a sensor of iron availability.[55] In effect, physiologic changes in iron availability regulate the aconitase activity reciprocally (increased with iron repletion) and RNA-binding affinity (increased with iron depletion) of the IRE-BP. As shown in Figure 39-2, the IRE-BP seems to exist in three states[51]: (1) the (oxidized) [4Fe-4S] cluster form of the IRE-BP is active as an aconitase and has a low affinity for the IRE, (2) the (reduced) [3Fe-4S] state lacks aconitase activity but still has a low affinity for the iron-responsive element, and (3) the IRE-BP with high affinity for the IRE (and without aconitase activity). The high affinity form of the IRE-BP seems to be the product of a further, marked structural change, possibly destruction of the Fe-S cluster.[56–58] Within a cell, a decrease in the availability of iron would increase the proportion of the IRE-BP in the high-affinity state (without aconitase activity), enhancing the binding between the IRE-BPs and iron-responsive elements. Conversely, an increase in available cellular iron would increase the fraction of the IRE-BP in the low-affinity [4Fe-4S] state (with aconitase activity), decreasing binding between IRE-BPs and iron-responsive elements. In this manner, the IRE-BP seems to function as a sensor of intracellular iron availability.

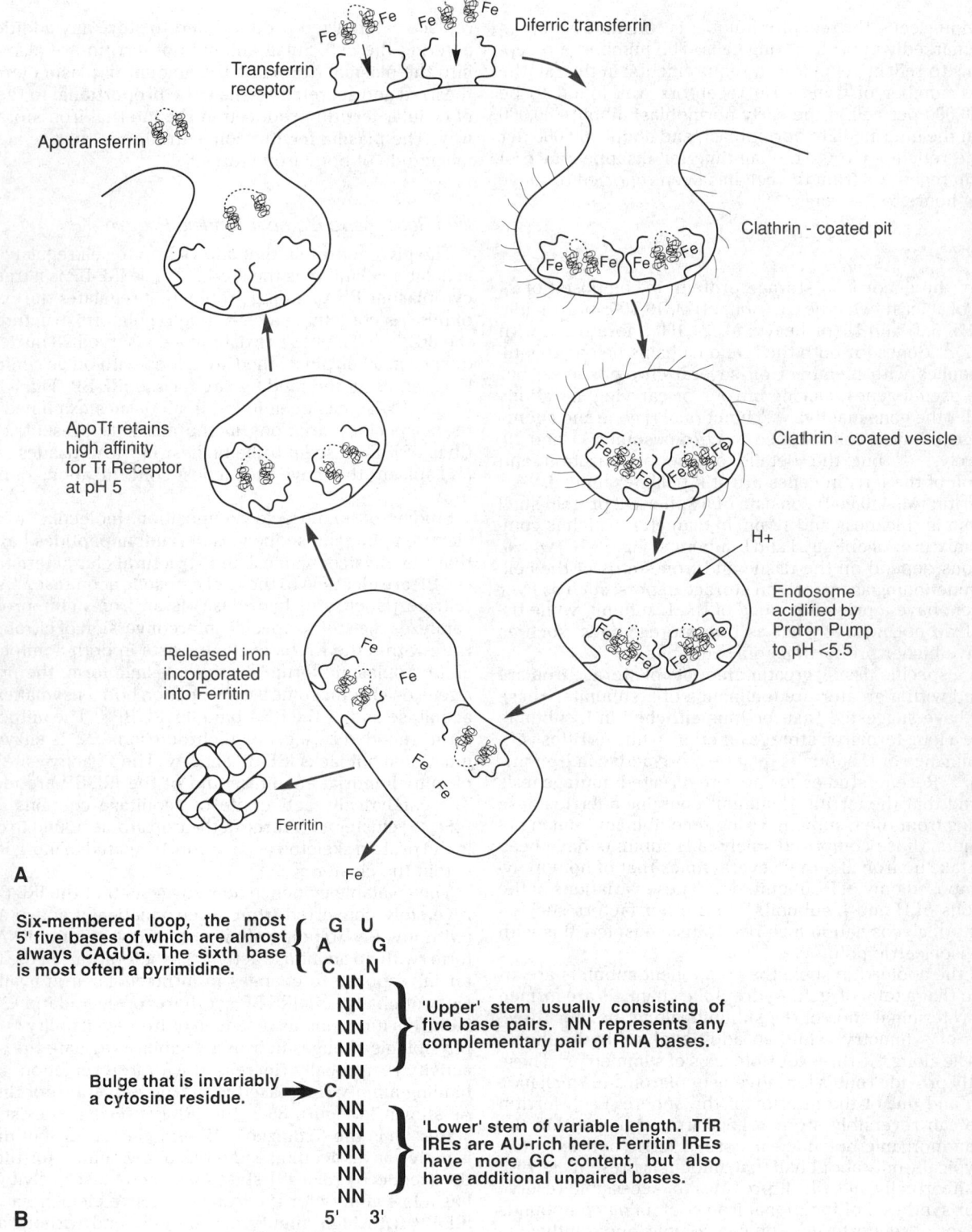

Transferrin receptor

Diferric transferrin

Apotransferrin

Clathrin - coated pit

ApoTf retains high affinity for Tf Receptor at pH 5

Clathrin - coated vesicle

H+

Endosome acidified by Proton Pump to pH <5.5

Released iron incorporated into Ferritin

Ferritin

Fe

A

Six-membered loop, the most 5' five bases of which are almost always CAGUG. The sixth base is most often a pyrimidine.

G U
A   G
C   N
NN
NN   'Upper' stem usually consisting of
NN   five base pairs. NN represents any
NN   complementary pair of RNA bases.
NN

Bulge that is invariably a cytosine residue. → C

NN
NN   'Lower' stem of variable length. TfR
NN   IREs are AU-rich here. Ferritin IREs
NN   have more GC content, but also
NN   have additional unpaired bases.

5' 3'

B

Fig. 38-2. Cellular iron supply and storage. **(A)** Schematic representation of the process of cellular iron uptake and transferrin-receptor recycling. Iron delivery to the cell begins with the binding of up to two molecules of mono- or diferric transferrin to a transferrin receptor in an energy- and temperature-dependent process. Once bound, the iron-bearing transferrin/receptor complex rapidly clusters with other transferrin/receptor complexes in a clathrin-coated pit, which seals over and fuses to form an internal vesicle or endosome. Moving to the interior of the cell, the endosome then fuses with an acidic vesicle whose internal pH is <5.5. In this acidic environment iron is released from transferrin and is then made available for cellular use or storage. Acidification within the endosome also increases the affinity of the now iron-free apotransferrin for the transferrin receptor, with the result that the apotransferrin-receptor bond remains intact as the complex within the endosome is transported back to the cell surface. On exposure to the neutral pH of the plasma, the apotransferrin loses its affinity for the transferrin receptor and is released from the membrane, which makes both the apotransferrin and the receptor available for neutralization. (Adapted from Irie and Tavassoli,[397] with permission.) **(B)** Structure of an IRE. The consensus structure for an IRE is shown, as derived from sequences and possible secondary structures of IREs from ferritin and transferrin receptor mRNAs. (From Klausner et al.,[88] with permission.) *(Figure continues.)*

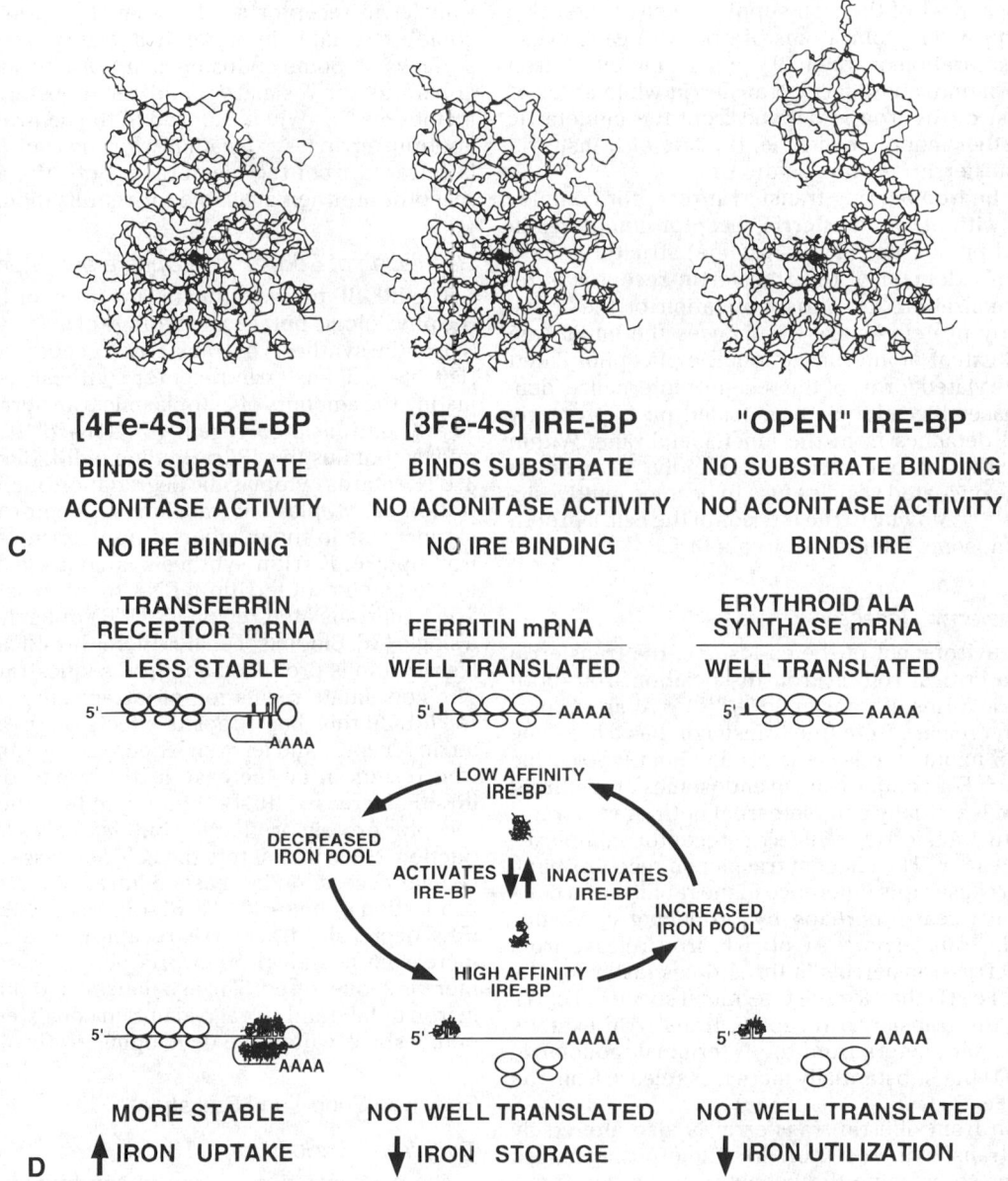

[4Fe-4S] IRE-BP

BINDS SUBSTRATE

ACONITASE ACTIVITY

C   NO IRE BINDING

[3Fe-4S] IRE-BP

BINDS SUBSTRATE

NO ACONITASE ACTIVITY

NO IRE BINDING

"OPEN" IRE-BP

NO SUBSTRATE BINDING

NO ACONITASE ACTIVITY

BINDS IRE

TRANSFERRIN
RECEPTOR mRNA

LESS STABLE

FERRITIN mRNA

WELL TRANSLATED

ERYTHROID ALA
SYNTHASE mRNA

WELL TRANSLATED

LOW AFFINITY
IRE-BP

DECREASED
IRON POOL

ACTIVATES   INACTIVATES
IRE-BP   IRE-BP

INCREASED
IRON POOL

HIGH AFFINITY
IRE-BP

MORE STABLE

D   ↑ IRON UPTAKE

NOT WELL TRANSLATED

↓ IRON STORAGE

NOT WELL TRANSLATED

↓ IRON UTILIZATION

Fig. 38-2 *(Continued).* **(C)** Proposed model for forms of the IRE-BP. The [4Fe-4S] IRE-BP binds substrate, is enzymatically active as an aconitase but has no RNA binding activity. The [3Fe-4S] IRE-BP binds substrate but is not enzymatically active and has no RNA binding activity. The (apoenzyme) IRE-BP mRNA-binding form does not bind substrate, has no aconitase activity, but binds to mRNA iron-responsive elements. In this form, a conformational change is shown schematically in which the Fe-S cluster has been disassembled by widening the intermolecular cleft. [From Klausner et al.,[88] with permission.] **(D)** Schematic representation of the coordinate regulation of transferrin receptor, ferritin and erythroid-specific δ-aminolevulinic acid synthase [eALAS] synthesis by the IRE-BP. Transferrin receptor synthesis is controlled by adjusting the amounts of cytoplasmic transferrin receptor mRNA. The 3' untranslated region (3' UTR) of transferrin receptor mRNA contains five IREs. Binding of IRE-BPs to the IREs in the 3' UTR retards cytoplasmic degradation, increasing the concentration of cytoplasmic transferrin receptor mRNA and the rate of transferrin receptor synthesis. With an increased number of cellular transferrin receptors, iron uptake is enhanced.[398] By contrast, ferritin[31] and eALAS[399,400] synthesis is controlled without changes in the amount of ferritin or eALAS mRNA present by repressing translation of ferritin or eALAS mRNA. The 5' untranslated regions (5' UTRs) of both ferritin and eALAS mRNA contain a single IRE. Binding of an IRE-BP to the IRE in the 5' UTR (1) arrests translation of ferritin mRNA so less ferritin is produced and iron sequestration is diminished, and (2) stops translation of eALAS mRNA, decreasing production of eALAS and diminishing utilization of iron in the heme biosynthetic pathway.

Cellular Iron Supply and Storage

The coordinate roles of transferrin, transferrin receptor, and ferritin in cellular iron supply and storage are shown schematically in Figure 38-2. Iron delivery to the cell begins with the binding of one or two molecules of mono- or diferric transferrin to a transferrin receptor in an energy- and temperature-dependent process[59,60] that is complete within 2–3 minutes. At the neutral pH of plasma, the iron-transferrin complex is further stabilized by the binding of transferrin to the transferrin receptor, both for monoferric and diferric transferrin.[61–63]

The efficiency of iron delivery to the cell depends on the amounts of mono- and diferric plasma transferrin available. With normal erythropoiesis and a normal transferrin saturation of about 33%, the higher affinity of the receptor for diferric transferrin causes most of the iron supply to cells to devolve from this form, providing four atoms of iron with each cycle. At a transferrin saturation of about 19%, equal amounts of iron are provided by mono- and diferric transferrin while at lower saturations, most of the iron is derived from the monoferric form.[20,64,65] Whether mono- or diferric, the fate of transferrin bound to the transferrin receptor is the same.

Once bound, the iron-bearing transferrin/receptor complex rapidly clusters with other transferrin/receptor complexes in a clathrin-coated pit; a YXRF (Tyr-X-Arg-Phe) structural motif in the cytoplasmic domain of the transferrin receptor is required for internalization.[66,67] Phosphorylation of the transferrin receptor by protein kinase C enhances the initial rate but not the final extent of internalization; the phosphorylated and nonphosphorylated forms of the receptor internalize identically.[68] Once assembled the clathrin-coated pit is promptly internalized and detaches from the inner membrane. Within the cytoplasm, the coated vesicle is rapidly stripped of clathrin[69] and the uncoated vesicles fuse to become multivesicular endosomes.[70–73] Moving to the interior of the cell, a proton pump lowers endosome internal pH to about 5.6.[74–80]

Role of the Transferrin Receptor

In the acidic environment of the endosome, the transferrin receptor plays a critical role in iron dissociation from both mono- and diferric forms of transferrin.[61–63,81,82] At an endosomal pH of 5.6, iron release from free transferrin has a half-time of release of >15 minutes; release is predominantly from the N-terminal site.[61,82] For comparison, in endosomes of erythroid cells, iron release is virtually complete from both sites of transferrin bound into transferrin/transferrin receptor complexes within 2–3 minutes.[61,83] The effect of transferrin receptor binding to transferrin causes this difference in the rapidity and completeness of iron release, perhaps by producing conformational changes in transferrin.[62] At pH 5.6, iron release from unbound monoferric transferrins is three times faster for the N-terminal form (Fe_NTf) than for the C-terminal species (Fe_cTf). When bound to the transferrin receptor, transferrin exhibits the same release parameters from the N-terminal monoferric transferrin (Fe_NTf) but substantially increases release from the C-terminal site (Fe_cTf).[61,62]

Release of iron from diferric transferrin is also altered by binding to the transferrin receptor. In studies using mixed metal transferrins to examine the behavior of the two transferrin iron-binding sites when both are occupied (iron at one site and inert cobalt at the other), iron bound at the N-terminal site was found to be six times more available than that at the C-terminal site when transferrin was unbound.[63] By contrast, transferrin binding to the transferrin receptor, facilitated iron release from the C-terminal site by a factor of four, while release at the N-terminal site was retarded by a factor of two. Binding to the transferrin receptor at pH 5.6 alters site-site cooperative interactions between the two sites of doubly occupied transferrin: iron at the N-terminal lobe is stabilized, while iron at the C-terminal lobe is labilized.[63] Overall, transferrin receptor binding at endosomal pH enhances both the rate and completeness of iron release from transferrin, while minimizing differences between the N- and C-terminal sites.

After release, the iron must then be transported across the endosomal membrane.[84] Kinetic studies have suggested that ferric iron is released from transferrin, reduced to the ferrous form within the endosome, and then transported through the endocytic vesicle membrane by a concentration gradient-driven process.[85] The exact form and fate of the iron derived from the endosome are still unknown,[86] but the newly released iron presumably is available to mitochondria for heme synthesis or to ferritin for storage. Acidification within the endosome increases the affinity of the now iron-free apotransferrin for the transferrin receptor so that that the apotransferrin/receptor complex remains intact as it is transported back to the cell surface.[87,88] Some endosomes are briefly shunted to the Golgi apparatus for resialation and repair before returning to the membrane.[89,90] When exposed to the neutral pH of the plasma, apotransferrin loses its affinity for the transferrin receptor and is released from the membrane. Both the apotransferrin and receptor are then available for reutilization.[74,75]

Regulation of Cellular Iron Uptake and Storage

The IRE-BP provides the means for coordinate regulation of the physiologic uptake and storage of iron by translational control of the synthesis of transferrin receptor and ferritin[31,46,88,91] (Fig. 38-2). Transferrin receptor synthesis is controlled by adjusting the amounts of cytoplasmic transferrin receptor mRNA. The 3' untranslated region (3' UTR) of transferrin receptor mRNA contains five IREs. Binding of IRE-BPs to the IREs in the 3' UTR retards cytoplasmic degradation, increasing the concentration of cytoplasmic transferrin receptor mRNA. The resulting increase in the number of transferrin receptors enhances iron uptake. Ferritin synthesis is controlled without changes in the amount of ferritin mRNA by repressing its translation. The 5' untranslated region (5' UTR) of ferritin mRNA contains a single IRE. Binding of an IRE-BP to this IRE arrests translation; less ferritin is produced and iron sequestration is diminished. The coordinate regulation of intracellular iron availability by the IRE-BP thus has opposite effects on the synthesis of transferrin receptor and ferritin. A decrease in intracellular available iron results in an increase in the proportion of high-affinity IRE-BP. Increased IRE-BP binding to IREs increases transferrin receptor protein production but decreases ferritin protein production. More iron enters the cell, and less is sequestered from cellular access. An increase in intracellular iron decreases the proportion of high-affinity IRE-BP. Fewer IRE-BPs are bound to IREs, decreasing transferrin receptor protein production while increasing ferritin protein production. Less iron enters, and more is sequestered. These balanced and opposing alterations in iron uptake and storage maintain consistent physiologic iron homeostasis within the developing erythroid cell.

Body Iron Supply and Storage

Body Iron Distribution

The concentration of iron in the human body is normally about 40–50 mg Fe/kg body weight; women typically have lower amounts than men.[92–95] (Table 38-2). Most of this iron is contained in compounds required for normal metabolic activity. The functional iron compartment includes about 30 mg Fe/kg as hemoglobin iron contained within circulating red cells and an additional 6–7 mg Fe/kg that is present in many tissues in myoglobin, in a variety of heme enzymes (cytochromes, cata-

Table 38-2. Distribution of Iron in the Audit

	Concentration (mg/kg)	
Type of Iron	Men	Women
Functional iron		
Hemoglobin	31	28
Myoglobin	5	4
Heme enzymes	1	1
Nonheme enzymes	1	1
Transport iron		
Transferrin	<1 (0.2)	<1 (0.2)
Storage iron		
Ferritin	8	4
Hemosiderin	4	2
Total	50	40

lases, peroxidases), and in nonheme enzymes (ribonucleotide reductase, metalloflavoproteins, iron/sulfur proteins). Transport iron consists of the small fraction (<0.5%) of the total body iron that is in transit to supply tissue iron needs. It is bound to the protein transferrin in the plasma and extracellular fluid. The remainder of the iron (5–6 mg Fe/kg in women, 10–12 mg Fe/kg in men) is storage iron in the form of ferritin and hemosiderin, principally in hepatocytes and in macrophages in the liver, bone marrow, spleen, and muscle, available as a readily available reserve in the event of blood loss.

Iron Balance: Iron Absorption and Loss

The major pathways for absorption, loss, internal exchange, and storage of iron are shown schematically in Figure 38-3. Iron balance is the difference between the amounts of iron entering and leaving the body. Humans are unique in their lack of any effective means to excrete excess iron.[96,97] Iron balance is thus physiologically regulated by controlling iron absorption: iron stores and absorption are reciprocally related, so that as stores decline, absorption increases.[98,99] Normally, iron exchange with the environment is extremely limited. Less than 0.05% of the total body iron is acquired or lost each day, making humans unique among animals in the effectiveness with which iron is conserved.

Iron is absorbed as both heme iron and nonheme iron through the brush border of the upper small intestine.[98] The iron content of the diet is a function of caloric intake; typical diets in the United States contain about 7 mg/1,000 kcal. The availability of dietary iron for absorption is determined by the amount and form of the iron, the composition of the diet, and gastrointestinal factors.[2] Heme iron is usually only a small portion of the dietary iron but is highly available for absorption (≥20–30% absorbable) and is little affected by other components in the diet. Most dietary iron (often >90%) is nonheme iron, which enters a common intraluminal pool, whose avail-

IRON REQUIREMENTS

Overall, the iron requirement for an individual includes not only that iron needed to replenish physiologic losses and to meet the demands of growth and pregnancy but also any additional amounts needed to replace pathologic losses. Physiologic iron losses are generally restricted to the small amounts of iron contained in the urine, bile, and sweat; the shedding of iron-containing cells from the intestine, urinary tract, and skin; occult gastrointestinal blood loss; and, in women, uterine losses during menstruation and pregnancy.[97] In normal men, the daily basal iron loss is slightly <1.0 mg/day, and in normal menstruating women it is about 1.5 mg/day. The median total iron loss with pregnancy is about 500 mg, or almost 2 mg/day over the 280 days of gestation.[272]

ability is determined by the balance between inhibitors (e.g., phytates, tannates, phosphates) and enhancers (amino acids, ascorbic acid) of absorption.[98] Frequently, <5% of the nonheme iron is available for absorption. Iron availability is also influenced by gastrointestinal factors such as gastric secretion, intestinal motility, and the consequences of surgery or bowel disease.

The absorption of available iron is regulated by the mucosal cells of the proximal small intestine. Mucosal regulation of iron absorption might occur by controlling one or more of the following steps: (1) mucosal uptake of iron across the brush border membrane, (2) retention of iron in storage form within the mucosal cell, and (3) transfer of the iron from the mucosal cell to the plasma.[98,100] The molecular route of iron uptake has not been established with certainty, although a number of iron-binding proteins have been identified in the mucosa.[101–110] Physiologically, the major determinants of mucosal iron absorption are the amount of body iron stores and the level of erythropoiesis—absorption increases with diminished storage iron and increased erythropoietic activity.[111] Hypoxia may independently increase iron absorption.[112] Practically, a maximum of about 3.5 mg Fe/day may be absorbed from the diet, even with an abundance of bioavailable iron and the enhanced level of absorption found in the iron-deficient individual.[113]

Internal Iron Exchange

Once absorbed, iron is bound to plasma transferrin. The daily disposition of this transferrin-bound iron is summarized in Figure 38-3.[114] In an iron-replete 70-kg man, the amount of transferrin iron in the plasma at any given time is only about 3 mg, but >30 mg of iron moves through this transport compartment each day.[94]

The erythron consists of the aggregate of all erythroid elements, including cells at all stages of development, immature and mature, and at all sites within the body, in the marrow, circulation, and extravascular space. Iron is required by every human cell, but most of the iron in the body is found within the erythron. Most of its daily movement cycles through the erythron. About 80% of the iron in transit (about 24 mg Fe/day) is taken up by erythroid precursors in the marrow. Most of this iron (17 mg Fe/day) becomes hemoglobin iron in circulating red cells. Red cells are eventually catabolized by specialized macrophages in the marrow, spleen, and liver, which release iron from the hemoglobin and return it to plasma transferrin. Some of the erythroid marrow iron (7 mg Fe/day) arrives at the macrophage more directly because of phagocytosis of defective erythroid precursors or removal of erythrocyte ferritin. Thus, the macrophage can return to the plasma trans-

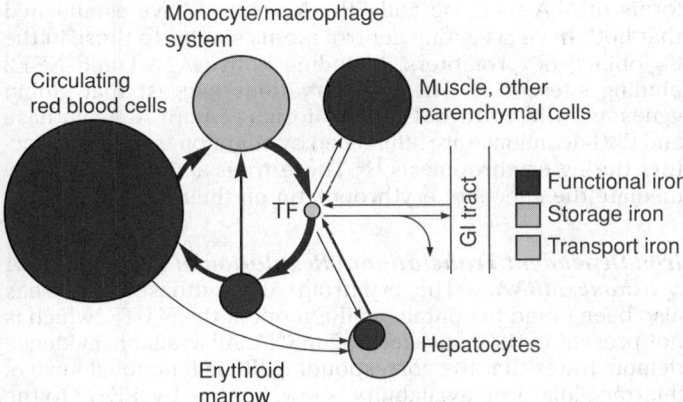

Fig. 38-3. Body iron supply and storage. Schematic representation of the routes of iron movement. The major pathway of internal iron exchange is a unidirectional flow from plasma transferrin (TF) to the erythron to the macrophage and back to plasma transferrin. Storage iron in the macrophages of the liver, bone marrow, and spleen is derived almost entirely from phagocytosis of senescent erythrocytes or defective developing red cells. The macrophage is virtually unable to take up iron from plasma transferrin while the hepatocyte may either donate iron to, or receive iron from, plasma transferrin. Normally, the overall magnitude of iron exchange by hepatocytes is only about one-fifth that of macrophages. Other pathways of iron movement involve approximately equal exchanges for iron absorption and losses, for transfer between the plasma and extravascular transferrin compartments, and for movement between extravascular transferrin and parenchymal tissues. In a pregnant woman, iron is taken up via placental transferrin receptors and unidirectionally passed to fetal transferrin for utilization by fetal tissues. (Adapted from Finch and Huebers,[95] with permission.)

Figure labels: Monocyte/macrophage system; Circulating red blood cells; Muscle, other parenchymal cells; GI tract; TF; Functional iron; Storage iron; Transport iron; Erythroid marrow; Hepatocytes

ferrin an amount of iron (22 mg Fe/day) almost equivalent to that donated to the erythron.

The remainder of daily erythron iron turnover is derived from some of the newly absorbed iron from the gastrointestinal tract and from the minor fraction (2 mg Fe/day) of hemoglobin iron that is lost into the plasma on enucleation of normoblasts or from intravascular hemolysis. This iron is bound to haptoglobin or hemopexin and delivered to the hepatocyte for eventual return to plasma transferrin.

The remaining 20% of iron carried by transferrin includes (1) iron exchange with hepatocytes (5 mg Fe/day), (2) movement between the plasma and extravascular transferrin compartments (about 3 mg Fe/day), (3) exchange between extravascular transferrin and parenchymal tissues (about 2 mg Fe/day), and (4) limited external exchange of iron through obligatory losses and absorption of iron from the gastrointestinal tract (about 1 and 1.5 mg Fe/day for men and women, respectively). The successive movement of iron through the major pathway of internal iron exchange—from plasma transferrin to the erythron to the macrophage and back to plasma transferrin—is summarized below with particular attention to those factors that regulate the flow of iron through the cycle.[114]

Movement of Iron from Transferrin to the Erythron. The movement of iron from transferrin to the erythron is determined by (1) the aggregate number of transferrin receptors on erythroid and nonerythroid cells and (2) the amounts of apo-, mono-, and diferric plasma transferrin. The number of transferrin receptors is a prime determinant of cellular iron supply. Because the number of transferrin receptors in nonerythroid tissues is stable under normal circumstances, the rate of erythropoiesis is the major determinant of the number of transferrin receptors in the erythron. As the rate of erythropoiesis increases, greater numbers of erythroid precursors with transferrin receptors are produced, increasing the rate of iron uptake.

Iron Uptake by Erythroid Cells. The acquisition, utilization, and storage of iron by erythroid cells is controlled differently during different phases of erythropoiesis. While the available evidence is fragmentary and incomplete, studies of human bone marrow and of erythroid cell lines in culture have suggested that erythropoietin acts as an indirect inducer for the transcription of mRNA for the erythroid-specific enzymes δ-aminolevulinic acid (ALA)-synthase and porphobilinogen (PBG)-deaminase in the heme biosynthetic pathway[115,116] and of α- and β-globin mRNA.[117] Repression of heme oxygenase, the enzyme responsible for heme degradation, has been proposed as an initiating event in the differentiation of erythroid progenitors.[116] Heme enhances the transcription of globin mRNA and acts to increase the translatability of globin mRNA.[118] Studies of early erythroid progenitors from chick embryos, have shown that the transferrin receptor gene is hyperexpressed at the transcriptional level by mechanisms not responsive to the availability of intracellular iron.[119] Mouse burst-forming unit-erythroid have few transferrin receptors; the number is higher in colony-forming unit-erythroid,[120] progressively increasing to about 300,000 per cell at the proerythroblast stage and peaking at 800,000 per cell in basophilic erythroblasts in which maximal iron uptake occurs.[23,121] Terminal maturation is associated with a fall in the number of receptors to about 100,000 in the circulating reticulocyte.

The rate of iron uptake from transferrin during erythroid cell development correlates closely with the number of transferrin receptors, suggesting that the level of transferrin receptors is the major factor that determines the rate of iron uptake during erythroid cell development.[23,121] Increased transferrin receptor expression thus succeeds the increase in the expression

of erythropoietin receptors but precedes the onset of heme synthesis.[122] In Friend erythroleukemia cells undergoing erythroid differentiation, heme synthesis is required for maximum transcription of mRNA for the transferrin receptor[123,124] and the H subunit of ferritin.[125] Other studies using the same model have suggested that an increase in heme during erythroid differentiation is required for the optimal transcription of mRNA for globin chains, transferrin receptor, and ferritin.[123,124] After hemoglobin synthesis is fully established in late erythroblasts and reticulocytes, translational control of the expression of transferrin receptor, ferritin, and heme seems to become the more important regulatory mechanism.

Use of Iron for Heme Synthesis in Erythroid Cells. Almost all the iron taken up by the erythron is used for the synthesis of heme. Small amounts are reserved for use in iron-containing enzymes in erythroid cells or sequestered within ferritin. In the adult, the erythron produces >85% of the total heme synthesized in the body.

The enzymes of the heme biosynthetic pathway must be expressed during the life of each cell in the body to provide for cytochrome and other vital heme enzymes (see Ch. 39). In addition to these constitutive or "housekeeping enzymes" produced during the life of all cells, erythroid-specific isozymes have been identified for ALA-synthase, which catalyzes the first step in the heme biosynthetic pathway, and for PBG-deaminase, which catalyzes the third. In humans, the two isozymes for ALA-synthase are encoded by different genes. The gene for the constitutive or "housekeeping" isozyme is on chromosome 3p21; that for the erythroid-specific form is on the X chromosome (Xp21-q21).[126-128] Only a single gene for PBG-deaminase exists in the human genome but it has two overlapping transcription units.[129-131] The upstream promoter is active in all cells; the downstream promoter is erythroid specific.[132] Alternative splicing produces two mRNAs that encode the PBG-deaminase isozymes.[133,134]

Studies of the promoter regions for the erythroid-specific forms of ALA-synthase and PBG-deaminase have established that both have cis-acting control motifs similar to those in the β-globin gene promoters, including both GATA-1 and NF-E2 binding sites.[132-136] These observations suggest that globin genes and the erythroid-specific forms of both ALA-synthase and PBG-deaminase are influenced by common trans-acting factors during erythropoiesis.[136] These trans-acting factors may mediate the effects of erythropoietin on their transcription.

Iron-Dependent Translational Regulation of Erythroid ALA Synthase mRNA. The erythroid ALA-synthase mRNA has also been found to contain an IRE motif in the 5' UTR, which is not present in the housekeeping mRNA. All available evidence demonstrates that the corresponding IRE is functional in vivo: if intracellular iron availability is low, binding by IRE-BP to the erythroid-specific ALA-synthase mRNA[136,137] will prevent translation (Fig. 38-2). This IRE may, therefore, help coordinate iron uptake and heme synthesis in erythroid cells.[137] The observation that erythroid ALA-synthase activity is decreased in erythroblasts from patients with iron deficiency[138] is consistent with translational regulation of erythroid ALA-synthase mRNA.

A reduction in erythroid ALA-synthase activity in iron deficiency anemia could be a protective mechanism to prevent the accumulation of porphyrins and porphyrin precursors and the stigmata of acquired porphyria.[138] Red cell protoporphyrin concentrations do increase with iron-deficiency anemia but the magnitude of the increase is restricted by translational regulation of erythroid ALA-synthase activity. The experimental data seem to exclude any involvement of the IRE in the feedback inhibition of erythroid ALA-synthase by heme. Hemin (ferric protoporphyrin IX) has been reported to inactivate the IRE-

BP,[139–142] but both the specificity of this effect and the physiologic relevance of this observation are uncertain.[143,144] Release of iron from heme into the intracellular iron pool may affect iron-regulated systems but this is an effect of the heme-derived iron rather than a direct effect of heme itself.[144,145] Altogether, the available evidence suggests that regulation of the activity of erythroid-specific ALA-synthase and, thereby, of the rate of heme synthesis in erythroid cells, involves (1) developmental transcriptional control by erythroid-specific trans-acting factors, (2) feedback inhibition by heme through a still undefined mechanism that does not influence the function of the mRNA, and (3) intracellular iron availability through IRE-BP control of the translation of the erythroid-specific ALA synthase mRNA.

Ferritin in Erythroid Cells. Iron delivered to developing red cells in excess of that required for heme synthesis is sequestered within ferritin. The more immature erythroid precursors contain higher concentrations of intracellular ferritin than mature forms and also have greater proportions of the H-type subunit.[146–148] The physiologic role of the iron contained in the H-rich ferritin in erythroid cells has not been established. Early studies suggested that iron within H-rich ferritin is stored temporarily before use in heme synthesis,[149] while the L-rich ferritin has been postulated to be a more stable reservoir for excess iron.[146–148] Other investigations using radiolabelled iron have been unable to demonstrate that erythroid ferritin iron functions as a donor for heme synthesis.[150,151] In any event, the major determinants of the ferritin content of the erythroid cell appear to be the plasma transferrin saturation (reflecting the iron supply to the erythroblast) and the rate of hemoglobin synthesis (an indicator of the erythroid iron requirement). Erythroid cell ferritin is decreased in patients with iron deficiency or with severe inflammatory disorders, but increased in other conditions in which hemoglobin synthesis is reduced, such as thalassemic disorders or sideroblastic anemias, or with iron overload.[152]

Other Regulatory Functions of Intracellular Iron Availability. Iron availability in erythroid cells can specifically alter the rates of production of heme, transferrin receptor, and ferritin through the IRE-BP; it also has more general effects on the metabolism of the developing erythroid cell. Although not yet reported for erythroid cells, the finding of an IRE in the 5′ UTR of (pig heart) mitochondrial aconitase mRNA[137] and the demonstration that the IRE-BP can bind to this site[153] raises the possibility of a further role in the regulation of cellular metabolism by coupling iron availability and the activity of the Krebs cycle.

Movement of Iron from the Erythron to the Macrophage.
The major pathway of iron movement from the erythron is into a specialized population of macrophages in the bone marrow, liver, and spleen when red cells reach the end of their lifespan (Fig. 38-3). The developing erythroid cell is dedicated to the acquisition of iron from transferrin. These select macrophages are devoted to the extraction of iron from hemoglobin for prompt return to transferrin or, if necessary, for storage for future use. In contrast to the detailed information available about red cell production, little is known about determinants of the fate of the senescent red cell and its contents. Less is known about the molecular mechanisms underlying the disposition of iron by the macrophage than about any other aspect of iron metabolism.[154]

Removal and Catabolism of Senescent or Damaged Erythrocytes. Senescent or damaged erythrocytes are selectively recognized and removed from the bloodstream by a specialized population of macrophages in the bone marrow, liver, and, especially, in the spleen. Marrow macrophages are also responsible for culling defective immature erythroid cells, to prevent their release into the circulation, and for removing some deposits of erythrocyte ferritin from developing red cells. During their life within the bloodstream, red cells undergo oxidant damage, alterations of membrane proteins and lipids, loss of surface sialic acid and electrostatic charge, decreases in ion gradients, and metabolic depletion of glycolytic and other enzymes.[155–157] Hemichrome formation with oxidative damage to membrane transport proteins may produce increased membrane permeability and defective volume regulation.[158] Cross-linking by hemoglobin or hemichromes of membrane band-3 molecules and the formation of "senescent" antigens have been reported.[158–160] Aged erythrocytes become dehydrated and lose surface area, with a decrease in cell volume and an increase in intracellular hemoglobin concentration making the cells less deformable.[161] Which one or which combination of these derangements forms the proximate stimulus for the removal from the circulation remains unknown. Under normal circumstances, billions of red cells are eliminated each day without any evidence of overt erythrophagocytosis within macrophages. Some form of erythrocyte fragmentation may thus occur before ingestion by macrophages.[162]

The overall pattern of the metabolism of catabolized hemoglobin in humans has been examined using heat-damaged erythrocytes labeled with radioactive iron.[163] Appearance of radioiron in the plasma occurs about 40 minutes after injection, presumably representing the time needed for phagocytosis of the cell and catabolism of heme. Radioiron is then released in a biphasic manner, a pattern that has also been observed in dogs[164] and in macrophages in culture.[165–167] In normal human volunteers, two-thirds of the administered radioiron re-emerges in an early rapid phase of iron release with a $t_{1/2}$ of about 30 minutes; the remaining one-third is incorporated into macrophage stores. It reappears in a late slow-phase $t_{1/2}$ of about 6 days.[163] In iron deficiency, iron release is derived entirely from the recently catabolized erythrocyte. With replete iron stores, the proportion of the radioiron derived from ingested red cells declines, especially during the early, rapid phase of iron output. The rate of late release is also influenced by the magnitude of iron stores; the greater the amount of storage iron, the longer the delay in release. In these studies, the macrophage seemed unable to retain >80% of the administered radioiron in storage form, even when plasma transferrin was fully saturated.[163] Inflammation[163,168,169] and ascorbic acid deficiency[170] increase the proportion of catabolized erythrocyte iron retained within macrophages.

The catabolism of red cells after phagocytosis by macrophages in vitro has been examined ultrastructurally in studies of the processing of IgG-coated red blood cells by Kupffer cells.[171–173] Each macrophage is able to fully process at least one ingested erythrocyte per hour.[174] Ingested antibody-coated erythrocytes are surrounded by projections of the plasma membrane and moved to the perinuclear area. Macrophage lysosomes fuse with the vacuole containing the phagocytzed red cell, forming a network of interconnecting channels that fragment the erythrocyte as its components are digested.[173] The erythrocyte membrane is lysed and the hemoglobin within oxidatively precipitated. Almost all the hemoglobin is rapidly catabolized with the globin proteolytically processed to amino acids, releasing heme. The heme is somehow transported to the endoplasmic reticulum of the macrophage to be degraded by heme oxygenase. Erythrophagocytosis has been shown to induce synthesis of heme oxygenase.[175]

Catabolism of Hemoglobin Iron. Heme oxygenase is a microsomal enzyme that catalyzes the rate-limiting step in the oxidative catabolism of heme. Two isoforms (or isozymes) of heme oxygenase have been recognized in rat liver and testis, and designated as HO-1 and HO-2,[176] but the form(s) present in macrophages have not been delineated. The two forms of heme oxygenase may be different gene products[177,178]; only HO-1 seems to be substrate inducible by heme.

The process of heme degradation by heme oxygenase has been characterized as a series of autocatalytic oxidations with the reaction intermediates as cofactors.[179] A total of three oxygen molecules and six reducing equivalents is required to degrade one heme molecule to biliverdin IXa. One iron and one carbon monoxide molecule are released. The precise reaction sequence has not been established. Conversion of the α-methane carbon to carbon monoxide is the sole physiologic source of carbon monoxide in the body. Iron release from the biliverdin/iron complex generates the linear tetrapyrrole biliverdin IXα, which is then reduced by biliverdin reductase to bilirubin IXα.[179]

The disposition of the iron released from heme is incompletely understood. It presumably enters an intracellular reservoir where the IRE-BP monitors iron availability. While peripheral blood monocytes have few transferrin receptors, cultured monocytes and macrophages of a variety of types express surface transferrin receptors and take up iron by this route.[180–182] (Ferrokinetic investigations in humans have found no evidence for movement of iron from transferrin to the macrophage in vivo,[183] but these studies may be less sensitive than studies of individual cells.) Maturation of monocytes to macrophages was associated with marked increases in active (reduced, high-affinity) IRE-BP and in both mRNA and protein for transferrin receptor and ferritin, probably as a result of increased gene transcription.[184,185] Most importantly, iron salts stimulated IRE-BP activity in cultured macrophages and was associated with a translationally mediated increase in both transferrin receptor and ferritin synthesis; treatment with the iron chelator desferrioxamine decreased transferrin receptor synthesis.[184,185]

These results should be contrasted with the findings in erythroid cells where an increase in iron exposure diminishes IRE-BP activity with a resultant decrease in transferrin receptor synthesis and an increase in ferritin synthesis; treatment with an iron chelator increases transferrin receptor synthesis. The consequences of these contrasting patterns of response to iron loading would apparently be to maintain a constant and consistent supply of bioavailable iron for utilization in heme synthesis in the erythroid cell but to increase both iron acquisition and storage in the macrophage. The net effect would be to move iron to the erythron from the macrophage in times of iron lack but to store iron within the macrophage system when iron stores are replete. The molecular bases for the difference in macrophage regulation of transferrin receptor and ferritin synthesis, as opposed to the erythroid cell pattern have not yet been determined.

Storage of Iron Within the Macrophage. Under normal circumstances, macrophages dedicated to reprocessing hemoglobin iron maintain an equilibrium between iron storage and release. Whatever the molecular mechanisms involved, synthesis of ferritin is induced in response to erythrophagocytosis. In the absence of iron deficiency, a portion of the iron derived from the ingested erythrocyte is retained within the macrophage as ferritin iron. No data are available to indicate whether incorporation into ferritin is an obligatory step during the passage of all iron through the macrophage or whether only that fraction to be stored is incorporated into ferritin. Studies of heat-damaged erythrocytes found that the fraction of radioiron sequestered within the macrophage can vary from virtually none in association with iron deficiency to a maximum of almost 80% in the presence of marrow aplasia and a fully saturated plasma transferrin.[163] Under no circumstances, is the macrophage able to retain more than approximately 80% of

the iron derived from the catabolized erythrocyte. Within the macrophage, this iron is stored predominantly in ferritin-rich L subunits.[149]

No turnover data are available for macrophage ferritin, but the half-life of hepatic ferritin is about 60 hours.[35] Catabolism of cellular ferritin may involve digestion of the protein shell, with reutilization of the iron core, or conversion to hemosiderin, an amorphous water insoluble storage compound with a higher iron content and slower turnover than ferritin. Hemosiderin is suitable for long-term storage of iron.[36,37] Both ferritin and hemosiderin iron in the macrophage remain available for mobilization in time of need. As storage iron within the macrophage increases, the proportion of iron stored within hemosiderin progressively increases. Ascorbic acid seems to retard ferritin degradation by reducing lysosomal autophagy of the protein,[38,39] thereby increasing the amount of iron stored in cytoplasmic ferritin.

Movement of Iron from the Erythron to the Hepatocyte. Hemoglobin iron that is released into the plasma during the enucleation of erythroblasts, or in states of intramedullary or intravascular hemolysis, is delivered to the hepatocyte for eventual return to plasma transferrin (Fig. 38-3). During normal erythropoiesis, this portion of the total iron flux is minor. It can increase substantially in disorders with increased ineffective erythropoiesis or intravascular hemolysis. Delivery of hemoglobin iron from the plasma to hepatocytes depends primarily on two glycoproteins: (1) haptoglobin for the binding and transport of αβ-dimers of hemoglobin; and (2) hemopexin for the binding and transport of heme, assisted, if needed, by albumin.

Haptoglobin Binding and Transport of Hemoglobin. At the low plasma concentration of hemoglobin produced by erythrocyte enucleation or normal levels of ineffective erythropoiesis, most of the hemoglobin dissociates into αβ dimers. Pairs of αβ dimers are then quickly bound in a symmetric fashion to a single molecule of haptoglobin. The half-life of apohaptoglobin is about 5 days, but that of the hemoglobin/haptoglobin complex is only about 10–30 minutes; the complexes are cleared by specific hepatocyte receptors.[186] The hemoglobin/haptoglobin complex (M_r 150,000) is too large to be filtered by the kidneys, a feature that helps restrict the renal loss of iron. After binding to the haptoglobin receptor of the hepatocyte, the hemoglobin/haptoglobin/receptor complex is internalized and dissociated symmetrically by limited proteolysis into two subunits of M_r 82,000 having intact hemes. Unlike the transferrin/transferrin receptor complex, the haptoglobin/haptoglobin receptor is degraded and cannot be recycled. The hemes are released to an unidentified carrier and catabolized by heme oxygenase, releasing iron within the hepatocyte.[186,187] Consumption of haptoglobin does not induce increased hepatic production, so that sustained hemoglobinemia produces hypo- or ahaptoglobinemia. Haptoglobin is a positive acute phase reactant, so inflammatory or infectious episodes may increase plasma concentrations.

Hemopexin Binding and Transport of Heme. Plasma hemoglobin that is not bound to haptoglobin is quickly oxidized to ferrihemoglobin (methemoglobin) that in turn can dissociate into globin and ferriheme (metheme). Ferriheme can then be bound by hemopexin; a single hemopexin binds a single ferriheme.[188] The half-life of apohemopexin is about 7 days, but that of the heme/hemopexin complex is 7–8 hours; these complexes are also cleared by specific hepatocyte receptors.[189,190] After binding, the heme/hemopexin/receptor complex is internalized within clathrin-coated pits. Receptor-mediated endocytosis results in catabolism of heme but not of the hemopexin or hemopexin receptor. They are recycled to the cell surface for reutilization in a manner analogous to the transferrin/transferrin receptor complex.[189] Delivery of heme into the hepatocyte results in induction of heme oxygenase, which releases the iron into the cell.[191,192]

Despite recycling, hemopexin may become depleted in patients with hemolysis. Each molecule of human albumin contains two binding sites for ferriheme, but these have a much lower affinity than that of the binding site of hemopexin. Binding of ferriheme produces methemalbumin which, after a delay of several days, ultimately also delivers the heme to the hepatocyte where the iron is liberated for reuse.[193]

Movement of Iron from the Macrophage to Transferrin.

The final step in the movement of iron through the cycle shown in Figure 38-2 requires the return of iron derived from the catabolism of senescent erythrocytes to plasma transferrin for delivery to the erythroid marrow. The outpouring of iron to plasma apotransferrin from macrophages in the bone marrow, liver, and spleen normally constitutes the largest single flux of iron from cells in the body. Despite the importance and magnitude of this flow, the mechanisms permitting the exit of iron from the macrophage remain an almost complete mystery. Virtually no definite information is available about (1) the form of iron within the cell before its departure, (2) the manner in which the iron is able to pass through the plasma membrane, (3) the form of the iron on its emergence from the cell, (4) the site and manner of delivery of the iron to plasma apotransferrin, or (5) the importance of iron release involving ferritin or carriers other than transferrin.

Release of Iron from Macrophages to Plasma.

Studies with radiolabelled, heat-damaged erythrocytes in normal volunteers have found a biphasic pattern of release of iron from the macrophage, with an early, rapid ($t_{1/2}$ about 30 minutes) phase and a late, slow phase ($t_{1/2}$ about 6 days).[163] Variations in iron release from the macrophage have been considered to be responsible for diurnal variations in the plasma iron concentration. The amount of the iron released is a function, in part, of the amount delivered to the macrophage. In some manner, iron release from the macrophage also seems to be influenced by erythroid marrow requirements. In iron deficiency, all the iron derived from hemoglobin catabolism is promptly returned to the plasma. None is diverted to macrophage stores.[163] During increased erythropoiesis associated with acute blood loss, macrophage iron stores are mobilized but the maximal rate of release from this source in the adult is limited to about 40-60 mg/day of iron.[194] When erythroid activity is increased in association with a sustained hemolytic state as much as 80-160 mg/day of iron may be released from macrophages to transferrin.[194] Decreased erythropoiesis can be matched by a reduction in macrophage iron release, but a minimum of about 20% of the iron presented to the macrophage must be returned to the plasma daily.[92,163] Iron release from macrophages may be inadequate to meet erythroid marrow needs in ascorbate deficiency,[171] and copper deficiency. In copper deficiency, hypoferremia is corrected by the administration of ceruloplasmin but not by copper itself.[195,196]

The overall patterns of iron release from macrophages have been described but the underlying mechanisms are almost entirely obscure. The release of iron is temperature dependent,[167,174] implying that macrophage processing and release of iron are energy-dependent processes. Export is not affected by iodoacetate, chloroquine, colchicine, cytochalasin B, or cylcohexamide, suggesting the lack of any role in the release process for glycolysis, acidification of an intracellular compartment, microtubule function, microfilament function, or protein synthesis.[167,174] Inflammatory states are associated with delayed processing and release of iron.[197] The exact mediators of this response are uncertain; no influence on the course of iron release from the Kupffer cell was found with interleukin (IL)-1, interferon-γ or tumor necrosis factor.[174] In other studies of peritoneal macrophages from mice, incubation with tumor necrosis factor in vitro decreased iron release.[198,199]

Apotransferrin Is Not Required for the Release of Iron from Macrophages.

Transferrin acts as the sole physiologic means for transport of iron to the erythroid marrow, but a requirement for unsaturated transferrin for release of iron from the macrophage has not been established. Apotransferrin does not enter the macrophage; it accepts iron only after the release of iron from the cell.[174,200] Release of iron derived from heat-damaged red cells was unaffected in vivo by transferrin saturation.[164,169,201] Injection of apotransferrin did not increase iron release.[168,202] The presence of apotransferrin was repeatedly shown to exert little or no effect on the magnitude of iron release in vitro,[166,174,200,203] although an enhanced release was observed in some studies.[204,205] The explanation for these apparently discrepant findings is not evident. Apotransferrin may not be required for the exit of iron from the macrophage, but much of the released iron is nonetheless available for binding by transferrin.[166,200,205]

Release of Iron from Macrophages in Ferritin.

Several studies have now found that much of the iron released from macrophages is in the form of ferritin,[174,200,205] but the physiologic fate of this released ferritin and its iron remain uncertain.[154] Iron-loaded ferritin, released by Kupffer cells after erythrophagocytosis in vitro, has been shown to be readily ingested by hepatocytes,[174,206] possibly by specific hepatocyte ferritin receptors.[207] These results have suggested the possibility that ferritin released by Kupffer cells may serve as an intrahepatic carrier of iron to the hepatocyte. Such a mechanism would protect the hepatocyte against iron deficiency but would also create the risk of iron loading with chronic hemolysis.[154]

Other Pathways of Iron Movement.

Ferrokinetic studies have suggested that the macrophage takes up little if any iron from plasma transferrin. By contrast, the hepatocyte may either donate iron to or receive iron from plasma transferrin. At high transferrin saturations, iron moves from the plasma to the liver, while at low saturations, iron is mobilized from hepatocyte stores and supplied to plasma transferrin. Normally, the overall magnitude of iron exchange by hepatocytes is only about one-fifth that by macrophages. Other pathways of iron movement involve approximately equal exchanges: about 1 mg Fe/day is absorbed and lost, about 3 mg Fe/day is transferred between the plasma and extravascular transferrin and parenchymal tissues.

In a pregnant woman the placenta is amply provided with transferrin receptors; these can successfully compete with the erythroid marrow for transferrin iron, which is taken up and unidirectionally passed to fetal transferrin for utilization by fetal tissues. Lactoferrin is a glycoprotein that is structurally similar to transferrin with a single polypeptide chain and two reversible binding sites for iron.[1,208-213] Lactoferrin has no established role in iron transport and is found principally in neutrophils and in external secretions.

Laboratory Evaluation of Iron Status

Figure 38-4 summarizes the continuum of changes in iron stores and distribution in the presence of increased or decreased body iron content. Characteristic values for clinically available indicators of iron status are also shown. The general

PLASMA FERRITIN CONCENTRATIONS

Decreased plasma ferritin concentrations are of great value in the detection of iron deficiency. Plasma ferritin concentrations decline with storage iron depletion; a plasma ferritin concentration of <12 μ/L is virtually diagnostic of absent iron stores. The only known conditions that may lower the plasma ferritin concentration independent of a decrease in iron stores are hypothyroidism and ascorbate deficiency.[234] These conditions would only rarely cause problems in clinical interpretation. Increased plasma ferritin concentrations may indicate increased iron stores, but a number of disorders may raise the plasma ferritin independently of the body iron. Plasma ferritin is an acute-phase reactant, increased ferritin synthesis being a nonspecific response that is part of the general pattern of the systemic effects of inflammation. Thus, fever, acute infections, rheumatoid arthritis, and other chronic inflammatory disorders elevate the plasma ferritin. Both acute and chronic damage to the liver, as well as to other ferritin-rich tissues, may increase plasma ferritin as an inflammatory process or by releasing tissue ferritins from damaged parenchymal cells. These tissue ferritins are not glycosylated.

TRANSFERRIN CONCENTRATION

An indicator of body iron stores that is much less sensitive than plasma ferritin is the transferrin concentration, usually measured in the clinical laboratory as the total iron-binding capacity. Transferrin may increase with storage iron depletion and decrease with iron overload but is not a consistently reliable index because of the degree to which levels are altered by other factors.[7,67,93] Inflammation, infection, malignancy, liver disease, nephrotic syndrome, and malnutrition all depress transferrin levels, while pregnancy and oral contraceptives produce elevations.

PLASMA IRON AND TRANSFERRIN SATURATION

Plasma iron and the transferrin saturation, which equals the ratio of plasma iron to total iron-binding capacity, provide a measure of current iron supply to tissues.[2] After storage iron is depleted, the serum iron falls; a transferring saturation of <16% is often used as the criterion for iron-deficient erythropoiesis. By contrast plasma iron and transferrin saturation are not reliably elevated with increased iron stores within macrophages, as occurs initially with transfusional iron overload, although the transferrin saturation may increase with parenchymal iron loading. Interpretation of the transferrin saturation is complicated by the substantial circadian fluctuations in plasma iron, as well as by day-to-day variations of ≥30%. Furthermore, the plasma iron is decreased by infection, inflammation, malignancy, and ascorbate deficiency but increased by iron ingestion, aplastic and sideroblastic anemia, ineffective erythropoiesis, and liver disease.

usefulness of these measures is considered here. Their specific application in the diagnosis of iron deficiency and iron overload is described below. Body iron supply and stores may be evaluated by both direct and indirect means, but no single indicator or combination of indicators is ideal in all clinical circumstances.[93] As body iron content decreases from the iron-replete normal to the amounts found in iron-deficiency anemia, or increases to the magnitudes found in iron overload, each available measure reflects in a different manner the continuum of changes shown in Figure 38-4. In addition, each indicator may be affected by other conditions, including infection, inflammation, liver disease, malignancy, or malnutrition. Each parameter must be interpreted with an awareness of the potential influence of such coexisting disorders.

Direct measures of body iron status yield quantitative, specific, and sensitive determinations of body or tissue iron stores. Quantitative phlebotomy provides a direct measure of total mobilizable storage iron.[93,214-216] Repeated venesection to remove about 500 ml of blood weekly is performed until the hemoglobin concentration falls below 10 g/dl for 2 weeks without further phlebotomy. Mobilizable storage iron may then be calculated as the amount of hemoglobin iron removed, with corrections for the hemoglobin deficit and estimated gastrointestinal iron absorption during the course of phlebotomy. Quantitative phlebotomy is primarily a research tool. It is not applicable to most anemic disorders but is occasionally useful in the diagnostic evaluation of some forms of iron overload.

Bone marrow aspiration and biopsy provide information about (1) macrophage storage iron, by semiquantitative grading of marrow hemosiderin stained with Prussian blue or, if needed, by chemical measurement of nonheme iron; (2) iron supply to erythroid precursors by determining the proportion and morphology of marrow sideroblasts (i.e., normoblasts with visible aggregates of iron in the cytoplasm); and (3) the general morphologic features of hematopoiesis.[93,217-219] Bone marrow aspiration and biopsy are useful in studies of iron deficiency but of limited applicability in the evaluation of iron overload because no information about the extent of parenchymal iron deposition is provided. In the evaluation of iron overload, liver biopsy is the best direct test for assessing iron deposition, permitting quantitative measurement of the nonheme iron concentration and histochemical examination of the pattern of iron accumulation in hepatocytes and Kupffer cells.[93,217,220,221]

These direct methods for assessing iron status have the disadvantages of being invasive procedures, with their attendant discomfort, lack of acceptability to patients, and, in the case of liver biopsy, risk. Several noninvasive means of measuring tissue iron stores are under development, including determination of hepatic magnetic susceptibility,[222] computed tomography,[223,224] and magnetic resonance imaging,[224-229] but as yet none is clinically available.[224,230,231]

Indirect measures of body iron status offer the advantages of ease and convenience but are subject to extraneous influences. Each lacks specificity or sensitivity, or both. The measurement of plasma ferritin provides the most useful indirect estimate of body iron stores.[40,93,231] Ferritin is secreted into the plasma in small amounts. While intracellular ferritin is produced by the smooth endoplasmic reticulum, plasma ferritin is synthesized by the rough endoplasmic reticulum and glycosylated by the Golgi apparatus. Under normal circumstances, the amount of plasma ferritin synthesized and secreted seems to be proportional to the amount of cellular ferritin produced in the internal iron storage pathway. Thus, the plasma ferritin concentration is related to the magnitude of body iron stores.[41]

The small amounts of ferritin secreted into the circulation can be measured by immunoassay and have been found to

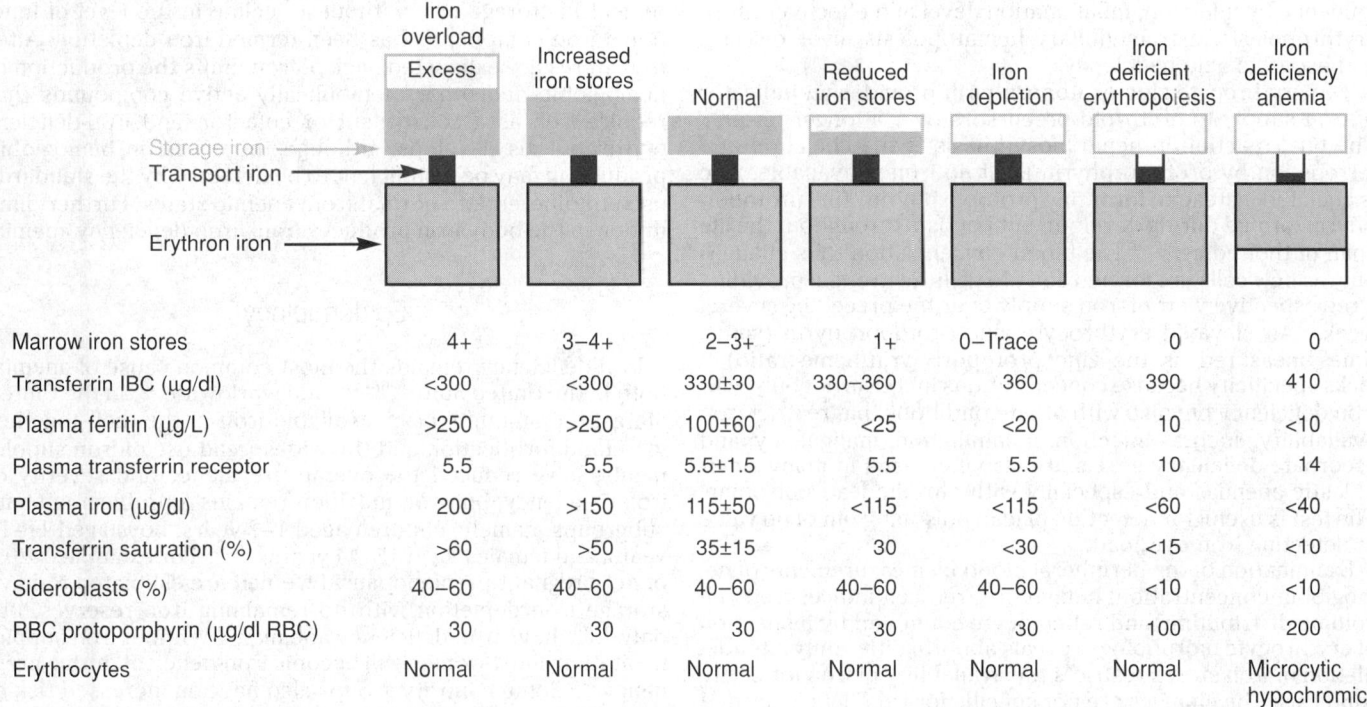

	Iron overload Excess	Increased iron stores	Normal	Reduced iron stores	Iron depletion	Iron deficient erythropoiesis	Iron deficiency anemia
Marrow iron stores	4+	3–4+	2–3+	1+	0–Trace	0	0
Transferrin IBC (µg/dl)	<300	<300	330±30	330–360	360	390	410
Plasma ferritin (µg/L)	>250	>250	100±60	<25	<20	10	<10
Plasma transferrin receptor	5.5	5.5	5.5±1.5	5.5	5.5	10	14
Plasma iron (µg/dl)	200	>150	115±50	<115	<115	<60	<40
Transferrin saturation (%)	>60	>50	35±15	30	<30	<15	<10
Sideroblasts (%)	40–60	40–60	40–60	40–60	40–60	<10	<10
RBC protoporphyrin (µg/dl RBC)	30	30	30	30	30	100	200
Erythrocytes	Normal	Normal	Normal	Normal	Normal	Normal	Microcytic hypochromic

Fig. 38-4. Continuum of changes in iron stores and distribution in the presence of increased or decreased body iron content. Abnormalities indicating the onset of specific stages of negative iron balance are enclosed in boxes. (From Herbert,[401] with permission.)

have a logarithmic relationship to body iron stores in normal individuals.[42,43,232] In the absence of complicating factors, plasma ferritin concentrations decrease with depletion of storage iron and increase with storage iron accumulation. A maximum glycosylated plasma ferritin concentration of about 4,000 µg/L has been postulated,[233] perhaps representing an upper physiologic limit of the rate of synthesis; higher concentrations are believed to be due to the release of intracellular ferritin from damaged cells.

Interpretation of plasma ferritin concentration is complicated by conditions that alter the relationship of plasma ferritin to body iron stores. Ascorbate deficiency may lower the plasma ferritin concentration independently of a decrease in iron stores.[234] Plasma ferritin is an "acute phase reactant." Increased synthesis is a nonspecific response that is part of the general pattern of the systemic effects of inflammation.[235] Consequently, fever, acute infections, and chronic inflammatory disorders elevate the plasma ferritin. Acute or chronic damage to the liver, as well as to other ferritin-rich tissues, may increase plasma ferritin by an inflammatory process or by releasing tissue ferritins from damaged parenchymal cells, or both.[233] Hepatic dysfunction may also raise the plasma ferritin by impeding clearance of circulating ferritin. Hemolysis and ineffective erythropoiesis are associated with elevations of plasma ferritin that are unrelated to an increase in body iron stores. Finally, malignancy may elevate plasma ferritin concentrations by inflammatory effects, by release of ferritin from damaged cells (especially with chemotherapy), by associated hepatic dysfunction impeding clearance, or by direct synthesis of ferritins by tumor cells.[40]

Measurement of the plasma transferrin receptor concentration provides a useful new means of detecting iron deficiency.[236] The soluble transferrin receptor is a truncated form (M_r 85,000) of the tissue transferrin receptor. It consists of the N-terminal cytoplasmic domain that has probably been proteolytically released from the cell membrane.[237–239] Immunoassays for the soluble truncated form in human plasma are becoming clinically available.[240] Much remains to be learned

about the origin and fate of plasma transferrin receptors. Most are derived from the erythroid marrow. The concentration of circulating soluble receptor is primarily determined by erythroid marrow activity.[240–244] Decreased levels are found in patients with erythroid hypoplasia (aplastic anemia, chronic renal failure), while increased levels are present in patients with erythroid hyperplasia (thalassemia major, sickle cell anemia, chronic hemolytic anemia). Iron deficiency also increases soluble transferrin receptor concentrations. It is not clear to what extent this increase is due to increased transferrin receptor expression by individual erythroblasts or simply an appropriate response to the degree of anemia and associated erythropoietin stimulation.

Initial clinical experience indicates that the plasma transferrin receptor concentration reflects the total body mass of tissue receptor. In the absence of other conditions causing erythroid hyperplasia, an increased concentration provides a sensitive, quantitative measure of tissue iron deficiency.[236,245] In particular, measurement of the plasma transferrin receptor concentration may help in the task of differentiating between the anemia of iron deficiency and the anemia associated with chronic inflammatory disorders. Plasma ferritin may be disproportionately elevated in relationship to iron stores in patients with inflammation or liver disease, but the plasma transferrin receptor concentration seems to be unaffected by these disorders.[246] It could provide a more reliable laboratory indicator of iron deficiency. Measurement of plasma transferrin receptor concentration is of no use in the detection of iron overload.

The measurement of urinary iron excretion with chelating agents, such as desferrioxamine[247] or diethylenetriamine penta-acetate,[248] offers another means of assessing body iron stores.[94] This test is not helpful in the detection of iron deficiency because of the overlap between values in individuals with normal and decreased iron stores; it is applied primarily to the evaluation of iron overload. The usefulness of the measurement of chelated iron in the urine is limited. The results do not correlate well with quantitative phlebotomy in states of parenchymal iron overload and are susceptible to extraneous influence by infection, inflammation, level and effectiveness of erythropoiesis, extramedullary hematopoiesis, liver disease, and ascorbic acid deficiency.

The erythrocyte zinc protoporphyrin provides an indicator of iron supply to erythroid precursors over a longer term.[249] The final reaction in heme biosynthesis is the chelation of a ferrous ion by protoporphyrin IX. If no iron is available, zinc is chelated instead to form zinc protoporphyrin. Zinc protoporphyrin formed during development persists throughout the life span of the red cell.[250] The blood concentration thus changes only as new cells are formed and old cells destroyed, providing a retrospective view of iron supply over the preceding several weeks. An elevated erythrocyte zinc protoporphyrin (sometimes measured as the zinc protoporphyrin/heme ratio)[251] lacks specificity because concentrations increase not only with iron deficiency but also with other conditions that restrict iron availability, such as infection, inflammation, malignancy, and ascorbate deficiency; levels are also increased in many sideroblastic anemias and especially with chronic lead poisoning. The test is useful for detection of lead poisoning but of no value in detecting iron overload.

Examination of the peripheral blood by measurements of hemoglobin concentration, hematocrit, red cell indices, red cell volume distribution, and reticulocyte count and by inspection of erythrocyte morphology reveals abnormalities only after depletion of iron stores restricts the availability of iron for erythropoiesis. The changes are not specific for iron deficiency and may be found in other conditions with defective hemoglobin synthesis, such as thalassemia, infection, inflammation, liver disease, and malignancy.[93,94,252] Iron overload does not produce any diagnostic abnormalities in the peripheral blood smear.

Future Directions

The molecular basis of cellular iron metabolism is beginning to be deciphered.[38] More detailed structural studies should clarify how the IRE-BP recognizes and binds to the IRE. Recently, Cys 437 in the IRE-BP has been identified as the target of regulation in vitro of RNA binding.[58] Definitive identification of ligands for intracellular low-molecular-weight iron is still needed, along with an understanding of their interrelationship with the IRE-BP. Differences in the IRE-BP in specific tissues[185] are likely to continue to emerge. Other proteins whose mRNA contains an IRE will almost surely be identified. A link between translational regulation through IREs and the nitric oxide/nitric oxide-synthase pathway has recently been reported[253,254] and needs to be more fully explored.

The interconnection of translational regulation through IREs and cytokines will be examined more thoroughly.[255–257]

Further understanding of the regulation of iron absorption may be imminent. Recently, studies of the mouse microcytic anemia *mk* have suggested that a single hematopoietic transcription factor, NF-E2, may link the control of erythropoeisis and of intestinal iron absorption.[258] NF-E2 is involved in the erythroid enhancer activity of the α- and β-globin locus control regions.[259] Homozygous *mk* mice have a severe hypochromic, microcytic anemia that is the result of diminished globin synthesis, defective erythroid iron uptake, and impaired intestinal iron absorption. The *mk* allele was found to carry a missense mutation while p45 NF-E2 mRNA was detected in both erythroid and duodenal tissue. These results suggested that NF-E2 is a nuclear regulator that links intestinal iron absorption and heme biosynthesis in erythroid cells, the major site of iron utilization within the body.[258]

IRON DEFICIENCY

Iron deficiency denotes a deficit in total body iron, resulting from iron requirements that exceed iron supply. Three successive stages of iron lack may be distinguished (Fig. 38-3). A decrement in storage iron without a decline in the level of functional iron compounds has been termed iron depletion. After iron stores are exhausted, lack of iron limits the production of hemoglobin and other metabolically active compounds that require iron as a constituent or cofactor, and iron-deficient erythropoiesis develops, although the effect on hemoglobin production may be insufficient to be detected by the standards used to differentiate normal from anemic states. Further diminution in the body iron produces frank iron-deficiency anemia.

Epidemiology

Iron deficiency remains the most common cause of anemia, both in the United States[260–262] and worldwide.[263] In the United States, the amounts of bioavailable iron in the diet, together with food fortification and the widespread use of iron supplements, have reduced the overall prevalence and severity of iron deficiency, but iron nutrition remains a problem in some subgroups, namely, children aged 1–2 years, boys aged 11–14 years, and females aged 15–44 years.[260,262] For example, >20% of nonpregnant premenopausal women are estimated to have storage iron depletion with no remaining iron reserves, but only 2.6% have iron-deficiency anemia.[264] Without iron supplementation, most women will become iron-deficient during pregnancy.[265] Some minority groups also have an increased risk of iron deficiency.[266] Globally, about 30% of the estimated world population of almost 4.5 billion are anemic, and at least one-half of these, or 500–600 million people, are believed to have iron-deficiency anemia.[263] Populations who have diets low in bioavailable iron or who suffer from chronic gastrointestinal blood loss due to helminthic infection, or both, have the highest prevalences of iron deficiency.

Etiology and Pathogenesis

The foremost task in the evaluation of a patient with iron deficiency is to identify and treat the underlying cause of the imbalance between iron requirements and supply (Table 38-3). The most common cause of increased iron requirements leading to iron deficiency is blood loss; in men and postmenopausal women, iron deficiency almost inevitably signifies gastrointestinal blood loss.[267] Within the gastrointestinal tract, any hemorrhagic lesion may be responsible for blood loss, including hiatal hernia, esophageal varices, gastritis, duodenitis, peptic ulcer, cholelithiasis, intrahepatic bleeding, inflammatory bowel disease, diverticulosis, hemorrhoids, and adenomatous polyps. Iron deficiency is often the first sign of an occult gastrointestinal malignancy. Chronic ingestion of drugs such as alcohol, salicylates, steroids, and nonsteroidal anti-inflammatory agents may cause or contribute to blood loss.

The most frequent cause of gastrointestinal blood loss world-

Table 38-3. Causes of Iron Deficiency

Increased iron requirements
Blood loss
Gastrointestinal tract
Genitourinary tract
Respiratory tract
Blood donation
Growth
Pregnancy and lactation
Inadequate iron supply
Diets with insufficient amounts of bioavailable iron
Impaired absorption of iron
Intestinal malabsorption
Gastric surgery

wide is hookworm—about 1 billion people are believed to be infected. Other helminthic infections, such as *Schistosoma mansoni, Schistosoma japonicum,* and severe *Trichuris trichiura* infection, may also cause gastrointestinal blood loss. Less common causes of gastrointestinal bleeding must also be considered in individual patients, including vascular purpura with scurvy, aberrant pancreas, Meckel's diverticulum, hereditary hemorrhagic telangiectasia, other vascular ectasia of the bowel, and colonic polyposis.

In women of childbearing age, genitourinary blood loss with menses is often responsible for increased iron requirements.[268] Menstrual losses tend to be decreased with the use of oral contraceptives but are increased with intrauterine devices. Other causes of genitourinary bleeding include uterine malignancies or fibroids; stones, infarction, infection with *Schistosoma haematobium,* inflammatory disease, or malignancy of the urinary tract; and, rarely, chronic hemoglobinuria or hemosiderinuria resulting from paroxysmal nocturnal hemoglobinuria or chronic intravascular hemolysis.

Respiratory tract blood loss resulting from chronic recurrent hemoptysis of any cause may rarely produce iron deficiency. In two uncommon conditions, idiopathic pulmonary siderosis[269] and Goodpasture syndrome,[270] hemoptysis and intrapulmonary bleeding may be inapparent but lead to the sequestration of iron in pulmonary macrophages. This sequestered iron is still within the body, but it is "lost" for systemic utilization. Severe iron deficiency anemia can develop. Recurrent blood donation may lead to iron deficiency, particularly in menstruating women.[271]

In infants, children, and adolescents, iron needed for growth may exceed the supply available from diet and stores. At birth, the iron endowment of the infant is primarily determined by the birthweight and hemoglobin concentration. Mild maternal iron deficiency does not usually restrict iron delivery to the fetus, but moderate to severe iron-deficiency anemia in the mother can cause both a decreased hemoglobin concentration and lower birthweight in the neonate.[272] Premature infants, with a lower birthweight and a more rapid postnatal rate of growth, have a high risk of iron deficiency. Rapid growth during the first year of life normally triples the body weight. Iron requirements (expressed as micrograms iron per kilogram body weight) are at a high level. Iron requirements decline as growth slows during the second year of life and into childhood but rise again during the adolescent growth spurt.

Without supplemental iron, pregnancy entails the net loss of the equivalent of 1,200–1,500 ml blood. On the average, 270 mg of iron is donated to the fetus, an additional 90 mg is contained in the cord and placenta, and 150 mg is present in the lochia and blood lost at delivery, a total of slightly >500 mg of iron.[94] During pregnancy, the red cell mass increases by more than one-third, requiring almost another 500 mg of iron. This iron is returned to stores after delivery and is not included in the net cost of a pregnancy. The resumption of menstruation after delivery is usually delayed for some months, but if the infant is breast-fed, lactation requires about 0.5–1.0 mg Fe/day.

An inadequate supply may contribute to or, under special circumstances, account for the development of, iron deficiency. In infants[273] or women who have experienced heavy menstrual losses or multiple pregnancies, the risk of iron deficiency will be further increased by the habitual consumption of diets with insufficient amounts of bioavailable iron, such as those with little or no heme iron or with small amounts of enhancers or large amounts of inhibitors of nonheme iron absorption. For older children, men, and postmenopausal women, the restricted availability of dietary iron is almost never the sole explanation for iron deficiency and other causes, especially blood loss, must be considered.

Impaired iron absorption infrequently produces iron deficiency. Intestinal malabsorption of iron may occur as a manifestation of more generalized syndromes, such as steatorrhea of various causes, sprue, celiac disease, or diffuse enteritis. Atrophic gastritis and the attendant achlorhydria may impair iron absorption. In all ages and sexes, but particularly in pregnant women and children, pica, the compulsive chewing or ingestion of food or nonfood substances, may contribute to iron deficiency if the material consumed inhibits iron absorption. Iron deficiency frequently complicates gastric surgery (e.g., partial or total gastric resection or gastroenterostomy for bypass of the duodenum).[274] Poor absorption is due to the loss of gastric acid production and to the decreased time available for iron absorption; the latter is a consequence of the increased rate of intestinal transit. Recurrent bleeding at the surgical site may also contribute. Despite impaired absorption of dietary iron, therapeutic preparations of iron salts are usually well absorbed.

Increased iron requirements and an inadequate supply of iron often work in concert to produce iron deficiency. Infants fed cow's milk receive iron in inadequate amounts with low bioavailability; moreover, this diet also increases iron losses by causing gastrointestinal bleeding.[275,276] Menstruating women, who exhibit the highest iron requirements, may consume diets that have a low content of iron and that also contain inhibitors of iron absorption, such as calcium.[277] Patients with ulcer disease and increased gastrointestinal blood loss may be treated with antacids, which diminish dietary iron absorption.

Clinical Presentation

Patients with iron deficiency may present (1) with no signs or symptoms, coming to medical attention only because of abnormalities in laboratory tests; (2) with the features of the underlying disorder responsible for the development of iron deficiency; and (3) with the manifestations common to all anemias. Patients may, but often do not, exhibit one or more of the few signs and symptoms considered highly specific for iron deficiency: pagophagia, koilonychia, and blue sclerae. No signs or symptoms have been ascribed to uncomplicated depletion of storage iron, although patients without iron reserves will not respond as rapidly to an increased need for iron resulting from blood loss, growth, or pregnancy.

Deficits in body iron, sufficient to restrict the synthesis of functional iron compounds and cause anemia may be either asymptomatic or may produce a variety of clinical manifestations. Iron-deficiency anemia exhibits the signs and symptoms common to all anemias: pallor, palpitations, tinnitus, headache, irritability, weakness, dizziness, and easy fatiguability. The prominence of these signs depends on both the degree and the rate of development of the anemia.[92] Because iron deficiency is often of insidious onset and prolonged duration, adaptive circulatory and respiratory responses may minimize these manifestations, permitting surprising tolerance of low hemoglobin concentrations. With greater severity, anemia becomes increasingly debilitating as work capacity and tolerance of physical exertion are restricted. Severe anemia can eventually produce cardiorespiratory failure and even death.

Iron deficiency can produce clinical manifestations independent of anemia. These result from the depletion of functional iron compounds in nonerythroid tissues, resulting in impaired proliferation, growth, and function.[273,280] Epithelial tissues have high iron requirements due to rapid rates of growth and turnover and are thus affected in many patients with chronic iron deficiency. Glossitis, angular stomatitis, postcricoid esophageal web or stricture (which may become malignant), and gastric atrophy may develop; the combination of glossitis, a sore or burning mouth, dysphagia, and iron deficiency is called the Plummer-Vinson or Patterson-Kelly syndrome. The prevalence of these abnormalities seems to vary geographically, which suggests that environmental or genetic factors may also be involved.[94]

Determining whether gastric atrophy is the cause or consequence of iron deficiency may be difficult, particularly in older patients; in some, pernicious anemia and iron deficiency coexist. Changes in the lingual or buccal mucosa have been suggested as factors causing or contributing to the pica that develops in many patients with iron deficiency. Pagophagia, a variant of pica in which ice is the substance obsessively consumed, is a behavioral abnormality that is considered to be a highly specific symptom of iron deficiency, resolving within a few days to 2 weeks after the beginning of iron therapy.[279-282] Other types of pica, with a variety of nonfoods, such as clay, starch, paper, or dirt, or with an assortment of foods, may occur, but these are not as clearly linked to a lack of iron or as frequently responsive to iron therapy.

Koilonychia (fingernails that are thin, friable, and brittle, with the distal half in a concave or "spoon" shape resulting from impaired nailbed epithelial growth) are virtually pathognomonic of iron deficiency, but present in a small minority of patients. Blue sclerae, or sclerae with a definite or striking bluish hue, were recognized in 1908 by Osler[283] as associated with iron deficiency and have been reported to be both highly specific and sensitive as an indicator of iron deficiency. The bluish tinge is thought to result from thinning of the sclera, which makes the choroid visible; the thin sclera has been postulated to be the result of impairment of collagen synthesis by iron deficiency. In one series of patients with iron deficiency anemia, mucosal pallor was found in 30%, glossitis in 17%, and koilonychia in 4%, while blue sclerae were present in 87% of patients, with a 94% specificity.[284] Iron deficiency has also been postulated to cause other nonhematologic derangements, involving impaired immunity and resistance to infection, diminished exercise tolerance and work performance, and behavioral and neuropsychological abnormalities.[278,285-289]

Laboratory Evaluation

There is a characteristic sequence of changes in the indicators of iron status that occur as body iron decreases from normal iron-replete levels to those found in iron-deficiency anemia (Fig. 38-4). The patterns shown are those developing in the absence of complicating factors, such as infection, inflammation, liver disease, malignancy, or other disorders. Any of the diatheses listed in Table 38-3 will initially cause iron requirements to exceed the available supply. Iron is mobilized from body stores and absorption is increased. If these combined amounts are inadequate, depletion of storage iron follows. At this stage, bone marrow examination shows absent, or nearly absent, hemosiderin iron. The serum ferritin falls, while the total iron-binding capacity rises.

Exhaustion of iron reserves results in an inadequate supply of iron to the developing erythroid cell. Iron-deficient erythropoiesis commences. Plasma transferrin receptor concentrations increase as the total body mass of tissue receptor expands. The plasma ferritin decreases to <12 μg/L, reflecting the absence of storage iron; the total iron-binding capacity continues to rise. The plasma iron declines, and in combination with the increase in total iron-binding capacity, the transferrin saturation falls to $<16\%$. As a result, most iron is derived from mono- rather than diferric transferrin, and most ferric transferrin/transferrin receptor complexes provide only one or two atoms of iron with each intracellular delivery cycle. Marrow examination begins to show a decrease in the proportion of sideroblasts because too little iron is available to support siderotic granule formation. The erythrocyte zinc protoporphyrin progressively increases as the amount of iron available for heme formation declines.

As hemoglobin production becomes restricted, frank iron-deficiency anemia finally develops. The normocytic, normochromic red cells previously formed under iron-replete circumstances are gradually replaced by a microcytic hypochromic population. Both the time needed to replace the normal population and the extent of the disparity between erythroid needs and available iron supply determine the rate and degree of change in erythrocyte morphology and red cell indices, such as the mean corpuscular volume, mean corpuscular hemoglobin, and measures of the distribution of red cell volumes (e.g., red cell volume distribution width). Chronic, long-standing iron-deficiency anemia may produce severe microcytosis and hypochromia, with very pale, distorted red cells and dramatic reductions in the mean corpuscular volume and mean corpuscular hemoglobin. By contrast, some patients with mild iron-deficiency anemia may have erythrocyte morphology and indices indistinguishable from those found in normal, iron-replete individuals.[290] Nonetheless, laboratory evaluation of uncomplicated iron deficiency in otherwise healthy individuals is usually not difficult. The characteristic patterns of indicators of body iron status shown in Figure 38-4 will typically be diagnostic.

Differential Diagnosis

Iron deficiency is the only microcytic hypochromic disorder in which mobilizable iron stores are absent; in all others, storage iron is normal or increased (Table 38-4). Thus the diagnosis of iron deficiency can almost always be verified by direct assessment of body iron stores using bone marrow examination: if no iron stores are present, the diagnosis of iron deficiency is established; if hemosiderin is found, iron deficiency is excluded. In addition, with iron deficiency sideroblasts will be absent or greatly decreased to $<10\%$ of normoblasts.[291] Rarely, previous parenteral iron therapy can complicate interpretation because of the presence of aggregates of iron that are effectively unavailable. Technical errors due to sampling or artifacts can usually be avoided by the examination of biopsy cores and of both stained and unstained aspirates containing ample amounts of stroma.

Difficulties in the evaluation of microcytic hypochromic disorders usually arise when direct assessment of marrow iron is

---

THERAPEUTIC TRIAL OF IRON THERAPY

The diagnosis of iron deficiency is often confirmed by the outcome of a therapeutic trial of iron therapy. A specific orderly response to, and only to, treatment with iron constitutes the final, definitive proof that a lack of iron is the cause of an anemia. The unequivocal diagnostic response consists of (1) a reticulocytosis, which begins about 3–5 days after adequate iron therapy is instituted, reaching a maximum on the eight to tenth day and then declining; and (2) a significant increase in the hemoglobin concentration, which should begin shortly after the reticulocyte peak, is invariably present by 3 weeks after iron therapy is begun, and persists until the hemoglobin concentration is restored to normal.[92] The result of a therapeutic trial of iron must be evaluated with due regard for possible confounding factors, such as poor compliance with iron therapy, malabsorption of therapeutic iron, continuing blood loss, and the effects of coexisting conditions, especially infectious, inflammatory, or malignant disorders.

Table 38-4. Differential Diagnosis of Microcytic Hypochromic Anemia

With decreased body iron stores
    Iron deficiency anemia
With normal or increased body iron stores
    Impaired iron metabolism
        Anemia in chronic disease
        Defective absorption, transport, or utilization of iron
    Disorders of globin synthesis
        Thalassemia
        Microcytic hemoglobinopathies
    Disorders of heme synthesis: sideroblastic anemias
        Hereditary
        Acquired

unavailable or inadvisable and the diagnosis depends on indirect indicators of iron status. In otherwise healthy individuals, these indirect measures are often helpful, but in the presence of infection, inflammation, malignancy, malnutrition, alcoholism, or liver disease, their interpretation is often problematic. Of the indirect indicators, the plasma ferritin is most useful if the concentration is <12 µg/L. In the absence of hypothyroidism or ascorbate deficiency, such a low ferritin is highly specific for iron deficiency. By contrast, a plasma ferritin within the normal range does not necessarily indicate the presence of storage iron, for ferritin concentrations may be increased independently of iron status by the aforementioned states.

Measurement of the plasma transferrin receptor concentration may be useful in differentiating the anemia of iron deficiency from the anemia associated with chronic inflammatory disorders. While serum ferritin may be disproportionately elevated in relationship to iron stores in patients with inflammation or liver disease, the plasma transferrin receptor concentration seems to be unaffected by these disorders and to provide a more reliable laboratory indicator of iron-deficiency anemia.[246] Disorders that restrict the cellular iron supply may further complicate interpretation by lowering the plasma iron and transferrin saturation, increasing the erythrocyte zinc protoporphyrin, and in the peripheral blood by producing reticulocytopenia, microcytosis, hypochromia, and anemia. Because of the lack of sensitivity and specificity of the indirect indicators of iron status, the most reliable means of diagnosing iron deficiency in some patients may be to resort to bone marrow examination or to undertake a therapeutic trial of iron.

Specific entities to be considered in the differential diagnosis of hypochromic microcytic disorders are listed in Table 38-4; in all of these body iron stores are normal or increased. In some, the hematologic abnormalities are associated with impaired iron metabolism. The anemia of chronic disease is the most common cause of anemia in hospitalized patients,[292] typi-

IRON DEFICIENCY AND COEXISTING DISORDERS

Detection of iron deficiency in the presence of chronic infectious, inflammatory, or malignant disorders is more problematic. Even if iron lack contributes to the anemia of chronic disease, the transferrin concentration will be decreased and the plasma ferritin concentration increased. Under these circumstances, bone marrow examination is definitive: if iron deficiency is present, iron stores are absent; if the anemia of chronic disease is alone responsible, iron stores are present and typically increased. A therapeutic trial of iron therapy may also be helpful in determining whether a lack of iron contributes to the anemia of chronic disease.

cally developing over several weeks in those with chronic infectious, inflammatory, or malignant disorders.[293] The anemia is usually mild to moderate, the severity being approximately proportional to that of the chronic illness. Erythrocytes are normocytic or slightly microcytic and variably hypochromic. The underlying disorders impair iron release from macrophages; iron accumulates within these cells. The plasma iron falls, and iron supply to tissue diminishes. Within the bone marrow is found the diagnostic combination of increased iron sequestered in macrophage stores with decreased sideroblasts, reflecting the inadequate supply of iron to developing erythroid cells. While in uncomplicated iron deficiency the transferrin concentration (total iron-binding capacity) increases, in the anemia of chronic disease the transferrin concentration decreases, a characteristic feature useful in distinguishing between the two causes of anemia. The plasma ferritin may also be diagnostically helpful: concentrations fall to <12 µg/L in uncomplicated iron deficiency but rise in the anemia of chronic disease. The plasma transferrin receptor concentration will remain within the normal range with the anemia of chronic disorders but will increase with iron deficiency.[246] These indirect indicators of iron status usually allow differentiation of the anemia of chronic disease from uncomplicated iron deficiency.

Microcytosis and hypochromia resulting from defective absorption, transportation, or utilization of iron occur rarely. Congenital atransferrinemia is an autosomal recessive disorder in which plasma transferrin is nearly absent.[294-296] A severe microcytic hypochromic anemia, present from birth, is refractory to iron therapy but responds to transferrin infusion. Iron absorption is normal or increased. Iron deposits are found in the liver and other parenchymal tissues but are scant or absent in the bone marrow. Patients die without transferrin infusion[295] or blood transfusions and are at risk of the complications of iron overload.

Several rare congenital defects characterized by microcytic hypochromic anemias in combination with parenchymal iron overload have also been reported. Defective uptake of iron by erythroid precursors was suggested by the findings in two siblings with a severe hypochromic anemia in conjunction with increased plasma iron, marked hepatic iron deposition, and fibrosis, but no definite etiology was established.[297] A single patient has been reported to have an acquired microcytic hypochromic anemia resulting from an IgM autoantibody against the transferrin receptor, causing diminished iron incorporation by erythroid precursors. In this patient serum iron was increased, but marrow iron stores were absent.[298] Three siblings with microcytic hypochromic anemia apparently due to isolated malabsorption and defective utilization of iron have been described.[299] The effect of copper deficiency on iron metabolism and erythropoiesis is still under investigation.[300]

Microcytic hypochromic anemias resulting from disorders of globin synthesis (thalassemias, microcytic hemoglobinopathies) and from disorders of heme synthesis (sideroblastic anemias, congenital and acquired) are discussed in Chapters 40 and 42. In general, the plasma iron, transferrin saturation, plasma ferritin concentration, and bone marrow iron stores are normal or increased in these disorders, and their differentiation from iron deficiency is not difficult.

Therapy

The goal of therapy for iron deficiency anemia is to supply sufficient iron to repair the hemoglobin deficit and replenish storage iron. Oral iron is the treatment of choice for almost all patients because of its effectiveness, safety, and economy. Local and systemic adverse reactions restrict the use of parenteral iron to those few patients unable to absorb or tolerate adequate amounts of oral iron. Rarely, red cell transfusions are needed to prevent cardiac or cerebral ischemia in severe

ORAL IRON THERAPY

Oral iron therapy should begin with a ferrous iron salt, taken apart from meals in three or four divided doses and supplying a daily total of 150–200 mg elemental iron in adults or 3 mg iron per kilogram body weight in children. Simple ferrous preparations are the best absorbed and least expensive; ferrous sulfate is the most widely used, either as tablets containing 60–70 mg iron for adults or as a liquid preparation for children. Administration between meals maximizes absorption. In patients with a hemoglobin concentration of <10 g/dl, this regimen will initially provide about 40–60 mg iron per day for erythropoiesis, permitting red cell production to increase to two to four times normal and the hemoglobin concentration to rise by about 0.2 g/dl/day.[195] An increase in the hemoglobin concentration of ≥2 g/dl after 3 weeks of therapy is generally used as the criterion for an adequate therapeutic response.[94] For milder anemia, a single daily dose of about 60 mg iron per day may be adequate. After the anemia has been fully corrected, oral iron should be continued to replace storage iron, either empirically for an additional 4–6 months or until the plasma ferritin concentration exceeds about 50 μg/L.[252]

anemia or to support patients whose chronic rate of iron loss exceeds the rate of replacement possible with parenteral therapy.

Most patients are able to tolerate oral iron therapy without difficulty; 10–20% may have symptoms attributable to iron.[252] The most common side effects are gastrointestinal. The development of either diarrhea or constipation can usually be treated symptomatically; alterations in bowel habits do not appear to be related to the dose of iron and seldom necessitate a change in the oral regimen.

Upper gastrointestinal symptoms do seem to be dose related, reflecting the concentration of ferrous iron in the stomach and duodenum. These side effects occur within about 1 hour of iron ingestion and may be mild, with nausea and epigastric discomfort, or severe, with abdominal pain and vomiting. Often upper gastrointestinal side effects can be managed by administering the iron with or immediately after meals. If symptoms persist, reductions in the amount of iron in each dose may be helpful, either by changing to tablets that contain smaller amounts of iron or by using a liquid preparation of ferrous sulfate. Decreasing the amount of iron in each dose is usually effective in controlling side effects, but if symptoms persist, a reduction in frequency to a single dose per day may be helpful. After a time at lower doses, patients may subsequently be able to tolerate more iron.

With patience and persistence, an acceptable oral iron regimen can be devised for virtually all patients. Costly iron preparations with other additives, with enteric coating, or in sustained-release form do not appear to offer any advantages that cannot be achieved by simply reducing the dose of plain ferrous salts.[301] Administering iron with food and decreasing the dose will diminish the amount of iron absorbed daily and thereby prolong the period of treatment, but haste in the correction of iron deficiency is rarely needed.

Parenteral iron therapy, with the risk of adverse reactions, should be reserved for the exceptional patient who (1) remains intolerant of oral iron despite repeated modifications in dosage regimen, (2) has iron needs that cannot be met by oral therapy because of chronic uncontrollable bleeding, or (3) malabsorbs iron. A screening test for iron malabsorption is the administra-

PARENTERAL IRON THERAPY

The most widely used parenteral iron preparation is an iron dextran,[402] containing about 50 mg/ml of elemental iron in a dark brown colloidal suspension of ferric oxyhydroxide and low-molecular-weight dextran. The iron dextran may be given either intramuscularly or intravenously in a dose calculated from the deficit in body iron, with allowance both for iron to correct the hemoglobin deficit and for iron to rebuild stores.[252] Immediate life-threatening anaphylactic reactions constitute the most serious risk associated with the use of either intramuscular or intravenous iron dextran, occur in 0.5–1% of patients[403,404] and may have a fatal outcome, even with treatment.[405–407] Delayed but severe serum sickness-like reactions may develop in a substantial proportion of patients, with fever, urticaria, adenopathy, myalgias, and arthralgias.[403,404,408] Iron dextran may exacerbate arthritis in patients with ankylosing spondylitis[409] and rheumatoid arthritis.[410,411] With intramuscular administration, local reactions include skin staining (which may be minimized by using a Z technique for injection), muscle necrosis, phlebitis, and persistent pain at the injection site. In animals given massive doses of iron dextran, sarcomas have developed at the injection site, but no conclusive evidence of a carcinogenic risk in humans has been presented.[412] Before every intramuscular or intravenous injection of iron dextran, the manufacturer recommends a 0.5-ml test dose to be given ≥1 hour before the therapeutic injection.[402] The value of this precaution is limited because anaphylaxis is not dose dependent and can occur with the test dose, so iron dextran should be administered parenterally only if the facilities and medical expertise for managing anaphylactic reactions are available.[403] In the past, repeated intravenous or intramuscular injections of iron dextran were considered less convenient and more hazardous than administration of the total dose of iron dextran in a single intravenous infusion.[403] At present, however, the manufacturer stipulates that the *maximum* intravenous or intramuscular daily dose should not exceed 2 ml undiluted iron dextran, the equivalent of 100 mg of iron, and warns of an increased incidence of adverse effects with larger doses.[402] This 2-ml/day limit may be compared with the total dose of 40 ml iron dextran, the equivalent of 2,000 mg of iron, suggested by the manufacturer for an iron-deficient 70-kg individual with a hemoglobin level of 7 g/dl. Despite these risks and restrictions, parenteral iron therapy is still preferred for those patients who cannot be managed with oral iron, for the hazards and expense of chronic red cell transfusion are even greater.

tion to the fasting patient of 100 mg elemental iron as ferrous sulfate in a liquid preparation, followed by measurements of the plasma iron 1 and 2 hours later. In an iron-deficient patient with an initial plasma iron of <50 μg/dl, an increase of 200–300 μg Fe/dl is expected; an increase in plasma iron of <100 μg/dl suggests malabsorption and is an indication for a small bowel biopsy.[252]

Prognosis

The prognosis for iron deficiency itself is excellent, and the response to either oral or parenteral iron is similar. Frequently, both clinical and subjective impressions of constitutional improvement are present within the first few days of treatment, with an enhanced sense of well-being and increased vigor and appetite. Pica may resolve and soreness and burning of the mouth abate. Hematologically, mild reticulocytosis begins within 3–5 days, is maximal by the eighth to tenth day, and then declines. The hemoglobin concentration begins to increase after the first week and has generally returned to normal within 6 weeks. Complete recovery from microcytosis may take ≤4 months. With oral iron dosage totaling ≤200 mg/day, the plasma ferritin remains at <12 μg/dl until the anemia is corrected, gradually rising as storage iron is replaced over the next several months.[302] Although epithelial abnormalities begin to improve promptly with treatment, resolution of glossitis and koilonychia may take several months. The overall prognosis depends on the underlying disorder responsible for the iron deficiency. Treatment with lower iron doses may prolong the recovery period.

Failure to obtain a complete and characteristic response to iron therapy necessitates a review and reevaluation of the patient. A common problem is an incorrect diagnosis, with the anemia of chronic disease mistaken for the anemia of iron deficiency. Coexistent conditions, such as other nutritional deficiencies, hepatic or renal disease, or infectious, inflammatory, or malignant disorders, may impede recovery. It is especially important to remember that occult blood loss may be responsible for an incomplete response. With oral iron therapy, the adequacy of the form and dose of iron used should be reconsidered, compliance with the treatment regimen reviewed, and finally, the possibility of malabsorption considered.

Future Directions

Future progress is anticipated in further understanding of the effects of iron deficiency apart from anemia, both at the cellular level and more generally in terms of the effects of lack of iron on immunity and resistance to infection, exercise and work performance, and behavior and development, particularly in the infant and child.[274,289] Diagnostically, the development of an immunoassay for plasma transferrin receptor should be clinically useful in distinguishing the anemia of iron deficiency from the anemia associated with chronic disorders.[236,246] Therapeutically, carbonyl iron[271] may offer an effective means of preventing and treating iron deficiency that avoids the risk of accidental iron poisoning in children. Alternatively, a recent report of the use of a gastric delivery system (GDS) for supplemental iron during pregnancy provided evidence that a single iron-GDS tablet daily (total of 50 mg Fe) was as effective as two tablets of ferrous sulfate daily (total of 100 mg Fe) while virtually eliminating side effects.[303] The iron/GDS preparation may be especially useful in patients who have difficulty tolerating other iron preparations. Although iron nutrition has improved in the United States and other developed countries, iron deficiency remains a widespread problem in the rest of the world, and effective methods of iron fortification still represent an important need.[263]

IRON OVERLOAD

Iron overload denotes an excess in total body iron resulting from an iron supply that exceeds iron requirements. Because requirements are limited and humans lack a physiologic means of excreting excess iron, any sustained increase in intake may eventually result in accumulation of iron. The continuum of increase is shown in Figure 38-4. In adults and children, iron overload may be caused by an increased absorption of dietary iron, by parenteral administration of iron, or by a combination of the two. In the neonate and infant, iron overload is a rare disorder, apparently resulting from an abnormality in iron balance between mother and fetus. Focal iron overload may result from sequestration of iron, as in pulmonary hemosiderosis. Whatever the source of excess iron, when the accumulation overwhelms the body's capacity for safe storage, potentially lethal tissue damage is the result. The toxic manifestations of iron overload depend in part on the amount of excess iron, the rate of iron accumulation, and the partition of the iron burden between relatively benign sites in the macrophage and more hazardous deposits in parenchymal cells.

Epidemiology

The most common form of iron overload in the United States is a genetically determined disorder, the homozygous state for hereditary hemochromatosis, occurring in as much as 0.5% of the population or as many as 1 million individuals.[220,304] Similar frequencies of an iron-loading gene have been found elsewhere.[305–308] In the United States, other forms of iron overload are less frequent but affect several thousand patients with iron-loading or transfusion-dependent anemias such as thalassemia major and acquired refractory anemias. Globally, thalassemia major and other iron-loading anemias are an important public health problem in countries bordering the Mediterranean and in an area extending from southwest Asia and the Indian subcontinent to southeast Asia.[309] Dietary iron overload resulting from intake of iron in brewed beverages is a common problem affecting many populations in sub-Saharan Africa and may also have a genetic component.[310] The various forms of neonatal iron overload and the syndromes associated with focal sequestration of iron are all rare disorders.

Genetic Aspects

The forms of iron overload known to be genetically determined include hereditary hemochromatosis and certain of the iron-loading anemias. Hereditary hemochromatosis has an autosomal recessive mode of inheritance; the hemochromatosis locus is tightly linked to the HLA-A locus on the short arm of chromosome 6.[311–314] Only homozygotes are at risk of symptomatic iron overload. The hemochromatosis gene has been found to have a frequency of 5–7% in various countries, suggesting that ≥10% of their populations are heterozygous and that 0.25–0.5% are homozygous for the gene.[304–307] The iron-loading anemias with established genetic components include the inherited sideroblastic anemias (see Ch. 40) as well as some of the hereditary disorders of globin synthesis (thalassemias) (see Chs. 40 and 44).

Etiology and Pathogenesis

Iron overload is caused by conditions that alter or bypass the normal control of body iron content by regulation of intestinal iron absorption. In hereditary (HLA-linked) hemochromatosis, a genetic abnormality results in an inappropriately elevated iron absorption, with a chronic progressive increase in body iron stores.[315] Iron absorption is also increased in the iron-loading anemias, apparently as the result of erythroid hyperplasia with ineffective erythropoiesis. In dietary iron overload of the type found in sub-Saharan Africa, control of iron absorption is overwhelmed by the large amounts of bioavailable iron in the upper small intestine; a genetic component, not linked to the HLA-A locus, may be involved.[310] The iron contained in transfused red cells given to patients with refractory anemias such as thalassemia major circumvents intestinal regulation of body iron content and also produces progressive iron loading.

With each of these causes of systemic iron overload, the timing of the onset of toxic manifestations, the pattern of the organs affected, and the severity of tissue damage are known to be influenced by a variety of factors. These include (1) the magnitude of the body iron burden; (2) the rate of loading; (3) the distribution of the iron load between apparently innocuous storage deposits in tissue macrophages and potentially injurious accumulations in parenchymal cells; (4) ascorbate status, which helps determine the allocation of iron between macrophage and parenchymal cells; and (5) the extent of internal redistribution of iron between macrophage and parenchymal sites. In general, the amount and rate of iron accumulation within parenchymal cells of the liver, heart, pancreas, and other organs seem to be the principal determinants of tissue injury. The exact mechanisms whereby iron produces cellular injury have not been established, but lipid peroxidation of membrane lipids of subcellular organelles or iron-induced lysosomal disruption, or both, may be involved. Tissue damage may also be produced by plasma iron not complexed with transferrin (i.e., non-transferrin-bound iron) that appears in the circulation of patients with iron overload.[316–318]

Iron overload as a result of increased iron absorption may result either from an abnormality in the control of iron absorption with a diet containing normal amounts of bioavailable iron or from consumption of such excessive amounts of bioavailable iron that a normal regulatory mechanism is overridden. In homozygotes for hereditary (HLA-linked) hemochromatosis, an inappropriately elevated iron absorption occurs at any level of body iron and produces progressive parenchymal iron accumulation, initially in the liver but later in the pancreas, heart, and other organs.[319–327] Despite marked parenchymal iron deposition, macrophage iron in the bone marrow may be scant or even absent.[328] Symptoms of parenchymal damage do not usually develop until middle or late life, when body iron stores have increased from the normal range of ≤1 g to ≥15–20 g.[320,321,324,329,330] Further increases in the body iron burden may be lethal, although the total iron accumulation may reach 40–50 g in some patients.[324]

Clinical manifestations of the disease are influenced by environmental factors such as dietary iron content and especially by alcohol use. The disorder typically becomes apparent in patients who are middle aged or older, but hemochromatosis may also develop in younger patients.[331–333] About 25% of heterozygotes develop evidence of minor, apparently harmless increases in body iron stores.[305,319] The risk of iron loading in heterozygotes who inherit or acquire certain other disorders, is not well established. Iron overload has been reported in heterozygotes for hemochromatosis with coexisting hereditary spherocytosis,[334,335] but the effect of an allele for hemochromatosis on iron loading is uncertain in idiopathic sideroblastic anemia[336,337] and sporadic porphyria cutanea tarda.[338–340] Heterozygotes for hemochromatosis and β-thalassemia trait do not seem to develop iron overload.[341]

Excessive absorption of dietary iron may also produce severe iron overload in the iron-loading anemias. These refractory disorders, characterized by erythroid hyperplasia with marked ineffective erythropoiesis, include thalassemia major and intermedia, hemoglobin E-β thalassemia, congenital dyserythropoietic anemia, pyruvate kinase deficiency, a variety of sideroblastic anemias, and other anemias associated with impaired incorporation of iron into hemoglobin. The rate of iron loading is not related to the severity of the anemia, and patients with nearly normal hemoglobin concentrations may develop massive iron overload.[111,342,343] Any red cell transfusions will add to the iron burden. The amount and distribution of iron deposits resemble those found in hereditary hemochromatosis. Excess iron localizes predominantly in parenchymal

cells, initially in the hepatocyte, but later also in the pancreas, heart, and other organs.

Mild iron overload may follow increased absorption of dietary iron in some patients with chronic liver disease, including those with alcoholic cirrhosis and portacaval shunting. More patients with alcoholic liver disease are iron deficient from repeated episodes of gastrointestinal blood loss, but storage iron is increased in a few.[344] The gene for hereditary hemochromatosis is not responsible.[305,345] The cause of increased absorption is unknown; alcohol-induced folate deficiency and sideroblastic abnormalities due to deranged pyroxidine biochemistry with ineffective erythropoiesis and hyperferremia may contribute.[346] Storage iron is usually only 2–4 g. In contrast to hereditary hemochromatosis, iron deposition is predominantly in Kupffer, rather than parenchymal, cells.

Mild iron overload from increased iron absorption is also found in patients with porphyria cutanea tarda, a hepatic porphyria (see Ch. 40) in which the liver produces excessive amounts of photosensitizing porphyrins, which circulate to the skin.[347] In symptomatic patients hepatic iron stores characteristically are increased modestly to 2–4 g. Alcoholic cirrhosis coexists in some patients, but more often no cause for increased iron absorption is found. The importance of iron for these clinical manifestations is shown by the dramatic effect of iron removal by phlebotomy, producing clinical and biochemical remission of the disease. Conversely, reaccumulation of iron results in recrudescence of symptoms.

Rare congenital defects associated with iron overload have been reported. In atransferrinemia, dietary iron is readily absorbed, but little can be used for red cell production. Instead, iron is deposited predominantly in the liver, pancreas, heart, thyroid, and kidneys. Little iron is found in the spleen and virtually none in the marrow. Another rare congenital defect, ascribed to defective uptake of iron by red cell precursors, is also associated with marked hepatic iron deposition and fibrosis.[297]

African dietary iron overload, associated with increased iron absorption from the excessive amounts of iron contained in brewed beverages, occurs in at least nine countries in sub-Saharan Africa.[348] A traditional fermented maize beverage, home brewed in steel drums from locally grown crops, is the source of the increased amount of bioavailable iron. Beverage consumption may supply as much as 50–100 mg of iron daily, many times the 10–20 mg of iron in typical American diets. Moreover, much of this iron is in the highly bioavailable ferrous form, which is readily absorbed in the upper small intestine.

The form of iron overload common in sub-Saharan Africa has previously been thought to result solely from increased dietary iron. New evidence that a non-HLA-linked gene may be involved[310] suggests that such a gene might be common in populations of African derivation. Iron burdens as great as or greater than those in patients with hereditary hemochromatosis develop and may reach an estimated ≥40–50 g. Initially, iron is deposited both in hepatocytes and in Kuppfer cells. Later, when the liver is cirrhotic, iron progressively accumulates in the pancreas, heart, and endocrine organs.

The role of protracted medicinal iron ingestion as a cause of iron overload remains indeterminate. Equivocal evidence is found in case reports of apparently normal individuals who have taken medicinal iron chronically. The issue is complicated by the possible influence of an unrecognized allele for hemochromatosis in these case reports. Medicinal iron ingestion is undoubtedly harmful to patients with iron-loading disorders.

Parenteral iron overload is usually the result of repeated red cell transfusions in patients with chronic anemia, but occasionally it is unintentionally produced by repeated injections of iron dextran or other parenteral iron preparations in patients with anemias unresponsive to iron therapy. Transfusional iron overload progressively develops in patients with chronic refractory anemia who require red cell support. In patients with severe congenital anemias, such as thalassemia major (Cooley's anemia) or the Blackfan-Diamond syndrome, transfusional iron loading begins in infancy.[349] Severe iron loading may also develop in transfusion-dependent anemias that appear later in life,[350] namely, aplastic anemia, pure red cell aplasia, hypoplastic or myelodysplastic disorders, and the anemia of chronic renal failure. If ineffective erythropoiesis and erythroid hyperplasia complicate the underlying anemia, increased absorption may contribute to the iron burden. An adequate transfusion regimen will help suppress erythropoiesis and may reduce dietary iron absorption to near normal levels. Patients with sickle cell anemia or sickle cell-β-thalassemia are also at risk of iron overload if chronically given transfusions for the prevention of recurrent complications such as central nervous system disorders, severe infections, and incapacitating painful crises.[351]

Each unit of transfused red cells contains 200–250 mg of iron. Most patients with severe refractory anemia require 200–300 ml/kg/yr of blood,[349] or the equivalent of 6–10 g iron per year in a 70-kg adult. Without chelation therapy to remove iron, cardiac iron deposition develops in patients who have received ≥100 U of blood (≥20 g of iron)[352] and is often accompanied by other evidence of iron-induced damage to the liver, pancreas, and endocrine organs. Inadvertent iron overload from inappropriate therapeutic injections of iron may make an unnecessary contribution to the iron burden in patients with anemias unresponsive to iron, particularly those with refractory microcytic anemias. At one time injectable iron was recommended for the replacement of iron losses in chronically hemodialyzed patients, but it was later recognized[353] that routine use of parenteral supplementation could lead to potentially dangerous iron overload. The practice has been abandoned in favor of supplemental oral iron.

Perinatal iron overload develops in some rare metabolic disorders of the newborn, presumably as the result of disturbances in the regulation of fetal or maternal-fetal iron balance. In hereditary tyrosinemia (hypermethioninemia), moderate iron deposition is restricted to the liver, which is typically cirrhotic; renal abnormalities and hyperplasia of the pancreatic islet cells are also present.[354] The cerebrohepatorenal syndrome, or Zellweger syndrome, is a fatal disorder with an autosomal recessive mode of inheritance, characterized by abnormal facies, hypotonia, and polycystic kidneys. Parenchymal iron deposits are found in the liver, spleen, kidney, and lungs.[355] Perinatal hemochromatosis,[356–360] also known as neonatal hemochromatosis or neonatal iron storage disease, is a usually fatal disorder of the newborn of unknown etiology, characterized by hepatic cirrhosis and iron deposition in parenchymal cells of the liver, heart, and endocrine organs but not in bone marrow or spleen. A three- to fourfold increase in the hepatic iron concentration has been found.[359]

Focal sequestration of iron in other rare disorders produces various patterns of localized iron deposition. In idiopathic pulmonary hemosiderosis, repeated episodes of alveolar hemorrhage are followed by the uptake and sequestration of iron in pulmonary macrophages. This excess iron is not available for use elsewhere, and iron stores in the liver and bone marrow may be decreased or absent. In conditions with chronic hemoglobinuria, renal hemosiderosis may develop. Renal iron deposits are harmless and have no apparent effect on kidney structure or function. The Hallervorden-Spatz syndrome is a rare degenerative neurologic disease with an autosomal recessive mode of inheritance, characterized by the juvenile onset of progressive motor abnormalities, dementia, dysarthria, and dysphagia, with optic nerve atrophy.[361] The role of iron in the disorder has not been determined, but marked iron deposition is found in the globus pallidus and reticular zone of the substantia nigra.

Clinical Manifestations

Clinical manifestations of iron toxicity generally develop only when the magnitude of iron accumulation is sufficient to produce tissue damage. At risk are homozygotes for hereditary hemochromatosis and patients with iron-loading anemias, congenital defects in iron metabolism, African dietary iron overload, chronic medicinal iron ingestion, and parenteral iron loading. Heterozygotes for hereditary hemochromatosis and patients with chronic liver disease or porphyria cutanea tarda are usually spared because of the limited extent of the iron excess. Whatever the etiology of systemic iron overload, similar clinical features eventually develop. Symptomatic patients may present with any of the characteristic manifestations: increased skin pigmentation, hepatic disease, diabetes mellitus, gonadal insufficiency or other endocrine disorders, abdominal pain, cardiac dysfunction, arthropathy, or, occasionally, neurologic and psychological abnormalities. The classic clinical tetrad, appearing in middle age in homozygotes for hereditary hemochromatosis, consists of skin pigmentation, liver disease, diabetes mellitus, and gonadal failure.[322,325] In younger patients with hereditary hemochromatosis, cardiac abnormalities and gonadal failure may be the presenting features.[331,333]

Adequately transfused patients with thalassemia major or other congenital refractory anemias grow and develop normally during the first decade of life. Thereafter, without treatment for iron excess, growth fails, sexual maturation is delayed or absent, and liver disease, diabetes mellitus, and other endocrine abnormalities develop; patients usually die of heart disease in adolescence.[349] Transfusion-dependent forms of refractory anemia acquired later in life, such as aplastic, myelodysplastic, or sideroblastic anemias, ultimately follow a similar course.[350]

Characteristic manifestations of iron toxicity are found in specific organ systems. Increased skin pigmentation, with a bronze hue in some patients and a slate-gray coloration in others, often accompanies iron overload, although the change in pigment may be too slight to be readily evident clinically. Increased melanin is responsible for the bronzing, while the slate-gray appearance is attributed to iron deposition in sweat glands and in the basal layers of the epidermis. Massive iron overload sometimes produces "reverse freckling," with small pigment-free areas scattered over a conspicuous slate-gray discoloration of the skin.[350]

Liver disease is the most common complication of iron overload. Hepatocyte iron deposition produces hepatomegaly, functional abnormalities, fibrosis, and eventually cirrhosis. Iron accumulates first in the periportal hepatocytes. Later, perilobular fibrosis appears, with deposition of iron in fibrous septa, bile duct epithelium, and Kupffer cells. Cirrhosis of the macronodular or mixed macro- and micronodular pattern eventually develops.[362] Hepatocellular carcinoma can be an ultimate complication. Liver cancers rarely develop in noncirrhotic patients.

The development and severity of hepatic damage is closely correlated with the magnitude of hepatocyte iron deposition in all varieties of iron overload.[330,363–365] In both hereditary hemochromatosis and African dietary iron overload, fibrosis or cirrhosis usually develop only after the concentration of hepatic iron is >4,000–5,000 μg Fe/g of liver (wet weight; normal 50–500).[366,368] In unchelated patients with thalassemia major, aplastic anemia, or red cell aplasia, the apparent threshold concentration for the development of fibrosis seems to be higher, about 10,000 μg Fe/g of liver, perhaps because of differences in the duration of exposure to the iron load or in the distribution of the excess iron between macrophage and parenchymal cells.[365]

Diabetes mellitus is a common complication of all forms of systemic iron overload[349,368]; the risk may be greater in patients with a family history of diabetes. Virtually all the secondary manifestations of diabetes may develop, including retinopathy, nephropathy, neuropathy, and vascular disease. Gonadal insufficiency and other endocrine abnormalities also occur.[349,368] Hypogonadism may result from primary testicular failure or may be hypogonadotrophic in origin. In hereditary hemochromatosis, impotence may be the presenting symptom. Abnormalities in pituitary and end-organ function may develop[369,370]; hypothyroidism, hypoparathyroidism, and adrenal insufficiency are infrequent complications. During the second decade of life, both growth and sexual maturation are usually retarded in untreated patients with transfusional iron overload.[349] Abdominal pain of unknown origin may be part of the initial complex of symptoms in ≤25% of patients with hereditary hemochromatosis.[322,324,329]

Iron-induced cardiac disease, occurring as a cardiomyopathy with heart failure or as arrhythmias, or as both, may be a fatal complication of all varieties of systemic iron overload. Heart disease is the most frequent cause of death in patients with transfusional iron overload.[349] About 10–15% of patients with untreated hereditary hemochromatosis develop congestive heart failure.[321,324] Particularly severe cardiac disease may be the presenting symptom in young patients with hereditary hemochromatosis.[331–333]

Chondrocalcinosis and other forms of arthropathy are common complications of hereditary hemochromatosis and may be the presenting feature.[321,329,371] The pathogenesis of the joint changes is unknown. In transfusional iron overload, arthropathy occurs but is uncommon.[372] Osteoporosis is found in some patients with hereditary hemochromatosis. Ascorbate acid deficiency occurs in transfusional siderosis and may play a protective role in some patients because a lack of ascorbate prevents the redistribution of iron from macrophage to parenchymal cells.[373] The combination of ascorbic acid deficiency and osteoporosis is particularly common in African dietary iron overload.[94]

The effect of iron excess on the risk of infection remains uncertain. Infection is not a frequent complication of any of the iron overload syndromes, but clinical reports have suggested that an increased availability of iron might be pathogenetically related to infections with certain organisms, including *Vibrio vulnificus*, *Listeria monocytogenes*, *Yersinia enterocolitica*, *Escherichia coli*, and *Candida* spp.[286,374,375]

Laboratory Evaluation

The characteristic sequence of changes in clinically useful indicators of iron status as body iron increases from the iron-replete normal to the amounts found in iron overload is shown in Figure 38-4. The most useful of the indirect measures of body iron status are plasma ferritin and plasma iron and iron-binding capacity. In the absence of complicating factors, plasma ferritin rises to a maximum concentration of about 4,000 μg/L as the body iron burden increases.[233] Under some circumstances, the relationship between plasma ferritin and body iron stores is distorted—the plasma ferritin may greatly underestimate the extent of iron accumulation or even be normal despite a considerable increase in body iron in a small number of patients with hereditary hemochromatosis. The explanation for this disproportion is unknown.[40,376,377] The plasma ferritin may also underestimate the body iron burden in a small number of patients with transfusional iron overload; ascorbate deficiency may be responsible in some of these cases.[378] Conversely, coexistent liver disease, inflammation, infection, or malignancy may increase plasma ferritin concentrations and complicate the assessment of patients with iron-related hepatotoxicity, hepatitis, hepatoma, or other disorders.

The plasma iron, total iron-binding capacity, and transferrin

---

TESTING FOR IRON OVERLOAD

A direct measure of body iron avoids the uncertainties inherent in the interpretation of indirect indicators of iron status. Liver biopsy is the definitive direct test for assessing iron deposition and tissue damage in iron overload, permitting measurement of the nonheme iron concentration, histochemical determination of the cellular distribution of iron between hepatocytes and Kupffer cells, and pathologic examination of the extent of tissue injury. In patients with hereditary hemochromatosis who are undergoing therapeutic venesection, quantitative phlebotomy provides an accurate retrospective determination of the amount of storage iron that can be mobilized for hemoglobin formation. When liver biopsy is contraindicated in patient, quantitative phlebotomy is occasionally useful in establishing the diagnosis of hereditary hemochromatosis. Bone marrow aspiration and biopsy provide no information about the extent of parenchymal iron loading and are of limited value in the evaluation of iron overload. Iron overload produces no specific abnormalities in the peripheral blood.

---

saturation provide indications of the current iron supply to the tissues. An increased plasma iron and transferrin saturation and a decreased total iron-binding capacity suggest parenchymal iron loading but provide no measure of its magnitude. The transferrin saturation may be normal despite increased iron stores within macrophages, as is found in early transfusional iron loading; it is also affected by coexistent disorders such as liver disease, inflammation, or malignancy.

Differential Diagnosis

The detection and diagnosis of iron overload are most problematic in those conditions resulting from an increased absorption of iron (Table 38-5). Hereditary hemochromatosis is potentially detectable either genetically or phenotypically. Since the gene for hemochromatosis remains unidentified, direct analy-

Table 38-5. Causes of Iron Overload

Increased iron absorption
　From diets with normal amounts of bioavailable iron
　　Hereditary (HLA-linked) hemochromatosis
　　Iron-loading anemias (refractory anemias with hypercellular erythroid marrow)
　　Chronic liver disease (cirrhosis, portacaval shunt)
　　Porphyria cutanea tarda
　　Congenital defects (atransferrinemia and other disorders)
　From diets with increased amounts of bioavailable iron
　　African dietary iron overload (may have genetic component)
　　Medicinal iron ingestion(?)
Parenteral iron overload
　Transfusional iron overload
　Inadvertent iron overload from therapeutic injections
Perinatal iron overload
　Hereditary tyrosinemia
　Cerebrohepatorenal syndrome
　Perinatal hemochromatosis
Focal sequestration of iron
　Idiopathic pulmonary hemosiderosis
　Renal hemosiderosis
　Hallervorden-Spatz syndrome

sis of genomic DNA is not yet feasible as a means of identifying homozygotes. Because the hemochromatosis locus is closely linked to the HLA-A locus, HLA typing can be used to identify the genotypes of the first-degree relatives of a proband with hereditary hemochromatosis as normal, heterozygous, or homozygous. In such families, HLA type permits identification of those at risk of iron overload but does not indicate the extent of iron loading.

Although helpful within a family in which an affected individual has been identified, HLA typing is of no use as a population screening device. HLA haplotypes linked to the hemochromatosis locus differ in different families. Linkage with HLA-A3 has been found in some populations, but no HLA haplotype is a certain marker of hemochromatosis. Typing is of no help in ascertaining whether an isolated individual is homozygous. No abnormal gene product has been identified to permit phenotypic identification of affected individuals. As a result, screening procedures must rely on detection of the disordered iron metabolism. The most characteristic abnormality is the increase in body iron stores.

The best indirect means of identifying homozygotes for hereditary hemochromatosis is a combination of measurements of the plasma ferritin and of the plasma iron and transferrin saturation. If any of these measurements is abnormal, definitive diagnosis can be attempted by liver biopsy, biochemical measurement of the hepatic nonheme iron concentration, histochemical evaluation of the pattern of iron deposition, and pathologic determination of the extent of tissue injury. If the diagnosis of hemochromatosis is established, screening of family members at risk of the disease is mandatory, including siblings and—because of the possibility of homozygous-heterozygous matings—parents and children. HLA typing may be useful in these family studies. Plasma ferritin and transferrin saturations should be determined; in younger individuals, these measurements should be repeated periodically—some affected individuals do not manifest iron burdens until well into adult life.

In patients with iron-loading anemias who are not transfusion dependent, the severity of anemia provides no indication of the risk of iron loading from increased dietary iron absorption. Patients with only minor anemia may accumulate major iron loads.[111,343] Examination of the peripheral blood may show changes of the underlying hematologic disorders. Either morphologic or ferrokinetic techniques may be used to estimate the extent of ineffective erythropoiesis in order to assess the risk of iron loading. Plasma ferritin and transferrin saturations provide the best direct means of screening for iron overload.

A liver biopsy is the direct and definitive means of determining the extent of parenchymal iron accumulation. Differentiation of the iron overload associated with chronic liver disease, especially of alcoholic origin, from hereditary hemochromatosis may require special study. The presence of liver disease complicates the interpretation of plasma ferritin and transferrin saturation. In this circumstance the results of liver biopsy are again definitive. Histochemically, in chronic liver disease iron is deposited principally in Kupffer cells, whereas in hereditary hemochromatosis the iron is found predominantly within hepatocytes. The hepatic iron concentration, corrected for the age of the patient, can also be used to distinguish between patients with alcoholic liver disease with iron loading and those with the heterozygous and homozygous forms of hereditary hemochromatosis.[367]

The differential diagnosis of the remaining causes of iron overload (Table 24-5) poses few problems. Porphyria cutanea tarda is discussed more fully in Chapter 39 and is readily diagnosed by measurement of urinary porphyrins. The source of the iron overload in patients with parenteral iron loading is evident, whether from transfusion or from repeated injections of therapeutic iron. The various causes of perinatal iron overload are clearly distinguished by clinical and pathologic find-

ings. The diagnosis of idiopathic pulmonary hemosiderosis should be considered whenever iron deficiency anemia develops with coexistent pulmonary abnormalities. Previously, demonstration of iron deposits in the basal ganglia of patients with the Hallervorden-Spatz syndrome was possible only at autopsy, but magnetic resonance imaging now provides a means of detecting the localized brain iron during life.[379,380]

Therapy

The goal of therapy for iron overload is the reduction and maintenance of the body iron at normal or near normal amounts. When possible, phlebotomy is the treatment of choice for hereditary hemochromatosis,[323] for iron-loading anemia if the hemoglobin concentration is high enough to permit venesection, for porphyria cutanea tarda, and for African dietary iron overload. Once the diagnosis of iron overload is established, phlebotomy therapy should begin promptly, for any delay extends exposure to potentially toxic iron accumulations. For most patients phlebotomy should remove 500 ml of blood, containing 200–250 mg of iron, once weekly, until storage iron is depleted. The regimen should be individualized; for patients with iron-loading anemia, smaller amounts of blood will need to be withdrawn weekly, while for heavily loaded patients with hereditary hemochromatosis, an even more vigorous program of phlebotomy twice weekly has been advocated.[381] The hematocrit or hemoglobin concentration should be measured before each phlebotomy. After an initial fall in the hemoglobin as erythropoiesis accelerates to keep pace with venesection, the hemoglobin will remain within about 10% of its initial value. The progress of iron removal can be followed by periodic measurements of plasma ferritin, iron, and transferrin saturation. The plasma ferritin declines progressively as iron is removed, but the plasma iron and transferrin saturation remain elevated until iron stores near depletion. In a patient with porphyria cutanea tarda, a few weeks of phlebotomy will suffice, while in hereditary hemochromatosis and an initial body iron burden of 25 g, removal of the iron burden may require ≥2 years.

Occasionally, plasma iron falls and hemoglobin regeneration is temporarily delayed despite incomplete removal of excess iron, as indicated by continued elevation of the plasma ferritin. A brief halt in the phlebotomy regimen, presumably to permit mobilization of the remaining iron, is usually all that is needed before resuming weekly venesection. Eventually, when iron stores are exhausted, the ferritin will decline to <12 µg/L, the

---

TIMING OF CHELATION THERAPY

In patients who are transfusion-dependent from early infancy (thalassemia major and other congenital refractory anemias), chelation therapy is best started after about 10–20 transfusions, usually around 3 years of age.[387,391] In older patients with acquired refractory anemias who become transfusion dependent, it seems advisable to begin chelation early, after transfusion of 10–20 U of blood.[413] In patients with iron-loading anemias and those with sickle cell disease who are chronically transfused for prevention of complications, early therapy also seems prudent, beginning when the hepatic iron concentration or the serum ferritin increases to about two or three times the upper limit of normal. In each of these disorders, delay in beginning chelation therapy only exposes the patient to a greater risk of iron toxicity.

plasma iron and transferrin saturation will be decreased, and the hemoglobin concentration will fall to <10 g/dl for 2 weeks without further phlebotomy. After complete removal of the iron load, lifelong maintenance therapy is needed, usually requiring phlebotomy of 500 ml every 3–4 months. Maintenance phlebotomy should preserve a normal transferrin saturation and a plasma ferritin of <50 µg/L. Phlebotomy is not generally recommended for patients with the modest iron overload that sometimes develops with chronic liver disease; removal of the iron load in these cases seems to have no clinical benefit.[382]

For patients with transfusion-dependent refractory anemias, most patients with iron-loading anemias, and the rare patients with hereditary hemochromatosis in whom phlebotomy is impossible, treatment with the iron chelator desferrioxamine is the only means of preventing or removing toxic accumulations of iron.[383] In patients with hereditary hemochromatosis and cardiac failure, a combination of phlebotomy and chelation therapy has been recommended.[324] Unfortunately, desferrioxamine given orally is poorly absorbed; to be effective the drug must be administered by subcutaneous or intravenous infusion with a small portable syringe pump, ideally for 9–12 hours each day.[384] Compliance with this regimen may be difficult, but a number of studies have now shown that regular chelation therapy with desferrioxamine can remove tissue iron, prevent organ damage, and prolong survival.[385–389]

In patients with modest iron loads and no evidence of iron toxicity, slow subcutaneous infusion of desferrioxamine for 9–12 hr/day usually provides adequate therapy. In severely iron-loaded patients and in patients with evidence of iron toxicity, particularly those with cardiac complications, chronic slow intravenous infusions through an indwelling central venous catheter may permit more rapid reduction of the body iron burden.[387] Administration of ascorbic acid can enhance desferrioxamine-induced iron excretion but carries the risk of an internal redistribution of iron from relatively benign storage sites in macrophages to a potentially toxic pool in parenchymal cells. Although the evidence is circumstantial, large doses of ascorbic acid should be regarded as hazardous in patients with iron overload.[373,383] Ascorbate supplementation is probably not needed by patients whose diets regularly include ascorbate-rich foods.

Desferrioxamine is a generally safe and nontoxic drug in the iron-loaded patient, but systemic complications have been reported, including allergic anaphylactoid reactions, infectious complications,[383] visual abnormalities, auditory dysfunction,[390] and growth retardation.[391,392] The risk of many of these complications may be minimized by adjusting the desferrioxamine dose to the magnitude of the body iron load. Adequate desferrioxamine therapy should produce a progressive decrease in the body storage iron of almost any patient with iron overload. If no decline is observed, blood and desferrioxamine use, compliance, ascorbate status, and other features of the therapeutic regimen should be thoroughly reassessed.

Prognosis

The prognosis in patients with iron overload is influenced by many factors, including the magnitude, rate, and route of iron loading; the distribution of iron deposition between macrophage and parenchymal sites; the amount and duration of exposure to circulating non-transferrin-bound iron; ascorbate status; and coexisting disorders, especially alcoholism. The magnitude of iron accumulation seems crucial. In hereditary hemochromatosis the minor iron load found in some heterozygotes seems innocuous.[180,184,305,320] Equal numbers of male and female homozygotes are expected, but symptomatic expression is ≤10 times as common in men, presumably be-

cause iron losses during menstruation and pregnancy leave women with lower iron burdens.[319,330]

The hepatic iron concentration is a major determinant of the risk of cirrhosis of the liver[367] and in turn of hepatocellular carcinoma, now the two major causes of death in hereditary hemochromatosis. Without coexistent alcoholic liver disease, fibrosis or cirrhosis usually does not develop until the hepatic storage iron reaches a concentration of 4,000–5,000 µg Fe/g of liver, wet weight[367] (normal range about 50–500 µg/g, wet weight). The development of cirrhosis increases the risk of hepatocellular carcinoma by >200-fold. Hepatomas, the ultimate cause of death in 20–30% of patients with hemochromatosis, occurs almost exclusively in patients with hepatic cirrhosis.[324,329,330] Conversely, if the disease is diagnosed before tissue injury has occurred, phlebotomy therapy to remove the excess iron can prevent all the complications of hemochromatosis, including cirrhosis, and return the patient's life expectancy to normal.[329,330]

Even in the presence of organ damage, further progression is prevented by phlebotomy, and amelioration of some features of the disease is possible.[329,330] Skin pigmentation diminishes; hepatic function may improve, while fibrosis is arrested or may sometimes regress; and cardiac abnormalities or even failure may resolve. Diabetes and other endocrine abnormalities usually improve only slightly, if at all, although reversal of hypogonadism has occurred. Arthropathy is usually not improved and may even continue to progress despite phlebotomy. In patients with iron overload who cannot be treated by phlebotomy, chelation therapy is effective in reducing the body iron burden and improving the prognosis. Chronic infusion of parenteral desferrioxamine decreases the hepatic iron concentration, improves hepatic function, promotes growth and sexual maturation, and helps protect against cardiac disease and early death. In all forms of iron overload the most effective means of avoiding complications is to prevent iron accumulation, either by early identification and phlebotomy treatment of homozygotes for hereditary hemochromatosis or by early institution of chelation therapy in patients with iron-loading or transfusion-dependent anemias.

Future Directions

Future progress is expected toward a better understanding of the basic pathophysiology of iron overload, especially of the role of iron-induced peroxidation as a mechanism of tissue injury and of the molecular mechanisms responsible for iron absorption and its control. The techniques of molecular biology are being used to attempt to identify the abnormal gene(s) responsible for hereditary hemochromatosis[311,314]; success in this endeavor would lead to major advances in the understanding and diagnosis of this genetic disease. Perinatal iron overload is receiving increased attention, and further insights into this disorder are anticipated. Several methods for the noninvasive diagnosis and measurement of iron overload are under development that would be most useful in the detection and management of patients with iron overload. Therapeutically, substantial progress has been made toward the development of iron chelators that remain active when administered orally.[393–396] The development of a safe, effective, and inexpensive oral chelating agent would be a major advance in the treatment of iron overload, which could substantially improve both the quality and length of life of affected patients in the United States and provide important public health benefits worldwide.

REFERENCES

1. Baker EN, Lindley PF: New perspectives on the structure and function of transferrins. J Inorg Biochem 47:147, 1992
2. Huebers HA, Finch CA: The physiology of transferrin and transferrin receptors. Physiol Rev 67:520, 1987

3. Huerre C, Uzan G, Grzeschik K et al: The structural gene for transferrin (TF) maps to 3q21-qter. Ann Genet 27:5, 1984
4. Rabin M, McClelland A, Kuhn L et al: Regional localization of the human transferrin receptor gene to 3q26-qter. Am J Hum Genet 37:1112, 1985
5. Park I, Schaeffer E, Sidoli A et al: Organization of the human transferrin gene: direct evidence that it originated by gene duplication. Proc Natl Acad Sci USA 82:3149, 1985
6. Bailey S, Evans RW, Garratt RC et al: Molecular structure of serum transferrin at 3.3-Å resolution. Biochemistry 27:5804, 1988
7. Welch S, Langmead L: A comparison of the structure and properties of normal human transferrin and a genetic variant of human transferrin. Int J Biochem 22:275, 1990
8. Aisen P, Leibman A, Zweier J: Stoichiometric and site characteristics of the binding of iron to human transferrin. J Biol Chem 253:1930, 1978
9. Zak O, Aisen P: Evidence for functional differences between the two sites of rabbit transferrin: effects of serum and carbon dioxide. Biochim Biophys Acta 1052:24, 1990
10. van Eijk HG, van Noort WI: A non-random distribution of transferrin iron in fresh human sera. Clin Chim Acta 157:299, 1986
11. Williams J, Moreton K: The distribution of iron between the metal-binding sites of transferrin in human serum. Biochem J 185:483, 1980
12. de-Jong G, van-Eijk HG: Microheterogeneity of human serum transferrin: a biological phenomenon studied by isoelectric focusing in immobilized pH gradients. Electrophoresis 9:589, 1988
13. Aisen P: Transferrin metabolism and the liver. Semin Liver Dis 4:192, 1984
14. Awai M, Brown EB: Clinical and experimental studies of the metabolism of I[131]-labeled human transferrin. J Lab Clin Med 61:363, 1963
15. Enns CA, Suomalaninen H, Gebhardt J et al: Human transferrin receptor: expression of the receptor is assigned to chromosome 3. Proc Natl Acad Sci USA 79:3241, 1982
16. Miller YE, Jones C, Scoggin C et al: Chromosome 3q(22-ter) encodes the human transferrin receptor. Am J Hum Genet 35:573, 1983
17. McClelland A, Kuhn LC, Ruddle FH: The human transferrin receptor gene: genomic organization and the complete primary structure of the receptor deduced from a cDNA sequence. Cell 39:267, 1984
18. Trowbridge IS, Newman RA, Domingo DL et al: Transferrin receptors: structure and function. Biochem Pharmacol 33:925, 1984
19. Huebers HA, Csiba E, Huebers E et al: Competitive advantage of diferric transferrin in delivering iron to reticulocytes. Proc Natl Acad Sci USA 80:300, 1983
20. Klausner RD, Ashwell G, Van RJ et al: Binding of apotransferrin to K562 cells. Proc Natl Acad Sci USA 80:2263, 1983
21. Morgan EH: Effect of pH and iron content of transferrin on its binding to reticulocyte receptors. Biochim Biophys Acta 762:498, 1983
22. Cotner T, Das GA, Papayannopoulou T et al: Characterization of a novel form of transferrin receptor preferentially expressed on normal erythroid progenitors and precursors. Blood 73:214, 1989
23. Iacopetta BJ, Morgan EH, Yeoh G: Transferrin receptors and iron uptake during erythroid cell development. Biochim Biophys Acta 687:204, 1982
24. Trowbridge IS, Omary MB: Human cell surface glycoprotein related to cell proliferation is the receptor for transferrin. Proc Natl Acad Sci USA 78:3039, 1981
25. Ward JH, Jordan I, Kushner JP et al: Heme regulation of HeLa cell transferrin receptor number. J Biol Chem 259:13235, 1984
26. Harrison PM, Andrews SC, Artymiuk PJ et al: Ferritin. p. 81. In Ponka P, Schulman HM, Woodworth RC (eds): Iron Transport and Storage. CRC Press, Boca Raton, FL, 1990
27. Jain SK, Barrett KJ, Boyd D et al: Ferritin H and L chains are derived from different multigene families. J Biol Chem 260:11762, 1985
28. Caskey JH, Jones C, Miller YE et al: Human ferritin gene is assigned to chromosome 19. Proc Natl Acad Sci USA 80:482, 1983
29. Hentze MW, Keim S, Papadopoulos P et al: Cloning, characterization, expression and chromosomal location of a human ferritin heavy chain gene. Proc Natl Acad Sci USA 83:7226, 1986
30. Worwood M, Brook JD, Cragg S et al: Assignment of human ferritin genes to chromosomes 11 and 19q13. 3:371, 1985
31. Munro H: The ferritin genes: their response to iron status. Nutr Rev 51:65, 1993
32. Levi S, Luzago A, Cesarni G et al: Mechanism of ferritin iron uptake: activity of the H-chain and deletion mapping of the ferro-oxidase site A. J Biol Chem 263:18086, 1988
33. Levi S, Luzzago A, Franceschinelli F et al: Mutational analysis of the channel and loop sequences of human ferritin H-chain. Biochem J 264:381, 1989
34. Santambrogio P, Levi S, Cozzi A et al: Production and characterization of recombinant heteropolymers of human ferritin H and L chains. J Biol Chem 268:12744, 1993
35. Treffry A, Lee PJ, Harrison PM: The effect of iron on ferritin turnover. FEBS Lett 165:243, 1984
36. Richter GW: Studies of iron overload. Rat liver siderosome ferritin. Lab Invest 50:26, 1984
37. Wixom RL, Prutkin L, Munro HN: Hemosiderin: nature, formation and significance. Int Rev Exp Pathol 22:193, 1980
38. Bridges KR, Hoffman KE: The effects of ascorbic acid on the intracellular metabolism of iron and ferritin. J Biol Chem 61:14273, 1986
39. Bridges KR: Ascorbic acid inhibits lysosomal autophagy of ferritin. J Biol Chem 262:1, 1987
40. Finch CA, Bellotti V, Stray S et al: Plasma ferritin determination as a diagnostic tool. West J Med 145:657, 1986
41. Jacobs A, Worwood M: Ferritin in serum. Clinical and biochemical implications. N Engl J Med 292:951, 1975
42. Jacobs A: Ferritin. Curr Top Hematol 5:25, 1985
43. Lipschitz DA, Cook JD, Finch CA: A clinical evaluation of serum ferritin as an index of iron stores. N Engl J Med 290:1213, 1974
44. Theil EC: Ferritin. Annu Rev Biochem 56:289, 1987
45. Walters GO, Miller FM, Worwood M: Serum ferritin concentration and iron stores in normal subjects. J Clin Pathol 26:770, 1973
46. Theil EC: The IRE (iron regulatory element) family: structures which regulate mRNA translation or stability. Biofactors 4:87, 1993
47. Bettany AJ, Eisenstein RS, Munro HN: Mutagenesis of the iron-regulatory element further defines a role for RNA secondary structure in the regulation of ferritin and transferrin receptor expression. J Biol Chem 267:16531, 1992
48. Dix DJ, Lin PN, Kimata Y et al: The iron regulatory region of ferritin mRNA is also a positive control element for iron-independent translation. Biochemistry 31:2818, 1992
49. Dix DJ, Lin PN, McKenzie AR et al: The influence of the base-paired flanking region on structure and function of the ferritin mRNA iron regulatory element. J Mol Biol 231:230, 1993
50. Kennedy MC, Mende-Mueller L, Blondin GA et al: Purification and characterization of cytosolic aconitase from beef liver and its relationship to the iron-responsive element binding protein. Proc Natl Acad Sci USA 89:11730, 1992
51. Klausner RD, Rouault TA: A double life: cytosolic aconitase as a regulatory RNA binding protein. Mol Biol Cell 4:1, 1993
52. Rouault TA, Stout CD, Kaptain S et al: Structural relationship between an iron-regulated RNA-binding protein IRE-BP and aconitase: functional implications. Cell 64:881, 1991
53. Lauble H, Kennedy MC, Beinert H et al: Crystal structures of aconitase with isocitrate and nitroisocitrate bound. Biochemistry 31:2735, 1992
54. Tang CK, Chin J, Harford JB et al: Iron regulates the activity of the iron-responsive element binding protein without changing its rate of synthesis or degradation. J Biol Chem 267:24466, 1992
55. Constable A, Quick S, Gray NK et al: Modulation of the RNA-binding activity of a regulatory protein by iron in vitro: switching between enzymatic and genetic function? Proc Natl Acad Sci USA 89:4554, 1992
56. Emery-Goodman A, Hirling H, Scarpellino L et al: Iron regulatory factor expressed from recombinant baculovirus: conversion between the RNA-binding apoprotein and Fe-S cluster containing aconitase. Nucleic Acids Res 21:1457, 1993
57. Haile DJ, Rouault TA, Tang CK et al: Reciprocal control of RNA-binding and aconitase activity in the regulation of the iron-responsive element binding protein: role of the iron-sulfur cluster. Proc Natl Acad Sci USA 89:7536, 1992
58. Philpott CC, Haile D, Rouault TA et al: Modification of a free Fe-S cluster cysteine residue in the active iron-responsive element-binding protein prevents RNA binding. J Biol Chem 268:17655, 1993
59. Zaman Z, Heynen M, Verwilghen RL: Studies on the mechanism of transferrin iron uptake by rat reticulocytes. Biochim Biophys Acta 632:553, 1980
60. Jandl JH, Katz JH: The plasma-to-cell cycle of transferrin. J Clin Invest 42:314, 1963
61. Bali PK, Aisen P: Receptor-modulated iron release from transferrin: differential effects on N- and C-terminal sites. Biochemistry 30:9947, 1991
62. Bali PK, Zak O, Aisen P: A new role for the transferrin receptor in the release of iron from transferrin. Biochemistry 30:324, 1991
63. Bali PK, Aisen P: Receptor-induced switch in site-site cooperativity during iron release by transferrin. Biochemistry 31:3963, 1992
64. Huebers H, Huebers E, Csiba E et al: Iron uptake from rat plasma transferrin by rat reticulocytes. J Clin Invest 62:944, 1978
65. Huebers H, Csiba E, Huebers E et al: Molecular advantage of diferric transferrin in delivering iron to reticulocytes: a comparative study. Proc Soc Exp Biol Med 179:222, 1985
66. Collawn JF, Stangel M, Kuhn LA et al: Transferrin receptor internalization sequence YXRF implicates a tight turn as the structural recognition motif for endocytosis. Cell 63:1061, 1990

67. Miller K, Shipman M, Trowbridge IS et al: Transferrin receptors promote the formation of clathrin lattices. Cell 65:621, 1991

68. Eichholtz T, Vossebeld P, van OM et al: Activation of protein kinase C accelerates internalization of transferrin receptor but not of major histocompatibility complex Class I. independent of their phosphorylation status. J Biol Chem 267:22490, 1992

69. Hansen SH, Sandvig K, van Deurs B: Internalization efficiency of the transferrin receptor. Exp Cell Res 199:19, 1992

70. Choe HR, Moseley ST, Glass J et al: Rabbit reticulocyte coated vesicles carrying the transferrin-transferrin receptor complex. I. Purification and partial characterization. J Biol Chem 70:1035, 1987

71. Egyed A, Fodor I, Lelkes G: Coated pit formation: a membrane function involved in the regulation of cellular iron uptake. Br J Haematol 64:263, 1986

72. Hanover JA, Beguinot L, Willingham MC et al: Transit of receptors for epidermal growth factor and transferrin through clathrin-coated pits. Analysis of the kinetics of receptor entry. J Biol Chem 260:15938, 1985

73. Harding C, Heuser J, Stahl P: Receptor-mediated endocytosis of transferrin and recycling of the transferrin receptor in rat reticulocytes. J Cell Biol 97:329, 1983

74. Dautry-Varsat A, Ciechanover A, Lodish HF: pH and the recycling of transferrin during receptor-mediated endocytosis. Proc Natl Acad Sci USA 80:2258, 1983

75. Dautry-Varsat A, Lodish HF: How receptors bring proteins and particles into cells. Sci Am 250:52, 1984

76. Adachi I, Puopolo K, Marquez-Sterling N et al: Dissociation, cross-linking, and glycosylation of the coated vesicle proton pump. J Biol Chem 265:967, 1990

77. Adachi I, Arai H, Pimental R et al: Proteolysis and orientation on reconstitution of the coated vesicle proton pump. J Biol Chem 265:960, 1990

78. Arai H, Pink S, Forgac M: Interaction of anions and ATP with the coated vesicle proton pump. Biochemistry 28:3075, 1989

79. Arai H, Terres G, Pink S et al: Topography and subunit stoichiometry of the coated vesicle proton pump. J Biol Chem 263:8796, 1988

80. Perin MS, Fried VA, Stone DK et al: Structure of the 116-kDa polypeptide of the clathrin-coated vesicle/synaptic vesicle proton pump. J Biol Chem 266:3877, 1991

81. Aisen P: Entry of iron into cells: a new role for the transferrin receptor in modulating iron release from transferrin. Ann Neurol 32:S62, 1992

82. Sipe DM, Murphy RF: Binding of cellular receptors results in increased iron release from transferrin. J Biol Chem 266:8002, 1991

83. Bomford A, Young SP, Williams R: Release of iron from the two iron-binding sites of transferrin by cultured human cells: modulation by methylamine. Biochemistry 24:3472, 1985

84. Bakkeren DL, de JJN, Kroos MJ et al: Release of iron from endosomes is an early step in the transferrin cycle. Int J Biochem 19:179, 1987

85. Nunez MR, Gaete V, Abra WJ et al: Mobilization of iron from endocytic vesicles: the effects of acidification and reduction. J Biol Chem 265:6688, 1990

86. Richardson DR, Baker E: Intermediate steps in cellular iron uptake from transferrin. J Biol Chem 30:21384, 1992

87. Klausner RD: From receptors to genes—insights from molecular iron metabolism. Clin Res 36:494, 1988

88. Klausner RD, Rouault TA, Harford JB: Regulating the fate of mRNA: the control of cellular iron metabolism. Cell 72:19, 1993

89. Eskelinen S, Kok JW, Sormunen R et al: Coated endosomal vesicles: sorting and recycling compartment for transferrin in BHK cells. Eur J Cell Biol 56:210, 1991

90. Robertson BJ, Park RD, Snider MD: Role of vesicular traffic in the transport of surface transferrin receptor to the Golgi complex in cultured human cells. Arch Biochem Biophys 292:190, 1992

91. Kuhn LC, Hentze MW: Coordination of cellular iron metabolism by post-transcriptional gene regulation. J Inorg Biochem 47:183, 1992

92. Harris JW, Kellermeyer RW: The Red Cell. Production, Metabolism, Destruction: Normal and Abnormal. Harvard University Press, Cambridge, MA, 1970

93. Brittenham GM, Danish EH, Harris JW: Assessment of bone marrow and body iron stores. Semin Hematol 18:194, 1981

94. Bothwell TH, Charlton RW, Cook JD et al: Iron Metabolism in Man. Blackwell Scientific, Oxford, 1979

95. Finch CA, Huebers H: Perspectives in iron metabolism. N Engl J Med 306:1520, 1982

96. Finch CA, Ragan HA, Dyer IA et al: Body iron loss in animals. Proc Soc Exp Biol Med 159:335, 1978

97. Green R, Charlton R, Seftel H et al: Body iron excretion in man. Am J Med 45:336, 1968

98. Cook JD, Skikne BS: Intestinal regulation of body iron. Blood Rev 1:267, 1987

99. Kuhn IN, Monsen ER, Cook JD et al: Iron absorption in man. J Lab Clin Med 71:715, 1968

100. McLaren GD, Nathanson MH, Jacobs A et al: Control of iron absorption in hemochromatosis. Mucosal iron kinetics in vivo. Ann NY Acad Sci 526:185, 1988

101. Conrad ME, Umbreit JN, Moore EG: Rat duodenal iron-binding protein mobilferrin is a homologue of calreticulin. Gastroenterology 104:1700, 1993

102. Conrad ME, Umbreit JN, Peterson RD et al: Function of integrin in duodenal mucosal uptake of iron. Blood 81:517, 1993

103. Teichmann R, Stremmel W: Iron uptake by human upper small intestine microvillous membrane vesicles. Indication for a facilitated transport mechanism mediated by a membrane iron-binding protein. J Clin Invest 86:2145, 1990

104. Conrad ME, Umbreit JN, Moore EG et al: A newly identified iron binding protein in duodenal mucosa of rats. Purification and characterization of mobilferrin. J Biol Chem 265:5273, 1990

105. Conrad ME, Umbreit JN, Moore EG: A role for mucin in the absorption of inorganic iron and other metal cations. A study in rats. Gastroenterology 100:129, 1991

106. Conrad ME: Regulation of iron absorption. Prog Clin Biol Res 380:203, 1993

107. Raja KB, Simpson RJ, Peters TJ: Ferric iron reduction and uptake by mouse duodenal mucosa. Biochem Soc Trans 19:3165, 1991

108. Simpson RJ, Peters TJ: Forms of soluble iron in mouse stomach and duodenal lumen: significance for mucosal uptake. Br J Nutr 63:79, 1990

109. Snape S, Simpson RJ, Peters TJ: Subcellular localization of recently-absorbed iron in mouse duodenal enterocytes: identification of a basolateral membrane iron-binding site. Cell Biochem Funct 8:107, 1990

110. Stremmel W, Riedel HD, Niederau C et al: Pathogenesis of genetic haemochromatosis. Eur J Clin Invest 23:321, 1993

111. Pootrakul P, Kitcharoen K, Yansukon P et al: The effect of erythroid hyperplasia on iron balance. Blood 71:1124, 1988

112. Raja KB, Simpson J, Pippard MJ et al: In vivo studies of the relationship between intestinal iron (Fe^{3+}) absorption, hypoxia and erythropoiesis in the mouse. Br J Haematol 68:373, 1988

113. Finch CA, Cook JD, Labbe RF et al: Effect of blood donation on iron stores as evaluated by serum ferritin. Blood 50:441, 1977

114. Brittenham GM: Iron in the red cell cycle. p. 31. In Brock J, Pippard M, Halliday J, Powell L (eds): Iron Metabolism in Health and Disease. Academic Press, London, 1994

115. Abraham NG, Nelson JC, Ahmed T et al: Erythropoietin controls heme metabolic enzymes in normal human bone marrow culture. Exp Hematol 17:908, 1989

116. Abraham NG: Molecular regulation—biological role of heme in hematopoiesis. Blood Rev 5:19, 1991

117. Nijhof W, Wierenga PK, Sahr K et al: Induction of globin mRNA transcription by erythropoietin in differentiating erythroid precursor cells. Exp Hematol 15:779, 1987

118. Bonanou-Tzedaki SA, Sohi MK, Arnstein HR: The effect of haemin on RNA synthesis and stability in differentiating rabbit erythroblasts. Eur J Biochem 144:589, 1984

119. Chan L, Gerhardt EM: Transferrin receptor gene is hyperexpressed and transcriptionally regulated in differentiating erythroid cells. J Biol Chem 267:8254, 1992

120. Lesley J, Hyman R, Schulte R et al: Expression of transferrin receptor on murine hematopoietic progenitors. Cell Immunol 83:14, 1984

121. Iacopetta BJ, Morgan EH: Transferrin endocytosis and iron uptake during erythroid cell development. Biomed Biochim Acta 42:S182, 1983

122. Cox TM, Ponka P, Schulman HN: Erythroid cell iron metabolism and heme synthesis. p. 263. In Ponka P, Schulman HM, Woodworth RC (eds): Iron Transport and Storage. CRC Press, Boca Raton, FL, 1990

123. Battistini A, Marziali G, Albertini R et al: Positive modulation of hemoglobin, heme, and transferrin receptor synthesis by murine interferon-alpha and -beta in differentiating Friend cells. J Biol Chem 266:528, 1991

124. Battistini A, Coccia EM, Marziali G et al: Intracellular heme coordinately modulates globin chain synthesis, transferrin receptor number, and ferritin content in differentiating Friend erythroleukemia cells. Blood 78:2098, 1991

125. Coccia EM, Profita V, Fiorucci G et al: Modulation of ferritin H-chain expression in Friend erythroleukemia cells: transcriptional and translational regulation by hemin. Mol Cell Biol 12:3015, 1992

126. Sutherland GR, Baer E, Callen DF et al: 5-Aminolevulinate synthase is a 3p21 and thus not the primary defect in X-linked sideroblastic anemia. Am J Human Genet 43:331, 1988

127. Fujita H, Yamamoto M, Yamagami T et al: Erythroleukemia differentiation. Distinctive responses of the erythroid specific and the nonspecific delta aminolevulinate synthase mRNA 266:17494, 1991

128. Bishop DF, Henderson AS, Astrim KM: Human delta-aminolevulinate syn-

thase: assignment of the housekeeping gene to 3p21 and the erythroid specific gene to the X-chromosome. Genomics 7:207, 1990

129. Grandchamp B, De VH, Beaumont C et al: Tissue-specific expression of porphobilinogen deaminase. Two isoenzymes from a single gene. 162:105, 1987

130. Grandchamp B, Picat C, de-Rooij F et al: A point mutation Eur J Biochem A in exon 12 of the porphobilinogen deaminase gene results in exon skipping and is responsible for acute intermittent porphyria. Nucleic Acids Res 17: 6637, 1989

131. Beaumont C, Porcher C, Picat C et al: The mouse porphobilinogen deaminase gene. Structural organization, sequence, and transcriptional analysis. J Biol Chem 264:14829, 1989

132. Chretien S, Dubart A, Beaupain D, et al: Alternative transcription and splicing of the human porphobilinogen deaminase gene result either in tissue-specific or in housekeeping expression. Proc Natl Acad Sci USA 85:6, 1988

133. Mignotte V, Eleouet JF, Raich N et al: Cis- and trans-acting elements involved in the regulation of the erythroid promoter of the human porphobilinogen deaminase gene. Proc Natl Acad Sci USA 86:6548, 1989

134. Raich N, Mignotte V, Dubart A et al: Regulated expression of the overlapping ubiquitous and erythroid transcription units of the human porphobilinogen deaminase PBG-D gene introduced into non erythroid and erythroid cells. J Biol Chem 264:10186, 1989

135. Mignotte V, Wall L, deBoer E et al: Two tissue-specific factors bind the erythroid promoter of the human porphobilinogen deaminase gene. Nucleic Acids Res 17:37, 1989

136. Cox TC, Bawden MJ, Martin A et al: Human erythroid 5-aminolevulinate synthase: promoter analysis and identification of an iron-responsive element in the mRNA. EMBO J 10:1891, 1991

137. Dandekar T, Stripecke R, Gray NK et al: Identification of a novel iron-responsive element in murine and human erythroid delta-aminolevulinic acid synthase mRNA. EMBO J 10:1903, 1991

138. Houston T, Moore MR, McColl KE et al: Erythroid 5-aminolaevulinate synthase activity during normal and iron deficient erythropoiesis. Br J Haematol 78:561, 1991

139. Lin JJ, Daniels-McQueen S, Gaffield L et al: Specificity of the induction of ferritin synthesis by hemin. Biochim Biophys Acta 1050:146, 1990

140. Lin JJ, Daniels-McQueen S, Patino MM et al: Derepression of ferritin messenger RNA translation by hemin in vitro. Science 247:74, 1990

141. Lin JJ, Patino MM, Gaffield L et al: Crosslinking of hemin to a specific site on the 90-kDa ferritin repressor protein. Proc Natl Acad Sci USA 88:6068, 1991

142. Goessling LS, Daniels-McQueen S, Bhattacharyya-Pakrasi M et al: Enhanced degradation of the ferritin repressor protein during induction of ferritin messenger RNA translation. Science 256:670, 1992

143. Haile DJ, Rouault TA, Harford JB et al: The inhibition of the iron responsive element RNA-protein interaction by heme does not mimic in vivo iron regulation. J Biol Chem 265:12786, 1990

144. Eisenstein RS, Garcia-Mayol D, Pettingell W et al: Regulation of ferritin and heme oxygenase synthesis in rat fibroblasts by different forms of iron. Proc Natl Acad Sci USA 88:688, 1991

145. Rouault T, Rao K, Harford J et al: Hemin, chelatable iron, and the regulation of transferrin receptor biosynthesis. J Biol Chem 260:14862, 1985

146. Cazzola M, Dezza L, Bergamaschi G et al: Biologic and clinical significance of red cell ferritin. Blood 62:1078, 1983

147. Hodgetts J, Peters SW, Hoy TG et al: The ferritin content of normoblasts and megoloblasts from human bone marrow. Br J Haematol 70:47, 1986

148. Invernizzi R, Cazzola M, De FP et al: Immunocytochemical detection of ferritin in human bone marrow and peripheral blood cells using monoclonal antibodies specific for the H and L subunit. Br J Haematol 76:427, 1990

149. Speyer BE, Fielding J: Ferritin as a cytosol iron transport intermediate in human reticulocytes. Br J Haematol 42:255, 1979

150. Ponka P, Wilczynska A, Schulman HM: Iron utilization in rabbit reticulocytes. A study using succinylacetone as an inhibitor of heme synthesis. Biochim Biophys Acta 720:96, 1982

151. Adams ML, Ostapiuk I, Grasso JA: The effect of inhibitors of heme synthesis on the intracellular localization of iron in rat reticulocytes. Biochim Biophys Acta 1012:243, 1989

152. Cazzola M, Ascari E: Red cell ferritin as a diagnostic tool. Br J Haematol 62: 209, 1986

153. Zheng L, Kennedy MC, Blondin GA et al: Binding of cytosolic aconitase to the iron responsive element of porcine mitochondrial aconitase mRNA. Arch Biochem Biophys 299:356, 1992

154. Aisen P: Iron metabolism in the reticuloendothelial system. p. 281. In Ponka P, Schulman HM, Woodworth RC (eds): Iron Transport and Storage. CRC Press, Boca Raton, FL, 1990

155. Clark MR: Senescence of red blood cells: progress and problems. Physiol Rev 68:503, 1988

156. Danon D, Marikovsky Y: The aging of the red blood cell. A multifactor process. Blood Cells 14:07, 1988

157. Thorburn DR, Beutler E: The loss of enzyme activity from erythroid cells during maturation. Adv Exp Med Biol 307:15, 1991

158. Low PS, Waugh SM, Zinke K et al: The role of hemoglobin denaturation and band 3 clustering in red cell aging. Science 227:531, 1985

159. Kay M, Sorensen K, Wong P et al: Antigenicity: storage and aging. Physiologic autoantibodies to cell membrane and serum proteins and the senescent cell antigen. Mol Cell Biochem 49:65, 1982

160. Lutz HU, Fasler S, Stammler P et al: Naturally occurring anti-band 3 antibodies and complement in phagocytosis of oxidatively-stressed and in the clearance of senescent red cells. Blood Cells 14:175, 1988

161. Waugh RE, Narla M, Jackson CW et al: Rheologic properties of sensecent erythrocytes: loss of surface area and volume with red blood cell age. Blood 79:1351, 1992

162. Jandl JH: Blood: Textbook of Hematology. Little, Brown, Boston, 1987

163. Fillet G, Beguin Y, Baldelli L: Model of reticuloendothelial iron metabolism in humans: abnormal behavior in idiopathic hemochromatosis and in inflammation. Blood 74:844, 1989

164. Fillet G, Cook JD, Finch CA: Storage iron kinetics. VII. A biologic model for reticuloendothelial iron transport. J Clin Invest 53:1527, 1974

165. Bassett ML, Halliday JW, Powell LW: Ferritin synthesis in peripheral blood monocytes in idiopathic hemochromatosis. J Lab Clin Med 100:137, 1982

166. Brock JH, Esparza I, Logie AC: The nature of iron released by resident and stimulated mouse peritoneal macrophages. Biochim Biophys Acta 797:105, 1984

167. Custer G, Balcerzak S, Rinehart J: Human macrophage hemoglobin-iron metabolism in vitro. Am J Hematol 13:23, 1982

168. Lipschitz DA, Simon MO, Lynch SR et al: Some factors affecting the release of iron from reticuloendothelial cells. Br J Haematol 20:155, 1971

169. Noyes WD, Bothwell TH, Finch CA: The role of the reticuloendothelial cell in iron metabolism. Br J Haematol 6:43, 1960

170. Lipschitz DA, Bothwell TH, Seftel HC et al: The role of ascorbic acid in the metabolism of storage iron. Br J Haematol 20:155, 1971

171. Munthe-Kaas AC, Kaplan G, Sleljelid R: On the mechanism of internalization of opsonized particles by rat Kupffer cells in vitro. Exp Cell Res 103:201, 1976

172. Munthe-Kaas AC: Phagocytosis in rat Kupffer cells in vitro. Exp Cell Res 99: 319, 1976

173. Edwards VD, Simon GT: Ultrastructural aspects of red cell destruction in the normal rat spleen. J Ultrastruct Res 3:187, 1970

174. Kondo H, Saito K, Grasso JP et al: Iron metabolism in the erythrophagocytosing Kupffer cell. Hepatology 8:32, 1988

175. Clerget M, Polla BS: Erythrophagocytosis induces heat shock protein synthesis by human monocytes-macrophages. Proc Natl Acad Sci USA 87:1081, 1990

176. Maines MD, Trakshel GM, Kutty RK: Characterization of two constitutive forms of rat liver microsomal heme oxygenase. Only one molecular species of the enzyme is inducible. Lab Invest 261:411, 1986

177. Cruse I, Maines MD: Evidence suggesting that the two forms of heme oxygenase are products of different genes. J Biol Chem 263:3348, 1988

178. McCoubrey WK, Ewing JF, Maines MD: Human heme oxygenase-2: characterization and expression of a full-length cDNA and evidence suggesting that the two HO-2 ranscripts may differ by choice of polyadenylation signal. Arch Biochem Biophys 295:13, 1992

179. Abraham NG, Lin J, Schwartzman ML et al: The physiological significance of heme oxygenase. Int J Biochem 20:543, 1988

180. MacSween R, MacDonald RA: Iron metabolism by reticuloendothelial cells. In vitro uptake of transferrin bound iron by rat and rabbit cells. Lab Invest 21:230, 1969

181. Nishisato T, Aisen P: Uptake of transferrin by rat peritoneal macrophages. Br J Haematol 52:631, 1982

182. Hirata T, Bitterman PB, Mornex JF et al: Expression of the transferrin receptor gene during the process of mononuclear phagocyte maturation. J Immunol 136:1339, 1986

183. Finch CA, Ceubelbeiss K, Cook JD et al: Ferrokinetics in man. J Clin Invest 43:17, 1970

184. Testa U, Petrini M, Quaranta MT et al: Iron up-modulates the expression of transferrin receptors during monocyte-macrophage maturation. J Biol Chem 264:13181, 1989

185. Testa U, Petrini M, Quaranta MT et al: Differential regulation of iron-responsive element-binding protein in activated lymphocytes versus monocytes-macrophages. Curr Stud Hematol Blood Transfus 58:158, 1991

186. Oshiro S, Nakajima H: Intrahepatocellular site of the catabolism of heme and globin moiety of hemoglobin-haptoglobin after intravenous administration to rats. J Biol Chem 263:16032, 1988

187. Okuda M, Tokunaga R, Taketani S: Expression of haptoglobin receptors in human hepatoma cells. Biochim Biophys Acta 1136:143, 1992
188. Muller-Eberhard U: Hemopexin. N Engl J Med 283:1090, 1970
189. Smith A, Hunt RC: Hemopexin joins transferrin as representative members of a distinct class of receptor-mediated endocytic transport systems. Eur J Cell Biol 53:234, 1990
190. Smith A, Farooqui SM, Morgan WT: The murine haemopexin receptor. Evidence that the haemopexin binding site resides on a 20 kDa subunit. Biochem J 276:417, 1991
191. Alam J, Smith A: Receptor-mediated transport of heme by hemopexin regulates gene expression in mammalian cells. J Biol Chem 264:17637, 1989
192. Taketani S, Kohno H, Sawamura T et al: Hemopexin-dependent down-regulation of expression of the human transferrin receptor. J Biol Chem 23:13981, 1990
193. Bunn HF, Jandl JH: Exchange of heme among hemoglobins and between hemoglobin and albumin. J Biol Chem 243:465, 1968
194. Hillman RS, Henderson PA: Control of marrow production by relative iron supply. J Clin Invest 48:454, 1969
195. Osaki S, Johnson DA, Frieden L: The mobilisation of iron from the perfused mammalian liver by a serum copper enzyme ferrioxidase. J Biol Chem 46:3018, 1971
196. Ragan HA, Nacht S, Lee GR et al: Effect of ceruloplasmin on plasma iron in copper-deficient swine. Am J Physiol 217:1320, 1969
197. Deiss A: Iron metabolism in reticuloendothelial cells. Semin Hematol 20:81, 1983
198. Alvarez-Hernandez X, Licéaga J, McKay IC et al: Induction of hypoferremia and modulation of macrophage iron metabolism by tumor necrosis factor. Lab Invest 61:319, 1989
199. Brock JH, Alvarez-Hernandez X: Modulation of macrophage iron metabolism by tumour necrosis factor and interleukin 1. FEMS Microbiol Immunol 1:309, 1989
200. Saito K, Nishisato T, Grasso JA et al: Interaction of transferrin with iron-loaded rat peritoneal macrophages. Br J Haematol 1986;62:275
201. Siegenberg D, Baynes RD, Bothwell TH et al: Factors involved in the regulation of iron transport through reticuloendothelial cells. Proc Soc Exp Biol Med 193:65, 1990
202. Finch CA: Erythropoiesis, erythropoietin and iron. Blood 60:1241, 1982
203. Esparza I, Brock JH: Release of iron by resident and stimulated mouse peritoneal macrophages following ingestion and degradation of transferrin-anti-transferrin immune complexes. Br J Haematol 49:603, 1981
204. Fedorko ME: Loss of iron from mouse peritoneal macrophages in vitro after uptake of ^{55}Fe ferritin and ^{55}Fe ferritin rabbit antiferritin complexes. J Cell Biol 62:802, 1974
205. Ramón R, Sánchez J, Octave JN: Iron mobilization from cultured rat bone marrow macrophages. Biochim Biophys Acta 968:51, 1988
206. Sibille JC, Kondo H, Aisen P: Interactions between isolated hepatocytes and Kupffer cells in iron metabolism. Hepatology 8:296, 1988
207. Adams PC, Powell LW, Halliday JW: Isolation of a human hepatic ferritin receptor. Hepatology 8:719, 1988
208. Day CL, Anderson BF, Tweedie JW et al: Structure of the recombinant N-terminal lobe of human lactoferrin at 2.0 Å resolution. J Mol Biol 232:1084, 1993
209. Day CL, Stowell KM, Baker EN et al: Studies of the N-terminal half of human lactoferrin produced from the cloned cDNA demonstrate that interlobe interactions modulate iron release. J Biol Chem 267:13857, 1992
210. Day CL, Norris GE, Anderson BF et al: Preliminary crystallographic studies of the amino terminal half of human lactoferrin in its iron-saturated and iron-free forms. J Mol Biol 228:973, 1992
211. Anderson BF, Baker HM, Dodson EJ et al: Structure of human lactoferrin at 3.2-Å resolution. Proc Natl Acad Sci USA 84:1769, 1987
212. Anderson BF, Baker HM, Norris GE et al: Apolactoferrin structure demonstrates ligand-induced conformational change in transferrins (see comments). Nature 344:784, 1990
213. Baker EN, Anderson BF, Baker HM et al: Structure, function and flexibility of human lactoferrin. Int J Biol Macromol 13:122, 1991
214. Birgegard G, Hogman C, Killander A: Serum ferritin and erythrocyte 2,3-DPG during quantitated phlebotomy and iron treatment. Scand J Haematol 19:327, 1977
215. Conrad M, Crosby W: The natural history of iron deficiency induced by phlebotomy. Blood 20:173, 1962
216. Haskins D, Stevens AR Jr, Finch SC et al: Iron metabolism: iron stores in man as measured by phlebotomy. J Clin Invest 31:543, 1952
217. Weinfeld A: Storage iron in man. J Intern Med Suppl 427:1, 1964
218. Trubowitz S, Miller WL, Zamora JC: The quantitative estimation of non-heme iron in human marrow aspirates. Am J Clin Pathol 54:70, 1970
219. Gale E, Torrance J, Bothwell TH: The quantitative estimation of total iron stores in human bone marrow. J Clin Invest 42:1076, 1963
220. Edwards CQ, Kushner JP: Screening for hemochromatosis. N Engl J Med 328:1616, 1993
221. Weinfeld A, Lundin P, Lundvall O: Significance for the diagnosis of iron overload of histochemical and chemical iron in the liver of control subjects. J Clin Pathol 21:35, 1968
222. Brittenham GM, Farrell DE, Harris J et al: Magnetic susceptibility measurement of human iron stores. N Engl J Med 307:1671, 1982
223. Leighton DM, de CJ, Matthews R et al: Dual energy CT estimation of liver iron content in thalassemic children. Australas Radiol 32:214, 1988
224. Bonkovsky HL, Slaker DP, Bills EB et al: Usefulness and limitations of laboratory and hepatic imaging studies in iron-storage disease. Gastroenterology 99:1079, 1990
225. Stark DD, Moseley ME, Bacon B et al: Magnetic resonance imaging and spectroscopy of hepatic iron overload. Radiology 154:137, 1985
226. Andersen PB, Birgegärd G, Nyman R et al: Magnetic resonance imaging in idiopathic hemochromatosis. Eur J Haematol 47:174, 1991
227. Bartzokis G, Aravagiri M, Oldendorf WH et al: Field dependent transverse relaxation rate increase may be a specific measure of tissue iron stores. Magn Reson Med 29:459, 1993
228. Guyader D, Gandon Y, Robert JY et al: Magnetic resonance imaging and assessment of liver iron content in genetic hemochromatosis. J Hepatol 15:304, 1992
229. Kaltwasser JP, Gottschalk R, Schalk KP et al: Non-invasive quantitation of liver iron-overload by magnetic resonance imaging. Br J Haematol 74:360, 1990
230. Brittenham GM: Noninvasive methods for the early detection of hereditary hemochromatosis. Ann NY Acad Sci 526:199, 1988
231. Borgna-Pignatti C, Castriota-Scanderbeg A: Methods for evaluating iron stores and efficacy of chelation in transfusional hemosiderosis. Haematologica 76:409, 1991
232. Addison GM, Beamish MR, Hales CN et al: An immunoradiometric assay for ferritin in the serum of normal subjects and patients with iron deficiency and iron overload. J Clin Pathol 25:326, 1972
233. Worwood M, Cragg SJ, Jacobs A: Binding of serum ferritin to concanavalin A of patients with homozygous thalassemia and transfusional overload. Br J Haematol 46:409, 1980
234. Roeser HP, Halliday JW, Sizemore D et al: Serum ferritin in ascorbic acid deficiency. Br J Haematol 45:457, 1980
235. Baynes R, Bezwoda W, Bothwell T et al: The non-immune inflammatory response: serial changes in plasma iron, iron-binding capacity, lactoferrin, ferritin and C-reactive protein. Scand J Clin Lab Invest 46:695, 1986
236. Cook JD, Skikne BS, Baynes RD: Serum transferrin receptor. Annu Rev Med 44:63, 1993
237. Shih YJ, Baynes RD, Hudson BG et al: Characterization and quantitation of the circulating forms of serum transferrin receptor using domain-specific antibodies. Blood 81:234, 1993
238. Baynes RD, Shih YJ, Hudson BG et al: Production of the serum form of the transferrin receptor by a cell membrane-associated serine protease. Proc Soc Exp Biol Med 204:65, 1993
239. Shih YJ, Baynes RD, Hudson BG et al: Serum tranferrin receptor is a truncated form of tissue receptor. J Biol Chem 265:19077, 1990
240. Flowers CH, Skikne BS, Covell AM et al: The clinical measurement of serum transferrin receptor. J Lab Clin Med 114:368, 1989
241. Huebers HA, Beguin Y, Pootrakul P et al: Intact transferrin receptors in human plasma and their relation to erythropoiesis. Blood 75:102, 1990
242. Kohgo Y, Nishisato T, Kondo H et al: Circulating transferrin receptor in human serum. Br J Haematol 64:277, 1986
243. Kohgo Y, Niitsu Y, Kondo H et al: Serum transferrin receptor as a new index of erythropoiesis. Blood 70:1955, 1987
244. Beguin Y, Huebers HA, Josephson B et al: Transferrin receptors in rat plasma. Proc Natl Acad Sci USA 85:637, 1988
245. Skikne BS, Flowers CH, Cook JD: Serum transferrin receptor: a quantitative measure of tissue iron deficiency. Blood 75:1870, 1990
246. Ferguson BJ, Skikne BS, Simpson KM et al: Serum transferrin receptor distinguishes the anemia of chronic disease from iron deficiency anemia. J Lab Clin Med 119:385, 1992
247. Balcerzak SP, Westerman MP, Heinle EW et al: Measurement of iron stores using desferrioxamine. Ann Intern Med 68:518, 1968
248. Barry M, Cartel G, Sherlock S: Quantitative measurement of iron stores with diethylenetriamine penta-acetic acid. Gut 11:891, 1970
249. Labbe RF, Rettmer RL: Zinc protoporphyrin. Semin Hematol 26:40, 1989
250. Sandberg S, Brun A, Hovding G: Light-induced release of protoporphyrin, but not of zinc protoporphyrin, from erythrocytes in a patient with greatly elevated erythrocyte protoporphyrin. Blood 62:846, 1983
251. Rettmer RL, Fernandez-Cano P, Sayers M: The zinc protoporphyrin/heme ratio in laboratory diagnosis. Clin Chem 31:1026, 1985

252. Cook JD: Iron deficiency anemia. Curr Ther Hematol Oncol 3:9, 1987
253. Weiss G, Goossen B, Doppler W, et al: Translational regulation via iron-responsive elements by the nitric oxide/NO-synthase pathway. EMBO J 12:3651, 1993
254. Drapier J-C, Hirling H, Wietzerbin J et al: Biosynthesis of nitric oxide activates iron regulatory factor in macrophages. EMBO J 12:3643, 1993
255. Seiser C, Teixeira S, Kuhn LC: Interleukin-2-dependent transcriptional and post-transcriptional regulation of transferrin receptor mRNA. J Biol Chem 268:13074, 1993
256. Rogers JT, Bridges KR, Durmowicz GP et al: Translational control during the acute phase response. Ferritin synthesis in response to interleukin-1. J Biol Chem 265:14572, 1990
257. Lissoni P, Cazzaniga M, Ardizzoia A et al: Cytokine regulation of iron metabolism: effect of low-dose interleukin-2 subcutaneous therapy on ferritin, transferrin and iron blood concentrations in cancer patients. J Biol Regul Homeost Agents 7:31, 1993
258. Peters LL, Andrews NC, Eicher EM et al: Mouse microcytic anemia caused by a defect in the gene encoding the globin enhancer-binding protein NF-E2. Nature 362:768, 1993
259. Raich N, Romeo PH: Erythroid regulatory elements. Stem Cells 11:95, 1993
260. Pilch SM, Senti FR (eds): Assessment of the Iron Nutritional Status of the U.S. Population Based on Data Collected in the Second National Health and Nutrition Examination Survey. Life Sciences Research Office, Federation of American Societies for Experimental Biology, Bethesda, 1984, p. 1
261. Dallman PR, Yip R, Johnson C: Prevalence and causes of anemia in the United States. Am J Clin Nutr 39:437, 1984
262. Group ESW: Summary of a report on assessment of the iron nutritional status in the United States. Am J Clin Nutr 42:1318, 1985
263. DeMaeyer E, Adiels-Tegman M: The prevalence of anemia in the world. World Health Stat Q 38:305, 1985
264. Cook JD, Skikne BS, Lynch SR et al: Estimates of iron sufficiency in the U.S. population. Blood 68:726, 1986
265. Life Sciences Research Office, Federation of American Societies for Experimental Biology (eds): Guidelines for the assessment and management of iron deficiency in women of childbearing age. Department of Health and Human Services Publication No. (PHS) 91-2146, 1991
266. Looker AC, Johnson CL, McDowell MA et al: Iron status: prevalence of impairment in three Hispanic groups in the United States. Am J Clin Nutr 49:553, 1989
267. Beveridge BR, Bannerman RM, Evanson JM et al: Hypochromic anemia. A retrospective study and follow up of 378:145, 1965
268. Gilles HM: Selective primary health care. XVII. Hookworm infection and anemia. Rev Infect Dis 7:111, 1985
269. Yeager H, Powell D, Weinberg R et al: Idiopathic pulmonary hemosiderosis. Arch Intern Med 136:11145, 1976
270. Proskey AJ, Weatherbee L, Easterling R et al: Goodpasture's syndrome. Am J Med 48:162, 1970
271. Devasthali SD, Gordeuk VR, Brittenham GM et al: Bioavailability of carbonyl iron: a randomized, double-blind study. Eur J Haematol 46:272, 1991
272. Institute of Medicine Subcommittee on Dietary Intake and Nutrient Supplements During Pregnancy. Iron nutrition during pregnancy. In: Nutrition During Pregnancy. Part 2. Dietary intake and nutrient supplements. National Academy Press, Washington, DC, 1990
273. Oski FA: Iron deficiency in infancy and childhood. N Engl J Med 329:190, 1993
274. Hines JD, Hoffbrand AV, Mollin DL: The hematologic complications following partial gastrectomy. Am J Med 43:555, 1967
275. Saarinen UM, Siimes MA: Iron absorption from breast milk, cow's milk and iron-supplemented formula. Pediatr Res 13:143, 1979
276. Formon SJ, Zeiegler EE: Cow milk feeding in infancy. J Pediatr 98:540, 1981
277. Barton JC, Conrad ME, Parmley RT: Calcium inhibition of inorganic iron absorption in rats. Gastroenterology 84:90, 1983
278. Cook JD, Lynch SR: The liabilities of iron deficiency. Blood 68:803, 1986
279. Brown WD, Dyment PG: Pagophagia and iron deficiency anemia in adolescent girls. Pediatrics 49:766, 1972
280. Coltman CA Jr: Pagophagia and iron lack. JAMA 207:516, 1969
281. McDonald R, Marshall SR: The value of iron therapy in pica. Pediatrics 34:558, 1964
282. Reynolds RD, Binder HJ, Miller M et al: Pagophagia and iron deficiency anemia. Ann Intern Med 69:435, 1968
283. Osler W: Primary or Essential Anemia. In: The Principles and Practice of Medicine. Appleton, New York, 1908, p. 721
284. Kalra L, Hamlyn AN, Jones B: Blue sclerae: a common sign of iron deficiency. Lancet 2:1267, 1986
285. Dallman PR: Manifestations of iron deficiency. Semin Hematol 19:19, 1982
286. Hershko C, Peto T, Weatherall DJ: Iron and infection. Br Med J 296:660, 1988
287. Walter T: Impact of iron deficiency on cognition in infancy and childhood. Eur J Clin Nutr 47:307, 1993
288. Lozoff B, Jimenez E, Wolf AW: Long-term developmental outcome of infants with iron deficiency (see comments). N Engl J Med 325:687, 1991
289. Dallman PR: Iron deficiency: does it matter? J Intern Med 226:367, 1989
290. McLaren CE, Brittenham GM, Gordeuk VR: Statistical modelling of the distribution of red blood cell volumes in iron deficiency anemia using the expectation-maximisation algorithm. Statistician 35:135, 1986
291. Bainton DF, Finch CA: The diagnosis of iron deficiency anemia. Am J Med 37:62, 1964
292. Yip R, Dallman PR: The roles of inflammation and iron deficiency as causes of anemia. Am J Clin Nutr 45:1295, 1988
293. Means RT, Krantz SB: Progress in understanding the pathogenesis of the anemia of chronic disease. Blood 80:1639, 1992
294. Von Heilmeyer L, Keller W, Vivell O et al: Kongenitale atransferrin; anamie bei einem sieben Jahre alten Kind. Dtsch Med Wochenschr 86:1745, 1961
295. Schwick HG, Cap J, Goya N: Therapy of atransferrinemia with transferrin. J Clin Chem 16:75, 1978
296. Goya N, Miyazaki S, Kodate S et al: A family of congenital atransferrinemia. Blood 40:239, 1972
297. Shahidi NT, Nathan DG, Diamond LK: Iron deficiency anemia associated with an error of iron metabolism in two siblings. J Clin Invest 43:510, 1964
298. Larrick JW, Hyman ES: Acquired iron-deficiency anemia caused by an antibody against the transferrin receptor. N Engl J Med 311:214, 1984
299. Buchanan GR, Sheehan RG: Malabsorption and defective utilization of iron in three siblings. J Pediatr 98:723, 1981
300. Williams DM: Copper deficiency in humans. Semin Hematol 20:118, 1983
301. Callender ST: Treatment of iron deficiency. Clin Haematol 11:327, 1982
302. Wheby MS: Effect of iron therapy on serum ferritin levels in iron-deficient anemia. Blood 56:138, 1980
303. Simmons WK, Cook JD, Bingham KC et al: Evaluation of a gastric delivery system for iron supplementation in pregnancy. Am J Clin Nutr 58:622, 1993
304. Edwards CQ, Griffen LM, Goldgar D et al: Prevalence of hemochromatosis among 11,065 presumably healthy blood donors. N Engl J Med 318:1355, 1988
305. Bassett ML, Halliday JW, Powell LW: HLA typing in idiopathic hemochromatosis: distinction between homozygotes and heterozygotes with biochemical expression. Hepatology 1:120, 1981
306. Beaumont C, Simon M, Fauchet R et al: Serum ferritin as a possible marker for the hemochromatosis allele. N Engl J Med 301:169, 1979
307. Borwein ST, Ghent CN, Flanagan P et al: Genetic and phenotypic expression of hemochromatosis in Canadians. Clin Invest Med 6:171, 1983
308. Olsson KS, Ritter B, Rosen U et al: Prevalence of iron overload in central Sweden. J Intern Med 213:145, 1983
309. Group WW: Community control of hereditary anemia: memorandum from a WHO meeting. Bull WHO 61:63, 1983
310. Gordeuk V, Mukiibi J, Hasstedt SJ et al: Iron overload in Africa. Interaction between a gene and dietary iron content (see comments). N Engl J Med 326:95, 1992
311. Jazwinska EC, Lee SC, Webb SI et al: Localization of the hemochromatosis gene close to D6S105. Am J Hum Genet 53:347, 1993
312. Gasparini P, Borgato L, Piperno A et al: Linkage analysis of 6p21 polymorphic markers and the hereditary hemochromatosis: localization of the gene centromeric to HLA-F. Hum Mol Genet 2:571, 1993
313. el-Kahloun A, Chauvel B, Mauvieux V et al: Localization of seven new genes around the HLA-A locus. Hum Mol Genet 2:55, 1993
314. Gruen JR, Goei VL, Summers KM et al: Physical and genetic mapping of the telomeric major histocompatibility complex region in man and relevance to the primary hemochromatosis gene (HFE). Genomics 14:232, 1992
315. Weintraub LR, Edwards CQ, Krikker M (eds): Hemochromatosis: Proceedings of the First International Conference. Ann NY Acad Sci 526:1, 1988
316. Grootveld M, Bell JD, Halliwell B et al: Non-transferrin-bound iron in plasma or serum from patients with idiopathic hemochromatosis. Characterization by high performance liquid chromatography and nuclear magnetic resonance spectroscopy. J Biol Chem 264:4417, 1989
317. Hershko C, Peto T: Non-transferrin plasma iron. Br J Haematol 66:149, 1987
318. Singh S, Hider RC, Porter JB: A direct method for quantification of non-transferrin-bound iron. Anal Biochem 186:320, 1990
319. Cartwright GE, Edwards CQ, Kravitz K et al: Hereditary hemochromatosis: phenotypic expression of the disease. N Engl J Med 301:175, 1979
320. Dadone MM, Kushner JP, Edwards CQ et al: Hereditary hemochromatosis: analysis of the laboratory expression of the disease by genotype in 18 pedigrees. J Clin Pathol 78:196, 1982
321. Edwards CQ, Cartwright GE, Skolnick MH et al: Homozygosity for hemochromatosis: clinical manifestations. Ann Intern Med 93:515, 1980
322. Finch SC, Finch CA: Idiopathic hemochromatosis, an iron storage disease. Iron metabolism in hemochromatosis. Medicine 34:381, 1955
323. Finch CA: Iron metabolism in hemochromatosis. J Clin Invest 28:780, 1949

324. Milder MS, Cook JD, Stray S et al: Idiopathic hemochromatosis: an interim report. Medicine 59:34, 1980

325. Sheldon JH: Haemochromatosis. Oxford University Press, London, 1935

326. Valberg LS, Simon JB, Manley P et al: Distribution of storage iron as body iron stores expand in patients with hemochromatosis. J Lab Clin Med 86:479, 1975

327. Walters GO, Jacobs A, Woorwood M et al: Iron absorption in normal subjects and patients with idiopathic hemochromatosis. Gut 16:188, 1975

328. Brink B, Disler P, Lynch S et al: Patterns of iron storage in dietary iron overload and idiopathic hemochromatosis. J Lab Clin Med 88:725, 1977

329. Strohmeyer C, Niederau C, Stremmel W: Survival and causes of death in hemochromatosis. Ann NY Acad Sci 526:245, 1988

330. Niederau CR, Fisher R, Sonnenberg A et al: Survival and causes of death in cirrhotic and noncirrhotic patients with primary hemochromatosis. N Engl J Med 313:1256, 1985

331. Cazzola M, Ascari E, Barosi G: Juvenile idiopathic hemochromatosis. Hum Genet 65:149, 1983

332. Haddy TB, Castro OL, Rana SR: Hereditary hemochromatosis in children, adolescents and young adults. Am J Pediatr Hematol Oncol 10:23, 1988

333. Lamon JM, Marynick SP, Rosenblatt R et al: Idiopathic hemochromatosis in a young female. A case study and review of the syndrome in young people. Gastroenterology 76:178, 1979

334. Mohler DN, Wheby MS: Case report: hemochromatosis heterozygotes may have significant iron overload when they also have hereditary spherocytosis. Am J Med Sci 292:320, 1986

335. Fargion S, Cappellini D, Piperno A: Association of hereditary spherocytosis and idiopathic hemochromatosis. Am J Clin Pathol 86:645, 1986

336. Simon M, Beaumont C, Briere J: Is the HLA-linked haemachromatosis allele implicated in idiopathic sideroblastic anemia? Br J Haematol 60:75, 1985

337. Cartwright GE, Edwards CQ, Skolnick MH et al: Association of HLA-linked hemochromatosis with idiopathic sideroblastic anemia. J Clin Invest 65:989, 1980

338. Kushner JP, Edwards CQ, Dadone MM et al: Heterozygosity for HLA-linked hemochromatosis as a likely cause of the hepatic siderosis associated with sporadic porphyria cutanea tarda. Gastroenterology 88:1232, 1985

339. Kushner JP, Edwards CQ, Dadone MM et al: HLA-linked hemochromatosis and sporadic porphyria cutanea tarda. Gastroenterology 90:801, 1986

340. Beaumont C, Nordmann Y: HLA-linked hemochromatosis and sporadic porphyria cutanea tarda. Gastroenterology 90:800, 1986

341. Edwards CQ, Skolnick MH, Kushner JP: Coincidental nontransfusional iron overload and thalassemia minor. Blood 58:84, 1981

342. Cazzola M, Barosi G, Bergamaschi G et al: Iron loading in congenital dyserythropoietic anemias and congenital sideroblastic anemias. Br J Haematol 54:649, 1983

343. Peto T, Pippard MJ, Weatherall DJ: Iron overload in mild sideroblastic anemia. Lancet 1:375, 1983

344. Jakobvits AW, Morgan MY, Sherlock S: Hepatic siderosis in alcoholics. Dig Dis Sci 24:305, 1979

345. Simon M, Bourel M, Fauchet R et al: Association of HLA-A3 and HLA-B14 antigens with idiopathic hemochromatosis. Gut 17:332, 1976

346. Conrad M, Barton JC: Anemia and iron kinetics in alcoholism. Blood 17:149, 1980

347. Grossman ME, Bickers DR, Poh-Fitzpatrick MB et al: Porphyria cutanea tarda: clinical features and laboratory findings in 40 patients. Am J Med 67:277, 1979

348. Gordeuk VR, Boyd RD, Brittenham GM: Dietary iron overload persists in rural sub-Saharan Africa. Lancet 1:1310, 1986

349. Model B, Berdoukas V: The Clinical Approach to Thalassemia. Grune & Stratton, London, 1984

350. Schaefer AI, Cheron RG, Dluhy R et al: Clinical consequences of acquired transfusional iron overload in adults. N Engl J Med 304:319, 1981

351. Porter JB, Huehns ER: Transfusion and exchange transfusion in sickle cell anemias, with particular reference to iron metabolism. Acta Haematol 78:198, 1987

352. Buja LM, Roberts WC: Iron in the heart, etiology and clinical significance. Am J Med 51:209, 1971

353. Gokal R, Millard PR, Weatherall D et al: Iron metabolism in haemodialysis patients. A study of the management of iron therapy and iron overload. Q J Med 48:369, 1979

354. Perry TL, Hardwick DF, Dixon G et al: Hypermethioninemia. Pediatrics 36:236, 1965

355. Volpe JJ, Adams RD: Cerebro-hepato-renal syndrome of Zellweger. Acta Neuropathol 20:175, 1972

356. Hardy L, Hansen JL, Kushner JP et al: Neonatal hemochromatosis. Genetic analysis of transferrin-receptor, H-apoferritin, and L-apoferritin loci and of the human leukocyte antigen class I region. Am J Pathol 137:149, 1990

357. Knisely AS: Neonatal hemochromatosis. Adv Pediatr 39:383, 1992

358. Hayes AM, Jaramillo D, Levy HL et al: Neonatal hemochromatosis: diagnosis with MR imaging. AJR 159:623, 1992

359. Silver MM, Beverley DW, Valberg L et al: Perinatal hemochromatosis. Clinical, morphologic and quantitative iron studies. Am J Pathol 128:538, 1987

360. Goldfischer S, Grotsky HW, Chang C et al: Idiopathic neonatal iron storage involving the liver, pancreas, heart, and endocrine and exocrine glands. Hepatology 1:58, 1981

361. Dooling EC, Schoene WC, Richardson EP: Hallervorden-Spatz syndrome. Arch Neurol 30:70, 1974

362. Scheuer P, Williams R, Muir AR: Hepatic pathology in relatives of patients with hemochromatosis. J Pathol 84:53, 1962

363. Bomford A, Williams R: Long-term results of venesection therapy in idiopathic hemochromatosis. Q J Med 45:611, 1976

364. Isaacson C, Seftel H, Keeley KJ et al: Siderosis in the Bantu. The relationship between iron overload and cirrhosis. J Lab Clin Med 58:845, 1961

365. Risdon RA, Barry M, Flynn DM: Transfusional iron overload: the relationship between tissue iron concentration and hepatic fibrosis in thalassemia. J Pathol 116:83, 1975

366. Bothwell TH, Isaacson C: Siderosis in the Bantu. A comparison of the incidence in males and females. Br Med J 1:522, 1962

367. Bassett ML, Halliday JW, Powell LW: Value of hepatic iron measurements in early hemochromatosis and determination of the critical iron level associated with fibrosis. Hepatology 6:24, 1986

368. Stremmel W, Niederau C, Berger M et al: Abnormalities in estrogen, androgen and insulin metabolism in idiopathic hemochromatosis. Ann NY Acad Sci 526:209, 1988

369. McNeil LW, McKee LC, Lorber P et al: The endocrine manifestations of hemochromatosis. Am J Med Sci 285:7, 1983

370. Walton C, Kelly WF, Laing I et al: Endocrine abnormalities in idiopathic hemochromatosis. Q J Med 52:99, 1983

371. Schumacher HR, Straka PC, Krikker MA et al: The arthropathy of hemochromatosis. Recent studies. Ann NY Acad Sci 526:224, 1988

372. Abbott DF, Gresham GA: Arthropathy in transfusional siderosis. Br Med J 1:1418, 1972

373. Cohen A, Cohen IJ, Schwartz E: Scurvy and altered iron stores in thalassemia major. N Engl J Med 304:158, 1981

374. Boyce N, Wood C, Holdsworth S et al: Life-threatening sepsis complicating heavy metal chelation therapy with desferrioxamine. Aust NZ J Med 15:654, 1985

375. Karp JE, Mertz WG: Association of reduced iron-binding capacity and fungal infections in leukemic granulocytopenic patients. J Clin Oncol 4:216, 1986

376. Feller ER, Pout A, Wands JR et al: Familial hemochromatosis. Physiologic studies in the precirrhotic stage of the disease. N Engl J Med 296:1422, 1977

377. Wands JR, Rowe JA, Mezey S et al: Normal serum ferritin concentrations in precirrhotic hemochromatosis. N Engl J Med 294:302, 1976

378. Chapman R, Hussain N, Gorman A: Effect of ascorbic acid deficiency on serum ferritin concentration in patients with β-thalassemia major and iron overload. J Clin Pathol 35:487, 1982

379. Mutoh K, Okuno T, Ito M et al: MR imaging of a group I case of Hallervorden-Spatz disease. J Comput Assist Tomogr 5:851, 1988

380. Drayer B, Burger P, Darwin R et al: MRI of brain iron. AJR 147:103, 1986

381. Crosby WH: Treatment of hemochromatosis by energetic phlebotomy. One patient's response to the letting of 55 litres of blood in 11 months. Br J Haematol 4:82, 1958

382. Grace ND, Greenberg MS: Phlebotomy in the treatment of iron overload. A controlled trial. Gastroenterology 60:744, 1971

383. Hershko C, Weatherall DJ: Iron-chelating therapy. CRC Crit Rev Lab Sci 26:303, 1988

384. Propper RD, Shurin SB, Nathan DG: Reassessment of the use of desferrioxamine B in iron overload. N Engl J Med 294:1421, 1976

385. Brittenham GM, Griffith PM, Nienhuis AW: Desferrioxamine (DFO) use protects against heart disease and death from transfusional iron overload in thalassemia major. Blood 72:56a, 1988

386. Cohen A, Martin M, Schwartz E: Depletion of excessive liver iron stores with desferrioxamine. Br J Haematol 58:369, 1984

387. Cohen A: Management of iron overload in the pediatric patient. Hematol Oncol Clin North Am 1:521, 1987

388. Wolfe L, Oliveri W, Sallan D et al: Prevention of cardiac disease by subcutaneous desferrioxamine in patients with thalassemia major. N Engl J Med 312:1600, 1985

389. Hoffbrand AV, Gorman A, Laulicht M et al: Improvement in iron status and liver function in patients with transfusional iron overload with long-term subcutaneous desferrioxamine. Lancet 1:947, 1979

390. Oliveri NF, Buncic JR, Chew E et al: Visual and auditory neurotoxicity in patients receiving subcutaneous desferrioxamine infusions. N Engl J Med 314:869, 1986

391. De Virgiliis S, Congia M, Frau F et al: Deferoxamine-induced growth retardation in patients with thalassemia major. J Pediatr 113:661, 1988

392. Olivieri NF, Koren G, Harris J et al: Growth failure and bony changes induced by deferoxamine. Am J Pediatr Hematol Oncol 14:48, 1992

393. Olivieri NF, Matsui D, Liu PP et al: Oral iron chelation with 1,2-dimethyl-3-hydroxypyrid-4-one (L1) in iron loaded thalassemia patients. Bone Marrow Transplant 1:9, 1993

394. al-Refaie FN, Wonke B, Hoffbrand AV et al: Efficacy and possible adverse effects of the oral iron chelator 1,2-dimethyl-3-hydroxypyrid-4-one (L1) in thalassemia major (see comments). Blood 80:593, 1992

395. Bergeron RJ, Brittenham GM (eds): The Development of Iron Chelators for Clinical Use. 1st Ed. CRC Press, Boca Raton, FL, 1994, p. 416

396. Brittenham GM: Development of iron-chelating agents for clinical use, editorial comment. Blood 80:569, 1992

397. Irie S, Tavassoli M: Transferrin-mediated cellular iron uptake. Am J Med Sci 293:103, 1987

398. Leibold EA, Guo B: Iron-dependent regulation of ferritin and transferrin receptor expression by the iron-responsive element binding protein. Annu Rev Nutr 12:345, 1992

399. Bhasker CR, Burgiel G, Neupert B et al: The putative iron-responsive element in the human erythroid 5-aminolevulinate synthase mRNA mediates translational control. J Biol Chem 268:12699, 1993

400. Melefors O, Goossen B, Johansson HE et al: Translational control of 5-aminolevulinate synthase mRNA by iron-responsive elements in erythroid cells. J Biol Chem 268:5974, 1993

401. Herbert V: Anemias. p. 593. In Paige DM (ed): Clinical Nutrition. 2nd Ed. CV Mosby, St. Louis, 1988

402. Corporation F: Imferon. p. 1005. In Zurich DB (ed): Physicians' Desk Reference. Medical Economics Data, Montvale, NJ, 1993

403. Auerbach M, Witt D, Toler W et al: Clinical use of the total dose intravenous infusion of iron dextran. J Lab Clin Med 111:566, 1988

404. Hamstra RD, Block MH, Schocket AL: Intravenous iron dextran in clinical medicine. JAMA 243:1726, 1980

405. Becker CE, MacGregor RR, Walker KS et al: Fatal anaphylaxis after intramuscular iron-dextran. Ann Intern Med 65:745, 1966

406. Clay B, Rosenberg B, Sampson N et al: Reactions to total dose intravenous infusion of iron dextran (Imferon). Br Med J 1:29, 1965

407. Jacobs J: Death due to iron parenterally. South Med J 62:216, 1969

408. Wallerstein RO: Intravenous iron-dextran complex. Blood 32:690, 1968

409. Cantor RI, Downs GE, Abruzzo JL: Acute exacerbation of ankylosing spondylitis after an iron dextran infusion. Ann Intern Med 77:933, 1972

410. Blake DR, Lunec J, Ahern M et al: Effect of intravenous iron dextran on rheumatoid arthritis. Ann Rheum Dis 44:183, 1985

411. Winyard PG, Chirico S, Blake D et al: Mechanism of exacerbation of rheumatoid synovitis by total-dose iron-dextran infusion. Lancet 1:69, 1987

412. Weinbren K, Salm R, Greenberg G: Intramuscular injections of iron compounds and oncogenesis in man. Br Med J 1:683, 1978

413. Brittenham GM: Iron-chelating agents. Curr Ther Hematol Oncol 3:149, 1987

414. Newman R, Schneider C, Sutherland R et al: The transferrin receptor. Trends Biochem Sci 7:397, 1982

Heme Biosynthesis and Its Disorders: Porphyrias and Sideroblastic Anemias

39

Robert J. Desnick and Karl E. Anderson

HEME BIOSYNTHETIC PATHWAY

Heme Biosynthetic Enzymes

The heme biosynthetic pathway is shown in Figure 39-1. The first and last three enzymes function in the mitochondrion, whereas the other four function in the cytosol. Each of the eight heme biosynthetic enzymes is encoded by a nuclear gene. The full-length human cDNAs for seven enzymes have been isolated and sequenced[1-9] and the genomic structures and/or the entire genomic sequences for five of the enzymes have been characterized.[10-14] Only the cDNA encoding protoporphyrinogen oxidase has not been cloned. The chromosomal locations of the seven cloned heme biosynthetic cDNAs have been assigned to six different chromosomes by somatic cell or in situ hybridization techniques[15-23] (Table 39-1). Each of the enzymes in the pathway is briefly described.

ALA-Synthase

The first enzyme in the pathway is ALA-synthase, which catalyzes the condensation of glycine, activated by pyridoxal phosphate, and succinyl coenzyme A to form δ-aminolevulinic acid (ALA). ALA-synthase is the rate-limiting enzyme for the pathway, particularly in liver, where it is inducible by a variety of drugs, steroids, and other chemicals.[24] Distinct erythroid-specific and nonerythroid housekeeping forms of ALA-synthase, encoded by separate genes, have been identified and their respective full-length cDNAs have been cloned and sequenced.[5,6] The human nonerythroid housekeeping gene is expressed in all tissues. It has been assigned to the chromosomal region 3p21 by in situ hybridization techniques.[20,21] The gene encoding the human erythroid-specific isozyme has been isolated, its genomic structure characterized,[12] and its chromosomal location assigned to Xp11.[21] These findings provide a basis for the tissue-specific regulation of this pathway. Expression of erythroid-specific ALA-synthase appears essential for supplying the large amounts of heme required for hemoglobin formation. Induction of the housekeeping form in the liver supplies heme for the hepatic cytochrome P-450 enzymes.[25,26]

Two isoforms of the erythroid-specific enzyme are produced by an alternative splicing mechanism that differs among various species.[27] The regulatory implications of these isoforms are unknown. Since the erythroid-specific and housekeeping isozymes have remarkably short intracellular half-lives (ap-

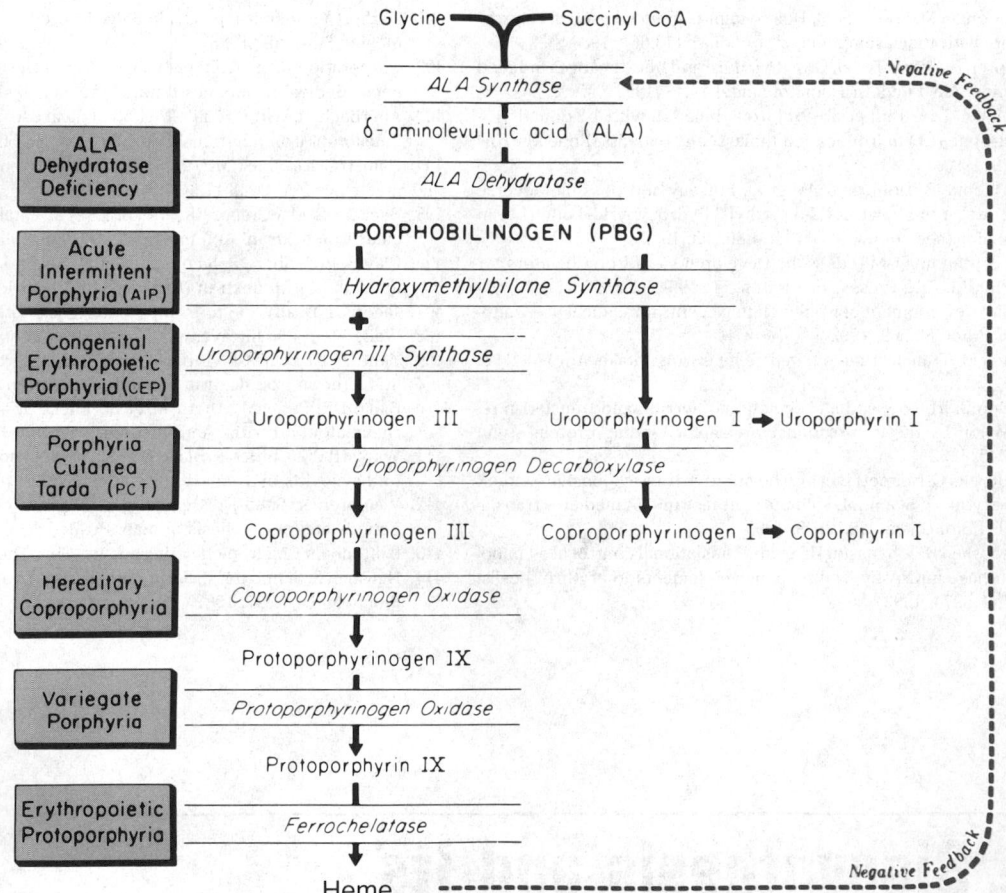

Fig. 39-1. The human heme biosynthetic pathway and the inherited porphyrias.

proximately 30 minutes), limited information is available on the physical and kinetic properties of the human isozymes. The recent expression of the full-length human cDNAs in *Escherichia coli*[28] portends the availability of recombinant isozymes for analysis of their respective properties.

Families with an X-linked, pyridoxine-responsive sideroblastic anemia have been described,[29–33] including some with chromosomal rearrangement breakpoints at Xp13.[34] Recently, specific mutations in the erythroid-specific gene at Xp11 have been identified in patients with X-linked sideroblastic anemias that were pyridoxine responsive[35,36] (see Ch. 40).

Table 39-1. Chromosomal Localization of the Heme Biosynthetic Genes

Structural Gene	Chromosomal Assignment	Method	Reference
ALA-synthase			
Housekeeping	3p21	cDNA	Bishop et al.[21]; Sutherland et al.[20]
Erythroid	Xp21–q22	cDNA	Bishop et al.[21]
ALA-dehydratase	9q34	cDNA	Potluri et al.[19]
HMB synthase	11q23–qter	SCH	Wang et al.[15]
		cDNA	Namba et al.[16]
URO-synthase	10q25.2 → q26.3	SCH	Astrin et al.[22]
URO-decarboxylase	1p34	cDNA	Romeo et al.[18]
COPRO-oxidase	9	SCH	Grandchamp et al.[17]
Ferrochelatase	18q22	cDNA	Whitcombe et al.[23]

Abbreviations: cDNA, in situ hybridization with cDNA probe; SCH, analysis of somatic cell hybrids.

ALA-Dehydratase

The second enzymatic reaction in the pathway, catalyzed by ALA-dehydratase, is the condensation of two molecules of ALA to form a cyclic compound, the pyrrole derivative porphobilinogen (PBG). Purified human ALA-dehydratase is composed of eight identical 31-kd subunits and eight atoms of zinc.[35] The zinc atoms are required for both stability and catalytic activity.[38] In 1986, isolation of the full-length cDNA encoding human ALA-dehydratase was reported.[4] Sequence analysis revealed that the zinc atoms are bound to each subunit by a typical zinc finger domain consisting of four cysteine and two histidine residues. The zinc atoms protect essential sulfhydryl groups of the enzyme and can be displaced by lead or other heavy metals. In fact, the measurement of erythrocyte ALA-dehydratase activity is used as a highly sensitive index of lead exposure.[39] The gene for human ALA-dehydratase has been assigned by in situ hybridization to the 9q34 chromosomal region.[19] Erythroid and housekeeping promoter regions in the gene have been identified that generate alternative transcripts but have the same coding sequence.[14]

The ALA-dehydratase locus has two common alleles: ALAD-1 and ALAD-2. This accounts for the occurrence of three electrophoretically distinguishable ALA-dehydratase enzyme forms[40,41] designated 1–1, 1–2, and 2–2. The frequencies of the corresponding phenotypes in white populations are about 80%, 18%, and 1%, respectively, giving gene frequencies of 0.9 and 0.1 for the ALAD-1 and ALAD-2 alleles, respectively. In Hispanics and American blacks, the gene frequency of the ALAD-2 allele was lower,[41] and in a Liberian population the ALAD-2 allele was not detected.[42] The occurrence of this common polymorphism in the white population has been hypothesized to be associated with a difference in susceptibility to lead poisoning.[41] A recessively inherited hepatic porphyria due to deficient ALA-dehydratase activity has been described,[41,42] and specific mutations in its genes have been reported.[45,46]

Hydroxymethylbilane Synthase (PBG-Deaminase)

The formation of uroporphyrinogen III from four molecules of PBG occurs by a two-step process catalyzed by the third and fourth enzymes in the pathway, hydroxymethylbilane (HMB)-synthase (formerly known as PBG-deaminase or uroporphyrinogen I synthase) and uroporphyrinogen III synthase (URO-synthase) (Fig. 39-1). HMB-synthase catalyzes the head-to-tail condensation of four PBG molecules by a series of deaminations to form the linear tetrapyrrole HMB. HMB can slowly cyclize nonenzymatically to form uroporphyrinogen I. Because HMB-synthase activity is almost as low as ALA-synthase activity in most normal tissues, it may become rate-limiting when the enzyme is partially deficient and when there is an excess supply of PBG. The half-normal activity of HMB-synthase is the enzymatic defect in acute intermittent porphyria.[47]

HMB-synthase, purified from human erythrocytes, has been separated into multiple forms (designated A, B, C, D, and E).[48] These represent the native enzyme (A) and enzyme/substrate complexes of the mono- (B), di- (C), tri- (D), and tetrapyrrole (E) intermediates. A unique dipyrromethane cofactor is made by the enzyme from porphobilinogen and binds the pyrrole intermediate at the active site until formation of HMB is complete.[49] Two tissue-specific isoenzymes of HMB-synthase are produced by a single gene,[2] which has been mapped to the chromosomal region 11q24.1→q24.2.[15,16] Both the erythroid and non-erythroid or housekeeping forms are monomeric proteins; the molecular weight of the erythroid-specific form is approximately 38,000, while that of the housekeeping form is approximately 40,000.[2]

The human cDNAs and the entire genomic sequence encoding the erythroid and housekeeping forms have been cloned and sequenced.[1,2,13] The 10-kb chromosomal gene for HMB-synthase has 15 exons. Tissue specificity for this enzyme results from alternative splicing of exons 1 and 2.[50] In erythroid cells, the erythroid-specific transcript is encoded by exons 2–15. Intron 1 contains the erythroid promoter. In nonerythroid cells, the HMB-synthase housekeeping transcript is encoded by exons 1 and 3–15. The 5′ flanking region contains the housekeeping promoter. The erythroid promoter functions only in erythroid cells, whereas the housekeeping promoter functions in all cell types. Therefore, both enzyme forms can be expressed in erythroid cells.[50] The erythroid-specific promoter contains cis-acting regions that bind the NF-E1 and NF-E2 trans-acting erythroid-specific factors. These factors are required for transcriptional regulation of the HMB-synthase erythroid promoter.[50,51]

Uroporphyrinogen III Synthase

URO-synthase (or cosynthase) catalyzes the rearrangement of HMB (by inversion of the pyrrole D ring) and rapid cyclization to form the asymmetric and physiologic uroporphyrinogen type III isomer (Fig. 39-1). In the absence of URO-synthase, HMB nonenzymatically cyclizes to form the uroporphyrinogen I isomer. This nonphysiologic compound can be metabolized to coproporphyrinogen I, but further metabolism cannot proceed because the next enzyme is stereospecific for the III isomer. Human URO-synthase has been purified from erythrocytes, and its physical and kinetic properties have been characterized.[52] The enzyme is a monomer with a subunit molecular weight of 29,500. In 1988, Tsai et al.[7] reported cloning and sequencing of the full-length cDNA encoding this enzyme and production of large amounts of the enzyme by expression of the cDNA in E.

coli. The erythroid and hepatic forms of the enzyme appear to be identical. The chromosomal location of the URO-synthase gene has been assigned to the narrow region 10q25.2→q26.3 by analysis of somatic cell hybrids containing portions of chromosome.[22] HMB-synthase and URO-synthase are both cytosolic enzymes and may exist as an enzyme complex, possibly in association with the other two cytosolic enzymes of the pathway.[7] URO-synthase activity is markedly deficient, but not absent, in congenital erythropoietic porphyria (CEP).[53,54]

Uroporphyrinogen Decarboxylase

Uroporphyrinogen III is an octacarboxylate porphyrinogen. In comparison with other uroporphyrinogen isomers, it is the preferred substrate for uroporphyrinogen decarboxylase (URO-decarboxylase), the fifth enzyme in the pathway. This cytosolic enzyme catalyzes the sequential removal of the four carboxyl groups from the acetic acid side chains of uroporphyrinogen III (clockwise, starting with ring D) to form the four methyl groups of coproporphyrinogen III, a tetracarboxylate porphyrinogen. URO-decarboxylase, purified from human erythrocytes, is a monomeric protein with a molecular weight of 42,000,[55] which catalyzes all four decarboxylations. The full-length cDNA for the human enzyme has been isolated and sequenced.[3] The chromosomal gene encoding URO-decarboxylase, which is about 3 kb in length, contains 10 exons[10] and has been localized to the chromosomal region 1p34.[18] Evidence for two isoenzymes in human erythrocytes has been presented by some investigators[56] but not by others.[57] A single species of mRNA for URO-decarboxylase has been found in various tissues, suggesting that there are no tissue-specific isoenzymes.[3] Deficiencies of this enzymatic activity cause the metabolic defects in porphyria cutanea tarda and hepatoerythropoietic porphyria.[58,59]

Coproporphyrinogen Oxidase

The mitochondrial enzyme coproporphyrinogen oxidase catalyzes the decarboxylation of two of the four proprionic acid groups of coproporphyrinogen III (on rings A and B) to form the two vinyl groups of protoporphyrinogen IX, a dicarboxylate porphyrinogen. Coproporphyrinogen oxidase (COPRO-oxidase) is functional in mitochondria between the inner and outer membranes.[60,61] It requires molecular oxygen for its activity. A 3-carboxylate porphyrinogen (termed harderoporphyrinogen because the corresponding porphyrin was first isolated from the rodent harderian gland) is an intermediate in the two-step decarboxylation. Coproporphyrinogen I, which is formed by decarboxylation of uroporphyrinogen I, is not a substrate for this enzyme, and therefore is not metabolized to heme. Although human COPRO-oxidase has not been isolated, the bovine liver enzyme has been purified and shown to be a monomer with a molecular weight of 71,600.[62] Recently, the bovine and human cDNAs have been isolated.[9,63] The locus for the human gene encoding COPRO-oxidase has been assigned to chromosome 9.[17] The half-normal activity of COPRO-oxidase is the metabolic defect in hereditary coproporphyria (HCP).[64] Homozygous forms of HCP and harderoporphyria (a variant of HCP) are associated with more severe deficiencies of COPRO-oxidase activity.[65,66]

Protoporphyrinogen Oxidase

The seventh enzyme in the pathway, protoporphyrinogen oxidase (PROTO-oxidase), catalyzes the oxidation of protoporphyrinogen IX to protoporphyrin IX by the removal of six hydrogen atoms. The product of the reaction is a porphyrin (oxidized form), in contrast to the preceding several substrates, which are porphyrinogens (reduced forms). This oxidation occurs readily under aerobic conditions in vitro in the absence of the enzyme. PROTO-oxidase, an integral protein of the mitochondrial inner membrane,[67] has not been purified from human sources, nor has the cDNA been isolated. The murine enzyme has been purified and shown to be a monomer of 65 kd[68] whose activity is inhibited by bilirubin.[69] Presumably the human enzyme also is inhibited by bilirubin, accounting for the decreased levels of PROTO-oxidase activity in Gilbert disease.[70] The half-normal activity of this enzyme is the enzymatic defect in variegate porphyria.[71] Linkage analysis suggests localization of the gene for this disease on chromosome 14.[72]

Ferrochelatase

The final step in heme biosynthesis is the insertion of ferrous iron into protoporphyrin IX to form heme. This reaction is catalyzed by ferrochelatase, an enzyme also known as heme synthetase or protoheme ferrolyase. Ferrochelatase is associated with the inner side of the inner mitochondrial membrane,[73,74] is specific for the reduced form of iron (Fe^{2+}) but can use other metals (e.g., Zn^{2+} and Co^{2+}) and other dicarboxylate porphyrins. The enzyme in mammals has a monomeric molecular weight of about 40,000 and aggregates to a 240-kd form at low salt concentrations.[73,74] It may function as a dimer in intact mitochondria.[77] The bovine enzyme first binds iron, then the porphyrin; arginyl residues are involved in porphyrin binding.[75] Iron binding is mediated by two vicinal sulfhydryl groups. The human ferrochelatase gene has been assigned to chromosome 18q22.[23] Recently, full-length cDNAs encoding the enzyme were isolated from several species including humans.[8,78,79] Ferrochelatase activity is deficient in erythropoietic protoporphyria (EPP)[80,81] and is also sensitive to inhibition by lead.[82]

Regulation of Heme Biosynthesis

In humans about 85% of heme is synthesized in erythroid cells to provide heme for hemoglobin (see Ch. 38), while most of the remaining heme is produced in the liver, where it is used primarily as the prosthetic group in cytochrome P-450 enzymes and other hemoproteins. In the liver, the heme biosynthetic pathway is under negative feedback control by the concentration of "free" heme. Heme represses the synthesis of mRNA for ALA-synthase in liver and can also interfere with the transport of a cytosolic form of the enzyme into mitochondria.[83–85] ALA-synthase is inducible by many of the same chemicals that induce cytochrome P-450, a family of hemoproteins in the endoplasmic reticulum of the liver and other tissues.[25] Because most of the heme synthesized in the liver is used for the synthesis of the cytochrome P-450 enzymes, the induction of hepatic ALA-synthase and the cytochrome P-450s occurs in a coordinated fashion.[25] When the regulatory "free" heme pool becomes depleted (which may occur, for example, when more heme is required for synthesis of hemoproteins), the synthesis of ALA-synthase is increased. Conversely, repression of ALA-synthase synthesis results from augmentation of the regulatory heme pool. The evidence that ALA-synthase functions as a rate-controlling enzyme, at least in the liver, includes its relatively low V_{max} value (compared with most other enzymes in the pathway), its inducibility and short half-life, and its great sensitivity to repression by cellular heme (at concentrations of $<10^{-6}$ M). Low affinity of the enzyme for glycine suggests that the intracellular glycine concentration also determines the rate of ALA formation.

Control of heme biosynthesis in tissues other than the liver and erythroid cells has not been the subject of intensive investigation. The existence of erythroid-specific forms of ALA-synthase and HMB synthase suggests that the regulation of this pathway is distinct in erythroid cells. These enzymes make

REGULATORY MECHANISMS FOR ERYTHROID HEME PRODUCTION

Erythroid cells have novel regulatory mechanisms for the production of the very large amounts of heme needed for hemoglobin synthesis. For example, there are erythroid-specific forms of ALA-synthase[5,6] and HMB-synthase,[1,2,27] the first and third enzymes of the heme biosynthetic pathway. The erythroid-specific gene for ALA-synthase on the X chromosome is expressed at high levels during erythroid differentiation, providing sufficient ALA-synthase to produce the required amounts of heme. Transcriptional control of erythroid ALA-synthase is exerted by erythroid-specific promoter elements in the 5′-flanking region of the gene.[12] Translational control results from an iron-responsive element in the 5′-untranslated region of the mRNA. Transcription of the housekeeping ALA-synthase gene on chromosome 3 may be down-regulated during erythroid differentiation.[87] In contrast to liver, erythroid ALA-synthase gene transcription is not negatively regulated by heme. A conserved heme regulatory motif may confer inhibition by heme of the transport of a precursor form of the erythroid enzyme into mitochondria.[88] More distal enzymes, such as HMB-synthase and ferrochelatase, may also have rate-limiting functions during erythroid differentiation and heme formation. The HMB-synthase gene has a separate erythroid-specific promoter (in addition to its housekeeping promoter) that provides the means to increase expression in erythroid cells.[13,51] Similarly, the ALA-dehydratase gene has unique erythroid-specific and housekeeping promoters that generate transcripts encoding the identical polypeptide.[14] Sequential increases in the enzymes of the heme biosynthetic pathway, probably due to transcriptional activation of the corresponding genes, precede the accumulation of newly synthesized heme in differentiating erythroid cells.[87,89] In addition, heme regulates the rate of its synthesis in erythroid cells by controlling the transport of iron (required for ferrochelatase) into reticulocytes.[90]

heme for cytochromes and other hemoproteins in all cells. However, it is possible that neurons may depend in part on surrounding non-neural cells for heme or heme precursors.[86]

CLASSIFICATION AND DIAGNOSIS OF PORPHYRIAS

Diagnosis

For medical management and genetic counseling, it is important to establish which porphyria is present in a given patient (Table 39-2). Because many of the symptoms of the various porphyrias are nonspecific and can mimic those of other more common diseases, diagnosis is often delayed. Incorrect diagnoses of porphyria are not uncommon in patients with symptoms due to other diseases. When porphyria is suspected clinically, proper laboratory testing is important to confirm or exclude the diagnosis. Tests for porphyria may be difficult to interpret because abnormal porphyrin results can occur in some disorders other than porphyrias, and minimally elevated levels of porphyrins or their precursors may have little or no diagnostic significance.

Intermediates of the heme biosynthetic pathway that accumulate in the porphyrias may be excreted unchanged or may

Table 39-2. Classification of the Human Porphyrias

Type/Porphyria	Deficient Enzyme	Inheritance	Photosensitivity	Neurovisceral Symptoms
Hepatic				
ALA-dehydratase deficiency	ALA-dehydratase	AR	−	+
Acute intermittent porphyria (AIP)	HMB-synthase	AD	−	+
Hereditary coproporphyria (HCP)	COPRO-oxidase	AD	+	+
Variegate porphyria (VP)	PROTO-oxidase	AD	+	+
Porphyria cutanea tarda (PCT)	URO-decarboxylase	AD	+	−
Erythropoietic				
Congenital erythropoietic porphyria (CEP)	URO-synthase	AR	+++	−
Erythropoietic protoporphyria (EPP)	Ferrochelatase	AD	+	−

Abbreviations: AR, autosomal recessive; AD, autosomal dominant.

undergo chemical modifications prior to excretion. ALA and PBG are colorless and nonfluorescent compounds; they are largely excreted unchanged but may degrade to colored products. Porphyrinogens are colorless, nonfluorescent, and subject to auto-oxidation to the corresponding porphyrins outside the cell. Porphyrins are reddish in color and fluoresce when exposed to long-wavelength ultraviolet light. Porphyrins are progressively less water soluble the fewer the number of carboxylate groups in their molecules. Excess ALA, PBG, uroporphyrin I and III, and 7-, 6-, and 5-carboxylate porphyrins are excreted mostly in the urine. Coproporphyrins are excreted partly in urine and partly in bile, whereas harderoporphyrin and protoporphyrin are excreted almost entirely in the bile and feces. Evidence shows that coproporphyrin I is more readily excreted in bile than is coproporphyrin III, which may explain the increase in the ratio of these isomers that occurs when hepatobiliary function is impaired.[91]

Table 39-3 summarizes the major metabolites that accumulate in each porphyria. Urinary ALA and PBG are easily quantitated by chemical methods.[92] The individual porphyrins in urine and feces can be separated and quantitated by high-performance liquid chromatography.[93] If carried out properly, especially in the presence of symptoms, these studies should identify a diagnostic profile of accumulated precursors and/or porphyrins.[94] However, the definitive diagnosis of a particular porphyria requires the demonstration of the specific enzymatic defect. Assays are described in the literature for each of the eight heme biosynthetic enzymes using erythrocytes,

lymphocytes, cultured lymphoblasts, or cultured fibroblasts, although some are not widely available for diagnostic purposes.[95]

INBORN AND ACQUIRED ERRORS OF HEME BIOSYNTHESIS

ALA-Dehydratase-Deficient Porphyria

ALA-dehydratase-deficient porphyria is the most recently described type of porphyria. It is inherited as an autosomal recessive trait. To date it has been identified in only four unrelated males in Europe. The affected homozygotes had <5% of normal activity in their erythrocytes, whereas their parents and heterozygous relatives had about half-normal levels of activity.

Biochemical and Molecular Aspects

ALA-dehydratase-deficient porphyria is characterized by markedly increased urinary excretion of ALA and coproporphyrin III and increased erythrocyte protoporphyrin. The markedly reduced erythrocyte ALA-dehydratase activity in these patients was not restored to normal by the in vitro addi-

Table 39-3. Major Metabolites Accumulated in Human Porphyrias

Type/Porphyria	Increased Erythrocyte Porphyrins	Porphyrin Excretion	
		Urine	Stool
Hepatic			
ALA-dehydratase deficiency	PROTO IX	ALA, COPRO III	−
Acute intermittent porphyria (AIP)	−	ALA, PBG	−
Hereditary coproporphyria (HCP)	−	ALA, PGB, COPRO III	COPRO III
Variegate porphyria (VP)	−	ALA, PBG, COPRO III	COPRO III, PROTO IX
Porphyria cutanea tarda (PCT)	−	URO I, 7-carboxylate	ISOCOPRO
Erythropoietic			
Congenital erythropoietic porphyria (CEP)	URO I	URO I	COPRO I
Erythropoietic protoporphyria (EPP)	PROTO IX	−	PROTO IX

Abbreviations: ALA, δ-aminolevulinic acid; PBG, porphobilinogen; COPRO I, coproporphyrin I; COPRO III, coproporphyrin III; ISOCOPRO, isocoproporphyrin; URO I, uroporphyrin I; URO III, uroporphyrin III; PROTO, protoporphyrin IX.

CLASSIFICATION OF HUMAN PORPHYRIAS

Classification of the porphyrias is now based on an understanding of specific deficiencies (usually inherited) of enzymes in the heme biosynthetic pathway. The porphyrias have been classified as hepatic or erythropoietic, according to whether the excess production of porphyrin precursors and/or porphyrins takes place primarily in the liver or in the erythron. Neurologic symptoms and elevated plasma and urinary concentrations of the porphyrin precurors ALA and PBG are characteristic of the four acute porphyrias. The excess intermediates originate in the liver in at least three of the acute porphyrias. By contrast, individuals affected with erythropoietic porphyrias have elevated bone marrow and erythrocyte porphyrins. Plasma porphyrins increase and become deposited in the skin and lead to cutaneous photosensitivity in erythropoietic and several hepatic porphyrias. Autosomal dominant hepatic porphyrias may have erythropoietic features (e.g., increased erythrocyte porphyrins) in homozygous patients. Patients with dual porphyria have deficiencies of more than one heme pathway enzyme.

tion of sulfhydryl reagents such as dithiothreitol. Immunologic studies in three cases revealed the presence of nonfunctional enzyme proteins, which cross-reacted with anti-ALA-dehydratase antibodies.[96,97] Differences from normal in size or charge of the mutant enzymes were not detected.[96] The presence of cross-reactive immunologic material (CRIM) indicated that the mutant genes were transcribed and translated but that the resultant CRIM-positive proteins had markedly altered catalytic properties and somewhat decreased stabilities. Molecular studies in three patients have demonstrated point mutations resulting in single amino acid substitutions.[45,46] The parents in each case were nonconsanguinous, and the index cases had inherited a different ALA-dehydratase mutation from each parent.

Genetic Aspects

ALA-dehydratase-deficient porphyria is inherited as an autosomal recessive trait. Its frequency is unknown. Onset and severity of the disease are variable, presumably depending on the amount of residual ALA-dehydratase activity. Heterozygotes are clinically asymptomatic, do not excrete increased levels of ALA, and can be detected by demonstration of intermediate levels of erythrocyte ALA-dehydratase activity. To date, the prenatal diagnosis of this disorder has not been made but should be possible by determination of the ALA-dehydratase activity or the specific molecular lesions in cultured chorionic villi or amniocytes.

Clinical Manifestations

The clinical presentations of the four unrelated homozygotes with ALA-dehydratase deficiency have been remarkably different, presumably due to the genetic heterogeneity in this disorder. The first reported patients were adolescents with symptoms resembling those of acute intermittent porphyria (AIP), including abdominal pain and neuropathy.[43] The third patient was an infant, who had more severe disease, including failure to thrive.[44] Presumably, the earlier age of onset and more severe manifestations in this patient reflect a more significant deficiency of ALA-dehydratase activity. The fourth patient was essentially normal until age 63, when an acute motor polyneuropathy developed.[98] Diagnostic studies showed elevated plasma and urine ALA concentrations and deficient ALA-dehydratase activity; the patient also had polycythemia. It is unclear whether this porphyria should, like the other acute porphyrias, be classified as hepatic. The third reported patient underwent liver transplantation, with only marginal clinical improvement.[99] ALA and porphyrins did not decrease after transplantation in this case, suggesting that the excess intermediates originated in tissues other than the liver, and possibly the bone marrow.

Differential Diagnosis

Lead, styrene, and succinylacetone (which accumulates in hereditary tyrosinemia and is structurally similar to ALA) inhibit ALA-dehydratase, causing increased urinary excretion of ALA and clinical manifestations that resemble those of the acute porphyrias.[100–103] Therefore, lead intoxication, other environmental chemical exposures, and hereditary tyrosinemia (fumarylacetoacetase deficiency) should be considered in the differential diagnosis of ALA-dehydratase-deficient porphyria. Idiopathic acquired ALA-dehydratase deficiency has been reported.[104]

Acute Intermittent Porphyria

AIP is an autosomal dominant ecogenetic condition resulting from half-normal levels of HMB-synthase activity.[47] Although the enzymatic deficiency occurs in all individuals who inherit a mutant allele, clinical expression of this hepatic porphyria is highly variable. Activation of the disease is clearly related to ecogenic factors, which can precipitate the disease manifestations. Symptomatic patients always have increased urinary excretion of the porphyrin precursors ALA and PBG. However, the great majority of heterozygotes with HMB-synthase deficiency remain clinically asymptomatic ("latent") and may never have increased urinary ALA and PBG excretion.

Biochemical and Molecular Aspects

The metabolic defect in AIP results from the half-normal activity of HMB-synthase. Four major classes of mutations have been identified, demonstrating genetic heterogeneity at the HMB-synthase locus.[105] Most AIP heterozygotes had no CRIM produced by the mutant allele (designated CRIM-negative type I). The CRIM-negative type I mutations are heterogeneous at the molecular level and may include complete or partial gene deletions or insertions, mutations that alter splicing or stability of the mRNA, chain-terminating codons, or missense mutations that alter the activity, conformation, or stability of the mutant protein. A much less common CRIM-negative mutation (designated CRIM-negative type II) results in a deficient enzyme in nonerythroid tissues but normal enzymatic activity in erythrocytes. This variant form of AIP was first well described in Finland.[106] Subsequent molecular studies have shown that the molecular lesions causing the CRIM-negative type II AIP are mutations that impair splicing of exon 1 to exon 3, precluding the formation of the housekeeping transcript. These tissue-specific splicing mutations provide an explanation for the deficient activity in the liver and other nonerythroid tissues and normal levels of activity in erythrocytes.[107,108]

Two types of CRIM-positive mutations (designated types 1 and 2) have been characterized[105,109]; in both of which the mutant alleles are expressed but the enzyme proteins have altered kinetic or stability properties (or both). Presumably the CRIM-positive mutations result from single-base substitutions in the coding region of the HMB-synthase gene. For example, the first point mutation in a CRIM-positive type I family, resulted in exon skipping, yielding a shortened transcript, and a noncatalytic but immunoreactive enzyme protein.[110]

Genetic Aspects

AIP is inherited as an autosomal dominant trait. It is an excellent example of an ecogenic disorder, since its expression is usually precipitated by hormonal, metabolic, dietary, or environmental factors. The disease occurs in all ethnic groups but may be more common in Scandinavia, Britain, and Ireland.[111] One severely affected child was found to be homozygous for AIP.[112] The gene encoding HMB-synthase has been localized to 11q24.1→q24.2.[15,16] Molecular cloning revealed the presence of two cDNAs for HMB-synthase, one encoding the housekeeping form and the other erythroid specific.[1,2] The occurrence of erythroid and housekeeping forms was suggested initially by biochemical studies.[2] Subsequent isolation and characterization of the chromosomal gene revealed that two transcripts were encoded by a single gene, which had two promoters, one responsible for the expression of the transcript for the housekeeping form of the enzyme probably found in all tissues and the other for the erythroid-specific transcript.[13,113] When enzymatic assays for HMB-synthase are diagnostically inconclusive, heterozygotes can be confirmed by restriction fragment length polymorphism studies in informative families using several polymorphic sites in the HMB-synthase gene.[13,114–116] A prenatal diagnosis of an affected heterozygous fetus has been made by enzymatic analysis.[117] The future identification of the specific mutation in an at-risk family will permit the more accurate molecular diagnosis of fetuses carrying the defective gene (see the section Laboratory Evaluation).

FACTORS THAT PRECIPITATE PORPHYRIC ATTACKS

Endogenous steroid hormones are probably the most important precipitating factors of porphyric attacks. This is indicated by a number of clinical features of AIP, including (1) the rarity of symptoms and excess porphyrin precursor excretion before puberty; (2) more frequent clinical expression women than in men; (3) premenstrual attacks of the disease in some women and their prevention by the administration of gonadotropin-releasing hormone analogues[131]; (4) exacerbation of AIP due to exogenous steroids, including oral contraceptive preparations; and (5) the presence of more subtle abnormalities in steroid hormone metabolism, such as a deficiency of hepatic steroid 5α-reductase activity that can predispose to the excess production of steroid hormone metabolites that are inducers of ALA-synthase in the liver.[123]

Although attacks of porphyria can occur during pregnancy, pregnancy is usually well tolerated.[132] Earlier reports of worsening symptoms during pregnancy may have been due to the use of barbiturates and perhaps to reduce caloric intake. Thus, clinical experience and experimental data indicate that pregnancy is not contraindicated in AIP if harmful drugs are avoided and if attention is given to proper nutrition.

Drugs are a key cause of AIP attacks; many patients with AIP do well because they avoid harmful drugs. Most porphyrinogenic drugs induce ALA-synthase and heme synthesis in the liver. Induction of ALA-synthase is closely associated with induction of cytochrome P-450, a process that increases the demand for heme synthesis in the liver.[70] Some drugs can also increase heme turnover by promoting the destruction of cytochrome P-450, at least in experimental systems.[133] Sulfonamide antibiotics inhibit HMB-synthase.[134] An attack following ingestion of a harmful drug in an HMB-synthase-deficient heterozygote may not be due to the drug alone. Rather, other predisposing factors such as endogenous hormones and nutritional factors probably play a role as well. Drugs are only rarely reported to cause acute symptoms in children with HMB-synthase deficiency. A large retrospective study of risk from anesthetic use in AIP concluded that barbiturates or other inducing drugs are quite frequently detrimental in patients who already have porphyric symptoms but that they seldom exacerbate latent disease.[135] HMB-synthase-deficient heterozygotes who require long-term anticonvulsants for epilepsy do not always suffer exacerbations of porphyria. However, it is recommended that exposure to porphyrinogenic drugs be avoided in all HMB-synthase-deficient heterozygotes, including children. The major drugs known or strongly suspected to be harmful in AIP, HCP, or VP, as well as drugs known to be safe, are listed in the table below. Other reviews and more extensive lists of drugs that are harmful, safe, or in intermediate categories are available.[123,124] The choice of anesthetic agents also has been studied in animal models and reviewed.[133,136] Smoking results in exposure to chemicals that induce cytochrome P-450 enzymes and heme synthesis in the liver and may increase the risk of attacks of porphyria.[137]

Categories of Safe and Unsafe Drugs in AIP, HCP, and VP	
Unsafe	Safe
Barbiturates	Narcotic analgesics
Sulfonamide antibiotics	Aspirin
Meprobamate	Acetaminophen
Glutethimide	Phenothiazines
Methyprylon	Penicillin and
Ethchlorvynol	derivatives
Mephenytoin	Streptomycin
Phenytoin	Glucocorticoids
Succinimides	Bromides
Carbamazepine	Insulin
Valproic acid	Atropine
Pyrazolones	
Griseofulvin	
Ergots	
Synthetic estrogens and progestins	
Danazol	
Alcohol	

Etiology and Pathogenesis

Most of the factors known to precipitate acute porphyric attacks have the potential to induce the synthesis of hepatic ALA-synthase and cytochrome P-450, thereby increasing the levels of ALA, PBG, other heme pathway intermediates. Normally, the amount of HMB-synthase, particularly in the liver, is low but sufficient to avoid any accumulation of PBG. However, when certain environmental, metabolic, and hormonal factors increase the flux of ALA, PBG, and porphyrinogens through the pathway, the 50% of normal enzymatic activity that is present may be insufficient to metabolize the increased levels of PBG that result from the influence of these precipitating factors.

A number of hypotheses have been proposed to explain neural damage in AIP and related disorders, but none has been satisfactorily substantiated.[118,119] The possibility that ALA or PBG might be neurotoxic is favored by the increased production of porphyrin precursors during acute porphyric attacks.[120] ALA is taken up by most tissues. It can be further metabolized more readily than PBG, which appears to cross the blood-brain barrier more efficiently.[121] These intermediates may be converted in vivo to other substances that may have neurotoxic potential. That AIP, HCP, variegate porphyria (VP), ALA-D-deficient porphyria, plumbism, and hereditary tyrosinemia are all associated with increased ALA and similar neurologic manifestations favors a neuropathic role for ALA. ALA is structurally analogous to γ-aminobutyric acid (GABA) and can interact with GABA receptors. Alternatively, the deficiency of HMB-synthase might lead to a functional heme deficiency in the nervous system or predispose to unsaturation of hepatic tryptophan pyrrolase, leading to altered tryptophan delivery to nervous tissue.[122] Possible mechanisms for neurologic dysfunction in the acute porphyrias are reviewed in more detail elsewhere.[123,124]

Clinical Manifestations

The neurovisceral and circulatory disturbances that characterize this disease rarely occur before puberty, are often nonspecific, and require a high index of suspicion to suggest the proper diagnosis. The disease can be disabling but is only occasionally fatal. Abdominal pain, the most common symptom, is usually steady and poorly localized but may be cramping. Signs of ileus, including abdominal distension and decreased bowel sounds, are common. However, increased bowel sounds and diarrhea may occur. The abdominal manifestations are neurologic rather than inflammatory; therefore tenderness, fever, and leukocytosis are generally absent or mild. Other manifestations include nausea, vomiting, constipation, tachycardia, hypertension, mental symptoms, limb, head, neck, or chest pain, muscle weakness, and sensory loss. Tachycardia, hypertension, restlessness, fine tremors, and excess sweating may be due to sympathetic overactivity. Dysuria and bladder dysfunction may occur, and urinary retention may require catheterization.

Peripheral neuropathy in AIP is primarily motor and appears to result from axonal degeneration, rather than from demyelinization.[125–127] Fortunately, significant neuropathy does not develop in all patients with acute attacks, even when abdominal symptoms are severe. Weakness most commonly begins in the proximal muscles, in the arms more often than in the legs. The course and degree of involvement are variable. Tendon reflexes may be little affected or hyperactive in early stages but are usually decreased or absent in advanced neuropathy. Paresis can be asymmetric and focal. Cranial nerves, most commonly the tenth and seventh, can be affected. Rarely, involvement of the optic nerves or occipital lobes may produce blindness. Sensory involvement with areas of paresthesia and loss of sensation may be noted. Muscle weakness can progress to respiratory and bulbar paralysis and death, but this seldom occurs unless the porphyria is not recognized, harmful drugs are not discontinued, and appropriate treatment is not instituted. Sudden death, presumably due to cardiac arrhythmia, may also occur. Even advanced neuropathy is potentially reversible.

The central nervous system also may be involved. Anxiety, insomnia, depression, disorientation, hallucinations, and paranoia, which can be especially severe during acute attacks, may suggest a primary mental disorder. Some patients have been mistakenly regarded as hysterical. Depression and other mental symptoms may be chronic in AIP patients. Surveys of psychiatric patients suggest that the disease is often unrecognized in such individuals.[128] It has not been proved, however, that the prevalence of AIP is higher in psychiatric patients than in the general population. Seizures may occur as part of the acute neurologic manifestations of AIP or as a result of hyponatremia or of causes unrelated to porphyria. Hyponatremia may be due to inappropriate antidiuretic hormone secretion or may result from vomiting, diarrhea, and poor intake or from excess renal sodium loss. An acute attack may resolve quite rapidly. Abdominal pain disappears within a few hours and paresis within a few days. After a severe attack, motor function and mental health may continue to improve for several years but may leave some residual weakness.

Morbidity and mortality in AIP and other acute porphyrias have improved markedly during the past 20–30 years.[129] This may be attributed in part to earlier detection, less use of barbiturates, and better treatment of acute attacks. AIP is commonly associated with mild abnormalities in liver function.[130] In rare cases, more advanced liver disease and hepatocellular carcinoma may complicate the disease. AIP may also predispose to chronic hypertension and impaired renal function.[129]

A low caloric intake, usually instituted in an effort to lose weight, is a common contributing cause of acute attacks. Metabolic ward studies have shown that caloric or carbohydrate restriction can precipitate acute symptoms of AIP and increase porphyrin precursor excretion.[138] Therefore, even brief periods of starvation during weight reduction, postoperative periods, or intercurrent illnesses should be avoided in patients with this disease.

Attacks of porphyria can be provoked by intercurrent infections and other illnesses and by major surgery. The mechanisms are not understood but may involve metabolic stress, impaired nutrition, and the increased production of steroid hormones and their ALA-synthase-inducing metabolites.

Laboratory Evaluations

Urinary excretion of porphyrin precursors is markedly increased during acute attacks of AIP, with PBG excretion generally ranging from approximately 50–200 mg/day. Excretion of ALA is usually about half that of PBG. If monitored, increased ALA and PBG excretion can often be demonstrated in an AIP heterozygote for some time before an attack. It is useful to follow ALA and PBG excretion in a symptomatic patient because the concentrations of these compounds generally decrease with clinical improvement. Such decreases are particularly dramatic after hematin infusions.

A normal result of a quantitative test for urinary PBG virtually excludes acute porphyria as a cause for concurrent symptoms. An exception is the rare form of acute porphyria due to ALA-dehydratase deficiency, in which there is an increase in ALA but not PBG.[43,44,98] Once AIP has become clinically expressed, it is distinctly unusual for excretion of these precursors to decrease to normal levels unless the disease becomes clinically latent for a prolonged period. However, these levels may decrease to normal soon after acute attacks of HCP and VP.

ALA and PBG are colorless. The reddish urine in AIP is due to increased porphyrins, which can form nonenzymatically from PBG. Brownish discoloration may be due to porphobilin, a degradation product of PBG, or dipyrrylmethenes. Fecal porphyrins are usually normal or minimally increased in AIP, which can help distinguish this disorder from HCP and VP. HMB-synthase is about half-normal in erythrocytes in most cases and should be measured in family members to identify other AIP heterozygotes.[139]

The diagnosis of AIP heterozygotes, particularly asymptomatic heterozygotes who usually have normal levels of urinary ALA and PBG, has been problematic by enzymatic assay, primarily due to the significant overlap between high heterozygote and low normal values.[140–142] Moreover, the identification of asymptomatic heterozygotes for the variant (CRIM-negative type II) AIP is not possible, since they exhibit normal erythrocyte enzymatic activity.[106] Thus, the recent identification of the full-length HMB-synthase cDNAs[1,2] and entire genomic sequence[13] has facilitated the identification of the specific molecular lesions causing AIP. To date, >20 mutations have been identified (Fig. 39-2) in the HMB-synthase gene.[107,108,143–149] Each of these mutations was found in single families or only a few unrelated families, emphasizing the heterogeneity of the molecular lesions causing AIP.

Congenital Erythropoietic Porphyria

CEP also known as Günther disease, is due to markedly deficient activity of URO-synthase. Uroporphyrinogen I and other porphyrinogens accumulate in erythroid cells and are oxidized to porphyrins, which are transported to other tissues of individuals affected with this autosomal recessive trait.

Biochemical and Molecular Aspects

Affected homozygotes have markedly deficient URO-synthase in erythrocytes, cultured lymphoblasts, or cultured fibroblasts.[159] It is notable that URO-synthase activity is not totally deficient in homozygotes, and that sufficient enzyme is present to produce uroporphyrinogen III for normal or even increased rates of heme production. The human enzyme has been purified from erythrocytes and has been shown to be a 29.5-kd monomer.[52] Recently, the chromosomal localization of the gene for human URO-synthase has been assigned to the narrow region q25.3→q26.3 of chromosome 10.[22] The full-length cDNA

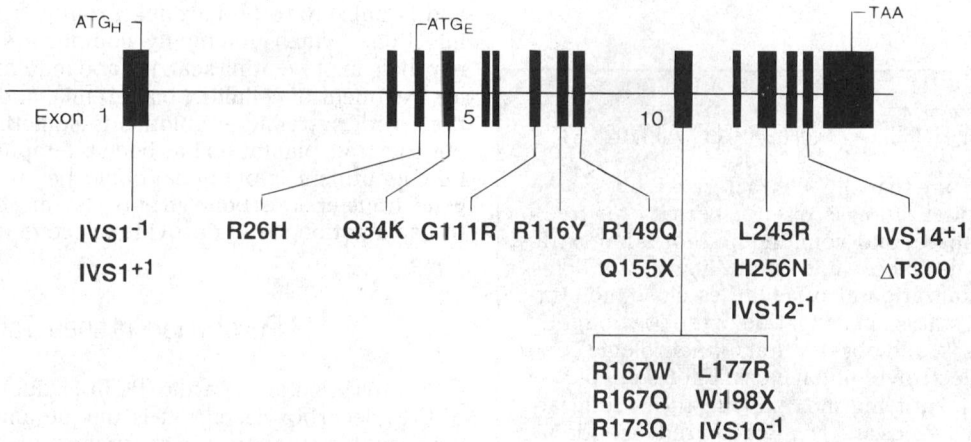

Fig. 39-2. Molecular lesions in the HMB-synthase gene responsible for AIP. Coding exons are shown as solid rectangles. ATG_H and ATG_E are the initiation of translation codons of the housekeeping and erythroid transcripts, respectively. TAA is the stop codon. Missense and nonsense mutations are indicated by the one-letter amino acid code and codon position. Q155X, glutamine codon (Q) at position 155 replaced by termination codon (X). Splicing mutations are indicated by intervening sequence (IVS) position; Δ, deletion.

encoding the human enzyme has been cloned, sequenced, and expressed in large quantities in *E. coli.*[7] The isolation of the full-length cDNA and the characterization of the gene's intron-exon boundaries[160] have permitted the identification of the molecular lesions causing CEP. More than 15 mutations have been detected in unrelated CEP families (Fig. 39-3) including missense mutations, a small exonic deletion, and a small exonic insertion.[161-165] One missense mutation (P53L) occurred in about 20% of mutant alleles, while the other lesions were found mostly in single families.[161]

Genetic Aspects

To date about 100 cases of CEP have been reported. The deficient activity of URO-synthase is the enzymatic defect in CEP and is inherited as an autosomal recessive trait.[53,159,166] Affected fetuses can be detected in utero by measuring porphyrins in amniotic fluid[167] and URO-synthase activity in cultured amniotic fluid cells.[168] In families whose URO-synthase mutations are known, prenatal diagnosis can be accomplished by molecular techniques. Genetic heterogeneity in this disease accounts at least in part for the considerable variation in the severity of symptoms. For example, a clinically mild case of CEP has been described in which an URO-synthase missense mutation encodes an enzyme polypeptide with significant residual activity,[169] thereby resulting in lower levels of accumulated uroporphyrin I in erythrocytes and urine.

Clinical Manifestations

Severe cutaneous photosensitivity usually begins in early infancy and is manifested by increased friability and blistering of the epidermis on the hands and face and other sun-exposed areas. Bullae and vesicles contain serous fluid and are susceptible to rupture and infection. The skin may be thickened, with areas of hypo- and hyperpigmentation. Hypertrichosis of the face and extremities is often prominent. Sunlight, other sources of ultraviolet light, and minor skin trauma increase the severity of the cutaneous manifestations. Recurrent vesicles and secondary infection can lead to cutaneous scarring and deformities, as well as to loss of digits and facial features such as eyelids, nose, and ears. Corneal scarring can lead to blindness. Porphyrins deposited in the teeth produce a reddish brown color in natural light, termed erythrodontia. The teeth may fluoresce on exposure to long wavelength ultraviolet light. Porphyrin deposition in bone also occurs, and bone demineralization has been described.[170] Later-onset adult patients have

been described. Life expectancy may be shortened by infection or hematologic complications.

A number of factors cause the phenotypic variability in CEP. These include (1) the amount of residual URO-synthase activity,[169] (2) the resultant degree of hemolysis and consequent stimulation of erythropoiesis, and (3) exposure to ultraviolet light. Therefore, as in other porphyrias, an interplay of environmental factors with the deficient enzymatic activity determines clinical expression of disease.

Laboratory Evaluation

Uroporphyrin I accumulation in bone marrow, erythrocytes, plasma, and urine is the biochemical hallmark of the disease. Reddish urine is usually noted shortly after birth. Urinary porphyrins are primarily uroporphyrin I and coproporphyrin I, the intermediate 7-, 6-, and 5-carboxylate porphyrins being excreted in excess as well. There is a great predominance of type I isomers, although type III isomers also are in excess. Urinary excretion of ALA and PBG is not increased. Fecal porphyrins are markedly increased with a predominance of coproporphyrin I. By contrast, the urine porphyrins in erythropoietic protoporphyria are normal. Hepatoerythropoietic porphyria (HEP), which recently has been shown to be a disease distinct from CEP, represents the homozygous deficiency of URO-decarboxylase. It is distinguishable from CEP by the presence of high levels of isocoproporphyrin in feces and urine and decreased URO-decarboxylase activity in erythrocytes. Very rare homozygous forms of VP and HCP also may be characterized by photosensitivity in childhood and increased erythrocyte porphyrins.

Therapy

For homozygotes with severe manifestations, blood transfusions given in sufficient amounts to suppress erythropoiesis significantly can be effective. For example, Piomelli et al.[170] have described a case in which frequent transfusions designed to maintain the hematocrit at >32% completely suppressed the symptoms of CEP. Deferoxamine administration, in conjunction with the transfusion regimen, reduced iron overload to some degree, and splenectomy substantially reduced the transfusion requirements in that patient.[170] Oral charcoal is sometimes effective.[173] This approach may be useful for patients who are not transfusion dependent and who have milder disease. For all CEP homozygotes, protection of the skin from sunlight and minor trauma is highly important. Sunscreen lotions may be helpful. β-Carotene may be of some value in CEP[174]

THERAPY FOR ACUTE PORPHYRIC ATTACKS

Acute attacks are usually characterized by severe symptoms. Hospitalization is often necessary for treatment of pain, nausea, and vomiting and for administration of intravenous glucose and heme (hematin or heme arginate). Hospitalization also facilitates close monitoring of nutritional status, investigation of the precipitating causes of an attack, and observation for neurologic complications and electrolyte imbalances. Efforts should be directed toward identifying and removing the inciting factors. Narcotic analgesics are usually required for abdominal pain. Nausea, vomiting, anxiety, and restlessness generally respond well to chlorpromazine or other phenothiazines. Large doses of phenothiazines are usually not required and may produce unpleasant side effects in AIP patients. Chloral hydrate can be employed for insomnia. Diazepam in low doses is probably safe if a minor tranquilizer is required. Although treatment with intravenous glucose ($\geq$300 g/day) has been recommended for patients hospitalized with attacks of porphyria,[138] a more complete nutritional regimen, including intravenous vitamins, lipids, and amino acids, might be beneficial, particularly if oral feeding is not possible for a prolonged period. However, the safety and efficacy of parenteral nutrition regimens in AIP patients have not been studied.

Intravenous infusion of heme is more effective than glucose in reducing excretion of porphyrin precursors.[121,150] Advanced neurologic damage and subacute or chronic symptoms are unlikely to respond.[151,152] Although the recommended dose is 3 mg/kg body weight infused intravenously once or twice daily, lower-dose regimens (e.g., 1–1.5 mg/kg once daily) may be equally effective.[152] The pharmacokinetics for the drug and the duration of response of porphyrin precursor excretion[153] suggest that once-daily treatment should be effective. Heme arginate has been reported to produce neither phlebitis nor an anticoagulant effect and is more stable than hematin.[154] Similar advantages have been described for hematin reconstituted with human albumin.[155] Diagnosis of AIP is more difficult during, and for several days after, heme therapy because of the capacity of this treatment to normalize porphyrin precursor excretion. A clinical response to heme therapy is dependent on the degree of neuronal damage and may not be observed for $\geq$48 hours. An investigational approach is to combine heme therapy with an inhibitor of heme breakdown, such as Sn-protoporphyrin, to prolong the efficacy of the administered heme.[156]

Manipulation of endogenous hormones by administration of analogues of gonadotropin-releasing hormone (GnRH) is clearly effective for women with frequent premenstrual attacks of porphyria.[131] Women who respond to GnRH analogue administration are unlikely to require this treatment for a major portion of their reproductive years and after several years may no longer require ovulatory suppression.[157,158] Estrogen/progestin combinations have been given safely to some women with AIP.[129] However, the risk of exacerbating the disease is greater than with a GnRH analogue.

and is unlikely to be harmful. Prompt treatment of bacterial infections, which commonly complicate cutaneous blisters, may help in preventing scarring and mutilation. Hospitalization for treatment of cellulitis, bacteremia, and other severe infections with systemic antibiotics is sometimes required. Bone marrow transplantation has been attempted[175] and, if successful engraftment is obtained, could be curative. In the future, gene transfer into bone marrow stem cells and autologous transplantation should provide effective therapy.

Porphyria Cutanea Tarda

Porphyria cutanea tarda (PCT) is due to reduced activity of URO-decarboxylase.[176] It is unique among the porphyrias because this cutaneous porphyria occurs in sporadic (type I) and familial (types II and III) forms, as well as forms induced by exposure to certain environmental chemicals. All types of PCT are characterized by a marked deficiency of URO-decarboxylase in the liver. In type I PCT, URO-decarboxylase activity is normal in erythrocytes and other nonhepatic cells. In type II PCT, the enzymatic activity is half-normal in the liver and in all nonhepatic tissues. Type III PCT, which may be a familial form, since family members are affected, is characterized by normal erythrocyte URO-decarboxylase activity and deficient activity only in the liver.[176] In addition, hepatic URO-decarboxylase deficiency and a biochemical pattern resembling PCT can be produced by exposure to a number of halogenated aromatic hydrocarbons. The most notable case of environmentally induced PCT was an outbreak in Turkey due to ingestion of wheat treated with the fungicide hexachlorobenzene. HEP is due to a homozygous deficiency of URO-decarboxylase with disease manifestations usually beginning in childhood. Type II PCT can be distinguished by the finding of low URO-decarboxylase activity in erythrocytes. Types I and III PCT and PCT due to toxic exposures are difficult to distinguish from each other unless adequate family studies can be carried out or there is clearly an outbreak of toxic porphyria in many unrelated individuals.

Biochemical and Molecular Aspects

In type I PCT, URO-decarboxylase is deficient only in liver. Although an unidentified genetic disposition cannot be excluded, the hepatic enzymatic deficiency appears to be acquired as follows. First, the amount of hepatic URO-decarboxylase protein, as measured immunochemically, is normal in this condition, suggesting either the presence of an inhibitor or that the enzyme has been inactivated. With treatment by phlebotomy, enzymatic activity gradually increases.[176] Second, no evidence has been found to demonstrate the presence of tissue-specific isoenzymes of URO-decarboxylase. Therefore, a mutation of the gene for this enzyme is unlikely to lead to a tissue-specific enzymatic deficiency. Third, mutations at the URO-decarboxylase locus have not been found in type I PCT.[57]

In type II PCT, URO-decarboxylase activity in nonhepatic tissues such as erythrocytes and cultured skin fibroblasts is approximately 50% of normal in clinically affected individuals and in family members with latent disease.[58] Erythrocyte immunoreactive enzyme is also reduced approximately 50% in familial PCT.[177] Thus, most cases of familial PCT are CRIM negative, suggesting that the mutant allele does not express detectable enzyme protein. URO-decarboxylase is not a rate-limiting enzyme for heme biosynthesis, and therefore, most type II PCT heterozygotes do not develop porphyria. Moreover, type I and II PCT are clinically very similar, and the same precipitating factors are involved in both types. These precipitating factors (iron, alcohol, estrogens, and hepatitis C) are generally different from those important in the acute porphyrias and do not

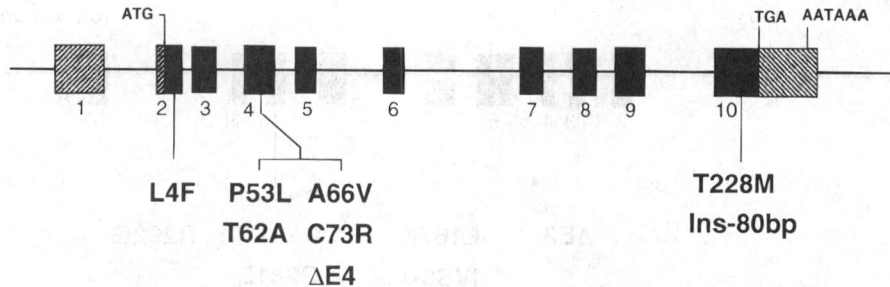

Fig. 39-3. Molecular lesions in the URO-synthase gene responsible for CEP. Hatched exons show 5' and 3' untranslated regions; Ins, insertion; see also Figure 30-2 legend.

act primarily by inducing hepatic ALA-synthase and heme synthesis. Therefore, the degree of enzymatic deficiency in the liver is presumed to be about half-normal when type II PCT is latent and considerably lower when the disease is active due to the same processes that inhibit or inactivate hepatic URO-decarboxylase in type I PCT.

Type III PCT is rare and resembles type I in that URO-decarboxylase activity is normal in extrahepatic tissues such as erythrocytes. It is presumed to be inherited because multiple family members are affected.[176,178] Because the only feature of type III PCT that is different from type I is a positive family history, these conditions can be difficult to differentiate. The genetic basis for this type of PCT is not yet understood. The same factors that reduce hepatic URO-decarboxylase to a significantly low level of activity in type I and II PCT are probably operative in type III.

HEP can be regarded as the homozygous form of type II PCT.[59] However, the mutations at the URO-decarboxylase locus in HEP often do not lead to complete loss of the enzyme activity and some are CRIM positive.[179,180] In 16 reported HEP cases URO-decarboxylase activity has been within the range of 3–28% of normal.[181]

Genetic Aspects

Considerable evidence shows that type I PCT is an acquired condition. The decreased hepatic URO-decarboxylase activity is not accompanied by a decrease in the concentration of the

enzyme protein.[182] Activity returns to normal following a prolonged remission. However, it is possible that a genetic defect, transmitted as an autosomal recessive trait, might be the underlying cause of some sporadic cases of PCT and that the additional presence of hepatic siderosis might be required for clinical expression.[183] Although recent studies did not reveal mutations in the URO-decarboxylase coding sequence or in the upstream promoter region in cases of type I PCT, mutations may occur in uncharacterized promoter regions or at other loci that may predispose to the development of this disorder.[55] Kinetic data reported by Mukerji and Pimstone[184] suggest that PCT may be associated with an intrinsically abnormal erythrocyte enzyme with altered chemical properties. Others have not found evidence for more than one form of the enzyme.[57]

The deficient activity of URO-decarboxylase in type II PCT is clearly inherited as an autosomal dominant trait. Molecular characterization of type II heterozygotes have revealed a 5' donor splice site mutation (IVS6^{+1}), and several missense mutations[185–187] (Fig. 39-4).

Type III PCT has been studied in four Spanish families, in which at least two relatives had clinically manifest PCT with decreased URO-decarboxylase activity in liver but normal levels in erythrocytes and other tissues. These observations certainly suggest that PCT associated with normal erythrocyte URO-decarboxylase activity has a genetic basis in some families.[176,187] To our knowledge, mutations of the URO-decarboxylase locus have not been demonstrated in type III PCT. It seems unlikely that a mutation at the URO-decarboxylase locus can result in the selectively decreased activity of the enzyme in the liver, since human URO-decarboxylase is encoded by a single gene and transcript.[3,10] The existence of only one mRNA is consistent with the observation that the erythroid and hepatic enzymes are physically and kinetically indistinguishable.[188] However, a mutation that alters URO-decarboxylase in such a manner as to make it selectively susceptible to inactivation in the liver could be present in these families.[189]

The specific molecular defect that caused HEP in two related patients from Tunisia has been determined (Fig. 39-4). A missense mutation in exon 8 at codon 860 of the URO-decarboxylase gene (G281Q) has been identified that alters the stability of the enzyme protein.[190] This mutation has also been found in two unrelated Spanish HEP patients, but not in two unrelated patients from Italy and Portugal, nor in 13 unrelated heterozygotes with familial PCT.[191]

Thus, of the three types of PCT, only type II has been shown to have mutations in the URO-decarboxylase gene. Clearly, the inherited mutations in themselves are not sufficient to cause porphyria, except perhaps in patients with HEP and severe homozygous deficiencies of URO-decarboxylase activity. Other factors are important in all types of PCT and these predispose to inactivation of URO-decarboxylase activity in the liver. In inbred mice the development of hepatic URO-decarboxylase deficiency after treatment with certain polyhalogenated aromatic hydrocarbons is influenced by levels of hepatic iron

---

HEMOLYSIS IN CONGENITAL ERYTHROPOIETIC PORPHYRIA

Hemolysis is a feature of CEP. The more severely affected homozygotes may be transfusion dependent. Anemia due to hemolysis can be severe but can be minimal or absent if compensation by the bone marrow is adequate. Splenomegaly is found in most cases. Affected individuals who are not transfusion dependent typically have a milder form of the disease.

Hemolysis in CEP is often accompanied by anisocytosis, poikilocytosis, polychromasia, basophilic stippling, reticulocytosis, increased nucleated red cells, absence of haptoglobin, increased unconjugated bilirubin, increased fecal urobilinogen, and increased plasma iron turnover. Hemolysis probably results from the accumulated uroporphyrin I in erythrocytes, and secondary splenomegaly develops in response to the increased uptake of abnormal erythrocytes from the circulation. Splenic enlargement may contribute to the anemia and also result in leukopenia and thrombocytopenia. The latter is sometimes associated with significant bleeding[171,172]; splenectomy may be beneficial in such cases.

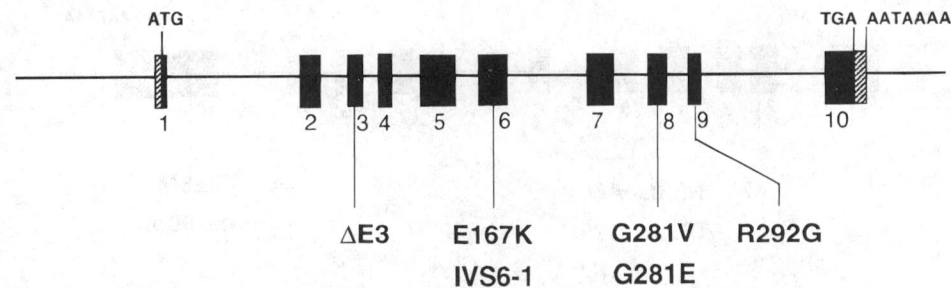

Fig. 39-4. Molecular lesions in the URO-decarboxylase gene responsible for PCT. Hatched exons show 5′ and 3′ untranslated regions; see also Figure 30-2 legend.

stores and by the inherited inducibility of certain forms of cytochrome P-450.[192] Thus, development of PCT probably involves both acquired and genetic factors. These are capable of increasing hepatic iron stores, modulating cytochrome P-450 induction and the production of reactive metabolites from exogenous or endogenous chemicals, leading to hepatic URO-decarboxylase inhibition.

Clinical Manifestations

Cutaneous photosensitivity is the major clinical feature of PCT. Neurologic manifestations are not observed. Skin lesions develop on sun-exposed areas such as the face, dorsa of the hands and feet, forearms, and legs. Fluid-filled vesicles and bullae are more common in the summer than in the winter. Sun-exposed skin becomes friable. Minor trauma may precede the formation of bullae or may cause denudation of the skin. Small white plaques, termed milia, are also common and may precede or follow vesicle formation. Bullae and denuded areas of skin tend to heal slowly. Lesions can become infected especially when severe and recurrent. Other cutaneous manifestations include hypertrichosis and hyperpigmentation, especially of the face, which can present in the absence of vesicles. Thickening, scarring, and calcification of affected areas of skin is sometimes striking and has been termed pseudoscleroderma because it can mimic the cutaneous changes of systemic sclerosis. The skin lesions in PCT are generally indistinguishable from those in VP and HCP. The lesions of CEP and HEP are also similar but more severe.

PCT is commonly associated with evidence of chronic liver disease and sometimes with cirrhosis. Patients with PCT are also at risk of the development of hepatocellular carcinoma; in several series, the incidence has been within the range of 4–47%.[193–195] These tumors appear as a complication of PCT and do not themselves contain or produce porphyrins in large amounts.[194] Their cause is unknown but could be related to long-standing liver damage, hemosiderosis, exposure to halogenated chemicals that are also carcinogenic, or to the effects of porphyrin deposition in the liver. Recent reports that, at least in some locations, PCT is commonly associated with chronic infection with hepatitis C virus[196–199] or human immunodeficiency syndrome infection,[200,201] or both[202] suggests that chronic viral infections can contribute to inactivation of hepatic URO-decarboxylase activity. Hepatitis C virus infection may sometimes explain chronic, progressive liver disease or the development of hepatocellular carcinoma in PCT patients.

HEP, the homozygous form of familial PCT,[59] is a rare condition that resembles CEP clinically. The disease presents in infancy or childhood with onset of blistering skin lesions, hypertrichosis, scarring, and red urine. HEP is genetically heterogeneous; unusually mild cases have been described.[179–181]

Laboratory Evaluation

In patients with PCT, porphyrins are increased in the liver, plasma, urine, and stool. Except for a slight increase in ALA in some patients, porphyrin precursor excretion is normal. Urinary porphyrins consist mostly of uroporphyrin and 7-carboxylate porphyrin, with lesser amounts of coproporphyrin and 5- and 6-carboxylate porphyrin.[209] The excess urinary uroporphyrin in PCT is predominantly isomer I; 7- and 6-carboxylate porphyrin are mostly isomer III; and 5-carboxylate porphyrin and coproporphyrin are approximately equal mixtures of isomers I and III. Plasma porphyrins also are increased in PCT[210]; the distribution pattern is similar to that in urine.

The major fecal porphyrins in PCT are often of the isocoproporphyrin series. Isocoproporphyrins also may be present in plasma and urine.[211] The finding of increased isocoproporphyrins is diagnostic for a deficiency of hepatic URO-decarboxylase. These unusual 4-carboxylate porphyrins are produced when hepatic URO-decarboxylase is deficient, because 5-carboxylate porphyrinogen III, which accumulates in PCT, can be metabolized by COPRO-oxidase to yield dehydroisocoproporphyrinogen. This porphyrinogen is excreted in bile. It undergoes autooxidation and side chain modification by bacterial enzymes in the intestine to give isocoproporphyrin and de-ethylisocoproporphyrin, the major representatives of the isocoproporphyrin

---

FACTORS THAT CONTRIBUTE TO PORPHYRIA CUTANEA TARDA

Patients with PCT often have a history of alcohol abuse. Other important contributing factors are liver damage (sometimes due to hepatitis C virus), excess iron, and intake of estrogens. While liver histopathology is almost always evident, it is usually not diagnostic of alcoholic liver disease. PCT can also be induced by exposure to various chemicals. An extensive outbreak of PCT occurred in eastern Turkey in 1955–1958 as a result of ingestion of wheat treated with the fungicide hexachlorobenzene.[203] Subsequently, hexachlorobenzene was shown to produce a porphyria similar to PCT and hepatic URO-decarboxylase deficiency in animals.[204] Cases of PCT in humans have also been reported after exposure to other chemicals, including di- and trichlorophenols and 2,3,7,8-tetrachlorodibenzo-*p*-dioxin (TCDD, dioxin).[205,206] PCT sometimes occurs in patients with end-stage renal disease.[207] PCT in this setting is often more severe and intractable than PCT occurring in the absence of advanced renal disease. Recombinant erythropoietin is likely to be an effective treatment and can support phlebotomy in such patients.[208]

series in feces of PCT patients.[209] Levels of porphyrin in the skin are increased. The highest concentrations occur in areas that have not been exposed to light, which suggests that light destroys porphyrins in the skin.[212] Increased liver porphyrins are composed mostly of uroporphyrin and 7-carboxylate porphyrin. The biochemical findings in HEP are similar to those in other forms of PCT. In addition, the erythrocyte protoporphyrin concentration is increased.

Therapy

The diagnosis of PCT should be firmly established before treatment is initiated, because VP and HCP can produce similar cutaneous lesions but are unresponsive to measures that are highly effective in PCT. Imaging studies are advisable to exclude complicating hepatocellular carcinoma and to serve as a baseline for follow-up. It is reasonable to screen for hepatitis C and human immunodeficiency virus infections which, as noted above, are prevalent in association with PCT in some parts of the world. Patients should abstain from alcohol, estrogens, iron supplements, or other exogenous agents that may exacerbate the disease.

Drugs such as barbiturates, phenytoin, and sulfonamides, which are harmful to patients with acute porphyrias, are seldom reported to contribute to the clinical expression of PCT, but should be avoided as a precaution. Improvement after the cessation of alcohol can be dramatic[213]; however, the results are generally unpredictable or slow.[214]

Phlebotomy can produce remissions in almost all patients and remains the standard therapy for PCT.[213] The aim is to gradually reduce excess hepatic iron, which contributes to activation of PCT. About 500 ml of blood can be removed at intervals of 1–2 weeks. Remission of photosensitivity due to PCT usually begins as plasma ferritin and porphyrin levels decrease. These levels are valuable guides to efficacy of phlebotomy therapy.[215,216] The intervals between phlebotomies can be lengthened as the ferritin nears the lower limit of normal. Hemoglobin or hematocrit levels should be followed closely to prevent the course of phlebotomies from leading to a symptomatic degree of anemia. After a remission is obtained, continued phlebotomies may not be needed, even if ferritin levels later return to normal. However, it is advisable to follow porphyrin levels and reinstitute phlebotomies if porphyrin levels begin to rise. Even cutaneous scarring and pseudoscleroderma can improve with phlebotomies.[214] Abnormal liver function tests may also improve.[217] Liver histologic abnormalities may not completely resolve.

Small doses of chloroquine or hydroxychloroquine are effective in producing remissions of PCT.[218] The drug complexes with the excess porphyrin and promotes its excretion. Especially at standard antimalarial doses, the excess porphyrins are removed rapidly from the liver and accumulate in plasma prior to urinary excretion. This can be associated with a transient increase in photosensitivity and abnormalities in liver function. Such side effects are minimal or absent with low doses (e.g., 125 mg of chloroquine phosphate twice weekly), which remove porphyrins from the liver gradually. Thus, a low-dose chloroquine regimen is a useful alternative when repeated phlebotomies are contraindicated.[219]

Hereditary Coproporphyria

HCP, a hepatic porphyria, results from the deficient activity of COPRO-oxidase.[64] It is inherited as an autosomal dominant trait whose clinical expression is influenced by ecogenic and metabolic factors. HCP has been reported mostly in Britain, Europe, and North America and is less frequent than AIP. Two biochemically distinguishable forms of HCP have been reported in homozygous affected individuals. One form, harderoporphyria, is characterized by about 10% residual COPRO-oxidase activity and the accumulation of primarily harderoporphyrin, whereas the other form results from a more marked enzymatic deficiency (residual level approximately 2% of normal) and the accumulation primarily of coproporphyrin III.

Biochemical and Molecular Aspects

Activity of the mitochondrial enzyme COPRO-oxidase is about 50% of normal in cultured fibroblasts, circulating lymphocytes, and leukocytes of HCP heterozygotes.[64,220] Assays for COPRO-oxidase are not readily available. No evidence that the enzyme can be assayed in erythrocytes, which do not contain mitochondria, has been published, although such an assay is offered commercially. For screening of family members, measurement of fecal porphyrins is advisable; however, children with the enzymatic deficiency may not excrete excess porphyrins.[65]

Genetic Aspects

The enzyme defect is inherited as an autosomal dominant trait. Homozygous patients with a much more profound enzyme deficiency have been described.[66,221] Human COPRO-oxidase has not been purified to homogeneity for characterization of its physical and genetic properties. The chromosomal locus of the gene encoding COPRO-oxidase has however, been assigned to human chromosome 9 by somatic cell genetic techniques.[222]

In one case of homozygous HCP the residual COPRO-oxidase activity (approximately 2% of normal) had a normal K_m value.[221] By contrast, three cases in a family with harderoporphyria provided evidence for a different COPRO-oxidase defect. The mutant enzyme exhibited increased thermostability and reduced affinity for both harderoporphyrinogen and coproporphyrinogen III, consistent with a structurally altered enzyme.[66] A single active site on the normal enzyme is believed to carry out both decarboxylations, and most of the harderoporphyrinogen formed from coproporphyrinogen III is not released before being further decarboxylated to protoporphyrinogen IX. The reduced affinity of the mutant enzyme for both substrates in this family may cause harderoporphyrinogen to dissociate from the enzyme more readily than normal and to be excreted in feces as harderoporphyrin. The heterozygous parents of these patients had intermediate harderoporphyrin excretion. Thus, at least two different types of mutations producing different abnormalities of COPRO-oxidase can lead to HCP and its more severe homozygous forms.

CLINICAL MANIFESTATIONS OF HEREDITARY COPROPORPHYRIA

HCP is clinically very similar to AIP, although generally somewhat milder. Photosensitivity similar to that in PCT sometimes occurs. HCP can be exacerbated by many of the same factors that cause attacks in AIP, including barbiturates and other drugs, and endogenous or exogenous steroid hormones.[222] The disease is latent before puberty. Symptoms are more common in women than in men. Neurovisceral symptoms are virtually identical to those of AIP but are less severe. Only a few patients have been reported to expire from respiratory paralysis.

Hepatitis and other superimposed liver diseases in an HCP patient can increase porphyrin retention and photosensitivity.[64] Several cases of homozygous HCP, with cutaneous lesions beginning in early childhood, have been documented.[221,222]

Laboratory Evaluation

Coproporphyrin III is markedly increased in the urine and feces of symptomatic heterozygotes with HCP as well as in some asymptomatic (or latent) heterozygotes. Increased urinary excretion of ALA, PBG, and uroporphyrin is observed during acute attacks. With resolution of symptoms, ALA and PBG levels revert to normal more readily than in AIP. Porphyrin excretion patterns in homozygous HCP resemble those observed in heterozygotes but reflect a more profound enzymatic deficiency. Harderoporphyria is characterized by a marked increase in fecal excretion of harderoporphyrin as well as coproporphyrin.

Therapy

Acute attacks of HCP are treated in the same manner as AIP attacks. Cholestyramine may be of some value for the photosensitivity that occurs with liver dysfunction.[223] Phlebotomy and chloroquine are not effective.

Variegate Porphyria

VP, inherited as an autosomal dominant trait, is an hepatic porphyria. It results from deficient activity of PROTO-oxidase. The disorder is described as variegate because it can present with neurologic manifestations or photosensitivity, or both.

Biochemical and Molecular Aspects

PROTO-oxidase activity is approximately half-normal in cultured skin fibroblasts and lymphocytes from VP patients.[69] However, the assay of PROTO-oxidase activity in cultured cells is difficult to perform and is not widely available for diagnosis and family screening. Measurement of fecal porphyrins in relatives of known VP patients is recommended to detect latent cases; levels may not be increased in all heterozygotes, especially children and elderly subjects.[224] Since it is likely that a significant number of adults with inherited PROTO-oxidase deficiency excrete normal amounts of porphyrins in urine and feces, more of these individuals would be identified if assays for this enzyme were more readily available for family screening.[225] The isolation of the cDNA encoding this enzyme would permit the development of molecular diagnostics.

Protoporphyrinogen IX, the substrate for PROTO-oxidase, accumulates in patients with VP and undergoes auto-oxidation to protoporphyrin IX, which is characteristically increased in VP. A close functional association between PROTO-oxidase in the inner mitochondrial membrane and COPRO-oxidase in the intermembrane space may relate to the excess excretion of both protoporphyrin and coproporphyrin in this disease.[67] HMB-synthase activity has been reported to be somewhat decreased in some VP patients when compared to controls, although it usually remains within the normal range.[215]

Genetic Aspects

PROTO-oxidase deficiency, which is transmitted as an autosomal dominant trait, is the underlying genetic defect in VP. Although the cDNA encoding this enzyme has not been cloned, pedigree analysis of several large South African families has established the synteny of PROTO-oxidase with α_1-antitrypsin; the gene has been provisionally assigned to chromosome 14 on this basis.[72] In most countries, VP is less common than AIP, with the notable exception of South Africa, where 3 of every 1,000 white persons have inherited VP.[226] Most cases can be traced to a couple who emigrated from Holland and who were married in South Africa in 1688.

Several cases of homozygous VP with marked reductions in PROTO-oxidase have been documented.[224,227] The heterozy-

gous parents of the patients had approximately half-normal enzymatic activity, as expected. Photosensitivity, and in some cases neurologic symptoms and developmental disturbances, including growth retardation, were noted in infancy or childhood. All patients had increased erythrocyte zinc protoporphyrin levels, a characteristic finding in all homozygous porphyrias so far described.

In a large family from Britain, some individuals had acute porphyric attacks and evidence of deficiencies of both PROTO-oxidase and HMB-synthase.[228] The disease in this family has been termed Chester porphyria. Photosensitivity was not observed. It is unclear whether the porphyria in this lineage should be considered a variant of VP or of AIP.

Laboratory Evaluation

Fecal protoporphyrin and coproporphyrin and urinary coproporphyrin are markedly increased in clinically expressed VP. Urinary and fecal coproporphyrin is mostly type III. Urinary ALA, PBG, and uroporphyrin are increased during acute attacks but may be normal or only slightly increased during remission. Plasma porphyrins, consisting in part of a dicarboxylate porphyrin tightly bound to plasma proteins, are increased, especially when photosensitivity is present in VP.[229] The neutral fluorescence spectrum of plasma porphyrins in VP is characteristic and can distinguish this disease from other types of porphyria; the emission maximum occurs at 626 nm in VP, 619 nm in PCT, CEP, HCP, and AIP, and 634 nm in EPP.[231]

Therapy

Glucose, hematin, and other measures employed in AIP are usually effective for the treatment of acute attacks of VP. Other therapies such as propranolol, D-penicillamine, hemodialysis, alkalization of urine, and β-carotene are of little or no benefit. Repeated venesections and chloroquine are highly effective in PCT but not in VP.[232] Measures to protect the skin from sunlight with appropriate clothing, including gloves and a broad-brimmed hat, as well as with opaque sunscreen preparations, are useful. Exposure to short wavelength ultraviolet light, which does not excite porphyrins, may provide some protection by increasing skin pigmentation.[233]

CLINICAL MANIFESTATIONS OF VARIEGATE PORPHYRIA

Clinical expression of VP before puberty is rare. The neurovisceral manifestations of VP are indistinguishable from those of AIP or HCP. Skin manifestations are very similar to those of PCT and HCP, are usually of longer duration, and occur apart from the neurovisceral symptoms. Photosensitivity is more common than in HCP. Drugs, steroids, and nutritional factors that are detrimental in AIP also can provoke exacerbations of VP.[229] In a survey of 300 patients in South Africa,[230] the most common clinical features include abdominal pain, tachycardia, vomiting, constipation, hypertension, neuropathy, back pain, confusion, bulbar paralysis, psychiatric complaints, fever, urinary frequency, and dysuria. Skin manifestations were present in 85% of the patients studied. Photosensitivity may be less commonly associated with VP in more northern countries, where sunlight is less intense.[225]

Erythropoietic Protoporphyria

EPP, which is due to the partially deficient activity of ferrochelatase, is inherited as an autosomal dominant trait. Excess protoporphyrin is found in erythroid cells, plasma, bile, and feces of heterozygotes in whom EPP is clinically expressed. EPP also has been termed *erythrohepatic protoporphyria* and *protoporphyria*. EPP is the most common form of erythropoietic porphyria and after PCT is perhaps the second most common porphyria. Well over 300 cases having been reported.[234] Although the disease seems most common in whites, it does occur in persons of other races, including blacks.[235]

Biochemical and Molecular Aspects

Ferrochelatase is probably partially deficient in all tissues, including bone marrow, marrow reticulocytes,[81] liver, cultured fibroblasts,[80,236] and blood or leukocytes from patients with EPP.[81,237,238] The deficient enzymatic activity becomes rate-limiting for protoporphyrin conversion to heme, primarily in bone marrow reticulocytes. Because normal erythrocyte protoporphyrin content is less than the optimal concentration for heme formation, substrate concentration as well as enzymatic activity may influence the rate of heme formation by ferrochelatase in vivo. Substrate concentration might increase sufficiently to increase the rate of heme formation even with partially deficient ferrochelatase activity.[81] Ferrochelatase activity in tissue lysates of EPP patients has been reported to be only 10–25% of normal.[80,238,239] Kinetic data have suggested an inhibitor or a reduced K_m for a porphyrin substrate.[240] Altered heat stability of the enzymatic activity in EPP bone marrow preparations and the inability of EPP fibroblasts to incorporate zinc into protoporphyrin have been interpreted as indications of a structurally altered enzyme.[241] Immunochemical studies have shown no decrease in ferrochelatase protein in both human and bovine protoporphyria, suggesting point mutations in the ferrochelatase gene.[239]

The recent availability of the full-length cDNA encoding ferrochelatase[8] has facilitated the identification of the molecular lesions causing EPP. Molecular studies of a patient with homozygous EPP revealed two missense mutations in the ferrochelatase gene, each inherited from a parent.[242] In heterozygous patients, two missense mutations and a splicing mutation in the ferrochelatase gene have been identified,[243,244] demonstrating the molecular heterogeneity of the defects causing EPP.

Genetic Aspects

EPP is inherited as an autosomal dominant trait[245] with considerable variation in phenotypic expression. Some obligate heterozygotes by lineage and/or enzyme assay have little or no increase in erythrocyte protoporphyrin. The cause of the considerable variability in protoporphyrin levels and clinical severity among individuals who are heterozygotes for this enzyme deficiency is not clear. A case of homozygous EPP (with a lymphocyte ferrochelatase activity of 6% of normal) has been documented by demonstration of the specific molecular lesions.[242] However, there are heterozygous patients with EPP that have ferrochelatase activities considerably <50% of normal, suggesting a dominant-negative effect. The suggestion that ferrochelatase might function as a dimer[77] is one possible explanation for both autosomal dominant inheritance and markedly decreased enzymatic activity in EPP heterozygotes. In the future, the identification of the specific mutations and their effect on ferrochelatase activity will provide further insight into the biochemical pathology of EPP. EPP with autosomal recessive inheritance has been described in cattle and in mice.[239,247]

Etiology and Pathogenesis

Porphyrins absorb light maximally at wavelengths near 400 nm (the Soret band). They enter an excited energy state that is manifested by fluorescence and, in the presence of molecular oxygen, by the formation of singlet oxygen and other oxygen species that can produce tissue damage.[248] As might be expected, the skin is maximally sensitive to 400-nm light in EPP. Light-induced tissue damage may be accompanied by lipid peroxidation,[249] oxidation of amino acids, and cross-linking of proteins in cell membranes.[250] Histologic changes, predominantly in the upper dermis, may include amorphous material deposited around blood vessels and may resemble the findings in PCT. Immediate light-induced damage to capillary endothelial cells in the upper dermis has been described in EPP.[251] Histamine, kinins, photoactivation of the complement system, and release of chemotactic factors have been proposed as mediators of skin damage.[252,253]

Circulating erythrocytes are an insufficient source for the excess protoporphyrin produced and excreted in EPP. Reticulocytes in the bone marrow presumably are the primary source. During erythroid differentiation, protoporphyrin accumulation begins in this disease just before loss of the cell nuclei. As a result, bone marrow fluorescence is almost entirely in reticulocytes rather than nucleated erythroid cells.[81,254,255] Although the liver may be an important source of protoporphyrin in EPP,[256–258] quantitation of its contribution relative to that of the erythron has not been possible.[257]

Erythrocyte protoporphyrin in EPP is free and not complexed with zinc. It declines much more rapidly with red cell age than it does in conditions in which erythrocyte zinc protoporphyrin is increased.[254,255] Excess erythrocyte zinc protoporphyrin in lead poisoning and iron deficiency is bound to hemoglobin and persists in the red cell as long as it circulates. Free protoporphyrin in EPP binds less readily to hemoglobin than does zinc protoporphyrin and diffuses more rapidly into the plasma. Moreover, ultraviolet light may cause free protoporphyrin to photodamage its hemoglobin binding site and thus be released from the red cell even without disruption of the cell membrane. Protoporphyrin may then diffuse into the plasma, where it is bound to albumin.[259,260] This light-mediated mechanism for the release of free protoporphyrin from hemoglobin in EPP may be important because binding of excess free protoporphyrin to hemoglobin is usually greater than binding to plasma proteins. Most of the protoporphyrin in erythrocytes is found in a small percentage of cells. The rate of protoporphyrin leakage from these cells is proportional to their protoporphyrin content.[261] The capacity of the liver to take up and excrete protoporphyrin into bile may also influence the flux of protoporphyrin from erythroid cells to the plasma.[235]

Although there is little evidence for impaired erythropoiesis or abnormal iron metabolism,[81,234,256,262] depletion of iron stores may be relatively common, even in the absence of iron deficiency anemia in EPP.[262] Iron accumulation in erythroblasts and ring sideroblasts occur in some EPP patients.[263] Hemolysis is uncommon or very mild in uncomplicated cases. However, mild anemia with hypochromia and microcytosis[81,234,264] or mild anemia with reticulocytosis is sometimes noted.[265] Patients with EPP seem predisposed to develop gallstones that are fluorescent and composed at least in part of protoporphyrin.

Liver function is usually normal in EPP, sometimes even when protoporphyrin in the liver appears to be considerably increased. A few EPP patients develop chronic liver disease, which can progress rapidly and lead to death from liver failure.[266] EPP sometimes presents with advanced liver disease as the major clinical manifestation.[267] Upper abdominal pain may suggest biliary obstruction. Unnecessary laparotomy to exclude this possibility can be detrimental.[266]

Concurrent factors impairing liver function or the metabolism of protoporphyrin to heme, such as viral hepatitis, alcohol, iron deficiency, fasting, or oral contraceptive steroids, have played a modulating role in some patients.[268,269] An enterohepatic circulation of protoporphyrin may favor its retention in the liver, especially when liver function is impaired. Liver damage probably results at least in part from protoporphyrin accumulation itself, as this porphyrin is insoluble, tends to form crystalline structures in liver cells, can impair mitochondrial functions in liver cells, and can decrease hepatic bile formation and flow.[266,270,271] In one patient hepatic complications and hemolysis were both considerably improved by splenectomy,[272] which suggests that the bone marrow had been the major source of excess protoporphyrin.

Laboratory Evaluation

Protoporphyrin concentrations are increased in the bone marrow, circulating erythrocytes, plasma, bile, and feces of EPP patients. However, an increased erythrocyte protoporphyrin concentration is not a specific indication of EPP. Erythrocyte protoporphyrin concentrations are increased in conditions such as lead poisoning, iron deficiency, anemia of chronic disease[274] and various hemolytic disorders.[275] The increased protoporphyrin in conditions other than EPP is in the form of zinc protoporphyrin. However, many assays for erythrocyte protoporphyrin or "free erythrocyte protoporphyrin" measure both the zinc and free protoporphyrins. As already noted, erythrocyte zinc protoporphyrin is increased in all homozygous forms of porphyria and may be somewhat increased in AIP. Plasma porphyrins are seldom significantly increased in conditions other than EPP and other porphyrias with cutaneous manifestations. Other heme pathway intermediates do not accumulate in EPP. Thus, urinary porphyrin and porphyrin precursor concentrations are normal.

Unfortunately, it is difficult to predict the potentially life-threatening hepatic complications of EPP by laboratory tests.

However, these complications are commonly preceded by increased photosensitivity and by increasing erythrocyte and plasma protoporphyrin levels, abnormal liver function tests, and marked deposition of protoporphyrin in liver cells and bile canaliculi. An increasing ratio of erythrocyte to fecal protoporphyrin and an increasing ratio of biliary protoporphyrin to biliary bile acids also may suggest impending hepatic complications.[266,276,277]

A partial deficiency of ferrochelatase activity has been found in bone marrow, reticulocytes, liver, cultured fibroblasts, and leukocytes from patients with EPP.[80,81] A deficiency of this enzyme also was demonstrated by increased protoporphyrin accumulation after ALA loading of cultured skin fibroblasts and mitogen-stimulated lymphocytes.[236] These assays are not yet generally available for diagnostic purposes.

Therapy

β-Carotene was developed primarily as a drug for treating EPP. Tolerance to sunlight is improved, sometimes considerably, in most patients. This has been substantiated in large series of patients.[278,279] Doses of 120–180 mg/day in adults are usually required to maintain serum carotene levels within the recommended range of 600–800 μg/dl. Improvement is noted 1–3 months after initiation of treatment. When pure preparations of β-carotene have been used, no side effects other than a mild and dose-related skin discoloration due to carotenemia have been noted.[278]

The mechanism of action of β-carotene is not fully established but may involve quenching of singlet oxygen or free radicals. The drug appears less effective in other forms of porphyria associated with photosensitivity, such as CEP and PCT. Dihydroxyacetone and lawsone (napthoquinone), which darken the skin when applied topically, may thereby partially block exposure of the dermis to light and be of some benefit in EPP.[234,280] Cholestyramine, which may interrupt the enterohepatic circulation of protoporphyrin and promote its fecal excretion, has been reported to reduce liver protoporphyrin and improve cutaneous symptoms in some EPP patients.[266] Treatment of hepatic complications is difficult and must be individualized. However, cholestyramine and other porphyrin absorbents such as activated charcoal should be considered, especially in patients with complicating hepatic dysfunction. Oral bile acid supplementation has shown benefit in some animal models but has been the subject of only one report in EPP patients.[281] Splenectomy may be beneficial when EPP is complicated by hemolysis and splenomegaly.

Caloric restriction, and drugs or hormone preparations that impair hepatic excretory function should be avoided.[282] Iron deficiency should be corrected if present.[283] Resolution of hepatic complications may occur spontaneously, especially if another reversible cause of liver dysfunction, such as viral hepatitis or alcohol, is contributing.[268,269] Other therapeutic options include transfusions and intravenous hematin to suppress erythroid and hepatic protoporphyrin production, as well as liver transplantation.[276] Unexplained increased photosensitivity and neuropathy have been observed in some EPP patients with liver disease after blood transfusions[284] or liver transplantation.[285]

Dual Porphyria

Patients with porphyria and deficiencies of more than one heme biosynthetic enzyme are classified as having dual porphyria. For example, kindreds with individuals having both VP and familial PCT have been described.[233,286] Patients with deficiencies of both HMB-synthase and URO-decarboxylase may develop symptoms of AIP or PCT or both.[287] An infant with severe porphyria was found to have inherited COPRO-oxidase deficiency from one parent and URO-synthase deficiency from both parents.[288]

Sideroblastic Anemias

Sideroblastic anemias are a heterogeneous group of hypoproliferative anemias. They share in common the morphologic feature of ringed sideroblasts in the bone marrow,[33,289-295] which are pathologic erythroid precursors that contain iron-laden mitochondria. These mitochondria encircle the nucleus and form a Prussian blue positive-staining ring, accounting for the ringed appearance. It is commonly thought that sideroblastic anemias share in common one or more defects in the biosynthesis of heme.

Classification, Etiology, and Nomenclature

Sideroblastic anemias are classified as inherited or acquired. The inherited sideroblastic anemias are usually transmitted as X-linked traits; however, rare forms of autosomal recessive disease have been documented. Acquired sideroblastic anemias are designated as primary or secondary. Primary sideroblastic anemias are frequently myelodysplastic disorders,[292,293] considered in more detail in Chapters 40 and 147. In patients with these disorders, the ringed sideroblasts are merely a phenotypic manifestation of an underlying stem cell disorder, which affects multiple hematopoietic lineages. Secondary acquired sideroblastic anemias arise by the toxic effect of various substances on the bone marrow, notably alcohol, the antituberculosis drug isoniazid, and drugs such as cycloserine, pyrazinamide, isonicotinic acid hydrazide, or chloramphenicol. They may also be due to infection or chronic inflammation.[289,295-307]

Pathophysiology and Clinical Features

The major mechanism responsible for anemia in patients with sideroblastic anemia is ineffective erythropoiesis, which leads to secondary iron overload.[308-312] In this respect, sideroblastic anemias behave similarly to other inherited and acquired defects of hemoglobin synthesis (e.g., iron deficiency and thalassemia). Thus, one frequently encounters normal or hyperplastic erythroid activity in the bone marrow in the face of a low reticulocyte count. The hypochromia and microcytosis associated with hemoglobin-deficient red cells is not always encountered in a straightforward way, however. In primary acquired sideroblastic anemia, the morphology is frequently normocytic or even macrocytic. Presumably, this reflects selective intramedullary destruction of the clone of sideroblastic cells, with persistence of the remaining clones of more nearly hemoglobinized cells, including megablastoid sublines in many cases.

In inherited and secondary forms of sideroblastic anemia, one frequently encounters a hypochromic and microcytic cell population. The anemia is frequently dimorphic; that is, hypochromic microcytic cells coexist with normally hemoglobinized erythrocytes. This is especially true in female carriers of the X-linked form, in whom the phenomenon presumably reflects Lyonization of the defective X chromosome. The mechanism underlying secondary acquired sideroblastic anemia is presumed to be direct toxicity to mitochondria (e.g., alcohol) or inhibition of one or more steps of heme biosynthesis (e.g., isoniazid). The role of pyridoxine (vitamin B_6) metabolism has been explored by several investigators attempting to decipher the mechanisms responsible for sideroblastic anemia.[307,313,314] The active cofactor of pyridoxine, pyridoxal-5-phosphate, is essential for the first step in heme biosynthesis mediated by

ALA synthetase (see earlier discussion in this chapter). Numerous attempts to document deficiency or diminished bioavailability of this cofactor in various forms of sideroblastic anemia, especially that mediated by alcohol intoxication, have been unsuccessful.[305,315-317] However, well documented examples of clinical response to pharmacologic doses of pyridoxine have been reported.[303-305,315] Moreover, co-administration of pyridoxine with isoniazid greatly reduces the incidence of sideroblastic anemia induced by this drug.

Recently, mutations in the gene encoding erythroid ALA-synthase were shown to cause pyridoxine-responsive sideroblastic anemia.[35,36] The enzyme defects in the unrelated patients studied were responsive to pyridoxine and required increased amounts of pyridoxine for maximal activation. Additional mutations in this gene are likely to be identified, providing insight into the pyridoxine-responsive and unresponsive forms of sideroblastic anemia.

Diagnosis and Therapy

Sideroblastic anemias are usually identified by examination of Prussian blue-stained bone marrow aspirate specimens obtained during the evaluation of anemia or pancytopenia. Ring sideroblasts are not specific and are sometimes found in other disorders, including EPP.[250] X-linked sideroblastic anemia frequently presents during the second decade of life with symptoms due to a falling hematocrit. A dimorphic peripheral blood smear is often encountered as evidence of a hypochromic microcytic subpopulation in maternal and female sibling blood. An appropriate clinical setting and family history are other diagnostic criteria.

Management of the primary acquired form is usually directed toward maintenance of the hematocrit with transfusions, if needed; removal of the offending drug or toxin in secondary acquired forms is usually curative. Inherited forms may be sufficiently severe to require transfusion, but, paradoxically, some patients actually benefit from slow, carefully controlled *phlebotomy* until an iron-unloaded state is achieved. When performed judiciously, phlebotomy causes improved efficiency of erythropoiesis via iron unloading of the marrow; this effect seems to be sufficient to offset the loss of red cells, and the hematocrit remains stable, or may even increase by 3–5 points.[318-320] Alternatively, deferoxamine may be used to remove excessive iron. Pyridoxine in doses of 50–200 mg/day is usually given to these patients, but only a few respond.

ACKNOWLEDGMENT

This work was supported in part by grants from the National Institutes of Health, including research grant 5 R01 DK26824, grant 5 P30 HD28822 for the Mount Sinai Child Health Research Center, grants 5 M01 RR00071 and 2 M01 RR00073 for the Mount Sinai and University of Texas Medical Branch General Clinical Research Centers from the National Center for Research Resources, as well as grant FD-R-00710-01 from the U.S. Food and Drug Administration Office of Orphan Product Development.

REFERENCES

1. Raich N, Romeo PH, Dubart A et al: Molecular cloning and complete primary sequence of human erythrocyte porphobilinogen deaminase. Nucleic Acids Res 14:5955, 1986
2. Grandchamp B, de Verneuil H, Beaumont C et al: Tissue-specific expression of porphobilinogen deaminase: two isozymes from a single gene. Eur J Biochem 162:105, 1987
3. Romeo PH, Raich N, Dubart A: Molecular cloning and nucleotide sequence of a complete human uroporphyrinogen decarboxylase cDNA. J Biol Chem 261:9825, 1986
4. Wetmur JG, Bishop DF, Cantelmo S et al: Human δ-aminolevulinate dehydratase. Nucleotide sequence of a full-length cDNA clone. Proc Natl Acad Sci USA 83:7703, 1986

5. Bawden MJ, Borthwick IA, Healy HM et al: Sequence of human 5-aminolevulinate synthase cDNA. Nucleic Acids Res 15:8563, 1987

6. Bishop DF: Two different genes encode δ-aminolevulinate synthase in humans: nucleotide sequences of cDNAs for the housekeeping and erythroid genes. Nucleic Acids Res 18:7187, 1990

7. Tsai SF, Bishop DF, Desnick RJ: Human uroporphyrinogen III synthase: molecular cloning, nucleotide sequence and expression of a full-length cDNA. Proc Natl Acad Sci USA 85:7049, 1988

8. Nakahashi YN, Taketani ST, Okuda MO et al: Molecular cloning and sequence analysis of cDNA encoding human ferrochelatase. Biochem Biophys Res Commun 173:745, 1990

9. Martasek P, Camadro JM, Delfau-Larue M-H et al: Molecular cloning, sequencing and functional expression of a cDNA encoding human coproporphyrinogen oxidase. Proc Natl Acad Sci USA 91:3024, 1994

10. Romana M, Dubart A, Beaupain D et al: Structure of the gene for human uroporphyrinogen decarboxylase. Nucleic Acids Res 15:7345, 1987

11. Taketani S, Inazawa J, Nakahashi Y et al: Structure of the human ferrochelatase gene: exon/intron gene organization and location of the gene to chromosome 18. J Biochem 205:217, 1992

12. Conboy JG, Cox TC, Bottomley SS et al: Human erythroid 5-aminolevulinate synthase. Gene structure and species-specific differences in alternate RNA splicing. J Biol Chem 267:18753, 1992

13. Yoo HW, Warner CA, Chen C-H, Desnick RJ: Hydroxymethylbilane synthase: complete genomic sequence and amplifiable polymorphisms in the human gene. Genomics 15:21, 1993

14. Kaya AH, Plewinska M, Wong DM et al: Human δ-aminolevulinate dehydratase: genomic structure and alternative splicing of the erythroid and housekeeping transcripts. Genomics 19:242, 1994

15. Wang AL, Arrendondo-Vega FX, Giampietro PF et al: Regional gene assignment of human porphobilinogen deaminase and esterase A4 to chromosome 11q23-11qter. Proc Natl Acad Sci USA 78:5734, 1981

16. Namba H, Narahara K, Tsuji K et al: Assignment of human porphobilinogen deaminase to 11q24.1→q24.2 by in situ hybridization and gene dosage studies. Cyto Cell Genet 57:105, 1991

17. Grandchamp B, Weil D, Nordmann Y et al: Assignment of the human coproporphyrinogen oxidase gene to chromosome 9. Hum Genet 64:180, 1983

18. Romeo PH, Raich N, Dubart A et al: Molecular cloning and tissue-specific expression analysis of human porphobilinogen deaminase and uroporphyrinogen decarboxylase. p. 25. In Nordmann Y (ed): Porphyrins and Porphyrias. Colloque INSERM. John Libbey Eurotext, Paris, 1986

19. Potluri VR, Astrin KH, Wetmur JG et al: Chromosomal localization of the structure gene for human ALA-dehydratase to 9q34 by in situ hybridization. Hum Genet 76:236, 1987

20. Sutherland GR, Baker E, Callen DF et al: 5-Aminolevulinate synthase is at 3p21 and thus not the primary defect in X-linked sideroblastic anemia. Am J Hum Genet 43:331, 1988

21. Bishop DF, Henderson AS, Astrin KH: Human δ-aminolevulinate synthase. Assignment of the housekeeping gene to 3p21 and the erythroid gene to the X chromosome. Genomics 7:207, 1990

22. Astrin KH, Warner CA, Yoo H-W et al: Regional assignment of the human uroporphyrinogen III synthase (UROS) gene to chromosome 10q25.2→q26.3. Hum Genet 87:18, 1991

23. Whitcombe DM, Carter NP, Albertson DG et al: Assignment of the human ferrochelatase gene (FECH) and a locus for protoporphyria to chromosome 18q22. Genomics 11:1152, 1991

24. Granick S: The induction in vitro of the synthesis of δ-aminolevulinic acid synthetase in chemical porphyria. A response to certain drugs, sex hormones, and foreign chemicals. J Biol Chem 241:1359, 1966

25. Anderson KE, Freddara U, Kappas A: Induction of hepatic cytochrome P-450 by natural steroids: relationship to the induction of δ-aminolevulinate synthase and porphyrin accumulation in the avian embryo. Arch Biochem Biophys 217:597, 1982

26. Yomogida K, Yamamoto M, Yamagami T et al: Structure and expression of the gene encoding rat nonspecific form δ-aminolevulinate synthase. J Biochem Tokyo 113:364, 1993

27. Conboy JG, Cox TC, Bottomley SS et al: Human erythroid 5-aminolevulinate synthase: gene structure and species-specific differences in alternative RNA splicing. J Biol Chem 267:18753, 1992

28. Ferreira GC, Dailey HA: Expression of mammalian 5-aminolevulinate synthase in Escherichia coli. Overproduction, purification and characterization. J Biol Chem 268:584, 1993

29. Aoki Y, Muranaka S, Nakabayashi K et al: δ-Aminolevulinic acid synthetase in erythroblasts of patients with pyridoxine-responsive anemia. Hypercatabolism caused by the increased susceptibility to the controlling protease. J Clin Invest 64:1196, 1979

30. Bottomley SS, Healy HM, Brandenburg MA, May BK: δ-Aminolevulinate synthase in sideroblastic anemias: messenger RNA and enzyme activity levels in bone marrow cells. Am J Hematol 41:76, 1992

31. Bishop RC, Bethel FH: Hereditary hypochromic anemia with transfusion hemosiderosis treated with pyridoxine. N Engl J Med 261:486, 1959

32. Lee GR, MacDiarmid WD, Cartwright GE et al: Hereditary, X-linked, sideroachrestic anemia. The isolation of two erythrocyte populations differing in Xg(A) blood type and porphyrin content. Blood 32:59, 1968

33. Prasad AS, Tranchida L, Konno ET et al: Hereditary sideroblastic anemia and glucose-6-phosphate dehydrogenase deficiency in a Negro family. J Clin Invest 47:1415, 1968

34. Dewald DW, Pierre RV, Phyliky RL: Three patients with structurally abnormal X chromosomes, each with Xq13 breakpoints and a history of idiopathic acquired sideroblastic anemia. Blood 59:100, 1985

35. Cotter PD, Baumann M, Bishop DF: Enzymatic defect in X-linked sideroblastic anemia: molecular evidence for erythroid δ-aminolevulinate synthase deficiency. Proc Natl Acad Sci USA 89:4028, 1992

36. Cotter PD, Bishop DF: Congenital sideroblastic anemia: correlation of the microcytic, pyridoxine-responsive phenotype with coding region mutations in the erythroid δ-aminolevulinate synthase gene. Am J Hum Genet 53:145A, 1993

37. Anderson PM, Desnick RJ: Purification and properties of δ-aminolevulinic acid dehydratase from human erythrocytes. J Biol Chem 254:6924, 1979

38. Jaffe EK, Salowe SP, Chen NT et al: Porphobilinogen synthase modification with methylmethanethiosulfonate. A protocol for the investigation of metalloproteins. J Biol Chem 259:5032, 1984

39. Morgan JM, Burch HB: Comparative tests for the diagnosis of lead poisoning. Arch Intern Med 130:335, 1972

40. Battistuzzi G, Petrucci R, Silvagni L: δ-Aminolevulinate dehydrase: a new genetic polymorphism in man. Ann Hum Genet 45:223, 1981

41. Astrin KH, Bishop DF, Kaul B et al: Human δ-aminolevulinate dehydrogenase isozymes and lead toxicity. Ann NY Acad Sci 514:23, 1987

42. Benkmann HG, Bogdanski P, Goedde WH: Polymorphism of delta aminolevulinic acid dehydratase in various populations. Hum Hered 33:62, 1983

43. Doss M, Von Tiepermann R, Schneider J: Acute hepatic porphyria syndrome with porphobilinogen synthase defect. Int J Biochem 12:823, 1980

44. Thunell S, Holmberg L, Lundgren J: Aminolevulinate dehydrase porphyria in infancy. A clinical and biochemical study. J Clin Chem Clin Biochem 25:5, 1987

45. Plewinska M, Thunell S, Holmberg L et al: δ-Aminolevulinate dehydratase deficient porphyria: identification of the molecular lesions in a severely affected homozygote. Am J Hum Genet 49:167, 1991

46. Ishida N, Fujita H, Fukuda Y et al: Cloning and expression of the defective genes from a patient with δ-aminolevulinate dehydratase porphyria. J Clin Invest 89:1431, 1992

47. Strand LJ, Felsher BF, Redeker AG et al: Decreased red cell protoporphyrinogen I synthetase activity in intermittent acute porphyria. J Clin Invest 51:2530, 1972

48. Anderson PM, Desnick RJ: Purification and properties of uroporphyrinogen I synthase from human erythrocytes. Identification of stable enzyme-substrate intermediates. J Biol Chem 255:1993, 1980

49. Jordan PM: The biosynthesis of 5-aminolevulinic acid and its transformation into coproporphyrinogen in animals and bacteria. p. 55. In Dailey HA (ed): Biosynthesis of Heme and Chlorophylls. McGraw-Hill, New York, 1990

50. Raich N, Mignotte V, Dubart A et al: Regulated expression of the overlapping ubiquitous and erythroid transcription units of the human porphobilinogen deaminase (PBG-D) gene introduced into non-erythroid and erythroid cells. J Biol Chem 264:10186, 1989

51. Mignotte V, Elequet JF, Raich N et al: Cis- and trans-acting elements involved in the regulation of the erythroid promoter of the human porphobilinogen deaminase gene. Proc Natl Acad Sci USA 86:6548, 1989

52. Tsai SF, Bishop DF, Desnick RJ: Purification and properties of uroporphyrinogen III synthase from human erythrocytes. J Biol Chem 262:1268, 1987

53. Romeo G, Levin EY: Uroporphyrinogen III cosynthetase in human congenital erythropoietic porphyria. Proc Natl Acad Sci USA 63:856, 1969

54. Tsai SF, Bishop DF, Desnick RJ: Coupled-enzyme and direct assays for uroporphyrinogen III synthase activity in human heterozygotes and homozygotes with congenital erythropoietic porphyria. Anal Biochem 166:120, 1987

55. de Verneuil H, Sassa S, Kappas A: Purification and properties of uroporphyrinogen decarboxylase from human erythrocytes. J Biol Chem 258:2454, 1983

56. Mukerji SK, Pimstone NR: Evidence for two uroporphyrinogen decarboxylase isoenzymes in human erythrocytes. Biochem Biophys Res Commun 146:1196, 1987

57. Garey JR, Franklin KF, Brown DA et al: Analysis of uroporphyrinogen decarboxylase complementary DNAs in sporadic porphyria cutanea tarda. Gastroenterology 105:165, 1993

58. de Verneuil H, Aitken G, Nordmann Y: Familial and sporadic porphyria cutanea tarda. Two different diseases. Hum Genet 44:145, 1978

59. Elder GH, Smith SG, Herrero C et al: Hepatoerythropoietic porphyria: a new uroporphyrinogen decarboxylase defect or homozygous porphyria cutanea tarda? Lancet 1:916, 1981

60. Elder GH, Evans JO: Evidence that the coproporphyrinogen oxidase activity of rat liver is situated in the intermembrane space of mitochondria. Biochem J 172:345, 1978

61. Grandchamp B, Phung N, Nordmann Y: The mitochondrial localization of coproporphyrinogen III oxidase. Biochem J 176:97, 1978

62. Yoshinaga T, Sano S: Coproporphyrinogen oxidase. II. Reaction mechanism and role of tyrosine residues on the activity. J Biol Chem 255:4727, 1980

63. Kohno H, Furukawa T, Yoshinage T et al: Coproporphyrinogen oxidase: purification, molecular cloning and induction of mRNA during erythroid differentiation. J Biol Chem 268:21359, 1993

64. Elder GH, Evans JO, Thomas N et al: The primary enzyme defect in hereditary coproporphyria. Lancet 2:1217, 1976

65. Grandchamp B, Nordmann Y: Decreased lymphocyte coproporphyrinogen III oxidase activity in hereditary coproporphyria. Biochem Biophys Res Commun 74:1089, 1977

66. Nordmann Y, Grandchamp B, de Verneuil H et al: Harderoporphyria: a variant hereditary coproporphyria. J Clin Invest 72:1139, 1983

67. Deybach JC, da Silva V, Grandchamp B et al: The mitochondrial location of protoporphyrinogen oxidase. Eur J Biochem 149:431, 1985

68. Dailey HA, Karr SW: Purification and properties of murine protoporphyrinogen oxidase. Biochemistry 26:2697, 1987

69. Ferriera GC, Dailey HA: Mouse protoporphyrinogen oxidase: kinetic parameters and demonstration of inhibition by bilirubin. Biochem J 250:597, 1988

70. McColl KEL, Thompson GG, Moore MR et al: Abnormal haem biosynthesis in Gilbert's syndrome. Gut 26:1985

71. Brenner DA, Bloomer JR: The enzymatic defect in variegate porphyria: studies with human cultured skin fibroblasts. N Engl J Med 302:765, 1980

72. Bissbort S, Hitzeroth HW, du Wertzel DP: Linkage between the variegate porphyria (VP) and the alpha-1-antitrypsin (PI) genes on human chromosome 14. Hum Genet 79:289, 1988

73. Jones MS, Jones OTG: The structural organization of heme synthesis in rat liver mitochondria. Biochem J 113:507, 1969

74. McKay R, Druyan R, Getz GS et al: Intramitochondrial localization of δ-aminolevulate synthetase and ferrochelatase in rat liver. Biochem J 114:455, 1969

75. Dailey HA, Fleming JE: The role of arginyl residues in porphyrin binding to ferrochelatase. J Biol Chem 261:7902, 1986

76. Bloomer JR, Hill HD, Morton KO: The enzyme defect in bovine protoporphyria. J Biol Chem 262:7902, 1987

77. Straka JG, Bloomer JR, Kempner ES: The functional size of ferrochelatase determined *in situ* by radiation inactivation. J Biol Chem 266:24637, 1991

78. Taketani S, Nakahashi Y, Osumi T, Tokunaga R: Molecular cloning, sequencing, and expression of mouse ferrochelatase. J Biol Chem 265:19377, 1990

79. Brenner DA, Frasier F: Cloning of murine ferrochelatase. Proc Natl Acad Sci USA 88:849, 1991

80. Bonkowsky HL, Bloomer JR, Ebert PS: Heme synthetase deficiency in human protoporphyria: demonstration of the defect in liver and cultured skin fibroblasts from patients with protoporphyria. J Clin Invest 56:1139, 1975

81. Bottomley SS, Tanaka M, Everett MA: Diminished erythroid ferrochelatase activity in protoporphyria. J Lab Clin Med 86:126, 1975

82. Taketani S, Tokunaga R: Rat liver ferrochelatase. Purification, properties and stimulation by fatty acids. J Biol Chem 256:12748, 1981

83. Hayashi N, Yoda B, Kikuchi G: Mechanism of allylisopropylacetamide-induced increase of δ-aminolevulinate synthetase in liver mitochondria. IV. Accumulation of the enzyme in the soluble fraction of rat liver. Arch Biochem Biophys 131:83, 1969

84. Whiting, MJ: Synthesis of δ-aminolaevulinate synthase by isolated liver polyribosomes. Biochem J 158:391, 1976

85. Ades IZ, Stevens TM, Drew PD: Biogenesis of embryonic chick liver δ-aminolevulinate synthase: regulation of the level of mRNA by hemin. Arch Biochem Biophys 253:297, 1987

86. Whetsell WO Jr, Kappas A: Protective effect of exogenous heme against lead toxicity in organotypic cultures of mouse dorsal root ganglia (DRG): electron microscopic observations, abstracted. J Neuropathol Exp Neurol 40:334, 1981

87. Fujita H, Yamamoto M, Yamagami T et al: Sequential activation of genes for heme pathway enzymes during erythroid differentiation of mouse Friend virus-transformed erythroleukemia cells. Biochim Biophys Acta 1090:311, 1991

88. Lathrop JT, Timko MP: Regulation by heme of mitochondrial protein transport through a conserved amino acid motif. Science 259:522, 1993

89. Beru N, Goldwasser E: The regulation of heme biosynthesis during erythropoietin-induced erythroid differentiation. J Biol Chem 260:9251, 1985

90. Neuwirt J, Ponka P: Regulation of Haemoglobin Synthesis. Martinus Nijhoff Medical Division, The Hague, 1977

91. Kaplowitz N, Javitt N, Kappas A: Coproporphyrin I and III excretion in bile and urine. J Clin Invest 51:2895, 1972

92. Mauzerall D, Granick S: The occurrence and determination of delta-aminolevulinic acid and porphobilinogen in urine. J Biol Chem 219:435, 1956

93. Lim CK, Peters TJ: Urine and faecal porphyric profiles by reversed-phase high performance liquid chromatography in the porphyrias. Clin Chim Acta 139:55, 1984

94. Elder GH, Smith SG, Jane Smyth S: Laboratory investigation of the porphyrias. Ann Clin Biochem 27:395, 1990

95. Bishop DF, Desnick RJ: Assays of the heme biosynthetic enzymes. Enzyme 28:91, 1982

96. de Verneuil H, Doss M, Brusco N et al: Hereditary hepatic porphyria with delta aminolevulinate dehydrase deficiency: immunologic characterization of the non-catalytic enzyme. Hum Genet 69:174, 1985

97. Fujita H, Sassa S, Lundgren J et al: Enzymatic defect in a child with hereditary hepatic porphyria due to homozygous δ-aminolevulinic acid dehydratase deficiency: immunochemical studies. Pediatrics 80:880, 1987

98. Hassoun A, Verstraeten L, Mercelis R et al: Biochemical diagnosis of an hereditary aminolevulinate dehydratase deficiency in a 63-year-old man. J Clin Chem Clin Biochem 27:781, 1989

99. Thunell S, Henrichson A, Floderus Y et al: Liver transplantation in a boy with acute porphyria due to aminolaevulinate dehydratase deficiency. Eur J Clin Chem Clin Biochem 30:599, 1992

100. Sassa S, Kappas A: Hereditary tyrosinemia and the heme biosynthetic pathway. J Clin Invest 71:625, 1983

101. Anderson KE, Fischbein A, Kestenbaum D et al: Plumbism from airborne lead in a firing range. An unusual exposure to a toxic heavy metal. Am J Med 63:306, 1977

102. Lindblad B, Lindstedt S, Steen G: On the enzymatic defects in hereditary tyrosinemia. Proc Natl Acad Sci USA 74:4641, 1977

103. Fujita H, Koizumi A, Furusawa T, Ikeda M: Decreased erythrocyte δ-aminolevulinate dehydratase activity after styrene exposure. Biochem Pharmacol 36:711, 1987

104. Akagi R, Prchal JT, Eberhart CE, Sassa S: An acquired acute hepatic porphyria: a novel type of δ-aminolevulinate dehydratase inhibition. Clin Chim Acta 212:79, 1992

105. Anderson PM, Reddy RM, Anderson KE et al: Characterization of the PBG-deaminase deficiency in acute intermittent porphyria. I. Immunologic evidence for heterogeneity of the genetic defect. J Clin Invest 68:1, 1981

106. Mustajoki P, Tenhunen R: Variant of acute intermittent porphyria with normal erythrocyte uroporphyrinogen-I-synthase activity. Eur J Clin Invest 15:281, 1985

107. Grandchamp B, Picat C, Mignotte V et al: Tissue-specific splicing mutation in acute intermittent porphyria. Proc Natl Acad Sci USA 86:661, 1989

108. Grandchamp B, Picat C, Kauppinen R et al: Molecular analysis of acute intermittent porphyria in a Finnish family with normal erythrocyte porphobilinogen deaminase. Eur J Clin Invest 19:415, 1989

109. Desnick RJ, Ostasiewicz LT, Tishler PA et al: Acute intermittent porphyria: characterization of a novel mutation in the structural gene for porphobilinogen deaminase. J Clin Invest 76:865, 1985

110. Grandchamp B, Picat C. de Rooij F et al: A point mutation G→A in exon 12 of the porphobilinogen deaminase gene results in exon skipping and is responsible for acute intermittent porphyria. Nucleic Acids Res 17:6637, 1989

111. Wetterberg L: A Neurophyschiatric and Genetical Investigation of Acute Intermittent Porphyria. Svenska Bokfolaget. Scandinavian University Books, Norstedts, Sweden, 1967, p. 175

112. Beukeveld GJJ, Wolthers BG, Nordmann Y et al: A retrospective study of a patient with homozygous form of acute intermittent porphyria. J Inher Metab Dis 13:673, 1990

113. Chretien S, Dubart A, Beaupain D et al: Alternative transcription and splicing of the human porphobilinogen deaminase gene results either in tissue-specific or in housekeeping expression. Proc Natl Acad Sci USA 85:6, 1988

114. Llewellyn DH, Kalsheker NA, Elder GH et al: A *Msp*I polymorphism for the human porphobilinogen gene. Nucleic Acids Res 15:1342, 1987

115. Lee JS, Anvret M, Lindsten J et al: DNA polymorphisms within the porphobilinogen deaminase gene in two Swedish families with acute intermittent porphyria. Hum Genet 79:379, 1988

116. Schreiber WE, Jamani A, Ritchie B: Detection of a T/C polymorphism in the porphobilinogen deaminase gene by polymerase chain reaction amplification of specific alleles. Clin Chem 38:2153, 1992

117. Sassa S, Solish G, Levese RD et al: Studies in porphyria. IV. Expression of the gene defect of acute hepatic intermittent porphyria in cultured human skin fibroblasts and amniotic cells: prenatal diagnosis of the porphyric trait. J Exp Med 142:722, 1975

118. Bonkowsky HL, Schady W: Neurologic manifestations of acute porphyria. Semin Liver Dis 2:108, 1982

119. Yeung Laiwah AC, Moore MR, Goldberg A: Pathogenesis of acute porphyria. Q J Med 241:377, 1987

120. Becker DM, Kramer S: The neurological manifestations of porphyria: a review. Medicine 56:411, 1977

121. Bonkowsky HL, Tschudy DP, Collins A et al: Repression of the overproduction of porphyrin precursors in acute intermittent porphyria by intravenous infusions of hematin. Proc Natl Acad Sci USA 8:2725, 1971

122. Litman DA, Correia MA: Elevated brain tryptophan and enhanced 5-hydroxytryptamine turnover in acute hepatic heme deficiency: clinical implications. J Pharmacol Exp Ther 232:337, 1985

123. Kappas A, Sassa A, Anderson KE: The Porphyrias. p. 1301. In Stanbury JB, Wyngaarden JB, Frederickson DS et al (eds): The Metabolic Basis of Inherited Disease. 5th Ed. McGraw-Hill, New York, 1983

124. Moore MR, McColl KEL, Rimington C, Goldberg A: Disorders of Porphyrin Metabolism. Plenum, New York, 1987, p. 374

125. Cavanagh JB, Mellick RS: On the nature of the peripheral nerve lesions associated with acute intermittent porphyria. J Neurol Neurosurg Psychiatry 28:320, 1965

126. Sweeney VP, Pathak MA, Asbury AK: Acute intermittent porphyria: increased ALA-synthetase activity during an acute attack. Brain 93:369, 1970

127. Ridley A: Porphyric neuropathy. p. 942. In Dyck PJ, Thomas PK, Lambert EH (eds): Peripheral Neuropathy. Vol. 2. WB Saunders, Philadelphia, 1975

128. Tishler PV, Woodward B, O'Connor J et al: High prevalence of intermittent acute porphyria in a psychiatric patient population. Am J Psychiatry 142:1430, 1985

129. Kauppinen R, Mustajoki P: Prognosis of acute porphyria: occurrence of acute attacks, precipitating factors, and associated diseases. Medicine 71:1, 1992

130. Ostrowski J, Kostrzewska E, Michalak T et al: Abnormalities in liver function and morphology and impaired aminopyrine metabolism in hereditary hepatic porphyrias. Gastroenterology 85:1131, 1983

131. Anderson KE, Spitz IM, Sassa S et al: Intranasal luteinizing hormone-releasing hormone agonist for prevention of cyclical attacks of acute intermittent porphyria. p. 225. In Nordmann Y (ed): Porphyrins and Porphyrias. Colloque INSERM, John Libbey Eurotext, Paris, 1986

132. Milo R, Neuman M, Klein C et al: Acute intermittent porphyria in pregnancy. Obstet Gynecol 73:450, 1989

133. Marks GS: Exposure to toxic agents: the heme biosynthetic pathway and hemoproteins as indicator. CRC Crit Rev Toxicol 15:151, 1985

134. Peters PG, Sharma ML, Hardwicke DM, Piper WN: Sulfonamide inhibition of rat hepatic uroporphyrinogen I synthetase activity and the biosynthesis of heme. Arch Biochem Biophys 201:88, 1980

135. Mustajoki P, Heinonen J: General anesthesia in "inducible" porphyrias. Anesthesiology 53:15, 1980

136. Blekkenhorst GH, Harrison GG, Cook ES: Screening of certain anaesthetic agents for their ability to elicit acute porphyric phases in susceptible patients. Br J Anaesth 52:759, 1980

137. Lip GYH, McColl KEL, Goldberg A, Moore MR: Smoking and recurrent attacks of acute intermittent porphyria. Br Med J 302:507, 1991

138. Tschudy DP, Lamon JM: Porphyrin metabolism and the porphyrias. p. 939. In Bondy PK, Rosenberg LE (eds): Duncan's Diseases of Metabolism. 8th Ed. WB Saunders, Philadelphia, 1980

139. Pierach CA, Weimer MK, Cardinal RA et al: Red blood cell porphobilinogen deaminase in the evaluation of acute intermittent porphyria. JAMA 7:60, 1987

140. Lamon JM, Frykholm BC, Tschudy DP: Family evaluations in acute intermittent porphyria using red blood cell uroporphyinogen-1-synthase. J Med Genet 16:134, 1979

141. McColl KEL, Morre MR, Thompson GG, Goldberg A: Screening for latent acute intermittent porphyria: the value of measuring both leukocyte δ-aminolevulinate acid synthase and erythrocyte uroporphyrinogen-I-synthase activities. J Med Genet 19:271, 1982

142. Pierach CA, Weimer MK, Cardinal RA et al: Red blood cell porphobilinogen deaminase in the evaluation of acute intermittent porphyria. JAMA 257:60, 1987

143. Delfau MH, Picat C, de Rooij FWM et al: Two different point G to A mutations in exon 10 of the porphobilinogen deaminase gene are responsible for acute intermittent porphyria. J Clin Invest 86:1511, 1990

144. Scobie GA, Llewellyn DH, Urquhart AJ et al: Acute intermittent porphyria caused by a C→T mutation that produces a stop codon in the porphobilinogen deaminase gene. Hum Genet 85:631, 1990

145. Delfau MH, Picat C, de Rooij F et al: Molecular heterogeneity of acute intermittent porphyria: identification of four additional mutations resulting in the CRIM-negative subtype of the disease. Am J Hum Genet 49:421, 1991

146. Lee J-S, Anvret M: Identification of the most common mutation within the porphobilinogen deaminase gene in Swedish patients with acute intermittent porphyria. Proc Natl Acad Sci USA 88:10912, 1991

147. Gu X-F, de Rooij F, Voortman G et al: High frequency of mutations in exon 10 of the porphobilinogen deaminase gene in patients with a CRIM-positive subtype of acute intermittent porphyria. Am J Hum Genet 51:660, 1992

148. Mgone CS, Lanyon WG, Moore MR, Connor JM: Detection of seven point mutations in the porphobilinogen deaminase gene in patients with acute intermittent porphyria, by direct sequencing of in vitro amplified cDNA. Hum Genet 90:12, 1992

149. Chen C-H, Astrin KH, Lee G et al: Acute intermittent porphyria: identification and expression of exonic mutations in the hydroxymethylbilane synthase gene. J Clin Invest (in press)

150. Yeung Laiwah AC, McColl KEL: Management of attacks of acute porphyria. Drugs 34:604, 1987

151. Lamon JM, Frykholm BC, Hess RA et al: Hematin therapy for acute porphyria. Medicine 58:252, 1979

152. Bissell DM: Treatment of acute hepatic porphyria with hematin. J Hepatol 6:1, 1988

153. Petryka ZJ, Dhar GJ, Bossenmaier I: Hematin clearance in porphyria. p. 259. In Doss M (ed): Porphyrins in Human Disease. S Karger, Basel, 1976

154. Mustajoki P, Tenhunen R, Pierach C, Volin L: Heme in the treatment of porphyrias and hematological disorders. Semin Hematol 26:1, 1989

155. Bonkovsky HL, Healey BS, Lourie AN, Gerron GG: Intravenous heme-albumin in acute intermittent porphyria: evidence for repletion of hepatic hemoproteins and regulatory heme pools. Am J Gastroenterol 86:1050, 1991

156. Dover SB, Graham A, Fitzsimons E et al: Tin protoporphyrin prolongs the biochemical remission produced by heme arginate in acute hepatic porphyria. Gastroenterology 105:500, 1993

157. Anderson KE: LHRH analogues for hormonal manipulation in acute intermittent porphyria. Semin Hematol 26:10, 1989

158. Anderson KE, Spitz IM, Bardin CW, Kappas A: A GnRH analogue prevents cyclical attacks of porphyria. Arch Intern Med 150:1469, 1990

159. Tsai S-F, Bishop DF, Desnick RJ: Coupled-enzyme and direct assays for uroporphyrinogen III synthase. Enzymatic diagnosis of homozygotes and heterozygotes with congenital erythropoietic porphyria. Anal Biochem 166:120, 1987

160. Warner CA, Yoo H-W, Tsai SF et al: Congenital erythropoietic porphyria: characterization of the genomic structure and identification of mutations in the uroporphyrinogen III synthase gene. Am J Hum Genet, suppl. 47:A83, 1990

161. Deybach J-C, de Verneuil H, Boulechfar S et al: Point mutations in the uroporphyrinogen III synthase gene in congenital erythropoietic porphyria. Blood 75:1763, 1990

162. Warner CA, Yoo H-W, Roberts AG, Desnick RJ: Congenital erythropoietic porphyria: identification and expression of exonic mutations in the uroporphyrinogen III synthase gene. J Clin Invest 89:693, 1992

163. Boulechfar S, Da Silva V, Deybach J-C et al: Heterogeneity of mutations in the uroporphyrinogen III synthase gene in congenital erythropoietic porphyria. Hum Genet 88:320, 1992

164. Yoo H-W, Warner CA, Xu W, Desnick RJ: Identification of a novel splicing defect and a missense mutation in the uroporphyrinogen III synthase gene causing congenital erythropoietic porphyria. Pediatr Res 31:137A, 1992

165. Xu W, Warner CA, Desnick RJ: Congenital erythropoietic porphyria: identification and expression of new mutations in the uroporphyrinogen III synthase gene. Am J Hum Genet 53:156, 1993

166. Deybach JC, de Verneuil H, Phung N et al: Congenital erythropoietic porphyria (Gunther's disease): enzymatic studies on two cases of late onset. J Lab Clin Med 97:551, 1981

167. Kaiser IH: Brown amniotic fluid in congenital erythropoietic porphyria. Obstet Gynecol 56:383, 1980

168. Deybach JC, Grandchamp B, Grelier M et al: Prenatal exclusion of congenital erythropoietic porphyria (Gunther's disease) in a fetus at risk. Hum Genet 53:217, 1980

169. Warner CA, Poh-Fitzpatrick MB, Zaider EF et al: Congenital erythropoietic porphyria—a mild variant with low uroporphyrin-I levels due to a missense mutation (A66V) encoding residual uroporphyrinogen-III synthase activity. Arch Dermatol 128:1243, 1992

170. Piomelli S, Poh-Fitzpatrick MB, Seaman C et al: Complete suppression of the symptoms of congenital erythropoietic porphyria by long-term treatment with high-level transfusions. N Engl J Med 314:1029, 1986

171. Pain RW, Welch FW, Woodruffe AJ et al: Erythropoietic uroporphyria of Gunther first presenting at 58 years with positive family studies. Br Med J 3:621, 1975

172. Weston MJ, Nicholson DC, Lim CK et al: Congenital erythropoietic uroporphyria (Gunther's disease) presenting in a middle aged man. Int J Biochem 9: 921, 1978

173. Tishler PV, Winston SH: Rapid improvement in the chemical pathology of congenital erythropoietic porphyria with treatment with superactivated charcoal. Methods Find Exp Clin Pharmacol 12:645, 1990

174. Mathews-Roth MM: Beta-carotene in congenital porphyria. Arch Dermatol 115:641, 1979

175. Kauffman L, Evans D, Stevens R, Weinkove C: Bone-marrow transplantation for congenital erythropoietic porphyria. Lancet 337:1510, 1991

176. Elder GH: Human uroporphyrinogen decarboxylase defects. p. 857. In Orfanos CE (ed): Dermatology in Five Continents. Springer-Verlag, Berlin, 1988

177. Elder GH, Sheppard DM, Tovey JA et al: Immunoreactive uroporphyrinogen decarboxylase in porphyria cutanea tarda. Lancet 1:1301, 1983

178. Held JL, Sassa S, Kappas A, Harber LC: Erythrocyte uroporphyrinogen decarboxylase activity in porphyria cutanea tarda: a study of 40 consecutive patients. J Invest Dermatol 93:332, 1989

179. Fujita H, Sassa S, Toback AC et al: Immunochemical study of uroporphyrinogen decarboxylase in a patient with mild hepatoerythropoietic porphyria. J Clin Invest 79:1533, 1987

180. de Verneuil H, Beaumont C, Deybach JC et al: Enzymatic and immunological studies of uroporphyrinogen decarboxylase in familial porphyria cutanea tarda and hepatoerythropoietic porphyria. Am J Hum Genet 36:613, 1984

181. Toback AC, Sassa S, Poh-Fitzpatrick MB et al: Hepatoerythropoietic porphyria: clinical, biochemical, and enzymatic studies in a three-generation family lineage. N Engl J Med 316:645, 1987

182. Elder GH, Urquhart AJ, de Salamanca RE et al: Immunoreactive uroporphyrinogen decarboxylase in the liver in porphyria cutanea tarda. Lancet 1:229, 1985

183. Kushner JP, Edwards CQ, Dadone MM et al: Heterozygosity for HLA-linked hemochromatosis as a likely cause of the hepatic siderosis associated with sporadic porphyria cutanea tarda. Gastroenterology 88:1232, 1985

184. Mukerji SK, Pimstone NR: Reduced substrate affinity for human erythrocyte uroporphyrinogen decarboxylase constitutes the inherent biochemical defect in porphyria cutanea tarda. Biochem Biophys Res Commun 127:517, 1985

185. Garey JR, Hansen JL, Lyle M: A point mutation in the coding region of uroporphyrinogen decarboxylase associated with familial porphyria cutanea tarda. Blood 73:892, 1989

186. Garey JR, Harrison LM, Franklin KF et al: Uroporphyrinogen decarboxylase: a splice site mutation causes the deletion of exon 6 in multiple families with porphyria cutanea tarda. J Clin Invest 86:1416, 1990

187. Roberts AG, Elder GH, Newcombe RG et al: Heterogeneity of familial porphyria cutanea tarda. J Med Genet 25:669, 1988

188. Elder GH, Urquhart AJ: Human uroporphyrinogen decarboxylase. Do tissue specific isoenzymes exist? Biochem Soc Trans 12:661, 1984

189. Kushner JP: The enzymatic defect in porphyria cutanea tarda. N Engl J Med 306:799, 1982

190. de Verneuil H, Grandchamp B, Beaumont C et al: Uroporphyrinogen decarboxylase structural mutant (Gly^{281}→Glu) in a case of porphyria. Science 234:732, 1986

191. de Verneuil H, Hansen J, Picat C et al: Prevalence of the 281 (gly→glu) mutation in hepatoerythropoietic porphyria and porphyria cutanea tarda. Hum Genet 78:101, 1986

192. Smith A, Francis J: Synergism of iron and hexachlorobenzene inhibits hepatic uroporphyrinogen decarboxylase in inbred mice. Biochem J 214:909, 1983

193. Kordac V: The frequency of occurrence of hepatocellular carcinoma in patients with porphyria cutanea tarda in long-term follow-up. Neoplasia 19: 135, 1982

194. Cortes JM, Oliva H, Paradinas FJ et al: The pathology of the liver in porphyria cutanea tarda. Histopathology 4:471, 1980

195. Salata H, Cortes JM, de Salamanca RE et al: Porphyria cutanea tarda and hepatocellular carcinoma. J Hepatol 1:477, 1985

196. Fargion S, Piperno A, Cappellini MD et al: Hepatitis-C virus and porphyria cutanea tarda—evidence of a strong association. Hepatology 16:1322, 1992

197. Herrero C, Vicente A, Bruguera M et al: Is hepatitis-C virus infection a trigger of porphyria cutanea tarda? Lancet 341:788, 1993

198. Lacour JP, Bodokh I, Castanet J et al: Porphyria cutanea tarda and antibodies to hepatitis-C virus. Br J Dermatol 128:121, 1993

199. DeCastro M, Sanchez J, Herrera JF et al: Hepatitis-C virus antibodies and liver disease in patients with porphyria cutanea tarda. Hepatology 17:551, 1993

200. Wissel PS, Sordillo P, Anderson KE et al: Porphyria cutanea tarda associated with the acquired immune deficiency syndrome. Am J Hematology 25:107, 1987

201. Cohen PR: Porphyria cutanea tarda in human immunodeficiency virus-seropositive men: case report and literature review. J Acq Immun Defic Syndrome 4:1112, 1991

202. Gafa S, Zannini A, Gabrielli C: Porphyria cutanea tarda and HIV infection—effect of zidovudine treatment on a patient. Infection 20:373, 1992

203. Schmid R: Cutaneous porphyria in Turkey. N Engl J Med 263:397, 1960

204. Taljaard JJF, Shanley BC, Deppe WM et al: Porphyrin metabolism in experimental hepatic siderosis in the rat. II. Combined effect of iron overload and hexachlorobenzene. Br J Haematol 23:513, 1972

205. Lynch RE, Lee GR, Kushner JP: Porphyria cutanea tarda associated with disinfectant misuse. Arch Intern Med 135:549, 1975

206. Doss M, Sauer H, Von Tiepermann R et al: Development of chronic hepatic porphyria (porphyria cutanea tarda) with inherited uroporphyrinogen decarboxylase deficiency under exposure to dioxin. Int J Biochem 16:369, 1984

207. Praga M, Enriquez de Salamanca R, Andres A et al: Treatment of hemodialysis-related porphyria cutanea tarda with deferoxamine. N Engl J Med 316: 547, 1987

208. Anderson KE, Goeger DE, Carson RW et al: Treatment of hemodialysis-associated porphyria cutanea tarda with erythropoietin. N Engl J Med 322:315, 1990

209. Elder GH: Porphyrin metabolism in porphyria cutanea tarda. Semin Hematol 14:227, 1977

210. Moore MR, Thompson GG, Allen BR et al: Plasma porphyrin concentrations in porphyria cutanea tarda, short communication. Clin Sci 45:711, 1973

211. Day RS, Eales L, Pimstone NR: Familial symptomatic porphyria in South Africa. S Afr Med J 56:909, 1979

212. Malina L, Miller VL, Magnus IA: Skin porphyrin assay in porphyria. Clin Chim Acta 83:55, 1978

213. Ramsay CA, Magnus IA, Turnbull A et al: The treatment of porphyria cutanea tarda by venesection. Q J Med 43:169, 1974

214. Topi GC, Amantea A, Griso D: Recovery from porphyria cutanea tarda with no specific therapy other than avoidance of hepatic toxins. Br J Dermatol 3:75, 1984

215. Rocchi E, Gibertini P, Cassanelli M et al: Serum ferritin in the assessment of liver iron overload and iron removal therapy in porphyria cutaneda tarda. J Lab Clin Med 107:36, 1986

216. Ratnaike S, Blake D, Campbell D et al: Plasma ferritin levels as a guide to the treatment of porphyria cutanea tarda by venesection. Australas J Dermatol 29:3, 1988

217. Adjarov D, Ivanov E: Clinical value of serum γ-glutamyl transferase estimation in porphyria cutanea tarda. Br J Dermatol 102:541, 1980

218. Tsega E, Besrat A, Damtew B et al: Chloroquine in the treatment of porphyria cutanea tarda. Trans R Soc Trop Med Hyg 75:401, 1981

219. Ashton RE, Hawk JLM, Magnus IA: Low-dose oral chloroquine in the treatment of porphyria cutanea tarda. Br J Dermatol 3:609, 1984

220. Nordmann Y, Grandchamp B: Hereditary coproporphyria: demonstration of a genetic defect in coproporphyrinogen metabolism. Monog Hum Genet 10:217, 1978

221. Grandchamp B, Phung N, Nordmann Y: Homozygous case of hereditary coproporphyria. Lancet 2:1348, 1977

222. Brodie MJ, Thompson GG, Moore MR et al: Hereditary coproporphyria. Demonstration of the abnormalities in haem biosynthesis in peripheral blood. Q J Med 46:229, 1977

223. Eschbach JW, Egrie JC, Downing MR et al: Correction of the anemia of end-stage renal disease with recombinant human erythropoietin. N Engl J Med 316:73, 1987

224. Mustajoki P, Tenhunen R, Niemi KM et al: Homozygous variegate porphyria. Clin Genet 32:300, 1987

225. Muhlbauer JE, Pathak MA, Tishler PV et al: Variegate porphyria in New England. JAMA 247:3095, 1982

226. Dean G: The Porphyrias: A Study of Inheritance and Environment. 2nd Ed. Pitman Medical, London, 1971

227. Murphy GM, Hawk JLM, Magnus IA et al: Homozygous variegate porphyria: two similar cases in unrelated families. J R Soc Med 79:361, 1986

228. McColl KEL, Thompson GG, Moore MR et al: Chester porphyria: biochemical studies of a new form of acute porphyria. Lancet 2:796, 1985

229. Perlroth MG, Tschudy DP, Ratner A et al: The effect of diet in variegate porphyria. Metabolism 71:10, 1968

230. Eales L, Day RS, Blekkenhorst GH: The clinical and biochemical features of variegate porphyria: an analysis of 300 cases studied at Groote Schuur Hospital, Cape Town. Int J Biochem 12:837, 1980

231. Poh-Fitzpatrick MB: A plasma porphyrin fluorescence marker for variegate porphyria. Arch Dermatol 116:543, 1980

232. Cramers M, Jepsen LV: Porphyria variegata: failure of chloroquin treatment. Acta Derm Venered (Stockh) 60:89, 1980

233. Day RS: Variegate porphyria. Semin Dermatol 5:138, 1986

234. De Leo VA, Poh-Fitzpatrick M, Mathews-Roth M et al: Erythropoietic protoporphyria. 10 years experience. Am J Med 60:8, 1976

235. Poh-Fitzpatrick MB: Erythropoietic porphyrias: current mechanistic, diagnostic, and therapeutic considerations. Semin Hematol 14:211, 1977

236. Sassa S, Zalar GL, Poh-Fitzpatrick MB et al: Studies in porphyria X: functional evidence for a 50% deficiency of ferrochelatase activity in mitogen-stimulated lymphocytes from patients with erythropoietic protoporphyria. J Clin Invest 69:809, 1982

237. Brodie MJ, Thompson GG, Moore MR et al: Haem biosynthesis in peripheral blood in erythropoietic protoporphyria. Clin Exp Dermatol 2:381, 1978

238. De Goeij AFPM, Christianse K, Van Steveninck J: Decreased haem synthetase activity in blood cells of patients with erythropoietic protoporphyria. Eur J Clin Invest 5:397, 1975

239. Straka JG, Hill HD, Krikava JM et al: Immunochemical studies of ferrochelatase protein: characterization of the normal and mutant protein in bovine and human protoporphyria. Am J Hum Genet 48:72, 1991

240. Bloomer JR: Characterization of deficient heme synthase activity in protoporphyria with cultured skin fibroblasts. J Clin Invest 65:321, 1980

241. Kramer S, Viljoen JD: Erythropoietic protoporphyria: evidence that it is due to a variant ferrochelatase. Int J Biochem 12:925, 1980

242. Lamoril J, Boulechfar S, de Verneuil H et al: Human erythropoietic protoporphyria: two point mutations in the ferrochelatase gene. Biochem Biophys Res Commun 181:594, 1991

243. Nakahashi Y, Fujita H, Taketani S et al: The molecular defect of ferrochelatase in a patient with erythropoietic protoporphyria. Proc Natl Acad Sci USA 89:281, 1992

244. Wang X, Poh-Fitzpatrick M, Carriero D et al: A novel mutation in erythropoietic protoporphyria: an aberrant ferrochelatase mRNA caused by exon skipping during RNA splicing. Biochim Biophys Acta 1181:198, 1993

245. Donaldson EM, Donaldson AD, Rimington C: Erythropoietic protoporphyria: a family study. Br Med J 1:659, 1967

246. Brenner DA, Didier JM, Frasier F et al: A molecular defect in human protoporphyria. Am J Hum Genet 50:1203, 1992

247. Tutois S, Montagutelli X, Dasilva V et al: Erythropoietic protoporphyria in the house mouse: a recessive inherited ferrochelatase deficiency with anemia, photosensitivity, and liver disease. J Clin Invest 88:1730, 1991

248. Sandberg S, Romslo I: Porphyrin-induced photodamage at the cellular and the subcellular level as related to the solubility of the porphyrin. Clin Chim Acta 109:193, 1981

249. Goldstein BD, Harber LC: Erythropoietic protoporphyria: lipid peroxidation and red cell membrane damage associated with photohemolysis. J Clin Invest 51:892, 1972

250. De Goeij AFPM, Van Steveninch J: Photodynamic aspects of protoporphyrin on cholesterol and unsaturated fatty acids in erythrocyte membranes in protoporphyria and in normal red blood cells. Clin Chim Acta 68:115, 1976

251. Schnait FG, Wolff K, Konrad K: Erythropoietic protoporphyria—submicroscopic events during the acute photosensitivity flare. Br J Dermatol 92:545, 1975

252. Lim HW, Poh-Fitzpatrick MB, Gigli I: Activation of the complement system in patients with porphyrias after irradiation in vivo. J Clin Invest 74:1961, 1984

253. Magnus IA: The cutaneous porphyrias. Semin Hematol 5:380, 1968

254. Clark KGA, Nicholson DC: Erythrocyte protoporphyrin and iron uptake in erythropoietic protoporphyria. Clin Sci 41:363, 1971

255. Piomelli S, Lamola AA, Poh-Fitzpatrick MB et al: Erythropoietic protoporphyria and Pb intoxication: the molecular basis for difference in cutaneous photosensitivity. I. Different rates of disappearance of protoporphyrin from the erythrocytes, both in vivo and in vitro. J Clin Invest 56:1519, 1975

256. Gray CH, A Kulczycka DC, Nicholson IA et al: Isotope studies on a case of erythropoietic protoporphyria. Clin Sci 26:7, 1964

257. Nicholson DC, Cowger ML, Kalivas J et al: Isotopic studies of the erythropoietic and hepatic components of congenital porphyria and "erythropoietic" protoporphyria. Clin Sci 44:135, 1973

258. Scholnick P, Marver HS, Schmid R: Erythropoietic protoporphyria: evidence for multiple sites of excess protoporphyrin formation. J Clin Invest 50:203, 1971

259. Sandberg S, Brun A: Light-induced protoporphyrin release from erythrocytes in erythropoietic protoporphyria. J Clin Invest 70:693, 1982

260. Sandberg S, Talstad I, Hovding G et al: Light-induced release of protoporphyrin, but not of zinc protoporphyrin, from erythrocytes in a patient with greatly elevated erythrocyte protoporphyrin. Blood 62:846, 1983

261. Sassaroli M, Dacosta R, Vaananen H et al: Distribution of erythrocyte free porphyrin content in erythropoietic protoporphyria. J Lab Clin Med 120:614, 1992

262. Turnbull A, Baker H, Vernon-Roberts B et al: Iron metabolism in porphyria cutanea tarda and in erythropoietic protoporphyria. Q J Med 42:341, 1973

263. Rademakers LHPM, Koningsberger JC, Sorber CWJ et al: Accumulation of iron in erythroblasts of patients with erythropoietic protoporphyria. Eur J Clin Invest 23:130, 1993

264. Mathews-Roth MM: Anemia in erythropoietic protoporphyria. JAMA 230:824, 1974

265. Suurmond D: Some aspects of erythropoietic protoporphyria in the Netherlands. Dermatologica 138:303, 1969

266. Bloomer JR: The liver in protoporphyria. Hepatology 8:402, 1988

267. Singer JA, Plaut AG, Kaplan MM: Hepatic failure and death from erythropoietic protoporphyria. Gastroenterology 74:588, 1978

268. Bonkowsky HL, Schned AR: Fatal liver failure in protoporphyria: synergism between ethanol exess and the genetic defect. Gastroenterology 90:191, 1986

269. Poh-Fitzpatrick MB, Whitlock RT, Lefkowitch JH: Changes in protoporphyrin distribution dynamics during liver failure and recovery in a patient with protoporphyria and Epstein-Barr viral hepatitis. Am J Med 80:943, 1986

270. Avner DL, Lee RG, Berenson MM: Protoporphyrin-induced cholestasis in the isolated in situ perfused rat liver. J Clin Invest 67:385, 1981

271. Berenson MM, Kimura R, Samowitz W, Bjorkman D: Protoporphyrin overload in unrestrained rats: biochemical and histopathologic characterization of a new model of protoporphyric hepatopathy. Int J Exp Pathol 73:665, 1992

272. Porter FS, Lowe BA: Congenital erythropoietic protoporphyria. I. Case reports, clinical studies and porphyrin analyses in two brothers. Blood 22:521, 1963

273. Eales L: Liver involvement in erythropoietic protoporphyria (EPP). Int J Biochem 12:915, 1980

274. Hastka J, Lasserre JJ, Schwarzbeck A et al: Zinc protoporphyrin in anemia of chronic disorders. Blood 81:1200, 1993

275. Anderson KE, Sassa S, Peterson CM, Kappas A: Increased erythrocyte uroporphyrinogen-I-synthetase, δ-aminolevulinic acid dehydratase and protoporphyrin in hemolytic anemias. Am J Med 63:359, 1977

276. Morton KO, Schneider F, Weiner MK et al: Hepatic and bile porphyrins in patients with protoporphyria and liver failure. Gastroenterology 94:1488, 1988

277. Poh-Fitzpatrick MB: Protoporphyrin metabolic balance in human protoporphyria. Gastroenterology 88:1239, 1985

278. Mathews-Roth MM, Pathak MA, Fitzpatrick TB et al: Beta-carotene therapy for erythropoietic protoporphyria and other photosensitivity diseases. Arch Dermatol 113:1229, 1977

279. Thomsen K, Schmidt H, Fischer A: Beta-carotene in erythropoietic protoporphyria: 5 years' experience. Dermatologica 159:82, 1979

280. Fusaro RM, Runge WJ: Erythropoietic protoporphyria. IV. Protection from sunlight. Br Med J 1:730, 1970

281. Van Hattum J, Baart de la Faille H, Van den Berg JWO et al: Chenodeoxycholic acid therapy in erythrohepatic porphyria. J Hepatol 3:407, 1986

282. Bloomer JR: Pathogenesis and therapy of liver disease in protoporphyria. Yale J Biol Med 52:39, 1979

283. Gordeuk VR, Brittenham GM, Hawkins CW et al: Iron therapy for hepatic dysfunction in erythropoietic protoporphyria. Ann Intern Med 105:27, 1986

284. Todd DJ, Callender ME, Mayne EE et al: Erythropoietic protoporphyria, transfusion therapy and liver disease. Br J Dermatol 127:534, 1992

285. Nordmann Y: Erythropoietic protoporphyria and hepatic complications. J Hepatol 16:4, 1992

286. Day RS, Eales L, Meissner D: Coexistent variegate porphyria and porphyria cutanea tarda. N Engl J Med 307:36, 1982

287. Doss M: Dual porphyria in double heterozygotes with porphobilinogen deaminase and uroporphyrinogen decarboxylase deficiencies. Clin Genet 35:146, 1989

288. Nordmann Y, Amram D, Deybach JC et al: Coexistent hereditary coproporphyria and congenital erythropoietic porphyria (Günther disease). J Inherit Metab Dis 13:687, 1990

289. Mollin DL: Sideroblasts and sideroblastic anemia. Br J Haematol 11:41, 1965

290. Dacie JV, Doniach I: The basophilic properties of the iron containing granules in siderocytes. J Pathol 59:684, 1947

291. McFadzean AJS, Davis LJ: Iron staining erythrocyte inclusions with special reference to acquired hemolytic anemia. Glasgow Med J 28:237, 1947

292. Bjorkman SE: Chronic refractory anaemia with sideroblastic bone marrow, a study of four cases. Blood 11:250, 1956

293. Dacie JV, Smith MD, White JC, Mollin DL: Refractory normoblastic anaemia. A clinical and haematological study of seven cases. Br J Haematol 5:56, 1959

294. Heilmeyer L, Emmrich J, Hennemann HH: Uber eine chronische hypochrome

Anaemie bei zwei Geschwistern auf der Grundlage ein Eisenverwertungs-störung (anaemia hypochromische sideroachrestica bei iteria). Folia Haematol (Frankfurt) 2:61, 1958

295. Bernard J, Lortholary P, Levy JP: Les anémies normochromes sidéroblas-tiques primitives. Nouv Rev Fr Hematol 3:723, 1961
296. MacGibbon BH, Mollin DL: Sideroblastic anemia in man: observations of seventy cases. Br J Haematol 11:59, 1965
297. Verwilghen R, Reybrouck G, Callens L, Cosemans J: Antituberculous drugs and sideroblastic anemia. Br J Haematol 11:92, 1965
298. Hines JD, Grasso JA: The sideroblastic anemias. Semin Hematol 7:86, 1970
299. Bessis MC, Jensen WN: Sideroblastic anaemia, mitochondria, and erythro-blastic iron. Br J Haematol 11:49, 1965
300. Jensen WN, Moreno G: Les ribosomes et les ponctuations basophiles des érythrocytes dans l'intoxication par le plomb. C R Acad Sci III 258:3596, 1964
301. Jensen WN, Moreno GD, Bessis MC: An electron microscopic description of basophilic stippling in red cells. Johns Hopkins Med J 25:933, 1965
302. Griggs RC: Lead poisoning: hematologic aspects. Prog Hematol 4:117, 1964
303. Harris JW, Whittington RM, Weissman RJ, Horrigan DL: Pyridoxine respon-sive anemia in the human adult. Proc Soc Exp Biol Med 91:427, 1956
304. Horrigan DL, Harris JW: Pyridoxine responsive anemia in man. Vitam Horm 26:549, 1968
305. Gehrman G: Pyridoxine responsive anemias. Br J Haematol 11:86, 1965
306. Bessis MC: Living Blood Cells and Their Ultrastructure. Springer-Verlag, New York, 1973
307. Hammond E, Deiss A, Carnes WH, Cartwright GE: Ultrastructural character-istics of siderocytes in swine. Lab Invest 21:292, 1969

308. Horrigan DL, Harris JW: Pyridoxine-responsive anemia: analysis of 62 cases. Adv Intern Med 12:103, 1964
309. Bell RE, Schewchuk HW: Refractory normoblastic anemia with sideroblasts in the bone marrow. Am J Clin Pathol 35:338, 1961
310. Barry WE, Day HJ: Refractory sideroblastic anemia: clinical and hematologic study of ten cases. Ann Intern Med 61:1029, 1964
311. Bernard J, Bessis M, Boiron M et al: Anémie hypochromie hypersidérémique sans anomalie de l'hémoglobine. Étude du métabolisme du fer. Effêt de la pyridoxine. Nouv Rev Fr Hematol 15:318, 1960
312. Singh AK, Shinton NK, Williams JDF: Ferrokinetic abnormalities and their significance in patients with sideroblastic anemia. Br J Haematol 18:67, 1970
313. Harris EB, MacGibbon BH, Mollin DL: Experimental sideroblastic anemia. Br J Haematol 11:99, 1965
314. Deiss A, Kurth D, Cartwright GE, Wintrobe MM: Experimental production of siderocytes. J Clin Invest 45:353, 1966
315. Vavra JD, Poff SA: Heme and porphyrin synthesis in sideroblastic anemia. J Lab Clin Med 69:904, 1967
316. Mason DY, Emerson PM: Primary acquired sideroblastic anaemia: response to treatment with pyridoxal-5-phosphate. Br Med J 1:389, 1973
317. Chillar RK, Johnson CS, Beutler E: Erythrocyte pyridoxine kinase levels in patients with sideroblastic anemia. N Engl J Med 295:881, 1976
318. Vogler WR, Mingioli ES: Porphyrin synthesis and heme synthetase activity in pyridoxine-responsive anemia. Blood 32:979, 1968
319. Weintraub LR, Conrad ME, Crosby WH: Iron-loading anemia. Treatment with repeated phlebotomies and pyridoxine. N Engl J Med 275:169, 1966
320. French TJ, Jacobs P: Sideroblastic anaemia associated with iron overload treated by repeated phlebotomy. S Afr Med J 50:594, 1976

Sideroblastic Anemias

40

James S. Wiley

INTRODUCTION

Sideroblastic anemias are a heterogeneous group of disor-ders characterized by anemia of varying severity and diag-nosed by finding ring sideroblasts in the bone marrow aspirate. The peripheral blood shows hypochromic red cells, which are microcytic in the hereditary forms (Fig. 40-1A), but are often macrocytic in the acquired forms of the disease. The red cell parameters from automated cell counting may show bimodal volume distribution curves (Fig. 40-1B); however, this dimor-phic size distribution is not always present. Tiny inclusions may be visible in the red cells; these can be confirmed as iron-containing Pappenheimer bodies by Prussian blue staining of the blood smear. The diagnostic test is bone marrow examina-tion together with Prussian blue staining of the bone marrow smears. The presence of ring sideroblasts (Fig. 40-1C) is defined as erythroblasts containing iron-positive (siderotic) granules arranged in a perinuclear collar distribution around one-third or more of the nucleus. Electron microscopic examination has shown that these siderotic granules are mitochondria contain-ing amorphous deposits of ferric phosphate and ferric hy-droxide.

Iron overload is a common clinical feature of refractory sider-oblastic anemia and, in severe cases, may lead to complications that characterize secondary hemosiderosis (e.g., diabetes, car-diac failure). Marrow examination shows prominent erythroid

hyperplasia, which is a sign of the ineffective erythropoiesis and is responsible for increased iron absorption. The sider-oblastic anemias have diverse etiologies but have in common an impaired biosynthesis of heme in the erythroid cells of the marrow. Most sideroblastic anemias are acquired as a clonal disorder of erythropoiesis, with varying degrees of myelodys-plastic features (Table 40-1). The inherited forms are uncom-mon and occur predominantly in males with an X-linked pattern of inheritance. A number of drugs have been associated with a reversible sideroblastic anemia, while ring sideroblasts may be found in patients with alcohol abuse (Table 40-1). The first descriptions of ring sideroblasts in association with chronic refractory anemias appeared in the late 1950s[1,2] following an earlier description of familial X-linked hypochromic microcytic anemia.[3] Heme synthesis and its disorders have been the sub-ject of recent reviews.[4-6]

HEREDITARY SIDEROBLASTIC ANEMIA

Biologic and Molecular Aspects

Erythroid cells account for the largest production of heme in the body while lesser amounts are produced in the liver and other organs for the synthesis of cytochrome P-450 and various hemoproteins. The first step in the heme synthetic pathway is

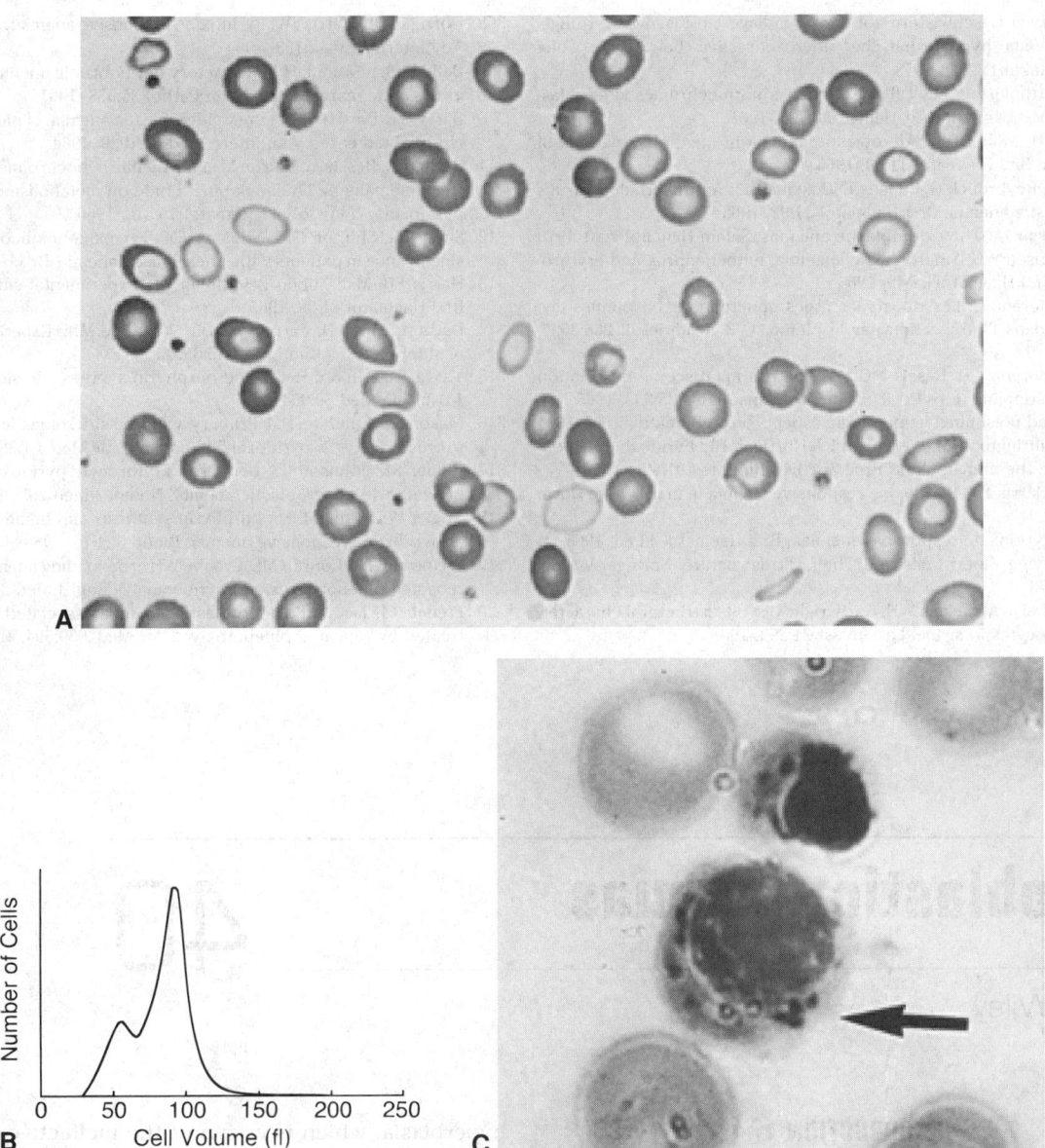

Fig. 40-1. (A) Peripheral blood smear in hereditary sideroblastic anemia showing a population of hypochromic and microcytic erythrocytes.
(B) Erythrocyte volume distribution curve in a patient with hereditary sideroblastic anemia. A dimorphic size distribution is evident. **(C)**
Bone marrow smear stained with Prussian blue, showing ring sideroblasts (arrow).

the condensation of glycine and succinyl coenzyme A catalyzed by δ-aminolevulinic acid synthase (ALA-S). ALA-S exists as two isoenzymes: a ubiquitous type expressed in all tissues, but particularly in liver; and a tissue-specific isoform expressed exclusively in erythroid cells.[4] The ubiquitously expressed ALA-S gene is localized on chromosome 3, whereas the erythroid-specific ALA-S gene is on the X-chromosome.[7,8] Enzyme levels of ubiquitous and erythroid isoenzymes of ALA-S are controlled by different mechanisms. Ubiquitous ALA-S levels in liver are regulated by negative feedback by heme, which represses transcription of the gene and inhibits transport of ALA-S from the cytosol into the mitochondrial matrix. While heme does not affect transcription of the erythroid ALA-S gene, it does inhibit transport of the erythroid ALA-S into the mitochondrial matrix[9] and possibly the accumulation of intracellular iron (Fig. 40-2). Levels of intracellular iron may in turn regulate the translation of mRNA for erythroid-specific ALA-S. A specific repressor protein interacts with an iron-responsive element in the erythroid

ALA-S mRNA and prevents translation, but this repression is relieved by high iron levels.[5] Thus, iron uptake by erythroid cells has a positive effect on the enzymatic step catalyzed by ALA-S. This effect ensures that protoporphyrin synthesis is coupled to iron availability.

Erythroid cells from patients with X-linked forms of hereditary sideroblastic anemia generally exhibit low activity of ALA-S.[4,10–13] A defect in this enzyme is firmly established in those patients whose anemia responds to pyridoxine therapy, since pyridoxal phosphate is an essential cofactor for ALA-S. However, even affected females with moderate anemia unresponsive to pyridoxine have been documented to have low levels of ALA-S in bone marrow lysates.[12,14] In some male patients with X-linked pyridoxine-responsive sideroblastic anemia, the low ALA-S activity in bone marrow increased to levels above the normal range when the patient took pyridoxine supplements and recovered from the anemia.[11,12,15] There are several possible explanations for this enhancement of ALA-S activity

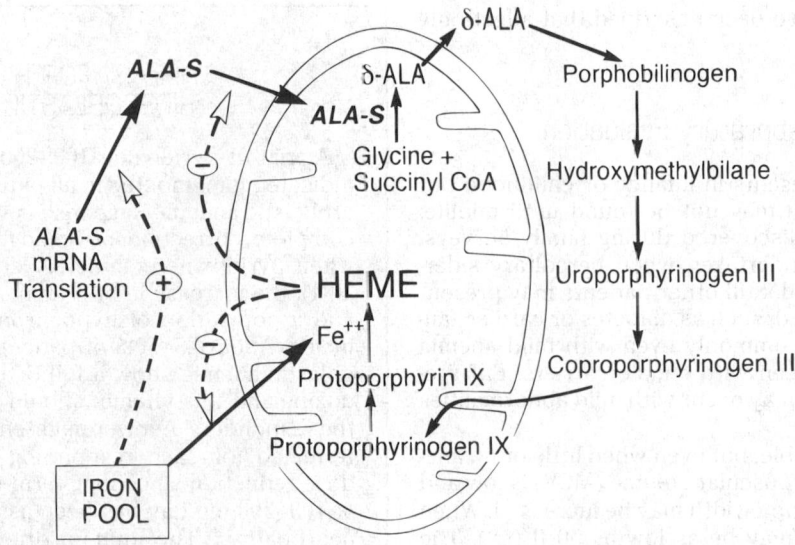

Fig. 40-2. Pathway and regulation of heme synthesis in erythroblasts. The first step in the pathway is catalyzed by ALA-S and occurs within the mitochondrion, using pyridoxal phosphate as a cofactor. The product of the last step, heme inhibits translocation of ALA-S into the mitochondrion as well as inhibiting the uptake of iron from transferrin into the cytosol. Cytosolic iron enhances the translation of mRNA for ALA-S by inhibiting the interaction of a repressor protein with an iron-responsive element in the mRNA. Decreased activity of ALA-S is found in X-linked hereditary sideroblastic anemias.

by dietary pyridoxine supplements. First, pyridoxine (or its phosphate) may stabilize the ALA-S during folding of the enzyme following its synthesis.[15] Second, pyridoxine may protect a mutant ALA-S from degradation by mitochondrial protease.[11] Finally, the mutant enzyme may have a higher Michaelis constant (K_m) for pyridoxal phosphate so that increased amounts of its cofactor are required for normal activity.[12]

In members of a kindred with X-linked pyridoxine-responsive sideroblastic anemia, a single base alteration C → G has been identified that results in an amino acid change from threonine to serine at residue 388 of ALA-S.[15] In an unrelated single, male patient with pyridoxine-responsive sideroblastic anemia, a single base alteration T → A has been reported resulting in an isoleucine → asparagine substitution at residue 471 of the erythroid ALA-S structure.[16] Both mutations result in an erythroid ALA-S with reduced catalytic activity, probably by altering ALA-S structure in the vicinity of the lysine residue that binds pyridoxal phosphate. As most of the hereditary sideroblastic anemias are unresponsive to pyridoxine supplementation, it is clear that there will be a variety of different mutations in the

erythroid ALA-S gene, and perhaps elsewhere, responsible for sideroblastic anemia in different families.

Genetic Aspects

In the great majority of families with hereditary sideroblastic anemia, males are affected with an X-linked pattern of inheritance (Fig. 40-3). Thus, the assignment of the gene for erythroid ALA-S to the X-chromosome[7,8] provides support for the concept of a mutation in erythroid ALA-S as the underlying defect in X-linked hereditary sideroblastic anemia.[4,5] In several families, co-inheritance of other X-linked traits (e.g., glucose-6-phosphate dehydrogenase [G6PD] deficiency or ataxia with sideroblastic anemia) has been described.[17,18] There are well-documented families in which the sideroblastic anemia was inherited as an autosomal dominant trait[19,20]; both sporadic

Table 40-1. Classification of Sideroblastic Anemias

Hereditary
    X-linked[a]
    Autosomal dominant or recessive[a]

Acquired
    Idiopathic acquired[a] (refractory anemia with ring sideroblasts)
    Associated with previous chemotherapy, irradiation, or in "transitional" myelodysplasia/myeloproliferative diseases

Drugs
    Alcohol
    Isoniazid
    Chloramphenicol

Rare causes
    Pearson syndrome
    Siderblastic anemia associated with increased erythrocyte protoporphyrin
    Copper deficiency or zinc overload
    Hypothermia

[a] Trial of pyridoxine indicated.

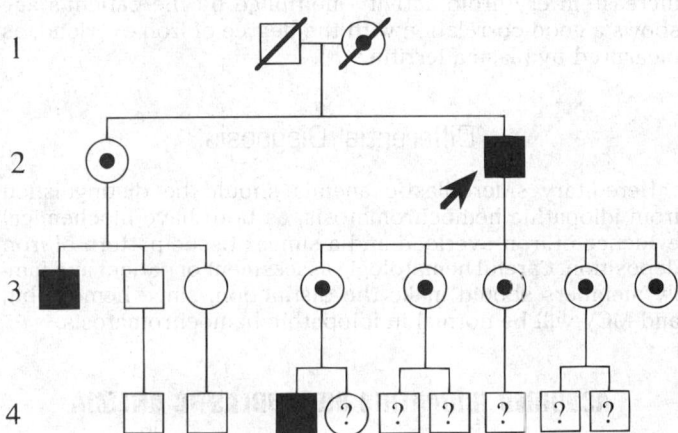

Fig. 40-3. Pedigree of a family with pyridoxine-responsive sideroblastic anemia showing X-linked recessive inheritance. ■, affected; ⊙ carrier, ?, unknown status. Diagonal lines indicate deceased members. This pedigree[15] has been abbreviated to show only the affected branches of the family. The arrow indicates the proband.

as well as familial cases have been described that affect only females.[10,21,22]

Clinical and Laboratory Evaluation

Typically, the anemia presents in infancy or childhood but the milder forms of anemia may not be found until midlife. Some cases may only be discovered during family surveys, which should always be undertaken when hereditary sideroblastic anemia is diagnosed. Still other patients may present with features of iron overload, such as diabetes or cardiac failure. Iron overload occurs commonly even with mild anemia and may occasionally be seen with female carriers. Enlargement of the liver and spleen may occur with mild abnormalities of liver function tests.

Anemia is extremely variable, but even when little or no anemia is present, the mean corpuscular volume (MCV) is low and the red cell volume distribution width may be increased. When anemia is severe the MCV may be as low as 50 fl (μ^3). The blood smear shows a population of cells with hypochromic, microcytic morphology (Fig. 40-1A), which contrasts with the other normochromic, normocytic cells (dimorphism). Anisocytosis, poikilocytosis, elongated cells and siderocytes may also be seen. The characteristic erythrocyte dimorphism is most prominent in patients with milder anemia, in female carriers, or in those patients in whom pyridoxine has corrected the anemia but not restored the MCV to normal. Leukocyte values are normal, whereas the platelet count is normal or increased.

Serum iron concentration is increased and transferrin shows an increased percentage of saturation with iron. Serum ferritin levels are invariably increased. Ineffective erythropoiesis can be confirmed by ferrokinetic measurements showing that plasma iron clearance is rapid with subnormal retention of the iron isotope in erythrocytes after 10–14 days. Some other features of ineffective erythropoiesis may be variably present: mild increase in bilirubin, decrease in haptoglobin, mild increase in lactate dehydrogenase, and normal or slight increase in reticulocyte numbers. The magnitude of iron overload correlates poorly with the degree of anemia in patients who are not transfused. The degree of ineffective erythropoiesis is a better predictor of the degree of iron overload. Where ferrokinetics are unavailable, the extent of erythroid hyperplasia relative to normal acts as a rough measure of the magnitude of ineffective erythropoiesis. Several studies have shown that the relative increase in erythroid activity multiplied by the patient's age shows a good correlation with the degree of iron overload, as measured by plasma ferritin.[22,23]

Differential Diagnosis

Hereditary sideroblastic anemia should be distinguished from idiopathic hemochromatosis, as both have biochemical evidence of iron overload and a similar tissue pattern of iron deposition. Careful hematologic assessment of patient and family members should make the distinction, since hemoglobin and MCV will be normal in idiopathic hemochromatosis.

ACQUIRED IDIOPATHIC SIDEROBLASTIC ANEMIA

Acquired sideroblastic anemia may either be idiopathic or occur following chemotherapy or irradiation (Table 40-1). Nearly all cases show evidence of dyserythropoiesis in the marrow and there may also be dysplastic changes in either the myeloid precursors or megakaryocytes, or both. Acquired idiopathic sideroblastic anemia falls within the diagnostic category

---

THERAPY FOR HEREDITARY SIDEROBLASTIC ANEMIA

A trial of pyridoxine 100–200 mg/day taken orally is indicated for 3 months in all patients with hereditary sideroblastic anemia. Response is variable and ranges from complete correction of hemoglobin to no effect. Even when pyridoxine completely corrects the anemia (Fig. 40-4), the increase in MCV may not reach normal values and a population of hypochromic, microcytic cells remains. About 25–50% of patients with hereditary sideroblastic anemia show a full or partial response to pyridoxine and this vitamin should be continued lifelong in the responders. A lower maintenance dose should be determined for each responding patient by progressive dose reduction since long-term therapy with pyridoxine at 100–200 mg/day has been associated with peripheral neuropathy.[24] The adult nutritional requirement for pyridoxine is 1–2 mg/day and some patients have been maintained on as little as 4 mg/day as supplement.[15] Folic acid supplements should also be administered because the erythroid hyperplasia increases demand for this vitamin. There has been one report of hereditary sideroblastic anemia responding to parenteral pyridoxal-5′-phosphate after failing oral pyridoxine.[25]

Transfusions are the mainstay of treatment for severe anemia that is unresponsive to pyridoxine. Regular administration of packed red cells using white cell filters should be given to relieve symptoms and permit normal childhood development. Iron overload and secondary hemosiderosis rapidly progress after transfusions begin, chelation therapy with desferrioxamine should be initiated from the outset.

Iron removal may be of great benefit for patients who have mild or moderate anemia and evidence of iron overload.[22,23] These patients often can tolerate intermittent phlebotomy, which is preferable to chelation therapy for iron removal and should be continued to reduce ferritin levels to <500 ng/ml. All patients with iron overload should avoid ingestion of ascorbic acid supplements, which not only enhance iron absorption but also increase the tissue toxicity of elemental iron. Splenectomy is contraindicated in this disease.

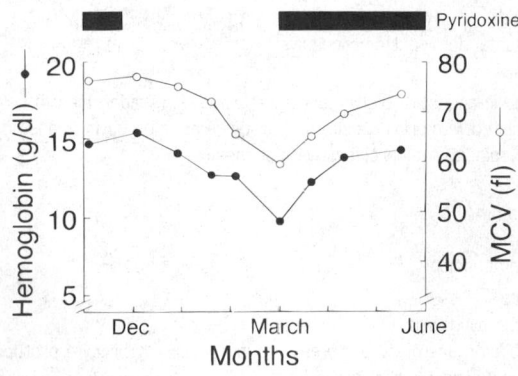

Fig. 40-4. Response of the hemoglobin and MCV to withdrawal and reinstitution of pyridoxine in a responsive hereditary sideroblastic anemia.

of refractory anemia with ring sideroblasts as defined by the French-American-British group.[26] Acquired sideroblastic anemia has also been described as a rare finding in myeloproliferative disorders such as idiopathic myelofibrosis (see Chs. 71 and 76). However distinction between idiopathic myelofibrosis and myelodysplasia is sometimes difficult and some of the reported cases may represent disease that is intermediate or transitional between these two entities.[27–29]

Biologic and Molecular Aspects

Clonal hematopoiesis has been demonstrated in acquired idiopathic sideroblastic anemia as well as in the related myelodysplastic syndromes. Specific evidence was first provided by finding a single G6PD isoenzyme in erythrocytes, granulocytes, platelets and B lymphocytes in a woman who was heterozygous for G6PD and thus carried two isoenzymes in her skin and T lymphocytes.[30,31] This technique is applicable only to the few women who have G6PD heterozygosity, but restriction fragment length polymorphism analysis (see Ch. 1) can now be applied to most women using probes directed at other X-chromosome genes such as phosphoglycerate kinase or to an X-linked variable copy number tandem repeat sequence (see Ch. 1).[32,33] The results show uniform monoclonality of hematopoiesis in acquired sideroblastic anemia either with or without associated myelodysplastic features. Initial reports of low levels of ALA-S in bone marrow of acquired idiopathic sideroblastic anemia have not been confirmed[13,34] and the cause of the defective heme synthesis in the abnormal clone is unclear. Some indirect evidence exists for a primary mitochondrial lesion that may impair heme synthesis as a secondary event.[6,34]

Etiology

Clonal chromosomal changes are found in bone marrow cells in approximately 60% of patients with acquired sideroblastic anemia. Characteristic changes are monosomy 7, trisomy 8, deletions involving chromosomes 5, 7, 11, or 20 and a number of balanced translocations.[35] When sideroblastic anemia is acquired secondary to chemotherapy or irradiation, chromosomal changes are nearly always found and tend to be multiple.[35] Among these changes, the loss of an entire chromosome (5 and/or 7), deletion of a long arm [(del)5 or (del)7] or an unbalanced translocation are typical.[36] Indeed, when karyotype shows loss of material from chromosomes 5 and/or 7, a detailed occupational history may show exposure to potentially mutagenic chemical agents in a proportion of patients.[37] However, the development of visible chromosomal changes is probably a late event in acquired sideroblastic anemia and may be preceded by the expansion of a clone of genetically unstable stem cells.[31] This concept is in accord with the view that multiple genetic events underlie the pathogenesis of other myelodysplastic syndromes as well as acute myeloid leukemia.[31,38,39]

Clinical and Laboratory Evaluation

Typically this anemia develops insidiously in a middle-aged or elderly patient with normal or increased MCV and a blood smear showing a population of hypochromic red cells. Hepatosplenomegaly may be present. Leukocyte and platelet counts are usually normal, but some patients have thrombocytosis that occasionally exceeds 1,000,000/mm³.[40] If leukopenia or thrombocytopenia is present, a careful search should be made for myelodysplastic features, which are often associated with these cytopenias. An iron stain of the bone marrow smear shows ring sideroblasts, which should total more than 15% of

---

THERAPY FOR ACQUIRED SIDEROBLASTIC ANEMIA

Transfusions are indicated for relief of symptomatic anemia. A trial of pyridoxine at 100–200 mg/day for 3 months is worthwhile in those patients with anemia but displaying no neutropenia or thrombocytopenia. Only a small proportion of patients with acquired idiopathic sideroblastic anemia respond to this vitamin. If any response is achieved, maintenance therapy with pyridoxine at lower dosage is indicated.

---

all erythroblasts to make the diagnosis of acquired sideroblastic anemia.[26,41–43] The bone marrow also shows erythroid hyperplasia; although mild dyserythropoiesis (multinuclearity, nuclear budding) and megaloblastoid changes are present, both myelopoiesis and megakaryopoiesis are usually normal. Concomitant dysplasia of myelo- or megakaryopoietic elements is suggested by the following features: Pelger-Hüet-like anomaly, hypersegmentation or hypogranularity of neutrophils, micromegakaryocytes, large mononuclear megakaryocytes, and megakaryocytes with multiple small nuclei.[41] Dysmegakaryopoiesis is more easily detected in trephine biopsies than in marrow smears, while the trephine may also show unsuspected islands of myeloblasts characteristic of myelodysplasia.[44] The overall blast count in marrow smears is, by definition, <5%. Cytogenetic analysis of marrow aspirates provides important information, since a normal karyotype predicts long survival in any type of acquired sideroblastic anemia.[45]

Differential Diagnosis

Ring sideroblasts are not limited to acquired sideroblastic anemia, as they also occur in other myelodysplastic conditions, such as refractory anemia with excess blasts, in which the blast count is >5%.[46] Careful examination of peripheral blood and bone marrow will distinguish acquired idiopathic sideroblastic anemia from these related myelodysplastic conditions. Family surveys are very useful in distinguishing acquired from hereditary forms of sideroblastic anemia, as the latter may present in late adult life.

Prognosis

Acquired idiopathic sideroblastic anemia and the related entity of refractory anemia have the most favorable outlook among the myelodysplastic syndromes, with a median survival of 50 months and 8–12% incidence of leukemic progression.[35] The prognosis can be correlated with three factors. First is the severity of the anemia, since repeated transfusions markedly increase iron overload and invariably lead to the organ dysfunction characteristic of secondary hemosiderosis (e.g., heart and liver failure, diabetes). The second factor is whether neutropenia or thrombocytopenia, or both, are associated with the anemia. These cytopenias form the basis of a simple prognostic scoring system in which two or more of the following place the patient in a poor prognostic category[47,48]: (1) hemoglobin <10 g/dl, (2) neutrophils <2,500/mm³, (3) platelets <100,000/mm³, and (4) blasts >5%. Finally, karyotypic analysis of marrow aspirates provides valuable information, since a normal karyotype carries a more favorable prognosis. Conversely, monosomy 7 or a partial loss of the long arm of chromosome 7 as a single defect imparts a high probability of transformation to acute myeloid leukemia. Multiple chromosomal abnormalities or del(20q) are also associated with an increased risk of progression to leukemia; by contrast, trisomy 8 has no adverse prognostic significance.[35] Evolution of acquired idiopathic sideroblastic anemia to other myelodysplastic conditions, such as refractory anemia with excess blasts, has been described.[49]

SIDEROBLASTIC ANEMIA SECONDARY TO DRUGS

Alcohol

Ring sideroblasts may be found in the bone marrow of malnourished anemic alcoholics, usually in the presence of associated folate deficiency.[50-52] By contrast, binge drinking or chronic alcohol ingestion in subjects with good nutrition is not associated with sideroblastic abnormality. Sideroblastic change is never the sole cause for the anemia of alcoholism. Alcohol has a direct toxic effect on hematopoiesis.[53,54] An increased or high normal MCV and vacuolation of red cell precursors is often seen in addition to the ring sideroblast abnormality. Red cells show dimorphic morphology; evidence in the marrow of folate deficiency is present in one-half of the cases.[54] Transferrin saturation and marrow iron stores tend to be increased but may be low if gastrointestinal bleeding is present. The ring sideroblasts gradually disappear over 4–12 days when alcohol is withdrawn[52]; during this period, there may be a rebound erythroid hyperplasia, reticulocytosis, and thrombocytosis. Folic acid should be given for the associated megaloblastic changes after blood is taken for vitamin B_{12} and folate assays.

Alcohol consumption lowers the plasma concentration of pyridoxal phosphate, a cofactor for ALA-S, the first step in heme synthesis.[55,56] Conversion of ethanol to acetaldehyde is necessary for this effect and it has been shown that acetaldehyde acts by accelerating the degradation of intracellular pyridoxal phosphate in the liver, thus lowering plasma levels of this coenzyme.[57] In one study, the alcohol-induced sideroblastic changes responded to parenteral pyridoxal phosphate, but not to a combination of pyridoxine with folic acid.[55] Although alcohol may reduce the supply of coenzyme for erythroid ALA-S, there is evidence that other steps in the pathway of heme synthesis may also be inhibited.[58]

Isoniazid

Administration of the antituberculous drug isoniazid has been uncommonly associated with development of a sideroblastic anemia after 1–10 months of therapy. The anemia is both hypochromic and microcytic with a dimorphic blood smear and ring sideroblasts in the marrow. This complication is thought to occur only in slow acetylators of isoniazid, allowing this drug to react nonenzymatically with pyridoxal and to form a hydrazone that is rapidly excreted in the urine. The anemia can be fully reversed by co-administration of pyridoxine, 25–50 mg/day with isoniazid or by withdrawing the latter drug.[59-61]

Chloramphenicol

Chloramphenicol is an antibiotic that produces a reversible suppression of erythropoiesis after several days of therapy (plasma levels 10–15 μg/ml). This effect is both predictable and separate from the rare idiosyncratic side effect of aplastic anemia in about 1 of 20,000 exposed persons. Nearly all patients given >2 g/day develop vacuolation of the erythroid precursors, as well as ring sideroblasts. These effects are thought to arise from suppression of mitochondrial respiration. Chloramphenicol inhibits mitochondrial protein synthesis and reduces cytochrome a + a_3 and b levels.[62,63] It is unclear why the erythroid precursors are so vulnerable to the toxic action of chloramphenicol; the higher concentrations of serine and glycine in erythroid cell mitochondria may play a role.[64] Serum iron concentrations are increased and reticulocyte numbers are subnormal, but these changes revert on stopping the antibiotic.

PRESENTATIONS ASSOCIATED WITH SIDEROBLASTIC ANEMIA

Pearson Syndrome

Pearson syndrome is a rare entity that presents in early infancy with anemia and exocrine pancreatic dysfunction. The anemia is normocytic or macrocytic, reticulocytes are low, and variable neutropenia and thrombocytopenia is present. The bone marrow shows a striking vacuolation, as well as ring sideroblasts.[65] Although usually fatal, milder forms of the anemia are consistent with survival into adult life. The syndrome is thought to result from deletions or rearrangements of mitochondrial DNA affecting multiple tissues of the body.[66,67]

Increased Erythrocyte Protoporphyrin

There have been three reports of idiopathic sideroblastic anemia associated with marked increase in erythrocyte protoporphyrin.[68-70] Dermal photosensitivity was present in two of these cases suggesting similarities to erythropoietic protoporphyria, an inherited disorder with reduced activity of heme synthase. In one of the cases, the patient developed fatal liver disease with raised hepatic protoporphyrins, a complication that has also been described in erythropoietic protoporphyria.[70]

Copper Deficiency or Zinc Overload

Copper is widely distributed in foods. Copper deficiency has been described only in malnourished premature infants[71] or in patients receiving long-term parenteral hyperalimentation.[72,73] The syndrome of copper deficiency consists of sideroblastic anemia with hypochromic cells in the blood smear, accompanied by ring sideroblasts and vacuolated erythroid and myeloid precursors in the marrow and of neutropenia with an absence of late myeloid forms in the marrow. Additional features may also be seen in infants, namely, osteoporosis and long bone changes, depigmentation of skin and hair, and central nervous system abnormalities. Platelet counts remain normal. Serum copper and ceruloplasmin levels are low while serum iron and transferrin saturation are normal. Prompt reversal of the hematologic changes follows therapy with 2–5 mg/day copper sulfate taken orally or 100–500 μg/day copper supplement to the intravenous alimentation formula.

Large quantities of ingested zinc interfere with copper absorption and produce the neutropenia and sideroblastic anemia characteristic of copper deficiency.[74,75] Zinc sulfate is freely available from health food stores, and as little as 450 mg/day for 2 years is sufficient for this effect. Serum zinc levels are high, while serum copper and ceruloplasmin levels are low. Zinc must be discontinued for 9–12 weeks for full reversal of the anemia and neutropenia.

Hypothermia

Thrombocytopenia, erythroid hypoplasia, and ring sideroblasts have been described in patients with hypothermia associated with neurologic disease.[76] These changes reverse slowly as body temperature returns to normal.

REFERENCES

1. Bjorkman SE: Chronic refractory anemia with sideroblastic bone marrow. A study of four cases. Blood 11:250, 1956
2. Dacie JV, Smith MD, White JC, Mollin DL: Refractory normoblastic anaemia: a clinical and haematological study of seven cases. Br J Haematol 5:56, 1959
3. Cooley TB: A severe type of hereditary anemia with elliptocytosis. Interesting sequence of splenectomy. Am J Med Sci 209:561, 1945
4. Bottomley SS, Muller-Eberhard U: Pathophysiology of heme synthesis. Semin Hematol 25:282, 1988
5. May BK, Bhasker CR, Bawden MJ, Cox TC: Molecular regulation of 5-aminolevulinate synthase. Diseases related to heme synthesis. Mol Biol Med 7:405, 1990
6. Jacobs A: Primary acquired sideroblastic anaemia. Br J Haematol 64:415, 1986
7. Cox TC, Bawden MJ, Abraham NG et al: Erythroid 5-aminolevulinate synthase is located on the X-chromosome. Am J Human Genet 46:107, 1990
8. Bishop DF, Henderson AS, Astrin KH: Human δ-aminolevulinate synthase: assignment of the housekeeping gene to 3p21 and the erythroid-specific gene to the X chromosome. Genomics 7:207, 1990
9. Lathrop JT, Timko MP: Regulation by heme of mitochondrial protein transport through a conserved amino acid motif. Science 259:522, 1993
10. Lee GR, McDiarmid WD, Cartwright GE, Wintrobe MM: Hereditary, X-linked, sideroachrestic anemia. The isolation of two erythrocyte populations differing in Xg^a blood type and porphyrin content. Blood 32:59, 1968
11. Aoki Y, Muranaka S, Nakabayashi K, Ueda Y: δ-Aminolevulinic synthetase in erythroblasts of patients with pyridoxine-responsive anemia. J Clin Invest 64:1196, 1979
12. Konopka L, Hoffbrand AV: Haem synthesis in sideroblastic anaemia. Br J Haematol 42:73, 1979
13. Bottomley SS, Healy HM, Brandenburg MA, May BK: 5 Aminolevulinate synthase in sideroblastic anemias: mRNA and enzyme activity levels in bone marrow cells. Am J Hematol 41:76, 1992
14. Buchanan GR, Bottomley SS, Nitschke R: Bone marrow delta-aminolevulinate synthase deficiency in a female with congenital sideroblastic anemia. Blood 55:109, 1980
15. Cox TC, Bottomley SS, Wiley JS et al: X-linked pyridoxine-responsive sideroblastic anemia due to a THR^{388}-to-SER substitution in erythroid 5-aminolevulinate synthase. N Eng J Med 330:675, 1994
16. Cotter PD, Bauman M, Bishop DF: Enzymatic defect in "X-linked" sideroblastic anemia: molecular evidence for erythroid δ-aminolevulinate synthase deficiency. Proc Natl Acad Sci USA 89:4028, 1992
17. Prasad AS, Tranchida L, Konno ET et al: Hereditary sideroblastic anemia and glucose-6-phosphate dehydrogenase deficiency in a Negro family. J Clin Invest 47:1415, 1968
18. Pagon RA, Bird TD, Detter JC, Pierce I: Hereditary sideroblastic anaemia and ataxia: an X-linked recessive disorder. J Med Genet 22:267,1985
19. Soslan G, Brodsky I: Hereditary sideroblastic anemia with associated platelet abnormalities. Am J Hematol 32:298, 1989
20. van Waveren Hogervorst GD, van Roermund HPC, Snijders PJ: Hereditary sideroblastic anaemia and autosomal inheritance of erythrocyte dimorphism in a Dutch family. Eur J Haematol 38:405, 1987
21. Pasanen AVO, Salmi M, Tenhunen R, Vuopio P: Haem synthesis during pyridoxine therapy in two families with different types of hereditary sideroblastic anaemia. Ann Clin Res 14:61, 1982.
22. Peto TEA, Pippard MJ, Weatherall DJ: Iron overload in mild sideroblastic anaemias. Lancet 1:375, 1983
23. Cazzola M, Barosi G, Bergamaschi G et al: Iron loading in congenital dyserythropoietic anaemias and congenital sideroblastic anaemias. Br J Haematol 54:649, 1983
24. Parry GJ, Bredesen DE: Sensory neuropathy with low-dose pyridoxine. Neurology 35:1466, 1985
25. Mason DY, Emerson PM: Primary acquired sideroblastic anaemia: response to treatment with pyridoxal-5-phosphate. Br Med J 1:389, 1973
26. Bennett JM, Catovsky D, Daniel MT et al: Proposals for the classification of the myelodysplastic syndromes. Br J Haematol 51:189, 1982
27. Kushner JP, Lee GR, Wintrobe MM, Cartwright GE: Idiopathic refractory sideroblastic anemia. Clinical and laboratory investigation of 17 patients and review of the literature. Medicine 50:139, 1971
28. Pagliuca A, Layton DM, Manoharan A et al: Myelofibrosis in primary myelodysplastic syndromes: a clinico-morphological study of 10 cases. Br J Haematol 71:499, 1989
29. Reilly JT, Dolan G: Proposed classification for the myelodysplasia/myelofibrosis syndromes. Br J Haematol 79:653, 1991
30. Prchal JT, Throckmorton DW, Carroll AJ et al: A common progenitor for human myeloid and lymphoid cells. Nature 274:590, 1978
31. Raskind WH, Tirumali N, Jacobson R et al: Evidence for a multistep pathogenesis of a myelodysplastic syndrome. Blood 63:1318, 1984
32. Young NS: The problem of clonality in aplastic anemia: Dr. Dameshek's riddle, restated. Blood 79:1385, 1992
33. Janssen JWG, Buschle M, Layton M et al: Clonal analysis of myelodysplastic syndromes: evidence of multipotent stem cell origin. Blood 73:28, 1989
34. Aoki Y: Multiple enzymatic defects in mitochondria in hematological cells of patients with primary sideroblastic anemia. J Clin Invest 66:43, 1980
35. Third MIC Cooperative Study Group: Recommendations for a morphologic, immunological, and cytogenetics (MIC) working classification of the primary and therapy-related myelodysplastic disorders. Cancer Genet Cytogenet 32: 1, 1988
36. Neuman WL, Rubin C, Rios RB et al: Chromosomal loss and deletion are the most common mechanisms for loss of heterozygosity from chromosomes 5 and 7 in malignant myeloid disorders. Blood 79:1501, 1992
37. Golomb HM, Alimena G, Rowley JD et al: Correlation of occupation and karyotype in adults with acute nonlymphocytic leukemia. Blood 60:404, 1982
38. Fialkow PJ, Janssen JWG, Bartram CR: Clonal remissions in acute nonlymphocytic leukemia: evidence for a multistep pathogenesis of the malignancy. Blood 77:1415, 1991
39. Gale RE, Wheadon H, Goldstone AH et al: Frequency of clonal remission in acute myeloid leukaemia. Lancet 341:138, 1993
40. Streeter RR, Presant CA, Reinhard E: Prognostic significance of thrombocytosis in idiopathic sideroblastic anemia. Blood 50:427, 1977
41. Gattermann N, Aul C, Schneider W: Two types of acquired idiopathic sideroblastic anaemia (AISA). Br J Haematol 74:45, 1990
42. Cazzola M, Barosi G, Gobbi PG et al: Natural history of idiopathic refractory sideroblastic anemia. Blood 71:305, 1988
43. May SJ, Smith SA, Jacobs A et al: The myelodysplastic syndrome: analysis of laboratory characteristics in relation to the FAB classification. Br J Haematol 59:311, 1985
44. Tricot G, De Wolf-Peeters C, Hendrickx B, Verwilghen RL: Bone marrow histology in myelodysplastic syndromes. I. Histological findings in myelodysplastic syndromes and comparison with bone marrow smears. Br J Haematol 57:423, 1984
45. Yunis J, Rydell RE, Oken MM et al: Refined chromosome analysis as an independent prognostic indicator in de novo myeloplastic syndromes. Blood 67: 1721, 1986
46. Juneja SK, Imbert M, Sigaux F et al: Prevalence and distribution of ringed sideroblasts in primary myeloplastic syndromes. J Clin Pathol 36:566, 1983
47. Mufti GJ, Stevens JR, Oscier DG et al: Myeloplastic syndromes: a scoring system with prognostic significance. Br J Haematol 59:425, 1985
48. Vallespi T, Torrabadella M, Julia A et al: Myelodysplastic syndromes: a study of 101 cases according to the FAB classification. Br J Haematol 61:83, 1985
49. Hussein KK, Salem Z, Bottomley SS, Livingston RB: Acute leukemia in idiopathic sideroblastic anemia: response to combination chemotherapy. Blood 59:652, 1982
50. Hines JD: Reversible megaloblastic and sideroblastic marrow abnormalities in alcoholic patients. Br J Haematol 16:87, 1969
51. Pierce HI, McGuffin RG, Hillman RS: Clinical studies in alcoholic sideroblastosis. Arch Intern Med 136:283, 1976
52. Eichner ER, Hillman RS: The evolution of anemia in alcoholic patients. Am J Med 50:218, 1971
53. Jandl JH: The anemia of liver disease: observations on its mechanism. J Clin Invest 34:390, 1955
54. Savage D, Lindenbaum J: Anemia in alcoholics. Medicine 65:322, 1986
55. Hines JD, Cowan DH: Studies on the pathogenesis of alcohol-induced sideroblastic bone-marrow abnormalities. N Engl J Med 283:441, 1970
56. Lumeng L, Li T-K: Vitamin B$_6$ metabolism in chronic alcohol abuse. Pyridoxal phosphate levels in plasma and the effects of acetaldehyde on pyridoxal phosphate synthesis and degradation in human erythrocytes. J Clin Invest 53:693, 1974
57. Veitch RL, Lumeng L, Li T-K: Vitamin B$_6$ metabolism in chronic alcohol abuse. The effect of ethanol oxidation on hepatic pyridoxal 5'-phosphate metabolism. J Clin Invest 55:1026, 1975
58. Ali MAM, Sweeney G: Erythrocyte coproporphyrin and protoporphyrin in ethanol-induced sideroblastic erythropoiesis. Blood 43:291, 1974
59. Roberts PD, Hoffbrand AV, Mollin DL: Iron and folate metabolism in tuberculosis. Br Med J 2:198, 1966

60. Haden HT: Pyridoxine-responsive sideroblastic anemia due to antituberculous drugs. Arch Intern Med 120:602, 1967

61. McCurdy PR, Donohoe RF: Pyridoxine-responsive anemia conditioned by isonicotinic acid hydrazide. Blood 27:352, 1966

62. Martelo OJ, Manyan DR, Smith US, Yunis AA: Chloramphenicol and bone marrow mitochondria. J Lab Clin Med 74:927, 1969

63. Firkin FC: Mitochondrial lesions in reversible erythropoietic depression due to chloramphenicol. J Clin Invest 51:2085, 1972

64. Abou-Khalil S, Abou-Khalil WH, Whitney PL, Yunis AA: Importance of the mitochondrial amino acid pool in the sensitivity of erythroid cells to chloramphenicol. Role of glycine and serine. Phramacology 35:308, 1987

65. Pearson HA, Lobel JS, Kocoshis SA et al: A new syndrome of refractory sideroblastic anemia with vacuolization of marrow precursors and exocrine pancreatic dysfunction. J Pediatr 95:976, 1979

66. Rotig A, Cormier V, Blanche S et al: Pearson's marrow-pancreas syndrome: a multisystem mitochondrial disorder in infancy. J Clin Invest 86:1601, 1990

67. McShane MA, Hammans SR, Sweeney M et al: Pearson syndrome and mitochondrial encephalomyopathy in a patient with a deletion of mtDNA. Am J Hum Genet 48:39, 1991

68. Rothstein G, Lee R, Cartwright GE: Sideroblastic anemia with dermal photo-

sensitivity and greatly increased erythrocyte protoporphyrin. N Engl J Med 280:587, 1969

69. Romslo I, Brun A, Sandberg S et al: Sideroblastic anemia with markedly increased free erythrocyte protoporphyrin without dermal photosensitivity. Blood 59:628, 1982

70. Scott AJ, Ansford AJ, Webster BH, Stringer HCW: Erythropoietic protoporphyria with features of a sideroblastic anemia terminating in liver failure. Am J Med 54:251, 1973

71. Ashkenazi A, Levin S, Djaldetti M et al: The syndrome of neonatal copper deficiency. Pediatrics 52:525, 1973

72. Dunlap WM, James GW, Hume DM: Anemia and neutropenia caused by copper deficiency. Ann Intern Med 80:470, 1974

73. Zidar BL, Shadduck RK, Zeigler Z, Winkelstein A: Observations on the anemia and neutropenia of human copper deficiency. Am J Hematol 3:177, 1977

74. Patterson WP, Winkelmann M, Perry MC: Zinc-induced copper deficiency: megamineral sideroblastic anemia. Ann Intern Med 103:385, 1985

75. Ramadurai J, Shapiro C, Kozloff M, Telfer M: Zinc abuse and sideroblastic anemia. Am J Hematol 42:227, 1993

76. O'Brien H, Amess JAL, Mollin DL: Recurrent thrombocytopenia, erythroid hypoplasia and sideroblastic anaemia associated with hypothermia. Br J Haematol 51:451, 1982

Megaloblastic Anemias

41

Aśok C. Antony

INTRODUCTION

The term megaloblastic anemia is used to describe a group of disorders characterized by a distinct morphologic pattern in hematopoietic cells. A common biochemical feature is a defect in DNA synthesis, with lesser alterations in RNA and protein synthesis, leading to a state of unbalanced cell growth and impaired cell division. The cell cycle of normal cells involves a coordinated series of events in DNA, RNA, and protein synthesis; a resting phase is followed by rapid doubling of cellular DNA in the S phase, followed by mitosis and division into two cells. Therefore, at any given time, most cells have DNA values of 2N, while a few have DNA values of 4N (where N is the amount of DNA in the haploid genome). By contrast, most megaloblastic cells are not resting but are vainly engaged in attempting to double their DNA, with frequent arrest in the S phase and lesser arrest in other phases of the cell cycle. Thus, an increased percentage of these cells have DNA values of 2–4N because of delayed cell division. This increased DNA content in megaloblastic cells is morphologically expressed as larger than normal "immature" nuclei with finely particulate chromatin, whereas the relatively unimpaired RNA and protein synthesis result in large cells with greater "mature" cytoplasm and cell volume. The net result of megaloblastosis is a cell whose nuclear maturation is arrested (immature), while its cytoplasmic maturation proceeds normally independently of the nuclear events. The microscopic appearance of this nuclear/cytoplasmic asynchrony (or dissociation) is morphologically described as megaloblastic. Each cell lineage has a limited but unique repertoire of expression of defective DNA synthesis. This is significantly influenced by the normal patterns of maturation of the affected cell line. Additional variables that affect RNA and protein synthesis can lead to the attenuation or modification of megaloblastic expression.

Megaloblastic hematopoiesis commonly presents as anemia, but this feature is only a manifestation of a more global defect in DNA synthesis that affects all proliferating cells. The peripheral blood picture is characteristic and reflective of megaloblastic hematopoiesis within the bone marrow. The diagnosis is therefore usually fairly simple. However, since any condition that specifically perturbs DNA synthesis can lead to megaloblastosis, determination of the precise etiology is necessary before therapy is instituted. Inappropriate therapy can lead to disastrous consequences for the patient. Therefore, the biochemical basis for megaloblastosis needs to be understood within the context of evaluation of potential and real variables affecting DNA, RNA, and protein synthesis in a given patient. The most common causes of megaloblastosis are true cellular deficiencies of vitamin B_{12} (cobalamin) or folate, vitamins essential for DNA synthesis. The pathophysiology of cellular deficiency is most readily discerned by the clinician who approaches megaloblastosis with a clear understanding of the physiology of these vitamins. A detailed discussion of cobalamin (Cbl) and folate follows.

COBALAMIN

The term cobalamin (Cbl) refers to a family of compounds with the structure shown in Figure 41-1; Cbl itself lacks a ligand in the cobalt β-position. Vitamin B_{12} is called cyano-Cbl because when it was originally isolated from liver, this position

Structure of cobalamin
(components and substitutions)

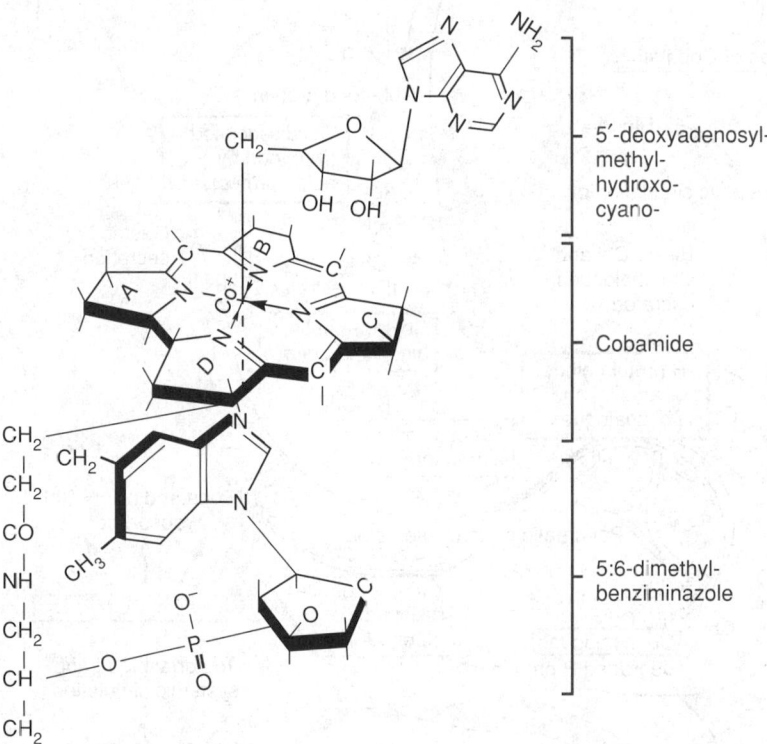

Fig. 41-1. Cobalamin chemistry and nomenclature. Vitamin B_{12}, cyanocobalamin (CN-Cbl), is a complex molecule consisting of two major portions. A planar group consisting of four reduced pyrrole rings (the corrin nucleus) is attached at right angles to an unusual nucleotide. Three of the four reduced pyrrole rings (designated A–D) are connected to one another by methylene carbon bridges; the α-carbons of rings A and D are, however, directly linked. The pyrrole rings are linked to a central cobalt atom. One coordinate position of cobalt (above the plane of the corrin nucleus) occupied by CN in CN-Cbl can be occupied by various anionic group ligands (−R) in vitro and in vivo. Substitution at this position forms the basis for the specificity of the molecule as a coenzyme in vivo. The second coordination position of the central cobalt atom (below the plane of the corrin nucleus and nearly perpendicular to it) is a linkage with the glyoxalinium nitrogen atom of the imidazole ring of the nucleotide. The nucleotide consists of a base, 5,6-dimethylbenziminazole, attached to ribose phosphate by α-glycoside linkages. The ribose is phosphorylated at C-3; the nucleotide is connected to the ring D of the corrin nucleus through an ester linkage. A compound containing a corrin nucleus is given the generic name corrinoid. The addition of cobalt to the corrin nucleus containing standard side chains gives rise to cobyrinic acid. Additional substitutions in terminal carboxyl groups or modified carboxyl groups (designated a–g) gives rise to various compounds such as cobamic acid, cobinic acid, cobamide, and cobamide. Cobamide is found in vitamin B_{12}, whose systematic name is therefore α-(5,6-dimethylbenziminazolyl)cobamide cyanide.[2,3] (From Chanarin,[2] with permission.)

was occupied by a cyano group (an artifact generated in vitro). Details of the chemistry, nomenclature, and in vivo substitutions of Cbl are shown in Figures 41-1 to 41-3 (see also Fig. 41-7), and excellent reviews are available on the history, chemistry, and biology of Cbl.[1-6] Cbl is synthesized and used by some microorganisms (e.g., bacteria, fungi).[6a] Some strains produce Cbl in excess of their requirements, making them excellent commercial sources for Cbl used in therapy (cost is approximately $60/yr/patient requiring Cbl replacement in the United States). Cbl analogues with Cbl- or anti-Cbl-like effects (due to alterations in the corrin nucleus or the nucleotide portion) are produced by microbes or pure chemical interactions of Cbl in nature or as by-products of Cbl metabolism in vivo.[5-11]

Nutrition

Cbl is produced in nature only by Cbl-producing microorganisms.[6a] Humans receive Cbl solely from the diet. Herbivores obtain their dietary quota of Cbl from plants contaminated with Cbl-producing bacteria that grow in roots and nodules of leg-

umes. Exogenous contamination of plants by feces (manure used in fertilization) may also be a source of Cbl. The ingested Cbl is used by animals for Cbl-dependent reactions in muscular and parenchymal tissues. Carnivores obtain their Cbl supply by ingesting these tissues. Cbl is produced by bacteria in the large bowel of humans, but at a site too distal for physiologic Cbl absorption.

While food Cbl is stable to high-temperature cooking processes, it can readily be converted to inactive analogues by ascorbic acid. Animal protein is the major dietary Cbl source.[12] Meats from parenchymal organs are richest in Cbl (>10 μg Cbl/100 g wet weight), while fish and animal muscle, milk products, and egg yolk have 1–10 μg/100 g wet weight. An average Western diet contains 5–7 μg/day of Cbl, which adequately sustains normal Cbl equilibrium.[13,14]

Cbl is exceptionally well stored in tissues in its coenzyme forms. Of the total body content of 2–5 mg in adults, approximately 1 mg is in the liver.[15,16] Regardless of total body Cbl content, the obligatory loss is 0.1%/day (1.3 μg).[14] It takes about 3–4 years to deplete Cbl stores when dietary Cbl is abruptly malabsorbed, but it may take longer to develop nutri-

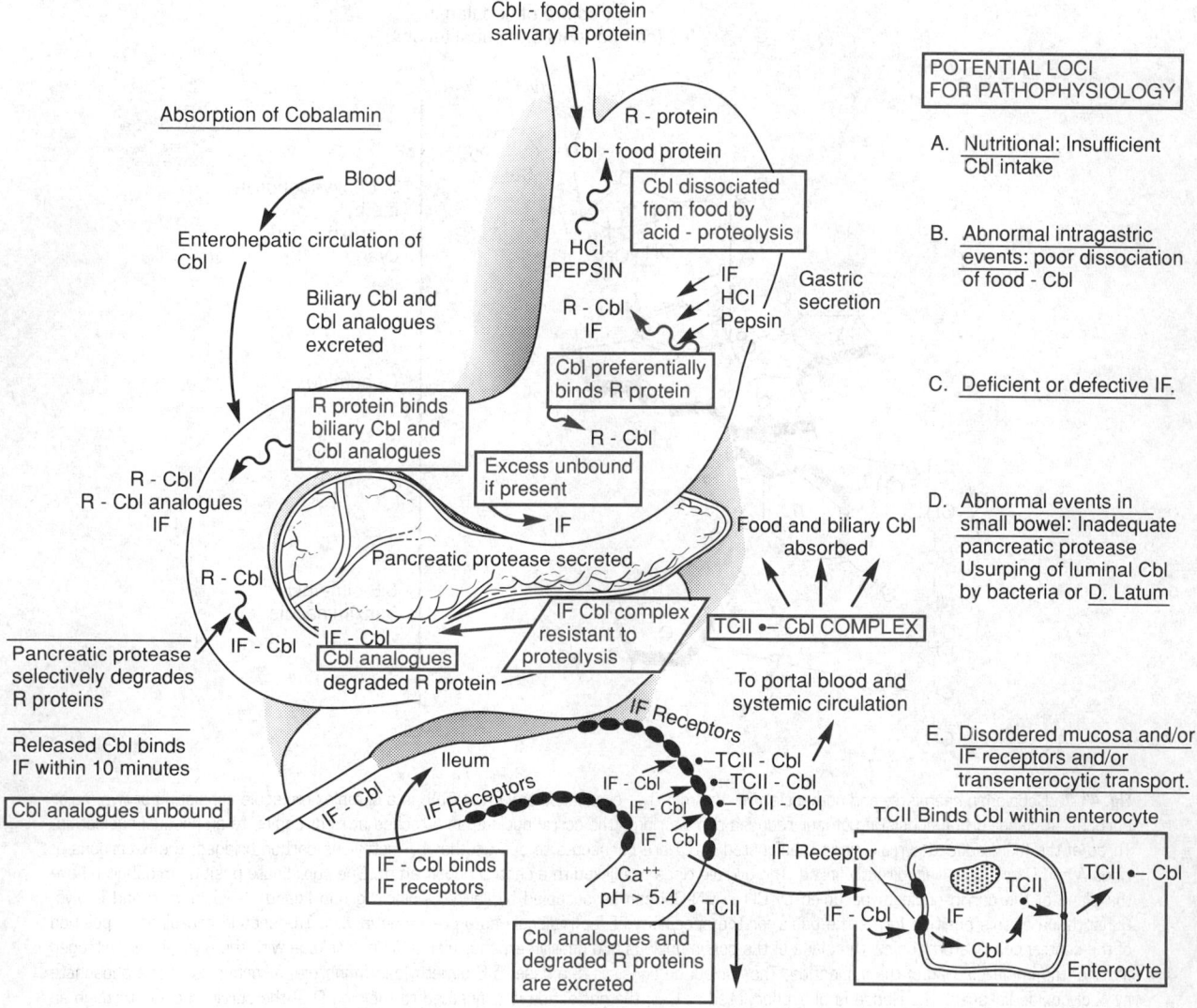

Fig. 41-2. Components and mechanism of cobalamin absorption (see text for details).

tional Cbl deficiency, owing to an efficient enterohepatic circulation,[17] which accounts for a turnover of 5–10 μg/day of Cbl.

Absorption

Cbl in food is usually in coenzyme form (5'-deoxyadenosyl Cbl [Ado-Cbl] and methylcobalamin [Me-Cbl]), nonspecifically bound to proteins (Fig. 41-2). In the stomach, peptic digestion at low pH is a prerequisite for Cbl release from food protein.[18] This is of clinical significance in the 70–80-year-old population, among whom achlorhydria is frequently present (in 25–50%), leading to inadequate release of protein-bound Cbl through proteolysis with pepsin (pepsin requires a low pH for optimum activity). While these individuals can absorb crystalline CN-Cbl[57] Co, they may be unable to absorb CN-Cbl[57] Co incorporated in vitro or in vivo into food protein.[19–22] This forms the basis for use of a modified "food Cbl" absorption test to define the mechanism of food-Cbl malabsorption in this cohort of individuals.

Once released by proteolysis, Cbl preferentially binds a high-affinity Cbl-binding protein called R protein, which migrates more rapidly on electrophoresis than the gastric Cbl-binding protein, intrinsic factor (IF).[23] Gastric juice and salivary R proteins (150-kd) have higher affinity than IF for Cbl at both acidic

and neutral pH (50-fold higher at pH 2 and 3-fold higher at pH 8). Thus, R protein (also called haptocorrin) is the preferred binding protein once Cbl is released from food.[24] Research on the cloned porcine R protein cDNA will likely reveal the structural basis for its high Cbl binding ability.[25]

The Cbl-R protein (holo-R protein) complex together with excess unbound (apo)-R protein and IF pass through into the second part of the duodenum, where pancreatic proteases degrade both holo-R and apo-R proteins, but not IF. The degradation of holo-R and apo-R proteins results in a 150-fold decrease in affinity for Cbl, with a consequent transfer of Cbl to IF within 10 minutes. Failure to degrade holo-R proteins by pancreatic protease will preclude involvement of IF in Cbl absorption, since ileal IF/Cbl receptors are specific for IF-bound Cbl and not R-bound Cbl. Indeed, 30% of patients with pancreatic insufficiency malabsorb Cbl.[24,26] This transfer of Cbl from R protein to IF is a physiologic event; once released from R protein, Cbl binds to the 45-kd glycoprotein IF with high affinity ($K_a = 1.5 \times 10^{10}$ M^{-1}), 1:1 molar stoichiometry, stability, and resistance to proteolysis over a pH range of 3–9.[23,27–29] While R proteins bind both Cbl and most Cbl analogues with comparably high affinity, IF only binds Cbl. The production of IF has been localized to the parietal (oxyntic) cells in the fundus and cardia of the stomach[27,28] in the rough endoplasmic reticulum, IF release from these cells involves membrane-associated vesicular transport, as opposed to release from secretory granules.[30] IF has two binding sites: one for Cbl and another for the ileal IF/Cbl receptor. The IF/Cbl receptor-binding site is located in the N-terminal domain of IF (at amino acid 25–62 out of 399 amino acids), while the Cbl-binding site is at the C-terminal end; glycosylation is apparently not necessary for the integrity of either of the two binding sites.[31,32] IF is produced in far greater excess than is actually required for absorption,[33] and the IF in 2–4 ml of normal gastric juice is all that is necessary to reverse Cbl deficiency in adults who lack IF. In the absence of IF, <2% of ingested Cbl is absorbed, whereas in its presence, approximately 70% is absorbed.

IF is secreted in response to food in the stomach in a manner analogous to the secretion of acid (i.e., by vagal and hormonal stimulation). There is however an unexplained subtle discordance between IF and acid secretion, since IF release is inhibited by long-term intake of H_2 blockers, but not by the alternative H^+/K^+-ATPase antagonist (gastric acid-pump inhibitor) omeprazole.[34,35] Nevertheless, omeprazole can lead to malabsorption of food Cbl through the induction of achlorhydria.[35a] IF binds both biliary Cbl and newly ingested Cbl on their transfer from R protein.[36,37] Biliary Cbl analogues are not transferred from R protein to IF, resulting in an efficient method for fecal excretion of analogues, while allowing for reabsorption of biliary Cbl. The stable IF/Cbl complex, in the form of oligomers and dimers, passes through the jejunum to the ileum, where there are membrane-associated IF/Cbl receptors for the IF/Cbl complex on microvilli of mucosal cells of the distal ileum.[38–43]

The IF/Cbl receptors from several species have been isolated. The canine IF/Cbl receptor, 220-kd, is composed of two pairs of subunits of 62-kd and 48 kd.[44] It requires Ca^{2+} for binding at pH >5.4 and does not bind free IF, Cbl, or R-Cbl and is therefore highly specific for IF/Cbl (K_a approximately 10^9 M^{-1}). This receptor contains no carbohydrate, is immunologically distinct from IF, and orients itself in artificial bilayers[45] with its ligand-binding site (for IF/Cbl) oriented to the luminal surface. The native hydrophobic species can be digested by papain to a hydrophilic form of 180–190 kd, which retains its ligand-binding site. The remaining fragment probably represents the membrane anchor of the receptor.[46] This topology differs from that of porcine and human IF/Cbl receptors, which are believed to be composed of several pairs of two types of subunit[47]; a hydrophilic pair (α) faces the lumen and is enclosed by a pair of membrane-anchored hydrophobic (β) subunits, which are attached to α-subunits by disulfide bonds. The IF/Cbl complex in dimer form apparently binds to the luminal portion of the receptor. The human ileum contains enough IF/Cbl receptors to bind ≤1 μg of IF-bound Cbl; this is the rate-limiting factor in Cbl absorption.

The events following binding of IF/Cbl to IF/Cbl receptors on enterocytes have not been fully delineated.[27,28] While transport into the cells requires energy,[48] some studies suggest that the IF/Cbl complex is first internalized by endocytosis and IF is then released from Cbl by lysosomal digestion, whereas others suggest that only Cbl, but not IF, is internalized.[48–50] Human colon adenocarcinoma cells[51] exhibit many features common to human enterocytes; they express a 280-kd IF/Cbl receptor on the apical brush border, as well as transcobalamin II (TC II) intracellularly. TC II is secreted unidirectionally across the basolateral surface, and Cbl apparently binds TC II within or at the basal surface of the ileal enterocyte.[52–54] Thus, Cbl bound to IF is transcytosed from the apical to basal direction; during transcytosis, a transfer to TC II is accomplished.[55] After a delay of 3–5 hours, Cbl appears in the portal blood largely (>90%) bound to TC II. While some of the Cbl in the enterocyte is converted to Ado-Cbl, the major portion is destined for the portal blood and reaches peak levels in about 8 hours.

Cbl in large doses can also passively diffuse through buccal, gastric, and jejunal mucosa, so that <1% of a large (>1-mg) dose appears in the circulation within minutes; this property is used to advantage in some individuals in lieu of parenteral replacement.[56,57]

Transport

More than 90% of recently absorbed or injected Cbl is bound to TC II, which is a specific transport protein for delivery of Cbl to tissues. TC II, a 38-kd polypeptide synthesized in many tissues, binds Cbl with a 1:1 molar stoichiometry and high affinity ($K_a = 1 \times 10^{11}$ M^{-1}).[23,27,28,58–62] Unlike IF, it will also bind a variety of Cbl analogues (as does R protein). It does not, however, belong to the R protein family and is immunologically distinct from two other plasma Cbl-binding R proteins, TC I and TC III. The TC II/Cbl complex is cleared so rapidly from the circulation (half-life 6–9 minutes)[63–65] that 98% of TC II in plasma is unsaturated. TC II/Cbl is rapidly bound to specific surface receptors for TC II that are present on several cells.[66–68] High-affinity TC II/Cbl binding to TC II receptors is specific only for holo- and apo-TC II ($K_a = 2$–5×10^{10} M^{-1}). (Since some Cbl analogues can bind TC II with high affinity, these also have the same potential for cellular uptake as Cbl.[69]) Once bound to TC II receptors, TC II/Cbl is internalized by receptor-mediated endocytosis.[70,71] At the low pH extant in lysosomes, TC II dissociates from Cbl; it is then degraded, while the Cbl is reduced and converted to coenzyme forms (Fig. 41-3). The importance of the transport function of TC II is underscored by the fact that TC II deficiency leads to life-threatening cellular Cbl deficiency.[72]

Cbl is not found free in plasma. Binding to TC II accounts for 10–30% of the total serum Cbl, with most of the remaining Cbl bound to the R protein TC I. TC I has an N-terminal amino acid sequence similar to that of TC III but differs from TC III by a higher content of sialic acid residues, resulting in significant differences in their rates of clearance.[23,73] Even though TC I binds 75% of the circulating Cbl (present predominantly as Me-Cbl) in fasting plasma, about one-half of the total TC I is in apo form. TC I is not a transport protein and Cbl-bound TC I has a slow clearance rate (half-life of 9–12 days).

Neither the origin nor the physiologic importance of TC I in blood has been defined. Indeed, hereditary deficiency of TC I is apparently of no clinical consequence.[74] TC I may be a plasma storage form of Cbl, since it accounts for <0.5% of total cellular Cbl uptake. With the recent molecular cloning of the TC I cDNA, new functional data should be forthcoming.[75] TC I is found in secondary granules of mature polymorphonuclear leukocytes with expression restricted to later stages of myeloid development.[76] TC III appears to have a transport function, as it is cleared from plasma within 3 minutes exclusively by hepatic asialoglycoprotein receptors, a mechanism common to a variety of asialoglycoproteins whose terminal β-galactosyl end groups are intact.[77] Conversely, desialation of TC I results in hepatic clearance identical to that of TC III. TC III is derived from specific granules of granulocytes and is released during clotting. Because of its rapid clearance, it is predominantly unsaturated. Functionally, TC III binds a wide spectrum of Cbl analogues, which are rapidly cleared by the liver into bile for fecal excretion.[23,36,37] By contrast, 0.5–9 μg of Cbl taken up by hepatic TC II receptors is secreted into bile, of which approximately 75% is reabsorbed, analogous to food Cbl.

Cellular Processing

Following TC II receptor-mediated endocytosis (Fig. 41-3) into lysosomes, the release of Cbl by lysosomal degradation of TC II is an obligatory process for further intracellular metabolism.[70,71,78,79] Following specific transport across the lysosome into the cytoplasm through a newly identified specific transport system,[80] >95% of intracellular Cbl is then bound to

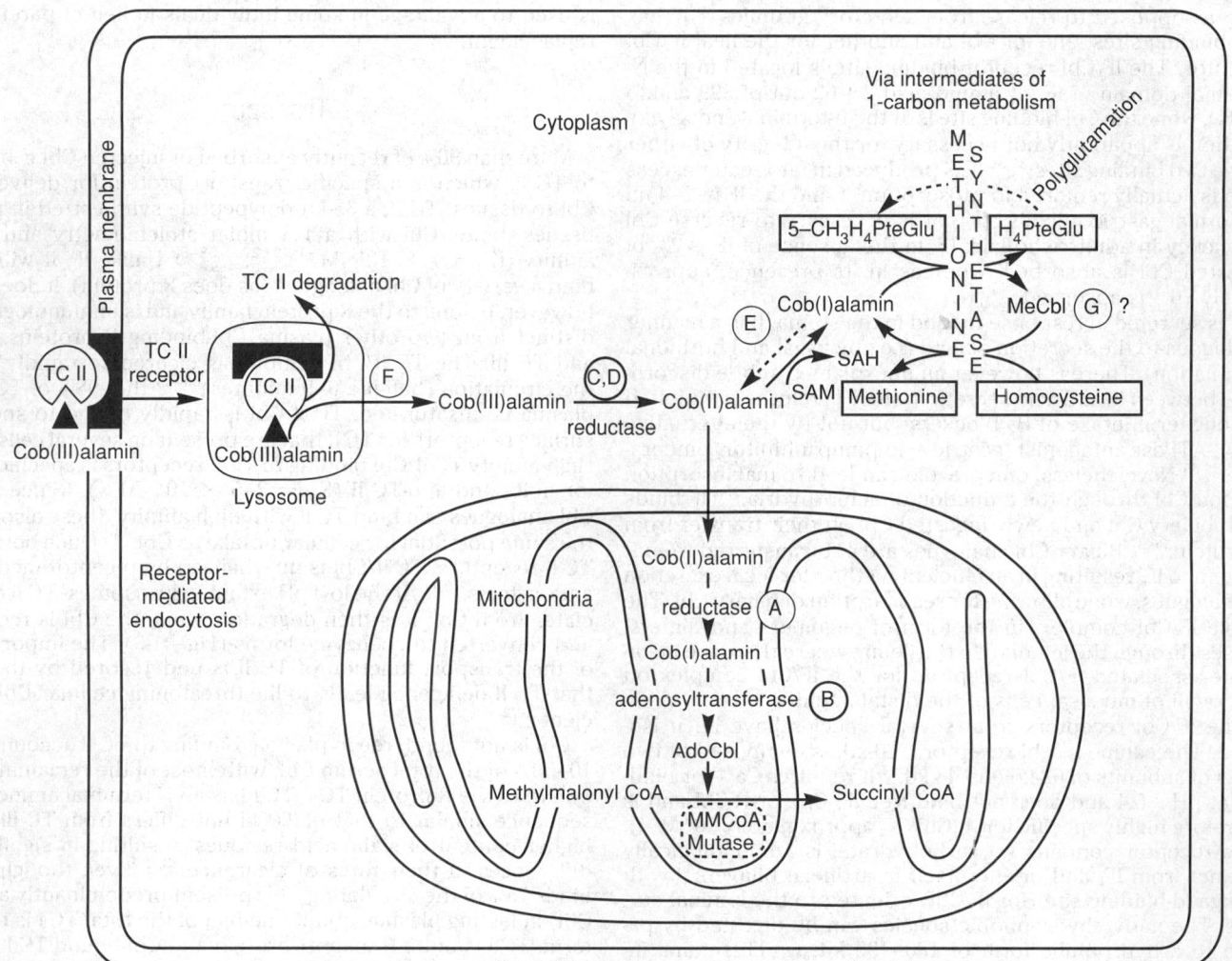

Fig. 41-3. Cellular uptake and intracellular reactions involving Cbl. A large family of natural and synthetic cobalamins can be generated when the CN moiety (the upper axial ligand in CN-Cbl) is replaced.[2,3] On exposure to light, CN is gradually lost from CN-Cbl with the production of hydroxocobalamin (hydroxo-Cbl). Another intermediate reaction is the replacement of the hydroxo group by water, resulting in the formation of aquo-Cbl. In vivo substitutions include the replacement of hydroxo-Cbl or CN-Cbl by a 5'-deoxyadenosyl group attached by a covalent bond, giving rise to Ado-Cbl. Me-Cbl is the main form in plasma. In vivo, 5-methyltetrahydrofolate readily donates its methyl group to Cob(II)alamin in a reaction involving methionine synthase to form Me-Cbl. The loci for defects in Cbl mutants *cblA–cblG* are indicated by circled letters A–G. Recent studies which indicate that Me-Cbl must be converted to Cob(II) alamin before binding and activation of human methionine synthase and other studies with the bacterial enzyme indicate that this diagram is an oversimplification.[88–90]

the two intracellular enzymes: methylmalonyl-CoA mutase and methionine synthase.[81] Studies of human cells in culture, biosynthetic studies, and inborn errors of Cbl metabolism[82–84] all suggest that Cob(III)alamin, the most "oxidized" form of Cbl, must be converted to Cob(II)alamin and Cob(I)alamin by two sequential reductase steps (Fig. 41-3).

In mitochondria, Cob(I)alamin is subsequently converted to its coenzyme form Ado-Cbl,[85] which acts as a coenzyme in the intramolecular exchange of a hydrogen attached to one carbon atom with a group attached to an adjacent carbon atom. Methylmalonyl-CoA mutase in the presence of Ado-Cbl thus converts methylmalonyl-CoA to succinyl-CoA,[86,87] thereby converting the products of propionate metabolism, (i.e., methylmalonyl-CoA) into easily metabolized products.

In the cytoplasm Cbl, as Me-Cbl, functions as a coenzyme for the reaction involving methionine synthase, which catalyzes the transfer of methyl groups from Me-Cbl to homocysteine (HCYS) to form methionine.[88–90] In this process Me-Cbl is converted to Cob(I)alamin. The methyl group of 5-methyltetrahy-

drofolate (5-Me-H₄PteGlu) is donated to Cob(I)alamin, thereby regenerating Me-Cbl; 5-Me-H₄PteGlu is thus converted to tetrahydrofolate (H₄PteGlu). Folates and Cbl are thus required together for normal one-carbon metabolism. Spontaneous oxidation of Cob(I)alamin to Cob(II)alamin requires reduction back to Cob(I)alamin before it can accept a methyl group, since the cobalt atom in Me-Cbl has a 1+ valence. Methionine synthase also catalyzes the conversion of S-adenosylmethionine to S-adenosylhomocysteine, during which the methyl group of S-adenosylmethionine may also be used for re-methylation of Cob(I)alamin. Human methionine synthase binds Cob(II)alamin with a 1:1 molar ratio and contains 2 mol of iron/1 mol of enzyme. Since Cob(II)alamin must somehow be reduced to Cob(I)alamin before a methyl group can be added to form Me-Cbl, methionine synthase and S-adenosylmethionine/S-adenosylhomocysteine together with a reducing system, may be involved in this process.[91] The physiologic importance of the key cofactor roles of the two forms of Cbl (Ado-Cbl and Me-Cbl) in methylmalonyl CoA mutase and methionine synthase, respectively, is that the products and by-products of these enzymatic reactions are critical, as discussed later, for DNA, RNA and protein biosynthesis.

FOLATES

Nutrition

Folates (Fig. 41-4), are widely distributed in nature in reduced and polyglutamated forms.[92] They are synthesized by microorganisms and plants. Leafy vegetables (spinach, lettuce, broccoli, beans), fruits (bananas, melons, lemons), yeast, mushrooms, and animal protein (liver, kidney) are rich sources of folate.[93,94] Folates are extremely thermolabile; prolonged cooking (>15 minutes) in large quantities of water in the absence of reducing agents destroys folates. Oxidation of food folate by nitrites reduces its bioavailability.[95] Since some organisms require exogenous folate for growth, bacteriologic methods (using *Lactobacillus casei*) have been a mainstay for measuring the folate content of food and tissues. The minimum daily requirement of folate is 50 μg; the recommended daily intake for folate is 3 μg/kg/day (approximate intakes: adults 100 μg,

children 50 μg, pregnancy 500 μg, and lactation 300 μg).[96] A balanced Western diet contains adequate amounts of folate, but the net dietary intake of folate in the developing countries is often insufficient to sustain folate balance.[97]

Absorption

Pteroylpolyglutamates (PteGlu$_n$) are absorbed less efficiently than pteroylmonoglutamate (PteGlu). Although folates in some foods (cabbage, lettuce, orange) are not well absorbed,[98–100] most other dietary folates are nutritionally available (bioavailable). Pteroylpolyglutamates are hydrolyzed to their pteroylmonoglutamate derivatives by the enzyme pteroylpolyglutamate hydrolase in the brush-border membranes of small intestinal cells.[101] This enzyme, composed of two polypeptides of 145 and 115 kd, displays maximal exopeptidase activity at pH 5.5 in the presence of zinc, with equal affinity for pteroylpolyglutamates of different glutamate chain lengths, and is essential for hydrolyzing dietary folates before absorption.[102]

Luminal pteroylglutamate interacts with brush-border membrane-associated folate-binding moieties,[103] vaguely resembling folate-binding proteins and folate receptors that mediate cellular folate uptake (discussed below); however, their pre-

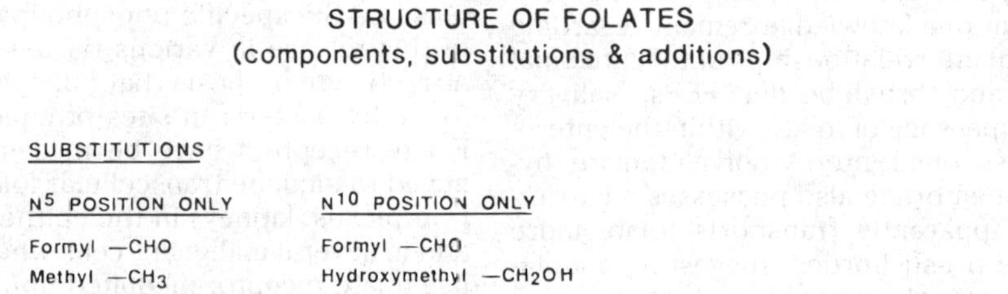

STRUCTURE OF FOLATES
(components, substitutions & additions)

Fig. 41-4. Folate chemistry and nomenclature. Folic acid (PteGlu) is the commercially available parent compound for >100 compounds collectively referred to as folates.[2,304] PteGlu consists of three basic components: (1) a pteridine derivative, (2) a *p*-aminobenzoic residue and, (3) an L-glutamic acid residue. Before PteGlu can play a role as a coenzyme, it must first be reduced at positions 7 and 8 to dihydrofolic acid (H$_2$PteGlu) and then to 5,6,7,8-tetrahydrofolic acid (H$_4$PteGlu); one to six additional glutamic acid residues must then be added via γ-peptide bonds to the L-glutamate moiety. Folate coenzymes either donate or accept 1-carbon units in numerous reactions in amino acid and nucleotide metabolism. The various substitutions in H$_4$PteGlu$_{(n)}$ occur either at positions 5 or 10, or both; thus, position 5 can be substituted by methyl (CH$_3$), formyl (CHO), or formimino (CHNH), while position 10 can be substituted by formyl or hydroxymethyl (CH$_2$OH). Positions 5 and 10 can be bridged by methylene (—CH$_2$—) or methenyl (—CH—).

cise role in mediating transport through intestinal cells is still unclear. They exhibit rapid equilibrium binding (<5 minutes), pH dependency (pH 5 optimal), high affinity (K_d approximately 0.08 μM), and saturability. There is broad specificity for binding pteroyltriglutamate, 5-Me-H_4PteGlu, and other folate derivatives, and binding capacity is enhanced by physiologic (luminal) concentrations of zinc,[104–110] and transport of reduced-folates occurs within seconds in human brush-border membrane vesicles.[136] Jejunal transport sharply increases with decreasing extravesicular pH from 7 to 5 while intravesicular pH is still 7, supporting its physiologic relevance. The pH effect is probably multifactorial, involving the transporting carrier and PteGlu$^-$:OH$^-$ exchange or PteGlu$^-$:H$^+$ transport; it is not observed in the ileum.

Ingested human milk, which contains specific folate-binding proteins (FBPs),[111] probably regulates the nutritional bioavailability of ingested folate in neonates by binding with, and thereby decreasing, folate transport in the jejunum.[112] In the ileum, however, there is no alteration in transport between FBP-bound folate relative to free folate. The net result is a more gradual rise in plasma folate level, leading to slower urinary excretion. This finding was borne out by a clinical study that indicated that breast-fed infants had higher tissue folate levels at 6 months than those weaned at <2 months of age.[113] Another effect of milk FBPs may be to withhold folate uptake by folate-requiring intestinal bacteria. Although FBP-bound folate appears to be transported by the same transport system as free folate, considerable gaps in our knowledge remain regarding the structure and functional interrelationships of the intestinal folate transport carrier and brush-border FBPs, salivary FBPs,[114] the mechanism of passage of folate within the enterocyte, and the role of lysosomal pteroylpolyglutamate hydrolases. The basolateral membrane also possesses a carrier-mediated system, which apparently transports folate more efficiently than that in the brush border, suggesting adaptation for eventual transport into the portal blood.[115]

Passive diffusion of folate (M_r 441) across the intestinal mucosa is probably the primary mechanism of folate absorption at high pharmacologic concentrations.[116,117] Within this context, the small intestine has a large capacity to absorb folate; a substantial enterohepatic circulation amounts to approximately 90 μg/day of folate.[118] Peak folate levels in plasma are achieved 1–2 hours after oral administration. While therapeutically administered PteGlu enters the portal blood unchanged, food PteGlu$_{(n)}$ is hydrolyzed before transport into the enterocyte, where they are completely reduced to H_4PteGlu and methylated to 5-Me-H_4PteGlu before release into plasma.

Transport and Enterohepatic Circulation

The normal serum folate level is maintained by dietary folate and an intact enterohepatic circulation.[118] Folates are rapidly cleared from plasma (≤95% in 3 minutes) by tissues, including the liver. Transport of 5-Me-H_4PteGlu into isolated hepatocytes and basolateral membrane vesicles is through a concentrative process via co-transport with H$^+$ ions and is electroneutral and inhibited by other natural folates.[119] Biliary drainage results in a dramatic fall in serum folate (approximately 30% of basal levels within 6 hours), while abrupt interruption of dietary folate leads to a fall in serum folate levels within about 3 weeks. In the plasma, one-third of the folate is free, while two-thirds is nonspecifically and loosely bound to serum proteins such as albumin. A small amount of folate is specifically bound to high-affinity intrinsically soluble hydrophilic 40-kd FBPs; the physiologic significance of this interaction is not clear.[120,121] In contrast to Cbl uptake, no specific serum transport protein has been found to enhance cellular folate uptake.

Cellular Folate Uptake

Serum 5-Me-H_4PteGlu specifically interacts with a family of cell-surface membrane-associated 44-kd folate receptors before transport into the cell. The biologic chemistry of folate receptors has recently been reviewed.[122] These externally oriented hydrophobic glycoproteins are attached to the plasma membrane by either a short hydrophobic polypeptide tail or a glycosylphosphatidylinositol (GPI) anchor.[123,124] They bind folate with 1 : 1 molar stoichiometry and high affinity with dissociation constants K_d (in the nanomolar range), in the range needed for binding serum folates. Folate receptors are true receptors[122] in that they first bind and then transport folate intracellularly into both malignant[125,126] and normal hematopoietic progenitor cells.[127–129] GPI-anchored folate receptors transfer folate intracellularly by a mechanism involving non-clathrin-coated pits known as caveolae.[130] Folate is believed to be dissociated from folate receptors at acid pH generated within caveolae by a proton pump and is transported through a putative folate transporter into the cytoplasm, while apo-folate receptors recycle back to the surface to bind more folate (Figs. 41-5 and 41-6). In other cells, folate receptor-mediated endocytotic mechanisms have been documented as well.[131,132]

Folate receptors are precursors to the small amounts of soluble (40-kd) hydrophilic FBPs released extracellularly.[111,133–138] Conversion to hydrophilic FBPs is mediated by a specific endogenous hydrophobic folate receptor-directed metalloprotease or GPI-specific phospholipases C/D.[122] The significance of this release in various tissues remains to be defined. The attractive hypothesis that FBPs assist in preventing uptake of folate by bacteria in sites of infection remains to be proved. Folate receptors have been identified in several tissues believed to mediate transcellular folate transport (placenta, choroid plexus, kidney) in the epithelial cells of secretory glands and in several malignant cells where these tissues presumably use folate receptor-mediated uptake mechanisms for intracellular folate delivery.[122,139–144] Folate receptors are up- and down-regulated in response to extra- and intracellular folate concentrations in some cells,[145] but the precise mechanism(s) underlying regulation in most other tissues remain(s) unclear. The functional role of folate receptors in mediating folate uptake has been shown extensively in vitro[122]; while they probably play an important role in vivo, this remains to be shown directly.

A second mechanism for folate uptake, primarily demonstrated in malignant cells, appears to be due to a carrier-mediated pH- and energy-dependent process, which transports reduced folates equally efficiently at higher than physiologic concentrations[146–148] (Fig. 41-5). The relative importance of folate receptors and of this other reduced-folate carrier-mediated transport system and their interrelationship in mediating physiologic folate uptake requires further clarification (Fig. 41-5).

Findings of several recent studies merit mention: (1) folate receptor overexpression allows cells to tolerate growth in low folate medium[149,150]; (2) distinct isoforms of folate receptors have been identified with subtle differences in binding of various folates, including the newest generation of antifolates, which enter cells through folate receptors, targeting several of the enzymes involved in one-carbon metabolism (Fig. 41-6) (the implication is that manipulation of cellular expression of folate receptor isoforms may influence specificity of antifolate uptake and achieve greater therapeutic effect while reducing toxicity in normal cells[151]); (3) in malignant cells, the folate receptor-mediated and reduced-folate carrier neither interact with nor influence the uptake of folate through the other system (i.e., cross-talk is lacking)[152]; (4) folate receptor overexpression increases the sensitivity of some malignant cells to antifolates[153]; and (5) one of the mechanisms of antifolate resistance is a transport defect mediated by reduced-folate receptor expression on the cell surface.[154] Collectively, these interesting stud-

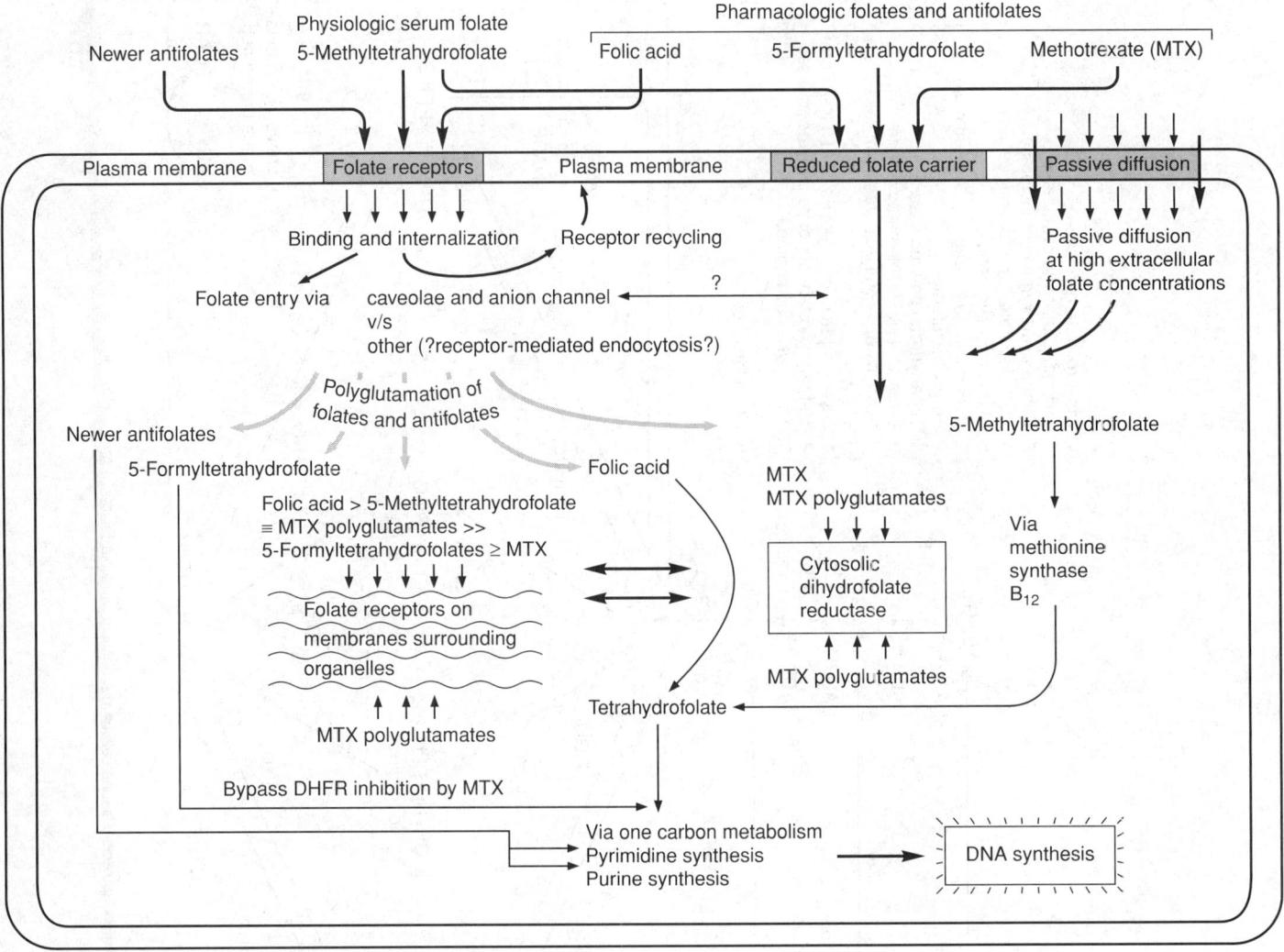

Fig. 41-5. Pathways for the entry and intracellular disposition of physiologic and pharmacologic folates and antifolates. The participation of each of the components involved in folate uptake is distinct in different cells, depending on (1) the relative efficiency of folate receptor-mediated and reduced-folate carrier-mediated mechanisms, (2) the basal intracellular content of folate receptors and folates, as well as (3) the extracellular concentration of folates and antifolates. The reduced-folate carrier has not been definitively shown to exist in normal human cells. (From Antony,[122] with permission.)

ies indicate that folate receptor-mediated uptake will be exploited in future therapy with antifolates.[122] Moreover, folate receptor cDNAs have been cloned from several tissues,[155–159] and studies aimed at cloning the reduced-folate carrier gene (transporter)[160,160a] promise to clarify the biochemical basis for several of these and related issues.

Cellular Retention and Excretion

Polyglutamation of folate is the major factor for intracellular retention,[161–163] and the interaction of these forms with intracellular membrane-associated folate receptors may also play a role[122,133,164] (Fig. 41-5). As a corollary, human malignant cells with reduced folyl polyglutamate synthase are resistant to antifolates, which cannot be (polyglutamated and) retained intracellularly.[165] In the human erythrocyte, folate is accumulated at earlier stages within the marrow by folate receptors[128]; on maturation, >90% of PteGlu(n) molecules interact with hemoglobin, which, due to its high capacity, assists in intracellular folate retention.[166] Red blood cell (RBC) folates are not significantly influenced by the serum folate level; therefore, RBC folate levels provide a measure of folate stores, which correlate

with hepatic folate stores.[2,6,167,168] Intracellular folate receptors probably influence intracellular folate metabolism by binding 5-Me-H_4PteGlu, as well as by competing with dihydrofolate reductase for binding polyglutamates (Fig. 41-5). The attenuating effect on methotrexate cytotoxicity in vitro by high pre-existing extracellular folate concentrations[164] is attributed to the fact that folates can also passively diffuse into cells.[129] This is potentially significant for protocols involving high-dose (suprapharmacologic) folate analogue therapy.[169]

INTRACELLULAR METABOLISM AND COBALAMIN/FOLATE INTERRELATIONSHIPS

Pteroylpolyglutamates are the natural substrates for the various enzymes involved in one-carbon metabolism (Figs. 41-5 and 41-6). Thus, pteroylmonoglutamates must be polyglutamated by folyl polyglutamate synthase before they participate in one-carbon metabolism.[161] This is best appreciated in mutant Chinese hamster ovary cells, which lack folyl polyglutamate synthase.[162] As a consequence of failure in polyglutamation, these cells have <10% of the intracellular folate content of wild-type cells, as well as an inability to generate reactions

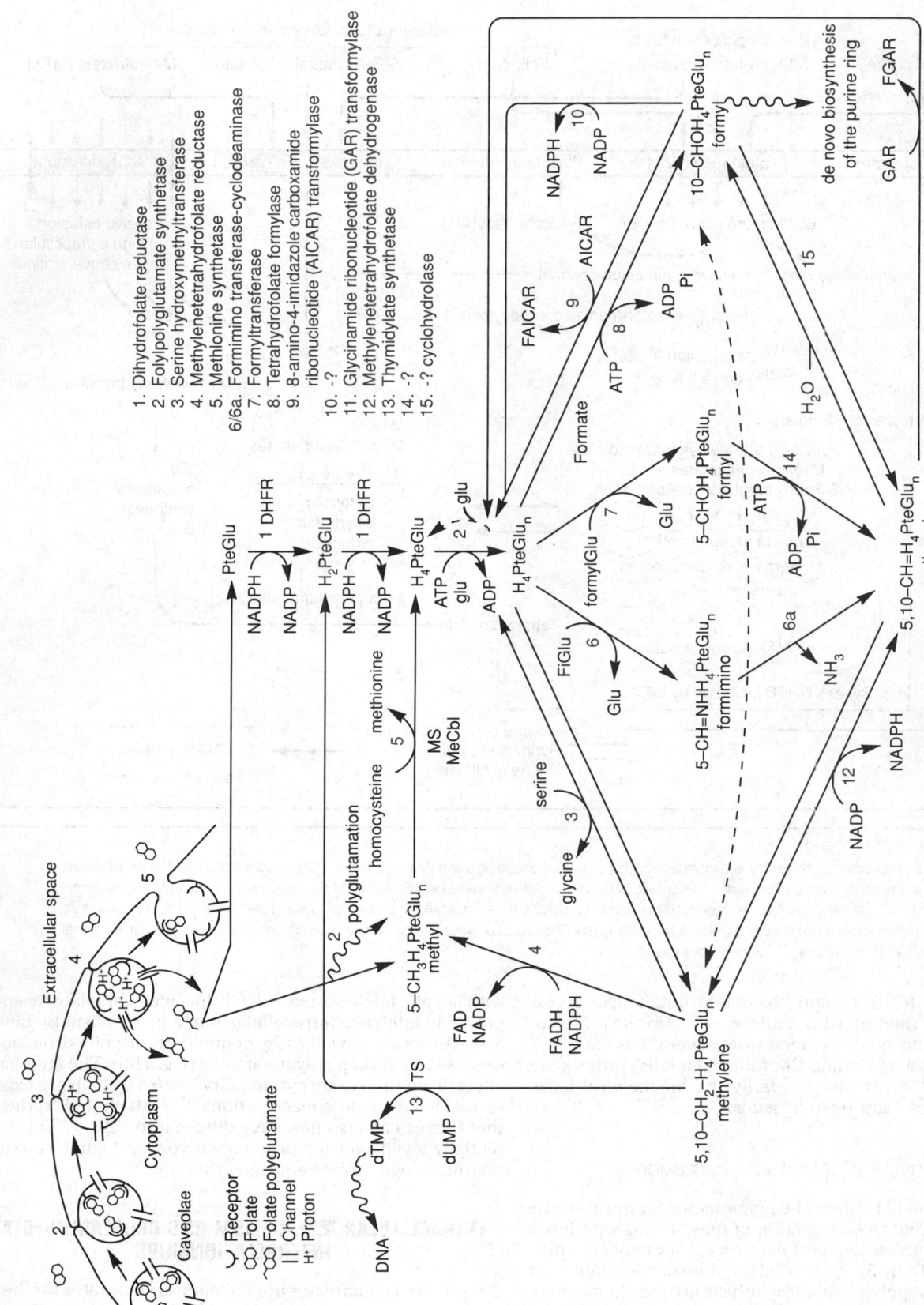

Fig. 41-6. Folate receptor-coupled folate uptake and intracellular one-carbon metabolism involving folates. (See text for details.) [Data from Shane and Stokstad[163] and from Rothberg et al.[442]]

1. Dihydrofolate reductase
2. Folylpolyglutamate synthetase
3. Serine hydroxymethyltransferase
4. Methylenetetrahydrofolate reductase
5. Methionine synthetase
6/6a. Formimino transferase-cyclodeaminase
7. Formyltransferase
8. Tetrahydrofolate formylase
9. 8-amino-4-imidazole carboxamide ribonucleotide (AICAR) transformylase
10. -?
11. Glycinamide ribonucleotide (GAR) transformylase
12. Methylenetetrahydrofolate dehydrogenase
13. Thymidylate synthetase
14. -?
15. -? cyclohydrolase

of one-carbon metabolism. The mutant cells therefore require that the products of one-carbon metabolism (methionine, glycine, purines, and thymidine) be exogenously supplied. By contrast, wild-type cells can grow as long as adequate folate, Cbl, and HCYS are available, since they can synthesize their own folate polyglutamates, which then participate in one-carbon metabolism and generate these substances intracellularly.

$H_4PteGlu$ is the preferred substrate for folyl polyglutamate synthase; the polyglutamal form of tetrahydrofolate ($H_4PteGlu_n$) plays a central role in one-carbon metabolism.[163] Thus, factors that either limit the supply of $H_4PteGlu$ or that regulate folyl polyglutamate synthase would influence polyglutamation and cellular retention of folates. As the physiologic substrate for folyl polyglutamate synthase, $H_4PteGlu_n$ can be converted to (1) formate as 10-formyl-$H_4PteGlu$ (used in de novo biosynthesis of purines), and (2) formaldehyde as 5,10-methylene-$H_4PteGlu$ (for synthesis of thymidylate). Furthermore, 5,10-methylene-$H_4PteGlu$ and 10-formyl-$H_4PteGlu$ can be interconverted by intermediates.

In order to understand the functions of folate coenzymes (Figs. 41-4 and 41-6), it is important to recognize at the outset that 5,10-methylene-$H_4PteGlu$ can be used in either (1) the thymidylate cycle by means of thymidylate synthase for thymidine and DNA synthesis, or (2) the methylation cycle to form 5-Me-$H_4PteGlu$, which, by means of methionine synthase, leads to formation of methionine and $H_4PteGlu$. Both methionine and $H_4PteGlu$ are essential (1) for polyglutamate formation (hence for retention of folates and perpetuation of normal one-carbon metabolism), and (2) for the interconversion to 5,10-methylene-$H_4PteGlu$ (essential for DNA synthesis). Thus, perturbation of either pathway, directly or indirectly, affects DNA synthesis. Thymidylate synthase- and methionine synthase-catalyzed reactions, coupled with the factors that control them through product inhibition, are central issues in protection from megaloblastosis. Additional reactions catalyzed by folate coenzymes involve amino acid interconversions and purine synthesis.[1,2,163,170]

Pteroylmonoglutamate (PteGlu, folic acid) is not a biologically active form of folate; when given therapeutically, it requires reduction to $H_4PteGlu$ by dihydrofolate reductase (M_r 20,000) in a two-step reaction (pteroylglutamate [PteGlu] → dihydropteroylglutamate [$H_2PteGlu$] → tetrahydropteroylglutamate [$H_4PteGlu$]). The major form of folate transported into the cell by folate receptors is 5-methyl-$H_4PteGlu$ (Figs. 41-5 and 41-6). The details of intracellular 5-methyl-$H_4PteGlu$ movement in the cytoplasm and the precise order of channeling of folate along reactions by enzymes involved in one-carbon metabolism are not entirely clear. However, evidence suggests that folate-mediated one-carbon metabolism is indeed compartmentalized among intracellular organelles, leading to substrate channeling along folate coenzymes; this has been reviewed recently.[171] For example, some of the enzymes "distal" to $H_4PteGlu$ are multifunctional, permitting sequential channeling of folate coenzyme forms (e.g., $H_4PteGlu$ → 5-CHNH-$H_4PteGlu$ → 5,10-CH = $H_4PteGlu$). Thymidylate synthase catalyzes the transfer of the formaldehyde from 5,10-methylene-$H_4PteGlu$ to the 5-position of deoxyuridylate; in this process, 5,10-methylene-$H_4PteGlu$ is also reduced to dihydrofolate, which inhibits 5,10-methylene-$H_4PteGlu$ reductase (Fig. 41-7). Methionine, the product of the methionine synthase reaction, also inhibits this enzyme, illustrating that modulation of 5,10-methylene-$H_4PteGlu$ reductase by levels of dihydrofolate and methionine can determine the degree of channeling of 5,10-methylene-$H_4PteGlu$ into the methylation and thymidylate cycle[163,171] (Figs. 41-6 and 41-7).

The mechanism whereby Cbl deficiency produces its megaloblastic effects is not precisely known. It is generally agreed that Cbl deficiency causes a functional intracellular deficiency of 5,10-methylene-$H_4PteGlu$ (Fig. 41-7). The "methylfolate trap"[172,173] hypothesis centers around the excess buildup (trapping) of 5-methyl-$H_4PteGlu$ due to inhibition of the Cbl-dependent methionine synthase; the result is that 5-methyl-$H_4PteGlu$ leaks out of the cell, causing an intracellular folate deficiency. The "formate starvation" hypothesis centers around the relatively greater merit of formate (in the form of 10-formyl-$H_4PteGlu$) and the precursor of formate, methionine, which is also decreased when methionine synthase is inhibited by cobalamin deficiency.[174] When methionine is in excess intracellularly, its methyl group is oxidized to formate, which can be used to generate 5-formyl- and 10-formyl-$H_4PteGlu$ (reactions 7 and 8, Fig. 41-6). Excellent articles are available supporting either hypothesis.[163,168,170,172–178]

CONSEQUENCES OF PERTURBED ONE-CARBON METABOLISM

Thymidylate and DNA Synthesis

In either Cbl or folate deficiency, a net decrease in 5,10-methylene-$H_4PteGlu$ interrupts the reaction mediated by thymidylate synthase, which converts deoxyuridine monophosphate (dUMP) to deoxythymidine monophosphate (dTMP).[181,182] Although a salvage pathway via thymidine kinase normally accounts for 5–10% of thymidine synthesis,[183,184] this pathway cannot meet the remaining 90% demand for dTMP generation. (Salvage pathways for purine synthesis can be activated to compensate for diminished generation of purines through folate coenzyme-mediated reactions.) The resulting thymidine deficiency leads to a marked increase in the dUMP/dTMP ratio. Because of the decrease in dTMP, and eventually deoxythymidine triphosphate (dTTP), the result is an increase in dUMP, and thereby deoxyuridine triphosphate (dUTP). Since DNA polymerase cannot distinguish between dUTP and dTTP, this elevated dUTP promotes misincorporation of uridine residues into DNA. An editorial enzyme, DNA uracil glycosylase, recognizes this faulty misincorporation. It excises dUTP, but the inadequate supply of dTTP leads to a failure to repair the break in this DNA strand. Repeated DNA strand breaks lead to significant fragmentation of DNA, with consequent leakage of DNA fragments out of the cell.[185–191]

The foregoing considerations form the basis for the deoxyuridine (dU) suppression test, which is employed clinically.[184] When cells containing normal dUMP/dTMP ratios are incubated with [^{3}H]thymidine and excess unlabeled dU, <10% of [^{3}H]thymidine is incorporated into DNA (by the salvage thymidine kinase pathway), since most of the unlabeled dU is used by thymidylate synthase to form dTMP. If the dUMP/dTMP ratio is increased (as in Cbl deficiency), unlabeled dU will not be used, and >10% of [^{3}H]thymidine is incorporated into DNA. The addition of Cbl (but not 5-Me-$H_4PteGlu$) to another aliquot of these cells will lead to conversion of endogenous (and unlabeled) dUMP to dTMP; the net result is less [^{3}H]thymidine incorporation into DNA through the salvage pathway. The addition of 5-Me-$H_4PteGlu$ will facilitate conversion of dUMP to dTMP in folate-deficient cells but will have no effect in Cbl deficiency. Although this method of testing does not simply represent thymidylate synthase-catalyzed pathways but affects additional pathways involving nucleotide metabolism,[192] the reduction of previously increased [^{3}H]thymidine incorporation in Cbl- or folate-deficient cells by the addition of exogenous Cbl or folate, respectively, has been useful in differentiating Cbl deficiency from folate deficiency; this is the principle of the diagnostic dU suppression test.[184] The modified diagnostic dU suppression test is useful in the clinical setting of suspected inborn errors of Cbl/folate metabolism or when coincident iron deficiency or thalassemia masks the megaloblastic expression,[6,193]

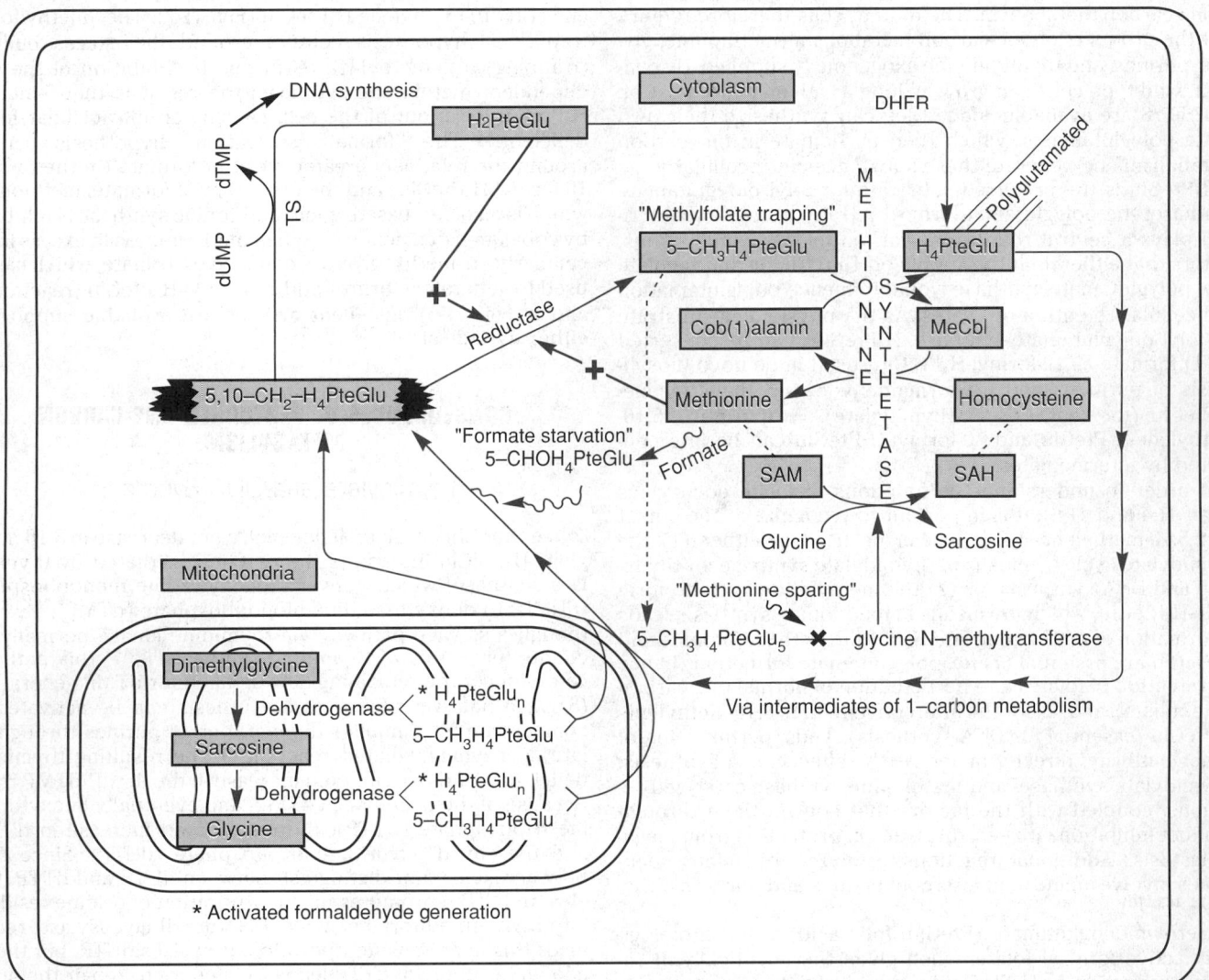

Fig. 41-7. Major pathways involving Cbl/folate interrelationships. Intramitochondrial dehydrogenases[179] that preferentially bind $H_4PteGlu_5$ provide activated formaldehyde (via dimethylglycine → sarcosine → glycine). The activated formaldehyde reacts nonenzymatically with the enzyme-bound $H_4PteGlu_5$ to form $5,10\text{-}CH_2\text{-}H_4PteGlu$ for methionine synthase and thymidylate synthase. Another cytosolic dehydrogenase (glycine N-methyltransferase) that synthesizes sarcosine in the presence of S-adenosylmethionine from glycine (with conversion of S-adenosylmethionine to S-adenosylHCYS) is activated on phosphorylation but is allosterically inhibited by (trapped and polyglutamated) $5\text{-}CH_3H_4PteGlu_5$ in Cbl deficiency. This effect of $5\text{-}CH_3H_4PteGlu_5$ may lead to methionine sparing; the methionine could in turn inhibit the formation of more $5\text{-}CH_3H_4PteGlu$ from $5,10\text{-}CH_2H_4PteGlu$ and channel the latter for DNA synthesis. Alternatively, phosphorylation of glycine N-methyltransferase itself may provide a mechanism for modulation of enzymatic activity.[180] Nevertheless, this is an area in which the methylfolate trap and formate starvation hypotheses are conceivably closely interrelated.

although measurement of metabolites indicative of Cbl/folate deficiency are now available for routine clinical use (see below) and may supplant the dU suppression test.

Chromosomal and Cell-Cycle Defects

Defective DNA synthesis[194] is reflected by numerous chromosomal abnormalities. Excessive chromosomal elongation with despiralization is present, associated with random breaks and exaggerated centromere constriction, expression of folate-sensitive fragile sites in hematopoietic cells, as well as reduced biosynthesis, acetylation, and methylation of arginine-rich histone.[182,195-200] This leads to perturbation of the cell cycle with an increased proportion of cells in prophase of the mitotic cycle and G_2. This arrest in various stages of DNA synthesis causes many cells to have DNA contents of 2–4N.[201-204]

Morphologic Expression of Megaloblastosis

Widening disparity in nuclear/cytoplasmic asynchrony is displayed as a Cbl- or folate-deficient cell divides, until the more mature generations of daughter cells either die in the marrow or are arrested (as megaloblastic cells) at various stages in the cell cycle.[202-206] In fact, the plethora of bone marrow morphologic changes may lead the untrained observer to entertain the diagnosis of acute leukemia.[207] All proliferating cells exhibit megaloblastosis, including epithelial cells lining the gastrointestinal tract (buccal mucosa, tongue, small intestine), cervix, vagina, and uterus.[208-212] However, megaloblastic changes are most striking in the blood and bone marrow. Ineffective hematopoiesis extends into the long bones, and the bone marrow aspirate (which is superior to the biopsy for observing megaloblastosis) exhibits trilineal hypercellularity, especially in the erythroid series. In contrast to what appears as exuberant cell

---

MORPHOLOGY IN MEGALOBLASTOSIS FROM Cbl AND FOLATE DEFICIENCY IS THE SAME

Peripheral smear
   Increased MCV with macroovalocytes ($\leq$14 μm)[a]
   Nuclear hypersegmentation of PMNs (1 PMN with 6 lobes or 5% with 5 lobes)
   Thrombocytopenia (mild to moderate)
   Leukoerythroblastic morphology (from extramedullary hematopoiesis)
Bone marrow aspirate
   General increase in cellularity of all three major hematopoietic elements
   Abnormal erythropoiesis—orthochromatic megaloblasts
   Abnormal leukopoiesis—giant metamyelocytes and "band" forms (pathognomonic), hypersegmented PMNs
   Abnormal megakaryocytopoiesis—pseudohyperdiploidy

---

[a] Associated with varying anisocytosis and poikilocytosis.

---

proliferation with numerous mitotic figures, the cells are actually very slowly proliferating. However, megaloblastosis induced in vitro by antifolate receptor antibodies causes a true increase in cell proliferative capacity initiated at the level of cell-surface folate receptors, suggesting a constitutive control of folate receptors in hematopoietic cell proliferation.[122,128,129,213] Erythroid hyperplasia reduces the myeloid/erythroid ratio from 3:1 to 1:1. Proerythroblasts are not as obviously abnormal as later forms; they may simply be larger (promegaloblasts). Megaloblastic changes are most strikingly displayed in intermediate and orthochromatic stages, which are larger than their normoblastic counterparts. In contrast to the normally dense chromatin of comparable normoblasts, megaloblastic erythroid precursors have an open, finely stippled, reticular, sieve-like pattern. The orthochromatic megaloblast, with its hemoglobinized cytoplasm, continues to retain its large sieve-like immature nucleus, in sharp contrast to the clumped chromatin of orthochromatic normoblasts. The nucleus is often eccentrically placed in these large oval or oblong cells; lobulation or indentation of nuclei with bizarre karyorrhexis is often seen. In those cells destined for the circulation as macroovalocytes, the nucleus occasionally is not completely extruded. Of the potential progeny of proerythroblasts that develop into later megaloblastic forms, 80–90% die in the bone marrow. Marrow macrophages effectively scavenge dead/partially disintegrated megaloblasts. This is the basis for ineffective erythropoiesis (intramedullary hemolysis).

Leukopoiesis is also abnormal. There is an absolute increase in these cells, which are large and have similar sieve-like chromatin. Spectacular giant (20–30-μm) metamyelocytes and "band" forms are often seen; these are pathognomonic for megaloblastosis. Bizarre nucleoli with small cytoplasmic vacuoles may be seen. It is probable that giant metamyelocytes cannot easily traverse marrow sinuses and their maturation into circulating hypersegmented polymorphonuclear neutrophils (PMNs) is unlikely. Granulation of the cytoplasm remains unaffected.

Megakaryocytes may be normal or increased in numbers and may exhibit additional complexities in megaloblastic expression.[214] The process of complex hypersegmentation (pseudohyperdiploidy) is associated with liberation of fragments of cytoplasm and giant platelets into the circulation. The net output of platelets is invariably decreased in severe megaloblastosis and abnormal, but reversible platelet dysfunction has been documented.[215]

In early Cbl or folate deficiency, normoblasts may dominate the marrow, with only a few megaloblasts seen. Complete transformation to megaloblastic hematopoiesis is observed in florid cases and is reflected by pancytopenia of varying degrees. The earliest manifestation of megaloblastosis is an increase in mean corpuscular volume (MCV) with macro-ovalocytes ($\leq$14 μm). Since these cells have adequate hemoglobin, the central pallor, which normally occupies about one-third of the cell, is decreased. In severe anemia, poikilocytosis and anisocytosis are evident. Cells containing remnants of DNA (Howell-Jolly bodies), arginine-rich histone, and nonhemoglobin iron (Cabot rings) may be observed. Extramedullary megaloblastic hematopoiesis may also result in a leukoerythroblastic picture.

Ineffective use of iron results in an increased percentage saturation of transferrin and increased iron stores. If there is associated iron deficiency, the MCV may be normal; only iron therapy will unmask the megaloblastic manifestations in the peripheral blood. In thalassemia, the entire erythrocyte morphology normally expected in megaloblastosis is masked[216,217]; however, megaloblastic leukopoiesis is still observed. Significant intramedullary hemolysis (ineffective erythropoiesis) involving >90% of megaloblastic precursors is reflected by a lowered absolute reticulocyte count, increased bilirubin ($\leq$2 mg/dl), decreased haptoglobin, and increased lactate dehydrogenase (LDH), often >1,000 U/ml. Circulating RBCs also show a modest decrease in life span.

Nuclear hypersegmentation of DNA in PMNs strongly suggests megaloblastosis when associated with macro-ovalocytosis. Normally, <5% of PMNs have more than five lobes, and no cells have more than six lobes in the peripheral blood. If megaloblastosis is suspected (>5% PMNs with more than five lobes or a single PMN with more than six lobes), a formal lobe count per PMN (lobe index) of >3.5 may be obtained.[5] Megaloblastosis in rapidly proliferating cells of the gastrointestinal tract leads to a variable degree of morphologic changes and atrophy of the epithelial cells of the luminal lining. This leads to functional defects, which include a failure in secretion of IF and malabsorption of Cbl and folate in certain subsets of patients, establishing a vicious circle whereby megaloblastosis begets more megaloblastosis. It can only be interrupted by specific therapy with Cbl or folate. This fact must be recognized when interpreting diagnostic tests involving Cbl absorption (discussed below). Similar hematopoietic changes have been induced in a folate-deficient mouse model recently.[218]

Neurologic Dysfunction with Cobalamin Deficiency

Since megaloblastosis due to either folate or Cbl deficiency leads to a functional folate coenzyme deficiency, the morphologic manifestations of both deficiencies are understandably indistinguishable. However, only Cbl deficiency results in a patchy demyelination process, which is expressed clinically as cerebral abnormalities and subacute combined degeneration of the spinal cord.[219]

The precise role of Cbl in maintaining the integrity of the central nervous system has not been completely defined. Early studies of the Cbl-dependent enzyme, methylmalonyl-CoA mutase, demonstrated that the inability to metabolize propionate adequately results in accumulation of propionyl CoA, which can compete with acetyl CoA in pathways of fatty acid synthesis. Thus, fatty acids with odd numbers of carbon atoms can be incorporated into lipids[220]; although this has been demonstrated in nerve biopsies from patients with Cbl deficiency,[221] cause and effect have not been proved. Nitrous oxide was later

CLUES TO DISTINGUISHING COBALAMIN AND FOLATE DEFICIENCIES

Although the megaloblastic manifestations of Cbl and folate deficiencies are clinically indistinguishable, certain distinct patterns in mode of presentation can give a clue to the type and etiology of deficiency. In general, the cause of folate deficiency will be found in the fairly recent past (within 6 months) primarily from the history and physical examination. By contrast, the cause of Cbl deficiency will be obscure until specific tests (e.g., Schilling test) to define the etiology are carried out. In bygone days, by the time anemia was symptomatic, >80% of patients had neurologic manifestations; in 50% of cases, this led to some incapacity. Perhaps as a result of the widespread use of multivitamins containing folic acid among patients (and even in the food given livestock in the West), the hematologic expression of Cbl deficiency is often substantially attenuated, leading to pure neurologic presentations. Recent studies highlight the apparent inverse correlation between hematologic and neurologic presentations such that in one-third of patients with Cbl deficiency, the earliest signs are often purely neurologic, with symptoms related to paresthesias and diminished proprioception bringing the patient to the physician. Based on the multiple potential etiologies giving rise to megaloblastic anemias, the truism that "what the mind does not know, the eyes do not see" is a caveat that cannot be taken lightly; failure to recognize Cbl deficiency as the etiology of neurologic disease and treatment of Cbl deficiency with folate or misdiagnosis of megaloblastosis as erythroleukemia represent significant extremes of deviation from the dictum primum non nocere. Areas of overlap in symptomatology in Cbl/folate deficiency are related to megaloblastosis (e.g., common cardiopulmonary and some gastrointestinal manifestations). While pure folate deficiency in the alcoholic with thiamin deficiency (Wernicke's encephalopathy) and peripheral neuropathy is almost indistinguishable from and may mimic Cbl deficiency, the remainder of the neurologic manifestations are uniquely due to Cbl deficiency.

tion of nitrous oxide-induced Cbl deficiency occurs when hematologic abnormalities are absent.[223,231,232] This was recently verified clinically in humans where there appears to be no correlation between the Cbl levels and neurologic dysfunction; in fact, there is an apparent inverse correlation between the extent of neurologic defects versus hematologic abnormalities.[233,234] Recent studies also highlight the greater sensitivity of human glial cells in culture to short-term Cbl deprivation.[235] The demyelinating process involves patchy swelling of the myelin sheath, followed by its breakdown (demyelination), leading to axonal degeneration. Microscopic foci coalesce with one another, giving the surface of the spinal cord (on cross section) a spongy appearance; later, the long tracts undergo secondary wallerian degeneration. Patchy demyelination usually begins in the dorsal columns in the thoracic segments of the spinal cord and then spreads contiguously to involve corticospinal tracts. These lesions spread throughout the length of the cord and ultimately involve spinothalamic and spinocerebellar tracts. Degeneration of the dorsal root ganglia, celiac ganglia, and Meissner's and Auerbach's plexus also occur. Although demyelination may extend to the white matter of the brain, it is unclear whether the peripheral neuropathy is due to a distinct lesion or is secondary to spinal cord disease; thus, the clinical manifestations may be extremely varied.[10,219,236]

Other Effects of Cobalamin and Folate Deficiency

Cbl more often than folate deficiency can also result in sterility from the effects on the gonads. A curious unexplained finding is generalized melanin pigmentation, which is reversible by specific nutrient replenishment. The mechanism of defective bactericidal activity in Cbl deficiency also remains unexplained. Since Cbl deficiency is associated with an inordinately high incidence of tuberculosis, and *Mycobacterium tuberculosis* has been shown to use methylmalonyl-CoA as a substrate for synthesis of tetramethyl-branched C_6–C_{20} mycocerosic acids,[237] it has been hypothesized that this milieu (i.e., of MMA-emia in Cbl deficiency) may favor the growth of the tubercle bacillus. In folate deficiency, other effects include a reduction in lymphocyte subsets,[238] enhanced predisposition to chemical-induced gastrointestinal carcinogenesis,[239] which may have a clinical correlate in patients with ulcerative colitis with low folate status,[240] and delayed tumor growth.[241]

BIOCHEMICAL INDICATORS OF EVOLVING DEFICIENCY

Abrupt induction of nutritional folate deficiency causes a decline in the serum folate level; within 3 weeks, it falls below the normal range.[242,243] It is therefore a sensitive indicator of negative folate balance. Tissue folate deficiency develops only when hepatic folate stores are depleted (after about 4 months) and is marked by a decrease in RBC folate levels. Early manifestations of negative Cbl balance are increased serum MMA and HCYS levels[227–229] and a decrease in percentage of saturation of TC II.[244] This occurs when the total Cbl in serum is still normal, when approximately 80% of serum Cbl is bound to TC I, while only about 20% is bound to TC II. Only later does negative Cbl balance lead to an absolute decrease in serum Cbl level. Negative nutrient balance (decreased serum folate or decreased percentage of saturation of TC II) thus seems to precede evidence of decreased intracellular nutrient availability (decreased RBC folate or serum Cbl levels), as well as biochemical evidence of abnormal thymidylate synthesis (impaired conversion of dUMP to dTMP), morphologic expression of perturbed DNA in PMNs (lobe index), macro-ovalocytosis, and anemia.[6] The biochemical basis for selective nutrient deficiency

recognized as an inducer of functional Cbl coenzyme deficiency in vivo, because individuals exposed to this gas developed both hematologic and neurologic manifestations similar to those of Cbl deficiency. Since methionine (required in numerous methylation reactions, including those in nerve tissue) also ameliorates the neurologic dysfunction in monkeys, this led to a focus on the methionine synthase-catalyzed reaction and on the potential importance of lack of methionine in Cbl deficiency. The potential etiologic role of some natural Cbl analogues[222] that have anti-Cbl effects and that have been shown to accumulate in the brains of nitrous oxide-treated/Cbl-deficient fruit bats[223] is also under investigation. Since elevated levels of both serum methylmalonic acid (MMA) and HCYS are positively correlated with Cbl-dependent neurologic dysfunction in humans, perturbation of the activity of both Cbl-dependent enzymes may be important.[224–229] Conversely, hereditary defects in methionine synthase-catalyzed reactions are associated with neurologic dysfunction,[230] while methylmalonyl-CoA mutase deficiency is not. Nitrous oxide also inhibits methionine synthase much more than methylmalonyl-CoA mutase, elevating the importance of methionine synthase in maintaining the integrity of myelin in humans.

Curiously, in fruit bats and monkeys, the neurologic dysfunc-

in various tissues (e.g., hematopoietic but not gastrointestinal cells) is unclear.[5,6]

Biochemical Evaluation of Cobalamin/Folate Deficiency

Serum Homocysteine and Methylmalonic Acid Levels

Cellular nutrient deficiency of either Cbl or folate is reflected by decreased intracellular concentrations. By contrast, defective utilization of Cbl/folate due to intracellular Cbl/folate-dependent enzyme deficiency may allow normal intracellular coenzyme levels. Deficient coenzyme and enzyme levels are both reflected by perturbation of the major Cbl/folate-dependent enzyme-catalyzed reactions. Thus, reduced activity of methionine synthase leads to substrate buildup and to elevated serum levels of HCYS, which can be measured by a sensitive assay.[226] In a 1988 study, 77 of 78 patients with clinically confirmed Cbl deficiency had elevated values of HCYS, correlating with clinical parameters of Cbl deficiency.[227] In the same patient group, 74 of the 78 also had increased serum MMA levels,[227] indicating reduced activity of the second Cbl-dependent enzyme, methylmalonyl-CoA mutase, and reduced conversion of methylmalonyl-CoA to succinyl-CoA.[224,225] Similarly, 18 of 19 patients with folate deficiency had elevated levels of HCYS due to reduced activity of the methionine synthase-catalyzed reaction.[227]

The combined use of serum HCYS and MMA can distinguish between Cbl and folate deficiency, since most patients with folate deficiency have normal levels of MMA the rest have only mild elevations.[227-229] Normal MMA levels rule out Cbl deficiency with nearly 100% confidence, provided the patient is not dehydrated and does not have renal dysfunction.[245] These two tests are now clinically available; they are useful diagnostically as well as in following the patient's response to replacement therapy, since the abnormally high metabolites will only return to normal when replaced with the appropriate (deficient) vitamin.[227,229,236] Thus, a positive response to Cbl, documented by falling levels of HCYS and MMA, is evidence of Cbl deficiency. Conversely, therapy with folate results in a decrease in the isolated HCYS level if folate deficiency is present.

Serum Cobalamin Levels

Serum Cbl levels previously measured by microbiologic assay using the Cbl-dependent organism *Lactobacillus leichmannii*[245a] have been replaced by a simpler assay method that relies on the competitive inhibition by serum Cbl of the binding of CN-[[57]Co]Cbl to IF (rather than R protein, which falsely measured Cbl analogues as well).[10,246,247] For the most part, serum Cbl is an established biochemical indicator of Cbl deficiency.[248,249] However, a recent report of neuropsychiatric disorders attributed to Cbl deficiency in some patients, despite both the absence of anemia and normal or minimally depressed Cbl levels, underscores the caution that clinicians should observe in interpreting this test.[233,234,250,251]

The serum Cbl level may be occasionally low in the absence of true Cbl deficiency. This phenomenon is seen in one-third of patients with folate deficiency and also in multiple myeloma, TC I deficiency, megadose vitamin C therapy, and for no apparent cause.[168,248,249] A low serum Cbl is not synonymous with Cbl deficiency, and several associated diseases/conditions can falsely raise or lower Cbl levels (Table 41-1). However, recent studies have also identified patients with true Cbl deficiency who have Cbl levels in the low-normal range (see below).

Serum and RBC Folate Levels

Microbiologic assays of folate using *L. casei*[252-256] suffer from the same limitations as assays for Cbl. These too, have been supplanted by various radioisotope dilution assays[257,258] without adequate documentation, in many cases, of clinical validity.

Table 41-1. Serum Cbl: False-Positive Tests[a] and False-Negative Tests[b]

Falsely low serum Cbl in the absence of true Cbl deficiency
　　Folate deficiency (one-third of patients)
　　Multiple myeloma
　　TC I deficiency
　　Megadose vitamin C therapy
　　Patient's serum contains other radioisotopes (^{99m}Tc or ^{67}Ga used in organ scanning)
Falsely raised Cbl levels in the presence of a true deficiency
　　Cbl binders (TC I and II) increased (myeloproliferative states, hepatomas, and fibrolamellar hepatic tumors)
　　TC II-producing macrophages are activated (autoimmune diseases, monocytic leukemias, and lymphomas)
　　Release of Cbl from hepatocytes (active liver disease)

[a] Although a low serum Cbl is not synonymous with Cbl deficiency, 5% of patients with true Cbl deficiency will have low-normal Cbl levels.
[b] A potentially serious problem, since the patient's underlying Cbl deficiency will progress if uncorrected.

Moreover, there is a significant discrepancy in folate levels when a variety of kits are used on the same sample. It is also uncertain whether these assays are better than microbiologic assays.[259-261] It remains to be confirmed whether new improved versions of the latter assays can be standardized for widespread clinical use without the existing disadvantages.[262]

Serum folate level is highly sensitive to folate intake. A single hospital meal may normalize it in a patient with true folate deficiency. Moreover, it can be low in the absence of megaloblastosis in patients with anorexia, alcoholism, or normal pregnancy and in those receiving anticonvulsant therapy.[168,248,249] In these instances, the serum folate level (low in one-third of hospitalized patients) simply represents the state of negative folate balance, which, if continued, would lead to true deficiency. The intracellular RBC folate level is 30 times as high as the serum folate.[254] Thus, slight hemolysis can falsely raise the serum folate level. Reduced RBC folate levels (in pure folate deficiency) provide a good indicator of tissue folate deficiency and correlate well with hepatic folate stores and megaloblastic changes.[2,5,6,254] In Cbl deficiency, however, the trapped Cbl leaks out of the cell resulting in low RBC folate and in normal to increased serum folate levels. Recognition of these variables forms the basis for the use of all three tests (serum folate, serum Cbl, and RBC folate) to differentiate isolated deficiency of Cbl or folate from combined Cbl/folate deficiency (Fig. 41-2).

Summary of the Clinical Value of Tests for Cbl and Folate Deficiency

Conventionally, the results for both serum Cbl and folate are generated from one sample. The assay for RBC folate is run separately. None of the older tests (serum and RBC folate, serum Cbl) used to diagnose Cbl/folate deficiency are infallible.[168,248] They may be abnormal in some situations in which no deficiency is present, or they may be normal in the face of nutrient deficiency. Knowledge of the variables that influence these tests is necessary to interpret the results in the clinical context.

Approximately 5% of patients with true Cbl deficiency associated with either hematologic or neurologic abnormalities, or both, have serum Cbl levels in the lower end of the normal scale; that is, this result will detract from the fact that such a patient is Cbl deficient. However, the metabolite levels (MMA and HCYS) are elevated under such circumstances.[229] Since the incidence of falsely elevated levels is negligible, assuming no renal dysfunction/dehydration, this fact alone highlights the increased value and sensitivity of measuring metabolite levels when the clinical picture is suggestive, but the Cbl level is within the low normal range. The sensitivity of the measurement of MMA and HCYS is again illustrated in those patients

Table 41-2. Differentiating Pure Cbl/Folate Deficiency from Combined Folate and Cbl Deficiency Using Blood Tests[a]

	Serum Folate	RBC Folate	Serum Cbl	Serum HCYS[c]	Serum MMA[c]
Negative folate balance[b]	Low	Normal	Normal	Normal	Normal
Folate deficiency	Low	Low	Normal	High	Normal
Cbl deficiency	Normal	Normal/low	Low	High	High
Folate plus Cbl deficiency	Low	Low	Low	High	High

[a] Normal values suggest macrocytosis without megaloblastosis or nonfolate/Cbl responsive megaloblastosis.

[b] If untreated, true folate deficiency will ensue when hepatic stores are exhausted.

[c] False-positive increases of serum HCYS and MMA will be seen with volume depletion and renal failure. Perform these tests of Cbl is in the low normal range.

with pernicious anemia who are on replacement therapy with Cbl. When these patients do not receive Cbl for some time, the level of MMA and HCYS progressively increase much earlier than the drop in Cbl levels; this too indicates that measurement of metabolite levels are a much more sensitive, and also a more specific, reflection of true tissue deficiency than that obtained from serum Cbl analysis.[229] Another report also independently confirms these data.[263] The combined used of measurements of MMA and HCYS also helps differentiate Cbl from folate deficiency (Table 41-2), but cannot distinguish pure Cbl deficiency from combined Cbl and folate deficiency.

An important recent study conclusively demonstrates that overlooking true Cbl deficiency is highly unlikely when the two metabolites are measured, since one or both metabolites were increased in 99.8% of >400 patients with proven Cbl deficiency.[245] These data collectively indicate that these serum tests (MMA and HCYS) are the now the "gold standard" for the diagnosis of Cbl deficiency. Thus, the use of serum HCYS and MMA tests, which are routinely done together, can confirm Cbl deficiency when Cbl levels are in the low normal range (<300 pg/ml; normal >200 pg/ml) or when a defect in Cbl utilization is suspected.[236]

PATHOGENESIS OF COBALAMIN DEFICIENCY

Nutritional Cobalamin Deficiency

Insufficient Cobalamin Intake

Among 138 vegetarian Indians residing in the United Kingdom (13–80 years of age) with megaloblastic hematopoiesis, 95 had nutritional Cbl deficiency, some with early neuropsychiatric manifestations.[264] The sole Cbl source for these individuals, who abstain from consuming meats, eggs, and cheese, was boiled milk and yogurt. One-third had evidence of intestinal malabsorption with osteomalacia, associated iron deficiency (attributable to the low bioavailability of iron in these diets) and an inordinately high incidence of tuberculosis (see above). In Northwest India, three-fourths of 136 consecutive cases of nutritional megaloblastic anemia[265] had Cbl deficiency, with 60% presenting in the second and third decade with pancytopenia, mild hepatomegaly (46%), mild splenomegaly (34%), fever (42%), thrombocytopenic bleeding (80%), and neutropenia (43%). The hemorrhagic diathesis frequently encountered with thrombocytopenia was reversed with 12–24 hours of replacement with Cbl.[215,265]

Food faddists may also develop nutritional Cbl deficiency when they practice strict lacto-ovovegetarianism for "health" reasons. However, owing to an efficient enterohepatic circulation, Cbl deficiency normally develops very slowly (over >10 years). Since the "staying power" of fads is often of shorter duration, this complication is rarely seen. Long-term mainte-

nance therapy requires oral 5-µg aqueous hydroxo-Cbl or 50-µg Cbl tablets; this approach allows for continued vegetarianism. The breast-fed offspring of strict vegans (or mothers with tropical sprue and subclinical Cbl deficiency) are also recognized as being at high risk of the development of nutritional Cbl deficiency.[266–269]

Intragastric Events Leading to Cobalamin Malabsorption

Inadequate Dissociation of Cobalamin from Food Protein

Dietary Cbl is bioavailable only following proteolytic digestion of food by gastric acid and pepsin. Thus, failure to release Cbl from food protein can present as Cbl deficiency, even though gastric analysis shows the presence of IF.[19–21] Some older patients (>50 years old) with atrophic gastritis or partial gastrectomy with hypochlorhydria have low serum Cbl levels and normal absorption of crystalline Cbl but poor absorption of CN-Cbl[57] Co, which is incorporated into food as a "food-Cbl absorption" test.[19–22,270] Some of these patients may progress to overt clinical manifestations of Cbl deficiency. They may also represent a cohort in an early stage in the natural history of pernicious anemia. Geriatric patients with low Cbl levels, abnormal food-Cbl absorption tests and increased metabolite levels consistent with Cbl deficiency have been encountered[271,272]; recent estimates measure the prevalence of these findings in ≥14.5% of geriatric outpatients.

Congenital Intrinsic Factor Deficiency

Congenital IF deficiency, transmitted as an autosomal recessive trait and expressed in homozygotes by the age of 2 years, is characterized by a pure IF deficiency without other gastric abnormalities. Only 40 or so cases have been described; affected children present with irritability, vomiting, diarrhea, and loss of weight with megaloblastic anemia. Except for the absence of IF in gastric juice, gastric histology/function are normal.[273–275]

Atrophy of Gastric Oxyntic Mucosa

Total gastrectomy, which results in removal of IF-producing cells, invariably leads to Cbl deficiency within about 5 years (range 2–10 years), often associated with iron deficiency (dimorphic anemia).[276,277] IF deficiency arising from atrophy of gastric parietal (oxyntic) mucosal cells must be associated with parallel insufficient HC1 secretion and can be caused by (1) partial gastrectomy; (2) autoimmune destruction as observed in adult addisonian pernicous anemia (PA) or, rarely, in a similar disease in children (juvenile PA); and (3) destruction of gastric mucosa by caustic (lye) ingestion.

Partial Gastrectomy

Cbl deficiency is observed in only 10–20% of patients 8 years after partial gastrectomy, although 30% have Cbl malabsorption[278]; ≤6% of these Cbl-deficient patients will develop frank clinical manifestations of Cbl deficiency with megaloblastic anemia. The etiology is multifactorial—contributing factors include decreased IF secretion, hypochlorhydria (from atrophy of residual oxyntic mucosal cells), intestinal bacterial overgrowth of Cbl-consuming organisms, associated nutritional folate deficiency in 20%, and iron deficiency in about 50% of cases. The degree of Cbl deficiency depends on the size of the remaining gastric remnant. It is more common in Billroth II than in Billroth I surgery, in subtotal than in partial gastrectomy, and in gastric rather than duodenal peptic ulcer disease.[277–281] Morbidly obese patients treated surgically with gastric bypass also have more food Cbl malabsorption than do those patients treated with vertical banded gastroplasty.[282]

Absent IF Secretion

The most common cause of Cbl malabsorption is PA, a disease of unknown origin in which the fundamental defect is atrophy of the gastric (parietal cell) oxyntic mucosa eventually leading to the absence of IF and HC1 secretion. Since Cbl can only be absorbed by binding to IF and uptake by ileal IF/Cbl receptors, the net consequence is severe Cbl malabsorption leading to Cbl deficiency.

The incidence of PA is approximately 25 new cases/yr/ 100,000 persons >40 years. While the average age of onset is at about 60 years,[2] it is being increasingly encountered in persons 5–10 years younger.[283] PA is not a respecter of age, race, or ethnic origin.[284–286] The predisposition to developing PA may have a genetic basis, but neither the mode of inheritance nor the initiating events or primary mechanism is precisely understood. About 30% of patients have a positive family history,[287] among whom the risk of familial PA is 20 times as high as in the general population; approximately 20% of siblings are projected to develop PA by the age of 90 years. PA developing concordantly in identical twins has been documented.[287–289]

There is a significant association of PA with other autoimmune diseases.[2,290–295] PA is associated with Graves disease (30%), Hashimoto thyroiditis (11%), and vitiligo (8%), as well as Addison disease, idiopathic hypoparathyroidism, and adult-onset hypogammaglobulinemia. The histologic appearance of the gastric mucosa (infiltration with plasma cells and lymphocytes) is also strongly reminiscent of autoimmune-type lesions. There is also a high incidence of anti-parietal cell IgG antibodies in the serum of 90% of patients with PA.[296,297] These antiparietal cell IgG antibodies are cytotoxic to canine gastric parietal cells in vitro.[298] When chronically injected into rats, these antibodies decrease gastric HCl, IF, and pepsin secretion and lead to gastric atrophy.[299] The major antigen to which antibodies from patients with autoimmune gastritis and PA are directed is the acid-producing enzyme H^+, K^+-ATPase (a 92-kd protein), found on the membrane of parietal cells.[300] The precise interplay of the various mechanisms for antiparietal cell IgG-mediated dysfunction of parietal cells remains to be shown in vivo. It is not clear whether the target antigen of antiparietal cell IgG found in ≤8% of the normal 30–60-year-old population, 20% of women >60 years old, and 50–60% of patients with simple atrophic gastritis, is also H^+, K^+-ATPase or another antigen. Anti-IF antibodies are found in the serum of approximately 60% of patients with PA and in the gastric juice of 75%; approximately 90% of patients with PA have anti-IF antibodies in either serum or gastric juice.[283–285,301–304] Similar IF antibodies are quite rare in the general population; anti-IF antibodies are thus highly specific and confirmatory for PA.

There are two types of IF antibodies. Type I are directed to the Cbl-binding site on IF and are usually of IgG subclass in the serum. In gastric secretions, they may be both IgG and secretory IgA subclass. Type II IF antibodies bind to the IF/Cbl complex and prevent binding to ileal IF/Cbl receptors. Type II antibodies, usually not seen in the absence of type I antibodies, are found in approximately 35% of patients with PA, although recent studies using a technique that detects both antibodies indicates a higher prevalence than previously documented.[305] Owing to their functional properties, these intraluminal anti-IF antibodies may hasten the development of PA and interfere with tests for Cbl absorption.[306] Patients with anti-IF antibodies also have a higher T_4/T_8 cell ratio than that of patients without anti-IF antibodies or controls. The significance of this is unclear, nor is the reason that patients with PA have an increased frequency of antibodies in serum directed against antigens

from thyroid acinar cells, lymphocytes, renal collecting duct cells, and altered cellular immunity.[290–300]

The corticosteroid responsiveness in some patients with PA (regeneration of atrophic gastric mucosa and increased IF secretion antedating a decrease in anti-IF antibodies) also implicates an autoimmune pathogenesis of PA.[307,308] The clustering of parietal cell dysfunction among first-degree relatives of patients with PA in inbred populations, that some individuals (96% of black women with PA) have high titers of blocking anti-IF antibodies but lack antiparietal cell antibodies,[283–285] and that neither antibody may be detected in patients with PA and acquired agammaglobulinemia all suggest that the pathogenesis of PA is heterogeneous. Juvenile PA presents in the second decade with severe Cbl deficiency in conjunction with many of the associated endocrinopathies and autoantibodies observed in adults[309]; why these patients present so much earlier with a seemingly identical disease is unknown. Taken together, these facts suggest that while there is a genetic predisposition to PA, the full expression of the disease, which appears to have an autoimmune basis, may be modified by acquired environmental influences.

Abnormal IF Molecules

A defective IF molecule was identified by age 2 years in three siblings that was identical to IF in all but one respect—it was markedly susceptible to acid and proteolytic enzyme (pepsin or trypsin) digestion resulting in defective Cbl absorption by ileal IF/Cbl receptors and megaloblastic anemia.[310] In another case, an abnormal IF molecule having a 60-fold lower binding affinity for ileal IF/Cbl receptors resulted in lower (but not absent) Cbl absorption, probably accounting for the delayed clinical presentation with Cbl deficiency at the age of 13 years.[311,312]

Abnormal Events in the Small Bowel Lumen

Impaired Transfer of Cobalamin from R Protein to Intrinsic Factor

Insufficient Pancreatic Protease

Since approximately 30% of patients with severe pancreatic insufficiency fail to degrade R proteins, there is no transfer of food Cbl to IF and consequent Cbl malabsorption (R-Cbl does not bind ileal IF/Cbl receptors). R proteins are highly susceptible to proteolysis by even small quantities of pancreatic protease released in response to food. Thus, in partial insufficiency there is abnormal absorption of CN-Cbl[57]Co on an empty stomach but normal absorption when the CN-Cbl[57]Co is given with food. Administration of pancreatic extract completely normalizes Cbl malabsorption in those with complete pancreatic insufficiency.[313,314]

Inactivation of Pancreatic Protease

Pancreatic protease can be inactivated by the massive gastric hypersecretion arising from a gastrinoma in Zollinger-Ellison syndrome.[315] The continued low pH of the luminal contents reaching the ileum can also conceivably perturb interaction of the IF/Cbl complex with IF/Cbl receptors for which a pH of >5.4 is required.

Usurpation of Luminal Cobalamin

The near sterile conditions of the small bowel are maintained by a combination of the mechanical cleansing action of peristalsis and the chemical action of gastric acid. Disorders conducive to relative stasis, impaired motility, and hypogammaglobulinemia are predisposing factors favoring colonization by bacteria. Many of these bacteria take up free Cbl, while the uptake of

IF-bound Cbl is markedly diminished. However, if colonization extends proximally to the locus at which IF and Cbl interact, significant Cbl may be usurped before it can bind to IF.[316-318] Possible absorption of inert Cbl analogues produced by these bacteria may permit competition with normal Cbl to produce an additional anti-Cbl effect.[319] This Cbl malabsorption can be corrected to some extent by a 7–10-day course of antibiotic therapy; definitive surgical correction is indicated if the patient has significant symptoms (weight loss and diarrhea) that are only partially relieved by antibiotics. Recently the malabsorption of food Cbl in patients with atrophic gastritis has also been normalized with antibiotics, thereby incriminating bacterial usurpation of food Cbl at a very proximal level.[320]

Approximately 3% of individuals infested with the fish tapeworm *Diphyllobothrium latum* develop frank Cbl deficiency. Humans become infected when they eat partially cooked or raw fish or fish roe containing pleroceroids.[321] In a given patient, the degree of Cbl deficiency is probably related to the number of worms and the extent to which they lodge proximal to ileal IF/Cbl receptors. They are commonly found in the jejunum; poised in this strategic location, they avidly usurp Cbl for growth.[322,323] In fact, worm extracts are so rich in Cbl that they have been used successfully to replenish Cbl in Cbl-deficient states.[324] Once ova have been identified in the stools, expulsion of the worms with niclosamide and Cbl replenishment is invariably curative.

Disorders of Ileal Intrinsic Factor/Cobalamin Receptors or Mucosa

Absence of IF/Cbl Receptors

The distal ileum has the greatest density of IF/Cbl receptors, and removal of only 1–2 ft of terminal ileum via resection or bypass can reduce ileal IF/Cbl receptor numbers or interaction with IF/Cbl, respectively, to result in Cbl malabsorption.[43,325-327] Thus, ileal bypass or diseased ileal architecture may lead to reduction in transenterocytic transport of Cbl (and folate), which is treatable with parenteral Cbl replacement.

Defective IF/Cbl Receptors or Post-IF/Cbl Receptor Defects

A heterogeneous group of congenital disorders in children involving selective Cbl malabsorption leading to megaloblastic anemias associated with mild, persistent, benign, nonspecific proteinuria (in 90% of cases) is collectively known as Immerslund-Gräsbeck syndrome.[328-330] These patients are heterogeneous with respect to precise biochemical abnormalities involving Cbl malabsorption. In one case, an abnormality in ileal IF/Cbl receptors was demonstrated,[320] but most appear to involve a postreceptor defect; parenteral therapy with Cbl bypasses the defect and reverses Cbl deficiency.[331-333]

Drug-Induced Defects

H_2 antagonists, but not omeprazole, inhibit IF secretion.[34,334] Biguanides appear to decrease IF and acid secretion in healthy volunteers; they also probably inhibit transenterocytic transport of Cbl.[335] Other drugs (e.g., slow K, cholestyramine, colchicine, neomycin, para-aminosalicylate) probably also impair transepithelial transport of Cbl,[2,27,28] manifested by a decrease in serum Cbl levels with mild to insignificant Cbl deficiency; these drugs also commonly interfere with the Schilling test.

Disorders of Plasma Cobalamin Transport

Absence of Transcobalamins I and III

Congenital R-protein deficiency is not associated with cellular Cbl deficiency. However, since 80% of serum Cbl is bound to TC I, the serum Cbl levels will invariably be low. Two of six patients in one study, however, have developed a biochemically uncharacterized neurologic syndrome, which has led to speculation that TC III deficiency may result in inability to clear Cbl analogues that may have a pathogenic role in the neurologic dysfunction.[23]

Deficiency of Transcobalamin II

Megaloblastic anemia in infancy associated with normal Cbl levels is the characteristic clinical presentation when TC II is absent or markedly deficient.[336,337] (Cbl levels are normal due to the TC I-bound Cbl, but this Cbl is unavailable for physiologic cellular uptake.) The impairment in intestinal absorption of Cbl in such patients is also due to the absence of TC II, which plays an important role in binding Cbl within the enterocyte before entering the circulation. In all, approximately 30 patients have been described.[331-333] They can be successfully treated by exploiting the property of passive intracellular diffusion of Cbl by daily/biweekly injections of 1 mg Cbl, which ensures Cbl delivery into cells.

Defective Transcobalamin II

Defective TC II, also presenting with Cbl deficiency, can be diagnosed when the amount of TC II, measured by radioimmunoassay, is normal concomitant with a qualitative abnormality based on its inability to bind Cbl.[338,339] Conversely, in another patient with normal amounts of TC II by radioimmunoassay, the TC II was functionally active in binding Cbl but was unable to facilitate the uptake of Cbl into cells.[340]

Disorders of Intracellular Cobalamin Utilization

Congenital Metabolic Defects (Inborn Errors) of Cbl Metabolism, Cbl mutants A–F

The combination of megaloblastic anemia with increased HCYS and/or MMA in serum and urine despite normal Cbl and folate levels should suggest an inborn error of Cbl metabolism.[84,263,331-333] The inherited defects of Cbl utilization (Fig. 41-3) are heterogeneous and are empirically defined as Cbl mutations A–G (*cblA–cblG*) through the use of complementation studies involving in vitro fusion of cultured mutant fibroblasts obtained from skin biopsies. Mutants involving the synthesis of Ado-Cbl within the mitochondria involve defects in the reduction of Cob(II)alamin to Cob(I)alamin (*cblA*) and of Cob(I)alamin to Ado-Cbl by Ado-Cbl transferase (*cblB*). These defects result in an accumulation of excess MMA. The clinical picture in infancy is dominated by acidosis and ketosis associated with lethargy, failure to thrive, vomiting, dehydration, respiratory distress, hepatomegaly, and coma. Biochemical evidence of MMAemia, ketonemia, and ketonuria without megaloblastosis is found. Since some of these defects are incomplete, treatment with large doses of Cbl may alleviate the defect.[331-333]

Cloning of methylmalonyl-CoA mutase cDNA from fibroblasts of a patient with *mut⁻* phenotype in whom residual enzymatic activity is evident in cultured cells exposed to high concentrations of OH-Cbl has identified a single base substitution (Gly 717 → Val) as the basis for this mutant at the molecular level; moreover, this identifies that Ado-Cbl binds to determinants in the C-terminal portion of the enzyme.[341] Defects involving conversion of Cob(III)alamin to Cob(II)alamin (*cblC, cblD*) present with combined evidence of reduced activity of methylmalonyl-CoA mutase and methionine synthase (i.e., with increased HCYS and MMA in blood and urine).[331-333] These patients have prominent neuropsychiatric problems with mental retardation, microcephaly, psychosis, delirium, and retinopathy with megaloblastosis. *cblC* mutants have hemolytic uremic syndrome as an integral manifestation of the spectrum of this disorder.[342] While the disorder usually presents in infancy, some patients do present with problems in later childhood. Hydroxo-Cbl [Cob(III)alamin] appears to be more effective than CN-Cbl in these patients. *cblE* (distinguished by the absence of increased MMA) is thought to be a defect arising from the inability to maintain Cbl bound to methionine synthase in its reduced state.[343,344] *cblF* is due to the inability of Cbl to be transported from the lysosome into the cytoplasm[345]; this has recently been visualized by quantitative electron microscopic radiography.[346] Among patients with mutant *cblG* defects, one case presenting at the age of 21 years with a multiple sclerosis-like syndrome was initially undiagnosed simply because the serum Cbl level and studies of Cbl absorption were normal.[230] This suggests that even adults presenting with cerebral, myelopathic, or neuropathic disturbances (occasionally masquerading as multiple sclerosis) should be screened for such defects using the dU suppression test or serum HCYS and MMA levels which may reflect the biochemical disorder.

Acquired Disorder of Cbl Utilization: Nitrous Oxide Exposure

Nitrous oxide inactivates coenzyme forms of Cbl by oxidizing the fully reduced Cob(I)alamin to Cob(III)alamin; this results in a state of functional intracellular Cbl deficiency. This syndrome was first identified in patients with tetanus given nitrous oxide for ≤6 days[347,348]; subsequently, patients exposed to nitrous oxide for open heart surgery, and through chronic (surreptitious/accidental/occupational) exposure have been recognized as high-risk individuals for the development of megaloblastosis and Cbl-deficient neuromyelopathy.[349–351] While megaloblastosis develops within 24 hours and lasts <1 week after a single exposure, the neurologic syndrome is usually seen with chronic intermittent exposure. The integrity of the methionine synthase-catalyzed reaction can be tested by measuring serum HCYS even after 75 minutes of exposure during surgery.[352] Reduced enzymatic activity explains the metabolic block and can be bypassed by 5-formyl-H₄PteGlu (leucovorin).

CLINICAL EVALUATION OF Cbl ABSORPTION

Schilling Test

Nutritional deficiency and hereditary enzymatic defects of intracellular Cbl utilization account for the minority of cases of Cbl deficiency. Most patients with clinical Cbl deficiency have impaired Cbl absorption. If Cbl absorption is intact, CN-[⁵⁷Co]Cbl administered orally will first bind R protein in the stomach. In the duodenum, the R protein of the R-CN-[⁵⁷Co]Cbl complex will be degraded by pancreatic protease resulting in rapid transfer of released CN-[⁵⁷Co]Cbl to the patient's own IF. The CN-[⁵⁷Co]Cbl/IF complex will travel down to the ileum, where it interacts with specific IF/Cbl receptors. Once taken up by the enterocyte, CN-[⁵⁷Co]Cbl will be transported into the portal blood while bound to TC II. If the blood contains an excess of Cbl (from a "flushing" injection of exogenously administered Cbl), >8% of CN-[⁵⁷Co]Cbl will be excreted in the urine within 24 hours (stage I test). If there is a decrease in endogenous IF (as in PA), <8% will ultimately be excreted; however, if IF is given exogenously with the CN-[⁵⁷Co]Cbl, this abnormality will be corrected[353] (stage II test). In situations involving usurption of CN-[⁵⁷Co]Cbl by bacterial overgrowth, resulting in decreased absorption of CN-[⁵⁷Co]Cbl + IF, prior therapy with antibiotics for 7–10 days will correct Cbl malabsorption[316–320] (stage III test); however, antibiotics will not correct Cbl malabsorption due to fish tapeworm infestation or defects involving net deficiency of IF/Cbl receptors, such as ileal resection, fistulas, or diseases of the ileal mucosa (including TC II deficiency).

ETIOPATHOPHYSIOLOGIC CLASSIFICATION OF COBALAMIN DEFICIENCY

Nutritional Cbl deficiency (insufficient Cbl intake)
  Vegetarians, vegans, breast-fed infants of mothers with pernicious anemia
Abnormal intragastric events (inadequate proteolysis of food Cbl)
  Atrophic gastritis, partial gastritis with hypochlorhydria
Loss/atrophy of gastric oxyntic mucosa (deficient IF molecules)
  Total or partial gastrectomy, pernicious anemia, caustic destruction (lye)
Abnormal events in small bowel lumen
  Inadequate pancreatic protease (R-Cbl not degraded, Cbl not transferred to IF)
    Insufficient pancreatic protease—pancreatic insufficiency
    Inactivation of pancreatic protease—Zollinger-Ellison syndrome
  Usurping of luminal Cbl (inadequate Cbl binding to IF)
    By bacteria—stasis syndromes (blind loops, pouches of diverticulosis, strictures, fistulas, anastomoses); impaired bowel motility (scleroderma, pseudo-obstruction), hypogammaglobulinemia
    By *Diphyllobothrium latum* (fish tapeworm)
Disorders of ileal mucosa/IF/Cbl receptors (IF/Cbl not bound to IF/Cbl receptors)
  Diminished or absent IF/Cbl receptors—ileal bypass/resection/fistula
  Abnormal mucosa architecture/function—tropical/nontropical sprue, Crohn disease, tuberculosis ileitis, infiltration by lymphomas, amyloidosis
  IF-/post-IF/Cbl receptor defects—Immerslund-Gräsbeck syndrome, TC II deficiency
  Drug-induced effects (slow K, biguanides, cholestyramine, colchicine, neomycin, para-aminosalicylate)
Disorders of plasma Cbl transport (TC II/Cbl not delivered to TC II receptors)
  Congenital TC II deficiency, defective binding of TC II/Cbl to TC II receptors (rare)
Metabolic disorders (Cbl not used by cell)
  Inborn enzyme errors (rare)
  Acquired disorders: Cbl functionally inactivated by irreversible oxidation; nitrous oxide inhalation

In pancreatic protease deficiency, CN-[⁵⁷Co]Cbl remains bound to R protein and will not be transferred to IF; the result is diminished absorption and overall urinary excretion,[24,26] an effect that is correctable by simultaneous administration of pancreatin (Creon) or by carrying out the test while the patient's pancreas is optimally stimulated with a meal or Secretin. In the rare syndrome in which IF is unusually susceptible to degradation by acid and pepsin, the abnormal Schilling test can be partially corrected by administration of sodium bicarbonate.[301,302] Those patients with hypochlorhydria and an inability to release food Cbl proteolytically with consequent low serum Cbl with or without clinical manifestations of Cbl deficiency will have a normal stage I Schilling test, since they have no problem in absorbing crystalline CN-[⁵⁷Co]Cbl. The appropriate test to order under these circumstances is the oval-

Table 41-3. Results of Schilling Tests

Condition	CN-[^{57}Co]Cbl plus H$_2$O Stage I Test	CN-[^{57}Co]Cbl plus IF Stage II Test	CN-[^{57}Co]Cbl after 7–10 Days of Antibiotics Stage III Test	CN-[^{57}Co]Cbl Plus Pancreatic Extract	CN-[^{57}Co]Cbl-Food Cbl Absorption Test
Normal	N^a				
Lack of IF	Low^a	N			
Usurping of Cbl by bacteria	Low	Low	N		
Pancreatic insufficiency	Low	Low	Low	N	
Lack/bypass of ileal IF/Cbl receptors/defective transenterocytic Cbl transport	Low	Low	Low	Low	
Inadequate dissociation of Food Cbl	N				Low

^{a} N means the results indicate normal absorption; low means the results indicate less than normal absorption.

bumin-CN-[^{57}Co]Cbl absorption test, in which the capacity of the patient to release the CN-[^{57}Co]Cbl that is bound to food protein is specifically examined. Such individuals usually have malabsorption of food-bound CN-[^{57}Co]Cbl (incorporated into an egg or mixed with chicken serum in vitro).[19–22,270]

The most common cause of an abnormal Schilling test[248,354] is incomplete collection of urine. Patients with renal impairment will also excrete less than normal amounts of radioactive Cbl.[355] While this potential pitfall can be avoided by sampling plasma after administration of CN-[^{57}Co]Cbl, results between patients with true PA and normal individuals show significant overlap; ideally, this requires the use of equipment for whole body counting,[356] which is not widely available.

The "flushing" dose of unlabeled Cbl administered during the Schilling test will invalidate further testing of serum Cbl and initiate a hematologic response in Cbl-deficient patients. Technical difficulties (resulting in diagnosis of Cbl malabsorption in the face of normal Cbl status) include (1) renal failure; (2) incomplete urine collection; (3) failure to give either the test or flushing dose; (4) use of decomposed CN-[^{57}Co]Cbl or inert IF; and (5) simultaneous ingestion of drugs that impair Cbl absorption. False-normal values in the presence of true Cbl deficiency can arise from contamination of urine with stool containing unabsorbed CN-[^{57}Co]Cbl and the presence of another isotope used in diagnostic tests (^{99m}Tc or ^{67}Ga).[248] It is therefore crucial to be alert to the timing of the Schilling test relative to other nuclear imaging studies. Furthermore, it should be re-emphasized that because Cbl/folate deficiency causes megaloblastosis of intestinal cells, the stage I Schilling test (with CN-[^{57}Co]Cbl alone) may be abnormal in folate deficiency, or a patient with IF deficiency (e.g., PA) may be diagnosed as having an abnormal stage II test from an intestinal cause.[357,358] This phenomenon occurs often enough (25–75% of cases) to warrant a repeat stage II Schilling test in patients diagnosed as having Cbl malabsorption (from an intestinal cause) after 2 months of Cbl replacement; only patients with PA will correct in the stage II test (Table 41-3).

Gastric Analysis

A significant titer of IF antibodies of the blocking type in gastric juice will lead to an abnormal stage II Schilling test. This is overcome by using an augmented stage II test with a higher dose of IF. Moreover, a clue as to whether these patients have gastric IF antibodies will be found in the serum, which may contain IF antibodies. Gastric analysis for achlorhydria in adults is valuable only in the single situation in which the presence of gastric acidity in response to maximal stimulation (e.g., Histalog) helps exclude the diagnosis of PA. In children, however, gastric analysis for IF and acid can differentiate between congenital IF deficiency (acid present), juvenile PA (acid and

IF absent), and Immerslund-Gräsbeck syndrome (acid and IF present).

The assay for anti-IF blocking antibodies depends on the displacement of CN-[^{57}Co]Cbl binding to IF in vitro. This can be significantly affected by prior injection of Cbl (as given with a Schilling test) or by radioactive isotopes from other diagnostic tests (^{99m}Tc, ^{67}Ga).

PATHOGENESIS OF FOLATE DEFICIENCY

Folate deficiency is usually recognized in the course of certain clinical presentations that predispose to negative folate balance and subsequent deficiency. It is therefore instructive to conceptualize cellular folate deficiency as arising from etiologic categories of decreased supply (reduced intake/absorption/transport/utilization), or increased requirement (metabolic consumption/destruction/excretion). However, in the same patient more than one mechanism may result in net folate deficiency. The precise contribution of one mechanism over the other is often not obvious. Specific tests designed to define each mechanism are not routinely available for clinical use.

Manifestations of folate deficiency may be hematologic (pancytopenia with megaloblastic marrow), cardiopulmonary, gastrointestinal (megaloblastosis with or without malabsorption), dermatologic (skin pigmentation), genital (megaloblastosis of cervical epithelium), infertility (sterility), and psychiatric (Table 41-4). These manifestations are discussed within the context of the history and physical examination. Cases of neuropathy attributed to folate deficiency are rarely encountered; when they are, the possibility of alcoholism with thiamine deficiency must be considered. In any case, every patient with neuropathy, myelopathy, or psychiatric manifestations associated with megaloblastosis must be investigated in detail to rule out Cbl deficiency. It must be remembered that gastrointestinal megaloblastosis leads to further folate malabsorption, which propagates a vicious circle of folate deficiency in the short term and Cbl deficiency in the long term. With the exception of drug-induced defects or inborn errors of folate metabolism that result in decreased utilization of intracellular folates, all etiologies, irrespective of mechanism, result in reduced net delivery of folates to normal proliferating cells. In pursuing the causes of folate deficiency in a given patient, efforts should be directed toward obtaining positive evidence for all possible conditions predisposing to negative folate balance and deficiency.

Nutritional Causes of Folate Deficiency

Decreased Intake and/or Increased Requirements

The body stores of folate are adequate for only about 4 months.[6,12,242,243] The requirement for folate is 100 μg/day in adults and approximately 50 μg/day in children, which is about

Table 41-4. Megaloblastic Sequelae of Folate and Cbl Deficiency and Several Clinical Manifestations are the same[a]

Hematologic	Pancytopenia with megaloblastic marrow
Cardiopulmonary	Congestive heart failure
Gastrointestinal	Beefy-red tongue and added stigmata of broad spectrum malabsorption in folate deficiency[b]
Dermatologic	Melanin pigmentation and premature graying
Genital	Cervical/uterine dysplasia
Reproductive	Infertility/sterility
Psychiatric	Depressed affect/cognitive dysfunction
Neuropsychiatric[c]	Unique to Cbl deficiency with cerebral, myelopathic or peripheral neuropathic disturbances, including optic and autonomic nerve dysfunction

[a] However, the neurologic spectrum of dysfunction with Cbl deficiency is distinct. Inadequate hemoglobinization (from inadequate iron stores and/or globin synthesis) will mask the expected erythroid megaloblastic morphology in the bone marrow and peripheral smear; only specific therapy (e.g., iron) will unmask classic megaloblastic manifestations (masked megaloblastosis). Megaloblastic leukopoiesis will be unchanged.

[b] If folate deficiency is uncorrected for >2–3 years, Cbl deficiency will supervene.

[c] Dorsal tract involvement is earliest manifestation in >70% patients with Cbl deficiency. Neuropsychiatric manifestations are not associated with megaloblastosis in ≤30% patients.

five times the adult requirement on a weight-for-weight basis. Folate stores are probably depleted much earlier in individuals who are chronically in negative folate balance or who have additional conditions "tipping" them into true folate deficiency. The incidence of folate deficiency in the setting of general malnutrition in the developing countries is very high and is invariably a problem of multiple vitamin deficiencies when associated with protein-calorie malnutrition (about 38,000 children die every day of hunger and starvation-related illness).[359] Decreased availability of folate-rich foods (more frequent in winter months, or the wet season in central Africa), poverty, various cultural/ethnic diets (consisting of maize, rice, or well-cooked beans and vegetables), and cooking techniques that destroy food folate, coupled with the anorexia that accompanies chronic illnesses, are just a few of the reasons for rapid development of folate deficiency.[2,5,97,360,361]

The rapidly proliferating tissues in children have an absolute requirement for exogenously supplied folate. Although human or cow's milk is barely adequate to maintain folate balance in breast-fed infants, superimposition of associated illnesses that lead to anorexia or folate malabsorption readily shifts them into negative folate balance. Infants fed powdered milk formulas, goat's milk (6 µg/L folate), or milk that has been boiled (>50% of folate may be destroyed) are at high risk in this regard, as are those on restricted formulas for phenylketonuria and maple syrup urine disease. In Western countries, food faddism, alcoholism, and slimming diets usually lead to decreased folate intake in young to middle-aged individuals.[2,180,362–365] Although beer has a higher folate content than that of other alcoholic beverages, alcoholism may lead to neglect of normal dietary practices in favor of the high calories and "high" of alcohol. The edentulous, infirm, or neglected elderly who are too ill to prepare their meals, and psychiatric patients are particularly at risk of nutritional folate deficiency.[2,97,182]

Pregnancy and Infancy

Except for malnutrition in children, pregnancy with poor folate intake is the commonest cause of megaloblastic anemia in the world. Pregnancy and lactation are associated with significantly higher folate requirements (300–400 µg/day) for the growth of the fetus, placenta, breast, and other maternal tissues; recent studies have identified increased catabolism of folate during pregnancy as yet another cause predisposing to

deficiency.[366] This demand for folate must be met by adequate dietary intake.[2,97,182] The placenta has a large number of folate receptors,[124,367] which probably facilitate binding and transport of folates to the developing fetus. Preferential delivery of folate to the fetus can cause or aggravate folate deficiency in the mother. This fact is commonly observed clinically when a mother with severe folate deficiency gives birth to a baby who has normal folate stores.[2] Folate deficiency in the pregnant mother can nevertheless lead to decreased placental weight and premature, low birth weight infants.[182,368,369] There is now unambiguous evidence that periconceptional folate supplementation (800 µg/day) for normal women reduces the incidence of neural tube defects (spina bifida, meningocoele, anencephaly).[370] The recent recognition that folate consumption may not be optimal in adolescent girls is a matter for concern, given the importance of optimizing folate status in women of childbearing age in the prevention of neural tube defects.[371] The Food and Drug Administration may recommend the addition of folic acid to certain foods to ensure adequate folate intake to prevent folate-responsive neural tube defects in normal women. In addition, periconceptional folic acid in higher doses (4 mg/day) also protects nearly 75% of those fetuses of women at risk (women at risk include those who have previously given birth to a child with neural tube defects; these women have a 10-fold increased risk of delivering a subsequent child with the same disorder).[372,373] In addition, unconfirmed data suggest that folic acid administered periconceptionally in high doses (10 mg/day) may reduce the incidence of cleft lip.[374] These provocative studies highlight the importance of folic acid during human development, a subject that is under active investigation. The issue of folate supplementation has been extended to the animal sciences, where the dramatic increase in conception rate, live births, and overall reproductive performance achieved[375,376] verifies many of the clinical observations discussed above.

The incidence of megaloblastic marrows in the United States, Canada, and the United Kingdom during late pregnancy is approximately 25%[2] but in Southern India it is approximately 55%.[377] Folate deficiency is eight times as high in twin pregnancies. Multiparity (multiple, frequent pregnancies with prolonged states of negative folate balance) and hyperemesis gravidarum commonly lead to folate deficiency. However, since the anemia of pregnancy is most frequently due to iron deficiency, the picture of combined iron and folate deficiency (dimorphic anemia) is the more frequent clinical presentation. Increased utilization of folates in newborns leads to a drop in folate levels by approximately 6 weeks. This drop is markedly exaggerated in premature infants, who because of feeding difficulties, infection, or hemolytic disease often develop pure folate deficiency.[2,97,182]

Intrinsic Hematologic Disease

Since folate is necessary for hematopoiesis, folate requirements are increased when there is (1) significant compensatory erythropoiesis in response to peripheral red blood cell destruction, (2) abnormal hematopoiesis, or (3) infiltration by abnormal cells in marrow. The recognition that folate deficiency developing in hemolytic disorders can lead to an acute aplastic crisis has led to routine prophylactic administration of folate. An unexpected increase in transfusional requirement or a fall in platelets should also suggest folate deficiency.[2,97,182]

Folate Malabsorption with Normal Intestinal Mucosa

Inhibition of brush-border pteroylpolyglutamate hydrolase has been suggested but not documented as a mechanism whereby some drugs cause folate deficiency. The recent purification of this enzyme,[102] should clarify the issue.

Congenital Folate Malabsorption

Patients with this disorder (usually the progeny of consanguineous marriages) present in the first 3 months with failure to thrive, diarrhea, sore mouth, megaloblastic anemia with low serum folate, RBC and cerebrospinal fluid folates, normal Cbl levels, progressive mental retardation, seizures, cerebral calcification, athetosis, and ataxia. They do not respond to oral folate or 5-formyl-H_4PteGlu (5 mg), owing to specific intestinal folate malabsorption, as well as to defective folate transport through the choroid plexus into the central nervous system.[116,378-381] Parenteral therapy in high concentrations is necessary to ensure passive folate transport. These "experiments of nature" are the best evidence for (1) a specific, single transport system for folates in the gut and central nervous system, and (2) the occurrence in vivo of passive folate transport at high extracellular folate concentrations. While the details of the former are incompletely understood, the latter has been experimentally demonstrated in vitro,[129] and in vivo during high-dose antifolate protocols.[169] The precise biochemical defect remains to be characterized. Furthermore, the mental retardation and peripheral neuropathy in some of these individuals suggest a role for folates in maintenance of normal functioning of the nervous system. To establish the diagnosis, it is necessary to document that the patient has normal gastrointestinal absorption of other nutrients, intact pancreatic function, and normal mucosa on small intestinal biopsy. The differential diagnosis includes congenital IF deficiency, Immerslund-Gräsbeck syndrome, TC II deficiency, and inborn errors of Cbl metabolism.

Folate Malabsorption with Intestinal Mucosal Abnormalities

Tropical Sprue

Residents of, and visitors to, endemic areas in the tropics can acquire a disorder of unknown etiology characterized by small intestinal malabsorption.[2,182,382,383] Generalized nonspecific small bowel malabsorption leads to a wide spectrum of clinical manifestations arising from defective absorption of fat, carbohydrate, albumin, calcium, folate, and in later stages, Cbl.[384,385] The endemic nature in the tropics (and in certain households)[386,387] and the beneficial response to antibiotics,[388,389] all suggest an infectious etiology. However, the dramatic response to folate, which is curative in the first year in approximately 60% of cases (cited to be almost diagnostic of the disease) has not been explained.[2,182,390] It is unlikely that pure folate deficiency is the primary cause, since nutritional folate deficiency does not result in tropical sprue; the clinical response to antibiotics suggests a close interplay between a pathogenic infectious agent, endogenous flora, and the folate status of the enterocyte.

Tropical sprue shows varying degrees of villous atrophy and loss of intestinal functional surface. Although less severe than in nontropical sprue, it is more extensive, involving the entire small intestine. The clinical picture is one of abrupt onset of explosive, intermittent or continuous diarrhea, abdominal distension and pain associated with anorexia, vomiting, and extreme fatigue. Stools are fluid or semisolid and frequently contain mucus and blood. This stage is followed weeks to months later by nutrient deficiency. Later, as steatorrhea continues, megaloblastosis dominates the clinical picture. In the short term malabsorption leads to folate deficiency, but later in the chronic (>3-year) phase of the disease, Cbl malabsorption contributes additional clinical manifestations of Cbl neuropathy.[2,182,391]

Coexisting iron deficiency (common in these areas) leads to a dimorphic blood picture; pellagra and beri-beri may also coexist in these patients. Treatment of the chronic phase with folate will cure the hematologic manifestations but exacerbate Cbl-deficient neurologic disease. In Southern India, among 64% of patients with megaloblastic anemia from tropical sprue, 21% were due to Cbl deficiency, 33% to folate deficiency alone, and 44% to combined Cbl and folate deficiency.[387] After investigations for associated iron, Cbl, and folate deficiency, therapy with folate and a broad-spectrum antibiotic is indicated together with symptomatic treatment of diarrhea, vomiting, fluid, mineral and electrolyte imbalance, and associated additional nutritional deficiency.[384-391]

Nontropical Sprue (Celiac Disease, Gluten-Induced Enteropathy)

Nontropical sprue is the commonest cause of intestinal malabsorption in temperate zones. It is due to a possibly inherited sensitivity to gluten (a glutamine-rich protein found in wheat and other grains) and to a related substance, gliadin.[392-398] The precise mechanism for induction of sensitivity is unknown. The intestinal lesion (villous atrophy with hypertrophied crypts and lymphocytic and plasma cell infiltrate of the lamina propria) is more florid than that seen in tropical sprue but occurs to a greater extent in the proximal small intestine with relative ileal sparing; as a result, Cbl malabsorption is less common. The consequences of malabsorption are otherwise the same. Patients present at 30–50 years of age with intermittent or persistent diarrhea (abrupt in 20%), weight loss, abdominal distension with discomfort, glossitis, and megaloblastic anemia. Diagnosis is established by tests for malabsorption, characteristic radiographic findings ("moulage" sign), and jejunal biopsy. The symptoms will be exacerbated following a challenge with gluten. Institution of a gluten-free diet not only is curative but also decreases the risk of subsequent malignancy (small intestinal lymphoma/gastrointestinal carcinoma, especially of the esophagus). Evidence of iron deficiency may be prominent in children. The megaloblastosis responds well to folate therapy.[2,182]

Regional Enteritis and Other Small Intestinal Disorders

The distal small intestine is involved in 80% of individuals with Crohn disease, but folate is efficiently absorbed in other more proximal areas. Thus, only with extensive involvement or fistulas do these patients develop folate deficiency. Even in this case, the blood picture is more that of an iron deficiency or anemia of chronic disease. Frank pure megaloblastic anemia occurs rarely enough in this setting to suggest another etiology for folate or Cbl malabsorption.[2,182] Human immunodeficiency virus infection results in an enteropathy, in the absence of opportunistic infection, which leads to the malabsorption of folates.[399]

Defective Cellular Folate Uptake

A rare syndrome of familial aplastic anemia thought to be due to defective cellular folate uptake is presumed to reflect a defect in the physiologic membrane transporter for folates.[400] Although the precise biochemical defect is uncertain, patients with this syndrome only respond to suprapharmacologic doses of folates (which enters cells by passive diffusion). The disorder presents in young adulthood. The diagnosis should be entertained when serum Cbl and folate are normal and the RBC folate is low (Cbl metabolic defects must be excluded) in a patient who has megaloblastosis with an aplastic marrow associated with pancytopenia.[400,401]

Drugs that Perturb Folate Metabolism

Ethanol

Ethanol in amounts of >80 g/day is toxic to hematopoietic precursors and can directly lead to megaloblastosis with abnormal vacuolization of normoblasts as well as to sideroblastic anemias; these toxic changes seen in severe alcoholics are usually associated with significantly higher alcohol consumption and revert to normal with alcohol withdrawal. Patients who have one nutritious meal each day tend to stave off the eventual development of folate deficiency. Alcohol consumption leads to a relatively rapid (2–4-day) fall in serum folates. This is due to the combined effects[182] of increased urinary folate excretion; interruption of the enterohepatic circulation, due to an effect on hepatic pteroylpolyglutamate synthesis and reduced release of tissue folates into plasma and/or bile; formation of acetaldehyde/$H_4PteGlu$ adducts (5,10-(CH_3-CH)-$H_4PteGlu$); increased catabolism of 5-Me$H_4PteGlu$ > folinic acid > folic acid by ethanol → acetaldehyde/xanthine oxidase-generated superoxide[402]; malabsorption of folate by inhibition of jejunal folate pteroylpolyglutamate hydrolase[403]; slight decrease in methionine synthase activity; and increased urinary excretion of formate, which is normally metabolized via folate-requiring enzymes.[404–414] The relative degree to which each of these mechanisms contributes to folate deficiency remains to be determined. Alcohol is probably the most common cause of folate deficiency in the United States.

Trimethoprim and Pyrimethamine

Trimethoprim and pyrimethamine bind to bacterial and parasitic dihydrofolate reductase with much greater affinity than to human dihydrofolate reductase but patients with underlying folate deficiency appear to be more susceptible to the drug. The ensuing megaloblastosis can be reversed by 5-formyl-$H_4PteGlu$.[251]

Methotrexate

Methotrexate binds to human dihydrofolate reductase (K_i approximately 7×10^{-10} M) and leads to trapping of folate as a metabolically inert form ($H_2PteGlu$). This leads to a true depletion of $H_4PteGlu$ within hours and consequently to functional deficiency of 5,10-methylene-$H_4PteGlu$ and reduced thymidylate synthesis. Although megaloblastosis can develop rapidly, the toxic effects of methotrexate can be avoided by administration of 5-formyl-$H_4PteGlu$ within 1–2 hours. However, the effects of repletion on tumor 5,10-methylene-$H_4PteGlu$ represent a problem. Folate receptors take up methotrexate at lower doses, but reduced-folate carrier-mediated and/or passive diffusion appears to be the main route of cellular uptake at high doses (Fig. 41-5). Once in the cell, methotrexate will be polyglutamated, and this determines its cytotoxicity. The maintenance of a gradient between the extracellular and intracellular compartment appears to determine polyglutamation and thus efficiency of cytotoxicity. Although data suggest that intracellular membrane-associated folate receptors bind methotrexate polyglutamates with affinity equally as high as that of dihydrofolate reductase, the clinical and therapeutic significance and interplay of intracellular polyglutamates, dihydrofolate reductase and folate receptors remains to be explored.[122]

Sulfasalazine

Sulfasalazine produces megaloblastosis in ≤67% of patients taking full doses (>2g/day) by decreasing absorption of PteGlu, decreasing conversion of $H_4PteGlu_{(n)}$ to $H_4PteGlu$, and induction of Heinz body hemolytic anemia (increased requirements).

Oral Contraceptives

It is unclear whether cases in which megaloblastic anemia develops while patients are receiving oral contraceptives represent a cause and effect relationship. They may increase folate catabolism (metabolic consumption) or may weakly interfere with DNA synthesis. The megaloblastosis of cervical epithelium often reverses with folate therapy alone.[182]

Anticonvulsants

The mechanism whereby anticonvulsants can lead to impaired absorption of folate has not been established.[415,416] These drugs induce folate-requiring enzyme pathways, leading to increased utilization (consumption) of folates accompanied by increased catabolic products of folate in the urine. There is also a dose-related impairment in thymidine incorporation into DNA, although the precise nature of perturbation is unclear, because abnormal dU suppression is unrelated to the patient's folate/Cbl status. How folates provoke a return of seizures in patients receiving anticonvulsants is unclear, but this effect may be mediated by glutamate (or related) receptors.[417]

Inborn Errors of Folate Metabolism

Knowledge of the intracellular metabolic pathways involving folates can help predict the net effect of deficiency of a single enzyme (Fig. 41-6). Substrate buildup or product deficiency leads to the clinical manifestations. The precise biochemical defects can be proved by specific enzyme assays of the patient's fibroblasts. Deficiency of 5,10-methylenetetrahydrofolate reductase is the most frequent of these rare disorders. It presents with excess HCYS in the serum and urine and with hypomethionineemia. The disease is recognized in infancy because of developmental delay/mental retardation, with motor abnormalities and disturbance in gait. Occasionally, it has remained undiagnosed until adolescence. Serum folates are normal or low, but Cbl is normal. There is no megaloblastosis, TC II levels are normal, and there is often a poor response to PteGlu. Despite a variety of treatments administered, no consistent pattern of response has emerged (which may reflect significant genetic heterogeneity within this disorder). Excellent reviews of these and other inborn errors of folate metabolism are available.[116,332]

Acute Folate Deficiency

The cause of acute folate deficiency in some patients in intensive care units is unknown. Clinically, the presentation is acute megaloblastic arrest of hematopoiesis with thrombocytopenia. These patients are often acutely ill and in subclinical negative folate balance. The combination of additional insults (decreased intake, total parenteral nutrition containing ethanol, dialysis, surgery, sepsis, drugs) appears to provoke frank folate deficiency. Remarkably, the serum folate is often normal in the face of megaloblastosis in the bone marrow without obvious peripheral blood abnormalities. No data on MMA and HCYS levels in this condition have been reported. The dU suppression test has documented intracellular folate deficiency, but is not widely available to confirm the diagnosis. Empirical therapy with 5-formyl-$H_4PteGlu$ (leucovorin) is recommended. Exposure to nitrous oxide[348] should be considered in the differential diagnosis.[182]

MEGALOBLASTIC ANEMIA NOT DUE TO FOLATE OR COBALAMIN DEFICIENCY

In Western countries, megaloblastic anemias induced by chemotherapeutic agents may be more common than those caused by folate or Cbl deficiency. Several chemotherapeutic

ETIOPATHOPHYSIOLOGIC CLASSIFICATION OF FOLATE DEFICIENCY

Nutritional causes
  Decrease dietary intake
    Poverty and famine, institutionalized individuals (psychiatric/nursing homes)/chronic debilitating disease/goats milk (low in folate), cultural/ethnic cooking techniques (food folate destroyed) or special slimming diets or food fads (folate-rich foods not consumed)
  Decreased diet and increased requirements
    Physiologic
      Pregnancy and lactation, prematurity, hyperemesis gravidarum, infancy
    Pathologic
      Intrinsic hematologic diseases involving hemolysis with compensatory erythropoiesis, abnormal hematopoiesis, or bone marrow infiltration with malignant disease
      Dermatologic—psoriasis
Folate malabsorption
  With normal intestinal mucosa
    Some drugs (controversial)
    Congenital folate malabsorption (rare)
  With mucosal abnormalities
    Tropical and nontropical sprue, regional enteritis
Defective cellular folate uptake
  Familial aplastic anemia (rare)
Inadequate cellular utilization
  Folate antagonists (methotrexate)
  Hereditary enzyme deficiencies involving folate
Drugs (multiple effects on folate metabolism)
  Alcohol, sulfasalazine, triamterine, pyrimethamine, trimethoprim-sulfamethoxazole, diphenylhydantoin, barbiturates
Acute folate deficiency (intensive care unit setting, uncertain etiology)

MISCELLANEOUS MEGALOBLASTIC ANEMIAS NOT DUE TO COBALAMIN OR FOLATE DEFICIENCY

Congenital disorders of DNA synthesis
  Orotic aciduria
  Lesch-Nyhan syndrome
  Congenital dyserythropoietic anemia
Acquired disorders of DNA synthesis
  Deficiency—thiamine responsive (DIDMOAD)
  Malignancy—erythroleukemia
    Refractory sideroblastic anemias
    All antineoplastic drugs that inhibit DNA synthesis (including antinucleosides used against human immunodeficiency virus and other viruses)
Toxic—alcohol

agents (e.g., antimetabolites, alkylating agents) kill malignant cells primarily by interfering with DNA synthesis; megaloblastosis is therefore an expected side effect. Hereditary orotic aciduria usually presents in the first year of life, due to deficiency or absence of enzymes that convert orotic acid to uridine monophosphate via orotidine monophosphate. The net cellular deficiency of uridine monophosphate leads to perturbed synthesis of DNA as well as RNA.[418] Thiamine deficiency in the DIDMOAD syndrome (*d*iabetes *i*nsipidus, *d*iabetes *m*ellitus, *m*egaloblastosis, *o*ptic *a*trophy, and sensorineural *d*eafness) due to an inability to transport physiologic thiamine is another rare cause for megaloblastosis in childhood.[419]

CLINICAL PRESENTATIONS AND EVALUATION FOR FOLATE AND Cbl DEFICIENCY

Interview

The patient's general demeanor and answers to questions may reveal a blunted affect with evidence of depression, irritability, forgetfulness, and sleep deprivation (common in pure folate deficiency). Alternatively, Cbl deficiency may present with paranoid ideation (mimicking paranoid schizophrenia),

dementia, cognitive dysfunction, delusions, or lack of energy manifested by slowed responses (Table 41-4). Hallucinations or even obtundation may preclude obtaining an adequate history. The family may indicate the progressive evolution of a marked personality change and may be able to help trace the evolution of symptoms and deviations from the time when the patient was last well. Intermittent therapy with multivitamins, liver pills, and/or injections (often given by a well-meaning family member or unregistered practitioner) is a common "quick-fix" remedy in many cultures. The family is a good source for details on the patient's dietary habits (e.g., food faddism, vegetarianism, alcohol intake), and family history of medical problems (e.g., blood diseases, gluten sensitivity, autoimmune diseases).

A past medical history of epilepsy or alcoholism with seizure disorder (anticonvulsant therapy) is important. Rarely, patients with autoimmune hemolytic anemias may be lost to follow-up and return with acute aplastic crises when they run out of folate. A past surgical history of total or partial gastrectomy and/or anastomosis, fistula, or bowel resection will demonstrate the potential for perturbation of physiologic absorption (loss of IF, bypassing or loss of absorptive surface, blind loop syndromes). Surreptitious or accidental inhalation of nitrous oxide in an occupational setting (dental or anesthesiology professionals) and deliberate inhalation of nitrous oxide (cartridges attached to whipped cream dispensers or visits to "houses of laughter," where nitrous oxide can be inhaled for a small fee) will be revealed only on direct questioning. Visits to tropical countries and the development of intermittent episodic diarrhea may give a clue to tropical sprue; prolonged (>3 years) chronic gastrointestinal symptoms followed by insidious development of neurologic problems predicts a combined (folate followed by Cbl) deficiency.

Systemic review of symptoms may range from none (incidental increased MCV and/or PMN hypersegmentation) to severe (unstable angina from severe anemia). With slow development of anemia, the patient will often not develop cardiopulmonary symptoms until there is a 50% reduction in hemoglobin concentration, which leads to dyspnea on exertion, palpitation and generalized fatigue or lethargy. Only when hemoglobin is <5 g/dl will the patient develop dyspnea at rest and angina on modest exertion or even at rest. Congestive heart failure is heralded by pedal edema, nocturia, orthopnea, and tender hepatomegaly.

Upper gastrointestinal symptoms with anorexia associated with intrinsic gastrointestinal disease or anemia with heart failure must be distinguished from symptoms due to glossitis. The latter may lead to an inability to wear dentures, tolerate hot drinks or spicy foods because of burning, and even odynophagia, which may compromise further food intake (seen in both Cbl and folate deficiency). The patient may volunteer that glossitis is relieved by multivitamin ingestion, at which time the interviewer should remember to ask questions related to the subsequent evolution of neurologic symptoms. Weight loss in Cbl deficiency is not as severe as in folate deficiency arising from intrinsic gastrointestinal disease. Episodic or chronic diarrhea with steatorrhea is commonly due to tropical sprue, although it may be brought on by gluten-containing foods. While these symptoms may be accompanied by abdominal pain, pain in the absence of diarrhea could be due to tabetic crisis (vomiting, abdominal rigidity, absence of leukocytosis, or fever) accompanying spinothalamic involvement in Cbl-deficient myelopathy.

The patient with PA may have two or three semisolid bowel movements per day; although this may be construed as a normal pattern, it may in fact represent a change since the last time the patient was well. Constipation may be related to obstipation arising from involvement of Meissner's and Auerbach's plexus within the gastrointestinal tract. Similarly, incipient loss of bladder or bowel control due to Cbl myelopathy may present with urgency or nocturia.

In contrast to musculoskeletal symptoms (arthralgia or frank arthritis) of autoimmune diseases, nocturnal cramps or pain in upper and lower extremities may indicate spinothalamic tract involvement. Hypoparathyroidism or systemic lupus erythematosus, alone or associated with PA, leads to significant overlap of cerebral, musculoskeletal, and neurologic presentations.

A review of skin symptoms may elicit a history of increased diffuse or blotchy generalized brownish skin pigmentation, especially of nailbeds and skin creases. This is common in Cbl and folate deficiency; associated vitiligo suggests autoimmune disease.

Although symptoms related to neurologic dysfunction may be volunteered, a complete detailed questionnaire should be formulated during the interview. Questions should be directed to perversions in taste or smell, decreased visual acuity, color vision or eye pain (neuritis), tinnitus, or headache. Dizziness with orthostatic hypotension and "blacking out" may be related to severe anemia. Vertigo or difficulty in walking in the dark (loss of proprioception and position sense), difficulty in ambulation (which may feel like "walking on cotton wool"), stiffness of extremities (corticospinal tracts), or ataxia (spinocerebellar tracts) may be indicative of a serious Cbl myelopathy. Early symptoms are symmetric tingling ("pins and needles"), extending from the tips of the toes to a glove and stocking distribution in later stages. "Burning feet" syndrome or, more commonly, complaints of difficulty in performing simple tasks such as buttoning clothes, may also be a presenting symptom. When loss of bladder and bowel control brings the patient to the physician, advanced neurologic dysfunction is invariably present.

Other genitourinary symptoms such as recurrent cystitis from bladder dysfunction, impotence (Cbl neuropathy) or a recent Papanicolaou smear indicative of cervical dysplasia may, rarely, be presenting symptoms. Multiple pregnancies with short intervals between delivery and conception predispose to a high risk of overt folate deficiency. (Cbl deficiency is more often associated with infertility.)

Physical Examination

The physical examination may indicate different features in well-nourished patients (Cbl-deficient vegetarians or PA patients) and poorly nourished (folate-deficient) individuals. The latter will show evidence of significant weight loss or other stigmata of multiple deficiency due to "broad-spectrum" malabsorption. Thus, associated deficiency of vitamins A, D, and K and/or protein-calorie malnutrition may give rise to angular cheilosis, bleeding mucous membranes, dermatitis, osteomalacia, and chronic infections. Varying degrees of pallor with lemon-tint icterus (a combination of pallor and icterus best observed in fair-skinned individuals) are common features of megaloblastosis.

When anemia is severe, the patient may have a low-grade fever. The skin may show either a diffuse brownish pigmentation or abnormal blotchy tanning. Special emphasis should be given to pigmentation of skin creases and nailbeds. In contrast to Addison disease, mucous membrane pigmentation will not be noted. Premature graying is observed in both light- and dark-haired individuals.

A blunted mask-like facies is extremely common in folate deficiency. Alternatively, the patient may show evidence of classic hyper- or hypothyroid facies (associated with PA). Special attention should be given to the eyes and eyebrows for signs of thyroid dysfunction.

Examination of the mouth may reveal glossitis with a smooth (depapillated), beefy red tongue with occasional ulceration of the lateral surface. The neck may show thyromegaly (diffuse or with nodules) in the case of associated disease. Increased jugular venous distension should alert the examiner to cardiovascular failure, with its attendant gallop, cardiomegaly (with or without pericardial effusions), pulmonary basal crepitations, and pleural effusion, tender hepatomegaly and pedal edema. Nontender hepatomegaly, but more often mild splenomegaly, may rarely be due to extramedullary hematopoiesis in severe anemia, but a mid-epigastrium mass raises the ominous possibility of gastric carcinoma (three times as likely as in PA).

No correlation has been found between the extent of anemia and neurologic dysfunction. Patients with normal CBC values will often have neurologic signs and symptoms. In prolonged Cbl deficiency, neurologic examination will demonstrate clear-cut evidence of involvement of posterior and pyramidal, spinocerebellar, and spinothalamic tracts. Among the earliest signs of posterior column dysfunction are loss of position sense in the index toes (before great toe involvement), which is elicited by passive movement, and loss of the ability to discern vibration of a high-pitched (256-cps) tuning fork (a very early elicitable, objective sign) that invariably precedes by many months the loss of ability to sense the vibration of a lower-pitched (128-cps) tuning fork. Usually the patient loses vibration sense to 256 cps from toe to hip before loss of 128 cps vibration sense even begins. Owing to the slow coalescence of contiguous spinal cord lesions, a constellation of elicitable signs may be obtained. Upper motor neuron disease is indicated by weakness and progressive spasticity with increased muscle tone, exaggerated deep tendon reflexes with clonus, extensor plantar response, and incoordinate or scissor gait, which may progress to spastic paraplegia. The involvement of peripheral nerves may markedly modify these signs to include flaccidity and the absence of deep tendon reflexes. A positive Romberg sign is not uncommon, and a positive Lhermitte sign may be elicited. Loss of sphincter and bowel control; altered cranial nerve dysfunction with altered taste, smell, and visual acuity or color perception; and optic neuritis, with an unexplained predominance in males, may be other physical signs indicative of Cbl deficiency. Inability to carry out serial subtraction of 7 from 100 is a valuable test to document reduced cerebral function (the electroencephalogram often indicates slow wave frequency) in PA.

Diagnostic Issues Related to Using Macrocytosis as an Indicator of Megaloblastosis

A recent study that analyzed the significance of macrocytosis in 109 patients identified that only 55% of patients with an MCV of >105 fl had vitamin deficiency.[420] Since macrocytosis per

Table 41-5. Clinical Conditions Not to Be Confused with Megaloblastosis

Macrocytosis[a] without megaloblastosis
    Reticulocytosis
    Liver disease
    Aplastic anemia
    Myelodysplastic syndromes (especially 5q⁻)
    Multiple myeloma
    Hypoxemia
    Smokers
Spurious increases in MCV without macro-ovalocytosis[b]
    Cold agglutinin disease
    Marked hyperglycemia
    Leukocytosis
    Older individuals

[a] The central pallor that normally occupies about one-third of the normal red blood cell is decreased in macro-ovalocytes. This contrasts with the finding of thin macrocytes, where the central pallor is increased.

[b] When the Coulter counter readings of a high MCV are not confirmed by looking at the peripheral smear.

se is not associated with megaloblastosis in nearly one-half of all cases (Table 41-5); additional tests are necessary for complete diagnosis. It should be appreciated that while megaloblastosis implies that a bone marrow test has been performed, with the recent addition of highly sensitive tests for the specific diagnosis of Cbl and folate deficiency, the need for a bone marrow test is often dictated by the urgency to make the diagnosis (see below). In the case of florid hematologic/neurologic disease suggestive of Cbl/folate deficiency, a bone marrow aspiration carried out as soon as possible is invaluable in assisting in rapid diagnosis of megaloblastosis.

Recent Insights into the Changing Spectrum of Cbl Deficiency

The biochemical and clinical spectrum of presentations of Cbl deficiency in the West has changed fairly dramatically compared with that of the developing countries and to earlier descriptions. For instance, in the developing countries, most patients with nutritional Cbl deficiency presented in the second and third decade with pancytopenia, mild hepatosplenomegaly, fever, and thrombocytopenic bleeding, all in keeping with the concept of ineffective hematopoiesis of megaloblastosis.[265,421,422] However, other reports pointed out that the expected findings of anemia and macrocytosis in Cbl deficiency were often absent.[251] When the clinical spectrum and diagnosis of Cbl deficiency was reevaluated among a cohort of unselected consecutive patients in New York and Colorado who fulfilled criteria for unambiguous Cbl deficiency, normal values in hematocrit, MCV, and LDH were found in more than one-third of patients, and approximately 80% had normal white blood cell counts and platelet and serum bilirubin levels.[423] Strikingly, 33% of the patients' blood smears were not identified as diagnostic when evaluated by laboratory personnel, as compared with 94% when evaluated by the investigators themselves. The latter is important, since most physicians in general practice rely heavily on laboratory personnel to "flag" an abnormal blood smear. Equally striking was the important finding that neuropsychiatric abnormalities were noted in nearly one-third of patients, often in the absence of anemia or macrocytosis, or both.[233] These data formed the basis for reevaluating the diagnostic sensitivity and specificity of serum HCYS and MMA in clear-cut Cbl deficiency (406 patients) or folate deficiency (119 patients), the largest cohort of patients reported thus far.[245] In patients with Cbl deficiency, serum MMA levels were elevated in 98.4% and serum HCYS in 95.9%; both metabolites were normal in only one patient (0.2%). For pa-

tients with folate deficiency, the serum HCYS was increased in 91% and MMA was elevated in 12.2% in all but one case, this was attributed to renal insufficiency or dehydration, conditions known to falsely raise concentrations of this metabolite. These data allowed for the conclusion that "normal levels of both MMA and total HCYS rule out clinically significant Cbl deficiency with virtually 100% certainty."[245]

The changing pattern of neurologic presentations deserves special mention. A recent classic review of 153 episodes of Cbl deficiency involving the nervous system uncovered the following facts[234]: most importantly, more than one-fourth of these patients, showed no reduction in the hematocrit despite neurologic disease, and only a few patients had combined hematologic and neurologic disease. The inclusion of anemic and nonanemic patients who were Cbl deficient led to the dramatic conclusion that the higher the hematocrit, the more severe the neurologic disorder. This has its experimental correlates in monkeys and fruit bats, which have severe neurologic disease in the absence of anemia.[219,223,231,232] Profoundly anemic patients frequently had no neurologic deficits, and the level of Cbl had no correlation with either the existence or severity of neurologic disease. Although simultaneous consumption of folate may have negated the development of potential hematologic abnormalities in Cbl, this could not be documented. Among the patients studied, neurologic deficits were mild in 65%, moderate in approximately 25%, and severe in approximately 10% of cases. Paresthesias or ataxia were most commonly the first symptoms, and diminished vibratory sensation and proprioception in the lower extremities were the most common objective early signs. While multiple neurologic syndromes were often seen in the same patient, the spectrum of objective signs could include loss of fine/coarse touch, decreased or increased deep tendon reflexes with spasticity or muscle weakness, urinary or fecal incontinence, orthostatic hypotension, amaurosis, dementia, psychosis, or mood disturbances.[234] Overall, although the neurologic deficits were mild in most cases, severity was related to the duration of symptoms before diagnosis; not unexpectedly, those with shorter duration responded most to appropriate replacement. The recent demonstration of cognitive improvement in 11 of 18 geriatric subjects with low Cbl and quantitative cognitive dysfunction treated with Cbl, as well as the observation of a limited window of opportunity for effective intervention also highlights the importance of early diagnosis for this population.[424]

APPROACH TO DIAGNOSIS OF AND THERAPY FOR MEGALOBLASTOSIS

In general, there are three stages in approaching a patient: (1) recognizing that megaloblastic anemia is present; (2) distinguishing whether folate, Cbl, or combined folate and Cbl deficiencies have led to the anemia; and (3) diagnosing the underlying disease and mechanism responsible for the deficiency. Establishing that the patient does have megaloblastosis is theoretically straightforward. This is easily done by evaluating the CBC, MCV, and peripheral smear, followed by a bone marrow aspiration. Clues to whether Cbl or folate deficiency is responsible for megaloblastosis can be obtained by serum Cbl, serum folate, and RBC folate levels; additional testing of serum MMA and HCYS will define the true nature of the deficiency.[425]

This ideal and orderly work up is not always feasible in clinical practice, where the patient may (1) present for the first time with megaloblastosis with or without associated neurologic disease; (2) be referred after a variable workup has already been initiated for possible megaloblastosis; (3) present with symptoms primarily attributed to a disease predisposing to Cbl or folate deficiency, in which case anemia or neurologic dysfunction may only be a minor symptom; (4) present with isolated neurologic disease in the absence of anemia; or (5) be referred after empiric therapy has been given for presumed Cbl and or folate deficiency.

The immediate question therefore pertains to the overall status of the patient. *If the patient is decompensated or decompensation is imminent,* serum and RBC folate and serum Cbl levels should be obtained and bone marrow aspiration performed to confirm megaloblastosis. The next step is to proceed with transfusion of 1 U of packed RBCs slowly, with vigorous diuretic therapy and/or simultaneous phlebotomy (from the other arm) to obviate further congestive heart failure from fluid overload. Both Cbl and folate should be administered simultaneously in full doses. Tests for Cbl absorption can be deferred until the patient is more stable. Transfusion does not apparently alter serum folate/Cbl levels but will alter red cell folate levels.[426]

If the patient is moderately symptomatic, but not in heart failure, the strong likelihood of a dramatic response (in the sense of well-being and relief of sore tongue) within 2–3 days before hematologic improvement argues against immediate blood transfusion.[427] Therefore, one should proceed with appropriate diagnostic workup as for the well-compensated patient.

If the patient is well compensated, and in the outpatient setting, the physician has time to develop an orderly sequence of diagnostic tests. First, the peripheral smear should be checked and other macrocytic anemias (thin macrocytes with a normoblastic marrow in contrast to macro-ovalocytes) ruled out. Blood should be drawn for Cbl and folate levels. The serum and red cell folate and serum Cbl (drawn before the patient's first hospital meal) will be useful to sort out whether the problem is due to (1) negative folate balance (low serum folate only), (2) pure folate deficiency (low serum and RBC folate only), (3) pure Cbl deficiency (normal serum folate, low serum Cbl, low RBC folate), or (4) combined Cbl and folate deficiency (low serum and RBC folate with low serum Cbl). Assuming that there is no urgency to make the diagnosis, the physician can elect to wait for the results of these tests before proceeding with the next test in the diagnostic workup. If the diagnosis of the presence of absence of megaloblastosis *is urgently* needed, a cost-effective test is the bone marrow aspirate, the results of which will be available within 1 hour. If bone marrow aspiration is performed, samples should be sent for special stains (periodic acid-Schiff positivity for erythroleukemia) and for chromosomal analysis (i.e., myelodysplastic syndromes can exhibit some megaloblastic changes in the erythroid series, but megaloblastic granulopoiesis will not be seen). If the marrow is not obviously megaloblastic, but the iron stain indicates absent stores, the morphology should be reviewed again, with special emphasis on granulocytic precursors and promegaloblasts.

If the patient refuses a bone marrow aspiration and/or Cbl deficiency is suspected but Cbl levels are normal, a strong case can be made to test for serum HCYS and MMA. Serum MMA and HCYS are ordered together (the same sample remaining from the serum sent for Cbl and folate may be used if they were stored frozen). The results of the serum HCYS and MMA, which will be available after ≥1 week, will distinguish pure Cbl deficiency from pure folate deficiency. However, pure Cbl deficiency cannot be distinguished from combined Cbl and folate deficiency (increased MMA and HCYS in both) (Table 41-2). A normal MMA and HCYS level eliminates Cbl deficiency with 100% confidence. Normal HCYS suggests that megaloblastic anemia is not due to folate deficiency. These tests are particularly useful if (1) the patient has pure neurologic disease (i.e., no hematologic manifestations from Cbl deficiency), or (2) associated conditions such as iron deficiency or thalassemia are masking the megaloblastosis. It should be noted that administration of folate or Cbl immediately invalidates the diagnostic value of the serum folate and Cbl levels; also, since the elevated serum HCYS and MMA levels begin to drop and normalize after

only about 1 week, a little <1 week after administration of folate/Cbl is left to clinch the diagnosis. (The lack of a validated commercial kit precludes the usefulness of the dU suppression test in routine diagnostic workup. Serum MMA and HCYS can theoretically substitute for this test. Nevertheless, in the rare situations in which a defect in utilization of Cbl or folate is suspected, arrangements should be made with any of the handful of research laboratories in the country [see reference list] where the dU suppression test can be performed on a sample of bone marrow aspirate.)

A reticulocyte count, which will indicate a hypoproliferative state, will be useful to follow the patient's response to appropriate replacement therapy. Additional supporting studies to document increased serum LDH, haptoglobin, and bilirubin (evidence for intramedullary hemolysis) may be performed. Subsequent studies to define the mechanism for Cbl malabsorption with the Schilling test can then be carried out.

Once the megaloblastic state is established, an attempt should be made to determine the underlying mechanism of Cbl/folate deficiency. The etiology of folate deficiency is usually sorted out by this time from the history, physical examination, and clinical setting. If pure folate deficiency has been prolonged, associated Cbl deficiency is expected to ensue, giving special emphasis to the identification of subtle manifestations of neurologic disease. If Cbl deficiency is present, one should proceed with the Schilling test (Table 41-3) and test for serum anti-IF antibodies (specific for PA). This will assist in differentiating PA from other conditions that cause Cbl deficiency. It should be noted that the Schilling test per se will initiate a reticulocytosis by the second or third day in pure Cbl deficiency and may also give a partial response in pure folate deficiency. By this time, additional tests for associated autoimmune diseases should be made, if indicated. If serum IF antibodies are negative, gastric analysis for Histalog-fast achlorhydria need not be performed, except in children for whom it is necessary to distinguish congenital IF deficiency from juvenile PA and Imerslund-Gräsbeck syndrome. In adults, a strong presumptive diagnosis of PA can usually be made with the Schilling test (Table 41-3).

A therapeutic trial can be invaluable. A hematologic response to physiologic doses of Cbl (1–2 μg/day) or folate (100–200 μg/day), manifested by appropriate reticulocytosis, constitutes a positive response. If subnormal responses are obtained to either vitamin, the other can be added. If in doubt, the patient should be treated with full doses of Cbl and folate until further diagnostic tests can be carried out at another facility. Serum HCYS and MMA levels are particularly useful: elevated MMA levels will not return to normal until Cbl is correctly administered; conversely, the elevated HCYS will not return to normal until folic acid is correctly administered.

Therapy

Routine treatment with full doses of parenteral Cbl (1 mg/day) and oral folate (folic acid) (1–5 mg/day) before knowledge of the type of vitamin deficiency is established should only be reserved for the severely ill patient. An appropriate regimen for conditions in which Cbl replenishment will correct cellular Cbl deficiency, but will not correct the underlying problem that led to the deficiency (e.g., PA) is 1 mg/day IM of CN-Cbl (week 1), 1 mg twice weekly (week 2), 1 mg/wk for 4 weeks, and then 1 mg/mo for life (approximately 15% or 150 μg will be retained 48 hours after each 1-mg Cbl injection).

Since the doses of Cbl are much greater than that required physiologically, any theoretical advantage of OH-Cbl over CN-Cbl (greater binding to Cbl-binding proteins, greater serum levels, and less renal excretion) is of little significance in general clinical practice. For patients who refuse monthly parenteral therapy or who prefer daily oral therapy, 1-mg/day tablets are recommended for those with Cbl malabsorption, where Cbl is passively absorbed at high doses.[56,57] This approach is applicable for patients with PA and for patients with an inability to absorb food Cbl. The important issue is to ensure that the patient is compliant and demonstrates adequate Cbl levels and resolution of hematologic and neurologic abnormalities on follow-up examination. For nutritional Cbl deficiency in which the entire circuitry in Cbl absorption is intact, oral tablets or a syrup of Cbl (50 μg/day for life) will suffice. This is a popular form of therapy for Cbl-deficient vegetarians and for patients with disorders of hemostasis; nasal sprays of Cbl may replace this form in the future.

Oral folate (folic acid) at doses of 1–5 mg/day results in adequate absorption, even when intestinal malabsorption of physiologic food folate is present. Therapy should be continued until complete hematologic recovery is documented. If the underlying cause leading to folate deficiency is not corrected, folate may be continued. Folinic acid (5-formyl-H$_4$PteGlu [leucovorin]) should be reserved only for rescue protocols involving antifolates (methotrexate/trimethoprim-sulfamethoxazole, 5-fluorouracil modulation protocols) and in the rare acute folate deficiency syndrome. It is too expensive for conventional repletion in folate-deficient states.

Response to Replenishment

The response of the patient to appropriate replacement is reversion of megaloblastic hematopoiesis to normal hematopoiesis, probably initiated at the stem cell level, within the first 12 hours; by 48 hours, normal hematopoiesis is re-established, and the only evidence for a prior megaloblastic state may be the persistence of a few giant metamyelocytes. Delay of a diagnostic bone marrow aspirate is to be avoided for this reason. Clinically, the first 36–48 hours are often highlighted by the awakening of an occasional semistuporous individual whose "chief complaint" is amazement at the remarkably improved sense of well-being experienced, with increased alertness and appetite, and reduced soreness of the tongue. The ongoing normoblastic hematopoiesis is evidenced by decreases in plasma iron and potassium (1–2 mEq/dl drop in 48 hours), MMA, HCYS, and phosphate excretion. The patient must be given supplemental potassium if borderline or low potassium levels are found before therapy is initiated to obviate potentially fatal arrhythmias. The elevated serum MMA and HCYS levels will return to normal by the end of the first week.

Accelerated turnover of normal DNA in erythroid precursors is associated with an increase in serum urate, which usually peaks by the fourth day, and with increased cellular phosphate uptake for nucleotide synthesis. This may precipitate an attack of gout if the patient has a "gouty predisposition." The reticulocyte count increases by the second to third day and peaks by the fifth to eighth day, with the peak reticulocyte count directly proportional to the degree of pre-existing anemia. This is followed by a rise of RBC count, hemoglobin, and hematocrit by the end of the first week, which eventually normalizes by about 2 months regardless of the initial degree of anemia. By the end of the third week, the RBC count should be above 3×10^6/mm^3; if it is not, additional causes of underlying iron deficiency, hemoglobinopathy, chronic disease, or hypothyroidism should be entertained (Table 41-6).

Table 41-6. Causes of Nonresponsiveness of Megaloblastosis to Therapy with Cbl or Folate

Wrong diagnosis
Combined folate/Cbl deficiency being treated with only one vitamin
Associated iron deficiency
Associated hemoglobinopathy (sickle cell disease/thalassemia)
Associated anemia of chronic disease
Associated hypothyroidism

Hypersegmented PMNs continue to remain in the blood for 10–14 days; however, the number of normal PMNs and platelets rises and normalizes within the first week. During this process, there may be a transient left shift to include myeloid precursors. The reduced intramedullary hemolysis caused by normalized hematopoiesis leads to a gradual reduction in the serum bilirubin by the end of the first week, and LDH levels will drop concomitantly.

In response to Cbl, progression of neurologic damage and dysfunction is inhibited. In general, the degree of functional recovery (reversal of neurologic damage) is inversely related to the extent of disease and duration of signs and symptoms. As a rough estimate, signs and symptoms that have been present for <3 months are usually completely reversible; with longer duration, invariable residual neurologic dysfunction occurs. The reversibility of neurologic damage is slow (a maximal response may take 6 months). Substantial increments in recovery are unlikely to be gained after the first 12 months of appropriate therapy, which indicates irreversibility at this point. However, most neurologic abnormalities have improved in ≤90% of patients with documented subacute combined degeneration.

Follow-up

Patients with neurologic dysfunction from Cbl deficiency have traditionally been given more frequent doses of Cbl (biweekly rather than monthly therapy for the first 6 months), despite the lack of evidence that this form of therapy is more beneficial. Nevertheless, this approach serves a purpose in that improvement in neurologic status can be carefully documented. Once maximal responses have been established and patients are deemed capable of administering Cbl independently, they can be given vials of Cbl with appropriate instructions for lifelong monthly injections. Follow-up outpatient visits every 6 months should be instituted to ensure adequate maintenance of hematopoiesis, as well as early diagnosis of other diseases commonly associated with the Cbl/folate-deficient state.

Although patients with PA have a two-fold increase in proximal femur and vertebral fractures and a threefold increase in distal forearm fractures, it is unclear whether this is reduced by therapy with Cbl. However, because of the excess risk of gastric cancer and carcinoid tumors in patients with PA,[428] the value of endoscopic surveillance was studied prospectively; in 56 patients, 2 patients each with early gastric cancer and gastric carcinoids were identified. This suggests that routine surveillance of all patients with PA every 3 years may be a cost-effective strategy.

Routine Supplementation of Cbl and folate

Routine periconceptional supplementation of folate (1) for normal women,[370] and (2) in higher doses for those women at risk at delivering babies with neural tube defects[372,373] provides effective prophylaxis against the development of neural tube defects. Supplementation with folate throughout pregnancy also helps prevent premature delivery of low-birthweight infants[368,369]; routine supplementation for premature infants and lactating mothers is also recommended. In addition to hematologic diseases leading to increase folate requirements (e.g., autoimmune hemolytic anemia, β-thallasemia), folic acid supplements appear to reduce the toxicity of methotrexate in rheumatoid arthritis and psoriasis.[429–431] The conditions that warrant routine folate/Cbl supplementation are summarized in Table 41-7. However, the beneficial role of Cbl in somatic and autonomic symptoms of diabetic neuropathy,[432] persistent sleep/wake schedule disorders,[433,434] the role of folate/Cbl in reversing vitiligo,[435] aphthous stomatitis,[436] the role of Cbl in

Table 41-7. Indications for Prophylaxis with Cbl/Folate

Prophylaxis with Cbl
    Infants of mothers with PA[a]
    Infants on specialized diets[a]
    Lacto-ovo-vegetarians/vegans[a]
    Total gastrectomy[b]
Prophylaxis with folic acid[c]
    All women contemplating pregnancy ($\geq$400 μg/day)
    Pregnancy and lactation, premature infants
    Mothers at risk of delivery of infants with neural tube defects[d,e]
    Hemolytic anemias/hyperproliferative hematologic states
    Patients with rheumatoid arthritis or psoriasis on therapy with methotrexate[f]

[a] In food Cbl malabsorption secondary to an inability to cleave food Cbl by acid and pepsin, replacement therapy should be 50 μg tablets/day. In all other conditions involving abnormality of Cbl absorption, 1,000 μg/day should be administered to ensure Cbl transport via passive diffusion across the intestine.

[b] Consider late development of Cbl deficiency and iron malabsorption (prophylaxis with oral Cbl and iron).

[c] Ensure that the patient does not have symptoms of Cbl deficiency (commonest: paresthesias/numbness) before initiating folate prophylaxis.

[d] Previous delivery of a child with neural tube defects (spina bifida, encephalocele, meningocele) gives a 10-fold greater risk of subsequent neural tube defects.

[e] Folic acid (4 mg/day) administered periconceptionally and throughout first trimester.

[f] To reduce toxicity of the antifolate.

preventing experimental testicular toxicity,[437] as well as the role of high-dose folate for psychiatric disease[438,439] require further study. Finally, that increased serum HCYS is a risk factor for occlusive arterial disease[440,441] indicates that future intervention trials related to early reversal of Cbl/folate deficiency-related increase in serum HCYS will be forthcoming.

REFERENCES

1. Beck WS: The metabolic functions of vitamin B_{12}. N Engl J Med 266:708, 765, 814, 1962
2. Chanarin I: The Megaloblastic Anemias. 1st & 2nd Eds. Blackwell Scientific, Oxford, 1969 & Edinburgh, 1979
3. International Union for Pure and Applied Chemistry/International Union: The nomenclature of corrinoids. Biochemistry 13:1555, 1974
4. Beck WS: Cobalamin as coenzyme: a twisting trail of research. Am J Hematol 34:83, 1990
5. Herbert V: Biology of disease. Megaloblastic anemias. Lab Invest 52:3, 1985
6. Herbert V: The 1986 Herman Award Lecture. Nutrition Science as a continually unfolding story: the folate and vitamin B_{12} paradigm. Am J Clin Nutr 46:387, 1987
6a. Battersby AR: How nature builds the pigments of life: the conquest of vitamin B_{12}. Science 264:1551, 1994
7. Kondo H, Binder MJ, Kolhouse JF et al: Presence and formation of cobalamin analogues in multivitamin-mineral pills. J Clin Invest 70:889, 1982
8. Herbert V, Drivas G, Foscaldi R et al: Multivitamin/mineral food supplements containing vitamin B_{12} may also contain analogues of B_{12}. N Engl J Med 307:255, 1982
9. Brandt LJ, Bernstein IH, Wagle A: Production of vitamin B_{12} analogues in patients with small bowel overgrowth. Ann Intern Med 87:546, 1977
10. Kondo H, Kolhouse JF, Allen RH: Presence of cobalamin analogues in animal tissues. Proc Natl Acad Sci USA 77:817, 1980
11. Stabler SP, Brass EP, Marcell PD, Allen RH: Inhibition of cobalamin-dependent enzymes by cobalamin analogues in rats. J Clin Invest 87:1422, 1991
12. Rothenberg S, Cotter R: Nutrient deficiencies in man: vitamin B_{12}. In Rechcigl M Jr (ed): CRC Handbook Series in Nutrition and Food. Section E. Nutritional Disorders. CRC Press, Boca Raton, FL, 1978
13. Sullivan LW, Herbert V: Studies on the minimum daily requirement for vitamin B_{12}. N Engl J Med 272:340, 1965
14. Hall CA: Long term excretion of $Co^{57}B_{12}$ and turnover within the plasma. Am J Clin Nutr 14:156, 1964
15. Hsu JM, Kawin B, Minor P, Mitchell JA: Vitamin B_{12} concentrations in human tissues. Nature 210:1264, 1966
16. Herbert V: Recommended dietary intakes (RDI) of vitamin B_{12} in humans. Am J Clin Nutr 45:671, 1987
17. Kanazawa S, Herbert V, Herzlich B et al: Removal of cobalamin analogue in bile by enterohepatic circulation of vitamin B_{12}. Lancet 1:707, 1983
18. Cooper BA, Castle WB: Sequential mechanisms in the enhanced absorption of vitamin B_{12} by intrinsic factor in the rat. J Clin Invest 39:199, 1960
19. Doscherholmen A, McMahon J, Ripley J: Inhibitory effect of eggs on vitamin B_{12} absorption: description of a simple ovalbumin ^{57}Co-vitamin B_{12} absorption test. Br J Haematol 33:261, 1976
20. Carmel R: Subtle and atypical cobalamin deficiency states. Am J Hematol 34:108, 1990
21. Del Corral A, Carmel R: Transfer of cobalamin from the cobalamin-binding protein of egg yolk to R binder of human saliva and gastric juice. Gastroenterology 98:1460, 1990
22. Scarlett JD, Read H, O'Dea K: Protein-bound cobalamin absorption declines in the elderly. Am J Hematol 39:79, 1992
23. Allen RH: Human vitamin B_{12} transport proteins. Prog Hematol 9:57, 1975
24. Allen RH, Seetharam B, Podell E, Alpers DH: Effect of proteolytic enzymes on the binding of cobalamin to R protein and intrinsic factor. In vitro evidence that a failure to partially degrade R protein is responsible for cobalamin malabsorption in pancreatic insufficiency. J Clin Invest 61:47, 1978
25. Hewitt JE, Seetharam B, Leykam J, Alpers DH: Isolation and characterization of a cDNA encoding porcine gastric haptocorrin. Eur J Biochem 189:125, 1990
26. Marcoullis G, Parmentier Y, Nicolas JP et al: Cobalamin malabsorption due to nondegradation of R protein in the human intestine. Inhibited cobalamin absorption in exocrine pancreatic dysfunction. J Clin Invest 66:430, 1980
27. Seetharam B, Alpers DH: Absorption and transport of cobalamin (vitamin B_{12}). Annu Rev Nutr 2:343, 1983
28. Kapadia CR, Donaldson RM: Disorders of cobalamin (vitamin B_{12}) absorption and transport. Annu Rev Med 36:93, 1985
29. Allen RH, Mehlman CS: Isolation of gastric vitamin B_{12}-binding proteins using affinity chromatography. I. Purification and properties of human intrinsic factor. J Biol Chem 248:3660, 1973
30. Levine JS, Nakane PK, Allen RH: Human intrinsic factor secretion: immunocytochemical demonstration of membrane associated vesicular transport in parietal cells. J Cell Biol 90:644, 1981
31. Tang LH, Chokshi H, Hu CB, Gordon MM, Alpers DH: The intrinsic factor (IF)-cobalamin receptor binding site is located in the amino-terminal portion of IF. J Biol Chem 267:22982, 1992
32. Gordon MM, Hu C, Chokshi H et al: Glycosylation is not required for ligand or receptor binding by expressed rat intrinsic factor. Am J Physiol 260: G736, 1991
33. Jeffries GH, Sleisenger MH: The pharmacology of intrinsic factor secretion in man. Gastroenterology 48:444, 1965
34. Festen HP: Intrinsic factor secretion and cobalamin absorption. Physiology and pathophysiology in the gastrointestinal tract. Scand J Gastroenterol 188:1, 1991
35. Koop H, Bachem MG: Serum iron, ferritin, and vitamin B_{12} during prolonged omeprazole therapy. J Clin Gastroenterol 14:288, 1992.
35a. Marcuard SP, Albernez L, Khazanie PG: Omeprazole therapy causes malabsorption of cyanocobalamin (vitamin B_{12}). Ann Intern Med 120:211, 1994
36. Green R, Jacobsen DW, Van Tonder SV et al: Enterohepatic circulation of cobalamin in the non human primate. Gastroenterology 81:773, 1981
37. el Kholty S, Gueant JL, Bressler L et al: Portal and biliary phases of enterohepatic circulation of corrinoids in humans. Gastroenterology 101:1399, 1991.
38. Herbert V: Mechanism of intrinsic factor action in everted sacs of rat small intestine. J Clin Invest 38:102, 1959
39. Donaldson RM, Mackenzie IL, Trier JS: Intrinsic factor-mediated attachment of vitamin B_{12} to brush borders and microvillous membranes of hamster intestine. J Clin Invest 46:1215, 1967
40. MacKenzie IL, Donaldson RM: Effect of divalent cations and pH on intrinsic factor-mediated attachment of vitamin B_{12} to intestinal microvillous membranes. J Clin Invest 51:2465, 1972
41. Mathan VI, Babior BM, Donaldson RM: Kinetics of the attachment of intrinsic factor-bound cobamides to ileal receptors. J Clin Invest 54:598, 1974
42. Hooper DC, Alpers DH, Mehlman CS, Allen RH: Characterization of ileal vitamin B_{12} binding using homogeneous human and hog intrinsic factors. J Clin Invest 52:3074, 1973
43. Hagedorn CH, Alpers DH: Distribution of human intrinsic factor-vitamin B_{12} receptors in human intestine. Gastroenterology 73:1019, 1977
44. Seetharam B, Alpers DH, Allen RH: Isolation and characterization of the ileal receptor for intrinsic factor-cobalamin. J Biol Chem 256:3785, 1981
45. Seetharam B, Bagur SS, Alpers DH: Interaction of ileal receptor for intrinsic factor-cobalamin with synthetic and brush border lipids. J Biol Chem 256: 9813, 1981
46. Seetharam B, Bagur SS, Alpers DH: Isolation and characterization of proteolytically derived ileal receptor for intrinsic factor-cobalamin. J Biol Chem 257:183, 1981
47. Kouvonen I, Gräsbeck R: Topology of the hog intrinsic factor receptor in the intestine. J Biol Chem 256:154, 1981
48. Kapadia CR, Serfilippi D, Voloshin K, Donaldson RM: Intrinsic factor me-

diated absorption of cobalamin by guinea pig ileal cells. J Clin Invest 71: 440, 1983

49. Rothenberg SP, Weisberg H, Ficarra A: Evidence for the absorption of immunoreactive intrinsic factor into the intestinal epithelial cell during vitamin B_{12} absorption. J Lab Clin Med 79:587, 1972

50. Levine JS, Nakane PK, Allen RH: Immunocytochemical localization of intrinsic factor-cobalamin bound to the guinea pig ileum in vitro. Gastroenterology 82:284, 1982

51. Ramanujam KS, Seetharam S, Ramasamy M, Seetharam B: Expression of cobalamin transport proteins and cobalamin transcytosis by colon adenocarcinoma cells. Am J Physiol 260:G416, 1991.

52. Chanarin I, Muir M, Hughes A, Hoffbrand AV: Evidence for intestinal origin of transcobalamin II during vitamin B_{12} absorption. Br Med J 1:1453, 1978

53. Rothenberg SP, Weiss JP, Cotter R: Formation of transcobalamin II-vitamin B_{12} complex by guinea pig mucosa in organ culture after in vivo incubation with intrinsic factor vitamin B_{12}. Br J Haematol 40:401, 1978

54. Peters TJ, Linnell JC, Matthews DM, Hoffbrand AV: Absorption of vitamin B_{12} in the guinea pig. III. The forms of vitamin B_{12} in ileal mucosa and portal plasma in the fasting state and during absorption of cyanocobalamin. Br J Haematol 20:299, 1971

55. Ramasamy M, Alpers DH, Tiruppathi C, Seetharam B: Cobalamin release from intrinsic factor and transfer to transcobalamin II within the rat enterocyte. Am J Physiol 257:G791, 1989.

56. Berlin R, Berlin H, Brante G: Oral treatment of pernicious anemia with high doses of vitamin B_{12} without intrinsic factor. J Intern Med 184:247, 1968

57. Berlin R, Berlin H, Brante G, Pilbrant A: Vitamin B_{12} body stores during oral and parental treatment of pernicious anaemia. Acta Med Scand 204:81, 1978

58. Green PD, Savage CR, Hall CA: Mouse transcobalamin II biosynthesis and uptake by L 929 cells. Arch Biochem Biophys 176:683, 1976

59. Carmel R, Neely SM, Francis RB Jr: Human umbilical vein endothelial cells secrete transcobalamin II. Blood 75:251, 1990

60. Quadros EV, Rothenberg SP, Jaffe EH: Endothelial cells from human umbilical vein secrete functional transcobalamin II. Am J Physiol 255:C296, 1989

61. Platica O, Janeczko R, Quadros EV et al: The cDNA sequence and the deduced amino acid sequence of human transcobalamin II show homology with rat intrinsic factor and human transcobalamin I. J Biol Chem 266:7860, 1991

62. Allen RH, Majerus PW: Isolation of vitamin B_{12}-binding proteins using affinity chromatography. III. Purification and properties of human plasma transcobalamin II. J Biol Chem 247:7709, 1972

63. Rappazzo ME, Hall CA: Transport function of transcobalamin II. J Clin Invest 51:1915, 1972

64. Hall CA: Transcobalamins I and II as natural transport proteins of vitamin B_{12}. J Clin Invest 56:1125, 1975

65. Schneider RJ, Burger RL, Mehlman CS, Allen RH: The role and fate of rabbit and human transcobalamin II in the plasma transport of vitamin B_{12} in the rabbit. J Clin Invest 56:27, 1976

66. Retief FP, Gottlieb CW, Herbert V: Mechanism of vitamin B_{12} uptake by erythrocytes. J Clin Invest 45:1907, 1966

67. Friedman PA, Shia MA, Wallace JK: A saturable high affinity binding site for transcobalamin II-vitamin B_{12} complexes in human placental membrane preparations. J Clin Invest 59:51, 1977

68. Seligman PA, Allen RH: Characterization of a receptor for transcobalamin II isolated from human placenta. J Biol Chem 253:1766, 1978

69. Kolhouse JF, Allen RH: Absorption, plasma transport, and cellular retention of cobalamin analogues in the rabbit. Evidence for the existence of multiple mechanisms that prevent the absorption and tissue dissemination of naturally occurring cobalamin analogues. J Clin Invest 60:1381, 1977

70. Youngdahl-Turner P, Rosenberg LE, Allen RH: Binding and uptake of transcobalamin II by human fibroblasts. J Clin Invest 61:133, 1978

71. Youngdahl-Turner P, Mellman IS, Allen RH, Rosenberg LE: Protein mediated vitamin uptake. Absorptive endocytosis of the transcobalamin II-cobalamin complex by cultured human fibroblasts. Exp Cell Res 118:127, 1979

72. Hakami N, Neiman PE, Canellos GP, Lazerson J: Neonatal megaloblastic anemia due to inherited transcobalamin II deficiency in two siblings. N Engl J Med 285:1163, 1971

73. Burger RL, Mehlman CS, Allen RH: Human plasma R-type vitamin B_{12} binding proteins. I. Isolation and characterization of transcobalamin I, transcobalamin III and the normal granulocyte vitamin B_{12} binding protein. J Biol Chem 250:7700, 1975

74. Carmel R: R binder deficiency. A clinically benign cause of cobalamin pseudodeficiency. JAMA 250:1886, 1983

75. Johnston J, Bollekens J, Allen RH, Berliner N: Structure of the cDNA encoding transcobalamin I, a neutrophil granule protein. J Biol Chem 264:15754, 1989

76. Johnston J, Yang-Feng T, Berliner N: Genomic structure and mapping of the chromosomal gene for transcobalamin I (TCNI): comparison to human intrinsic factor. Genomics 12:459, 1992 (Erratum: 14:208, 1992)

77. Ashwell G, Morell AG: The role of surface carbohydrates in the hepatic recognition and transport of circulating glycoproteins. Adv Enzymol 41:99, 1974

78. Newmark P, Newman GE, O'Brien JRP: Vitamin B_{12} in the rat kidney. Evidence for an association with lysosomes. Arch Biochem Biophys 141:121, 1970

79. Pletch QA, Coffey JW: Properties of proteins that bind vitamin B_{12} in subcellular fractions of rat liver. Arch Biochem Biophys 151:157, 1972

80. Idriss JM, Jonas AJ: Vitamin B12 transport by rat liver lysosomal membrane vesicles. J Biol Chem 266:9438, 1991

81. Kolhouse JF, Allen RH: Recognition of two intracellular cobalamin binding proteins and their identification as methylmalonyl-CoA mutase and methionine synthetase. Proc Natl Acad Sci USA 74:921, 1977

82. Fenton WA, Rosenberg LE: Mitochondrial metabolism of hydroxocobalamin: synthesis of adenosylcobalamin by intact rat mitochondria. Arch Biochem Biophys 189:441, 1978

83. Fenton WA, Rosenberg LE: Genetic and biochemical analyses of human cobalamin mutants in cell culture. Annu Rev Genet 12:223, 1978

84. Rosenberg LE: Disorders of propionate and methylmalonate metabolism. p. 821. In Scriver CR, Beaudet AL, Sly WS, Valle (eds); Stanbury JB, Wyngaarden JB, Fredrickson DS (consulting eds): The Metabolic Basis of Inherited Disease. Vol. 1. 6th Ed. McGraw-Hill, New York, 1989

85. Peterkofsky A, Weissbach H: Release of inorganic tripolyphosphate from adenosine triphosphate during vitamin B_{12} coenzyme biosynthesis. J Biol Chem 238:1491, 1963

86. Beck WS, Flavin M, Ochoa S: Metabolism of propionic acid in animal tissues. III. Formation of succinate. J Biol Chem 229:997, 1957

87. Beck WS, Ochoa S: Metabolism of propionic acid in animal tissues. IV. Further studies on the enzymatic isomerization of methylmalonyl coenzyme A. J Biol Chem 232:931, 1958

88. Banerjee RV, Frasca V, Balou DP, Matthews RG: Participation of cob(I)alamin in the reaction catalyzed by methionine synthase from Escherichia coli: a steady-state and rapid reactino kinetic analysis. Biochemistry 29:11101, 1990

89. Kolhouse JF, Utley C, Stabler SP, Allen RH: Mechanism of conversion of human apo- to holomethionine synthase by various forms of cobalamin. J Biol Chem 266:23010, 1991

90. Banerjee RV, Matthews RG: Cobalamin-dependent methionine synthase. FASEB J 4:1450, 1990

91. Utley CS, Marcell PD, Allen RH et al: Isolation and characterization of methionine synthetase from human placenta. J Biol Chem 260:13656, 1985

92. IUPAC-IUB Joint Commission on Biochemical Nomenclature: Nomenclature and symbols for folic acid and related compounds. Recommendations 1986. J Biol Chem 263:605, 1988

93. Butterworth CE, Santini R, Frommeyer WB: The pteroylglutamate components of American diets as determined by chromatographic fractionation. J Clin Invest 42:1929, 1963

94. Butterworth CE: The availability of food folate. Br J Haematol 14:339, 1968

95. Hoppner K, Lampi B: Effect of nitrite ingestion on the bioavailability of folate in the rat. Int J Vit Nutr Res 62:244, 1992

96. Herbert V: Recommended dietary intakes (RDI) of folate in humans. Am J Clin Nutr 45:661, 1987

97. Cooper BA: Folate nutrition in man and animals. p. 49. In Blakley R, Whitehead VM (eds): Folates and Pterins. Nutritional Pharmacological and Physiological Aspects. Vol. 3. Wiley-Interscience, New York, 1986

98. Rosenberg IH: Folate absorption and malabsorption. N Engl J Med 293:1303, 1975

99. Godwin HA, Rosenberg IH: Comparative studies of the intestinal absorption of [^{3}H]pteroylmonoglutamate and [^{3}H]pteroylheptaglutamate in man. Gastroenterology 69:364, 1975

100. Butterworth CE, Baugh CM, Krumdieck CL: A study of folate absorption and metabolism in man using carbon-14-labelled polyglutamates synthesized by the solid phase method. J Clin Invest 48:1131, 1969

101. Reisenauer AM, Krumdieck CL, Halsted CH: Folate conjugase: two separate activities in human jejunum. Science 198:196, 1977

102. Chandler CJ, Wang TT, Halsted CH: Pteroylpolyglutamate hydrolase from human jejunal brush borders. Purification and characterization. J Biol Chem 261:928, 1986

103. Reisenauer AM, Chandler CJ, Halsted CH: Folate binding and hydrolysis by pig intestinal brush border membranes. Am J Physiol 251:G481, 1986

104. Selhub J, Rosenberg IH: Folate transport in isolated brush border membrane vesicles from rat intestine. J Biol Chem 256:4489, 1981

105. Said HM, Ghishan FK, Redha R: Folate transport by human intestinal brush-border membrane vesicles. Am J Physiol 252:G229, 1987

106. Schron CM, Washington C, Blitzer B: The transmembrane pH gradient drives uphill folate transport in rabbit jejunum. J Clin Invest 76:2030, 1985
107. Schron CM: pH modulation of the kinetics of rabbit jejunal, brush-border folate transport. J Membr Biol 120:192, 1991
108. Zimmerman J: Drug interactions in intestinal transport of folic acid and methotrexate. Further evidence for the heterogeneity of folate transport in the human small intestine. Biochem Pharmacol 44:1839, 1992
109. Said HM, Mohammadkhani R: Folate transport in intestinal brush border membrane: involvement of essential histidine residue(s). Biochem J 290:237, 1993
110. Reisenauer AM: Affinity labelling of the folate-binding protein in pig intestine. Biochem J 267:249, 1990
111. Antony AC, Utley CS, Marcell PD, Kolhouse JF: Isolation characterization and comparison of the solubilized particulate and soluble folate binding proteins from human milk. J Biol Chem 257:10081, 1982
112. Said HM, Horne DW, Wagner C: Effect of human milk folate binding protein on folate intestinal transport. Arch Biochem Biophys 251:114, 1986
113. Olivares M, Hertrampf E, Llaguno S, Stekel A: Nutritional intake of folic acid in breast-fed infants. Bol Oficina Sanit Panam 106:185, 1989
114. Verma RS, Antony AC: Immunoreactive folate-binding proteins from human saliva. Isolation and comparison of two distinct species. Biochem J 286:707, 1992 [Erratum: 289:927, 1993]
115. Said HM, Redha R: A carrier-mediated transport for folate in basolateral membrane vesicles of rat small intestine. Biochem J 247:141, 1987
116. Rowe PB: Inherited disorders of folate metabolism. p. 498. In Stanbury JB, Wyngaarden JB, Fredrickson DS (eds): Metabolic Basis of Inherited Disease. 5th Ed. McGraw-Hill, New York, 1983
117. Rosenberg IH, Selhub J: Intestinal absorption of folates. p. 148. In Blakley RL, Whitehead VM (eds): Folates and Pterins. Nutritional, Pharmacological and Physiological Aspects. Vol. 3. Wiley-Interscience, New York, 1986
118. Steinberg SE, Campbell CL, Hillman RS: Kinetics of the normal folate enterohepatic cycle. J Clin Invest 64:83, 1979
119. Horne DW: Transport of folates and antifolates in liver. Proc Soc Exp Biol Med 202:385, 1993
120. Waxman S: Folate binding proteins. Br J Haematol 29:23, 1975
121. Henderson GB: Folate binding proteins. Annu Rev Nutr 10:319, 1990
122. Antony AC: The biological chemistry of folate receptors. Blood 79:2807, 1992
123. Luhrs CA, Slomiany BL: A human membrane-associated folate binding proteins is anchored by a glycosyl-phosphatidylinositol tail. J Biol Chem 264:21446, 1989
124. Verma RS, Gullapalli S, Antony AC: Evidence that the hydrophobicity of isolated, in situ, and de novo synthesized native human placental folate receptors is a function of glycosyl-phosphatidylinositol anchoring to membranes. J Biol Chem 267:4119, 1992
125. Antony AC, Kane MA, Elwood PC et al: Studies of the role of a particulate folate-binding protein in the uptake of 5-methyltetrahydrofolate by cultured malignant human KB cells. J Biol Chem 260:14911, 1985
126. Kamen BA, Capdevila A: Receptor-mediated folate accumulation is regulated by the cellular folate content. Proc Natl Acad Sci USA 83:5983, 1986
127. Antony AC, Kincade RS, Verma RS, Krishnan SR: The identification of high affinity folate binding proteins in human erythrocyte membranes. J Clin Invest 80:711, 1987
128. Antony AC, Bruno E, Briddell RA et al: Effect of perturbation of specific folate receptors during in vitro erythropoiesis. J Clin Invest 80:1618, 1987
129. Antony AC, Kane MA, Krishnan SR et al: Folate (pteroylglutamate) uptake in human red blood cells, erythroid precursors and KB cells at high extracellular folate concentrations. Evidence against a role for specific folate-binding and transport proteins. Biochem J 260:401, 1989
130. Anderson RGW, Kamen BA, Rothberg KG, Lacey SW: Potocytosis: sequestration and transport of small molecules by caveolae. Science 255:410, 1992
131. Hjelle JT, Christensen EI, Carone FA, Selhub J: Cell fractionation and electron microscope studies of kidney folate-binding protein. Am J Physiol 260:C338 1991
132. Leamon CP, Low PS: Cytotoxicity of momordin-folate conjugates in cultured human cells. J Biol Chem 267:24966, 1992
133. Elwood PC, Kane MA, Portillo RM, Kolhouse JF: The isolation, characterization and comparison of the membrane-associated and soluble folate binding proteins from human KB cells. J Biol Chem 261:15416, 1986
134. Kane MA, Elwood PC, Portillo RM et al: The interrelationship of the soluble and membrane-associated folate binding proteins in human KB cells. J Biol Chem 261:15625, 1986
135. Antony AC, Verma RS: Hydrophobic erythrocyte folate binding proteins are converted by hydrophilic forms by trypsin in vitro. Biochim Biophys Acta 979:62, 1989
136. Antony AC, Verma RS, Unune AR, LaRosa JA: Identification of a Mg²⁺-dependent protease in human placenta which cleaves hydrophobic folate binding proteins to hydrophilic forms. J Biol Chem 264:1911, 1989
137. Verma RS, Antony AC. Kinetic analysis, isolation, and characterization of hydrophobic folate-binding proteins released from chorionic villi cultured under serum-free conditions. J Biol Chem 266:12522, 1991
138. Elwood PC, Deutsch JC, Kolhouse JF: The conversion of the human membrane-associated folate binding protein (folate receptor) to the soluble folate binding protein by a membrane-associated metalloprotease. J Biol Chem 266:2346, 1991
139. Holm J, Hansen SI, Hoier-Madsen M, Bostad L: High-affinity folate binding in human choroid plexus. Characterization of radioligand binding, immunoreactivity, molecular heterogeneity and hydrophobic domain of the binding protein. Biochem J 280:267, 1991
140. Lee HC, Shoda R, Krall JA et al: Folate binding protein from kidney brush border membranes contains components characteristic of a glycoinositol phospholipid anchor. Biochemistry 31:3236, 1992
141. Selhub J, Franklin WA: The folate-binding protein of rat kidney. Purification, properties and cellular distribution. J Biol Chem 259:6601, 1984
142. Selhub J, Nakamura S, Carone FA: Renal folate absorption and the kidney folate binding protein. II. Microperfusion studies. Am J Physiol 252:F757, 1986
143. McMartin KE, Morshed KM, Hazen-Martin DJ, Sens DA: Folate transport and binding by cultured human proximal tubule cells. Am J Physiol 263:F841, 1992
144. Weitman SD, Weinberg AG, Coney LR et al: Cellular localization of the folate receptor: Potential role in drug toxicity and folate homeostasis. Cancer Res 52:6708, 1992
145. Kane MA, Elwood PC, Portillo RM et al: Influence on immunoreactive folate binding proteins of extracellular folate concentrations in cultured human cells. J Clin Invest 81:1398, 1988
146. Goldman ID, Lichtenstein WS, Oliverio VT: Carrier mediated transport of the folic acid analogue methotrexate in the L 1210 cell. J Biol Chem 243:5007, 1968
147. Henderson GB: Transport of folate compounds into cells. p. 207. In Blakley RL, Whitehead VM (eds): Folates and Pterins. Nutritional Pharmacological and Physiological Aspects. Vol. 3. Wiley-Interscience, New York, 1986
148. Fan J, Vitols K, Huennekens FM: Biotin derivatives of methotrexate and folate. Synthesis and utilization for affinity purification of two membrane associated folate transporters from L1210 cells. J Biol Chem 266:14862, 1991
149. Luhrs Ca, Raskin CA, Durbin R et al: Transfection of a glycosylated phosphatidylinositol-anchored folate-binding protein complementary DNA provides cells with the ability to survive in low folate medium. J Clin Invest 90:840, 1992
150. Matsue H, Rothberg KG, Takashima A et al: Folate receptor allows cells to grow in low concentrations of 5-methyltetrahydrofolate. Proc Natl Acad Sci USA 89:6006, 1992
151. Wang X, Shen F, Freisheim JH, et al: Differential stereospecificities and affinities of folate receptor isoforms for folate compounds and antifolates. Biochem Pharmacol 44:1898, 1992
152. Dixon KH, Mulligan T, Chung KN et al: Effects of folate receptor expression following stable transfection into wild type and methotrexate transport-deficient ZR-75-1 human breast cancer cells. J Biol Chem 267:24140, 1992
153. Chung N-K, Saikawa Y, Paik T-H et al: Stable transfectants of human MCF-7 cancer cells with increased levels of human folate receptor exhibit an increased sensitivity to antifolates. J Clin Invest 91:1289, 1993
154. Saikawa Y, Knight CB, Saikawa T et al: Decreased expression of the human folate receptor mediates transport-defective methotrexate resistance in KB cells. J Biol Chem 268:5293, 1993
155. Sadasivan E, Rothenberg SP: The complete amino acid sequence of a human folate binding protein from KB cells determined from the cDNA. J Biol Chem 264:5806, 1989 (Erratum: 265:1821, 1990)
156. Elwood PC: Molecular cloning and characterization of the human folate-binding protein cDNA from placenta and malignant tissue culture (KB) cells. J Biol Chem 264:14893, 1989
157. Lacey SW, Sanders KG, Rothberg KG et al: Complementary DNA for the folate binding protein correctly predicts anchoring to the membrane by glycosyl-phosphatidylinositol. J Clin Invest 84:715, 1989
158. Ratnam M, Marquardt H. Duhring JL, Freisheim JH: Homologous membrane folate binding proteins in human placenta: cloning and sequence of a cDNA. Biochemistry 28:8249, 1989
159. Ragoussis J, Senger G, Trowsdale J, Campbell IG: Genomic organization of the human folate receptor genes on chromosome 11q13. Genomics 14:423, 1992
160. Underhill TM, Williams FM, Murray RC, Flintoff WF: Molecular cloning of a gene involved in methotrexate uptake by DNA-mediated gene transfer. Somat Cell Mol Genet 18:337, 1992
160a. Dixon KH, Lanpher BC, Chiu J et al: A novel cDNA restores reduced folate carrier activity and methotrexate sensitivity to transport deficient cells. J Biol Chem 269:17, 1994

161. Shane B: Folylpolyglutamate synthesis and role in the regulation of one-carbon metabolism. Vitam Horm 45:263, 1989

162. Taylor RT, Hanna ML: Folate-dependent enzymes in cultured Chinese hamster cells. Folylpolyglutamate synthetase and its absence in mutants auxotrophic for glycine + adenosine + thymidine. Arch Biochem Biophys 181: 331, 1977

163. Shane B, Stokstad ELR: Vitamin B_{12}-folate interrelationships. Annu Rev Nutr 5:115, 1985

164. Kane MA, Portillo RM, Elwood PC et al: The influence of extracellular folate concentration on methotrexate uptake by human KB cells. J Biol Chem 261: 44, 1986

165. McCloskey DE, McGuire JJ Russell CA et al: Decreased folylpolyglutamate synthetase activity as a mechanism of methotrexate resistance in CCRF-CEM human leukemia sublines. J Biol Chem 266:6181, 1991

166. Benesch RE, Kwong S, Benesch R, Baugh C: The binding of folyl and antifolylpolyglutamates to hemoglobin. J Biol Chem 260:14653, 1985

167. Hoffbrand AV, Newcombe BFA, Mollin DL: Method of assay of red cell folate activity and the value of the assay as a test for folate deficiency. J Clin Pathol 19:178, 1966

168. Chanarin I: Megaloblastic anemia, cobalamin and folate. J Clin Pathol 40: 978, 1987

169. Evans WE, Crom WR, Abromovitch M et al: Clinical pharmacodynamics of high-dose methotrexate in acute lymphocytic leukemia. Identification of a relationship between concentration and effect. N Engl J Med 314:471, 1986

170. Chanarin I, Deacon R, Lumb M et al: Cobalamin-folate interrelations: a critical review. Blood 66:479, 1985

171. Appling DR. Compartmentation of folate-mediated one-carbon metabolism in eukaryotes. FASEB J 5:2645, 1991

172. Herbert V, Zalusky R: Interrelation of vitamin B_{12} and folic acid metabolism: clearance studies. J Clin Invest 41:1263, 1962

173. Noronha JM, Silverman M: On folic acid, vitamin B_{12}, methionine and formiminoglutamic acid metabolism. p. 728. In Heinrich HC (ed): Vitamin B_{12} und Intrinsic Faktor 2. Eur Symp Enke, Hamburg, 1962

174. Chanarin I, Deacon R, Lumb M, Perry J: Vitamin B_{12} regulates folate metabolism by supply of formate. Lancet 2:505, 1980

175. Perry J, Chanarin I, Deacon R, Lumb M: Chronic cobalamin inactivation impairs folate polyglutamate synthesis in the rat. J Clin Invest 71:1183, 1983

176. Lumb M, Chanarin I, Perry J, Deacon R: Turnover of the methyl moiety of 5-methyltetrahydropteroylglutamic acid in the cobalamin-inactivated rat. Blood 66:1171, 1985

177. Chanarin I, Deacon R, Lumb M, Perry J: Cobalamin and folate: recent developments. J Clin Pathol 45:277, 1992

178. Hoffbrand AV, Jackson BFA: Correction of the DNA synthesis defect in vitamin B_{12} deficiency by tetrahydrofolate: evidence in favour of the methylfolate trap hypothesis as the cause of megaloblastic anaemia in vitamin B_{12} deficiency. Br J Haematol 83:643, 1993

179. Wagner C: Proteins binding pterins and folates. p. 251. In Blakely RL, Whitehead VM (eds): Folates and Pterins. Nutritional, Pharmacological and Physiological Aspects. Wiley-Interscience, New York, 1986

180. Wagner C, Decha-Umphai W, Corbin J: Phosphorylation modulates the activity of glycine N-methyltransferase, a folate binding protein. In vitro phosphorylation is inhibited by the natural folate ligand. J Biol Chem 264:9638, 1989

181. Beck WS: Metabolic features of cobalamin deficiency in man. p. 403. In Babior BM (ed): Cobalamin: Biochemistry and Pathophysiology. Wiley-Interscience, New York, 1975

182. Chanarin I: Folate deficiency. p. 75. In Blakley RL, Whitehead VM (eds): Folates and Pterins. Nutritional, Pharmacological and Physiological Aspects. Vol. 3. Wiley-Interscience, New York, 1986

183. Killman S-A: Effect of deoxyuridine on incorporation of tritiated thymidine: difference between normoblasts and megaloblasts. J Intern Med 175:483, 1964

184. Metz J: The deoxyuridine suppression test. CRC Crit Rev Clin Lab Sci 20: 205, 1984

185. Goulian M, Bleile B, Tseng BY: The effect of methotrexate on levels of dUTP in animal cells. J Biol Chem 225:10630, 1980

186. Goulian M, Bleile B, Tseng BY: Methotrexate induced uracil misincorporation of uracil into DNA. Proc Natl Acad Sci USA 77:1956, 1980

187. Lindahl T: New class of enzymes acting on damaged DNA. Nature 259:64, 1976

188. Rogers JC: Characterization of DNA excreted from phytohemagglutinin-stimulated lymphocytes. J Exp Med 143:1249, 1976

189. Matthews JH, Armitage J, Wickramasinghe SN: Thymidylate synthesis and utilization via the de novo pathway in normal and megaloblastic human bone marrow cells. Eur J Haematol 42:396, 1989

190. Curtin NJ, Harris AL, Aherne GW: Mechanism of cell death following thymidylate synthase inhibition: 2-deoxyuridine 5'-triphosphate accumulation. DNA damage, and growth inhibition following exposure to CB3717 and dipyridamole. Cancer Res 51:2346, 1991

191. Matthews JH, Shiels S, Wickramasinghe SN. The effects of folate deficiency on thymidylate synthase activity, deoxyuridine suppression, cell size and doubling time in a cultured human myeloid cell line. Eur J Haematol 45:43, 1990

192. Pelliniemi T-T, Beck WS: Biochemical mechanisms in the Killman experiment. Critique of the deoxyuridine suppression test. J Clin Invest 65:449, 1980

193. Carmel R: Reversal by cobalamin therapy of minimal defects in the deoxyuridine suppression test in patients without anemia: further evidence for a subtle metabolic cobalamin deficiency. J Lab Clin Med 119:240, 1992

194. Waxman S, Metz J, Herbert V: Defective DNA synthesis in human megaloblastic bone marrow: effects of homocysteine and methionine. J Clin Invest 48:284, 1969

195. Health CW: Cytogenetic observations in vitamin B_{12} and folate deficiency. Blood 27:800, 1966

196. Menzies RC, Crossen PE, Fitzgerald PH, Gunz FW: Cytogenetic and cytochemical studies on marrow cells in B_{12} and folate deficiency. Blood 28:581, 1966

197. Vance GH, Moncino M, Heerema N: Cytogenetic findings of a child with transcobalamin II deficiency. Am J Med Genetics 46:615, 1993

198. Kass L: Acetylation and methylation of histones in pernicious anemia. Blood 44:125, 1974

199. Lawler SD, Roberts PD, Hoffbrand AV: Chromosome studies in megaloblastic anemia before and after treatment. Scand J Haematol 8:309, 1971

200. Wickremasinghe RG, Hoffbrand AV: Reduced rate of DNA replication fork movement in megaloblastic anemia. J Clin Invest 65:26, 1980

201. Nathan DG, Gardner FH: Erythroid cell maturation and hemoglobin synthesis in megaloblastic anemia. J Clin Invest 41:1086, 1962

202. Myhre E: Studies on megaloblasts in vitro. Scand J Clin Lab Invest 16:307, 320, 1964

203. Rondanelli EG, Gorini P, Magliulo E, Fiori GP: Differences in proliferative activity between normoblasts and pernicious anemia megaloblasts. Blood 24:542, 1964

204. Wickramasinghe SN, Chalmers DG, Cooper EH: Disturbed proliferation of erythropoietic cells in pernicious anemia. Nature 215:189, 1967

205. Wickramasinghe SN, Bush V: Electron microscope and high resolution autoradiographic studies of megaloblastic erythropoiesis. Acta Haematol 57:1, 1977

206. Wickramasinghe SN, Pratt JR: Myelocyte proliferation in pernicious anemia. Acta Haematol 44:37, 1970

207. Cacoub P, Gatfosse M, Derbel A et al: Vitamin deficiency-induced pancytopenia mimicking leukemia. Three cases. Presse Med 20:1603, 1991

208. Boddington MM: Changes in buccal cells in the anemias. J Clin Pathol 12: 222, 228, 1959

209. Graham RM, Rheault MH: Characteristic cellular changes in cells of non hematopoietic origin in pernicious anemia. J Lab Clin Med 43:235, 1954

210. Lloyd HED, Garry J: Atypical cells in vaginal smears in pernicious anemia. Am J Obstet Gynecol 85:408, 1963

211. Whitehead N, Reyer F, Lindenbaum J: Megaloblastic changes in the cervical epithelium. JAMA 226:1421, 1973

212. Massey BW, Rubin CE: The stomach in pernicious anemia. Am J Med Sci 227:481, 1954

213. Epstein RD: Cells of the megakaryocyte series in pernicious anemia. Am J Pathol 25:239, 1949

214. Antony AC, Briddell, Brandt JE et al: Megaloblastic hematopoiesis in vitro: interaction of anti-folate receptor antibodies with hematopoietic progenitor cells leads to a proliferative response independent of megaloblastic changes. J Clin Invest 87:313, 1991

215. Terade H, Niikura H, Mori H et al: Megaloblastic anemia and platelet function—a qualitative platelet defect in pernicious anemia. Rinsho Ketsueki 31:254, 1990

216. Green R, Kuhl J, Jacobsen R et al: Masking of macrocytosis by α-thalassemia in blacks with pernicious anemia. N Engl J Med 307:1322, 1982

217. Das KC, Herbert V, Colman N, Longo D: Unmasking covert folate deficiency in iron deficient subjects with neutrophil hypersegmentation: dU suppression tests on lymphocytes and bone marrow. Br J Haematol 39:357, 1978

218. Bills ND, Koury MJ, Clifford AJ, Dessypris EN: Ineffective hematopoiesis in folate-deficient mice. Blood 79:2273, 1992

219. Agamanolis D, Green R, Harris JW: Neuropathology of vitamin B_{12} deficiency. p. 293. In Dreosti IE, Smith RM (eds): Neurobiology of the Trace Elements. Humana Clifton, NJ, 1983

220. Cardinale GJ, Carty J, Abeles RH: Effect of methylmalonyl coenzyme A, a

metabolite which accumulates in vitamin B_{12} deficiency, on fatty acid synthesis. J Biol Chem 247:4270, 1972

221. Frenkel EP: Abnormal fatty acid metabolism in peripheral nerves of patients with pernicious anemia. J Clin Invest 52:1237, 1973

222. Kondo H, Osborne ML, Kolhouse JF et al: Nitrous oxide has multiple deleterious effects on cobalamin metabolism and causes decreases in activities of both mammalian cobalamin-dependent enzymes in rats. J Clin Invest 67: 1270, 1981

223. Green R, van Tonder SV, Oettle GJ et al: Neurological changes in fruit bats deficient in vitamin B_{12}. Nature 254:148, 1975

224. Marcell PD, Stabler SP, Allen RH: Quantitation of methylmalonic acid and other dicarboxylic acids in normal serum and urine using capillary gas chromatography-mass spectrometry. Anal Biochem 150:158, 1985

225. Stabler SP, Marcell PD, Podell ER, Allen RH: Assay of methylmalonic acid in the serum of patients with cobalamin deficiency using capillary gas chromatography-mass spectrometry. J Clin Invest 77:1606, 1986

226. Stabler SP, Marcell PD, Podell ER, Allen RH: Quantitation of total homocysteine, total cysteine and methionine in normal serum and urine using capillary gas chromatography-mass spectrometry. Anal Biochem 162:185, 1987

227. Stabler SP, Marcell PD, Podell ER et al: Elevation of total homocysteine in the serum of patients with cobalamin or folate deficiency detected by capillary gas chromatography-mass spectrometry. J Clin Invest 81:466, 1988

228. Allen RH, Stabler SP, Savage D, Lindenbaum J: Diagnosis of cobalamin deficiency. I. Usefulness of serum methylmalonic acid and total homocysteine concentrations. Am J Hematol 34:90, 1990

229. Lindenbaum J, Savage D, Stabler SP, Allen RH: Diagnosis of cobalamin deficiency. II. Relative sensitivities of serum cobalamin, methylmalonic acid and total homocysteine concentrations. Am J Hematol 34:99, 1990

230. Carmel R, Watkins D, Goodman SI, Rosenblatt DS: Hereditary defect of cobalamin metabolism (*Cbl* G mutation) presenting as a neurologic disorder in adulthood. N Engl J Med 318:1738, 1988

231. Agamanolis DP, Chester EM, Victor M et al: Neuropathology of experimental vitamin B_{12} deficiency in monkeys. Neurology 26:905, 1976

232. Weir DG, Keating S, Molloy A et al: Methylation deficiency causes vitamin B_{12}-associated neuropathy in the pig. J Neurochem 51:1949, 1988

233. Lindenbaum J, Healton EB, Savage DG et al: Neuropsychiatric disorders caused by cobalamin deficiency in the absence of anemia or macrocytosis. N Engl J Med 318:1720, 1988

234. Healton EB, Savage DG, Brust JCM et al: Neurologic aspects of cobalamin deficiency. Medicine 70:229, 1991.

235. Pezacka EH, Jacobsen DW, Luce K, Green R: Glial cells as a model for the role of cobalamin in the nervous system: impaired synthesis of cobalamin coenzymes in cultured human astrocytes following short-term cobalamin-deprivation. Biochem Biophys Res Commun 184:832, 1992

236. Allen RH: Megaloblastic anemia. p. 846. In Wyngaarden JB, Smith LH Jr, Bennett JC (eds): Cecil Textbook of Medicine. 19th Ed. WB Saunders, Philadelphia, 1992

237. Rainwater DL, Kalattukudy PE: Fatty acid biosynthesis in *Mycobacterium tuberculosis var bovis* bacillus Calmette-Guérin. J Biol Chem 260:616, 1985

238. Dhur A, Galan P, Christides JP et al: Effect of folic acid deficiency upon lymphocyte subsets from lymphoid organs in mice. Comp Biochem Physiol 98:235, 1991

239. Cravo ML, Mason JB, Dayal Y et al: Folate deficiency enhances the development of colonic neoplasia in dimethylhydrazine-treated rats. Cancer Res 52:5002, 1992

240. Lashner BA, Heidenreich PA, Su GL et al: Effect of folate supplementation on the incidence of dysplasia and cancer in chronic ulcerative colitis. A case-control study. Gastroenterology 97:255, 1989

241. Bills ND, Hinrichs SH, Morgan R, Clifford AJ: Delayed tumor onset in transgenic mice fed a low-folate diet. J Natl Cancer Inst 84:332, 1992

242. Herbert V: Experimental nutritional folate deficiency in man. Trans Assoc Am Physicians 75:307, 1962

243. Altman L: Who Goes First. The Story of Self Experimentation in Medicine. Random House, New York, 1987

244. Herzlich B, Herbert V: Depletion of serum holo-transcobalamin. II. An early sign of negative vitamin B_{12} balance. Lab Invest 58:332, 1988

245. Savage D, Lindenbaum J, Stabler SP, Allen RH: Sensitivity of serum methylmalonic acid and total homocysteine determinations for diagnosing cobalamin and folate deficiencies. Am J Med 96:239, 1994

245a. Thompson HT, Dietrich LS, Elvehjem CA: The use of *Lactobacillus leishmannii* in the estimation of vitamin B_{12} activity. J Biol Chem 184:175, 1950

246. Kolhouse JF, Kondo H, Allen NC et al: Cobalamin analogues are present in human plasma and can mask cobalamin deficiency because current radioisotope dilution assays are not specific for true cobalamin. N Engl J Med 299:785, 1978

247. Cooper BA, Whitehead VM: Evidence that some patients with pernicious anemia are not recognized by radiodilution assay for cobalamin in serum. N Engl J Med 299:816, 1978

248. Shojania AM: Problems in the diagnosis and investigation of megaloblastic anemia. Can Med Assoc J 122:999, 1980

249. Lindenbaum J: Status of laboratory testing in the diagnosis of megaloblastic anemia. Blood 61:624, 1983

250. Herbert V: Don't ignore low serum cobalamin (vitamin B_{12}) levels. Arch Intern Med 148:1705, 1988

251. Carmel R: The expected findings of very low serum cobalamin levels, anemia and macrocytosis are often lacking. Arch Intern Med 148:1712, 1988

252. Baker H, Herbert V, Frank O et al: A microbiologic method for detecting folic acid deficiency in man. Clin Chem 5:275, 1959

253. Herbert V: The assay and nature of folic acid activity in human serum. J Clin Invest 40:81, 1961

254. Hoffbrand AV, Newcombe BFA, Mollin DL: Method of assay of red cell folate activity and the value of the assay as a test for folate deficiency. J Clin Pathol 19:17, 1966

255. Goulian M, Beck WS: Modification in the *Lactobacillus casei* assay of serum folate activity. Am J Clin Pathol 46:390, 1966

256. Herbert V: Aseptic addition method for *Lactobacillus casei* assay of folate activity in human serum. J Clin Pathol 19:12, 1966

257. Waxman S, Schreiber C: Measurement of serum folate levels and serum folic acid-binding proteins by 3HPGA radioassay. Blood 42:281, 1973

258. Longo DL, Herbert V: Radioassay for serum and red cell folate. J Lab Clin Med 87:138, 1976

259. Dawson DW, Fish DI, Frew IDO et al: Laboratory diagnosis of megaloblastic anemia: current methods assessed by external quality assurance trials. J Clin Pathol 40:393, 1987

260. Arnaud J, Cotisson A, Meffre G et al: Comparison of different methods for serum folate assay. Ann Biol Clin (Paris) 50:25, 1992

261. Brown RD, Jun R, Hughes W et al: Red cell folate assays: some answers to current problems with radioassay variability. Pathology 22:82, 1990

262. O'Broin S, Kelleher B: Microbiological assay on microtitre plates of folate in serum and red cells. J Clin Pathol 45:344, 1992

263. Hall CA, Chu RC: Serum homocysteine in routine evaluation of potential vitamin B12 and folate deficiency. Eur J Haematol 45:143, 1990

264. Chanarin I, Malkowska V, O'Hea AM et al: Megaloblastic anemia in a vegetarian Hindu community. Lancet 2:1168, 1985

265. Sarode R, Garewal G, Marwaha N, Marwaha RK: Pancytopenia in nutritional megalobastic anaemia. A study from northwest India. Trop Geogr Med 41: 331, 1989

266. Higginbottom MC, Sweetman L, Nyhan WL: A syndrome of methylmalonic aciduria, homocystinuria, megaloblastic anemia and neurologic abnormalities in a vitamin B_{12} deficient breast-fed infant of a strict vegetarian. N Engl J Med 299:317, 1978

267. Johnson PR, Roloff JS: Vitamin B_{12} deficiency in an infant strictly breast-fed by a mother with latent pernicious anemia. J Pediatr 100:917, 1982

268. Doyle JJ, Langevin AM, Zipursky A: Nutritional vitamin B12 deficiency in infancy: three case reports and a review of the literature. Pediatr Hematol Oncol 6:161, 1989

269. Miller DR, Specker BL, Ho ML, Norman EJ: Vitamin B-12 status in a macrobiotic community. Am J Clin Nutr 53:524, 1991

270. King CE, Liebach J, Toskes PP: Clinically significant vitamin B_{12} deficiency secondary to malabsorption of protein-bound vitamin B_{12}. Dig Dis Sci 24: 397, 1979

271. Pennypacker LC, Allen RH, Kelly JP et al: High prevalence of cobalamin deficiency in elderly outpatients. J Am Geriatr Soc 40:1197, 1992

272. Norman EJ, Morison JA: Screening elderly populations for cobalamin (vitamin B_{12}) using the urinary methylmalonic acid assay by gas chromatography mass spectrometry. Am J Med 94:589, 1993

273. Waters AH, Murphy MEB: Familial juvenile pernicious anemia. A study of the hereditary basis of pernicious anemia. Br J Haematol 9:1, 1963

274. Miller DR, Bloom GE, Streiff RR et al: Juvenile "congenital" pernicious anemia: clinical and immunologic studies. N Engl J Med 274:978, 1966

275. Carmel R: Gastric juice in congenital pernicious anemia contains no immunoreactive intrinsic factor molecule: study of three kindreds with variable ages at presentation including a patient first diagnosed in adulthood. Am J Hum Genet 35:67, 1983

276. Paulson M, Harvey JC: Hematological alterations after total gastrectomy: evolutionary sequences over a decade. JAMA 156:1556, 1954

277. MacLean LD, Sunberg RD: Incidence of megaloblastic anemia after total gastrectomy. N Engl J Med 254:885, 1956

278. Lous P, Schwartz M: The absorption of vitamin B_{12} following partial gastrectomy. J Intern Med 164:407, 1959

279. Deller DJ: Megaloblastic and transitional megaloblastic anemia following partial gastrectomy: study of 27 cases. Aust NZ J Med 2:235, 1969

280. Hines JD, Hoffbrand AV, Mollin DL: The hematologic complications following partial gastrectomy. A study of 292 patients. Am J Med 43:555, 1967

281. Miller A, Furlong D, Burrows BA, Slingerand DW: Bound vitamin B_{12} absorption in patients with low serum B_{12} levels. Am J Hematol 40:163, 1992

282. Yale CE, Gohdes PN, Schilling RF: Cobalamin absorption and hematologic status after two types of gastric surgery for obesity. Am J Hematol 42:63, 1993

283. Carmel R, Johnson CS: Racial patterns in pernicious anemia: early age of onset and increased frequency of intrinsic factor antibody in black women. N Engl J Med 298:647, 1978

284. Metz J, Randal TW, Kniep CH: Addisonian pernicious anemia in young Bantu females. Br Med J 1:178, 1961

285. Solanki DL, Jacobsen RJ, Green R et al: Pernicious anemia in blacks. Am J Clin Pathol 75:96, 1981

286. Sievers ML: Pernicious anemia in southwestern American Indians. Blood 41:309, 1973

287. Mosbeck J: Heredity in Pernicious Anemia. Munksgaard, Copenhagen, 1953

288. Varis K, Ihamaki T, Harkonen M et al: Gastric morphology, function and immunology in first-degree relatives of probands with pernicious anemia and controls. Scand J Gastroenterol 14:129, 1979

289. Girdwood RH, Eastwood MS, Finlayson NDC, Graham GS: Pernicious anemia as a cause of infertility in twins. Lancet 1:528, 1971

290. Jeffries GH, Hoskins DW, Sleisenger MH: Antibody to intrinsic factor in serum from patients with pernicious anemia. J Clin Invest 41:1106, 1962

291. Fisher JM, Taylor KB: A comparison of autoimmune phenomena in pernicious anemia and chronic atrophic gastritis. N Engl J Med 272:499, 1965

292. Goldberg LS, Fudenberg H: The autoimmune aspects of pernicious anemia. Am J Med 46:489, 1969

293. Irvine WJ: Immunologic aspects of pernicious anemia. N Engl J Med 273:432, 1965

294. Castle WB: Current concepts of pernicious anemia. Am J Med 48:541, 1970

295. Ardeman S, Chanarin I, Krafchik B, Singer W: Addisonian pernicious anemia and intrinsic factor antibodies in thyroid disorders. Q J Med 35:421, 1966

296. Goldberg LS, Cunningham JE, Terasaki PI: Lymphocytotoxins and pernicious anemia. Blood 39:862, 1972

297. Gardner, PI, Heier HE: A human autoantibody to renal collecting ducts associated with thyroid and gastric autoimmunity and possible renal tubular acidosis. Clin Exp Immunol 51:29, 1983

298. DeAizpura HJ, Cosgrove IH, Ungar B, Toh BH: Autoantibodies cytotoxic to gastric parietal cells in serum of patients with pernicious anemia. N Engl J Med 309:625, 1983

299. Inada M, Glass GBJ: Effect of prolonged administration of homologous and heterologous intrinsic factor antibodies on the parietal and peptic cell masses and the secretory function of the rat gastric mucosa. Gastroenterology 69:396, 1975

300. Karlsson FA, Burman P, Loof L, Mardh S: Major parietal cell antigen in autoimmune gastritis with pernicious anemia in the acid-producing H^+, K^+ adenosine triphosphatase of the stomach. J Clin Invest 81:475, 1988

301. Schade SG, Abels J, Schilling RF: Studies on antibody to intrinsic factor. J Clin Invest 46:615, 1967

302. Bradhan KD, Hall Jr, Spray GH, Callendar STE: Blocking and binding autoantibodies to intrinsic factor. Lancet 2:62, 1968

303. Schade SG, Feick P, Muckerheide M, Schilling RF: Occurrence in gastric juice of antibody to a complex of intrinsic factor and vitamin B_{12}. N Engl J Med 275:528, 1966

304. Rose MS, Chanarin I, Donaich D et al: Intrinsic-factor antibodies in absence of pernicious anemia. 3–7 year follow up. Lancet 2:9, 1970

305. Waters HM, Dawson DW, Howarth JE, Geary CG: High incidence of type II autoantibodies in pernicious anemia. J Clin Pathol 46:45, 1993

306. Rose MS, Chanarin I: Intrinsic factor antibody and absorption of vitamin B_{12} in pernicious anemia. Br Med J 1:25, 1971

307. Ardeman S, Chanarin I: Steroids and addisonian pernicious anemia. N Engl J Med 273:1352, 1965

308. Jeffries GH, Todd JE, Sleisenger MH: The effect of prednisolone on gastric mucosal histology, gastric secretion, and vitamin B_{12} absorption in patients with pernicious anemia. J Clin Invest 45:803, 1966

309. McIntyre OR, Sullivan LW, Jeffries GJ, Silver RH: Pernicious anemia in childhood. N Engl J Med 272:981, 1965

310. Yang Y, Ducos R, Rosenberg AJ et al: Cobalamin malabsorption in three siblings due to an abnormal intrinsic factor that is markedly susceptible to acid and proteolysis. J Clin Invest 76:2057, 1985

311. Katz M, Lee SK, Cooper BA: Vitamin B_{12} malabsorption due to a biological inert intrinsic factor. N Engl J Med 287:425, 1972

312. Katz M, Mehlman CS, Allen RH: Isolation and characterization of an abnormal human intrinsic factor. J Clin Invest 53:1274, 1974

313. Veeger W, Abels J, Hellermans N, Nieweg HO: Effects of sodium bicarbonate and pancreatin on the absorption of vitamin B_{12} and fat in pancreatic insufficiency. N Engl J Med 267:1341, 1962

314. Toskes PP, Deren JJ, Conrad ME: Trypsin-like nature of pancreatic factor that corrects vitamin B_{12} malabsorption associated with pancreatic dysfunction. J Clin Invest 52:1660, 1973

315. Shimoda SS, Saunders DR, Rubin CE: The Zollinger-Ellison syndrome with steatorrhoea. Mechanisms of fat and vitamin B_{12} malabsorption. Gastroenterology 55:705, 1968

316. Cameron DG, Watson GM, Witts LJ: The clinical association of macrocytic anemia with intestinal stricture and anastomosis. Blood 4:793, 1949

317. Giannella RA, Broitman SA, Zamcheck N: Vitamin B_{12} uptake by intestinal microorganisms. Mechanism and relevance to syndromes of bacterial overgrowth. J Clin Invest 50:1100, 1971

318. Giannella RA, Broitman SA, Zamcheck N: Competition between bacteria and intrinsic factor for vitamin B_{12}. Implications for vitamin B_{12} malabsorption in intestinal bacterial overgrowth. Gastroenterology 62:255, 1972

319. Murphy MF, Sourial NA, Burman JF et al: Megaloblastic anemia due to vitamin B_{12} deficiency caused by small intestinal bacterial overgrowth. Possible role of vitamin B_{12} analogues. Br J Haematol 62:7, 1986

320. Suter PM, Golner B, Godin BR et al: Reversal of protein-bound vitamin B12 malabsorption with antibiotics in atrophic gastritis. Gastroenterology 101:1039, 1991

321. Nyberg W: Absorption and excretion of vitamin B_{12} in subjects infected with *Diphyllobothrium latum* and in non-infected subjects following oral administration of radioactive B_{12}. Acta Haematol 19:90, 1958

322. Nyberg W: *Diphyllobothrium latum* and human nutrition, with particular reference to vitamin B_{12} deficiency. Proc Nutr Soc 22:8, 1963

323. Scudamore HH, Thompson JH, Owen CA: Absorption of Co^{60}-labelled vitamin B_{12} in man and uptake by parasites, including *Diphyllobothrium latum*. J Lab Clin Med 57:240, 1961

324. Von Bonsdorff B, Gordin B: Treatment of pernicious anemia with intramuscular injections of tapeworm extracts. J Intern Med 144:263, 1953

325. Allcock E: Absorption of vitamin B_{12} in man following extensive resection of the jejunum, ileum and colon. Gastroenterology 40:81, 1961

326. Steinberg F: The megaloblastic anemia of regional ileitis. N Engl J Med 264:186, 1961

327. Buchwald H: Vitamin B_{12} absorption deficiency following bypass of the ileum. Dig Dis Sci 9:755, 1964

328. Immerslund O: Idiopathic chronic megaloblastic anemia in children. Acta Paediatr Scand, suppl. 49:1, 1960

329. Gräsbeck R, Gordin R, Kantero I, Kuhlback B: Selective vitamin B_{12} malabsorption and proteinuria in young people: syndrome. J Intern Med 167:289, 1960

330. Mackenzie IL, Donaldson RM, Trier JS, Mathan VI: Ileal mucosa in familial selective vitamin B_{12} malabsorption. N Engl J Med 286:1021, 1972

331. Cooper BA, Rosenblatt DS: Inherited defects of vitamin B_{12} metabolism. Annu Rev Nutr 7:291, 1987

332. Erbe RW: Inborn errors of folate metabolism. p. 413. In Blakley RL, Whitehead VM (eds): Folates and Pterins. Nutritional Pharmacological and Physiological Aspects. Vol. 3. Wiley-Interscience, New York, 1986

333. Rosenblatt DS, Cooper BA: Inherited defects of vitamin B_{12} utilization. Bioessays 12:331, 1990

334. Festen HP, Tuynman HA, Den Hollander W, Meuwissen SG: Repeated high oral doses of omeprazole do not affect intrinsic factor secretion: proof of a selective mode of action. Aliment Pharmacol Ther 3:375, 1989

335. Adams JF, Clark JS, Ireland JT et al: Malabsorption of vitamin B_{12} and intrinsic factor secretion during biguanide therapy. Diabetalogia 24:16, 1983

336. Hitzig WH, Dohman V, Pluss HJ, Vischer D: Hereditary transcobalamin II deficiency: clinical findings in a new family. J Pediatr 85:622, 1974

337. Burman JF, Mollin DL, Sourial NA, Sladden RA: Inherited lack of transcobalamin II in serum and megaloblastic anemia: a further patient. Br J Haematol 43:27, 1979

338. Haurani FI, Hall CA, Rubin RN: Megaloblastic anemia due to an abnormal transcobalamin II. Blood 48:964, 1976

339. Seligman PA, Steiner LL, Allen RH: Studies of a patient with megaloblastic anemia and an abnormal transcobalamin II. N Engl J Med 303:1209, 1980

340. Haurani FI, Hall CA, Rubin R: Megaloblastic anemia as a result of an abnormal transcobalamin II (Cardeza). J Clin Invest 64:1253, 1979

341. Crane AM, Jansen R, Andrews ER, Ledley FD: Cloning and expression of a mutant methylmalonyl coenzyme A mutase with altered cobalamin affinity that causes mut methylmalonic aciduria. J Clin Invest 89:385, 1992

342. Geraghty MT, Perlman EJ, Martin LS et al: Cobalamin C defect associated with hemolytic-uremic syndrome. J Pediatr 120:934, 1992

343. Rosenblatt DS, Cooper BA, Pottier A et al: Altered vitamin B_{12} metabolism in fibroblasts from a patient with megaloblastic anemia and homocysteinuria due to a new defect in methionine biosynthesis. J Clin Invest 74:214

344. Schuh S, Rosenblatt DS, Cooper BA et al: Homocysteinuria and megaloblastic anemia responsive to vitamin B_{12} therapy. An inborn error of metabolism due to a defect in cobalamin metabolism. N Engl J Med 310:686, 1984

345. Rosenblatt DS, Hosack A, Matiaszuk NV, Cooper BA: Defect in vitamin B_{12} release from lysosomes: newly described inborn error of vitamin B_{12} metabolism. Science 228:1319, 1985

346. Vassiliadis A, Rosenblatt DS, Cooper BA, Bergeron JJM: Lysosomal cobalamin accumulation in fibroblasts from a patient with an inborn error of cobalamin metabolism (*CblF* complementation group): Visualization by electron microscope radioautography. Exp Cell Res 195:295, 1991

347. Lassen JCA, Henrickson E, Neukirch F, Kristensen HS: Treatment of tetanus. Severe bone marrow depression after prolonged nitrous-oxide anaesthesia. Lancet 1:527, 1956

348. Amess JAL, Burman JF, Nancekievill DG, Mollin DL: Megaloblastic haemopoiesis in patients receiving nitrous oxide. Lancet 2:339, 1978

349. Salienk Z, Mendel Jr, Coun D, Nachtman J: Polyneuropathy from inhalation of N_2O cartridges through a whipped cream dispenser. Neurology 28:485, 1978

350. Schilling RF: Is nitrous oxide a dangerous anesthetic for vitamin B_{12} deficient subjects? JAMA 255:1605, 1986

351. Sweeney B, Bingham RM, Amos RJ et al: Toxicity of bone marrow in dentists exposed to nitrous oxide. BMJ 291:567, 1985

352. Ermens AA, Refsum H, Rupreht J et al: Monitoring cobalamin inactivation during nitrous oxide anesthesia by determination of homocysteine and folate in plasma and urine. Clin Pharmacol Ther 49:385, 1991

353. Schilling R: Intrinsic factor studies II. The effect of gastric juice on the urinary excretion of radioactivity after the oral administration of radioactive vitamin B_{12}. J Lab Clin Med 42:860, 1953

354. Chanarin I, Waters DAW: Failed Schilling tests. Scand J Haematol 12:245, 1974

355. Rath CE, McCurdy PR, Duffy BJ: Effect of renal disease on the Schilling test. N Engl J Med 256:111, 1956

356. Callendar ST, Witts LJ, Warner GT, Oliver R: The use of a simple whole body counter for haematological investigations. Br J Haematol 12:276, 1966

357. Carmel R, Herbert V: Correctable intestinal defect of vitamin B_{12} absorption in pernicious anemia. Ann Intern Med 67:1201, 1967

358. Lindenbaum J, Pezzimenti JF, Shea N: Small intestinal function of vitamin B_{12} deficiency. Ann Intern Med 80:326, 1974

359. Grant JP (ed): The State of the Worlds Children—1988. Oxford University Press, New York, 1988

360. Ramalingaswami V, Menon PS: Folic acid in nutritional macrocytic anemia. Indian J Med Res 37:471, 1949

361. Mukiibi JM, Paul B, Mandisodza A: Megaloblastic anaemia in Zimbabwe. 1. Seasonal variation. Central Afr J Med 35:310, 1989

362. Ballard HS, Lindenbaum J: Megaloblastic anemia complicating hyperalimentation therapy. Am J Med 56:740, 1974

363. Luhby AL: Megaloblastic anemia in infancy: clinical considerations and analysis. J Pediatr 54:617, 1959

364. Royston NJW, Parry TE: Megaloblastic anemia complicating dietary treatment of phenylketonuria in infancy. Arch Dis Child 37:430, 1962

365. Strelling MK, Blackledge GD, Goodall HB, Walker CHM: Megaloblastic anemia and whole blood folate levels in premature infants. Lancet 1:898, 1966

366. McPartlin J, Halligan A, Scott JM et al: Accelerated folate breakdown in pregnancy. Lancet 341:148, 1993

367. Antony AC, Utley CS, van Horne KC, Kolhouse JF: Isolation and characterization of a folate receptor from human placenta. J Biol Chem 256:9684, 1981

368. Baumslag N, Edelstein T, Metz J: Reduction of incidence of prematurity by folic acid supplementation in pregnancy. Br Med J 1:16, 1970

369. Iyengar L, Rajalakshmi K: Effect of folic acid supplement on birth weights of infants. Am J Obstet Gynecol 122:332, 1975

370. Cziezel AE, Dudas I: Prevention of the first occurrence of neural tube defects by periconceptional vitamin supplementation. N Engl J Med 327:1832 and editorial, 1992

371. Tsui JC, Nordstrom JW: Folate status of adolescents: effects of folic acid supplementation. J Am Diet Assoc 90:1551, 1990

372. MRC Vitamin Study Research Group: Prevention of neural tube defects. Results of the Medical Research Council Vitamin Study. Lancet 338:131 and editorial p. 153, 1991

373. Vergel RG, Sanchez LR, Heredero BL et al: Primary prevention of neural tube defects with folic acid supplementation: Cuban experience. Prenat Diagn 10: 149, 1990

374. Tolarova M: Periconceptional supplementation with vitamins and folic acid to prevent recurrence of cleft lip. Lancet 2:217, 1982

375. Lindemann MD: Supplemental folic acid: a requirement for optimizing swine reproduction. J Animal Sci 71:239, 1993

376. Mooij PN, Wouters MG, Thomas CM et al: Disturbed reproductive performance in extreme folic acid deficient golden hamsters. Eur J Obstet Gynecol Reprod Biol 43:71, 1992

377. Karthigaini S, Gnanasundaram R, Baker SJ: Megaloblastic erythropoiesis and serum vitamin B_{12} and folic acid levels in pregnancy in South Indian women. Br J Obstet Gynaecol 71:115, 1964

378. Luhby AL, Eagle FJ, Roth E, Cooperman JM: Relapsing megaloblastic anemia and mental retardation as defect in gastrointestinal absorption of folic acid. Am J Dis Child 102:482, 1961

379. Santiago-Borrero PJ, Santini R, Perez-Santiago E, Maldonado N: Congenital isolated defect of folic acid absorption. J Pediatr 82:450, 1973

380. Poncz M, Colman N, Herbert V et al: Therapy of congenital folate malabsorption. J Pediatr 98:76, 1981

381. Corbeel L, VandenBerghe G, Jaeken J et al: Congenital folate malabsorption. Eur J Pediatr 143:284, 1985

382. Stefanini M: Clinical features and pathogenesis of tropical sprue. Medicine 27:379, 1948

383. O'Brien W: Acute military tropical sprue in Southeast Asia. Am J Clin Nutr 21:1007, 1968

384. Gardner FH: Tropical sprue. N Engl J Med 258:791, 835, 1958

385. Klipstein FA: Progress in gastroenterology: tropical sprue. Gastroenterology 54:275, 1968

386. Mathan VI, Ignatius M, Baker SJ: A household epidemic of tropical sprue. Gut 7:490, 1966

387. Baker SJ, Mathan VI: Tropical sprue in southern India. In Wellcome Trust Collaborative Study, Tropical Sprue and Megaloblastic Anemia. Churchill, London, 1971

388. Guerra R, Wheby MS, Bayless TM: Long term antibiotic therapy in tropical sprue. Ann Intern Med 63:619, 1965

389. Klipstein FA, Schenk EA, Samloff IM: Folate repletion associated with oral tetracycline therapy in tropical sprue. Gastroenterology 51:317, 1966

390. Swanson VL, Wheby MS, Bayless TM: Morphological effects of folic acid and vitamin B_{12} on the jejunal lesion of tropical sprue. Am J Pathol 49:167, 1966

391. Baker SJ: Vitamin B_{12} and tropical sprue. Br J Haematol, suppl. 23:135, 1972

392. Cooke WT, Peeney ALP, Hawkins CF: Symptoms, signs and diagnostic features of idiopathic steatorrhoea. Q J Med 22:59, 1953

393. Kowlessar OD, Sleisenger MH: The role of gliadin in the pathogenesis of adult celiac disease. Gastroenterology 44:357, 1963

394. Benson GD, Kowlessar OD, Sleisenger MH: Adult celiac disease with emphasis upon response to gluten-free diet. Medicine 43:1, 1964

395. McCrae WM: Inheritance of coeliac disease. J Med Genet 6:129, 1969

396. French JM, Hawkins CF, Cooke WT: Clinical experience with the gluten-free diet in idiopathic steatorrhoea. Gastroenterology 38:592, 1960

397. Cooke WT, Foue DJ, Cox EV et al: Adult celiac disease. Gut 4:279, 1963

398. Pollock DJ, Nagle RE, Jeejeebhoy KN, Coghill NF: The effect on jejunal mucosa of withdrawing and adding dietary gluten in cases of idiopathic steatorrhoea. Gut 11:567, 1970

399. Revell P, O'Doherty MJ, Tang A, Savidge GF: Folic acid absorption in patients infected with the human immunodeficiency virus. J Intern Med 230:227, 1991

400. Branda RF, Muldow CF, MacArthur JR et al: Folate-induced remission in aplastic anemia with familial defect of cellular folate uptake. N Engl J Med 298:469, 1978

401. Howe RB, Branda RF, Douglas SD, Brunning RD: Hereditary dyserythropoiesis with abnormal membrane folate transport. Blood 54:1080, 1979

402. Shaw S, Jayatilleke E, Herbert V, Colman N: Cleavage of folates during ethanol metabolism. Role of acetaldehyde/xanthine oxidase-generated superoxide. Biochem J 257:277, 1989

403. Naughton CA, Chandler CJ, Duplantier RB, Halsted CH: Folate absorption in alcoholic pigs: in vitro hydrolysis and transport at the intestinal brush border membrane. Am J Clin Nutr 50:1436, 1989

404. Lindenbaum J: Aspects of vitamin B_{12} and folate metabolism in malabsorption syndromes. Am J Med 67:1037, 1979

405. Jandl JH: Anemia of liver disease: observations on its mechanisms. J Clin Invest 34:390, 1955

406. Herbert V, Zalusky R, Davidson CS: Correlation of folate deficiency with alcoholism and associated macrocytosis, anemia and liver disease. Ann Intern Med 58:977, 1963

407. Klipstein FA, Lindenbaum J: Folate deficiency in chronic liver disease. Blood 25:443, 1965

408. Halsted CH, Robles EA, Mezey E: Intestinal malabsorption in folate deficient alcoholics. Gastroenterology 64:526, 1973

409. Cherrick GR: Observations on hepatic avidity for folate in Laennec's cirrhosis. J Lab Clin Med 66:446, 1965

410. Eichner ER: The hematologic disorders of alcoholism. Am J Med 54:621, 1973

411. Eichner ER, Hillman RS: Effect of alcohol on serum folate level. J Clin Invest 52:584, 1973

412. Hillman RS, Steinberg SE: The effects of alcohol on folate metabolism. Annu Rev Med 33:345, 1982

413. Herbert V (ed): Hematologic complications of alcoholism. Semin Hematol 17:83, 1980

414. Lindenbaum J: Folate and vitamin B$_{12}$ deficiencies in alcoholism. Semin Hematol 17:119, 1980

415. Dansky LV, Rosenblatt DS, Andermann E: Mechanism of teratogenesis: folic acid and antiepileptic therapy. Neurology 42:32, 1992

416. Porras Tejero E, Lluch Fernandez MD: Folic acid and vitamin B12 in children under long-term anticonvulsant therapy. An Esp Pediatr 38:113, 1993

417. Van Rijn CM, Van der Velden TJ, Rodrigues de Miranda JF et al: Folates: epileptogenic effects and enhancing effects on [3H]TBOB binding to the GABA-receptor complex. Epilepsy Res 5:199, 1990

418. Kelley WM: Hereditary orotic aciduria. p. 1202. In Stanbury JB, Wyngaarden JB, Fredrickson DS (eds): Metabolic Basis of Inherited Disease. 5th Ed. McGraw-Hill, New York, 1983

419. Rindi G, Casirola D, Poggi V et al: Thiamine transport by erythrocytes and ghosts in thiamine-responsive megalobastic anaemia. J Inher Metab Dis 15: 231, 1992

420. Outeirino Perez JJ, Sanchez Fayos J, Outeirino Hernanz J et al: Hematologic significance of erythrocytic macrocytosis: prospective analysis of 109 successively studied cases. Sangre 34:32, 1989

421. Mukiibi JM, Makumbi FA, Paul B et al: Megaloblastic anemia in Zimbabwe: the pernicious anaemias. East Afr Med J 67:501, 1990

422. Mukiibi JM, Makumbi FA, Gwanzura C: Megaobastic anaemia in Zimbabwe: spectrum of clinical and haematological manifestations. East Afr Med J 69: 83, 1992

423. Stabler SP, Allen RH, Savage DG et al: Clinical spectrum and diagnosis of cobalamin deficiency. Blood 76:871, 1990

424. Martin DC, Francis J, Protetch J, Huff FJ: Time dependency of cognitive recovery with cobalamin replacement: report of a pilot study. J Am Geriatr Soc 40:168, 1992

425. Beck WS: Diagnosis of megaloblastic anemias. Annu Rev Med 42:311, 1992

426. Ho CH: The effects of blood transfusion on serum ferritin, folic acid, and cobalamin levels. Transfusion 32:764, 1992

427. Carmel R. Shulman IA: Blood transfusion in medically treatable chronic anemia. Pernicious anemia as a model for transfusion overuse. Arch Pathol Lab Med 113:995, 1989

428. Sjoblom SM, Sipponen P, Jarvinen H: Gastroscopic follow up of pernicious anemia patients. Gut 34:28, 1993

429. Leung CF, Lao TT, Chang AM: Effect of folate supplement on pregnant women with beta-thalassaemia minor. Eur J Obstet Gynecol Reprod Biol 33: 209, 1989

430. Morgan SL, Baggott JE, Vaughn WH et al: The effect of folic acid supplementation on the toxicity of low-dose methotrexate in patients with rheumatoid arthritis. Arthritis Rheum 33:9, 1990

431. Duhra P: Treatment of gastrointestinal symptoms associated with methotrexate therapy for psoriasis. J Am Acad Dermatol 28:466, 1993

432. Yaqub BA, Siddique A, Sulimani R: Effects of methylcobalamin on diabetic neuropathy. Clin Neurol Neurosurg 94:105, 1992

433. Ohta T, Ando K, Iwata T, Ozaki N et al: Treatment of persistent sleep-wake schedule disorders in adolescents with methylcobalamin (vitamin B$_{12}$) Sleep 14:414, 1991

434. Honma K, Kohsaka M, Fukuda N et al: Effects of vitamin B$_{12}$ on plasma melatonin rhythm in humans: increased light sensitivity phase-advances for circadian clock? Experientia 48:716, 1992

435. Montes LF, Diaz ML, Lajous J, Garcia NJ: Folic acid and vitamin B$_{12}$ in vitiligo: a nutritional approach. Cutis 50:39, 1992

436. Porter S, Flint S, Scully C, Keith O: Recurrent aphthous stomatitis: the efficacy of replacement therapy in patients with underlying hematinic deficiencies. Ann Dent 51:14, 1992

437. Mori K, Kaido M, Fujishiro K et al: Preventive effects of methylcobalamin on the testicular damage induced by ethylene oxide. Arch Toxicol 65:396, 1991

438. Procter A: Enhancement of recovery from psychiatric illness by methylfolate. Br J Psychiatry 159:271, 1991

439. Bottiglieri T, Hyland K, Laundy M et al: Enhancement of recovery from psychiatric illness by methylfolate. Lancet 336:1579, 1990

440. Brattstrom L, Israelsson B, Norrving B et al: Impaired homocysteine metabolism in early-onset cerebral and peripheral occlusive arterial disease. Effects of pyridoxine and folic acid treatment. Atherosclerosis 81:51, 1990

441. Clarke R, Daly L, Robinson K et al: Hyperhomocysteinemia: an independent risk factor for vascular disease. N Engl J Med 324:1149, 1991

442. Rothberg KG, Ying Y, Kolhouse JF et al: The glycophospholipid-linked folate receptor internalizes folate without entering the clathrin-coated pit endocytic pathway. J Cell Biol 110:637, 1990

Thalassemia Syndromes

42

Elias Schwartz, Edward J. Benz, Jr.,
and Bernard G. Forget

INTRODUCTION

The thalassemia syndromes are a heterogeneous group of inherited anemias characterized by defects in the synthesis of one or more of the globin chain subunits of the hemoglobin tetramer. The clinical syndromes associated with thalassemia arise from the combined consequences of inadequate hemoglobin accumulation and unbalanced accumulation of globin subunits. The former causes hypochromia and microcytosis; the latter leads to ineffective erythropoiesis and hemolytic anemia. Clinical manifestations are diverse, ranging from asymptomatic hypochromia and microcytosis to profound anemia, which is fatal in utero or in early childhood if untreated. This heteroge-

neity arises from the variable severity of the primary biosynthetic defects and co-inherited modulating factors, such as accelerated synthesis of fetal globin subunits. Palliative treatment of the severe forms by blood transfusion is eventually defeated by the concomitant problems of iron overload, alloimmunization, and blood-borne infections.

Taken as a group, the thalassemias represent the most common single gene disorder known. In many parts of the world, they constitute major public health problems. Laboratory analysis of these disorders has been one of the most productive and enlightening endeavors of biomedical research. Study of the molecular defects underlying the thalassemia syndromes has led to fundamental advances in our understanding of eukaryotic gene structure and function. For each of these reasons, a thorough understanding of thalassemia and its related disorders is essential to the hematologist. This chapter surveys the major features of these syndromes. Readers wishing more detailed information than can be included here are referred to the comprehensive monographs and chapters written by Weatherall and Clegg,[1] Bunn and Forget,[2] Weatherall,[3] and McDonagh and Nienhuis.[4]

The classification, genetic basis, and pathophysiology of the thalassemia syndromes are based on thorough understanding of the human hemoglobins, their biosynthesis, their encoding globin gene families, and their function as soluble oxygen-carrying pigments. Therefore, the readers of this chapter should first familiarize themselves with the material presented in Chapters 17 and 35. The material presented in this chapter is also substantially clarified by prior reading of Chapter 38, since the principles underlying the pathophysiology of, and therapy for, thalassemia draw heavily on knowledge of iron metabolism.

DEFINITIONS AND NOMENCLATURE

The term thalassemia is derived from a Greek term, which, loosely translated, means "the sea" (Mediterranean) in the blood.[1] It was first applied to the anemias encountered frequently in people of the Italian and Greek coasts and nearby islands.[5-7] The term is now used to refer to inherited defects in globin chain biosynthesis. Individual syndromes are named according to the globin chain whose synthesis is adversely affected. Thus, α-globin synthesis is reduced in α-thalassemia, β-globin synthesis in β-thalassemia, δ and β synthesis in $\delta\beta$-thalassemia, and so forth. In some contexts it is also useful to subclassify the syndromes according to whether synthesis of the affected globin chain is totally absent (i.e., β^0-thalassemia) or only partially reduced (i.e., β^+-thalassemia).

The most common forms of thalassemia arise from the total absence or the partial reduction in the synthesis of structurally normal globin chains. In contrast to the "structural" hemoglobinopathies (e.g., sickle cell anemia), characterized by the production of normal amounts of mutant globin chains having deranged physical or chemical properties, thalassemias are "quantitative" disorders—the primary lesion lies in the amount of globin produced. However, some rare forms of thalassemia are characterized by the production of structurally abnormal globin chains in reduced amounts. These thalassemic hemoglobinopathies share features of both thalassemia and structural hemoglobinopathies.[8]

Some mutations alter the patterns of fetal to adult hemoglobin switching. These conditions, called hereditary persistence of fetal hemoglobin (HPFH), are not generally associated with clinical symptoms; nonetheless, they merit consideration in this chapter. Their importance lies in their role as modulating factors when co-inherited with other hemoglobinopathies, and their usefulness both as models for investigating the molecular basis for globin gene regulation during human development and as paradigms for rational therapy for the major β-chain hemoglobinopathies, namely, sickle cell anemia and β-thalassemia.

ETIOLOGY, EPIDEMIOLOGY, AND PATHOPHYSIOLOGY

The thalassemias are inherited as pathologic alleles of one or more of the globin genes located on chromosomes 11 and 16 (see Ch. 35). These lesions range from total deletion or rearrangement of the loci to point mutations that impair transcrip-

tion, processing, or translation of globin mRNA. The precise nature of the defects is summarized in a later section.

Thalassemias have been encountered in virtually every ethnic group and geographic location. They are most common in the Mediterranean basin and equatorial or near-equatorial regions of Asia and Africa. The "thalassemia belt" extends along the shores of the Mediterranean and throughout the Arabian peninsula, Turkey, Iran, India, and southeastern Asia, especially Thailand, Cambodia, and southern China.[9-12] Gene frequencies in these regions are within the range of 2.5–15%. Like sickle cell anemia and many other hemoglobinopathies, thalassemias are most common in those areas historically afflicted with endemic malaria. Malaria seems to exert heterozygote selection on genes for these hemoglobinopathies. Infection of heterozygotes with the malaria parasite is thought to result in milder disease and less impact on reproductive fitness.[1,2,13] Therefore, the genes for the hemoglobinopathies tend to become fixed and abundant in populations exposed to malaria.

PATHOPHYSIOLOGY—GENERAL PRINCIPLES

The pathophysiology and molecular genetics of individual forms of thalassemia are closely intertwined. Therefore, detailed consideration of these syndromes is best deferred to their individual subsections. This section considers only mechanisms common to the pathogenesis of all these syndromes.[1,4,14]

The primary lesion in all forms of thalassemia is reduced or absent production of one or more globin chains. For all practical purposes, the major impact on clinical well-being occurs only when these lesions affect the α- or β-globin chains necessary for the synthesis of hemoglobin A ($\alpha_2\beta_2$). (Severe impairment of γ-, ϵ-, or ζ-globin production is presumably lethal in utero.) One consequence of reduced globin chain production is immediately apparent: reduced production of functioning hemoglobin tetramers. As a result, hypochromia and microcytosis are characteristic of virtually all patients with thalassemia. In the milder forms of the disease, this phenomenon may be barely detectable.

The second consequence of impaired globin biosynthesis is unbalanced synthesis of the individual α- and β-subunits. Hemoglobin tetramers are highly soluble and have reversible oxygen-carrying properties exquisitely adapted for both oxygen transport and delivery under physiologic conditions. Free or "unpaired" α-, β-, and γ-globin chains are either highly insoluble or incapable of releasing oxygen normally, or both. For poorly understood reasons, no compensatory regulatory mechanism exists whereby impaired synthesis of one globin subunit leads to a compensatory downward adjustment in the production of the other (partner) globin chain of the hemoglobin tetramer. Thus, useless unpaired α-globin chains continue to accumulate in β-thalassemia and β-globin chains in α-thalassemia. (During uterine development, unpaired γ-globin chains accumulate in α-thalassemic individuals.)

The abnormal solubility or oxygen-carrying properties of these chains lead to a variety of physiologic derangements. Indeed, in the severe forms of thalassemia, it is the behavior of the unpaired globin chains accumulating in relative excess that dominates the pathophysiology of the syndrome, rather than the mere underproduction of functioning hemoglobin tetramers. The precise complications of this pathophysiologic phenomenon are rather diverse, depending on both the amount and the identity of the globin chain accumulating in excess. For the moment, the fundamental principle that must be appreciated is that thalassemias cause symptomatology both by underproduction of hemoglobin and by accumulation of unpaired globin subunits. The unpaired subunits are usually the major source of morbidity and mortality.

The predominant circulating hemoglobin at the moment of birth is fetal hemoglobin (Hb F [$\alpha_2\gamma_2$]) (see Ch. 25). Although the switch from γ- to β-globin biosynthesis begins before birth, the composition of hemoglobin in the peripheral blood changes much later because of the long life span of normal circulating red cells. Hb F is thus slowly replaced by adult hemoglobin (Hb A), so that infants do not depend heavily on normal amounts and function of Hb A until they are 4–6 months of age. The pathophysiologic consequences of these considerations are that α-chain hemoglobinopathies tend to be symptomatic in utero and at birth, whereas individuals with β-chain abnormalities are asymptomatic until 4–6 months of age. These differences in the onset of phenotypic expression arise because α-chains are needed to form both Hb F and Hb A, whereas β-chains are required only for Hb A.

β-THALASSEMIA SYNDROMES

Nomenclature

Many different mutations cause β-thalassemia and its related disorders such as $\delta\beta$-thalassemia and the silent carrier state. They are inherited in a multitude of genetic combinations responsible for a heterogeneous group of clinical syndromes. β-Thalassemia major, also known as Cooley's anemia or homozygous β-thalassemia, is a clinically severe disorder due to inheritance of two β-thalassemia alleles, one on each copy of chromosome 11. As a consequence of diminished Hb A synthesis, the circulating red cells are small, thin, and distorted; they contain markedly reduced amounts of hemoglobin. Accumulation of free α-globin chains leads to the deposition of precipitated aggregates of these chains to the detriment of the erythrocyte and its precursor cells in the bone marrow. The hypochromic anemia of thalassemia major is so severe that chronic blood transfusions are usually required.

The term β-thalassemia intermedia is applied to a less severe clinical phenotype in which significant anemia occurs but chronic transfusion therapy is not absolutely required. It is usually due to inheritance of two β-thalassemia mutations, one mild and one severe; inheritance of two mild mutations; or occasionally, inheritance of complex combinations, such as a single β-thalassemia defect and an excess of normal α-globin genes, or two β-thalassemia mutations co-inherited with heterozygous α-thalassemia (in this last form, known as $\alpha\beta$-thalassemia, the α-thalassemia allele reduces the burden of unpaired α-chains).[15–17] Simple heterozygosity for certain forms of β-thalassemic hemoglobinopathies can also be associated with a thalassemia intermedia phenotype.[18,19]

Thalassemia minor, also known as β-thalassemia trait or heterozygous β-thalassemia, is due to the presence of a single β-thalassemia mutation and a normal β-globin gene on the other chromosome. It is characterized by profound microcytosis with hypochromia but mild or minimal anemia.

β-Thalassemia is also called by several other names, including Cooley's anemia, von Jaksch's anemia,[1] target cell anemia, erythroblastic anemia, and familial microcytosis.

Molecular Pathology

Forms of β-thalassemia arise from mutations that affect every step in the pathway of globin gene expression: transcription, processing of the mRNA precursor, translation of mature mRNA, and post-translational integrity of the β-polypeptide

Table 42-1. Common β-Thalassemia Mutations in Different Racial Groups

Racial Group	Description
Mediterranean	IVS-1, position 110 (G → A)
	Codon 39, nonsense (CAG → TAG)
	IVS-1, position 1 (G → A)
	IVS-2, position 745 (C → G)
	IVS-1, position 6 (T → C)
	IVS-2, position 1 (G → A)
Black	−29, (A → G)
	−88, (C → T)
	Poly(A), (AATAAA → AACAAA)
Southeast Asian	Codons 41/42, frameshift (−CTTT)
	IVS-2, position 654 (C → T)
	−28, (A → G)
Asian Indian	IVS-1, position 5 (G → C)
	619-bp deletion
	Codons 8/9, frameshift (+G)
	Codons 41/42, frameshift (−CTTT)
	IVS-1, position 1 (G → T)

(Data from Kazazian and Boehm[21] and personal communication, 1993.)

chain (Fig. 42-1 and Table 42-1). Large deletions removing two or more non-α-genes are found in rare cases, as are smaller partial or total deletions of the β-gene alone (Fig. 42-1). Most types of β-thalassemia are due to point mutations affecting one or a few bases. (The original literature for this section is massive; it is summarized in several reviews.[2–4,20–24]) Of the >125 point mutations causing β-thalassemia, about 15 account for the vast majority of affected patients, with the remainder responsible for the disorder in only relatively few patients. It has been determined that 5 or 6 mutations usually account for >90% of the cases of β-thalassemia in a given ethnic group or geographic area[21,22] (Table 42-1).

Transcription

Several mutations alter promoter regions upstream of the β-globin mRNA sequence, impairing mRNA synthesis, whereas mutations that derange the sequence used as the signal for addition of the poly-(A) tail (polyadenylation signal, see Ch. 35) have been shown to result in abnormal cleavage and polyadenylation of the nascent mRNA precursor, with resulting reduced accumulation of mature mRNA.[20–23]

Processing

Many forms of β-thalassemia are due to mutations that impair splicing of the mRNA precursor into mature mRNA in the nucleus or that prevent translation of the mRNA in the cytoplasm. The molecular pathology of splicing mutations is complex (Fig. 42-1). Some base substitutions ablate the donor (GT) or acceptor (AG) dinucleotides (see Ch. 36), which are absolutely required at the intron-exon boundaries for normal splicing, and thereby completely block production of mature functional mRNA. Thus, no β-globin can be synthesized (β^0-thalassemia). Other mutations alter the consensus sequences that surround the GT- and AG-invariant dinucleotides and decrease the efficiency of normal splicing signals by 70–95%, resulting in β^+-thalassemia; some consensus mutations even abolish splicing completely, causing η^0-thalassemia. A third type of splicing aberration results from mutations that are not in the immediate vicinity of a normal splice site. These alter regions within the gene, called cryptic splice sites, which resemble consensus splicing sites but do not normally sustain splicing (Fig. 42-2). The mutations activate the site by supplying a critical GT or AG nucleotide or by creating a sufficiently strong consensus signal to stimulate splicing at that site 60–100% of the time. The activated cryptic sites generate an

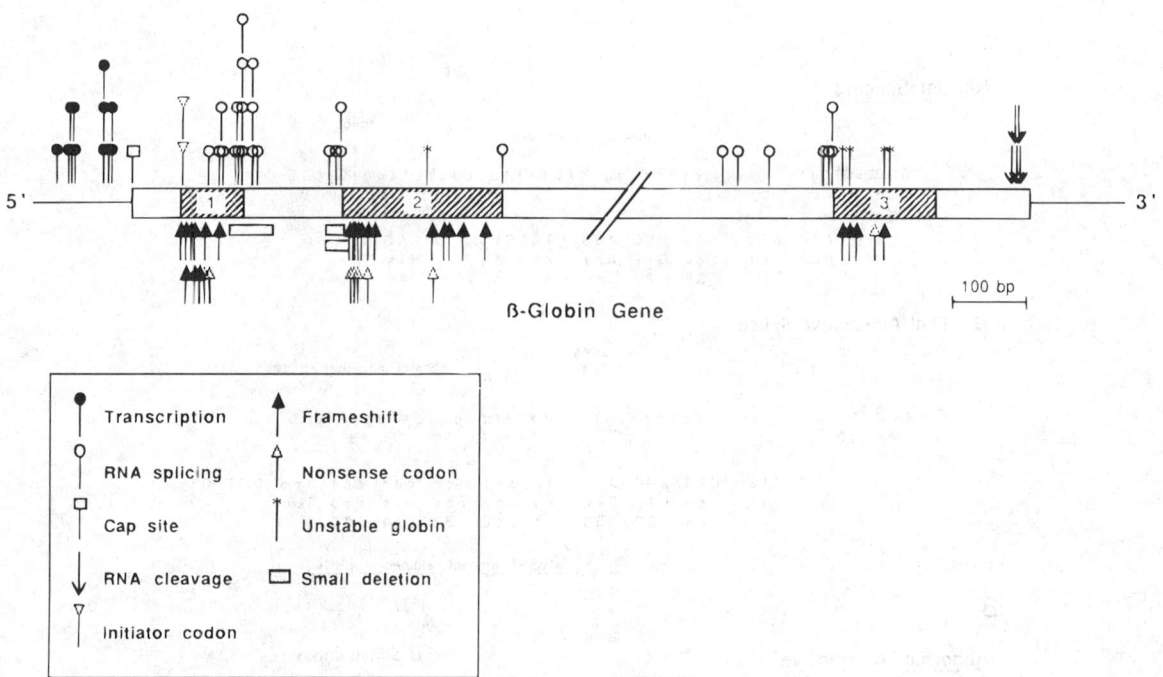

Fig. 42-1. Model of human β-globin gene showing sites and types of various mutations causing β-thalassemia. (From Kazazian,[22] with permission.)

abnormally spliced, untranslatable mRNA species. Only 10–40% of the mRNA precursors are thus spliced at the normal sites, which causes β⁺-thalassemia of varying severity. The mutation responsible for the most common form of β-thalassemia among Greeks and Cypriots (Fig. 42-2) activates a cryptic splice site near the 3′ end of the first intron (position 110).[25,26] The determinants that dictate the degree to which each mutation alters splice site utilization remain largely unknown.

Translation

Mutations that abolish translation occur at several locations along the mature mRNA and are very common causes of β⁰-thalassemia (Fig. 42-1 and Table 42-1). The most common form of β⁰-thalassemia in Sardinians results from a base substitution in the gene that changes the codon encoding the thirty-ninth amino acid of the β-globin chain from CAG, which encodes glutamine, to TAG, whose equivalent (UAG) in mRNA specifies termination of translation[27,28] (Fig. 42-3). A premature termination codon totally abrogates the ability of the mRNA to be translated into normal β-globin. Premature translation termination also results indirectly from frameshift mutations[28] (i.e., small insertions or deletions of a few bases, other than multiples of 3, that alter the phase or frame in which the nucleotide sequence is read during translation). An in-phase premature termination codon is always encountered within the next 50 bases downstream from a frameshift.

Other Sites

Rare mutations that affect gene function by intriguing mechanisms have been described. An extremely large deletion of the β-globin gene cluster has been described that removes the ε-, γ-, and δ-genes.[29] The patient has a severe β-thalassemia phenotype, but the β-globin gene and 500 bases of adjacent 5′ and 3′ DNA have an entirely normal nucleotide sequence. The β-gene functions normally in surrogate cells. The critical aspect of this deletion is that it removes the critical locus control region (LCR)[30] (see Ch. 35) located thousands of bases upstream from the beginning of the globin gene cluster at the 5′

end of the ε-globin gene; loss of this region severely impairs β-gene expression. A number of additional deletions involving the LCR and various portions of the β-gene cluster, but sparing the β-gene itself, have the same phenotype.[30] In other cases of β-thalassemia, the β-gene and adjacent DNA are structurally normal, and the basis of abnormal gene expression is unknown.[22]

The relationship between an individual mutation and the clinical severity of the β-thalassemia phenotype associated with that particular mutation is complex.[21,22] For example, the A→G mutation at position −29 of the β-gene promoter commonly encountered in blacks is associated with a different clinical severity than that found in Chinese patients inheriting the same mutation.[31] Clearly, the genetic "context" of the mutation is different in the two populations. The mutant β-globin gene in the two different racial groups probably arose in different chromosomal backgrounds that have different potentials for γ-gene expression, as discussed in the following paragraph.

Multiple forms or haplotypes of normal non-α-globin gene clusters exist in various human populations. These are defined by the patterns of restriction fragment length polymorphisms[32] (see Ch. 1) detected when DNA is digested with restriction endonucleases and analyzed by Southern gene blotting for the fragments bearing the non-α-globin genes. Haplotypes differ according to whether each restriction site is present along the gene cluster. More than 12 haplotypes have been defined by examination of several restriction sites located along the cluster that are present or absent in a polymorphic manner in normal individuals.[32] The clinical variability encountered in two different groups bearing identical primary mutations correlates best with the haplotype or fragments on which the mutation is inherited. The differences in physiologically important functions among haplotypes that modulate severity remain unknown, but a possible explanation lies in the varying ability of the γ-globin genes in different individuals to respond to severe erythroid stress (see Ch. 17) by increased expression during postnatal life. The γ-globin genes carried on some haplotypes differ in the degree to which they can respond in this manner.[33] Since Hb F synthesis reduces the severity of β-chain hemoglobinopathies,[1] this factor can play an important modulating role.

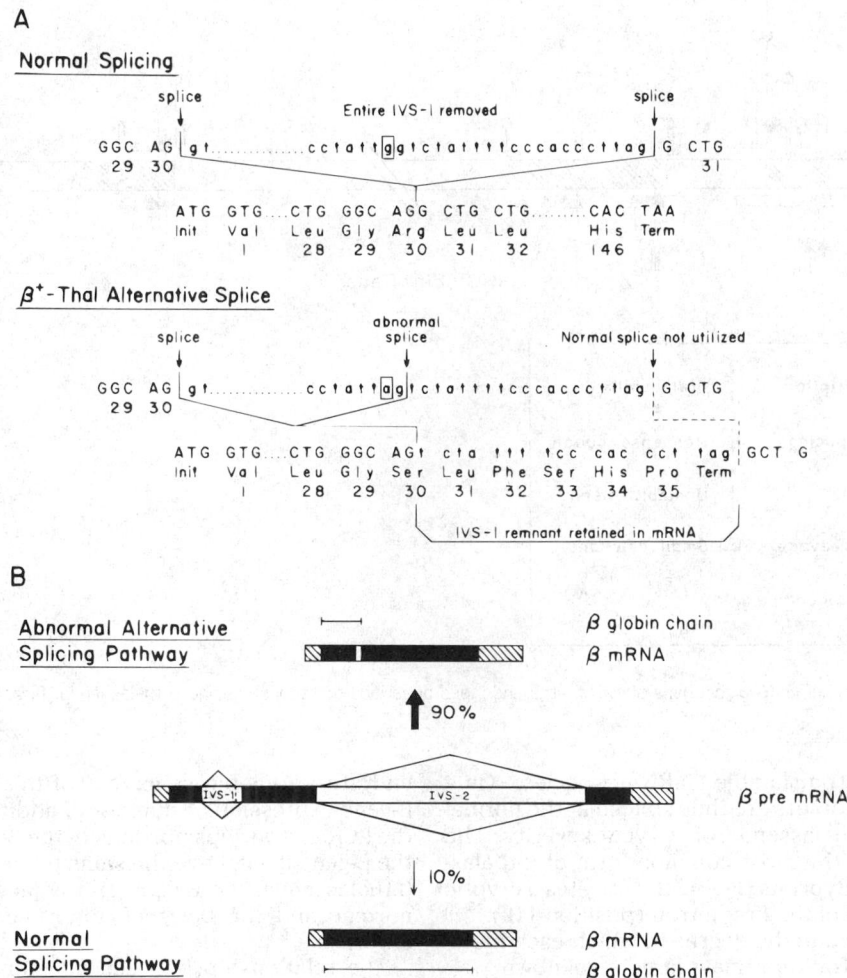

Fig. 42-2. β+-Thalassemia arising from alternative mRNA splicing due to a mutation activating a cryptic splicing site. **(A)** The g → a mutation is shown enclosed in squares, located near the 3' end of intron 1 (IVS-I); it creates a sequence motif closely mimicking a pre-mRNA acceptor splice site. The product of the alternative splicing event is also shown. Note that use of the activated cryptic site generates a mature mRNA that contains an in-frame termination codon and therefore does not encode a functional β-globin chain. (From Benz,[20] with permission). **(B)** Diagram of the means by which use of the cryptic splice site 90% of the time (the observed value) causes only 10% of the mRNA precursor molecules to be spliced normally into translatable mature mRNA, thus causing β+-thalassemia. (From Bunn and Forget,[2] with permission.)

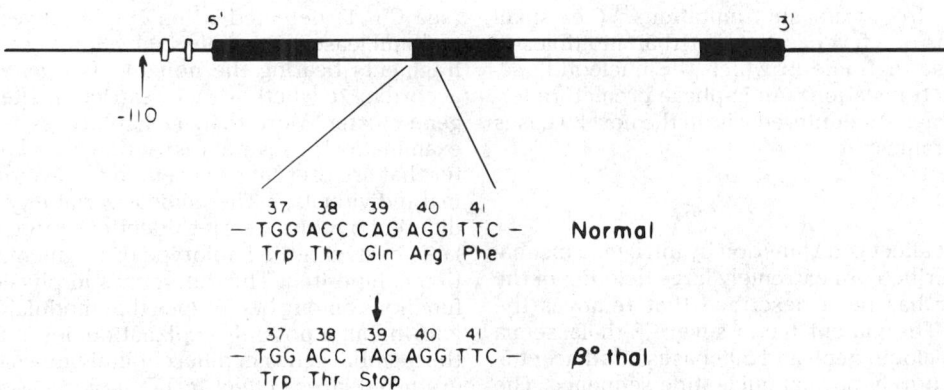

Fig. 42-3. β0-Thalassemia arising from a mutation changing an amino acid codon to a termination codon (nonsense mutation). (From Takeshita et al.,[249] with permission.)

Pathophysiology

The biochemical hallmark of β-thalassemia is reduced biosynthesis of the β-globin subunit of Hb A ($\alpha_2\beta_2$). In β-thalassemia heterozygotes, β-globin synthesis is about half-normal (β/α synthetic ratio 0.5–0.7). In homozygotes for β^0-thalassemia, who account for about one-third of patients, β-globin synthesis is absent. β-Globin synthesis is reduced to 5–30% of normal levels in β^+-thalassemia homozygotes or β^+/β^0-thalassemia compound heterozygotes, who together account for about two-thirds of cases.[1]

Since synthesis of Hb A ($\alpha_2\beta_2$) is markedly reduced or absent, the red cells are hypochromic and microcytic. γ-Chain synthesis is partially reactivated, so that the hemoglobin of the patient contains a relatively large proportion of Hb F.[1] However, these γ-chains are quantitatively insufficient to replace β-chain production.

In heterozygotes (with β-thalassemia trait), relatively little α-globin accumulation occurs. Output from the single normal β-globin gene supports substantial Hb A formation, thus preventing harmful accumulation of excess α-globin chains. Thus, one encounters hypochromia with microcytosis but relatively little evidence of anemia or erythroid stress.

Individuals inheriting two β-thalassemic alleles experience a more profound deficit of β-chain production. Little or no Hb A is produced; more importantly, the imbalance of α- and β-globin production is far more severe (Fig. 42-4). The limited capacity of red cells to proteolyze the excess α-globin chains, a capacity that probably exerts a protective effect in heterozygous β-thal-

assemia, is overwhelmed in homozygotes. Free α-globin accumulates, and unpaired α-chains aggregate and precipitate to form inclusion bodies, which cause oxidative membrane damage within the red cell[34] and destruction of immature developing erythroblasts within the bone marrow (ineffective erythropoiesis).[35] Consequently, very few of the proerythroblasts beginning erythroid maturation in the bone marrow survive long enough to be released into the blood as erythrocytes. The occasional erythrocytes that survive erythropoiesis bear a burden of inclusion bodies. These abnormal cells are removed prematurely by the reticuloendothelial cells in the spleen, liver, and bone marrow, producing hemolytic anemia.

Defective β-globin synthesis exerts at least three distinct yet interlocking effects on the generation of oxygen-carrying capacity for the peripheral blood (Fig. 42-4): (1) ineffective erythropoiesis, which impairs production of new red cells; (2) hemolytic anemia, which shortens the survival of the few red cells produced; and (3) hypochromia with microcytosis, which reduces the oxygen-carrying capacity of those few red cells that do survive. In the most severe forms of the disorder, these three factors conspire to produce a catastrophic anemia, complicated by the stigmata of exuberant hemolysis.

The profound deficit in the oxygen-carrying capacity of the blood stimulates production of high levels of erythropoietin in an attempt to promote compensatory erythroid hyperplasia. Unfortunately, the ability of the marrow to respond is sabotaged by ineffective erythropoiesis. Massive bone marrow expansion does occur, but very few erythrocytes are actually supplied to the circulation. The marrow becomes choked with

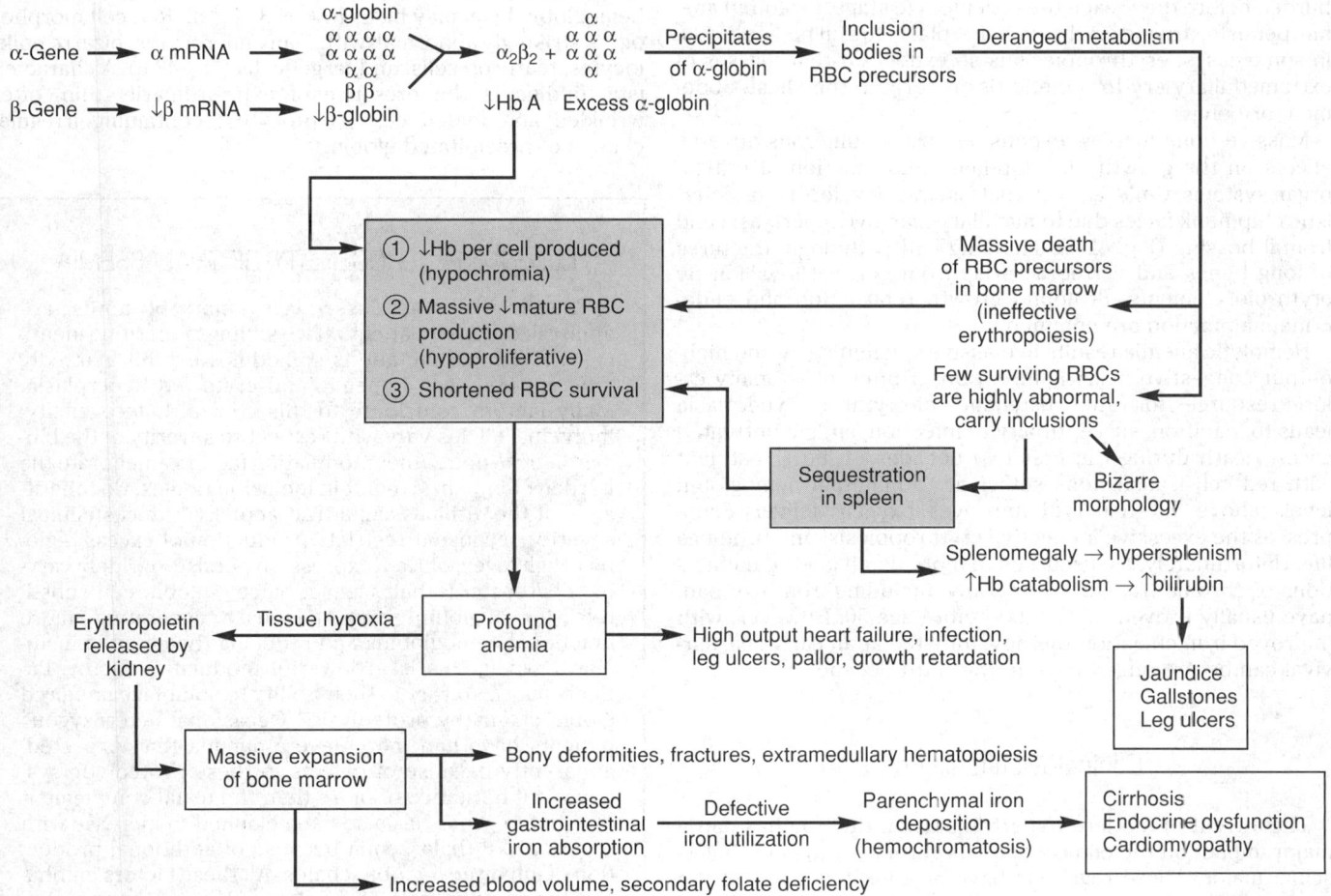

Fig. 42-4. Pathophysiology of severe forms of β-thalassemia. The diagram outlines the pathogenesis of clinical abnormalities resulting from the primary defect in β-globin chain synthesis.

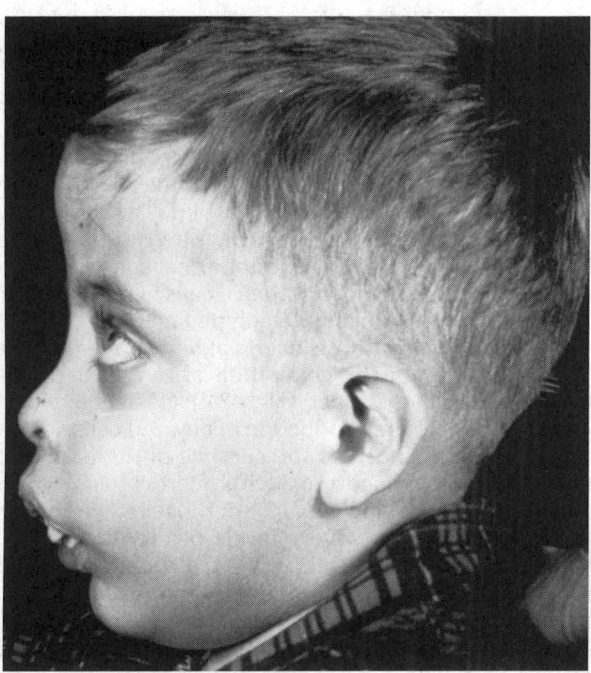

Fig. 42-5. Thalassemic facies. See text for description. (From Jurkiewicz et al.,[198] with permission.)

immature erythroid progenitors, which die from their α-globin burden before they reach the reticulocyte stage. Profound anemia persists, driving erythroid hyperplasia to still higher levels. In some cases, erythropoiesis is so exuberant that masses of extramedullary erythropoietic tissue form in the chest, abdomen, or pelvis.

Massive bone marrow expansion exerts numerous adverse effects on the growth, development, and function of critical organ systems. Children with thalassemia develop a characteristic chipmunk facies due to maxillary marrow hyperplasia and frontal bossing (Fig. 42-5). Thinning and pathologic fractures of long bones and vertebrae arise from cortical invasion by erythroid elements. Profound growth retardation and endocrine malfunction are common.

Hemolytic anemia results in massive splenomegaly and high-output congestive heart failure. Conscription of so many caloric resources for futile sustenance of erythroid hyperplasia leads to inanition, susceptibility to infection, and, in untreated cases, death during the first two decades of life. Treatment with red cell transfusions sufficient to maintain hemoglobin levels above 9.0–10.0 g/dl improves oxygen delivery, suppresses the excessive ineffective erythropoiesis, and prolongs life. Unfortunately, as discussed in more detail later, complications of chronic transfusion therapy, including iron overload, have usually proven to be fatal before age 30. However, with improved iron chelation therapy, initiated at an early age, survival can be prolonged beyond the third decade.

Clinical Manifestations

The advent of modern hypertransfusion therapy has had a major impact on the clinical and laboratory features of thalassemia major. These regimens have ameliorated many of the most striking manifestations of the disease. The disastrous symptom constellation so prevalent in the past is now, at least in the North America, England, and most European countries,

of largely historical importance. Nonetheless, it is the symptoms of untreated β-thalassemia major that best illustrate the principles of the pathophysiology just outlined. We include features of the untreated disease in this section. These descriptions apply to the disease as it was seen before 1965 and is still prevalent in many parts of the world. The clinical features of thalassemia treated with modern hypertransfusion and chelation are also discussed.

Protected by prenatal Hb F production, the infant with Cooley's anemia is born free of significant anemia, although deficient β-chain synthesis can be demonstrated at birth. Quantitative Hb A determinations of cord blood reveal that thalassemia homozygotes have <2% Hb A, heterozygotes have 6.8–9.9%, and normals have 20%.[36] Clinical manifestations usually emerge by the second 6 months of life. The diagnosis is almost always evident by 2 years of age.[37] Pallor, irritability, growth retardation, abdominal swelling due to enlargement of the liver and spleen, and jaundice are the usual presenting features.[38] Facial and skeletal changes develop later. Untreated victims die in late infancy or early childhood as a consequence of severe anemia. In a retrospective review from Italy, the average survival of children with untreated thalassemia major was <4 years; ≥80% died in the first 5 years of life.[39]

Clinical and Laboratory Evaluation
Blood

The anemia of thalassemia major is characterized by severe hypochromia and microcytosis. No anemia is present at birth, but the hemoglobin level decreases progressively during the first months of life. When the child becomes symptomatic, the hemoglobin level may be as low as 3–4 g/dl. Red cell morphology is strikingly abnormal, with many microcytes, bizarre poikilocytes, teardrop cells, and target cells (Fig. 42-6). A characteristic finding is the presence of extraordinarily thin, often wrinkled and folded cells (leptocytes) containing irregular clumps of precipitated globin.

CLINICAL HETEROGENEITY OF THALASSEMIA

The severity of β-thalassemia is remarkable for its variability in different patients. Two siblings inheriting identical thalassemia mutations sometimes exhibit markedly different degrees of anemia and erythroid hyperplasia. Many factors contribute to this clinical heterogeneity. Individual alleles vary with respect to severity of the biosynthetic lesion. Other modulating factors ameliorate the burden of unpaired α-globin inclusion bodies. Co-inheritance of the α-thalassemia trait actually reduces clinical severity because it restricts production of excess α-globin. High levels of Hb F expression persist to widely varying degrees in β-thalassemia. Since γ-globin can substitute for β-globin, simultaneously generating more functional hemoglobins and reducing the α-globin inclusion burden, this is a powerful modulating factor. Patients may also vary in their ability to solubilize unpaired globin chains by proteolysis.[1] Occasional heterozygous patients have had more severe anemia than expected, apparently because of defects in these proteolytic systems.[1,2] Inheritance of more than the usual complement of α-globin genes has also been claimed to increase with severity of β-thalassemia because of additional production of unpaired α-globin chains. All these factors emphasize the essential role of α-globin inclusions in the pathophysiology of β-thalassemia.

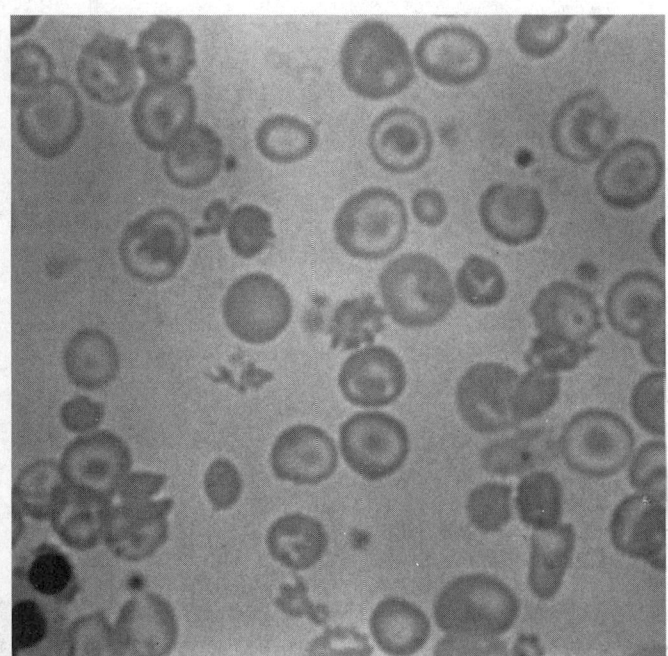

Fig. 42-6. Morphology of the peripheral blood film in severe β-thalassemia. Note the many bizarre cells, the hypochromia, nucleated RBCs, target cells, and leptocytes. (From Pearson and Benz,[248] with permission.)

Nucleated red cells are abundant. The reticulocyte count is 2–8%, lower than would be expected in view of the extreme erythroid hyperplasia and hemolysis. The low count reflects the severity of intramedullary erythroblast destruction. The white blood cell count is elevated. A moderate polymorphonuclear leukocytosis and normal platelet count are typical unless hypersplenism has developed. The bone marrow exhibits marked hypercellularity consequent to normoblastic hyperplasia. These red cell precursors also show defective hemoglobinization and reduced amounts of cytoplasm. Prodigious elevations of circulating nucleated red blood cells, increased white count, and thrombocytosis all occur after splenectomy.

The osmotic fragility is strikingly abnormal. The red cells are so markedly resistant to hemolysis in hypotonic sodium chloride solution that some are not entirely hemolyzed, even in distilled water. The serum iron is increased, and iron-binding proteins are fully saturated.[40]

The hemoglobin profile reveals predominantly Hb F. In patients with homozygous β^0-thalassemia, no Hb A is found. In the newborn with β^+-thalassemia, about 90% is Hb F; with advancing age Hb F slowly decreases, but it is always considerably higher than normal (10–90%). Transfusions will confound the estimation of the true Hb F level. The Hb A_2/Hb A ratio, which in the normal person is about 1:40, is increased to above 1:20 in thalassemia trait, but Hb A_2 levels in thalassemia major are variable, probably because of increased numbers of F cells that have a decreased Hb A_2 content.[1] Other biochemical abnormalities of the red cell in thalassemia major include a postnatal persistence of the i antigen and a decrease of red cell carbonic anhydrase; these findings are probably also due to the elevated levels of circulating F cells.

The intraerythrocytic inclusions in the peripheral blood cells, first described by Fessas,[41] are especially prominent after splenectomy. These inclusions, best seen by supravital staining with methyl violet or by phase microscopy, are aggregates of precipitated, denatured α-chains.[42] They are also found in large numbers within erythroid precursors in the bone marrow.

The serum is icteric; unconjugated bilirubin levels fall within 2.0–4.0 mg/dl. Hepatitis, obstruction from gallstones, or cho-

langitis should be considered if the value is higher. Red cell survival in thalassemia major is variable but usually markedly decreased. The ^{51}Cr half-life falls within 6.5–19.5 days, in contrast to the normal half-life of 25–35 days.[35] Increased plasma iron turnover and poor radio-iron utilization indicate ineffective erythropoiesis.[35] Serum SGOT and SGPT are frequently increased, reflecting hepatic damage secondary to hemosiderosis or viral hepatitis. Lactate dehydrogenase levels are quite elevated as a consequence of ineffective erythropoiesis. Haptoglobin and hemopexin are reduced or absent.[43]

Low levels of serum zinc are present. A relationship between this finding and growth failure has been postulated but not established.[44,45] Low levels of serum and leukocyte ascorbic acid are common in thalassemic patients because increased metabolism of the vitamin to oxalic acid occurs in the presence of iron overload.[46] Biochemical evidence of folic acid deficiency, presumably on the basis of excessive consumption, has been described.[47,48] Daily supplementation with 1.0 mg of folic acid is therefore reasonable, especially if the diet is not optimal. The large amounts of iron present in patients with thalassemia major, coupled perhaps with malabsorption secondary to pancreatic and hepatic fibrosis, may lead to decreased levels of vitamin E. Serum levels of α-tocopherol are often reduced to <0.5 mg/dl, and evidence of increased red cell membrane lipid peroxidation has been described.[49,50] Unfortunately, therapy with large doses of vitamin E neither improves survival of transfused red cells nor decreases transfusion requirements.[51]

Coagulation abnormalities similar to those found in patients with liver disease of any etiology (i.e., lowered levels of factors II, V, VII, IX, X, and XI) occur, particularly in older patients. Only rarely are the abnormalities sufficient to require specific therapy. A general correlation exists between the coagulation status and the other parameters of hepatic function. Both deteriorate in patients with massive iron overload.[52] Six of nine thalassemia patients studied for platelet function had slightly prolonged bleeding times and abnormal platelet aggregation.[53] Although these changes are probably not of great clinical significance, salicylates should be used with caution.

Skeletal Changes

Skeletal abnormalities (Fig. 42-7) result primarily from hypertrophy and expansion of the erythroid marrow.[54] These cause widening of the marrow space and thinning of the cortex, with consequent osteoporosis.[55] Striking changes in the skull and facial bones include thickening of the frontal bone with prominent frontal bossing. The thickened membranous bones of the skull do not expand adjacent to the sutures, resulting in a "hot cross bun" configuration of the skull. Radiographs reveal the diploic spaces to be widened. At first the skull has a granular appearance, but later perpendicular bony trabeculae appear, giving the classic "hair on end" or crew cut appearance (Fig. 42-7).

The maxilla is regularly involved. Pneumatization of the sinusoids is markedly delayed; marked overgrowth of the maxilla results in severe malocclusion, jumbling of the upper incisors, and prominence of the malar eminences.[56] These bone changes produce the classic facies. The earliest skeletal changes are observed in the metacarpals, metatarsals, and phalanges, where expanded medullary cavities produce a rectangular and then a convex shape (Fig. 42-7). Marked osteoporosis and cortical thinning may predispose to pathologic fractures of the extremities; compression fractures of the vertebrae may also occur (Fig. 42-8). Premature fusion of the epiphyses of the long bones is common in patients who are >10 years old. Irregular fusion of the epiphyses of the proximal humerus results in characteristic shortening of the upper arms.[57,58]

Several abnormalities in the ribs may occur, including notching and osteolytic lesions.[54,59] The ribs are very broad, especially at the point of attachment to the vertebral column. They may expand to the extent that they resemble paravertebral

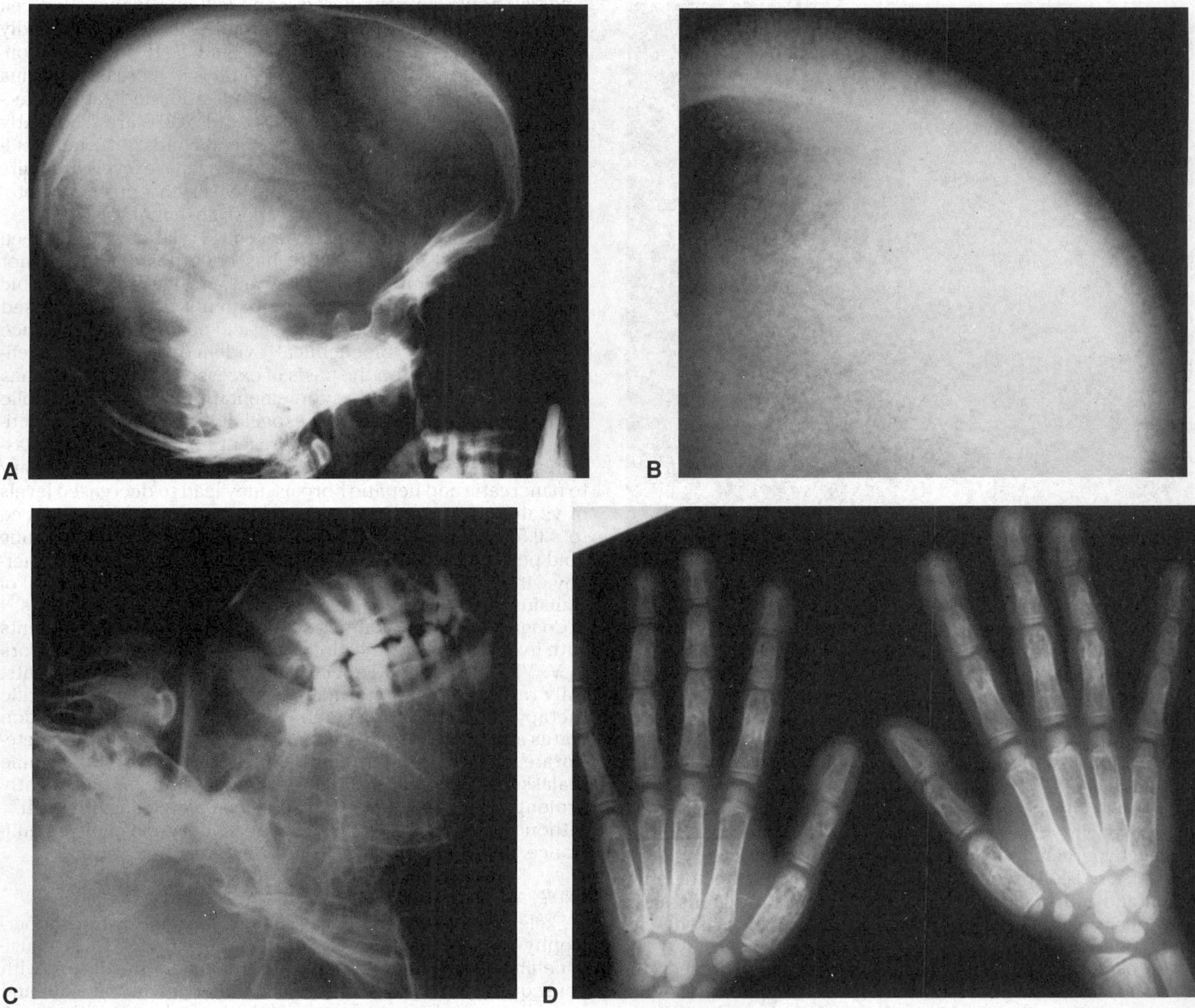

Fig. 42-7. Bony abnormalities in severe β-thalassemia. **(A & B)** "Hair-on-end" appearance of the skull, especially obvious in the closeup view shown in Fig. B. **(C)** Distortion of the maxillary bones, as well as poor development of the sinus cavities due to opaque masses of extramedullary erythropoiesis. **(D)** Squaring and convexity abnormalities of the hands. (From Pearson and Benz,[248] with permission.)

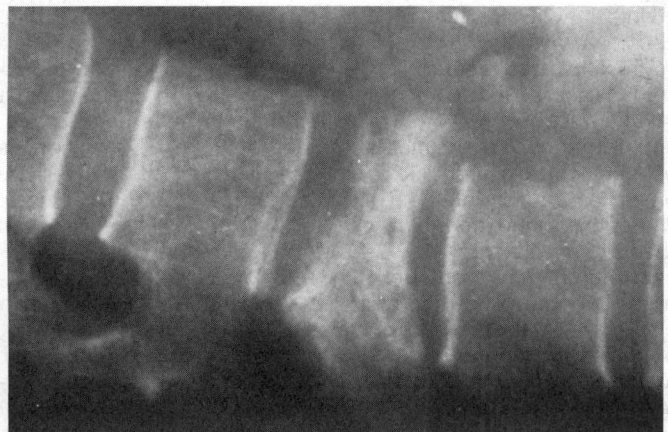

Fig. 42-8. Compression fracture of L2 vertebra in a patient with severe β-thalassemia. (From Pearson and Benz,[248] with permission.)

masses (Fig. 42-9). An unusual complication is expansion of paravertebral hematopoietic tissue into the spinal canal with resultant cord compression.[60] Decompressive laminectomy or radiation therapy may be necessary to prevent permanent paralysis.[61,62]

The character and degree of the bone lesions change significantly with age. In older children, the bone lesions regress in the more distal portions of the skeleton (hands, arms, and legs), a feature correlating with the normal developmental replacement of red marrow by fatty marrow. The characteristic changes of the hands and other peripheral areas are thus diminished and may disappear in later life.[63,64] However, in the skull, spine, and pelvis (which are sites of active, persistent erythropoiesis) the radiographic changes become more conspicuous.[63]

Liver and Gallbladder

Hepatomegaly is prominent in severely affected patients. This is a consequence of extramedullary hematopoiesis initially, so that early hepatomegaly can be reduced by hyper-

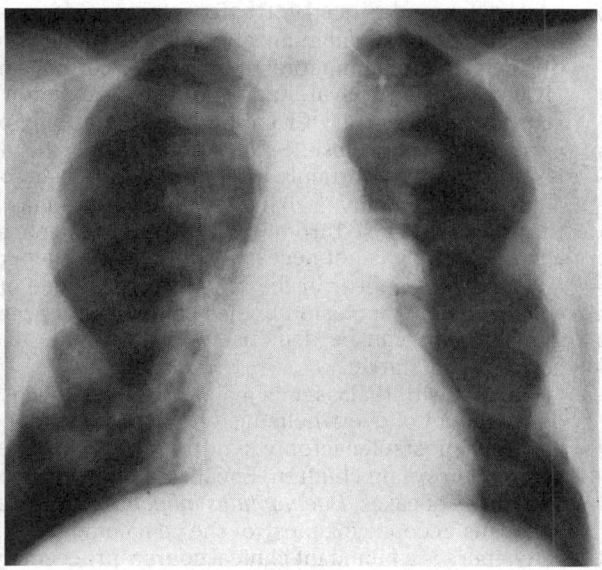
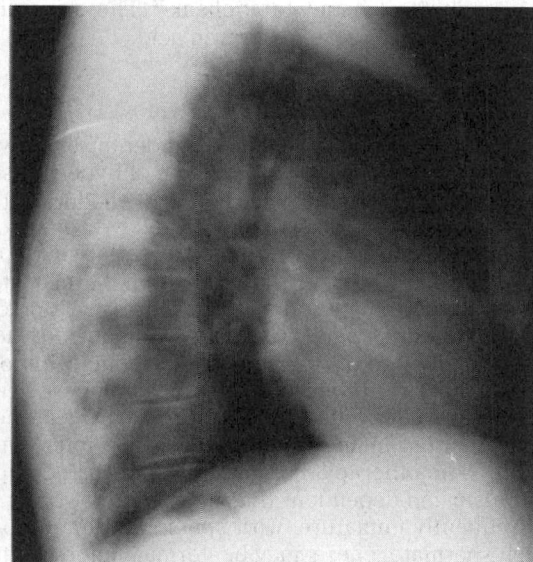

Fig. 42-9. Chest radiograph typical of severe β-thalassemia. Note the thickening of the rib ends, as well as cardiac dilation. (From Pearson and Benz,[248] with permission.)

transfusion.[65] Later in the course of the disease, hepatomegaly is associated with extensive cirrhosis. Iron deposition, first present in the Kupffer cells, ultimately engorges the parenchymal cells, resulting in an appearance that is indistinguishable from that of idiopathic hemochromatosis.[66,67] The hepatocellular injury of iron overload may be due to the liberation of hydrolases resulting from initiation by the ferrous form of iron of peroxidative damage of lysosomal membrane lipids.[68]

Many patients have had viral hepatitis, which may augment liver damage. In Italy, a high incidence of hepatitis B surface markers (HBsAg) and hepatitis B core antigen (anti-HBc) and anti-HBs antibodies was found in a group of 253 children.[69] In other reports, a high frequency of chronic active hepatitis was observed. Multiply transfused patients also have a high prevalence of seropositivity for antihepatitis C antibody, indicating a likely additional factor contributing to chronic liver disease. It has also been postulated that liver iron overload may facilitate persistence of virus-induced progressive liver diseases.[70] The most important abnormalities of liver function include hypergammaglobulinemia, hypoalbuminemia, moderate decreases in the coagulation factors that are synthesized in the liver, and increased levels of transaminases.[52]

Pigmentary gallstones due to high rates of bilirubin generation are found in an increasing number of patients >4 years old. Two-thirds of patients have multiple calcified bilirubinate calculi after the age of 15.[71] Gallbladder surgery is not usually indicated unless biliary colic or obstructive jaundice has occurred. However, if gallstones are detected at splenectomy, simultaneous cholecystectomy or stone removal may be considered.

Heart

Cardiac abnormalities are important causes of morbidity and mortality in patients with thalassemia major. Cardiac dilation secondary to anemia is almost always present in untreated young children (Fig. 42-9). Unless intensive chelation therapy is started in the first decade of life, myocardial hemosiderosis is inevitable during the second decade, when serious cardiac disorders become frequent. Early electrocardiographic abnormalities include a prolonged PR interval, first-degree heart

block, and premature atrial contractions.[72] Later, ST-segment depression and ventricular ectopic beats constitute ominous indicators of myocardial damage. Periodic evaluation of cardiac function is essential. Echocardiographic estimation of left ventricular function may reveal abnormalities before there are any symptoms. The left ventricular end systolic pressure-dimension relationship (ejection fraction), as determined by echocardiography, provides a noninvasive measure of ventricular contractility.[73] Sterile pericarditis occurs in many patients with massive iron overload, but cardiac tamponade has not been observed.[74] Although pericarditis is most often attributed to hemosiderosis, an association with β-hemolytic streptococcal infection has also been suggested.[75] Therapy is symptomatic: bed rest, treatment of infection, management of superimposed congestive heart failure, and salicylates or corticosteroids for pain.

Cardiomegaly and left ventricular deterioration progress to chronic refractory congestive heart failure. In addition to standard therapy for failure, one must maintain the hemoglobin level at >10–12 g/dl and institute or continue intensive chelation therapy. The iron-overloaded myocardium has little capacity to improve its performance, unless excess iron is removed. Arrhythmias may cause sudden death. Supraventricular tachycardia and atrial fibrillation may necessitate the use of antiarrhythmic agents even though these agents can further depress ventricular function. These complications are the usual cause of death in patients with thalassemia major.

Lungs

Mild abnormalities of pulmonary function are common. Some patients exhibit primarily restrictive defects[76,77]; others experience mild-to-moderate small airway obstruction and hyperinflation.[78,79] Most patients have a decreased maximal oxygen uptake and anaerobic threshold; these do not normalize after transfusion.[80]

Kidneys

The kidneys are frequently enlarged, owing in part to extramedullary hematopoiesis and in part to marked dilation of the renal tubules.[81] The urine is often dark brown, reflecting the excretion of products of heme catabolism.[82] The urine also contains large amounts of urates and uric acid.

Growth and Endocrine Status

Growth retardation, including skeletal and dental age,[83] was common even in young children until the use of hypertransfusion regimens restored relatively normal growth during the first decade. The adolescent growth spurt is delayed or absent without intensive chelation therapy; most patients, even those well maintained by transfusion, do not attain normal stature.[37,84] Menarche is frequently delayed. Breast development may be poor, and many female patients are oligomenorrheic or amenorrheic. Induction of cyclic uterine bleeding with low-dose estrogen and progesterone may be of psychological benefit. Pregnancy may occur even in patients who have been transfusion dependent from infancy if they have been intensively treated with chelation therapy. Pregnancy has occurred in patients with transfusion-dependent thalassemia.[85,86]

Boys are frequently immature, with sparse facial and body hair. Although spermatogenesis may be normal, libido is often decreased. When lack of secondary sexual characteristics is emotionally disturbing, small doses of androgen may be used to produce phallic enlargement, deepening of the voice, and growth of facial and body hair.

A multicenter study of 250 adolescent patients in northern Italy showed that despite hypertransfusion and 7–10 years of iron chelation therapy, two-thirds of males and one-third of females >14 years old were ≥2 SD below the mean for height.[87] Many adolescents aged 12–18 years old lacked any secondary sexual changes of puberty. However, the mean serum ferritin level in the entire group was 3,500 ng/ml, indicating persistence of a high level of excess iron burden in most of this group. More intensive chelation therapy started in the first decade of life frequently will allow normal onset of puberty and development of secondary sexual changes.

Growth retardation and hypogonadism are also found in association with zinc deficiency. Because urinary excretion of zinc is increased by hemolysis, a clinical trial of zinc supplementation was conducted in Turkey[88]; it showed enhanced growth velocity in the treated group. Since these patients did not receive adequate transfusion or chelation therapy, the applicability of these findings to intensively treated patients is uncertain.

Abnormal carbohydrate metabolism is common in older patients with thalassemia major. Prepubertal children usually have normal insulin-stimulated glucose metabolism, but pubertal patients exhibit impaired responses despite normal steady-state blood glucose levels. Impaired oral glucose tolerance and higher than normal insulin levels in response to hyperglycemia are also encountered.[89] The defect in these patients appears to be related to insulin resistance, with insulin deficiency developing later in the progression to diabetes. Multiple endocrine abnormalities such as hypoparathyroidism,[90,91] hypothyroidism,[92] and hypothalamic pituitary insufficiency[93] are usually detectable only by provocative tests.

Spleen and Splenectomy

Massive splenomegaly is unusual in hypertransfused patients. Thrombocytopenia and neutropenia may result from hypersplenism in untreated patients, although infection and bleeding are unusual. The usual indication for splenectomy is a progressive shortening of the survival rate of transfused blood cells, as evidenced by an increased transfusion requirement. The transfusion requirements of splenectomized patients are considerably less than those of patients whose spleens are intact.[94,95] A transfusion requirement >180–200 ml/kg/yr of packed red blood cells usually represents excessive red cell

breakdown and a need for splenectomy. Occasionally, serologic evidence of isoimmunization may be documented, permitting selection of compatible donor cells that have normal survival. Red cell survival studies and determination of splenic sequestration by the ^{51}Cr method are not usually of value for prediction of response. Splenectomy should be deferred as long as possible, certainly until after 5 or 6 years of age.

After splenectomy, striking thrombocytosis may occur, but this does not cause thromboembolic phenomena, and anticoagulant therapy is not necessary. Increased numbers of nucleated red cells appear in the blood; the presence of many red cells containing inclusion bodies composed of precipitated α-globin chains can be demonstrated. The urine may become considerably darker.

Patients with thalassemia major are at significant risk of the development of overwhelming, often fatal, infection after splenectomy (postsplenectomy syndrome). The problem is most common in young children. Encapsulated pneumococci cause two-thirds of cases; *Haemophilus influenzae* type B and meningococcus account for most of the remaining infections. Typically, there is a fulminant clinical course, proceeding from mild fever and headache to hyperpyrexia, prostration, shock, and death within 6–12 hours; in one study, 10–30% of splenectomized children with thalassemia major developed this complication,[96] but antipneumococcal vaccine and prophylaxis with antibiotics have dramatically reduced the incidence.

Removal of the spleen impairs immunity in many ways. The monocyte/macrophage tissues of the spleen are uniquely suited for clearance of bacteria from the blood in the absence of specific antibody.[97] The spleen may actively participate in antibody formation, especially in the early hours of an infection,[98] and is probably crucial to the alternate complement pathway needed for opsonization when specific antibody is lacking. Levels of IgM are also low in splenectomized patients.[99] A role for high levels of serum iron and saturation of iron-binding protein, which may predispose to infection, has been suggested but remains controversial.[100] When bacteria gain entrance to the bloodstream of a splenectomized patient, they are not cleared but proliferate rapidly in the circulation. Enormous numbers accumulate in a relatively short time, causing hyperpyrexia, shock, disseminated intravascular coagulation, adrenal hemorrhage, and, potentially, death.

Splenectomy should clearly be deferred as long as possible. Patients are more likely to have developed humoral immunity to a broad range of bacteria of the spleen is present until ≥3 years of age. Oral penicillin therapy, used as prophylaxis against postsplenectomy infection, is now generally given to patients with thalassemia. Following splenectomy, the patient's parents should be instructed to seek medical attention immediately if significant fever (>102°F) develops. Polyvalent antipneumococcal and anti-*H. influenzae* vaccines should be administered before splenectomy.[101] In addition to postsplenectomy sepsis, *Yersinia enterocolitica* or pseudotuberculosis infections have been noted in patients with thalassemia major receiving the iron chelator deferoxamine.[102–104]

Transfusion Therapy

Transfusion therapy for thalassemia was once regarded as a palliative measure.[105] If palliation is defined as the prevention of discomfort and the maintenance of as nearly normal a life as possible, the transfusion programs then in general use were unsatisfactory even for these limited purposes. Symptoms of anemia and the cosmetic and other consequences of overgrowth of erythropoietic tissue rendered life unpleasant and uncomfortable. Because many of the problems of children with thalassemia major could be related to anemia, several centers initiated chronic, more aggressive transfusion programs designed to ameliorate these symptoms. The programs were designed to maintain hemoglobin levels at >9–10 g/dl. These more vigorous regimens have been designated hypertransfusion.

The clinical benefits of hypertransfusion programs were dramatic. The growth of younger children returned to normal percentiles for height and weight.[106] Erythropoiesis was substantially, albeit partially, suppressed, as evidenced by decreased numbers of reticulocytes and normoblasts and marked reduction of the level of Hb F. Enlargement of the liver and spleen receded. Abnormal facies and osteoporosis of long bones either did not develop or regressed. Cardiac dilation improved, and normal age-appropriate activities were possible.[64,107]

Hypertransfusion programs require an increase of ≥25% in the amount of administered blood. Fears that this would result in accelerated iron overload, more rapid development of complications, and death at an earlier age were fortunately not realized. The life expectancy of children maintained by hypertransfusion programs has not been shortened, probably because the amelioration of severe anemia is associated with significant reduction of gastrointestinal iron absorption; this offsets to some degree the increased transfusional iron load. The clinical superiority of hypertransfusion has led most treatment centers in developed countries to adopt it as standard management. Complications of anemia and erythropoietic hypertrophy have thus become uncommon.

More vigorous transfusional programs (supertransfusion) aimed at keeping hemoglobin levels at >12.0 g/dl have been used to suppress erythropoiesis further. After a transient increase in blood consumption during the first several months,[108] the blood requirements are not increased in splenectomized β^0-thalassemia patients during these regimens, although they commonly do increase in β^+-thalassemia and in unsplenectomized children. A significant reduction in blood volume can be documented.[109,110] This probably reflects the blood volume needed to support the expanded marrow tissues at lower levels of transfusion. The long-term effect of this more aggressive transfusion strategy on well-being or prognosis has not been determined.

An experimental transfusion program has been designed to reduce transfusion requirements by using a young population of red blood cells (neocytes) prepared by differential centrifugation or cell separators.[110,111] These neocyte preparations should circulate longer in the recipient because they have a mean cell age of 30 days, compared with the 60 days of unfractionated blood. However, in two prospective clinical trials, blood requirements were reduced only by means of 13% and 16%.[112,113] Neocyte preparations are two to four times more expensive than ordinary packed or glycerol-frozen red blood cells. Their use also entails greater risks of isoimmunization and viral infections owing to the increased number of donor units needed.[112] An even more complicated procedure involving the use of neocyte/gerocyte exchange transfusions has been suggested as a method for further reducing iron overload.[110,114] The method attempts to remove nearly senescent red cells before they are catabolized, thereby adding their iron to the body stores. Unfortunately, these methods are extraordinarily expensive.

Before the first blood transfusion is given to an infant with thalassemia major, a complete genotype of the red blood cells should be obtained. This precaution applies to all patients facing long-term transfusion therapy. This information is valuable for identifying minor blood group incompatibility if isoimmunization develops later. In an Italian cooperative study of 1,435 patients, 5.2% had significant red cell alloantibodies (136 antibodies in 74 patients).[115] Group- and type-specific red cells that are compatible as determined by the indirect antiglobulin reaction should be used. Blood should be as fresh as possible, preferably before 2,3-diphosphoglycerate levels decline (4–5 days).[116]

Febrile reactions are frequent in patients who have had multiple transfusions. Pretransfusion therapy with acetaminophen and diphenhydramine or prior treatment of cells by freezing in glycerol, thawing, and washing may reduce the severity of the reaction. Glycerol-frozen red cell preparations contain very few leukocytes and produce few febrile reactions[117]; filtered blood is equally effective in preventing reactions.[118] Isoimmunization and transfusion reactions may still occur even with scrupulous techniques.[119] A superimposed autoimmune hemolytic process with circulating autoantibodies has been described in thalassemia patients.[120] A syndrome of post-transfusional hypertension, convulsions, and cerebral hemorrhage of uncertain etiology has also been reported.[121]

In practice, it is usually most efficient to give one to three donor units of red cells every 3–5 weeks, depending on the size of the patient and the destruction rate of transfused cells. Except for very young patients, those with hypersplenism, and those with thalassemia intermedia, a regularly scheduled transfusion every 3 weeks is both possible and convenient without the need of extra visits for measurement of hemoglobin levels. In more severely anemic patients, several initial transfusions may be necessary to increase the hemoglobin level to 12–14 g/dl, but no more than 15 ml/kg of packed red cells should be given within a 24-hour period. Patients receiving chronic transfusion therapy are at particular risk of acquiring viral infections from blood products, including hepatitis B and C viruses, cytomegalovirus, and human immunodeficiency virus (HIV). Immunization against hepatitis B should be given early to thalassemia major patients, particularly in areas where the virus is common.[122] The availability of serologic screening of donor blood for anti-hepatitis C antibodies should greatly reduce the risk of infection in the future. In a 1987 study of patients in Europe who received transfusions for hemoglobinopathy, 1.6% were shown to be HIV-positive, including two patients with the clinical acquired immunodeficiency syndrome (AIDS).[123] In New York, where there is a higher incidence of AIDS than in Europe, a 1987 study of 70 chronically transfused thalassemia patients indicated that 17.1% were positive for HIV antibody, three had AIDS-related complex, or ARC, and one had clinical AIDS.[123] In Philadelphia, only 2 of 60 similar patients were HIV positive; none have developed AIDS.[124]

Hemosiderosis and Chelation Therapy

Iron accumulation in thalassemia major depends directly on both the number of blood transfusions received and the age of the patient. Transfusional hemosiderosis is the major cause of late morbidity and mortality in thalassemia major. Establishment of a more favorable iron balance should lead to improved survival; this belief has motivated detailed study of several iron unloading maneuvers.

The calculated daily acquisition of iron in the transfusion-dependent child averages 8–16 mg of iron, given a dose of 250–500 ml of red blood cells every month.[126] Excessive gastrointestinal absorption of iron adds to this burden, although absorption is reduced when a hemoglobin level of >9 g/dl is maintained.[127] No physiologic way to induce significant excretion has been found. Phlebotomy, the most efficient method of removing iron in other situations, is obviously precluded in this disease. A pharmacologic approach using specific iron-chelating agents has thus been adopted.

Several drugs with chelating properties have been synthesized or recovered from microorganisms. Many lack iron specificity or are inefficient; others cause significant toxicity. Only one has achieved clinical utility. Deferoxamine mesylate (Desferal, DFO) a siderophore isolated from cultures of *Streptomyces pilosus*, was introduced in 1960; it is a nearly specific iron-chelating agent (i.e., no other ions are chelated) with low toxicity.[128]

Increased iron excretion following administration of DFO is proportional to body iron stores. To offset the amount of iron received by way of transfusions and attain negative iron balance, the chelating agent must effect the daily urinary excretion of ≥15 mg of iron. In the case of DFO, this was initially achieved in a British controlled study by daily intramuscular injections of 0.5 g/day for several years and led to a reduced rate of hepatic iron accumulation and hepatic fibrosis in thalassemic patients.[129] An Australian study using an injection of 1.0 g/day showed decreases in cardiac and hepatic size and improved cardiac function in a small group of patients treated for 2–10 years.[130] These studies were valuable in that they demonstrated potential efficacy, but lifelong daily intramuscular injection is clearly impossible as a method for dispensing the drug. The observation that iron excretion induced by DFO is markedly enhanced by slow intravenous or subcutaneous injection of the drug provided an important advance.[131] A prolonged infusion period permits a longer exposure of the drug to a relatively small "chelatable" iron pool present at any given time in equilibrium with a nearly nonchelatable pool. In iron-overloaded ascorbic acid-replete patients, >300 mg of daily urinary iron excretion can be accomplished with large continuous intravenous doses.[132]

Slow infusion of DFO will achieve negative iron balance in many transfusion-dependent patients over 4–5 years of age.[133-138] This involves daily 10–12-hour subcutaneous injections of about 2.0 g of DFO using a small battery-driven pump. The pump impels a syringe that infuses an aqueous solution of DFO through a #25 "butterfly" needle placed under the skin of the abdomen or thigh. Most patients use the pump during sleeping hours. In patients who are poorly compliant with subcutaneous therapy or in those with severe iron overload, home administration of DFO in high doses can be accomplished intravenously via a central venous catheter. The injection site is either a totally implantable reservoir or in the external end of the catheter. Intravenous DFO may also be useful for rapidly lowering the total iron burden and even for reversal of short-term cardiac morbidity.

Measurement of serum ferritin levels is a convenient way to assess efficacy.[135] In compliant patients, a clear drop in ferritin should occur after 1 year of treatment, with continued decline to a level of <1,000 ng/ml in 3–5 years.[133,135] Although urinary measurements are usually used to evaluate excreted iron, an approximately equal amount of iron is lost in the stool during long-term therapy.

The optimal age for starting this program has not been established. Some reports describe success in children as young as 2–4 years,[139] but there may be an adverse effect on growth. Many centers wait until the patient is 5–6 years of age, when significant iron excretion can be accomplished and patient cooperation is better. The hard painful "lumps" that occur at the injection sites from time to time are usually avoided by careful placement of the needle for subcutaneous rather than intradermal injection.

Infections, hypersensitivity, and tachyphylaxis are rare. After 10 years of use, results with DFO protocols are very encouraging, especially in younger patients.[133-135,138,140] Children begun on chelation before 8–10 years of age show significant decreases in serum ferritin levels and may attain normal levels after 3–5 years of use. With persistence of DFO administration, the onset of cardiac disease may be prevented, particularly in children started on treatment in the first decade of life.[141] Results in older patients have not been as promising. Many patients begun on chelation therapy after 10 years of age have developed evidence of the progressive cardiac dysfunction associated with hemosiderosis. Nonetheless, severe cardiac disease, either congestive heart failure or ventricular arrhythmias, has been reversed in some patients by intensive high-dose (15 mg/kg/hr for 10 hr/day) intravenous DFO treatment.[134,142] The

treatment may be self-administered nightly at home through a central venous catheter.

A relationship between iron overload and ascorbic acid depletion (first suggested by the epidemiology of scurvy among the Bantu) exists in thalassemia major.[143,144] Enhancement by ascorbic acid treatment of DFO-induced urinary iron excretion in thalassemia major has been well documented. Administration of 100–200 mg/kg/day of oral ascorbic acid results in an approximate doubling of DFO-induced urinary iron excretion. However, cardiotoxicity manifested as arrhythmias and decreased ventricular contractility has been attributed to vitamin C therapy.[145] Ascorbic acid should only be used while DFO is being administered and only in patients who are ascorbate depleted. As ferritin levels decrease toward normal, the efficacy of vitamin C for augmenting iron excretion disappears.

In general, DFO is well tolerated. Chronic administration of >100 mg/kg/day of DFO has caused cataracts in dogs, but this has not been observed in thalassemic patients. The most serious current concern regarding toxicity is decreasing visual and auditory acuity. Some clinics have found that many patients experience impaired sight and hearing, which is partially or completely reversible on discontinuing DFO[146]; others have encountered a lower incidence.[147] Any patient receiving chronic DFO treatment should undergo periodic tests of vision and hearing. DFO should be discontinued if abnormalities arise, with cautious re-initiation when abnormalities reverse. DFO may rarely cause acute pulmonary disease, which is reversible with discontinuation of the drug.

Existing chelation protocols are highly imperfect, expensive, and inconvenient. Chronic infusion requires a great deal of dedication and persistence on the part of the patient and family; noncompliance is frequent. These realities have stimulated a search for oral chelators. 2,3-Dihydrobenzoic acid, another iron-chelating agent, enhances iron excretion when given orally. However, it is not very effective; iron excretion is increased to only about 4.5 mg/day.[148] A more promising source for a long-awaited effective oral iron chelator consists of the 1-alkyl-3-hydroxy-2-methylpyrid-4-ones, which can be easily synthesized from the inexpensive natural plant product, maltol.[149-153] One compound, 1,2-dimethyl-3-hydroxypyrid-4-one (L1), has not been toxic in mice or rabbits at doses effective in humans for oral chelation.[151] Initial clinical trials in London on eight iron-loaded patients, four with β-thalassemia major (13–26 years old) and four with myelodysplasia (47–65 years old), showed maximal 24-hour urinary iron excretions of 46–99 mg in thalassemia patients with 2–3-g/day doses of L1; these results are comparable to those of urinary iron excretion induced by DFO in the same patients.[152] However, L1 does not increase fecal iron excretion,[154] whereas DFO induces substantial fecal iron excretion in addition to the urinary excretion.

The effectiveness of L1 in reducing body iron burden and serum ferritin is still under investigation. One short-term study showed unchanged serum ferritin levels following L1 therapy.[154] However, other studies showed significant decreases in hepatic iron as well as serum ferritin.[155,156] Both mild adverse reactions, including musculoskeletal pain and stiffness, as well as infrequent more serious side effects, including agranulocytosis, have been reported with L1 therapy.[156-158] Longer clinical trials with L1 will be necessary to determine both efficacy and safety.

There are a number of other classes of orally effective iron chelating drugs that are being developed and tested.[153] However, DFO is the only Food and Drug Administration-approved, effective, iron-chelating agent for use in patients with transfusional hemosiderosis.

Bone Marrow Transplantation

Since 1982, when bone marrow transplantation (BMT) in thalassemia major was first successfully accomplished,[159] much additional experience has been gained, particularly in

THERAPY FOR β-THALASSEMIA MAJOR

Current therapy for thalassemia major consists of regular red cell transfusions to maintain a baseline hemoglobin level >9 g/dl, coupled with intensive parenteral chelation therapy with deferoxamine. Splenectomy is appropriate when transfusion requirements increase considerably more than expected for growth; these patients should also receive immunization against pneumococcal and *Haemophilus influenzae* B infections, as well as penicillin prophylaxis. Folic acid supplements may be added to meet the needs of increased erythropoiesis. Specific endocrine deficiencies associated with iron overload may require appropriate interventions. Psychosocial problems are common,[146] as is true for many children with chronic disease; early intervention is necessary. Better treatment, screening and genetic counseling, and accurate prenatal diagnosis have shifted the age distribution of patients, a higher proportion of cases now occurring in adolescents and adults.[147]

Italy.[160-168] Procedure-related deaths and nonengraftment have occurred; the currently reported mortality of 10–20% and disease-free survival after 3–5 years of 75–90% depend on age and iron status at the time of the procedure. Impressive recent results of early BMT suggest that it be considered seriously when feasible; however, the persistent 10–25% mortality rate at most centers, coupled with the improving efficacy of conventional treatment, make decisions regarding bone marrow transplantation very difficult on both clinical and ethical grounds.[169-171]

The largest experience has been reported by Guido Lucarelli and associates in Pesaro, Italy.[162,163,165-167] This group has performed >500 BMTs for thalassemia major. They have reported that when BMT was performed early in life, using an HLA-matched donor relative, there is a 90% probability of cure. The best prognostic category of patients (class 1) consisted of those who lacked hepatomegaly and portal fibrosis and who were receiving adequate iron chelation therapy.

These remarkable results have led some authorities to recommend that BMT should be strongly considered in any young thalassemia major patient who has a compatible donor.[169,170,172] This opinion is probably justified on the basis of the high cure rate, great expense of lifelong conventional transfusion-chelation therapy, and the high prevalence of noncompliance with chronic iron chelation therapy using DFO. Nevertheless, there are dissenting views and certain reservations.[169-171]

At this time, a decision to recommend or not to recommend BMT in a young thalassemia major patient who has a suitable donor is controversial. Families should be apprised of the risks and potential benefits of the procedure and helped to make an informed decision. If an HLA-compatible donor is not available, BMT is not considered an acceptable option.

BMT in older children and adults, many of whom have significant hepatic hemosiderosis and fibrosis, has been less extensively attempted and usually has not been very successful. Nevertheless, Lucarelli et al.[166] recently described excellent results of BMT in older patients who were iron overloaded and had significant hepatic abnormalities. Eighty percent of his adult patients had long-term disease-free survival. These results will lead to a re-evaluation of the use of BMT in older thalassemia major patients.

Experimental Therapies

Gene Manipulation and Replacement

Much recent effort has focused on stimulation of γ-globin gene expression or replacement of defective β-globin genes. Enhanced γ-gene expression would ameliorate the unbalanced globin chain synthesis. Normal β-genes, if introduced into stem cells in such a way as to allow them to function normally, would directly correct the β-globin chain deficit.

Active γ-genes are hypomethylated in utero (see Ch. 35) but are methylated and inactive after birth. Hypomethylation of the γ-genes can be induced by the drug 5-azacytidine; indeed, this drug produced the predicted effect in vivo, but the effect was transient.[173] Despite much subsequent experimental work, it remains unclear whether the effect was due to direct stimulation of fetal genes or to recruitment of earlier burst-forming unit-erythroid (BFU-E), which have greater potential to produce Hb F.[174-176] Hydroxyurea has an effect on BFU-E similar to that of 5-azacytidine and may perhaps be a safe drug for long-term use. Short-term as well as longer trials with both agents have been reported in a number of patients with thalassemia or sickle cell disease[174-180]; Hb F levels do rise in some patients with thalassemia intermedia, but toxicity is frequent and long-term efficacy remains unproven. The combination of hydroxyurea with recombinant hematopoietic growth factors such as erythropoietin is also being tested for possible additional potentiating effects on Hb F production.[176,181] Recombinant erythropoietin alone has also been administered, to patients with β-thalassemia intermedia and resulted in a sustained increase in total production of red blood cells, but without a specific or selective effect on Hb F production.[182]

Butyrate is another compound that has been demonstrated to augment Hb F production in various animal model systems.[174,183] It is thought to act by altering chromatin configuration. Short-term treatment with intravenous infusions of arginine butyrate in a limited number of patients resulted in increased levels of γ-globin chain production that were quite striking in some cases and resulted in a marked increase in γ/α-globin chain synthetic ratio as well as marked improvement in the degree of anemia.[184] Orally absorbable compounds also resulted in an increase in F cell and γ-globin chain production, but the effect was not as sustained or quantitatively important as was intravenous arginine butyrate.[185] Although no severe toxic side effects were observed in these short-term trials in humans, the infusion of high doses of butyrate into baboons did result in significant neurologic toxicity.[186] Further studies will be required to assess the long-term safety and efficacy of therapy with butyrate.

Successful gene replacement in thalassemia remains a goal for the future despite intensive investigation in this area. Techniques for isolating specific human genes and inserting them into the DNA of other cells have been developed.[187] However, formidable problems must be solved before it becomes routinely possible to place genes in a human stem cell, ensure their safe and active expression at effective levels, and preserve normal growth, differentiation, and proliferation of the genetically transformed stem cell.[188]

Thalassemia Intermedia

Approximately 10% of patients with homozygous β-thalassemia exhibit a phenotype characterized by intermediate hematologic severity.[1-4] The hemoglobin patterns and the β/α ratios of globin synthesis may be similar to those found in thalassemia major or somewhat higher, indicating a less severe defect in β-chain synthesis. For example, homozygous β-thalassemia in blacks, Portuguese, and others may be relatively mild, at least for the first two decades.[189,190] Homozygotes or mixed heterozygotes for forms of β-thalassemia associated with normal Hb A_2 and normal Hb F (silent carrier state) also tend to have mild to moderate disease.[191,192] Certain patients have a milder clinical phenotype because they have co-inherited a form of α-thalassemia,[15–17] or carry one (or two) β-thalassemia chromosome(s) with a higher than usual potential for high levels of γ-gene expression.

Individuals with thalassemia intermedia do not require regular blood transfusions and usually develop only moderate degrees of splenomegaly. The ability to maintain a hemoglobin level compatible with comfortable survival in the absence of regular transfusion is the generally accepted criterion for diagnosis of thalassemia intermedia. Some of these patients can survive well into adult life, frequently with normal maturation and sexual development. However, some patients with thalassemia intermedia develop cardiomegaly, osteoporosis, fractures, arthritis, and splenomegaly. Complications of extramedullary hematopoiesis in the thorax, skull, and pelvis may occur, including spinal cord compression and growths resembling tumors or abscesses.[193] Disfiguring facial changes may result in a grotesque appearance, which causes considerable emotional and psychological distress. Complications can be prevented by a transfusion program designed to suppress erythropoiesis by maintaining normal hemoglobin levels, in which case the patients must be reclassified as having thalassemia major.

These patients pose a therapeutic dilemma. If transfusions are begun, progressive hemosiderosis will develop. However, failure to institute transfusions may be associated with unacceptable morbidity. Each patient's treatment must be individualized with consideration of the patient's clinical condition, not just the hemoglobin level. An index of the degree of abnormal bone expansion may be useful,[194] but risks of transfusion and iron overload must also be considered. The further availability of more effective oral chelation therapy may make the therapeutic decision easier.

Whether these patients receive regular transfusions, they ultimately develop progressive iron overload because of increased absorption of dietary iron induced by hemolytic anemia and marrow hyperactivity. By the third or fourth decade, the total iron burden may attain the levels seen in transfusion-dependent patients.[195] Regular consumption of tea with meals to reduce iron absorption is advisable (the tannins in tea chelate iron in the gut).[196] Chelation therapy with DFO is indicated when patients become significantly iron loaded.[197] Reconstruction of the maxilla may be needed to provide cosmetic improvement of facial asymmetry and malocclusion.[198] Gallstones regularly occur by the second decade of life. Leg ulcers often occur in late adolescence or afterward, potentially necessitating transfusions until they heal. Folic acid supplementation is particularly important because of the marked marrow hyperplasia. Aplastic crises associated with parvovirus or other infections may result in life-threatening anemia. Splenectomy usually is required in cases of secondary hypersplenism, a state that can worsen the degree of anemia in the absence of transfusions.

Some patients with heterozygous β-thalassemia will have a moderately severe clinical disorder, with anemia, hemolysis, and splenomegaly. Some of these patients carry a greater than normal number of α-globin genes, owing to triplication of one of the α-gene loci: ααα/αα.[199,200] However, most heterozygous patients with triplicated α-loci are clinically similar to those with simple β-thalassemia trait. Most cases of severe heterozygous β-thalassemia are due to the inheritance of a gene for a β-thalassemia hemoglobinopathy due to a structurally abnormal, unstable, β-globin chain that may form inclusion bodies.[18,19] For those heterozygotes with unusual clinical severity, splenectomy may be beneficial.

β-Thalassemia Minor (Thalassemia Trait)

Inheritance of a single β-thalassemia allele results in a mild hypochromic microcytic anemia. The hemoglobin level averages 1 or 2 g/dl lower than that seen in normal persons of the same age and sex. Elevations in Hb A_2 and Hb F occur during the early years of life.[201–203] Hb F levels decline more slowly than normal; the diagnostic elevated Hb A_2 levels are established by about 6 months of age. Strong intrafamilial correlations of both Hb A_2 and mean corpuscular volume (MCV) are noted.[201] Osmotic fragility is decreased; indeed, a one-tube osmotic fragility test has been used for mass screening.[204] The red cell count is increased or normal. The red cells are characteristically hypochromic (mean corpuscular hemoglobin [MCH] <26 pg) and microcytic (MCV <75 fl). The smear shows varying numbers of target cells, poikilocytes, ovalocytes, and basophilic stippling (Fig. 42-10). The reticulocyte count is normal or slightly elevated. Red cell survival is normal, iron utilization is decreased, and slight ineffective erythropoiesis is present.[205] Most patients are asymptomatic.

During pregnancy the anemia of thalassemia trait often becomes more severe, and transfusions are sometimes necessary. Because iron deficiency may occur during pregnancy, iron supplementation has been advised to avoid a compounding of causes of anemia.[206,207] In many instances, iron deficiency anemia is erroneously diagnosed, and iron therapy is given without significant improvement.

Microcytic anemia refractory to iron therapy should always suggest the possibility of thalassemia trait. Although a variety of indices calculated from blood count parameters have been suggested to differentiate thalassemia from iron deficiency, each has some degree of inaccuracy; most are no better than the MCV alone.[208] Direct tests for iron deficiency are preferable. In general, the MCV is rarely >75, or the hematocrit <30 in β-thalassemia trait. In iron deficiency, the hematocrit usually falls to <30 before the MCV falls to <80. Free erythrocyte porphyrin levels are normal in thalassemia trait but are elevated in iron deficiency.[1]

There may be characteristic racial differences in the hematologic severity of β-thalassemia trait. In blacks, the condition is invariably milder, red cell morphologic abnormalities less marked, and β/α synthetic ratios higher than in whites and Asians with the trait.[209]

The diagnosis of β-thalassemia trait is established in most instances by the demonstration of altered proportions of Hb A_2. The level of Hb A_2 in β-thalassemia trait averages 5.1% (range 3.5–7.0%), approximately twice the normal level (1.5–3.5%); the Hb A_2/HbA$_1$ ratio is 1:20 instead of the normal 1:40. This increase is probably due to a post-translational (assembly) phenomenon with increased opportunity for δ-chains to combine with α-chains is in the face of β-chain deficiency.[2] If concomitant severe iron-deficiency anemia occurs, Hb A_2 levels may fall, sometimes into the normal range.[210]

Hb F levels are inconsistently elevated in β-thalassemia. In about one-half of cases, Hb F is within the normal range (<2.0%); in the remainder they are moderately elevated (2.1–5.0%). However, in almost every instance, a minor population of red cells (F cells) containing substantial amounts of Hb F can be demonstrated by the Kleihauer technique.[1] Rarely, an individual with heterozygous thalassemia, as evidenced by a reduced β/α synthetic ratio or by virtue of having a child with thalassemia intermedia or major, has normal Hb A_2, Hb F, and hemoglobin electrophoresis, without (silent carrier) or with (quiet carrier) minor hematologic changes.[192] Rare individuals have been encountered who exhibit characteristically abnormal red cell morphology but normal levels of Hb A_2 and Hb F.[1–4] Such individuals are probably carriers of γδβ-thalassemia.[1–4] They require exclusion of iron deficiency and globin chain synthesis or gene mapping studies to establish a diagnosis with certainty.

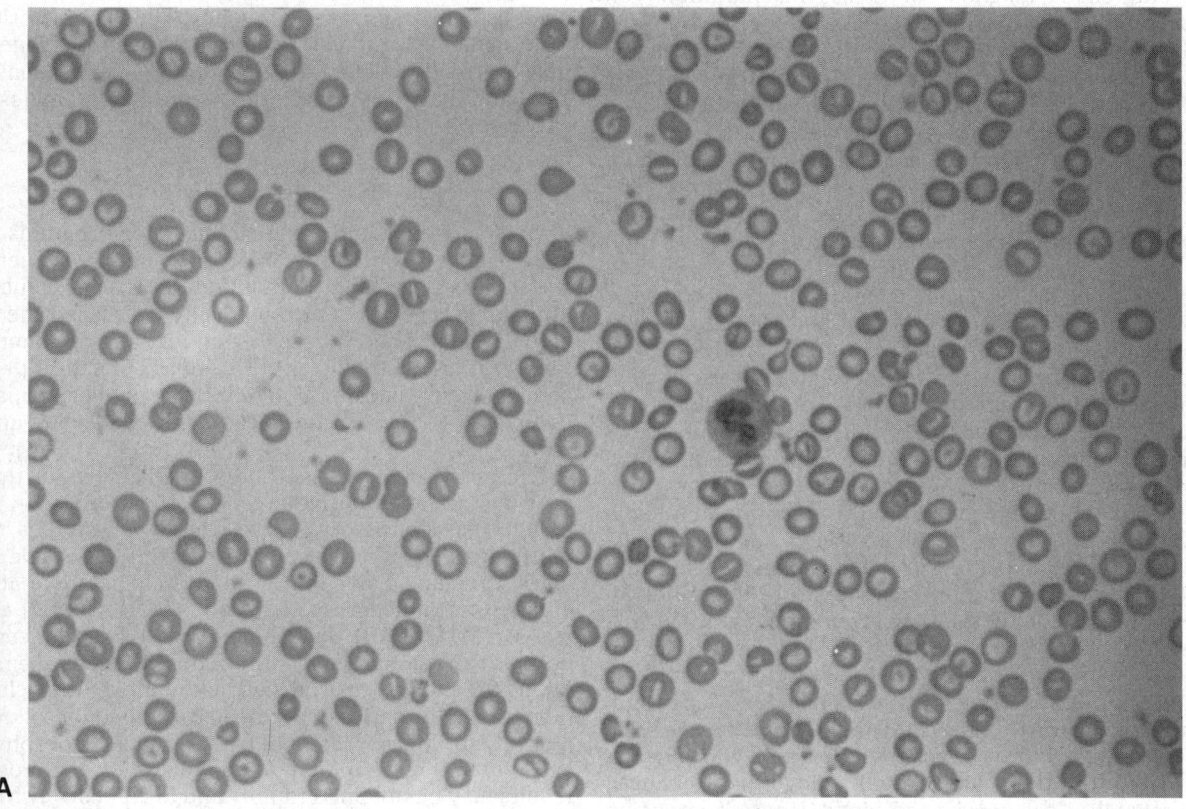

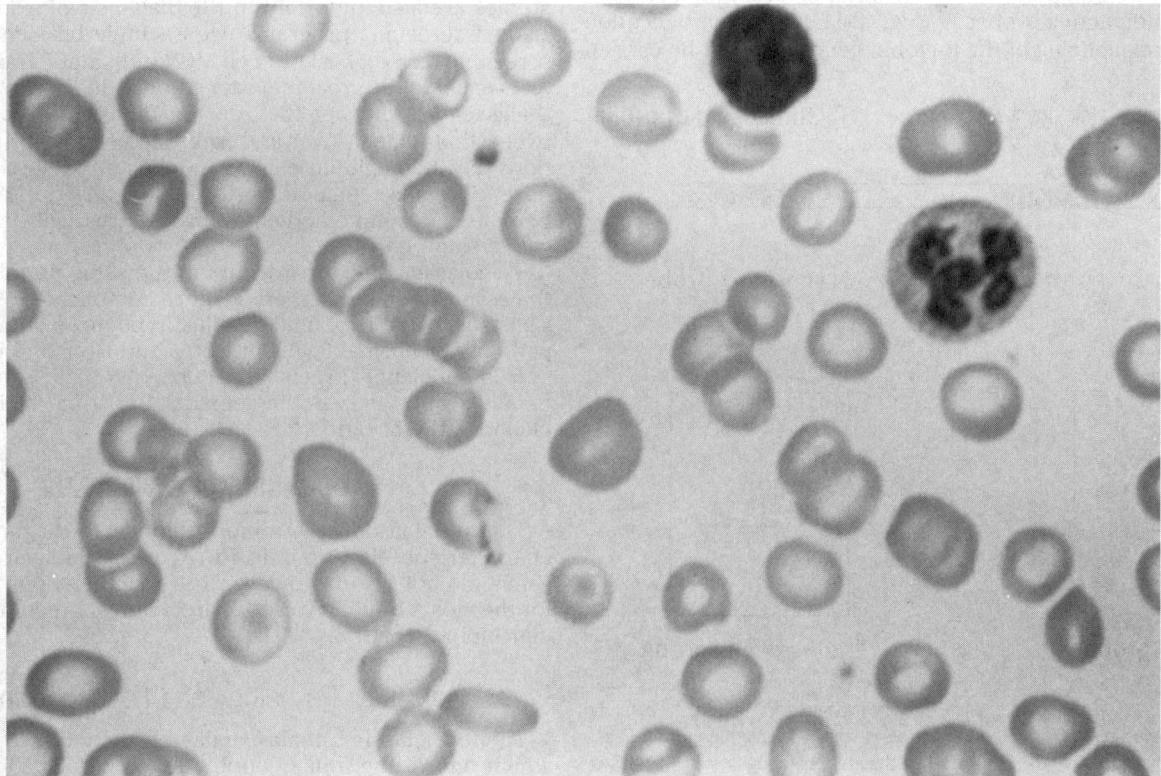

Fig. 42-10. Morphology of the peripheral blood film in **(A)** heterozygous β-thalassemia and **(B)** heterozygous α-thalassemia. Note the profound hypochromia and microcytosis and the many target cells. (From Pearson and Benz,[248] with permission.)

Prenatal Diagnosis

Routine and reliable diagnosis of thalassemia mutations can now be accomplished by using fetal DNA obtained between the eighth and eighteenth week of gestation. The most reliable methods are based on identification of the abnormal gene by direct DNA analysis.[21,22] Both amniocentesis and chorionic villus biopsy have been used with success. In experienced hands, the latter method is preferable because adequate amounts of DNA can be obtained safely at an earlier gestational age. The DNA is analyzed by a variety of PCR-based or other methods for the presence of the thalassemia mutation (see Chs. 1 and 164).

The heterogeneity of thalassemia mutations complicates the approach to antenatal diagnosis. More than 125 independent mutations can cause β-thalassemia.[24] Until recently, this required complicated and somewhat indirect analyses of DNA polymorphisms in both parents, multiple Southern blot analyses of fetal DNA (requiring larger specimens), and a considerable time lag. The final results were only 70–80% predictive of the genotype of the fetus.

Three major factors have improved the efficacy and reliability of DNA diagnosis. First, extensive surveys of most populations in which these alleles are frequent have revealed that about 15 β-thalassemia mutations account for >90% of individuals afflicted worldwide. Within any given ethnic group, three to five mutations usually account for the vast majority of severe cases.[21,22] One can thus "customize" the search for mutations according to the ethnic origins of the family at risk. Second, the polymerase chain reaction (PCR) and exquisitely precise oligonucleotide hybridization assays (allele-specific oligonucleotide or hybridization), which detect single base changes with great reliability, can now be combined to permit screening of minute DNA samples for several mutations very rapidly, even with nonradioactive probes[211] (Fig. 42-11). Third, amplification and even sequencing of the β-globin genes can now be carried

out by use of the PCR in about the time formerly required to culture amniocytes and perform Southern blot analysis.

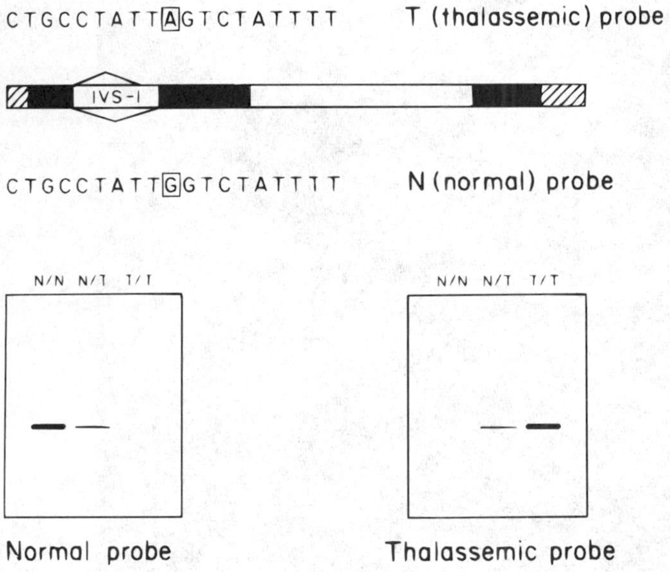

Diagnosis of most cases of severe α-thalassemia can be accomplished by similar approaches. The vast majority of clinically significant α-thalassemia cases arise from gene deletions that are readily detected. Therefore, genetic counseling and antenatal diagnosis should be offered to all families at risk of either severe α- or β-thalassemia.

Screening for Thalassemia Trait

Mass screening and genetic counseling programs are active in Italy, Greece, and other areas in which the frequency of thalassemia is very high. Population screening, combined with prenatal diagnosis, has dramatically decreased the incidence of thalassemia major births in sections of these countries.[212,213] These programs require a critical mass of expert professional and laboratory backup. Voluntary informed participation, confidentiality of results, and meaningful counseling must be ensured.

The most definitive methods for diagnosis of thalassemia trait include quantitative determinations of Hb A_2, Hb F, and globin chain synthetic ratios, as well as DNA studies for specific mutations. These are accurate but too expensive for initial mass screening. Since thalassemia is almost invariably associated with significant hypochromia (MCH <26 pg) and microcytosis (MCV <75 fl), determination of red cell indices has been used as a preliminary indicator of possible thalassemia trait.[214] Microcytosis due to iron deficiency must be excluded.[215] A number of alternatives have been described for follow-up diagnostic tests. Measurement of free erythrocyte porphyrin levels is useful in the evaluation of individuals with microcytosis, as results may be obtained rapidly and inexpensively from a drop of blood.[1] Serum ferritin and iron and iron-binding capacity studies are also important in the diagnosis of iron deficiency.

Most screening programs use a simple but sensitive initial screening test such as red cell MCV or osmotic fragility. These tests exclude the great majority of individuals who do not have thalassemia trait, but they do not differentiate precisely between thalassemia trait and iron deficiency. Hb F determinations and hemoglobin electrophoresis are necessary to diagnose δβ-thalassemia and Hb Lepore traits in microcytic persons. No simple screening procedures will detect the so-called silent carrier.

α-Thalassemia, which occurs in the same populations as β-thalassemia, makes screening more complicated. This diagnosis is suggested by a mild, familial hypochromic microcytosis, with low or normal levels of Hb A_2 and Hb F and no evidence of iron deficiency. Precise diagnosis of α-thalassemia requires demonstration of α-globin gene deletions or a high β/α-globin chain synthetic ratio.

α-THALASSEMIA SYNDROMES

The α-thalassemias are more difficult to diagnose because characteristic elevations in Hb A_2 or Hb F, seen in β-thalassemia, do not occur. However, the gene deletions responsible for the most common varieties are readily detectable by molecular biology methods.[216,217]

Molecular Pathology and Pathophysiology

The four classic α-thalassemias are α-thalassemia-2 trait, in which one of the four α-globin gene loci fails to function; α-thalassemia-1 trait, with two dysfunctional loci; Hb H disease, with three loci affected; and hydrops fetalis with Hb Bart's, in which all four loci are defective. These syndromes are usually due to deletion of one, two, three, or all four of the α-genes, respectively (Fig. 42-12). Nondeletion forms of α-thalassemia, which account for 15–20% of patients, arise from mutations

C T G C C T A T T [A] G T C T A T T T T   T (thalassemic) probe

IVS-I

C T G C C T A T T [G] G T C T A T T T T   N (normal) probe

Normal probe   Thalassemic probe

Fig. 42-11. Example of the use of allele-specific probes for diagnosis of a common form of β-thalassemia. The mutation shown is that discussed in Fig. 42-2 and the text. Two oligonucleotide probes are synthesized, differing only at the position of the mutation. When hybridized under sufficiently stringent conditions, each probe will anneal only to the gene that is perfectly complementary by Watson-Crick basepairing. Thus, a homozygous normal fetal DNA sample (N/N) will anneal only to the normal probe, homozygous β-thalassemic DNA (T/T) only to the thalassemic probe, and DNA from a heterozygote (N/T) to both probes, but with a reduced intensity to each. (From High and Benz,[250] with permission.)

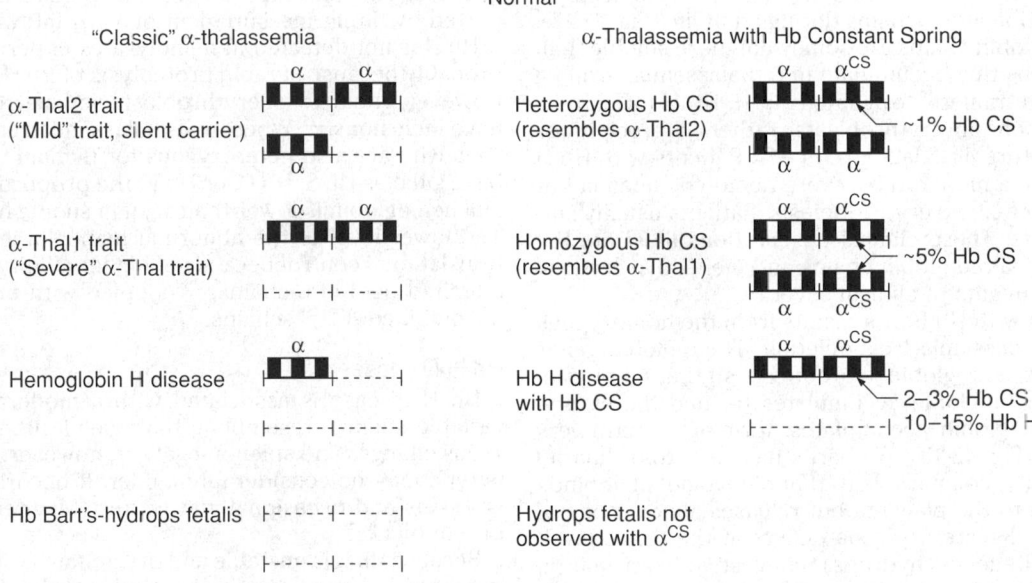

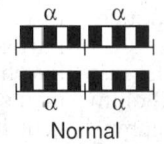

Fig. 42-12. Genetic origins of the "classic" α-thalassemia syndromes due to gene deletions in α-globin gene cluster. Hb Constant Spring (Hb CS) is an α-chain variant synthesized in such small amounts (1–2% of normal) that it has the phenotypic impact of a severe nondeletion α-thalassemia allele; however, the α^{CS} allele is always linked to a functioning α-globin gene, so that it has never been associated with hydrops fetalis.

similar to those described for β-thalassemia.[216,217] Figure 42-13 illustrates the different α-thalassemia mutations and phenotypes. Structurally abnormal hemoglobins have been associated with α-thalassemia. The Quong Sze α-globin chain ($\alpha^{125\ Leu \rightarrow Pro}$) is an exceedingly labile α-chain destroyed so rapidly after its synthesis that no hemoglobin tetramers can be formed.[218]

α-Thalassemia-2 trait is an asymptomatic silent carrier state,

commonly associated with the deletion of a single α-globin gene. Offspring of an individual with α-thalassemia-2 whose spouse has α-thalassemia-1 trait can inherit a form of α-thalassemia more severe than either of these, namely Hb H disease.

α-Thalassemia-1 trait results from deletion or nonfunction of two α-globin alleles. In Asian and Mediterranean populations, a deletion that removes both loci from the same chromosome (cis deletion) is common,[216,217] as is homozygosity for α-thalas-

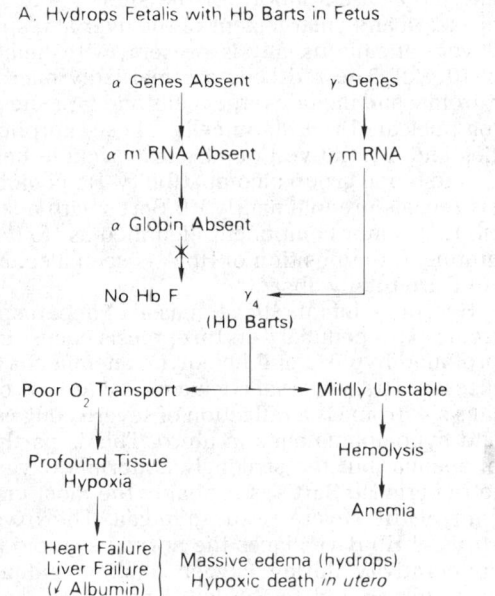

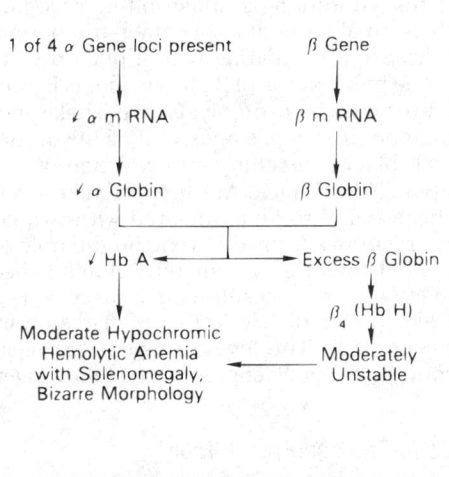

Fig. 42-13. Pathophysiology of Hb H disease and hydrops fetalis with Hb Bart's. (From Benz,[20] with permission.)

semia-2 (trans deletion). In blacks, both α-globin genes are only rarely deleted in cis, whereas homozygosity for α-thalassemia-2 (trans deletion) is quite common.[219] Both genotypes produce asymptomatic hypochromia and microcytosis.

Hb H disease usually results from co-inheritance of the cis α-thalassemia-1 deletion and α-thalassemia-2 trait. α-Globin chain production is only 25–30% of normal; γ-chains accumulate during gestation and β-chains during adult life (Fig. 42-13). The unpaired β-globin chains are somewhat more soluble than the α-globin chains that accumulate in β-thalassemia, forming recognizable β_4 tetramers designated Hb H. Hb H forms relatively few inclusions in erythroblasts; rather, it precipitates slowly within mature circulating red cells. Patients with Hb H disease thus have a moderately severe hemolytic anemia but relatively little ineffective erythropoiesis. Patients usually survive into adult life. These clinical observations illustrate the central role of unpaired globin chains and ineffective erythropoiesis as determinants of clinical severity.

Hydrops fetalis with Hb Bart's results from the homozygous state for the α-thalassemia-1 cis deletion. The α-globin genes are totally absent; no α-globin is produced, so that no physiologically useful hemoglobin accumulates beyond the embryonic stage. Free γ-globin accumulates, forming γ_4 tetramers called Hb Bart's (Fig. 42-13). Hb Bart's has an extraordinarily high oxygen affinity, comparable to that of myoglobin. It binds oxygen delivered to the placenta but releases almost none of it to fetal tissues. Severe asphyxia occurs at the tissue level, causing profound edema (hydrops), congestive heart failure, and death in utero. These fatal complications do not occur in fetuses with Hb H disease because enough Hb F is made to sustain life. α-Thalassemia-2 trait is very common in blacks, having a gene frequency of 20–30% in some populations. However, the cis α-thalassemia-1 deletion is rare in blacks. Thus, even though α-thalassemia-2 trait and the trans deletion form of α-thalassemia-1 are very common, Hb H disease is rarely encountered, and hydrops fetalis has not yet been reported in blacks.[219,220]

Clinical Manifestations

Silent Carrier (α-Thalassemia-2 Trait)

α-Thalassemia-2 trait has no consistent hematologic manifestations. The red cells are not microcytic, and Hb A_2 and Hb F are normal. During the newborn period, small amounts (≤3%) of Hb Bart's (γ_4) may be seen by electrophoresis or column chromatography. This condition is most often recognized when an apparently normal individual becomes the parent of a child with Hb H disease after mating with a person with α-thalassemia-1 trait. The mild excess of β-globin chains is probably removed in erythroblasts by proteolysis.[221] α-Thalassemia-2 is particularly common in Melanesia, as well as in southeast Asia and in American blacks, reaching a prevalence of >80% in north coastal Papua, New Guinea. At the molecular level, α-thalassemia-2 has been found to be associated with two common gene deletions resulting from different nonhomologous crossing over events between the two linked α-globin genes: a 3.7-kb rightward deletion ($-\alpha^{3.7}$) resulting in a fused $\alpha_2\alpha_1$-globin gene, and a 4.2-kb leftward deletion ($-\alpha^{4.2}$) resulting in loss of the 5' (α_2) gene.[216,217] The level of α-gene expression differs in the two conditions, as discussed in the following section.

α-Thalassemia Trait (α-Thalassemia-1 Trait)

α-Thalassemia-1 trait is characterized by levels of Hb A_2 in the low to low-normal range (1.5–2.5%) and β/α synthetic ratios averaging 1.4:1. During the perinatal period, elevated amounts of Hb Bart's are noted (3–8%). Microcytosis is present in cord blood erythrocytes.

Studies of newborns from the archipelago of Vanuatu in the southwest Pacific and from Papua, New Guinea, indicate that homozygotes for the rightward $-\alpha^{3.7III}$ deletion (where only a fused $\alpha_2\alpha_1$ gene mostly of the α_2 type remains) have lower Hb Bart's levels (3.5 ± 0.8%) than those of infants homozygous for the leftward $-\alpha^{4.2}$ deletion (where only the α_1-gene remains) (6.0 ± 1.4%). These results suggest that the 5' α_2-globin gene has a higher output than the 3' α_1-gene, a conclusion supported by direct measurement of α_2/α_1 mRNA ratios.[223,224]

Hb H is not detected in hemolysates of peripheral red cells, probably because of rapid proteolysis of Hb H or free β-chains. However, about 1% of erythroblasts and marrow reticulocytes have inclusions.[221] When an α-thalassemia gene occurs in persons who are also heterozygous for β-chain variant hemoglobins, such as Hb S, Hb C, or Hb E, the proportion of the abnormal hemoglobin is lower than seen in simple heterozygotes.[225] The lower level of the abnormal hemoglobin is due to post-translational control because of higher affinity of β^A chains for a limited pool of α-chains,[226] coupled with proteolysis of the uncombined $\beta^{variant}$-chains.

Hb H Disease

Hb H disease is associated with a moderately severe but variable anemia, resembling thalassemia intermedia with osseous changes and splenomegaly[227]; however, the clinical phenotype may be considerably milder. It occurs predominantly in Asians and occasionally in whites (Mediterraneans) but is rare in blacks.

Because Hb H is unstable and precipitates within the circulating red cell, hemolysis occurs. Hb H can be demonstrated by incubation of blood with supravital oxidizing stains such as 1% brilliant cresyl blue. Multiple small inclusions form in the red cells (Fig. 31-13). Electrophoresis of a freshly prepared hemolysate at alkaline or neutral pH demonstrates a fast-moving component amounting to 3–30% of the total hemoglobin. Concomitant iron deficiency may reduce the amount of Hb H in the patient's red cells.[228] A syndrome of Hb H disease associated with mental retardation, other congenital anomalies, and large deletions on chromosome 16 have been noted in several white families.[216,217]

Hydrops Fetalis with Hb Bart's

Hydrops fetalis with Hb Bart's occurs almost exclusively in southeastern Asians, especially Chinese, Cambodians, Thais, and Filipinos. Affected fetuses usually are born prematurely and either are stillborn or die shortly after birth.[1–4] Marked anascara and enlargement of the liver and spleen are present. Severe anemia usually is present, with hemoglobin levels of 3–10 g/dl. The red cells are markedly microcytic and hypochromic and include target cells and large numbers of circulating nucleated red blood cells. These morphologic abnormalities and a negative Coombs test exclude hemolytic diseases due to blood group incompatibility. Hemoglobin electrophoresis reveals predominantly Hb Bart's with a smaller amount of Hb H. A minor component identified as Hb Portland ($\zeta_2\gamma_2$) migrating in the position of Hb A is seen also. Normal Hb A and Hb F are totally absent.[229]

Hydropic infants have massive hepatosplenomegaly. Extreme extramedullary erythropoiesis occurs in response to the profound hypoxia and hemolytic anemia characteristic of this disease. The universal edema characteristic of the hydrops fetalis syndrome is a reflection of severe congestive heart failure and hypoalbuminemia in utero. This is partly a consequence of anemia, but the strikingly abnormal oxygen affinity of the tetrameric Hb Bart's is probably the most important determinant of the severe tissue hypoxia. The oxygen dissociation curve of Hb Bart's lacks the normal sigmoid form due to noncooperativity during oxygen loading and unloading and is markedly shifted to the left. The shift is so great that little oxygen is released under conditions of low oxygen concentration in the tissues.

Infants with this syndrome do not die in an earlier trimester of pregnancy because of the presence of Hb Portland ($\zeta_2\gamma_2$). This hemoglobin does display cooperativity in a manner similar to that of Hb F and therefore, has a much more favorable oxygen dissociation pattern than that of Hb Bart's. A high incidence of toxemia of pregnancy has been described in women carrying severely affected infants, providing an increased rationale for prenatal diagnosis of this condition.

Prenatal Diagnosis

Using molecular hybridization technology, Kan and associates[230] detected the complete absence of α-genes in fetal fibroblasts obtained by amniocentesis in a pregnancy at risk of homozygous α-thalassemia-1 and the hydrops fetalis syndrome. The presence of hydrops can also be detected by ultrasonography. DNA studies or globin synthesis evaluation may be used to confirm the diagnosis in utero. PCR-based assays are available for the detection of the common α-thalassemia-1 deletions.[231]

Therapy

Fetuses with homozygous α-thalassemia-1 usually die in utero because of severe hydrops fetalis and are stillborn. One infant was born alive after cesarean section but survived only a few hours despite vigorous exchange transfusion therapy.[229] Others have had successful blood exchange immediately after birth and were maintained by chronic transfusion therapy afterward.[232–234] It is also theoretically possible to salvage affected fetuses by in utero blood transfusions.

Patients with Hb H disease usually require neither red cell transfusions nor splenectomy. Splenectomy can result in a clinically important rise in hemoglobin level and should thus be considered in patients with marked anemia. Oxidant drugs can accelerate precipitation of Hb H and exacerbate hemolysis; it should therefore be avoided.

Infants with heterozygous α-thalassemia-1 trait lose their Hb Bart's during the first few months of life and are left with the hematologic findings of α-thalassemia trait, a mild hypochromic microcytosis that persists throughout life.[1] The degree of morphologic abnormality varies greatly among different individuals. That α-thalassemia can be easily diagnosed by hemoglobin electrophoresis at birth gives some impetus to cord blood screening studies.

THALASSEMIC STRUCTURAL VARIANTS

Certain structural hemoglobin variants are characterized by the presence of a biosynthetic defect as well as abnormal structure.[8] Thalassemic hemoglobinopathies are unusual forms of thalassemia caused by such structural variants.

Hb Lepore

Hb Lepore ($\alpha_2[\gamma\delta\gamma\beta_2]$) is the prototype of a group of hemoglobinopathies characterized by fused globin chains.[1–4] The chains begin with a normal δ-chain sequence at their N terminus and end with the normal β-chain sequence at their C terminus. These hemoglobinopathies arise by unequal or nonhomologous crossover or recombination events that fuse the proximal end of one gene with the distal end of a closely linked structurally homologous gene (Fig. 42-14). During meiosis, mispairing and crossover of the highly homologous δ- and β-genes can occur, resulting in a Lepore chromosome, which contains (in addition to γ-genes) only the fused δβ gene, and an anti-Lepore chromosome, which contains the reciprocal fusion product (βδ), as well as intact δ- and β-globin genes.[1–4]

Lepore globin is synthesized in low amounts presumably because it is under the control of the δ-globin gene promoter, which normally sustains transcription at only 2.5% the level of the β-globin gene.[235] Patients with Hb Lepore have the phenotype of β-thalassemia, distinguished by the added presence of 5–15% Hb Lepore. By contrast, the anti-Lepore globin (Miyada) is not associated with a β-thalassemia phenotype because of the presence of an intact and functionally normal β-gene on the same chromosome.

Heterozygotes for Hb Lepore have the clinical phenotype of β-thalassemia trait; homozygotes are usually similar to patients with homozygous β-thalassemia. Compound heterozygotes for Hb Lepore and a "classic" β-thalassemia allele usually have severe thalassemia. Hb Lepore thus interacts with thalassemia in the same way as a severe β-thalassemia gene does, although occasional cases have a milder phenotype of the thalassemia intermedia variety, perhaps due to an associated higher than usual level of γ-globin gene expression. The presence of Hb

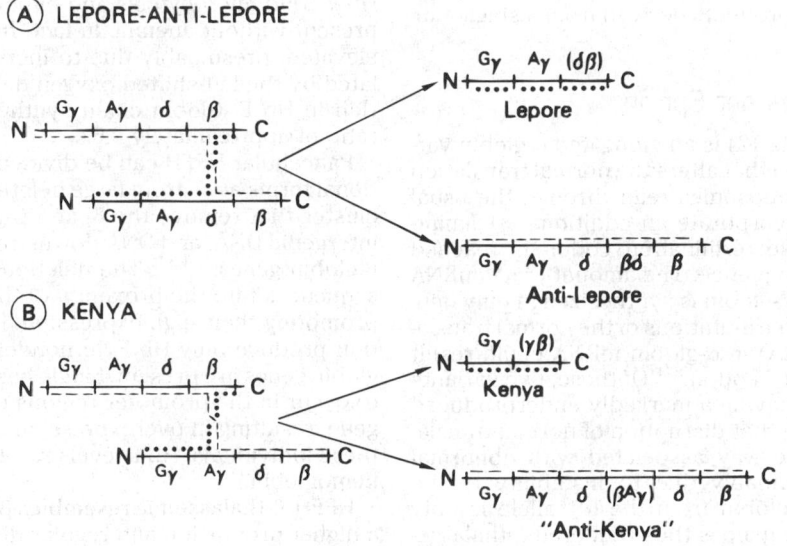

Fig. 42-14. Genetic origins of Hb Lepore, anti-Lepore Hb, and Hb Kenya. (From Benz,[20] with permission.)

Lepore should be suspected in hypochromic microcytic individuals who also have a small amount of an abnormal hemoglobin migrating in the position of Hb S on routine electrophoretic gels. Hb Lepore accounts for 5–10% of the β-thalassemias seen in Greek and Italian populations. Several forms of Hb Lepore have been described, which differ in the position at which the transition from δ to β DNA and amino acid sequence occurs.

An analogous variant, Hb Kenya ($\alpha_2[^A\gamma\beta]_2$), arises from nonhomologous crossing over between the $^A\gamma$- and β-globin genes[236] (Fig. 42-14) and is associated with the phenotype of $^G\gamma$ HPFH. It is now clear that a DNA sequence about 600 bases downstream from the β-globin gene acts as a strong enhancer, promoting the erythroid-specific expression of the β-globin genes in adult cells.[3,4,23] The fused $^A\gamma\beta$ gene as well as the linked upstream $^G\gamma$-gene are thought to come under the influence of the enhancer, because of its abnormal proximity, and thus are expressed at high levels in adult life. Hb Kenya is rare.

Hb E

Hb E ($\alpha_2\beta_2^{26Glu\rightarrow Lys}$) is a common variant (15–30% of the population) in Cambodia, Thailand, parts of China, and Vietnam. Hb E trait resembles very mild β-thalassemia trait. Homozygotes exhibit more microcytosis but are still asymptomatic.[237] Compound heterozygotes for Hb E and a β-thalassemia gene (Hb E-β-thalassemia) resemble patients with β-thalassemia intermedia or β-thalassemia major. Hb E is very mildly unstable, but this instability does not alter red cell life span significantly. The high frequency of the Hb E gene is due to the thalassemia phenotype associated with its inheritance.

The only nucleotide sequence abnormality found in the β^E gene is a base change in codon 26 that causes the amino acid substitution. This mutation, which occurs in a potential cryptic RNA splice region, alters the consensus sequence surrounding a potential GT donor splice site and thus activates the cryptic site. Alternative splicing at this position occurs approximately 40–50% of the time, generating a structurally abnormal globin mRNA, which cannot be translated appropriately.[238] The other mRNA precursors are spliced at the normal site, generating functionally normal mRNA, which is translated into β^E-globin because the mature mRNA retains the base change that encodes lysine at codon 26.

Hb E is important because it is so common in Southeast Asian populations. Genetic counseling of these individuals should emphasize the potential consequences of the interaction of Hb E with β-thalassemia. Hb E is also an instructive example of the pleiotropic effects that point mutations may have on the amounts and types of gene products derived from a single mutant gene.

Hb Constant Spring

Hb Constant Spring (Fig. 42-12) is an elongated α-globin variant resulting from a mutation that alters the normal translation termination codon.[239] Polyribosomes read through the usual translation stop site and incorporate an additional 31 amino acids until another in-phase termination codon is reached within the 3′ untranslated sequence. The amount of α^{cs} mRNA is markedly reduced, and α^{cs}-globin is synthesized in only minute amounts.[223,240] Six possible mutations of the normal translation termination codon (UAA) in α-globin mRNA could result in the generation of a "sense" codon.[241] Of these, five variants have been identified, each having a markedly underproduced abnormal variant, indicating that disruption of normal translation termination is in some way associated with abnormal mRNA accumulation, presumably due to instability of the mRNA.[223] The output of α-globin from the α^{cs} allele is only about 1% of normal, and the gene is thus rendered α-thalassemic. The α^{cs} allele has been identified only on chromosomes containing a cis-linked functionally normal α_1-globin gene.[1-4]

Thus, α-thalassemia-2 trait and Hb H disease ($--/\alpha^{cs}\alpha$) associated with Hb Constant Spring are common, but hydrops fetalis cannot occur in association with this variant. Homozygosity for the variant is associated with a relatively severe form of Hb H disease.[1-4]

Extraordinarily Unstable Hemoglobins

Rare cases of α-thalassemia (e.g., Hb Quong Sze[218]) and β-thalassemia (e.g., Hb Indianapolis, recently renamed Hb Terre Haute[242,243]) arise from mutations that produce extremely labile globin chains. The chains fail to pair with the complementary chain, or they precipitate and are degraded so rapidly that they never form tetramers. These post-translational lesions have the same pathophysiologic effects on hemoglobin biogenesis as reduction of globin mRNA production or function. Another group of β-chain variants, usually due to mutations in exon 3 of the β-globin gene, are associated with inclusion body formation and a phenotype of dominant β-thalassemia intermedia.[18,19]

HEREDITARY PERSISTENCE OF FETAL HEMOGLOBIN

HPFH consists of a group of rare conditions characterized by continued synthesis of high levels of Hb F in adult life.[1-4,244] No deleterious effects on patients are observed, even when 100% of the hemoglobin produced in HPFH homozygotes is Hb F. These patients thus demonstrate convincingly that prevention or reversal of the Hb F to Hb A switch would provide efficacious therapy for sickle cell anemia and β-thalassemia.

Two major types of HPFH have been described. Pancellular HPFH is characterized by very high levels of fetal hemoglobin synthesis and uniform distribution of Hb F among all red cells. Heterocellular HPFH results from inherited increases in the number of F cells (see Chs. 17 and 35).

HPFH shows ethnic differences. In blacks with heterozygous pancellular deletional HPFH, the Hb F is within a range of 15–35% and contains $^G\gamma$- and $^A\gamma$-chains in a ratio of 2:3. In Greeks with pancellular nondeletional HPFH, Hb F levels are lower, 10–20%, and the Hb F is 90% of the $^A\gamma$ type. Hb A$_2$ levels are lower than normal, but there are no other hematologic abnormalities in these persons, although β/α-globin chain synthesis ratios may be decreased in some black heterozygotes.

A few black patients have been described with homozygous HPFH. All hemoglobin within the red cells of these patients is Hb F. Mild microcytosis and hypochromia of the red cells are present without anemia. In fact, hemoglobin levels are mildly elevated, presumably due to increased erythropoiesis stimulated by the left-shifted oxygen dissociation curve of red cells rich in Hb F. Globin chain synthesis reveals a γ/α synthetic ratio of approximately 0.5.

Pancellular HPFH can be divided into two classes. The deletional forms arise from large deletions within the β-globin gene cluster that remove the δ- and β-globin genes, part of the γδ intergenic DNA, and DNA downstream (to the 3′ side) from the β-globin genes.[1-4,244] The deletions appear to bring enhancer sequences into the proximity of the remaining γ-globin genes, promoting their high expression. Homozygotes for this condition produce only Hb F. In nondeletional HPFH, the β- and δ-globin genes are present. Single base changes have been shown to occur in the promoter regions of either the $^A\gamma$- or $^G\gamma$-globin gene, resulting in overexpression of that form of Hb F.[1-4,244] In these individuals, Hb F levels rarely account for >20% of total hemoglobin.

HPFH/β-thalassemia resembles β-thalassemia trait except for a higher proportion and regular distribution of Hb F in the red cells.[1-4]

In both δβ-thalassemia and HPFH, persistence of Hb F after

the period of perinatal Hb F to Hb A switching is more marked than in the "classic" (high Hb A_2) forms of thalassemia. Indeed, $\delta\beta$-thalassemia and HPFH represent varying degrees of the same genetic phenomenon. Both conditions frequently arise from deletions of DNA, which remove or inactivate the β-globin gene.[1-4,244]

Heterocellular HPFH appears to result in many cases from mutations outside the β-globin gene cluster. One controlling locus resides on the X chromosome.[245,246] Patients with these conditions probably represent the extreme end of a distribution of polymorphic capacities to produce F cells in adult life. Hb F levels are usually much lower than in the pancellular forms. In some situations, elevated levels of Hb F are seen in otherwise normal individuals. In others, the high levels of Hb F become apparent only when other factors producing erythroid stress are present.

ACKNOWLEDGMENT

Portions of this chapter have been modified and updated from previous chapters we have written.[20,23,247,248]

REFERENCES

1. Weatherall DJ, Clegg JB: The Thalassemia Syndromes. 3rd Ed. Blackwell Scientific, Oxford, 1981
2. Bunn HF, Forget BG: Hemoglobin: Molecular, Genetic and Clinical Aspects. WB Saunders, Philadelphia, 1986
3. Weatherall DJ: The thalassemias. p. 157. In Stamatoyannopoulos G, Nienhuis AW, Majerus PW, Varmus HE (eds): Molecular Basis of Blood Diseases. 2nd Ed. WB Saunders, Philadelphia, 1993
4. McDonagh KT, Nienhuis AW: The thalassemias. p. 783. In Nathan DG, Oski FA (eds): Hematology of Infancy and Childhood. 4th Ed. WB Saunders, Philadelphia, 1993
5. Cooley TB, Lee P: A series of cases of splenomegaly in children with anemia and peculiar bone changes. Trans Am Pediatr Soc 37:29, 1925
6. Cooley TB, Witwer ER, Lee P: Anemia in children with splenomegaly and peculiar changes in bones: report of cases. Am J Dis Child 34:347, 1927
7. Whipple GH, Bradford WL: Mediterranean disease-thalassemia (erythroblastic anemia of Cooley): associated pigment abnormalities simulating hemochromatosis. J Pediatr 9:279, 1932
8. Adams JG III, Coleman MB: Structural hemoglobin variants that produce the phenotype of thalassemia. Semin Hematol 27:229, 1990
9. Barrai I, Rosity A, Cappellozza G et al: Beta-thalassemia in the Po delta: selection, geography and population structure. Am J Hum Genet 36:1121, 1984
10. Livingston FB: Abnormal Hemoglobins in Human Populations. Aldine, Chicago, 1967
11. Malamos B, Fessas P, Stamatoyannopoulos G: Types of thalassemia-trait carriers as revealed by a study of their incidence in Greece. Br J Haematol 8:5, 1962
12. Pearson HA, Guiliotis DK, O'Brien RT et al: Thalassemia in Greek Americans. J Pediatr 86:917, 1975
13. Nagel RL, Roth EF Jr: Malaria and red cell genetic defects. Blood 74:1213, 1989
14. Nathan DG, Gunn RB: Thalassemia: the consequences of unbalanced hemoglobin synthesis. Am J Med 41:815, 1966
15. Kanavakis E, Wainscoat JS, Wood WG et al: The interaction of α-thalassemia with heterozygous β-thalassemia. Br J Haematol 52:465, 1982
16. Rosatelli C, Falchi AM, Scalas MT et al: Hematological phenotype of the double heterozygous state for alpha and beta thalassemia. Hemoglobin 8:25, 1984
17. Wainscoat JS, Kanavakis E, Wood WG et al: Thalassaemia intermedia in Cyprus: the interaction of α- and β-thalassaemia. Br J Haematol 53:411, 1983
18. Thein SL: Dominant β-thalassemia: molecular basis and pathophysiology. Br J Haematol 80:273, 1992
19. Kazazian HH Jr, Dowling CE, Hurwitz RL et al: Dominant thalassemia-like phenotypes associated with mutations in exon 3 of the β-globin gene. Blood 79:3014, 1992
20. Benz EJ Jr: The hemoglobinopathies. p. 1423. In Kelly WN, DeVita VT (eds): Textbook of Internal Medicine. JB Lippincott, Philadelphia, 1988
21. Kazazian HH Jr, Boehm CD: Molecular basis and prenatal diagnosis of β-thalassemia. Blood 72:1107, 1988
22. Kazazian HH Jr: The thalassemia syndromes: molecular basis and prenatal diagnosis in 1990. Semin Hematol 27:209, 1990
23. Forget BG, Pearson HA: Hemoglobin synthesis and the thalassemias. In Handin RE, Lux SE, Stossel T (eds): Blood: Principles and Practice of Hematology. JB Lippincott, Philadelphia, 1994 (in press)
24. Huisman THJ: The β- and δ-thalassemia repository. Hemoglobin 17:479, 1993
25. Westaway D, Williamson R: An intron nucleotide sequence variant in a cloned β^+-thalassemia globin gene. Nucleic Acids Res 9:1777, 1981
26. Spritz RA, Jagadeeswaran P, Choudary PV et al: Base substitution in an intervening sequence of a β^+-thalassemic human globin gene. Proc Natl Acad Sci USA 78:2455, 1981
27. Trecartin RF, Liebhaber SA, Chang JC et al: β^0-thalassemia in Sardinia is caused by a nonsense mutation. J Clin Invest 68:1012, 1981
28. Orkin SH, Goff SC: Nonsense and frameshift mutations in β-thalassemia detected in cloned β-globin genes. J Biol Chem 256:9782, 1981
29. Van der Ploeg LHT, Konings A, Oort M et al: $\gamma\beta$-Thalassaemia studies showing that deletion of the γ and δ genes influences β globin gene expression in man. Nature 283:637, 1980
30. Townes TM, Behringer RR: Human globin locus activation region (LAR): role in temporal control. Trends Genet 6:219, 1990
31. Huang S-Z, Wong C, Antonarakis SE et al: The same TATA box β-thalassemia mutation in Chinese and US blacks: another example of independent origins of mutations. Hum Genet 74:152, 1986
32. Antonarakis SE, Kazazian HH Jr, Orkin SH: DNA polymorphism and molecular pathology of the human globin gene clusters. Hum Genet 69:1, 1985
33. Gilman JG, Huisman THJ: DNA sequence variation associated with elevated $^G\gamma$ globin production. Blood 66:783, 1985
34. Shinar E, Rachmilewitz EA: Oxidative denaturation of red blood cells in thalassemia. Semin Hematol 27:70, 1990
35. Sturgeon P, Finch CA: Erythrokinetics in Cooley's anemia. Blood 12:64, 1957
36. Cossu G, Manca M, Pirastu MG et al: Neonatal screening of beta thalassemia by thin layer isoelectric focusing. Am J Hematol 13:149, 1982
37. Logothetis J, Loewenson RB, Augoustaki O et al: Body growth in Cooley's anemia (homozygous beta-thalassemia) with a correlative study as to other aspects of the illness in 138 cases. Pediatrics 50:92, 1972
38. Baty JM, Blackfan KD, Diamond LK: Blood studies in infants and in children. I. Erythroblastic anemia: a clinical and pathologic study. Am J Dis Child 43:665, 1932
39. Silvestroni E, Bianco I: Screening for microcytemia in Italy: analysis of data collected in the past 30 years. Am J Hum Genet 27:198, 1975
40. Smith CH, Sisson TRC, Floyd WH Jr et al: Serum iron and iron-binding capacity of the serum in children with severe Mediterranean (Cooley's) anemia. Pediatrics 5:799, 1950
41. Fessas P: Inclusions of hemoglobin in erythroblasts and erythrocytes of thalassemia. Blood 21:21, 1963
42. Fessas P, Loukopoulos D, Kaltsoya A: Peptide analysis of the inclusions of erythroid cells in β-thalassemia. Biochim Biophys Acta 124:439, 1966
43. Cutello S, Meloni T: Serum concentration of haptoglobin and hemopexin in favism and thalassemia. Acta Haematol 52:65, 1974
44. Arcasoy A, Cavdar AO: Changes of trace minerals (serum iron, zinc, copper and magnesium) in thalassemia. Acta Haematol 53:341, 1975
45. Prasad AS, Diwany M, Gabr M et al: Biochemical studies in thalassemia. Ann Intern Med 62:87, 1965
46. Propper RD, Nathan DG: Desferrioxamine and the pump. In Zaino EC, Roberts RH (eds): Chelation Therapy in Chronic Iron Overload. Symposia Specialists, Miami, FL, 1977
47. Jandl JH, Greenberg MS: Bone marrow failure due to relative nutritional deficiency in Cooley's hemolytic anemia. N Engl J Med 266:461, 1959
48. Luhby AL, Cooperman JM: Folic acid deficiency in thalassemia major. Lancet 2:490, 1961
49. Hyman CB, Landing B, Alfin-Slater R et al: dl-α-Tocopherol, iron and lipofuscin in thalassemia. Ann NY Acad Sci 232:211, 1974
50. Rachmilewitz EA, Lubin BH, Shohet SB: Lipid membrane peroxidation in β-thalassemia major. Blood 47:495, 1976
51. Rachmilewitz EA, Shifter A, Kahane I: Vitamin E deficiency in β-thalassemia major. Changes in hematological and biochemical parameters following a therapeutic clinical trial with alpha-tocopherol. Am J Clin Nutr 32:1850, 1979
52. Hilgartner MW, Smith CH: Coagulation studies as a measure of liver function in Cooley's anemia. Ann NY Acad Sci 119:631, 1964
53. Stuart MJ: Platelet dysfunction in homozygous beta thalassemia. Pediatr Res 13:1345, 1992
54. Lawson JP, Ablow RC, Pearson HA: The ribs in thalassemia. II. The pathogenesis of the changes. Radiology 140:673, 1981
55. Caffey J: Cooley's anemia: a review of the roentgenographic findings in the skeleton. AJR 78:381, 1957

56. Asbell MB: Orthodontic aspects of Cooley's anemia. Ann NY Acad Sci 119: 662, 1964

57. Currarino G, Erlandson ME: Premature fusion of epiphyses in Cooley's anemia. Radiology 83:656, 1964

58. Lawson JP, Ablow RC, Pearson HA: Premature fusion of the primal humeral epiphyses in thalassemia. AJR 140:239, 1983

59. Lawson JP, Ablow RC, Pearson HA: The ribs in thalassemia. I. The relationship of therapy. Radiology 140:656, 1981

60. Spinal cord compression in thalassemia, editorial. Lancet 1:664, 1982

61. Isseragrisil HC, Piankigagum A, Wasi P: Spinal cord compression in thalassemia: report of 12 cases and recommendations for treatment. Arch Intern Med 141:1033, 1981

62. Papavasilou C, Sandilos P: Effect of radiotherapy on symptoms due to heterotopic marrow in β-thalassaemia. Lancet 1:13, 1987

63. Caffey J: Cooley's erythroblastic anemia: some skeletal findings in adolescents and young adults. AJR 65:547, 1951

64. Piomelli S, Danoff SJ, Becker MH et al: Prevention of bone malformation and cardiomegaly in Cooley's anemia by early hypertransfusion regimen. Ann NY Acad Sci 165:427, 1969

65. O'Brien RT, Pearson HA, Spencer RP: Transfusion induced decrease in spleen size in thalassemia major. J Pediatr 81:105, 1972

66. Ellis JT, Schulman I, Smith CH: Generalized siderosis with fibrosis of liver and pancreas in Cooley's (Mediterranean) anemia. Am J Pathol 30:287, 1954

67. Fink H: Transfusion hemochromatosis in Cooley's anemia. Ann NY Acad Sci 119:680, 1964

68. Mak IT, Weglicki WB: Characterization of iron-mediated peroxidative injury in isolated hepatic lysosomes. J Clin Invest 75:58, 1985

69. DeVirgillis S, Fiorelli G, Fargion S et al: Chronic liver disease in transfusion-dependent thalassemia: hepatitis B virus marker studies. J Clin Pathol 33: 949, 1980

70. DeVirgillis S, Carnacchia G, Sanna G et al: Chronic liver disease in transfusion-dependent thalassemia: liver iron content and distribution. Acta Haematol 65:32, 1981

71. Dewey KW, Grossman H, Canale VC: Cholelithiasis in thalassemia major. Radiology 96:385, 1970

72. Engle MA: Cardiac involvement in Cooley's anemia. Ann NY Acad Sci 119: 694, 1964

73. Borow KM, Propper R, Bierman FZ et al: The left ventricular end-systolic pressure dimension relation in patients with thalassemia major. Circulation 66:980, 1982

74. Stanfield JB: Acute benign pericarditis in thalassemia major. Proc R Soc Med 55:236, 1962

75. Wasi P: Streptococcal infection leading to cardiac and renal involvement in thalassemia. Lancet 1:949, 1971

76. Cooper DM, Mansell AL, Weiner MA et al: Low lung capacity and hypoxemia in children with thalassemia major. Am Rev Respir Dis 121:639, 1980

77. Secchi GC, Scotti PG, Cambiagli G et al: Respiratory function tests in adolescents with β-thalassemia major. Haematologica 67:23, 1982

78. Hoyt RW, Scarpa N, Wilmott RW et al: Pulmonary function abnormalities in homozygous β-thalassemia. J Pediatr 109:452, 1986

79. Keens TG, O'Neal MH, Ortega JA et al: Pulmonary function abnormalities in thalassemia patients on a hypertransfusion program. Pediatrics 65:1013, 1980

80. Cooper DM, Hyman CB, Weiler-Ravell D et al: Gas exchange during exercise in children with thalassemia major and Diamond-Blackfan anemia. Pediatr Res 19:1215, 1985

81. Grossman H, Dischl MR, Winchester PH, Canali V: Renal enlargement in thalassemia major. Radiology 100:645, 1971

82. Kreimer-Birnbaum M, Pinkerton PH, Bannerman RN: Urinary dipyrroles: their occurrence and significance in thalassemia and other disorders. Blood 28:933, 1966

83. Laor E, Garfunkel A, Koyoumdjisky-Kaye E: Skeletal and dental retardation in β-thalassemia major. Hum Biol 54:85, 1982

84. Johnston FE, Krogman WM: Patterns of growth in children with thalassemia major. Ann NY Acad Sci 119:667, 1964

85. Afifi AM: High transfusion regimen in the management of reproduction wastage and maternal complications of pregnancy in thalassemia major. Acta Haematol 52:331, 1974

86. Thomas RM, Skalicka AE: Successful pregnancy in transfusion-dependent thalassemia. Arch Dis Child 55:572, 1980

87. Borgna-Pignatti C, DeStefano P, Zonta MS et al: Growth and sexual maturation in thalassemia major. J Pediatr 106:150, 1985

88. Arcasoy A, Cavdar A, Cin S et al: Effects of zinc supplementation on linear growth in beta-thalassemia (a new approach). Am J Hematol 24:127, 1987

89. Merkel PA, Simonson DC, Amiel S et al: Insulin resistance and hyperinsulinemia in patients with thalassemia major treated by hypertransfusion. N Engl J Med 318:809, 1988

90. Gertner JM, Broadus AE, Anast CS et al: Impaired parathyroid response to induced hypocalcemia in thalassemia major. J Pediatr 95:210, 1979

91. Masala A, Meloni T, Gallisai D et al: Endocrine functioning in multitransfused prepubertal patients with homozygous β-thalassemia. J Clin Endocrinol Metab 58:667, 1984

92. deLuca F, Melluso R, Sobbrio G et al: Thyroid function in thalassemia major. Arch Dis Child 55:389, 1980

93. Pintor C, Cella SG, Manso P et al: Impaired growth hormone (GH) response to GH-releasing hormone in thalassemia major. J Clin Endocrinol Metab 62: 263, 1986

94. Cohen A, Markenson AL, Schwartz E: Transfusion requirements and splenectomy in thalassemia major. J Pediatr 97:100, 1980

95. Modell B: Total management of thalassemia major. Arch Dis Child 52:489, 1977

96. Singer DB: Postsplenectomy sepsis. Perspect Pediatr Pathol 1:285, 1973

97. Schulkind ML, Ellis EF, Smith RJ: Effect of antibody or clearance of I[125]-labeled pneumococci by the spleen and liver. Pediatr Res 1:178, 1967

98. Hosea SW, Burch CG, Brown EJ, Berg RA: Impaired immune response in splenectomized patients to polyvalent pneumococcal vaccine. Lancet 1:804, 1981

99. Schumacker MJ: Serum immunoglobulin and transferrin level after childhood splenectomy. Arch Dis Child 45:114, 1970

100. Baltimore R, Shedd DG, Pearson HA: Effect of iron saturation on the bacteriostasis of human serum. J Pediatr 101:519, 1982

101. Amman AJ, Addiego J, Wara DW et al: Polyvalent pneumococcal-polysaccharide immunization of patients with sickle cell anemia and patients with splenectomy. N Engl J Med 297:897, 1977

102. Gallant T, Freedman M, Vellend H et al: *Yersinia* sepsis in patients with iron overload treated with deferoxamine. N Engl J Med 314:1643, 1986

103. Gordts B, Rummens E, deMeirleir L et al: *Yersinia* pseudotuberculosis septicaemia in thalassaemia major. Lancet 1:41, 1984

104. Robins-Browne RM, Prpic JK: Desferrioxamine and systemic yersiniosis. Lancet 2:1372, 1983

105. Wolman IJ: Transfusion therapy in Cooley's anemia: growth and health as related to long range hemoglobin levels: a progress report. Ann NY Acad Sci 119:736, 1964

106. Kattamis C, Touliatis N, Chaidis S, Matsaniotis N: Growth of children with thalassemia and effect of different transfusion regimens. Arch Dis Child 45: 502, 1970

107. Piomelli S, Karpatkin MH, Arzanian M et al: Hypertransfusion regimen in patients with Cooley's anemia. Ann NY Acad Sci 232:186, 1974

108. Masera G, Terzoli S, Avanzini A et al: Evaluation of the supertransfusion regimen in homozygous beta-thalassaemia children. Br J Haematol 52:111, 1982

109. Gabutti V, Piga A, Nicola P et al: Haemoglobin levels and blood requirement in thalassemia. Arch Dis Child 57:156, 1982

110. Propper RD, Button LN, Nathan DG: New approaches to the transfusion management of thalassemia. Blood 55:55, 1980

111. Bracey AW, Klein HG, Chambers S et al: Ex vivo selective isolation of young red blood cells using the IBM-2991 cell washer. Blood 61:1068, 1983

112. Cohen AR, Schmidt JM, Martin MB et al: Clinical trial of young red cell transfusions. J Pediatr Res 104:865, 1984

113. Marcus RE, Wonke B, Bantock HM et al: A prospective trial of young red cells in 48 patients with transfusion-dependent thalassemia. Br J Haematol 60:153, 1985

114. Propper RD: Neocytes and neocyte-gerocyte exchange. Prog Clin Biol Res 88:227, 1982

115. Sirchia G, Zanella A, Parravicini A et al: Red cell alloantibodies in thalassemia major. Transfusion 25:110, 1985

116. DeFuria FG, Miller DR, Canale VC: Red blood cell metabolism and function in transfused β-thalassemia. Ann NY Acad Sci 232:323, 1974

117. Avanzi G, Bacigalupo A, Strada P et al: Frozen red blood cell transfusion in patients with Cooley's disease. Haematologica 68:646, 1983

118. Sirchia G, Rebulla P, Parravicini A et al: Leucocyte depletion of red cell units at the bedside by transfusion through a new filter. Transfusion 27:402, 1987

119. Coles SM, Klein HG, Holland PV: Alloimmunization in two multitransfused patient populations. Transfusion 21:462, 1981

120. Cividalli G, Sandler SG, Yatziv S et al: β[0]-thalassemia complicated by autoimmune hemolytic anemia. Acta Haematol 63:37, 1980

121. Constantopoulos A, Matsaniotis N: Hypertension, convulsion and cerebral hemorrhage in thalassemic patients after multiple blood transfusions. Helv Paediatr Acta 35:269, 1980

122. Matsaniotis N, Kattamis C, Laskari S et al: When should at-risk patients with thalassaemia be boosted with hepatitis B vaccine? Lancet 1:1321, 1987

123. Lefrere JJ, Girot R: HIV infection in polytransfused thalassaemic patients. Lancet 2:686, 1987
124. Hilgartner MW: AIDS in the transfused patient. Am J Dis Child 141:1984, 1987
125. Ohene-Frempong K, Rappaport E, Schwartz E: Thalassemia syndromes: recent advances. Hematol Oncol Clin North Am 1:503, 1987
126. Modell CB, Beck J: Long-term desferrioxamine therapy in thalassemia. Ann NY Acad Sci 323:201, 1974
127. Erlandson ME, Walden B, Stern G et al: Studies on congenital haemolytic syndromes. IV. Gastrointestinal absorption of iron. Blood 19:359, 1962
128. Keberle H: The biochemistry of desferrioxamine and its relation to iron metabolism. Ann NY Acad Sci 119:758, 1964
129. Barry M, Flynn DM, Letsky EA, Rison RA: Long-term chelation therapy in thalassemia major: effect on iron concentration, liver histology, and clinical progress. Br Med J 1:16, 1974
130. Seshadri R, Colebatch JH, Gordon P: Long-term administration of desferrioxamine in thalassemia major. Arch Dis Child 49:8, 1974
131. Propper RD, Cooper B, Rufo RR et al: Continuous subcutaneous administration of deferoxamine in patients with iron overload. N Engl J Med 297:418, 1977
132. Cohen A, Witzleben C, Schwartz E: Treatment of iron overload. Semin Liver Dis 4:228, 1984
133. Cohen A, Martin M, Schwartz E: Depletion of excessive liver iron stores with desferrioxamine. Br J Haematol 58:369, 1984
134. Cohen A, Mizanin J, Schwartz E: Rapid removal of excessive iron using daily high-dose chelation therapy through in-dwelling central venous catheters. J Pediatr 115:151, 1989
135. Cohen A, Mizanin J, Schwartz E: Treatment of iron overload in Cooley's anemia. Ann NY Acad Sci 445:274, 1985
136. Modell B, Berdoukas V: The Clinical Approach to Thalassaemia. Grune & Stratton, Orlando, FL, 1984
137. Propper RD, Shurin SB, Nathan DG: Reassessment of the use of desferrioxamine B in iron overload. N Engl J Med 294:1421, 1976
138. Fosburg MT, Nathan DG: Treatment of Cooley's anemia. Blood 76:435, 1990
139. Fargion S, Taddei MT, Gabulti V et al: Early iron overload in beta thalassemia major: when to start chelation therapy. Arch Dis Child 57:929, 1982
140. Weatherall DJ, Pippard MJ, Callender ST: Editorial retrospective: iron loading in thalassemia—5 years with the pump. N Engl J Med 308:456, 1983
141. Wolfe L, Olivieri N, Sallan D et al: Prevention of cardiac disease by subcutaneous deferoxamine in patients with thalassemia major. N Engl J Med 312:16, 1985
142. Olivieri NF, Berriman AM, Tyler BJ et al: Reduction in tissue iron stores with a new regimen of continuous ambulatory intravenous deferoxamine. Am J Hematol 41:61, 1992
143. Cohen A, Cohen IJ, Schwartz E: Scurvy and altered iron stores in thalassemia major. N Engl J Med 304:158, 1981
144. Wapnick AA, Lynch SR, Krawitz P et al: Effects of iron overload on ascorbic acid metabolism. Br Med J 3:704, 1968
145. Nienhuis AW: Safety of intensive chelation therapy. N Engl J Med 296:114, 1977
146. Olivieri N, Raymond-Buncic J, Chow E: Visual and auditory neurotoxicity in patients receiving subcutaneous deferoxamine infusions. N Engl J Med 314:869, 1986
147. Cohen A, Martin M, Mizanin J et al: Vision and hearing during deferoxamine therapy. J Pediatr 117:326, 1990
148. Peterson CM, Graziano JH, Grady RW et al: Chelation studies with 2,3-dihydrobenzoic acid in patients with β-thalassemia major. Br J Haematol 33:477, 1976
149. Kontoghiorghes GJ, Sheppard L: Simple synthesis of the potent iron chelators 1-alkyl-3-hydroxy-2-methylpyrid-4-ones. Inorg Chim Acta 136:111, 1987
150. Kontoghiorghes JG: Dose response studies using desferrioxamine and orally active chelators in a mouse model. Scand J Haematol 37:63, 1986
151. Kontoghiorghes GJ, Hoffbrand AV: Orally active α-ketohydroxypyridine iron chelators intended for clinical use: in vivo studies in rabbits. Br J Haematol 62:607, 1986
152. Kontoghiorghes GJ, Aldouri MA, Hoffbrand AV et al: Effective chelation of iron in β-thalassemia with the oral chelator 1,2-dimethyl-3-hydroxypyrid-4-one. Br J Med 295:1509, 1987
153. Brittenham GM: Development of iron-chelating agents for clinical use. Blood 80:569, 1992
154. Kontoghiorghes GJ, Bartlett AN, Hoffbrand AV et al: Long-term trial with the oral iron chelator 1,2-dimethyl-3-hydroxypyrid-4-one. I. Iron chelation and metabolic studies. Br J Haematol 76:295, 1990
155. Olivieri NF, Koren G, Matsui D et al: Reduction of tissue iron stores and normalization of serum ferritin during treatment with the oral iron chelator L1 in thalassemia intermedia. Blood 79:2741, 1992
156. Al-Refaie FN, Wonke B, Hoffbrand AV et al: Efficacy and possible adverse effects of the oral iron chelator 1,2-dimethyl-3-hydroxypyrid-4-one (L1) in thalassemia major. Blood 80:593, 1992
157. Bartlett AN, Hoffbrand AV, Kontoghiorghes GJ: Long-term trial with the oral iron chelator 1,2-dimethyl-3-hydroxypyrid-4-one. II. Clinical observations. Br J Haematol 76:301, 1990
158. Al-Refaie FN, Veys PA, Wilkes S et al: Agranulocytosis in a patient with thalassemia major during treatment with the oral iron chelator, 1,2-dimethyl-3-hydroxypyrid-4-one. Acta Haematol 89:86, 1993
159. Thomas ED, Buckner CD, Sanders JE et al: Bone marrow transplantation for thalassaemia. Lancet 2:227, 1982
160. Brochstein JA, Kirkpatrick D, Giardina PJ et al: Bone marrow transplantation in two multiply transfused patients with thalassemia major. Br J Haematol 63:445, 1986
161. Delfini C, Polchi P, Izzi T et al: Bone marrow donors other than HLA genotypically identical siblings for patients with thalassemia. Exp Hematol 13:1197, 1985
162. Lucarelli G, Polchi P, Galimberti M et al: Marrow transplantation for thalassaemia following busulphan and cyclophosphamide. Lancet 1:1355, 1985
163. Lucarelli G, Galimberti M, Polchi P et al: Marrow transplantation in patients with advanced thalassemia. N Engl J Med 316:1050, 1987
164. Shaw PJ, Poynton CH, Barrett AJ: Timing of bone-marrow transplantation in thalassemia major. Lancet 2:153, 1985
165. Lucarelli G, Galimberti M, Polchi P et al: Bone marrow transplantation in patients with thalassemia. N Engl J Med 322:417, 1990
166. Lucarelli G, Galimberti M, Polchi P et al: Bone marrow transplantation in adult thalassemia. Blood 80:1603, 1992
167. Lucarelli G, Galimberti M, Polchi P et al: Marrow transplantation in patients with thalassemia responsive to iron chelation therapy. N Engl J Med 329:840, 1993
168. Borgna-Pignatti C: Bone marrow transplantation for the hemoglobinopathies. p. 151. In Greleaven J, Barrett J (eds): Bone Marrow Transplantation in Practice. Churchill Livingstone, Edinburgh, 1992
169. Lucarelli G, Weatherall DJ: For debate: bone marrow transplantation for severe thalassaemia. (1) The view from Psaro. (2) To be or not to be. Br J Haematol 78:300, 1991
170. Weatherall DJ: Bone marrow transplantation for thalassemia and other inherited disorders of hemoglobin. Blood 80:1379, 1992
171. Weatherall DJ: The treatment of thalassemia—slow progress and new dilemmas. N Engl J Med 329:877, 1993
172. Giardina PJ, Hilgartner MW: Update on thalassemia. Pediatr Rev 13:55, 1992
173. Ley TJ, DeSimone J, Anagnou NP et al: 5-Azacytidine selectively increases γ-globin synthesis in a patient with β$^+$-thalassemia. N Engl J Med 307:1469, 1982
174. Ley TJ: The pharmacology of hemoglobin switching: of mice and men. Blood 77:1146, 1991
175. Kaufman RE: Hydroxyurea: specific therapy for sickle cell anemia? Blood 79:2503, 1992
176. Stamatoyannopoulos G, Veith R, Al-Khatti A, Papayannopoulou T: Induction of fetal hemoglobin by cell-cycle-specific drugs and recombinant erythropoietin. Am J Pediatr Hematol/Oncol 12:21, 1990
177. Veith R, Galanello R, Papayannopoulou T et al: Stimulation of F-cell production in patients with sickle cell anemia treated with cytarabine or hydroxyurea. N Engl J Med 313:1571, 1985
178. Rodgers GP, Dover GJ, Noguchi CT et al: Hematologic responses of patients with sickle cell disease to treatment with hydroxyurea. N Engl J Med 322:1037, 1990
179. Charache S, Dover GJ, Moore RD et al: Hydroxyurea: effects on hemoglobin F production in patients with sickle cell anemia. Blood 79:2555, 1992
180. Lowrey CH, Nienhuis AW: Treatment with azacitidine of patients with end-stage β-thalassemia. N Engl J Med 329:845, 1993
181. Rodgers GP, Dover GJ, Uyesaka N et al: Augmentation by erythropoietin of the fetal-hemoglobin response to hydroxyurea in sickle cell disease. N Engl J Med 328:73, 1993
182. Rachmilewitz EA, Goldfarb A, Dover G: Administration of erythropoietin to patients with β-thalassemia intermedia: a preliminary trial. Blood 78:1145, 1991
183. Bunn HF: Reversing ontogeny. N Engl J Med 328:129, 1993
184. Perrine SP, Ginder GD, Faller DV et al: A short-term trial of butyrate to stimulate fetal-globin gene expression in the β-globin disorders. N Engl J Med 328:81, 1993
185. Dover GJ, Brusilow S, Samid D: Increased fetal hemoglobin in patients receiving sodium 4-phenylbutyrate. N Engl J Med 327:569, 1992
186. Blau AC, Constantoulakis P, Shaw CM, Stamatoyannopoulos G: Fetal hemoglobin induction with butyric acid: efficacy and toxicity. Blood 81:529, 1993
187. Mulligan RCP: The basic science of gene therapy. Science 260:926, 1993
188. Forget BG: Gene therapy. In Embury SE, Hebbel RP, Narla M, Steinberg MH

(eds): The Sickle Hemoglobinopathies: Science and Medicine. Raven, New York, 1994 (in press)

189. Friedman S, Hamilton RW, Schwartz E: β-Thalassemia in the American Negro. J Clin Invest 52:1453, 1973

190. Tamagnini GP, Lopes MC, Castanheira ME et al: β⁺-Thalassaemia-Portuguese type: clinical haematological and molecular studies of a newly defined form of β-thalassaemia. Br J Haematol 54:189, 1983

191. Aksoy M, Bermek E, Almis G et al: β-Thalassemia intermedia homozygous for normal hemoglobin A₂β-thalassemia. Study in four families. Acta Haematol 67:57, 1982

192. Schwartz E: The silent carrier of β-thalassemia. N Engl J Med 281:1327, 1969

193. Newton KL, McNeeley G, Novick M: Extramedullary hematopoiesis presenting as a pelvic mass in a patient with β-thalassemia intermedia. JAMA 205: 2178, 1983

194. Sbyrakis S, Karagiorga-Lagana M, Voskaki I et al: A simple index for initiating transfusion treatment in thalassaemia intermedia. Br J Haematol 67:479, 1987

195. Pippard MJ, Callender ST, Warner GT, Weatherall DJ: Iron absorption and loading in beta thalassemia intermedia. Lancet 2:819, 1979

196. de Alarcon D, Donovan ME, Forbes GB et al: Iron absorption in the thalassemia syndromes and its inhibition by tea. N Engl J Med 300:5, 1979

197. Cossu P, Toccafondi D, Vardau F et al: Iron overload and desferioxamine chelation therapy in beta thalassemia intermedia. Eur J Pediatr 137:267, 1981

198. Jurkiewicz MJ, Pearson HA, Furlow LY: Reconstruction of the maxilla in thalassemia. Ann NY Acad Sci 165:437, 1969

199. Camaschella C, Bertero MJ, Serra A et al: A benign form of thalassemia may be determined by the interaction of triplicated α locus and heterozygous β-thalassemia. Br J Haematol 66:103, 1987

200. Kulozik AE, Thein SL, Wainscoat JS et al: Thalassaemia intermedia: interaction of the triple α-globin gene arrangement and heterozygous β-thalassaemia. Br J Haematol 66:109, 1987

201. Berman BW, Ritchey AK, Jeckel JF et al: Hematology of beta thalassemia trait: age related developmental aspects and intrafamilial correlations. J Pediatr 97:901, 1980

202. Metaxatou-Mavromati AD, Antonopoulou HK, Laskani SS et al: Developmental changes in Hb F levels during the first two years of life in normal and heterozygous beta thalassemia infants. Pediatrics 69:734, 1982

203. Wood WG, Weatherall DJ, Hart GM et al: Hematologic changes and hemoglobin analysis of beta thalassemia heterozygotes during the first year of life. Pediatr Res 16:286, 1982

204. Silvestroni E, Bianco I: A highly cost effective method of mass screening for thalassemia. Br Med J 286:1007, 1983

205. Pippard MJ, Wainscoat JS: Erythrokinetics and iron status in heterozygous β-thalassemia and the effect of interaction with α-thalassemia. Br J Haematol 66:123, 1987

206. Hedge UM, Klumda S, Marsh GW et al: Thalassemia, iron and pregnancy. Br Med J 13:509, 1975

207. Schuman JB, Taiser CL, Peloquin R et al: The erythropoietic response to pregnancy in β thalassemia minor. Br J Haematol 25:249, 1973

208. Borgna-Pignatti C, Zonta L, Bongo I et al: Red blood cell indices in adults and children with heterozygous beta-thalassemia. Haematologica 68:149, 1983

209. Weatherall DJ: Biochemical phenotypes of thalassemia in the American Negro population. Ann NY Acad Sci 119:450, 1964

210. Wasi P, Disthasongchan P, Na-Nakorn S: The effect of iron deficiency on the levels of hemoglobins A₂ and E. J Lab Clin Med 71:85, 1968

211. Saiki RK, Chang CA, Levenson CH et al: Diagnosis of sickle cell anemia and β-thalassemia with enzymatically amplified DNA and nonradioactive allele-specific oligonucleotide probes. N Engl J Med 319:537, 1988

212. Cao A, Rosatelli MC, Leoni GB et al: Antenatal diagnosis of β-thalassemia in Sardinia. Ann NY Acad Sci 612:215, 1990

213. Loukopoulos D, Hadji A, Papadakis M et al: Prenatal diagnosis of thalassemia and of the sickle cell syndromes in Greece. Ann NY Acad Sci 612:226, 1990

214. Pearson HA, O'Brien RT, McIntosh S: Screening for thalassemia trait by electronic measurements of mean corpuscular volume. N Engl J Med 288: 351, 1973

215. Mentzer WG Jr: Differentiation of iron deficiency from thalassemia trait. Lancet 1:882, 1973

216. Higgs DR, Vickers MA, Wilkie AOM et al: A review of the molecular genetics of the human α-globin gene cluster. Blood 73:1081, 1989

217. Higgs DR: α-Thalassemia. Balliere's Clin Hemat 6:117, 1993

218. Liebhaber SA, Kan YW: α-Thalassemia caused by an unstable α-globin mutant. J Clin Invest 71:461, 1983

219. Dozy AM, Kan YW, Embury SH: α-Globin gene organization in blacks precludes the severe form of α-thalassemia. Nature 280:605, 1979

220. Schwartz E, Atwater J: Alpha thalassemia in the American Negro. J Clin Invest 51:412, 1972

221. Wickramasinghe SN, Hughes M, Fucharoen S et al: The fate of excess β-globin chains within erythropoietic cells in α-thalassaemia 2 trait, α-thalassaemia 1 trait, haemoglobin H disease and haemoglobin Q-H disease: an electron microscope study. Br J Haematol 56:473, 1984

222. Bowden DK, Hill AVS, Higgs DR et al: Different hematologic phenotypes are associated with the leftward (−α⁴·²) and rightward (−α³·⁷), α⁺-thalassemia deletions. J Clin Invest 79:39, 1987

223. Liebhaber SA, Kan YW: Differentiation of the mRNA transcripts originating from the α₁- and α₂-globin loci in normals and α-thalassemia. J Clin Invest 68:439, 1981

224. Orkin SH, Goff SC: The duplicated human α-globin genes: their relative expression as measured by RNA analysis. Cell 24:345, 1981

225. Weatherall DJ: The genetics of the thalassemias. Br Med Bull 25:24, 1969

226. Liebhaber SA, Cash FE, Cornfield DB: Evidence for post-translational control of Hb C synthesis in an individual with Hb C trait and α-thalassemia. Blood 71:502, 1988

227. Koler RD, Rigas DA: Genetics of haemoglobin H. Ann Hum Genet 25:95, 1961

228. O'Brien RT: The effect of iron deficiency on the expression of hemoglobin H. Blood 41:853, 1973

229. Weatherall DJ, Clegg JB, Wong HB: The haemoglobin constitution of infants with the haemoglobin Bart's hydrops foetalis syndrome. Br J Haematol 18: 357, 1970

230. Dozy AM, Kan YW, Forman EN et al: Antenatal diagnosis of homozygous α-thalassemia. JAMA 241:1610, 1979

231. Bowden DK, Vickers MA, Higgs DR: A PCR-based strategy to detect the common severe determinants of α-thalassaemia. Br J Haematol 81:104, 1992

232. Beaudry MA, Ferguson DJ, Pearse K et al: Survival of a hydropic infant with homozygous α-thalassaemia-1. J Pediatr 108:713, 1986

233. Bianchi DW, Beyer EC, Stark AR et al: Normal long-term survival with α-thalassemia. J Pediatr 108:716, 1986

234. Li CK, Chan HB, Chiu WK, Chow CB: Survival of an infant with homozygous α-thalassemia, abstracted. Pediat Res 27:266A, 1990

235. Humphries RK, Ley T, Turner P et al: Differences in human α-, β-, and δ-globin gene expression in monkey kidney cells. Cell 30:173, 1982

236. Ojwang PJ, Nakatsuji T, Gardiner MB et al: Gene deletion as the molecular basis for the Kenya-Gγ-HPFH condition. Hemoglobin 7:115, 1983

237. Fairbanks VF, Oliveros R, Brandabur JH et al: Homozygous hemoglobin E mimics β-thalassemia minor without anemia or hemolysis: hematologic, functional, and biosynthetic studies of first North American cases. Am J Hematol 8:109, 1980

238. Orkin SH, Kazazian HH Jr, Antonarakis SE et al: Abnormal RNA processing due to the exon mutations of βᴱ-globin gene. Nature 300:768, 1982

239. Milner PF, Clegg JB, Weatherall DJ: Haemoglobin H disease due to a unique haemoglobin variant with elongated α-chain. Lancet 1:729, 1971

240. Kan JW, Todd D, Dozy AM: Haemoglobin Constant Spring synthesis in red cell precursors. Br J Haematol 28:103, 1974

241. Weatherall DJ, Clegg JB: The α-chain termination mutants and their relation to the α-thalassemias. Philos Trans R Soc Lond Biol 271:411, 1975

242. Adams JG III, Boxer LA, Baehner RL et al: Hemoglobin Indianapolis (β 112 [G14] arginine): an unstable β-chain variant producing the phenotype of severe β-thalassemia. J Clin Invest 63:931, 1979

243. Coleman MB, Steinberg MH, Adams JG III: Hemoglobin Terre Haute arginine β¹⁰⁶: a posthumous correction to the original structure of hemoglobin Indianapolis. J Biol Chem 266:5798, 1991

244. Bollekens JA, Forget BG: δβ-Thalassemia and hereditary persistence of fetal hemoglobin. Hematol Oncol Clin North Am 5:399, 1991

245. Miyoshi K, Kaneto Y, Kawai H et al: X-Linked dominant control of F-cells in normal adult life: characterization of the Swiss type as hereditary persistence of fetal hemoglobin regulated by gene(s) on X chromosome. Blood 72:1854, 1988

246. Dover GJ, Smith KD, Chang YE et al: Fetal hemoglobin levels in sickle cell disease and normal individuals are partially controlled by an X-linked gene located at Xp22.2. Blood 80:816, 1992

247. Schwartz E, Benz EJ Jr: Thalassemia syndromes. p. 428. In Miller DR, Baehner RL (eds): Smith's Blood Diseases of Infancy and Childhood. 6th Ed. CV Mosby, St. Louis, 1989

248. Pearson HA, Benz EJ Jr: Thalassemia syndromes. p. 439. In Miller DR, Baehner RL, McMillan CW (eds): Smith's Blood Diseases of Infancy and Childhood. 5th Ed. CV Mosby, St. Louis, 1984

249. Takeshita K, Forget BG, Scarpa A, Benz EJ Jr: Intranuclear defects in β-globin mRNA accumulation due to a premature translation termination codon. Blood 64:13, 1984

250. High KA, Benz EJ Jr: The ABCs of molecular genetics: a haematologist's introduction. p. 25. In Hoffbrand AV (ed): Recent Advances in Haematology. Churchill Livingstone, New York, 1985

Sickle Cell Disease

43

Stephen H. Embury

INTRODUCTION

Sickle cell disease is an inherited multisystem disorder. Its cardinal features, chronic hemolytic anemia and recurrent painful episodes, relate to the presence of mutant sickle cell hemoglobin (Hb S) within red blood cells. The illness affects most organ systems and the psychosocial adjustment of those affected. Owing to the complexity of the illness, a comprehensive, combined-modality approach offers the best method of management.[1,2] The further exigency of living with a chronic, painful, life-threatening disease in an ethnically complex society provides additional challenges to the psychosocial aspects of this illness.[3] Traditional concepts of sickle cell pathophysiology ascribe all features of disease to sequential effects of the A→T nucleotide substitution in the sixth codon of the β-globin gene, substitution of valine for glutamic acid on the outer surface of the Hb S molecule, reduced solubility and polymerization of Hb S when deoxygenated, sickling and poor deformability of polymer-containing erythrocytes, and occlusion by sickle red cells of the microvasculature[1,2,4–9] (Fig. 43-1). While polymerization remains the sine qua non of sickle cell disease,[6,7] a contemporary understanding of pathophysiology requires an integrated perspective derived from physical chemistry, molecular and cellular biology, biochemistry, coagulation, and genetics.[8–12]

The syndromes (and genotypes) that comprise sickle cell disease are mainly sickle cell anemia (Hb SS), sickle cell-β°-thalassemia (Hb S-β°-thal), Hb SC disease (Hb SC), and sickle cell-β⁺-thalassemia (Hb S-β⁺-thal). Sickle cell trait (Hb AS) is not associated with either anemia or recurrent pain. This chapter presents the history, epidemiology, genetics, pathophysiology, clinical manifestations, laboratory diagnosis, and treatment of the sickle cell syndromes. Normal hemoglobin synthesis, structure, and function are described in Chapter 35; the thalassemias are considered in Chapter 42; and the properties of Hb S are presented in Chapter 44.

BACKGROUND

The chronicle of sickle cell anemia began in 1910 with a report by James Herrick[13] of Chicago on the clinical manifestations and sickled appearance of the red blood cells of a student with recurrent pain and anemia[14] (Fig. 43-2). Disease manifestations had been recognized long before in Africa, where different tribes had bestowed on the malady various onomatopoetic appellations that evoked the basic nature of recurrent pain.[15] The importance of deoxygenation of sickle red cells was first appreciated in 1927 when Hahn and Gillespie[16] demonstrated that oxygen deprivation induced a sickle-like deformation that was both enhanced by acidic pH and reversible on reoxygenation. Later studies showed that the bulk viscosity of sickle cell suspensions rose dramatically and reversibly on deoxygenation.[17] Evidence that the unique pathologic properties of sickle red cells were due to an abnormal hemoglobin was provided in 1940 by Sherman,[18] who discovered that sickle but not normal erythrocytes exhibited optical birefringence when deoxygenated. The same year, Ham and Castle[19] proposed the celebrated "vicious cycle of erythrostasis" hypothesis—a logical synthesis of the combined knowledge regarding the interactions of deoxygenation, acidic pH, and viscosity of sickle cells. The abnormality of hemoglobin was confirmed in 1949 when Pauling and colleagues[20] reported the different electrophoretic mobilities of Hb S and normal adult hemoglobin (Hb A). In 1950 the importance of Hb S to the pathobiology of sickle red cells was established by Harris' description of reversible sol-gel transformation of deoxygenated Hb S solutions[21] and by Perutz and Mitchison's report[22] of the insolubility of deoxygenated Hb S solutions. Unification of the electrophoretic and solubility abnormalities of Hb S was provided by a series of experiments published between 1956 and 1958 in which Ingram[23–25] identified the substitution of valine for glutamic acid as the sixth amino acid of the β-globin chain. While the polymerization-sickling doctrine had come full circle, the earlier observation by Diggs and Bibb[26] of a population of irreversibly sickled cells (ISCs) that would not revert to discocytes with reoxygenation forewarned that sickle cell pathophysiology was too complex to be explained by polymerization alone.

GENETICS, EVOLUTION, MALARIA, AND G6PD DEFICIENCY

Genetics

The first evidence that sickle cell anemia is inherited derived from the finding by Huck[27] that red blood cells from unaffected parents and relatives could be made to sickle, a phenomenon that led Sydenstricker and colleagues[28] to propose "active" and "latent" varieties of sickle cell disease. In 1949, the conclusion that sickle cell anemia results from homozygous inheritance of a genetic determinant from heterozygous parents was reached independently by Beet,[29] Neel,[30] and Pauling and colleagues,[20] who found that patients with sickle cell anemia have all Hb S, but their parents have both Hb S and Hb A. Before these reports, Silvestroni and Bianco[31] had described a variety of sickle cell disease with small sickle cells, now known as sickle cell-β-thalassemia, which was inherited from one parent carrying the sickling disorder and another with constitutional microcytic anemia. This was the first evidence that the sickle cell and β-thalassemia genes are alleles.

Near the β-globin gene on chromosome 11 are restriction fragment length polymorphisms[32] distinct constellations of which define β-globin haplotypes having specific ethnogeographic origins.[33] The association of the sickle cell gene with different haplotypes constitutes evidence that the sickle cell mutation has arisen at least five times throughout the course of evolution, four times within Africa—the Senegal, Benin, Bantu, and Cameroon haplotypes—and once without—the Arab-Indian haplotype[34] (Fig. 43-3A). Despite rigorous scrutiny,[34,35] no evidence has been obtained to suggest that haplotypes have provided selective evolutionary pressures on the sickle cell gene.[34]

Malaria Hypothesis

The gene for sickle cell hemoglobin has persisted despite its devastating clinical effects in homozygotes because of "heterozygous advantage." In any population, the much greater number of individuals heterozygous for a particular gene compared

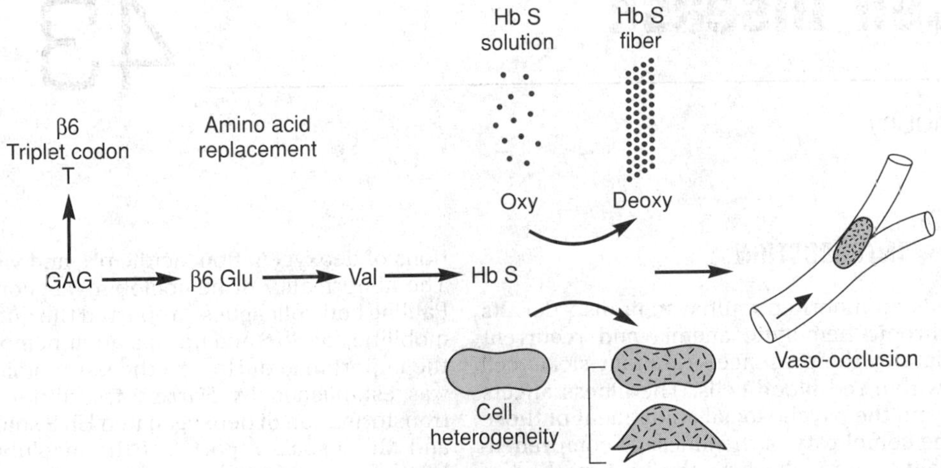

Fig. 43-1. Schematic view of the pathophysiology of sickle cell disease. The GAG→GTG mutation in the sixth codon of the β-globin gene results in the substitution of valine for glutamic acid as the sixth amino acid of β-globin. The presence of mutant β^S chains in the tetramer creates the variant Hb S. The insolubility of deoxygenated Hb S results in its polymerization and in both the loss of deformability and sickling of deoxygenated sickle erythrocytes. Vessels become occluded as a result of several processes, including the poor deformability of polymer-containing sickle cells. (Modified from Bunn and Forget,[5] with permission.)

with those homozygous creates a positive evolutionary pressure, provided the heterozygous condition offers some selective advantage. Allison[36] found that the stable frequency of the sickle cell gene existing in areas of hyperendemic falciparum malaria was the result a balance between gene exclusion from the premature death of homozygotes and gene selection from the resistance of heterozygotes against death from malaria, thereby defining the concept of genetic polymorphism. Children with sickle cell trait have lower rates of parasitemia and cerebral malaria.[37] In Africa, selection of the sickle cell gene relates to the introduction 2,000 years ago of slash-and-burn agriculture. This destroyed the root structure of tropical jungles that had drained standing water and introduced sunlight into these previously shadowy areas, provided a breeding ground for the mosquito vector *Anopheles gambiae*.[38,39] As a result of its selective advantage against death from malaria, the worldwide distribution of the sickle cell gene parallels that

of falciparum malaria, its highest frequencies occurring in the "malaria belt"[40] (Fig. 43-3B).

The mechanism by which the sickle cell gene protects against malaria is not understood.[34,38] Although rigid sickle cell trait red cells may repel parasitic invasion,[41] the equal rates of infection of sickle cell trait and nonsickle red cells[42] suggests that the inhospitable nature of the sickle cell trait erythrocyte is manifest at some later stage.[43] Consistent with this hypothesis is the retarded parasite replication in sickle cell trait red cells at low oxygen tension.[44] Other disruptive influences on the symbiosis of malarial parasite in sickle trait red cell include the more rapid sickling and removal from the circulation of parasitized sickle cell trait erythrocytes (related to intracellular oxygen consumption by parasites[45]); reduced intraerythrocytic pH levels[46]; oxidation of parasite and red cells as a consequence of iron released from denatured sickle cell hemoglobin[47]; cellular potassium loss that inhibits parasite growth[46]; poor nutrition provided parasites by Hb S[48]; and physical disruption of parasite membranes by Hb S polymer.[49] Notions regarding the mechanisms of protection against malaria must be interpreted within the context of evidence showing that protection from severe malaria is related to the common West African HLA class I antigen HLA-Bw53,[50] which provides the ability to present liver-stage-specific malarial antigens to cytotoxic T cells as part of the immune response.[51]

G6PD Deficiency

The influence of glucose-6-phosphate dehydrogenase (G6PD) deficiency, another common African polymorphism, on the epidemiology, expression, and frequency of the sickle cell gene has been a matter of debate. G6PD deficiency was reported to have greater frequency among patients with sickle cell disease.[52] More recent reports have emphasized that the detection of G6PD deficiency is easily confounded by the young age of circulating sickle erythrocytes and have not confirmed a higher frequency of the mutant G6PD gene.[53,54] Neither greater hemolysis nor more frequent pain were found among male subjects having both sickle cell disease and G6PD deficiency.[55]

Prevalence

The clinical challenge posed by sickle cell disease is inherent in the distribution and frequency of the sickle cell gene, as influenced by evolutionary pressures[34] and transmission via

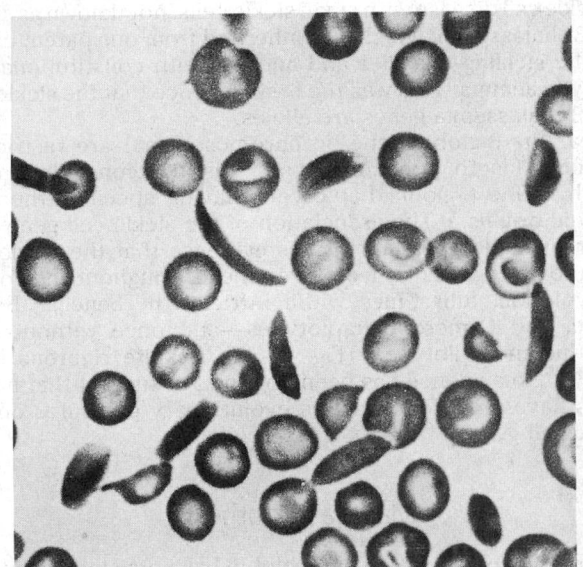

Fig. 43-2. Peripheral blood smear showing the "peculiar elongated forms of the red corpuscles." (From van Assendelft,[571] with permission.)

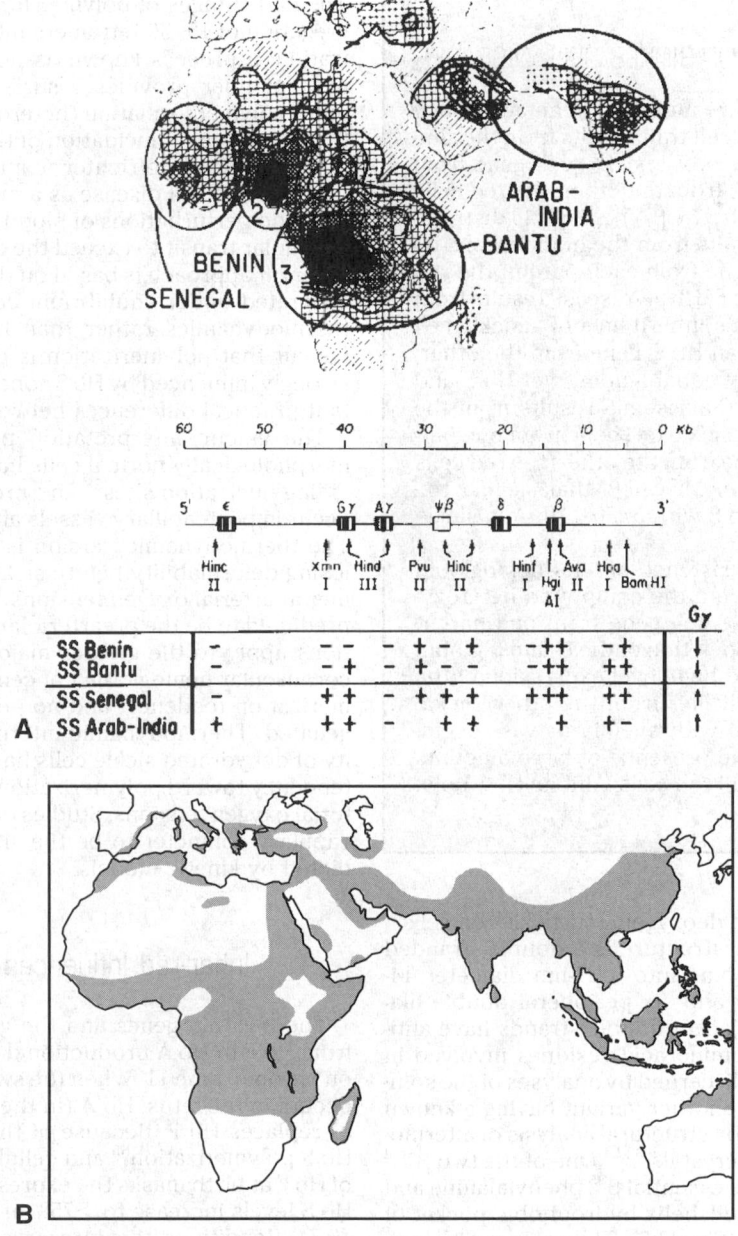

Fig. 43-3. (A) Origins of the sickle cell gene mutations. **(Above)** World map showing the incidence of Hb S in the African continent with the approximate locations where the sickle cell mutations occurred independently—Benin, Senegal, Bantu, and Arab-Indian. **(Middle)** β-Globin gene cluster with polymorphic restriction sites identified by arrows. **(Below)** Restriction fragment length polymorphism combinations that dictate the four major haplotypes. (Adapted from Nagel and Fleming,[34] with permission.) **(B)** Distribution of falciparum malaria in the Old World approximately 150 years ago. (From Boyd,[572] with permission.)

trade routes and slave trade.[56] While the prevalence of sickle cell trait is 8–10% among African-American newborns,[57] its prevalence is as high as 25–30% in western Africa.[58] Calculations based on the frequency among African-Americans of the sickle cell (0.045), Hb C (0.015), and β-thalassemia (0.004) genes[57] suggest that in the United States, 4,000–5,000 pregnancies a year are at risk of sickle cell disease.[59] This figure gains perspective from the estimate that in Africa 120,000 babies are born every year with sickle cell disease.[58]

PATHOPHYSIOLOGY

The striking influence of deoxygenation on Hb S polymerization, cellular sickling, and blood viscosity enunciates the pathophysiology of sickle cell disease—each of the manifestations

of sickle cell disease is ultimately attributable to Hb S polymerization.[6,7] Despite the apparent sufficiency of this interpretation, a more complete appreciation of the several processes involved in sickle cell pathophysiology provides a more thorough understanding.[1,2,4,5,8,9]

Hb S Polymer

Oxygenated Hb S is as soluble as Hb A. The increased surface hydrophobicity of Hb S tetramers, resulting from valine rather than glutamic acid as the sixth amino acid of the β^s chain, results in decreased solubility of the deoxygenated molecule.[60] Intermolecular bonding of deoxy-Hb S tetramers forms polymer filaments that associate into bundles, which can be identified

INHERITANCE PATTERN OF SICKLE CELL DISEASES

The sickle cell diseases are inherited in an autosomal codominant manner. Sickle cell trait results from the simple heterozygous inheritance of a sickle cell gene from one parent and a Hb A gene from the other; the red cells contain Hb A ($\alpha_2\beta^A_2$) and Hb S ($\alpha_2\beta^S_2$) in a 60:40 distribution. Sickle cell anemia results from the homozygous inheritance of a sickle cell gene from each parent; the red cells contain virtually all Hb S. Hb SC disease results from the compound heterozygous inheritance of a sickle cell gene from one parent and an Hb C gene from the other; the red cells contain nearly equal amounts of Hb S and Hb C ($\alpha_2\beta^C_2$). Sickle cell-β-thalassemia results from the compound inheritance of a sickle cell gene from one parent and a β-thalassemic gene from the other; the red cells contain virtually all Hb S in sickle cell-β°-thalassemia; the red cells contain mostly Hb S with 5–30% Hb A in sickle cell β^+-thalassemia.

Sickle cell-hereditary persistence of fetal hemoglobin (sickle cell-HPFH) results from the compound heterozygous inheritance of a sickle cell gene from one parent and an HPFH "gene" (i.e., a deletion of the δ- and β-globin genes that allows continued high level expression of the fetal γ-globin genes in adult life) from the other. Sickle cell-HPFH is not associated with anemia or vaso-occlusive symptoms, because the presence of large amounts (25–35%) of Hb F ($\alpha_2\gamma_2$) in all red cells inhibits Hb S polymerization.

by electron microscopy within deoxygenated sickle red cells[61] (Fig. 43-4). The basic polymer structure is a double-stranded filament. Seven of these combine into a 21-nm diameter 14-strand fiber having one inner and six peripheral double filaments organized such that adjacent double strands have antiparallel orientation.[61,62] The amino acid residues involved in intermolecular bonding were discerned by analyses of the solubility of mixtures of Hb S and another variant having a known amino acid substitution[63] and by structural analysis of intermolecular contact points in Hb S crystals.[62,64] One of the two β^{6val} forms a lateral contact with the essential β^{85} phenylalanine and β^{88} leucine residues within the F-helix hydrophobic pocket of an adjacent Hb S tetramer[62,64] (Fig. 43-5). The second β^{6val} residue does not participate in intermolecular bonding. This fact is relevant to considerations of the degree to which $\alpha_2\beta^s\gamma$ mixed tetramers participate in polymerization when both Hb S and fetal hemoglobin (Hb F) are present.[65] Intermolecular bonds form axial and lateral contacts within the double filament and lateral contacts between double filaments.[62,64,66] Critical residues include additional lateral contacts—$\beta6$, $\beta73$, $\beta66$, $\beta83$, $\beta87$; axial contacts—$\beta121$, $\beta16$, $\beta17$, $\beta19$, $\beta22$, $\alpha16$, $\alpha116$; and interpair contacts—$\alpha54$, $\alpha47$, $\alpha75$, $\alpha78$, $\alpha6$, $\alpha11$, $\alpha68$.

Polymerization

The solubility of deoxy-Hb S is approximately 17 g/dl, a level far below the intraerythrocytic concentration of hemoglobin of approximately 34 g/dl; deoxygenation results in supersaturation of deoxy-Hb S solutions, aggregation, and polymer formation.[60] Studies of the polymerization process rely on separation of the two-phases of deoxy-Hb S solutions—sol and gel. The delay time to polymer formation is inversely proportional of the deoxy-Hb S concentration with 15th–30th-order kinetics.

The early stages of polymer formation most likely involve aggregation of 15–30 tetramers into a single nucleus of polymerization, a process known as homogeneous nucleation.[60] The nascent fiber provides a surface that constitutes nuclei for more polymer formation (heterogeneous nucleation)[67] (Fig. 43-6). In an elegant elucidation of the kinetics of Hb S polymerization, Eaton and Hofrichter[6] explained the entire pathophysiology of sickle cell disease as a function of polymerization, sickling, and perturbations of blood flow that prolong the duration of cellular transit to exceed the delay time to polymerization. A different approach is based on the maximal amount of polymer generated under equilibrium conditions, a system driven by thermodynamics rather than kinetics.[7] Both interpretations concur that polymerization is detrimental to sickle cells and strongly influenced by Hb S concentration, but there are important practical differences between the two.

The kinetic interpretation presupposes that oxygenated, morphologically normal cells have no persistent polymer providing nucleation sites[68] and predicts that vaso-occlusion will occur in postcapillary vessels after a delay time for nucleation. The thermodynamic version is based on deoxygenated cells losing deformability before sickling[69] and persistence of polymer at arterial oxygen tensions.[70] The site of vaso-occlusion is predicted to be the prearteriolar sphincter.[7] Kinetic considerations apply to the greater majority of cells with lower mean corpuscular hemoglobin concentration (MCHC), a lesser polymerization tendency, and no persistent polymer when reoxygenated. Thermodynamic interpretations describe the minority of dehydrated sickle cells having very high MCHC, a strong tendency toward polymerization, and persistent polymer at arterial oxygen tensions. Studies of flow ex vivo showed the postcapillary sphincter to be the site of vaso-occlusion,[71] as predicted by kinetic models.

Inherited Influences on Polymerization

The β-globin genes and the genes that regulate the switch from Hb F to Hb A production during development are located on chromosome 11. When the switch from γ- to β-globin chains occurs in the fetus, Hb A (in the case of sickle cell anemia, Hb S) replaces Hb F. Because of the inhibitory effect of Hb F on Hb S polymerization[65] and cellular sickling,[72] the high fraction of Hb F at birth masks the expression of sickle cell disease until Hb S levels increase to >75% at about 6 months of age[2,5] (Fig. 43-7). Conditions that preserve elevated levels of Hb F into adulthood modulate the course of sickle cell disease.[73] The compound heterozygous conditions, sickle-hereditary persistence of Hb F (Hb S-HPFH) and sickle cell-β-thalassemia, both have higher Hb F levels and milder clinical courses than are characteristic of sickle cell anemia.[5,74] Additional mitigating influences in sickle cell-β-thalassemia are elevated levels of Hb A_2[6] and, in sickle cell-β^+-thalassemia, levels of Hb A of ≤30%, both of which affect the solubility and polymerization of Hb S.

Hb F is a more active inhibitor of polymerization than Hb A. Hb S solutions with 15–30% Hb A (resembling sickle cell-β^+-thalassemia) have delay times 10–100 times longer than pure Hb S solutions; Hb S solutions with 20–30% Hb F (resembling Hb S-HPFH) have delay times 1,000–1,000,000 times longer.[75,76] The greater activity of Hb F than Hb A in increasing Hb S solubility is related to an important molecular difference—Hb A is excluded, but $\alpha_2\beta^A\gamma$ hybrid tetramers are included in Hb S polymer, while both Hb F and $\alpha_2\beta^s\gamma$ hybrid tetramers are excluded.[65,77,78] Hematologic values for sickle cell anemia, the sickle cell-β-thalassemias, and Hb S-HPFH are found in Table 43-1.

α-Thalassemia also modulates the clinical expression of sickle cell disease in part by reducing the MCHC.[79] Prevalences

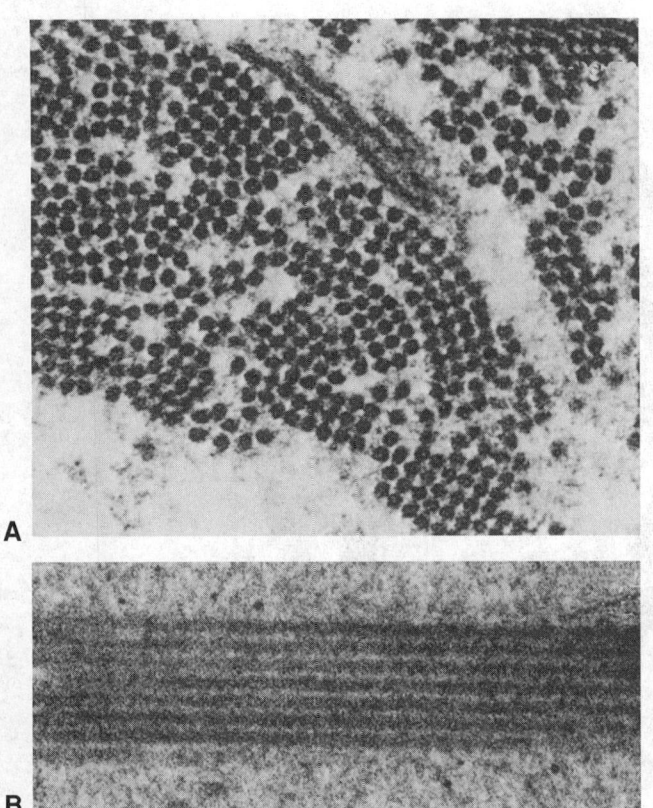

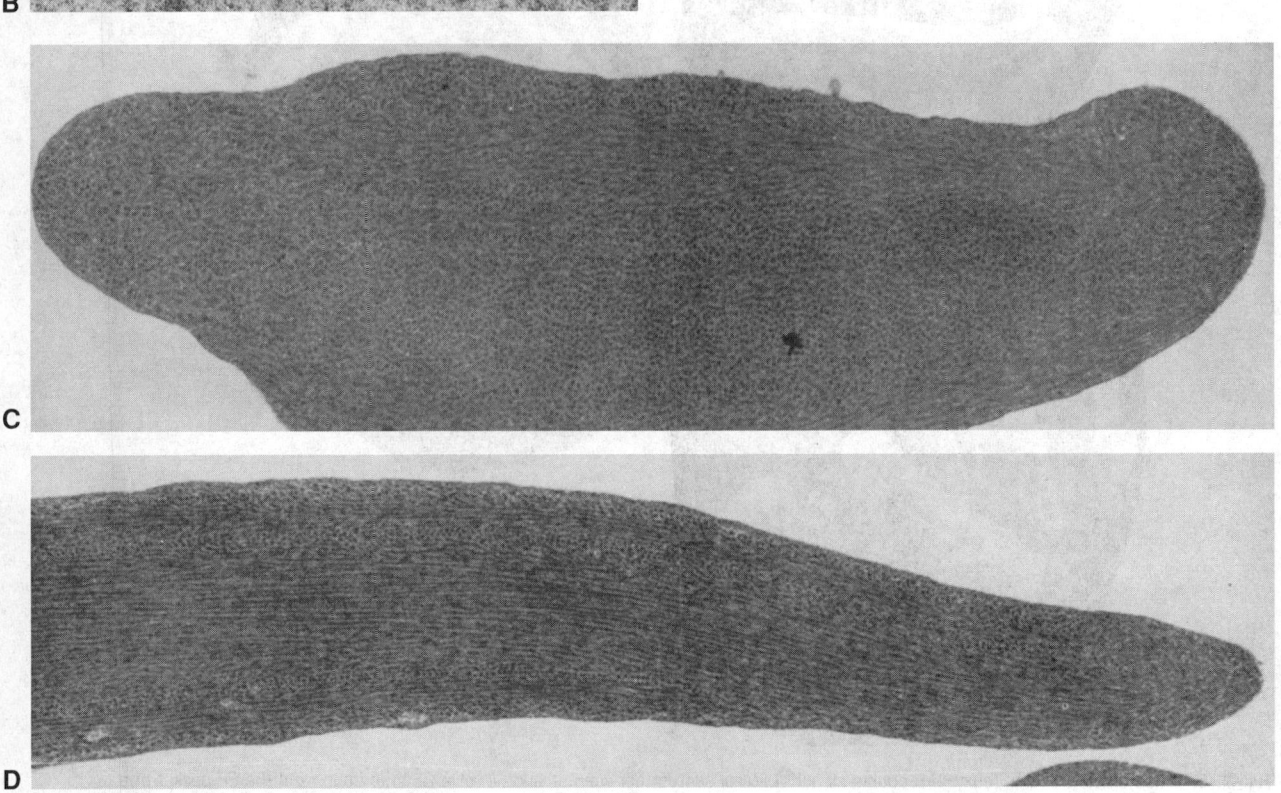

Fig. 43-4. (A & B) Electron micrographs of a centrifuge pellet of deoxyHb S. (× 325,000.) **(A)** Transfer section showing bundles of Hb S fibers. **(B)** Longitudinal section showing aligned fibers. (From Finch et al.[554] with permission.) **(C & D)** Electron micrograph of deoxygenated SS erythrocyte. **(C)** Cross section. **(D)** Longitudinal section. (From Bertles and Döbler,[573] with permission.)

of the silent carrier of α-thalassemia syndrome (genotype–α/ αα) and α-thalassemia trait (genotype–α/–α) among African-Americans are approximately 30% and 2%, respectively.[80] The lower intraerythrocytic concentrations of Hb S associated with α-thalassemia modulate the hematologic, pathophysiologic, and clinical manifestations of disease,[79,81–86] particularly the severity of anemia, which is diminished after the age of 7 years with either the–α/αα or the–α/–α genotype[87,88] (Table 43-2).

Cellular Sickling

Sickled-appearing red cells are rigid, as demonstrated by the dramatic increase in bulk viscosity of sickle cell suspensions on deoxygenation.[17] Within 0.5 seconds, these cells accumulate Hb S aggregates and lose deformability despite having normal morphology; by 3 seconds, the biconcave discs contain short linear polymer; by 15 seconds, the discs acquire protuberances

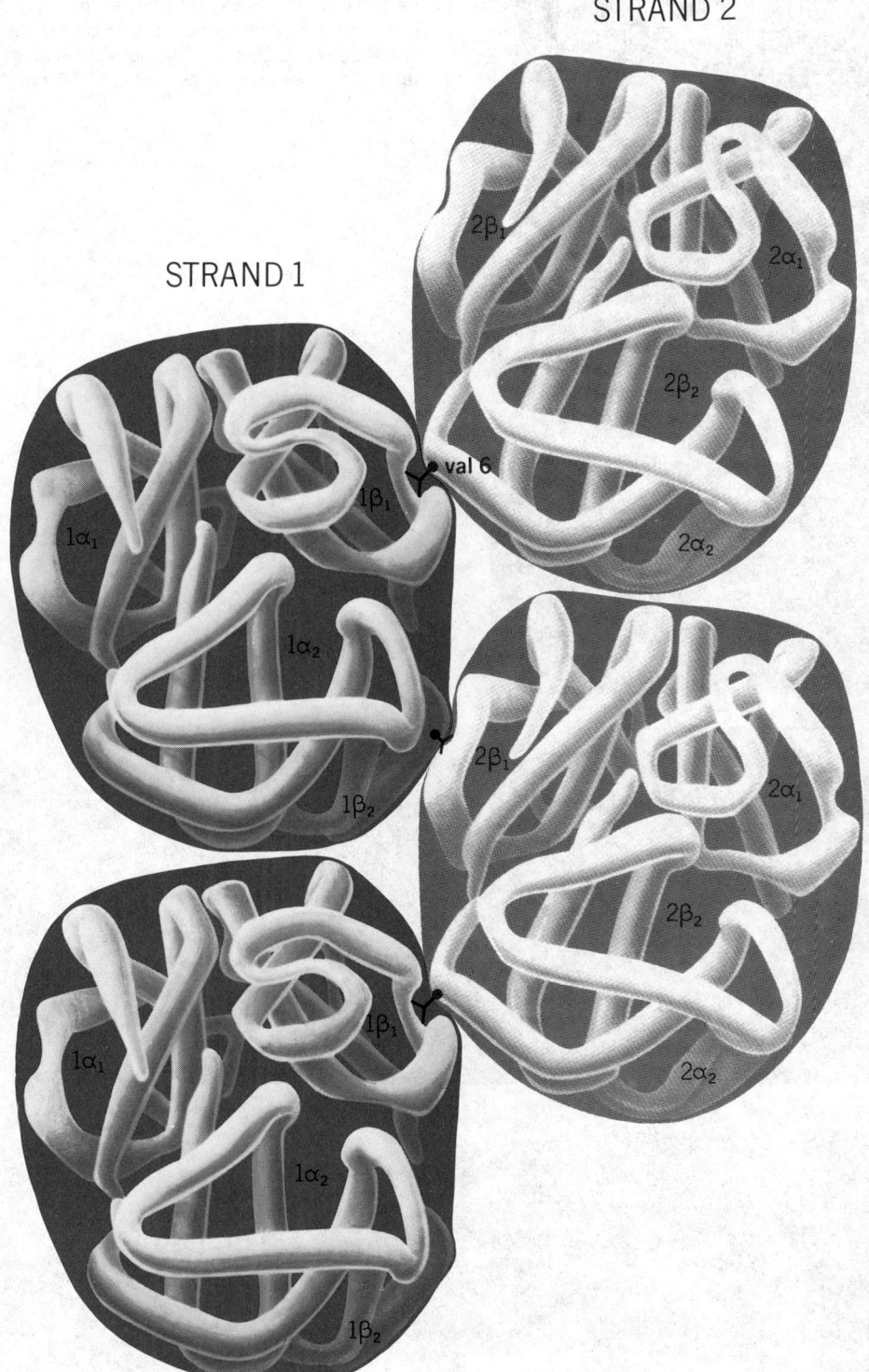

STRAND 2

STRAND 1

Fig. 43-5. Close up view of the deoxyHb S double strand. Lateral contact between strands involve β^{6val} as donor and the EF pocket of a molecule on the adjoining strand as acceptor. Axial contacts connect molecules vertically along the same strand. (From Dickerson and Geis,[62] with permission.)

and longer linear polymer; and by 30 seconds, the cells have a holly-leaf shape and considerable amounts of polymer.[69,89] Reoxygenation results in loss of much polymer within 3 seconds; deformation persists despite very little polymer at 5 seconds; no polymer or cell deformation remains after 10 seconds. Viscosity parallels the presence of polymer in both deoxygenated and reoxygenated cells. The poor deformability of re-

versibly sickled cells has been confirmed using laser diffraction viscosimetry and filtration methods.[90–92]

Deoxygenation rate and shear stress both influence the alignment of intracellular polymer domains, which may affect the rheologic properties of sickle cells and blood. The earliest reports of sickle cells described heterogeneous morphologic changes—classic sickle forms, holly-leaf shapes, and granular

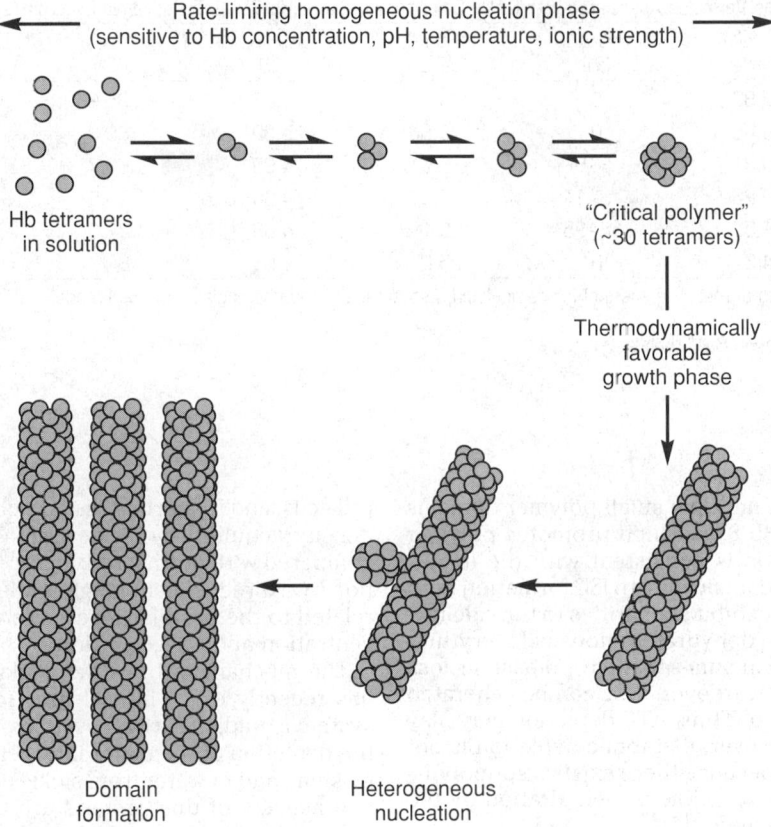

Fig. 43-6. Model for the polymerization and alignment of deoxyHb S showing homogeneous and heterogeneous nucleation. (Data from Hofrichter et al.[60] and Ferrone et al.[67])

deformities.[13] Subsequent physical studies[93,94,95] documented a correlation between sickle cell morphology and pattern of intraerythrocytic polymer domains: archetypal crescents have a single domain of highly aligned polymer that seems to have arisen by homogeneous nucleation from a single nucleus; holly leaves have a few less-well-aligned domains that appear to have arisen by heterogeneous nucleation from a limited number of nuclei; and granular cells have multiple poorly aligned domains that apparently have arisen by heterogeneous nucleation from many nuclei (Fig. 43-8). The rate of deoxygenation influenced

the formation of polymer domains; slower deoxygenation was associated with homogeneous nucleation, and rapid deoxygenation favored heterogeneous nucleation.[96,97] Shear stress also influenced polymer formation: shear applied during the delay period accelerated the onset of polymerization and increased viscosity, perhaps by creating more nucleation sites; shear applied after polymerization diminished viscosity by breaking the solid polymer phase.[98,99] The impact of deoxygenation rate and shear remains speculative, because there is little knowledge of the effect of domain patterns on rheologic properties of sickle cells or blood.

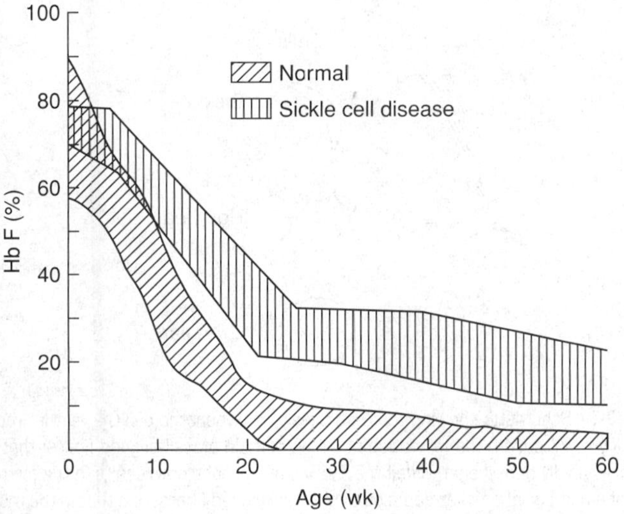

Irreversibly Sickled Cells

Some of the pathophysiologic events in the sickling process are not directly oxygen dependent, since a fraction of red cells remain sickled despite reoxygenation. The preponderance of ISCs among the most dense sickle cells[100,101] suggested to many that the common pathway of sickle cell destruction is via dehydration. However, Bertles and Milner[102] found among the densest cells a group of younger cells having unexpectedly low Hb F content—cells apparently predestined to early destruction by lacking the protective effect of Hb F.[65,72] The relative youth of the most dense cell fraction was confirmed using glycosylated hemoglobin as a measure of cell age.[103]

The rheologic disadvantage of ISCs is demonstrated by their poor deformability[104] and short circulatory survival.[105] The mechanisms responsible for their generation are not completely understood. Although membrane skeletal protein shells from ISCs have characteristically elongated shapes,[106] their poor cellular deformability is substantially improved by reducing MCHC with osmotic manipulation,[107,108] a fact incompatible with rigid membranes causing their rheologic impairment. Alternatively, the elongated (rather than crescentic) shape of

Fig. 43-7. Hb F decline in children with Hb AA and SS. (From O'Brien et al.,[478] with permission.)

Table 43-1. Hematologic Variables Associated with Sickle Cell Anemia, the Sickle Cell-β-Thalassemia Syndromes, and Sickle Cell-HPFH

Genotype	Hb[a]	Hb A[b] (%)	Hb F[b] (%)	Hb A$_2$[a] (%)	MCV[a]	Reticulocytes[a]	No.
Hb SS[c]	7.83	0	4.56	2.87	85.9	10.18	~123
Hb S-β°-thal[c]	8.85	0	5.86	5.02	69.3	7.2	~41
Hb S-β⁺-thal, type I[d]	8.37	3–5	6.8	4.90	63.7	9.7	3
Hb S-β⁺-thal, type II[d]	10.28	8–14	5.2	4.68	70.0	6.6	14
Hb S-β⁺-thal, type III[e]	11.55	18–25	5.1	4.66	73.3	1.27	76
Hb S-HPFH[f]	14.6	0	25.8	1.95	81.7	2.4	4

[a] Mean data for each variable. Units of measure are g/dl for hemoglobin, percentage of total hemoglobin for Hb F and A$_2$, fl for MCV, and percentage of total red cells for reticulocytes.
[b] Percentage Hb A that defines the Hb S-β⁺-thalassemia type.[451]
[c] Data from Sergeant et al.[454]
[d] Data from Christakis et al.[453]
[e] Data from Sergeant et al.[455]
[f] Data from Eaton et al.[567]

ISCs is probably the result of multiple small polymer domains within highly concentrated Hb S,[108] which promotes polymer formation.[6] This interpretation is consistent with the importance of recurrent sickling and unsickling to ISC formation both in vitro[109] and in vivo.[110] ISCs exhibit similarities to the calcium-loaded, potassium-depleted, dehydrated nonsickle erythrocytes that have undergone calcium-sensitive potassium loss by the Gardos phenomenon. Moreover, ISCs can be generated by metabolic depletion in vitro. Thus, ATP depletion may play a role in their genesis.[111] However, metabolic depletion is not essential for ISC production, because there exists a subpopulation of sickle cells that are susceptible to dehydration by the Gardos effect while energy replete.[112,113]

The clinical importance of ISCs relates to their presence as sickled forms on the peripheral blood smear; reversibly sickled cells, by definition, become morphologically normal when exposed to ambient oxygen tensions. The ISC number is generally constant in individual patients and correlates mainly with the degree of anemia.[114] The number of ISCs on the peripheral smear does not change with episodic complications of disease and is not a reliable indicator of events such as the acute painful episode.[115] However, painful episodes have been reported following artificial perturbation of their numbers to exceed steady-state levels.[110] The primary clinical use of detecting ISCs on the peripheral smear is in diagnosing sickle cell syndromes—ISCs are seen in all sickle cell disease genotypes but not in sickle cell trait.

Cation Homeostasis and Cell Dehydration

During their brief circulatory sojourn, sickle cells become profoundly dehydrated,[102] a process critically important for the generation of ISCs, for the unique pathobiology of Hb SC

red cells, and for certain disease complications. The far greater density acquired by sickle cells (MCHC ranging to ≤50 g/dl) compared with normal red cells[6,107] promotes Hb S polymerization by a direct effect of higher MCHC[7] and by an indirect effect related to the peculiar inverse relationship between Hb S concentration and oxygen affinity.[116]

The mechanism by which sickle cells become dehydrated has recently come into clearer focus. Several energy driven systems, gradient driven systems, and pathways contribute to the depletion of the major intracellular monovalent cation, potassium, and of water from sickle erythrocytes.[117,118] While certain aspects of this process are the result of deoxygenation, polymerization, and sickling, others are induced by the mere presence of mutant hemoglobin within the cell. A deoxygenation-induced passive cation leak results in balanced potassium efflux and sodium influx. The ion fluxes exceed by an order of magnitude those of normal erythrocytes and oxygenated sickle cells. The fixed stoichiometry of 3 sodium ions pumped out for every 2 potassium ions pumped into the cell during reparative attempts by Na⁺/K⁺ ATPase[119,120] results in a net depletion of cellular monovalent cation and water.[121] Mathematical modeling of sickle cell volume regulation indicates that the major effectors of cell dehydration are actually potassium/chloride co-transport and calcium-dependent potassium loss (the Gardos pathway), acting interdependently.[112] A population of calcium-sensitive reticulocytes preferentially lose potassium by the Gardos effect, thereby developing intracellular acidosis,

Table 43-2. Effect of α-Thalassemia on the Level of Anemia in Sickle Cell Anemia

Sources	αα/αα[a]	–α/αα	–α/–α
Data mainly from older subjects[83,84,86]	7.9[b] (n = 186)[c]	8.7 (n = 101)	9.0 (n = 61)
Data from subjects age 5 years[87]	8.6 (n = 88)	8.4 (n = 52)	8.3 (n = 50)
Data from subjects age 11 years[87]	7.9 (n = 40)	8.5 (n = 34)	9.6 (n = 2)

[a] The different α-globin genotypes indicate the presence of four (αα/αα), three (–α/αα), or two (–α/–α) α-globin genes.
[b] The mean hemoglobin level (g/dl) for each group is shown.
[c] The number of subjects in each group is denoted by n.

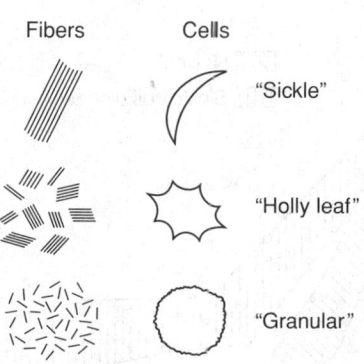

Fig. 43-8. Schematic showing that in a slowly deoxygenated cell the "sickle" morphology results from the formation of single domain of well-aligned fibers; that in a more rapidly deoxygenated cell the "holly leaf" morphology results in the formation of a number of smaller domains of shorter aligned fibers; and that in the most rapidly deoxygenated cells the "granular" morphology results from the formation of a large number of very small domains of randomly oriented short fibers. (Adapted from Eaton and Hofrichter,[565] with permission.)

which potentiates further potassium loss through potassium/chloride co-transport.[113] The calcium content of sickle cells is also elevated, particularly in ISCs.[122] Although most calcium is sequestered in vesicles,[123] it appears that free calcium is sufficiently available to participate in the Gardos phenomenon.[113] Factors that contribute to potassium loss include shape transformation[124] and oxidation of membrane transport proteins.[125]

Among the clinical consequences most directly attributable to cell dehydration are the renal complications of sickle cell trait. The loss of urinary concentrating ability combined with the hematuria exhibited in these individuals demonstrate that even Hb AS cells can cause vaso-occlusion when severely dehydrated by the hypertonic environment of the renal medulla.[126,127] Another demonstration of the clinical impact of cellular dehydration is the clinical morbidity in Hb SC disease. Although sickle cell trait and Hb SC red cells each contain "heterozygous" proportions of Hb S and another hemoglobin that does not participate in polymerization,[128] individuals with sickle cell trait are asymptomatic carriers, while those with Hb SC disease have anemia and painful vaso-occlusion.[5] This key difference is the result of higher Hb S concentrations within Hb SC cells due to greater fractional content of Hb S (50% versus 40%)[128] and to the cellular dehydration[128,129] mediated by Hb C-induced potassium/chloride co-transport activity.[129,130]

A third clinical correlate of red cell hydration, the interaction of α-thalassemia and sickle cell anemia, is perhaps more important for broadening the perspective of sickle cell pathophysiology than for reaffirming the importance of polymerization. Clearly, the less severe anemia associated with coexistent α-thalassemia[79,83,84] (Table 43-2) is accompanied by findings that emphasize the importance of polymerization: the lower MCHC[83,84] retards polymerization[6,7;] the fewer dense cells and ISCs[82,84,131] extend the known relationship between severity of anemia and number of ISCs[114]; and the diminished deoxygenation-induced cation leak[81] is consistent with the better hydration[132] and greater deformability of α-thalassemic sickle cells.[82,133] Despite the internal consistency of this synthesis,[134] exceptions to its strict interpretation demonstrate the need for a pathophysiologic understanding that extends beyond polymerization. The lack of α-thalassemia effect on anemia before age 7 years[87,88] (Table 43-2) suggests an age-dependent effector proximate to the influence of MCHC on polymerization. In this regard, it has been suggested[79] that persistent splenic conditioning in early childhood may deprive α-thalassemic sickle cells of their fundamental advantage—the greater degree of membrane redundancy[135]—which protects them against deformation-induced cation loss[124] during polymerization. The limitations of polymerization-based interpretations are further demonstrated by the detrimental clinical effects associated with α-thalassemia—that is, an increased incidence of osteonecrosis,[79,136,137] and higher hemoglobin levels associated with a greater frequency of pain, which after the age of 20 years is associated with a higher mortality rate.[138] Coexistent beneficial and detrimental influences of α-thalassemia demonstrate the doubtful validity of using polymerization equations to predict disease severity[74] and the need for pathophysiologic interpretations that include polymerization-independent mechanisms of cell pathobiology[10] and the detrimental rheologic effects of higher hematocrit and viscosity.[104,133]

Some experimental therapeutic strategies have used methods for improving cellular hydration. Inducing hyponatremia in patients was reported to swell red cells osmotically, lower MCHC, and ameliorate painful episodes.[139] Pharmacologic preservation of sickle cell hydration by cetiedil citrate (Cetiedil), an agent that inhibits the Gardos phenomenon and induces passive sodium influx, has shown therapeutic potential.[140] Im-

idazole inhibitors of Gardos pathway also provide a therapeutic option for maintaining cell hydration.[141] Future therapeutic options directed at improving cell hydration are anticipated.

Oxidative Damage

In addition to its abnormal electrophoretic mobility and solubility, Hb S is unstable.[142-145] Consequences of Hb S instability are the increased generation of methemoglobin[146] and release of heme,[147] processes that contribute to the increased generation of oxidative radicals by sickle red cells.[147,148] In addition, the normal physiologic processes of hemoglobin oxygenation and deoxygenation generate methemoglobin S (metHb S) and oxidative radicals continuously[149] (Fig. 43-9). These processes perpetuate an oxidative stress within sickle red cells that has major pathophysiologic importance to metabolism, membrane lipids, membrane proteins, and the integrity of the Hb S molecule itself.[10,150]

Oxidative stress on red cell metabolism is particularly important to sickle cell pathophysiology. Impaired reductive defense mechanisms potentiate other sources of oxidative damage to the cell. The presence of free heme within sickle red cells inhibits the activity of several enzymes needed to generate NADH and NADPH for protection against oxidation.[148] Sickle cells have been found to have decreased NADH redox potential,[151] hexomonophosphate shunt activity,[152,153] and GSH content.[153] The metabolic disadvantages of sickled red cells represent underappreciated contributions to sickle cell pathobiology.

The lipids and proteins of the erythrocyte membranes are targets of oxidative damage. The impaired metHb S reduction and absence of metHb S from sickle erythrocytes, despite increased generation of metHb S,[154] suggest the rapid conversion of metHb S to another form. This is consistent with the generation of hemichrome from which heme is liberated to cause oxidant damage of cytoplasmic and membrane components.[155,156] Both heme and nonheme iron have been found in

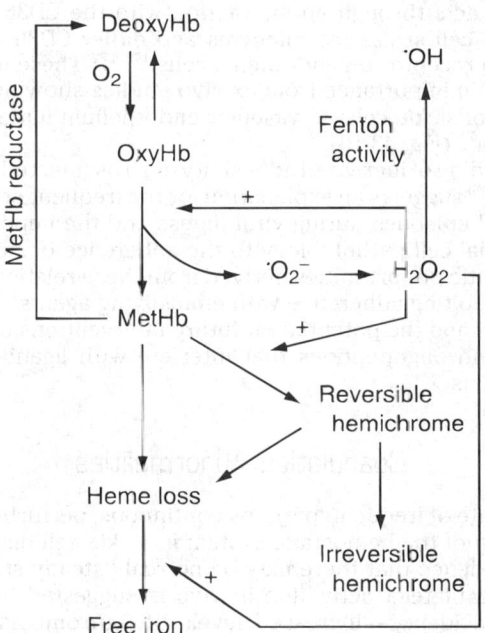

Fig. 43-9. Schematic diagram showing the generation of oxidative radicals by physiologic oxygenation and deoxygenation, the auto-oxidation of hemoglobin, and the impact of these processes on the liberation of hemichrome, heme, and free iron and on the self-perpetuation of oxidative processes. (Kindly provided by RP Hebbel.)

increased amounts on sickle cell membranes.[150] The accumulation of hemichrome aggregates on the cytoplasmic portion of band 3 initiates co-clustering of band 3 molecules in the membrane and assembly of IgG and complement on the extracellular domains of band 3 molecules.[157,158] These promote sickle cell recognition by macrophages[159] and adherence to endothelial cells.[160] The uneven distribution of band 3 and of another transmembrane protein, glycophorin A,[161] demonstrates that the membrane skeletons of sickle cells are disrupted. Abnormalities of skeletal proteins are apparent from the impaired association of the major membrane skeletal protein, spectrin, into sickle cell membranes.[162] There is also direct evidence for oxidative damage to the membrane skeletal proteins spectrin, ankyrin, band 3, and band 4.1.[163]

There is also oxidative damage to sickle cell membrane lipids.[164] It is probable that similar abnormalities of membrane lipids are related to their reduced lateral mobility in sickle cell membranes[165] and to the loss of phosphatidylinositol-anchored membrane proteins such as DAF and MIRL[166] (see the section Mechanisms of Hemolysis).

Sickle Cell Adherence

The discovery that sickled red cells are more adherent to cultured vascular endothelial cells[161,167] has contributed greatly to our understanding of sickle cell pathophysiology.[10] The importance of sickle cell adherence gained perspective from the observation that the vaso-occlusive severity of individual patients was directly related to the adhesivity of their sickle cells.[168] Subsequent studies have revealed that adherence differs according to subpopulation of sickle cells, source of endothelial cells, cytoadhesive ligands, and cell membrane receptors.[10] In general, the least dense reticulocyte-enriched fraction of sickle cells is most adherent[71,169] Cytoadherence ligands reported to mediate adherence include unusually high-molecular-weight von Willebrand factor,[169] immunoglobulin,[160] fibronectin,[169] fibrinogen,[170] and thrombospondin.[171,172] Thrombospondin, the most potent mediator of sickle cell adherence, acts through an interaction with the CD36 receptor on sickle cell stress reticulocytes and either CD36 or the vitronectin receptor on endothelial cells.[171,172] These molecular details gain importance from ex vivo studies showing that adherence of sickle cells to vascular endothelium initiates vaso-occlusion[71] (Fig. 43-10).

The finding of increased adhesivity of virus-infected endothelial cells[160] suggests an explanation for the frequent occurrence of painful episodes during viral illness and the importance of endothelial cell pathobiology to the adherence of sickle cells. Therapeutic opportunities derived from these relationships include inhibiting adherence with emulsifying agents[173] such as RheothRx and the potential for future interventions using antibodies and oligopeptides that interfere with ligand-receptor interactions.

Coagulation Abnormalities

The state of frequent, perhaps continuous, perturbation and activation of the hemostatic system in sickle cell disease provides evidence that there may be no real "steady state."[11,174] Increased platelet activation in vivo is suggested by several lines of evidence—increased levels of β-thromboglobulin[175] and platelet factor 4,[176] increased activation-associated antigens on platelet membranes,[177] reduced amounts of thrombospondin in circulating platelets,[177] and increased urinary levels of thromboxane.[178] Reduced platelet count and shortened platelet survival during acute painful episodes suggest that platelet activation occurs during these events, as does the re-

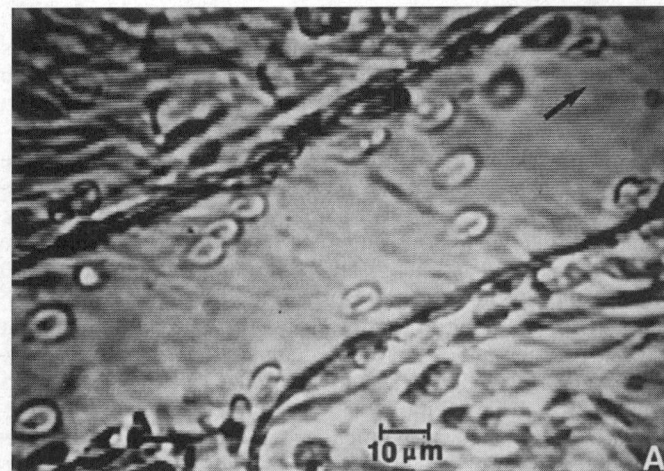
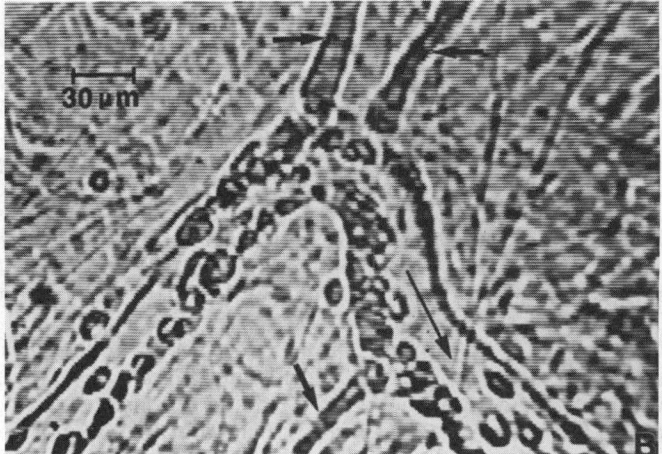

Fig. 43-10. Adhesion of sickle erythrocytes in venules. **(A)** Adherent discocytic sickle cells tethered to the endothelial wall of a venule and aligned in the direction of the flow (arrow). **(B)** Increased adherence of sickle cells at venule or bending and at junctions of smaller diameter post capillary venules. The post capillary vessels (small arrows) are totally blocked. Large arrow indicates flow direction. (From Kaul et al.,[71] with permission.)

cent finding of thrombospondin release from platelets during pain crises.[179,180]

Steady-state levels of procoagulants and of the natural anticoagulants, protein C, protein S, and antithrombin III are not consistently abnormal.[11] During acute painful episodes, fibrinogen levels rise.[181] It is unclear whether fibrinolytic system is abnormal, but increased levels of fibrin degradation product suggest ongoing fibrinolysis.[11]

A source of hemostatic activation specific for sickle cell disease is the red cell itself. Both ISCs and deoxygenated reversibly sickled cells express abnormal amounts of phosphatidylserine on the outer membrane leaflet, which may activate the coagulation cascade.[182] In addition, cellular sickling results in exovesiculation of phosphatidylserine-rich membrane vesicles[183] that can activate coagulation.[184]

Perturbation of vascular endothelial cells is yet another source of hemostatic activation.[185] Evidence of increased thrombin activity found in sickle cell disease[180] suggests that endothelial cells may be stimulated to release von Willebrand factor, prostacyclin, plasminogen activators, and platelet activating factor, to express tissue factor and cytoadhesive molecules on the cell membrane, to promote vasoconstriction, and to activate thrombomodulin. Endothelial cell abnormalities are also emerging as important to sickle cell pathophysiology (see the section Sickle Cell Adherence and Vaso-occlusion).

Pathophysiology of Vaso-occlusion

Sickle cell vaso-occlusion is not solely ascribable to polymerization of Hb S and sickling of red cells containing Hb S, even though these processes are fundamentally necessary for vaso-occlusion.[12,186] "Sickling" is a chronic, ongoing process rather than a sudden cataclysmic one. Sickle cells are deoxygenated on an average of four times per minute. There is no reason to believe that the recurrent vaso-occlusive events in the lives of sickle cell patients are related to systemic deoxygenation. Moreover, certain of the processes related to vascular occlusion are chronically activated, suggesting that there may be no real "steady state" in sickle cell blood circulation.[174]

While the clinical morbidity associated with high intraerythrocytic concentrations of Hb S in Hb SC disease,[128] the clinical benignity associated with the high amounts and pancellular distribution of Hb F in sickle cell-HPFH,[187] and the clinical complications caused by specific circumstances known to enhance polymerization[188-190] confirm the importance of polymerization, there are sufficient exceptions to this association that polymerization and sickling should probably be regarded as necessary but not sufficient for vaso-occlusion. The argument that polymerization tendency is the major determinant of clinical severity[74] is only valid as it pertains to the severity of anemia. This proviso is further exemplified by the interaction of α-thalassemia with sickle cell anemia. The lower MCHC and polymerization tendency improves the level of anemia,[84] but the higher blood viscosity[133] is detrimental to vaso-occlusive severity.[138] The major influence of Hb F on polymerization[65] and sickling[72] has only small effects on the frequency of pain.[191] The profound effect of Hb S concentration on polymerization is most important to cells having high MCHC (ISCs). However, the frequency of pain not only fails to correlate with the fraction of ISCs in the circulation[115] but also appears to have an inverse relationship.[192,193] Ex vivo studies of sickle cell blood flow indicate that vaso-occlusion is initiated by the vascular adherence of younger cells with lower MCHC (Fig. 43-10), and that the role of poorly deformable, polymerization-prone ISCs is to propagate but not initiate the process.[71]

Increasing evidence for the importance of sickle cell-endothelial cell adherence, hemostatic activation, vascular reactivity, and leukocyte participation suggest that polymerization considerations provide a first approximation of the severity of sickle cell disease.[74] Moment-to-moment vaso-occlusive changes are better understood by considering a wider variety of processes.[12,186] It has been suggested that the apparent lack of predictability in the periodic vaso-occlusion of sickle cell disease may not be random but chaotic, and thereby dictated by specific internal deterministic parameters.[194] Vaso-occlusion may be better understood as chaos than as the result of any one deterministic process or factor.[12]

Mechanisms of Hemolysis

Premature destruction of sickle erythrocytes occurs both extravascularly and intravascularly.[195] Extravascular hemolysis results from abnormalities of the sickle cell that permit its recognition and phagocytosis by macrophages[196] and from impaired deformability of sickle red cells, enabling their physical entrapment.[197] Changes in sickle cell membranes from oxidative damage by unstable Hb S and from recurrent sickling promote binding to the membrane of increased amounts of IgG, which mediates recognition by macrophages.[196,198] Oxidatively denatured hemoglobin binds to the cytosolic portion of the transmembrane protein, band 3, which signals adherence of IgG and complement to the band 3 exterior.[157,158] Impaired complement inactivation on sickle cell membranes[199] permits the presence of complement, which facilitates the recognition

and phagocytosis of sickle cells by macrophages.[159] Mechanical trapping of poorly deformable ISCs also contributes to extravascular hemolysis, as evidenced by the poor deformability of ISCs,[104] their brief circulatory survival,[105] and correlation of their numbers with severity of anemia.[114] The declining fraction of dense cells and slight worsening of anemia during painful episodes,[200,201] and the selective trapping of dense cells in ex vivo flow systems[197] suggests further that mechanical trapping contributes to extravascular hemolysis.

Elevations of free plasma hemoglobin in patients suggest that one-third the total hemolysis in sickle cell anemia is intravascular.[195] One mechanism of intravascular hemolysis is sickling-associated exovesiculation[183,202] of vesicles rich in phosphatidylinositol-anchored membrane proteins[203] depleting the cell of the complement regulatory proteins DAF and MIRL and leaving the cells susceptible to complement-mediated intravascular lysis.[166] Another component of intravascular hemolysis is increased mechanical fragmentation of sickle cells,[204] which accounts for the accelerated hemolysis of sickle cell patients during exercise.[204]

Immune Deficit

The propensity of children with sickle cell disease to *Streptococcus pneumoniae* infection is related to impaired splenic function[205] and diminished serum opsonizing activity.[206] Even before the eventual autoinfarction of the spleen in patients with sickle cell anemia,[207] defective splenic function is demonstrable by Howell-Jolly bodies on the peripheral blood smear,[205] visible "pits" on the surface of red blood cells, and abnormal results of radionuclide spleen scanning.[208] Splenic function is restorable by transfusion before the second decade of life.[209] The greater the rate of hemolysis of specific syndromes, the earlier the age at which splenic function is lost—sickle cell anemia > Hb SC disease > sickle cell-β+-thalassemia.[208]

Opsonization defects and abnormalities of the alternate complement pathway coexist in patients with sickle cell disease,[210] but evidence of a causal relationship is lacking.[211] Rather, the opsonic defect is the result of an abnormality in natural antibody response that impairs the effector arm of opsonization assays.[211] The variable opsonic defects for different bacteria may depend on selective antibody requirements for opsonization of the different microbes.

The decreased titer of antibody against *S. pneumoniae* antigens following splenectomy in individuals without sickle cell disease[212] suggests that splenic hypofunction may mediate the opsonic deficiency of sickle cell disease. This conclusion is consistent with the earlier loss of splenic function in genotypes characterized by more rapid hemolysis,[208] the correlation between free plasma hemoglobin levels and the rate of consumption of alternate complement pathway components,[213] and the suppression of B-lymphocyte activity by phosphatidylserine-rich vesicles.[214,215]

CLINICAL MANIFESTATIONS

The clinical manifestations of sickle cell disease vary tremendously between and among the major genotypes. Even within the genotype regarded as being most severe—sickle cell anemia—some entirely asymptomatic patients are detected only incidentally, whereas others are disabled by recurrent pain and chronic complications. Patients are typically anemic but lead an asymptomatic life punctuated by painful episodes. Virtually every organ system in the body is subject to vaso-occlusion, which accounts for the characteristic acute and chronic multisystem failure of this disease. Important clinical features less directly related to vaso-occlusion are growth retardation, psychosocial problems, and susceptibility to infection. This section describes the systemic manifestations of disease and those of specific organ systems. Specific therapeutic recommendations are included. For detailed discussions, the reader is referred to the versions presented by Serjeant,[2] Mankad and Moore,[216] and Embury et al.[1] Practical monographs recommended include *Management and Therapy of Sickle Cell Disease*,[217] and a review of pediatric therapy by Vichinsky and Lubin.[218]

Life Expectancy

In 1973 Diggs[219] reported that the mean survival of patients with sickle cell disease was 14.3 years; in 1994 Platt et al.[220] reported a life expectancy of 42 years for men and of 48 years for women with sickle cell anemia. Prolonged survival over the past 20 years is more the result of improved general medical care than of successful antisickling therapy. The ability of prophylactic penicillin therapy to prevent mortality from pneumococcal sepsis[221] may now be having an impact on survival.

Chronic Anemia

Chronic hemolytic anemia is a hallmark of sickle cell disease. Sickle erythrocytes are destroyed randomly with a mean life span of 17 days.[222] The survival of ISCs is much shorter than of other sickle cells[102]; the overall hemolytic rate reflects the number of ISCs.[114] Anemia is most severe in sickle cell anemia and Hb S-β°-thalassemia, milder in Hb S-β+-thalassemia and Hb SC disease,[223] and, among patients with sickle cell anemia, less severe in those who have coexistent α-thalassemia[79] (Tables 43-1 and 43-2). In addition, erythropoietin levels are inappropriately low,[224] more severely so in adults than in children,[224] suggesting the presence of subclinical renal disease. The lower erythropoietin levels may reflect the retardant effect of increased blood viscosity on erythropoietin production.[225]

Exacerbations of Anemia

Hemolytic anemia may be exacerbated by any of several events: aplastic crises and acute splenic sequestration or, less commonly, sequestration in other organs, chronic renal disease, bone marrow necrosis, deficiency of folic acid or iron, and hyperhemolysis.

Aplastic and Hypoplastic Crises

Aplastic crises are transient arrests of erythropoiesis characterized by abrupt falls in hemoglobin levels, reticulocyte number, and red cell precursors in the marrow. Although these episodes typically last only a few days, the level of anemia may be severe because the hemolysis continues unabated in the absence of red cell production. The mechanisms that impair erythropoiesis in inflammation are operative in infections of all types[226] (see Ch. 152). Human parvovirus B19, which specifically invades proliferating erythroid progenitors,[227] is very important in these syndromes[228] (see Ch. 23). Parvovirus B19 accounts for 68% of aplastic crises in children with sickle cell disease,[229] but the high incidence of protective antibodies in adults[230] makes parvovirus a less frequent cause of aplasia in older patients. Other reported causes of transient aplasia are infections by *S. pneumoniae, Salmonella,* other *streptococci,* and Epstein-Barr virus. Bone marrow necrosis, an event characterized by fever, bone pain, reticulocytopenia, and a leukoerythroblastic response, also causes aplastic crisis.[231] This may also be the result of parvovirus infection.[232] Inhaled oxygen therapy can cause transient red cell hypoproduction; su-

praphysiologic oxygen tensions curtail erythropoietin production promptly and suppress reticulocytosis within 2 days.[110]

The mainstay of treating aplastic crises is red cell transfusion. When transfusion is necessitated by the degree of anemia or cardiorespiratory symptoms, a single transfusion usually will suffice, since reticulocytosis resumes spontaneously within a few days. Transfusion may be avoided by keeping severely anemic patients at bed rest to prevent symptoms and by avoiding supraphysiologic oxygen tensions.

Splenic Sequestration and Hyperhemolytic Crises

Acute splenic sequestration is characterized by acute exacerbation of anemia, persistent reticulocytosis, a tender, enlarging spleen, and sometimes hypovolemia.[233] Patients susceptible to this complication are those whose spleen has not undergone fibrosis—young patients with sickle cell anemia and adults with Hb SC disease or sickle cell-β+-thalassemia.[234] Sequestration may occur as early as a few weeks of age[235] and may cause death before sickle cell disease is diagnosed.[236] In one study, 30% of children had splenic sequestration over a 10-year period, and 15% of the attacks were fatal.[233,237] The basis of therapy is to restore blood volume and red cell mass. Because splenic sequestration recurs in 50% of cases,[233] splenectomy is recommended after the event has abated. Alternatively, chronic transfusion therapy can be used in young children to delay splenectomy until it can be tolerated safely.[238] Because recurrence may occur during the course of transfusion therapy,[238] parents should be trained to detect a rapidly enlarging spleen and to seek immediate medical attention in this event. Less common sites of acute sequestration include the liver[239] and possibly the lung.[240]

Hyperhemolytic crisis is defined as the sudden exacerbation of anemia with increased reticulocytosis and bilirubin level. It has been argued that many diagnoses of hyperhemolytic crisis are actually occult splenic sequestration or aplastic crises detected during the resolving reticulocytosis. In one report, seven of the eight children with hyperhemolysis had G6PD deficiency.[241] In the presence of hyperhemolysis, it is probable that many cases are related to some complicating etiology such as G6PD deficiency or immune hemolysis.

Chronic worsening of anemia may be due to developing renal insufficiency (see Ch. 148) or deficiency of folic acid or iron (see Chs. 41 and 38). Inadequate erythropoietin production in renal failure[242] results in deficient compensation for sickle cell hemolysis. Administration of recombinant human erythropoietin may improve this situation,[243] but caution must be exer-

---

SPLENIC SEQUESTRATION CRISIS

Splenic sequestration crisis may cause rapid severe worsening of anemia accompanied by persistent reticulocytosis and a tender enlarging spleen. Hypovolemic shock is a risk, particularly in children. Young children with sickle cell anemia (Hb SS) have a 30% incidence of this complication, and patients of all ages with Hb SC disease (Hb SC) and sickle cell-β-thalassemia (Hb S-β-thal) are at risk. The mortality rate is 15%. Sequestration is recurrent in 50% of cases, so splenectomy is recommended after the acute event remits. In young children, chronic transfusion can be used to prevent recurrence until splenectomy can be performed safely. These episodes often occur concomitant with a viral illness, so parents are trained to palpate enlarging spleens during viral illnesses to detect this complication in its early stages.

THERAPY FOR PAIN

The object of analgesic therapy in patients with acute painful episodes is to relieve pain rapidly and safely. The most successful approach to this end has been achieved by comprehensive centers that provide individualized therapy in setting apart from the emergency department. A helpful approach to dealing with the patient in pain is to provide psychosocial support by teams composed of physicians, social workers, and nurses who are known to the patient. Parents and extended family of pediatric patients should be included. Some programs are successful using oral medication, but often parenteral narcotics are necessary. (See Table 43-6 for recommended agents, doses, schedules, and drug combinations.) After initial control of pain using aggressive narcotic regimens, patient-controlled analgesia is useful for maintenance inpatient management. The use of constant intravenous infusion of narcotics must be monitored closely because of the risk of respiratory depression, which is particularly dangerous for patients with sickle cell disease. The switch from parenteral to oral analgesics may be problematic because of inadequate dosing of oral drugs and their variable absorption. Following discharge of children from the clinic, emergency department, or hospital, it may be helpful to provide school reentry liaison services. Patients should be discharged from the hospital with a limited supply of analgesics to avoid fostering drug-seeking behavior that may become detrimental to future pain management. Narcotic addiction is no more frequent in sickle cell patients than in any others requiring analgesia and is more related to societal issues than to problems specific to sickle cell disease.

cised not to elevate the hematocrit to levels that result in hyperviscosity. Chronic hemolysis results in increased utilization of folic acid stores,[244] and megaloblastic crises from folic acid deficiency have been reported.[245] Despite increased intestinal absorption of iron in sickle cell disease,[246] the combination of nutritional deficiency[247] and urinary iron losses[248] result in iron deficiency in 20% of children with sickle cell disease.[247] The diagnosis of iron deficiency may be obscured by the elevated serum iron levels associated with chronic hemolysis, necessitating the detection of a low serum ferritin or an elevated serum transferrin for the diagnosis.

Acute Painful Episode

An episode of acute pain was originally called a "sickle cell crisis" by Diggs, who used the expression "crisis" to refer to any new rapidly developing syndrome in the life of a patient with sickle cell disease. In modern parlance, the term acute painful episode is favored over crisis.

Acute pain is the first symptom of disease in more than one-fourth of patients, the most frequent symptom after age 2 years,[249] and the complication for which patients with sickle cell disease most commonly seek medical attention.[250] Although a general correlation of vaso-occlusive severity and genotype has been posited,[74] tremendous variability occurs within genotypes and in the same patient over time. In one large study of patients with sickle cell anemia, one-third rarely had pain, one-third were hospitalized for pain approximately two to six times per year, and one-third had more than six pain-related hospitalizations per year.[251] The frequency of pain

peaks between the ages of 19 and 39 years. After the age of 19, more frequent pain is associated with higher mortality rate.[138] Over a 5-year period in the National Cooperative Study of Sickle Cell Disease, 40% of patients had no painful episodes, 5% of patients accounted for one-third of the emergency department visits, and pain frequency correlated with high total hemoglobin levels and low Hb F levels.[138] Medical personnel who see patients only in the emergency department gain a biased view of sickle cell disease skewed by a frequently afflicted few whose severe disease is the result of specific hematologic determinants.[252]

Pain may be precipitated by events such as cold, dehydration, infection, stress, menses, and alcohol consumption, but most painful episodes have no identifiable cause.[253] It can affect any area of the body (most commonly the back, chest, extremities, and abdomen), may vary from trivial to excruciating, and is usually endured at home without a visit to the emergency department. There are often premonitory symptoms.[254] The duration averages a few days.[255] Painful episodes are biopsychosocial events[253] caused by vaso-occlusion in an area of the body having nociceptors and nerves.[256] Pain is an affect, and, as such, consists of sensory, perceptual, cognitive, and emotional components.[253] Frequent pain generates feelings of despair, depression, and apathy, which interfere with everyday life and promote an existence that revolves around pain. This scenario may lead to a chronic debilitating pain syndrome, which, fortunately, is rare. The management of pain is discussed below in the section Therapy.

Approximately one-half of episodes present with objective clinical signs, such as fever, swelling, tenderness, tachypnea, hypertension, nausea, and vomiting.[193] Numerous laboratory tests have been found to lack specificity as indicators of acute vaso-occlusion—leukocytosis,[257] D-dimer fragments of fibrin,[258] and markers of platelet activation.[259] The most promising laboratory indicators of acute vaso-occlusion are changes in the distribution of sickle cell subpopulations and rheologic properties of the blood.[201,260] Just before the onset of pain, the fraction of dense cells increases and maximum deformability of sickle cells decreases; during the evolution of pain, the dense cell fraction declines and the overall red cell deformability increases. The evolution of pain is also associated with changes in the levels of acute-phase reactants,[174,261] serum lactate dehydrogenase,[262] interleukin-1, tumor necrosis factor,[263] and serum viscosity.[181] These tests are of limited clinical value.

Psychosocial Issues

Modern insights into the psychosocial adjustment of patients with sickle cell disease are beginning to provide a level of understanding that permits interventional therapy.[264–266] While most patients with sickle cell disease are generally well adjusted,[267] the disorder is associated with risks of depression, low self-esteem, social isolation, poor family relationships, and withdrawal from normal daily living.[267–269] Specific stressors include recurrent pain and the response to it,[270] curtailed activity due to pain,[271] misinterpretation of the meaning of pain,[272] and depression leading to learned helplessness.[273] Some patients with sickle cell disease become addicted to narcotics, but this is uncommon[274] and is usually the result of social influences, rather than pain therapy.[217] Well-adjusted patients have active coping strategies,[275] family support,[276] and support from the extended family unit common in African-American society.[277] Interventional approaches should emphasize recognizing and reinforcing individual strengths, confronting pathologic behavior, and establishing coping skills through reinterpreting pain, diverting attention from pain, and using support systems. Attention to psychosocial concerns is vitally important to the well-being and integration into society of patients with sickle cell disease.[276]

Growth and Development

By 2 years of age, children with sickle cell disease have detectable growth retardation, which affects weight more than height and has no clear gender difference.[278] Normal height is achieved by adulthood, but weight remains lower than that of controls. More severe growth delay is noted in children with sickle cell anemia and sickle cell-$\beta°$-thalassemia; Hb SC disease is associated with a less severe growth delay. Skeletal maturation is also delayed.[279] Girls with sickle cell disease have retarded sexual maturation that is greater in those with sickle cell anemia and sickle cell-$\beta°$-thalassemia than in those with Hb SC disease and sickle cell-β^+-thalassemia,[278] and is associated with elevated gonadotropin levels for the stage of sexual development[280] and with delayed menarche.[281] Boys also have delayed sexual maturation that is more severe in those with sickle cell anemia than in those with Hb SC disease.[278] Retarded sexual maturation in males can be due to primary hypogonadism,[282] hypopituitarism,[283] or hypothalamic insufficiency.[284] Delayed growth and sexual maturation correlate with the degree of hemolysis due to the increased basal metabolic requirements of a patient with hemolysis.[285] It has been possible to restore normal growth by nutritional supplementation.[286] There have been reports of responses to folic acid[287] and zinc supplementation,[288] but these approaches are not recommended as standard care.

Infections

Infectious complications of sickle cell disease are a major cause of morbidity and mortality.[289,290] The type of infection caused by particular organisms are shown in Table 43-3; the specific organisms affecting different target organs are shown in Table 43-4.[291]

S. pneumoniae is the most common cause of bacteremia in children with sickle cell disease,[290,292,293] accounting for 5–10 episodes per 100 patient-years in infants.[289] This event is accompanied by leukocytosis, a "left shift," aplastic crisis, sometimes disseminated intravascular coagulation, and a 20–50% mortality rate.[289] The second most common organism responsible for bacteremia in these children, *Haemophilus influenzae* type b, has accounted for 10–25% of episodes.[294,295] *H. influenzae* bacteremia affects older children. It is less fulminant than *S. pneumoniae* bacteremia, but it can be fatal.[289,296] While pneumococcal vaccination has been disappointing,[221,297,298] the use of vaccination against *H. influenzae* type b,[299] prophylactic penicillin,[221] and the long-acting broad-spectrum antibiotic ceftriaxone[300,301] has greatly ameliorated the impact of childhood bacteremia. Conjugated *H. influenzae* type b vaccines produce excellent antibody responses in children with sickle cell disease[299] and are now administered in early infancy. Prophylactic penicillin beginning in infancy has reduced the incidence of *S. pneumoniae* bacteremia in children <3 years of age by 84%,[221,297] and its use is currently recommended[292] (see the section Therapy). A disadvantage of this approach relates to the impaired anti-*S. pneumoniae* antibody production and resulting uncertainty regarding the safety of discontinuing prophylaxis. The efficacy of ceftriaxone therapy for *S. pneumoniae* and *H. influenzae* infection[300,301] has led to new treatment algorithms that recommend outpatient therapy for most patients (see the section Therapy). Bacteremia in older patients is more likely due to *Escherichia coli* and other gram-negative organisms, as are urinary tract infections.[289,293]

Meningitis in sickle cell anemia is primarily a problem of

Table 43-3. Bacteria and Viruses that Most Frequently Cause Serious Infection in Patients with Sickle Cell Disease

Microorganism	Type of Infection	Comments
Streptococcus pneumoniae	Septicemia	Common despite prophylactic penicillin and pneumococcal vaccine
	Meningitis	Less frequent than in years past
	Pneumonia	Rarely documented except in infants and young children
	Septic arthritis	Uncommon
Haemophilus influenzae type b	Septicemia Meningitis Pneumonia	Much less common in recent years because of immunization with conjugate vaccine
Salmonella sp.	Osteomyelitis Septicemia	Most common cause of bone and joint infection
Escherichia coli and other gram-negative enteric pathogens	Septicemia Urinary tract infection Osteomyelitis	Focus sometimes inapparent
Staphylococcus aureus	Osteomyelitis	Uncommon
Mycoplasma pneumonia	Pneumonia	Pleural effusions; multilobe involvement
Chlamydia pneumoniae	Pneumonia	
Parvovirus B19	Bone marrow suppression (aplastic crisis)	High fever common; rash and other organ involvement infrequent
Hepatitis viruses (A, B, C)	Hepatitis	Marked hyperbilirubinemia

(From Buchanan,[291] with permission.)

infants and young children, is caused most frequently by *S. pneumoniae,* and occurs in the setting of bacteremia.[290] Rapid administration of antibiotics has resulted in a lower incidence of meningitis among bacteremic patients compared with 20 years ago when the incidence was 50%.[293,302] *H. influenzae* type b is a less common cause of meningitis.[290] (see the section Therapy for a discussion of antibiotic therapy.)

Bacterial pneumonia may be the cause of the acute chest syndrome. Patients with any combination of dyspnea, cough, chest pain, fever, tachypnea, or leukocytosis should be evaluated by chest radiography, arterial blood gases, blood and sputum culture, cold agglutinins, and serologic study for *Mycoplasma pneumoniae* and *Chlamydia. S. pneumoniae* and *H. influenzae* type b are uncommon causes of acute chest syndrome even in children.[303] *M. pneumoniae* and *Chlamydia pneumoniae* account for approximately 20% of cases.[303,304] Antibiotic therapy for the acute chest syndrome should cover these four agents (see the section Therapy). Respiratory viruses are common causes of pulmonary infection. General therapy for the acute chest syndrome is discussed in the section Pulmonary Complications.

Osteomyelitis occurs more commonly in sickle cell disease than in normal individuals,[290] probably as a result of infection of infarcted bone. In this patient population, osteomyelitis is commonly caused by caused by *Salmonella* species.[305] *Staphylococcus aureus,* the most common etiology in patients without sickle cell disease, accounts for <25% of sickle cell disease cases.[306] Infection usually affects long bones, often at multiple sites.[307] Diagnosis is confirmed by culture of blood or infected bone, before parenteral antibiotics covering *Salmonella* and *S. aureus* are begun[305] (see the section Therapy). Articular infection is less common and often due to *S. pneumoniae.*[305]

Table 43-4. Organ-Related Infection in Sickle Cell Disease

Primary Sites of Infection	Most Common Pathogen(s)	Other Pathogens	Pathophysiology	Prevention	Management
Septicemia	*Streptococcus pneumoniae*	*Haemophilus influenzae* *Escherichia coli* *Salmonella* sp.	Defective splenic function; deficiency of opsonic antibody	Vaccines[a] Prophylactic penicillin	Empirical intravenous antibiotics for fever
Meningitis	*S. pneumoniae*		———————— Same as for septicemia ————————		
Osteomyelitis and septic arthritis	*Salmonella* sp. *S. pneumoniae*	*E. coli* *Proteus* sp. *Staphylococcus aureus*	Ischemic or infarcted tissue	—	Surgical drainage, prolonged course intravenous antibiotics
Pneumonia	*Mycoplasma pneumoniae* Respiratory viruses	*Chlamydia pneumoniae* *S. pneumoniae*	Concomitant infection and intrapulmonary vaso-occlusion leading to infarction and/or sequestration	Vaccines[a]	See the sections Pulmonary and Therapy, for management of acute chest syndrome

[a] Against *S. pneumoniae* and *H. influenzae* type b.
(From Buchanan,[291] with permission.)

Neurologic Complications

The neurologic complications occurring in 25% of patients with sickle cell disease[308] include transient ischemic attacks, cerebral infarction, cerebral hemorrhage, seizures, unexplained coma, spinal cord infarction or compression, central nervous system infections, vestibular dysfunction, and sensory hearing loss.[309,310]

The most common signs of cerebrovascular accident (CVA) in patients with sickle cell disease are hemiparesis, seizures, coma, speech defects, and visual impairment. CVA may occur spontaneously or intercurrently with other complications, such as pneumonia, aplastic crisis, painful episodes, or dehydration.[311] Hematologic indicators of CVA risk are more severe anemia,[312] higher reticulocyte counts,[312] lower Hb F levels,[313] higher white cell counts,[314] and sickle cell anemia (rather than Hb SC disease or sickle cell-β-thalassemia). Genetic markers of

increased risk are the Central African Republic haplotype[315] and the absence of α-thalassemia.[315] Cerebral thrombosis, which accounts for 70–80% of all CVA in sickle cell disease,[308,316,317] results from large vessel occlusion[318–320] (Fig. 43-11), rather than the more typical microvascular occlusion of sickle cell disease. CVAs are heralded by focal seizures in 10–33% of cases[308,309,312] and by transient ischemic attacks in 10%.[308,311,317] CVAs are fatal in approximately 20% of initial cases, recurrent within 3 years in nearly 70%, and the cause of motor and cognitive impairment in the most.[308] Thrombosis occurs in all age groups; hemorrhage is confined to older patients.[308]

Intracranial hemorrhage results in the same signs as thrombosis, but neck stiffness, photophobia, severe headache, vomiting, and altered consciousness are more common. Coma suggests hemorrhage, rather than thrombosis.[312] A typical presentation is coma and seizures without hemiparesis. Although the mortality rate may be as high as 50%,[321–324] the

ACUTE CENTRAL NERVOUS SYSTEM EVENTS

Both children and adults with sickle cell disease have an increased risk of CVA. Patients with hemiparesis, seizures, coma, speech defects, or visual impairment should be evaluated for CVA. Cerebral thrombosis accounts for 70–80% of all CVA in sickle cell disease, causes death in approximately 20%, recurs within 3 years in 70%, and causes motor and cognitive impairment in the majority. Thrombosis occurs in all age groups, but hemorrhage is far more common in older patients. Intracranial hemorrhage results in the same signs as thrombosis, but neck stiffness, photophobia, severe headache, vomiting, and coma are more common. The mortality rate may be as high as 50%, but the morbidity of survivors is low.

Patients presenting with symptoms and signs of CVA should be evaluated immediately by CT scanning or MRI to distinguish cerebral thrombosis and hemorrhage. In patients with thrombosis, prompt partial exchange transfusion is performed, and chronic transfusion is begun to maintain the Hb S level <30% and prevent recurrent thrombosis. Those with hemorrhage should have angiography after partial exchange transfusion is performed to avoid complications associated with injected contrast material. Those hemorrhages due to ruptured aneurysm are particularly amenable to surgical intervention.

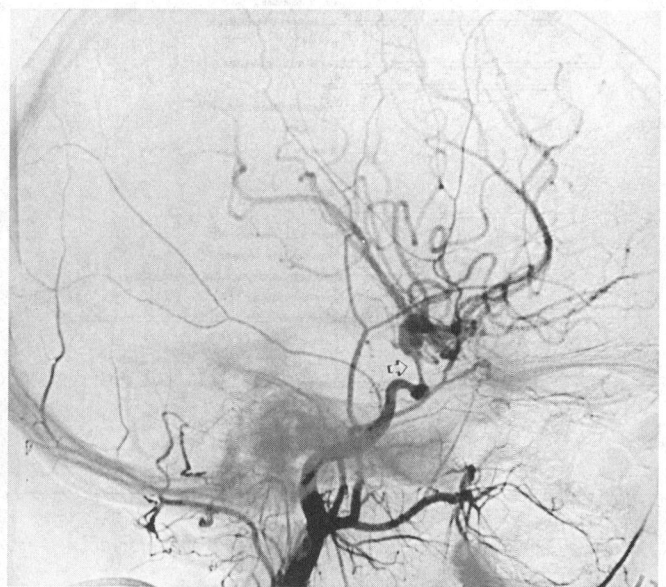

Fig. 43-11. Left common carotid arteriogram taken in lateral projection demonstrating high-grade stenosis of distal internal carotid artery (open arrow). This is a study of a 6-year-old boy with sickle cell disease who developed right-sided weakness and had extensive MRI evidence of prior cerebral infarction at the time of his first clinical symptoms. (Kindly provided by RJ Adams.)

morbidity of survivors is low.[325] Hemorrhage may be subarachnoid, intraparenchymal, or intraventricular, which can be differentiated by angiography.[322,323] In 30% of patients with sickle cell disease, major vessel stenosis results in the formation of friable collateral vessels that appear as puffs of smoke ("moyamoya" in Japanese) on angiography.[326] These pseudomoyamoya are vulnerable to both thrombosis and hemorrhage. The favorable neurosurgical outcome in subarachnoid hemorrhage due to ruptured aneurysm justifies an aggressive approach to diagnosis, transfusion, vasodilatory therapy, and surgery.[322,323,327]

Patients presenting with symptoms and signs of CVA should be evaluated immediately using computed tomography (CT) scanning or magnetic resonance imaging (MRI) to distinguish transient ischemic attacks, cerebral thrombosis, and hemorrhage. In those with hemorrhage, angiography is indicated, after partial exchange transfusion is performed to avoid complications associated with injected contrast material. In those with thrombosis, prompt partial exchange transfusion is performed and chronic direct transfusion to maintain the Hb S level <30% is instituted to prevent recurrent thrombosis[311,319] and promote resolution of arterial stenoses.[311,328] Although recurrent CVAs during chronic transfusion have been reported,[329] this therapeutic modality provides the current best means of preventing recurrence[319] (Fig. 43-12). After 5 years of red cell transfusion, clinical response and blood flow[328,330] are reassessed to guide the decision regarding discontinuing therapy. Transfusion therapy may be required indefinitely in those with persistent flow abnormalities. For those who recur soon after discontinuing therapy, indefinite transfusion is reinstituted.[331]

The occurrence of subclinical cerebral infarction has been detected by MRI, positron emission tomography, transcranial Doppler flow studies, and autopsy[332–336]; certain of these mo-

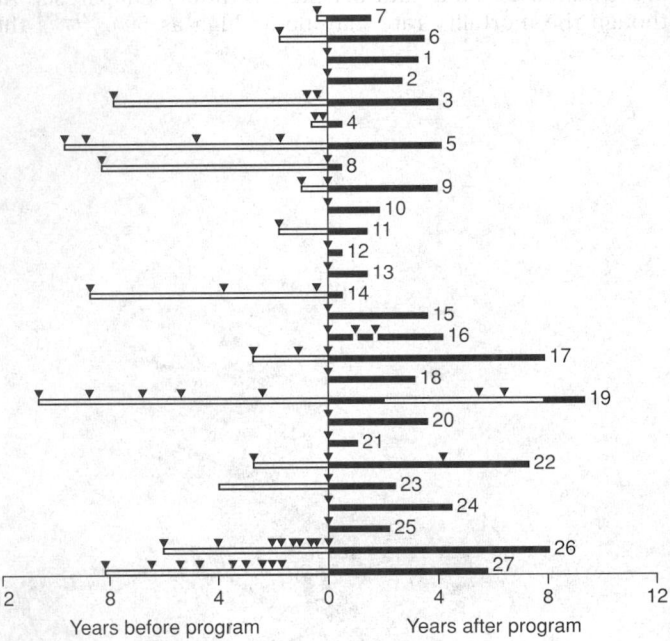

Fig. 43-12. Distribution of central nervous system episode in 27 patients with relationship to transfusion program (Tx). Empty bars indicate periods when no transfusions were given, filled bars indicate periods of chronic transfusion program, and arrow heads indicate central nervous system episodes. The central vertical line separates the untransfused from the transfused periods. (Adapted from Sarnaik et al.,[319] with permission.)

ACUTE CHEST SYNDROME

Symptoms and signs of the acute chest syndrome include dyspnea, cough, chest pain, less commonly abdominal pain, fever, tachypne, leukocytosis, and a pulmonary infiltrate on the chest radiograph. This event that has an approximate 10% risk of mortality. The process is usually due to infection or vaso-occlusion, but it may also be the result of noncardiogenic pulmonary edema or of pulmonary embolization from a distant thrombus or bone marrow infarction. Responsible infectious agents include *S. pneumoniae, H. influenzae, Mycoplasma, Chlamydia, Legionella,* and viruses. Infection with pyogenic bacteria is more common in children than in adults, and the urgency to initiate therapy is greater in the pediatric population. In adults, the decision to initiate antibiotics is a matter of clinical judgment. Antibiotic coverage include *S. pneumoniae, H. influenzae* type b, *M. pneumoniae,* and *C. pneumoniae* (e.g., cefuroxime and erythromycin.)

Whatever the etiology, the major danger of the acute chest syndrome is hypoxemia and its attendant widespread sickling and vaso-occlusion, which create a risk of multiorgan failure. The tachypneic patient should be evaluated with arterial blood gas measurements to distinguish metabolic acidosis, hypoxemia, and anxiety. Thereafter, hypoxemia can be followed by pulse oximetry. If a paO_2 >70 mmHg cannot be maintained by oxygen inhalation, the patient is transferred to an intensive care unit, where an emergency partial exchange transfusion is performed. Again, there is a greater sense of urgency regarding hypoxemia in children than in adults, and many pediatricians elect partial exchange transfusion at the first sign of the acute chest syndrome. After transfusion, oxygenation is often rapidly improved despite continued radiographic abnormalities. Severe episodes may not respond to this therapy and require support with artificial ventilation or even extracorporeal membrane oxygenation while awaiting recovery.

dalities may be useful in predicting CVA.[336] Neurodevelopmental abnormalities resulting in poor school performance may be the outcome of silent cerebral infarcts.[337] It remains to be determined whether transfusion therapy should be instituted when premorbid lesions are detected.

Pulmonary Complications

Sickle cell disease has both acute and chronic pulmonary manifestations. The acute chest syndrome consists of dyspnea, chest pain, fever, tachypnea, pulmonary infiltrate on radiograph, and leukocytosis. It affects approximately 30% of patients with sickle cell disease and may be life-threatening.[303,338] The usual etiology is vaso-occlusion or infection, or both simultaneously.[339] Antibiotics are often indicated as therapy. Microbial pathogens are more commonly identified in children.[339] Many episodes in which common pathogens are not cultured are due to "atypical" agents, *Mycoplasma, Legionella,* and *Chlamydia,*[303,304] suggesting a role for erythromycin therapy. Less common etiologies are marrow embolus following bone marrow necrosis[340] and noncardiogenic pulmonary edema.[341] Some patients have a rapidly progressive course associated with a precipitous decrease in arterial oxygen tension, which may require intensive care.[339] When arterial oxygen tension cannot be maintained at >70 mmHg with inhaled oxygen, par-

RIGHT UPPER QUADRANT SYNDROME

An acute complication manifest by some or all of the following features—hyperbilirubinemia, abdominal pain, fever, right upper quadrant abdominal tenderness, hepatomegaly, abnormal liver function tests, and hepatic failure—has been called the right upper quadrant syndrome. Possible etiologies include cholelithiasis, viral hepatitis, biliary cholestasis, and hepatic ischemia. Hemoglobin levels usually do not change greatly. An asymptomatic syndrome of benign cholestasis associated with severe hyperbilirubinemia that resolves within 7–10 days has been reported in children. A syndrome more common in adults is associated with fever, leukocytosis, abdominal pain, and deteriorating liver function tests. This hepatic crisis usually progresses to hepatic failure, coagulopathy, and death. This syndrome appears to be caused by hepatic ischemia, but viral hepatitis may produce the same clinical picture. Because of the nearly uniform mortality of this type of hepatic crisis, exchange transfusion and plasmapheresis have been used as therapy. No control data are available to support this approach.

tial exchange transfusion is indicated.[306] Under extreme circumstances, artificial ventilation and cardiopulmonary bypass have been used.[342]

Evaluation of pulmonary status in patients with sickle cell anemia indicates chronic restrictive lung disease, hypoxemia, and pulmonary hypertension singly or in combination, not restricted to those with past history of acute chest syndrome.[343-345] Etiologies unrelated to prior acute episodes may relate to chronic vascular insufficiency[174] or to oxidative damage mediated by free plasma Hb S.[346] Blood gas and pulmonary function measurements should be established as baseline data for all patients.

Hepatobiliary Complications

The prevalence of pigmented gallstones in sickle cell disease is directly related to the rate of hemolysis.[347] In sickle cell anemia, gallstones occur in children as young as 3–4 years of age[348] and are eventually found in approximately 70% of patients.[349] Some have recommended the surgical removal of asymptomatic gallstones to avoid subsequent difficulty in distinguishing gallbladder pain from acute painful episodes.[350] This approach has become more feasible with the availability of laparoscopic cholecystectomy.[351]

The common hepatomegaly and liver dysfunction in sickle cell disease is related to intrahepatic trapping of sickle cells, transfusion-acquired infection, and transfusional hemosiderosis.[352] Histologic examination of the liver shows centrilobular parenchymal atrophy, bile pigment, periportal fibrosis, hemosiderosis, and cirrhosis. In addition to infection with hepatitis viruses, acute hepatic episodes are unique to sickle cell disease. In all these cases, the combination of hemolysis, hepatic dysfunction, and renal tubular defects result in strikingly high serum bilirubin levels, sometimes >100 mg/dl.[353] One of these syndromes, benign cholestasis of sickle cell disease, results in severe asymptomatic hyperbilirubinemia without fever, pain, leukocytosis, hepatic failure, or mortality.[354] A far graver event is the "hepatic crisis," in which hepatic ischemia results in fever, pain, leukocytosis, severe hyperbilirubinemia, and abnormal liver function tests.[355] Crisis may progress to liver failure, which has a dismal prognosis.[356,357]

Obstetric and Gynecologic Issues

Although gynecologic complications delayed menarche, dysmenorrhea, ovarian cysts, pelvic infection, and fibrocystic disease of the breast are more frequent in women with sickle cell disease,[358] the major reproductive concern in these patients is pregnancy. The fetal complications of pregnancy, most of which are related to compromised placental blood flow, are the increased incidence of spontaneous abortion, intrauterine growth retardation, pre-eclampsia, low birthweight, and mortality; maternal complications include increased rates of painful episodes, severe anemia, infections, and mortality.[359-362] The course of pregnancy is more benign in Hb SC disease than in sickle cell anemia.[360,361] Better fetal and maternal outcomes in recent years are largely due to generally improved antenatal and obstetric care.[362] An unresolved specific issue pertains to the role of transfusions in pregnancy.[363] On the basis of personal experience, some experts recommend prophylactic transfusion,[364] but a large controlled study showed no improvement in fetal outcome from this management option.[365] The type of delivery does not appear to represent a problem. Both spontaneous delivery and cesarean section are well tolerated.

Some experts advise that hypertonic saline injections are contraindicated for elective termination of pregnancy, because of the risk of sickling-induced vaso-occlusion. However, most methods of abortion are well tolerated. The very high incidence of acute painful episodes following therapeutic abortion (personal observation) supports the use of inpatient intravenous hydration before and for the 24 hours after the procedure.

Oral contraceptives containing low-dose estrogen are a safe and recommended method of birth control.[366] The choice of barrier methods, oral contraception, and injections of medroxyprogesterone every 3 months for birth control must weigh the risk versus benefit of each.

Renal Complications

The kidney is particularly vulnerable to complications in sickle cell disease because of its hypoxic, acidotic, and hypertonic microenvironment.[189,367] Clinical manifestations result from medullary and distal tubular, proximal tubular, and glomerular abnormalities. Occlusion of the vasa rectae compromises flow to the medulla (Fig. 43-13), resulting in an inability to concentrate the urine, as well as papillary infarction with hematuria, incomplete renal tubular acidosis, and abnormal potassium metabolism. Isosthenuria, reversible with red cell transfusion at ≤15 years of age, accounts for a propensity to dehydration when fluid intake is insufficient.[368,369]

A common complication is hematuria from papillary infarction, which is usually unilateral from the left kidney, may be massive, and appears more common in sickle cell trait than disease because of the much greater frequency of the heterozygous condition.[370] Patients with sickle cell disease or trait who have hematuria must be evaluated to exclude life-threatening etiologies. This can be accomplished using ultrasonography, which obviates the risks associated with contrast material in intravenous pyelography. Therapy with hydration, alkalinization of the urine, and diuresis is standard,[371,372] but ε-aminocaproic acid,[373] triglycyl vasopressin,[374] intravenous distilled water,[371] and nephrectomy[375] have been required.

Patients with sickle cell disease are unable to excrete acid and potassium normally. They usually do not develop systemic acidosis or hyperkalemia without an additional acid load such as renal insufficiency.[376] Abnormal proximal tubular function, partly related to chronic use of analgesics, results in increased clearance of uric acid[377] and creatinine and reabsorption of phosphate.[378]

Glomerular abnormalities result from vaso-occlusion, hyper-

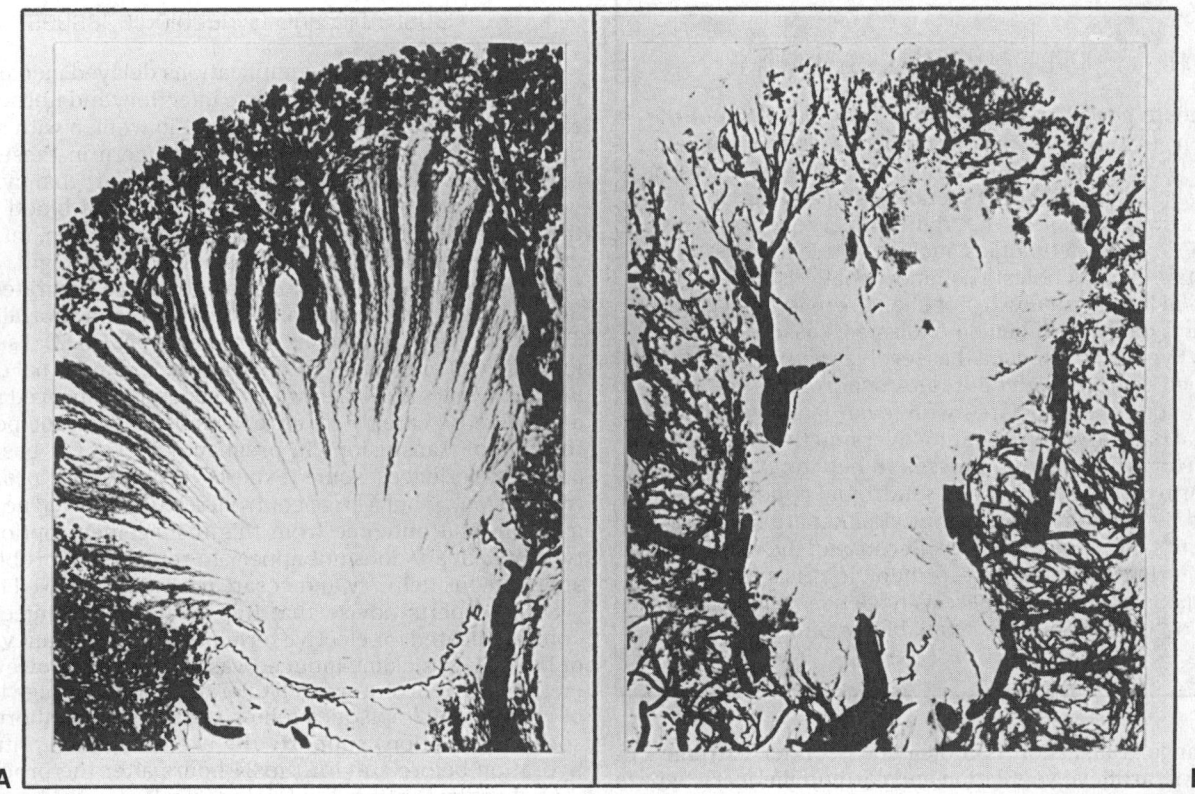

Fig. 43-13. Postmortem microangiographic studies of the vasa recta. **(A)** Normal individual. **(B)** Patient with sickle cell anemia. (From Statius van Eps et al.,[566] with permission.)

perfusion, and immune complex nephropathy. Chronic renal insufficiency may be preceded by hypertension, proteinuria, hyperkalemia, or worsening anemia. The average age of onset is 23 years in sickle cell anemia and 50 years in Hb SC disease.[379] Therapy with an inhibitor of angiotensin-converting enzyme was used to diminish hyperperfusion and was found to diminish proteinuria, but not to improve glomerular filtration rate.[380] Renal transplantation is effective therapy for end-stage renal disease in sickle cell syndromes.[381]

Priapism

Priapism has been defined as an unwanted painful erection. It affects nearly two-thirds of males with sickle cell disease,[382] peak frequencies are at ages 5–13 years and at 21–29 years,[383] and it is most likely to develop in patients with lower Hb F levels and reticulocyte counts, increased platelet counts, and the Hb SS genotype. Onset can be acute, recurrent, chronic, acute on chronic, or "stuttering."[384] The engorgement in priapism affects the corpora cavernosum but spares the glans penis and corpus spongiosum.[385] As a result of recurrent priapism, sickle cell patients have abnormal nocturnal penile tumescence and scarred fibrotic corpora,[386] which may eventuate in impotence. In some patients, generally those who are postpubertal, the engorgement also affects the corpus spongiosum and glans[387]; tricorporal priapism can be diagnosed by means of nuclear scanning of the penis.[388] Impotence is more frequent in tricorporal priapism.[387]

One successful approach to therapy[389] entails monitoring responses to therapy by intercavernous pressure measurements and to transfusion therapy by quantitative hemoglobin electrophoresis. First-line therapy is conservative consisting of intravenous hydration and analgesia. If priapism persists for 12 hours, partial exchange transfusion[390] is performed to reduce the Hb S level to <30%. If no resolution ensues within 12 hours of transfusion, corporal aspiration with saline and α-adrenergic agents is recommended.[391] If there is still no response within 12 hours of irrigation, surgery is recommended.[392] The procedure of choice is the Winter procedure, creating a fistula between the glans penis and the corpora cav-

PRIAPISM

Priapism affects nearly two-thirds of males with sickle cell disease. It is typically bicorporal, affecting the corpora cavernosum and sparing the glans penis and corpus spongiosum. Tricorporal priapism is less common, also affects the corpus spongiosum and glans, and more frequently results in impotence. Recommended management includes monitoring response to therapy by intercavernous pressure measurements and to transfusion therapy by quantitative hemoglobin electrophoresis. Initial therapy consists of intervenous hydration and analgesia. If priapism persists for 12 hours, partial exchange transfusion intended to reduce the Hb S level to <30% is performed. If there is no resolution within 12 hours of transfusion, corporal aspiration with saline and α-adrenergic agents is recommended. If there is no response within 12 hours of irrigation, surgery is recommended. The Winter procedure of creating a fistula between the glans penis and the corpora cavernosum by inserting a large-bore needle through the glans under general anesthesia is the procedure of choice. If the problem does not resolve after the Winter procedure, the Grayhack saphenous vein bypass shunt is recommended.

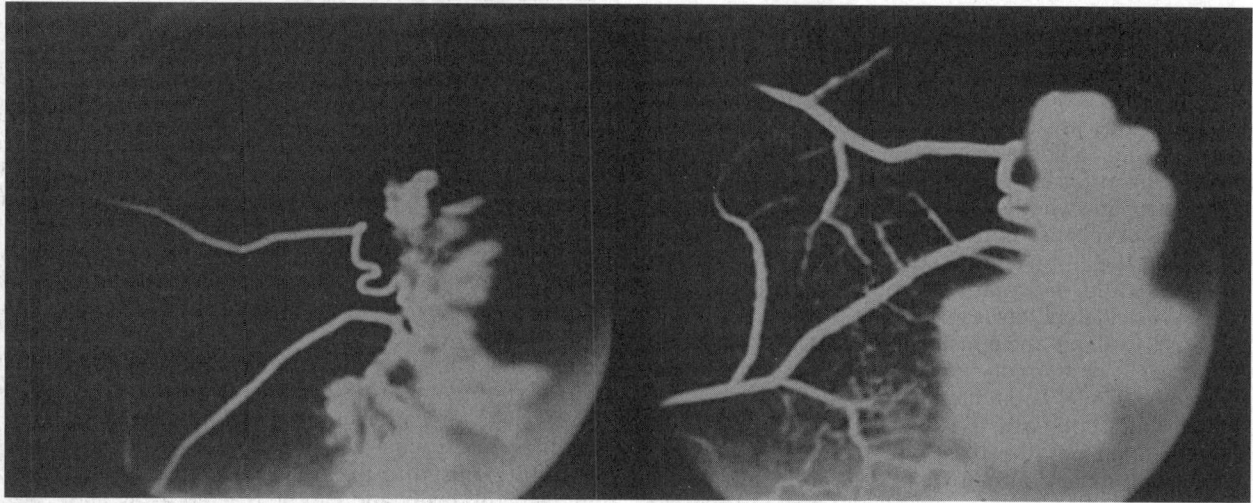

Fig. 43-14. Flourescein angiography demonstrating a "sea fan" appearance of sickle proliferative retinopathy. (Kindly provided by WC Mentzer.)

ernosum by insertion of a large-bore needle through the glans under general anesthesia.[393] If this is unsuccessful, the creation of a more formal shunt, such as the Grayhack saphenous vein bypass, may be attempted.[394] Whether conservative or aggressive therapy is used, 45% of patients who have priapism will develop some degree of impotence. When impotence persists for 12 months, implantation of a semirigid penile prosthesis may be considered.[395]

Ocular Complications

Ophthalmologic complications can include anterior chamber ischemia, tortuosity of conjunctival vessels, retinal artery occlusion, angioid streaks, proliferative retinopathy, and retinal detachment and hemorrhage.[396,397] The retina is particularly vulnerable to vaso-occlusion. Routine retinal examination is part of routine health care maintenance for patients with sickle cell disease. Superficial retinal hemorrhages have a pink "salmon patch" appearance that resolves into an iridescent schisis cavity. Deeper retinal hemorrhages have a "black sunburst" appearance. The retinopathy is often seen best using fluorescein angiography (Fig. 43-14). The earlier onset and greater frequency of proliferative retinopathy in Hb SC disease and sickle cell-β^+-thalassemia than in sickle cell anemia and sickle cell-β°-thalassemia[398] suggest that retinal vessels are more susceptible to occlusion by more viscous blood than by more rigid individual cells. Peripheral sickle retinopathy may require vision-saving therapy with laser photocoagulation.[399]

Bone Complications

Chronic tower skull, bossing of the forehead, and fishmouth deformity of vertebrae are the result of extended hematopoietic marrow causing widening of the medullary space, thinning of the trabeculae and cortices, and osteoporosis.[400] Osteonecrosis may cause a step-like depression of vertebrae, selected shortening of the cuboidal bones of the hands and feet, and acute "aseptic or avascular necrosis."[401] The excruciating pain of bone infarction in the "hand-foot syndrome" that occurs around the age of 2 years is often the first symptom of

sickle cell disease[402] (Fig. 43-15). This dactylitis resolves spontaneously and is treated with hydration and analgesia. Bone infarcts are demonstrable using nuclear medicine scintigraphy or MRI.[403–405] Serial scans specific for bone osteoclasts, bone marrow macrophages, and inflammatory cells may be useful adjuncts for distinguishing bone marrow infarction from osteomyelitis,[403] but it is essential to obtain cultures directly from the affected tissue before starting antibiotics. Treatment of osteomyelitis is addressed in the sections Infection and Therapy.

Infarction of bone trabeculae and marrow cells causing osteonecrosis occurs in all sickle cell disease genotypes, but most frequently in sickle cell anemia with coexistent α-thalassemia.[136,406] The process is associated with increased intraosseous pressure[407] and is most sensitively detected by MRI.[408]

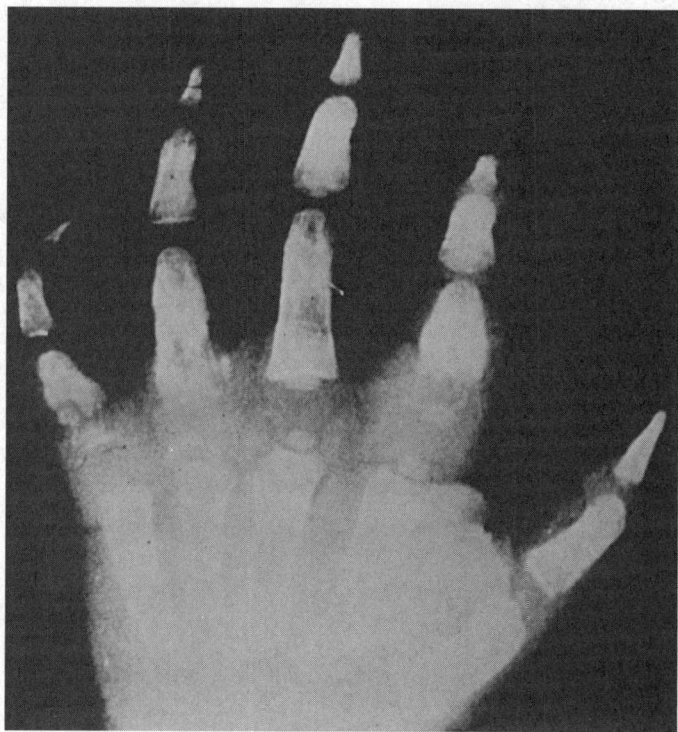

Fig. 43-15. Radiogram showing the bone infarctions in the hands of a child with hand-foot syndrome dactylitis. (Kindly provided by WC Mentzer.)

Necrosis occurs with equal frequency in the femoral and humeral heads, but the femoral heads more commonly undergo progressive joint destruction, as a result of chronic weight bearing.[136,137,409] Core decompression surgery to relieve increased intraosseous pressure can be used in early-stage osteonecrosis (i.e., no radiographic evidence of bone collapse) to prevent disease progression.[407] In more advanced disease, a choice must be made whether to accept limited joint mobility or to attempt major reconstructive therapy. This decision must take into account the 30% likelihood that a second hip revision will be required within 4–5 years of prosthetic hip placement in patients with sickle cell disease.[136]

Arthritic pain, swelling, and effusion may be related to periarticular infarction[410] or to gouty arthritis.[411] Appropriate therapy is with nonsteroidal anti-inflammatory agents.

Bone marrow infarction causes reticulocytopenia, exacerbation of anemia, a leukoerythroblastic picture, and sometimes pancytopenia. Pulmonary fat embolism is a rare complication of marrow infarction.[412] It is associated with fat globules in the sputum[412] and refractile bodies visible in the optic fundi.[413] This life-threatening event may require prompt exchange transfusion, and perhaps the use of heparin and corticosteroids.[412]

Dermatologic Complications

Leg ulcers are a major cause of morbidity in sickle cell disease as a result of their frequency, chronicity, and resistance to therapy. Most occur near the medial or lateral malleolus (Fig. 43-16); they are frequently bilateral.[414,415] They may begin spontaneously or as a result of trauma and may become infected, most commonly by *S. aureus Pseudomonas, Streptococcus,* or *Bacteroides*.[416] Systemic infection, osteomyelitis, and tetanus are rare complications.[414] Ulcers are resistant to healing[417] and tend to be recurrent in well over one-half of cases.[416] Their incidence has been reported to vary from 0%[418] to 75%.[414] Ulcers rarely occur before 10 years of age and are most common in sickle cell anemia, less common in sickle cell-β^{0}-thalassemia, and nonexistent in Hb SC disease and sickle cell-β^{+}-thalassemia.[415] The incidence in sickle cell anemia patients declines substantially in those who have coexistent α-thalassemia.[415] Males have a threefold greater risk of developing leg ulcers than that of females.[414,415]

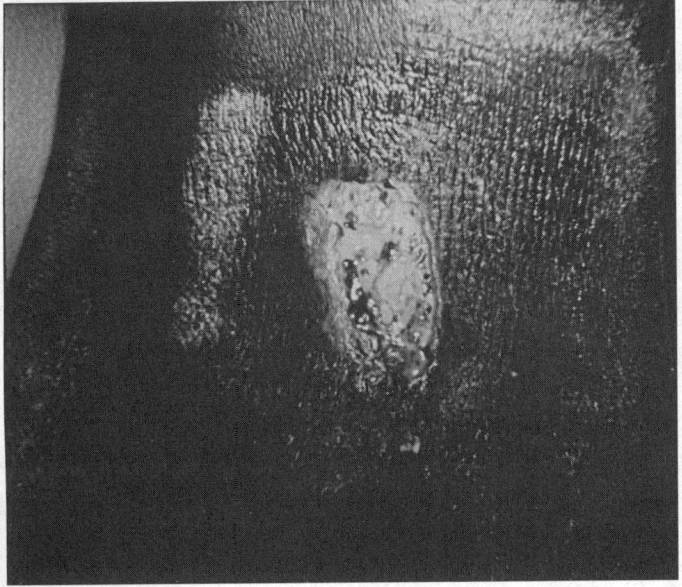

Fig. 43-16. Chronic leg ulcer near the medial malleolus. (Kindly provided by WC Mentzer.)

SKIN ULCERS

Leg ulcers occur in patients with sickle cell disease beginning in the adolescent years. They usually occur near the lateral or medial malleoli and may become chronic and debilitating. Their pathogenesis presumably is related to vaso-occlusion in the skin microvasculature leading to tissue necrosis. It occurs most commonly in males, those with more severe anemia, and those with lower Hb F levels. Treatment of leg ulcers begins with cleansing, debridement, and topical antibiotics. Gentle debridement to remove nonviable, superficial tissue from more vital areas can be achieved using wet-to-dry dressings or Duoderm hydrocolloid dressings. Once debridement is complete, zinc oxide-impregnated Unna boots are used to promote healing. Leg edema retards healing of ulcers and can be treated using elastic wraps or leg elevation. Trauma to the area is to be minimized, and shoes must be selected accordingly. Transfusions may be required. Skin grafting has been successful in the most recalcitrant cases.

Treatment of leg ulcers requires persistence and patience; healing usually requires weeks. Therapy begins with gentle debridement to remove nonviable superficial tissue from more vital areas. Wet to dry dressings and Duoderm hydrocolloid dressings facilitate devitalization. Once debridement is complete, zinc oxide-impregnated Unna boots are used to promote healing. Bed rest speeds healing[419] and topical antibiotics may be required.[420] It may be necessary to use elastic wraps or leg elevation to control edema. Oral zinc, local hyperbaric oxygen, chronic transfusion, recombinant erythropoietin, hydroxyurea, skin grafts, and pentoxifylline are unproven modalities that may be tried.

Myofascial syndromes consist of soft tissue swelling in subcutaneous edema that may have a peau d'orange appearance. These may be large or discrete lesions of a few centimeters in diameter. These lesions are probably the result of dermal or subdermal vaso-occlusion. Treatment is symptomatic.

Cardiac Complications

Despite the lack of convincing evidence for a specific cardiomyopathy in sickle cell disease, there are important cardiac considerations in the management of these patients. The chronic anemia of sickle cell disease is compensated by high cardiac output,[421] which results in chronic chamber enlargement and cardiomegaly,[422] even in young children.[423] While exercise capacity of sickle cell patients is diminished,[424] congestive heart failure is uncommon,[425] and restriction of activity is seldom necessary. An age-dependent loss of cardiac reserve[426] creates a greater risk of heart failure in adult patients during fluid overload, transfusion, reduced oxygen-carrying capacity, or hypertension.[422] Cardiac function can be improved by transfusion.[427] The electrocardiogram shows evidence of left ventricular hypertrophy and less often first-degree block and nonspecific ST-T wave changes.[428] Acute myocardial infarction in the absence of coronary disease has been reported,[429] and in one autopsy series 17% of 70 consecutive patients with sickle cell disease had had myocardial infarction.[430] It appears that when increased oxygen demand exceeds a limited oxygen carrying capacity, there is a risk of myocardial infarction despite normal coronary arteries.

VARIANT SICKLE CELL SYNDROMES

The sickle cell syndromes that result from inheritance of the sickle cell gene in simple heterozygosity or in compound heterozygosity with other mutant β-globin genes are sickle cell trait, Hb SC disease, and sickle cell-β-thalassemia. These and sickle cell anemia with coexistent α-thalassemia are reviewed in this section.

Sickle Cell Trait

The prevalence of sickle cell trait is approximately 8–10% in African-Americans[57] and as high as 25–30% in certain areas of western Africa.[58] Approximately 2.5 million people in the United States and 30 million in the world are heterozygous for the sickle cell gene. Sickle cell trait is a benign carrier condition[126] with no hematologic manifestations—red cell morphology, red cell indices, and the reticulocyte count are normal, and sickle forms (ISCs) are not seen on the peripheral blood smear. The usual partition of Hb A and Hb S in sickle cell trait is 60:40 due to a greater post-translational affinity of α-chains for β^A than for β^S chains.[431] When α-thalassemia is co-inherited with sickle cell trait, this preferential affinity for a limiting pool of free α-chains results in a decreasing percentage of hemoglobin S according to the number of α-globin genes deleted (i.e., αα/αα, 40% Hb S;–α/αα, 35% Hb S;–α/–α, 29% Hb S;––/–α, 21% Hb S).[79]

Few clinical complications of sickle cell trait have been reported.[126] Splenic infarction occurs at high altitude,[432] curiously more commonly in whites than in those of African ancestry.[433] It must be remembered that sickle cell trait is a common cause of hematuria among African-Americans.[434] Impaired urinary concentrating ability is directly related to the intraerythrocytic concentration of Hb S and, therefore, to the number of α-globin genes inherited.[127] The degree of hyposthenuria in children progresses with age, and up to a certain age is reversed by transfusion.[435] The frequency of urinary tract infection may be increased in sickle cell trait.[436,437] The incidence of anesthetic complications is not increased.[438] The 30-fold increased incidence of unexplained sudden death during basic training of military recruits with sickle cell trait was apparently related to exercise-induced vaso-occlusion and rhabdomyolysis.[439]

Despite the known complications, past experience with discrimination in the employment market and health insurance industry provides reminders that the rare clinical events in sickle cell trait provide no real justification for regarding it as anything but a benign carrier condition.[440] Newborn screening programs detect a large number of infants with sickle cell trait for whose parents genetic counseling is essential. Parents should understand that their child has a benign hereditary condition not a disease but that there is a risk of a subsequent child being born with sickle cell disease.

In individuals who appear to have sickle cell trait but who are symptomatic, the laboratory diagnosis must be verified. Hemoglobins other than S can polymerize. These may account for reports of "sickle cell trait" associated with clinical problems. Examples are heterozygous Hb S^Antilles[441] and Hb Quebec-CHORI[442] In the latter case, the hemoglobin variant was distinguished from Hb A using mass spectroscopy.

Hb SC Disease

The allele for Hb C is approximately one-fourth as frequent among African-Americans as the sickle cell allele,[57] accounting for correspondent prevalences of Hb SC disease and sickle cell anemia. Although oxygenated Hb C forms crystals,[443] Hb C does not participate in polymerization with deoxy-Hb S.[128] The red cell desiccation that results from the altered potassium-chloride co-transport due to the presence of Hb C[129,130] raises the intraerythrocytic concentration of Hb S[128,129] to levels that support polymerization, sickling, and clinical symptoms (see the section Cationic Homeostasis and Cell Dehydration).

Compound heterozygosity for Hb S and C results in a disease that is generally less severe than sickle cell anemia.[444,445] Splenomegaly may be the only physical finding, and clinical complications may be less frequent than in sickle cell anemia. As a result of a longer circulatory survival of Hb SC red cells compared to Hb SS cells (i.e., 27 versus 17 days),[222] the degree of anemia and reticulocytosis is frequently milder, with three-fourths of patients having a milder level of anemia (hematocrit level >28%) than is usually seen in sickle cell anemia.[223] The predominant red cell abnormality on the peripheral smear is an abundance of target cells; folded (pita bread) cells, ISCs, "billiard ball" cells, and crystal-containing cells also may be seen.[446]

The great clinical heterogeneity within this genotype notwithstanding, its clinical course is generally milder than that of sickle cell anemia. The frequency of acute painful episodes is approximately one-half that of sickle cell anemia.[138] Life expectancy is two decades longer.[220] The incidence of fatal bacterial infection is less than in sickle cell anemia,[289] but there is still an increased risk of *S. pneumoniae* and *H. influenzae* infection.[447] Leg ulcers are uncommon.[415] The incidence of peripheral retinopathy in Hb SC disease is higher than in sickle cell anemia,[398] but the higher incidence of osteonecrosis reported[448] has been disproven.[136]

Sickle Cell-β-Thalassemia

The gene frequency of β-thalassemia among African-Americans is 0.004, one-tenth that of the sickle cell gene.[57] This population displays commensurately one-tenth the prevalence of compound heterozygous sickle cell-β thalassemia. Sickle cell-β-thalassemia is divided into sickle cell-β⁺-thalassemia and sickle cell-β°-thalassemia, in which, respectively, no or reduced amounts of Hb A is present.[449,450] Most β-thalassemia mutations among African-Americans result in β⁺-thalassemia.[451,452] Sickle cell-β⁺-thalassemia is subclassified according to the percentage of Hb A present: type I has 3–5%, type II has 8–14%, and type III has 18–25%.[451,453] Eighty percent of African-American β-thalassemia mutations are due to the promoter region mutations (−88 [C→T] and −29 [A→G]) that result in a type III phenotype.[451,452] Compound heterozygous sickle cell-β°-thalassemia occurs infrequently.

The hematologic and clinical severity is a function of the amount of Hb A inherited.[453,454] In sickle cell-β-thalassemia, the red cells are hypochromic and microcytic. The ISCs present on the peripheral blood smear are more numerous in sickle cell-β°-thalassemia than in sickle cell-β⁺-thalassemia. The hematologic severity is an inverse function of the amount of Hb A inherited, as demonstrated in Table 43-1.

The more benign clinical nature of sickle cell-β⁺-thalassemia compared to sickle cell-β°-thalassemia is reflected by its three-fold higher incidence of incidental diagnosis (26% versus 9%), later mean age of presentation (8.2 years versus 3.2 years), approximately threefold less frequent leg ulcers (8% versus 23%), approximately one-half as frequent acute chest syndrome (14% versus 24%), priapism in 0 of 27 versus 4 of 28, and aplastic crises in 0 versus 2.[455] Splenomegaly occurred in approximately one-third of both groups. There was a higher incidence of proliferative retinopathy in sickle cell-β⁺-thalassemia (18% versus 10%), consistent with the notion that those sickle cell syndromes having higher hematocrits are more likely to be associated with ocular complications. Growth and development was more retarded in sickle cell-β°-thalassemia than in sickle cell-β⁺-thalassemia.[278]

Sickle Cell Anemia with Coexistent α-Thalassemia

The use of restriction endonuclease mapping to detect the α-globin gene deletions responsible for α-thalassemia[456,457] demonstrated a gene frequency of 0.16 for the α-thalassemia-2 haplotype (–α) among African-Americans—nearly one in three are silent carriers of α-thalassemia (genotype–α/αα), and 2% have α-thalassemia trait due to homozygous α-thalassemia-2 (genotype–α/–α).[80] This high frequency combined with the powerful effect of Hb S concentration on the kinetics[6] and extent[7] of Hb S polymerization suggested that the lower MCHC of thalassemia would influence the pathophysiology in a large number of patients with sickle cell anemia. This prediction was substantiated by the finding of milder anemia in subjects with sickle cell anemia who had the deletion of either one (genotype–α/αα) or two (genotype–α/–α) α-globin genes[83,84,86] (Table 43-2). This effect was related to a diminished hemolytic rate[85] and was not demonstrable until approximately 7 years of age[87,88] (Table 43-2). The mechanisms by which α-thalassemia benefits the hematologic aspects of sickle cell anemia are discussed in the section Cation Homeostasis and Cell Dehydration.

Besides milder anemia, α-thalassemia is associated with fewer reticulocytes[83,84,86] and ISCs.[82,84] The peripheral blood smear contains less polychromasia, fewer sickle forms, and more hypochromia and microcytosis, commensurate with the numbers of α-globin genes deleted. Increased Hb A₂ levels are associated with increasing α-globin gene deletions; the Hb F levels are not consistently affected.[83,84,86] The prediction of higher affinity of α- for γ-chains resulting in greater levels of Hb F when α-chains are limiting is not consistently realized, apparently because of the selective survival of α-thalassemic sickle cells which obscures the Hb F effect.[458]

The documented clinical effects of this epistatic interaction are not consistently beneficial. The reported decreased incidence of acute chest syndrome[84] was not substantiated in another study.[86] The incidence of leg ulcers is decreased,[84,415] but the incidence of osteonecrosis is increased.[136,137] The original suggestion of increased incidence of peripheral retinopathy[396] was related to the higher hemoglobin, mean corpuscular volume (MCV), and MCHC levels.[459] The frequency of retinal vessel closure is higher, but not the incidence of retinopathy.[460] A large multicenter study demonstrated a higher incidence of acute painful episodes associated with higher hemoglobin levels, but the influence of α-thalassemia did not extend beyond its influence on level of anemia.[138] While one group reported longer life expectancy in subjects having sickle cell anemia and α-thalassemia,[131,461] a large multi-institutional national study documented an increased mortality rate associated higher hemoglobin levels in patients >20 years of age.[138] The mixed effects of α-thalassemia on sickle cell anemia demonstrate the inadvisability of extrapolating broadly from polymerization formulas to assumptions of disease severity.[74]

Sickle Cell-δβ°-Thalassemia

δβ-Thalassemia usually results from large deletion of the δ- and β-globin genes that fail to retard the switch from Hb F to Hb A production, thereby allowing an attempted switch from the expression of γ-globin to that of deleted genes (see Chs. 35 and 42). This uncommon compound heterozygous condition is associated with Hb S, F, and A₂ with the 15–25% Hb F distrib-

uted in a heterocellular fashion. Anemia and reticulocytosis are mild and clinical complications infrequent.[462]

Sickle Cell-Hereditary Persistence of Fetal Hemoglobin

HPFH results from one of several large deletions of the δ- and β-globin genes that retard the switch from the production of Hb F to Hb A (see Chs. 35 and 42). A more recently discovered variety of HPFH is not due to a deletion, but to one of many point mutations that up-regulate the expression of the γ-globin gene. The clinical expression of deletional and nondeletional HPFH differs in that the 15–35% Hb F in the former is distributed in a pancellular fashion, the 1–5% Hb F in the latter is distributed in a heterocellular fashion. Certain mild types of nondeletional HPFH express high Hb F levels only in conditions of erythropoietic stress, such as compound heterozygosity with the sickle cell gene. It is likely that many cases of apparent sickle cell anemia with unexplained elevations of Hb F are the result of a nondeletion HPFH mutation.

The gene frequency of the deletional HPFH locus is 0.0005 among African-Americans,[463] resulting in a calculated incidence for compound heterozygous sickle cell-deletional HPFH of 1/100 that of sickle cell anemia. Sickle cell-deletional HPFH provided the first evidence that Hb F was a potent inhibitor of Hb S polymerization—individuals with pancellular distribution of 25% Hb F were generally neither anemic nor afflicted with vaso-occlusive manifestations[187] (Table 43-1). Hemoglobin electrophoresis revealed only Hb S, F, and A₂, which resembles sickle cell anemia, sickle cell-β°-thalassemia, and sickle cell-δβ°-thalassemia. Distinguishing features of sickle cell-HPFH are the pancellular distribution of 15–35% Hb F, Hb A₂ levels of <2.5%, and the absence of anemia.[464] The generally benign course of sickle cell-deletional HPFH is uncommonly associated with vaso-occlusive complication.[187]

Sickle Cell-Hb Lepore Disease

The Hb Lepore gene is a crossover fusion product of the δ- and β-globin genes, the product of which, in the case of Hb Lepore Boston, has the same alkaline electrophoretic mobility as Hb S. Because of the thalassemic expression of the fusion gene, individuals with simple heterozygosity for Hb Lepore Boston resemble on hemoglobin electrophoresis sickle cell trait with only 12% Hb S. Compound heterozygous Hb S-Hb Lepore Boston resembles sickle cell anemia or sickle cell-β°-thalassemia electrophoretically, but has less severe anemia, resembling that of sickle cell-β⁺-thalassemia. The combination of predominantly Hb S with microcytosis suggests sickle cell-β-thalassemia, but this diagnosis is suggested by the low to low-normal Hb A₂ levels that result from the incapacitation of one δ-globin gene by the crossover. Hb F levels vary. The peripheral smear shows microcytosis, hypochromia, and ISCs. Vaso-occlusive complications occur, and splenomegaly is common.[465]

Sickle Cell-Hb D Disease

Because Hb D Punjab, also called Hb D Los Angeles ($\alpha_2\beta_2^{121\text{-}Glu\rightarrow Gln}$), has a similar electrophoretic mobility to Hb S under alkali conditions, Hb SD disease was first reported as an unusual case of sickle cell anemia.[466] Hb D can be distinguished from Hb S by acid electrophoresis or isoelectric focusing. There is moderately severe hemolytic anemia, and the peripheral smear shows marked anisocytosis and poikilocytosis, target cells, and ISCs. The clinical manifestations of this syndrome are similar to those of sickle cell anemia.[467]

Sickle Cell-Hb O Arab Disease

Although Hb O Arab ($\alpha_2\beta_2^{121Glu\rightarrow Lys}$) was first described in an Israeli Arab family,[468] its distribution is widespread. Sickle cell-O Arab disease resembles Hb SC disease on alkaline electrophoresis, but Hb O Arab can be distinguished from Hb C by either acid electrophoresis or isoelectric focusing. This syndrome is associated with moderately severe hemolytic anemia, and the peripheral smear shows anisocytosis, poikilocytosis, and ISCs.[469]

Sickle Cell-Hb E Disease

Hb E ($\alpha_2\beta_2^{26Glu\rightarrow Lys}$) is a β-thalassemic hemoglobinopathy found predominantly in southeast Asia (see Chs. 42 and 44). The structural mutant has an electrophoretic mobility similar to Hb C under alkaline conditions[470,471] but can be resolved by acid electrophoresis or isoelectric focusing. The GAG→AAG mutation in codon 26 activates a cryptic splice site within the first intron of the β^E gene causing alternate splicing and decreased expression of the structural mutant.[472] As a result, Hb E comprises only 30% of the total hemoglobin in compound heterozygosity for the sickle cell and Hb E genes. Hb SE disease is reported to cause mild hemolysis, no vaso-occlusive complications, and no remarkable abnormality of red blood cell morphology.[473–475] However, one report documented hematuria and a probable splenic infarct during air travel[476] and another described moderately severe hemolysis, jaundice, bone pain, splenic infarction, recurrent pneumonia and ISCs on the peripheral blood smear. Those patients with Hb SE disease having vaso-occlusive complications justify the inclusion of this syndrome among the sickle cell diseases.

DIAGNOSIS

Both the methods of diagnosing sickle cell syndromes and the goals of diagnostic programs vary depending on the developmental stage of the subject. Characterization of adult hemoglobins is challenging in the fetal and newborn periods because of the predominance of Hb F, which confounds reliable detection of Hb S by solubility testing. In infancy, the diagnosis of sickle cell disease is also influenced by the absence of anemia. As Hb S increases and Hb F declines during the first months of life (Fig. 43-7), the clinical manifestations of sickle cell disease emerge.[478] ISCs can be seen in the peripheral blood of children with sickle cell anemia at 3 months of age, and by 4 months of age moderately severe hemolytic anemia is evident. Useful diagnostic methods include those that separate hemoglobin species according to amino acid composition (i.e., hemoglobin electrophoresis or thin-layer isoelectric focusing) (Fig. 43-17), solubility testing, and examination of the peripheral blood smear[5,479,480] (Fig. 43-2).

Older Children and Adults

The purpose of correct diagnosis in this age group is to identify those who need therapy for sickle cell disease and counseling for the disease or the trait. Cellulose acetate electrophoresis at pH 8.4 is a standard method of separating Hb S from other variants. However, Hb S, G, and D have the same electrophoretic mobility with this method. Using citrate agar electrophoresis at pH 6.2, Hb S has a different mobility than Hb D and G, which co-migrate with Hb A in this system. A solubility test such as the Sickledex also distinguishes Hb D and G from Hb S—only Hb S precipitates. Thus, the combination of cellulose acetate electrophoresis with either citrate agar electro-

---

SICKLE CELL DISEASE DIAGNOSIS

Diagnosis of sickle cell syndromes (genotypes) employs examination of the peripheral smear, solubility testing, and hemoglobin electrophoresis (or thin-layer isoelectric focusing).

The peripheral smear is normal in sickle cell trait (Hb AS), but sickle cells are seen in each of the major sickle cell disease syndromes—sickle cell anemia (Hb SS), Hb SC disease (Hb SC), and sickle cell-β-thalassemia (Hb S-β-thal).

Solubility tests are abnormal in all syndromes having at least one sickle cell gene—sickle cell trait (Hb AS), sickle cell anemia (Hb SS), Hb SC disease (Hb SC), and sickle cell-β-thalassemia (Hb S-β-thal).

Hemoglobin electrophoresis (or thin-layer isoelectric focusing) provides definitive diagnostic information.

Newborns with sickle cell anemia (Hb SS) and sickle cell-β°-thalassemia (Hb S-β°-thal) have Hb F and S (FS pattern); older patients have predominantly Hb S (SS pattern).

Newborns with Hb SC disease (Hb SC) have Hb F, S, and C (FSC pattern); older patients have Hb S and C (SC pattern).

Both sickle cell trait (Hb AS) and sickle cell-β+-thalassemia (Hb S-β+-thal) have Hb S and A, but in different proportions. In the former, Hb A >S; in the latter, Hb S >A.

Newborns with sickle cell trait (Hb AS) have Hb F, A, and S (FAS pattern); older patients have Hb A and S (AS pattern).

Newborns with sickle cell-β+-thalassemia (Hb S-β+-thal) have Hb F, S, and A (FSA pattern); older patients have Hb S and A (SA pattern)

---

phoresis or a solubility test permits a definitive diagnosis of a sickle cell syndrome. Alternatively, thin-layer isoelectric focusing will separate Hb S, D, and G and can replace the two electrophoretic methods. Even with thin-layer isoelectric focusing, it is still necessary to use a confirmatory solubility test for Hb S. It should be noted that the "sickle cell preparation" using metabisulfite or dithionite is not in routine clinical use at this time and is of historical interest only.

Results from electrophoresis or thin-layer isoelectric focusing are similar in sickle cell anemia and sickle cell-β°-thalassemia—nearly all the hemoglobin consists of Hb S. While differences in the Hb F and Hb A_2 levels may be useful in distinguishing these syndromes, the presence of microcytosis or one parent without sickle cell trait are useful indicators of sickle cell-β°-thalassemia. The diagnosis of Hb SC disease is straightforward; nearly equal amounts of Hb S and Hb C are detected. Sickle cell-β⁻-thalassemia and sickle cell trait both have substantial amounts of Hb A and Hb S. Sickle cell trait is associated with neither anemia nor microcytosis and has an Hb A fraction that exceeds 50%.[431] Sickle cell-β⁺-thalassemia is associated with anemia, microcytosis, and an Hb A fraction in a range of only 5–30%.[5] Solubility tests are positive in both sickle cell disease and sickle cell trait, but sickled forms (ISCs) occur on the peripheral smear only in the sickle cell diseases and not in sickle cell trait. In sickle cell anemia, ISCs predominate and target cells may be few; in either variety of sickle cell-β-thalassemia ISCs, target cells, and hypochromic microcytic discocytes are prominent; in Hb SC disease, target cells predominate and ISCs are rare.

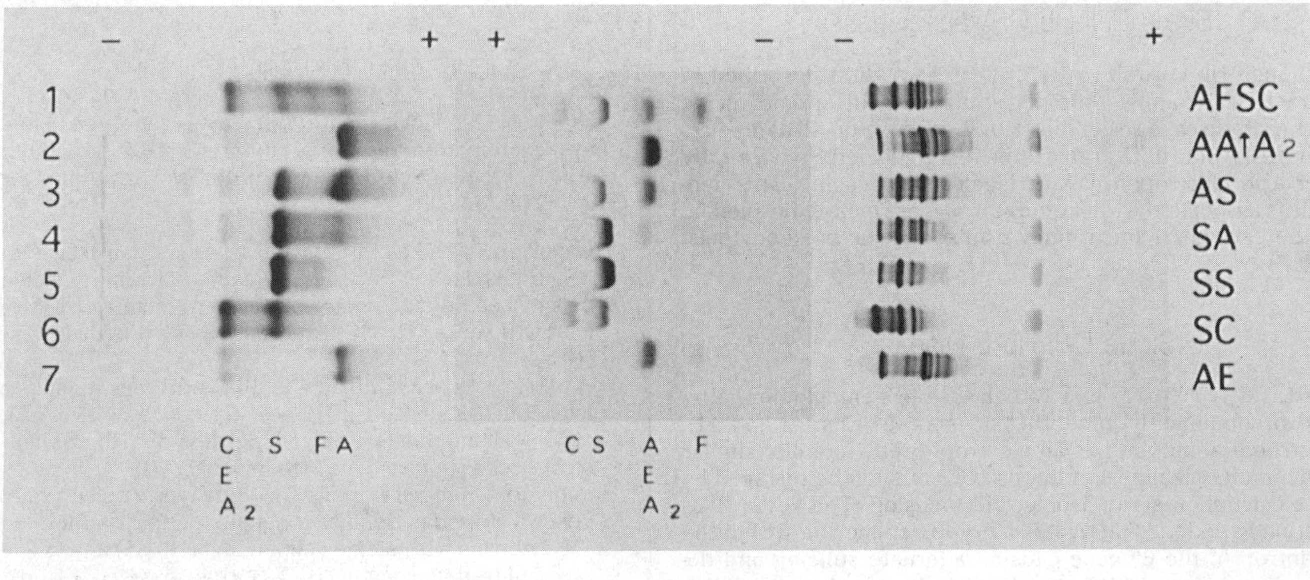

Fig. 43-17. Comparative analyses of several mutant hemoglobins using alkaline electrophoresis, acid electrophoresis, and thin-layer isoelectric focusing. On the right are shown the components of the standard (at the top) and the phenotypes of the other six samples. Their analyses are shown by **(left)** alkaline hemoglobin electrophoresis, **(center)** acid electrophoresis and **(right)** thin-layer isoelectric focusing. Location of the various hemoglobin bands are shown below the left and center panels. (Kindly provided by MH Steinberg.)

Newborn Screening

The use of prophylactic penicillin[221] and the provision of comprehensive medical care during the first 5 years of life have reduced mortality from approximately 25% to <3%, providing impetus for early identification of infants with sickle cell disease.[294] On the basis of its economy and superiority of detection, universal screening of all newborns is recommended[481] over ethnically targeted approaches.[482] Blood samples for testing are obtained by heel stick and spotted onto filter paper for stable transport and subsequent electrophoresis or thin-layer isoelectric focusing.[483,484] The results of solubility testing may be invalid due to the large amount of Hb F present.

A requirement for tests used in newborn screening is the capability to distinguish Hb F, S, A, and C. According to convention, the patterns of hemoglobins present are described in descending order according to the quantities detected. Newborns with sickle cell anemia have predominantly Hb F with a small amount of Hb S and no Hb A (FS pattern). An FS pattern is obtained also in newborns who have sickle cell-β°-thalassemia, sickle cell-HPFH, and sickle cell-Hb D or sickle cell-Hb G (i.e., Hb D and G have the same electrophoretic mobility as Hb S). Family studies are helpful; in the newborn with sickle cell-β°-thalassemia, one parent has sickle cell trait and the other β-thalassemia minor. When family members are not available, the diagnosis is established by DNA-based testing or repeat hemoglobin analysis at age 3–4 months.

The newborn with sickle cell trait will have Hb F, Hb A, and Hb S (FAS pattern). The quantity of Hb A is greater than that of Hb S. If the quantity of Hb S exceeds that of Hb A, the presumptive diagnosis is sickle cell-β⁺-thalassemia (FSA pattern). It may not be possible to distinguish FAS and FSA patterns in newborns, so DNA-based testing or repeat hemoglobin testing at age 3–6 months is recommended. In the future, polymerase chain reaction (PCR)-based diagnosis from blood spotted onto a filter paper may be used to detect sickle cell genes directly.[485]

Prenatal Diagnosis

The limited efficacy of available treatment options for sickle cell disease accounts for the importance of prenatal diagnosis to its overall management. This endeavor is best performed by a team of obstetricians, geneticists, counselors, and support staff that provides a comprehensive approach.[486] In one large survey, it was found that parents at risk of having a child with sickle cell disease were interested in prenatal diagnosis and would consider termination of pregnancy for an affected fetus.[487]

The first successful prenatal diagnoses relied on obtaining fetal blood samples for analysis of globin chain synthesis.[488] Discovery of a restriction fragment length polymorphism in linkage disequilibrium with the sickle cell gene established DNA-based testing, a method not influenced by the presence of Hb F, and spurred the development of second-trimester amniocentesis for obtaining fetal DNA for testing.[489] Direct detection of the GAG→GTG mutation responsible for the sickle cell gene employed allele-specific hybridization with labeled synthetic DNA probes[490] or restriction endonuclease analysis to determine whether the cleavage site of the enzyme Mst II was ablated by the mutation.[491] The development of the PCR for amplifying DNA sequences of interest in vitro allowed testing of minute quantities of DNA and motivated the development of several new methods for detecting the sickle cell gene—restriction analysis[492,493] (Fig. 43-18), allele-specific hybridization,[494] reverse dot-blotting[495] and allele-specific fluorescence PCR.[496] PCR-based diagnosis for Hb SC disease is possible using specific molecular methods for detecting the Hb C gene,[497,498] and the diagnosis of sickle cell-β-thalassemia can be made using reverse dot-blot methodology to screen the many African-American β-thalassemia mutations,[451,452,499] as well as the Hb S and Hb C mutations, with a single hybridization reaction.[500] Currently, fetal DNA samples are obtained by chorionic villus sampling at 10–12 weeks' gestation.[489] Preimplantation diagnosis and testing fetal cells isolated from the maternal circulation are under development.[486]

Other Laboratory Testing

The chronic hemolytic anemia of sickle cell disease is usually associated with mildly to moderately low PCV, hemoglobin, and red cell levels, reticulocytosis of approximately 3–15% (accounting for high or high-normal MCV), unconjugated hyperbilirubinemia, and elevated lactate dehydrogenase and low hapto-

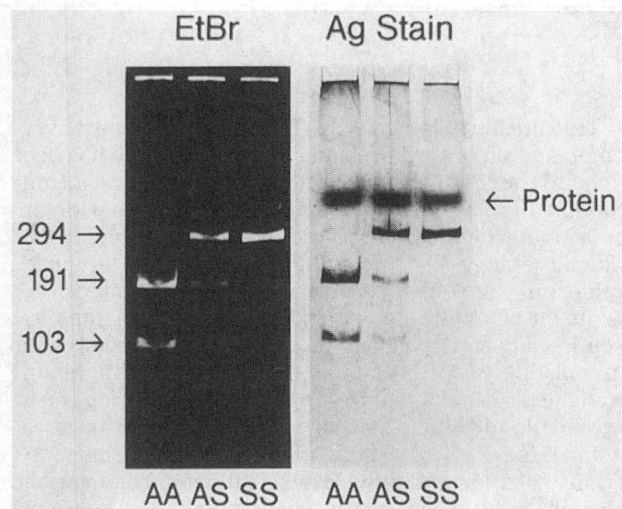

Fig. 43-18. PCR-based restriction analysis for the sickle cell gene. The genotypes of the DNA samples tested are shown below. The size in base pairs for the undigested PCR product and the products resultant from *OxaNI* are shown at the left in base pairs. The fragments from normal β-globin DNA (AA) shows complete *OxaNI* cleavage, from sickle cell trait DNA (AS), shows partial cleavage, and from sickle cell anemia (SS) shows no cleavage. (Adapted from Chehab et al.,[493] with permission.)

globin levels. The blood smear may show polychromasia indicative of reticulocytosis and Howell-Jolly bodies demonstrating hyposplenia. The red cells are normochromic unless there is coexistent thalassemia or iron deficiency. If the age-adjusted MCV is not elevated, the possibility of sickle cell-β-thalassemia, coincident α-thalassemia, or iron deficiency must be considered.

The Hb F level is usually slightly to moderately elevated. The amount of elevation varies among patients. The amount of Hb F present is a function of the number of reticulocytes that contain Hb F, the extent of selective survival of Hb F-containing reticulocytes to become mature Hb F-containing erythrocytes (F cells), and the amount of Hb F/F cell.[501] The β-globin cluster haplotypes[502] (see the section Pathophysiology) appear to be related to factors that regulate production of Hb F. The Arab-Indian and Senegal haplotypes are associated with higher levels of Hb F than the others[502] probably as a result of linkage with important γ-globin regulatory sequences in the locus control region.[503]

A comprehensive analysis of the clinical laboratory data collected from 2,600 subjects with sickle cell disease provides a background for interpreting laboratory abnormalities in this patient group.[223] In particular, normal ranges were established according to genotype, age, and gender. White blood cell counts are higher than normal in sickle cell anemia, particularly in those <10 years of age. Mean white cell counts were not elevated in Hb SC disease or sickle cell-β+-thalassemia. Mean platelet counts are elevated in sickle cell anemia, particularly in those <18 years of age, but are normal in those with Hb SC disease and sickle cell-β+-thalassemia.

Serum bilirubin is higher in sickle cell anemia than in Hb SC disease or sickle cell-β+-thalassemia as a result of a greater hemolytic rate. The level rises after the first decade, possibly as a result of chronic hepatobiliary dysfunction. SGOT and SGPT levels are often elevated, particularly in adult patients with sickle cell anemia, but mean levels are normal. Alkaline phosphatase levels are elevated in all genotypes until puberty, which occurred later in males and in those with homozygous Hb S.

Serum creatinine levels are low in all genotypes until age 18 years, when males experience a rise apparently related to increasing muscle mass. Creatinine levels increase with age in all genotypes, presumably due to declining renal function.

THERAPY

Treatment recommendations specific for sickle cell disease can be divided into general health care maintenance and specific indications or modalities for therapy.[217]

Health Care Maintenance

Patients with sickle cell disease should have routine office appointments to establish baseline physical findings, laboratory values, and relationships with health care professionals. These steady-state values provide standards for comparison at times of clinical exacerbations. Red cell phenotyping is performed, and individualized blood bank files instituted during chronic phase visits. Education regarding the nature of disease, genetic counseling, and psychosocial assessments of patients and their families are best accomplished during these routine visits. Parents of small children are instructed regarding early detection of infection and palpating enlarging spleens. Children are immunized against *S. pneumoniae, H. influenzae,*[297-299] hepatitis B, and influenza. For children <5 years of age, prophylactic penicillin recommendations are for 125 mg penicillin V PO bid until the age of 2–3 years and 250 mg thereafter.[292] The age at which penicillin may be discontinued safely is under investigation. Folic acid (1 mg/day PO) is administered.[244] Retinal evaluation is begun at school age and continued routinely, more frequently in the event of retinopathy. Sexually active women should receive routine pelvic examinations and instruction about birth control. Oral contraception with low-dose estrogen can be safely administered.[366]

Infections

The most critical aspect of infectious illness in sickle cell disease is the evaluation and treatment of the febrile child. Routine evaluation includes a physical examination, a complete blood count, blood and urine cultures, a lumbar puncture if meningitis is suspected, and a chest radiograph to evaluate for pneumonia. Results of the complete blood count are compared to baseline values. A left shift in the differential count suggests bacterial infection. Because of the high mortality rate of bacteremia, hospitalization, obtaining blood and cerebrospinal fluid cultures, and administration of parenteral antibiotics has been the standard of care for children with fevers of >38.5°C.[504,505] However, the recent demonstration of the efficacy of ceftriaxone[300,301] has led to a different set of guidelines. Those with sickle cell anemia or sickle cell-β°-thalassemia who appear toxic, have temperatures of >40°C, or are not receiving prophylactic penicillin are hospitalized for administration of intravenous ceftriaxone 75 mg/kg. For those with sickle cell anemia or sickle cell-β°-thalassemia who have temperatures of <40°C and who are compliant with prophylactic penicillin and those with Hb SC disease or sickle cell-β+-thalassemia who have temperatures of >38.5°C, the recommended approach is to obtain blood cultures, administer intramuscular ceftriaxone 75 mg/kg up to a maximum dose of 2 g, observe for several hours in the emergency department before discharge, and follow closely with outpatient follow-up evaluation. For those with Hb SC disease or sickle cell-β+-thalassemia who have temperatures of <38.5°C, therapy is as indicated symptomatically.[300,301] Therapy for documented *S. pneumoniae* bacteremia is with parenteral penicillin or ceftriaxone for several days.

THE CHILD WITH A HIGH FEVER

The most critical infectious disease consideration of sickle cell disease is the child with a high fever. Evaluation includes a physical examination, complete blood count, blood and urine cultures, lumbar puncture if meningitis is suspected, and a chest radiograph. A left shift in the differential count suggests bacterial infection. In the past the standard of care has been hospitalization, blood and cerebrospinal fluid cultures, and administration of parenteral antibiotics for children with fevers of >38.5°C. Recently, however, a new set of guidelines has emerged. Only those with sickle cell anemia or sickle cell-β°-thalassemia who appear toxic, have temperatures of >40°C, or are not receiving prophylactic penicillin are hospitalized for administration of ceftriaxone (75 mg/kg IV up to a maximum dose of 2 g). Those with sickle cell anemia or sickle cell-β°-thalassemia who have temperatures of <40°C and are compliant with prophylactic penicillin and those with Hb SC disease or sickle cell-β⁺-thalassemia who have temperatures of >38.5°C are administered ceftriaxone (75 mg/kg IM) up to a maximum dose of 2 g) after blood cultures are obtained, observed for several hours prior to discharge, and followed up closely as outpatients. For those with Hb SC or sickle cell-β⁺-thalassemia who have temperatures of <38.5°C, therapy is as indicated symptomatically.

Therapy for documented *S. pneumoniae* bacteremia is with parenteral penicillin or ceftriaxone for several days.

TRANSFUSION THERAPY

Transfusion of red cells has been used for almost every complication of sickle cell disease, but its value has been demonstrated for few. Indications for transfusion include the need for oxygen carrying capacity (i.e., aplastic crisis), blood volume (i.e., splenic sequestration), improved blood rheology (i.e., prevent CVA recurrences, leg ulcers, priapism), and protection from imminent danger (i.e., acute chest syndrome with PaO_2 <70 mmHg, acute CVA, septicemia, metabolic acidosis). The routine acute painful episode is not an indication for transfusion. Simple transfusion is sufficient to supply oxygen-carrying capacity and blood volume. Partial exchange transfusion is recommended for acute indications and for chronic programs where avoiding hyperviscosity and iron overload are important. Hemoglobin levels much >10 g/dl must be avoided during transfusion, because they may result in hyperviscosity and vaso-occlusive complications. A formula useful for manual partial exchange transfusion in adults is to phlebotomize 500 ml whole blood, infuse 300 ml normal saline, phlebotomize another 500 ml whole blood, and infuse 4–5 U packed red blood cells. In typical patients with sickle cell anemia having hemoglobin levels of 8 g/dl, this generally results in hemoglobin levels of approximately 10 g/dl with <50% Hb S.

Preoperative transfusion is recommended, although neither its clearcut efficacy in preventing complications nor the desired post-transfusion hemoglobin or Hb S levels have been established.

Each patient should be characterized according to red blood cell antigen phenotype, and this record maintained in the blood bank. Alloimmunization is diminished by transfusing extended-matched red cells or racially compatible units.

Meningitis therapy should cover *S. pneumoniae* and probably *H. influenzae* type b[302] and be continued for ≥2 weeks.

When antibiotics are used to treat the acute chest syndrome, they should cover *S. pneumoniae, H. influenzae* type b, *M. pneumoniae,* and *C. pneumoniae.* The combination of cefuroxime and erythromycin is recommended.

Management of osteomyelitis is to confirm the diagnosis by culture of blood or infected bone, administer parenteral antibiotics that cover *Salmonella* and *S. aureus,* and tailor antibiotic therapy using culture results. Parenteral antibiotics are continued for 2–6 weeks.[305] Surgical drainage or sequestrectomy may be required. Most patients are cured by this approach, but there may be recurrences.[305]

Transfusion Therapy

Patients with sickle cell disease have some of the same indications for transfusion as do those with without hemoglobinopathies, that is, oxygen-carrying capacity and blood volume replacement (e.g., aplastic crisis, splenic sequestration), as well as indications that are unique to the special needs of their disease, protection from imminent danger (e.g., acute chest syndrome, septicemia, metabolic acidosis) and improved rheologic properties of blood (e.g., prevention of recurrent cerebral thrombosis, priapism, probably preoperatively).[506,507] The routine painful episode is not an indication for transfusion. Transfusion complications include alloimmunization, iron overload, and transmission of viral illness. The 30% incidence of alloimmunization in transfused sickle cell patient is due in part to minor blood group incompatibilities in racially mismatched blood.[508,509] Accordingly, antibodies against the Rh (E, C), Kell (K), Duffy (Fya, Fyb), and Kidd (Jk) antigens present the greatest problem in transfusing this patient group.[508,509] Approaches to minimizing this complication include transfusing extended-matched, phenotypically compatible blood,[510] and using racially matched donors.[511]

Despite impressions to the contrary,[512] as sickle cell patients live longer iron overload has become a problem in a subset of patients who are chronically transfused.[513] Chelation with deferoxamine is recommended when the total body iron is elevated.[514] Chelation guidelines for patients with sickle cell disease are similar to those for other chronically transfused iron-overloaded patients; serum ferritin levels should not be allowed to exceed 2,000 µg/ml.[515] This therapy is inconvenient and expensive, and the development of oral chelating agents[516,517] will provide a tremendous advantage to these patients.

Transfusion transmission of human immunodeficiency virus, hepatitis B and C, and human T-cell leukemia/lymphoma virus-1 has diminished with improved screening of banked units[518] but remains a problem in patients with sickle cell disease.[506,507] In addition to better screening programs, the use of leukocyte-depleted red cell transfusions may be of value in reducing this hazard.[519]

The necessity of preoperative transfusion of patients with sickle cell disease is controversial.[520,521] A multicenter cooperative study designed to determine the relative merits of simple transfusion to Hb S <60% and aggressive partial exchange transfusion to Hb S <30% found that a nonrandomized untransfused control group had a 13% incidence of perioperative acute chest syndrome, a frequency significantly higher than either of the transfused arms.[522] The suggestion that transfusion protects against perioperative morbidity remains to be confirmed in a controlled study.

Table 43-5. Transfusion Formulas[a]

A. Simple transfusion

$$\text{PRBC volume (PRBCV) (ml)} = \frac{(\text{Hct}_d - \text{Hc}_i) \times \text{TBV}}{\text{Hct}_{rp}}$$

B. Dilutional effects of transfusion on Hb S

$$\text{Hb S}_f = \left[1 - \frac{(\text{PRBCV} \times \text{Hct}_{rp})}{(\text{TBV} \times \text{Hct}_i) + (\text{PRBCV} \times \text{Hct}_{rp})} \right] \times \text{Hb S}_i$$

C. Manual partial exchange transfusion[b]

$$\text{Exchange volume (ml)} = \frac{(\text{Hct}_d - \text{Hct}_i) \times \text{TBV}}{\text{Hct}_{rp} - \dfrac{(\text{Hct}_i + \text{Hct}_d)}{2}}$$

D. Automated exchange transfusion

$$\text{Red cell volume (ml)} = \text{Hct}_i \times \text{TBV}$$

Abbreviations: TBV, estimated total blood volume in milliliters (children 80 ml/kg, adults 65 ml/kg, nomograms are available)[c]; Hct_d, desired hematocrit; Hct_i, initial hematocrit; Hct_{rp}, hematocrit of replacement cells (usually 0.75); Hb S_i, initial Hb S; Hb S_f, final Hb S.

[a] Hct and Hb S are fractions (e.g., 40% = 0.4)
[b] From Nieburg and Stockman,[568]
[c] From Linderkamp et al.[569]
(Modified from Wayne et al.,[506] with permission.)

Simple transfusion can be used to restore oxygen-carrying capacity or blood volume when anemia or volume depletion is severe, but partial exchange transfusions are usually recommended for both acute emergencies and chronic transfusion because of the improved viscosity effects and reduced iron burden of this approach.[506,507] Volume guidelines for simple and exchange transfusions (Table 43-5) are particularly important for transfusing children. For normal-size adults, the general rule is that each unit of red cells infused will increase the hemoglobin level approximately 1 g/dl. Partial exchange transfusion in adults is accomplished by phlebotomizing 500 ml, infusing 300 ml normal saline, phlebotomizing another 500 ml, and infusing 4–5 U packed red cells.[512]

Pain Management

The acute painful episode is the most frequent cause of patients with sickle cell disease seeking medical attention. When a patient presents complaining of pain, the physician is charged with ruling out etiologies other than vaso-occlusion (e.g., an infectious cause); maintaining optimal hydration by oral or intravenous fluid resuscitation (particularly in children); and aggressive relief of pain using narcotics, other analgesics, or other modalities.[523,524] Neither red blood cell transfusion nor oxygen inhalation is indicated for treating the routine acute painful episode, but oxygen administration may be required for patients who have become hypoxemic. Patients are often undertreated for pain, because many physicians and other health care providers are unfamiliar with the pharmacology of analgesia and overly concerned with the potential for addiction. Consequently, the duration of painful episodes may be prolonged, a "drug-seeking" ("pain-relieving"?) behavior pattern is encouraged, and a pain-oriented personality may evolve. Prompt administration of appropriate doses of analgesia will diminish this potential.

Table 43-6 describes analgesics and presents recommendations for their use in the treatment of the painful episodes of sickle cell disease.[523,524] Patients in pain are treated optimally in a familiar ambulatory setting that avoids the hectic environment of the emergency department. Hospitalization and intravenous administration of fluid and narcotics are often required for the treatment of severe pain. Intravenous morphine is recommended for prompt pain relief, and patient-controlled analgesia is an excellent means of subsequent pain control.[525] When patients do not respond to conventional doses of analgesia, the rapid metabolism of narcotics in patients with sickle cell disease must be considered.[526] Comprehensive management of the biopsychosocial pain experience includes the use of psychosocial support systems, local anesthetics, epidural anesthetics, combinations of nonsteroidal anti-inflammatory agents and narcotics, and antidepressive drugs.[524,527] The rare chronic sickle cell pain syndrome may require therapy similar to that used for the management of the pain of terminal cancer,[528] such as long-acting morphine and fentanyl patches.

NEW THERAPEUTIC MODALITIES

The cure of sickle cell disease has been an elusive goal. Many agents have been proposed and tested, but no cure has been found. As new therapies are developed, it is important to offer cautious optimism but not false hope to patients with sickle cell disease. Table 43-7 lists therapeutic modalities according to hemoglobin liganding, membrane active, vasoactive, anticoagulant, and antioxidant activities.

Agents that Decrease Hb S Polymerization

The fundamental importance of Hb S polymerization is focused attention on agents that acted on the hemoglobin molecule to increase its solubility, either directly or indirectly by increasing its oxygen affinity. The hemoglobin ligands react with the hemoglobin molecule noncovalently or covalently and can be classified as having stereospecific (S), left-shifting (L), right-shifting (R), hydrophobic bond-breaking (H), and electrostatic bond-breaking (E) activities. In general, treatment with these drugs has not been successful as a result of untargeted delivery to cells other than the red cell and attendant toxicity, inefficient transport across the red cell membrane, and modification of the red cell membrane enhancing hemolysis. Extracorporeal treatment of red cells has proven impractical.

Membrane Active Agents

Membrane-active agents that improve sickle cell hydration and deformability, such as Ceteidil[140] and imidazole compounds, such as clotrimazole,[141] have shown promise. Ceteidil has shown limited therapeutic success in a controlled clinical trial,[140] and clinical study of clotrimazole is planned. Compounds that improve membrane deformability are not effective.[529]

The nonionic block copolymer Pluronic F-68 or Poloxamer 188, the emulsifying agent in the perfluorochemical blood substitute Fluosol DA, improves the rheological properties of sickle red cells and inhibits their adherence to endothelial cells as a result of a "lubricating" effect on cell surfaces.[173] Clinical trials are currently underway to determine whether an intravenous bolus of the agent will terminate or shorten a painful episode.

Vasoactive Compounds

Vasodilating agents that improve membrane deformability have not been found effective.[530]

Antioxidant Agents

A systematic study of antioxidant agents intended to counter the detrimental effects of oxidation on sickle cells has not been accomplished. Such a study would be complicated by the relative redox potentials of participants in the auto-oxidative

Table 43-6. Recommended Dose and Interval of Analgesics for Treating the Acute Painful Episode

	Dose/Rate	Comments
Severe/moderate pain		
Morphine	0.15 mg/kg q3–4h (IV, SC, IM, PCA)[a] 0.6 mg/kg q4h (PO)	Drug of choice for pain; lower doses in aged, liver failure, and impaired ventilation
Meperidine (Demerol)	1.5 mg/kg q2–4h (IM, IV) 1.5 mg/kg q4h (PO)	Increased incidence of seizures, avoid in patients with renal or neurologic disease or who receive monoamine oxidase inhibitors
Hydromorphone (Dilaudid)	0.02 mg/kg q3–4h (IM, IV) 0.04 mg/kg q4h (PO)	
Oxycodone (Percodan)	5–10 mg q4h (PO)	
Mild pain[b]		
Codeine	1.0 mg/kg q4h (PO)	Drug of choice for mild-to-moderate pain not relieved by aspirin or acetaminophen
Propoxyphene (Darvon)	65 mg q4h (PO) (100 mg as napsylate)	Not recommended for children, a narcotic with addiction potential, toxic metabolites accumulate with repetitive dosing
Aspirin	0.3–0.6 g (PO) q4h (adults 8 mg/kg (children)	Often given with a narcotic to enhance analgesia, can cause gastric irritation
Acetaminophen (Tylenol)	0.3–0.6 g (PO) q5h (adults 8 mg/kg (children)	Often given with a narcotic to enhance analgesia
Ibuprofen (Advil, Motrin)	300–400 mg q4h (PO)	Not FDA-approved for children, can cause gastric irritation
Naproxen (Naprosyn)	250 mg q12h (PO)	Long duration of action, can cause gastric irritation
Indomethacin (Indocin)	25 mg q4–8h (PO)	Contraindicated in psychiatric, neurologic, renal diseases, can cause gastric irritation; useful in gout
Tolmetin (Tolectin)	400 mg q8h (PO)	Approved for children

[a] Continuous intravenous infusion, patient-controlled analgesic (PCA) devices, and continuous subcutaneous infusion are useful in pain control but should be performed only by institutions familiar with their use. Because of their risk of respiratory depression, vital signs should be monitored carefully.
[b] Other useful mild analgesics: piroxicam, sulindac.
(Adapted from Vichinsky and Lubin,[218] with permission.)

process—Hb S, oxidative radicals, free heme, hemichromes, nonheme iron, membrane lipid, membrane protein, and intermediate metabolites. An agent capable of reducing one component may oxidize another, and a clinical study would have to be carefully controlled to dissect the complex interdependence of oxidation-reduction substrates.

Induction of Hb F Synthesis

A logical therapeutic approach based on the inhibitory effect of Hb F on Hb S polymerization[65] and cellular sickling[72] is the pharmacologic induction of Hb F.[531] Based on the observed rise in maternal Hb F levels in the second trimester of pregnancy, the therapeutic effect of human chorionic gonadotropin and progesterone was tested[532,533] but not widely adopted as treatment. 5-Azacytidine was shown to increase Hb F production four- to eightfold[534] but because of concerns regarding its potential carcinogenicity attention turned to alternative agents. Hydroxyurea is an inhibitor of ribonucleotide reductase without known carcinogenicity that also induces therapeutically significant increases in Hb F synthesis,[535,536] an effect that is potentiated by conjoint administration of recombinant human erythropoietin.[537] A poorly understood effect of hydroxyurea is the improved rheologic properties of sickle cells[538,539] and diminished hemolysis[536] that occur independently of Hb F changes. The effect of hydroxyurea on incidence of pain is currently being evaluated in a multicenter double-blind placebo-controlled study.

Butyric acid appears to impede the switch from fetal to adult hemoglobin,[540] but enthusiasm for its apparent ability to induce increased numbers of Hb F-containing reticulocytes[541] is tempered by concerns regarding uncertain efficacy,[542,543] neurologic toxicity,[542] and unacceptably severe nausea and vomiting.[544]

Bone Marrow Transplantation

Successes in β-thalassemia encouraged the use of bone marrow transplantation (BMT) for sickle cell disease (see Chs. 28–30). To date there have been 57 reported BMTs for sickle

cell anemia, with four deaths.[545–552] A major challenge to expanded use of BMT in this setting is identification of appropriate recipients. The extremely poor prognosis of sickle cell disease in Africa supports the widespread use of BMT in that setting,[547,548] but decisions in better-developed countries hinge on less absolute considerations. The comparative costs of $150,000–200,000 for an uncomplicated BMT in the United States versus ≤$112,000 annually for conventional medical care[553] suggest that BMT may be the more cost-effective approach. The increasing life-expectancy[220] and large fraction of asymptomatic patients[138,251] in sickle cell disease suggest that BMT be reserved for those with severe disease. Current methods for identifying BMT candidates are unsatisfactory; awaiting serious complications allows the potential for serious disability prior to BMT,[554,555] and transplanting those predicted by genetic polymorphisms to be severe may subject the misidentified to unnecessary risks of BMT.[227] Another obstacle is the limited availability of suitable donors. The usual one compatible donor per three siblings is further reduced by the existence of sickle cell disease among family members. Solutions for this problem include broadening the ethnic composition of the registry donor pool, improving BMT using partially matched donors, and correcting the sickle cell gene in autologous marrow erythroid precursors.

Gene Therapy

Recent advances in gene therapy technology provide promise for the future of sickle cell disease[556,557] (see Ch. 31). The seminal importance of a single nucleotide substitution to a disease so thoroughly understood renders the sickle cell gene an ideal candidate for this technology. Efficient gene transfer has been accomplished using replicative defective retroviral vectors.[558] High-level expression is attained by including in the vector regulatory sequences from the locus control region[559] and by inserting the normal gene into its native environment by homologous recombination (an approach that offers the additional advantage of knocking out the mutant gene by inserting the normal).[560] Sustained expression of the corrected gene is gained by transfer into self-replicating stem cells.[561] Success-

Table 43-7. Therapeutic Agents for Sickle Cell Disease

Hemoglobin ligands
  Noncovalent ligands
    Phenylalanine derivatives (S)
    Clofibrate (S)
    Urea (H)
    Quinine (S)
    Chloraquine (S)
    Quinaquine (S)
    Tryptophan derivatives (S)
    5-Bromotryptophan (S)
    Alkylureas (H)(S)
    Oligopeptides (S)
    Lyotropic salts (E)
    Benzyloxy acids (S)
    Phenoxy acids (S)
  Covalent ligands
    Carbon monoxide (L)
    12C79 (L)
    Cyanate (L)
    Vanillin (L)(S)
    Acetyl phosphates (S)(R)
    Pyridoxal phosphate (S)(R)
    Ethacrynic acid (S)(L)
    Aspirin (S)
    Fumarate (L)
    Cystamine (L)
    Dimethyl adipimidate (L)
    Nitrogen mustard (S)
Membrane active drugs
  Transport
    Cetiedil
    Monensin
    Okadaic acid
    Quinine
    Charybdotoxin
    Clotrimazole
    Hemisodium
    Ouabain
    Stilbene disulfonates
    Dihydroindenyl oxyalkanoic acid
    Nitrendipine
    Fendiline
    Bepridil
  Rheologic properties
    Ticlopidine
    Pentoxyfylline (Oxpentifylline)
    Tellurite
    Pluronic F-68 (Poloxamer or RheothRx)
    Fluosol
    Zinc
Vascular-active drugs
  Nifedipine
Anticoagulants
  Heparin
  Ticlopidine
  Aspirin
  Dipyridamole
  Coumadin
Antoxidants
  α-Tocopherol
  Ascorbic acid
  Lawsone

Abbreviations: S, stereospecific; L, left-shifting agents; R, right-shifting agents; H, hydrophobic bond breakers; E, electrostatic bond breakers.

(Adapted from Orringer et al.,[570] with permission.)

ful expression of the human sickle gene in transgenic mice demonstrates the feasibility of this approach.[562] Its safety remains to be determined.[563]

ACKNOWLEDGMENTS

This work was partially supported by grant HL 20985 from the National Institutes of Health. I am grateful to Margaret Venables for providing editorial assistance and to Miriam Hirsch for extending the resources of the Barnett-Briggs Library in the preparation of this manuscript.

REFERENCES

1. Embury SH, Hebbel RP, Mohandas N, Steinberg MH: Sickle Cell Disease: Basic Principles and Clinical Practice. Raven Press, New York, 1994
2. Serjeant GR: Sickle Cell Disease. Oxford University Press, Oxford, 1992
3. Treadwell MJ, Gil KM: Psychosocial aspects. p. 517. In Embury SH, Hebbel RP, Mohandas N, Steinberg MH (eds): Sickle Cell Disease: Basic Principles and Clinical Practice. Raven Press, New York, 1994
4. Bunn HF: Sickle hemoglobin and other hemoglobin mutants p. 207. In Stamatoyannopoulos G, Nienhuis AW, Majerus PW, Varmus H (eds): The Molecular Basis of Blood Disease, WB Saunders, Philadelphia, 1993
5. Bunn HF, Forget BG: Hemoglobin: Molecular, Genetic and Clinical Aspects. WB Saunders, Philadelphia, 1986
6. Eaton WA, Hofrichter J: Sickle cell hemoglobin polymerization. Adv Protein Chem 40:63, 1990
7. Noguchi CT, Schechter AN: The intercellular polymerization of sickle hemoglobin and its relevance to sickle cell disease. Blood 59:1057, 1981
8. Embury SH: The clinical pathophysiology of sickle cell disease. Annu Rev Med 37:361, 1986
9. Wagner GM, Vichinsky EP, Lande WM, Pennathur-Das R: Sickling syndromes and unstable hemoglobin disease. p. 145. In Mentzer WC, Wagner GM (eds): The Hereditary Hemolytic Anemias. Churchill Livingstone, New York, 1989
10. Hebbel RP: Beyond hemoglobin polymerization: the red blood cell membrane sickle cell disease pathophysiology. Blood 77:214, 1991
11. Francis RB, Johnson CS: Vascular occlusion in sickle cell disease: current concepts unanswered questions. Blood 77:1405, 1991
12. Embury SH, Hebbel RP, Mohandas N, Steinberg MH: Pathogenisis of Vasoocclusion. p. 311. In Embury SH, Hebbel RP, Mohandas N, Steinberg MH (eds): Sickle Cell Disease: Basic Principles and Clinical Practice. Raven Press, New York, 1994
13. Herrick JB: Peculiar elongated and sickle-shaped red blood corpuscles in a case of severe anemia. Arch Intern Med 6:517, 1910
14. Savitt TL, Goldberg MF: Herrick's 1910 case report of sickle cell anemia. The rest of the story. JAMA 261:266, 1989
15. Konotey-Ahulu FI: The sickle cell diseases: clinical manifestations including the "sickle crisis." Arch Intern Med 133:611, 1974
16. Hahn EV, Gillespie EB: Sickle cell anemia. Report of a case greatly improved by splenectomy. Experimental study of sickle cell formation. Arch Intern Med 39:233, 1927
17. Harris JW, Brewster HH, Ham TH, Castle WB: Studies on the destruction of red blood cells. X. The biophysics and biology of sickle-cell disease. Arch Intern Med 97:145, 1956
18. Sherman IJ: The sickling phenomenon, with special reference to the differentiation of sickle cell anemia from the sickle cell trait. Bull Johns Hopkins Hosp 67:309, 1940
19. Ham TH, Castle WB: Relationship of increased hypotonic fragility of erythrostasis to the mechanisms of hemolysis in certain anemias. Trans Assoc Am Physicians 55:127, 1940
20. Pauling L, Itano HA, Singer SJ, Wells IC: Sickle cell anemia, a molecular disease. Science 110:543, 1949
21. Harris JW: Studies on the destruction of red blood cells. VIII. Molecular orientation in sickle cell hemoglobin solutions. Proc Soc Exp Biol 75:197, 1950
22. Perutz MF, Mitchison JM: State of haemoglobin in sickle cell anaemia. Nature 166:677, 1950
23. Ingram VM: A specific chemical difference between the globins of normal human and sickle-cell anemia haemoglobin. Nature 178:792, 1956
24. Ingram VM: Gene mutations in human haemoglobin: the chemical difference between normal and sickle cell haemoglobin. Nature 180:326, 1957
25. Ingram VM: How do genes act? Sci Am 198:68, 1958
26. Diggs LW, Bibb J: The erythrocyte in sickle cell anemia. Morphology, size, hemoglobin content, fragility and sedimentation rate. JAMA 112:695, 1939
27. Huck JG: Sickle cell anemia. Bull Johns Hopkins Hosp 34:335, 1923
28. Sydenstricker VP, Mulherin WI, Houseal RW: Sickle cell anemia: report of 2 cases in children, with necropsy in one case. Am J Dis Child 26:132, 1923

29. Beet EA: The genetics of the sickle-cell trait in a Bantu tribe. Ann Eugen 14: 279, 1949

30. Neel JV: The inheritance of sickle cell anemia. Science 110:64, 1949

31. Silvestroni E, Bianco I: Una nuova entità nosologica: "La malattia microdrepanocytica." Haematologica 29:455, 1946

32. Orkin SH, Kazazian HH, Antonarakis SE et al: Linkage of β-thalassaemia mutations β-globin gene polymorphisms with DNa polymorphisms in human β-globin gene cluster. Nature 296:627, 1982

33. Pagnier J, Mears GJ, Dunda-Belkhodja O et al: Evidence for the multicentric origin of the sickle cell hemoglobin gene in Africa. Proc Natl Acad Sci USA 81:1771, 1984

34. Nagel RL, Fleming AF: Genetic epidemiology of the beta^S gene. Baillieres Clin Haematol 5:331, 1992

35. Powars D, Chan LS, Schroeder WA: The variable expression of sickle cell disease is genetically determined. Semin Hematol 27:360, 1990

36. Allison AC: Notes on sickle-cell polymorphism. Ann Hum Genet 19:39, 1954

37. Raper AB: Sickling in relation to morbidity from malaria and other diseases. Br Med J 1:965, 1956

38. Eaton J: Malaria and the selection of the sickle gene. p. 13. In Embury SH, Hebbel RP, Mohandas N, Steinberg MH (eds): Sickle Cell Disease: Basic Principles and Clinical Practice. Raven Press, New York, 1994

39. Livingstone FB: Anthropological implications of sickle cell gene distribution in West Africa. Am Anthropol 60:533, 1958

40. Huehns ER, Shooter EM: Human haemoglobins. J Med Genet 2:48, 1965

41. Pavsol G, Weatherall DJ, Wilson RJM: Cellular mechanism for the protective effect of hemoglobin S against *P. falciparum* malaria. Nature 274:701, 1978

42. Beutler E, Dern RJ, Flanagan CL: Effect of sickle-cell trait on resistance to malaria. Br Med J 1:1189, 1955

43. Roth EF Jr, Friedman M, Ueda Y et al: Sickling rates of human AS red cells infected in vitro with *Plasmodium falciparum* malaria. Science 202:650, 1978

44. Friedman MJ: Erythrocytic mechanism of sickle-cell resistance to malaria. Proc Natl Acad Sci USA 75:1994, 1978

45. Luzzatto L, Nwachuku-Jarrett ES, Reddy S: Increased sickling of parasitised erythrocytes as mechanism of resistance against malaria in the sickle-cell trait. Lancet 1:319, 1970

46. Friedman MJ, Roth EF, Nagel RL, Trager W: *Plasmodium falciparum:* physiological interactions with the human sickle cell. Exp Parasitol 47:73, 1979

47. Hershko C, Peto TEA: Deferoxamine inhibition of malaria is independent of host iron status. J Exp Med 168:375, 1988

48. Etkin NL, Mahoney JR, Eaton JW: Hemoglobin S: molecular basis for antimalarial effect. Am J Phys Anthropol 54:217, 1981

49. Friedman MJ: Ultrastructural damage to the malarial parasite in the sickled cell. J Protozol 26:195, 1979

50. Hill AVS, Allsopp CEM, Kwiatkowski D et al: Common West African HLA antigens are associated with protection from severe malaria. Nature 352: 595, 1991

51. Hill AVS, Elvin J, Willis AC et al: Molecular analysis of the association of HLA-B53 and resistance to severe malaria. Nature 360:434, 1992

52. Piomelli S, Reindorf CA, Arzanian MT, Corash LM: Clinical and biochemical interactions of G6PD deficiency and sickle-cell anemia. N Engl J Med 287: 213, 1972

53. Beutler E, Johnson C, Powars D, West C: Prevalence of glucose-6-phosphate dehydrogenase deficiency in sickle cell disease. N Engl J Med 290:826, 1974

54. Steinberg MH, Dreiling BJ: Glucose-6-phosphate dehydrogenase deficiency in sickle cell anemia. Ann Intern Med 80:217, 1974

55. Steinberg MH, West S, Gallagher D, Mentzer W, the Cooperative Study of Sickle Cell Disease: Effects of glucose-6-phosphate dehydrogenase deficiency upon sickle cell anemia. Blood 71:748, 1988

56. Nagel RL: The origin of the Hemoglobin S gene: clinical genetic. Einstein Q J Biol Med 2:53, 1984

57. Motulsky AG: Frequency of sickling disorders in U.S. blacks. N Engl J Med 288:31, 1972

58. Fleming AF: The presentation, management and prevention of crisis in sickle cell disease in Africa. Blood Rev 1:18, 1989

59. Embury SH: Prenatal diagnosis. p. 485. In Embury SH, Hebbel RP, Mohandas N, Steinberg MH (eds): Sickle Cell Disease: Basic Principles and Clinical Practice. Raven Press, New York, 1994

60. Hofrichter J, Ross PD, Eaton WA: Supersaturation in sickle cell hemoglobin solutions. Proc Natl Acad Sci USA 73:3035, 1976

61. Dykes GW, Crepeau RH, Edelstein SJ: Three-dimensional reconstruction of the 14-filament fibers of hemoglobin S. J Mol Biol 130:451, 1979

62. Dickerson RE, Geis I: Abnormal Human Hemoglobins. p. 117. In: Hemoglobin: Structure, Function, Evolution, and Pathology. Benjamin-Cummings, Menlo Park, CA, 1983

63. Bookchin RM, Nagel RL: Interactions between human hemoglobins: sickling and related phenomena. Semin Hematol 11:577, 1974

64. Wishner BC, Ward KB, Lattman EE, Love WE: Crystal structure of sickle-cell deoxyhemoglobin as 5 Å resolution. J Mol Biol 98:179, 1975

65. Goldberg MA, Husson MV, Bunn HF: Participation of hemoglobins A and F in polymerization of sickle hemoglobin J Biol Chem 252:3414, 1977

66. Edelstin SJ: Molecular topology in crystals and fibers of hemoglobin S. J Mol Biol 150:557, 1981

67. Ferrone FA, Hofrichter J, Eaton WA: Kinetics of sickle hemoglobin polymerization. II. A double nucleation mechanism. J Mol Biol 183:611, 1985

68. Coletta M, Hofrichter J, Ferrone F, Eaton WA: Kinetics of sickle haemoglobin polymerization in single red cells. Nature 300:194, 1982

69. Messer MJ, Hahn JA, Bradley TB: The kinetics of sickling and unsickling of red cells under physiologic conditions: rheologic and ultrastructural correlations. p. 225. In Proceedings of a Symposium on the Molecular and Cellular Aspects of Sickle Cell Disease. DHEW (NIH) Publ. No. 76-1007. National Institutes of Health, Bethesda, 1976

70. Noguchi CT, Torchia DA, Schechter AN: Determination of deoxyhemoglobin S polymer in sickle erythrocytes upon deoxygenation. Proc Natl Acad Sci USA 77:5487, 1980

71. Kaul DK, Fabry ME, Nagel RL: Microvascular sites and characteristics of sickle cell adhesion to vascular endothelium in shear flow conditions: pathophysiological implications. Proc Natl Acad Sci USA 86:3356, 1989

72. Sewchand LS, Johnson CS, Meiselman HJ: The effect of fetal hemoglobin on the sickling dynamics of SS erythrocytes. Blood Cells 9:147, 1983

73. Blau AC, Stamatoyannopoulos G: Regulation of fetal hemoglobin production. p. 247. In Embury SH, Hebbel RP, Mohandas N, Steinberg MH (eds): Sickle Cell Disease: Basic Principles and Clinical Practice. Raven Press, New York, 1994

74. Brittenham GM, Schechter AN, Noguchi CT: Hemoglobin S polymerization: primary determination of the hemolytic and clinical severity of the sickling syndromes. Blood 65:283, 1985

75. Sunshine HR, Hofrichter J, Eaton WA: Requirements for therapeutic inhibition of sickle hemoglobin gelation. Nature 275:238, 1978

76. Behe MJ, Englander SW: Mixed gelation theory. Kinetics, equilibrium and gel incorporation in sickle hemoglobin mixtures. J Mol Biol 133:137, 1979

77. Sunshine HR: Effects of other hemoglobins on gelation of sickle cell hemoglobin. Tex Rep Biol Med 40:233, 1981

78. Nagel RL, Bookchin RM, Johnson J et al: Structural bases of the inhibitory effects of hemoglobin F and hemoglobin A$_2$ on the polymerization of hemoglobin S. Proc Natl Acad Sci USA 76:670, 1979

79. Steinberg MH, Embury SH: α-Thalassemia in blacks: genetic clinical aspects and interactions with the sickle hemoglobin gene. Blood 68:985, 1986

80. Dozy AM, Kan YW, Embury SH et al: Alpha globin gene organization in blacks precludes the severe form of alpha thalassemia. Nature 280:605, 1979

81. Embury SH, Backer K, Glader BE: Monovalent cation changes in sickle erythrocytes: a direct reflection of α-globin gene number. J Lab Clin Med 106:75, 1985

82. Embury SH, Clark MR, Monroy GM, Mohandas N: Concurrent sickle cell anemia and α-thalassemia: effect on pathological properties of sickle red cells. J Clin Invest 73:116, 1984

83. Embury SH, Dozy AM, Miller J et al: Concurrent sickle-cell anemia and α-thalassemia: effect on severity of anemia. N Engl J Med 306:270, 1982

84. Higgs DR, Aldridge BE, Lamb J et al: The interaction of α-thalassemia and homozygous sickle-cell disease. N Engl J Med 306:1441, 1982

85. de Ceulear D, Higgs DR, Weatherall DJ et al: α-Thalassemia reduces the hemolytic rate in homozygous sickle cell disease. N Engl J Med 309:189, 1983

86. Steinberg MH, Rosenstock W, Coleman MB et al: Effects of thalassemia and microcytosis on the hematologic and vasoocclusive severity of sickle cell anemia. Blood 63:1353, 1984

87. Felice AE, McKie KM, Cleek MP et al: Effects of α-thalassemia-2 on the developmental changes of hematological values in children with sickle cell disease from Georgia. Am J Hematol 25:389, 1987

88. Stevens MCG, Maude GH, Beckford M et al: α-Thalassemia and the hematology of homozygous sickle cell disease in childhood. Blood 67:411, 1986

89. Hahn JA, Messer MJ, Bradley TB: Ultrastructure sickling and unsickling in the time-lapse studies. Br J Haematol 34:559, 1976

90. Schmalzer EA, Manning RS, Chien S: Filtration of sickle cells: recruitment into a rigid fraction as a function of density and oxygen tension. J Lab Clin Med 113:727, 1989

91. Nash GB, Johnson CS, Meiselman HJ: Influence of oxygen tension on the viscoelastic behavior of red blood cells in sickle cell disease. Blood 67:110, 1986

92. Sorette MP, Lavenant MG, Clark MR: Ektacytometric measurement of sickle cell deformability as a continuous function of oxygen tension. Blood 69:316, 1987

93. White JG: The fine structure of sickled hemoglobin in situ. Blood 31:561, 1968

94. Finch JT, Perutz MF, Bertles JF, Dobler J: Structure of sickled erythrocytes and of sickle-cell hemoglobin fibers. Proc Natl Acad Sci USA 70:719, 1973

95. Mickols W, Maestre MF, Tinoco I: Visualization of oriented hemoglobin S in erythrocytes by differential extinction of polarized light. Proc Natl Acad Sci USA 82:6527, 1985

96. Mickols WE, Corbett JD, Maestre MF et al: The dependence of the percentage of aligned hemoglobin in sickle cell anemia on the speed of deoxygenation by using linear dichroism microscopy. J Biol Chem 263:4338, 1988

97. Asakura T, Mayberry J: Relationship between morphologic characteristics of sickle cells and method of deoxygenation. J Lab Clin Med 104:987, 1984

98. Briehl RW, Mann ES: Hemoglobin polymerization fiber lengths, rheology and pathogenesis. Ann NY Acad Sci 565:295, 1989

99. Kaul DK, Xue H: Rate of deoxygenation and rheologic behavior of blood in sickle cell anemia. Blood 77:1353, 1991

100. Glader BE, Lux SE, Muller-Sayano A et al: Energy reserve and cation composition of irreversibly sickled cells in vivo. Br J Haematol 40:527, 1978

101. Clark MR, Morrison CE, Shohet SB: Monovalent cation transport in irreversibly sickled cells. J Clin Invest 61:329, 1978

102. Bertles JF, Milner PFA: Irreversibly sickled erythrocytes: a consequence of the heterogeneous distribution of hemoglobin types in sickle-cell anemia. J Clin Invest 47:1731, 1968

103. Noguchi CT, Dover GJ, Rodgers GP et al: α-Thalassemia changes erythrocyte heterogeneity in sickle cell disease. J Clin Invest 75:1632, 1985

104. Chien S: Rheology of sickle cells and erythrocyte content. Blood Cells 3:283, 1977

105. McCurdy PR, Sherman HS: Irreversibly sickled cells red cell survival in sickle cell anemia: a study with both DF^{32}P and ^{51}CR. Am J Med 64:253, 1978

106. Lux SE, John KM, Karnovsky MJ: Irreversible deformation of the spectrin-actin lattice in irreversibly sickled cells. J Clin Invest 58:955, 1976

107. Clark MR, Mohandas N, Shohet SB: Deformability of oxygenated irreversibly sickled cells. J Clin Invest 65:189, 1980

108. Clark MR, Guatelli JC, Mohnadas N, Shohet SB: Influence of red cell water content on the morphology of sickling. Blood 55:823, 1980

109. Ohnishi ST, Horiuchi KY, Horiuchi K et al: Nitrendipine, nifedipine, and verapamil inhibit the in vitro formation of irreversibly sickled cells. Pharmacology 2:248, 1986

110. Embury SH, Garcia JF, Mohandas N et al: Oxygen inhalation by subjects with sickle cell anemia. Effects on endogenous erythropoietin kinetics erythropoiesis. N Engl J Med 311:291, 1984

111. Jensen M, Shohet SB, Nathan DG: The role of red cell energy metabolism in the generation of irreversibly sickled cells in vitro. Blood 42:835, 1973

112. Lew VL, Freeman CJ, Ortiz OE, Bookchin RM: A mathematical model of the pH, volume and ion content regulation in reticulocytes. Application to the pathophysiology of sickle cell dehydration. J Clin Invest 87:100, 1991

113. Bookchin RM, Ortiz OE, Lew VL: Evidence for a direct reticulocyte origin of dense red cells in sickle cell anemia. J Clin Invest 87:113, 1991

114. Serjeant GR, Serjeant BE, Milner PF: The irreversibly sickled cell: a determinant of haemolysis in sickle cell anemia. Br J Haematol 17:527, 1969

115. Serjeant GR, Serjeant BE, Desai P et al: The determinants of irreversibly sickled cells in homozygous sickle cell disease. Br J Haematol 40:431, 1978

116. Seakins M, Gibbs WN, Milner PF: Erythrocyte Hb-S concentration: an important factor in the low oxygen affinity of blood in sickle cell anemia. J Clin Invest 52:422, 1973

117. Canessa M: Red cell volume-related ion transport systems in hemoglobinopathies. Hematol Oncol Clin North Am 5:495, 1991

118. Brugnara C: Cation homeostasis. p. 173. In Embury SH, Hebbel RP, Mohandas N, Steinberg MH (eds): Sickle Cell Disease: Basic Principles and Clinical Practice. Raven Press, New York, 1994

119. Tosteson DC, Carlsen E, Dunham ET: The effects of sickling on ion transport. I. Effect of sickling on potassium transport. J Gen Physiol 39:31, 1955

120. Glader BE, Nathan DG: Cation permeability alterations during sickling: relationship to cation composition and cellular hydration of irreversibly sickled cells. Blood 51:983, 1978

121. Joiner CH, Platt OS, Lux SEIV: Cation depletion by the sodium pump in red cells with pathologic cation leaks. Sickle cells and xerocytes. J Clin Invest 78:1487, 1986

122. Eaton J, Skelton TD, Swolford HS et al: Elevated erythrocyte calcium in sickle cell disease. Nature 246:105, 1973

123. Lew VL, Hockaday A, Sepulveda M-I et al: Compartmentalization of sickle cell calcium in endocytic inside-out vesicles. Nature 315:586, 1985

124. Mohandas N, Rossi ME, Clark MR: Association between morphologic distortion of sickle cells and deoxygenation-induced cation permeability increase. Blood 69:450, 1986

125. Ney PA, Christopher MM, Hebbel RP: Synergistic effects of oxidation and deformation on erythrocyte monovalent cation leak. Blood 75:1192, 1990

126. Sears DA: The morbidity of sickle cell trait: a review of the literature. Am J Med 64:1021, 1978

127. Gupta AK, Kirchner KA, Nicholson R et al: Effects of α-thalassemia and sickle polymerization tendency on the urine-concentrating defect of individuals with sickle cell trait. J Clin Invest 88:1963, 1991

128. Bunn HF, Noguchi CT, Hofrichter J et al: Molecular and cellular pathogenesis of Hb SC disease. Proc Natl Acad Sci USA 79:7527, 1982

129. Fabry ME, Kaul DK, Raventos-Saurez C et al: SC erythrocytes have an abnormally high intracellular hamoglobin concentration. J Clin Invest 70:1315, 1982

130. Brugnara C, Kopin AS, Bunn HF, Tosteson DC: Regulation of cation content and cell volume in hemoglobin erythrocytes from patients with homozygous hemoglobin C disease. J Clin Invest 75:1608, 1985

131. Fabry ME, Mears JG, Patel P et al: Dense cells in sickle cell anemia: the effects of gene interaction. Blood 64:1042, 1984

132. Fabry ME, Nagel RL: The effect of deoxygenation of red cell density: significance for the pathophysiology of sickle cell anemia. Blood 60:1370, 1982

133. Serjeant BE, Mason KP, Kenny KW et al: Effect of alpha thalssemia on the rheology of homozygous sickle cell disease. Br J Haematol 55:479, 1983

134. Embury SH: Alpha thalassemia: a modifier of sickle cell disease. Ann NY Acad Sci 565:213, 1989

135. Embury SH, Oliver M, Kropp J: The beneficial effect of α-thalassemia on sickle cell anemia (SCA) is related to increased membrane redundancy. Blood, suppl. 1. 66:58A, 1985

136. Milner PF, Kraus AP, Sebes JI et al: Sickle cell disease as a cause of osteonecrosis of the femoral head. N Engl J Med 325:1476, 1991

137. Milner PF, Kraus AP, Sebes JI et al: Osteonecrosis of the humeral head in sickle cell disease. Clin Orthop 289:136, 1993

138. Platt OS, Thorington BD, Brambilla DJ et al: Pain in sickle cell disease: rates and risk factors. N Engl J Med 325:11, 1991

139. Rosa RM, Brirer BE, Thomas R et al: A study of induced hyponatremia in the prevention and treatment of sickle cell crisis. N Engl J Med 303:1138, 1980

140. Benjamin LJ, Berkowitz LR, Orringer E et al: A collaborative, double-blind randomized study of cetiedil citrate in sickle cell crisis. Blood 67:1442, 1986

141. Brugnara C, de Franceschi L, Alper SL: Inhibition of Ca(2$^+$)-dependent K$^+$ transport and cell dehydration in sickle erythrocytes by clotrimazole and other imidazole derivatives. J Clin Invest 92:520, 1993

142. Bender JW, Adachi K, Asakura T: Precipitation of oxyhemoglobins A and S by isopropanol. Hemoglobin 5:463, 1981

143. Adachi K, Kinney TR, Schwartz E, Asakura T: Molecular stability and function of Hb C-Harlem. Hemoglobin 4:1, 1980

144. Asakura T, Agarwal PL, Relman DA et al: Mechanical instability of the oxy-form of sickle haemoglobin. Nature 244:437, 1973

145. Macdonald VW, Charache S: Drug-induced oxidation and precipitation of hemoglobins A, S, and C. Biochim Biophys Acta 701:39, 1982

146. Waugh SM, Willardson BM, Kannan R et al: Heinz bodies induce clustering of band 3, glycophorin and ankyrin in sickle erythrocytes. J Clin Invest 78:1155, 1986

147. Hebbel RP, Morgan WT, Eaton JW, Hedlund BE: Accelerated autoxidation and heme loss due to instability of sickle hemoglobin. Proc Natl Acad Sci USA 85:237, 1988

148. Hebbel RP, Eaton JW, Balasingam M, Steinberg MH: Spontaneous oxygen radical generation by sickle erythrocytes. J Clin Invest 70:1253, 1982

149. Misra HP, Fridovich R: The generation of superoxide radical during the autoxidation of hemoglobin. J Biol Chem 247:6960, 1972

150. Hebbel RP: The sickle erythrocyte in double jeopardy: autoxidation and iron decompartmentalization. Semin Hematol 27:51, 1990

151. Zerez CR, Lachant NA, Lee SJ, Tanaka KR: Decreased erythrocyte nicotinamide adenine dinucleotide redox potential and abnormal pyridine nucleotide content in sickle cell disease. Blood 71:512, 1988

152. Schrader MC, Simplaceanu V, Ho C: Measurement of fluxes through the pentose phosphate pathway in erythrocytes from individuals with sickle cell anemia by carbon-13 nuclear magnetic resonance spectroscopy. Biochim Biophys Acta 1182:179, 1993

153. Lachant NA, Davidson WD, Tanaka KR: Impaired pentose phosphate shunt function in sickle cell disease: a potential mechanism for increased Heinz body formation and membrane lipid peroxidation. Am J Hematol 15:1, 1983

154. Zerez CR, Lachant NA, Tanaka KR: Impaired erythrocyte reduction in sickle cell disease: dependence of methemoglobin reduction on reduced nicotinamide adenine dinucleotide content. Blood 76:1008, 1990

155. Chiu D, Lubin B: Oxidative hemoglobin denaturation and RBC destruction: the effect of heme on red cell membranes. Semin Hematol 26:128, 1989

156. Hebbel RP, Eaton JW: Pathobiology of heme interaction with the erythrocyte membrane. Semin Hematol 26:136, 1989

157. Corbett JD, Golan DE: Band 3 and glycophorin are progressively aggregated in density-fractionated sickle and normal red blood cells. Evidence from rotational and lateral mobility studies. J Clin Invest 91:208, 1993

158. Low PS, Waugh SM, Zinke K, Drenckhahn D: The role of hemoglobin denaturation and band 3 clustering in red blood cell aging. Science 227:531, 1985

159. Turrini F, Arese P, Yuan J, Low PS: Clustering of integral membrane proteins of the human erythrocyte membrane stimulates autologous IgG binding, complement deposition and phagocytosis. J Biol Chem 266:23611, 1991

160. Hebbel RP, Visser MR, Goodman JL et al: Potentiated adherence of sickle erythrocytes to endothelium infected by virus. J Clin Invest 80:1503, 1987

161. Hebbel RP, Yamada O, Moldow CF et al: Abnormal adherence of sickle erythrocytes to cultured vascular endothelium. Possible mechanism for microvascular occlusion in sickle cell disease. J Clin Invest 65:154, 1980

162. Platt OS, Falcone JF, Lux SE: Molecular defect in the sickle erythrocyte skeleton: abnormal spectrin binding to inside-out vesicles. J Clin Invest 75: 266, 1985

163. Rank BH, Carlsson J, Hebbel RP: Abnormal redox status of membrane-protein thiols in sickle erythrocytes. J Clin Invest 75:1531, 1985

164. Jain SK, Shohet SB: A novel phospholipid in irreversibly sickled cells: evidence for in vivo peroxidative damage in sickle cell disease. Blood 63:362, 1984

165. Boullier JA, Brown BA, Bush JCJ, Barisas BG: Lateral mobility of a lipid analog in the membrane of irreversible sickle erythrocytes. Biochim Biophys Acta 856:301, 1986

166. Test ST, Kleman K, Lubin B: Characterization of the complement sensitivity of density-fractionated sickle cells. Blood, suppl. 1. 78:202a, 1991

167. Hoover R, Rubin R, Wise G, Warren R: Adhesion of normal sickle erythrocytes to endothelial monolayer cultures. Blood 54:872, 1979

168. Hebbel RP, Boogaerts MAB, Eaton JW, Steinberg MH: Erythrocyte adherence to endothelium in sickle-cell anemia. N Engl J Med 302:992, 1980

169. Wick TM, Moake JL, Udden MM et al: Unusually large von Willebrand factor multimers increase adhesion of sickle erythrocytes to human endothelial cells under controlled flow. J Clin Invest 80:905, 1987

170. Hebbel RP, Moldow CF, Steinberg MH: Modulation of erythrocyte-endothelial interactions the vasocclusive severity of sickling disorders. Blood 58: 947, 1981

171. Sugihara K, Sugihara T, Mohandas N, Hebbel RP: Thrombospondin mediates adherence of CD 36+ sickle reticulocytes to endothelial cells. Blood 80: 2634, 1992

172. Brittain HA, Eckman JR, Swerlick RA et al: Thrombospondin from activated platelets promotes sickle erythrocyte adherence to human microvascular endothelium under physiologic flow: a potential role for platelet activation in sickle cell vaso-occlusion. Blood 81:2137, 1993

173. Smith CMII, Hebbel RP, Tukey DP et al: Pluronic F-68 reduces the endothelial adherence and improves the rheology of liganded sickle erythrocytes. Blood 69:1631, 1987

174. Akinola NO, Stevens SME, Franklin IM et al: Subclinical ischaemic episodes during the steady state of sickle cell anemia. J Clin Pathol 45:902, 1992

175. Green D, Scott JP: Is sickle cell crisis a thrombotic event? Am J Hematol 23:317, 1986

176. Kaplan KL, Owen J: Plasma Levels of beta-thromboglobulin and platelet factor 4 as indicies of platelet activation in vivo. Blood 57:199, 1981

177. Sugihara K, Sugihara T, Mohandas N et al: Thrombospondin at pathophysiologic levels mediates adherence of CD36-positive sickle reticulocytes to endothelial cells, abstracted. Blood 80:334a, 1992

178. Ibe BO, Kurantsin-Mills J, Raj JU et al: Urinary levels of thromboxane metabolites in sickle cell disease reflects activated platelets in vivo, abstracted. In Proceedings of the Eighteenth Annual Meeting of the National Sickle Cell Disease, Program 76a, 1993

179. Haut MJ, Cowan DH, Harris JW: Platelet function and survival in sickle cell disease. J Lab Clin Med 82:44, 1973

180. Hebbel RP, Steinberg MH, Mosher D: Plasma and platelet thrombospondin levels in sickle disease, abstracted. Clin Res 41:762A, 1993

181. Richardson SGN, Matthews KB, Stuart J et al: Serial changes in coagulation and viscosity during sickle-cell crisis. Br J Haematol 41:95, 1979

182. Lubin B, Chiu D, Bastacky J et al: Abnormalities in membrane phospholipid organization in sickled erythrocytes. J Clin Invest 67:1643, 1981

183. Allan D, Limbrick AR, Thomas P, Westerman MP: Release of spectrin-free spicules on reoxygenation of sickled erythrocytes. Nature 295:612, 1982

184. Zwaal RFA: Membrane and lipid involvement in blood coagulation. Biochim Biophys Acta 515:163, 1978

185. Rodgers GM: Hemostatic properties of normal and perturbed vascular cells. FASEB J 2:116, 1988

186. Nagel RL: Pathophysiologic Aspects of Sickle Cell Vaso-occlusion. Alan R Liss, New York, 1987

187. Conley CL, Weatherall DJ, Richardson SN et al: Hereditary persistence of fetal hemoglobin: a study of 79 affected persons in 15 negro families in Baltimore. Blood 21:261, 1963

188. Claster S, Godwin MJ, Embury SH: The risk of altitude exposure in sickle cell disease. West J Med 135:364, 1981

189. Alleyne GEO, Statius van Eps LW, Addar SK et al: The kidney in sickle cell anemia. Kidney Int 7:371, 1975

190. Richards D, Nulsen FE: Angiographic media and the sickling phenomenon. Surg Forum 22:403, 1971

191. Nagel RL: Sickle cell anemia is a multigene disease: sickle painful crises, a case in point. Am J Hematol 42:96, 1993

192. Lande WM, Andrews DL, Clark MR et al: The incidence of painful crisis in homozygous sickle cell disease: correlation with red cell deformability. Blood 72:2056, 1988

193. Ballas SK, Larner J, Smith ED et al: Rheologic predictors of the severity of the painful sickle cell crisis. Blood 72:1216, 1988

194. Denton TA, Diamond GA, Helfant RH et al: Fascinating rhythm: a primer on chaos theory and its application to cardiology. Am Heart J 120:1419, 1990

195. Crosby WH: The metabolism of hemoglobin and bile pigment in hemolytic disease. Am J Med 18:112, 1955

196. Hebbel RP, Miller WJ: Phagocytosis of sickle erythrocytes: immunologic oxidative determinants of hemolytic anemia. Blood 64:733, 1984

197. Kaul DK, Fabry ME, Nagel RL: Vaso-occlusion by sickle cells: evidence for selective trapping of dense cells. Blood 68:1162, 1986

198. Hebbel RP, Miller WJ: Unique promotion of erythrophagocytosis by malondialdehyde. Am J Hematol 29:222, 1988

199. Test ST, Woolworth VS: Multiple defects in the regulation of membrane attack complex (MAC) assembly by sickle erythrocytes. Blood, suppl. 1. 80: 75a, 1992

200. Fabry ME, Benjamin L, Lawrence C, Nagel RL: An objective sign in painful crisis in sickle cell anemia. The concomitant reduction of high density red cells. Blood 64:559, 1984

201. Ballas SK, Smith ED: Red blood cell changes during the evolution of the sickle cell painful crisis. Blood 79:2154, 1992

202. Padlia F, Bromberg PA, Jensen WA: The sickle-unsickle cycle: a cause of cell fragmentation and deformation. Blood 41:653, 1973

203. Butikofer P, Kuypers FA, Xu CM et al: Enrichment of two clycosylphosphatidylinositol-anchored proteins, acetylcholine esterase and decay accelerating factor, in vesicles released from human red blood cells. Blood 74:1481, 1989

204. Platt OS: Exercise-induced hemolysis in sickle cell anemia: shear sensitivity and erythrocyte dehydration. Blood 59:1055, 1982

205. Pearson HT, Spencer RD, Cornelius EA: Functional asplenia in sickle cell anemia. N Engl J Med 281:923, 1969

206. Winkelstein JA, Drachman RH: Deficiency of pneumococcal serum opsonizing activity in sickle-cell disease. N Engl J Med 279:459, 1966

207. Diggs LW: Siderfibrosis of the spleen in sickle cell anemia. JAMA 104:539, 1935

208. Pearson HA, Gallagher R, Chilcote E: Developmental pattern of splenic dysfunction in sickle cell disorders. Pediatrics 76:392, 1985

209. Pearson HT, Cornelius RA, Schwartz AD: Transfusion reversible functional asplenia in young children with sickle cell anemia. N Engl J Med 283:334, 1970

210. Johnston RB Jr, Newman SL, Struth AG: An abnormality of the alternate pathway of complement activation in sickle-cell disease. N Engl J Med 288: 803, 1973

211. Bjornson AB, Lobel JS: Direct evidence that decreased serum opsonization of *Streptococcus pneumoniae* via the alternative complement pathway in sickle cell disease is related to antibody deficiency. J Clin Invest 79:388, 1987

212. Hosea SW, Burch CG, Brown EJ et al: Impaired immune response of splenectomised patients to polyvalent pneumococcal vaccine. Lancet 1:804, 1981

213. De Ceulaer K, Wilson WA, Morgan AG, Serjeant GR: Haemoglobinaemia and activation of the complement system in homozygous sickle cell disease. J Clin Lab Immunol 6:57, 1981

214. Carr DJJ, Guarcello V, Blalock JE: Phosphatidulserine suppresses antigenspecific IgM production by mice orally administered sheep red blood cells. Proc Soc Exp Biol Med 200:548, 1992

215. Franck PFH, Bevers EM, Lubin BH et al: Uncoupling of the membrane skeleton from the lipid bilayer. The cause of accelerated phospholipid flip-flop leading to an enhanced procoagulant activity of sickled cells. J Clin Invest 75:183, 1985

216. Mankad VN, Moore RB: Sickle Cell Disease: Pathophysiology, Diagnosis and Management. Praeger, Westport, CT, 1992

217. Charache S, Lubin B, Reid C: Management and Therapy of Sickle Cell Disease. NIH Publ. 89-2117 1. National Institutes of Health, Bethesda, MD, 1989

218. Vichinsky E, Lubin B: Suggested guidelines for treatment of children with sickle cell anemia. Hematol Oncol Clin 1:483, 1987

219. Diggs LM: Anatomic lesions in sickle cell disease. p. 189. In Abramson H, Bertles JF, Wethers DL (eds): Sickle Cell Disease Diagnosis. Management, Education, and Research. CV Mosby, St. Louis, 1973

220. Platt OS, Brambilla DJ, Rosse WF et al: The Cooperative Study of Sickle Cell Disease: mortality in sickle cell disease: life expectancy and risk factors for early death. N Engl J Med 330:1639, 1994

221. Gaston MH, Verter JI, Woods G et al: Prophylaxis with oral penicillin in children with sickle cell anemia. N Engl J Med 314:1593, 1986

222. McCurdy PR: ^{32}DFP and ^{51}Cr for measurement of red cell life span in abnormal hemoglobin syndromes. Blood 33:214, 1969

223. West MS, Wethers D, Smith J, Steinberg M, the Cooperative Study of Sickle Cell Disease: Laboratory profile of sickle cell disease: a cross-sectional analysis. J Clin Epidemiol 45:893, 1992

224. Sherwood JB, Goldwasser E, Chilcote R et al: Sickle cell anemia patients have low erythropoietin levels for their degree of anemia. Blood 67:46, 1986

225. Singh A, Eckhardt KU, Zimmerman A et al: Increased plasma viscosity as a reason for inappropriate erythropoietin formation. J Clin Invest 91:251, 1993

226. Means RT Jr, Dessypris EN, Krantz SB: Inhibition of human colony-forming-unit erythroid by tumor necrosis factor requires accessory cells. J Clin Invest 86:538, 1990

227. Mortimer PP, Humphries RK, Moore JG et al: A human parvovirus-like virus inhibits haematopoietic colony formation in vitro. Nature 302:426, 1983

228. Pattison JR, Jones SE, Hodgson J et al: Parvovirus infections and hypoplastic crisis in sickle cell anaemia. Lancet 1:664, 1981

229. Rao SP, Miller ST, Cohen BJ: Transient aplastic crisis in patients with sickle cell disease. Am J Dis Child 146:1328, 1992

230. Anderson LJ: The role of human parvovirus B19 in human disease. J Pediatr Infect Dis 6:711, 1987

231. Pardoll DM, Rodeheffer RJ, Smith RRL, Charache S: Aplastic crisis due to extensive bone necrosis in sickle cell disease. Arch Intern Med 142:2223, 1982

232. Conrad ME, Studdard H, Anderson LJ: Case report: aplastic crisis in sickle cell disorders: bone marrow necrosis and human parvovirus infections. Am J Med Sci 295:212, 1988

233. Topley JM, Rogers DW, Stevens MCG, Serjeant GR: Acute splenic sequestration and hypersplenism in the first five years in homozygous sickle cell disease. Arch Dis Child 56:765, 1981

234. Orringer EP, Fowler VG, Owens CM et al: Case report: splenic infarction and acute splenis sequestration in adults with hemoglobin SC disease. Am J Med Sci 302:374, 1991

235. Pappo A, Buchanan GR: Acute splenic sequestration in a 2-month-old infant with sickle cell anemia. Pediatr 84:578, 1989

236. Jenkins ME, Scott RB, Baird RL: Studies in sickle cell anemia. J Pediatr 56:30, 1960

237. Emond AM, Collis R, Darvill D et al: Acute splenic sequestration in homozygous sickle cell disease: natural history and management. J Pediatr 107:201, 1985

238. Kinney TR, Ware RE, Schultz WH, Filston HC: Long-term management of splenic sequestration in children with sickle cell disease. J Pediatr 117:194, 1990

239. Hatton CSR, Bunch C, Weatherall DJ: Hepatic sequestration in sickle cell anaemia. Br Med J 190:215, 1985

240. Davies SC, Win AA, Luce PJ et al: Acute chest syndrome in sickle cell disease. Lancet 1:36, 1984

241. Smits HL, Oski FA, Brody JI: The hemolytic crisis of sickle cell disease: the role of glucose-6-phosphate dehydrogenase deficiency. J Pediatr 74:544, 1969

242. Morgan AG, Gruber CA, Serjeant GR: Erythropoietin and renal function in sickle cell disease. Br Med J 285:1686, 1982

243. Steinberg MH: Erythropoietin for anemia of renal failure in sickle cell disease. N Engl J Med 324:1369, 1991

244. Pearson HA, Cobb WT: Folic acid studies in sickle cell anemia. J Lab Clin Med 64:913, 1964

245. Lopez R, Shimizu N, Cooperman JM: Recurrent folic acid deficiency in sickle cell disease. Am J Dis Child 122:48, 1971

246. O'Brien RT: Iron burden in sickle cell anemia. J Pediatr 1978:579, 1978

247. Lanzkowsky P: Iron deficiency anemia. Pediatr Ann 3:6, 1974

248. Vichinsky E, Kleman K, Embury SH: The diagnosis of iron deficiency anemia in sickle cell disease. Blood 58:963, 1981

249. Bainbridge R, Higgs DR, Maude GH, Serjeant GR: Clinical presentation of homozygous sickle cell disease. J Pediatr 1067:881, 1985

250. Brozovic M, Davles S, Brownell A: Acute admissions of patients with sickle cell disease who live in Britain. Br Med J 294:1206, 1987

251. Powars DR: The natural history of sickle cell disease—the first ten years. Semin Hematol 12:267, 1975

252. Baum FK, Dunn DT, Maude GH, Serjeant GR: The painful crisis of homozygous sickle cell disease. A study on the risk factors. Arch Intern Med 47:1231, 1987

253. Shapiro BS, Ballas SK: The acute painful episode. p. 531. In Embury SH, Hebbel RP, Mohandas N, Steinberg MH (eds): Sickle Cell Disease: Basic Principles and Clinical Practice. Raven Press, New York, 1994

254. Murray N, May A: Painful crises in sickle cell disease—patients' perspectives. Br Med J 297:452, 1988

255. Shapiro BS, Dinges DF, Orne EC et al: Recording of crisis pain in sickle cell disease. p. 313. In Tyler DC, Krane EJ (eds): Pediatric Pain. Advances in Pain Research Therapy. Raven Press, New York, 1990

256. Benjamin LJ: Sickle cell disease. In Max M, Portenoy R, Laska E (eds): Advances in Pain Research and Therapy. Raven Press, New York, 1991

257. Diggs LW: The blood picture in sickle cell anemia. South Med J 25:615, 1932

258. Devine DV, Kinney TR, Thomas PF et al: Fragment D-dimer levels: an objective marker of vaso-occlusive crisis and other complications of sickle cell disease. Blood 68:317, 1986

259. Buchanan GR, Holtkamp CA: Evidence against increased platelet activity in sickle cell anaemia. Br J Haematol 54:595, 1983

260. Akinola NO, Stevens SME, Franklin IM et al: Rheological changes in the prodromal and established phases of sickle cell vaso-occlusive crisis. Br J Haematol 81:598, 1992

261. Becton DL, Raymond L, Thompson C: Acute-phase reactants in sickle cell disease. J Pediatr 115:99, 1989

262. Neely CL, Wajima T, Kraus AP et al: Lactic acid dehydrogenase activity and plasma hemoglobin elevations in sickle cell disease. Am J Clin Pathol 52:167, 1969

263. Shreeniwas R, Koga S, Karakurum M et al: Hypoxia mediated induction of endothelial cell interleukin-la. J Clin Invest 90:2333, 1992

264. Whitten CF, Fischoff J: Psychosocial effects of sickle cell disease. Arch Intern Med 133:681, 1974

265. Drotar D: Psychological perspectives in chronic childhood illness. J Pediatr Psychol 6:211, 1981

266. Alleyne SI, Wint E, Serjeant GR: Psychological aspects of sickle cell disease. Health Social Work 1:105, 1976

267. Kumar S, Powars D, Haywood LJ: Anxiety, self-concept and personal and social adjustment in children with sickle cell anemia. J Pediatr 88:859, 1976

268. Conyard S, Krishnamurthy M, Dosik H: Psychological aspects of sickle cell anemia in adolescents. Health Social Work 5:20, 1980

269. Barrett DH, Wisotzek IE, Rouleau JL et al: Assessment of psychosocial functioning of patients with sickle cell disease. South Med J 81:745, 1988

270. Vichinsky EP, Johnson R, Lubin BH: Multidisciplinary approach to pain management in sickle cell disease. Am J Pediatr Hematol Oncol 4:328, 1982

271. Gil KM, Williams DA, Thompson RJ, Kinney TR: Sickle cell disease in children and adolescents: the relation of child and parent pain coping strategies to adjustment. J Pediatr Psychol 16:643, 1991

272. Ross DM, Ross SA: Childhood Pain. Urban & Schwarzenberg, Baltimore, 1988

273. Seligman MEP: Depression and learned helplessness. In Friedman RJ, Katz MM (eds): The Psychology of Depression: Contemporary Theory and Research. John Wiley & Sons, New York, 1974

274. Rosse W: Diagnosis and treatment of painful episode in sickle cell disease. N C Med J 44:419, 1983

275. Gil KM, Abrams MR, Phillips G, Williams DA: Sickle cell disease pain. 2. Predicting health care use and activity level at 9-month follow-up. J Cons Clin Psychol 60:267, 1992

276. Thompson RJ Jr, Gil KM, Abrams MR, Phillips G: Stress, coping and psychological adjustment of adults with sickle cell disease. J Consult Clin Psychol 60:433, 1992

277. Slaughter DT, Dilworth-Anderson P: Care of black children with sickle cell disease: fathers, maternal support and esteem. Fam Rel 37:281, 1988

278. Platt OS, Rosenstock W, Espeland MA: Influence of sickle hemoglobinopathies on growth and development. N Engl J Med 311:7, 1984

279. Stevens MCG, Maude GH, Cupidore L et al: Prepubertal growth and skeletal maturation in children with sickle cell disease. Pediatrics 78:124, 1986

280. Olambiwonnu NO, Penny R, Frasier SD: Sexual maturation in subjects with sickle cell anemia: studies of serum gonadotropin concentration, height, weight, and skeletal age. J Pediatr 87:459, 1975

281. Alleyne SI, D'Hereux Rauseo R, Serjeant GR: Sexual development and fertility of Jamaican female patients with homozygous sickle cell disease. Arch Intern Med 141:1295, 1981

282. Abbasi AA, Prasad AS, Ortega J et al: Gonadal function abnormalities in

sickle cell anemia: studies in adult male patients. Ann Intern Med 85:601, 1976

283. Dada OA, Nduka EU: Endocrine function and haemoglobinopathies: relation between the sickle cell gene and circulating plasma levels of testosterone, LH, and FSH in adult males. Clin Chim Acta 105:269, 1980

284. Landefeld S, Shambelan M, Kaplan S, Embury SH: Clomiphene-responsive hypogonadism in sickle cell anemia. Ann Intern Med 99:480, 1983

285. Badaloo A, Jackson AA, Jahoor F: Whole body protein turnover and resting metabolic rate in homozygous sickle cell disease. Clin Sci 77:93, 1989

286. Heyman MB, Vichinsky E, Katz R et al: Growth retardation in sickle-cell disease treated by nutritional support. Lancet 1:903, 1985

287. Watson-Williams EJ: Folic acid deficiency in sickle cell anemia. East Afr Med J 39:213, 1962

288. Prasad AS, Cossack ZT: Zinc supplementation and growth in sickle cell disease. Ann Intern Med 100:367, 1984

289. Zarkowsky HS, Gallagher D, Gill FM et al: Bacteremia in sickle hemoglobinopathies. J Pediatr 109:579, 1986

290. Barrett-Connor E: Bacterial infection and sickle cell anemia. An analysis of 250 infections in 106 patients and a review of medicine. Medicine 50:97, 1971

291. Buchanan GR: Infection. p. 567. In Embury SH, Hebbel RP, Mohandas N, Steinberg MH (eds): Sickle Cell Disease: Basic Principles and Clinical Practice. Raven Press, New York, 1994

292. Wong W-Y, Powars DR, Chan L et al: Polysaccharide encapsulated bacterial infection in sickle cell anemia: a thirty year epidemiologic experience. Am J Hematol 39:176, 1992

293. Overturf GD, Powars D, Baraff LJ: Bacterial meningitis and septicemia in sickle cell disease. Am J Dis Child 131:784, 1977

294. Vichinsky E, Hurst D, Earles A et al: Newborn screening for sickle cell disease: effect on mortality. Pediatrics 81:749, 1988

295. Ward J, Smith AL: *Hemophilus influenzae* bacteremia in children with sickle cell disease. J Pediatr 88:261, 1976

296. Powars D, Overturf G, Turner E: Is there an increased risk of *Haemophilus influenzae* in children with sickle cell anemia? Pediatrics 71:927, 1983

297. John AB, Ramlal A, Jackson H et al: Prevention of pneumococcal infection in children with homozygous sickle cell disease. Br Med J 288:1567, 1984

298. Buchanan GR, Vedro D, Morrison R, Schiffman G: Antibody response to polyvalent pneumococcal vaccine in children with sickle cell anemia. Pediatr Res 27:139A, 1990

299. Marcinak JF, Frank AL, Labotka RL et al: Immunogenicity of *Haemophilus influenzae* type b polysaccharide-diptheria toxoid conjugate vaccine in 3- to 17-month old infants with sickle cell diseases. J Pediatr 118:69, 1991

300. Rogers ZR, Morrison RA, Vedro DA, Buchanan GR: Outpatient management of febrile illness in infants and young children with sickle cell anemia. J Pediatr 117:736, 1990

301. Wilimas JA, Flynn PM, Harris S et al: A randomized study of outpatient treatment with ceftriaxone for selected febrile children with sickle cell disease. N Engl J Med 329:472, 1993

302. Robinson MG, Watson RJ: Pneumococcal meningitis in sickle cell anemia. N Engl J Med 274:923, 1966

303. Poncz M, Kane E, Gill F: Acute chest syndrome in sickle cell disease: etiology and clinical correlates. J Pediatr 107:861, 1985

304. Miller ST, Hammerschlag MR, Chirgwin K et al: Role of *Chlamydia pneumoniae* in acute chest syndrome of sickle cell disease. J Pediatr 118:30, 1991

305. Syrogiannopoulos GA, McCracken GH Jr, Nelson JD: Osteoarticular infections in children with sickle cell disease. Pediatrics 78:1090, 1986

306. Givner LB, Luddy RE, Schwartz AD: Etiology of osteomyelitis in patients with major sickle hemoglobinopathies. J Pediatr 99:411, 1981

307. Adeyokunnu AA, Hendrickse RG: *Salmonella* osteomyelitis in childhood. A report of 63 cases seen in Nigerian children of whom 57 had sickle cell anaemia. Arch Dis Child 55:175, 1980

308. Powars D, Wilson B, Imbus C et al: The natural history of stroke in sickle cell disease. Am J Med 65:416, 1978

309. Sarnaik AS, Lusher JM: Neurological complications of sickle cell anemia. Am J Pediatr Hematol Oncol 4:386, 1982

310. Merkel KH, Ginsberg PL, Parker JC et al: Cerebrovascular disease in sickle cell anemia: a clinical, pathological and radiological correlation. Stroke 9:45, 1978

311. Russell MO, Goldberg HI, Reis L et al: Effect of transfusion therapy on the arteriographic abnormalities and on the recurrence of stroke in sickle cell disease. Blood 63:162, 1984

312. Wood DH: Cerebrovascular complications of sickle cell anemia. Stroke 12:73, 1977

313. Powars DR, Schroeder WR, Weiss JN et al: The lack of influence of fetal hemoglobin levels or red cell indices on the severity of sickle cell anemia. J Clin Invest 65:732, 1980

314. Balkaran B, Char G, Morris JS et al: Stroke in a cohort or patients with homozygous sickle cell disease. J Pediatr 120:360, 1992

315. Powars DR: Sickle cell anemia: β^S-Gene cluster haplotypes as prognostic indicators of vital organ failure. Semin Hematol 28:202, 1991

316. Pavlakis SG: Neurologic complications of sickle cell disease. Adv Pediatr 36:247, 1989

317. Frempong KO: Stroke in sickle cell disease: demographic, clinical and therapeutic considerations. Semin Hematol 28:213, 1991

318. Gerald B, Sebes JI, Langston JW: Cerebral infarction secondary to sickle cell disease: arteriographic findings. AJR 134:1209, 1980

319. Sarnaik S, Soorya D, Kim J et al: Periodic transfusion for sickle cell anemia and CNS infarction. Am J Dis Child 133:1254, 1979

320. Stockman JA, Nigro MA, Mishkin MM, Oski FA: Occlusion of large cerebral vessels in sickle cell anemia. N Engl J Med 287:846, 1972

321. Van Hoff J, Ritchey K, Shaynitz B: Intracranial hemorrhage in children with sickle cell disease. Am J Dis Child 139:1120, 1985

322. Oyesiku NM, Barrow DL, Eckman JR et al: Intracranial aneurysms in sickle-cell anemia: clinical features and pathogenesis. J Neurosurg 75:356, 1991

323. Anson NM, Koshy M, Ferguson L, Crowell RM: Subarachnoid hemorrhage in sickle-cell disease. J Neurosurg 75:552, 1991

324. Overby MC, Rothman AS: Multiple intracranial aneurysms in sickle cell anemia. J Neurosurg 62:430, 1985

325. Boros L, Wiener WJ: Sickle cell anemia and other hemoglobinopathies. p. 33. In Vicken PJ, Bruyn GW (eds): Handbook of Clinical Neurology. Elsevier, Amsterdam, 1978

326. Suzuki J, Takaku A: Cerebrovascular Moyamoya disease. Disease showing abnormal net-like vessels in base of brain. Arch Neurol 20:288, 1969

327. Allen GS, Ahn HS, Preziosi TJ et al: Cerebral arterial spasm—a controlled trial of nimodipine in patients with subarachnoid hemorrhage. N Engl J Med 308:619, 1983

328. Russell MO, Goldberg HI, Reis L et al: Transfusion therapy for cerebrovascular abnormalities in sickle cell disease. J Pediatr 88:382, 1976

329. Buchanan GR, Bowman WP, Smith SJ: Recurrent cerebral ischemia during hypertransfusion therapy in sickle cell anemia. J Pediatr 103:921, 1983

330. Huttenlocher PR, Moohr JW, Johns L, Brown FD: Cerebral blood flow in sickle cell cerebrovascular disease. Pediatrics 73:615, 1984

331. Wang WC, Kovnar EH, Tonkin IL et al: High risk of recurrent stroke after discontinuance of five to twelve years of transfusion therapy in patients with sickle cell disease. J Pediatr 118:377, 1991

332. Song J: Pathology of Sickle Cell Disease. Charles C Thomas, Springfield, IL, 1971

333. Zimmerman RA, Gill F, Goldberg HI et al: MRI of sickle cell cerebral infarction. Neuroradiology 29:232, 1987

334. Pavlakis SG, Bello J, Prohovnik I et al: Brain infarction in sickle cell anemia: magnetic resonance imaging correlates. Ann Neurol 23:125, 1987

335. Rodgers GP, Clark CM, Larsen SM et al: Brain glucose metabolism in neurologically normal patients with sickle cell disease. Arch Neurol 45:78, 1987

336. Adams R, McKie V, Nichols F et al: The use of transcranial ultrasonography to predict stroke in sickle cell disease. N Engl J Med 326:605, 1992

337. Wasserman AL, Williams JA, Fairclough DL et al: Subtle neuropsychological defects in children with sickle cell disease. Am J Pediatr Hematol Oncol 3:14, 1991

338. Charache S, Scott JC, Charache P: Acute chest syndrome in adults with sickle cell disease. Arch Intern Med 139:67, 1984

339. Barrett-Connor E: Acute pulmonary disease and sickle cell anemia. Am Rev Respir Dis 104:159, 1971

340. Diggs LW, Pulliam HN, King JC: The bone changes in sickle cell anemia. South Med J 30:249, 1937

341. Haynes JJr, Allison RC: Pulmonary edema. Complication in the management of sickle cell pain crisis. Am J Med 80:833, 1986

342. Gillett DS, Gunning KEJ, Sawicka EH et al: Life threatening sickle chest syndrome treated with extracorporeal membrane oxygenation. Br Med J 294:81, 1987

343. Powars D, Weidman JA, Odom-Maryon T et al: Sickle cell chronic lung disease: prior morbidity and the risk of pulmonary failure. Medicine 67:66, 1988

344. Wall MA, Platt OS, Streider DJ: Lung function in children with sickle cell anemia. Am Rev Respir Dis 129:219, 1979

345. Collins FFS, Orringer EP: Pulmonary hypertension and cor pulmonale in the sickle hemoglobinopathies. Am J Med 73:814, 1982

346. Seibert AF, Taylor AE, Bass JB, Haynes J Jr: Hemoglobin potentiates oxidant injury in isolated rat lungs. Am J Physiol 260:H1980, 1991

347. Rennels MB, Dunne MG, Grossman NJ, Schwartz AD: Cholelithiasis in patients with major sickle hemoglobinopathies. Am J Dis Child 138:66, 1984

348. Webb KDH, Darby JS, Dunn DT et al: Gall stones on Jamaican children with homozygous sickle cell disease. Arch Dis Child 64:693, 1989

349. Sarnaik S, Slovis TL, Corbett DP et al: The choleliothiasis in sickle cell anemia using the ultrasonic gray scale technique. J Pediatr 96:1005, 1980

350. Malone BS, Werlin SL: Cholecystitis and cholelithiasis in sickle cell anemia. Am J Dis Child 142:799, 1988

351. Ware RE, Kinney TR, Casey JR et al: Laparoscopic cholecystectomy in young patients with sickle hemoglobinopathies. J Pediatr 120:58, 1992

352. Bauer TW, Moore GW, Hutchins GM: The liver in sickle cell disease: a clinical copathologic study of 70 patients. Am J Med 69:833, 1980

353. Barrett-Connor E: Sickle cell disease and viral hepatitis. Ann Intern Med 69: 517, 1968

354. Buchanan GR, Glader BE: Benign course of extreme hyperbilirubinemia in sickle cell anemia: analysis of six cases. J Pediatr 91:21, 1977

355. Rosenblate HJ, Eisenstein R, Holmes AW: The liver in sickle cell anemia: a clinical-pathologic study. Arch Pathol Lab Med 90:235, 1970

356. Sheehy TW, Law DE, Wade BH: Exchange transfusion for sickle cell intrahepatic cholestasis. Arch Intern Med 140:1364, 1980

357. Owen DM, Aldridge JE, Thompson RB: An unusual hepatic sequela of sickle cell anemia: a report of five cases. Am J Med Sci 249:175, 1965

358. Wagner G, Johnson R, Claster S et al: Gynecological and obstetrical complications in sickle cell disease. p. 26A. In Sickle Cell Disease: Progress and Prospects. National Sickle Cell Disease Program, Boston, 1986

359. Pritchard JA, Scott DE, Whalley PJ et al: The effects of maternal sickle cell hemoglobinopathies and sickle cell trait on reproductive performance. Am J Obstet Gynecol 117:662, 1973

360. Charache S, Scott JC, Niebyl J, Bonds D: Management of sickle cell disease in pregnant patients. Obstet Gynecol 55:407, 1980

361. Milner PF, Jones BR, Döbler J: Outcome of pregnancy in sickle cell anemia and sickle cell hemoglobin C disease. Am J Obstet Gynecol 138:239, 1980

362. Powars DR, Sandhu M, Niland Weiss JN et al: Pregnancy in sickle cell disease. Obstet Gynecol 67:217, 1986

363. Morrison JC, Propst MC, Blake PG: Sickle hemoglobin and the gravid patient: a management controversy. Clin Perinatol 7:273, 1980

364. Morrison JC, Whybrew WD, Bucovaz ET: Use of partial exchange transfusion preoperatively in patients with sickle hemoglobinopathies. Am J Obstet Gynecol 132:59, 1978

365. Koshy M, Burd L, Wallace D et al: Prophylactic red cell transfusions in pregnant patients with sickle cell disease. N Engl J Med 319:1447, 1988

366. Freie HMP: Sickle cell disease and hormonal contraception. Acta Obstet Gynecol Scand 62:211, 1983

367. Strauss J, Zilleruelo G, Abitbol C: The kidney and hemoglobin S. Nephron 43:241, 1986

368. Statius van Eps LW, Shouten H et al: The influence of red blood cell transfusions on the hyposthenuria and renal hemodynamics of sickle cell anemia. Clin Chim Acta 17:449, 1967

369. Statius van Eps LW, Shouten H, Ter Haar Romeny-Wachter, La Porte-Wijsman LW: The relation between age and renal concentrating capacity in sickle cell disease and hemoglobin C disease. Clin Chim Acta 27:501, 1970

370. Lucas WM, Bullock WH: Hematuria in sickle cell disease. J Urol 83:733, 1960

371. Knochel JP: Hematuria in sickle cell trait. Arch Intern Med 123:160, 1969

372. McInnes BK III: The management of hematuria associated with sickle hemoglobinopathies. J Urol 124:171, 1980

373. Immergut MA, Stevenson T: The use of epsilon-amino caproic acid in the control of hematuria associated with hemoglobinopathies. J Urol 93:110, 1965

374. John EG, Schade SG, Spigos DG et al: Effectiveness of triglycyl vasopressin in persistent hematuria associated with sickle cell hemoglobin. Arch Intern Med 140:1589, 1980

375. Harrison FG, Harrison FG Jr: Hematuria with sickle cell disease. J Urol 68: 942, 1952

376. DeFronzo RA, Taufield PA, Black H et al: Impaired renal tubular potassium excretion in sickle cell disease. Ann Intern Med 90:310, 1979

377. Diamond HS, Meisel A, Sharon E et al: Hyperurocosuria and increased tubular secretion of urate in sickle cell anemia. Am J Med 59:796, 1975

378. de Jong PE, de Jong-Van Den Berg LTW, Statius van Eps LW: The tubular reabsorption of phosphate in sickle-cell nephropathy. Clin Sci Mol Med 55: 429, 1978

379. Powars DR, Elliott-Mills DD, Chan L et al: Chronic renal failure in sickle cell disease: risk factors, clinical course, and mortality. Ann Intern Med 115:614, 1991

380. Falk RJ, Scheinman J, Phillips G et al: Prevalence and pathologic features of sickle cell nephropathy and response to inhibition of angiotension converting enzyme. N Engl J Med 326:910, 1992

381. Chatterjee SN: National study on the natural history of renal allografts in sickle cell disease or trait. Nephron 25:199, 1980

382. Tarry WF, Duckett JW Jr, Snyder HM III: Urological complications of sickle cell disease in a pediatric population. J Urol 138:592, 1987

383. Hamre MA, Harmon EP, Kirkpatrick DV et al: Priapism as a complication of sickle cell disease. J Urol 145:1, 1991

384. Hashmat AI, Rehman JU: Priapism. In Hashmat AI, Das S (eds): The Penis. Lea & Febinger, Baltimore, 1993

385. Tripe JW: Case of continued priapism. Lancet 2:8, 1845

386. Allen RP, Burnett AL, Tempany CM et al: Evaluation of erectile function in men with sickle cell disease. J Urol 149:277A, 1993

387. Sharpsteen JR, Powars D, Johnson C et al: Multisystem damage associated with tricorporal priapism in sickle cell disease. Am J Med 94:289, 1993

388. Hashmat AI, Raju S, Singh I, Macchia RJ: 99mm-Tc penile scan: an investigative modality in priapism. Urol Radiol 9:58, 1989

389. Hakim LS, Hashmat AI, Macchia RJ: Priapism. p. 633. In Embury SH, Hebbel RP, Mohandas N, Steinberg MH (eds): Sickle Cell Disease: Basic Principles and Clinical Practice. Raven Press, New York, 1994

390. Hanno PM: Priapism. American Urological Association (AUA) Update Series Lesson 20. 3:1, 1984

391. Dittrich A, Albrecht K, Bar-Moshe O, Vandendris M: Treatment of pharmacological priapism with phenylephrine. J Urol 146:323, 1991

392. Hashmat AI, Horowitz M, Macchia RJ: Surgery in priapism. p. 891. In Droller MJ (ed): Surgical Management of Urologic Disease: An Anatomic Approach. CV Mosby-Year Book, St Louis, 1992

393. Winter CC: Priapism cured by creation of fistulas between glans penis and corpora cavernosa. J Urol 119:227, 1978

394. Grayhack JT, McCullough W, O'Connor VL, Trippel O: Venous bypass to control priapism. Invest Urol 1:509, 1964

395. Bertram RA, Carson CC, Webster GD: Implantation of penile prosthesis in patients impotent after priapism. Urology 26:325, 1985

396. Hayes RJ, Condon PI, Serjeant GR: Haematologic factors associated with proliferative retinopathy in homozygous sickle cell disease. Br J Ophthalmol 65:29, 1981

397. Nagpal K, Goldberg M, Rabb M: Ocular manifestations of sickle hemoglobinopathies. Surv Ophthalmol 21:391, 1977

398. Condon PI, Hayes RJ, Serjeant GR: Retinal and choroidal neovascularization in sickle cell disease. Trans Ophthalmol Soc UK 100:434, 1980

399. Goldberg MF, Acacio I: Argon laser photocoagulation of proliferative sickle retinopathy. Arch Ophthalmol 90:35, 1973

400. Diggs LW: Bone and joint lesions in sickle-cell disease. Clin Orthop 52:119, 1967

401. Bohrer SP: Bone Ischemia and Infarction in Sickle Cell Disease. Warren H Green, St Louis, 1981

402. Stevens MCG, Padwick M, Serjeant GR: Observations on the natural history of dactylitis in homozygous sickle cell disease. Clin Pediatr (Phila) 20:311, 1981

403. Lutzker LG, Alavi A: Bone and marrow imaging on sickle cell disease: diagnosis of infarction. Semin Nucl Med 6:83, 1976

404. Alavi A, Heyman K, Kim HC: Scintigraphic examination of bone and marrow infarcts in sickle cell disorders. Semin Roentgenol 23:213, 1987

405. Mankad VN, Williams JP, Harpen MD et al: Magnetic resonance imaging of bone marrow in sickle cell disease: clinical hematologic and pathologic correlations. Blood 75:274, 1990

406. Ballas SK, Talacki CA, Rao VM, Steiner RM: The prevalence of avascular necrosis in sickle cell anemia: correlation with α-thalassemia. Hemoglobin 13:649, 1989

407. Arlet J, Ficat P: Forage-biopsie de la tête fémoral dans l'osteonécrose primitive: observations histo-pathologiques portant sur huit forages. Rev Rhum Mal Osteoartic 31:257, 1964

408. Mitchell DG, Steinberg ME, Dalinka MK et al: Magnetic resonance imaging of the ischemic hip. Alterations within the osteonecrotic, viable and reactive zones. Clin Orthop 244:60, 1989

409. Steinberg ME, Steinberg DR: Evaluation and staging of avscular necrosis. Semin Arthroplasty 2:175, 1991

410. Schumacher HR, Dorwart BB, Bond J et al: Chronic synovitis with early cartilage destruction in sickle cell disease. Ann Rheum Dis 36:413, 1977

411. Hanissian AS, Silverman A: Arthritis of sickle cell anemia. South Med J 67: 28, 1974

412. Hutchinson RM, Merrick MV, White JM: Fat embolism in sickle cell disease. J Clin Pathol 26:620, 1973

413. Chmel H, Bertles JF: Hemaoglobin Hb SC disease in pregnant woman with crisis and fat embolism syndrome. Am J Med 58:563, 1975

414. Serjeant GR: Leg ulceration in sickle cell anemia. Arch Intern Med 133:690, 1974

415. Koshy M, Entsuah R, Koranda A et al: Leg ulcers in patients with sickle cell disease. Blood 74:1403, 1989

416. Sehgal SC, Arunkumar BK: Microbial flora and its significance in the pathology of sickle cell disease leg ulcers. Infection 20:86, 1992

417. Ankra-Badu GA: Sickle cell leg ulcers in Ghana. East Afr Med J 69:366, 1992

418. Perrine RP, Pembrey ME, John P et al: Natural history of sickle cell anemia in Saudi Arabs. A study of 270 subjects. Ann Intern Med 88:1, 1978

419. Keidan AJ, Stuart J: Rheological effects of bed rest in sickle cell disease. J Clin Pathol 40:1187, 1987

420. Baum KF, MacFarlane DE, Maude GH, Serjeant GR: Topical antibiotics in chronic sickle cell leg ulcers. Trans R Soc Trop Med Hyg 81:847, 1987

421. Varat MA, Adolph RJ, Fowler NO: Cardiovascular effects of anemia. Am Heart J 83:415, 1972

422. Gerry JL, Bulkley BH, Hutchins GM: Clinical analysis of cardiac dysfunction in 52 patients with sickle cell anemia. Am J Cardiol 42:211, 1978

423. Balfour IC, Covitz W, Davis H et al: Cardiac size and function in children with sickle cell anemia. Am Heart J 108:345, 1984

424. Covitz W, Eubig C, Balfour IC et al: Exercise induced cardiac dysfunction in sickle cell anemia. Am J Cardiol 61:395, 1988

425. Karayalcin G, Rosner F, Kim KY et al: Sickle cell anemia—clinical manifestations in 100 patients and review of the literature. Am J Med Sci 269:51, 1975

426. Val-Mejias J, Lee WK, Weisse AB, Regan TJ: Left ventricular performance during and after sickle cell crisis. Am J Heart 97:585, 1979

427. Miller DM, Winslow RM, Klein HG et al: Improved exercise performance after exchange transfusion in subjects with sickle cell anemia. Blood 56:1127, 1980

428. Ng ML, Leibman J, Anslovar J, Gross S: Cardiovascular findings in children with sickle cell anemia. Dis Chest 52:788, 1967

429. Martin CR, Cobb C, Tatter D et al: Acute myocardial infarction in sickle cell disease. Arch Intern Med 143:830, 1983

430. Martin C, Cobb C, Tatter D, Johnson C: Cardiovascular pathology in sickle cell disease. J Am Coll Cardiol 1:723, 1983

431. Bunn HF: Subunit assembly of hemoglobin: an important determinant of hematologic phenotype. Blood 69:1, 1987

432. Lane PA, Githens JH: Splenic syndrome at mountain altitudes in sickle cell trait. JAMA 253:2251, 1985

433. Castro O, Finch SC: Splenic infarction in sickle-cell trait: are whites more susceptible? N Engl J Med 291:630, 1974

434. Atkinson DW: Sickling and hematuria. Blood 34:736, 1969

435. Keital HG, Thompson D, Itano HA: Hyposthenuria in sickle cell anemia. A reversible defect. J Lab Clin Med 88:389, 1976

436. Ashcroft MT, Miall WE, Milner PF: A comparison between the characteristics of Jamaican adults with normal hemoglobin and those with sickle cell trait. Am J Epidemiol 90:236, 1969

437. Tuck SM, Studd JWW, White JM: Pregnancy in women with sickle cell trait. Br J Obstet Gynaecol 90:112, 1983

438. Altas SA: The sickle cell trait and surgical complications. A matched-pair patient analysis. JAMA 229:1078, 1974

439. Kark JA, Posey DM, Schumacher HR, Ruehle CV: Sickle cell trait as a risk factor for sudden death in physical training. N Engl J Med 317:781, 1987

440. Heller P: Risk in sickle-cell trait. Ann Intern Med 78:613, 1973

441. Monplaisir N, Mérault G, Poyart C et al: Hemoglobin S-Antilles ($\alpha_2^A\beta_2^{6Glu-Val, 23 Val-Ileu}$): a new variant with solubility lower than Hb S and producing sickle cell disease in heterozygotes. Proc Natl Acad Sci USA 83:9363, 1986

442. Witkowska HE, Lubin BH, Beuzard Y et al: Sickle cell disease in a patient with sickle cell trait and compound heterozygosity for hemoglobin S and hemoglobin Quebec-Chori. N Engl J Med 325:1150, 1991

443. Hirsch RE, Raventos-Suarez C, Olson JA, Nagel RL: Ligand state in intraerythrocytic circulating Hb C crystal in homozygous CC patients. Blood 74:1823, 1989

444. Ballas SK, Lewis CN, Noone AM et al: Clinical, hematological and biochemical features of Hb SC disease. Am J Hematol 13:37, 1982

445. River GL, Robbins AB, Schwartz SO: SC hemoglobin: a clinical study. Blood 18:385, 1961

446. Lawrence C, Fabry M, Nagel RL: The unique red cell heterogeneity of SC disease: crystal formation, dense reticulocytes, and unusual morphology. Blood 78:2104, 1991

447. Buchanan GR, Smith SJ, Koltcamp CA, Fuseler JP: Bacterial infections and splenic reticuloendothelial function in children with hemoglobin SC disease. Pediatrics 72:93, 1983

448. Barton CJ, Cockshott WP: Bone changes in Hb SC disease. AJR 88:523, 1962

449. Singer K, Singer L, Goldberg SR: Studies on abnormal hemoglobins. XI. Sickle cell-thalassemia disease in the Negro. The significance of the S+A+F and S+A patterns obtained by hemoglobin analysis. Blood 10:405, 1955

450. Smith EW, Conley CL: Clinical features of the genetic variants of sickle cell disease. Bull Johns Hopkins Hosp 94:289, 1954

451. Gonzalez-Redondo JM, Stoming TA, Lanclos KD et al: Clinical genetic heterogeneity in black patients with homozygous β-thalassemia from the southeastern United States. Blood 72:1007, 1988

452. Gonzalez-Redondo JM, Kutlar A, Kutlar F et al: Molecular characterization of Hb S(C) β-thalassemia in American blacks. Am J Hematol 38:9, 1991

453. Christakis J, Vavatsi N, Hassapopoulou H et al: A comparison of sickle cell syndromes in northern Greece. Br J Haematol 77:386, 1991

454. Serjeant GR, Sommereux AM, Stevenson M et al: Comparison of sickle cell-β° thalassemia and homozygous sickle cell disease. Br J Haematol 41:83, 1979

455. Serjeant GR, Serjeant BE: Comparison of sickle cell-β° thalassemia and sickle cell-β + thalassemia in black populations. p. 233. In Cao A, Carcassi U, Rowley PT (eds): Thalassemia: Advances in Detection and Treatment. Birth Defects Original Article Series. Alan R Liss, New York, 1982

456. Embury SH, Lebo RV, Dozy AM, Kan YW: Organization of the α-globin genes in the Chinese α-thalassemia syndromes. J Clin Invest 63:1307, 1979

457. Embury SH, Miller JA, Dozy AM et al: Two different molecular organizations account for the single α-globin gene in the α-thalassemia genotype. J Clin Invest 66:1319, 1980

458. Dover GJ, Chang VT, Boyer SH et al: The cellular basis for different fetal hemoglobin levels among sickle cell individuals with two, three or four alpha-globin genes. Blood 69:341, 1987

459. Fox PD, Higgs DR, Serjeant GR: Influence of α thalassemia on the retinopathy of homozygous sickle cell disease. Br J Ophthalmol 77:89, 1993

460. Fox PD, Dunn DT, Morris JS, Serjeant GR: Risk factors for peripheral sickle retinopathy. Br J Ophthalmol 74:172, 1990

461. Mears JG, Lachman HM, Labie D, Nagel RL: Alpha thalassemia is related to prolonged survival in sickle cell anemia. Blood 62:286, 1983

462. Kinney TR, Friedman SH, Cifuentes E et al: Variations in globin synthesis in delta-beta-thalassemia. Br J Haematol 38:15, 1978

463. Bradley TB, Brawner JN, Conley CL: Further observations on an inherited anomaly characterized by persistence of fetal hemoglobin. Bull Johns Hopkins Hosp 108:242, 1961

464. Murray N, Serjeant BE, Serjeant GR: Sickle cell-hereditary persistence of fetal hemoglobin and its differentiation from other sickle cell syndromes. Br J Haematol 69:89, 1988

465. Stevens MCG, Lehmann H, Mason KP et al: Sickle cell-Hb Lepore Boston syndrome. Uncommon differential diagnosis to homozygous sickle cell disease. Am J Dis Child 136:19, 1982

466. Cooke JV, Mack JK: Sickle-cell anemia in a white American family. J Pediatr 5:601, 1934

467. Sturgeon P, Itano HA, Bergren WR: Clinical manifestations of inherited abnormal hemoglobin. I. The interaction of hemoglobin-S with hemoglobin-D. Blood 10:389, 1955

468. Ramot R, Fisher S, Remex D et al: Haemoglobin O in an Arab family. Sickle cell-haemoglobin O Arab. Br Med J 2:1262, 1960

469. Milner PF, Miller C, Grey R et al: Hemoglobin O Arab in four Negro families and its interaction with hemoglobin S and hemoglobin C. N Engl J Med 283:1417, 1970

470. Itano HA, Bergren WR, Sturgeon P: Identification of a fourth abnormal human hemoglobin. Am Chem Soc 76:2278, 1954

471. Chernoff AI, Minnich V, Congchareonsuk S: Hemoglobin E, a hereditary abnormality of human hemoglobin. Science 120:605, 1954

472. Orkin SH, Kazazian HH, Antonarakis SE et al: Abnormal RNA processing due to the exon mutation of β^E-globin gene. Nature 300:768, 1982

473. Aksoy M, Lehmann H: The first observation of sickle-cell haemoglobin E disease. Nature 179:1248, 1957

474. Aksoy M: The hemoglobin E syndromes. II. Sickle-cell-hemoglobin E disease. Blood 15:610, 1960

475. Altay C, Naizei GA, Huisman THJ: A combination of Hb F and Hb E in a black female. Hemoglobin 1:100, 1976

476. Schroeder WA, Powars D, Reynolds RD, Fisher JI: Hb-E in combination with Hb S and Hb-C in a black family. Hemoglobin 1:287, 1976

477. Rosenberg MR: In vivo and in vitro interactions of human haemoglobins A, S, and C with a variant haemoglobin E. Nature 219:1040, 1968

478. O'Brien RT, McIntosh S, Aspnes GT, Pearson HA: Prospective study of sickle cell anemia in infancy. J Pediatr 89:205, 1976

479. Huisman THJ, Jonxis JHP: Methods. In: The Hemoglobinopathies: Techniques of Identification. Marcel Dekker, New York, 1977

480. Honig GR, Adams JGIII: Laboratory identification, screening, education, and counseling for abnormal hemoglobins and thalassemias. p. 251. In Human Hemoglobin Genetics. Springer-Verlag, Vienna, 1986

481. National Institutes of Health Consensus Development Panel: Newborn screening for sickle cell disease and other hemoglobinopathies. JAMA 258:1205, 1987

482. Tsevat J, Wong JB, Pauker SG, Steinberg MH: Neonatal screening for sickle cell disease: a cost-effectiveness analysis. J Pediatr 118:546, 1991

483. Schneider RG: Laboratory identification of hemoglobin variants in the newborn. p. 137. In Carter TP, Wiley AM (eds): Genetic Disease—Screening and Management. Alan R Liss, New York, 1986

484. National Committee for Clinical Laboratory Standards: Blood Collection on

Filter Paper for Neonatal Screening Programs. Vol 5, No. 14. publication LA4-T. National Committee for Laboratory Standards, Villanova, PA, 1988

485. Jinks DC, Minter M, Tarver DA et al: Molecular genetic diagnosis of sickle cell disease using dried blood specimens on blotters used for newborn screening. Hum Genet 81:363, 1989

486. Goldberg JD (ed): Fetal medicine. West J Med 159:259, 1993

487. Jones S, Shickle DA, Goldstein AR, Serjeant GR: Acceptability of antenatal diagnosis for sickle-cell disease among mothers and female patients. West Indian Med J 37:12, 1988

488. Kan YW, Golbus MS, Trecartin R: Prenatal diagnosis of sickle-cell anemia. N Engl J Med 294:1039, 1976

489. Shulman LP, Elias S: Amniocentesis and chorionic villus sampling. West J Med 159:260, 1993

490. Conner BJ, Reyes AA, Morin C et al: Detection of sickle cell β^S-globin allele by hybridization with synthetic oligonucleotides. Proc Natl Acad Sci USA 80:278, 1983

491. Geever RF, Wilson LB, Nallaseth FS et al: Direct identification of sickle cell anemia by blot hybridization. Proc Nat Acad Sci USA 78:5081, 1981

492. Embury SH, Scharf SJ, Saiki RK et al: Rapid prenatal diagnosis of sickle cell anemia by a new method of DNA analysis. N Engl J Med 316:656, 1987

493. Chehab FF, Doherty M, Cai S et al: Detection of sickle cell anaemia and thalassaemias. Nature 329:293, 1987

494. Saiki RK, Bugawan TL, Horn GT et al: Analysis of enzymatically amplified β-globin HLA-DQα DNA with allele-specific oligonucleotide probes. Nature 324:163, 1986

495. Saiki RK, Walsh PS, Levenson CH, Erlich HA: Genetic analysis of amplified DNA with immobilized sequence-specific oligonucleotide probes. Proc Natl Acad Sci USA 86:6230, 1989

496. Chehab FF, Kan YW: Detection of sickle cell anaemia mutation by colour DNA amplification. Lancet 335:15, 1990

497. Fischel-Ghodsian N, Hirsch PC, Bohlman MC: Rapid detection of the hemoglobin C mutation by allele-specific polymerase chain reaction. Am J Hum Genet 47:1023, 1990

498. Kropp GL, Cornett PA, Leavitt AD et al: Resolution of complex genotypes containing hemoglobin C genes using the allele-specific fluorescence polymerase chain reaction. Blood, suppl. 1. 76:257a, 1990

499. Antonarakis SE, Orkin SH, Cheng T-C et al: β-Thalassemia in American blacks: novel mutations in the "TATA" box and an acceptor splice site. Proc Natl Acad Sci USA 81:1154, 1984

500. Embury SH, Saiki R, Erlich H, Sutcharitchan P: Detecting African-American β-thalassemia mutations with a single, rapid reverse dot blot hybridization, abstracted. In Proceedings of the Twenty-fifth Congress of the International Society of Hematology, Cancun, 1994

501. Dover GJ, Boyer SH, Charache S, Heintzelman K: Individual variation in the production and survival of F cells in sickle-cell disease. N Engl J Med 299:1428, 1978

502. Nagel RL, Ranney HM: Genetic epidemiology of structural mutations of the β-globin gene. Semin Hematol 27:342, 1990

503. Öner Ç, Dimovski AJ, Altay C et al: Sequence variations in the 5' hypersensitive site-2 of the locus control region of β^S chromosomes are associated with different levels of fetal globin in hemoglobin S homozygotes. Blood 79:813, 1992

504. Powars D, Overturf G, Weiss J et al: Pneumococcal septicemia in children with sickle cell anemia. JAMA 245:1839, 1981

505. Kravis E, Fleisher G, Ludwig S: Fever in children with sickle cell hemoglobinopathies. Am J Dis Child 136:1075, 1986

506. Wayne AS, Kevy SV, Nathan DG: Transfusion management of sickle cell disease. Blood 81:1109, 1993

507. Vichinsky E: Transfusion. p. 791. In Embury SH, Hebbel RP, Mohandas N, Steinberg MH (eds): Sickle Cell Disease: Basic Principles and Clinical Practice. Raven Press, New York, 1994

508. Vichinsky EP, Earles A, Johnson RA et al: Alloimmunization in sickle cell anemia and transfusion of racially unmatched blood. N Engl J Med 322:1617, 1990

509. Rosse WF, Gallagher D, Kinney TR et al: Transfusion and alloimmunization in sickle cell disease. Blood 76:1431, 1990

510. Carangelo J, Otis OM: Sickle cell anemia in pregnancy. South Med J 40:1016, 1947

511. Beattie KM, Shafer AW: Broadening the base of a rare donor program by targeting minority populations. Transfusion 26:401, 1986

512. Charache S: Treatment of sickle cell anemia. Annu Rev Med 32:195, 1981

513. Cohen AR: Transfusion therapy for disorders of hemoglobin. p. 52. In Kasprisin DO, Luban NLC (eds): Pediatric Transfusion Medicine. Vol. II. CRC Press, Boca Raton, FL, 1987

514. Cohen A, Schwartz E: Excretion of iron in response to deferoxamine in sickle cell anemia. J Pediatr 92:659, 1978

515. Porter JB, Herhns ER: Transfusion and exchange transfusion in sickle cell anemias with particular reference to iron metabolism. Acta Haematol 78:198, 1987

516. Olivieri N, Koren G, Hermann C et al: Comparison of oral chelator L1 and desferrioxamine in iron-loaded patients. Lancet 336:1275, 1990

517. Brittenham G: Development of iron-chelating agents for clinical use. Blood 80:569, 1992

518. Dodd RY: The risk of transfusion-transmitted infection. N Engl J Med 327:419, 1992

519. Klein HG, Dzik WH, Strauss RG, Busch MP: Leukocyte-reduced blood component therapy. p. 76. In MacArthur JR, Menitove JE (eds): Hematology 1992: Education Program of the American Society of Hematology. American Society of Hematology, Anaheim, CA, 1992

520. Bischoff RJ, Williamson A, Dalali MJ et al: Assessment of the use of transfusion therapy perioperatively in patients with sickle cell hemoglobinopathies. Ann Surg 207:434, 1988

521. Ware R, Filston HC, Schultz WH, Kinney TR: Elective cholecystectomy in children with hemoglobinopathies: successful outcome using a preoperative transfusion regimen. Ann Surg 208:17, 1988

522. National SCA Preoperative Transfusion Study Group: Preoperative transfusion in sickle cell anemia. Blood, suppl. 1. 74:184A, 1989

523. Payne R: Pain management in sickle cell disease, rationale and techniques. Ann NY Acad Sci 565:189, 1989

524. Ballas SK: Treatment of pain in adults with sickle cell disease. Am J Hematol 34:49, 1990

525. McPherson E, Perlin E, Finke H et al: Patient-controlled analgesia in patients with sickle cell vaso-occlusive crisis. Am J Med Sci 299:10, 1990

526. Abbuhl S, Jacobson S, Murphy JG, Gibson G: Serum concentration of meperidine in patients with sickle cell crises. Ann Emerg Med 15:433, 1986

527. Shapiro BS: The management of pain in sickle cell disease. Pediatr Clin North Am 36:1029, 1989

528. Brookoff D, Polomano R: Treating sickle cell pain like cancer pain. Ann Intern Med 116:364, 1992

529. Cummings DM, Ballas SK, Ellison MJ: Lack of effect of pentoxifylline on red blood cell deformability. J Clin Pharmacol 32:1050, 1992

530. Rodgers GP, Roy MS, Noguchi CT, Schechter AN: Is there a role for selective vasodilation in the management of sickle cell disease? Blood 71:597, 1988

531. Stamatoyannopoulos JA, Nienhuis AW: Therapeutic approaches to hemoglobin switching in treatment of hemoglobinopathies. Annu Rev Med 43:497, 1992

532. Beutler E: The effect of methemoglobin formation in sickle cell disease. J Clin Invest 40:1856, 1961

533. De Ceulaer K, Gruber C, Hayes RJ, Serjeant GR: Medroxyprogesterone acetate and homozygous sickle cell disease. Lancet 2:229, 1982

534. Ley TJ, DeSimone J, Noguchi CT et al: 5-Azacytidine increases γ-globin synthesis and reduces the proportion of dense cells in patients with sickle cell anemia. Blood 62:370, 1993

535. Charache S, Dover GJ, Moore RD et al: Hydroxyurea: effects on hemoglobin F production in patients with sickle cell anemia. Blood 79:2555, 1992

536. Goldberg MA, Brugnara C, Dover GJ et al: Treatment of sickle cell anemia with hydroxyurea and erythropoietin. N Engl J Med 323:366, 1990

537. Rodgers GP, Dover GJ, Vyesaka N et al: Augmentation by erythropoietin of the fetal-hemoglobin response to hydroxyuria in sickle cell disease. N Engl J Med 328:73, 1993

538. Orringer EP, Blythe DS, Johnson AE et al: Effects of hydroxyurea on HbF and water content in red blood cells of dogs and of patients with sickle cell anemia. Blood 78:212, 1991

539. Ballas SK, Dover GJ, Charache S: Effect of hydroxyurea on the rheological properties of sickle erythrocytes in vivo. Am J Hematol 32:104, 1989

540. Perrine SP, Rudolph A, Faller DV et al: Butyrate infusions in the ovine fetus delay the biologic clock for globin gene switching. Proc Natl Acad Sci USA 85:8540, 1988

541. Perrine SP, Miller BA, Faller DV et al: Sodium butyrate enhances fetal globin expression in erythroid progenitors of patients with HbSS and beta-thalassemia. Blood 74:454, 1989

542. Blau AC, Constanttoulakis P, Shaw CM, Stamatoyannopoulos G: Fetal hemoglobin induction with butyric acid: efficacy and toxicity. Blood 81:529, 1993

543. Sher GD, Entsuah B, Ginder G et al: Intravenous (IV) infusion of arginine butyrate (AB) increases γ-globin mRNA expression and F-reticulocytes in patients (PTS) with homozygous β-thalassemia (HBT) and sickle cell disease (SCD). Blood, suppl. 1. 82:1233A, 1993

544. Perrine S, Dover G, Costin D et al: Correction of globin chain imbalance in thalassemia major by arginine butyrate therapy. Blood, suppl. 1. 82:1232A, 1993

545. Johnson FL, Look AT, Gockerman J et al: Bone-marrow transplantation in a patient with sickle-cell anemia. N Engl J Med 311:780, 1984

546. Mentzer WC, Packman S, Wara W, Cowan M: Successful bone marrow trans-

plant in a child with sickle cell anemia and Morquio's disease. Blood, suppl. 1. 76:69a, 1990

547. Vermylen C, Fernandez-Robles E, Ninane J, Cornu G: Bone marrow transplantation in five children with sickle cell anaemia. Lancet 2:1427, 1988

548. Vermylen C, Cornu G, Philippe M et al: Bone marrow transplantation on sickle cell anemia. Arch Dis Child 66:1195, 1991

549. Ferster A, De Valek C, Azzi N et al: Bone marrow transplantation for severe sickle cell anaemia. Br J Haematol 80:102, 1992

550. Vermylen C, Cornu G, Ferster A et al: Bone marrow transplantation in sickle cell disease: the Belgian experience. Bone Marrow Transplant, suppl. 1. 12:116, 1993

551. Bernaudin F, Souillet G, Vannier JP et al: Bone marrow transplantation (BMT) in 14 children with severe sickle cell disease (SCD): the French experience. Bone Marrow Transplant, suppl. 1. 12:118, 1993

552. Galimberti C, Galimberti M, Lucarelli G et al: Bone marrow transplantation in sickle-cell anemia in Pesaro. Bone Marrow Transplant, suppl. 1. 12:122, 1993

553. Ballas SK: Bone marrow transplantation in sickle-cell anaemia: why so few so late? Lancet 340:1226, 1992

554. Nagel RL: The dilemma of marrow transplantation in sickle cell anemia. Semin Hematol 28:233, 1991

555. Kodish E, Lantos J, Stocking C et al: Bone marrow transplantation for sickle cell disease: a study of parent's decisions. N Engl J Med 325:1349, 1991

556. Nienhuis AW, McDonagh KT, Bodine DM: Gene therapy into hematopoietic stem cells. Cancer 67:2700, 1991

557. Miller AD: Human gene therapy comes of age. Nature 357:455, 1992

558. Miller AD: Progress toward human gene therapy. Blood 76:271, 1990

559. Townes TM, Behringer RR: Human globin locus activation region (LAR): role in temporal control. Trends Genet 6:219, 1990

560. Smithies O, Gregg RG, Boggs SS et al: Insertion of DNA sequences into the human chromosomal β-globin locus by homologous recombination. Nature 317:230, 1985

561. Bodine DM, McDonagh KT, Brandt SJ et al: Development of a high titer retrovirus producer cell line capable of gene transfer into rhesus monkey hematopoietic stem cells. Proc Natl Acad Sci USA 87:3738, 1990

562. Fabry ME, Nagel RL, Pachnis A et al: High expression of human β^S and α-globin in transgenic mice: hemoglobin composition and hematologic consequences. Proc Natl Acad Sci USA 89:12150, 1992

563. Cornetta K: Safety aspects of gene therapy. Br J Haematol 80:421, 1992

564. Finch JT, Perutz MF, Bertles JF, Dobler J: Structure of sickled erythrocytes and of sickle-cell hemoglobin fibers. Proc Natl Acad Sci USA 70:718, 1973

565. Eaton WA, Hofrichter J: Hemoglobin S gelation sickle cell disease. Blood 70:1245, 1987

566. Statius van Eps LW, Pinedo-Veels C, De Vries GH, De Konig J: The relation between age and renal concentrating capacity in sickle cell disease and hemoglobin C disease. Lancet 1:450, 1970

567. Friedman S, Schwartz E, Ahern E, Ahern V: Variations in globin chain synthesis in hereditary persistence of fetal hemoglobin. Br J Haematol 32:357, 1976

568. Nieburg PI, Stockman JA: Rapid correction of anemia with partial exchange transfusion. Am J Dis Child 131:60, 1977

569. Linderkamp O, Versmold HT, Riegel KP, Betke K: Estimation and prediction of blood volume in infants and children. Eur J Pediatr 125:227, 1977

570. Orringer EP, Abraham DJ, Parker JC: Development of drug therapy. p. 861. In Embury SH, Hebbel RP, Mohandas N, Steinberg MH (eds): Sickle Cell Disease: Basic Principles and Clinical Practice. Raven Press, New York, 1994

571. van Assendelft OW: Interpretation of the quantitative blood cell count. p. 61. In Koepke JA (ed): Practical Laboratory Hematology. Churchill Livingstone, New York, 1991

572. Boyd MF (ed): Malariology. WB Saunders, Philadelphia, 1949

573. Bertles JF, Döbler J: Reversible and irreversible sickling: a distinction by electron microscopy. Blood 33:884, 1969

Hemoglobin Variants Associated with Hemolytic Anemia, Altered Oxygen Affinity, and Methemoglobinemias

44

Edward J. Benz, Jr.

INHERITED DISEASES

Hemoglobinopathies are inherited diseases due primarily to mutations affecting the globin genes. Nearly 1,000 mutations that alter the structure, expression, or developmental regulation of individual globin genes, and the hemoglobins they encode, have been described. Most of these mutations do not produce clinical disease. Many hemoglobin variants are highly instructive for students of gene structure, function, and regulation, but further consideration of most is not warranted in a clinically oriented textbook. Sickle cell anemia and the thalassemia syndromes are by far the most important mutations that cause clinical morbidity, in terms of both the complexity of the clinical syndromes they cause and the number of patients affected. These conditions are considered in detail in other chapters (see Chs. 42 and 43). This chapter reviews other abnormalities of the hemoglobin molecule that produce clinical syndromes. Each variant is uncommon. In the aggregate, however, hemoglobinopathies represent important problems for hematologists because they must be considered as possible

Table 44-1. Classification of Hemoglobinopathies

Structural hemoglobinopathies—hemoglobins with altered amino acid sequences that result in deranged function or altered physical or chemical properties
    Abnormal hemoglobin polymerization—Hb S
    Altered oxygen affinity
        High affinity—polycythemia
        Low affinity—cyanosis, pseudoanemia
    Hemoglobins that oxidize readily
    Unstable hemoglobins, hemolytic anemia, jaundice
    M hemoglobins—methemoglobinemia, cyanosis

Thalassemias—defective production of globin chains
    α-Thalassemias
    β-Thalassemias
    $\delta\beta$-, $\gamma\delta\beta$-, $\alpha\beta$-Thalassemias

Structural hemoglobinopathies—structurally abnormal Hb associated with co-inherited thalassemia phenotype
    Hb E
    Hb Constant Spring
    Hb Lepore

Hereditary persistence of fetal hemoglobin—persistence of high levels of Hb F into adult life
    Pancellular—all red cells contain elevated Hb F levels
        Nondeletion forms
        Deletion forms
        Hb Kenya
    Heterocellular—only specific subpopulation of red cells contain elevated levels of Hb F
    Acquired (see below)

Acquired hemoglobinopathies
    Methemoglobin due to toxic exposures
    Sulfhemoglobin due to toxic exposures
    Carbonoxyhemoglobin
    Hb H in erythroleukemia
    Elevated Hb F in states of erythroid stress and bone marrow dysplasia, usually heterocellular

etiologies for conditions about which hematologists are often consulted: hemolytic anemia, cyanosis, polycythemia, rubor, splenomegaly, or reticulocytosis.

The major hemoglobinopathies producing clinical symptoms, other than sickle cell anemia and thalassemias, can be classified as those hemoglobins exhibiting altered solubility (unstable hemoglobins), hemoglobins with increased oxygen affinity, hemoglobins with decreased oxygen affinity, and methemoglobins, (Table 44-1). A few acquired conditions, in which toxic modifications of the hemoglobin molecule are important (e.g., carbon monoxide poisoning), are also considered briefly.

The sections that follow emphasize hemoglobinopathies that produce the most severe or dramatic alterations in clinical phenotype and those in which a single clinical abnormality (e.g., hemoglobin precipitation) predominates. However, it is important to emphasize at the outset that of the >100 mutations altering globin chain structure that have been shown to affect solubility or affinity, or both, only a few are clinically important. The abnormal functional properties of most mutant hemoglobins can be detected readily in sophisticated research laboratories, but do not produce laboratory or clinical abnormalities relevant to clinical practice. Moreover, many mutations are pleiotropic, affecting several functional properties of the hemoglobin molecule. Thus, a single mutation can increase oxygen affinity and reduce solubility or produce both methemoglobinmenia and reduce solubility.

Table 44-2 summarizes the major forms of structurally abnormal hemoglobin, with examples. This table serves as a point of reference for the remaining sections of the chapter.

"UNSTABLE" HEMOGLOBINS

The term "unstable" hemoglobins has been applied to hemoglobins exhibiting reduced solubility or higher susceptibility to oxidation of amino acid residues within the individual globin chains. More than 100 structurally different unstable hemoglobin mutants have been documented. Most exhibit only mild instability in in vitro laboratory tests and do not generate significant clinical manifestations. Both α- and β-globin variants can cause this condition; about 75% of the mutations described, however, are β-globin variants. This probably reflects the potential for α-globin variants to exert pathologic effects in utero. Clinical symptomatology of unstable hemoglobins also depends in part on the quantitative proportion of the abnormal hemoglobin. Since the α-globin genes are duplicated, mutations in an individual locus will generally produce only 25–35% abnormal globin. By contrast, a simple heterozygote at the single β-globin locus will produce 50% of the abnormal variant.

The mutations that impair hemoglobin solubility usually disrupt hydrogen bonding and/or hydrophobic interactions that retain either the heme moiety within the heme binding pockets or hold the tetramer together (Fig. 44-1). Some alter the helical segments (Hb Geneva [$\beta^{28\text{Leu}\rightarrow\text{Pro}}$]), others weaken contact points between the α- and β-subunits (Hb Philadelphia [$\beta^{35\text{Tyr}\rightarrow\text{Phe}}$]), while still others derange interactions of the hydrophobic pockets of the globin subunits with heme (e.g., Hb Köln, ($\beta^{98\text{Val}\rightarrow\text{Met}}$]).The common pathway to reduced solubility ultimately leads to weakening of the binding of heme to globin. An actual loss of heme groups can occur, for example, in Hb Gun Hill, in which five amino acids, including the F8 histidine, are deleted. In other cases, this results from mutations that introduce prolines into helical segments, disrupting the helices and interfering with normal folding of the polypeptide around the heme group. Another feature of these mutations is disruption of the integrity of the tetrameric structure of globin chains. It is only the intact hemoglobin tetramer that can remain dissolved at the high concentrations that must be achieved within the circulating red cell (see Ch. 35).

Pathophysiology of Unstable Hemoglobin Disorders

The mechanisms by which unstable hemoglobin mutations produce hemoglobin precipitation remain incompletely understood. However, the major outlines of the process have been described (Fig. 44-2). The fundamental step in the pathogenesis appears to be derangement of the normal linkages between heme and globins. Loss of appropriate globin chain folding and interaction may ultimately destabilize the heme/globin linkage or lead to partial proteolysis of the chain, thereby releasing heme from that linkage. Once freed from its cleft, heme probably binds nonspecifically to other regions of the globin molecule, forming precipitated hemichromes, which lead to further denaturation and aggregation of the globin subunits to form a precipitate containing α- and β-globin chains, globin fragments, and heme, called the Heinz body.

Heinz bodies interact with delicate red cell membrane components (see Ch. 43), thereby reducing red cell deformability. These cells tend to be trapped in the splenic microcirculation and "pitted," reflecting attempts by the splenic macrophages to remove the Heinz bodies. Red cell damage may be aggravated by the release of free heme into the red cell. Several biochemical perturbations correlate with the presence of free heme, such as generation of reactive oxidants (hydrogen peroxide, superoxide, and hydroxyl radicals). The end result of this process is premature destruction of the red cell, producing the hemolytic anemia.

Individual unstable hemoglobins vary considerably in their propensity to generate Heinz bodies and hemolysis. For example, Hb Zurich exhibits relatively mild insolubility. Hemolysis is virtually absent in patients with this variant. Hemolysis may become clinically apparent only in the presence of additional oxidant stresses, such as infection and fever, or the ingestion

Table 44-2. Mutations Producing Abnormal Hemoglobin Molecules[a]

Residue	Mutation	Common Name(s)	Molecular Pathology
Abnormal solubility			
β6	Glu → Val	S	Polymerization
β6	Glu → Lys	C	Crystallization
β121	Glu → Gln	D-Los Angeles, D-Punjab	Increases polymer in S/D heterozygote
β121	Glu → Lys	O-Arab	Increases polymer in S/O heterozygote
Increased oxygen affinity			
α92	Arg → Gln	J-Capetown	Stabilizes R state
α141	Arg → His	Suresnes	Eliminates bond to Asn 126 in T state
β89	Ser → Asn	Creteil	Weakens bonds in T state
β99	Asp → Asn	Kempsey	Breaks T state intersubunit bonds
Decreased oxygen affinity			
α94	Asp → Asn	Titusville	Alters R state intersubunit bonds
β102	Asn → Thr	Kansas	Breaks R state intersubunit bond
β102	Asn → Ser	Beth Israel	Breaks R state intersubunit bond
Methemoglobin			
α58	His → Tyr	M-Boston, M-Osaka	Heme liganded to Tyr not His
α87	His → Tyr	M-Iwate	Heme liganded to both His and Tyr
β28	Leu → Gln	St. Louis	Opens heme pocket
β63	His → Tyr	M-Saskatoon	Tyr ligand stabilizes ferri-heme
β67	Val → Glu	M-Milwaukee-I	Negative charge stabilizes ferri-heme
β92	His → Tyr	M-Hyde Park	Bond of His to heme disrupted
Unstable			
α43	Phe → Val	Torino	Loss of heme contact
α94	Asp → Tyr	Setif	Alters subunit contacts
β28	Leu → Gln	St. Louis	Polar group in heme pocket
β35	Tyr → Phe	Philly	Loss of dimer bond favors precipitation
β42	Phe → Ser	Hammersmith	Loss of heme
β63	His → Arg	Zürich	Opens heme pocket
β88	Leu → Pro	Santa Ana	Disrupts helix
β91	Leu → Pro	Sabine	Disrupts helix
β91–95	Deletion	Gun Hill	Shortens F helix
β98	Val → Met	Köln	Alters heme contact

[a] Includes some of the most widely studied hemoglobin structural mutations.
(Adapted from Dickerson and Geis,[3] with permission.)

of oxidant drugs. Because of the propensity of these molecules to be hypersensitive to oxidation, some patients with unstable hemoglobins can exhibit episodic hemolysis in response to the same oxidative stressors as those exacerbating the clinical phenotype of glucose-6-phosphate dehydrogenase (G6PD)-deficient patients.

Patterns of Inheritance and Clinical Manifestations

Unstable hemoglobins are usually inherited as autosomal dominant disorders. However, the rate of spontaneous mutation appears to be high, so that the absence of affected parents or sibs does not rule out the presence of an unstable hemoglobin in an individual family. Nonetheless, the presence of a positive family history can be a useful adjunct to diagnosis, and should provoke consideration of an unstable hemoglobin as the cause of the familial hemolytic diathesis.

The clinical syndrome associated with unstable hemoglobin disorders is often called congenital Heinz body hemolytic anemia. This term derives its origins from the fact that only the most severe cases were detected before the widespread availability of sophisticated methods for detecting and characterizing abnormal hemoglobins. Clinical manifestations are highly variable, ranging from a virtually asymptomatic state in the absence of environmental stressors to severe hemolytic anemia presenting at birth. Patients suffering from chronic hemolysis present with variable degrees of typical symptoms, including anemia, reticulocytosis, hepatosplenomegaly, jaundice, leg ulcers, and propensity to premature biliary tract disease.

For hemoglobin variants with a given degree of reduced solubility, the degree of anemia may vary because some of these variants also exhibit altered oxygen affinity. Thus, Hb Köln has increased oxygen affinity, resulting in relatively higher levels of tissue hypoxia and erythropoietin stimulation at any given level of hematocrit (see next section); thus, patients with Hb Köln tend to have higher hematocrits than expected on the basis of hemolytic severity because of increased erythropoietin stimulation. By contrast, Hb Hammersmith exhibits decreased oxygen affinity, improving oxygen delivery and allowing patients to function at a lower hematocrit. Hb Zurich possesses, for complex molecular reasons, a higher-than-normal affinity for carbon monoxide. Patients with Hb Zurich who also smoke develop a high carbon monoxide hemoglobin level. Binding of carbon monoxide protects Hb Zurich from denaturation, thus reducing hemolysis so that these individuals tend to exhibit lesser degrees of hemolytic anemia than do nonsmoking relatives.

Diagnosis

The presence of an unstable hemoglobin should be suspected in patients with one or more stigmata of accelerated red cell destruction: chronic or intermittent hemolytic anemia and/or jaundice, premature development of bilirubin gallstones or biliary tract disease (due to accelerated red cell turn-

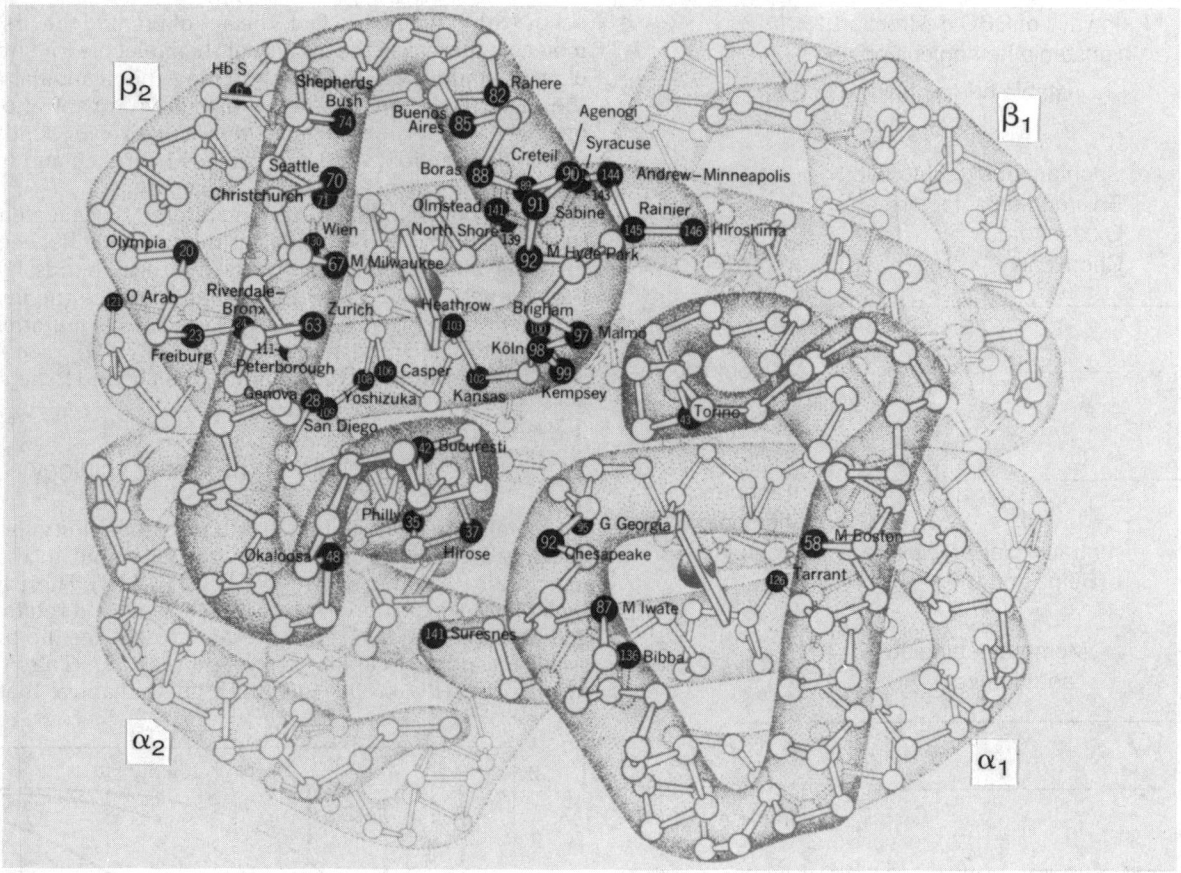

Fig. 44-1. Hemoglobin tetramer showing the position of the more common, clinically significant hemoglobin mutants. Most of those that have been described occur on the β-chain at invariant residue sites, near critical intermolecular contacts, or in proximity to the prosthetic heme-binding site. (Modified from Dickerson and Geis,[3] with permission.)

over), unexplained reticulocytosis, or bouts of intermittent symptoms that can be related to exposure to oxidant drugs or infections. Other suggestive symptoms include dark urine, transient jaundice, or leg ulcers.

Laboratory diagnosis depends on identification of a mutant hemoglobin that precipitates more easily than normal hemoglobin. The peripheral blood smear may or may not show evidence of hemolysis, (i.e., poikilocytosis, polychromasia, or shift cells). The morphologic evidence for precipitated hemoglobin is the Heinz body, the intraerythrocytic inclusion body detected by staining the peripheral blood smear with a supravital dye, such as brilliant cresyl blue or new methylene blue. The spleen removes Heinz bodies efficiently, especially if hemolysis is not particularly acute or brisk. Thus, Heinz bodies may not be demonstrable at all times. Two provacative laboratory maneuvers are employed to aid detection. Both unmask the tendency of unstable hemoglobins to precipitate: the heat instability test (heating of a hemoglobin solution to 50°C) or the isopropanol instability test (insolubility in 17% isopropanol).

Hemoglobin electrophoresis should be performed but should not be relied on as the major diagnostic criterion for ruling in or ruling out a hemoglobinopathy. Many amino acid substitutions that have a profound effect on solubility do not change the overall charge on the hemoglobin molecule. For example, Hb Köln, the most common of the unstable hemoglobin mutations, arises from a mutation changing the valine at position 98 to a methionine; this mutation is electrically neutral. It does not alter electrophoretic mobility. Therefore, these variants will not form an abnormal band on an electrophoresis gel. Demonstration of an abnormal band would clearly add

strong evidence in support of the diagnosis. A normal electrophoretogram, however, should never be regarded as strong evidence against the presence of a mutant hemoglobin, especially if the clinical picture or family history otherwise support the diagnosis.

Sophisticated analyses of hemoglobin can be obtained from reference laboratories if detailed characterization seems warranted. For example, abnormal hemoglobin or globin bands migrating to novel positions on an isoelectric focusing gel can result from hemoglobin or globin moieties lacking heme in groups. When heme is added to the sample and the proteins are reanalyzed, these bands disappear. This behavior is nearly diagnostic of an unstable variant.

Detection of unstable hemoglobins is occasionally compromised by the selective precipitation of the unstable variant into Heinz bodies. Since most patients are heterozygotes, this phenomenon greatly reduces the *apparent* percentage of the variant in soluble form. Thus, even a variant possessing altered electrophoretic mobility may be very difficult to detect. Indeed, some unstable hemoglobins, such as Hb Geneva or Hb Terre Haute, are so unstable that no mutant gene product can be detected in the steady state. These abnormal hemoglobins actually produce a thalassemic phenotype (see Ch. 42). They are detectable only by isotope labeling studies or direct analysis of the globin genes.

The differential diagnosis of unstable hemoglobin variants is usually straightforward if the general category of hemolytic disorders is suspected. The most common form of G6PD deficiency can also present with bouts of intermittent or chronic hemolysis exacerbated by oxidant drugs or infection (see Ch. 134). This diagnosis should be considered, as should other

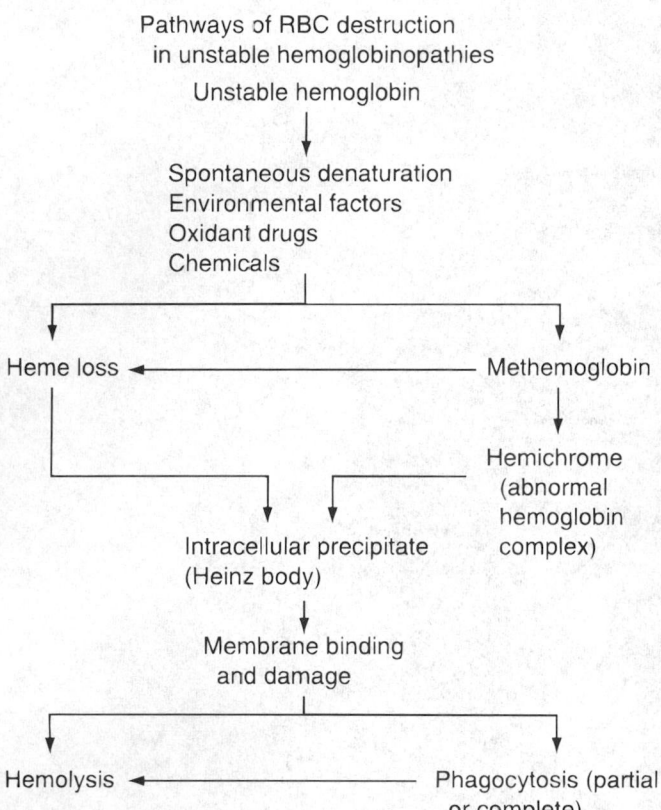

Pathways of RBC destruction
in unstable hemoglobinopathies

Unstable hemoglobin

↓

Spontaneous denaturation
Environmental factors
Oxidant drugs
Chemicals

Heme loss ←——————— Methemoglobin

↓

Hemichrome
(abnormal
hemoglobin
complex)

Intracellular precipitate
(Heinz body)

↓

Membrane binding
and damage

Hemolysis ←——————— Phagocytosis (partial
or complete)

Fig. 44-2. Presumed mechanisms by which denaturation of hemoglobin leads to erythrocyte destruction are outlined. The rate of travel through the various pathways probably differs for different hemoglobin variants and for a variety of stresses to which the protein is subjected. (From Wyngaarden et al.,[9] with permission.)

causes of chronic or intermittent hemolytic anemia, such as red cell membrane disorders (e.g., hereditary spherocytosis) or immune hemolytic anemias. Spherocytes are relatively rare in unstable hemoglobin disorders; this is sometimes a useful discriminant.

Management

The severity of the clinical complications of unstable hemoglobins varies enormously. Many patients can be managed adequately by observation and education to avoid drugs provoking hemolysis. Some patients may require transfusions during bouts of severe acute hemolytic anemia. Individuals who suffer significant morbidity because of chronic anemia or repeated episodes of severe hemolysis should be considered candidates for splenectomy, especially if hypersplenism has developed. Children with severe hemolysis may require transfusion support until they are old enough (age 3 or 4 years) to undergo splenectomy without unacceptable immunologic compromise. Splenectomy is usually effective for abolition or reduction of symptoms. Infection will often exacerbate hemolysis. Fever should therefore prompt close monitoring of patients for evidence of hemolysis or anemia.

HEMOGLOBINS WITH INCREASED OXYGEN AFFINITY

Oxygen transport by hemoglobin depends on the sigmoidal shape of the hemoglobin/oxygen affinity curve. During the transition from the fully deoxygenated (tense, or T) to the fully oxygenated (relaxed, or R) state, the initial oxygenation steps

occur with difficulty. In fact, the act of binding the first oxygen molecule increases the affinity of the molecule for subsequent oxygen binding events, thus creating the sigmoidal shape of the curve. The necessary intramolecular reorganization occurs only when the proper arrangement of hydrogen bonds, hydrophobic interactions, and salt bridges is broken and formed in the proper sequence during R-T transitions.

Mutant hemoglobins exhibiting altered oxygen affinity arise from amino acid substitutions at the interface between α- and β-chains or in regions affecting the hydrogen bonds, hydrophobic interactions, or salt bridges that influence the interaction of heme with oxygen. A second major class of mutations alters binding to 2,3-diphosphoglycerate (2,3-DPG) (see Ch. 35), which in turn alters oxygen affinity when bound to hemoglobin.

Pathogenesis and Pathophysiology

High-affinity hemoglobins exhibit higher avidity for oxygen, causing the oxygen dissociation curve to shift to the left; an example is Hb Kempsey ($\beta^{99Asp \to Asn}$) (Fig. 42-3). These hemoglobins bind oxygen more readily than normal and retain the oxygen at lower PO_2 levels but are able to deliver the oxygen to tissues at normal capillary oxygen pressures. The PO_2 in the normal lung ($PO_2 = 90–100$ mmHg) is well above that needed

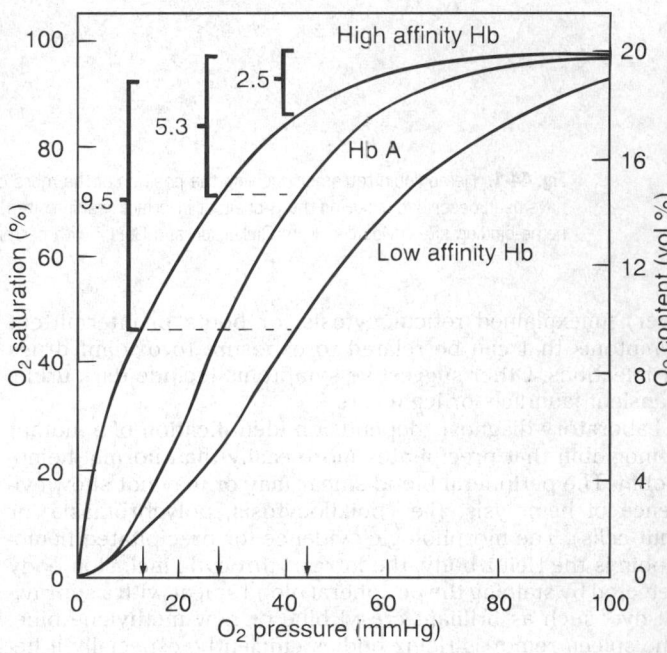

Fig. 44-3. Hemoglobin/oxygen dissociation curves are illustrated for normal hemoglobin (Hb A) and for model abnormal hemoglobins with high and low oxygen affinities. On the abscissa, the partial pressure of oxygen is indicated in millimeters of mercury. On the left ordinate, the saturation of hemoglobin with oxygen is indicated as a percentage; on the right ordinate the oxygen content of the hemoglobin is expressed as volumes percent. The three inverted arrows show the P_{50} for the three hemoglobins (the partial pressure of oxygen at which the hemoglobin is 50% saturated). This value is lowest for the high-affinity hemoglobin. As the partial pressure of oxygen drops from 100 (arterial) to 40 (tissues), hemoglobin desaturates, giving up a portion of its bound oxygen; the numbers on the brackets indicate the amount of oxygen unloaded by the three hemoglobin types expressed in volumes percent. Note that the high-affinity hemoglobin delivers less than one-half the oxygen that Hb A gives to the tissues, resulting in tissue anoxia, increased erythropoietin secretion, and erythrocytosis. Conversely, the low-affinity hemoglobin is even more efficient than Hb A in supplying the tissues with oxygen, resulting in diminished erythropoietin production and anemia. (From Wyngaarden et al.,[9] with permission.)

to saturate hemoglobin fully with oxygen (60 mmHg). These variant hemoglobins cannot acquire any additional oxygen in the lung despite their higher affinity. They cannot carry significantly more oxygen to the tissues. At capillary PO_2 (35–45 mmHg), however, high-affinity hemoglobins deliver less oxygen. At normal hematocrits, a mild tissue hypoxia results; this stimulates erythropoietin release, causing elevated red cell production and polycythemia. In extreme cases, hematocrits of 60–65% can be encountered.

Many types of mutations can increase oxygen affinity. Some alter interactions within the heme pocket, others disrupt the Bohr effect or the salt-bond site, and still others impair the binding of Hb A to 2,3-DPG. Loss of 2,3-DPG binding results in increases in oxygen affinity (see Ch. 35). These and numerous other examples that have been analyzed at the molecular level have greatly aided our understanding of the molecular basis for reversible oxygen binding.

Diagnosis

High-affinity hemoglobins cause unexplained erythrocytosis, especially if there is a positive family history (see Ch. 142). Functional testing of the hemoglobin is the key to diagnosis. Oxygen affinity is usually measured as P_{50}, the partial pressure of oxygen at which hemoglobin is 50% saturated with oxygen (Fig. 44-3). The hemoglobin preparation is exposed to increasing oxygen pressures and the relative percentages of oxyhemoglobin and deoxyhemoglobin are determined. The values are plotted on a curve with which the 50% saturation point is determined. A shift to the left means that the hemoglobin reaches 50% saturation at a lower partial pressure of oxygen. High-affinity variants are thus associated with a lower-than-normal P_{50} value. Hemoglobin electrophoresis can, but may not, reveal an abnormal band.

The most common etiology of a low P_{50} value is carbon monoxide. Carbon monoxyhemoglobin has an extremely left-shifted oxygen-affinity curve. Carbon monoxide stabilizes hemoglobin in the R state without the need for oxygen binding. The clinical consequences are the same as those seen with high-affinity hemoglobin variants. The most common cause of carbon monoxide toxicity is cigarette smoking, although chronic carbon monoxide exposure can elevate the hematocrit in individuals such as caisson workers or tunnel toll collectors.

Management

Most patients with high-affinity hemoglobins have mild erythrocytosis; they do not require intervention. Very rarely, the hematocrit is very high (>55–60). The blood viscosity is then sufficiently elevated to require therapeutic phlebotomy.

HEMOGLOBINS WITH DECREASED OXYGEN AFFINITY

Pathogenesis

Low-affinity hemoglobin variants, such as Hb Kansas ($\beta^{102Asn\rightarrow Thr}$), arise from mutations that impair hemoglobin/oxygen binding or reduce cooperativity. In Hb Kansas, the threonine position β^{102} cannot form a hydrogen bond with aspartic acid at position α^{94}. This residue stabilizes the R (oxy) state; therefore, Hb Kansas binds oxygen less well and exhibits a right-shifted P_{50} value (Fig. 44-3).

Most low-affinity variants possess enough oxygen affinity to become fully saturated in the normal lung. At the low capillary PO_2 in other tissues, these hemoglobins deliver higher-than-normal amounts of oxygen. They become more desaturated than normal hemoglobins. Two abnormalities result from this high level of oxygen delivery. First, since tissue oxygen delivery is so efficient, normal oxygen requirements can be met by lower than normal hematocrits. This situation produces a state of pseudo-anemia, in which the low hematocrit is deceiving because both oxygen delivery—and the patients—are completely normal. Second, the amount of desaturated hemoglobin circulating in capillaries and veins can be >5 g/dl. Cyanosis may thus be associated with these variants. This usually ominous finding is entirely misleading in these individuals, since it reflects no morbidity.

Diagnosis

Patients with unexplained anemia or cyanosis who appear to be entirely well in all other respects should be evaluated, especially if there is a positive family history. Testing for the abnormal variant follows the same reasoning as that just described for high-affinity variants. The P_{50} value will be shifted to the right; the numerical value of the P_{50} will be higher than normal.

Management

Patients with low-affinity hemoglobins are invariably asymptomatic. No treatment is required. It is important to document that a low-affinity hemoglobin is the cause of an apparent anemia or cyanosis in order to preempt inappropriate workups and provide reassurance to the patient. Cyanosis in some patients can pose a cosmetic problem, but correction with transfusions is rarely justified.

METHEMOGLOBINEMIAS

Methemoglobin results from oxidation of the iron moieties in hemoglobin from the ferrous (Fe^{2+}) to the ferric (Fe^{3+}) state. Normal oxygenation of hemoglobin causes a partial transfer of an electron from the iron to the bound oxygen. Iron in this state thus resembles ferric iron and the oxygen resembles superoxide (O_2^-). Deoxygenation returns the electron to the iron, with release of oxygen. Methemoglobin forms if the election is not returned. Methemoglobin constitutes ≤3% of the total hemoglobin in normal humans. Methemoglobin levels in humans are in fact maintained at ≤1% by the methemoglobin reductase enzyme system (nicotinamide adenine dinucleotide [NADH]-dehydratase, NADH-diaphorase, erythrocyte cytochrome b_3). This enzyme reduces hemoglobin iron by transfer of an electron from NADH to oxidize cytochrome b_3; cytochrome b_3 then converts ferric to ferrous iron by direct interaction with hemoglobin. The generation of NADH depends on the glycolytic pathway.

A second reducing enzyme, nicotinamide adenine dinucleotide phosphate (NADPH)-dependent methemoglobin reductase, does not normally function in erythrocytes because no electron carrier is available in erythrocytes to interact with NADPH. Exogenous electron carriers, such as methylene blue, can provide the missing activity. Agents such as methylene blue can therefore serve as pharmacologic agents for the treatment of methemoglobinemia. Reduced glutathione and ascorbic acid reduce methemoglobin directly, but these nonenzymatic reactions are considerably slower than the reductase pathways.

Pathogenesis and Clinical Manifestations

Methemoglobinemias of clinical interest arise by one of three distinct mechanisms: (1) globin chain mutations that result in increased formation of methemoglobin; (2) deficiencies of

Table 44-3. Types of Methemoglobinemia

Congenital
   Defective enzymatic reduction of Fe^{3+}-hemoglobin to Fe^{2+}-hemoglobin
      NADH-methemoglobin reductase (cytochrome b_5 reductase) deficiency
      Cytochrome b_5 deficiency
      Abnormal hemoglobins resistant to enzymatic reduction (M hemoglobins)
Acquired
   Excessive (toxic) oxidation of Fe^{2+}-hemoglobin
      Environmental chemicals
      Drugs

methemoglobin reductase; and (3) "toxic" methemoglobin-emia, in which normal red cells are exposed to substances that oxidize hemoglobin iron such that normal reducing mechanisms are subverted or overwhelmed (Table 44-3).

Abnormal hemoglobins producing methemoglobinemia (M hemoglobins) arise from mutations that stabilize the heme iron in the ferric state. Classically, a histidine in the vicinity of the heme pocket is replaced by a tyrosine; the hydroxyl group of the tyrosine forms a complex that stabilizes the iron in the ferric state (Fig. 44-4). The oxidized heme iron is relatively resistant to reduction by the methemoglobin reductase system.

Methemoglobin has a brownish to blue color that does not revert to red on exposure to oxygen. These individuals thus appear to be cyanotic. In contrast to truly cyanotic individuals, however, PaO_2 values are normal. Patients with these hemoglobins are otherwise asymptomatic, as methemoglobin is rarely >30–50%, the levels at which symptomatology becomes apparent.

Hereditary methemoglobinemia resulting from methemoglo-

bin reductase deficiency is very rare; 100–200 cases have been described. Numerous recessive mutations cause a variety of abnormalities of enzymatic activity or amount, including catalytic activity, electrophoretic mobility, and structural stability. Hispanic, Inuit, and Native American groups are more frequently affected. Some individuals also exhibit neurologic defects. The mutation might thus affect isoforms of the enzyme common to both erythrocytes and other tissues, including brain. Other individuals exhibit only the methemoglobin abnormality.

Like patients with M hemoglobins, patients with methemoglobin reductase deficiency exhibit slight gray "pseudocyanosis." Even homozygotes, however, rarely accumulate >25% methemoglobin, a level compatible with absence of symptoms. Heterozygotes can have normal methemoglobin levels but are especially sensitive to agents cause methemoglobinemia.

A third toxic form of methemoglobinemia is caused by exposure to certain chemical agents and drugs that accelerate the oxidation of methemoglobin (Table 44-4). Nitrite compounds are especially notorious and common. Some of these compounds also have a propensity to exacerbate G6PD deficiency and exacerbate the precipitation of unstable hemoglobins.

Nitrates are a frequent environmental cause of toxic methemoglobinemia. Nitrates do not directly interact with either hemoglobin or the reductase pathway but are converted to nitrites in the gut. Well water is a frequently encountered source of excessive nitrates. In general, substantial intake of these agents is required before significant amounts of methemoglobin are generated. Very young infants are more susceptible to these agents than are adults, but all age groups are at risk given sufficient exposure.

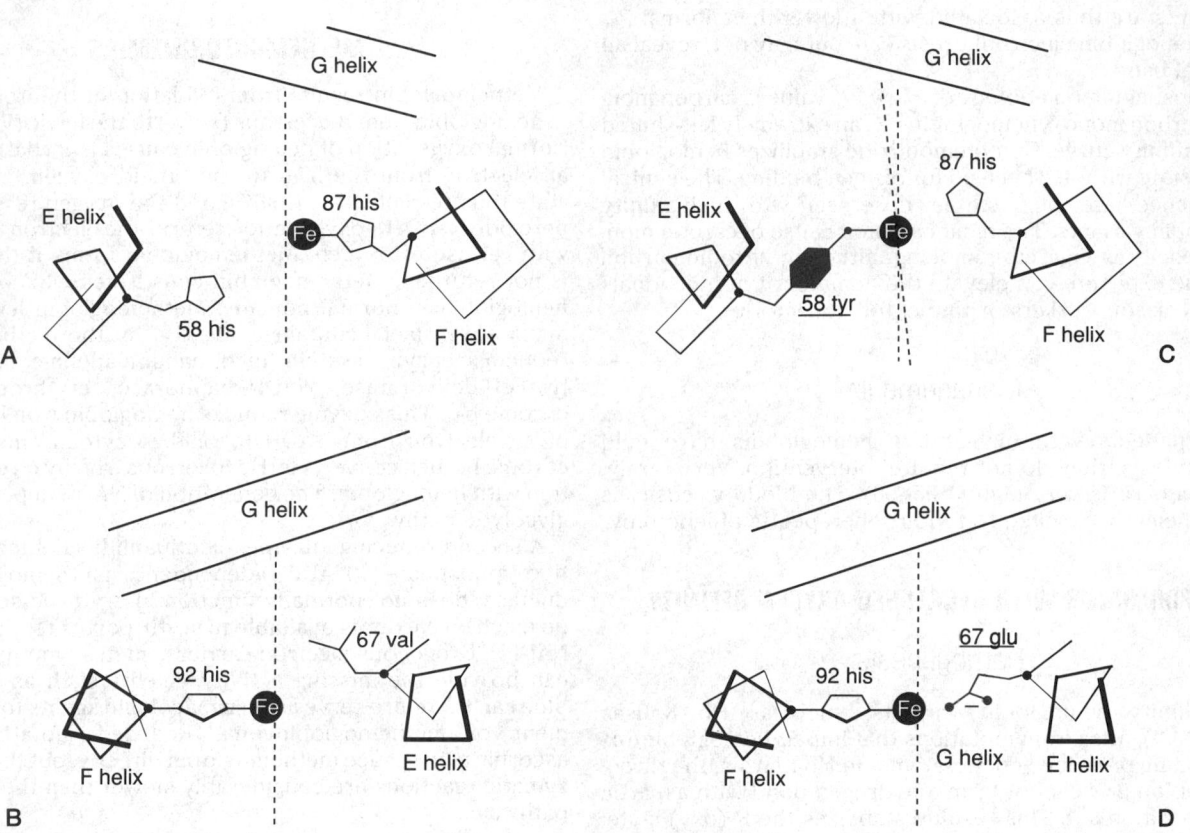

Fig. 44-4. Modifications of the heme and its environment accounting for two common M hemoglobins. **(A)** Hemoglobin A has a His residue at the α58(E7) position. **(B)** Hemoglobin M-Boston, the histidine is replaced by a tyrosine, the phenolic side chain of which is capable of covalently binding to the heme iron, resulting in a stabilization in the oxidized form. **(C)** Hb A has a Val residue at position β67(E11). **(D)** Hb M-Milwaukee has a glutamic acid substitution for the β67 valine. The carboxylic side chain of the Glu forms a bond with iron, shifting the equilibrium toward the ferric state. (Modified from Dickerson and Geis,[3] with permission.)

Table 44-4. Drugs and Chemicals Having Toxic Effect on Hemoglobin Molecule

Agent	Hemoglobin-Derivative Observed	
	Methemoglobin	Sulfhemoglobin
Acetanilid, phenacetin	+	+
Nitrites (amyl, sodium, potassium, nitroglycerin)	+	+
Trinitrotoluene, nitrobenzene	+	+
Aniline, hydroxylamine dimethylamine	+	+
Sulfanilamide	+	+
p-Aminosalicylic acid	+	
Dapsone	+	
Primaquine, chloroquine	+	
Prilocaine, benzocaine, lidocaine	+	
Menadione, naphthoquinone	+	
Naphthalene	+	
Resorcinol	+	
Phenylhydrazine	+	+

Acquired methemoglobinemia is virtually the only situation in which life-threatening amounts of methemoglobin accumulate. In general, the only symptom produced when methemoglobin comprises <30% of total hemoglobin is the cosmetic effect of cyanosis. As levels of methemoglobin rise to >30%, however, patients begin to exhibit symptoms of oxygen deprivation, such as malaise, giddiness, and other alterations of mental status. The symptoms reflect a true lack of oxygen availability at the tissue level. Methemoglobin is a markedly left-shifted hemoglobin that delivers little oxygen to the tissues. When methemoglobin is >50% of total hemoglobin, loss of consciousness, coma, and death can rapidly ensue. At this level, the blood is chocolate brown.

Diagnosis

Methemoglobinemia should be suspected in patients with unexplained cyanosis. It is obviously a medical emergency when any patient has cyanosis and altered mental status; a normal PaO_2 should trigger a consideration of methemoglobinemia. The ingestion of nitrites as a suicide gesture, especially in individuals knowledgeable with respect to chemistry, medicine, or pharmacology, should be considered. Methemoglobinemia can be suspected from the brownish color of blood when it is drawn. Laboratory detection is simple; methemoglobin exhibits characteristic peaks of absorption at 630 and 502 nm, rendering it easily distinguishable from normal hemoglobin. The inherited M hemoglobin mutants are frequently detectable by altered electrophoretic mobility, especially if ferricyanide treatment in vitro is used to convert all the hemoglobin solution to methemoglobin.

In the case of toxic methemoglobinemia, recognition of exposure to an appropriate agent provides the most important historical clue. Acute poisoning can represent a life-threatening emergency; therefore, laboratory evaluation for methemoglobin should be requested for any individual displaying atypical cyanosis or cyanosis occurring along with normal blood gas values. Methemoglobin due to deficiencies of the reductase system can be further evaluated in reference laboratories by direct analysis of these enzymes.

Management

Patients with M hemoglobins are usually asymptomatic and require no management. The secondary cyanosis can present a cosmetic problem. The cyanosis is not reversible, as ascorbic acid and methylene blue (see below) are generally ineffective.

Patients with deficiency of the reductase system generally do not require treatment. Cyanosis in these cases can be improved by treatment with oral methylene blue, 100–300 mg/day, or 500 mg/day of oral ascorbic acid. Riboflavin (20 mg/day) has also been reported to be effective and may be the preferred agent, because methylene blue produces discolored (blue) urine, and ascorbic acid can cause sodium oxalate stones.

Emergency treatment of high levels of toxic methemoglobinemia begins with 1–2 mg/kg of intravenous methylene blue, as a 1% solution in saline. It is usually infused rapidly (10–15 minutes). The dose may be repeated if necessary. This treatment is usually effective. Methylene blue acts via the NADPH reductase system, which in turn requires G6PD activity. The method is therefore ineffective in patients who also have G6PD deficiency. These patients, or patients who are severely affected, may require exchange transfusion. Oral ascorbic acid is not useful for emergency situations because it acts too slowly. Follow-up maintenance management, however, can be accomplished with either ascorbic acid or oral methylene blue.

Mild cases of methemoglobin intoxication do not require treatment. The patient can be monitored for 1–3 days, during which time methemoglobin levels will gradually return to normal if the offending agent is eliminated. The most important follow-up therapy for patients with toxic methemoglobinemia involves a thorough search for the offending agent and its removal from the environment.

SUGGESTED READINGS

1. Bunn HF: Sickle hemoglobin and other hemoglobin mutants. In Stamatoyannopoulos G, Nienhuis AW, Majcrus PO, Varmus H (eds): The Molecular Basis of Blood Disease. WB Saunders, Philadelphia, 1993
2. Bunn HF, Forget BG: Hemoglobin: Molecular, Cellular and Clinical Aspects. WB Saunders, Philadelphia, 1985
3. Dickerson RE, Geis I: Hemoglobin: Structure, Function, Evolution, and Pathology. Benjamin-Cummings, Menlo Park, CA, 1983
4. Fermi G, Pertuz MF: Atlas of Molecular Structures in Biology. Vol. 2: Hemoglobin and Myoglobin. Oxford University Press, Oxford, 1981
5. Ho C (ed): Hemoglobin and Oxygen Binding. Elsevier Biomedical, New York, 1982
6. Park CM, Nagel RL: Sulfhemoglobinemia: clinical and molecular aspects. N Engl J Med 310:1579, 1984
7. Pertuz MF: Molecular anatomy, physiology, and pathology of hemoglobin. p. 127. In Stamatoyannopoulos G, Nienhuis AW, Leder P, Majerus PW (eds): The Molecular Basis of Blood Diseases. WB Saunders, Philadelphia, 1987
8. Smith RP, Olson MV: Drug-induced methemoglobinemia. Semin Hematol 10: 253, 1973
9. Wynngaarden JB, Smith LH Jr, Bennett JC (eds): Cecil Textbook of Medicine. WB Saunders, Philadelphia, 1992
10. Wishner BC, Ward KB, Lattman EE, Love WE: Crystal structure sickle-cell deoxyhemoglobin at 5Å resolution. J Mol Biol 98:179, 1975

Enzymopathies

45

Donald E. Paglia

INTRODUCTION

Normal physiologic function and longevity of mature circulating erythrocytes are critically dependent on the fulfillment of small but distinct energy needs (see Ch. 33). The biochemical capacity of these cells, however, is restricted to a very few functional metabolic pathways, with little or no redundancy. Anaerobic glycolysis via the Embden-Meyerhof pathway, oxidative glycolysis through the hexose monophosphate shunt, and certain nucleotide salvage pathways are essentially all that the mature red cell can rely on for energy generation.

Hereditary or acquired enzyme defects may or may not have perceptible effects on red cell function or survival, depending on the physiologic importance of the affected reactions and on the availability of alternate metabolic pathways. Those enzymopathies that do have adverse clinical consequences frequently fall into two patterns. Defects that occur in the hexose monophosphate shunt and in those reactions normally responsible for maintenance of reduced glutathione (antioxidative mechanisms) are generally associated with periodic hemolytic episodes induced by oxidant food or drugs, the duress of surgery or infections, or other physiologic stresses. By contrast, deficiency states in the Embden-Meyerhof pathway and certain enzymes concerned with nucleotide metabolism are generally expressed by shortened red cell survival and consequent chronic hemolytic anemia. The common denominator among the latter diverse conditions is an inability to generate sufficient ATP to fulfill cellular energy needs. This is presumed to be the pathophysiologic basis for premature hemolysis.[1]

The relationships between inheritance of one or more mutant alleles for a red cell enzyme and clinical phenotype are far more complex than initially appreciated. Historically, hereditary enzymopathies were first detected as in vitro activity decrements measured in optimized assay systems with hemolysates as the source of the enzymes. Observed activities were <10-20% of those found in normal control hemolysates, and such enzymopathies have come to be termed quantitative or classic deficiency states. Affected individuals were presumed to be homozygotes because intermediate (about 40-60%) levels of enzymatic activities, consistent with heterozygous deficiency states, were often found in parents and other relatives. Such inheritance patterns could be explained by the presence of mutuant genes that coded for the production of an abnormal, catalytically inactive, enzyme protein or by null genes that failed to produce appropriate amounts of otherwise normal enzyme protein.

As more cases of different enzymopathies were detected and studied, no consistent correlation emerged between the severity of enzyme decrements and their clinical expression. It soon became apparent that a number of different abnormalities in biochemical characteristics of affected enzymes could result in functional deficiencies, even though optimal activities observed in vitro were minimally decreased, normal, or even increased.

Broad polymorphism in genetic expression is now understood to pertain to most of the known erythroenzymopathies.[2-10] Mutant genes may code for production of enzyme protein that is catalytically impotent, unstable, kinetically aberrant, or altered in terms of its response to physiologic activators, inhibitors, cofactors, and allosteric modifiers. Alternatively, it may exhibit diverse combinations of any of these characteristics. Any of these parameters may be further manifested by such factors as altered pH optima and electrophoretic migration rates. In the absence of consanguinity, therefore, affected individuals often represent compound heterozygous states rather than true homozygosity. Nonetheless, sex-linked and dominant patterns with variable penetrance have also been observed. A few instances of molecular identity between mutant variants identified in unrelated kindreds have been documented.[2]

The pathophysiology of red cell enzymopathies is further complicated by the erythrocyte's unique handicap, its inability to replace degraded or inactivated enzymes by biosynthesis of new enzyme molecules. Studies of normal and variant enzymes must take into account the effects of red cell aging and the possibility of superimposed activities of multiple isoenzymes. As will be seen in the following account of specific enzymopathies, many mammalian enzymes exist as multiple tissue-specific isoenzymes. Some of these may undergo post-translational modifications that further alter their characteristics, while others may be dominant in erythroid precursors, including reticulocytes, and become progressively less active as the cells age in the circulation. Finally, since the mature erythrocyte is unable to synthesize new protein components, each enzyme appears to have a characteristic decay rate in the aging cell that is presumably a function of its inherent biochemical stability, its susceptibility to ambient oxidative stresses, and its resistance to intracellular protease activity. The resultant effect is an enzyme profile that may vary significantly as the reticulocyte matures and as the erythrocyte progresses toward senescence. This spectrum of enzyme alterations is further reflected by variations in intracellular concentrations of various intermediates and metabolites, including ATP, many of which have been postulated as ultimately responsible for the finite life span of the erythrocyte.

ENZYMOPATHIES ASSOCIATED WITH HEMOLYTIC SYNDROMES

Defects in Anaerobic Glycolysis

Hexokinase

Because hexokinase is responsible for priming the glycolytic pump (see Ch. 33), it has been generally assumed that serious hereditary defects in this enzyme would likely be lethal mutations. That might well be true in many instances, but a small heterogeneous group of deficient patients who survive into adulthood has been detected.[11-26]

As many as four distinct tissue-specific isoenzymes of hexokinase have been identified (the number obtained depending on methods of separation and purification), and these have been accordingly designated HK-1–HK-4.[27] Several heterogeneous subtypes of HK-1 have been identified in erythrocytes,[28-30] including one that predominates in reticulocytes,[31] and are presumably responsible for the steep biphasic decay curve observed as reticulocytes mature and erythrocytes age. HK-1 is also found in brain but differs from the isoenzymes found in other blood cells and tissues.

MAJOR FEATURES OF GLYCOLYTIC ENZYME DEFECTS

Deficiencies of red cell glycolytic enzymes usually produce hemolytic anemia of variable severity. These are often called nonspherocytic hemolytic anemias because the red cell morphology is minimally altered. (Notable exceptions include the poikilocytosis and xerocytosis seen in pyruvate kinase deficiency.) The final common pathway of the biochemical defect is ATP deficiency leading to inadequate homeostasis of Na^+, K^+, Ca^{2+}, and water. However, a few enzyme deficiencies, as noted in the table below, lead to decreased 2,3-DPG concentra-

tions. This in turn causes increased hemoglobin/oxygen affinity (left shift) and may lead to erythrocytosis.

Enzymopathies other than G6PD deficiency are very rare. PK deficiency accounts for 95% of all cases; it has been reported to be present in only a few hundred patients. These defects are thus unlikely causes in most patients with hemolytic anemia unless a positive family history or associated muscle, neurologic, or psychiatric abnormalities are present.

Defects of Red Cell Glycolytic Enzymes

Enzyme	Inheritance	Red Cell Abnormality	Abnormality of Other Systems	Comment
Hexokinase (HK)	AR	HA (moderate)	None	Rarely autosomal dominant
Glucose phosphate isomerase	AR	HA (moderate)	None	Second most common defect
Phosphofructokinase	Complex autosomal	HA erythrocytosis	Myopathy	Multiple genes; complex inheritance Tauri's disease
Fructose diphosphate aldolase	AR	HA	Mental retardation	Very rare
Triose phosphate isomerase	AR	HA moderate–severe	Severe neuromuscular abnormalities	Splenectomy not helpful
Phosphoglycerate kinase	X-linked	HA (variable)	Neurologic and mental impairment	—
Diphosphoglyceratemutase and diphosphoglycerate phosphatase	AR	Erythrocytosis	—	Decreased 2,3-DPG supply
Enolase	—	None described ?HA	None described	—
Pyruvate kinase	AR	HA (variable)	—	Accounts for 90% of glycolytic defects; splenectomy often beneficial in severe cases

Abbreviations: AR, autosomal recessive; AD, autosomal dominant; X, X-linked.

HK-1 is a cytosolic enzyme formed in monomers of approximately 10-kd molecular weight. Its structural gene is located at gene locus 10q. Inheritance of defects generally conforms to an autosomal recessive mode, although some cases appear to follow a dominant transmission pattern, perhaps with variable penetrance.[21,22] A wide range of molecular heterogeneity among the variant HK-1 isoenzymes has been reported. These are reflected by variations in optimal activities, thermostability, electrophoretic migrations, kinetics for glucose and/or Mg^{2+} ATP, and regulatory responses to glucose-6-phosphate (G6P), glucose-1,6-diphosphate, 2,3-diphosphoglycerate (2,3-DPG), and inorganic phosphate. The principal clinical manifestation of severe HK-1 deficiency is confined to erythroid elements in the form of chronic mild-to-severe hemolytic anemia. Heterozygous deficiency states are without apparent effect on red cell function or longevity. In severe cases with heavy transfusion requirements, splenectomy may offer some benefit.[11–14,24] Erythrocyte hexokinase deficiency may also be included among such multisystem abnormalities as Fanconi syndrome. Hemolysis due to an acquired form of HK deficiency occurs in Wilson disease, due to inhibition of HK by the high levels of copper.

Glucosephosphate Isomerase

Deficiencies of glucosephosphate isomerase comprise the second most common erythroenzymopathy of anaerobic glycolysis after pyruvate kinase deficiency. A single dimeric enzyme of approximately 134-kd, encoded by a gene on autosome 19, is present in humans. Some slight differences, originally thought to represent tissue-specific isoenzymes, most likely represent slight post-translational modifications, rather than distinct isoenzymes.[33]

Curiously, virtually all the mutant gene products thus far reported have been characterized by marked instability. Cells capable of protein synthesis may compensate for this lability by increased enzyme production, but erythrocytes do not share this capacity and consequently die prematurely. Thus, hemolytic anemia may be the only clinical manifestation of this multisystem disorder, although neuromuscular and mental changes may sometimes accompany the anemia.[34–36] Autosomal recessive inheritance is the rule, but rare cases have been thought to result from a single copy of a mutant gene.

A broad spectrum of molecular heterogeneity also characterizes these variant isoenzymes. In addition to instability, alterations have been observed in optimal catalytic activity, electrophoretic migration rates, pH optima, and varying combinations of these parameters.[34–44] Biochemical changes induced by the defective enzyme are also frequently demonstrable. These include increased intracellular concentrations of G6P, decreased concentrations of glycolytic intermediates distal to the point of blockade, altered ATP/ADP concentrations and ratios (both increased and decreased), and severely impaired ability (<1–10% of normal) to recycle fructose-6-phosphate back through the hexose monophosphate shunt,[39–41] even though shunt activity itself may be increased significantly as G6P diversion occurs.

Clinical expression of the anemia of glucosephosphate isomerase deficiency varies from mild to severe in homozygotes or compound heterozygotes, while simple heterozygotes are hematologically normal. Severe homozygous deficiency has been documented as a rare cause of hydrops fetalis.[43] Therapeutic attempts to stimulate glycolysis with ascorbic acid, methylene blue, or inorganic phosphate have not been rewarding. Splenectomy in severe cases has been followed by variably positive responses in terms of increased hemoglobin levels and decreased transfusion requirements.[44]

Phosphofructokinase

If the relative importance of any single step in such a complex metabolic process as glycolysis can be assessed, a strong case can be made that the role of phosphofructokinase deserves the highest distinction. It occupies a key rate-limiting position in the earliest stage of glycolysis. Its activity is subject to complex and subtle modulations by a number of key metabolites and ions, including ATP, ADP, AMP, 2,3-DPG, and fructose-1,6-diphosphate.[45-50] Additionally, fructose-1,6-diphosphate, the product of this essentially irreversible reaction, is the principal allosteric activator of pyruvate kinase, another crucial rate-limiting enzyme in terminal glycolysis.

Human phosphofructokinase is a tetramer composed of three dissimilar subunits, designated L, M, and P (or F) according to their occurrence in liver and leukocytes, muscle, and platelets (or fibroblasts).[47-52] Each is encoded by separate genes residing respectively on autosomes 21, 1, and 10. As pointed out by Vora,[53] M subunits tend to predominate in tissues that rely heavily on glycolysis, such as skeletal and cardiac muscle and brain tissues, whereas L subunits seem to be associated with tissue reliance on gluconeogenesis, such as liver and adipose tissue. The red cell contains approximately equal amount of the L and M subunits arranged in all five possible tetramers: L_4, L_3M_1, L_2M_2, L_1M_3, and M_4.

Phosphofructokinase deficiency states are multiple and various, depending on which subunit is affected. Defects of the M subunit, for example, are clinically expressed as myopathies, since the skeletal muscle isoenzyme is the homotetramer M_4. The red cells in such patients must rely complete on the L_4 homotetramer; the resultant decrease in phosphofructokinase activity may impair glycolysis sufficiently to result in clinically detectable hemolysis.[54-57] Other forms of phosphofructokinase deficiency include some with hemolysis but no myopathy and others without either myopathy or hemolysis despite severe reductions in activity.

In the classic form of Tarui disease, red cell phosphofructokinase activities are reduced to about half-normal in the absence of the M subunit. This results in decreased concentrations of distal glycolytic intermediates, including 2,3-DPG, which alters the oxyhemoglobin dissociation curve sufficiently to induce erythrocytosis. The hemolytic process may therefore be well compensated by erythrocytosis, and such patients may be hematologically asymptomatic.[58-60]

Fructose Diphosphate Aldolase

Aldolase reversibly catalyzes the equilibrium between fructose-1,6-diphosphate and its component trioses, dihydroxyacetone phosphate and glyceraldehyde-3-phosphate. It is a tetrameric enzyme of approximately 158-kd. Three tissue-specific isoenzymes have been described.[61,62] Severe deficiency states have been reported in two unrelated families conforming to an autosomal recessive mode of inheritance. In one case, moderately severe hemolysis with multiple malformations and possible mental retardation were present in an uncertain association[63]; in another family, hemolysis alone was observed.[64] In the latter, the residual erythrocyte enzyme exhibited decreased affinity for its substrate, fructose-1,6-diphosphate, and decreased stability.

Triosephosphate Isomerase

The interconversion of dihydroxyacetone phosphate and glyceraldehyde-3-phosphate is catalyzed by triosephosphate isomerase, a dimeric enzyme with a molecular weight of 26,750. Its identical subunits of 248 amino acids are structurally encoded by a single gene on autosome 12. All tissues share a common enzyme; therefore, all are affected to some degree by deficiency states. Null alleles have been detected in a number of subjects, who exhibit half-normal activities coupled with comparable amounts of immunologically cross-reacting protein.[65,66] Clinically, significant deficiencies have been documented in approximately 25 patients, most of whom exhibited 5-20% of the triosephosphate isomerase activity present in normal control erythrocytes. These cases also encompass a broad range of molecular heterogeneity in regard to their residual enzymes, which is principally manifested as stability, kinetic, and electrophoretic abnormalities.[67-78] A single amino acid substitution has been observed to render the enzyme protein unstable.[79] Transmission of the genetic defect follows an autosomal recessive pattern. Clinically affected individuals are homozygotes or compound heterozygotes; simple heterozygotes are devoid of hematologic, neuromuscular, or other abnormalities.

A prominent biochemical consequence of severe isomerase impairment is the accumulation of dihydroxyacetone phosphate, which may have cytotoxic effects. In affected red cells, this triose may be present in concentrations as high as 50 times normal. Other tissues in which the enzyme has been quantitatively measured also show markedly reduced enzyme activities.

The clinical consequences of severe triosephosphate isomerase deficiency are dominated by the severity of the neuromuscular abnormalities that invariably accompany the disorder. These usually become apparent within the first year and inexorably progress in severity, with few children surviving to adulthood. A subjective impression of increased susceptibility to infections may reflect leukocyte involvement, but distinct functional abnormalities in phagocytic and bactericidal processes have not been identified. Arrhythmias and sudden death occur presumably as a consequence of cardiac muscle involvement. The hemolytic anemia associated with triosephosphate isomerase deficiency is also moderate to severe and is not effectively ameliorated by splenectomy.

Phosphoglycerate Kinase

Phosphoglycerate kinase is the only enzyme of anaerobic glycolysis known to be encoded by a gene on the X chromosome. All tissues contain the same enzyme, which exists as a monomer of 416 amino acids totaling about 45 kd. This enzyme catalyzes the first ATP-generating step of glycolysis, transferring the high-energy phosphate of 1,3-DPG to ADP. That substrate may also be converted to a low-energy state and stored as 2,3-DPG by irreversible mutation into the Rapoport-Luebering shunt. The direction of substrate flow is determined primarily by intracellular pH and the ATP/ADP ratio. As expected, deficiencies of phosphoglycerate kinase usually result in decreased concentrations of ATP and increased concentrations of 2,3-DPG, with a consequent right shift in the oxyhemoglobin dissociation curve. Increased intracellular sodium concentrations have also been observed. These can be ascribed to alterations in Na^+/K^+ pump activity secondary to decreased ATP production from this reaction.[80]

Phosphoglycerate kinase deficiency states are rare. Those that have been studied have shown considerable polymorphism. Several variants have been sequenced and shown to be due to single amino acid substitutions.[81-84] Other variants have exhibited abnormal kinetics for substrates and/or cofactors as well as decreased optimal activities and instability.[81-83,85-94] Although some variants are silent, about one-half are associated with hemolytic anemia of variable severity and with neurologic and mental abnormalities in affected males. Females exhibit mosaicism with variably sized populations of normal and enzyme-deficient erythrocytes and may have slight to moderate hemolytic manifestations.

Phosphoglycerate kinase deficiency has also been demonstrable in assays of other tissues, including skeletal and cardiac muscle, brain, liver, leukocytes, and platelets.[95] Phagocytosis by deficient leukocytes may be ineffective because of impaired bactericidal processes.[96] Hemolysis without neuromuscular disease[94] and isolated myopathy have also been reported.[92,93] If severe, the anemia of phosphoglycerate kinase deficiency may be ameliorated by splenectomy, but the response rate has been inconsistent. Aplastic crises occasionally occur, but progressive neurologic complications usually dominate the clinical picture.

Pyruvate Kinase

Mammalian pyruvate kinase is a homotetrameric enzyme composed of 50–60-kd subunits. The gene determinant of liver pyruvate kinase resides on chromosome 1. That for the muscle isoenzyme is on chromosome 15. Variations in the primary structure of tissue-specific isoenzymes may be induced by gene rearrangements, by alternative RNA splicing, by differences in mRNA, or by post-translational proteolytic modifications.[97-103]

The dominant isoenzymic forms present in adult liver (L), muscle (M_1), leukocytes and platelets (M_2), and erythrocytes (R) all have features in common but are identifiable by distinct biochemical differences. M_2 is the dominant form in fetal tissues. There are very close similarities between L and R isoenzymes, and the liver has been shown to have decreased pyruvate kinase activity (partially compensated by ongoing synthesis) in cases of erythrocyte enzyme deficiency. Partially purified red cell pyruvate kinase is electrophoretically separable into two bands, R_1 and R_2, both of which migrate apart from the L form, even though all three are antigenically identical. The M_2 fetal form in erythroid precursors is normally replaced by R_1 in normoblasts and reticulocytes and eventually by R_2, the dominant form in mature erythrocytes. In some human and ca-

nine deficiency states, R forms fail to develop, and the M_2 isoenzyme persists.[104-106]

Pyruvate kinase catalyzes the second crucial ATP-generative step in glycosis, which is necessary if there is to be any net gain in ATP. It requires magnesium and potassium for optimal activity and is sensitive to a number of regulatory influences. All the isoenzymes except M_1 are subject to allosteric regulation by substrate or cofactors. In particular, the product of the phosphofructokinase reaction, fructose-1,6-diphosphate, converts the sigmoidal kinetic curve of pyruvate kinase to the hyperbolic curve of Michaelis-Menten kinetics. Additionally, potassium concentration influences enzyme affinity for ADP, and increasing concentrations of APT inhibit activity.

Genetic defects that result in alterations of these various regulatory properties, as well as those that result in significantly decreased stability of catalytic activity (Fig. 45-1), may show identical phenotypic expression in a chronic hemolytic syndrome of variable severity. Pyruvate kinase deficiency was the first enzymopathy of the Embden-Meyerhof pathway to be recognized as a cause of hereditary nonspherocytic hemolytic anemia.[107,108] Along with class 1 deficiencies of glucose-6-phosphate dehydrogenase (G6PD), pyruvate kinase defects comprise the most common erythroenzymopathy responsible for chronic hemolysis. Well over 300 cases have been reported,[2,4,109] and internationally standardized procedures for their evaluation have been adopted.[110] People of northern European and peri-Mediterranean heritage are most commonly affected, but the deficiency state has been observed in persons of a wide range of ethnic and geographic origins.

In consanguineous families, homozygosity for the defect results in chronic hemolysis, whereas virtually all heterozygotes are hematologically normal. Because of the broad range of molecular heterogeneity among pyruvate kinase variants and the relative infrequency of consanguinity, most affected individuals are compound heterozygotes whose red cells often contain mixtures of at least two mutant isoenzymic forms. Because of its tetrameric nature, dissimilar subunit assembly could produce as many as five isoenzymes.[111,112] Although this complicates their biochemical characterization, it appears clear that most clinically significant deficiency states are associated with enzyme variants that have either markedly reduced specific activity, decreased affinity for the substrate phosphoenolpyruvate, reduced stability, or an impaired capacity to respond to allosteric activation by fructose-1,6-diphosphate or to inhibition by ATP. Other alterations, such as decreased affinity for

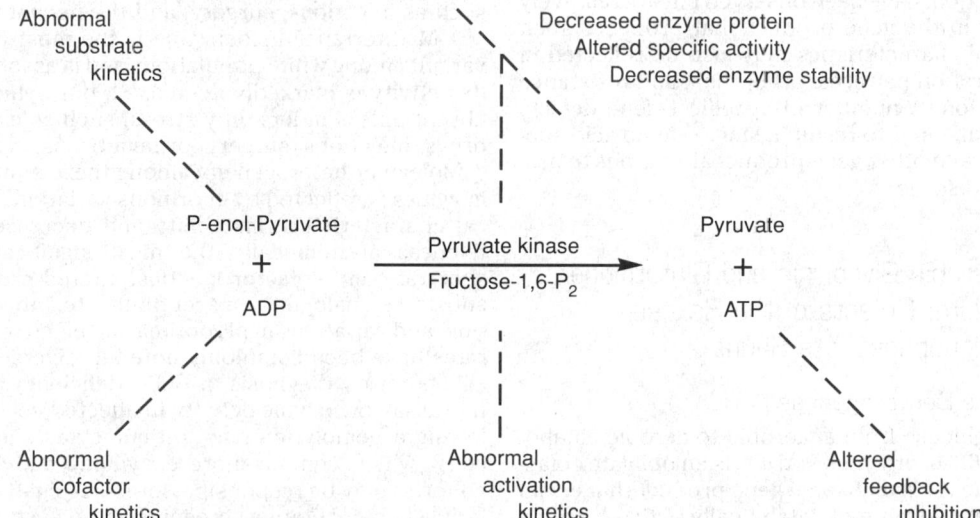

Fig. 45-1. Components of the pyruvate kinase reaction that have been found defective with various mutant erythrocyte isoenzymes.

PYRUVATE KINASE DEFICIENCY

Regardless of the molecular mechanism involved, impairment of glycolysis at the pyruvate kinase step results in decreased intracellular concentrations of total adenine nucleotides, decreased ATP generation, elevated concentrations of glycolytic intermediates above the blockade (particularly 2,3-DPG), and decreased total NAD$^+$/NADH concentrations with altered ratios. The concentration of 2,3-DPG may increase two- or threefold, shifting the oxyhemoglobin dissociation curve sufficiently to help compensate for the anemia by favoring tissue oxygenation.

The clinical consequence of pyruvate kinase deficiency is chronic hemolysis that can vary from completely compensated asymptomatic cases to severe, transfusion-dependent, life-threatening anemia. The latter are often apparent during the neonatal period, when exchange transfusions may be required. Severe deficiency may also be manifested as hydrops fetalis.

Clinical and laboratory findings are no more distinctive in pyruvate kinase deficiency than in any other chronic hemolytic process. One distinct feature of this condition is the peripheral blood smear, which may show striking numbers of acanthocytes, echinocytes and sperocytes, as well as xerocytes (see Ch. 46); the latter reflect cellular dehydration due to markedly low ATP levels, and reduced Na$^+$,K$^+$-ATPase pump activity. The dehydrated cells also have markedly elevated mean corpuscular hemoglobin concentration. Splenomegaly, icterus, indirect hyperbilirubinemia, decreased haptoglobin, and reticulocytosis with marrow erythroid hyperplasia are commonly observed in direct proportion to the severity of the anemia. The stresses of surgery, infections, and pregnancy have all been associated with acute exacerbations of the chronic hemolytic process, and aplastic crises may occur particularly in association with parvovirus or related infections. In severe cases, especially in young children, splenectomy has often resulted in increased erythrocyte and reticulocyte counts and hemoglobin concentrations and has frequently reduced or eliminated transfusion requirements.

the cofactor ADP, increased substrate affinity, or decreased enzyme protein production, have been observed but are relatively rare. Any alteration in the gene product that produces such variable biochemical characteristics may also be reflected in electrophoretic migration patterns, pH optima, and resistance to thermal inactivation. A number of specific L-gene defects have now been documented to result in single amino acid substitutions, deletions, and other gene-product alterations to produce the hemolytic disorder.[2]

Defects in Aerobic Glycolysis and Glutathione Metabolism: Defects of the Hexose Monophosphate Shunt

Glucose-6-Phosphate Dehydrogenase

The diversion of glucose from anaerobic to aerobic catabolism is initiated by G6PD, for which NADP$^+$ is an obligate cofactor. This enzyme is an X chromosome gene product that exists in a pH-dependent equilibrium of catalytically active homodimers and homotetramers with subunits of about 59 kd. Activity is strongly influenced by intracellular concentrations of substrate, cofactor, products, hydrogen ions, and metal cations, and its catalytic rate is normally only a small fraction of its potential fully stimulated capacity. Both NADPH and ATP serve as inhibitors, competitive with NADP$^+$ and G6P, respectively. These regulatory properties are physiologically important because they permit appropriate production of NADPH in response to variable oxidative stresses. This pyridine cofactor is crucial to peroxide detoxification via cyclic glutathione peroxidase and reductase activities; additionally, NADPH is avidly bound as a structural component of catalase. The ability of the red cell to survive assaults by ambient oxidants is therefore crucially dependent on effective hexosemonophosphate shunt activity. This in turn requires adequate G6PD activity.

Deficiencies of G6PD comprise the single most common human enzymopathy, hematologic or otherwise, and affect nearly one-tenth the world's population. They are by far the most common red cell enzymopathy, accounting for millions of affected persons; the next most common deficiency, pyruate kinase deficiency occurs in only a few hundred patients. The geographic distribution coincides with that of tropical malaria, and the hypothesis that deficient erythrocytes might be more resistant to *Plasmodium falciparum* parasitization has support from a number of studies.

An enormous number of deficient variants continues to expand the literature on G6PD deficiency, and international standards for evaluating and designating them have been adopted.[113,114] Mutant isoenzymes are classified according to the association of severe enzyme deficiency with chronic hemolytic anemia (class I) or with syndromes of acute episodic hemolysis associated with severely or moderately decreased activity (class II and III, respectively), normal activity (class IV), or increased activity (class V). The A-minus and Mediterranean isoenzymes are thus categorized as class III variants.

The normal G6PD enzyme, traditionally designed G6PD B, is common to all human cells, but post-translational modifications may alter its properties slightly from one tissue to another. A normal African isoenzyme, designated G6PD A, results from a single amino acid substitution. Its catalytic activity and other biochemical properties are similar or identical to those of G6PD B, except for altered electrophoretic migration. An A-minus variant differs by an additional amino acid substitution, which significantly decreases its stability, alters other biochemical properties, and has clinical manifestations. The A and A-minus isoenzymes are common among black Americans (30 and 11%, respectively), Hemizygosity for A-minus is responsible for an intermittent acute hemolytic syndrome associated with administration of certain drugs or with other stresses, such as infections, surgery, and the neonatal period.

A Mediterranean isoenzyme is the most common defective variant among white populations and is associated with favism. Its activity is markedly decreased, but hemolysis is generally absent unless induced by stress, such as exposure to certain drugs, infections, surgery, or fava beans.

Molecular heterogeneity among these numerous mutant isoenzymes is reflected by enormous variations in their biochemical characteristics. Instability and decreased catalytic effectiveness are clinically the most significant, but impaired substrate and cofactor kinetics, altered cross-reactivity with substrate analogues, susceptibility to inhibition or inactivation, and variations in pH optima and electrophoretic migration rates have been commonly noted in diverse combinations.

Laboratory diagnosis of G6PD deficiency requires quantitative assay of enzyme activity in affected cells. Immediately following a hemolytic crisis, reticulocytes and surviving young cells (which contain more enzymatic activity than do older cohorts) may be responsible for false-negative results, particularly when qualitative screening assay systems are used. Similarly, heterozygosity may be difficult to detect because of mosaicism. Abnormal production of Heinz bodies is a frequent

CLINICAL ASPECTS OF GLUCOSE-6-PHOSPHATE DEHYDROGENASE DEFICIENCY

Because G6PD deficiency is a sex-linked disorder, clinical manifestations appear principally in male hemizygotes or female homozygotes. Heterozygous females exhibit mosaicism, with dual populations of erythrocytes containing either the normal or the mutant isoenzymes. Heterozygotes are usually asymptomatic but may be susceptible to hemolytic crises, depending on the size of the population of defective cells, which varies because of the randomness of X chromosome inactivation (Lyonization).[115] Female homozygosity is rare but must be considered. X-linkage of this common enzyme deficiency has also provided the basis for establishing neoplastic monoclonality for a number of benign and malignant tumors.[116]

Two major types of clinical syndromes result for G6PD deficiency. The first, by far the most common, is that exemplified by the A-minus variant that is highly prevalent in the African population. Since this enzyme exhibits some reduction in catalytic activity and some reduction in stability, its activity becomes more severely deficient as the red cell ages. Reticulocytes and younger red cells actually possess sufficient activity to cope with normal oxidative stresses. However, increased oxidative stress, such as that occurring in the presence of fever, infection, diabetic ketoacidosis, exposure to certain drugs, and toxins (see table below), and, perhaps, the perinatal period can overwhelm the red cell's compromised ability to resist oxidation. Consequently, G6PD activity is reduced to insufficient levels, oxidized glutathione accumulates at the expense of reduced glutathione, and reacts with hemoglobin, resulting in loss of heme and precipitation to form Heinz bodies. The end stage is generation of a Heinz-body hemolytic anemia not unlike that seen in unstable hemoglobin disorders (see Ch. 44). If the oxidative stress is especially severe, intravascular hemolysis with hemoglobinuria may occur. Usually, however, hemolysis is self-limited, because it is only the older red cells that are destroyed. The younger red cells, which still possess more adequate levels of the enzyme, frequently survive the challenge.

The second common G6PD-deficient syndrome is characterized by moderate-to-severe chronic hemolysis exacerbated to potentially fatal levels by exposure to oxidants. The most common example of this syndrome is the G6PD deficiency encountered in 3–5% of individuals of Mediterranean ancestry, Ashkenazi Jews, and some Asians. These individuals inherit extremely unstable variants that survive in the red cell for only a few hours. Most of their red cells are thus highly compromised in their ability to deal with normal or increased oxidative stresses. The syndrome of favism is characterized by profound hemolysis after the ingestion of fava beans; it occurs in individuals with the Mediterranean isoenzyme variant.

A characteristic cell seen on peripheral blood smears of patients with G6PD deficiency is the "bite" cell. The cytoplasm of these erythrocytes contains a coagulum of precipitated hemoglobin that, when sustained, often separates from the membrane, leaving a rim of nonstaining material. The membrane cresent surrounding this rim is often not visible, giving the cells the appearance of having had a bite removed from them.

The G6PD A-minus variant accounts for the vast majority of patients. Hemolysis in these individuals is usually self limited, followed within 7–10 days by stabilization of the hematocrit and reticulocytosis. Therapy is usually conservative. The use of offending drugs, or exposure to offending agents, should clearly be avoided. The hemolysis itself usually does not require intervention; indeed, if the offending drug must be continued because discontinuance or substitution of a nonoxidative alternative is not possible, the hematocrit usually stabilizes and can even increase toward normal. This occurs because of the resistance of the remaining younger cells to the oxidative stress, and the replacement of the previously destroyed older cells by reticulocytes.

Patients with severely defective variants and chronic hemolysis should be treated by avoidance of offending agents, and prompt intervention by transfusion or exchange transfusion in the face of life-threatening hemolysis. Splenectomy has proved beneficial in selected cases.

Some Agents That Provoke Hemolytic Episodes in G6PD-Deficient Individuals

Acetanilide	Primaquine
Methylene blue	Sulfacetamide
Nalidixic acid	Sulfamethoxazo e
Naphthalene (mothballs)	Sulfanilamide
Niridazole	Sulfapyridine
Nitrofurantoin	Thiazole sulfone
Pamaquine	Toluidine blue
Pentaquine	Trinitrotoluene
Phenylhydrazine	

but nonspecific feature of the deficiency. DNA-based diagnosis is also available to identify specific aminoacid substitutions.

Glutathione Peroxidase and Glutathione Reductase

Clinical syndromes involving other enzymes of aerobic glycolysis have been described only for glutathione reductase and glutathione synthesis. Free-radical formation mediates many of the deleterious cellular effects of diverse pathologic processes, including radiation and chemical injury, inflammation, and aging. Sophisticated mechanisms to neutralize free radicals have evolved to protect cell membranes, enzymes, and other cellular components from the destructive structural and functional consequences of lipid peroxidation, altered redox states, and protein denaturation.

Human erythrocytes contain a dismutase that inactivates superoxide free radicals by conversion to hydrogen peroxide, which can then be decomposed by catalase or reduced to water by glutathione peroxidase in a coupled oxidation of reduced glutathione. The latter is regenerated by the action of glutathione reductase with NADPH as hydrogen donor.

Defects in any of these enzymes or in the synthesis and maintenance of glutathione itself could theoretically compromise antioxidant defenses, potentially rendering such cells susceptible to stress-induced hemolysis. Acatalasemia, however, is associated with oral ulcers rather than a hemolytic syndrome, and significant deficiencies of superoxide dismutase have not been observed.

Partial deficiencies of glutathione peroxidase have been seen

DRUGS AND AGENTS THAT DO AND DO NOT CAUSE HEMOLYSIS IN G6PD-DEFICIENT INDIVIDUALS

Hematologists are sometimes asked to give opinions about the safety of certain compounds in G6PD-deficient individuals or persons in whom this condition is a concern. Among many agents (see previous box) that cause hemolysis in these individuals, certain commonly used agents are prominent: most (but not all) antimalarial agents, some sulfa drugs, some urinary antibiotics (e.g., nalidixic acid, nitrofurantoin), mothballs, and some dyes. It is also helpful to know that some agents are safe in usual doses: chloroquine, aspirin, acatominophen, vitamin C, quinidine, colchichine, isoniazid procainamide, and vitamin K, among others, are often questioned as hemolytic agents, but are probably safe.

in association with hemolytic disorders.[117–122] but a cause-and-effect relationship has not been established. A wide range of red cell activities has been observed among certain populations on the basis of heredity or of dietary deficiency of selenium, an essential enzyme component, but these have not been accompanied by premature hemolysis.

It was recently shown that NADPH is a tightly bound component of mammalian catalase and necessary for its resistance to inactivation by hydrogen peroxide. Contrary to earlier studies, it appears that both catalase and glutathione peroxidase are of comparable importance in the physiologic detoxification of peroxidase.

Similarly, deficiency states of glutathione reductase have been observed in uncertain association with hemolytic syndromes.[123–125] Many of these resulted from inadequate riboflavin conversion to flavin adenine dinucleotide, which is a cofactor for the enzyme.[126,127] The encoding gene for glutathione reductase resides on chromosome 8. A family with heterozygous and homozygous deficiencies of both erythrocyte and leukocyte enzymes that were not dependent on the flavin cofactor has been observed.[128] Glutathione instability and a hemolytic episode induced by fava bean consumption in one of these cases suggest a probable cause and effect relation between severe reductase deficiency and susceptibility to oxidant-induced hemolysis.

Glutathione Synthesis

Inability to synthesize glutathione from three constituent amino acids in separate ATP-dependent reactions results in virtual absence of the tripeptide and a moderate chronic hemolytic syndrome.

The first step in glutathione synthesis is mediated by γ-glutamylcysteine synthetase. Hereditary deficiency of this enzyme is transmitted as an autosomal recessive disorder.[129] Heterozygotes have no clinical manifestations, but homozygotes exhibit chronic hemolysis with barely detectable concentrations of erythrocyte glutathione. Decreased concentrations of glutathione in other tissues, such as skeletal muscle (25%) and leukocytes (50%), have not been accompanied by apparent dysfunction. This may be a result of continued production of a catalytically functional but unstable enzyme in those tissues capable of ongoing protein synthesis. Although a spinocerebellar degenerative process was present in the first cases studied, another case of severe deficiency with hemolytic anemia was devoid of neurologic features.[130]

The second step in glutathione synthesis adds glycine to the dipeptide γ-glutamylcysteine and is catalyzed by glutathione synthetase. Severe deficiencies of this enzyme are accompanied by a hemolytic disorder and in many cases by a variety of other clinical manifestations, including neurologic and metabolic abnormalities.[131–133] Heterozygotes with intermediate synthetase activities have normal cellular concentrations of glutathione and are clinically and hematologically normal. The apparent clinical heterogeneity may again relate to ongoing synthesis of an unstable isoenzyme or to tissue-specific protease activity.[134] The loss of feedback inhibition of γ-glutamylcysteine production by glutathione itself allows this dipeptide to accumulate and to affect concentrations of related metabolites. Severe 5-oxoprolinemia and metabolic acidosis requiring bicarbonate therapy are common sequences. In addition to chronic hemolysis, subjects with severe deficiencies of either glutathione synthetic enzyme are susceptible to acute episodes of stress-induced hemolysis with Heinz-body production.

Defects in Nucleotide Metabolism

Abnormalities in erythrocyte nucleotide metabolism have been observed in association with hyperactive as well as deficient enzymes. Those that appear to have clinical relevance include hyperactivity of ADA and deficiencies of adenylate kinase and pyrimidine nucleotidase. A number of other deficiency states (e.g., those involving ADA, purine nucleoside phosphorylase, and the phosphoribosyltransferases of adenine and hypoxanthine guanine) and hyperactivity of ribose-phosphate pyrophosphokinase are apparently unaccompanied by adverse effects on red cells.

Adenosine Deaminase

Marked elevations in ADA activity, approaching two orders of magnitude, have been associated with compensated hemolytic processes in four unrelated families from the United States, Japan, and France.[135–138] The abnormality is transmitted as a genetic dominant trait. All tissues share a common enzyme protein, a gene product of a single locus on chromosome 20, but post-translational modifications may result in apparent tissue-specific isoenzymes. The hyperactive enzyme is structurally and biochemically normal. Its overproduction is isolated to erythroid elements by a defect in mRNA translation.[139,140]

Affected individuals may have subclinical hemolytic anemia well compensated by a brisk reticulocytosis. ATP and total adenine nucleotides are deficient; they are present at about half the normal erythrocyte concentrations. This presumably results from the rapid deamination of plasma adenosine, which reduces or eliminates it as a potential substrate for an essential nucleotide salvage pathway in erythrocytes catalyzed by adenosine kinase.[136–141] The converse situation is seen in cases of immunodeficiency disease due to severely deficient ADA: an increase in erythrocyte concentrations of adenine and deoxyadenine nucleotides reflects increased availability of the nucleosides as substrates for phosphorylation by adenosine kinase.

The disorder is accompanied by prominent elevations in activity of another erythrocyte enzyme, pyrimidine nucleotidase, but the significance of this linkage is unknown. The nucleotidase appears to be biochemically normal and does not show any increased ability to dephosphorylate AMP to account for the diminished adenine nucleotide pool.[136–141]

Adenylate Kinase

The rapidly reversible equilibrium existing among components of the erythrocyte adenine nucleotide pool is mediated by an active adenylate kinase. The importance of this enzyme to normal cell function and longevity remains uncertain. Four families with variably severe adenylate kinase deficiency have been studied.[142-146] Among those with moderate-to-severe hemolytic anemia, residual activities ranged from 44% to <10% of normal controls. Partial deficiency of G6PD coexisted in one subject, and psychomotor retardation was present in another in uncertain associations. Genetic transmission appeared consistent with autosomal recessive or dominant with variable penetrance. Parental adenylate kinase was electrophoretically identical to the common AK-1 phenotype. Heterozygosity was thought to exist in some nonanemic relatives because of half-normal enzymatic activity.

Two siblings in a black American family displayed widely disparate clinical findings.[146] Both had virtually undetectable adenylate kinase activities, but only one had hemolytic anemia, the other appearing entirely normal. The reason for this difference remains unexplained, and the possibility of compound defects remains. Salvage reactions that generate AMP from adenine or adenosine theoretically require adenylate kinase activity to provide the diphosphates and ultimately the triphosphates to maintain the balance of the adenine nucleotide pool. It may be that adenylate kinase activities reduced by two or even three orders of magnitude below normal are still adequate to serve that purpose, since erythrocyte concentrations of all adenine nucleotides were minimally altered, if at all, in either child.

Pyrimidine 5'-Nucleotidase

Nucleotidases are common enzymes that catalyze the hydrolytic dephosphorylation of nucleoside monophosphates to yield nucleosides and inorganic phosphate. The isoenzyme found in erythrocytes is unique, particularly in regard to specificity, since it is essentially restricted to pyrimidine substrates. During reticulocyte maturation, this permits clearance of pyrimidine components of RNA degradation by diffusion while simultaneously protecting AMP from a similar fate.[147-149] Another normal erythrocyte isoenzyme appears to react principally with deoxyribonucleotides and may serve as a complementary system with pyrimidine nucleotidase to clear erythroid elements of both DNA and RNA degradation products.[150,151] This deoxyribonucleotidase has yet to be found deficient in any form.

By contrast, deficiencies of pyrimidine nucleotidase appear to be almost as common as those of pyruvate kinase, particularly among people of peri-Mediterranean, African, and Jewish heritage. Defects are transmitted as autosomal recessive traits, with heterozygotes hematologically and biochemically normal except for half-normal enzymatic activities. Severe deficiency states usually are associated with residual activities around 5–10% of normal and variably severe hemolytic anemia.

Impairment in hydrolysis of uridine and cytidine monophosphates by the defective enzyme allows accumulation of numerous pyrimidine compounds, most of which are normally undetectable in erythrocytes. This is reflected morphologically by aggregation of undegraded or partially degraded ribosomal nucleoprotein, producing the distinctive basophilic stippling characteristic of this disorder[147,149] (Fig. 45-2). Biochemically, the accumulating pyrimidine compounds often include conjugates, such as cytidine diphosphate-choline, cytidine diphosphate-ethanolamine, and uridine diphosphate-glucose. As much as 80% of the intracellular nucleotides in affected erythrocytes may be pyrimidine compounds. This provides a simple and useful screening test for the deficiency, since acid extracts of the cells exhibit ultraviolet absorption spectra in the region of 265–270 nm that grossly depart from the sharp adenine absorption peak at 258 nm characteristic of normal erythrocytes.[147,149] Several procedures are available to assay the enzyme directly. Recent recommendations for evaluating nucleotidase deficiencies have been formulated by an international panel.[152,153]

Twofold elevations in erythrocyte glutathione concentrations have been consistently observed in severe deficiency states, as has reduction in ribosephosphate pyrophosphokinase activity to about 25% of normal. The mechanisms underlying these changes and their hematologic significances remain speculative. They are currently regarded as epiphenomena with no demonstrable roles in the hemolytic process.

An acquired form of pyrimidine nucleotidase deficiency can

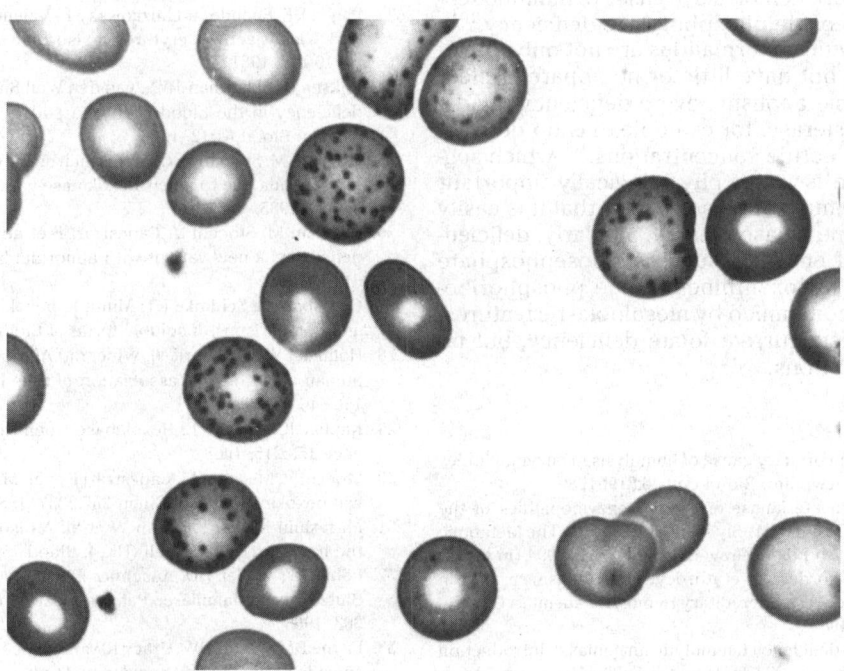

Fig. 45-2. Pronounced basophilic stippling apparent in Wright-stained peripheral erythrocytes with severe deficiency of pyrimidine 5'-nucleotidase.

be induced by lead and possibly by other heavy metals to which the enzyme has extraordinary susceptibility for inactivation.[47] Chronic exposure to low levels of lead reduces pyrimidine nucleotidase activities significantly, with negligible effects on glycolytic and many other erythrocyte enzymes. At lead concentrations in the region of 200 μg/dl packed red cells, nucleotidase activities are decreased to approximate those seen in severe hereditary deficiencies. At that point, pyrimidine compounds begin to accumulate, the absorption spectra shift, and affected erythrocytes may show the characteristic basophilic stippling.[154,155] In some cases, the complete hereditary deficiency syndrome has been reproduced by lead toxicity, including the epiphenomena involving glutathione and ribose-phosphate pyrophosphokinase.[156]

As with several other enzymopathies accompanied by severe anemia, splenectomy has been occasionally but inconsistently beneficial in terms of reducing transfusion dependence and elevating peripheral hemoglobin concentration and red cell counts.

ENZYMOPATHIES DEVOID OF PREMATURE HEMOLYSIS

A number of erythrocyte enzymes have been found sufficiently defective to result in detectable biochemical alterations but not in hemolytic anemia. Severe deficiency of 2,3-diphosphoglyceromutase, for example, was found to result in a virtual absence of intracellular 2,3-DPG. The consequent shift in the oxyhemoglobin dissociation curve induced a compensatory erythrocytosis but no evidence of hemolysis or other clinical problems.[157] Similarly, defects in the H subunit of lactate dehydrogenase resulting in severely deficient activities may alter $NAD^+/NADH$ ratios but are unaccompanied by hemolysis.[158-160]

Markedly reduced activities of 6-phosphogluconate dehydrogenase have been observed without evidence of adverse effects on red cell function or survival.[161-163] Severe deficiency of ADA found in some cases of combined immunodeficiency disease causes pronounced elevations in erythrocyte adenine nucleotide concentrations, particularly the deoxy forms, but no hemolysis. Nor is there premature hemolysis in cases of immunodeficiency disease with nucleoside phosphorylase deficiency.[164]

Other erythrocyte enzyme abnormalities are not only free of hemolytic consequences but have little or no apparent effect on other aspects of cell metabolism Severe deficiency of adenine phosphoribosyltransferase, for example, has no detectable effect on adenine nucleotide concentrations,[165] which suggests either that adenine is not a physiologically important substrate for erythrocyte nucleotide salvage or that it is easily compensated by adenosine kinase activity. Similarly, deficiencies or hyperactivities of enzymes such as ribosephosphate pyrophosphokinase and hypoxanthine-guanine phosphoribosyltransferase may be accompanied by megaloblastic features, perhaps on the basis of concurrent folate deficiency, but no other demonstrable alterations.

REFERENCES

1. Valentine WN, Paglia DE: The primary cause of hemolysis in enzymopathies of anaerobic glycolysis: a viewpoint. Blood Cells 6:819, 1980
2. Tanaka KR, Paglia DE: Pyruvate kinase and other enzymopathies of the erythrocyte. In Scriver CR, Beaudet AL, Sly WS, Valle D (eds): The Metabolic Basis of Inherited Disease. 7th Ed. McGraw-Hill, New York, 1994 (in press)
3. Mentzer WC, Glader BE: Disorders of erythrocyte metabolism. p. 267. In Mentzer WC, Wagner GM (eds): The Hereditary Hemolytic Anemias. Churchill Livingstone, New York, 1989
4. Dacie J: Hereditary enzyme-deficiency haemolytic anaemias. I. Introduction and pyruvate-kinase deficiency. p. 282. In Dacie J (ed): The Haemolytic Anaemias. Churchill Livingstone, London, 1985
5. Dacie J: Hereditary enzyme-deficiency haemolytic anaemias. II. Deficiencies of enzymes of the Embden-Meyerhoff (EM) pathway other than pyruvate

kinase and of enzymes involved in purine and pyrimidine metabolism. p. 321. In Dacie J (ed): The Haemolytic Anaemias. Churchill Livingstone, London, 1985
6. Valentine WN, Tanaka KR, Paglia DE: Hemolytic anemias and erythrocyte enzymopathies. Ann Intern Med 103:249, 1985
7. Miwa S, Fujii H: Molecular aspects of erythroenzymopathies associated with hereditary hemolytic anemia. Am J Hematol 19:293, 1985
8. Beutler E: Hemolytic anemia in disorders of red cell metabolism. p. 199. In Wintrobe MM (ed): Topics in Hematology. Plenum, New York, 1978
9. Sullivan DW, Glader BE: Erythrocyte enzyme disorders in children. Pediatr Clin North Am 27:449, 1980
10. Miwa S: Hereditary disorders of red cell enzymes in the Embden-Meyerhof pathway. Am J Hematol 14:381, 1983
11. Valentine WN, Oski FA, Paglia DE et al: Hereditary hemolytic anemia with hexokinase deficiency. Role of hexokinase in erythrocyte aging. N Engl J Med 276:1, 1967
12. Valentine WN, Oski FA, Paglia DE et al: Erythrocyte hexokinase and hereditary hemolytic anemia. p. 288. In Beutler E (ed): Hereditary Disorders of Erythrocyte Metabolism. Grune & Stratton, Orlando, FL, 1968
13. Keitt AS: Hemolytic anemia with impaired hexokinase activity. J Clin Invest 48:1997, 1969
14. Necheles TF, Rai US, Cameron D: Congenital nonspherocytic hemolytic anemia associated with an unusual erythrocyte hexokinase abnormality. J Lab Clin Med 76:593, 1970
15. Moser K, Ciresa M, Schwarzmeier J: Hexokinasemangel bei hämolytischer Anämie. Med Welt 46:1977, 1970
16. Goebel KM, Gassel WD, Gebel FD, Kafarnik H: Hemolytic anemia and hexokinase deficiency associated with malformations. Klin Wochenschr 50:349, 1972
17. Rijksen G, Staal GEJ: Human erythrocyte hexokinase deficiency: characterization of a mutant enzyme with abnormal regulatory properties. J Clin Invest 62:294, 1978
18. Gilsanz F, Meyer E, Paglia DE, Valentine WN: Congenital hemolytic anemia due to hexokinase deficiency. Am J Dis Child 132:637, 1978
19. Board PG, Trueworthy R, Smith JE, Moore K: Congenital nonspherocytic hemolytic anemia with an unstable hexokinase variant. Blood 51:111, 1978
20. Beutler E, Dyment PG, Matsumoto F: Hereditary nonspherocytic hemolytic anemia and hexokinase deficiency. Blood 51:935, 1978
21. Siimes MA, Rahiala E-L, Leisti J: Hexokinase deficiency in erythrocytes: a new variant in 5 members of a Finnish family. Scand J Haematol 22:214, 1979
22. Newman P, Muir A, Parker AC: Non-spherocytic haemolytic anaemia in mother and son associated with hexokinase deficiency. Br J Haematol 46:537, 1980
23. Paglia DE, Shende A, Lanzkowsky P, Valentine WN: Hexokinase "New Hyde Park": a low activity erythrocyte isozyme in a Chinese kindred. Am J Hematol 10:107, 1981
24. Rijksen G, Akkerman JWN, van den Wall Bake AWL: Generalized hexokinase deficiency in the blood cells of a patient with nonspherocytic hemolytic anemia. Blood 61:12, 1983
25. Magnani M, Stocchi V, Cucchiarini L et al: Hereditary nonspherocytic hemolytic anemia due to a new hexokinase variant with reduced stability. Blood 66:690, 1985
26. Magnani M, Stocchi V, Canestrari F et al: Human erythrocyte hexokinase deficiency: a new variant with abnormal kinetic properties. Br J Haematol 61:41, 1985
27. Grossbard L, Schimke RT: Multiple hexokinases of rat tissues. Purification and comparisons of soluble forms. J Biol Chem 244:3546, 1966
28. Holmes EW Jr, Malorie JI, Winegrad AI, Oski FA: Hexokinase isoenzymes in human erythrocytes: association of type II with fetal hemoglobin. Science 156:646, 1967
29. Kaplan JC, Beutler E: Hexokinase isoenzymes in human erythrocytes. Science 159:215, 1968
30. Stocchi V, Magnani M, Canestrari F et al: Multiple forms of human red blood cell hexokinase. J Biol Chem 257:2357, 1982
31. Murakami K, Blei F, Tilton W et al: An isozyme of hexokinase specific for the human red blood cell (HK_R). Blood 75:770, 1990
32. Löhr GW, Waller HD, Anschütz F, Knopp A: Biochemische Defekte in den Blutzellen bei familiärer Panmyelopathie (Typ Fanconi). Humangenetik 1:383, 1965
33. Payne DM, Porter DW, Gracy RW: Evidence against the occurrence of tissue-specific variants and isoenzymes of phosphoglucose isomerase. Arch Biochem Biophys 151:122, 1972
34. Van Biervliet JPGM: Glucosephosphate isomerase deficiency in a Dutch family. Acta Pediatr Scand 64:868, 1975

35. Zanella A, Izzo C, Rebulla P et al: The first stable variant of erythrocyte glucosephosphate isomerase associated with severe hemolytic anemia. Am J Hematol 9:1, 1980

36. Schröter W, Eber SW, Bardosi A et al: Generalised glucosephosphate isomerase (GPI) deficiency causing haemolytic anaemia, neuromuscular symptoms and impairment of granulocyte function: a new syndrome due to a new stable GPI variant with diminished specific activity (GPI Homberg). Eur J Pediatr 144:301, 1985

37. Welch SG: Qualitative and quantitative variants of human phosphoglucose isomerase. Hum Hered 21:467, 1971

38. Arnold H, Hasslinger K, Witt I: Glucosephosphate-isomerase type Kayserslautern. A new variant causing congenital nonspherocytic hemolytic anemia. Blut 46:271, 1983

39. Baughan MA, Valentine WN, Paglia DE et al: Hereditary hemolytic anemia associated with glucosephosphate isomerase (GPI) deficiency—a new enzyme defect of human erythrocytes. Blood 32:236, 1968

40. Paglia DE, Paredes R, Valentine WN et al: Unique phenotypic expression of glucosephosphate isomerase deficiency. Am J Hum Genet 27:62, 1975

41. Oski F, Fuller E: Glucose-phosphate isomerase (GPI) deficiency associated with abnormal osmotic fragility and spherocytes. Clin Res 19:427, 1971

42. Paglia DE, Holland P, Baughan MA, Valentine WN: Occurrence of defective hexosephosphate isomerization in human erythrocytes and leukocytes. N Engl J Med 280:66, 1969

43. Ravindranath Y, Paglia DE, Warrier I et al: Glucosephosphate isomerase deficiency as a cause of hydrops fetalis. N Engl J Med 316:258, 1987

44. Paglia DE, Valentine WN: Hereditary glucosephosphate isomerase deficiency. A review. Am J Clin Pathol 62:740, 1974

45. Layzer RB, Rowland LP, Bank WJ: Physical and kinetic properties of human phosphofructokinase from skeletal muscle and erythrocytes. J Biol Chem 244:3823, 1969

46. Staal GEJ, Koster JF, Banziger CJM, van Milligen-Boersma L: Human erythrocyte phosphofructokinase: its purification and some properties. Biochim Biophys Acta 276:113, 1972

47. Karadsheh NS, Uyeda K, Oliver RM: Studies on the structure of human erythrocyte phosphofructokinase. J Biol Chem 252:3515, 1977

48. Cottreau D, Levin MJ, Kahn A: Purification and partial characterization of different forms of phosphofructokinase in man. Biochim Biophys Acta 586:183, 1979

49. Kahn A, Meienhofer M-C, Cottreau D et al: Phosphofructokinase (PFK) isozymes in man. 1. Studies of adult human tissue. Hum Genet 48:93, 1979

50. Meienhofer M-C, Lagrange J-L, Cottreau D et al: Phosphofructokinase in human blood cells. Blood 54:389, 1979

51. Vora S, Seaman C, Durham S, Piomelli S: Isozymes of human phosphofructokinase: identification and subunit structural characterization of a new system. Proc Natl Acad Sci USA 77:62, 1980

52. Kahn A, Cottreau D, Meienhofer M-C: Purification of F_4 phosphofructokinase from human platelets and comparison with the other phosphofructokinase forms. Biochim Biophys Acta 611:114, 1980

53. Vora S: Isoenzymes of phosphofructokinase. p. 119. In Rattazzi MC, Scandalios JG, Whitt GS (eds): Isozymes: Current Topics in Biological and Medical Research. Vol. 6. Alan R Liss, New York, 1982

54. Etiemble J, Kahn A, Boivin P et al: Hereditary hemolytic anemia with erythrocyte phosphofructokinase deficiency. Studies of some properties of erythrocyte and muscle enzyme. Hum Genet 31:83, 1976

55. Miwa S, Sato T, Murao H et al: A new type of phosphofructokinase deficiency, hereditary nonspherocytic hemolytic anemia. Acta Haematol Jpn 35:113, 1972

56. Etiemble J, Picat C, Simeon J et al: Inherited erythrocyte phosphofructokinase deficiency: molecular mechanism. Hum Genet 55:383, 1980

57. Waterbury L, Frankel EP: Hereditary nonspherocytic hemolysis with erythrocyte phosphofructokinase deficiency. Blood 39:415, 1972

58. Tarui S, Okuno G, Ikura Y et al: Phosphofructokinase deficiency in skeletal muscle: a new type of glycogenosis. Biochem Biophys Res Commun 19:517, 1965

59. Tarui S, Kono N, Nasu T, Nishikawa M: Enzymatic basis for the coexistence of myopathy and hemolytic disease in inherited muscle phosphofructokinase deficiency. Biochem Biophys Res Commun 34:77, 1969

60. Layzer RB, Rowland LP, Ranney HM: Muscle phosphofructokinase deficiency. Arch Neurol 17:512, 1967

61. Penhoet E, Rajkumar T, Rutter WJ: Multiple forms of fructose diphosphate aldolase in mammalian tissues. Proc Natl Acad Sci USA 56:1275, 1966

62. Lebherz HG, Ruller WJ: Distribution of fructose diphosphate aldolase variants in biological systems. Biochemistry 8:109, 1969

63. Buetler E, Scott S, Bishop A et al: Red cell aldolase deficiency and hemolytic anemia: a new syndrome. Trans Assoc Am Physicians 86:154, 1974

64. Miwa S, Fujii H, Tani K et al: Two cases of red cell aldolase deficiency associated with hereditary hemolytic anemia in a Japanese family. Am J Hematol 11:425, 1981

65. Neel JV, Mohrenweiser HW, Meisler MH: Rate of spontaneous mutation at human loci encoding protein structure. Proc Natl Acad Sci USA 77:6037, 1980

66. Gracy RW: Glucosephosphate and triosephosphate isomerases: significance of isozyme structural differences in evolution, physiology, and aging. p. 183. In Rattazzi MC, Scandalios JG, Whitt GS (eds): Isozymes. Current Topics in Biological and Medical Research. Vol. 6. Alan R Liss, New York, 1982

67. Schneider AS, Valentine WN, Hattori M, Heins HL Jr: Hereditary hemolytic anemia with triosephosphate isomerase deficiency. N Engl J Med 272:229, 1965

68. Valentine WN, Schneider AS, Baughan MA et al: Hereditary hemolytic anemia with triosephosphate isomerase deficiency. Studies in kindreds with coexistent sickle cell trait and erythrocyte glucose-6-phosphate dehydrogenase deficiency. Am J Med 41:27, 1966

69. Schneider AS, Valentine WN, Baughan MA et al: Triosephosphate isomerase deficiency. A. A multi-system inherited enzyme disorder. Clinical and genetic aspects. p. 265. In Beutler E (ed): Hereditary Disorders of Erythrocyte Metabolism. Grune & Stratton, Orlando, FL, 1968

70. Schneider AS, Dunn I, Ibsen KH, Weinstein IM: Triosephosphate isomerase deficiency. B. Inherited triosephosphate isomerase deficiency. Erythrocyte carbohydrate metabolism and preliminary studies of the erythrocyte enzyme. p. 273. In Beutler E (ed): Hereditary Disorders of Erythrocyte Metabolism. Grune & Stratton, Orlando, FL, 1968

71. Kaplan JC, Teeple L, Shore NA, Beutler E: Electrophoretic abnormality in triosephosphate isomerase deficiency. Biochem Biophys Res Commun 31:768, 1968

72. Harris SR, Paglia DE, Jaffé ER et al: Triosephosphate isomerase deficiency in an adult. Clin Res 18:529, 1970

73. Angelman H, Brain MC, MacIver JE: A case of triosephosphate isomerase deficiency with sudden death. p. 122. In Abstracts of the Thirteenth International Congress of Hematology, Munich, 1970

74. Freycon F, Lauras B, Bovier-LaPierre F et al: Anémie hémolytique congénitale par deficit en triosephosphate isomerase. Pediatrie 30:55, 1975

75. Skala H, Dreyfus J-C, Vives-Corrons JL et al: Triosephosphate isomerase deficiency. Biochem Med Metab Biol 18:226, 1977

76. Vives-Corrons J-L, Rubinson-Skala H, Matep M et al: Triosephosphate isomerase deficiency with hemolytic anemia and severe neuromuscular disease: familial and biochemical studies of a case found in Spain. Hum Genet 42:171, 1978

77. Eber SW, Dunnwald M, Belohradsky BH et al: Hereditary deficiency of triosephosphate isomerase in four unrelated families. Eur J Clin Invest 9:195, 1979

78. Rosa R, Prehu M-O, Calvin MC et al: Hereditary triosephosphate isomerase deficiency: seven new homozygous cases. Hum Genet 71:235, 1985

79. Daar IO, Artymiuk PJ, Phillips DC, Maquat LE: Human triosephosphate isomerase deficiency: a single amino acid substitution results in a thermolabile enzyme. Proc Natl Acad Sci USA 83:7903, 1986

80. Segel GB, Feig SA, Glader BE et al: Energy metabolism in human erythrocytes: the role of phosphoglycerate kinase in cation transport. Blood 46:271, 1975

81. Yoshida A, Watanabe S, Chen S-H et al: Human phosphoglycerate kinase. II. Structure of a variant enzyme. J Biol Chem 247:446, 1972

82. Fujii H, Yoshida A: Molecular abnormality of phosphoglycerate kinase-Uppsala associated with chronic nonspherocytic hemolytic anemia. Proc Natl Acad Sci 77:5461, 1980

83. Fujii H, Krietsch WKG, Yoshida A: A single amino acid substitution (Asp → Asn) in a phosphoglycerate kinase variant (PGK München) associated with enzyme deficiency. J Biol Chem 255:6421, 1980

84. Fujii H, Chen S-H, Akatsuka J et al: Use of cultured lymphoblastoid cells for the study of abnormal enzymes: molecular abnormality of a phosphoglycerate kinase variant associated with hemolytic anemia. Proc Natl Acad Sci USA 78:2587, 1981

85. Valentine WN, Hsieh H-S, Paglia DE et al: Hereditary hemolytic anemia: association with phosphoglycerate kinase deficiency in erythrocytes and leukocytes. Trans Assoc Am Physicians 81:49, 1968

86. Valentine WN, Hsieh H-S, Paglia DE et al: Hereditary hemolytic anemia associated with phosphoglycerate kinase deficiency in erthrocytes and leukocytes. A probable X-chromosome-linked syndrome. N Engl J Med 280:528, 1969

87. Cartier P, Habibi B, Leroux J-P, Marchand J-C: Anémie hémolytique congénitale associée à un déficit en phosphoglycérate kinase dans les globules rouges, les polynucléaires et les lymphocytes. Nouv Rev Fr Hematol 11:565, 1971

88. Konrad PN, McCarthy DJ, Mauer AM et al: Erythrocyte and leukocyte phos-

phoglycerate kinase deficiency with neurologic disease. J Pediatr 82:456, 1973

89. Boivin P, Hakim J, Mandereau J et al: Deficit en 3-phosphoglycerate kinase érythrocytaire et leucocytaire. Étude des propriétés de l'enzyme, de la fonction phagocytaire des polynucléaires et revue de la littérature. Nouv Rev Fr Hematol 14:495, 1974

90. Yoshida A, Miwa S: Characterization of a phosphoglycerate kinase variant associated with hemolytic anemia. Am J Hum Genet 26:378, 1974

91. Dodgson SJ, Lee CS, Holland RAB et al: Erythrocyte phosphoglycerate kinase deficiency: enzymatic and oxygen binding studies. Aust NZ J Med 10:614, 1980

92. Rosa R, George C, Fardeau M et al: A new case of phosphoglycerate kinase deficiency: PGK Creteil associated with rhabdomyolysis and lacking hemolytic anemia. Blood 60:84, 1982

93. Dimauro S, Dalakas M, Miranda AF: Phosphoglycerate kinase deficiency: another cause of recurrent myoglobinuria. Ann Neurol 13:11, 1983

94. Guis MS, Karadsheh N, Mentzer WC: Phosphoglycerate kinase San Francisco, a new variant associated with hemolytic anemia but not with neuromuscular manifestations. Am J Hematol 25:175, 1987

95. Svirklys LG, O'Sullivan WJ: Tissue levels of glycolytic enzymes in phosphoglycerate kinase deficiency. Clin Chim Acta 108:309, 1980

96. Baehner RL, Feig SA, Segel GB et al: Metabolic, phagocytic, and bactericidal properties of phosphoglycerate kinase deficient (PGK) polymorphonuclear leukocytes (PMN). Blood 38:833, 1971

97. Etiemble J, Picat C, Boivin P: A red cell pyruvate kinase mutant with normal L-type PK in the liver. Hum Genet 61:256, 1982

98. Noguchi T, Inque H, Tanaka T: The M_1 and M_2-type isozymes of rat pyruvate kinase are produced from the same gene by alternative RNA splicing. J Biol Chem 261:13807, 1986

99. Marie J, Simon M-P, Dreyfus J-C, Kahn A: One gene, but two messenger RNAs encode liver L and red cell L' pyruvate kinase subunits. Nature 292:70, 1981

100. Noguchi T, Tanaka T: The M_1 and M_2 subunits of rat pyruvate kinase are encoded by different messenger RNAs. J Biol Chem 257:1110, 1982

101. Marie J, Garreau H, Kahn A: Evidence for a postsynthetic proteolytic transformation of human erythrocyte pyruvate kinase into L-type enzyme. FEBS Lett 78:91, 1977

102. Kahn A, Marie J, Garreau H, Sprengers ED: The genetic system of the L-type pyruvate kinase forms in man. Subunit structure, interrelation and kinetic characteristics of the pyruvate kinase enzymes from erythrocytes and liver. Biochim Biophys Acta 523:59, 1978

103. Marie J, Kahn A: Proteolytic processing of human erythrocyte pyruvate kinase: study of normal and deficient enzyme. Biochem Biophys Res Commun 91:123, 1979

104. Miwa S, Nakashima K, Ariyoshi K et al: Four new pyruvate kinase (PK) variants and a classical type PK deficiency. Br J Haematol 29:135, 1975

105. Takegawa S, Miwa S: Change of pyruvate kinase (PK) isozymes in classical type PK deficiency and other PK deficiency cases during red cell maturation. Am J Hematol 16:53, 1984

106. Black JA, Rittenberg MB, Standerfer RJ, Peterson JS: Hereditary persistence of fetal erythrocyte pyruvate kinase in the Basenji dog. Prog Clin Biol Res 21:275, 1978

107. Valentine WN, Tanaka KR, Miwa S: A specific erythrocyte glycolytic enzyme defect (pyruvate kinase) in three subjects with congenital non-spherocytic hemolytic anemia. Trans Assoc Am Physicians 74:100, 1961

108. Tanaka KR, Valentine WN, Miwa S: Pyruvate kinase (PK) deficiency hereditary non-spherocytic hemolytic anemia. Blood 19:267, 1962

109. Tanaka KR, Paglia DE: Pyruvate kinase deficiency. Semin Hematol 8:367, 1971

110. Miwa S, Boivin P, Blume KG et al: Recommended methods for the characterization of red cell pyruvate kinase variants. International Committee for Standardization in Haematology. Br J Haematol 43:275, 1979

111. Valentine WN, Herring WB, Paglia DE et al: Pyruvate kinase Greensboro. A four-generation study of a high $K_{0.5s}$ (phosphoenolpyruvate) variant. Blood 72:1054, 1988

112. Valentine WN, Paglia DE: Erythroenzymopathies and hemolytic anemia. The many faces of inherited variant enzymes. J Lab Clin Med 115:12, 1990

113. World Health Organization Scientific Group: Standardization of Procedures for the Study of Glucose-6-Phosphate Dehydrogenase. WHO Tech Rep Ser: 366, 1967

114. Beutler E: The molecular biology of enzymes of erythrocyte metabolism. In Stamatoyannopoulos G, Nienhus AW, Majerus PW, Varmus H (eds): The Molecular Basis of Blood Disease. WB Saunders, Philadelphia, 1993

115. Gartier SM, Riggs AD: Mammalian x-chromosome inactivation. Annu Rev Genet 17:155, 1983

116. Woodruff MFA: Tumor clonality and its biologic significance. Adv Cancer Res 50:197, 1988

117. Boivin P, Galand C, Hakim J et al: Anémie hémolytique avec déficit en glutathion-peroxidase chez un adulte. Enzyme 10:6B, 1969

118. Necheles TF, Maldonado N, Barquet-Chediale A, Allen DM: Homozygous erythrocyte glutathione-peroxidase deficiency. Clinical and biochemical studies. Blood 33:164, 1969

119. Necheles TF, Steinberg MH, Cameron D: Erythrocyte glutathione-peroxidase deficiency. Br J Haematol 19:605, 1970

120. Steinberg M, Brauer MJ, Necheles TF: Acute hemolytic anemia associated with erythrocyte glutathione-peroxidase deficiency. Arch Intern Med 125: 302, 1970

121. Steinberg M, Necheles TF: Erythrocyte glutathione peroxidase deficiency. Am J Med 50:542, 1971

122. Hopkins J, Tudhope GR: Glutathione peroxidase in human red cells in health and disease. Br J Haematol 25:563, 1973

123. Blume KG, Gottwik M, Löhr GW, Rudiger HW: Familienintersuchungen zum Glutathionreducktase-Mangel menschlicher Erythrocyten. Hum Genet 6: 163, 1968

124. Beutler E: Drug induced hemolytic anemia. Pharmacol Rev 21:73, 1969

125. Frischer H, Ahmad T: Consequences of erythrocyte glutathione reductase deficiency. J Lab Clin Med 109:583, 1987

126. Beutler E: Effect of flavin compounds on glutathione reductase activity: in vivo and in vitro studies. J Clin Invest 48:1957, 1969

127. Beutler E: Glutathione reductase: stimulation in normal subjects by riboflavin supplementation. Science 165:613, 1969

128. Loos H, Roos D, Weening R, Houwerzijl J: Familial deficiency of glutathione reductase in human blood cells. Blood 48:53, 1976

129. Konrad PN, Richards F II, Valentine WN, Paglia DE: γ-Glutamylcysteine synthetase deficiency. A cause of hereditary hemolytic anemia. N Engl J Med 286:557, 1972

130. Beutler E, Moroose R, Kramer L et al: Gamma-glutamylcysteine synthetase deficiency and hemolytic anemia. Blood 75:271, 1990

131. Jellum E, Kluge T, Borrensen HC et al: Pyroglutamic aciduria—a new inborn error of metabolism. Scand J Clin Lab Invest 26:327, 1970

132. Wellner VP, Sekura R, Meister A, Larsson A: Glutathione synthetase deficiency, an inborn error of metabolism involving the τ-glutamyl cycle in patients with 5-oxprolinuria (pyroglutamic aciduria). Proc Natl Acad Sci USA 71:2505, 1984

133. Spielberg SP, Garrick MD, Corash LM et al: Biochemical heterogeneity in glutathione synthetase deficiency. J Clin Invest 61:1417, 1978

134. Beutler E: Selectivity of proteases as a basis for tissue distribution of enzymes in hereditary deficiencies. Proc Natl Acad Sci USA 80:3767, 1983

135. Valentine WN, Paglia DE, Tartaglia AP, Gilsanz F: Hereditary hemolytic anemia with increased red cell adenosine deaminase (45- to 70-fold) and decreased adenosine triphosphate. Science 195:783, 1977

136. Paglia DE, Valentine WN, Tartaglia AP et al: Control of red blood cell adenine nucleotide metabolism. Studies of adenosine deaminase. Prog Clin Biol Res 21:319, 1978

137. Miwa S, Fujii H, Matsumoto N et al: A case of red-cell adenosine deaminase overproduction associated with hereditary hemolytic anemia found in Japan. Am J Hematol 5:107, 1978

138. Perignon JL, Hamet M, Buc HA et al: Biochemical study of a case of hemolytic anemia with increased (85-fold) red cell adenosine deaminase. Clin Chim Acta 124:205, 1982

139. Chottiner EG, Cloft HJ, Tartaglia AP, Mitchell BS: Elevated adenosine deaminase activity and hereditary hemolytic anemia. Evidence for abnormal translational control of protein synthesis. J Clin Invest 79:1001, 1987

140. Chottiner EG, Ginsburg D, Tartaglia AP, Mitchell BS: Erythrocyte adenosine deaminase overproduction in hereditary hemolytic anemia. Blood 74:448, 1989

141. Paglia DE, Valentine WN: Haemolytic anaemia associated with disorders of the purine and pyrimidine salvage pathways. Baillieres Clin Haematol 10: 81, 1981

142. Szeinberg A, Gavendo S, Cahane D: Erythrocyte adenylate-kinase deficiency. Lancet 1:315, 1969

143. Szeinberg A, Kahana D, Gavendo S et al: Hereditary deficiency of adenylate kinase in red blood cells. Acta Haematol 42:111, 1969

144. Boivin P, Galand C, Hakim J et al: Une nouvelle érythroenzymopathie. Anémie hémolytique congénitale non spherocytaire et déficit héréditaire en adenylate-kinase érythrocytaire. Presse Med 79:215, 1971

145. Miwa S, Fujii H, Tani K et al: Red cell adenylate kinase deficiency associated with hereditary nonspherocytic hemolytic anemia: clinical and biochemical studies. Am J Hematol 14:325, 1983

146. Beutler E, Carson D, Dannawi H et al: Metabolic compensation for profound erythrocyte adenylate kinase deficiency. A hereditary defect without hemolytic anemia. J Clin Invest 72:648, 1983

147. Valentine WN, Fink K, Paglia DE et al: Hereditary hemolytic anemia with

human erythrocyte pyrimidine 5'-nucleotidase deficiency. J Clin Invest 54: 866, 1974

148. Paglia DE, Valentine WN: Characteristics of a pyrimidine-specific 5'-nucleotidase in human erythrocytes. J Biol Chem 250:7973, 1975

149. Paglia DE, Valentine WM: Hereditary and acquired defects in the pyrimidine nucleotidase of human erythrocytes. Curr Top Hematol 3:75, 1980

150. Paglia DE, Valentine WN, Brockway RA: Identification of thymidine nucleotidase and deoxyribonucleotidase activities among normal isozymes of 5'-nucleotidase in human erythrocytes. Proc Natl Acad Sci USA 81:588, 1984

151. Paglia DE, Valentine WN, Brockway RA, Nakatani M: Substrate specificity and pH sensitivity of deoxyribonucleotidase and pyrimidine nucleotidase activities in human hemolysates. Exp Hematol 15:1041, 1987

152. Miwa S, Luzzatto L, Rosa R et al: Recommended screening test for pyrimidine 5'-nucleotidase deficiency. Clin Lab Haematol 11:55, 1989

153. Miwa S, Luzzatto L, Rosa R et al: Recommended methods for an additional red cell enzyme (pyrimidine 5'-nucleotidase) assay and the determination of red cell adenosine-5'-triphosphate, 2,3-diphosphoglycerate and reduced glutathione. Clin Lab Haematol 11:131, 1989

154. Paglia DE, Valentine WN, Dahlgren JG: Effects of low-level lead exposure on pyrimidine 5'-nucleotidase and other erythrocyte enzymes. Possible role of pyrimidine 5'-nucleotidase in the pathogenesis of lead-induced anemia. J Clin Invest 56:1164, 1975

155. Paglia DE, Valentine WN, Fink K: Lead poisoning. Further observations on erythrocyte pyrimidine-nucleotidase deficiency and intracellular accumulation of pyrimidine nucleotides. J Clin Invest 60:1362, 1977

156. Valentine WN, Paglia DE, Fink K, Madokoro G: Lead poisoning. Association with hemolytic anemia, basophilic stippling, erythrocyte pyrimidine 5'-nucleotidase deficiency, and intraerythrocytic accumulation of pyrimidines. J Clin Invest 58:926, 1976

157. Rosa R, Prehic M-P, Beuzaid Y, Rosa J: The first case of a complete deficiency of diphosphoglycerate mutase in human erythrocytes. J Clin Invest 62:907, 1978

158. Miwa S, Nishina T, Kakehashi Y et al: Studies on erythrocyte metabolism in a case with hereditary deficiency of H-subunit of lactate dehydrogenase. Acta Haematol Jpn 34:228, 1971

159. Kitamura M, Iijima N, Hashimoto F, Hiratsuka A: Hereditary deficiency of subunit H of lactate dehydrogenase. Clin Chim Acta 34:419, 1971

160. Kanno T, Sudo K, Takeuchi I et al: Hereditary deficiency of lactate dehydrogenase M-subunit. Clin Chim Acta 108:267, 1980

161. Brewer GJ, Dern RJ: A new inherited enzymatic deficiency of human erythrocytes: 6-phosphogluconate dehydrogenase deficiency. Am J Hum Genet 16: 472, 1964

162. Dern RJ, Brewer GJ, Tashian RE, Shows TB: Hereditary variation of erythrocytic 6-phosphogluconate dehydrogenase. J Lab Clin Med 67:255, 1966

163. Parr CW, Fitch LJ: Inherited quantitative variations of human phosphogluconate dehydrogenase. Ann Hum Genet 30:339, 1967

164. Giblett ER, Ammann AJ, Sandman R et al: Nucleoside-phosphorylase deficiency in a child with severely defective T-cell immunity and normal B-cell immunity. Lancet I:1010, 1975

165. Van Acker KJ, Simmonds HA, Potter C, Cameron JS: Complete deficiency of adenine phosphoribosyltransferase. Report of a family. N Engl J Med 297: 127, 1977

Red Cell Membrane Disorders

46

Jiri Palek and Petr Jarolim

INTRODUCTION

Recent progress in the characterization of the structure, function, and assembly of the red cell membrane proteins and their genes (Table 46-1) has improved our understanding of the molecular pathology of red cell membrane disorders considerably, enabling us to define mutations of many membrane proteins as a cause of hereditary hemolytic disease. Likewise, our knowledge of the molecular mechanisms underlying changes in red cell deformability, structural integrity, and shape has advanced. Importantly, red cell shape abnormalities often provide a clue to the pathobiology and diagnosis of the underlying disorder. Consequently, this chapter categorizes red cell membrane disorders according to the following morphologic and clinical phenotypes: (1) dominantly or recessively inherited spherocytosis (HS); (2) hereditary elliptocytosis and a related disorder, pyropoikilocytosis (HE and HPP), (3) Southeast Asian ovalocytosis (SAO); (4) hereditary and acquired acanthocytosis; and (5) hereditary and acquired stomatocytosis. Below, we outline some hypothesis attempting to explain the molecular basis of these shape abnormalities.

Vertical and Horizontal Interactions of Membrane Proteins, Spherocytosis, and Elliptopoikilocytosis

This hypothesis[45,46] divides membrane protein-protein and protein-lipid interactions into two categories (Fig. 46-1): (1) vertical interactions, which are perpendicular to the plane of the membrane and which stabilize the lipid bilayer membrane, involve the spectrin-ankyrin-band 3 interaction, the protein 4.1-glycophorin C linkage and the weak interactions between the skeletal proteins and the negatively charged lipids of the inner half of the membrane lipid bilayer; and (2) horizontal interactions, which are parallel to the plane of the membrane and which support the structural integrity of the cells after their exposure to shear stress. These involve the spectrin heterodimer contact, whereby spectrin heterodimers assemble to tetramers, the principal building blocks of the skeleton, and the contacts of the distal ends of spectrin heterodimers with actin and protein 4.1 within the junctional complex (Fig. 46-1).

According to this hypothesis, we consider HS a disorder of vertical interactions. Although the primary molecular defects in HS are heterogeneous (including deficiencies or dysfunc-

Table 46-1. Major Red Cell Membrane Proteins and Their Involvement in Hereditary Hemolytic Anemias

Band	Protein	MW (gel) (kd)	MW (calc) (kd)	Copies per Cell (10^{-3})	Total[a] (%)	Gene Symbol	Chromosomal Localization	Amino Acids	Gene Size (kb)	No. of Exons	Involvement in Hemolytic Anemias	References
1	α-Spectrin	240	280	240	16	SPTA1	1	q22–q23	2,429	80	52	HE, HS	1,2
2	β-Spectrin	220	246	240	14	SPTB	14	q23–q24.2	2,137	>100	~32	HE, HS	3,4
2.1	Ankyrin, 2.1 isoform[b]	210	206	120	4.5	ANK1	8	p11.2	1,881	>100	40	HS	5,6
	α-Adducin[c]	103	81	30	2		4					N	7
	β-Adducin[c]	97	80	30	2							N	7
3	Anion exchanger 1	90–100	102	1,200	27	EPB3	17	q21–qter	911	17	20	HS, SAO, HAc	8,9
4.1	Protein 4.1	80	66[d]	200	5	EL1 1	1	p33–p34.2	588[d]	>100		HE	10,11
4.2	Pallidin	72	77	200	5	EB42	15	q15–q21	691	20	13	HS[e]	12–15
4.9[f]	Dematin	48 + 52	43[k]	40[i]	1				383[k]			N	16–19
4.9[f]	p55	55	53	80		MPP1	X	q28	466			N	20
5	β-Actin	43		400–500	5.5	ACTB	7	pter–q22				N	21–23
	Tropomodulin	43	41	30		TMOD	9	q22	359			N	24,25
6	G3PD	35	37		3.5[g]	GAPD	12	p13.31–p13.1				N	26
7	Stomatin	31	32		2.5					12	6	HSt	27
	Tropomyosin	27 + 29		80	1	TPM3	1	q31				N	28–30
PAS-1	Glycophorin A[j]	36		500–1,000	85	GYPA	4	q28–q31	131	>40	7	N	31–35
PAS-2	Glycophorin C[j]	32	14	50–100	4	GYPC[h]	2	q14–q21	128	14	4	HE	36–38
PAS-3	Glycophorin B[j]	20		100–300	10	GYPB	4	q28–q31	72	>30	5	N	31,39
	Glycophorin D[j]	23		20	1	GYPC[h]	2	q14–q21	107			N	36,40
	Glycophorin E[j]	—		—	—	GYPE	4	q28–q31	59	>30	4	N	31,41

Abbreviations: HS, hereditary spherocytosis; HE, hereditary elliptocytosis; HPP, hereditary pyropoikilotcytosis; SAO, Southeast Asian ovalocytosis; HAc hereditary acanthocytosis; HSt, hereditary stomatocytosis; G3PD, glyceraldehyde-3-phosphate dehydrogenase; N, no hematologic abnormalities reported; SDS-PAGE, sodium dodecyl sulfate-polyacrylamide gel electrophoresis.

[a] Quantitation based on scanning of SDS-PAGE gels of red cell membranes prepared from healthy blood donors (this laboratory).

[b] Bands 2.1, 2.2, 2.3, and 2.6 are protein isoforms of erythroid ankyrin, at least some of which are produced by alternative splicing of ankyrin mRNA.

[c] Since adducin comigrates with band 3, no numerical band designation is available.

[d] Numerous erythroid and nonerythroid isoforms of protein 4.1 produced by alternative splicing have been described.[42,43] The values correspond to the major erythroid protein 4.1 isoform.

[e] Recent study demonstrated association of the pallidin gene with murine platelet storage pool disorder.[44]

[f] Both dematin and p55 migrate within the 4.9 band.

[g] Variable amounts of band 6 are detected in red cell membranes.

[h] Glycophorins C and D are likely synthesized from the same mRNA.[36]

[i] 40,000 of dematin trimers are present in one red cell.

[j] Detectable on PAS-stained gels only.

[k] Encodes the 48-kd subunit of dematin.

(From Palek and Jarolim,[45] with permission.)

tions of spectrin, ankyrin, band 3, and 4.2 proteins; see below), the common feature of HS red cells is a weakening of the vertical contacts between the skeleton and the overlying lipid bilayer membrane together with its integral proteins. Consequently, the lipid bilayer membrane is destabilized, leading to release of bilayer lipids from the cells in the form of skeleton-free lipid vesicles.[47,48] This lipid loss, in turn, results in membrane surface area deficiency and spherocytosis.[49]

In most patients with HE, and in a closely related disorder, HPP, characterized by a severe hemolytic anemia with marked microspherocytosis, poikilocytosis, and fragmentation, the principal lesion involves horizontal membrane protein associations, namely, the spectrin dimer-dimer contact. In a smaller subset of HE patients with a deficiency or a dysfunction of the 4.1 protein this horizontal defect resides in the junctional complex, where the distal ends of spectrin tetramers connect to actin, with the aid of the 4.1 protein.[50,51] In patients carrying severely dysfunctional spectrin mutations, the weakened spectrin dimer-dimer self-association disrupts the skeletal lattice, leading to a marked skeletal instability and cell fragmenta-tion.[48] In patients carrying mildly dysfunctional spectrins, red cell shape is that of biconcave elliptocytes. We speculate that elliptocytes are permanently deformed cells because the weakened horizontal interactions facilitate a shear stress-induced rearrangement of skeletal proteins, precluding recovery of the normal biconcave shape (for details, see the section Hereditary Elliptocytosis). This hypothesis is not applicable to all forms of elliptocytosis, for example, in SAO, the ovalocytic cells containing mutant band 3 protein are rigid and "hyperstable" rather than unstable.[52–55] Further details are discussed below.

Acanthocytosis, Stomatocytosis, and the Bilayer Couple Hypothesis

The mechanism of acanthocytosis and stomatocytosis associated with defects of membrane proteins is considerably less clear. Most forms of acanthocytosis are associated with either acquired or inherited abnormalities of membrane lipids (e.g., acanthocytosis in end-stage liver disease and abetalipopro-

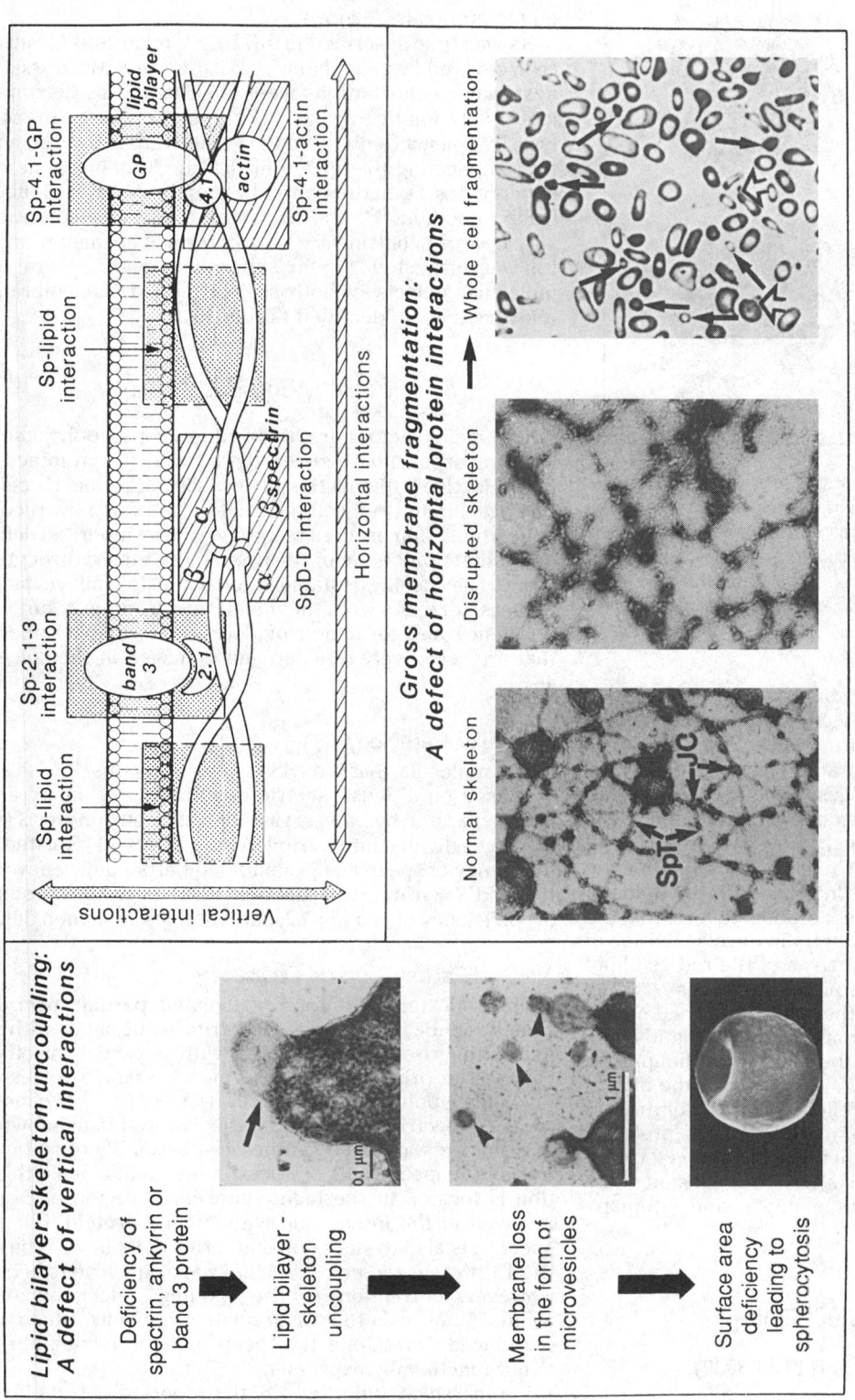

Fig. 46-1. (Upper right panel) Vertical and horizontal interactions of membrane proteins and the pathobiology of the red cell lesion in hereditary spherocytosis and ellipto-poikilocytosis. **(Left panel)** A defect of vertical interactions as exemplified by the red cell membrane lesion in hereditary spherocytosis. Partial deficiencies of spectrin, ankyrin, or band 3 protein lead to uncoupling of the membrane lipid bilayer from the underlying skeleton (arrow) followed by a formation of spectrin-free microvesicles of about 0.2–0.5 μm in diameter (arrowheads). These vesicles can be visualized by transmission electron microscopy but they are not seen during examination of a peripheral blood film. The subsequent loss of cell surface area and a decrease in the surface/volume ratio leads to spherocytosis. For further details, see Figs. 46-3, and 46 4. **(Bottom right panel)** Defect of horizontal interactions of skeletal proteins as exemplified by the membrane lesion in hemolytic forms of hereditary elliptocytosis associated with a defect of spectrin heterodimer self-association. The molecular lesion involving a weakened self-association of spectrin heterodimers to tetramers represents a horizontal defect of the shear stress-resisting protein interactions. It leads to a disruption of the membrane skeletal lattice and, consequently, to destabilization of the whole cell followed by cell fragmentation as seen on peripheral blood films. [Modified from Palek and Jarolim,[45] with permission.]

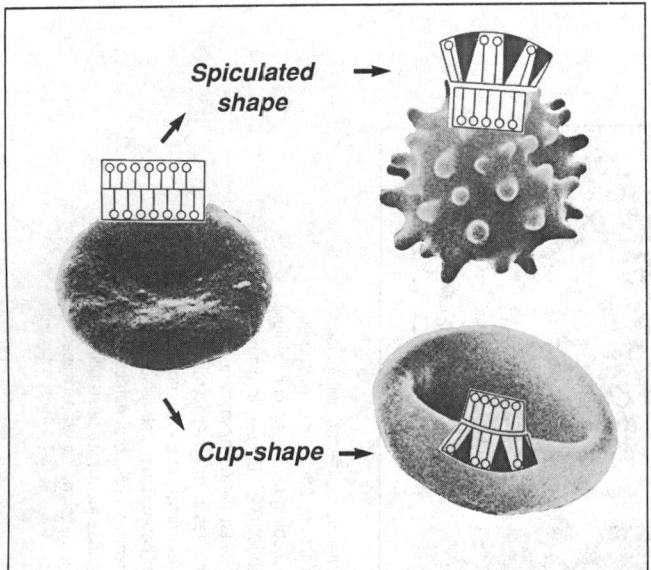

Fig. 46-2. Bilayer couple hypothesis and the discocyte/echinocyte/stomatocyte transformation. Red cell shape is determined by the ratio of the surface areas of the two hemileaflets of the lipid bilayer. Compounds (black triangles) that preferentially accumulate in the outer hemileaflet produce its expansion followed by red cell crenation (echinocytosis or acanthocytosis). By contrast, expansion of the inner lipid bilayer leaflet leads to cup shape (stomatocytosis) and surface invaginations.

teinemia).[56] In rare subjects with acanthocytosis, membrane protein abnormalities have been detected, but the mechanism whereby they lead to acanthocyte formation is unknown. These include the McLeod phenotype characterized by a deficiency of the Kx and, consequently, K antigen,[57] the chorea-acanthocytosis syndrome,[56] and the rare example of acanthocytosis associated with abnormalities of the band 3 protein.[58,59] In all forms of acanthocytosis studied to date, the acanthocytic shape is normalized by agents that interact with the lipids of the inner lipid bilayer leaflet.[57,60] These studies suggest that the shape abnormalities reflect an asymmetry in the distribution of membrane lipids between the two halves of the red cell lipid bilayer as predicted by the bilayer couple hypothesis[61–64] (Fig. 46-2). This hypothesis is based on the well-established notion that the lipid bilayer is highly asymmetric: phosphatidylcholine and sphingomyelin constitute the main phospholipids of the outer face of the bilayer leaflet.[65] According to the bilayer couple hypothesis, red cell shape reflects the ratio of the surface areas of the two hemileaflets of the bilayer. The preferential expansion of the outer hemileaflet leads to red cell crenation (echinocytosis or acanthocytosis), while expansion of the inner lipid bilayer leaflet produces a cup shape (stomatocytosis) and surface invaginations.

HEREDITARY SPHEROCYTOSIS

Definition, Prevalence, and History

The typical diagnostic features of HS include a dominantly inherited hemolytic anemia of mild to moderate severity, spherocytosis on the peripheral blood film, and a favorable response to splenectomy. However, the clinical spectrum of HS is variable,[66–69] including both mild and asymptomatic forms that may be first diagnosed late in life,[70] as well as severe forms that are often inherited as an autosomal recessive disorder.[71–75] The previously reported HS prevalence in the Western

population, 1 per 5,000,[76] may be an underestimation, since mild forms of HS may be asymptomatic, detected only by osmotic fragility testing.[77,78] HS has also been reported in Japanese and African populations,[79–82] but its prevalence in these ethnic groups is unknown.

HS was first described in 1871 by Vanlair and Masius[83] and rediscovered 20 years later by Wilson[84] and Minkowski.[85] The next major contributions were (1) Chauffard's description of increased osmotic fragility,[86] (2) reports of correction of hemolysis by splenectomy,[87,88] and (3) the studies by Ham and Castle[89] implicating the spleen in the conditioning of hereditary spherocytes. Soon thereafter, HS membranes were found to be leaky to sodium[90,91] and to exhibit a loss of lipids leading to surface area deficiency.[92,93] An abnormality of membrane skeleton was suspected[94]; in the subsequent years, several distinct molecular defects of both skeletal and transmembrane proteins have been identified (Table 46-2).

Etiology and Pathobiology

Two major factors are involved in HS pathophysiology: (1) an intracorpuscular red cell defect, and (2) an intact spleen that selectively retains the intrinsically abnormal HS cells.[95–97] The accelerated red cell destruction in HS is now recognized to be a multistep process resulting from an inherited deficiency or dysfunction of one of the proteins of the erythrocyte membrane. The ensuing destabilization of the lipid bilayer facilitates a release of lipids from the membrane, leading to surface area deficiency and formation of poorly deformable spherocytes that are selectively retained and damaged in the spleen (Fig. 46-3).

Molecular Pathology

The molecular basis of HS is heterogeneous[98–101] (Table 46-1). Based on a densitometric quantitation of membrane proteins separated by polyacrylamide gel electrophoresis (PAGE), HS can be divided into the following subsets: (1) isolated partial deficiency of spectrin, (2) combined partial deficiency of spectrin and ankyrin, (3) partial deficiency of band 3 protein and, (4) deficiency of protein 4.2, and other less common defects.[102]

Isolated Partial Spectrin Deficiency

The reported mutations of isolated partial spectrin deficiency include both α- and β-spectrin. In one family with a dominantly inherited HS associated with a partial spectrin deficiency, the primary defect has been assigned to β-spectrin, involving a point mutation of 202 Trp → Arg.[103] The molecular basis of spectrin deficiency in this kindred is unknown and it may involve a reduced synthesis or assembly of mutant spectrin on the membrane, or spectrin instability. Since this mutation is located in the highly conserved region of β-spectrin involved in the interaction with the 4.1 protein, this mutant spectrin is also dysfunctional in terms of its in vitro binding to the 4.1 protein and hence, the linkage of spectrin to actin.[104,105] However, correction of the binding defect by reducing agents[106] suggests that in circulating red cells, which are rich in reduced glutathione, the spectrin/4.1 protein-binding defect is not functionally expressed.

In recessively inherited HS, the reported defects involve α-spectrin. A point mutation 969 Ala → Asp in repetitive segment α9 was detected in one kindred[107]; however, it is not clear whether this point mutation reflects the primary lesion or merely a linked polymorphism. In a report of a lethal HS associated with a dramatic (26% of normal) spectrin deficiency, the pulse label studies of burst-forming unit-erythroid-derived erythroblasts revealed a marked decrease in α-spectrin synthesis.[108] Although the underlying molecular basis of this defect

Table 46-2. Molecular Defects of Red Cell Membrane Proteins Associated with Hereditary Spherocytosis

Protein	Biochemical phenotype[a]	Defect of structure/function	Molecular defect	Inheritance	References
α-Spectrin					
	Severe spectrin deficiency	Abnormal tryptic digest of the αII domain	Linked to an α-spectrin polymorphism 969Ala → Asp (GCT → GAT)	Recessive	107
β-Spectrin					
Kissimmee	Partial spectrin deficiency	Weak interaction of spectrin with protein 4.1	202Trp → Arg (TGG → CGG)	Dominant	103
	Normal SDS-PAGE	Unstable β-spectrin		Recessive	116
Ankyrin					
	Partial deficiency of spectrin and ankyrin		Approximate 50% reduction in ankyrin mRNA		74,113
	Partial deficiency of spectrin and ankyrin		Deletion of one copy of ankyrin gene due to deletion of 8p11–p21.1		112
Prague	Partial deficiency of spectrin and ankyrin	Deficiency of ankyrin 2.1; additional ankyrin band of 174 kd (2.2')	Insertion of 201 nucleotides into 2.1 and 2.2 mRNA between exons 36 and 37	Dominant	115,117
Rakovnik	Partial deficiency of spectrin and ankyrin 2.1	55% of ankyrin 2.1 105% of ankyrin 2.2 58% of spectrin	Decreased stability of 2.1 mRNA due to 669 Glu → Ter (GAA → TAA) mutation	Dominant	115
Unnamed 1			2-nt deletion (GGTGAG → GGAG) in exon 1—72/73 nt from the translation start site	Recessive[b]	118
Unnamed 2			T → C in the potential promoter (CCTGG → CCCGG)—108 nt from the translation start site	Recessive[b]	118
Stuttgart	Partial deficiency of spectrin and ankyrin		2-nt deletion (GCA → A) in codon 329	Dominant	118
Walsrode			463 Val → Ile (GTC → ATC)		118
Einbeck	Partial ankyrin deficiency	97% of spectrin, 86% of ankyrin	1-nt insertion (CCC → CCCC) in codon 572	Dominant	118,614
Marburg	Partial spectrin and ankyrin deficiency	64% of spectrin, 71% of ankyrin	4-nt deletion (TTAGTC → TC) from codons 797–798	Dominant	118,614
Bovenden	Partial spectrin and ankyrin deficiency		1436Arg → Ter (CGA → TGA)	Dominant	118
Düsseldorf	Partial spectrin and ankyrin deficiency		1592Asp → Asn (GAC → AAC)	Recessive	118
Band 3					
Montefiore	Severe protein 4.2 deficiency (88%)	30% decrease in binding of protein 4.2 to inside-out vesicles	40Glu → Lys (GAG → AAG)	Recessive	119
Tuscaloosa	Partial protein 4.2 deficiency (30%)	30% decrease in binding of protein 4.2 to inside-out vesicles	327Pro → Arg (CCC → CGC) and a linked polymorphism 56Lys → Glu (AAG → GAG) (Band 3 Memphis)	Dominant	120
Coimbra	Partial band 3 deficiency (18–24%)		488Val → Met(GTG → ATG)	Dominant	121
Hradec Kralove	Partial band 3 deficiency (30–40%)		760Arg → Trp (CGG → TGG)	Dominant	122
Prague II	Partial band 3 deficiency (30–40%)		760Arg → Gln (CGG → CAG)	Dominant	122
Jablonec	Partial band 3 deficiency (30–40%)		808Arg → Cys (CGC → TGC)	Dominant	122
Prague I	Partial band 3 deficiency (30–40%)	Decreased density of intramembrane particles, decreased lateral and rotational mobility of band 3	Duplication of 10 bases (CACCCAGATG) following codon 818	Dominant	123
Prague III	Partial band 3 deficiency (30–40%)		870Arg → Trp (CGG → TGG)	Dominant	122
Protein 4.2					
Lisboa			1-nt deletion in exon 2		(J. Delaunay, personal communication)
Nippon	Doublet of 72 and 74 kd detected by immunoblotting, complete absence by Coomassie blue staining		142Ala → Thr (GCT → ACT)		124
Tozeur			310 Arg → Gln (CGA → CAA)		(J. Delaunay, personal communication)

[a] SDS-PAGE or a quantitation by radioimmunoassay.[75]
[b] With the exception of compound heterozygosity for the ankyrin Walsrode and the ankyrin unnamed 2, the nature of the second defect is unknown.

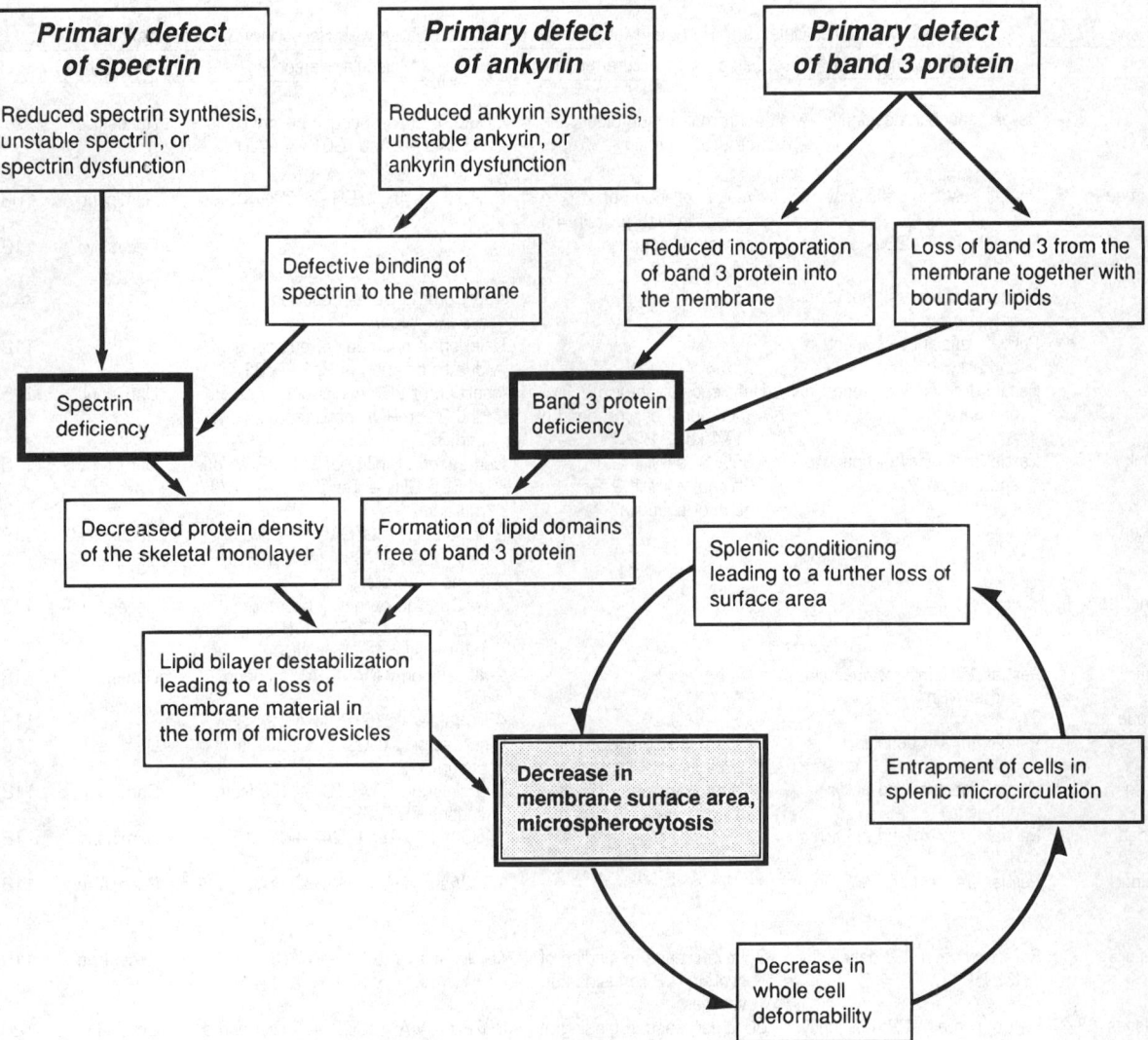

Fig. 46-3. Pathobiology of red cell lesion in hereditary spherocytosis. The principal abnormality of hereditary spherocytes is the deficiency of membrane surface area leading to microspherocytosis. Three distinct pathways produce surface area deficiency. A partial deficiency of spectrin, resulting either from a primary defect of spectrin or a primary defect of ankyrin, leads to a reduced density of the skeletal monolayer (see Fig. 46-5). As a result, the lipid bilayer is destabilized as manifested by a release of membrane lipids in the form of microvesicles. The second pathway involves a primary defect of band 3, which leads to band 3 protein deficiency and, consequently, a decrease in the number of band 3-containing intramembrane particles. As a result, particle-free lipid regions are formed that subsequently bleb off in the form of microvesicles. In the third pathway, a primary defect of band 3 protein (or possibly of ankyrin) leads to a loss from the cells of band 3 together with lipids that surround this protein ("boundary" lipids). Each of the three pathways ultimately results in the loss of membrane material and, hence, surface area deficiency. The resulting decrease in whole red cell deformability predisposes red cells to splenic entrapment. Subsequent splenic conditioning of hereditary spherocytes inflicts additional damage thereby amplifying the vicious circle of red cell injury. For further details, see Figs. 46-4 and 46-5.

is unknown, a family history of a mild dominantly inherited HS in the mother and the finding of slightly increased osmotic fragility in the hematologically normal father suggest that the proband inherited two genetic defects that in a simple heterozygote have either minimal or no adverse consequences. It is of interest that in both reports, the putative α-spectrin defect was either recessively inherited,[107] or, in the case of lethal HS with a markedly decreased α-spectrin synthesis, one parent had a mild dominantly inherited HS, while the other parent was asymptomatic.[108] This is in accord with the finding that in normal erythroid cells, α-spectrin is synthesized in a large excess of β-spectrin.[109] Consequently, subjects carrying one normal and one synthetically inactive α-spectrin allele are expected to be asymptomatic, because α-spectrin production remains in excess of β-spectrin synthesis and normal amounts

of spectrin heterodimers can be assembled on the membrane.[110]

Combined Partial Deficiency of Spectrin and Ankyrin

The biochemical phenotype of combined partial deficiency of spectrin and ankyrin, originally described by Coetzer et al.,[74] is probably the most common.[111] In one patient, the underlying molecular defect involved an absence of the entire ankyrin gene on chromosome 8 due to a large interstitial deletion.[112] In a subsequent study of one of the originally reported patients,[74] the ankyrin mRNA levels and ankyrin synthesis were markedly reduced due to an unknown molecular defect.[113] Since ankyrin represents the principal binding site for spectrin on the membrane, it is not surprising that the deficiency of this protein was found to be accompanied by a proportional decrease in spectrin assembly on the membrane in spite of normal spectrin synthesis.[113] A primary defect of ankyrin has also been implicated by restriction fragment length polymorphism (RFLP) linkage study in a large family with autosomal dominant HS,[114] but the underlying molecular lesion remains unknown. Abnormal alternative splicing in the regulatory domain of ankyrin has recently been described in two kindred with autosomal dominant HS with mild ankyrin 2.1 and spectrin deficiency.[115] Two abnormal alternative splices were detected in one family (ankyrin[PRAGUE]) and an altered proportion of normal alternative splices encoding ankyrin isoforms 2.1 and 2.2 was found in the other kindred (ankyrin[RAKOVNIK]).[115] In a recent study of 34 German patients, several ankyrin mutations have been revealed by a single-strand conformational polymorphisms of the genomic DNA.[118] Most of these mutations are small deletions and insertions causing frameshift and premature termination of translation (Table 46-2).

Partial Deficiency of Band 3 Protein

Partial deficiency of band 3 protein is found in a subset of HS[125,126] that presents with a phenotype of a mild to moderate dominantly inherited HS with mushroom-shaped "pincered" red cells.[102,125] In three kindred, RFLP excluded linkage to α-spectrin, β-spectrin, and ankyrin genes and suggested linkage to the band 3 gene.[127,128] Indeed, several mutations residing near the C terminus of the band 3 protein were recently detected[122,123] (Table 46-2).

In some of the band 3-deficient HS subjects, the deficiency is considerably greater in the dense reticulocyte-poor cells, than in the light reticulocyte-rich cells.[125] This finding, in conjunction with the report of normal band 3 synthesis and normal mRNA levels in one patient,[129] is consistent with the idea that in some patients the band 3 protein is unstable, susceptible to accelerated release from the cells. The mechanism of such accelerated band 3 loss is unknown, and the hypothetical molecular mechanisms include a weakened binding of band 3 protein to ankyrin, due to a primary defect of either the band 3 protein or ankyrin, or a defective assembly of band 3 on the membrane. In some band 3-deficient HS patients, the band 3 gene expression may be reduced or a band 3 mutation of highly conserved amino acids in the transmembrane domain of band 3 may interfere with the proper co-translational insertion of band 3 into membranes of the endoplasmic reticulum or translocation of band 3 to the plasma membrane.[123]

Deficiency of Protein 4.2

Deficiency of protein 4.2 is relatively common in Japan.[79,80] A mutation 142 Ala → Thr has recently been identified,[124] but the cause-and-effect relationship between this mutation and the clinical phenotype is unknown. Two recent reports found the protein 4.2 deficiency to be caused by reduced binding of the normal 4.2 protein to the membrane due to substitutions 327 Pro → Arg and 40 Glu → Lys within the cytoplasmic domain of band 3.[119,120]

Molecular Basis of Surface Area Deficiency

Hereditary spherocytes are intrinsically unstable, releasing lipids under a variety of in vitro conditions,[49] including ATP depletion or exposure of cells to shear stress. The loss of membrane material occurs through the release of 0.2–0.5-μm vesicles containing integral proteins but are devoid of spectrin.[47,130,131] During in vitro incubation, the loss of membrane material is of a sufficient magnitude to augment the surface area deficiency as evidenced by increased osmotic fragility of the cells after incubation.[93,132,133] It is generally assumed that a similar process takes place in vivo, but its experimental verification is yet to be provided.

Considering that the molecular basis of HS is heterogeneous, it is likely that the surface area deficiency is a consequence of several distinct molecular mechanisms that all share a weakening of the vertical connections between the skeleton and the lipid bilayer membrane. Three distinct hypothetical pathways that may lead to surface area deficiency are depicted in Fig. 46-4. In patients with isolated spectrin deficiency or a combined deficiency of spectrin and ankyrin, the surface area deficiency may involve an uncoupling of the lipid bilayer membrane from the underlying skeleton. In normal red cells, the skeleton forms a nearly monomolecular submembrane layer occupying more than one-half of the inner surface of the membrane.[48] Consequently, spectrin deficiency leads to a decreased density of this network (Fig. 46-5). As a result, areas of the lipid bilayer membrane that are not directly supported by the skeleton are susceptible to release from the cells in the form of microvesicles.

In HS associated with the deficiency of band 3 protein, two hypothetical pathways may lead to a loss of surface area (Fig. 46-4). One such mechanism may involve a loss of band 3 protein from the cells.[125,129] Since band 3 protein spans the lipid bilayer membrane many times,[99] it is likely that a substantial amount of "boundary" lipids are released together with the band 3 protein, thus leading to surface area deficiency. Another possible mechanism may involve a formation of band 3 free domains in the membrane, followed by formation of membrane blebs, which are subsequently released from the cells as microvesicles.[123] Such hypothesis is based on the observations that aggregation of intramembrane particles (composed principally of the band 3 protein[134]) in ghosts leads to a formation of particle-depleted domains from which membrane lipids bleb off as microvesicles.[135]

Alterations in Cation Content and Permeability

HS red cells, particularly those collected from the spleen, are somewhat dehydrated.[136,137] This contrasts with findings of increased influx of sodium into the cells in vitro,[91,138] presumably as a consequence of the underlying skeletal defect. The cellular dehydration may be due to activation of pathways causing a selective loss of potassium and water such as the K^+, Cl^- co-transport, which may be stimulated by the relatively low pH of the spleen (see below) or by oxidative damage,[139,140] possibly in sites at which red cells are in contact with macrophages producing oxygen radicals. Furthermore, the Na^+/K^+ pump that regulates the intracellular sodium and potassium content is hyperactive in HS cells,[91] compensating for the increased sodium leak into the cells. Increased activity of this pump could lead to red cell dehydration, since for every two atoms of potassium transported inward, three sodium atoms are extruded from the cell.[141]

Entrapment of Nondeformable Spherocytes in the Spleen

The importance of the spleen in the pathophysiology of hemolysis in HS has already been appreciated in the original description of the disease[83] and substantiated by subsequent studies.[89,95–97] Two factors participate in the selective destruction of the HS cell in the spleen: (1) a poor HS red cell deformability,[142–144] and (2) the unique anatomy of the splenic vasculature that acts as a "microcirculation filter."[145,146]

The poor red cell deformability is principally a consequence of a decreased cell surface/cell volume ratio, resulting from the loss of surface material.[142,147] In contrast to normal discocytes, which have an abundant surface allowing the cells to deform and pass through narrow microcirculation openings, the HS red cells lack this extra surface. Their poor deformability may be further impaired by cellular dehydration.[142,148,149] By con-

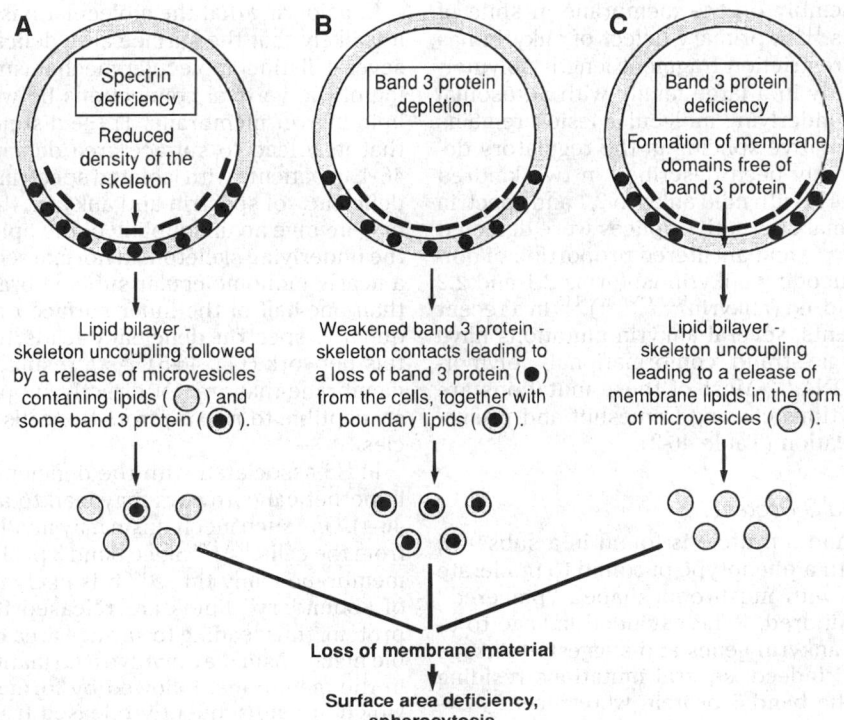

Fig. 46-4. Schematic model of hypothetical mechanisms of membrane lipid loss that underlies surface area deficiency of hereditary spherocytes. **(A)** Proposed mechanism of membrane lipid loss in HS associated with a partial deficiency of spectrin. Since spectrin (solid rectangles) constitutes the major protein of the skeleton, the deficiency of spectrin leads to a decrease in the density of this monomolecular skeletal layer. In normal red cells, the skeleton occupies most of the inner membrane surface. In addition, spectrin and protein 4.1 bind to the negatively charged lipids, thereby stabilizing the lipid bilayer. Consequently, decreased density of the skeletal layer in spectrin-deficient HS cells facilitates uncoupling of the bilayer from the underlying skeleton followed by a release of skeleton-free microvesicles (shaded circles) from the cells. Some of these vesicles contain band 3 protein (solid circles), because only a fraction of this protein is associated with the membrane skeleton. This loss of membrane material leads to surface area deficiency with spherocytosis. **(B)** One of the proposed mechanisms of surface area deficiency in HS associated with a partial deficiency of the band 3 protein. This hypothesis proposes that HS red cells are depleted of the band 3 protein due to its release from the cells in vivo, presumably because of weakened binding of the band 3 protein to the underlying skeleton (such as a weakened band 3-ankyrin linkage). Since band 3 protein traverses the lipid bilayer multiple times, the loss of the band 3 protein is accompanied by a concomitant loss of the "boundary" lipids that surround this protein. The ensuing loss of membrane material leads to surface area deficiency with spherocytosis. **(C)** The second proposed mechanism of the loss of surface area of HS red cells deficient in band 3 protein involves a reduced band 3 synthesis or a diminished incorporation of band 3 into the membrane. As a result of the band 3 deficiency, membrane domains are formed that are devoid of band 3 protein. We propose that this process is analogous to membrane blebbing of ghosts treated with agents that aggregate intramembrane particles (that contain band 3 protein). In such ghosts, membrane domains that are depleted in the band 3 protein bleb off as vesicles that are free of band 3 protein and spectrin. As with the two previous mechanisms, this membrane loss causes surface area deficiency and spherocytosis. Further details and references are given in the text. (From Palek and Jarolim,[45] with permission.)

trast, the deformability of the HS red cell membrane is normal or even increased.[142,150]

The principal sites of red cell entrapment in the spleen are fenestrations in the wall of splenic sinuses, where blood from the splenic cords of the red pulp enters the venous circulation.[145,146] In the rat spleen, the length and width of these fenestrations (2–3 μm and 0.2–0.5 μm, respectively) are about one-half the red cell diameter.[146] Electron microscopic micrographs of spleen specimens show that very few HS red cells traverse these slits.[151,152] Consequently, the nondeformable spherocytes accumulate in the red pulp, which becomes grossly engorged, as evidenced on the anatomic sections of the spleen taken after splenectomy.[151–154]

Splenic Conditioning and Destruction

Once trapped in the spleen, HS red cells undergo additional damage manifested by further loss of surface area and increase in cell density, as evident in cells removed from the spleen at splenectomy.[89,96,155,156] In part, these conditioned red cells re-enter the systemic circulation, as revealed by the "tail" of the

osmotic fragility curve (see below), indicating the presence of a subpopulation of cells with a markedly reduced surface area.[96,155–157] After splenectomy, this red cell population disappears.

Earlier studies attempted to simulate splenic conditioning of HS red cells by in vitro incubation.[71,153] The possible conditioning factors may include a relatively low pH in the spleen,[158,159] as well as in the sequestered red cells,[160] that may further compromise the poor HS red cell deformability,[158,159] and a contact of red cells with macrophages that may inflict additional damage to the red cell membrane.[139,161,162] Glucose deprivation and the ensuing intracellular ATP depletion does not appear to be a significant factor, since cells collected from the spleen at splenectomy have a normal ATP content.[137]

The conditioning effect of the spleen appears to represent a cumulative injury: the average residence time of HS red cells in the splenic cords is about 10–100 minutes and only 1–10% of blood entering the spleen is temporarily sequestered in the congested cords, while the remaining 90% of blood flow is rapidly shunted into the venous circulation.[145]

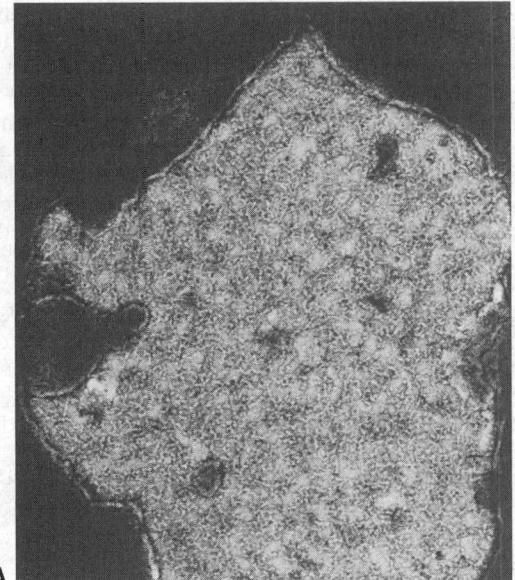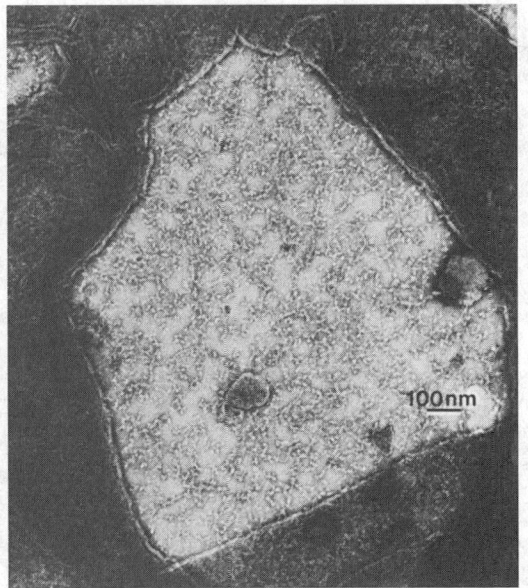

Fig. 46-5. Ultrastructure of the membrane skeleton in normal red cells and in red cells from a patient with severe HS associated with a combined deficiency of spectrin and ankyrin. Hemoglobin-free ghosts were sonicated to open a "window" that allows us to see the intact skeleton at the inner membrane surface. The ghosts were fixed and negatively stained. The skeleton is preferentially stained under these conditions. **(A)** In ghosts from normal red cells, the individual skeletal proteins are in close apposition to each other and form a monomolecular layer. **(B)** By contrast, the HS skeleton is considerably less dense with the individual proteins separated by skeleton-free areas. (Courtesy of S.C. Liu.)

Although most HS red cells are eventually sequestered and destroyed in the spleen, HS cells that have been most severely damaged in the spleen can be destroyed outside of this organ as well.[157] The HS red cell surface alterations that trigger red cell phagocytosis by tissue macrophages are unknown. One possible pathway may involve alterations in phospholipid distribution within the two bilayer leaflets, leading to the exposure in the external hemileaflet of phosphatidylserine that promotes red cell attachment to macrophages and phagocytosis in vitro.[163] Although the distribution of phospholipids in the two bilayer hemileaflets is normal in most HS patients,[164] altered phospholipid distribution has been demonstrated in red cells from patients with severe forms of HS.[165] It is possible, but not proven, that similar changes in phospholipid asymmetry take place in the end-stage HS cells that are repeatedly conditioned in the spleen. Unlike senescent normal red cells and some abnormal erythrocytes, HS red cells have normal amounts of surface-associated IgG.[166] Thus, it is unlikely that the HS erythrocytes undergo surface alterations leading to an exposure of new antigenic sites on their surface (the "senescent red cell" antigen).[167]

Involvement of Nonerythroid Tissues in HS and the Relationship to the Underlying Generic Defects

In most HS cases, the clinical manifestations are confined to the erythroid lineage, principally because many of the nonerythroid counterparts of the red cell membrane proteins are encoded by separate genes (e.g., spectrin, ankyrin and the anion-exchange protein[98–100]) or because some proteins (e.g., protein 4.1) are subject to tissue specific alternative splicing.[50] However, there are notable exceptions. Several HS kindred have been reported, in whom HS coexisted with a degenerative disorder of the spinal cord,[168] cardiomyopathy,[169] or mental retardation.[168] Although the molecular basis of the nonerythroid involvement is unknown, these reports are noteworthy, in light of the recent studies of the mouse model of HS called the *nb* mutation.[170,171] The *nb/nb* homozygotes have a severe HS with spectrin and ankyrin deficiencies attributable to a primary mo-

lecular defect of ankyrin.[171] They develop a neurologic syndrome, the progression of which coincides with the degeneration of Purkinje cells in the cerebellum.[170] Purkinje cells normally express erythroid ankyrin, which is absent in *nb/nb* mice.[170,172]

Inheritance

Because of the heterogeneous molecular basis of HS, the "HS genes" can be assigned to several chromosomes, including chromosome 1 (α-spectrin), chromosome 8 (ankyrin), chromosome 14 (β-spectrin), and chromosome 17 (band 3 protein) (Table 46-1). The inheritance is both autosomal dominant (most HS patients)[66–68] and autosomal recessive.[68,173]

While the clinical severity of HS is highly variable among different kindreds, it is relatively uniform within a given family in which HS is typically inherited as an autosomal dominant disorder.[68,76] However, HS has been identified in one or more siblings whose parents had no identifiable abnormalities or only slightly abnormal osmotic fragility after incubation.[66,67, 69,174] In some cases, this may reflect a variable penetrance of the genetic defect. Another explanation of such sporadic HS is a de novo mutation or possibly a mild form of recessively inherited HS.

Only a few cases of homozygous HS have been reported. These patients have a severe hemolytic anemia, while their parents have a very mild form of the disease.[72,73] By contrast, the homozygous state for the more typical hemolytic form of HS appears to be lethal; in one such kindred, both consanguineous parents and three offspring (presumable HS heterozygotes) had moderately severe HS, one offspring was normal, and there were two miscarriages, a frequency consistent with the predicted homozygosity for the HS gene.[175]

While HS is dominantly inherited in most patients, several cases of recessively inherited HS manifesting with severe hemolytic anemia have been reported. All such cases were found to be severely deficient in red cell spectrin, and the putative defect has been assigned to the α-chain of spectrin heterodimer.[107,173] The second condition, characterized by a recessive inheritance pattern is hereditary deficiency of the 4.2 protein.[101,119] This deficiency is associated with relatively mild hemolysis, and the red cell morphology reveals the presence of stomatocytes and ovalocytes that are not seen in other patients with HS.

Clinical Manifestations

Typical Forms

A typical HS patient is relatively asymptomatic. As already noted in one of the first descriptions of the disorder,[85] mild jaundice may be the only symptom of the disease. Splenomegaly is present in most patients,[66,69] occasionally reaching large dimensions. Anemia is usually mild or even absent due to compensatory bone marrow hyperplasia as manifested by reticulocytosis.

Mild Forms and HS Carrier State

In some patients, anemia is absent, reticulocyte count is normal or only minimally elevated, laboratory evidence of hemolysis is either minimal or absent,[66–68] and the changes in red cell shape may be mild escaping detection on the peripheral blood film.[68] The presence of HS is detected only by osmotic fragility testing (see below) or during evaluation of another relative with a more symptomatic form of the disease. Some patients are first diagnosed during pregnancy,[176] during transient infections such as infectious mononucleosis[177] or parvovirus infection,[178,179] or, occasionally, the diagnosis is made even in the seventh to ninth decades of life.[70]

Severe and Atypical Forms

The relatively rare patients with autosomal recessive form of HS present with a severe life-threatening hemolysis early in life.[71–74] In one report, the parents, who were distant cousins, were asymptomatic HS carriers and their offsprings (presumed HS homozygotes) presented with a life-threatening hemolytic anemia that was only partially improved by splenectomy.[72]

Laboratory Evaluation

Most HS patients either have a very mild anemia or normal red cell counts and hemoglobin and hematocrit values, reflecting the fact that the hemolytic rate is often very mild and that the hemolysis is fully compensated by increased red cell production, as evidenced by reticulocytosis. In spite of increased percentage of reticulocytes, which have a larger volume than mature red cells, the mean corpuscular volume of HS red cells is often low normal or even slightly decreased, a finding that together with slight increase in mean corpuscular hemoglobin concentration reflects mild cellular dehydration. Some patients, however, particularly those with recessive HS, are severely anemic, with hemoglobin concentration ≥4 g/dl. Evidence of accelerated red cell destruction, as indicated by increased lactate dehydrogenase, unconjugated bilirubin, decreased haptoglobin, as well as reticulocytosis, is present in most patients. However, these abnormalities may be absent in subjects with a mild form of the disease.

Blood Film

In typical HS, spherocytes are readily identified by their characteristic shape on the peripheral blood film (Fig. 46-6A). They lack central pallor, their mean cell diameter is decreased, and they appear more intensely hemoglobinized. The latter reflects both altered red cell geometry and increased cell density.[68] In a three-dimensional view, some spherocytes have a spherostomatocytic shape[180] that is occasionally appreciated on the peripheral blood film. In a mild form of the disease, the peripheral blood smear may appear normal since the loss of surface area may be too small to be appreciated by blood smear evaluation; the cells appear as "fat" discs rather than as true spherocytes.

Additional morphologic features have been described in some HS patients. A subset of HS patients whose red cells are deficient in band 3 protein have some pincered red cells (Fig. 46-6B, arrows) on the peripheral blood film,[125,129] a finding that is both sensitive and specific for this HS subset. However, pincered cells disappear after splenectomy.[102] Cells with irregular contour were found in two patients with severe combined spectrin and ankyrin deficiency[74] (Fig. 46-6C), and surface spiculation was described in a family with HS with a defect of β-spectrin leading to abnormal interaction of spectrin with protein 4.1[104] (Fig. 46-6D). Another atypical phenotype involves the presence of sphero-ovalocytes and stomatocytes, as reported in Japanese patients with protein 4.2 deficiency.[124]

Osmotic Fragility

The osmotic fragility test (Fig. 46-7) measures an in vitro lysis of red cells suspended in solutions of decreasing osmolarity. Normal red cell membrane is unstretchable and is virtually freely permeable to water.[181] Hence, the cell behaves as a nearly perfect osmometer, in that it increases its volume in hypotonic solutions progressively until a "critical hemolytic volume" is reached. At this point, the red cell membrane ruptures and hemoglobin escapes into the supernatant solution through a single hole.[182] As a result of the loss of membrane material and the ensuing surface area deficiency, the critical hemolytic volume of spherocytes is considerably lower than that of normal red cells. Consequently, these cells hemolyze more than normal red cells when suspended in hypotonic NaCl solutions. However, a finding of increased osmotic fragility is not unique to HS and is also present in other conditions associated with spherocytosis on the peripheral blood film (see below).

The slight dehydration of hereditary spherocytes (which in other conditions is associated with decreased osmotic fragility) has no appreciable effect on HS osmotic fragility because of the overriding effect of the markedly diminished cell-surface area. In fact, the densest, most dehydrated, cells exhibit the greatest increase in osmotic fragility.[66,183] The relative contributions of cell dehydration and surface area deficiency can be accurately determined by osmotic gradient ectacytometry.[148] The osmotic fragility curve often reveals uniformly increased osmotic fragility (Fig. 46-7). In addition, in nonsplenectomized HS subjects, a "tail" of the osmotic fragility curve may be present indicating a subpopulation of particularly fragile red cells conditioned by splenic stasis.[66,96] This subpopulation of cells disappears after splenectomy. In subjects with mild HS, osmotic fragility may be normal and abnormalities can be found only after incubation that further augments the loss of surface area[66]; however, the sensitivity of incubated osmotic fragility may be outweighed by a loss of its specificity.[184]

Autohemolysis and Other Tests

Red cell autohemolysis, the spontaneous hemolysis of red cells incubated under sterile conditions without glucose, was previously advocated as a sensitive test for the detection of HS.[71] This test is being used less frequently and is probably no more sensitive than the incubated osmotic fragility. Other tests have also been described in the literature (i.e., the "glycerol lysis test,"[78,185–187] the "pink test,"[188,189] and the "skeleton gelation test").[190,191] The former two tests, which employ glycerol to retard the osmotic swelling of red cells, are preferred

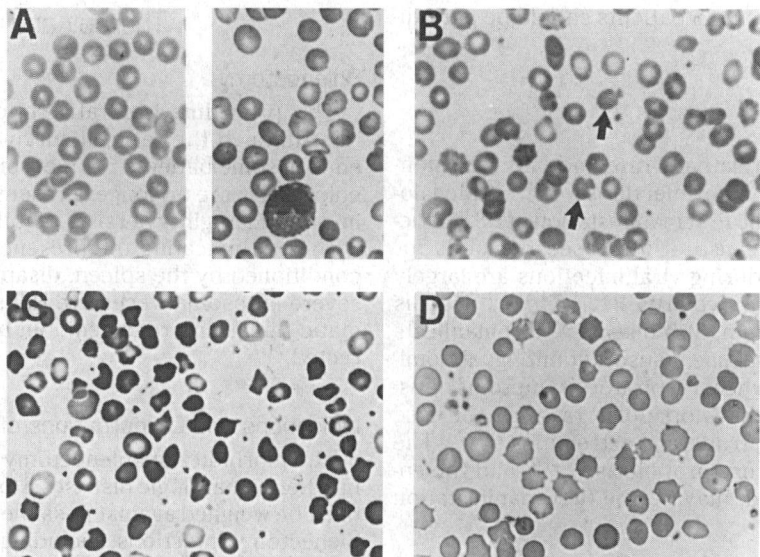

Fig. 46-6. Blood films from patients with HS of varying severity. **(A)** Two blood films of typical moderately severe HS with a mild deficiency of red cell spectrin and ankyrin. Although many cells have spheroidal shape, some retain a central concavity. **(B)** HS with pincered red cells (arrows), as typically seen in HS associated with band 3 deficiency. Occasional spiculated red cells are also present. **(C)** Severe atypical HS due to a severe combined spectrin and ankyrin deficiency. In addition to spherocytes, many cells have irregular contour. **(D)** HS with isolated spectrin deficiency due to a β-spectrin mutation.[105,106] Some of the spherocytes have prominent surface projections resembling spheroacanthocytes. (Blood film D was provided courtesy of D.L. Wolfe.)

in some laboratories because they are easy to perform and can be adapted to microsamples.[78]

Detection of the Underlying Molecular Defect

Since the most common finding in patients with HS is a deficiency of one or more of the membrane proteins, the initial study should include PAGE of sodium dodecyl sulfate-solubilized red cell membrane proteins (SDS-PAGE) in gel systems of Laemmli[192] and Fairbanks et al.,[193] followed by densitometric quantitation. This technique reveals abnormalities in about 70–80% of patients, defining four distinct biochemical phenotypes discussed under Molecular Pathology. Direct quantitation of membrane proteins by classic radioimmunoassay[75] is more sensitive than the densitometric quantitation and permits accurate measurement of the copy number of the individual proteins per red cell. The importance of the latter approach is heightened by the fact that densitometry may underestimate spectrin and ankyrin deficiencies[73] because it involves a normalization to the band 3 protein (i.e., spectrin/band 3 ratio), the loss of which, together with membrane lipids, may spuriously normalize the spectrin/band 3 ratio. Consequently, the spectrin/band 3 ratio is lower after splenectomy.[73]

The subsequent strategy to search for the underlying defect is complex. Studies of protein function, which remain the gold standard in the detection of putative spectrin mutations in HE and HPP have been disappointing in detecting abnormalities in HS, with the exception of HS characterized by a weakened β-spectrin-protein 4.1 interaction.[104] Studies of membrane protein synthesis and assembly, using either reticulocytes, or erythroblasts derived from peripheral blood burst-forming units in vitro,[108,110] were previously used to detect two defects: (1) a marked decrease in α-spectrin synthesis in a lethal HS,[108] and (2) a primary defect involving reduced synthesis and expression of ankyrin in HS with a combined spectrin and ankyrin deficiency.[113] However, these are likely to be insensitive to detect mild to moderate abnormalities in membrane protein synthesis and assembly.

Several laboratories have focused on linkage studies, employing RFLP, either for linkage exclusion or, in large families, linkage verification.[114,127,128] This approach led to the detection of ankyrin as the primary defect in a large HS kindred with spectrin deficiency,[114] and it excluded the defect of α-spectrin, β-spectrin, and ankyrin in two families with band 3 deficiency, raising the possibility that the primary defect may involve the band 3 protein.[127,128] RFLP linkage may be substituted by mutation scanning techniques,[194] among which the single-strand conformational polymorphism technique appears to be most promising, followed by sequencing of the abnormal segment of the cDNA or genomic DNA.

Complications

Gallstones

Bilirubin stones are found in approximately 50% of patients with HS, often even in those presenting with a very mild form of the disease. They are rarely found in children and their incidence increases with age.[66,195] However, gallstones have been occasionally detected as early as in the third year of life.[196,197]

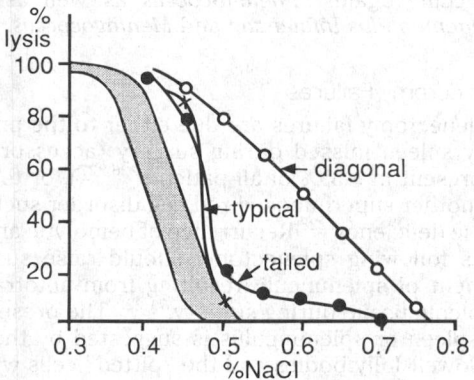

Fig. 46-7. Characteristic osmotic fragility curves in hereditary spherocytosis. The typical curve of increased osmotic fragility is the most common finding. The tailed curve reveals a second population (a tail) of very fragile erythrocytes. The diagonal curve is seen in patients with severe HS. (Modified from Dacie,[71] with permission.)

Because of their high incidence, HS patients should be periodically examined by ultrasound.

Crises

True hemolytic crises are relatively rare and only occasionally reported in association with infections.[177,196,197] Megaloblastic crisis may represent the first manifestation of HS, particularly during pregnancy, because of increased demands for folic acid.[176] Aplastic crises during viral infections are largely attributable to infection by parvovirus B19.[178,179,198-202] This infection (erythema infectiosum, fifth disease[200,202]) manifests with fever, chills, lethargy, malaise, nausea, vomiting, abdominal pain with occasional diarrhea, respiratory symptoms, muscle and joint pains, and a maculopapular rash on the face ("slapped cheek syndrome"), trunk, and extremities.[198-201] The virus selectively suppresses erythropoiesis,[199-201] and the ensuing anemia, often profound, may be the first manifestation of HS.[178,179]

Other Complications

In patients with more severe forms of HS, other complications include leg ulcers and/or dermatitis that heal after splenectomy[71,203] and symptoms of expanded erythroid space, including paravertebral masses of extramedullary hematopoiesis, which may raise a possibility of an underlying neoplasm.[204,205] Several cases of hemochromatosis in HS patients have been reported. In some hemochromatosis resulted from repeated transfusions[206]; in others, the patients had two genetic defects, one involving HS and the other involving a hemochromatosis carrier state.[207-210]

Differential Diagnosis

Because of the relatively asymptomatic presentation of HS, this diagnosis should be considered during evaluation of unexplained splenomegaly, unconjugated hyperbilirubinemia of unknown cause, gallstones at a young age, anemia during pregnancy that can worsen the severity of hemolysis in HS,[211,212] or transient anemia during acute infections, some due to parvovirus B19.[179] The diagnosis of HS can be missed in mild forms of the disease, because spherocytosis may not be apparent on the peripheral blood film. However, an osmotic fragility test of incubated red cells usually provides a diagnostic answer. It should be noted that spherocytosis is transiently improved and both the osmotic fragility and hemolysis are normalized in patients in whom obstructive jaundice develops.[213] This is due to an expansion of red cell surface area that follows an increased uptake of phospholipids and cholesterol from the abnormal plasma lipoproteins. In normal red cells, this leads to target cell formation; in HS, spherocytes are transformed to discocytes. Spherocytosis and increased osmotic fragility of HS red cells are likewise improved by iron deficiency, but the red cell life span remains shortened.[214] In addition, a coexistence of β-thalassemia trait and HS partially corrects the HS phenotype.[215]

More typical forms of HS, characterized by relatively uniform spherocytosis with increased mean corpuscular hemoglobin concentration are usually easily distinguished from other disorders manifesting with spherocytosis, such as immunohemolytic anemias and unstable hemoglobins; in some patients, the spherostomatocytes in the rare Rh deficiency syndrome and the intermediate syndromes of hereditary stomatocytosis may be confused with HS red cells.

Therapy and Prognosis

Splenectomy

This procedure is curative in patients with typical forms of HS. Although the red cell survival may remain slightly shortened in some patients,[216] hyperbilirubinemia, anemia, and reticulocytosis are no longer present. Spherocytosis and increase in osmotic fragility persists, but the "tail" of the osmotic fragility curve, indicating the presence of a subpopulation of cells conditioned by the spleen, disappears.[66,96,157] In patients with severe autosomal recessive HS, splenectomy produces a dramatic clinical improvement, but hemolysis is only partially corrected.[71,73,74]

Indications and Complications of Splenectomy

The morbidity of splenectomy is generally lower in HS than in other hematologic diseases. However, the benefits of surgery must be weighed against possible complications, such as postsplenectomy infections, including the postsplenectomy sepsis syndrome.[217-220] Although these complications are rare and their frequency is likely to diminish further with appropriate vaccinations, these investigators do not support recommendations of indiscriminate use of splenectomy in all HS patients with splenomegaly.[221,222] The risk/benefit ratio and the changing trends in indications of splenectomy have been analyzed in a recent review.[195] In the opinion of these and other investigators,[223,224] unequivocal indications for splenectomy include either growth retardation and a symptomatic hemolytic disease or even a mild HS associated with a presence of gallstones or the history of gallstones in other relatives with a similar severity of hemolytic disease. The latter recommendation may be questioned considering that, in general population with gallstones, the reported incidence of symptoms or complications is low (18%).[195] Although no data are available comparing the natural history of cholesterol stones in the general population and bilirubin stones in HS, it is likely that the latter are more symptomatic, justifying the above recommendation. Because of increased frequency of postsplenectomy infection in young children, splenectomy should not be performed earlier than at 3–5 years of age.[223] Occasionally a child with severe HS and growth retardation or skeletal deformities may require splenectomy earlier. Based on the recent finding that partial splenectomy improved hemolytic rate, while maintaining the splenic phagocytic function, this procedure has been proposed for consideration in transfusion-dependent HS infants.[225] Considering the high regenerative potential of splenic tissue, the long-term benefits of this procedure are uncertain. Several weeks prior to splenectomy, patients should be immunized with polyvalent vaccine against *Pneumococcus* as well as vaccines against *Haemophilus influenzae* and *Meningococcus*.

Postsplenectomy Failures

Postsplenectomy failures are due either to the presence of accessory spleen missed during surgery (accessory spleens may be present in ≤39% of all patients[226,227]), or to the presence of another superimposed red cell disorder such as pyruvate kinase deficiency.[228] Recurrence of hemolytic anemia several years following splenectomy should raise suspicion of development of splenunculi, resulting from autotransplantation of splenic tissue during surgery.[71,229] The presence of accessory spleen or splenunculus is suggested by the absence of both Howell-Jolly bodies and the "pitted" cells with crater-like surface indentations readily seen by interference contrast microscopy.[230,231] A definitive confirmation of splenosis is made by a radiocolloid liver/spleen scan or a scan using [95]Cr-labeled-heated red cells taken up by the ectopic splenic tissue.[232,233] A spontaneous regression of HS, presumably as a result of development of hyposplenic state, has been observed in two family members who had both HS and sickle cell trait.[234]

HEREDITARY ELLIPTOCYTOSIS AND RELATED DISEASES

Definition, Prevalence, and History

HE designates a group of inherited disorders that have in common the presence of elliptical red cells on peripheral blood films. Elliptocytosis was first described by Dresbach[235] in 1904 and its heritability was firmly established by Hunter.[236,237] Subsequent reports have revealed a considerable heterogeneity of clinical expression and have defined several distinct syndromes, including HPP[238] and SAO.[239–241]

In the U.S. population, the prevalence of HE is about 3–5 per 10,000.[242–244] By contrast, in areas of endemic malaria, HE is considerably more frequent. In equatorial Africa, the prevalence of common HE is $\geq 0.6\%$.[245] In the U.S. population, HE appears to be more common among blacks. The prevalence of SAO is as high as 30%.[239,246–248]

The molecular basis of HE remained obscure until approximately 15 years ago, when a defect of skeletal proteins was suggested by several studies.[249–255] Subsequently, many skeletal protein defects have been described, some characterized at the level of amino acid and DNA sequence (Table 46-3).

On the basis of red cell morphology, HE can be divided into three major groups. Common HE, a dominantly inherited condition, is morphologically characterized by biconcave elliptocytes and, in some patients, rod-shaped cells. The clinical severity of common HE is highly variable, ranging from an asymptomatic condition to a severe recessively inherited hemolytic anemia designated HPP in which the blood film reveals numerous red cell fragments, microspherocytes, and poikilocytes. Spherocytic HE, also called hemolytic ovalocytosis, is a rare condition in which both round "fat" ovalocytes and spherocytes are present on the blood film. SAO, a disorder highly prevalent in malaria-infested belt of Southeast Asia and Pacific, is characterized by rigid spoon shaped cells that have either a longitudinal slit or a transverse ridge[306] (Fig. 46-8).

Common Hereditary Elliptocytosis

A possibility that the primary lesion of HE and HPP erythrocytes resides in the proteins of the red cell membrane skeleton was first raised by findings of thermal instability of HPP spectrin,[249,250] retention of the elliptical shape in HE membrane skeletons,[251] disintegration of membrane skeletons after exposure to shear stress, defective self-association of spectrin dimers to tetramers,[252,253] altered susceptibility of spectrin to tryptic digestion,[254] and a deficiency of skeletal protein 4.1.[307] Subsequently, a large number of reports followed documenting either dysfunction or deficiencies of several skeletal proteins. In many cases, the underlying genetic defect has now been defined (Table 46-3).

Etiology

Spectrin Mutations

The most common defects in HE, found in about 60% of all patients, are mutations of α- or β-spectrin.[308,309] Most of these subjects are black, but these mutations have also been detected in whites, Arabs,[46,306,310] and Melanesians (Jarolim P, Palek J et al., unpublished observations).

Both α- and β-spectrin are elongated flexible molecules consisting of triple helical repeats connected by nonhelical segments.[304,305] These polypeptides are associated side to side in an antiparallel position forming a flexible rod-like αβ hetero-

dimer (Fig. 46-9), in which the N-terminal end of α-spectrin and the C terminus of β-spectrin form the head region of the heterodimer. Spectrin heterodimers are associated head to head to form spectrin tetramers, the major structural subunits of the membrane skeleton. Spectrin tetramers, in turn, are interconnected into a highly ordered two-dimensional lattice through binding, at their distal ends, to actin oligomers with the aid of protein 4.1.[306,311,312]

The contact site between the α- and β-spectrin chains of the opposed heterodimers is a combined triple helical repetitive segment in which the first two helices are contributed by the C terminus of β-spectrin, while the helix 3 is the first helical segment of α-spectrin[51] (Fig. 46-10). The spectrin dimer-tetramer interconversion is governed by a simple thermodynamic equilibrium that under physiologic conditions strongly favors spectrin tetramers.[313]

Most α-spectrin defects described to date reside at or near the N-terminal end of α-spectrin, which is involved in the heterodimer contact (the so-called αI domain defined by limited tryptic peptide mapping, see the section Laboratory Evaluation and Fig. 46-9). Consequently, these mutations impair the self-association of spectrin into tetramers.[51] Most α-spectrin mutations reported to date are point mutations (Table 46-3 and Fig. 46-10). These mutations create abnormal proteolytic cleavage sites that typically reside in the third helix of a repetitive segment and give rise to abnormal tryptic peptides on two-dimensional tryptic peptide maps of spectrin, which provides the basis for their designation[51] (Table 46-3) (see also the section Laboratory Evaluation).

Most of the reported elliptocytogenic β-spectrin mutations are C-terminal truncations[51] (Table 46-3 and Fig. 46-10), which disrupt the formation of the combined αβ triple-helical repetitive segment and consequently, the self-association of spectrin heterodimers to tetramers. Only three point mutations have been detected to date, all residing in helices 1 or 2 of the combined αβ repetitive segment.[280,281,314] All these mutations open a proteolytic cleavage site residing in the third helix of the combined repetitive segment, which gives rise to the 74-kd αI peptide.[51]

Although most spectrin mutations reside in the vicinity of the αβ spectrin heterodimer contact, several mutations residing in the αII domain have been found.[276,277] These mutations are asymptomatic in the simple heterozygous state but cause elliptocytic hemolytic anemia with a mild increase in spectrin heterodimers in homozygous subjects.

Protein 4.1 Mutations

Another group of elliptocytogenic mutations, although less common than spectrin mutations, are deficiencies and dysfunctions of the 4.1 protein. Protein 4.1 is a multifunctional protein that contains two important functional sites: the spectrin-binding domain, where 4.1 binds to the distal end of the spectrin αβ heterodimer, markedly increasing the binding of spectrin to oligomeric actin; and the basic N-terminal domain, where 4.1 interacts with glycophorin C, phosphatidylinositol, and phosphatidylserine, facilitating the attachment of the distal end of spectrin to the membrane.[311,315–322]

Studies of 4.1 mRNA from normal red cells revealed multiple 4.1 isoforms resulting from alternate mRNA splicing.[50] On SDS-PAGE, according to Laemmli,[192] protein 4.1 is resolved into two bands of different size: 4.1a and 4.1b. The larger band, 4.1a, is typically found in normal red cells while the shorter one, 4.1b, represents the major isoform of reticulocytes.[323] The 4.1b isoform is converted into 4.1a isoform by deamidation of Asn 502.[324]

A partial deficiency of protein 4.1 is associated with mild dominantly inherited HE,[308,325–328] while a complete deficiency (a homozygous state) leads to a severe hemolytic dis-

Table 46-3. Red Cell Membrane Mutations in Hereditary Elliptocytosis and Pyropoikilocytosis

Designation[a]	Abnormal Function	Limited Proteolysis or Other Studies[b,c]	Primary Structure[b,c]	DNA Defect[d]	Heterozygote	Homozygote or Double Heterozygote	Prevalence and Comments	References
α-Spectrin								
Sp α^I/78 Tunis	SpD-SpD contact	78-kd peptide cleaved at 16 Lys	41 Arg → Trp (repetitive segment α', helix 3)	41 CGG → TGG (exon 2 of α-Sp)	Mild HE		One report	256
	SpD-SpD contact	78-kd peptide cleaved at 16 Lys	45 Arg → Ser (repetitive segment α', helix 3)	45 AGG → AGT (exon 2 of α-Sp)	Mild HE		One report	257
Sp α^I/74	SpD-SpD contact	74-kd peptide cleaved at 48 Lys	28 Arg → Cys (repetitive segment α', helix 3)	28 CGT → TGT (exon 2 of α-Sp)	Mild to moderately	HPP	A common group of α-spectrin	258,259
	SpD-SpD contact	74-kd peptide cleaved at 48 Lys	28 Arg → Leu (repetitive segment α', helix 3)	28 CGT → CTT (exon 2 of α-Sp)	Severe HE or asymptatic	HPP	Mutations found in whites, blacks, Arabs, Melanesians	258,260
	SpD-SpD contact	74-kd peptide cleaved at 48 Lys	28 Arg → Ser (repetitive segment α', helix 3)	28 CGT → AGT (exon 2 of α-Sp)	Severe HE or asymptomatic	HPP		258,260
	SpD-SpD contact	74-kd peptide cleaved at 48 Lys	28 Arg → His (repetitive segment α', helix 3)	28 CGT → CAT (exon 2 of α-Sp)	Severe HE or asymptomatic	HPP		258,261,262
Genova	SpD-SpD contact	74-kd peptide cleaved at 48 Lys	34 Arg → Trp (repetitive segment α', helix 3)	34 CGG → TGG (exon 2 of α-Sp)	Mild HE		One report	263
Culoz	SpD-SpD contact	74-kd peptide cleaved at 48 Lys	46 Gly → Val (repetitive segment α', helix 3)	46 GGT → GTT (exon 2 of α-Sp)			One report	264
	SpD-SpD contact	74-kd peptide cleaved at 48 Lys	48 Lys → Arg (repetitive segment α', helix 3)	48 AAG → AGG (exon 2 of α-Sp)			One report	260
Lyon	SpD-SpD contact	74-kd peptide cleaved at 45 Arg	49 Leu → Phe (repetitive segment α', helix 3)	49 CTT → TTT (exon 2 of α-Sp)			One report	264
Sp α^I/65	SpD-SpD contact	65-kd peptide cleaved at 137 Arg	Duplication of 154 Leu (repetitive segment α1, helix 3)	154 TTG duplication (exon 4 of α-Sp)	Mild HE	Moderately severe HE	Relatively common in blacks	265–267
Ponte de Sor	Normal		151 Gly → Asp (repetitive segment α1, helix 3)	151 GGT → GAT (exon 4 of α-Sp)	Asymptomatic	Severe HE	One report	268
Sp α^I/46	SpD-SpD contact	46-kd peptide cleaved at 258 Lys, shortened spectrin band α'	Deletion of amino acids 178–226 from repetitive segment α2	Skipping of exon 5 associated with ~1 kb insertion into the intron following exon 5	Mild HE		One report	269
Sp α^I/50a	SpD-SpD contact	50-kd peptide cleaved at 256 Arg of 258 Lys	207 Leu → Pro (repetitive segment α2, helix 2)	207 CTG → CCG (exon 5 of α-Sp)	Mild HE or asymptomatic HPP carrier	HPP	Relatively common in blacks	270,271

Variant	Functional defect	Protein abnormality	Amino acid change	DNA mutation	Clinical phenotype	Severe phenotype	Comment	Reference
	SpD-SpD contact	50-kd peptide cleaved at 256 Arg of 258 Lys	260 Leu → Pro (repetitive segment α2, helix 3)	260 CTG → CCG (exon 6 of α-Sp)				265,270
Sp α^I/50a	SpD-SpD contact	50-kd peptide cleaved at 256 Arg of 258 Lys	207 Leu → Pro (repetitive segment α2, helix 2)	207 CTG → CCG (exon 5 of α-Sp)	Mild HE or asymptomatic HPP carrier	HPP	Relatively common in blacks	270,271
	SpD-SpD contact	50-kd peptide cleaved at 256 Arg of 258 Lys	260 Leu → Pro (repetitive segment α2, helix 3)	260 CTG → CCG (exon 6 of α-Sp)				265,270
	SpD-SpD contact	50-kd peptide cleaved at 256 Arg of 258 Lys	261 Ser → Pro (repetitive segment α2, helix 3)	261 TTC → CCC (exon 6 of α-Sp)				265,270
Sp α^I/36 Sfax	SpD-SpD contact	36- and 33-kd peptides cleaved from the αI domain	Deletion of amino acids 363–371 from repetitive segment α3, helix 3	Deletion of 27 bases due to activation of a cryptic splice donor site in exon 8 of α-Sp	Asymptomatic HE		One report	272
Sp α^I/50b	SpD-SpD contact	50-kd peptide cleaved at 468 Arg or 470 Arg	469 His → Arg (repetitive segment α4, helix 3)	469 CAT → CGT (exon 11 of α-Sp)			Apparently rare	270,273
	SpD-SpD contact	50-kd peptide cleaved at 468 Arg or 470 Arg	471 Glu → Pro (repetitive segment α4, helix 3)	471 CAG → CCG (exon 11 of α-Sp)			One report	265,270
Barcelona	SpD-SpD contact	50-kd peptide cleaved at 468 Arg or 470 Arg	469 His → Pro (repetitive segment α4, helix 3)	469 CAT → CCT			One report	274
Alexandria	SpD-SpD contact	50-kd peptide cleaved at 468 Arg or 470 Arg	Deletion of 469 His	Deletion of codon 469			One black family	275
Sp α^II/31 Jendouba	SpD-SpD contact and another unknown defect	Abnormal peptides of 31, 26, 21, and 18 kd, cleavage after Lys 788	791 Asp → Glu (repetitive segment α7, helix 3)	791 GAC → GAA	Asymptomatic HE		Probably rare	276
Sp α^II/21 Oran	Slight impairment of the SpD-SpD contact	Abnormal 21- and 16-kd peptides derived from the αII domain	Deletion of amino acids 822–862 from repetitive segment α8	A → G(−1) in the acceptor splice site upstream of exon 18 leading to skipping of exon 18	Asymptomatic HE	Severe HE	One report	277,278
β-Spectrin								
Sp α^I/74 Cagliari	SpD-SpD contact	Increase in the 74-kd fragment cleaved from αI domain	2018 Ala → Gly (repeat β17)	2018 GCC → GGC (exon X of β-Sp)	Mild HE	Severe HPP	One report	279
Providence	SpD-SpD contact	Increase in the 74-kd fragment cleaved from αI domain	2019 Ser → Pro (repeat β17)	2019 TCT → CCT (exon X of β-Sp)	Mild HE	Lethal hydrops fetalis	One report	280
	SpD-SpD contact	Increase in the 74-kd fragment cleaved from αI domain	2053 Ala → Pro (repeat β17)	2053 GCT → CCT (exon X of β-Sp)	Asymptomatic	Severe HPP	One report	281

(Table continues)

Table 46-3. *(Continued)*

Designation[a]	Abnormal Function	Limited Proteolysis or Other Studies[b]	Primary Structure[b,c]	DNA Defect[d]	Heterozygote	Homozygote or Double Heterozygote	Prevalence and Comments	References
Sp β[220/330] Detroit	Nearly normal function	Spectrin β' chain of 330 kD, 25% of total, probably unstable			Asymptomatic HE caused by coexisting α I/65 mutation		One report	282
Sp β[220/218] Rouen	SpD-SpD contact	Spectrin β' chain of 218 kd with reduced phosphorylation	Abnormal and truncated C terminus	G → T(+3) in donor splice site leading to skipping of exon Y and frameshift with premature chain termination			One report	283,284
Sp β[220/216] Tandil	SpD-SpD contact	Truncated spectrin β' band with absence of phosphorylation	Abnormal and truncated C terminus	Deletion of 7 bp at codon 2041 in exon X of β-Sp	Hemolytic HE			285
Tokyo	SpD-SpD contact	Truncated spectrin β' band with absence of phosphorylation	Truncated C terminus due to premature chain termination	Deletion of C in codon 2059	Mild hemolytic HE		One report	286
Nice	SpD-SpD contact	Truncated spectrin β' band with absence of phosphorylation.	Truncated C terminus due to premature chain termination	AG duplication at codons 2045/2046 in exon X leading to frameshift and premature chain termination			One report, new mutation	287
Sp β[220/214] Göttingen	SpD-SpD contact	Truncated spectrin β' band with absence of phosphorylation	Truncated C terminus due to premature chain termination	T → A(+2) in the donor splice site of intron following exon X leading to skipping of exon X and a frameshift A → G(+4) in the donor splice site of inton following exon C leading to skipping of exon X and a frameshift			One report	288
LePuy	SpD-SpD contact	Truncated spectrin β' band with absence of phosphorylation	Truncated C terminus due to premature chain termination				One report	289

Protein / Variant[a]	Deficiency / defect	Protein mutation[b]	DNA mutation	Phenotype (heterozygote)	Phenotype (homozygote)	Comments	Ref
Protein 4.1							
4.1(−)	HE group involving partial or complete deficiency of protein 4.1	Complete protein 4.1 deficiency in the homozygote, 50% deficiency in heterozygotes	318-nt deletion encompassing the downstream (erythroid-specific) initiation codon ATG → AGG in the downstream initiation codon	Mild HE	Severe HE	Heterozygous state is relatively frequent in North Africa	290
Madrid		Complete 4.1 deficiency in the homozygote. Also marked reduction of glycophorin C and a decrease in spectrin and actin			Asymptomatic elliptocytosis	Severe HE	Molecular basis probably heterogeneous	291
4.1(+)	Membrane instability due to abnormal spectrin-actin interaction, incompletely studied	Protein 4.1-derived peptides of abnormal sizes						
4.1 80/95			Duplication of 407 Lys through 529 Gln	Duplication of 3 exons (63 + 177 + 129nt)			One report	292,293
4.1 80/76–78			Deletion of 407 Lys through 427 Glu	Deletion of 1 exon (63 nt)			One report[e]	294
4.1 80/65–68			Deletion of 407 Lys through 486 Gly	Deletion of 2 exons (63 + 177 nt)			One report	292,293
4.1 80/73,74 Presles			Deletion of 34 amino acids	Preferential skipping of one exon (102 nt)	Asymptomatic		One report	295
Glycophorin C							
Leach		Absence of glycophorin C	Deletion of exons 3 and 4	7-kb gene deletions encompassing exons 3 and 4	Asymptomatic	Mild HE	Rare	296–298
			Mutations in codons 44 and 45	TGGCCG → TTGCCG in codons 44, 45 resulting in frameshift and premature termination	Asymptomatic	Mild HE	One case	296

[a] Skeletal protein deficiencies are designated in parentheses following the disease state in which they have been described. Superscripts − and □ indicate a partial or complete protein deficiency, respectively. Spectrin mutations are designated by indicating in the superscript the most prominent tryptic peptide which is generated instead of the normal 80-kd peptide representing the αI domain. Elongated or truncated proteins are designated in the superscript by indicating the molecular weight of the normal and the mutant allele.

[b] The numbering of amino acids and the respective codons of α-spectrin is based on the cDNA sequence,[1] including the first six amino acids that were not detected by protein sequencing.[299,300] Position of β-spectrin mutation is marked according to Winkelmann et al.[3]

[c] The designation of the α-spectrin repetitive segments is based on the proposed spatial arrangement of helices 1, 2, and 3[301-303] and not on the sequence homology as originally proposed.[299,300,304,305] According to the conformation phasing,[302] the combined αβ triple helical segment is composed of repeat 17 of β-spectrin and repeat α′ (helix 3) from the N-terminal portion of α-spectrin and the first repetitive segment of α-spectrin begins with helix 1 (see also Fig. 4G-4).

[d] Position of the mutations in individual exons of the α-spectrin gene is designated according to Kotula et al.[2] Abnormal membrane proteins in which the mutation has not been defined at the DNA level are not included in this table.

[e] This mutation was detected in dog erythrocytes.[294]

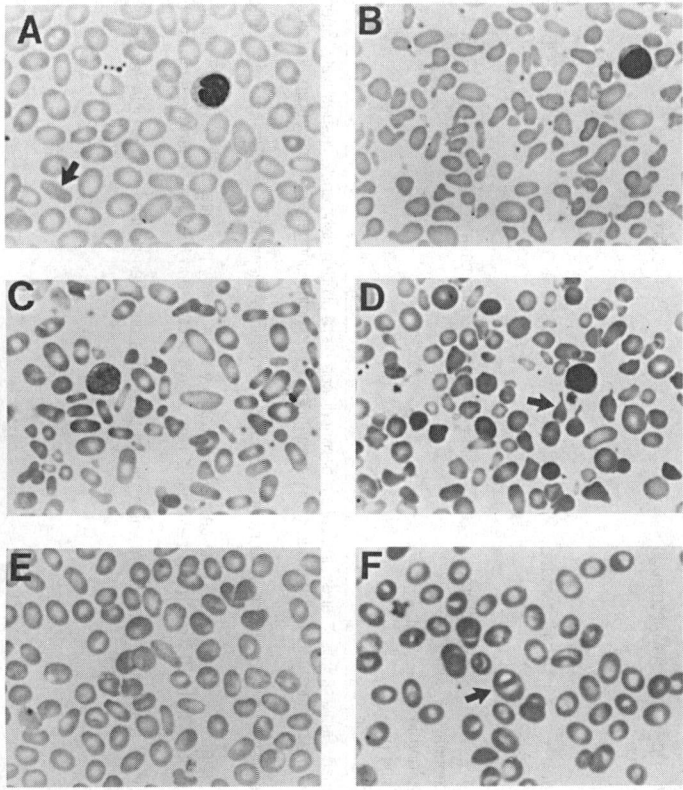

Fig. 46-8. Blood films of subjects with various forms of HE. **(A)** Simple heterozygote with mild common HE Sp α^{I/65}. Note the predominant elliptocytosis with some rod-shaped cells (arrow) and virtual absence of poikilocytes. **(B)** Simple heterozygote with severe common hemolytic elliptocytosis (HE Sp α^{I/74}). Note the numerous small fragments and poikilocytes. **(C)** "Homozygous" common HE due to doubly heterozygous state for two mutant α-spectrins, Sp α^{I/74} and Sp α^{I/65}. Both parents have mild HE. Again, note the many elliptocytes as well as numerous fragments and poikilocytes. **(D)** HPP, Sp α^{I/74}. The patient is a double heterozygote for mutant α-spectrin (Sp α^{I/74}) and a presumed synthetic defect of this protein. Note the prominent microspherocytosis, micropoikilocytosis, and fragmentation. Only few elliptocytes are present. Some poikilocytes are in the process of budding (arrow). **(E)** Spherocytic HE (hereditary ovalocytosis). Most red cells are oval rather than truly elliptical. Many oval cells are "fat," lacking a central concavity, the feature distinguishing spherocytic HE from common HE. **(F)** SAO (Melanesian). Most cells are oval, some containing either a longitudinal slit or a transverse ridge (arrow). All blood smears were photographed at the same magnification. (×1,000.) The molecular defects are designated as described in Table 46-3.

ease.[255,328,329] Most patients with protein 4.1 deficiency are of North African descent.[308,330] The protein 4.1 deficiencies defined to date involve a deletion that includes the exon encoding the erythroid transcription start size,[290] a mutation of the transcription initiation codon,[291] and other defects.[50] The dysfunctions of the 4.1 protein include deletions and duplications of the exons encoding the spectrin-binding domain, leading either to truncated or elongated forms of protein 4.1.[50]

Glycophorin C Deficiency

Glycophorin C has been found absent due to a variety of molecular defects.[36] In contrast to other forms of HE, which are dominantly inherited, heterozygous carriers are asymptomatic with normal red blood cell morphology while homozygous subjects have no anemia, with only mild elliptocytosis as shown on the peripheral blood film.[36]

Glycophorin C deficiency with elliptocytosis (the so-called Leach phenotype[331,332]), caused by reduced expression of glycophorin C, should be distinguished from the immunochemically defined phenotypes Gerbich and Yus, in which abnormal

glycoproteins are formed that can functionally substitute for normal glycophorin C and preserve the normal red cell shape.[36,333,334]

Glycophorin C-deficient subjects are also partially deficient in the 4.1 protein. In addition, glycophorin C is decreased in patients with protein 4.1 deficiency, presumably because the two proteins form a complex and recruit or stabilize each other on the membrane.[335,336] By contrast, subjects deficient in glycophorin A, the major transmembrane glycoprotein, are asymptomatic.[337]

Pathobiology of the Red Cell Lesion

Most of the elliptocytogenic mutations of spectrin reside within, or in the vicinity of, the spectrin heterodimer contact site disrupting this site, consequently disrupting the two-dimensional integrity of the membrane skeleton. These "horizontal" defects are readily detected by ultrastructural examination

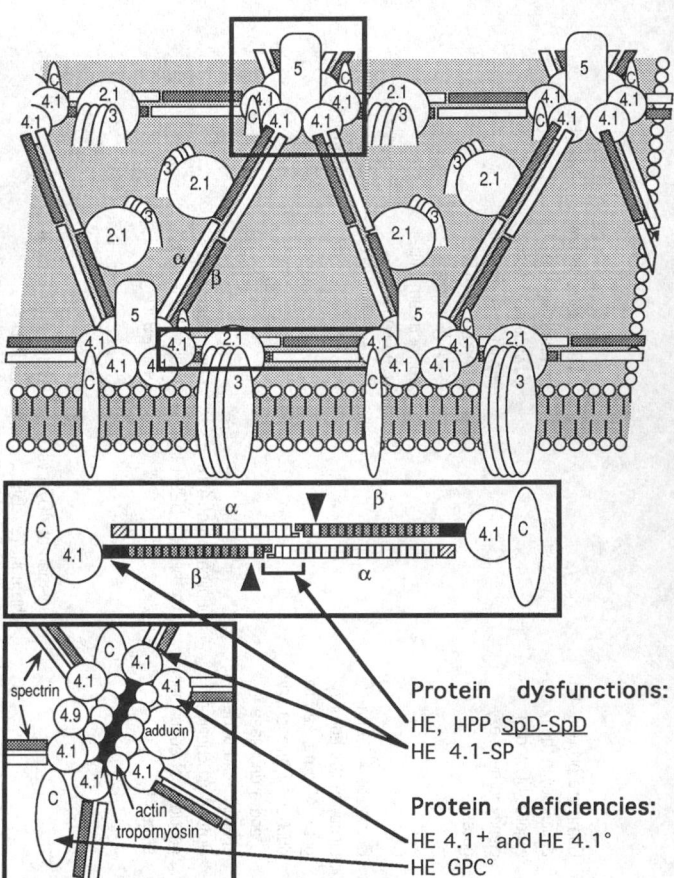

Fig. 46-9. Schematic representation of the molecular assembly of the membrane skeleton and the molecular defects in HE and HPP. Spectrin is composed of α-spectrin and β-spectrin heterodimers (SpD) that associate in their head regions into tetramers. At their distal ends, SpD bind to the junctional complexes of oligomeric actin (band 5) and protein 4.1. Additional proteins found in the junctional complex, such as adducin, tropomyosin, and protein 4.9, are shown in the lower enlarged area. Membrane skeleton is attached to transmembrane proteins by interactions of β-spectrin with ankyrin (protein 2.1, black arrow designates the ankyrin-binding site in β-spectrin), which in turn binds to the cytoplasmic domain of band 3, and by linkage of protein 4.1 to glycophorin C. The known protein dysfunctions in HE and HPP include (1) defects of the SpD head region due to a mutation of either α- or β-spectrin, causing impaired assembly of SpD into tetramers; or (2) an abnormality of protein 4.1, which binds weakly to spectrin. The known protein deficiencies include those of protein 4.1 and glycophorin C. The clinical expression of these defects and the underlying genetic lesions are shown in Table 46-3.

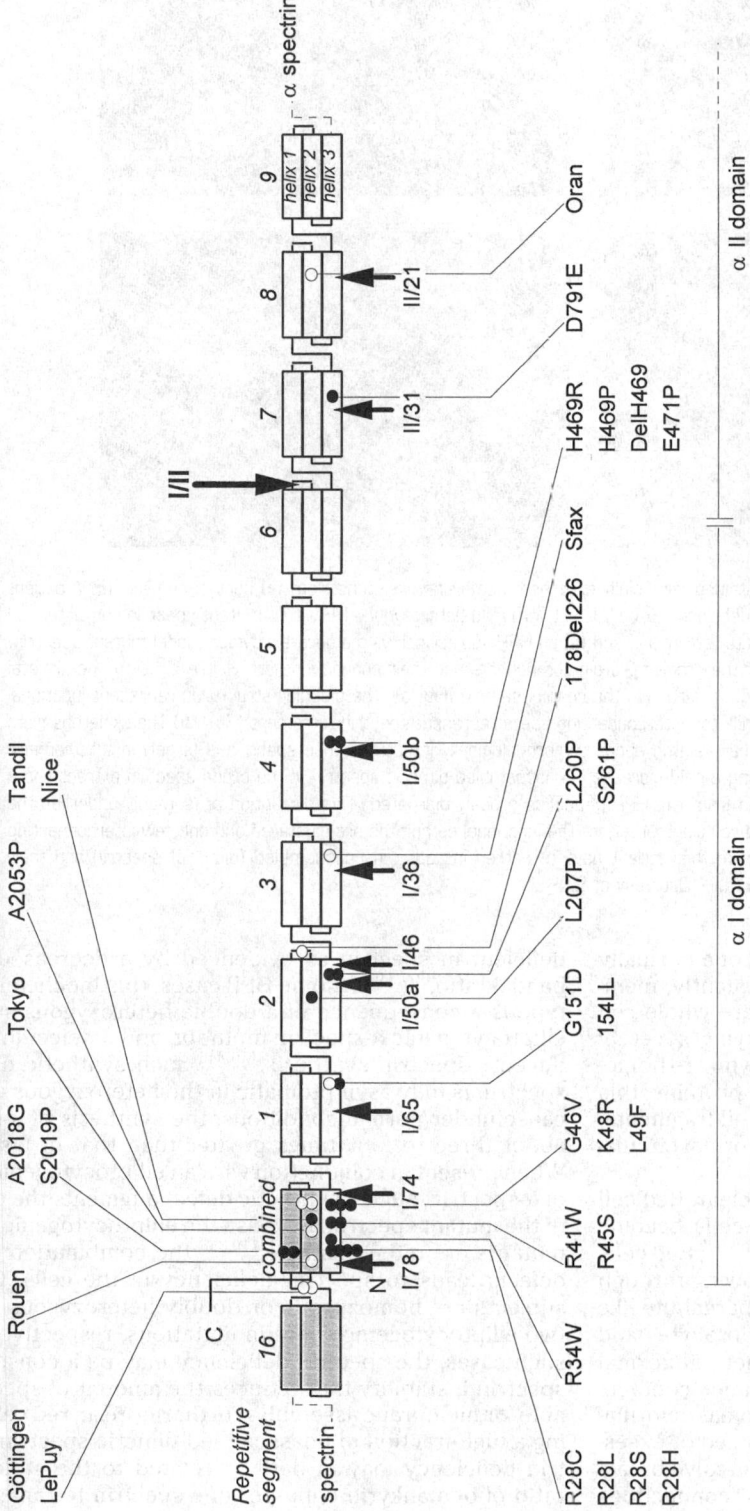

Fig. 46-10. Mutations of α- and β-spectrin affecting association of spectrin dimers into tetramers. Schematic representation of the contact site between the α- and β-spectrin chanins of the opposite heterodimers. Full circles denote point mutations and open circles designated protein deletions and insertions, all of which affecting self-association of spectrin heterodimers into tetramers. The position of open circles corresponds to the last normal amino acid preceding the mutation. We use the abbreviated designation of point mutations (e.g., A2053P being 2053 Ala → Pro, R28C 28 Arg → Cys, 178Del226 deletion of amino acids 178 to 226, 154LL duplication of leucine 154). For protein deletions, we use their designation from the original reports whenever available. The numbering of amino acids and the respective codons of α-spectrin is based on the cDNA sequence,[1] including the first six amino acids not detected by protein sequencing.[299,300] Most mutations either increase trypsin cleavage at normal sites or open new trypsin cleavage sites (short arrows) giving rise to abnormal tryptic peptides. Their sizes are indicated next to the short arrows. The size of these abnormal peptides provides a basis for designation of some of these mutations (e.g., Sp α[I/46], see Table 46-3). Trypsin cleavage site creating the normal 80-kd αI peptide is denoted by the long arrow. The spectrin repetitive segments are phased according to conformation, rather than sequence homology.[302] Correspondingly, the combined repeat contains α-spectrin repeat α′ (helix 3) and β-spectrin repeat 17. Repetitive segment, αI is then formed by helices 1, 2, and 3. Note that most spectrin mutations are located within helix 3 of each repetitive segment. For more detailed description of individual mutations, see Table 46-3. [From Palek and Jarolim,[45] with permission.]

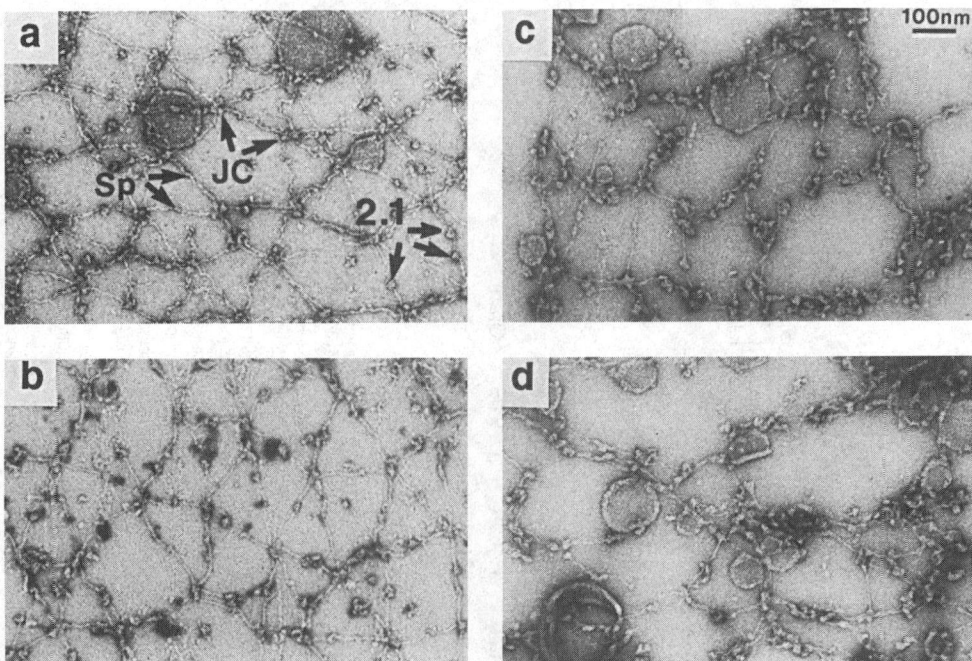

Fig. 46-11. Electron micrographs of negatively stained, artificially extended membrane skeletons from **(a)** control subject, **(b)** a patient with moderately severe HS with partial spectrin deficiency, **(c)** a subject with mild heterozygous HE with a mutant spectrin characterized by a defective self-association of spectrin dimers to tetramers, and **(d)** an HPP subject carrying a severely dysfunctional mutant spectrin. The skeletons were uniformly stretched so that their major protein components and their connections are visible.[312] Only one skeletal layer is exposed. Note the uniform, largely hexagonal lattice in the control sample (Fig. a). The globular structures represent junctional complexes (JC) composed of oligomeric actin, while the interconnecting fibers represent spectrin tetramers (Sp). **(b)** The skeletons from an HS patient with a spectrin deficiency. The skeleton appears morphologically intact, because spectrin is largely in a tetrameric form. **(c)** A carrier of the spectrin mutation having a mild increase in unassembled dimeric spectrin in the crude spectrin extract and a mildly disrupted skeletal lattice. **(d)** The skeleton from the HPP patient is grossly disrupted. This disruption presumably underlies the marked membrane instability of red cells and red cell fragmentation. The junctional complexes are clustered and only few interconnecting spectrin tetramers can be seen. Membranes from this patient have a marked increase in unassembled (dimeric) spectrin and their spectrin content is reduced to about 70% of normal. (Courtesy of S.C. Liu.)

of membrane skeleton, which reveals disruption of a normally uniform hexagonal lattice[338] (Fig. 46-11). Consequently, membrane skeletons are mechanically unstable, as are whole cell membranes and the cells.[48,339] In patients carrying severely dysfunctional spectrin mutations, or in subjects who are homozygous or doubly heterozygous for such mutant proteins, this membrane instability is sufficient to cause red cell fragmentation with hemolytic anemia under conditions of normal circulatory shear stress.

The pathobiology of elliptocytic shape is less clear. Red cell precursors in common HE are round, and the cells become progressively more elliptical as they age in vivo.[340–342] Red cells subjected to shear stress in vitro, or red cells flowing through microcirculation in vivo, have an elliptical or parachute-like shapes, respectively.[143,343] It is possible that elliptocytes and poikilocytes are permanently stabilized in their abnormal shape because the weakened spectrin heterodimer contacts facilitate skeletal reorganization, which follows axial deformation of cells resulting from application of a prolonged or excessive shear stress. This reorganization is likely to involve breakage of the unidirectionally stretched protein connections followed by a formation of new protein contacts that preclude the recovery of normal biconcave shape.[339] This process has been recently shown to account for permanent deformation of irreversibly sickle cells.[344]

In HPP, the recessively inherited form of HE characterized by severe hemolysis, red cells have two abnormalities. They contain a mutant spectrin that characteristically disrupts spectrin heterodimer self-association, and they are also partially deficient in spectrin as evidenced by a decreased spectrin/band 3 ratio.[309,345] In some HPP cases, this biochemical phenotype is a consequence of a double heterozygous state for an elliptocytogenic α-spectrin mutation and a defect involving reduced α-spectrin synthesis.[110,346] Such synthetic defect of α-spectrin is fully asymptomatic in the heterozygous carrier, because under normal conditions, the synthesis of α-spectrin is about three to four times greater than that of β-spectrin.[113] When present in conjunction with an elliptocytogenic mutation of α-spectrin, such a synthetic defect augments the expression of the mutant spectrin. Because the elliptocytogenic α-spectrin mutants are often unstable,[110,345] the combination of the two defects leads to spectrin deficiency in the cells. Other HPP subjects are homozygous or doubly heterozygous for one or two elliptocytogenic spectrin mutations, respectively.[110,347] In such cases, the spectrin deficiency may be a consequence of spectrin instability that reduces the amount of spectrin available for membrane assembly. Furthermore, in red cells containing a high fraction of unassembled dimeric spectrin, the spectrin deficiency may in part be related to the stoichiometric ratio of one ankyrin copy per one spectrin tetramer (i.e., two spectrin heterodimers). Consequently, only about one-half of spectrin heterodimers succeed in attaching to the ankyrin binding sites. The phenotype of HPP, characterized by the presence of fragments and elliptocytes, together with evidence of red cell surface area deficiency (as reflected by the presence of microspherocytes on the peripheral blood film), suggests that the membrane dysfunction involves both the vertical interactions (a consequence of spectrin deficiency, see above) and the horizontal interactions involving the elliptocytogenic spectrin mutation.

The red cell lesion in 4.1 deficiency shows similarities in regard to cell shape and membrane stability to the above elliptocytogenic mutations of spectrin,[339] suggesting that the deficiency principally affects the spectrin-actin contact (i.e., a horizontal interaction) rather than the skeleton attachment to glycophorin C via the 4.1 protein (a vertical interaction).

The molecular basis of elliptocytosis and mechanical instability of glycophorin C deficient red cells is not fully understood. However, recent studies suggest that the deficiency of glycophorin C is not directly responsible for the altered mechanical properties.[348] Instead, the mechanical instability appears to be related to a concomitant partial deficiency of protein 4.1, as evidenced by a full correction of membrane instability by introduction into the cells of protein 4.1 or its spectrin-binding peptide, which facilitates the contact of β-spectrin to actin. The superimposed deficiency of protein 4.1 is likely to be related to the fact that the glycophorin C serves as an attachment site for protein 4.1 to the membrane, recruiting protein 4.1 to the red cell membrane.[36,50] The effects of the above defects on the mechanical stability of glycophorin C deficient cells appear relatively minor, because glycophorin C deficient subjects have no detectable hemolytic anemia and the mechanical properties of the red cells are normal when tested by micropipette aspiration.[349]

Previous studies of HE red cells revealed increased utilization of ATP and 2,3-diphosphoglycerate,[350] presumably due to increased transmembrane sodium movements.[351] As a result of the underlying skeletal defect, HE and HPP red cells also exhibit an abnormally increased Na, K, and Ca permeability.[351,352] The latter defect was proposed to represent the primary molecular lesion in a case of severe microcytic hemolytic anemia associated with thermal instability of red cells, but subsequent studies of this patient identified a spectrin mutation.[352,353]

Inheritance

In most patients, HE is inherited as an autosomal dominant disorder. The clinical severity is highly variable both among different kindred (reflecting heterogeneous molecular lesions[46,310,354]) and, to a lesser extent in a given kindred, presumably because of other genetic or acquired defects that modify disease expression.[355–357] Occasionally, HE is inherited as an autosomal recessive condition from an asymptomatic parent who carries the same molecular defect of spectrin as the HE offspring.[46] HE is linked to blood group antigens Rh and Duffy, the genes of which are located on chromosome 1; the Duffy blood group locus being close to the gene for α-spectrin,[358,359] while the Rh gene locus (1p 33) is close to the gene for protein 4.1[244,290,360,361] (Table 46-1).

The inheritance of HPP, a disorder closely related to HE, is autosomal recessive: one of the parents carries the α-spectrin mutation and either is asymptomatic or has mild HE, while the other parent is fully asymptomatic and has no detectable abnormalities by current biochemical approaches.[46,310] However, several HPP patients have been recently studied who were doubly heterozygous for two α-spectrin mutations; in the heterozygous parents, these mutations were either silent or expressed as mild HE.[362]

Clinical Manifestations

In view of the striking molecular heterogeneity of common HE, it is not surprising that the clinical spectrum of this disorder is variable ranging from an asymptomatic trait without hemolysis to a life-threatening hemolytic anemia.

Mild Hereditary Elliptocytosis and Asymptomatic Carrier State

In most of these subjects, HE is found accidentally during evaluation of the peripheral blood film. While some HE subjects have a mild compensated hemolytic anemia,[169,357,363] others do not have any evidence of hemolysis, their red cell survival is normal,[364] and the peripheral blood film may reveal only modest ($\geq 15\%$) elliptocytosis[46,310]; they even may be blood donors.[365] The molecular basis of mild HE is heterogeneous, and the reported molecular defects include both α- and β-spectrin mutations, partial deficiency of the 4.1 protein, and the absence of glycophorin C (Table 46-3). Some individuals carrying the spectrin mutation are fully asymptomatic, including normal red cell morphology; this is often the case in one of the parents of a patient with HPP.[46,310,354,366]

Hereditary Elliptocytosis with Sporadic Hemolysis

Worsening of hemolysis together with appearance of poikilocytes on the peripheral blood film has been reported in patients with hypersplenism, infections, vitamin B_{12} deficiency,[46] as well as microangiopathic hemolysis such as disseminated intravascular coagulation, or thrombotic thrombocytopenic purpura.[367] In the latter two conditions, worsening hemolysis may be due to microcirculatory damage superimposed on the underlying mechanical instability of red cells.

Hereditary Elliptocytosis with Neonatal Poikilocytosis

Neonate offsprings of parents with mild HE present with symptomatic hemolytic anemia and a marked poikilocytosis. During the first year of life, the hemolysis and poikilocytosis abate, and the clinical picture transforms into that of mild HE.[368–370] Such patients typically carry one mutant α-spectrin allele.[46,310] The severity of the molecular defect, in terms of the percentage of spectrin dimers and the amount of mutant spectrin in the cells, is the same in the neonatal period as it is later in life. The worsening of hemolysis in the neonatal period has been attributed to the presence of fetal hemoglobin, which binds poorly to 2,3-diphosphoglycerate (2,3-DPG).[371] The ensuing elevation of free 2,3-DPG levels has a marked destabilizing effect on the spectrin-protein 4.1-actin interaction,[371,372] thereby further destabilizing the membrane skeleton.

Hereditary Elliptocytosis with Chronic Hemolysis

Patients with HE with chronic hemolysis present with moderate to severe hemolytic anemia with elliptocytes and poikilocytes on peripheral blood film; some require splenectomy.[355–357,373,374] In some of the kindred, the hemolytic HE has been transmitted through several generations.[375,376] In two families, the afflicted individuals carried a severely dysfunctional Sp α[I/74].[258] In some kindred, not all the HE subjects have chronic hemolysis; some of them have a mild hemolysis only, presumably because of another genetic factor modifying the disease expression.[355,357]

Homozygous and Doubly Heterozygous Hereditary Elliptocytosis

Several HE individuals have been reported who were apparent homozygotes for the HE gene.[46,310,377] More recently, these cases were found to be either homozygotes or double heterozygotes for one or two α- or β-spectrin mutations[347,378–380] (Table 46-3). The clinical severity is variable, depending on the severity of the underlying molecular defect; patients homozygous for the mildly dysfunctional Sp α[I/65] have a relatively mild hemolytic anemia that does not require splenectomy, while other homozygous or doubly heterozygous patients, such as those with the Sp $\alpha^{I/74}$ mutation have a severe life-threatening disease.[347,378] In addition, peripheral blood films of some homozygous HE subjects (e.g., Sp $\alpha^{I/74}$) contain numerous very small microspherocytes, and their red cells are partially deficient in spectrin.[347] Thus, their clinical presentation is indistinguishable from HPP.

Hereditary Pyropoikilocytosis

Under the term HPP, Zarkowsky et al.[238] described an autosomal recessive severe hemolytic anemia with striking micropoikilocytosis and thermal instability of red cells. It is now established that HPP represents a subtype of common HE as evidenced by the coexistence of both HE and HPP in the same family and the presence of the same molecular defect of spectrin (Sp $\alpha^{I/74}$, Sp $\alpha^{I/46}$, or Sp $\alpha^{I/78}$) (Table 46-3). Unlike HE subjects carrying the spectrin mutation, red cells of the HPP subjects are also partially deficient in spectrin.[309,345] Typically, one parent of the HPP offspring carries an α-spectrin mutation, while the other parent is fully asymptomatic and has no detectable biochemical abnormality. In many such patients, the asymptomatic parent carries a silent "thalassemia-like" defect of spectrin synthesis, enhancing the expression of the spectrin mutant and leading to a superimposed spectrin deficiency in the HPP offspring.[46,310] Some HPP subjects inherited two α-spectrin mutations; their parents were either hematologically normal, or one of them had mild HE.[310,347,362] In these HPP patients, spectrin deficiency may be related to instability of the mutant spectrin.[381] In one such doubly heterozygous proband,[382] these red cell spectrin content (spectrin/band 3 ratio) was normal, the hemolysis was mild, and the peripheral blood smear resembled hemolytic HE (poikilocytes and elliptocytes) rather than HPP, further highlighting the overlap between these two disorders. The thermal instability of spectrin originally reported as diagnostic of HPP is not unique for this disorder, and it is also found in HE subjects carrying this α-spectrin mutation, both in the homozygous and the heterozygous state.[347] HPP is seen predominantly in black subjects, but it has also been diagnosed in Arabs and whites.[308,383–385]

Molecular Determinants of Clinical Severity

The severity of hemolysis in common HE often varies not only among different kindred but within a given family as well. The two principal determinants of severity of hemolysis are the spectrin content of the cells and the percentage of dimeric spectrin in the crude spectrin extract.[49] The fraction of dimeric spectrin in such extract, in turn, depends on several factors. The first of them is the degree of dysfunction of the mutant spectrin. Typically, mutations that are either within or near the combined $\alpha\beta$ triple helical repetitive segment representing the spectrin heterodimer self-association site produce a more severe clinical phenotype and more severe defect of spectrin function than are seen with point mutations in the more distant triple helical repeats.[51] Second, the percentage of the dimeric spectrin depends on the fraction of the mutant spectrin in the cells, which, in turn, is determined by the gene dose (e.g., simple heterozygote versus homozygote or double heterozygote) or the presence of other genetic defects such as the presence, in trans, of a defect leading to a reduced α-spectrin synthesis in some subjects with HPP. Another determinant of the fraction of the mutant spectrin in the cells and, consequently, the severity of hemolysis is an additional α-spectrin mutation either in cis or in trans, located within the site at which spectrin monomers assemble into heterodimers (the spectrin heterodimer nucleation site).[51,301,386] The presence of such mutation in trans diminishes the propensity of the otherwise normal allele to associate with the corresponding β-chain, favoring the attachment of the elliptocytogenic α-spectrin allele. Conversely, the coexistence of the α-spectrin mutation in cis together with the mutation involving the α-spectrin nucleation site diminishes the propensity of the mutant allele to be incorporated into the spectrin heterodimer, thereby ameliorating the clinical severity of this mutation.[51,386]

Certain acquired factors affect the clinical severity of HE. In neonatal red cells, the weak binding of 2,3-DPG by fetal hemoglobin leads to an increase in free 2,3-DPG, which in turn induces a superimposed destabilization of the spectrin-actin-protein 4.1 interaction.[371,372] Lastly, hemolytic anemia can be worsened by several acquired conditions, including those that alter the microcirculatory stress to the cells.[367]

Laboratory Evaluation

Blood Film and Laboratory Evidence of Hemolysis

A careful blood smear evaluation is essential both for the diagnosis of HE and the classification of the disorder into three major subtypes outlined above (Fig. 46-8). In patients in whom elliptocytosis is the only morphologic abnormality, hemolysis is characteristically minimal or absent, with the exception of spherocytic elliptocytosis, in which the presence of round "fat" ovalocytes is associated with accelerated red cell destruction (see below). In patients with hemolytic forms of common HE, poikilocytosis is characteristically found on the blood film. In severe forms of HE, particularly in homozygous HE, many red cells circulate as cell fragments, producing a marked decrease in mean cell volume. Finding of red cell fragments together with a striking microspherocytosis, and often only occasional elliptocytes is characteristic of HPP (Fig. 46-8).

Osmotic, Thermal, and Mechanical Fragility

Osmotic fragility is increased in HPP, in spherocytic elliptocytosis, and in those HE patients who have poikilocytosis on their peripheral blood film.[46,71,197] In patients with a mild common HE without poikilocytosis on the peripheral blood film, osmotic fragility is normal.[71]

Thermal instability of red cells has been originally reported by Zarkowsky et al.[238] as a characteristic feature of HPP. It reflects thermal instability of the mutant spectrin: in normal red cells, spectrin is denatured and red cell fragment at 49°C. HPP red cells fragment and their spectrin denatures at 46°C. However, the diagnostic value of this test is limited, since thermal instability of red cells is also noted in HE red cells containing mutant spectrin.[347] By contrast, an occasional patient with otherwise typical HPP may have a normal thermal stability of both red cells and spectrin.[387] Red cells in common HE have unstable membranes and membrane skeletons when subjected to shear stress.[46,388]

Electrophoretic Separation of Solubilized Membrane Proteins

In HE and HPP, the SDS-PAGE approach may reveal proteins of abnormal mobility, the origin of which can be subsequently identified by Western blotting (e.g., truncated β- or α-spectrins in HE and HPP, or elongated or truncated forms of the 4.1 protein, and a partial or, rarely, complete deficiency of the 4.1 protein in HE) (Fig. 46-12A and Table 46-3). In HPP, SDS-PAGE reveals a partial deficiency of spectrin, as indicated by a decreased spectrin/band 3 ratio.[309,345] Spectrin deficiency, in conjunction with an elliptocytogenic spectrin mutation affecting the spectrin heterodimer contact, is invariably found in HPP.

In a rare subject with a mild recessive HE, it is useful to stain the gels with the periodic acid-Schiff reagent. This approach may reveal a deficiency of glycophorin C. Glycophorin C deficiency is also found in patients deficient in the 4.1 protein,

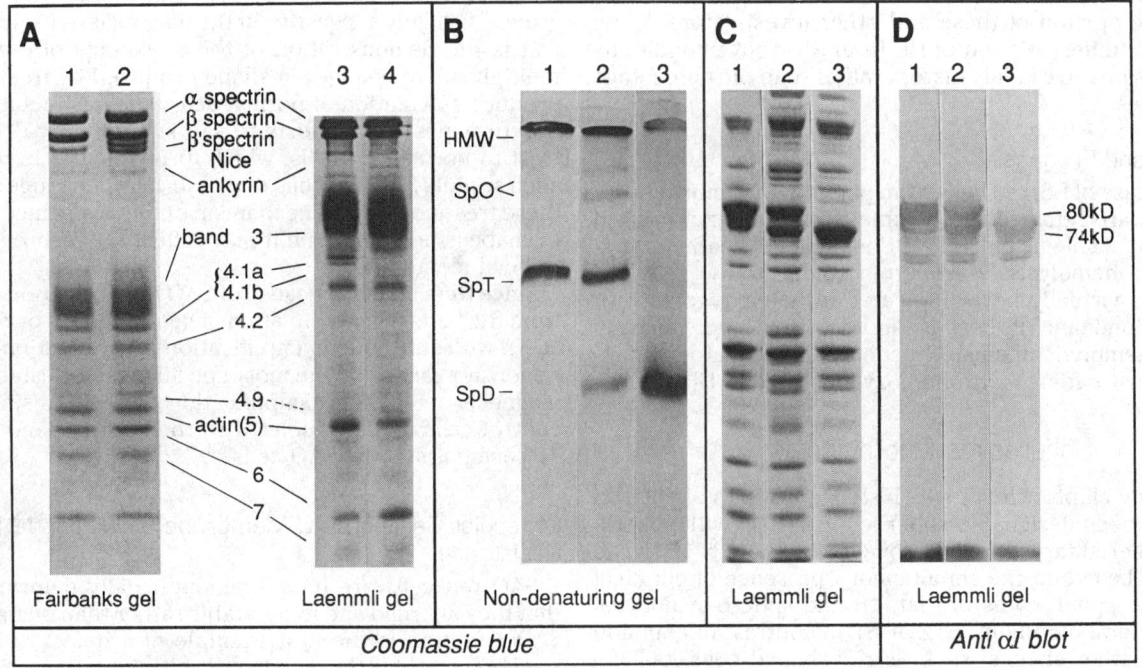

Fig. 46-12. Evaluation of a defect of the membrane skeleton in HE and HPP. **(A)** Identification of β-spectrin mutant with abnormal mobility (Spectrin Nice; gel 2) and the deficiency of protein 4.1 (gel 4) in HE. Membrane proteins from control red cells (gels 1 and 3) and red cells of the two patients (gels 2 and 4) were solubilized in sodium dodecylsulfate and electrophoresed in a Fairbanks nonlinear 3.5–17% polyacrylamide gradient gel[193] (first two gels) and Laemmli gel[192] (last two gels). Note excellent resolution of α-spectrin β-spectrin, and ankyrin bands, as well as the β-spectrin mutant (Spectrin Nice) in the modified Fairbanks system. In the Laemmli system, β-spectrin and ankyrin bands overlap. However, the Laemmli system resolves band 4.1 into two bands (4.1a, 4.1b). Both bands are absent in the HE 4.1° (gel 4). **(B)** Nondenaturing polyacrylamide gels of crude Sp extracts: 1 is a control, 2 is one of the two parents who both have common HE, and 3 is a homozygous HE offspring. Red cells of the HE parent, who is heterozygous for the Sp $\alpha^{1/74}$, contain both dimeric (SpD) and tetrameric (SpT) Sp. In the homozygous offspring, Sp is almost exclusively in a dimeric state. **(C & D)** SDS-PAGE of tryptic digests of Sp and the corresponding immunoblots with anti-α I antibody (Fig. D) from the members of the same family. Note that the gel from the HE parent contains both the normal 80,000-dalton and the abnormal 74,000-dalton peptides, implying that the parent is a simple heterozygote for the Sp $\alpha^{1/74}$ mutant. In the gel from the homozygous offspring, only the abnormal 74,000-dalton peptide is seen. (From Palek and Lambert,[49] with permission.)

possibly because the latter protein plays a role in the recruitment of glycophorin C on the membrane.[36,50]

Nondenaturing Gel Electrophoresis of Low Ionic Strength Spectrin Extract

Analysis of the ratio of tetrameric and dimeric spectrin in the low ionic strength extracts reveals the most common functional abnormality in HE (i.e., weakened self-association of spectrin heterodimers into tetramers) (Fig. 46-12B). Because the spectrin dimer-tetramer interconversion has a high activation energy, it is kinetically immobilized at near 0°C.[389] Consequently, the percentage of spectrin dimers and tetramers in the 0°C crude spectrin extract reflects the relative distribution of these species in the red cell membrane in situ.[390] Mutations of α- or β-spectrin residing within or near the αβ spectrin heterodimer contact site invariably lead to increase in the fraction of dimeric spectrin (normal range 5 ± 5%) in the crude 0°C spectrin extract[51,391] (Table 46-3).

Tryptic Peptide Mapping of Spectrin and the Detection of the Underlying DNA Defect

As reviewed,[51,98,391] tryptic digestion of spectrin under controlled conditions followed by electrophoretic separation gives rise to highly reproducible tryptic peptide patterns (Fig. 46-12C & D). Among these peptides, the 80-kd αI domain peptide representing the self-association site of the normal α-spectrin

is the most prominent one. Virtually all α- or β-spectrin mutations reported to date are associated with a formation of tryptic peptides of abnormal size and mobility that are generated instead of the normal 80-kd αI domain peptide. The cleavage sites of the most common abnormal tryptic peptides were mapped[51] and found to reside in the third helix of a given triple helical repetitive segment (Fig. 46-10). The reported mutations reside in the vicinity of these cleavage sites either in the same helix or, less commonly, in helix 1 or 2 of a given repetitive segment[51] (Fig. 46-10). Consequently, tryptic peptide mapping remains a powerful tool with which to map the site of the underlying spectrin mutation, which can be subsequently defined by polymerase chain reaction amplification and sequencing of the respective region of the genomic DNA or cDNA.

Differential Diagnosis

Various acquired and inherited conditions can be associated with elliptocytosis and poikilocytosis, including iron deficiency, thalassemias, megaloblastic anemias, myelofibrosis, myelophthisic anemias, myelodysplastic syndromes, and pyruvate kinase deficiency. The percentage of elliptocytes in these conditions is seldom >60%.[340,392,393] However, this is not diagnostically useful, since some HE subjects may have a relatively low percentage of elliptocytes.[46,310] In normal subjects, the percentage of elliptocytes is not >5%,[46,394] although in earlier reports, it was listed as high as 15%.[341,363] Previous diagnostic criteria of HE, based on the percentage of elliptocytes, such as

25%,[244] 33%,[395] or 40%,[341] and their axial ratio[356] do not appear useful in the opinion of these and other investigators.[71] The most reliable differentiation of HE from the above conditions is based on a positive family history rather than the percentage of elliptocytes.[71]

Treatment and Prognosis

As in the case of HS, red cells from patients with more severe forms of HE are retained by the spleen, producing a marked engorgement of splenic pulp.[396,397] Consequently, patients with symptomatic hemolysis benefit from splenectomy.[71,197] This procedure is virtually never indicated in heterozygotes with autosomal dominant HE because most do not have clinically significant hemolytic anemia. By contrast, splenectomy is required in most patients with homozygous HE and HPP.

Spherocytic Elliptocytosis

Spherocytic elliptocytosis, which shares features of both HS and HE, has been designated spherocytic HE, HE with spherocytosis, or hereditary hemolytic ovalocytosis.[49,310,398,399] The diagnosis is based on the simultaneous presence of elliptical red cells and spherocytes or "fat," round sphero-ovalocytes in the peripheral blood film (Fig. 46-8). In contrast to common HE, cells of other shapes, such as rod-shaped cells, poikilocytes, and fragments, are absent. Importantly, the presence of hemolysis, in spite of relatively mild alterations in red cell morphology, together with increased osmotic fragility, are the main diagnostic features distinguishing this disorder from common HE. The molecular basis of this rare condition is unknown.

Southeast Asian Ovalocytosis

SAO is characterized by the presence of oval red cells, many containing one or two transverse ridges or a longitudinal slit (Fig. 46-8). The condition is widespread in certain ethnic groups of Malaysia, Papua New Guinea, the Philippines, and Indonesia.[239,240,400–402] Numerous functional abnormalities of ovalocytes have been reported, including increased red cell rigidity,[403,404] decreased osmotic fragility,[241] increased thermal stability,[405,406] resistance to shape change by echinocytic agents,[53,404,406] and a reduced expression of many red cell antigens.[407] A remarkable feature of ovalocytes is their resistance to in vitro invasion by several strains of malaria parasites, including *Plasmodium falciparum* and *Plasmodium knowlesi*.[405,406,408] Moreover, in areas of endemic malaria, the ovalocytic subjects contain reduced numbers of intracellular parasites in vivo.[409]

The finding of a tight linkage of the abnormal proteolytic digest of erythrocyte band 3 protein to the SAO phenotype has led to the detection of the underlying molecular defect.[53] All carriers of the SAO phenotype were found to be heterozygotes, with one band 3 allele normal and the other containing two mutations in cis: the deletion of 9 colons encoding amino acids 400–408 from the boundary of the cytoplasmic and membrane domains of band 3 and the 56 Lys → Glu substitution.[52,54,55] The 56 Lys → Glu substitution represents an asymptomatic polymorphism known as the band 3 Memphis.[410–412] SAO phenotype is associated with a tighter binding of band 3 to ankyrin,[53] increased tyrosine phosphorylation of the band 3 protein,[413–415] inability to transport sulfate anions,[416,417] and a markedly restricted lateral and rotational mobility of the band 3 protein in the membrane.[53,54]

Laboratory Evaluation

The finding of ≥30% of oval red cells on the peripheral blood film, some containing a central slit or a transverse ridge, together with a notable absence of clinical and laboratory evidence of hemolysis in a subject from the above-noted ethnic groups, is highly suggestive of the diagnosis. A useful screening test is the demonstration of the resistance of ovalocytes or their ghosts to changes in shape produced by treatments that produce spiculation in normal cells, such as metabolic depletion or exposure of ghosts to salt solutions.[52,53,404,406] In contrast to normal red cells, which form spicules in response to such stimuli, SAO red cells or ghosts do not change shape after these treatments. The mechanism of this resistance to changes in shape is not clear, and it may reflect the high rigidity of the red cell membrane.

Since the underlying cause of SAO is the deletion of 27 bases from the band 3 gene, isolation of genomic DNA or reticulocyte cDNA with subsequent amplification of the deletion-containing region appears to be the most specific test for establishing the diagnosis of SAO. This amplification produces a single band in control cells and a doublet with the second band shorter by 27 base pairs in the SAO cells.[52,54,418]

Molecular Basis of SAO Membrane Rigidity and Malaria Resistance

SAO red cells are unique among axially deformed cells in that they are rigid and hyperstable rather than unstable.[403] The SAO mutation is the first example of a defect of an integral membrane protein leading to red cell membrane rigidity, which has been previously attributed to properties of the membrane skeleton.[143] Exposure of red cells to various ligands that bind to glycophorin A has been found to decrease membrane deformability.[419,420] In both conditions, conformational changes of the cytoplasmic domain of the respective proteins may preclude lateral movement (extension) of the skeletal network during deformation.[143] Another putative mechanism of the high SAO membrane rigidity is increased binding of band 3 to ankyrin and thus to the underlying skeleton[53] or increased propensity of the band 3 protein to aggregate into higher oligomers with increased band 3-ankyrin stoichiometry, which, in turn, can facilitate band 3 attachment to ankyrin.[421] Yet another proposed mechanism involves a nonspecific adherence of the SAO band 3 to the skeleton, possibly due to denaturation of the membrane spanning domain.[422]

The molecular basis of malaria resistance of SAO red cells is likely related to altered properties of the band 3 protein, which serves as one of the malaria receptors as evidenced by the inhibition of in vitro invasion by band 3-containing liposomes.[423] In normal red cells, the invasion process is associated with a marked membrane remodeling, which involves redistribution of intramembrane particles that contain band 3 protein.[424] Such particles cluster at the site of parasite invasion forming a ring around the orifice through which the parasite enters the cell. The invaginated red cell membrane, which surrounds the invading parasite, is free of intramembrane particles. The reduced lateral mobility of band 3 protein in SAO red cells[53,54] may preclude band 3 receptor clustering, thereby preventing the attachment of the parasites to the cells. Decreased exchange of anions across the red cell membrane has also been proposed to contribute to the resistance of ovalocytes to malaria invasion.[416,417] In addition, SAO red cells also consume ATP at a higher rate than normal cells, and the partial depletion of ATP levels in ovalocytes has been suggested to account, at least in part, for the resistance of these cells to malaria invasion in vitro.[425]

ACANTHOCYTOSIS AND RELATED CONDITIONS

Acanthocytes (from Greek *acantha* "thorn") or spur cells are red cells with prominent thorn-like surface protrusions, which vary in width, length, and surface distribution. Spur cells must

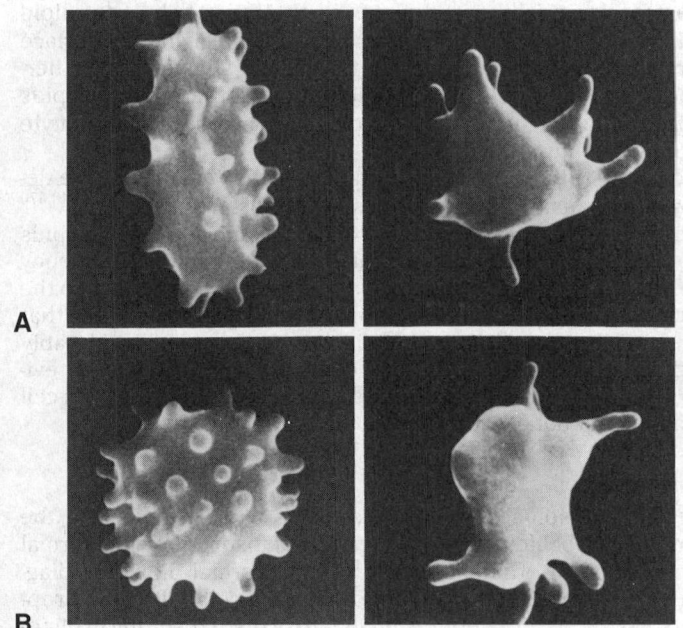

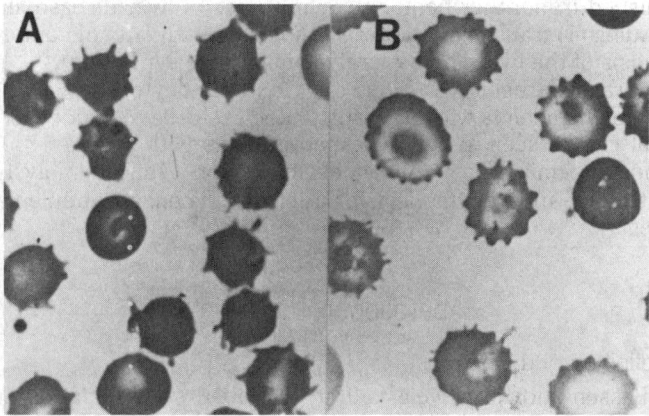

Fig. 46-14. Blood film of a patient with liver cirrhosis and spur cell anemia **(A)** before and **(B)** after splenectomy. The latter smear demonstrates the effect of cholesterol acquisition leading to both targeting (indicating increase in surface area) and irregularities in cell contour. The conditioning effect of the spleen (smear A) is demonstrated by the spheroidal shape of the cells and the remodeling of the spicules. (From Cooper et al.,[443] with permission.)

Fig. 46-13. Morphologic differences between **(A)** acanthocytes and **(B)** echinocytes as demonstrated by scanning electron microscope. (Adapted from Bessis,[426] with permission).

be distinguished from echinocytes (Greek *echinos* "urchin") or burr cells, characterized by multiple small projections that are uniformly distributed throughout the cell surface[426] (Fig. 46-13). Acanthocytes should be also distinguished from keratocytes ("horn" red cells) that have few massive protuberances (see below).

Acanthocytosis has been first described in abetalipoproteinemia[427,428] and subsequently in severe liver disease,[429,430] chorea-acanthocytosis syndrome,[431,432] McLeod blood group phenotype,[433] as well as other conditions.[434–438] In severe liver disease and abetalipoproteinemia, the molecular mechanisms leading to acanthocytosis have been extensively studied and have been attributed to changes in composition of membrane lipids and their altered distribution between the two hemileaflets of the lipid bilayer.

Spur Cell Hemolytic Anemia of Severe Liver Disease

Spur cell hemolytic anemia is an uncommon ominous complication of severe liver disease, manifested by rapidly progressive hemolytic anemia together with the presence of acanthocytes on the peripheral blood smear.[429,430,439,440]

Pathobiology

Human red cell membrane contains nearly equal amounts of free (unesterified) cholesterol and phospholipids. The plasma free cholesterol readily equilibrates with the red cell membrane cholesterol pool,[441] in contrast to esterified cholesterol that cannot be transferred from plasma into the red cell membrane. The plasma of patient's with severe liver disease contains abnormal lipoproteins that have a high free cholesterol/phospholipid ratio.[440] The excess free cholesterol readily partitions into the red cell membrane, leading to a marked increase in free cholesterol in the cells.[440,441] Consequently, spur cell shape can be produced in normal cells after their transfusion to a patient with severe liver disease,[439] incubation with patient's plasma, or with cholesterol-enriched liposomes.[442] Spur cell

formation involves two steps (Fig. 46-14). The first step is evident in red cells of splenectomized subjects with spur cell hemolytic anemia: red cells have an expanded surface area with irregular contour and targeting,[443] reflecting accumulation of free cholesterol in the membrane. This extra cholesterol accumulates preferentially in the outer bilayer leaflet, as suggested by findings of increased accessibility of cholesterol to cholesterol oxidase and a selective decrease in lipid fluidity of the outer hemileaflet of the lipid bilayer.[60,417,444]

The second step in acanthocyte formation involves red cell remodeling by the spleen.[443] As a result, red cells become spheroidal and the surface projections are considerably longer and more irregular (Fig. 46-14). The end result of this process are poorly deformable red cells with long bizarre projections[430,443,445] that are readily trapped in the spleen,[443] which is often markedly enlarged because of passive congestion due to underlying portal hypertension. Cholesterol also alters membrane permeability[446] and interacts with several membrane skeletal proteins,[447] but the role of these changes in spur cell lesions is unclear.

Clinical Manifestions

Most patients with chronic liver disease have a mild to moderate anemia related to gastrointestinal blood loss, iron and folic acid deficiencies, hemodilution, or direct effect of alcohol on red cell precursors.[441,448–450] Peripheral blood smears from these patients often reveal target cells that are particularly prominent in obstructive jaundice (see below).

In some patients, particularly those with end-stage liver disease, anemia rapidly worsens and a large percentage of spur cells appears on the blood film.[429,430,439,442] This is accompanied by a worsening jaundice, rapid deterioration of liver functions, hepatic encephalopathy, and hemorrhagic diathesis. A similar clinical syndrome has been described in patients with advanced metastatic liver disease, cardiac cirrhosis, Wilson disease, fulminant hepatitis, and infantile cholestatic liver disease.[451] The development of spur cell hemolytic anemia is an ominous sign in most patients, predicting a survival seldom exceeding weeks to months.[441] In theory, splenectomy could provide a marked improvement, since the spleen is the major sequestration site of nondeformable acanthocytes; in reality, splenectomy is seldom considered because of severity of the underlying liver disease.[443]

Spur cell hemolytic anemia of liver disease must be distinguished from other hemolytic syndromes of liver disease, including (1) transient hemolysis associated with fatty metamorphosis of the liver and hyperglycemia (Zieve syndrome),[441,452] (2) transient hemolytic anemia with stomatocytosis,[453,454] (3) hemolytic anemia with rigid spiculated red cells (echinocytes) that can be seen in malnourished patients with severe hypophosphatemia and hypomagnesemia,[455] or a mild hemolysis with some spherocytes seen in patients with congestive splenomegaly.[441]

Abetalipoproteinemia

Definition and History

Bassen and Kornzweig[427] first described an association of acanthocytosis with atypical retinitis pigmentosa, hepatic encephalopathy, and a "celiac disease" later attributed to fat malabsorption.[428] Subsequently, several investigators reported a congenital absence of β-lipoprotein, accounting for the diverse manifestations of the disorder.[456]

Pathobiology

This autosomal recessive disorder has been detected in people of diverse ethnic background.[456] The primary molecular defect involves a congenital absence of B apolipoprotein in plasma.[456-458] The B apoproteins (B100 and B48) are generated by alternate transcription of a single gene residing on the short arm of chromosome 2.[456] The deficiency is secondary to defective cellular secretion of the apoprotein by liver cells, caused either by aberrant post-translational processing or by defective aposecretion, as indicated by a significant increase in mRNA, as well as normal to increased amounts of hepatocyte apolipoprotein.[459] As a result, apoprotein B is absent in plasma as are the individual lipoprotein fractions that contain this apoprotein.[428,457,458] These include chylomicrons and very-low-density lipoproteins that transport triglycerides as well as low-density lipoproteins that are products of very-low-density lipoproteins and transport cholesterol. Consequently, preformed triglycerides are not transported from the intestinal mucosa,[457,460] and they are nearly absent in the plasma. Plasma cholesterol and phospholipids are markedly reduced with a relative increase in sphingomyelin at the expense of lecithin.[461-463]

As is the case in acanthocytosis of liver disease, the acanthocytic lesion is acquired from the plasma: red cell precursors have a normal shape and the acanthocytic lesion develops as the cells mature and age in the circulation.[457,464] Normal cells acquire this shape when transfused to the recipient.

The most striking abnormality of red cell membrane lipids involves a net increase in sphingomyelin. Since the plasma lipids readily exchange with the lipids of the red cell membrane,[446] it is likely that this change simply mirrors the alterations in plasma lipid composition. In contrast to red cells in spur cell anemia of severe liver disease, the content of membrane cholesterol is either normal or only slightly increased.[445,457,462,465]

The role of membrane lipids in the acanthocyte shape transformation has been first established by findings of restoration of biconcave shape after extraction of lipids from the cell membrane by detergents.[466] The molecular basis of acanthocytic shape is unknown, but several indirect observations suggest that it is related to an increase of the surface area of the outer hemileaflet of the lipid bilayer relative to the inner leaflet. In normal red cells, sphingomyelin is present predominantly in the outer bilayer leaflet[467]; thus, it is likely that the extra sphingomyelin is located in the same leaflet. This conclusion is supported by finding of shape transformation of acanthocytes to discocytes by incubation with chlorpromazine, a compound that preferentially accumulates in the inner half of the lipid bilayer, leading to its expansion, thus normalizing the surface area asymmetry between the two bilayer halves.[468] Furthermore, sphingomyelin is less fluid than the other phospholipids presumably accounting for the overall decrease in acanthocyte membrane fluidity.[469]

Several other abnormalities have been noted, including a decrease in plasma lecithin cholesterol transferase activity,[440,470] and an increased susceptibility of membrane and plasma lipids to oxidation, resulting from malabsorption-induced deficiency of vitamin E.[471] The contributions of these abnormalities to the acanthocyte red cell lesions is unknown. It should be noted that the membrane lesion in abetalipoproteinemia is considerably milder than that in spur cells of severe liver disease, as evidenced by only mild anemia and moderately shortened red cell half-life of abetalipoproteinemic acanthocytes.[457,461]

Clinical Manifestations

This autosomal recessive disease is usually evident in the first month of life, manifested by fat malabsorption with normal absorption of other nutrients.[457,460] Intestinal biopsy is diagnostic, revealing engorgement of mucosal cells with lipid droplets.[428,457,460,472,473] Retinitis pigmentosa often resulting in blindness; a progressive ataxia with intention tremors usually develops at 5–10 years of age, progressing to death in the second or third decade.[473,474] Occasionally, the ocular manifestations are absent.[475]

The hematologic manifestations are relatively mild and include mild normocytic anemia with acanthocytosis (50–90%) and normal or slightly elevated reticulocyte counts.[427,428,456,457,464] Occasional patients may have more severe anemia resulting from nutritional deficiencies (iron and folate) that accompany fat malabsorption.[456,457] The treatment includes dietary restriction of triglycerides and supplementation of lipid soluble vitamins A, K, D, and E. Vitamin E may stabilize, or even improve, both the retinal and neuromuscular abnormalities.[457]

Autosomal recessive abetalipoproteinemia should be distinguished from the homozygous form of familiar hypobetalipoproteinemia.[456,457] Although the clinical presentation of both disorders is similar, the latter disorder is milder and the parents have occasional acanthocytes on the peripheral blood film and their plasma low-density lipoproteins are decreased. The molecular lesions in familial hypobetalipoproteinemia involve a variety of apoprotein B gene mutations, leading to aberrant apoprotein B gene transcription or translation, including a formation of truncated forms.[456,476-480]

Variable degree of acanthocytosis without anemia has been also described in an isolated deficiency of apoprotein B100.[479,480] One of two reported patients was ataxic while the other had some degree of fat malabsorption. None had evidence of retinopathy and plasma triglycerides were normal.

Chorea-Acanthocytosis Syndrome

Reports largely published in the neurologic literature described an autosomal recessive syndrome of adult onset, manifested by multiple neurologic abnormalities, including limb chorea, progressive orofacial dyskinesia with ticks, and tongue-biting neurogenic muscle hypotonia and atrophy.[431,432,481-484] The hematologic manifestations are minimal, including a variable percentage of acanthocytes on the peripheral blood film without anemia and with normal or only slightly decreased red cell survival.[431,485]

Some subjects developed parkinsonism[486] or pigmentary retinopathy.[487] One patient with acanthocytosis had a stroke-like syndrome due to encephalopathy, chronic lactic acidosis (possibly related to mitochondrial abnormalities of the muscle), and pellagra-like changes on neuropathologic examination.[488]

The mechanism of acanthocytosis in this syndrome is unknown. Studies of plasma and red cell membrane lipids revealed no abnormalities[431,481,485,489] except for a high content of unsaturated fatty acids,[490] presumably accounting for a reduced red cell membrane fluidity.[489,490] Additional abnormalities of uncertain significance include an uneven distribution of intermembrane particles,[491] an impaired phosphorylation of the erythrocyte actin-bundling protein dematin,[492] and in one recent report, altered function and structure of the erythrocyte anion-exchange protein.[493]

McLeod Phenotype

The McLeod syndrome is characterized by a decreased expression of the Kell antigen on the red cell surface and a mild compensated hemolytic anemia with a variable percentage of acanthocytes in the peripheral blood (8–85%, better appreciated in wet preparation).[433,494,495] The McLeod syndrome was reported in association with chronic granulomatous disease of childhood,[496,497] retinitis pigmentosa, and Duchenne muscular dystrophy.[498] This association is due to the close proximity of the genetic loci for the above disorders in the p21 region of the X chromosome (Xp21); its deletion leads to the above diseases.[497–500] It is possible that the close linkage of the McLeod phenotype to that of the Duchenne muscular dystrophy gene (coding for skeletal protein dystrophin that is abnormal in this disease[501]) may explain occasional findings of either echinocytes or stomatocytes in Duchenne dystrophy,[502] or a choreiform disorder in some subjects with McLeod phenotype.[503,504] Because of the red cell mosaicism predicted by the Lyon hypothesis of X chromosome inactivation, female heterozygote carriers may have occasional acanthocytes on the peripheral blood film.[495,496]

The molecular basis of acanthocytosis in the McLeod syndrome is unknown. The Kell antigen appears to consist of two protein components: 37-kd protein, which carries the Kx antigen, a precursor molecule necessary for the Kell antigen expression, and a 93-kd protein, which carries the Kell blood group antigen.[505,506] Red cells with the McLeod phenotype have no detectable Kx antigen, and they have a marked deficiency of the 93-kd protein that carries the Kell antigen. McLeod red cells should be distinguished from Kell null (Ko) red cells, which have a normal shape. In Ko cells, only the Kell antigen carrying 93-kd glycoprotein is absent, while these cells have twice the amount of the Kx antigen.[506] As in the other acanthocytic disorders, the surface projections of acanthocytes may be related to asymmetry of the surface area of the two lipid bilayer hemileaflets, as indicated by correction of acanthocytosis by agents expanding the inner lipid layer,[507,508] as well as findings of an increased rate of exchange of phosphatidylcholine (localized preferentially in the outer lipid hemileaflet[467,509]) with an exogenous source.[510] Studies of membrane lipid and protein composition, membrane fluidity, intracellular enzyme and ATP levels were all normal.[511,512] By contrast, abnormalities were found in phosphorylation of certain membrane proteins and phospholipids,[512] density of intramembrane particles,[513] water permeability,[510] as well as reduced deformability and mechanical stability of red cells,[514] but the contribution of these abnormalities to the cell lesion is unknown.

Acanthocytosis in Other Conditions

Two of eight subjects carrying the In phenotype, characterized by a dominant inherited decreased expression of the Lutheran Pl, I, and Aua blood group antigens were reported to have acanthocytosis on their peripheral blood smear.[515] In a recent report, a dominantly inherited acanthocytosis has been found in association with structural alterations of the anion channel protein involving increased molecular size, restricted rotational diffusion, and a decrease in high affinity binding site for ankyrin.[58]

Acanthocytes have also been noted in malnourished patients, including anorexia nervosa and cystic fibrosis[434,436,445] in whom the red cell shape normalizes after restoration of the nutritional status.[434] Likewise, a small number of cells with long spicules resembling acanthocytes are found in hypothyroidism,[437] after splenectomy,[438] and in myelodysplasia.[407]

Differentiation of Acanthocytes from Other Spiculated Red Cells

Echinocytes

In contrast to acanthocytes, echinocytes, also called burr cells, have rather uniform surface projections. While early echinocytic forms have a regularly scalloped cell contour, advanced forms of echinocytes have spheroidal shape and the surface projections appears as short, narrow spikes (Fig. 46-13).

Although findings of echinocytes on peripheral blood film is often an artifact related to blood storage, contact with glass or elevated pH,[394,438] several hemolytic anemias have been reported in association with echinocytosis on peripheral blood films. These include mild hemolytic anemia in long-distance runners,[516] patients with hypomagnesemia and hypophosphatemia (presumably because of decreased intracellular ATP stores),[455] uremia due to an unknown plasma factor,[517] and pyruvate kinase deficiency.[438]

Inspection of wet blood preparations (but not dried blood films) reveals echinocytosis in most patients with liver disease.[518] In contrast to spur cells in patients with severe liver disease, these echinocytes have a normal cholesterol content and the molecular abnormality may be related to the binding of abnormal echinocytogenic high-density lipoproteins to the red cell surface.[518]

The mechanisms of echinocytosis in these diverse disorders are likely to be heterogenous as suggested by findings that many diverse factors, such as exposure of red cells to certain drugs,[518] loading by calcium,[519] or ATP depletion,[520,521] can induce the transformation of discocytes to echinocytes in vitro. However, in vitro studies of the discocyte-echinocyte-stomatocyte equilibrium have suggested a possible common denominator. As discussed in the Introduction, the lipid bilayer of normal red cells is asymmetric in lipid composition: the outer half of the lipid bilayer is relatively enriched in sphingomyelin and phosphatidylcholine, whereas the inner half is preferentially enriched in the negatively charged phosphatidylserine and phosphatidylethanolamine.[467,509] Agents that preferentially bind to one or another class of these phospholipids dramatically influence red cell shape. Consequently, agents that preferentially accumulate in the outer half of the red cell lipid bilayer, expanding this lipid bilayer produce an echinocytic shape presumably by creating an asymmetry between the two surface areas of the two halves of the lipid bilayer (Fig. 46-2). Conversely, agents which asymmetrically expand the inner half of the lipid bilayer, such as chlorpromazine, lead to stomatocytic shape transformation.[64] In the case of echinocytes produced by ATP depletion or calcium loading, the altered phospholipid distribution between the two bilayer hemileaflets may be a consequence of calcium-induced phospholipid scrambling or a decrease in the activity of aminophopholipid translocase, and ATP-dependent enzyme that actively translocates aminophospholipids from the outer leaflet to the inner hemileaflet.[65]

Keratocytes, Bizarre Poikilocytes, and Schistocytes

Occasionally, mechanical trauma of circulating red cells produced bizarre shapes resembling acanthocytes such as cells with horny projections (keratocytes). Some acanthocyte-like cells are also seen in splenectomized HE and HS subjects. Similar shape changes are seen in heated red cells, in which spectrin has been damaged by thermal denaturation,[250] suggesting that these cells are bizarre poikilocytes rather than true acanthocytes. Similar shape abnormalities have been described as an asymptomatic trait (Woronet trait).[522]

RED CELL MEMBRANE LIPID DISORDERS MANIFESTING BY TARGET CELL FORMATION

The common feature of target cells is an increase in the ratio of the cell surface area to cell volume. In microcytic red cells of patients with various forms of thalassemia and hemoglobinopathies, the increased surface to volume ratio, and consequently, the target cell shape reflects, at least in part, the *relative* abundance of cell surface area. In liver disease and other disorders discussed below, the target cell formation reflects an *absolute* expansion of the cell-surface area because of a net accumulation of membrane phospholipids and cholesterol.

Liver Disease

The presence of target cells in association with either normal or slightly increased cell volume is characteristically found in patients with obstructive jaundice, including various forms of liver disease associated with intrahepatic cholestasis.[441,446] These target cells have a normal survival in circulation.

The target cell formation is a consequence of a net uptake of both free cholesterol and phospholipids into the red cell membrane from the plasma because of abnormalities in the cholesterol/phospholipid/protein ratios of low density lipoproteins.[441,446] Target cells have a decreased osmotic fragility as the excess of membrane surface area leads to increase of the critical hemolytic volume.

Lecithin Cholesterol Acyltransferase Deficiency

The lecithin cholesterol acyltransferase (LCAT) enzyme catalyzes the transfer of fatty acids from phosphatidylcholine to cholesterol.[523] It circulates in plasma as a complex with components of high-density lipoproteins. The deficiency of this enzyme is a rare autosomal dominant disorder manifested by premature atherosclerosis, mild anemia, and the presence of target cells on the blood film. The anemia is due to mild hemolysis together with a diminished compensatory erythropoiesis.[523] As in obstructive jaundice, the target cells in LCAT deficiency have a marked increase in both cholesterol and phospholipids. In addition, the membrane phosphatidylcholine is increased at the expense of sphingomyelin and phosphatidylethanolamine.[523,524] Bone marrow aspiration and biopsy reveals the presence of sea blue histiocytes. Analysis of plasma lipoproteins reveals multiple abnormalities secondary to the underlying enzyme deficiency. Inherited LCAT deficiency should be distinguished from an acquired deficiency of this enzyme, which is found in patients with severe liver disease.[440,470]

STOMATOCYTOSIS AND RELATED DISORDERS SYNDROMES

Stomatocytes were first described in a girl with dominantly inherited hemolytic anemia.[525] On blood films, her red cells contained a wide transverse slit or stoma (Fig. 46-15). In a three-dimensional view, these cells have a shape of a cup or a bowl.[526] The slit-like appearance is an artifact, resulting from folding of the cells during blood smear preparation.

Stomatocytes are seen in a variety of acquired and inherited disorders. The latter are often associated with abnormalities in red cell cation permeability leading to changes in red cell volume that may be either increased (hence the designation hydrocytosis)[527,528] or decreased (dessicocytosis or xerocytosis)[529] or, in some cases, near normal.

There is no unifying theory to explain this morphologic abnormality. In vitro, stomatocytes can be produced by drugs that preferentially intercalate into the inner half of the asymmetric lipid bilayer, expanding its surface area relative to that of the outer half of the bilayer.[64]

Hereditary Stomatocytosis

Hereditary stomatocytosis (hydrocytosis) designates a seemingly heterogeneous group of hereditary hemolytic anemias that are transmitted in an autosomal dominant mode in most patients.[527,530–532] The disorder is characterized by a

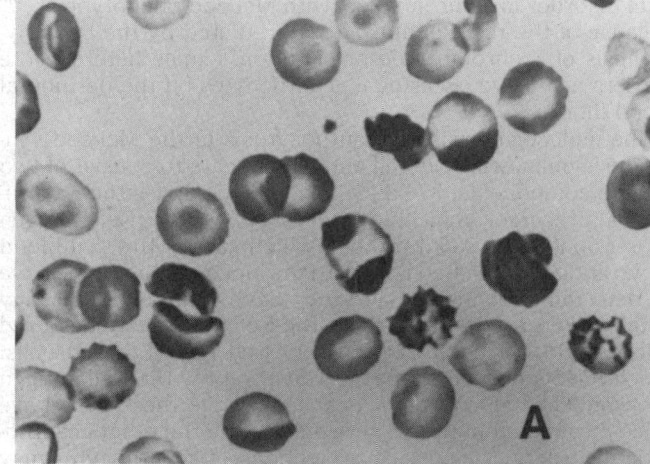

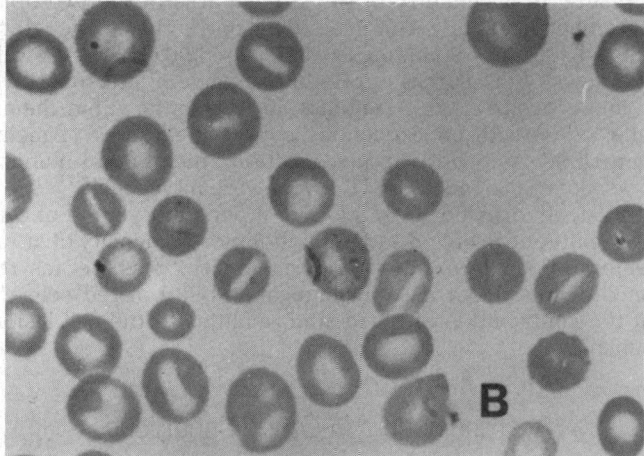

Fig. 46-15. Peripheral blood smear of a patient with hereditary **(A)** xerocytosis (dessicocytosis) and **(B)** stomatocytosis (hydrocytosis). (From Lande and Mentzer,[533] with permission.)

moderate to severe hemolytic anemia with 10–30% stomatocytes, an elevated mean corpuscular volume, and a reduced mean corpuscular hemoglobin concentration. Osmotic fragility of red cells is markedly increased, since some of the swollen red cells approach their critical hemolytic volume. For unexplained reasons, red cell membrane lipids and, consequently, membrane surface area are also increased,[533] but this increase in surface area is insufficient to correct the osmotic fragility of the red cells. Red cell deformability is decreased.[528,534] Hemolytic anemia is improved, although not fully corrected, by splenectomy.[528,534,535]

The principal cellular lesion involves a marked increase in intracellular sodium and water content with a mild decrease in intracellular potassium, resulting from a marked sodium influx into the red cells.[528,530–534] In spite of a marked compensatory increase of active transport of sodium and potassium by the Na^+/K^+-ATPase (which normally maintains the low sodium and high concentrations in the cells), and an ensuing increase in glycolysis, the pump hyperactivity is unable to compensate for the vastly increased sodium leak.[528,530–537] The molecular basis of this permeability defect is unknown. In vitro, the defect is corrected by a bifunctional cross-linking agent,[538,539] suggesting an involvement of a membrane protein. Analysis of membrane protein was normal in some patients,[528,530–534] while in others the presence of a 25-kd protein of an unknown function was reported.[540] However, this protein was also present in subjects with other disorders who have undergone splenectomy and who had elevated reticulocyte counts.[541] In some patients, a protein migrating in the band 7 region was reported missing.[541,542] This protein has now been cloned and sequenced, but no mutations have been found in two unrelated patients deficient in this protein.[27,30,543,544]

Hereditary Xerocytosis and the Intermediate Syndromes

Hereditary xerocytosis or dessicocytosis describes rare subjects with an autosomal dominant hemolytic anemia characterized by red cell dehydration and decreased osmotic fragility.[545–547] These patients have characteristically moderate to severe hemolysis with an increased mean corpuscular hemoglobin concentration, reflecting cellular dehydration. The mean corpuscular volume is slightly increased, principally reflecting the increase in reticulocyte count.[547] Peripheral blood film reveals stomatocytes (which are more prominent on wet films), target cells, and spiculated cells. In some of the cells, hemoglobin is concentrated ("puddled") in discrete areas on the cell periphery (Fig. 46-15). Hemolysis is improved but not fully corrected by splenectomy.[547]

The mechanism of cellular dehydration is unclear and complex, involving a net potassium loss from the cells that is not accompanied by a proportional gain of sodium.[545–548] Consequently, the net intracellular cation content and cell water are decreased. In some reports, a decrease in red cell 2,3-DPG has been also noted.[549,550] Analysis of membrane lipids and proteins failed to detect any abnormalities, except for an increase of membrane-associated glyceraldehyde-3-phosphate dehydrogenase.[551] This enzyme binds to the band 3 protein.[552]

Some of the reported cases of hereditary stomatocytosis share features of both hereditary stomatocytosis and xerocytosis. Lux and Glader[553] categorized these disorders as "intermediate syndromes." These patients have characteristically both stomatocytes and some target cells on the peripheral blood smear. Their osmotic fragilities are either normal or slightly increased. Their sodium and potassium permeability is somewhat increased, but the intracellular cation concentration and the red cell volume are either normal or slightly reduced. These cells were reported to have subnormal glutathione con-

tent.[554,555] In two other reported patients, red cells underwent in vitro hemolysis at 5°C[555,556]; hence, the disorder was designated cryohydrocytosis. In one patient, hemolysis was worsened by swimming and the red cells hemolyzed when exposed to shear stress.[557]

Several investigators have also reported a dominantly inherited hemolytic anemia with stomatocytosis, occasional target cells, and spherocytes, as well as a decreased osmotic fragility, in which the main red cell membrane abnormality involved a near 50% increase in phosphatidylcholine and a corresponding decrease in phosphatidylethanolamine.[533,558–560] In wet preparations, about 30% of the cells were stomatocytes.[559] The molecular basis of this syndrome in unclear. Since abnormalities in membrane phospholipid composition have not been systematically investigated, it is uncertain whether the disorder represents a distinct disease entity.[561] For additional details on this rare group of disorders, the reader is referred to several reviews.[533,560]

The results of splenectomy in this group of disorders are variable. In some patients, hemolytic anemia is improved, although often not fully corrected, by splenectomy,[528,534–536,547] while in others, the severity of hemolysis is unchanged.[562]

Rh Deficiency Syndrome

Rh deficiency syndrome designates rare individuals who have either absent (Rh_{null}) or markedly reduced (Rh_{mod}) Rh antigen expression, mild to moderate hemolytic anemia associated with the presence of stomatocytes and occasional spherocytes on the peripheral blood film.[503,563]

The Rh antigens are present in about 20,000–30,000 copies per cell and reside on minor transmembrane proteins with an electrophoretic mobility of 28–33 kd on SDS-PAGE.[564] Immunoprecipitation of Rh polypeptides by c, D, and E antigen-specific antibodies followed by two-dimensional mapping of the iodine-labeled chymotryptic peptides indicates that these proteins are distinct but closely related, a conclusion further verified by analysis of their cDNA. Furthermore, recent studies of the Rh gene locus are consistent with the existence of two closely linked genes, one encoding the D polypeptide and the other encoding the Cc, Ee proteins, the antigenic expression of which is a consequence of alternate splicing of their pre-mRNA.[565–567] Prediction of their structure from hydropathy plots revealed that the Rh proteins span the lipid bilayer multiple times, with the C and N termini located at outer and inner surfaces, respectively.[565] The Rh proteins are heavily palmitoylated, forming dimers or oligomers in solutions and, presumably, in the membrane as well. They are linked to the red cell membrane skeleton,[568,569] but their function is unknown. A previous suggestion that Rh proteins may be involved in the translocation of aminophospholipids across the membrane has been excluded by finding of normal phosphatidylserine transport in these cells.[570] In Rh_{null} human red cells, two proteins (32 kd and 34 kd) containing extracellular thiol groups are absent.

The genetic basis of the Rh deficiency syndrome is heterogeneous, and at least two groups can be defined. The two most common types are a "regulatory type," resulting from a homozygosity for the autosomal recessive suppressor gene, which is genetically distinct from the Rh locus. The second type, referred to as "amorph type" is related to a gene defect involving an RhD gene, but its detailed molecular basis is unknown.[565,571,572]

Red cells of some patients have increased osmotic fragility reflecting a marked reduction of membrane surface area.[573] These cells are also dehydrated, as indicated by decreased cell cation and water content and increased cell density.[573] The potassium transport and the Na^+/K^+ pump activity are increased, possibly because of reticulocytosis.[574,575] Hemolytic

BLOOD FILM EVALUATION: A CLUE TO PATHOPHYSIOLOGY AND DIAGNOSIS OF A RED CELL MEMBRANE DISORDER

Recent advances in our understanding of the structure and function of red cell membrane have highlighted the importance of blood film evaluation in the diagnosis of a red cell membrane disorder. Red cell shape abnormalities may provide clues both to disease pathobiology and to diagnosis (see table below).

Microspherocytes

Finding of microspherocytes indicates a deficiency of red cell surface area. In autoimmune hemolytic anemia caused by warm (IgG) autoantibodies, the IgG-coated red cells attach to macrophages, which remove parts of the membrane material from the cells. In hemolytic anemias associated with the presence of Heinz bodies, membrane material is removed together with the membrane-associated Heinz bodies as a result of the pitting function of the spleen. In a setting of a lifelong hemolytic anemia and/or a positive family history, finding of spherocytes leads to the diagnosis of hereditary spherocytosis. Since the surface area deficiency of HS red cells reflects a lipid loss resulting from the underlying deficiency of spectrin or other major membrane proteins, the molecular investigation should begin with the quantitation of spectrin, ankyrin, or band 3 protein.

Elliptocytes, Poikilocytes, and Fragments

Elliptocytes and poikilocytes are found both in HE and in many acquired conditions, including iron deficiency, megaloblastic anemias, myelofibrosis, myelophthisic anemias, and myelodysplastic syndromes. The molecular basis of acquired elliptocytosis is unclear; in our experience, laboratory evaluation of the underlying molecular defect yields negative results. By contrast, many molecular defects have been detected in HE, and the laboratory evaluation is useful both in establishing the diagnosis and in detecting asymptomatic carriers. In more severe forms of the disorder, elliptocytosis is invariably associated with the presence of poikilocytes and red cell fragments. Such findings indicate that the membrane is markedly unstable, as in hemolytic forms of HE or HPP, in which a skeletal protein defect alters the two-dimensional integrity of membrane skeleton. Accordingly, in a patient with elliptocytes on the peripheral blood film and a positive family history, the molecular evaluation should focus on (1) a defect of spectrin, involving the site at which spectrin $\alpha\beta$ heterodimers assemble into tetramers, the major structural subunits of the skeleton (the most common group of molecular defects in HE), or (2) a possible deficiency or dysfunction of protein 4.1 that promotes the attachment of spectrin to actin. In severe hemolytic forms of HE and in HPP, the mean corpuscular volume is markedly reduced since many red cells circulate in the form of fragments, which implies a severe defect in the stress-supporting horizontal interactions of the membrane skeleton due to the underlying spectrin mutation. The red cell size distribution index is high, indicating a considerable size heterogeneity of the circulating red cell fragments. Such fragments differ from schisto-cytes produced by a mechanical trauma to the red cells: the former fragments are round, often seen budding from the red cell membrane, whereas schistocytes appear as "cuts" with sharp edges and often bizarre shapes, while the remaining red cells are relatively intact.

Echinocyte/Discocyte/Stomatocyte Equilibrium

Echinocytes, cells with fine, multiple, and uniform spicules are found in many conditions, including malnutrition associated with mild hemolysis due to hypomagnesemia and hypophosphatemia, uremia, and hemolytic anemia in long-distance runners. They are also a common artifact of elevated pH, blood storage, or contact with glass. Although the mechanism of echinocyte formation in vivo is not clear, studies in vitro suggest that echinocytosis is caused by an expansion of the outer hemileaflet of the lipid bilayer, relative to the inner bilayer hemileaflet. By contrast, expansion of the inner lipid bilayer leaflet, relative to the outer leaflet, leads to cup shape formation (stomatocytosis) and surface invaginations. Stomatocytosis is seen either as an inherited hemolytic anemia associated with cell volume changes or as an acquired condition, particularly in alcoholism.

Acanthocytes

In contrast to echinocytes, acanthocytes contain long, irregular protrusions that suggest both a net accumulation of lipids in the red cell membrane and an asymmetry between the two lipid bilayer hemileaflets with a preferential expansion of the outer hemileaflet. In the spur cell hemolytic anemia associated with severe liver disease, these "spurs" reflect a net gain of free (unesterified) cholesterol that preferentially accumulates in the outer half of the lipid bilayer. Because of the conditioning effect of the spleen, the cells are also spheroidal, indicating a secondary loss of surface area; yet their surface protuberances are very prominent. In abetalipoproteinemia, acanthocytes contain excess sphingomyelin in the outer lipid bilayer hemileaflet. The mechanisms of acanthocytosis in other conditions (choreacanthocytosis syndrome, malnutrition, hypothyroidism, and McLeod phenotype) are unknown.

Target Cells

In contrast to spherocytes, target cells have either a relative or an absolute excess of surface for a given red cell volume. A relative excess of the surface area is typically found in microcytic red cells in most patients with thalassemia minor and some hemoglobinopathies (hemoglobin C, D, E). In red cells having normal or even slightly increased volume, targeting indicates an absolute excess of surface area. For example, in a patient with liver disease or obstructive jaundice, red cell surface area is expanded because both phospholipids and cholesterol are transferred from the abnormal plasma lipoproteins into the red cell membrane.

BLOOD FILM EVALUATION: *Continued*

Dehydrated Red Cells

Changes in red cell density, as reflected by increased mean corpuscular hemoglobin concentration, can likewise be appreciated on the blood film. The staining intensity of intracellular hemoglobin of spherocytes, regardless of mechanism of their formation, is greater than that of normal discocytes, since the hemoglobin layer that is in the optical path between the light source and the observer's eye is thicker than in the normal discocyte. However, the staining intensity of intracellular hemoglobin and, hence, the density of hereditary spherocytes is typically greater than that of spherocytes in autoimmune hemolytic anemia, since hereditary spherocytes are also somewhat dehydrated. In some inherited disorders associated with cellular dehydration (xerocytosis), cells may be either stomatocytic or appear as bizarre targets with intracellular hemoglobin puddled into distinct clumps.

Peripheral Blood Film Evaluation in a Patient With Red Cell Membrane Disorder

Shape	Pathobiology	Diagnosis
Microspherocytes	Loss of membrane lipids leading to a reduction of surface area resulting from deficiencies of spectrin, ankyrin or band 3 protein	HS
	Removal of membrane material from antibody coated red cells by macrophages	Immunohemolytic anemias
	Removal of membrane associated Heinz bodies, with the adjacent membrane lipids, by the spleen	Heinz body hemolytic anemias
Elliptocytes	Permanent red cell deformation resulting from a weakening of skeletal protein interactions (such as the spectrin dimer-dimer contact). This facilitates disruption of existing protein contacts during shear stress induced elliptical deformation. Subsequently, new protein contacts are formed that stabilize elliptical shape	Mild common HE
	Unknown	Iron deficiency, megaloblastic anemias, myelofibrosis, myelophthisic anemias, myelodysplastic syndrome, thalassemias
Poikilocytes/fragments	Weakening of skeletal protein contacts resulting from skeletal protein mutations	Hemolytic HE HPP
	Unknown	Iron deficiency, megaloblastic anemias, myelofibrosis, myelophthisic anemias, myelodysplastic syndrome, thalassemias
Schistocytes, fragmented red cells	Red cells "torn" by mechanical trauma (fibrin strands, turbulent flow)	"Microangiopathic" hemolytic anemia associated with disseminated intravascular coagulation, thrombotic thrombocytopenic purpura, vasculitis, heart valve prostheses
Acanthocytes	Uptake of cholesterol and its preferential accumulation in the outer leaflet of the lipid bilayer	Spurr cell hemolytic anemia in severe liver disease
	Selective accumulation of sphingomyelin in the outer lipid leaflet	Abetalipoproteinemia
	Unknown	Chorea-acanthocytosis syndrome, malnutrition, hypothyroidism McLeod phenotype

(Continues)

Peripheral Blood Film Evaluation in a Patient With Red Cell Membrane Disorder		
Shape	Pathobiology	Diagnosis
Echinocytes	Expansion of the surface area of the outer hemileaflet of lipid bilayer relative to the inner hemileaflet	Hemolytic anemia associated with hypomagnesemia and hypophosphatemia in malnourished patients, pyruvate kinase deficiency; in vitro artifact of low blood storage (ATP) depletion), contact with glass or elevated pH
	Unknown	Hemolysis in long-distance runners, renal failure
Stomatocytes	Expansion of the surface area of the inner hemileaflet of the bilayer relative to the outer leaflet	Exposure of red cells to cationic anesthetics in vitro; in vivo, the drug concentrations may not be sufficient to produce similar effect
	Unknown	Alcoholism, inherited disorders of membrane permeability (hereditary stomatocytosis)
Target cells	Absolute excess of membrane lipids (both cholesterol and phospholipids: "symmetric" lipid gain), followed by an increase of cell surface area	Obstructive jaundice, liver disease with intrahepatic cholestasis
	Relative excess of surface area because of a decrease in cell volume	Thalassemias and some hemoglobinopathies (C, D, E)

anemia is improved by splenectomy.[563] Additional serologic aberrations involve a weakened expression of Ss and U antigens[576,577] that, unlike the Rh antigen system, reside on one of the transmembrane glycoproteins, glycophorin B,[578] the level of which is reduced in Rh null cells by about 30%, possibly because glycophorin B is, in part, present as a complex with the Rh proteins.

Familial Deficiency of High-Density Lipoproteins

Severe deficiency or absence of high-density lipoproteins leads to accumulation of cholesteryl esters in many tissues, leading to clinical findings of large orange tonsils and hepatosplenomegaly.[524] The reported hematologic manifestations include a moderately severe hemolytic anemia with stomatocytosis.[579] Membrane lipid analysis revealed a low free cholesterol content, leading to a decreased cholesterol to phospholipid ratio and a relative increase in phosphatidylcholine at the expense of sphingomyelin.[579]

Acquired Stomatocytosis

Stomatocytes have been noted in diverse acquired conditions, including neoplasms, cardiovascular and hepatobiliary disease, alcoholism, and therapy with drugs some of which are known to be stomatocytogenic in vitro.[580,581] In some of these conditions, the percentage of stomatocytes on peripheral blood smear exceeded 50%. However, the clinical significance of the above observation is unclear because stomatocytes are absent in most patients with the above conditions. Furthermore, some stomatocytes are often found in normal individuals (3–5%).[453,454] The most consistent association is that of stomatocytosis and heavy alcohol consumption.[453,454] Stomato-

cytosis has also been reported in Mediterranean immigrants in Australia. Its cause is unknown, but it may be related to alcoholism.[582,583]

MEMBRANE ALTERATIONS IN OTHER HEMOLYTIC ANEMIAS

Abnormalities of Membrane Proteins and Lipids

Abnormalities of both membrane proteins and lipids have been described in red cells in sickle cell anemia, unstable hemoglobins, and thalassemias, as well as deficiencies or glucose-6-phosphate dehydrogenase and related enzymes.[584–592] These abnormalities include cross-linking of membrane and skeletal proteins, clustering of transmembrane proteins in areas in which denatured hemoglobin attaches to the membrane,[592,593] lipid peroxidation, and formation of lipid-protein adducts,[589,594] as well as destabilization of membrane-protein interactions.[584,585,588] The molecular mechanisms involved in these changes include oxidative damage[587,595–599] and release from the denatured hemoglobin of hemin that, in addition to its oxidative effect, has striking detergent-like effects resulting in destabilization of membrane-protein interactions.[600–603] As discussed in the chapters dealing with these diseases, as well as several reviews,[587,594,595,604] these alterations may play an important role in an accelerated destruction of the abnormal red cells.

Cation Permeability Defects

Secondary defects of cation permeability are found in a variety of disorders, including hereditary spherocytosis,[91,136–138,183] hereditary pyropoikilocytosis,[351,352] sickle cell disease,[604] and other hemoglobinopathies, as well as disorders characterized by impaired maintenance of intracellular ATP stores, such as pyruvate kinase deficiency.[605] Depending on the underlying permeability defect, the net defect is either a cellular dehydration or swelling.

Dehydrated Red Cells

Varying degrees of red cell dehydration are found in several hemolytic anemias, such as sickle cell disease and other hemoglobinopathies,[604,606] or hereditary spherocytosis.[136,137] Such cells have a reduced cell water content, increased cell potassium, and decreased cell sodium content and increased cell density. The dehydration is principally related to a loss of potassium together with water from the cells. The causes of a preferential potassium loss leading to cellular dehydration include a calcium-mediated increase in potassium leak from the cells (the so-called Gardos phenmonenon), increase in the K^+ Cl^- co-transport pathway (which exports both ions from the cells), activated by acidification or cell swelling, as well as other mechanisms.[139,141,161,548,607,608]

Swollen Red Cells

Colloid osmotic swelling followed by lysis represents the principal pathway of red cell destruction during complement activation on the cell surface.[609,610] The cells swell as a result of an insertion into the lipid bilayer of a multimolecular complex of the terminal components of the complement pathway (the membrane attack complex) that forms a cation channel, allowing a free passage of sodium and potassium according to their concentration gradients.[609-612] Because of the net negative charge of intracellular hemoglobin, sodium influx into the cells exceeds the potassium loss, leading to gain in cell water, swelling, and cell lysis. The formation of only one such membrane attack complex per cell is considered sufficient to produce cell lysis.[613]

REFERENCES

1. Sahr KE, Laurila P, Kotula L et al: The complete cDNA and polypeptide sequences of human erythroid α-spectrin. J Biol Chem 265:4434, 1990
2. Kotula L, Laury-Kleintop LD, Showe L et al: The exon-intron organization of the human erythrocyte α-spectrin gene. Genomics 9:131, 1991
3. Winkelmann JC, Chang JC, Tse WT et al: Full length sequence of the cDNA for human erythroid β spectrin. J Biol Chem 265:11827, 1990
4. Amin KM, Scarpa AL, Winkelmann JC et al: The exon-intron organization of the human erythroid beta-spectrin gene. Genomics 18:118, 1993
5. Lux SE, John KM, Bennett V: Analysis of cDNA for human erythrocyte ankyrin indicates a repeated structure with homology to tissue-differentiation and cell cycle control proteins. Nature 344:36, 1990
6. Lambert S, Yu H, Prchal JT et al: cDNA sequence for human erythrocyte ankyrin. Proc Natl Acad Sci USA 87:1730, 1990
7. Joshi R, Gilligan DM, Otto E et al: Primary structure and domain organization of human α-adducin and β-adducin. J Cell Biol 115:665, 1991
8. Lux SE, John KM, Kopito RR, Lodish HF: Cloning and characterization of band 3, the human erythrocyte anion exchange protein (AE1). Proc Natl Acad Sci USA 86:9089, 1989
9. Tanner MJA, Martin PG, High S: The complete amino acid sequence of the human erythrocyte membrane anion-transport protein deduced from the cDNA. Biochem J 256:703, 1988
10. Conboy J, Kan YW, Shohet SB, Mohandas N: Molecular cloning of protein 4.1, a major structural element of the human erythrocyte membrane skeleton. Proc Natl Acad Sci USA 83:9152, 1986
11. Tang CJC, Tang TK: Rapid localization of membrane skeletal protein 4.1 (EL1) to human chromosome 1p33-p34.2 by nonradioactive in situ hybridization. Cytogenet Cell Genet 57:119, 1991
12. Korsgren C, Cohen CM: Organization of the gene for human erythrocyte membrane protein 4.2: structural similarities with the gene for the a subunit of factor XIII. Proc Natl Acad Sci USA 88:4840, 1991
13. Korsgren C, Lawler J, Lambert S et al: Complete amino acid sequence and homologies of human erythrocyte membrane protein band 4.2. Proc Natl Acad Sci USA 87:613, 1990
14. Najfeld V, Ballard SG, Menninger J et al: The gene for human erythrocyte protein 4.2 maps to chromosome 15q15. Am J Hum Genet 50:71, 1992
15. Sung LA, Chien S, Chang L-S et al: Molecular cloning of human protein 4.2: a major component of the erythrocyte membrane. Proc Natl Acad Sci USA 87:955, 1990
16. Husain-Chishti A, Faquin W, Wu CC, Branton D: Purification of erythrocyte dematin (protein 4.9) reveals an endogenous protein kinase that modulates actin-bundling activity. J Biol Chem 264:8985, 1989
17. Husain-Chishti A, Levin A, Branton D: Abolition of actin-bundling by phosphorylation of human erythrocyte protein 4.9. Nature 334:718, 1988
18. Siegel DL, Branton D: Partial purification and characterization of an actin-bundling protein, band 4.9, from human erythrocytes. J Cell Biol 100:775, 1985
19. Rana AP, Ruff P, Maalouf GJ et al: Cloning of human erythroid dematin reveals another member of the villin family. Proc Natl Acad Sci USA 90:6651, 1993
20. Ruff P, Speicher DW, Husain-Chisti A: Molecular identification of a major palmitoylated erythrocyte membrane protein containing the src homology 3 motif. Proc Natl Acad Sci USA 88:6595, 1991
21. Cohen CM, Jackson PL, Branton D: Actin-membrane interactions: association of G-actin with the red cell membrane. J Supramol Structure 9:113, 1978
22. Nakashima K, Beutler E: Comparison of structure and function of human erythrocyte and human muscle actin. Proc Natl Acad Sci USA 76:935, 1979
23. Pinder JC, Gratzer WB: Structural and dynamic states of actin in the erythrocyte. J Cell Biol 96:768, 1983
24. Fowler VM: Identification and purification of a novel Mr 43,000 tropomyosin-binding protein from human erythrocyte membranes. J Biol Chem 262:12792, 1987
25. Sung LA, Fowler VM, Lambert K: Molecular cloning and characterization of human fetal liver tropomodulin—a tropomyosin-binding protein. J Biol Chem 267:2616, 1992
26. Hanauer A, Mandel JL: The glyceraldehyde-3-phosphate dehydrogenase gene family: structure of a human cDNA and of an X chromosome linked pseudogene; amazing complexity of the gene family in mouse. EMBO J 3:2627, 1984
27. Hiebl-Dirschmied CM, Entler B, Glotzmann C et al: Cloning and nucleotide sequence of cDNA encoding human erythrocyte band 7 integral membrane protein. Biochim Biophys Acta 1090:123, 1991
28. Gallagher PG, Upender M, Ward DC, Forget BG: The gene for human erythrocyte membrane protein band-7.2 (EPB72) maps to 9q33-q34 centromeric to the Philadelphia chromosome translocation breakpoint region—brief report. Genomics 18:167, 1993
29. Fowler VM, Bennett V: Erythrocyte membrane tropomyosin. J Biol Chem 259:5978, 1984
30. Stewart GW, Hepworth-Jones BE, Keen JN et al: Isolation of cDNA coding for an ubiquitous membrane protein deficient in high Na+, low K+ stomatocytic erythrocytes. Blood 79:1593, 1992
31. Fukuda M: Molecular genetics of the glycophorin A gene cluster. Semin Hematol 30:138, 1993
32. Kudo S, Fukuda M: Structural organization of glycophorin A and B genes: glycophorin B gene evolved by homologous recombination at Alu repeat sequences. Proc Natl Acad Sci USA 86:4619, 1989
33. Siebert PD, Fukuda M: Isolation and characterization of human glycophorin A cDNA clones by a synthetic oligonucleotide approach: nucleotide sequence and mRNA structure. Proc Natl Acad Sci USA 83:1665, 1986
34. Tomita M, Furthmayr H, Marchesi VT: Primary structure of human erythrocyte glycophorin A. Isolation and characterization of peptides and complete amino acid sequence. Biochemistry 17:4756, 1978
35. Tomita M, Marchesi VT: Amino-acid sequence and oligosaccharide attachment sites of human erythrocyte glycophorin. Proc Natl Acad Sci USA 72:2964, 1975
36. Cartron J-P, Le Van Kim C, Colin Y: Glycophorin C and related glycoproteins. Structure, function and regulation. Semin Hematol 30:152, 1993
37. Colin Y, Rahuel C, London J et al: Isolation of cDNA clones for human erythrocyte glycophorin C. J Biol Chem 261:229, 1986
38. Mattei MG, Colin Y, Le Van Kim C: Localization of the gene for human erythrocyte glycophorin C to chromosome 2, q14-21. Hum Genet 74:420, 1986
39. Siebert PD, Fukuda M: Molecular cloning of a human glycophorin B cDNA: nucleotide sequence and genomic relationship to glycophorin A. Proc Natl Acad Sci USA 84:6735, 1987
40. El-Maliki B, Blanchard D, Dahr W et al: Structural homology between glycophorins C and D of human erythrocytes. Eur J Biochem 183:639, 1989
41. Kudo S, Fukuda M: Identification of a novel human glycophorin, glycophorin E, by isolation of genomic clones and complementary cDNA clones utilizing polymerase chain reaction. J Biol Chem 265:1102, 1990
42. Conboy JG, Chan J, Mohandas N, Kan YW: Multiple protein 4.1 isoforms

produced by alternative splicing in human erythroid cells. Proc Natl Acad Sci USA 85:9062, 1988

43. Tang TK, Qin Q, Leto T et al: Heterogeneity of mRNA and protein products arising from the protein 4.1 gene in erythroid and nonerythroid tissues. J Cell Biol 110:617, 1990

44. White RA, Peters LL, Adkison LR et al: The murine pallid mutation is a platelet storage pool disease associated with the protein 4.2 (pallidin) gene. Nature Genet 2:80, 1992

45. Palek J, Jarolim P: Clinical expression and laboratory detection of red cell membrane protein mutations. Semin Hematol 30:258, 1993

46. Palek J: Hereditary elliptocytosis and related disorders. Baillieres Clin Haematol 14:45, 1985

47. Liu SC, Derick L, Duquette MA, Palek J: Separation of the lipid bilayer from the membrane skeleton during discocyte-echinocyte transformation of human erythrocyte ghosts. Eur J Cell Biol 49:358, 1989

48. Liu S-C, Derick LH: Molecular anatomy of the red blood cell membrane skeleton. Structure-function relationships. Semin Hematol 29:231, 1992

49. Palek J, Lambert S: Genetics of the red cell membrane skeleton. Semin Hematol 27:290, 1990

50. Conboy JG: Structure, function and molecular genetics of erythroid membrane skeletal protein 4.1 in normal and abnormal red blood cells. Semin Hematol 30:58, 1993

51. Delaunay J, Dhermy D: Mutations involving the spectrin heterodimer contact site: clinical expression and alterations in specific function. Semin Hematol 30:21, 1993

52. Jarolim P, Palek J, Amato D et al: Deletion in erythrocyte band 3 gene in malaria-resistant Southeast Asian ovalocytosis. Proc Natl Acad Sci USA 88:11022, 1991

53. Liu SC, Zhai S, Palek J et al: Molecular defect of the band 3 protein in Southeast Asian ovalocytosis. N Engl J Med 323:1530, 1990

54. Mohandas N, Winardi R, Knowles D et al: Molecular basis for membrane rigidity of hereditary ovalocytosis—a novel mechanism involving the cytoplasmic domain of band-3. J Clin Invest 89:686, 1992

55. Schofield AE, Tanner MJA, Pinder JC et al: Basis of unique red cell membrane properties in hereditary ovalocytosis. J Mol Biol 223:949, 1992

56. Palek J: Acanthocytosis, stomatocytosis, and related disorders. p. 582. In Williams WJ, Beutler E, Erslev AJ, Lichtman MA (eds): Hematology. McGraw-Hill, New York, 1990

57. Redman CM, Marsh WL: The Kell blood group system and the McLeod phenotype. Semin Hematol 30:1, 1993

58. Kay MMB, Bosman GJCGM, Lawrence C: Functional topography of band 3: specific structural alteration linked to functional aberrations in human erythrocytes. Proc Natl Acad Sci USA 85:492, 1988

59. Kay MMB, Goodman J, Lawrence C et al: Membrane channel protein abnormalities and autoantibodies in neurological disease. Brain Res Bull 24:105, 1990

60. Lange Y, Cutler HB, Steck TL: The effect of cholesterol and other interrelated amphipaths on the contour and stability of the isolated red cell membrane. J Biol Chem 255:9331, 1980

61. Daleke DL, Huestis WH: Erythrocyte morphology reflects the transbilayer distribution of incorporated phospholipids. J Cell Biol 108:1375, 1989

62. Evans E: Bending resistance and chemically induced moments in membrane bilayers. Biophys J 14:923, 1974

63. Mohandas N, Greenquist AC, Shohet SB: Bilayer balance and regulation of red cell shape changes. J Supramol Struct 9:453, 1978

64. Sheetz MP, Singer SJ: Biological membranes as bilayer couples: a molecular mechanism of drug-erythrocyte interactions. Proc Natl Acad Sci USA 71:4457, 1974

65. Devaux PF: Protein involvement in transmembrane lipid asymmetry. Annu Rev Biophys Biomol Struct 21:417, 1992

66. Young LE, Izzo MJ, Platzer RF: Hereditary spherocytosis. I. Clinical, haematologic and genetic features in 28 cases, with particular reference to the osmotic and mechanical fragility of incubated erythrocytes. Blood 6:1073, 1951

67. Jensson O, Jonasson JL, Magnusson S: Studies on hereditary spherocytosis in Iceland. J Intern Med 201:187, 1977

68. McKinney AA Jr, Morton NE, Kosower NS et al: Ascertaining genetic carriers of hereditary spherocytosis by statistical analysis of multiple laboratory tests. J Clin Invest 41:554, 1962

69. McKinney AA: Hereditary spherocytosis: clinical family studies. Arch Intern Med 116:257, 1965

70. Friedman EW, Williams JC, Van Hook L: Hereditary spherocytosis in the elderly. Am J Med 84:513, 1988

71. Dacie J: The Haemolytic Anaemias. 3rd Ed. Churchill Livingstone, Edinburgh, 1985, p. 114

72. Agre P, Orringer EP, Bennett V: Deficient red-cell spectrin in severe, recessively inherited spherocytosis. N Engl J Med 306:1155, 1982

73. Agre P, Asimos A, Casella JF, McMillan D: Inheritance pattern and clinical response to splenectomy as a reflection of erythrocyte spectrin deficiency in hereditary spherocytosis. N Engl J Med 315:1579, 1986

74. Coetzer TL, Lawler J, Liu SC et al: Partial ankyrin and spectrin deficiency in severe, atypical hereditary spherocytosis. N Engl J Med 318:230, 1988

75. Agre P, Casella JF, Zinkham WH: Partial deficiency of erythrocyte spectrin in hereditary spherocytosis. Nature 314:380, 1985

76. Morton NE, MacKinney AA, Kosower N: Genetics of spherocytosis. Am J Hum Genet 14:170, 1962

77. Godal HC, Heist H: High prevalence of increased osmotic fragility of red blood cells among Norwegian blood donors. Scand J Haematol 27:30, 1981

78. Eber SW, Pekrun A, Neufeldt A, Schroter W: Prevalance of increased osmotic fragility of erythrocytes in German blood donors—screening using a modified glycerol lysis test. Ann Hematol 64:88, 1992

79. Nozawa Y, Noguchi T, Iida H et al: Erythrocyte membrane of hereditary spherocytosis: alteration in surface ultrastructure and membrane proteins, as inferred by scanning electron microscopy and SDS-disc gel electrophoresis. Clin Chim Acta 55:81, 1974

80. Hayashi S, Koomoto R, Yano A et al: Abnormality in a specific protein of the erythrocyte membrane in hereditary spherocytosis. Biochem Biophys Res Commun 57:1038, 1974

81. Kline AH, Holman GH: Hereditary spherocytosis in the Negro. Am J Dis Child 94:609, 1957

82. Metz J: Hereditary spherocytosis in the Bantu. S Afr Med J 33:1034, 1959

83. Vanlair CF, Masius JB: De la microcythémie. Bull R Acad Med Belg 5:515, 1871

84. Wilson C: Some cases showing hereditary enlargement of the spleen. Trans Clin Soc (Lond) 23:162, 1890

85. Minkowski O: Ueber eine hereditare, unter dem bilde eines chronischen ikterus mit Urobilinurie, Splenomegalie und Nierensiderosis verlaufende Affektion. Verh Dtsch Kongr Inn Med 18:316, 1900

86. Chauffard MA: Pathogène del'ictère congénital del'adulte. Semin Med 27:25, 1907

87. Sutherland GA, Burghard FF: The treatment of splenic anemia by splenectomy. Lancet 2:1819, 1910

88. Wynter WE: Case of acholuric jaundice after splenectomy. Proc R Soc Med Clin Sect 6:80, 1912

89. Ham TH, Castle WB: Studies on destruction of red blood cells. Relation of increased hypotonic fragility and erythrostasis to the mechanism of hemolysis in certain anemias. Proc Am Philos Soc 82:411, 1940

90. Bertles JE: Sodium transport across the surface membrane of red blood cells in hereditary spherocytosis. J Clin Invest 36:816, 1957

91. Jacob HS, Jandl JH: Cell membrane permeability in the pathogenesis of hereditary spherocytosis (HS). J Clin Invest 43:1704, 1964

92. Reed CF, Swisher SN: Erythrocyte lipid loss in hereditary spherocytosis. J Clin Invest 45:777, 1966

93. Cooper RA, Jandl JH: The role of membrane lipids in the survival of red cells in hereditary spherocytosis. J Clin Invest 48:736, 1969

94. Jacob HS, Ruby A, Overland ES, Mazia D: Abnormal membrane protein of red blood cells in hereditary spherocytosis. J Clin Invest 50:1800, 1971

95. Dacie JV, Mollison PL: Survival of normal erythrocytes after transfusion to patients with familial haemolytic anaemia (acholuric jaundice). Lancet 1:550, 1943

96. Emerson CP Jr, Shen SC, Ham TH et al: The mechanism of blood destruction in congenital hemolytic jaundice. J Clin Invest 26:1180, 1947

97. Young LE, Platzer RI, Ervin DM, Izzo MJ: Hereditary spherocytosis. II. Observations on the role of the spleen. Blood 6:1099, 1951

98. Gallagher PG, Forget BG: Spectrin genes in health and disease. Semin Hematol 30:4, 1993

99. Tanner MJA: Molecular and cellular biology of the erythrocyte anion exchanger (AE1). Semin Hematol 30:34, 1993

100. Peters LL, Lux SE: Ankyrins: structure and function in normal cells and hereditary spherocytes. Semin Hematol 30:85, 1993

101. Cohen CM, Dotimas L, Korsgren C: Human erythrocyte membrane protein band 4.2 (pallidin). Semin Hematol 30:119, 1993

102. Jarolim P, Brabec V, Ballas SK et al: Biochemical heterogeneity of the hereditary spherocytosis syndrome, abstracted. Presented at the Twenty-fourth Congress of the International Society of Haematology, 1992, p. 35

103. Becker PS, Tse WT, Lux SE, Forget BG: β Spectrin Kissimmee—a spectrin variant associated with autosomal dominant hereditary spherocytosis and defective binding to protein 4.1. J Clin Invest 92:612, 1993

104. Wolfe LC, John KM, Falcone JC et al: A genetic defect in binding of protein 4.1 to spectrin in a kindred with hereditary spherocytosis. N Engl J Med 307:1367, 1982

105. Becker PS, Tse WT, Lux SE, Forget BG: Identification of the molecular defect of β spectrin in autosomal dominant hereditary spherocytosis (HS) associated with defective binding of protein 4.1, HS (Sp-4.1), abstracted. Blood, suppl. 1. 76:25a, 1990

106. Becker PS, Morrow JS, Lux SE: Abnormal oxidant sensitivity and β-chain structure of spectrin in hereditary spherocytosis associated with defective spectrin-protein 4.1 binding. J Clin Invest 80:557, 1987

107. Marchesi SL, Agre PA, Speicher DW et al: Mutant spectrin αII domain in recessively inherited spherocytosis, abstracted. Blood, suppl. 1. 74:182a, 1989

108. Whitfield CF, Follweiler JB, Lopresti-Morrow L, Miller BA: Deficiency of α-spectrin synthesis in burst-forming units-erythroid in lethal hereditary spherocytosis. Blood 78:3043, 1991

109. Hanspal M, Palek J: Biogenesis of normal and abnormal red blood cell membrane skeleton. Semin Hematol 29:305, 1992

110. Hanspal M, Hanspal J, Fibach E, Palek J: Molecular basis of spectrin deficiency in hereditary pyropoikilocytosis (HPP). Blood 82:1652, 1993

111. Savvides P, Shalev O, John KM, Lux SE: Combined spectrin and ankyrin deficiency is common in autosomal dominant hereditary spherocytosis, abstracted. Clin Res 39:313A, 1991

112. Lux SE, Tse WT, Menninger JC et al: Hereditary spherocytosis associated with deletion of human erythrocyte ankyrin gene on chromosome 8. Nature 345:736, 1990

113. Hanspal M, Yoon S-H, Yu H et al: Molecular basis of spectrin and ankyrin deficiencies in severe hereditary spherocytosis: evidence implicating a primary defect of ankyrin. Blood 77:165, 1991

114. Costa FF, Agre P, Watkins PC et al: Linkage of dominant hereditary spherocytosis to the gene for the erythrocyte membrane-skeleton protein ankyrin. N Engl J Med 323:1046, 1990

115. Jarolim P, Rubin HL, Brabec V, Palek J: Abnormal alternative splicing of erythrocyte ankyrin mRNA in two kindred with hereditary spherocytosis (ankyrin^PRAGUE and ankyrin^RAKOVNIK), abstracted. Blood, suppl. 1. 82:5a, 1993

116. Marchesi SL, Benoit L, Beardsley D et al: Two families with spherocytosis and unstable β spectrin, abstracted. Blood, suppl. 1. 80:276a, 1992

117. Jarolim P, Brabec V, Lambert S et al: Ankyrin Prague: a dominantly inherited mutation of the regulatory domain of ankyrin associated with hereditary spherocytosis, abstracted. Blood, suppl. 1. 76:37a, 1990

118. Eber SW, Lux ML, Gonzalez JM et al: Discovery of 8 ankyrin mutations in hereditary spherocytosis (HS) indicates that ankyrin defects are a major cause of dominant and recessive HS, abstracted. Blood, Suppl. 1. 82:3089, 1993

119. Rybicki AC, Qiu JJH, Musto S et al: Human erythrocyte protein 4.2 deficiency associated with hemolytic anemia and a homozygous ⁴⁰glutamic acid → lysine substitution in the cytoplasmic domain of band 3 (band 3^Montefiore). Blood 81:2155, 1993

120. Jarolim P, Palek J, Rubin HL et al: Band 3 Tuscaloosa: Pro³²⁷ → Arg³²⁷ substitution in the cytoplasmic domain of erythrocyte band 3 protein associated with spherocytic hemolytic anemia and partial deficiency of protein 4.2. Blood 80:523, 1992

121. Alloisio N, Texier P, Forissier A et al: Band 3 coimbra: a variant associated with dominant hereditary spherocytosis and band 3 deficiency, abstracted. Blood, suppl. 1. 82:4a, 1993

122. Jarolim P, Rubin HL, Brabec V, Palek J: Clustered arginine substitutions in the membrane domain of erythroid band 3 protein in hereditary spherocytosis with band 3 deficiency, abstracted. Blood, suppl. 1. 82:3089, 1993

123. Jarolim P, Rubin HL, Liu S-C et al: Duplication of 10 nucleotides in the erythroid band 3 (AE1) gene is a kindred with hereditary spherocytosis and band 3 protein deficiency (band 3^PRAGUE). J Clin Invest 93:121, 1994

124. Bouhassira EE, Schwartz RS, Yawata Y et al: An alanine-to-threonine substitution in protein 4.2 cDNA associated with a Japanese form of hereditary hemolytic anemia (protein 4.2^NIPPON). Blood 79:1846, 1992

125. Jarolim P, Ruff P, Coetzer TL et al: A subset of patients with dominantly inherited hereditary spherocytosis has a marked deficiency of the band 3 protein, abstracted. Blood, suppl. 1. 76:37a, 1990

126. Packman CH, Leddy JP: Acquired hemolytic anemia due to warm reacting autoantibodies. p. 666. In Williams WJ, Beutler E, Erslev AJ, Lichtman MA (eds): Hematology McGraw-Hill, New York, 1990

127. Prchal JT, Guan Y, Jarolim P et al: Hereditary spherocytosis in a large family is linked with the band 3 gene and not with α-spectrin, β-spectrin or ankyrin, abstracted. Blood, suppl. 1. 78:81a, 1991

128. Jarolim P, Rubin HL, Brabec V, Palek J: Band 3 Prague: a duplication of 10 bases in the erythroid band 3 gene in a kindred with hereditary spherocytosis with band 3 deficiency, abstracted. Blood, suppl. 1. 80:277a, 1992

129. Saad STO, Liu SC, Golan D et al: Mechanism underlying band 3 deficiency in a subset of patients with hereditary spherocytosis (HS), abstracted. Blood, suppl. 1. 78:81a, 1991

130. Liu S-C, Derick LH, Duquette MA: Surface area density of membrane skeleton (MS) in normal red cells and severe hereditary spherocytosis (HS): role in lipid bilayer destabilization, abstracted. Blood, suppl. 1. 72:31a, 1988

131. Liu S-C, Derick LH, Palek J: Molecular anatomy of erythrocyte membrane skeleton in health and disease. p. 171. In Cohen CM, Palek J (eds): Cellular and Molecular Biology of Normal and Abnormal Erythroid Membranes. Wiley-Liss, New York, 1990

132. Cooper RA, Jandl JH: The selective and conjoint loss of red cell lipids. J Clin Invest 48:906, 1969

133. Wiley JS: Red cell survival studies in hereditary spherocytosis. J Clin Invest 49:666, 1970

134. Edwards HH, Mueller TJ: Distribution of transmembrane polypeptides in freeze fracture. Science 203:54, 1979

135. Elgsaeter A, Shotton DM, Branton D: Intramembrane particle aggregation in erythrocyte ghosts II. The influence of spectrin aggregation. Biochim Biophys Acta 426:101, 1976

136. Maizels M: The anion and cation contents of normal and anaemic bloods. Biochem J 30:821, 1936

137. Mayman D, Zipursky A HS: The metabolism of erythrocytes in peripheral blood and the splenic pulp. Br J Haematol 27:201, 1974

138. Bertles JE: Sodium transport across the surface membrane of red blood cells in hereditary spherocytosis. J Clin Invest 36:816, 1957

139. Orringer EP: A further characterization of the selective K movements observed in human red blood cells following acetylphenylhydrazine exposure. Am J Hematol 16:355, 1984

140. Lauf PK, Bauer J, Adragna NC et al: Erythrocyte K-Cl cotransport: properties and regulation. Am J Physiol 263:C917, 1992

141. Clark MR, Guatelli JC, White AT, Shohet SB: Study of dehydrating effect of the red cell Na⁺/K⁺ pump in nystatin-treated cells with varying Na⁺ and water content. Biochim Biophys Acta 646:422, 1981

142. Mohandas N, Clark MR, Jacobs MS, Shohet SB: Analysis of factors regulating erythrocyte deformability. J Clin Invest 66:563, 1980

143. Mohandas N, Chasis JA, Shohet SB: The influence of membrane skeleton on red cell deformability, membrane material properties, and shape. Semin Hematol 20:225, 1983

144. Reinhart WH, Chien S: Roles of cell geometry and cellular viscosity in red cell passage through narrow pores. Am J Physiol 248:473, 1985

145. Weiss L: The red pulp of the spleen: structural basis of blood flow. Baillieres Clin Haematol 12:375, 1983

146. Chien LT, Weiss S: The role of the sinus wall in the passage of erythrocytes through the spleen. Blood 41:529, 1973

147. Nakashima K, Beutler E: Erythrocyte cellular and membrane deformability in hereditary spherocytosis. Blood 53:481, 1979

148. Clark MR, Mohandas N, Shohet SB: Osmotic gradient ektacytometry: comprehensive characterization of red cell volume and surface maintenance. Blood 61:899, 1983

149. Erslev AJ, Atwater J: Effect of mean corpuscular hemoglobin concentration on viscosity. J Lab Clin Med 62:401, 1963

150. Waugh RE, Agre P: Reductions of erythrocyte membrane viscoelastic coefficients reflect spectrin deficiencies in hereditary spherocytosis. J Clin Invest 81:133, 1988

151. Barnhart MT, Lusher JM: The human spleen as revealed by scanning electron microscopy. Am J Hematol 1:243, 1976

152. Molnar Z, Rappaport H: Fine structure of red pulp of the spleen in hereditary spherocytosis. Blood 39:81, 1972

153. Ferrant A: The role of spleen in haemolysis. Baillieres Clin Haematol 12:489, 1983

154. Jensen OM, Kristensen J: Red pulp of the spleen in autoimmune haemolytic anaemia and hereditary spherocytosis: morphometric light and electron microscopy studies. Scand J Haematol 36:263, 1986

155. Emerson CP Jr, Shen SC, Ham TH et al: Studies on the destruction of red blood cells. IX. Quantitative methods for determining the osmotic and mechanical fragility of red cells in the peripheral blood and splenic pulp: the mechanism of increased hemolysis in hereditary spherocytosis (congenital hemolytic jaundice) as related to the function of the spleen. Arch Intern Med 97:1, 1956

156. Prankerd T: Studies on the pathogenesis of haemolysis in hereditary spherocytosis. Q J Med 29:199, 1960

157. Griggs RC, Weisman R Jr, Harris JW: Alteration in osmotic and mechanical fragility related to in vivo erythrocyte aging and splenic sequestration in hereditary spherocytosis. J Clin Invest 39:89, 1960

158. LaCelle PL: pH in the mouse spleen and its effect on erythrocyte flow properties. Blood 44:910, 1974

159. Murphy JR: The influence of pH and temperature on some physical properties of normal erythrocytes from patients with hereditary spherocytosis. J Lab Clin Med 69:758, 1967

160. Palek J, Mircevová L, Brabec V: 2,3-Diphosphoglycerate metabolism in hereditary spherocytosis. Br J Haematol 17:59, 1969

161. Maridonneau I, Braquet P, Garay RP: Na⁺ and K⁺ transport damage induced by oxygen free radicals in human red cell membranes. J Biol Chem 258:3107, 1983

162. Vercellotti GM, van Asbeck BS, Jacob HS: Oxygen radical-induced erythrocyte hemolysis by neutrophils. Critical role of iron and lactoferrin. J Clin Invest 76:956, 1985

163. Schroit AJ, Madsen JW, Tanaka Y: In vivo recognition and clearance of red blood cells containing phosphatidylserine in their plasma membranes. J Biol Chem 260:5131, 1985

164. Kuypers FA, Lubin BH, Yee M et al: The distribution of erythrocyte phospholipids in hereditary spherocytosis demonstrates a minimal role for erythrocyte spectrin on phospholipid diffusion and asymmetry. Blood 81:1051, 1993

165. Lubin B, Chiu D, Schwartz RS: Abnormal membrane phospholipid organization in spectrin deficient human red cells, abstracted. Blood, suppl. 1. 62:34a, 1983

166. Szymanski IO, Odgren PR, Fortier NL, Snyder LM: Red blood cell associated IgG in normal and pathologic states. Blood 55:48, 1980

167. Clark MR, Shohet SB: Red cell senescence. Baillieres Clin Haematol 14:223, 1985

168. McCann SR, Jacob HS: Spinal cord disease in hereditary spherocytosis: report of two cases with hypothesized common mechanism for neurologic and red cell abnormalities. Blood 48:259, 1976

169. Moiseyev VS, Korovina EA, Polotskaya EL: Hypertrophic cardiomyopathy associated with hereditary spherocytosis in three generations of one family. Lancet 2:853, 1987

170. Peters LL, Birkenmeier CS, Bronson RT et al: Purkinje cell degeneration associated with erythroid ankyrin deficiency in nb/nb mice. J Cell Biol 114:1233, 1991

171. White RA, Birkenmeier CS, Lux SE, Barker JE: Ankyrin and the hemolytic anemia mutation, nb, map to mouse chromosome 8: presence of the nb allele is associated with truncated erythrocyte ankyrin. Proc Natl Acad Sci USA 87:3117, 1990

172. Peters LL, Turtzo CL, Birkenmeier CS, Barker JE: Distinct fetal Ank-1 and Ank-2 related proteins and mRNAs in normal and nb/nb mice. Blood 81:2144, 1993

173. Marchesi SL, Agre PA, Speicher DW: Abnormal spectrin αII domain in recessive spherocytosis, abstracted. J Cell Biochem, suppl. 13B:213, 1989

174. Stevens RF, Evans DIK: Congenital spherocytosis is often not hereditary. Clin Pediatr 20:47, 1981

175. Race RR: On the inheritance and linkage relations of acholuric jaundice. Ann Eugen 11:365, 1942

176. Kohler HG, Meynell MJ, Cooke WT: Spherocytic anaemia complicated by megaloblastic anaemia of pregnancy. BMJ 1:779, 1960

177. Taylor JJ: Haemolysis in infectious mononucleosis: inapparent congenital spherocytosis. BMJ 4:525, 1973

178. Conklin GT, George JN, Sears DA: Transient erythroid aplasia in hemolytic anemia: a review of the literature with two case reports. Tex Rep Biol Med 32:391, 1974

179. Lefrere JJ, Courouce AM, Girot R et al: Six cases of hereditary spherocytosis revealed by human parvovirus infection. Br J Haematol 62:653, 1986

180. LeBlond PF, DeBoisfleury A, Bessis M: La forme des erythrocytes dans la sphérocytose héréditaire. Etude au microscope à balayage: rélation avécleur déformabilité. Nouv Rev Fr Hematol 13:873, 1973

181. Rand RP, Burton AC: Mechanical properties of the red cell membrane. Membrane stiffness and intracellular pressure. Biophys J 4:115, 1964

182. Rand RP, Burton AC: Area and volume changes in hemolysis of single erythrocytes. J Cell Comp Physiol 61:245, 1963

183. Joiner CH, Lux SE: Cation permeability is increased in spectrin deficient mouse red cells, abstracted. Blood, suppl. 1. 60:21a, 1982

184. Godal HC, Gjonnes G, Ruyter R: Does preincubation of the red blood cells contribute to the capability of the osmotic fragility test to detect very mild forms of hereditary spherocytosis? Scand J Haematol 29:89, 1982

185. Zanella A, Izzo C, Rebulla P et al: Acidified glycerol lysis test: a screening test for spherocytosis. Br J Haematol 45:481, 1980

186. Gottfried EL, Robertson NA: Glycerol lysis time of incubated erythrocytes in the diagnosis of hereditary spherocytosis. J Lab Clin Med 84:746, 1974

187. Rutherford CJ, Postlewaight BF, Hallowes M: An evaluation of the acidified glycerol lysis test. Br J Haematol 63:119, 1986

188. Judkiewicz L, Bartosz G, Oplatowska A: Modified osmotic fragility test for the laboratory diagnosis of hereditary spherocytosis. Am J Hematol 31:136, 1989

189. Vettore L, Zanella A, Molaro GL et al: A new test for the laboratory diagnosis of spherocytosis. Acta Haematol Pol 72:258, 1984

190. Armbrust R, Eber SW, Schroter W: Absence of phosphorylation-induced gelation of erythrocyte membrane skeletons—a diagnostic tool for hereditary spherocytosis. Ann Hematol 64:93, 1992

191. Pinder JC, Dhermy D, Baines AJ et al: Phenomenological difference between cytoskeletal protein complexes isolated from normal and hereditary spherocytosis erythrocytes. Br J Haematol 55:455, 1983

192. Laemmli UK: Cleavage of structural proteins during the assembly of the head of bacteriophage T4. Nature 227:680, 1970

193. Fairbanks G, Steck TL, Wallach DFH: Electrophoretic analysis of the major polypeptides of the human erythrocyte membrane. Biochemistry 10:2606, 1971

194. Grompe M: The rapid detection of unknown mutations in nucleic acids. Nature Genet 5:111, 1993

195. Hurst D, Vichinsky EP: Splenectomy indications in childhood. p. 407. In Pochedly C, Sills RH, Schwartz AD (eds): Disorders of Spleen. Pathophysiology and management. Marcel Dekker, New York, 1989

196. Krueger HC, Burgert EO: Hereditary spherocytosis in 100 children. Mayo Clin Proc 41:821, 1966

197. Lux SE: Disorders of the red cell membrane skeleton: hereditary spherocytosis and hereditary elliptocytosis. p. 1581. In Stanbury JB, Wyngaarden JB, Frederickson DS, Goldstein JL, M Brown (eds): The Metabolic Basis of Inherited Disease. 5th Ed. McGraw-Hill, New York, 1983

198. Kelleher JF, Luban NLC, Mortimer PP, Kamimura T: Human serum parvovirus: a specific cause of aplastic crisis in children with hereditary spherocytosis. J Pediatr 102:720, 1983

199. Saarinen UM, Chorba TL, Tattersall P et al: Human parvovirus B19-induced epidemic acute red cell aplasia in patients with hereditary hemolytic anemia. Blood 67:1411, 1986

200. Young N: Hematologic and hematopoietic consequences of B19 parvovirus infection. Semin Hematol 25:159, 1988

201. Mortimer PP, Humphries RK, Moore JG et al: A human parvovirus-like virus inhibits haematopoietic colony formation in vitro. Nature 302:426, 1983

202. Davidson RF, Brown T, Wiseman D: Human parvovirus infection and aplastic crisis in hereditary spherocytosis. J Infect Dis 9:298, 1984

203. Taylor ES: Chronic ulcer of the leg associated with congenital jaundice. JAMA 112:1574, 1939

204. Hanford RB, Schneider GF, MacCarthy FD: Massive thoracic extramedullary hemopoiesis. N Engl J Med 263:120, 1960

205. Vetrani A, Cecere C, Fulciniti F, Ferrante G: Intrathoracic extramedullary hematopoiesis. Report of case in a patient with hereditary spherocytosis. Pathologica 76:733, 1984

206. Barry M, Scheuer PS, Sherlock S et al: Hereditary spherocytosis with secondary haemochromatosis. Lancet 2:481, 1968

207. Edwards CQ, Skolnick MH, Dadone MM, Kushner JP: Iron overload in hereditary spherocytosis: association with HLA-linked hemochromatosis. Am J Hematol 13:101, 1982

208. Mohler DN, Wheby MS: Hemochromatosis heterozygotes may have significant iron overload when they also have hereditary spherocytosis. Am J Med Sci 292:320, 1986

209. Fargion S, Cappellini MD, Piperno A et al: Association of hereditary spherocytosis and idiopathic hemochromatosis. A synergistic effect in determining iron overload. Am J Clin Pathol 86:645, 1986

210. Zimelman AP, Miller A: Primary hemochromatosis with hereditary spherocytosis. Arch Intern Med 140:983, 1980

211. Ho-Ten DO: Hereditary spherocytosis presenting in pregnancy. Acta Haematol 72:29, 1984

212. Ventura CS: Hereditary spherocytosis with haemolytic crisis during pregnancy. Aust NZ J Obstet Gynaecol 22:50, 1982

213. Cooper RA, Jandl JH: The role of membrane lipids in the survival of red cells in hereditary spherocytosis. J Clin Invest 49:666, 1970

214. Crosby WH, Conrad ME: Hereditary spherocytosis: observation on hemolytic mechanisms and iron metabolism. Blood 15:662, 1960

215. Miraglia del Giudice E, Perrotta S, Nobili B et al: Coexistence of hereditary spherocytosis (HS) due to band 3 deficiency and β-thalassaemia trait: partial correction of HS phenotype. Br J Haematol 85:553, 1993

216. Chapman RG: Red cell life span after splenectomy in hereditary spherocytosis. J Clin Invest 47:2263, 1968

217. Van dyck DB: Overwhelming postsplenectomy infection: the clinical syndrome. Lymphology 16:107, 1987

218. Brigden ML: Postsplenectomy sepsis syndrome. How to identify and manage patients at risk. Postgrad Med 77:215, 1985

219. Schwartz AD: Physiology of the spleen and the consequences of hyposplenism. p. 145. In Pochedly C, Sills RH, Schwartz AD (eds): Disorders of Spleen. Pathophysiology and management. Marcel Dekker, New York, 1989

220. Lortan JE: Management of asplenic patients. Br J Haematol 84:566, 1993

221. Croom RD III, McMillan CW, Sheldon GF, Orringer EP: Hereditary spherocy-

tosis: recent experience and current concepts of pathophysiology. Ann Surg 203:34, 1986

222. Wiley JS: Hereditary spherocytosis, elliptocytosis, and related disorders. p. 21. In Brain MC, Carbonne PC (eds): Current Therapy. Hematology-Oncology. BC Decker, Toronto, 1988

223. Lux SE: Disorders of the red cell membrane. p. 489. In Nathan DG, Oski FA (eds): Hematology of Infancy and Childhood. WB Saunders, Philadelphia, 1987

224. Palek J: Hereditary spherocytosis. p. 558. In Williams WJ, Beutler E, Ersler AJ, Lichtman MA (eds): Hematology. McGraw-Hill, New York, 1989

225. Tchernia G, Gauthier F, Mielot F et al: Initial assessment of the beneficial effect of partial splenectomy in hereditary spherocytosis. Blood 81:2014, 1993

226. Lawrie GM, Ham M: The surgical treatment of hereditary spherocytosis. Surg Gynecol Obstet 139:208, 1974

227. Rutkow IM: Twenty years of splenectomy for hereditary spherocytosis. Arch Surg 116:306, 1981

228. Brook J, Tanaka KR: Combination of pyruvate kinase (PK) deficiency and hereditary spherocytosis (HS). Clin Res 18:176A, 1970

229. Dacie J: The Haemolytic Anaemias. 3rd Ed. Churchill Livingstone, Edingburgh, 1985, p. 119

230. Buchanan GR, Holtkamp CA: Pocked erythrocyte counts in patients with hereditary spherocytosis before and after splenectomy. Am J Hematol 25: 253, 1987

231. Kvindesdal BB, Jensen MK: Pitted erythrocytes in splenectomized subjects with congenital spherocytosis and in subjects splenectomized for other reasons. Scand J Haematol 37:41, 1986

232. Bart B, Appel MF: Recurrent hemolytic anemia secondary to accessory spleens. South Med J 71:608, 1978

233. Satou S, Yokota E, Sugihara J et al: Relapse of hereditary spherocytosis following splenectomy. Acta Haematol Jpn 48:1337, 1985

234. Babiker MA, ElSeed FAA: A family with sickle cell trait and hereditary spherocytosis. Scand J Haematol 33:54, 1984

235. Dresbach M: Elliptical human red corpuscles. Science 19:469, 1904

236. Hunter WC, Adams RB: Hematologic study of three generations of a white family showing elliptical erythrocytes. Ann Intern Med 2:1162, 1929

237. Hunter WC: Further study of a white family showing elliptical erythrocytes Ann Intern Med 6:775, 1932

238. Zarkowsky HS, Mohandas N, Speaker CB, Shohet SB: A congenital haemolytic anaemia with thermal sensitivity of the erythrocyte membrane. Br J Haematol 29:537, 1975

239. Amato D, Booth PB: Hereditary ovalocytosis in Melanesians. P N G Med J 20:26, 1977

240. Lie-Injo LE: Hereditary ovalocytosis and haemoglobin E-ovalocytosis in Malayan aborigines. Nature 208:1329, 1965

241. Honig GR, Lacson PS, Maurer HS: A new familial disorder with abnormal erythrocyte morphology and increased permeability of the erythrocytes to sodium and potassium. Pediatr Res 5:159, 1971

242. Wyandt H, Bancroft PM, Winship TO: Elliptic erythrocytes in man. Arch Intern Med 68:1043, 1941

243. McCarty SH: Elliptical red blood cells in man. J Lab Clin Med 19:612, 1934

244. Bannerman RM, Renwick JH: The hereditary elliptocytosis: clinical and linkage data. Ann Hum Genet 26:23, 1962

245. Lecomte MC, Dhermy D, Gautero H et al: L'elliptocytose héréditaire en Afrique de l'Ouest. Fréquence et repartition des variants de la spectrine. C R Acad Sci III 306:43, 1988

246. Cattani JA, Gibson FD, Alpers MP, Crane GG: Hereditary ovalocytosis and reduced susceptibility to malaria in Papua New Guinea. Trans R Soc Trop Med Hyg 81:705, 1987

247. Lie-Injo LE, Fix A, Bolton JM, Gilman RH: Haemoglobin E-hereditary elliptocytosis in Malayan aborigines. Acta Haematol 47:210, 1972

248. Ganesan J, George R, Lie-Injo LE: Abnormal haemoglobins and hereditary ovalocytosis in the Ulu Jempul district of Kuala Pilah, West Malaysia. Southeast Asian J Trop Med Public Health 7:430, 1976

249. Chang K, Williamson JR, Zarkowsky H: Effect of heat on the circular dichroism of spectrin in hereditary pyropoikilocytosis. J Clin Invest 64:326, 1979

250. Palek J, Liu SC, Liu PY et al: Altered assembly of spectrin in red cell membranes in hereditary pyropoikilocytosis. Blood 57:130, 1981

251. Tomaselli MB, John KM, Lux SE: Elliptical erythrocyte membrane skeletons and heat sensitive spectrin in hereditary elliptocytosis. Proc Natl Acad Sci USA 78:1911, 1981

252. Liu SC, Palek J, Prchal J: Defective membrane skeleton assembly in hereditary elliptocytosis. p. 157. In Kruckeberg W, Eaton J, Breuer G (eds): Erythrocyte Membranes. Vol. 2: Recent Clinical and Experimental Advances. Alan R Liss, New York, 1981

253. Liu SC, Palek J, Prchal JT, Castleberry P: Altered spectrin dimer-dimer asso-

ciation and instability of erythrocyte membrane skeletons in hereditary pyropoikilocytosis. J Clin Invest 68:597, 1981

254. Coetzer T, Zail SS: Tryptic digestion of spectrin in variants of hereditary elliptocytosis. J Clin Invest 67:1241, 1981

255. Feo CJ, Fischer S, Piau JP et al: Premier observation de l'absence d'une proteine de la membrane érythrocyaire familiale. Nouv Rev Fr Hematol 22: 315, 1980

256. Morlé L, Morlé F, Roux AF et al: Spectrin Tunis (Sp $\alpha^{I/78}$), an elliptocytogenic variant, is due to the CGG → TGG codon change (Arg → Trp) at position 35 of the αI domain. Blood 74:828, 1989

257. Lecomte MC, Garbarz M, Grandchamp B et al: Sp $\alpha^{I/78}$: a mutation of the αI spectrin domain in a white kindred with HE and HPP phenotypes. Blood 74:1126, 1989

258. Coetzer TL, Sahr K, Prchal J et al: Four different mutations in codon 28 of α spectrin are associated with structurally and functionally abnormal spectrin $\alpha^{I/74}$ in hereditary elliptocytosis. J Clin Invest 88:743, 1991

259. Lorenzo F, Miraglia del Giudice E, Alloisio N et al: Severe poikilocytosis associated with a de novo α28 Arg → Cys mutation in spectrin. Br J Haematol 83:152, 1993

260. Floyd PB, Gallagher PG, Valentino LA et al: Heterogeneity of the molecular basis of hereditary pyropoikilocytosis and hereditary elliptocytosis associated with increased levels of the spectrin $\alpha^{I/74}$-kilodalton tryptic peptide. Blood 78:1364, 1991

261. Garbarz M, Lecomte MC, Féo C et al: Hereditary pyropoikilocytosis and elliptocytosis in a white French family with the spectrin $\alpha^{I/74}$ variant related to a CGT to CAT codon change (Arg to His) at position 22 of the spectrin αI domain. Blood 75:1691, 1990

262. Baklouti F, Maréchal J, Morlé L et al: Occurrence of the αI 22 Arg → His (CGT → CAT) spectrin mutation in Tunisia: potential association with severe elliptopoikilocytosis. Br J Haematol 78:108, 1991

263. Miraglia del Giudice E, Perrotta S, Sciarratta G et al: αI/74 spectrin Genova: a new elliptocytogenic variant due to Arg → Trp substitution at position 34 of α spectrin, abstracted. Blood, suppl. 1. 80:277a, 1992

264. Morlé L, Roux A-F, Alloisio N et al: Two elliptocytogenic $\alpha^{I/74}$ variants of the spectrin αI domain. Spectrin Culoz (GGT → GTT; αI 40 Gly → Val) and spectrin Lyon (CTT → TTT; αI 43 Leu → Phe). J Clin Invest 86:548, 1990

265. Sahr K, Tobe T, Scarpa A et al: Sequence and exon-intron organization of the DNA encoding the αI domain of human spectrin. Application to the study of mutations causing hereditary elliptocytosis. J Clin Invest 84:1243, 1989

266. Roux AF, Morlé F, Guetarni D et al: Molecular basis of Sp$\alpha^{I/65}$ hereditary elliptocytosis in North Africa: insertion of a TTG triplet between codons 147 and 149 in the α-spectrin gene from five unrelated families. Blood 73: 2196, 1989

267. Miraglia del Giudice E, Ducluzeau MT, Alloisio N et al: αI/65 hereditary elliptocytosis in Southern Italy: evidence for an African origin. Hum Genet 89: 553, 1992

268. Dhermy D, Boulanger L, Silva CJ et al: Spectrin Ponte de Sôr (Gly151Asp): a mutation of the spectrin (Sp) α gene associated with Sp $\alpha^{I/65}$ hereditary elliptocytosis (HE), abstracted. p. 143. Presented at the Twenty-Fourth Congress of the International Society of Haematology, 1992

269. Hassoun H, Coetzer TL, Sahr KE et al: An insertion within the α spectrin gene leading to exon skipping in a family with hereditary elliptocytosis (HE) and pyropoikilocytosis (HPP), abstracted. Blood, suppl. 1. 80:19a, 1992

270. Marchesi SL, Letsinger JT, Speicher DW et al: Mutant forms of α-spectrin in hereditary elliptocytosis. J Clin Invest 80:191, 1987

271. Gallagher PG, Tse WT, Coetzer T et al: A common type of the spectrin αI 46–50a-kD peptide abnormality in hereditary elliptocytosis and pyropoikilocytosis is associated with a mutation distant from the proteolytic cleavage site—evidence for the functional importance of the triple helical model of spectrin. J Clin Invest 89:892, 1992

272. Baklouti F, Meréchal J, Wilmotte R et al: Elliptocytogenic $\alpha^{I/36}$ spectrin Sfax lacks nine amino acids in helix 3 repeat 4. Evidence for the activation of a cryptic 5'-splice site in exon 8 of spectrin α-gene. Blood 79:2464, 1992

273. Gallagher PG, Marchesi SL, Forget BG: A new point mutation associated with αI/50b kDa hereditary elliptocytosis (HE) and hereditary pyropoikilocytosis (HPP), abstracted. Clin Res 39:313a, 1991

274. Dalla Venezia N, Alloisio N, Forissier A et al: Elliptopoikilocytosis associated with the α469 His → Pro spectrin barcelona ($\alpha^{I/50-46b}$). Blood 82:1661, 1993

275. Gallagher PG, Roberts WE, Benoit L et al: Poikilocytic hereditary elliptocytosis associated with spectrin Alexandria: an αI/50b Kd variant that is due to a single amino acid deletion. Blood 82:2210, 1993

276. Alloisio N, Wilmotte R, Morlé L et al: Spectrin Jendouba: an $\alpha^{II/31}$ spectrin variant that is associated with elliptocytosis and carries a mutation distant from the dimer self-association site. Blood 80:809, 1992

277. Alloisio N, Morlé L, Pothier B et al: Spectrin Oran ($\alpha^{II/21}$), a new spectrin

variant concerning the αII domain and causing severe elliptocytosis in the homozygous state. Blood 71:1039, 1988

278. Alloisio N, Wilmotte R, Marechal J et al: A splice site mutation of α-spectrin gene causing skipping of exon 18 in hereditary elliptocytosis. Blood 81:2791, 1993

279. Sahr KE, Coetzer TL, Moy LS et al: An ALA to GLY substitution in helix 1 of β spectrin repeat 17 that severely disrupts the structure and self-association of the erythrocyte spectrin heterodimer. J Biol Chem 268:22656, 1993

280. Gallagher PG, Tse WT, Mohandas N et al: Spectrin Providence: a defect of erythrocyte beta spectrin ($\beta^{2109Ser-Pro}$) homozygosity for which is associated with fatal hydrops fetalis, abstracted. Blood, suppl. 1. 80:145a, 1992

281. Tse WT, Lecomte MC, Costa FF et al: Point mutation in the β-spectrin gene associated with αI/74 hereditary elliptocytosis. Implications for the mechanism of spectrin dimer self-association. J Clin Invest 86:909, 1990

282. Johnson RM, Ravindranath Y, Brohn F, Hussain M: A large erythroid spectrin β-chain variant. Br J Haematol 80:6, 1992

283. Garbarz M, Tse WT, Gallagher PG et al: Spectrin Rouen ($\beta^{220-218}$), a novel shortened β-chain variant in a kindred with hereditary elliptocytosis—characterization of the molecular defect as exon skipping due to a splice site mutation. J Clin Invest 88:76, 1991

284. Lecomte MC, Gautero H, Bournier O et al: Ellyptocytosis-associated spectrin Rouen ($\beta^{220/218}$) has a truncated but still phosphorylatable β chain. Br J Haematol 80:242, 1992

285. Garbarz M, Boulanger L, Pedroni S et al: Spectrin β^{Tandil}, a novel shortened β-chain variant associated with hereditary elliptocytosis is due to a deletional frameshift mutation in the β-spectrin gene. Blood 80:1066, 1992

286. Kanzaki A, Rabodonirina M, Yawata Y et al: A deletional frameshift mutation of the β-spectrin gene associated with elliptocytosis in spectrin Tokio ($\beta^{220/216}$), abstracted. Blood 80:2115, 1992

287. Tse WT, Gallagher PG, Pothier B et al: An insertional frameshift mutation of the β-spectrin gene associated with elliptocytosis in spectrin Nice ($\beta^{220/216}$). Blood 78:517, 1991

288. Yoon SH, Yu H, Eber S, Prchal JT: Molecular defect of truncated β-spectrin associated with hereditary elliptocytosis. β-Spectrin Göttingen. J Biol Chem 266:8490, 1991

289. Gallagher PG, Tse WT, Costa F et al: A splice site mutation of the β-spectrin gene causing exon skipping in hereditary elliptocytosis associated with a truncated β-spectrin chain. J Biol Chem 266:15154, 1991

290. Conboy J, Mohandas N, Tchernia G, Kan YW: Molecular basis of hereditary elliptocytosis due to protein 4.1 deficiency. N Engl J Med 315:680, 1986

291. Dalla Venezia N, Gilsanz F, Alloisio N et al: Homozygous 4.1 (−) hereditary elliptocytosis associated with a point mutation in the downstream initiation codon of protein 4.1 gene. J Clin Invest 90:1713, 1992

292. Conboy J, Marchesi S, Kim R et al: Molecular analysis of insertion/deletion mutations in protein 4.1 in elliptocytosis. II. Determination of molecular genetic origins of rearrangements. J Clin Invest 86:524, 1990

293. Marchesi SL, Conboy J, Agre P et al: Molecular analysis of insertion/deletion mutations in protein 4.1 in elliptocytosis. I. Biochemical identification of rearrangements in the spectrin/actin binding domain and functional characterizations. J Clin Invest 86:516, 1990

294. Conboy JG, Shitamoto R, Parra M et al: Hereditary elliptocytosis due to both qualitative and quantitative defects in membrane skeletal protein 4.1. Blood 78:2438, 1991

295. Feddal S, Hayette S, Baklouti F et al: Prevalent skipping of an individual exon accounts for shortened protein 4.1 Presles. Blood 80:2925, 1992

296. Telen MJ, Le Van Kim C, Chung A et al: Molecular basis for elliptocytosis associated with glycophorin C and glycophorin D deficiency in the Leach phenotype. Blood 78:1603, 1991

297. High S, Tanner MJA, MacDonald EB, Anstee DJ: Rearrangements of the red cell membrane glycophorin C (sialoglycoprotein β) gene. Biochem J 262:47, 1989

298. Tanner MJA, High S, Martin PG et al: Genetic variants of human red cell membrane sialoglycoprotein β. Study of the alterations occuring in the sialoglycoprotein β gene. Biochem J 250:407, 1988

299. Speicher DW, Davis G, Marchesi VT: Structure of human erythrocyte spectrin. II. The sequence of the α-I domain. J Biol Chem 258:14938, 1983

300. Speicher DW, Davis G, Yurchenco PD, Marchesi VT: Structure of the human erythrocyte spectrin. I. Isolation of the α-I domain and its cyanogen bromide peptides. J Biol Chem 258:14931, 1983

301. Speicher DW, Weglarz L, DeSilva TM: Properties of human red cell spectrin heterodimer (side-to-side) assembly and identification of an essential nucleation site. J Biol Chem 267:14775, 1992

302. Speicher DW, DeSilva TM, Speicher KD et al: Location of human red cell spectrin tetramer binding site and detection of a related "closed" hairpin loop dimer using proteolytic footprinting. J Biol Chem 268:4227, 1993

303. Winograd E, Hume D, Branton D: Phasing the conformational unit of spectrin. Proc Natl Acad Sci USA 88:10788, 1991

304. Speicher DW, Marchesi VT: Erythrocyte spectrin is comprised of many homologous triple helical segments. Nature 311:177, 1984

305. Speicher DW: The present status of erythrocyte spectrin structure: the 106-residue repetitive structure is a basic feature of an entire class of proteins. J Cell Biochem 30:245, 1986

306. Palek J: Hereditary elliptocytosis, spherocytosis and related disorders: consequences of a deficiency or a mutation of membrane skeletal proteins. Blood Rev 1:147, 1987

307. Féo CJ, Fischer S, Piau JP et al: Première observation de l'absence d'une protéine de la membrane érythrocytaire (bande 4₁) dans un cas d'anémie elliptocytaire familiale. Nouv Rev Fr Hematol 22:315, 1980

308. Dhermy D, Garbarz M, Lecomte MC et al: Hereditary elliptocytosis. Clinical, morphological and biochemical studies of 38 cases. Nouv Rev Fr Hematol 28:129, 1986

309. Coetzer T, Lawler J, Prchal JT, Palek J: Molecular determinants of clinical expression of hereditary elliptocytosis and pyropoikilocytosis. Blood 70:766, 1987

310. Palek J: Hereditary elliptocytosis, spherocytosis and related disorders: consequences of a deficiency of a mutation of membrane skeletal proteins. Blood 1:147, 1987

311. Marchesi VT: Stabilizing infrastructure of cell membranes. Ann Rev Cell Biol 1:531, 1985

312. Liu SC, Derick LH, Palek J: Visualization of the hexagonal lattice in the erythrocyte membrane skeleton. J Cell Biol 104:527, 1987

313. Ungewickell E, Gratzer W: Self-association of human spectrin. A thermodynamic and kinetic study. Eur J Biochem 88:379, 1978

314. Sahr KE, Coetzer TL, Moy LS et al: An Ala to Gly substitution in β spectrin associated with spectrin $\alpha^{I/74}$ in hereditary elliptocytosis (HE) and hereditary pyropoikilocytosis (HPP), abstracted. Blood, suppl. 1. 80:276a, 1992

315. Cohen C: The molecular organization of the red cell membrane skeleton. Semin Hematol 20:141, 1983

316. Bennett V: The molecular basis for membrane-cytoskeleton association in human erythrocytes. J Cell Biochem 18:49, 1982

317. Correas I, Leto TL, Speicher DW, Marchesi VT: Identification of the functional site of erythrocyte protein 4.1 involved in spectrin-actin associations. J Biol Chem 261:3310, 1986

318. Pasternack GR, Anderson RA, Leto TL, Marchesi VT: Interactions between protein 4.1 and band 3. J Biol Chem 260:3676, 1985

319. Anderson RA, Lovrien RE: Glycophorin is linked by band 4.1 protein to the human erythrocyte membrane skeleton. Nature 307:655, 1984

320. Rybicki AC, Heath R, Lubin B, Schwartz RS: Human erythrocyte protein 4.1 is a phosphatidylserine binding protein. J Clin Invest 82:255, 1988

321. Cohen AM, Liu SC, Lawler J et al: Identification of the protein 4.1 binding site to phosphatidylserine vesicles. Biochemistry 27:614, 1988

322. Bennett V: The spectrin-actin junction of erythrocyte membrane skeletons. Biochim Biophys Acta 988:107, 1989

323. Sauberman N, Fortier N, Fairbanks G, O'Connor RJ, Snyder LM: Red cell membrane in hemolytic disease studies on variables affecting electrophoretic analysis. Biochim Biophys Acta 556:292, 1979

324. Inaba M, Gupta KC, Kuwabara M et al: Deamidation of human erythrocyte protein 4.1: Possible role in aging. Blood 79:3355, 1992

325. Lambert S, Conboy J, Zail S: A molecular study of heterozygous protein 4.1 deficiency in hereditary elliptocytosis. Blood 72:1926, 1988

326. Lambert S, Zail S: Partial deficiency of protein 4.1 in hereditary elliptocytosis. Am J Hematol 26:263, 1987

327. McGuire M, Smith BL, Agre P: Distinct variants of erythrocyte protein 4.1 inherited in linkage with elliptocytosis and Rh type in three white families. Blood 72:287, 1988

328. Tchernia G, Mohandas N, Shohet SB: Deficiency of skeletal membrane protein band 4.1 in homozygous hereditary elliptocytosis: implications for erythrocyte membrane stability. J Clin Invest 68:454, 1981

329. Mueller TJ, Morrison M: Cytoskeletal alterations in hereditary elliptocytosis. J Supramol Struct 5:131, 1981

330. Alloisio N, Morlé L, Dorléc E et al: The heterozygous form of 4.1 (−) hereditary elliptocytosis [the 4.1 (−) trait]. Blood 65:46, 1985

331. Anstee DJ, Parsons SF, Ridgwell K et al: Two individuals with elliptocytic red cells apparently lack three minor erythrocyte membrane sialoglycoproteins. Biochem J 218:615, 1984

332. Daniels GL, Shaw M-A, Judson PA et al: A family demonstrating inheritance of the Leach phenotype: a Gerbich-negative phenotype associated with elliptocytosis. Vox Sang 50:117, 1986

333. Anstee DJ, Ridgwell K, Tanner MJA et al: Individuals lacking the Gerbich blood-group antigen have alterations in the human erythrocyte membrane sialoglycoproteins β and α. Biochem J 221:97, 1984

334. Reid ME, Anstee DJ, Jensen RH, Mohandas N: Normal membrane function of abnormal β-related erythrocyte sialoglycoproteins. Br J Haematol 67:467, 1987

335. Mueller T, Morrison M: Glycoconnectin (PAS 2) a membrane attachment site for the human erythrocyte cytoskeleton. p. 95. In Kruckeberg W, Eaton J, Brewer G (eds): Erythrocyte Membranes. Vol. 2: Recent Clinical and Experimental Advances. In: Progress in Clinical and Biological Research. Alan R Liss, New York, 1981

336. Alloisio N, Morlé L, Bachir D et al: Red cell membrane sialoglycoprotein in homozygous and heterozygous 4.1 (−) hereditary elliptocytosis. Biochim Biophys Acta 816:57, 1985

337. Gahmberg CG, Myllyla G, Leikola J et al: Absence of the major sialoglycoprotein in the membrane of human En (a −) erythrocyte and increased glycosylation of band 3. J Biol Chem 251:6108, 1976

338. Liu SC, Derick LH, Agre P, Palek J: Alteration of the erythrocyte membrane skeletal ultrastructure in hereditary spherocytosis, hereditary elliptocytosis, and pyropoikilocytosis. Blood 76:198, 1990

339. Mohandas N, Chasis JA: Red blood cell deformability, membrane material properties and shape: regulation by transmembrane, skeletal and cytosolic proteins and lipids. Semin Hematol 30:171, 1993

340. Florman AL, Wintrobe MM: Human elliptical red corpuscles. Bull Johns Hopkins Hosp 63:209, 1938

341. Wyandt H, Bancroft PM, Winship TO: Elliptic erythrocytes in man. Arch Intern Med 68:1043, 1941

342. Rebuck JW, van Slyck EJ: An unsuspected ultrastructural fault in human elliptocytes. Am J Clin Pathol 49:19, 1968

343. Bessis M: The erythrocytic series. p. 85. In: Living Blood Cells and Their Ultrastructure. Springer-Verlag, New York, 1973

344. Liu S-C, Derick LH, Palek J: Dependence of the permanent deformation of red blood cell membranes on spectrin dimer-tetramer equilibrium: implication for permanent membrane deformation of irreversibly sickled cells. Blood 81:522, 1993

345. Coetzer TL, Palek J: Partial spectrin deficiency in hereditary pyropoikilocytosis. Blood 67:919, 1986

346. Gallagher PG, Tse WT, Marchesi VT: A defect in α spectrin accumulation in hereditary pyropoikilocytosis, abstracted. Clin Res 39:313, 1991

347. Coetzer T, Palek J, Lawler J et al: Structural and functional heterogeneity of α spectrin mutations involving the spectrin heterodimer self-association site: relationships to hematologic expression of homozygous hereditary elliptocytosis and hereditary pyropoikilocytosis. Blood 75:2235, 1990

348. Discher D, Knowles D, McGee S: Mechanical linkage between red cell skeleton and plasma membrane is not a demonstrated function of protein 4.1. Blood 82:309a, 1993

349. Nash GB, Parmar J, Reid ME: Effects of deficiencies of glycophorins C and D on the physical properties of the red cell. Br J Haematol 76:282, 1990

350. DeGruchy GC, Loder PB, Hennessy IV: Haemolysis and glycolytic metabolism in hereditary elliptocytosis. Br J Haematol 8:168, 1962

351. Peters JC, Rowland M, Israels LG, Zipursky A: Erythrocyte sodium transport in hereditary elliptocytosis. Can J Physiol Pharmacol 44:817, 1966

352. Wiley JS, Gill FM: Red cell calcium leak in congenital hemolytic anemia with extreme microcytosis. Blood 47:197, 1976

353. Lawler J, Palek J, Liu SC et al: Molecular heterogeneity of hereditary pyropoikilocytosis: identification of a second variant of the spectrin alpha-subunit. Blood 62:1182, 1983

354. Palek J, Lux SE: Red cell membrane skeletal defects in hereditary and acquired hemolytic anemias. Semin Hematol 20:189, 1983

355. Weiss HJ: Hereditary elliptocytosis with hemolytic anemia. Report of six cases. Am J Med 35:455, 1963

356. Penfold JB, Lipscomb JM: Elliptocytosis in man, associated with hereditary hemorrhagic telangiectasia. Q J Med 36:157, 1942

357. Jensson O, Jonasson TH, Olafsson O: Herediary elliptocytosis in Iceland. Br J Haematol 13:844, 1967

358. Keats BJB: Another elliptocytosis locus on chromosome 1? Hum Genet 50:227, 1979

359. Huebner K, Palumbo AP, Isobe M et al: The α-spectrin gene is on chromosome 1 in mouse and man. Proc Natl Acad Sci USA 82:3790, 1985

360. Morton NE: The detection and estimation of linkage between the genes for elliptocytosis and the Rh blood type. Am J Hum Genet 8:80, 1956

361. Cook PJL, Noades JE, Newton MS, de Mey R: On the orientation on the Rh: EL, linkage group. Ann Hum Genet 41:157, 1977

362. Lawler J, Coetzer TL, Mankad VN et al: Spectrin-α^{I/61}: A new structural variant of α-spectrin in a double-heterozygous form of hereditary pyropoikilocytosis. Blood 72:1412, 1988

363. Geerdink RA, Hellman PW, Verloop MC: Hereditary elliptocytosis and hyperhaemolysis: a comparative study of 6 families with 145 patients. J Intern Med 179:715, 1966

364. Motulsky AG, Singer K, Crosby WH, Smith V: The life span of the elliptocyte in hereditary elliptocytosis and its relationship to other familial hemolytic diseases. Blood 9:57, 1954

365. Kruskall MS, Messier DS, Doherty BV, Pacini DG: Elliptocytosis in blood donors. Transfusion 27:113, 1987

366. Mentzer WC, Turetsky T, Mohandas N et al: Identification of the hereditary pyropoikilocytosis carrier state. Blood 63:1439, 1984

367. Jarolim P, Palek J, Coetzer TL et al: Severe hemolysis and red cell fragmentation caused by the combination of a spectrin mutation with a thrombotic microangiopathy. Am J Hematol 32:50, 1989

368. Austin RF, Desforges JF: Hereditary elliptocytosis: an unusual presentation of hemolysis in the newborn associated with transient morphologic abnormalities. Pediatrics 44:196, 1969

369. Carpentieri U, Gustavson LP, Haggard ME: Pyknocytosis in a neonate: an unusual presentation of hereditary elliptocytosis. Clin Pediatr 16:76, 1977

370. Zarkowsky HS: Heat-induced erythrocyte fragmentation in neonatal elliptocytosis. Br J Haematol 29:537, 1979

371. Mentzer WC, Iarocci TA, Mohandas N et al: Modulation of erythrocyte membrane mechanical stability by 2,3-diphosphoglycerate in the neonatal poikilocytosis/elliptocytosis syndrome. J Clin Invest 79:943, 1987

372. Sheetz MP, Casaly J: 2,3-Diphosphoglycerate and ATP dissociate erythrocyte membrane skeletons. J Biol Chem 255:9955, 1980

373. Pearson HA: The genetic basis of hereditary elliptocytosis with hemolysis. Blood 32:972, 1968

374. Letman H: Hereditary haemolytic elliptocytosis. J Intern Med 151:41, 1955

375. Baker SJ, Jacob E, Rajan KT, Gault EW: Hereditary haemolytic anaemia associated with elliptocytosis: a study of three families. Br J Haematol 7:210, 1961

376. Dugla-Siares A, Parreira F: Anémie élliptocytique familiale. Le Sang 29:33, 1958

377. Haddy TB, Rana SR: Homozygous hereditary elliptocytosis with hemolytic anemia. South Med J 77:631, 1984

378. Dhermy D, Lecomte MC, Garbarz M et al: Molecular defect of spectrin in the family of a child with congenital hemolytic poikilocytic anemia. Pediatr Res 18:1005, 1984

379. Evans JPM, Baines AJ, Hann IM et al: Defective spectrin dimer-dimer association in a family with transfusion dependent homozygous hereditary elliptocytosis. Br J Haematol 54:163, 1983

380. Garbarz M, Lecomte MC, Dhermy D et al: Double inheritance of an α^{I/65} spectrin variant in a child with homozygous elliptocytosis. Blood 67:1661, 1986

381. Hanspal M, Hanspal J, Palek J: Molecular basis of spectrin deficiency in hereditary pyropoikilocytosis (HPP) associated with mutant spectrin α^{I/46}, abstracted. Blood, suppl. 1.72:43a, 1988

382. Iarocci TA, Wagner GM, Mohandas N et al: Mild hereditary pyropoikilocytosis assiciated with the co-inheritance of two α spectrin abnormalities. Blood 71:1390, 1989

383. Peterson LC, Dampier C, Coetzer T et al: Clinical and laboratory study of two Caucasian families with hereditary pyropoikilocytosis and hereditary elliptocytosis. Am J Clin Pathol 88:58, 1987

384. Mallouh A, Sadi AR, Ahmad MS, Salamah M: Hereditary pyropoikilocytosis: report of two cases from Saudi Arabia. Am J Med Genet 18:413, 1984

385. Lecomte MC, Dhermy D, Garbarz M et al: Hereditary pyropoikilocytosis and elliptocytosis in a Caucasian family. Transmission of the same molecular defect in spectrin through three generations with different clinical expression. Hum Genet 77:329, 1987

386. Alloisio N, Morlé L, Maréchal J et al: Sp α^{V/41}: a common spectrin polymorphism at the αIV-αV domain junction. Relevance to the expression level of hereditary elliptocytosis due to α-spectrin variants located in trans. J Clin Invest 87:2169, 1991

387. Ravindranath Y, Johnson RM: Altered spectrin association and membrane fragility without abnormal spectrin heat sensitivity in a case of congenital hemolytic anemia. Am J Hematol 20:53, 1985

388. Mohandas N, Clark MR, Health BP et al: A technique to detect reduced mechanical stability of red cell membranes: relevance to elliptocytic disorders. Blood 59:768, 1982

389. Ungewickell E, Gratzer WB: Self-association of human spectrin. A thermodynamic and kinetic study. Eur J Biochem 88:379, 1987

390. Liu SC, Windisch P, Kim S, Palek J: Oligomeric states of spectrin in normal erythrocyte membranes: biochemical and electron microscopic studies. Cell 37:587, 1984

391. Palek J, Sahr KE: Mutations of the red blood cell membrane proteins: from clinical evaluations to detection of the underlying genetic defect. Blood 80:308, 1992

392. Djaldetti M, Cohen A, Hart J: Elliptocytosis preceding myelofibrosis in a patient with polycythemia vera. Acta Haematol 72:26, 1984

393. Rummens JL, Verfaillie C, Criel A et al: Elliptocytosis and schistocytosis in myelodysplasia: report of two cases. Acta Haematol 75:174, 1986
394. Bessis M: General pathology of erythrocytes. p. 197. In: Living Blood Cells and Their Ultrastructure. Springer-Verlag, New York, 1973
395. Goodall HB, Hendry DW, Lawler SD, Stephen SA: Data on linkage in man: elliptocytosis and blood groups II. Family 3. Ann Eugen 17:272, 1952
396. Lusher JM, Barnhart MI: The role of the spleen in the pathophysiology of hereditary spherocytosis and hereditary elliptocytosis. Am J Pediatr Hematol Oncol 2:31, 1980
397. Shneidman D, Kiessling P, Onslad J et al: Red pulp of the spleen in hereditary elliptocytosis. Virchows Arch A Pathol Anat Histo Pathol 372:337, 1977
398. Lux SE, Becker PS: Disorders of the membrane skeleton: hereditary spherocytosis and hereditary elliptocytosis. p. 2367. In Scriver CR, Baudet AB, Sly WS, Valle D (eds): The Metabolic Basis of Inherited Diseases. McGraw-Hill, New York, 1989
399. Dacie J: Hereditary elliptocytosis (HE). p. 216. In: The Haemolytic Anaemias. Churchill Livingstone, Edinburgh, 1985
400. Serjeantson S, Bryson K, Amato D, Babona D: Malaria and hereditary ovalocytosis. Hum Genet 37:161, 1977
401. Holt M, Hogan PF, Nurse GT: The ovalocytosis polymorphism on the western border of Papua New Guinea. Hum Biol 53:23, 1981
402. Fix AG, Baer AS, Lie-Injo LE: The mode of inheritance of ovalocytosis/elliptocytosis in Malaysian Orange Asli families. Hum Genet 61:250, 1982
403. Mohandas N, Lie-Injo LE, Friedman M, Mak JW: Rigid membranes of Malayan ovalocytes: a likely genetic barrier against malaria. Blood 63:1385, 1984
404. Saul A, Lamont G, Sawyer WH, Kidson C: Decreased membrane deformability in Melanesian ovalocytes from Papua New Guinea. J Cell Biol 98:1348, 1984
405. Kidson C, Lamont G, Saul A, Nurse GT: Ovalocytic erythrocytes from Melanesians are resistant to invasion by malaria parasites in culture. Proc Natl Acad Sci USA 78:5829, 1981
406. Castelino D, Saul A, Myler P et al: Ovalocytosis in Papua New Guinea: dominantly inherited resistance to malaria. Southeast Asian J Trop Med Public Health 12:549, 1981
407. Booth PB, Serjeantson S, Woodfield DG, Amato D: Selective depression of blood group antigens associated with hereditary ovalocytosis among Melanesians. Vox Sang 32:99, 1977
408. Hadley T, Saul A, Lamont G et al: Resistance of Melanesian elliptocytes (ovalocytes) to invasion by *Plasmodium knowlesi* and *Plasmodium falciparum* malaria parasites in vitro. J Clin Invest 71:780, 1983
409. Cattani JA, Gibson FD, Alpers MP, Crane GG: Hereditary ovalocytosis and reduced susceptibility to malaria in Papua New Guinea. Trans R Soc Trop Med Hyg 81:705, 1987
410. Mueller TJ, Morrison M: Detection of a variant of protein 3, the major transmembrane protein on the human erythrocyte. J Biol Chem 252:6573, 1977
411. Yannoukakos D, Vasseur C, Driancourt C et al: Human erythrocyte band 3 polymorphism (band 3 Memphis): characterization of the structural modification (Lys56 → Glu) by protein chemistry methods. Blood 78:1117, 1991
412. Jarolim P, Rubin HL, Zhai S et al: Band 3 Memphis: a widespread polymorphism with abnormal electrophoretic mobility of erythrocyte band 3 protein caused by substitution AAG → GAG (Lys → Glu) in codon 56. Blood 80: 1592, 1992
413. Jones GL, McLemore-Edmundson H, Wesche D, Saul A: Human erythrocyte band 3 has an altered N-terminus in malaria-resistant Melanesian ovalocytosis. Biochim Biophys Acta 1096:33, 1991
414. Husain-Chishti A, Andrabi K, Palek J et al: Altered tyrosine phosphorylation of the red cell band 3 protein in malaria resistant Southeast Asian ovalocytosis (SAO), abstracted. Blood, suppl. 1. 78:80a, 1991
415. Jones GL: Red cell membrane proteins in Melanesian ovalocytosis autophosphorylation and proteolysis, abstracted. Proc Aust Biochem Soc 16:34, 1984
416. Schofield AE, Reardon DM, Tanner MJA: Defective anion transport activity of the abnormal band 3 in hereditary ovalocytic red blood cells. Nature 355: 836, 1992
417. Tanner MJA, Bruce L, Groves JD et al: The defective red cell anion transporter (band 3) in hereditary Southeast Asian ovalocytosis and the role of glycophorin A in the expression of band 3 anion transport activity in *Xenopus* oocytes. Biochem Soc Trans 20:542, 1992
418. Tanner MJA, Bruce L, Martin PG et al: Melanesian hereditary ovalocytes have a deletion in red cell band 3. Blood 78:2785, 1991
419. Chasis JA, Mohandas N, Shohet SB: Erythrocyte membrane rigidity induced by glycophorin A-ligand interaction. Evidence for a ligand-induced association between glycophorin A and skeletal proteins. J Clin Invest 75:1919, 1985
420. Chasis JA, Reid ME, Jensen RH, Mohandas N: Signal transduction by glycophorin A: role of extracellular and cytoplasmic domains in a modulatable process. J Cell Biol 107:1351, 1988
421. Liu S-C, Yi SJ, Derick LH et al: Characterization of the band 3 protein in Southeast Asian ovalocytosis (SAO): interrelationships among band 3 self-association, ankyrin binding, rotational and lateral mobilities, abstracted. Clin Res 41:135A, 1993
422. Moriyama R, Ideguchi H, Lombardo CR et al: Structural and functional characterization of band 3 from Southeast Asian ovalocytes. J Biol Chem 267: 25792, 1992
423. Okoye VCN, Bennett V: *Plasmodium falciparum* malaria. Band 3 as a possible receptor during invasion of human erythrocytes. Science 227:169, 1985
424. Dluzewski AR, Fryer PR, Griffiths S et al: Red cell membrane protein distribution during malarial invasion. J Cell Sci 92:691, 1989
425. Dluzewski AR, Nash GB, Wilson RJM et al: Invasion of hereditary ovalocytes by *Plasmodium falciparum* in vitro and its relation to intracellular ATP concentration. Mol Biochem Parasitol 55:1, 1992
426. Bessis M: Red cell shapes: an illustrated classification and its rationale. p. 1. In Bessis M, Weed RI, Leblond PF (eds): Red Cell Shape: Physiology and Ultrastructure. Springer-Verlag, New York, 1973
427. Bassen FA, Kornzweig AL: Malformation of the erythrocytes in a case of atypical retinitis pigmentosa. Blood 5:381, 1950
428. Salt HB, Wolff OH, Lloyd JK et al: On having no betalipoprotein: a syndrome comprising abetalipoproteinemia, acanthocytosis, and steatorrhoea. Lancet 2:325, 1960
429. Smith JA, Lonergan ET, Sterling K: Spur-cell anemia: hemolytic anemia with red cells resembling acanthocytes in alcoholic cirrhosis. N Engl J Med 271: 396, 1964
430. Cooper RA: Anemia with spur cells: a red cell defect acquired in serum and modified in the circulation. J Clin Invest 48:1820, 1969
431. Estes JW, Morely TJ, Levine IM, Emerson CP: A new hereditary acanthocytosis syndrome. Am J Med 42:868, 1967
432. Critchley EMR, Betts JJ, Nicholston JT, Weatherall D: Acanthocytosis, normolipidemia and multiple tics. Postgrad Med J 46:698, 1970
433. Allen FH, Krabbe SMR, Corcoran PA: A new phenotype (McLeod) in the Kell blood group system. Vox Sang 6:555, 1961
434. Mant MJ, Faragher BS: The hematology of anorexia nervosa. Br J Haematol 23:737, 1972
435. Monzon CM, Woodruff CW: Anemia and edema as presenting signs in cystic fibrosis: case report. J Med Clin Exp Theor 17:135, 1986
436. Gracey M, Hilton HB: Acanthocytosis and hypobetalipoproteinemia. Lancet 1:679, 1973
437. Wardrop C, Hutchisen HE: Red cell shape in hypothyroidism. Lancet 1:1243, 1969
438. Bessis M: Blood Smears Reinterpreted. Springer-Verlag, Berlin, 1977
439. Silber R, Amorosi E, Lhowe J, Kayden HJ: Spur-shaped erythrocytes in Laennec's cirrhosis. N Engl J Med 275:639, 1966
440. Cooper RA, Diloy-Puray M, Lando P, Greenberg MS: An analysis of lipoproteins, bile acids and red cell membranes associated with target cells and spur cells in patients with liver disease. J Clin Invest 51:3182, 1972
441. Cooper RA: Hemolytic syndromes and red cell membrane abnormalities in liver disease. Semin Hematol 17:103, 1980
442. Cooper RA, Arner EC, Wiley JS, Shattil SJ: Modification of red cell membrane structure by cholesterol-rich lipid dispersions. J Clin Invest 55:115, 1975
443. Cooper RA, Kimball DB, Durocher JR: The role of the spleen in membrane conditioning and hemolysis of spur cells in liver disease. N Engl J Med 290: 1279, 1974
444. Vanderkooi J, Fischkoff S, Chance B, Cooper RA: Fluorescent probe analysis of the lipid architecture of natural and experimental cholesterol-rich membranes. Biochemistry 13:1589, 1974
445. McBride JA, Jacob HS: Abnormal kinetics of red cell membrane cholesterol in acanthocytosis: studies in genetic and experimental abetalipoproteinemia and in spur cell anemia. Br J Haematol 18:383, 1970
446. Cooper RA: Abnormalities in red cell membrane lipids: clinical-biophysical correlates. p. 69. In Silber R, LoBue J, Gordon AS (eds): The Year in Hematology. Plenum, New York, 1978
447. Mühlebach T, Cherry RJ: Influence of cholesterol on the rotation and self-association of band 3 in the human erythrocyte membrane. Biochemistry 21:4225, 1982
448. Conrad ME, Barton JC: Anemia and iron kinetics in alcoholism. Semin Hematol 17:149, 1980
449. Lindenbaum J: Folate and vitamin B_{12} deficiencies in alcoholism. Semin Hematol 17:119, 1980
450. Colman N, Herbert V: Hematologic complications of alcoholism: overview. Semin Hematol 17:164, 1980
451. Becker PS, Lux SE: Disorders of the red cell membrane. p. 529. In Nathan DG, Oski FA (eds): Hematology of Infancy and Childhood. WB Saunders, Philadelphia, 1992
452. Zieve L: Jaundice, hyperlipemia and hemolytic anemia: a heretofore unrec-

ognized syndrome associated with alcoholic fatty liver and cirrhosis. Ann Intern Med 48:471, 1968

453. Douglass CC, Twomey JJ: Transient stomatocytosis with hemolysis: a previously unrecognized complication of alcoholism. Ann Intern Med 72:159, 1970

454. Wisloff F, Boman D: Acquired stomatocytosis in alcoholic liver disease. Scand J Haematol 23:43, 1979

455. Jacob HS, Amsden T: Acute hemolytic anemia with rigid red cells in hypophosphatemia. N Engl J Med 285:1446, 1971

456. Kane JP, Havel RJ: Disorders of the biogenesis and secretion of lipoproteins containing the B apolipoproteins. p. 1139. In Scriver CR, Beaudet AL, Sly WS, Valle D (eds): The Metabolic Basis of Inherited Disease. 6th Ed. McGraw-Hill, New York, 1989

457. Herbert PN, Assmann G, Gotto AM Jr, Frederickson DS: Familial lipoprotein deficiency: abetalipoproteinemia, hypobetalipoproteinemia and Tangier disease. p. 589. In Stanbury JB, Wyngaarden JB, Frederickson DS (eds): The Metabolic Basis of Inherited Disease. McGraw-Hill, New York, 1983

458. Gotto AM Jr, Levy RI, John K, Frederickson DS: On the protein defect in abetalipoproteinemia. N Engl J Med 284:813, 1971

459. Blackhart BD, Ludwig EM, Pierolti BR et al: Structure of the apolipoprotein B gene. J Biol Chem 261:15364, 1986

460. Isselbacher KJ, Scheif R, Plotkin GR, Caulfield JB: Congenital betalipoprotein deficiency: an hereditary disorder involving a defect in the absorption and transport of lipids. Medicine 43:347, 1964

461. Ways P, Reed CF, Hanahan DJ: Red cell and plasma lipids in acanthocytosis. J Clin Invest 42:1248, 1963

462. Levy RI, Fredrickson DS, Laster L: The lipoproteins and lipid transport in abetalipoproteinemia. J Clin Invest 45:531, 1966

463. Jones JW, Ways P: Abnormalities of high density lipoproteins in abetalipoproteinemia. J Clin Invest 46:1151, 1967

464. Simon ER, Ways P: Incubation hemolysis and red cell metabolism in acanthocytosis. J Clin Invest 43:1311, 1964

465. Philips GB: Quantitative chromatographic analysis of plasma and red blood cell lipids in patients with acanthocytosis. J Lab Clin Med 59:357, 1962

466. Switzer S, Eder HA: Interconversion of acanthocytes and normal erythrocytes with detergents. J Clin Invest 41:1404, 1962

467. Zwaal RFA, Roelofsen B, Comfurius P, Van Deenen LLM: Organization of phospholipids in human red cell membranes as detected by the action of various purified phospholipases. Biochim Biophys Acta 406:83, 1975

468. Lange Y, Steck TL: Mechanism of red blood cell acanthocytosis and echinocytosis in vivo. J Membr Biol 77:153, 1984

469. Cooper RA, Durocher JR, Leslie M: Decreased fluidity of red cell membrane lipids in abetalipoproteinemia. J Clin Invest 60:115, 1977

470. Cooper RA, Gulbrandsen CL: The relationship between serum lipoproteins and red cell membranes in abetalipoproteinemia: deficiency of lecithin: cholesterol acyltransferase. J Lab Clin Med 78:323, 1971

471. Dodge JT, James T, Cohen G et al: Peroxidative hemolysis of red blood cells from patients with abetalipoproteinemia (acanthocytosis). J Clin Invest 46: 357, 1967

472. Sperling MA, Hengstenberg F, Yunis E et al: Abetalipoproteinemia: metabolic and electron-microscopic investigations. Pediatrics 48:91, 1971

473. Ways PO, Parmentier CM, Kayden HJ et al: Studies on the absorptive defect for triglyceride in abetalipoproteinemia. J Clin Invest 46:35, 1967

474. Mier M, Schwartz SO, Boshes B: Acanthocytosis, pigmentary degeneration of the retina and ataxic neuropathy: a genetically determined syndrome with associated metabolic disorder. Blood 16:1586, 1960

475. Akamatsu K, Sakaue M, Tada M et al: A case report of abetalipoproteinemia (Bassen-Kornzweig syndrome), the first case in Japan. Jpn J Med 22:231, 1983

476. Welty FK, Hubl ST, Pierotti VR, Young SG: A truncated species of apolipoprotein B (B67) in a kindred with familial hypobetalipoproteinemia. J Clin Invest 87:1748, 1991

477. Young SG, Hubl ST, Chappell DA et al: Familial hypobetalipoproteinemia associated with a mutant species of apolipoprotein B (B-46). N Engl J Med 320:1604, 1989

478. Ross RS, Gregg RE, Law SW et al: homozygous hypobetalipoproteinemia: a disease distinct from abetalipoproteinemia at the molecular level. J Clin Invest 81:590, 1988

479. Takashima Y, Kodama T, Lida H et al: Normotriglyceridemic abetalipoproteinemia in infancy: an isolated apolipoprotein B-100 deficiency. Pediatrics 75:541, 1985

480. Malloy MJ, Kane JP, Hardman DA et al: Normotriglyceridemic abetalipoproteinemia: absence of the B-100 apoprotein. J Clin Invest 67:1441, 1981

481. Gross KB, Skrivanek JA, Carlson KC, Kaufman DM: Familial amyotrophic chorea with acanthocytosis. New clinical and laboratory investigations. Arch Neurol 42:753, 1985

482. Aminoff MJ: Acanthocytosis and neurological disease. Brain 95:749, 1972

483. Sotaniemi KA: Chorea-acanthocytosis: neurological disease with acanthocytosis. Acta Neurol Scand 68:53, 1983

484. Serra S, Xerra A, Arena A: Amyotrophic choreo-acanthocytosis: A new observation in southern Europe. Acta Neurol Scand 73:481, 1986

485. Critchey EMR, Clark DB, Winkler A: Acanthocytosis and a neurological disorder without abetalipoproteinemia. Arch Neurol 18:134, 1968

486. Spitz MC, Jankovic J, Killian JM: Familial tic disorder, parkinsonism, motor neuron disease, and acanthocytosis: a new syndrome. Neurology 35:366, 1985

487. Luckenbach MW, Green WR, Miller NR et al: Ocular clinicopathologic correlation of Hallervorden-Spatz syndrome with acanthocytosis and pigmentary retinopathy. Am J Ophthalmol 95:369, 1983

488. Mukoyama M, Kazui H, Sunohara N et al: Mitochondrial myopathy, encephalopathy, lactic acidosis, and stroke-like episodes with acanthocytosis: a clinicopathological study of a unique case. J Neurol 233:228, 1986

489. Villegas A, Moscat J, Vazquez A et al: A new family with hereditary choreoacanthocytosis. Acta Haematol 7:215, 1987

490. Oshima M, Osawa Y, Assano K, Saito T: Erythrocyte membrane abnormalities in patients with amyotrophic chorea with acanthocytosis. Part 1. Spin labeling studies and lipid analyses. J Neurol Sci 68:147, 1985

491. Ueno E, Oguchi K, Yanaqisawa N: Morphological abnormalities of erythrocyte membrane in the hereditary neurological disease with chorea, areflexia and acanthocytosis. J Neurol Sci 56:89, 1982

492. Cianci CD, Mische SM, Morrow JS: Impaired cAMP dependent phosphorylation of erythrocyte protein 4.9 in patients with hereditary spheroacanthocytosis and neurodegenerative disease. J Cell Biol 107:469a, 1988

493. kay MMB: Band 3 in ageing and neurological disease. Ann NY Acad Sci 621: 179, 1991

494. Taswell HF, Lewis JC, Marsh WL et al: Erythrocyte morphology in genetic defects of the Rh and Kell blood group systems. Mayo Clin Proc 52:157, 1977

495. Wimer BM, Marsh VL, Taswell HF, Galey WR: Haematological changes associated with the McLeod phenotype of the Kell blood group system. Br J Haematol 36:219, 1977

496. Symmans WA, Shepherd CS, Marsh WL et al: Hereditary acanthocytosis associated with the McLeod phenotype of the Kell blood group system. Br J Haematol 42:575, 1979

497. Frey D, Mächler M, Seger R et al: Gene deletion in a patient with chronic granulomatous disease and McLeod syndrome: fine mapping of the Xk gene locus. Blood 71:252, 1988

498. Francke V, Ochs HD, De Martinville B et al: Minor Xp21 chromosome deletion in a male associated with expression of Duchenne muscular dystrophy, chronic granulomatous disease, retinitis pigmentosa and McLeod's syndrome. Am J Hum Genet 37:250, 1985

499. de Saint-Basile G, Bohier MC, Fischer A et al: Xp21 DNA microdeletion in a patient with chronic granulomatous disease, retinitis pigmentosa and MacLeod phenotype. Hum Genet 42:703, 1988

500. Bertelson CJ, Pogo AO, Chaudhuri A et al: Localization of the McLeod Locus (XK) within Xp21 by deletion analysis. Am J Hum Genet 42:703, 1988

501. Koenig M, Monaco AP, Kunkel LM: The complete sequence of dystrophin predicts a rod shaped cytoskeletal protein. Cell 53:219, 1988

502. Vasiljevic ZM, Polic DD: Morphological changes of erythrocytes in patients and carriers of Duchenne disease. Acta Neurol Scand 67:242, 1983

503. Marsh WL: Deleted antigen of the Rhesus and Kell blood groups: association with cell membrane defects. p. 165. In Garraty G (ed): Blood Group Antigens and Diseases. American Association of Blood Banks, Washington, DC, 1983

504. Swash M, Schwartz MS, Carter ND et al: Benign X-linked myopathy with acanthocytes (McLeod syndrome): its relationship to X-linked muscular dystrophy. Brain 106:717, 1983

505. Marsh WA: Molecular defects associated with the McLeod blood group phenotype. p. 17. In Salmon C (ed): Blood Groups and Other Red Cell Surface Markers in Health and Disease. Masson, New York, 1982

506. Redman CM, Marsh WL, Scarborough A et al: Biochemical studies on Markers in Health McLeod phenotype red cells and isolation of Kx antigen. Br J Haematol 68:131, 1988

507. Khodadad JK, Weinstein RS, Steck TL: Quantitation of intramembrane particles of McLeod red cells. p. 218. In the Proceedings of the Forty-fourth Annual Meeting of Electron Microscopy Society of America. Bailey W (ed): Claitor's, Baton Rouge, 1984

508. Redman CM, Robbins TH, Lee S, Marsh WL: Effect of phosphatidylserine on the shape of McLeod red cell acanthocytes. Blood 74:1826, 1989

509. Schwartz RS, Tsun-Yee Chiu D, Lubin B: Plasma membrane phospholipid organization in human erythrocytes. Curr Top Hematol 5:63, 1985

510. Kuypers FA, Van Linde-Sibenius Trip M, Roelofsen B et al: The phospholipid

organization in the membranes of McLeod and Leach phenotype erythrocytes. FEBS Lett 184:20, 1985

511. Galey WR, Evan AP, Van Nice PS et al: Morphology and physiology of the McLeod erythrocyte. I. Scanning electron microscopy and electrolyte and water transport properties. Vox Sang 34:152, 1978

512. Tang LL, Redman CM, Williams D, Marsh WL: Biochemical studies on McLeod phenotype erythrocytes. Vox Sang 40:17, 1981

513. Glaubensklee CS, Evan AP, Galey WR: Structure and biochemical analysis of the McLeod erythrocyte membrane. I. Freeze-fracture and discontinuous polyacrylamide gel electrophoresis analysis. Vox Sang 42:262, 1982

514. Ballas SK, Smith ED: Decreased red cell and membrane deformability in McLeod syndrome. Blood 72:23a, 1988

515. Udden MM, Umeda M, Hirano Y, Marcus DM: New abnormalities in the morphology, cell surface receptors, and electrolyte metabolism of In (Lu) erythrocytes. Blood 69:52, 1987

516. Selby GB, Frame DC, Eichner LK, Eichner ER: Athlete's echinocytes: new cause of exertional hemolysis? Blood, suppl. 1. 70:56a, 1987

517. Cooper RA: Pathogenesis of burr cells in uremia, abstracted. J Clin Invest 49:22a, 1974

518. Owen JS, Brown DJC, Harry DS, McIntyre N: Erythrocyte echinocytosis in liver disease. J Clin Invest 76:2275, 1985

519. White JG: Effects of an ionophore, A23187, on the surface morphology of normal erythrocytes. Am J Pathol 77:507, 1974

520. Nakao M, Nakao T, Yamazoe S: Adenosine triphosphate and maintenance of shape of the human red cells. Nature 187:945, 1960

521. Seigneuret M, Devaux PF: ATP-dependent asymmetric distribution of spin-labeled phospholipids in the erythrocyte membrane: relation to shape changes. Proc Natl Acad Sci USA 81:3751, 1984

522. Beutler E, West C, Tavassoli M, Grahn E: The Woronets trait: a new familial erythrocyte anomaly. Blood 6:281, 1980

523. Glomset JA, Norum KR, Glone E: Familial lechithin-cholesterol acyltransferase deficiency. p. 643. In Stanbury JB, Wyngaarden JB, Frederickson DS (eds): The Metabolic Basis of Inherited Disease. 5th Ed. McGraw-Hill, New York, 1983

524. Jain SK, Mohandas N, Sensabaugh GF et al: Hereditary plasma lecithin-cholesterol acyl transferase deficiency. J Lab Clin Med 99:816, 1982

525. Lock SP, Sephton-Smith R, Hardisty RM: Stomatocytosis: a hereditary red cell anomaly associated with haemolytic anaemia. Br J Haematol 7:303, 1961

526. Bessis M: Experimental changes in the shape of erythrocytes. p. 146. In: Living Blood Cells and Their Ultrastructure. Springer-Verlag, New York, 1973

527. Nathan DG, Shohet SB: Erythrocyte iron transport defects and hemolytic anemia: "hydrocytosis" and "desicocytosis." Semin Hematol 7:381, 1970

528. Mentzer WC, Smith WB, Goldstone J, Shohet SB: Hereditary stomatocytosis: membrane and metabolism studies. Blood 46:659, 1975

529. Synder LM, Lutz HU, Sauberman N et al: Fragmentation and myelin formation in hereditary xerocytosis and other hemolytic anemias. Blood 53:750, 1978

530. Nathan DG, Oski FA, Shaafi RI, Shohet SB: Congenital hemolytic anemia with extensive cation permeability. Blood 28:976, 1966

531. Zarkowsky HS, Oski FA, Shaafi R et al: Congenital hemolytic anemia with high sodium, low potassium red cells. I. Studies of membrane permeability. N Engl J Med 278:573, 1968

532. Oski FA, Naiman JL, Blum SF et al: Congenital hemolytic anemia with high-sodium, low potassium red cells: study of three generations of a family with a new variant. N Engl J Med 280:909, 1969

533. Lande WM, Mentzer WC: Haemolytic anaemia associated with increased cation permeability. Baillieres Clin Haematol 14:89, 1985

534. Mentzer WC, Smith WB, Goldstone J, Shohet SB: Role of the spleen in hereditary stomatocytosis. Blood 42:980a, 1973

535. Mutoh S, Sasaki R, Takaku R et al: A family of hereditary stomatocytosis associated with normal level of Na$^+$-K$^+$-ATPase activity of red blood cells. Am J Hematol 14:113, 1983

536. Schröter W, Ungefehr K, Tillmann W: Role of the spleen in congenital stomatocytosis associated with high sodium low potassium erythrocytes. Klin Wochenschr 59:173, 1981

537. Bienzle U, Niethammer D, Kleeberg U et al: Congenital stomatocytosis and chronic haemolytic anaemia. Scand J Haematol 15:339, 1975

538. Mentzer WC, Lubin BH, Emmons S: Correction of the permeability defect in hereditary stomatocytosis by dimethyl adipimidate. N Engl J Med 294:1200, 1976

539. Mentzer WC, Lubin BH: The effect of crosslinking agents on red cell shape. Semin Hematol 16:115, 1979

540. Bienzle U, Bhadki S, Knuffermann H et al: Abnormality of erythrocyte membrane in a case of congenital stomatocytosis. Klin Wochenschr 55:569, 1977

541. Lande WM, Thiemann PVW, Mentzer WC: Missing band 7 membrane protein

542. Morlé L, Pothier B, Alloisio N et al: Reduction of membrane band 7 and activation of volume stimulated (K$^+$, Cl$^-$)-cotransport in a case of congenital stomatocytosis. Br J Haematol 71:141, 1989

543. Gallagher PG, Segel G, Marchesi SL, Forget BG: The gene for erythrocyte band 7.2b in hereditary stomatocytosis, abstracted. Blood, suppl. 1. 80:276a, 1992

544. Wang D, Turetsky T, Perrine S, Johnson RM, Mentzer WC: Further studies on RBC membrane protein 7.2b deficiency in hereditary stomatocytosis, abstracted. Blood, suppl. 1. 80:275a, 1992

545. Glader BE, Fortier NL, Snyder LM: Hereditary hemolytic anemia associated with RBC K-loss and dehydration: A family study. Clin Res 24:309a, 1976

546. Snyder LM, Lutz HU, Sauberman N et al: Fragmentation and myelin formation in hereditary xerocytosis and other hemolytic anemias. Blood 52:750, 1978

547. Glader BE, Fortier N, Albala MA, Nathan DG: Congenital hemolytic anemia associated with dehydrated erythrocytes and increased potassium loss. N Engl J Med 291:491, 1974

548. Joiner CH, Platt OS, Lux SE: Cation depletion by the sodium pump in red cells with pathologic cation leaks: sickle cells and xerocytes. J Clin Invest 78:1487, 1986

549. Albala MM, Fortier NL, Glader BE: Physiologic features of hemolysis associated with altered cation and 2,3-diphosphoglycerate content. Blood 52:135, 1978

550. Wiley JS, Ellory JC, Shuman M et al: Characteristics of the membrane defect in the hereditary stomatocytosis syndrome. Blood 46:337, 1975

551. Fairbanks G, Dino JE, Fortier NL, Snyder LM: Membrane alterations in hereditary xerocytosis: elevated binding of glyceraldehyde-3-phosphate dehydrogenase. p. 173. In Kruckeberg WC, Eaton JW (eds): Erythrocyte Membranes: Recent Clinical and Experimental Advances. Alan R Liss, New York, 1978

552. Kliman HJ, Steck TL: Association of glyceraldehyde-3-phosphate dehydrogenase with the human red cell membrane. J Biol Chem 255:6314, 1980

553. Lux SE, Glader BE: Disorders of the red cell membrane. p. 525. In Nathan DG, Oski FA (eds): Hematology of Infancy and Childhood. WB Saunders, Philadelphia, 1981

554. Lo SS, Marti HR, Hitzig WH: Hemolytic anemia associated with decreased concentration of reduced glutathione in red cells. Acta Haematol 46:14, 1971

555. Miller G, Townes PL, MacWhinney JB: A new congenital hemolytic anemia with deformed erythrocytes (? "stomatocytes") and remarkable susceptibility of erythrocytes to cold hemolysis in vitro. I. Clinical and hematologic studies. Pediatrics 35:906, 1965

556. Lande W, Cerrone K, Mentzer W: Congenital hemolytic anemia with abnormal cation permeability and cold hemolysis in vitro, abstracted. Blood, suppl. 1. 54:29a, 1979

557. Platt OS, Lux SE, Nathan DG: Exercise-induced hemolysis in xerocytosis: erythrocyte dehydration and shear sensitivity. J Clin Invest 68:631, 1981

558. Jaffe ER, Gottfried EL: Hereditary nonspherocytic hemolytic disease associated with an altered phospholipid composition of the erythrocytes. J Clin Invest 47:1375, 1968

559. Godin DV, Gray GR, Frohlich J: Study of erythrocytes in a hereditary hemolytic syndrome (HHS): comparison with erythrocytes in lecithin cholesterol acyltransferase (LCAT) deficiency. Scand J Haematol 24:122, 1980

560. Nolan GR: Hereditary xerocytosis: a case history and review of the literature. Pathology 16:151, 1984

561. Clark MR, Shohet SB, Gottfried EL: Hereditary hemolytic disease with increased red blood cell phosphatidylcholine and dehydration: one, two, or many disorders? Am J Hematol 42:25, 1993

562. Otsuka A, Sugihara T, Yawata Y: No beneficial effect of splenectomy in hereditary high red cell membrane phosphatidylcholine hemolytic anemia: clinical and membrane studies of 20 patients. Am J Hematol 34:8, 1990

563. Nash R, Shojania AM: Hematological aspect of Rh deficiency syndrome: a case report and a review of the literature. Am J Hematol 24:267, 1987

564. Agre P, Saboori AM, Asimos A, Smith BL: Purification and partial characterization of the M, 30,000 integral membrane protein associated with the erythrocyte Rh(D) antigen. J Biol Chem 262:17497, 1984

565. Cartron J, Agre P: Rh blood group antigens: protein and gene structure. Semin Hematol 30:1, 1993

566. Agre P, Cartron J-P: Biochemistry and molecular genetics of Rh antigens. Baillieres Clin Haematol 4:793, 1991

567. Agre P, Cartron J-P: Molecular biology of the Rh antigens. Blood 78:551, 1991

568. Rigwell K, Tanner MJ, Anstee DJ: The Rhesus (D) polypeptide is linked to the human erythrocyte cytoskeleton. FEBS Lett 174:7, 1984

569. Gahmberg CG, Karhi KK: Association of the Rho (D) polypeptides with the

membrane skeleton in Rho (D) positive human red cells. J Immunol 133: 334, 1984

570. Smith RE, Daleke DL: Phosphatidylserine transport in Rh$_{null}$ erythrocytes. Blood 76:1021, 1990

571. Tippett P: Regulator genes affecting red cell antigens. Transfus Med Rev 4: 56, 1990

572. Chérif-Zahar B, Raynal V, Le Van Kim C et al: Structure and expression of the Rh locus in Rh-deficiency syndrome. Blood 82:656, 1993

573. Ballas SK, Clark MR, Mohandas N et al: Red cell membrane and cation deficiency in Rh Null syndrome. Blood 63:1046, 1984

574. Lanz PK, Joiner CH: Increased potassium transport and ouabain binding in human Rh Null red cells. Blood 48:457, 1976

575. Wiley JS: Cation fluxes in Rh Null red cells. Blood 51:555, 1978

576. Schmidt PJ, Lostumbo MM, English CT, Hunter OB Jr: Aberrant U blood group accompanying Rh$_{null}$. Transfusion 7:33, 1967

577. Sturgeon P: Hematological observations on the anemia associated with blood type Rh Null. Blood 36:310, 1970

578. Huang CH, Johe K, Moulds JJ et al: Delta glycophorin (glycophorin B) gene deletion in two individuals homozygous for the S-s-U blood group phenotype. Blood 70:1830, 1987

579. Assmann G, Schmitz G, Brewer HB Jr: Familial high density lipoprotein deficiency: Tangier disease. p. 1267. In Scriver CR, Beaudet AL, Sly WS, Valle D (eds): The Metabolic Basis of Inherited Disease. 6th Ed. McGraw-Hill, New York, 1989

580. Davidson RJ, How J, Lessels S: Acquired stomatocytosis: its prevalence and significance in routine haematology. Scand J Haematol 19:47, 1977

581. Neville AJ, Rand CA, Barr RD, Mohan Pai KR: Drug-induced stomatocytosis and anemia during consolidation chemotherapy of childhood acute leukemia. Am J Med Sci 287:3, 1984

582. Lauder H: More maladies in Mediterranean migrants: stomatocytosis and macrothrombocytopenia. Med J Aust 1:438, 1971

583. von Behrenz WE: Splenomegaly, macrothrombocytopenia and stomatocytosis in healthy Mediterranean subjects. Scand J Haematol 14:258, 1975

584. Platt OS, Falcone JF: Membrane protein lesions in erythrocytes with Heinz bodies. J Clin Invest 82:1051, 1988

585. Platt OS, Falcone JF, Lux SE: Molecular defect in the sickle erythrocyte skeleton, abnormal spectrin binding to sickle inside-out vesicles. J Clin Invest 75:266, 1985

586. Rank BH, Carlsson J, Hebbel RP: Abnormal redox status of membrane-protein thiols in sickle erythrocytes. J Clin Invest 75:1531, 1985

587. Hebbel RP, Eaton JW: Pathobiology of heme interaction with the erythrocyte membrane. Semin Hematol 26:136, 1989

588. Shinar E, Rachmilewitz EA, Lux SE: Differing erythrocyte membrane skeletal protein defects in alpha and beta thalassemia. J Clin Invest 83:404, 1989

589. Flynn TP, Allen DW, Johnson GJ, White JG: Oxidant damage of the lipids and proteins of the erythrocyte membranes in unstable hemoglobin disease. Evidence for the role of lipid peroxidation. J Clin Invest 71:1215, 1983

590. Johnson GJ, Allen DW, Fairbanks VF et al: Red cell membrane polypeptide aggregates in glucose-6-phosphate dehydrogenase mutants with chronic hemolytic disease. N Engl J Med 301:522, 1979

591. Lorand L, Michalska M, Murthy SNP et al: Cross-linked polymers in the red cell membranes of a patient with Hb-Koln Disease. Biochem Biophys Res Commun 147:602, 1987

592. Waugh SM, Willardson BM, Kannan R et al: Heinz bodies induce clustering of band 3, glycophorin, and ankyrin in sickle cell erythrocytes. J Clin Invest 78:1155, 1986

593. Waugh SM, Walder JA, Low PS: Partial characterization of the copolymerization reaction of erythrocyte membrane band 3 with hemichromes. Biochemistry 26:1777, 1987

594. Rachmilewitz E, Oppenheim A, Shale O: The red blood cell in thalassemia. In RL Nagel (ed): Genetically Abnormal Red Cells. CRC Press, Boca Raton, FL, 1988

595. Chiu D, Lubin B: Oxidative hemoglobin denaturation and RBC destruction: the effect of heme on red cell membranes. Semin Hematol 26:128, 1989

596. Sadrzadeh SMH, Graf E, Panter SS et al: Hemoglobin. A biologic Fenton reagent. J Biol Chem 259:14354, 1984

597. Hebbel RP, Eaton JW, Balasingam M, Steinberg MH: Spontaneous generation of oxygen radicals by sickle erythrocytes. J Clin Invest 70:1253, 1982

598. Johnson GJ, Allen DW, Flynn TP et al: Decreased survival in vivo of diamide-incubated dog erythrocytes. A model of oxidant-induced hemolysis. J Clin Invest 66:955, 1980

599. Snyder LM, Fortier NL, Trainor J, Jacobs J et al: Effects of hydrogen peroxide exposure on normal human erythrocyte deformability, morphology, surface characteristics, and spectrin-hemoglobin crosslinking. J Clin Invest 76:1971, 1985

600. Jacob HS, Winterhalter KH: The role of hemoglobin heme loss in Heinz body formation: studies with a partially heme-deficient hemoglobin and with genetically unstable hemoglobins. J Clin Invest 49:2008, 1970

601. Liu SC, Zhai S, Lawler J, Palek J: Hemin-mediated dissociation of erythrocyte membrane skeletal proteins. J Biol Chem 260:12234, 1985

602. Kirschner-Zilber I, Rabizadeh E, Shaklai N: The interaction of hemin and bilirubin with the human red cell membrane. Biochim Biophys Acta 690:20, 1982

603. Jarolim P, Lahav M, Liu S-C, Palek J: Effect of hemoglobin oxidation products on the stability of red cell membrane skeletons and the associations of skeletal proteins: correlation with a release of hemin. Blood 76:2125, 1990

604. Nagel RL, Fabry ME: The HbS containing cell. p. 1. In Nagel RL (ed): Genetically Abnormal Red Cells. CRC Press, Boca Raton, FL, 1988

605. Nathan DG, Oski FA, Sedel VW, Diamond LK: Extreme hemolysis and red cell distortion in erythrocyte pyruvate kinase deficiency. II. Measurements of erythrocyte glucose consumption, potassium flux and adenosine triphosphate stability. N Engl J Med 272:118, 1965

606. Fabry ME, Nagel RL: Hemoglobin CC and SC Red Cells. In RL Nagel (ed): Genetically Abnormal Red Cells. CRC Press, Boca Raton, FL, 1988

607. Bookchin RM, Ortiz OE, Lew VL: Activation of calcium-dependent potassium channels in deoxygenated sickled red cells. Prog Clin Biol Res 240:193, 1987

608. Joiner CH: Cation transport and volume regulation in sickle red blood cells. Am J Physiol 264:C251, 1993

609. Mayer MM, Hammer CH, Michaels DW, Shin ML: Immunologically mediated membrane damage: the mechanism of complement action and the similarity of lymphocyte-mediated cytotoxicity. Immunochemistry 15:813, 1979

610. Müller-Eberhard HJ: The membrane attack complex of complement. Annu Rev Immunol 4:503, 1986

611. Müller-Eberhard HJ: Molecular organization and function of the complement system. Annu Rev Biochem 57:321, 1988

612. Malinski JA, Nelsestuen GL: Membrane permeability to macromolecules mediated by the membrane attack complex. Biochemistry 28:61, 1989

613. Borsos T, Rapp HJ, Mayer MM: Studies on the second complement component. J Immunol 87:310, 1961

614. Eber SW, Sho M, Brugnara C et al: Increased band 3 mobility and decreased anion transport in ankyrin deficient hereditary spherocytes, abstracted. Blood, suppl. 1, 82:175a, 1993

Autoimmune Hemolytic Anemias

47

Robert S. Schwartz, Leslie E. Silberstein,
and Eugene M. Berkman

INTRODUCTION

The autoimmune hemolytic anemias are a group of disorders in which autoantibodies against antigens on the erythrocyte membrane cause a shortened red blood cell (RBC) life span. The antierythrocyte autoantibodies of these diseases fall into three generic types, each of which has distinctive serologic properties: (1) cold agglutinins, almost always of the IgM isotype, clump RBCs at cold temperatures; (2) the IgG Donath-Landsteiner antibody fixes to RBC membranes in the cold and activates the hemolytic complement cascade when the cells are warmed to 37°C; and (3) IgG warm autoantibodies bind to erythrocytes at 37°C but fail to agglutinate the cells. Each of these three categories of autoantibodies delineates one or more characteristic clinical disorders, known collectively as autoimmune hemolytic anemia. Autoimmune hemolytic anemia can occur as a primary (idiopathic) disorder, coexist with another disease (secondary autoimmune hemolytic anemia), or follow administration of certain drugs (Table 47-1). The nomenclature of these conditions is imprecise and sometimes confusing. This chapter refers to the hemolytic diseases associated with warm-reactive IgG autoantibodies as autoimmune hemolytic anemia, to the hemolytic anemias caused by cold-reactive IgM autoantibodies as cold agglutinin disease, and to the syndromes associated with the Donath-Landsteiner antibody as paroxysmal cold hemoglobinuria.

HISTORICAL BACKGROUND

Any reader interested in the origins of hematology should seek out Dacie's[1] superb review of the history of autoimmune hemolytic anemia. Much of this section follows his scholarly account. An earlier historical analysis by Dameshek and Schwartz[2] is a classic. Rosenfield's[3] personal narrative of the history of immunohematology is also strongly recommended.

Paroxysmal cold hemoglobinuria was the first recognized form of hemolytic anemia, probably because its clinical manifestations are so graphic; the principal sign of the disease, the passage of black urine after exposure to the cold, can hardly be ignored. Descriptions of patients with attacks of hemoglobinuria after exposure to cold temperatures, including the case of a 10-year-old boy with *chromaturie*,[4] began to appear between 1854 and 1865 in the medical literature.[4-6] In 1879, Rosenbach[7] reported how he had induced hemoglobinuria by immersing his patient's feet in ice water; 2 years later, Paul Ehrlich[8] reported his observation of hemolysis and erythrophagocytosis in blood obtained from a chilled finger of a patient with the disease.

The association of paroxysmal cold hemoglobinuria with syphilis was first noted in 1884 by Götze,[9] but nothing else was known of the cause of the disease until 1904, when Donath and Landsteiner[10] published their landmark work. They described three cases of paroxysmal cold hemoglobinuria in which (1) an autolysin bound to the patient's RBCs in the cold, and (2) a heat-labile serum factor (now known to be hemolytic complement components) lysed the sensitized erythrocytes when the temperature was raised to 37°C. This classic paper presents the first description of an autoimmune disease.

Less obvious forms of hemolytic anemia were not identified until the end of the nineteenth century, when Le Gendre[11] and Hayem[12] distinguished a form of jaundice with bile in the plasma, but not in the urine (acholuric jaundice). Widal and Abrami[13] were among the first to recognize congenital and acquired forms of hemolytic anemia; in 1907 they reported the presence of autoagglutination of erythrocytes in their patients with *l'ictère hémolytique acquis*. The following year, Chauffard and Troisier[14] described cases of severe hemolytic anemia with serum hemolysins, but progress in delineating autoimmune hemolytic anemia ceased until 1938, when Dameshek and Schwartz[15] revived interest in the topic with their report of similar cases. Dameshek and Schwartz[16] also demonstrated that injection of heterologous antierythrocyte antibodies into guinea pigs induced hemolytic anemia, with spherocytosis and increased osmotic fragility of RBCs, establishing the first experimental model of immune hemolytic anemia. Even so, the idea of an autoimmune form of hemolytic anemia was resisted for several reasons, not the least of which was the difficulty in diagnosis. Only cold-reactive antibodies, which directly agglutinate erythrocytes, and rare forms of lytic autoantibodies could be recognized in the laboratory. In 1918, the first example of cold agglutinin disease was described,[17] but the validity of such cases was suspect because cold-reactive autoantibodies were also found in normal serum, an observation made 15 years earlier by Landsteiner.[18] Not until 1937 was it recognized that the serum of patients with cold agglutinin disease had markedly elevated titers of cold agglutinins.[19]

The antiglobulin test, designed to detect nonagglutinating antierythrocyte antibodies, was introduced into clinical medicine by Coombs et al.[20] in 1945. The Coombs test revolutionized immunohematology; within 1 year it was applied to the diagnosis of autoimmune hemolytic anemia.[21] Ironically, essentially the same procedure, developed in 1908 by Moreschi,[22] was ignored for almost 40 years, perhaps because Moreschi's report dealt with animal RBCs.

In 1954, autoimmune hemolytic anemia in dogs was reported,[23] and in 1958, the first easily bred animal model of the disease, the NZB mouse, was described.[24] This discovery was a turning point in the development of the scientific basis for the study of autoimmunization.

The first recorded attempt to treat acquired hemolytic anemia with splenectomy was carried out in 1911[25]; and in 1950 the beneficial effect of corticotropin on autoimmune hemolytic anemia in two patients with lymphoma was reported by Dameshek[26] and in a 5-year-old girl by Gardner.[27]

IMMUNOLOGIC MECHANISMS OF RED CELL DESTRUCTION

Immunologic Tolerance

Regardless of their underlying cause, autoimmune hemolytic anemias, ultimately result from derangement of the mechanism of immunologic tolerance. An understanding of this mechanism

Table 47-1. Classification of Autoimmune
Hemolytic Anemia

Warm autoimmune hemolytic anemia
Primary (idiopathic)
Secondary
    Lymphoproliferative diseases
    Connective tissue diseases
    Miscellaneous diseases
    Drugs
        Hapten type
        Immune complex type
        Autoantibody type
Cold autoimmune hemolytic anemia
Primary (idiopathic)
Secondary
    Lymphoproliferative diseases
    Infections
        Mycoplasma pneumoniae
        Infectious mononucleosis
        Other
    Miscellaneous diseases
Paroxysmal cold hemoglobinuria
Associated with tertiary syphyllis
Postviral infection (self-limited)

is essential. At the end of its life, when it transforms from a biconcave disc to a sphere, the RBC undergoes the initial steps required to trigger an immune response, namely, phagocytosis and proteolysis by a macrophage. There is no reason to doubt that macrophages produce potentially immunogenic peptide fragments from those worn-out spheres and offer them to lymphocytes. This, after all, is a major function of macrophages, and it applies to virtually any particle or molecule they can ingest and digest. However, the lymphocytes of the immune system specifically ignore the numerous self-antigenic determinants on the RBC membrane. Those same antigens would nonetheless engender an immune response if injected into another person with a different constellation of blood groups. The complex mechanisms that prevent autoimmunization, while simultaneously permitting alloimmunization, are known collectively as immunologic tolerance. The rules governing immunologic tolerance are essential aspects of the mechanisms of immune recognition of erythrocytes.

Owen's[28] classic study of the RBCs of dizygotic cattle twins, published in 1945, was the first to uncover evidence of this remarkable aspect of the immune system. Owen observed that such twins had in their circulation a mixture of erythrocytes, some with self-blood groups and others with blood groups of the allogeneic twin. These cattle twins were erythrocyte chimeras, a condition caused by the exchange of hematopoietic stem cells through the vascular anastomoses of the common placenta that nourished both fetuses in utero. The immunologic consequences of chimerism did not escape Owen, who emphasized the lack of any alloantibodies in the twins despite the presence of "foreign" erythrocytes in their blood.

Owen's work was a key element in the theory of immunologic tolerance advanced 4 years later by Burnet and Fenner.[29] Their sweeping new idea was that contact with any antigen during embryonic life would result in immunologic tolerance (their original term), and they attributed self-tolerance to clonal deletion—the lethal consequence to an embryonic lymphocyte that contacts an antigen. One of the main predictions of this theory was substantiated in 1953 by Billingham et al.,[30] who showed that fetal mice injected with foreign cells would later "tolerate" skin grafts from the donors of those cells. The principle established by that historic experiment has been reaffirmed by recent experiments with transgenic mice, which carry a foreign gene implanted in their germline DNA. A foreign protein

encoded by the gene, if expressed early in embryonic life, fails to induce any immune response in the transgenic animal.[31]

The thymus is an important seat of this mechanism (see Ch. 8). There is now convincing evidence that the fetal thymus inactivates T cells with the potential to respond to self-antigens.[32] The fetal thymus contains macrophages, epithelial cells, and dendritic cells that not only ingest and degrade (process) antigenic material but that also bind the resulting peptide fragments to class II MHC molecules.[33] The latter are membrane glycoproteins required for antigen recognition by T cells; the T-cell receptor for antigen recognizes a configuration consisting of an immunogenic peptide and a portion of the class II MHC glycoprotein[34] (Fig. 47-1). Intrathymic antigen-presenting cells can, for example, ingest and digest RBCs within the thymus and bind degraded fragments of self-hemoglobin to their class II MHC molecules.[35]

Each T-cell clone arising within the thymus expresses its own unique receptor, the result of random recombinations of V_α and V_β or V_δ and V_γ gene segments.[32] This stochastic mechanism will inevitably yield clones with receptors capable of recognizing a self-peptide/class II MHC complex. Such clones are destined for deletion from the immune repertoire; the fetal thymus eliminates any thymocyte whose receptor binds with high affinity to an antigen-presenting cell.[36]

Tolerance of Blood Group Antigens

The immune system's solution to the problem of distinguishing self from foreign requires an about-face late in fetal development. The dominant function of the immune system during early embryonic life is the acquisition of immunologic tolerance of the antigens bathing its milieu but, as birth approaches, the fetus begins to acquire the capacity to respond to immunogens. This principle is clearly evident in the case of the ABO blood group antigens, oligosaccharides not only expressed on the membranes of erythrocytes and many other kinds of cells, but also circulating in soluble form in the plasma. The immunodominant sugar of the A antigen is *N*-acetylglucosamine; the B determinant, galactose, differs from the A sugar only by a single acetyl group. The core of transfusion therapy is the infallible ability of the immune system to recognize that minute difference. The extreme rarity of autoimmune hemolytic anemia due to anti-A or anti-B antibodies attests to the deletion from the immune repertoire of lymphocytes with the capacity to produce such autoantibodies. Such clones are probably eliminated or inactivated very early in ontogeny, since the embryo begins to synthesize A or B substances within 5 weeks of its implantation in the uterine wall.[37]

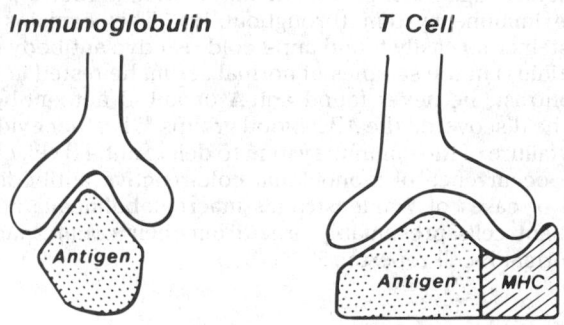

Immunoglobulin   **T Cell**

Antigen   Antigen MHC

Fig. 47-1. Antigen-specific receptors. Antigen recognition by immunoglobulin-variable regions and T cell receptors. The antibody molecule typically recognizes a three-dimensional configuration on the antigen, whereas the T-cell receptor binds to a compound structure consisting of a peptide fragment of the antigen (produced as the result of antigen processing by macrophages) and a portion of a MHC structure. CD4+ T cells recognize an antigen fragment plus a class II MHC structure; CD8+ T cells bind to processed peptides plus a class I MHC structure.

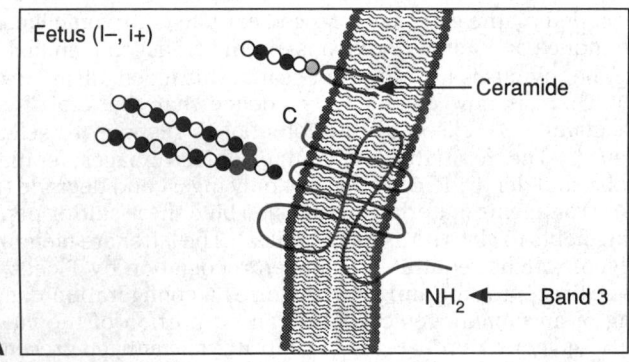

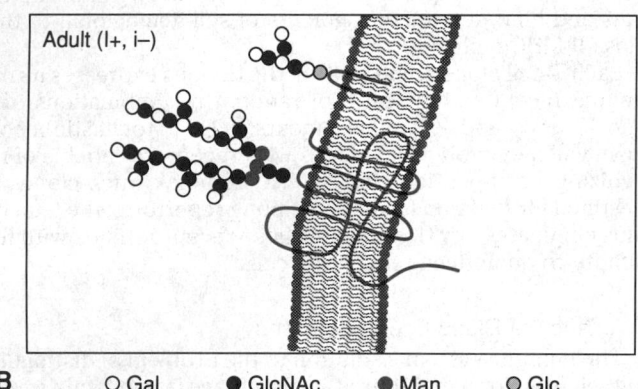

Fig. 47-2. The I/i blood group system in **(A)** the fetus and **(B)** the adult. The fetus lacks the enzymes (branching enzymes) required to produced the branched forms of ceramide and the I antigen. The unbranched (fetal) and branched (adult) variants of the I antigen are immunochemically distinct structures. Shaded structure represents the erythrocyte membrane. The modified N-terminus of band 3 faces the interior of the RBC. (From Hakomori,[40] with permission.)

Another telling example of the fetal acquisition of immunologic tolerance is the I/i blood group system, originally discovered by Wiener et al.[38] in a case of cold-reactive autoimmune hemolytic anemia. The serum of their patient contained high titers of an autoantibody with a specificity they denoted I. Its counterpart antigen, i, is typical of fetal erythrocytes[39] (Fig. 47-2). The fetus with I−/i+ erythrocytes presumably lacks the enzymatic capacity to convert the unbranched i oligosaccharide to the antigenically different branched oligosaccharide structure of I.[40] Thus, the fetus has no opportunity to acquire immunologic tolerance of the branched I ganglioside, and B-cell clones capable of producing anti-I autoantibodies persist in the immune system throughout life. This explains why Landsteiner so easily found anti-I cold-reactive antibody (cold agglutinins) in the samples of normal serum he tested in 1903. By contrast, he never found anti-A or anti-B autoantibodies when he discovered the ABO blood groups.[41] Further evidence of the failure of the immune system to delete anti-I B cell clones is the occurrence of monoclonal cold-reactive antibodies in ≤10% of cases of Waldenström's macroglobulinemia[42]; such malignant cells presumably arise from their counterparts in the normal B-cell repertoire.

Self-reactive Lymphocytes

It is highly unlikely that the fetal thymus can purge all self-reactive lymphocytes from the immune system. In the first place, B cells do not differentiate in the thymus and their receptors for antigen—surface immunoglobulins—do not depend on recognition of an antigen/MHC complex. Indeed, self-reactive B cells occur in a surprisingly high frequency; about 1 in 10⁴ B cells from healthy young mice produce anti-DNA antibodies.[43]

B cells from normal humans, when activated by mitogens in vitro, also produce autoantibodies.[44,45] Furthermore, it is improbable that all the body's different proteins, estimated at 100,000 in number,[32] find their way into the fetal thymus. Some, like the I antigen, are expressed only after birth; others are sequestered in the brain and other internal organs. The peripheral lymphocyte population must therefore, contain at least some antiself-T cells and B cells. The existence of such cells accounts for the success of the classic experiment of Rose and Witebsky,[46] who were able to induce autoimmune thyroiditis in rabbits by immunization with rabbit thyroglobulin. If all lymphocytes capable of responding to self-thyroglobulin had been deleted, the animals would have been unresponsive to the injected thyroglobulin.

Immunoregulation

Growing evidence shows that the antiself-immune repertoire is normally constrained by suppressor T cells. In humans, the mature T-cell population consists of CD4+ helper cells, which augment the activity of B cells, and CD8+ cytotoxic and suppressor cells. Two subsets of CD4+ cells have been identified: helper-inducer T cells, identified by the 4B4 membrane glycoprotein, and suppressor-inducer T cells, marked by the 2H4 (or CD45R) glycoprotein.[47] The latter regulate a subset of CD8+ T cells that have been shown to suppress antibody formation in vitro.[48] An imbalance in suppressor (or suppressor-inducer) T cells is a plausible explanation of the origins of some autoimmune diseases.[49] How such an impairment occurs in the first place is enigmatic, but clinical and experimental findings support the concept. Two children with autoimmune hemolytic anemia and a profound deficiency of suppressor cells, probably due to a thymic defect, have been reported.[50] Removal of the thymus from mice within a few days after birth can result in a variety of T-cell-mediated organ-specific autoimmune diseases. The thymectomy apparently prevents entrance of newly formed suppressor cells into the periphery; administration of T cells from intact mice prevents the autoimmune process.[51] Cyclosporine, a potent immunosuppressive drug, can have the paradoxical effect of causing autoimmune diseases,[52–55] presumably by disrupting immunoregulatory T-cell populations.

Antigen-independent polyclonal activation of self-reactive B cells, another possible mechanism of autoimmunization, could result from an inherent abnormality of B cells, as has been demonstrated in some patients with systemic lupus erythematosus (SLE),[56] or from the excessive production of B-cell-stimulatory lymphokines (e.g., interleukin [IL]-6) by T cells. The case of a patient with an IL-6-secreting atrial myxoma who produced large amounts immunoglobulins and autoantibodies[57] is instructive, as is the development of thyroiditis and antithyroglobulin autoantibodies in cancer patients treated with large doses of IL-2.[58,59] The hypergammaglobulinemia and production of autoantibodies in parasitic diseases[60] and in patients with human immunodeficiency virus infection[61–64] probably also originate as a consequence of polyclonal B-cell activation.

ANIMAL MODELS OF AUTOIMMUNE HEMOLYTIC ANEMIA

Evidence for Genetic Factors

NZB Mice

The inbred NZB mouse is genetically programmed to develop autoimmune hemolytic anemia around the age of 6–8 months (the life span of a normal mouse is about 2 years). Antierythrocyte autoantibodies begin to appear around the age of 3 months, and by 9 months the direct antiglobulin test (DAT) is positive in 60–80% of the animals. Typical signs of hemolytic anemia develop, with reticulocytosis, spherocytosis, a shortened RBC survival time, and splenomegaly[65] (Fig. 47-3). The autoantibodies are of two types: anti-X, an IgG autoantibody, reacts with the X antigen exposed on the erythrocyte membrane and causes the hemolytic anemia; anti-HB, an IgM autoantibody, reacts with a hidden phosphorylcholine erythrocyte antigen revealed by in vitro enzyme (bromelain) treatment of the RBCs. Both the X and the HB antigens circulate in the plasma.[66] Anti-HB antibodies, found in virtually all normal strains of mice, are not pathogenic. They are produced by CD5+ B cells[67]; their high levels in NZB serum undoubtedly stem from the marked increase of CD5+ B cells in NZB mice.[68] Other antierythrocyte autoantibodies in NZB mice include an IgG antibody with probable specificity for spectrin[69], and cold-reactive antibodies with a resemblance to anti-I autoantibodies in humans.[70]

The F_1 progeny of crosses between NZB and NZW mice or between NZB and SWR mice do not develop autoimmune hemolytic anemia, and the antiglobulin test is negative. Instead, lupus nephritis and high levels of anti-DNA antibodies dominate the disease in these animals.[71] Mice of the SWR strain are normal—they never develop any evidence of SLE or any other autoimmune disease. Yet in the (NZB × SWR) cross, a substantial fraction of the anti-DNA antibodies arises from genes inherited from the SWR parent.[72] In the (NZB × SWR)F_1 hybrid, therefore, the inherent immunologic abnormalities of the NZB strain[65] can induce pathogenic autoantibodies that originate from the genome of a normal animal. The shift from autoimmune hemolytic anemia in the NZB parent to nephritis in the F_1 hybrid demonstrates that genetic factors influence not only susceptibility to autoimmunization but also its clinical manifestations.

Graft-Versus-Host Disease: the Graft-Versus-Host Model

Conditions are ripe for a graft-versus-host reaction when foreign lymphocytes are injected into hosts that cannot reject them. In the classic graft-versus-host reaction, the grafted T lymphocytes respond to MHC antigens of the host. A chronic graft-versus-host reaction can occur in F_1 hybrid mice following injection of lymphocytes from one of the parental strains: A → (A × B)F_1. The strain A T cells respond to class II MHC antigens inherited by the F_1 animal from its B parent.

Several different autoimmune diseases can develop in mice

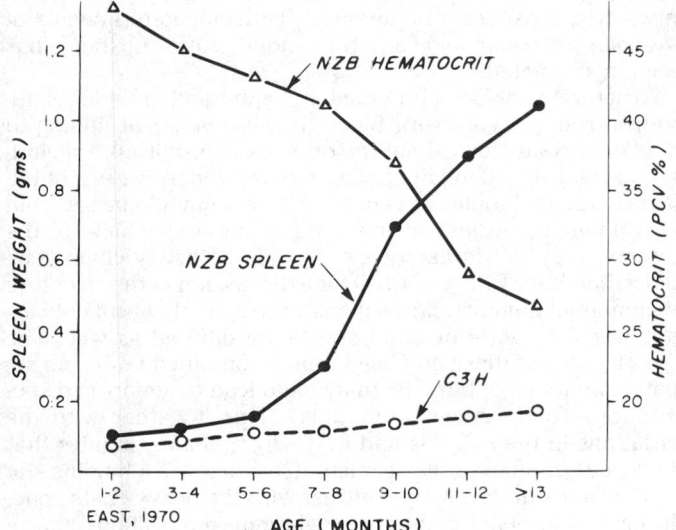

Fig. 47-3. Development of autoimmune hemolytic anemia in NZB mice. Splenic enlargement is due to the effects of the hemolytic anemia and also to marked polyclonal proliferation of CD5+ B cells. As the animals age, the polyclonal population of CD5+ B cells converts to a monoclonal population (see text).

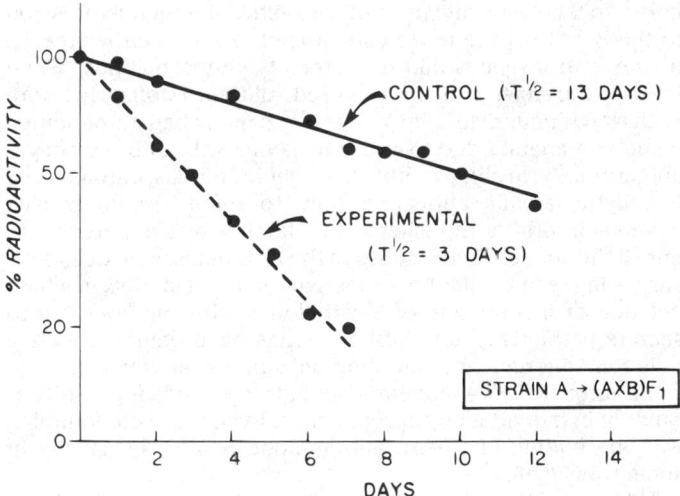

Fig. 47-4. Autoimmune hemolytic anemia in F_1 hybrid mice, (A × B)F_1, injected with parental strain (A) T cells. The two graphs compare survival of ^{51}Cr-tagged syngenic erythrocytes in control and experimental animals. Red cell life span is markedly reduced, and the antiglobulin tests are positive, in animals with the chronic graft-versus-host reaction.

or rats as a result of a chronic graft-versus-host reaction. The particulars of the outcome depend on the donor → host combination.[72] For example, when lymphocytes from BALB/c mice are injected into (BALB/c × A/J)F_1 animals, the recipients develop typical autoimmune hemolytic anemia[73] (Fig. 47-4). If, however, DBA/2 lymphocytes are injected into (DBA/2 × C57Bl/6)F_1 mice, the result is severe glomerulonephritis of the type seen in SLE.[74] In each of these examples, both the donors and the F_1 recipients are normal strains of mice.

The principal requirement for triggering the autoimmune disease is a difference in class II MHC antigens between the donor and the recipient.[75] This intense immunogenic stimulus causes a marked activation of the donor's T cells, which release large amounts of IL-4 and IL-6, potent polyclonal activators of B cells.[76] The host's B cells can respond in two ways: by the production of autoantibodies and, in some cases, by a persistent lymphoproliferative reaction that culminates in malignant lymphoma.[77] The graft-versus-host model provides ample evidence of the importance of polyclonal B-cell activation in autoimmunization, but the genetic factors that determine the particulars of disease a given F_1 hybrid develops are unknown.

Several complications of chronic graft-versus-host disease in humans, including immune thrombocytopenia,[78] the sicca syndrome, and scleroderma,[79] may arise on a similar basis, but since bone marrow transplantation is rarely carried out when there is a class II HLA mismatch, other factors are probably involved. The development of autoimmune hemolytic anemia in recipients of renal allografts could be associated with a graft-versus-host reaction caused by donor lymphocytes in the organ graft.[80] However, the role of cyclosporine, which has been associated with the induction of autoimmunization, cannot be discounted in these cases.[81–83]

Autoimmune Hemolytic Anemia in Transgenic Mice

Okamoto et al.[84] developed transgenic mice by inserting the V_H or V_L genes for an NZB antierythrocyte autoantibody into the germline of a normal strain of mice.* The NZB V genes were

---

* The DNA constructs for either the heavy or light chain genes were microinjected into fertilized eggs of C57Bl/6 mice; the eggs were then transferred to pseudopregnant mice. The presence of the transgenes in the newborn animals was verified by Southern blot analysis.

linked to B-cell-specific promoters, restricting their expression to the B cells of the new hosts. Mice harboring either the V_H or the V_L transgenes had no detectable abnormalities. When these two trangenic lines were bred, all their F_1 offspring bore both NZB immunoglobulin V genes, and many had autoimmune hemolytic anemia due to the transgenic NZB antierythrocyte autoantibody. In some double transgenic animals, autoimmune hemolytic anemia appeared, only to remit spontaneously, whereas in others the anemia was fatal. It was apparent that not all the antiself B-cell clones in the F_1 animals were deleted, a surprising result in light of other experimental models in which deletion or inactivation of B-cell clones with the potential to secrete pathogenic autoantibodies has been demonstrated.[85] Deletion, anergy, and autoimmunization—all involving the same autoantibody—appeared and disappeared, apparently at random in individual transgenic mice. Even more confounding was the finding of severe autoimmune hemolytic anemia in some transgenics.

This interesting model shows some of the features of autoimmune hemolytic anemia in humans; the tendency toward spontaneous remissions and relapses in the F_1 transgenic mice is noteworthy. In subsequent work, Murakami et al.[86] found that the CD5+ B-cell is the main source of the hemolytic autoantibody in the F_1 transgenic (see Ch. 13 for a discussion of CD5+ B cells). In adult mice, CD5+ B cells reside mainly in the peritoneal cavity. The peritoneal fluid contains many CD5+ B cells, but only a few erythrocytes. The transgenic CD5+ B cells in the peritoneum would be thus be isolated from "self" RBC, and not susceptible to clonal deletion by autoantigen. However, death of those antiself CD5+ B cells occurs within 12 hours of an intraperitoneal injection of autologous red cells.[86] It is plausible that the erratic course of autoimmune hemolytic anemia in the F_1 transgenics was due to the chance entrance of red cells into the peritoneal cavity—perhaps as the result of casual injury when the animals were handled by the investigators. This model emphasizes the importance of antigen in maintaining self-tolerance: no antigen, no tolerance.

Origins of Antierythrocyte Autoantibodies

The vast improvement in our understanding of what prevents autoimmunization has not yet informed us of the mechanism that causes autoimmunization. Virtually nothing is known of the origins of warm-reactive IgG antierythrocyte autoantibodies, despite the availability of a thoroughly investigated, spontaneous animal model of the disease (the NZB mouse) and stocks of pathogenic autoantibodies, readily obtained from patients with the disease. A major impediment to advances in our perceptions of how autoimmune hemolytic anemia originates is that the autoantigen(s) are for the most part unknown. Even in those cases in which blood group specificity of the autoantibodies has been identified, the relevant structures have not been elucidated. Leddy et al.[87] have succeeded in identifying four proteins on the red cell membrane that bind to antierythrocyte autoantibodies: the band 3 anion transporter, glycophorin A, and two polypeptides probably related to the Rh family of antigens. Various combinations of those four autoantibody specificities were found in a group of 20 patients with autoimmune hemolytic anemia.

The association of autoimmune hemolytic anemia with systemic lupus and with immune thrombocytopenia (Evans syndrome, see below), the induction of the disease by drugs which seem to perturb immune regulation (see below), and the graft-versus-host model of autoimmune hemolytic anemia all suggest that at least in some cases there is antigen-independent activation of clones of B cells with the capacity to produce IgG anti-RBC autoantibodies. Such polyclonal B-cell activation may account for the production of antierythrocyte autoantibodies in

patients with acquired immunodeficiency syndrome[88,89]—hypergammaglobulinemia and other signs of nonspecific activation of B cells are prominent in human immunodeficiency virus infection.[90]

The immunologic basis of autoimmune hemolytic anemia in patients with chronic lymphocytic leukemia (CLL) or a B-cell lymphoma is equally obscure.[91] In CLL, the autoantibodies are IgG and often polyclonal,[92] whereas the malignant CD5+ B cells of that disease generally produce only IgM antibodies that are monoclonal. It is therefore likely that B cells other than those constituting the leukemia produce the autoantibodies. The large mass of CD5+ B cells in CLL might induce non-neoplastic CD5− B cells to produce IgG autoantibodies, perhaps by a disturbance of immunoregulatory idiotypic networks (Fig. 47-5). The demonstration of the simultaneous presence of autoantibodies and anti-idiotypic antibodies on red cells in autoimmune hemolytic anemia[93] suggests that such networks may indeed have a role in the disease.

By contrast with the autoantigens that bind to warm-reactive autoantibodies, the structures of the autoantigens of cold agglutinin disease, the I/i system, are known[40] (Fig. 47-2); this has clarified our thinking about the immunology of this group of disorders. There is little reason to doubt that the very high levels of monoclonal cold agglutinins found in some patients with B-cell neoplasms are produced by the malignant cells. The demonstration that an idiotypic marker on monoclonal cold agglutinins could be detected not only on the patients' neoplastic B cells but also on 3–10% of normal B cells[94] supports the view that these autoantibodies are part of the normal immune repertoire; malignant transformation of a cold agglutinin-producing B cell results in a lymphoma complicated by chronic cold agglutinin disease.

The basis of the association of paroxysmal cold hemoglobinuria with syphilis may be antigenic mimicry, in which structural similarities between a microbial antigen and a self-antigen trigger an autoantibody response. In the case of paroxysmal cold hemoglobinuria, the infecting organism, *Treponema pallidum,* should possess two antigenic determinants (epitopes): one recognized by T cells (the foreign epitope), the other by self-reactive B cells (the mimicking epitope). Donath-Landsteiner antibodies would be produced only by syphilitic patients whose class II MHC glycoproteins can present the foreign epitope in an immunogenic form to T cells (Fig. 47-6). A similar mechanism could apply to postinfectious acute cold agglutinin disease, in which a cross-reaction involving antigenic determinants of *Mycoplasma pneumoniae* and the I blood group substance has been incriminated.[95]

Structural analyses of monoclonal anti-I and anti-i autoantibodies from patients with B-cell neoplasms are beginning to yield important clues about the origins of chronic cold agglutinin disease. A striking observation is the repetitive use of the same immunoglobulin V_H gene, $V_H4.21$, in monoclonal IgM cold agglutinins, regardless of the anti-I or anti-i specificty of the autoantibody.[96,97] In each case, the $V_H4.21$ heavy chain gene had a different CDR3 (see Ch. 9 for a discussion of the structure of immunoglobulin-coding regions); the light chains of cold agglutinins with anti-I or anti-i specificity differed as well. The $V_H4.21$ genes of these cold agglutinins contained few or no somatic mutations of the type that would lead to amino acid substitutions (replacement mutations). This, together with the variations in their CDR3s and in the light chains, implies that the $V_H4.21$ germline gene segment itself encodes a binding site for the I and i antigens. By contrast with the heavy chain gene, the light chain genes of the cold agglutinins did contain replacement mutations, especially in their hypervariable regions.[97]

It appears from these results that (1) the germline $V_H4.21$ heavy chain encodes the dominant specificity of monoclonal cold agglutinins; (2) the somatic mutations of the light chain genes of the cold agglutinins are the result of an immune re-

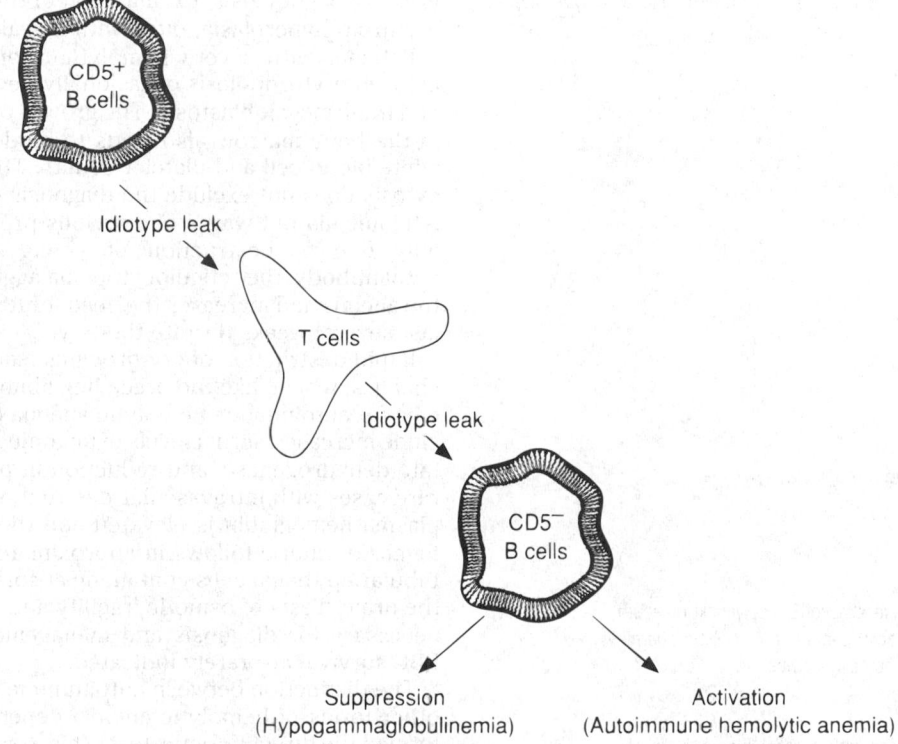

Fig. 47-5. Hypothetical link between CD5⁺ B cells and the immunologic complications of CLL. The idiotype displayed by the IgM surface immunoglobulins of the large mass of monoclonal CD5⁺ B cells stimulates a population of T cells with a complementary anti-idiotype. In turn, the anti-idiotypic T cells affect normal CD5⁻ B cells, either by inducing suppression (with resulting hypogammaglobulinemia) or polyclonal activation (resulting in autoimmune hemolytic anemia due to IgG autoantibodies).

sponse; (3) the V_H CDR3 and the light chain confer fine specificity (e.g., for I or i) on the cold agglutinin and influence its affinity. These data make a convincing case that monoclonal cold agglutinins arise as the result of an immune response, perhaps an autoimmune response to an autoantigen on erythrocytes. The results of these molecular studies of cold agglutinins complement other evidence favoring a role for antigen-mediated

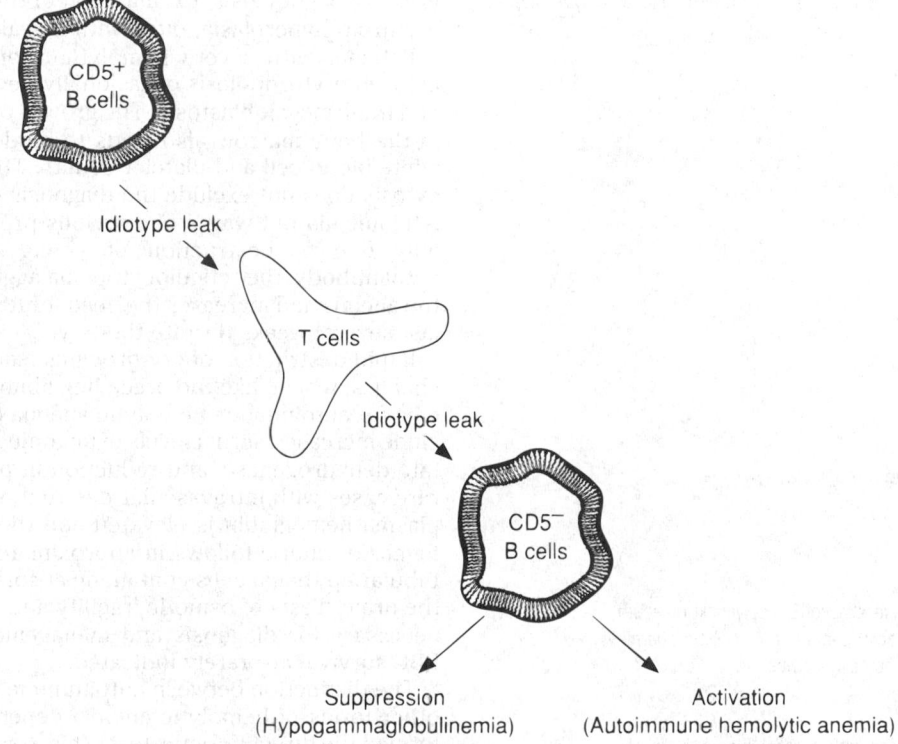

Fig. 47-6. Induction of autoimmunization by antigenic mimicry. **(A)** The usual foreign antigen contains antigenic determinants (epitopes) recognized by both T cells and B cells. The result is a cooperative interaction between helper T cells and B cells. **(B)** A self-antigen may be recognized by B cells, but T/B collaboration does not occur because of the deletion from the immune repertoire of T cells with receptors for the autoantigen. **(C)** A microbe with a self-mimicking epitope could engender T/B collaboration because T cells would recognize the foreign epitope and B cells would bind to the self-mimicking structure.

clonal selection in some types of B-cell neoplasms (see Ch. 77 for a discussion of clonal selection in B-cell neoplasms).

By contrast with monoclonal cold agglutinins associated with chronic cold agglutinin disease, the naturally occurring IgM cold agglutinins that are present in low titers in normal serum are not restricted to the $V_H4.21$ gene segment. They are associated with different genes of the V_H3 family as well as the $V_H4.21$ gene.[98] It therefore appears that B-cell neoplasia is an important, but not exclusive, element in the association between $V_H4.21$ and cold agglutinins. The correlation with lymphomas has added interest because $V_H4.21$ has been independently linked to B-cell lymphomas that do not secrete cold agglutinins.[99] Both kinds of $V_H4.21$-related B-cell tumors may originate from an uncontrolled autoimmune response against I or i RBC antigens; one type lacking the capacity for secreting the cold agglutinin, the other able to secrete it as a monoclonal IgM immunoglobulin.

AUTOIMMUNE HEMOLYTIC ANEMIA

Clinical Manifestations

The incidence of autoimmune hemolytic anemia is estimated to be approximately 10 cases per million population; for comparison, the incidence of acute myeloid leukemia is about 50 cases per million.[100] Autoimmune hemolytic anemia is more common in women than in men; it occurs at all ages, but usually in midlife. About one-half of cases are idiopathic (i.e., they are unassociated with any other disease). Some cases are induced by drugs, and others occur simultaneously, with another autoimmune disease, especially SLE. That disorder may begin with Evans syndrome, a rare combination of autoimmune hemolytic anemia and immune thrombocytopenia.[101] A substantial proportion of cases develop in patients with B-cell lymphomas or

Table 47-2. Diseases Rarely Associated with Autoimmune Hemolytic Anemia

Collagen vascular disease
    Rheumatoid Arthritis
    Scleroderma
    Polyarteritis Nodosa
    Serum sickness
    Sjögren syndrome
Lymphoreticular malignancy
    Macroglobulinemia
    Hodgkin disease
    Multiple myeloma
    Mycosis fungoides
Other malignancy
    Acute leukemia
    Thymoma
    Carcinoma: colon, kidney, lung, ovary
Miscellaneous diseases
    Myelofibrosis with myeloid metaplasia
    Ulcerative colitis
    Pernicious anemia
    Thyroid disease
    Ovarian cysts
    Mucocutaneous lymph node syndrome (Kawasaki disease)
    Evans syndrome (thrombocytopenia and hemolytic anemia)
    Congenital immunodeficiency syndromes
    Guillain-Barré syndrome
    Primary biliary cirrhosis
    Multiply transfused patients with hemoglobinopathies

CLL. A number of other diseases have also been complicated by autoimmune hemolytic anemia, but only as unusual exceptions[102] (Table 47-2).

Clinical Findings in Autoimmune Hemolytic Anemia

The clinical findings in autoimmune hemolytic anemia are variable. They include jaundice (usually mild) and symptoms and signs of anemia. The spleen may be palpable 2–8 cm below the costal margin, especially after several months of unremitting hemolytic anemia. The spleen is enlarged in about one-third of patients. The disease can make its appearance acutely, with symptoms due to rapidly developing anemia, or it can develop gradually in a relatively asymptomatic form. Occasionally, the blood bank provides the diagnosis in a patient referred for transfusion therapy by discovering a positive antiglobulin test. The physical examination may reveal only pallor or slight jaundice, but signs of congestive heart failure are not unusual in patients with rapidly developing severe autoimmune hemolytic anemia. Lymphadenopathy, fever, hypertension, renal failure, a rash, petechiae, or ecchymoses should alert the physician to the possibility of an underlying disease.

Laboratory Evaluation

Laboratory findings reflect the intensity of the hemolytic process and the bone marrow's response to the anemia. In fulminant cases, with a RBC life span of <5 days, the anemia is severe and erythropoiesis increases 8–10-fold. As a result, the reticulocyte count rises, sometimes to levels >40%. In less severe cases, the regenerative capacity of the bone marrow lags only slightly behind the rate of RBC destruction; hence a mild anemia but an elevated reticulocyte count. Between these extremes are many variations. Inspection of the blood smear in a typical case will reveal polychromatophilia, spherocytes, a few fragmented RBCs, and nucleated RBCs, and occasionally erythrophagocytosis. Examination of the bone marrow shows erythroid hyperplasia, often with megaloblastoid features.

Patients with severe hemolytic anemia and markedly increased erythropoiesis occasionally develop folate deficiency and frank megaloblastosis. The growth of hematopoietic tissue in the bone marrow also leads to moderate increases in the white blood cell and platelet counts. The absence of reticulocytosis does not exclude the diagnosis of autoimmune hemolytic anemia but warns of a serious prognosis.[103–106] Presumably due to destruction of young erythrocytes by the autoantibody, the reticulocytopenia aggravates the severity of the anemia and increases the need for RBC transfusions; it may last several weeks despite therapy.

Rapid destruction of erythrocytes leads to other laboratory changes, which, like the preceding abnormalities, are not specific for autoimmune hemolytic anemia (see Ch. 36). These include increased serum levels of unconjugated bilirubin and lactate dehydrogenase, and reduction in plasma haptoglobin. In rare cases with intravascular destruction of erythrocytes, the plasma hemoglobin is elevated and there is hemoglobinuria; hemosiderinuria follows in approximately 7 days, when renal tubular epithelial cells containing absorbed iron defoliate into the urine. Tests of osmotic fragility and autohemolysis are unnecessary for diagnosis and management; measurements of RBC survival are rarely indicated.

The distinction between autoimmune hemolytic anemia and other forms of hemolytic anemia depends on the DAT, often termed the direct Coombs test. This assay detects the sine qua non of autoimmune hemolytic anemia: the presence of IgG or complement bound to the RBC membrane (Fig. 47-7). It is performed by washing the patient's RBCs free of plasma, adding the antiglobulin reagent, centrifuging, and reading for the presence or absence of agglutination. The DAT thus tests for the presence of immunoglobulin or complement on the patient's RBCs. In patients with severe autoimmune hemolytic anemia, the DATs are usually strongly positive, but the titer of the autoantibody and the strength of the reaction do not always predict the severity of disease.

The IgG autoantibodies in autoimmune hemolytic anemia are predominantly of the IgG1 and IgG3 subclasses, both of which are capable of activating complement. In most cases, either IgG

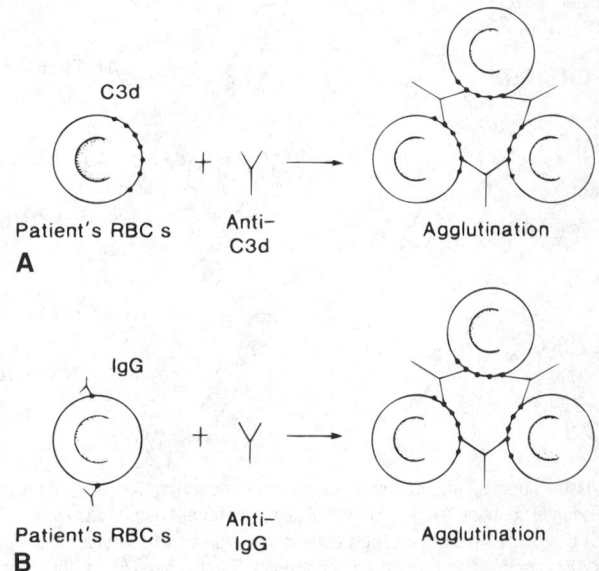

Fig. 47-7. DAT for detection of **(A)** erythrocyte-bound C3d or **(B)** IgG. Hemagglutination occurs when anti-C3d or anti-IgG can create a lattice structure by bridging sensitized RBCs.

or C3d (a proteolytic fragment of C3; see below) is bound to the RBC membrane. Therefore, the screening antiglobulin reagent, made by immunizing rabbits or by blending murine monoclonal antibodies, must contain antibodies against IgG (including IgG1 and IgG3 subclasses) and C3d.[107-114] Broad-spectrum antiglobulin test reagents may also contain antibodies against other serum proteins that can bind nonspecifically to RBCs. Therefore, when the routine antiglobulin test is positive, it should be repeated using reagents specific for IgG and C3d. IgA and IgM autoantibodies are rare causes of warm autoimmune hemolytic anemia[115-118] and need not be considered in usual routine tests.[119]

A positive antiglobulin test, confirmed with a specific anti-IgG reagent, is occasionally found in normal people; approximately 1 in 10,000 blood donors has a positive antiglobulin test without anemia or evidence of increased hemolysis.[120] A positive antiglobulin test with a monospecific anti-C3d reagent is also seen occasionally in normal subjects,[121] but such a result almost always points to either warm or cold-reactive autoantibodies. In about 10% of cases of autoimmune hemolytic anemia, erythrocyte-bound C3d occurs in the absence of erythrocyte-bound IgG, whereas in all cases of cold agglutinin disease erythrocyte-bound C3d is detected. SLE should be suspected in cases of autoimmune hemolytic anemia in which both IgG and C3d are detected. By contrast, α-methyldopa-induced autoimmune hemolytic anemia is rarely associated with erythrocyte-bound C3d—only IgG is present.

The unexpected report of a negative antiglobulin test in a patient suspected of having autoimmune hemolytic anemia, although uncommon, may have several explanations. Technical error is infrequent, but it can occur. Other rare causes are IgA autoantibodies or low-affinity IgG autoantibodies.[122] More commonly, the test is not sensitive enough to detect small numbers of erythrocyte-bound IgG molecules; this occurs most often in autoimmune hemolytic anemia associated with a lymphoma or CLL. Manual antiglobulin tests detect 200–500 molecules of IgG per cell; amounts below this level, although undetectable, may be clinically important. In such cases, sensitive assays such as the antiglobulin consumption[123] or tests with ^{125}I-staphylococcal protein A, which binds avidly to IgG, can reveal the autoantibodies.[124]

Like any other laboratory test, DAT requires interpretation. We have already seen that a positive antiglobulin test can occur in healthy subjects and that patients with autoimmune hemolytic anemia can have a negative antiglobulin test. It is equally important that a positive antiglobulin test does not always signify erythrocyte-bound IgG antibody or complement, nor does a positive result necessarily imply that the patient has hemolytic anemia. The frequency of false-positive tests in hospitalized patients can be as high as 15%.[125] They can stem from tests on clotted blood,[126] silicone gel tubes,[127] collection of samples from intravenous lines containing low-ionic-strength solutions,[128] medications (e.g., cephalin) that cause nonspecific attachment of plasma protein to the RBC surface,[129,130] and hypergammaglobulinemia.[131,132] If the DAT is positive, specific reagents are required to identify the erythrocyte-bound protein.

In about 80% of patients with autoimmune hemolytic anemia, the autoantibodies are present in the serum as well as on the red cell membrane.[133] The indirect antiglobulin test (indirect Coombs test) detects the presence of these serum antibodies in the patient's serum (Fig. 47-8). The procedure entails incubating the test serum and normal RBCs, usually at 37°C for 1 hour, washing the cells free of serum, adding the antiglobulin reagent, and reading for agglutination. The antibodies detected by the indirect antiglobulin test may be autoantibodies in a patient with autoimmune hemolytic anemia, or they may be alloantibodies induced by blood transfusion or maternal/fetal incompatibility. Alloantibodies, present only in the serum, have specificity for RBC antigen(s) not present on the patient's erythrocytes. The DAT is therefore negative in alloimmunization; exceptions may occur if the alloantibodies bind to recently transfused RBCs.

The specificity of the antibodies detected by the indirect antiglobulin test can be assessed by reacting the test serum with a panel of erythrocytes of known antigenic composition. Alloantibodies have definable specificities, whereas the serum autoantibodies of autoimmune hemolytic anemia usually react with all RBCs except those that contain no Rh antigens, the so-called Rh null RBCs.[134] Even so, the identity of the Rh-associated determinant implied by the lack of reactivity of the autoantibodies with Rh null cells is unknown. Occasionally (1–2% of cases), relative specificity within the Rh system can be demonstrated, and RBCs lacking the corresponding Rh antigen survive better in vivo than those which express the antigen.[135-138] Specificities of IgG autoantibodies for other blood groups have been described.[139-147] Specificity for different subunits of the RBC membrane has recently been reported.[148-152] In Evans syndrome in patients with the lupus anticoagulant (antiphospholipid antibody syndrome), the erythrocyte-bound autoantibody can react with phospholipids.[153-157] An important practical point is that, with rare exceptions, the autoantigens are present on all normal erythrocytes; in practice, all RBCs are incompatible (see the section, Therapy, Transfusion).

Pathophysiology

Immune Clearance of Erythrocytes

The autoantibodies that cause RBC destruction in autoimmune hemolytic anemia and the antierythrocyte autoantibodies in healthy persons with no discernible signs of abnormal hemolysis may have the same isotype and even identical serologic specificities. Therefore, the pathogenicity of anti-red cell autoantibodies must depend on additional considerations. The amount of the autoantibody, its avidity for the erythrocyte

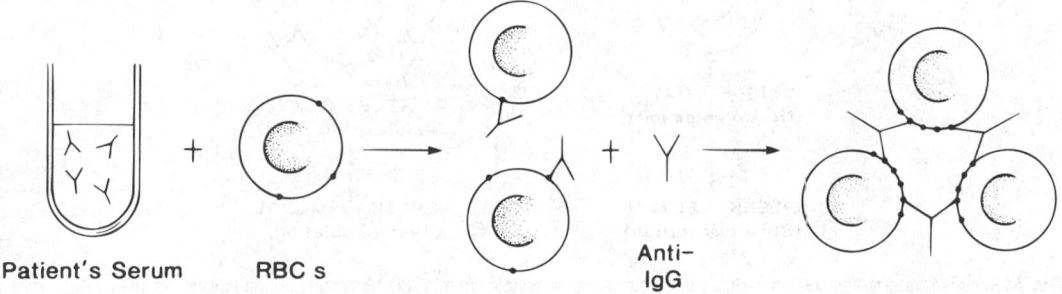

Patient's Serum   RBCs   Anti-IgG

Fig. 47-8. Indirect antiglobulin test for detection of antierythrocyte antibodies in serum. The patient's serum is mixed with a panel of normal RBCs, some (or all) of which express the antigen(s) recognized by the serum antibodies. After the antibody-coated erythrocytes are washed, an anti-IgG reagent is added. Hemagglutination occurs, as in Figure 47-7.

autoantigen, and its ability to fix complement are of particular importance.[158] Each of these factors probably contributes independently and cumulatively to the erythrocyte lesion.

Immune hemolysis in vivo begins with opsonization by autoantibodies. The terminal effect can be destruction of the RBC directly within the circulation (intravascular hemolysis) or removal of the cell from the circulation by tissue macrophages (extravascular hemolysis), or both. Opsonized RBCs are recognized and cleared from the circulation by macrophages located primarily in the spleen, and to a lesser extent in the liver.[159] The interaction of macrophages with RBCs coated with IgG or C3b (or both) occurs through receptors specific for the Fc portion of IgG (especially IgG1 and IgG3) and for C3b.[160,161] Initiation of the events that culminate in the deposition of C3b on the erythrocyte surface requires at least two IgG molecules bound in close proximity on the RBC membrane. Furthermore, the subclass of the IgG autoantibodies is important not only for binding to macrophage Fc receptors (IgG3 > IgG1) but also for complement activation. The potency of subclasses for complement activation is as follows: IgG1 > IgG3 > IgG2 > IgG4.[159–164]

The presence on the erythrocyte membrane of both IgG and C3b accelerates immune clearance,[165–167] suggesting that the Fc and C3b macrophage receptors act synergistically. Sequential studies in one subject of the clearance of RBCs coated in vitro with different amounts of the same antibody showed that the amount of erythrocyte-bound IgG is another factor influencing the rate of hemolysis. Little information is available on the minimum number of erythrocyte-bound IgG molecules required for interaction with macrophages; in some cases of autoimmune hemolytic anemia, <200 IgG molecules per erythrocyte (too few for detection by the DAT) is sufficient to cause in vivo hemolysis.[163]

The splenic environment is especially conducive to immune clearance. IgG-coated RBCs are efficiently trapped from the hemoconcentrated circulation within the spleen. The relatively low plasma concentration in splenic sinusoids tends to alleviate competition between plasma IgG and IgG-coated RBCs for Fc receptors, thus providing optimal interactions between opsonized erythrocytes and macrophages.[160,166]

Red Blood Cell Lesion

The macrophage may ingest an opsonized RBC entirely; more likely, proteolytic ectoenzymes on its surface digest away bits of the erythrocyte membrane, producing a spherocyte, a RBC with the lowest possible surface area/volume ratio.[161] Spherocytes are less deformable and more susceptible to osmotic lysis than disc-shaped red cells, so they are especially susceptible to hemolysis during their traversals through the sluggish circulation of the splenic sinusoids. This is why the predominant mechanism of destruction of erythrocytes coated with IgG with or without C3b occurs extravascularly in autoimmune hemolytic anemia (Fig. 47-9). By contrast, intravascular hemolysis is rare because regulatory proteins of the complement system (C3b inactivator and β_1 H globulin) limit completion of the complement cascade on the surface of the opsonized erythrocyte.[168] The C3b inactivator system contributes to the local arrest of the complement cascade by degrading C3b to C3d; spontaneous elution of the autoantibody (a measure of its avidity for the RBC) leaves an erythrocyte coated only with C3d.

Macrophage-mediated mechanisms predominate in causing the lesion of autoimmune hemolytic anemia, but the participation of cytotoxic lymphocytes (natural killer cells), which cause antibody-dependent cell lysis, has not been excluded. The efficiency of reticuloendothelial function probably also contributes to the degree of immune clearance, and may account for exacerbations of autoimmune hemolytic anemia by viral or bacterial infections. In vitro assays of the ability of blood monocytes from patients with viral infections to phagocytose Ig-coated RBCs have shown marked deviations from normal.[169,170]

Therapy

General Principles

Since the severity of autoimmune hemolytic anemia may range from the indolent to the life-threatening, the impetus to initiate treatment must begin with a thorough appraisal of

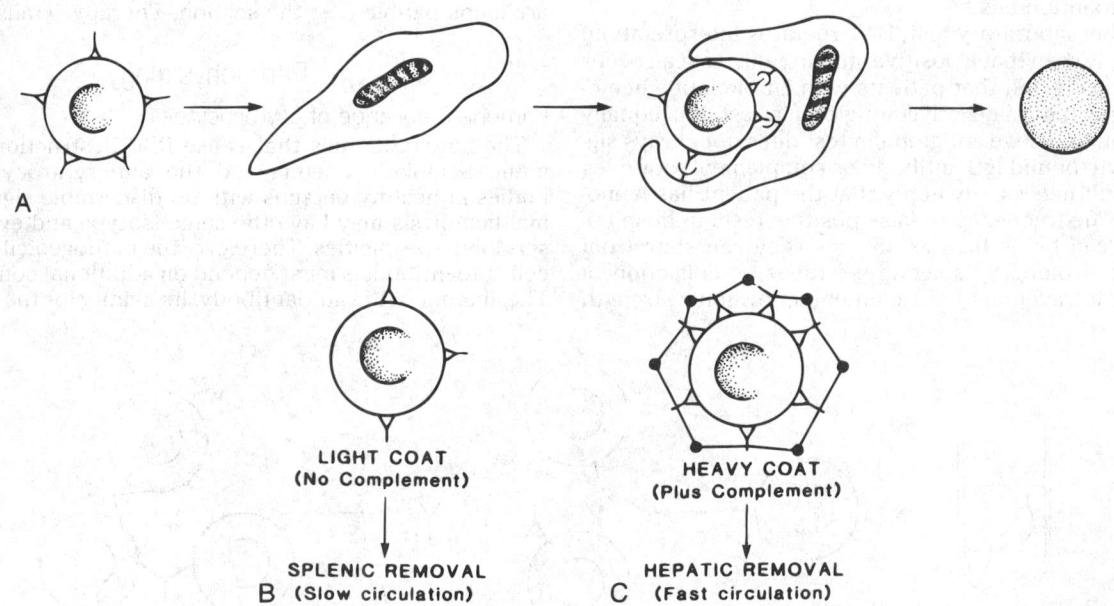

Fig. 47-9. Mechanism of extravascular hemolysis in autoimmune hemolytic anemia. **(A)** Macrophage encounters an IgG-coated erythrocyte and binds to it via its Fc receptors. Thus entrapped, the RBC loses bits of its membrane as a result of digestion by the macrophage's ectoenzymes. The discoid erythrocyte transforms into a sphere. **(B)** RBC lightly coated with IgG (and therefore incapable of activating the complement cascade) is preferentially removed in the sluggish circulation of the spleen. **(C)** RBC with a heavy coat of IgG; thus, C3b (black circles) can be removed both by the spleen and the liver.

HAZARDS OF TRANSFUSION THERAPY

The idea that transfusion therapy represents a special hazard in patients with autoimmune hemolytic anemia[179-182] has been overemphasized; nevertheless, transfusions are not to be undertaken lightly in such patients. The decision to transfuse requires that the clinician and the blood bank work together. The clinician must supervise the transfusions and insist on close observation of the patient. An adverse reaction dictates additional laboratory tests, but even sophisticated serologic techniques do not ensure uneventful transfusions; acute intravascular hemolysis can occur with no evidence of serologic incompatibility. In vivo compatibility testing with ^{51}Cr-tagged RBCs is of no value in the management of most patients.

Transfusion is warranted without delay and, if necessary, before all the serologic tests are completed when cardiac or cerebral function is threatened. Alleviation of signs and symptoms of anemia can usually be accomplished with relatively small quantities of RBCs—as little as 0.5 to 1 U of RBCs. Overtransfuction in the presence of high-output cardiac failure can easily lead to circulatory overload, another reason to justify careful observation of the patient during the transfusion.

symptoms and the extent of the damage. Rapidly developing anemia with a hematocrit of <20 requires urgent management, but in the less aggressive forms of the disease, especially in the elderly, it may be more prudent to allow the patient to tolerate mild anemia than to institute risky treatment.

The management of autoimmune hemolytic anemia depends in part on whether the disease is primary or whether it is secondary to such disorders as B-cell malignancies or SLE.[171,172] This too demands a careful assessment before any treatment begins. In some cases of autoimmune hemolytic anemia secondary to lymphoma or CLL, the pathogenic autoantibody (usually monoclonal) is secreted by the neoplastic B cells. Combination chemotherapy or irradiation of the underlying malignancy often brings the hemolytic anemia under control.[173-175] In other cases, however, the autoantibodies (usually polyclonal) do not originate from the B-cell neoplasm but probably result from abnormal immune regulation instigated by the neoplastic B cells. Treatment of the latter type of secondary autoimmune hemolytic anemia with immunosuppressive agents may improve the anemia, but it may also actually trigger an exacerbation.[176]

The ultimate goal of therapy is control of B-cell populations that secrete pathogenic autoantibodies. However, so little is known about such cells[177,178] that the currently available therapy is, by default, nonspecific. The desired therapeutic effect is eradication of the abnormal hemolytic process, and not reversal of the serologic abnormalities. Indeed, the DAT often remains positive in the face of a hematologic response.

Transfusion

Severe anemia may cause pulmonary edema (in the setting of high-output cardiac failure), somnolence, and even obtundation. These manifestations occur when the hemoglobin falls to <4 g/dl. They are life-threatening and necessitate transfusion with RBCs. The persistence of tachycardia, postural hypotension, dyspnea, and angina also call for transfusion. Oxygen therapy may be prescribed, but it is no substitute for transfusion.

Alloantibodies, usually with specificity for the Rh or Kell blood group systems, occur in approximately 30% of patients

with autoimmune hemolytic anemia who have a history of blood group immunization by maternal/fetal incompatibility or previous transfusions.[183-185] These alloantibodies can escape notice in a patient with a positive indirect antiglobulin test because of the concomitant presence in the serum of autoantibodies that react with virtually all normal RBCs. Nevertheless, several techniques may help detect suspected alloantibodies.[186-188] Absorption of the autoantibodies with the patient's own RBCs can permit recognition of residual alloantibodies. Before absorption, the autoantibody must be eluted from the patient's RBCs; enzyme treatment of the patient's cells increases autoantibody absorption. Another method involves absorption of the patient's serum with normal RBCs of selected phenotypes and then retesting of the absorbed serum.

The above techniques should not be required as pretransfusion tests in patients with autoimmune hemolytic anemia. Transfusions should never be delayed if the tests are not readily available. However, standard antibody detection and identification tests with both the patient's serum and an eluate prepared from the patient's cells should be performed whenever possible. Titration of the eluate and the serum against RBCs of various Rh phenotypes can indicate an autoantibody specificity (or preference) within the Rh system. Any such specificity should be respected in selecting donor's units.[189,190]

Corticosteroids

Corticosteroids are the mainstay of treatment for patients with symptomatic, unstable autoimmune hemolytic anemia of either the idiopathic or the secondary forms. The clinical response to prednisone results primarily from its ability to disable macrophages from clearing IgG- or C3b-coated erythrocytes. Corticosteroids interfere with both the expression and function of macrophage Fc receptors. This is probably the earliest, and perhaps even the primary, mechanism of the ability of steroids to diminish the immune clearance of blood cells.[191-194] Prednisone can also reduce autoantibody production, but only after several weeks of therapy.

Splenectomy

Indications for splenectomy in autoimmune hemolytic anemia include failure to respond to prednisone, dependence on prednisone dosages that are >10–20 mg/day, or intractable side effects of the corticosteroid. The procedure can be highly effective because along with the removal of the spleen go its phagocytosing macrophages and autoantibody-producing B cells. In most young adults with primary autoimmune hemolytic anemia, the question of splenectomy arises almost inevitably. However, in an elderly patient with a stable but incomplete remission, maintenance therapy with prednisone at a dose of 10 mg/day for an indefinite period may be the better alternative. There is a slight risk of developing overwhelming sepsis syndrome immediately following splenectomy, but systemic bacterial infections can occur long after the postoperative period as well.[195] These risks are lessened by immunization with pneumococcal and meningococcal vaccines, always given preoperatively, and by the prompt use of antibiotics for febrile illness.

The response to splenectomy does not correlate with the age of the patient, the presence or absence of an underlying B-cell disorder, the strength of the antiglobulin test, prior response to prednisone, or pattern of sequestration of ^{51}Cr-labeled red cells; these criteria cannot be used to predict the response to splenectomy.[196] About 50–60% of patients with classic autoimmune hemolytic anemia will have a good to excellent initial response to splenectomy. They will require <15 mg/day of prednisone to maintain an adequate level of hemoglobin.[197] Information regarding the clinical implications of an

PREDNISONE THERAPY

Therapy can begin with prednisone (there is no clear advantage to alternative forms of corticosteroids) in a dose of 1–2 mg/kg/day in divided doses, depending on the severity of the disease. The physician can consider beginning with a lower dose (e.g., 0.6 mg/kg/day) in elderly patients, especially those who are immobilized or who already have osteoporosis, or when faced with infection or other mitigating complications. Whatever the amount selected, it should be continued until a response becomes evident, usually within 3 weeks, by a rise in the hematocrit and a fall in the reticulocyte count.

Autoimmune hemolytic anemia in children is likely to respond to prednisone with a durable remission. By contrast, permanent remissions are infrequent in adults. Therapy for adults therefore requires a plan to manage (or avoid) relapse. Essential elements to consider in formulating the long-term management of a patient with autommune hemolytic anemia are the duration of treatment with the initial dose of prednisone and the rate of dosage reduction after a response has been achieved. The tapering schedule depends, in part, on the severity of the initial presentation and on the prominence of side effects of the treatment. In the absence of contraindications, prednisone is continued at the initial dose until the hemoglobin reaches a level of ≥10 g/dl, by which time transfusions should no longer be necessary. Thereafter, gradual reduction in the dose can begin, usually at a rate of 5–10 mg/wk. During this second phase of treatment, the divided daily prednisone dose can be consolidated into a single daily dose. If the remission remains stable after a dose of 10 mg/day is reached, further tapering over a 3–4-month period can proceed cautiously. Some hematologists will continue treatment for many months, at low doses (e.g., 10 mg every other day), but the efficacy of this practice has not been investigated.

CYTOTOXIC DRUG THERAPY

The administration of cytotoxic drugs is best reserved for refractory cases: symptomatic patients who have not responded to splenectomy, those in whom splenectomy is an unacceptable medical risk, those who refuse the operation, or patients who have serious side effects from corticosteroids. Cyclophosphamide (2 mg/kg/day) or azathioprine (1.5 mg/kg/day) should be continued for ≥3 months to ensure maximal inhibition of autoantibody synthesis. Less than one-half of patients treated with these drugs will respond with a rise in the hemoglobin that can be maintained in the face of substantially reduced doses of prednisone. Indeed, this estimate may be overly optimistic, since negative or unfavorable results seldom reach publication. Unfortunately, no controlled clinical trials of cytostatic agents in the treatment of autoimmune hemolytic anemia have been conducted.

accessory spleen in autoimmune hemolytic anemia is meager. Faced with such a rare finding in a relapsed patient, many hematologists would recommend its removal. The role of splenectomy in patients with mixed IgG, IgM, or mixed cold- and warm-reactive IgG antibodies is unclear.

Immunosuppressive Therapy

Most experience with immunosuppressive drugs in the treatment of autoimmune hemolytic anemia has been with alkylating agents (cyclophosphamide and chlorambucil) and thiopurines (azathioprine and 6-mercaptopurine).[198] The basis for the clinical use of these drugs is their inhibitory effect on the immune system, possibly affecting both B cells and T cells.[199,200]

Cyclophosphamide and azathioprine, like prednisone, can induce numerous side effects. Some of these occur concomitant with their use; others become evident only after sustained administration. The early side effects include bone marrow suppression and impairment of the immune response (particularly T-cell-mediated immunity). In addition, cyclophosphamide damages ovarian function, inhibits spermatogenesis,[201–204] and causes bladder fibrosis.[205] Acute myeloid leukemia can develop years after sustained use.[199] By contrast, the prolonged use of azathioprine has not been associated with a statistically significant increase in malignant diseases. All these considerations demand careful monitoring of any patient treated with either cyclophosphamide or azathioprine.

Plasma Exchange

In a normal person, plasma exchange of 1–1.5 plasma volumes is effective in lowering the serum level of IgG by ≥50%. However, continuous antibody production and the large extravascular distribution of IgG limit the efficacy of plasma exchange in autoimmune hemolytic anemia. On cessation of the therapy, the rate of return of pretreatment levels of autoantibody depends on the rate of autoantibody production.[206] Occasional dramatic responses have been reported in patients being prepared for surgery or when plasma exchange was a temporizing measure following the initiation of immunosuppressive therapy.[207,208]

Vinca Alkaloids

Responses in a few patients with autoimmune hemolytic anemia have been reported following infusion with vincristine-laden IgG-coated platelets; the platelets serve the drug directly to macrophages, presumably interfering with the ability of the macrophages to bind or ingest IgG-coated RBCs. Reported responses have been of long duration and associated with a delayed fall in the titer of the DAT. Therapeutic effects of vinca alkaloids alone in autoimmune hemolytic anemia have not been systematically investigated.[209]

Danazol

An attenuated synthetic androgen, danazol, is useful in patients with autoimmune thrombocytopenic purpura when given in a dose of 400–600 mg/day PO. It has benefited a limited number of patients with refractory autoimmune hemolytic anemia. Remissions of ≤1 year have been reported.[210] In view of the relatively low risk of long-term side effects (the drug can cause abnormal liver function), danazol may find a secure place in the management of prednisone-dependent patients.

Intravenous γ-Globulin

Intravenous γ-globulin has been found effective in managing selected cases of autoimmune thrombocytopenia. The recommended dose is 400 mg/kg/day for 5 days. The soluble IgG in the material may increase the life span of IgG-coated RBCs by saturating Fc receptors on macrophages. In a recent study of patients with autoimmune hemolytic anemia associated with lymphoproliferative disorders, a long-term benefit was observed with a maintenance dose schedule of intravenous IgG every 21 days. A decrease in antiglobulin titer was found in these patients, suggesting a mechanism other than blockade of Fc receptors by intravenous IgG.[211]

COLD AGGLUTININ DISEASE

Cold agglutinin disease refers to a group of disorders caused by antierythrocyte autoantibodies (e.g., cold agglutinins) that preferentially bind RBCs at cold temperatures (4°–18°C). Virtually all sera from healthy individuals contain low-titer cold agglutinins regarded as benign/harmless RBC autoantibodies and considered polyclonal. Similarly, cold agglutinins that arise following certain infections are also polyclonal and usually benign; in rare cases, a transient form of cold agglutinin disease ensues (see below). By contrast, monoclonal cold agglutinins are generally pathogenic and are derived from clonal B-cell expansions (as in idiopathic/chronic cold agglutin disease), which may progress to frank lymphoma (Table 47-3).

Chronic Cold Agglutinin Disease

The most common type of cold agglutinin disease, a chronic form characterized principally by a stable anemia of moderate severity and attacks of acrocyanosis precipitated by exposure to cold, constitutes about one-third of all cases of immunohemolytic anemia. Cold agglutinins cause the cardinal abnormalities of the disease. The acrocyanosis stems from intra-arteriolar agglutination of erythrocytes in the relatively cool tips of the fingers, feet, earlobes, and nose. The hemolytic anemia depends on the capacity of the cold agglutinins to initiate activation of the complement cascade on the surface of the RBC (see the section Pathophysiology). Most patients with chronic cold agglutinin disease are in the fifth to eighth decade of life, and many of them have a B-cell neoplasm—lymphoma, Waldenström's macroglobulinemia, or CLL. The cold agglutinin in those latter cases is monoclonal, almost always IgM-κ, and may show up as a monoclonal band in the γ-region of the serum protein electrophoretic pattern. In the absence of a B-cell neoplasm, the spleen and lymph nodes are rarely enlarged; such findings warrant a search for the neoplasm.

Laboratory Evaluation

The usual laboratory findings of hemolytic anemia (i.e., anemia, reticulocytosis, polychromatophilia, spherocytosis, erythroid hyperplasia in the bone marrow, and elevations of serum bilirubin and lactate dehydrogenase) are generally not striking in chronic cold agglutinin disease. Hemagglutination may be visible to the unaided eye in blood drawn from a patient with cold agglutinin disease and can interfere with automated blood counts. The anemia is often mild and stable because the C3b inactivator in serum limits the extent of cold agglutinin-induced complement activation on the erythrocyte membrane. However, exposure to cold may greatly augment the binding of cold agglutinins, exceeding the restraints of the inactivator system. This can result in a sudden drop in hematocrit, with comple-

Table 47-3. Classification of Cold Agglutinin Disease

Monoclonal[a]
   Idiopathic/chronic
   B-cell lymphoma
Polyclonal
   Benign/natural
   Postinfectious (e.g., *Mycoplasma pneumoniae*, Epstein-Barr virus, human immunodeficiency virus), collagen vascular disorders

[a] Monoclonal cold agglutinins are derived from a spectrum of clonal B-cell expansions ranging from preneoplastic (e.g., no evidence of malignancy) to frank lymphoma.

ment-mediated intravascular hemolysis and renal failure. In a distinctive subset of patients with aggressive cold agglutinin disease, the cold agglutinin titer is relatively low, but the autoantibody has a high thermal amplitude. Recognition of patients with this variant of cold agglutinin disease is important because they can respond to prednisone,[212] whereas patients with high-titer cold agglutinin disease usually do not.

In typical cases of chronic cold agglutinin disease, the cold agglutinin titer is very high ($>1:10^5$, and occasionally $>1:10^6$). The antibodies are most reactive in the cold, and hemagglutination disappears as the temperature rises toward 37°C. In some cases, however, the antibody is reactive at relatively high temperatures, and occasionally even at 37°C. The reactivity of the cold agglutinin at high temperatures (i.e., its thermal amplitude), and not the titer of the antibody, most accurately predicts the severity of the disease. The DAT is positive because of erythrocyte-bound C3d (see the section Pathophysiology), but tests with anti-IgG reagents are negative. The indirect antiglobulin test, conducted at 37°C, is negative. In addition to monoclonal IgM cold agglutinins, IgG/IgM mixed cold agglutins have been reported.[213–215] Besides the usual high titers of IgM cold agglutinins, some cases of cold agglutinin disease have low titers of IgG and IgA cold agglutinins.

Cold agglutinins are not cryoglobulins. The latter are most often monoclonal IgM immunoglobulins that, in the cold, either self-associate and precipitate from solution (type I cryoglobulinemia) or precipitate as complexes with polyclonal IgG molecules (type II cryoglobulinemia, often due to a monoclonal IgM rheumatoid factor). Type III cryoglobulins consist of a mixture of polyclonal IgM and polyclonal IgG immunoglobulins. The clinical manifestations of the cryoglobulinemic syndromes are highly variable: types I and II cryoglobulinemia occur in B-cell neoplasms (Waldenström's macroglobulinemia, multiple myleoma, lymphoma, and CLL); type II and III cryoglobulinemia can produce a picture of immune complex-mediated vasculitis, with vascular purpura, arthritis, and nephritis as the dominant complications. In occasional patients, the cryoglobulin can also be a cold agglutinin.[216–219]

Transient Cold Agglutinin Disease

A second type of cold agglutinin disease, usually acute and always self-limited, occurs as a rare complication of several infectious diseases, most notably *M. pneumoniae* infection and infectious mononucleosis. Patients with this form of cold agglutinin disease are therefore much younger than those with chronic cold agglutinin disease. The onset is abrupt, appearing as the infection wanes, and the anemia can be severe. Cold agglutinin titers are moderately elevated, and the cold agglutinins are polyclonal.

Targets of Cold Agglutinin Disease

The antigenic specificity of cold agglutinins is usually identified by their degree of reactivity with RBCs from adults (blood group I) and cord blood (blood group i). The cold-reactive autoantibody produced after some cases of *M. pneumoniae* infection has anti-I specificity,[89] whereas the antibody in infectious mononucleosis frequently, (but not always), has anti-i specificity.[220,221] Additional specificities have been identified by tests with rare adult RBCs that lack the I antigen, or with enzyme-treated erythrocytes. Cold agglutinins with these antigenic specificities (I^T, I^F, Pr, Gd, Sa, Lud, F1) have no distinguishing clinical features.[222–230]

Pathophysiology

The pathogenic IgM autoantibody in cold agglutinin disease is highly efficient in activating the classic complement pathway on the erythrocyte membrane.[231,232] However, the thermal de-

TRANSFUSIONS AND COLD AGGLUTININ DISEASE

Transfusion in a patient with cold agglutinin disease requires the same prudent safeguards observed with transfusions in autoimmune hemolytic anemia. All compatibility tests must be carried out at 37°C and with IgG-specific antiglobulin reagents to avoid confusion with the serum cold agglutinin and the erythrocyte-bound C3d. The use of "inline" blood warmers is advisable, and more elaborate measures to perform the entire transfusion process at 37°C are occasionally required.[243] Hypothermia must be avoided during cardiac surgery, and special techniques must be used to avoid lowering the temperature of blood in the coronary arteries.[244]

pendency of the antibody constrains its pathogenic effects. The autoantibody rapidly elutes off red cells at the 37°C temperature of the visceral circulation, but in the cool peripheral circulation of the hands and feet the cold agglutinin remains on the erythrocyte membrane for at least a few seconds. That amount of time is sufficient to activate the complement cascade to the stage of C3b, which adheres to the RBC after it re-enters the central circulation. In the hepatic circulation, $C3b^+$ RBCs encounter macrophages with receptors specific for C3b[158,166,229]; however, C3b sensitization is only a weak signal for the activation of phagocytosis—hepatic clearance of C3b-coated RBCs requires 500–800 C3b molecules/RBC. As a result, many $C3b^+$ RBCs escape unharmed into the systemic circulation, where they come under the influence of the regulatory proteins of the complement system. The C3b inactivator system degrades C3b into C3dg or C3d, or both. The result is a cohort of erythrocytes coated with C3d, but not with the IgM autoantibody.[159] Since macrophages bind to C3d with even lower avidity than to C3b, the $C3d^+$ erythrocytes tend to have a near-normal survival in vivo despite a heavy coating with that degradation product of C3.[163,233]

These limits on the pathogenicity of cold agglutinins account for the subdued hematologic picture in most patients with cold agglutinin disease. If, however, the regulatory C3b inactivator proteins are impaired, limiting cleavage of RBC-bound C3b, or the production of IgM autoantibodies with a high thermal amplitude are impaired, permitting completion of the complement cascade in the visceral circulation, severe extravascular hemolysis can occur. Several patients with high titers of IgA cold agglutinins have been reported. These cases are not associated with cold agglutinin disease, which may relate to the lack of complement activation by IgA antibodies.[234–242]

Therapy

Chronic Cold Agglutinin Disease

Therapy for the cold agglutinin syndromes depends on the gravity of the symptoms, the serologic characteristics of the autoantibody, and any underlying disease. In the idiopathic, or primary, form of chronic cold agglutinin disease, prolonged survival and spontaneous remissions and exacerbations are not unusual. The anemia is generally mild, and the simple measure of avoiding exposure to cold temperatures can avoid exacerbations, especially when the cold agglutinin has a low thermal amplitude. Prednisone has been beneficial in rare cases showing relatively low titers of cold agglutinins of a high thermal amplitude or in which an IgG cold-reactive antibody is produced. However, prednisone is not useful therapy in most patients with primary IgM-induced cold agglutinin disease, and

its administration should not be undertaken lightly, given the chronicity of the disease. Plasma exchange may help as a temporary measure in acute situations.[207] Splenectomy is usually ineffective because the liver is the dominant site of sequestration of red cells heavily sensitized with C3b. However, rare cases with an enlarged spleen have responded to splenectomy; in some of these patients, a localized splenic lymphoma was found, whereas in others only lymphoid hyperplasia was evident.

It is essential to seek evidence of a B-cell neoplasm before initiating therapy for chronic cold agglutinin disease. Oral alkylating agents (chlorambucil or cyclophosphamide) help many patients with the secondary form of cold agglutinin disease because of their effect on the B-cell neoplasm, but only occasionally do they benefit patients with the primary form of the disease.[245,246] When cold agglutinin disease is part of an established B-cell malignancy, the severity of hemolysis often waxes and wanes in parallel with the activity of the neoplasm.

Transient Cold Agglutinin Disease

Transient cold agglutinin disease is a rare form that is always self-limited. Supportive measures, including transfusions and avoidance of cold, may suffice to tide the patient over the bout of hemolysis. Corticosteroids are usually not helpful, and splenectomy is almost never indicated.

PAROXYSMAL COLD HEMOGLOBINURIA

Clinical Manifestations

There are two clearly divisible groups of patients with paroxysmal cold hemoglobinuria: persons with tertiary or congenital syphilis, and children or young adults who develop the disease after a viral illness. The syphilitic variant is rarely seen today. Although the Donath-Landsteiner antibody often occurs in tertiary or congenital syphilis, it generally does not cause hemolytic disease. On exposure to cold, an occasional patient develops paroxysms of hemoglobinuria and constitutional symptoms: fever, back pain, leg pain, abdominal cramps, and rigors followed by hemoglobinuria. The infrequent postviral form of paroxysmal cold hemoglobinuria[247–249] is characterized by constitutional symptoms with fulminant intravascular hemolysis and its associated signs of hemoglobinemia, hemoglobinuria, jaundice, severe anemia, and sometimes renal failure. The disease is self-limited, usually lasting 2–3 weeks.

Laboratory Evaluation

The IgG antibody responsible for paroxysmal cold hemoglobinuria is found in the patient's serum by incubation of normal erythrocytes, fresh normal serum as a source of complement, and the patient's serum, first at 4°C and then at 37°C, with appropriate controls. The Donath-Lansteiner antibody fixes the first two components of complement in the cold and completes the cascade on warming to 37°C.[250] The DAT is almost always negative, but occasionally weak reactions for erythrocyte-bound complement are manifested. The indirect antiglobulin test is negative. Most Donath-Landsetiner antibodies have specificity for the P blood group system,[251,252] but other specificities have been described.[253–255] The diagnosis depends on recognition of the clinical picture, since tests for the Donath-Landsteiner antibody are not routinely performed.

Therapy

No specific treatment for paroxysmal cold hemoglobinuria has been found. Prednisone is not useful. The best approach is supportive care transfusions to alleviate symptoms and avoidance of cold temperatures.

DRUG-INDUCED IMMUNE HEMOLYTIC ANEMIA

Drug-induced immune hemolytic anemia was commonly seen when penicillin was administered in large doses (i.e., >20 million U/day) and when α-methyldopa was widely used in the treatment of hypertension.[256,257] However, the disease is unusual in present-day clinical practice.[258]

Three distinct mechanisms are associated with the disorder. In the first, the patient makes antibodies against a drug (e.g., penicillin) that can bind to the RBC membrane, exposing its haptenic determinant. The antidrug antibodies combine with the erythrocyte-bound drug, opsonizing and preparing the RBC for destruction. In the case of penicillin,[259] hemolytic anemia occurs only when large amounts are administered; in patients treated with lower doses, a positive DAT without hemolytic anemia is not unusual because the production of low-avidity IgG antipenicillin antibodies is a common event. Discontinuation of the drug brings the hemolytic anemia to a rapid halt. Clues to the diagnosis are the appropriate clinical setting: a positive DAT, a negative indirect antiglobulin test, and failure of antibodies eluted from the patient's RBCs to bind to normal erythrocyte. The diagnosis is established when both the eluate and the patient's serum react with penicillin-coated cells.

The second mechanism involves immune complexes. The offending drug, or drug metabolite, binds to a plasma protein, forming an immunogenic conjugate. The resulting antidrug antibody binds to the drug/plasma protein conjugate, forming an immune complex that adheres to RBCs. The antidrug antibody, usually IgM, causes a clinical picture of intravascular hemolysis, hemoglobinemia, hemoglobinuria, and even renal failure by efficiently activating complement on the erythrocyte membrane. This chain of events accounts for most reported examples of drug-induced immune hemolytic anemia.

Serologic findings with erythrocyte-bound immune complexes are similar to those of the first mechanism, except that the DAT reveals complement only bound to the RBC; the IgM antibody is presumed to be no longer present after complement activation. The patient's serum reacts with RBCs (lacking antidrug antibody) in the presence of the offending drug, and the eluate from the patient's RBCs generally does not react with normal erythrocytes.

The third mechanism involves in vivo sensitization to drugs by the formation of immunogenic drug/RBC complexes. In these cases, the specificity of the drug-induced antibodies is contributed not only by the drug (or its metabolites), but also by defined RBCs antigens, particularly of the Rhesus and I/i systems.[260]

The fourth mechanism involves the induction of authentic autoantibodies against RBCs by a drug. α-Methyldopa is the classic example[261] (Fig. 47-10). As many as 20% of patients treated with α-methyldopa develop a positive DAT, but few develop hemolytic anemia. The antiglobulin test may take several months or >1 year after the start of drug therapy to become positive. In patients with hemolytic anemia, discontinuation of the drug results in the gradual cessation of the hemolytic anemia and disappearance of the autoantibody. Curiously, the autoantibody is usually specific for antigens of the Rh system. The serologic findings are indistinguishable from those of primary autoimmune hemolytic anemia; they include a positive DAT, usually a positive indirect antiglobulin test, and an eluate that reacts with normal erythrocytes. In contrast to the preceding examples, in this case the drug is not required in the test system to demonstrate the presence of the antibodies. Patients taking α-methyldopa often have antinuclear antibodies, rheumatoid factor, and antibodies to gastric parietal cells in addition to the RBC autoantibodies. The mechanism by which α-methyldopa induces autoantibodies is unknown but may involve effects on immunoregulatory T cells.

DRUGS REPORTED TO CAUSE HEMOLYTIC ANEMIA

Mechanism and serologic findings are summarized.

Mechanism	Hapten	Immune Complex	Autoantibody
Example	Penicillin	Stibophen	Methyldopa
DAT	Positive	Positive	Positive
Anti-IgG	Positive	Rarely positive	Positive
Anti-C3d	Rarely positive	Positive	Negative
Indirect antiglobulin test (drug not present in test system)	Negative	Negative	Negative or positive
Indirect antiglobulin test (drug in test system)	Positive	Positive	No change due to drug
Other drugs	Cephalothin Cephaloridine Ampicillin Methicillin Carbenicillin Akfluor 25% Cefotaxine	Qinine Quinidine Phenacetin Hydrochlorothiazide Rifampin p-Aminosalicylic acid Antihistamines Sulfonamides Isoniazid Chlorpromazine Pyramidon Dipyrone Melphalan Insulin Tetracyline Acetaminophen Streptomycin Hydralazine Probenecid Carbimazole Sulfonylurea derivative Chlorinated hydrocarbon insecticides Cianidanol Cephalosporin Nomifensine 5-Fluorouracil Tolmetin Fenoprofen Sulindac Cefotaxine Ceftriaxone Radiographic contrast medium	Mefenamic acid L-dopa Procainamide Ibuprofen Diclofenac Thioridazine Interferon-α

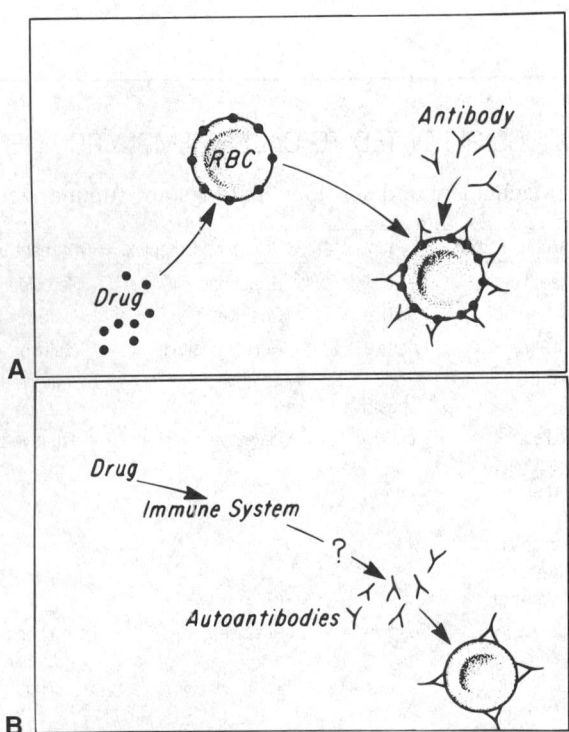

Fig. 47-10. Drug-induced hemolytic anemia. **(A)** The "planted antigen" mechanism, of which penicillin-induced hemolytic anemia is the paradigm, entails binding of a drug to the RBC membrane, followed by binding of antidrug antibody to the "planted" antigen. **(B)** By contrast, in the autoimmune mechanism, the patient produces authentic antierythrocyte autoantibodies.

UNUSUAL FORMS OF IMMUNE HEMOLYTIC ANEMIA

Hemolytic anemia due to heteroantibodies or alloantibodies may be confused with autoimmune hemolytic anemia in certain cases. Some lots of antithymocyte globulin contain heterologous antihuman RBC antibodies, which can precipitate attacks of immune hemolysis[262]; anti-A alloantibodies in some preparations of intravenous human γ-globulin have resulted in RBC destruction[263,264,] and the synthesis of alloantibodies by B cells in transplanted livers and kidneys may cause a hemolytic anemia that masquarades as autoimmune hemolytic anemia.[265]

FUTURE DIRECTIONS

The lifelong symbiotic relationship between the immune system and erythrocytes begins to unfold during the early stages of embryonic life. Lymphocytes and macrophages supply immature erythrocytes with growth-promoting lymphokines and with iron; in return, mature RBCs furnish the immune system with oxygen. Old erythrocytes, no longer discs but spheres, end their lives within antigen-presenting macrophages. Even so, lymphocytes ignore virtually all the proteins, glycoproteins, and glycolipids on the RBC membrane. Those same components can trigger the production of antibodies with a lethal potential when injected into another person with a different constellation of blood groups, even if the difference is but a single sugar molecule. The molecular biology of this striking aspect of lymphocyte physiology—immunologic tolerance—is not understood, nor are the mechanisms responsible for its induction and maintenance. The developmental immunology of structurally defined human blood groups is an untapped mine of information with considerable relevance to the phenomenon of immunologic tolerance in humans. The advantages

of such studies over experiments on specially bred transgenic mouse for immunologic investigations should be self-evident.

Virtually nothing is known about how the immunologic tolerance of erythrocyte autoantigens breaks down—the cause of autoimmune hemolytic anemia. Research on this question needs to focus on three topics: the structures of the autoantibodies, molecular identification of the autoantigens, and elucidation of the networks of lymphocytes and idiotypes that enforce unresponsiveness to erythrocyte autoantigens. Modern techniques of molecular biology (gene analysis, protein microsequencing, and cell cloning, in particular) are ripe for application to the problem. A particularly fruitful line for future investigations is the mechanism of the production of IgG warm-reactive antierythrocyte autoantibodies in CLL. This is one of the few cases in which a monoclonal population of B cells with obvious relevance to polyclonal autoantibodies can be cloned in vitro and analyzed with the armamentarium of molecular immunology.

The present classification of the autoimmune hemolytic anemias does not accommodate all variants of these disorders, but it is generally useful. Our terminology reflects current practice: most clinicians recognize that the unembellished term *autoimmune hemolytic anemia* refers to hemolytic anemia due to warm-reactive IgG autoantibodies and that cold agglutinin disease means hemolytic anemia associated with cold-reactive IgM autoantibodies. Not all cases fit into these neat categories, however. The thermal behavior of the autoantibody, or its isotype, may not correspond to arbitrary rules, and some patients produce mixtures of IgG, IgM, and even IgA autoantibodies. Furthermore, the serologic specificity of the autoantibody in autoimmune hemolytic anemia is highly variable. Some autoantibodies bind to well-defined blood group antigens, whereas others show much broader patterns of reactivity. Still others bind to structural membrane proteins or phospholipids with no known relationship to blood group antigens. Additional contributions to the heterogeneity of the autoimmune hemolytic anemias include the complement-fixing ability of the autoantibody and its avidity for the erythrocyte autoantigen. A realistic classification of the autoimmune hemolytic anemias would take this extensive heterogeneity into account, but it might prove too cumbersome for practical application.

The physician encounters additional layers of complexity in deciding about treatment. Is the disorder primary or secondary? Does the patient have SLE or a lymphoma? Could a drug be involved? Are transfusions warranted if a compatible donor cannot be identified? Management of the patient with autoimmune hemolytic anemia in relapse remains a major problem. None of the available tests accurately predicts the efficacy of splenectomy in an individual case. This research problem has a useful potential, not only in the autoimmune hemolytic anemias but in other immune-mediated cytopenias as well. Despite the plausible and detailed description of the in vivo mechanism of antibody-mediated destruction of RBCs, effective therapeutic advances based on this knowledge have made slow progress.

Every patient with an autoimmune hemolytic anemia tests the knowledge, skill, and art of the physician. These qualities are, to be sure, of singular importance, but common sense and good judgment count above all. They make the difference in any rare disease for which the outcome is unpredictable.

REFERENCES

1. Dacie JV: The Hemolytic Anemias. Part II. The Auto-immune Haemolytic Anemias. Grune & Stratton, Orlando, FL, 1962
2. Dameshek W, Schwartz SO: Acute hemolytic anemia (acquired hemolytic icterus, acute type). Medicine 19:231, 1940
3. Rosenfield RE: The past and future of immunohematology. Am J Clin Pathol 64:569, 1975

4. Dressler DR: Ein Fall von intermittirender Albuminurie und Chromaturie. Arch Pathol Anat Physiol 6:264, 1854

5. Harley G: Notes of two cases of intermittent haematuria: with remarks upon their pathology and treatment. Lancet 1:568, 1865

6. Hassall AH: On intermittent or winter haematuria. Lancet 2:368, 1865

7. Rosenbach O: Zur Lehre von der periodischen Hämoglobinurie. Dtsch Med Wochenschr 5:613, 1879

8. Ehrlich P: Über paroxysmale Hämoglobinurie. Z Klin Med 3:383, 1881

9. Götze L: Beitrag zur Lehre von der paroxysmalen Hämoglobinurie. Berl Klin Wochenschr 21:716, 1884

10. Donath J, Landsteiner K: Über paroxysmale Hämoglobinurie. Munch Med Wochenschr 51:1590, 1904

11. Le Gendre P: Ictère urobilinique chronique (durant depuis douze ans) chez un jeune homme de dix-huit ans. Bull Soc Med Hop Paris 14:407, 1897

12. Hayem G: Sur une variété particulière d'ictère chronique. Ictère infectieux chronique splénomégalique. Presse Med 6:121, 1898

13. Widal F, Abrami P: Types divers d'ictères hémolytiques non congénitaux, avec anémie. A la recherche de la résistance globulaire par le procédé des hématies déplasmatisées. Bull Soc Med Paris 24:1127, 1907

14. Chauffard MA, Troisier J: Anémie grave avec hémolysine dans le sérum; ictère hémolysinique. Semin Med (Paris) 28:345, 1908

15. Dameshek W, Schwartz SO: The presence of hemolysins in acute hemolytic anemia; preliminary note. N Engl J Med 218:75, 1938

16. Dameshek W, Schwartz SO: Hemolysins as the cause of clinical and experimental hemolytic anemias, with particular reference to the nature of spherocytosis and increased fragility. Am J Med Sci 196:769, 1938

17. Clough MC, Richter IM: A study of an autoagglutinin occurring in a human serum. Johns Hopkins Hosp Bull 29:86, 1918

18. Landsteiner K: Über Beziehungen zwischen dem Blutserum und den Körperzellen. Munch Med Wochenschr 50:1812, 1903

19. McCombs RP, McElroy JS: Reversible autohemagglutination with peripheral vascular symptoms. Arch Intern Med 59:107, 1937

20. Coombs RRA, Mourant AE, Race RR: A new test for the detection of weak and incomplete Rh agglutinins. Br J Exp Pathol 26:255, 1945

21. Boorman KE, Dodd BE, Loutit JF: Hemolytic icterus (acholuric jaundice) congenital and acquired. Lancet 1:812, 1946

22. Moreschi C: Neue tatsachen uber die blutkorperchen agglutinationen. Zentralbe Bakteriol 46:49, 1908

23. Lewis RM, Henry WB, Thornton GW et al: A syndrome of autoimmune hemolytic anemia and thrombocytopenia in dogs. Proc J Am Vet Med Assoc 1:140, 1963

24. Bielschowsky M, Helyer BJ, Howie JB: Spontaneous hemolytic anemia in mice of the NZB/Bl strain. Proc Univ Otago Med Sch 37:9, 1959

25. Micheli F: Unmittelbare Effekte der Splenektomie bei einem Fall von erworbenen hamolytischen splenomegalischen Ikterus, Typus Hayem-Widal. Wien Klin Wochenschr 24:1269, 1911

26. Dameshek W: ACTH in leukemia, abstracted. Blood 5:791, 1950

27. Gardner F: ACTH in leukemia, abstracted. Blood 5:791, 1950

28. Owen RD: Immunogenetic consequences of vascular anastomoses between bovine twins. Science 102:400, 1945

29. Burnet FM, Fenner F: The Production of Antibodies. Macmillan, London, 1949

30. Billingham RE, Brent L, Medawar PB: "Actively acquired tolerance" of foreign antigens. Nature 172:603, 1953

31. Cuthbertson A, Klintworth GK: Transgenic mice—a gold mine for furthering knowledge in pathobiology. Lab Invest 58:484, 1988

32. Marrack P, Kappler J: The T cell receptor. Science 238:1073, 1987

33. Lo D, Sprent J: Identity of cells that imprint H-2 restricted T-cell specificity in the thymus. Nature 319:672, 1986

34. Unanue ER, Allen PM: The basis for the immunoregulatory role of macrophages and other accessory cells. Science 236:551, 1987

35. Lorenz RG, Allen PM: Thymic cortical epithelial cells can present self-antigens in vivo. Nature 337:560, 1989

36. Von Boehmer H, Teh HS, Kisielow P: The thymus selects the useful, neglects the useless and destroys the harmful. Immunol Rev 10:57, 1989

37. Szulman AE: The histologic distribution of blood group substances in man as disclosed by immunofluorescence. III. The A, B, and H antigens in embryos and fetuses from 18 mm in length. J Exp Med 119:503, 1964

38. Wiener AS, Unger LJ, Cohen L, Feldman J: Type-specific cold auto-antibodies as a cause of acquired hemolytic anemia and hemolytic transfusion reactions: biologic test with bovine red cells. Ann Intern Med 44:221, 1956

39. Marsh WL, Jenkins WJ: Anti-i: a new cold antibody. Nature 188:753, 1960

40. Hakomori S: Blood group ABH and Ii antigens of human erythrocytes: chemistry, polymorphism and their developmental changes. Semin Hematol 18:39, 1981

41. Landsteiner K: Zur Kenntnis der antifermentativen, lytischen und agglutinierenden Wirkungen des Blutserums und der Lymphe. Zentralbl Bakteriol 27:357, 1900

42. Merlini G, Farhangi M, Osserman EF: Monoclonal immunoglobulins with antibody activity in myeloma, macroglobulinemia and related plasma cell dyscrasias. Semin Oncol 13:350, 1986

43. Souroujon M, White-Scharf ME, André-Schwartz J et al: Preferential autoantibody reactivity of the preimmune B cell repertoire in normal mice. J Immunol 140:4173, 1988

44. Levinson AI, Dalal NF, Haidar M et al: Prominent IgM rheumatoid factor production by human cord blood lymphocytes stimulated in vitro with Staphylococcus aureus, Cowan I. J Immunol 139:2237, 1987

45. Cairns E, St. Germain J, Bell DA: The in vitro production of anti-DNA antibody by cultured peripheral blood or tonsillar lymphoid cells from normal donors and SLE patients. J Immunol 135:3839, 1985

46. Rose NR, Witebsky E: Studies on organ specificity. V. Changes in the thyroid glands of rabbits following acute immunization with rabbit thyroid extracts. J Immunol 76:417, 1956

47. Morimoto C, Letvin NL, Distaso JA et al: The isolation and characterization of the human suppressor inducer T cell subset. J Immunol 134:1508, 1985

48. Takeuchi T, Schlossman SF, Morimoto C: Development of an antigen-specific CD8 suppressor effector clone in man. J Immunol 141:3010, 1988

49. Schwartz RS, Miller KB: Autoimmunity and suppressor T lymphocytes. Adv Intern Med 27:281, 1982

50. Horowitz SD, Borcherding W, Hong R: Autoimmune hemolytic anemia as a manifestation of T-suppressor cell deficiency. Clin Immunol Immunopathol 33:313, 1984

51. Taguchi O, Nishizuka Y: Self tolerance and localized autoimmunity. Mouse models of autoimmune disease that suggest tissue-specific suppressor T cells are involved in self tolerance. J Exp Med 165:146, 1987

52. Glazier A, Tutschka PJ, Farmer ER et al: Graft-versus-host disease in cyclosporin A-treated rats after syngeneic and autologous bone marrow reconstitution. J Exp Med 158:1, 1983

53. Sorokin R, Kimura H, Schroder K et al: Cyclosporine-induced autoimmunity. Conditions for expressing disease, requirement for intact thymus, and potency estimates of autoimmune lymphocytes in drug-treated rats. J Exp Med 164:1615, 1986

54. Jenkins MK, Schwartz RH, Pardoll DM: Effects of cyclosporine A on T cell development and clonal deletion. Science 241:1655, 1988

55. Sakaguchi S, Sakaguchi N: Transplantation of the thymus from cyclosporin A-treated mice caused organ-specific autoimmune disease in athymic nude mice. J Exp Med 167:1479, 1988

56. Suzuki N, Sakane T: Induction of excessive B cell proliferation and differentiation by an in vitro stimulus in culture in human systemic lupus erythematosus. J Clin Invest 83:937, 1989

57. Hirano T, Taga T, Yasukawa K et al: Human B-cell differentiation factor defined by an anti-peptide antibody and its possible role in autoantibody production. Proc Natl Acad Sci USA 31:228, 1987

58. Atkins MB, Mier JW, Parkinson DR et al: Hypothyroidism after treatment with interleukin-2 and lymphokine-activated killer cells. N Engl J Med 318:1557, 1988

59. Perez R, Padavic K, Kreigel R, Weiner L: Antierythrocyte autoantibody formation after therapy with interleukin-2 and gamma-interferon. Cancer 67:2512, 1991

60. McGregor IA: The significance of parasitic infections in terms of clinical disease. Parasitology 94:5159, 1987

61. Ammann AJ, Abrams D, Conant M et al: Acquired immune dysfunction in homosexual men: immunologic profiles. Clin Immunol Imunopathol 27:315, 1983

62. Kopelman R, Zolla-Pazner S: Association of human immunodeficiency virus infection and autoimmune phenomena. Am J Med 84:82, 1988

63. Toy P TCY, Reid ME, Burns M: Positive direct antiglobulin test associated with hyperglobulinemia in acquired immunodeficiency syndrome (AIDS). Am J Hematol 19:145, 1985

64. Bloom EJ, Abrams DI, Rogers G: Lupus anticoagulant in the acquired immunodeficiency syndrome. JAMA 256:491, 1986

65. Theofilopoulos AN, Dixon FJ: Murine models of systemic lupus erythematosus. Adv Immunol 37:269, 1985

66. Linder E, Edgington TS: Immunobiology of the autoantibody response. I. Circulating analogues of erythrocyte autoantigens and heterogeneity of the autoimmune response of NZB mice. J Immunol 13:279, 1973

67. Mercolino TJ, Arnold LW, Hawkins LA, Haughton G: Normal mouse peritoneum contains a large population of Ly-1+ (CD5) B cells that recognize phosphatidyl choline. J Exp Med 168:687, 1988

68. Stall AM, Fariñas MC, Tarlinton DM et al: Ly-1 B cell clones similar to human chronic lymphocytic leukemias routinely develop in older normal mice and

young autoimmune (New Zealand Black-related) animals. Proc Natl Acad Sci USA 85:7312, 1988

69. Linder E: Autoantibodies against the inner aspect of erythrocyte membranes in NZB mice. Clin Exp Immunol 27:531, 1977

70. Costea N, Yakulis V, Heller P: Cold reactive antibody in NZB/Bl mice. Blood 35:583, 1970

71. Gavalchin J, Nicklas JA, Eastcott JW et al: Lupus prone (SWR×NZB) F_1 mice produce potentially nephritogenic autoantibodies inherited from the normal SWR parent. J Immunol 134:885, 1985

72. Datta SK, Schwartz RS: Autoimmunization and graft versus host reactions. Transplant Rev 31:44, 1976

73. Oliner H, Schwartz RS, Dameshek W: Studies in experimental autoimmune disorders. I. Clinical and laboratory features of autoimmunization (runt disease) in the mouse. Blood 17:20, 1961

74. Lewis RM, Armstrong MYK, André-Schwartz J et al: Chronic allogeneic disease. I. Development of glomerulonephritis. J Exp Med 128:653, 1968

75. Gleichmann H, Gleichmann E, André-Schwartz J, Schwartz RS: Chronic allogeneic disease. III. Genetic requirements for the induction of glomerulonephritis. J Exp Med 135:516, 1972

76. Dobashi K, Ono S, Murakami S et al: Polyclonal B cell activation by a B cell differentiation factor, B151-TRF2 III. B151-TRF2 as a B cell differentiation factor closely associated with autoimmune disease. J Immunol 138:780, 1987

77. Schwartz RS, Beldotti L: Malignant lymphomas following allogeneic disease: transition from an immunologic to a neoplastic disorder. Science 149:1511, 1965

78. Anasetti C, Rybka W, Sullivan KM et al: Graft-v-host disease is associated with autoimmune-like thrombocytopenia. Blood 73:1054, 1989

79. Sullivan KM, Shulman HM: Graft versus host disease: allo-and autoimmunity after bone marrow transplantation. Concepts Immunopathol 6:141, 1988

80. Bevan PC, Seaman M, Tolliday B, Chalmers DG: ABO haemolytic anemia in transplanted patients. Vox Sang 49:42, 1985

81. Bapat AR, Schuster SJ, Dahlke M, Ballas SK: Thrombocytopenia and autoimmune hemolytic anemia following renal transplantation. Transplantation 44: 157, 1987

82. Albrechtsen D, Solheim BG, Flatmark A et al: Autoimmune hemolytic anemia in cyclosporine-treated organ allograft recipients. Transplant Proc 20:959, 1988

83. Mangal AK, Growe GH, Sinclair M et al: Acquired hemolytic anemia due to "auto"-anti-A or "auto"-anti-B induced by blood group O homograft in renal transplant recipients. Transfusion 24:201, 1985

84. Okamoto M, Murakami M, Shimizu A et al: A transgenic model of autoimmune hemolytic anemia. J Exp Med 175:71, 1992

85. Goodnow CC: Transgenic mice and analysis of B-cell tolerance. Annu Rev Immunol 10:489, 1992

86. Murakami M, Tsubata T, Okamoto M et al: Antigen-induced apoptotic death of Ly-1 B cells responsible for autoimmune disease in transgenic mice. Nature 357:77, 1992

87. Leddy JP, Falany JL, Passador ST: Erythrocyte membrane proteins reactive with warm (warm-reacting) anti-red cell autoantibodes. J Clin Invest 91: 1672, 1993

88. Bloy C, Blanchard D, Lambin P et al: Human monoclonal antibody against Rh(D) antigen: partial characterization of the Rh(D) polypeptide from human erythrocytes. Blood 69:1491, 1987

89. Rapoport AP, Rowe JM, McMican A: Life-threatening autoimmune hemolytic anemia in a patient with the acquired immune deficiency syndrome. Transfusion 28:190, 1988

90. Lane HC, Masur H, Edgar LC et al: Abnormalities of B cell activation and immunoregulation in patients with the acquired immunodeficiency syndrome. N Engl J Med 309:453, 1983

91. Kipps DJ, Carson DA: Autoantibodies in chronic lymphocytic leukemia and related systemic autoimmune disease. Blood 81:2475, 1993

92. Leddy JP, Bakemeier RF: Structural aspects of human erythrocyte autoantibodies. J Exp Med 121:1, 1965

93. Masouredis SP, Branks MJ, Victoria EJ: Antiidiotypic IgG crossreactive with Rh alloantibodies in red cell autoimmunity. Blood 70:710, 1987

94. Stevenson FK, Smith GJ, North J et al: Identification of normal B-cell counterparts of neoplastic cells which secrete cold agglutinins of anti-I and anti-i specificity. Br J Haematol 72:9, 1989

95. Costea N, Yakulis VJ, Heller P: Inhibition of cold agglutinins (anti-I) by *M. pneumoniae* antigens. Proc Soc Exp Biol 139:476, 1972

96. Pascual V, Victor K, Lelz D et al: Nucleotide sequence analysis of the V regions of two IgM cold agglutinins. J Immunol 146:4385, 1991

97. Silberstein LE, Jefferies LC, Goldman J et al: Variable region gene analysis of pathologic human autoantibodies to the related i and I red blood cell antigens. Blood 78:2372, 1991

98. Jeffries LC, Carchidi CM, Silberstein LE: Naturally occurring anti-i/I cold

agglutinins may be encoded by different V_H3 genes as well as the $V_H4.21$ gene segment. J Clin Invest 92:2821, 1993

99. Stevenson FK, Spellerberg MB, Treasure J et al: Differential usage of an Ig heavy chain variable region gene by human B-cell tumors. Blood 82:224, 1993

100. National Cancer Institute: Surveillance, Epidemiology, and End Results. Monograph 57. U.S. Department of Health and Human Services, Bethesda, MD, 1981

101. Evans RS, Takahashi K, Duane RT et al: Primary thrombocytopenic purpura and acquired hemolytic anemia. Evidence for a common etiology. Arch Intern Med 87:48, 1951

102. Pirofsky B: Autoimmunization and the Autoimmune Hemolytic Anemias. Williams & Wilkins, Baltimore, 1969

103. Crosby WH, Rappaport H: Reticulocytopenia in autoimmune hemolytic anemia. Blood 11:929, 1956

104. Conley CL, Lippman SM, Ness PM et al: Autoimmune hemolytic anemia with reticulocytopenia and erythroid marrow. N Engl J Med 306:281, 1982

105. Conley CL, Lippman SM, Ness PM: Autoimmune hemolytic anemia with reticulocytopenia: a medical emergency. JAMA 244:1688, 1980

106. Mangan KF, Besa EC, Shadduck RK et al: Demonstration of two distinct antibodies in autoimmune hemolytic anemia with reticulocytopenia and red cell aplasia. Exp Hematol 12:788, 1984

107. Petz LD, Garraty G: Antiglobulin sera—past, present and future. Transfusion 18:257, 1978

108. Voak D, Downie DM, Moore BPL, Engelfriet CP: Anti-human globulin reagent specification: the European and ISBT/ICSH view. Biotest Bull 1:7, 1986

109. Recommended methods for anti-human globulin evaluation. Division of Blood and Blood Products, Office of Biologics Research and Review Center for Drugs and Biologics, Food and Drug Administration. Docket 84S-0182:6, 1984

110. Stratton F, Rawlinson VI: C3 components on red cells under various conditions. p. 113. In: International Symposium on the Nature and Significance of Complement Activation. Ortho Research Institute of Medical Science, Raritan, NJ, 1976

111. Beck ML, Marsh WL: Complement and the antiglobulin test. Transfusion 17: 529, 1977

112. Petz LD, Garratty G: Complement in immunohematology. Prog Clin Immunol 2:175, 1974

113. Moore JA, Chaplin H Jr: Anti-C3d antiglobulin reagents. II. Preparation of an antiglobulin serum monspecific for C3d. Transfusion 14:416, 1974

114. Chaplin H Jr, Monroe MC: Comparisions of pooled polyclonal rabbit antihuman C3d with four monoclonal mouse anti-human C3ds. II. Quantitation of RBC-bound C3d, and characterization of antiglobulin agglutination reactions against RBC from 27 patients with autoimmune hemolytic anemia. Vox Sang 50:87, 1986

115. Stratton F, Rawlinson VI, Chapman SA et al: Acquired hemolytic anemia associated with IgA anti-e. Transfusion 12:157, 1972

116. Reusser P, Osterwalder B, Burri H, Speck B: Autoimmune hemolytic anemia associated with IgA-diagnostic and therapeutic aspects in a case with long-term follow-up. Acta Haematol 77:53, 1987

117. Shirey RS, Kickler TS, Bell W et al: Fatal immune hemolytic anemia and hepatic failure associated with a warm-reacting IgM autoantibody. Vox Sang 52:219, 1987

118. Freedman J, Wright J, Lim FC, Garvey MB: Hemolytic warm IgM autoagglutinins in autoimmune hemolytic anemia. Transfusion 27:464, 1987

119. Gottsche B, Salama A, Mueller-Eckhardt C: Autoimmune hemolytic anemia associated with an IgA autoanti-Gerbich. Vox Sang 58:211, 1990

120. Gorst DW, Rawlinson VI, Merry AH, Stratton F: Positive direct antiglobulin test in normal individuals. Vox Sang 38:99, 1980

121. Merry AH, Thomson EE, Rawlinson VI, Stratton F: The quantification of C3 fragments on erythrocytes: estimation of C3 fragments on normal cells, acquired haemolytic anaemia cases and correlation with agglutination of sensitized cells. Clin Lab Haematol 5:387, 1983

122. Unger LJ: A method for detecting Rh_o antibodies in extremely low titer. J Lab Clin Med 37:825, 1951

123. Gilliland BC, Baxter E, Evans RS: Red-cell antibodies in acquired hemolytic anemia with negative antiglobulin serum tests. N Engl J Med 285:252, 1971

124. Salama A, Mueller-Eckhardt C, Bhakdi S: A two stage immunorandiometric assay with ^{125}I-Staphylococcal protein A for the detection of antibodies and complement on human blood cells. Vox Sang 48:239, 1985

125. Judd WJ, Butch SH, Oberman HA et al: The evaluation of a positive direct antiglobulin test in pretransfusion testing. Transfusion 20:17, 1980

126. Freedman J, Massey A: Complement components detected on normal red blood cells taken into EDTA and CPD. Vox Sang 37:1, 1979

127. Geisland JR, Milam JD: Spuriously positive direct antiglobulin tests caused by silicone gel. Transfusion 20:711, 1980

128. Grindon AJ, Wilson MJ: False-positive DAT caused by variables in sample procurement. Transfusion 21:313, 1981

129. Molthan L, Reidenberg MM, Eichman MF: Positive direct Coombs test due to cephalothin. N Engl J Med 277:123, 1967

130. Lutz P, Dzik W: Very high incidence of a positive direct antiglobulin test (+ DAT) in patients receiving Unasyn®. Transfusion, suppl. 32:23S, 1992

131. Garratty G: The significance of IgG on the red cell surface. Transfusion Med Rev 1:47, 1987

132. Heddle NM, Kelton JG, Turchyn KL, Ali MAM: Hypergammaglobulinemia can be associated with a positive direct antiglobulin test, a nonreactive eluate, and no evidence of hemolysis. Transfusion 28:29, 1988

133. Issitt PD, Pavone BG, Goldfinger D et al: Anti-Wr^b and other autoantibodies responsible for positive direct antiglobulin tests in 150 individuals. Br J Haematol 34:5, 1976

134. Weiner W, Vos GH: Serology of acquired hemolytic anemias. Blood 22:606, 1963

135. Weiner W, Battey DA, Cleghorn TE et al: Serological findings in a case of haemolytic anaemia with some general observations on the pathogenesis of this syndrome. BMJ 2:125, 1953

136. Dacie JV, Cutbush M: Specificity of auto-antibodies in acquired haemolytic anaemia. J Clin Pathol 7:18, 1954

137. Hogman C, Killander J, Sjolin S: A case of idiopathic auto-immune haemolytic anaemia due to anti-e. Acta Paediatr 49:270, 1960

138. Sachs, V: Anti-C as a sole autoantibody in autoimmune hemolytic anemia. Transfusion 25:587, 1985

139. Dube VE, House RF, Moulds J, Polesky HF: Hemolytic anemia caused by auto anti-N. Am J Clin Pathol 63:828, 1975

140. Marsh WL, Oyen R, Alicea E et al: Autoimmune hemolytic anemia and the Kell blood groups. Am J Hematol 7:155, 1979

141. Reynolds MV, Vengelen-Tyler V, Morel PA: Autoimmune hemolytic anemia associated with autoanti-Ge. Vox Sang 41:61, 1981

142. Ellisor SS, Reid ME, O'Day T et al: Autoantibodies mimicking anti-Jkb plus anti-Jk3 associated with autoimmune hemolytic anemia in a primipara who delivered an unaffected infant. Vox Sang 45:53, 1983

143. Alessandrino EP, Costamagna L, Pagani A, Coronelli M: Late appearance of autoantibody-anti S in autoimmune hemolytic anemia. Transfusion 24:369, 1984

144. Becton DL, Kinney TR: An infant girl with severe autoimmune hemolytic anemia: apparent anti-Vel specificity. Vox Sang 51:108, 1986

145. O'Brien DA, Mullahy DE, Garvey MA, Jackson JF: Cold autoimmune haemolytic anaemia in a 3-year-old infant due to anti-Rx (previously anti-Sdx). Clin Lab Haematol 10:105, 1988

146. Owen I, Chowdhury V, Reid ME et al: Autoimmune hemolytic anemia associated with anti-Sc1. Transfusion 32:173, 1992

147. Shulman IA, Vengelen-Tyler V, Thompson JC et al: Autoanti-Ge associated with severe autoimmune hemolytic anemia. Vox Sang 59:232, 1990

148. Marsh WL, DiNapoli J, Oyen R et al: "New" autoantibody specificity in autoimmune hemolytic anemia defined with red cells treated with 2-aminoethylisothiouronium bromide and a dithiothreitol-papain solution. Transfusion 25:364, 1985

149. Roelcke D, Dahr W, Kalden JR: A human monoclonal IgM kappa cold agglutinin recognizing oligosaccharides with immunodominant sialyl groups preferentially at the blood group M-specific peptide backbone of glycophorins: anti-Prm. Vox Sang 51:207, 1986

150. Kajii E, Miura Y, Ueki J, Ikemoto S: Acquired glycophorin-like antigens associated with autoimmune hemolytic anemia. Acta Haematol Jpn 50:175, 1987

151. Reid ME, Vengelen-Tyler V, Shulman I, Reynolds MV: Immunochemical specificity of autoanti-Gerbich from two patients with autoimmune haemolytic anaemia and concomitant alteration in the red cell membrane sialoglycoprotein beta. Br J Haematol 69:61, 1988

152. Wakui H, Imai H, Kobayashi R et al: Autoantibody against erythrocyte protein 4.1 in a patient with autoimmune hemolytic anemia. Blood 72:408, 1988

153. Deleze M, Oria CV, Alarcon-Segovia D: Occurrence of both hemolytic anemia and thrombocytopenic purpura (Evans' syndrome) in systemic lupus erythematosus. Relationship to antiphospholipid antibodies. J Rheumatol 15:611, 1988

154. Hazeltine M, Rauch J, Danoff D et al: Antiphospholipid antibodies in systemic lupus erythematosus: evidence of an association with positive Coombs' and hypocomplementemia. J Rheumatol 15:80, 1988

155. Miescher PA, Tucci A, Beris P, Favre H: Autoimmune hemolytic anemia and/or thrombocytopenia associated with lupus parameters. Semin Hematol 29,1:13, 1992

156. Fong KY, Loizou S, Boey ML, Walport MJ: Anticardiolipin antibodies, haemolytic anaemia and thrombocytopenia in systemic lupus erythematosus. Br J Rheumatol 31:453, 1992

157. Arvieux J, Schweizer B, Roussel B, Colomb P: Autoimmune haemolytic anaemia due to anti-phospholipid antibodies. Vox Sang 61:190, 1991

158. Borsos T, Rapp, HJ: Complement fixation on cell surfaces by 19S and 7S antibodies. Science 150:505, 1965

159. Sokol RJ, Booker DJ, Stamps R: The pathology of autoimmune hemolytic anemia. J Clin Pathol 45:1047, 1992

160. Huber H, Polley MJ, Linscott WD, Muller-Eberhard HJ: Human monocytes: distant receptor sites for the third component of complement and for immunoglobulin G. Science 162:1281, 1962

161. LoBuglio AF, Cotran RS, Jandl JH: Red cells coated with immunoglobulin G: binding and sphering by mononuclear cells in man. Science 158:1582, 1967

162. Huber H, Douglas SD, Nusbacher J et al: IgG subclass specificity of human monocyte receptor sites. Nature 229:419, 1971

163. Abramson N, Gelfand EW, Jandl JH, Rosen FS: The interaction between human monocytes and red cells. Specificity for IgG subclasses and IgG fragments. J Exp Med 132:1207, 1970

164. Red cell antigens and antibodies and their interactions. p. 258. In Mollison PL, Engelfriet CP, Conteras M (eds): Blood Transfusion in Clinical Medicine. Blackwell Scientific, London, 1988

165. Schreiber AD, Frank MM: Role of antibody and complement in the immune clearance and destruction of erythrocytes. I. In vivo effects of IgG and IgM complement-fixing sites. J Clin Invest 51:575, 1972

166. Fleer A, van der Meulen FW, Linthout E et al: Destruction of IgG sensitized erythrocytes by human blood monocytes: modulation of inhibition by IgG. Br J Hematol 39:425, 1978

167. Schreiber AD, Frank MM: Role of antibody and complement in the immune clearance and destruction of erythrocytes. II. Molecular nature of IgG and IgM complement-fixing sites and effects of their interaction with serum. J Clin Invest 51:583, 1972

168. Schreiber AD, McDermott PB: Effect of C3b inactivator on monocyte-bound C3-coated human erythrocytes. Blood 52:896, 1978

169. Munn LR, Chaplin H Jr: Rosette formation by sensitized human red cells—effects of source of peripheral leukocyte monolayers. Vox Sang 33:129, 1977

170. Brown DL, Lachmann PJ, Dacie JV: The in vivo behavior of complement-coated red cells: studies in C6-deficient, C3-depleted and normal rabbits. Clin Exp Immunol 7:401, 1970

171. Pruzanski W, Shumack KH: Biologic activity of cold-reacting antibodies (second of two parts). N Engl J Med 297:583, 1977

172. Frank MM, Schreiber AD, Atkinson JP, Jaffe CJ: Pathophysiology of immune hemolytic anemia. Ann Intern Med 87:210, 1977

173. Silberstein LE, Robertson GA, Hannam-Harris AC et al: Etiologic aspects of cold agglutinin disease: evidence for cytogenetically defined clones of lymphoid cells and the demonstration that an anti-Pr cold autoantibody is derived from a chromosomally aberrant B cell clone. Blood 67:1705, 1986

174. Silberstein LE, Goldman J, Kant JA, Spitalnik SL: Comparative biochemical and genetic characterization of clonally related human B-cell lines secreting pathogenic anti-Pr₂ cold agglutinins. Arch Biochem Biophys 264:244, 1988

175. Crisp D, Pruzanski W: B-cell neoplasma with homogeneous cold-reacting antibodies (cold agglutinins). Am J Med 72:915, 1982

176. Rosenthal MC, Pisciotta AV, Komninos et al: The auto-immune hemolytic anemia of malignant lymphocytic disease. Blood 10:197, 1955

177. Hamblin TJ, Oscier DG, Young BY: Autoimmunity in chronic lymphocytic leukaemia. J Clin Pathol 39:713, 1986

178. Sikora K, Krikorian J, Levy R: Monoclonal immunoglobulin rescue from a patient with chronic lymphocytic leukemia and autoimmune hemolytic anemia. Blood 54:513, 1979

179. Rosenfield RE, Jagathambal K: Transfusion therapy for autoimmune hemolytic anemia. Semin Hematol 13:311, 1976

180. Petz LD: Transfusing the patient with autoimmune hemolytic anemia. Clin Lab Med 2:193, 1982

181. Plapp FV, Beck ML: Transfusion support in the management of immune haemolytic disorders. Clin Haematol 13:167, 1984

182. Sokol RJ, Hewitt S, Booker DJ, Morris BM: Patients with red cell autoantibodies: selection of blood for transfusion. Clin Lab Haematol 10:257, 1988

183. Wallhermfechtel MA, Polhl BA, Chaplin H: Alloimmunization in patients with warm autoantibodies. Transfusion 24:482, 1984

184. Laine ML, Beattie KM: Frequency of alloantibodies accompanying autoantibodies. Transfusion 25:545, 1985

185. James P, Rowe GP, Tozzo GG: Elucidation of alloantibodies in autoimmune haemolytic anaemia. Vox Sang 54:167, 1988

186. Widmann FK (ed): Technical Manual. 9th Ed. American Association of Blood Banks, Washington, DC, 1981

187. Edwards JM, Moulds JJ, Judd WJ: Chloroquine dissociation of antigen-antibody complexes. A new technique for typing red blood cells with a positive direct antiglobulin test. Transfusion 22:59, 1982

188. Branch DR, Petz LD: A new reagent (ZZAP) having multiple applications in immunohematology. Am J Clin Pathol 78:161, 1982

189. Mollison PL: Measurement of survival and destruction of red cells in haemolytic syndromes. Br Med Bull 15:59, 1959

190. Petz LD, Garratty G: Acquired Immune Hemolytic Anemias. Churchill Livingstone, New York, 1980

191. Atkinson JP, Schreiber AD, Frank MM: Effects corticosteroids and splenectomy on the immune clearance and destruction of erythrocytes. J Clin Invest 52:1509, 1975

192. Schreiber AD, Parsons J, McDermott P, Cooper RA: The effect of corticosteroids on the human monocyte IgG and complement receptors. J Clin Invest 56:1189, 1975

193. Schreiber AD: Clinical Immunology of the corticosteroids. Prog Clin Immunol 3:103, 1977

194. Fries LF, Brickman CM, Frank MM: Monocyte receptors for the Fc portion of IgG increase in number in autoimmune hemolytic anemia and other hemolytic states and are decreased by glucocorticoid therapy. J Immunol 131:1240, 1983

195. Schwartz SI, Bernard RP, Adams JT, Bauman AW: Splenectomy for hematologic disorders. Arch Surg 101:338, 1970

196. Jandl JH, Kaplan ME: The destruction of red cells by antibodies in man. III. Quantitative factors influencing the pattern of hemolysis in vivo. J Clin Invest 39:1145, 1960

197. Parker AC, MacPherson AIS, Richmond J: Value of radiochromium investigation in autoimmune hemolytic anemia. BMJ 1:308, 1977

198. Murphy S, LoBuglio AF: Drug therapy of autoimmune hemolytic anemia. Semin Hematol 13:323, 1976

199. Fauci AS, Dale DC, Wolff SM: Cyclophosphamide and lymphocyte subpopulations in Wegener's granulomatosis. Arthritis Rheum 17:355, 1974

200. Steinberg, AD, Plotz PH, Wolff SM et al: Cytotoxic drugs in treatment of nonmalignant disease. Ann Intern Med 76:619, 1972

201. Floersheim GL: A comparative study of the effects of anti-tumor and immunosuppressive drugs on antibody forming and erythropoeitic cells. Clin Exp Immunol 6:861, 1970

202. Fahey JL: Cancer in the immunosuppressed patient. Ann Intern Med 75:310, 1971

203. Miller JJ, III, Williams GF, Leissring JC: Multiple late complications of therapy with cyclophosphamide, including ovarian destruction. Am J Med 50:530, 1971

204. Qureshi MSA, Goldsmith HJ, Pennington JH, Cox PE: Cyclophosphamide therapy and sterility. Lancet 2:1290, 1972

205. Johnson WW, Meadows DC: Urinary-bladder fibrosis and telangiectasia associated with long-term cyclophosphamide therapy. N Engl J Med 284:290, 1971

206. Orlin JB, Berkman EM: Partial plasma exchange using albumin replacement: removal and recovery of normal plasma constituents. Blood 56:1055, 1980

207. Silberstein LE, Berkman EM: Plasma exchange in autoimmune hemolytic anemia (AIHA). J Clin Apheresis 1:238, 1983

208. Kutti J, Wadenvik H, Safai-Kutti S et al: Successful treatment of refractory autoimmune hemolytic anemia by plasmapheresis. Scand J Haematol 32:149, 1984

209. Ahn, YS, Harrington WJ, Byrnes JJ et al: Treatment of autoimmune hemolytic anemia with Vinca-loaded platelets. JAMA 249:2189, 1983

210. Ahn YS, Harrington WJ, Mylvaganam R et al: Danazol therapy for autoimmune hemolytic anemia. Ann Intern Med 102:298, 1985

211. Besa EC: Rapid transient reversal of anemia and long-term effect of maintenance intravenous immunoglobulin for autoimmune hemolytic anemia in patients with lymphoproliferative disorders. Am J Med 84:691, 1988

212. Schreiber AD, Herskovitz BS, Goldwein M: Low-titer cold-hemagglutinin disease: mechanism of hemolysis and response to corticosteroids. N Engl J Med 296:1490, 1977

213. Szymanski IO, Teno R, Rybak ME: Hemolytic anemia due to a mixture of low-titer IgG lambda and IgM lambda agglutinins reacting optimally at 22°C. Vox Sang 51:112, 1986

214. Silberstein LE, Shoenfeld Y, Schwartz RS, Berkman EM: A combination of IgG and IgM autoantibodies in chronic cold agglutinin disease: immunologic studies and response to splenectomy. Vox Sang 48:105, 1985

215. Tschirhart DL, Kunkel L, Shulman IA: Immune hemolytic anemia associated with biclonal cold autoagglutinins. Vox Sang 59:222, 1990

216. Umlas J, Kaufman M, MacQueston C et al: A cryoglobulin with cold agglutinin and erythroid stem cell suppressant properties. Transfusion 31:361, 1991

217. Tsai CM, Zopf DA, Yu RK et al: A Waldenstrom macroglobulin that is both a cold agglutinin and a cryoglobulin because it binds N-acetylneuraminosyl residues. Immunology 74:4591, 1977

218. Deutsch HF: Properties and modifications of a cryomacroglobulin possessing cold agglutinin activity. Biopolymers 7:21, 1969

219. Kuenn JW, Weber R, Teague PO, Keitt AS: Cryopathic gangrene with an IgM lambda cryoprecipitating cold agglutinin. Cancer 42:1826, 1978

220. Capra JD, Dowling PM, Cook S, Kunkel HG: An incomplete cold γG antibody with i specificity in infectious mononucleosis. Vox Sang 16:10, 1969

221. Rosenfield RE, Schmidt PJ, Calvo RC, McGinniss MH: Anti-i, a frequent cold agglutinin in infectious mononucleosis. Vox Sang 10:631, 1965

222. Roelcke D, Anstee DJ, Jungfer H et al: IgG-type cold agglutinins in children and corresponding antigens: detection of a new Pr antigen: Pr$_a$. Vox Sang 20:218, 1971

223. Roelcke D, Ebert W, Geisen HP: Anti-Pr$_3$: serological and immunochemical identification of a new anti-Pr subspecificity. Vox Sang 30:122, 1976

224. Roelcke D, Riesen W, Geisen HP, Ebert W: Serological identification of the new cold agglutinin specificity anti-Gd. Vox Sang 33:304, 1977

225. Roelcke D, Pruzanski W, Ebert W et al: A new human monoclonal cold agglutinin Sa recognizing terminal N-acetylneuraminyl groups on the cell surface. Blood 55:677, 1980

226. Roelcke D: The Lud cold agglutinin: a further antibody recognizing N-acetyl neuraminic acid-determined antigens not fully expressed at birth. Vox Sang 41:316, 1981

227. Roelcke D: A further cold agglutinin. F1, recognizing a N-acetylneuraminic acid-determined antigen. Vox Sang 41:98, 1981

228. Roelcke D, Weber MT: Simultaneous occurrence of anti-F1 and anti-I cold agglutinins in a patient's serum. Vox Sang 47:122, 1984

229. Konig AL, Kather H, Roelcke D: Autoimmune hemolytic anemia by coexisting anti-I and anti-F1 cold agglutinins. Blut 49:363, 1984

230. Hidajat M, Van Hoff A, Van Besien K et al: Acute hemolysis due to IgG cold reactive anti-Pr antibodies in three patients. Transfusion, suppl. 32:24S, 1992

231. Pruzanski W, Shumack KH: Biologic activity of cold-reacting autoantibodies. I. N Engl J Med 297:538, 1977

232. Ruddy S, Gigli I, Austen KF: The complement system of man. I. N Engl J Med 287:489, 1972

233. Atkinson JP, Frank MM: Studies on the in vivo effects of antibody: interaction of IgM antibody and complement in the immune clearance and destruction of erythrocytes in man. J Clin Invest 54:339, 1974

234. Silberstein LE, Berkman EM, Schreiber AD: Cold hemagglutinin disease associated with IgG cold-reactive antibody. Ann Intern Med 106:238, 1987

235. Garratty G, Petz LD, Brodsky I, Fundenberg HH: An IgA high-titer cold agglutinin with an unusual blood group specificity within the Pr complex. Vox Sang 25:32, 1973

236. Pruzanski W, Cowan DH, Parr DM: Clinical and immunochemical studies of IgM cold agglutinins with lambda type light chains. Clin Immunol Immunopathol 2:234, 1974

237. Tonthat H, Rochant H, Henry A et al: A new case of monoclonal IgA kappa cold agglutinin with anti-Pr$_1$d specificity in a patient with persistent HB antigen cirrhosis. Vox Sang 30:464, 1976

238. Angevine CD, Andersen BR, Barnett EV: A cold agglutinin of the IgA class. J Immunol 96:578, 1966

239. Dellagi K, Brouet JC, Schenmetzler C. Praloran V: Chronic hemolytic anemia due to monoclonal IgG cold agglutinin with anti-Pr specificity. Blood 57:189, 1981

240. Moore JA, Chaplin H Jr: Autoimmune hemolytic anemia associated with an IgG cold incomplete antibody. Vox Sang 24:236, 1973

241. Ambrus M, Bajtain G: A case of an IgG-type cold agglutinin disease. Haematologia 3:225, 1969

242. Shulman I, Branch DR, Nelson JM et al: Autoimmune hemolytic anemia with both cold and warm autoantibodies. JAMA 253:1746, 1985

243. Andrzejewski C, Gault E, Briggs M, Silberstein LE: The benefit of a 37°C extracorporeal circuit in plasma exchange therapy for selected cases with cold agglutinin disease. J Clin Apheresis 4:13, 1988

244. Park JV, Weiss CI: Cardiopulmonary bypass and myocardial protection: management problems in cardiac surgical patients with cold autoimmune disease. Anesth Analg 67:75, 1988

245. Hippe E, Jenson KB, Olesen H et al: Chlorambucil treatment of patients with cold agglutinin syndrome. Blood 35:68, 1970

246. Schubothe H: The cold hemagglutinin disease. Semin Hematol 3:27, 1966

247. Nordhagen R, Stensvold K, Winsnes A et al: Paroxysmal cold haemoglobinuria: the most frequent acute autoimmune haemolytic anaemia in children? Acta Paediatr Scand 73:258, 1984

248. Heddle NM: Acute paroxysmal cold hemoglobinuria. Trans Med Rev 3:219, 1989

249. Gottsche B, Salama A, Mueller-Eckhardt C: Donath-Landsteiner autoimmune hemolytic anemia in children. Vox Sang 58:281, 1990

250. Hinz CF, Picken ME, Lepow IH: Studies on immune human hemolysis. II. The Donath-Landsteiner reaction as a model system for studying the mechanism of action of complement and the role of C1 and C1 esterase. J Exp Med 113:193, 1961

251. Levine P, Celano MJ, Falkowski F: The specificity of the antibody in paroxysmal cold hemoglobinuria (P.C.H.). Transfusion 3:278, 1963
252. Worlledge SM, Rousso C: Studies on the serology of paroxysmal cold haemoglobinuria (P.C.H.) with special reference to its relationship with the P blood group system. Vox Sang 10:293, 1965
253. Engelfriet CP, von dem Borne AEGK, Moes M, van Loghem JJ: Serological studies in autoimmune haemolytic anaemia. Bibl Haematol 29:473, 1968
254. Weiner W, Gordon EG, Rowe D: A Donath-Landsteiner antibody (non-syphilitic type). Vox Sang 9:684, 1964
255. Judd WJ, Wilkinson SL, Issitt PD et al: Donath-Landsteiner hemolytic anemia due to an anti-Pr-like biphasic hemolysin. Transfusion 26:423, 1986
256. Worlledge SM: Immune drug induced hemolytic anemias. Semin Hematol 10:327, 1973
257. Petz LD: Drug-induced immune haemolytic anaemia. Clin Haematol 9:455, 1980
258. Danielson DA, Douglas SW III, Herzog P et al: Drug-induced blood disorders. JAMA 252:3257, 1984
259. Petz LD, Fudenberg HH: Coombs-positive hemolytic anemia caused by penicillin administration. N Engl J Med 274:171, 1966
260. Salama A, Mueller-Eckhardt C: On the mechanisms of sensitization and attachment of antibodies to RBC in drug-induced immune hemolytic anemia. Blood 69:1006, 1987
261. Carstairs KC, Breckenridge A, Dollery CT, Worlledge SM: Incidence of a positive direct Coombs test in patients on α-methyldopa. Lancet 2:133, 1966
262. Prchal JT, Huang ST, Court WS, Poon MC: Immune hemolytic anemia following administration of antithymocyte globulin. Am J Hematol 19:95, 1985
263. Copelan EA, Strohm PL, Kennedy MS, Tutschka PJ: Hemolysis following intravenous immunoglobulin therapy. Transfusion 26:410, 1986
264. Hillyer CD, Schwenn MR, Fulton DR et al: Autoimmune hemolytic anemia in Kawasaki disease: a case report. Transfusion 30:738, 1990
265. Albrechtsen D, Solheim BG, Flatmark et al: Autoimmune hemolytic anemia in cyclosporene-treated organ allograft recipients. Transplant Proc 20:959, 1988

Extrinsic Nonimmune Hemolytic Anemias

48

Stanley Schrier

INTRODUCTION

By definition, extrinsic causes of hemolysis are abnormalities in the environment in which the red cells circulate. These abnormalities may occur acutely or may be chronic in nature and may be due to either congenital or acquired lesions, but mostly the latter. The decision that a patient has an anemia belonging to this category is made by using the approaches described in Chapter 36 and determining that hemolysis with varying levels of compensation is the cause of the anemia. It should be emphasized that important forms of extrinsic hemolytic anemia are those caused by immune mechanisms (see Ch. 47). On the basis of the clinical and morphologic information available from the patient, one can list the misfortunes that can befall red cells in their travels. They can be trapped in an abnormal marrow stroma network, sheared by jets in an abnormal heart, cut and fragmented by fibrin strands stretched across damaged areas in the microvasculature, or attacked by parasites. They also can undergo stasis and perhaps metabolic depletion in giant hemangiomas or in an enlarged spleen. An abnormally functioning liver or kidney can cause a buildup of materials in plasma that can alter red cell shape and metabolism. Drugs can cause oxidation or other metabolic damage, whereas toxins, venoms, heat, and mechanical trauma can directly destroy the membrane. In general, except for the devastating destruction that leads to intravascular hemolysis, the initial damage leads eventually to a change in the external portion of the red blood cell (RBC) membrane. That change, in turn, causes macrophages to retard, hold, remove, or otherwise modify these RBCs. Sometimes these RBC surface changes are accompanied by decreases in RBC deformability, which retards flow and thereby facilitates the action of macrophages

on the affected RBC. These changes lead to extravascular hemolysis.

FRAGMENTATION HEMOLYSIS—MICROANGIOPATHY

Clinical Manifestations

Patients present with varying degrees of hemolytic anemia and compensation, with evidence of red cell fragmentation on smear (Plate 48-1). Red cell removal is generally extravascular, with minimal or moderately decreased levels of haptoglobin, but if red cell damage is severe, signs of intravascular hemolysis may also be present. Because of the underlying pathology, some of the syndromes may show evidence of platelet removal, leading to thrombocytopenia. Occasionally the underlying cause may also produce procoagulant activation and depletion with consequent activation of the fibrinolytic system, consistent with disseminated intravascular coagulation (DIC) (Table 48-1).

Pathophysiology

Brain et al.[1] saw a possible relationship of vascular lesions to cases of RBC fragmentation and postulated that the lesions either produced shearing forces sufficiently strong to fragment the red cells or led to inflammation of small vessel walls, which in turn generated the fibrin strands that literally cut the passing red cell into irregular pieces. The red cell membrane is viscoelastic and has self-sealing properties (see Chs. 4 and 32), so that little hemoglobin leaks out as the cell is being cut. However, prolonged distortion of the membrane produces a plastic

Table 48-1. Causes of Red Blood Cell Fragmentation Hemolysis

Damaged microvasculature
   TTP-HUS
   Associated with pregnancy: pre-eclampsia/eclampsia, HELLP
   Associated with malignancy: with or without mitomycin C
   Vasculitis: polyarteritis, Wegener's granulomatosis, acute glomerulonephri-
     tis, *Rickettsia*-like infections
   Abnormalities of renal vasculature: malignant hypertension, acute glomerulo-
     nephritis, scleroderma, allograft rejection with or without cyclosporine
   Disseminated intravascular coagulation
Atrioventricular malformations
   Kasabach-Merritt syndrome
   Hemangioendotheliomas
   Atrioventricular shunts, congenital and acquired
Cardiac abnormalities
   Replaced valve, prosthesis, grafts, patches
   Aortic stenosis, regurgitant jets as in ruptured sinus of Valsalva

Abbreviations: TTP/HUS, thrombotic thrombocytopenic purpura/hemolytic uremic syndrome; HELLP, hemolysis + elevated liver enzymes + low platelet count.

change; therefore, the smaller red cell fragments do not usually become microspheres or microdiscs but continue to display the evidence of the shearing event or the distortion in the form of the typical irregular shapes. These irregular shapes and the rigidity that they reflect subsequently interferes with the ability of red cells to fold, elongate, and deform sufficiently to pass through 3-μm capillaries and even smaller slits in the walls of the sinusoids of the reticuloendothelial system. This sequence leads to their destruction.

Differential Diagnosis

Generally, the differential diagnosis of fragmentation hemolysis can be deduced from the clinical setting. The presence of a prosthetic heart valve (Waring blender syndrome) is a readily appreciated source of this entity. The clinical picture of thrombotic thrombocytopenic pupura/hemolytic uremic syndrome (TTP/HUS) is generally dramatic and acute (see Ch. 127). Atrioventricular malformations may be associated with DIC and platelet removal. The presence of pre-eclampsia in a pregnant patient with microangiopathic hemolysis is usually obvious, but the HELLP syndrome (hemolysis + elevated liver enzymes + low platelet count) is a serious complication of pregnancy, which can occur without other signs of pre-eclampsia or hypertension.[2] This syndrome can produce hepatic rupture, visual failure, DIC, seizures, and congestive heart failure and needs to be treated by prompt delivery of the fetus (see Ch. 149). Vessels supplying malignant tumors are thought to be structurally abnormal. They exhibit the same sort of fibrin stranding that produces fragmentation hemolysis in DIC and TTP/HUS.

It now appears that some drugs can produce microangiopathic hemolysis. Cyclosporine[3] and mitomycin C have been implicated as causing an HUS picture. However, for mitomycin C, at least, it is frequently difficult to distinguish the action of the drug from that of the cancer being treated.[4] The new antiplatelet agent ticlopidine also seems to be capable of producing a TTP-like syndrome. There are a few preliminary reports and the incidence is probably quite low.[5]

Therapy

Management is primarily directed at the underlying disease or event. In addition, one should optimize compensation of red cell production by replacing iron or folic acid if the patient is deficient in these nutrients. Occasionally it is necessary to remove or replace a prosthetic heart valve because the hemoly-

---

DIFFERENTIAL DIAGNOSIS OF EXTRINSIC NONIMMUNE HEMOLYTIC ANEMIAS

There is no simplistic approach to differential diagnosis of this type of hemolysis; one must rely very heavily on the clinical setting. Useful clues come from a determination of whether red cell breakdown is predominantly extravascular or intravascular. However, most important in the analysis is the observation of red cell morphology, because an accurate appreciation of morphology focuses and limits the differential diagnosis. This is the place to discard nonhelpful terms such as *aniso* and *poik*. The RBCs are spherocytic, stomatocytic, fragmented, echinocytic, acanthocytic, spurred, or bite cells, or mixtures of these. When necessary, I strongly recommend supplementing the standard Wright-Giemsa-sustained peripheral blood smear with a wet preparation in which 10 to 20 μl of freshly drawn heparinized whole blood is added to 200 μl of 1% glutaraldehyde in phosphate buffered saline. After several moments to allow for fixation, the RBCs are examined under phase microsocpy (phase 2, $\times$ 400 or phase 3 $\times$ 1,000), and the three-dimensional appearance of the cells can be appreciated. Subtle degrees of stomatocytosis (spherocytes are really stomatocytes), red cell budding, and acanthocytosis become apparent, and artifacts in smear preparation are avoided.

---

sis produces a disabling transfusion requirement. The HUS of mitomycin C/adenocarcinoma is said to respond reasonably well to use of the staphylococcal protein A immunoperfusion column[6] or to infusion of vincristine,[4] but it may be necessary to proceed to apheresis with fresh frozen plasma replacement (see Ch. 127).

OTHER FORMS OF MECHANICAL DAMAGE TO RED CELLS

Heat Denaturation

Normal RBCs will undergo budding and fragmentation when exposed to a temperature of 49°C in vitro. In some of the hereditary hemolytic anemias this occurs at temperatures as low as 46°C (see Ch. 46). Isolated circumstances have been identified in which temperatures sufficient to cause heat denaturation of RBCs have been generated. Occasionally, cell warmers used to bring transfused red cells to body temperature before infusion in treatment of cold agglutinin disease have malfunctioned and cooked the red cells about to be transfused. In one case, a patient's mother decided to warm red cells with a hot water bottle, reasoning that such cells would cause less vein irritation to her child. Such transfusion was followed by evidence of both intra- and extravascular hemolysis, and the peripheral smear showed red cell budding and fragmentation (Fig. 48-1). Presumably, similar events can lead to hemolysis in patients who have sustained very extensive burns. In patients suffering from heatstroke, the temperature is usually below 42°C, and at this temperature little RBC denaturation occurs.

Mechanical Trauma

The classic example of red cell damage due to mechanical trauma is march hemoglobinuria, which occurs in soldiers after a long march, joggers after running on a hard road, or karate or conga drumming enthusiasts following practice. Anemia is

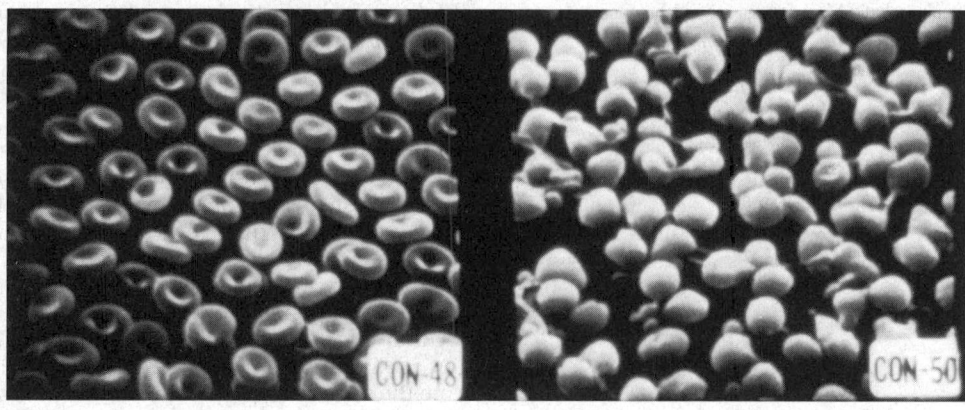

Fig. 48-1. Change in RBC morphology produced by heating normal RBCs at the indicated temperatures. Note the budding that begins abruptly at 50°C, leading eventually to spherocytosis.

rare, and reticulocytosis is uncommon. Evidence of typical intravascular red cell destruction is present, which is thought to be caused by direct trauma to the red cells in vessels of the feet or hands, because switching the jogging path or using better footwear relieves the problem. In some cases, there appears to be evidence of an underlying red cell membrane abnormality.[7] Occasionally, malfunction of the cell savers used during abdominal or thoracic surgery can mechanically injure red cells.

Cardiopulmonary Bypass

The postperfusion syndrome occurs in some patients following cardiopulmonary bypass and includes acute intravascular hemolysis and leukopenia as part of a febrile inflammatory clinical picture. Some of these patients go on to develop pulmonary distress and even adult respiratory distress syndrome. Visible hemoglobinemia occurs, with rising plasma hemoglobin levels, associated with an increase of lysed red cell ghosts seen in the whole blood and plasma. These ghosts have been shown to be coated with the complement complex C5b–C9 (see Ch. 12). Presumably, the complement pathway is activated as the blood is passed through the oxygenator. Why the complement activation has resulted in lytic attack on red cells (and also granulocytes) is not known. Treatment involves knowledge of the process and requisite support[8] until the situation corrects itself.

Osmotic Attack

Abrupt changes in osmolality can also cause hemolysis. Freshwater drowning may be associated with so much water in the lungs that the red cells swell as they undergo an in vivo osmotic fragility test in the lung vessels. Saltwater drowning, conversely, can cause profound dehydration of red cells, producing a situation analogous to xerocytosis (see Ch. 46). Very rarely, acute hemolysis may occur from mistaken infusion or exposure to concentrated hypertonic solutions such as those used in hemodialysis. To manage such an event, one must recognize its cause, appreciate the shrunken RBCs on peripheral smear, and restore isotonicity as quickly as possible. The use of a hemodialysis device, if available, may be helpful in this regard.[9]

HYPERSPLENISM

In all organs of the monocyte/macrophage system, blood cells leaving the arterial bed are generally unloaded into channels such that they must pass through the wall of the sinus to reenter the circulation. The sinusoidal wall has slits 1–3 μm in size and is usually endothelialized on one side and has a macrophagic lining on the other (see Chs. 15 and 50). The spleen is somewhat more complicated in that the afferent arterioles pass through lymphoid nodules (the white pulp) and then terminate in the cords of Billroth (the red pulp), into which the blood cells are discharged. In the slow flow of the cords of Billroth, the blood cells are selectively attacked by macrophages and are in direct contact with several classes of lymphocytes. The blood cells must then pass through the cordal walls before they can approach the sinus wall, which they must pass through to reenter the circulation. Thus, the spleen provides a double filter, the blood cells must be remarkably deformable to pass through it. Furthermore, this slow passage permits highly selective action on the blood cells by the macrophages, which have receptors that can detect several sorts of alterations in these blood cells. These receptors include the Fc receptor for the appropriate portion of the immunoglobulin molecule, receptors for complement components such as C3b, and perhaps receptors that detect alterations in the outer portion of the phospholipid bilayer or in the externally oriented glycopeptides. The macrophage then holds, retards, modifies ("pits" function), or removes ("culls" function) the blood cells so identified. Normally, the pitting function of the spleen allows it to remove Howell-Jolly bodies and normally occurring endocytic vacuoles (called pocks because of their appearance on phase interference or Nomarski microscopy). The normal culling function of the spleen is exemplified by its removal of senescent RBCs.[10]

All the activities of the spleen are presumably markedly accentuated in a large spleen, and if the increased activity is extensive enough, the clinical picture called *hypersplenism* ensues. It is the size of the spleen, not the portal pressure, that is important in determining the degree of red cell sequestration that occurs.[11] Other factors that may play a role are the state of activation of the splenic macrophages and the size of the small slits between the splenic cords and sinuses. Both macrophages and slits seem to be under a degree of control, as evidenced by variations in splenic removal of red cells in patients infected with malaria.[12,13]

The clinical picture of hypersplenic hemolysis is dominated by the specific cause of the splenomegaly. Although causes of splenomegaly are legion, there are several general mechanisms (Table 48-2). Generally, there is a varying degree of anemia, with varying evidence of a compensatory increase in red cell production. Because stasis and trapping in the spleen are associated with macrophagic attack and remodeling of the red cell surface, the reduction in surface area/volume ratio leads to spherocytosis. If the red cells undergo a prolonged period of

Table 48-2. Pathophysiologic Mechanisms for Splenomegaly

Mechanisms	Examples
Neoplasia	Lymphoma, hairy cell leukemia
Infections	Bacterial endocarditis
	Malaria, schistosomiasis
	Tuberculosis
Portal bed obstruction	Alcoholic cirrhosis
	Splenic vein thrombosis
Collagen-vascular disease	Systemic lupus erythematosus, rheumatoid arthritis-malignant phase
Chronic inflammatory disease	Rheumatoid arthritis
Chronic hereditary or acquired hemolytic anemias	Severe β-thalassemia
	Autoimmune hemolytic anemia
Miscellaneous disorders	
Lipoidosis	Gaucher disease
Amyloidosis	AL and AA types

distortion in traversing the cordal-sinus barrier, then tailed red cells will be present as the red cell membranes undergo a plastic change (Plate 48-2) (see Ch. 32). Presumably, the enlarged spleen can also trap and remove platelets and white blood cells (WBCs), so that variable thrombocytopenia and leukopenia may occur. The bone marrow may show normal to increased cellularity, with erythroid hyperplasia.

Management depends on the etiology of the splenic enlargement. Generally, the anemia or pancytopenia is not very profound, but if the anemia is very severe, splenectomy may be contemplated. It is worth recalling that massive splenomegaly is frequently associated with expansion of the plasma compartment so that measurement of hemoglobin, hematocrit, or red cell count may give a falsely low value of the actual red cell mass present. In that circumstance the true RBC mass can be determined by a ^{51}Cr determination (see Ch. 34).

INFECTION

Pathophysiologically, there are several mechanisms by which infection can cause hemolytic anemia (Table 48-3).

Direct Parasitization

The classic example of direct parasitization is *Plasmodium falciparum, P. vivax,* or *P. malariae* infection. In each of the malarias, sporozoites injected by the mosquito in its saliva make their way to liver cells, where after 1–2 weeks they become merozoites, which burst out of the liver cells and into the bloodstream. Then, in a remarkable process, the parasite via its apical end and related organelles called *rhopteries* attaches to a specific receptor on the red cell surface. For *P. vivax,* the Duffy blood group antigen appears to be involved.

Table 48-3. Mechanisms by which Infection Can Cause Hemolysis

Direct parasitization of red cells
  Examples: malaria, babesiosis
Immune mechanisms
  Example: cold agglutinin hemolysis following infectious mononucleosis or mycoplasmal pneumonia (see see Ch. 47)
Induction of hypersplenism
  Examples: malaria, schistosomiasis
Altered red cell surface topology
  Example: Haemophilus influenzae
Release of toxins and enzymes
  Example: clostridial infection

P. falciparum binds to sialic acid residues on the red cell surface that are not on glycophorin A, B, or C. Following specific attachment a convulsive movement occurs, during which the red cell engulfs the parasite by a process resembling receptor-mediated endocytosis. The parasite then immediately co-opts the red cell's metabolic machinery, degrades and ingests hemoglobin, and grows, eventually bursting out of the red cell, so that the cycle can begin again. The red cells are lysed both intravascularly as a consequence of direct parasitic destruction and extravascularly as a consequence of changes in the splenic microvasculature and in the activation state of the monocyte/macrophage system noted above.

Other infections that have somewhat similar pathophysiologies include Carrión disease (bartonellosis), in which a bite from the sandfly injects *Bartonella bacilliformis,* which attaches to the red cell surface and somehow causes lysis; and babesiosis, a disorder found mostly on Nantucket Island, in which the parasite is transmitted by ticks and directly invades red cells. In addition, there are sporadic reports indicating that acquired chronic toxoplasmosis can occasionally be associated with hemolytic anemia.[14]

An example of an infection that may produce hemolysis by altering the red cell surface is that caused by *Haemophilus influenzae* type b.[15] Severely affected patients, particularly those with meningitis, have developed hemolytic anemias requiring red cell transfusions. The capsular polysaccharide of the bacterium, composed of polyribosyl ribosyl phosphate (PRP) is released during infection and binds to the red cell surface. Infected patients develop antibodies to PRP. When the balance between PRP-coated RBCs and anti-PRP antibodies is correct, an immune sort of hemolysis, requiring complement, occurs. Red cell destruction is thought to be both intra- and extravascular.

Bacterial Products Causing Hemolysis

The most dramatic example of hemolysis due to bacterial action is clostridial infection, during which the organism releases enzymes that acutely degrade the phospholipids of the membrane bilayer and the structural membrane proteins. The setting can be any infection, but my personal experience is limited to acute cholecystitis, surgery of the biliary tree, and infections surrounding an obstetric event, including criminal or self-induced abortion or other infection of the gravid uterus. The signs of infections may be obvious, but fever may be unimpressive.[16,17] Signs of collapse appear acutely, and the clue is profound intravascular hemolysis, with a spherocytic anemia developing with shocking suddenness. A clue to the severity of the process may be the inability of the laboratory to perform chemical determinations or type and cross-match the blood because the sample is hemolyzed. With even the slightest suspicion, one immediately starts full doses of a penicillin, evaluates the patient for DIC (see Ch. 116), and prepares to support the patient for shock, DIC, acute renal failure, and hemolytic anemia. In the case of septic abortion it is not clear that hysterectomy is life-saving.[17]

HEMOLYSIS ASSOCIATED WITH LIVER DISEASE

Hemolysis in liver disease is usually not of overwhelming clinical importance by itself but might contribute to the severity of anemia when coupled with RBC production defects and the type of gastrointestinal blood loss that occurs in several sorts of liver disease. There are several causes of hemolysis in patients with liver disease. The spleen can be enlarged as a consequence of portal hypertension[18] and produce a hypersplenic picture, a phenomenon seen quite commonly in hepatic cirrhosis.

Considerable literature has developed concerning red cell shape change in liver disease. The target cell in cirrhosis has an increased surface area/volume ratio, which appears to be a consequence of an increase in both the cholesterol and phospholipid content of the membrane bilayer. The cholesterol increase is usually proportionately greater, resulting in an increase in the cholesterol/phospholipid ratio. It is this increase in lipid that probably accounts for the increase in RBC surface area, which means that there is more membrane than usual for the cellular contents. These red cells probably circulate as bell-shaped RBCs called codocytes, but on dried blood films they assume the appearance of target cells. Target cells per se do not have a shortened RBC survival.[18,19] The RBCs of patients with liver disease are frequently echinocytes when wet preparations are examined, but these echinocytes are not easily apparent on dried blood smears.[19] The echinocytes seem to be produced by a material in a patient's plasma that causes normal red cells to become echinocytic; this material is an abnormal echinocytogenic high-density lipoprotein. Echinocytes per se do not necessarily have a shortened red cell survival. Some forms of echinocytosis are normally deformable when studied in the ektacytometer or rheoscope.

A brisk, clinically important hemolysis can occur in some patients with severe liver disease. The peripheral smear in these individuals usually shows acanthocytes (distorted RBCs), extreme forms of which are called spur cells. Spur cells are probably acanthocytes additionally remodeled by an enlarged spleen (Plate 48-3) and are considerably enriched in cholesterol.[18] They are rapidly removed in the spleen, which is usually enlarged. It may be that increased red cell membrane proteolytic activity is a partial explanation of the differences between acanthocytosis and spur cells.[20] On occasion, spur cell hemolytic anemia is severe enough to necessitate consideration of splenectomy. The operative morbidity in such cases is considerable, because the underlying alcoholism usually produces problems with thrombocytopenia and leukopenia, while the severity of the liver disease can cause problems with procoagulants and intolerance to anesthesia.

Acute alcoholism can be associated with hypophosphatemia, defined as levels <0.2 mg/dl. Such hypophosphatemia presumably interferes with red cell intermediary metabolism (see Ch. 45), and the RBC ATP levels fall; very low ATP levels are associated with RBC rigidity. This rigidity leads to fragmentation, loss of surface area, and spheroidicity. These RBCs are then further trapped in the spleen. This hypophosphatemia syndrome also can cause neuromuscular disorders, including weakness, paresthesias, tremors, and seizures, and should be treated aggressively with oral and intravenous phosphate supplements. Hypophosphatemia also occurs in cirrhotic patients, patients on total parenteral nutrition whose phosphate intake is not carefully monitored, and patients taking large amounts of phosphate binding antacids.[21,22]

Stomatocytosis can occur in severe liver disease and is also thought to be a sign of acute alcoholic intoxication. This change in RBC shape can also be seen in acute pancreatitis. The stomatocyte is a cell well on its way to becoming a spherocyte. The reduction in surface area/volume ratio leads to trapping in the microvasculature of the spleen and other organs of the monocyte/macrophage system, producing varying degrees of hemolysis.

RENAL DISEASE

Disease of the small renal arterioles can produce fragmentation hemolysis of the sort seen in TTP/HUS, pre-eclampsia, and malignant hypertension (Table 48-1). In the past, some patients on chronic hemodialysis were exposed to unusual concentrations of chloramine in the tap water and underwent acute oxidative hemolysis[23] (see below). This occurrence has become very rare, if it still exists. Otherwise it is not clear that uremia per se produces significant shortening of red cell survival.

VENOMS, BITES, STINGS, AND TOXINS

The best known example of toxin-caused hemolysis is discussed above under clostridial sepsis.

Insect, Spider, and Snake Bites

Instances of hemolysis have occurred following bee and wasp stings, snake bites, and spider bites. Isolated cases of acute intravascular hemolysis have been reported after bee and wasp stings. Two kinds of dangerous spiders live in the United States: the southern black widow and the brown recluse spider. Both sexes of the black widow produce the venom, but only the female has fangs capable of penetrating human skin. Black widow spider bites produce generalized muscle pain and muscular rigidity. Hemolysis, if it occurs at all, is not common. Brown recluse spider bites cause a considerable local reaction, called the volcano lesion. Both DIC and hemolysis may occur after a 24–48-hour lag period. Corticosteroids may be beneficial.

In other parts of the world, cobra bites can cause intravascular hemolysis because the venom contains phospholipases, while in the United States the two classes of venomous snakes are pit vipers (rattlesnakes, cottonmouths, moccasins, and copperheads) and coral snakes. Pit viper venom effects hemostasis and may produce DIC with bleeding but rarely hemolysis. Coral snake venom produces severe neurologic impairment. Therapy consists of support and of the appropriate antivenin and prophylactic antimicrobials and tetanus injections.

Drugs and Chemicals (Exclusive of Those Producing Oxidative Hemolysis)

Potassium Chlorate

Potassium chlorate ingestion is listed as a cause of hemolysis, but this compound is no longer available in hospital pharmacies and has no currently recognized medical use. Arsine gas (AsH_3) is generated in industrial plants that engage in lead plating, galvanizing, etching, and soldering. Inhalation of a toxic amount produces a severe intravascular hemolysis[24] of unknown pathogenesis.

Copper

The idea that copper can produce human hemolytic disease is best supported by observations of episodes of severe hemolysis in patients with Wilson disease. The patient is usually a child, adolescent, or young adult in whom the diagnosis of Wilson disease has not yet been made.[25,26] The initial clinical presentation usually is dominated by the hemolytic anemia, accompanied by weakness and dark urine. RBC morphology has not been well described, but reticulocytosis is present, with an increased serum bilirubin partly attributable to the underlying liver disease. Because of the hereditary deficiency in the copper-binding protein ceruloplasmin, serum and urine copper levels in patients with hemolysis are very high. Curiously, in one report hemoglobin A_2 levels were also elevated.[25] Free copper can interfere with glucose metabolism by hexokinase inhibition and alternatively, can generate oxidative hemolysis, perhaps by acting as a Fenton reagent. It is important to establish the diagnosis promptly by considering the possibilities, looking for the Kayser-Fleischer rings on physical examination, and measuring serum and urine copper and ceruloplasmin levels. Treatment with penicillamine reduces the serum copper level and stops the hemolysis. Presumably other forms of copper poisoning also may cause hemolysis in patients who do not have underlying Wilson disease, but the amount of copper ingested would have to exceed the normal copper-binding capacity of normal ceruloplasmin.

Lead Poisoning

There are at least two general forms of lead intoxication. Occupational exposure is an example of chronic, slow cumulative poisoning (saturnism). The symptoms are predominantly neurologic and nephrologic, with variable degrees of anemia, which may be due to a production defect combined with hemolysis. Relatively acute poisoning occurs when lead inadvertently finds its way into a food source[27] or is consumed as part of an exotic medication. Such subacute lead poisoning leads to central nervous system symptoms, hepatitis, nephrotoxicity, hypertension, and abdominal colic, along with seizures and severe hemolytic anemia. Physical examination may reveal the lead line on the gums. The peripheral smear shows extensive coarse basophilic stippling and reticulocytosis; however, red cell morphology is not otherwise characteristic. Some authors state that intravascular destruction occurs, but no proof has been provided. Bilirubin is not significantly elevated.

The diagnosis of lead-related hemolysis can be made by the history, noticing the gingival lead line, and then observing the coarse basophilic stippling on red cells, which reflects the pathologic aggregation of ribosomes. The diagnosis is confirmed by measurement of blood and urine lead levels. The level of acuity determines the therapy.

The cause of the anemia is complex; lead interferes with several steps in heme synthesis, particularly those involving heme synthetase and δ-aminolevulinic acid dehydratase (see Ch. 39). The inhibition of heme synthetase probably accounts for the elevation in free erythrocyte protoporphyrin, which provides a useful corroborative diagnostic test for lead toxicity. Inhibition of heme synthesis also probably accounts for the elevated urinary levels of δ-aminolevulinic acid and coproporphyrin. Lead poisoning mimics the basophilic stippling and accumulation of pyrimidines seen in hereditary deficiency of the enzyme pyrimidine 5′-nucleotidase,[28] probably because lead attacks the enzyme (see Ch. 45).

DRUG-INDUCED OXIDATIVE HEMOLYSIS
General Concepts

The potential for normal RBCs to undergo autooxidative destruction is great because the cell is loaded with 20 mM hemoglobin, most of which is bonded to oxygen at the iron(II) atom in heme. The bond that allows the reversible association and dissociation of oxygen from the heme moiety of hemoglobin involves partial transfer of an electron from iron(II) to oxygen. That oxygen now has an extra electron, which makes it a superoxide radical. Ordinarily, when oxygen leaves hemoglobin, it returns the electron but, if it does not, a highly reactive superoxide ion is released, leaving behind it an iron(III) moiety otherwise called methemoglobin.

$$Hb\ Fe^{+2}\ O_2 \rightarrow Hb\ Fe^{+3} + O_2^{-1} \tag{1}$$

Methemoglobin cannot reversibly bind oxygen. It is not in itself harmful to red cells, but if the oxidative assault persists, methemoglobin is converted to hemichromes, which are variably denatured hemoglobin intermediates in which the distal histidine unit binds to the oxidized heme. This step is associated with conversion of a high to a low spin state, as measured by electron spin resonance. Continued oxidation leads to irreversibility of the hemichrome oxidation, to precipitation, and eventually to the formation of Heinz bodies. Hemichromes and Heinz bodies can destroy membrane function directly or can cause oxidation of membrane proteins and lipids.[29] It is estimated that each day about 3% of hemoglobin is converted to methemoglobin, but since only 1% of hemoglobin normally is in the form of methemoglobin, this indicates that a mechanism that prevents oxidation in red cells is in effect. This mechanism involves the NADH and NADPH-dependent reducing systems, catalase, glutathione, and the glutathione reductase and peroxidase systems. Defects in this defense system against oxidation lead to an enhanced (see Ch. 45) tendency to oxidative hemolysis. An example is the several glucose-6-phosphate dehydrogenase (G6PD) deficiency states. Any agent or event that interferes with the smooth off-loading of oxygen will enhance the generation of O_2^{-1} and methemoglobin (equation 1). If the reducing power of the red cell is inadequate, hemichromes and Heinz bodies will subsequently be generated. In fact, many agents appear to cause oxidative hemolysis by interfering with the smooth functioning of the heme cleft.

Pathophysiology

Once the oxidative attack has been initiated, the sequence proceeds along a recognizable track. The oxidative attack is directed at hemoglobin and the red cell membrane. However, these are not clearly separable because the precipitated hemichrome and Heinz bodies come to lie against the cytosol face of the membrane. Methemoglobinemia may be detectably elevated, with levels as high as 50–60% of total hemoglobin. The hemichromes by themselves, or their iron portions acting as a Fenton reagent, mediate the generation of hydroxyl free radicals, which add their effect to that of superoxide and hydrogen peroxide. Lipid peroxidation may take place, membrane proteins may be cross-linked, and adducts between spectrin

Table 48-4. Agents that Cause Oxidative Hemolysis

Therapeutic agents	Recreational drugs
Nitrofurantoin (Furadantin)	Isobutyl nitrate
Sulfasalaine (Azulfidine)	Amyl nitrite
p-Aminosalicylic acid	Miscellaneous
Phenazopyridine (Pyridium)	Naphthalene mothballs
Phenacetin	Paraquat
Dapsone and other sulfones	Hydrogen peroxide

and denatured globin may form.[30] Such red cells are rigid and are susceptible to trapping in sinusoidal structures whether or not they have Heinz bodies lying against the membrane. In addition, in vitro evidence suggests that such oxidized red cells are increasingly susceptible to phagocytosis by macrophages. These features may account for the extravascular destruction. The oxidative lesions can be so severe as to cause intravascular destruction as well, with hemoglobinemia and hemoglobinuria.

The smear may show bite cells (Plate 48-4), which look as if a macrophage had taken a bite, removing a Heinz body-containing segment of membrane. Red cell rigidity may result in irregularly shaped cells, since these undeformable cells are unable to undergo elastic recoil after fighting their way through the sinus wall. Recurrent loss of membrane material may produce spherocytes. Severe hemolysis may produce the kind of circulating ghost or hemighost called a blister cell or bite cell. These red cells have an empty veil of membrane on one side and puddled hemoglobin on the other.[31,32] A Heinz body preparation may be positive.

The clinical picture is determined by the specific agent used. It may be useful to screen for G6PD deficiency or a related disorder by using an enzyme assay or the ascorbate cyanide test. The agents that can cause such episodes of oxidative hemolysis are listed in Table 48-4.

Paraquat ingestion has occurred inadvertently and in suicide attempts.[33] Profound cyanosis with methemoglobinemia can occur within hours, with levels of $\geq 20\%$. This can be succeeded by hemolysis, with Heinz bodies seen in appropriate preparations of red cells.

Nitrites have been used in suicide attempts,[34] and there have been industrial exposures as well. More recently nitrites have also been used as inhaled or swallowed recreational agents.[35,36] The nitrite may be sold in sex shops under the name "Locker Room," "Sweat," or "Rush." Methemoglobinemia may be so profound as to produce coma. If methylene blue infusion does not quickly turn the chocolate color of blood back to normal, one must consider the possibility that the patient is G6PD deficient and therefore unable to generate adequate amounts of NADPH (see above). In that case, exchange transfusion may be life-saving.[37]

Pyridium can cause oxidative hemolysis,[38] even in the absence of renal disease.[39] I have recently seen a case of almost fatal oxidative hemolysis in which a patient with the acquired immunodeficiency syndrome (AIDS) injected hydrogen peroxide directly into his Hickman catheter. (Some persons infected with the human immunodeficiency virus [HIV] are circulating a pamphlet suggesting that hydrogen peroxide can be used therapeutically to control the HIV infection.)

It has been recognized for ≥ 30 years that therapy with dapsone causes oxidative hemolysis.[40] In the past, dapsone was used primarily to treat leprosy and dermatitis herpetiformis and thus was not encountered very often as a cause of oxidative hemolysis. More recently, dapsone has come into more widespread use in some communities as a very effective prophylatic agent against *Pneumocytsis carinii* pneumonia in patients with AIDS. In some clinics it is the practice to screen potential recipients for the G6PD deficiency (see Ch. 45) and if negative proceed with dapsone therapy. However, dapsone can cause

oxidative attack on RBCs, leading sequentially to methemoglobinemia, then Heinz bodies, and finally hemolysis, all at generally accepted standard doses.[41] We are now seeing AIDS patients with dapsone-induced methemoglobinemia and hemolytic anemia. The methemoglobinemia if severe is treated as described above and in Chapter 44. One study suggests that the severity of the oxidative attack can be partially ameliorated by administration of 800 U/day of vitamin E, an agent that has antioxidant action.[42]

REFERENCES

1. Brain MC, Dacie JV, Hourihane DOB: Microangiopathic haemolytic anemia. The possible role of vascular lesions in pathogenesis. Br J Haematol 8:358, 1962
2. Baca L, Gibbons RB: The HELLP syndrome: a serious complication of pregnancy with hemolysis, elevated levels of liver enzymes, and low platelet count. Am J Med 85:590, 1988
3. Bonser RS, Adu D, Franklin I, McMaster P: Cyclosporin-induced haemolytic uraemic syndrome in liver allograft recipient. Lancet 2:1337, 1984
4. Grem JL, Merritt JA, Carbone PP: Treatment of mitomycin-associated microangiopathic hemolytic anemia with vincristine. Arch Intern Med 146:566, 1986
5. Page Y, Tardy B, Zeni F et al: Thrombotic thrombocytopenic purpura related to ticlopidine. Lancet 337:774, 1991
6. Korec S, Schein PS, Smith FP et al: Treatment of cancer-associated hemolytic uremic syndrome with staphylococcal protein A immunoperfusion. J Clin Oncol 4:210, 1986
7. Banga JP, Pinder JC, Gratzer WB et al: An erythrocyte membrane-protein anomaly in march haemoglobinuria. Lancet 2:1048, 1979
8. Salama A, Hugo F, Heinrich D et al: Deposition of terminal C5b-9 complement complexes on erythrocytes and leukocytes during cardiopulmonary bypass. N Engl J Med 318:408, 1988
9. Mulligan I, Parfrey P, Phillips ME et al: Acute haemolysis due to concentrated dialysis fluid. Br Med J 284:1151, 1982
10. Rosse WF: The spleen as a filter. N Engl J Med 317:704, 1987
11. Holzbach RT, Shipley RA, Clark RE, Chudniz EB: Influence of spleen size and portal pressure on erythrocyte sequestration. J Clin Invest 43:1125, 1964
12. Looareesuwan S, Ho M, Wattanagoon Y et al: Dynamic alteration in splenic function during acute falciparum malaria. N Engl J Med 317:675, 1987
13. Looareesuwan S, Merry AH, Phillips RE et al: Reduced erythrocyte survival following clearance of malarial parasitaemia in Thai patients. Br J Haematol 67:473, 1987
14. Kalderon A, Kikkawa Y, Bernstein J: Chronic toxoplasmosis associated with severe hemolytic anemia. Arch Intern Med 114:95, 1964
15. Shurin SB, Anderson P, Zollinger J, Rathbun RK: Pathophysiology of hemolysis in infections with *Hemophilus influenzae* type b. J Clin Invest 77:1340, 1986
16. Bennett JM, Healey PJM: Spherocytic hemolytic anemia and acute cholecystitis caused by *Clostridium welchii*. N Engl J Med 268:1070, 1963
17. Pritchard JA, Whalley PJ: Abortion complicated by *Clostridium perfringens* infection. Am J Obstet Gynecol 111:484, 1971
18. Cooper RA: Hemolytic syndromes and red cell membrane abnormalities in liver disease. Semin Hematol 17:103, 1980
19. Owen JS, Brown DJC, Harry DS et al: Erythrocyte echinocytosis in liver disease. J Clin Invest 76:2275, 1985
20. Olivieri O, Guarini P, Negri M et al: Increased proteolytic activity of erythrocyte membrane in spur cell anaemia. Br J Haematol 70:483, 1988
21. Jacob HS, Amsden T: Acute hemolytic anemia with rigid red cells in hypophosphatemia. N Engl J Med 285:1446, 1971
22. Martin DW Jr, Watts HD: Hypophophatemia. West J Med 122:482, 1975
23. Yawata Y, Howe R, Jacob HS: Abnormal red cell metabolism causing hemolysis in uremia. Ann Intern Med 79:362, 1973
24. Fowler BA, Weissberg JB: Arsine poisoning. N Engl J Med 291:1171, 1974
25. Robitaille GA, Piscatelli RL, Majeski EJ, Gelehrter TD: Hemolytic anemia in Wilson's disease. JAMA 237:2402, 1977
26. Forman SJ, Kumar KS, Redeker AG, Hochstein P: Hemolytic anemia in Wilson disease: clinical findings and biochemical mechanisms. Am J Hematol 9:269, 1980
27. Carton JA, Maradona JA, Arribas JM: Acute-subacute lead poisoning. Arch Intern Med 147:697, 1987
28. Valentine WN, Paglia DE, Fink D et al: Lead poisoning: association with hemolytic anemia, basophilic stippling, erythrocyte pyrimidine-5' nucleotidase and intraerythrocytic accumulation of pyrimidines. J Clin Invest 58:926, 1976
29. Hebbel RP, Eaton JW: Pathobiology of heme interaction with the erythrocyte membrane. Semin Hematol 26:136, 1989

30. Chiu D, Lubin B: Oxidative hemoglobin denaturation and RBC destruction: the effect of heme on red cell membranes. Semin Hematol 26:128, 1989

31. Chan TK, Chan WC, Weed RI: Erythrocyte hemighosts: a hallmark of severe oxidative injury in vivo. Br J Haematol 50:575, 1982

32. Yoo D, Lessin LS: Drug-associated "bite cell" hemolytic anemia. Am J Med 92:243, 1992

33. Ng LL, Naik RB, Polak A: Paraquat ingestion with methaemoglobinaemia treated with methylene blue. Br Med J 284:1445, 1982

34. Smith M, Stair T, Rolnick MA: butyl nitrite and a suicide attempt. Ann Intern Med 92:719, 1980

35. Wason S, Detsky AS, Platt OS, Lovejoy FH Jr: Isobutyl nitrite toxicity by ingestion. Ann Intern Med 92:637, 1980

36. Sharp CW, Stillman RC: Blush not with nitrites. Ann Intern Med 92:700, 1980

37. Brandes JC, Bufill JA, Pisciotta AV: Amyl nitrite-induced hemolytic anemia. Am J Med 86:252, 1989

38. Nathan DM, Siegel AJ, Bunn HF: Acute methemoglobinemia and hemolytic anemia with phenazopyridine. Arch Intern Med 137:1636, 1977

39. Fincher ME, Campbell HT: Methemoglobinemia and hemolytic anemia after phenazopyridine hydrochloride (pyridium) administration in end-stage renal disease. South Med J 82:372, 1989

40. Pengelly CDR: Dapsone-induced haemolysis. Br Med J 2:662, 1963

41. Spriggs AI, Smith RS, Griffith H, Truelove SC: Heinz-body anaemia due to salicylazosulphapyridine. Lancet 2:1039, 1958

42. Prussick R, Ali MAM, Rosenthal D, Guyatt G: The protective effect of vitamin E on the hemolysis associated with dapsone treatment in patients with dermatitis herpetiformis. Arch Dermatol 128:210, 1992

WHITE BLOOD CELLS

Part V

Neutrophil Structure and Function

49

Peter E. Newburger and Richard T. Parmley

INTRODUCTION

Neutrophils are the rapid deployment and effector arm of the immune system. They are present in large numbers in the circulation, through which they rapidly transit en route to tissue, where they form the first line of cellular defense against invading microorganisms. As potent agents of the inflammatory response, they also play a major role in the inflammation and tissue damage of a wide variety of noninfectious diseases, such as arthritis and inflammatory bowel disease.

This chapter considers in turn (1) the production of neutrophils, including both the kinetics of myelopoiesis and the structure of the cells at each stage of differentiation; and (2) the function of the mature cells. Much of our knowledge of normal neutrophil production and operation derives from kinetic and functional disorders, so important complementary material may be found in Chapters 52 and 54.

NEUTROPHIL PRODUCTION AND KINETICS

The neutrophil life cycle can be divided into bone marrow, blood, and tissue phases. Within the bone marrow is a mitotic compartment and a nonmitotic storage compartment consisting of relatively mature cells.[1] Transit time through the marrow compartment is approximately 14 days, with 6 of those days spent in the mitotic compartment. As determined by [^{32}P]-diisopropylfluorophosphate labeling studies, the bone marrow produces approximately $60–400 \times 10^7$ neutrophils/day.[2] A variety of hematopoietic growth factors drive neutrophil production and include colony-stimulating factor-granulocyte (CSF-G), colony-stimulating factor-granulocyte/macrophage (CSF-GM), interleukin-3 (IL-3), and Steel factor (also called stem cell factor or c-kit ligand).[3,4] Most of these cytokines have been shown to promote proliferation and differentiation of a stem cell compartment, comprising <0.1% of bone marrow cells, identified by their expression of the CD34 antigen and the absence of HLA and other antigens.[5,6] For a detailed treatment of growth factors and hematopoiesis, see Chapter 16.

The bone marrow storage compartment in adults contains approximately 8.8×10^9 cells, whereas blood neutrophils comprise the circulating granulocyte pool and the marginating granulocyte pool and contain 0.7×10^9 cells.[1,2] Thus, most of the neutrophils in the body reside in the bone marrow; peripheral blood counts measure <10% of total body neutrophils. Peripheral neutrophil counts vary significantly with age. During the first few days of life leukocytosis is present, with generally >10,000 neutrophils/mm^3 of blood.[7] The number rapidly falls to an average of approximately 3,000–4,000 neutrophils/mm^3, which is maintained throughout life. Absolute neutrophil counts can fall to as low as 1,000 cells/mm^3 during the first year of life; however, after that time neutrophil counts are generally >1,500 cells/mm^3. Lymphocytes generally outnumber neutrophils in children ≤2 years of age, after which neutrophils comprise >50% of peripheral blood counts.

Granulocytes from the bone marrow are released as a result of complex interactions between the mature leukocyte membrane, the endothelial lining, and the basement membrane, under the influence of a number of stimulating or releasing factors.[3,8] Once released into the blood, neutrophils have a half-life of 6–9 hours and reversibly move from circulating to marginating pools,[1,2] the latter consisting of cells attached to endothelial cells and not measured in peripheral blood neutrophil counts. The granulocytes irreversibly leave the blood by diapedesis between endothelial cells and penetration of the basement membrane (for detailed treatment of this process, see the section Neutrophil Function). Neutrophil death is generally believed to occur through apoptosis or programmed cell death.[9] Several microbial products and cytokines (including CSF-G, CSF-GM, and interferons [IFNs]) can block this process, prolonging neutrophil survival, and can presumably enhance their effectiveness at sites of inflammation.[9]

The following sections describe the development of neutrophil structure in each of its individually identifiable bone marrow precursors.

NEUTROPHIL STRUCTURE

Myeloblasts

Myeloblasts, which give rise to neutrophils as well as eosinophils and basophils, comprise ≤3% of bone marrow cells. These cells represent the earliest stage of the mitotic myeloid compartment, with a transit time of approximately 18 hours as determined by ^{32}P-labelling studies.[2] Myeloblasts vary from 10 to 15 μm in diameter and often lack morphologic features that predict their differentiation into one of the granulocytic lines. The single round nucleus contains abundant dispersed chromatin and one to four distinct nucleoli averaging 1.5 μm in diameter. The cytoplasm appears gray-blue in Wright-stained preparations and circumferentially surrounds the nucleus. Ultrastructurally, numerous polyribosomes and some segments of endoplasmic reticulum are present (Fig. 49-1). There is a variably prominent Golgi region from which the formation of the first cytoplasmic granules allows definitive identification of differentiation of myeloblasts into neutrophilic leukocytes. Ultrastructurally, peroxidase can frequently be identified in these granules or in the Golgi complex and endoplasmic reticulum.[10]

Promyelocytes

Early neutrophilic leukocytes or promyelocytes comprise approximately 2–4% of marrow cells and include a morphologic spectrum of cells involved in synthesis of lysosomal granules termed primary or azurophilic granules.[10–12] This cell is in the midstage of the mitotic compartment, with a transit time of approximately 24 hours. In Wright-stained smears, the cells average 13–18 μm in diameter, with a single round nucleus that contains predominantly dispersed nuclear chromatin and one to two nucleoli. The cytoplasm is abundant and contains numerous segments of dilated rough endoplasmic reticulum and polyribosomes, accounting for the basophilia seen in light

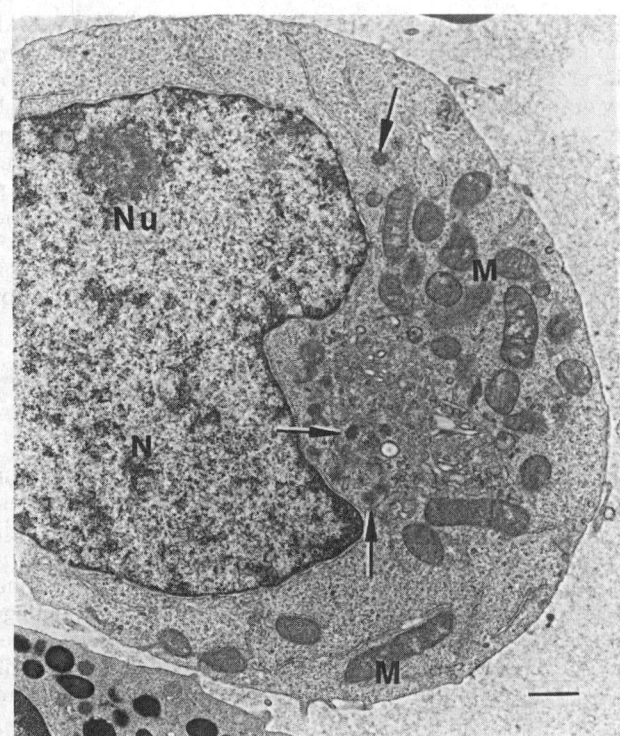

Fig. 49-1. Electron micrograph of a typical human bone marrow myeloblast. The single nucleus (N) features dispersed nuclear chromatin and a prominent nucleolus (Nu). The cytoplasm contains large mitochondria (M), sparse endoplasmic reticulum, a central Golgi region, and occasional characteristic small primary granules (arrows). Human bone marrow, stained with uranyl acetate and lead citrate. Bar = 1 μm.

have similarly demonstrated $^{35}SO_4$ incorporation into Golgi lamellae and primary granules of promyelocytes. Cationic proteins[22] and vicinal glycol-containing glycoconjugates, which include glycoprotein enzymes, can also be demonstrated ultrastructurally in immature primary granules.[23] Staining of sulfate, cations, vicinal glycols, and acid phosphatase is decreased in mature primary granules, possibly reflecting continued modification of granule contents during maturation, and results from either removal, complexing, or masking of granule components. The cytochemical observation of a similar intragranular distribution and masking of anionic glycoconjugates and acid phosphatase, together with the biochemical observation that glycosaminoglycans inhibit lysosomal enzymes, has

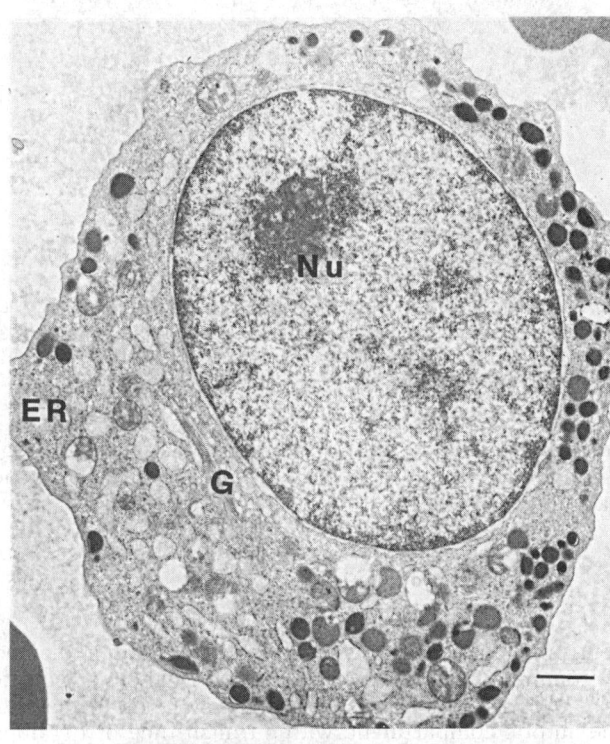

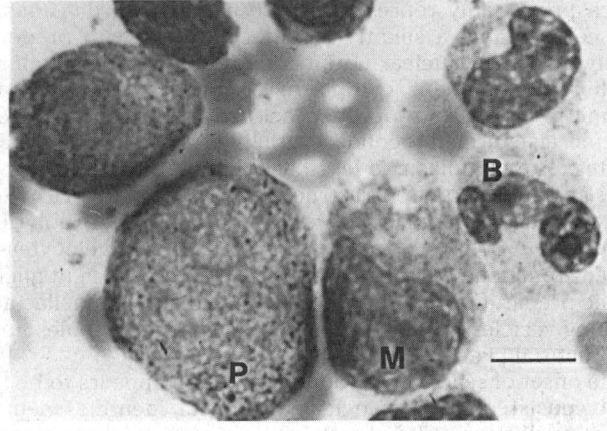

Fig. 49-2. Electron micrograph **(upper panel)** and light micrograph **(lower panel)** of human bone marrow promyelocytes. **(Upper panel)** A promyelocyte with a moderate number of cytoplasmic primary or azurophilic granules, endoplasmic reticulum (ER), and a central Golgi region (G). The large round nucleus contains dispersed nuclear chromatin and a prominent nucleolus (Nu). Electron micrograph from human bone marrow stained with uranyl acetate and lead citrate. Bar = 1 μm. **(Lower panel)** For comparison, a Wright-stained promyelocyte (P) with numerous azurophilic granules, a myelocyte (M), and a band neutrophil (B). The latter cell contains numerous secondary or specific granules that lack affinity for cationic dyes; primary granules are less prominent. Bar = 10 μm.

microscopic preparations (Fig. 49-2). Ultrastructurally, the Golgi apparatus is prominent and appears as a clear perinuclear zone in light microscopic preparations. Numerous vesicles can be observed budding from the Golgi apparatus and coalescing to form condensing vacuoles or granule precursors. Variable numbers of primary granules in different stages of maturation or condensation, or both, can be observed throughout the cytoplasm. Secondary or specific granules are not observed at the promyelocyte stage of development.

In ultrastructural preparations, primary granules vary from 0.2 to 0.4 μm in diameter. Ultrastructural cytochemistry[11,12] and biochemical studies[13–16] have identified peroxidase as the most consistent marker of this granule population (Fig. 49-3). Several biochemically distinct forms of myeloperoxidase appear to be differentially distributed in primary granule "subpopulations" and are under separate secretory control.[17] Ultrastructural studies have distinguished two types of myeloperoxidase-containing granules: one is a functionally distinct, low-density, glycoprotein-rich microgranule population[18]; the other is a physically dense, large, rim-stained granule that is poor in glycoproteins and contains increased amounts of defensins, a group of antimicrobial cationic polypeptides[19] (see the section Neutrophil Function). Acid phosphatase, β-glucuronidase, aryl sulfatase, elastase, and various proteases have also been identified in endoplasmic reticulum, Golgi vesicles, and primary granules of promyelocytes[10–12,20] or in isolated primary granules.[13–15]

Primary granules vary from deeply azurophilic to neutral in Wright-stained preparations, with the most intense staining observed in the immature granules (Fig. 49-3). This affinity for cationic dyes is reflected at the ultrastructural level by intense staining of sulfate, contained in glycosaminoglycans, including chondroitin and heparan sulfate.[21] Autoradiographic studies

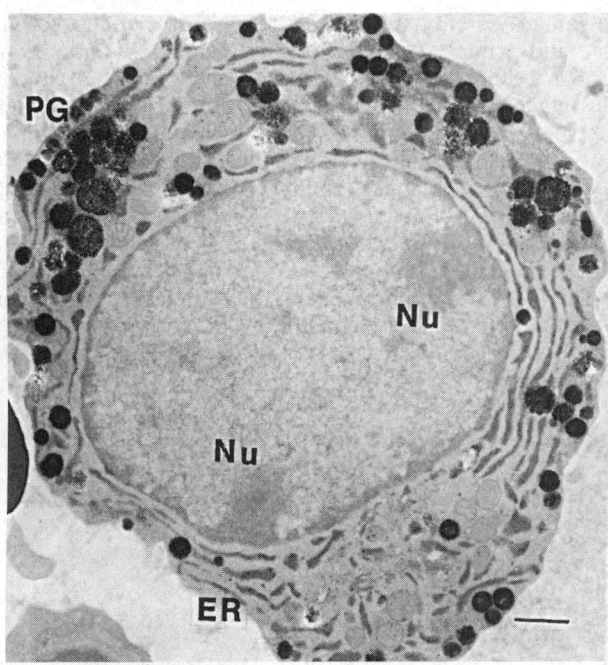

Fig. 49-3. Human bone marrow promyelocyte, stained with diaminobenzidine to show myeloperoxidase in the endoplasmic reticulum (ER) and primary granules (PG). The cell contains a single round nucleus with two nucleoli (Nu). Thin section, not counterstained. Bar = 1 μm.

resulted in speculation that primary granule glycosaminoglycans function to inactivate some enzymes and to facilitate their storage in lysosomes.[24]

Myelocytes

Neutrophilic myelocytes vary from 10 to 15 μm in diameter and comprise approximately 13% of marrow nucleated cells.[10,25] Myelocytes represent the last stage of development in the mitotic compartment, with a transit time of 104 hours, which presumably represents three to four cell divisions.[1,2] The cells contain a slightly indented nucleus with predominantly dispersed nuclear chromatin and one or two small nucleoli. The abundant cytoplasm contains numerous cytoplasmic granules, some of which lack azurophilia and represent specific, also termed secondary, granules not found in promyelocytes. The cytoplasm is less basophilic than the promyelocytes and corresponds ultrastructurally to the presence of less dilated rough endoplasmic reticulum and fewer polyribosomes. The Golgi apparatus of neutrophilic myelocytes is rather prominent, corresponding to a clear zone in light microscopic preparations, and to an area with distinct lamellae and budding vesicles forming secondary or specific granules in ultrastructural preparations.

The onset of secondary granule formation appears to be the most consistent morphologic feature that identifies neutrophilic myelocytes. Ultrastructurally, human secondary granules vary from 0.1 to 0.3 μm in diameter, are moderately dense, and may be elongated in appearance (Fig. 49-4). Although in humans the granules overlap in size with primary granules, they appear to have less osmiophilia and less affinity for metal counterstains in morphologic preparations. In most species, secondary granules outnumber primary granules by a ratio of 3:1 in late myeloid cells.

Secondary granules are recognized by their content of lactoferrin and vitamin B$_{12}$-binding protein, plus a part of the intracellular store of phagocyte cytochrome b$_{558}$.[23,26–29] In sucrose

and Percoll gradients, secondary or specific granules generally demonstrate less physical density than most primary or azurophilic granules,[13–15] although some overlap in density with primary granules does occur.[29] Secondary granules appear to be heterogeneous in that subpopulations with different contents of lactoferrin and vitamin B$_{12}$-binding protein exhibit different responses to cytosolic free calcium.[30] In fact, Rice[29] has reported the isolation of 13 distinct granule fractions from human neutrophils. Secondary granules lack peroxidase (Fig. 49-5), acid phosphatase, elastase, acidic glycoproteins, sulfated glycosaminoglycans, cations, and cationic proteins found in primary granules.

Late Neutrophils

Metamyelocytes as well as band and segmented neutrophils represent nondividing cells in which a progressive condensation of nuclear chromatin occurs and nucleoli become indistinct. In fully developed cells, an average of three nuclear lobes with fully condensed nuclear chromatin may be identified (Figs. 49-3 to 49-5). In females, distinct drumstick appendages corresponding to the inactivated X chromosome may be seen, although these may be confused with less distinct club-like appendages seen in both males and females. The Golgi appara-

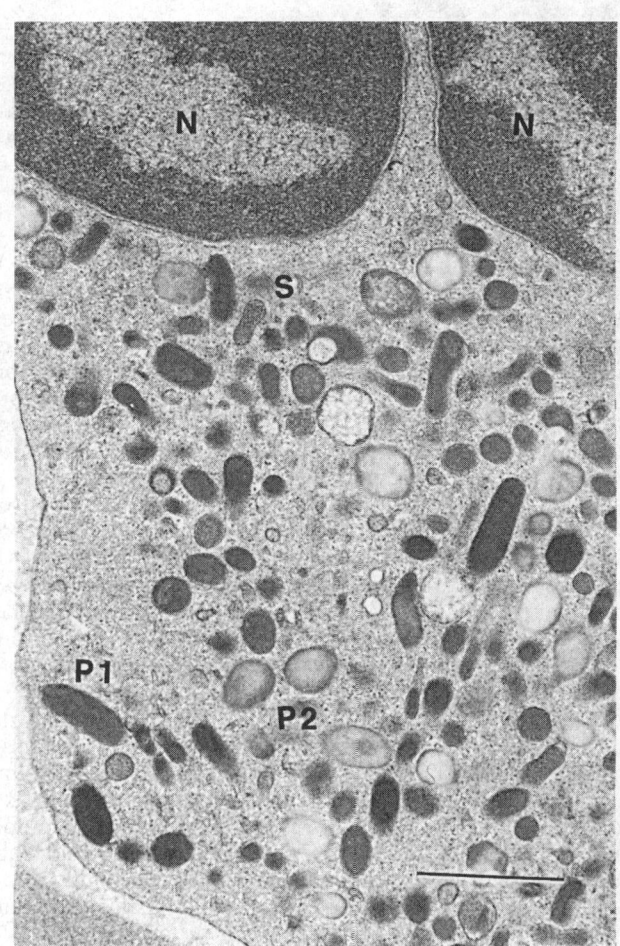

Fig. 49-4. Enlarged portion of human neutrophil cytoplasm, demonstrating nuclei (N) and a variety of cytoplasmic granules. Primary granules are generally larger and tend to have a uniformly dense (P1) or rim density (P2) type of staining. Presumed secondary granules (S) tend to be smaller and are moderately dense, often overlapping in size with primary granules. Peripheral blood stained with uranyl acetate and lead citrate. Bar = 1 μm.

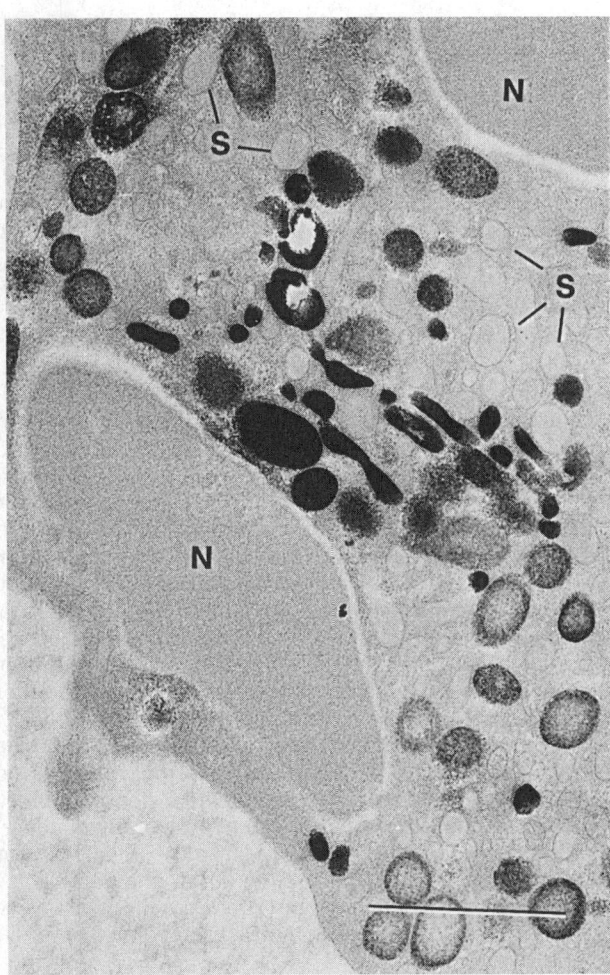

Fig. 49-5. Human peripheral blood neutrophil. Intense diaminobenzidine staining of myeloperoxidase is evident in primary granules, whereas more numerous secondary (S) granules lack staining. Peroxidase may also be found in a microgranule population (M) and in larger uniformly stained (P1) and rim stained (P2) granules. Portions of two nuclear lobes (N) are evident. Bar = 1 μm.

tus is much less prominent than in early and midmyeloid cells, and the cytoplasm contains very little endoplasmic reticulum. Mitochondria are fewer and no large increase in granules occurs in segmented neutrophils as compared with metamyelocytes. Glycogen is prominent in late (Fig. 49-6), in contrast to early, myeloid cells.

Tertiary granules are found in late neutrophils, where they appear to be actively synthesized. These granules are smaller than most primary and secondary granules, varying from 0.1 to 0.2 μm in diameter in humans. Ultrastructurally, they are moderately electron-dense and stain for acid phosphatase, aryl sulfatase, and sulfated glycosaminoglycans,[21] but lack peroxidase. Electron microscopy with cytochemical stains has resulted in the identification of an average of three to four granules for each cell section, although some studies have suggested a higher frequency for this granule type. Consistent with the active synthesis of these granules in late neutrophils, the Golgi apparatus stains for acid phosphatase and sulfated glycosaminoglycans; sulfate incorporation into the Golgi region, and eventually into tertiary granules, has been demonstrated using cytochemical and radioautographic methods.

The size, density distribution, and biochemical, cytochemical, and functional properties of neutrophil granules are not entirely consistent with a simple two- or three-granule model. Heterogeneity of both primary and secondary granules has been demonstrated,[16–19,29,31] and variable descriptions of ter-

tiary granules exist in the literature.[21,32] While some, if not all, of this heterogeneity appears to be related to maturation and continued programmed or environmental modification of preformed granules, further studies are required to determine whether more than three de novo granule types are produced by neutrophils.

In addition to cytoplasmic granules, a variety of vesicles are present in late neutrophils. Some of these contain hydrolases being transported from the Golgi region to nascent tertiary granules.[21] Some vesicles appear to be derived from the plasmalemma and may contain endocytosed material or nicotinamide adenine dinucleotide phosphate (NADPH) oxidase.[26,28] Other vesicles appear to contain elastase-like enzymes. Alkaline phosphatase, which stains strongly in late neutrophils, is confined to vesicles that are translocated to the cell surface on neutrophil activation[26,30] (see the section Neutrophil Function). Lipid droplets may also be identified within the neutrophil cytoplasm.

The neutrophil cytoskeleton is composed primarily of microfilaments and microtubules that function in formation of cell shape, locomotion, attachment, phagocytosis, and exocytosis.[33] Microtubules measuring approximately 20–25 nm in diameter are arranged in a stellate configuration around centrioles generally located in the perinuclear cytoplasm near the Golgi region. The centriole appears to function in organizing the microtubules and consists of nine sets of triplet microtubules (Fig. 49-7). Microfilaments corresponding to actin are distributed throughout the cytoplasm and average 7 nm in diameter. Circulating neutrophils have a spherical appearance, with

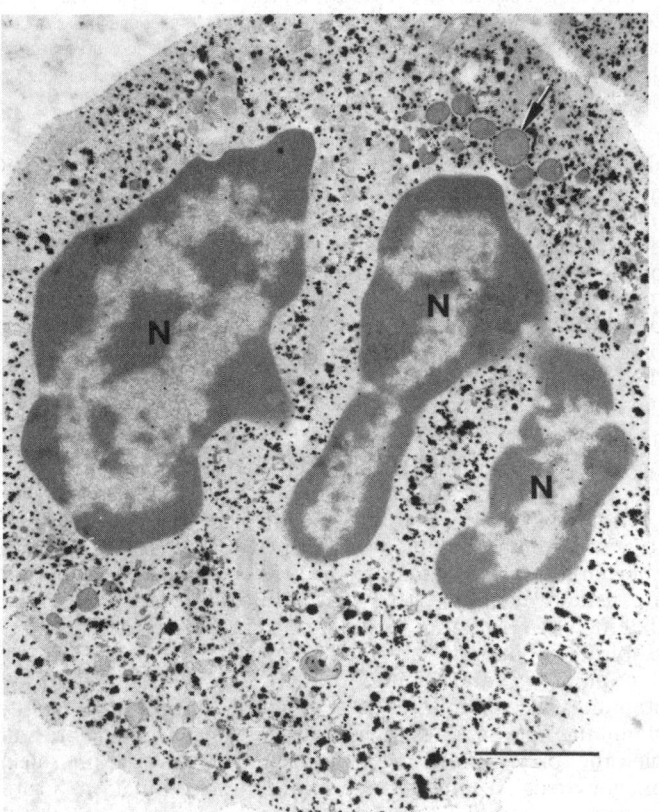

Fig. 49-6. Segmented neutrophil. Intense staining of particulate glycogen is scattered throughout the cytoplasm and corresponds to the intense periodic acid-Schiff (PAS) staining seen in neutrophils at the light microscope level. Finer staining of glycoprotein is evident in cytoplasmic granules (arrow). Nuclear lobes (N) are evident. Thin section stained with periodate-thiocarbohydrazide-silver proteinate. Bar = 1 μm.

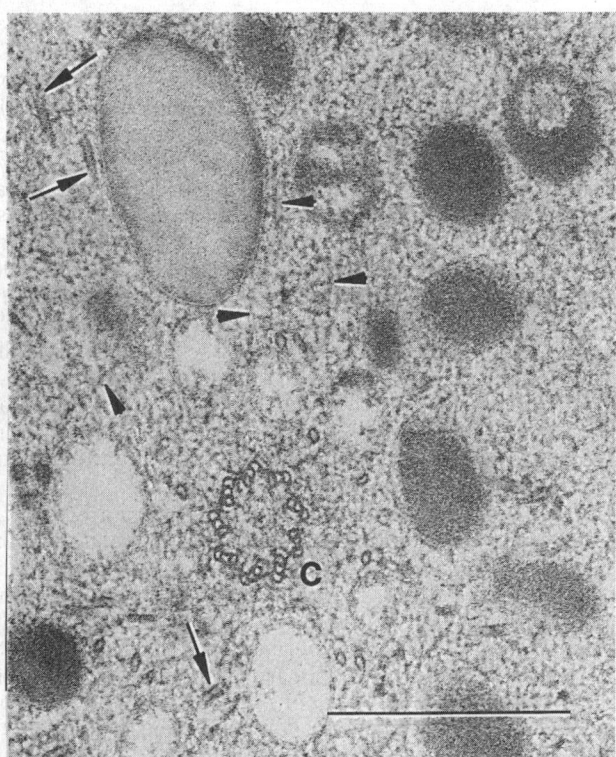

Fig. 49-7. Electron micrograph of a neutrophil prepared by freeze substitution. A centriole cut in cross-section illustrates nine sets of triplet microtubules (C). At a further distance from the centriole are more longitudinally sectioned microtubules (arrows). Smaller (7-nm diameter) actin filaments (arrowheads) are scattered through the cytoplasm. Thin section stained with uranyl acetate and lead citrate. Bar = 0.5 μm.

some cytoplasmic projections and surface ruffles (Fig. 49-8); however their shape changes dramatically with attachment, migration, and phagocytosis. After neutrophil activation, the distribution of microfilaments appears more peripheral and becomes asymmetric, and the cell shape changes from round to polar.[34] Particle phagocytosis involves transitions of actin between filamentous and soluble forms to permit extension of pseudopodia and invagination of the phagocytic vesicle (see the following section).

NEUTROPHIL FUNCTION

The essential function of the neutrophil is to move rapidly to a site of microbial invasion and then to engulf and kill the microorganism. The complex processes of phagocytic function are usually divided, somewhat artificially, into components that include (1) migration and ingestion, (2) degranulation, (3) respiratory burst activity, and (4) cytokine response and production. However, it is important to keep in mind that many stimuli evoke multiple effector functions that proceed either simultaneously or in rapidly overlapping succession. For example, the process evocatively termed "regurgitation during phagocytosis" frequently occurs when degranulation, a rapid response to stimulation, begins prior to closure of a phagocytic vacuole, thus releasing granule contents into the surrounding environment as well as into the nascent vacuole. Furthermore, a single receptor may be involved in more than one part of the neutrophil response; for example, the CD11b/CD18 integrin (see below) serves both as an adhesion molecule that mediates adherence to blood vessel walls and as a receptor for the complement component C3bi that induces neutrophil activation.

Migration and Ingestion

The earliest recognized distinguishing features of phagocytes, classically described by Metchnikoff,[35] are directed movement (i.e., chemotaxis) and ingestion. These related activities result from adhesive interactions between paired adhesion molecules on the neutrophil and endothelium and from active changes in the organization and assembly of the neutrophil actin and cytoskeletal networks.

The first step in neutrophil recruitment to a site of inflammation is the detection of the inflammatory process, either by perception of a gradient of chemoattractant molecules or by binding to adhesion molecules presented to circulating leukocytes by activated endothelial cells. Neutrophils respond to chemotactic stimuli of diverse origins and chemical structures. The root term *chemotaxis* refers to the process in which neutrophils, or other motile cells, detect a ligand (often at levels as low as 10^{-9}mol/L) and then follow the concentration gradient toward its origin.[36] At higher concentrations, most of the chemoattractants also stimulate the neutrophil to generate a brief respiratory burst (see the section Respiratory Burst Activity).

Neutrophils possess an array of chemotactic receptors, and identification of additional receptor molecules and genes is rapidly expanding at this time.[37,38] Table 49-1 presents the characteristics of several receptors that have a known functional importance. Peptide chemoattractants originate at sites of inflammation, from both complement activation and the release of bacterial products, including the formyl oligopeptides unique to prokaryotes and their intracellular descendants, the mitochondria. The formyl peptide receptor is also known as the FMLP receptor, based on its best known ligand, formylmethionyl-leucyl-phenylalanine. The lipid chemoattractants are generated by cytokine-activated endothelial cells as well as by neutrophils themselves in a positive feedback loop. They

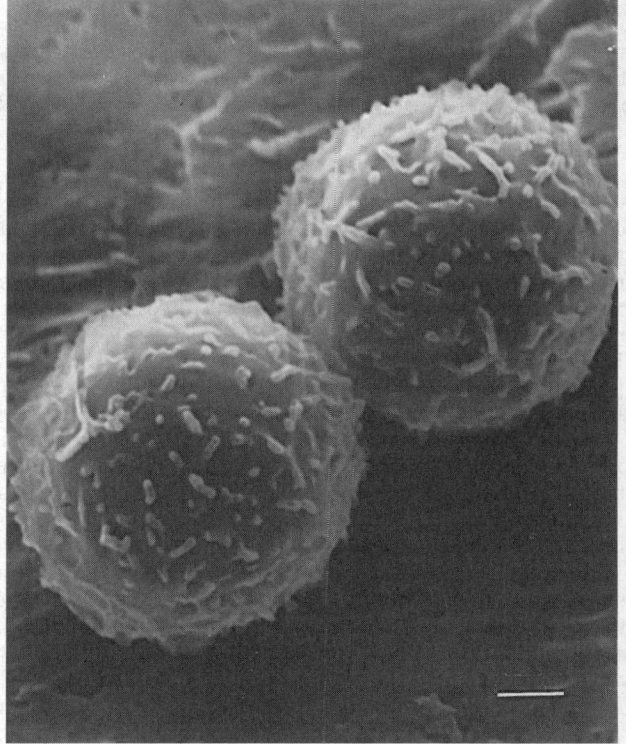

Fig. 49-8. Scanning electron micrograph of two peripheral blood neutrophils. The isolated neutrophils were fixed in suspension resulting in a spherical shape as seen for circulating neutrophils. The surface contains numerous cytoplasmic projections and occasional ruffles. Bar = 1 μm.

Table 49-1. Neutrophil Chemotactic Receptors

Receptor (Chemoattractant)	Ligand	Source of Ligand	Function
	Peptides		
C5aR	C5a	Complement activation	Chemotaxis, activation
FPR	N-formyl peptides	Bacteria, mitochondria	Chemotaxis, activation
	Lipids		
—	Leukotriene B₄	Neutrophils, monocytes, endothelial and other cells	Chemotaxis, activation
PAFR	Platelet-activating factor	Neutrophils, monocytes, endothelial and other cells	Chemotaxis, activation
	α-Chemokines		
IL-8RA, IL-8RB	IL-8	Monocytes, endothelial and other cells	Chemotaxis, activation
	GRO-α	Monocytes, endothelial and other cells	Chemotaxis, activation
	NAP-2	Platelets	Activation

Abbreviations: FPR, N-formyl peptide receptor. IL-8RA and -B, interleukin-8 receptors A and B; NAP-2, neutrophil-activating protein-2; PAFR, platelet-activating factor receptor.

mediate both local inflammatory activities and recruitment of neutrophils into sites of inflammation.[39,40]

Unlike the other, highly specific, chemoattractant receptors, the two forms of high-affinity IL-8 receptor (IL-8RA and IL-8RB) also bind other members of the α-chemokine family with varying affinities.[38] The α-chemokine family includes IL-8; GROα, GROβ, and GROγ; and neutrophil-activating protein-2 (NAP-2). The β-chemokines (such as MCP-1 and RANTES) do not interact with neutrophils. These intercellular signaling proteins, named for their combined *chemo*tactic and cyto*kine* properties, recruit neutrophils and mononuclear phagocytes to sites of inflammation. IL-8 and the GRO cytokines are generated by monocytes, macrophages, and mesenchymal cells (including endothelial cells, fibroblasts, epithelial cells, and hepatocytes) on stimulation by other inflammatory cytokines such as IL-1 and tumor necrosis factor (TNF).[41,42] NAP-2 is generated through the cleavage of platelet secretory products by cathepsin G from neutrophil or monocyte granules.[43]

The primary structures for all of these chemoattractant receptor molecules, except that for leukotriene B₄, have been determined by molecular cloning of their cDNA.[37,38] Despite the great diversity of their ligands, all of the receptors share the structural and functional features that define the seven transmembrane-domain receptor family. As the name implies, all members of the family have seven segments of the hydrophobic amino acid sequence; these are highly conserved within the seven transmembrane-domain receptor superfamily, which also includes receptors involved in signal transduction for vision, olfaction, hormone action, cell proliferation, and neurotransmission.[44] All members of the receptor superfamily accomplish signal transduction for neutrophil activation by association with heterotrimeric G proteins (see Ch. 6).

Most neutrophil locomotion and phagocytic activity takes place in tissues. In order to exit the circulation and enter the tissues, neutrophils must adhere to the vessel walls and migrate through the vascular endothelium. The transmigration process involves multiple stages of interaction between the surface receptors and enzymes of the neutrophil with molecules on endothelial cells and in the basement membrane (Fig. 49-9). The circulating neutrophil (Fig. 49-9, left) possesses che-

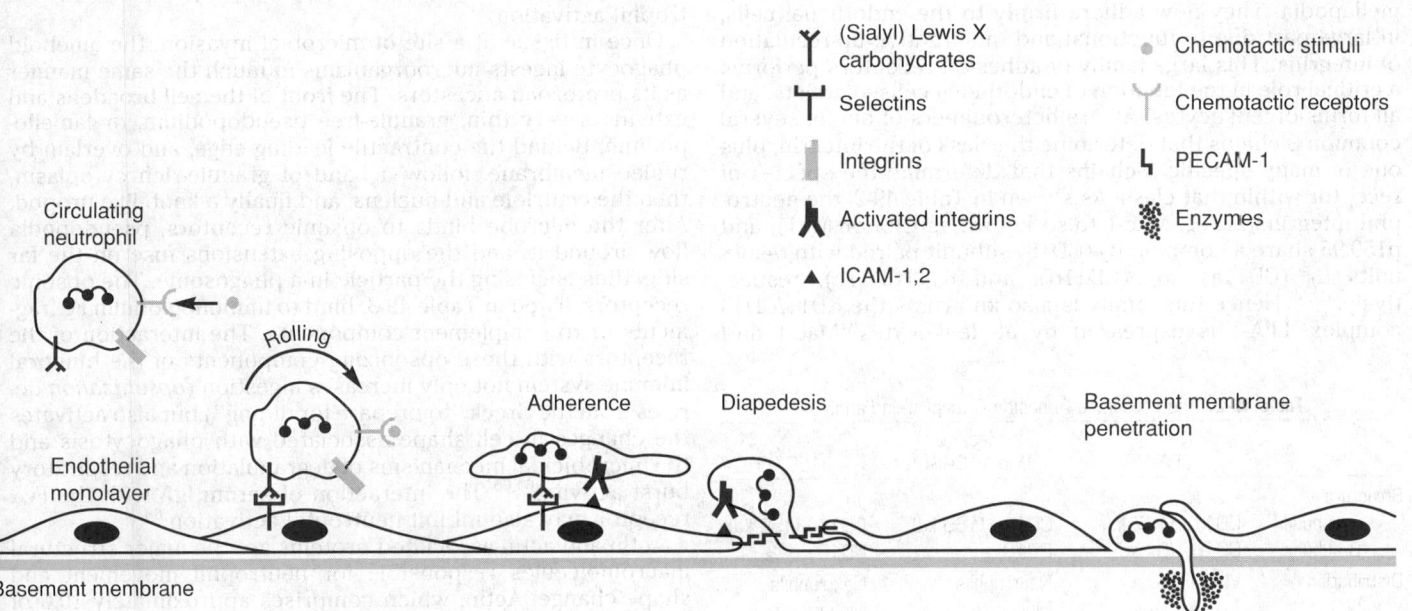

Fig. 49-9. Schematic diagram of neutrophil interactions with vascular endothelium. Starting from the left: (1) circulating neutrophil, with representative surface molecules: unoccupied chemotactic receptor, (sialyl) Lewis X carbohydrate, and unactivated integrin; (2) rolling neutrophil, with loose adherence to endothelium mediated by selectin binding to (sialyl) Lewis X; (3) adherent neutrophil, with strong adhesion mediated by binding of activated integrin to endothelial cell ICAM; (4) diapedesis of neutrophil between endothelial cells, mediated by binding of neutrophil PECAM-1 to its endothelial homologue; and (5) penetration of the basement membrane, mediated by secreted hydrolytic enzymes.

motactic receptors that respond to corresponding chemotactic factors, here illustrated as a soluble molecule in the blood plasma. It also has surface carbohydrates and adhesion molecules, the latter in an unactivated form.

The next step in transmigration is a weak, reversible, rolling interaction with the endothelial lining of blood vessels, particularly in postcapillary venules.[45,46] At any time, a small percentage of neutrophils leaves the central stream of flowing blood to roll along the endothelium and then return to the stream; this shifting subpopulation, although located in the margins of blood vessels, is not the same as the marginating pool of neutrophils discussed above (see the section Neutrophil Production and Kinetics). Transition of neutrophils to the rolling state is stimulated by endothelial surface IL-8 and other chemotactic factors; the weak adherence is mediated by the interactions of selectins with their carbohydrate ligands.[45,46] The selectin family of leukocyte adhesion molecules comprises glycoproteins that bind specific carbohydrates[47,48] and mediate leukocyte adhesion and homing. P-selectin (CD62), the most important member for neutrophil adhesion, is located in α-granules of platelets and Weibel-Palade bodies of endothelial cells. Activation of endothelia by inflammatory cytokines (such as IFN-γ, IL-1, and TNF-α) causes rapid P-selectin expression on the cell surface, where it binds the neutrophil surface carbohydrates Lewis X (CD15; $Gal\beta1{\rightarrow}4(Fuc\alpha1{\rightarrow}3)GlcNac{\rightarrow}R$) and sialyl-Lewis^X, which are present on multiple glycoproteins and glycolipids.[49] Other members of the selectin family include L-selectin, constitutively present on neutrophils and monocytes, and E-selectin, present on endothelial cells and up-regulated by inflammatory cytokines with a 1–8 hour lag for de novo protein synthesis. L-selectin can mediate neutrophil rolling in vivo,[46] but the severe compromise of neutrophil rolling and delayed recruitment to peritoneal inflammation in P-selectin-deficient mice produced by gene "knock-out"[50] demonstrates the relative primacy of attachment via P-selectin.

Rolling neutrophils may detach and return to the circulation, or may undergo the changes depicted in the third panel of Figure 49-9. Activated neutrophils shed L-selectin and undergo a shape change from rounded to flattened, with extending lamellapodia. They now adhere firmly to the endothelial cells, in large part due to functional and quantitative up-regulation of integrins. This large family of adhesion receptors performs a critical role in the function of endothelial cells, platelets, and all forms of leukocytes. All are heterodimers of one of several common β-chains that determine the class of the integrin, plus one of many specific α-chains that determine the species of receptor within that class. As shown in Table 49-2, the neutrophil integrins LFA-1, Mac-1 (also known as CR3 or Mo1), and p150,95 share a common β_2-(CD18) subunit paired with α-subunits α_L (CD11a), α_M (CD11b), and α_X (CD11c), respectively.[51–53] Hence this family is also known as the CD11/CD18 complex. LFA-1 is expressed by all leukocytes; Mac-1 and p150,95 are expressed by neutrophils, monocytes, and some lymphocytes. The major endothelial counter-receptors for the neutrophil integrins include intercellular adhesion molecules (ICAMs), members of the immunoglobulin supergene family.[52,54,55] Evidence exists for at least one additional, as yet unidentified, endothelial counter-receptor for p150,95 and possibly for Mac-1.[52] ICAM-1, but not ICAM-2, undergoes up-regulation at sites of inflammation due to the activation of endothelial cells by inflammatory cytokines.[56] The leukocyte adhesion proteins are stored in secretory vesicles in resting cells, and then expressed on the surface membrane on neutrophil activation.[57–59] In addition to this increase in the number of surface receptors, integrins in activated neutrophils undergo a conformational change to an increased affinity state.[53] The severe recurrent infections that occur in patients with leukocyte adhesion deficiency (see Ch. 54) demonstrate the physiologic importance of integrin-mediated adhesion to host defense. Blockade of integrin binding to counter-receptors has shown promise for the reduction of tissue damage from inflammation and ischemia-reperfusion injury.[60,61]

The last two steps of transmigration are diapedesis between endothelial cells and penetration of the basement membrane (Figs. 49-9 and 49-10). Neutrophils actively move between endothelial cells in a process dependent on (1) loosening of intercellular junctions in the endothelium, (2) adhesion of Mac-1 and LFA-1 to endothelial ICAM-1, and (3) homologous association of neutrophil and endothelial PECAM-1 (CD31; platelet and endothelial cellular adhesion molecule), another member of the immunoglobulin supergene family.[62] Figure 49-10 presents an electron micrograph of neutrophil diapedesis. The leading edge has migrated between endothelial cells and lies sandwiched between the endothelial and basement membrane layers of a postcapillary venule. To make the final step of the journey from blood to tissue, the neutrophil must digest a hole in the basement membrane by release of lytic enzymes from secretory granules (for details, see the section Degranulation). These products include collagenase, elastase, gelatinase, and other hydrolases; they are released in response to chemotactic factors, generally at lower levels than are required for full neutrophil activation.[63]

Once in tissue at a site of microbial invasion, the ameboid phagocyte ingests microorganisms in much the same manner as its protozoan ancestors. The front of the cell broadens and extends a very thin, granule-free pseudopodium, or lamellopodium. Behind the contractile leading edge, and overlain by ruffled membrane, follow a band of granule-rich cytoplasm, then the centriole and nucleus, and finally a knob-like uropod. After the microbe binds to opsonic receptors, pseudopodia flow around it, and the opposing extensions fuse on the far side, thus enclosing the particle in a phagosome. The opsonic receptors, listed in Table 49-3, bind to immunoglobulin Fc fragments or to complement components. The interaction of the receptors with these opsonizing components of the humoral immune system not only increases ingestion (*opsonization* derives from the Greek "to prepare for dining") but also activates the changes in cell shape associated with phagocytosis and the microbicidal mechanisms of degranulation and respiratory burst activity.[64,65] The interaction of serum IgA with the Fcα receptor may also inhibit neutrophil activation.[66]

Actin and actin-associated proteins are the major structural macromolecules responsible for neutrophil movement and shape change. Actin, which comprises approximately 10% of the neutrophil protein content, exists in soluble form as a globular 42.5 kd monomer and in gel form as double helical filaments.[67] The filaments align in parallel bundles when purified, but in the intracellular environment they form a highly branched network due to angled junctions formed by actin-binding protein and other actin cross-linkers.[68,69] Actin-binding protein and a rapidly expanding array of other proteins also

Table 49-2. The Leukocyte Adhesion Glycoprotein Family

	LFA-1	Mac-1 (Mo-1, CR3)	p150,95
Structure			
α-subunit	CD11a (177 kd)	CD11b (165 kd)	CD11c (150 kd)
β-subunit	CD18 (94 kd)	CD18	CD18
Distribution	Virtually all leukocytes	Neutrophils Monocytes Large granular lymphocytes	Neutrophils Monocytes Large granular lymphocytes Some T cells
Ligands	ICAM-1, ICAM-2, ICAM-3	ICAM-1, C3bi, matrix proteins	C3bi, ?other endothelial ligands

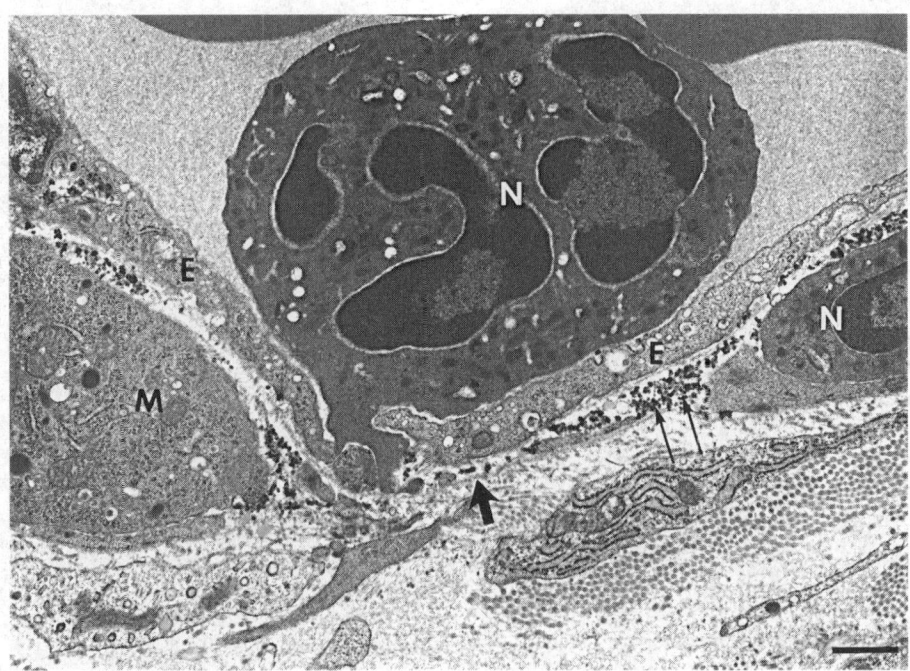

Fig. 49-10. Rat neutrophil (N) performing diapedesis across the venular wall between endothelial cells (E). Another neutrophil and a macrophage (M) are temporarily arrested in the venular wall between the endothelial cells and the basement membrane (thick arrow). Rat cremasteric muscle 2 hours after subcutaneous injection of histamine and an intravenous injection of carbon black to demonstrate the potential space between the endothelium and basement membrane. Histamine induces venular endothelial cells to contract and to form gaps; carbon black (thin arrows) has exited the blood vessel but is retained by the basement membrane. Bar = 1 μm. (Photomicrograph by I. Joris and J. M. Underwood.)

contribute to the connections of the actin lattice to the cell membrane. Some of these connections (such as those involving integrins, talin, vinculin, and others) provide strong anchors through the membrane to neighboring cells or the extracellular matrix and thus provide the necessary "traction" for movement. Others are important for the regulation of cell shape, such as the connection via actin-binding protein to FcγRI, which releases on binding of ligand to the receptor.

The regulation of actin filament length involves a large group of proteins that specifically interact with actin monomers or filaments; under the influence of intracellular second messengers, they promote the assembly or disassembly of filaments.[68,69] A dynamic cycle of actin assembly and disassembly (Fig. 49-11) continually remodels the actin network at the leading lamella of motile cells. The filaments exhibit polarity, with the "barbed" end growing more rapidly due to higher affinity for monomers. Calcium and diacylglycerol inhibit filament assembly and promote disassembly by increasing the affinity of binding proteins (including gelsolin and many others) that fragment actin filaments and cap the barbed ends. In addition,

these "second messengers" of receptor activation increase sequestration of actin monomers by other escort proteins (including profilin and others) and thus further inhibit assembly. On the other side of the cycle, second messenger polyphosphoinositides (PIP and PIP$_2$) switch on actin assembly by decreasing the affinity of the escort proteins, resulting in uncapping of barbed filament ends and desequestration of monomers. During chemotaxis, the activation of chemotactic receptors promotes actin assembly at the leading edge of the moving cell, while net disassembly occurs at the rear of the lamella. The growth of filaments in the network helps direct the flow of escort-bound monomers and filament fragments toward the front to provide material for further extension, as well as endocytic vesicles that recycle chemotactic and adhesion receptors back to the leading edge to provide signaling and traction, respectively.

The source for generation of force by the neutrophil actin remodeling remains controversial.[69] Movement of membrane-bound myosin I along the actin filaments may push the membrane forward,[70] but the means of attachment of myosin to the

Table 49-3. Neutrophil Opsonic Receptors

Receptor	Ligands	Source of Ligand	Function
Fc fragment of immunoglobulin			
FcγR I	Monomeric IgG	IgG + antigen (high-affinity)	Opsonic adherence
FcγR II	Complexed IgG	IgG-antigen complex (low-affinity)	Phagocytosis
FcγR IIIB	Complexed IgG	IgG-antigen complex (low-affinity)	Opsonic adherence, activation, antibody-dependent cytotoxicity
FcαR	IgA	Polymeric IgA	Phagocytosis, activation, inhibition, antibody-dependent cytotoxicity
Complement components			
CR1	C3b, C4b	Complement activation	Phagocytosis
CR3[a]	C3bi	Complement activation	Phagocytosis, activation

[a] CR3 (CD11b/CD18) also serves as an adhesion receptor (see Table 49-2).

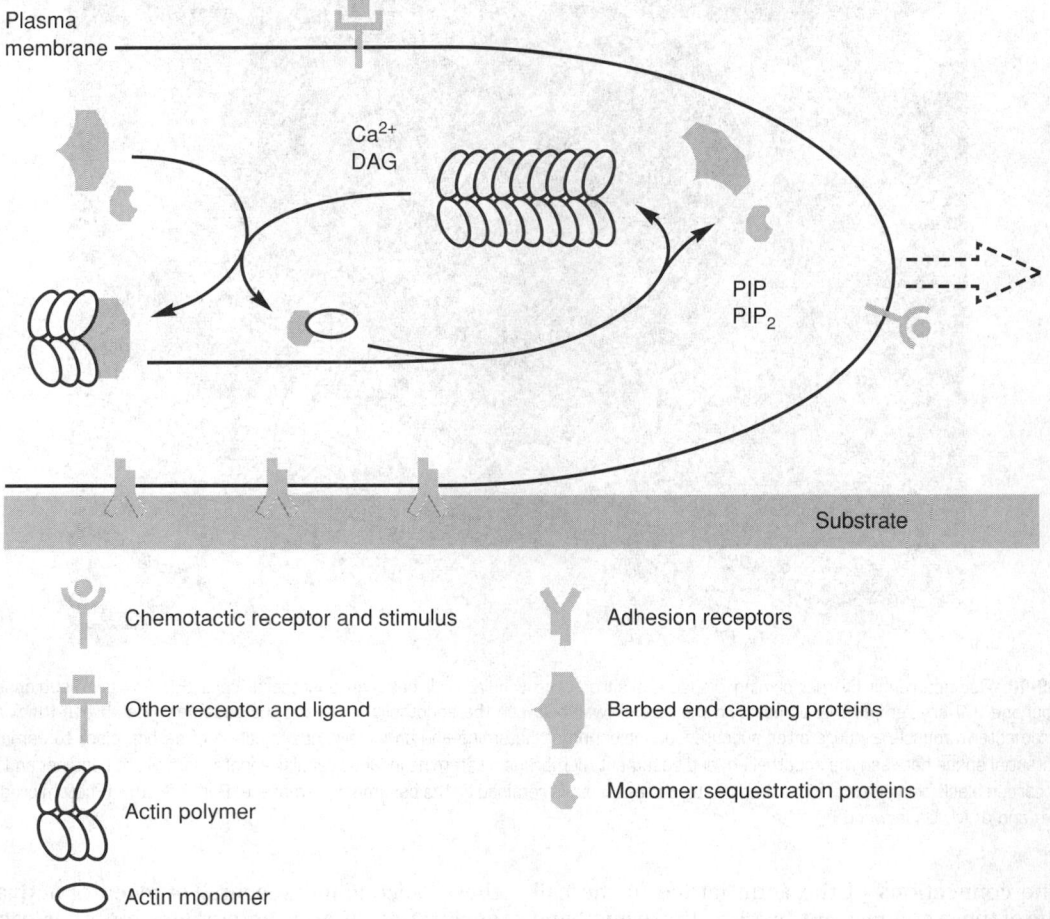

Plasma membrane

Ca²⁺
DAG

PIP
PIP₂

Substrate

Y	Chemotactic receptor and stimulus		Y	Adhesion receptors
T	Other receptor and ligand			Barbed end capping proteins
Actin polymer				Monomer sequestration proteins
Actin monomer				

Fig. 49-11. Schematic diagram of the actin cycle in the leading lamella of a moving neutrophil. Receptor-mediated signal transduction by Ca²⁺ and diacylglycerol (DAG) inhibit filament assembly and promote disassembly by increasing the affinity of binding proteins that (1) fragment actin filaments and cap the barbed ends and (2) sequester actin monomers. On the other side of the cycle, chemotactic receptor activation generates polyphosphoinositides (PIP and PIP₂) that switch on actin assembly by decreasing the affinity of the actin-binding proteins, resulting in actin filament growth by addition of free monomers to the uncapped barbed filament ends. Activated adhesion receptors provide traction by adherence to the underlying endothelium or extracellular matrix. (Adapted from Stossel et al.,[68] with permission.)

membrane remain unknown, and the actin-myosin interaction certainly differs from that of muscle cells. Other possibilities are localized osmotic swelling at sites of actin solvation and brownian motion of actin filaments, with net forward motion due to addition of actin monomers to the leading end of the fiber whenever space is provided by either mechanism.

Degranulation

Granule populations are classically subdivided histochemically into peroxidase-positive primary or azurophilic granules and peroxidase-negative secondary or specific granules. However, subcellular fractionation studies indicate the presence of at least two additional forms of packaging for secretion and probably considerable heterogeneity within each group. Table 49-4 shows a current classification of neutrophil secretory organelles and their contents.[63] Many proteins localize to more than one type of granule, and, conversely, all granules of a given population may not contain exactly the same array of ingredients. Granule matrix contents are the true secretory products that diffuse into the surrounding medium on degranulation. Most are synthesized in the cell during myeloid development; however, the secretory vesicles,[26] which are probably similar in appearance but are probably distinct from endocytic

vesicles, also contain accumulated plasma proteins. The contents of the granule membrane generally remain in the neutrophil plasma membrane after granules fuse during exocytosis, so the secondary granules and secretory vesicles in particular serve as an intracellular pool for the addition of important membrane components such as Mac-1 and cytochrome b₅₅₈ (a component of the respiratory burst apparatus).

Neutrophils mobilize the secretory organelles as a part of the receptor-mediated activation response that also includes shape change, movement, and respiratory burst activity. The azurophilic granules, which contain proteins used primarily for microbial killing and digestion, discharge into phagosomes in response to the same stimuli (mediated by Fc and complement receptors) that initiate phagocytosis. The other compartments also respond to chemotactic stimuli, mediated by localized increases in intracellular calcium concentration. As the calcium level rises, the organelles mobilize in order of increasing size and density, so first the secretory vesicles fuse with the plasma membrane and discharge their contents, followed by the gelatinase-containing granules, and then the secondary granules as receptor stimulation and calcium concentration continue to ascend.[63]

Gelatinase (also termed tertiary)[71] and secondary granules overlap somewhat in their contents, but the shared proteins are generally distributed largely in one compartment or the

Table 49-4. Neutrophil Secretory Organelles: Major Classes and Contents[a]

Primary (Azurophilic)	Secondary (Specific)	Gelatinase (Tertiary)	Secretory Vesicle
Membrane	Membrane	Membrane	Membrane
CD63	CD15 (Lewis X)	Formyl peptide receptor	Alkaline phosphatase
CD68	Cytochrome b_{558}	[Mac-1]	CD10 (CALLA)[b]
	Formyl peptide receptor		[Cytochrome b_{558}]
	Fibronectin receptor		?FcγRIII
	G proteins (Rap1,2; G_α subunits)		Formyl peptide receptor
	Laminin receptor		Mac-1
	[Mac-1]		
	Thrombospondin receptor		
	Tumor necrosis factor receptor		
	Vitronectin receptor		
Matrix	Matrix	Matrix	Vesicle contents
α_1-antitrypsin	Collagenase	Acetyltransferase	Plasma proteins
α-mannosidase	[Gelatinase]	Gelatinase	
Bacteriocidal/permeability-increasing agent	Heparanase		
β-glucuronidase	Histaminase		
β-glycerophosphatase	Lactoferrin		
Cathepsins B, D, and G	Lysozyme		
Cationic proteins	Plasminogen activator		
Defensins	B_{12}-binding protein		
Elastase			
Lysozyme			
Myeloperoxidase			
N-acetyl-β-glucosaminidase			
Proteinase 3			

[a] Brackets indicate a relatively minor part of the distribution of the indicated component.

[b] Common acute lymphocytic leukemia antigen, a neutral endopeptidase that cleaves biologically active peptides, including formyl peptide chemoattractants, angiotensins I and II, enkephalins, bradykinin, neurotensin, oxytocin, and substance P.

(Adapted from Borregaard et al.,[63] with permission.)

other, indicated in Table 49-4 by brackets around each entry that represents the minor portion. They represent two ends of a spectrum of heterogeneous peroxidase-negative granule packaging, with several mixed populations in between, sharing multiple components.[71] Secondary granules are classically defined by their content of lactoferrin, an iron-binding protein that has direct bacteriocidal activity and helps catalyze iron-dependent oxygen free radical reactions (see the section Respiratory Burst Activity).[72,73] However, they also contain a part of the intracellular store of cytochrome b_{558}, collagenase, and an array of integrins and other adhesive proteins (including receptors for laminin, fibrinogen, fibronectin, and vitronectin) that have led to the alternate name of *adhesosome*.[58] However, recent recognition of rapidly mobilized secretory vesicles[59,74] has led to reassignment of part or all of the adhesive protein reserve to the vesicle compartment. Patients with secondary granule deficiency, who fail to mobilize the specific granules to the cell surface, show decreased chemotaxis but do not have as severe a defect in host defense as those without CD11/CD18 integrins (see Ch. 54).

Azurophilic granules are histochemically defined by their content of myeloperoxidase, an important part of the respiratory burst microbicidal system. They also possess several proteins capable of oxygen-independent microbicidal activity.[75] Bactericidal/permeability-increasing agent is a 58-kd, highly cationic, lysine-rich protein capable of killing certain strains of gram-negative bacteria by increasing membrane permeability, as the name implies.[76] Cathepsin G, a neutral protease with chymotrypsin-like activity, kills both gram-positive and -negative bacteria as well as yeast forms of *Candida* spp.[77] The defensins are a group of small (M_r 30,000–40,000) cystine-rich cyclic polypeptides that make up approximately 5% of the neutrophil total protein by weight. They are cytotoxic to metabolically active bacteria and fungi, enveloped viruses, and even

some normal and transformed human cells in vitro.[78,79] Lysozyme has long been known as a bactericidal agent[80]; the enzyme hydrolyzes the glycosidic bonds of cell wall peptidoglycans containing acetylmuramic acid, leading directly to lysis of susceptible bacteria.[81]

The molecular mechanisms of granule membrane fusion and matrix release have attracted considerable attention. Much of the research has used secretory granule systems from other cell types, but the findings are probably applicable to neutrophils. Cytosolic fusogenic proteins identified in chromaffin cells and neurons include a large class of annexins.[82] Three of them have also been found in neutrophils, where they bind to phospholipid membranes and promote membrane fusion and granule aggregation in response to calcium and diacylglycerol.[83] The secretory granule matrix may also play an active role in product release by rapidly swelling in response to negative electrical potential.[84]

Respiratory Burst Activity

Neutrophils and other phagocytes kill microorganisms by generating reactive oxygen species with potent microbicidal activity. The severity of infections when this system is defective, such as in chronic granulomatous disease, demonstrates the prime importance of the oxygen-dependent microbicidal system in host defense. The oxygen-dependent killing mechanism is inactive in resting cells, but on activation rapidly generates a set of oxygen-consuming metabolic reactions termed the respiratory burst of phagocytosis.[85–87] The burst usually terminates within 2–20 minutes, depending on the nature of the stimulus.[88] The first, essential reaction of the pathway is the 1-electron reduction of molecular oxygen to superoxide

(O_2^-), a free radical anion, by the multicomponent enzyme system NADPH oxidase:

$$NADPH + 2O_2 \rightarrow NADP^+ + 2O_2^-$$

NADPH is then regenerated by the hexosemonophosphate shunt pathway. Superoxide is a reducing agent with mild direct bactericidal activity. However, it undergoes a dismutation reaction, either spontaneously or with catalysis by superoxide dismutase, to produce hydrogen peroxide and molecular oxygen:

$$2H^+ + O_2^- + O_2^- \rightarrow H_2O_2 + O_2$$

Hydrogen peroxide not only possesses direct microbicidal activity but also serves as a source of even more potent reactive oxygen species. It reacts with superoxide in an iron-catalyzed Haber-Weiss reaction to produce hydroxyl radical (HO·), the most reactive of the oxygen products, and possibly singlet oxygen, a high-energy form of molecular oxygen.[89]

$$H_2O_2 + O_2^- \xrightarrow{Fe^{+++}} HO\cdot + OH^- + O_2$$

Hydrogen peroxide also combines with halides (such as bromide and chloride ions) in the presence of myeloperoxidase (MPO) to generate hypobromous or hypochlorous acid.[90,91]

$$H_2O_2 + Cl^- \xrightarrow{MPO} HOCl + OH^-$$

Neutrophils also generate complex, long-lived chloramine (nitrogen- and chloride-containing) radicals by mechanisms that are still not entirely elucidated but that are also dependent on myeloperoxidase activity.[92] Mouse macrophages also generate nitric oxide, a radical species with both cytocidal and intercellular signaling functions.[93,94] Nitric oxide synthetase has not yet been detected in neutrophils, but indirect evidence suggests that they too may generate reactive nitrogen intermediates.[95]

The reactive oxygen products are toxic to normal cells surrounding the activated neutrophil and thus constitute important mediators of inflammatory tissue damage. Even the neutrophil itself is subject to auto-oxidation. Normal cells are protected in part by antioxidant defense pathways such as the glutathione cycle and by free radical and peroxide quenching molecules such as α-tocopherol (vitamin E).[96,97]

The NADPH oxidase enzyme system responsible for superoxide generation forms a small electron transport chain that follows the probable order: NADPH → flavoprotein → cytochrome b → oxygen. For a detailed model of the oxidase structure and activation, see Figure 54-2. The identification of the components of this system has greatly benefited from the analysis of its defects, which produce the various forms of chronic granulomatous disease (see Ch. 54). The terminal electron donor to oxygen is a unique, low-mid-point-potential cytochrome b, termed cytochrome b_{558} for its spectral peak of light absorbance at 558 nm. The heterodimeric molecule combines a 91-kd glycoprotein (termed gp91-*phox*) and a 22-kd nonglycosylated polypeptide (termed p22-*phox*).[98–100] The gene for gp91-*phox* was one of the first to be identified by positional cloning.[98] In the initial stages of activation, a cytosolic oxidase component, p47-*phox,* is phosphorylated and then translocated to the membrane along with a second cytosolic component, p67-*phox,* and possibly a third (as yet unidentified) species.[101,102] The active membrane-bound complex also includes small G-protein species that may regulate respiratory burst activity.[103,104] The orientation of the transmembrane electron transport system results in the oxidation of NADPH on the cytoplasmic surface and the generation of superoxide on the outer surface of the membrane, which forms the inner surface of the phagosome on invagination during phagocytosis. Thus the reactive oxygen species are concentrated at the site of the ingested microorganism.

Cytokine Response and Production

Cytokines such as the IFNs, CSFs, and TNF-α regulate the production and activity of neutrophils. Chapter 16 describes their control of granulocytopoiesis, which at first appeared to be the sole avenue of CSF effector function. However, mature neutrophils possess receptors for both CSF-G and CSF-GM. These agents act on the terminally differentiated cells to up-regulate respiratory burst activity[105,106]; CSF-GM also increases expression of adhesion receptors, with a consequent decrease in chemotactic activity that may help retain neutrophils at sites of inflammation.[69] Neutrophils also modulate activity in response to IL-1, -4, and -8, IFN-γ, and TNF-α.[42,107–111]

A widespread, but incorrect, view of the neutrophil portrays it as a terminally differentiated cell with a condensed nucleus, hence incapable of induced gene expression and protein synthesis. However, in spite of its dense chromatin and paucity of ribosomes, the neutrophil also up-regulates genes involved in respiratory burst activity[112] and serves as an effector cell of the cytokine network.[113] Stimulation with lipopolysaccharide induces neutrophils not only to synthesize IL-1γ and -1β,[114,115] which augment acute phase responses and activate T, B, and endothelial cells, but also to secrete IL-1 receptor antagonist,[113] the complementary anti-inflammatory regulator. Neutrophils also contribute to B-cell activation by production of IL-6 in response to CSF-GM.[116] TNF-α expression by neutrophils occurs in response to lipopolysaccharide, CSF-G and CSF-GM,[117] serving immunomodulatory functions similar to IL-1 and creating a feedback loop for further neutrophil recruitment and activation. In another autoregulatory loop, neutrophils stimulated by CSF-GM synthesize both CSF-G and CSF-M,[115] leading not only to attraction of more neutrophils, but also to recruitment of monocytes to form the second wave of the inflammatory response. In another feedback loop, neutrophils augment their own recruitment by up-regulation of expression of IL-8,[118] a major chemoattractant.

REFERENCES

1. Boggs DR: The kinetics of neutrophilic leukocytes in health and disease. Semin Hematol 4:359, 1967
2. Warner HR, Athens JW: An analysis of granulocyte kinetics in blood and bone marrow. Ann NY Acad Sci 113:523, 1964
3. Lieschke GJ, Burgess AW: Granulocyte colony-stimulating factor and granulocyte-macrophage colony-stimulating factor. N Engl J Med 327:28, 1992
4. Witte ON: Steel locus defines a new multipotent growth factor. Cell 63:1112, 1990
5. Ema H, Suda T, Nagayoshi K et al: Target cells for granulocyte colony-stimulating factor, interleukin-3, and interleukin-5 in differentiation pathways of neutrophils and eosinophils. Blood 76:1956, 1990
6. Ogawa M: Differentiation and proliferation of hematopoietic stem cells. Blood 81:2844, 1993
7. Lubin BH: Reference Values in Infancy and Childhood. WB Saunders, Philadelphia, 1987
8. Harlan JM: Leukocyte-endothelial interactions. Blood 65:513, 1985
9. Colotta R, Re F, Polentarutti N et al: Modulation of granulocyte survival and programmed cell death by cytokines and bacterial products. Blood 80:2012, 1992
10. Bainton DF, Ullyot JL, Farquhar MG: The development of neutrophilic polymorphonuclear leukocytes in human bone marrow. Origin and content of azurophil and specific granules. J Exp Med 134:907, 1971
11. Dunn WB, Hardin JH, Spicer SS: Ultrastructural localization of myeloperoxidase in human neutrophil and rabbit heterophil and eosinophil leukocytes. Blood 32:935, 1968
12. Ackerman GA, Clark MA: Ultrastructural localization of peroxidase activity in normal human bone marrow cells. Z Zellforsch Mikrosk Anat 117:463, 1971
13. Bretz U, Baggiolini M: Biochemical and morphological characterization of

azurophil and specific granules of human neutrophilic polymorphonuclear leukocytes. J Cell Biol 63:251, 1974

14. Spitznagel JK, Dalldorf FG, Leffell MS et al: Character of azurophil and specific granules purified from human polymorphonuclear leukocytes. Lab Invest 30:774, 1974

15. West BC, Rosenthal AS, Gelb NA, Kimball HR: Separation and characterization of human neutrophil granules. Am J Pathol 77:41, 1974

16. Gilbert CS, Parmley RT, Rice WG, Kinkade JMJ: Heterogeneity of peroxidase-positive granules in normal human and Chédiak-Higashi neutrophils. J Histochem Cytochem 41:837, 1993

17. Pember SO, Kinkade JM Jr: Differences in myeloperoxidase activity from neutrophilic polymorphonuclear leukocytes of differing density: relationship to selective exocytosis of distinct forms of the enzyme. Blood 61:1116, 1983

18. Parmley RT, Rice WG, Kinkade JM Jr et al: Peroxidase-containing microgranules in human neutrophils: physical, morphological, cytochemical, and secretory properties. Blood 70:1630, 1987

19. Rice WG, Ganz T, Kinkade JM Jr et al: Defensin-rich dense granules of human neutrophils. Blood 70:757, 1987

20. Clark JM, Vaughan DW, Aiken BM, Kagan HM: Elastase-like enzymes in human neutrophils localized by ultrastructural cytochemistry. J Cell Biol 84:102, 1980

21. Parmley RT, Hurst RE, Takagi M et al: Glycosaminoglycans in human neutrophils and leukemic myeloblasts: ultrastructural, cytochemical, immunologic, and biochemical characterization. Blood 61:257, 1983

22. Dunn WB, Spicer SS: Histochemical demonstration of sulfated mucosubstances and cationic proteins in human granulocytes and platelets. J Histochem Cytochem 17:668, 1969

23. Fittschen C, Parmley RT, Austin RL, Crist WM: Vicinal glycol-staining identifies secondary granules in human normal and Chédiak-Higashi neutrophils. Anat Rec 205:301, 1983

24. Avila JL: The influence of the type of sulphate bond and degree of sulphation of glcyosaminoglycans on their interaction with lysosomal enzymes. Biochem J 171:489, 1978

25. Ackerman GA: The human neutrophilic myelocyte: a correlated phase and electron microscopic study. Z Zellforsch Mikrosk Anat 121:153, 1971

26. Borregaard N, Miller LJ, Springer TA: Chemoattractant-regulated mobilization of a novel intracellular compartment in human neutrophils. Science 237:1204, 1987

27. Pryzwansky KB, Rausch PG, Spitznagel JK, Herion JC: Immunocytochemical distinction between primary and secondary granule formation in developing human neutrophils: correlation with Romanowsky stains. Blood 53:179, 1979

28. Jesaitis AJ, Beuscher ES, Harrison D et al: Ultrastructural localization of cytochrome b in the membranes of resting and phagocytosing human granulocytes. J Clin Invest 85:821, 1990

29. Rice WG: High resolution of heterogeneity among human neutrophil granules. Physical, biochemical, secretory and ultrastructural features of newly identified granule types. Doctoral dissertation, Emory University, Atlanta, 1986

30. Kobayashi T, Robinson JM: A novel intracellular compartment with unusual secretory properties in human neutrophils. J Cell Biol 113:743, 1991

31. Perez HD, Marder S, Elfman F, Ives HE: Human neutrophils contain subpopulations of specific granules exhibiting different sensitivities to changes in cytosolic free calcium. Biochem Biophys Res Commun 145:976, 1987

32. Dewald B, Bretz U, Baggiolini M: Release of gelatinase from a novel secretory compartment of human neutrophils. J Clin Invest 70:518, 1982

33. Hoffstein S, Weissmann G: Microfilaments and microtubules in calcium ionophore induced secretion of lysosomal enzymes from human polymorphonuclear leukocytes. J Cell Biol 78:769, 1978

34. Coates TD, Watts RG, Hartman R, Howard TH: Relationship of F-actin distribution to development of polar shape in human polymorphonuclear neutrophils. J Cell Biol 117:765, 1992

35. Metchnikoff E: Untersuchungen über die intracellulare Verdauung bei wirbellosen Thieren. Arb Zoologischen Inst Univ Wien 5:141, 1883

36. Zigmond SH: The ability of polymorphonuclear leukocytes to orient in gradients of chemotactic factors. J Cell Biol 75:606, 1977

37. Baggiolini M, Boulay F, Badwey JA, Curnutte JT: Activation of neutrophil leukocytes: chemoattractant receptors and respiratory burst. FASEB J 7:1004, 1993

38. Murphy PM: The family of leukocyte chemoattractant receptors. Annu Rev Immunol 1994 (in press)

39. Gay J, Beckman J, Zaboy K, Lukens J: Modulation of neutrophil oxidative responses to soluble stimuli by platelet activating factor. Blood 67:931, 1986

40. Goetzl EJ, Sherman JW, Ratnoff WD et al: Receptor-specific mechanisms for the responses of human leukocytes to leukotrienes. Ann NY Acad Sci 524:345, 1988

41. Oppenheim JJ, Zachariae CO, Mukaida N, Matsushima K: Properties of the novel proinflammatory supergene "intercrine" cytokine family. Annu Rev Immunol 9:617, 1991

42. Baggiolini M, Walz A, Kunkel SL: Neutrophil-activating peptide-1/interleukin 8, a novel cytokine that activates neutrophils. J Clin Invest 84:1045, 1989

43. Walz A, Baggiolini M: Generation of neutrophil-activating peptide NAP-2 from platelet basic protein or connective tissue peptide III through monocyte proteases. J Exp Med 171:449, 1990

44. Caterina MJ, Devreotes PN: Molecular insights into eukaryotic chemotaxis. FASEB J 5:3078, 1991

45. Lawrence MB, Springer TA: Leukocytes roll on a selectin at physiologic flow rates: distinction from and prerequisite for adhesion through integrins. Cell 65:859, 1991

46. Doré M, Korthuis RJ, Granger DN et al: P-selectin mediates spontaneous leukocyte rolling in vivo. Blood 82:1308, 1993

47. Lorant DE, Topham MK, Whatley RE et al: Inflammatory roles of P-selectin. J Clin Invest 92:559, 1993

48. Springer TA: Adhesion receptors of the immune system. Nature 346:425, 1990

49. Springer TA, Lasky LA: Cell adhesion. Sticky sugars for selectins. Nature 349:196, 1991

50. Mayadas TN, Johnson RC, Rayburn H et al: Leukocyte rolling and extravasation are severely compromised in P selectin-deficient mice. Cell 74:541, 1993

51. Kishimoto TK, O'Connor K, Lee A et al: Cloning the β subunit of the leukocyte adhesion proteins: homology to an extracellular matrix receptor defines a novel supergene family. Cell 48:681, 1987

52. Smyth SS, Joneckis CC, Parise LV: Regulation of vascular integrins. Blood 81:2827, 1993

53. Hynes RO: Integrins: versatility, modulation, and signaling in cell adhesion. Cell 69:11, 1992

54. Smith CW, Marlin SD, Rothlein R et al: Cooperative interactions of LFA-1 and Mac-1 with intercellular adhesion molecule-1 in facilitating adherence and transendothelial migration of human neutrophils in vitro. J Clin Invest 83:2008, 1989

55. Staunton DE, Dustin ML, Springer TA: Functional cloning of ICAM-2, a cell adhesion ligand for LFA-1 homologous to ICAM-1. Nature 339:61, 1989

56. Osborn L: Leukocyte adhesion to endothelium in inflammation. Cell 62:3, 1990

57. Petrequin PR, Todd RF, Devall LJ et al: Association between gelatinase release and increased plasma membrane expression of the Mo1 glycoprotein. Blood 69:605, 1987

58. Singer II, Scott S, Kawka DW, Kazazis DM: Adhesomes: specific granules containing receptors for laminin, C3bi/fibrinogen, fibronectin, and vitronectin in human polymorphonuclear leukocytes and monocytes. J Cell Biol 109:3169, 1989

59. Sengelov H, Kjeldsen L, Diamond MS et al: Subcellular localization and dynamics of Mac-1 ($\alpha_m\beta_2$) in human neutrophils. J Clin Invest 92:1467, 1993

60. Lefer AM, Lefer DJ: Pharmacology of the endothelium in ischemia-reperfusion and circulatory shock. Annu Rev Pharmacol Toxicol 33:71, 1993

61. Wu X, Pippin J, Lefkowith JB: Attenuation of immune-mediated glomerulonephritis with an anti-CD11b monoclonal antibody. Am J Physiol 264:F715, 1993

62. Muller WA, Weigl SA, Deng X, Phillips DM: PECAM-1 is required for transendothelial migration of leukocytes. J Exp Med 178:449, 1993

63. Borregaard N, Lollike K, Kjeldsen L et al: Human neutrophil granules and secretory vesicles. Eur J Haematol 51:187, 1993

64. Baggiolini M, Wymann MP: Turning on the respiratory burst. Trends Biochem Sci 15:69, 1990

65. Fischer A, Lisowska-Grospierre B, Anderson DC, Springer TA: Leukocyte adhesion deficiency: molecular basis and functional consequences. Immunodefic Rev 1:39, 1988

66. Fanger MW, Goldstine SN, Shen L: Cytofluorographic analysis of receptors for IgA on human polymorphonuclear cells and monocytes and the correlation of receptor expression with phagocytosis. Mol Immunol 20:1019, 1983

67. Southwick FS, Stossel TP: Contractile proteins in leukocyte function. Semin Hematol 20:305, 1983

68. Stossel TP, Chaponnier C, Ezzell RM et al: Nonmuscle actin-binding proteins. Annu Rev Cell Biol 1:353, 1985

69. Yong K, Addison IE, Johnson B et al: Role of leucocyte integrins in phagocytic responses to granulocyte-macrophage colony-stimulating factor (GM-CSF): in vitro and in vivo studies on leucocyte adhesion deficient neutrophils. Br J Haematol 77:150, 1991

70. Adams RJ, Pollard TD: Binding of myosin I to membrane lipids. Nature 340:565, 1989

71. Kjeldsen L, Bainton DF, Sengelov H, Borregaard N: Structural and functional heterogeneity among peroxidase-negative granules in human neutrophils: identification of a distinct gelatinase containing granule subset by combined immunocytochemistry and subcellular fractionation. Blood 82:3183, 1993

72. Ambruso DR, Johnston RB Jr: Lactoferrin enhances hydroxyl radical production by human neutrophils, neutrophil particulate fractions, and an enzymatic generating system. J Clin Invest 67:352, 1981

73. Ellison RT III, Giehl TJ: Killing of gram-negative bacteria by lactoferrin and lysozyme. J Clin Invest 88:1080, 1991

74. Borregaard N, Christensen L, Bjerrum OW et al: Identification of a highly mobilizable subset of human neutrophil intracellular vesicles that contains tetranectin and latent alkaline phosphatase. J Clin Invest 85:408, 1990

75. Lehrer RI, Ganz T: Antimicrobiol polypeptides of human neutrophils. Blood 76:2169, 1990

76. Gray PW, Flaggs G, Leong SR et al: Cloning of the cDNA of a human neutrophil bactericidal protein. Structural and functional correlations. J Biol Chem 264:9505, 1989

77. Odeberg H, Olsson I: Antibacterial activity of cationic proteins from human granulocytes. J Clin Invest 56:1118, 1975

78. Lehrer RI, Ganz T, Selsted ME: Oxygen-independent bactericidal systems. Mechanisms and disorders. Hematol Oncol Clin North Am 2:159, 1988

79. Selsted ME, Harwig SSL, Ganz T et al: Primary structures of three human neutrophil defensins. J Clin Invest 76:1436, 1985

80. Fleming A: On a remarkable bacteriolytic element found in tissues and secretions. Proc R Soc Lond [Biol] 93:307, 1922

81. Strominger JL, Tipper DJ: Structure of bacterial cell walls: the lysozyme substrate. p. 169. In Osserman E, Canfield W, Beckok C (eds): Lysozyme. Academic Press, San Diego, 1984

82. Creutz CE: The annexins and exocytosis. Science 258:924, 1992

83. Francis JW, Balazovich KJ, Smolen JE et al: Human neutrophil annexin I promotes granule aggregation and modulates Ca^{2+}-dependent membrane fusion. J Clin Invest 90:537, 1992

84. Nanavati C, Fernandez JM: The secretory granule matrix: a fast-acting smart polymer. Science 259:963, 1993

85. Iyer GYN, Islam DMF, Quastel JH: Biochemical aspects of phagocytosis. Nature 192:535, 1961

86. Sbarra AJ, Karnovsky ML: The biochemical basis of phagocytosis. I. Metabolic changes during the ingestion of particles by polymorphonuclear leukocytes. J Biol Chem 234:1355, 1959

87. Babior BM: The respiratory burst oxidase. Trends Biochem Sci 12:241, 1987

88. Whitin JC, Cohen HJ: Disorders of respiratory burst termination. Hematol Oncol Clin North Am 2:289, 1988

89. Fridovich I: The biology of oxygen radicals. Science 201:875, 1978

90. Klebanoff SJ: Iodination of bacteria: a bactericidal mechanism. J Exp Med 126:1063, 1967

91. Clark RA: Modulation of the inflammatory response by the neutrophil myeloperoxidase system. Adv Exp Med Biol 141:207, 1982

92. Test ST, Lampert MB, Ossanna PJ et al: Generation of nitrogen-chlorine oxidants by human phagocytes. J Clin Invest 74:1341, 1984

93. Xie Q, Cho HJ, Calaycay J et al: Cloning and characterization of inducible nitric oxide synthase from mouse macrophages. Science 256:225, 1992

94. Stamler JS, Singel DJ, Loscalzo J: Biochemistry of nitric oxide and its redox-activated forms. Science 258:1898, 1992

95. Malawista SE, Montgomery RR, Van Blaricom G: Evidence for reactive nitrogen intermediates in killing of staphylococci by human neutrophil cytoplasts. A new microbicidal pathway for polymorphonuclear leukocytes. J Clin Invest 90:631, 1992

96. Flohe L: The glutathione peroxidase reaction: molecular basis of the antioxidant function of selenium in animals. Curr Top Cell Regul 27:473, 1985

97. Lubin B, Machlin LJ: Vitamin E: biochemical, hematological, and clinical aspects. Ann NY Acad Sci 393:1, 1982

98. Royer-Pokora B, Kunkel LM, Monaco AP et al: Cloning the gene for an inherited disorder—chronic granulomatous disease—on the basis of its chromosomal location. Nature 322:32, 1986

99. Parkos CA, Dinauer MC, Walker LE et al: The primary structure and unique expression of the 22 kilodalton light chain of human neutrophil cytochrome b. Proc Natl Acad Sci USA 85:3319, 1988

100. Curnutte JT: Chronic granulomatous disease: the solving of a clinical riddle at the molecular level. Clin Immunol Immunopathol 67:S2, 1993

101. Heyworth PG, Curnutte JT, Nauseef WM et al: Neutrophil nicotinamide adenine dinucleotide phosphate oxidase assembly. Translocation of p47-*phox* and p67-*phox* requires interaction between p47-*phox* and cytochrome b$_{558}$. J Clin Invest 87:352, 1991

102. Babior BM, Kuver R, Curnutte JT: Kinetics of activation of the respiratory burst oxidase in a fully soluble system from human neutrophils. J Biol Chem 263:1713, 1988

103. Abo A, Pick E, Hall A et al: Activation of the NADPH oxidase involves the small GTP-binding protein p21^{racl}. Nature 353:668, 1991

104. Bokoch GM, Quilliam LA, Bohl BP et al: Inhibition of Rap1A binding to cytochrome b$_{558}$ of NADPH oxidase by phosphorylation of Rap1A. Science 254:1794, 1991

105. Weisbart RH, Golde DW, Clark SC et al: Human granulocyte-macrophage colony-stimulating factor is a neutrophil activator. Nature 314:361, 1985

106. Roilides E, Walsh TJ, Pizzo PA, Rubin M: Granulocyte colony-stimulating factor enhances the phagocytic and bactericidal activity of normal and defective human neutrophils. J Infect Dis 163:579, 1991

107. Ferrante A: Activation of neutrophils by interleukins-1 and -2 and tumor necrosis factors. Immunol Ser 57:417, 1992

108. Le J, Vilcek J: Tumor necrosis factor and interleukin 1: cytokines with multiple overlapping biological activities. Lab Invest 56:234, 1987

109. Boey H, Rosenbaum R, Castracane J, Borish L: Interleukin-4 is a neutrophil activator. J Allergy Clin Immunol 83:978, 1989

110. Shalaby MR, Aggarwal BB, Rinderknecht E et al: Activation of human polymorphonuclear neutrophil functions by interferon gamma and tumor necrosis factors. J Immunol 135:2069, 1985

111. Beutler B, Cerami A: The biology of cachectin/TNF—A primary mediator of the host response. Annu Rev Immunol 7:625, 1989

112. Newburger PE, Dai Q, Whitney C: *In vitro* regulation of human phagocyte cytochrome b heavy and light chain gene expression by bacterial lipopolysaccharide and recombinant human cytokines. J Biol Chem 266:16171, 1991

113. Lloyd AR, Oppenheim JJ: Poly's lament: the neglected role of the polymorphonuclear neutrophil in the afferent limb of the immune response. Immunol Today 13:169, 1992

114. Lord PC, Wilmoth LM, Mizel SB, McCall CE: Expression of interleukin-1 alpha and beta genes by human blood polymorphonuclear leukocytes. J Clin Invest 87:1312, 1991

115. Lindemann A, Riedel D, Oster W et al: Granulocyte-macrophage colony-stimulating factor induces cytokine secretion by human polymorphonuclear leukocytes. J Clin Invest 83:1308, 1989

116. Melani C, Mattia GF, Silvani A et al: Interleukin-6 expression in human neutrophil and eosinophil peripheral blood granulocytes. Blood 81:2744, 1993

117. Dubravec DB, Spriggs DR, Mannick JA, Rodrick ML: Circulating human peripheral blood granulocytes synthesize and secrete tumor necrosis factor alpha. Proc Natl Acad Sci USA 87:6758, 1990

118. Bazzoni F, Cassatella MA, Rossi F et al: Phagocytosing neutrophils produce and release high amounts of the neutrophil-activating peptide 1/interleukin 8. J Exp Med 173:771, 1991

Monocyte and Macrophage Development and Function

50

Douglas V. Faller and Steven J. Mentzer

INTRODUCTION

The functional macrophage was first described approximately 130 years ago when large cells with unsegmented nuclei were observed in acutely damaged tissues and areas of inflammation. In chronic inflammation, these cells were more frequent and appeared larger, suggesting that the cells were capable of ingesting demolished cells and inflammatory debris. Because these cells appeared to be capable of ingesting large particles, they were termed macrophages. This scavenger function was long thought to be their principal role until in 1882 Robert Koch noted that these inflammatory phagocytic cells could engulf tubercle bacilli. Metchnikoff concluded that the "epithelioid-like" cells making up tuberculous granulomas were actually derived from monocytoid cells of the blood. The monocyte was established as a distinct cell type by 1913. Even then, many pathologists were convinced that monocytes and macrophages were cells of different ontogeny. Much later, cells were identified that represented intermediate forms between typical monocytes in the circulating blood and tissue macrophages, and the connection between these two cell types was established.

In the 1960s, the critical role played by monocytes and macrophages in the eradication of certain intracellular microorganisms was discovered. The macrophages in the skin, lung, and gut appeared to provide a first line of defense against microbial and parasitic infections.[1-4] Exposure to environmental pathogens caused macrophages to enlarge, to increase their number of lysosomes, and to become more phagocytic. Furthermore, macrophages developed strong resistance to these microorganisms with repeated challenge. This altered state was termed activation.

An additional observation was that even after the acute macrophage-mediated inflammation subsided, rechallenge with the same exogenous microorganism would result in rapid reaccumulation and activation of macrophages. This reactivation appeared to be an antigen-specific event triggered by memory lymphocytes. These results indicated an important interaction between lymphocytes and macrophages. Subsequent studies have implicated macrophages in all steps of the host's encounter with microbial pathogens: the initial processing of exogenous antigens, their presentation to lymphocytes, and their own subsequent activation by these lymphocytes. Thus, it appears that macrophages play an active role in regulating both the afferent and the efferent arms of the immune system. Finally, the role of monocytes and macrophages in the host response to tumors is an active area of research that is only now being elucidated. The activities of monocytes and macrophage can be divided into three broad categories (Table 50-1), as described below.

Tissue Maintenance

Tissue maintenance includes repair and remodeling activities, for example, the osteoclast remodeling of bone after injury and the osteoclast mobilization of bone in calcium homeostasis.[5-8] Splenic macrophages mediate phagocytosis of senescent red blood cells.[9] Langerhans cells control keratinization of the skin epidermis,[9] and Kupffer cells in the liver manage gut-absorbed endotoxin as well as red blood cell phagocytosis in the neonate.[11,12]

Immune Regulation

Monocytes and macrophages play a central role in immune regulation by coordinating the interaction of T and B cells during antigen presentation.[13-15] The macrophage not only processes antigens, but releases cytokines that modulate lymphocyte function. Immune regulatory function may also include monocyte- or macrophage-mediated suppressor activities such as suppression of lymphocyte proliferation[16,17] and inhibition of lymphocyte cytokine production.[18]

Pathogen Control

The antimicrobial properties of monocytes and macrophages may be antibacterial,[19,20] antiparasitic,[21] antifungal,[22] and antiviral.[23] Monocytes and macrophages may have multiple roles in a single area of inflammation. For example, macrophages may infiltrate an area of damaged tissue, debride the wound, direct fibroblast and connective tissue regrowth, participate in angiogenesis, and destroy invading pathogens.[24-29] The versatile role that migratory monocytes and tissue macrophages play in areas of inflammation demands that they have the capacity to express a wide range of morphologic, functional, and biochemical phenotypes. Furthermore, the interaction of monocytes and macrophages with immune, hematopoietic, endothelial, or connective tissue cells appears to require cellular communication mediated both by cell-cell contact as well as the elaboration of cytokines and growth factors (Table 50-2).

ORIGINS OF MONOCYTES AND MACROPHAGES

Monocytes appear in the fetal circulation at approximately the fifth month of gestation and increase in number during the third trimester.[30] The monocyte count reaches a peak at approximately 12 hours of age and remains high during the first 2 weeks of life. Monocytes develop from progenitor cells in the bone marrow.[31] This progenitor cell can commit along both granulocytic and monocytic lineages. The signals responsible for the commitment to the monocytic lineage are not known, although colony-stimulating factor-1 (CSF-1), interleukin-3 (IL-3), and colony-stimulating factor-granulocyte/macrophage (CSF-GM) have been shown to mediate differentiation of monocytic cells both in vitro and in vivo.[32,33] CSF-GM is produced by T cells, endothelial cells, and fibroblasts; CSF-1 is

Table 50-1. Spectrum of Monocyte and Macrophage Activity

Tissue maintenance
    Regulation of proliferation
        Fibroblasts
        Smooth muscle cells
        Endothelium
        Lymphoid, myeloid, erythroid cells
    Scavenger function
        Phagocytosis
        Detoxification
        Removal of senescent cells
    Secretory function
        Cytokines
        Proteases and antiproteases
        Complement components
        Coagulation factors
        Arachidonic acid metabolites, prostaglandins
    Wound repair
        Debridement and phagocytosis
        Angiogenesis
        Remodeling
    Calcium metabolism
    Iron storage
Immune regulation
    Antigen processing and presentation
    Accessory functions for humoral and cellular immunity
Pathogen control
    Antiviral activity
    Antimicrobial activity
    Antitumor activity

Table 50-2. Monocyte/Macrophage Macromolecular Secretory Products

Interleukin-1 (IL-1) family
    IL-1α
    IL-1β
    IL-1 receptor
    IL-1 receptor antagonist
Platelet-derived growth factor (PDGF) family
    PDGF-A
    PDGF-B/c-*sis*
    PDGF-related vasculatory permeability factor
Transforming growth factor-β (TGF-β) family
    TGF-β1
    TGF-β2
    Activin
Immediate-response gene growth factor family
    Macrophage inflammatory proteins (MIP)-1α, MIP-1β, MIP-2
    Monocyte chemoattractant proteins (MCP)-1/JE, MCP-2, MCP-3
    Mig
    Interleukin-6
    Colony-stimulating factor-monocyte
    KC (MGSA, Gro)
    Inflammatory protein-10
    Inflammatory protein-8
Proteases
    Plasminogen activator
    Collagenase
    Elastase
    Angiotensin convertase
    Acid protease
Coagulation factors
    Factors V, VII, IX, and X and prothrombin
    Prothrombinase
    Plasminogen activator
    Plasminogen inhibitor
    Plasmin inhibitor
    Lipoprotein lipase
Adhesion/matrix factors
    Thrombospondin
    Proteoglycans
    Fibronectin
Miscellaneous polypeptide factors
    Tumor necrosis factor-α
    Colony-stimulating factor-granulocyte/macrophage
    Colony-stimulating factor-granulocyte
    Leukemia inhibitory factor/DIA
    Erythropoietin
    Transforming growth factor-α
    Basic fibroblast growth factor
    Insulin-like growth factor-I
    Denfensins
    Thymosin
    Bombesin
    Corticotropin
    Interferon-α and -β
    Lysozyme
    Neutrophil-activating factor (interleukin-8)
    Complement factors: C1, C2, C3, and C5
    Alternate pathway factors: factors B and D, properidin
Other reguatory products
    Prostaglandin E$_2$
    Acidic isoferritin
    Nitric oxide
    Respiratory burst products
    Nitrates

produced by monocytes, endothelial cells, and fibroblasts.[34] Bone marrow precursors exposed to CSF-GM produce mixed granulocyte-monocyte/macrophage colonies (CFU-GM); CSF-1 produces colonies that are primarily monocytic (CFU-M).

A current concept for the development of the monocyte lineage emphasizes the close relationship between the origins of monocytes and granulocytes (Fig. 50-1). Once the progenitor cell has committed to the monocyte lineage, the cell develops through morphologically distinct monoblast and promonocyte stages. The mature monocyte is released into the peripheral circulation in the G$_1$ phase of the cell cycle. Blood monocytes rapidly partition between the marginating and circulating pools in the peripheral circulation. Although the marginating pool is approximately 3.5 times greater than the circulating pool,[35] the factors regulating monocyte margination are unclear. The monocyte remains in the peripheral circulation for 8–72 hours before migrating into peripheral tissues.[35,36]

Circulating blood monocytes are 12–15 μm in diameter, with a highly convoluted surface and a lobulated (kidney-shaped or folded) foamy nucleus. A Wright-stained smear of peripheral blood monocytes typically demonstrates indistinct nucleoli as well as gray and variably vacuolated cytoplasm.[37] Monocytes contain a single type of granule with staining characteristics suggestive of lysosomes. Monocytes may be further identified by the presence of a fluoride-sensitive nonspecific esterase. After the monocyte has migrated into the extravascular tissues, the cell becomes larger and acquires the cytologic appearance of a tissue macrophage. The cell nucleus appears oval and euchromatic, with more prominent nucleoli. The cytoplasm stains blue, reflecting an increase in RNA. More ribosomes, lysosomes, mitochondria, endoplasmic reticulum, open vesicles, and electron-dense inclusions of varying sizes and shapes appear. Mature macrophages also have increased levels of pinocytic as well as phagocytic activity.

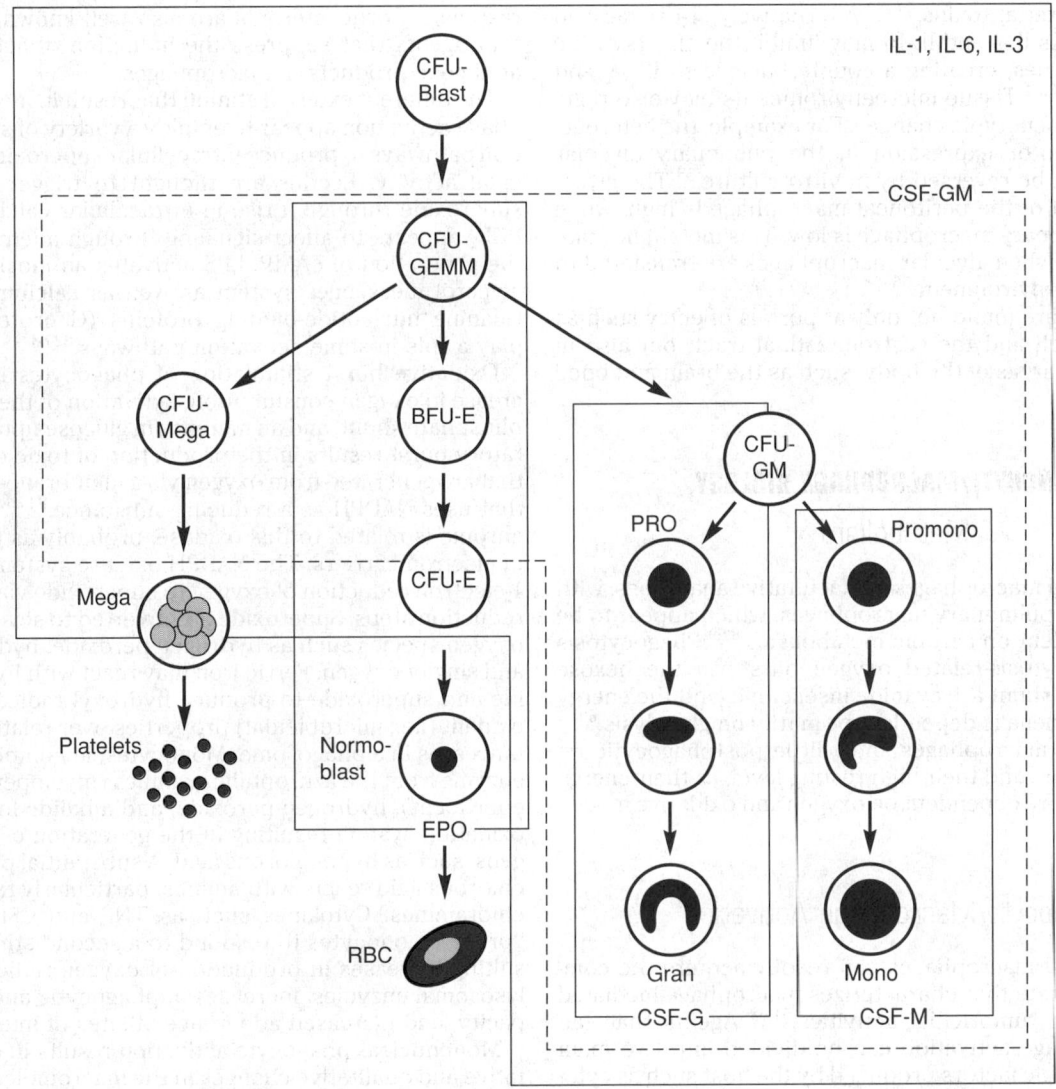

Fig. 50-1. Hematopoietic cell development. (From Gabrilove,[208] as adapted from Griffin,[209] with permission.)

TRANSITION OF MONOCYTES TO MACROPHAGES

The number of circulating and extravasating monocytes produced is controlled at a number of levels. Active inflammation can affect the generation and circulating time of peripheral blood monocytes. The production of monocytes from promonocytes can increase up to four-fold within 12 hours after an inflammatory stimulus.[38,39] In this setting, the average circulation time of monocytes in the peripheral blood may fall to as low as 30 minutes.[35] The young monocyte is capable of producing growth factors that can act in an autocrine manner, including CSF-1 and CSF-GM.[40–42] Monocytes contain the intracellular enzymes elastase and cathepsin but have little capacity for production of metaloproteases. As monocytes differentiate into macrophages, they begin to produce predominantly metaloproteases and metaloprotease inhibitors.[43] The movement of the peripheral blood monocyte into the extravascular tissue produces a tissue-specific macrophage.[44–46] Although the specific differentiation signals are unknown, the tissue microenvironment appears to play an important role in determining the tissue-specific maturation of the macrophage.

Tissue macrophages are a heterogeneous population with different morphologic and functional properties depending on the tissue where they reside.[47,48] Alveolar macrophages, Kupffer cells, osteoclasts, peritoneal macrophages, and synovial type-A cells all belong to the resident mononuclear phagocyte system (or reticuloendothelial system). Mature resident macrophages in tissues have a relatively long life and are generally quiescent. These cells perform homeostatic functions rather than antipathogen activities. Tissue macrophages retain some propensity for chemotaxis and have full capacity for phagocytosis and oxygen-dependent microbicidal activity. In inflammatory infiltrates, mononuclear phagocytes also comprise a heterogeneous group. They consist of macrophages already residing in the tissue before the onset of inflammation (resident macrophages), as well as mononuclear phagocytes recruited from the circulation (exudate macrophages). The differentiation from circulating monocyte into resident macrophage may include a transitional form called the exudate-resident macrophage.

Once extravasation has occurred, it is likely that the microenvironment plays a critical role in determining the cell's maturation. The tissue-specific levels of lymphokines, monokines, hormones, and toxins may act as microenvironmental mediators of maturation. Macrophages achieve a spectrum of functional phenotypes depending on these microenvironmental signals. Interferon (IFN)-γ-treated macrophages are more bactericidal and tumoricidal, express increased levels of MHC class II for antigen presentation to lymphocytes, and are primed for the release of cytokines such as tumor necrosis factor-α (TNF-α) in response to bacterial toxins.[49-52] Alternatively, T-cell-derived cytokines such as IL-4 and IL-10 may inhibit the effects of the activating cytokines, creating a counterbalance to IFN-γ and CSF-GM effects.[53,54] Tissue microenvironments may also regulate reversible phenotypic changes. For example, the heterogeneity in Fc-receptor expression in the pulmonary alveolar macrophage can be reversed by in vitro culture.[55] The glycolytic metabolism of the peritoneal macrophage is high, while that of the pulmonary macrophage is low. This metabolic state can be reversed when alveolar macrophages are transfered to an oxygen-poor environment.[56-58]

Macrophages are found not only at portals of entry such as pulmonary alveoli and the gastrointestinal tract, but also in generally sterile areas of the body, such as the brain and bone marrow.

MONOCYTE/MACROPHAGE BIOLOGY

Metabolism

Monocytes and macrophages are facultative anaerobes, with the exception of pulmonary macrophages, which appear to be uniquely dependent on aerobic metabolism.[58,59] Phagocytosis and the phagocytosis-related oxygen burst via the hexose monophosphate shunt are cyanide insensitive, and the energy for these phenomena is dependent primarily on glycolysis.[60,61] Only pulmonary macrophages show little postphagocytic respiratory burst beyond their high resting level, as their energy metabolism is more dependent on oxygen and oxidative metabolism.[62]

Monocyte/Macrophage Activation

Monocytes and macrophages can readily acquire the complex metabolic state that characterizes macrophage-mediated microbicidal and tumoricidal activities.[51,63] Agents that can trigger macrophage activation can be divided into two main classes: physiologic factors produced by the host such as cytokines and metabolites; and environmental factors derived from viruses, bacteria, or chemical synthesis. Although both classes of activators can stimulate the macrophage, combinations of stimuli may be synergistic in activating macrophages. Furthermore, the activation process in vivo is likely to be a multistep, multipathway process involving a defined sequence of events. A plausible sequence for macrophage activation in situ may include the priming of the macrophage with one agent (e.g., a physiologic macrophage-activating factor), with synergistic cellular activation on exposure to a second agent.[64,65] This sequence provides an explanation for the combination of physiologic (e.g., IFN-γ) and environmental (lipopolysaccharide [LPS] or phorbol esters [e.g., phorbol myristate acetate]) signals required to activate macrophage tumoricidal activity. It is likely that different combinations of the stimuli are responsible for the multiple activation phenotypes.

A soluble factor produced by T lymphocytes was the first cytokine identified as a stimulus of the macrophage activation process. It was termed macrophage-activating factor (MAF)[51,63,66,67] and was later identified as IFN-γ.[68-70] More recently, additional, noninterferon forms of MAF activity have been identified, including T-cell products such as IL-2 and IL-4, hematopoietic growth factors, including CSF-1 and CSF-GM, and a variety of other products.[71-81] The combination of MAF plus bacterial LPS appears to be sufficient for antitumor activity. Inhibitors of macrophage function or activation have been identified and include prostaglandin E$_2$ (PGE$_2$).[51,63,66,67] The synthesis and release of PGE$_2$ by macrophages is likely to provide a negative feedback loop for the modulation of the immune response. Corticosteroids are also well known anti-inflammatory agents that suppress the induction of activation-associated gene products in macrophages.

The different external stimuli that result in monocyte/macrophage activation appear to employ a variety of signal transduction pathways to produce intracellular superoxide and microbicidal activity. Lectins are thought to trigger production of superoxide through a rise in intracellular calcium,[82] whereas PGE$_2$ appears to affect signaling through adenyl cyclase with the generation of cAMP. LPS activates an inositol and diacylglycerol messenger system as well as calcium mobilization. Guanine nucleotide-binding proteins (G proteins) may also play a role in some activation pathways.[82,83]

Oxidative burst stimulation of phagocytes leads to an increase in oxygen consumption, activation of the hexose monophosphate shunt, and an increase in glucose uptake. This respiratory burst results in the production of toxic oxygen species that are generated from oxygen via a membrane-bound oxidase that uses NADPH as a reducing substance.[84,85] A B-type cytochrome is related to this oxidase, probably as part of a chain of electron carriers. The NADPH oxidase system catalyses the 1-electron reduction of oxygen to superoxide via oxidation and reduction steps. Superoxide is converted to several other toxic oxygen species such as hydrogen peroxide, hydroxyl radicals, and singlet oxygen. Ferric iron may react with hydrogen peroxide and superoxide to produce hydroxyl radicals with strong oxidant (i.e., microbicidal) properties over relatively short distances, as in a phagosome. Monocytes, in combination with an enzyme from the azurophilic granules (myeloperoxidase, or an equivalent), hydrogen peroxide, and a halide form a powerful oxidation system resulting in the generation of oxidized halogens, such as hypochlorous acid. A substantial portion of hypochlorous acid reacts with amines, particularly taurine, to yield chloramines. Cytokines such as TNF and CSFs are able to "prime" monocytes to respond to a second stimulus, with resulting increases in production of oxygen radicals, release of lysosomal enzymes, increases in phagocytic and cytotoxic capacity, and increased adherence at sites of infection.[86]

Mononuclear phagocyte activation results in certain quantitative and qualitative changes in the macromolecular composition of the macrophage cell membrane. These changes include the increased expression of Fc receptors, class II MHC antigens, IL-2 receptors, the MO-3 antigen,[87] and membrane-associated TNF. By contrast, macrophage activation results in decreased expression of other receptors such as transferrin, mannose-fucose, and C3bi (complement receptor [CR] 3).

Movement

Extravasation

Monocytes constitute 1–6% of nucleated blood cells under normal conditions. Resident tissue macrophages derived from monocytes are recruited, in the absence of inflammation, by unknown mechanisms. Inflammation induces the rapid egress of monocytes from the circulation. Factors responsible for inflammatory cell recruitment include N-formyl-methionyl-capped bacterial proteins, complement products, fibrinopeptides, and a large number of growth factors and cytokines such as transforming growth factor-β (TGF-β), platelet-derived growth factor (PDGF), IL-1, TNF, and IL-2.[88] Factors selectively chemotactic for monocytes or T cells, or both, have been recently characterized. Monocyte chemotactic protein-1 (MCP-1) and RANTES are chemotactic for monocytes alone or for monocytes and T lymphocytes of the memory phenotype. These factors may provide an explanation for the macrophage predominance in chronic inflammatory lesions such as tuberculous granulomas. Two other monocyte chemotactic proteins, MCP-2 and MCP-3, have also recently been identified.[89]

Macrophage inflammatory protein-1α (MIP-1α), MIP-1β, and MIP-2 induce mixed phagocyte recruitment.[90-92]

A number of agents appear to facilitate extravascular transmigration by inducing endothelial cell adhesivity to circulating monocytes. These factors include IL-1, TNF-α, LPS, IFN-γ, thrombin, and viral infections, including herpes simplex type 1 and cytomegalovirus.[93] Conversely, stimulation of monocytes with the cytokines IL-3 or CSF-GM, with complement chemotactic factors, with phorbol esters, or with the bacterial product f-met-leu-phe increase adhesion of monocytes to the endothelium through monocyte activation.[93-95] Monocytes selectively transmigrate through endothelial junctions during inflammatory states.[96] Monocyte migration into the subendothelial space may also occur in response to chemoattractants present in the intima or media of the vessel wall.[97]

Adhesive/Receptor Characteristics

Macrophage have abundant cell adhesion receptors and ligands, including three leukocyte-restricted integrins, leukocyte function-associated antigen-1 (LFA-1), Mac-1, and p150,95. These leukocyte integrins belong to the integrin superfamily of molecules and consist of heterodimers of a unique α- and a shared β-chain. LFA-1 (CD11a/CD18) and one of its many ligands, intercellular adhesion molecule-1 (ICAM-1), are both present on monocytes and mediate homotypic cell-cell interactions,[98,99] as well as the attachment of monocytes to endothelial cells and monocyte contact with lymphocytes bearing the corresponding receptor/ligand, facilitating antigen presentation.[95,98-100] Mac-1 (CD11b/CD18) appears to have a major role in the attachment and possibly extravasation of monocytes through activated endothelia.[94] Inflammatory cytokines such as TNF and IL-1 induce the expression of ICAM-1, vascular cell adhesion molecule-1 (VCAM-1), and endothelial leukocyte adhesion molecule-1 (ELAM-1) on endothelial cells. VLA-4 and other ligands on monocyte plasma membranes mediate binding to endothelial VCAM-1 and ELAM-1, facilitating monocyte recruitment into inflammatory sites. Adhesion molecules, such as the integrin β-chain, may also have a transmembrane signaling function. Cellular activation appears to be triggered by macrophage binding to the extracellular matrix proteins type IV collagen and fibronectin.[101]

Pinocytosis/Phagocytosis

Macrophage activation results in increased membrane adhesiveness and the simultaneous invagination of membrane and extension of pseudopodia that cause the formation of endocytic vacuoles. Small or soluble molecules are taken up by the process known as pinocytosis. Pinocytosis may be "bulky" (the molecules are in solution around the cell and are taken up into pinocytic vesicles), or may be "adsorptive" (the molecules adhere to the monocyte plasmalemma and enter the vesicles attached to it). If the attachment of these molecules is to a specific receptor, the internalization process is termed receptor-mediated endocytosis.

The uptake of larger objects is termed phagocytosis. Cytoplasmic granules and Golgi-derived vesicles fuse with the plasmalemma at the site of recognition and subsequently discharge their granular contents across the membrane barrier in a process called degranulation. Degranulation results in discharge of granule contents into the extracellular fluids. The granules can also fuse with phagocytic vesicles containing ingested objects. The resulting phagolysosome plays an important role in the digestion of internalized particles. Macrophage phagocytosis is important to host defenses against many potential pathogens such as *Mycobacterium*, *Leishmania*, and *Salmonella* spp. Some of these organisms may prevent phagosome-lysosome

fusion and are able to grow within the resident alveolar macrophages in the absence of macrophage activation.

At least three types of plasma membrane phagocytic receptors exist on macrophage. These include Fc receptors,[102] complement receptors CR1 and CR3, and carbohydrate receptors, such as the macrophage mannose receptor. Fc receptors mediate uptake of immunoglobulin-opsonized particles and immune complexes. FcRI is expressed only on mononuclear phagocytes and binds free monomeric IgG, in contrast to the other Fc receptors. FcRII is expressed on both neutrophils and mononuclear phagocytes. Ligand binding to the Fc receptor induces the release of numerous products from the macrophage, including TNF and plasminogen activator, and triggers the respiratory burst. Complement receptors bind many solid-phase complement ligands. CR3, for example, binds particles coated with C3bi.[103] Complement fragments may not only identify potential pathogens, but may facilitate their phagocytosis. The mannose receptor is found on mature nonactivated macrophages; it binds mannosylated proteins and mediates the ingestion of yeast wall particles (such as zymosan) and *Pneumocystis carinii*.[104-106]

Monocytes and macrophages also express receptors for coagulation factors VII and VIIA,[107,108] β-endorphin,[67,109] low-density lipoprotein (LDL), and very-low-density lipoprotein (VLDL).[110-113]

Synthesis and Secretion of Cytokines and Growth Factors

Macrophages are capable of secreting >100 well-defined molecules, which fall into a broad number of categories[66,87] (Table 50-2). These categories include cytokines, growth factors, eicosenoids, enzymes and enzyme inhibitors, clotting factors and complement components, plasma-binding proteins, and low-molecular-weight reactive oxygen and nitrogen products.

Macrophage-derived cytokines (monokines) can be grouped in to several classes based on similarities in structure or biologic activities, or both. TNF-α, IL-1α, and IL-1β, although structurally quite distinct, have broadly overlapping activity profiles.[52,114] In addition, there are distinct families of secreted products that are structurally related by virtue of four positionally conserved cysteine residues. These families include IL-8, KC (melanocyte growth stimulating activity [MGSA, GN, JE]), inflammatory protein-10, MCP-1 (JE), and the macrophage inflammatory proteins (MIP)-1, -2, and -3.[115-120] Although some of these factors have been reported to exhibit growth or chemoattractant activity, or both, the exact function for each family member has not been clearly defined. The varied activity of these factors can be shown by the cytokines MIP-1 and MIP-2, which are chemotactic for neutrophils in vitro and elicit a marked inflammatory response when injected in vivo.[121]

Additional cytokines are associated with the inflammatory stimulation of mononuclear phagocytes. These include PDGFs, fibroblast growth factors (FGFs), TGFs, CSF-GM, CSF-1, the IFNs (α and β), and IL-6.[67,122-126] All these cytokines are produced early after stimulation, are expressed only transiently, and do not appear to depend on the synthesis of any other gene products for their expression. Many of these factors are made in response to the lipid A component of LPS[127] or to cytokines made by other cells.[128] The process is calcium dependent[129] and requires the synthesis and increased stability of specific mRNAs,[130] and protein synthesis, processing, and secretion.[131] Of these secreted proteins, only IL-1 is not made with a signal peptide.[132,133] Some of the TNF produced is attached to the monocyte membrane,[134] but most is secreted into the medium.[135] These factors, which are likely to contribute to the inflammatory and hematopoietic effects of macrophages, may also play a role in effecting and regulating macrophage cytotoxic activity.[63,66,67,81] For example, TNF-α induces the expression of IL-1 and IL-6.[80,136] Conversely, IL-1 stimulates the synthesis of TNF-α, IL-6, CSF-1, CSF-GM, and IL-1 itself.[80,137,138] The IFNs are potent inducers of a number of monokines. Combinations of cytokines can have additive, synergistic, or antagonistic regulatory effects on monokine production by macrophage.

Monokines may have interrelated functions that affect specific cells involved in inflammation as well as the general process of host metabolism. For example, monokines can alter endothelial cell function.[139] IL-1 and TNF can cause fever,[132,133,140,141] muscle breakdown,[141] and changes in liver metabolism.[142] IL-1 and TNF both appear to be involved in the cachexia associated with chronic infection and malignancy.[143] TNF may play a role in the anemia of chronic disease.[144] IL-1 indirectly results in the synthesis of acute-phase reactants, through stimulation of IL-6 synthesis and secretion. These acute-phase reactants are secreted into the circulation; they include C-reactive protein, fibrinogen, α₁-antitrypsin, haptoglobin, and serum amyloid A. In addition, IL-6 causes a decrease in the synthesis of albumin, fibrinectin, and transferrin.[145] The latter is responsible for the decrease in total iron-binding capacity associated with inflammation. The CSFs synthesized and secreted by monocytes and macrophages stimulate the appropriate progenitor cells in the bone marrow to make neutrophils and monocytes in response to infection. The interactions of these factors appear to play an important role in the regulation of cell growth, protein synthesis, cell movement, and cell-cell interactions.

PATHOGEN CONTROL

Macrophages have microbiostatic or microbicidal effects on the facultative and obligate intracellular bacteria, protozoa, and fungi. After activation, macrophages synthesize an array of proteins that regulate and catalyze the production of toxic oxygen intermediates.[146,147] Toxic oxygen intermediates appear in the phagolysosome and kill microorganisms, primarily those that produce pyogenic infections. Intracellular killing in macrophages, as in granulocytes, is mediated by an oxygen-dependent system that uses hydrogen peroxide, a halide, and a myeloperoxidase-like enzyme.[148] Macrophages, in contrast to monocytes, lack the myeloperoxidase enzyme but may have a similar alternative enzyme. Alternatively, microbicidal activity may be related to the direct activity of reactive oxygen species.[149,150] Highly reactive oxygen radicals, including superoxide, hydrogen peroxide, singlet oxygen, and hydroxyl radical, are produced by a membrane-associated NADPH oxidase and associated reactions. These reactive oxygen species are available for the microbicidal process. The initial bacteriocidal reagent in these reactions is hypochlorous acid.[148] Ferric ion may react with hydrogen peroxide and superoxide to produce hydroxyl radicals with strong oxidant properties over relatively short distances as in a phagosome. Lysosome activity has not conclusively been shown to kill ingested bacteria directly and may be limited to degrading dead organisms.

Oxygen-independent bactericidal mechanisms also exist, as evidenced by bacterial killing under anaerobic conditions, and antimicrobial activity by phagocytes with impaired oxidative metabolism as in chronic granulomatous disease. Oxygen-independent mechanisms include perforin or perforin-like activities[151] as well as cationic proteins that may kill bacteria and fungi through their action on the microbial plasma membrane.[152] Numerous bactericidal secretory products, lysosomal enzymes, and other factors from macrophages have also been described.[153] These microbicidal proteins include lysozyme, lactoferrin, cathepsin G, and defensin.[154] Oxygen-independent cytocidal mechanisms may be more selective in their expression than oxygen-dependent mechanisms.[148] Although in vitro evidence for cytocidal activity against bacteria, fungi, and some viruses exists,[155] no comprehensive studies of human monocyte and macrophage oxygen-independent cytocidal mechanisms have been done. The biologic importance of oxygen-independent cytocidal mechanisms thus remains unclear.

In addition to microbicidal capacity, macrophages possess microbiostatic activity for a variety of intercellular organisms.[153,156–159] The capacity for macrophages to inhibit the growth of intracellular microorganisms depends on previous exposure to the activating agent and, in some cases, to chemical signals originating from the microbe itself.[158–160] An important contribution to microbiostasis appears to be the synthesis of nitric oxide by the macrophage. An inducible enzyme that catalyzes the production of nitric oxide (nitric oxide synthase) has recently been identified in cells of monocytic origin and is inducible by cytokines and LPS.[161,162] Killing of *Leishmania* amastigotes by IFN-γ-activated macrophage and macrophage fungistasis are both mediated by nitric oxide.[163,164]

The originally identified macrophage-activating factor, IFN-γ, enhances macrophage killing of intracellular pathogens, including *Candida, Toxoplasma gondii,* and mycobacteria.[165] Therapeutic activation of the circulating blood monocyte has been achieved following intravenous, intradermal, intramuscular, and subcutaneous administration of IFN-γ in patients with cancer, lepromatous leprosy, acquired immunodeficiency syndrome, and chronic granulomatous disease. Activation of the alveolar macrophage has also been induced in a compartmentalized fashion by aerosolized IFN-γ.[166]

Monocytes and macrophages express the CD4 membrane molecule and can serve as a reservoir for the human immunodeficiency virus (HIV). The predominant infected cell found in cerebrospinal fluid from patients with HIV meningoencephalitis is a macrophage. The brain macrophage, the microglia cell, and macrophage-derived multinucleate giant cells have all been found to be infected by HIV.[167–170] HIV can also be found in pulmonary macrophages, epidermal Langerhans cells, and lymph node macrophages. Not all macrophages, however, appear to be susceptible to HIV infection; Kupffer cells, for example, cannot be infected. The reason for this resistance to HIV is unknown.

IMMUNOLOGIC FUNCTIONS

Antigen Presentation

The monocyte lineage gives rise to cells involved in the processing of antigen, which is required for the development of an immune response. Langerhans cells of the skin, interdigitating cells of the thymus, reticular cells of the spleen, and dendritic cells of lymph nodes have all been implicated in the processing of exogenous antigen. The process involved in antigen presentation is poorly understood, but appears to involve the association of antigenic peptides with MHC class II molecules. This molecular association appears to occur within lysosomes prior to being expressed on the cell surface.[171] T-lymphocyte interaction with antigen presented by mononuclear cells in the context of class II MHC molecules appears to involve direct cell-cell contact. The activation of the T lymphocytes may be enhanced by the elaboration of monokines such as IL-1. Subsequent T- and B-lymphocyte collaboration results in immunoglobulin production. Antigen-presenting cells in certain tissues, such as lung, are not phagocytic and may internalize antigen by pinocytosis[172]; nonetheless, these cells retain Fc and C3b receptors on their surface for interaction with T lymphocytes and antigen. Macrophages can also present processed antigen to B cells to elicit a humoral response.[173,174]

Cellular Cytotoxicity

Toxicity by monocytes and macrophages to tumor cells can be divided into two types.

Antibody-Dependent Cellular Cytotoxicity

Antibody-coated target cells are recognized by the Fc receptor on monocytes. This recognition enables the monocyte to kill selected target cells with efficiencies determined by the immunoglobulin class, the density of immunoglobulin bound to the target cell, and the Fc receptor type involved on the effector cell. This process is termed antibody-dependent cell-mediated cytotoxicity (ADCC) and such tumoricidal activity has been demonstrated on a number of tumor cell lines in culture.[175-177] Monocyte tumoricidal activity may be induced by a variety of agents, including endotoxin, IFN-γ, ILs, TNF, phorbol esters[106] and CSF-GM.[178] This antitumor activity appears to be markedly enhanced by CSF-1.[175,176,178]

In vivo, the importance of tumor-associated macrophages in tumor rejection remains unclear. Tumor-associated macrophages have the potential to inhibit tumor growth and destroy neoplastic cells, as illustrated by MCP-1 gene transfer studies.[179-181] Conversely, macrophages can produce growth factors and promote angiogenesis, thus resulting in a possible paracrine stimulation of neoplastic cells. The clinical importance of ADCC is suggested by regression of neuroblastoma and melanoma in culture when murine monoclonal antibodies were added.[182,183] Studies of human cells engrafted into nude mice also indicate that ADCC may be an important mechanism for tumoricidal activity.[175]

Antibody-Independent Cellular Cytotoxicity

Recognition of specific target cell structures alone by monocytes and macrophages is a possible stimulus for spontaneous cellular cytotoxicity. The ability of monocytes that have not been previously activated to kill tumor target cells remains controversial.[142] Induction of non-receptor-mediated cytotoxicity can be achieved in monocytes using various soluble and particulate mediators. Phorbol esters, zymosan-activated serum, and aggregated IgG are capable of stimulating monocyte-mediated target cell lysis and the oxidative burst.[100,184] The maturation of monocytes to macrophages in long-term culture enhances tumoricidal activity.[185]

Mechanisms of Cellular Cytotoxicity

The mechanism of tumor cell lysis appears to involve cell-cell contact[186] and the secretion of a variety of cytotoxic mediators.[187,188] The cytocidal mechanisms for macrophages may differ from those of their monocyte progenitors because myeloperoxidase is absent,[189] and the energy for killing may depend more heavily on oxidative phosphorylation[190] than on glycolysis. Arginine-derived nitric oxide is also a major mediator of tumor cytostasis by activated macrophages.[191,192] Potential cellular targets of nitric oxide in tumor cells include the oxidoreductases in the electron transport chain, the Krebs cycle enzyme aconitase, and ribonucleotide reductase.[161,162,191-193] Nitric oxide-independent mechanisms apparently also exist that facilitate tumor cell destruction by activated macrophages and may include TNF production.[194] The production of TNF by activated monocytes appears to play an important role in some cytotoxicity,[177,178] although TNF may not be essential in all systems.[175]

TISSUE MAINTENANCE

Resident tissue macrophages are capable of playing a wide variety of roles because of their ability to develop specialized functions upon extravasation into certain tissues.

Waste Management

Littoral Macrophages

Resident tissue macrophages were formerly referred to as histiocytes. In organs that act as filters for blood and lymph, such as the spleen, liver, lungs, and lymph nodes, the macrophages (littoral macrophages) are located in specific sites to facilitate the clearance of pathogenic organisms and senescent cells. This filtering role of the littoral mononuclear phagocyte system led to the older designation of reticuloendothelial system. The recognition of the monocyte/macrophage lineage as well as the phagocytic function of these cells has led to the newer mononuclear phagocyte system nomenclature.

Spleen

Macrophages are found in all parts of the spleen, including in association with lymphocytes and germinal centers, and in the red pulp and sinuses, where intimate contact occurs between red blood cells and macrophages during the sluggish percolation of blood through this circulation.

Liver

The portal circulation of the liver flows through the spaces of Disse before entering the hepatic venous system. These spaces are lined with liver macrophages, also known as Kupffer cells, again allowing for intimate contact of the elements of blood with these phagocytic cells.

Lymph Nodes

Macrophages exist in all areas of the lymph node and are especially abundant in the medullary zones, close to efferent lymphatic and blood capillaries. Antigen presentation by macrophages to T lymphocytes is likely to occur in these areas.[195]

Bone Marrow

Macrophages are found throughout the bone marrow, in hematopoietic islands, and on the walls of the marrow sinuses, where they probably have a clearance function, especially in states of ineffective hematopoiesis.[196] In lysosomal storage diseases such as Gaucher disease, large inclusions build up within marrow macrophages (as well as hepatic and splenic macrophages) because of the inability of the cells to break down their lysosomal contents.[197]

Lung

Inhaled foreign material such as asbestos or particulates from smoking may be found in pulmonary alveolar macrophages. Hemosiderin-laden alveolar macrophages may be diagnostic of recurrent pulmonary hemorrhage, such as in idiopathic hemosiderosis or Goodpasture syndrome, in which iron is sequestered in lung tissue. In the lung, macrophages reside both in the interstitium of alveolar sacs and freely within the spaces. These cells have a role in the clearance of inhaled microorganisms and particulate matters.[198]

Other Tissues

Mononuclear phagocytes are also found throughout the alimentary tract, particularly in the submucosal tissues and villi of the small intestine. Monocytes are also present in the central nervous system, especially after injury. Mammary gland macrophages appear in the milk during lactation and have been implicated as a potential source of postnatal transmission of the HIV virus.[199]

Lipid Metabolism

Monocytes take up denatured LDL and native VLDL by receptor-mediated endocytosis.[110-113] The LDL enters the lysosomal compartments. Free cholesterol is liberated in the lysozome and esterified in the cytoplasm. Cells exposed to sufficient quantities of denatured LDL can acquire the appearance of foam cells, possibly contributing to the accepted role of monocytes in atherogenesis.[110] Plasma LDL that has undergone minor chemical oxidative modification can potently stimulate MCP-1 expression in cultured vascular cells.[200] Lipoproteins in the blood may facilitate adhesion of circulating monocytes to endothelium. The monocyte-derived macrophage plays a role throughout all stages of arteriosclerotic plaque formation. From the initial events in atherogenesis (increased vascular permeability, increased monocyte adherence, and intimal recruitment) to the advanced disease (monocyte/macrophage-derived foam cells, cell necrosis, and formation of a necrotic plaque), atherosclerotic pathogenesis appears to involve a strong monocyte/macrophage inflammatory component. Although the macrophage has usually been considered to be a terminally differentiated cell, proliferation of macrophages in atherosclerotic lesions has been observed.[201]

Clearance of Senescent or Damaged Cells

Senescent and defective red blood cells (such as those formed in hereditary spherocytosis) may be sequestered in the spleen and removed from the circulation by splenic macrophages. Subsequent degradation of cellular material returns of iron to the storage iron pool. The presence of antibody or complement components on red blood cells enhances macrophage erythrophagocytosis in the spleen and the bone marrow and plays a central role in the pathophysiology of immune-mediated hemolytic anemias.

Macrophages have the ability to recognize circulating proteins or cell-associated proteins that have been modified by nonenzymatic reactions with extracellular glucose over time. These glycosylated proteins are taken up through a specific cell-surface receptor designated the advanced glycosylation end-product receptor.[202] Binding to this receptor results in activation of the macrophage with release of cytokines. Macrophages are able to recognize certain sugar residues on tumor cells by specific cell-surface lectins. An N-acetyl galactosamine/galactose-specific receptor on liver macrophages mediates the attachment of desialylated cells to liver macrophages.[203]

Tissue Growth and Repair

Wound Healing

Macrophages are required for angiogenesis and wound healing.[28] They secrete large amounts of fibroblast and epithelial cell growth factors such as TGF-β, FGF, epidermal growth factors, PDGF, and insulin-like growth factors. Many of these growth factors have overlapping angiogenic activities. In addition, macrophages secrete several complement inhibitors such as α_2-macroglobulin, α_1-protease inhibitor, and C3 inhibitor, as well as a wide range of proteases and neutral or metaloprotease inhibitors that facilitate reduction of inflammation and tissue remodeling, respectively.[88] Macrophages are able to induce neovascularization, angiogenesis, and endothelial cell mitogenesis.[204] Macrophages can be activated by the low oxygen pressure and high lactate concentrations within inflamed or wounded tissue.

Hematopoiesis

In the adult bone marrow and fetal liver, resident tissue macrophages express cell-surface receptors that bind developing myeloid and erythroid cells without causing phagocytosis.[205,206] Monocytes and macrophage are capable of secreting a number of hematopoietic growth factors, including CSF-GM, CSF-G, IL-1, and CSF-1.[88]

Bone Metabolism

The osteoclast, which is responsible for bone resorption, remodeling, and calcium homeostasis, is likely derived from a monocyte precursor if not from the monocyte itself. In addition, monocytes release factors such as IL-1 that are potent stimulators of bone resorption through the osteoclast.

Nerve Regeneration

Macrophages appear to play a critical role in nerve regeneration. In addition to the "path clearing" achieved by removal of axonal and myelin debris, macrophages also appear to have a direct effect on regrowth of neurites and Schwann cells, resulting in the production of nerve growth factor and insulin-like growth factor.[207]

REFERENCES

1. Allison AC: On the role of mononuclear phagocytes in immunity against viruses. Prog Med Virol 18:15, 1974
2. Cohn Z: The activation of mononuclear phagocytes: fact, fancy, future. J Immunol 121:813, 1978
3. Fidler IJ, Poste G: Macrophage-mediated destruction of malignant tumor cells and new strategies for the therapy of metastatic disease. Springer Semin Innumopathol 5:161, 1982
4. Karnovsky ML, Lazdins JK: Biochemical criteria for activated macrophages. J Immunol 121:809, 1978
5. Fishman DA, Hay ED: Origin of osteoclasts from mononuclear leukocytes in regenerating new limbs. Anat Rec 143:329, 1962
6. Loutit JF, Nisbet NW: The origin of osteoclasts. Immunobiology 161:193, 1982
7. Junqueira LC, Carneiro J, Contopoulos A: Bone cells. p. 120. In: Basic Histology. 2nd Ed. Lange, Los Altos, 1977
8. Kahn AJ, Stewart CC, Teitelbaum SL: Contact-mediated bone resorption by human monocytes in vitro. Science 199:988, 1978
9. Simon GT, Burke JS: Electron microscopy of the spleen. III. Erythroleukophagocytosis. Am J Pathol 58:451, 1970
10. Potten CS, Allen TD: A model implicating the Langerhans cell in keratinocyte proliferation control. Differentiation 5:443, 1976
11. Wisse E: On the fine structure and function of rat liver Kupffer cells. p. 361. In Carr I, Daems WT (eds): The Reticuloendothelial System, A Comprehensive Treatise. Vol 1. Morphology. Plenum Press, New York, 1980
12. Liehr H, Grun M: Clinical aspects of Kupffer cell failure in liver diseases. p. 427. In Wisse E, Knook DL (eds): Kupffer Cells and Other Liver Sinusoidal Cells. Elsevier, Amsterdam, 1977
13. Unanue ER, Allen PM: The basis for the immunoregulatory role of macrophages and other accessory cells. Science 236:551, 1987
14. Rosenthal AS: Determinate selection and macrophage function in genetic control of the immune response. Immunol Rev 40:136, 1978
15. Unanue ER: The regulation of lymphocyte functions by the macrophage. Immunol Rev 40:227, 1978
16. Kirchner H, Herberman RB, Glaser M, Lavrin DH: Suppression in vitro lymphocyte stimulation in mice bearing primary Moloney sarcoma virus-induced tumors. Cell Immunol 13:32, 1974
17. Kirchner H, Muchmore AW, Chused TM et al: Inhibition of proliferation of lymphoma cells and T lymphocytes by suppressor cells from spleens of tumor-bearing mice. J Immunol 114:206, 1975
18. Varesio L, Herberman RB, Gerson JM, Holden HT: Suppression of lymphokine production by macrophages infiltrating murine virus-induced tumors. Int J Cancer 24:97, 1979
19. Collins FM: Cellular mechanisms of anti-mycobacterial immunity. Host defense to intracellular pathogens. Adv Exp Med 162:157, 1983
20. Sbarra AJ, Paul BB, Jacobs AA et al: Role of phagocyte in host-parasite interactions. XXXVII. Metabolic activities of the phagocyte as related to antimicrobial action. J Reticuloendothel Soc 12:109, 1972
21. Trischmann TM: Natural and acquired resistance to *Trypanosoma cruzi*. Host defenses to intracellular pathogens. Adv Exp Med 162:365, 1983
22. Domer JE, Carrow EW: Immunity to fungal infections. Host defenses to intracellular pathogens. Adv Exp Med 162:383, 1983
23. Rager-Zisman B, Brosnan CF, Bloom BR: Macrophage oxidative metabolism:

a defense against viral infection. Host defenses to intracellular pathogens. Adv Exp Med 162:489, 1983

24. Glen KC, Ross R: Human monocyte-derived growth factor(s) for mesenchymal cells: activation of secretion by endotoxin and concanavalin A. Cell 25:603, 1981

25. Nelson M, Nelson DS, Hopper KE: Inflammation and tumor growth. I. Tumor growth in mice with depressed capacity to mount inflammatory response: possible role of macrophages. Am J Pathol 104:114, 1981

26. Averbach R: Angiogenesis-inducing factors; a review. Lymphokines 4:68, 1981

27. Kenyon AJ, Michaels EB: Modulation of early cellular events in wound-healing in mice. Am J Vet Res 44:340, 1983

28. Liebovich SD, Ross R: The role of macrophage in wound repair. Am J Pathol 78:71, 1975

29. Clar RA, Store RD, Leung DYK et al: Role of macrophages in wound-healing. Surg Forum 27:16, 1976

30. Mills EL: Mononuclear phagocytes in the newborn: their relation to the state of relative immunodeficiency. Am J Pediatr Hematol Oncol 5:189, 1983

31. Volkman A, Gowans JL: The origin of macrophages from the bone marrow of the rat. Br J Exp Pathol 46:62, 1965

32. Ralph P, Warren MK, Landner MB et al: Molecular and biological properties of human macrophage growth factor. CSF-1. Cold Spring Harbor Symp Quant Biol 43:679, 1986

33. Shadduck RK, Garsten AL, Chikkappa G et al: Inhibition of diffusion chamber (DC) granulopoiesis by anti-CSF serum. Proc Soc Exp Biol Med 158:542, 1979

34. Heberman RB: Cetus Immunoprimer Series. Part 3. Cetus Publishing, Emeryville, CA, 1989

35. Meuret G, Hoffman G: Monocyte kinetic studies in normal and disease states. Br J Haematol 24:275, 1973

36. Whitelaw DM: Observations on human monocyte kinetics after pulse labeling. Cell Tissue Kinet 5:311, 1972

37. Douglas SD, Musson RA: Phagocytic defects—monocytes/macrophages. Clin Immunol Immunopathol 40:62, 1986

38. Meuret G, Detel U, Kilz HP et al: Human monocytopoiesis in acute and chronic inflammation. Acta Haematol 54:328, 1975

39. Meuret G, Batara E, Furste HO: Monocytopoiesis in normal man: pool size, proliferative activity and DNA synthesis time of promocytes. Acta Haematol 54:261, 1975

40. Piacibello W, Lu L, Wachter M et al: Release of granulocyte-macrophage colony factors from major histocompatibility complex class II antigen-positive monocytes is enhanced by human gamma interferon. Blood 66:1343, 1985

41. Horiguchi J, Warren MK, Ralph P, Kufe D: Expression of the macrophage specific colony-stimulating factor (CSF-1) during human monocyte differentiation. Biochem Biophys Res Commun 141:924, 1986

42. van Waarde DE, Hulsing-Hesselink DE, van Furth R: Properties of a factor increasing monocytopoiesis (FIM) occurring in serum during the early phase of an inflammatory reaction. Blood 50:727, 1977

43. Shapiro SD, Campbell EJ, Senior RM, Welgus HG: Proteinases secreted by human mononuclear phagocytes. J Rheumatol 18:95, 1991

44. Lewis MR: The formation of macrophages, epitheloid cells and giant cells from leukocytes in incubated blood. Am J Pathol 1:91, 1925

45. Ebert RH, Florey HN: The extravascular development of the monocyte observed in vivo. Br J Exp Pathol 20:342, 1938

46. Reeves DL: A study of the in vivo and in vitro behavior of monocytes of the blood stream and connective tissue. Bull Johns Hopkins Hosp 55:245, 1934

47. Johnston RB Jr: Monocytes and macrophages. N Engl J Med 318:574, 1986

48. van Furth R: Development of mononuclear phagocytes. p. 3. In Forster O, Landy O (eds): Heterogeneity of Mononuclear Phagocytes, Academic Press, San Diego, 1981

49. Gordon S: The Biology of the macrophage. J Cell Sci, suppl. 4:267, 1986

50. Kaplan G, Cohn Z: Leprosy and cell-mediated immunity. Curr Opin Immunol 3:91, 1991

51. Adams DO, Hamilton TA: The cell biology of macrophage activation. Annu Rev Immunol 2:283, 1984

52. Beutler B, Cerami A: The biology of cachectin/TNF—a primary mediator of the host response. Annu Rev Immunol 7:625, 1989

53. Hudson MM, Markowitz AB, Gutterman JU et al: Effect of recombinant human interleukin 4 on human monocyte activity. Cancer Res 50:3154, 199.

54. Fiorentino DF, Bond MW, Mosmann TR: Two types of mouse T helper cell. IV. Th2 clones secrete a factor that inhibits cytokine production by Th1 clones. J Exp Med 170:2081, 1989

55. Bar-Eli M, Territo ML, Cline MS: The progeny of a single progenitor cell can

56. Oren R, Farnham AE, Saito K et al: Metabolic patterns in three types of phagocytizing cells. J Cell Biol 17:487, 1963

57. Cohn Z: The structure and function of monocytes and macrophages. Adv Immunol 9:163, 1968

58. Simon LM, Robin ED, Phillips JR et al: Enzymic basis of bioenergenic differences of alveolar versus peritoneal macrophages and enzyme regulation by molecular O_2. J Clin Invest 59:443, 1977

59. Sharra AJ, Karnovsky ML: The biochemical basis of phagocytosis. II. Incorporation of C14-labeled building blocks into lipid, protein and glycogen of leukocytes during phagocytosis. J Biol Chem 235:2224, 1960

60. Cline MJ, Lehrer RL: Phagocytosis by human monocytes. Blood 32:423, 1968

61. Cline MJ: Drug potentiation of macrophage function. Infect Immunol 2:601, 1970

62. Cohen AB, Cline MJ: The human alveolar macrophage: isolation, cultivation in vitro, and studies of morphologic and functional characteristics. J Clin Invest 50:1390, 1971

63. Hamilton TA: Molecular mechanisms in the activation of mononuclear phagocytes. p. 213. In Rogers TJ, Gilman SC (eds): Immunopharmacology. Telford Press, Princeton, NJ, 1988

64. Hamilton TA, Adams DO: Molecular mechanisms of signal transduction in macrophages. Immunol Today 8:151, 1987

65. Adams DO, Johnson SP, Uhing RJ: Early gene expression in the activation of mononuclear phagocytes. p. 587. In Grinstein S, Rothstein OD (eds): Mechanisms of Leukocyte Activation. Academic Press, New York, 1990

66. Nathan CF, Cohn ZA: Cellular components of inflammation: monocytes and macrophages. p. 346. In Kelly W, Harris E, Ruddy S, Hedge R (eds): Textbook of Rheumatology. WB Saunders, Philadelphia, 1984

67. Nathan CF: Secretory products of macrophages. J Clin Invest 79:319, 1987

68. Pace JL, Russell SW, Torres BA et al: Recombinant mouse interferon gamma induces the priming step in macrophage activation for tumor cell killing. J Immunol 130:2011, 1983

69. Schreiber RD, Pace JL, Russell SW et al: Macrophage activating to gamma interferon. J Immunol 131:283, 1983

70. Schultz RM, Kleinschmidt WJ: Functional identity between murine gamma interferon and macrophage activating factor. Nature 305:259, 1983

71. Grabstein KH, Urdal DL, Tushinki RJ et al: Induction of macrophage tumoricidal activity of granulocyte-macrophage colony stimulating factor. Science 232:506, 1986

72. Numerof RP, Aronson FR, Mier JW: IL-2 stimulates the production of IL-1 alpha and IL-1 beta by human peripheral blood mononuclear cells. J Immunol 141:4250, 1988

73. Kovacs EJ, Brock B, Varesio L, Young HA: IL-2 induction of IL-1beta mRNA expression in monocytes. Regulation by agents that block second messenger pathways. J Immunol 143:3532, 1989

74. Narumi S, Finke JH, Hamilton TA: Interferon and interleukin 2 synergize to induce selective monokine expression in murine peritoneal macrophages. J Biol Chem 265:7036, 1990

75. Hart PH, Vitt GF, Burgess DR et al: Potential antiinflammatory effects of interleukin 4: suppression of human monocyte tumor necrosis alpha, interleukin 1, and prostaglandin E_2. Proc Natl Acad Sci USA 86:3803, 1989

76. Hart PH, Burgess DR, Vitti GF, Hamilton JA: Interleukin-4 stimulates human monocytes to produce tissue-type plasminogen activator. Blood 74:1222, 1989

77. Cao H, Wolff RG, Meltzer MS, Crawford RM: Differential regulation of class II MHC determinants on macrophages by IFN-γ and IL-4. J Immunol 143:3523, 1989

78. Essner R, Rhoades K, McBride WH et al: IL-4 down-regulates IL-1 and TNF gene expression in human monocytes. J Immunol 142:3857, 1989

79. Geissler K, Harrington M, Srivastava C et al: Effects of recombinant human colony stimulating factors (CSF) (granulocyte-macrophage CSF, and CSF-1) on human monocyte/macrophage differentiation. J Immunol 143:140, 1989

80. Aderka D, Le J, Vilcek J: IL-6 inhibits lipopolysaccharide-induced tumor necrosis factor production in cultured human monocytes, U937 cells, and in mice. J Immunol 143:3517, 1989

81. Mace KF, Ehrke MJ, Hori K et al: Role of tumor necrosis factor in macrophage activation and tumoricidal activity. Cancer Res 48:5427, 1988

82. Scully SP, Segel GB, Lichtman MA: The relationship of superoxide production to cytoplasmic free calcium in human monocytes. J Clin Invest 77:1349, 1986

83. Verghese MW, Smith CD, Charles LA et al: A guanine nucleotide regulatory protein controls polyphosphoinositide metabolism. Ca^{2+} mobilization, and cellular responses to chemoattractants in human monocytes, J Immunol 137:271, 1986

56. develop characteristics of either a tissue or an alveolar macrophage. Blood 57:95, 1980

84. Babior BM: Oxidants from phagocytes: agents of defense and destruction. Blood 64:959, 1984

85. Klebanoff SJ: Oxygen-dependent cytotoxic mechanisms of phagocytes. p. 111. In Gallin JL, Fauci AS (eds): Advances in Host Defense Mechanisms. Vol. 1. Raven Press, New York, 1982

86. Steinbech MJ, Roth JA: Neutrophil activation by recombinant cytokines. Rev Infect Dis 11:549, 1989

87. Todd RF III, Ikuko F, Mizukami IF et al: Human mononuclear phagocyte activation antigens. Blood Cells 16:167, 1990

88. Rappolee DA, Werb Z: Macrophage-derived growth factors. p. 87. In Russell SW, Gordon S (eds): Macrophages and Macrophage Activation. Current Topics in Microbiology and Immunology. Springer-Verlag, Berlin, 1992

89. Van Damme J, Proost P, Lenaerts JP, Opdenakker G: Structural and functional identification of two human tumor-derived monocyte chemotactic proteins (MCP-2 and MCP-3) belonging to the chemokine family. J Exp Med 176:59, 1992

90. Stein M, Keshav M: The versatility of macrophages. Clin Exp Allergy 22:19, 1992

91. Leonard EJ, Yoshimura T: Human monocyte chemoattractant protein-1 (MCP-1). Immunol Today 11:97, 1990

92. Schall T, Bacon K, Toy KJ, Goeddel DV: Selective attraction of monocytes and T-lymphocytes of the memory phenotype by cytokine RANTES. Nature 347:669, 1990

93. Faruqi RM, DiCorleto PE: Mechanisms of monocyte recruitment and accumulation. Br Heart J, suppl. 69:S19, 1993

94. Arnaout A, Lanier LL, Faller DV: The relative contribution of the leukocyte molecules Mo1, LFA-1, p150,95 (Leu M5) in adhesion of granulocytes and monocytes to vascular endothelium is tissue- and stimulus-specific. J Cell Physiol 137:305, 1988

95. Mentzer SJ, Crimmins MAV, Burakoff SJ, Faller DV: Alpha and beta subunits of the LFA-1 membrane molecule are involved in human monocyte-endothelial cell adhesion. J Cell Physiol 130:410, 1987

96. Pawloski NA, Kaplan G, Abraham E, Cohn ZA: The selective binding and transmigration of monocytes through the junctional complexes of human endothelium. J Exp Med 168:1865, 1988

97. Schwartz CJ, Sprague EA, Kelly JL et al: Aortic intimal monocyte recruitment in the normo- and hypercholesterolemic baboon (Papio cynocephalus). An ultrastructural study: implications in atherogenesis. Virchows Arch A Pathol Anat Histopathol 405:175, 1985

98. Mentzer SJ, Burakoff SJ, Guyre PM, Faller DV: Spontaneous aggregation as a mechanism for human monocyte purification. Cell Immunol 101:101, 1986

99. Mentzer SJ, Burakoff SJ, Faller DV: Interferon-γ induction of LFA-1 mediated homotypic adhesion of human monocytes. J Immunol 137:108, 1986

100. Mentzer SJ, Burakoff SJ, Faller DV: CDw18 regulation of phorbol ester-induced human monocyte-mediated cytotoxicity. Cell Immunol 115:66, 1988

101. Haskill S, Yurochko AD, Isaacs KL: Regulation of macrophage infiltration and activation in sites of chronic inflammation. Ann NY Acad Sci 664:93, 1992

102. Anderson CL, Shen L, Eicher DM et al: Phagocytosis mediated by three distinct Fc gamma receptor classes on human leukocytes. J Exp Med 171:1333, 1990

103. Brown EJ: Complement receptors and phagocytosis. Curr Opin Immunol 3:76, 1991

104. Stahl P, Schlesinger PH, Sigardson E et al: Receptor-mediated pinocytosis of mannose glycoconjugates by macrophages: characterization and evidence for receptor recycling. Cell 79:207, 1980

105. Ezekowitz RA, Stahl PD: The structure and function of vertebrate mannose lectin-like proteins. J Cell Sci, suppl. 9:121, 1988

106. Hoppe CA, Lee YC: The binding and processing of mannose-bovine serum albumin derivatives by rabbit alveolar macrophages. Effect of sugar density. J Biol Chem 258:14193, 1983

107. Broze G: Binding of human factor VII and VIIa to monocytes. J Clin Invest 70:526, 1992

108. Bar-Shavit R, Kahn A, Wilner GD, Fenton JW II: Monocyte chemotaxis: stimulation by specific exosite region in thrombin. Science 220:728, 1983

109. Lolait SJ, Lim ATW, Toh BH, Funder JW: Immunoreactive beta-endorphin in a subpopulation of mouse spleen macrophages. J Clin Invest 73:277, 1984

110. Brown MS, Goldstein JL: Lipoprotein metabolism in the macrophage: implications for cholesterol deposition in atherosclerosis. Annu Rev Biochem 52:223, 1983

111. Fogelman AM, Shecter I, Seager J et al: Malondialdehyde alteration of low density lipoproteins leads to cholesterol ester accumulation in human monocyte-macrophages. Proc Natl Acad Sci USA 77:2214, 1980

112. Gianturco SH, Bradley WA, Gotto AM Jr et al: Hypertriglyceridenic very low density lipoproteins induce tryglyceride synthesis and accumulation in mouse peritoneal macrophages. J Clin Invest 70:168, 1982

113. Kraemer FB, Chen YD, Lopez RD, Reaven GM: Characterization of the binding site on thioglycolate-stimulated mouse peritoneal macrophages that mediates uptake of very low density lipoproteins. J Biol Chem 258:1219, 1983

114. Mizel SB: The interleukins. FASEB J 3:2379, 1989

115. Baggiolini M, Walz A, Kunkel SL: Neutrophil-activating peptide-1/interleukin 8, a novel cytokine that activates neutrophils. J Clin Invest 84:1045, 1989

116. Luster AD, Unkeless JC, Ravetech JB: Gamma interferon transcriptionally regulates an early response gene containing homology to platelet proteins. Nature 315:672, 1985

117. Oquendo P, Albertas J, Wen D et al: The platelet derived growth factor-inducible KC gene encodes a secretory protein related to platelet alpha granules. J Biol Chem 264:4133, 1989

118. Anisowicz A, Bardwell L, Sager R: Constitutive overexpression of a growth-regulated gene in transformed chinese hamster and human cells. Proc Natl Acad Sci USA 84:7188, 1987

119. Graves DT, Jiang YL, Williamson MJ, Valente AJ: Identification of monocyte chemotactic activity produced by malignant cells. Science 254:1490, 1989

120. Ohmori Y, Hamilton TA: A macrophage LPS-inducible early gene encodes the murine homologue IP-10. Biochem Biophys Res Commun 168:1261, 1990

121. Sherry B, Horii Y, Manogue KR et al: Macrophage Inflammatory Proteins 1 and 2: An Overview. Cytokines. Vol. 4. Karger, Basel, 1992

122. Singh JP, Bonin PD: Purification and biochemical properties of a human monocyte-derived growth factor. Proc Natl Acad Sci USA 85:6374, 1988

123. Martinet Y, Bitterman PB, Mornex JF et al: Activated human monocytes express the c-sis-proto-oncogene and release a mediator showing PDGF like activity. Nature 319:158, 1986

124. Blair A, Mormede P, Bohlen P: Immunoreactive fibroblast growth factor in cells of peritoneal exudate suggests its identity with macrophage-derived growth factor. Biochem Biophys Res Commun 126:358, 1985

125. Shimokada K, Raines EW, Madtes DK et al: A significant part of macrophage derived growth factor consists of at least two forms of PDGF. Cell 43:277, 1985

126. Navarro S, Debili N, Bernaudin J-F et al: Regulation of the expression of IL-6 in human monocytes. J Immunol 142:4339, 1989

127. Sayers TJ, Macher I, Chung J et al: The production of tumor necrosis factor by mouse bone marrow-derived macrophages in response to bacterial lipopolysaccharide and chemically synthesized monosaccharide precursor. J Immunol 136:2935, 1987

128. Fibbe WE, Van Damme J, Billiau A et al: Interleukin 1 induces release of granulocyte-macrophage colony-stimulating activity from human mononuclear phagocytes. Blood 68:1316, 1986

129. Simon PL: Calcium mediates one of the signals required for interleukin-1 and 2 production by murine cell lines. Cell Immunol 87:720, 1984

130. Beutler B, Krochin N, Milsark IW et al: Control of cachectin (tumor necrosis factor) synthesis: mechanisms of endotoxin resistance. Science 232:977, 1986

131. Burchett SK, Weaver WM, Westall JA et al: Regulation of tumor necrosis factor/cachectin and IL-1 secretion in human mononuclear phagocytes. J Immunol 140:3473, 1988

132. Dinarello CA: Biology of interleukin 1. FASEB J 2:108, 1988

133. Dinarello CA: Interleukin-1. Ann NY Acad Sci 546:122, 1988

134. Kriegler M, Perez C, DeFay K et al: A novel form of TNF/cachectin is a cell surface cytotoxic transmembrane protein: ramifications for the complex physiology of TNF. Cell 53:45, 1988

135. Beutler B, Milsark IW, Cerami A: Cachectin/tumor necrosis factor: production, distribution, and metabolic fate in vivo. J Immunol 135:3972, 1985

136. Turner M, Chantry D, Buchan G et al: Regulation of expression of human IL-1alpha and IL-1beta genes. J Immunol 143:3556, 1989

137. Dinarello CA, Ikejim T, Warner SJC et al: Interleukin 1 induces interleukin 1. Induction of circulating interleukin 1 in rabbits in vivo in human mononuclear cells in vitro. J Immunol 139:1902, 1987

138. Nishizawa M, Nagata S: Regulatory elements responsible for inducible expression of granulocyte colony-stimulating factor gene in macrophages. Mol Cell Biol 10:2022, 1990

139. Bevilacqua MP, Pober JS, Najeau GR et al: Recombinant tumor necrosis factor induces procoagulant activity in cultured human vascular endothelium: characterization and comparison with the actions of interleukin 1. Proc Natl Acad Sci USA 83:4533, 1986

140. Dinarello CA, Cannon JG, Wolff SM et al: Tumor necrosis factor (cachectin) is an endogenous pyrogen and induces production of interleukin-1. J Exp Med 163:1433, 1986

141. Hasselgren PO, Pedersen P, Sax HC et al: Current concepts of protein turnover and amino acid transport in liver and skeletal muscle during sepsis. Arch Surg 123:992, 1988

142. Mackiewicz A, Ganapathi MK, Schultz D et al: Regulation of rabbit acute phase protein biosynthesis by monokines. Biochem J 253:851, 1988

143. Moldawer LL, Georgieff M, Lundholm K: Interleukin 1, tumor necrosis factor-alpha (cachectin) and the pathogenesis of cancer cachexia. Clin Physiol 7: 263, 1987

144. Moldawer LL, Marano MM, Wei H et al: Cachectin/tumor necrosis factor-alpha alters red blood cell kinetics and induces anemia in vivo. FASEB J 3: 1637, 1989

145. Castell JV, Gomez-Lechon MJ, David M et al: Interleukin-6 is the major regulator of acute phase protein synthesis in adult human hepatocytes. FEBS Lett 242:237, 1989.

146. Mackaness GB: Resistance to intracellular infection. J Infect Dis 123:439, 1971

147. Nathan CF: Secretion of oxygen intermediates: role in effector functions of activated macrophages, Fed Proc 41:2206, 1982

148. Klebanoff SJ: Oxygen-dependent antimicrobial systems in mononuclear phagocytes. p. 487. In Reichard S, Kojima M (eds): Macrophage Biology. Alan R Liss, New York, 1985

149. Territo MC, Cline MJ: Monocyte function in man. J Immunol 118:187, 1977

150. Cline MJ, Lehrer RI, Territo MC, Golde DW: Monocytes and macrophages: functions and diseases. Ann Intern Med 88:78, 1978

151. Young LH, Liu CC, Joag S et al: How lymphocytes kill. Annu Rev Med 41:45, 1990

152. Ganz T, Selsted ME, Szklarek D et al: Defensins: natural peptide antibiotics of human of human neutrophils. J Clin Invest 76:1427, 1985

153. Elsbach P, Weiss J: A reevaluation of the roles of the O_2-dependent and O_2-independent microbiocidal systems of phagocytes. J Clin Invest 5:843, 1983

154. Lehrer RI, Ganz T, Selsted ME et al: Neutrophils and host defense. Ann Intern Med 109:127, 1988

155. Ganz T, Sherman MP, Selsted ME, Lehrer RI: Newborn rabbit alveolar macrophages are deficient in two microbicidal cationic peptides, MCP-1 and MCP-2. Am Rev Respir Dis 132:901, 1986

156. Jones TC: Interactions between murine macrophages and obligate intracellular protozoa. Am J Pathol 102:127, 1981

157. Brummer E, Morozumi PA, Philpott DE, Stevens DA: Virulence of fungi: correlation of virulence of *Blastomyces dermatitidis* in vivo with escape from macrophage inhibition of replication in vitro. Infect Immun 32:864, 1981

158. Wu-Hsieh B, Howard DH: Inhibition of growth of *Histoplasma capsulatum* by lymphokine-stimulated macrophages. J Immunol 132:2593, 1984

159. Gentry LO, Remington JS: Resistance against cryptococus conferred by intracellular bacteria and protozoa. J Infect Dis 123:22, 1971

160. Green S, Meltzer MS, Crawford RM, Nacy CA: *Leishmania major* amastigotes initiate L-arginine-dependent killing activity in IFN-gamma-stimulated macrophages by induction of INF-alfa. J Leukoc Biol 1:92, 1990

161. Stuehr DJ, Kwon NS, Gross SS et al: Synthesis of nitrogen oxides from L-arginine by macrophage cytosol: requirement for inducible and constitutive components. Biochem Biophys Res Commun 161:420, 1989

162. Stuehr DJ, Nathan CF: Nitric oxide, a macrophage product responsible for cytostasis and respiratory inhibition in tumor target cells. J Exp Med 169: 1543, 1989

163. Nacy CA, Green SJ, Leiby DA et al: Macrophages, cytokines, and leishmania. p. 100. In Lopez-Berestein G, Klostergaard J (eds): Mononuclear Phagocytes in Cell Biology. CRC Press, Boca Raton, FL, 1992

164. Granger DL, Lee-See K, Hibbs JB Jr: Role of macrophage-derived nitrogen oxide in antimicrobial function. p. 304. In Lopez-Berestein G, Klostergaard J (eds): Mononuclear Phagocytes in Cell Biology. CRC Press, Boca Raton, FL, 1992

165. Nathan CF, Murray HW, Wiebe ME, Rubin BY: Identification of interferon-γ as the lymphokine that activates human macrophage oxidative metabolism and antimicrobial activity. J Exp Med 158:670, 1983

166. Murray HW: The interferons, macrophage activation, and host defense against nonviral pathogens. J Interferon Res 12:319, 1992

167. Gendelman HE, Orenstein JM, Weiser B et al: The macrophage in the persistence and pathogenesis of HIV infection. AIDS 3:475, 1989

168. Meltzer MS, Skillmam DS, Gomatos PJ et al: Role of mononuclear phagocytes in the pathogenesis of human immunodeficiency virus infection. Annu Rev Immunol 8:169, 1990

169. Stoler MH, Eskin TA, Benn S et al: Human T cell lymphotropic virus type III infection of the central nervous system. Preliminary in situ analysis. JAMA 256:2360, 1986

170. Koenig S, Gendelman HE, Orenstein JM et al: Detection of AIDS virus in macrophages in brain tissue from AIDS patients with encephalopathy. Science 233:1089, 1986

171. Peters PJ, Neefjes JJ, OOrschot V et al: Segregation of MHC class II molecules from MHC class molecules in the Golgi complex for transport to lysosome compartments. Nature 349:669, 1991

172. Grey HM, Chestnut RW: The role of macrophages and B cells in antigen processing and presentation to T cells. p. 125. In Reichard S, Kojima M (eds): Macrophage Biology. Alan R Liss, New York, 1985

173. Kosco MH: Antigen presentation to B cells. Curr Opin Immunol 3:336, 1991

174. Rizvi N, Chaturvedi UC, Mathur A: Obligatory role of macrophages in dengue virus antigen presentation to B lymphocytes. Immunology 67:38, 1989

175. Mufson RA, Aghajanian J, Wong G et al: Macrophage colony-stimulating factor enhances monocyte and macrophage antibody-dependent cell-mediated cytotoxicity. Cell Immunol 119:182, 1989

176. Munn DH, Cheung NKV: Antibody-dependent antitumor cytotoxicity by human monocytes cultured with recombinant macrophage colony-stimulating factor: induction of efficient antibody-mediated antitimor cytotoxicity not detected by isotope release assays. J Exp Med 170:511, 1989

177. Peck R, Brockhaus M, Frey JR: Cell surface tumor factor (TNF) accounts for monocyte and lymphocyte-mediated killing of TNF-resistant target cells. Cell Immunol 122:1, 1989

178. Sampson-Johannes A, Carlino JA: Enhancement of human monocyte tumoricidal activity by recombinant M-CSF. J Immunol 141:3680, 1989

179. Mantovani A, Bottazzi B, Colotta F et al: The origin and function of tumor-associated macrophages. Immunology Today 13:265, 1992

180. Rollins BJ, Sunday ME: Suppression of tumor formation in vivo by expression of the JE gene in malignant cells. Mol Cell Biol 11:3125, 1991

181. Bottazzi B, Walter S, Govoni D et al: Monocyte chemotactic gene transfer modulates macrophage infiltration, growth, and susceptibility to IL-2 therapy of a murine melanoma. J Immunol 148:1280, 1992

182. Houghton AN, Mintzer D, Cordon-Cordo C et al: Mouse monoclonal IgG3 antibody detecting GD3 ganglioside: a phase I trial in patients with malignant melanoma. Proc Natl Acad Sci USA 82:1242, 1985

183. Cheung NK, Lazarus H, Miraldi FD et al: Ganglioside GD2 specific monoclonal antibody 3F8: a phase I study in patients with neuroblastoma and malignant melanoma. J Clin Oncol 5:1430, 1987

184. Mentzer SJ, Faller DV: Soluble and surface bound immunoglobulin triggers human monocyte activation and hydrogen peroxide release. Exp Hematol 18:812, 1990

185. Sagone AL, Rinehart JJ: Human monocyte to macrophage differentiation in vitro: characterization and mechanisms of the increased antibody-dependent cytotoxicity associated with differentiation. J Leukoc Biol 35:217, 1984

186. Adams DO, Nathan CF: Molecular mechanisms in tumor cell killing by activated macrophages. Immunol Today 4:166, 1983

187. Pace JL, Russel SW: Activation of mouse macrophages for tumor cell killing. Quantitative analysis of interactions between lymphokine and lipopolysaccharide. J Immunol 126:1863, 1981

188. Meltzer MS: Macrophage activation for tumor cytotoxicity: characterization of priming and trigger signals during lymphokine activation. J Immunol 127: 179, 1981

189. Simmons SR, Karnovsky ML: Iodinating ability of various leukocytes and their bactericidal activity. J Exp Med 138:44, 1973

190. Miller TE: Metabolic event involved in the bactericidal activity of normal mouse macrophages. Infect Immunol 3:390, 1971

191. Hibbs JB Jr, Vavrin Z, Taintor RR: L-arginine is required for expression of the activated macrophage effector mechanism causing selective metabolic inhibition in target cells. J Immunol 138:550, 1987

192. Hibbs JB Jr, Taintor RR, Vavrin Z, Rachlin EM: Nitric oxide: a cytotoxic activated macrophage effector molecule. Biochem Biophys Res Commun 157:87, 1988

193. Lepoivre M, Chenais B, Yapo A et al: Alterations of ribonucleotide reductase activity following induction of the nitrate-generating pathway in adenocarcinoma cells. J Biol Chem 265:14143, 1990

194. Higuchi M, Higashi N, Taki H, Osawa T: Cytolytic mechanisms of activated macrophages: tumor necrosis factor and L-arginine-dependent mechanisms act synergistically as the major cytolytic mechanisms of activated macrophages. J Immunol 144:1425, 1990

195. Unanue ER, Beller DI, Lu CY, Allen PM: Antigen presentation: comments on its regulation and mechanism. J Immunol 732:1, 1984

196. Tavassoli M: Intravascular phagocytosis in the rabbit bone marrow: a possible fate of normal senescent red cells. Br J Haematol 36:323, 1977

197. Johnston RB Jr: Monocytes and macrophages. N Engl J Med 318:747, 1988

198. Holian A, Scheule RK: Alveolar macrophage biology. Hosp Pract 25:53, 1990

199. Friedland GH, Klein, RS: Transmission of the human immunodeficiency virus. N Engl J Med 317:278, 1987

200. Cushing SD, Berliner JA, Valente AJ et al: Minimally modified low density lipoprotein induces monocyte chemotactic protein-1 in human endothelial cells and smooth muscle cells. Proc Natl Acad Sci USA 87:5134, 1990

201. Rosenfeld ME, Ross R: Macrophage and smooth muscle cell proliferation in atherosclerotic lesions of WHHL and comparably hypercholesterolemic fat-fed rabbits. Arteriosclerosis 10:680, 1990

202. Radoff S, Cerami A, Vlassara H: Isolation of surface binding protein specific

for advanced glycosylation end products from mouse macrophage-derived cell line RAW 264.7. Diabetes 39:1510, 1990

203. Kolb-Bachofen V, Schlepper-Schafer J, Roos P et al: GalNAc/Gal-specific rat liver lectins: their role in cellular recognition. Biol Cell 51:219, 1984

204. Sunderkotter C, Goebeler M, Schulze-Osthoff K et al: Macrophage-derived angiogenesis factors. Pharmacol Ther 51:195, 1991

205. Crocker PR, Gordon S: Isolation and characterization of resident stromal macrophages and haematopoietic cell clusters from mouse bone marrow. J Exp Med 162:993, 1985

206. Perry HV, Brown MC: Macrophages and nerve regeneration. Curr Opin Neurobiol 2:679, 1992

207. Morris L, Crocker PR, Gordon S: Murine foetal liver macrophages bind developing erythroblasts by a divalent cation-dependent haemagglutinin. J Cell Biol 104:649, 1988

208. Gabrilove JL: Introduction and overview of hematopoietic growth factors. Semin Hematol, suppl. 2, 26:1, 1989

209. Griffin JD: Clinical applications of colony stimulating factors. Oncology 2: 15, 1988

Eosinophil and Basophil Structure and Function

51

Susan B. Shurin

INTRODUCTION

Eosinophils and basophils are cells that originate from myeloid stem cells, develop in the bone marrow, and spend most of their lives within tissues, rather than in the blood or bone marrow. They enter the province of hematology because of their myeloid origin and because increased numbers of these cells in the peripheral blood are important clues to the existence of systemic diseases, including bone marrow dysfunction. Many of the intricacies of their function and pathology are detailed in the disciplines of pathology, immunology, allergy, and parasitology. Eosinophils and basophils share the developmental characteristics as well as many of the functional characteristics of their first cousins, neutrophils and monocytes. They are terminally differentiated cells, incapable of cell division, but are more long-lived than neutrophils. Their granule contents are responsible for many stimulatory and inhibitory effects on acute inflammation. Their cell bodies express surface receptors for immunoglobulins and complement that dramatically affect their function. The temptation to draw precise parallels between the physiologic function of eosinophils and basophils and those of neutrophils and monocytes/macrophages has been accentuated by their scarcity in peripheral blood, the difficulties in isolating viable, intact cells from tissues, and their altered functional status in circumstances in which their increased numbers make them more accessible. Nonetheless, much is known about their structure, the contents of their granules, and their surface membrane receptors. Their function in pathologic states is better understood than is their role in normal homeostasis.

Eosinophils and basophils appear to interact in mediating allergic and inflammatory reactions. They stimulate and inactivate each other's functions and share some unusual granule contents (major basic protein [MBP] and Charcot-Leyden crystal [CLC] protein). Patients lacking both eosinophils and basophils have been described, and both eosinophils and basophils tend to be elevated in conditions in parasitic infections. Mixed eosinophil and basophil colonies occur in vitro, and basophils often appear in clonally derived eosinophilic colonies (Table 51-1).

EOSINOPHILS

Eosinophils are capable of both enhancing and suppressing acute inflammatory reactions.[1] Eosinophils are involved in mediating or responding to helmintic infection, allergy, and certain tumors. They are capable of phagocytosis, like neutrophils, but are primarily secretory cells. Most of their functions require the release of granule contents or reactive species generated by the cell membrane when the membrane is activated by particulate or soluble stimuli. Eosinophils respond to unique chemotactic agents and growth factors, permitting their accumulation in sites of inflammatory reactions. Their nuclei are bilobed and are often obscured by the prominent granules that overlie them. The cells are somewhat larger than neutrophils and appear to be quite fragile, often fragmenting when blood smears are made.

Eosinophilic Structure

Eosinophil Granules

The granules of eosinophils, their most distinctive morphologic feature, were first described in 1879 by Paul Ehrlich. The strongly basic proteins within the granules stain intensely with acid dyes. They also have a striking and unique appearance under the electron microscope.[2] Three types of eosinophil granules are recognized at different stages of cell maturation.[3] The primary granules are round, uniform, and noted at the stage of eosinophilic promyelocyte in the bone marrow. As eosinophils differentiate, they develop cores, later recognized as secondary or specific granules. These granules consist of an electron-dense core and a relatively radiolucent matrix surrounding the core. Eosinophil peroxidase (EPO) activity is located in the granule matrix. The dense core has a crystalloid structure with periodicity in both its longitudinal and cross-sectional axis. The dense core contains MPB,[4] while the matrix surrounding it contains eosinophil cationic proteins (ECPs),[5] eosinophil-derived neurotoxin (EDN), and a variety of enzymes. The third type of granule contains acid phosphatase and arylsulfatase.

Table 51-1. Comparison of Eosinophils and Basophils

	Eosinophils	Basophils
Chemoattractants	C5a	Eosinophil chemotactic factor
	FMLP	of anaphylaxis
	LTB$_4$	LTB$_4$
	PAF	
	Histamine	
	IL-3	
Stimulants for degranulation	LTB$_4$	IgE
	ECFA	C3a, C5a
	Tumor necrosis factor	IL-1, IL-5
		Insect venoms
	PAF	Cold exposure
	IgG, IgA, IgE	Some drugs
	IL-3, IL-5	Some hormones
	Histamine	CSF-GM
	CSF-GM	
Arachidonic acid products produced by cells	LTB$_4$	LTC$_4$
	LTC$_4$	LTD$_4$ (SRS-A)
		PAF
Colony-stimulating factors for cells	IL-3	IL-1
	IL-5	IL-3
	CSF-GM	CSF-GM
Granule contents	MBP (dense core)	Histamine
	EPO (matrix)	Kallikrein
	EDN	TAME-esterase
	Arginine-rich cationic proteins	Sulfated glycosaminoglycans (heparin, chondroitin sulfate)
	Acid phosphatase	MBP
	Aryl sulfatase	Trypsin
		Chymotrypsin
Membrane	NADPH-dependent oxidase	Fcε receptor
		Lysophospholipase
	Fcα, -γ, -ε	
	C3b receptor	
	C5a receptor	
	FMLP receptor	

MBP is a relatively small protein (11,000 MW) with an isoelectric point of ≥pH 10. It comprises >50% of the total granule protein. The molecule has a pronounced tendency to aggregate in solution. Antibodies raised to MBP have permitted localization of the protein to the dense, crystalloid core of the granule.[4,6,7] Purified MBP is capable of inflicting considerable damage on schistosomules of *Schistosoma mansoni* by binding tightly to the membrane of the parasite and disrupting the membrane.[8,9] Eosinophils bind to schistosomules opsonized with IgG antibody and degranulate on their surfaces, depositing large amounts of MBP.[10] MBP on the surface of schistosomules increases the adherence of both eosinophils and neutrophils to the schistosomules, thereby enhancing cytotoxicity. MBP is also released into the culture supernatant of degranulating eosinophils.[11,12] Incubation in medium containing released MBP damages the larvae of *Trichinella spiralis,* as well as several varieties of murine tumor cells. MBP also induces histamine release from basophils and mast cells.[12]

ECPs are a group of granule proteins with molecular weights ranging from 21,000 to 29,000 and isoelectric points greater than pH 11. They are rich in arginine and cystine.[5,6,14] ECPs comprise about 30% of the granule protein. While they are similar in physicochemical properties, and thus tend to co-purify, the proteins are immunologically distinct. ECPs bind to hepa-

rin, neutralize its anticoagulant activity, and have complex relationships with both contact factors and fibrinolytic proteins in human plasma. They are also toxic to the schistosomules of *S. mansoni,* in a manner similar to MBP, but they are less extensively studied. EDN is a powerful neurotoxin that acts against myelinated nerve fibers.[5,14] The initial demonstration of this effect in experimental animals in 1933 was one of the earliest demonstrations of host tissue damage by eosinophils and is known as the Gordon phenomenon, for its discoverer, M. H. Gordon. The molecular weight of EDN is about 18,000.[15] EDN is an extremely potent neurotoxin; intrathecal administration of microgram quantities to rabbits and guinea pigs produces a characteristic syndrome of ataxia, weakness, and movement disorders, without evidence of impairment of intellectual function or level of consciousness. The Purkinje cells disappear from the cerebellum, and the white matter of cerebellum, brain stem, and spinal cord are damaged, while the gray matter is intact. EDN is thought to play a role in the neurologic abnormalities occasionally encountered in patients with idiopathic hypereosinophilic syndrome and in conditions with cerebrospinal fluid eosinophilia.

EPO is located in the matrix of the eosinophil granule.[16,17] The peroxidase activity of eosinophils is 2.5 times as great as that of neutrophils on a per cell basis. EPO consists of a single polypeptide chain of 75,000 MW that also exists as a dimer. EPO is a different enzyme biochemically, immunochemically, and genetically from myeloperoxidase (MPO) of neutrophils. Patients with neutrophil MPO deficiency have normal EPO activity. However, the biochemical effects of EPO are similar to those of MPO. Using hydrogen peroxide and a halide, EPO generates reactive oxygen species, such as hypochlorous acid, capable of killing a wide variety of targets, including bacteria, fungi, viruses, *Mycoplasma,* helminths, and tumor cells. EPO is a sticky protein that tends to adhere both to host cells (eosinophils that have secreted EPO and to mast cells in the neighborhood) and target cells, enhancing the cytotoxic effect of even small amounts of hydrogen peroxide in the presence of physiologic amounts of halide ions, especially chloride and iodide. EPO plays a major role in antihelmintic activities of eosinophils, although some cytotoxic capability against schistosomules and *Trypanosoma cruzi* is retained without EPO. It is also released in human mucous membranes with degranulation of eosinophils during allergic reactions. EPO deficiency has been described and appears to have no clinical significance. Five EPO-deficient subjects were identified from 131,000 peripheral blood samples examined for automated analysis.[18] The cells of these subjects contain ECP and EDN, and display an increased ratio of the granule core volume to the total granule volume.

Neutrophil-specific granule deficiency is a rare disorder in which the secondary or specific granules are lacking in polymorphonuclear leukocytes. The eosinophils of patients with specific granule deficiency are also deficient in their specific granule contents.[19] The eosinophil granule contains both primary and secondary granule contents. CLC protein and EPO can both be found in these eosinophils. However, ECP, EDN, and MBP cannot be detected in cells that contain EPO. The characteristic staining pattern of eosinophils is determined by the proteins that are missing, so eosinophils are not readily identified morphologically in patients with specific granule deficiency. mRNA transcripts for these three proteins are found in these cells, so the global defect appears to be in granule formation rather than in the absence of genetic material for the proteins themselves. These granules are formed from the Golgi apparatus in both cell types. The precise defect is not known.

Plasma Membrane Activities

NADPH-dependent membrane-bound oxidase is similar or identical in kinetics and behavior to that of the neutrophil oxidase but appears to be present in much larger quantities in the eosinophil. Thus, eosinophils generate considerably greater quantities of superoxide when stimulated by either soluble or particulate stimuli than do neutrophils.[20-23] A substantial component of the antihelmintic activity of eosinophils is oxygen dependent and is eliminated by incubation of the cells in anaerobic environments. Eosinophils from patients with chronic granulomatous disease (CGD) are unable to generate superoxide or other reactive oxygen species; they have biochemical deficits identical to those seen in CGD neutrophils, but their antiparasitic and antitumor activities are not eliminated.[24] Oxygen-independent mechanisms of cytotoxicity are capable of inflicting substantial damage.

Lysophospholipase (CLC protein) was first described morphologically in patients with leukemia and asthma.[25] It is only expressed in eosinophils and basophils, in approximately equivalent amounts. The bipyramidal hexagons in tissues and body fluids are pathologic fingerprints of the eosinophil. The molecular weight of reduced lysophospholipase is 13,000, but it normally exists as a dimer and readily polymerizes to form CLCs. Lysophospholipase catalyzes the hydrolysis and inactivation of lysophospholipids, which in turn are formed by the action of phospholipase A_2. The biologic effect of lysophospholipase is to prevent the generation of a wide variety of arachidonic acid metabolites, effectively dampening the inflammatory process. The enzyme activity appears to be located primarily in the plasma membrane of the eosinophil and basophils, and it co-purifies with the plasma membrane fractions. Granule fractions show no lysophospholipase activity, but ultrastructurally, CLC protein is found in a crystalloid-free granule population of mature eosinophils. This may be a granule protein that is transferred to the plasma membrane.[26] cDNA for CLC protein encodes a sequence that does not resemble prokaryotic or eukaryotic lysophospholipases but has substantial sequence homology with C-terminal domains of four IgE-binding proteins, including Mac-2.[27] It is not clear whether CLC protein exhibits lectin carbohydrate-binding activity. A functional CLC promoter has been identified and exhibits similarities to other leukocyte-specific promoters.[28]

Plasma membrane receptors respond to, and interact with, IgG, IgA, IgE (Fcγ, Fcα, and Fcε), C3b, and antigens identified by antieosinophilic antibodies that are not characterized.[29,30] These receptors mediate both phagocytosis and degranulation. Also present are receptors that enable the cells to respond to a variety of chemotactic stimuli, such as f-met-leu-phe (FMLP) and C5a,[31] as well as specific receptors for platelet-activating factor (PAF).[32,33] These PAF receptors are involved in signal transduction via G proteins, analogous to identical processes in neutrophils.[34] Eosinophils, unlike neutrophils, express the ligand (VLA-4) that mediates adhesion to vascular cell adhesion molecule-1.[35] Expression of these receptors is crucial for the intercellular interactions that control neutrophil function.[36]

Eosinophilic Function

Eosinophils respond to a variety of chemotactic factors that enable them to enter inflammatory sites to perform their various functions. These chemotactic factors include several shared with neutrophils, such as C5a, N-formyl-methionyl peptides, and leukotriene B_4 (LTB$_4$).[37] Several chemotactic stimuli are highly specific for eosinophils. These include PAF, which is produced by a wide variety of cells involved in acute inflammation such as neutrophils, platelets, monocytes, and eosinophils themselves, and eosinophil stimulation promoter, which is produced by T lymphocytes. Basophils and tissue mast cells release histamine, eosinophil chemotactic factor of anaphylaxis (ECFA), and LTB$_4$ that are chemotactic for the eosinophil.[38] A variety of parasite-derived factors are chemotactic for

eosinophils in much the same way that bacterial factors are chemotactic for neutrophils.

Some of the same factors that attract eosinophils are capable of activating them—enhancing cell-surface receptors, inducing degranulation, activating the NADPH-dependent oxidase, and inducing release of arachidonic acid metabolites. These factors include LTB$_4$, histamine, and ECFA from mast cells and basophils[39]; tumor necrosis factor and eosinophil-activating factor from monocytes; parasite-derived factors; and colony-stimulating factors (CSFs), which also induce eosinophil production. The dense and α-granules of platelets secrete chemotactic activity for eosinophils not released by completely degranulated platelets and decreased in amount in storage pool defect.[40] When stimulated, eosinophils release significant amounts of the inflammatory mediators leukotriene C_4 (LCT$_4$) and 15-HETE, as well as LTB$_4$, thus contributing to ongoing inflammation.[41] Secretion of the basic proteins in specific granules appears to have some selectivity, depending on the specific stimulus.[42] For instance, IgG and IgG antibodies induce release of ECP and EDN, which IgE antibodies do not. By contrast, IgE induces release of EPO, but not ECP. IgA induces release of EPO, but IgG does not. These findings suggest that each of the immunoglobulin receptors may be linked to a different signal transduction pathway.[43]

PAF is one of the most important activators of normal eosinophils.[33] Specific receptors are coupled to the pertussis toxin-sensitive G_i protein.[44,45] Phosphoinositide turnover and generation of the second messengers diacylglycerol and inositol triphosphate are stimulated by activation of PAF receptors. Responses to PAF include chemotaxis, adherence to endothelial cells, enhanced binding of IgE, production and release of superoxide, release of granule proteins, decrease in cell density, and synthesis of prostanoids.[46] PAF is also synthesized and released by activated eosinophils.[47]

Both the numbers of cells developing in the bone marrow and the physiologic activity of eosinophils are enhanced by the effects of CSF-granulocyte/macrophage (CSF-GM), interleukin (IL)-5, and IL-3.[48,49] In vitro growth of colony-forming unit-eosinophil (CFU-Eo), mature cell-surface receptor expression, degranulation, and reactive oxygen radical production can be enhanced by exposure of these cells to CSF-GM, IL-5, and IL-3, in precise analogy to the effects on neutrophils and monocytes by cytokines.[50-54] Exposure to low doses of IL-5 specifically primes eosinophils for later actions of other stimulants, and exposure to IL-3 and CSF-GM primes both eosinophils and neutrophils.[54] Doses of IL-3 and CSF-GM required to induce eosinophil production in vitro are 10-fold higher than the doses needed to induce production of neutrophils or macrophages. Priming effects of cytokines are probably responsible for the altered physiology of eosinophils in states of eosinophilia. While both IL-3 and CSF-GM enhance eosinophil production, they do so to a much lesser extent than the enhancement of neutrophil and macrophage production. IL-1 and IL-6 do not appear to induce CFU-Eo growth in vitro and do not enhance the effects of IL-5, IL-3, or CSF-GM.[48]

IL-5 has a specific and potent effect on eosinophil growth in culture, with virtually no stimulation of other myeloid colony growth in vitro.[50-57] Administration of anti-IL-5 antibody to mice infected with a variety of parasites completely prevents eosinophilia.[58] Transgenic mice expressing IL-5 show long-lasting eosinophilia.[59] High levels of IL-5 are found in with idiopathic eosinophilia and eosinophilia associated with known disorders.[60-62] The recruitment of eosinophils to Hodgkin disease granulomata appears to result from production of IL-5 by Reed-Sternberg cells, in which mRNA for IL-5 has been identified.[63] IL-5 also enhances eosinophil function, by increasing CD11b/CD18-mediated adhesion and priming cells for the effects of other cell activators to a greater extent than other cytokines prime eosinophils.[64] While IL-5 activates and enhances production of eosinophils, it is only weakly chemotactic for eosinophils. Enhanced tissue migration of eosinophils when IL-5 is increased appears to be mediated by up-regulation of adhesion molecules. IL-5 increases expression of CD11b and enhances adherence to endothelial cells, which can be blocked by antibody to CD11b or CD18. With even weak chemotactic activity induced by IL-5, increased adherence of long-lived cells would be expected to increase their tissue numbers.

The metabolism and behavior of eosinophils vary under different circumstances. The pathologic states associated with eosinophilia are also associated with alterations in eosinophil function.[65-67] "Activated" eosinophils have enhanced generation of reactive oxygen species, enhanced glucose utilization and transport, increased oxygen consumption, reduced cell surface charge, and activation of acid phosphatase in specific granules. Accompanying these changes is a reduction in cell density. Eosinophils are normally more dense than neutrophils and can be separated from them in normal blood on density gradients that are hypertonic (metrizamide) or isotonic (Percoll).[65] In hypereosinophilic states, the cells tend to be substantially lower in density than are normal eosinophils and may be less dense than normal neutrophils.[67] Low-density eosinophils have significantly higher protein kinase C activity than high-density eosinophils.[68] Protein kinase C is important for mediating signal transduction, and its elevation appears to correlate with the enhanced reactivity of low-density eosinophils. Eosinophils may be involved in killing tumor cells in vivo. Patients with colon or breast carcinoma and those with Hodgkin disease, who have peripheral eosinophilia or eosinophil infiltration of their tumors, appear to have a better prognosis than do those without.[69-74]

Eosinophils perform an immunoenhancing function in the defense against helmintic infections.[75] They are able to perform these functions by binding to the surface of helminths, both larval and adult forms; by damaging the target cells with oxygen-dependent mechanisms similar to those of neutrophils, including generation of reactive oxygen species and peroxidation of the surface of larvae and tumor cells via EPO; and by damaging the surface of larval, tumor, and host cells with granule proteins such as MBP and ECP.[76-78] Mice rendered eosinophilopenic with antieosinophil serum are far more susceptible to extensive, invasive infection with a variety of helminths.[79] Eosinophils are capable of producing extensive damage to helminths in vitro. Eosinophil granule proteins, especially MBP and ECP, and reactive oxygen species generated by the membrane oxidase and EPO are capable of killing helminths both alone and in concert. Eosinophil membranes possess Fc receptors and complement receptors; in the presence of specific antibody and complement, they recognize and bind to even large, extracellular, and uningestible multicelled helminths very effectively.[78] In fact, in close apposition with parasites, the eosinophil membrane tends to extend along, and fuse with, the helminth. As a result, the helminth may acquire surface characteristics of the host eosinophil, in addition to its own antigenic characteristics.[77] Although neutrophils, monocytes, and macrophages are capable of many of the functions of the eosinophil, it appears that the eosinophil defends against certain parasitic infections more effectively than do other phagocytic or secretory cells with cytotoxic activity.

The interaction of eosinophils with tumor cells is less well understood. The localization of eosinophils in Hodgkin disease appears to be a function of production of IL-5 by Reed-Sternberg cells.[63] Eosinophils contribute to the fibrosis in nodular sclerosis Hodgkin disease by producing transforming growth factor-β1 (TGF-β1).[78] A positive correlation exists between survival time and eosinophilia in carcinoma of the cervix[70,72] and Hodgkin disease.[73] Tumor infiltration of eosinophils has been associated with a survival advantage in several diseases,[69,71]

but whether this is a cause-and-effect relationship remains unclear.

Eosinophils perform an immunosuppressive function in immediate hypersensitivity reactions.[80] These complex reactions require both phagocytic activity and secretory activity of the cells. The major phagocytic activity is ingestion of granules released from mast cells.[81] Prostaglandins E_1 and E_2 (PGE$_1$ and PGE$_2$) are released from the membrane of activated eosinophils and are capable of suppressing basophil degranulation.[82] Other granule contents are capable of inactivating inflammatory mediators. These include histaminase, which inactivates histamine; phospholipase B, which inactivates PAF of mast cells; MBP, which inactivates mast cell heparin; plasminogen, which reduces local thrombin activity; arylsulfatase, which oxidizes the slow-reacting substance of anaphylaxis (SRS-A)[83]; and lysophospholipase, which prevents the generation of arachidonic acid metabolites.

Fibrosis as a part of inflammatory tissue damage is due to fibroblast growth and collagen synthesis. TGF-β and TGF-α are produced by eosinophils.[84] Eosinophils appear to be the primary source of TGF-β in nodular sclerosing Hodgkin disease.[85] mRNA for TGF-β is detected in eosinophils in nodular sclerosis Hodgkin disease, but not in the eosinophils in other histologic types of Hodgkin disease without fibrosis.

Eosinophils also mediate tissue damage through the effects of MBP, ECP, superoxide, and other reactive oxygen species enhanced by the EPO-peroxide-halide system.[86] The damage to tracheal epithelium mediated by purified MBP is similar to that seen in bronchial asthma. The cardiac and hepatic fibrosis seen in hypereosinophilic syndromes appears to be due to release of toxic components from circulating, activated eosinophils. IL-5 is intimately involved in the cardiac disease induced by eosinophils; it appears to be produced by the cells, and to contribute to their activation.[87]

The balance between the stimulation and inhibition of inflammation by eosinophils is a delicate one. The eosinophils that circulate in states of eosinophilia are qualitatively as well as quantitatively different from normal resting eosinophils. The cells are markedly different in density from normal eosinophils, having already released their dense granule contents. Surface receptor expression is enhanced when the cells are activated. Since the release of granule contents and reactive oxygen species does not occur in normal tissues when eosinophils are not activated, eosinophils are probably more important in inactivating inflammatory mediators in normal conditions than in pathologic conditions, in which they are increased in number and altered in function.

BASOPHILS

Basophils are key mediators of immediate hypersensitivity reactions: asthma, urticaria, allergic rhinitis, and anaphylaxis. They may participate in delayed cutaneous hypersensitivity, and they mediate some of the late-phase responses of anaphylaxis, occurring 3–11 hours after exposure to a stimulus. Basophils are stimulated by soluble mediators, primarily IgE, and degranulate with the release of both granule contents and arachidonic acid metabolites from their plasma membrane. Their relationship to mast cells, which have morphologic and some functional similarities, remains unclear. Increasing information about control of mast cell development, derived from the mast cell-deficient mouse W/Wv, and the involvement of stem cell factor and c-kit ligand, have made these questions increasingly relevant, but they remain unanswered.

Basophilic Structure

Basophils are the least common of the human granulocytes, both in the bone marrow and in the peripheral blood. They normally constitute <0.5% of the nucleated bone marrow cells and peripheral blood leukocytes. Less is known about the basophil than about any other leukocyte. Mast cells are related to, but different from, basophils. Basophils are bilobed, with larger and fewer granules, while mast cells are mononuclear. Labeled basophils appear 2.5–7 days after administration of tritium-labeled thymidine and are gone by 2 weeks. By contrast, mast cells are not labeled by this technique and are long-lived in the tissues, where they are capable of division even after undergoing degranulation.[88] Human mast cells differ phenotypically from basophils. Basophils express receptors for IL-2, IL-3, and CD11b/CD18 that are not expressed on mast cells. Intercellular adhesion molecule-1 receptors and the c-kit product are expressed on mast cells but not basophils.[89] Nevertheless, biochemical similarities exist. Both cells participate in immediate and cutaneous hypersensitivity. They are secretory cells whose cell-surface receptors and granule contents are responsible for their biologic effects.[90] Both cells are derived from a common hematopoietic progenitor cell in the bone marrow.[91] Unlike monocytes and macrophages, transformation between the circulating and tissue forms of these close relatives has not been observed. Both cell types release histamine, kinins, and specific esterases, but only mast cells release PGD_2.

Basophil Granules

The cytoplasmic granules of basophils and mast cells contain sulfated glycosaminoglycans. In normal basophils this is predominantly heparin, but in leukemic basophils it mostly consists of chondroitin sulfate. The heparin of basophils and mast cells appears to have poor anticoagulant activity. The sulfated glycosaminoglycans are the major granule contents responsible for the intense metachromatic staining with basic dyes and for the striking morphologic identifying feature of the basophil.

Basophil granules are the source of most or all circulating histamine. Histamine is synthesized by basophils and is stored within the granule. Many of the immediate hypersensitivity effects are mediated by histamine release. In addition to interacting with histamine receptors in tissues (thus mediating many of the vascular and tissue changes seen in allergic reactions), histamine is a potent eosinophil chemoattractant. Other eosinophil chemotactic factors are contained within the basophil granule that, on release, attract eosinophils to the site of basophil degranulation. Basophils contain about 3% of the MBP present in eosinophils. No other phagocytic cells are thought to possess MBP.

Trypsin and chymotrypsin-like enzymes similar to those identified in neutrophils are also present in basophil granules. These enzymes are responsible for some tissue damage and leakage of capillaries in chronic inflammation.

Basophil kallikrein, which participates in immediate hypersensitivity and particularly in anaphylactic reactions, is present in the basophil granule. The kinins released by degranulated basophils act directly on tissue integrity as well as in stimulating blood coagulation and complement activation.

Basophil Plasma Membrane

A variety of arachidonic acid metabolites are released by basophils when they degranulate; the most important is LTC_4. Perhaps even more important to function are the high-affinity IgE receptors in the basophil membrane that mediate degranulation. The numbers and specificity of IgE receptors vary under different physiologic conditions and tend to be increased in allergic persons. Even at basal levels, the IgE receptors on basophil membranes are notable for their high affinity for ligands.

Basophils express plasma membrane receptors for IL-2, -3, -4, -5, and -8,[92–94] CD11b/CD18, and nerve growth factor.[95] IL-3 is the principal cytokine inducing basophil growth and differentiation in humans, but CSF-GM, IL-4, and IL-5 also participate.[89] It is common to find some basophils among eosinophil colonies

in vitro under the influence of IL-5. Eosinophils and basophils share a common committed stem cell.[96] Most prominent from a functional standpoint is the presence of high-affinity receptors for IgE on the surface of basophils.

Basophilic Function

Interaction between IgE receptors and IgE, with di- or multivalent antigens bridging the receptors, leads to anaphylactic degranulation.[97] Antibodies to the receptors may also directly trigger degranulation.[98] Other stimuli, including C5a and C3,[99] some neutrophil lysosomal proteins, insect venoms, cold, calcium ionophores, some hormones, and some drugs (narcotics, muscle relaxants, radiocontrast dyes) may also directly stimulate basophil degranulation.[100]

When the IgE receptors are brought together after interacting with any appropriate stimulus, the membranes that limit the cytoplasmic granules fuse with the external plasma membrane of the cell, leading to almost immediate release of granule contents.[101,102]

Release of heparin rarely results in significant systemic anticoagulation, perhaps because of the poor anticoagulant activity of the heparin/chondroitin sulfate present in these granules. Clinically significant symptoms derive from the release of histamine and kallikrein, with their multitude of biologic effects.

Other inflammatory mediators released from stimulated basophils are the slow-reacting substance of anaphylaxis (SRS-A also termed LTD_4), PAF-acether, and ECFA, all of which are chemoattractants for eosinophils.[103] Release of ECFAs attracts eosinophils into the area of basophil degranulation. This enables the eosinophils to perform their "damping down" reactions (i.e., inactivation of SRS-A and oxidation of histamine) as well as to contribute to elimination of parasites. As for other granulocytes, physiologic activity and growth (in vitro, and in vivo) of basophils are affected by lymphokines, especially IL-3, but also IL-1 and CSF-GM.[104–106]

Basophils may have a very important role in the late-phase reaction (manifestations of allergic reaction occurring in skin and lung hours after the antigen challenge). Corticosteroids inhibit basophil histamine and LTC_4 release but have no effect on mast cell mediator release. Only IgE-mediated stimuli are active on all mast cells in vitro, while IgE immune complexes, C5a, C3a, FMLP, PAF, and a variety of cytokines, as well as histamine-releasing factor, will degranulate basophils.[107,108]

SUMMARY

Eosinophils and basophils are myeloid cells that are closely related in their bone marrow development and that share several biochemical, functional, and anatomic features (Table 51-1). Both are present in relatively low numbers, except in pathologic conditions, and they tend to be elevated in similar circumstances. Both have bilobed nuclei and highly characteristic granules. Both normally secrete their granule contents and release inflammatory mediators extracellularly, although eosinophils are capable of phagocytosis. Both affect vascular permeability via their inflammatory mediators and express IgE receptors that mediate their degranulation. Basophils contain several mediators that attract and stimulate eosinophils; eosinophils contain compounds that inactivate the inflammatory substances of basophils. Complex interactions between the two cell types and other components of the immune system—monocytes, macrophages, mast cells, platelets, and lymphocytes—are involved in normal immunologic responses to infections, tumors, and parasites. The most unique and apparently specific roles of both eosinophils and basophils are as mediators of hypersensitivity reactions, but they also play major roles as mediators of chronic inflammation, wound healing, fibrosis, neoplasia, and parasitic and allergic diseases.

Recent advances in understanding of the processes of

growth and differentiation of eosinophils and basophils have led to a better appreciation of cytokine biology, cell-cell interactions, and elucidation of key questions in hematopoiesis. Gene transcription in eosinophils and basophils appears to be controlled by GATA-binding proteins,[109] which is easier to appreciate in cells that express proteins not seen in any other myeloid cell lineage. The places where stem cells converge and diverge in development may be easier to identify with studies on eosinophils, basophils and mast cells, since mast cell-deficient mice and rats have basophils and are able to mount normal basophil responses to parasitic infections.[110] The small number of these cells in the blood limits the number of studies, but not the biologic importance of such investigations.

REFERENCES

1. Gleich GJ, Loegering DA: Immunobiology of eosinophils. Annu Rev Immunol 2:429, 1984
2. Archer GT, Hirsch JG: Isolation of granules from eosinophil leukocytes and study of their enzyme content. J Exp Med 118:277, 1963
3. Bainton DF, Farquhar GM: Segregation and packaging of granule enzymes in eosinophilic leukocytes. J Cell Biol 45:54, 1970
4. Lewis DM, Lewis JC, Loegering DA et al: Localization of the guinea pig eosinophil major basic protein to the core of the granule. J Cell Biol 77:702, 1978
5. Ackerman SJ, Loegering DA, Venge P et al: Distinctive cationic proteins of the human eosinophil granule: major basic protein, eosinophil cationic protein and eosinophil-derived neurotoxin. J Immunol 131:2977, 1983
6. Olsson I, Venge P, Spitznagel JK et al: Arginine-rich cationic proteins of human eosinophil granules. Lab Invest 36:493, 1977
7. Peters MS, Schroeter AL, Kephart GM et al: Localization of eosinophil granule major basic protein in chronic urticaria. J Invest Dermatol 81:39, 1983
8. Gleich FJ, Loegering DA, Mann KG et al: Comparative properties of the Charcot-Leyden crystal protein and the major basic protein from human eosinophils. J Clin Invest 57:633, 1976
9. Butterworth AE, Vadas MA, Wassom DL et al: Interactions between human eosinophils and schistosomules of *Schistosoma mansoni*. II. The mechanisms of irreversible eosinophil adherence. J Exp Med 150:1456, 1979
10. Gleich GJ, Frigas E, Loegering DA et al: Cytotoxic properties of the eosinophil major basic protein. J Immunol 123:2925, 1979
11. Wassom DL, Loegering DA, Solley GO et al: Elevated serum levels of the eosinophil granule major basic protein in patients with eosinophilia. J Clin Invest 67:651, 1981
12. Frigas F, Loegering DA, Solley GO et al: Elevated levels of the eosinophil granule major basic protein in the sputum of patients with bronchial asthma. Mayo Clin Proc 56:345, 1981
13. O'Donnell MC, Ackerman SJ, Gleich GJ et al: Activation of basophil and mast cell histamine release by eosinophil granule major basic protein. J Exp Med 157:1981, 1983
14. Filley WV, Ackerman SJ, Gleich GJ: An immunofluorescent method for specific staining of eosinophil granule major basic protein. J Immunol Methods 47:227, 1981
15. Durack DT, Ackerman SJ, Loegering DA et al: Purification of human eosinophil-derived neurotoxin. Proc Natl Acad Sci USA 78:5165, 1981
16. Jong EC, Henderson WR, Klebanoff SJ: Bactericidal activity of eosinophil peroxidase. J Immunol 124:1378, 1980
17. Migler R, DeChatelet LR, Bass DA: Human eosinophil peroxidase: role in bactericidal activity. Blood 51:445, 1978
18. Zabucci G, Soranzo MR, Menegazzi R et al: Eosinophil peroxidase deficiency: morphological and immunocytochemical studies of the eosinophil-specific granules. Blood 80:2903, 1992
19. Rosenberg HF, Gallin JI: Neutrophil-specific granule deficiency includes eosinophils. Blood 82:268, 1993
20. DeChatelet LR, Shirley PS, McPhail L et al: Oxidative metabolism of the human eosinophil. Blood 50:525, 1977
21. DeChatelet LR, Migler RA, Shirley PS et al: Enzymes of oxidative metabolism in the human eosinophil. Proc Soc Exp Biol Med 158:537, 1978
22. Tauber AI, Goetzl EJ, Babior MM: Unique characteristics of superoxide production by human eosinophils in eosinophilic states. Inflammation 3:261, 1979
23. Pincus SH, Schooley WR, DiNapoli AM, Broder S: Metabolic heterogeneity of eosinophils from normal and hypereosinophilic patients. Blood 58:1176, 1981
24. Roberts RL, Ohno Y, Gallin JI: Staining of eosinophils with nitroblue tetrazolium in patients with chronic granulomatous disease. Pediatr Res 20:373, 1986
25. Weller PF, Bach D, Austen KF: Human eosinophil lysophospholipase: the sole protein component of Charcot-Leyden crystals. J Immunol 128:1346, 1982
26. Dvorak AM, Letourneau L, Login GR et al: Ultrastructural localization of the Charcot-Leyden crystal protein (lysophospholipase) to a distinct crystalloid-free granule population in mature human eosinophils. Blood 72:150, 1988
27. Ackerman SJ, Corrette SE, Rosenberg HF et al: Molecular cloning and characterization of human eosinophil Charcot-Leyden crystal protein (lysophospholipase): similarities to IgE-binding proteins and the S-type animal lectin superfamily. J Immunol 150:456, 1993
28. Gomolin HI, Yamaguchi Y, Paulpillai AV et al: Human eosinophil Charcot-Leyden crystal protein: cloning and characterization of a lysophospholipase gene promoter. Blood 82:1868, 1993
29. Abu-Ghazaleh RI, Fujisawa T, Mastecky J et al: IgA-induced eosinophil degranulation. J Immunol 142:2393, 1989
30. Capron M. Eosinophils: receptors and mediators in hypersensitivity. Clin Exp Allergy, suppl. 1. 19:3, 1989
31. Gerard NP, Hodhes MK, Drazen JM et al: Characterization of a receptor for C5a anaphylatoxin on human eosinophils. J Biol Chem 264:1760, 1989
32. Kroegel C, Ykawa T, Dent G et al: Stimulation of degranulation from human eosinophils by platelet-activating factor. J Immunol 142:3518, 1989
33. Hwang SB: Specific receptors of platelet-activating factor, receptor heterogeneity, and signal transduction mechanisms. J Lipid Mediat 2:123, 1990
34. Agrawal DK, Ali N, Numao T: PAF receptors and G-proteins in human blood eosinophils and neutrophils. J Lipid Mediat 5:101, 1992
35. Weller PF, Rand TH, Goelz SE et al: Human eosinophil adherence to vascular endothelium mediated by binding to VCAM-1 and ELAM-1. Proc Natl Acad Sci USA 88:7430, 1991
36. Weller PF: Intercellular interactions in the recruitment and functions of human eosinophils. Int Arch Allergy Immunol 99:178, 1992
37. Anwar ARE, Kay AB: The ECF-A tetrapeptides and histamine selectivity enhance human eosinophil complement receptors. Nature 269:522, 1977
38. Jones DG: The eosinophil. J Comp Pathol 108:317, 1993
39. Weller PF, Lee CW, Foster DW et al: Generation and metabolism of 5-lipoxygenase pathway leukotrienes by human eosinophils: predominant production of leukotriene C4. Proc Natl Acad Sci USA 80:7621, 1983
40. Burgers JA, Schweizer RC, Koenderman L et al: Human platelets secrete chemotactic activity for eosinophils. Blood 81:49, 1993
41. Jorg A, Henderson WR, Murphy RC et al: Leukotriene generation by eosinophils. J Exp Med 155:390, 1982
42. Tomassini M, Tsicopoulos A, Tai P-C et al: Release of granule proteins by eosinophils from allergic and non-allergic patients with eosinophilia on immunoglobulin-dependent activation. J Allergy Clin Immunol 88:365, 1991
43. Shute J: Signal transduction mechanisms in human eosinophils. Clin Exp Allergy 23:713, 1993
44. Kroegel C, Matthys H: Platelet-activating factor-induced human eosinophil activation. Generation and release of cyclooxygenase metabolites in human blood eosinophils from asthmatics. Immunology 78:279, 1993
45. Tool ATJ, Koenderman L, Kok PTM et al: Release of platelet-activating factor is important for the respiratory burst induced in human eosinophils by opsonised particles. Blood 79:2729, 1992
46. Kroegel C, Yukawa T, Dent G et al: Simulation of degranulation from human eosinophils by platelet activating factor. J Immunol 142:3518, 1989
47. Kay AB: Biological properties of eosinophils. Clin Exp Allergy 21:23, 1991
48. Clutterbuck EJ, Hirst EM, Sanderson CJ: Human interleukin-5 (IL-5) regulates the production of eosinophils in human bone marrow cultures: comparison and interaction with IL-1, IL-3, IL-6, and GMCSF. Blood 73:1504, 1989
49. Clutterbuck EJ, Sanderson CJ: Human eosinophil hematopoiesis studied in vitro by means of murine eosinophil differentiation factor (IL5): production of functionally active eosinophils from normal human bone marrow. Blood 71:646, 1988
50. Rothenberg ME, Owen WF Jr, Silberstein DS et al: Human eosinophils have prolonged survival, enhanced functional properties, and become hypodense when exposed to human interleukin 3. J Clin Invest 81:1986, 1988
51. Lopez AF, Sanderson CJ, Gamble JR et al: Recombinant human interleukin 5 is a selective activator of human eosinophil function. J Exp Med 167:219, 1988
52. Warren DJ, Moore MA: Synergism among interleukin 1, interleukin 3, and interleukin 5 in the production of eosinophils from primitive hematopoietic stem cells. J Immunol 140:94, 1988
53. Shurin SB: Pathologic states associated with activation of eosinophils. Hematol Oncol Clin North Am 2:171, 1988
54. Carlson M, Peterson C, Venge P: The influence of IL-3, IL5, and GM-CSF on normal human eosinophil and neutrophil C3b-induced degranulation. Allergy 48:437, 1993

55. Johnson GR, Gonda TJ, Metcalf D et al: A lethal myeloproliferative syndrome in mice transplanted with bone marrow cells infected with a retrovirus expressing granulocyte-macrophage colony stimulating factor. EMBO J 8: 441, 1989

56. Chang JM, Metcalf D, Lang RA et al: Nonneoplastic hematopoietic myeloproliferative syndrome induced by dysregulated multi-CSF (IL-3) expression. Blood 73:1487, 1989

57. Sanderson CJ: Interleukin-5, eosinophils, and disease. Blood 79:3101, 1992

58. Coffman RL, Seymour BW, Hudak S et al: Antibody to interleukin-5 inhibits helminth-induced eosinophilia in mice. Science 245:308, 1989

59. Dent LA, Strath M, Mellor AL et al: Eosinophilia in transgenic mice expressing interleukin 5. J Exp Med 172:1425, 1990

60. Limaye AP, Abrams JS, Silver JE et al: Regulation of parasite-induced eosinophilia: selectively increased interleukin 5 production in helminth-infected patients. J Exp Med 172:399, 1990

61. Owen WF, Rothenberg ME, Petersen J et al: Interleukin 5 and phenotypically altered eosinophils in the blood of patients with the idiopathic hypereosinophilic syndrome. J Exp Med 170:343, 1989

62. Owen WFJ, Petersen J, Sheff DM et al: Hypodense eosinophils and interleukin 5 activity in the blood of patients with the eosinophilia-myalgia syndrome. Proc Natl Acad Sci USA 87:8647, 1990

63. Samoszuk M, Nansen L: Detection of interleukin-5 messenger RNA in Reed Sternberg cells of Hodgkin's disease with eosinophilia. Blood 75:13, 1990

64. Walsh GM, Hartnell A, Wardlaw AJ et al: IL-5 enhances the in vitro adhesion of human eosinophils, but not neutrophils, in a leucocyte integrin (CD11/18)-dependent manner. Immunology 71:258, 1990

65. Vadas MA, David JR, Butterworth AE et al: A new method for the purification of human eosinophils and neutrophils, and a comparison of the abilities of these cells to damage schistosomula of *Schistosoma mansoni.* J Immunol 122:1228, 1979

66. Peters MS, Gleich GJ, Cunnette SL, Fukuda T: Ultrastructural study of eosinophils from patients with the hypereosinophilic syndrome: a morphological basis of hypodense eosinophils. Blood 71:780, 1988

67. Caufield JP, Hein A, Rothenberg ME et al: A morphometric study of normodense and hypodense eosinophils that are derived *in vivo* and *in vitro.* Am J Pathol 137:27, 1990

68. Bates ME, Bertics PJ, Calhoun WJ et al: Increased protein kinase C activity in low density eosinophils. J Immunol 150:4486, 1993

69. Pretlow TP, Keith EF, Cryar AK et al: Eosinophil infiltration of human colonic carcinomas as a prognostic indicator. Cancer Res 43:2997, 1983

70. Lowe D, Jorizzo J, Hutt MSR: Tumour-associated eosinophilia: a review. J Clin Pathol 34: 1343, 1981

71. Pasternak A, Jansa P: Local eosinophilia in stroma of tumors related to prognosis. Neoplasma 31:323, 1984

72. Iwasaki K, Torisu M, Fujimura T: Malignant tumor and eosinophils. Cancer 58:1321, 1986

73. Vaughan-Hudson B, Linch DC, Macintyre EA et al: Selective peripheral blood eosinophilia associated with survival advantage in Hodgkin's disease (BNLI Report No 31). J Clin Pathol 40:247, 1987

74. Butterworth AE, Remold HG, Houba V et al: Antibody-dependent eosinophil-mediated damage to 51Cr-labeled schistosomula of *Schistosoma mansoni:* mediation by IgG, and inhibition by antigen-antibody complexes. J Immunol 118:2230, 1977

75. Grove DI, Mahmoud AAF, Warren KS: Eosinophils in resistance to *Trichinella spiralis.* J Exp Med 145:755, 1977

76. Butterworth AE, David JR, Franks D et al: Antibody-dependent eosinophil-mediated damage to 51Cr-labeled schistosomula of *Schistosoma mansoni:* damage by purified eosinophils. J Exp Med 145:136, 1977

77. Caulfield JP, Korman G, Butterworth A et al: The adherence of human neutrophils and eosinophils to schistosomula: evidence for membrane fusion between cells and parasites. J Cell Biol 86:46, 1980

78. Vadas MA, Butterworth AE, Sherry B et al: Interactions between human eosinophils and schistosomules of *Schistosoma mansoni.* II. Stable and irreversible antibody-dependent eosinophil adherence. J Immunol 124:1441, 1980

79. Mahmoud AAF, Warren KS, Peters PA: A role for the eosinophil in acquired resistance to *Schistosoma mansoni* infection as determined by antieosinophil serum. J Exp Med 142:805, 1975

80. Gleich GJ, Olson GM, Loegering DA: The effect of ablation of eosinophils on immediate-type hypersensitivity. Arch Pathol Lab Med 99:1, 1975

81. O'Donnell MC, Ackerman JS, Gleich SJ et al: Activation of basophil and mast cell histamine release by eosinophil granule major basic protein. J Exp Med 157:1981, 1983

82. Hubscher T: Role of the eosinophil in the allergic reactions. II. Release of prostaglandins from human eosinophilic leukocytes. J Immunol 114:1389, 1975

83. Wasserman SI, Goetzl EJ, Austen KF: Inactivation of slow-reacting substance of anaphylaxis by human eosinophil arylsulfatase. J Immunol 114:645, 1975

84. Wong DT, Weller PF, Galli SJ et al: Human eosinophils express transforming growth factor-alpha. J Exp Med 172:673, 1990

85. Capron M, Tomassini M, Torpier G et al: Selectivity of mediators released by eosinophils. Int Arch Allergy Appl Immunol 88:54, 1989

86. Dri P, Cramer R, Spessotto P et al: Eosinophil activation on biological surfaces: production of O_2^- in response to physiologic stimuli is differently modulated by extracellular matrix components and endothelial cells. J Immunol 147:613, 1991

87. Desreumaux P, Janin A, Dubucquoi S et al: Synthesis of interleukin-5 by activated eosinophils in patients with eosinophilic heart disease. Blood 82:1553, 1993

88. Kuriu A, Sonoda S, Kanakura Y et al: Proliferative potential of degranulated murine peritoneal mast cells. Blood 74:925, 1989

89. Denburg JA: Basophil and mast cell lineages *in vitro* and *in vivo.* Blood 79:846, 1992

90. Hatanaka K, Kitamura Y, Nishimune Y: Local development of mast cells from bone marrow-derived precursors in the skin of mice. Blood 53:142, 1979

91. Patterson R, Pruzansky JJ, Dykewicz MS, Lawrence ID: Basophil-mast cell response syndromes: a unified clinical approach. Allergy Proc 9:611, 1988

92. Mayer P, Valent P, Schmidt G et al: The *in vivo* effects of recombinant human interleukin-3: demonstration of basophil differentiation factor, histamine producing activity, and priming of GM-CSF responsive progenitors in nonhuman primates. Blood 74:613, 1989

93. Valent P, Majdic O, Bodger M et al: Further characterization of surface membrane structures expressed on human basophils and mast cells. Int Arch Allergy Appl Immunol 91:198, 1990

94. Stain C, Stockinger H, Scharf M et al: Human blood basophils display a unique phenotype including activation-linked membrane structures. Blood 70:1872, 1987

95. Matsuda H, Switzer J, Coughlin MD et al: Human basophilic cell differentiation promoted by 2.5 S nerve growth factor. Int Arch Allergy Appl Immunol 86:453, 1988

96. Denberg JA, Telizyn S, Messner H et al: Heterogeneity of human peripheral blood eosinophil-type colonies: evidence for a common basophil-eosinophil progenitor. Blood 66:312, 1985

97. Malveaux FJ, Conroy MC, Adkinson NF, Lichtenstein LM: IgE receptors on human basophils. J Clin Invest 62:176, 1978

98. Pruzansky JJ, Patterson R: Limiting concentrations of human basophil-bound IgE antibody required for histamine release. Immunology 64:307, 1988

99. Schulman ES, Post TJ, Henson PM, Giclas PC: Differential effects of the complement peptides, C5a and C5a Des Arg on human basophil and lung mast cell histome release. J Clin Invest 81:918, 1988

100. Marone G, Casolaro V, Cirillo R et al: Pathophysiology of human basophils and mast cells in allergic disorders. Clin Immunol Immunopathol 50:524, 1989

101. Marone G: Control mechanisms of mediator release in human basophils and mast cells. Immunol Invest 17:707, 1988

102. White KN, Metzger H: Translocation of protein kinase C in rat basophilic leukemia cells induced by phorbol ester or by aggregation of IgE receptors. J Immunol 141:942, 1988

103. Lewis RA, Goetzl EJ, Wasserman SI et al: The release of four mediators of immediate hypersensitivity from human leukemic basophils. J Immunol 114:87, 1975

104. Haak-Frendscho M, Dinarello C, Kaplan AP: Recombinant human interleukin-1 beta causes histamine release from human basophils. J Allergy Clin Immunol 82:218, 1988

105. Haak-Frendscho M, Arai N, Arai K et al: Human recombinant granulocyte-macrophage colony-stimulating factor and interleukin 3 cause basophil histamine release. J Clin Invest 82:17, 1988

106. Kirshenenbaum AS, Goff JP, Dreskin SC et al: IL-3-dependent growth of basophil-like cells and mastlike cells from human bone marrow. J Immunol 142:2424, 1989

107. Massey WA, Lichtenstein LM: Role of basophils in human allergic disease. Int Arch Allergy Immunol 99:184, 1992

108. Charlesworth EN, Kagey-Sobotka A, Schleimer RP et al: Prednisone inhibits the appearance of inflammatory mediators and the influx of eosinophils and basophils associated with the cutaneous late-phase response to allergen. J Immunol 146:671, 1991

109. Zon LI, Yamaguchi Y, Yee K et al: Expression of mRNA for the GATA-binding proteins in human eosinophils and basophils: potential role in gene transcription. Blood 81:3234, 1993

110. Kasugai T, Okada M, Morimoto M et al: Infection of *Nippostrongylus brasiliensis* induces normal increase of basophils in mast cell-deficient Ws/Ws rats with a small deletion at the kinase domain of c-kit. Blood 81:2521, 1993

Leukocytosis and Leukopenia

52

Thomas D. Coates and Robert Baehner

INTRODUCTION

Changes in the number of circulating leukocytes can represent a primary disorder of leukocyte production, or it may reflect a secondary response to a disease process or toxin. Leukocytosis or leukopenia should be defined on the basis of the respective population means for age of neutrophils, lymphocytes, monocytes, or eosinophils. The distribution of leukocytes or "differential," undergoes specific developmental changes as well as changes that reflect disease states. In the neonate, a predominance of neutrophils persists until the second or third week of life, when lymphocytes begin to predominate. At about 5 years of age, the neutrophil again becomes the predominant leukocyte. Abnormalities in lymphocytes, monocytes, and eosinophils are considered elsewhere in this book. This chapter focuses on abnormal elevation or depression of mature neutrophils.

Regulation of Granulocyte Counts

The peripheral neutrophil count reflects the equilibrium of several compartments. The bone marrow contains a mitotic pool, a maturation pool, and a storage pool. Outside the marrow are found a circulating pool, a marginated pool of neutrophils adherent to vascular endothelium, and a tissue pool. The clinical assay for the number of neutrophils, the white blood cell (WBC) count and differential, only measures neutrophils in the circulating pool during a brief 3–6-hour period of transit from marrow to tissue. A complex interplay of factors regulates the production of granulocytes and their movement from one pool to another, but the movement is always from marrow to blood to tissue.

Granulocytes are derived from a common progenitor that also gives rise to erythrocytes, megakaryocytes, eosinophils, basophils, and monocytes. Proliferation of the common progenitor is stimulated by interleukin-3 (IL-3), while latter differentiation is regulated by colony-stimulating factors-granulocyte (CSF-G).[1,2] Some of these cytokines, along with components of complement,[3-6] cause the release of granulocytes from the marrow storage pool. This can result in a two- to threefold increase in the granulocyte count within 4–5 hours.[3,7] More than one-half the granulocytes in the peripheral circulation at a given time are attached to the vascular endothelium.[8] These "marginated" neutrophils can be released almost immediately at times of stress. Epinephrine in part mediates this effect.[9] Clear evidence now exists that margination is mediated by specific receptor interactions. L-selectin is constitutively expressed on the neutrophil surface and tethers the cell to the vessel, probably by binding to sulfated glycoconjugates on the endothelium. E-selectin and P-selectin may also be involved in this process. Some experimental evidence supports a feedback inhibition loop in the regulation of neutrophil production. Lactoferrin, which is contained in neutrophil-specific granules, suppresses the production of CSFs by monocytes, resulting in a decrease in neutrophil production when granulocyte counts rise. Acidic isoferritins may also participate in this down-regulation.[10,11]

Of the 1.2×10^9 granulocytes/kg, approximately 20% are in the myeloid precursor pool, 75% in the marrow storage pool, 3% in the marginated pool, and 2% in the circulating blood.[8,12] Normally, 1.5×10^9 granulocytes/kg body weight are produced per day. Production can be increased in the presence of an inflammatory stimulus. Granulocytes spend about 9 days in marrow, 3–6 hours in blood, and 1–4 days in the tissues.[8] Thus, the total granulocyte count, as measured from peripheral blood, represents a sample of a population that comprises only 5% of the total pool sampled during a fleeting 2% of the total transit time.

In assessing neutrophilia and neutropenia, one must consider the movement of neutrophils from one compartment to another, as well as changes in production. Thus, neutrophilia can be due to increased production as in infection or myeloproliferative disorders of inhibition of egress from the blood as in certain chemotactic disorders or steroid therapy.[7] Neutropenia may be due to decreased production; to increased margination and egress, as in systemic complement activation of burns[13,14]; or to destruction, as in immune neutropenia.

Practically, evaluation of these processes is limited to an examination of the peripheral blood and bone marrow. The existing radiotracer techniques, albeit sophisticated, are not of much clinical use. Similarly, clinical tests such as hydrocortisone (or prednesone) challenge or epinephrine stimulation, which reflect a releasable marrow storage pool or marginated pool, have limited differentiating power.

Leukocytosis

Leukocytosis refers to elevation of the WBC count to >2 SD above the mean of one or more subsets of circulating WBCs. Neutrophilia refers specifically to elevation of the absolute neutrophil count. The latter is calculated by multiplying the percentage of neutrophilic granulocytes by the total WBC count. The usual explanation for leukocytosis is neutrophilia. Abnormal elevations of eosinophils and lymphocytes are considered elsewhere in this text.

Neutrophil counts show considerable variability during the neonatal period, with a mean of 11,000/mm^3 and a range of 6,000 to 26,000/mm^3. Total WBC counts may be as high as 38,000/mm^3 at 12 hours of age.[15] The count drops after 12 hours, reaching a mean neutrophil count of 5,500/mm^3 (1,500–10,000) at 1 week. The differential in the first week of life resembles that of the adult, with approximately 60% neutrophils. From 1 week until 5–6 years, however, lymphocytes predominate. Thereafter, neutrophils increase to about 60%. The mean adult total leukocyte count is 7,500/mm^3 (4,500–11,000) and the mean neutrophil count is 4,400/mm^3 (1,800–7,700).[15] Total leukocyte counts of premature infants are about 30% lower than in term infants. The sequential changes noted after birth also occur in premature infants but with greater variability.[16]

Leukemoid Reaction

Leukocytosis exceeding 50,000/mm^3 is referred to as a leukemoid reaction,[17] characterized by a significant increase in early neutrophil precursors in the peripheral blood. The differential count has a marked "left shift," evidenced by the presence of myelocyte, metamyelocyte, and band forms. Progranulocytes and myeloblasts may be observed in severe reactions. In contrast to acute leukemia, proliferation of all normal myeloid elements is observed in the bone marrow. Chronic myeloid leukemia (CML) may be distinguished from a leukemoid reaction by the finding of a low leukocyte alkaline phosphatase (LAP) score and the presence of the Philadelphia chromosome on karyotypic analysis of the bone marrow. Leukemoid reactions to infections may be accompanied by toxic granulation, Döhle bodies, and cytoplasmic vacuoles in the neutrophils.[17]

Newborns have unique responses to stress and infection. The relative number of band forms and of less mature granulocyte precursors in the differential of newborn infants has been correlated with sepsis and with depletion of the marrow neutrophil storage pool.[18,19] In the normal infant, the band/neutrophil ratio is <0.11–0.14 in the first 48 hours, irrespective of birthweight or gestational age.[20] An immature/total neutrophil ratio exceeding 0.8 in the peripheral blood indicates that marrow reserves are depleted and the risk of death in septic infants is significantly increased.[18]

When the marrow is directly invaded by tumor or in cases of marrow fibrosis or in granuloma reactions, neutrophilia associated with immature granulocytes, nucleated red cells, and teardrop-shaped erythrocytes may be seen, often accompanied by thrombocytosis. This is called a leukoerythroblastic response. A bone marrow biopsy performed to look for granuloma, or a marrow culture for fungus, may be helpful in these instances.

Pelger-Huët Anomaly

A benign dominantly inherited defect of terminal neutrophil differentiation with a frequency at birth of 1:6,000, called the Pelger-Huët anomaly, can give rise to apparent bandemia, often confused with a left shift. Most of these neutrophils have bilobate nuclei and excessively coarse clumping of nuclear chromatin. The two lobes are joined by a thin bridge that is much thinner than that seen in a normal band. The function of these cells is normal.[21] Interestingly, Pelger-Huët cells can develop multiple lobes during states of vitamin B$_{12}$ or folate deficiency but return to their bilobate state once the vitamin deficiency is corrected.[22] Colchicine and sulfonamides can induce the anomaly reversibly.[23,24] This so-called pseudo-Pelger cell has also been reported transiently during certain acute infections, in acute myeloid leukemia and in myelofibrosis. The homozygous state results in neutrophils that contain a single round eccentric nucleus with clumped chromatin. Eosinophils and basophils may be involved as well. An unusual case of Pelger-Huët anomaly has been reported in association with four generations of one family with late-onset progressive proximal muscular dystrophy.[25]

NEUTROPHILIA

Neutrophilia and a left shift can be indicative of disease or may be totally benign. The major primary and acquired causes of neutrophilia are outlined in Table 52-1. The causes of neutrophilia have been divided into two groups: those that seem to be due to intrinsic problems with the neutrophil or regulation of neutrophil production, and those that are secondary to some other disease process.

Table 52-1. Classification of Neutrophilia

Primary (no other evident associated disease)
    Hereditary neutrophilia
    Chronic idiopathic neutrophilia
    Chronic myeloid leukemia and other myeloproliferative diseases
    Familial myeloproliferative disease
    Congenital anomalies and leukemoid reaction
    Down syndrome
    Leukocyte adhesion factor deficiency
    Familial cold urticaria and leukocytosis
Secondary
    Infection
    Stress neutrophilia
    Myocardial infarction
    Drug-induced
    Nonhematologic malignancy
    Heatstroke
    Generalized marrow stimulation (as in hemolysis)
    Asplenia and hyposplenism

Primary Neutrophilia

Hereditary Neutrophilia

A family of four was described in 1974[26] with leukocyte counts that were chronically in the 20,000–70,000/mm^3 range, splenomegaly, and widened diploe of the skull. No apparent propensity to bacterial infection was reported. The defect seemed to be dominantly inherited. Subsequent follow-up (W. Herring, personal communication, 1989) demonstrates that two more children have been born to the same mother, and both have chronic leukocytosis. The LAP scores were high in all affected subjects. To date, none of the family members has had any serious medical problems other than a bleeding diathesis related to platelet dysfunction.[26] Neutrophil function and surface CD18/CD11b expression in one member of this family are normal, so this is not a variant of leukocyte adhesion deficiency (W. Herring, T.D. Coates, unpublished data). In a second family with this syndrome, the father had marked leukocytosis and splenomegaly and eventually had his spleen removed. His son had similar problems, with neutrophil counts at times in the 100,000/mm^3 range, as well as massive splenomegaly. The neutrophil function and CD18/CD11b expression in the affected father and son are also normal (D. Powars and T. D. Coates, unpublished data).

Chronic Idiopathic Neutrophilia

Chronic leukocytosis can occur in patients who are otherwise well. A series of 34 patients with leukocyte counts of 11,000–40,000/mm^3 were followed for ≤20 years without associated clinical problems. Bone marrow aspirations were generally normal, and LAP scores were normal. The remainder of the blood counts were normal, except for occasional thrombocytosis.[27] These data point out that certain normal subjects fall outside the normal range with respect to WBC count and should be considered normal, sparing them frequent and extensive evaluations.

Chronic Myeloid Leukemia

The major differential diagnosis of leukemoid reaction is CML. This topic is considered in detail in Chapter 66. It can be difficult to distinguish between leukemoid reactions and CML. The classic differentiating features are the presence of a low LAP score and presence of the Philadelphia chromosome in CML. The LAP score is also low in familial myeloproliferative disease[28] and paroxysmal nocturnal hemoglobinuria.[29] The LAP score can be normal in CML, and the Philadelphia chromosome is absent in juvenile CML. Juvenile CML can be distinguished from the usual adult form by the ability of circulating stem cells to form monocyte colonies in vitro.[30] Leukocyte counts in CML can be extremely high, occasionally >500,000/mm³. Patients with granulocyte counts of >200,000–300,000/mm³ require emergent intervention to prevent the vaso-occlusive complications of hyperviscosity related to the markedly elevated WBCs.

Familial Myeloproliferative Disease

A syndrome of growth retardation, hepatosplenomegaly, anemia, and leukocytosis has been described.[28] Some affected children died in early life, while others remained stable or improved. All of these subjects had low LAP scores. Furthermore, several other members, in four generations of the family, had low LAP scores but no other findings. Chromosomal analysis showed no significant consistent abnormalities, and no subject had a Philadelphia chromosome.

Congenital Anomalies and Leukemoid Reaction

Leukemoid reactions have been associated with amegakaryocytic thrombocytopenia and with congenital deformities such as tetralogy of Fallot, dextrocardia and absent radii, and rudimentary little toes.[31,32]

Down Syndrome

Infants with Down syndrome may have a transient leukemoid reaction that resembles congenital leukemia.[33] Affected children can also have an exaggerated leukemoid response to stress.[34] A transient leukemoid reaction has been seen in a phenotypically normal child who expressed trisomy 21 mosaicism in myeloid cells but not in skin fibroblasts. The chromosomal abnormality disappeared after the leukemoid reaction resolved.[35,36]

Leukocyte Adhesion Factor Deficiency

Since the 1970s, several patients have been described with persistent leukocytosis, delayed separation of the umbilical cord, recurrent infections, and a stimulus-dependent activation defect of the neutrophils. These children have impaired neutrophil chemotaxis and an inability to phagocytose opsonized particles. There is a defect in adherence as well. Neutrophils from these patients lack the surface receptor for the inactivated third component of complement (C3bi).[37]

Clinically, these patients can be classified as having severe (totally lacking the adhesion receptor) or moderate (1–10% expression) leukocyte adhesion factor deficiency). The patients who manifest severe recurrent infection in infancy often progress to death during the first years of life. They have severe skin and mucosal infections, poor wound healing and a notable lack of pus at the sites of infection, and delayed separation of the umbilical cord. Patients with the moderate phenotype may survive into young adulthood. Surviving patients have problems with chronic infections such as sinusitis, otitis, and severe periodonitis leading to loss of teeth.[37]

The laboratory hallmark of these disorders is leukocytosis. WBC counts may be only mildly elevated (10,000–12,000/mm³) but are often in the 18,000–30,000/mm³ range and may be as high as 150,000/mm³ during infection.[37,38] No specific morphologic abnormalities are seen in the granulocytes. The diagnosis is established by the demonstration of absence or marked reduction (<10% of control) in the CR3 receptor on granulocytes. Studies of the patients' granulocytes show defects in chemotaxis, adherence, and phagocytosis of C3bi-coated particles.

The respiratory burst, including nitroblue tetrazolium reduction, is absent in response to C3bi-coated particles and is generally, but not always, normal in response to soluble stimuli.

Neutrophil functions that depend on opsonization by C3bi, such as phagocytosis or respiratory burst stimulated by zymosan, are decreased. These functions are normal when stimulated by unopsonized latex particles.[39] In general, polymorphonuclear neutrophils (PMNs) from these patients respond normally to soluble stimuli such as phorbol myristate acetate (PMA) or the chemotactic tripeptide formyl-methionyl-leucyl-phenylalanine (FMLP), although exceptions have been reported. Superoxide production was diminished in response to PMA and enhanced in response to FMLP in three patients with LAD.[38–40]

Enhanced oxidative response to FMLP and impaired chemotaxis has been seen in lactoferrin deficiency.[41] Interestingly, one patient with documented LAD[39] had been evaluated independently[10] and was found to have 1–10% of normal lactoferrin in her PMNs. Extensive studies of her granulopoiesis showed that her lactoferrin did not inhibit colony-stimulating factor-granulocyte/macrophage (CSF-GM) production by normal monocytes and furthermore, production of CSF-GM by her mononuclear cells was not inhibited by normal lactoferrin,[10] suggesting a possible mechanism for the neutrophilia in this patient with LAD. The only curative therapy is bone marrow transplantation. This should be considered in patients with the severe phenotype who have HLA-identical matches.[37]

A second type of LAD (LAD II) has recently been described[42,43] in two patients with psychomotor retardation, Bombay blood group, and severe recurrent infections. These children had leukocytosis in the range of 30,000–150,000/mm³ and lack sialyl-Lewis X, the ligand for E-selectin, an endothelial adhesion receptor that directs early attachment of PMNs to the vessel wall. This receptor is believed to mediate neutrophil rolling on endothelium and is probably involved in part in neutrophil margination.

Familial Cold Urticaria and Leukocytosis

A very interesting syndrome of leukocytosis, fever, urticaria, rash, and muscle and skin tenderness on exposure to cold has been reported. This syndrome appears to be dominantly inherited. The onset of symptoms occurs during infancy, and symptoms have been provoked by exposure to cold in the delivery room. Urticaria followed by fever starts about 7 hours after cold exposure. Leukocytosis, sometimes ≤34,000/mm³, starts about 10 hours after cold exposure and begins to subside 12–14 hours later.[44,45] In contrast to other causes of urticaria, the skin rash in these patients is characterized histologically by a marked infiltration of neutrophils. The leukocytosis and urticaria were blocked in patients infused with endotoxin prior to cold exposure. This has been related to "cold activation of clotting system," as it is associated with a transient decrease in levels of C1 esterase inhibitor.[46,47]

Secondary Neutrophilia

Acute Infection

Modest leukocytosis with a left shift is commonly seen in association with many acute bacterial infections. Certain bacteria, such as *Pneumococcus* or *Staphylococcus,* may cause particularly high leukocyte counts. Leukocytosis is seen in association with acute otitis media, with 9% of patients having a WBC count of >20,000/mm³,[48] while 27% of culture proven positive acute otitis media cases have WBC counts below the mean for age.[48] The predictive value of leukocytosis and increased bandforms (WBCs >15 × 10⁹/L immature/total >0.2) in detecting bacterial disease was increased from 32% to 71% when associated with depressed fibronectin levels (1 SD below mean for age). This finding is of particular interest, in view of the role of fibronectin in promoting phagocytosis by PMNs and monocytes.[49]

Chronic Inflammation

Acute changes in the neutrophil count are due to release from the marrow storage pool and the marginated pool. Cases of overwhelming infection can lead to marrow depletion, resulting in neutropenia rather than neutrophilia. Chronic inflammatory processes result in stimulation of granulocyte production, they are usually more modest in degree and may be associated with an increase in monocytes.

Stress Neutrophilia

Modest elevation in the neutrophil count has been associated with many types of "stress." Neutrophilia can occur within minutes of exercise[50] or stress[51] or epinephrine injection[9] and is presumed to be related to movement of neutrophils from the marginated pool into the circulating pool. The neutrophilia secondary to catecholamine injection has been related to reduced neutrophil adherence. The neutrophilia as well as the adherence-inhibiting ability of plasma can be blocked by pretreatment of the subject with propranolol, or in vitro treatment of the adherence assay system by antibody to cAMP.[9]

Studies on exercise-induced neutrophilia failed to show blockade by propranolol, despite measurable increases in plasma epinephrine.[52] The neutrophilia was directly related to the workload and cardiac output, suggesting a larger role for mechanical and flow-related effects on dislodgment of the leukocytes sequestered in the lung, than possible direct effects of catecholamines on the neutrophils. Other studies show no effect of exercise on circulating colony-forming unit-granulocyte/macrophage or -granulocyte/crythrocyte/macrophage/megakaryocyte (CFU-GM or CFU-GEMM),[50] although it has been suggested that the delayed leukocytosis (≤235% increase at 5 hours postexercise) may be related to marrow release of leukocytes.[53]

Mild neutrophilia and lymphopenia have been associated with unipolar depression but may be related to the use of antidepressants.[54] Neutrophilia is also seen during the postoperative period. The leukocyte count doubles approximately 3 hours after surgery. This does not seem to be related to the type of anesthesia.[55,56]

Leukocytosis in the 12,000–20,000/mm³ range has been reported in the postictal state. This can be associated with fever or pulmonary edema and resolves within a few hours to days.[57]

An interesting association between leukocyte count and myocardial infarction has been noted. Subjects with a leukocyte count of >9,000 had a 4.5-fold higher incidence of myocardial infarction than that of patients with a leukocyte count of <6,000.[58] This may have been related to smoking. It is also not clear whether the WBC count is a risk factor or merely an indicator of chronic stress.[59]

Drug-Induced Neutrophilia

Leukocytosis has been seen in association with a number of drugs and drug reactions. Steroids are well known to induce release of neutrophils from the bone marrow[7] and result in a chronic low-grade neutrophilia. β-Agonists produce an acute neutrophilia by releasing neutrophils from the marginated pool.[60] Lithium is well known to produce leukocytosis by increasing production of CSF and has been used with varying success to treat several neutropenic states.[61]

Nonhematologic Malignancy

Leukocytosis is frequently seen in large cell lung cancer.[62] The leukocytosis seen with solid tumors is usually modest, in the 12,000–30,000/mm³ range,[62-64] although it can be as high as 100,000/mm³ in the absence of marrow metastasis.[65] Leukemoid reactions have been seen in patients with marrow involvement with tumor from lung, stomach, or breast or with neuroblastoma in children.[65] In some instances, solid tumors have been shown to secrete substances with colony-stimulating activity.[66]

Heatstroke

WBC counts of ≤30,000/mm³ have been seen in heatstroke. Up to 50% of the neutrophils may have botryoid nuclei, with nuclear segments smaller than usual, resembling a clustering of grapes around a central stem.[67,68]

Marrow Stimulation

Significant leukocytosis can be seen in states of chronic stimulation of the bone marrow, such as hemolytic anemia or immune thrombocytopenia.[69] For example, patients with sickle cell anemia commonly have leukocyte counts in the 12,000–15,000/mm³ range and with infection have an exaggerated elevation in WBC counts. This response may be further augmented by functional asplenia seen in sickle cell disease. Likewise, significant rebound leukocytosis can occur in the recovery phase of marrow suppression.[70,71] These reactions can last several weeks. In one instance 90% myeloblasts were found in the marrow and as many as 20% myeloblasts in the peripheral blood.[72]

Asplenia

Moderate neutrophilia can be associated with congenital disease-related asplenia (e.g., dextrocardia and sickle cell anemia) or surgical asplenia.[73,74]

Approach to Evaluation of Neutrophilia

One of the considerations that must be included in the evaluation of isolated neutrophilia or neutropenia is laboratory error. Current technology, has removed much of the human error factor,[75] although some clinicians continue to believe that manual counts are more accurate. Blood counts that do not make sense within the context of the clinical findings should be repeated before extensive evaluation is undertaken. Automatic cell counters are widely used for measurement of the WBC count. These instruments count cells based on size distribution of particles moving through an aperture. Newer instruments can differentiate types of leukocytes based on light-scattering properties and size distribution, and can provide "three part differentials" that are generally very accurate, except in hematologic malignancies. The histograms of cell size provided by these instruments may add new insights into subpopulation changes in leukocytes that may occur in disease states.[76]

Factitious leukocytosis can be seen due to blood sampling problems or certain primary disease states. Inadequate anticoagulation of the specimen can result in platelet clumps being counted as leukocytes by automated cell counters. The WBC count is rarely increased >10% and is usually associated with spurious thrombocytopenia.[77,78] In cryoglobulinemia, a temperature-dependent increase in leukocyte and platelet counts occurs at about 30°C and can result in WBC counts of ≤50,000/mm³ and a doubling of the platelet count, attributed to various sizes of precipitated cryoglobulin particles.[79] This effect is increased if the sample is allowed to cool to lower temperatures.

The general approach to the evaluation of the patient with neutrophilia will depend on the degree of neutrophilia and on the signs and symptoms of the associated diseases. Neutrophilia is most commonly seen secondary to some acute or chronic inflammatory processes, and the diagnosis and treatment are dictated by the nature of the primary illness. Examination of the bone marrow is of little help, except in certain instances of leukemoid reactions or leukoerythroblastosis, in which direct invasion of the marrow must be excluded. Bone marrow biopsy should be included in these situations, as well as fungal cultures. The biopsy may reveal granulotoma, which may intensify the search for fungus, or metastatic tumor that is missed in a marrow aspirate. The LAP score, which is high in infection and low in CML, is also of help. It must be kept in mind, however, that the LAP score can be normal in CML, particularly juvenile CML, making this diagnosis difficult at times.

A number of factors contribute to the wide variability in granulocyte counts in normal populations. Particularly in the asymptomatic patient with persistent mild neutrophilia, one must remember that, by definition, the WBC count in 2.5% of the normal population must be >2 SD above the mean. Since regulation of granulocyte production is genetically controlled,[27,80–82] examination of the parents' or siblings' blood counts may be of help in these situations.

LEUKOPENIA

Causes of neutropenia are fewer than those of neutrophilia. Since most clinicians are looking for increased WBC counts, the diagnosis of neutropenia is often overlooked. Neutropenia is defined as a neutrophilic granulocyte count of <1,500/mm³. This definition can be used for all ages and races, although, strictly speaking, separate standards should be used for certain groups. For example, newborn infants have elevated granulocyte counts during the first few days of life,[15,16] and certain populations of blacks and Yemenite Jews normally have lower granulocyte counts.[80,81]

The absolute neutrophil count (ANC) is calculated by multiplying the total WBC count by the percentage of bands and mature neutrophils:

$$ANC = WBC \times (\% \text{ bands} + \% \text{ mature neutrophils}) \times 0.01$$

Granulocytes less mature than bands are not included in the calculation.

Relationship of Absolute Neutrophil Count to Propensity to Infection

Propensity to infection in neutropenic patients is related to the ANC (Table 52-2). The relationship holds particularly well in situations in which neutrophil production and marrow reserve pools of neutrophils are decreased. In patients with peripheral destruction or margination of neutrophils, such as seen in immune neutropenias, the degree of neutropenia does not correlate as well with a propensity to infection.

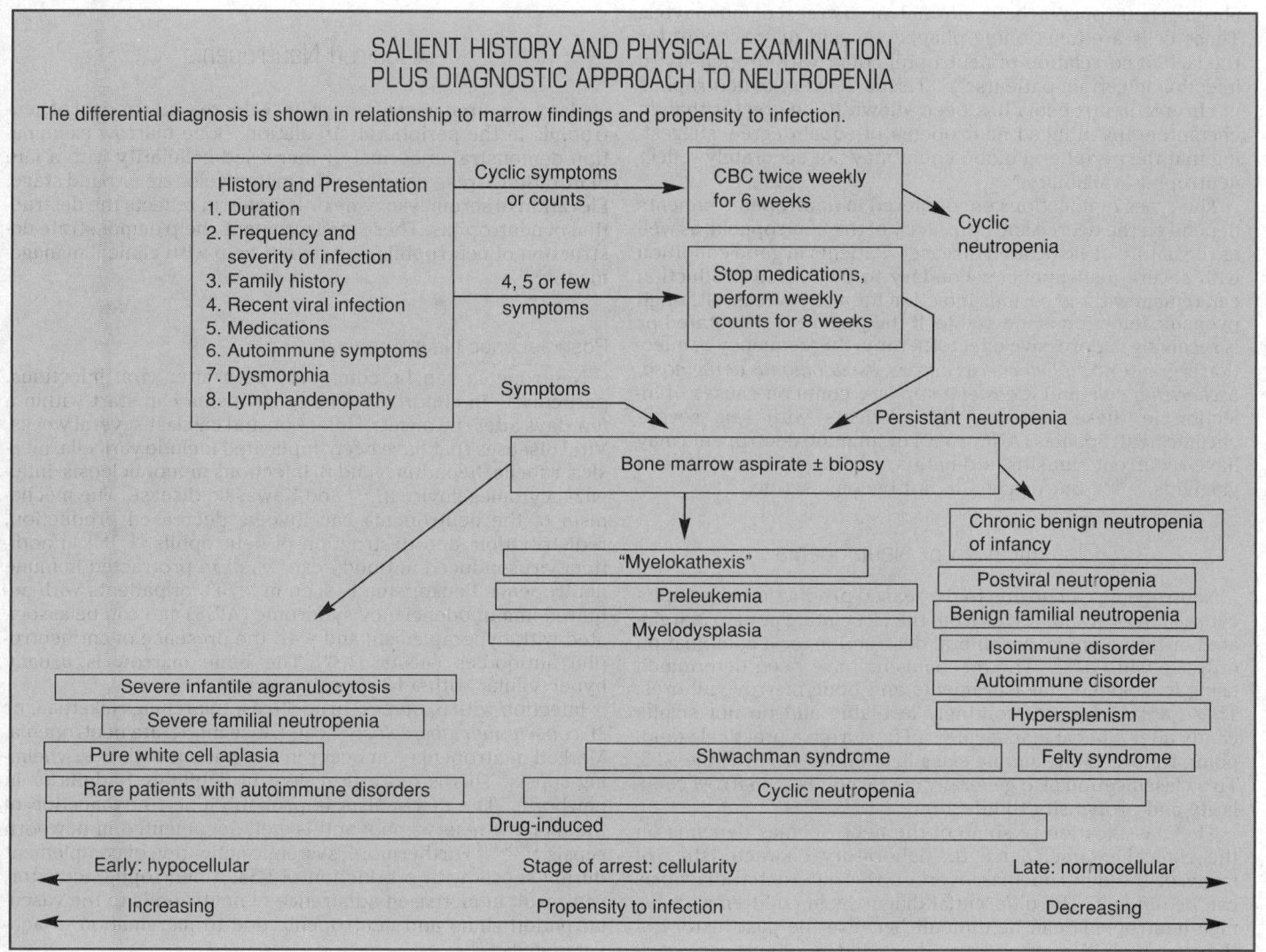

SALIENT HISTORY AND PHYSICAL EXAMINATION
PLUS DIAGNOSTIC APPROACH TO NEUTROPENIA

The differential diagnosis is shown in relationship to marrow findings and propensity to infection.

Table 52-2. Clinically Significant Neutrophil Counts[a]

Count	Significance
>1,500/mm³	Normal
1,000–>1,500	No significant propensity to infection; fevers can be managed on an outpatient basis
500–1,000	Some propensity to infection; occasionally fever can be managed on an outpatient basis
<500	Significant propensity to infection fever; should always be managed on an inpatient basis with parenteral antibiotics; few clinical signs of infection

[a] These rules apply strictly for neutropenia with hypoplastic marrow or early myeloid arrest. There is more latitutde for neutropenias with normocellular marrows. The only regular exception is documented chronic benign neutropenia of childhood.

Patients with neutropenia secondary to chemotherapy, marrow failure, or marrow exhaustion are at great risk of overwhelming bacterial infection.[18,19,83] By contrast, children with chronic benign neutropenia of infancy and childhood may have neutrophil counts of <200/mm³ for months or years and have no serious infectious problems.[83] Similarly, some adults with immune neutropenia may have severe depression of their neutrophil counts and suffer no serious episodes of infection.[84] Both entities are characterized by neutropenia and cellular marrow. The marrow differential usually shows normal early granulocyte precursors but no mature neutrophils. This maturation block is called a maturation arrest. Many patients with chronic neutropenia have normal or increased monocytes. These cells are functioning phagocytes and may account for the lack of correlation of neutrophil count with propensity to infection in certain patients.[85,86] Tissue delivery of neutrophils in chronic neutropenia has been shown to be greater than in chemotherapy-induced neutropenia of equal degree, suggesting that the peripheral blood count may not accurately reflect neutrophil availability.[87]

The types of infections encountered in neutropenic patients depend on the degree and chronicity of the neutropenia, as well as the nature of associated diseases. Patients in good condition with severe neutropenia secondary to decreased production can remain without serious infection for many weeks, although pyogenic infection is inevitable. If the patient is debilitated or is receiving suppressive chemotherapy, the frequency of infection is greater. *Staphylococcus aureas, Pseudomonas aeruginosa, Escherichia coli,* and *Klebsiella* spp. are common causes of infection in these patients.[85,86,88] Patients with less severe chronic neutropenias (ANC >300) or immune neutropenia may have recurrent sinusitis, stomatitis, perirectal infections, and gingivitis,[85,86,89] but usually do not become septic.

Classification of Neutropenia

Neutropenia can be due to decreased production of granulocytes, shift of granulocytes from the circulating pool to marginated or tissue pools, peripheral destruction, or a combination of these causes.[86,90] The mechanisms have been determined using leukokinetic measurements and bone marrow cultures. These assays are not routinely available and do not significantly alter clinical management. Thus, from a practical standpoint, we prefer the simple classification shown in Table 52-3. This classification also generally corresponds to marrow cellularity and propensity to infection.

The classification of some of the neutropenias depends on the clinical course. Since the laboratory characteristics of many of the neutropenias overlap, the differential diagnosis can be difficult. The differential diagnosis in children with benign neutropenia can be difficult because the past history of the young child may be very short and is often negative. If

Table 52-3. Classification of Neutropenias

Acquired neutropenia
    Postinfectious neutropenia
    Drug-induced neutropenia
    Benign familial neutropenia
    Chronic benign neutropenia of childhood
    Chronic idipathic neutropenia
    Autoimmune neutropenia
    Isoimmune neutropenia
    Neutropenia associated with immunologic abnormalities
    Neutropenia associated with metabolic diseases
    Neutropenia due to increased margination
    Nutritional deficiency
Intrinsic defects
    Severe infantile agranulocytosis
    Myelokathexis/neutropenia with tetraploid leukocytes
    Cyclic neutropenia
    Shwachman-Diamond-Oski syndrome
    Chediak-Higashi syndrome
    Reticular dysgenesis
    Dyskeratosis congenita

there is no family history of neutropenia, and the bone marrow is normocellular or hypercellular, there is no certain way to differentiate the various neutropenias other than to follow the patient clinically.

Acquired Neutropenia

Many acquired neutropenias have decreased survival of neutrophils in the peripheral circulation. Bone marrow examination demonstrates normal or increased cellularity with a late maturation arrest, usually at the metamyelocyte or band stage. Elevation of serum lysozyme or lactoferrin reflects the destruction of neutrophils. These measurements help demonstrate destruction of neutrophils, but do not help with clinical management.[13,91]

Postinfectious Neutropenia

Neutropenia can be commonly seen after viral infections, particularly in children.[92] The neutropenia can start within a few days after the onset of infection and can last several weeks. Viral diseases that have been implicated include varicella, measles, rubella, hepatitis A and B, infectious mononucleosis, influenza, cytomegalovirus,[93,94] and Kawasaki disease. The mechanism of the neutropenia can involve decreased production, redistribution, and destruction of neutrophils.[90,95–97] In addition, virus-induced antibody can result in protracted immune neutropenia. Leukopenia is seen in >70% of patients with acquired immunodeficiency syndrome (AIDS) and can be associated with hypersplenism and with the presence of antineutrophil antibodies (ANAs).[98–101] The bone marrow is usually hypercellular with a late myeloid arrest.

Infection with *S. aureus,* brucellosis, tularemia, rickettsia, or *Mycobacterium tuberculosis*[90] can cause moderate neutropenia. Marked neutropenia can occur in any patient with overwhelming sepsis. This is more prevalent in debilitated adults or in newborns. The mechanism is probably due to exhaustion of the marrow reserve pool and is well documented in newborn sepsis.[18,19,102] Furthermore, systemic activation of complement during sepsis with production of C5a, a neutrophil activator, can result in increased adherence of neutrophils to the vascular endothelium and neutropenia due to margination of activated cells.[103]

Drug-Induced Neutropenia

A number of therapeutic agents have been shown to cause neutropenia.[104] The mechanism can involve direct bone marrow suppression, as seen with antineoplastic agents, antibody and complement-mediated damage to precursor cells,[105,106] or peripheral destruction and clearance of neutrophils.[50,84,107,108] Most drug-related neutropenias are due to dose-dependent marrow suppression. Phenothiazines, semisynthetic penicillins, nonsteroidal anti-inflammatory drugs, aminopyrine derivatives, and antithyroid medications are the most common offenders. Recovery usually starts within a few days of stopping the drug, and is preceded by the appearance of monocytes and immature neutrophils in the peripheral blood.[107] Rebound leukocytosis with marrow and peripheral blasts has been reported and can simulate a leukemic state.[71,72]

Benign Familial Leukopenia

Benign familial leukopenia is characterized by neutrophil counts in the 2100–2600/mm^3 range and no propensity to infection. The disorder has dominant inheritance and is not associated with any propensity to infection. The bone marrow is normocellular.[82,109] This has been seen in several ethnic populations as well, including American and African blacks, Yemenite Jews, and West Indians.[80–82] The observation of low leukocyte counts in these families and ethnic groups does not represent a disease entity but underscores genetically controlled differences in the regulation of neutrophil proliferation.

Chronic Benign Neutropenia of Infancy and Childhood

Chronic benign neutropenia of infancy and childhood[110,111] is a "chronic state of mature neutrophil depletion with a compensatory increase in immature granulocytes in the bone marrow analogous to erythroid hyperplasia in hemolytic anemia."[111] The median age of detection is 8 months. Although it can present any time in the first 3 years of life, 90% of cases are detected before 14 months of age. There is a slight female predominance (3:2) and no correlation with birth order. Neutrophil counts are usually very low at presentation, although these counts are normal at birth. No family history of neutropenia has been demonstrated.[83,110,111]

Antineutrophil surface antibodies have been detected in 98% of patients when both immunofluorescent and agglutination assays are used. Agglutinins were present in 78%, and the immunofluorescent assay was positive in 88%. The antibodies are primarily of the IgG type, with a small percentage of patients having both IgG and IgM detectable.[83] The antibodies react mainly with neutrophils, although there is some reactivity with subpopulations of lymphocytes.[112] While the precise mechanism of the neutropenia is unclear, that ANAs are frequently no longer detectable late in the course of the disease[83] and that anti-immune therapy is effective[83,113,114] suggest an immune mechanism. Circulating immune complexes have been detected in about one-half of patients as well. Their role is unclear, although they may be related to chronic infection.[83] Serum colony-stimulating activity is normal, and marrow from these patients grows normally in culture without exogenous addition of CSF-G.[115]

Children with chronic benign neutropenia of childhood present with fever and infection. A few patients have been seen with hepatosplenomegaly.[83] Pyogenic skin infection, oral ulceration, otitis, or sinusitis is seen but is not common. It is probably more accurate to say that the neutropenia is an incidental finding on a blood count obtained during the course of a febrile episode. These patients commonly have neutrophil counts of <200/mm^3 and for several months have no febrile episodes. Although these patients probably have a slightly increased incidence of pyogenic infection, it is most often not due to the usual

organisms associated with severe neutropenia. The infections that do occur, respond well to antibiotic therapy. The ANC may increase during infection or remain low. A few children do have symptomatic oral, rectal, or vaginal ulcers. These ulcers do cause discomfort, but they do not progress, and deep pyogenic infections do not develop. It is interesting to speculate as to whether these patients have a mild vasculitis or antibody-mediated neutrophil functional defect, as has been seen in adults with immune neutropenia.[116]

The median duration of neutropenia has been estimated at 20 months, with 95% of the patients recovering by 4 years of age.[83] Some patients remain neutropenic into adulthood.

The laboratory hallmark of this disorder is neutropenia, usually with an ANC of <500/mm^3. The neutropenia is frequently associated with a mild eosinophilia or monocytosis.[83,111,117] The bone marrow is normocellular or hypercellular, with a late-stage maturation arrest, usually at the band or metamyelocyte stage. Many patients may demonstrate an increase in neutrophils in response to a hydrocortisone (or prednisone) challenge, but some do not. Assays for ANAs are of some help in confirming this diagnosis, although the absence of detectable antibody does not exclude the diagnosis. Some of these patients have measurable defects in neutrophil movement and have been described as having the so-called lazy leukocyte syndrome.[117] Evaluation of T-cell function and immunoglobulins may identify patients with neutropenia associated with other immunodeficiency syndromes.

This disorder must be differentiated from other neutropenias with normocellular marrows. We consider the diagnosis of chronic benign neutropenia of infancy and childhood to be established if (1) presentation is within the first 2 years of life, (2) there is no history of severe infections over a 2–3-month observation period, (3) neutrophil morphology is normal, (4) the bone marrow is normocellular of hypercellular with a late-stage myeloid arrest or no arrest, and (5) the process resolves by 4 years of age. The clinical aspects of this definition are very important. If the child has sepsis or other severe pyogenic infections, the diagnosis is not benign neutropenia, and other lines of investigation must be pursued. Forms of severe combined immunodeficiency may present with neutropenia and have the same marrow findings as benign neutropenia of infancy.

The primary treatment of this disorder is management of infections. We require a 2–3-month observation period with no infection or excellent response to treatment of infections before we will add the word "benign" to the diagnosis of neutropenia. When these patients are first encountered, febrile episodes should be treated very aggressively with parenteral antibiotics to cover gram-negative and gram-positive pathogens. Once the first four diagnostic criteria have been met, infectious episodes may be managed the same as for any other child. If the child is toxic or is not responding to treatment within the unusual time period, parenteral antibiotics should be considered.

High-dose γ-globulin has been used successfully to raise the neutrophil counts in these patients,[83,113] as have steroids. γ-Globulin in a regimen similar to that used in idiopathic thrombocytopenic purpura should be considered in severe infections such as pneumonia or osteomyelitis.[113] Treatment with CSF-G has been successful in these patients as well.[118] Since the prognosis is excellent, even if the child remains neutropenic, and since the disease remits spontaneously, treatment directed at chronically raising the neutrophil count is rarely indicated.

Chronic Idiopathic Neutropenia

Chronic idiopathic neutropenia is the term that can be applied to those patients who do not fit into one of the other categories of neutropenia. Onset can occur from infancy to late adulthood. The clinical findings and presentation are quite variable.[85,86] Neutrophil counts are commonly 200–500/mm[3], and the bone marrow examination usually reveals normal to increased numbers of myeloid precursors with an arrest at a late stage of maturation. Often peripheral monocytosis is present. Some affected patients may have moderately hypocellular marrows.[86] Hepatosplenomegaly is not seen, and no other infectious, inflammatory, or malignant disease is present to which the neutropenia can be attributed. Frequently these patients have a benign course despite the degree of neutropenia. This may be because they have some marrow reserve, as demonstrated by the response of their neutrophil count to a hydrocortisone (or prednisone) stimulation test.[86] These patients are also able to mobilize more neutrophils to the tissue than are patients with acute drug-induced suppression of equal degree.[87] ANAs, as well as other immunologic abnormalities, have been seen in some patients, although these studies are usually normal.[86,119–121] The lack of strong evidence for ANAs in these patients does not preclude the possibility that antibodies against myeloid precursors are present. Antibodies against the promyelocytic leukemic line, HL-60, were detected in sera from three patients with idiopathic neutropenia with no detectable antibody to mature neutrophils.[121] Bone marrow cytogenetic studies are normal, as is CSF-G concentration.[86,115]

Corticosteroids, splenectomy, and cytotoxic agents have been successful in increasing neutrophil counts.[86] CSF-G has recently been used successfully to treat a patient with idiopathic neutropenia.[122] This patient's course was benign for several years until his marrow became hypocellular. Since the clinical course of this disease may be benign, treatment intended to increase the neutrophil count should be reserved for those patients with significant recurrent infectious complications.

Autoimmune Neutropenia

Autoimmune neutropenia has been seen as an isolated phenomenon,[84,123] secondary to other known autoimmune diseases,[84,123,124] related to infections,[95] and related to administration of drugs.[84] Furthermore, with increasing sophistication of immunologic evaluations, immunologic mechanisms are being seen in cases of neutropenia that have been classified as "idiopathic."[83,84,121,124] Immune neutropenia can be seen in association with idiopathic thrombocytopenic purpura and immune hemolytic anemia as well.[84] In the neutropenia associated with Rh hemolytic disease, however, evidence exists of down-regulation of neutrophil production associated with an increase in erythropoiesis.[125]

Patients with autoimmune neutropenia have moderate to severe neutropenia, usually accompanied by monocytosis. Marrow cellularity is increased with a late maturation arrest. The propensity to infection is related to the degree of neutropenia, but the correlation is not good.[84,124,126] Hepatosplenomegaly has been seen in about one-half of patients. The age of presentation is wide, ranging from early childhood to old age.

Neutrophil-specific antibodies to the neutrophil antigens NA1, NA2, ND1, ND2, and NB1 as well as to antigens shared by erythrocytes and to HLA antigens have been detected.[112] They are detected by a variety of assays, including leukoagglutination,[112,127] opsonization,[60,124] immunochemical assays,[84] direct antibody binding,[123] complement activation,[84,128] and various modifications of these techniques.[129] The antibodies are usually of IgG and IgM type. The lack of a good, readily available, panel of known neutrophil antigens, limits most assays to the detection of only the presence of neutrophil-associated antibody. Detection of ANAs is helpful in establishing the diagnosis of immune neutropenia, although a negative assay does not exclude the diagnosis.[84,112] This may be due to antibody specificity for neutrophil progenitors, rather than mature neutrophils.[105,106,121] The degree of neutropenia is related to the speci-

ficity of the antibody as well as the titer. This probably accounts for the variability of success in correlating amount of antibody with severity of disease.[84,123,124] In addition to neutrophil-associated antibodies, circulating immune complexes have been detected in about one-third of patients with immune neutropenia[124] and in patients with chronic idiopathic neutropenia.[130] While immune complexes can produce a positive indirect immunofluorescent test (L. L. Beyer, J. Church, T. D. Coates, unpublished data), patients with immune complexes and negative immunofluorescence ANA tests have been reported.[124]

ANAs of the IgG type have been reported in systemic lupus erythematosus (SLE). These antibodies have been seen both before and after correction of neutropenia by therapy.[84,131] Approximately 50% of patients with SLE are neutropenic, although few have severe enough neutropenia to result in increased in susceptibility to infection.[131] Neutropenia in SLE may also be related to decreased myelopoiesis.[132]

The neutropenia of Felty syndrome (rheumatoid arthritis, splenomegaly, and neutropenia) has also been related to the presence of ANAs. In this complex autoimmune disorder, decreased granulocyte survival as well as decreased production have been reported.[132–134] Immune complexes have also been associated with this disorder.[133,134] More recently, suppressor T cells have been implicated in mediation of the neutropenia.[135,136] Improvement in neutropenia and a decrease in ANA levels with methotrexate treatment provides further evidence that an immune mechanism may play a role in the etiology of this neutropenia.[137]

Treatment of autoimmune neutropenia depends on the severity of the neutropenia-related symptoms and on the nature of the underlying disease. Since many of these patients have a benign course, therapy designed solely to increase the neutrophil count is not indicated. If the patient has significant neutropenia (ANC <500/mm[3]) and recurrent or severe infections, high-dose γ-globulin[113,114,138] or steroids may be used. Splenectomy provides only transient correction of the neutropenia and results in a subsequent propensity to infection. Other cytotoxic therapy may be considered, particularly in SLE or rheumatoid arthritis.[131,137]

Isoimmune Neutropenia

Moderate to severe neutropenia can occur in newborn infants secondary to IgG antibodies transferred from mother to infant. The pathogenesis of this disorder is identical to that of Rh hemolytic disease, with prenatal sensitization to neutrophil antigens resulting in production of antibodies that then cross the placenta.[108,112,139] The incidence has been estimated at 2 in 1,000 live births.[139]

The infant may present with sepsis or may be asymptomatic. Since neutropenia is frequently associated with sepsis in infants, it is difficult to determine whether the neutropenia resulted in sepsis or visa versa. Bone marrow examination shows normal cellularity with a late myeloid arrest, although antibody-mediated early arrests have been seen. ANAs can be detected in infant and maternal serum and may show specificity for the father's neutrophils, rather than the mother's.[112,139] Recovery is usually uneventful, with no episodes of serious infection. The neutropenia resolves within 12–15 weeks, although prolonged neutropenia for 24 weeks has been seen (T. D. Coates, unpublished data).

Treatment initially involves antibiotics, as neutropenia can be a sign of sepsis in the neonate.[18–20,102] Steroids are of little value. Intravenous γ-globulin has been successfully used in one infant.[140] We usually do not proceed with marrow aspiration in these instances but prefer to watch the peripheral blood counts. The neutropenia is usually noted in an otherwise normal infant. These patients are usually treated with antibiotics and do well with no culture proof of infection. If the infant is clearly septic or if subsequent episodes of fever that are clinically considered pyogenic occur, marrow aspiration should be performed. If there is early arrest or storage pool depletion, treatment with granulocyte transfusions should be considered. The safety of CSFs in newborns is unproven but is likely to be a viable approach in the future.[141]

Pure White Cell Aplasia

Pure white cell aplasia (PWCA) is a rare syndrome characterized by severe pyogenic infections and neutropenia. Many of these patients (70%) have an associated thymoma. In some instances, PWCA occurs years after thymoma removal. Bone marrow examination shows almost complete absence of myeloid precursors with normal erythroid precursors and megakaryocytes. This is in contrast to Tγ neutropenia or Kostmann syndrome (infantile agranulocytosis), in which early myeloid precursors are seen. Marrow inhibitory activity is seen in both IgG and IgM fractions of patients' sera and disappears as the marrow recovers. In some instances, the inhibitory activity is in lymphocyte fractions, and not in the plasma. PWCA has been seen with ibuprofen therapy. In vitro serum inhibitory activity required the presence of the drug and complement. The clinical syndrome resolved when ibuprofen was discontinued. Removal of the thymoma is indicated but may not be sufficient. Cyclophosphamide, steroids, and Cyclosporin A have been effective in treatment of PWCA, as has intravenous IgG.[142]

Neutropenia Associated with Immunologic Abnormalities

Neutropenia has been seen in association with a number of immunologic abnormalities. Affected patients usually present in childhood with frequent bacterial infections, hepatosplenomegaly, and failure to thrive. Some of these children die within the first few years of life. Hypergammaglobulinemia or hypogammaglobulinemia,[143-145] T-cell defects,[146,147] natural killer (NK) cell abnormalities,[121] and autoimmune phenomena[147,148] have been seen. Many reported patients have had a positive family history of neutropenia.[143-145] Chronic diarrhea, skin rashes, and recurrent viral infections may also be seen in these children. Treatment of these disorders depends on the constellation of immunologic abnormalities present. Some of these patients have been treated with bone marrow transplantation.[146]

It is important to distinguish these patients from patients with the much more common syndrome of idiopathic benign neutropenia. In contrast to benign neutropenia, children with global immune defects associated with neutropenia have manifestations of recurrent or unusual infections. If the child demonstrates failure to thrive, frequent hospitalizations for pneumonia or sepsis, an immunologic evaluation is indicated. Furthermore, live-virus vaccines must be withheld and any blood products irradiated, until the possibility of a T-cell defect has been eliminated.

Most patients with AIDS have neutropenia as well as anemia. About 30% have thrombocytopenia.[149] Neutropenia has been seen in ≤8% of asymptomatic human immunodeficiency virus (HIV) carriers. The bone marrow is usually hypercellular and has lymphoid aggregates and plasmacytosis. Dysplastic changes are commonly seen in the granulocytes. The neutropenia is believed to be due to ineffective hematopoiesis. The immunoglobulin fraction of HIV-positive serum inhibits CFU-GM and burst-forming unit-erythroid in vitro and thus may contain antibodies to progenitors.

Tγ Lymphocytosis and Neutropenia

Approximately 80% of patients with Tγ lymphocytosis present with neutropenia during the course of evaluation for recurrent infections.[150] The median age of onset is 55–65 years, although it has been seen in children. There may also be a history of rheumatoid arthritis. Splenomegaly occurs in many of the patients, although an enlarged liver or lymphadenopathy is not common. The peripheral blood shows lymphocytosis, rarely >20,000. Most of the lymphocytes are large granular lymphocytes. The bone marrow in these disorders is normocellular with an arrest at the myelocyte stage and an increase in lymphocytes. The lymphocytes may show CD2, CD3, Fc, or HNK-1 but lack CD5.[151] They may also show the myeloid marker M1. NK cells are a subpopulation of these cells, making this syndrome of particular interest. Most patients have a benign course for many years. The longest survival is 20 years. Patients die of progressive lymphoproliferation or of sepsis related to neutropenia.[147,148,151] Although the course may be relatively protracted and benign, the lymphocytosis does represent a clonal proliferation and is thought by some to be malignant.[148,152,153] A decrease in suppressor cell and NK cell activity concomitant with improvement in neutropenia after treatment with intravenous γ-globulin[114,138] supports laboratory data[11,136] suggesting that these cells play a role in the regulation of myelopoiesis and in the pathophysiology of neutropenia.

Metabolic Diseases

Neutropenia can be associated with ketoacidosis in patients with hyperglycemia, hyperglycinuria, orotic aciduria, and methylmalonic aciduria.[154-157] Neutropenia is also commonly seen in association with glycogen storage disease type Ib, but not with glycogen storage disease type Ia. Recurrent infections are a major source of morbidity in these patients. The degree of neutropenia is variable, but commonly counts may be <500/mm^3. The bone marrow is normocellular or hypercellular. Variable functional defects have been seen in neutrophils from these patients.[158,159] Patients with glycogen storage disease Ib have been treated with CSF-G and CSF-GM.[160] Two patients with severe symptoms were helped by treatment with CSF-GM.[160] Interestingly, both patients had hypercellular marrow with no evidence of arrest. CSF-GM was required twice daily to maintain granulocyte counts, suggesting a role of this cytokine in promoting release of granulocytes from the marrow storage pool.

Neutropenia Due to Increased Margination

Both acute and chronic neutropenia can occur as a result of complement activation.[91,92,103,161-163] The mechanism was first recognized in patients undergoing hemodialysis and is associated with pulmonary dysfunction.[162,163] Generation of C5a activates neutrophils, resulting in increased adherence and aggregation and subsequent entrapment in the pulmonary vasculature.[92,103] Similar activation of complement and neutropenia has been seen with the use of membrane oxygenators.[164] Complement-mediated neutropenia due to shifts in the neutrophil pools has also been seen with burns[13] and transfusion reactions.[91] Since lung dysfunction and pulmonary infiltrates have been seen in some of these processes, the neutrophil has been implicated in the pathophysiology of adult respiratory distress syndrome.[13,91,92] However, the occurrence of adult respiratory distress syndrome and severe neutropenia, with no neutrophilic infiltration of the lungs, suggests that mechanisms other than direct damage by neutrophils are possible.[165] Neutropenia may be related to complement-mediated destruction of neutrophils, as seen in paroxysmal nocturnal hemoglobinuria[166,167] or due to similar destruction of granulocyte precursors.[105,106,128]

Hypersplenism

Neutropenia can be seen in association with hypersplenism. The neutropenia is usually not severe enough to cause symptoms, unless associated antineutrophil surface antibodies are present. Anemia and thrombocytopenia are usually present as well. Improvement in the hypersplenism-induced leukopenia in a patient with AIDS was obtained by splenic embolization.[168]

Nutritional Deficiency

Neutropenia has been seen in association with anemia in nutritional deficiency of vitamin B_{12}, folate, and copper.[169–171] All these neutropenias are characterized by ineffective myelopoiesis and megaloblastic changes in the bone marrow. Similar findings have been seen in the inherited deficiency of transcobalmin II.[172] Neutropenia and megaloblastosis have also been seen in association with sideroblastic anemia in the DIDMOAD syndrome (diabetes insipidus, diabetes mellitus, optic atrophy, deafness). The hematologic abnormalities were responsive to thiamin.[172]

Intrinsic Defects

Infantile Agranulocytosis

Severe infantile agranulocytosis was described by Kostmann in 1956.[173] This is one of several similar disorders that present in early infancy with severe, recurrent infections and neutropenia. This entity has been reported as having an autosomal dominant or autosomal recessive[165] type of inheritance. Bone marrow examination usually indicates myeloid hypoplasia with an arrest at the promyelocyte stage. Ultrastructural examination shows abnormalities in granule production in some patients.[165] Bone marrow culture studies generally show colony growth,[115,174] which is dependent on exogenous CSFs. This previously fatal disorder responds well to CSF-G,[175,176] and therapy with CSF-G should be seriously considered in all patients in whom the diagnosis is confirmed.

Myelokathexis/Neutropenia with Tetraploid Leukocytes

Several cases of severe recurrent infections, neutropenia, and dysmyelopoieic features have been described. Many affected patients display neutrophil mobility abnormalities as well.[165,177–179] Although they have been reported as separate diseases, many of the infantile neutropenia syndromes overlap considerably.[165,173,177,178] While these symptoms usually present in childhood, a patient with "myelokathexis" presented at 34 years of age.[180]

One patient had neutrophil counts in the 100–450/mm³ range with binucleate and tetraploid-nucleated neutrophils, bands, and metamyelocytes in the bone marrow. All mature neutrophils, 64% of the bands, and 42% of the metamyelocytes were binucleate. By contrast, early precursors were normal, and only rare abnormal neutrophils were found in the peripheral blood. The cellularity and structure of the marrow were normal, except for the binucleate cells. This child had a history of severe recurrent infections. Chemotaxis of neutrophils obtained from the marrow was markedly decreased compared with that of controls.[178]

Similar abnormalities have been seen in patients with "myelokathexis." One of the first reported patients had abnormal chemotaxis, as assessed by Rebuck skin window.[177] Some of these patients have nuclear abnormalities in peripheral blood neutrophils as well. Abnormalities in phagocytosis, chemotaxis, and the respiratory burst were seen in another patient with multiple congenital anomalies, neutropenia, and abnormally hypersegmented neutrophil nuclei.[179] These patients have been helped by treatment with CSF-G.[181]

Cyclic Neutropenia

Cyclic neutropenia is a dominantly inherited disorder with variable expression characterized by neutropenia that recurs every 15–35 days. The patients have associated recurrent

fever, pharyngitis, stomatitis, and other bacterial infections. The severity of the infections parallel the severity of the neutropenia and can be variable. While the disease tends to be benign, several patients have died of infection.[182] Most of these patients present in childhood, but an adult-onset form has been reported. The disorder can persist for many years but tends to decrease in severity with time. The bone marrow during times of neutropenia is usually hypoplastic, with a myelocyte arrest.[182–184]

Cyclic neutropenia is thought to represent a stem cell regulatory defect. In an animal model it can be cured by bone marrow transplantation[182] and has been transferred from an affected human donor to a recipient during bone marrow transplantation.[185]

The disorder must be differentiated from cyclic fevers without neutropenia[186] and from other causes of neutropenia. The diagnosis is established by documentation of periodic neutropenia. This requires monitoring of the neutrophil count at least twice a week for 6–8 weeks. The nadir of the neutropenia can be missed if the patient is monitored less frequently.

Treatment is largely supportive and should include regular and aggressive dental care. Antibacterial mouthwashes, such as Peridex, are useful in decreasing gingivitis. Patients with severe infections should be considered for treatment with CSF-G.[187]

Shwachman-Diamond-Oski Syndrome

The combination of neutropenia, metaphyseal dysplasia, and pancreatic insufficiency is known as Shwachman-Diamond-Oski syndrome.[188] Affected patients present in the first 10 years of life with steatorrhea and infections. Severe or fatal infections occur in more than one-half of patients, but many have relatively few problems with infection despite the neutropenia. Although pancreatic insufficiency can be detected by fecal fat determination or by trypsin or lipase measurement, some patients have minimal problems with steatorrhea; therefore, the absence of a clear history of bowel problems does not rule out the diagnosis. Short stature and a variety of other physical anomalies, including strabismus, cleft palate, syndactyly, and microcephaly, are noted at physical examination. Metaphyseal dysplasia occurs in 25% of patients.

Neutrophil counts are usually <500/mm³. Thrombocytopenia may be present in 70% of patients, and a mildly megaloblastic prednisone-responsive anemia is seen in 10% of patients.[188] In addition to neutropenia, a neutrophil-capping and chemotactic defect is present. A partial chemotactic defect may be seen in the parents,[11] consistent with the presumed recessive inheritance. The reported functional defects have been corrected by injection with thiamin in some patients.[189] The mechanism for this response is unknown. The bone marrow is usually hypoplastic, although it can be normal. Sweat chloride determination is normal.

The steatorrhea responds to pancreatic enzyme replacement and resolves by 5 or 10 years of age, although the pancreatic insufficiency remains. Treatment consists of management of infections and bleeding episodes. The anemia may respond to treatment with prednisone. The neutropenia has responded to CSF-G. Since not all patients have problems with infection, it is unnecessary to treat all of these patients with CSF-G. However, if any serious infection related to neutropenia develops, CSF-G should be started. The overall expected survival is approximately 50%. As with other constitutional marrow failure syndromes, Shwachman-Diamond-Oski syndrome is associated with an increased incidence of malignancy. Both lymphocytic and nonlymphocytic leukemias have been reported,[190,191] accounting for some of the mortality seen with this syndrome.

Chédiak-Higashi Syndrome

Chédiak-Higashi syndrome is a rare inherited disorder characterized by oculocutaneous albinism, progressive neurologic impairment, and giant granules in many cells, including neutrophils. Severe neutropenia, develops as well, believed to be due to ineffective granulopoiesis.[192]

Reticular Dysgenesis

The syndrome known as reticular dysgenesis is characterized by agranulocytosis, lymphoid hypoplasia, and thymic dysplasia with normal megakaryocyte and erythroid precursors.[193,194] Affected patients have low IgM and IgA concentrations, and abnormal lymphocytes.[194] The marrow is hypoplastic with very few neutrophilic or lymphocytic precursors. The few early myeloid cells present display decreased granule formation.[194] As patients with reticular dysgenesis die in infancy, early bone marrow transplantation should be considered.

Dyskeratosis Congenita

Dyskeratosis congenita is an X-linked disorder involving abnormalities of integument and mild neutropenia.[195] Some patients have pancytopenia.[196,197] The marrow can be hypocellular, and some studies suggest an immunologic mechanism for the neutropenia.[196]

Other Neutropenias

Isolated neutropenia can be part of the presentation of other marrow failure syndromes, such as myelodysplasia, preleukemia, Fanconi anemia, and aplastic anemia. Usually other characteristic features are associated with the neutropenia.

Management of Neutropenia

The clinical management of neutropenic states depends on the cause and degree of the neutropenia and on associated disease states. The key problem is management of infectious complications. Patients with severe neutropenia and little marrow reserve have acute severe pyogenic infections, while patients with hypercellular marrow tend to have chronic infections or no infectious problems at all.

Table 52-2 presents the relationship between the ANC and propensity for infection. These guidelines should be used in patients with chemotherapy-induced neutropenia and in neutropenia associated with granulocyte hypoplasia such as aplastic anemia, infantile agranulocytosis, or familial severe neutropenia. These patients have no marrow reserve and tend to have decreased marrow cellularity with an early myeloid arrest. Since these patients are unable to respond to infection, many of the inflammatory signs of infection may be absent. For example, radiographs may not demonstrate pneumonia, or the patient may not exhibit abdominal tenderness with an early ruptured viscus. The organisms that cause infections come from the gastrointestinal tract or skin and can result in overwhelming sepsis very quickly. Thus, febrile patients with neutropenia related to marrow suppression should be treated immediately with broad-spectrum parenteral antibiotics. Antibiotics should be continued for several days after the fever has subsided. If fever and neutropenia persist for >1 week, consideration should be given to the empirical use of amphotericin B. Granulocyte transfusions are effective in certain instances of culture-proven gram-negative sepsis. They should be used in patients with severe neutropenia with culture-proven gram-negative sepsis who have not shown a clinical response to antibiotics within 24–48 hours. Enthusiasm for the use of granulocyte transfusions has waned in recent years due in part to difficul-

---

DIAGNOSTIC APPROACH TO NEUTROPENIA

The approach to the diagnostic evaluation of a patient with neutropenia can be largely guided by the clinical history and physical examination and does not always require an extensive laboratory evaluation at the onset (see previous box). If the patient is asymptomatic and has no significant history or physical findings to warrant immediate further evaluation, clinical observation is the best approach. Examination of the oral cavity is important in the evaluation of a patient with chronic neutropenia. The presence of gingivitis, tooth abscess, or tooth loss suggests the presence of clinically significant neutropenia. Isolated neutropenia is an unusual presentation of malignancy, so there is usually time to follow the course of the neutropenia before proceeding with extensive evaluations. This is particularly true in young children, in whom the most common neutropenias are benign. If the ANC is >500–1,000/mm^3, it is unlikely that anything will be gained by bone marrow aspiration. If anemia, particularly normocytic or macrocytic anemia, or thrombocytopenia is present, bone marrow aspiration should be performed immediately. If there is a recent history of a viral infection or if the patient is on a medication known to be associated with neutropenia, several weeks of observation, and discontinuation of the medication may reveal resolution of the neutropenia and avoid a bone marrow aspiration. If the neutropenia is persistent, bone marrow aspiration with biopsy, immunologic evaluation, marrow chromosomes, assay of ANAs, repeated collagen vascular workup, or other tests (see later box) may be useful in determining the cause of the neutropenia. Bone marrow culture, epinephrine stimulation test, and hydrocortisone stimulation tests are often discussed but are of little discriminatory value and do not alter the approach to treatment.

On the basis of the history plus marrow cellularity and morphology, most of these patient's can be classified as having a secondary neutropenia or a primary marrow defect and management can be determined.

In summary, asymptomatic patients with isolated neutropenia can be observed clinically for several weeks. Patients with infections attributable to their neutropenia, or other clinical manifestations of serious diseases associated with neutropenia should be evaluated.

---

ties in procurement and to better antibiotics. Routine reverse isolation procedures are of no benefit[198,199] and serve to decrease contact with medical personnel. While empirical antibiotics are clearly indicated in the case of fever, prophylactic antibiotics should not be routinely used.

Patients with late marrow arrests and normocellular marrows may be able to handle infections reasonably well. Children in whom the diagnosis of chronic benign neutropenia of infancy has been confirmed can be treated like normal children. In older patients with evidence of marrow reserve and a several month history of severe neutropenia without serious infections, less aggressive therapy may be reasonable as well. When these patients are first encountered, however, they should be treated like other patients with more severe forms of neutropenia.

All patients with chronic neutropenia should receive regular dental care. Chronic gingivitis and recurrent stomatitis can be major sources of morbidity. Antibiotic mouthwashes, such as Peridex, can be very helpful in preventing gingivitis.

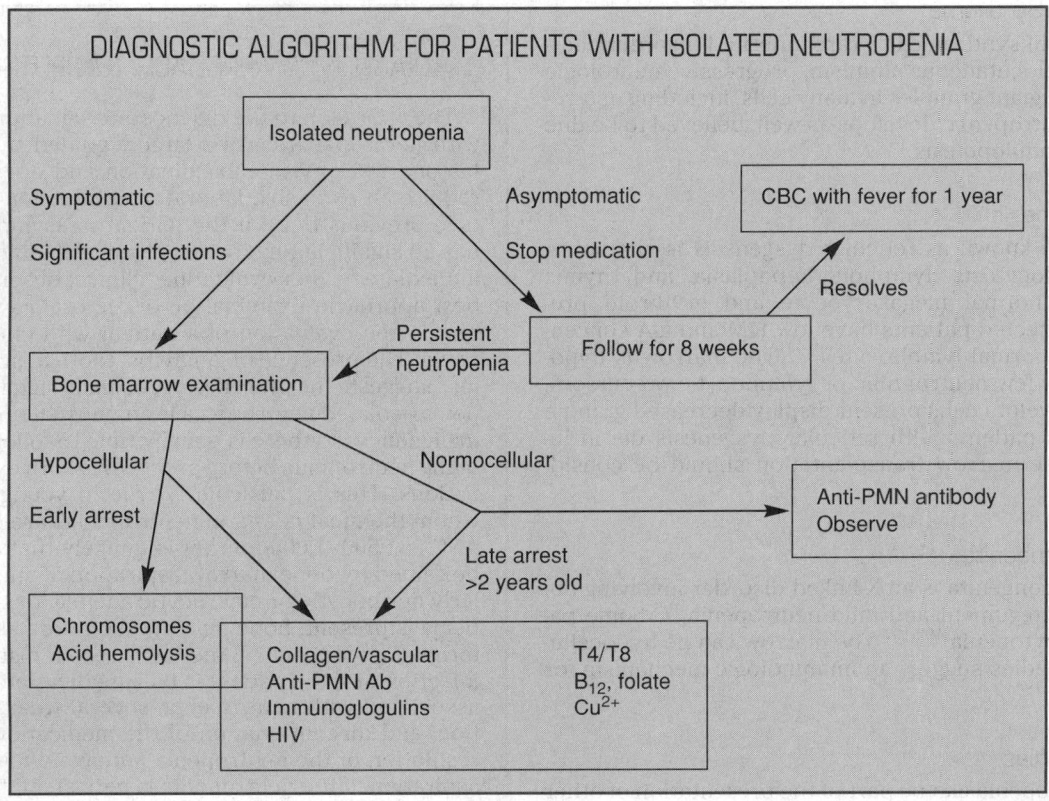

DIAGNOSTIC ALGORITHM FOR PATIENTS WITH ISOLATED NEUTROPENIA

Until recently, therapy designed to increase the neutrophil count has had only variable success. Corticosteroids have been effective in some instances of immune-mediated neutropenia,[86,91,108] as has intravenous γ-globulin. Recombinant CSF-G has been effective in correcting neutropenia in cyclic neutropenia and severe infantile agranulocytosis and should be considered in symptomatic patients.[160,175,176,187] The use of CSF-G has met with enthusiasm, however, it is not indicated for all instances of neutropenia. CSF-G is most likely to be helpful in patients with neutropenia associated with early myeloid arrest. As some patients with primary neutropenia have relatively little problem with infection, and these cytokines are very expensive, this therapy should be reserved for patients with demonstrated infectious morbidity related to their neutropenia, and not for treatment of the blood count. Bone marrow transplantation has been used successfully in certain instances of severe neutropenia and should be considered if an appropriate donor is available.

MONOCYTOPENIA AND MONOCYTOSIS

Alterations in the number of circulating monocytes are seen in a number of clinical situations (Table 52-4), although generally, the disorders are less well defined than those of granulocytes. Production of monocytes is regulated by IL-3 and CSF-GM produced by T lymphocytes and by CSF-M produced by endothelial cells and by monocytes themselves. IL-3 and CSF-GM selectively induce CSF-M production by monocytes, suggesting one mechanism for production of the monocytosis associated with certain chronic infections associated with enhanced T-lymphocyte activity.[200] Monocytes comprise 1–9% of peripheral leukocytes, although the total monocyte count is higher during the first 2 weeks of life.[201,202]

The blood monocyte and tissue monocyte/macrophage undoubtedly play an important role in defense against bacteria and fungal invasion. However, no clear association has been found between circulating numbers of monocytes and propensity to infection, as exists with granulocytes. Decreases in the number of monocytes have been seen with endotoxemia and with glucocorticoid administration.[203] Noncirculating monocytes appear to be relatively resistant to radiation and cytotoxic chemotherapy.[204]

Monocytosis is generally seen in association with chronic inflammatory processes, whether infectious or immune. Monocytosis has been seen with tuberculosis,[205] subacute bacterial

Table 52-4. Disorders Associated with Monocytosis

Inflammatory diseases
    Infectious diseases
        Tuberculosis
        Syphilis
        Subacute bacterial endocarditis
        Fever of unknown origin
    Autoimmune/granulomatous
        Systemic lupus erythematosus
        Rheumatoid arthritis
        Temporal arteritis
        Myositis
        Polyarteritis
        Ulcerative colitis
        Regional enteritis
        Sarcoidosis
Malignant disorders
    Preleukemia
    Acute myeloid leukemia
    Histiocytoses
    Hodgkin disease
    Non-Hodgkin lymphoma
    Carcinomas
Miscellaneous
    Chronic neutropenia
    Postsplenectomy

endocarditis, syphilis, and fevers of unknown origin.[205,206] Collagen vascular diseases, such as rheumatoid arthritis, SLE, myositis, periarteritis, and temporal arteritis, have been associated with monocytosis as well as with granulomatous diseases, such as sarcoid, regional enteritis, and ulcerative colitis.[205,207]

Monocytosis has been seen with several primary neutropenic syndromes, including cyclic neutropenia, chronic idiopathic neutropenia, and infantile agranulocytosis.[109,111,173,182] An increase in monocytes usually heralds recovery from agranulocytosis. Monocytosis is commonly seen in a number of primary hematologic malignancies. Increased promonocytes and monocytes are seen in patients with chronic and acute myeloid leukemias as well as in preleukemic states.[168,208,209] In many of these instances, the monocytes may be malignant but are indistinguishable from normal by light microscopy.[209] In addition to leukemia, monocytosis has been seen in both Hodgkin and non-Hodgkin lymphomas and in histiocytoses as well as nonhematologic malignancies.[210–212]

REFERENCES

1. Dinarello C, Mier J: Lymphokines. N Engl J Med 317:940, 1987
2. Clark S, Kamen R: The human hematopoietic colony-stimulating factors. Science 236:1229, 1987
3. Ghebrehiwet B, Mueller-Eberhard H: C3e: an acidic fragment of human C3 with leukocytosis-inducing activity. J Clin Immunol 123:616, 1979
4. Hosprich PD Jr, Dahinden C, Lachmann P et al: A synthetic nonapeptide corresponding to the NH_2-terminal sequence of C3d-k causes leukocytosis in rabbits. J Biol Chem 260:2597, 1985
5. Ulich T, Del-Castillo J, Keys M, et al: Kinetics and mechanisms of recombinant human interleukin 1 and tumor necrosis factor-alpha-induced changes in circulating numbers of neutrophils and lymphocytes. J Immunol 139:3406, 1987
6. Sobrado J, Moldawer L, Bistrian B et al: Effect of ibuprofen on fever and metabolic changes induced by continuous infusion of leukocytic pyrogen (interleukin 1) or endotoxin. Infect Immun 42:997, 1983
7. Dale D, Fauci A, Guerry D, Wolff S: Comparison of agents producing a neutrophilic leukocytosis in man. J Clin Invest 56:808, 1975
8. Ho-Yen D, Martin K: The relationship between atypical lymphocytosis and serological tests in infectious mononucleosis. J Infect 3:324, 1981
9. Boxer L, Allen J, Baehner R: Diminished polymorphonuclear leukocyte adherence. Function dependant upon release of cyclic AMP by endothelial cells after stimulation of beta receptors by epinephrine. J Clin Invest 66:268, 1980
10. Broxmeyer H, Gentile P, Cooper S et al: Functional activities of acidic isoferritins and lactoferrin in vitro and vivo. Blood Cells 10:397, 1984
11. Broxmeyer H, Lu L, Bognacki J: Transferrin, derived from an OKT8-positive subpopulation of T-lymphocytes, suppresses the production of granulocyte-macrophage colony-stimulating factors from mitogen-activated T lymphocytes. Blood 62:37, 1983
12. Goldberg L: Amphetamines and leukocytosis. A possible association. Postgrad Med 73:113, 1983
13. Wolach B, Coates T, Hugli T et al: Plasma lactoferrin reflects granulocytes activation via complement in burn patients. J Lab Clin Med 103:284, 1984
14. Craddock C: Granulocyte kinetics. p. 593. In Williams WJ, Buetler E, Erslev AS, Rundles NW (eds): Hematology. McGraw-Hill, New York, 1972
15. Nathan D, Oski F: Hematology of Infancy and Childhood. WB Saunders, Philadelphia, 1987, p. 1688
16. Xanthou M: Leukocyte blood picture in healthy full term and premature babies during the neonatal period. Arch Dis Child 45:242, 1970
17. Jandl J: Blood Textbook of Hematology. Little, Brown, Boston, 1987, p. 462
18. Christensen R, Bradley P, Rothstein G: The leukocyte left shift in clinical and experimental neonatal sepsis. J Pediatr 98:101, 1981
19. Manroe B, Rosenfeld C, Weinberg A, Browne R: The differential leukocyte count in the assessment and outcome of early-onset group B streptococcal disease. J Pediatr 91:632, 1977
20. Manroe B, Browne R, Weinberg A et al: Leukocyte count in streptococcal disease. Pediatr Res 10:428, 1976
21. Johnson C, Bass D, Trillo A et al: Functional and metabolic studies of polymorphonuclear leukocytes in congenital Pelger-Huët anomaly. Blood 55:466, 1980
22. Taylor R: Pelger-Huët anomaly in megaloblastic anemia. Am J Clin Pathol 60:932, 1973
23. Dorr A, Moloney W: Acquired pseudo Pelger anomaly of granulocytic leukocytes. N Engl J Med 261:742, 1959
24. Kaplan J, O'Barrett N: Reversible pseudo Pelger anomaly related to sulfisoxazole therapy. N Engl J Med 277:421, 1967
25. Schneiderman L, Sampson W, Schoene W, Haydon G: Genetic studies of a family with two unusual autosomal dominant conditions: muscular dystrophy and Pelger-Huët anomaly. Clinical, pathologic and linkage considerations. Am J Med 46:380, 1969
26. Herring W, Smith L, Walker R, Herion J: Hereditary neutrophilia. Am J Med 56:729, 1974
27. Ward H, Reinhard E: Chronic idiopathic leukocytosis. Ann Intern Med 75:193, 1971
28. Randall DL, Reiquam C, Githens J, Robinson A: Familial myeloproliferative disease. Am J Dis Child 110:479, 1965
29. Lewis S, Dacie J: Neutrophil leukocyte alkaline phosphatase in paroxysmal nocturnal haemoglobinuria. Br J Haematol 11:549, 1965
30. Altman A, Palmer C, Baehner R: Juvenile "chronic granulocytic" leukemia: a panmyelopathy with prominent monocytic and circulating monocyte colony forming cells. Blood 43:341, 1974
31. Emery J, Gordon R, Rendle-Short J et al: Congenital amegakaryocytic thrombocytopenia with congenital deformities and a leukemoid blood picture in the newborn. Blood 12:567, 1957
32. Dignan P, Mauer A, Frantz C: Phocomelia with congenital hypoplastic thrombocytopenia and myeloid leukemoid reactions. J Pediatr 70:561, 1967
33. Weinstein H: Congenital leukemia and the neonatal myeloproliferative disorders associated with Down's syndrome. Clin Hematol 7:147, 1978
34. Rubins J and Wakem C: Hypoglycemia and leukemoid reaction with hypernephroma. NY State J Med 77:406, 1977
35. Brodeur G, Dahl G, Williams D et al: Transient leukemoid reaction and trisomy 21 mosaicism in a phenotypically normal newborn. Blood 55:691, 1980
36. Jones G, Weaver M, Laug W: Transient blastemia in phenotypically normal newborns. Am J Pediatr Hematol Oncol 9:153, 1987
37. Fischer A, Lisowska-Grospierre B, Anderson D, Springer T: Leukocyte adhesion deficiency: molecular basis and functional consequences. Immunodefic Rev 1:39, 1988
38. Torres M, Caldwell SE, Coates TD et al: MO1 deficiency and protein kinase C. J Cell Biol 103:509a, 1986
39. Weisman S, Berkow R, Plautz G et al: Glycoprotein-180 deficiency: genetics and abnormal neutrophil activation. Blood 65:696, 1985
40. Nauseef W, De Alarcon P, Bale J, Clark R: Aberrant activation and regulation of the oxidative burst in neutrophils with Mo1 glycoprotein deficiency. J Immunol 137:636, 1986
41. Boxer L, Coates T, Haak R et al: Lactoferrin deficiency associated with altered granulocyte function. N Engl J Med 307:404, 1982
42. Frydman M, Etzioni A, Eidlitz Markus T et al: Rambam-Hasharon syndrome of psychomotor retardation, short stature, defective neutrophil motility, and Bombay phenotype. Am J Med Genet 44:297, 1992
43. Etzioni A, Frydman M, Pollack S et al: Brief report: recurrent severe infections caused by a novel leukocyte adhesion deficiency. N Engl J Med 327:1789, 1992
44. Tindall John P, Beeker Sharon K, Rosse Wendell F: Familial cold urticaria. A generalized reaction involving leukocytosis. Arch Intern Med 124:129, 1969
45. Hendrik M, Doeglas M, Bleumink E: Familial cold urticaria. Clinical findings. Arch Dermatol 110:382, 1974
46. Martens BP, Berrens L: Enzyme activation and inhibition induced by cold provocation in a patient with cold urticaria. Acta Derm Venereol (Stockh) 55:121, 1975
47. Nilsson T: Aspects of C1-inhibitor biochemistry and pathophysiology. Clin Rheumatol 6:332, 1987
48. Schwartz R, Hayden G, Rodriguez W et al: Leukocyte counts in children with acute otitis media. Pediatr Emerg Care 2:10, 1986
49. Koenig J, Patterson L, Rench M, Edwards M: Role of fibronectin in diagnosing bacterial infection in infancy. Am J Dis Child 142:884, 1988
50. Christensen R, Hill H: Exercise-induced changes in the blood concentration of leukocyte populations in teenage athletes. Am J Pediatr Hematol Oncol 9:140, 1987
51. Christensen R, Rothstein G: Pitfalls in the interpretation of leukocyte counts of newborn infants. Am J Clin Pathol 72:608, 1979
52. Foster N, Martyn J, Rangno R et al: Leukocytosis of exercise: role of cardiac output and catecholamines. J Appl Physiol 61:2218, 1986
53. McCarthy D, Perry J, Melsom R, Dale M: Leucocytosis induced by exercise. Br Med J Clin Res 295:636, 1987
54. Darko D, Rose J, Gillin J et al: Neutrophilia and lymphopenia in major mood disorders. Psychiatry Res 25:243, 1988
55. Jakobsen B, Pedersen J, Egeberg B: Postoperative lymphocytopenia and leucocytosis after epidural and general anaesthesia. Anaesthesiol Scand 30:668, 1986

56. Nanji A, Freeman J, Nair G: Postoperative leukocytosis in morbidity obese patients: relationship to serum cholesterol. Am J Hematol 20:417, 1985

57. Mulroy J, Mickell J, Tong T, Pellock J: Postictal pulmonary edema in children. Neurology 35:403, 1985

58. Zalokar J, Richard J, Claude J: Leukocyte count, smoking and myocardial infarction. N Engl J Med 304:465, 1981

59. Fava M: Leukocytes and the risk of ischemic diseases. JAMA 258:907, 1987

60. Boxer L, Stossel T: Effects of anti-human neutrophil antibodies in vitro. J Clin Invest 53:1534, 1974

61. Boggs D, Joyce R: The hematopoietic effects of lithium. Semin Hematol 20:129, 1983

62. Ascensao J, Oken M, Ewing S et al: Leukocytosis and large cell lung cancer. A frequent association. Cancer 60:903, 1987

63. Shoenfeld Y, Tal A, Berliner S, Pinkhas J: Leukocytosis in nonhematological malignancies—a possible tumor-associated marker. J Cancer Res Clin Oncol 111:54, 1986

64. Riddle P, Dincsoy H: Primary squamous cell carcinoma of the thyroid associated with leukocytosis and hypercalcemia. Arch Pathol Lab Med 111:373, 1987

65. Eichenhorn M, Van-Slyck E: Marked mature neutrophilic leukocytosis: a leukemoid variant associated with malignancy. Am J Med Sci 284:32, 1982

66. Obara T, Ito Y, Kodama T et al: A case of gastric carcinoma associated with excessive granulocytosis. Production of a colony-stimulating factor by the tumor. Cancer 56:782, 1985

67. Anonymous: Medical Staff Conference: Heat stroke. West J Med 121:305, 1974

68. Hernandez J, Aldred S, Bruce J et al: "Botryoid" nuclei in neutrophils of patients with heat stroke. Lancet 2:642, 1980

69. Rochant H: Hemolyse retardée post-transfusionnelle, syndrome leucémoide, anémie hémolytique auto-immune. Comité de coordination pour l'Exploration Spécifique des Anémies (CESA) sous la responsabilité de H. Rochant. Nouv Rev Fr Hematol 29:425, 1987

70. Michaelson A: Severe leukemoid reaction after promazine-induced agranulocytosis. J Fla Med Assoc 45:1418, 1959

71. Rudvic R, Jelic S: Haematologic aspects of drug-induced agranulocytosis. Scand J Haematol 9:18, 1972

72. Levine P, Weintraub L: Pseudo-leukemia following recovery from dapsone-induced agranulocytosis. Ann Intern Med 68:1060, 1968

73. McBride J, Dacie J, Shapley R: The effect of splenectomy on the leukocyte count. Br J Haematol 14:225, 1968

74. Spencer R, McPhedran P, Finch S, Morgan W: Persistent neutrophilic leukocytosis associated with idiopathic functional asplenia. J Nucl Med 13:224, 1972

75. Rappaport E, Helbert B, Beissner R, Trowbridge A: Automated hematology: where we stand. South Med J 81:365, 1988

76. Walters J, Garrity P: Case Studies in the New Morphology. American Scientific Products, McGaw Park, IL, 1987, p. 5

77. Solanki D, Blackburn B: Spurious leukocytosis and thrombocytopenia. A dual phenomenon caused by clumping of platelets in vitro. JAMA 250:2514, 1983

78. Savage R: Pseudoleukocytosis due to EDTA-induced platelet clumping. Am J Clin Pathol 81:317, 1984

79. Patel K, Hughes C, Parapia L: Pseudoleucocytosis and pseudothrombocytosis due to cryoglobulinemia. J Clin Pathol 40:120, 1987

80. Caramihai E, Karayalcin G, Aballi A, Lanzkowsky P: Leukocyte count differences in healthy white and black children 1 to 5 years of age. J Pediatr 86:252, 1975

81. Shoenfeld Y, Weinberger A, Avishar R et al: Familial leukopenia among Yemenite Jews. Isr J Med Sci 14:1271, 1978

82. Shoenfeld Y, Ben-Tal O, Berliner S, Pinkhas J: The outcome of bacterial infections in subjects with benign familial neutropenia. Biomed Pharamacother 39:23, 1985

83. Lalezari P, Khorshidi M, Petrosova M: Autoimmune neutropenia of infancy. J Pediatr 109:764, 1986

84. Logue G, Shimm D: Autoimmune granulocytopenia. Annu Rev Med 31:191, 1980

85. Kyle R: Natural history of chronic idiopathic neutropenia. N Engl J Med 302:908, 1980

86. Dale D, Guerry D, Wewerka J et al: Chronic neutropenia. Medicine 58:128, 1979

87. Wright D, Meierovics A, Foxley J: Assessing the delivery of neutrophils to tissues in neutropenia. Blood 67:1023, 1986

88. Bodey G, Buckley M, Sathe Y, Freireich E: Quantitative relationships between circulating leukocytes and infection in patients with acute leukemia. Ann Intern Med 64:328, 1966

89. Howard M, Strauss R, Johnston R: Infections in patients with neutropenia. Am J Dis Child 131:788, 1977

90. Murdock J, Smith C: Hematologic aspects of systemic disease: infection. Clin Hematol 1:619, 1972

91. Weetman R, Boxer L: Childhood neutropenia. Pediatr Clin North Am 27:361, 1980

92. Jacob H: Granulocyte-complement interaction. Arch Intern Med 138:461, 1978

93. Ivarsson S, Ljung R: Neutropenia and congenital cytomegalovirus infection. Pediatr Infect Dis J 7:436, 1988

94. Avanzini A, Colombo T, Santucci S: Neutropenia in a cytomegalovirus (CMV) infected VVLBW infant. Acta Paediatr Scand 80:738, 1991

95. Stevens D, Everett E, Boxer L, Landstein R: Infectious mononucleosis with severe neutropenia and opsonic antineutrophil activity. South Med J 72:519, 1979

96. Calabro J, Williamson P, Lowe E et al: Kawasaki syndrome. N Engl J Med 306:237, 1982

97. Habib M, Babka J, Burningham R: Profound granulocytopenia associated with infectious mononucleosis. Am J Med Sci 265:339, 1973

98. Fronteira M, Myers A: Peripheral blood and bone marrow abnormalities in the acquired immunodeficieincy syndrome. West J Med 147:157, 1987

99. Church J, Beyer L, Coates T: Serum neutrophil antibodies in children with HIV infection. Presented at the Fifth International Conference on AIDS, Montreal (Quebec) Canada. 1989

100. Lobut J, Reinert P, Kohout G et al: [Autoimmune neutropenia disclosing AIDS in a child.] Ann Med Intern (Paris) 138:416, 1987

101. McCance-Katz E, Hoecker J, Vitale N: Severe neutropenia associated with anti-neutrophil antibody in a patient with acquired immunodeficiency syndrome-related complex. Pediatr Infect Dis 6:417, 1987

102. Christianson R, Rothstein G: Exhaustion of mature marrow neutrophils in neonates with sepsis. J Pediatr 96:316, 1980

103. Craddock P, Hammerschmidt D, Moldow C et al: Granulocyte aggregation as a manifestation of membrane interactions with complement: possible role in leukocyte margination, microvascular occlusion and endothelial damage. Semin Hematol 16:140, 1979

104. Finch S: Neutropenia. p. 777. In Williams WJ, Beutler E, Erslev AJ, Lichtman MA (eds): Hematology. McGraw-Hill, New York, 1983

105. Levitt L: Pure white-cell aplasia. Antibody-mediated autoimmune inhibition of granulopoiesis. N Engl J Med 308:1141, 1983

106. Mamus S, Burton J, Groat J et al: Ibuprofen-associated pure white cell aplasia. N Engl J Med 314:624, 1986

107. Heimpel H: Drug-induced agranulocytosis. Med Toxicol Adverse Drug Exp 3:449, 1988

108. Boxer L: Immune neutropenias: clinical and biological implications. Am J Pediatr Hematol Oncol 3:89, 1981

109. Cutting H, Lang J: Familial benign chronic neutropenia. Ann Intern Med 61:876, 1964

110. Stahlie T: Chronic benign neutropenia in infancy and early childhood. J Pediatr 48:710, 1956

111. Zeulzer W, Bajoghli M: Chronic granulocytopenia in childhood. Blood 23:359, 1964

112. Lalezari P: Neutrophil antigens: immunology and clinical implications. p. 209. In Greenwalt TJ, Jamieson GA (eds): The Granulocyte: Function and Clinical Utilization. 1977

113. Bussel J, Lalezari P, Fikrig S: Intravenous treatment with γ-globulin of auto-immune neutropenia of infancy. J Pediatr 112:298, 1988

114. Ikeda H, Ozawa T, Takahashi H et al: Immunological and hematological changes during high-dose immunoglobulin therapy in an infant with autoimmune neutropenia. Eur J Pediatr 146:412, 1987

115. Kawaguchi Y, Kobayashi M, Tanabe A et al: Granulopoiesis in patients with congenital neutropenia. Am J Hematol 20:223, 1985

116. Hartman KR, Wright DG: Identification of autoantibodies specific for the neutrophil adhesion glycoproteins CD11b/CD18 in patients with autoimmune neutropenia. Blood 78:1096, 1991

117. Miller M, Oski F, Harris M: Lazy-leukocyte syndrome. A new disorder of neutrophil function. Lancet 1:665, 1971

118. Komiyama A, Ishiguro A, Kubo T et al: Increases in neutrophil counts by purified human urinary colony-stimulating factor in chronic neutropenia of childhood. Blood 71:41, 1988

119. Komiyama A, Kawai H, Yamada S et al: Impaired natural killer cell recycling in childhood chromic neutropenia with morphological abnormalities and defective chemotaxis of neutrophils. Blood 66:99, 1985

120. Van-Der-Veen J, Hack C, Englefriet C et al: Chronic idiopathic and secondary neutropenia: clinical and serological investigations. Br J Haematol 63:1988

121. Currie M, Weinberg J, Rustagi P, Logue G: Antibodies to granulocyte precursors in selective myeloid hypoplasia and other suspected autoimmune neutropenia: use of HL-60 cells as targets. Blood 69:529, 1987

122. Jakubowski A, Souza L, Kelly F et al: Effects of human granulocyte colony-stimulating in a patient with idiopathic neutropenia. N Engl J Med 320:38, 1989

123. Cines D, Passero F, Guerry D et al: Granulocyte-associated IgG in neutropenic disorders. Blood 59:124, 1982

124. Hadley A, Holburn A, Bunch C, Chapel H: Anti-granulocyte opsonic activity and autoimmune neutropenia. Br J Haematol 63:581, 1986

125. Koenig J, Christensen R: Neutropenia and thrombocytopenia in infants with Rh hemolytic disease. J Pediatr 114:625, 1989

126. Greenberg P, Mara B, Steed S, Boxer L: The chronic idiopathic neutropenia syndrome: correlation of clinical features with in vitro parameters of granulocytopoiesis. Blood 55:915, 1980

127. Ducos R, Madyastha P, Warrier R et al: Neutrophil agglutinins in idiopathic chronic neutropenia of early childhood. Am J Dis Child 140:65, 1986

128. Rustagi P, Currie M, Logue G: Activation of human complement by immunoglobulin G antigranulocyte antibody. J Clin Invest 70:1137, 1982

129. McCullough J, Clay M, Priest J et al: A comparison of methods for detecting leukocyte antibodies in autoimmune neutropenia. Transfusion 21:483, 1981

130. van der Veen JP, Hack C, Engelfriet C et al: Chronic idiopathic and secondary neutropenia: clinical and serological investigations. Br J Haematol 63:161, 1986

131. Starkebaum G, Price T, Lee M, Arend W: Autoimmune neutropenia in systemic lupus erythematosus. Arthritis Rheum 21:504, 1978

132. Duckham D, Rhyne R, Smith F, Williams R: Retardation of colony growth of in vitro bone marrow culture using serum from patients with Felty's syndrome, disseminated lupus erythematosus, rheumatoid arthritis, and other disease states. Arthritis Rheum 18:323, 1975

133. Cryer P, Kissane J: Rheumatoid arthritis with Felty's syndrome, hyperviscosity, and immunologic hyperreactivity. Am J Med 70:89, 1981

134. Spivak J: Felty's syndrome. Johns Hopkins Med J 141:156, 1977

135. Abdou N, Na Pombejara C, Balentine L: Suppressor-cell mediated Felty's syndrome. J Clin Invest 61:738, 1978

136. Bagby J, Gabourel J: Neutropenia in three patients with rheumatic disorders: suppression of granulopoiesis by cortisol-sensitive thymus-dependent lymphocytes. J Clin Invest 64:72, 1979

137. Fiechtner J, Miller D, Starkebaum G: Reversal of neutropenia with methotrexate treatment in patients with Felty's syndrome. Correlation of response with neutrophil-reactive IgG. Arthritis Rheum 32:194, 1989

138. Engelhard D, Warner J, Kapoor N, Good R: Effect of intravenous immune globulin on natural killer cell activity: possible association with autoimmune neutropenia and idiopathic thrombocytopenia. J Pediatr 108:77, 1986

139. Levine D, Madyastha P: Isoimmune neonatal neutropenia. Am J Perinatol 3:231, 1986

140. Hanada T, Shin R, Hosio M et al: Intravenous gammaglobulin in treatment of isoimmune neonatal neutropenia. Eur J Pediatr 148:218, 1988

141. Cairo MS, Plunkett JM, Mauss D, Van de ven C: Seven-day administration of recombinant human granulocyte colony-stimulating factor to newborn rats: modulation of neonatal neutrophilia, myelopoiesis, and group B *Streptococcus* sepsis. Blood 76:1788, 1990

142. Marinone G, Roncoli B, Marinone M Jr: Pure white cell aplasia. Semin Hematol 28:298, 1991

143. Lonsdale D, Deohar S, Mercer R: Familial granulocytopenia associated with immunoglobulin abnormality. Report of three cases in young brothers. J Pediatr 71:790, 1967

144. Webster A, Slavin G, Strelling M, Asherson G: Combined immunodeficiency with hyperimmunoglobulinemia. Arch Dis Child 50:486, 1975

145. Bjorksten B, Lundmark K: Recurrent bacterial infections in for siblings with neutropenia, eosinophilia, hyperimmunoglobinemia A and defective neutrophil chemotaxis. J Infect Dis 133:63, 1976

146. Perreault C, Bonny Y, Gyger M et al: Congenital T cell deficiency with neutropenia and erythroblastopenia. Transplantation 39:321, 1985

147. Herrod H, Wang W, Sullivan J: Chronic T-cell lymphocytosis with neutropenia. Am J Dis Child 139:405, 1985

148. Loughran TP Jr, Kadin M, Starkebaum G et al: Leukemia of large granular lymphocytes: association with clonal chromosomal abnormalities and autoimmune neutropenia, thrombocytopenia, and hemolytic anemia. Ann Intern Med 102:169, 1985

149. Zon L, Groopman J: Hematologic manifestations of the human deficiency virus (HIV). Semin Hematol 25:208, 1988

150. Berliner N: T gamma lymphocytosis and T cell chronic leukemias. Hematol Oncol Clin North Am 4:473, 1990

151. Chan W, Gu L, Masih A et al: Large granular lymphocyte proliferation with the natural killer-cell phenotype. Am J Clin Pathol 97:353, 1992

152. Okabe M, Tanaka M, Uehara Y et al: Immunological functions and T-cell receptor gene rearrangement of proliferating lymphocytes in a case of T gamma lymphocytosis with neutropenia. Tohoku J Exp Med 151:105, 1987

153. Miedema F, Terpstra F, Smit J et al: T gamma lymphocytosis is clinically non-progressive but immunologically heterogeneous. Clin Exp Immunol 61:440, 1985

154. Childs B, Borden W, Bard M, Cooke R: Idiopathic hyperglycinemia and hyperglycinuria: a new disorder of amino acid metabolism. Pediatrics 27:522, 1961

155. Soriano J, Taitz L, Finberg L, Edelmann C: Hyperglycinemia with ketoacidosis and leukopenia. Metabolic studies on the nature of the defect. Pediatrics 38:818, 1967

156. Huguley C, Bain J, Rivers S, Scroggins R: Refractory megaloblastic anemia associated with excretion of orotic acid. Blood 14:615, 1959

157. Rosenberg L, Lilljequist A, Hsia Y: Methylmelonic aciduria: an inborn error leading to metabolic acidosis, long-chain ketonuria, and intermittent hyperglycinemia. N Engl J Med 278:1319, 1968

158. Ambruso D, McCabe R, Anderson D et al: Infectious and bleeding complications in patients with glycogenesis Ib. Am J Dis Child 139:691, 1985

159. di Rocco M, Borrone C, Dallergri F et al: Neutropenia and impaired neutrophil function in glycogenosis type Ib. J Inherit Metab Dis 151, 1984

160. Roe T, Coates TD, Thomas DW et al: Treatment of chronic inflammatory bowel disease in glycogen storage disease type 1b with colony stimulating factors. N Engl J Med 326:1666, 1992

161. Joyce R, Boggs D, Chervenick P, Lalezari P: Neutrophil kinetics in Felty's syndrome. Am J Med 69:695, 1980

162. Craddock P, Fehr J, Brigham K et al: Complement and leukocyte-mediated pulmonary dysfunction in hemodialysis. N Engl J Med 296:769, 1977

163. Craddock P, Fehr J, Dalmasso A et al: Hemodialysis leukopenia. Pulmonary vascular leukostasis resulting from complement activation by dialyzer cellophane membranes. J Clin Invest 59:879, 1977

164. Cavarocchi N, Pluth J, Schaff H et al: Complement activation during cardiopulmonary bypass. Comparison of bubble and membrane oxygenators. J Thorac Cardiovasc Surg 91:252, 1986

165. Parmley R, Crist W, Ragab A et al: Congenital dysgranulopoietic neutropenia: clinical, serologic, ultrastructural, and in vitro proliferative characteristics. Blood 56:465, 1980

166. Burroughs S, Devine D, Browne G, Kaplin M: The population of paroxysmal nocturnal hemoglobinuria neutrophils deficient in decay-accelerating factor is also deficient in alkaline phosphatase. Blood 71:1086, 1988

167. Davita M, Low M, Nussenzweig V: Release of decay-accelerating factor (DAF) from the cell membrane by phosphatidylinositol-specific phospholipase (PIPLC). Selective modification of a complement regulatory protein. J Exp Med 163:1150, 1986

168. Shaw R, Mahour GH, Ford EG, Stanley P: Partial splenic embolism, an effective alternative to splenectomy for hypersplenism. Am Surg 56:774, 1990

169. Becton D, Schultz W, Kinney T: Severe neutropenia caused by copper deficiency in a child receiving continuous ambulatory peritoneal dialysis. J Pediatr 108:735, 1986

170. Zidar B, Shadduck R, Ziegler Z, Winkelstein A: Observations on the anemia and neutropenia of human copper deficiency. Am J Hematol 3:177, 1977

171. Perillie P, Kaplin S, Finch S: Significance of changes in serum muramidase activity in megaloblastic anemia. N Engl J Med 227:10, 1967

172. Sacher M, Paky F, Frater-Schroder M: Inherited transcobalamin-II deficiency: clinical, genetic studies and diagnosis using cultured fibroblasts. Helv Paediatr 45:1, 1956

173. Kostmann R: Infantile genetic agranulocytosis. Acta Paediatr 45:1, 1956

174. Parmley R, Ogawa M, Darby C, Spicer S: Congenital neutropenia: neutrophil proliferation with abnormal maturation. Blood 46:723, 1975

175. Bonilla M, Gillio A, Ruggiero M et al: In vivo recombinant human granulocyte colony stimulating factor corrects neutropenia in patients with congenital agranulocytosis. Blood, suppl. 74:110a, 1988

176. Dale DC, Bonilla MA, Davis MW et al: A randomized controlled phase III trial of recombinant human granulocyte colony-stimulating factor (filgrastim) for treatment of severe chronic neutropenia. Blood 81:2496, 1993

177. O'Regan S, Newman A, Grahm R: "Myelokathexis" neutropenia with marrow hyperplasia. Am J Dis Child 131:655, 1977

178. Mamlok R, Juneja H, Elder FF et al: Neutropenia and defective chemotaxis associated with binuclear, tetraploid myeloid-monocytic leukocytes. J Pediatr 111:555, 1987

179. Plebani A, Cantu-Rajnoldi A, Collo G et al: Myelokathexis associated with multiple congenital malformation: immunological study on phagocytic cells and lymphocytes. Eur J Haematol 40:12, 1988

180. Rassam S, Roderick P, Al-Hakim I, Hoffbrand A: A myelokathexix-like variant of myelodysplasia. Eur J Haematol 42:99, 1989

181. Weston B, Axtell RA, Todd RF et al: Clinical and biologic effects of granulocyte colony stimulating factor in treatment of myelokathexis. J Pediatr 118:229, 1991

182. Lange R, Jones J: Cyclic neutropenia: review of clinical manifestations and management. Am J Pediatr Hematol Oncol 3:363, 1981

183. Leale M: Recurrent furunculosis in an infant showing unusual blood picture. JAMA 54:1854, 1910

184. Rutledge B, Hansen-Pruss O, Thayer W: Recurrent agranulocytosis. Bull Johns Hopkins Hosp 46:369, 1930

185. Krance R, Spruce W, Forman S et al: Human cyclic neutropenia transferred by allogeneic bone marrow grafting. Blood 60:1263, 1982

186. Marshall G, Edwards K, Butler J, Lawton A: Syndrome of periodic fever, pharyngitis, and aphthous stomatitis. J Pediatr 110:43, 1987

187. Hammond W, Price T, Souza L, Dale D: Treatment of cyclic neutropenia with granulocyte colony-stimulating factor. N Engl J Med 320:1306, 1989

188. Aggett P, Cavangh N, Matthew D et al: Shwachman's syndrome. A review of 21 cases. Arch Dis Child 55:331, 1980

189. Szuts P, Katona Z, Ilyes M et al: Correction of defective chemotaxis with thiamine in Shwachman-Diamond syndrome. Lancet 8385:1072, 1984

190. Stevens M, Lilleyman J, Williams RB: Shwachman's syndrome and acute lymphoblastic leukemia. Br Med J 2:18, 1978

191. Woods WG, Roloff JS, Lukews SN et al: The occurrence of leukemia in patients with the Shwachman syndrome. J Pediatr 99:425, 1981

192. Boxer L, Baehner R: Defects in neutrophil-leukocyte function. In Ammann AJ (ed): Clinical Immunology Update. Medcom, Garden Grove, CA, 1983

193. De Vaal O, Seynhaeve V: Reticular dysgenesis. Lancet 2:1123, 1959

194. Roper M, Parmley R, Crist W et al: Severe congenital leukopenia (reticular dysgenesis). Immunologic and morphologic characterizations of leukocytes. Am J Dis Child 139:832, 1985

195. Bryan H, Nixon R: Dyskeratosis congenita and familial pancytopenia. JAMA 192:203, 1965

196. Hanada T, Abe T, Nakazawa M et al: Bone marrow failure in dyskeratosis congenita. Scand J Haematol 32:496, 1984

197. Jacobs P, Saxe N, Gordon W, Nelson M: Dyskeratosis congenita. Haematologic, cytogenetic, and dermatologic studies. Scand J Haematol 32:461, 1984

198. Gurwith M, Brunton J, Lank B et al: Granulocytopenia in hospitalized patients. I. Prognostic factors and etiology of fever. Am J Med 64:121, 1978

199. Newman S, Sweet D: Single protective isolation in patients with granulocytopenia. N Engl J Med 304:1493, 1981

200. Cannistra S, Griffin J: Regulation of the production and function of granulocytes and monocytes. Semin Hematol 25:173, 1988

201. Kato K: Leukocytes in infancy and childhood a statistical analysis of 1081 total and differential counts from birth to 15 years. J Pediatr 7:7, 1935

202. Munan L, Kelly A: Age-dependent changes in monocyte populations in man. Clin Exp Immunol 35:161, 1979

203. Thompson J, van Furth R: The effect of glucocorticoids on the proliferation and kinetics of promonocytes and monocytes of the bone marrow. J Exp Med 137:10, 1973

204. Valkmann A, Gowans J: The production of macrophages in the rat. Br J Exp Pathol 46:50, 1965

205. Maldonado J, Hanlon D: Monocytosis: a current appraisal. Mayo Clin Proc 40:248, 1965

206. Hill R, Bayrd E: Phagocytic reticuloendothelial cells in subacute bacterial endocarditis with negative cultures. Ann Intern Med 47:968, 1960

207. Goodwin J, DeHoratius R, Israel H et al: Suppressor cell function in sarcoidosis. Ann Intern Med 90:169, 1980

208. Saarni M, Liman J: Preleukemia: the hematologic syndrome preceding acute leukemia. Am J Med 55:38, 1973

209. Shaw M: The distinctive features of acute monocytic leukemia. Am J Hematol 4:97, 1978

210. Hurst D, Meyer O: Giant follicular lymphoblastoma. Cancer 14:753, 1961

211. Levinson B, Walter B, Wintrobe M, Cartwright G: A clinical study of Hodgkin's disease. Arch Intern Med 99:519, 1957

212. Warnke R, Kim H, Dorfman R: Malignant histiocytosis (histiocytic medullary reticulosis). Clinicopathologic study of 29 cases. Cancer 35:215, 1975

Eosinophilia and the Hypereosinophilic Syndrome

53

David P. Schenkein and Sheldon M. Wolff

INTRODUCTION

The evaluation of a patient with eosinophilia involves many of the medical subspecialties and is often a frustrating endeavor for both the physician and the patient, as the list of diagnostic possibilities is long and diverse (Table 53-1). Regardless of the underlying cause, when disease occurs the pathophysiology is the same: tissue deposition of eosinophils and the release of eosinophil granule products that cause the tissue and organ damage.[1] Even after a thorough evaluation some patients are left without an explanation. The term hypereosinophilic syndrome (HES) is used for such instances of chronic eosinophilia.[2] The defining feature of HES is persistent eosinophilia with evidence of tissue infiltration by eosinophils. The criteria that distinguish HES patients from other patients with a clear underlying cause for their eosinophilia, are (1) >1,500 eosinophils/mm³ for >6 months, (2) a lack of other diagnoses to explain the eosinophilia, and (3) presumptive signs or symptoms bof organ infiltration by eosinophils.[3] These criteria, established by Chusid and colleagues[3] (including one of us) at the National Institutes of Health (NIH), were developed to help define a relatively small group of patients with a clinical syndrome that is distinct from the secondary eosinophilias with respect to both treatment and prognosis.

This chapter focuses on patients who meet the diagnostic criteria for HES. We delineate the clinical features and mechanisms of the syndrome that help the hematologist to distinguish it from secondary eosinophilia. HES likely represents a heterogenous collection of diseases. The complex and controversial relationship between HES and other hematologic disorders such as myelodysplasia and acute leukemia associated with eosinophilia are also reviewed.

HISTORICAL BACKGROUND, ETIOLOGY, AND PATHOPHYSIOLOGY

Descriptions of patients with intense eosinophilia in the blood and tissues have been reported for >80 years under a variety of eponyms.[2-7] The interrelationship, if any, between

Table 53-1. Secondary Causes of Eosinophilia

Allergic disorders
    Allergic rhinitis
    Asthma
    Atopic dermatitis
    Acute urticaria
    Drug reactions: eosinophilia-myalgia syndrome associated with L-tryptophan
Parasitic diseases
    Tissue-invasive helminthiasis
        Filariasis
        Schistosomiasis
        Strongyloidiasis
        Trichinosis
        Toxocariasis
        Ascariasis
        Hookworm, echinococcus, cysticercus (uncommon) infection
Other infections
    Coccidiomycosis
    Tuberculosis
    Cat scratch disease
    Convalescent phase of many infections
Dermatologic diseases
    Bullous pemphigoid
    Herpes gestationis
    Recurrent granulomatous dermatitis
    Scabies
    Eosinophilic lymphofolliculosis
    Subcutaneous angiolymphoid hyperplasia with eosinophilia (Kimura disease)
    Episodic angioedema and eosinophilia
Pulmonary diseases
    Transient pulmonary eosinophilic infiltrates (Löffler syndrome)
    Hypersensitivity pneumonitis
    Allergic bronchopulmonary aspergillosis
    Tropical eosinophilia
    Pulmonary infiltrates with eosinophilia (PIE syndrome)
Collagen vascular disorders
    Allergic angiitis and granulomatosis (Churg-Strauss syndrome)
    Angiitis with hepatitis B antigenemia
    Rheumatoid arthritis (severe)
    Eosinophilic fascitis
    Sjögren syndrome
Neoplastic diseases
    Solid tumors
        Mucin-secreting
        Epithelial cell origin
    Lymphomas
        T cell type
        Hodgkin disease
    Leukemias
        T-cell lymphocytic leukemia
        Myelomonocytic leukemia with eosinophilia (M4Eo)
    Histiocytosis X (eosinophilic granuloma)
Immunodeficiency diseases
    Selective IgA deficiency
    Swiss-type and sex-linked combined immunodeficiency
    Nezelof syndrome
    Wiskott-Aldrich syndrome
    Hyper-IgE syndrome (Job syndrome)
    Graft-versus-host disease
Uncommon causes
    Eosinophilic gastroenteritis
    Inflammatory bowel disease
    Chronic active hepatitis
    Chronic dialysis
    Acute pancreatitis
    Postirradiation
    Hypopituitarism

(Modified from Bass,[79] with permission.)

these syndromes still remains a source of controversy. Löffler endocarditis, a diffuse infiltration of eosinophils into the endocardium with fibrosis and recurrent pericarditis, was first reported in 1936.[6] Löffler also described a syndrome characterized by a productive cough with eosinophilic crystals in the sputum, pulmonary infiltrates, and blood eosinophilia. This disorder, Löffler syndrome, which is often self-limited, has been associated with a variety of infectious, and noninfectious etiologies.[5,8] In 1968, Hardy and Anderson[2] introduced the term hypereosinophilic syndrome to denote many syndromes characterized by prolonged blood eosinophilia with organ infiltration. They included disorders such as Löffler pulmonary syndrome,[5] pulmonary infiltration with eosinophilia syndrome[9,10] Löffler endomyocarditis[6] disseminated eosinophilic vasculitis (Churg-Strauss syndrome), and eosinophilic leukemia.[7]

Although Hardy and Andersen[2] considered eosinophilic leukemia as a terminal event in the clinical spectrum of the HES, its inclusion in the current definition of HES remains problematic. The term "eosinophilic leukemia" has not been recognized by the French-American-British leukemia group as a subtype of acute myeloid leukemia (AML).[12] Several key pieces of information need to be reviewed to help address the possible link between HES, the myeloproliferative disorders, and acute leukemia:

1. Eosinophilia can be associated with a variety of malignant disorders, including acute leukemia,[13] Hodgkin disease,[14] T-cell lymphoma,[15] and several solid tumors.[8] In these instances, the eosinophilia is likely a secondary phenomenon, related to the production of growth factors (e.g., interleukin-5 [IL-5]) by the malignant cell.[16,17] There is no evidence that the eosinophils are part of the malignant clone.

2. The M4Eo variant of AML is characterized by myelomonocytic blasts with eosinophilia.[12] The eosinophils in M4Eo are abnormal by both morphologic and histochemical criteria; however, the malignant clonal population of cells is clearly the myelomonocyte.[13] The presence of the inverted 16 chromosomal abnormality in the eosinophils in a patient with M4Eo has been reported,[18] but others have demonstrated that the eosinophils in AML are not part of the population of malignant cells.[19] The inverted 16 chromosomal abnormality that characterizes M4Eo[13] has not been associated with HES or other conditions associated with eosinophilia.[3]

3. Several patients with HES whose disease evolved into lymphoproliferative or myeloproliferative states have been reported.[3,20] There is no evidence directly linking the preceding HES to the supervening malignant syndrome.

4. T lymphocytes cultured from HES patients secrete high levels of the eosinophilopoeitin IL-5, which probably plays a major role in the pathogenesis of the disease.[21] These T lymphocytes are polyclonal when examined by T-cell-receptor gene rearrangement analysis, thus suggesting a reactive rather than a malignant etiology of HES.

5. Reports of patients with clinical features of HES and chromosomal abnormalities support a clonal and malignant pathogenic mechanism.[22–24] No translocations or chromosomal aberrations that are shared between HES patients have been noted, although some unique translocations have been reported. Although the chromosomal defects have not been demonstrated directly in the eosinophils, their presence does suggest an overlap between HES and the myeloproliferative syndromes.

HES can usually be distinguished from malignant disorders associated with eosinophilia, in particular acute leukemia. However, there are patients with an aggressive clinical picture, with or without a chromosomal abnormality, whose disease may be difficult to distinguish from a myeloproliferative state.[22,25,26] The term eosinophilic leukemia[7] should be avoided for patients with elevated blast counts, since this probably represents variants of either AML or chronic myeloid leukemia associated with eosinophilia.

In 1975, Chusid et al.[3] described >60 HES patients gathered from the literature and 14 patients treated at the NIH. Their paper provided the current definition of HES and documented the dismal prognosis for these patients if left untreated. This series of patients still stands as the largest published collection of HES patients; it also provides a detailed clinical analysis of the syndrome. As discussed below, this report also suggested that aggressive treatment could improve the prognosis.

A better understanding of the factors that control eosinophil proliferation and maturation has provided insight into the clinical manifestations of secondary eosinophilia and HES.[27] Several eosinophil granule products have been implicated in the tissue destruction associated with these disorders.[1] Although several colony-stimulating factors (CSFs) influence eosinophil maturation and proliferation, IL-5 appears to be the dominant and most distinct eosinophilopoietin.[21,28,29] IL-5 is also involved in eosinophil activation and serves as an eosinophil chemoattractant.[30,31] Additional evidence for the central role played by IL-5 in eosinophil biology comes from studies on transgenic mice bearing a T-cell gene that drives IL-5 production.[32] In this transgenic model, IL-5 is sufficient to produce and regulate eosinophils. From other studies, IL-5 appears to maintain eosinophil survival in vitro by inhibiting apoptosis.[33]

Despite a lack of direct evidence to explain the pathophysiology underlying HES, one can postulate a mechanism that involves overexpression of IL-5 or related cytokines (Fig. 53-1). Several groups have examined the role that IL-5 plays in the pathogenesis of HES and secondary eosinophilia.[34–38] Cultured T cells isolated from patients with HES produce IL-5 at higher levels than T cells cultured from normal subjects.[21,34] The IL-5-producing T-cell clones (CD4+, CD8−) derived from these patients are polyclonal rather than monoclonal.[34] Elevated serum IL-5 levels have been detected in some patients with HES, in comparison with healthy control subjects.[35,36] Similarly, elevated IL-5 levels have been detected in patients with the syndrome of episodic angioedema and eosinophilia[37] and in patients with active parasitic infections associated with eosinophilia.[39] IL-5 expression has been documented within Reed-Sternberg cells by in situ hybridization in cases of Hodgkin disease associated with eosinophilia.[17] The eosinophilia associated with IL-2 therapy also appears to be mediated by overexpression of IL-5.[40,41] The diversity of disorders associated with overexpression of IL-5 suggests a common mechanism for the increase in eosinophils seen in HES and the secondary eosinophilias. Other CSFs that contribute to the control of eosinophil development and that may play a role in the pathogenesis of HES are IL-3 and CSF-granulocyte/macrophage.[42,43] Elevated serum IL-2 receptor levels have been detected in patients with HES or lymphoproliferative disorders associated with eosinophilia but not in patients with eosinophilia secondary to parasitic infections.[44]

The characteristic features of HES are the tissue deposition of eosinophils and tissue destruction.[45] Eosinophils in HES can infiltrate any organ, although certain organs such as the heart appear to be particularly susceptible.[3,46] Eosinophil-mediated tissue damage is related to the release of at least four proteins that constitute the bulk of the eosinophil granules.[1] These proteins, major basic protein (MBP), eosinophil peroxidase (EPO), eosinophil cationic protein (ECP), and eosinophil-derived neurotoxin (EDN), mediate tissue destruction by a variety of mechanisms[1,47] (Fig. 53-1).

In patients with HES and cardiac damage, elevated serum levels of MBP and circulating degranulated eosinophils have been noted.[48,49] Cardiac biopsies from HES patients reveal endocardial and endothelial deposition of MBP, ECP, and EPO.[50] Recently Slungaard and colleagues[51] have shown that three of the cationic eosinophil proteins (MBP, EPO, and ECP) accumulate on endocardial and endothelial surfaces and inhibit the function of the natural anticoagulant protein C and the cell-surface receptor thrombomodulin. This inhibition may promote the endocardial thrombosis that occurs frequently in HES

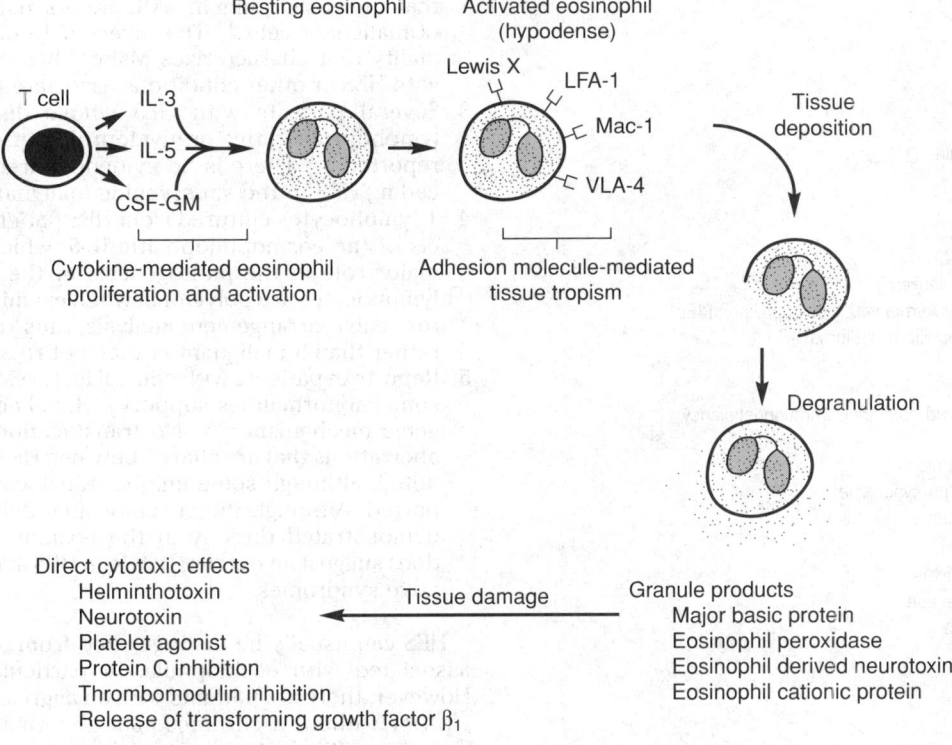

Fig. 53-1. Proposed mechanism of eosinophil-mediated tissue damage in HES.

patients.[46] Other effects of the eosinophil granule proteins on the coagulation and fibrinolytic pathways have been described.[45] Another contributor to the development of mural thrombi is endothelial cell damage mediated by MBP, which is likely to result in recruitment of platelets. Eosinophils from patients with HES have been show to produce both transforming growth factor-α (TGF-α[52]) and TGF-β_1.[53] By contrast, TGF-β_1 was not expressed by the eosinophils from normal donors.[53] TGF-β_1 may contribute to the fibrosis in the cardiopulmonary lesions of HES patients and in the dermal fibrosis in patients with onchocerciasis. TGF-β_1 is known to promote extracellular matrix formation and has been noted in other diseases associated with excessive fibrosis.[54]

The apparent tropism of eosinophils to certain tissues and organs in HES is probably related to adhesion molecules[27,55] (Fig. 53-1). Eosinophils, like other granulocytes, express the sialyated Lewis X antigen and thus bind to selectins on endothelial cells[56,57] and platelets.[58] When eosinophils become activated, principally through the action of platelet activation factor and IL-5, they express additional adhesion molecules such as leukocyte function-associated antigen-1 (LFA-1), Mac-1, and VLA-4, of the integrin family.[59] The mechanism by which the activated eosinophil homes to cardiac tissue is not understood, although it is highly likely that the adhesion molecules play a major role.

DIFFERENTIAL DIAGNOSIS

A large number of diseases have been associated with secondary eosinophilia, and the clinical presentation will therefore vary widely. These disorders, listed in Table 53-1, need to be distinguished from HES. While it is beyond the scope of this chapter to review the clinical presentation of all the secondary causes of eosinophilia, it is important to discuss the two most common causes, allergic reactions and parasitic infections.

When evaluating a patient with eosinophilia, the exclusion of an allergic response is usually based on the history, physical examination, and review of current medications. Some respiratory allergic diseases are associated with eosinophilia, presumably in response to the release of eosinophilia chemotactic peptides from degranulating mast cells and basophils.[60] Patients with these diseases are likely to present with an elevated IgE level, but some patients with HES may also have elevated IgE levels. A myriad of drugs may generate an allergic reaction accompanied by eosinophilia, a rash, and fever. All nonessential medications should be discontinued when evaluating such patients.

Invasive parasitic infections frequently present with eosinophilia. These are most commonly the tissue-invasive helminths such as strongyloides, trichinella, schistosomia, filaria, and toxocara.[61] Multiple stool samples and a small bowel aspirate are recommended to rule out such infectious disorders, particularly in patients with diarrhea or a particular risk factor such as travel outside the United States or animal exposure, or a concomitant immunodeficiency state (e.g., acquired immunodeficiency syndrome).[62] Serologic assays for strongyloides, trichinella, and toxocara are available and should be performed.[61] Hypereosinophilia with tissue invasion and eosinophilic granuloma formation has been reported in patients with visceral larvae migrans secondary to *Toxocara canis;* such patients can be confused with HES patients.[63] Pulmonary findings suggestive of the Churg-Strauss syndrome have also been mimicked by *Toxocara* infestations.[63] The role played by the eosinophil in eliminating the pathogenic parasite is currently under scrutiny. Several of the eosinophil granule proteins are potent helminthotoxins,[60] but mice treated with monoclonal antibodies to IL-5, and thus unable to develop eosinophilia, overcome parasitic infections as well as mice treated with control antibodies.[64]

CLINICAL MANIFESTATIONS

A thorough evaluation is necessary to meet the diagnostic criteria for HES (eosinophils >1,500/mm^3 for 6 months, lack of another etiology, and evidence for tissue involvement by eosinophils). HES should be viewed as a diagnosis of exclusion. Following a complete history and physical examination, the evaluation should include serologic assays for connective tissue diseases; radiologic tests to exclude an occult lymphoproliferative syndrome or solid tumor; multiple stool examinations, serologic assays, and duodenal aspirate to exclude a parasitic infection; careful examination of the peripheral blood smear and bone marrow to exclude a malignant hematologic disorder; and immunoglobulin levels to exclude an underlying immunodeficiency state.[3,45]

In the largest published series of patients meeting the criteria for HES, the mean age of onset was 33 years, with a range from 5 to 80 years.[3] Although the age range was broad, the greatest incidence was in the fourth decade of life. A striking predominance of male patients (91%) was noted. Most patients presented with nonspecific symptoms, and in 12% the eosinophilia was found on routine laboratory evaluation. In this series, 46% were febrile during their illness, and 40% had significant weight loss. Eighty percent of patents had hepatomegaly or splenomegaly, but adenopathy was found in only 20%.

Hematologic Findings

The blood smear in patients with HES usually reveals normal mature eosinophils with typical morphology, although hypogranulation and cytoplasmic vacuoles have been reported.[45] Hypodense eosinophils (light density) have been isolated from HES patients and from patients with secondary eosinophilia.[65] They represent "activated" eosinophils and contain smaller granules. The total leukocyte count is typically between 10,000 and 30,000/mm^3, of which 30–70% are eosinophils. Progressive leukocytosis with eosinophilia should raise the possibility of HES. Occasionally, primitive eosinophil precursors have been noted in the peripheral blood film. The presence of myeloblasts or dysplastic findings, or both, in the peripheral blood suggests an alternative diagnosis, such as AML or one of the myelodysplastic syndromes. In contrast to the eosinophils in HES, the eosinophils in acute myelomonocytic leukemia (M4Eo) have monocytic nuclei and basophilic granules that stain with periodic acid-Schiff, Sudan black, and the nonspecific esterases—features that are typical for eosinophilic granules. Myeloid and erythroid forms are typically normal in HES, although dysplastic findings may be present.

The bone marrow in HES patients is usually hypercellular, with eosinophilia ranging from 25% to 75% of the marrow elements.[3] Fibrosis is rare. This marrow picture is not specific. Examination of the marrow is used to exclude a myelo- or lymphoproliferative disorder. An increased number of blasts shifts the diagnosis from HES to acute leukemia.[12] Other hematologic manifestations associated with HES include anemia of chronic disease, thrombocytopenia, and an elevated sedimentation rate (68% of patients). Progressive leukocytosis with eosinophilia and a hypercellular bone marrow without an increased number of blasts is a pattern that is often difficult to differentiate from a myeloproliferative syndrome.

Cardiovascular Findings

Cardiac changes dominate the clinical abnormalities associated with HES. They are the leading causes of morbidity and mortality in this disorder.[3,45,46] However, the cardiac findings in HES resemble those in patients with prolonged eosinophilia from a defined secondary cause and are thus more likely related to the degree and duration of the eosinophilia rather than the underlying diagnosis. As originally described by Löffler, patients may develop chronic congestive heart failure, valvular abnormalities, and distinctive fibrous biventricular endocardial thickening with mural thrombi. Löffler termed this disorder fibroplastic parietal endocarditis with blood eosinophilia; other terms commonly used include endomyocardial fibrosis, Löffler endocarditis, and endomyocardial fibroelastosis.[8]

The clinical features of cardiac disease in HES and secondary eosinophilia include congestive heart failure, mitral regurgitation, cardiomegaly, systemic embolization, and nonspecific electrocardiographic changes. Parrillo and colleagues[46] have reviewed the cardiac manifestations of HES in >80 patients. Congestive heart failure was noted in 50–75% of patients, and mitral regurgitant murmurs were detected in 50%. Dyspnea and chest pain were the commonest presenting symptoms, although 42% of the NIH patients were asymptomatic. Aortic valvular abnormalities were uncommon. Systemic embolization occurred in only 4% of patients.

The echocardiogram is the most sensitive method for detecting cardiac abnormalities in these patients. Eighty-two percent of HES patients seen at the NIH had echocardiographic abnormalities, of which thickening of the left ventricular free wall was the most common (68%). The left ventricular ejection fraction was normal in all patients, a finding consistent with a restrictive cardiomyopathy. These features are characteristic of HES cardiomyopathy, but the diagnosis must be established in the appropriate clinical setting and not on the basis of the echocardiogram alone. Electrocardiographic changes were common (65%) but were not specific.

Pathologic analysis of the heart of HES patents reveals four dominant features:

1. Endocardial fibrosis and thickening with frequent extension into, and involvement of, the mitral valve and its supporting structures, leading to poor leaflet movement and regurgitation
2. Mural thrombosis of the endocardium with infiltration by eosinophils
3. Involvement of the small intramural coronary vessels by fibrosis, thrombosis, and inflammatory cells
4. Eosinophilic infiltration of the endocardium and myocardium (not present in all cases)

There is evidence to suggest a stepwise progression of disease, from an early stage manifested by eosinophilic infiltrates in the myocardium and focal necrosis, to the next stage characterized by mural endocardial thrombosis, to a final stage of diffuse fibrosis.[45] It is important to note that the echocardiogram may be normal in the early stage of the disease, as ventricular thickening has not yet occurred.[66]

To some extent, the pathologic changes in HES may be reversible. In patients who received aggressive treatment with steroids or cytotoxic agents, or both, echocardiographs showed a decrease in the thickness of the ventricular free wall.[46,67] Treatment with diuretics and digitalis remains standard for patients with signs of congestive heart failure. Mitral and aortic valve replacements have been reported in small numbers of patients; they may be complicated by a high incidence of thrombotic complications.[68] No firm recommendation on the type of replacement valve can be made. Control of the underlying eosinophilia appears to be critical in maintaining valve patency. Some patients require surgical stripping of the endocardium to relieve symptoms related to chronic pericarditis.[45]

Pulmonary Findings

Pulmonary involvement in HES is common. However, pulmonary syndromes with secondary eosinophilia need to be excluded. Some of these primary pulmonary disorders, such as

Löffler pulmonary syndrome, may be closely related to HES.[8] Since Löffler syndrome is self-limited and presents with transient pulmonary infiltrates that resolve spontaneously, it is important to distinguish it from HES. Only time can reveal the diagnosis. The pulmonary infiltration with eosinophilia syndrome was described by Reeder and Goodrich[10] in 1952, and additional patients were reviewed by Carrington et al.[9] in 1969. In this severe, and sometimes chronic, illness patients present with peripherally located pulmonary infiltrates, fever, cough, weight loss, and eosinophilia. Wheezing occurs in 50–60% of the patients. While the response to steroids is often dramatic, some patients may develop chronic eosinophilia and progress to HES with additional organ involvement (e.g. cardiac).[66] The distinction between pulmonary infiltrates with eosinophilia and HES may be artificial, as the mechanism of tissue destruction is certainly the same. Another disorder related to HES is the Churg-Strauss syndrome (allergic angiitis and granulomatosis), a form of systemic vasculitis that includes, in addition, asthma, pulmonary infiltrates, and eosinophilia.[11] The histologic documentation of vasculitis helps to distinguish this condition from HES.

Other Clinical Findings

Neurologic manifestations in patients with HES or chronic secondary eosinophilia include peripheral neuropathies, focal deficits related to embolic phenomena, and global central nervous system dysfunction.[3,25,45] A presentation with peripheral neuropathy requires nerve biopsy to exclude a vasculitis such as Churg-Strauss syndrome or polyarteritis nodosa. Skin involvement is common; over two-thirds of patients in the NIH series had skin changes.[69] The most common were either an erythematous, pruritic, maculopapular eruption, or urticaria associated with angioedema. In some patients, skin changes may be the only clinical manifestation. The typical histopathologic picture is a dermal perivascular infiltrate of eosinophils and mononuclear cells. This pattern helps to distinguish HES from other skin diseases with eosinophilia, such as eosinophilic lymphofolliculosis and subcutaneous angiolymphoid hyperplasia with eosinophilia.[69] In 1984, Gleich and colleagues[69a] described a syndrome of angioedema, urticaria, fever, weight gain, and eosinophilia with eosinophilic infiltration of the dermis. These patients do not appear to develop cardiac abnormalities despite the eosinophilia; the clinical syndrome responds to brief treatment with prednisone.

Chronic active hepatitis with infiltration of the portal triads by eosinophils has been reported and may be the sole manifestation of HES.[45] In vitro studies have demonstrated deposition of one of the major eosinophilic basic proteins in liver biopsy specimens from affected patients.[70] Although liver disease is frequent at autopsy, its presence does not usually lead to overt clinical manifestations.[71] Gastrointestinal tract involvement may occur, and some authors speculate that eosinophilic gastroenteritis is a clinical manifestation of HES.[72] Charcot-Leyden crystals are frequently noted in stool samples of HES patients.[45] Renal involvement with hematuria, proteinuria, and renal failure, is uncommon.[3,45] Ocular complications with episcleritis and keratoconjunctivitis have been reported.[73] The rapid development of adult respiratory distress syndrome in two patients with HES undergoing general anesthesia supports the preoperative use of steroids in patients with HES.[74]

THERAPY AND PROGNOSIS

To a great extent, the therapy and prognosis of patients with eosinophilia depends on the diagnosis. Here we focus on the prognosis and therapeutic strategies for patients who fulfill the

PREFERRED TREATMENT APPROACH: DIAGNOSIS AND TREATMENT

Patients evaluated at the New England Medical Center for eosinophilia undergo a thorough clinical and laboratory investigation that consists of the following:

Complete history and physical examination
Complete blood count with total eosinophil count and review of the peripheral blood smear
Hepatic and renal function tests, urine analysis
Serologic assays: erythrocyte sedimentation rate, antinuclear antibody, rheumatoid factor, anti-ssDNA, anti-dsDNA, human immunodeficiency virus
Quantitative IgE level
Stool for ova, parasites ×3, duodenal aspirate
Serologic assays for stronglyoides, trichinella, and toxocara
Bone marrow aspirate and biopsy (with cytogenetics)
Chest radiograph, computed tomograph scan of chest, abdomen, and pelvis

Electrocardiogram and echocardiogram

Patients who meet the diagnostic criteria for HES: (1) >1,500 eosinophils/mm^3 for >6 months; a lack of other diagnoses to explain the eosinophilia; and (3) presumptive signs or symptoms of organ infiltration by eosinophils are managed according to the strategy in the algorithm below (adapted from Schooley et al.,[25] with permission). Patients without evidence for organ dysfunction or severe symptoms are observed without treatment. Periodic reinvestigation into the etiology of the eosinophilia is appropriate every 3 months to reaffirm the diagnosis of HES.

The treatment for hypereosinophilia secondary to a defined etiology should be directed at the underlying cause. In patients who fail to respond to these measures a trial of corticosteroids to halt progressive organ dysfunction secondary to the eosinophilia is warranted.

TREATMENT STRATEGY

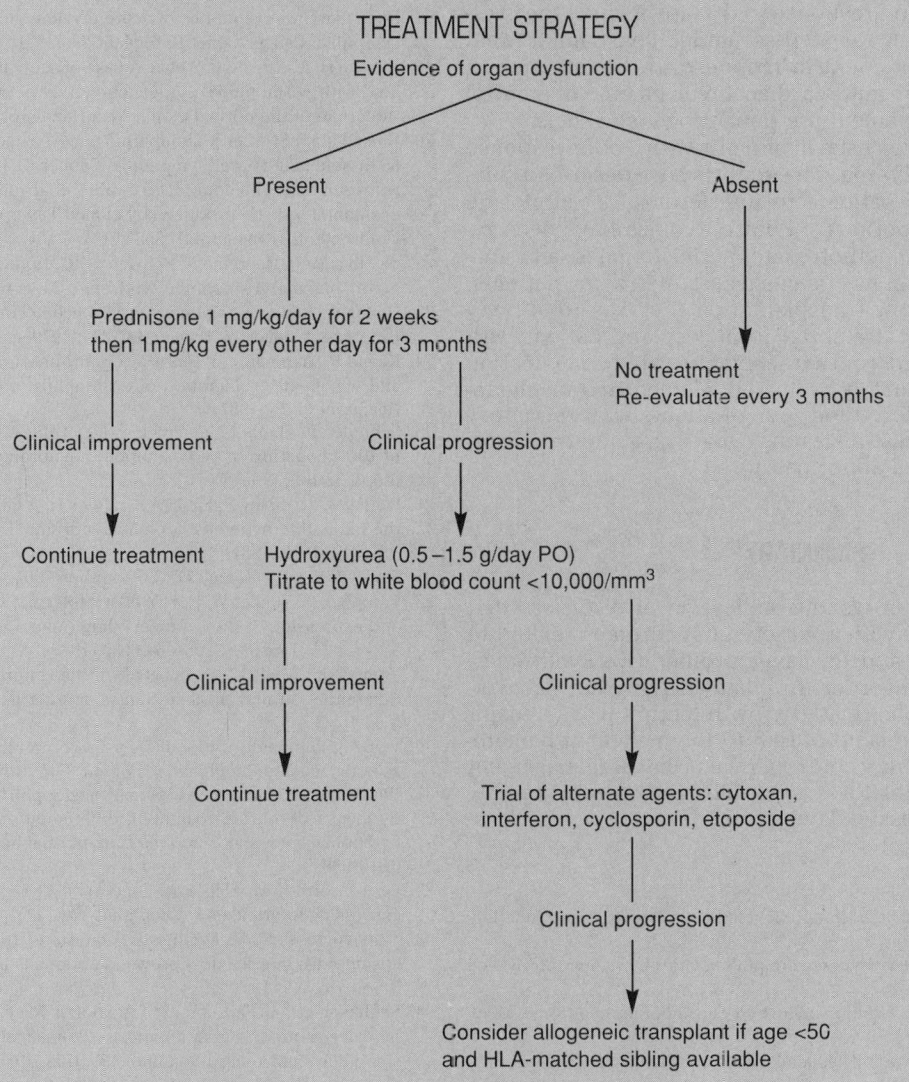

Evidence of organ dysfunction

Present — Absent

Prednisone 1 mg/kg/day for 2 weeks then 1mg/kg every other day for 3 months

Absent → No treatment / Re-evaluate every 3 months

Clinical improvement → Continue treatment

Clinical progression → Hydroxyurea (0.5–1.5 g/day PO) Titrate to white blood count <10,000/mm^3

Clinical improvement → Continue treatment

Clinical progression → Trial of alternate agents: cytoxan, interferon, cyclosporin, etoposide

Clinical progression → Consider allogeneic transplant if age <50 and HLA-matched sibling available

classic criteria for HES. Treatment for the secondary eosino-philias is directed against the underlying disease rather than the eosinophilia.

In all the published series of HES patients reported before 1978, the prognosis was dismal. The median survival was <1 year, and the 3-year survival was approximately 12%.[3] To some extent, this poor prognosis may have been influenced by the lack of firm diagnostic criteria for HES. Many of these earlier reports describe patients with myeloblasts in the peripheral blood, who probably had acute leukemia with eosinophilia rather than HES.

Corticosteriods have been and remain the mainstay of ther-apy in HES. The indication for treatment is evidence of progres-sive organ involvement or symptoms (excluding skin only). The 1978 NIH protocol[67] utilized prednisone at 1 mg/kg/day for 1 week followed by 1 mg/kg every other day for 3 months. If an adequate response was noted, then alternate-day steroids (1 mg/kg) were continued for 1 year. In patients not responding to steroids, hydroxyurea (1–2 g/day) was given to maintain the white blood count within the normal range. With this approach, along with aggressive medical and surgical treatment for car-diac complications, the 5-year survival was approximately 70% for all patients, and 90% for patients without cardiac disease.

Therapy should be withheld from asymptomatic patients with stable disease. In them, careful and frequent follow-up (every 3 months) is warranted. Several prognostic features that appear to predict a good response to therapy include the pres-ence of angioedema, an elevated serum IgE level, and a rapid drop in the eosinophil count in response to the initiation of steroids.[25,26] Splenomegaly, cardiac involvement, or central nervous system involvement are poor prognostic signs.

Other drugs have been used in patients with a poor response to steroids and hydroxyurea. Case reports have described clini-cal responses in HES patients to interferon-α_{2b},[75] etoposide (VP-16),[76] and Cyclosporin A.[77] Poor outcomes have been re-ported with busulfan, methotrexate, antihistamines, and ana-bolic steroids.[3] Cytoxan has been successful in some patients. Allogeneic bone marrow transplantation (cytoxan/total body irradiation) has been attempted in at lest one patient with HES.[78] However, he died from a transplant-related complication and could not be adequately evaluated. Allogeneic transplanta-tion should be considered for young patients with refractory HES and clinical features suggesting a myeloproliferative disor-der (e.g., chromosomal abnormality).

SUMMARY

The HESs are a heterogenous collection of disorders that share clinical features with a variety of syndromes related to both the vasculitides and the myeloproliferative syndromes. The etiology of these disorders is unknown; however, the over-expression of eosinophil-related growth factors plays a major role. The actual relationship of HES to the malignant hemato-poietic disorders remains controversial. Clinical management is directed at controlling the eosinophilia and thereby limiting eosinophil-mediated tissue damage.

REFERENCES

1. Gleich G, Adolphson C: The eosinophilic leukocyte: structure and function. Adv Immunol 39:177, 1986
2. Hardy W, Anderson R: The hypereosinophilic syndromes. Ann Intern Med 68:1220, 1968
3. Chusid M, Dale D, West B, Wolff SM: The hypereosinophilic syndrome. Medi-cine 54:1, 1975
4. Stillman R: A case of myeloid leukemia with predominance of eosinophil cells. Med Rec 81:594, 1912
5. Löffler W: Die fluchtigen Lungeninfiltrate mit eosinoplie. Schweiz Med Wo-chenschr 66:1069, 1936
6. Löffler W: Endocarditis parietalis fibroplastica mit Bluteosinoplihila. Schweiz Med Wochenschr 66:817, 1936
7. Evans T, Nesbitt R: Eosinophilic leukemia. Report of a case with autopsy confirmation; review of the literature. Blood 4:603, 1949
8. Beeson P, Bass D: The eosinophil. In Smith LH (ed): The Eosinophil. WB Saunders, Philadelphia, 1977
9. Carrington C, Addington W, Goff A et al: Chronic eosinophilic pneumonia. N Engl J Med 280:787, 1969
10. Reeder W, Goodrich B: Pulmonary infiltration with eosinophilia. Ann Intern Med 36:1217, 1952
11. Churg J, Strauss L: Allergic granulomatosis, allergic angiitis, and periarteritis nodosa. Am J Pathol 27:277, 1951
12. Bennett J, Catovsky D, Daniel M: Proposed revised criteria for the classifica-tion of acute myeloid leukemia. A report of the French-American-British co-operative group. Ann Intern Med 103:626, 1985
13. Le Beau M, Larson R, Bitter M et al: Association of an inversion of chromo-some 16 with abnormal marrow eosinophils in acute myelomonocytic leuke-mia. A unique cytogenetic-clinicopathological association. N Engl J Med 309: 630, 1983
14. Fuggle W, Crocker J, Smith P: A quantitative study of eosinophil polymorphs in Hodgkin's disease. J Clin Pathol 37:267, 1984
15. Murata K, Yamada Y, Kamihira S et al: Frequency of eosinophilia in adult T-cell leukemia/lymphoma. Cancer 69:966, 1992
16. Slungaard A, Ascensao J, Zanjini E, Jacob H: Pulmonary carcinoma with eosin-ophilia: demonstration of a tumor derived eosinophilic factor. N Engl J Med 309:778, 1983
17. Samoszuk M, Nansen L: Detection of interleukin-5 messenger RNA in Reed-Sternberg cells of Hodgkin's disease with eosinophilia. Blood 75:13, 1990
18. Nakamura H, Sadimori N, Tagawa M et al: Inversion of chromosome 16 in bone marrow eosinophils of acute myelomonocytic leukemia (M4) with eo-sinophilia. Cancer Genet Cytogenet 29:327, 1987
19. Kimura H, Abe R, Shiga Y et al: A case of acute myelogenous leukemia associ-ated with eosinophilia: cytogenetic study of eosinophilic colonies showing the origin of the normal clone. Acta Haematol 77:15, 1987
20. Kim CJ, Park SH, Chi JG: Idiopathic hypereosinophilic syndrome terminating as disseminated T-cell lymphoma. Cancer 67:1064, 1991
21. Schrezenmeier H, Thome SD, Tewald F et al: Interleukin-5 is the predominant eosinophilopoietin produced by cloned T lymphocytes in hypereosinophilic syndrome. Exp Hematol 21:358, 1993
22. da Silva MAP, Heerema N, Schwenk GRJ, Hoffman R: Evidence for the clonal nature of hypereosinophilic syndrome. Cancer Genet Cytogenet 32:109, 1988
23. Huang C, Gomez G, Kohno S et al: Chromosomes and causation of human cancer and leukemia. Cancer 44:1284, 1979
24. Keene P, Mandelow B, Pinto M et al: Abnormalities of chromosome 12p13 and malignant proliferation of eosinophils: a nonrandom association. Br J Haematol 67:25, 1987
25. Schooley R, Flaum M, Gralnick A, Fauci HR: A clinicopathologic correlation of the idiopathic hypereosinophilic syndrome. II. Clinical manifestations. Blood 58:1021, 1981
26. Flaum M, Schooley R, Fauci A, Gralnick H: A clinicopathologic correlation of the idiopathic hypereosinophilic syndrome. I. Hematologic manifestations. Blood 58:1012, 1981
27. Spry CJ, Kay AB, Gleich GJ: Eosinophils 1992. Immunol Today 13:384, 1992
28. Campbell H, Tucker W, Hort Y et al: Molecular cloning, nucleotide sequence, and expression of the gene encoding human eosinophil factor (interleukin-5). Proc Natl Acad Sci USA 84:6629, 1987
29. Yamaguchi Y, Suda T, Suda J et al: Purified interleukin-5 supports the terminal differentiation and proliferation of murine eosinophilic precursors. J Exp Med 167:43, 1988
30. Wang J, Rambaldi A, Biondi A et al: Recombinant human interleukin-5 is a selective eosinophil chemoattractant. Eur J Immunol 19:701, 1989
31. Clutterbuck E, Sanderson C: Human eosinophil hematopoiesis studies in vitro by means of murine eosinophil differentiation factor (IL-5): production of functionally active eosinophils from normal human bone marrow. Blood 71: 646, 1988
32. Dent L, Strath M, Mellor A, Sanderson C: Eosinophilia in transgenic mice expressing interleukin-5. J Exp Med 172:1425, 1990
33. Yamaguchi Y, Suda T, Ohta S: Analysis of the survival of mature human eosinophils: interleukin-5 prevents apoptosis in mature human eosinophils. Blood 78:2542, 1991
34. Raghavachar A, Fleischer S, Frickhofen N et al: T lymphocyte control of human eosinophilic granulopoiesis. Clonal analysis in an idiopathic hypereo-sinophilic syndrome. J Immunol 139:3753, 1987
35. Enokihara H, Kajitani H, Nagashima S: Interleukin-5 activity in sera from pa-tients with eosinophilia. Br J Haematol 75:458, 1990
36. Owen WF, Rothenberg ME, Petersen J et al: Interleukin 5 and phenotypically

altered eosinophils in the blood of patients with the idiopathic hypereosinophilic syndrome. J Exp Med 170:343, 1989

37. Butterfield JH, Leiferman KM, Abrams J et al: Elevated serum levels of interleukin-5 in patients with the syndrome of episodic angioedema and eosinophilia. Blood 79:688, 1992
38. Coffman R, Seymour B, Hudak S et al: Antibody to interleukin-5 inhibits helmith-induced eosinophilia in mice. Science 245:308, 1989
39. Limaye A, Abrams J, Awadzi K et al: Interleukin-5 and the posttreatment eosinophilia in patients with onchocerciasis. J Clin Invest 88:1418, 1991
40. Lotze MT, Matory YL, Rayner AA et al: Clinical effects and toxicity of interleukin-2 in patients with cancer. Cancer 58:2764, 1986
41. Macdonald D, Gordon AA, Kajitani H et al: Interleukin-2 treatment-associated eosinophil is mediated by interleukin-5 production. Br J Haematol 76:168, 1990
42. Warren D, Moore M: Synergism among interleukin-1, interleukin-3, and interleukin-5 in the production of eosinophils from primitive hemopoietic stem cells. J Immunol 140:94, 1988
43. Clutterbuck E, Sanderson C: Regulation of a human eosinophil precursor by cytokines: a comparison of recombinant human interleukin-1 (rhIL-1), rhIL-3, rhIL-5, rhIL-6, and rh granulocyte-macrophage colony stimulating factor. Blood 75:1774, 1990
44. Prin L, Plumas J, Gruart V et al: Elevated serum levels of soluble interleukin-2 receptor: a marker of disease activity in the hypereosinophilic syndrome. Blood 78:2626, 1991
45. Fauci A, Harley J, Roberts W et al: The idiopathic hypereosinophilic syndrome. Ann Intern Med 97:78, 1982
46. Parrillo J, Borer J, Henry W et al: The cardiovascular manifestations of the hypereosinophilic syndrome. Am J Med 67:572, 1979
47. Gleich G, Frigas E, Loegering D et al: Cytotoxic properties of the eosinophil major basic protein. J Immunol 123:2925, 1979
48. Spry C, Tai P: Studies on blood eosinophils. II. Patients with Löffler's cardiopathy. Clin Exp Immunol 24:423, 1976
49. Wassom D, Leogering D, Solley G et al: Elevated serum levels of the eosinophil major basic protein in patients with eosinophilia. J Clin Invest 67:651, 1981
50. Tai PC, Ackerman SJ, Spry CJ et al: Deposits of eosinophil granule proteins in cardiac tissues of patients with eosinophilic endomyocardial disease. Lancet 1:643, 1987
51. Slungaard A, Vercellotti GM, Tran T et al: Eosinophil cationic granule proteins impair thrombomodulin function. A potential mechanism for thromboembolism in hypereosinophilic heart disease. J Clin Invest 91:1721, 1993
52. Wong DT, Weller PF, Galli SJ et al: Human eosinophils express transforming growth factor alpha. J Exp Med 172:673, 1990
53. Wong DT, Elovic A, Matossian K et al: Eosinophils from patients with blood eosinophilia express transforming growth factor beta 1. Blood 78:2702, 1991
54. Barnard J, Lyons R, Moses HL: The cell biology of transforming growth factor beta. Biochim Biophys Acta 1032:79, 1990
55. Weller PF: Intercellular interactions in the recruitment and functions of human eosinophils. Ann NY Acad Sci 664:116, 1992
56. Dobrina A, Menegazzi R, Carlos TM et al: Mechanisms of eosinophil adherence to cultured vascular endothelial cells. Eosinophils bind to the cytokine-induced ligand vascular cell adhesion molecule-1 via the very late activation antigen-4 integrin receptor. J Clin Invest 88:20, 1991
57. Weller PF, Rand TH, Goelz SE et al: Human eosinophil adherence to vascular endothelium mediated by binding to vascular cell adhesion molecule 1 and

58. de Bruijne-Admiraal L, Modderman P, Von dem Borne A, Sonnenberg A: P-selectin mediates Ca^{2+} dependent adhesion of activated platelets to many different types of leukocytes: detection by flow cytometry. Blood 80:134, 1993
59. Neeley SP, Hamann KJ, White SR: Selective regulation of expression of surface adhesion molecules Mac-1, L-selectin, and VLA-4 on human eosinophils and neutrophils. Am J Respir Cell Mol Biol 8:633, 1993
60. Sur S, Adolphson C, Gleich G: Eosinophils. In Middleton E, Reed CE, Ellis EF et al (eds): Allergy: Principles and Practice. CV Mosby, St Louis, 1993
61. Warren K: Diseases due to helminths: introduction. p. 2134. In Mandell GL, Douglas RG, Bennet JE (eds): Principles and Practice of Infectious Diseases. 3rd Ed. Churchill Livingstone, New York, 1992
62. Pearson R, Guerrant R: Enteric fever and other causes of abdominal symptoms and fever. In Mandell GL, Bennett JE, Dolin R (eds): Principles and Practice of Infectious Diseases. 4th Ed. Churchill Livingstone, New York, 1995
63. Feldman GJ, Parker HW: Visceral larva migrans associated with the hypereosinophilic syndrome and the onset of severe asthma. Ann Intern Med 116:838, 1992
64. Sher A, Coffman R, Hieny S et al: Ablation of eosinophil and IgE responses with anti-IL5 or anti-IL4 antibodies fails to affect immunity against *Schistosoma mansoni* in the mouse. J Immunol 145:3911, 1990
65. Winquist I, Olofsson T, Olsson I et al: Altered density, metabolism and surface receptors of eosinophils in eosinophilia. Immunology 47:531, 1982
66. Wolff S, Fallon J: Case records of the Massachussetts General Hospital. N Engl J Med 302:1077, 1980
67. Parrillo J, Fauci A, Wolff S: Therapy of the hypereosinophilic syndrome. Ann Intern Med 89:167, 1978
68. Boustany CWJ, Murphy GW, Hicks GLJ: Mitral valve replacement in idiopathic hypereosinophilic syndrome. Ann Thorac Surg 51:1007, 1991
69. Kazmierowski J, Chusid M, Parrillo J et al: Dermatologic manifestations of the hypereosinophilic syndrome. Arch Dermatol 114:531, 1978
69a. Gleich GJ, Schroeter AL, Marcoux JP et al: Episodic angioedema associated with eosinophilia. N Engl J Med 310:1621, 1984
70. Foong A, Scholes JV, Gleich GJ et al: Eosinophil-induced chronic active hepatitis in the idiopathic hypereosinophilic syndrome. Hepatology 13:1090, 1991
71. Croffy B, Kopelman R, Kaplan M: Hypereosinophilic syndrome. Association with chronic active hepatitis. Dig Dis Sci 33:233, 1988
72. Scheurlen M, Mork H, Weber P: Hypereosinophilic syndrome resembling chronic inflammatory bowel disease with primary sclerosing cholangitis. J Clin Gastroenterol 14:59, 1992
73. Bozkir N, Stern GA: Ocular manifestations of the idiopathic hypereosinophilic syndrome, letter. Am J Ophthalmol 113:456, 1992
74. Samsoon G, Wood ME, Knight GAB, Britt RP: General anaesthesia and the hypereosinophilic syndrome: severe postoperative complications in two patients. Br J Anaesth 69:653, 1992
75. Zielinski RM, Lawrence WD: Interferon-alpha for the hypereosinophilic syndrome [see comments]. Ann Intern Med 113:716, 1990
76. Smit AJ, van Essen LH, de Vries EGE: Successful long-term control of idiopathic hypereosinophilic syndrome with etoposide. Cancer 67:2826, 1991
77. Zabel P, Schlaak M: Cyclosporin for hypereosinophilic syndrome. Ann Hematol 62:230, 1991
78. Archimbaud E, Guyotat D, Guillaume C et al: Hypereosinophilic syndrome with multiple organ dysfunction treated by allogeneic bone marrow transplantation. Am J Hematol 27:302, 1988
79. Bass DA: Eosinophilic syndromes. p. 1011. In Wyngaarden JB, Smith LH (eds): Cecil Textbook of Medicine. 17th Ed. WB Saunders, Philadelphia, 1985

endothelial leukocyte adhesion molecule 1. Proc Natl Acad Sci USA 88:7430, 1991

Disorders of Phagocyte Function

54

John T. Curnutte

INTRODUCTION

The defense of the host against pathogenic microbes is the critical responsibility of the immune system. Unfortunately for the host, these microbes are diverse in nature—viruses, bacteria, fungi, or uni- or multicellular parasites—and many have evolved an impressive array of mechanisms to penetrate the host, evade immune surveillance, and even neutralize the antimicrobial "poisons" generated by the host defense systems. In light of this diversity, and the evolutionary "cat and mouse game" played between pathogens and the immune system, it is not surprising that the immune system has evolved into a complex defense system comprising a variety of cell types and humoral mediators. The branch of the immunologic defense mechanism that is responsible for the first line of protection against invading bacteria, fungi, and parasites is the phagocytic system. As reviewed in Chapters 49 to 51, phagocytes perform their critical functions either as resident cells in a variety of tissues or as circulating marauders in the bloodstream capable of traveling into any infected tissue. Members of the former category include such well-studied cells as the alveolar, hepatic, peritoneal, and splenic macrophages. The circulating phagocytes, on the other hand, are dominated by neutrophils but also include monocytes and eosinophils.

A complex series of cellular regulatory phenomena are involved in the phagocyte's role as a primary defender of the host. These are most acute in the case of the circulating granulocytes, which must be able to sense exceedingly weak chemotactic signals from infected tissues, transduce this information rapidly into purposeful movement toward the source of the signals, engulf the target microbes on arrival at the infected tissue, and then destroy the pathogens with extremely potent and effective agents while sparing surrounding normal tissues. Microbial killing is accomplished by two types of mechanisms: (1) de novo synthesis of highly toxic and often unstable derivatives of molecular oxygen by an enzyme known as the respiratory burst oxidase, and (2) delivery into the phagocytic vacuoles containing the ingested microbes of preformed polypeptide "antibiotics" and proteases stored within several types of lysosomal granules.[1-6]

Congenital and acquired disorders of each of the steps in phagocyte function have been described. As would be predicted, these disorders are manifested clinically by recurrent bacterial and fungal infections. Interestingly, the converse of this is only rarely observed. Most patients with recurrent infections do not have any identifiable abnormality in their phagocytes. There are at least two explanations for the clinical rarity of phagocyte disorders. First, given their critical role in host defense, nature may be quite intolerant of major abnormalities in phagocytes. Prior to the modern antibiotic era, patients afflicted with severe disorders probably did not survive into their childbearing years. As discussed below, chronic granulomatous disease (CGD) and leukocyte adhesion deficiency (LAD) are often fatal in early childhood, unless aggressive medical management is provided. Second, there is a remarkable redundancy in the antimicrobial machinery of the phagocytes that permits one system to compensate for a defect in another. For

example, the host does not rely on a single chemotactic signal or neutrophil membrane receptor to ensure that phagocytes accumulate at sites of infection. Instead, multiple chemotactic signals and receptors are employed. A similar phenomenon is seen in the reactions that kill microbes as both oxidative and nonoxidative systems are employed.

This chapter reviews the major functional disorders of phagocytes and is organized according to the cellular functions outlined above: disorders of the respiratory burst microbicidal pathway, abnormalities of phagocyte adhesion and chemotaxis, and defects in the structure and function of lysosomal granules. The chapter is not meant to be an encyclopedic review of the many papers published on phagocyte abnormalities. It is important to note that in many of these reports the observed in vitro abnormalities are marginal, with little evidence that they are responsible for a clinical problem. This chapter focuses on these disorders for which such a correlation does exist, with particular emphasis on those that are best understood at the molecular level. Many comprehensive reviews are available to the reader who is interested in the less well-characterized phagocyte disorders that are of unclear clinical significance.[2,7-20]

DISORDERS OF THE RESPIRATORY BURST PATHWAY

The unstimulated human neutrophil consumes relatively little oxygen and relies primarily on glycolysis for energy.[21-23] Within seconds after contact with suitably opsonized microorganisms or a variety of soluble stimuli, the rate of oxygen consumption abruptly increases, usually by a factor >100, a metabolic event known as the respiratory burst.[24] This oxygen is consumed in a nonmitochondrial reaction in which it is reduced with a gain of one electron to form superoxide (as the O_2^- ion) by a plasma membrane-bound NADPH oxidase referred to as the respiratory burst oxidase (Fig. 54-1, reaction 1).[25] NADPH is the preferred substrate for this enzyme, and O_2^- appears to be the sole metabolite of oxygen in most instances.[22,25] NADPH oxidase, along with those enzymes and reactions that are directly involved in the production or metabolism of O_2^-, constitute the respiratory burst pathway as depicted in Figure 54-1.[22] Five clinically significant defects have been identified in this pathway. They involved the following enzymes: NADPH oxidase[25] (reaction 1), leukocyte glucose-6-phosphate dehydrogenase (G6PD)[26] (reaction 8), myeloperoxidase[27,28] (reaction 4), glutathione reductase[13,29] (reaction 7), and glutathione synthetase[13] (reaction 9). These reactions are involved in the production of O_2^- (reactions 8 and 1), in the conversion of O_2^- and hydrogen peroxide to other toxic derivatives (reaction 4), or in the detoxification of excess hydrogen peroxide needed to protect the phagocyte during the respiratory burst (reactions 7, 8, and 9).

Chronic Granulomatous Disease

Biology

CGD comprises a heterogeneous group of defects, that share in common the failure of neutrophils, monocytes, macrophages, and eosinophils to undergo a respiratory burst and

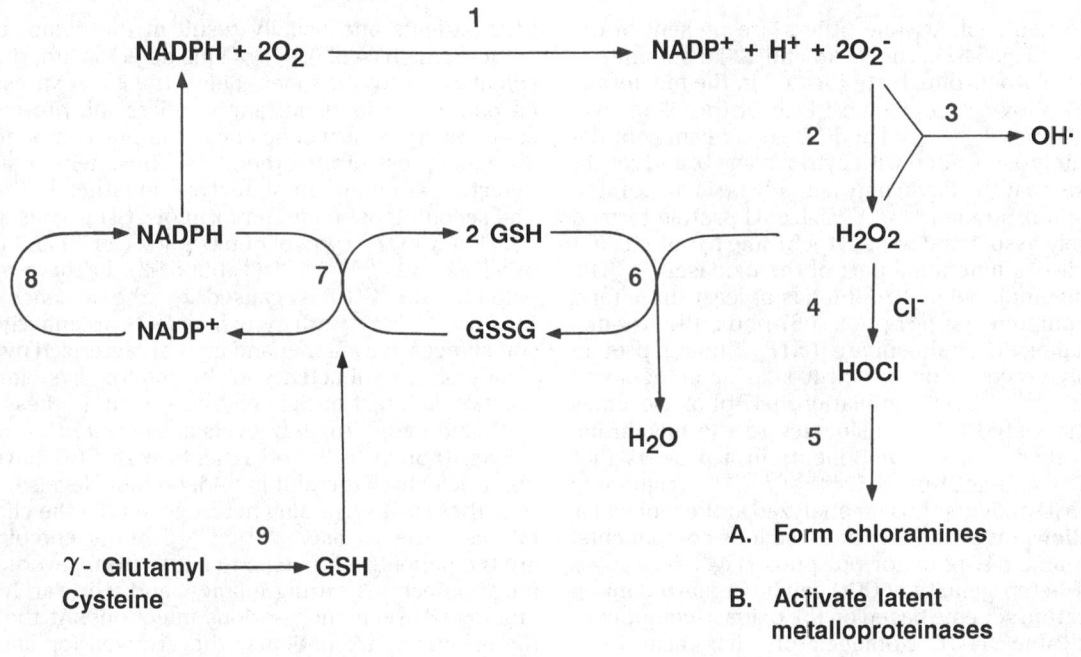

Fig. 54-1. Reactions of the respiratory burst pathway. The enzymes responsible for reactions 1–9 are as follows: (1) the respiratory burst oxidase (NADPH oxidase); (2) superoxide dismutase or spontaneous; (3) nonenzymatic, Fe^{2+} catalyzed; (4) myeloperoxidase; (5) spontaneous; (6) glutathione peroxidase; (7) glutathione reductase; (8) glucose-6-phosphate dehydrogenase; and (9) glutathione synthetase.

generate O_2^-.[7,19,30–35] The disorder is relatively rare; approximately 1 in 750,000 individuals are affected, based on unpublished estimates from large urban populations. Because of the central role of superoxide and other respiratory burst products in microbial killing, patients with CGD suffer from recurrent bacterial and fungal infections, which are often severe.[32,36] The disease was first described in 1957 in two independent reports by Good and colleagues[37] and Landing and Shirley,[38] both of which describe severe recurrent infections associated with visceral granulomas containing pigmented histiocytes. The disease was termed fatal granulomatous disease owing to this distinguishing histologic feature and the grim clinical course in most patients.[37,39,40] It was not until the late 1960s and early 1970s that the defect in oxygen consumption and O_2^- production was identified and a convenient diagnostic assay, the nitroblue tetrazolium (NBT) test, was developed.[41–45] During that time it also became apparent that CGD is a heterogeneous disorder. While most patients were male and had inherited the disease in an X-linked manner,[46] a few females with CGD were discovered in whom the mode of inheritance appeared to be autosomal recessive.[31,47–49] By 1975 it was clear that most, if not all, instances of CGD were caused by defects in the activity (or activation) of NADPH oxidase[50] (Fig. 54-1, reaction 1).

Our current understanding of CGD was reached with the aid of two major findings. The first was that a unique, low-potential cytochrome b was undetectable in nearly all patients with X-linked disease.[35,51] The second was the discovery of a method by which NADPH oxidase could be activated in a cell-free system in the presence of negatively charged lipids such as arachidonic acid.[52–55] These studies disclosed that both cytosolic and membrane proteins were required for oxidase activation and that all patients had defects involving either the membranes or the cytosol.[52,56,57] Table 54-1 demonstrates this point. If cytosol and membranes from a normal individual are combined in the cell-free system and activated with arachidonic acid, large fluxes of O_2^- are generated. In experiment 1, cytosol

and membranes from a patient with X-linked CGD (who was missing cytochrome b) were combined, and virtually no O_2^- was produced following arachidonate stimulation. The cross-mixing experiment indicated that the patient's membranes, but not cytosol, were defective. In experiment 2, a female patient with autosomal recessive CGD associated with a normal level of cytochrome b was studied. In contrast to the patient with X-linked CGD, her cytosol was severely defective while her membranes were normal.

It is now appreciated that NADPH oxidase is a complex enzyme consisting of multiple catalytic and regulatory subunits and that the activity of the oxidase appears to be regulated by controlling the assembly of these components.[25,57–66] Perhaps as a fail-safe mechanism to prevent inadvertent activation, some of these components are localized in the membrane in

Table 54-1. Cell-Free Activation of NADPH Oxidase in Two Genetic Forms of Chronic Granulomatous Disease

Source of Subcellular Fraction		Superoxide Generation[a,b]	
Cytosol	Membrane	Experiment 1	Experiment 2
Normal	Normal	73.2	58.5
Patient	Patient	0.1	0.3
Normal	Patient	0.1	50.1
Patient	Normal	68.7	4.1
50% patient/50% normal	Normal	65.3	24.4

[a] Numerical data represent nanomoles of O_2^-/min/10^7 cell-equivalent of membrane.

[b] The rate of superoxide generation was used to measure the extent of activation of dormant NADPH oxidase in a cell-free activation system using arachidonic acid (82 μM) as the stimulus. Experiment 1 was performed with membranes and cytosol from a normal individual and a patient with X-linked cytochrome b-negative CGD, the most common type of CGD. Experiment 2 was performed with a different normal donor and a patient with autosomal recessive, cytochrome b-positive CGD lacking the p47-phox cytosol oxidase component, the second most common type of CGD. Oxidase activation was performed as described in Curnutte et al.[56]

the unstimulated neutrophil, while others are present in the cytosol (left side of Fig. 54-2). The 91-kd and 22-kd subunits of the heterodimeric cytochrome b are located in the membrane and termed gp91-phox (glycoprotein 91 kd of the phagocyte oxidase) and p22-phox.[51,65,67–74] The FAD redox center of the oxidase is intimately associated with cytochrome b, and recent evidence suggests that the flavin may actually be incorporated within the gp91-phox subunit.[75,76] A ras-like G protein termed rap1 is also closely associated with cytochrome b, but it is not known whether it is a functional part of the oxidase.[77–79] The cytosol of the unstimulated neutrophil has at least three (and possibly four) components: p47-phox, p67-phox, the low-molecular-mass guanosine triphosphate (GTP)-binding protein rac2, and possibly a recently described 40-kd protein (depicted as α in Fig. 54-2).[64,80–100] On stimulation, p47-phox becomes partially phosphorylated and translocates to the membrane along with the other cytosol components in a process that requires both GTP and gp21-phox[58,59,64,81,82,101–107] (right side of Fig. 54-2). All CGD patients thus far analyzed at the molecular level have mutations involving one of these four components: gp91-phox, p22-phox, p47-phox, or p67-phox (Fig. 54-2).

The molecular heterogeneity of CGD can be organized into a modern classification scheme based on the oxidase component affected[108–110] (Table 54-2). Nomenclature has also been adopted for an abbreviated designation for each subtype of CGD, as outlined in Table 54-2. Defects in gp91-phox are all inherited in an X-linked fashion and account for approximately 65% of all CGD patients.[110] In most X-linked CGD, gp91-phox is completely absent and there is no measurable cytochrome b, NBT reduction, or intact cell superoxide production (the X91⁰ subtype). In about 10% of X-linked patients, gp91-phox can be present in normal levels but can be nonfunctional (X91⁺), partially deficient (X91⁻), or mutated in such a way that the Michaelis constant (K_m) for NADPH is abnormal (X91⁻).[35,111–118] Mutations involving p22-phox occur in approximately 5–7% of

CGD patients and usually result in the complete absence of cytochrome b (A22⁰).[119–123] This defect is inherited in an autosomal recessive manner. Since the full expression of cytochrome b in the membrane requires the production of both subunits, a primary deficiency of either component leads to a secondary loss of the other.[67,124] Thus, neither subunit can be detected on immunoblot analysis in either X91⁰ or A22⁰ CGD. The second most common form of CGD is caused by a severe deficiency in the cytosol of p47-phox (A47⁰) and is seen in 25% of all patients[56,83,84,86,87] (Table 54-2). In the remaining 5% of patients, the CGD is caused by the absence of p67-phox (A67⁰).[56,83,84,86,87] Both cytosol defects are inherited in an autosomal recessive manner and are characterized by a severe deficiency of cytosol activity in the cell-free system.[56] Membrane function is intact in the cell-free system in these two types of CGD, and cytochrome b levels are normal.[56]

Even though >90% of patients with CGD have respiratory burst defects that result in undetectable levels of O_2^- production, there is a surprising heterogeneity in the clinical manifestations of the disease.[7,14,31,36,109,125] At one end of the spectrum are the patients who begin to suffer from severe bacterial and fungal infections during infancy, and who rarely have >4–12 months between such serious infections. At the other end of the spectrum are patients who are well for many years and then unexpectedly develop a highly unusual infection such as a staphylococcal hepatic abscess or *Aspergillus* pneumonia. After their first major infection, some of these patients may be relatively healthy again for another 3–10 years before the next severe infection occurs. Based on my experience with >70 CGD patients, those with X91⁰ and A22⁰ CGD tend to have a more severe clinical course, while patients with A47⁰ CGD often enjoy the milder clinical phenotype despite the severity of their respiratory burst defect.[125] Those individuals with A67⁰ CGD, or partial respiratory burst activity <10% of normal (most X91⁻ patients) tend to have disease of intermediate severity. Be-

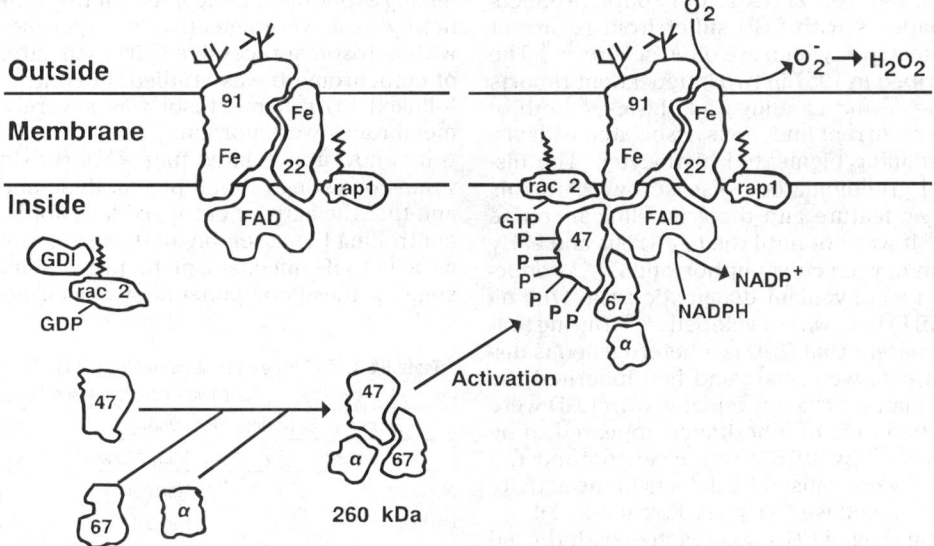

Fig. 54-2. Hypothetical model of NADPH oxidase activation. Current knowledge of the oxidase suggests that in its dormant state (left), it is composed of both membrane-bound and cytosolic components. The former include the gp91-phox and p22-phox subunits of cytochrome b_{558} (and possibly rap 1A). Recent evidence suggests that the flavin adenine dinucleotide (FAD) redox center is bound to gp91-phox,[75,76] but since this has not been conclusively established, the FAD is shown bound to a distinct oxidase subunit in the membrane. The cytosolic components include p47-phox and p67-phox, which appear to exist in a preformed complex of 260 kd.[57] It is likely that this complex contains at least one other additional component (possibly a recently described 40-kd protein), labeled in this model as α. The low-molecular-mass GTP-binding protein rac2 is also present in the cytosol in its inactive state (with GDP bound), presumably complexed with a GDP dissociation inhibitor (GDIs) that serves to keep rac 2 in its inactive state. Upon stimulation, the p47-phox/p67-phox complex translocates to the membrane. This process may be under control of the active (GTP-bound) form of rac 2 and further regulated by phosphorylation of p47-phox. In its active state, the FAD redox center accepts electrons from NADPH and passes them on to molecular oxygen via the heme groups in cytochrome b_{558}. Two heme groups are believed to be present in each cytochrome b_{558} heterodimer.[74]

Table 54-2. Classification of Chronic Granulomatous Disease

Component Affected	Gene Locus	Inheritance	Subtype Designation[a]	NBT Score (% positive)	O_2^- Production (% normal)	Cytochrome b Spectrum (% normal)	Defect in Cell-Free System	Families Evaluated Scripps[b]	Families Evaluated Europe[c]	Frequency (% of cases)
gp91-*phox*	Xp21.1	X	X91⁰	0	0	0	Membrane	33	35	56
			X91⁻	80–100 (weak)	3–30	3–30	Membrane	4	2	5
			X91⁻	5–10	5–10	5–10	Membrane	2	0	2
			X91⁺	0	0	100	Membrane	2	0	2
p22-*phox*	16p24	AR	X22⁰	0	0	0	Membrane	4	3	6
			A22⁺	0	0	100	Membrane	1	0	1
p47-*phox*	7q11.23	AR	A47⁰	0	0–1	100	Cytosol	15	13	23
p67-*phox*	1q25	AR	A67⁰	0	0–1	100	Cytosol	4	3	6

Abbreviations: X, X-linked inheritance; AR (or A), autosomal recessive inheritance; NBT, nitroblue tetrazolium.

[a] In this nomenclature, the first letter represents the mode of inheritance (X-linked [X] or autosomal recessive [A]), while the number indicates the *phox* component that is genetically affected. The superscript symbols indicate whether the level of protein of the affected component is undetectable (⁰), diminished, (⁻), or normal (⁺) as measured by immunoblot analysis.

[b] This group represents 65 kindreds with 71 total patients followed at Scripps Clinic in La Jolla, CA.

[c] Cooperative study reported in 1992[110] represents 56 kindreds and 61 patients.

(From Curnutte,[109] with permission.)

cause of this heterogeneity, the diagnosis of CGD should be entertained, not only in young children with recurrent severe infections, but also in adolescents and young adults who experience exceptionally severe or unusual infections.

Molecular Genetics

All the subtypes of X-linked CGD are caused by mutations in the gene encoding the gp91-phox subunit of cytochrome b[67,71, 72,126] (Table 54-2). This gene, termed CYBB, contains 13 exons and spans approximately 30 kb in the Xp21.1 region of the X chromosome.[127–130] Based on our analysis of >50 X-linked CGD kindreds and those published in the literature, there is a striking heterogeneity in the mutations seen; most are family specific. There are roughly equal numbers of deletions, frameshifts, splice site, nonsense, and missense mutations distributed more or less randomly throughout the gp91-*phox* gene[71,116,118,128,129,131–139] (Table 54-3). Two putative regulatory mutations have been identified to date.[139] Thus it appears that most instances of X-linked CGD arise from mutations in the structural portion of CYBB and not from defects in the regulation of the gene. Most of these mutations affect either the stability of the mRNA or the protein (or both), usually to the extent that no measurable cytochrome b is expressed in the phagocytes (Table 54-2).

The diversity of the mutations in gp91-*phox* parallels the clinical heterogeneity seen in X-linked CGD and in many cases provides an explanation for the phenotype observed. For example, the large interstitial deletion in patient 1 (Table 54-3) affects not only CYBB, but also the flanking gene loci for Duchenne muscular dystrophy, X-linked retinitis pigmentosa, and the McLeod hemolytic anemia syndrome (absence of the Kell erythrocyte antigen, Kx) and thus accounts for the constellation of clinical problems seen in this unfortunate patient.[128] Since the McLeod locus is closer to CYBB than the Duchenne locus,[140] it is more common to see McLeod hemolytic anemia in conjunction with CGD, as evidenced by patients 3 and 4 in Table 54-3, in whom the deletions are smaller.[71,131,132,134] The "variant" forms of X-linked CGD (X91⁻), in which some residual cytochrome b and respiratory burst activity are retained, can also be explained at the molecular genetic level. In patient 8 in Table 54-3, an in-frame nucleotide triplet deletion predicts the loss of a single amino acid (K315), a change that is apparently well tolerated in this putative extracellular domain of gp91-phox since the patient has approximately 25% normal O_2^- production. Similarly, in patient 40, a single point mutation (A 494→G) predicts a conservative amino acid substitution (K161→R) that allows the patient's neutrophils to still generate low levels of O_2^- (2–4% of normal)—an amount sufficient to

confer a milder phenotype on the patient. In other instances, missense mutations predicting less conservative changes result in either absent (e.g., patient 36) or nonfunctional (e.g., patients 37 and 49) cytochrome b and a more severe clinical picture. The severe phenotype is also more frequently seen in those patients with either nonsense or frameshift mutations since these predict stop codons at either the site of mutation or slightly downstream (in the case of a frameshift). Truncated forms of gp91-phox are apparently highly unstable, as these patients all have undetectable levels of cytochrome b and respiratory burst activity.

As mentioned above, mutations in the regulatory regions of the gp91-phox gene are relatively uncommon. The two that have been described are from unrelated kindreds that involve point mutations 55 and 57 base pairs (bp) upstream (5′) of exon 1.[139] Interestingly, three patients from the two families exhibited the same, highly unusual biochemical phenotype. By both NBT testing and flow cytometric analysis of hydrogen peroxide production (using the dichlorofluorescin assay[141]), 5–10% of each patient's neutrophils had full respiratory burst activity, while the remaining cells were devoid of activity. Cytochrome b expression and O_2^- production were also 5–10% of normal, presumably expressed only in the small clone of cells with full respiratory burst activity. It has been hypothesized that these putative regulatory mutations adversely affect cytochrome b expression in most, but not all, of the circulating, neutrophils and that this reflects some type of underlying heterogeneity in the way certain subpopulations regulate gp91-phox expression.

Mutations in the gene for the p22-phox subunit of cytochrome b cause one of the three forms of autosomal recessive CGD and account for about 6% of all CGD (Table 54-2). The p22-phox gene, termed CYBA, resides at chromosome 16q24 and contains six exons that span 8.5 kb.[120] As in the case of X-linked CGD, the mutations identified thus far in the seven kindreds studied (six females and three males) are heterogeneous and family specific[44,47,120,122,123] (Table 54-4). In all but one of the instances listed in Table 54-4 (kindred 2), the patients are homozygous for the mutant allele due to consanguinity of the parents. The mutations in general predict either major defects in p22-phox (e.g., kindred 1) or nonconservative amino acid substitutions. Not surprisingly, then, these patients fail to express p22-phox, are devoid of cytochrome b, cannot generate O_2^-, and have clinically more severe disease. The one exception is kindred 6, which has a nonfunctional, yet spectrally normal cytochrome b expressed at normal levels. There is a predicted structural defect in the intracytoplasmic C-terminal domain due to the substitution of a glutamine for proline at

Table 54-3. Summary of gp91-*phox* Mutations in 51 Patients with CGD

Patient No. and Type of Mutation	Exon(s) Affects	Nucleotide Change[a]	Predicted Amino Acid Change	CGD Type[b]	Comments	References
Deletion						
1	1–13+	~5,000 kb deletion	No gp91-*phox*	X91⁰	Severe with DMD, RP, McLeod	128
2	1–13+	~4,000 kb deletion	No gp91-*phox*	X91⁰	Severe with DMD and McLeod	71, 129, 131
3	1–13+	~1,000 kb deletion	No gp91-*phox*	X91⁰	Severe with McLeod. Seen in ≥5 kindreds	132, 133
4	1–13+	Not known	No gp91-*phox*	X91⁰	Severe with McLeod and RP	134
5	1–13+	≥30 kb deletion	No gp91-*phox*	X91⁰	No McLeod	135
6	11–13	>4 kb deletion	Deletion of I 439–F 570	X91⁰	—	133
7	13	~1 kb deletion	Deletion of ~T 530–F 570	X91⁰	Severe CGD	71
8	9	Deletion of G 954, A 955, A 956	Deletion of K 315	X91⁻	In-frame deletion; clinically mild	133
Frameshift						
9	3	Insert G 207	Stop in exon 4	X91⁰	Severe	133
10	3	Delete C 263	Stop in exon 4	X91⁰	Multiple abnormally spliced mRNA	133
11	5	Insert A 455	Stop in exon 5	X91⁰	—	133
12	7	Delete A 713 and G 714	Stop in exon 7	(X91⁰)	—	133
13	7	Delete A 728–T 732	Stop in exon 7	X91⁰	Severe CGD	133
14	7	Insert A 754	Stop in exon 8	X91⁰	Seen in 3 unrelated kindreds; severe CGD	133
15	7	Insert A 772	Stop in exon 8	X91⁰	Severe CGD	133
16	9	Delete G 975	Stop in exon 9	(X91⁰)	—	133
Splice						
17	Intron 11 (3′)	ag → gg	Delete A 488–E 497	X91⁺	Cryptic splice site with in-frame deletion; mild CGD	118
18	Intron 7 (5′)	gt → ga	Delete exon 7 then frameshift	X91⁰	—	136
19	Intron 5 (5′)	gta → gtt	Delete exon 5 then stop	X91⁰	—	136
20	Intron 3 (5′)	gtaag → gtaaa	Delete exon 3	X91⁰	In-frame deletion	136
21	Intron 1 (3′)	ag → aa	Delete exon 2	X91⁰	In-frame deletion	136
22	Intron 2 (5′)	gt → tt	Delete exon 2	X91⁰	Severe CGD	133
23	Intron 2 (3′)	ag → gg	Delete exon 3	X91⁰	Severe CGD	133
24	Intron 5 (5′)	gt → gc	Not determined	(X91⁰)	—	133
25	Intron 9 (5′)	gtgc deleted	Not determined	X91⁰	Severe CGD	133
Nonsense						
26	3	C 229 → T	R 73 → stop	X91⁰	2 kindreds	133, 137
27	4	C 283 → T	R 91 → stop	X91⁰	2 kindreds	133
28	5	C 454 → T	Q 148 → stop	(X91⁰)	—	133
29	5	C481 → T	R 157 → stop	X91⁰	2 kindreds	133
30	7	C 688 → T	R 226 → stop	X91⁰	Heterozygous female with severe CGD	138
31	8	C 880 → T	R 290 → stop	X91⁰	Severe CGD	133
32	9	G 1,018 → T	E 336 → stop	X91⁰	Severe CGD	133
33	11	C 1,332 → A	Y 440 → stop	(X91⁰)	—	133
34	11	G 1,341 → A	W 443 → stop	X91⁰	—	133
35	12	C 1,531 → T	Q 507 → stop	X91⁰	Severe CGD	133
Missense						
36	2	G 70 → C	G 20 → R	X91⁰	Severe CGD	133
37	3	G 173 → C	R 54 → S	X91⁺	Nonfunctional cytochrome	133
38	4	A 314 → G	H 101 → R	X91⁰	—	137
39	5	G 478 → A	A 156 → T	X91⁰	2 kindreds	133, 137
40	5	A 494 → G	K 161 → R	X91⁻	Low levels O₂⁻; mild CGD	133
41	6	C 637 → T	H 209 → Y	X91⁰	Same residue as patient 42	137
42	6	T 639 → A	H 209 → Q	X91⁰	See patient 41	133
43	7	T 742 → C	C 244 → R	(X91⁰)	Same residue as patient 44	133
44	7	G 743 → C	C 244 → S	X91⁻	See patient 43	137
45	9	C 937 → A	E 309 → K	X91⁻	Low levels O₂⁻; mild CGD	133
46	9	T 1,009 → C	S 333 → P	(X91⁰)	—	133
47	9	G 1,151 → A	W 380 → R	X91⁰	Mild CGD	133
48	10	G 1,178 → C	G 389 → A	X91⁻	—	137
49	10	C 1,256 → A	P 415 → H	X91⁺	Nonfunctional cytochrome	116
Regulatory						
50	5′ Regulatory	−57a → c	Not applicable	X91⁻	5–10% of cells NBT positive	139
51	5′ Regulatory	−55t → c	Not applicable	X91⁻	Similar to patient 50	139

Abbreviations: DMD, Duchenne muscular dystrophy; RP, X-linked retinitis pigmentosa; McLeod, McLeod hemolytic anemia syndrome.
[a] Nucleotide residues are numbered according to the cDNA sequence described by Orkin.[428]
[b] CGD types in parentheses are inferred from the mutation, since biochemical data regarding cytochrome b levels are missing in these patients. See Table 54-2 for explanation of CGD types.
(From Forehand et al.[429] with permission.)

Table 54-4. Summary of p22-*phox* Mutations in Seven Kindreds with CGD

Kindred No. and Type of Mutation	Exon(s) Affected	Nucleotide Change[a]	Predicted Amino Acid Change	CGD Type[b]	Comments	References
Deletion						
1	1–6+	>10 kb deletion	No p22-*phox*	A22⁰	Homozygous[c]; severe CGD	44, 120
Frameshift						
2	4	Delete C 272	Stop in exon 6	A22⁰	See kindred 3 for mutation in other allele	47, 120
Missense						
3	4	G 297 → A	R 90 → Q	A22⁰	Homozygous in one kindred[b]; heterozygous in a second kindred (see 2)	47, 120, 122
4	4	A 309 → G	H 94 → R	A22⁰	Homozygous[c]	122
5	5	C 382 → A	S 118 → R	A22⁰	Homozygous[c]	120
6	6	C 495 → A	P 156 → Q	A22⁺	Homozygous[c]; nonfunctional cytochrome	123
Splice						
7	Intron 4	gt → at	Delete exon 4	A22⁰	Homozygous[c]	122

[a] Nucleotide residues are numbered according to the cDNA sequence described in Orkin.[428]
[b] See Table 54-2 for explanation of CGD types.
[c] In these cases, homozygosity of the mutant allele was due to consanguinity in the parents.
(From Forehand et al.,[429] with permission.)

residue 156.[123] Analogous to the X91⁺ patients described above, this mutant nonfunctional cytochrome b is unable to support a respiratory burst and results in severe disease.

The gene for p47-phox, termed NCF1, resides on chromosome 7 at q11.23[142] and contains nine exons spanning 18 kb.[143] Mutations at this locus cause autosomal recessive CGD and account for about 25% of all CGD (Table 54-2). In contrast to the diversity of mutations seen in patients with cytochrome b defects, only three different mutations have been reported thus far in the nine unrelated patients studied[143,144] (Table 54-5). Six of the nine patients are homozygous for a mutant allele with a GT deleted at the beginning of exon 2 that predicts a premature stop codon later in that same exon.[144] The other three patients are compound heterozygotes with one allele containing the GT deletion in exon 2 and the second, one of two missense mutations.[143]

Mutations in the gene for p67-phox account for the remaining 5% of CGD patients (Table 54-2). This gene, referred to as NCF2, is located on the long arm of chromosome 1 at position q25[142] and contains 16 exons that span 40 kb.[145] To date, mutations in the p67-phox gene have only been reported in one patient with this type of autosomal recessive CGD. The patient was found to be homozygous for a point mutation in exon 3 (G 233→A) that predicts a Gly 78→Gln replacement.[146]

Clinical Manifestations

In approximately two-thirds of patients, the first symptoms of CGD appear during the first year of life with the onset of recurrent, purulent bacterial and fungal infections. Table 54-6 summarizes the types of infections and infecting organisms most frequently encountered in CGD.[7,36,147–153] The most common types of infections are those that involve sites in contact with the outside world—consistent with the role of neutrophils as the first line of defense against infection. *Staphylococcus aureus*, enteric gram-negative bacteria, *Serratia marcescens*, *Pseudomonas cepacia* (usually not *aeruginosa*), and *Aspergillus* spp. represent the most frequently encountered pathogens. Most CGD pathogens share the property of catalase positivity; as such, they are unable to "lend" hydrogen peroxide metabolically generated within the microbes to the peroxide-starved CGD phagocyte. For catalase-negative organisms, the CGD phagocytes use the bacteria-generated peroxide (once converted to hypochlorous acid (HOCl) by myeloperoxidase [Fig. 54-1]) to kill the microbe.[154] It also appears that at least some

Table 54-5. Summary of p47-*phox* Mutations in Nine Patients with A 47 CGD

Patient No./Sex	Mutation Type	O₂⁻	p47-*phox* Protein	mRNA	Nucleotide Change[a]	Amino Acid Change	CGD Type[b]	References
1–3/M	Deletion/frameshift (homozygous)	NR	0	N	Deletion of G 95 and T 96 at beginning of exon 2	Frameshift with substitution of 25 incorrect amino acids (residues 26–50) before premature stop codon	A47⁰	144
4–6/two M, one F	Deletion/frameshift (homozygous)	0	0	N	Same as patients 1–3		A47⁰	143
7/F	1) Deletion/frameshift 2) Missense	0–1%	0	N	1) Same as patients 1–3 2) A 179 → G	Thr 53 → Ala	A47⁰	143
8, 9/M	1) Deletion/frameshift 2) Missense	0–1%	0	N	1) Same as patients 1–3 2) A 425 → G	Lys 135 → Glu	A47⁰	143

Abbreviations: N, normal; NR, not reported.
[a] Nucleotide residues are numbered according to Casimir et al.[144] beginning with the 5′ and of the p47-*phox* cDNA.
[b] See Table 54-2 for explanation of CGD types.
(From Curnutte,[32] with permission.)

Table 54-6. Infections in Chronic Granulomatous Disease[a]

Infection	Relative Frequency (%)	Infecting Organism	Isolates (%)
Pneumonia	70–80	*Staphylococcus aureus*	30–50
Lymphadenitis[b]	60–80	*Aspergillus* spp.	10–20
Cutaneous infections/ impetigo[b]	60–70	*Escherichia coli*	5–10
Hepatic/perihepatic abscesses[b]	30–40	*Klebsiella* spp.	5–10
Osteomyelitis	20–30	*Salmonella* spp.	5–10
Perirectal abscesses/ fistulae[b]	15–30	*Pseudomonas cepacia* and *aeruginosa*	5–10
Septicemia	10–20	*Serratia marcescens*	5–10
Otitis media[b]	≈20	*Staphylococcus epidermidis*	5
Conjunctivitis	≈15	*Streptococcus* spp.	4
Enteric infections	≈10	*Enterobacter* spp.	3
Urinary tract infections/ pyelonephritis	5–15	*Proteus* spp.	3
Sinusitis	<10	*Candida* spp.	3
Renal/perinephric abscesses	<10	*Nocardia* spp.	2
Brain abscesses	<5	*Haemophilus influenzae*	1
Pericarditis	<5	*Pneumocystis carinii*	<1
Meningitis	<5	*Mycobacterium fortuitum*	<1
		Chromobacterium violaceum	<1
		Francisella philomiragia	<1
		Torulopsis glabrata	<1

[a] The relative frequencies of different types of infections in CGD are estimated from data pooled from several large series of patients in the United States, Europe, and Japan.[7,36,148–153] These series encompass approximately 550 patients with CGD after accounting for overlap between reports. The list of infecting organisms is also arranged according to the data in these reports and is not paired with the entities in the first column.

[b] Those infections most frequently seen at the time of presentation.
(From Curnutte,[32] with permission.)

of the CGD pathogens are resistant to the nonoxidative killing mechanisms of the phagocyte and thus can proliferate relatively unchecked.[155] In my experience, it is somewhat surprising how often one fails to identify the infecting organism in CGD—perhaps more than half the time despite aggressive culturing. In this situation, the antibiotic that ought to work is used empirically; if failure ensues, then more invasive diagnostic procedures are aggressively pursued, looking for one (or more) of the less commonly seen microbes such as *Nocardia* spp., *Candida,* and a host of other bacteria and fungi[153,156–175] (Table 54-6).

Pneumonia is the most common type of infection seen in CGD; *S. aureus, Aspergillus* spp., *P. cepacia,* and enteric gram-negative bacteria are the major pathogens. It is noteworthy that in the past 8 years *P. cepacia* has emerged as one of the most lethal pneumonias.[176–180] Often it is not covered with the first line of antibiotics used for *S. aureus* and most gram-negative bacteria and can quietly proliferate (with persistent fevers) to the point of collapse due to endotoxic shock. Intravenous trimethoprim sulfamethoxazole has been most effective in treating patients if given before widespread dissemination of the infection. An open lung biopsy is often needed to establish the diagnosis. *Aspergillus* pneumonia is also difficult to treat, but usually responds to 3–6 *months* of daily (then thrice weekly) amphotericin B therapy (with interferon-γ [IFN-γ]). Surgery has generally not been needed except for biopsy or resection of large cavitary lesions.

Lymphadenitis is the second most common infection and is

usually caused by gram-negative organisms, *S. aureus,* or *S. marcescens* (Table 54-6). Incision and drainage should be performed if the lesion fails to respond to parenteral antibiotics. Cutaneous abscesses should be similarly managed. Recurrent impetigo, frequently in the parinasal area, often requires months of therapy (mostly oral antibiotics) to clear. Hepatic (and perihepatic) abscesses are also quite common in CGD and are usually caused by *S. aureus.*[181,182] Most lesions require drainage (needle or surgical) to permit efficient healing to occur. Bone infections are particularly problematic in CGD; they arise from either hematogenous or contiguous spread (as often is the case when *Aspergillus* infections in the lung invade the ribs, vertebral bodies, or diaphragm).[183–186] Perirectal abscesses are difficult to treat, even with months of therapy, and can lead to fistula formations.[181]

Many of the more problematic complications of CGD result from imperfectly controlled infections in which stalemates develop between the pathogen and the patients' leukocytes. These lesions become granulomas as the host employs lymphocytes and histiocytes to aid the failing neutrophils in containing the pathogens. As a result of this chronic inflammatory stimulation, CGD patients can suffer from a variety of more chronic complications (Table 54-7). Lymphadenopathy, hepatosplenomegaly, eczematoid dermatitis,[187] and anemia of chronic disease (hemoglobin levels usually 8–10 g/dl) are common manifestations of this process and are most prominent in the first 5–10 years of life in CGD. A chronic ileocolitis resembling Crohn disease is seen in about 10% of patients and can range from mild diarrhea to a debilitating syndrome of bloody diarrhea and malabsorption that can necessitate a colectomy.[188–191] Throughout the body, granuloma formation can lead to dysfunction and obstruction in the esophagus,[192] stomach,[181,193,194] intestine,[195] and urinary bladder and kidneys.[196–204] In the stomach, gastric antral narrowing can be severe enough in infants and children to resemble pyloric ste-

Table 54-7. Chronic Conditions Associated with CGD

Condition	Relative Frequency[a] (%)
Lymphadenopathy	98
Hypergammaglobulinemia	60–90
Hepatomegaly	50–90
Splenomegaly	60–80
Anemia of chronic disease	Common*
Underweight	70
Chronic diarrhea	20–60
Short stature	50
Gingivitis	50
Dermatitis	35
Hydronephrosis	10–25
Ulcerative stomatitis	5–15
Pulmonary fibrosis	<10*
Esophagitis	<10*
Gastric antral narrowing	<10
Granulomatous ileocolitis	<10
Granulomatous cystitis	<10
Chorioretinitis	<10
Glomerulonephritis	<10
Discoid lupus erythematosus	<10

[a] The relative frequencies of the chronic conditions associated with CGD were estimated from the series of reports listed in Table 54-6. In some instances (asterisks), the incidence is estimated from the 40 cases of CGD followed at Scripps Clinic and Research Foundation (unpublished data).
(From Curnutte,[32] with permission.)

nosis. Granulomatous lesions and inflammatory cell infiltrates in the urinary system can lead to chronic cystitis, dysuria, and hydronephrosis. Other types of chronic inflammation include gingivitis,[205] chorioretinitis,[206] destructive white matter lesions in the brain,[207,208] and glomerulonephritis.[198,209] In rare circumstances, patients may develop either discoid or systemic lupus erythematosus by a mechanism that is unknown.[210–213]

Carriers of CGD, whether of the X-linked form or any one of the autosomal recessive forms, are usually asymptomatic, with two important exceptions. First, X-linked carriers are at risk of developing mild to moderately severe discoid lupus erythematosus characterized by discoid skin lesions and photosensitivity.[212,214,215] A few will also suffer from arthralgias, polyarthritis, and Raynaud's phenomenon. The frequency of discoid lupus in X-linked carriers is not known, but based on my experience, about one-fourth of women are symptomatic, with onset usually in the second decade of life. The disease does not progress to systemic lupus erythematosus nor does one find serologic evidence of even subclinical disease. Severe discoid lupus can be treated with hydroxychloroquine. The second important complication of the CGD carrier state is infection in those X-linked carriers who have an unusually high degree of inactivation of the normal X chromosome in their myeloid cells. If the circulating neutrophil population is skewed to the point that <10% of the cells function, then the carrier has an increased risk of infections. Fortunately these infections are usually mild.[138,216–218]

Diagnosis

The diagnosis of CGD is usually suggested by the unusual clinical histories outlined above, or by a family history of CGD. The diagnosis is most easily confirmed using the NBT slide test.[44] A typical result is shown in Figure 54-3. Figure 54-3A shows the normal positive staining of a group of seven neutrophils and one monocyte. Figure 54-3B shows the complete absence of NBT staining in a patient with X91^0 CGD, the classic X-linked form of the disease. Figure 54-3C shows the mixed population of NBT-positive and NBT-negative cells observed in that patient's mother. Because of random X-chromosome inactivation, some of the female carrier's cells are NBT positive and others negative.[216,217,219] Because in this test nearly 100% of the normal cells are positive, we are able to detect reliably the carrier state in X-linked CGD, when as few as 5% of the cells are NBT negative. This test also permits detection of diffuse populations of weakly positive cells such as those seen in X91$^-$ CGD, which are characterized by a partial deficiency of cytochrome b. Since X-linked CGD can arise by new mutations in the germlines of the mothers (in approximately 25% of all my cases), one does not always see NBT negative cells in the mother.[22,133]

The diagnosis of CGD can also be established by measuring respiratory burst activity directly as oxygen consumption, O_2^- production, or hydrogen peroxide production.[108,141] The subtyping of CGD also requires measurement of the cytochrome b content in the patient's (and parents') neutrophils, usually by a spectrophotometric assay.

Also required in many instances is the measurement of activity of the patient's neutrophil membranes and cytosol in the cell-free oxidase activation system, as depicted in Table 54-1. Once a cytosol defect is suspected, the determination of which component is defective can be made by either immunoblot analysis or complementation studies in the cell-free system using known cytosols deficient in either p47-phox or p67-phox.[84] These latter tests are best performed by laboratories specializing in neutrophil biochemistry.

Molecular genetic analysis of either myeloid cell cDNA[116] or genomic DNA[133,220] can be used to confirm the genetic subtype and define further the molecular properties of the mutant oxidase. Moreover, the molecular genetic data can be used for genetic counseling in identifying carriers and (if genomic se-

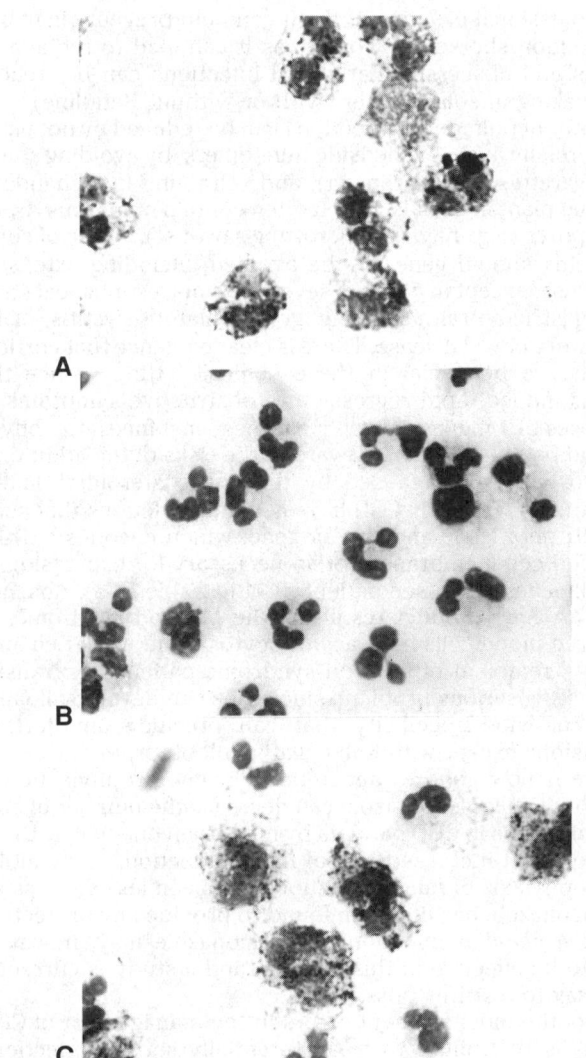

Fig. 54-3. NBT slide test. Peripheral blood neutrophils and monocytes from a drop of fresh whole blood were made adherent to glass slides and stimulated with phorbol myristate acetate. **(A)** Normal neutrophils and monocytes, all of which are NBT positive. **(B)** Neutrophils and monocytes from an X-linked CGD patient, which are all NBT negative. **(C)** A mixture of NBT-positive and NBT-negative neutrophils from the X-linked carrier mother of the patient in Fig. B.

quencing can be used) for prenatal diagnosis using fetal DNA from the chorionic villus or amniocytes.[220,221] Alternatively, potentially informative polymorphisms exist in the genes for gp91-phox and p67-phox that can be used for fetal DNA analysis.[135,145,220,222,223] In the absence of a molecular genetic approach, prenatal diagnosis can be performed using the NBT test and a small sample of fetal blood obtained by percutaneous umbilical sampling.[224–229]

Therapy

The four cornerstones of therapy in CGD are (1) prevention and early treatment of infections; (2) aggressive use of parenteral antibiotics for most infections; (3) use of prophylactic trimethoprim sulfamethoxazole (5 mg/kg/day of trimethoprim) or dicloxacillin (25–50 mg/kg/day) for sulfa-allergic patients; and (4) use of prophylactic recombinant human IFN-γ. Several approaches can be used to prevent infections. Patients with CGD should receive all their routine immunizations on schedule, with the influenza vaccine administered each year as well. Cuts and skin abrasions should be cleansed promptly with soap and water and a topical antiseptic applied (2% hydrogen peroxide or Betadine ointment). Frequent brushing, flossing, and professional cleaning of teeth can help prevent gingivitis. Constipation should be avoided, as it can lead to rectal/anal fissures and abscesses. Early anal infections can be treated with soaking in soapy water (with or without Betadine). The frequency of pulmonary infections can be reduced by not using commercially available bedside humidifiers, by avoiding smoking (cigarettes and marijuana), and refraining from handling decaying plant materials, which often contain numerous *Aspergillus* spores (e.g., hay, mulch, rotting sawdust).[230] Use of corticosteroids should generally be avoided, including extensive topical use, except in cases of severe asthma, esophageal strictures, gastric antral narrowing, granulomatous cystitis, or inflammatory bowel disease. There is clear evidence that corticosteroids are beneficial in these clinical settings, since the steroids induce rapid regression of obstructive symptoms at oral doses of 1 mg/kg/day.[231–233] In these instances, the physician and patient should be aware of the risks of the additional immunosuppression caused by the corticosteroids. Finally, rare patients with X91⁰ CGD have genomic deletions that span the gp91-phox gene and the *Xk* gene, which encodes a 37-kd red blood cell membrane protein necessary for expression of the Kell genes[234,235] (see patients 1–4 in Table 54-3). Absence of the *Xk* gene product results in the McLeod syndrome, in which red blood cells have acanthocytosis and weak Kell antigens.[234] Treatment of McLeod syndrome patients by transfusion poses a serious problem, since they can develop alloantibodies of wide specificity that can preclude any further transfusions except with Kell-negative blood products.

There is now good evidence that chronic prophylactic trimethoprim sulfamethoxazole can decrease the number of bacterial infections in CGD patients by more than one-half, without a concomitant increased risk of fungal infection.[150,236] Antibiotic prophylaxis of fungal infections has been less successful, as ketoconazole has not been found to provide any protection against *Aspergillus* infections.[150] Itraconazole may, however, prove to be effective in this context, and a study is currently underway to test this possibility.

One of the most frequent errors in the management of CGD patients is the failure to treat potentially serious infections promptly and aggressively with appropriate parenteral antibiotics. Even the best antibiotics can be rendered ineffective if given too late in the course of an infection in CGD. Therefore, early intervention is advisable. While many of the minor infections and low-grade fevers in CGD patients can be managed on an outpatient basis, episodes of consistently high fever over a 24-hour period or clearly established infections (such as pneumonia or lymphadenitis) should be treated with parenteral antibiotics that cover *S. aureus* and enteric gram-negative organisms. Reasonable attempts to define the source of the infection and the responsible microbe should also begin promptly. If the infection fails to respond, then more aggressive diagnostic procedures should be instituted (computed tomography, bone, and gallium scans; open biopsies if indicated); empirical changes should also be made in the antibiotics used to broaden coverage to *P. cepacia*. If fungus is identified or strongly suspected, amphotericin B is the drug of choice. Even when appropriate antibiotics are used, certain types of infections respond slowly and may require months of therapy, particularly *Aspergillus* infections. For *Aspergillus* infections 4–12 months of amphotericin B (given daily for 2–3 months and then thrice weekly) followed by a 1–3-year course of daily oral itraconazole has been effective in clearing most infections and preventing recurrence. It is important to note that surgical drainage or resection can sometimes play a key role in accelerating healing of certain types of infection such as lymphadenitis, osteomyelitis, and abscesses of visceral organs such as the liver. Finally, granulocyte transfusions may be of benefit in the treatment of stubborn or extremely serious infections.[152,237–240] In my experience, bone marrow transplant is rarely indicated when balanced against the effectiveness of aggressive medical management.

Table 54-8. Summary of the Phase III Study Data Establishing the Efficacy of IFN-γ for Infection Prophylaxis in CGD[a]

Variable	Treatment Group		P Value
	IFN-γ	Placebo	
No. of patients	63	65	
Age ± SD (yr)	14.3 ± 10.1	15.0 ± 9.6	
No. of patients with at least one serious infection (%)	14 (22%)	30 (46%)	0.0006
Total no. of serious infections	20	56	<0.0001
Total hospital days	497	1,493	0.02
Average hospital stay (days)	32	48	
Percentage without serious infection[b]			
Age			
<10 yr (52 patients)	81	20	
≥10 yr (76 patients)	73	34	
Inheritance			
X-linked (86 patients)	79	33	
Autosomal (42 patients)	71	39	
Prophylactic antibiotics			
Yes (111 patients)	78	33	
No (17 patients)	69	28	

[a] The table shows a summary of the final results of a phase III randomized, double-blind, placebo-controlled study in which 128 patients with CGD received either IFN-γ (50 μg/m²/dose) or placebo by subcutaneous injections three times per week for an average duration of 8.9 months.[241] The major end points of the study were the time to the first serious infection and the number of such infections. A serious infection was defined as an event requiring hospitalization and parenteral antibiotics.

[b] The bottom portion of the table shows the Kaplan-Meier estimates of the cumulative proportion of patients free of serious infections at 12 months (after randomization) with adjustment for stratification factors.

A multicenter trial was completed in 1990 in which 128 patients were randomized in a double-blind fashion to receive either placebo or IFN-γ (0.05 mg/m² three times per week).[241] The results from this study, summarized in Table 54-8, showed a substantial decrease in the number of serious infections in the INF arm—a 70% reduction in risk compared with placebo. Side effects were observed in some patients, but these were minimal (mild headaches and low-grade fevers). The highly significant clinical improvements were not accompanied by improvements in phagocyte function, as measured by O_2^- production or in vitro *S. aureus* killing. A few patients with rare variant forms of X91⁻ CGD have shown modest-to-dramatic increases in O_2^- production.[242–244] It now appears that IFN-γ augments host defense in the vast majority of patients by means other than reversing the respiratory burst defect.[245,246] This interpretation is consistent with the observation that IFN-γ was comparably effective in both X-linked and autosomal recessive types of CGD across a broad range of mutations that would preclude the synthesis of a functional oxidase. I have now treated a group of >30 CGD patients with IFN-γ for 3–5 years without interruption of their thrice weekly regimen. No additional adverse reactions have been noted, and the patients continue to show a substantial benefit, with fivefold fewer serious infections compared with the placebo group in the phase III study in Table 54-8. On average, this group of patients is averaging one serious infection for each patient every 4–5 years.

Neutrophil Glucose-6-Phosphate Dehydrogenase Deficiency

NADPH, the primary substrate for the respiratory burst oxidase, is generated by the first two reactions of the hexose monophosphate shunt pathway, for which the responsible en-

Table 54-9. Summary of Neutrophil CGPD Deficiency

Incidence	Extremely rare
Inheritance	X-linked
Molecular defect	Poorly characterized family of mutations that cause congenital nonspherocytic hemolytic anemia (CNSHA) in erythrocytes and functional failure of G6PD in neutrophils (possibly kinetic mutants); other rare mutants may also be responsible
Pathogenesis	Severe functional failure of neutrophil G6PD (<5% of normal), leading to an extremely low steady-state concentration of NADPH, which serves as the substrate for NADPH oxidase.
Clinical manifestations	CNSHA (hemolytic anemia that occurs even in the absence of redox stress) CGD-like syndrome with recurrent bacterial infections.
Laboratory evaluation	Neutrophil G6PD activity <5% of normal Severely diminished respiratory burst and abnormal NBT test Associated CNSHA with elevated reticulocyte count and diminished erythrocyte G6PD activity
Differential diagnosis	CGD Glutathione reductase or synthetase deficiency
Therapy	Prophylactic trimethoprim sulfamethoxazole Aggressive use of parenteral antibiotics Transfusion support for severe anemia
Prognosis	Not clear, since too few patients have been reported May be as severe as CGD

zymes are G6PD (Fig. 54-1, reaction 8) and 6-phosphogluconate dehydrogenase (6PGD).[22,26,247] As would be expected, a severe deficiency of G6PD in neutrophils results in a greatly attenuated respiratory burst and a clinical picture that can resemble CGD.[22,248-253] The key features of this extremely rare X-linked disorder are summarized in Table 54-9. In light of the relatively high frequency of G6PD mutations in the American black and Mediterranean populations,[26,247] as well as that leukocyte and erythrocyte G6PD are encoded by the same gene,[247] it might be expected that clinically significant neutrophil G6PD deficiency would occur more often than it does. One of the reasons it does not is the short life span of the neutrophil. Since most G6PD mutations cause the enzyme to decay over a period of days and weeks, levels in the short-lived neutrophil usually do not become critically low, even in some of the most unstable G6PD variants. It appears that only those rare and poorly understood mutations that cause congenital nonspherocytic hemolytic anemia are associated with extremely low (<5% of normal) levels of G6PD in the neutrophil.[247,249-252] Thus, a CGD-like syndrome due to neutrophil G6PD deficiency has only been observed in patients who also have congenital nonspherocytic hemolytic anemia (hemolysis that occurs in the absence of redox stress). This unique clinical association, coupled with the laboratory demonstration of extremely low G6PD levels in neutrophils and erythrocytes, serves to distinguish this disease from CGD.[248] The treatment for neutrophil G6PD deficiency is the same as for CGD except that the efficacy of IFN-γ has not been demonstrated in the former. The chronic hemolytic anemia is treated by supportive means, including transfusions.[247]

Disorders of Glutathione Metabolism

As depicted in Figure 54-1 (reaction 6), the reduced form of glutathione (GSH) serves to protect the neutrophil from the deleterious effects of hydrogen peroxide on NADPH oxidase and other neutrophil proteins such as microtubules.[254,255] Ade-

quate intracellular levels of reduced glutathione are maintained by recycling oxidized glutathione to GSH by glutathione reductase (Fig. 54-1, reaction 7) as well as by de novo synthesis of glutathione by glutathione synthetase (Fig. 54-1, reaction 9). Severe deficiencies in either of these enzymes have been observed to cause mild phagocytic defects.[254-256] The key features of these disorders are outlined in Table 54-10. Both are extremely rare and are apparently inherited in an autosomal recessive manner. The precise mutations for the individual disorders have not been established. In the case of glutathione reductase deficiency, the respiratory burst terminates prematurely, presumably owing to the toxic effects of accumulating hydrogen peroxide on NADPH oxidase.[29] This brief burst of O_2^-, however, appears to be sufficient for adequate microbial killing, since the few patients reported have not had problems with recurrent infections.[256] They do have a congenital hemolytic anemia due to diminished levels of glutathione reductase in erythrocytes.[256] This hemolysis becomes clinically evident during periods of oxidant stress.

In glutathione synthetase deficiency the respiratory burst proceeds normally.[255] The patients have some problems with recurrent infections and have a severe metabolic acidosis due to elevated levels of 5-oxoproline. This metabolite is the product of the first step in glutathione synthesis and is present in

Table 54-10. Disorders of Glutathione Metabolism

Disease Aspect	Glutathione Reductase Deficiency	Glutathione Synthetase Deficiency
Incidence	One family: three siblings	Several reported cases
Inheritance	Autosomal recessive	Autosomal recessive
Molecular defect	Diminished glutathione reductase levels in neutrophils (10–15% of normal) and erythrocytes; mutation not known	Severe deficiency of glutathione synthetase activity (5–10% normal); precise mutation(s) not known
Pathogenesis	Brief respiratory burst truncated by toxic accumulation of hydrogen peroxide in neutrophil caused by diminished catabolism of hydrogen peroxide by glutathione	Same as with glutathione reductase deficiency; elevated 5-oxoproline due to lack of feedback inhibition by glutathione
Clinical manifestations	No history of repeated infection Hemolysis with oxidant stress	Metabolic acidosis due to elevated 5-oxoproline Otitis media Intermittent neutropenia Hemolysis with oxidant stress
Laboratory evaluation	Glutathione reductase level diminished Premature cessation of O_2^- production by neutrophils	Severe decrease in glutathione synthetase level Normal respiratory burst
Differential diagnosis	CGD G6PD deficiency	Glutathione reductase deficiency
Therapy	None required	Vitamin E for hemolysis and infections Treatment of metabolic acidosis
Prognosis	Benign disorder	Relatively benign disorder

increased levels because of a lack of feedback of GSH on the synthetic pathway. Patients with glutathione synthetase deficiency also have intermittent neutropenia[257] (perhaps caused by the acidosis) as well as oxidant-induced hemolysis.[255] Therapy with vitamin E (400 IU/day) has been found to be beneficial in patients with severe glutathione synthetase deficiency suffering from hemolysis and infections.[257] Patients with less severe deficiencies usually do not require therapy.

Myeloperoxidase Deficiency

Myeloperoxidase (MPO) deficiency is the most common inherited disorder of phagocytes.[258] Complete deficiency is seen in approximately 1 in 4,000 individuals, and partial deficiency is even more common (1 in 2,000 persons).[27,259] The key features of MPO deficiency are summarized in Table 54-11. The disorder is inherited in an autosomal recessive[260–264] manner, although variable expression of the defect has been observed.[265] Acquired forms of MPO deficiency are also seen. Interestingly, the gene that encodes for MPO is located on chromosome 17 at q22-q23 near the breakpoint for the 15-17 translocation of promyelocytic leukemia.[266–269] Subpopulations of MPO-deficient cells can be seen not only in the M3 (promyelocytic) form of acute myeloid leukemia but also in the M2 and M4 forms.[27] MPO-deficient cells are also seen in approximately 25% of patients with chronic myeloid leukemia and myelodysplastic syndromes.[270–272]

A growing understanding of the molecular basis of congenital MPO deficiency has been made possible by the isolation of both cDNA and genomic clones for MPO[27,273–278] and gives us insights on how MPO gene expression is regulated.[279,280] In the few patients thus far studied, several different types of genetic lesions have been observed.[281,282] These generally appear to affect the post-translational processing of a precursor polypeptide for MPO (proMPO).[27,258,283,284] While the levels of MPO are

severely deficient in neutrophils and monocytes as a result of these mutations, the level of eosinophil peroxidase is normal in MPO-deficient patients, since it is encoded for by a separate gene.[285] (A series of 21 patients with eosinophil peroxidase deficiency has been reported.[286] As with MPO deficiency, these patients were asymptomatic.)

One of the most curious features of MPO deficiency is the remarkable lack of clinical symptoms in affected persons. As shown in Figure 54-1 (reaction 4), MPO catalyzes a key reaction—the production of a potent antimicrobial agent, HOCl.[22,287] HOCl in turn reacts with a variety of primary and secondary amines to form chloramines, some of which can be toxic. Moreover, HOCl is capable of activating latent metalloproteinases (e.g., collagenase) and inactivating antiproteinases.[22,27,28,258] Thus, one might predict that severe MPO deficiency would cripple important antimicrobial reactions catalyzed by hypochlorous acid. In vitro, an impressive defect in killing *Candida albicans* and hyphal forms of *Aspergillus fumigatus* is observed.[258,259,263] Bacterial killing in vitro is also abnormal (somewhat slower than normal), but eventually it is complete.[259–263,265,288] These in vitro abnormalities, however, are rarely manifested in patients, except for rare individuals who also suffer from diabetes mellitus.[259,260,263] In these individuals disseminated fungal infections (usually candidiasis) are seen.

The discrepancy between the in vitro and in vivo manifestations of MPO deficiency in most patients can be explained in several ways. First, the respiratory burst in MPO-deficient neutrophils is substantially augmented in terms of velocity and duration, presumably owing to the absence of the toxic effects of HOCl on NADPH oxidase.[27,29,258] Second, other products of the respiratory burst besides HOCl, together with the oxygen-independent antibacterial proteins, appear to have sufficient potency to compensate for the loss of MPO-dependent reactions.[27] Finally, residual amounts of MPO coupled with the normal levels of eosinophil peroxidase may provide at least some degree of peroxidative activity at the sites of infection.

Treatment is usually not required for MPO deficiency except in those individuals suffering from fungal infections. In these patients aggressive use of antifungal antibiotics is indicated. The prognosis is excellent in most patients with MPO deficiency.

DISORDERS OF PHAGOCYTE ADHESION AND CHEMOTAXIS

Since 1970 numerous investigators have found in vitro chemotactic abnormalities in neutrophils from patients suffering from a wide variety of clinical disorders associated with increased susceptibility to bacterial and fungal infections.[10,15,16] In most circumstances the chemotactic abnormality identified was only marginal and not always clearly related to the clinical status of the patient. In other instances, however, clear and major defects were identified in vitro that correlated with the in vivo propensity for infection. Extensive classification systems have been devised to categorize the numerous acquired defects in chemotaxis,[10] and several reviews are available on this subject.[10,15,289,290] The problem in many of these reports is that it is unclear whether the infections were caused by the in vitro chemotactic abnormality or by the multiple medical complications of the underlying disorder (e.g., acidosis, malnutrition, or exposure to nosocomial infections). A further complicating factor is that there are inherent limitations in the in vitro chemotaxis assays. Abnormal migration of purified neutrophils through filter discs in response to in vitro generated chemotactic gradients is difficult to quantify and is subject to laboratory artifacts. Furthermore, the extent to which these in vitro chemotactic assay systems faithfully reflect prevailing in vivo conditions is not known. Our understanding of chemotactic disorders has been hampered by the limitations of these assays,

Table 54-11. Summary of MPO Deficiency

Incidence	1 in 2,000 (partial deficiency)
	1 in 4,000 (total deficiency)
Inheritance	Autosomal recessive with variable expression; MPO gene on chromosome 17 at q22–q23
Molecular defect	Defective post-translational processing of an abnormal MPO precursor polypeptide due to at least four genetic lesions; eosinophil peroxidase encoded by a different gene and levels normal
Pathogenesis	Partial or complete MPO deficiency leads to diminished production of HOCl and HOCl-derived chloramines; MPO products are necessary for rapid killing of microbes (especially *Candida*) but not absolutely required
Clinical manifestations	Usually clinically silent
	Rarely, disseminated candidiasis/fungal disease (usually in conjunction with diabetes mellitus); acquired deficiency in M2, M3, and M4 acute myeloid leukemias (AML) and myelodysplasia
Laboratory evaluation	Deficiency of neutrophil/monocyte peroxidase by histochemical analysis (eosinophil peroxidase normal)
	Delayed, but eventually normal, killing of bacteria *in vitro*
	Failure to kill *C. albicans* and hyphal forms of *A. fumigatus* in vitro
Differential diagnosis	Acquired partial MPO deficiency seen in M2, M3, and M4 AML, and myelodysplastic syndromes
Therapy	None in asymptomatic patients
	Aggressive treatment of fungal infections when they occur
	Control of blood glucose levels in diabetics
Prognosis	Usually excellent

just as the elucidation of respiratory burst defects was obscured when the major available assay was in vitro bacterial killing. In this section the most important and best characterized of the chemotactic disorders, LAD, is discussed in detail. A brief discussion of several other clinically significant chemotactic disorders is also provided.

Leukocyte Adhesion Deficiency

Biology

LAD is a relatively rare disorder of leukocyte adhesion and chemotaxis that results in severe and sometimes fatal bacterial infections.[15,291–293] Approximately 20 patients were described in the literature in the 1970s who, in retrospect, probably had LAD and shared the clinical phenotype of recurrent infections, decreased neutrophil motility, and abnormal particle-stimulated respiratory burst activity.[291] Many also had persistent leukocytosis and delayed umbilical cord separation. The molecular basis for LAD was first suggested by Crowley and colleagues,[294] who found that neutrophils from a patient with this clinical syndrome lacked a high-molecular-weight membrane glycoprotein. The molecular weight was originally thought to be 110,000 but was subsequently found to be approximately 95,000. The variability was likely due to the erratic electrophoretic mobility of glycoproteins. The patient's neutrophils could not be made to adhere to plastic surfaces or to respond to serum-opsonized particles in terms of ingestion and respiratory burst activity.[294] It was hypothesized that the missing glycoprotein was responsible for cell-surface adhesion and for cell-particle interactions. Several other reports quickly followed, which described other patients in whom a similar glycoprotein was missing.[295,296] In 1984 it was found that the missing glycoprotein was actually a group of closely related glycoproteins (ranging from 95 kd [β_2 subunit] to 150–180 kd [three distinct α-subunits]) that form three types of $\alpha\beta$ heterodimers. The dominant heterodimer in phagocytes was designated Mol (or Mac-1)[297,298]; it functions as the C3bi receptor (CR3) of human neutrophils and monocytes.[298–302]

The molecular basis of LAD has now been proved to involve this group of three leukocyte glycoproteins, which are part of the integrin superfamily of adhesion molecules.[298,301–309] Integrins are noncovalently linked heterodimeric glycoproteins consisting of an α- and a β-subunit.[292] Within each of the eight known integrin subfamilies the β-subunit is identical (and defines the subfamily), while the α-subunit varies and confers the functional specificity on the integrin.[292,304,305] To date, a total of 22 distinct integrin subunits have been defined (14 α- and 8 β-chains) that give rise to about 20 different integrins; these integrins function as mediators of adhesion (cell-cell and cell-extracellular matrix) and receptors for C3bi and a group of coagulation factors (factor X, fibrinogen, and von Willebrand factor) (Table 54-12). The molecular defect in LAD involves all three members of the β_2 integrin subfamily: $\alpha_L\beta_2$ (CD11a/CD18), $\alpha_M\beta_2$ (CD11b/CD18), and $\alpha_X\beta_2$ (CD11c/CD18).[292,298,301,302] The molecular weights of these subunits are α_L, 180,000; α_M, 170,000; α_X, 150,000; and β_2, 95,000. CD11a/CD18 is often referred to as LFA-1, while CD11b/CD18 is called Mol or Mac-1. In the dozens of patients with LAD who have been studied thus far at the molecular level, an absent, diminished, or structurally abnormal β_2-subunit (CD18) has been identified. In the absence of a normal β-subunit, the three types of α-chains in the β_2 integrin subfamily cannot assemble into normal $\alpha\beta$ heterodimers. Thus, all three β_2 integrins are moderately to severely deficient in all leukocytes in LAD. As summarized in Table 54-12, the β_2 integrins serve as receptors for the opsonic complement fragment C3bi, the intercellular adhesion molecules-1 and -2, and fibrinogen.[292]

In all of the LAD patients reported to date who have been analyzed at the molecular genetic level, mutations have been identified in the gene encoding the β_2 (CD18) subunit. Mutations in the α-subunits have not been found thus far in patients with LAD. The gene encoding CD18 is located on the long arm of chromosome 21 at position q22.3 (the genes for β_2 integrin α-subunits are clustered on chromosome 16p11.1-p13).[310–317] CD18 is synthesized as a 747-amino acid polypeptide with a 22-amino acid signal sequence that is subsequently cleaved. The glycoprotein has a single transmembrane domain with a 46-residue cytoplasmic tail. Near the N terminus of the large extracellular domain is a stretch of 250 conserved amino acids, and it is in this region that most LAD mutations are found.[292,310,318–325] Table 54-13 summarizes the CD18 mutations found in LAD. As with X-linked CGD, LAD mutations are heterogeneous in nature, family specific, and can lead to either undetectable or low (9–20% of normal) levels of $\alpha\beta$ dimer expression that correlates with the clinical severity of the disease. Among the 12 different mutant alleles identified, there are 8 missense mutations, 2 splice defects, 1 interstitial deletion of 230 bp (patient 19), and 1 frameshift due to a single bp deletion (patient 18) (Table 54-13).

An example of a mutation leading to low levels of CD18 expression and a moderate clinical phenotype is patient 14. Two different missense mutations are present, one in the conserved region of the extracellular domain (Lys 196→Thr) and the other in a cysteine-rich area (Arg 593→Cys).[323] It is not clear which allele permits the expression of 10–20% normal levels of the β_2 integrins (or whether both do). A similar moderate phenotype is seen in the three related patients (8–11) in Table 54-13. These patients have a third-position mutation in a 5′ splice site (gtga→gtca) that results in aberrant splicing in 97% of the mRNA with the in-frame loss of 90 nucleotides.[319–321] The β_2-subunit precursor translated from this defective mRNA was abnormally small and apparently unable to associate normally with the α-subunit precursors. Roughly 3% of the CD18 mRNA, however, was found to be normally spliced and was probably responsible for the low level of $\alpha\beta$ dimer expression in the patient's leukocytes and the moderate phenotype. Severe LAD, with undetectable β_2 integrins, is seen in patient 18. The one mutant allele identified has a frameshift due to a single nucleotide deletion that predicts a premature stop codon and the loss of the last 56 amino acids that encompass the entire cytoplasmic domain and part of the transmembrane region.[324] Nor surprisingly, this mutation fails to permit the synthesis of $\alpha\beta$ dimers. The other mutant allele (not identified) must also have a severe mutation.

The diminished or absent expression of all three β_2 integrins in LAD leukocytes results in the failure of phagocytes to emigrate from the bloodstream to sites of infection.[307] The early stages of phagocyte-endothelial cell interactions, termed *rolling*, is mediated by selectins[326] and occurs normally in LAD.[307] It is the tight adherence of neutrophils and monocytes to cytokine-activated endothelium that is severely defective in LAD, since these interactions are mediated by the β_2 integrins. Transendothelial migration is also impaired. The other major functional defect in LAD is the failure of phagocytes to bind C3bi-opsonized microbes. Since CD11b/CD18 is the predominant C3bi receptor for the neutrophil, those phagocytic functions dependent on this opsonin receptor (i.e., C3bi-mediated ingestion, degranulation, and respiratory burst activity) are severely affected in LAD.[291–293] Thus, LAD neutrophils are not able to ingest and kill microbes opsonized with C3bi efficiently, a defect that contributes to the propensity of these patients to become infected. Despite the absence of CD11a/CD18, patients with LAD rarely have clinical manifestations of impaired lymphocyte function.[15,292] It is now believed that the role CD11a/CD18 plays in lymphoid cell function can be compensated by other adhesion proteins (CD2, CD4, CD8, and so forth).[292]

Table 54-12. Integrin Family of Adhesion Receptors[a]

Integrin Subunits β	α	Other Designations for the Integrin Complex	Ligands and Counter-receptors	Binding Site[b]	Cell Distribution of Integrin
β₁ (CD29)	α₁ (CD49a)	VLA-1	Collagens, LN	—	
	α₂ (CD49b)	VLA-2, GPIa/IIa	Collagens, LN	DGEA	
	α₃ (CD49c)	VLA-3	FN, LN, collagens	RGD (?)	
	α₄ (CD49d)	VLA-4	FN, VCAM-1	EILDV	
	α₅ (CD49e)	VLA-5, GPIc/IIa, FN receptor	FN	RGD	Fibroblasts
					Lymphocytes
					Platelets
	α₆ (CD49f)	VLA-6, GPIc/IIa	LN	—	Endothelium
	α₇	—	LN	—	Monocytes (VLA-4)
	α₈	—	?	—	
	αᵥ (CD51)	VN receptor-β₁	VN, FN (?)	RGD	
β₂ (CD18)	αL (CD11a)	LFA-1	ICAM-1 (CD54), ICAM-2	—	B cells, T cells, monocytes, macrophages, granulocytes, NK cells
	αM (CD11b)	Mac-1, Mol, CR3	C3bi, ICAM-1, Factor X, FB	—	Monocytes, macrophages, granulocytes, NK cells
	αx (CD11c)	p150,95 CR 4	FB, C3bi (?)	GPRP	Monocytes/macrophages, granulocytes, NK cells, some activated lymphocytes
β₃ (CD61)	αIIb (CD41b)	GPIIb/IIIa	FB, FN, vWF, VN, TSP	RGD	Platelets Endothelium
	αᵥ (CD51)	VN receptor-β₃	VN, FB, vWF, TSP, FN, collagen	RGD	Endothelium
β₄	α₆ (CD49f)	—	LN (?)	—	Epithelial cells
β₅	αᵥ (CD51)	VN receptor-β₅	VN	RGD	Epithelial cells
β₆	αᵥ (CD51)	—	FN	RGD	—
β₇	α₄ (CD49d)	—	FN, VCAM-1	EILDV	Lymphocytes
β₈	αᵥ (CD51)	—	?	—	—

Abbreviations: CR3 (and -4), complement receptor 3 (and 4); C3bi, complement fragment C3bi; FB, fibrinogen; FN, fibronectin; ICAM-1 (and -2), intercellular adhesion molecule-1 (and -2); LFA-1, lymphocyte function-related antigen-1; LN, laminin; NK, natural killer cells; TSP, thrombospondin; VCAM-1, vascular cell adhesion molecule-1; VLA, very late activation antigen; VN, vitronectin; vWF, von Willebrand factor.

[a] Data from references 292, and 303-309.

[b] Recognition sequences are given using the single-letter amino acid code.

(From Curnutte et al.,[430] with permission.)

Clinical Manifestations

The key features of LAD are summarized in Table 54-14. Approximately 60 patients have been described in the literature to date.[292] The mode of inheritance is autosomal recessive, consistent with the location of the CD18 gene on chromosome 21.[292,293] The clinical presentation of LAD is heterogeneous and is related to the severity of the deficiency of the β₂ integrins. The severe clinical phenotype is associated with <0.3% of the normal amount of these glycoproteins on the leukocyte surface, while the moderate phenotype has 2.5–6% of normal levels.[15,293] In both the severe and moderate forms of the disease, persistent granulocytosis (neutrophil count of 12,000–100,000/mm³) is a constant finding, as are recurrent cutaneous abscesses and periodontal infections and/or gingivitis.[15,291–293] Additional clinical features seen more often in the severe clinical phenotype include delayed umbilical cord separation, perirectal cellulitis, severe ulcerative stomatitis, and bacterial sepsis. Since neutrophils are unable to emigrate to tissues, abscesses and other sites of infections are devoid of pus despite the marked neutrophilia.

Diagnosis

The diagnosis of LAD is made by flow cytometric measurement of surface CD11b (or CD18) in unstimulated and stimulated neutrophils using monoclonal antibodies directed against CD11b (or CD18).[15,291] Neutrophils contain an intracellular pool of CD11b/CD18 in their secondary (specific) and tertiary granules, which can be mobilized to the cell surface during stimulation.[292,327,328] Therefore, the deficiency of CD11b can be more dramatically demonstrated by using stimulated neutrophils. Carriers of LAD can be identified by this method, since they have been found to express approximately 50% of normal levels of CD11b on the surface of their stimulated neutrophils.[293,327]

Therapy

Treatment for LAD depends on the clinical severity of the disorder. In those patients with the moderate clinical phenotype, cutaneous and oral infections can be managed as they occur. The use of prophylactic antibiotics such as trimethoprim sulfamethoxazole appears to be beneficial, as does aggressive prophylactic treatment of periodontal disease. It is important to note that even patients with the moderate phenotype can die of overwhelming infection, as evidenced in several recent reviews and by the absence of any known patients >40 years of age.[15,291–293] In patients with severe LAD, aggressive management is indicated because of the high incidence of death <2 years of age.[15,291,292] At present, bone marrow transplantation is recommended for these patients and has been reported to be successful in several cases.[291,319,329,330] In theory, LAD should be amenable to gene replacement therapy. The technical feasibility of this approach has now been demon-

Table 54-13. β_2-Subunit (CD18) Mutations in Leukocyte Adhesion Deficiency

Patient No.	Mutation Type[a]	mRNA Levels	Protein Expression		Clinical Severity	Mutations Identified[a]		References
			β Precursor	αβ Dimer		Nucleotide	Amino Acid Change[b]	
1–3	NR	0	0	0	Severe	Not reported		319, 320
4–7	NR	Low	0–trace	0–low	Moderate	Not reported		319, 320
8–11	Splice/ deletion (homozygous)	Normal	Abnormally small	Low	Moderate	g → c at position 3 of 5' splice site of intron following exon containing nt 1,066–1,155 causing 90 nt deletion in 97% of mRNA	30 AA deletion (residues 332–361)	319–321
12	NR	Normal	Abnormally large	0	Severe	Not identified; appears to cause an extra N-glycosylation site		319, 320
13	1) Missense 2) NR	Normal	Normal	0	Severe	1) G 577 → A 2) Not identified (? homozygous)	1) Gly 169 → Arg 2) Not expressed	322
14	1) Missense 2) Missense	Normal	Normal	10–20%	Moderate	1) A 659 → C 2) C 1,849 → T	1) Lys 196 → Thr 2) Arg 593 → Cys	323
15	1) Missense 2) NR	Normal	Normal	Low	Moderate	1) T 517 → C 2) Not identified (probably after nt 965)	1) Leu 149 → Pro 2) Not identified	322
16	1a) Splice/ insertion 1b) Missense 2) Missense	Normal	Normal	10–20%	Moderate	1a) c → a in intron 6 forming aberrant splice site and insertion of 12 nt after nt 813 1b) C 1,828 → T (? polymorphism) 2) A 1,124 → G	1a) In-frame insertion of PSSQ after Pro 247 1b) Arg 586 → Trp 2) Asn 351 → Ser	318
17	1) Missense 2) Deletion	Low	Low	9%	Moderate	1) T 74 → A (initiation codon) 2) Deletion T 2,142	1) Delete Met 1; low-level initiation at codon 2 (Leu) 2) Frameshift with premature stop codon predicting loss of last 56 AA	324
18	1) Deletion 2) NR	NR	NR	0	Severe	1) Deletion T 2,142 2) Not identified	1) Frameshift with premature stop codon predicting loss of last 56 AA 2) Not identified	324
19	1) Missense 2) Deletion	Normal	NR	NR	NR	1) C 605 → T 2) Deletion nt 1,729–1,959	1) Pro 170 → Leu 2) Loss of 78 AA (residues 553–630) and then frameshift	325

Abbreviations: 0, undetectable level; AA, amino acid; NR, not reported.
[a] The two alleles are indicated by numbers 1 and 2.
[b] Predicated from nucleotide change. Nucleotides are numbered according to Kishimoto et al.[310] beginning with the 5' end of the β_2 subunit cDNA.
(From Curnutte et al.,[430] with permission.)

strated by two groups using Epstein-Barr virus (EBV)-transformed lymphocyte lines from LAD patients.[331,332]

Actin Polymerization Defect Associated with Leukocyte Adhesion Deficiency

A subset of patients with severe LAD may suffer from an additional biochemical abnormality characterized by defective neutrophil actin polymerization.[333] An infant boy who suffered from extremely severe infections associated with profound defects in neutrophil chemotaxis/ingestion was described in 1974 by Boxer and colleagues.[334] The underlying defect appeared to reside in the neutrophil actin, since it failed to polymerize normally in vitro in response to 0.6 M KCl. This index patient was subsequently diagnosed as having LAD on the basis of intermediate levels of CD11b found in neutrophils from surviving family members. A 1989 report by Southwick et al.[333] has established that LAD is not generally associated with defective

actin filament assembly. In rare patients with LAD, however, actin polymerization is abnormal and presumably reflects a functional link between the cell-surface integrins and the cytoskeleton. There is good evidence that the cytoplasmic domains of the integrin α- and β-chains associate with cytoskeletal proteins such as talin, vinculin, and α-actinin.[305,335,336] Given the heterogeneity of the mutations in LAD (Table 54-13), it is possible that only certain types of mutations lead to an associated defect in actin function.

Leukocyte Adhesion Deficiency Due to a Deficiency in Sialated-Lewis[X] Moieties (LADII)

A clinical syndrome closely related to LAD, but caused by a defect in selectin-mediated adhesion events, has been reported in two unrelated boys of Moslem Arab origin and has been termed LADII.[337] The disease appears to be inherited in an autosomal recessive manner since both patients were products of

Table 54-14. Summary of Leukocyte Adhesion Deficiency

Incidence	Approximately 60 patients described in literature
Inheritance	Autosomal recessive
Molecular defect	An absent, diminished, or structurally abnormal β-subunit (CD18) caused by one of several types of mutations in the β-gene; in the absence of a normal β-subunit, the three types of α-chains in the β₂ integrin subfamily (CD11a,-b,-c) cannot assemble into normal αβ heterodimers
Pathogenesis	All three β₂ integrins (CD11a/CD18, CD11b/CD18, and CD11c/CD18) are deficient on all leukocytes, causing multiple abnormalities in cell function: adherence, chemotaxis, and C3bi-mediated ingestion/degranulation/respiratory burst
Clinical manifestation	Persistent granulocytosis (neutrophil count of 12,000–100,000/mm³) Severe or moderate phenotypes depending on severity of deficiency Recurrent pyogenic infections with absent neutrophil infiltration Delayed umbilical cord separation Severe gingivitis/periodonitis
Laboratory evaluation	Flow cytometric measurements of surface CD11b (or CD18) in stimulated neutrophils with monoclonal anti-CD11b (or CD18)
Differential diagnosis	CGD May be associated with severe neutrophil actin dysfunction
Therapy	Bone marrow transplant in clinically severe patients (CD11b <0.3% of normal) Aggressive use of parenteral antibiotics Possible benefit of prophylactic trimethoprim sulfamethoxazole
Prognosis	Severe: high incidence of death before 2 years Moderate: can survive into twenties and thirties but with recurrent infections

consanguineous matings. Like LAD patients, the patients had marked neutrophilia, recurrent bacterial infections, and periodontitis yet their neutrophils expressed normal levels of CD18. A clue as to the molecular cause of LADII came from the observation that the patients had the rare Bombay (hh) erythrocyte phenotype and were Lewis antigen negative as well. These antigenic defects share in common the failure to form certain fucose carbohydrate linkages, raising the possibility that the patients had a generalized defect in fucose metabolism leading not only to the erythrocyte defects, but also to a failure to synthesize critical sialated-Lewis^X moieties on E-selectin and P-selectin counter-receptors on neutrophils. As predicted, neutrophils from both boys were devoid of immunoreactive sialated-Lewis^X structures and were unable to adhere to human umbilical cord endothelial cells activated with interleukin-1β to induce E-selectin expression. The precise defect in fucose metabolism is still under investigation.

Hyperimmunoglobulin E Syndrome

Biology

The hyperimmunoglobulin E syndrome is a complex disorder characterized by markedly elevated serum IgE levels, serious recurrent infections, and chronic dermatitis.[11,338–342] While technically not a phagocyte defect per se, neutrophils from patients with this syndrome exhibit a variable and at times profound chemotactic defect.[11,338,339,343–345] Therefore, this disorder is briefly reviewed in this chapter. The hyper-IgE syndrome was first described in 1966 and was called Job syndrome, in reference to the biblical description of Job who was afflicted with "sore boils from the soles of his feet unto his crown."[338] The skin abscesses in patients with hyper-IgE syndrome lack the erythema typical of such lesions and are referred to as cold abscesses. The key features of the hyperimmunoglobulin E syndrome are described in Table 54-15.

The disease is extremely rare and its mode of inheritance has not been firmly established, although familial occurrence has been noted.[11,339,341] Both males and females have been affected, which suggests autosomal inheritance. The molecular basis for the syndrome is not known. The extremely high serum IgE level is believed to reflect a T-lymphocyte imbalance, leading to abnormal regulation of IgE production, as well as decreased production of IFN-γ and tumor necrosis factor.[11,342,346–348] Further evidence for a more broad-based immune disorder is the finding that hyper-IgE patients mount abnormal antibody responses to vaccines.[349] The recurrent bacterial infections are thought to arise by two mechanisms: (1) excessive production of IgE directed against *S. aureus* that occurs at the expense of protective antistaphylococcal IgG[350]; and (2) a variable neutrophil chemotactic defect that occurs independently of fluctuations in the serum IgE level.[11,351,352] The underlying T-cell defect may be responsible for this chemotactic defect, as it may cause the release of chemotactic inhibitors from mononuclear cells.[11]

Clinical Manifestations

The clinical manifestations of the hyper-IgE syndrome are at times dramatic.[11] Onset is generally in the first 2 months of life and is manifested by chronic dermatitis. By 5 years of age,

Table 54-15. Summary of Hyper-IgE Syndrome

Incidence	Approximately 50 cases have been reviewed in the literature; single institution series of 6, 13, and 23 cases have been described
Inheritance	Autosomal (? dominant) with incomplete penetrance
Molecular defect	Unknown; putative T-lymphocyte defect, in part manifested by diminished production of IFN-γ, which affects regulation of IgE production as well as other immune functions
Pathogenesis	The following may contribute to the increased risk of infection: high levels of antistaphylococcal IgE and low levels of antistaphylococcal IgG; fluctuating neutrophil chemotactic defect possibly due to an inhibitor from mononuclear cells; poor antibody response in some patients
Clinical manifestations	Staphylococcal pneumonia Pneumatoceles Fungal superinfection of lung cysts "Cold" cutaneous skin abscesses and furuncles Chronic eczematoid dermatitis Mucocutaneous candidiasis Course facies, growth retardation, osteopenia Sinusitis, keratoconjunctivitis
Laboratory evaluation	Serum IgE >2,500 IU/ml Peripheral blood eosinophilia
Differential diagnosis	Atopic dermatitis Wiskott-Aldrich syndrome, DiGeorge syndrome Hypergammaglobulinemia CGD
Therapy	Prophylactic anti-*S. aureus* antibiotics Aggressive treatment of acute infections with parenteral antibiotics Surgical drainage of deep infections and resection of lung cysts Plasmapheresis in severe cases (experimental) IFN-γ (experimental)
Prognosis	Generally good if managed aggressively Some patients develop lymphoid malignancies

patients have a history of recurrent skin abscesses, pneumonias, chronic otitis media, and sinusitis. As patients grow older, recurrent staphylococcal pneumonia is a common problem and can be complicated by the formation of pneumatoceles.[353,354] Septic arthritis, cellulitis, and osteomyelitis are also observed with the offending microbe, usually *S. aureus*, although other bacterial pathogens have also been found. Patients can have chronic mucocutaneous candidiasis and occasionally exhibit keratoconjunctivitis, sometimes complicated by corneal scarring. Osteopenia of unknown etiology is observed in most patients and results in increased risk of fractures to the long bones and vertebral bodies.[341] One feature noted in most patients is the presence of coarse facial features (broad nasal bridge, prominent nose).

Diagnosis

The diagnosis of hyper-IgE syndrome should be entertained in any child or young adult who has the clinical picture described above or simply a history of recurrent infections. The hallmark laboratory finding is a marked elevation of serum IgE, almost always >2,500 IU/ml.[11] Levels can be as high as 150,000 IU/ml.[11] Despite the impressive elevations in serum IgE seen in the syndrome, this laboratory finding alone is not diagnostic, since comparably high serum levels of IgE can be seen in patients with atopic dermatitis.[11] Since many patients with this latter disorder are also afflicted with eczema and superficial skin infections, atopic dermatitis must be considered in the differential diagnosis of hyper-IgE syndrome. The two can be distinguished because of the severe and recurrent nature of the staphylococcal furuncles and pneumonias seen in hyper-IgE syndrome. Patients with other primary immunodeficiency syndromes such as CGD may also manifest elevated IgE levels[11] (Table 54-15).

Therapy

The therapy for hyper-IgE syndrome is largely supportive as there is no known curative treatment. Prophylactic antibiotics (e.g., dicloxacillin or trimethoprim sulfamethoxazole) can be effective in preventing *S. aureus* infections.[11] Dermatitis can be treated with topical steroids. Intravenous antibiotics are used for deep-seated infections or for resistant cutaneous infections. Surgical resection of persistent pneumatoceles is sometimes indicated to prevent superinfection by fungal and gram-negative organisms. Plasmapheresis has been reported to be effective in treating patients who have not responded to the above-mentioned therapies.[11]

Treatment of hyper-IgE syndrome with recombinant human IFN-γ has been investigated based on the observations that this cytokine can suppress the synthesis of IgE[355,356] and that IFN-γ production in this disease is diminished.[346,347] In uncontrolled studies, patients treated with IFN-γ (50 μg/m² SC thrice weekly) reported that they felt better; they also exhibited improved in vitro chemotaxis[357,358] and occasional decreases in IgE levels.[359] In light of the results observed with IFN-γ in CGD discussed above, there may be a role for IFN-γ in preventing infections in hyper-IgE syndrome.

Miscellaneous Chemotactic Disorders

One of the most consistently observed chemotactic abnormalities is seen in neonatal neutrophils.[15,289,358,360–364] These cells exhibit impaired chemotaxis in vitro in response to a wide variety of chemotactic factors.[15] This abnormality may be partly due to defects in cellular adhesion as a result of diminished mobilization of intracellular adhesion-promoting molecules to the cell surface.[10,360,365] Defective neutrophil chemotaxis can be seen in normal neonates between birth and 5 days of age.[15] In severely ill infants, the defect may persist for a

longer time. As with hyper-IgE syndrome, IFN-γ may be helpful, as this cytokine has been found to increase the chemotactic activity of neonate neutrophils in vitro.[358,362]

Localized juvenile periodontitis (LJP) is a heterogeneous disorder of unknown etiology characterized by chronic and recurrent periodontal infections and severe alveolar bone loss with onset at the time of puberty. Nearly three-fourths of patients with LJP have been reported to have defective neutrophil chemotaxis in vitro.[15,366–374] The molecular basis for the chemotactic defect is poorly understood. A number of reports suggest that cellular products derived from certain periodontal bacteria can alter leukocyte function and may be responsible for the diminished chemotactic activity.[375,376] These inhibitors cannot entirely explain the disorder, however, since neutrophils from patients with LJP exhibit abnormal chemotaxis in vitro even in the presence of normal serum.[15,367,368,370,371] At present it appears that LJP is an acquired disorder in some patients and a genetic disorder in others. It may also be a combination of both in certain patients, as they may inherit an unusual sensitivity to the chemotactic inhibitors released by certain periodontal microorganisms. The diagnosis of the disorder is made on the basis of severe periodontal disease and destructive alveolar bone loss involving the first molars and incisors developing during adolescence. It is important to note that many qualitative and quantitative neutrophil disorders are also associated with severe periodontal disease.[15,377] Therefore, the differential diagnosis should include neutropenia (both chronic and cyclic), LAD, CGD, and Chédiak-Higashi syndrome.

DEFECTS IN THE STRUCTURE AND FUNCTION OF LYSOSOMAL GRANULES

Two major disorders of neutrophil granules have been described: Chédiak-Higashi syndrome and specific granule deficiency. While the molecular lesions responsible for both have

Table 54-16. Summary of Chédiak-Higashi Syndrome

Incidence	Approximately 200 cases described
Inheritance	Autosomal recessive
Molecular defect	A putative defect in granule morphogenesis resulting in abnormally large granules in multiple tissues
Pathogenesis	Giant coalesced azurophil/specific granules in neutrophils, resulting in ineffective granulopoiesis and neutropenia, delayed and incomplete degranulation, and defective chemotaxis
Clinical manifestations	Partial oculocutaneous albinism Recurrent severe bacterial infections (usually *S. aureus*) Cranial and peripheral neuropathies (muscle weakness, ataxia, sensory loss) Hepatosplenomegaly and complications of pancytopenia in the accelerated phase
Laboratory evaluation	Giant granules in peripheral blood granulocytes and in bone marrow myeloid progenitor cells Widespread lymphohistiocytic infiltrates in accelerated phase
Differential diagnosis	Other genetic forms of partial albinism Giant granules can be seen in acute and chronic myelogenous leukemias
Therapy	Prophylactic trimethoprim sulfamethoxazole Parenteral antibiotics for acute infections Ascorbic acid (200 mg/day for infants; 6 g/day for adults) Bone marrow transplant at beginning of accelerated phase
Prognosis	Most patients die from infection or complications of the accelerated phase during the first or second decade of life; a few patients have survived into their thirties

yet to be identified, a great deal has been learned about the structural and functional abnormalities of neutrophils from patients with these conditions. Both disorders are exceedingly rare but are obligatory components in the differential diagnosis for any patient with recurrent bacterial/fungal infections.

Chédiak-Higashi Syndrome

Biology

The Chédiak-Higashi syndrome is a rare autosomal recessive, multisystem disease characterized by partial oculocutaneous albinism, frequent (and sometimes fatal) bacterial infections, giant lysosomes in leukocytes, a mild bleeding diathesis, and peripheral as well as cranial neuropathies associated with decussation defects at the optic chiasm.[10,12,378–381] Giant granules are also present in melanosomes, Schwann cells, and certain cells in the liver, kidney, and spleen.[381] Those who survive the recurrent infections develop an "accelerated phase" of the disease—a progressive lymphoproliferative syndrome that is eventually fatal due to the profound pancytopenia that develops.[10,379]

The underlying molecular disorder in Chédiak-Higashi syndrome is not known. The presence of dysmorphic granules in multiple tissues suggests an underlying global defect in granule morphogenesis.[15,379–387] The oculocutaneous albinism characteristic of Chédiak-Higashi syndrome, for example, is caused by imperfect pigment dilution in melanocytes due to the giant melanosomes.[379] The most dramatic lysosomal defects, however, are manifested in the various blood cells. Phagocytes contain a highly inhomogeneous population of giant granules,[388] which appear to be derived from both azurophilic and specific granules.[382,383,389,390] Certain granule constituents such as cathepsin G and elastase are surprisingly absent,[147] providing further evidence for an underlying defect in granule mor-

phogenesis. The giant granules are often more prominent in the bone marrow than in the peripheral blood, since many of the abnormal myeloid precursors are apparently destroyed before they leave the marrow, resulting in moderate neutropenia with white blood counts ranging from 2,000 to 3,000 cells/mm^3.[379,391] The neutropenia also contributes to the propensity of Chédiak-Higashi patients to develop infections, although it is not the only cause. Phagocyte function is also impaired. Not surprisingly, degranulation is delayed and incomplete in Chédiak-Higashi neutrophils.[392–395] Moreover, chemotaxis is defective, perhaps owing to the presence of the giant granules, which interfere with the ability of the phagocyte to travel through narrow passages (e.g., between endothelial cells).[378,396] Making matters worse, the granules are markedly deficient in antimicrobial proteins such as cathepsin G.[147] Monocytes and macrophages exhibit similar giant cytoplasmic granules,[389] with resultant abnormalities in their phagocytic functions.[12] Giant granules are also seen in lymphocytes and are associated with diminished antibody-dependent cell-mediated cytolysis of tumor cells.[397–399] Natural killer cell function is also markedly abnormal in Chédiak-Higashi syndrome.[397] Eosinophils contain large granules, the functional significance of which is not known.[400] Platelets in this disorder have a storage pool deficiency of ADP and serotonin, presumably due to the abnormal granule morphogenesis in the megakaryocytes,[387,401–404] leading to a defect in platelet aggregation that manifests as easy bruising and epistaxis.

Clinical Manifestations

The key features of Chédiak-Higashi syndrome are summarized in Table 54-16. The disease usually manifests in infancy or early childhood, with infections involving the lungs, skin, and mucous membranes being most commonly encoun-

CLINICAL APPROACH TO PATIENTS WITH DISORDERS OF PHAGOCYTE FUNCTION

All the disorders of granulocyte function discussed in this chapter present with recurrent bacterial and fungal infections. The major diagnostic problem faced by the clinician is that patients with recurrent bacterial and fungal infections seldom have an identifiable granulocyte or monocyte defect. Given this low yield and the relative unavailability of laboratories capable of evaluating phagocyte defects, the physician is faced with the difficult question of deciding which patients with recurrent infections merit a complete evaluation. An excellent discussion of this problem has been published by Johnston.[17] Guidelines are not well defined, and the following comments should be viewed as suggestions.

Our approach at Scripps Clinic is to consider four aspects of each patient's infection history: frequency, severity, location, and responsible pathogen. When considering frequency, the patient's age and associated medical conditions must be taken into account. For example, recurrent otitis media in a 2-year-old patient is far less worrisome than a similar history in a 40-year-old patient. Another recommendation is that the more unusual the infection, the less frequently it has to occur before a phagocyte evaluation is indicated (see below). Similarly, as few as two or three infections of unusual severity might warrant an evaluation. Infections in unexpected anatomic locations should also alert the clinician to a possible underlying immune disorder. Hepatic, pulmonary, and rectal abscesses, as well as disseminated candidal infections, may be indicative of an underlying phagocyte defect. Finally, the identification of certain pathogens (e.g., *S. marcescens*, *Aspergillus* spp., *Nocardia* spp., and *Pseudomonas cepacia*) in children and young adults can provide the strongest indications for pursuing further studies. Certain unusual clinical findings can also be helpful in determining which patients warrant further testing. For example, an infant with a history of delayed separation of the umbilical cord who has also had several bouts of pneumonia should be evaluated for LAD, and a child with nystagmus, fair skin, and recurrent staphylococcal infections should be evaluated for Chédiak-Higashi syndrome.

Once the physician has decided that a phagocyte evaluation is warranted, what is the appropriate sequence of tests to perform? A useful algorithm is presented below for approaching patients with recurrent infections regardless of the immune defect responsible. The algorithm should be used in conjunction with the published literature relevant to these disorders, and each laboratory finding must always be interpreted in the clinical context of the patient under examination. Not shown in the algorithm are tests for HIV infection, an important element in the differential diagnosis of a patient with recurrent or unusual infections.*

---

* (From Lehrer et al.,[18] with permission.)

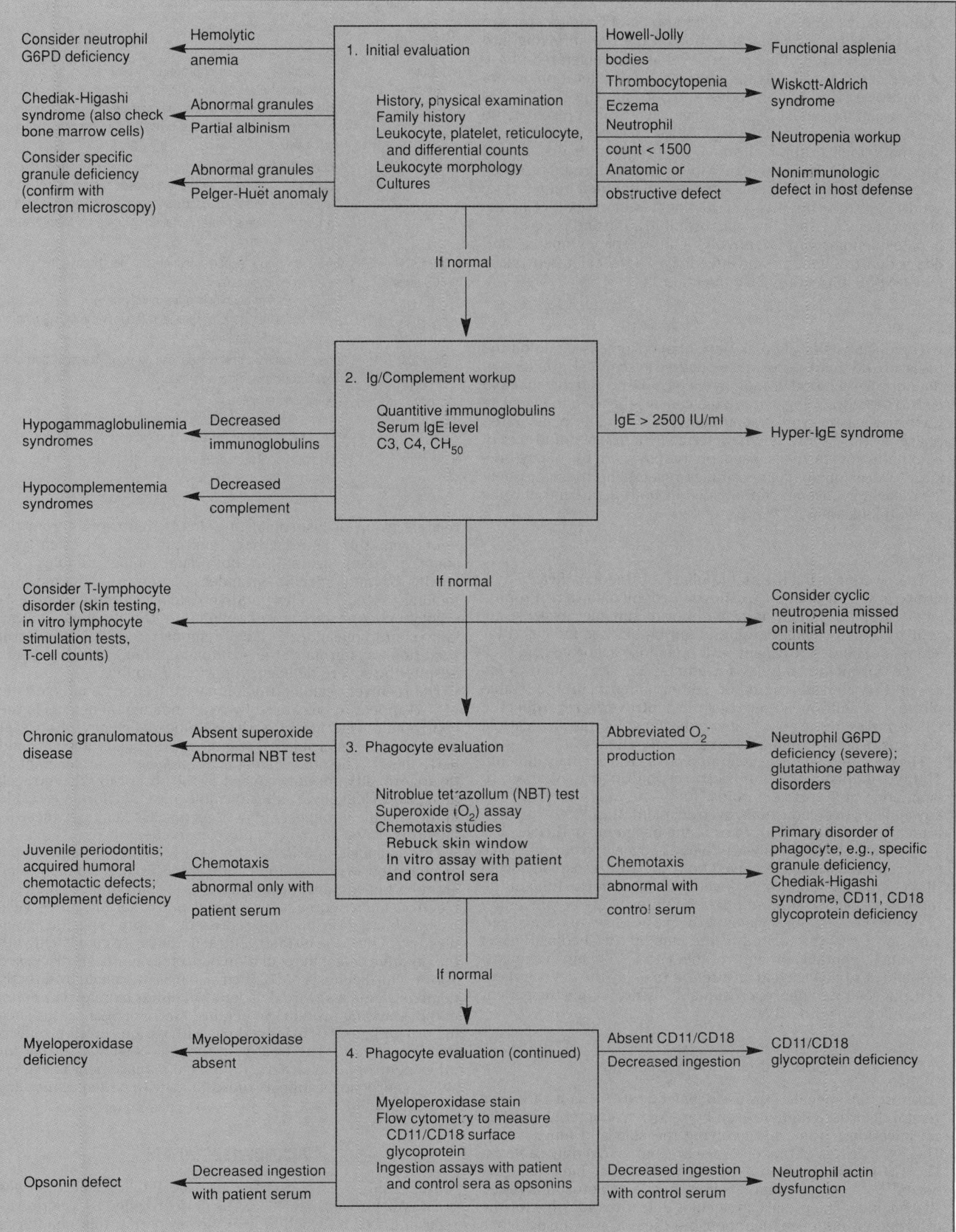

Consider neutrophil G6PD deficiency ← Hemolytic anemia — **1. Initial evaluation** — Howell-Jolly bodies → Functional asplenia

1. Initial evaluation

- History, physical examination
- Family history
- Leukocyte, platelet, reticulocyte, and differential counts
- Leukocyte morphology
- Cultures

Chediak-Higashi syndrome (also check bone marrow cells) ← Abnormal granules / Partial albinism

Consider specific granule deficiency (confirm with electron microscopy) ← Abnormal granules / Pelger-Huët anomaly

Thrombocytopenia / Eczema → Wiskott-Aldrich syndrome

Neutrophil count < 1500 → Neutropenia workup

Anatomic or obstructive defect → Nonimmunologic defect in host defense

If normal

2. Ig/Complement workup

- Quantitive immunoglobulins
- Serum IgE level
- C3, C4, CH$_{50}$

Hypogammaglobulinemia syndromes ← Decreased immunoglobulins

Hypocomplementemia syndromes ← Decreased complement

IgE > 2500 IU/ml → Hyper-IgE syndrome

If normal

Consider T-lymphocyte disorder (skin testing, in vitro lymphocyte stimulation tests, T-cell counts) ← → Consider cyclic neutropenia missed on initial neutrophil counts

3. Phagocyte evaluation

- Nitroblue tetrazollum (NBT) test
- Superoxide (O$_2$) assay
- Chemotaxis studies
  - Rebuck skin window
  - In vitro assay with patient and control sera

Chronic granulomatous disease ← Absent superoxide / Abnormal NBT test

Juvenile periodontitis; acquired humoral chemotactic defects; complement deficiency ← Chemotaxis abnormal only with patient serum

Abbreviated O$_2^-$ production → Neutrophil G6PD deficiency (severe); glutathione pathway disorders

Chemotaxis abnormal with control serum → Primary disorder of phagocyte, e.g., specific granule deficiency, Chediak-Higashi syndrome, CD11, CD18 glycoprotein deficiency

If normal

4. Phagocyte evaluation (continued)

- Myeloperoxidase stain
- Flow cytometry to measure CD11/CD18 surface glycoprotein
- Ingestion assays with patient and control sera as opsonins

Myeloperoxidase deficiency ← Myeloperoxidase absent

Opsonin defect ← Decreased ingestion with patient serum

Absent CD11/CD18 / Decreased ingestion → CD11/CD18 glycoprotein deficiency

Decreased ingestion with control serum → Neutrophil actin dysfunction

tered.[379] The most frequent offending organism is *S. aureus.*[12] Gram-negative bacteria, *Aspergillus* spp., and *Candida* spp. are also responsible for many infections. Children surviving into the second decade of life often develop an accelerated phase of the disease in which lymphohistiocytic proliferation occurs in the liver, spleen, lymph nodes, and bone marrow.[379,384] Occasionally children with Chédiak-Higashi syndrome present in the accelerated phase. The cellular infiltration is not neoplastic by histopathologic criteria, although the prognosis is dismal—all patients die unless curative therapy is administered. The accelerated phase resembles the virus-associated hemophagocytic syndrome, since the invading histiocytes often exhibit hemophagocytosis.[384] The bone marrow infiltration and progressive hepatosplenomegaly eventually lead to pancytopenia and death due to infection and bleeding. The accelerated phase may be precipitated by EBV infection.[405]

Diagnosis

The diagnosis of Chédiak-Higashi syndrome is made on the basis of the giant peroxidase-positive lysosomal granules in the peripheral blood granulocytes or in bone marrow myeloid cells. This morphologic approach can also be used to diagnose Chédiak-Higashi syndrome prenatally.[406,407] The accelerated phase of the disease is characterized by diffuse infiltrates of lymphohistiocytic cells seen on biopsy and by pancytopenia.[384] Occasionally giant granules resembling those of Chédiak-Higashi syndrome can be seen in both acute and chronic myeloid leukemias.[408–410]

Therapy

The treatment for the stable phase of Chédiak-Higashi syndrome is similar to that for other neutrophil disorders. Prophylactic antibiotics such as trimethoprim sulfamethoxazole appear to be beneficial. Parenteral antibiotics are indicated for acute infections. Treatment with high-dose ascorbic acid (200 mg/day for infants, 6 g/day for adults) has been found to improve the clinical status of some patients in the stable phase.[411,412] Although there is some controversy regarding the efficacy of ascorbic acid,[413] given the safety of this medication, it seems prudent to administer it to all patients.

The treatment of the accelerated phase is extremely difficult. The lymphohistiocytic infiltrates respond poorly, if at all, to vincristine and corticosteroids.[379,384] The only curative therapy appears to be bone marrow transplantation,[12,414–418] which is ideally performed prior to or at the beginning of the accelerated phase. Six patients with Chédiak-Higashi syndrome have been reported to have received bone marrow transplants from HLA-compatible donors; five were still alive at the time of the reports.[12] The accelerated phase could possibly be prevented or delayed by vaccines against EBV.[12] The onset of the accelerated phase may be related to the inability of Chédiak-Higashi patients to contain and control this virus.[384,405] Intravenous γ-globulin has been used in an attempt to delay the development of the accelerated phase, presumably by protecting the patient from infection with EBV.

Specific Granule Deficiency

Neutrophil-specific granule deficiency (SGD) is a rare congenital disorder characterized by recurrent bacterial and fungal infections, primarily involving the skin and lungs.[12,15,419] The key features of this disorder are summarized in Table 54-17. SGD is quite rare, but the five cases that have been reported[419–421] suggest that it is inherited in an autosomal recessive manner. The precise molecular defect responsible for the disorder has not been identified, but there is growing evidence of an abnormality in the regulation of the synthesis of a closely

Table 54-17. Summary of Neutrophil Specific Granule Deficiency

Incidence	Five cases reported
Inheritance	Autosomal recessive
Molecular defect	Deficiencies in lysosomal proteins in both azurophil granules (defensins) and specific granules (lactoferrin, vitamin B_{12}-binding protein) suggest a common defect in the regulation of the production of these proteins; the precise defect is unknown.
Pathogenesis	Recurrent infections result from the combined effect of deficiencies in microbicidal granule proteins, such as defensins and lactoferrin, and abnormal chemotaxis, perhaps due to a failure to up-regulate surface β_2 integrins from specific granule stores
Laboratory evaluation	Absent or empty specific granules in neutrophils by light or electron microscopy Bilobed nuclei in neutrophils frequently seen Severe deficiency of neutrophil lactoferrin, vitamin B_{12}-binding protein, and defensins
Differential diagnosis	Acquired specific granule deficiency (e.g., thermal burns or myeloproliferative syndromes)
Therapy	Prophylactic antibiotics Parenteral antibiotics for acute infections Surgical drainage of refractory infections
Prognosis	With appropriate medical management, patients can survive into their adult years

related group of lysosomal proteins.[12] Neutrophils from patients with this disorder have multiple deficiencies in lysosomal proteins present in both azurophilic granules (defensins)[147] and specific granules (lactoferrin, vitamin B_{12}-binding protein).[421] The putative defect in protein synthesis regulation appears to be confined to the myeloid lineage. Lomax and colleagues[422] have demonstrated that lactoferrin secretion was normal in the glandular epithelia of SGD patients despite the severe deficiency in the neutrophils.

The recurrent skin and pulmonary infections characteristic of SGD appear to be caused by two fundamental defects in the neutrophils. One defect is the marked deficiency of at least two important microbicidal granule proteins, lactoferrin[421] and defensins.[147] The other defect is a relatively severe chemotactic abnormality possibly caused by the absence of the intracellular pool of leukocyte adhesion molecules that normally reside in the specific granules.[420,423–425] As discussed above, these β_2 integrins play a key role in phagocyte chemotaxis.

The diagnosis of SGD can be readily made by microscopic examination. Wright-stained neutrophils are devoid of specific granules but contain normal numbers of azurophilic granules.[12] Electron microscopy reveals small peroxidase-negative vesicles, which presumably represent empty specific granules.[12,426] Thus, the ultrastructural findings are consistent with the putative defect in regulation of protein synthesis discussed above. The diagnosis of SGD can also be established by directly demonstrating a severe deficiency in either lactoferrin or vitamin B_{12}-binding protein. An acquired form of SGD can be seen in burn patients[12] or in individuals with various myeloproliferative disorders.[427] The treatment for SGD is similar to that for other neutrophil disorders. If medical management is aggressive, the prognosis appears quite good, with patients surviving into their adult years.

ACKNOWLEDGMENTS

This study was supported by U.S. Public Health Service grants AI24838 and RR00833. The help provided by Valerie Moreau and Deborah Schiff, M.D., in preparing this chapter is gratefully acknowledged.

REFERENCES

1. Gabay JE, Scott RW, Campanelli D et al: Antibiotic proteins of human polymorphonuclear leukocytes. Proc Natl Acad Sci USA 86:5610, 1989
2. Lehrer RI, Ganz T, Selsted ME: Oxygen-independent bactericidal systems: mechanisms and disorders. Hematol Oncol Clin North Am 2:159, 1988
3. Lehrer RI, Ganz T, Selsted ME: Defensins: endogenous antibiotic peptides of animal cells. Cell 64:229, 1991
4. Spitznagel JK: Antibiotic proteins of human neutrophils. J Clin Invest 86:1381, 1990
5. Lehrer RI, Ganz T: Antimicrobial polypeptides of human neutrophils. Blood 76:2169, 1990
6. Elsbach P, Weiss J: Oxygen-independent antimicrobial systems of phagocytes. p. 603. In Gallin JI, Goldstein IM, Snyderman R (eds): Inflammation: Basic Principles and Clinical Correlates. 2nd Ed. Raven Press, New York, 1992
7. Tauber AI, Borregaard N, Simons E et al: Chronic granulomatous disease: a syndrome of phagocyte oxidase deficiencies. Medicine 62:286, 1983
8. Malech HL, Gallin JI: Current concepts: immunology. Neutrophils in human diseases. N Engl J Med 317:687, 1987
9. Lomax KJ, Malech HL, Gallin JI: The molecular biology of selected phagocyte defects. Blood Rev 3:94, 1989
10. Brown CC, Gallin JI: Chemotactic disorders. Hematol Oncol Clin North Am 2:61, 1988
11. Leung DYM, Geha RS: Clinical and immunologic aspects of the hyperimmunoglobulin E syndrome. Hematol Oncol Clin North Am 2:81, 1988
12. Boxer LA, Smolen JE: Neutrophil granule constituents and their release in health and disease. Hematol Oncol Clin North Am 2:101, 1988
13. Whitin JC, Cohen HJ: Disorders of respiratory burst termination. Hematol Oncol Clin North Am 2:289, 1988
14. Forehand JR, Nauseef WM, Johnston RB Jr: Inherited disorders of phagocyte killing. p. 2779. In Scriver CR, Beaudet AL, Sly WS, Valle D (eds): The Metabolic Basis of Inherited Disease. 6th Ed. McGraw-Hill, New York, 1989
15. Anderson DC, Smith CW, Springer TA: Leukocyte adhesion deficiency and other disorders of leukocyte motility. p. 2751. In Scriver CR, Beaudet AL, Sly WS, Valle D (eds): The Metabolic Basis of Inherited Disease. 6th Ed. McGraw-Hill, New York, 1989
16. Gallin JI: Disorders of phagocytic cells. p. 859. In Gallin JI, Goldstein IM, Snyderman R (eds): Inflammation: Basic Principles and Clinical Correlates. 2nd Ed. Raven Press, New York, 1992
17. Johnston RB: Recurrent bacterial infections in children. N Engl J Med 310:1237, 1984
18. Lehrer RI, Ganz T, Selsted ME et al: Neutrophils and host defense. Ann Intern Med 109:127, 1988
19. Malech HL: Phagocyte oxidative mechanisms. Curr Opin Hematol 123, 1993
20. Rotrosen D, Gallin JI: Disorders of phagocyte function. Annu Rev Immunol 5:127, 1987
21. Sbarra AJ, Karnovsky ML: The biochemical basis of phagocytosis. I. Metabolic changes during the ingestion of particles by polymorphonuclear leukocytes. J Biol Chem 234:1355, 1959
22. Curnutte JT, Babior BM: Chronic granulomatous disease. p. 229. In Harris H, Hirschhorn K (eds): Advances in Human Genetics. Plenum, New York, 1987
23. Curnutte JT, Babior BM: Effects of anaerobiosis and inhibitors of O_2^- production by human granulocytes. Blood 45:851, 1975
24. Curnutte JT, Tauber AI: Failure to detect superoxide in human neutrophils stimulated with latex particles. Pediatr Res 17:281, 1983
25. Babior BM: The respiratory burst oxidase. Adv Enzymol 65:49, 1992
26. Beutler E: Glucose-6-phosphate dehydrogenase: new perspectives. Blood 73:1397, 1989
27. Nauseef WM: Myeloperoxidase deficiency. Hematol Oncol Clin North Am 2:135, 1988
28. Weiss SJ: Tissue destruction by neutrophils. N Engl J Med 320:365, 1989
29. Cohen HJ, Tape EH, Novak J et al: The role of glutathione reductase in maintaining human granulocyte function and sensitivity of exogenous H_2O_2. Blood 69:493, 1987
30. Smith RM, Curnutte JT: Molecular basis of chronic granulomatous disease. Blood 77:673, 1991
31. Curnutte JT: Molecular basis of the autosomal recessive forms of chronic granulomatous disease. Immunodefic Rev 3:149, 1992
32. Curnutte JT: Disorders of granulocyte function and granulopoiesis. p. 904. In Nathan DG, Oski FA (eds): Hematology of Infancy and Childhood. 4th Ed. WB Saunders, Philadelphia, 1992
33. Babior BM, Woodman RC: Chronic granulomatous disease. Semin Hematol 27:247, 1990
34. Dinauer MC, Orkin SH: Chronic granulomatous disease. Annu Rev Med 43:117, 1992
35. Bohler M-C, Seger RA, Mouy R et al: A study of 25 patients with chronic granulomatous disease: a new classification by correlating respiratory burst, cytochrome b, and flavoprotein. J Clin Immunol 6:136, 1986
36. Forrest CB, Forehand JR, Axtell RA et al: Clinical features and current management of chronic granulomatous disease. Hematol Oncol Clin North Am 2:253, 1988
37. Berendes H, Bridges RA, Good RA: Fatal granulomatosus of childhood: clinical study of new syndrome. Minn Med 40:309, 1957
38. Landing BH, Shirkey HS: A syndrome of recurrent infection and infiltration of viscera by pigmented lipid histiocytes. Pediatrics 20:431, 1957
39. Johnston RB Jr, McMurry JS: Chronic familial granulomatosis: report of five cases and review of the literature. Am J Dis Child 114:370, 1967
40. Bridges RA, Berendes H, Good RA: A fatal granulomatous disease of childhood. The clinical, pathological, and laboratory features of a new syndrome. Am J Dis Child 97:387, 1959
41. Quie PG, White JG, Holmes B et al: In vitro bactericidal capacity of human polymorphonuclear leukocytes: diminished activity in chronic granulomatous disease of childhood. J Clin Invest 46:668, 1967
42. Holmes B, Page AR, Good RA: Studies of the metabolic activity of leukocytes from patients with a genetic abnormality of phagocytic function. J Clin Invest 46:1422, 1967
43. Curnutte JT, Whitten DM, Babior BM: Defective superoxide production by granulocytes from patients with chronic granulomatous disease. N Engl J Med 290:593, 1974
44. Baehner RL, Nathan DG: Quantitative nitroblue tetrazolium test in chronic granulomatous disease. N Engl J Med 278:971, 1968
45. Briggs RT, Karnovsky ML, Karnovsky MJ: Hydrogen peroxide production in chronic granulomatous disease. J Clin Invest 59:1088, 1977
46. Windhorst DB, Page AR, Holmes B et al: The pattern of genetic transmission of the leukocyte defect in fatal granulomatous disease of childhood. J Clin Invest 47:1026, 1968
47. Quie PG, Kaplan EL, Page AR et al: Defective polymorphonuclear-leukocyte function and chronic granulomatous disease in two female children. N Engl J Med 278:976, 1968
48. Azimi PH, Bodenbender JG, Hintz RL et al: Chronic granulomatous disease in three female siblings. JAMA 206:2865, 1968
49. Chandra RK, Cope WA, Soothill JF: Chronic granulomatous disease. Evidence for an autosomal mode of inheritance. Lancet 2:71, 1969
50. Curnutte JT, Kipnes RS, Babior BM: Defect in pyridine nucleotide dependent superoxide production by a particulate fraction from the granulocytes of patients with chronic granulomatous disease. N Engl J Med 293:628, 1975
51. Segal AW, Cross AR, Garcia RC et al: Absence of cytochrome b_{-245} in chronic granulomatous disease: a multicenter European evaluation of its incidence and relevance. N Engl J Med 308:245, 1983
52. Curnutte JT: Activation of human neutrophil nicotinamide adenine dinucleotide phosphate, reduced (triphosphopyridine nucleotide, reduced) oxidase by arachidonic acid in a cell-free system. J Clin Invest 75:1740, 1985
53. Bromberg Y, Pick E: Unsaturated fatty acids stimulate NADPH-dependent superoxide production by cell-free system derived from macrophages. Cell Immunol 88:213, 1984
54. McPhail LC, Shirley PS, Clayton CC et al: Activation of the respiratory burst enzyme from human neutrophils in a cell-free system. J Clin Invest 75:1735, 1985
55. Heyneman RA, Vercauteren RE: Activation of a NADPH oxidase from horse polymorphonuclear leukocytes in a cell-free system. J Leukoc Biol 36:751, 1984
56. Curnutte JT, Berkow RL, Roberts RL et al: Chronic granulomatous disease due to a defect in the cytosolic factor required for nicotinamide adenine dinucleotide phosphate oxidase activation. J Clin Invest 81:606, 1988
57. Curnutte JT, Kuver R, Scott PJ: Activation of neutrophil NADPH oxidase in a cell-free system. Partial purification of components and characterization of the activation process. J Biol Chem 262:5563, 1987
58. Clark RA, Volpp BD, Leidal KG et al: Two cytosolic components of the human neutrophil respiratory burst oxidase translocate to the plasma membrane during cell activation. J Clin Invest 85:714, 1990
59. Heyworth PG, Curnutte JT, Nauseef WM et al: Neutrophil nicotinamide adenine dinucleotide phosphate oxidase assembly. Translocation of p47-phox and p67-phox requires interaction between p47-phox and cytochrome b_{558}. J Clin Invest 87:352, 1991
60. Curnutte JT, Erickson RW, Ding J et al: Reciprocal interactions between protein kinase C and components of the NADPH oxidase complex may regulate superoxide production by neutrophils stimulated with a phorbol ester. J Biol Chem 269:10813, 1994
61. Woodman RC, Ruedi JM, Jesaitis AJ et al: Respiratory burst oxidase and three of four oxidase-related polypeptides are associated with the cytoskeleton of human neutrophils. J Clin Invest 87:1345, 1991
62. Rotrosen D, Kleinberg ME, Nunoi H et al: Evidence for a functional cyto-

plasmic domain of phagocyte oxidase cytochrome b$_{558}$. J Biol Chem 265: 8745, 1990

63. Kleinberg ME, Mital D, Rotrosen D, Malech HL: Characterization of a phagocyte cytochrome b$_{558}$ 91-kilodalton subunit functional domain: identification of peptide sequence and amino acids essential for activity. Biochemistry 31:2686, 1992

64. Uhlinger DJ, Tyagi SR, Inge KL et al: The respiratory burst oxidase of human neutrophils. Guanine nucleotides and arachidonate regulate the assembly of a multicomponent complex in a semirecombinant cell-free system. J Biol Chem 268:8624, 1993

65. Segal AW, Nugent JHA: Composition and function of the NADPH oxidase of phagocytic cells with particular reference to redox components located within the membrane. p. 1. In Cochrane CG, Gimbrone MA Jr (eds): Cellular and Molecular Mechanisms of Inflammation. Vol. 4. Biological Oxidants: Generation and Injurious Consequences. 1st Ed. Academic Press, San Diego, 1992

66. Heyworth PG, Peveri P, Curnutte JT: Cytosolic components of NADPH oxidase: identity, function and role in regulation of oxidase activity. p. 43. In Cochrane CG, Gimbrone MA Jr (eds): Cellular and Molecular Mechanisms of Inflammation. Vol. 4. Biological Oxidants: Generation and Injurious Consequences. 1st Ed. Academic Press, San Diego, 1992

67. Segal AW: Absence of both cytochrome b$_{-245}$ subunits from neutrophils in X-linked chronic granulomatous disease. Nature 326:88, 1987

68. Parkos CA, Allen RA, Cochrane CG et al: Purified cytochrome b from human granulocyte plasma membrane is comprised of two polypeptides with relative molecular weights of 91,000 and 22,000. J Clin Invest 80:732, 1987

69. Parkos CA, Dinauer MC, Walker LE et al: Primary structure and unique expression of the 22-kilodalton light chain of human neutrophil cytochrome b. Proc Natl Acad Sci USA 85:3319, 1988

70. Parkos CA, Allen RA, Cochrane CG et al: The quaternary structure of the plasma membrane b-type cytochrome of human granulocytes. Biochim Biophys Acta 932:71, 1988

71. Royer-Pokora B, Kunkel LM, Monaco AP et al: Cloning the gene for an inherited human disorder—chronic granulomatous disease—on the basis of its chromosomal location. Nature 322:32, 1986

72. Dinauer MC, Orkin SH, Brown R et al: The glycoprotein encoded by the X-linked chronic granulomatous disease locus is a component of the neutrophil cytochrome b complex. Nature 327:717, 1987

73. Jesaitis AJ, Buescher ES, Harrison D et al: Ultrastructural localization of cytochrome b in the membranes of resting and phagocytosing human granulocytes. J Clin Invest 85:821, 1990

74. Quinn MT, Mullen ML, Jesaitis AJ: Human neutrophil cytochrome b contains multiple hemes. Evidence for heme associated with both subunits. J Biol Chem 267:7303, 1992

75. Segal AW, West I, Wientjes F et al: Cytochrome b$_{-245}$ is a flavocytochrome containing FAD and the NADPH-binding site of the microbicidal oxidase of phagocytes. Biochem J 284:781, 1992

76. Rotrosen D, Yeung CL, Leto TL et al: Cytochrome b$_{558}$: the flavin-binding component of the phagocyte NADPH oxidase. Science 256:1459, 1992

77. Quinn MT, Parkos CA, Walker L et al: Association of a Ras-related protein with cytochrome b of human neutrophils. Nature 342:198, 1989

78. Quinn MT, Mullen ML, Jesaitis AJ et al: Subcellular distribution of the Rap1A protein in human neutrophils: colocalization and cotranslocation with cytochrome b$_{559}$. Blood 79:1563, 1992

79. Quinn MT, Curnutte JT, Parkos CA et al: Reconstitution of defective respiratory burst activity with partially purified human neutrophil cytochrome B in two genetic forms of chronic granulomatous disease: possible role of Rap1A. Blood 79:2438, 1992

80. Babior BM, Kuver R, Curnutte JT: Kinetics of activation of the respiratory burst oxidase in a fully soluble system from human neutrophils. J Biol Chem 263:1713, 1988

81. Okamura N, Curnutte JT, Roberts RL et al: Relationship of protein phosphorylation to the activation of the respiratory burst in human neutrophils. Defects in the phosphorylation of a group of closely related 48-kDa proteins in two forms of chronic granulomatous disease. J Biol Chem 263:6777, 1988

82. Okamura N, Malawista SE, Roberts RL et al: Phosphorylation of the oxidase-related 48K phosphoprotein family in the unusual autosomal cytochrome-negative and X-linked cytochrome-positive types of chronic granulomatous disease. Blood 72:811, 1988

83. Curnutte JT, Scott PJ, Mayo LA: Cytosolic components of the respiratory burst oxidase: resolution of four components, two of which are missing in complementing types of chronic granulomatous disease. Proc Natl Acad Sci USA 86:825, 1989

84. Clark RA, Malech HL, Gallin JI et al: Genetic variants of chronic granulomatous disease: prevalence of deficiencies of two cytosolic components of the NADPH oxidase system. N Engl J Med 321:647, 1989

85. Lomax KJ, Leto TL, Nunoi H et al: Recombinant 47 kD cytosol factor restores NADPH oxidase in chronic granulomatous disease. Science 245:409, 1989

86. Nunoi H, Rotrosen D, Gallin JI et al: Two forms of autosomal chronic granulomatous disease lack distinct neutrophil cytosol factors. Science 242:1298, 1988

87. Volpp BD, Nauseef WM, Clark RA: Two cytosolic neutrophil oxidase components absent in autosomal chronic granulomatous disease. Science 242:1295, 1988

88. Volpp BD, Nauseef WM, Donelson JE et al: Cloning of the cDNA and functional expression of the 47-kilodalton cytosolic component of the human neutrophil respiratory burst oxidase. Proc Natl Acad Sci USA 86:7195, 1989

89. Leto TL, Lomax KJ, Volpp BD et al: Cloning of a 67-kD neutrophil oxidase factor with similarity to a noncatalytic region of p60^{c-src}. Science 248:727, 1990

90. Bolscher BGJM, van Zwieten R, Kramer IM et al: A phosphoprotein of Mr 47,000, defective in autosomal chronic granulomatous disease, copurifies with one of two soluble components required for NADPH:O$_2$ oxidoreductase activity in human neutrophils. J Clin Invest 83:757, 1989

91. Kramer IJM, Verhoeven AJ, van der Bend RL et al: Purified protein kinase C phosphorylates a 47 kDa protein in control neutrophil cytoplasts but not in neutrophil cytoplasts from patients with the autosomal form of chronic granulomatous disease. J Biol Chem 263:2352, 1988

92. Caldwell SE, McCall CE, Hendricks CL et al: Coregulation of NADPH oxidase activation and phosphorylation of a 48-kD protein(s) by a cytosolic factor defective in autosomal recessive chronic granulomatous disease. J Clin Invest 81:1485, 1988

93. Abo A, Pick E, Hall A et al: Activation of the NADPH oxidase involves the small GTP-binding protein p21^{rac1}. Nature 353:668, 1991

94. Knaus UG, Heyworth PG, Evans T et al: Regulation of phagocyte oxygen radical production by the GTP-binding protein Rac 2. Science 254:1512, 1991

95. Heyworth PG, Knaus UG, Xu X et al: Requirement for posttranslational processing of rac GTP-binding proteins for activation of human neutrophil NADPH oxidase. Mol Biol Cell 4:261, 1993

96. Abo A, Boyhan A, West I et al: Reconstitution of neutrophil NADPH oxidase activity in the cell-free system by four components: p67-phox, p47-phox, p21rac1, and cytochrome b$_{-245}$. J Biol Chem 267:16767, 1992

97. Kwong CH, Malech HL, Rotrosen D et al: Regulation of the human neutrophil NADPH oxidase by rho-related G-proteins. Biochemistry 32:5711, 1993

98. Wientjes FB, Hsuan JJ, Totty NF et al: p40phox, a third cytosolic component of the activation complex of the NADPH oxidase to contain src homology 3 domains. Biochem J 296:557, 1993

99. Ando S, Kaibuchi K, Sasaki T et al: Post-translational processing of rac p21s is important both for their interaction with the GDP/GTP exchange proteins and for their activation of NADPH oxidase. J Biol Chem 267:25709, 1992

100. Uhlinger DJ, Inge KL, Kreck ML et al: Reconstitution and characterization of the human neutrophil respiratory burst oxidase using recombinant p47-phox, p67-phox and plasma membrane. Biochem Biophys Res Commun 186:509, 1992

101. Heyworth PG, Shrimpton CF, Segal AW: Localization of the 47 kDa phosphoprotein involved in the respiratory-burst NADPH oxidase of phagocytic cells. Biochem J 260:243, 1989

102. Uhlinger DJ, Burnham DN, Lambeth JD: Nucleoside triphosphate requirements for superoxide generation and phosphorylation in a cell-free system from human neutrophils. Sodium dodecyl sulfate and diacylglycerol activate independently of protein kinase C. J Biol Chem 266:20990, 1991

103. Tyagi SR, Neckelmann N, Uhlinger DJ et al: Cell-free translocation of recombinant p47-phox, a component of the neutrophil NADPH oxidase: effects of guanosine 5'-O-(3-thiotriphosphate), diacylglycerol, and an anionic amphiphile. Biochemistry 31:2765, 1992

104. Peveri P, Heyworth PG, Curnutte JT: Absolute requirement for GTP in the activation of the human neutrophil NADPH oxidase in a cell-free system. Role of ATP in regenerating GTP. Proc Natl Acad Sci USA 89:2494, 1992

105. Ding J, Badwey JA: Effects of antagonists of protein phosphatases on superoxide release by neutrophils. J Biol Chem 267:6442, 1992

106. Ding J, Badwey JA, Erickson RW et al: Protein kinases potentially capable of catalyzing the phosphorylation of p47-phox in normal neutrophils and neutrophils of patients with chronic granulomatous disease. Blood 82:940, 1993

107. Rotrosen D, Leto TL: Phosphorylation of neutrophil 47-kDa cytosolic oxidase factor: translocation to membrane is associated with distinct phosphorylation events. J Biol Chem 265:19910, 1990

108. Curnutte JT: Classification of chronic granulomatous disease. Hematol Oncol Clin North Am 20:241, 1988

109. Curnutte JT: Chronic granulomatous disease: the solving of a clinical riddle at the molecular level. Clin Immunol Immunopathol 67:S2, 1993

110. Casimir C, Chetty M, Bohler M-C et al: Identification of the defective NADPH-

oxidase component in chronic granulomatous disease: a study of 57 European families. Eur J Clin Invest 22:403, 1992

111. Lew PD, Southwick FS, Stossel TP et al: A variant of chronic granulomatous disease: deficient oxidative metabolism due to a low-affinity NADPH oxidase. N Engl J Med 305:1329, 1981

112. Newburger PE, Luscinskas FW, Ryan T et al: Variant chronic granulomatous disease: modulation of the neutrophil defect by severe infection. Blood 68: 914, 1986

113. Borregaard N, Johansen KS, Esmann V: Quantitation of superoxide production in human polymorphonuclear leukocytes from normals and 3 types of chronic granulomatous disease. Biochem Biophys Res Commun 90:214, 1979

114. Seger RA, Tiefenauer L, Matsunaga T et al: Chronic granulomatous disease due to granulocytes with abnormal NADPH oxidase activity and deficient cytochrome-b. Blood 61:423, 1983

115. Roos D, de Boer M, Borregaard N et al: Chronic granulomatous disease with partial deficiency of cytochrome b_{558} and incomplete respiratory burst: variants of the X-linked, cytochrome b_{558}-negative form of the disease. J Leukoc Biol 51:164, 1992

116. Dinauer MC, Curnutte JT, Rosen H et al: A missense mutation in the neutrophil cytochrome b heavy chain in cytochrome-positive X-linked chronic granulomatous disease. J Clin Invest 84:2012, 1989

117. Azuma H, Oomi H, Ueda D et al: Cytochrome b positive X-linked chronic granulomatous disease: a normal cell surface expression of cytochrome b. Eur J Pediatr 151:279, 1992

118. Schapiro BL, Newburger PE, Klempner MS et al: Chronic granulomatous disease presenting in a 69-year-old man. N Engl J Med 325:1786, 1991

119. Weening RS, Corbeel L, de Boer M et al: Cytochrome b deficiency in an autosomal form of chronic granulomatous disease. A third form of chronic granulomatous disease recognized by monocyte hybridization. J Clin Invest 75:915, 1985

120. Dinauer MC, Pierce EA, Bruns GAP et al: Human neutrophil cytochrome b light chain (p22-$phox$): gene structure, chromosomal location, and mutations in cytochrome-negative autosomal recessive chronic granulomatous disease. J Clin Invest 86:1729, 1990

121. Ohno Y, Buescher ES, Roberts R et al: Reevaluation of cytochrome b and flavin adenine dinucleotide in neutrophils from patients with chronic granulomatous disease and description of a family with probable autosomal recessive inheritance of cytochrome b deficiency. Blood 67:1132, 1986

122. de Boer M, de Klein A, Hossle J-P et al: Cytochrome b_{558}-negative, autosomal recessive chronic granulomatous disease: two new mutations in the cytochrome b_{558} light chain of the NADPH oxidase (p22-$phox$). Am J Hum Genet 51:1127, 1992

123. Dinauer MC, Pierce EA, Erickson RW et al: Point mutation in the cytoplasmic domain of the neutrophil p22-$phox$ cytochrome b subunit is associated with a nonfunctional NADPH oxidase and chronic granulomatous disease. Proc Natl Acad Sci USA 88:11231, 1991

124. Parkos CA, Dinauer MC, Jesaitis AJ et al: Absence of both the 91kD and 22kD subunits of human neutrophil cytochrome b in two genetic forms of chronic granulomatous disease. Blood 73:1416, 1989

125. Weening RS, Adriaansz LH, Weemaes CMR et al: Clinical differences in chronic granulomatous disease in patients with cytochrome b-negative or cytochrome b-positive neutrophils. J Pediatr 107:102, 1985

126. Teahan C, Rowe P, Parker P et al: The X-linked chronic granulomatous disease gene codes for the beta-chain of cytochrome b_{-245}. Nature 327:720, 1987

127. Francke U: Random X inactivation resulting in mosaic nullisomy of region Xp21.1→p21.3 associated with heterozygosity for ornithine transcarbamylase deficiency and for chronic granulomatous disease. Cytogenet Cell Genet 38:298, 1984

128. Francke U, Ochs HD, De Martinville B et al: Minor Xp21 chromosome deletion in a male associated with expression of Duchenne muscular dystrophy, chronic granulomatous disease, retinitis pigmentosa, and McLeod syndrome. Am J Hum Genet 37:250, 1985

129. Baehner RL, Kunkel LM, Monaco AP et al: DNA linkage analysis of X chromosome-linked chronic granulomatous disease. Proc Natl Acad Sci USA 83: 3398, 1986

130. Skalnik DG, Dorfman DM, Perkins AS et al: Targeting of transgene expression in monocyte/macrophages by the gp91-$phox$ promoter and consequent histiocytic malignancies. Proc Natl Acad Sci USA 88:8505, 1991

131. Kousseff B: Linkage between chronic granulomatous disease and Duchenne's muscular dystrophy? Am J Dis Child 135:1149, 1981

132. Frey D, Machler M, Seger R et al: Gene deletion in a patient with chronic granulomatous disease and McLeod syndrome: fine mapping of the Xk gene locus. Blood 71:252, 1988

133. Hopkins PJ, Kuruto R, Curnutte JT: Molecular genetic analysis of X-linked chronic granulomatous disease, abstracted. Am J Hum Genet 51:A37, 1992

134. de Saint-Basile G, Bohler MC, Fischer A et al: Xp21 DNA microdeletion in a patient with chronic granulomatous disease, retinitis pigmentosa, and McLeod phenotype. Hum Genet 80:85, 1988

135. Pelham A, O'Reilly M-AJ, Malcolm S et al: RFLP and deletion analysis for X-linked chronic granulomatous disease using the cDNA probe: potential for improved prenatal diagnosis and carrier determination. Blood 76:820, 1990

136. de Boer M, Bolscher BGJM, Dinauer MC et al: Splice site mutations are a common cause of X-linked chronic granulomatous disease. Blood 80:1553, 1992

137. Bolscher BGJM, de Boer M, de Klein A et al: Point mutations in the β-subunit of cytochrome b_{558} leading to X-linked chronic granulomatous disease. Blood 77:2482, 1991

138. Curnutte JT, Hopkins PJ, Kuhl W et al: Studying X inactivation. Lancet 339: 749, 1992

139. Hopkins PJ, Skalnik DG, Eklund EA et al: Mutations in the gp91-$phox$ gene promoter region result in clonal expression of cytochrome b_{558} and symptomatic chronic granulomatous disease, abstracted. Blood 80:251a, 1992

140. Ho MF, Monaco AP, Blonden LA et al: Fine mapping of the McLeod locus (XK) to a 150–380-kb region in Xp21. Am J Hum Genet 50:317, 1992

141. Bass DA, Parce JW, Dechatelet LR et al: Flow cytometric studies of oxidative product formation by neutrophils: a graded response to membrane stimulation. J Immunol 130:1910, 1983

142. Francke U, Hsieh C-L, Foellmer BE et al: Genes for two autosomal recessive forms of chronic granulomatous disease assigned to 1q25 (NCF2) and 7q11.23 (NCF1). Am J Hum Genet 47:483, 1990

143. Chanock SJ, Barrett DM, Curnutte JT et al: Gene structure of the cytosolic component, $phox$-47 and mutations in autosomal recessive chronic granulomatous disease, abstracted. Blood 78:165a, 1991

144. Casimir CM, Bu-Ghanim HN, Rodaway ARF et al: Autosomal recessive chronic granulomatous disease caused by deletion at a dinucleotide repeat. Proc Natl Acad Sci USA 88:2753, 1991

145. Kenney RT, Malech HL, Epstein ND et al: Characterization of the p67-$phox$ gene: genomic organization and restriction fragment length polymorphism analysis for prenatal diagnosis in chronic granulomatous disease. Blood 82: 3739, 1993

146. de Boer M, Hilarius-Stokman PM, Hossle J-P et al: Autosomal recessive chronic granulomatous disease with absence of the 67-kD cytosolic NADPH oxidase components: identification of mutation and detection of carriers. Blood 83:531, 1994

147. Ganz T, Metcalf JA, Gallin JI et al: Microbicidal/cytotoxic proteins of neutrophils are deficient in two disorders: Chédiak-Higashi syndrome and "specific" granule deficiency. J Clin Invest 82:552, 1988

148. Johnston RB Jr, Newman SL: Chronic granulomatous disease. Pediatr Clin North Am 24:365, 1977

149. Hitzig WH, Seger RA: Chronic granulomatous disease, a heterogeneous syndrome. Hum Genet 64:207, 1983

150. Mouy R, Fischer A, Vilmer E et al: Incidence, severity, and prevention of infections in chronic granulomatous disease. J Pediatr 114:555, 1989

151. Hayakawa H, Kobayashi N, Yata J: Chronic granulomatous disease in Japan: a summary of the clinical features of 84 registered patients. Acta Paediatr Jpn 27:501, 1985

152. Gallin JI, Buescher ES, Seligmann BE et al: Recent advances in chronic granulomatous disease. Ann Intern Med 99:657, 1983

153. Cohen MS, Isturiz RE, Malech HL et al: Fungal infection in chronic granulomatous disease. The importance of the phagocyte in defense against fungi. Am J Med 71:59, 1981

154. Mandell GL, Hook EW: Leukocyte bactericidal activity in chronic granulomatous disease: correlation of bacterial hydrogen peroxide production and susceptibility in intracellular killing. J Bacteriol 100:531, 1969

155. Odell EW, Segal AW: Killing of pathogens associated with chronic granulomatous disease by the non-oxidative microbicidal mechanisms of human neutrophils. J Med Microbiol 34:129, 1991

156. Phillips P, Forbes JC, Speert DP: Disseminated infection with *Pseudallescheria boydii* in a patient with chronic granulomatous disease: response to gamma-interferon plus antifungal chemotherapy. Pediatr Infect Dis 10:536, 1991

157. White CJ, Kwon-Chung KJ, Gallin JI: Chronic granulomatous disease of childhood. An unusual case of infection with *Aspergillus nidulans* var. *echinulatus*. Am J Clin Pathol 90:312, 1988

158. Kenney RT, Kwon-Chung KJ, Witebsky FG et al: Invasive infection with *Sarcinosporon inkin* in a patient with chronic granulomatous disease. Am J Clin Pathol 94:344, 1990

159. Washburn RG, Bryan CS, DiSalvo AF et al: Visceral botryomycosis caused

by *Neisseria mucosa* in a patient with chronic granulomatous disease. J Infect Dis 151:563, 1985

160. Chusid MJ, Parrillo JE, Fauci AS: Chronic granulomatous disease: diagnosis in a 27-year-old man with *Mycobacterium fortuitum.* JAMA 233:1295, 1975

161. Schwartz DA: *Sporothrix* tenosynovitis—differential diagnosis of granulomatous inflammatory disease of the joints. J Rheumatol 16:550, 1989

162. Sorensen RU, Jacobs MR, Shurin SB: *Chromobacterium violaceum* adenitis acquired in the northern United States as a complication of chronic granulomatous disease. Pediatr Infect Dis 4:701, 1985

163. Macher AM, Casale TB, Fauci AS: Chronic granulomatous disease of childhood and *Chromobacterium violaceum* infections in the southeastern United States. Ann Intern Med 97:51, 1982

164. Bujak JS, Kwon-Chung KJ, Chusid MJ: Osteomyelitis and pneumonia in a boy with chronic granulomatous disease of childhood caused by a mutant strain of *Aspergillus nidulans.* Am J Clin Pathol 61:361, 1974

165. Bujak JS, Ottesen EA, Dinarello CA et al: Nocardiosis in a child with chronic granulomatous disease. J Pediatr 83:98, 1973

166. Southwick FS: Case records of the Massachusetts General Hospital. Weekly clinicopathological exercises, case 26-1981. N Engl J Med 304:1592, 1981

167. Wenger JD, Hollis DG, Weaver RE et al: Infection caused by *Francisella philomiragia* (formerly *Yersinia philomiragia*). A newly recognized human pathogen. Ann Intern Med 110:888, 1990

168. Pedersen FK, Johansen KS, Rosenkvist J et al: Refractory *Pneumocystis carinii* infection in chronic granulomatous disease: successful treatment with granulocytes. Pediatrics 64:935, 1979

169. Adinoff AD, Johnston RB Jr, Dolen J et al: Chronic granulomatous disease and *Pneumocystis carinii* pneumonia. Pediatrics 69:133, 1982

170. Fleischmann J, Church JA, Lehrer RI: Case report: primary *Candida* meningitis and chronic granulomatous disease. Am J Med Sci 291:334, 1986

171. Ephros M, Engelhard D, Maayan S et al: *Legionella gormanii* pneumonia in a child with chronic granulomatous disease. Pediatr Infect Dis 8:726, 1989

172. Kaplan A, Israel F: *Corynebacterium aquaticum* infection in a patient with chronic granulomatous disease. Am J Med Sci 296:57, 1988

173. Kenney RT, Kwon-Chung KJ, Waytes AT et al: Successful treatment of systemic *Exophiala dermatididis* infection in a patient with chronic granulomatous disease. Clin Infect Dis 14:235, 1992

174. Silliman CC, Lawellin DW, Lohr JA et al: *Paecilomyces lilacinus* infection in a child with chronic granulomatous disease. J Infect 24:191, 1992

175. Williamson PR, Kwon Chung KJ, Gallin JI: Successful treatment of *Paecilomyces varioti* infection in a patient wtih chronic granulomatous disease and a review of *Paecilomyces* species infections. Clin Infect Dis 14:1023, 1992

176. O'Neil KM, Herman JH, Modlin JF et al: *Pseudomonas cepacia:* an emerging pathogen in chronic granulomatous disease. J Pediatr 108:940, 1986

177. Clegg HW, Ephros M, Newburger PE: *Pseudomonas cepacia* pneumonia in chronic granulomatous disease. Pediatr Infect Dis 5:111, 1986

178. Styrt B, Klempner MS: Late-presenting variant of chronic granulomatous disease. Pediatr Infect Dis J 3:556, 1984

179. Goldmann DA, Klinger JD: *Pseudomonas cepacia:* biology, mechanisms of virulence, epidemiology. J Pediatr 108:806, 1986

180. Sieber OF, Fulginiti VA: *Pseudomonas cepacia* pneumonia in a child with chronic granulomatous disease and selective IgA deficiency. Acta Paediatr Scand 65:519, 1976

181. Mulholland MW, Delaney JP, Simmons RL: Gastrointestinal complications of chronic granulomatous disease: surgical implications. Surgery 94:569, 1983

182. Garel LA, Pariente DM, Nezelof C et al: Liver involvement in chronic granulomatous disease: the role of ultrasound in diagnosis and treatment. Radiology 153:117, 1984

183. Sponsellar PD, Malech HL, McCarthy EF Jr et al: Skeletal involvement in children who have chronic granulomatous disease. J Bone Joint Surg 73a: 37, 1991

184. Wolfson JJ, Kane WJ, Laxdal SD et al: Bone findings in chronic granulomatous disease of childhood: a genetic abnormality of leukocyte function. Surgery 51:1573, 1969

185. Heinrich SD, Finney T, Craver R et al: Aspergillus osteomyelitis in patients who have chronic granulomatous disease. J Bone Joint Surg 73-a:456, 1991

186. Kawashima A, Kuhlman JE, Fishman EK et al: Pulmonary *Aspergillus* chest wall involvement in chronic granulomatous disease of childhood. CT and MRI findings. Skeletal Radiol 20:487, 1991

187. Windhorst DB, Good RA: Dermatologic manifestations of fatal granulomatous disease of childhood. Arch Dermatol 103:351, 1971

188. Ament ME, Ochs HD: Gastrointestinal manifestations of chronic granulomatous disease. N Engl J Med 288:382, 1973

189. Fisher JE, Khan AR, Heitlinger L et al: Chronic granulomatous disease of childhood with acute ulcerative colitis: a unique association. Pediatr Pathol 7:91, 1987

190. Sty JR, Chusid MJ, Babbitt DP et al: Involvement of the colon in chronic granulomatous disease of childhood. Radiology 132:618, 1979

191. Isaacs D, Wright VM, Shaw DG et al: Case report: chronic granulomatous disease mimicking Crohn's disaease. J Pediatr Gastroenterol Nutr 4:498, 1985

192. Renner WR, Johnson JF, Lichtenstein JE et al: Esophageal inflammation and stricture: complication of chronic granulomatous disease of childhood. Radiology 178:189, 1991

193. Dickerman JD, Colletti RB, Tampas JP: Gastric outlet obstruction in chronic granulomatous disease of childhood. Am J Dis Child 140:567, 1986

194. Griscom NT, Kirkpatrick JA Jr, Girdany BR et al: Gastric antral narrowing in chronic granulomatous disease of childhood. Pediatrics 54:456, 1974

195. Elliot GR, Clay ME, Mills EL et al: Granulocyte transfusion kinetics measured by chemiluminescence, nitroblue tetrazolium reduction, and recovery of indium-111-labeled granulocytes. Transfusion 27:23, 1987

196. Walther MM, Malech H, Berman A et al: The urological manifestations of chronic granulomatous disease. J Urol 147:1314, 1992

197. Kontras SB, Bodenbender JG, McClave CR et al: Interstitial cystitis in chronic granulomatous disease. J Urol 105:575, 1971

198. Frifelt JJ, Schonheyder H, Valerius NH et al: Chronic granulomatous disease associated with chronic glomerulonephritis. Acta Paediatr Scand 74:152, 1985

199. Bloomberg SD, Ehrlich RM, Neu HC et al: Chronic granulomatous disease of childhood with renal involvement. Urology 4:193, 1974

200. Aliabadi H, Gonzalez R, Quie PG: Urinary tract disorders in patients with chronic granulomatous disease. N Engl J Med 321:706, 1989

201. Bauer SB, Kogan SJ: Vesical manifestations of chronic granulomatous disease in children. Its relation to eosinophilic cystitis. Urology 37:463, 1991

202. Cyr WL, Johnson H, Balfour J: Granulomatous cystitis as a manifestation of chronic granulomatous disease of childhood. J Urol 110:357, 1973

203. Young AK, Middleton RG: Urologic manifestations of chronic granulomatous disease in infancy. J Urol 123:119, 1980

204. Southwick FS, van der Meer JWM: Recurrent cystitis and bladder mass in two adults with chronic granulomatous disease. Ann Intern Med 109:118, 1988

205. Cohen MS, Leong PA, Simpson DM: Phagocytic cells in periodontal defense: periodontal status of patients with chronic granulomatous disease of childhood. J Periodontol 56:611, 1985

206. Martyn LJ, Lischner HW, Pileggi AJ et al: Chorioretinal lesions in familial chronic granulomatous disease of childhood. Am J Ophthalmol 73:403, 1972

207. Hadfield MG, Ghatak NR, Laine FJ et al: Brain lesions in chronic granulomatous disease. Acta Neuropathol 81:467, 1991

208. Walker DH, Okiye G: Chronic granulomatous disease involving the central nervous system. Pediatr Pathol 1:159, 1983

209. van Rhenen DJ, Koolen MI, Feltkamp-Vroom TM et al: Immune complex glomerulonephritis in chronic granulomatous disease. Acta Med Complex 206:233, 1979

210. Stalder JF, Dreno B, Bureau B et al: Discoid lupus erythematosus-like lesions in an autosomal form of chronic granulomatous disease. Br J Dermatol 114: 251, 1986

211. Smitt JHS, Bos JD, Weening RS et al: Discoid lupus erythematosus-like skin changes in patients with autosomal recessive chronic granulomatous disease. Arch Dermatol 126:1656, 1990

212. Manzi S, Urbach AH, McCune AB et al: Systemic lupus erythematosus in a boy with chronic granulomatous disease: case report and review of the literature. Arthritis Rheum 34:101, 1991

213. Strate M, Brandrup F, Wang P: Discoid lupus erythematosus-like skin lesions in a patient with autosomal recessive chronic granulomatous disease. Clin Genet 30:184, 1986

214. Schaller J: Illness resembling lupus erythematosus in mothers of boys with chronic granulomatous disease. Ann Intern Med 76:747, 1972

215. Yeaman GR, Froebel K, Galea G et al: Discoid lupus erythematosus in an X-linked cytochrome-positive carrier of chronic granulomatous disease. Br J Dermatol 126:60, 1992

216. Mills EL, Rholl KS, Quie PG: X-linked inheritance in females with chronic granulomatous disease. J Clin Invest 66:332, 1980

217. Johnston RB, Harbeck RJ, Johnston RB Jr: Recurrent severe infections in a girl with apparently variable expression of mosaicism for chronic granulomatous disease. J Pediatr 106:50, 1985

218. Cazzola M, Sacchi F, Pagani A et al: X-linked chronic granulomatous disease in an adult woman. Evidence for a cell selection favoring neutrophils expressing the mutant allele. Haematologica 70:291, 1985

219. Buescher ES, Alling DW, Gallin JI: Use of an X-linked human neutrophil marker to estimate timing of lyonization and size of the dividing stem cell pool. J Clin Invest 76:1581, 1985

220. Hopkins PJ, Bemiller LS, Curnutte JT: Chronic granulomatous disease: diagnosis and classification at the molecular level. Clin Lab Med 12:277, 1992
221. de Boer M, Bolscher BGJM, Sijmons RH et al: Prenatal diagnosis in a family with X-linked chronic granulomatous disease with the use of the polymerase chain reaction. Prenat Diagn 12:773, 1992
222. Battat L, Francke U: Nsi I RFLP at the X-linked chronic granulomatous disease locus (CYBB). Nucleic Acids Res 17:3619, 1989
223. Muhlebach TJ, Robinson W, Seger RA et al: A second NsiI RFLP at the CYBB locus. Nucleic Acids Res 18:4966, 1990
224. Newburger PE, Cohen HJ, Rothchild SB et al: Prenatal diagnosis of chronic granulomatous disease. N Engl J Med 300:178, 1979
225. Newburger PE: Superoxide generation by human fetal granulocytes. Pediatr Res 16:573, 1982
226. Linch DC, Levinsky RJ: Prenatal diagnosis of immunodeficiency disorders. Br Med Bull 39:399, 1983
227. Matthay KK, Golbus MS, Wara DW et al: Prenatal diagnosis of chronic granulomatous disease. Am J Med Genet 17:731, 1984
228. Levinsky RJ, Harvey BAM, Nicolaides K et al: Antenatal diagnosis of chronic granulomatous disease. Lancet 1:504, 1986
229. Huu TP, Dumez Y, Marquetty C et al: Prenatal diagnosis of chronic granulomatous disease (CGD) in four high risk male fetuses. Prenat Diagn 7:253, 1987
230. Conrad DJ, Warnock M, Blanc P et al: Microgranulomatous aspergillosis after shoveling wood chips: report of a fatal outcome in a patient with chronic granulomatous disease. Am J Ind Med 22:411, 1992
231. Chin TW, Stiehm ER, Falloon J et al: Corticosteroids in treatment of obstructive lesions of chronic granulomatous disease. J Pediatr 111:349, 1987
232. Collman RJ, Dickerman JD: Corticosteroids in the management of cystitis secondary to chronic granulomatous disease. Pediatrics 85:219, 1990
233. Danziger RN, Goren AT, Becker J et al: Outpatient management with oral corticosteroid therapy for obstructive conditions in chronic granulomatous disease. J Pediatr 122:303, 1993
234. Marsh WL, Redman CM: Recent developments in the Kell blood group system. Trans Med Rev 1:4, 1987
235. Marsh WL, Redman CM: The Kell blood group system: a review. Transfusion 30:158, 1990
236. Margolis DM, Melnick DA, Alling DW et al: Trimethoprim-sulfamethoxazole prophylaxis in the management of chronic granulomatous disease. J Infect Dis 162:723, 1990
237. Quie PG: The white cells: use of granulocyte transfusions. Rev Infect Dis 9:189, 1987
238. Raubitschek AA, Levin AS, Stites DP et al: Normal granulocyte infusion therapy for Aspergillosis in chronic granulomatous disease. Pediatrics 51:230, 1973
239. Fanconi S, Seger R, Gmur J et al: Surgery and granulocyte transfusions for life-threatening infections in chronic granulomatous disease. Helv Paediatr Acta 40:277, 1985
240. Depalma L, Leitman SF, Carter CS et al: Granulocyte transfusion therapy in a child wtih chronic granulomatous disease and multiple red cell alloantibodies. Transfusion 29:421, 1989
241. Gallin JI, Malech HL, Weening RS et al: A controlled trial of interferon gamma to prevent infection in chronic granulomatous disease. N Engl J Med 324:509, 1991
242. Ezekowitz RAB, Orkin SH, Newburger PE: Recombinant interferon gamma augments phagocyte superoxide production and X-chronic granulomatous disease gene expression in X-linked variant chronic granulomatous disease. J Clin Invest 80:1009, 1987
243. Ezekowitz RAB, Dinauer MC, Jaffe HS et al: Partial correction of the phagocyte defect in patients with X-linked chronic granulomatous disease by subcutaneous interferon gamma. N Engl J Med 319:146, 1988
244. Newburger PE, Ezekowitz RAB: Cellular and molecular effects of recombinant interferon gamma in chronic granulomatous disease. Hematol Oncol Clin North Am 2:267, 1988
245. Woodman RC, Erickson RW, Rae J et al: Prolonged recombinant interferon-gamma therapy in chronic granulomatous disease: evidence against enhanced neutrophil oxidase activity. Blood 79:1558, 1992
246. Muhlebach TJ, Gabay J, Nathan CF et al: Treatment of patients with chronic granulomatous disease with recombinant human interferon-gamma does not improve neutrophil oxidative metabolism, cytochrome b558 content or levels of four anti-microbial proteins. Clin Exp Immunol 88:203, 1992
247. Valentine WN, Tanaka KR, Paglia DE: Hemolytic anemias and erythrocyte enzymopathies. Ann Intern Med 103:245, 1985
248. Mamlok RJ, Mamlok V, Mills GC et al: Glucose-6-phosphate dehydrogenase deficiency, neutrophil dysfunction and Chromobacterium violaceum sepsis. J Pediatr 111:852, 1987
249. Baehner RL, Johnston RB, Nathan DG: Comparative study of the metabolic and bactericidal characteristics of severely glucose-6-phosphate dehydrogenase deficient polymorphonuclear leukocytes and leukocytes from children with chronic granulomatous disease. J Reticuloendothel Soc 12:150, 1972
250. Cooper MR, Dechatelet LR, McCall CE et al: Complete deficiency of leukocyte glucose-6-phosphate dehydrogenase with defective bactericidal activity. J Clin Invest 51:769, 1972
251. Gray GR, Stamatoyannopoulos G, Naiman SC et al: Neutrophil dysfunction, chronic granulomatous disease, and non-spherocytic haemolytic anaemia caused by complete deficiency of glucose-6-phosphate dehydrogenase. Lancet 2:530, 1973
252. Vives Corrons JL, Feliu E, Pujades MA et al: Severe glucose-6-phosphate dehydrogenase (G6PD) deficiency associated with chronic hemolytic anemia, granulocyte dysfunction, and increased susceptibility to infections: description of a new molecular variant (G6PD Barcelona). Blood 59:428, 1982
253. Mamlok RJ, Mills GC, Goldblum RM et al: Glucose-6-phosphate dehydrogenase Beaumont: a new variant with severe enzyme deficiency and chronic nonspherocytic hemolytic anemia. Enzyme 34:15, 1985
254. Roos D, Weening RS, Voetman AA et al: Protection of phagocytic leukocytes by endogenous glutathione: studies in a family with glutathione reductase deficiency. Blood 53:851, 1979
255. Spielberg SP, Boxer LA, Oliver JM et al: Oxidative damage to neutrophils in glutathione synthetase deficiency. Br J Haematol 42:215, 1979
256. Loos JA, Roos D, Weening RS et al: Familial deficiency of glutathione reductase in human blood cells. Blood 48:53, 1976
257. Boxer LA, Oliver JM, Spielberg SP et al: Protection of granulocytes by vitamin E in glutathione synthetase deficiency. N Engl J Med 301:901, 1979
258. Nauseef WM: Myeloperoxidase deficiency. Hematol Pathol 4:165, 1990
259. Parry MF, Root RK, Metcalf JA et al: Myeloperoxidase deficiency: prevalence and clinical significance. Ann Intern Med 95:293, 1981
260. Cech P, Stalder H, Widmann JJ et al: Leukocyte myeloperoxidase deficiency and diabetes mellitus associated with Candida albicans liver abscess. Am J Med 66:149, 1979
261. Cramer R, Soranzo MR, Dri P et al: Incidence of myeloperoxidase deficiency in an area of northern Italy: histochemical, biochemical and functional studies. Br J Haematol 51:81, 1982
262. Larrocha C, deCastro MF, Fontan G et al: Hereditary myeloperoxidase deficiency: a study of 12 cases. Scand J Haematol 29:389, 1982
263. Lehrer RI, Cline MJ: Leukocyte myeloperoxidase deficiency and disseminated candidiasis: the role of myeloperoxidase in resistance to Candida infection. J Clin Invest 48:1478, 1969
264. Salmon SE, Cline MJ, Schultz J et al: Myeloperoxidase deficiency. Immunological study of a genetic leukocyte defect. N Engl J Med 282:250, 1970
265. Kitahara M, Eyre HJ, Simonian Y et al: Hereditary myeloperoxidase deficiency. Blood 57:888, 1981
266. Van Tuinen P, Johnson KR, Ledbetter SA et al: Localization of myeloperoxidase to the long arm of human chromosome 17: relationship to the 15,17 translocation of acute promyelocytic leukemia. Oncogene 1:319, 1987
267. Chang KS, Schroeder W, Siciliano MJ et al: The localization of the human myeloperoxidase gene is in close proximity to the translocation breakpoint in acute promyelocytic leukemia. Leukemia 1:458, 1987
268. Inazawa J, Inquie K, Nishigaki H et al: Assignment of the human myeloperoxidase gene (MPO) to bands q21.3→q23 of chromosome 17. Cytogenet Cell Genet 50:135, 1989
269. Liang JC, Chang KS, Schroeder WT et al: The myeloperoxidase gene is translocated from chromosome 17 to 15 in a patient with acute promyelocytic leukemia. Cancer Genet Cytogenet 30:103, 1988
270. Bendix-Hansen K: Myeloperoxidase-deficient polymorphonuclear leukocytes (VII): incidence in untreated myeloproliferative disorders. Scand J Haematol 36:8, 1986
271. Bendix-Hansen K, Kerndrup G: Myeloperoxidase-deficient polymorphonuclear leukocytes (V): relation to FAB classification and neutrophil alkaline phosphatase activity in primary myelodysplastic syndromes. Scand J Haematol 35:197, 1985
272. Bendix-Hansen K, Kerndrup G, Pedersen B: Myeloperoxidase-deficient polymorphonuclear leukocytes (VI): relation to cytogenetic abnormalities in primary myelodysplastic syndromes. Scand J Haematol 36:3, 1986
273. Chang KS, Trujillo JM, Cook RG et al: Human myeloperoxidase gene: molecular cloning and expression in leukemic cells. Blood 68:1411, 1986
274. Morishita K, Kubota N, Asano S: Molecular cloning and characterization of cDNA for human myeloperoxidase. J Biol Chem 262:3844, 1987
275. Weil SC, Rosner GL, Reid MS et al: cDNA cloning of myeloperoxidase—decrease in myeloperoxidase mRNA upon maturation of HL-60 cells. Proc Natl Acad Sci USA 84:2057, 1987

276. Taylor KL, Uhlinger DJ, Kinkade JM Jr: Expression of recombinant myeloperoxidase using a baculovirus expression system. Biochem Biophys Res Commun 187:1572, 1992

277. Moguilevsky N, Garcia-Quintana L, Jacquet A et al: Structural and biological properties of human recombinant myeloperoxidase produced by Chinese hamster ovary cell lines. Eur J Biochem 197:605, 1991

278. Jacquet A, Deby C, Mathy M et al: Spectral and enzymatic properties of human recombinant myeloperoxidase: comparison with the mature enzyme. Arch Biochem Biophys 291:132, 1991

279. Meier RW, Chen T, Friss RR et al: Myeloperoxidase is a primary response gene in HL60 cells, directly regulated during hematopoietic differentiation. Biochem Biophys Res Commun 176:1345, 1991

280. Lubbert M, Miller CW, Koeffler HP: Changes of DNA methylation and chromatin structure in the human myeloperoxidase gene during myeloid differentiation. Blood 78:345, 1991

281. Nauseef WM: Aberrant restriction endonuclease digests of DNA from subjects with hereditary myeloperoxidase deficiency. Blood 73:290, 1989

282. Tobler A, Selsted ME, Miller CW et al: Evidence for a pretranslational defect in hereditary and acquired myeloperoxidase deficiency. Blood 73:1980, 1989

283. Miller ME, Nilsson UR: A familial deficiency of the phagocytosis enhancing activity of serum related to a dysfunction of the 5th component of complement (C5). N Engl J Med 282:354, 1970

284. Selsted ME, Miller CW, Novotny MJ et al: Molecular analysis of myeloperoxidase deficiency shows heterogeneous patterns of complete deficiency state manifested at the genomic, mRNA, and protein levels. Blood 82:1317, 1993

285. Shurin SB: Pathologic states associated with activation of eosinophils and with eosinophilia. Hematol Oncol Clin North Am 2:171, 1988

286. Cappelletti P, Doretto P, Signori D et al: Eosinophilic peroxidase deficiency. Cytochemical and ultrastructural characterization of 21 new cases. Am J Clin Pathol 98:615, 1992

287. Nauseef WM, Metcalf JA, Root RK: Role of myeloperoxidase in the respiratory burst of human neutrophils. Blood 61:483, 1983

288. Lehrer RI, Hanifin J, Cline MJ: Defective bactericidal activity in myeloperoxidase-deficient human neutrophils. Nature 223:78, 1969

289. Hill HR: Biochemical, structural, and functional abnormalities of polymorphonuclear leukocytes in the neonate. Pediatr Res 22:375, 1987

290. Gallin JI: Abnormal phagocyte chemotaxis: pathophysiology, clinical manifestations, and management of patients. Rev Infect Dis 3:1196, 1981

291. Todd RF III, Freyer DR: The CD11/CD18 leukocyte glycoprotein deficiency. Hematol Oncol Clin North Am 2:13, 1988

292. Arnaout MA: Structure and function of the leukocyte adhesion molecules CD11/CD18. Blood 75:1037, 1990

293. Anderson DC, Schmalstieg FC, Finegold MJ et al: The severe and moderate phenotypes of heritable Mac-1, LFA-1 deficiency: their quantitative definition and relation to leukocyte dysfunction and clinical features. J Infect Dis 152:668, 1985

294. Crowley CA, Curnutte JT, Rosin RE et al: An inherited abnormality of neutrophil adhesion: its genetic transmission and its association with a missing protein. N Engl J Med 302:1163, 1980

295. Arnaout MA, Pitt J, Cohen HJ et al: Deficiency of a granulocyte-membrane glycoprotein (gp150) in a boy with recurrent bacterial infections. N Engl J Med 306:693, 1982

296. Bowen TJ, Ochs HD, Altman LC et al: Severe recurrent bacterial infections associated with defective adherence and chemotaxis in two patients with neutrophils deficient in a cell-associated glycoprotein. J Pediatr 101:932, 1982

297. Dana N, Todd RF III, Pitt J et al: Deficiency of a surface membrane glycoprotein (Mo1) in man. J Clin Invest 73:153, 1984

298. Springer TA, Thompson WS, Miller LJ et al: Inherited deficiency of the Mac-1, LFA-1, p150,95 glycoprotein family and its molecular basis. J Exp Med 160:1901, 1984

299. Beller DI, Springer TA, Schreiber RD: Anti-Mac-1 selectively inhibits the mouse and human type three complement receptor. J Exp Med 156:1000, 1982

300. Wright SD, Rao PE, van Voorhis WC et al: Identification of the C3bi receptor of human monocytes and macrophages by using monoclonal antibodies. Proc Natl Acad Sci USA 80:5699, 1983

301. Anderson DC, Schmalstieg FC, Kohl S et al: Abnormalities of polymorphonuclear leukocyte function associated with a heritable deficiency of high molecular weight surface glycoproteins (GP138): common relationship to diminished cell adherence. J Clin Invest 74:563, 1984

302. Springer TA, Miller LJ, Anderson DC: p150,95, the third member of the Mac-1, LFA-1 human leukocyte adhesion glycoprotein family. J Immunol 136:240, 1986

303. Springer TA: Adhesion receptors of the immune system. Nature 346:425, 1990

304. Larson RS, Springer TA: Structure and function of leukocyte integrins. Immunol Rev 114:181, 1990

305. Hynes RO: Integrins: Versatility, modulation, and signaling in cell adhesion. Cell 69:11, 1992

306. Ruoslahti E: Integrins. J Clin Invest 87:1, 1991

307. Carlos TM, Harlan JM: Membrane proteins involved in phagocyte adherence to endothelium. Immunol Rev 114:5, 1990

308. Schwartz BR, Harlan JM: Consequences of deficient granulocyte-endothelium interactions. p. 231. In Gordon JL (ed): Vascular Endothelium: Interactions with Circulating Cells. Elsevier Science Publishing, New York, 1991

309. Albelda SM, Buck CA: Integrins and other cell adhesion molecules. FASEB J 4:2868, 1990

310. Kishimoto TK, O'Connor K, Lee A et al: Cloning of the β subunit of the leukocyte adhesion proteins: homology to an extracellular matrix receptor defines a novel supergene family. Cell 48:681, 1987

311. Law SKA, Gagnon J, Hildreth JEK et al: The primary structure of the β-subunit of the cell surface adhesion glycoproteins LFA-1, CR3 and p150,95 and its relationship to the fibronectin receptor. EMBO J 6:915, 1987

312. Corbi AL, Garcia-Aguilar J, Springer TA: Genomic structure of an integrin alpha subunit, the leukocyte p150,95 molecule (erratum JBC 265:12750, 1990). J Biol Chem 265:2782, 1990

313. Corbi AL, Kishimoto TK, Miller LJ et al: The human leukocyte adhesion glycoprotein Mac-1 (complement receptor type 3, CD11b) alpha subunit: cloning, primary structure, and relation to the integrins, von Willebrand factor and factor B. J Biol Chem 263:12403, 1988

314. Corbi AL, Larson RS, Kishimoto TK et al: Chromosomal location of the genes encoding the leukocyte adhesion receptors LFA-1, Mac-1, and p150,95. Identification of a gene cluster involved in cell adhesion. J Exp Med 167:1597, 1988

315. Corbi AL, Miller LJ, O'Connor K et al: cDNA cloning and complete primary structure of the alpha subunit of a leukocyte adhesion glycoprotein, p150,95. EMBO J 6:4023, 1987

316. Larson RS, Corbi AL, Berman L et al: Primary structure of the LFA-1 alpha subunit: an integrin with an embedded domain defining a protein superfamily. J Cell Biol 108:703, 1989

317. Marlin SD, Morton CC, Anderson DC et al: LFA-1 immunodeficiency disease: definition of the genetic defect and chromosomal mapping of alpha and beta subunits by complementation in hybrid cells. J Exp Med 164:855, 1986

318. Nelson C, Rabb H, Arnaout MA: Genetic cause of leukocyte adhesion molecule deficiency. Abnormal splicing and a missense mutation in a conserved region of CD18 impair cell surface expression of β2 integrins. J Biol Chem 267:3351, 1992

319. Fischer A, Lisowska-Grospierre B, Anderson DC et al: Leukocyte adhesion deficiency: molecular basis and functional consequences. Immunodefic Rev 1:39, 1988

320. Kishimoto TK, Hollander N, Roberts TM et al: Heterogeneous mutations in the β subunit common to the LFA-1, Mac-1, and p150,95 glycoproteins cause leukocyte adhesion deficiency. Cell 50:193, 1987

321. Kishimoto TK, O'Connor K, Springer TA: Leukocyte adhesion deficiency: aberrant splicing of a conserved integrin sequence causes a moderate deficiency phenotype. J Biol Chem 264:3588, 1989

322. Wardlaw AJ, Hibbs ML, Stacker SA et al: Distinct mutations in two patients with leukocyte adhesion deficiency and their functional correlates. J Exp Med 172:335, 1990

323. Arnaout MA, Dana N, Gupta SK et al: Point mutations impairing cell surface expression of the common β subunit (CD18) in a patient with leukocyte adhesion molecule (Leu-CAM) deficiency. J Clin Invest 85:977, 1990

324. Sligh JE Jr, Hurwitz MY, Zhu C et al: An initiation codon mutation in CD18 in association with the moderate phenotype of leukocyte adhesion deficiency. J Biol Chem 267:714, 1992

325. Back AL, Hickstein DD: Two different CD18 mutations in a child with severe leukocyte adhesion deficiency (LAD), abstracted. Blood 76:176a, 1990

326. Lawrence MB, Springer TA: Leukocytes roll on a selectin at physiologic flow rates: distinction from and prerequisite for adhesion through integrins. Cell 65:859, 1991

327. Arnaout MA, Spits H, Terhorst C et al: Deficiency of a leukocyte surface glycoprotein (LFA-1) in two patients with Mol deficiency. Effects of cell activation of Mo1/LFA-1 surface expression in normal and deficient cells. J Clin Invest 74:1291, 1984

328. Miller LJ, Bainton DF, Borregaard N et al: Stimulated mobilization of monocyte Mac-1 and p150,95 adhesion proteins from an intracellular vesicular compartment to the cell surface. J Clin Invest 80:535, 1987

329. Fischer A, Descamps-Latscha B, Gerota I et al: Bone marrow transplantation for inborn error of phagocytic cells associated with defective adherence, chemotaxis, and oxidative response during opsonised particle phagocytosis. Lancet 2:473, 1983

330. Le Deist F, Blanche S, Keable H et al: Successful HLA nonidentical bone marrow transplantation in three patients with the leukocyte adhesion deficiency. Blood 74:512, 1989

331. Back AL, Kwok WW, Adam M et al: Retroviral-mediated gene transfer of the leukocyte integrin CD18 subunit. Biochem Biophys Res Commun 171:787, 1990

332. Wilson JM, Ping AJ, Krauss JC et al: Correction of CD18-deficient lymphocytes by retrovirus-mediated gene transfer. Science 248:1413, 1990

333. Southwick FS, Howard TH, Holbrook T et al: The relationship between CR3 deficiency and neutrophil actin assembly. Blood 73:1973, 1989

334. Boxer LA, Hedley-Whyte ET, Stossel TP: Neutrophil actin dysfunction and abnormal neutrophil behavior. N Engl J Med 291:1093, 1974

335. Horwitz A, Duggan E, Buck C et al: Interaction of plasma membrane fibronectin receptor with talin—a transmembrane linkage. Nature 320:531, 1986

336. Marcantonio EE, Guan JL, Trevithick JE et al: Mapping of the functional determinants of the integrin β_1 cytoplasmic domain by site-directed mutagenesis. Cell Regul 1:597, 1990

337. Etzioni A, Frydman M, Pollack S et al: Brief report: recurrent severe infections caused by a novel leukocyte adhesion deficiency. N Engl J Med 327:1789, 1992

338. Davis SD, Schaller J, Wedgwood RJ: Job's syndrome: recurrent, "cold," staphylococcal abscesses. Lancet 1:1013, 1966

339. Donabedian H, Gallin JI: The hyperimmunoglobulin E recurrent-infection (Job's) syndrome. A review of the NIH experience and the literature. Medicine 62:195, 1983

340. Buckley RH, Wray BB, Belmaker EZ: Extreme hyperimmunoglobulinemia E and undue susceptibility to infection. Pediatrics 49:59, 1972

341. Buckley RH: Immunodeficiency, hyper IgE type. p. 953. In Buyse ML (eds): Birth Defects Encyclopedia. Blackwell Scientific Publications, Cambridge, 1990

342. Buckley RH, Becker WG: Abnormalities in the regulation of human IgE synthesis. Immunol Rev 41:288, 1978

343. Hill HR, Ochs HD, Quie PG et al: Defect in neutrophil granulocyte chemotaxis in Job's syndrome of recurrent "cold" staphylococcal abscesses. Lancet 2:617, 1974

344. Hill HR, Estensen RD, Hogan NA et al: Severe staphylococcal disease associated with allergic manifestations, hyperimmunoglobulinemia E, and defective neutrophil chemotaxis. J Lab Clin Med 88:796, 1976

345. Mawhinney H, Killen M, Fleming WA et al: The hyperimmunoglobulin E syndrome: a neutrophil chemotactic defect reversible by histamine H2 receptor blockade? Clin Immunol Immunopathol 17:483, 1980

346. Matricardi PM, Capobianchi MR, Paganelli R et al: Interferon production in primary immunodeficiencies. J Clin Immunol 4:388, 1984

347. Del Prete G, Tiri A, Maggi E et al: Defective in vitro production of gamma interferon and tumor necrosis factor-alpha by circulating T cells from patients with the hyper-immunoglobulin E syndrome. J Clin Invest 84:1830, 1989

348. Geha RS, Reinherz E, Leung D et al: Deficiency of suppressor T cells in hyperimmunoglobulin E syndrome. J Clin Invest 68:783, 1981

349. Sheerin KA, Buckley RH: Antibody responses to protein, polysaccharide, and phi X174 antigens in the hyperimmunoglobulinemia E (hyper-IgE) syndrome. J Allergy Clin Immunol 87:803, 1991

350. Dreskin SC, Goldsmith PK, Gallin JI: Immunoglobulins in the hyperimmunoglobulin E and recurrent infection (Job's) syndrome: deficiency of anti-Staphylococcus aureus immunoglobulin A. J Clin Invest 75:26, 1985

351. Donabedian H, Gallin JI: Mononuclear cells from patients with the hyperimmunoglobulin E-recurrent infection syndrome produce an inhibitor of leukocyte chemotaxis. J Clin Invest 69:115, 1982

352. Donabedian H, Gallin JI: Two inhibitors of neutrophil chemotaxis are produced by hyperimmunoglobulin E recurrent infection syndrome mononuclear cells exposed to heat-killed staphylococci. Infect Immun 40:1030, 1983

353. Merten DF, Buckley RH, Pratt PC et al: Hyperimmunoglobulinemia E syndrome: radiographic observations. Radiology 132:71, 1979

354. Shamberger RC, Wohl ME, Perez-Atayde A et al: Pneumatocele complicating hyperimmunoglobulin E syndrome (Job's syndrome). Ann Thorac Surg 54:1206, 1992

355. Snapper CM, Paul WE: Interferon-gamma and B cell stimulatory factor-1 reciprocally regulate Ig isotype production. Science 236:944, 1987

356. Coffman RL, Carty J: A T cell activity that enhances polyclonal IgE production and its inhibition by interferon-gamma. J Immunol 136:949, 1986

357. Jeppson JD, Jaffe HS, Hill HR: Use of recombinant human interferon gamma to enhance neutrophil chemotactic responses to Job syndrome of hyperimmunoglobulinemia E and recurrent infections. J Pediatr 118:383, 1991

358. Hill HR: Modulation of host defenses with interferon-gamma in pediatrics. J Infect Dis 167:S23, 1993

359. King CL, Gallin JI, Malech HL et al: Regulation of immunoglobulin production

360. in hyperimmunoglobulin E recurrent-infection syndrome of interferon gamma. Proc Natl Acad Sci USA 86:10085, 1989

360. Anderson DC, Hughes BJ, Smith CW: Abnormal mobility of neonatal polymorphonuclear leukocytes: relationship to impaired redistribution of surface adhesion sites by chemotactic factor or colchicine. J Clin Invest 68:863, 1981

361. Anderson DC, Hughes BJ, Wible LJ et al: Impaired motility of neonatal PMN leukocytes: relationship to abnormalities of cell orientation and assembly of microtubules in chemotactic gradients. J Leukoc Biol 36:1, 1984

362. Hill HR, Augustine NH, Jaffe HS: Human recombinant interferon gamma enhances neonatal polymorphonuclear leukocyte activation and movement, and increases free intracellular calcium. J Exp Med 173:767, 1991

363. Klein RB, Fischer TJ, Gard SE et al: Decreased mononuclear and polymorphonuclear chemotaxis in human newborns, infants, and young children. Pediatrics 60:467, 1977

364. Wilson CB: Immunologic basis for increased susceptibility of the neonate to infection. J Pediatr 108:1, 1986

365. Anderson DC, Becker Freeman KL, Heerdt B et al: Abnormal stimulated adherence of neonatal granulocytes: impaired induction of surface MAC-1 by chemotactic factors or secretagogues. Blood 70:740, 1987

366. Van Dyke TE, Schweinebraten M, Cianciola LJ et al: Neutrophil chemotaxis in families with localized juvenile periodontitis. J Periodont Res 20:503, 1985

367. Van Dyke TE: Role of the neutrophil in oral disease: receptor deficiency in leukocytes from patients with juvenile periodontitis. Rev Infect Dis 7:419, 1985

368. Van Dyke TE, Zinney W, Winkel K et al: Neutrophil function in localized juvenile periodontitis. Phagocytosis, superoxide production and specific granule release. J Periodontol 57:703, 1986

369. Cianciola LJ, Genco RJ, Patters MR et al: Defective polymorphonuclear leukocyte function in a human periodontal disease. Nature 265:445, 1977

370. Perez HD, Kelly E, Elfman F et al: Defective polymorhonuclear leukocyte formyl peptide receptor(s) in juvenile periodontitis. J Clin Invest 87:971, 1991

371. Clark RA, Page RC, Wilde G: Defective neutrophil chemotaxis in juvenile periodontitis. Infect Immun 18:694, 1977

372. Suzuki JB, Colison C, Falker WF et al: Immunologic profile of juvenile periodontitis. II. Neutrophil chemotaxis, phagocytosis and spore germination. J Periodontol 55:461, 1984

373. Van Dyke TE, Horoszewicz HU, Cianiola LJ et al: Neutrophil chemotaxis dysfunction in human periodontitis. Infect Immun 27:124, 1980

374. Agarwal S, Suzuki JB: Altered neutrophil function in localized juvenile periodontitis: intrinsic cellular defect or effect of immune mediators? J Periodont Res 26:276, 1991

375. Shurin SB, Socransky SS, Sweeney E et al: A neutrophil disorder induced by capnocytophaga, a dental micro-organism. N Engl J Med 301:849, 1979

376. Tsai C-C, McArthur WP, Baehni PC et al: Extraction and partial characterization of a leukotoxin from a plaque-derived gram-negative microorganism. Infect Immun 25:427, 1979

377. Van Dyke TE, Peshoff CM: Periodontal manifestations of immune disorders. Immunol Allergy Pract 6:418, 1984

378. Wolff SM, Dale DC, Clark RA et al: The Chédiak-Higashi syndrome: studies of host defenses. Ann Intern Med 76:293, 1972

379. Blume RS, Wolff SM: The Chédiak-Higashi syndrome: studies in four patients and a review of the literature. Medicine 51:247, 1972

380. Windhorst DB, Padgett G: The Chédiak-Higashi syndrome and the homologous trait in animals. J Invest Dermatol 60:529, 1973

381. Witkop CJ Jr, Quevedo WC Jr, Fitzpatrick TB et al: Albinism. p. 2905. In Scriver CR, Beaudet AL, Sly WS, Valle D (eds): The Metabolic Basis of Inherited Disease. 6th Ed. McGraw-Hill, New York, 1989

382. Rausch PG, Pryzwansky KB, Spitznagel JK: Immunocytochemical identification of azurophilic and specific granule markers in the giant granules of Chédiak-Higashi neutrophils. N Engl J Med 298:693, 1978

383. White JG, Clawson CC: The Chédiak-Higashi syndrome: the nature of the giant neutrophil granules and their interactions with cytoplasm and foreign particulates. I. Progressive enlargement of the massive inclusions in mature neutrophils. II. Manifestations of cytoplasmic injury and sequestration. III. Interactions between giant organelles and foreign particulates. Am J Pathol 98:151, 1980

384. Rubin CM, Burke BA, McKenna RW et al: The accelerated phase of Chédiak-Higashi syndrome. An expression of the virus-associated hemophagocytic syndrome? Cancer 56:524, 1985

385. Padgett GA, Reiquam CW, Gorham JR et al: Comparative studies of the Chédiak-Higashi syndrome. Am J Pathol 51:553, 1967

386. Ito J, Tokumaru M, Okazaki T. Chédiak-Higashi syndrome: report of a case with autopsy and electron microscopic studies. Acta Pathol Jpn 22:755, 1972

387. Sjaastad OV, Blom AK, Stormorken H et al: Adenine nucleotides, serotonin

and aggregation properties of the platelets of blue foxes (Alopex lagopus) with the Chédiak-Higashi syndrome. Am J Med Genet 35:373, 1990

388. Gilbert CS, Parmley RT, Rice WG et al: Heterogeneity of peroxidase-positive granules in normal human and Chédiak-Higashi neutrophils. J Histochem Cytochem 41:837, 1993

389. Davis WC, Spicer SS, Greene WB et al: Ultrastructure of cells in bone marrow and peripheral blood of normal mink and mink with the homologue of the Chédiak-Higashi trait of humans. II. Cytoplasmic granules in eosinophils, basophils, mononuclear cells and platelets. Am J Pathol 63:411, 1971

390. Davis WC, Douglas SD: Defective granule formation and function in the Chédiak-Higashi syndrome in man and animals. Semin Hematol 9:431, 1972

391. Blume RS, Bennett JM, Yankee RA et al: Defective granulocyte regulation in the Chédiak-Higashi syndrome. N Engl J Med 279:1009, 1968

392. Root RK, Rosenthal AS, Balestra DJ: Abnormal bactericidal, metabolic, and lysosomal functions of Chédiak-Higashi syndrome leukocytes. J Clin Invest 51:649, 1972

393. Stossel TP, Root RK, Vaughn M: Phagocytosis in chronic granulomatous disease and Chediak-Higashi syndrome. N Engl J Med 286:120, 1972

394. Padget GA: Neutrophilic function in animals with Chediak-Higashi syndrome. Blood 29:906, 1967

395. Clawson CC, Repine JE, White JG: The Chédiak-Higashi syndrome. Quantitation of a deficiency in maximal bactericidal capacity. Am J Pathol 94:539, 1979

396. Clark RA, Kimball HR: Defective granulocyte chemotaxis in the Chédiak-Higashi syndrome. J Clin Invest 50:2645, 1971

397. Klein M, Roder J, Haliotis T et al: Chédiak-Higashi gene in humans. II. The selectivity of the defect in natural-killer and antibody-dependent cell-mediated cytotoxicity function. J Exp Med 151:1049, 1980

398. Nair MPN, Gray RH, Boxer LA et al: Deficiency of inducible suppressor cell activity in the Chédiak-Higashi syndrome. Am J Hematol 26:55, 1987

399. Holcombe RF, van de Griend R, Ang S-L et al: Gamma-delta T cells in Chédiak-Higashi syndrome. Acta Haematol 83:193, 1990

400. Hamanaka SC, Gilbert CS, White DA et al: Ultrastructural morphology, cytochemistry, and morphometry of eosinophil granules in Chédiak-Higashi syndrome. Am J Pathol 143:618, 1993

401. Boxer GJ, Holmsen H, Robkin L et al: Abnormal platelet functions in Chédiak-Higashi syndrome. Br J Haematol 35:521, 1977

402. Buchanan GB, Handin RI: Platelet function in the Chédiak-Higashi syndrome. Blood 47:941, 1976

403. Bell TG, Meyers KM, Prieur DJ et al: Decreased nucleotide and serotonin storage associated with defective function in Chédiak-Higashi syndrome cattle and human platelets. Blood 48:175, 1976

404. Novak EK, McGarry MP, Swank RT: Correction of symptoms of platelet storage pool deficiency in animal models for Chédiak-Higashi syndrome and Hermansky-Pudlak syndrome. Blood 66:1196, 1985

405. Merino F, Henle W, Ramirez Duque P: Chronic active Epstein-Barr virus infection in patients with Chédiak-Higashi syndrome. J Clin Immunol 6:299, 1986

406. Durandy A, Berton-Gorius J, Guy-Grand D et al: Prenatal diagnosis of syndromes associating albinism and immune deficiencies (Chédiak-Higashi syndrome and variant). Prenat Diagn 13:13, 1993

407. Diukman R, Tanigawara S, Cowan MJ et al: Prenatal diagnosis of Chédiak-Higashi syndrome. Prenat Diagn 12:877, 1992

408. Van Slyck EJ, Rebuck JW: Pseudo-Chédiak-Higashi anomaly in acute leukemia. Am J Clin Pathol 62:673, 1974

409. Gorman AM, O'Connell LG: Letter to the editor. Pseudo-Chédiak-Higashi anomaly in acute leukemia. Am J Clin Pathol 65:1030, 1976

410. Tulliez M, Vernant JP, Brenton-Gorius J et al: Pseudo-Chédiak-Higashi anomaly in a case of acute myeloid leukemia: electron microscopic studies. Blood 54:863, 1979

411. Boxer LA, Watanabe AM, Rister M et al: Correction of leukocyte function in Chédiak-Higashi syndrome by ascorbate. N Engl J Med 295:1041, 1976

412. Weening RS, Schoorel EP, Roos D et al: Effect of ascorbate on abnormal neutrophil, platelet, and lymphocyte function in a patient with the Chédiak-Higashi syndrome. Blood 57:856, 1981

413. Gallin JI, Elin RJ, Hubert RT et al: Efficacy of ascorbic acid in Chédiak-Higashi syndrome (CHS): studies in humans and mice. Blood 53:226, 1979

414. Virelizier J-L, Lagrue A, Durandy A et al: Reversal of natural killer defect in a patient with Chédiak-Higashi syndrome after bone-marrow transplantation. N Engl J Med 306:1055, 1982

415. Kazmierowski JA, Elin RJ, Reynolds HY et al: Chédiak-Higashi syndrome: reversal of increased suceptibility to infection by bone marrow transplantation. Blood 47:555, 1976

416. Fischer A, Friedrich W, Levinsky R et al: Bone-marrow transplantation for immunodeficiencies and osteopetrosis: European survey, 1968–1985. Lancet 2:1080, 1986

417. Griscelli C, Virelizier J-L: Bone marrow transplantation in a patient with Chédiak-Higashi syndrome. p. 333. In Wedgwood RJ, Rosen F et al (eds): Primary Immunodeficiency Diseases. Alan R Liss, New York, 1983

418. Colgan SP, Hull-Thrall MA, Gasper PW et al: Restoration of neutrophil and platelet function in feline Chédiak-Higashi syndrome by bone marrow transplantation. Bone Marrow Transplant 7:365, 1991

419. Gallin JI: Neutrophil specific granule deficiency. Annu Rev Med 36:263, 1985

420. Gallin JI, Fletcher MP, Seligmann BE et al: Human neutrophil-specific granule deficiency: a model to assess the role of neutrophil-specific granules in the evolution of the inflammatory response. Blood 59:1317, 1982

421. Boxer LA, Coates TD, Haak RA et al: Lactoferrin deficiency associated with altered granulocyte function. N Engl J Med 307:404, 1982

422. Lomax KJ, Gallin JI, Rotrosen D et al: Selective defect in myeloid cell lactoferrin gene expression in neutrophil specific granule deficiency. J Clin Invest 83:514, 1989

423. Yoon PS, Boxer LA, Mayo LA et al: Human neutrophil laminin receptors: activation-dependent receptor expression. J Immunol 138:259, 1987

424. Parmley RT, Tzeng DY, Baehner RL et al: Abnormal distribution of complex carbohydrates in neutrophils of a patient with lactoferrin deficiency. Blood 62:538, 1983

425. Petrequin PR, Todd RF III, Smolen JE et al: Expression of specific granule markers on the cell surface of neutrophil cytoplasts. Blood 67:1119, 1986

426. Parmley RT, Gilbert CS, Boxer LA: Abnormal peroxidase-positive granules in "specific granule" deficiency. Blood 73:838, 1989

427. Kuriyama K, Tomonaga M, Matsuo T et al: Diagnostic significance of detecting pseudo-Pelger-Huët anomalies and micro-megakaryocytes in myelodysplastic syndrome. Br J Haematol 63:665, 1986

428. Orkin SH: Molecular genetics of chronic granulomatous disease. Annu Rev Immunol 7:277, 1989

429. Forehand JR, Nauseef WM, Curnutte JT et al: Inherited disorders of phagocyte killing. In Scriver CR, Beaudet AL, Sly WS, Valle D (eds): The Metabolic Basis of Inherited Disease. 7th Ed. McGraw-Hill, New York, 1994

430. Curnutte JT, Orkin SH, Dinauer MC: Genetic disorders of phagocyte function. p. 493. In Stamatoyannopoulos G, Nienhuis AW, Majerus PW, Varmus H (eds): The Molecular Basis of Blood Disorders. 2nd Ed. WB Saunders, Philadelphia, 1994

Disorders of Lymphocyte Function

55

Richard A. Insel

INTRODUCTION

Disorders of lymphocyte function may be categorized as either primary defects of secondary to, or associated with, some underlying disorder. This chapter emphasizes primary lymphocyte defects[1-6] (Table 55-1) and briefly summarizes secondary disorders[7] (Table 55-2), many of which are detailed in other chapters of this textbook. The secondary immunodeficiency diseases, which include malnutrition and acquired immunodeficiency syndrome (Chs. 86 and 155) are far more numerous both in the United States and worldwide. Immunodeficiency secondary to Epstein-Barr virus (EBV) is discussed in Chapter 58 and that secondary to bone marrow transplantation (BMT) in this chapter and in Chapters 27 to 30.

The primary immunologic defects can be divided into those giving rise to immunodeficiency diseases involving primarily antibody production and those that have combined defects in both antibody production and T-lymphocyte function. Excluding IgA deficiency, primary immunodeficiency disorders have a frequency of approximately 1 in 10,000 and most commonly present in the first 6 years of life. The immunodeficiency diseases are characterized by an increased frequency or severity of infections or by infections with unusual, relatively avirulent opportunistic organisms. Antibody deficiency diseases, which are more common than T-cell disorders, are most frequently characterized by recurrent pyogenic infections. T-cell deficiency is associated with difficulty in handling intracellular pathogens—viral, fungal, or parasitic—on the basis of abnormal T-cell function, as well as pyogenic bacteria, because of impaired production of antibody by lymphocytes due to the T-cell deficiency. Diarrhea, malabsorption, autoimmune disorders, and malignancies frequently occur in primary immunodeficiency diseases. Most malignancies are observed in patients with ataxia-telangiectasia (AT), Wiskott-Aldrich syndrome, and common variable immunodeficiency (CVID).[8,9]

The immunodeficiency diseases reflect defects of lymphocyte development along a maturational pathway, detailed in Chapter 20, or in the function and cooperative interaction of mature lymphoid cells, as described in Chapters 10 and 13. Primary defects of lymphocyte function are usually inherited; the chromosomal map locations of several of the congenital defects[10-12] and the molecular basis for some of these disorders have been demonstrated and are discussed.

ANTIBODY DEFICIENCIES

X-Linked Agammaglobulinemia

Etiology and Pathophysiology

The defect in X-linked agammaglobulinemia (XLA) is characterized by the failure of B cells to develop from pre-B cells. Mature B cells are absent or markedly decreased in the peripheral blood, plasma cells are absent in lymphoid tissues, and functional antibody is not produced. Pre-B cells, which express cytoplasmic IgM heavy (H) chain ($C\mu$) but not light (L) chain or surface immunoglobulin, are in low-normal numbers or absent in the bone marrow.[13] When present, a smaller proportion of these $C\mu^+$ pre-B cells than control pre-B cells are proliferating. Pro-B cells ($C\mu^-$, TdT^+, $CD19^+$, $CD10^+$) are present in normal numbers,[13] suggesting a block at the $C\mu^+$ pre-B-cell stage of B-cell development. The B cells from patients with this disease do not usually undergo immunoglobulin gene rearrangement, and any $C\mu$ detected may result from expression of a germline IgM transcript composed of a leader sequence spliced to the IgM constant region or of a $D\mu$ protein product of DJ_H recombination.[14] These represent minor products of normal immunoglobulin gene rearrangement found in healthy persons.[15] Rare B cells can be detected in the circulation of patients and, when present, have an immature surface phenotype with a high ratio of surface IgM and IgD and low levels of HLA class II gene products.[16] Occasionally, circulating mature B cells and serum IgG levels higher than observed in typical XLA are detected in patients, but deficiency of antibody production persists.[17]

By genetic linkage analysis using restriction fragment length polymorphisms,[12,18-20] the XLA gene was mapped to Xq21.3–q22 on the proximal portion of the long arm of the X chromosome. There is, however, a degree of nonallelic genetic heterogeneity of the disease, and about 10% of families are not linked to this locus.[20,21] Variability in expression of the XLA defect, however, does not seem to be explained by genetic heterogeneity but appears to reflect variability in gene expression, which can occur in a pedigree or in siblings.[17,22,23] The defect that maps to Xq21.3–q22 is intrinsic to the B cell. In B cells of female carriers of XLA, only the normal X chromosome, and not the XLA-affected X chromosome, is used as the active X chromosome.[12,24,25] Presumably, pre-B cells that use the active X chromosome with the XLA defective gene fail to develop into mature B cells because of decreased proliferation or survival compared with cells expressing the normal X chromosome. The genetic defect at this locus has been shown to be due to defective gene expression of a B-cell specific, cytoplasmic protein tyrosine kinase, termed BPK (B-cell progenitor kinase) or ATK (agammaglobulinemia tyrosine kinase).[26,27] Reduction in, or absence of, the tyrosine kinase transcript or protein and kinase activity has been observed in XLA pre-B and B-cell lines. The precise function of this cytoplasmic tyrosine kinase is under investigation.

Clinical Manifestations

Affected boys have the onset of recurrent pyogenic infections during the latter half of the first year of life as maternal antibody disappears. The initial manifestation is usually chronic or recurrent otitis media, pneumonitis, or pyoderma.[28] Invariably, infections occur at more than one anatomic site and are usually caused by pyogenic bacteria such as pneumococci, streptococci, and *Haemophilus influenzae*. On physical examination, patients with XLA are found to have a paucity of tonsils, adenoids, and peripheral lymph nodes. Mono- or oligoarticular arthritis of large joints with, not uncommonly, sterile effusions may be the presenting problem.[29] The sterile effusion may be caused by infection with an enterovirus or a nonpathogenic

Table 55-1. Primary Immunodeficiencies

Disorder	Inheritance	Locus	Presumed Pathogenesis	Associated Features
Predominantly antibody deficiencies				
X-linked agammaglobulinemia	XL	Xq21.3–q22	Defect of pre-B-cell differentiation secondary to abnormality of a B-cell lineage tyrosine kinase	
X-linked hypogammaglobulinemia with growth hormone deficiency	XL	Xq21.3–q22	Unknown	Short stature
Ig deficiency with hyper-IgM (hyper-IgM syndrome)	XL,AR,?	Xq26.3–q27.1	Failure in isotype switching secondary to abnormal expression of T-cell CD40 ligand	Autoimmune hematologic diseases
CVID (predominant antibody deficiency, predominant CMI defect)	AR,AD,?	?6p21.3	Defect of B-cell maturation/differentiation with intrinsic B-cell defect, decreased B-cell numbers, defective T-helper cell function, antibodies to B cells, or augmented suppressor function	Autoimmunity, malignancy
IgA deficiency	XL,AR,?	?6p21.3	Failure of deletional isotype switching to, and differentiation of, IgA-secreting B cells	Autoimmunity, allergy
Selective deficiency of IgG subclasses	?	?	Defects of isotype differentiation	
Ig heavy chain deletion	AR	14q32.3	Chromosomal deletion at Ig heavy chain gene locus	
κ-chain deficiency	AR	2p11	Point mutation at κ light chain gene locus	
Transient hypogammaglobulinemia of infancy	?	?	Defect of B-cell differentiation	Frequent in families with ID
Combined immunodeficiencies				
SCID				
X-linked	XL	Xq13.1–q13.3	Defect of lymphocyte development secondary to abnormal expression of T-cell IL-2 receptor γ-chain	
Autosomal	AR		Defect of T- and B-cell development	
ADA deficiency	AR	20q13–ter	Defect of T- and B-cell development secondary to toxic metabolites due to deficiency of ADA	Cartilage abnormalities in some
MHC class II deficiency	AR		Defect of transcription of MHC class II molecules	
Reticular dysgenesis	AR		Defect of maturation of lymphoid and myeloid cells	Pancytopenia
PNP deficiency	AR	14q13.1	Defect of T-cell development and function secondary to toxic metabolites due to deficiency of PNP	Anemia, neurologic syndrome
T-cell activation defects				
CD3γ or ε deficiency	AR		Defect of CD3γ or ε transcription	
Defective response to cytokines or expression of cytokine receptors	?		Defect of IL-2 or IL-2 receptor	
Omenn syndrome	AR		?Leaky autosomal SCID	Rash, lymphadenopathy, hepatosplenomegaly, eosinophilia
Other immunodeficiencies				
WAS	XL	Xp11.22–p11.3	Defect of hematopoietic cells	Thrombocytopenia, eczema, malignancies
AT	AR	11q22.3–q23	Defect of DNA repair	Ataxia-telangiectasia, malignancies
DiGeorge syndrome (3rd and 4th pharyngeal pouch/arch syndrome)	AR,?	22q11.21–q11.23	Embryopathy with thymic hypoplasia or aplasia secondary to chromosomal abnormality	Hypoparathyroidism, abnormalities of cardiac outflow tract, and abnormal facies

Abbreviations: CVID, common variable immunodeficiency; SCID, severe combined immunodeficiency; PNP, purine nucleoside phosphorylase; WAS, Wiskott-Aldrich syndrome; AT, ataxia-telangiectasia; ID, immunodeficiency; XL, X-lined; AR, autosomal recessive; ?, unknown; Ig, immunoglobulin; IL, interleukin; CMI, cell-mediated immunity.

(Modifed from WHO Classification of Immunodeficiency Diseases.)

Table 55-2. Associated or Secondary Lymphocyte Disorders with Other Diseases

Secondary Disorder	Immunologic Abnormalities	Associated Features
Chromosomal abnormalities		
Bloom syndrome	Decreased Ig and T-cell function	Chromosomal instability, retarded growth, photosensitivity, malignancy
Fanconi anemia	Decreased IgA and T-cell function	Anemia, neutropenia, skeletal abnormalities
Down syndrome	Decreased Ab and T-cell function	Physical stigmata of trisomy 21
Centromeric instability in chromosomes 1,9,16	Decreased Ig	Malabsorption, dysmorphic facies, developmental delay
Multiple organ system abnormalities		
Partial albinism	Decreased Ig and T-cell function	Albinism, cerebral atrophy
Cartilage hair hypoplasia/short limb dwarfism	Decreased T-cell number and/or T-cell function	Short-limb dwarfism, megacolon
Chédiak-Higashi syndrome	Defective NK cell activity	Granules in nucleated cells
Hereditary metabolic defects		
Transcobalamin 2 deficiency	Decreased Ig and Ab	Vitamin B_{12} deficiency, diarrhea, failure to thrive, megaloblastic pancytopenia
Acrodermatitis enteropathica	Decreased Ig and T-cell function	Skin rash, diarrhea, malabsorption, zinc deficiency
Type 1 hereditary orotic aciduria	Decreased T cells and function	Diarrhea, poor growth, megaloblastic anemia
Biotin-dependent carboxylase deficiency	Decreased IgA and T cells	Acidosis, neurologic abnormalities, dermatitis, alopecia
Other—some examples		
Malnutrition	Thymic and lymphoid atrophy Decreased T-cell number and function	Marasmus, kwashiorkor
Intestinal lymphogiectasia	Decreased Ig and T cells	Edema, ascites
Uremia	Decreased T-cell function	Renal failure
Immunosuppressive agents (radiation, steroids, cytotoxic drugs, chemotherapy)	Decreased lymphocyte number and function	
Infectious disease		
HIV-1 infection, AIDS	Decreased CD4 T-cell number and function	HIV-positive serology, opportunistic infections, malignancy
X-linked lymphoproliferative syndrome	Decreased Ig and Ab	Severe EBV infection, aplastic anemia, lymphoma
Malignancy		
Thymoma	Decreased B and pre-B cells, Ab, and T-cell function	Absent pre-B and B cells, aregenerative anemia, eosinopenia, cytopenia, autoantibodies
Infiltrative and hematologic diseases	Decreased Ab and T-cell function	
Bone marrow transplantation	Decreased B- and T-cell function	GVHD

Abbreviations: Ig, immunoglobulin; Ab, antibody; NK, natural killer; GVHD, graft-verus-host disease; HIV, human immunodeficiency virus; AIDS, acquired immunodeficiency virus; EBV, Epstein-Barr virus.

commensal strain of *Mycoplasma*.[30] Diarrhea from infection with organisms such as *Giardia lamblia* or rotavirus is a common problem. Vaccine-associated poliomyelitis is a potential complication of immunization of these children and is caused by the persistence and mutation of the attenuated poliovirus vaccine strain to a more virulent neurotropic form.[31] Neutropenia may occur during an infection, and leukemia and lymphoma are seen at increased frequency.[7,8] There may be a family history of death at an early age from infection in maternal male relatives.

Infectious diseases can cause significant morbidity. Chronic infections of the upper and lower respiratory tract with otitis media, pneumonitis, and sinusitis may occur despite immunoglobulin replacement therapy. Chronic pulmonary disease develops in almost one-half of XLA patients, and hearing loss, as a result of chronic otitis media or meningoencephalitis, occurs in about one-third of patients.[28] Chronic disseminated enterovirus infection, especially from echovirus, is a potentially fatal complication that may be associated with meningoencephalitis, hepatitis, pneumonitis, or vasculitis, as well as with a dermatomyositis-like syndrome with rash, brawny edema of the subcutaneous tissues, and muscle weakness.[32,33] These complications, as well as other serious infections, have accounted for a mortality rate of about 15% by the age of 20.[28] Earlier diagnosis and more effective intravenous immunoglobulin replacement therapy should lower this mortality rate.

Laboratory Evaluation

Absent antibody responses after immunization or natural antigenic exposure, low levels of serum immunoglobulins, and absent or very low levels of peripheral blood B lymphocytes are characteristic of the disease. The IgG level is usually <200 mg/dl, but exceptions do occur. The other immunoglobulin isotypes are usually low or absent. T-lymphocyte numbers and function are intact. Neutropenia, accompanied by a maturation arrest of granulocytes in the bone marrow occurs not uncommonly as a presenting feature.[34] Lymph nodes show absence of plasma cells, lymphoid follicles, and germinal centers. The definitive diagnosis, prenatal diagnosis, and diagnosis of the carrier state will be facilitated by genetic analysis now that the gene defect has been defined.

Therapy

Immunoglobulin replacement therapy is the mainstay of therapy and should be started once the diagnosis is made, preferably before repetitive infections have caused irreversible pulmonary damage.[35,36] Intravenous immunoglobulin replacement therapy should be employed to provide high doses of immunoglobulin, especially if the volume required for administration by the intramuscular route is excessive. The higher amounts of IgG that can be administered by the intravenous route appear to be better than intramuscular therapy at preventing chronic pulmonary disease and chronic enteroviral meningoencephalitis, but the latter has occurred even with intra-

WHEN TO SUSPECT IMMUNODEFICIENCY STATES

Laboratory studies should be used to confirm a diagnosis of an immunodeficiency disease after performing a thorough history and physical examination to exclude a localized anatomic or physiologic defect that might predispose to recurrent infections. An immunodeficiency should be suspected with the occurrence of infections of an unusual frequency, type, or severity. Recurrent infections may occur at multiple sites and infections may be caused by unusual or opportunistic organisms such as *Pneumocystis carinii, Candida, Mycobacterium avium, Pseudomonas, Serratia,* and cytomegalovirus. There is often a lack of history of exposure, as well as excessive severity or complication of infections and poor response to treatment. With immunodeficiency diseases, organisms may disseminte more widely, multiply to greater numbers, or remain alive in phagocytes. Patients with immunodeficiency diseases often fail to recover to normal health between infections and may have weight loss or poor weight gain. Autoimmune diseases may accompany antibody deficiency states.

Recurrent pyogenic infections, such as otitis media, sinusitis, pneumonia, meningitis, arthritis, and osteomyelitis from encapsulated bacteria (e.g., *Streptococcus pneumoniae, Haemophilus influenzae type b, Neisseria meningitidis, Staphylococcus aureus*) suggest a deficiency of antibody or, less commonly, an abnormality of white blood cells or serum complement. Low numbers or poor function of polymorphonuclear white blood cells is also commonly associated with abscesses and infections with nonencapsulated, nonpathogenic bacteria that reside at the skin or mucosal surfaces. Recurrent infection from viruses, fungi, or intracellular bacteria suggests a deficiency of T-cell function. Infection with *Pneumocystis* suggests T-cell deficiency. Combined deficiency of T- and B-cell function is characterized by bacterial or viral infections. Recurrent systemic *Neisseria* infections suggest deficiency of a terminal complement component. Antibody deficiency in the young child does not predispose to infections until the latter half of the first year of life due to the passive protection provided by maternal antibody. T-cell immunity, however, is not present at birth.

Laboratory evaluation should initially be directed to the type of deficiency suspected on the basis of history and physical examination. Studies should begin with the less expensive and more readily available tests. Results must be compared to age-related normal values. Examination of the CBC and peripheral blood smear may suggest the diagnosis. Live viral immunization should be withheld, and blood products should be irradiated before administration to prevent graft-versus-host disease in patients with T-cell deficiency.

LABORATORY EVALUATION FOR SUSPECTED IMMUNODEFICIENCY DISEASE

General
  CBC
  Chest radiograph
  Serology, culture, and polymerase chain reaction or antigen detection for human immunodeficiency virus
Antibody deficiency
  Initial
    Quantitative immunoglobulins
    Antibody titers before and after immunization: tetanus toxoid, diphtheria toxoid, *Haemophilus influenzae* type b or pneumococcal capsular polysaccharides
    Isohemagglutinins
  Later
    Quantitation of B cells
    IgG subclasses
    In vitro immunoglobulin isotype switching and synthesis
    B-cell XLA-related tyrosine kinase expression
    T-cell CD40 ligand expression
T-lymphocyte deficiency
  Initial
    Absolute lymphocyte count
    Quantitation of T cells and T-cell subsets
    Delayed hypersensitivity skin tests: *Candida,* mumps, *Trichophyton,* tuberculin
  Later
    Lymphocyte proliferative response to mitogens, antigens, and allogeneic cells
    Quantitation of enzymatic activity: ADA, nucleoside phosphorylase
    IL-2 receptor γ-chain, MHC class I and II expression
    In vitro T-cell activation studies
Complement deficiency
  Initial
    Total hemolytic complement (CH_{50})
  Later
    Quantitation and functional analysis of individual components
Polymorphonuclear leukocyte and macrophage deficiency
  Initial
    Polymorphonuclear count and morphology
    Howell-Jolly bodies
    IgE level
    Nitroblue tetrazolium reduction test
  Later
    Rebuck skin window
    Assays for chemotaxis, random migration, phagocytosis, killing, oxidative metabolism, enzymatic activity
    CD11/CD18 expression
    Spleen scan
Other
  α-Fetoprotein
  Skin biopsy and genetic analysis for graft-versus-host disease

venous therapy.[33,37,38] Patients with persistent enterovirus infections have been treated successfully with immunoglobulin preparations containing high titers of antibody specific for the infecting enterovirus.[32,39] For the treatment of enteroviral meningoencephalitis, immunoglobulins may have to be administered directly into the ventricles of the brain to obtain high levels at that site,[40] but even with this therapeutic approach, infection has not always been cleared.[33] Pyogenic infections that occur should be treated vigorously with antibiotics to prevent organ damage.[41] Chronic or recurrent infection of the upper and lower respiratory tracts may require continual prophylactic antibiotic therapy.

IMMUNOGLOBULIN REPLACEMENT THERAPY

Replacement therapy with γ-globulins or immunoglobulins is indicated for patients with recurrent infections with an inability to make antibody responses. The cost of immunoglobulin replacement therapy is quite high and, therefore, should not be used indiscriminately. Ideally, antibody titers before and after immunization with protein and polysaccharide antigens should be evaluated to assess the need for replacement therapy (see previous sidebar). The usual indications include X-linked agammaglobulinemia, common variable immunodeficiency, severe combined immunodeficiency disease, hyper-IgM syndrome, and the Wiskott-Aldrich syndrome. Replacement therapy should not be given to patients with IgG subclass deficiency unless they have been shown to have a deficiency of antibody production and have not responded to antibiotic prophylaxis. Immunoglobulin replacement therapy is not usually indicated for IgA deficiency because IgA is not transported from serum into mucosal surfaces, where it is deficient, and the half-life of transfused serum IgA is very short. In addition, severe or fatal anaphylactic reactions from anti-IgA antibodies of the IgE isotype can occur with the intravenous administration of IgA-containing blood products to IgA-deficient patients. Some patients with IgA deficiency, concomitant deficiency of IgG antibody production, and severe recurrent infections, who also had sustained anaphylactic reactions to the administration of blood products with IgA, have been successfully treated with intravenous immunoglobulin replacement therapy using immunoglobulin preparations containing low levels of IgA.

Development of safe intravenous γ-globulin formulations allows high doses to be given without the pain, side effects, and tissue loss experienced with intramuscular γ-globulin replacement. Intramuscular γ-globulin (16% solution of Cohn fraction II) may still be useful, however, in small infants in whom chronic complications of infections have not occurred and for whom there is difficulty with access to a center where intravenous γ-globulin can be administered. Contraindications to intramuscular γ-globulin include thrombocytopenia, inadequate muscle mass, and poor control of infections. A dose of 100 mg/kg/mo is given, after loading the patient with the same dose administered three times over a 1–2-week period.

Multiple intravenous preparations are approved by the Food and Drug Administration (FDA). All preparations are safe, contain roughly comparable and consistent IgG antibody titers, and are therapeutically equivalent. The FDA-licensed γ-globulins do not carry a risk of transmitting hepatitis or human immunodeficiency virus. Patients vary in their half-life of administered IgG. The optimal amount, frequency of infusion of immunoglobulin, and the serum level of IgG to be achieved need to be individualized to render the patient asymptomatic, but it is recommended that a trough serum level be attained before the next injection ≥200–400 mg/dl higher than the pretherapy level. An initial IgG dose of 400 mg/kg is usually given, followed by a dose of 200–400 mg/kg/mo. These high doses of immunoglobulin, which are more easily provided by the intravenous route, appear better at preventing chronic pulmonary disease or enteroviral meningoencephalitis, but the latter has not been an invariable finding. If patients complain of fatigue, upper respiratory infection, or conjunctivitis during the week before the next infusion, or if other infections occur, the frequency of infusion or the dose should be increased to increase the trough serum level to >500 mg/dl. During intercurrent infections, extra infusions are required because the catabolic rate of the γ-globulin increases. Home infusion therapy is now being practiced widely in the United States.

Adverse reactions to intravenous γ-globulin include flushing, chest tightness, flank or abdominal pain, nausea/vomiting, chills, fever, headache, myalgias, dyspnea, diaphoresis, or hypotension. These reactions can usually be controlled by decreasing the infusion rate. In general, reactions are more common with the first infused dose and in the presence of an intercurrent infection. Infusions should therefore be slower and more cautiously administered in these situations. Repeated severe reactions that fail to respond to a decrease in the rate or volume of the infusion may, in some patients, be averted by pretreatment with aspirin, antihistamines, or steroids. In rare cases, anaphylactic reactions occur. This may be caused by production of IgE antibodies to IgA in patients with IgA deficiency or CVI with absent IgA. In the event of an anaphylactic reaction, the infusion must be stopped and replaced with immediate administration of epinephrine, steroids, and antihistamines, as well as respiratory and circulatory support. Anti-IgA antibodies should be quantitated following an anaphylactic reaction and, if these antibodies are present, intravenous immunoglobulin preparations with low levels of IgA used with caution.

All male siblings and maternal male cousins of an affected boy should be screened for B-cell number, immunoglobulin levels, or the genetic defect during the first several months of life. The carrier state can be detected by analysis of X chromosome inactivation patterns in B cells, by restriction fragment length polymorphism linkage studies in a kindred, or by genetic screening for the X chromosome-encoded tyrosine kinase gene.[10–12]

X-Linked Hypogammaglobulinemia with Growth Hormone Deficiency

X-linked hypogammaglobulinemia with growth hormone deficiency is a rare disorder in which males have marked hypogammaglobulinemia and isolated growth hormone deficiency.[42–44] It should be noted that most patients with growth hormone deficiency have a normal immune system. Absent or decreased numbers of B cells and poor antibody responses with preserved T-cell responses are found. The B-cell defect resembles that observed in XLA and the syndrome maps to a position on the X chromosome similar to XLA, suggesting a contiguous gene deletion syndrome involving the gene for XLA or an allelic variant of this gene.[45]

Immunoglobulin Deficiency with Hyper-IgM

Etiology and Pathophysiology

Immunoglobulin deficiency with increased IgM, termed an immunodeficiency with hyper-IgM (HIM) or the hyper-IgM syndrome, is associated with recurrent infections, increased serum levels of polyclonal IgM and, at times, IgD, and low levels of other immunoglobulin isotypes.[46] The only isotypes expressed on the surface of B cells from these patients are usually IgM and IgD, and when B cells are stimulated in vitro or immortalized with EBV, they secrete only IgM, and not IgG or IgA. Plasmacytoid cells spontaneously secreting IgM are present in the circulation and in lymphoid tissues.[47] Rarely, cells expressing surface IgM and IgG can be detected, but this may result from alternative splicing of a long germline-encoded C_H region sequence RNA transcript that has not undergone isotype switch recombination.[48]

The disease may be acquired or congenital and may be inherited in an X-linked (HIGMX-1) or autosomal recessive manner. HIGMX-1 maps to Xq24–q27, a locus distinct from the XLA locus.[49] T cells were implicated to be the site of the defect with the demonstration that a malignant human T-cell line from a patient with Sézary syndrome could isotype switch B cells from patients with HIM.[50] The defect in HIGMX-1 is due to failure of activated T cells to express a functional CD40 ligand.[51-55] Interaction between the CD40 ligand on activated T cells and CD40 on B cells provides a signal to the B cell to proliferate and mature to allow the B cells to undergo deletional isotype switching in the presence of particular cytokines or interleukins (e.g., IL-4, IL-10). Both point mutations and deletions in the T-cell CD40 ligand gene, which maps to Xq26.3–q27.1, have been described. Cross-linking of CD40 on B cells from patients with HIGMX-1 with antibody or a functional CD40 ligand and stimulation with the appropriate cytokines overcome the defect and activates normal isotype switching and IgG secretion. An acquired form of this syndrome has been described in both sexes, and has been associated with congenial rubella infection or anticonvulsant (phenytoin) therapy. However, the etiology of the acquired form is unknown.

Clinical Manifestations

Recurrent pyogenic bacterial infections begin during the first or second year of life, as observed in XLA, with primarily recurrent otitis media, upper respiratory tract infections, and pneumonia. In contrast to other primary humoral immunodeficiencies, HIM is associated with an unusual susceptibility to *Pneumocystis carinii* pneumonia. Diarrhea and malabsorption are common. Lymphoid hyperplasia with lymphadenopathy, tonsillar enlargement, and hepatosplenomegaly occur. Neutropenia, hemolytic anemia, and thrombocytopenia result from the production of autoantibodies. Another form of neutropenia, which is usually cyclic, can also result from defective myeloid differentiation. Stomatitis and recurrent oral ulcers are complications of the neutropenia. Surface IgM+ non-Hodgkin and Hodgkin lymphoma with gastrointestinal tract involvement may develop as well.

Laboratory Evaluation

Serum levels of IgM and, at times, IgD, are markedly elevated, and the other isotypes are low or absent. The IgM is polyclonal, and antibody responses, when they occur, are restricted to the IgM isotype. In addition to the normally occurring 19S IgM molecules, a 7S IgM fraction may be produced and lead to overestimation of levels of immunoglobulins quantitated by radial immunodiffusion. Peripheral blood B lymphocytes express IgM and IgD, but cells with surface IgG or IgA are usually, but not invariably,[48] absent. In vitro stimulation of peripheral blood B lymphocytes with anti-CD40 in the presence of IL-10 or IL-4 will activate IgG isotype switching to, and secretion of, IgG or IgE, respectively. Definitive diagnosis of the HIGMX-1 is made by demonstrating the lack of binding of soluble forms of CD40 to the CD40 ligand on activated T cells. Female carriers of HIGMX-1 can be diagnosed by demonstrating binding of CD40 to only one-half their activated T cells. Lymph nodes lack follicles and

germinal centers in the primary HIM syndrome, probably secondary to defective signaling to CD40 on B cells by the T-cell CD40 ligand. This signal is required to prevent apoptosis, or programmed cell death, of germinal center B cells.

Therapy

As in XLA, immunoglobulin therapy is indicated. With treatment, the IgM level sometimes decreases, presumably on the basis of feedback inhibition, and lymphoid hyperplasia and neutropenia may be reversed.[56]

Common Variable Immunodeficiency

Etiology and Pathophysiology

CVID, the most frequent type of primary specific immunodeficiency other than IgA deficiency, includes a group of heterogeneous disorders associated with recurrent infections, poor antibody responses, and hypogammaglobulinemia. CVID includes both congenital and acquired defects that have variable ages of onset, clinical symptoms, immunologic defects, and underlying basic defects.[57-59]

Decreased numbers of B lymphocytes are found in few patients. In most patients, B cells are normal in number but fail to differentiate into antibody-secreting plasma cells after stimulation.[59] Failure of B-cell maturation and differentiation are usually thought to be primarily due to an intrinsic B-cell defect and, less frequently, secondary to a T-cell defect.[57-60] Intrinsic B-cell defects include a failure of B-cell proliferation or maturation and differentiation after appropriate stimuli or an inability to secrete immunoglobulins synthesized in a B-cell that has differentiated.[57-62] The basis for the former defect is unknown but is sometimes associated with an immature B-cell surface phenotype.[61,63,64] The surface IgG-bearing cells in CVID more commonly co-express surface IgM than do B cells from normal controls. The failure to secrete immunoglobulins has been associated with abnormal glycosylation of immunoglobulins.[65] The literature on in vitro stimulation of B cells has been reviewed; a classification of patients based on the ability of B cells from patients with CVID to secrete IgM or IgG after stimulation with anti-IgM and IL-2 or EBV distinguishes five subgroups of CVID.[59,66] Isolated defects of helper/inducer T lymphocytes or increased numbers of circulating activated suppressor/cytotoxic T cells that inhibit B-cell differentiation and antibody production are occasionally found as the primary defect.[57-61,67] Some patients show decreased T-cell production of IL-2, IL-4, and IL-5 after stimulation through the CD3/T-cell receptor complex.[60] Circulating antilymphocyte antibodies or inhibitors that block in vivo B-cell activation and differentiation have also been demonstrated in some patients.[68,69]

Occasionally, the disorder can be familial, with or without a clear-cut pattern of inheritance. First-degree relatives may have selective IgA deficiency or autoimmune diseases such as systemic lupus erythematosus, hemolytic anemia, or idiopathic thrombocytopenic purpura.[70-72] A CVID susceptibility gene has been proposed to lie within or near the MHC class III region on chromosome 6. This is based on common expression of particular extended haplotypes with deletions in the complement C4 locus in patients with either CVID or IgA deficiency, suggesting a common genetic predisposition underlying both disorders.[73-75] Viral infections, including congenital rubella and EBV, have been incriminated in the etiology of some instances of CVID. By contrast, HIV and hepatitis virus infections have been reported to restore IgG and antibody production in some patients with CVID.[76-79]

Clinical Manifestations

CVID occurs in both sexes. The clinical spectrum is variable, with the age of onset varying from childhood to late adulthood. Recurrent pyogenic infections resulting in otitis media, sinusitis, bronchitis, and pneumonia, often caused by pneumococci, staphylococci, *H. influenzae,* or *Mycoplasma pneumoniae,* occur.[58,80-82] Bronchiectasis is a frequent complication and may even be the presenting abnormality. Cor pulmonale and respiratory failure on the basis of chronic lung disease are common causes of death. In contrast to XLA, lymphoid tissue is normal or enlarged as a result of B-cell proliferation and prominent germinal center formation. Splenomegaly occurs in approximately 25% of patients and may be associated with neutropenia and thrombocytopenia from hypersplenism. Noncaseating granulomas resembling sarcoidosis, in the spleen, liver, or lung, may be observed. Arthritis and arthralgia are common. Chronic gastritis and achlorhydria, diarrhea, a sprue-like syndrome with malabsorption, lactose deficiency, or protein-losing enteropathy may complicate the clinical course.[83] *G. lamblia* or *Campylobacter* infection of the gastrointestinal tract may contribute to these gastrointestinal symptoms.[77] Pernicious anemia develops in some patients because of atrophic gastritis and absence of intrinsic factor. Hepatitis may occur. Autoimmune diseases, including autoimmune hemolytic anemia, thrombocytopenia or neutropenia, rheumatoid arthritis, chronic active hepatitis, or thyroiditis, are frequently seen.

Overall there is a 5-fold increase in the incidence of cancer in CVID, with a 47-fold increase in gastric cancer and a 30-fold increase in lymphomas.[7,84-86] This increased incidence of gastric cancer may be related to the high frequency of achlorhydria, decreased gastric secretion, and atrophic gastritis.[87] A nonmalignant lymphoproliferation with follicular hyperplasia of the lymph nodes or nodular lymphoid hyperplasia of the intestine and splenomegaly may also occur and must be distinguished from malignant lymphoma.[88]

Laboratory Evaluation

Serum immunoglobulins, especially IgG and IgA, are decreased, and antibody responses are impaired. The peripheral blood B-cell number is normal in about three-fourths of patients, but the surface phenotype may be immature, and the cells fail to differentiate to antibody-secreting cells after appropriate stimuli. T-cell numbers may be decreased and a reversal of the helper/suppressor (CD4/CD8) T-cell ratio may be present. Some patients have expanded numbers of activated CD8+/CD57+ circulating T cells.[60,89] Depressed T-cell function and absent delayed hypersensitivity skin test reactivity may be found, especially in older patients, and in those patients with lymphopenia.

Therapy

Immunoglobulin replacement and aggressive antibiotic therapy are indicated. After immunoglobulin replacement therapy is instituted, pulmonary radiographic and functional changes may stabilize.[38,90] Serial pulmonary function tests need to be followed. Acute infections, however, may still occur and require prolonged antibiotic treatment to prevent deterioration of lung function. Parenteral therapy with vitamin B$_{12}$ is required for pernicious anemia. A small bowel biopsy may be required to diagnose *Giardia* infestation.

Selective IgA Deficiency

Etiology and Pathogenesis

Deficiency of serum IgA, defined as a serum IgA concentration of <5 mg/dl, is found at a frequency of approximately 1 in 600 persons of European descent.[91-96] Most are asymptomatic, but some patients suffer from recurrent sinopulmonary infections because of the deficiency of IgA in mucosal secretions. Autoimmune and allergic diseases are relatively common with this disorder. These disorders occur as a result of either absorption of environmental and dietary antigens into the systemic circulation due to the lack of secretory IgA at mucosal surfaces or on the basis of an underlying broader immunologic defect with poor regulation of autoantibody production due to common susceptibility genes in IgA deficiency and autoimmunity.[73,74,97,98]

IgA deficiency may be primary or secondary. It occurs in a sporadic form or with autosomal dominant or recessive patterns of inheritance.[99] Particular fixed haplotypes of MHC genes, so-called supratypes reflecting conserved ancestral haplotypes, are associated with IgA deficiency.[72-74,100] An important locus for regulation of IgA production appears to be present in the MHC class III gene cluster, an 1,100-kb region of DNA located between the class I and II gene clusters. The gene(s) appear(s) to be affected by deletions, duplications, or rearrangements that also involve the complement protein C4 or the 21-hydroxylase enzyme genes. IgA deficiency may be found in relatives of patients with hypogammaglobulinemia, and family members of patients with IgA deficiency may have altered immunoglobulin levels or CVID.[70,72-74] The presence of an MHC class II susceptibility gene has also been suggested.[97,98] These putative MHC gene(s) may be necessary but not sufficient for the development of the immunodeficiency; they may also increase susceptibility to the autoimmune diseases observed in IgA deficiency. Congenital infections with rubella, cytomegalovirus, or *Toxoplasma gondii* and acquired EBV infection have been associated with IgA deficiency. IgA deficiency may also occur after use of the drugs penicillamine, phenytoins, sodium aurothiomalate, captopril, sulfasalazine, or antimalarial agents. The underlying genetic predisposition to IgA deficiency may also increase susceptibility to these drug reactions, which usually resolve when the drug is withdrawn. At times, IgA deficiency is transitory both in adults and in children, especially when the serum IgA is moderately decreased, but concomitant IgG2 deficiency and abnormal antibody responses may still persist.[101]

Most patients with IgA deficiency have intact structural IgA immunoglobulin heavy chain genes.[102] Surface IgA-bearing B cells are present in normal to slightly decreased number, but the cells may display an immature phenotype in some patients with co-expression of surface IgM.[103] The primary defect appears to be failure of B cells to differentiate to mature isotype-switched surface IgA positive B cells and IgA-secreting plasma cells with appropriate stimuli.[95,96,104,105] Defective in vitro T-helper cells and excessive suppressor T-cell activity for IgA production are occasionally but not usually present.[95,96,104-107] Most patients lack both serum and secretory IgA and have a deficiency of both the IgA1 and IgA2 subclasses. Patients with IgA deficiency who lack serum IgA but express IgA2 secretory plasma cells in the gastrointestinal tract have been described. Rarely, IgA deficiency is associated with a deficiency of the secretory component, the protein that is required for secretion of IgA into the mucosa. The susceptibility to infection in IgA deficiency may not be secondary to IgA deficiency per se, but either to a concomitant deficiency of IgG2 and IgG4 subclass immunoglobulins or to defective production of antibody to bacterial antigens, especially bacterial polysaccharides, or both.[94,108-111] Thus, IgA deficiency in some patients may represent a manifestation of a more widely based immunologic defect with similarities to CVID, which also is an arrest in B-cell differentiation, and occurs in family members and shares common MHC haplotypes with IgA deficiency.[96,111] IgA deficiency may in fact evolve into CVID and is also frequently found in AT, which is also associated with T-cell abnormalities and IgG subclass deficiency, as detailed below.

Clinical Manifestations

Most people with IgA deficiency are healthy, but many exhibit variable clinical symptoms.[93-96] An increased frequency of upper and lower respiratory tract infections occurs. Infections are more commonly seen when low levels of IgA occur with a deficiency of IgG subclasses.[108] Some patients have recurrent sinusitis, otitis media, bronchitis, and even bronchiectasis. An increased incidence of autoimmune diseases, especially rheumatoid arthritis and systemic lupus erythematosus, may occur in 5% of IgA-deficient patients.[112] Other autoimmune diseases may be observed, and autoantibodies may be present without symptoms. Allergic diseases, including rhinitis, urticaria, eczema, and asthma, occur at increased frequency. Gastrointestinal and hepatic complications in IgA deficiency include malabsorption, celiac disease, giardiasis, nodular lymphoid hyperplasia, pernicious anemia, atrophic gastritis, primary biliary cirrhosis, and chronic active hepatitis.[83] Gastric and colonic carcinoma are found at increased frequency.[113] Production of antibodies to food antigens, such as cow's milk, may cause immune complexes that may be pathogenic.[114]

Laboratory Evaluation

The serum concentration of IgA is <5 mg/dl, and the levels of IgG and IgM are normal. Secretory IgA is also decreased. Approximately one-fourth of patients have decreased levels of IgE. Some patients, especially those with recurrent sinopulmonary infections, have a concomitant deficiency of the IgG2 and IgG4 subclasses or defective antibody responses to polysaccharides, or both.[108,109] IgA and IgG levels should be repeated after a period of time to determine whether the deficiency of IgA is persistent[101] or whether the immunologic disorder has become more extensive and begun to resemble CVID. A high incidence of autoantibodies (to nuclear proteins, immunoglobulins, thyroglobulin, or adrenal, parietal, smooth muscle, or pancreatic cells) or to food antigens such as cow's milk proteins is found. Serum antibodies to IgA occur in 30–40% of patients with IgA deficiency but are not predictive of adverse reactions to blood products containing IgA.[15] Exposure to blood products with IgA may, however, induce IgE anti-IgA antibodies that can cause anaphylactic reactions.[116]

Therapy

Treatment should be directed to the associated infections, allergic, autoimmune, and gastrointestinal diseases. Precipitating drugs should be discontinued. Antibiotic therapy is indicated for bacterial infections. If infections are severe or cause significant sequelae, prophylactic antibiotics should be considered. Immunoglobulin replacement therapy is not usually indicated for IgA deficiency[35] (see the sidebar Immunoglobulin Replacement Therapy). Severe or fatal anaphylactic reactions can occur with the intravenous administration of IgA-containing blood products to IgA-deficient patients.[116,117] This may be caused by anti-IgA antibody of the IgE isotype that may increase after immunoglobulin replacement therapy.[116] Some patients with anaphylactic reactions to IgA and with severe recurrent infections and concomitant deficiency of IgG subclasses and antibody production, however, have benefited clinically from treatment with intravenous immunoglobulin replacement therapy with immunoglobulin preparations with low levels of IgA.[116,117] Blood products should be washed prior to transfusion of IgA-deficient patients or obtained from IgA-deficient donors, including the recipient, prior to surgery. Plasma for transfusion should be collected from other IgA-deficient patients. Oral administration of γ-globulin has improved chronic diarrhea in some patients.

Selective Deficiency of Immunoglobulin Isotypes

Selective deficiency of an immunoglobulin isotype is not usually associated with structural gene abnormalities. Rarely, deletions of the immunoglobulin constant-region genes have been described and may involve several or single constant-region gene segments.[118-120] Most patients with these partial deletions, however, are healthy.

Selective IgM deficiency is a rare immunodeficiency disorder characterized by a low level of serum IgM and severe or life-threatening recurrent infections.[121,122] Pneumococcal and meningococcal sepsis or meningitis may occur. IgM antibodies are not produced, and IgG antibody responses are usually decreased, despite the normal IgG level. Defects of T-cell helper and excessive suppressor T-cell activity have been described.[122] In some cases, CVID may subsequently develop.

The absence of either κ or λ light chains associated with hypogammaglobulinemia or IgA deficiency and recurrent respiratory tract infections, pernicious anemia, diarrhea, or malabsorption have been reported in rare instances. In one patient with κ light chain deficiency, a point mutation was found in the Ck gene involving amino acid residues required for the formation of intrachain disulfide bonds and protein folding.[123]

IgG Subclass Deficiency

Recurrent upper and lower respiratory tract bacterial infections, sinusitis, and otitis media may occur in patients with normal total IgG levels and low levels of an IgG subclass.[111] The most common symptomatic IgG subclass deficiency in childhood is IgG2 subclass deficiency. This subclass represents approximately 20–25% of the total IgG.[111,124-127] IgG subclass defects may occur alone or with concomitant IgG4 subclass or IgA deficiency[108,111,127] and may be associated with the inability to generate antibodies to polysaccharides.[111,126] The subclass deficiency does not represent the primary etiology for the poor antibody responses to polysaccharide antigens. IgG2 subclass deficiency, poor antibody responses, and IgA deficiency may reflect an underlying broader immunoregulatory defect in these patients. Recurrent infections with decreased antibody responses to polysaccharide antigen may, in fact, occur with either normal or low IgG subclass levels. The poor antibody responses to polysaccharide antigens may contribute, however, to a low IgG2 subclass level. In most patients, the structural IgG heavy chain genes on chromosome 14 are normal.[111,118] Rarely, patients who lack one or more IgG subclasses on the basis of a homozygous deletion of heavy chain IgG constant-region genes have been described,[118] but such patients are usually asymptomatic. Antibody deficiency and not isolated IgG subclass deficiency per se is therefore the cause of recurrent infections. Isolated IgG subclass deficiency may be associated with IgA deficiency as noted above,[108,111] or with AT.[128] Although IgG2 subclass deficiency predominates in children, symptomatic isolated IgG3 deficiency is more commonly detected in adults.[87-89]

Interpretation of IgG subclass values must be approached with attention to the wide range of normal age-related values. The finding of a low IgG subclass level should lead to quantifying the antibody response to a polysaccharide vaccine, such as the H. influenzae type b or pneumococcal capsular polysaccharide vaccine.[129] In children with recurrent sinopulmonary infections, quantitation of antibody responses to protein and polysaccharide antigens (see the sidebar Laboratory Evaluation for Suspected Immunodeficiency Disease) is preferable to quantitating IgG subclass levels. Immunization with polysaccharide-protein conjugate vaccines can overcome the unresponsiveness to polysaccharide antigens in IgG2 subclass deficiency[130] and may be of therapeutic value. If the frequency of infections in patients with symptomatic IgG subclass deficiency is not decreased with prophylactic antibiotics, immunoglobulin replacement therapy may be used, but caution must be exercised in the face of concomitant IgA deficiency. In some children, the IgG subclass deficiency spontaneously disappears with time.

Transient Hypogammaglobulinemia of Infancy

Transient hypogammaglobulinemia of infancy is characterized by a prolongation of the physiologic hypogammaglobulinemia normally observed in infants at 3–6 months of age resulting from the catabolism of maternally derived IgG.[131–133] Low levels of serum IgG are observed during the first 2 years of life because of decreased IgG synthesis. These levels then slowly increase to normal. Circulating B lymphocytes are normal in number, and antibody responses to protein antigens are preserved. The serum IgM and IgA may also be decreased. Intrinsic B-cell defects or T-cell helper defects have been incriminated in the disorder.[134] Two groups of patients should be distinguished.[131] In one group, young infants have relatives with immunodeficiency diseases and are relatively asymptomatic.[131–133,135] The other group, without immunodeficient relatives, suffers from frequent sinopulmonary infections. The disorder must be distinguished from primary immunodeficiency diseases by careful immunologic evaluation and follow-up. Because the affected infants spontaneously outgrow their susceptibility to infection, immunoglobulin replacement therapy is rarely indicated, except for those patients with severe recurrent infections. Although immunoglobulin levels usually return to normal, persistent IgA deficiency or borderline low levels of serum IgG may be observed for a prolonged period in some patients.[131–133]

COMBINED IMMUNODEFICIENCIES

Severe Combined Immunodeficiency-X-Linked, Autosomal Recessive, Adenosine Deaminase Deficiency, MHC Class II Deficiency, T-Cell Activation Defects

Etiology and Pathophysiology

Severe combined immunodeficiency (SCID) is a heterogeneous disorder characterized by profound T- and B-lymphocyte deficiency that may have an autosomal recessive or X-linked inheritance.[136] About 80% of affected patients are boys, and only about one-third of SCID patients have a positive family history. In SCID, there is a defect in T- or T- and B-cell development. Because bone marrow transplantation can completely correct the defect, a thymic defect is not thought to be the underlying basis of the disease in most patients. The thymus is secondarily affected with defective epithelial cell differentiation and absence of lymphoid cells and Hassall's corpuscles.

The X-linked form of SCID (X-SCID), thought to be the most common form, maps to Xq13.1–q21.1 and is characterized by absence of mature T cells and the presence of B cells.[10–12,137] The molecular basis of X-SCID is a mutation in the IL-2 receptor γ-chain (IL-2Rγ), a component of the high- and intermediate-affinity IL-2 receptors, and a component of the IL-7 and IL-4 receptors.[138,139] The gene for IL-2Rγ maps to human chromosome Xq13. IL-2Rγ is constitutively expressed in T cells. Mutations of the γ-chain will interfere with T-cell development in the thymus, clonal proliferation, and signal transduction. Although the number of B cells in X-SCID may be normal, the B cells are not functional. The B cells have an immature phenotype and fail to differentiate or produce IgG after in vitro stimulation.[140,141] B-cell dysfunction is secondary to a lack of T-cell help, and possibly to a subtle intrinsic B-cell defect. The latter

is demonstrated by the delay in establishing normal B-cell function after BMT and by the finding of nonrandom X chromosome inactivation patterns in mature differentiated B cells of carriers.[10–12] Female carriers are immunologically normal. T cells as well as mature B cells of carriers show nonrandom X chromosome inactivation patterns, with the X chromosome bearing the X-SCID mutation consistently being inactive.[142,143] These findings suggest that both T-cell and mature B-cell development are affected by the X-linked gene defect.

Approximately 30–40% of patients with the autosomal recessive form of SCID have deficiencies of the enzyme ADA, an enzyme of the purine salvage pathway that deaminates adenosine and deoxyadenosine to inosine and deoxyinosine.[144–146] The pathophysiologic mechanisms whereby ADA deficiency causes lymphocyte abnormalities have not been conclusively established. Although ADA is expressed by all cell types, ADA deficiency preferentially affects the lymphoid system and interferes with lymphoid development in the thymus (these sites contain the highest level of ADA activity in the body). ADA deficiency is characterized by an accumulation of the toxic metabolites of purine metabolism, dATP and 2'-deoxyadenosine. Deoxyadenosine is generated in high amounts in the thymus from the extensive lymphocyte death that occurs with lymphoid development at that site. Deoxyadenosine is freely transported out of cells but is converted intracellularly by deoxyadenosine kinase into dATP that is not in equilibrium with the extracellular space. These metabolites preferentially accumulate in lymphocytes because of their high expression of deoxyadenosine kinase. dATP inhibits T-cell proliferation by affecting DNA synthesis through inhibition of ribonucleotide reductase. Accumulation of *S*-adenosylhomocysteine, which occurs from inactivation of the enzyme *S*-adenosylhomocysteine hydrolase by 2-deoxyadenosine, interferes with methylation reactions and may also contribute to the lymphocyte defect. The accumulation of these metabolites may also block endogenous DNA repair, leading to chromosomal breaks. ADA deficiency, which may be complete or partial, is usually due to point mutations of the ADA gene, located on the long arm of chromosome 20, giving rise to a nonfunctional protein because of alteration in enzymatic activity, stability, or structure.[144] Splicing defects and chromosomal deletions of the ADA gene have also been described. The immunodeficiency is progressive and variable in age of presentation, depending on the amount of residual ADA activity.[147] In contrast to other forms of SCID, in ADA deficiency the thymus may develop with production of Hassall's corpuscles but then involutes with increasing age during infancy.

In another autosomal recessive form of the disease, so-called Swiss-type SCID, ADA activity is normal with the failure of maturation of T and B lymphocytes, resulting in lymphopenia. Natural killer (NK) cells are present and functional. The molecular basis of this form of SCID is unknown. The possibility that this form of SCID is due to defective DNA repair, which is required during the normal rearrangement of immunoglobulin and T-cell receptor (TCR) genes, has been suggested by the finding of aberrant D-J$_H$ joining in bone marrow pre-B cells from patients with SCID.[148] Additional support for a DNA repair defect comes from the finding of increased radiosensitivity of colony-forming unit-granulocyte/macrophage and skin fibroblasts from patients with ADA$^+$ autosomal recessive SCID.[149]

A related entity is Omenn syndrome, an autosomal recessive combined immunodeficiency disorder with dermatitis, generalized lymphadenopathy, eosinophilia, hepatosplenomegaly, and failure to thrive. The syndrome clinically resembles graft-versus-host disease (GVHD),[150–152] but the cells infiltrating the skin and organs are autologous activated self-reactive cells. These activated cells (HLA-DR$^+$, CD45 R0$^+$, CD29$^+$) have restricted heterogeneity and spontaneously produce high levels of IL-5, which may explain the eosinophilia. Families in which one offspring had Omenn syndrome and another offspring had typical lymphopenic SCID have been described. Cells from patients with Omenn syndrome also show the increased radiosensitivity described above. Both findings suggest that Omenn syndrome may be a "leaky" Swiss-type SCID.[136,149,152] Treatment with either cyclosporine[151] or interferon-γ (IFN-γ)[153] have improved the clinical condition and even the eosinophilia, but BMT is required to correct the syndrome permanently.

MHC class II deficiency is an autosomal recessive disorder characterized by failure of expression of HLA class II (HLA-DR, -DQ, and -DP) surface molecules on bone marrow-derived cells, enterocytes, and endothelial cells.[154] B lymphocytes, monocytes, and activated T lymphocytes fail to express class II molecules. MHC class II recognition is required for the positive selection of T cells in the thymus and for interaction of T cells with antigen-presenting cells (see Chs. 10 and 20). Antigen recognition by CD4+ T cells requires the presentation and recognition of antigen with HLA class II molecules on the surface of the antigen-presenting cell. The defect in this disease results from defective transcription of the HLA class II α- and β-chains.[154–156] The protein transactivating regulatory factor, termed RF-X, fails to bind to a 5′-regulatory sequence common to HLA class II promoters, hence the failure of induction of HLA class II molecule transcription. This failure to bind could reflect the lack of another normal transcriptional factor required for cooperative binding or needed to bind prior to RF-X binding. An alternative possibility is that the mutation affects the configuration of the promoter.[157–160] Recent data suggest that the factor(s) defective in some patients with MHC class II deficiency control(s) the accessibility of the class II promoter within the native environment of the MHC.[160] The gene affected demonstrates heterogeneity, with at least four distinct genetic defects.[158] This syndrome differs from another subtype of the bare lymphocyte syndrome, characterized by inconstant and incomplete abnormal expression of HLA class I antigens that is always corrected by IFN.[161] Normal numbers of T and B lymphocytes are found in MHC class II deficiency, but CD4 lymphocytes are commonly decreased and CD8 lymphocytes increased. Lymphocyte function is abnormal, with absent in vitro and in vivo T-cell responses to specific antigens. This is because antigen must be presented within the context of MHC class II molecules. Mitogen and allogeneic in vitro responses may be preserved, although class II molecules are not expressed after T-cell activation. Macrophages fail to present antigens to normal T cells. Normal immunoglobulin levels may be present, but antibody responses after immunization are usually absent. Patients with MHC class II deficiency present with a clinical picture typical of SCID with recurrent, severe bacterial and viral infections, chronic diarrhea, and failure to thrive.[154]

T-cell defects that impair T-cell activation through the TCR and CD3 complex may lead to SCID in the presence of normal numbers of T lymphocytes.[162,163] Different defects can lead to impairment of early events in T cell-signaling and signal transduction.[162–165] In some of these defects, the TCR/CD3 complex is poorly expressed on T cells because of mutations in the genes encoding one of the protein constituents of the CD3 receptor. Mutations in the genes encoding the CD3γ- or ε-chains lead to an autosomal recessive form of SCID with defective expression of, and signaling through, the TCR/CD3 complex.[166,167] Occasional cases of SCID have been attributed to defective production of IL-2.[168–170] The defect causing IL-2 deficiency may be heterogeneous. IL-2 deficiency in one patient was accompanied by deficiency of other cytokines (IL-3, IL-4, IL-5, and IFN-γ).[169] In the latter situation, a defect was present in binding activity of the T lymphocyte nuclear factor of activated T cells, a T-cell specific transfactor that binds a response element in the regulatory region of IL-2.[171] Exogenous IL-2 has been shown in some patients to achieve partial correction of the impaired T-cell function in vitro, and in vivo trials with IL-2 and polyethylene glycol-modified IL-2 are currently under way.[168,172] Abnormal responses to IL-1,[173] and IL-2,[174] have also been associated with SCID.

Another autosomal recessive form of SCID is termed reticular dysgenesis, characterized by the absence of both B and T lymphocytes and granulocytes in the peripheral blood and bone marrow.[175,176] Both B cell and myeloid lineage cells in the bone marrow demonstrate defective maturation. The molecular basis of this defect is unknown. Overwhelming infections ensue unless the defect is corrected by bone marrow transplantation.[177]

Clinical Manifestations

The different forms of SCID are generally clinically indistinguishable.[136] SCID usually presents in early infancy with recurrent severe infections or persistent infections with low-virulence opportunistic organisms, such as *Candida albicans*, which give rise to chronic thrush, or *Pneumocystis carinii*, which give rise to chronic interstitial pneumonitis. Chronic diarrhea and failure to thrive usually occur. Recurrent otitis media, skin infections, and chronic severe viral infections are frequent.

In contrast to other forms of SCID, patients with partial ADA deficiency may have symptoms delayed until the latter half of the first or second year of life or even at 3–8 years. The progression of immunity deterioration is slower with partial ADA deficiency because of the time required to accumulate the toxic metabolites. About one-half of children with ADA deficiency may have radiologic anomalies of the rib cage, with flared costochondral junctions, and of the scapula and skeleton, but these abnormalities are not specific for ADA deficiency. Neurologic abnormalities have been observed with ADA deficiency.

GVHD may arise from transfusion of nonirradiated blood products or, more rarely, from maternal/fetal transfer of lymphocytes in utero or at delivery, manifested by fever, rash, diarrhea, and hepatosplenomegaly.[178–180] Although engraftment with maternal lymphocytes occurs in ≤50% of children with SCID, GVHD usually does not ensue, probably because the maternal lymphocyte cells are immature, represent a limited repertoire, and have suboptimal responses to activation.[181,182]

Laboratory Evaluation

In an effort to offer the best therapy, the diagnosis of SCID should be established at the earliest age possible. The total lymphocyte count is often low, but normal lymphocyte counts do not exclude the diagnosis of SCID. T-cell numbers, and especially CD4+ T cells, are usually markedly decreased, and those present may display an immature phenotype.[183] If substantial numbers of T cells are present, they may be derived from engraftment of maternal lymphocytes or may reflect the presence of a T-cell activation defect or MHC class II deficiency. B-cell numbers may be decreased, normal, or elevated. Swiss-type SCID is associated with decreased T and B lymphocytes. In vitro T-cell responses to mitogens and allogeneic cells are absent or very poor, and responses to antigens are absent. Cutaneous delayed-type hypersensitivity reactions are absent. Immunoglobulin levels are usually decreased and antibody responses absent, but exceptions have been observed in some patients with partial ADA deficiency. NK cells may be increased in number. Infection with human immunodeficiency virus must be ruled out as a cause of this type of immunodeficiency.

Special studies that may be necessary include quantitation of ADA, dATP, and deoxyadenosine, purine nucleoside phosphorylase (PNP) activity, dGTP, and deoxyguanosine (see below) in blood; examination of cells for the presence of class

I and class II MHC surface molecules; and skin biopsy of rashes to establish the diagnosis of GVHD.

Therapy

If the immunodeficiency is not corrected, SCID invariably proves fatal. Transplantation of bone marrow cells from HLA genotypically identical family donors completely restores the immunologic function of patients with various forms (X-linked, autosomal recessive ADA$^-$ and ADA$^+$, PNP deficiency, reticular dysgenesis, MHC class II deficiency) of SCID without causing GVHD[184-190] (see Ch. 27). Pretransplant preparative cytoablation is not required for haploidentical transplants. The success rate of HLA identical BMT is now >90% with engraftment of both donor T and B lymphocytes.[136] Both lymphoid and hematopoietic stem cell engraftment are required to correct SCID from reticular dysgenesis, MHC class II deficiency, and IL-1 deficiency.[190] In the absence of matched related donors, T-cell-depleted haploidentical parental[186,188] or matched unrelated donor[189] BMTs are successful with relatively low frequencies of GVHD.[186,188] Mature T cells are depleted from the bone marrow by physical (rosetting with sheep erythrocytes and removal on lectin soybean agglutinin columns) or by immunologic (antibodies and complement) approaches to prevent GVHD from transferred mature donor T cells. Donor stem cells develop into T cells that undergo clonal deletion and anergy

in the host thymus, establishing a state of tolerance of the host.[190] Although T cells can engraft in the absence of GVHD with these purged bone marrow transplants, immunologic reconstitution is slower than that observed after HLA-identical BMT, probably because T cells are developing solely from donor lymphoid stem cells with recapitulation of immunologic ontogeny. B-cell engraftment may be extremely delayed or may fail to occur because of failure of cooperation between donor haploidentical T-helper cells and host B cells.[190-192] Failure of engraftment is correlated with preserved recipient NK cell function and absence of IL-1 production by monocytes.[186] Myeloablation and immunosuppression of the marrow transplant recipient with busulfan and cyclophosphamide increase T- and B-cell engraftment. The success rate of haploidentical BMT is now >70% and is approaching the success rate of genotypically identical BMT.[136,186-188]

All blood products should be irradiated before transfusion into patients with SCID in order to prevent GVHD. Immunoglobulin replacement therapy, nutritional support, and prophylaxis of infection (*P. carinii*) are usually required. Family members should be immunized with the inactivated poliovirus vaccine to prevent infection in patients.

In the absence of an HLA-identical bone marrow donor for correction of ADA-deficient SCID, enzyme replacement therapy by intramuscular injection of polyethylene glycol (PEG)-modified bovine ADA, which prolongs the circulating half-life of the enzyme and decreases its immunogenicity, can improve the immunologic and clinical status of patients with ADA deficiency.[193] The exogenous ADA lowers the level of the toxic metabolites in ADA-deficient lymphocytes by deaminating adenosine and 2'-deoxyadenosine. The overall efficacy of long-term regular infusions is under evaluation, and it is not clear whether exogenous ADA is as efficacious as ADA synthesized within lymphocytes. Haploidentical BMT is an alternative approach favored by some for treatment of ADA-SCID. The use of PEG-ADA prior to transplantation, however, may restore host immunologic function and may predispose to graft rejection. Similarly, ADA activity in the transplanted marrow may stimulate immunologic function of the recipient's T cells that prevent engraftment, which can be avoided by the use of pretransplant cytotoxic agents. Gene replacement therapy for permanent correction of ADA deficiency is under investigation.[194,195] Children have been treated with autologous peripheral blood T cells and with autologous CD34$^+$ pluripotent stem cells that expressed a normal human ADA gene after transduction with retroviral vectors containing a human ADA cDNA. The success of these attempts at somatic gene therapy has not been defined.

ADA-deficient-SCID and X-SCID can be diagnosed prenatally, and the carrier state can be identified. The prenatal diagnosis of ADA deficiency is performed by assaying ADA activity or dATP levels in cultured amniotic cells, fetal blood obtained by fetoscopy, or chorionic villi samples. Using midtrimester fetal blood samples, T-cell subsets can be quantitated, in vitro proliferative responses measured, and deoxynucleotides measured to help confirm the diagnosis of SCID. Some children have small amounts of residual ADA activity, posing difficulties in diagnosis. The prenatal diagnosis of X-SCID will be easier now that the genetic defect has been identified.

Purine Nucleoside Phosphorylase Deficiency

PNP deficiency is a rare autosomal recessive disease that results from a defect in the gene at chromosome 14q13 coding for the enzyme nucleoside phosphorylase in the purine metabolic pathway.[146,196] The immunodeficiency is progressive; the symptoms, which are variable, commonly begin in early infancy with enhanced susceptibility to opportunistic viral and fungal infection and failure to thrive. Death may result from an overwhelming viral infection from herpes zoster, measles, or cytomegalovirus. The immunodeficiency is thought, but not yet proven to be, due to failure of phosphorolysis of deoxyguanosine to guanine, which leads to its phosphorylation to deoxyguanylic acid (dGMP) in lymphoid tissue.[146,196] This leads to the accumulation of the toxic metabolite deoxyguanosine triphosphate (dGTP), which inhibits ribonucleotide reductase, resulting in an inhibition of DNA synthesis and proliferation of thymocytes. T-cell numbers are markedly decreased, commonly leading to a lymphopenia. The reasons for preferential toxicity for T cells compared with B cells, and the differences with respect to ADA deficiency, have not been completely elucidated. In vitro T-cell responses are abnormal with absent delayed cutaneous hypersensitivity, and a diminution in T-cell function occurs over time. By contrast, production of antibody and immunoglobulins in some patients is normal; in some cases, the antibody response may even be exaggerated. Autoantibodies, including rheumatoid factors, antinuclear antibodies, and antibodies to red blood cells, may be produced and autoimmune hemolytic anemia, idiopathic thrombocytopenic purpura, and systemic lupus erythematosus may ensue. A megaloblastic anemia or neurologic abnormalities with spastic paresis of the trunk and extremities, developmental delay, or mental retardation may be observed.

The diagnosis is made by quantitating PNP activity in erythrocytes, lymphocytes, or fibroblasts and levels of deoxyguanosine and dGTP in blood. A low serum uric acid level is a useful screening assay for this enzyme deficiency. Prenatal diagnosis is possible.

Attempts at enzyme replacement therapy have not altered the clinical course, and BMT is the preferred form of therapy.[196,197] Gene therapy will probably be tried in the future to correct the enzymatic abnormality.

OTHER IMMUNODEFICIENCIES

Wiskott-Aldrich Syndrome

Etiology and Pathophysiology

Wiskott-Aldrich is an X-linked recessive syndrome characterized by the triad of eczema, thrombocytopenia, and immunodeficiency.[198,199] The cell lineages affected by the defect include both lymphoid and hematopoietic lines. Although the molecular basis of Wiskott-Aldrich syndrome (WAS) has not been established, the Wiskott-Aldrich gene has been mapped to position Xp11.22–p11.3 on the X chromosome.[200,201] Carrier females are asymptomatic because of selection against cells that have as their active X chromosome the X chromosome carrying the mutant Wiskott-Aldrich gene. Nonrandom X chromosome inactivation patterns are observed in obligate carriers in T and B lymphocytes, monocytes, polymorphonuclear leukocytes, and platelets but not in fibroblasts.[202–205] Hereditary X-linked thrombocytopenia is characterized by thrombocytopenia and small platelets, similar to WAS, without the immunodeficiency or eczema.[206,207] This disorder also maps to the WAS locus on the proximal short arm of the X chromosome.[208,209]

The defective gene product and the basis for the immunodeficiency and the diverse clinical and hematologic defects in WAS have not been identified. The defect is intrinsic to the abnormal lymphoid and hematopoietic elements, since BMT can completely correct the defects. The most profound immunologic abnormality is defective antibody response to polysaccharide antigens. Using scanning electron microscopy, an increased percentage of peripheral blood lymphocytes or T-cell lines with decreased surface microvilli are observed.[210,211] The cell-surface glycoprotein CD43, termed leukosialin or sialophorin, a major component of the plasma membrane that contributes heavily to the surface charge on lymphocytes, has been re-

ported to be absent, decreased, or structurally altered in lymphocytes of patients with WAS.[212] The gene for leukosialin maps to chromosome 16, however, and not to the X chromosome. Whether and how this secondary defect in leukosialin expression explains the immunodeficiency in WAS has not been clarified. A defect in expression or regulation of glycosyltransferases and altered O-glycan synthesis in B and T cells in WAS have been described.[213,214] B-cell lines from WAS patients show defective signal transduction following ligation of B-cell surface immunoglobulin,[215] and defective expression and impaired proteolysis of surface CD23.[216] These defects do not appear, however, to reflect poor expression of CD43.[217]

The etiology of the thrombocytopenia, the most consistent finding of the triad, has also not been completely explained. Although abnormal thrombocytopoiesis makes a major contribution to the thrombocytopenia, increased platelet destruction due to an intrinsic platelet defect and to factors extrinsic to the platelet contributes to the thrombocytopenia.[218–220] The mean platelet volume is reduced, but there is a broad overlap with the normal range. After splenectomy, the platelet count usually increases, and the mean distribution of the platelet volume returns to normal.[221,222] Platelet-associated IgG is frequently present and disappears after splenectomy. Relapse of thrombocytopenia after splenectomy may be accompanied by autoimmune thrombocytopenia and redevelopment of platelet-associated IgG.[223] The platelet volume does not decrease to the presplenectomy size with relapse, but it fails to increase to the size observed in immune-mediated platelet destruction. The glycoproteins on the surface of platelets have also been investigated but have not shown any consistent defect.[224]

Clinical Manifestations

The incidence of WAS is approximately 4 per 1 million live births.[225] The initial symptoms are usually petechiae or bleeding from the gastrointestinal or urinary tract, or from the umbilical cord, beginning in the first several months of life. At that age, an eczematoid rash appears that is most prominent in the antecubital and popliteal fossae and tends to become petechial. Recurrent infections with bacteria, fungi, or viruses occur. Recurrent pneumonia and otitis media with chronic purulent drainage and perforated tympanic membranes are prominent. The thrombocytopenia and bleeding tendency are often worsened with infection. Chronic or recurrent herpes simplex or disseminated varicella may occur. Autoimmune disorders with arthritis, vasculitis, or hemolytic anemias are not uncommon.

The median survival in WAS is 6.5 years, with the cause of death being infection, usually from pneumonia or sepsis, in 59%, bleeding in 27%, or malignancy in 5% of patients.[225] A high incidence (18% of patients) of lymphoreticular tumors, especially non-Hodgkin lymphomas with B-cell immunoblastic sarcomas predominating, occurs in WAS. These lymphomas initially present at extranodal sites and are observed in children who survive to later childhood.[8,9,226]

Laboratory Evaluation

The serum IgM level is decreased, and the IgA and IgE levels are often increased. IgG paraproteins may be present. Poor to virtually absent antibody responses to polysaccharide antigens and defective antibody responses to protein antigens with low titers, lack of immunologic memory, and isotype switching occur. Titers of isohemagglutinin antibodies to the blood group polysaccharide antigens are low. Peripheral blood B lymphocytes may show a decreased number of CD23+ and an increased number of CD20+ and CD21− B cells, suggesting defective B-cell differentiation.[215,227] T-cell responses to nonspecific mitogens are normal to decreased, but T-cell responses to antigens and allogeneic cells are usually absent. Delayed hypersensitivity skin reactions are absent at an early age in WAS. Lymphocyte counts are usually initially normal, and then decrease as a result of a progressive decline in T-cell numbers. Peripheral lymphoid tissues gradually become depleted of lymphoid cells. The platelet count and volume are low, with the platelet count usually 50,000–100,000/mm^3. The bleeding time is more prolonged than would be predicted from the platelet count. The carrier state can be diagnosed by demonstrating nonrandom X-chromosome inactivation patterns in T cells, B cells, or polymorphonuclear leukocytes.[10–12,204,205,228] Prenatal diagnosis can sometimes, but not invariably, be made by decreased fetal platelet count and size.[229]

Therapy

BMT can correct all the defects of this otherwise fatal disorder, including the susceptibility to malignancy.[230–232] Successful engraftment requires preparative ablative or cytoreduction of the recipient's bone marrow. While the success rate with HLA-identical sibling or parental marrow is high, the success rate of haploidentical parental BMT has been disappointing and has been complicated by the occurrence of lymphomas or chronic GVHD during the post-transplantation period.[232] Matched unrelated donor BMT for WAS has had some success.[189] Splenectomy combined with regularly administered prophylactic antibiotics has been used to manage some patients with severe bleeding problems who could not undergo BMT. Splenectomy will increase the platelet count and decrease the bleeding tendency, but it may increase susceptibility to overwhelming sepsis.[222] Relapses of thrombocytopenia can occur after splenectomy. Prednisone- or vincristine-loaded platelets[223] have been used to treat such relapses. Intravenous immunoglobulin replacement therapy is indicated to decrease the risk of infection.

Ataxia-Telangiectasia

Etiology and Pathophysiology

AT is an autosomal recessive disorder characterized by progressive cerebellar ataxia, telangiectasias, recurrent sinopulmonary infections, combined immunodeficiency, increased incidence of malignancies, and premature aging.[233–236] Genetic linkage analysis has localized the gene defect to chromosome 11q22–q23.[236,237] The disease is not genetically homogeneous, however. Complementation analyses with AT fibroblast heterokaryons has demonstrated at least five complementation groups, three that map to 11q12–q23, but there are no consistent phenotypic differences between complementation groups. Although the frequency of AT is estimated to be only 1 in 100,000 live births,[238] the carrier state is relatively frequent (0.68–7.7%) in the population. Heterozygotes as well as homozygotes appear to be at increased risk of malignancy.[239,240]

The underlying defect in AT is unknown, but AT cells display abnormalities suggesting a defect of DNA metabolism, processing, repair, or defective responses to ionizing-radiation damage.[233–237,241] The fibroblasts and lymphocytes show hypersensitivity to γ-rays and x-rays, ionizing radiation, and radiomimetic chemicals such as bleomycin. Carriers of AT show a sensitivity intermediate between those of normal individuals and homozygotes. X-ray-induced chromosomal breaks are not rejoined as efficiently as in normal people, and AT cells do not reduce their rate of DNA synthesis after x-ray exposure as do normal cells. A high spontaneous rate of intrachromosomal recombination is observed in AT fibroblasts.[242]

Ionizing radiation-induced double-stranded breaks in DNA of normal cells leads to an arrest of the cell cycle at the G1-S boundary. This arrest requires induction of the transcription factor p53. Cells from patients with AT fail to cease to replicate DNA and express p53 after ionizing radiation and other DNA damaging agents.[243,244] The defect in AT may reflect failure or poor control of timing DNA double-stranded break repair and damage-sensitive cell cycle checkpoints. AT cells may then replicate DNA prior to complete repair of DNA damage. In AT the frequency of lymphocytes with chromosome translocations is high, resulting in a high frequency of aberrant interlocus TCR gene rearrangements.[245,246] This checkpoint defect may lead to the aberrant recombination of immunoglobulin and TCR genes and the occurrence of lymphoid tumors observed in AT. Chromosomal breaks, inversions, and translocations cluster at bands 7p13–p14, 7q32–q35, 14q11, and 14q32 in 5–10% of peripheral T lymphocytes in AT.[247–251] It is at these sites that the TCR and immunoglobulin receptor genes normally undergo DNA rearrangement to generate a functional gene. This may account for the T- and B-cell abnormalities and low number of α/β compared to γ/δ bearing TCR on peripheral blood lymphocytes in AT.[252] In approximately 10% of AT patients, expanded clonal populations of nonmalignant T lymphocytes, with translocations involving chromosome 7 or 14 at 14q32.1, centromeric to the immunoglobulin heavy chain locus and possibly the site of a putative oncogene, appear in the blood.[248–252] These clonal cells have a proliferative advantage and may increase in a quiescent fashion in the blood over a period of years; in some cases, they may evolve into a T-cell leukemia. It is possible that the nonrandom translocation confers a preactivated, premalignant state that progresses to malignant transformation after a secondary genetic event.

In AT, defects in tissue differentiation with failure of organ maturation are also present. The immunologic defect is characterized by absence of or production of only a small thymus that has an embryonic histologic appearance with lack of Hassall's corpuscles and sparse population with lymphoid cells. Both variable T- and B-cell defects occur.[253] Other evidence for tissue immaturity includes presence of elevated levels of serum α-fetoprotein and carcinoembryonic antigen.[254,255]

Clinical Manifestations

The usual first presentation of AT is a progressive cerebellar ataxia observed in the second year of life.[256] Other neurologic symptoms that occur later are choreoathetosis, nystagmus, strabismus, dysarthric speech, and decreased deep-tendon reflexes. Telangiectasias appear later in childhood and are most prominent on the bulbar conjunctivae, exposed areas of the skin, external ear, eyelids, face, flexor folds of the neck, extremities, and the dorsa of the hands and feet. Recurrent sinopulmonary infections occur in most patients and may become chronic, resulting in bronchiectasis and respiratory insufficiency. The overall risk of cancer is 60–180 times the normal rate, with ≤10% of patients developing cancer.[239,240] Most neoplasms occur before age 15. Non-Hodgkin lymphomas with histologic subtypes observed with chromosome 14 translocations, and Hodgkin lymphoma, mostly of the lymphocyte depletion type, T-cell leukemia, and epithelial carcinomas predominate. Heterozygotes for the AT gene have an approximately three- to fourfold increased risk of malignancy.[240] Heterozygous females, who have an approximately fivefold increased risk of breast cancer, account for an estimated 9–18% of all breast cancer in the United States. Caution must be exercised in the treatment of neoplasms because of the increased sensitivity of patients with AT to radiation therapy.[257] Endocrinologic abnormalities commonly occur. These abnormalities include delayed somatic growth, insulin resistance, delayed development of secondary sexual characteristics in females (secondary to absent or hypoplastic ovaries), hirsutism in females, and hypogonadism in males. In most cases, skin shows premature aging and the hair becomes diffusely gray. Clinical variation on the basis of genetic subtypes has not been described.

Laboratory Evaluation

Absence or deficiency of serum IgA, secretory IgA, and IgE is found in about 75% of patients. Low levels of IgG2[111] and IgG4 and decreased antibody responses to immunization are found. Anergy to delayed hypersensitivity skin testing, decreased T-cell numbers, CD4+ and CD4+/CD45 RA+ or naive CD4+ T cells and abnormal in vitro lymphocyte responses are commonly found. Serum α-fetoprotein levels are increased in 95% of patients and carcinoembryonic antigens may be elevated.[254,255] Nonrandom chromosomal breaks and translocation of chromosome 14 to the other chromosome 14, to chromosome 7, or to the X chromosome occur. The prenatal diagnosis of AT has been based on both spontaneous chromosomal breakage and a translocation involving chromosome 14 in cultured amniotic fluid cells.[258]

Therapy

No therapy can halt the disease, and treatment is symptomatic. Antibiotics are indicated for recurrent pulmonary infections, and immunoglobulin replacement therapy may be indicated. Exposure to excessive sunlight should be minimized to prevent skin changes. Malignancies in AT patients may require the use of lower doses of radiotherapy and chemotherapy.[257]

DiGeorge Syndrome

Etiology and Pathophysiology

DiGeorge syndrome (third and fourth pharyngeal pouch syndrome) is due to either an abnormality of or an insult to the third and fourth pharyngeal pouches, which contribute to development of the thymus, parathyroid glands, cardiac outflow tract, ear, and facial structures, occurring during the fourth to seventh week of fetal development.[259-261] Development of the thymus, which is formed from the endodermal epithelium of the third and four pharyngeal pouches, is interrupted. In the most severe form of this development defect, the thymus may be completely absent, but more frequently it is small, hypoplastic and ectopic in location because of lack of descent into the mediastinum. This variability in thymic development produces variable T-cell deficiency. Most patients have a partial T-cell deficiency with decreased T-cell number and function at birth, that corrects itself with time. More rarely, complete thymic aplasia (complete DiGeorge syndrome) is present with profound deficiency of T-cell number and function; when present, it is associated with susceptibility to viral and fungal infections. Parathyroid aplasia is present at birth and produces hypocalcemia.

The etiology of the DiGeorge syndrome is unknown. It has been suggested to be a developmental field defect, and the embryologic reactive unit affected is the cephalic neural crest mesenchymal population of cells.[262,263] The failure of the neural crest to contribute to the mesenchymal derivatives of the pharyngeal pouches may explain the heart lesions typically found in the syndrome—interrupted aortic arch type B and truncus arteriosus. Targeted disruption of the mouse homeobox gene *hox*-1.5 gives rise to a developmental field defect that resembles the DiGeorge syndrome.[264] The homeobox-1.5 gene maps, however, to chromosome 7 and not human chromosome 22, which commonly observed to undergo deletions or translocations in this anomaly. The anomaly is usually sporadic in nature and thought to represent an environmental insult. Although most cases are sporadic, an autosomal dominant inherited form of DiGeorge syndrome with monosomy chromosome 22q11 can occur.[265-267] Translocations and deletions involving chromosome 22q11, as well as 10p13, have been described. With molecular studies, $\geq$90% of patients have 22q11 microdeletions, although only 30% of prospectively studied patients had monosomy 22q11.21–q11.23 demonstrable by high-resolution cytogenetic binding studies.[268-271] The size of the deletion does not appear to correlate with the clinical phenotype. Patients with the velocardiofacial syndrome, an autosomal disorder characterized by cleft palate, cardiac defects, learning disability, and typical facies, may have manifestation of the DiGeorge syndrome and also display deletions of 22q11.2.[271] A few instances of this syndrome have been associated with maternal alcoholism, diabetes, or exposure to retinoids.[259,272]

Clinical Manifestations

A broad and variable spectrum of malformations may occur.[259,273,274] Affected infants usually present with hypocalcemic tetany in the newborn period. Cardiac malformations may include interrupted, right-sided, or double aortic arch, truncus arteriosus, patent ductus arteriosus, or ventricular septal defect. These defects give rise to cyanosis or cardiac murmurs.[275,276] A type B interrupted aortic arch or truncus arteriosus frequently occurs and is suggestive of the diagnosis. Facial dysmorphic features include hypertelorism, antimongoloid slant of the eyes, midline facial clefts, micrognathia, shortened philtrum of the lip, cleft palate, choanal atresia, low-set posteriorly rotated ears, and notched ear pinnae. If the T-cell deficiency is severe, which occurs in <25% of patients,[259,277-279] the infant may develop chronic or recurrent rhinitis, pneumonia, *Candida* infections, diarrhea, and failure to thrive. Moderate to severe mental retardation, development delay, and hearing loss may be present.

Laboratory Evaluation

Total T cells are low to markedly decreased, and B-cell numbers and total lymphocyte counts are usually normal.[259,277-279] At times, B-cell numbers are increased. In vitro T-cell responses to nonspecific mitogens or allogeneic lymphocytes may be normal or absent. Unless the T-cell defect is severe, levels of IgG, IgA, and IgM are usually normal or increased. Patients with CD4+ T-cell counts of <400/mm^3 and decreased in vitro T-cell responses to mitogens may have increased susceptibility to infection and a persistent immunodeficiency.[278] Profound T-cell deficiency results in defective antibody responses. Decreased serum calcium, increased phosphorus, and decreased parathyrin levels are present.

Therapy

The hypocalcemia should be treated with intravenous calcium replacement and may prove difficult to control. Long-term treatment with oral calcium replacement, vitamin D, and a low-phosphate formula is usually required. The cardiac abnormalities, which may be quite severe, must be evaluated. Therapy is not usually required for partial T-cell deficiency, as T-cell function improves spontaneously with increasing age. In patients with severe persistent T-cell deficiency with marked susceptibility to infections and failure to thrive, transplantation of fetal thymus, fetal thymic epithelium, cultured autologous thymic tissue, or bone marrow may be indicated.[259,280,281] The efficacy of thymic transplantation for complete DiGeorge syndrome has not been critically evaluated. Blood products should be used from cytomegalovirus negative donors and be irradiated before administration to prevent GVHD, a potential complication with severe T-cell deficiency. Antibiotic prophylaxis to prevent *P. carinii* pneumonia is also indicated in the face of T-cell deficiency. Prenatal diagnosis is possible and may be indicated if molecular evaluation is informative in a parent of an affected child.

Immunodeficiency Secondary to Bone Marrow Transplantation*

BMT is used to correct several congenital immunodeficiency diseases, including SCID, WAS, and severe DiGeorge syndrome, and is a major component of therapy for multiple hematologic malignancies (see Part VI, Hematologic Malignancies). A secondary immunodeficiency is a normal accompaniment of BMT.

Cytoablation therapy administered prior to allogeneic or haploidentical BMT is designed to produce near-complete destruction of the recipient's immune system; this approach is intended to permit the donor cells to re-establish an immunohematopoietic system. For autologous BMT, immunoablation is not a requirement. However, chemotherapy administered to achieve complete destruction of the patient's malignancy will still result in comparable injury to the immune system. Following BMT, virtually all components of the body's defense system are affected.[282] The first line of defense, the integument and mucosal surfaces are damaged. Neutrophils and monocytes are not generated in significant amounts for 2–4 weeks. Leukocyte chemotaxis and bactericidal activity may also be impaired for the first 2–4 months following BMT, and longer if GVHD develops.[178,283] The use of recombinant hematopoietic growth factors reduces the duration of neutropenia and its recumbent risks (see Ch. 16). The duration of lymphocyte function impairment is even longer. The initial deficits are related to the virtual absence of circulating lymphocytes (NK, T, and B cells). Subsequent deficits are attributable to the disorganized interaction of lymphocytes as the immune system undergoes regeneration.[186,190]

During most of the first year following transplantation, an altered CD4/CD8 cell ratio is commonly observed.[284] The relative deficiency of CD4 cells gradually corrects itself unless infection or GVHD[178] interferes with recovery. IL-2-producing cells are reduced during the first several months post-BMT (autologous as well as allogeneic), limiting immune reconstitution.[285] These cells can respond, however, to exogenous IL-2. This situation is analogous to one of the T-cell activation defects leading to SCID, previously described in this chapter, but the reduction in IL-2 production may blunt GVHD and promote host tolerance by the donor immune system. A trial of low-dose continuous-infusion IL-2 following BMT has shown that it is well tolerated, and efficacy studies are planned.[286] In the event that GVHD is established or a systemic infection develops, the production and release of inflammatory cytokines such as tumor necrosis factor, IL-1, or IFN-γ may further disrupt immune recovery.[287] An element of GVHD may also be due to defective thymic elimination of autoreactive T-cell clones.[178,190] Autoreactive T cells could further interfere with normal lymphoid development. Efforts to reduce the risk of GVHD have employed T-cell depletion of the donated bone marrow by physical and immunologic approaches. The kinetics of immune reconstitution are generally slowed even further in this situation, and the incidence of nonengraftment and leukemic relapse is greater.[186,190,286] Also, 10–20% of patients receiving T-depleted marrow may develop B-cell lymphomas if a mismatch is present,[288,289] a complication prominent in congenital immunodeficiency diseases that predispose to malignancy such as the WAS.[232]

---

* Contributed by Reggie Duerst, M.D., Associate Professor, Department of Pediatrics (Hematology/Oncology), University of Rochester School of Medicine, Rochester, NY.

Recovery of B-cell function is delayed the longest after BMT. Several months are required before IgG production returns and hypogammaglobulinemia may result if chronic GVHD is significant.[282,290] During the first year after transplantation, heterogeneity of immunoglobulins may be limited. In addition, recipients of T-cell-depleted marrow may have incomplete immunologic engraftment, persistent hypogammaglobulinemia, and split lymphoid chimerism with donor T and recipient B lymphocytes. Donor T cells and recipient B cells may fail to cooperate because of developmental immaturity or because of an underlying defect of the B cells.[186,190–192] Antibody subclass deficiencies may persist for long periods, even in the absence of GVHD.[291,292] Because of the delayed recovery of B-cell function, re-immunization is warranted but should not be pursued for 6–12 months from BMT (or 1 year from the end of immunosuppressive therapy/active chronic GVHD). Antibody responses to vaccines, and polysaccharide vaccines especially, may be defective even after this period. Good personal hygiene, immunoglobulin replacement therapy, and prophylactic antibiotics are prescribed to support the patient until adequate immunologic recovery has been achieved.

REFERENCES

1. Rosen FS, Cooper MD, Wedgwood RJP: The primary immunodeficiencies. N Engl J Med 311:235, 300, 1984
2. Stiehm ER (ed): Immunologic Disorders in Infants and Children. 3rd Ed. WB Saunders, Philadelphia, 1989
3. Hong R: Update on the immunodeficiency diseases. Am J Dis Child 144:983, 1990
4. Huston DP, Kavanaugh AF, Rohane PW, Huston MM: Immunoglobulin deficiency syndromes and therapy. J Allergy Clin Immunol 87:1, 1991
5. Primary immunodeficiency diseases. Report of a WHO Scientific Group. Immunodefic Rev 3:195, 1992
6. Buckley RH: Immunodeficiency diseases. JAMA 268:2797, 1992
7. Shearer WT, Anderson DC: The secondary immunodeficiencies. p. 400. In Stiehm ER (ed): Immunologic Disorders in Infants and Children. 3rd Ed. WB Saunders, Philadelphia, 1989
8. Filipovich AH, Heinitz KJ, Robison LL, Frizzera G: The Immunodeficiency Cancer Registry. Am J Pediatr Hematol Oncol 9:183, 1987
9. Filipovich AH, Mathur A, Kamat D, Shapiro RS: Primary immunodeficiencies: genetic risk factors for lymphoma. Cancer Res 52:5465s, 1992
10. Schwaber J, Rosen FS: X chromosome linked immunodeficiency. Immunodefic Rev 2:233, 1990
11. Hendriks RW, Schuurman RKB: Genetics of human X-linked immunodeficiency diseases. Clin Exp Immunol 85:182, 1991
12. Conley ME: Molecular approaches to analysis of X-linked immunodeficiencies. Annu Rev Immunol 10:215, 1992
13. Campana D, Farrant J, Inamdar N et al: Phenotypic features and proliferative activity of B cell progenitors in X-linked agammaglobulinemia. J Immunol 145:1675, 1990
14. Schwaber J: Evidence for failure of V(D)J recombination in bone marrow pre-B cells from X-linked agammaglobulinemia. J Clin Invest 89:2053, 1992
15. Schwaber J, Malone B: Germ line transcription of the immunoglobulin heavy chain locus directs production of μ chain without VDJ. J Clin Invest 89:2046, 1992
16. Conley ME: B cells in patients with X-linked agammaglobulinemia. J Immunol 34:3070, 1985
17. Conley ME, Puck JM: Carrier detection in typical and atypical X-linked agammaglobulinemia. J Pediatr 112:688, 1988
18. Kwan SP, Kunkel L, Bruns G et al: Mapping of the X-linked agammaglobulinemia locus by use of restriction fragment-length polymorphism. J Clin Invest 77:649, 1986
19. Malcolm S, de Saint Basile G, Arveiler B et al: Close linkage of random DNA fragments from Xq 21.3-22 to X-linked agammaglobulinaemia (XLA). Hum Genet 77:172, 1987
20. Mensink EJBM, Thompson A, Schot JDL et al: Mapping of a gene for X-linked agammaglobulinemia and evidence for genetic heterogeneity. Hum Genet 73:327, 1986
21. Mensink EJBM, Thompson A, Schot JDL et al: Genetic heterogeneity in X-linked agammaglobulinemia complicates carrier detection and prenatal diagnosis. Clin Genet 31:91, 1987
22. Goldblum RM, Lord RA, Cooper MD et al: X-linked B lymphocyte deficiency. J Pediatr 85:188, 1974
23. Landreth KS, Engelhard D, Anasetti C et al: Pre-B cells in agammaglobulin-

emia: evidence for disease heterogeneity among affected boys. J Clin Immunol 5:84, 1985

24. Conley ME, Brown P, Pickard AR et al: Expression of the gene defect in X-linked agammaglobulinemia. N Engl J Med 315:564, 1986

25. Fearon ER, Winkelstein JA, Civin CI: Carrier detection in X-linked agammaglobulinemia by analysis of X-chromosome inactivation. N Engl J Med 316:427, 1987

26. Tsukada S, Saffran DC, Rawlings DJ et al: Deficient expression of a B cell cytoplasmic tyrosine kinase in human X-linked agammaglobulinemia. Cell 72:279, 1993

27. Vetrie D, Vorechovsky I, Sideras P et al: The gene involved in X-linked agammaglobulinaemia is a member of the *src* family of protein-tyrosine kinases. Nature 361:226, 1993

28. Lederman HM, Winkelstein JA: X-linked agammaglobulinemia: an analysis of 96 patients. Medicine 64:145, 1985

29. Petty RE, Cassidy JT, Tubergen DG: Association of arthritis with hypogammaglobulinema. Arthritis Rheum 20:441, 1977

30. Stuckey M, Quinn PA, Gelfand EW: Identification of *Ureaplasma urealyticum* (T-strain *Mycoplasma*) in patient with polyarthritis. Lancet 2:917, 1978

31. Wyatt HV: Poliomyelitis in hypogammaglobulinemics. J Infect Dis 128:802, 1973

32. McKinney RE Jr, Katz SL, Wilfert CM: Chronic enteroviral meningoencephalitis in agammaglobulinemic patients. Rev Infect Dis 9:334, 1987

33. Misbah SA, Spickett GP, Ryba PCJ et al: Chronic enteroviral meningoencephalitis in agammaglobulinemia: Case report and literature review. J Clin Immunol 12:266, 1992

34. Kozlowski C, Evans DIK: Neutropenia associated with X-linked agammaglobulinemia. J Clin Pathol 44:388, 1991

35. Buckley RH, Schiff RI: The use of intravenous immunoglobulin in immunodeficiency diseases. N Engl J Med 325:110, 1991

36. Schwartz SA: Clinical use of immune serum globulin as replacement therapy in patients with primary immunodeficiency syndromes. Clin Rev Allergy 10:1, 1992

37. Liese JG, Wintergerst U, Tympner KD, Belohradsky BH: High- vs low-dose immunoglobulin therapy in the long-term treatment of X-linked agammaglobulinemia. Am J Dis Child 146:335, 1992

38. Roifman CM, Gelfand EW: Replacement therapy with high dose intravenous gamma-globulin improves chronic sinopulmonary disease in patients with hypogammaglobulinemia. Pediatr Infect Dis J 5:S92, 1988

39. Mease PJ, Ochs HD, Wedgwood RJ: Successful treatment of echovirus meningoencephalitis and myositis-fascitis with intravenous immune globulin therapy in a patient with X-linked agammaglobulinemia. N Engl J Med 304:1278, 1981

40. Erlendsson K, Swartz T, Dwyer JM: Successful reversal of echovirus encephalitis in X-linked hypogammaglobulinaemia by intraventricular administration of immunoglobulin. N Engl J Med 312:351, 1985

41. Fasth A: Management of infections in primary immunodeficiency syndromes. Ann Clin Res 19:305, 1987

42. Fleisher TA, White RM, Broder S et al: X-linked hypogammaglobulinemia and isolated growth hormone deficiency. N Engl J Med 302:1429, 1980

43. Sitz KV, Burks W, Williams LW et al: Confirmation of X-linked hypogammaglobulinemia with isolated growth hormone deficiency as a disease entity. J Pediatr 116:2, 1990

44. Monafo V, Maghnie M, Terracciano L et al: X-linked agammaglobulinemia and isolated growth hormone deficiency. Acta Paediatr Scand 80:563, 1991

45. Conley ME, Burks AW, Herrod HG, Puck JM: Molecular analysis of X-linked agammaglobulinemia with growth hormone deficiency. J Pediatr 119:392, 1991

46. Notarangelo L, Duse M, Ugazio AG: Immunodeficiency with hyper-IgM (HIM). Immunodefic Rev 1992;3:101–122

47. Geha RS, Hyslop N, Alami S et al: Hyperimmunoglobulin M immunodeficiency (dysgammaglobulinemia): presence of immunoglobulin M-secreting plasmacytoid cells in peripheral blood and failure of immunoglobulin M-immunoglobulin G switch in B-cell differentiation. J Clin Invest 64:385, 1979

48. Akahori Y, Kurosawa Y, Kamachi Y et al: Presence of immunoglobulin (Ig) M and IgG double isotype-bearing cells and defect of switch recombination in hyper IgM immunodeficiency. J Clin Invest 85:1722, 1990

49. Mensink EJBM, Thompson A, Sandkuyl LA et al: X-linked immunodeficiency with hyperimmunoglobulinemia M appears to be linked to the DXS42 restriction fragment length polymorphism locus. Hum Genet 76:96, 1987

50. Mayer L, Kwan S-P, Thompson C et al: Evidence for a defect in "switch" T cells in patients with immunodeficiency and hyperimmunoglobulinemia M. N Engl J Med 314:409, 1986

51. Allen RC, Armitage RJ, Conley ME et al: CD40 ligand gene defects responsible for X-linked hyper-IgM syndrome. Science 259:990, 1993

52. Aruffo A, Farrington M, Hollenbaugh D et al: The CD40 ligand, gp39, is defec-

tive in activated T cells from patients with X-linked hyper-IgM syndrome. Cell 72:291, 1993

53. DiSanto JP, Bonnefoy JY, Gauchat JF et al: CD40 ligand mutations in X-linked immunodeficiency with hyper-IgM. Nature 361:541, 1993

54. Fuleihan R, Ramesh N, Loh R et al: Defective expression of the CD40 ligand in X-chromosome-linked immunoglobulin deficiency with normal or elevated IgM. Proc Natl Acad Sci USA 90:2170, 1993

55. Korthäuer U, Graf D, Mages HW et al: Defective expression of T-cell CD40 ligand causes X-linked immunodeficiency with hyper-IgM. Nature 361:539, 1993

56. Ackerman BD: Dysgammaglobulinemia: report of a case with a family history of congenital gamma globulin disorder. Pediatrics 34:211, 1964

57. Geha RS, Schneeberger E, Merler E, Rosen FS: Heterogeneity of "acquired" or common variable agammaglobulinemia. N Engl J Med 291:1, 1974

58. Cunningham-Rundles C: Clinical and immunologic analyses of 103 patients with common variable immunodeficiency. J Clin Immunol 9:22, 1989

59. Spickett GP, Webster ADB, Farrant J: Cellular abnormalities in common variable immunodeficiency. Immunodefic Rev 2:199, 1990

60. Jaffe JS, Eisenstein E, Sneller MC, Strober W: T-cell abnormalities in common variable immunodeficiency. Pediatr Res 33:S24, 1993

61. de la Concha EG, Oldham G, Webster DB et al: Quantitative measures of T and B cell function in variable primary hypogammaglobulinemia: evidence for a consistent B-cell defect. Clin Exp Immunol 27:208, 1976

62. Saiki O, Ralph P, Cunningham-Rundles C et al: Three distinct stages of B cell defects in common variable immunodeficiency. Proc Natl Acad Sci USA 79:6008, 1982

63. Fiorilli M, Crescenzi M, Carbonari M et al: Phenotypically immature IgG-bearing B cells in patients with hypogammaglobulinemia. J Clin Immunol 6:21, 1986

64. Saxon A, Giorgi JV, Sherr EH, Kagan JM: Failure of B cells in common variable immunodeficiency to transit from proliferation to differentiation is associated with altered B cell surface-molecule display. J Allergy Clin Immunol 84:44, 1989

65. Ciccimarra F, Rosen FS, Schneeberger E et al: Failure of heavy chain glycosylation of IgG in some patients with common variable agammaglobulinemia. J Clin Invest 57:1386, 1976

66. Bryant A, Calver NC, Toubi E et al: Classification of patients with common variable immunodeficiency by B cell secretion of IgM and IgG in response to anti-IgM and interleukin-2. Clin Immunol Immunopathol 56:239, 1990

67. Waldmann TA, Durm M, Broder S et al: Role of suppressor T cells in pathogenesis of common variable hypogammaglobulinaemia. Lancet 2:609, 1974

68. Tursz R, Preud'home J-L, Labaume S et al: Autoantibodies to B lymphocytes in a patient with hypogammaglobulinemia: characterization and pathogenic role. J Clin Invest 60:405, 1977

69. Rodriguez MA, Bankhurst AD, Williams RC: Characterization of the suppressor activity in lymphocytes from patients with common variable hypogammaglobulinemia: evidence for an associated primary B-cell defect. Clin Immunol Immunopathol 29:35, 1983

70. Wollheim FA, Williams RC: Immunoglobulin studies in six kindreds of patients with adult hypogammaglobulinemia. J Lab Clin Med 66:433, 1965

71. Friedman JM, Fialkow PJ, Davis SD et al: Autoimmunity in the relatives of patients with immunodeficiency diseases. Clin Exp Immunol 28:375, 1977

72. Ashman RF, Schaffer FM, Kemp JD et al: Genetic and immunologic analysis of a family containing five patients with common-variable immune deficiency or selective IgA deficiency. J Clin Immunol 12:406, 1992

73. Schaffer FM, Palermos J, Zhu ZB et al: Individuals with IgA deficiency and common variable immunodeficiency share complex polymorphisms of major histocompatibility complex class III genes. Proc Natl Acad Sci USA 86:8015, 1989

74. Volanakis JE, Zhu Z-B, Schaffer FM et al: Major histocompatibility complex class III genes and susceptibility to immunoglobulin A deficiency and common variable immunodeficiency. J Clin Invest 89:1914, 1992

75. Howe HS, So AKL, Farrant J, Webster ADB: Common variable immunodeficiency is associated with polymorphic markers in the human major histocompatibility complex. Clin Exp Immunol 84:387, 1991

76. Morell A, Barandun S, Locher G: HTLV-III seroconversion in a homosexual patient with common variable immunodeficiency. N Engl J Med 315:456, 1986

77. Wright JJ, Birx DL, Wagner DK et al: Normalization of antibody responsiveness in a patient with common variable hypogammaglobulinemia and HIV infection. N Engl J Med 317:1516, 1987

78. Webster ADB, Lever A, Spickett G et al: Recovery of antibody production after HIV infection in "common" variable hypogammaglobulinaemia. Clin Exp Immunol 77:309, 1989

79. Osur SL, Lillie MA, Chen PB et al: Elevation of serum IgG levels and normal-

izization of T4/T8 ratio after hepatitis in a patient with common variable hypogammaglobulinemia. J Allergy Clin Immunol 79:969, 1987

80. Hermans PE, Diax-Buxo JA, Stobo JD: Idiopathic late onset immunoglobulin deficiency. Clinical observations in 50 patients. Am J Med 61:221, 1976

81. Yocum MW, Kelso JM: Common variable immunodeficiency: the disorder and treatment. Mayo Clin Proc 66:83, 1991

82. Hermaszewski RA, Webster ADB: Primary hypogammaglobulinaemia: a survey of clinical manifestations and complications. Q J Med 86:31, 1993

83. Ament ME, Ochs HD, Davis SD: Structure and function of the gastrointestinal tract in primary immunodeficiency syndromes: a study of 39 patients. Medicine 52:227, 1972

84. Cunninghm-Rundles C, Siegal FP, Cunningham-Rundles S, Lieberman P: Incidence of cancer in 98 patients with common varied immunodeficiency. J Clin Immunol 7:294, 1987

85. Frizzera G, Rosai J, Dehner LP et al: Lymphoreticular disorders in primary immunodeficiencies. Cancer 46:692, 1980

86. Kinlen LJ, Webster ADB, Bird AG et al: Prospective study of cancer in patients with hypogammaglobulinaemia. Lancet 1:263, 1985

87. den Hartog G, van der Meer JWM, Jansen JBMJ et al: Decreased gastrin secretion in patients with late-onset hypogammaglobulinemia. N Engl J Med 318:1563, 1988

88. Sander CA, Medeiros LJ, Weiss LM et al: Lymphoproliferative lesions in patients with common variable immunodeficiency syndrome. Am J Surg Pathol 16:1170, 1992

89. Baumert E, Wolff-Vorbeck G, Schlesier M, Peter HH: Immunophenotypical alternations in a subset of patients with common variable immunodeficiency (CVID). Clin Exp Immunol 90:25, 1992

90. Watts WJ, Watts MB, Dai W et al: Respiratory dysfunction in patients with common variable hypogammaglobulinemia. Am Rev Respir Dis 134:699, 1986

91. Ammann AJ, Hong R: Selective IgA deficiency: presentation of 30 cases and a review of the literature. Medicine 50:223, 1971

92. Burks WA Jr, Steele RW: Selective IgA deficiency. Ann Allergy 57:3, 1986

93. Morgan G, Levinsky RJ: Clinical significance of IgA deficiency. Arch Dis Child 63:579, 1988

94. Hanson LA, Bjorkander J, Carlsson B et al: The heterogeneity of IgA deficiency. J Clin Immunol 8:159, 1988

95. Strober W, Sneller MC: IgA deficiency. Ann Allergy 66:363, 1991

96. Schaffer RM, Monteiro RC, Volanakis JE, Cooper MD: IgA deficiency. Immunodefic Rev 3:15, 1991

97. Olerup O, Smith CIE, Hammarström L: Different amino acids at position 57 of the HLA-DQβ chain associated with susceptibility and resistance to IgA deficiency. Nature 347:289, 1990

98. Olerup O, Smith CI, Bjorkander J, Hammarström L: Shared HLA class II-associated genetic susceptibility and resistance related to the HLA-DQβ1 gene, in IgA deficiency and common variable immunodeficiency. Proc Natl Acad Sci USA 89:10653, 1992

99. Cunningham-Rundles C: Genetic aspects of immunoglobulin A deficiency. Adv Hum Genet 19:235, 1990

100. Wilton AN, Cobain TJ, Dawkins RL: Family studies of IgA deficiency. Immunogenetics 21:333, 1985

101. Plebani A, Ugazio AG, Monafo V, Burgio GR: Clinical heterogeneity and reversibility of selective immunoglobulin A deficiency in 80 children. Lancet 1:829, 1986

102. Hammarström L, Carlsson B, Smith CIE et al: Detection of IgA heavy chain constant region genes in IgA deficient donors: evidence against gene deletions. Clin Exp Immunol 60:661, 1985

103. Conley ME, Cooper MD: Immature IgA B cells in IgA-deficient patients. N Engl J Med 305:495, 1981

104. Shinomiya N, Yata J: In-vitro analysis of defective IgA production in selective IgA deficiency in childhood. Clin Exp Immunol 62:746, 1985

105. Klemola TK, Eskola J, Savilahti E: T- and B-cell functions in IgA-deficient patients. Scand J Immunol 28:301, 1988

106. Atwater JS, Tomasi TB Jr: Suppressor cells and IgA deficiency. Clin Immunol Immunopathol 9:379, 1978

107. King MA, Wells JW, Nelson DS: IgA synthesis by peripheral blood mononuclear cells from normal and selectively IgA deficient subjects. Clin Exp Immunol 38:306, 1979

108. Oxelius VA, Laurell A-B, Lindquist B et al: IgG subclasses in selective IgA deficiency. Common occurrence of IgG2-IgA deficiency. N Engl J Med 304:1476, 1981

109. Lane PJL, Maclennan ICM: Imparied IgG2 anti-pneumococcal antibody responses in patients with recurrent infection and normal IgG2 levels but no IgA. Clin Exp Immunol 65:427, 1986

110. DeGraeff PA, The TH, vanMunster PJ et al: The primary immune response in patients with selective IgA deficiency. Clin Exp Immunol 54:778, 1983

111. Preud'Homme J-L, Hanson LA: IgG subclass deficiency. Imunodefic Rev 2:129, 1990

112. Liblau RS, Bach JF: Selective IgA deficiency and autoimmunity. Int Arch Allergy Immunol 99:16, 1992

113. Cunningham-Rundles C, Pudifin DJ, Armstrong D, Good RA: Selective IgA deficiency and neoplasia. Vox Sang 38:61, 1980

114. Cunningham-Rundles C, Brandeis WE, Pudifin DJ et al: Autoimmunity in selective IgA deficiency: relationship to anti-bovine protein antibodies, circulating immune complexes and clinical disease. Clin Exp Immunol 45:299, 1981

115. Ferreira A, Rodriguez MCG, Lopez-Trascase M et al: Anti-IgA antibodies in selective IgA deficiency and in primary immunodeficient patients treated with gamma globulin. Clin Immunol Immunopathol 47:199, 1988

116. Burks AW, Sampson HA, Buckley RH: Anaphylactic reactions after gamma globulin administration in patients with hypogammaglobulinemia. N Engl J Med 314:560, 1986

117. Bjorkander J, Hammarström L, Smith CIE et al: Immunoglobulin prophylaxis in patients with antibody deficiency syndromes and anti-IgA antibodies. J Clin Immunol 7:8, 1987

118. Lefranc M-P, Hammarström L, Smith CIE, Lefranc G: Gene deletions in the human immunoglobulin heavy chain constant region locus: molecular and immunological analysis. Immunodefic Rev 2:265, 1991

119. Migone N, Oliviero S, de Lange G et al: Multiple gene deletions within the human immunoglobulin heavy-chain cluster. Proc Natl Acad Sci USA 81:5811, 1984

120. Bottaro A, de Marchi M, de Lange G et al: New types of multiple and single gene deletions in the human IgCH locus. Immunogenetics 29:44, 1989

121. Faulk WP, Kiyasu WS, Cooper MD, Fudenberg HH: Deficiency of IgM. Pediatrics 47:399, 1971

122. Ohno T, Inaba M, Kuribayashi K et al: Selective IgM deficiency in adults: phenotypically and functionally altered profiles of peripheral blood lymphocytes. Clin Exp Immunol 68:630, 1987

123. Stavnezer-Nordgren J, Kekish O: Molecular defects in a human immunoglobulin κ chain deficiency. Science 230:458, 1985

124. Schur PH, Borel H, Gelfand EW et al: Selective gamma-G globulin deficiencies in patients with recurrent pyogenic infections. N Engl J Med 283:631, 1970

125. Oxelius VA: IgG subclass pattern in primary immunodeficiency disorders. Monogr Allergy 19:156, 1986

126. Umetsu DT, Ambrosino DM, Quinti I et al: Recurrent sinopulmonary infection and impaired antibody resposne to bacterial capsular polysaccharide antigen in children with selective IgG-subclass deficiency. N Engl J Med 313:1247, 1985

127. Oxelius VA: Chronic infections in a family with hereditary deficiency of IgG2 and IgG4. Clin Exp Immunol 17:19, 1974

128. Oxelius VA, Berkel AI, Hanson LA: IgG2 deficiency in ataxia-telangiectasia. N Engl J Med 306:515, 1982

129. Insel RA: Use of *Haemophilus influenzae* b vaccines in evaluating immunodeficiency. Pediatr Asthma Allergy Immunol 5:297, 1991

130. Insel RA, Anderson P: Resposne to oligosaccharide-protein conjugate vacciens against *Hemophilus influenzae* b in two patients with IgG2 deficiency unresponsive to capsular polysaccharide vaccine. N Engl J Med 315:499, 1986

131. Tiller TL Jr, Buckley RH: Transient hypogammaglobulinemia of infancy: review of the literature, clinical and immunologic features of 11 new cases, and long-term follow-up. J Pediatr 92:347, 1978

132. Rieger CHI, Nelson LA, Peri BA et al: Transient hypogammaglobulinemia of infancy. J Pediatr 91:601, 1977

133. McGeady SJ: Transient hypogammaglobulinemia of infancy: need to reconsider name and definition. J Pediatr 110:47, 1987

134. Siegel RL, Issekutz T, Schwaber J et al: Deficiency of T helper cells in transient hypogammaglobulinemia of infancy. N Engl J Med 305:1307, 1981

135. Soothill JF: Immunoglobulins in first-degree relatives of patients with hypogammaglobulinaemia: transient hypogammaglobulinaemia: a possible manifestation of heterozygosity. Lancet 1:1001, 1968

136. Fischer A: Severe combined immunodeficiencies. Immunodefic Rev 3:83, 1992

137. de Saint Basile G, Arveiler B, Oberle I et al: Close linkage of the locus for X chromosome-linked severe combined immunodeficiency to polymorphic DNA markers in Xq11-q13. Proc Natl Acad Sci USA 84:7576, 1987

138. Noguchi M, Huafang Y, Rosenblatt HM et al: Interleukin-2 receptor γ chain mutation results in X-linked severe combined immunodeficiency in humans. Cell 73:147, 1993

139. Taniguchi T, Minami Y: The IL-2/IL-2 receptor system: a current overview. Cell 73:5, 1993

140. Gougeon M-L, Drean G, Le Deist F et al: Human severe combined immunode-

ficiency disease: Phenotypic and functional characteristics of peripheral B lymphocytes. J Immunol 145:2873, 1990

141. Small TN, Keever C, Collins N et al: Characterization of B cells in SCID. Hum Immunol 25:181, 1989

142. Puck JM, Nussbaum RL, Conley ME: Carrier detection in X-linked severe combined immunodeficiency based on patients of X chromosome inactivation. J Clin Invest 79:1395, 1987

143. Conley ME, Lavoie A, Briggs C et al: Nonrandom X chromosome inactivation in B cells from carriers of X chromosome-linked severe combined immunodeficiency. Proc Natl Acad Sci USA 85:3090, 1988

144. Hirschhorn R: Adenosine deaminase deficiency. Immunodefic Rev 2:175, 1990

145. Hirschhorn R: Overview of biochemical abnormalities and molecular genetics of adenosine deaminase deficiency. Pediatr Res 33:S35, 1993

146. Cardon DA, Carrera CJ: Immunodeficiency secondary to adenosine deaminase deficiency and purine nucleotide phosphorylation deficiency. Semin Hematol 27:260, 1990

147. Morgan G, Levinsky RJ, Hugh-Jones K et al: Heterogeneity of biochemical, clinical and immunological parameters in severe combined immunodeficiency due to adenosine deaminase deficiency. Clin Exp Immunol 70:491, 1987

148. Schwarz K, Hansen-Hagge TE, Knobloch C et al: Severe combined immunodeficiency (SCID) in man: B cell-negative (B−) SCID patients exhibit an irregular recombination pattern at the JH locus. J Exp Med 174:1039, 1991

149. Cavazzana-Calvo M, Le Deist F, De Saint Basile G et al: Increased radiosensitivity of granulocyte macrophage colony-forming units and skin fibroblasts in human autosomal recessive severe combined immunodeficiency. J Clin Invest 91:1214, 1993

150. Omenn GS: Familial reticuloendotheliosis with eosinophilia. N Engl J Med 273:427, 1965

151. Wirt DP, Brooks EG, Vaidy AS et al: Novel T-lymphocyte population in combined immunodeficiency with features of graft versus host disease. N Engl J Med 32:370, 1989

152. De Saint Basile G, Le Deist F, De Villartay JP et al: Restricted heterogeneity of T lymphocytes in combined immunodeficiency and hypereosinophilia (Omenn's syndrome). J Clin Invest 87:1352, 1991

153. Schandene L, Ferster A, Mascart-Lemone F et al: T helper type 2-like cells and therapeutic effects of interferon-gamma in combined immunodeficiency with hypereosinophilia (Omenn's syndrome). Eur J Immunol 23:56, 1993

154. Griscelli C, Lisowska-Grospierre B: Combined immunodeficiency with defective expression in MHC class II genes. Immunodefic Rev 1:135, 1989

155. Reith W, Satola S, Sanchez CH et al: Congenital immunodeficiency with a regulatory defect in MHC class II gene expression lacks a specific HLA-DR promoter binding protein, RF-X. Cell 53:897, 1988

156. Reith W, Satola S, Kobr M et al: Cloning of the major histocompatibility complex class II promoter binding protein affected in a hereditary defect in class II gene regulation. Proc Natl Acad Sci USA 86:4200, 1989

157. dePreval C, Hadam MR, Mach B: Regulation of genes for HLA class II antigens in cell lines from patients with severe combined immunodeficiency. N Engl J Med 318:1295, 1988

158. Seidl C, Saraiya C, Osterweil Z et al: Genetic complexity of regulatory mutants defective for HLA class II gene expression. J Immunol 148:1576, 1992

159. Kara CJ, Glimcher LH: In vivo footprinting of MHC class II genes: bare promoters in the bare lymphocyte syndrome. Science 252:709, 1991

160. Kara CJ, Glimcher LH: Promoter accessibility within the environment of the MHC is affected in class II-deficient combined immunodeficiency. EMBO J 12:187, 1993

161. Touraine JL: The bare-lymphocyte syndrome: report on the registry. Lancet 1:319, 1981

162. Alarcon B, Terhorst C, Arnaiz-Villana A et al: Congenital T-cell receptor immunodeficiencies in man. Immunodefic Rev 2:1, 1990

163. Arnaiz-Villena A, Timon M, Rodriguez-Gallego C et al: Human T-cell activation deficiencies. Immunol Today 13:259, 1992

164. Chatila T, Wong R, Young M et al: An immunodeficiency characterized by defective signal transduction in T lymphocytes. N Engl J Med 320:696, 1989

165. Le Deist F, de Saint Basile G, Mazerolles F et al: Primary membrane T cell immunodeficiency. Clin Immunol Immunopathol 61:S56, 1991

166. Arnaiz-Villena A, Timon M, Corell A et al: Brief report: primary immunodeficiency caused by mutations in the gene encoding the CD3-γ subunit of the T-lymphocyte receptor. N Engl J Med 327:529, 1992

167. Soudais C, de Villartay J-P, Le Deist F et al: Independent mutations of the human CD3-ε gene resulting in a T cell receptor/CD3 complex immunodeficiency. Nature Genet 3:77, 1993

168. Weinberg K, Parkman R: Severe combined immunodeficiency due to a specific defect in the production of interleukin-2. N Engl J Med 322:1718, 1990

169. Chatila T, Castigli E, Pahwa R et al: Primary combined immunodeficiency

resulting from defective transcription of multiple T-cell lymphokine genes. Proc Natl Acad Sci USA 87:10033, 1990

170. Disanto JP, Keever CA, Small TN et al: Absence of interleukin 2 production in a severe combined immunodeficiency disease syndrome with T cells. J Exp Med 171:1697, 1990

171. Castigli E, Pahwa R, Good RA et al: Molecular basis of a multiple lymphokine deficiency in a patient with severe combined immunodeficiency. Proc Natl Acad Sci USA 90:4728, 1993

172. Pahwa R, Chatila T, Pahwa S et al: Recombinant interleukin-2 therapy in severe combined immunodeficiency disease. Proc Natl Acad Sci USA 86:5069, 1989

173. Chu ET, Rosenwasser LJ, Dinarello CA et al: Immunodeficiency with defective T-cell response to interleukin 1. Proc Natl Acad Sci USA 81:4945, 1984

174. Weinberg KI, Parr T: Severe combined immunodeficiency (SCID) due to defective interleukin 2 receptor α (IL-2Rα) expression. Pediatr Res 25:170, 1989

175. Gitlin D, Vawter G, Craig MM: Thymic alymphoplasia and congenital aleukocytosis. Pediatrics 33:184, 1964

176. Roper M, Parmley RT, Crist WM et al: Severe congenital leukopenia (reticular dysgenesis). Immunologic and morphologic characterizations of leukocytes. Am J Dis Child 139:832, 1985

177. Levinsky RJ, Tiedeman K: Successful bone-marrow transplantation for reticular dysgenesis. Lancet 1:671, 1983

178. Parkman R: Human graft-versus-host disease. Immunodefic Rev 2:253, 1991

179. Pollack MS, Kirkpatrick D, Kapoor N et al: Identification by HLA typing of intrauterine derived maternal T cells in four patients with severe combined immunodeficiency. N Engl J Med 397:662, 1981

180. Geha RS, Reinherz E: Identification of circulating maternal T and B lymphocytes in uncomplicated severe combined immunodeficiency by HLA typing of subpopulations of T cells separated by the fluorescence-activated cell sorter and of Epstein-Barr virus-derived B cell lines. J Immunol 130:2493, 1983

181. Knobloch C, Goldmann SF, Friedrich W: Limited T cell receptor diversity of transplacentally acquired maternal T cells in severe combined immunodeficiency. J Immunol 146:4157, 1991

182. Thompson LF, O'Connor RD, Bastian JF: Phenotype and function of engrafted maternal T cells in patients with SCID. J Immunol 133:2513, 1984

183. Buckley RH, Gilbertsen RB, Schiff R et al: Heterogeneity of lymphocyte subpopulations in severe combined immunodeficiency: evidence against a stem cell defect. J Clin Invest 58:130, 1976

184. Buckley RH: Advances in the correction of immunodeficiency by bone marrow transplantation. Pediatr Ann 16:412, 1987

185. Good RA: Bone marrow transplantation for immunodeficiency diseases. Am J Med Sci 294:68, 1987

186. O'Reilly RJ, Keever CA, Small TN, Brochstein J: The use of HLA-non-identical T-cell-depleted marrow transplants for correction of severe combined immunodeficiency disease. Immunodefic Rev 1:273, 1989

187. Fischer A, Landais P, Friedrich W et al: European experience of bone-marrow transplantation for severe combined immunodeficiency. Lancet 2:850, 1990

188. Friedrich W, Goldmann SF, Ebell W et al: Severe combined immunodeficiency: treatment by bone marrow transplantation in 15 infants using HLA-haploidentical donors. Eur J Pediatr 144:125, 1985

189. Filipovich AH, Shapiro RS, Ramsay NK et al: Unrelated donor bone marrow transplantation for correction of lethal congenital immunodeficiencies. Blood 80:270, 1992

190. Parkman R: The biology of bone marrow transplantation for severe combined immune deficiency. Adv Immunol 49:381, 1991

191. Buckley RH, Schiff SE, Sampson HA et al: Development of immunity in human severe primary T cell deficiency following haploidentical bone marrow stem cell transplantation. J Immunol 136:2398, 1986

192. Wijnaendts SL, Le Deist F, Griscelli C, Fischer A: Development of immunologic functions after BMT in 33 patients with SCID. Blood 74:2212, 1989

193. Hershfield MS, Chaffee S, Sorensen RU: Enzyme replacement therapy with polyethylene glycol-adenosine deaminase in adenosine deaminase deficiency: overview and case reports of three patients, including two now receiving gene therapy. Pediatr Res 33:S42, 1993

194. Blaese RM, Culver KW: Gene therapy for primary immunodeficiency disease. Immunodefic Rev 3:329, 1992

195. Blaese RM: Development of gene therapy for immunodeficiency: adenosine deaminase deficiency. Pediatr Res 33:S49, 1993

196. Markert ML: Purine nucleoside phosphorylase deficiency. Immunodefic Rev 3:45, 1991

197. Staal GEJ, Stoop JW, Zegers BJM et al: Erythrocyte metabolism in purine nucleoside phosphorylase deficiency after enzyme replacement therapy by infusion of erythrocytes. J Clin Invest 65:103, 1980

198. Aldrich RA, Steinberg AC, Campbell DC: Pedigree demonstrating a sex-linked

recessive condition characterized by draining ears, eczematoid dermatitis and bloody diarrhea. Pediatrics 13:133, 1954

199. Cooper MD, Chase HP, Lowman JT et al: Wiskott-Aldrich syndrome: immunologic deficiency diseases involving the afferent limb of immunity. Am J Med 44:499, 1968

200. Peacocke M, Siminovitch KA: Linkage of the Wiskott-Aldrich syndrome with polymorphic DNA sequences from the human X chromosome. Proc Natl Acad Sci USA 84:3430, 1987

201. Kwan SP, Lehner T, Hagemann T et al: Localization of the gene for the Wiskott-Aldrich sydnrome between two flanking markers, TIMP and DXS255, on Xp11.22-Xp11.3. Genomics 10:29, 1991

202. Gealy WJ, Dwyer JM, Harley JB: Allelic exclusion of glucose-6-phosphate dehydrogenase in platelets and T lymphocytes from a Wiskott-Aldrich syndrome carrier. Lancet 1:63, 1980

203. Prchal JT, Carroll AJ, Prchal JF et al: Wiskott-Aldrich syndrome: cellular impairments and their implications for carrier detection. Blood 56:1048, 1980

204. Greer WL, Kwong PC, Peacocke M et al: X-chromosome inactivation in the Wiskott-Aldrich syndrome: a marker for detection of the carrier state and identification of cell lineages expressing the gene defect. Genomics 4:60, 1989

205. Goodship J, Carter J, Espanol T et al: Carrier detection in Wiskott-Aldrich syndrome: combined use of M27 beta for X-inactivation studies and as a linked probe. Blood 77:2677, 1991

206. Weiden PL, Blaese RM: Hereditary thrombocytopenia: relation to Wiskott-Aldrich syndrome with special reference to splenectomy. J Pediatr 80:226, 1972

207. Standen GR, Lillicrap DP, Matthews N, Bloom AL: Inherited thrombocytopenia, elevated serum IgA and renal disease: identification as a variant of the Wiskott-Aldrich syndrome. Q J Med 59:401, 1986

208. Donner M, Schwartz M, Carlsson KU, Holmberg L: Hereditary X-linked thrombocytopenia maps to the same chromosomal region as the Wiskott-Aldrich syndrome. Blood 72:1849, 1988

209. de Saint Basile G, Schlegel N, Caniglia M et al: X-linked thrombocytopenia and Wiskott-Aldrich syndrome: similar regional assignment but distinct X-inactivation pattern in carriers. Ann Hematol 63:107, 1991

210. Kenney D, Cairns L, Remold-O'Donnell E et al: Morphological abnormalities in the lymphocytes of patients with the Wiskott-Aldrich syndrome. Blood 68:1329, 1986

211. Molina IJ, Kenney DM, Rosen FS, Remold-O'Donnell E: T cell lines characterize events in the pathogenesis of the Wiskott-Aldrich syndrome. J Exp Med 176:867, 1992

212. Remold-O'Donnell E, Rosen FS: Sialophorin (CD43) and the Wiskott-Aldrich syndrome. Immunodefic Rev 2:151, 1990

213. Piller F, Le Deist F, Weinberg KI et al: Altered O-glycan synthesis in lymphocytes from patients with Wiskott-Aldrich syndrome. J Exp Med 173:1501, 1991

214. Higgins EA, Siminovitch KA, Zhuang DL et al: Aberrant O-linked oligosaccharide biosynthesis in lymphocytes and platelets from patients with the Wiskott-Aldrich syndrome. J Biol Chem 266:6280, 1991

215. Simon H-U, Mills GB, Hashimoto S, Siminovitch KA: Evidence for defective transmembrane signaling in B cells from patients with Wiskott-Aldrich syndrome. J Clin Invest 90:1396, 1992

216. Simon HU, Higgins EA, Demetriou M et al: Defective expression of CD23 and autocrine growth-stimulation in Epstein-Barr virus (EBV)-transformed B cells from patients with Wiskott-Aldrich syndrome (WAS). Clin Exp Immunol 91:43, 1993

217. Dragone L, Pallant A, Insel R, Frelinger JG: CD43 is expressed normally on Wiskott-Aldrich-derived lymphocytes. Exp Clin Immunogenet 9:130, 1992

218. Baldini MG: Nature of the platelet defect in the Wiskott-Aldrich sydnrome. Ann NY Acad Sci 201:437, 1972

219. Ochs HD, Slichter SJ, Harker LA et al: The Wiskott-Aldrich syndrome: studies of lymphocytes, granulocytes, and platelets. Blood 55:243, 1980

220. Pearson HA, Shulman NR, Oski FA, Eitzman DV: Platelet survival in Wiskott-Aldrich syndrome. J Pediatr 68:754, 1966

221. Corash L, Shafer B, Blaese RM: Platelet-associated immunoglobulin, platelet size, and the effect of splenectomy in the Wiskott-Aldrich syndrome. Blood 65:1439, 1985

222. Lum LG, Tubergen DG, Corash L, Blaese RM: Splenectomy in the management of the thrombocytopenia of the Wiskott-Aldrich syndrome. N Engl J Med 302:892, 1980

223. Knutsen AP, Rosse WF, Kinney TR, Buckley RH: Immunologic studies before and after splenectomy in a patient with the Wiskott-Aldrich syndrome. J Clin Immunol 1:13, 1981

224. Pidard D, Didry D, Le Deist F et al: Analysis of the membrane glycoproteins of platelets in the Wiskott-Aldrich syndrome. Br J Haematol 69:529, 1988

225. Perry GS, III, Spector BD, Schuman LM et al: The Wiskott-Aldrich syndrome in the United States and Canada (1892–1979). J Pediatr 97:72, 1980

226. Cotelingam JD, Witebsky FG, Hsu SM et al: Malignant lymphoma in patients with the Wiskott-Aldrich syndrome. Cancer Invest 3:515, 1985

227. Morio T, Takase K, Okawa H et al: The increase of non-MHC-restricted cytotoxic cells (gamma/delta-TCR-bearing T cells of NK cells) and the abnormal differentiation of B cells in Wiskott-Aldrich syndrome. Clin Immunol Immunopathol 52:279, 1989

228. Fearon ER, Kohn DB, Winkelstein JA et al: Carrier detection in the Wiskott-Aldrich syndrome. Blood 72:1735, 1988

229. Lorenz P, Bollmann R, Hinkel GK et al: False-negative prenatal exclusion of Wiskott-Aldrich syndrome by measurement of fetal platelet count and size. Prenat Diagn 11:819, 1991

230. Meuwissen HJ, Bortin MM, Bach FH et al: Long-term survival after bone marrow transplantation: a 15-year follow-up report of a patient with Wiskott-Aldrich syndrome. J Pediatr 105:365, 1984

231. Parkman R, Rappeport J, Geha R et al: Complete correction of the Wiskott-Aldrich syndrome by allogeneic bone-marrow transplantation. N Engl J Med 298:921, 1978

232. Brochstein JA, Gillio AP, Ruggiero M et al: Marrow transplantation from human leukocyte antigen-identical or haploidentical donors for correction of Wiskott-Aldrich syndrome. J Pediatr 119:907, 1991

233. Bridges BA, Harnden DG (eds): Ataxia-Telangiectasia: A Cellular and Molecular Link Between Cancer, Neuropathology and Immunodeficiency. Wiley, Chichester, 1982

234. Boder E: Ataxia-telangiectasia: an overview. p. 1. In Gatti RA, Swift M (eds): Ataxia-Telangiectasia: Genetics, Neuropathology, and Immunology of a Degenerative Disease of Childhood. Alan R Liss, New York, 1985

235. Gatti RA, Boder E, Vinters HV et al: Ataxia-telangiectasis: an interdisciplinary approach to pathogenesis. Medicine 70:99, 1991

236. Swift M: Genetic aspects of ataxia-telangiectasia. Immunodefic Rev 2:67, 1990

237. Gatti RA: Localizing the genes for ataxia-telangiectasis: a human model for inherited cancer susceptibility. Adv Cancer Res 56:77, 1991

238. Swift M, Morrell D, Cromartie E et al: The incidence and gene frequency of ataxia-telangiectasis in the United States. Am J Hum Genet 39:573, 1986

239. Swift M, Reitnauer PJ, Morrell D, Chase CL: Breast and other cancers in families with ataxia-telangiectasia. N Engl J Med 316:1289, 1987

240. Swift M, Morrell D, Massey RB, Chase CL: Incidence of cancer in 161 families affected by ataxia-telangiectasia. N Engl J Med 325:1831, 1991

241. McKinnon PJ: Ataxia-telangiectasia: an inherited disorder of ionizing-radiation sensitivity in man. Progress in the elucidation of the underlying biochemical defect. Hum Genet 75:197, 1987

242. Meyn MS: High spontaneous intrachromosomal recombination rates in ataxia-telangiectasia. Science 260:1327, 1993

243. Kastan MB, Zhan Q, El-Deiry WS et al: A mammalian cell cycle checkpoint pathway utilizing p53 and GADD45 is defective in ataxia-telangiectasia. Cell 71:587, 1992

244. Hartwell L: Defects in a cell cycle checkpoint may be responsible for the genomic instability of cancer cells. Cell 71:543, 1992

245. Lipkowitz S, Stern MH, Kirsch IR: Hybrid T cell receptor genes formed by interlocus recombination in normal and ataxia-telangiectasis lymphocytes. J Exp Med 172:409, 1990

246. Kobayashi Y, Tycko B, Soreng AL, Sklar J: Transrearrangements between antigen receptor genes in normal human lymphoid tissues and in ataxia telangiectasia. J Imunol 147:3201, 1991

247. Hecht F, Hecht BK: Chromosome changes connect immunodeficiency and cancer in ataxia-telangiectasia. Am J Pediatr Hematol Oncol 9:185, 1987

248. Davey MP, Bertness V, Nakahara K et al: Juxtaposition of the T-cell receptor IgA-chain locus (14q11) and a region (14q32) of potential importance in leukemogenesis by a 14;14 translocation in patient with T-cell chronic lymphocytic leukemia and ataxia-telangiectasia. Proc Natl Acad Sci USA 85:9287, 1988

249. Stern MH, Theodorou I, Aurias A et al: T-cell nonmalignant clonal proliferation in ataxia telangiectasia: a cytological, immunological, and molecular characterization. Blood 73:1285, 1989

250. Russo G, Isobe M, Gatti R et al: Molecular analysis of a t(14;14) translocation in leukemic T-cells of an ataxia telangiectasia patient. Proc Natl Acad Sci USA 86:602, 1989

251. Stern MH, Theodorou I, Aurias A et al: T-cell nonmalignant clonal proliferation in ataxia telangiectasia: a cytological, immunological and molecular characterization. Blood 73:1285, 1989

252. Carbonari M, Cherchi M, Paganelli R et al: Relative increase on T cells expressing the gamma/delta rather than the alpha/beta receptor in ataxia-telangiectasia. N Engl J Med 322:73, 1990

253. Waldmann TA, Broder S, Goldman CK et al: Disorders of B cells and helper

T cells in the pathogenesis of the immunoglobulin deficiency of patients with ataxia telangiectasia. J Clin Invest 71:282, 1983

254. Waldmann TA, McIntire KR: Serum alpha-fetoprotein levels in patients with ataxia-telangiectasia. Lancet 2:1112, 1972

255. Sugimoto T, Sawada T, Tozawa M et al: Plasma levels of carcinoembryonic antigen in patients with ataxia telangiectasia. J Pediatr 92:436, 1978

256. McFarlin DE, Strober W, Waldmann TA: ataxia-telangiectasia. Medicine 51:281, 1972

257. Abadir R, Hakami N: Ataxia-telangiectasia with cancer. An indication for reduced radiotherapy and chemotherapy doses. Br J Radiol 56:343, 1983

258. Shaham M, Voss R, Becker Y et al: Prenatal diagnosis of ataxia telangiectasia. J Pediatr 100:134, 1982

259. Hong R. The DiGeorge anomaly. Immunodefic Rev 3:1, 1991

260. Lischner HW, Punnett HH, DiGeorge AM: Lymphocytes in congenital absence of the thymus. Nature 214:580, 1967

261. Robinson HB: DiGeorge III–IV pharyngeal pouch syndrome: pathology and a theory of pathogenesis. Perspect Pediatr Pathol 2:173, 1975

262. Bockman DE, Kirby ML: Dependence of thymus development on derivatives of the neural crest. Science 223:498, 1984

263. Lammer EJ, Opitz JM: The DiGeorge anomaly as a developmental field defect. Am J Med Genet 2:113, 1986

264. Chisaka O, Capecchi MR: Regionally restricted developmental defects resulting from targeted disruption of the mouse homeobox gene hox-1.5. Nature 350:473, 1991

265. Rohn RD, Leffell MS, Leadem P et al: Familial third-fourth pharyngeal pouch syndrome with apparent autosomal dominant transmission. J Pediatr 105:47, 1984

266. Keppen LD, Fasules JW, Burks AW et al: Confirmation of autosomal dominant transmission of the DiGeorge malformation complex. J Pediatr 113:506, 1988

267. Greenberg F, Elder FFB, Haffner P et al: Cytogenetic findings in a prosepctive series of patients with DiGeorge anomaly. Am J Hum Genet 43:605, 1988

268. Carey AH, Kelly D, Halford S et al: Molecular genetic study of the frequency of monosomy 22q11 in DiGeorge syndrome. Am J Human Genet 51:964, 1992

269. Wilson DI, Cross IE, Goodship JA et al: A prospective cytogenetic study of 36 cases of DiGeorge syndrome. Am J Hum Genet 51:957, 1992

270. Driscoll DA, Budarf ML, Emanuel BS: A genetic etiology for DiGeorge syndrome: consistent deletions and microdeletions of 22q11. Am J Hum Genet 50:924, 1992

271. Driscoll DA, Spinner NB, Budarf ML et al: Deletions and microdeletions of 22q11.2 in velo-cardio-facial syndrome. Am J Med Genet 44:261, 1992

272. Cavdar AO: DiGeorge's syndrome and fetal alcohol syndrome. Am J Dis Child 137:806, 1983

273. Conley ME, Bechwith JB, Maner JFK et al: The spectrum of DiGeorge syndrome. J Pediatr 94:883, 1979

274. Muller W, Peter HH, Wilken M et al: The DiGeorge syndrome. I. Clinical evaluation and course of partial and complete forms of the syndrome. Eur J Pediatr 147:496, 1988

275. Marmon LM, Balsara RK, Chen R et al: Congenital cardiac anomalies associated with the DiGeorge syndrome: a neonatal experience. Ann Thorac Surg 38:146, 1984

276. Lodewyk HS, Van Mierop MD, Kutsche LM: Cardiovascular anomalies in DiGeorge syndrome and importance of neural crest as a possible pathogenetic factor. Am J Cardiol 58:133, 1986

277. Kiel EA, Drummond WH, Barrett DJ: Prevalence of T-lymphocyte abnormalities in infants with congenital heart disease. Am J Dis Child 138:143, 1984

278. Bastian J, Law S, Vogler L et al: Prediction of persistent immunodeficiency in the DiGeorge anomaly. J Pediatr 115:391, 1989

279. Muller W, Peter HH, Kallfelz HC et al: The DiGeorge sequence. II. Immunologic findings in partial and complete forms of the disorder. Eur J Pediatr 149:96, 1989

280. Borzy MS, Ridgway D, Noya FJ, Shearer WT: Successful bone marrow transplantation with split lymphoid chimerism in DiGeorge syndrome. J Clin Immunol 9:386, 1989

281. Goldsobel AB, Haas A, Stiehm ER: Bone marrow transplantation in DiGeorge syndrome. J Pediatr 111:40, 1987

282. Lenarsky C: Mechanisms in immune recovery after bone marrow transplantation. Management of post-transplant immune deficiency. Am J Pediatr Hematol Oncol 15:49, 1993

283. Zimmerli W, Zarth A, Gratwohl A, Speck B: Neutrophil function and pyogenic infections in bone marrow transplant recipients. Blood 77:393, 1991

284. Keever CA, Small TN, Flomenberg N et al: Immune reconstitution following bone marrow transplantation: comparison of recipients of T-cell depleted marrow with recipients of conventional marrow grafts. Blood 73:1340, 1989

285. Welte K, Ciobanu N, Moore MAS et al: Defective interleukin 2 production in patients after bone marrow transplantation and in vitro restoration of defective T lymphocyte proliferation by highly purified interleukin 2. Blood 64:380, 1984

286. Soiffer RJ, Murray C, Cochran K et al: Clinical and immunologic effects of prolonged infusion of low-dose recombinant interleukin-2 after autologous and T-cell-depleted allogeneic bone marrow transplantation. Blood 79:517, 1992

287. Antin JH and Ferrara LM: Cytokine dysregulation and acute graft-versus-host disease. Blood 80:2964, 1992

288. Shapiro RS, McClain K, Frizzera G et al: Epstein-Barr virus associated B cell lymphoproliferative disorders following bone marrow transplantation. Blood 71:1234, 1988

289. Skinner JC, Gilbert EF, Hong R et al: B cell lymphoproliferative disorders following T cell depleted allogeneic bone marrow transplantation. Am J Pediatr Hematol Oncol 10:112, 1988

290. Valardi A, Cucciaioni S, Terenzi A et al: Acquisition of Ig isotype diversity after bone marrow transplantation in adults. A recapitulation of normal B cell ontogeny. J Immunol 141:815, 1988

291. Aucouturier P, Barra A, Intrator L et al: Long lasting IgG subclass and antibacterial polysaccharide antibody deficiency after bone marrow transplantation. Blood 70:779, 1987

292. Sheridan JF, Tutschka PJ, Sedmak DD et al: Immunoglobulin G subclass deficiency and pneumococcal infection after allogeneic bone marrow transplantation. Blood 75:1583, 1990

Histiocytic Syndromes

56

Jeffrey M. Lipton

INTRODUCTION

The histiocytic syndromes comprise a broad grouping of hematologic disorders united only by the observation that a macrophage or histiocyte-like cell appears to be the principal pathologic protagonist. The ubiquitous nature of the macrophage, its extraordinary metabolic capabilities, its role as a regulator of hematopoiesis, and its prominence in the immune and inflammatory response (as well as uncertainty regarding monocyte, macrophage, histocyte, and dendritic cell ontogeny) all contribute to the confusion surrounding the nosology of these disorders. Reactive proliferations and metabolic disor-

Table 56-1. The Histiocytic Syndromes

Class I histiocytoses: Langerhans cell histiocytosis (equivalent to "histiocytosis X")

    Eosinophilic granuloma

    Letterer-Siwe disease

    Hand-Schüller-Christian disease

Class II histiocytoses: hemophagocytic syndromes (equivalent to non-Langerhans cell histiocytosis)

    Familial hemophagocytic lymphohistiocytosis

    Infection-associated hemophagocytic syndrome

    Sinus histiocytosis with massive lymphadenopathy

Class III histiocytoses: malignant histiocytosis syndromes

    Leukemia

        Acute monocytic leukemia

        Chronic monocytic leukemia

        Chronic myelomonocytic leukemia (CMML)

            Adult CMML

            Childhood CMML (also called juvenile chronic myeloid leukemia)

    Malignant histiocytosis (includes some cases originally called histiocytic medullary reticulosis)

    True histiocytic lymphoma

(From Komp and Perry,[3] with permission.)

ders can, however, be distinguished from the primary histiocyte disorders[1,2] and, as such, are covered in more appropriate sections of this text. Recently three classes of histiocytic syndromes have been defined.[3] The class I histiocytoses, which comprise the clinical syndromes termed Langerhans cell histiocytosis (LCH)[3,4] previously known as histiocytosis X, are the main focus of this chapter. The class II histiocytoses are also covered. This class includes three distinct non-Langerhans cell histiocytoses: familial hemophagocytic lymphohistiocytosis (FHL), previously known as familial erythophagocytic lymphohistiocytosis, infection-associated hemophagocytic syndrome, and sinus histiocytosis with massive lymphadenopathy (SHML). The class III histiocytoses, the malignant histiocytic syndromes, include the malignant proliferations of the monocyte/macrophage lineage, acute and chronic monocytic and myelomonocytic leukemia, juvenile chronic myeloid leukemia, and true histiocytic lymphoma. They are discussed in other chapters. However, as if to emphasize the difficulties in classification, the class III syndrome malignant histiocytosis (MH) (originally called histiocytic medullary reticulosis) is discussed in this chapter. Table 56-1 presents the currently accepted classification of the histiocytic syndromes.

EPIDEMIOLOGY

The Class I histiocytoses (LCH) were originally considered by many to be malignant neoplasms. That they have been treated with aggressive chemotherapy and radiotherapy has not resolved the difficulties in properly categorizing this class of disorders. Although these modalities are still used, there are clear differences between most instances of LCH and true malignant disease that suggest conservative management for many patients. The clinical course of malignant neoplasia is generally relentlessly progressive, with virtually no survival in untreated patients (stage IVS neuroblastoma being the notable exception). In LCH, however, even with multiple site involvement, spontaneous remissions have been described.[5] In addition, varying morbidity and mortality have been reported in untreated patients with LCH, depending on the extent of disease. Pathologically, the lesions of LCH appear as reactive infiltrates, possessing little of the cellular atypicality and homogeneity characteristic of most malignancies. Using flow cytometry, Rabkin et al.[6] examined 29 patients, 17 with solitary bone lesions and 12 with disseminated disease, and found no aneuploid cells in any of the lesions examined. Although the etiology of these phenomena is unknown, in most cases LCH appears to represent a reactive autoimmune disorder triggered by unknown stimuli.[1,7,8] Recent preliminary data suggest that some cases, particularly those in infants with multisystem involvement, may be clonal neoplasms.[9] However, as pointed out by Kannourakis and Tiong,[10] ". . . rare progenitor cells resident or attracted into lesions in response to cytokines . . . may produce a non-neoplastic clonal proliferation of histiocytes." Thus the exact nature of these disorders still remains in doubt.

Historically, the classical LCH syndromes comprise monostotic or solitary (SEG) or multifocal eosinophilic granuloma (MEG), localized lesion(s) confined to bone[11,12]; Hand-Schüller-Christian disease, protracted multiple-site involvement with the classic but rare triad of skull defects, diabetes insipidus, and exophthalmos[13-16]; and Letterer-Siwe disease, deeper visceral lesions involving skin, liver, lungs, bone marrow, lymph nodes, spleen, and other mononuclear/phagocyte system organs.[17,18] The total incidence of these syndromes is roughly estimated to be 1 in 2 million.[19] They predominantly affect infants and young children, although disease in adults, even elderly adults,[20] is well described. A male predominance has been widely reported.[21-26] Since there is a continuum of disease that frequently does not fit these rigid and arbitrary designations, a grouping system has been developed. Classification is best accomplished according to the criteria originally developed by Lahey[27] and refined by Komp and co-workers[28] and Osband et al.[8] (Table 56-2). Other systems are useful but are more complicated.[24] This staging system, described in more detail later, can be used to determine both therapy and prog-

Table 56-2. Grouping System for Histiocytosis

Factor	Points
Age	
≥2	0
<2	1
Extent of disease	
<4 organs	0
≥4 organs	1
Dysfunction[a] (1, 2, or 3)	
No	0
Yes	1

Group[a]	Total Points[b]
0	Monostotic eosinophilic granuloma
I	0
II	1
III	2
IV	3

[a] Dysfunction includes the following:

1. Hepatic dysfunction: one or more of the following—hypoproteinemia (total protein <5.5 mg/dl or albumin <2.5 mg/dl), hyperbilirubinemia (>1.5 mg/dl), edema, ascites.
2. Pulmonary dysfunction: one or more of the following—tachypnea, dyspnea, cyanosis, cough, pneumothorax, pleural effusion.
3. Hematopoietic dysfunction: one or more of the following—anemia in the absence of iron deficiency or significant infection (<10 g/dl hemoglobin), leukopenia (<4,000/ml), thrombocytopenia (<100,000/ml).

[b] By arbitrarily assigning either 0 or 1 point for the absence or presence of one of the three important prognostic variables, a number of total points is obtained and a patient is assigned a group.

(Modified from Osband et al.,[8] with permission.)

nosis. Patients in groups 0 to II (Table 56-2) do quite well, with little morbidity and no mortality. They frequently require little or no systemic therapy. Some patients in group II and most in group III require systemic therapy and generally do well, while significant morbidity and mortality are encountered in group IV regardless of therapy,[8] lending credence to the recent observation that these patients may represent a subgroup with a clonal proliferation, perhaps malignant, of Langerhans cells.[9,10]

The optimal management for the patient with LCH is one that balances therapeutic intervention, utilized to minimize both short-and long-term disease-related morbidities, with a relative therapeutic nihilism designed to reduce treatment-associated morbidity. Philosophically, the agents used should be thought of as immunosuppressive rather than antineoplastic. Patients are treated to obtain disease control, followed by tapering of drug doses to achieve the lowest dose that maintains control. Eventually almost all patients who respond will be able to discontinue treatment completely, although recurrences are common. This philosophy applies to those patients (generally in groups I–III) with relatively favorable prognoses. The goal must now be to find effective therapy for those patients whose disease does not respond to therapy. (predominantly group IV).[3] These patients should have HLA typing at diagnosis and be considered for bone marrow transplantation, cyclosporine, or experimental immunosuppressive or immunomodulatory therapy.[3]

BIOLOGIC ASPECTS

In order to understand the histiocytic disorders, it is important to review monocyte/macrophage differentiation, which is characterized by the developmental sequence shown in Figure 56-1.[2,29,30]

In the bone marrow this process begins with the pluripotent hematopoietic stem cell, which may give rise either to a lymphoid progenitor capable of T- or B-lymphocyte lineage commitment or to a multipotent myeloid progenitor capable of differentiation to either erythroid, megakaryocyte, eosinophil, basophil/mast cell, or granulocyte/macrophage cell lines. The granulocyte and the macrophage share a common progenitor, the colony-forming unit-granulocyte/macrophage (CFU-GM). The CFU-GM, capable of granulocyte or monocyte differentiation, gives rise to the monocyte/macrophage progenitor (CFU-M). The CFU-M gives rise to the monoblast, then to the bone marrow promonocyte (the first morphologically identifiable macrophage [histiocyte] precursor), and finally to the monocyte, a process that takes approximately 6 days.[29] The promonocyte ranges from 10 to 18 μm in diameter and has a well-developed Golgi apparatus as well as peroxidase-positive granules. The typical monocyte has a folded nucleus, lightly basophilic cytoplasm, and faint azurophilic granules.[31]

Bone marrow monocytes enter the circulation and migrate, apparently in a random fashion, into tissues where they transform into tissue-specific histiocytes under the influence of the local environment and become the cells of the mononuclear/phagocyte system (MPS).[29] Although they are not as clearly determined, the circulating dendritic or veiled cells arise either from the monocyte or from the CFU-M and give rise in a similar manner to the cells comprising the tissue-based dendritic cell system (DCS).[30]

The MPS, also known as the reticuloendothelial system, consists of a multitude of ordinary tissue histiocytes (fixed macrophages) that act to provide host defense by disposing of senescent or damaged blood cells, ingesting invading organisms, processing antigens for the immune system, and stimulating the inflammatory process through the production of a number of cytokines.[29,30,32] The most important of these cytokines are

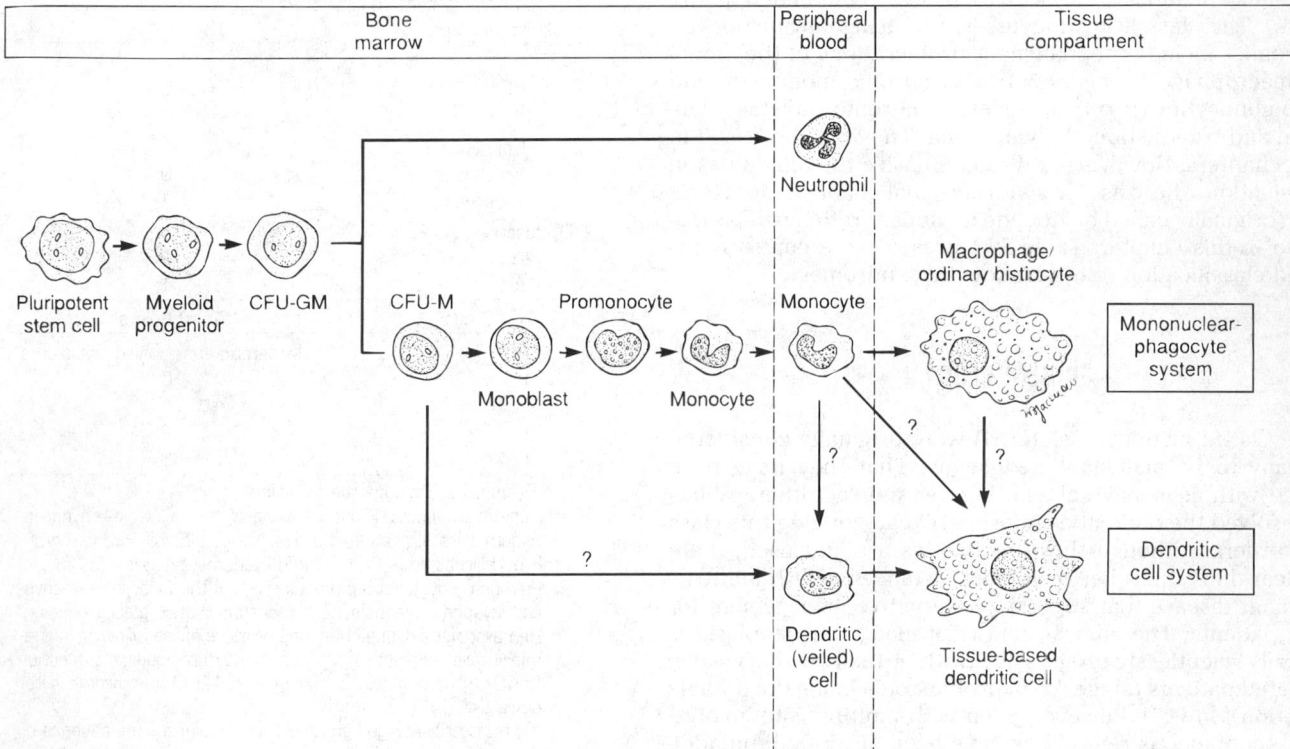

Fig. 56-1. Development of cells of the monocyte/macrophage lineage. CFU-GM, colony-forming unit-granulocyte/macrophage; CFU-M, colony-forming unit-macrophage.

interleukin-1 (IL-1) and tumor necrosis factor, which activate T lymphocytes as well as other macrophages.

The MPS system is a component of many organs. Specifically, these cells include splenic sinusoidal macrophages, hepatic Kupffer cells,[33] pulmonary alveolar macrophages,[34] bone osteoclasts,[35] pleural, peritoneal, and synovial macrophages, and microglial cells of the brain.[36,37]

As phagocytic cells, the ordinary tissue histiocytes have strong IgG Fc receptors, while tissue-based dendritic cells, which comprise the DCS, lack these strong receptors and are predominantly antigen-presenting cells.[30] The DCS consists of epidermal Langerhans cells,[38,46] which present antigen to T cells, and the paracortical or dendritic reticulum and interdigitating cells, which present antigen to B cells and T cells, respectively.[30,47] Thus LCH is a disorder of the DCS.

Hematopoietic differentiation is regulated by a family of glycoproteins termed colony-stimulating factors and ILS (see Ch. 16). A large family of these growth factors has been purified, cloned, and functionally characterized. Colony stimulating factor-granulocyte/macrophage (CSF-GM, IL-3 or multi-CSF, CSF-M, and CSF-G[48–51] exert a major influence on monocyte/macrophage differentiation.[48,52–54] CSF-GM and IL-3 have a broader range of activity, influencing differentiation of primitive as well as committed progenitors.[52,54] In addition, CSF-GM increases functional activity of mature granulocytes, eosinophils, and monocytes.[55–57] CSF-M and CSF-G, restricted in their activity, influence the discrete monocyte/macrophage and granulocyte pathways, respectively, as well as enhance granulocyte and monocyte/macrophage function.[58,59] Early work implicated T cells as a source of stimulating activity.[60] Since then, the monocyte/macrophage, the fibroblast, and other cells have also been shown to be involved in factor production.[61,62] In addition, the production of these factors by cells outside the bone marrow supports the finding that some factors have the dual functions of stimulating marrow progenitor differentiation and proliferation and of enhancing the function of mature myeloid cells.[63] Thus, there exists a complex regulatory network with activation by a wide variety of stimuli that control the proliferation and function of the MPS and the DCS as well as associated myeloid cells, whose presence characterizes the lesions of the histiocytic syndromes. The complexity of activation/inhibition, cellular transformation, proliferation, and phagocytosis, and the multitude of factors that modulate the DCS and MPS, contribute to the difficulty in understanding the histiocytic disorders described in this chapter. Since Nezelof et al.[41] first concluded that histiocytosis X was characterized by the proliferation of Langerhans cells, immunopathology, electron microscopy, and immunophenotyping have permitted an understanding of the pathobiology of what is now called LCH in the context of the developmental scheme described in Figure 56-1.

Johnston[29] summarizes the current state of knowledge when he says that the "term 'histiocyte' lacks precision", and ". . . has commonly been used to describe cells believed to be macrophages in fixed tissue preparations, but Langerhans cell histiocytosis (formerly called 'histiocytosis X') represents an . . . overgrowth of dendritic cells which are related to but different from macrophages." More strictly speaking, this histiocyte represents a "phenotypic transformation . . ." mediated by the "local tissue microenvironment,"[38] the progenitors of which arise from the bone marrow. In LCH the phenotype of this histiocyte may vary, reflecting a particular state of differentiation of a family of Langerhans-like cells not under the control of this tissue-specific microenvironment.[64]

CLINICAL MANIFESTATIONS

The signs and symptoms of LCH vary considerably depending on which organs are infiltrated by the Langerhans cells and other immunoreactive cells. Bone, skin, teeth, gingival tissue, ear, endocrine organs, lung, liver, spleen, lymph nodes, and bone marrow can all become involved and exhibit dysfunction secondary to cellular infiltration.[65] Although patients rarely fall into discrete categories defined by the classic designations of eosinophilic granuloma, Hand-Schüller-Christian disease, and Letterer-Siwe disease, this nomenclature remains valuable in order to catalog the clinical manifestations of LCH. In addition, these eponyms preserve the historical perspective of this enigmatic group of disorders.

The difficulty in diagnosis and the historically complex nomenclature have, as expected, made the true incidence and prevalence of these disorders difficult to ascertain.[38] Malone's[47] review reveals that most cases occur between 1 and 15 years of age.

SEG or MEG is found predominantly in older children, as well as in young adults, usually within the first three decades of life, the incidence peaking between 5 and 10 years of age.[66] SEG and MEG represent approximately 60–80% of all instances of histiocytosis.[66] Patients with systemic involvement frequently have similar bony lesions in addition to other manifestations of disease.[65] There is often an inability to bear weight, and a tender (sometimes warm) swelling due to tissue infiltrates overlying the bony lesions.[65,67] Radiographically, the lesions are sharply marginated, round, or oval, with a beveled edge that gives the appearance of depth.[65,68]

Hand-Schüller-Christian disease is described in younger children aged 2–5 years and represents 15–40% of patients.[66] Signs and symptoms include bony defects with exophthalmos due to tumor mass in the orbital cavity. This usually occurs from involvement of the roof and lateral wall of the orbital bones (although bony involvement is not necessary).[69] In addition, teeth are often lost due to gum infiltration and mandibular involvement. The most frequent sites of bony involvement are the flat bones of the skull, ribs, pelvis, and scapula.[65] There may be extensive involvement of the skull, with irregularly shaped lucent lesions, giving rise to the so-called geographic skull.[70] Somewhat less frequently, long bones and lumbosacral vertebral bones, usually the anterior portion of the vertebral body, are involved. In long bones, growth of lesions in the medullary cavity leads to pressure that may result in erosion through the cortex, stimulating the formation of periosteal new bone. A differential diagnosis, including Ewing and osteogenic sarcoma and osteomyelitis, must be considered in these instances. Only rarely are the wrists, hands, knees, feet, or cervical vertebrae involved.[65] Orbital involvement may result in vision loss or strabismus due to optic nerve or orbital muscle involvement, respectively. Oral involvement may begin in the gums or in the periapical regions of the teeth. Erosion of the lamina dura gives rise to the characteristic "floating tooth" seen on dental radiographs.[68] Erosion of gingival tissue causes premature eruption, decay, and tooth loss. Parents of affected children frequently report precocious eruption of teeth, when in fact, the gums are receding to expose immature dentition. The entire mandible may be involved, with loss of bone leading to diminished height of the mandibular rami.

Chronic otitis media, due to involvement of the mastoid and petrous portion of the temporal bone, and otitis externa are not uncommon. Fewer than one-third of children who ultimately develop diabetes insipious (DI) have polydypsia and polyuria as a presenting symptom of LCH.[71] Most children present within 4 years of diagnosis. DI affects 5–50% of patients with LCH.[71] Most occur in children who present with systemic disease and involvement of the orbit and skull.[71] DI is due to infiltration by Langerhans cells of the hypothalamus with or without involvement of the posterior pituitary gland.[72] Local tissue damage may be a consequence of IL-1 and prostaglandin E_2 production.[71] Polydipsia and polyuria may develop at presentation, during active disease (even when there is improvement in other areas), or after therapy is discontinued and there is no other active disease.

Short stature has been found in ≤40% of children with systemic LCH.[72] Chronic illness and steroid therapy play an important role in this phenomenon. Short stature has also been attributed to involvement of the anterior pituitary, but this theory has not been substantiated.[73,74] In fact, it is likely that growth hormone deficiency is not common in LCH, other than for those patients given substantial radiotherapy in the region of the anterior pituitary.[75] Other endocrine manifestations include hyperprolactinemia and hypogonadism due to hypothalamic infiltration.[73] Pancreatic and thyroid involvement have also been reported.[73,76]

Gastrointestinal tract disease has been identified[77–79] and is believed to be underestimated.[47] Intracranial lesions involving the cerebral hemispheres are rare.[80,81] Most intracranial lesions are extensions from the skull and do not penetrate the dura, although histiocytic infiltration of the leptomeninges has been described.[82]

The rarest (10% of cases) and most severe form of LCH is Letterer-Siwe disease.[66] Typically, an infant <2 years of age presents with a scaly seborrheic, eczematoid, sometimes purpuric rash involving the scalp, ear canals, abdomen, and intertriginous areas of the neck and face. The rash may be maculopapular or nodulopapular. Ulceration may result, especially in intertriginous areas. Ulcerated and denuded skin may serve as a portal of entry for microorganisms, leading to sepsis. Rarely, patients present with deep subcutaneous skin nodules only (Hashimoto-Pritzker syndrome).[38] Draining ears, lymphadenopathy, hepatosplenomegaly, and, in severe cases, hepatic dysfunction with hypoproteinemia and diminished synthesis of clotting factors can occur. Anorexia, irritability, failure to thrive, and significant pulmonary symptoms such as cough, tachypnea, and pneumothorax may occur as well. One of the most significant areas of involvement is that of the hematopoietic system; anemia and thrombocytopenia may manifest. The pathophysiology of hematopoietic dysfunction is not well understood, since an increase in bone marrow histiocytes and eosinophils is only occasionally noted, and significant marrow infiltrates are rare. Thrombocytopenia most frequently portends a fatal outcome.[21] Because of their physical appearance, these patients are frequently diagnosed as victims of abuse or neglect.

Three other presentations are seen. A nodal presentation, not to be confused with sinus histiocytosis showing massive lymphadenopathy, is characterized by massive enlargement of multiple lymph node groups, with little or no other signs of disease. In the pulmonary syndrome there is almost exclusive involvement of the lungs. This condition is usually seen in young adult men in their third or fourth decade (and occasionally in adolescents) and may follow an indolent, severe, and chronic debilitating course.[83] A relationship to cigarette smoking has been strongly suggested.[84] The pulmonary involvement in younger patients with systemic disease is frequently mild, although fulminant pulmonary disease may occur in this age group.[84,85] The chest radiograph may vary from a diffuse infiltrate consistent with bilateral interstitial pneumonia to a "honeycomb lung" appearance due to pulmonary fibrosis.[84,86] Finally, "pure" cutaneous disease with no evidence of dissemination has been described in children and adults.[87]

Thus, with such a vast spectrum of disease, adherence to strict labels such as Hand-Schüller-Christian or Letterer-Siwe disease cannot adequately describe a particular patient, and the development of the classification described above became necessary (Table 56-2).

NATURAL HISTORY AND PROGNOSIS

As originally proposed by Lahey,[27] the prognosis for patients with histiocytosis depends on three factors: age at onset, number of organs involved, and degree of dysfunction of specific organs. An adolescent or adult who presents with solitary bone eosinophilic granuloma has the best prognosis,[88] and an infant with multiple affected organs has the worst.[21–24,27,28] As already described, the classification allows us to discard the labels of eosinophilic granuloma, Hand-Schüller-Christian disease, Letterer-Siwe disease to group patients according to age at onset, localization, and severity of disease. Specifically, age >2 years is associated with a good prognosis, while patients <2 years tend to do more poorly (Table 56-3). When LCH presents at >65 years of age, regardless of site and extent of disease, the prognosis is usually poor.[47] Localized disease, with involvement of fewer than four organ systems, is a good prognostic sign (Table 56-4), and dysfunction of three organ systems (hepatic, pulmonary, and hematopoietic) is an extremely important adverse predictor of outcome (Table 56-3). In patients with multisystem disease, 20–30% enter sustained remission, and 10% die. The remaining 60–70% develop chronic disease.[47] Organ dysfunction, as described in Table 56-2, must be distinguished from involvement (e.g., hypoproteinemia, hyperbilirubinemia versus hepatomegaly), since involvement alone is not as adverse a prognostic sign as dysfunction. By arbitrarily assigning either 0 or 1 point for absence or presence of one of the three important prognostic variables, the grouping system described in Table 56-2 is defined. This classification is a reliable prognostic tool and also indicates which patients need systemic therapy. A review of 62 patients aged from birth to 14 years (median 18 months) confirms these observations, stressing the importance of two factors, age and localized disease. All but 1 of the 15 patients who died were <2 years of age at diagnosis. With regard to local involvement, the presence of bony involvement was a good prognostic sign, and skin involvement that was localized to the scalp predicted a considerably better outcome than generalized cutaneous involvement.[26]

PATHOLOGIC DIAGNOSIS

The typical histologic appearance of LCH varies with the age of the lesion examined. Early lesions are "cellular" and locally destructive, with a proliferation of essentially normal well-differentiated Langerhans cells.[47] Mitoses are usually not present.

Table 56-3. Survival Experience by Age and Organ Dysfunction

	Patients	Deaths	Median Survival (mo)	P Values for Survival
Age at diagnosis				
<2 yr	95	35	74+	0.002
>2 yr	56	9	147	
Organ dysfunction				
Present	59	27	43	0.002
Absent	92	17	145	

(From Komp et al.,[28] with permission.)

Table 56-4. Organ System Involvement as a Prognostic Indicator

Organ Systems Involved	Patients	Response to Therapy (CR + PR)[a]	Dead
1–2	13	8	0
3–4	20	15	4
5–6	22	12	9
7+	18	7	11

[a] Complete (CR) plus partial (PR) response.
(From Lahey,[27] with permission.)

Table 56-5. Criteria of the Writing Group of the Histiocyte Society (1987) for the Diagnosis of Langerhans Cell Histiocytosis (Formerly Histiocytosis X)

I	Presumptive diagnosis: study of conventionally stained biopsy material with findings that are "consistent" with those defined in the literature.
II	Diagnosis: an increased degree of diagnostic confidence with presumptive diagnosis plus presence of two or more features: positive stain for ATPase, S-100 protein, α-mannosidase, or peanut lectin.
III	Definitive diagnosis: requires the demonstration of Birbeck granules by electron microscopy or CD1 antigenic determinants (T6 positivity) on cryostat sections in the context of presumptive diagnosis or diagnosis.

(From Hall et al.,[94] with permission.)

When they are present, they are of no prognostic significance.[89] Multinucleated histiocytes are often present. Other inflammatory cells, such as granulocytes, eosinophils, macrophages, and occasionally lymphocytes and plasma cells, are present. The giant cells and macrophages may be phagocytic, but Langerhans cells are not.[89] With time the cells may accumulate cholesterol. The Langerhans cell is usually prominent in the histology of histiocytic lesions.[46] Occasionally there is necrosis, with only rare Langerhans cells, and as lesions mature there are fewer, and in some cases no, Langerhans cells. The pathologic diagnosis of histiocytosis is made on the basis of a biopsy demonstrating the characteristic histopathology.[44,89–92] The Langerhans cell is 15–25 μm in diameter, with a "central to slightly eccentric ovoid to uniform-shaped nucleus with a delicate chromatin network and inconspicuous nucleoli. An indentation or groove across the face of the nucleus is a feature of many cells."[90] The pathologic criteria for the diagnosis of LCH (Table 56-5) have recently been established.[47,89,93,94] The differential diagnosis of LCH is limited, and depends on the clinical presentation. It includes immunodeficiency syndromes with graft-versus-host disease, viral infections, infiltrative diseases such as leukemia or lymphoma, reticuloendothelial storage diseases, congenital infections, benign and malignant bone tumors and cysts, and papular xanthomas.

A careful evaluation of biopsy material will generally result in a diagnosis. However, one of the serious dilemmas in the evaluation of the histiocytic syndromes is that the histopathology of lesions from patients with single-site eosinophilic granuloma (group 0) is similar, if not identical, to that of Letterer-Siwe disease (groups III or IV).[65,91] Although patients are grouped in large part on extent of disease, untreated patients will not necessarily progress to a higher stage, as occurs with lymphoma patients. In fact, progression from a limited syndrome to diffuse systemic disease is virtually unheard of.[65] Within a few months after presentation it will become apparent that the bony lesions seen initially are limited to the skeleton or were the "heralding lesion(s)" of diffuse systemic involvement.[88] When cutaneous involvement is the only obvious presenting sign, 6–12 months may be required to determine the ultimate extent of disease.[65]

Newton and Hamoudi[92] have classified the histopathology of what is now termed LCH into types I and II in an attempt to distinguish an unfavorable from a favorable lesion, respectively. Type I histology is characterized by Langerhans cells that are noncohesive and that frequently occur as single cells. Nuclei of these cells contain basophilic clumped chromatin. Multinucleated giant cells, eosinophils, and necrosis are not prominent features of these lesions. Type II, or favorable histology, is characterized by Langerhans cells that orient themselves in cohesive, syncytial sheets with indistinct cell margins. These sheets are associated with eosinophils, lymphocytes, and neutrophils. Giant cells are prominent, and necrosis is often present. However, Favara[43] states that the histopathol-

ogy of skin lesions does not appear to correlate with prognosis. Thus, the association of histologic type with clinical outcome is controversial and not widely accepted. Methods of determining clonality may ultimately prove to be of greater prognostic value.[9,10] Additional diagnostic criteria beyond standard histopathology include immunochemical staining with ATPase, S-100 protein, α-mannosidase, peanut lectin, vimentin, and other markers.[64,89,94] These markers are quite sensitive, but less specific, and need to be evaluated in the context of histology. The definitive diagnosis requires the identification by electron microscopy of Langerhans cells based on the presence of Langerhans granules, also known as X bodies[41] or Birbeck granules,[42] as well as the presence of cell surface CD1. The immunophenotype of Langerhans cells has recently been established in some detail[47,64,89,94] (Table 56-6). It appears three distinct immunophenotypes of LCH exist, corresponding to the spectrum of differentiation, including Langerhans cells, interdigitating dendritic cells, and dendritic reticulum cells.[64] A variety of other antigens are being evaluated as new monoclonal reagents become available, and diagnostic guidelines may change with the availability of these probes.[47] Unfortunately, as with histopathology, the heterogeneity in immunophenotypes cannot be correlated with the clinical course or severity of disease. Considerable effort is currently being directed at understanding the role of the Langerhans cell in the pathophysiology of the histiocytosis syndromes.

THERAPY

The philosophy for treatment of LCH is to use the minimal amount of the least toxic therapy to control the disease. In patients with extremely morbid or life-threatening disease at presentation, or in those developing morbid or life-threatening disease during the course of treatment, more aggressive therapy should be considered. The primary caretaker should coordinate the care of these patients. Subspeciality consultation should be sought from dermatologists, dentists, orthopaedists, otolaryngologists, endocrinologists, and others experienced in managing histiocytosis. The goal of therapy for most patients must be to minimize loss of function and prevent cosmetic deformity.

Severely ill patients are hospitalized and given antibiotic, ventilatory, nutritional (including hyperalimentation), blood product, skin care, physical therapy, medical, and nursing support as required in addition to definitive treatment. Scrupulous hygeine is quite effective in limiting auditory canal, cutaneous, and dental lesions. Debridement, and even resection of severely affected gingival tissue, is used to limit oral involvement. The seborrhea-like dermatitis of the scalp may improve with the use of a selenium-based shampoo twice a week. Topical steroids are occasionally effective but should be used sparingly and only for short-term control of small areas. We do not advocate the use of topical nitrogen mustard lotion, as suggested by some authors.[95]

Surgery and Radiotherapy

After complete evaluation, those patients with disease involving a single bone and (in some cases) patients with disease involving multiple lesions and multiple bones are managed with local therapy. This involves surgical curettage for patients whose lesions are in easily accessible noncritical locations. Complete "cancer operation" resections are not necessary.

Table 56-6. Staining Characteristics of Histiocytes

	Mononuclear/Phagocyte System	Dendritic Cell System		
		LC	IDC	DRC
Enzyme histochemistry				
Frozen section				
Nonspecific esterase	+	−	−	−
Acid phosphatase	+	−	−	−
ATPase	−	+	+	−
5′ Nucleotidase	−	−	−	+
α-Mannosidase	−	+	−	−
Immunocytochemistry				
Paraffin section				
HLA-DR	+	+	+	+
KP-1 and KiM6 (CD68)	+	−	−	−
Mac-387	+	−	−	−
Lysozyme	+	−	−	−
α₁-antitrypsin	+	−	−	−
α₁-antichymotrypsin	+	−	−	−
S-100 protein	−	+	+	−
Peanut agglutinin	Diffuse	Halo + dot	Halo + dot	−
Frozen section				
CD14 (Leu M3/MY4)	+	+	+	+
CD11c (Leu M5)	+	+	+	+
CD68 (EBM11)	+	+	−	−
CD1	−	+	+	−
CD4	−	LCH only	−	−

Abbreviations: LC, Langerhans cell; IDC, interdigitating dendritic cell; DRC, dendritic reticulum cell; LCH, Langerhans cell histiocyte.
(Modified from Malone,[47] with permission.)

Surgical restraint must be exercised to avoid drastic cosmetic and orthopaedic deformities and loss of function. Localized radiotherapy (usually 600–900 cGy, with 450 cGy for small lesions and ≤1,500 cGy for large lesions) in 200-cGy fractions, utilizing only megavoltage equipment, is currently employed. Older patients may require slightly higher doses (2,000 cGy for large lesions). Structures such as the lens of the eye and the thyroid gland should be spared if at all possible. Patients at risk of skeletal deformity, visual loss secondary to exophthalmus, pathologic fractures, vertebral collapse, and spinal cord injury should receive radiotherapy. Those patients suffering from severe pain or symptomatic adenopathy, even when multiple lesions exist, should also receive radiotherapy to affected areas, if systemic therapy is not rapidly effective. Lesions in poorly accessible sites, such as the orbit or lesions recurring after curettage, should also be irradiated.[96,97] DI may occur at any time during the course of histiocytosis. Patients should be instructed to report signs of DI as soon as they develop, since dehydration and electrolyte imbalance may be quite serious. The results of hypothalamic and pituitary radiotherapy instituted early in the course of DI have been mixed, and the use of this modality is controversial.[97–99]

A review of 40 patients receiving radiotherapy between 1970 and 1984 indicates that patients with unifocal disease have a higher rate of response for individual lesions than patients with multifocal disease (two or more soft tissue sites). Thus, patients who appear to have an isolated lesion that do not respond to appropriate radiotherapy should be carefully re-evaluated for additional sites of disease. In this review, the complete plus partial response rate for bone lesions was 100% (35 of 35), with 24 complete responses. Soft tissue lesions adjacent to involved bone healed better than isolated soft tissue lesions. There was no response to irradiation for liver, spleen or lung lesions, and none of eight patients with DI responded.[98]

Chemotherapy

Historically, drugs used in the therapy of classic malignant diseases have been used systemically for LCH. Nitrogen mustard, chlorambucil, cyclophosphamide, steroids, procarbazine, methotrexate, vincristine, and vinblastine have been used singly or in combination, with variable success. Response to chemotherapy varies from 25% to 90%. An early study did show that treatment improves survival in patients <2 years of age (Table 56-7). Table 56-8 summarizes selected "best" controlled chemotherapeutic trials involving well-characterized patients.[100–110] Our current therapeutic approach to systemic therapy is to observe patients in group I (and some in group II) who respond to local (surgical, radiation) or nonsystemic therapy (i.e., topical steroids) and look for signs of spontaneous improvement. If there are symptomatic lesions or signs of failure to thrive, treatment should be pursued. The erythrocyte sedimentation rate is sometimes a useful indicator of disease activity. Patients in group III will benefit dramatically from chemotherapy, while there are poor responses and death in many group IV patients. A variety of experimental modalities, such as hemibody irradiation,[111] thymic hormone therapy,[8,112] and interferon-α have been explored at some centers for advanced or refractory disease. Currently the best results have been obtained with bone marrow transplantation[113–115] and Cy-

Table 56-7. Treatment[a] Versus No Treatment[b]

Patients	Treatment	Dead	Alive	Mean Age (mo)
27	No	27	0	10.5
64	Yes	40	24	15.0

[a] Variable chemotherapy (steroids, antimetabolites, and alkylating agents).
[b] Supportive care.
(Data from Lahey.[22])

Table 56-8. Comparison of Selected Chemotherapy Trials for Langerhans Cell Histiocytosis

Drug(s)[a]		Study Group		Patients	Response (CR + PR)
Single agents					
Vincristine	(VCR)	SWCCG	1972	6	50
Vinblastine	(VBL)	SWCCG	1972	20	55
	VBL	CCSG	1975	18	56
	VBL	Mayo	1980	18	77
Cyclophosphamide	(CTX)	SWCCG	1972	22	63
Procarbazine	(PCB)	SWOG	1974	10	50
Chlorambucil	(CMB)	SWOG	1980	32	56
	CMB	CCSG	1980	26	27
Etoposide	(VP-16)	Italy	1988	18	83
	VP-16	AIEOP (Italy)	1993	27	70
Combination therapy					
Methotrexate + prednisone	(MTX)				
	(PRED)	ALGB	1974	17	53
	VCR + PRED	ALGB	1974	11	64
	VBL + PRED	CCSG	1975	18	67
6-Mercaptopurine	(6MP) + PRED	CCSG	1975	25	48
	CTX + VCR + PRED + PCB	SWOG	1977	21	38
	CTX + VBL + PRED	SWOG	1977	25	25 <1 yr
					88 >1 yr
	MTX + CMB + VBL + PRED	Mexico	1988	68	75

Abbreviations: CR, complete response; PR, partial response in which there is resolution of >50% of the lesions.

[a] Pre-1972: anecdotal responses reported with antibiotics, corticosteroids, vincristine, vinblastine, methotrexate, cyclophosphamide, nitrogen mustard; 6-mercaptopurine, daunorubicin.

(Data from references 101–111.)

closporine A.[116] These therapies should be conducted in the context of controlled clinical trials.

The basic principle of systemic therapy is to begin with the most benign treatment and then add increasingly toxic agents, never making the treatment worse than the disease, while trying to prevent permanent disability. Table 56-9 outlines our current chemotherapeutic program. Adults seem to do better on the methotrexate, 6-mercaptopurine program, and we currently suggest starting with that regime in older patients.

Careful monitoring of blood counts and clinical status is important, since chemotherapeutic toxicity may cause severe complications in these already compromised patients. In the case of failure of both program I (vinblastine, prednisone) and program II (methotrexate, 6-mercaptopurine), individualized treatment plans are devised depending on the severity of disease. Recent results with etoposide in refractory patients warrant consideration of this agent.[109,110] An ongoing randomized trial essentially comparing etoposide with vinblastine should be helpful; however, reports of leukemia following etoposide treatment for LCH are worrisome. Alkylating agents, chlorambucil in particular, should be avoided due to the substantial risk of chemotherapy-induced malignancy. Group IV disease remains difficult to cure.

LONG-TERM FOLLOW-UP

Of 127 patients with histiocytosis reported by Greenberger and colleagues,[24] 84 received chemotherapy, and 6 developed late malignancies. Two patients who received radiotherapy developed an in-field tumor, and one received no chemotherapy. Table 56-10 briefly describes those patients. Late malignancy developed in 5 of 54 patients who received chlorambucil as a single agent or in combination and in 2 of 29 patients given nitrogen mustard as part of combination therapy, including chlorambucil, vincristine, procarbazine, and prednisone. The

risk of malignancy is similar to that reported following chlorambucil for the treatment of polycythemia vera. Thus, the judicious use of radiotherapy, significantly reduced chemotherapy, and good supportive care are highly recommended as a treatment philosophy. While patients with LCH could have an inherently increased risk of subsequent malignancy, the experience cited suggests an excess of malignancy associated with chlorambucil use. Also, the relatively poor outcome with this drug (Table 56-8) argues against its use in this disease.

Early reports of leukemia in LCH patients treated with etoposide as a single agent are appearing.[110,117] Depending on the true incidence, the use of this drug as a frontline agent in LCH may be precluded. Other sequelae of histiocytosis, such as chemotherapy-induced hepatic disease and growth retardation, may also be greatly reduced by a conservative treatment philosophy. A poorly characterized late occurring syndrome of severe cerebellar ataxia has been described in LCH patients treated with a variety of agents.[117] This may also be a consequence of therapy—a further justification for restraint. Better radiotherapy techniques, as described earlier, should reduce the incidence of in-field tumors.

All patients with systemic LCH should receive long-term follow-up. In addition to late malignancies, patients should be monitored for signs of long-term disabilities, including cosmetic and functional orthopaedic and cutaneous deformities that may lead to severe emotional disorders. Hearing impairment, loss of permanent dentition, pulmonary fibrosis, cor pulmonale, portal hypertension, cirrhosis, growth failure, and endocrinologic disorders, must all be carefully followed.

SINUS HISTIOCYTOSIS WITH MASSIVE LYMPHADENOPATHY

First described in 1969 and more recently reviewed by Rosai and Dorfman in 1990,[118,119] SHML is characterized clinically as a benign, frequently chronic, painless massive lymphadenopa-

Table 56-9. Current Mount Sinai School of Medicine Chemotherapeutic Treatment Program for Langerhans Cell Histiocytosis

Program I

1. Vinblastine (0.15 mg/kg/wk IV as a single weekly dose): If the patient is not improved after 2 weeks, increase the dose by 0.025–0.05 mg/kg/wk. The highest nonmyelosuppressive nonneurotoxic dose is used. In addition, if there is no or slow improvement, or if a more rapid response is required add:

2. Prednisone (2 mg/kg/day PO): With improvement taper to the smallest effective dose on an alternate-day schedule. With continued improvement or satisfactory control, a slow taper of prednisone is undertaken, but prednisone should be discontinued prior to the vinblastine taper. Vinblastine is tapered from weekly to every other week to every 3 or 4 weeks, and then the dosage is reduced to 0.15 mg/kg every 4 weeks prior to discontinuation. Reinstate lowest effective dose for disease rebound.

Program II—(if program I fails)

Methotrexate (10 mg/m² /wk IM, IV, or PO) and 6-mercaptopurine (6MP) (20 mg/m² /day PO) for 14 days of 21-day cycle. The highest nontoxic dose is used (toxicity: myelosuppression, mouth sores, hepatotoxicity). On improvement both drugs are slowly tapered. Mexthotrexate is tapered from weekly to every other week, to every 3 weeks. Oral therapy may be instituted. The 6MP schedule is maintained while the dose is reduced 10–15%/cycle. Reinstitute lowest effective dose for disease rebound.

thy usually involving cervical lymph nodes and (less frequently) axillary, hilar, peritracheal, and inguinal nodes.[120] Extranodal disease is present in 28% of patients.[121] The upper respiratory mucosa is involved in 20%,[118] bone in 25%,[122,123] and orbit or eyelid in 10% of patients.[124,125] Occasionally there is skin involvement,[126] as well as central nervous system, lung, liver, and kidney involvement.[119]

Although SHML is benign, significant morbidity and even death have been associated with massive tissue invasion of the liver, kidney, lung, and other critical structures.[119,127] In these instances the disease has a rapid downhill course.[38] Respiratory distress due to tracheal obstruction,[128] as well as paraplegia secondary to epidural involvement, is described.[129] Death in SHML has occurred as a consequence of severe hemolytic anemia.[127]

Eighty percent of patients are diagnosed in their first or second decade,[130,132] but the disorder can also affect the elderly.[128,132] Typically, patients are of African descent.[130,131] Males and females are equally affected.[47] Worldwide, the incidence of SHMC is greatest in Africa and the West Indies.[131]

Laboratory evaluation frequently reveals an elevated erythrocyte sedimentation rate, moderate polyclonal and (rarely) benign monoclonal hypergammaglobulinemia, anemia, and granulocytosis.[126,128]

Involved lymph nodes show marked sinusoidal dilation and follicular hyperplasia with proliferation of foamy histiocytes and multinucleated giant cells within the sinuses. There are no eosinophils, and abundant plasma cells are present.[118,120–122] Lymphocytes are often found in the cytoplasm of "histiocyte-

like" cells. This characteristic finding is referred to as emperipolesis.[128] The proliferating "histiocytes" share properties of histiocytes and interdigitating cells. These large pale cells are S-100 positive[133] but are morphologically distinguished from Langerhans cells found in the lymph nodes of patients with classic LCH by the absence of Langerhans granules[122] as well as by surface phenotype determined by monoclonal antibodies[126,134] and by the presence of α_1-antichymotrypsin.[128]

As with LCH, the etiology of this disorder is unknown; as in LCH, disordered immune regulation has been proposed.[126] It was originally thought that SHML represented an unusual response to a *Klebsiella* antigen or Epstein-Barr virus,[132] but recent studies do not support this contention.[126] Although patients are frequently febrile, infectious agents have not been implicated, and the fever is presumed to be a manifestation of systemic disease.

Treatment is usually both unnecessary and ineffective. Disease manifestations subside over several months to years. Of 215 cases in a patient registry, 21% had complete resolution of disease. However, 14 patients died. Five died from "immunologic" causes, such as severe hemolysis, three died from infections, and six probably died as a direct consequence of disease infiltration.[135] As the disease resolves, extranodal disease regresses prior to nodal disease. Radiation, corticosteroids, vinblastine, and low-dose cyclophosphamide are sometimes effective; however, the results with these agents have been inconsistent.[121,129,136,137] Attempts at treatment should be reserved for special circumstances, such as tracheal or epidural compression. Local excision may also be useful in selected patients.[122]

FAMILIAL HEMATOPHAGOCYTIC LYMPHOHISTIOCYTOSIS

FHL (formerly known as familial erythrophagocytic lymphohistiocytosis), is a rapidly fatal, inherited disorder characterized by peripheral pancytopenia with bone marrow hyperplasia, systemic lymphadenopathy, intermittent fevers, and severe liver dysfunction characterized by hepatosplenomegaly and increased serum enzymes.[138,139] Patients have a characteristic severe hypofibrinogenemia not attributable to disseminated intravascular coagulation, since plasma levels of all other clotting factors are normal, and no evidence of fibrinolysis is observed.[140] Hypertriglyceridemia is characteristic. Most affected children are infants (aged 2 weeks to 7 years), and two-thirds of them present within the first 3 months of life.[141] Patients usually present with pallor, irritability, anorexia, diarrhea, and failure to thrive. Occasionally there is a nonspecific, sometimes "sunburnt" appearing or maculopapular skin rash.[138,141] Pulmonary effusions are present in one-third of patients. The clinical course is usually progressive, lasting only an average of 6 weeks.[141] Most patients die as a consequence

Table 56-10. Late Malignancy Following Treatment of Langerhans Cell Histiocytosis

Patients	Treatment	Malignancy	Interval Between Histiocytosis and Malignancy (yr)
1	CMB	Hepatocellular carcinoma	14
2	CMB + RT	Thyroid carcinoma	16
3	CMB (CT) + RT	Acute leukemia	2
4	CMB, NM (CT) + RT	Acute leukemia	6.5
5	CMB, NM (CT) + RT	Acute leukemia	5
6	RT	Thyroid carcinoma	28

Abbreviations: CMB, chlorambucil; RT, radiotherapy; CT, combination therapy; NM, nitrogen mustard.

THERAPY FOR LANGERHANS CELL HISTIOCYTOSIS

Philosophy

The optimal management for the patient with LCH is one that balances therapeutic intervention (to minimize short- and long-term disease-related morbidities) with a relative therapeutic nihilism in order to reduce treatment-associated morbidity. One of the main goals of therapy is to prevent loss of function and minimize cosmetic deformity. Efforts should be made to identify and find effective therapy for those patients who disease is unlikely to respond to conservative management. The agents used should be thought of as immunosuppressive rather than antineoplastic. Patients are treated to obtain disease control, followed by tapering of drug doses to achieve the lowest dose that maintains control. Many patients will have recurrences but eventually almost all patients who respond will be able to discontinue treatment completely. However systemic treatment lasting in the range of 5 years is not uncommon and late recurrences do occur.

Prognostic Grouping

When patients are grouped using three prognostic variables—age, extent of disease, and presence of organ dysfunction—the prognosis, need for, and extent of treatment can be evaluated. By assigning either 0 to 1 point for the absence or presence of one of the three important prognostic variables, a patient may have from 0 points (group I) to 3 points (group IV) (Table 56-2). Patients in groups 0 and I and some in group II do quite well, with little morbidity and no mortality. They frequently need little or no systemic therapy. Patients in group III (and many in group II) require systemic therapy and generally do well, while significant morbidity and mortality are encountered in group IV patients. Group IV patients should have HLA typing and be considered for bone marrow transplantation, if a donor exists, or for cyclosporine or other experimental immunosuppressive therapy.

Supportive Care

Severely ill patients are hospitalized and given antibiotic, ventilatory, nutritional (including hyperalimentation), blood product, skin care, physical therapy, medical, and nursing support as required. Scrupulous hygiene is quite effective in limiting auditory canal, cutaneous, and dental lesions. Debridement, and even resection of severely affected gingival tissue, is used to limit oral involvement. The seborrhea-like dermatitis of the scalp may improve with the use of a selenium-based shampoo twice a week. If shampooing is not effective, topical steroids are used sparingly for short-term control of small areas. We do not advocate the use of topical nitrogen mustard lotion. Many patients require hormone replacement for DI or other manifestations of hypopituitarism.

Local Therapy (Surgery and Radiotherapy)

After complete evaluation, those patients with disease involving a single bone, and in some instances patients with disease involving multiple lesions and multiple bones, are managed with local therapy. This involves surgical curettage for patients whose lesions are in easily accessible, noncritical locations. Surgical restraint must be exercised to prevent drastic cosmetic and orthopaedic deformities and loss of function. Localized radiotherapy (usually 600–900 cGy, with 450 cGy for small lesions and $\leq$1,500 cGy for large lesions) in 200-cGy fractions, utilizing only megavoltage equipment, is employed. Older patients may require slightly higher doses (2,000 cGy for large lesions). Since individual lesions in patients with unifocal disease have a higher rate of response than those in patients with multifocal disease, patients who appear to have an isolated lesion and fail to respond to appropriate radiotherapy should be carefully re-evaluated for additional sites of disease.

Chemotherapy

Patients in group I and some in group II can be observed for signs of spontaneous improvement. If symptomatic lesions or failure to thrive are evident, treatment should be pursued. Patients in groups II and III will benefit dramatically from chemotherapy, while those in group IV will frequently die despite chemotherapy. Experimental modalities such as bone marrow transplantation are being pursued at specialized centers for group IV patients who are nonresponsive to conventional chemotherapy.

The basic principle for systemic therapy is to begin with the most benign treatment and then add increasingly toxic agents, never making the treatment worse than the disease, while trying to prevent permanent disability. Table 56-9 outlines our current chemotherapeutic treatment program. Other agents, including etoposide and cyclosporine in particular, are in use in ongoing clinical studies. We currently individualize therapy in those patients whose disease does not respond to programs I and II. Bactrim prophylaxis in patients for whom long-term immunosuppressive therapy is anticipated should be instituted.

Long-Term Follow-Up

All patients with systemic LCH should receive long-term follow-up. Patients are monitored for potential chronic disabilities such as cosmetic or functional orthopaedic and cutaneous disorders, neurotoxicity, and emotional problems that may arise from the disease or treatment. Patients having, or at risk of, hearing impairment, loss of permanent dentition, pulmonary fibrosis, cor pulmonale, portal hypertension, cirrhosis, DI, growth failure, and other endocrinologic disorders are followed closely by appropriate subspecialists.

of sepsis, bleeding, or a lymphocytic meningitis accompanied by refractory seizures. Approximately one-third of patients have central nervous system involvement.[141] Disease essentially confined to the central nervous system, leading to seizures, has been reported.[142] There is no sex predilection,[141] and the presence of the disorder in siblings and in cousins,[141] as well as the presence of parental consanguinity,[140] supports an autosomal recessive mode of inheritance.

There are no specific biologic markers of FHL, but laboratory evaluation consistently demonstrates hypofibrinogenemia, hyperlipidemia,[143] pancytopenia, hyperbilirubinemia, and increased serum liver enzymes.[138]

Pathology of the liver shows focal fatty changes, necrosis, and infiltration by lymphocytes and histiocytes. The infiltrate is periportal but extends into adjacent lobules. Erythrophagocytosis and hematophagocytosis are prominent and essential to the diagnosis. The spleen demonstrates similar focal necrosis and foci of lymphocytes and histiocytes with erythrophagocytosis. Involvement of the thymus and lymph nodes is similar, but later in the course of disease lymph nodes show significant lymphocytic depletion. Hematophagocytosis is also present. The lungs are infiltrated with lymphocytes and histiocytes, again with some erythrophagocytosis. The bone marrow is hyperplastic with increased numbers of hematophagocytic histiocytes.[138,141,144] The cellular infiltrate lacks features of malignant cells. The characteristic pathology and clinical presentation clearly distinguishes FHL from LCH and MH. However, FHL may be difficult to distinguish histopathologically from the so-called infection-associated hemophagocytic syndrome (IAHS), which was originally described in immunocompromised hosts as a consequence of an underlying viral infection[145] as well as bacterial and protozoal infections.[146,147] The clinical course of IAHS is variable, but a 40% mortality has been reported.[145] IAHS in the absence of an underlying immunodeficiency is difficult to distinguish from FHL.[147] Excellent diagnostic guidelines for the diagnosis of FHL have recently been published.[148] These diagnostic criteria should help remove doubt in the diagnosis of this confusing disorder.

Although the etiology remains obscure, immunodeficiency is a consistent finding in FHL. A recent report presents strong evidence that the disease is mediated by hypercytokinemia with elevated levels of interferon-γ, tumor necrosis factor, and in some instances IL-6.[149] The authors propose a genetic defect in cytokine regulation. There is depressed antigen-induced lymphocyte proliferation and decreased monocyte antibody-dependent cytotoxicity.[150] Removal of plasma by plasma exchange transiently corrects these abnormalities but does not improve prognosis.[128] Whether the disorder is due to a primary immunodeficiency, or whether the immune abnormalities are secondary to another underlying defect, is currently unknown.

Steroids and cytotoxic agents have generally been ineffective in the treatment of FHL. Etoposide has induced clinical remissions accompanied by resolution of the characteristic hyperlipidemia.[151] Although virtually all patients relapse, this agent may prove to be useful prior to more definitive therapy with bone marrow transplantation.[152]

MALIGNANT HISTIOCYTOSIS

MH differs from LCH, SHML, IAHS, and FHL in that, of this group, it is the only true malignant neoplasm. The pathology and clinical presentations of these disorders are not entirely distinct,[141] occasionally leading to confusion in diagnosis. The ubiquitous nature of the histiocyte and the lack of specific clinical or laboratory findings make careful analysis of tissue (using standard and immunologic techniques as well as electron microscopy) frequently necessary.

First described as histiocytic medullary reticulosis by Scott and Robb-Smith[153] in 1939, MH is characterized by fever, wasting, lymphadenopathy, abdominal pain, hepatosplenomegaly, progressive pancytopenia, disseminated intravascular coagulation, and the proliferation of atypical mature histiocytes[154,155] and their precursors.[156] The lymphadenopathy is most often supraclavicular and axillary. The adenopathy is frequently painful. Mediastinal, periaortic, and iliac lymphadenopathy are less common. In childhood, cutaneous lesions are characteristic, usually occurring as inflammatory nodules in the anterior chest wall. Yellow or red-purple, pruritic maculopapular or micronodular rashes are also reported. Pleural effusions, interstitial pulmonary infiltrates, and bone lesions are also described.[157]

Most patients are adults, with a male/female sex ratio of 2:1. In childhood, the disease is less common, and there is no sex predilection.[157]

Laboratory abnormalities are nonspecific and include hyperbilirubinemia, hypocholesterolemia, a positive Coombs test, leukocytosis or leukopenia, thrombocytopenia, and elevated lactate dehydrogenase. Abnormal circulating histiocytes can be seen in many cases.[157]

As stated, the histiocytic disorders previously described should not present difficulty in terms of a differential diagnosis. However, MH must be distinguished from lymphoma, in particular stage IV Hodgkin disease or diffuse "true histiocytic" lymphoma.

Lymph node pathology shows distortion of normal architecture with a diffuse infiltrate of pleomorphic, atypical naphthyl-ASD-acetate esterase-positive histiocytes. Sinusoidal patterns are partially maintained, and uninvolved residual lymphoid follicles are observed. Pericapsular soft tissue extension is occasionally present. There are frequent mitoses, and erythrophagocytosis is prominent. The atypical histiocytes have thick nuclear membranes, nuclei containing irregularly clumped chromatin, and irregular nucleoli with jagged borders. The atypical histiocytes, which may be multinucleated, are frequently S-100 positive, especially in children. Lysozyme and α1-antitrypsin staining is positive in some patients.[154,158,159] The concanavalin A receptor is found consistently. Thus, two immunophenotypes of MH may exist, perhaps distinguishing adult and pediatric cases. Bizarre giant cells resembling Reed-Sternberg cells may be present. In the liver, atypical histiocyte proliferation is found in portal and sinusoidal areas. In the spleen, the red pulp is frequently involved, and involvement may extend to the white pulp. Well-defined tumor nodules are rare in both the liver and spleen.[154] In skin lesions, normal as well as atypical histiocytes are present, with focal areas of necrosis and inflammation; erythrophagocytosis is rare.[155] Examination of the bone marrow may reveal atypical histiocytes with erythrophagocytosis.

The diagnosis of MH may be greatly facilitated in the future by the recent observation of a t(2;5)(p23;q35) translocation in the malignant histiocytes. It is of great interest that the CSF-M gene is located at 5q33 and that its receptor is coded for by the c-fms proto-oncogene assigned to 5q33-q34.[158]

Recent studies indicate that MH may be successfully treated in both children and adults with combination chemotherapy.[157,160–163] Most successful programs include doxorubicin. Although the numbers are not great, 5-year actuarial survival in the range of 40% can reasonably be expected.[160]

REFERENCES

1. Gotoff SP, Esterley NB: Histiocytosis. J Pediatr 85:592, 1974
2. Groopman JE, Golde DW: The histiocytic disorders: a pathophysiologic analysis. Ann Intern Med 94:95, 1981

3. Komp DM, Perry MC: Introduction: the histiocytic syndromes. Semin Oncol 18:1, 1991
4. Komp DM: Langerhans cell histiocytosis. N Engl J Med 316:747, 1987
5. Broadbent V, Davies EG, Heaf D et al: Spontaneous remission of multi-system histiocytosis X. Lancet 1:253, 1984
6. Rabkin MS, Wittwer CT, Kjeldsberg CR, Piepkorn MW: Flow-cytometric DNA content of histiocytosis X (Langerhans cell histiocytosis). Am J Pathol 131: 283, 1988
7. Vawter GF: Does Letterer-Siwe disease exist?: or, who's not afraid of infantile histiocytosis? p. 165. In Vuksanovic MM (ed): Clinical Pediatric Oncology: Research, Diagnosis, Treatment, and Prognosis of Malignant Tumors. Futura, Mt. Kisco, NY, 1972
8. Osband ME, Lipton JM, Lavin PL et al: Histiocytosis X. Demonstration of abnormal immunity, T-cell histamine H_2-receptor deficiency, and successful treatment with thymic extract. N Engl J Med 304:146, 1981
9. Willman CL, McClain KL, Griffith BB et al: Langerhans cell histiocytosis (LCH): a spectrum of clonal neoplastic and polyclonal reactive disorders. Meeting program, Histiocyte Society Ninth Annual Meeting, 1993
10. Kannourakis G, Tiong T: Studies on the clonality of FACS sorted CD 1a cells in Langerhans cell histiocytosis, using an X-linked polymorphic PCR method. Meeting Program, Histiocyte Society Ninth Annual Meeting, 1993
11. Otani S, Ehrlich JC: Solitary granuloma of bone simulating primary neoplasm. Am J Pathol 16:479, 1940
12. Lichtenstein L, Jaffe HL. Eosinophilic granuloma of bone. Am J Pathol 16: 595, 1940
13. Hand A: Polyuria and tuberculosis. Arch Pediatr 10:673, 1893
14. Schüller A: Uber Eingenartige Schadel defekte im Jugendalter. Fortschr Roentgenstr 23:12, 1915–1916
15. Christian HA: Defects in membranous bones, exophthalmos and diabetes insipidus, an unusual syndrome of dyspituitarism: a clinical study. Med Clin North Am 3:849, 1920
16. Hand A: Defects of membranous bones, exophthalmos and polyuria in childhood: is it dyspituitarism? Am J Med Sci 162:509, 1921
17. Letterer E: Aleukaemische Retikulose (ein Beitrag zu den proliferativen Erkrankungen des retikulo-endothelialen Panates) Frankfurt Z Pathol 30:377, 1924
18. Siwe SA: Die Reticuloendotheliose ein neives Krankheitschield unter den Hepatosplanomegalien. A Kinderheilk 55:212, 1933
19. Cheyne C: Histiocytosis X. J. Bone Joint Surg. 53B:366, 1971
20. Neumann C, Kolde G, Bonsmann G: Histiocytosis X in an elderly patient: ultrastructure and immunocytochemistry after PUVA photochemotherapy. Br J Dermatol 119:385, 1988
21. Lahey ME: Prognosis in reticuloendotheliosis in children. J Pediatr 60:664, 1962
22. Smith PJ, Ekert H, Campbell PE: Improved prognosis in disseminated histiocytosis. Med Pediatr Oncol 2:371, 1976
23. Nezelof C, Frileux-Herbet F, Cronier-Sachot J: Disseminated histiocytosis X. Analysis of prognostic factors based on a retrospective study of 50 cases. Cancer 44:1824, 1979
24. Greenberger JS, Crocker AC, Vawter G et al: Results of treatment of 127 patients with systemic histiocytosis (Letter-Siwe syndrome, Schuller-Christian syndrome and multifocal eosinophilic granuloma). Medicine 60:311, 1981
25. Matus-Ridley M, Raney RB, Thawerani H et al: Histiocytosis X in children: patterns of disease and results of treatment. Med Pediatr Oncol 11:99, 1983
26. Smith RJH, Evans JNG: Head and neck manifestations of histiocytosis X. Laryngoscope 94:395, 1984
27. Lahey ME: Histiocytosis X: an analysis of prognostic factors. J Pediatr 87: 184, 1975
28. Komp DM, Herson J, Starling KA et al: A staging system for histiocytosis X: a Southwest Oncology Group study. Cancer 47:798, 1981
29. Johnston RB Jr: Monocytes and macrophages. N Engl J Med 318:747, 1988
30. Favara BE: Langerhans' cell histiocytosis pathobiology and pathogenesis. Semin Oncol 18:3, 1991
31. Tenito MC, Clinc MJ: Monuclear phagocyte proliferation, maturation and function. Clin Haematol 4:685, 1975
32. Carr I. The biology of macrophages. Clin Invest Med 201:937, 1978
33. Gale RP, Sparkes RS, Golde DW: Bone marrow origin of hepatic macrophages (Kupffer cells) in humans. Science 201:937, 1978
34. Thomas ED, Ramberg RE, Sale GE et al: Direct evidence for a bone marrow origin of the alveolar macrophage in man. Science 192:1016, 1976
35. Ash P, Loutit JF, Townsend KMS: Osteoclasts derived from hematopoietic stem cells. Nature 283:669, 1980
36. Van Furth R: Mononuclear phagocytes. p. 11. In Van Furth R (ed): Infection, Inflammation, and Pathology. Blackwell Scientific Publications, London, 1976
37. LeFevre Me, Hammer R: Macrophages of the mammalian small intestine: a review. J Reticuloendothel Soc 26:553, 1979
38. Murphy GF, Messadi D, Fonferko E et al: Phenotypic transformation of macrophages to Langerhans cells in the skin. Am J Pathol 123:401, 1986
39. Katz SI, Tamaki K, Sachs DH: Epidermal Langerhans cells are derived from cells originating in bone marrow. Nature 282:324, 1979
40. Basset F, Nezelof C: Présence en microscopie électronique de structures filamenteuses originales dans les lesions pulmonaires et osseuses de l'histiocytoses X. Bull Soc Med Hosp Paris 117:413, 1966
41. Nezelof C, Basset F, Rousseau MF: Histiocytosis X: histogentic arguments for a Langerhans cell origin. Biomedicine 18:365, 1973
42. Birbeck MS, Breathnach AJ, Everall JD: An electron microscopic study of basal melanocytes and high level clear cells (Langerhans cells) in vitiligo. J Invest Dermatol 37:51, 1961
43. Favara BE: The pathology of 'histiocytosis.' Am J Pediatr Hematol Oncol 3: 45, 1981
44. Murphy GF, Bhan AK, Sato S et al: Characterization of Langerhans cells by the use of monoclonal antibodies. Lab Invest 45:465, 1981
45. Pierard GE, Franchimont C, Lapiere CM: Proliferation of the characteristic histiocyte of histiocytosis X in the skin. Am J Dermatopathol 4:215, 1982
46. Wolff K, Stingl G: The Langerhans cell. J Invest Dermatol 80:175, 1983
47. Malone M: The histiocytoses of childhood. Histopathology 19:105, 1991
48. Clark SC, Kamen R: The human hematopoietic colony stimulating factors. Science 236:1229, 1987
49. Wong GG, Witeck JS, Temple PA et al: Human GM-CSF: molecular cloning of the complementary DNA and purification of the natural and recombinant proteins. Science 228:810, 1985
50. Yang, Y-C, Ciarletta AG, Temple PA et al: Human IL-3 (multi-hemopoietic growth factor related to murine IL-3. Cell 47:3, 1986
51. Kawasaki ES, Ladner MB, Wang AM et al: Molecular cloning of a complementary DNA encoding human macrophage specific colony-stimulating factor (CSF-1). Science 230:291, 1985
52. Sieff CA, Emerson SG, Donahue RE et al: Human recombinant granulocyte-macrophage colony-stimulating factor: a multilineage hematopoietin. Science 230:1171, 1985
53. Sieff CA: Hematopoietic growth factors. J Clin Invest 79:1549, 1987
54. Suda T, Suda J, Splicer SS et al: Permissive role of interleukin 3 (IL-3) in proliferation and differentiation of multipotential hemopoietic progenitors in culture. J Cell Physiol 124:182, 1985
55. Gasson JC, Weisbart RH, Kaufman SE et al: Purified human granulocyte-macrophage colony-stimulating factor: direct action on neutrophils. Science 226:1339, 1984
56. Fleischmann J, Golde DW, Weisbart RH et al: Granulocyte macrophage colony-stimulating factor enhances phagocytosis of bacteria by human neutrophils. Blood 68:708, 1986
57. Weisbart RH, Golde DW. Clark SC et al: Human granulocyte-macrophage colony-stimulating factor is a neutrophil activator. Nature 314:361, 1985
58. Takaku F, Yuo A, Okabe T et al: Human recombinant granulocyte colony-stimulating factor stimulates alkaline phosphatase activity of neutrophilic granulocytes in patients with myelodysplastic syndrome. p. 113. In: First Conference on Differentiation Therapy, Sardinia, Italy, August 30–September 3, 1986
59. Nicola NA, Vadas M: Hemopoietic colony-stimulating factors. Immunol Today 5:76, 1984
60. Cline MJ, Golde DW: Production of colony stimulating activity by human lymphocytes. Nature 248:703, 1974
61. Linch DC, Lipton JM, Nathan DG: Identification of three accessory cell populations in human bone marrow with erythroid burst-promoting properties. J Clin Invest 75:1278, 1985
62. Tsai S, Emerson SG, Sieff CA et al: Isolation of a human stromal cell strain secreting hemopoietic growth factors. J Cell Psysiol 127:137, 1986
63. Burgess AW, Camakaris J, Metcalf D: Purification and properties of colony stimulating factor from mouse lung-conditioned medium. J Biol Chem 252: 1998, 1977
64. Groh V, Gadner H, Radaskiewicz T et al: The phenotypic spectrum of histiocytosis X cells. Soc Invest Dermatol 90:441, 1988
65. Vogel JM, Vogel P: Idiopathic histiocytosis: a discussion of eosinophilic granuloma, the Hand-Schüller-Christian syndrome, and the Letterer-Siwe syndrome. Semin Hematol 9:349, 1972
66. Mickelson MR, Bonfiglio M: Eosinophilic granuloma and its variations. Orthop Clin North Am 8:933, 1977

67. Bunch WG: Orthopedic and rehabilitation aspects of eosinophilic granuloma. Am J Pediatr Hematol Oncol 3:151, 1981

68. Mosely JE: Patterns of bone change in the reticuloendothelioses. J Mt Sinai Hosp 29:282, 1962

69. Nesbit ME, Wolfson JJ, Kieffem SA, Peterson HO: Orbital sclerosis in histiocytosis X. AJR 110:123, 1970

70. Arcomano JP, Barnett JC, Wunderlich HO: Histicytosis X. AJR 85:663, 1961

71. Dunger DB, Broadbent V, Yeoman E et al: The frequency and natural history of diabetes insipidus in children with Langerhans-cell histiocytosis. N Engl J Med 321:1157, 1989

72. McGavran MH, Spady HA: Eosinophillic granuloma of bone: a study of 28 cases. J Bone Joint Surg 42A:979, 1960

73. Braustein GD, Kohler PO: Endocrine manifestations of histiocytosis. Am J Pediatr Hematol Oncol 3:67, 1981

74. Bernard JD, Aguilan MJ: Localized hypothalamic histiocytosis X. Arch Neurol 20:368, 1968

75. Dean HJ, Bishop A, Winter JSD: Growth hormone deficiency in patients with histiocytosis X. J Pediatr 109:615, 1986

76. Lahey ME, Rallison ML, Hilding DA, Ater J: Involvement of the thyroid in histiocytosis X. Am J Pediatr Hematol Oncol 8:257, 1986

77. Egeler RM, Schipper ME, Heyman HS: Gastrointestinal involvement in Langerhans cell histiocytosis (histiocytosis X): a clinical report of three cases. Eur J Pediatr 149:325, 1990

78. Wada R, Yagihashi S, Konta R et al: Gastric polyposis caused by multifocal histiocytosis X. Gut 33:994, 1992

79. Lee RG, Braziel RM, Stenzel P: Gastrointestinal involvement in Langerhans cell histiocytosis (histiocytosis X): diagnosis by rectal biospy. Mod Pathol 3:154, 1990

80. Beers GJ, Manson J, Carter AP, Bell R: Intracranial histiocytosis X: a case report. CT 10:237, 1986

81. Enksen B, Janinis J, Variakojis D et al: Primary histiocytosis X of the parieto-occipital lobe. Hum Pathol 19:611, 1988

82. Elian M, Bornstein B, Matz S et al: Neurological manifestations of general xanthomatosis. Arch Neurol 21:115, 1969

83. Colby TV, Lombard C: Histiocytosis X in the lung. Hum Pathol 14:850, 1983

84. Carlson RA, Hattery RR, O'Connell EJ, Fontana RS: Pulmonary involvement by histiocytosis X in the pediatric age group. Mayo Clin Proc 51:542, 1976

85. Nandahl SR, Finlay JL, Farrell PM et al: A case report and literature review of primary pulmonary histiocytosis X of childhood. Med Pediatr Oncol 14:57, 1986

86. Case records of the Massachusetts General Hospital. Pulmonary eosinophilic granuloma. N Engl J Med 298:327, 1978

87. Wolfson SL, Botero F, Hurwitz S, Pearson HA: Pure cutaneous histiocytosis-X. Cancer 48:2236, 1981

88. Avery ME, McAfee JC, Guild HG: The course and prognosis of reticuloendotheliosis (eosinophilic granuloma, Schüller-Christian disease and Letterer-Siwe disease). A study of forty cases. Am J Med 12:636, 1957

89. Dehner LP: Morphologic findings in the histiocytic syndromes. Semin Oncol 18:8, 1991

90. Farber S: The nature of "solitary or eosinophilic granuloma" of bone. Am J Pathol 17:625, 1941

91. Lichtenstein L: Histiocytosis X. Integration of eosinophilic granuloma of bone, "Letterer-Siwe disease" and Schüller-Christian disease as related manifestations of a single nosologic entity. Arch Pathol 56:84, 1953

92. Newton WA Jr, Hamoudi AD: Histiocytosis: a histologic classification with clinical correlation. p. 251. In Rosenberg HS, Bolande RP (eds): Perspectives in Pediatric Pathology. Vol. 1. Year Book Medical Publishers, Chicago, 1973

93. Writing Group of the Histiocyte Society: Histiocytosis in children. Lancet 1:208, 1987

94. Hall PA, Doherty CJO, Levison DA: Langerhans cell histiocytosis: an unusual case illustrating the value of immunochemistry in diagnosis. Histopathology 11:1181, 1987

95. Zachariae H: Histiocytosis X in two infants treated with topical nitrogen mustard. Br J Dermatol 100:433, 1979

96. Smith DG, Nesbit ME, D'Angio GJ, Levitt SH: Histiocytosis X: to dose levels employed. Radiology 106:419, 1973

97. Greenberger JS, Cassady JR, Jaffe N et al: Radiation therapy in patients with histiocytosis. Management of diabetes insipidus and bone lesions. J Radiat Oncol Biol Phys 5:1749, 1979

98. Gramatovici R, D'Angio GJ: Radiation therapy in soft-tissue lesions in histiocytosis X (Langerhans cell histiocytosis). Med Pediatr Oncol 16:259, 1988

99. Kelly K, Yeomans E, Broadbent V: Is diabetes insipidus associated with LCH reversible? Meeting program, Histiocyte Society Ninth Annual Meeting, 1993.

100. Starling KA: Chemotherapy of histiocytosis. Am J Pediatr Hematol Oncol 3:157, 1981

101. Starling KA, Donaldson MH, Haggard ME et al: Therapy of histiocytosis X with vincristine, vinblastine, and cyclophosphamide. Am J Dis Child 123:105, 1972

102. Lahey ME: Histiocytosis X—comparison of three treatment regimens. J Pediatr 87:179, 1975

103. Komp DM, Trueworthy R, Hvizdala E, Sexauer C: Prednisolone, methotrexate and 6-mercaptopurine in the treatment of histiocytosis X. Cancer Treat Rep 63:2125, 1979

104. Jones B, Kung F, Chevalier L et al: Chemotherapy of reticuloendotheliosis. Comparison of methotrexate plus prednisone vs. vincristine plus prednisone. Cancer 34:1011, 1974

105. Komp DM, Vietti TJ, Berry DH et al: Combination chemotherapy in histiocytosis X. Med Pediatr Oncol 3:267, 1977

106. Starling KA, Iyer R, Silva-Sosa M et al: Chlorambucil in histiocytosis X: a Southwest Oncology Group study. J Pediatr 96:266, 1980

107. Lahey ME, Heyn RM, Newton WA et al: Histiocytosis X: clinical trial of chlorambucil: a report from Children's Cancer Study Group. Med Pediatr Oncol 7:197, 1979

108. Rivera-Luna R, Martinez-Guerra G, Altamirano-Alvarez E et al: Langerhans cell histiocytosis: clinical experience with 124 patients. Pediatr Dermatol 5:145, 1988

109. Ceci A, DeTerlizzi M, Colella R et al: Etoposide in recurrent childhood Langerhans cell histiocytosis: an Italian cooperative study. Cancer 62:2528, 1988

110. Ceci A, DeTerlizzi M, Colella R et al: Etoposide in disseminated children LCH. Results from the Italian protocol AIEOP ICL-89. Meeting program, Histiocyte Society North Annual Meeting, 1993

111. Griffin TW: The treatment of advanced histiocytosis X with sequential hemibody irradiation. Cancer 39:2435, 1977

112. Davies EG, Levinsky RJ, Butler M et al: Thymic hormone therapy for histiocytosis X. N Engl J Med 309:493, 1983

113. Ringdén O, Åhström L, Lönngvist B et al: Allogeneic bone marrow transplantation in a patient with chemotherapy-resistant histiocytosis X. N Engl J Med 316:733, 1987

114. Stoll M, Freund M, Schmid H et al: Allogeneic bone marrow transplantation for Langerhans cell histiocytosis. Cancer 66:284, 1990

115. Greenix HT, Storb R, Sanders JE, Peterson FB: Marrow transplantation for treatment of multisystem progressive Langerhans cell histiocytosis. Bone Marrow Transplant 10:39, 1992

116. Komp DM: Concepts in staging and clinical studies for treatment of Langerhans' cell histiocytosis. Semin Oncol 18:18, 1991

117. Haupt R, Fears TR, Rosso P et al: Secondary leukemia after Langerhans' cell histiocytosis. Meeting program, Histiocyte Society Ninth Annual Meeting, 1993

118. Rosai J, Dorfman RF: Sinus histiocytosis with massive lymphadenopathy: a newly recognized benign clinicopathological entity. Arch Pathol 87:63, 1969

119. Foucar E, Rosai J, Dorfman R: Sinus histiocytosis with massive lymphage (Rosai-Dorfman disease): reviews of the entity. Semin Diagn Pathol 7:19, 1990

120. Rosai J, Dorfman RF: Sinus histiocytosis with massive lymphadenopathy: a pseudolymphomatous benign disorder. Cancer 30:1174, 1972

121. Foucar E, Rosai J, Dorfman RF: Sinus histiocytosis with massive lymphadenopathy: ear, nose and throat manifestations. Arch Otolaryngol 104:687, 1978

122. Kessler E, Srulijes C, Toledo E, Shalit M: Sinus histiocytosis with massive lymphadenopathy and spinal epidural involvement: a case report and review of the literature. Cancer 38:1614, 1976

123. Walker PD, Rosai J, Dorfman RF: The osseous manifestations of sinus histiocytosis with massive lymphadenopathy. Am J Clin Pathol 75:131, 1981

124. Foucar E, Rosai J, Dorfman RF: The ophthalmologic manifestations of sinus histiocytosis with massive lymphadenopathy. Am J Opthalmol 87:354, 1979

125. Karcioglu ZA, Allam B, Insler MS: Ocular involvement in sinus histiocytosis with massive lymphadenopathy. Br J Ophthalmol 72:793, 1988

126. Olsen EA, Crawford JR, Vollmer RT: Sinus histiocytosis with massive lymphadenopathy: case report and review of a multisystemic disease with cutaneous infiltrates. J Am Acad Dermatol 18:1322, 1988

127. Foucar E, Rosai J, Dorfman RF, Eyman JM: Immunologic abnormalities and their significance in sinus histiocytosis with massive lymphadenopathy. Am J Clin Pathol 82:515, 1984

128. Miettinin M, Paljakka P, Haveri P, Saxen E: Sinus histiocytosis with massive lymphadenopathy: a nodal and extranodal proliferation of S-100 protein positive histiocytes? Am J Clin Pathol 88:270, 1987

129. Haas RJ, Helmig SE, Prechtel K: Sinus histiocytosis with massive lymphadenopathy and paraparesis: remission with chemotherapy: a case report. Cancer 42:77, 1978

130. Sanchez R, Rosai J, Dorfman RF: Sinus histiocytosis with massive lymphadenopathy: an analysis of 113 cases with special emphasis on its extranodal manifestations. Annu Meet Abstr 36:349, 1977

131. Thawerani H, Sanchez RL, Rosai J, Dorfman RF: The cutaneous manifestations of sinus histiocytosis with massive lymphadenopathy. Arch Dermatol 114:191, 1978

132. Lampert F, Lennert K: Sinus histiocytosis with massive lymphadenopathy: fifteen new cases. Cancer 37:783, 1976

133. Weisenburger DD, Grierson HLL, Daley DT et al: Immunologic studies of sinus histiocytosis with massive lymphadenopathy (SHML). Lab Invest 54: 68A, 1986

134. Eisen RN, Buckley PJ, Rosai J: Immunophenotypic characterization of sinus histiocytosis with massive lymphadenopathy (Rosai-Dorfman disease) Semin Diagn Pathol 7:74, 1990

135. Foucar E, Rosai J, Dorfman RF: Sinus histiocytosis with massive lymphadenopathy: an analysis of 14 deaths occurring in a patient registry. Cancer 54:1834, 1984

136. Suarez CR, Zeller WP, Silberman S et al: Sinus histiocytosis with massive lymphadenopathy: remission with chemotherapy. Am J Pediatr Hematol Oncol 3:235, 1983

137. Newman SB, Sweet DL, Vardiman JW: Sinus histiocytosis with massive lymphadenopathy: response to cyclophosphamide therapy. Cancer Treat Rep 68:901, 1984

138. Farquhar JW, Claireaux AE: Familial haemophagocytic reticulosis. Arch Dis Child 27:519, 1952

139. MacMahon HE, Bedizel M, Ellis CA: Familial erythrophagocytic lymphohistiocytosis. Pediatrics 32:868, 1963

140. McClure PD, Strachan P, Saunders EF: Hypofibrinogenemia and thrombocytopenia in familial hemophagocytic reticulosis. J Pediatr 85:67, 1974

141. Perry MC, Harrison EG, Burgert EO, Gilchrist GS: Familial erythrophagocytic lymphohistiocytosis: report of two cases and clinicopathologic review. Cancer 38:209, 1976

142. Price DL, Woolsey JE, Rosman NP, Richardson EP: Familial lymphohistiocytosis of the nervous system. Arch Neurol 24:270, 1971

143. Ansbacher LE, Singsen BH, Hosler MW et al: Familial erythrophagocytic lymphohistiocytosis: an association with serum lipid abnormalities. J Pediatr 2:270, 1983

144. Soffer D, Okon E, Rosen N et al: Familial hemophagocytic lymphohistiocytosis in Israel. II. Pathologic findings. Cancer 54:2423, 1984

145. Risdall RJ, McKenn RW, Nesbit ME et al: Virus associated hemophagocytic syndrome: a benign histiocytic proliferation distinct from malignant histiocytosis. Cancer 44:993, 1979

146. Arya S, Hong R, Gilbert EF: Reactive hemophagocytic syndrome. Pediatr Pathol 3:129, 1985

147. Suster S, Hilsenbeck S, Rywlin AM: Reactive histiocytic hyperplasia with hemophagocytosis in hemopoietic organs. Hum Pathol 19:705, 1988

148. Henter J-I, Elinder G, Ost A, and the FHL Study Group of the Histiocyte Society: Diagnostic Guidelines for Hemophagocytic lymphohistiocytosis. Semin Oncol 18:29, 1991

149. Henter J-I, Elinder G, Soder O et al: Hypercytokinemia in familial hemophagocytic lymphohistiocytosis. Blood 78:2918, 1991

150. Ladisch S, Ho W, Matheson D et al: Immunologic and clinical effects of repeated blood exchange in familial erythrophagocytic lymphohistiocytosis. Blood 4:814, 1982

151. Amruso DR, Hays T, Zwartjes WJ et al: Successful treatment of lymphohistiocytic reticulosis with phagocytosis with epipodophyllotoxin. VP 16-213. Cancer 45:2516, 1980

152. Ware R, Friedman HS, Kinney TR: Familial erythrophagocytic lymphohistiocytosis: late relapse despite continuous high-dose VP-16 chemotherapy. Med Pediatr Oncol 18:27, 1990

153. Scott RB, Robb-Smith AHT: Histiocytic medullary reticulosis. Lancet 2:194, 1939

154. Warnke RA, Kim H, Dorfman R: Malignant histiocytosis (histiocytic medullary reticulosis) I. Clinicopathologic study of 29 cases. Cancer 35:215, 1975

155. Robinowitz BN, Noguchi S, Bergfield WF: Tumor cell characterization of histiocytic medullary reticulosis. Arch Dermatol 113:927, 1977

156. Byrne GE, Rappaport H: Malignant histiocytosis. p. 145. In Akazaki K, Rappaport H, Berard CW et al (eds): Malignant Disease of the Hematopoietic Systems. University of Tokyo Press, Tokyo, 1973

157. Zucker JM, Caillaux JM, Vanel D, Gerard-Marchant R: Malignant histiocytosis in childhood. Clinical study and therapeutic results in 22 cases. Cancer 45: 2821, 1980

158. Benz-Lemoine E, Brizard A, Huret J-L et al: Malignant histiocytosis: a specific t(2;5)(p23;q35) translocation? Review of the literature. Blood 72:1046, 1988

159. Hibi S, Esumi N, Todo S, Imashuku S: Malignant histiocytosis in childhood: clinical, cytochemical and immunohistochemical studies of seven cases. Hum Pathol 19:713, 1988

160. Tseng A Jr, Coleman N, Cox RS et al: The treatment of malignant histiocytosis. Blood 64:48, 1984

161. Esumi N, Hashida T, Matsumura T et al: Malignant histiocytosis in childhood. Clinical features and therapeutic results by combination chemotherapy. Am J Pediatr Hematol Oncol 8:300, 1986

162. Esselline DW, DeLeeuw NKM, Berry GR: Malignant histiocytosis. Cancer 52: 1904, 1983

163. Simon JH, Tebbi CK, Freeman AI et al: Malignant histiocytosis: complete remission in two pediatric patients. Cancer 59:1566, 1987

Lysosomal Storage Diseases

57

Gregory A. Grabowski and Nancy Leslie

INTRODUCTION

The lysosome was first described by deDuve[1] as an acid phosphatase-containing unit-membrane-bounded organelle within the cytoplasm of eukaryotic cells. As the name implies, lysosomes participate in the lysis or breakdown of cellular material (i.e., the digestive tracts of cells or suicide packages). Furthermore, containment of hydrolytic enzymes within these organelles prevents autodigestion of cellular contents. Since then, the role of lysosomes has expanded to a variety of other cellular events, including degradation of other organelles within the cells. Several tissues have specialized lysosomal mechanisms that extrude hydrolytic enzymes into the extracellular microenvironment. Such cells and their lysosomal enzymes are critical to host defense, wound healing, and bone remodeling (e.g., osteoclasts and neutrophils). Implicit in deDuve's description[1] was the need for systems to sort and specifically localize proteins to lysosomes and the potential of replacing deficient enzymes.

The concepts of the lysosomes as hydrolytic sacs and the need for specific targeting of enzymes to the lysosome have provided a fertile milieu for research during the past three decades. Hers[2,3] was the first to delineate engorged lysosomes in patients with α-glucosidase deficiency and other lysosomal storage diseases. This description led to a pathophysiologic view that related the malfunction of these organelles to the architectural distortion of cells by stored materials. Recently, this passive process has been superseded by a more active role for toxic degradative products (e.g., lysosphingolipids) in altering normal cellular function.[4] Goldstein et al.,[5] Neufeld and collegues,[6] and others developed the concept of receptor-mediated endocytosis, and emphasized directed targeting and sorting of proteins from the extracellular space. This culminated in the Brown and Goldstein model of receptor-mediated endocytosis for the low-density lipoprotein (LDL) particle and its general implications for the uptake and targeting of proteins to cells.[5] Neufeld and collegues[7] described the phenomenon of cross-correction during co-culture of skin fibroblasts from patients with two different types of mucopolysaccharidoses (MPS). The subsequent loss of accumulated cellular deposits in each cell type suggested the presence of "specific corrective factors," which were secreted by one MPS cell type and internalized by the other cell type.[7] These factors were later identified as enzymes. Cross-correction required the secretion of a functional enzyme that contained a signal for receptor-mediated endocytosis by other cells. Since only one lysosomal hydrolase is usually defective in MPS variants, all other secretable lysosomal hydrolases would be normal and potentially able to correct a specific deficiency in other cells.

These investigations culminated in the characterization of the mannose-6-phosphate (M6P) receptor system by the groups of Sly,[8] Kornfeld,[9,10] von Figura,[11] and others. This ligand-mediated targeting system is central to selective sorting of most soluble lysosomal proteins within many, if not all cells, their uptake into cells, and their delivery to the lysosome.[10] In comparison, membrane-bound lysosomal proteins use different, poorly defined targeting systems.[12] These concepts of storage, cross-correction, and targeting have provided the foundation for the development of therapeutic interventions for lysosomal storage diseases such as enzyme reconstitution by transplanted tissue or enzyme replacement. Both approaches may stabilize or reverse the pathophysiologic process in selected lysosomal storage diseases. Comprehensive reviews of the lysosomal diseases are available (Table 57-1).

PHYSIOLOGY OF LYSOSOMES

Unlike mitochondria, lysosomes do not contain DNA and therefore cannot self-replicate. Consequently, lysosomal biogenesis is a continuous process that requires synthesis of lysosomal hydrolases, membrane constitutive proteins, and the surrounding membrane. Although not clearly defined, this process includes the fusion of vesicles from the trans-Golgi network (TGN) with late endosomes (multivesicular bodies)[13,14] (Fig. 57-1). The TGN vesicles contain lysosomal hydrolases. The maturation of TGN vesicular bodies to lysosomes and of endosomal vesicles from early to late compartments is accompanied by a progressive acidification of their internal environments. A gradient is established so that early endosomes have an internal pH of approximately 6.0–6.2, whereas late endosomes and lysosomes have a pH of approximately 5.5–6.0 and ≤5, respectively. The decreasing internal pH of these vesicles is necessary for the pH-determined dissociation of receptors and ligands (e.g., the M6P receptor and M6P-containing oligosaccharides) and the optimal functioning of lysosomal hydrolases.[15] Dissociation occurs in a functional compartment termed CURL (compartment of uncoupling of receptors and ligands). In comparison, formation and segregation of primary lysosomes with constitutive integral and associated membrane proteins are poorly understood.[16] These proteins are essential

for lysosomal integrity and function. In particular, the lysosomal membrane contains a proton pump needed for developing and maintaining the acidic internal environment for lysosomal hydrolases to function. The signals for the fusion of TGN vesicles with endosomal vesicles require the interaction of several membrane components, sorting of proteins destined for the lysosome, loss of the M6P receptors, and recycling of some of these receptors to the mid-Golgi bodies and plasma membrane.[15]

Post-translational modifications of lysosomal hydrolases are important for specific sorting/targeting of enzymes and their enzymatic activity. Lysosomal enzymes are glycoproteins that are synthesized on ribosomes of the rough endoplasmic reticulum (ER). As with all secretory proteins, lysosomal hydrolases are synthesized with an N-terminal hydrophobic leader, or signal peptide, that is required for penetration through the ER membrane and into the lumen of the ER. The detailed processes of these synthetic and transport systems have been unravelled during the past two decades. During penetration through the ER membrane, the lysosomal proteins are co-translationally glycosylated on selected N-glycosylation consensus sequences (Asp-X-Ser or Thr). This occurs by the en bloc transfer of antennerary mannosyl oligosaccharide chains from a dolicholphosphate lipid. It is unclear how N-glycosylation sequences are selected for occupancy except that Asp-Pro-Ser or Thr sites are not used, and the surrounding protein sequences may be important for transfer of the dolicholphosphate-oligosaccharide.[17]

Following complete synthesis and glycosylation, the lysosomal enzymes are incorporated into vesicles and transported to the cis-Golgi apparatus for further processing. At this stage, all proteins destined for the lysosomes contain only branched mannosyl chains that are terminated with short-chain α-glucosyl moieties. Most enzymes destined for the lysosome acquire complex oligosaccharide modifications during transport through the Golgi apparatus. A series of glycosylhydrolases and glycosyltransferases are localized within specific regions of the cis-, mid- or trans-Golgi for these sequential modifications. In the cis-Golgi network, α-glucosidases and α-mannosidases remove terminal glucose and mannose residues to produce mannose-terminated core oligosaccharides. For each branch point of the mannosyl chain there are specific α-mannosidases for cleavage.

Following mannosyl trimming, additional sugars, including β-N-acetylglucosamine and β-galactoside, are added in the mid-Golgi system to the short mannosyl core. The addition of terminal sialic acid residues occurs in the trans-Golgi. Each of these sugars is added by glycosyltransferases that are retained by specific signals in their respective Golgi compartments. Thus, the carbohydrate composition of the lysosomal proteins is indicative of its passage through regions of the Golgi system during the synthetic process. Prior to, or coincident with, ER or cis-Golgi modifications, is the attachment of an N-acetylglucosamine-1-phosphate to the sixth position on mannosyl residues of the mannosyl core oligosaccharide. This modification can be single or multivalent and is selective for various branches of the oligosaccharides on a specific lysosomal protein. An N-acetylglucosylaminyl-1-phosphotransferase is essential for this process, and its deficiency leads to a severe condition mucolipidosis II (I-cell disease), in which nearly all soluble lysosomal enzymes are lost by secretion out of the cell.[9,11] Shortly after the attachment of the phosphosugar group, a specific hydrolase cleaves the protecting N-acetylglucosamine from the phosphate to expose the M6P residue, the targeting signal for soluble lysosomal proteins.

At the end of these modification processes, most lysosomal enzymes have a series of oligosaccharide chains and each of the antennerary structures has different modifications. Some contain terminal sialic acids, and others have mannosyl termi-

Table 57-1. Selected Lysosomal Storage Diseases

Disease (Major Review)	Common Name	Enzyme Defect	Major Organs Involved—Phenotype Variation	Stored Substrate
Mucopolysaccharidoses (MPS)[105]				
MPS IH	Hurler syndrome	α-L-iduronidase	Liver, spleen, brain, heart, cornea, bone—mild and severe variants	Dermatan and heparan sulfate
MPS II	Hunter syndrome	Iduronate sulfatase	Liver, spleen, brain, heart, bone	Dermatan and heparan sulfate
MPS III	Sanfilippo A syndrome	Heparan N-sulfatase	Brain, liver, spleen, heart, bone	Heparan sulfate
	Sanfilippo B syndrome	N-acetylglucosaminidase	Brain, liver, spleen, heart, bones	Heparan sulfate
MPS IV	Morquio A syndrome	N-acetylgalactosamine 6-sulfatase	Bone, cornea	Keratan sulfate, chondroitin-6-sulfate
	Morquio B syndrome	β-Galactosidase	Bone, cornea	Keratan sulfate
MPS VI	Maroteaux-Lamy syndrome	N-acetylgalactosamine 4-sulfatase	Bone, cornea, liver, spleen, heart—moderate and severe variants	Dermatan sulfate
MPS VII	Sly syndrome	β-Glucuronidase	Brain, liver, spleen, bone, coronary arteries	Dermatan sulfate, heparan sulfate, chondroitin-4 and -6 sulfate
Glycoproteinoses[106]				
Mannosidosis		Lysosomal α-mannosidase	Brain, liver, spleen, bone—several variants	α-Mannose-rich oligosaccharides
Fucosidosis		Glycoprotein α-fucosidase	Brain, liver, spleen, heart, skin—several variants	Fucose-containing oligosaccharides
Aspartylglucosaminuria		Aspartylglucosaminidase	Brain, liver, spleen, bone, heart	Aspartylglucosamine-containing peptides
Sialidosis		Glycoprotein α-neuraminidase	Brain, liver, spleen, bone, retina—several variants	Sialylated glycopeptides
Galactosialidosis		Protector protein—combined α-neuraminidase/β-galactosidase deficiency	Brain, liver, spleen, bone—several variants	G_{M1}-ganglioside and sialylated glycopeptides
Mucolipidosis II[107]	I-cell disease	N-acetylglucosamine-1-phosphotransferase	Brain, bone, connective tissue	Glycoproteins, glycolipids
Mucolipidosis III	Pseudohurler polydystrophy	N-acetylglucosamine-1-phosphotransferase	Brain, bone, connective tissue	Glycoproteins, glycolipids
Sphingolipidoses				
Gaucher disease[49]	Gaucher disease type 1 (non-neuronopathic)	Acid β-glucosidase; glucocerebrosidase	Liver, spleen, bone, bone marrow—highly variable phenotype	Glucosylceramide
	Gaucher disease type 2 (acute neuronopathic)	Acid β-glucosidase; glucocerebrosidase	Brain, brainstem, liver, spleen, bone marrow, lung	Glucosylceramide; glucosylsphingosine
	Gaucher disease type 3 (subacute neuronopathic)	Acid β-glucosidase; glucocerebrosidase	Brain, liver, spleen, bone marrow, lung—variable phenotype	Glucosylceramide; glucosylsphingosine
Metachromatic leukodystrophy (MLD)[108]	Infantile MLD	Arylsulfatase A	Brain, peripheral nerves	Sulfatide
	Juvenile MLD	Arylsulfatase A	Brain, peripheral nerves	Sulfatide
	Adult MLD	Arylsulfatase A	Brain, peripheral nerves	Sulfatide
		Saposin B deficiency	Brain, peripheral nerves	Sulfatide
	Pseudodeficiency	Partial arylsulfatase A	Normal	None
Multiple sulfatase deficiency[108]		Unknown primary—multiple lysosomal and nonlysosomal sulfatase deficiencies	Brain, liver, spleen, bone	Sulfatide, dermatan and heparan sulfate
Gangliosidoses				
G_{M2} gangliosidoses[59]	Infantile Tay-Sachs disease (TSD)	β-Hexosaminidase A α-chain)	Brain	G_{M2} ganglioside
	Juvenile TSD	β-hexosaminidase A (α-chain)	Brain	G_{M2} ganglioside
	Adult TSD	β-Hexosaminidase A (α-chain)	Brain	G_{M2} ganglioside
	Activator deficiency	G_{M2} activator	Brain	G_{M2} ganglioside
	Sandhoff disease	β-Hexosaminidase B and A (β-chain)	Brain, liver, spleen, bone	G_{M2} ganglioside, globoside
G_{M1} gangliosidoses[59]	Landing disease	β-Galactosidase	Brain, liver, spleen, bone	G_{M1} ganglioside, keratan sulfate

(Table continues)

Table 57-1. *(Continued)*

Disease (Major Review)	Common Name	Enzyme Defect	Major Organs Involved—Phenotype Variation	Stored Substrate
Neutral Sphingolipisoses				
Fabry disease[35]		α-Galactosidase A	Kidney, vascular endothelial system, heart, central nervous system vessels	Globotriaosylceramide
Schindler disease[35]		α-N-acetylgalac-tosaminidase	Brain—probably several variants	N-acetylgalactose-linked oligosaccharides
Krabbe syndrome[109]		Galactocerebrosidase	Brain	Galactocerebroside
Niemann-Pick disease[110]	Niemann-Pick A disease (infantile)	Sphingomyelinase	Brain, liver, spleen, lung	Sphingomyelin
	Niemann-Pick B disease (late-onset)	Sphingomyelinase	Liver, spleen, lung	Sphingomyelin
Neutral lipid storage diseases				
Wolman disease[36]		Lysosomal acid lipase	Liver, spleen, adrenal glands, bone marrow	Cholesteryl esters, triglycerides
Cholesterol ester storage disease[36]		Lysosomal acid lipase	Liver, spleen, blood vessels	Cholesteryl esters
Farber disease[111]		Ceramidase	Brain, joints, tendon, skin, liver	Ceramide

nations. As a result, the lysosomal enzymes can have portions of the attached oligosaccharide tree with only mannose residues (high mannose modification), mannose residues as well as N-acetylglucosylamine, β-galactose- and sialic acid-containing oligosaccharides (mixed type modification), or only terminal sialic acid residues (complex type modification).[18,19]

Defective M6P targeting of soluble lysosomal proteins, as occurs in mucolipidosis II, has no effect on the integrity of the lysosome per se or its membrane. Lysosomal integral or associated membrane proteins (LIMPs or LAMPs) are sorted to the lysosomal membrane or to the interior of the lysosome via M6P-independent trafficking systems. Signals for trafficking have been identified as strategically located tyrosine residues near the C-terminal end of some LIMPs and LAMPs.[12] It is apparent that additional signals will be required for targeting of other lysosomal membrane components, particularly those that may be needed for lysosomal biogenesis. Importantly, for diseases involving LIMPs and LAMPs, cross-correction of co-cultured

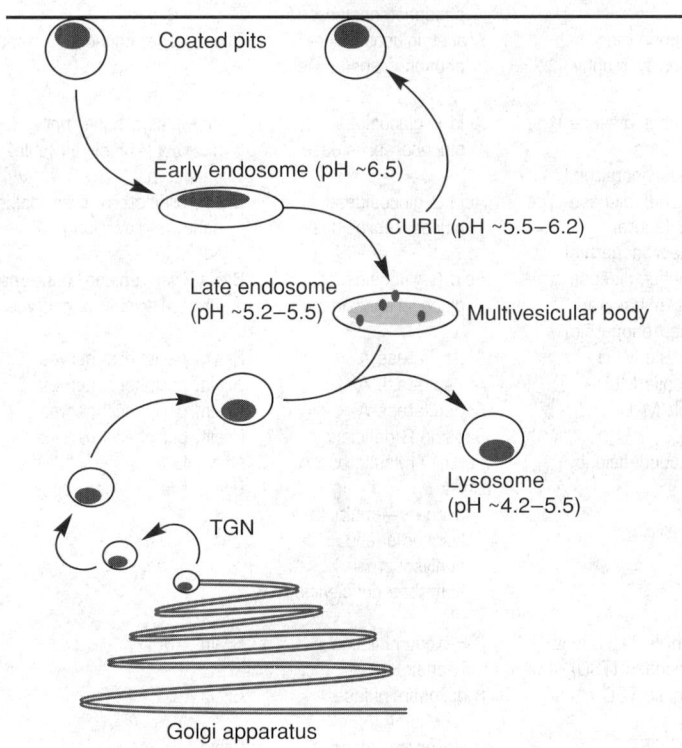

Fig. 57-1. Schematic diagram of lysosomal development from the trans-Golgi network (TGN) and the endosomal compartments developing from the plasma membrane clathrin-coated pits. The various endosomal compartments are distinguished by the progressive acidification of the vesicles from early to late endosomes and loss of the M6P receptors in the compartment of uncoupling of receptors and ligands (CURL). The multivesicular body is a compartment identified by electron microscopy containing multiple internal small vesicles that are derived from the plasma membrane. Vesicles that bud from the TGN fuse with the late endosomes or multivesicular bodies to form the lysosomal compartment. M6P receptors are recycled to the plasma membrane so that the multivesicular bodies and the lysosomes do not contain these receptors.

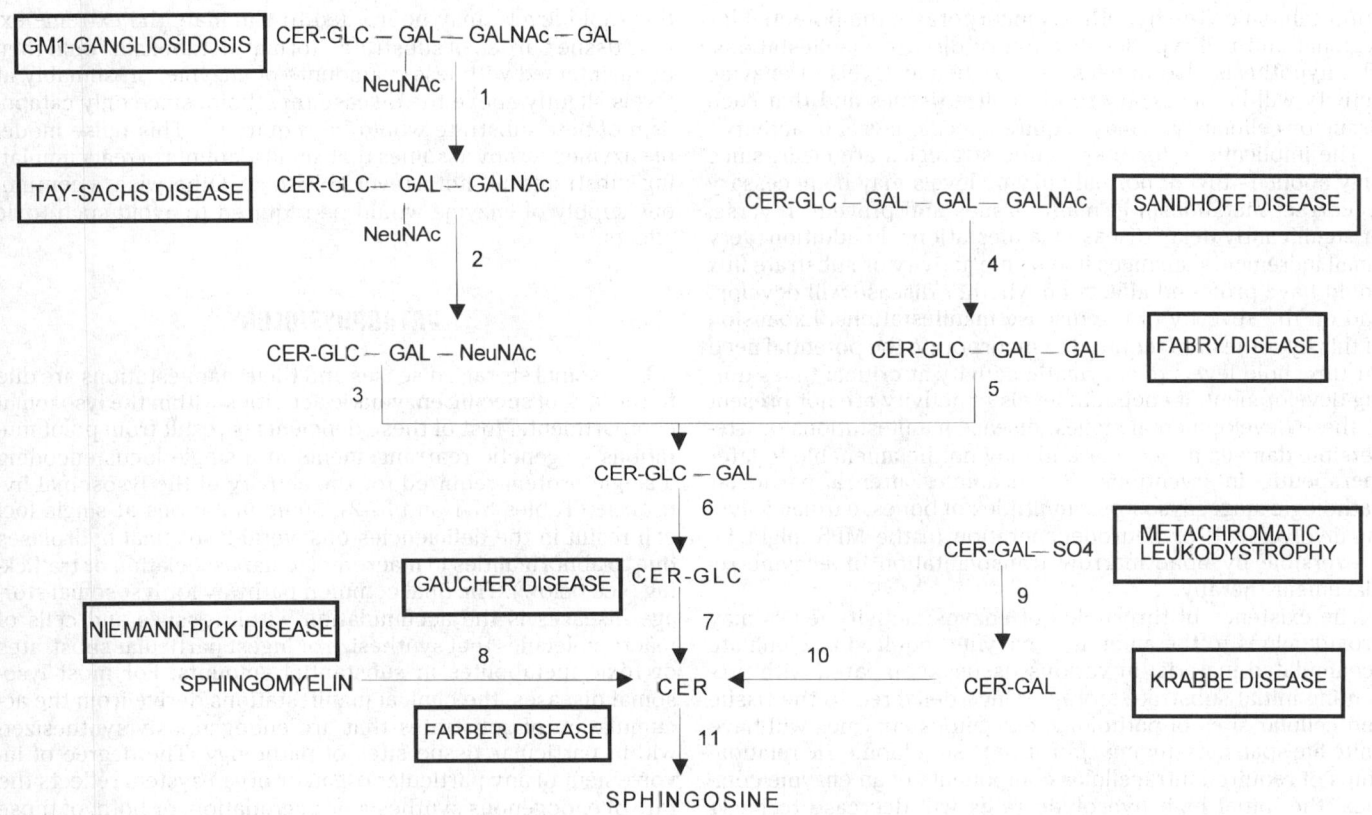

Fig. 57-2. Pathway of glycosphingolipid degradation and the diseases that result from specific enzyme deficiencies. The numbers refer to the following lysosomal hydrolases: (1) β-galactosidase, (2) β-hexosaminidase A, (3) ganglioside neuraminidase, (4) β-hexosaminidase B, (5) α-galactosidase A, (6) β-galactosidase for lactosylceramide, (7) acid β-glucosidase (glucocerebrosidase), (8) sphingomyelinase, (9) arylsulfatase A, (10) β-galactocerebrosidase, and (11) ceramidase. The deficiency of each of the respective enzymes leads to the accumulations of the substrate preceding the hydrolytic step. Diseases have yet to be described due to the deficiencies of either enzyme 3 or 6.

cells does not occur; this has significance for therapeutic strategies of such diseases.

In addition to glycosylation, some lysosomal proteins require proteolytic clipping, phosphorylation, or macromolecular assembly for the development of full function within the lysosomal environment. Proteolytic processing can occur at the N or C termini, or by clipping of single-peptide precursors into mature subunits or biologically active peptides. For example, prosaposin is cleaved into four biologically active saposins (A, B, C, and D) after reaching the lysosomal compartment[20–24] (Fig. 57-2). A "protector protein" precursor is involved in the disease galactosialidosis and is clipped from its zymogen form into two disulfide-linked subunits within the Golgi apparatus prior to its achieving proteolytic activity.[25,26] Some proteins may also acquire phosphorylation on serines or threonines, as well as sulfation of tyrosines. Macromolecular assembly is required for several heteromeric lysosomal proteins. The association of the β-hexosaminidase α- and β-chains occurs in the mid-Golgi as a necessary event in the synthesis of active hexosaminidase A (α- and β-heteromers) or hexosaminidase B (β-homomers). Macroassembly of the β-galactosidase/neuraminidase/protector protein complex probably occurs within the Golgi apparatus coincident with other processing required for the assembly of the active catalytic complex.[25]

Several tissues have distinct lysosomal functions and lysosomal hydrolase contents. Lysosomes of neutrophils contain a myeloperoxidase not present in fibroblast lysosomes.[27] Although the differential tissue expression of many lysosomal proteins has not been characterized, these differences do exist and may be important for understanding the pathophysiology of the lysosomal storage diseases. Variable phenotypes or expressions of lysosomal storage diseases may relate to the differential expression of hydrolases in particular tissues or cell types, although this hypothesis has not been proved. In most tissues, the constituent lysosomal hydrolases for degradation of macromolecules, such as mucopolysaccharides, glycoproteins, and glycosphingolipids, have similar relative compositions and therefore many lysosomal storage diseases involve most tissues to some degree. However, concordant levels of lysosomal hydrolase activities are not found in all tissues. For example, α-L-iduronidase and several other soluble lysosomal proteins are found at high levels in seminal fluid, whereas they exist at very low levels in plasma. α-L-iduronidase is also expressed at easily detectable levels in amniocytes and placental tissue, whereas it is nearly absent in early chorionic villus samples.[28] Acid β-glucosidase, which is deficient in Gaucher disease, is present at levels approximately 10-fold less in myeloid cells compared with fibroblastic cells.[29] This differential expression of selected lysosomal enzymes led Conzelmann and Sandhoff and their collegues[30,31] to propose a threshold hypothesis for the development of manifestations of specific lysosomal hydrolase deficiency diseases. This working hypothesis implies that, in the absence of alternative metabolic pathways, a certain level of residual enzymatic activity, or substrate flux, is necessary in tissues for the development of lysosomal disease manifestations. Above this threshold level of activity, disease manifestations in tissues or in a cell type will not occur, whereas below this level a phenotype will be expressed. In its simplest form this hypothesis formalizes the common-sense notion that less enzyme activity leads to more severe disease, and more enzyme activity results in fewer or delayed disease manifestations. This formalism is conceptually important since the hypothesis incorporates the potential for regional and cell type localization of disease manifestations. The hypothesis also implies that particular levels of enzyme activity will be necessary to normalize tissues and that each tissue or cellular type may require specific levels of activity.

The implications for therapeutic strategies are clear, since only about 1–10% of normal enzyme levels may be necessary to correct metabolism in many tissues and prevent, reverse, or significantly delay disease manifestations. In addition, very small incremental changes in enzyme activity or substrate flux could have profound affects on whether disease will develop, and on the severity of the disease manifestations. Expansion of this hypothesis is required to incorporate the potential need for threshold levels of enzymatic activity at critical times during development. If adequate levels of activity are not present at these developmental stages, disease manifestations or irreversible damage may occur and may not be amenable to later therapeutic interventions. For example, after a particular pathologic stage, dysostosis multiplex of bones, cardiac valvular involvement, or neurodegeneration in the MPS might be irreversible by bone marrow transplantation or enzyme replacement therapy.

The existence of thresholds of enzyme activity levels may provide clues to the amount of enzyme required to eliminate accumulated material in various tissues, compared with preventing initial substrate storage. Once delivered to the tissue and cellular sites of pathology, exogenous enzymes will have finite life spans. Assuming appropriate stoichiometric relationships of required intracellular components of an enzyme complex, the initial high hydrolytic rates will decrease to background levels over several half-lives of the supplied enzyme. Thus, large amounts of enzyme, potentially several-fold above threshold levels, may be needed to eliminate the extreme excess tissue burden of substrate. Normal metabolism could then be maintained with lesser amounts of enzyme, presumably at levels slightly above the disease threshold, since only catabolism of new substrate would be required.[31] This pulse model of enzyme therapy assumes that small amounts of reaccumulating substrates are not irreversibly toxic. Otherwise, a continuous supply of enzyme would be required to avoid such toxic effects.

PATHOPHYSIOLOGY

Lysosomal storage diseases and their manifestations are due to the lack of specific enzymatic activities within the lysosomal compartment. Most of these deficiencies result from point mutations or genetic rearrangements at a single locus encoding a single protein required for the activity of the lysosomal hydrolase (Tables 57-1 and 57-2). Some mutations at single loci can result in the deficiencies of several lysosomal hydrolases due to abnormalities in macromolecular association or trafficking (see below). The final common pathway for lysosomal storage diseases is the accumulation within tissues and cells of macromolecules that synthesize or ingest particular substrates or toxic metabolites in substantial amounts. For most lysosomal diseases, the clinical manifestations derive from the accumulation of substrates that are endogenously synthesized within particular tissue sites of pathology. The degree of involvement of any particular organ or organ system reflects the rate of endogenous synthesis or degradation, or both, of those specific compounds in the specific tissues. The stored substrates are macromolecules of mucopolysaccharides, glyco-

Table 57-2. Gene Mapping of Lysosomal Storage Diseases

Disease	Enzyme	Regional Mapping	cDNA Cloned
Mucopolysaccharidoses (MPS)			
MPS IH	α-L-iduronidase	4p16.3	Yes
MPS II	Iduronate sulfatase	Xq28.1	Yes
MPS IIIA	α-N-acetylglucoaminidase		
MPS IV	N-acetylgalacosamine 6-sulfatase	16q24.3	
MPS VI	N-acetylgalactosamine 4-sulfatase	12q14	Yes
MPS VII	β-Glucuronidase	5q11-q13	Yes
Glycoproteinoses			
Mannosidosis	α-Mannosidase	19p13-q13	
Fucosidosis	α-L-fucosidase	1p34	Yes
Aspartylglucosaminuria	Aspartylglucosaminidase	4q23-q27	Yes
Sialidosis	α-Neuraminidase	10pter-q23	
Galactosialidosis	Protector protein	20q13.1	Yes
Mucolipidosis II		4q21-q23	
Mucolipidosis III		4q21-q23	
Sphingolipidoses			
Gaucher disease	Acid β-glucosidase	1q21-23	Yes
Metachromatic leukodystrophy (MLD)	Arylsulfatase A	22q13.21	Yes
MLD	Saposin B deficiency	10q21-q22	Yes
G_{M2} gangliosidosis	β-Hexosaminidase α-chain	15q15.1-q22	Yes
G_{M2} gangliosidoses	β-Hexosaminidase β-chain	5q13	Yes
G_{M2} gangliosidoses	G_{M2} activator		Yes
G_{M1} gangliosidoses	β-Galactosidase	3p21-p14.2	Yes
Fabry disease	α-Galactosidase A	Xq21.33-q22	Yes
Schindler disease	N-Acetyl-α-galactosaminidase	22q11	Yes
Krabbe disease	Galactocerebrosidase	14q21-31	Yes
Niemann-Pick disease	Sphingomyelinase	11p15.1-15.4	Yes
Neutral Lipid Storage Diseases			
Wolman disease	Lysosomal acid lipase	10q23-q23.3	Yes
Cholesterol ester storage disease	Lysosomal acid lipase	10q23-q23.3	Yes
Farber disease	Ceramidase		Yes

proteins, or glycosphingolipids that require degradation through a pathway with the sequential removal of single components of the substrate molecules at each step in a catabolic cascade. Most of the enzymes are exohydrolases. The glycosphingolipid pathway is summarized in Figure 57-2.

Table 57-1 lists selected lysosomal storage diseases categorized according to substrate groups and indicates some of the tissues involved by the various diseases. Specific organ systems are involved by particular diseases to a greater or lesser extent and reflect the balance of endogenous and phagocytic substrate presentation. In Hurler syndrome (mucopolysaccharidosis IH), dermatan and heparan sulfate accumulate in a variety of tissues, including connective tissue, resulting in joint contractures and abnormal skin consistency. Tissue-specific pathology also applies to several other diseases. Galactocerebroside occurs with the greatest concentrations within the myelin sheaths of the central nervous system. Although the deficiency of galactocerebrosidase in Krabbe syndrome occurs in all tissues, the synthesis of galactocerebroside is much greater in the nervous system.[32,33] Consequently, the manifestations of the disease are localized to the nervous system. Similarly, in Tay-Sachs disease or Sandhoff disease, the deficiency of β-hexosaminidase A or β-hexosaminidase A and B, respectively, results in either primarily central nervous system disease or in combined central nervous system and visceral diseases due to the different accumulated substrates.[34] β-Hexosaminidase A cleaves the specific substrate G_{M2} ganglioside, whereas β-hexosaminidase B cleaves primarily sialogangliosides and globosides. G_{M2} ganglioside is synthesized in large amounts only in brain or other nervous tissues, and globoside is synthesized primarily in visceral tissues. Additional mechanisms, other than endogenous substrate synthesis, must be involved in pathologic substrate deposition in Fabry disease, Gaucher disease, and cholesterol ester storage disease (CESD). In Fabry disease, α-galactosidase A deficiency,[35] CESD,[36] and lysosomal acid lipase deficiency, result from an inability to catabolize globotriaosylceramide or cholesterol esters, respectively. Both of these compounds are carried in the plasma associated with LDL particles. These LDL particles are internalized via receptor-mediated endocytosis and presented to the lysosome for degradation. Consequently, major components of the pathophysiology, particularly endothelial cell involvement in these two disorders, relate to the LDL uptake of these substrates, synthesized at distant sites, and the inability to degrade them within the lysosomes of target cells. Since the endogenous synthesis of globotriaosylceramide as well as cholesterol esters is relatively low within most tissues, the vast majority of accumulated substrate is derived from sources external to the cells. The liver is the primary site of synthesis of the involved lipids in Fabry disease and CESD. In comparison, the visceral manifestations of Gaucher disease (acid β-glucosidase deficiency) derive from the storage of glucosylceramide, primarily in cells of monocyte/macrophage origin[37] (Fig. 57-3). The vast majority of the viscerally stored substrate probably derives from leukocyte membrane turnover due to the phagocytosis of aging leukocytes.[38] The inability to degrade the glucosylceramide from the membranes of these leukocytes results in storage in macrophage lysosomes. Thus, the major pathophysiology of visceral involvement disease relates to imported glycosphingolipid substrate rather than endogenously synthesized substrate within cells of the monocyte/macrophage system.

In comparison, Gaucher disease type 2 is a severe neurodegenerative disorder of infancy that results in death by about 2 years of age. The massive visceromegaly, particularly of the spleen and liver, as well as bone marrow infiltration by Gaucher cells in this disease, clearly results from the phagocytic pathway. However, this severe neurodegenerative disease appears to be related to the presence of toxic by-products derived from degradation of endogenously synthesized glucosylceramide

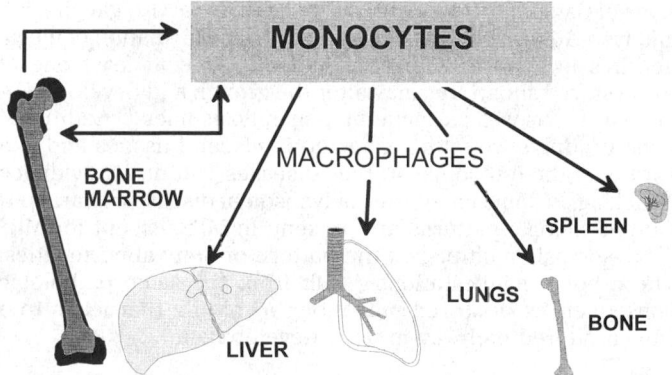

Fig. 57-3. Representation of the origin and major distribution of monocyte-derived tissue-bound macrophages. The major pathology in the non-neuronopathic forms of Gaucher disease results from the accumulation of glucosylceramide in these target sites of pathology. Most glucosylceramide deposited is thought to derive from membranes of senescent leukocytes and the inability of macrophages to degrade this sphingolipid completely due to the defective activity of acid β-glucosidase (glucoscerebrosidase). Pathologically, all the above organs are involved, but the bone marrow and spleen are nearly always severely involved by Gaucher disease. Greater variation of clinical involvement is observed in the liver, lungs, and bone.

within the central nervous system of affected patients. These endogenous toxic metabolites, as well as the importation of glucosylceramide from peripheral sources into the brain, contribute jointly to severe neurodegenerative disease. The role of transported and imported substrates in the pathophysiology of other diseases, such as metachromatic leukodystrophy, MPS, and some of the glycoproteinoses, are not fully understood and certainly would have an impact on therapeutic approaches to these diseases. It appears likely that several mechanisms—thresholds of enzyme activity, tissue or developmental specificity, substrate localization, and substrate importation—play specific roles in the pathophysiology of lysosomal storage diseases. The relative importance of each process varies among diseases and may explain differential organ involvement within a specific disease category.

The direct distortion of the lysosomal architecture (i.e., engorgement of lysosomes) probably has significant pathologic consequences, but the pharmacologic effects of the accumulated substrates or by-products are increasingly recognized as major components of the disease pathophysiology.[4,39,40] In the glycosphingolipidoses, the toxic metabolites of these complex lipids derive from their incomplete or improper degradation in the lysosome. The deacylated analogues of glycosphingolipids are known as sphingoid bases. These compounds are potent inhibitors of a variety of cellular enzymes, including protein kinase C isozymes and other membrane proteins.[40,41] Sphingoid bases (lyso-glycosphingolipids) accumulate in Tay-Sachs disease, Sandhoff disease,[42] Krabbe syndrome,[43] and Gaucher disease types 2 and 3.[44] The toxicity of sphingoid bases is most clear-cut in Krabbe syndrome and Gaucher disease type 2. The excessive accumulation of galactosylsphingosine and glucosylsphingosine in these diseases, respectively, leads to the destruction of neurons within the brains of affected individuals. Consequently, the central nervous system disease manifestations are the result of neuronal loss and death rather than the storage per se of galactosyl- or glucosylceramide.

In Gaucher disease type 1, glucosylsphingosine is known to accumulate in small amounts in visceral organs and may be related directly or via induced increases in cytokines[45,46] to the fibrosis that is seen in the liver, spleen, and bone marrow of affected patients.[47] This would provide a unifying pathophysiologic basis (i.e., cell death and scarring) for the manifestations of Gaucher disease. In Tay-Sachs disease, G_{M2} ganglioside and lyso-G_{M2} ganglioside accumulate.[42] The formation of mega-neurites in Tay-Sachs disease indicates that at least one of these stored substrates may alter the growth and development of neurons, as well as accumulating in lysosomes.[48] Additional toxic products would be expected in visceral tissues and in a variety of the lysosomal storage diseases, but direct evidence is lacking. In some categories of lysosomal diseases, characteristic pathologic patterns are present. In MPS, except for MPS IV, dysostosis multiplex is the pattern of bony abnormalities. These bony manifestations result from the same pathologic consequences of stored mucopolysaccharide that leads to a similar altered pathway in bony development.

MOLECULAR GENETIC MECHANISMS

The molecular mechanisms that result in the lysosomal storage diseases are as varied as the diseases themselves. These mechanisms must account for defects in single and multiple enzymes as well as the accumulation of specific substrates in the absence of the expected in vitro enzymatic deficiency. The vast majority of the lysosomal storage diseases result from mutations at single loci that involve a single gene product and are either point mutations or deletions/insertions in genes encoding subunits of a particular protein. Missense or nonsense mutations result in the production of proteins with abnormal catalytic function, stability, or processing of the enzyme. For many of these mutations, an abnormal protein with low enzyme activity is synthesized. For example, >30 mutations have been described in Gaucher disease or Tay-Sachs disease at the loci for acid β-glucosidase or β-hexosaminidase A α-chain, respectively.[49] These mutations have differential effects on enzyme stability, catalytic activity, and effector interactions.[50] Since these two diseases are found at high frequencies in the Ashkenazi Jewish population, a few common mutations would be expected in that population due to either founder effect or selective pressures. The summary in Tables 57-3 and 57-4 shows the frequencies of common mutations for these diseases. The phenotypic variation in these two diseases represents a continuum of degrees of involvement or age at onset of symptoms. In comparison, two completely different disease phenotypes appear to result from the same enzymatic deficiency due to mutations at the β-galactosidase locus: the G_{M1} gangliosidoses and Morquio syndrome type B (MPS IVB). In the former disease, G_{M1} ganglioside accumulates in the central nervous system and mucopolysaccharide metabolites build up in the visceral organs.[51] In Morquio syndrome type B disease, keratan sulfate accumulates in visceral organs; the central nervous system is not directly involved. These very different phenotypes result from mutations in the structural locus for β-galactosidase that affect different components of the same or overlapping active sites in the enzyme.[51,52] Thus, mutations in single lysosomal polypeptides can result in multiple disease variants.

Several lysosomal hydrolases are multimeric or occur as

Table 57-4. Common Mutations in G_{M2} Gangliosidosis (Tay-Sachs Disease Variants)

Enzyme Subunit	Mutation	Phenotype	Allele Frequency (%) Jewish	Non-Jewish
α-Chain	Exon 11 insertion	Tay-Sachs disease	73	16
α-Chain	Intron 12 splice site	Tay-Sachs disease	15	0
α-Chain	Gly 269 → Ser	Adult G_{M2} gangliosidosis	8	3

multienzyme complexes. A mutation in a common subunit or a component of the multienzyme structure could result in selective deficiencies of individual enzyme components or in all the components of the complex. Tay-Sachs disease and Sandhoff disease are typical examples of heteromeric proteins in which distinct phenotypes result from mutations in different subunits. β-Hexosaminidase A is composed of α- and β-chains, whereas β-hexosaminidase B is composed of only β-chains. Mutations at the α-chain locus result in Tay-Sachs disease (β-hexosaminidase A deficiency) whereas those in the β-chain result in Sandhoff disease (β-hexosaminidase A and B deficiency).[53] Since the substrates for β-hexosaminidase B occur in the viscera and the substrate for β-hexosaminidase A (G_{M2} ganglioside) occurs predominantly in brain, Sandhoff disease has manifestations in the central nervous system and in the viscera. The β-galactosidase/neuraminidase/protector protein complex is more complicated. Isolated deficiencies of each of these enzymatic components have been described.[51] Neuraminidase deficiency results in sialidosis (glycoprotein storage disease), and protector protein defects result in deficiencies of both β-galactosidase and neuraminidase. The protector protein is a protease that attaches to the neuraminidase/β-galactosidase complex some time during synthesis, and "protects" this complex from inactivation or degradation, or both.[25] Thus, point mutations in the protector protein can lead to galactosialidosis, a triple enzymatic deficiency producing extraordinarily variable phenotypes.[26]

Mutations in protein activators or cofactors necessary for the catalytic activity of a variety of glycosphingolipid hydrolases result in diseases that are phenocopies of the particular enzyme deficiency. For the glycosphingolipids these protein activators are termed saposins. Five different saposins have been described. Four saposins (A, B, C, and D) are encoded by a single locus on chromosome 10 (Fig. 57-4). The G_{M2} activator required for catabolism of G_{M2} ganglioside by β-hexosaminidase A is encoded by a different locus on chromosome 5.[54] The hallmark of saposin deficiency is the accumulation of specific lipid substrates for a suspected deficient enzyme activity, but normal in vitro activity of the associated enzyme. Gaucher-like diseases have been described due to the deficiency of saposin C and prosaposin.[55,56] A metachromatic leukodystrophy (MLD)-like disease results from a deficiency of saposin B,[57,58] and Tay-Sachs-like diseases have been described as due to G_{M2}-activator deficiency.[59] Of these saposin deficiencies, the defects in the prosaposin locus are particularly interesting. Each of the saposins A, B, C, and D participate in the hydrolysis of a variety of glycosphingolipids. It is thought that saposins A, B, and D and prosaposin are important in the presentation of glycosphingolipids to specific enzymes[60] and in ganglioside transport.[61] Saposin C is specifically required by acid β-glucosidase.[62] As expected, the deficiency of prosaposin leads to a complex disorder mimicking the deficiency of several glycosphingolipid hydrolases.[63] Importantly, the in vitro activities of the corresponding enzymes are nearly normal in tissues from patients with the saposin defects. It is anticipated that several other activator or cofactor molecules required for assistance

Table 57-3. Frequency of Alleles in Jewish Patients with Gaucher Disease Type 1

Mutation	Alleles (N)	%
N370S	369	71.2
84GG	60	11.58
L444P and XOVR[a]	23	4.44
IVS2^{+1}	11	2.12
V394L	4	0.9

[a] XOVR is a crossover fusion gene.
(Adapted from Grabowski,[71] with permission.)

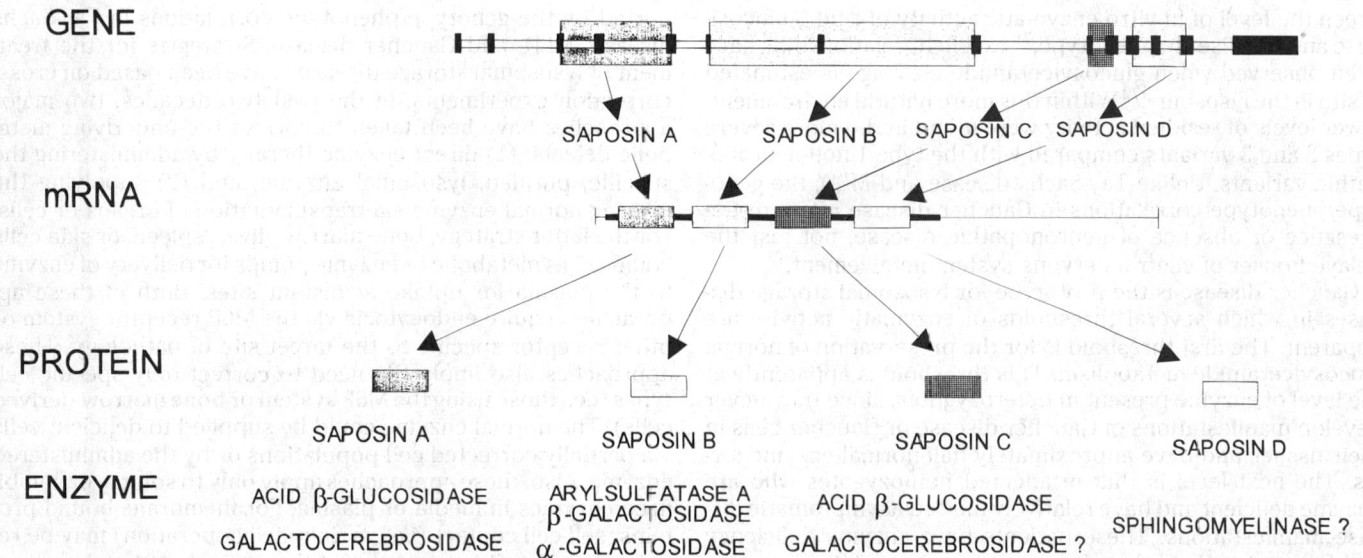

Fig. 57-4. Diagram of the processing of prosaposin from the chromosomal gene through mRNA to individual saposin proteins and their interactions with lysosomal enzymes. The chromosomal gene is >20 kb in length and is located on chromosome 10p. The most 5′ end of the gene is uncharacterized and the promotor structure is unknown. The mRNA contains four highly homologous, but not identical, domains that code for the saposins A, B, C, and D. In addition, interspersed coding sequences are cleaved by proteolysis. The individual saposins are produced by proteolytic cleavage within the lysosomes, where they interact with their respective lysosomal hydrolases.

in hydrolysis of complex macromolecules will be discovered in the future.

Mucolipidosis II exemplifies the impact on lysosomal enzymes of mutations at loci for nonlysosomal proteins. The enzyme N-acetylglucosamine-1-phosphotransferase is required for the attachment to many lysosomal proteins of the M6P ligand sorting signal.[9,11] Mutations at the loci for subunits encoding this enzyme result in the absence of the M6P ligand and the secretion into the media of most soluble lysosomal enzyme proteins. The lysosomes are nearly devoid of M6P receptor-targeted enzymes. Consequently, the phenotypes resemble a mixture of various mucopolysaccharide, glycoprotein, and glycosphingolipid degradation defects due to the loss of many enzymes and proteins involved in the respective catabolic pathways. Since some of the membrane-bound proteins of the lysosome are targeted via M6P-independent pathways, they are retained within the lysosomes. However, their catalytic activity may be affected by the loss of activator proteins and other lysosomal components that require M6P receptor-mediated sorting.

GENOTYPE/PHENOTYPE CORRELATIONS

Implicit in the threshold hypothesis is a relationship between the level of enzymatic activity in cells and the phenotype expressed in the patients' tissues. Consequently, for lysosomal storage diseases, as well as other inherited defects, investigators have attempted to relate the genetic mutations and the phenotypic manifestations in the patient. For three lysosomal storage diseases good correlations have been obtained: MLD, Tay-Sachs disease, and Gaucher disease. In each of these disorders, major variants include rapidly to slowly progressive onset types. In MLD, combinations of two mutant arylsulfatase A alleles account for most infantile, juvenile, and adult-onset variants.[64–66] The presence of two copies of a null allele (splicing defect in intron 2) results in an infantile disease. In comparison, a P426L substitution in its homozygous form leads to an adult-onset disease. Not unexpectedly, the combination of a null and P426L mutant alleles can lead to a juvenile-onset variant. These results correlate well with the measured in situ

lysosomal cleavage of exogenously supplied sulfatide substrate.[31] It is noteworthy that a very common "pseudodeficiency allele" at the arylsulfatase A locus results in deficient activity toward artificial substrates as measured in vitro, whereas the in vivo cleavage of sulfatide is low-normal in these cells. This mutant allele is due to an alteration in one of the polyadenylation signals in the 3′ untranslated region, leading to inefficient polyadenylation and a decrease in available mRNA for protein synthesis. In combination with the glycosylation or null alleles for MLD, individuals with a pseudodeficient allele appear to be deficient for arylsulfatase A activity and would be expected to develop MLD symptoms. This is an erroneous conclusion, and these individuals are asymptomatic. Since this pseudoallele is present in 10–15% of the population, it is important to exclude its presence in suspected MLD families, particularly prior to the institution of therapies.[65] Disease-causing mutations can occur on the background of the pseudodeficient allele. Thus, the detection of the pseudodeficient mutation does not exclude a disease mutation on the same allele. In situ measurement of sulfatide cleavage is required to ensure proper diagnosis, and interpretation can be difficult.[67] The "pseudodeficient" allele in non-Jewish Tay-Sachs disease raises similar concerns.[68]

In Tay-Sachs disease, combinations of null and missense mutations produce different onset forms of β-hexosaminidase A deficiency. The most common allele in the Ashkenazi Jewish population is a 4-base pair insertion that results in the production of a nonfunctional mRNA (i.e., a null allele resulting in the total lack of α-chains for β-hexosaminidase A synthesis)[53,69] (Table 57-4). In comparison, the missense mutation leading to a Gly 269→Ser (G269S) substitution allows for some hexosaminidase A activity and a more slowly progressive disease, with onset of neurodegeneration and dementia in adolescence to adulthood.[70] Similar to MLD, the combinations of null and partially functional mutations lead to the different ages of onset of the disease manifestations. In all of these disease variants, neuropathic manifestations are progressive, and the rate of deterioration is determined by the level of enzyme activity, from 0% to 5% of normal. In comparison, all Gaucher disease types are associated with residual enzymatic activity within cells. Although good correlations have not been obtained between the level of in vitro enzymatic activity of acid β-glucosidase and the disease phenotype,[71] excellent relationships have been observed when glucosylceramide cleavage is estimated in situ in the lysosome.[72] Within this more natural environment, lower levels of residual activity were found in the more severe types 2 and 3 variants compared with the type 1 non-neuronopathic variants. Unlike Tay-Sachs disease and MLD, the genotype/phenotype correlations in Gaucher disease relate to the presence or absence of neuronopathic disease, not just the delayed onset of central nervous system involvement.[73]

Gaucher disease is the prototype for lysosomal storage diseases in which several thresholds of enzymatic activity are apparent. The first threshold is for the preservation of normal glucosylceramide metabolism. This threshold is apparently at the level of enzyme present in heterozygotes, since they never develop manifestations of Gaucher disease or Gaucher cells in their tissues and have approximately half-normal enzyme levels. The next level is that in affected homozygotes who are enzyme deficient and have relatively mild-to-asymptomatic disease manifestations. These patients have enzyme deficiency and Gaucher cells in their bone marrow, but minimal disease involvement. The next threshold is for children, adolescents, or young adults with severe visceral manifestations and shortened life span. Within this group of type 1 individuals, the presence of the allele encoding N370S, together with other alleles, modifies the disease expression. Although the degree of involvement is highly variable, homozygotes for N370S are much less severely involved by the disease, and some are asymptomatic. In comparison, the N370S/null allele genotype usually leads to a severe disease course. The next threshold is for the development of neuronopathic disease. Within this group are the types 2 and 3 individuals, with the type 3 patients having later onset of neuronopathic manifestations. Among type 3 variants there is significant heterogeneity, with two different subtypes of neuronopathic disease, designated 3a and 3b.[74] From studies of in situ glucosylceramide metabolism, as well as genotype analysis among homozygotes for the L444P mutation, the type 3 patients appear to have significantly greater residual enzymatic activity than do the type 2 patients. The most severe type 2 patients may have one L444P mutation and an additional allele, which is null. These thresholds are relative, since even in normal individuals, the massive substrate load presented by acute myeloid leukemia (i.e. leukocyte membranes) results in the development of Gaucher disease-like cells associated with completely normal enzymatic activity. Thus, not unexpectedly, other factors or genes can modify the expression of the mutant enzyme activity and the disease phenotype even in patients with the same genotype. These factors or genes have yet to be identified, and the role of ethnic or racial background, or both, on disease expression requires definition.

From a practical view, the level of residual enzymatic activity could determine the eventual need for enzyme or gene therapy. In patients with substantial amounts of residual enzymatic activity (i.e., symptomatic Gaucher disease N370S homozygotes), less total enzyme may be needed than in patients who have the genotype N370S/null or other severely compromised alleles. For other lysosomal diseases, calculations based on in situ activity of enzymes indicate that very small differences in the quantity of enzyme in cells have major impacts on the phenotype.[31] Exogenously supplied enzyme might also influence the onset of specific organ, tissue, or cellular disease manifestations.

THERAPEUTIC APPROACHES AND IMPLICATIONS

The threshold hypothesis implies that small amounts of enzymatic activity may be sufficient for prevention of various disease manifestations in the lysosomal diseases. This is supported by the genotype/phenotype correlations in Tay-Sachs disease, MLD, and Gaucher disease. Strategies for the treatment of lysosomal storage diseases have been based on cross-correction experiments. In the past two decades, two major approaches have been taken to correct the underlying metabolic defects: (1) direct enzyme therapy by administering the specific, purified, lysosomal enzyme, and (2) supplying the missing normal enzyme via transplantation of organs or cells. For the latter strategy, bone marrow, liver, spleen, or skin cells could act as metabolic or enzyme pumps for delivery of enzyme to the plasma for uptake at distant sites. Both of these approaches require endocytosis via the M6P receptor system or other receptor specific to the target site of pathology. These approaches also imply the need to correct only specific cell types (i.e., those using the M6P system or bone marrow-derived cells). The normal enzyme could be supplied to deficient cells via partially corrected cell populations or by the administered enzyme. Also, these approaches apply only to soluble or solubilized enzymes in media or plasma. For membrane-bound proteins, cell-cell contact (i.e., metabolic cooperation) may be required for the direct transfer of the enzyme with subsequent targeting to the lysosome. In diseases in which the target sites of pathology may be distant from the sites of synthesis of a membrane-bound protein, delivery of enzymes via a secretory pathway will not work, and alternative strategies will be required for delivery of enzyme. Thus, the approach with enzyme therapy or cellular transplantation strategies is disease dependent and must be based on knowledge of the enzyme distribution and intra- and intercellular transport.

Substantial portions of the accumulated substrates in various tissues may be of exogenous origin (i.e., transported from distant sites and deposited in lysosomes within particular sites of pathology). Consequently, depletion of the plasma pool of these accumulating substrates may lead to a re-equilibration of previously stored material from tissue sources into the plasma. Although this is a hypothetical approach, it has been demonstrated in Fabry disease, in that previously stored substrate could be mobilized from tissue storage sites.[75] Similarly, if the accumulating substrates or toxic metabolites are transported into tissues from distant sites and the peripheral sites for accumulation can be depleted, significant impact might be obtained on pathophysiology. In the neuronopathic Gaucher disease phenotypes, some accumulating central nervous system substrate is derived from visceral sources.[76] Depletion of these visceral sources might lead to an alteration in the type or rate of central nervous system involvement in these diseases. This approach has not been exploited in many of the lysosomal storage diseases, since little is known about systemic mucopolysaccharide and glycopeptide trafficking. Additional information on the circulating pools of such metabolites will be required to determine the feasibility of this approach. However, if such depletion and re-equilibration can occur, the delivery of particular enzymes for specific diseases to the target site of pathology may not be required, and depletion of soluble (or at least transport of) toxic metabolites out of tissue sites might prove efficacious.

The implications for genetic therapeutic approaches to the treatment of lysosomal storage diseases are clear. If the deficient enzyme must be delivered directly to the target site of pathology, transplantation of the appropriate stem cell containing the appropriate genes may affect the visceral tissues. The macrophages/monocytes of liver, spleen, bone marrow, lungs, and other reticuloendothelial tissues can be replaced by bone marrow transplantation, and, thus, retroviral mediated gene transfer into bone marrow stem cells of the affected individuals should provide a cure for diseases involving these tissues. However, metabolites might not re-equilibrate out of brain rapidly enough to prevent manifestations of the disease in the central nervous system. Thus, the enzyme or cells would need to be delivered to the brain. The delivery of macromolecules and cells to the brain substance has proven to be particularly difficult and may present a significant barrier to the future development of gene therapy approaches for neurologic diseases, as it has for the treatment of neuronopathic diseases via enzyme therapy.

RESULTS AND LESSONS FROM THERAPY

The principal objective of cellular transplantation and enzyme therapy approaches has been to supply enzyme to various organs in the body via either cells or direct enzyme administration. The results and interpretations of these experiences are critically important to the development of future genetic engineering or gene therapy strategies for the lysosomal storage diseases. Based on the pluripotency of bone marrow stem cells, most transplantation studies have focused on these cells. The isolation and characterization of stem cells from other organs, including neuronal stem cells, have been encouraging and may provide pluripotent sources of enzyme in the future.[77,78] As indicated in Table 57-1, various lysosomal storage diseases have preferential sites of pathology. However, all cells in the body are involved with the enzyme deficiency, and most tissues can manifest symptoms and signs of these diseases. For bone marrow transplantation or other organ transplantations to be effective, the cells containing enzymes must be able to catabolize the substrate supplied. This ultimately depends on the mass of cells transplanted, since each cell can synthesize only a limited amount of enzyme for supply to the body. Such considerations are particularly relevant for organs like kidneys or liver, in which the cells do not migrate.

Transplantation

Bone marrow transplantation of a patient with Gaucher disease demonstrated the limitations of this strategy as an enzyme replacement approach.[79,80] Enzymatic reconstitution to about 40–50% of normal was achieved in the liver in the presence of full engraftment of the patient with normal donor bone marrow.[80] This level of enzyme corresponds to that expected with a fully reconstituted distribution space of Kupffer cells within the liver. Thus, enzymatic reconstitution did not occur in hepatocytes, since acid β-glucosidase is membrane bound and not secretable. In comparison, bone marrow transplantation of MPS (e.g., Hurler and Maroteaux-Lamy syndromes) has shown clearance of stored substrate in Kupffer cells and hepatocytes. These findings indicate that the normal, soluble enzymes (e.g., α-L-iduronidase and N-acetylgalactosamine-4-sulfatase) from the transplanted Kupffer cells can be transferred to hepatocytes and can degrade the accumulated substrate in those cells.

The results of animal and human experimentation identified a critical limitation to transplantation strategies for lysosomal storage diseases: the inability to get enzyme or sufficient bone marrow-derived cells (or both) into brain substance for metabolic correction. The delivery of the enzyme directly to the brain may not be necessary for central nervous system removal of cytotoxic substrates. However, it is theoretically desirable to deliver the enzyme to the involved cells and organs. Currently, insufficient data are available from autopsy or clinical material of transplanted humans to determine the extent of biochemical or clinical improvements in the brains of patients affected with each of the lysosomal storage diseases.

Animal models of lysosomal storage diseases have been studied extensively. The MPS I dog has a phenotype similar to humans with MPS IHS, although the central nervous system storage resembles the more severe MPS IH. Bone marrow trans-

plantation from unaffected littermates resulted in functional and pathologic improvement of bony deformity, cardiac abnormalities, corneal clouding, storage in lymphoid tissues, and hepatosplenomegaly.[81] The host hepatocytes were cleared of storage material, consistent with uptake of α-L-iduronidase from donor Kupffer cells. However, vertebral and joint changes continued to progress, although at a slower rate than untransplanted affected dogs. The central nervous system effect was difficult to evaluate from a functional level, but lysosomal distention was clearly decreased in glial cells, and there were varying improvements in neurons.

The MPS VII mouse (showing β-glucuronidase deficiency) has been used in intensive efforts to compare the effectiveness of various therapeutic regimens.[82–84] Bone marrow transplantation from syngeneic unaffected mice into irradiated MPS VII affected mice increased life span and cleared storage material from liver, spleen, kidney, and cornea. Leptomeningeal storage was improved, but neuronal lysosomal distention was identical to that of untransplanted control mice.[82] In further experiments, bone marrow stem cells from affected mice were harvested and infected with retrovirus containing β-glucuronidase sequences.[84] When transferred back into affected mice, expression of β-glucuronidase was present, and substrate clearance was achieved. Somewhat less of an effect was evident in bone, perhaps reflecting lower expression of the recombinant enzyme compared with the endogenous gene in bone marrow-derived normal cells. The effect of either therapy on the brain was difficult to detect. Measurement of enzyme activity in situ revealed almost no increase in enzyme activity in the central nervous system. Since phenotypic central nervous system manifestations of disease may be present or absent within the same range of detectable enzyme activity, it may be that the desired threshold in the central nervous system is below the level of detectable enzyme activity using current methodology.

A direct comparison of animal and human data is difficult. Histopathologic examination of tissues is much easier in animals, but the subtle effects of transplant on complex central nervous system functions can only be accomplished in humans. The effect of different genotypes at the disease-producing locus may be considerably greater in humans, in whom the genetic background is large compared with inbred animals. Nevertheless, responses to transplantation vary from animal to animal, as they do from human to human. The effect of cytoreductive therapy and graft-versus-host disease, and their interaction with the underlying disease, make the analysis of effectiveness even more complicated. If the objective of transplantation therapy for lysosomal storage disease is the complete elimination of disease, then this is rarely achieved. Preservation of function at a level below normal may be more readily achieved in selected diseases, such as MPS I. In animal model systems, particularly the MPS VII mouse model, bone marrow transplantation appears to be inferior to enzyme therapy for clearance of stored substrate from the central nervous system of affected mice.[83,85] Clearly, continued study of available animal models and rigorous evaluation of transplanted humans is necessary to determine the efficacy of these approaches for each lysosomal storage disease.

In humans the natural evolution of the tissue lesions in many of the lysosomal storage diseases and particularly in the brain are poorly documented. However, with time, these lesions probably become irreversible, and a window of opportunity may exist for achieving reversal of disease manifestations in each disease. Once the disease developmental threshold is passed, damage to the brain or other organs may continue to be progressive despite therapy. The results obtained in the Krabbe (human and murine) and Sanfilippo syndromes support this notion. Following bone marrow transplantation in the murine model of galactosylcerebrosidase deficiency (Krabbe syndrome), substantial improvements in peripheral nerve function were noted. The central nervous system manifestations continue to progress.[86] The results in the human Sanfilippo syndromes indicate an acceleration of the central nervous system disease following bone marrow transplantation. This occurred in patients who had significant central nervous system symptoms at the time of transplantation and suggests that either presymptomatic intervention is needed or that bone marrow transplantation will not be useful for treating this disease. Additional concerns relate to the partial tissue correction of an enzymatic or cellular defect. In Hurler syndrome, beneficial effects on visceral, bone marrow, and brain function were evident following bone marrow transplantation. The bony disease apparently progresses, and can become crippling in some long-term, fully engrafted patients.[87] In comparison, a patient with juvenile MLD had complete peripheral reconstitution of enzymatic activity. Although excellent central nervous system results were obtained in the short-term, progressive central nervous system deterioration began several years later in one patient who maintained full engraftment.

These results suggest that in particular organs (i.e., bone and central nervous system) transplantation may convert the disease from an earlier onset, severe abnormality to a later onset progressive disease. Transplantation with bone marrow will have its greatest beneficial effects in individuals who have primarily a single cell line involved in the disease process, which can be replaced by transplantation. This is exemplified by Gaucher disease, in which bone marrow transplantation cures the visceral lesions if instituted prior to irreversible damage in liver, spleen, lung, or bone marrow.[79,80,88,89] Clearly, bone marrow transplantation's effects on the resolution or progression of signs and symptoms have been disease and stage specific. Such transplantation is probably not warranted in patients with severe irreversible pathology. Careful baseline evaluation, selection, and follow-up of patients will be required to assess the therapeutic impact of bone marrow transplantation in the lysosomal storage diseases.

The results of transplantation of other organs in these diseases including the liver, kidney, and spleen, have been limited and less convincing. In those diseases that result from soluble enzyme defects, hepatic, splenic, or other solid organ transplantation may be beneficial, if sufficient amounts of enzyme can be synthesized and secreted for delivery to distant sources. In comparison, for diseases such as Gaucher disease, in which the enzyme is not secreted, transplantation of liver has resulted in the reaccumulation of Gaucher cells and redevelopment of pathology in transplanted livers.[90] These results indicate that hepatic transplantation alone is insufficient for preventing redevelopment of symptoms in such severely involved patients. Blood chimerism may develop following hepatic transplantation, since the donor liver may supply small amounts of enzyme and myeloid cells to recipient organs.[91] In the absence of concomitant enzyme replacement therapy, patients receiving hepatic transplantation and small amounts of donor bone marrow may become chimeric and develop two populations of bone marrow-derived cells in their body: those that are normal and those that are not. At a low level of chimerism, the storage cells would be expected to accumulate in tissues and in the absence of cross-correction eventually result in disease manifestations.

Enzyme Replacement

In comparison with the large number of diseases that have been subjected to organ transplantation, enzyme therapy has been extensively studied only in Gaucher disease. Enzyme therapy in this disease exploits the receptor for α-mannosyl-terminated oligosaccharide on the surface of cells of monocyte/macrophage origin for targeting the enzyme to these cells. The membrane-bound acid β-glucosidase is extracted from placental tissue, purified to homogeneity, treated with exoglycosidases to expose α-mannosyl groups, and intravenously administered to affected patients. Several independent studies have demonstrated the utility of this approach and, indeed, most patients have remarkable improvement following enzyme therapy.[92–98]

The population of reported patients is sufficiently varied to provide insight into the expected responses for individual patients during treatment. By 1 year of enzyme therapy (1) patients with hepatomegaly will have an approximately 20–30% decrease in liver volume, (2) patients with intact spleens will have an approximately 30–50% decrease in splenic volume, (3) anemic patients will have a 1.5 g% hemoglobin increase, with 33–50% of such patients achieving normal hemoglobin levels, and (4) mildly thrombocytopenic patients will normalize their platelet count, while those with lower platelet counts will double theirs. For liver and splenic volume decreases and hemoglobin increases, about 50% of patients met or exceeded these responses by 6 months. Patients on higher doses have somewhat better responses than those on smaller doses, but the dose/response relationships are not linear. In general, patients with massive splenic enlargement have poor hematologic responses until the spleen decreases below 20-fold greater than the expected volume (0.2% of body weight). These findings are sufficiently consistent to warrant additional evaluation for intercurrent illness if these guidelines are not met. The variation in response to enzyme therapy is great among patients and at different times during therapy in one patient. Consequently, insufficient data are available to conclude firmly greater efficacy of any dosing schedule or regimen.

Furthermore, the hepatic and splenic volume changes are more rapid, whereas the bony and pulmonary involvements are slow (as detected with current radiographic and pulmonary function tests). One cannot exclude the possibility that each tissue has a different dose-response threshold. This is of particular concern in light of the inability to discern bony or pulmonary changes during the period of rapid dose reduction, while maintaining hematologic, hepatic, and splenic improvement rates. However, few data are available on the tissue, cellular, and subcellular distribution or the half-lives of the enzyme administered. Data in mice suggest that the enzyme has relatively low uptake by monocyte/macrophage cells[99] and very different distinct uptake and survival patterns in bone marrow, liver, and lung.[94,100] In two treated patients, exogenous enzyme appeared to persist for a significant period in selected organs.[94] The paucity of such data continues to limit rational optimization of doses and dosing schedules.

In view of the high cost of enzyme therapy with all current infusion protocols, the timing of the initiation of therapy must be carefully evaluated. Highly symptomatic patients should begin therapy immediately. In addition, other patients with major hematologic and visceral organ involvement should receive high priority for therapy. Although bone disease appears to be the slowest to respond, patients with substantial bone involvement are candidates for treatment to recover bone integrity and to prevent irreversibility of some bony damage. More difficult questions are posed by presymptomatic patients, whose susceptibility to major disease manifestations can be anticipated by genotype analysis.[73] Clearly, the issue of the timing and use of an apparently universally effective therapy must be carefully considered and evaluated.

Using Gaucher disease as a prototype, several difficult scientific issues need to be resolved in an effort to promote optimal use of therapeutic strategies in the lysosomal storage diseases. There is extensive interpatient variability in dose response. What are the determinants of this variability? Will the effects of more easily accessed tissues be preferentially evaluated rather than those in more difficult, potentially more relevant, tissues?

THERAPEUTIC RECOMMENDATIONS FOR GAUCHER DISEASE

During the past several years, enzyme therapy for Gaucher disease has proved efficacious and safe for reversing the major signs and symptoms of affected patients. In >100 reported patients with Gaucher disease treated by the intravenous administration of α-mannosyl-terminated glucocerebrosidase (acid β-glucosidase), efficacy has been demonstrated in essentially all. The anemia, thrombocytpenia, and leukopenia were improved within the first 4–8 months of therapy in most patients. Substantial decreases of hepatic and splenic volumes have been documented in most patients within 6 months, and essentially in all patients by about 1 year. Symptomatic and architectural improvements in bony manifestations have been observed much more slowly, with responses requiring ≥2–3 years. The episodes of acute bony crises that some patients with Gaucher disease experience are lessened within the first year of therapy, long before architectural changes in bone can be detected. Clearly, the use of enzyme replacement therapy has become the standard of care for patients affected with Gaucher disease and is a critically important adjunct to therapy for all patients affected with this illness.

Although the vast majority of patients treated with enzyme therapy have been affected with non-neuronopathic or type 1 Gaucher disease, additional data on the neuronopathic variants (i.e., types 2 and 3) should become available within the next year. Anecdotal evidence in a patient with type 2 disease indicates a substantial improvement in both visceral and central nervous system involvement compared with a matched sibling. Enzyme therapy was initiated shortly after birth and prior to the onset of symptomatology. In this patient, substantial neurologic development has been achieved. Brain stem deficits have occurred, but at a rate that was much more slowly progressive than in her affected sibling. In addition type 2 patients treated with enzyme therapy following the onset of severe central nervous system involvement, no documentable improvement or effect on the central nervous system or visceral disease was obtained. Although several studies are ongoing to evaluate the efficacy of enzyme therapy in type 3 disease, no data are available. The effects in visceral organs are to be expected from the targeted delivery of enzyme to macrophage/monocyte-derived cells, whereas the effect on brain is not explicable by this mechanism. Studies in animals have indicated that intravenously administered α-mannose-terminated glucocerebrosidase does not enter the central nervous system. Consequently, the therapeutic results must derive from an indirect mechanism.

Current recommendations for baseline assessment prior to institution of enzyme therapy in patients with Gaucher disease type 1 include the following:

Establishment of the diagnosis of Gaucher disease by enzyme testing in suspected patients; bone marrow examination may be a useful adjunct but is insufficient to establish the diagnosis

Quantitative hepatic and splenic volume measurements by magnetic resonance imaging or computed tomography studies; ultrasound or physical examination assessments lack the needed precision for monitoring efficacy and can be misleading

Determination of the extent and types of bony involvement by skeletal radiographic surveys, quantitative com puted tomography, or densimetric assessments of bone calcium

Magnetic resonance imaging or technetium sulphur colloid scans of bone marrow to evaluate the extent and type of involvement by Gaucher disease

Pulmonary and liver function studies

Evaluation of cytopenias to exclude intercurrent causes

Endocrinologic and nutritional assessments in children with growth retardation or failure to thrive

Evaluation of coagulopathies

These studies should be conducted to assess patient changes during therapy about every 6 months for the first 18 months of therapy after this initial period. Depending on the rate of improvement, the time of restudy can be lengthened to 1 year. Lack of improvement should prompt evaluations for concomitant diseases. Every effort should be made to exclude intercurrent problems such as iron deficiency or its development while on enzyme therapy. The presence of malignancies, unrelated hepatic, renal, or pulmonary disease, and any nutritional deficiencies could blunt the effects of therapy.

Except in rare circumstances, splenectomy is not necessary for the treatment of Gaucher disease, since it is reversible by enzyme therapy. Total or partial splenectomy should be considered in patients in whom the organ size is sufficiently large to compromise cardiopulmonary function. Older individuals with severe thrombocytopenia or anemia, who are at substantial risk of internal hemorrhage or cardiac failure, may require the more immediate hematologic correction produced by splenectomy. The presence or absence of the spleen has no obvious influence on the efficacy of enzyme therapy.

All patients with significant involvement by Gaucher disease should be considered candidates for enzyme therapy. These will include patients with progressing mild disease, as well as individuals who are moderately to severely involved at initial evaluation. Individuals with substantial bony, hepatic, or splenic involvement, as well as cytopenia, should be considered for immediate institution of enzyme therapy. Individuals with documented Gaucher disease involvement of the lungs and pulmonary compromise should be given very high priority for the institution of enzyme therapy, since this is a highly lethal complication of Gaucher disease that is correctable. Irrespective of initial mildness of involvement, patients with progressive disease and worsening symptomatology should also be candidates for enzyme therapy. Older individuals who are documented to be asymptomatic, mildly affected, or have been serendipitously discovered to have acid β-glucosidase deficiency are not candidates for enzyme replacement therapy.

Nearly all the patients receiving enzyme therapy have been very symptomatic from their Gaucher disease. The potential to predict the future degree of involvement by Gaucher disease from genotype provides an opportunity for presymptomatic intervention. Since the vast majority of patients studied to date have massive organomegaly or severe cytopenias, the major efforts have been directed at reversal of symptomatology. By contrast, presymptomatic intervention could prevent the development of significant disease later in life. Recommendations for treating presymptomatic individuals hinges on the safety of enzyme replacement, but does provide a potential for a more cost-effective intervention compared with attempting reversal of gross pathology of the disease.

Several different dosing schedules and doses of Ceredase (alglucerase) have been used and demonstrated to be efficacious. Although the optimal regimen has not been established, an initial dose of 30–60 IU/kg body weight/mo has demonstrated efficacy. The dosing regimen can be either as biweekly infusions of one-half the monthly dose or more frequent administration (i.e., 3×/wk) to the aggregate monthly dose indicated above. The responses to specific doses of enzyme are highly individual and should be adjusted up or down depending on the particular patient's response. In some individuals, substantially more enzyme may be required to obtain therapeutic effects, and these individuals might benefit from more highly fractionated dosing regimens. These latter individuals are usually extraordinarily ill and have some of the most severe manifestations of Gaucher disease. In addition, the lowest effective doses for maintaining improvement or the state of improvement have not been established, but could be 10–20 IU/kg/mo as an aggregate dose.

Approximately 10–15% of patients develop antibodies to alglucerase. Of these about one-half become symptomatic with pruritus or urticaria (or both) or other vague symptoms during the infusion. Most of these adverse events are treatable by premedicating with appropriate H_1 and H_2 histamine receptor blockers. To date, all antibody reactions have been IgG mediated, and some patients have experienced complement activation. A few IgG-mediated anaphylactoid reactions have occurred, but these are rare. Non-antibody-mediated adverse events also have occurred. These include nausea, vomiting, diarrhea, chest pain, fever, exaggeration of existing bony pain, and transient decreases in blood pressure. These are poorly characterized and will require investigation to establish etiology, as well as methods of treatment. Since most patients who do develop antibodies do so within the the first 6–9 months, it is recommended that the enzyme be given under medical observation for about the first 9 months prior to initiation of home care.

Although enzyme therapy has clearly become the standard of care for the treatment of patients with Gaucher disease type 1, additional adjunct therapies and supportive care are also important in the overall treatment of these patients. These include transfusions, partial and total splenectomies in selected patients, joint replacement when indicated, and, in some patients organ transplantation for severe effects of terminal Gaucher disease. Furthermore, Gaucher disease is a life-long chronic illness with profound financial and psychological impact. Any comprehensive treatment program for affected patients must also include psychological, psychiatric, family, and social support.

Will certain tissues require specific doses of enzyme on cells that will determine overall efficacy of therapy? Is there a concomitant diminution in the need for intensive therapy for continued improvement as the tissues are healed? Most importantly, what is the window of opportunity for effective therapy? Is it more efficacious to prevent the disease manifestations than to attempt to return a very sick individual, with potentially irreversible tissue damage, to health? This is particularly relevant for those disorders that involve the central nervous system.

Gene Transfer

Lysosomal diseases that can be treated successfully by bone marrow transplantation should be amenable to permanent correction by gene therapy using hematopoietic stem cells carrying a copy of the normal gene. Following autologous transplantation with these corrected cells, somatic genetic reconstitution could be achieved by the repopulation of tissues with monocyte/macrophage-derived cells. For diseases due to defects of soluble enzymes, only a portion of stem cells would need to be corrected, since the corrected cells could supply enzyme to other tissues. For diseases that result from membrane-bound enzymes (e.g., Gaucher disease), all or most of the cells would need to be corrected, since the enzyme cannot cross-correct other cells, and tissue macrophage chimerism could have pathophysiologic effects. For either of these types of enzyme defects, the amount of enzyme supplied to tissues directly or via cellular replacement would be mass dependent, and insufficient amounts of enzyme or cells would lead to the redevelopment or only the delay in of symptoms and signs. In addition, stem cells that produce active lysosomal enzymes do not have any obvious proliferative advantage over those that do not. Thus, therapeutic effects would be expected only if the patient's untransformed cells were ablated by chemotherapy or irradiation. Rational strategy for the treatment of these diseases would include marrow ablation followed by autologous transplantation with transformed hematopoietic stem cells.[84] Considerable effort has been expended to develop the required efficient gene transfer technology and hematopoietic stem cell culture systems. Significant long-term expression of transgenes has been accomplished with several of these enzymes.[101–104] Protocols for somatic gene therapy of lysosomal diseases will be evaluated during the next few years.

DIAGNOSIS

The increasing elucidation of the molecular lesions causing the lysosomal storage diseases has provided insight into the great heterogeneity within each of these diseases. In addition, the proliferation of tests for the specific genetic lesions has led many investations to substitute molecular testing for enzyme-based diagnoses. The great specificity of molecular testing is its downfall, whereas the more generic nature of enzyme testing is a major strength. For any of the disease categories listed in Table 57-1, the diagnosis is established by detection of the specific enzyme defect. In experienced laboratories many of these assays are accurately performed and will establish a specific diagnosis. Once the diagnosis is established, additional molecular testing can provide supplementary information and, in some instances, prognostic insight. Because of the presence of "pseudodeficient alleles" in some lysosomal diseases, molecular testing and other adjunct investigations (e.g., sulfatide loading studies) are necessary to establish fully a phenotype and prognosis. Every effort should be made to characterize these patients thoroughly and completely at the clinical, biochemical, and molecular levels since such characterization is of utmost importance. Detailed neurologic and physical assessments by imaging and clinical examinations should be performed in all patients longitudinally so that the effects of intervention or the relationship of specific mutations to phenotype can be evaluated.

REFERENCES

1. deDuve C: Lysosomes revisited. Eur J Biochem 137:391, 1983
2. Hers HG: Inborn lysosomal diseases. Gastroenterology 48:625, 1965
3. Hers HG, Van Hoof F: The genetic pathology of lysosomes. Prog Liver Dis 3:185, 1970
4. Hannun YA, Bell RM: Lysosphingolipids inhibit protein kinase C: implications for the sphingolipidoses. Science 235:670, 1987
5. Goldstein JL, Brown MS, Anderson RGW et al: Receptor mediated endocytosis: concepts emerging from the LDL receptor system. Annu Rev Cell Biol 1:1, 1979
6. Rome LH, Weissmann B, Neufeld EF: Direct demonstration of binding of a lysosomal enzyme alpha-L-iduronidase, to receptors on cultured fibroblasts. Proc Natl Acad Sci USA 76:2331, 1979
7. Fratantoni JC, Hall CW, Neufeld EF: The defect in Hurler and Hunter syndromes. II: deficiency of specific factors involved in mucopolysaccharide degradation. Proc Natl Acad Sci USA 64:360, 1969
8. Fisher HD, Gonzalez-Noriega A, Sly WS, Morre DJ: Phosphomannosyl enzyme receptors in rat liver. J Biol Chem 255:9608, 1980
9. Varki A, Kornfeld A: Lysosomal enzyme targeting: N-acetylglucosaminylphosphotransferase selectively phosphorylated native lysosomal enzymes. J Biol Chem 256:11977, 1981
10. Kornfeld S, Mellman I: The biogenesis of lysosomes. Annu Rev Cell Biol 5: 483, 1989
11. Waheed S, Pohlmann R, Hasilik A, von Figura K: Subcellular location of two enzymes involved in the synthesis of phosphorylated recognition markers in lysosomal enzymes. J Biol Chem 256:4150, 1981
12. Braun M, Waheed A, von Figura K: Lysosomal acid phosphatase is transported to lysosomes via the cell surface. EMBO J 8:3633, 1989
13. Greenberg J, Howell KE: Membrane traffic in endocytosis: insights from cell free assays. Annu Rev Cell Biol 5:453, 1989
14. Pryer NK, Wuestehube LJ, Schekman R: Vesicle-mediated protein sorting. Annu Rev Biochem 61:471, 1992
15. Dahms NM, Lobel P, Kornfeld S: Mannose 6-phosphate receptors and lysosomal enzyme targeting. J Biol Chem 264:12115, 1989
16. Barriocanal JG, Bonifacino JS, Yuan L, Sandoval IV: Biosynthesis, glycosylation, movement through the Golgi system and transport to lysosomes by N-linked carbohydrate independent mechanism of three lysosomal integral membrane proteins. J Biol Chem 261:1604, 1986
17. Kornfeld R, Kornfeld S: Assembly of asparagine-linked oligosaccharides. Annu Rev Biochem 54:663, 1985
18. Gieselmann V, Schmidt B, von Figura K: In vitro mutagenesis of potential N-glycosylation sites of arylsulfatase A. Effects on glycosylation, phosphorylation, and intracellular sorting. J Biol Chem 267:13262, 1992
19. Dow KE, Riopelle RJ: Influence of N-linked oligosaccharides on the processing and neurite-promoting activity of proteoglycans released by neurons in vitro. Cell Tissue Res 268:553, 1992
20. Furst W, Machleidt W, Sandhoff K: The precursor of sulfatide activator protein is processed to three different proteins. Biol Chem Hoppe Seyler 369: 317, 1988
21. Nakano T, Sandhoff K, Stumper J et al: Structure of full-length cDNA coding for sulfatide activator, a Co-beta-glucosidase and two other homologous proteins: two alternate forms of the sulfatide activator. J Biochem 105:152, 1989
22. O'Brien JS, Kretz KA, Dewji N et al: Coding of two sphingolipid activator proteins (SAP-1 and SAP-2) by same genetic locus. Science 241:1098, 1988
23. Gavrieli-Rorman E, Grabowski GA: Molecular cloning of a human co-β-glucosidase cDNA: evidence the four sphingolipid hydrolase activator proteins are encoded by single genes in humans and rats. Genomics 5:486, 1989
24. Rorman EG, Scheinker V, Grabowski GA: Structure and evolution of the human prosaposin chromosomal gene. Genomics 13:312, 1992
25. Morreau H, Galjart NJ, Willemsen R et al: Human lysosomal protective protein. Glycosylation, intracellular transport, and association with beta-galactosidase in the endoplasmic reticulum. J Biol Chem 267:17949, 1992
26. Zhou XY, Galjart NJ, Willemsen R et al: A mutation in a mild form of galactosialidosis impairs dimerization of the protective protein and renders it unstable. EMBO J 10:4041, 1991
27. Nauseef W, Olsson I, Arnljots K: Biosynthesis and processing of myeloperoxidase: a marker for myeloid differentiation. Eur J Hematol 40:97, 1988
28. Young EP: Prenatal diagnosis of Hurler disease by analysis of alpha-iduronidase in chorionic villi. J Inherit Metab Dis 15:224, 1992
29. Grabowski GA, Dinur T, Gatt S, Desnick RJ: Gaucher type I (Ashkenazi) disease: a new method for heterozyote detection using a novel fluorescent natural substrate. Clin Chim Acta 124:123, 1982
30. Conzelmann E, Sandhoff K: Partial enzyme deficiencies: residual activities and the development of neurological disorders. Dev Neurosci 6:58, 1983
31. Leinekugel P, Michel S, Conzelman E, Sandhoff K: Quantitative correlation

between the residual activity of beta-hexosaminidase A and arylsulfatase A and the severity of the resulting lysosomal storage disease. Hum Genet 88:513, 1992
32. Inui K, Nishimoto J, Taniike M et al: Study of pathogenesis in twitcher mouse, an enzymatically authentic model of Krabbe's disease. J Neurol Sci 100:124, 1990
33. Thomas PK: Inherited neuropathies related to disorders of lipid metabolism. Adv Neurol 48:133, 1988
34. Suzuki K: Neuropathology of late onset gangliosidoses. A review. Dev Neurosci 13:205, 1991
35. Desnick RJ, Bishop DF: Fabry disease: alpha-galactosidase deficiency; Schindler disease: alpha-N-acetylgalactosaminidase deficiency. p. 1751. In Scriver CR, Beaudet AL, Sly WS, Valle D (eds): The Metabolic Basis of Inherited Disease. 6th Ed. McGraw-Hill, New York, 1989
36. Schmitz G, Assman G: Acid lipase deficiency. p. 1623. In Scriver CR, Beaudet AL, Sly WS, Valle D (eds): The Metabolic Basis of Inherited Disease. 6th Ed. McGraw-Hill, New York, 1989
37. Parkin JL, Brunning RD: Pathology of the Gaucher cell. Prog Clin Biol Res 95:151, 1982
38. Kattlove HE, Williams JC, Gaynor E et al: Gaucher cells in chronic myelocytic leukemia: an acquired abnormality. Blood 33:379, 1969
39. Sharratt GP, Price D, Curtis JA, Cornel G: Gaucher's disease with mitral valve calcification, letter. Pediatr Cardiol 13:127, 1992
40. van Echten G, Sandhoff K: Ganglioside metabolism: enzymology, topology and regulation. J Biol Chem 268:5341, 1993
41. Hakomori S-I: Bifunctional role of glycosphingolipids. J Biol Chem 265:18713, 1990
42. Kobayashi T, Goto I, Okada S et al: Accumulation of lysosphingolipids in tissues from patients with GM1 and GM2 gangliosidoses. J Neurochem 59: 1452, 1992
43. Sugama S, Eto Y, Yamamoto H, Kim SU: Psychosine cytotoxicity toward rat C6 glioma cells and the protective effects of phorbol ester and dimethylsulfoxide: implications for therapy in Krabbe's disease. Brain Dev 13:104, 1991
44. Nilsson O, Mansson JE, Hakansson G, Svennerholm L: The occurrence of psychosine and other glycolipids in spleen and liver from the three major types of Gaucher's disease. Biochim Biophys Acta 712:453, 1982
45. Gery I, Davies P, Derr J et al: Relationship between production and release of lymphocyte-activating factor (interleukin 1) by murine macrophages. 1. Effects of various agents. Cell Immunol 64:293, 1981
46. Gery I, Zigler JS Jr, Brady RO, Barranger JA: Selective effects of glucocerebroside (Gaucher's storage material) on macrophage cultures. J Clin Invest 68: 1182, 1981
47. Lee RE: The pathology of Gaucher disease. Prog Clin Biol Res 95:177, 1982
48. Uemura K-I, Sugiyama E, Taketomi T: Effects of an inhibitor of glucosylceramide synthase on glycosphingolipid synthesis and neurite outgrowth in murine neuroblastoma cell lines. J Biochem 110:96, 1991
49. Beutler E, Grabowski GA: Glucosylceramide lipidoses: Gaucher disease. In Scriver CR, Beaudet AL, Sly WS, Valle D (eds): The Metabolic Basis of Inherited Disease. 7th Ed. McGraw-Hill, New York, 1994
50. Grace ME, Newman KM, Scheinker V et al: Analysis of human acid beta-glucosidase by site-directed mutagenesis and heterologous expression. J Biol Chem 269:2283, 1994
51. O'Brien JS: The beta-galactosidase deficiencies. p. 1797. In Scriver CR, Beaudet AL, Sly WS, Valle D (eds): The Metabolic Basis of Inherited Disease. 6th Ed. McGraw-Hill, New York, 1989
52. Yoshida K, Oshima A, Sakuraba H et al: GM1 gangliosidosis in adults: clinical and molecular analysis of 16 Japanese patients. Ann Neurol 31:328, 1992
53. Mahuran DJ: The biochemistry of HEXA and HEXB gene mutations causing GM2 gangliosidosis. Biochim Biophys Acta 1096:87, 1991
54. Burg J, Conzelmann E, Sandhoff K et al: Mapping of the gene coding for the human GM2 activator protein to chromosome 5. Ann Hum Genet 49:41, 1985
55. Schnabel D, Schreoder M, Furst W et al: Simultaneous deficiency of sphingolipid activator proteins 1 and 2 is caused by a mutation in the initiation codon of their common gene. J Biol Chem 267:3312, 1992
56. Schnabel D, Schröder M, Sandhoff K: Mutation in the sphingolipid activator protein 2 in a patient with a variant of Gaucher disease. FEBS Lett 284:57, 1991
57. Holtschmidt H, Sandhoff K, Kwon HY et al: Sulfatide activator protein: alternative splicing that generates three mRNAs and a newly found mutation responsible for a clinical disease. J Biol Chem 266:7556, 1991
58. Rafi MA, Zhang X-L, DeGala G, Wenger DA: Detection of a point mutation in sphingolipid activator protein-1 mRNA in patients with a variant from metachromatic leukodystrophy. Biochem Biophys Res Commun 166:1017, 1990
59. Sandhoff K, Conzelmann E, Neufeld EF et al: The GM2-gangliosidoses. p.

1807. In Scriver CR, Beaudet AL, Sly WS, Valle D (eds): The Metabolic Basis of Inherited Disease. 6th Ed. McGraw-Hill, New York, 1989

60. Furst W, Sandhoff K: Activator proteins and topology of lysosomal sphingolipid catabolism. Biochim Biophys Acta 1126:1, 1992

61. Hiraiwa M, Soeda S, Kishimoto Y, O'Brien JS: Binding and transport of gangliosides by prosaposin. Proc Natl Acad Sci USA 89:11254, 1992

62. Berent SL, Radin NS: Beta-glucosidase activator protein from bovine spleen ("coglucosidase"). Arch Biochem Biophys 208:248, 1981

63. Harzer K, Paton BC, Poulos A et al: Sphingolipid activator protein deficiency in a 16-week-old atypical Gaucher disease patient and his fetal sibling: biochemical signs of combined sphingolipidoses. Eur J Pediatr 149:31, 1989

64. Gieselmann V, Polten A, Kreysing J et al: Molecular genetics of metachromatic leukodystrophy. Dev Neurosci 13:222, 1991

65. Gieselmann V, Fluharty AL, Tennesen T, von Figura K: Mutations in the arylsulfatase A pseudodeficiency allele causing metachromatic leukodystrophy. Am J Hum Genet 49:407, 1991

66. Kappler J, Pötter W, Gieselmann V et al: Phenotypic consequences of low arylsulfatase A genotypes (ASAp/ASAp and ASA-/ASAp): does there exist an association with multiple sclerosis? Dev Neurosci 13:228, 1991

67. Kreysing J, Bohne W, Bosenberg C et al: High residual arylsulfatase A (ASA) activity in a patient with late-infantile metachromatic leukodystrophy. Am J Hum Genet 53:339, 1993

68. Triggs-Raine BL, Mules EH, Kaback MM et al: A pseudodeficiency allele common in non-Jewish Tay-Sachs carriers: implications for carrier screening. Am J Hum Genet 51:793, 1992

69. Gravel RA, Triggs-Raine BL, Mahuran DJ: Biochemistry and genetics of Tay-Sachs disease. Can J Neurol Sci 18:419, 1991

70. Navon R: Molecular and clinical heterogeneity of adult GM2 gangliosidosis. Dev Neurosci 13:295, 1991

71. Grabowski GA: Gaucher disease: enzymology, genetics and therapy. p. 377. In Hirschhorn K, Harris H (eds): Advances in Human Genetics. 21st Ed. Plenum, New York, 1993

72. Agmon V, Cherbu S, Degan A et al: Synthesis of novel fluorescent glycosphingolipids: use in determining acid beta-glucosidase activity in situ and correlation with genotype in Gaucher disease. Biochim Biophys Acta 1170:72, 1993

73. Sibille A, Eng C, Kim S-G et al: Phenotype/genotype correlations in Gaucher disease type 1: clinical and therapeutic implications. Am J Hum Genet 52:1094, 1993

74. Brady RO, Barton NW, Grabowski GA: The role of neurogenetics in Gaucher disease. Arch Neurol 50:1212, 1993

75. Desnick RJ, Grabowski GA: Advances in the treatment of inherited metabolic diseases. Adv Hum Genet 11:281, 1981

76. Nilsson O, Svennerholm L: Accumulation of glucosylceramide and glucosylsphingosine (psychosine) in cerebrum and cerebellum in infantile and juvenile Gaucher disease. J Neurochem 39:709, 1982

77. Ryder EF, Snyder EY, Cepko CL: Establishment and characterization of multipotent neural cell lines using retrovirus vector-mediated oncogene transfer. J Neurobiol 21:356, 1990

78. Snyder EY, Deitcher DL, Walsh C et al: Multipotent neural cell lines can engraft and participate in development of mouse cerebellum. Cell 68:33, 1992

79. Starer F, Sargent JD, Hobbs JR: Regression of the radiological changes of Gaucher's disease following bone marrow transplantation. Br J Radiol 60:1189, 1987

80. Tsai P, Lipton JM, Sahdev I et al: Allogenic bone marrow transplantation in severe Gaucher disease. Pediatr Res 31:503, 1992

81. Breider MA, Shull RM, Constanopoulos G: Long-term effects of bone marrow transplantation in dogs with mucopolysaccharidosis I. Am J Pathol 134:677, 1989

82. Birkenmeier EH: Correction of murine mucopolysaccharidosis type VII (MPS VII) by bone marrow transplantation and gene transfer therapy. Hum Gene Ther 2:113, 1991

83. Birkenmeier EH, Barker JE, Vogler CA et al: Increased life span and correction of metabolic defects in murine mucopolysaccharidosis type VII after syngeneic bone marrow transplantation. Blood 78:3081, 1991

84. Wolfe JH, Sands MS, Barker JE et al: Reversal of pathology in murine mucopolysaccharidosis type VII by somatic cell gene transfer. Nature 360:749, 1992

85. Sands MS, Barker JE, Vogler C et al: Treatment of murine mucopolysacchar-

idosis type VII by syngeneic bone marrow transplantation in neonates. Lab Invest 68:676, 1993

86. Hoogerbrugge PM, Suzuki K, Poorthuis BJ et al: Donor-derived cells in the central nervous system of twitcher mice after bone marrow transplantation. Science 239:1035, 1988

87. Krivit W, Shapiro EG: Bone marrow transplantation for storage diseases. p. 203. In Desnick RJ (ed): Treatment of Genetic Diseases. Churchill Livingstone, New York, 1991

88. Svennerholm L, Erikson A, Groth CG et al: Norrbottnian type of Gaucher disease—clinical, biochemical and molecular biology aspects: successful treatment with bone marrow transplantation. Dev Neurosci 13:345, 1991

89. Erikson A, Groth CG, Mansson JE et al: Clinical and biochemical outcome of marrow transplantation for Gaucher disease of the Norrbottnian type. Acta Paediatr Scand 79:680, 1990

90. Carlson DE, Busuttil RW, Giudici TA, Barranger JA: Orthotopic liver transplantation in the treatment of complications of type 1 Gaucher disease. Transplantation 49:1192, 1990

91. Starzl T, Demetris AJ, Trucco M et al: Cell migration and chimerism after whole-organ transplantation: the basis of graft acceptance. Hepatology 17:1127, 1993

92. Grabowski GA, Barton N: Efficacy and safety of recombinant alglucerase for the therapy of Gaucher disease type 1. J Clin Invest 1993 (in preparation)

93. Barton NW, Brady RO, Dambrosia JM et al: Replacement therapy for inherited enzyme deficiency—macrophage-targeted glucocerebrosidase for Gaucher's disease. N Engl J Med 324:1464, 1991

94. Fallet S, Grace ME, Sibille A et al: Enzyme augmentation in moderate to life-threatening Gaucher disease. Pediatr Res 31:496, 1992

95. Pastores G, Sibille A, Grabowski GA: Enzyme therapy in Gaucher disease type 1: dosage efficacy and adverse effects in thirty-three patients treated for six to twenty-four months. Blood 82:408, 1993

96. Figueroa ML, Rosenbloom BE, Kay A et al: A less costly regimen of alglucerase to treat Gaucher's disease. N Engl J Med 327:1632, 1992

97. Beutler E, Kay A, Saven A et al: Enzyme replacement therapy for Gaucher disease. Blood 78:1183, 1991

98. Grabowski GA: The future of therapy in Gaucher disease. Horizons 1:3, 1992

99. Sato Y, Beutler E: Binding, internalization and degradation of mannose-terminated glucocerebrosidase by macrophages. J Clin Invest 91:1909, 1993

100. Xu Y-H, Leonova T, Ponce E, Grabowski GA: Tissue distribution and half-lives of intravenously administered alglucerase. (submitted)

101. Mulligan RC: The basic science of gene therapy. Science 260:926, 1993

102. Fink JK, Correll PH, Perry LK et al: Correction of glucocerebrosidase deficiency after retroviral-mediated gene transfer into hematopoietic progenitor cells from patients with Gaucher disease. Proc Natl Acad Sci USA 87:2334, 1990

103. Nolta JA, Yu XJ, Bahner I, Kohn DB: Retroviral-mediated transfer of the human glucocerebrosidase gene into cultured Gaucher bone marrow. J Clin Invest 90:342, 1992

104. Correl PH, Colilla S, Dave HPG, Karlsson S: High levels of human glucocerebrosidase activity in macrophages of long-term reconstitued mice after retroviral infection of hematopoietic stem cells. Blood 80:331, 1992

105. Neufeld EF, Muenzer J: The mucopolysaccharidoses. p. 1565. In Scriver CR, Beaudet AL, Sly WS, Valle D (eds): The Metabolic Basis of Inherited Disease. 6th Ed. McGraw-Hill, New York, 1989

106. Beaudet AL, Thomas GH: The glycoproteinoses: mannosidosis, fucosidosis, sialidosis and aspartylglucosaminuria. p. 1603. In Scriver CR, Beaudet AL, Sly WS, Valle D (eds): The Metabolic Basis of Inherited Disease. 6th Ed. McGraw-Hill, New York, 1989

107. Nolan CM, Sly WS: I-cell diseases and pseudohurler polydystrophy. p. 1589. In Scriver CR, Beaudet AL, Sly WS, Valle D (eds): The Metabolic Basis of Inherited Disease. 6th Ed. McGraw-Hill, New York, 1989

108. Kolodny EH: Metachromatic leukodystrophy and multiple sulfatase deficiency. p. 1721. In Scriver CR, Beaudet AL, Sly WS, Valle D (eds): The Metabolic Basis of Inherited Disease. 6th Ed. McGraw-Hill, New York, 1989

109. Suzuki K, Suzuki Y: Galactosylceramide lipidosis: globoid cell leukodystrophy (Krabbe disease). p. 1699. In Scriver CR, Beaudet AL, Sly WS, Valle D (eds): The Metabolic Basis of Inherited Disease. 6th Ed. McGraw-Hill, New York, 1989

110. Schuchman EH, Desnick RJ: Niemann-Pick disease: sphingomyelin storage diseases. In Scriver CR, Beaudet AL, Sly WS, Valle D (eds): The Metabolic Basis of Inherited Disease. 7th Ed. McGraw-Hill, New York, 1994

111. Moser HW, Moser AB, Chen WW, Schram AW: Ceramidase deficiency. p. 1699. In Scriver CR, Beaudet AL, Sly WS, Valle D (eds): The Metabolic Basis of Inherited Disease. 6th Ed. McGraw-Hill, New York, 1989

Infectious Mononucleosis and Other Epstein-Barr Virus-Associated Diseases

58

John L. Sullivan and Bruce A. Woda

INTRODUCTION

Knowledge of the association of Epstein-Barr virus (EBV) with diseases of lymphoreticular and hematopoietic tissue began in 1964 with the discovery of the virus.[1] Clinically apparent EBV infection was probably first described in 1885 by the Russian pediatrician Filatov as an idiopathic lymphadenopathy in childhood.[2] In 1885, Pfeiffer[3] described glandular fever, and the term *infectious mononucleosis* (IM) was first used in 1923 by Sprunt and Evans.[4] Paul and Bunnell[5] described the appearance of heterophile antibodies during the course of IM, and Davidsohn and Walker[6] devised the differential absorption test, which rendered the heterophile antibody test highly specific for IM.

A major advance in our understanding of EBV infection occurred in 1966, when Gertrude and Werner Henle[7,8] developed indirect immunofluorescent antibody assays that detected EBV-specific viral antigens. In 1968, the Henles[9] made a critical observation when they noted that seroconversion to EBV occurred during the course of acute IM. Furthermore, an immortalized EBV-carrying lymphoblastoid cell line was established from a peripheral blood leukocyte culture taken during the acute phase of the illness. The Henles followed up this observation with a study of a collection of sera. This collection consisted of sera obtained routinely from incoming college freshman, and later from individuals who had developed acute IM. This study, as well as others, revealed EBV-specific antibodies in the sera of all students who developed IM, thus confirming the association between EBV and IM.[10,11]

EPIDEMIOLOGY

Transmission and Persistence of EBV

EBV was reported in the early 1970s to be transmitted primarily through contact with oropharyngeal secretions.[12,13] Observations of EBV in the uterine cervix, reported by Sixbey et al.[14] in 1986, suggest a possible sexual mode of transmission as well. Usually, EBV infection is initiated following infection of oropharyngeal epithelial cells, and this infection leads to continued production and release of EBV into the oropharyngeal secretions and the infection of B cells in the lymphoid-rich areas of the oropharynx. The EBV-infected B cells disseminate the infection throughout the lymphoreticular system.

Distribution and Prevalence

Seroepidemiologic studies have demonstrated a wide variation in the age at which EBV infection is acquired.[15] Geographic and socioeconomic factors account for the differences in prevalence of EBV infection. In the New Hebrides, where large extended family units exist and the custom of mastication of food for infants by family members is practiced, nearly all infants are infected with EBV by the age of 1 year.[16] In the West Nile district in Africa, where Burkitt lymphoma is endemic, prospective studies have demonstrated that primary infection occurs in most infants between the ages of 4 months and 1 year.[17,18] By 2 years of age, 81% of children have had primary EBV infection. Most of these infections are asymptomatic.

These studies suggest that early widespread seroconversions to EBV and other herpesviruses during infancy are associated with intense interpersonal contact with many different individuals. EBV infections have been considered to be of low contagiousness, and true epidemics have not occurred. Spread of EBV within families has been studied by Fleisher et al.,[19] who demonstrated serologic evidence of transmission in 7 of 35 families. Each year in the college age population in the United States, approximately 10–15% of susceptible students will become infected, and 50–70% of the infections will be associated with a mononucleosis syndrome.

BIOLOGIC AND MOLECULAR ASPECTS OF EBV

Characteristics of EBV Infection

EBV is a ubiquitous virus infecting most (>90%) of the world's population. It is associated with both benign disorders (IM) and malignant diseases (African Burkitt lymphoma and nasopharyngeal carcinoma).[9,20,21] EBV is a 172-kilobase-pair guanine-cytosine-rich (60%) double-stranded DNA virus.[22,23] EBV is a member of the herpesvirus family, which also includes the human viruses herpes simplex, herpes zoster (varicella), and cytomegalovirus. The herpesvirus family, which contains >80 members, is clustered into three subfamilies, α-, β-, and γ-herpesviridae, based on host cell range, site of latent infection, cytopathology, and duration of the replicative cycle.[24] EBV is the prototype of the γ-herpesviridae, a subfamily characterized by tropism for B and T lymphocytes. Other members of the subfamily include herpesvirus saimiri, a monkey T-lymphotropic virus, and Marek disease herpesvirus, a chicken lymphotropic virus.[24]

Structurally, the EBV virion is composed of four elements: (1) a dense central genetic core composed of DNA coiled around protein; (2) a nucleocapsid with 162 capsomeres in an icosahedral shape; (3) a protein tegament; and (4) an outer membrane or envelope containing four major virus-encoded proteins, three glycosylated proteins (gp) of size 350, 220, and 85 kd (gp350, gp220, and gp85, respectively), and a nonglycosylated 140-kd protein (p140).[20,24,25] These proteins are incorporated into the host plasma membrane during virus assembly, as demonstrated by their identification on the plasma membrane of cells replicating the virus.[26,27] These proteins are acquired by the virion as it buds through the host cell membrane.

Virion Infectivity

The receptor for EBV is CD21,[28] the 140-kd complement receptor type 2, specific for the C3d/C3dg component of the complement cascade. The gp350 and gp220 components mediate EBV virion absorption by binding CD21.[29]

EBV is internalized into normal B cells by endocytosis into large, thin-walled vesicles that are distinct from the clathrin-receptosome-lysomal pathway used by other viruses.[30] These vesicles are different both in size (larger) and morphologic appearance (no electron-dense thickened appearance); they do not contain lysosomal enzymes and are not sensitive to weak bases, such as chloroquine, methylamine, or substituted ammonium chlorides.[30]

The mechanism of release of EBV nucleocapsids from vesicles into the cytoplasm is poorly understood. It is presumed to occur via virus-vesicle membrane fusion. The major glycoprotein mediating this fusion is probably gp85, since its amino acid sequence is similar to that of the glycoprotein of herpes simplex virus-1 (HSV-1), which is implicated in HSV-1 virus-vesicle membrane fusion.[31] Antibodies to gp85 do not inhibit virus adsorption or internalization but do inhibit virus-vesicle fusion and thereby inhibit release of EBV into the cytoplasm.[32]

Host Cell Range of EBV

EBV has traditionally been thought to have a very narrow host cell range, confined primarily to B lymphocytes and certain epithelial cells.[33,34] Recent descriptions of EBV infection of T cells in patients with peripheral T-cell lymphoma[35,36] and Reed-Sternberg cells in patients with Hodgkin disease[37,38] suggest a broader host cell range for EBV infection.

CD21 antigen expression is a specific feature of mature B lymphocytes[39] and either is not present or is present at very low density on pre-B and immature B cells. Activated B cells, but not plasma cells, also uniformly express CD21.[39] Although CD21 is necessary for infection, it is not sufficient. When B cells are fractionated by size only, the low-density, or resting B cells, are susceptible to infection.[40] These results suggest that prior activation of B cells may render cells refractory to EBV infection.[40] Susceptibility of B cells to EBV is apparently dependent on a number of factors, including CD21 expression and the physiologic state of the B cell.

It has long been recognized that a strict tropism for B cells is inconsistent with many experimental observations, including (1) the active shedding of virus into oropharyngeal secretions despite the presence of nonreplicating virus in B cells in vivo; (2) the association of EBV with nasopharyngeal carcinoma, an epithelial cell malignancy; and (3) a study demonstrating EBV viral genome in epithelial cells from a nasopharyngeal tumor.[41] Cytohybridization studies with oropharyngeal epithelial cells, reported in 1977, demonstrated the presence of EBV nucleic acid,[42] and subsequent work demonstrated EBV infection and replication in epithelial cells.[34]

Initial studies that focused on the mechanism of infection were unable to detect CD21 on the epithelial cell surface, which led to suggestions that infection resulted from infected lymphocytes.[43] The anti-CD21 monoclonal antibodies HB5 and anti-B2 have been shown to bind a 200-kd epithelial protein, which could be a homologue of CD21 and a receptor for EBV.[44] Epithelial cell expression of the CD21 homologue is concentrated in the microvilli, and a less dense expression of the CD21 homologue is present on epithelial cells compared with lymphoid cells.[44] Like CD21 expression on B cells, epithelial cell expression of CD21 homologue is dependent on differentiation; only the less differentiated epithelial cells demonstrate significant anti-CD21 monoclonal antibody staining. EBV has been detected in female cervical epithelium associated with active

shedding of EBV into the female genital tract.[14] Recent studies have shown that polymeric IgA specific to the EBV membrane glycoprotein gp350 can block immortalization of B lymphocytes while concurrently mediating virus entry into epithelium via the polymeric immunoglobulin receptor (secretory component).[45]

Latent Infection

EBV is associated with both latent and lytic infections. Infection of primary B lymphocytes is primarily a latent non-virus-producing infection, whereas infection of epithelial cells is believed to be primarily a lytic virus-producing infection. Latent infection of B lymphocytes by EBV causes activation and transformation, as evidenced by establishment of continuously growing B-lymphoblastoid cell lines.[46,47]

A limited number of viral genes are expressed during latent infection. At present 11 genes are known to be expressed: (1) six code for EBV nuclear antigens—EBNA 1, EBNA 2, EBNA 3A, 3B, and 3C (also termed EBNA 3, 4, and 6, respectively), and EBNA leader protein; (2) three code for latent membrane proteins (LMPs)—LMP1, LMP2A, and LMP2B (LMP2A and 2B are also referred to as terminal proteins, since they span the terminal region of the genome); and (3) two code for small nonpolyadenylated nuclear RNAs (EB-encoded RNAs [EBERs]). The EBERs are primarily transcribed by cellular RNA polymerase III and the latent genes by cellular RNA polymerase II.[56] Following infection, EBNA 2 and leader protein are expressed the earliest, with maximal levels obtained by 24 hours.[48,49] By 48 hours the remainder of the genes have reached maximal expression.[48,49]

PATHOGENESIS

EBV replicates in the lymphoreticular system and provokes an intense immunologic response, resulting in the immunopathology and clinical symptomatology that follows the initial infection. The virus remains latent in the lymphoreticular system following host recovery and can be reactivated during periods of immunosuppression. This reactivation leads to further disease manifestations. EBV is acquired by intimate contact of a susceptible person with a virus-containing secretion from a previously infected person. Saliva appears to be the most common vehicle of viral spread[41,50]; however, the recent demonstration of cell-free virus in female genital secretions raises the possibility of sexual transmission.[14] Infection of the host oropharyngeal tissue begins with the initial infection of the nasopharyngeal epithelial cells,[51] through which the virus gains access to the lymphoreticular system. EBV-infected B lymphocytes are disseminated throughout the lymphoid system, with EBV-infected B cells appearing in the circulation. Persistence of EBV in B lymphocytes has been demonstrated for the lifetime of an infected person. The incubation period from initial contact with a virus excreter to the appearance of large numbers of EBV-infected B cells in the circulation is approximately 30–50 days.[52]

IM is a self-limiting lymphoproliferative disease characterized by lymphadenopathy, splenomegaly, and lymphocytosis. The hallmark of acute IM is the presence in the peripheral blood of atypical lymphocytes. These are large lymphocytes with prominent cytoplasmic basophilia and azurophilic granules.[53] Atypical lymphocytes in IM result from the expansion of T cells, primarily those of the cytotoxic/suppressor (CD8) phenotype.[54,55] this expansion is believed to be the result of intense in vivo stimulation by EBV-infected and transformed B cells. The atypical CD8 T cells express predominantly the T-cell activation antigen HLA-DR, with little expression of CD25, the interleukin-2 receptor.[56,57] Even following complete resolution of IM, EBV is not completely eliminated, but the latent

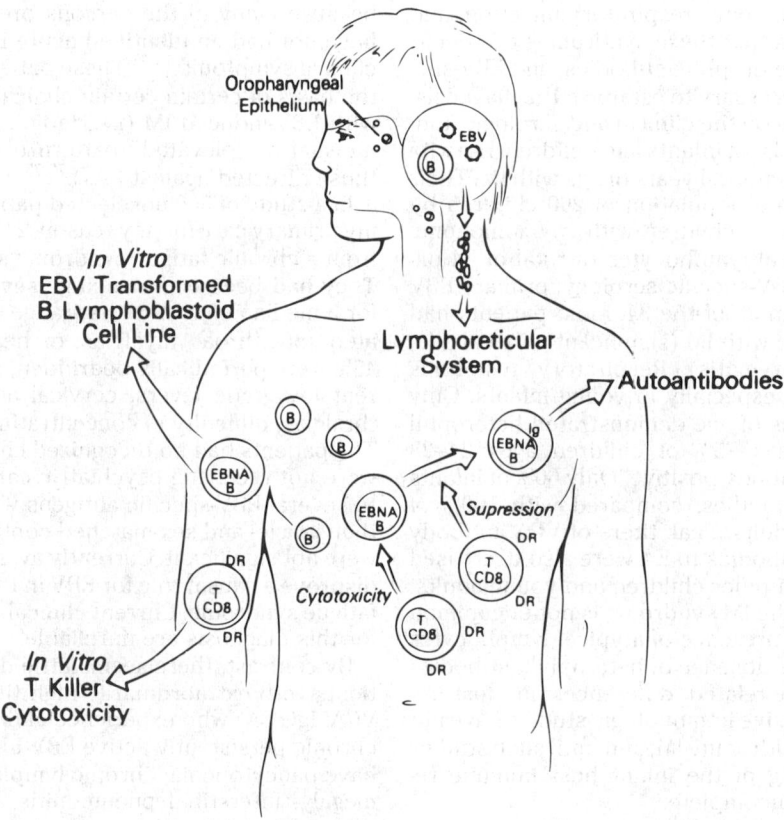

Fig. 58-1. Immunopathogenesis of acute EBV-induced infectious mononucleosis.

infection is generally a benign syndrome. This indicates the existence of highly efficient immunoregulatory mechanisms that can prevent EBV-induced lymphoproliferation.

Stimulation of both the humoral and cellular immune responses is evident during acute IM. The humoral response is characterized by non-EBV-specific (e.g., heterophil antibody and autoantibody responses) and EBV-specific responses directed against viral capsid antigen (VCA), early antigen (EA), membrane antigen (MA), and Epstein-Barr nuclear antigen (EBNA).[58,59] In addition to IgM and IgG isotypes, polymeric IgA specific to EBV-MA is transiently present in the serum.[45] The production of irrelevant antibodies is probably the product of polyclonal stimulation of B cells by EBV, a potent B-cell stimulator.[60] As demonstrated by the generation of many EBV-specific antibodies, a strong humoral response exists to EBV. However, it is the cellular immune response that is believed to be primarily responsible for controlling and preventing EBV-induced lymphoproliferative disorders.[61]

The specific cellular immune responses responsible for controlling EBV are not fully understood. The activated T-lymphocyte population exhibits both suppressor and cytotoxic functions.[62-64] The suppressor activity appears to be nonspecific in nature, as demonstrated by the ability of T cells in acute IM to suppress polyclonal immunoglobulin secretion by normal allogeneic B cells stimulated by pokeweed mitogen or EBV, and also to suppress lymphocyte proliferation stimulated by a variety of mitogens.[62]

The pathogenesis of acute EBV infection is summarized in Figure 58-1. Infection is initiated in the oropharynx following contact with infected secretions. Viral replication occurs first in epithelial cells and then in B lymphocytes, which disseminate virus throughout the lymphoreticular system. The cellular immune responses that occur following EBV infection are complex, and it is likely that these cellular events result in the immunopathology that accompanies acute infection. Although

humoral immune responses appear to be important in preventing recurrent infections, current evidence suggests that cellular mechanisms are responsible for the control of acute and reactivation infections with herpesviruses. Perturbations of these cellular immune responses may result in poorly controlled EBV infections or in immunologic disease clinically manifested as a lymphoproliferative disorder.

CLINICAL MANIFESTATIONS
Congenital and Neonatal Infections

The importance of EBV as a potential teratogen is as yet undefined. A few reports suggest that an embryopathy may occasionally occur as a result of intrauterine EBV infection.[65] If intrauterine infection with EBV is associated with an embryopathy, experience to date would indicate that this is a rare event. Chang and Seto[66] have evaluated >2,000 cord blood samples for evidence of in utero EBV infection and found only 1 to be positive. The EBV-positive infant demonstrated normal growth and development through the first 2 years of life. It is possible that EBV infection during pregnancy is associated with a high frequency of fetal wastage, and this could explain the difficulty in finding infants with congenital EBV infection.

Relatively little is known about the importance of EBV as a cause of perinatal infections. The description of a postnatal cytomegalovirus syndrome associated with blood transfusions in premature infants[67] highlights the importance of conducting similar studies to determine whether transfusion-acquired EBV infections pose a risk to the premature infant.

Primary EBV Infection in Infants and Children

Primary EBV infections in young infants and children are frequently asymptomatic. When symptoms do occur, a variety of syndromes have been observed, including otitis media, diarrhea, abdominal complaints, upper respiratory infection, and IM.[68,69] It is now appreciated that these syndromes can occur without the production of heterophil antibodies, and EBV-specific serologic studies are necessary to establish the diagnosis. Several studies have focused on the clinical and serologic findings that are associated with IM in infants and children. Horwitz et al.[68] have reported 32 patients <4 years of age with IM. Their patients were selected from a population of 200 children by review of blood smears. Those children with >50% mononuclear cells and >10% atypical lymphocytes (a total of 34 patients) were evaluated by EBV-specific serology; primary EBV infection was documented in 32 of the 34. Most patients had clinical evidence compatible with IM (significant cervical adenopathy and tonsillar pharyngitis). Respiratory symptoms were frequently prominent, especially in young infants. Only 25% of infants 10–24 months of age demonstrated heterophil antibody responses, whereas 75% of children ages 24–28 months were heterophil antibody positive. Only 60% of infants demonstrated VCA-IgM antibodies, compared with 100% of older children and young adults. Peak titers of VCA antibody and the development of antibodies to EA were also decreased in infants, as compared with older children and young adults.

This study suggests that the IM syndrome is not uncommon among young children. The presence of atypical lymphocytes and lymphadenopathy in the absence of heterophil antibodies further documents the age-related differences in host responses to EBV. Comprehensive immunologic studies have not been performed on infants with acute IM, and until such studies are available, understanding of the infant host immune response to EBV will remain incomplete.

Infectious Mononucleosis in the Young Adult

The IM syndrome appearing in young adults is characterized by fever, anterior and posterior cervical lymphadenopathy, exudative pharyngitis, and fatigue. The syndrome is self-limited, lasting on the average 2–3 weeks. It is estimated that 30–50% of students entering college in the United States are susceptible (seronegative) to EBV.[70] Approximately 10–15% of seronegative persons become infected each year, and most of those infected show signs and symptoms of classical IM.[70] Studies conducted at West Point have demonstrated an association of clinically apparent IM with the likelihood of being under stress.[70]

Individuals experiencing acute IM may develop morbilliform rashes when treated with ampicillin or penicillin during the acute phase of the disease.[70] Hepatosplenomegaly is commonly present and severe, but only rarely results in splenic rupture (following trauma) and fulminant hepatitis secondary to periportal necrosis. One of the most common causes of hospitalization during acute IM is severe pharyngitis with the possibility of airway obstruction. This complication, which usually resolves with in 24–72 hours, may be severe enough to warrant empirical treatment with intravenous steroids, although the efficacy of such treatment has not been proved.[72]

Chronic Active or Persistent EBV Infection

The use of the terms chronic mononucleosis,[73] active EBV,[74] and persistent EBV[75] has caused confusion and frustration for physicians investigating clinical disorders caused by EBV, as well as for those involved in day-to-day patient care. The major problem with these terms is the complete lack of proven objective criteria for applying them to a patient or group of patients. Their use to describe a syndrome characterized by chronic fatigue, fever, pharyngitis, myalgias, headaches, arthralgias, paresthesias, depression, and cognitive deficits is misleading,

because many of the persons presenting with the syndrome have not had an identified acute EBV infection at the start of clinical symptoms.[73,75] These patients have been diagnosed on the basis of certain certain clinical symptoms also associated with EBV-induced IM (i.e., fatigue, fever, pharyngitis) and an unusual or "elevated" pattern of EBV antibodies (especially those directed against EAs).[73,75]

In a study of 500 unselected patients aged 17–50 years seeking primary care for any reason, 21% were found to be suffering from a chronic fatigue syndrome suggestive of chronic EBV.[76] They had been experiencing "severe" fatigue, usually cyclic, for a median of 16 months (range 6–458 months), with associated sore throat, myalgias, or headaches. Of these patients, 45% were periodically bedridden, and 25–73% reported recurrent low-grade fevers, cervical adenopathy, paresthesia, arthralgias, difficulty in concentrating, and difficulty in sleeping. The patients had no recognized chronic "physical" illness and were not receiving psychiatric care. Although antibody titers to several EBV-specific antigens were higher in these patients than in age- and sex-matched control subjects, the differences were not significant. Currently available data neither prove nor disprove a causal role for EBV in the pathogenesis of a chronic fatigue syndrome. Current clinical and laboratory criteria used for this diagnosis are unreliable.

By contrast, there seems little doubt that there are rare patients with extraordinarily high titers of EBV antibodies (IgG-VCA, IgG-EA) who experience clinical symptoms in the face of chronic persistently active EBV infection. These patients may have pancytopenia, chronic lymphadenopathy, hepatosplenomegaly, interstitial pneumonitis, and chronic liver dysfunction.[76] Preliminary data suggest that an abnormal humoral immune response to EBV-EBNA antigens or infection with a variant EBV strain, or both, may be associated with chronic or persistent infection.[77] A relationship between these clinical syndromes and replication of EBV is suggested by apparent clinical responses to acyclovir therapy.[78]

Effects of EBV Infection on Hematopoietic Elements

The effects of EBV infection on the hematologic system have been reviewed in recent publications.[79,80] Patients with acute EBV infection present with lymphocytosis, and not uncommonly have an associated thrombocytopenia. Infrequently, patients develop more serious hematologic complications that may involve the erythroid, myeloid, or megakaryocytic lineages.

Neutropenia is seen in many patients with IM during the first month of disease,[81] but severe neutropenia is seen relatively infrequently. In a study performed by Sumaya and Ench,[82] it was shown that 8% of patients had an absolute neutrophil count of 500–1,000 cells/mm^3, and 8% had a neutrophil count of <500/mm^3. In most instances, the neutropenia resolved within 2 weeks. Fatal infections attributed to severe neutropenia have been reported.[83] Examination of the bone marrow may show left shifted myelopoiesis with a paucity of mature myeloid forms.[83] Neutrophil autoantibodies, which may be seen in a high proportion of patients with acute IM, may contribute to the neutropenia.[84] It has also been shown that T cells from patients with IM may decrease colony-forming unit-granulocyte/macrophage, suggesting that these T cells downregulate myelopoiesis.[85]

EBV infections in infants may rarely result in a clinical syndrome similar to juvenile chronic myeloid leukemia.[86] These patients present with hepatosplenomegaly, leukocytosis, and thrombocytopenia and have increased levels of fetal hemoglobin. This syndrome may be distinguished from juvenile chronic myeloid leukemia by evidence of acute or recent EBV infection. Clinical symptoms may persist for months or years, but usually resolve spontaneously. Immunoregulatory abnormalities have been described, but whether these are of primary or secondary importance in pathogenesis remains uncertain.

Erythropoiesis

Mild hemolysis is common in patients experiencing acute EBV infection; however, clinically significant anemia is uncommon, occurring in 1–3% of patients.[87] When hemolysis develops, it is usually seen within the first 2 weeks of illness. Patients usually have a positive direct Coombs test. Most frequently the autoantibody has anti-specificity.[88] Antibodies with anti-N,[89] anti-I,[90] and Dunath-Landsteiner antibodies[91] have also been described. In addition, patients with hereditary red cell defects may have an exaggerated rate of red blood cell destruction during acute EBV infection.[92] Pure red cell aplasia has been described following acute EBV infection and has been associated with persistently abnormal EBV serology over a 2-year period.[93]

Thrombopoiesis

Mild thrombocytopenia with platelet counts of 50,000–150,000/mm^3 is commonly seen in patients with acute EBV infection.[94,95] The thrombocytopenia usually occurs within the first 2 weeks following the onset of clinical symptoms. Severe thrombocytopenia may be seen in 1–3.5% of patients. The normalization of platelet counts may take ≤2 months.[95] Bone marrow examination shows normal or increased numbers of megakaryocytes, compatible with peripheral platelet destruction. It is thought that antiplatelet antibodies and sequestration with destruction in the spleen are responsible for the thrombocytopenia. Platelet counts usually return to normal within 2 months, and even the more chronic cases tend to resolve spontaneously.[95]

Bone Marrow Progenitors

Acute EBV infection rarely is complicated by pancytopenia and marrow hypoplasia compatible with aplastic anemia. This bone marrow complication is similar to that seen in patients with virus-associated hemophagocytic syndrome (VAHS) with pancytopenia. In a case report and review of the literature, Lazarus and Baehner[96] described six instances of aplastic anemia in which a bone marrow examination was performed; in four patients the findings met the criteria for severe aplastic anemia. The mean time from onset of symptoms of IM to the development of pancytopenia was 21 days, with recovery occurring by the end of the first week of bone marrow aplasia. Several mechanisms have been proposed for EBV-associated marrow aplasia, with experimental data to support some of them.[85] Suppressor T lymphocytes, which inhibit the growth of colony-forming unit-culture in vitro, have been described in some patients. A marked increase in T cells bearing the morphologic markers for the T-cytotoxic/suppressor cell population occurs during acute EBV infection and could play a role in marrow aplasia. It has also been postulated that cytotoxic cells may lyse hematopoietic stem cells. Autologous lymphocytotoxicity has been reported in patients with aplasia anemia.[85]

FATAL INFECTIOUS MONONUCLEOSIS

Virus-Associated Hemophagocytic Syndrome

The term VAHS was introduced by Risdall and co-workers[97] in 1979 to describe a disorder characterized by a benign generalized histiocytic proliferation, with marked hemophago-

Table 58-1. Infection-Associated Hemophagocytic Syndrome

Viral	Fungal
Epstein-Barr virus	*Histoplasma capsulatum*
Cytomegalovirus	*Candida albicans*
Herpes simplex virus	*Cryptococcus neoformans*
Varicella-zoster virus	Mycobacterial
Adenovirus	*Mycobacterium tuberculosis*
Parovirus B19	Rickettsia
Bacterial	*Coxiella burnetii*
Enteric gram-negative rods	Parasitic
Haemophilus influenzae	*Babesia microti*
Streptococcus pneumonia	*Leishmania donovani*
Staphylococcus aureus	
Brucella abortus	
Mycoplasma pneumoniae	

cytosis associated with a systemic virus infection. Since this initial description, the causes of a hemophagocytic syndrome have been expanded to include virtually any infectious agent, carcinomas, and hematologic malignancies.[98] Table 58-1 lists some of the infections associated with hemophagocytic syndrome. Thus far, EBV, cytomegalovirus, herpes simplex virus, varicella-zoster virus, adenovirus, and parvovirus B19 have been the viral agents implicated.[99–103]

The syndrome is characterized by fever and generalized constitutional symptoms with myalgias and malaise. Physical examination reveals an enlarged liver and spleen with generalized lymphadenopathy. Laboratory studies commonly demonstrate abnormal liver function tests with a coagulopathy that is more severe than that expected on the basis of the abnormal liver function. The VAHS patient is usually pancytopenic and may appear very toxic. Patients experiencing fatal EBV-induced IM frequent develop VAHS. In addition, this syndrome has been observed in persons with underlying immunosuppression. The mortality in patients experiencing VAHS has been high; however, it is likely that use of immunosuppressive agents in patients experiencing VAHS has contributed to this high mortality. The pathogenesis of EBV-associated hemophagocytic syndrome is poorly understood. Kawaguchi et al.[104] have recently reported the proliferation of EBV-infected T cells as a primary feature.

X-linked Lymphoproliferative Syndrome

The X-linked lymphoproliferative (XLP) syndrome is characterized by a selective immunodeficiency to EBV manifested by severe or fatal IM and acquired immunodeficiency.[105] Prospective studies in males prior to EBV infection have demonstrated normal cellular and humoral immunity.[106] During acute EBV infection, males with XLP demonstrate vigorous cytotoxic cellular responses, which predominantly involve polyclonally activated alloreactive cytotoxic T cells, but cytotoxic T cells that recognize EBV-infected autologous B cells have been demonstrated. Fatal EBV infections in males with XLP usually result from extensive liver necrosis, and those who survive acute EBV infection demonstrate global cellular immune defects with deficient T-cell, B-cell, and natural killer cell responses. It is hypothesized that uncontrolled alloreactive T-cell responses triggered by EBV-transformed B cells result in the immunopathology of XLP. Genetic studies have demonstrated XLP to be genetically linked to restriction fragment length polymorphisms detected with the DXS42 and DXS37 probes,[107,108] and studies of an affected male with a deletion of Xq25[109] have localized the XLP gene to the Xq25 region of the X chromosome. Genetic analysis allows for the detection of carrier females, and presymptomatic (EBV-seronegative) XLP males. Prenatal diagnosis of XLP has been performed.[110]

EBV and Post-Transplant Lymphomas

Allograft recipients are at increased risk of the development of EBV-induced lymphoreticular malignancies. The incidence of post-transplant lymphomas is 1–15%, depending on the allograft and the immunosuppressive regimen. The majority of the lymphomas are categorized as diffuse large cell lymphomas with most having immunoblastic features. Molecular probes specific for EBV have streamlined the diagnosis of EBV-associated post-transplant lymphomas. Studies employing molecular probes to analyze clonality of post-transplant lymphomas have demonstrated that most patients developing lymphomas have monoclonal tumors, but often the disease is multiclonal, with biopsy material from different anatomic sites showing different proliferating clones of tumor cells. Raab-Traub and Flynn[111] have developed a novel technique whereby tumor cell clonality as well as discrimination of replicating versus nonreplicating EBV may be ascertained in a single assay. The specific immune defect responsible for these lymphoproliferative disorders is unknown but is thought to be related to the loss of memory cytotoxic T lymphocytes specific for EBV-transformed B lymphocytes.

EBV and Human Immunodeficiency Virus Associated Non-Hodgkin Lymphoma

The incidence of non-Hodgkin lymphomas is 60–100 times that expected in human immunodeficiency virus (HIV)-infected individuals.[112] The incidence of lymphomas increased with the duration of infection. Pluda et al.[113] reported that 19% of patients with symptomatic HIV infection receiving antiretroviral therapy and surviving 3 years developed lymphoma.

Recent studies suggest that EBV is associated with most central nervous system lymphomas as well as systemic lymphomas developing in individuals with HIV infection. It appears that the combination of chronic B-lymphocyte stimulation in the setting of severe T-cell immunodeficiency in an individual with previous EBV infection is a set-up for the development of non-Hodgkin lymphoma.

Peripheral T-Cell Lymphoma and Hodgkin Disease

Recent studies suggest that peripheral T-cell non-Hodgkin lymphomas, which occur in individuals without global immune defects, are associated with EBV in 10–35% of patients.[35,36] Angioimmunoblastic lymphadenopathy and angiocentric polymorphous lymphoreticular infiltrates, known clinically as lethal midline granuloma, are T-cell lymphomas frequently associated with EBV. Both the A and B strains of EBV have been associated with EBV-associated T-cell lymphomas.

EBV is detectable in Reed-Sternberg cells in approximately 40% of patients with Hodgkin disease, particularly of the mixed cellularity subtype.[37,38] EBV is detectable in most instances of Hodgkin disease developing in HIV-infected individuals. The Reed-Sternberg cell has been shown to contain monoclonal EBV genomes with restricted expression (LMP I, EBER 1/2) of latent gene products. Recently Brousset et al.[38] have demonstrated EBV replication in Reed-Sternberg cells of Hodgkin disease. The role that EBV plays in the pathogenesis of these disorders remains poorly understood.

LABORATORY DIAGNOSIS

Serology

In 90–95% of young adults with clinical EBV-induced IM, atypical lymphocytosis and heterophil antibodies are present.[111] However, in young infants and children with primary EBV infec-

tion (whether or not associated with IM), heterophil antibody responses are frequently absent.[68] Primary EBV infection is usually suggested by the presence of atypical lymphocytes, but these may also be absent or present in small numbers.[69] Primary infection in childhood frequently requires EBV-specific serologic tests. Our approach to a patient suspected of having a primary EBV infection is first to perform a rapid slide test for heterophil antibodies. If this is positive (differential absorption with guinea pig kidney and beef red blood cell antigens should be performed), EBV-specific serology is unnecessary, but if the rapid slide test is negative, the serum sample should be tested for EBV-specific antibodies.

In individuals with negative Paul-Bunnell heterophil antibody tests (especially young infants and children) and patients with atypical primary EBV infections, specific antibodies for EBV should be determined. Antibodies to three specific EBV antigens have been thoroughly studied and found to be of diagnostic importance[114]: (1) VCA; (2) EAs (both of which may be expressed by certain EBV-infected B-lymphoblastoid cell lines); and (3) EBNAs, which are expressed by all cell lines. These antigens have been detected by the indirect immunofluorescence test using serum samples from patients with EBV-associated diseases. Individuals experiencing acute EBV-induced IM and the EBV-associated malignancies (Burkitt lymphoma and nasopharyngeal carcinoma) have been thoroughly studied, along with normal controls, and certain characteristic antibody patterns have been described.

Figure 58-2 shows the characteristic antibody patterns observed in young adults experiencing EBV-induced IM.[114] Prior to EBV infection, all three antibodies are absent but during the acute phase of infection, high titers of IgM and IgG antibodies to VCA are seen. IgM antibodies are transient and disappear after a few months. Most individuals develop transient IgG antibodies against early antigens, and these antibodies disappear after a few months. In 1985, it was reported that between 12% and 39% of normal persons will maintain moderate (1:20 to 1:40) antibody titers to EAs for years after primary infection.[115] Antibodies directed against the EBNA proteins are produced early in infection. However, detectable titers by indirect immunofluorescence are not usually found until 1–2 months following acute infection. This pattern of late appearance is probably a reflection of the insensitivity of the complement-dependent indirect immunofluorescent antibody (IFA) test, since sensitive enzyme-linked immunosorbant assay-based methods detect antibodies to the EBNAs early after infection. Healthy individuals who have had past infection with EBV show VCA-IgG antibodies. In young infants, VCA-IgM responses may be seen in only 60% and EA responses in approximately 50% of patients during acute EBV infection.[67]

In general, acute or recent primary infection is indicated by the following: (1) the presence of VCA-specific IgM antibodies, (2) high titers of VCA-specific IgG antibodies ($\geq 1:320$), (3) detection of anti-EA antibodies ($\geq 1:10$), and (4) the absence of anti-EBNA by IFA.[114] Convalescent serum samples should be obtained to demonstrate the disappearance of VCA-IgM and appearance of EBNA antibodies. EBV antibody titers should not be used to make a diagnosis of chronic IM or other EBV-associated syndromes on the basis of mild-to-moderate elevation of VCA (1:160 to 1:320) or EA (1:20 to 1:40) antibodies because normal individuals may show such titers years after uncomplicated infection.[115] Elevated EBV titers are also seen in patients with EBV-associated malignancies and those with virtually any condition associated with suppression of cellular immune function (i.e., allograft recipients, patients receiving chemotherapy, patients with HIV infection). Past infection is indicated by the presence of VCA-IgG and EBNA-IgG antibodies.

EBV cannot be cultured by routine viral culture methods that employ standard animal cell cultures, since it grows only in primate B lymphocytes. The presence of virus can be demon-

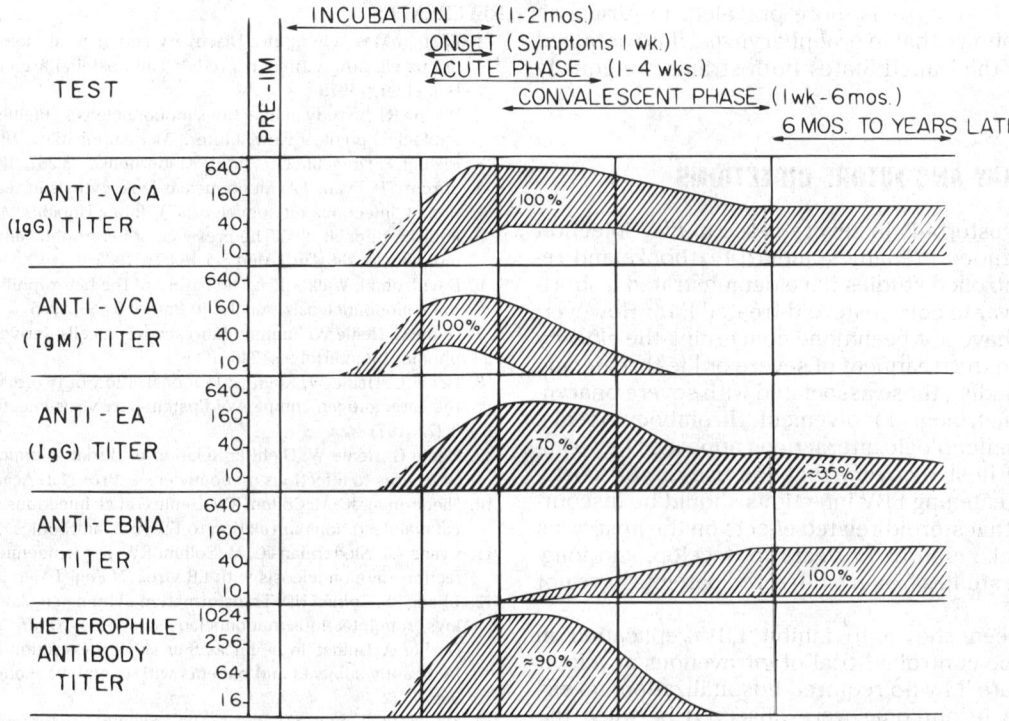

Fig. 58-2. Characteristic EBV-specific antibody responses observed in young adults with acute infectious mononucleosis. (Adapted from Henle et al.,[114] with permission.)

strated by inoculating human umbilical cord blood lymphocytes (EBV-nonimmune B lymphocytes) with throat washings or by establishing an EBNA-positive, spontaneous B-lymphoblastoid cell line from the peripheral blood of the infected person. However, both these methods will detect virus in persons with past infection, because EBV is a latent virus, and most healthy previously infected persons chronically shed virus in the oropharynx.[50] Because of the difficulties in making a serologic diagnosis in patients with unusual or rare manifestations of EBV infection, molecular diagnostic techniques must be employed.

Molecular Diagnostic Techniques

Molecular diagnostic techniques have contributed greatly to the identification of EBV in pathologic materials.[116] In situ hybridization (ISH), Southern blot analysis and the polymerase chain reaction (PCR) are useful techniques used alone and in combination.

In our own approach to these issues, we use Southern blot hybridization of DNA extracted from affected tissue when we do not need to identify infected cells morphologically or when we believe that sufficient cells within the lesion contain EBV. Such instances include entities such as HIV-associated lymphoma or Burkitt lymphoma. Southern blots are probed with a Bam W probe, which detects an internal repeat in the EBV genome.

The EBV genome contains terminal repeats that hybridize when the genome is in the circular or episomal form. When a clonal cell population is present, only one form of the genome with a single terminal repeat is present. When a Southern blot is probed with a terminal repeat probe such as Bam NJ, a single band is obtained.[111] Such results are found in Burkitt lymphoma or nasopharyngeal carcinoma. In a polyclonal infection, a heterogeneous collection of bands is found. This technique will also discriminate replicating from nonreplicating (latent) EBV infection.[111]

ISH using oligonucleotide probes complementary to the EBER genes has provided an extremely powerful technique for the identification of EBV-infected cells in tissue sections and smears.[117] The advantages of ISH for the detection of EBER-encoded RNA is that it is a relatively simple technique, uses cheap stable probes, can be used on archival material, does not require radioactivity, and provides a permanent morphologic end point. As latently infected cells may express millions of copies of EBER-RNA, ISH provides an extremely sensitive technique for the identification of even a few infected cells within a tissue. Not only does this technique provide morphologic information, it is more sensitive than Southern blotting and approaches the sensitivity of PCR. In our laboratory we use ISH when it is important to obtain morphologic information, when we only have access to paraffin-embedded archival material, when we would like to obtain information about what portion of cells may be infected, or when we need high sensitivity. This technique is now widely applied and has been extremely useful in identifying EBV in entities such as Hodgkin disease, T-cell lymphoma, VAHS, and nasopharyngeal carcinoma.

A third modality that is useful for the detection of EBV is PCR.[118–120] The advantages of PCR are its ability to detect rare infected cells on the order of 1 in 1×10^6 and its rapidity. DNA may be extracted from fresh material or from paraffin-embedded archival material. PCR is a relatively complex technique, and great care must be taken to ensure that positive signals are truly positive. Currently, we use a technique described by Shibata et al.,[118] which amplifies a portion of the EBNA 1 gene. We find this technique useful in screening materials that require high sensitivity, such as the determination of whether EBV may be found in novel lymph node diseases or carcinomas. Another utility of PCR is its ability to subtype EBV strains.[119,120] EBV strains are classifiable into two subtypes based on differences in genomic sequences, especially the EBNA 2 gene. The A subtype is prevalent in Western countries and Japan and has an enhanced ability to transform B lymphocytes in vitro. The B subtype is more prevalent in Africa, although it has been shown that in oral-pharyngeal fluid obtained from individuals in the United States both strains are equally distributed.

THERAPY AND FUTURE DIRECTIONS

The use of corticosteroids in severe cases of EBV infection and IM is recommended in many standard textbooks and review articles.[94] Controlled studies have demonstrated a shortened duration of fever in corticosteroid-treated IM.[72] However, controlled studies have not been done concerning the efficacy of corticosteroids in the treatment of severe or life-threatening EBV infections, including those associated with severe pharyngeal involvement, neurologic involvement, thrombocytopenia, and myocarditis. Immunologic interactions appear to be so important for normal host recovery that the use of corticosteroids in non-life-threatening EBV infections should be discouraged. It is possible that steroid-related effects on the host-virus relationship may take months or years to develop, and long-term epidemiologic studies of steroid-treated patients have not been reported.

Acyclovir has been shown to inhibit EBV replication in vitro.[121] In a placebo-controlled trial of intravenous acyclovir in patients with acute IM who required hospitalization, no significant differences in outcome were observed between the placebo- and acyclovir-treated groups.[122] A placebo-controlled trial of oral acyclovir in ambulatory college students experiencing acute IM also demonstrated no significant effects of acyclovir on clinical outcome.[123]

Various therapeutic agents have been tried unsuccessfully in XLP patients experiencing acute EBV infection. It is clear that high-dose immunosuppressive therapy predisposes these patients to fatal B-cell lymphoproliferative disorders. This effect has been observed with the use of high-dose corticosteroids and antithymocyte globulin. Acyclovir treatment of patients with the XLP syndrome has been reported,[124,125] with no objective evidence of clinical improvement apparent. Patients have died with disseminated EBV-infected B lymphocytes throughout the lymphoreticular organs despite a 2-week course of acyclovir (1,500 mg/m^2/day). Virologic studies have revealed that the virus in infected B lymphocytes was in a non-replicating state, and mature virus particles were not being produced. In view of these results, it is likely that acyclovir will prove to be efficacious only in those patients suffering syndromes associated with replicating EBV infection.

An anecdotal report of ganciclovir treatment in EBV-induced lymphoproliferative syndromes after organ transplantation suggests an efficacy similar to that of acyclovir.[126] In addition, there is one report of a patient with XLP unsuccessfully treated with interferon.[127] It is our current opinion that males with XLP experiencing primary EBV infection should be treated with broad-spectrum cytotoxic chemotherapy in an effort to eliminate the activated alloreactive cells and at the same time control the proliferation of the EBV-transformed B cells. Such therapy remains unproved but appears worthy of trial.

Correction of XLP syndrome by transplantation of bone marrow[128] and cord-blood stem cells[129] has been reported. The advent of a genetic diagnosis of presymptomatic (EBV-seronegative) XLP males makes it possible to correct the defect by transplantation before primary EBV infection has occurred. In the absence of a marrow or stem cell donor we are currently using high-dose (600 mg/kg/mo) intravenous γ-globulin containing high titers of EBV antibodies in an attempt to prevent primary infection. While this therapy is unproved, it is our hope to delay primary infection until such time as an EBV vaccine becomes available. It is likely that an experimental EBV vaccine will enter clinical trials before the end of the decade.

REFERENCES

1. Epstein MA, Achong BG: Discovery and general biology of the virus. p. 1. In Epstein MA, Achong BG (eds): The Epstein-Barr Virus. Springer-Verlag, Heidelberg, 1979
2. Wising RJ: A study of infectious mononucleosis (Pfeiffer's disease) from the etiological point of view. J Intern Med suppl 133:1, 1942
3. Pfeiffer E: Drusenfieber. Jahrb Kinderheilkd 23:257, 1885
4. Sprunt TP, Evans FA: Mononuclear leukocytosis in reaction to acute infections ("infectious mononucleosis"). Johns Hopkins Med J 374:410, 1923
5. Paul JR, Bunnell WW: The presence of heterophile antibodies in infectious mononucleosis. Am J Med Sci 183:91, 1932
6. Davidsohn I, Walker PH: The nature of the heterophilic antibodies in infectious mononucleosis. Am J Clin Pathol 5:455, 1935
7. Henle G, Henle W: Immunofluorescence in cells derived from Burkitt's lymphoma. J Bacteriol 91:1248, 1966
8. Henle G, Henle W, Klein G: Demonstration of two distinct components in the early antigen complex of Epstein-Barr virus-infected cells. Int J Cancer 8:272, 1971
9. Henle G, Henle W, Diehl F: Relation of Burkitt's tumor-associated herpestype virus to infectious mononucleosis. Proc Natl Acad Sci USA 59:94, 1968
10. Niederman, JC, McCollum RW, Henle G et al: Infectious mononucleosis: clinical manifestations in relation to EB virus antibodies. JAMA 203:204, 1968
11. Evans AS, Niederman JC, McCollum RW: Seroepidemiological studies of infectious mononucleosis with EB virus. N Engl J Med 279:1121, 1968
12. Chang RS, Golden HD: Transformation of human leukocytes by throat washings from infectious mononucleosis patients. Nature 234:359, 1971
13. Gerber A, Goldstein LI, Lucas S et al: Oral excretion of Epstein-Barr virus by healthy subjects and patients with infectious mononucleosis. Lancet 2:988, 1972
14. Sixbey JW, Lemon SM, Pagano JS: A second site for Epstein-Barr virus shedding: the uterine cervix. Lancet 2:1122, 1986
15. Evans AS, Niederman JC: Epstein-Barr virus. p. 309. In Evans AS (ed): Viral Infections of Humans. Plenum, New York, 1976
16. Lang DJ, Garruto RM, Gajdusek DC: Early acquisition of cytomegalovirus and Epstein-Barr virus antibody in several isolated Melanesian populations. Am J Epidemiol 105:480, 1977
17. Biggar RJ, Henle W, Fleisher G et al: Primary Epstein-Barr virus infections in African infants. I. Decline of maternal antibodies and time of infection. Int J Cancer 22:239, 1978
18. Biggar RJ, Henle G, Bocker J et al: Primary Epstein-Barr virus infections in African infants. II. Clinical and serological observations during seroconversion. Int J Cancer 22:244, 1978
19. Fleisher GR, Pasquariello PS, Warren WS et al: Intrafamilial transmission of Epstein-Barr virus infections. J Pediatr 98:16, 1981
20. Zur Hausen H, Schulte-Hothausen H, Klein G et al: EBV DNA in biopsies of Burkitt's tumor and anaplastic carcinomas of the nasopharynx. Nature 228:1056, 1970
21. Desgranges CH, Wolf H, de The G et al: Nasopharyngeal carcinoma: X. Presence of Epstein-Barr genomes in separated epithelial cells of tumors in patients from Singapore, Tunisia and Kenya. Int J Cancer 16:7, 1975
22. Given D, Kieff E: DNA of Epstein-Barr virus. IV. Linkage map for restriction enzyme fragments of the B95-8 and W91 strains of EBV. J Virol 21:524, 1978
23. Baer R, Bankier AT, Biggin MD et al: DNA sequence and expression of B95-8 Epstein-Barr virus genome. Nature 310:207, 1984
24. Roizman B. The family herpesviridae: general description, taxonomy and classification. p. 1. In Roizman B (ed): The Herpesviruses. Vol. 1. Plenum, New York, 1982
25. Pritchett RF, Haywood SD, Kieff E: Comparison of DNA of virus purified from HR-1 and B95-8 cells. J Virol 15:556, 1975
26. Strand B, Neubauer R, Rubin H et al: Correlation between Epstein-Barr virus membrane antigen and three large cell surface glycoproteins. J Virol 32:885, 1979
27. Thorley-Lawson DA: Characterization of cross-reacting antigens on the Epstein virus envelope and plasma membranes of producer cells. Cell 16:32, 1979
28. Nemerow G, Wolfert R, McNaughton M et al: Identification and characterization of the Epstein-Barr virus receptor on human B lymphocytes and its relationship to the C3d complement receptor CR2. J Virol 55:347, 1985
29. Nemerow G, Houghton R, Moore M et al: Identification of an epitope in the major envelope protein of Epstein-Barr virus that mediates viral binding to the B lymphocyte EBV receptor (CR2). Cell 56:369, 1989
30. Nemerow GR, Cooper NR: Early events in infection of B lymphocytes by Epstein-Barr virus: the internalization process. Virology 132:186, 1984
31. Heineman T, Gong M, Sample J et al: Identification of the Epstein-Barr virus gp85 gene. J Virol 62:1101, 1988
32. Miller N, Hutt-Fletcher LM: A monoclonal antibody to glycoprotein gp85

inhibits fusion but not attachment of Epstein-Barr virus. J Virol 62:2366, 1988

33. Jondal M, Klein G: Surface markers on human B and T lymphocytes. II. Presence of Epstein-Barr virus receptors on B lymphocytes. J Exp Med 138:1365, 1973

34. Sixbey JW, Vesterinen EH, Nedrud JG et al: Replication of Epstein-Barr virus in human epithelial cells infected in vitro. Nature 306:480, 1983

35. Jones JF, Shurin S, Abramowsky C et al: T-cell lymphoma containing Epstein-Barr viral DNA in patients with chronic Epstein-Barr virus infection. N Engl J Med 318:733, 1988

36. Chi-Long C, Sadler RH, Walling DM et al: Epstein-Barr virus (EBV) gene expression in EBV-positive peripheral T-cell lymphomas. J Virol 67:6303, 1993

37. Weiss LM, Strickler JG, Warnke RA et al: Epstein-Barr viral DNA in tissues of Hodgkin's disease. Am J Pathol 129:86, 1987

38. Brousset P, Knecht H, Rubin B et al: Demonstration of Epstein-Barr virus replication in Reed-Sternberg cells of Hodgkins disease. Blood 82:872, 1993

39. Tedder TF, Clement LT, Cooper MD: Expression of C3d receptors during human B cell differentiation: immunofluorescence analysis with the HB-5 monoclonal antibody. J Immunol 133:678, 1984

40. Aman P, Ehlin-Henriksson B, Klein G: Epstein-Barr virus susceptibility of normal human B lymphocytes populations. J Exp Med 159:208, 1984

41. Miller G, Niederman JC, Andrews L: Prolonged oropharyngeal excretion of EB virus following infectious mononucleosis. N Engl J Med 288:229, 1973

42. Lemon SM, Hutt IM, Shaw JE et al: Replication of EBV in epithelial cells during infectious mononucleosis. Nature 268:268, 1977

43. Shapiro IM, Volsky DJ: Infection of normal human epithelial cells by Epstein-Barr virus. Science 219:1225, 1983

44. Sixbey JW, Davis DS, Yung LS et al: Human epithelial cell expression of an Epstein-Barr virus receptor. J Gen Virol 68:805, 1987

45. Sixbey JW, Yao QY: Immunoglobulin A-induced shift of Epstein-Barr virus tissue tropism. Science 255:1578, 1992

46. Henle W, Diehl B, Kohn G et al: Herpes-type virus and chromosomal marker in normal leukocytes after growth with irradiated Burkitt cells. Science 157:1064, 1967

47. Pope JH, Horne MK, Scott W: Transformation of fetal human leukocytes in vitro by filtrates of a human leukemic cell line containing herpes-like virus. Int J Cancer 3:857, 1968

48. Moss DJ, Rickinson AB, Wallace LE et al: Sequential appearance of Epstein-Barr virus nuclear and lymphocyte-detected membrane antigens in B cell transformation. Nature 291:664, 1981

49. Moss DJ, Sculley T, Pope J: Induction of EBV nuclear antigens. J Virol 58:988, 1986

50. Yao QY, Rickinson AB, Epstein MA: A re-examination of the Epstein-Barr virus carrier state in healthy seropositive individuals. Int J Cancer 35:35, 1985

51. Sixbey JW, Nedrud JG, Raab-Traub N et al: Epstein-Barr virus replication in oropharyngeal epithelial cells. N Engl J Med 310:1225, 1984

52. Svedmyr E, Ernbert I, Seeley J et al: Virologic, immunologic and clinical observations on a patient during the incubation, acute, and convalescent phases of infectious mononucleosis. Clin Immunol Immunopathol 30:437, 1984

53. Shiftan TA, Mendelson J: The circulating atypical lymphocyte. Hum Pathol 9:51, 1973

54. Sheldon PJ, Papamichail M, Hemsfed EH et al: Thymic origin of atypical lymphoid cells in infectious mononucleosis. Lancet 2:53, 1973

55. Reinherz EL, O'Brien C, Rosenthal P et al: Cellular basis for viral-induced immunodeficiency: analysis by monoclonal antibodies. J Immunol 125:1296, 1980

56. Tomkinson BE, Wagner DK, Nelson DL et al: Activated lymphocytes during acute Epstein-Barr virus infection. J Immunol 139:3802, 1987

57. Tatsumi E, Kimura K, Takluchi V et al: T-lymphocytes expressing human IA-like antigens in infectious mononucleosis (IM). Blood 56:383, 1980

58. Henle G, Henle W, Horwitz CA: Antibodies to Epstein-Barr virus associated nuclear antigen in infectious mononucleosis. J Infect Dis 130:231, 1974

59. Pearson GR: The humoral response. p. 141. In Schlossberg D (ed): Infectious Mononucleosis. Praeger Monographs in Infectious Disease. Vol 1. Praeger Publishers, New York, 1983

60. Kirchner H, Tosato G, Blaise RM et al: Polyclonal immunoglobulin secretion by human B lymphocytes exposed to Epstein-Barr virus in vitro. J Immunol 122:1310, 1979

61. Rickinson AB: Cellular immunological responses to the virus infection. p. 75. In Epstein MA, Achong BG (eds): The Epstein-Barr Virus: Recent Advances. John Wiley & Sons, New York, 1986

62. Tosato G, Magrath I, Koski I et al: Activation of suppressor T-cells during Epstein-Barr virus induced infectious mononucleosis. N Engl J Med 301:1133, 1974

63. Svedmyr E, Jondal M: Cytotoxic effector cells specific for B-cell lines transformed by Epstein-Barr virus are present in patients with infectious mononucleosis. Proc Natl Acad Sci USA 72:1622, 1975

64. Royston I, Sullivan JL, Periman PO et al: Cell mediated immunity to Epstein-Barr virus transformed lymphoblastoid cells in acute infectious mononucleosis. N Engl J Med 293:1159, 1975

65. Goldberg GN, Fulginiti VA, Ray CG et al: In utero Epstein-Barr virus (infectious mononucleosis) infection. JAMA 246:1579, 1981

66. Chang RS, Seto DSY: Perinatal infection by Epstein-Barr virus. Lancet 2:201, 1979

67. Yaeger AS: Transfusion-acquired cytomegalovirus infection in newborn infants. Am J Dis Child 128:478, 1974

68. Horwitz C, Henle W, Henle G et al: Clinical and laboratory evaluation of infants and children with Epstein-Barr virus induced infectious mononucleosis: report of 32 patients (aged 10 months–48 months). Blood 57:933, 1981

69. Fleisher G, Paradise J, Lennette E: Leukocyte response in childhood infectious mononucleosis. Am J Dis Child 135:699, 1981

70. Evans AS, Niederman JC: Epstein-Barr virus. p. 253. In Evans AS (ed): Viral Infections of Humans. Plenum, New York, 1982

71. Pullen H, Wright N, Murdock JM: Hypersensitivity reactions to antibacterial drugs in infectious mononucleosis. Lancet 2:1176, 1967

72. Bolden KJ: Corticosteroids in the treatment of infectious mononucleosis. J R Coll Gen Pract 22:87, 1972

73. DuBois RE, Seeley JK, Brus I et al: Chronic mononucleosis syndrome. South Med J 77:1376, 1984

74. Jones JF, Ray CG, Minnich LL et al: Evidence for active Epstein-Barr virus infection in patients with persistent unexplained illnesses: elevated anti-early antigen antibodies. Ann Intern Med 102:1, 1985

75. Straus SE, Tosato G, Armstrong G et al: Persisting illness and fatigue in adults with evidence of Epstein-Barr virus infection. Ann Intern Med 102:7, 1985

76. Buchwald D, Sullivan JL, Komaroff AL: Frequency of "chronic active Epstein-Barr virus infection" in a general medical practice. JAMA 247:2303, 1987

77. Miller G, Grogan E, Rowe D et al: Selective lack of antibody to a component of EB nuclear antigen in patients with chronic active Epstein-Barr virus infection. J Infect Dis 156:26, 1987

78. Schooley RT, Carey RW, Miller G et al: Chronic Epstein-Barr virus infection associated with fever and interstitial pneumonia. Ann Intern Med 104:636, 1986

79. Sullivan JL: Hematologic consequences of Epstein-Barr virus infection. Hematol Oncol Clin North Am 1:397, 1987

80. Giller RH, Grose C: Epstein-Barr virus: the hematologic and oncologic consequences of virus-host interaction. Crit Rev Hematol Oncol 9:149, 1989

81. Carter RL: Granulocyte changes in infectious mononucleosis. J Clin Pathol 19:279, 1966

82. Sumaya CV, Ench Y: Epstein-Barr virus infectious mononucleosis in children. I. Clinical and general laboratory findings. Pediatrics 75:1003, 1988

83. Hammond WP, Harlan JM, Steinberg SE: Severe neutropenia in infectious mononucleosis. West J Med 131:92, 1979

84. Schooley RT, Densen P, Harmon D et al: Antineutrophil antibodies in infectious mononucleosis. Am J Med 76:85, 1984

85. Gardner RV, Grooms A, Simon M: The effect of T cells from patients with infectious mononucleosis on CFU-CGM proliferation: a preliminary report. Clin Immunol Immunopathol 39:61, 1986

86. Herrod HG, Dow LW, Sullivan JL: Persistant Epstein-Barr virus infection in two children with a syndrome mimicking juvenile chronic myelogenous leukemia. Blood 61:1098, 1983

87. Hoagland RJ: Infectious Mononucleosis. Grune & Stratton, Orlando, 1967, p. 132

88. Jenkins WJ, Koster GH, Marsh WL et al: Infectious mononucleosis: an unsuspected source of anti-i. Br J Haematol 11:480, 1965

89. Fernback DJ, Mahoney DH: The hematologic response. p. 127. In Schlossberg D (ed): Infectious Mononucleosis. Praeger Publishers, New York, 1983

90. Woodruff RK, McPherson AJ: Severe haemolytic anaemia complicating infectious mononucleosis. Aust NZ J Med 6:569, 1976

91. Wishart MM, Davey MG: Infectious mononucleosis complicated by acute haemolytic anemia with a positive Donath-Landsteiner reaction. J Clin Pathol 26:332, 1973

92. Chernoff AI, Josephson AM: Acute erythroblastopenia in sickle cell anemia and infectious mononucleosis. Am J Dis Child 82:310, 1951

93. Socinski MA, Ershler WB, Tosato G et al: Pure red blood cell aplasia associated with chronic Epstein-Barr virus infection: evidence for T-cell-mediated suppression of erythroid colony forming units. J Lab Clin Med 104:995, 1984

94. Chang RS: Complications, sequelae, prognosis. p. 60. In Infectious Mononucleosis.Hall Medical Publishers, Boston, 1980,

95. Radel EG, Schorr JB: Thrombocytopenic purpura with infectious mononucleosis. J Pediatr 63:46, 1963

96. Lazarus KH, Baehner RL: Aplastic anemia complicating infectious mononucleosis: a case report and review of the literature. Pediatrics 67:907, 1981

97. Risdall RJ, McKenna R, Nesbit ME et al: Virus associated hemophagocytic syndrome. A benign histiocytic proliferation distinct from malignant histiocytosis. Cancer 44:993, 1979

98. Reiner AP, Spivak JL: Hematophagic histiocytosis. Medicine 67:369, 1988

99. Liu Yin JA, Kumaran TO, Marsh GW et al: Complete recovery of histiocytic medullary reticulosis-like syndrome in a child with acute lymphoblastic leukemia. Cancer 51:200, 1983

100. McKenna RW, Risdall RJ, Nesbit ME et al: Virus associated hemophagocytic syndrome. Hum Pathol 12:395, 1981

101. Reisman RP, Greco MA: Virus associated hemophagocytic syndrome due to Epstein-Barr virus. Hum Pathol 15:290, 1984

102. Sullivan JL, Woda BA, Herrod HG et al: Epstein-Barr virus associated hemophagocytic syndrome: virological and immunopathological studies. Blood 65:1097, 1985

103. Boruchoff SE, Woda BA et al: Parvovirus B19-associated hemophagocytic syndrome. Arch Intern Med 150:897, 1990

104. Kawaguchi H, Miyashita T, Herbst H et al: Epstein-Barr virus-infected T lymphocytes in Epstein-Barr virus-associated hemophagocytic syndrome. J Clin Invest 92:1444, 1993

105. Sullivan JL, Byron KS, Brewster FE et al: X-linked lymphoproliferative syndrome. J Clin Invest 71:1765, 1983

106. Sullivan JL, Woda BA: X-linked lymphoproliferative syndrome. Immunodefic Rev 1:325, 1989

107. Skare JC, Milunsky A, Byron KS et al: Mapping of X-linked lymphoproliferative syndrome. Proc Natl Acad Sci USA 84:2015, 1987

108. Skare JC, Grierson HL, Sullivan JL et al: Linkage analysis of seven kindreds with the X-linked lymphoproliferative syndrome (XLP) confirms that the XLP locus is near DXS42 and DXS37. Hum Genet 82:354, 1989

109. Skare JC, Wu BL, Madan S et al: Characterization of three overlapping deletions causing X-linked lymphoproliferative disease. Genomics 16:254, 1993

110. Skare JC, Madan S, Glaser J et al: First prenatal diagnosis of X-linked lymphoproliferative disease. Am J Med Genet 44:79, 1992

111. Raab-Traub N, Flynn K: The structure of the termini of the Epstein-Barr virus as a marker of clonal cellular proliferation. Cell 47:883, 1986

112. Levine AM: AIDS-related malignancies: the emerging epidemic. J Natl Cancer Inst 85:1382, 1993

113. Pluda JM, Venzon DJ, Tosato G et al: Parameters affecting the development of non-Hodgkin's lymphoma in patients with severe human immunodeficiency virus infection receiving antiretroviral therapy. J Clin Oncol 11:1099, 1993

114. Henle W, Henle GE, Horwitz CA: Epstein-Barr virus specific diagnostic tests in infectious mononucleosis. Hum Pathol 5:551, 1974

115. Horwitz CA, Henle W, Henle GE et al: Long-term serological follow-up of patients for Epstein-Barr virus after recovery from infectious mononucleosis. J Infect Dis 151:1150, 1985

116. Pagano JS: Detection of Epstein-Barr virus with molecular hybridization techniques. Rev Infect Dis, suppl. 1. 13:S123, 1991

117. Chang KL, Chen YY, Shibata D et al: Description of an in situ hybridization methodology for detection of Epstein-Barr virus RNA in paraffin-embedded tissues, with a survey of normal and neoplastic tissues. Diagn Mol Pathol 1:246, 1992

118. Shibata D, Weiss LM, Nathwani BN et al: Epstein-Barr virus in benign lymph node biopsies from individuals infected with the human immunodeficiency virus is associated with concurrent or subsequent development of non-Hodgkin's lymphoma. Blood 77:1527, 1991

119. Borisch B, Finke J, Hennig I et al: Distribution and localization of Epstein-Barr virus subtypes A and B in aids-related lymphomas and lymphatic tissue of HIV-positive patients. J Pathol 168:229, 1992

120. Kunimoto M, Tamura S, Tabata T et al: One-step typing of Epstein-Barr virus by polymerase chain reaction: predominance of type 1 virus in Japan. J Gen Virol 73:455, 1992

121. Colby BM, Shaw JE, Elion GB et al: Effect of acyclovir [9-(2-hydroxyethoxymethyl)guanine] on Epstein-Barr virus DNA replication. J Virol 34:560, 1980

122. Andersson J, Britton S, Ernberg I et al: Effect of acyclovir on infectious mononucleosis: a double-blind, placebo-controlled study. J Infect Dis 153:283, 1986

123. VanderHorst CM, Joncas J, Ahronheim G et al: Lack of effect of peroral acyclovir for the treatment of acute infectious mononucleosis. J Infect Dis 164:788, 1991

124. Sullivan JL, Medveczky P, Forman SJ et al: Epstein-Barr virus induced lymphoproliferation: implications for anti-viral chemotherapy. N Engl J Med 311:1163, 1984

125. Sullivan JL, Byron KS, Brewster FE et al: Treatment of life-threatening Epstein-Barr virus infections with acyclovir. Am J Med 73:262, 1982

126. Pirsch JD, Stratta RJ, Sollinger HW et al: Treatment of severe Epstein-Barr virus-induced lymphoproliferative syndrome with ganciclovir: two cases after solid organ transplantation. Am J Med 86:241, 1989

127. Okano M, Thiele GM, Kobayashi RH et al: Interferon-gamma in a family with X-linked lymphoproliferative syndrome with acute Epstein-Barr virus infection. J Clin Immunol 9:48, 1989

128. Williams LL, Rooney CM, Conley ME et al: Correction of Duncan's syndrome by allogeneic bone marrow transplantation. Lancet 342:587, 1993

129. Vowels MR, Lam-Po-Tang R, Berdoukas V et al: Brief report: correction of X-linked lymphoproliferative disease by transplantation of cord-blood stem cells. N Engl J Med 329:1623, 1993

HEMATOLOGIC MALIGNANCIES

Part VI

Cytogenetics and Neoplasia 59

Michelle M. Le Beau and Richard A. Larson

INTRODUCTION

The malignant cells in many patients who have leukemia, lymphoma, or another hematologic neoplasm have acquired chromosomal abnormalities in a clonal fashion. A number of specific cytogenetic abnormalities have been recognized that are very closely, and sometimes uniquely, associated with morphologically and clinically distinct subsets of leukemia or lymphoma.[1,2] The detection of one of these recurring abnormalities can be quite helpful in establishing the correct diagnosis and can add information of prognostic importance. The appearance of new abnormalities in the karyotype of a patient under observation often signals a change in the pace of the disease, usually to a more aggressive disorder. Certainly, the detection of a cytogenetic abnormality clearly distinguishes between benign reactive lymphoid or myeloid hyperplasia and a monoclonal malignant proliferation.

This chapter focuses on the genetics of the leukemias and lymphomas from a primarily cytogenetic perspective. While these disorders do occasionally exhibit familial aggregation, this is for the most part uncommon and poorly defined and has resulted in few biologic insights or clinical recommendations. By contrast, the delineation of specific and reproducible cytogenetic abnormalities correlated with specific hematologic malignancies has helped delineate disorders with distinct prognoses and etiologies and, in combination with molecular biologic studies, has led to important insights into their pathogenesis. As should be apparent, this understanding of the relationship between cytogenetic abnormalities and the pathogenesis and natural history of cancer is much further advanced for the leukemias than for other malignancies. This is largely the result of the relative ease of obtaining and processing bone marrow or peripheral blood samples from leukemia patients. Nonetheless, recent improvements in cell culture and processing techniques have resulted in the identification of a number of recurring abnormalities in solid tumors. The analysis of these neoplasms promises to be an exciting area of cancer research during the next decade.

GENETIC CONSEQUENCES OF CHROMOSOMAL REARRANGEMENTS

During the past few years, the genes located at the breakpoints of a number of the recurring chromosomal translocations have been identified (Table 59-1). Molecular analysis has shown that alterations in expression of the genes or in the properties of the encoded proteins resulting from the rearrangement play an integral role in the process of malignant transformation.[3,4] The transforming genes involved in chromosomal translocations fall into several functional classes, including tyrosine protein kinases, serine protein kinases, cell-surface receptors, growth factors, and inner mitochondrial membrane proteins. However, the largest class of genes involved in translocations encode transcriptional regulatory factors.[3,4] Transcription factors are proteins involved in the initiation of gene transcription; they recognize and bind to target sequences located in the regulatory elements of genes, often functioning in a tissue-specific fashion. In this way, they play critical roles in differentiation and development in addition to

maintaining the function of differentiated cells. These genes have been implicated in the pathogenesis of T- and B-cell neoplasms, as well as some myeloid leukemias (Table 59-1). All the genes cloned to date from rearrangements in acute leukemia have been transcription factor genes. Many of these genes were first identified as a result of the molecular characterization of translocations in tumor cells.

Chromosomal translocations result in altered gene function by several mechanisms. The first is deregulation of gene expression. This mechanism is characteristic of the translocations in the lymphoid leukemias and lymphomas that involve the immunoglobulin genes in B-lineage tumors and the T-cell receptor genes in T-lineage tumors. These rearrangements result in inappropriate expression (either overexpression or aberrant expression in a tissue that does not normally express the gene) of the partner gene involved in the translocation, with no alteration in its protein structure.

The second mechanism is the expression of a novel fusion protein, resulting from the juxtaposition of coding sequences from two genes that are normally located on different chromosomes. Such fusion proteins are tumor-specific in that the fusion gene does not exist in nonmalignant cells; thus, the detection of such a fusion gene/protein can be important in diagnosing or detecting residual disease or relapse. Examples of chimeric proteins include the BCR/ABL protein or the PML/RARA protein, resulting from the t(9;22) in chronic myeloid leukemia (CML) or t(15;17) in acute myeloid leukemia (AML)-M3, respectively. All the translocations cloned to date in the myeloid leukemias result in a fusion mRNA and a chimeric protein (Table 59-1).

Chromosomal translocations result in the activation of genes in a dominant fashion. A number of human tumors, including retinoblastoma, Wilms tumor, and colon carcinoma, are believed to result from recessive mutations which, when present in a homozygous state, lead to tumor formation.[5] These mutations lead to the *absence* of the protein product, suggesting that these genes function as "suppressor" genes or "anti-oncogenes" whose normal role(s) are to limit cellular proliferation. The hallmark of tumor suppressor genes is the loss of genetic material. Such a loss may result from chromosomal loss or deletion, as well as by other genetic mechanisms, such as mitotic recombination. The identification of recurring chromosomal loss or deletions in the leukemias and lymphomas suggests that, as for a number of solid tumors, tumor suppressor genes may be involved in the pathogenesis of some hematologic malignant diseases.

METHODS

Cytogenetic analyses of malignant diseases must be based on the study of the tumor cells themselves. In leukemia, the specimen is usually obtained by bone marrow aspiration and is either processed immediately (direct preparation) or cultured for 24–48 hours. When a bone marrow aspirate cannot be obtained, a bone marrow biopsy (bone core specimen) can often be processed successfully. Alternatively, for patients who have a white blood cell (WBC) count >10,000/mm^3 with >10% immature myeloid or lymphoid cells, a sample of peripheral blood can be cultured without adding phytohemagglutinin. The

Table 59-1. Functional Classification of Transforming Genes at Translocation Junctions

SRC family (TYR protein kinases)			
ABL	9q34	t(9;22)	CML/ALL
LCK	1p34	t(1;7)	T-ALL
Serine protein kinase			
BCR	22q11	t(9;22)	CML/ALL
Cell-surface receptor			
TAN1	9q34	t(7;9)	T-ALL
Growth factor			
IL3	5q31	t(5;14)	Pre-B-ALL
Mitochondrial membrane protein			
BCL2	18q21	t(14;18)	NHL
Cell-cycle regulator			
CCND1 (BCL1;	11q13	t(11;14)	CLL/NHL
PRAD1)			
Unknown			
DEK	6p23	t(6;9)	AML-M2/M4
ETO	8q24	t(8;21)	AML-M2
Transcriptional regulatory factors			
BCL3	19q13	t(14;19)	B-CLL
LYT10	10q24	t(10;14)	B-NHL
AML1	21q22	t(8;21	AML-M2
CBFB	16q22	inv(16)	AML-M4Eo
Homeobox			
PBX1	1q23	t(1;19)	Pre-B-ALL
HOX11	10q24	t(10;14)/t(7;10)	T-ALL
Helix-loop-helix			
CAN	9q34	t(6;9)	AML
LYT1	19p13	t(7;19)	T-ALL
MYC[a]	8q24	t(8;14)	B-ALL/T-ALL
TAL1(SCL)	1p34	t(1;14)	T-ALL
TAL2	9q32	t(7;9)	T-ALL
TCF3(E2A)[a]	19p13	t(1;19)	Pre-B-ALL
Zinc finger			
MLL	11q23	t(11q23)	ALL/AML
PLZF	11q23.1	t(11;17)	APL
PML	15q22	t(15;17)	APL
RARA	17q11-12	t(15;17)	APL
LIM			
RBTN1(TTG1)	11p15	t(11;14)	T-ALL
RBTN2	11p13	t(11;14)	T-ALL
Leucine zipper			
HLF	17q22	t(17;19)	pro-B ALL

[a] Also leucine zipper.

karyotype of the dividing cells will be similar to that obtained from the bone marrow. Mitogens such as phytohemagglutinin are not added routinely to peripheral blood cultures in acute leukemia, since stimulation of division of normal lymphocytes may interfere with the analysis of spontaneously dividing malignant cells. An involved lymph node or tumor mass specimen may be processed similarly for the analysis of lymphomas. Some laboratories use amethopterin or fluorodeoxyuridine to synchronize dividing cells, combined with brief exposures to mitotic inhibitors such as colchicine or DNA-binding agents (ethidium bromide), to obtain elongated chromosomes that have an increased number of bands.

Cytogenetic studies are feasible only for specimens that contain viable dividing cells. For this reason, it is critical that the specimen be transported to the cytogenetics laboratory without delay. In some cases, analyses may be performed on specimens that have been transported by overnight delivery services; however, the shipment of specimens frequently results in loss of cell viability, and most laboratories experience a high proportion of inadequate analyses using such specimens. For

optimally handled specimens, 95–98% of all cases should be adequate for cytogenetic analysis.

Chromosomal abnormalities are described according to the International System for Human Cytogenetic Nomenclature[6] (see Appendices 59-1 and 59-2). The observation of at least two cells with the same structural rearrangement (e.g., translocations, deletions, or inversions) or gain of the same chromosome, or three hypodiploid cells, each showing loss of the same chromosome, is considered evidence for the presence of an abnormal clone. However, one cell with a normal karyotype is considered evidence for the presence of a normal cell line. Patients whose cells show no alteration or nonclonal (single cell) abnormalities are considered normal. That is, one abnormal cell generally does not constitute evidence for the presence of an abnormal clone, since occasional abnormalities (primarily numerical abnormalities) may result from technical artifact. An exception are single cells characterized by recurring abnormalities. In these cases, it is likely that this represents the karyotype of the malignant cells in that particular patient.

CHRONIC MYELOPROLIFERATIVE DISORDERS

The chronic myeloproliferative disorders are a group of diseases characterized by the neoplastic proliferation of hematopoietic stem cells and their differentiated progeny within the bone marrow and in extramedullary sites. Although each of these disorders has distinctive clinical and laboratory features, the clinical pathologic characteristics and natural history show considerable overlap. The clonal nature of each of these diseases has been demonstrated by cytogenetic and isoenzyme techniques. In each disorder, multiple cell lineages are quantitatively and qualitatively abnormal, providing evidence that the neoplastic transformation occurs in a multipotential hematopoietic stem cell.

Chronic Myeloid Leukemia

Chronic Phase

CML is a particularly important subtype of leukemia because it was in this disease that the first consistent chromosomal abnormality in a malignant disease was noted (Table 59-2). This abnormality, the Philadelphia (Ph) chromosome, was first described in 1960 by Nowell and Hungerford[7] as a deletion of part of the long arm of a G-group chromosome, and later with the use of quinacrine fluorescence banding techniques as a 22q−. The nature of the chromosomal aberration was clarified in 1973, when Rowley[8] reported that the Ph chromosome results from a reciprocal translocation involving chromosomes 9 (break at band q34) and 22 (break at band q11), rather than a terminal deletion, as many investigators had previously assumed (Fig. 59-1). Studies with chromosomal polymorphisms have shown that the same chromosome 9 (or 22) of each homologous pair in a particular patient is involved in the rearrangement in all the malignant cells. These observations confirm earlier work based on enzyme markers, indicating that the CML cells originated from a single cell and were therefore clonal in origin.

Historically, about 85% of patients diagnosed as having CML were found to have the Ph chromosome (Ph+).[9] Identification of patients as Ph+ or Ph negative (Ph neg) was found to be clinically significant in that Ph+ patients had a better prognosis than that of patients with Ph neg CML (42 versus 15 months survival). Patients with a Ph chromosome and additional chromosomal abnormalities (1–30% of patients examined at initial diagnosis during the chronic phase) have not had a substantially poorer survival rate in some series than

Table 59-2. Recurring Chromosomal Abnormalities in Malignant Myeloid Diseases

Disease	Chromosomal Abnormality	Frequency[a] (%)	Involved Genes[b]
CML	t(9;22)(q34;q11)	~98 (100)[c]	ABL-BCR
CML blast phase	t(9;22) with +8, +Ph, +19, or i(17q)	~70	ABL-BCR
AML-M2	t(8;21)(q22;q22)	18 (30)	ETO-AML1
APL-M3, M3V	t(15;17)(q22;q11-12)	14 (98)	PML-RARA
AMMoL-M4Eo	inv(16)(p13q22) or t(16;16)(p13;q22)	6 (~100)	MYH11-CBFB
AMMoL-M4, AMoL-M5	t(9;11)(p22;q23)	11 (30)	AF9-MLL
	t(10;11)(p11–p15; q23)		?-MLL
	t(11;17)(q23;q25)		MLL-?
	t(11;19)(q23;p13)		MLL-ENL
	other t(11q23)		MLL
	del(11)(q23)		
AML	+8	13	
	−7	9	
	−5 or del(5q)	10	
	t(6;9)(p23;q34)	1	DEK-CAN
	t(3;3)(q21;q26) or inv(3)(q21q26)	2	
	del(20q)	5	
	t(12p) or del(12p)	2	
Therapy-related AML	−7 or del(7q) and/or −5 or del(5q)	75	
	t(11)(q23)	3	MLL
	der(1;7)(q10;p10)	2	

Abbreviations: AML-M2, acute myeloid leukemia with maturation; AMMOL, acute myelomonocytic leukemia; AMMoL-M4Eo, acute myelomonocytic leukemia with abnormal eosinophils; AMOL, acute monoblastic leukemia; AML, acute myeloid leukemia; APL-M3, M3V, hypergranular (M3) and microgranular (M3V) acute promyelocytic leukemia; CML, chronic myeloid leukemia.

[a] The percentage refers to the frequency within the disease overall. The numbers in the parentheses refers to the frequency within the morphologic or immunologic subtype of the disease.[2]

[b] Genes are listed in order of citation in the karyotype (e.g., for CML, ABL is at 9q34 and BCR at 22q11).

[c] Some patients with CML have an insertion of ABL adjacent to BCR in a normal-appearing chromosome 22.

that of patients who have only a Ph chromosome.[9,10] A change in the karyotype, however, is considered a grave prognostic sign, indicating progression to the acute blast phase; the usual duration of survival after such a change is 2–5 months.[9]

Evidence has accumulated to suggest that CML should be defined by the presence of the Ph chromosome or its molecular consequence, the BCR-ABL fusion gene (see below), and that patients without this abnormality should be considered to have a different myeloproliferative disorder. Pugh et al.[11] reviewed 25 patients initially diagnosed as having CML but whose cells lacked the Ph chromosome and showed that most of these patients had some type of myelodysplastic syndrome, most commonly chronic myelomonocytic leukemia or refractory anemia with excess blasts (RAEB). The most common abnormality in these patients was trisomy 8. These observations have been confirmed by others,[12] suggesting that, with very few exceptions, Ph neg CML does not exist. The absence of the Ph chromosome thus raises the suspicion that the patient actually has a MDS or a myeloproliferative disorder other than CML. It is notable, however, that the leukemia cells in occasional individual cases that lack the Ph chromosome appear to contain a DNA rearrangement in which the molecular consequences are identical to that of the t(9;22) (described below).

The karyotypes of many patients with Ph + CML have been examined with banding techniques by a number of investigators; in a review of 1,129 Ph + patients, the 9;22 translocation was identified in 92% (1,036 patients).[13] The remaining patients had variant translocations, such as three-way translocations involving chromosomes 9 and 22, as well as a third chromosome. Recent data clearly demonstrate that chromosome 9 is affected in all variant translocations in CML.[14]

Molecular analysis of the DNA sequences located at the chromosomal breakpoints of both the standard and variant translocations in CML has revealed that the proto-oncogene ABL is consistently translocated adjacent to a region of a gene (BCR) on chromosome 22, known as the breakpoint cluster region (bcr)[15,16] (Fig. 59-1). This translocation results in the formation of a chimeric gene that contains protein coding sequences from both the ABL and BCR genes and the production of a fusion protein (210 kd), an activated form of the ABL protein tyrosine kinase.[17–19] A number of studies have examined whether the location of the breakpoint within the bcr is correlated with the clinical features of CML.[20] The initial observations suggested that patients who have 3′ breakpoints progress more rapidly to blast crisis than do those who have 5′ breakpoints. However, other investigators have not observed a difference in the distribution of breakpoints within the bcr; thus, no definitive conclusions can be drawn. Analysis of leukemia cells from rare patients with CML who lack the Ph chromosome has revealed a rearrangement involving ABL and BCR that is detectable only at the molecular level.[21] However, this rearrangement is not present in most patients who have been diagnosed as having "Ph neg CML," providing further evidence that the t(9;22) and subsequent fusion of the ABL and BCR genes is characteristic of all CML cases.

Perhaps the most compelling evidence suggesting that the BCR/ABL fusion protein plays a role in the transformation of myeloid cells is the observation of the development of various hematologic malignant diseases in mice transplanted with bone marrow cells infected with a retrovirus encoding the p210 fusion protein. Transplanted mice developed myeloproliferative disorders, similar to CML in humans. The essential role of the tyrosine kinase activity of the BCR/ABL oncogene in growth stimulation is clear; recent studies have shown that the BCR/ABL protein transmits mitogenic signals within a cell via the RAS pathway of signal transduction. Moreover, several studies have defined an essential role for the BCR portion of the chimeric protein and have demonstrated that interactions between the serine kinase domain of the BCR protein with the SH2 domain of the ABL protein within the chimeric protein are essential for altered function of this protein.

When patients with CML are treated with busulfan or hydroxyurea and a hematologic remission is achieved, the bone marrow morphology and leukocyte alkaline phosphatase score may return to normal. However, when such a "remission" bone marrow is analyzed cytogenetically, the Ph clone persists, and the percentage of Ph + cells in the bone marrow usually remains unchanged (the Ph chromosome is usually found in 100% of cells examined). Attempts have been made to eradicate the Ph + clone with aggressive cytotoxic therapy, but only rarely can this be achieved, and even then the benefit is transient. Studies using glucose-6-phosphate dehydrogenase isoenzyme techniques together with cytogenetic studies have shown that all three hematopoietic cell lines (myeloid, erythroid, and megakaryocytic) are involved in the malignant process as are lymphocytes of B-cell origin.[22,23] This finding suggests that the cell of origin of CML is a multipotential stem cell. Intensive chemoradiotherapy followed by allogeneic bone marrow transplantation has been successful in eradicating the Ph + cell line and restoring normal hematopoiesis of donor origin. Of great importance is recent evidence that daily use of interferon-α can induce complete cytogenetic remission in approximately 20% of patients with CML in the chronic phase.[24] The reappearance

t(9;22)(q34;q11)

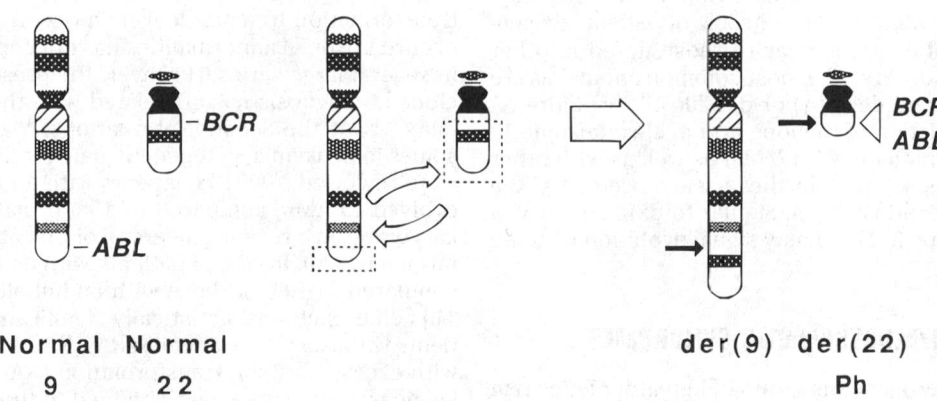

Normal Normal
9 22

der(9) der(22)
Ph

Fig. 59-1. Schematic diagram of a specific chromosomal abnormality, namely, the reciprocal translocation involving chromosomes 9 and 22, t(9;22)(q34;q11), which gives rise to the Ph chromosome in the malignant cells of patients with CML. Chromosomal breaks occur in bands q34 and q11 of chromosomes 9 and 22, respectively, followed by a reciprocal exchange of chromosomal material. This rearrangement results in the translocation of the *ABL* oncogene, normally located at 9q34, adjacent to the *BCR* gene on chromosome 22, giving rise to a chimeric *BCR-ABL* gene, whose protein product plays a role in the transformation of myeloid cells.

of cytogenetically normal marrow cells requires several months of treatment.[25] In most cases, molecular methods can still detect cells with the BCR/ABL fusion transcript. However, patients who have a cytogenetic complete response to interferon therapy have a longer survival than that of nonresponders or those treated only with hydroxyurea.

Blast Crisis

As they enter the terminal acute phase (blast crisis of CML), most patients (80%) show karyotypic evolution with the appearance of new chromosomal abnormalities in very distinct patterns, in addition to the Ph chromosome. For this reason, cytogenetic studies may be useful in confirming the clinical impression of the accelerated or acute phase of the disease. A change in the karyotype is considered a grave prognostic sign.[9] The available data suggest that, with the exception of an isochromosome of the long arm of chromosome 17 [i(17)(q10)], which is usually associated with a myeloid type of blast transformation, a particular karyotype has no association with the lymphoid or with the myeloid type of blast transformation, and these additional abnormalities are not correlated with the response to therapy during the acute phase.[13,26] The most common changes, a gain of chromosomes 8 or 19, or a second Ph (by gain of the first), or an i(17q), frequently occur in combination to produce modal chromosome numbers of 47-50.[13]

Polycythemia Vera

Polycythemia vera (PCV) is the second most extensively studied chronic myeloproliferative disorder.[13] Abnormalities are less common (about 14%) in untreated patients than in those treated with cytotoxic agents before their first cytogenetic examination (about 39%). An abnormal karyotype, frequently with multiple abnormalities, is detected in 85% of patients studied after they have developed leukemia. In PCV, the presence of cytogenetic abnormalities at diagnosis does not necessarily predict a short survival or the development of leukemia.[27-29] An evolutionary change in the karyotype during the disease course, however, may be an ominous sign.

In the polycythemic phase of PCV, the gain of chromosomes, which usually involves chromosomes 8 (15%) or 9 (20%), is

frequently observed. It is notable that a number of patients with PCV show gains of numbers 8 and 9; clones containing both +8 and +9 are seldom observed in other hematologic diseases and may therefore be unique to PCV. Structural rearrangements most often involve a deletion of chromosome 20 (q11.2q13.3) (30%) or a duplication of 1q (20%), especially bands 1q25–1q32. A deletion of 20q is not specific for PCV and has been noted in other malignant myeloid diseases; a deletion of 1q has been observed in other hematologic diseases, as well as in solid tumors.[30]

The cytogenetic pattern of the malignant cells in PCV patients who have developed AML shows some similarities to those observed in the polycythemic phase [e.g., +8, +9, del(20q)] but there are certain striking differences as well. For example, loss of number 7 is rarely observed in the polycythemic phase but is seen in 20% of patients in the leukemic phase. Rearrangements of chromosome 5, particularly a del(5q), are the most frequent changes noted in advanced disease (40% of patients).[13,31,32] As described in a later section, abnormalities of chromosomes 5 or 7, or both, are the most common abnormalities noted in therapy-related leukemia, suggesting that the leukemia in some patients with PCV may have a similar etiology. Chronic use of oral alkylating agents such as chlorambucil or the use of ^{32}P during the chronic phase of PCV has been shown to increase the rate of transformation to leukemia significantly.

Essential Thrombocythemia

One hundred-seventy cases of essential thrombocythemia (ET) were analyzed during the Third International Workshop on Chromosomes in Leukemia. Only 5% of patients had a definite chromosomal abnormality accepted by all the Workshop participants.[33] Moreover, no recurring abnormality could be identified in these patients. Previously, it had been reported that a del(21q) was a specific abnormality in ET; however, of 13 patients with del(21q) studied at the Workshop, 11 were from a single institution, and the absence of band 21q22 in these karyotypes was not uniformly accepted by the Workshop participants. Thus, currently available data do not reveal consistent karyotypic abnormalities in ET.

Myelofibrosis with Myeloid Metaplasia

Cytogenetic analysis of bone marrow cells of patients with myelofibrosis with myeloid metaplasia (MMM) has revealed the presence of clonal abnormalities in 35% of patients. In general, these abnormalities are similar to those noted in other malignant myeloid disorders. The most common anomalies are +8, −7 or a del(7q), and del(11q) or del(20q).[30,34,35] More recently, a recurring deletion of the long arm of chromosome 13 has been reported in patients with MMM as well as with other malignant myeloid disorders.[36] In these rearrangements, the consistently deleted band is 13q14. Similar to CML and PCV, a change in the karyotype in MMM may signal evolution to acute leukemia.

PRIMARY MYELODYSPLASTIC SYNDROMES

The MDSs are a heterogeneous group of hematopoietic stem cell disorders characterized by various combinations of anemia, neutropenia, or thrombocytopenia.[37,38] Several laboratories have reported that clonal chromosomal abnormalities can be detected in bone marrow cells in 40–70% of patients with primary MDS at diagnosis.[39–42] This contrasts with the 70–95% incidence of cytogenetic abnormalities detected in patients with AML de novo. Although trisomy 8 and loss of all or part of the long arm (q) of chromosomes 5 or 7 are common in both disorders, the specific structural rearrangements that are closely associated with distinct morphologic subsets of AML de novo (Table 59-2) are almost never seen in MDS (Table 59-3). With several exceptions (e.g., the 5q- syndrome), chromosomal abnormalities in MDS have not correlated with specific clinical or morphologic subsets using the criteria of the French-American-British (FAB) group.

Patients with MDS may have single or multiple chromosome changes (Table 59-3). A single chromosome change involves a single numerical change or a structural abnormality involving only one chromosome or a balanced translocation involving only two chromosomes. Occasionally, several unrelated abnormal clones may be detected (5% of cases); the frequency of such unrelated clones is higher than that observed in AML de novo (<1%). Additional chromosomal aberrations may evolve during the course of MDS or an abnormal clone may emerge in a patient with a previously normal karyotype; these changes appear to portend transformation to leukemia.

Table 59-3. Single Chromosome Changes in Primary MDS

−7

+8

del(5)(q13q33) and translocations involving 5q[a]

del(7q)

del(11q)[b]

del(12)(p11p13)

del(13q)[c]

del(20)(q11q13)

t(1;3)(p36;q21.2)

der(1;7)(q10;p10)

t(2;11)(p21;q23)

t(6;9)(p23;q34)

[a] Chromosomal breakpoints of the interstitial deletions of 5q are variable; proximal breakpoints frequently occur in bands 5q13–q15 and distal breakpoints frequently occur in bands q33–q35.

[b] q23 is always involved in either interstitial or terminal deletions.

[c] q14 is always involved in interstitial deletions of variable size.

The ability of cytogenetic analysis to predict the outcome for any individual patient with MDS is made more difficult because MDS is a life-threatening disorder due to persistent and profound pancytopenia (marrow failure), regardless of whether transformation to acute leukemia occurs. Thus, the presence of chromosomal abnormalities has not correlated with survival in several large series. However, the presence of an abnormal clone at diagnosis has correlated with the evolution of leukemia.[40–43] At the Second International Workshop on Chromosomes in Leukemia, cytogenetic data for 244 patients with MDS were reviewed.[42] Of 125 patients with an abnormal clone, 27% evolved to AML, compared to 15% of patients with a normal karyotype. In a recent University of Chicago report, MDS transformed to AML in 42% of patients with an abnormal karyotype, compared to 10% of those with an initially normal karyotype. This difference was statistically significant.[39] Among those patients with refractory anemia (RA), RAEB, or refractory anemia with excess blasts in transformation (RAEB-T), the risk of leukemic transformation was confined to those with an abnormal karyotype. In a series of 144 patients with RA or RAEB studied at the University of Pennsylvania, the presence of multiple chromosome changes was associated with shorter survival than that observed in MDS patients with a normal karyotype or with only single chromosomal abnormalities.[43] Eighty percent of the former group had died within 6 months, compared with about 30% in the latter two groups. Of note, the incidence of transformation to AML was similar among those with single (64%) or multiple chromosome changes (74%) and exceeded that observed in patients who had a normal karyotype (37%).

The 5q − syndrome is a distinctive hematologic disorder that occurs primarily in older women.[31,32] In contrast to other MDSs, in which males predominate, the male/female ratio here is 0.5. Eighty percent of patients with the 5q− syndrome are >50 years. Patients present with a refractory macrocytic anemia and normal or elevated platelet counts. The marrow is characterized by the presence of monolobulated and bilobulated megakaryocytes. Approximately two-thirds of patients have <5% blasts in the marrow (RA or RA with ringed sideroblasts) and the remainder have RAEB. Although 75% of patients have a del(5)(q13q33), other interstitial deletions [del(5)(q15q33) or del(5)(q22q33)] may be present. These patients can have a relatively benign course extending over several years.

ACUTE MYELOID LEUKEMIA DE NOVO

The acute leukemias are generally classified as either lymphocytic or myeloid. In either case, these result from neoplastic transformations of uncommitted or partially committed hematopoietic stem cells. Traditionally, classification of the acute leukemias has relied on morphology, reflecting the predominant cell type and relating that cell to its presumed normal counterpart.[44] In large part, the correlation of cytogenetic abnormalities with the morphologic features of the leukemia was made possible by the development of a classification system for the acute leukemias by the FAB Cooperative Group.[45,46]

Numerous reports have described cytogenetic analyses of relatively large series of unselected patients with AML as well as of single cases of selected patients.[13,30,47–49] In earlier series, abnormal karyotypes were reported in approximately 50% of all patients with AML de novo whose bone marrow cells were examined with banding techniques. At the Fourth International Workshop on Chromosomes in Leukemia held in Chicago in September 1982, 54% (354 of 660) of patients had chromosomal abnormalities.[50] The detection of cytogenetic abnormalities increases markedly when techniques for culturing leukemia cells and for obtaining prophase and prometaphase chromosomes are used. Currently, investigators are detecting an abnormal clone in 85% of AML patients. Initially, it appeared that AML patients with a normal karyotype had a significantly longer survival than that of patients with any detectable chromosomal abnormality. More recently, it has become clear that the prognostic importance resides within specific chromosome changes, several of which are associated with higher response rates and longer survival than the medians observed in AML patients who have no detectable abnormality.[48–51] This discussion emphasizes certain specific aberrations that occur frequently and that also appear to be of exceptional biologic interest (Table 59-2).

Chromosomal Gain and Loss

Although the karyotypes of patients with AML may be variable, both the nonrandom gain and loss of chromosomes and the involvement in structural rearrangements are evident. The number of chromosomes gained or lost in 354 patients with a clonal abnormality was examined at the Fourth International Workshop on Chromosomes in Leukemia.[50] With the exceptions of chromosome 16, which was never observed as a gain, and chromosome 1, which was never lost, each of the autosomes and sex chromosomes contributed to the numerical changes. Some chromosomes are clearly overrepresented as gains or losses, while others are underrepresented. Thus, a gain of chromosome 8, the most frequent abnormality seen in AML, was found in 13% (47 of 354) of patients. Loss of chromosome 7, another frequent numerical change, was observed in 9% (30 of 354) of patients, and loss of chromosome 5 was noted in 6% (20 of 354) of cases. A gain of either of these chromosomes is rarely observed. These abnormalities are seen in most subtypes of AML, although with some interesting differences in frequency.[52–54]

Loss of the Y chromosome, the second most frequent numerical change in the patients examined at this Workshop, or loss of the X chromosome often occurred in association with an 8; 21 translocation (80–90% of patients).[50] Loss of a Y chromosome as the sole abnormality has been described, but the sig-

nificance of this abnormality is uncertain because a missing Y chromosome has also been reported in bone marrow cells of hematologically normal males, particularly those >60 years old.[47] By contrast, the t(8;21) in AML-M2 is usually observed in younger adults.[13,42,48,50,51]

Erythroblastic Leukemia

In a recent analysis of 26 patients with acute erythroblastic leukemia (M6) at the University of Chicago, 77% were found to have clonal abnormalities, and 85% of these cases showed a loss of all or part of chromosome 5 or 7, or both.[55] In addition, the karyotypes were often complex with multiple abnormalities and subclones. These patients were older than those M6 patients with normal karyotypes or simple chromosomal changes, and they had a shorter survival. The former group had striking similarities to the biologic and clinical features of therapy-related AML (see below).

Specific Structural Rearrangements

The distribution of chromosomes involved in structural rearrangements in AML was examined at the Fourth International Workshop.[50] Translocations and deletions accounted for most of the rearrangements observed. The most frequently rearranged chromosome was 17; abnormalities of this chromosome were noted in 53 patients, 43 of whom had the t(15;17). Likewise, most cases with rearrangements of chromosomes 8, 15, or 21, the three next most frequently altered chromosomes, resulted from the two specific translocations: t(8;21) and t(15; 17). A deletion of 5q was identified in 25 patients, and rearrangements of 11q, primarily translocations, were also frequent. These specific rearrangements are described in further detail below.

8;21 Translocation in Acute Myeloid Leukemia

In 1973, Rowley[56] first described a balanced translocation between chromosomes 8 and 21 [t(8;21)(q22;q22)] (Fig. 59-2A). The t(8;21) is common, being observed in 18% of all AML cases

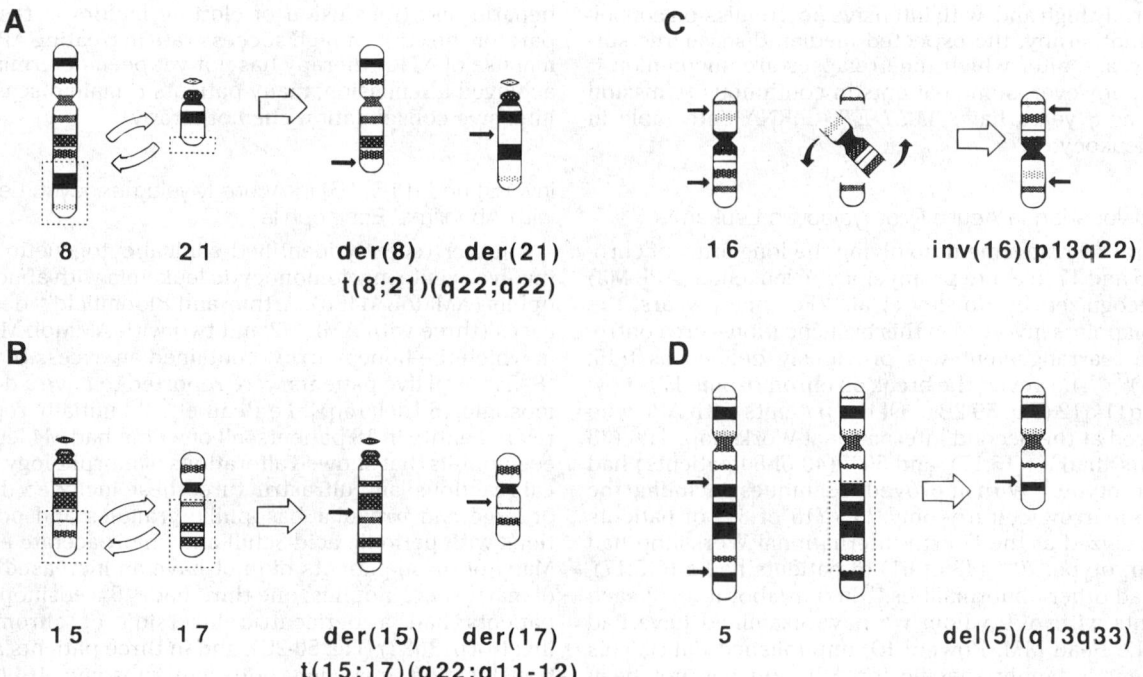

Fig. 59-2. Schematic diagram of four recurring chromosomal abnormalities characteristic of AML. **(A)** t(8;21)(q22;q22), AML-M2. **(B)** t(15;17)(q22;q11-12), APL-M3. **(C)** inv(16)(p13q22), AMMoL-M4Eo. **(D)** del(5)(q13q33), observed in MDS and AML. A del(5q) is frequently observed in t-MDS/t-AML.

with an abnormal karyotype and in 30% of M2 patients. This translocation is the most frequent abnormality in children with AML, reported in 17% (10 of 60) of karyotypically abnormal cases. This abnormality initially appeared to be restricted to patients with a diagnosis of M2 leukemia (AML with maturation) according to the FAB classification.[45] However, 7% (3 of 44) of patients analyzed at the Fourth International Workshop, who had a t(8;21) and had adequate bone marrow material available for morphologic review, had a diagnosis of acute myelomonocytic leukemia (M4).[50]

The t(8;21) interrupts two genes, *AML1* on chromosome 21, and *ETO* on chromosome 8, joining them to form a new chimeric gene on the der(8) chromosome.[57-59] The *AML1* gene encodes a protein with strong homology with the developmentally regulated segmentation gene, *runt,* in *Drosphila melanogaster.*[60] Recently, the AML1 protein has been demonstrated to be identical to CBFA, the α-subunit of a heterodimeric transcription factor (core binding factor [CBF]), which regulates gene expression in T cells. The nature of the ETO product is unknown; however, the chimeric protein containing the AML1 transcription factor sequences is likely to contribute to the development of this leukemia.

Although the M2 type of AML is heterogeneous, the presence of the t(8;21) identifies a morphologically and clinically distinct subset. In this disorder, blasts tend to have indented nuclei, and the cytoplasm is generally basophilic with a prominent paranuclear hof that may contain a few azurophilic granules.[61] Promyelocytes, myelocytes, and metamyelocytes are often quite prominent and may be large. Their cytoplasm has a waxy orange appearance and lacks a granular texture in Romanowski-stained specimens. Auer rods are easily identified, and several may be seen in a single cell. Bone marrow eosinophilia is also common.[61]

AML-M2 with the t(8;21) appears to have a favorable prognosis. The median age of these patients is approximately 25–30 years, significantly younger than that of patients with AML overall.[42,48,49] Some patients have <30% myeloblasts in the marrow at diagnosis and are therefore inappropriately classified as having MDS rather than AML. The complete remission rate is uniformly high and, with intensive postremission consolidation chemotherapy, the expected median disease-free survival is >2 years, after which time relapses are uncommon.[51] Remarkably, however, some patients in continuous remission for as long as 8 years have *AML1/ETO* mRNA detectable in circulating leukocytes.[62]

15;17 Translocation in Acute Promyelocytic Leukemia

A structural rearrangement involving the long arms of chromosomes 15 and 17 in acute promyelocytic leukemia (APL-M3) was first recognized by Rowley et al.[63] For many years, the precise breakpoints involved in this translocation were controversial. The rearrangement was previously defined as t(15;17)(q22;q21)[50,64]; however, the break on chromosome 17 is now designated q11-q12 (Fig. 59-2B).[1] Of the patients with APL who were reviewed at the Second International Workshop, 41% (33 of 80 patients) had a t(15;17), and 50% (40 of 80 patients) had a normal karyotype.[42] With improved techniques, including the use of bone marrow culture, only 25% (15 of 61) of patients with APL analyzed at the Fourth International Workshop had a normal karyotype; 70% (43 of 61) of patients had a t(15;17), and three had other abnormalities.[50] In our laboratory,[64] each of 90 patients with APL whom we have examined have had a t(15;17) (Le Beau MM, Rowley JD, unpublished data). This rearrangement is highly specific for APL and has not been found in patients with any other type of leukemia or solid tumor.

The breakpoint on chromosome 17 occurs within the first intron of the α-retinoic acid receptor gene *(RARA)* in most patients, whereas the break on chromosome 15 occurs within the *PML* gene.[65,66] *RARA* is a member of the steroid/thyroid hormone receptor superfamily. Retinoic acid is a ligand that binds to the nuclear receptor homodimer complex; this complex acts as a transcription factor (i.e., it activates transcription of other genes), inducing cellular differentiation. The *PML* gene encodes a DNA-binding protein; thus, this gene may also encode a transcription factor. The translocation results in a fusion *PML/RARA* gene that contains most of the *PML* coding sequences, as well as the DNA-binding and ligand-binding domains of the *RARA* gene. Although the precise mechanism is unknown, it appears that the fusion PML/RARA protein is integral to the sensitivity of APL cells to all-trans retinoic acid (ATRA).

APL is widely recognized as a unique clinicopathologic entity characterized by infiltration of the bone marrow by promyelocytes in association with a hemorrhagic diathesis. The characteristic folded, reniform (kidney-shaped), or bilobed nucleus is invariably found in some of the promyelocytes. Coarse azurophilic granules and multiple Auer rods are common.[61,64] The microgranular variant of APL differs from the more frequent hypergranular type only in that the cytoplasmic granules of the leukemia cells are smaller and sometimes beyond the limit of resolution of the light microscope.[64] Auer rods may also be fewer in number and the peripheral WBC count higher in the M3 microgranular variant, but the t(15;17) is similarly present.

Patients with APL and the t(15;17) are younger than other individuals who have AML.[48,50,64] Clinical or laboratory evidence of disseminated intravascular coagulation is almost invariably present at diagnosis and may worsen during the initial cytolytic response to chemotherapy. APL cells are exquisitely sensitive to the differentiating effect of ATRA, and evidence of disseminated intravascular coagulation rapidly resolves after starting this treatment.[67] Cases that lack the t(15;17) do not respond to ATRA. Patients with APL may enter complete remission without experiencing a period of marrow hypoplasia; the malignant promyelocytes are often slow to clear from the marrow even as normal hematopoiesis recovers.[51] Appropriate attention to the intravascular coagulation complication using heparin and transfusion of clotting factors is responsible in part for the current high success rate in treating APL. The optimal use of ATRA therapy has not yet been determined. Having achieved a remission, many patients remain disease-free after intensive consolidation chemotherapy.

Inv(16) and t(16;16) in Acute Myelomonocytic Leukemia with Abnormal Eosinophils

Another recently identified clinical/cytogenetic association involves acute myelomonocytic leukemia with abnormal eosinophils (AMMoL-M4Eo). Arthur and Bloomfield[68] described five cases (three with AML-M2 and two with AMMoL-M4 leukemia) in which the bone marrow contained an excess of eosinophils (8–54%); all five patients were reported to have a deleted chromosome 16 [del(16q)]. Le Beau et al.[69] initially reported on a related entity in 18 patients, all of whom had M4 leukemia with eosinophils that showed alterations of morphology, cytochemical reactions, and ultrastructure; these included the presence of large and irregular basophilic granules and positive reactions with periodic acid-Schiff and chloroacetate esterase.[69,70] Many of these patients did not have an increased percentage of marrow eosinophils; one-third had <5% eosinophils. Fifteen patients had a pericentric inversion of chromosome 16, inv(16)(p13q22) (Fig. 50-2C), and in three patients a reciprocal translocation involving both chromosome 16 homologues [t(16;16)(p13;q22)] was noted.[69-72] Among M4 patients in the University of Chicago series, 23% have had an inv(16) or t(16;16). This correlation between abnormal eosinophils and structural rearrangements of chromosome 16 was confirmed at the

Fourth International Workshop.[50] Of 25 patients with M4 and >5% marrow eosinophils, 10 had either a del(16) or an inv(16). Our experience suggests that breakpoints at both 16p13 and 16q22 are required for manifestation of the complete M4Eo syndrome, as patients with only del(16)(q22) have had different morphologic and clinical features.[72] Patients with inv(16) or t(16;16) have a good response to intensive chemotherapy. In our updated series, 78% (25 of 32) of treated patients entered complete remission.[72] The median survival for all 32 treated patients was >66 weeks, and the median survival for those 25 patients who had a complete remission was >104 weeks. This survival markedly exceeded the median of 29 weeks attained by 58 treated AMMoL patients who did not have this chromosomal rearrangement.

The inversion breakpoint at 16q22 occurs near the end of the coding region of the *CBFB* gene, also known as *PEBP2B*.[73] This gene encodes one subunit of a novel heterodimeric transcription factor (CBF); of note is that the α-subunit of CBF is encoded by *AML1*, at 21q22, the gene involved in the t(8;21) in AML-M2. A smooth muscle myosin heavy chain gene *(MYH11)* is interrupted by the breakpoint on 16p. A fusion protein containing the 5′ region of CBFB (165 of 182 amino acids) fused to the 3′ portion of MYH11 is produced. This portion of MYH11 contains a repeated α-helical structure involved in myosin filament interactions and, thus, may be important in dimerization of the fusion protein in M4 leukemia cells. The target genes of the CBF transcription factor are not yet known.

Rearrangements of the Long Arm of Chromosome 11 in Acute Monoblastic Leukemia

In 1980, Berger and co-workers first reported a higher than expected frequency of abnormalities of the long arm of chromosome 11 (11q) in 10 patients with acute monocytic leukemia (AMoL-M5). In an expanded series of cases, rearrangements of 11q were observed in 35% (12 of 34) of patients with M5, and the investigators emphasized an especially strong association between abnormalities of 11q and the poorly differentiated form of AMoL (M5a).[74] Rowley[75] noted that the association between 11q abnormalities and M5a was particularly strong in children. At the Fourth International Workshop on Chromosomes in Leukemia, the associations between 11q abnormalities, M5, and young age were confirmed.[50]

Recurring translocations involving chromosome 11, band q23, are of great interest in human acute leukemia for at least three reasons. First, >20 different recurring rearrangements involve 11q23 and, thus, along with band 14q32, 11q23 is one of the bands most frequently involved in rearrangements in human tumor cells.[1] The breakpoints in the 11q23 translocation partners include 1p32, 4q21, and 19p13.3 in acute lymphocytic leukemia (ALL) and 1q21, 2q21, 6q27, 9p22, 10p11, 17q25, 19p13.3, and 19p13.1 in AML, especially the monoblastic and myelomonocytic subtypes. Second, these translocations occur primarily in two morphologic types of leukemia that are different but that have similar features. One common translocation in infants, t(4;11)(q21;q23), usually has a lymphoblastic phenotype, although the leukemia cells may express some myeloid surface markers; in some cases, variable numbers of monocytoid blast cells have been identified.[61] A cell line with the 4;11 translocation (RS4;11) has rearranged immunoglobulin heavy chain and κ light chain genes, yet it can be induced to express monoblastic features on exposure to phorbol esters. Other translocations, such as the t(9;11) and t(11;19)(q23;p13.1), are common in monoblastic leukemias.[76] Abnormalities of 11q23 are seen in about 35% of M5 patients and in slightly less than one-half of the patients with M5a.[74,77,78] These data suggest that a gene at 11q23 may be involved in determining the differentiation of primitive hematopoietic stem cells into lymphoblasts or monoblasts or that it may be a gene that is active in both cell

lineages. Finally, translocations involving 11q23 have a very unusual age distribution; they comprise about two-thirds of chromosomal abnormalities in leukemia cells of children <1 year of age.[77,78] The t(4;11) in ALL and 11q23 abnormalities in AML are recognized cytogenetic subsets with a poor prognosis (described below).

Several groups of investigators have identified the gene located at the breakpoint at 11q23 in these recurring translocations.[79–82] The *MLL/TRX/ALL-1* gene is a very large gene with multiple large transcripts within the 11–12.5-kb range.[79] The encoded protein contains several motifs characteristic of transcription factors (e.g., A-T hooks, zinc finger domains), and the gene has homology to the *Drosophila* trithorax gene, which encodes a transcription factor involved in the developmental processes in this organism.[80,82] The genes on chromosomes 4, 9, and 19 (p13.3) have recently been identified. The translocations result in the production of a fusion gene; however, precisely how the *MLL* gene interacts with DNA sequences on these other chromosomes in the process of malignant transformation is unknown. It will be important to determine whether the genes on the partner chromosomes interact with *MLL* to affect the myeloid versus lymphoid phenotype of the corresponding leukemias or whether the cell lineage and stage at which the translocation occurs dictates the phenotype.

By molecular mapping of the region surrounding the breakpoint in the *MLL* gene, investigators have identified genomic DNA and *MLL* cDNA clones that detect the 11q23 translocations by Southern blot analysis.[83] These probes detect the rearrangements in all patients with the most common translocations, namely, t(4;11), t(9;11), t(6;11), t(11;19)(q23;p13.3), and t(11; 19)(q23;p13.1). In addition, rearrangements were detected in leukemia cells from patients with 16 other less common rearrangements affecting 11q23, including 11 translocations, 3 insertions, and 1 inversion.[83] In a recent study of infants with ALL, rearrangements were detected in 70% of cases, including some that were normal or inadequate by cytogenetic analysis.[84] Patients with 11q23 abnormalities had a significantly poorer outcome than that of patients who had no rearrangements of the *MLL* gene. Thus, rearrangements affecting *MLL* gene represent a major class of mutations in acute leukemia and identify patients with a poor outcome.

T(3;3) and inv(3) in AML with Thrombocytosis

Golomb et al.[85] initially reported on the presence of normal or elevated platelet counts in two patients with AML and structural abnormalities of the long arm of chromosome 3. These patients were found to have numerous micromegakaryocytes in their bone marrow. Additional patients who had identical or closely related cytogenetic abnormalities as well as thrombocytosis were subsequently reported by other investigators.[86]

We studied 14 patients with abnormalities of 3q and AML or MDS, and confirmed an association of certain cytogenetic abnormalities with thrombocytosis in AML patients.[87] The specific cytogenetic abnormalities associated with thrombocytosis in these patients involve bands 3q21 and 3q26 simultaneously and include the inv(3)(q21q26), t(3;3)(q21;q26), and the ins(5;3)(q14;q21q26) (insertion of chromosomal material from 3q into 5q). The t(3;3) and inv(3) comprise 3–4% of AML cases in our series. Seven of the eight patients in our series with these abnormalities had platelet counts of >100,000/mm³ before the initiation of cytoreductive therapy. Four patients had significant thrombocytosis with platelet counts as high as 1,731,000/mm³. This finding is quite striking when compared with the incidence of thrombocytosis in a large group of patients with AML studied at the Fourth International Workshop on Chromosomes in Leukemia.[50] At that workshop, only eight of 716 patients, including two with inv(3), had elevated platelet counts (unpublished data).

As might be expected, the most consistent bone marrow finding in these patients is an increase in the number of megakaryocytes, many of which are morphologically abnormal. In some of the patients, nearly all identifiable megakaryocytes are micromegakaryocytes. A few circulating megakaryoblasts were identified by the presence of platelet peroxidase activity in one of two patients we studied with this reaction.[87] These histopathologic findings are not indicative of acute megakaryoblastic leukemia.

6;9 Translocation in AML with Increased Basophils

A translocation involving chromosomes 6 and 9 [t(6;9)(p23; q34)] was first described in two patients by Rowley and Potter in 1976, and later in three patients by Vermaelen et al.[88] but no common features were detected. We have subsequently studied seven additional patients with this translocation.[89] Patients with a t(6;9) comprise about 2% of patients with AML in our series. Eight of these nine patients had an increase in the number of basophils in the bone marrow, within a range of 1.5–12%; the normal value is 0.2%. Because the marrow in all biopsy specimens was hypercellular, this represented a marked increase in the total basophil count. The basophils appeared to be morphologically normal. Only 5 of 163 AML patients whom we studied had increased numbers of marrow basophils (>1%) in the absence of the t(6;9). Of the nine t(6; 9) patients, five were classified as AML-M2, three as AMMoL-M4, and one as AML-M1. The median age was 38 years, lower than that for AML patients overall. As a group, patients with a t(6;9) have responded poorly to intensive remission induction therapy. Although the breakpoint in chromosome 9 is in the same band as the t(9;22) in CML, and a marked increase in basophils is a regular feature of CML, the t(6;9) involves the CAN gene, located >100 kb distal to the ABL gene.

Environmental Associations with Acute Myeloid Leukemia

Mitelman et al.[90] reported on a retrospective study of 162 Swedish patients with AML de novo; 52 of these patients gave a history suggesting occupational exposure to chemical solvents, insecticides, or petroleum products, whereas 110 patients had no such known exposure. Seventy-five percent of the exposed group had clonal chromosomal abnormalities, as compared to 32% in the nonexposed group. The exposed group had a distinctly nonrandom pattern of changes, with 79% of the chromosomally abnormal cases (60% of all patients) having at least one of four specific abnormalities: −5/del(5q), −7/del(7q), +8, or +21. Other investigators have found similar associations.[91,92] More recently, the Cancer and Leukemia Group B has reported on the association between smoking, irradiation, and exposure to solvents and hair dyes, and specific cytogenetic abnormalities and RAS oncogene activation in a prospective study of patients with AML or ALL.[93]

THERAPY-RELATED MYELODYSPLASTIC SYNDROMES AND ACUTE MYELOID LEUKEMIA

Of increasing interest have been characteristic chromosomal abnormalities found in patients who develop a therapy-related MDS or AML (t-MDS or t-AML) after chemotherapy and/or radiotherapy for an earlier disorder, such as Hodgkin disease, non-Hodgkin lymphoma (NHL), carcinoma, rheumatoid arthritis, or renal transplantation.[94,95] Two-thirds of these patients are first recognized by evidence of myelodysplasia, marrow

failure, and pancytopenia. Not uncommonly, the initial malignant disease is still present at the time of the secondary bone marrow dysfunction. Often, all three hematopoietic cell lines appear to be involved in the secondary malignancy.[95,96] One-half of patients diagnosed with t-MDS (<30% marrow blasts) will evolve to t-AML within a median of 6 months, but the other one-half will die of infectious or hemorrhagic complications of pancytopenia first.

Chromosomal abnormalities are found in most patients with t-MDS before the evolution of overt leukemia; these changes are often multiple and complex. Aberrations involving chromosomes 5 or 7 either alone or in combination with other changes account for most cytogenetic abnormalities in t-MDS.[97] In the University of Chicago series, 97% (47 of 48) of patients with t-MDS demonstrated a clonal chromosomal abnormality, and 87% had abnormalities of chromosome numbers 5 or 7, or both.[97] Thus, the detection of a clonal abnormality in a pancytopenic patient is convincing evidence of the existence of a malignant secondary neoplasm, even though the percentage of blasts in the marrow is not yet elevated.

More recently, a second variant of t-AML has been identified that is distinctly different from the more common leukemia that follows alkylating agents or irradiation.[98] This type of t-AML was first observed among patients receiving extremely high cumulative doses of etoposide for lung cancer but has also been seen in patients receiving other drugs known to inhibit topoisomerase II (e.g., teniposide, doxorubicin). These leukemias are characterized cytogenetically by abnormalities involving 11q23, such as t(9;11). The MLL gene is rearranged. Clinically, these patients have a short latency period (often only 1 or 2 years) and present with overt leukemia, usually with monocytic features. Other balanced rearrangements involving 21q21, such as t(8;21) and t(3;21), have been observed in t-AML following topo II inhibitors.[99]

Among those patients who present with frank AML and who have previously received cytotoxic therapy, some patients are likely to have developed their second neoplasm in a metachronous or completely unrelated fashion. Because causality cannot be definitively established, we prefer to designate these patients by the clinical term, t-AML. Occasionally, such a t-AML patient presenting with overt leukemia without a preleukemic phase will be found to have one of the specific chromosomal abnormalities closely linked with AML de novo, such as t(15; 17). This rare occurrence may in fact represent an unrelated second neoplasm, since these patients have a clinical response and outcome more like AML de novo than t-AML.

The following section summarizes the findings in the updated University of Chicago series of 129 patients with t-MDS/t-AML.[95,97] (unpublished data). Forty-seven had Hodgkin disease, 24 had NHL, 9 had multiple myeloma, one had hairy cell leukemia, 44 had various solid tumors, and 4 had had an organ transplant. Sixty-five patients had received both radiotherapy and chemotherapy before the development of their second malignancy, and 48 patients had had only chemotherapy. Sixteen patients had had only radiotherapy and, in most of these cases, major areas containing active marrow had been irradiated. The median time between the original diagnosis and the diagnosis of secondary bone marrow dysfunction was 56 months and did not vary significantly, depending on the primary disorder or the primary treatment.

Ninety-three percent (120 of 129) of patients with therapy-related malignancies were chromosomally abnormal[97] (unpublished data). More importantly, one or both of two consistent changes were noted in 81% (97 of 120) of patients with abnormalities. Among these 97 patients, 21 had loss of chromosome 5, 26 had a del(5q) (Fig. 59-2D), 8 had loss of 5q following unbalanced translocations, 51 had loss of chromosome 7, 11 had a del(7q), and 12 had loss of 7q as a result of an unbalanced translocation. Thirty-one patients had abnormalities of chro-

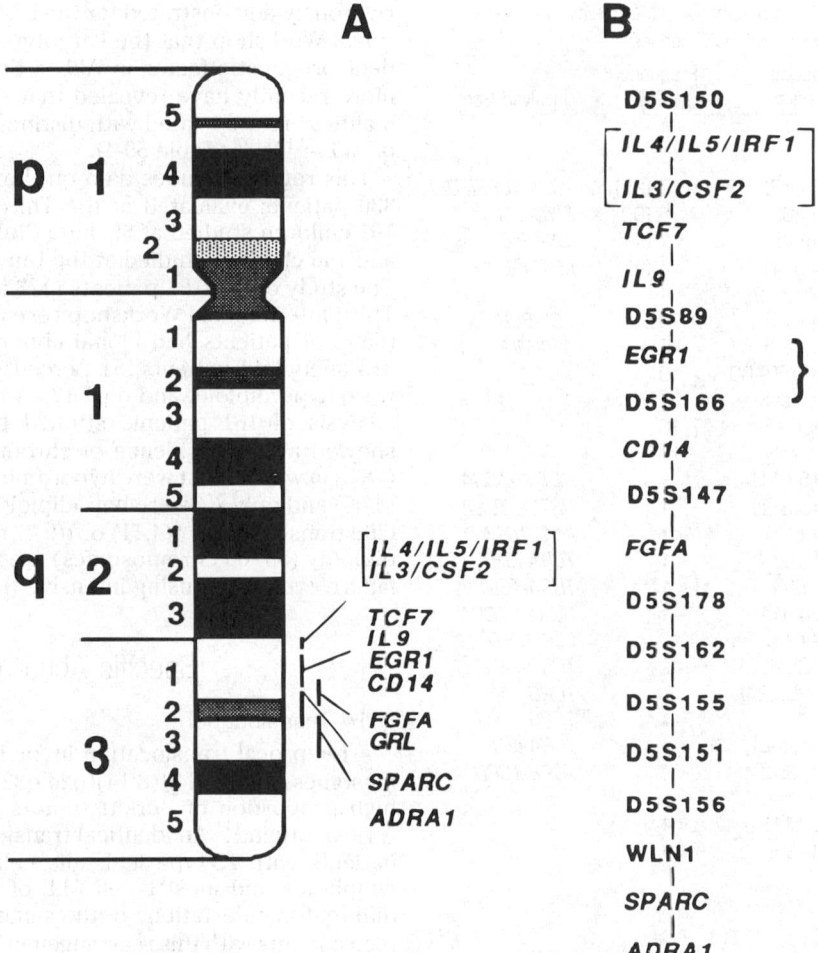

Fig. 59-3. Schematic diagram of the banding pattern of chromosome 5 illustrating the chromosomal localization and order of the *IL4/IL5/IRF1, IL3/CSF2, TCF7, IL9, EGR1, CD14, FGFA, GRL, SPARC,* and *ADRA1* genes determined by **(A)** FISH and **(B)** the physical order of cosmid and phage clones and genes and the relationship of loci on 5q to the critical region of 5q31 (brace). Brackets identify probes for which the order is unknown.

mosomes 5 and 7. Overall, 55 patients (43%) had abnormalities of chromosome 5. A del(5q) was the most common structural aberration in our series.

By analogy to retinoblastoma and Wilms tumor, one can propose that certain as yet unidentified critical genes located on 5q are related to leukemogenesis. By cytogenetic analysis of 135 patients with malignant myeloid diseases and a del(5q), we identified a small segment of 5q, consisting of band 5q31, that was deleted in each patient.[100,101] This segment has been termed the critical region. Distal 5q contains a number of genes encoding growth factors, hormone receptors, and proteins involved in signal transduction or transcriptional regulation.[101,102] These include several genes that are good candidates for a tumor suppressor gene as well as the genes encoding five hematopoietic growth factors (colony-stimulating factor-granulocyte/macrophage [CSF-GM; CSF-2] and several interleukins, [IL-3, IL-4, IL-5, and IL-9]) (Fig. 59-3). By fluorescence in situ hybridization analysis of probes to metaphase cells with overlapping deletions involving 5q31, we have narrowed the critical region to a small segment of 5q31 containing the *EGR1* gene.[101] The five hematopoietic growth factors genes and seven other genes are excluded from this region (Fig. 59-3). By physical mapping, the minimum size of the critical region is estimated to be 2.8 Mb. To date, no mutations of the remaining *EGR1* allele have been detected. The molecular characterization of the critical region will facilitate identification of a putative tumor suppressor gene in this band. With respect to

chromosome 7, cytogenetic analysis of the deletions of 7q noted in myeloid disorders suggests that there may be two different critical regions on 7q, namely, 7q22-q31 and 7q32-34 (Thangavelu M, Le Beau MM, unpublished observations). Recent studies, at the molecular level, provide further support for a critical region at 7q22-q31.2.[103,104] The identity of the relevant genes on this chromosome are unknown. The proto-oncogene *MET* is mapped to 7q31, and the genes encoding P-glycoprotein (*PGY1* and *PGY3*), proteins involved in the multidrug resistance phenotype, plasminogen activator inhibitor type 1 (*PLANHI*), and the erythropoietin gene (*EPO*), have been localized to 7q21-q22.[102] The *MET, PGY,* and *PLANHI* genes are deleted in cells with a del(7q); however, the *EPO* gene is not.[103,105] Moreover, the proximal breakpoints of the deletions may be located within a narrow segment of 7q22 between the *PLANHI* and *EPO* genes.[105] Neutrophil chemotactic factor is encoded by a gene on chromosome 7, and this activity may be deficient in patients with monosomy 7.

ACUTE LYMPHOCYTIC LEUKEMIA

The most useful prognostic indicators in ALL, the most frequent leukemia in children, are age, WBC count, and immunophenotype. Patients aged 3–7 years, with a WBC count of <10,000/ml, and whose leukemia cells express the common ALL antigen (CD10 [CALLA]) have the best prognosis. It was

Table 59-4. Cytogenetic-Imunophenotypic Correlations in Malignant Lymphoid Diseases

Phenotype	Chromosomal Abnormality	Frequency[a] (%)	Involved Genes[b]
Acute lymphocytic leukemia			
Pre-B	t(1;19)(q23;p13)	5 (25)	PBX1-TCF3(E2A)
B(SIg+)	t(8;14)(q24;q32)	5 (90)	MYC-IGH
	t(2;8)(p12;q24)	<1 (4)	IGK-MYC
	t(8;22)(q24;q11)	<1 (4)	MYC-IGL
	dic(9;12)(p11;p12)	1	
B or B-myeloid	t(9;22)(q34;q11)	10[c]	ABL-BCR
	t(4;11)(q21;q23)	5	AF4-MLL
Other	hyperdiploidy (50–60 chromosomes)	10	
	del(9p), t(9p)	10	
	del(12p), t(12p)	10	
T	t(11;14)(p15;q11)	1	RBTN1-TCRA
	t(11;14)(p13;q11)	1	RBTN2-TCRA
	t(8;14)(q24;q11)	<1	MYC-TCRA
	inv(14)(q11q32)	<1	TCRA-IGH
	inv(14)(q11q32)	<1	TCRA-TCL1
	t(10;14)(q24;q11)	1	HOX11-TCRA
	t(1;14)(p34;q11)	<1	LCK-TCRD
	t(7;9)(q34–35;q32)	<1	TCRB-TAL2
	t(7;9)(q34–35;q34)		TCRB-TAN1
	t(7;7)(p15;q11)		TCRG
	t(14;14)(q11;q32)		TCRA-IGH
	t(7;14)(q34–35; q11)		TCRB-TCRD
	t(7;14)(p15;q11)	<1	
	t(7;19)(q34–35; p13)	<1	
Non-Hodgkin lymphoma			
B(SIg+)	t(8;14)(q24;q32)	15 (30)	MYC-IGH
	t(2;8)(p12;q24)	1 (4)	IGK-MYC
	t(8;22)(q24;q11)	1 (4)	MYC-IGL
	t(14;18)(q32;q21)	25 (80)	IGH-BCL2
	t(11;14)(q13;q32)	5 (10)	CCND1-IGH
T or B(Ki1+)	t(2;5)(p23;q35)	2	
T	see T-cell ALL		
	t(4;16)(q26;p13.1)	>1	IL2-BCM
Chronic lymphocytic leukemia			
B	t(11;14)(q13;q32)	10	CCND1-IGH
	t(14;19)(q32;q13)	10	IGH-BCL3
	t(2;14)(p13;q32)	5	IGH
	t(14q)	20	
	+12	30	
T	t(8;14)(q24;q11)	5	MYC-TCRA
	inv(14)(q11q32)	5	TCRA/D-IGH
	inv(14)(q11q32)	5	TCRA/D-TCL1
Multiple myeloma			
B	t(11;14)(q13;q32)	10	CCND1-IGH
	t(14q)		
Adult T-cell leukemia			
	t(14;14)(q11;q32)		TCRA-IGH
	inv(14)(q11q32)		TCRA/D-IGH
	+3		

[a] The percentage refers to the frequency within the disease overall. The number in the parentheses refers to the frequency within the morphologic or immunologic subtype of the disease.

[b] Genes are listed in order of citation in karyotype (e.g., for pre-B-ALL, PBX1 is at 1q23 and TCF3 at 19p13).

[c] By cytogenetic analysis, the frequency in children is about 5%, and in adults is about 25%; this frequency is 30% in adults using molecular probes.

rigorously demonstrated for the first time at the Third International Workshop that the karyotype is an important independent prognostic factor in ALL.[33] Experimental data obtained more recently have revealed that several cytogenetic abnormalities are associated with distinct immunologic phenotypes of ALL.[33,106,107] (Table 59-4).

This review includes data on the chromosomal patterns of 330 patients evaluated at the Third International Workshop, 161 children studied at St. Jude Children's Research Hospital, and 146 children studied at the University of Chicago.[33,108–110] The study of 330 ALL patients (173 adults, 157 children) at the Third International Workshop revealed that a high proportion (65%) of patients had clonal abnormalities.[33,108] Also, of the 213 aneuploid patients, 51 percent were pseudodiploid, 37% were hyperdiploid, and only 12% were hypodiploid. Similarly, analysis of 161 patients studied by Williams et al.[109] also showed a high incidence of chromosomally abnormal cases (78%) in which most were hyperdiploid (49%) or pseudodiploid (44%) and only 7% were hypodiploid. The presence of the specific translocations t(4;11) or t(9;22) and the absence of hyperdiploidy (50–60 chromosomes) are associated with treatment failure even when using intensive therapy.[110]

Specific Abnormalities

8;14 Translocation

A reciprocal translocation involving the long arms of chromosomes 8 and 14 [t(8;14)(q24;q32)] has been detected in a high proportion of Burkitt tumors of both African and non-African origin.[111] An identical translocation is observed in ALL patients with L3-type leukemia cells, indicating that Burkitt lymphoma and most B-cell ALL of the L3 type are probably different manifestations of the same disease (Table 59-4). Sixteen patients with this rearrangement were studied at the Third International Workshop (7% of all cases with abnormalities).[33] This group included an excess of males over females and of adults over children. Most notable was the finding that, with one exception, all tested cases had B-cell markers and that all but one case were FAB type L3. In the exceptional patient, the leukemia cells had a pre-B-cell phenotype. This group of patients had a high incidence of central nervous system involvement at diagnosis and a poorer prognosis (complete remission rate: children 83%; adults 44%; median survival: 5 months) than that of any other group of patients classified according to chromosomal patterns.

Variant translocations have been reported in Burkitt lymphoma and B-cell ALL [t(2;8)(p12;q24) and t(8;22)(q24;q11)]. The first chromosomal abnormalities to be analyzed at the molecular level were the three translocations characteristic of L3 leukemia and Burkitt lymphoma (the outcome of these studies is described in the section Burkitt lymphoma).

4;11 Translocation

A translocation involving the long arms of chromosomes 4 and 11 [t(4;11)(q21;q23)] has been observed in patients with ALL, especially those with congenital leukemia.[112–115] Of 216 ALL patients with chromosomal abnormalities studied at the Third International Workshop, 8% (18 of 216 patients) had this rearrangement.[33] One-half of the patients were adults and the other half were children, most of whom were <1 year old. These patients had very high leukocyte counts (median WBC 183,000/mm³), itself a poor prognostic factor. The leukemia cells were L1 type in seven patients, L2 type in seven patients, and L3 type in one patient. Of eight patients in whom immunologic markers were tested, seven had non-T, non-B ALL, and one had T-cell ALL. These patients had a very poor outcome; although the complete remission rate was 67%, the median survival was only 7 months.[33,108] The association of the 4;11 translocation with neonatal or early-childhood ALL is particularly interesting in view of the low incidence of ALL in this age group (acute leukemias in this very young age group are usually of the myeloid type). The breakpoint (11q23) involves the *MLL* gene, a gene that is also involved in the t(9;11) associated with AMoL-M5a, and a number of other recurring translocations of 11q23.

Since the Workshop, a large number of patients with this translocation have been examined using a variety of experimental techniques. The most notable finding, first demonstrated by Parkin et al.[115] and later confirmed by others, is that acute leukemia associated with the 4;11 translocation may have both myeloid and lymphoid characteristics. Strong and associates[116] observed monocytic features (accentuated by maturation-inducing agents) as well as a clonal rearrangement of both immunoglobulin heavy and light chain genes in a cell line derived from a patient with acute leukemia in relapse, which had the 4;11 translocation. In another study, by Mirro and associates,[117] four of five patients had immunoglobulin heavy chain gene rearrangements; however, light chain gene rearrangements were demonstrated in only one of four patients tested.

In most cases of t(4;11) acute leukemia, blasts have been described as lymphoid in appearance and have been classified by light microscopy as L1 or L2 according to the FAB system.[114,116] In some leukemias that otherwise appear to be lymphoid, occasional blasts may appear monocytic; in some, populations of lymphoid and monocytoid blasts may occur in approximately equal proportion.[115] By ultrastructural examination, Parkin and associates confirmed the presence of a myeloid component in the leukemia of many of their patients. In addition to noting monocytoid blasts in some patients, they observed dysplasia of myeloid cells. Positive staining for myeloperoxidase or with Sudan Black B (myeloid cytochemical markers) may be present in some cases, and the nonspecific esterase reaction (granulocyte-monocyte cytochemical marker) may be positive in variable numbers of cells.[115,117] These leukemia cells are generally terminal deoxynucleotidyl transferase positive; they have expressed pan-B-cell antigens in most cases studied.[115,117] CD10 positivity has been observed in some instances. T-cell markers have consistently been negative.

9;22 Translocation

Ph+ leukemia occurs in two major forms, CML and ALL. Thirty-nine Ph+ ALL patients (18% of patients with abnormalities) were evaluated at the Third International Workshop; 30 were adults and 9 were children.[33,108] The incidence of Ph+ patients with ALL was 6% for children and 17% for adults. Thus, the Ph chromosome is the most frequent rearrangement in adult ALL. Thirty-six patients had the typical t(9;22), and the remaining three had variant translocations. The incidence of the variant form was 8%, similar to that observed in CML patients. About one-half of the patients showed abnormalities in addition to the Ph chromosome, a frequency substantially higher than that observed in CML in the chronic phase. With the exception of trisomy 8, which is seen occasionally, these abnormalities differ from those observed in the acute phase of CML. Monosomy 7 is a common secondary abnormality and is associated with a poorer outcome. A chromosomally normal cell line is frequently noted in the bone marrow of Ph+ ALL patients (70%), whereas normal cells are rarely observed in untreated CML patients.

The results of more recent studies using newer immunophenotyping techniques have suggested that Ph+ ALL is of pre-B-cell lineage; however, some cases have had both B-cell and myeloid markers.[118,119] In a recent prospective study of ALL patients conducted by the Cancer and Leukemia Group B, 23%

of adult ALL patients had the t(9;22); this frequency was 30% when molecular techniques were used to detect the *BCR/ABL* fusion.[119] Approximately one-half of B-lineage ALL patients were Ph+. These prospectively identified patients were no older than Ph-negative patients (median age 39 versus 37 years), nor was their complete remission rate significantly lower (71% versus 77%). However, median remission duration (10 versus 18 months) and survival (11 versus 22 months) were considerably shorter for Ph+ ALL patients.

Molecular studies of Ph+ ALL have revealed two distinct subgroups of patients. In the first group (about 30% of adults), the molecular rearrangement is identical to that observed in CML, in that the breaks occur within the *ABL* gene and within the bcr region of the *BCR* gene, giving rise to a chimeric gene and the production of an 8.5-kb message and a 210-kd fusion protein.[120] In the remaining patients, the breakpoint occurs upstream (5′) of bcr but still within the *BCR* gene,[121] giving rise to smaller fusion messages (6.5–7.4 kb)[122] and smaller proteins (185–190 kd).[123] The clinical outcome for both groups of patients appears to be similar. We do not know the protein substrates for the protein kinase activity of the abnormal *ABL* proteins in CML and ALL cells; it is possible, however, that the structural difference in the 210- and 185-kd proteins corresponds to an important functional difference in the leukemia cells. Such a functional difference might account for the biologic and clinical differences of Ph+ ALL, which, although characterized by the same chromosomal abnormality, is a disease entity distinct from CML.

1;19 Translocation

In 1978, pre-B-cell ALL was recognized as a distinct immunologic subtype of ALL that can be distinguished from null-cell and B-cell ALL by the presence of cytoplasmic immunoglobulin μ-chain (Cμ) expression.[124] Subsequently, it was recognized that pre-B leukemias have rearrangements of the immunoglobulin heavy chain genes, and occasionally of the light chain genes, and that patients with this form of leukemia have a less favorable response to therapy than that of patients who have common ALL (CD10 positive). In 1984, Williams et al.[109] described the association of a recurring chromosomal abnormality, namely, a reciprocal translocation involving chromosomes 1 and 19 [t(1;19)(q23;p13)] with pre-B cell ALL (Fig. 59-4A). Specifically, these investigators observed the t(1;19) in 30% (7 of 23) of patients with pre-B cell ALL whom they examined (6% of all ALL patients examined). This association was subsequently confirmed by other investigators, who also noted that children with pre-B ALL and a t(1;19) had low WBC counts and were CD10+[125] but experienced early treatment failure, suggesting that this translocation may distinguish a subgroup of patients with pre-B-cell ALL who have a poor prognosis.[126] The number of patients with this type of leukemia who have been treated is small, and the follow-up time is too short to determine definitively the prognosis associated with this cytogenetic abnormality. It should be noted that, in at least one series, patients with a t(1;19) did not appear to have a poor outcome.[125]

The t(1;19) involves the *E2A* gene at 19p13, which encodes two transcription factors (E12 and E47) that bind to enhancer elements in the *IGK* gene, as well as the regulatory elements of other genes.[127,128] The *E2A* gene is juxtaposed with *PBX1*, a homeobox gene on chromosome 1 (homeobox genes encode DNA-binding transcription factors that regulate developmental processes). *E2A/PBX1* fusion mRNAs are formed and code for chimeric proteins that consist of the transcriptional-activating domain of E12/E47, and the DNA-binding domain of *PBX1*[127,128] (Fig. 59-4B). *E2A* is expressed in all tissues, but the *PBX1* gene is not expressed in lymphoid cells (*PBX1* is expressed in many other fetal and adult tissues). Thus, the rearrangement results

A **t(1;19)(q23;p13)**

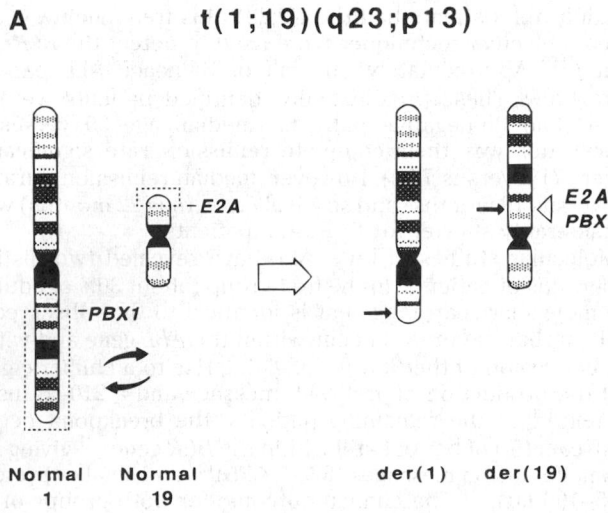

Normal 1   Normal 19   der(1)   der(19)

B PBX1   E2A

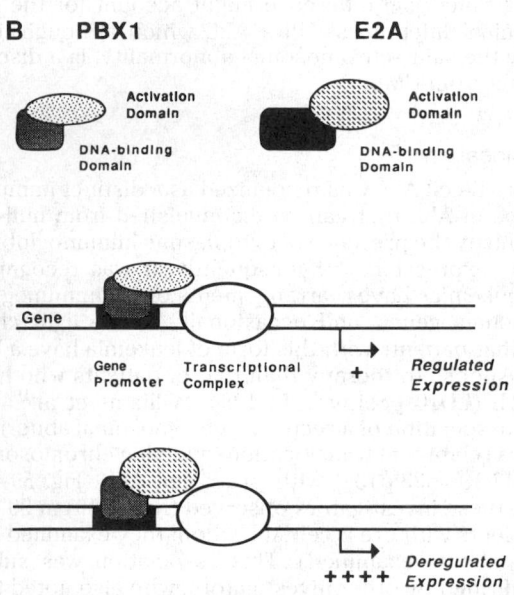

Fig. 59-4. (A) Schematic diagram of the t(1;19)(q23;p13) in pre-B ALL. The t(1; 19) results in the fusion of the *E2A* gene on chromosome 19, with the *PBX1* gene on chromosome 1. **(B)** Schematic model for the possible role of the E2A-PBX1 fusion proteins in the pathogenesis of pre-B-cell leukemias. Both the native E2A (basic helix-loop-helix domain) and PBX1 (homeodomain) proteins contain DNA-binding domains. The *E2A-PBX1* fusion gene encodes a fusion protein consisting of the transcriptional activation domain of E2A (5′ region of E2A), and the DNA-binding domain of PBX1 (3′ region of PBX1). This PBX1 DNA-binding domain binds to its target genes and activates expression. *PBX1* is not expressed in normal lymphoid cells; thus, the translocation may lead to deregulated expression of the *PBX1* gene as well as its target genes in lymphoid cells.

in the aberrant presence of the *PBX1* protein DNA-binding domain in lymphoid cells, which may result in the activation of expression of a cadre of genes not normally expressed in this tissue.

Hyperdiploidy with 50–60 Chromosomes

The leukemia cells of some patients with ALL are characterized by a gain of many chromosomes and relatively few structural abnormalities.[129] Chromosome numbers usually range

from 50 to 60, and a few patients may have ≤65 chromosomes. Certain additional chromosomes are commonly seen. Among 30 hyperdiploid patients (14% of patients with abnormalities), including 22 children and 8 adults, evaluated at the Third International Workshop, +21, +6, +18, +14, +4, or +10 were observed with decreasing frequency.[33]

The median age of the 22 children with this abnormal karyotype was 3 years and that of all 30 patients was 5 years, younger than that of patients with other abnormalities. The WBC count in patients with hyperdiploidy was low, with a median of 6,000/ mm³. The L1 and L2 types of leukemia cells were seen in about equal numbers, and all patients had non-T, non-B ALL. The complete remission rate was 86%, and the median survival time for these 30 patients was 34 months. Thus, in patients who have hyperdiploidy with >49 chromosomes, all the previously recognized clinical factors that indicate a good prognosis are present, including age of 3–7 years, low WBC count, and non-T, non-B markers. It should also be emphasized that the median survival time of the hyperdiploid patients, including both children and adults, is longer than that of ALL patients with a normal karyotype. Recent studies have suggested that structural rearrangements may occur in hyperdiploid ALL cells more frequently than was previously recognized, perhaps in as many as 50–70% of cases.[130] These patients appear to have a less favorable prognosis than that of patients who do not have structural rearrangements.[130]

T-Cell Acute Lymphocytic Leukemia

A distinct pattern of recurring karyotypic abnormalities has emerged.[1] Rearrangements involving the proximal bands of chromosome 14 (14q11) and two regions of chromosome 7 (7q34-q35 and 7p15) are particularly frequent in T-cell malignancies (Table 59-4). Most T-cell specific abnormalities involve 14q11. The first recurring abnormality to be defined was the reciprocal translocation involving chromosomes 8 and 14, t(8; 14)(q24;q11). Subsequently, other abnormalities involving 14q11 were recognized. Chromosome 7 is involved in six recurring abnormalities, two involving 7p15 [t(7;7)(p15;q11), t(7; 14)(p15;q11)] and four involving the distal long arm [t(7; 14)(q34-q35;q11), t(7;9)(q34-q35;q34), t(7;9)(q34-q35;q32), and t(7;19)(q34-q35;p13)].[1] In addition to their occurrence in T-cell leukemia, these T-cell-specific abnormalities have also been observed in lymphomas of T-cell origin. The genes located at the breakpoints of a number of these abnormalities have been identified and are described in a later section. Patients with T-ALL are most often young males and often have a mediastinal tumor mass, high WBC count, and leukemia cells in the cerebrospinal fluid. These same clinical characteristics are associated with lymphoblastic lymphoma, another T-cell malignancy.

MALIGNANT LYMPHOPROLIFERATIVE DISORDERS

Cytogenetic analyses of NHL have been reported in several large series.[131–136] These investigators have demonstrated that a high proportion of cases (>90%) are characterized by clonal chromosomal abnormalities and, more importantly, that many of these nonrandom abnormalities correlate with histology and immunologic phenotype[131,132,134] (Table 59-4). For example, the t(14;18)(q32;q21) is associated with follicular small cleaved B-cell neoplasms, whereas patients with a t(8;14)(q24;q32) have either small noncleaved cell (Burkitt or undifferentiated non-Burkitt) or diffuse large cell lymphomas. Band 14q32 is frequently involved in translocations in neoplasms of B-cell lineage. In a study of 94 patients with malignant lymphoma, Bloomfield and associates[131] noted that 70% (57 of 81) of patients with B-cell neoplasms had a structural abnormality involving

14q32. By contrast, a large proportion of neoplasms of T-cell origin are characterized by rearrangements that involve 14q11, 7q34-q35, or 7p15.[1,134,135,137]

Much less is known about the prognostic significance and clinical features associated with recurring chromosomal abnormalities in malignant lymphomas than in ALL. In large part, this is because cytogenetic analyses of lymphomas are more difficult than that of leukemias, the karyotypes tend to be more complex, access to involved tissue is more limited, and multiple morphologic subsets of lymphoma with different clinical features exist. However, the few studies that have correlated chromosomal abnormalities with outcome suggest that, as is the case in other hematologic malignancies, the karyotype in lymphoma may have important prognostic significance.

A number of karyotypic parameters have been reported to influence survival adversely; these include the absence of normal metaphase cells in the tumor tissue,[138,139] the presence of ring or marker chromosomes,[138] the complexity of the karyotype,[133] the presence of specific chromosomal abnormalities,[140,141] and the presence of abnormalities of chromosome 17.[142] Unfortunately, most of the studies reported to date have examined small numbers of patients and have included patients studied either at diagnosis or at relapse. Although histology remains the most important prognostic factor in both childhood and adult lymphoma, previous cytogenetic studies have not focused on specific histologies.[143,144] Thus, a major focus for future investigations will be to examine the clinical features of those subtypes of NHL with specific chromosomal abnormalities, the correlation of cytogenetic parameters with immunophenotype, and the prognostic significance of chromosomal abnormalities in NHL.

Burkitt Lymphoma

In 1972, Manolov and Manolova[145] identified a consistent abnormality (14q+) in the cells of fresh Burkitt lymphomas and in cultured cell lines. Several years later, Zech and associates[111] suggested that the rearrangement was a reciprocal translocation involving chromosomes 8 and 14, t(8;14)(q24;q32). The t(8;14) has also been observed in nonendemic Burkitt tumors from America, Europe, and Japan; this rearrangement is a highly characteristic anomaly in Burkitt tumors. This translocation was identified in Burkitt tumors that lacked any markers for the Epstein-Barr virus as well as in Epstein-Barr virus-positive tumors. It should be noted that the t(8;14) has also been observed in other lymphomas, particularly those of the small noncleaved cell (non-Burkitt) and large cell immunoblastic types as well as in B-cell ALL.[131,143]

As additional Burkitt tumors were examined, it became apparent that at least two other related translocations occur. All three translocations involved chromosome 8 with a break in the same band, 8q24. One variant translocation involved chromosome 2 with a break in the short arm [t(2;8)(p12;q24)], and the other involved chromosome 22 with a break in band q11 [t(8;22)(q24;q11)]. These same translocations have been seen in some patients with B-cell ALL.

In Burkitt lymphoma, *MYC* sequences are invariably juxtaposed with sequences from the immunoglobulin genes as a result of a chromosomal translocation involving chromosomes 14, 2, or 22, the sites of the immunoglobulin heavy chain, κ light chain, and λ light chain genes.[146,147] The result of these translocations is deregulated expression of the *MYC* gene. The product of the *MYC* gene is a member of the leucine-zipper and helix-loop-helix classes of transcription factors and is involved in the control of gene expression; thus, its constitutive expression may result in the unrestricted proliferation of the B cells that contain these chromosomal translocations. That altered *MYC* expression is important in the pathogenesis of these B-

cell neoplasms has been emphasized by the observation that transgenic mice, which carry DNA sequences from a breakpoint junction of an 8;14 translocation in their germline, frequently develop B-cell tumors.[148]

Other B-Cell Non-Hodgkin Lymphomas

Other recurring abnormalities in B-cell NHL include the t(14;18)(q32;q21), observed in 80% of adults with follicular (nodular) small cleaved cell lymphomas[131–133,149] and the t(11;14)(q13;q32), characteristic of mantle zone lymphomas and other B-cell lymphomas.[150] These translocations have been detected only in adult patients with NHL. With respect to B-cell NHL in children, the only available data are derived from the analysis of children with Burkitt lymphoma. In these cases, the t(8;14)(q24;q32) or one of the variant translocations [t(2;8) or t(8;22)] are always present.

Molecular analyses of the recurring chromosomal abnormalities that involve breaks at 14q32 within the immunoglobulin heavy chain *(IGH)* gene have resulted in the identification of the *CCND1* (PRAD1) sequences at the breakpoint on chromosome 11 in the t(11;14)(q13;q32),[150,151] and the *BCL2* gene at the breakpoint on chromosome 18 in the t(14;18)(q32;q21).[147,152–154] The *BCL2* gene encodes a 22-kd cytoplasmic protein; although the precise function of this protein is currently unknown, it appears to prolong cell survival by inhibiting programmed cell death (apoptosis) and to cooperate with the MYC protein in promoting cell proliferation.[153] The *CCND1* gene encodes cyclin D1, a protein involved in regulating the cell cycle.[151]

T-Cell Non-Hodgkin Lymphoma

A number of recurring chromosomal abnormalities have been recognized in lymphomas of T-cell origin (Table 59-4). These abnormalities are also observed in T-cell leukemias. Similar to B-cell neoplasms, in which rearrangements frequently involve the chromosomal bands containing the immunoglobulin gene loci, T-cell neoplasms often have rearrangements involving band q11 of chromosome 14, the site of the T-cell receptor α-chain and δ-chain genes *(TCRA, TCRD)*,[155] or, less often, one of two regions of chromosome 7 (7q34-q35 and 7p15) to which the T-cell receptor β-chain *(TCRB)* and γ-chain *(TCRG)* genes have been localized, respectively.[1] Molecular analysis of >11 recurring translocations has revealed that the break occurs within the corresponding T-cell receptor gene in each instance[146,156] (Table 59-4). With few exceptions, the involved gene on the partner chromosome encodes a transcription factor, whose expression is deregulated or activated in an aberrant tissue as a result of the rearrangement[3,4] (Table 59-1).

In summary, these studies indicate that, perhaps as a result of their capacity to be specifically rearranged, transcribed, and mutated in B cells or in T cells, the immunoglobulin and T-cell receptor gene loci are appropriate DNA sequences with which to mediate the activation of cellular oncogenes. A chromosomal rearrangement that brings an oncogene under the controlling influence of promoters or enhancers that are active for immunoglobulin synthesis in B cells or T-cell receptor synthesis in T cells may consequently impart a proliferative advantage to that cell and result in malignant clonal expansion.

Ki-1 Anaplastic Large Cell Lymphomas

A distinctive subtype of NHL, namely, Ki-1-positive anaplastic large cell lymphoma (Ki-1 + ALCL) has been characterized during the past few years. The Ki-1 antigen (CD30) is observed in nearly all cases of Hodgkin disease; however, this antigen is also expressed by a variable proportion of lymphoma cells in a variety of NHL subtypes. A subset of NHL with distinctive clinical and morphologic features is strongly Ki-1 positive. These patients tend to be young and they present with skin and/or lymph node infiltration by large, often bizarre lymphoma cells, which preferentially involve the paracortical areas and lymph node sinuses.[157,158] Most cases have T-cell phenotypes, but some appear to be B-cell lymphomas. The diagnosis may be confused with Hodgkin disease, anaplastic carcinoma, or a histiocytic disorder.

Recently, a reciprocal translocation involving the short arm of chromosome 2 (band p23) and the long arm of chromosome 5 (band q35), t(2;5)(p23;q35), has been associated with Ki-1+ ALCL.[159-161] This same rearrangement has also been reported in eight other patients, each of whom had a malignant hematologic disease designated as malignant histiocytosis.[1] Several of the cases reported by Agnarsson and Kadin[158] were referred initially to them in consultation as histiocytic disorders but were reclassified as Ki-1+ ALCL, suggesting that some or all of the previously reported cases with the t(2;5) may actually be Ki-1+ ALCL. Thus, the detection of a t(2;5) in a lymph node specimen may assist in the diagnosis of this neoplasm.

Other Lymphoproliferative Disorders

Less is known about the chromosomal abnormalities in malignant lymphoproliferative disorders other than those already discussed. In part, this is due to the low proliferative rate and mitotic index in these diseases and to the inability to stimulate mitoses in the malignant lymphoid cells without also stimulating cell division in the residual normal T or B lymphocytes. Thus, karyotypes have most often been reported to be normal in patients with chronic lymphocytic leukemia (CLL), multiple myeloma, or hairy cell leukemia, for example.

Trisomy 12 is the most common cytogenetic abnormality reported in patients with B-cell CLL (B-CLL); it is found in 21–62% of those with a cytogenetic abnormality.[162] Abnormalities involving band 14q32 are also common [e.g., t(14;19)(q32; q13)][163] (Table 59-4). Unfortunately, only one-half of patients with B-CLL will have an adequate number of metaphase cells in unstimulated cultures for thorough evaluation. Recently, Anastasi and co-workers[164] showed that fluorescence in situ hybridization (FISH) is a simple and sensitive method for detecting trisomy 12 in interphase CLL cells; 30% of patients had trisomy 12 and trisomy 12 was associated with a poorer survival.

T-cell CLL (T-CLL) is an uncommon disorder in which the malignant mature lymphocytes have a T-cell immunophenotype. Rearrangements involving bands 14q11 with or without an accompanying break in 14q32 have been reported in T-CLL as well as other T-cell lymphomas[1,165] (Table 59-4). Cutaneous T-cell lymphoma, a malignant proliferation of CD4+ (helper/inducer) cells involving skin (mycosis fungoides), blood (Sézary syndrome), and lymph nodes, has been reported to have a high incidence of random heteroploidy; less often, complex clonal abnormalities are present, sometimes involving chromosome 6.

Hairy cell leukemia is an uncommon B-cell disorder with a low proliferative rate. Recurring chromosomal abnormalities have been difficult to identify in hairy cell leukemia because of the low yield of mitotic cells. Del(6q), trisomy 3 and 12, and translocations involving 14q32 have been reported in several patients.[1] Unrelated structural abnormalities may also be present in individual patients.

Angioimmunoblastic lymphadenopathy with dysproteinemia is another rare lymphoproliferative disorder. Although it has been linked with drug hypersensitivity reactions, progres-

sion to a high-grade immunoblastic lymphoma of T-cell origin occurs in some cases. Clonal abnormalities involving trisomy 3 or 5 have been reported.[166] Although better understanding of these recurring abnormalities will no doubt increase our knowledge of malignant transformation, the greatest clinical importance of cytogenetic analyses in these disorders currently is to differentiate a reactive (polyclonal) lymphoid proliferation from a malignant (monoclonal) one. The identification of a clonal chromosomal abnormality in an enlarged lymph node or in peripheral blood cells provides convincing evidence of a neoplasm.

NEW TECHNIQUES TO DETECT CHROMOSOMAL ABNORMALITIES

Cytogenetic analysis of human tumors is often technically difficult due to the presence of multiple abnormal cell lines and the complexity of the chromosomal pattern, and requires highly skilled personnel. These factors have led investigators to seek alternative methods for identifying chromosomal abnormalities, such as Southern blot analysis of DNA or reverse transcription-polymerase chain reaction (RT-PCR) analysis of RNA from tumor cells (described below), or FISH.[167]

The technique of FISH is based on the same principle as Southern blot analysis, namely, the ability of single-stranded DNA to anneal to cDNA. In the case of FISH, the target DNA is the nuclear DNA of interphase cells, or the DNA of metaphase chromosomes affixed to a glass microscope slide (FISH can also be accomplished with bone marrow or peripheral blood smears or with fixed and sectioned tissue). The test probe is labeled with biotin- or digoxigenin-labeled nucleotides and detected with fluorescein isothiocyanate (FITC)-conjugated avidin or rhodamine-labeled antidigoxigenin antibodies. Probes directly labeled with fluorochrome are also available for hybridization, simplifying the technique by eliminating the probe detection steps. With the development of dual- and triple-pass filters, most laboratories now have the capacity to hybridize and detect two to three probes simultaneously.

Several types of probes can be used to detect chromosomal abnormalities by FISH. Hybridization of centromere-specific probes has been used to detect monosomy, trisomy, and other aneuploidies in both leukemias and solid tumors (Fig. 59-5). Chromosome-specific libraries, which paint the chromosomes, are particularly useful in identifying marker chromosomes (rearranged chromosomes of unidentified origin), or structural rearrangements, such as translocations. Chromosomal translocations can also be identified in interphase or metaphase cells by using probes (phage, cosmid, or yeast artificial chromosome probes) that are derived from the breakpoints of recurring translocations. Recently, investigators have demonstrated the use of FISH to detect allele loss in tumor cells, specifically the loss of the *RB1* gene in CLL.

FISH techniques have a number of applications (Table 59-5). In some cases, FISH analysis provides more sensitivity, in that cytogenetic abnormalities have been identified by FISH in samples that appeared to be normal by morphologic and conventional cytogenetic analyses. FISH is most powerful when the analysis is targeted toward those abnormalities known to be associated with a particular tumor or disease. An example of how FISH could be used in a clinical setting is as follows. Cytogenetic analysis could be performed at diagnosis to identify the chromosomal abnormalities in an individual patient's malignant cells. Thereafter, with the appropriate probes, FISH could be used to detect residual disease or early relapse and to assess the efficacy of therapeutic regimens.

Our new sophistication regarding the genetic changes in hematologic malignant diseases provides us with some very critical new diagnostic tools. Standard Southern blot analysis of

METAPHASE CELL   **INTERPHASE CELL**

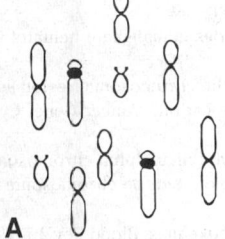 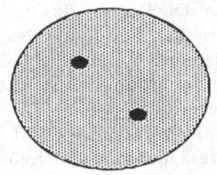

A

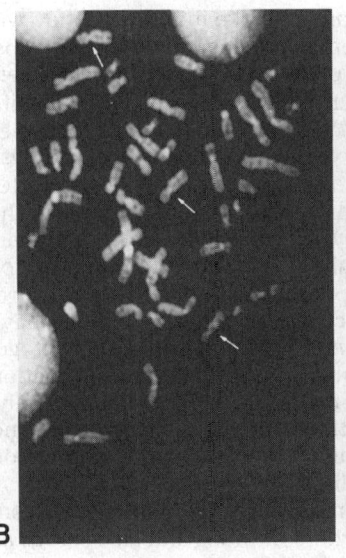 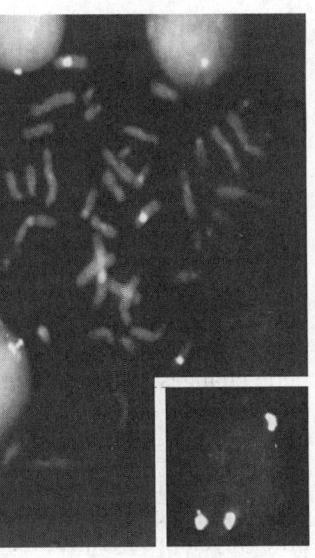

B

Fig. 59-5. **(A)** Schematic diagram of the hybridization pattern observed in metaphase cells or interphase cells hybridized with a centromere-specific repetitive probe. Centromere-specific probes hybridize to the repetitive DNA sequences that are present at the centromeres of human chromosomes. These probes result in two intense signals at the centromeres of the target chromosome in diploid metaphase cells or interphase nuclei. **(B)** Photomicrographs of metaphase cells and interphase cells following FISH. Hybridization of a chromosome-specific centromere probe for chromosome 8 to metaphase and interphase cells with trisomy 8 from a bone marrow sample of a patient with AML. The chromosome homologs are identified with arrows.

tumor DNA can reveal clonal rearrangements of genes (e.g., immunoglobulin or T-cell receptor genes), using the appropriate probes, as well as a number of recurring translocations. PCR can increase the sensitivity of detection of these aberrations; sometimes the sensitivity is too great to be clinically applicable. Translocations that result in fusion genes are especially suited for RT-PCR, a technique in which the fusion mRNA is copied into cDNA and then with appropriate primers from each gene, the fusion gene is amplified by PCR. Based on the position of the primers, the size(s) of the expected fusion product is known and can be compared with that actually obtained. The correctness of the amplified product can be confirmed using a smaller probe that contains the expected portion of the fusion gene. We and others have used this strategy to de-tect the rearranged genes in the t(8;21).[59] Using probes from *AML1* and *ETO* on standard Southern blot analysis, rearrangements can usually be detected in DNA from about 80% of patients known to have a t(8;21). With RT-PCR, the detection rate is 100%. We found positive signals of fusion mRNA in patients in complete remission who were negative on cytogenetic analysis and standard Southern blotting. More recently, we have detected the translocation in peripheral blood cells from three patients in unmaintained remission for 5–8 years.[62] This indicates that these patients have circulating t(8;21)-positive cells, even though they appear to be "cured" of their leukemia. The biologic significance of these observations remains to be determined; it seems clear, however, that decisions on whether to continue therapy cannot be based solely on a positive signal with RT-PCR methods. Other translocations routinely detected by RT-PCR include the t(9;22) and t(15;17).

This increasing precision in identifying the genetic changes in the malignant cells comes at a most opportune time, because physicians will soon be in a position to use targeted therapy aimed at the specific genetic defect in the malignant cells. Effective use of this targeted therapy requires a precise genotype of the malignant cells. Although a number of genes will be involved with various genetic changes, those reflected in chromosomal changes may be amongst the easiest to monitor.

Table 59-5. Applications and Advantages of FISH

Applications
   Detection of numerical and structural chromosomal abnormalities
   Identification of marker chromosomes (rearranged chromosomes of uncertain origin)
   Monitoring the effects of therapy, and detection of minimal residual disease or early relapse
   Identification of the origin of bone marrow cells following bone marrow transplantation
   Identification of the lineage of neoplastic cells
   Examination of the karyotypic pattern of nondividing or interphase cells
   Detection of gene amplification

Advantages
   Rapid technique
   The efficiency of hybridization and detection is high
   The sensitivity and specificity is very high
   Large numbers of cells can be analyzed in a short time
   Cytogenetic data can be obtained from nondividing or terminally differentiated cells, from tumors with a low mitotic index (e.g., CLL) or from poor samples that contain too few cells for routine cytogenetic studies
   Permits the direct correlation of cytogenetic and cytologic/morphologic features, which enables pathologists to differentiate malignant from benign conditions in equivocal cases
   Automated systems for analysis of hybridized slides are under development

CLINICAL IMPLICATIONS OF CYTOGENETICS

Cytogenetic analysis provides clinicians with a powerful tool for the diagnosis and classification of hematopoietic malignant diseases. The detection of an acquired somatic mutation establishes the diagnosis of a neoplastic disorder and rules out a reactive hyperplasia or morphologic changes due to toxic injury or vitamin deficiency. Given an equivocal pathologic diagnosis, the detection of a clonal chromosomal abnormality in a bone marrow specimen or in lymph node tissue provides sufficient justification to institute cytotoxic treatment with radiotherapy or chemotherapy.

Specific cytogenetic abnormalities identify homogeneous subsets of various malignant diseases and enable clinicians to predict their clinical course and the likelihood that they will respond to particular treatments. In many cases, the prognostic information derived from cytogenetic analysis is independent of that provided by other clinical features. Patients with favorable prognostic features benefit from standard therapies with well-known spectra of toxicities, whereas those with less favorable clinical or cytogenetic characteristics may be better treated with more intensive or investigational therapies. The disappearance of a chromosomal abnormality present at diagnosis is an important concomitant of complete remission following treatment, and its reappearance invariably heralds relapse of the disease. More recently, molecular methods have provided evidence of clonal remissions, suggesting that cytogenetic changes may be a late step in malignant transformation and not always present in the neoplastic stem cell. FISH analysis permits study of differentiated or nondividing cells, and molecular methods permit analysis of a whole population rather than just individual cells.

The presence of the Ph chromosome differentiates CML from other myeloproliferative disorders or MDSs and also serves as an important marker of persistent disease during interferon therapy or after allogeneic bone marrow transplantation. Karyotypic evolution in a patient with CML portends transformation to the acute phase and provides a useful signal to proceed, if possible, with bone marrow transplantation in higher-risk groups, such as older patients or those without HLA-identical sibling donors.

The optimal timing of marrow transplantation in the treatment of AML and ALL is controversial. Pretreatment cytogenetic analysis can be useful in choosing between postremission therapies that differ widely in cost, acute and chronic morbidity, and effectiveness.

Our own treatment results suggest that most patients with AML and favorable cytogenetic features [i.e. t(8;21), t(15;17), inv(16) or t(16;16)] can be cured with intensive consolidation chemotherapy, and hence should not undergo allogeneic transplantation in first remission.[51] Those who relapse can generally be salvaged with bone marrow transplantation in early relapse or second remission. Alternatively, AML patients with loss or deletion of chromosome 5 or ALL patients with t(9;22), or t(4; 11), or t(8;14) have relatively drug-resistant disease and are seldom cured with conventional chemotherapy alone, warranting the use of investigational agents or transplantation in first remission.

As molecular probes for the genes involved in recurring translocations become more readily available, it will be possible to evaluate marrow or blood samples of patients in clinical remission to determine the persistence of minimal residual disease at the level of 1 in 10^5 cells. It is too soon to know whether patients who are persistently positive by PCR methods are always destined to relapse. However, it seems likely that patients found negative by current PCR methods are most likely cured of their disease.

REFERENCES

1. Mitelman F, Kaneko Y, Trent JM: Report of the committee on chromosome changes in neoplasia. HGM11. Cytogenet Cell Genet 58:1053, 1991
2. Mitelman F, Heim S: Quantitative acute leukemia cytogenetics. Genes Chromosom Cancer 5:57, 1992
3. Rabbits TH: Translocations, master genes, and differences between the origins of acute and chronic leukemias. Cell 67:614, 1991
4. Nichols J, Nimer S: Transcription factors, translocations and leukemia. Blood 80:2953, 1992
5. Klein G: The approaching era of tumor suppressor genes. Science 238:1539, 1988
6. Mitelman F (ed): ISCN: Supplement to a International System for Human Cytogenetic Nomenclature. Guidelines for Cancer Cytogenetics. S Karger, Basel, 1991
7. Nowell PC, Hungerford DA: A minute chromosome in human chronic granulocytic leukemia. Science 132:1197, 1960
8. Rowley JD: A new consistent chromosomal abnormality in chronic myelogenous leukemia identified by quinacrine fluorescence and Giemsa staining. Nature 243:290, 1973
9. Whang-Peng J, Canellos GP, Carbone PP, Tjio JH: Clinical implications of cytogenetic variants in chronic myelocytic leukemia. Blood 32:755, 1968
10. Kantarjian HM, Smith TL, McCredie KB et al: Chronic myelogenous leukemia: a multivariate analysis of the associations of patient characteristics and therapy with survival. Blood 66:1326, 1985
11. Pugh WC, Pearson M, Vardiman JW, Rowley JD: Philadelphia chromosome-negative chronic myelogenous leukaemia: a morphological reassessment. Br J Haematol 60:457, 1985
12. Travis LB, Pierre RV, De Wald GW: Ph¹-negative chronic granulocytic leukemia: a nonentity. Am J Clin Pathol 85:186, 1986
13. Rowley JD, Testa JR: Chromosome abnormalities in malignant hematologic diseases. Adv Cancer Res 36:103, 1982
14. Hagemeijer A, Bartram CR, Smit EME et al: Is the chromosomal region 9q34 always involved in variants of the Ph¹ translocation? Cancer Genet Cytogenet 13:1, 1984
15. Groffen J, Stephenson JR, Heisterkamp N et al: Philadelphia chromosomal breakpoints are clustered within a limited region, bcr, on chromosome 22. Cell 36:93, 1984
16. Westbrook CA: The ABL oncogene in human leukemias. Blood Rev 2:1, 1988
17. Gale RP, Canaani E: An 8-kilobase abl RNA transcript in chronic myelogenous leukemia. Proc Natl Acad Sci USA 81:5648, 1984
18. Davis RL, Konopka JB, Witte ON: Activation of the c-abl oncogene by viral transduction or chromosomal translocation generates altered c-abl proteins with similar in vitro kinase properties. Mol Cell Biol 5:204, 1985
19. Witte ON: Functions of the abl oncogene. Cancer Surv 5:183, 1986
20. Birnie GD, Mills KI, Benn PA: Does the site of the breakpoint on chromosome 22 influence the duration of the chronic phase in chronic myelogenous leukemia? Leukemia 3:545, 1989
21. Ganesan TS, Rassool F, Guo A-P et al: Rearrangement of the bcr gene in Philadelphia chromosome-negative chronic myeloid leukemia. Blood 68:957, 1986
22. Fialkow PJ, Jacobson RJ, Papayannopoulou T: Chronic myelocytic leukemia: clonal origin in a stem cell common to the granulocyte, erythrocyte, platelet and monocyte/macrophage. Am J Med 63:125, 1977
23. Fitzgerald PH, Pickering AF, Eiby JR: Clonal origin of the Philadelphia chromosome and chronic myeloid leukaemia: evidence from a sex chromosome mosaic. Br J Haematol 21:473, 1971
24. Talpaz M, Kantarjian HM, McCredie K et al: Hematologic remission and cytogenetic improvement induced by recombinant human interferon alpha_A in chronic myelogenous leukemia. N Engl J Med 314:1065, 1986
25. Ozer H, George SL, Schiffer CA et al: Prolonged subcutaneous administration of recombinant α2b interferon in patients with previously untreated Philadelphia chromosome-positive chronic-phase chronic myelogenous leukemia. Blood 82:2975, 1993
26. Alimena G, De Cuia MR, Diverio D et al: The karyotype of blastic crisis. Cancer Genet Cytogenet 26:39, 1987
27. Westin J, Weinfeld A: The significance of clonal chromosome abnormalities in polycythemia vera (PV), abstracted. Int Cong Hematol 17:971, 1978
28. Testa JR, Kanofsky JR, Rowley JD et al: Karyotypic patterns and their clinical significance in polycythemia vera. Am J Hematol 11:29, 1984
29. Nowell P, Finan J: Chromosome studies in preleukemic states. IV. Myeloproliferative versus cytopenic disorders. Cancer 42:2254, 1978
30. Mitelman F: Catalog of Chromosome Aberrations in Cancer. Wiley-Liss, New York, 1991
31. Van den Berghe H, Vermaelen K, Mecucci C et al: The 5q– anomaly. Cancer Genet Cytogenet 17:189, 1985
32. Matthew P, Tefferi A, Dewald GW et al: The 5q– syndrome. A single-institution study of 43 consecutive patients. Blood 81:1040, 1993
33. Third International Workshop on Chromosomes in Leukemia. Cancer Genet Cytogenet 4:95, 1981
34. Miller BJ, Testa JR, Lindgren V, Rowley JD: The pattern and clinical significance of karyotypic abnormalities in patients with idiopathic and postpolycythemic myelofibrosis. Cancer 55:582, 1985
35. Demory JL, Dupriez B, Fenaux P et al: Cytogenetic studies and their prognostic significance in agnogenic myeloid metaplasia: a report on 47 cases. Blood 72:855, 1988
36. Johnson DD, Dewald GW, Pierre RV et al: Deletions of chromosome 13 in malignant hematologic disorders. Cancer Genet Cytogenet 18:235, 1985
37. Bennett JM, Catovsky D, Daniel MT et al: Proposals for the classification of the myelodysplastic syndromes. Br J Haematol 51:189, 1982
38. Larson RA: Management of myelodysplastic syndromes. Ann Intern Med 103:136, 1985
39. Jacobs RH, Cornbleet MA, Vardiman JW et al: Prognostic implications of

morphology and karyotype in primary myelodysplastic syndromes. Blood 67:1765, 1986

40. Gold EJ, Conjalka M, Pelus LM et al: Marrow cytogenetic and cell-culture analyses of the myelodysplastic syndromes: insights to pathophysiology and prognosis. J Clin Oncol 1:627, 1983

41. Third MIC Cooperative Study Group (1987): Morphologic, immunologic, and cytogenetic (MIC) working classification of the primary myelodysplastic syndromes and therapy-related myelodysplasias and leukemias. Cancer Genet Cytogenet 32:1, 1988

42. Second International Workshop on Chromosomes in Leukemia. Cancer Genet Cytogenet 2:89, 1980

43. Nowell PC, Besa EC, Stelmach T, Finan JB: Chromosome studies in preleukemic states: prognostic significance of single versus multiple abnormalities. Cancer 58:2571, 1986

44. Bennett JM: Classification of the acute leukemias: cytochemical and morphologic considerations. p. 169. In Wiernik PH, Canellos GP, Kyle RA, Schiffer CA (eds): Neoplastic Diseases of the Blood. 2nd Ed. Churchill Livingstone, New York, 1991

45. Bennett JM, Catovsky D, Daniel MT et al: Proposed revised criteria for the classification of acute myeloid leukemia: a report of the French-American-British Cooperative Group. Ann Intern Med 103:620, 1985

46. Koeffler HP: Syndromes of acute nonlymphocytic leukemia. Ann Intern Med 107:748, 1987

47. Sandberg AA: The Chromosomes in Human Cancer and Leukemia. 2nd Ed. Elsevier North-Holland, New York, 1990

48. Larson RA, Le Beau MM, Vardiman JW et al: The predictive value of initial cytogenetic studies in 148 adults with acute nonlymphocytic leukemia: a 12-year study (1970–1982). Cancer Genet Cytogenet 10:219, 1983

49. Schiffer CA, Lee EJ, Tomiyasu T et al: Prognostic impact of cytogenetic abnormalities in patients with de novo acute nonlymphocytic leukemia. Blood 73:263, 1989

50. Fourth International Workshop on Chromosomes in Leukemia. Cancer Genet Cytogenet 71:249, 1984

51. Samuels BL, Larson RA, Le Beau MM et al: Specific chromosomal abnormalities in acute nonlymphocytic leukemia correlate with drug susceptibility in vivo. Leukemia 2:79, 1988

52. Rowley JD, Alimena G, Garson OM et al: A collaborative study of the relationship of the morphologic type of acute nonlymphocytic leukemia with patient age and karyotype. Blood 59:1013, 1982

53. Le Beau MM, Rowley JD: Recurring chromosomal abnormalities in leukemia and lymphoma. Cancer Surv 3:371, 1984

54. Bloomfield CD, Arthur DC, Wurster-Hill D et al: Recurring chromosome abnormalities in de novo AML: a preliminary report of CALGB 8461, abstracted. Cytogenet Cell Genet 46:583, 1987

55. Olopade OI, Thangavelu M, Larson RA et al: Clinical, morphologic, and cytogenetic characteristics of 26 patients with acute erythroblastic leukemia. Blood 80:2873, 1992

56. Rowley JD: Identification of a translocation with quinacrine fluorescence in a patient with acute leukemia. Ann Genet 16:109, 1973

57. Miyoshi H, Shimizu K, Kozu T et al: The t(8;21) breakpoints on chromosome 21 in acute myeloid leukemia clustered within a limited region of a novel gene, AML1. Proc Natl Acad Sci USA 88:10431, 1991

58. Gao J, Erickson P, Gardiner K et al: Isolation of a yeast artificial chromosome spanning the 8;21 translocation breakpoint, t(8;21)(q22;q22.3) in acute myelogenous leukemia. Proc Natl Acad Sci USA 88:4882, 1991

59. Nucifora G, Birn DJ, Erickson P et al: Detection of DNA rearrangements in the AML1 and ETO loci and of an AML1/ETO fusion mRNA in patients with t(8;21) AML. Blood, 81:883, 1993

60. Erickson P, Gao J, Chang K-S et al: Identification of breakpoints in t(8;21) AML and isolation of a fusion transcript with similarity to Drosophila segmentation gene runt. Blood 80:1825, 1992

61. Bitter MA, Le Beau MM, Rowley JD et al: Associations between morphology, karyotype, and clinical features in myeloid leukemias. Hum Pathol 18:211, 1987

62. Nucifora G, Larson RA, Rowley JD: Persistence of the 8;21 translocation in patients with AML-M2 in long-term remission. Blood 82:712, 1993

63. Rowley JD, Golomb HM, Dougherty C: 15/17 Translocation, a consistent chromosomal change in acute promyelocytic leukemia. Lancet 1:549, 1977

64. Larson RA, Kondo K, Vardiman JW et al: Evidence for a 15;17 translocation in every patient with acute promyelocytic leukemia. Am J Med 76:827, 1984

65. De Thé H, Chomienne C, Lanotte M et al: The t(15;17) translocation of acute promyelocytic leukaemia fuses the retinoic acid receptor α gene to a novel transcribed locus. Nature 347:558, 1990

66. Borrow J, Goddard AD, Sheer D, Solomon E: Molecular analysis of acute promyelocytic leukemia breakpoint cluster region on chromosome 17. Science 249:1577, 1990

67. Castaigne S, Chomienne C, Daniel MT et al: All-trans retinoic acid as differentiation therapy for acute promyelocytic leukemia. Clinical results. Blood 76: 1704, 1990

68. Arthur DC, Bloomfield CD: Partial deletion of the long arm of chromosome 16 and bone marrow eosinophilia in acute nonlymphocytic leukemia: a new association. Blood 61:994, 1983

69. Le Beau MM, Larson RA, Bitter MA et al: Association of inv(16)(p13q22) with abnormal marrow eosinophils in acute myelomonocytic leukemia: a unique cytogenetic-clinicopathological association. N Engl J Med 309:630, 1983

70. Bitter MA, Le Beau MM, Larson RA et al: A morphologic and cytochemical study of acute myelomonocytic leukemia with abnormal marrow eosinophils associated with inv(16)(p13q22). Am J Clin Pathol 81:733, 1984

71. Testa JR, Hogge DE, Misawa S, Zandparsa N: Chromosome 16 rearrangement in acute myelomonocytic leukemia with abnormal eosinophils. N Engl J Med 310:468, 1984

72. Larson RA, Williams SF, Le Beau MM et al: Acute myelomonocytic leukemia with abnormal eosinophils and inv(16) or t(16;16) has a favorable prognosis. Blood 68:1242, 1986

73. Liu P, Tarlé S, Hajra A et al: Fusion between transcription factor CBFβ/PEBP2β and a myosin heavy chain in acute myeloid leukemia. Science 261: 1041, 1993

74. Berger R, Bernheim A, Sigaux F et al: Acute monocytic leukemia chromosome studies. Leuk Res 6:17, 1982

75. Rowley JD: Consistent chromosome abnormalities in human leukemia and lymphoma. Cancer Invest 1:267, 1983

76. Hagemeijer A, Hahlen K, Sizoo W, Abels J: Translocation (9;11)(p21;q23) in three cases of acute monoblastic leukemia. Cancer Genet Cytogenet 5:95, 1982

77. Kaneko Y, Maseki N, Takasaki N et al: Clinical and hematologic characteristics in acute leukemia with 11q23 translocations. Blood 67:484, 1986

78. Vermaelen K, Barbieri D, Michaux J et al: Anomalies of the long arm of chromosome 11 in human myelo- and lymphoproliferative disorders. I. Acute nonlymphocytic leukemia. Cancer Genet Cytogenet 10:105, 1983

79. Ziemin-van der Poel S, McCabe NR, Gill HJ et al: Identification of a gene, MLL, that spans the breakpoint in 11q23 translocations associated with human leukemias. Proc Natl Acad Sci USA 88:10735, 1991

80. Djabali M, Selleri L, Parry P et al: A trithorax-like gene is interrupted by chromosome 11q23 translocations in acute leukaemias. Nature Genet 2:113, 1992

81. Gu Y, Nakamura T, Alder H et al: The t(4;11) chromosome translocation of human acute leukemias fuses the ALL-1 gene, related to Drosophila trithorax, to the AF-4 gene. Cell 71:701, 1992

82. Tkachuk DC, Kohler S, Cleary ML: Involvement of a homolog of Drosophila trithorax by 11q23 chromosomal translocations in acute leukemias. Cell 71: 691, 1992

83. Thirman MJ, Gill HJ, Burnett RC et al: Rearrangement of the MLL gene in acute lymphoblastic and acute myeloid leukemias with 11q23 chromosomal translocations. N Engl J Med 329:909, 1993

84. Chen C-S, Sorenson PHB, Domer PH et al: Molecular rearrangements on chromosome 11q23 predominate in infant acute lymphoblastic leukemia and are associated with specific biologic variables and poor outcome. Blood 81:2386, 1993

85. Golomb HM, Vardiman JW, Rowley JD: Acute nonlymphocytic leukemia in adults: correlations with Q-banded chromosomes. Blood 48:9, 1976

86. Pintado T, Ferro MT, San Roman C et al: Clinical correlations of the 3q21; q26 cytogenetic anomaly: a leukemic or myelodysplastic syndrome with preserved or increased platelet production and lack of response to cytotoxic drug therapy. Cancer 55:535, 1985

87. Bitter MA, Neilly ME, Le Beau MM et al: Rearrangements of chromosome 3 involving bands 3q21 and 3q26 are associated with normal or elevated platelet counts in acute nonlymphocytic leukemia. Blood 66:1362, 1985

88. Vermaelen K, Michaux J, Louwagie A, Van den Berghe H: Reciprocal translocation t(6;9)(p21;q33): a new characteristic chromosome anomaly in myeloid leukemias. Cancer Genet Cytogenet 10:125, 1983

89. Pearson MG, Vardiman JW, Le Beau MM et al: Increased numbers of marrow basophils may be associated with a t(6;9) in ANLL. Am J Hematol 18:393, 1985

90. Mitelman F, Nilsson PG, Brandt L et al: Chromosome pattern, occupation, and clinical features in patients with acute nonlymphocytic leukemia. Cancer Genet Cytogenet 4:197, 1981

91. Golomb HM, Alimena G, Rowley JD et al: Correlation of occupation and karyotype in adults with acute nonlymphocytic leukemia. Blood 60:404, 1982

92. Crane MM, Keating MJ, Trujillo JM et al: Environmental exposures in cytogenetically defined subsets of acute nonlymphocytic leukemia. JAMA 262:634, 1989

93. Taylor JA, Sandler DP, Bloomfield CD et al: ras Oncogene activation and occupational exposures in acute myeloid leukemia. J Natl Cancer Inst 84: 1626, 1992

94. Koeffler HP, Rowley JD: Therapy-related acute nonlymphocytic leukemia. p. 357. In Wernick PH, Canellos GP, Kyle RA, Schiffer CA (eds): Neoplastic Diseases of the Blood. 1st Ed. Churchill Livingstone, New York, 1985

95. Rowley JD, Golomb HM, Vardiman JW: Nonrandom chromosome abnormalities in acute leukemia and dysmyelopoietic syndrome in patients with previously treated malignant disease. Blood 58:759, 1981

96. Vardiman JW, Golomb HM, Rowley JD, Variakojis D: Acute nonlymphocytic leukemia in malignant lymphoma: a morphologic study. Cancer 42:229, 1978

97. Le Beau MM, Albain KS, Larson RA et al: Clinical and cytogenetic correlations in 63 patients with therapy-related myelodysplastic syndromes and acute nonlymphocytic leukemia: further evidence for characteristic abnormalities of chromosomes no. 5 and 7. J Clin Oncol 4:325, 1986

98. Ratain MJ, Rowley JD: Therapy-related acute myeloid leukemia secondary to inhibitors of topoisomerase II. From the bedside to the target genes. Ann Oncol 3:107, 1992

99. Pedersen-Bjergaard J, Philip P: Balanced translocations involving chromosome bands 11q23 and 21q22 are highly characteristic of myelodysplasia and leukemia following therapy with cytostatic agents targeting at DNA-topoisomerase II. Blood 78:1147, 1991

100. Le Beau MM, Chandrasekharappa SC, Lemons RS et al: Molecular and cytogenetic analysis of chromosome 5 abnormalities in myeloid disorders: chromosomal localization and physical mapping of IL-4 and IL-5. Cancer Cells 7: 53, 1989

101. Le Beau MM, Espinosa R, Neuman WL et al: Cytogenetic and molecular delineation of the smallest commonly deleted region of chromosome 5 in malignant myeloid diseases. Proc Natl Acad Sci USA 90:5484, 1993

102. Cutticchia AJ, Pearson PL, Klinger HP (eds): Chromosome Coordinating Meeting 1992: Genome Priority Reports. Vol. 1. S Karger, Basel, 1993

103. Kere J, Ruutu T, Lahtinen R, de la Chapelle A: Molecular characterization of chromosome 7 long arm abnormalities in myeloid disorders. Blood 70: 1349, 1987

104. Shannon KM, Turham AG, Chang SSY et al: Familial bone marrow monosomy 7: evidence that the predisposing locus is not on the long arm of chromosome 7. J Clin Invest 84:984, 1989

105. Kere J, Ruutu T, Davies KA et al: Chromosome 7 long arm deletions in myeloid disorders: a narrow breakpoint region in 7q22 defined by molecular mapping. Blood 73:230, 1989

106. Raimondi SC: Current status of cytogenetic research in childhood acute lymphoblastic leukemia. Blood 81:2237, 1993

107. Pui CH, Crist WM, Look AT: Biology and clinical significance of cytogenetic abnormalities in childhood acute lymphoblastic leukemia. Blood 76:1449, 1990

108. Bloomfield CD, Goldman AI, Alimena G et al: Chromosomal abnormalities identify high-risk and low-risk patients with acute lymphoblastic leukemia. Blood 67:415, 1986

109. Williams DL, Harber J, Murphy SB et al: Chromosomal translocations play a unique role in influencing prognosis in childhood acute lymphoblastic leukemia. Blood 68:205, 1986

110. Rubin CM, Le Beau MM, Mick R et al: Impact of chromosomal translocations on prognosis in childhood acute lymphoblastic leukemia. J Clin Oncol 9: 2183, 1991

111. Zech L, Haglund V, Nilsson K, Klein G: Characteristic chromosomal abnormalities in biopsies and lymphoid cell lines from patients with Burkitt and non-Burkitt lymphomas. Int J Cancer 17:47, 1976

112. Prigogina EL, Fleischman EW, Puchkova GP et al: Chromosomes in acute leukemia. Hum Genet 53:5, 1979

113. Van den Berghe H, David G, Broeckaert-Van Orshoven A et al: A new chromosome anomaly in acute lymphoblastic leukemia. Hum Genet 46:173, 1979

114. Arthur DC, Bloomfield CD, Lindquist LL, Nesbit ME: Translocation 4;11 in acute lymphoblastic leukemia: clinical characteristics and prognostic significance. Blood 59:96, 1982

115. Parkin JL, Arthur DC, Abramson CS et al: Acute leukemia associated with the t(4;11) chromosome rearrangement: ultrastructural and immunologic characteristics. Blood 60:1321, 1982

116. Stong RC, Korsmeyer SJ, Parkin JL et al: Human acute leukemia cell line with the t(4;11) chromosomal rearrangement exhibits B lineage and monocytic characteristics. Blood 65:21, 1985

117. Mirro J, Kitchingman G, Williams D et al: Clinical and laboratory characteristics of acute leukemia with the 4;11 translocation. Blood 67:689, 1986

118. Ribeiro R, Abromowitch M, Raimondi SC et al: Clinical and biological hallmarks of the Philadelphia chromosome in childhood acute lymphoblastic leukemia. Blood 70:948, 1987

119. Westbrook CA, Hooberman AL, Spino C et al: Clinical significance of the BCR-ABL fusion gene in adult acute lymphoblastic leukemia. A Cancer and Leukemia Group B Study (8762). Blood 80:2983, 1992

120. de Klein A, Hagemeijer A, Bartram CR et al: bcr Rearrangement and translocation of the c-abl oncogene in Philadelphia positive acute lymphoblastic leukemia. Blood 68:1369, 1986

121. Rubin CM, Westbrook CA, Smith SD et al: Philadelphia chromosome-positive acute lymphoblastic leukemia: detection of a DNA rearrangement 50–250 kilobases proximal to BCR. p. 125. In Golde DW, Gale RP (eds): Recent Advances in Leukemia and Lymphoma. UCLA Symposium of Molecular and Cellular Biology. Alan R Liss, New York, 1987

122. Hermans A, Heisterkamp N, Von Lindern M et al: Unique fusion of bcr and c-abl genes in Philadelphia chromosome positive acute lymphoblastic leukemia. Cell 51:33, 1987

123. Clark SS, McLaughlin J, Crist WM et al: Unique forms of the abl tyrosine kinase distinguish Ph[1]-positive CML from Ph[1]-positive ALL. Science 235:85, 1987

124. Vogler LB, Crist WM, Bockman DE et al: Pre-B cell leukemia. A new phenotype of childhood lymphoblastic leukemia. N Engl J Med 298:872, 1978

125. Michael PM, Levin MD, Garson OM: Translocation 1;19—a new cytogenetic abnormality in acute lymphocytic leukemia. Cancer Genet Cytogenet 12: 333, 1984

126. Carroll AJ, Crist WM, Parmley MT et al: Pre-B cell leukemia associated with chromosome translocation 1;19. Blood 63:721, 1984

127. Mellentin JD, Murre C, Donlon TA et al: The gene for enhancer binding proteins E12/E47 lies at the t(1;19) breakpoint in acute leukemias. Science 246:379, 1989

128. Nourse J, Mellentin JD, Galili N et al: Chromosomal translocation t(1;19) results in synthesis of a homeobox fusion mRNA that codes for a potential chimeric transcription factor. Cell 60:535, 1990

129. Secker-Walker LM, Lawler SD, Hardisty RM: Prognostic implications of chromosomal findings in acute lymphoblastic leukemia at diagnosis. BMJ 2:1529, 1978

130. Pui C-H, Raimondi SC, Dodge RK et al: Prognostic importance of structural chromosomal abnormalities in children with hyperdiploid (>50 chromosomes) acute lymphoblastic leukemia. Blood 73:1963, 1989

131. Bloomfield CD, Arthur DC, Frizzera G et al: Nonrandom chromosome abnormalities in lymphoma. Cancer Res 43:2975, 1983

132. Levine EG, Arthur DC, Frizzera G et al: There are differences in cytogenetic abnormalities among histologic subtypes of the non-Hodgkin's lymphomas. Blood 66:1414, 1985

133. Yunis JJ, Frizzera G, Oken MM et al: Multiple recurrent genomic defects in follicular lymphoma: a possible model for cancer. N Engl J Med 316:79, 1987

134. Fifth International Workshop on Chromosomes in Leukemia-Lymphoma: Correlation of chromosome abnormalities with histologic and immunologic characteristics in non-Hodgkin's lymphoma and adult T-cell leukemia-lymphoma. Blood 70:1554, 1987

135. Koduru PRK, Fillipa DA, Richardson ME et al: Cytogenetic and histological correlations in malignant lymphoma. Blood 69:97, 1987

136. Kristoffersson U, Heim S, Mandahl N et al: Prognostic implications of cytogenetic findings in 106 patients with non-Hodgkin's lymphoma. Cancer Genet Cytogenet 25:55, 1987

137. Smith SD, Morgan R, Gemmill R et al: Clinical and biological characterization of T-cell neoplasias with rearrangements of chromosome 7 band q34. Blood 71:395, 1988

138. Kaneko Y, Abe R, Sampi K, Sakurai M: An analysis of chromosome findings in non-Hodgkin's lymphomas. Cancer Genet Cytogenet 5:107, 1982

139. Bloomfield CD, Arthur DC, Levine EG et al: Chromosome abnormalities in malignant lymphoma. Biologic and clinical correlations. Haematol Blood Transfus 29:145, 1985

140. Kaneko Y, Rowley J, Variakojis D et al: Prognostic implications of karyotype and morphology in patients with non-Hodgkin's lymphoma. Int J Cancer 32: 683, 1983

141. Fukuhara S, Nasu K, Kita K et al: Cytogenetic approaches to the clarification of pathogenesis in lymphoid malignancies: clinicopathologic characterization of 14q+ marker-positive non-T-cell malignancies. Jpn J Clin Oncol 13: 461, 1983

142. Levine EG, Arthur DC, Frizzera G: Cytogenetic abnormalities predict clinical outcome in non-Hodgkin lymphoma. Ann Intern Med 108:14, 1988

143. Yunis JJ, Oken MM, Kaplan ME et al: Distinctive chromosomal abnormalities in histologic subtypes of non-Hodgkin's lymphoma. N Engl J Med 307:1231, 1982

144. Offit K, Jhanwar SC, Ladanyi M et al: Cytogenetic analysis of 434 consecutively ascertained specimens of non-Hodgkin's lymphoma: correlations between recurrent aberrations, histology, and exposure to cytotoxic treatment. Genes Chromosom Cancer 3:189, 1991

145. Manolov G, Manolova Y: Marker band in one chromosome 14 from Burkitt lymphomas. Nature 237:33, 1972
146. Croce CM: Role of chromosome translocations in human neoplasia. Cell 49: 155, 1987
147. McKeithan TW: Molecular biology of non-Hodgkin's lymphoma. Semin Oncol 17:30, 1990
148. Adams JM, Harris AW, Pinkert CA et al: The c-*myc* oncogene driven by immunoglobulin enhancers induces lymphoid malignancy in transgenic mice. Nature 318:533, 1985
149. Fukuhara S, Rowley JD: Chromosome 14 translocations in non-Burkitt lymphomas. Int J Cancer 22:14, 1978
150. Tsujimoto Y, Yunis JJ, Onorato-Showe L et al: Molecular cloning of the chromosomal breakpoint of B-cell lymphomas and leukemias with the t(11;14) chromosome translocation. Science 224:1403, 1984
151. Motokura T, Bloom T, Goo KH et al: A novel cyclin encoded by a bcl-1 linked candidate oncogene. Nature 350:512, 1991
152. Tsujimoto Y, Yunis JJ, Onorato-Showe L et al: Molecular cloning of the chromosomal breakpoints of B-cell leukemias with the t(14;18) chromosomal translocation. Science 226:1097, 1984
153. Korsmeyer SJ: *BCL-2*: an antidote to programmed cell death. Cancer Surv 15:105, 1992
154. Rowley JD: Chromosome studies in non-Hodgkin's lymphomas: the role of the 14;18 translocation. J Clin Oncol 6:919, 1988
155. Erikson J, Williams DL, Finan J et al: Locus of the alpha-chain of the T-cell receptor is split by chromosome translocations in T-cell leukemia. Science 229:784, 1985
156. McGuire EA, Hockett RD, Pollack RM et al: The t(11;14) in a T-cell acute lymphoblastic leukemia cell line activates multiple transcripts including Ttg-1, a gene encoding a potential zinc finger protein. Mol Cell Biol 9:2124, 1989

157. Stein H, Mason DY, Gerdes J et al: The expression of the Hodgkin's disease associated antigen Ki-1 in reactive and neoplastic lymphoid tissue: evidence that Reed-Sternberg cells and histiocytic malignancies are derived from activated lymphoid cells. Blood 66:848, 1985
158. Agnarsson B, Kadin ME: Ki-1 positive large cell lymphoma: a morphologic and immunologic study of 19 cases. Am J Surg Pathol 12:264, 1988
159. Kaneko Y, Frizzera G, Edamura S et al: A novel translocation, t(2;5) (p23; q35), in childhood phagocytic large T-cell lymphoma mimicking malignant histiocytosis. Blood 73:806, 1989
160. Rimokh R, Magaud J-P, Berger F et al: A translocation involving a specific breakpoint (q35) on chromosome 5 is characteristic of anaplastic large cell lymphoma ("Ki-1 lymphoma"). Br J Haematol 71:31, 1989
161. Le Beau MM, Bitter MA, Larson RA et al: The t(2;5)(p23;q35): A recurring chromosomal abnormality in Ki-1 positive anaplastic large cell lymphoma. Leukemia 3:866, 1989
162. Han T, Henderson ES, Emrich LJ, Sandberg AA: Prognostic significance of karyotypic abnormalities in B-cell chronic lymphocytic leukemia: an update. Semin Hematol 24:257, 1987
163. McKeithan TW, Rowley JD, Shows TB, Diaz MO: Cloning of the chromosome translocation breakpoint junction of the t(14;19) in chronic lymphocytic leukemia. Proc Natl Acad Sci USA 84:9257, 1987
164. Anastasi J, Le Beau MM, Vardiman JW et al: Detection of trisomy 12 in chronic lymphocytic leukemia by fluorescence in situ hybridization to interphase cells: a simple and sensitive method. Blood 79:1796, 1992
165. Ueshima Y, Rowley JD, Variakojis D et al: Cytogenetic studies on patients with chronic T-cell leukemia/lymphoma. Blood 63:1028, 1984
166. Kaneko Y, Larson RA, Variakojis D et al: Nonrandom chromosome abnormalities in angioimmunoblastic lymphadenopathy. Blood 60:877, 1982
167. Le Beau MM: Fluorescence *in situ* hybridization in cancer diagnosis. p. 29. In De Vita VT, Hellman S, Rosenberg SA (eds): Important Advances in Oncology. JB Lippincott, Philadelphia, 1993

Appendix 59-1

Glossary of Cytogenetic Terminology*

Aneuploidy: An abnormal chromosome number due to either gain or loss of chromosomes.

Banded chromosomes: Chromosomes with alternating dark and light segments due to special stains or pretreatment of metaphase cells with enzymes before staining. Each chromosome pair has a unique pattern of bands.

Breakpoint: A specific site on a chromosome containing a DNA break that is involved in a structural rearrangement, such as a translocation or deletion.

Centromere: The constriction along the length of the chromosome that is the site of the spindle fiber attachment. The position of the centromere determines whether chromosomes are *metacentric* (X-shaped [e.g., chromosomes 1–3, 6–12, X, 16, 19, 20]) or *acrocentric* (inverted V-shaped [e.g., chromosomes 13–15, 21, 22, Y]). During mitosis, the two exact copies of the DNA in each chromosome are separated by shortening of the spindle fibers attached to opposite sides of the dividing cell.

Clone: In the cytogenetic sense, this is defined as two cells with the same additional or structurally rearranged chromosome or three cells with loss of the same chromosome.

Deletion: A segment of a chromosome is missing as a result of a single break (terminal deletion), or two breaks and loss of the intervening piece (interstitial deletion).

Diploid: Normal chromosome number and composition of chromosomes.

Haploid: Only one-half the normal complement (i.e., 23 chromosomes).

Hyperdiploid: Additional chromosomes; therefore, the modal number is ≥47.

Hypodiploid: Loss of chromosomes with a modal number of ≤45.

Inversion: Two breaks occur in the same chromosome with rotation of the intervening segment. If both the breaks were on the same side of the centromere, it is called a paracentric inversion. If they were on opposite sides, it is called a pericentric inversion.

Isochromosome: A chromosome that consists of identical copies of one chromosome arm with loss of the other arm. Thus, an isochromosome for the long arm of number 17 [i(17q)] contains two copies of the long arm (separated by the centromere) with loss of the short arm of the chromosome.

---

* Modified from Rowley JD: Chromosome abnormalities in human cancer. De Vita VT, Hellman S, Rosenberg S (eds): Practice and Principles of Oncology. 3rd Ed. JB Lippincott, Philadelphia, 1991.

Karyotype: Arrangement of chromosomes from a particular cell according to a well-established system such that the largest chromosomes are first and the smallest ones are last. A normal female karyotype is described as 46,XX and a normal male karyotype is 46,XY. An idiogram is an idealized representation (diagram) of the karyotype.

Pseudodiploid: A diploid number of chromosomes accompanied by structural chromosomal abnormalities.

Recurring abnormality: A numerical or structural abnormality noted in multiple patients who have a similar hematologic neoplasm. Such abnormalities are characteristic or diagnostic of distinct subtypes of leukemia and lymphoma that have unique morphologic or immunophenotypic features, or both. Recurring abnormalities represent genetic mutations involved in the pathogenesis of the corresponding diseases; many recurring abnormalities have prognostic significance.

Translocation: A break in at least two chromosomes with exchange of material. In a reciprocal translocation, there is no obvious loss of chromosomal material. Translocations are indicated by t; the chromosomes involved are noted in the first set of brackets and the breakpoints in the second set of brackets. The Ph translocation is t(9;22)(q34;q11).

Nomenclature symbols:

+: If before the chromosome, indicates a gain of a whole chromosome (e.g., +8) and if after the chromosome, indicates gain of part of the chromosome (e.g., 14q+, added material at the end of the long arm of number 14).

−: If before the chromosome, indicates a loss of a whole chromosome (e.g., −7), and if after the chromosome, indicates loss of part of the chromosome (e.g., 5q−, loss of part of the long arm of number 5)

?: Indicates uncertainty about the identity of the chromosome or band listed just after the question mark.

del: deletion
i: isochromosome
inv: inversion
mar: marker chromosome
p: Short arm
q: Long arm
r: ring chromosome
t: translocation

Appendix 59-2

Examples of Cytogenetic Nomenclature

46,XX or 46,XY: Nomenclature description of a normal female or male karyotype, respectively.

47,XX,+8,t(9;22)(q34;q11): Female with an extra chromosome 8 as well as a translocation affecting chromosome 9 with a break in the long arm, band q34, and chromosome 22 with a break in the long arm, band q11. The latter is the usual translocation seen in CML.

46,XX,t(9;22;10)(q34;q11;q24): Female with a variant (complex) Ph translocation affecting chromosome 9 with a break in band q34, chromosome 22 with a break in band q11, and chromosome 10 with a break in the long arm at band q24.

Chromosomal material from 9q is translocated to 22q, material from 22q is translocated to 10q, and material from 10q is translocated to 9q.

46,XY,inv(16)(p13q22): Male with a pericentric inversion of chromosome 16 resulting from breaks in the short arm in band p13, and in the long arm in band q22. The inv(16) is a recurring chromosomal abnormality associated with acute myelomonocytic leukemia with abnormal eosinophils.

46,XY,del(5)(q13q33): Deletion of part of the long arm of chromosome 5 including bands q13-q33.

Molecular Basis of Neoplasia

60

Naomi Rosenberg and Theodore G. Krontiris

INTRODUCTION

Malignant transformation involves both somatic and heritable changes in some of the genes that control normal cell growth and development. Genes of this type, generically referred to as oncogenes, are defined by their capacity to induce oncogenic growth when expressed in appropriate cell types. Most of these genes were initially discovered because of their presence in a variety of retroviruses that induce tumors in animals. Although retroviruses containing oncogenes are not known to be involved in human diseases, two discoveries focused attention on their role in human malignancy. First, the finding that retroviral oncogenes are derived from highly conserved normal cellular genes demonstrated that these genes are not unique to retroviruses. Second, the discovery that many oncogenes are altered in non-retrovirus-induced tumors cemented the relationship of these sequences to oncogenesis. Despite their involvement in a common process, malignant transformation, oncogenes are a diverse group, encoding proteins involved in more than one aspect of cellular growth and metabolism. While a clear definition of the mechanism by which even one of these genes induces transformation is lacking, proteins encoded by oncogenes function by mimicking the action of growth factors, growth factor receptors, signal transducers, and transcription factors that affect gene expression directly.

HISTORICAL PERSPECTIVE

Retroviruses—A Brief Introduction

Oncogenes originally came to light in experiments using retroviruses as model systems designed to understand tumorigenesis. Retroviruses are RNA viruses that contain two copies of their genome in each virion.[1] These viruses have the unique ability to transcribe these sequences into a double-stranded DNA copy, which is then integrated into the genome of the infected cell (Fig. 60-1). This occurs early in the infectious process within a capsid-like viral structure and is catalyzed by a virus-encoded enzyme called reverse transcriptase.[2] This enzyme uses both copies of the viral genome in a complex "jumping" process to generate a complete DNA copy called a provirus. Once integrated into the DNA of the host cell, the provirus behaves like any other cellular gene. It is expressed from a viral promoter by the cellular transcription machinery and is passed to daughter cells like other cellular sequences. RNA transcribed from the provirus can function either as mRNA, directing the synthesis of viral gene products, or as new retroviral genomes, packaged and released from the cell as virus particles.

Retroviruses that induce tumors in chickens were discovered in the early 1900s. One of these viruses, Rous sarcoma virus, became the subject of intense research in the succeeding years. These efforts demonstrated that induction of fibrosarcomas in chickens and transformation of chicken embryo fibroblasts in tissue culture required a viral gene[3] named src (pro-

nounced "sark"). The discovery in the mid-1970s that the src gene is homologous to a normal cellular gene present not only in birds but in many other eukaryotes, including Drosophila,[4,5] revolutionized the field. Soon thereafter, other work demonstrated that virtually all retroviruses that transformed tissue culture cells or that induced tumors with a short latency contained transforming genes that were distinct from src but also derived from normal cellular genes.[6] Indeed, by the early 1980s, >10 different oncogenes had been identified. The term proto-oncogene was introduced to distinguish the normal cellular form of these genes from their viral counterparts. Also, a three-letter designation was introduced to standardize the nomenclature of individual oncogenes; the three letter code is often preceded by a c- or a v- to denote the cellular or viral form, respectively.

Origin of Retroviral Oncogenes

Oncogenes found in retroviruses are derived from the cellular proto-oncogenes by a recombination process called transduction. Two basic models have been proposed to explain the steps in this process[6] (Fig. 60-2). In each case, one of the retroviruses in a cell integrates in the vicinity of the proto-oncogene. One scenario predicts that a portion of the retrovirus sequence is deleted; as a result, the retrovirus promoter expresses an RNA transcript that contains sequences from both the virus and the neighboring proto-oncogene. This RNA is processed and packaged into a virion along with a normal copy of the viral genome. After infection of a new cell, recombination between the genomes occurs during reverse transcription to generate the recombinant virus that contains sequences derived from the proto-oncogene.

The second transduction model predicts that hybrid RNAs containing virus and cellular sequences are a normal by-product of retroviral expression.[6] These RNAs are generated because a fraction of all retrovirus transcripts are not processed correctly and contain information derived from neighboring cellular sequences. As in the first model, the hybrid RNAs are packaged along with a normal viral RNA and recombination during reverse transcription occurs after infection of a new cell. The major difference between these two models is that the first predicts that rearrangement at the level of the DNA is required, while the second does not involve this step. Direct evidence that recombinant viruses can be generated using the pathway described in the second model has been presented,[7] but this may not be the only pathway by which oncogene-containing retroviruses are generated.

Differences Between Oncogenes and Proto-Oncogenes

Proto-oncogenes are highly conserved genes, which suggests that they play key roles in cellular metabolism and growth. This feature raises a fundamental question. How does a gene involved in a normal cellular process become a gene

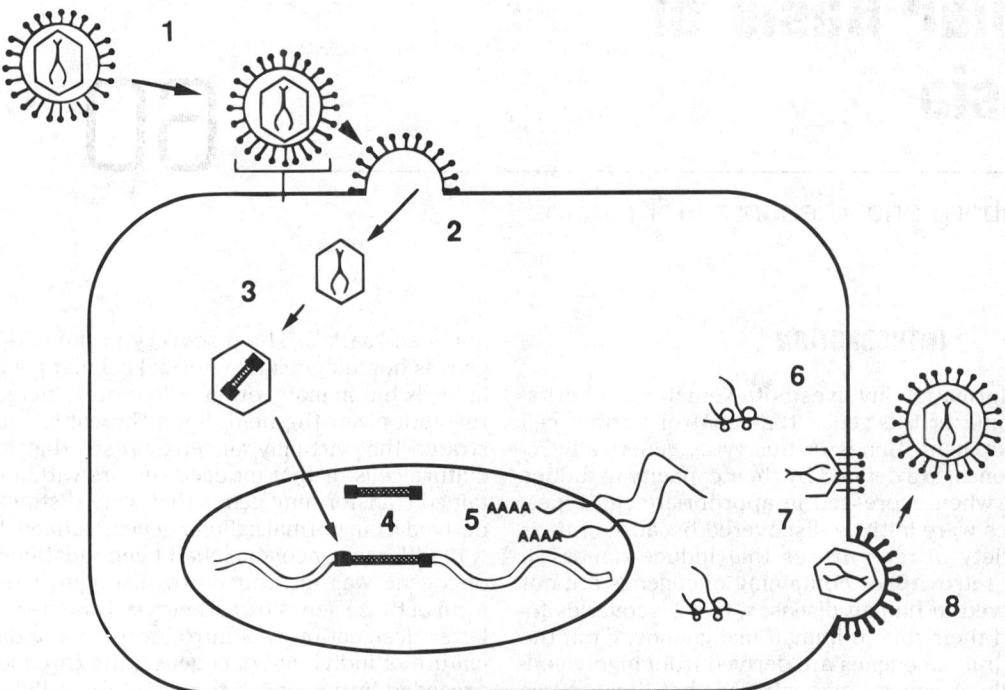

Fig. 60-1. Replication of retroviruses. Retroviruses interact with cells via specific receptors, a process called adsorption (1). Following binding to the receptor, the virus/receptor complex is taken up by the cell in a process of penetration (2). The virus core is released into the cytoplasm, and the RNA genomes are copied into a double-stranded DNA form (3). The core structure migrates to the nucleus, and the viral genome integrates into the cellular DNA (4). Cellular RNA polymerase transcribes the viral genes (5), and the RNA is processed and transported to the cytoplasm, where it is translated to give rise to viral proteins (6). Other transcripts serve as genomes for new virions, which are assembled (7) and bud from the cell (8).

that induces malignant growth? A single answer, beyond the obvious unifying feature of incorporation into retroviral genomes, cannot be found. Indeed, several types of alterations can occur as a consequence of the capture of these genes.[8] First, the cellular genes are removed from the elements that normally control their expression. In a retrovirus, expression of the gene is controlled by the viral promoter and enhancer elements located at the 5′ end of the integrated retrovirus in a structure called the long terminal repeat (LTR). Polyadenylation signals are contributed by LTR sequences located at the 3′ end of the viral genome. Second, because the gene is contained in an infectious element, it can be introduced into cell types that would not normally express the sequences. Finally, in most cases the coding sequence of the cellular gene is altered as a consequence of recombination with the viral genome. These alterations can result in expression of truncated proteins or of fusion proteins containing a portion specified by the cellular oncogene and a portion specified by a viral gene. Proteins that contain more subtle changes may also occur.

Insertional Mutagenesis and Oncogene Activation

Retroviral transduction of proto-oncogene sequences appears to be a relatively rare event. The recombination events must lead to a virus that can be expressed effectively and transmitted at a reasonable frequency. The first step in the process, integration of a provirus in the vicinity of a proto-oncogene, can have drastic effects on expression of the cellular gene, even in the absence of incorporation into a virus (Fig. 60-3). The simple disruption of a proto-oncogene by proviral integration may also lead to altered expression of the cellular gene. If a hybrid RNA similar to that formed during transduction is produced, an altered proto-oncogene product may be produced by the cell. The strong enhancer elements in the viral LTRs

can also activate the expression of proto-oncogenes if the provirus has integrated in the vicinity of the cellular gene. Any of these forms of aberrant expression may alter the growth of the infected cell. If the altered expression confers a distinct growth advantage or makes that cell malignant, a tumor can develop without production of a retrovirus that has acquired an oncogene. These changes, termed proviral insertional mutagenesis, have been shown to occur frequently subsequent to retroviral infection. Many oncogenes that have not been physically incorporated into retroviruses have been discovered because they are targets of insertional mutagenesis.[9–12] Given these considerations, it should not be surprising that mutational changes induced independent of retroviral infection can also activate proto-oncogenes. These latter events play an important role in spontaneous or carcinogen-induced tumors in animals, including humans.

ONCOGENE FUNCTIONAL GROUPS

The current list of known oncogenes exceeds 75. Indeed, new oncogenes or candidate oncogenes are still being identified with regularity. While some of these genes are clearly capable of inducing tumors and transforming cells in tissue culture, others have been identified as genes expressed in spontaneous tumors that are related by nucleic acid homology to known oncogenes. In the latter case, the actual role of the gene in the tumor and its potential to induce malignant transformation have not always been proved. This chapter does not attempt to cover all oncogenes but focuses on the major groups (Table 60-1), using examples that illustrate general mechanisms.

Oncogenes encode membrane-associated, cytoplasmic, or nuclear proteins that appear to affect virtually every aspect of cellular metabolism. Indeed, it is possible that any gene playing a key role in cellular growth has the potential to be an oncogene

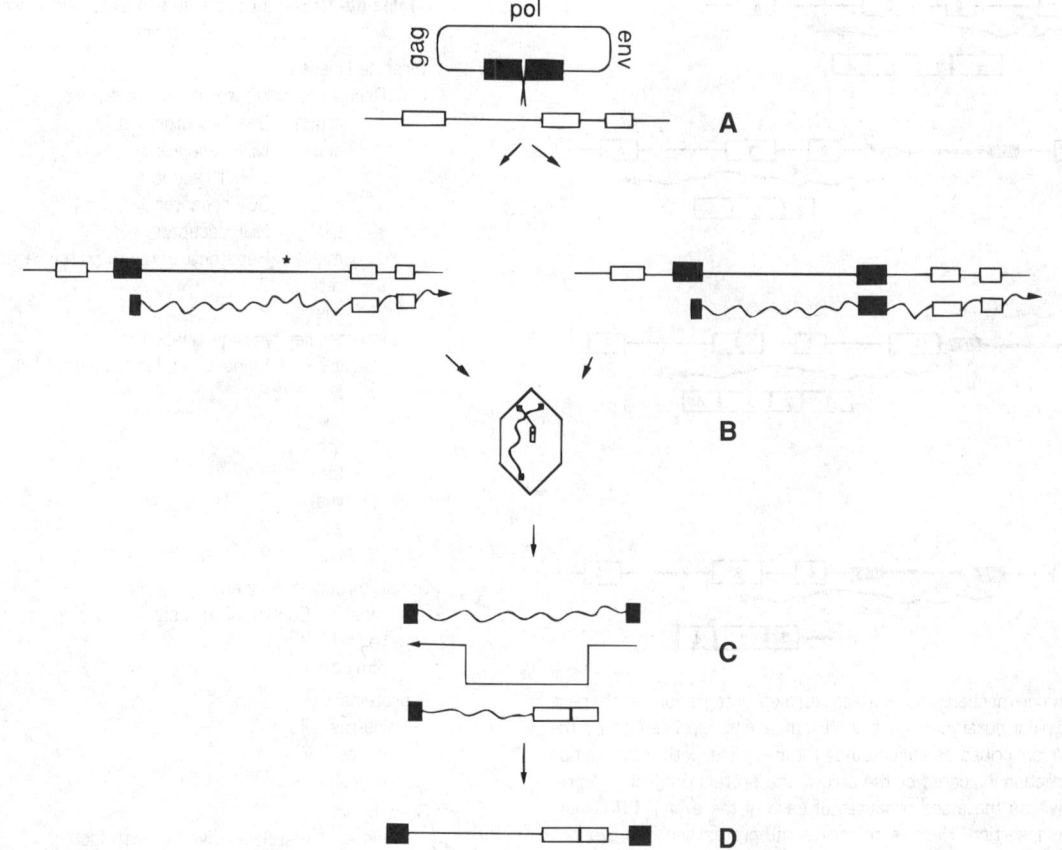

Fig. 60-2. Incorporation of oncogenes into viruses. **(A)** In the first step, a proviral form integrates into a cellular gene between two exons, represented by the open boxes. Following integration, two possible paths can be followed. On the left, a DNA deletion involving viral and cellular sequence occurs (*) and a fused virus and cell transcript is produced. On the right, a fraction of the normal viral transcripts fail to undergo normal processing and continue beyond the virus into flanking cellular sequences. **(B)** Either pathway can give rise to some virions that contain both a normal viral transcript and a hybrid transcript generated from viral and cellular sequences **(C).** When such a virion infects a new cell, recombination occurs during reverse transcription **(D)** and generates a recombinant virus containing the cellular sequences.

if mutated in the appropriate way. Most of the known oncogenes can be divided into groups based on their apparent mechanism of action and functional similarities. Oncogenes encoding proteins that appear to act through their association with the cellular membrane include growth factor receptors, membrane-bound intracellular proteins with tyrosine kinase activity, and membrane-bound intracellular proteins related to the signal-transducing G proteins. Oncogenes that encode nuclear proteins appear to function as transcriptional regulators. Other oncogenes encode proteins that are altered forms of growth factors, and still others encode proteins to which no function has yet been ascribed. Since oncogene products can act at multiple regulatory levels, it follows that some can complement the effects of others. Finally, some appear to share common signaling pathways.

PROTEIN TYROSINE KINASE ONCOGENES

The first oncogene protein to be assigned an enzymatic activity was src, a protein tyrosine kinase (PTK).[13,14] Before this discovery, a role for tyrosine phosphorylation in cellular growth had not even been proposed. Today, not only do PTKs comprise a major group of oncoproteins but tyrosine phosphorylation is recognized as one of the principal signaling

mechanisms in higher eukaryotic cells.[15] Although the actual pathways by which changes in tyrosine phosphorylation affect growth are not fully understood, it is likely that signals mediating cell division are regulated in part by phosphorylation and dephosphorylation of tyrosine residues. For example, the epidermal growth factor (EGF) receptor, the platelet-derived growth factor (PDGF) receptor, and the insulin receptor are tyrosine kinases that transmit the signal induced by ligand binding through tyrosine phosphorylation.[16–18] Proteins in this group all share the ability to phosphorylate themselves, in addition to other proteins, on the amino acid tyrosine (Fig. 60-4). This ability is required for the normal function of the cellular proto-oncogene, as well as for the transforming activity of the oncogenes. A central feature of any model explaining transformation induced by this class of proteins is that the normal controls regulating them are not operative, rendering them constitutively active.

Receptor Family of PTKs

One of the major types of PTK oncogenes encodes modified forms of growth factor receptors. Among this group are the oncogenes *erb*B, *kit, fms, neu, trk, met, ros,* and *ret.* The functions of the proto-oncogenes from which most of these were derived

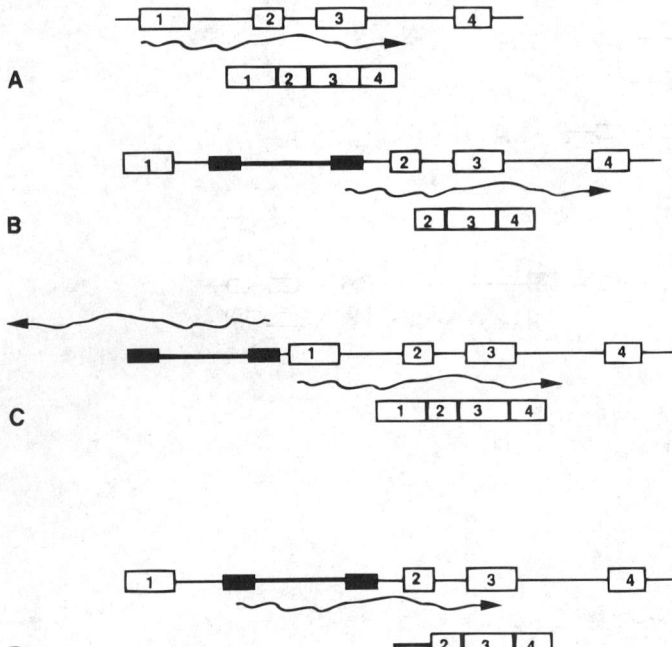

Fig. 60-3. Three common mechanisms by which retroviral integration affects gene expression. **(A)** A typical eukaryotic gene with four exons represented by the open boxes. RNA is transcribed as indicated by the wavy line, with transcription proceeding in the direction indicated by the arrow. The protein product is represented below the RNA as the fused products of each of the exons. **(B)** Consequences of promoter insertion. Here, a retrovirus integrates between exons 1 and 2 of the gene, and promoter sequences at the 3' end of the virus are used to direct synthesis of a truncated protein. **(C)** Consequences of enhancer insertion. Here, a retrovirus integrates near a cellular gene in the opposite transcriptional orientation. Enhancer sequences located in the retroviral LTR affect transcription from the normal promoter of the gene and elevate the level of expression. **(D)** Consequences of leader insertion. Here the retrovirus integrates within the gene as in Fig. B, but promoter sequences at the 5' end of the virus in concert with viral leader sequences lead to the translation of an altered form of the cellular gene product.

Table 60-1. Some Oncogene Products and Their Possible Functions

Tyrosine kinases		
Receptors with tyrosine kinase activity		
	erbB1	EGF receptor
	neu	NDF receptor
	fms	CSF-1 receptor
	kit	SCF receptor
	trk	NGF receptor
	met	Hepatocyte growth factor receptor
	ret	?
	ros	?
Intracellular tyrosine kinases		
	lck	Signal transduction from CD4
	fyn	?
	blk	?
	src	?
	fgr	?
	yes	?
	abl	?
	fes	?
Serine/threonine kinases		
	mos	Control of meiosis
	raf/mil	?
	pim1	?
G proteins		
	Ha-ras	?
	Ki-ras	?
	N-ras	?
Growth factor		
	sis	Platelet-derived growth factor
	hst	Basic fibroblast growth factor-like
	int-2	Basic fibroblast growth factor-like
Nuclear proteins		
Factors regulating gene transcription		
	erbA	Thyroid hormone receptor
	jun	Transcription factor, AP-1 component
	fos	Transcription factor, AP-1 component
	myb	Promoter-specific activation (PyAACG/TG)
	myc	Complexes with Max to bind CACGTG
	rel	NF-κB family member
	ski	?

Abbreviations: EGF, epidermal growth factor; CSF-1, colony-stimulating factor-1; NGF, nerve growth factor; SCF, stem cell factor; NDF, *neu* differentiation factor.

are known. The *erb*B gene, originally identified in a chicken virus that induces erythroblastosis, is an altered form of the EGF receptor gene.[19,20] The *fms* gene, isolated from a feline sarcoma virus,[21] was derived from the gene encoding the receptor for colony-stimulating factor-1, (CSF-1) which acts on myeloid cells.[22] The *kit* gene, first found in a feline sarcoma virus[23] arose from the gene encoding the receptor for stem cell factor, a cytokine directly involved in the development and maturation of hematopoietic, pigment, and germinal stem cells.[24–26] A combination of genetic and biochemical analyses revealed that *kit* was homologous to a known mouse locus called W, well known for its effects on hematopoiesis, fertility, and coat color.[27] The *trk* gene, originally isolated from human colon cancer,[28] is the receptor for nerve growth factor.[29,30] The *neu* oncogene, also called *her*-2 or *erb*B-2 because of its similarity to the EGF receptor, was first isolated from a rat neuroblastoma[31]; *neu* is prominently expressed in tumors of the breast and ovary[32] and interacts with a 44-kd protein called *neu* differentiation factor (NDF).[33] The *met* oncogene, originally isolated from a human osteogenic sarcoma cell line treated with carcinogen,[34] is the receptor for hepatocyte growth factor.[35] The *ret* oncogene was isolated from a human T-cell lymphoma,[36] and *ros* was first identified in a chicken sarcoma virus.[37] These genes encode proteins that resemble growth factor receptors, but their cognate ligands have not been identified.

Several different types of alterations have been found in the activated forms of these genes. In the case of *erb*B, activated forms of the gene express an altered protein that no longer interacts appropriately with its normal ligand.[38] This change results in constitutive activation of the kinase function of the protein. Other types of lesions can also affect receptor PTKs. For example, mutations altering the sequence of the extracellular portion of the fms protein outside the ligand-binding domain, as well as changes in the C terminus of the molecule, play a role in activating the oncogenic potential of this gene.[39] A point mutation resulting in a single amino acid change in the transmembrane portion of the neu protein activates the transforming potential of this oncogene,[40] perhaps by affecting aggregation of the receptor.[41]

Intracellular PTK Oncogene Products

A number of oncogenes encode PTKs that bind to the inner surface of the plasma membrane. These proteins share essential features with the membrane-associated PTKs in the region

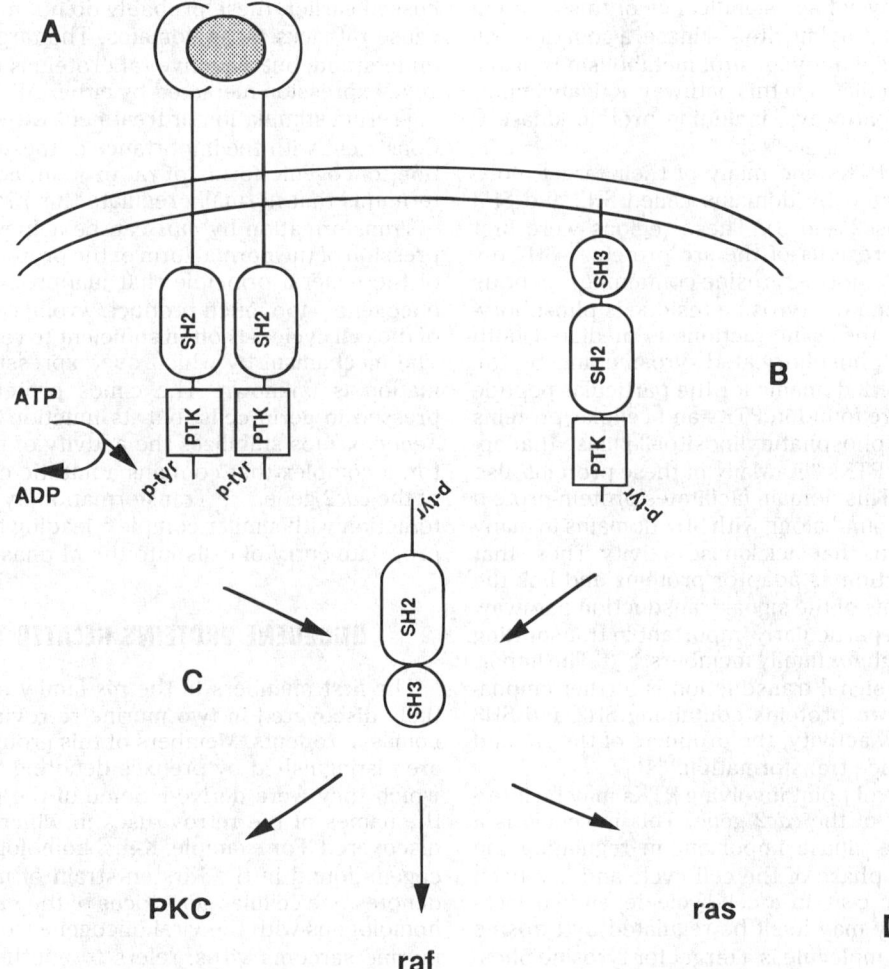

Fig. 60-4. Signaling mediated by protein tyrosine kinases. **(A)** Growth factor receptor protein tyrosine kinase that has bound ligand (filled circle). After binding ligand, kinase activity is stimulated and the molecule becomes phosphorylated on tyrosine. Oncogenic forms of the receptor are active constitutively and do not require interaction with ligand. **(B)** Cytoplasmic protein tyrosine kinase is illustrated. When the kinase is active and the molecule is phosphorylated on tyrosine, a signal can be transmitted. As for the receptors, a specific external signal is required for activation of the proto-oncogene product. Oncogenic forms are active constitutively. **(C)** Both receptor and cytoplasmic protein tyrosine kinases transmit signals via a number of different adaptor proteins that contain SH2 or SH2 and SH3 domains. This molecule could represent GAP, phospholipase C-γ, *crk*, phosphatidyl-inositol-3-kinase, or other proteins that interact with downstream signalling pathways. **(D)** Signals are transmitted from the adaptor proteins to different cellular pathways including those affected by protein kinase C (PKC), and the raf and ras proto-oncogene products.

of the molecule that is responsible for enzymatic activity, but they do not contain transmembrane or extracellular domains.[15,42] Oncogenes in this groups include *src, fgr, yes, abl*, and *fes.* All these genes were originally identified in retroviruses. The *src* and *yes* genes were obtained from independent isolates of chicken sarcoma virus,[43,44] the *fgr* and *fes* genes from cat sarcoma viruses,[45–47] and *abl* from a murine virus that induces pre-B-cell lymphoma.[48] As for oncoproteins in the tyrosine kinase receptor group, all the products of the oncogenic forms of these genes differ from the products specified by their normal cellular homologues. For most of these, the absence of a tyrosine residue that normally regulates the enzymatic activity of the molecule plays a key role in oncogenic activation.[15] In the case of the abl protein, changes near the N terminus of the molecule alter the localization of the protein.[49–51] The product of the proto-oncogene is localized to the nucleus, where it appears to interact with DNA[51,52]; the oncoprotein is found in the cytoplasm and can be associated with membranes.[53]

The actual mechanisms by which activated tyrosine kinases affect cell growth are still only partly understood. Normally,

these molecules appear tightly regulated and intimately involved in signal transduction within the cell.[15] In at least some cases, they transmit signals from cell-surface proteins to intracellular pathways that mediate growth (Fig. 60-4). For example, activation of T lymphocytes by means of the CD4 or CD8 receptor involves phosphorylation of the cellular PTK encoded by the *lck* gene.[54] The kinase activity of c-src protein is increased after interaction with PDGF receptors that have bound ligand.[55] If the PTK is the product of an oncogene and is constitutively active, the normal regulation provided by interaction with the cell-surface molecule is no longer operative, and growth stimulatory signals are continually transmitted.

A variety of cellular molecules, most of which are not oncogene products, are thought to transmit and amplify the signals received from the PTKs.[15] These include phosphatidylinositol-3-kinase, phospholipase C-γ, and the *ras*/GAP complex (Fig. 60-4). Many lines of evidence point to these interactions. For example, transformation by some PTKs can be blocked by antibodies to the ras oncoprotein,[56] a molecule related to signal-transducing G proteins (see below). GAP, a protein that regulates ras protein,[57] is phosphorylated on tyrosine by several

PTKs.[58] However, the physiologic significance of this reaction remains unclear. Phosphatidylinositol-3-kinase, a complex central to regulation of phosphatidylinositol metabolism is also a target for PTKs.[59] Intermediates in this pathway activate important limbs of signaling pathways, including protein kinase C and membrane calcium channels.[60]

Interactions between PTKs and many of their target molecules seem to be mediated by domains called SH2 and SH3 (src homologous regions 2 and 3). These regions were first identified as regulatory regions of the src protein.[61] SH2 domains interact with short tyrosine-containing peptide stretches in proteins when the tyrosine residue is phosphorylated.[62-64] Specificity in these interactions is mediated both by the presence of the phosphorylated tyrosine and by the preference of different SH2 domains for the particular peptide motifs.[63] SH2 domains are found in PTKs and cellular proteins such as PLC-γ, GAP and phosphatidylinositol-3-kinase that appear to be targets of the PTKs.[61,62] Many of these proteins also contain SH3 domains.[62] This domain facilitates protein-protein interaction and is often found along with SH2 domains in many PTKs and in some proteins that lack kinase activity. Those that lack kinase activity function as adaptor proteins and link the PTKs to downstream arms of the signal transduction pathway. These interactions seem particularly important in transmitting signals from PTKs through ras family members.[65-69] The importance of these motifs in signal transduction is further emphasized by the fact that two proteins containing SH2 and SH3 domains but lacking PTK activity, the products of the crk and vav oncogenes, can induce transformation.[70,71]

Another possible control point involving PTKs may be interaction with the product of the cdc2 gene. This molecule is a protein serine/threonine kinase important in regulating the entry of cells into the S phase of the cell cycle and has been shown to phosphorylate c-src in a cell-cycle-dependent fashion.[72,73] The cdc2 activity may itself be regulated by tyrosine phosphorylation, as this molecule is a target for tyrosine phosphorylation in vitro.[74] Therefore, a regulatory loop involving cdc2 and c-src may control cell division and may be disrupted when transformation occurs. The c-abl product is phosphorylated on serine during the M phase of the cell cycle; this modification seems to affect the ability of the molecule to bind DNA.[52] This feature and the observation that transformation of hematopoietic cells by v-abl involves stimulating early G_1 transit[75] reinforces the role of proto-oncogene and oncogene products in cell-cycle control.

PROTEIN SERINE/THREONINE KINASE ONCOGENES

Two oncogenes, mos and raf/mil, encode proteins that are protein serine/threonine kinases. The mos gene was first identified in a murine sarcoma virus,[76] while raf was first isolated from a murine virus that induces fibrosarcomas.[77] The mil gene, the avian homologue of the raf gene,[78] was isolated in an avian virus that induces myeloid leukemia. A third gene in this group, pim1, was identified because frequent proviral integrations were noted near this gene in murine thymic lymphomas.[79] Like the PTKs, the enzymatic activity of these molecules appears to be essential for transformation and aberrant regulation or overexpression of this activity is involved in oncogenic activation. These proteins are located primarily in the cytoplasm and, like the PTKs, function as key components of signal transduction pathways that mediate cell growth.

The mechanism by which the serine/threonine kinases affect growth is still being elucidated. Changes in the activity of the raf serine/threonine kinase occur after transformation by some PTKs, linking this molecule with others involved in PTK signal transduction. Complexes between PTKs and the raf protein seem to be involved.[80] However, unlike the complexes discussed earlier, these probably do not involve SH2 and SH3 because raf lacks these domains. The targets of raf are not well understood, but an active raf protein is required for increased gene expression mediated by either AP-1 or ets binding following serum stimulation or treatment with tumor promoters.[81,82] Consistent with the importance of these events in transformation, oncogenic forms of raf protein lack sequences at the N terminus that normally regulate this process.[81]

Transformation by mos can be achieved simply by overexpression of the normal form of the protein.[83] This is an example of the general principle that inappropriate expression of an oncogene—too much product, wrong cell type, or wrong time of the cell cycle—is often sufficient to result in transformation. The mechanism by which overexpression mediates transformation is unknown. The c-mos protein is prominently expressed in germ cells, but its function here is not clear.[84] In Xenopus, mos stabilizes the activity of mitosis promoting factor, a complex that contains a mitotic cyclin and the product of the cdc2 gene.[85,86] Transformation by v-mos may involve interaction with similar complex, leading to accelerated or inappropriate entry of cells into the M phase of the cell cycle.

ONCOGENE PROTEINS RELATED TO G PROTEINS

The first members of the ras family of oncogenes were initially discovered in two murine retroviruses that induce sarcomas in rodents. Members of this group are all called ras but are distinguished by prefixes denoting the cellular gene from which they were derived. Some of the prefixes are based on the names of the retroviruses in which the genes were first discovered. For example, K-ras, homologous with the viral oncogene found in the Kirsten strain of murine sarcoma virus, denotes one cellular gene locus of the ras family,[87] while H-ras, homologous with the viral oncogene isolated from the Harvey murine sarcoma virus, refers to another, distinct locus.[88] In addition to their presence in murine retroviruses, altered ras genes have been isolated from a variety of spontaneous tumors, including human tumors.[89]

Although each ras gene encodes a distinct product, all are proteins found on the inner surface of the plasma membrane, where they bind guanosine triphosphate (GTP) and hydrolyze it to the diphosphate.[90] These features demonstrate that ras proteins are one of a large group of molecules called G proteins. These proteins transmit signals to their cognate effectors when GTP is bound; activity is down-regulated by the hydrolysis of GTP (Fig. 60-5). Many signals from PTKs are transmitted by members of the ras protein family.

The targets of ras-mediated signaling remain to be fully elucidated. However, serine/threonine kinases such as the MAP kinases and the raf kinase are likely targets.[81,82,91] These interactions are probably indirect and mediated by adaptor proteins. One of these may be GAP. Although this protein clearly negatively regulates ras by enhancing the GTPase activity of the molecule,[57] there is some suggestion that it may transduce ras signals as well.[66,92] Oncogenic forms of ras usually contain point mutations that alter the sequence of the ras protein leading to a reduced ability to be converted to the inactive state. Either decreases in GTPase activity or increases in the rate of nucleotide exchange can be involved.[93,94] Thus, as with other oncoproteins, transformation by ras is a consequence of constitutive expression of the active or signal-transducing form of the molecule.

Two other members of the G protein family have been implicated in oncogenesis. One of these is the G_s α-protein, a molecule that regulates cAMP levels in the cell via adenyl cyclase. A point mutation in the gsp gene that encodes this molecule has been described that constitutively activates this gene in pituitary tumors.[95] Mutations in the gip gene that affect the

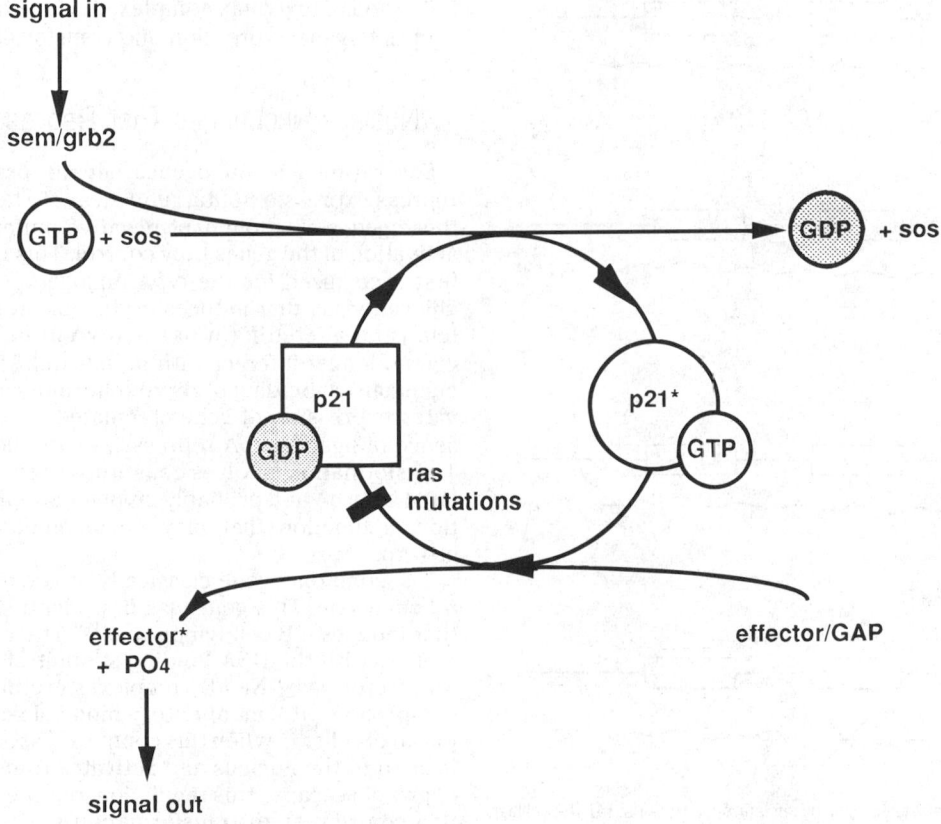

Fig. 60-5. ras G protein function. The p21 protein product of the *ras* gene family is inactive when bound to GDP. Signal input results in docking of *sem/grb* through their SH2 domains to receptor; activated *sem/grb* recruits *sos* through SH3 domains. *sos* interaction with *ras* p21 leads to the replacement of GDP with GTP and the consequent activation of the *ras* product. p21* then interacts with GAP/effector (see text), resulting in distal signal transduction. *ras* point mutations that lead to the transformed phenotype generally reduce GTP hydrolysis, keeping a greater proportion of cellular p21 molecules in the active state.

GTPase activity of its product, the G_i α-protein have also been detected in ovarian and adrenal tumors.[96]

GROWTH FACTOR ONCOGENES

Several oncogenes, including *sis*, *hst*, and *int2*, encode altered forms of growth factors. These genes came to light under diverse circumstances. The *sis* gene was discovered in a primate sarcomagenic virus,[97] while *int2* is a common site of proviral insertion in murine mammary carcinoma.[98] The *hst* gene was first isolated from a human gastric carcinoma.[99] The sis protein is an altered form of the β-chain of PDGF,[100,101] while *hst* and *int2* are related to basic fibroblast growth factor.[99,102] Oncogenes of this type appear to transform cells by direct autocrine stimulation. They are produced by the very cells they induce to grow. This stimulation does not necessarily require secretion of the growth factor. Recent evidence has shown that the interaction of the sis protein with its receptor occurs inside the cell.[103] Similar intracellular ligand-receptor interaction involving interleukin-3 has also been shown.[104] It is likely that this is a general mechanism by which growth factors can stimulate tumor growth.

NUCLEAR ONCOGENES

Unlike all the oncogene products previously discussed, one group of transforming genes encodes proteins that are primarily localized to the nucleus. The subcellular location of these proteins originally prompted speculation that these molecules are directly involved in regulating gene expression (Fig. 60-6). This hypothesis has now been proven for many of these genes.[105] Indeed, oncogene products that contain each of the motifs associated with DNA-binding proteins have been identified. For example, the myc proteins are members of the helix-loop-helix group, and the myb protein contains a helix-turn-helix motif.[106] The product of *erbA* contains a zinc finger and those of *fos* and *jun* contain leucine zippers. The product of the *rel* gene lacks these defined regions but is known to function as transcription factors. The ski product also probably belongs in this group. However, the function of this nuclear oncogene product, encoded by a chicken sarcoma virus,[107] is unknown.

Nuclear Oncogenes That Activate Transcription

As might be expected from the discussion of other oncogenes, the products of many oncogenes in this group activate gene expression constitutively. This ability leads to increased expression of some genes or invokes their expression at inappropriate times and is central to transformation by these oncogenes. However, exactly which genes are the critical targets of the transforming proteins and the way in which their products cause transformation is poorly defined. Oncogenes in this group include *myb*, originally identified in a chicken virus that induces myeloid leukemia,[108] *jun*, first identified in a chicken sarcoma virus,[109] and *fos*, first isolated in a murine retrovirus that induces osteosarcoma.[110] A final member of this group, the *myc* oncogene was first isolated in a chicken retrovirus that induces myeloid leukemias, carcinomas, and other tumors.[111] This gene is also a frequent target of proviral insertional mutagenesis in lymphomas in both birds and mice.[12]

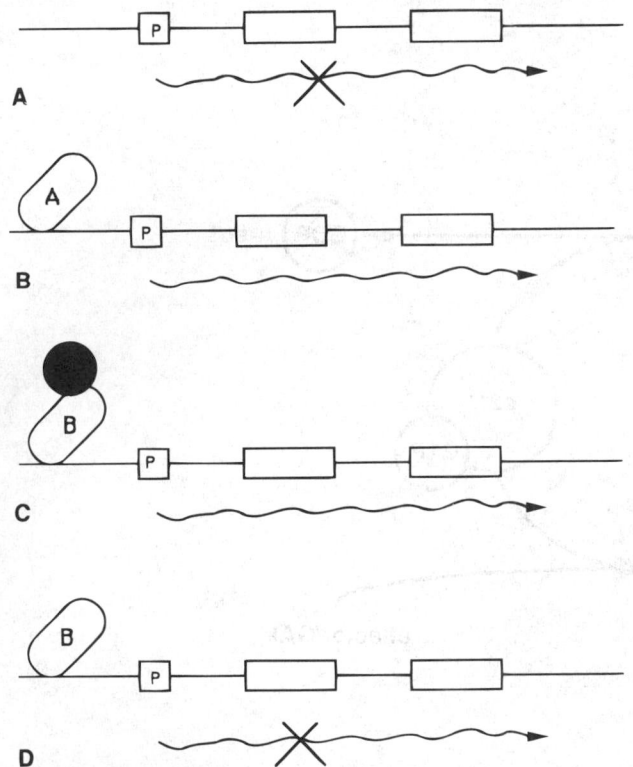

Fig. 60-6. Mechanisms of gene regulation by nuclear oncoproteins. **(A)** The cellular gene is not being expressed because no transcriptional activator protein complex is bound to enhancer elements upstream of the promoter (P). **(B)** The same gene with a transcriptional activator complex (A) bound upstream of P, a situation in which RNA, represented by the wavy line, is being transcribed. The situation in Figs. A and B represents the situation observed with positive regulators such as *fos*, *jun*, *myb*, and *myc*. **(C)** Diagram of a gene that is expressed if an activator complex (B) is bound in a complex with a second protein, represented by the dark circle. **(D)** The activator protein B binds in the absence of the second protein and causes repression of the gene. The situation diagrammed in Figs. C and D represents the situation observed for *erb*A and perhaps *rel*.

Mutations that result in loss of part of the coding sequence of the oncogene is a common way in which genes in this group have become activated. For example, the loss of either N- or C-terminal sequences of the myb protein renders the molecule oncogenic.[112] These mutations appear to affect the way in which the myb protein interacts with target DNA. Oncogenic activation of the *jun* also involves deletion of sequence that normally represses the function of the jun protein.[113,114] The jun protein is a component of the AP-1 transcription factor complex.[115,116] The product of the *fos* oncogene is also a component of this complex and interacts with the jun protein via the leucine zipper region present in both proteins.[117-119] Normally, expression of *fos* and *jun* is tightly controlled at the transcriptional and post-transcriptional levels. The oncogene homologues of these genes are expressed at high levels, a feature important for induction of transformation.

The myc protein is another oncoprotein that activates transcription. This protein is a member of the helix-loop-helix family of proteins.[120] Like most other nuclear oncogenes, the myc protein interacts with DNA. However, myc binds avidly only when complexed with another helix-loop-helix protein encoded by the *max* gene.[121] This interaction is required for transformation.[122] Normally myc is present in low amounts, limiting the amount of active myc/max complexes in the cell. A third protein, the product of *mad*, also regulates this complex by competing with myc for max.[123,124] When *myc* is overexpressed,

formation of myc/max complexes is facilitated, leading to inappropriate gene expression and transformation.

Nuclear Oncogenes That Repress Transcription

Several nuclear oncogenes encode proteins that normally repress expression of target genes.[105] The oncogenic forms of these genes are dominant negative mutants that prevent the activation of the genes they control. This type of alteration was first recognized for the *erb*A oncogene, originally found in a chicken virus that induces erythroblastosis.[125] The erbA protein is an altered form of the thyroid hormone receptor that can no longer interact with its ligand.[126,127] Under normal circumstances, binding of thyroid hormone to this molecule activates expression of genes regulated by the factor. In the absence of ligand, erbA represses expression of these genes.[128] Transformation involves constitutive repression of genes regulated by erbA and probably involves suppression of differentiation, a function that may be incompatible with continued growth.

A second oncogene classically included in this group is the *rel* oncogene. This gene was first identified in a chicken virus that induces a B-cell lymphoma.[129] The rel protein shares homology with the DNA binding subunit of the NF-κB transcription factor.[130,131] NF/κB complexes are normally regulated by complexing with an inhibitory molecule called IκB in the cytoplasm of cells.[132] When this complex dissociates, NF-κB is translocated to the nucleus and activates transcription. The *rel* oncoprotein escapes this regulation, but the precise way in which this contributes to transformation has yet to be discovered. Presumably, disrupted regulation of genes that prevent uncontrolled growth is involved. The importance of *rel*-related genes in regulating growth is emphasized by the observation that an altered form of the p65 subunit of NF-κB can induce transformation.[133] In addition, *Bcl-3*, a gene altered by translocation in some chronic B-cell leukemias[134] can associate with a *rel* family member and activate transcription.[135] This last observation has raised the possibility that at least some transforming events by members of this oncogene family involve transcriptional activation.

ACTIVATION OF CELLULAR PROTO-ONCOGENES

Proto-oncogenes normally play a role in controlling the cellular response to mitogenic signals as well as the passage through various compartments of the cell cycle. The initiation of DNA replication, cell division, and the commitment to cellular differentiation are all considered to be levels at which proto-oncogenes and their products may exert a regulatory influence. Consequently, proto-oncogenes represent obvious targets for processes that damage the growth control apparatus of the cell and lead to malignant transformation. This damage is often referred to as the "activation" of a proto-oncogene, resulting in the creation of an oncogene. In both leukemias and solid tumors, these processes have two basic effects. The first is to alter the protein product of the proto-oncogene, to produce a qualitative change in function. Mutation may lead to a protein with an enhanced catalytic activity or an activity no longer subject to the control of cognate regulatory factors. The second principal effect is to alter the regulation of proto-oncogene expression so that a quantitative effect on function results. The overproduction of an otherwise normal oncogene product is an example of this type of activation.

Damage to cellular proto-oncogenes that leads to their activation occurs by one of three mechanisms: genetic mutation, genetic rearrangement, or gene amplification. The first of these is usually associated with qualitative changes in function and the last with quantitative changes. Genetic rearrangement can have quite spectacular consequences, leading either to changes in the regulation of proto-oncogene transcription or to the creation of entirely new oncogene products.

Oncogene Mutation

The first defined alteration of a proto-oncogene to be discovered in a human tumor was the single-base mutation of a *ras* family member, Ha-*ras*1.[136,137] Point mutations affecting other *ras* genes (Ki-*ras*2 and N-*ras*) have subsequently been described in a wide variety of human leukemias and solid tumors.[90] The activating point mutations occur in quite specific locations—the bases of codons 12, 13, or 61—and yield single amino acid substitutions in what is now known to be the GTP-binding site of the *ras* gene product, p21. The biochemical phenotype of such mutations is the most prominent example of a qualitative change arising out of oncogene activation, namely, the p21-associated reduction of GTPase activity.[90] Since the GTP-bound form of p21 is considered the active one, the net effect of *ras* mutations is to increase the proportion of activated p21 molecules in the cell (Fig. 60-5). Given the previously described role of p21 as G protein in a signaling apparatus, the consequence of this shift toward the active form is presumably enhanced or constitutive transduction of mitogenic signals.

Although mutation was first detected in the Ha-*ras*1 gene, Ki-*ras*2 and N-*ras* are far more frequently the targets of somatic mutation in human tumors; Ha-*ras*1 mutations are, in fact, rarely observed. Interestingly, a pattern of tissue-specific mutation has emerged. For example, Ha-*ras* mutations are apparently limited largely to transitional epithelial tumors. Codon 13 mutations of the N-*ras* gene were found in 25–70% of acute myeloid leukemia (AML) samples examined.[138] Such observations have several important implications. First, the path traversed to produce, say, a specific leukemia subtype must be quite similar in most patients. This validates our observations on the nature of the pathogenetic lesions and gives us hope that the complexity of carcinogenesis will be resolved into a manageable number of combinatorial events. Second, despite this strong pattern of similarities, a significant fraction of tumors within a given class arise by a different path—different at least in the choice of *ras* substitutes. Finally, the specificity of these mutations hints at underlying functional attributes peculiar to each member of the *ras* gene family. In some experimental systems, for example, the introduction of a mutant Ha-*ras*1 gene may actually lead to differentiation rather than to unregulated proliferation.[139] Taking these disparate observations into account, we may speculate that each *ras* family member plays a role in signal transduction pathways with potentially distinct outcomes. Furthermore, the action of a given *ras* gene may be quite different from one cell type to another.

Evidently, *ras* mutations can occur before the transformation to frank malignancy takes place. There is abundant indirect evidence for this assertion in humans and direct evidence in animal tumor models. First, *ras* mutations may be detected in a significant proportion of myeloid cells present in a myelodysplastic bone marrow.[140] The mutations occur principally in patients destined to progress to AML but can occur in patients who remain free of leukemia. Second, the mutations can be demonstrated in a significant fraction of the precursor lesions to colon carcinoma (i.e., adenomatous polyps).[141] In the murine skin carcinoma model, benign epitheliomas generated by the application of chemical carcinogens uniformly contain Ha-*ras*1 mutations.[142] The epitheliomas may progress to invasive squamous carcinoma, or they may regress. Finally, transgenic mice bearing mutant *ras* genes are viable and develop normally but show a marked predisposition to the development of cancer.[143]

Although mutational activation in human tumors principally affects members of the *ras* family, several other candidate oncogenes have recently been described, somatic mutations of which are involved, rarely, in pathogenesis. In addition, six distinct oncogenes bearing mutations have been isolated from animal tumors. Each of these oncogenes has a human counterpart, although human mutations have not been observed. The most prominent of this set is the *neu* oncogene (lately *her* or *erb*B2), representing a transmembrane protein highly related to the EGF receptor.[31] This oncogene has been implicated in breast cancer (see below).

Oncogene Amplification

The expression of a given gene can be augmented in a variety of ways. Under normal circumstances, the complex interaction of control sequences located near genes with DNA-binding proteins that function as transcriptional regulatory factors leads to properly timed production of mRNA in a tissue- or cell-cycle-specific manner. Any disorganization of the plan of expression in genes responsible for the regulation of cell proliferation can, as described below, result in loss of growth control.

The first described occurrence of inappropriately elevated proto-oncogene expression in humans revealed activation by the mechanism of gene amplification. In this process, the initial duplication of a large chromosomal region by somatic recombination is followed by successive waves of replication and recombination to result in a large tandem array of DNA sequences not previously present in the normal cell genome. The array represents an increase in the number of copies of genes that happen to be present in the amplified DNA segment of the affected cell. This increase can be as large as several thousandfold. Recent evidence (see below) suggests that a propensity for gene amplication is conferred on cells in which certain tumor suppressor genes are functioning improperly.

Gene amplification in somatic cells was originally described for the dihydrofolate reductase gene, in which amplification led to methotrexate resistance.[144] In human tumors, the consequence of proto-oncogene amplification is usually a large increase in the level of transcribed mRNA and a corresponding increase in proto-oncogene protein product. Unlike dihydrofolate reductase amplification, in which a mutant enzyme is often the target of amplification, the product of an amplified proto-oncogene is usually qualitatively unchanged. Amplification most often involves genes whose transcripts have short half-lives. Therefore, the net result of amplification is the prolonged presence of mRNA and product, especially at inappropriate points in the cell cycle. This leads to a disruption of growth control since the product of the amplified gene, which would ordinarily be absent after a specified segment of the cell cycle passes, continues to provide the stimulus for cell DNA synthesis or cell division, or both.

The discovery of proto-oncogene (and drug resistance gene) amplification provides an explanation for two of the most prominent changes observed in tumor cell karyotypes. Double minutes (i.e., bipolar chromatin bodies without centrioles) commonly occur in malignant cells. The other chromosomal abnormality, known as the homogeneously staining region, appears when variable lengths of pale-staining chromatin are inserted into chromosomes. It is now recognized that these structures, which are apparently interchangeable within a given cell, represent the locations of gene amplification. Therefore, the amplification process can be so extensive that it results in grossly visible changes in chromosome structure.

The most prominent proto-oncogenes undergoing amplification in human tumors are members of the *myc* family. First observed in promyelocytic leukemia,[145] *myc* amplification has subsequently been documented in a broad range of cancers, including carcinomas of the lung, colon, and breast.[146] A consis-

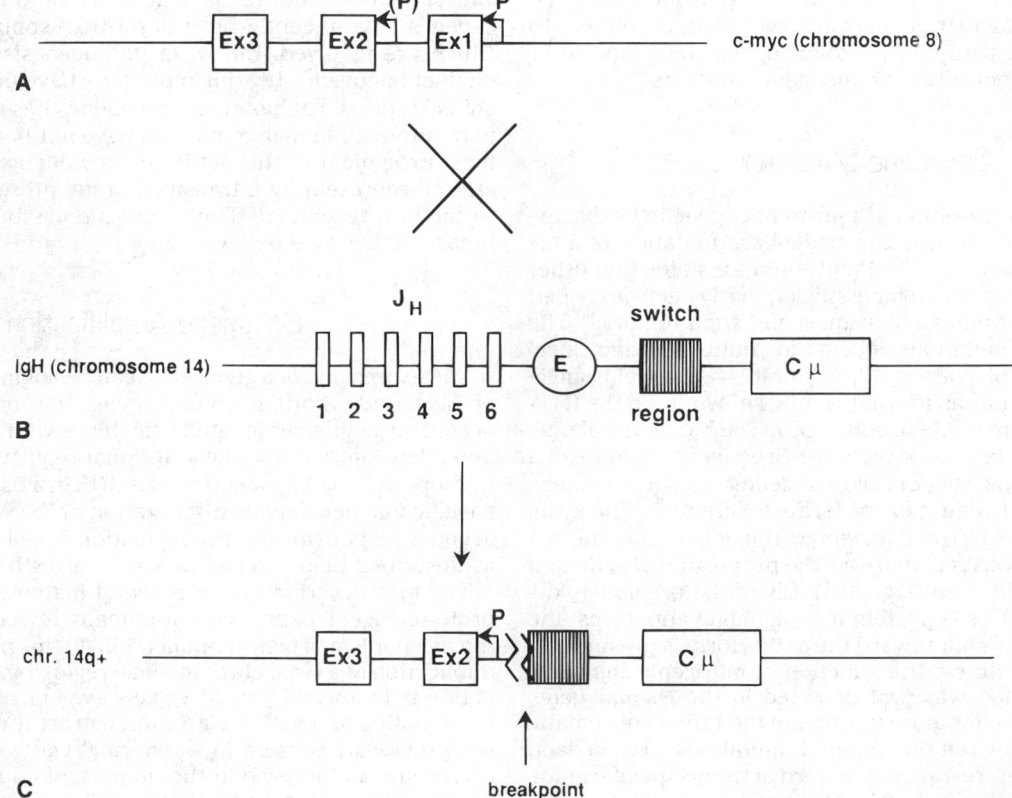

Fig. 60-7. Translocation of the c-*myc* oncogene. **(A)** Many c-*myc* translocations result from breakage of c-*myc* within intron 1, in which a cryptic promoter (P) is located. The c-*myc* chromosome 8 fragment is then joined to a C_H gene switch region. This creates the 14q + karyotypic anomaly noted in Burkitt lymphoma. **(B)** Translocation of C_γ. Translocation to distal (rightward) C_H genes also occurs. **(C)** Transcription of the translocated c-*myc* gene ensues from the cryptic promoter (now without parentheses) in the direction of the arrow. The boxes indicate c-*myc* exons.

tent pattern of *myc* amplification in a number of tumor subtypes has come to be associated with poor prognosis. For example, a particularly aggressive subset of small cell carcinoma of the lung, known to respond poorly to chemotherapy, consistently demonstrates amplification of one or another of the three *myc* genes.[147] Amplification of N-*myc* is a marker for poor prognosis in neuroblastoma.[148]

Overexpression of the c-*erb*B2 *(her/neu)* oncogene in breast cancer has recently been associated with poor prognosis.[149] The overexpression occasionally results from gene amplification, although excessive transcription of the gene can be seen in the absence of such amplification. This observation is potentially of great prognostic value, since *erb*B2 identifies individuals considered on the basis of other criteria, such as node status, to be at low risk of recurrence.

Oncogene Rearrangement

The most dramatic examples of proto-oncogene activation occur by genetic rearrangement, usually as a result of reciprocal chromosome translocations. These events are of particular pathogenetic significance in leukemias and lymphomas, for which specific translocations have been identified and analyzed in detail.

The significance of chromosome translocations, although long suspected to reflect the recruitment of genes important in carcinogenesis, was first demonstrated conclusively in human undifferentiated lymphoma and murine plasmacytoma.[150–152] In both instances, the cellular proto-oncogene, *myc,* was translocated from its normal position (in humans, chromosome 8)

to sites adjacent to or within the immunoglobulin heavy chain or Igκ or Igλ light chain constant region genes (Fig. 60-7). The resulting human translocations were t(8;14), t(2;8), and t(8;22), respectively. The mechanisms responsible for abnormal *myc* rearrangements are poorly understood; perhaps they represent errors in the normal rearrangement process that results in functional immunoglobulin genes.

The c-*myc* gene consists of three exons. The first exon does not encode protein and is thought to be one of the elements involved in regulating the level and timing of c-*myc* expression. In most translocations this exon is truncated from the remaining two, which are then transferred, for example, to the switch region of heavy chain constant region genes. In the minority of translocations in which all three exons of the gene are translocated to an immunoglobulin gene locus, somatic mutations are often observed to occur in exon 1. However, the DNA sequence of the protein product, encoded in exons 2 and 3, is nearly always unaffected.[153] Therefore, the c-myc protein produced by a translocated c-*myc* gene is usually identical to that produced by the normal gene. Finally, it has been observed that c-*myc* transcription from the translocated gene is constitutive, if not always elevated. Transcription from the normal gene ceases in a tumor with a c-*myc* translocation.

The picture that emerges from this set of observations, although not yet verified in significant details, is compelling. Moving a proto-oncogene away from resident influences that control the level and timing of transcription and into a locus that is actively expressed in a given state of differentiation (e.g., immunoglobulin genes in B lymphocytes) can result in oncogene activation and subsequent tumorigenesis. In the specific instance of c-*myc,* removal or mutational alteration of exon 1 seems critical to deregulation of transcription. Under circumstances in which the normal c-*myc* allele is silent, the translocated one continues to be expressed. This is an example of quantitative alteration of oncogene function.

Another prominent example of this type of activation is the t(14;18) translocation of human follicular lymphoma.[154] Once again, the immunoglobulin heavy chain gene is the recipient of a chromosome fragment bearing an oncogene from another chromosome, this time the *bcl*2 oncogene from the long arm of chromosome 18. As with c-*myc*, transcription of *bcl*2 is inappropriately constitutive in tumor cells as a result of the translocation.

This example also emphasizes the importance of chromosome translocations in finding new growth regulatory genes. The oncogene, *bcl*2, was unknown before the molecular analysis of t(14;18). It has subsequently been placed into a completely distinct class of genes: those that govern the onset of apoptosis, or programmed cell death.[155] Another gene discovered by cloning the breakpoint of a chromosome translocation, *bcl*3, has proved an inhibitor of particular transcriptional regulatory factors, probably belonging to the NF-κB family. *bcl*3 sequesters these factors in the cytoplasm, rendering them inactive.[156]

In addition to affecting the control of oncogene expression, translocations can alter the form of the oncogene product. In chronic myeloid leukemia (CML) the c-*abl* oncogene on chromosome 9 is moved into the *bcr* gene on chromosome 22 by t(9;22), the classic Philadelphia translocation.[157] Each translocation accomplishes the same result, truncating the N terminus of c-*abl*. The coding sequences responsible for the N terminus of the c-*abl* protein are replaced with coding sequences from *bcr*. Thus, an entirely new fusion protein is derived from two genes on two different chromosomes. Functionally, the translocation results in one certain and another possible outcome. The normal c-abl product is an intracellular tyrosine kinase. The activity of the enzyme is tightly regulated in vivo, however. Following translocation, the fusion product, which retains the tyrosine kinase domain of the original c-*abl* oncogene, has constitutively high kinase activity.[158] The second likely outcome of the translocation, although not yet proven, must be to alter some aspect of c-*abl* effector specificity or domain of action. This is inferred from (1) the regularity of the translocation (only *bcr* is involved), and the same region of the c-abl protein is affected; and (2) different portions of *bcr* are transferred to the N terminus of c-*abl*, depending on whether the Philadelphia translocation is observed in CML or ALL.

Two other translocations have been characterized in hematologic malignancies, which also create new genes by piecing together fragments of pre-existing genes. A t(1;19) translocation in acute pre-B-cell leukemia fuses the homeobox gene, *PBX1*, to the transcriptional regulatory factor, *E2A*.[159] Homeobox genes encode transcriptional regulatory products, which are important in development and differentiation, whereas the E2A protein is involved in the expression of genes in B cells. The chimeric product of t(1;19) redirects the activating potential of E2A to the gene targets of PBX1 regulation. In the t(15;17) translocation of acute promyelocytic leukemia, a new chimeric product is created from the fusion of the retinoic acid receptor locus, *RAR*α, and the *PML* gene, which interferes with the regulatory function of both parental products.[160]

TUMOR SUPPRESSOR GENES

We have shown that proto-oncogenes comprise a set of cellular genes that are involved at all levels of control of cell division and differentiation. In each of the genes discussed thus far, a somatic activating event results in a dominant change. A mutant *ras* gene has a dominant phenotype in the presence of the wild-type allele. A translocated c-*myc* gene is dominant over its unrearranged counterpart. In principle, however, genes that regulate growth and differentiation could demonstrate the opposite pattern: regulatory function preserving a normal pattern of growth would only be observed in the wild-type form (Fig. 60-8). Any mutation or rearrangement would tend to inactivate such genes, leading to loss of growth control. Since the wild-type allele could suppress these mutations, they would be recessive at the cellular level. Genes that display this property are called recessive oncogenes but, because of several additional properties described below, they have also come to be known as tumor suppressor genes, or anti-oncogenes.

Retinoblastoma Model

The childhood tumor retinoblastoma is one of the best characterized models for action of a recessive oncogene. In this cancer, which occurs in both inherited and sporadic forms, a "retinoblastoma" gene was proposed as the recessive oncogene, which normally suppresses the malignant transformation of retinoblasts. Individuals at risk of the familial form of the disease, according to a two-hit hypothesis advanced by Knudson,[161] inherit a damaged, nonfunctional gene. The second hit in such individuals would then be a somatic mutation, which inactivates the remaining normal allele. Individuals with sporadic retinoblastoma would suffer two independent somatic mutations damaging both alleles. More recent investigations have advanced this set of conjectures a considerable distance, culminating in the molecular cloning and characterization of the retinoblastoma gene, *Rb-1*.

Cytogenetic abnormalities in the form of interstitial deletions and a fortuitously observed linkage to the enzyme esterase D established the long arm of chromosome 13 as the probable site of a retinoblastoma gene.[162] Shortly thereafter, investigators were able to exploit the newly developed technique of restriction fragment length polymorphism to confirm an important prediction of the above-described model, namely, that loss of genetic material in the region of the putative *Rb-1* gene routinely occurred in tumors.[163] DNA probes identifying several polymorphic regions on chromosome 13 were used to compare patients' tumor DNA with their normal, or constitutional, DNA (Fig. 60-8). According to this approach, the polymorphic probes identify both maternal and paternal chromosomes on Southern blots; loss of genetic material is evident as a loss of heterozygosity (LOH). The results indicated a specific LOH at 13q. Furthermore, the chromosome (*Rb-1* allele) retained in each tumor of a patient with a familial retinoblastoma was from the affected parent. This was additional evidence for the supposition that somatic mutation (in this instance, gene loss) was required to advance the pathogenetic process in an individual inheriting one bad copy of the retinoblastoma gene. Subsequent work with DNA probes specific to 13q has demonstrated that chromosome loss and duplication, as well as mitotic recombination, are the somatic mechanisms by which loss of genetic material occurs.

Several groups have now reported molecular cloning of the human *Rb-1* gene.[164,165] The locus is quite large, extending over 200 kb of DNA and consisting of 27 exons. mRNA transcribed from this gene encodes a 110-kd phosphoprotein, described in more detail below. All cell types examined thus far express the *Rb-1* gene, and knowledge of its structure has enabled workers in the field to complete the molecular characterization of pathogenetic lesions in familial and sporadic retinoblastoma. First, *Rb-1* mRNA is either absent or of aberrant size in almost all tumors examined. In those tumors with grossly undetectable changes in mRNA, small deletions or mutations are observed, which either alter the reading frame of the mRNA or lead to abnormal splicing. Interestingly, similar lesions of the *Rb-1*

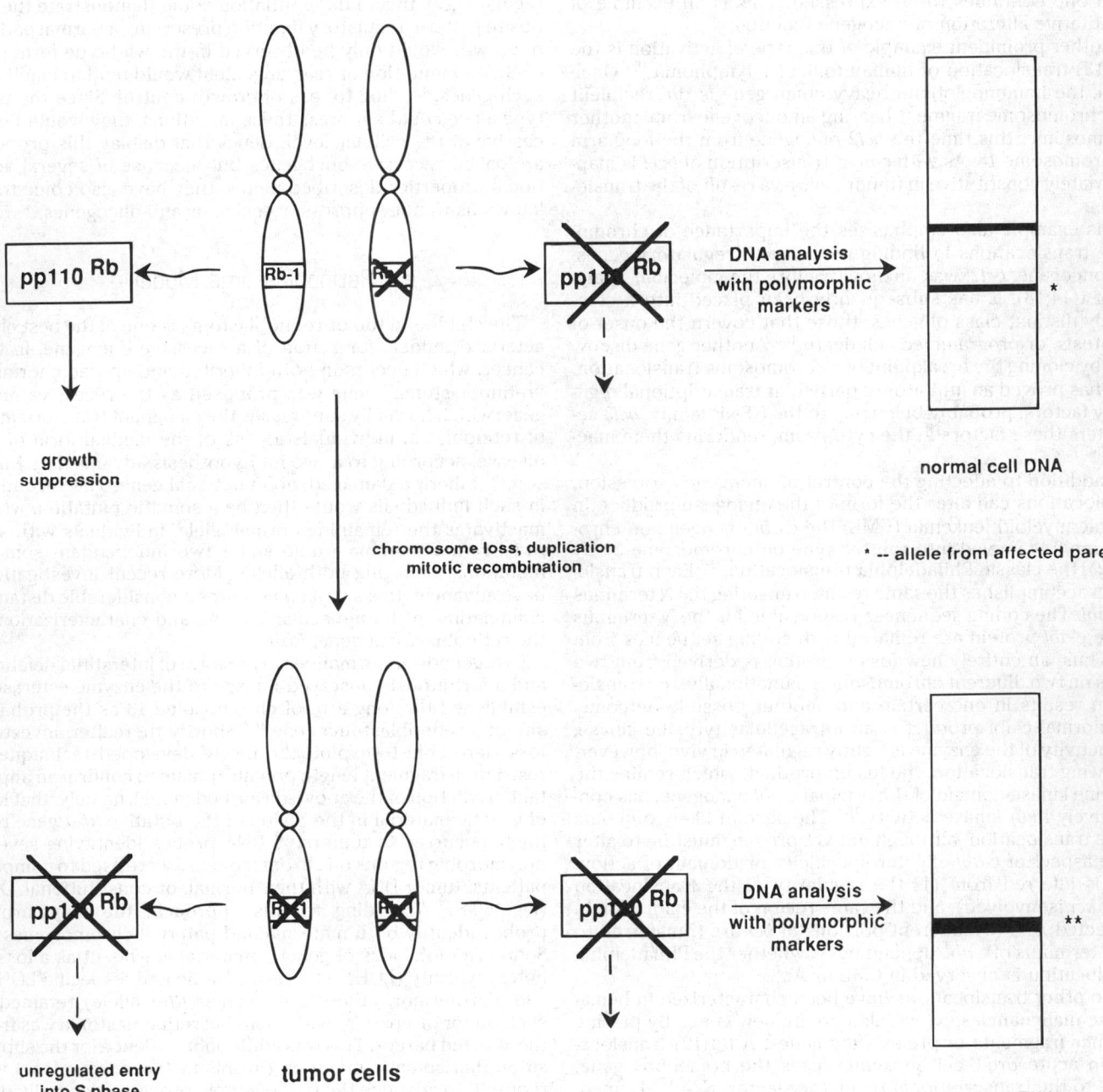

Fig. 60-8. (Left) Tumor progression in familial retinoblastoma. One damaged allele is inherited from an affected parent. (The allele could also represent a new mutation in the parent's germ cells.) Cells with one functioning (wild-type) copy of the *Rb-1* gene remain normal. As a result of somatic genetic damage (mutation, loss, mitotic recombination), the second allele may be inactivated, with malignant conversion resulting. This scenario is depicted for retinoblastoma but holds for most dominantly inherited familial cancer syndromes. In sporadic retinoblastoma, damage to the first allele occurs as a somatic event. **(Right)** Tumor loss of heterozygosity. If informative (heterozygous) polymorphic markers are used to analyze patients' normal and tumor DNA, a common accompaniment of damage to recessively acting oncogenes is loss of heterozygosity. Generally, one band (allele) on a Southern blot will disappear if the marker employed is close enough to the recessive oncogene locus, in this case, *Rb-1*. The allele retained in the tumor is inherited from the affected parent (*) and often occurs as a double copy (**).

locus occur in the osteosarcomas that arise frequently during adolescence in those patients who survive childhood retinoblastoma. The ability of the *Rb-1* gene to suppress tumorigenesis has been demonstrated directly by transferring a copy of the wild-type gene into cells of a retinoblastoma cell line.[166] Those cells that incorporate the normal *Rb-1* gene assume a slower growth rate in vitro and are no longer tumorigenic when injected into nude mice. Thus, the anti-oncogene or tumor suppressor gene phenotype of *Rb-1* is evident.

The *Rb-1* product, pp110^{RB}, is a zinc-finger protein that displays interesting behavior during the course of the cell cycle. In G$_1$, most molecules of pp110^{RB} are unphosphorylated.[167,168]

During S and G_2, all become phosphorylated, usually at multiple sites. Several DNA tumor viruses encode protein products that bind only the unphosphorylated form of pp110^{RB}.[169,170] It is probably through this binding of the cellular *Rb-1* gene product that transformation by these viruses is mediated. Thus far, this set of observations suggests that the unphosphorylated form of the Rb-1 protein is the active one and that pp110^{RB} probably functions as part of the barrier to entry into S phase.

The recent elucidation of the role of p53 in the pathogenesis of human cancer represents one of the signal achievements of basic cancer research. p53 was discovered >15 years ago because its 53-kd nuclear protein product bound simian virus 40 T antigen during viral transformation of host cells.[171] Following the cloning of this gene and its mapping to the short arm of chromosome 17, loss of heterozygosity in that region was noted in a large number of human tumor types. Ultimately, many investigators showed that this loss represented the frequent deletion of p53 genes. In several instances, particularly in colon cancer, the deletion of one allele was accompanied by mutation of the remaining allele. The frequent alteration of p53 genes has been detected in tumors of the colon, lung, breast, esophagus, urinary bladder, and brain; in sarcomas and hepatocellular carcinomas; and in tumors of the hematopoietic and lymphoreticular systems.[172] A germline mutation of p53 is the inherited cause of Li-Fraumeni syndrome, in which at-risk persons eventually develop multiple forms of cancer in the early to middle years of adulthood.[173]

The p53 product is a DNA-binding protein that binds a specific recognition site in the control regions of many genes.[174] Although its precise role in growth regulation has not yet been elucidated, p53 probably controls the transcription of a network of genes which, together, exert a dominant role in growth suppression. Simply replacing a wild-type p53 gene in a tumor cell line lacking it will often result in a loss of tumorigenicity.[175] Also, p53 may play a role in the G_1-S "checkpoint," the point in the cell cycle when the decision is made to proceed into S phase from G_1.[176] Cells apparently possess a mechanism that allows them to decide whether sufficient repairs have occurred to any damaged regions of the genome. If repairs have been adequate, the cells proceed on to DNA replication. A very interesting recent discovery related to this checkpoint function is the apparent correlation between loss of p53 and a high frequency of gene amplification.

Tumor Suppressor Genes in Other Familial Tumors

A pattern of similarity has emerged between familial retinoblastoma and nearly all the dominantly inherited cancer syndromes. During the past several years, many of the disease loci for these familial syndromes have been mapped, including several forms of multiple endocrine neoplasia,[177,178] polyposis coli,[179] neurofibromatosis types I[180] and II,[181] and Wilms tumor.[182] In each instance examined, tumor DNAs from such patients show LOH with markers near the appropriate family cancer gene. Each disease locus maps to a unique chromosome position, which strongly suggests the existence of multiple genes with the properties of *Rb-1*.

Three of the genes responsible for these familial cancer syndromes have been cloned. The Wilms tumor gene, *WT-1*,[183] encodes a transcriptional factor with zinc-finger motifs. It is probably not the only gene that can result in this syndrome. The gene responsible for neurofibromatosis I, *NF1*, encodes a protein highly homologous to rasGAP and, therefore, probably regulates the activity of some small G protein.[184] The *APC* gene, which is involved in familial polyposis, encodes a very large protein whose function is, as yet, completely unknown.[185]

Tumor Suppressor Genes in Sporadic Cancer

Although patients with dominantly inherited cancer syndromes do not form a large fraction of all cancer patients, the molecular genetics of these syndromes is highly relevant to sporadic cancer. First, specific patterns of LOH are observed in cancers of the breast, lung, colon, stomach, and kidney.[186-190] As we have shown, this molecular lesion is the hallmark of a recessive oncogene. Since each of these tumors displays different chromosomal sites for LOH, the existence of a large set of tumor suppressor genes is likely. Furthermore, in tumors such as colon cancer, sporadic cases sometimes show LOH of the same chromosome region (in this instance, 5q) as the familial form of the same cancer.[191] These findings imply that, like retinoblastoma, sporadic cancer can involve molecular lesions of the same genes, causing the familial form of the disease. Proof of this hypothesis for sporadic colon cancer has recently been obtained: most of these cancers display mutations of the *APC* gene.[192]

ONCOGENE COOPERATIVITY IN THE DEVELOPMENT OF CANCER AND LEUKEMIA

Given the relatively large number of oncogenes, what is the minimum number that must be activated to produce a malignant cell? Given the diversity of functional classes, what types of oncogenes must be activated? The answers to these questions are incomplete, but some conclusions may be drawn from the results of a variety of experimental approaches.[193] First, established cell lines that are nontumorigenic and that display relatively normal growth and morphology in vitro often require only one activated *ras* gene to become tumorigenic. This probably reflects genetic damage already undergone simply to obtain the immortalized state that cell lines, by definition, possess. Cells that have not been established permanently in culture and that have normal karyotypes are not significantly altered by the introduction of one activated oncogene. In this case, two activated oncogenes are required, one with a product located in the cytoplasm and one with a nuclear product.[194-196] Thus, the introduction of a mutant *ras* gene and a constitutively expressed *myc* gene (but not either alone) will transform a normal diploid fibroblast. Interestingly, cells transformed in this fashion will produce tumors when injected into recipient animals, but the tumors are generally small and often regress. Therefore, at least one other event must occur for the appearance of the fully malignant phenotype.

If tumorigenic cells bearing activated oncogenes are fused to normal cells, the tumorigenic phenotype is usually suppressed.[197] Such hybrid cells, injected into an animal host, will differentiate normally and remain quiescent. With prolonged passage in culture, however, tumorigenic segregants do arise rarely. This subset of the original population of hybrids maintains the activated oncogenes but now demonstrates specific chromosome loss or LOH, or both. The LOH is often specific to the cell types employed in the original fusions. Thus, somatic cell genetic experiments with activated oncogenes provide additional evidence for the class of tumor suppressor genes or anti-oncogenes discussed above and suggest that loss of such genes is required for progression of tumorigenesis. Furthermore, wild-type anti-oncogenes appear dominant over mutant (activated) proto-oncogenes of the *ras* and *myc* variety.

Once again, colon cancer has provided additional experimental support for this scenario. In a large study of colon tumors, ranging from small adenomas to invasive, poorly differentiated adenocarcinomas, Vogelstein and colleagues[198] detected the regular appearance of genetic lesions involving four different loci: K-*ras*, p53, a gene on chromosome 18 (*DCC*, which encodes a product with homology to adhesion molecules), and a gene on chromosome 5 (likely to be *APC;* another candidate is the nearby locus, *MCC*). The actual order in which these lesions appeared seemed less important than that, cumulatively, all were eventually present in the tumor. However, *ras* mutations tended to occur early, in adenomas, and p53 losses later, in the invasive carcinomas.

Finally, although malignant transformation apparently requires the complex interplay of oncogenes and anti-oncogenes, the evolution of cancer cells with metastatic potential may require the participation of further classes of genes not ordinarily included in the oncogene category. These include adhesion molecules and homing receptors expressed on the tumor cell surface, as well as specific proteases secreted by these same cells. Such products presumably enable a cell in which genetic changes are altering the mitogenic signal apparatus and program for cell division to invade local blood vessels and lymphatics, to travel to distant tissue targets, and to begin anew the expansion of a malignant cell population.

ACKNOWLEDGMENT

We thank Dr. John Coffin for his help with the illustrations.

REFERENCES

1. Coffin J: Genome structure. p. 17. In Weiss R, Teich N, Varmus H, Coffin J (eds): RNA Tumor Viruses. Cold Spring Harbor Laboratory Press, Cold Spring Harbor, NY, 1985
2. Varmus H, Swanstrom R: Replication of retroviruses. p. 75. In Weiss R, Teich N, Varmus H, Coffin J (eds): RNA Tumor Viruses. Cold Spring Harbor Laboratory Press, Cold Spring Harbor, NY, 1985
3. Martin GS: Rous sarcoma virus: a function required for the maintenance of the transformed state. Nature 227:1021, 1970
4. Stehelin D, Varmus H, Bishop JM, Vogt PK: DNA related to the transforming gene(s) of avian sarcoma viruses is present in normal avian DNA. Nature 260:170, 1976
5. Simon MA, Drees B, Kornberg T, Bishop JM: The nucleotide sequences and the tissue-specific expression of Drosophila c-src. Cell 42:831, 1985
6. Bishop JM, Varmus H: Functions and origins of retroviral transforming genes. p. 249. In Weiss R, Teich N, Varmus H, Coffin J (eds): RNA Tumor Viruses. Cold Spring Harbor Laboratory Press, Cold Spring Harbor, NY, 1985
7. Swain A, Coffin JM: Mechanism of transduction by retroviruses. Science 255:841, 1992
8. Benjamin T, Vogt P: Cell transformation by viruses. p. 317. In Fields BN, Knipe DM (eds): Virology. Raven Press, New York, 1990
9. Nilsen TW, Maroney PA, Goodwin RG et al: c-erbB activation in ALV-induced erythroblastosis: novel RNA processing and promoter insertion result in expression of an amino-truncated EGF receptor. Cell 41:719, 1985
10. Payne GS, Bishop JM, Varmus HE: Multiple arrangements of viral DNA and an activated host oncogene (c-myc) in bursal lymphomas. Nature 295:209, 1982
11. Hayward WS, Neel BG, Astrin SM: Activation of a cellular *onc* gene by promoter insertion in ALV-induced lymphoid leukosis. Nature 295:475, 1981
12. van Lohuizen M, Berns A: Tumorigenesis by slow-transforming retroviruses—an update. Biochim Biophys Acta 1032:213, 1990
13. Erikson RL, Collett MS, Erikson E, Purchio AF: Evidence that the avian sarcoma virus transforming gene product is a cyclic AMP-independent protein kinase. Proc Natl Acad Sci USA 76:6260, 1979
14. Hunter T, Sefton BM: Transforming gene product of Rous sarcoma virus phosphorylates tyrosine. Proc Natl Acad Sci USA 74:2011, 1980
15. Cantley LC, Auger KR, Carpenter C et al: Oncogenes and signal transduction. Cell 64:281, 1991
16. Chen WS, Lazar CS, Poenie M et al: Requirement for intrinsic protein tyrosine kinase in the immediate and late actions of the EGF receptor. Nature 328:820, 1987
17. Bishayee S, Ross AH, Werner R, Scher CD: Purified human platelet-derived growth factor receptor has ligand-stimulated tyrosine kinase activity. Proc Natl Acad. Sci USA 83:6756, 1986
18. Chou CK, Dull TJ, Russell DS et al: Human insulin receptors mutated at the ATP-binding site lack protein tyrosine kinase activity and fail to mediate post receptor effects of insulin. J Biol Chem 262:1842, 1987
19. Privalsky ML, Ralston R, Bishop JM: The glycoprotein encoded by the retroviral oncogene v-erbB is structurally related to tyrosine-specific protein kinases. Proc Natl Acad Sci USA 81:704, 1984
20. Downward J, Yarden Y, Mayes E et al: Close similarity of epidermal growth factor receptor and v-erbB oncogene protein sequences. Nature 307:521, 1984
21. Hampe A, Gobet M, Sherr CJ, Galibert F: Nucleotide sequence of the feline retroviral oncogene v-fms shows unexpected homology with oncogenes encoding tyrosine-specific protein kinases. Proc Natl Acad Sci USA 81:85, 1984
22. Sherr CJ, Rettenmier CW, Sacca R et al: The c-fms proto-oncogene product is related to the receptor for the mononuclear phagocyte growth factor, CSF-1. Cell 41:665, 1985
23. Besmer P, Murphy JE, George PC et al: A new acute transforming feline retrovirus and relationship of its oncogene v-kit with the protein kinase gene family. Nature 320:415, 1986
24. Zsebo KM, Williams DA, Geissler EN et al: Stem cell factor is encoded at the *SL* locus of the mouse and is the ligand for the c-kit tyrosine kinase receptor. Cell 63:213, 1990
25. Huang E, Nocka K, Beier DR et al: The hematopoietic growth factor KL is encoded at the *Sl* locus and is the ligand of the c-kit receptor, the gene product of the *w* locus. Cell 63:225, 1990
26. Anderson DM, Lyman SD, Baird A et al: Molecular cloning of mast cell growth factor, a hematopoietin that is active in both membrane bound and soluble forms. Cell 63:235, 1990
27. Geissler EN, Ryan MA, Housman DE: The dominant-white spotting (*W*) locus encodes the c-kit proto-oncogene. Cell 55:185, 1988
28. Pulciani S, Santos E, Lauver AV et al: Oncogenes in solid human tumors. Nature 300:539, 1982
29. Hempstead BL, Martin-Zanca D, Kaplan DR et al: High-affinity NGF binding requires coexpression of the *trk* proto-oncogene and the low-affinity NGF receptor. Nature 350:678, 1991
30. Kaplan DR, Hempstead BL, Martin-Zanca et al: The *trk* proto-oncogene product: a signal transducing receptor for nerve growth factor. Science 252:554, 1991
31. Schecter AL, Stern DF, Vaidyanathan L et al: The *neu* oncogene: an erbB-related gene encoding a 185,000 M_r tumor antigen. Nature 312:513, 1984
32. Slamon DJ, Godolphin W, Jones LA et al: Studies of the HER-2/neu protooncogene in human breast and ovarian cancer. Science 244:707, 1989
33. Peles E, Bacus SS, Koski RA et al: Isolation of the neu/HER-2 stimulatory ligand: a 44 kd glycoprotein that induces differentiation of mammary tumor cells. Cell 69:205, 1992
34. Cooper CS, Park M, Blair DG et al: Molecular cloning of a new transforming gene from a chemically transformed human cell line. Nature 311:229, 1984
35. Naldini L, Weidner KM, Vigna E et al: Scatter factor and hepatocyte growth factor are indistinguishable ligands for the *MET* receptor. EMBO J 10:2867, 1991.
36. Takahashi M, Ritz J, Cooper GM: Activation of a novel human transforming gene, *ret,* by DNA rearrangement. Cell 42:581, 1985
37. Feldman RA, Wang LH, Hanafusa H, Balduzzi PC: Avian sarcoma virus UR2 encodes a transforming protein which is associated with a unique protein kinase activity. J Virol 42:228, 1982
38. Ullrich A, Coussens L, Hayflick JS et al: Human epidermal growth factor receptor cDNA sequence and aberrant expression of the amplified gene in A431 epidermoid carcinoma cells. Nature 309:418, 1984
39. Roussel MF, Downing JR, Rettenmier CW, Sherr CJ: A point mutation in the extracellular domain of the human CSF-1 receptor (c-fms proto-oncogene product) activates its transforming potential. Cell 55:979, 1988
40. Bargmann CJ, Hung MC, Weinberg RA: Multiple independent activations of the *neu* oncogene by a point mutation altering the transmembrane domain of p185. Cell 45:649, 1986
41. Weiner DB, Liu J, Cohen JA et al: A point mutation in the *neu* oncogene mimics ligand induction of receptor aggregation. Nature 339:230, 1989
42. Hanks SK, Quinn AM, Hunter T: The protein kinase family: conserved features and deduced phylogeny of the catalytic domains. Science 241:42, 1988
43. Czernilofsky AP, Levinson AD, Varmus HE et al: Nucleotide sequence of an avian virus oncogene (src) and proposed amino acid sequence for the gene product. Nature 287:198, 1980
44. Kitamura N, Kitamura A, Toyoshima Y et al: Avian sarcoma virus Y73 genome sequence and structural similarity of its transforming gene product to that of Rous sarcoma virus. Nature 247:205, 1982
45. Naharro G, Robbins KC, Reddy EP: Gene product of v-fgr onc: hybrid protein containing a portion of actin and a tyrosine-specific protein kinase. Science 223:63, 1984
46. Hampe A, Laprevotte J, Galibert F et al: Nucleotide sequences of feline retroviral oncogenes (v-fes) provide evidence for a family of tyrosine-specific protein kinase genes. Cell 30:775, 1982
47. Shibuya M, Hanafusa H: Nucleotide sequence of Fujinami sarcoma virus: evolutionary relationship of its transforming gene with transforming genes of other sarcoma viruses. Cell 30:787, 1982

48. Witte ON, Dasgupta A, Baltimore D: Abelson murine leukemia virus protein is phosphorylated in vitro to form phosphotyrosine. Nature 283:826, 1980

49. Jackson P, Baltimore D: N-Terminal mutations activate the leukemogenic potential of the myristoylated form of c-abl. EMBO J 8:449, 1989

50. Franz WM, Berger P, Wang JYJ: Deletion of an N-terminal regulatory domain of the c-abl tyrosine kinase activates its oncogenic potential. EMBO J 8:137, 1989

51. Van Etten RA, Jackson P, Baltimore D: The mouse type IV cabl gene product is a nuclear protein, and activation of transforming ability is associated with cytoplasmic localization. Cell 58:669, 1989

52. Kipreos ET, Wang JYJ: Cell cycle-regulated binding of cabl tyrosine kinase to DNA. Science 256:382, 1992

53. Boss MA, Dreyfus G, Baltimore D: Localization of the Abelson murine leukemia virus protein in a detergent-insoluble subcellular matrix: architecture of the protein. J Virol 40:472, 1981

54. Veillette A, Bookman MA, Horak EM et al: Signal transduction through the CD4 receptor involves the activation of the internal membrane tyrosine-protein kinase p56^{lck}. Nature 338:257, 1989

55. Kypta RM, Goldberg Y, Ulug ET et al: Association between the PDGF receptor and members of the src family of tyrosine kinases. Cell 62:481, 1990

56. Smith MR, DeGudicibus SJ, Smith MR: Requirement for c-ras proteins during viral oncogene transformation. Nature 320:540, 1986

57. Trahey M, McCormick F: A cytoplasmic protein stimulates normal N-ras p21 GTPase but does not affect oncogenic mutants. Science 238:542, 1987

58. Ellis C, Moran M, McCormick F et al: Phosphorylation of GAP and GAP-associated proteins by transforming and mitogenic protein tyrosine kinases. Nature 343:377, 1990

59. Kaplan DR, Whitman M, Schaffhausen B et al: Common elements in growth factor stimulation and oncogenic transformation: 85 kd phosphoprotein and phosphatidylinositol kinase activity. Cell 50:1021, 1987

60. Berridge MJ, Irvine RF: Inositol phosphates and cell signalling. Nature 341: 197, 1989

61. Sadowski I, Stone JC, Pawson T: A noncatalytic domain conserved among cytoplasmic tyrosine kinases modifies the kinase activity and transforming function of Fujinami sarcoma virus p130$^{gap-fps}$. Mol Cell Biol 6:4396, 1986

62. Koch CA, Anderson D, Moran MF et al: SH2 and SH3 domains: elements that control interactions of cytoplasmic signaling proteins. Science 252:668, 1991

63. Songyang Z, Shoelson SE, Chaudhuri M et al: SH2 domains recognize specific phosphopeptide sequences. Cell 72:767, 1993

64. Waksman G, Shoelson SE, Pant N et al: Binding of a high affinity phosphotyrosyl peptide to the src SH2 domain: crystal structures of the complexed and peptide-free forms. Cell 72:779, 1993

65. Cicchetti P, Mayer BJ, Thiel G, Baltimore D: Identification of a protein that binds to the SH3 region of Abl and is similar to Bcl and GAP-rho. Science 257:803, 1992

66. Duchesne M, Scheighoffer F, Parker F et al: Identification of the SH3 domain of GAP as an essential sequence for RAS-GAP-mediated signalling. Science 259:525, 1993

67. Lowenstein EJ, Daly RJ, Batzer AG et al: The SH2 and SH3 domain-containing protein GRB2 links receptor tyrosine kinases to ras signalling. Cell 70:431, 1992

68. Simon MA, Dodson GS, Rubin GM: An SH3-SH2-SH3 protein is required for p21^{ras1} activation and binds to sevenless and sos proteins in vitro. Cell 73: 169, 1993

69. Olivier JP, Raabe T, Henkemeyer M et al: A drosophila SH2-SH3 adaptor protein implicated in coupling the sevenless tyrosine kinase to an activator of ras guanine nucleotide exchange, sos. Cell 73:179, 1993

70. Mayer BJ, Hamaguchi M, Hanafusa H: A novel viral oncogene with structural similarity to phospholipase C. Nature 332:272, 1988

71. Katzav S, Martin-Zanca D, Barbacid M: vav, a novel human oncogene derived from a locus ubiquitously expressed in hematopoietic cells. EMBO J 8:2283, 1989

72. Shenoy S, Choi J-K, Bagrudia S et al: Purified maturation promoting factor phosphorylates pp60c-src at the sites phosphorylated during fibroblast mitosis. Cell 57:763, 1989

73. Morgan DO, Kaplan JM, Bishop JM, Varmus HE: Mitosis-specific phosphorylation of pp60^{c-src} by p34^{cdc2}-associated protein kinase. Cell 57:775, 1989

74. Draetta G, Piwnica-Worms H, Morrison D et al: Human cdc2 protein kinase is a major cell cycle regulated tyrosine kinase substrate. Nature 236:738, 1988

75. Chen YY, Rosenberg N: Lymphoid cells transformed by Abelson virus require the v-abl protein tyrosine kinase only during early G1. Proc Natl Acad Sci USA 89:6683, 1992

76. Van Bevern C, Galleshaw JA, Jonas V et al: Nucleotide sequence and formation of the transforming gene of a mouse sarcoma virus. Nature 289:258, 1981

77. Jansen HW, Lurz R, Bister K et al: Homologous cell-derived oncogenes in avian carcinoma virus MH2 and murine sarcoma virus 3611-MSV. Nature 307:281, 1984

78. Jansen HW, Patschinsky T, Bister K: Avian oncovirus MH2: molecular cloning of proviral DNA and structural analysis of viral RNA and protein. J Virol 48:61, 1983

79. Selten G, Cuypers HT, Boelens W et al: The primary structure of the putative oncogene pim1 shows extensive homology with protein kinases. Cell 46: 603, 1986

80. Roberts TM: Raf-1: a kinase currently without a cause but not lacking in effects. Cell 64:479, 1991

81. Bruder JT, Heidecker G, Rapp UR: Serum-, TPA, and Ras-induced expression from Ap-1/Ets-driven promoters requires Raf-1 kinase. Genes Dev 6:545, 1992

82. Wood KW, Sarnecki C, Roberts TM, Blenis J: ras mediates nerve growth factor modulation of three signal-transducing protein kinases: MAP kinase, Raf-1 and RSK. Cell 68:1041, 1992

83. Blair DG, Oskarsson M, Wood TG et al: Activation of the transforming potential of a normal cell sequence: a molecular model for oncogenesis. Science 212:941, 1981

84. Goldman DS, Kiessling AA, Millette CF, Cooper GM: Expression of c-mos RNA in germ cells of male and female mice. Proc Natl Acad Sci USA 84:4509, 1987

85. Sagata N, Daar I, Oskarsson M et al: The product of the mos proto-oncogene as a candidate "initiator" for oocyte maturation. Science 245:643, 1989

86. Sagata N, Watanabe N, Vande Woude GF, Ikawa Y: The c-mos proto-oncogene product is a cytostatic factor responsible for meiotic arrest in vertebrate eggs. Nature 342:512, 1989

87. Ellis RW, DeFeo D, Shih TY et al: The p21 src genes of Harvey and Kirsten viruses originate from divergent members of a family of normal vertebrate genes. Nature 292:506, 1981

88. DeFeo D, Gonda MA, Young HA et al: Analysis of two divergent rat genomic clones homologous to the transforming gene of Harvey murine sarcoma virus. Proc Natl Acad Sci USA 78:3328, 1981

89. Marshall C: Human oncogenes. p. 487. In Weiss R, Teich N, Varmus H, Coffin J (eds): RNA Tumor Viruses. Cold Spring Harbor Laboratory Press, Cold Spring Harbor, NY, 1985

90. Barbacid M: ras genes. Annu Rev Biochem 56:779, 1987

91. Thomas SM, DeMarco M, D'Arcangelo G et al: Ras is essential for nerve growth factor-and phorbol ester-induced tyrosine phosphorylation of MAP kinases. Cell 68:1031, 1992

92. Farnsworth CL, Marshall MS, Gibbs JB et al: Preferential inhibition of the oncogenic form of ras^{H} by mutations in the GAP binding/"effector" domain. Cell 64:625, 1991

93. Gibbs JB, Sigal IS, Poe M, Scolnick EM: Intrinsic GTPase activity distinguishes normal and oncogenic Ras p21 molecules. Proc Natl Acad Sci USA 81:5704, 1984

94. Walter M, Clark SG, Levinson AD: The oncogenic activation of human p21 ras by a novel mechanism. Science 233:649, 1986

95. Landis CA, Masters SB, Spada A et al: GTPase inhibiting mutations activate the alpha chain of G$_s$ and stimulate adenyl cyclase in human pituitary tumors. Nature 340:692, 1989

96. Lyons J, Landis CA, Harsh G et al: Two G protein oncogenes in human endocrine tumors. Science 249:655, 1990

97. Devare SG, Reddy EP, Robbins KC et al: Nucleotide sequence of the transforming gene of simian sarcoma virus. Proc Natl Acad Sci USA 79:3179, 1982

98. Moore R, Casey G, Brookes S et al: Sequence, topography and protein coding potential of mouse int-2: a putative oncogene activated by mouse mammary tumor virus. EMBO J 5:919, 1986

99. Taira M, Yoshida T, Miyagawa K et al: cDNA sequence of human transforming gene hst and identification of the coding sequence required for transforming activity. Proc Natl Acad Sci USA 84:2980, 1987

100. Doolittle RF, Hunkapiller MW, Hood LE et al: Simian sarcoma virus onc gene, v-sis is derived from the gene (or genes) encoding a platelet-derived growth factor. Science 221:275, 1983

101. Waterfield MD, Scrace GJ, Whittle N et al: Platelet-derived growth factor is structurally related to the putative transforming protein p28^{sis} of simian sarcoma virus. Nature 304:35, 1983

102. Dickson C, Gordon P: Potential oncogene related to growth factors. Nature 326:833, 1987

103. Bejeck BE, Li DY, Deuel TF: Transformation by v-sis occurs by an internal autoactivation mechanism. Science 245:1496, 1989

104. Dunbar CE, Browder TM, Abrams JS, Nienhuis AW: COOH-terminal-modified interleukin-3 is retained intracellularly and stimulates autocrine growth. Science 245:1493, 1989

105. Lewin B: Oncogenic conversion by regulatory changes in transcription factors. Cell 64:303, 1991

106. Gabrielsen OS, Sentenac A, Fromageot P: Specific DNA binding by c-Myb: evidence for a double helix-turn-helix-related motif. Science 253:1140, 1991

107. Barkas AE, Brodeur D, Stavnezer E: Polyproteins containing a domain encoded by the v-*ski* oncogene are located in the nuclei of SKV-transformed cells. Virology 151:131, 1986

108. Roussel M, Saule S, Lagrou C et al: Three new types of viral oncogenes of cellular origin specific for hematopoietic cell transformation. Nature 281:452, 1979

109. Maki Y, Bos TJ, Davis C et al: Avian sarcoma virus 17 carries the *jun* oncogene. Proc Natl Acad Sci USA 84:2848, 1987

110. Van Beveren C, van Straaten F, Curran T et al: Analysis of FBJ-MuSV provirus and c-*fos* (mouse) gene reveals that viral and cellular *fos* gene products have different carboxy termini. Cell 32:1241, 1983

111. Bister K, Hayman MJ, Vogt PK: Defectiveness of avian myelocytomatosis virus MC29: isolation of long-term nonproducer cultures and analysis of virus-specific polypeptide synthesis. Virology 82:431, 1977

112. Klempnauer K-H, Arnold H, Biedenkapp H: Activation of transcription by v-*myb*: evidence for two different mechanisms. Genes Dev 3:1582, 1989

113. Bos TJ, Monetclaro FS, Mitsunobu F et al: Efficient transformation of chicken embryo fibroblasts by c-Jun requires structural modification in coding and noncoding sequences. Genes Dev 4:1677, 1990

114. Bohmann D, Tjian R: Biochemical analysis of transcriptional activation by Jun: differential activity of c- and v-Jun. Cell 59:709, 1989

115. Bohmann D, Bos TJ, Admon A et al: Human proto-oncogene c-*jun* encodes a DNA binding protein with structural and functional properties of transcription factor AP-1. Science 238:1386, 1987

116. Bos TJ, Bohmann D, Tsichie H et al: v-*jun* encodes a nuclear protein with enhancer binding properties of AP-1. Cell 52:705, 1988

117. Rauscher FJ III, Cohen DR, Curran T et al: Fos-associated protein p39 is the product of the *jun* proto-oncogene. Science 240:1010, 1988

118. Shverman M, Neuberg M, Hunter JB et al: The leucine repeat motif in fos proteins mediates complex formation with jun/AP1 and is required for transformation. Cell 56:507, 1989

119. Sassone-Corsi P, Ransone LJ, Lamph WW, Verma IM: Direct interaction between fos and jun nuclear oncoproteins: role of the "leucine zipper" domain. Nature 336:692, 1988

120. Murre C, McCaw PS, Baltimore D: A new DNA binding and dimerization motif in immunoglobulin enhancer binding, *daughterless, MyoD* and *myc* proteins. Cell 56:777, 1989

121. Blackwood EM, Eisenman RN: Max: a helix-loop-helix zipper protein that forms a sequence-specific DNA binding complex with Myc. Science 251:1211, 1991

122. Amati B, Brooks MW, Levy N et al: Oncogenic activity of the c-myc protein requires dimerization with max. Cell 72:233, 1993

123. Zervos AS, Gyuris J, Brent R: Mxi1, a protein that specifically interacts with max to bind myc-max recognition sites. Cell 72:223, 1993

124. Ayer DE, Kretzner L, Eisenman RN: Mad: a heterodimeric partner for max that antagonizes myc transcriptional activity. Cell 72:211, 1993

125. Graf T, Beug H: Role of the v-*erbA* and v-*erbB* oncogenes of avian erythroblastosis virus in erythroid cell transformation. Cell 34:7, 1983

126. Weinberger C, Hollenberg SM, Rosenfeld MG, Evans RM: Domain structure of human glucocorticoid receptor and its relationship to the v-*erbA* oncogene product. Nature 318:670, 1985

127. Sap J, Munoz A, Damm K et al: The c-*erbA* protein is a high affinity receptor for thyroid hormone. Nature 324:635, 1986

128. Damm K, Thompson CC, Evans RM: Protein encoded by erbA functions as a thyroid hormone receptor antagonist. Nature 339:593, 1989

129. Cohen RS, Wong TL, Lai MMC: Characterization of transformation- and replication-specific sequences of reticuloendotheliosis virus. Virology 113:672, 1980

130. Kieran M, Blank V, Logeat et al: The DNA binding subunit of NK-κB is identical to factor KBF1 and homologous to the *rel* oncogene product. Cell 62:1007, 1990

131. Ghosh S, Gifford A, Riviere LR et al: Cloning of the p50 DNA binding subunit of NF-κB: homology to *rel* and *dorsal*. Cell 62:1019, 1990

132. Baeuerle PA, Baltimore D: IκB: a specific inhibotr of the NF-κB transcription factor. Science 242:540, 1988

133. Narayanan R, Klement JF, Ruben SM et al: Identification of a naturally occurring transforming variant of the p65 subunit of NF-κB. Science 256:367, 1992

134. Ohno H, Takimoto G, McKeithan T: The candidate proto-oncogene *bcl-3* is related to genes implicated in cell lineage determination and cell cycle control. Cell 60:991, 1990

135. Bours V, Franzoso G, Azarenko V et al: The oncoprotein bcl-3 directly transcactivates through κB motifs via association with DNA-binding p50B homodimers. Cell 72:729, 1993

136. Tabin CJ, Bradley SM, Bargmann CI et al: Mechanism of activation of a human oncogene. Nature 300:143, 1982

137. Reddy EP, Reynolds RK, Santos E et al: A point mutation is responsible for the acquisition of transforming properties by the T24 human bladder carcinoma oncogene. Nature 300:149, 1982

138. Farr CJ, Saiki RK, Erlich HA et al: Analysis of RAS gene mutations in acute myeloid leukemia by polymerase chain reaction and oligonucleotide probes. Proc Natl Acad Sci USA 85:1629, 1988

139. Noda M, Ko M, Ogura A et al: Sarcoma viruses carrying *ras* oncogenes induce differentiation-associated properties in a neuronal cell line. Nature 318:73, 1985

140. Yunis JJ, Boot AJM, Mayer MG, Bos JL: Mechanisms of *ras* mutation in myelodysplastic syndrome. Oncogene 4:609, 1989

141. Vogelstein B, Fearon ER, Hamilton SR et al: Genetic alterations during colorectal-tumor development. N Engl J Med 319:525, 1988

142. Balmain A, Pragnell IB: Mouse skin carcinomas induced in vivo by chemical carcinogens have a transforming Harvey-*ras* oncogene. Nature 303:72, 1983

143. Sinn E, Muller W, Pattengale P et al: Coexpression of MMTV/v-Ha-ras and MMTV/c-myc genes in transgenic mice: synergistic action of oncogenes in vitro. Cell 49:465, 1987

144. Numberg JH, Kaufman RJ, Schimke RT et al: Amplified dihydrofolate reductase genes are localized to a homogeneously staining region of a single chromosome in a methotrexate-resistant Chinese hamster ovary cell line. Proc Natl Acad Sci USA 75:5553, 1978

145. Dalla-Favera R, Wong-Staal F, Gallo RC: Onc gene amplification in promyelocytic leukemia cell line HL-60 and primary leukemic cells of the same patient. Nature 299:61, 1982

146. Alitalo K, Schwab M: Oncogene amplification in tumor cells. Adv Cancer Res 47:235, 1986

147. Krystal G, Birrer M, Way J et al: Multiple mechanisms for transcriptional regulation of the *myc* gene family in small cell lung cancer. Mol Cell Biol 8:3373, 1988

148. Brodeur G, Seeger C, Schwab M et al: Amplification of N-myc in untreated human neuroblastomas correlates with advanced disease and stage. Science 224:1121, 1984

149. Slamon DJ, Clark GM, Wong SG et al: Human breast cancer: correlation of relapse and survival with amplification of the HER-2/*neu* oncogene. Science 235:177, 1987

150. Dalla-Favera R, Brogni M, Erikson J et al: Human c-myc oncogene is located on the region of chromosome 8 that is translocated in Burkitt lymphoma cells. Proc Natl Acad Sci USA 79:7824, 1982

151. Taub R, Kirsch I, Morton C et al: Translocation of the c-*myc* gene into the immunoglobulin heavy chain locus in human Burkitt lymphoma and murine plasmacytoma cells. Proc Natl Acad Sci USA 79:7837, 1982

152. Shen-Ong GLC, Keath EJ, Piccoli SP, Cole MD: Novel *myc* oncogene RNA from abortive immunoglobulin-gene recombination in mouse plasmacytomas. Cell 31:443, 1982

153. Showe LC, Croce CM: The role of chromosomal translocations in B- and T-cell neoplasia. Annu Rev Immunol 5:253, 1987

154. Tsujimoto Y, Finger LR, Yunis J et al: Cloning of the chromosome breakpoint of neoplastic B cells with the t(14;18) chromosome translocation. Science 226:1097, 1984

155. Hockenberry D, Nunez G, Milliman C et al: bcl-2 is an inner mitochondrial membrane protein that blocks programmed cell death. Nature 348:334, 1990

156. Franzoso G, Bours V, Park S et al: The candidate oncoprotein bcl-3 is an antagonist of p50/NF-kappa B-mediated inhibition. Nature 359:339, 1992

157. De Klein A, Guerts van Kessel A, Grosveld G et al: A cellular oncogene is translocated to the Philadelphia chromosome in chronic myeloid leukemia. Nature 300:765, 1982

158. Konopka JB, Watanabe SM, Witte ON: An alteration of the human c-*abl* protein in K562 unmasks associated tyrosine kinase activity. Cell 37:1035, 1984

159. Kamps MP, Baltimore D: E2A-Pbx1, the t(1,19) translocation protein of human pre-B-cell acute lymphocytic leukemia, causes acute myeloid leukemia in mice. Mol Cell Biol 13:351, 1993

160. Kakizuka A, Miller WH Jr, Umesono K et al: Chromosomal translocation t(15;17) in human acute promyelocytic leukemia fuses RAR alpha with a novel putative transcription factor, PML. Cell 66:663, 1991

161. Knudson AG: Mutation and cancer: statistical study of retinoblastoma. Proc Natl Acad Sci USA 68:820, 1971

162. Franke U, Kung F: Sporadic bilateral retinoblastoma and 13q- chromosomal deletions. Med Pediatr Oncol 2:379, 1976

163. Cavenee WK, Dryja TP, Phillips RA et al: Expression of recessive alleles by chromosomal mechanisms in retinoblastoma. Nature 290:261, 1983

164. Lee W-H, Bookstein R, Hong F et al: Human retinoblastoma susceptibility gene: cloning, identification and sequence. Science 235:1394, 1987

165. Friend SH, Bernards R, Rogelj S et al: A human DNA fragment with properties

of the gene that predisposes to retinoblastoma and osteosarcoma. Nature 323:643, 1986

166. Huang H-JS, Yee J-K, Shew J-Y et al: Suppression of the neoplastic phenotype by replacement of the RB gene in human cancer cells. Science 242:1563, 1988

167. Buchkovich K, Duffy LA, Harlow E: The retinoblastoma protein is phosphorylated during specific phases of the cell cycle. Cell 58:1097, 1989

168. Chen P-L, Scully P, Shew J-Y et al: Phosphorylation of the retinoblastoma gene product is modulated during the cell cycle and cellular differentiation. Cell 58:1193, 1989

169. DeCaprio JA, Ludlow JW, Figge J et al: SV40 large T antigen forms a specific complex with the product of the retinoblastoma susceptibility gene. Cell 54:275, 1988

170. Dyson N, Buchkovich K, Whyte P, Harlow E: The cellular 107K protein that binds to adenovirus E1A also associates with the large T antigens of SV40 and JC virus. Cell 58:249, 1989

171. Linzer DI, Levine AJ: Characterization of a 54K dalton cellular SV40 tumor antigen present in SV40-transformed cells and uninfected embryonal carcinoma cells. Cell 17:43, 1979

172. Hollstein M, Sidransky D, Vogelstein B, Harris C: p53 mutations in human cancer. Science 253:49, 1991

173. Malkin D, Li FP, Strong LC et al: Germ line p53 mutations in a familial syndrome of breast cancer, sarcomas, and other neoplasms. Science 250:1233, 1990

174. Kern SE, Kinzler KW, Bruskin A et al: Identification of p53 as a sequence-specific DNA-binding protein. Science 252:1708, 1991

175. Baker SJ, Markowitz S, Fearon ER et al: Suppression of human colorectal carcinoma cell growth by wild-type p53. Science 249:912, 1990

176. Kuerbitz SJ, Plunkett BS, Walsh WV, Kastan MB: Wild-type p53 is a cell cycle checkpoint determinant following irradiation. Proc Natl Acad Sci USA 89: 7491, 1992

177. Larsson C, Skogseid B, Nakamura Y, Nordenskjold M: Multiple endocrine neoplasia type 1 gene maps to chromosome 11 and is lost in insulinoma. Nature 332:85, 1988

178. Simpson NE, Kidd KK, Goodfellow PJ et al: Assignment of multiple endocrine neoplasia type 2A to chromosome 10 by linkage. Nature 328:528, 1987

179. Bodmer WF, Bailey CJ, Bodmer J et al: Localization of the gene for familial adenomatous polyposis on chromosome 5. Nature 328:614, 1987

180. Seizinger BR, Rouleau GA, Ozelius LJ et al: Genetic linkage of von Recklinghausen neurofibromatosis to the nerve growth factor gene. Cell 49:589, 1987

181. Rouleau GA, Haines JL, Bazanowski A et al: A genetic linkage map of the long arm of human chromosome 22. Genomics 4:1, 1989

182. Koufos A, Hansen MF, Lampkin BC et al: Loss of alleles at loci on human chromosome 11 during genesis of Wilm's tumor. Nature 309:170, 1984

183. Haber DA, Buckler AJ, Glaser T et al: An internal deletion within an 11p13 zinc finger gene contributes to the development of Wilms' tumor. Cell 61: 1257, 1990

184. Xu GF, OConnell P, Viskochil D et al: The neurofibromatosis type 1 gene encodes a protein related to GAP. Cell 62:599, 1990

185. Miyoshi Y, Ando H, Nagase H et al: Germ-line mutations of the APC gene in 53 familial adenomatous polyposis patients. Med Sci 89:4452, 1992

186. Chen LC, Dollbaum C, Smith HS: Loss of heterozygosity on chromosome 1q in human breast cancer. Proc Natl Acad Sci USA 86:7204, 1989

187. Mori N, Yokota J, Oshimura M et al: Concordant deletions of chromosome 3p and loss of heterozygosity for chromosomes 13 and 17 in small cell lung cancer. Cancer Res 49:5130, 1989

188. Vogelstein B, Fearon ER, Kern SE et al: Allelotype of colorectal carcinomas. Science 244:207, 1989

189. Motomura K, Nishisho I, Takai S et al: Loss of alleles on chromosome 13 in human primary gastric cancers. Genomics 2:180, 1988

190. Zbar B, Brauch H, Talmadge C, Lineham M: Loss of all loci on the short arm of chromosome 3 in renal cell cancer. Nature 327:721, 1987

191. Solomon E, Voss R, Hall V et al: Chromosome 5 allele loss in human colorectal carcinomas. Nature 328:616, 1987

192. Powell SM, Zilz N, Beazer-Barclay Y et al: APC mutations occur early during colorectal tumorigenesis. Nature 359:235, 1992

193. Weinberg RA: Oncogenes, anti-oncogenes and the molecular bases of multistep carcinogenesis. Cancer Res 49:3713, 1989

194. Land H, Parada LF, Weinberg RA: Tumorigenic conversion of primary embryo fibroblasts requires at least two cooperating oncogenes. Nature 304: 596, 1983

195. Ruley HE: Adenovirus early region 1A enables viral and cellular transforming genes to transform primary cells in culture. Nature 304:602, 1983

196. Thompson TC, Southgate J, Kitchener G, Land H: Multistage carcinogenesis induced by *ras* and *myc* oncogenes in reconstituted organ. Cell 56:917, 1989

197. Stanbridge EJ: Genetic analysis of human malignancy using somatic cell hybrids and monochromosome transfer. Cancer Surv 7:317, 1988

198. Vogelstein B. Fearon ER, Hamilton SR et al: Genetic alterations during colorectal-tumor development. N Engl J Med 319:525, 1988

Pharmacology of Antineoplastic Agents, Multidrug Resistance, and the Future

61

Sridhar Mani, Antonio C. Buzaid, and Edwin C. Cadman

INTRODUCTION

The vesicant properties of sulfur mustard have been known for >100 years. It was only in 1919, however, that Krumbhaar and Krumbhaar observed that poisoning by sulfur mustard produces leukopenia, aplasia of the bone marrow, marked decrease in lymphoid tissue, and ulceration of the gastrointestinal tract. These findings prompted Goodman and associates to test whether nitrogen mustard could be used therapeutically.[1] Following successful animal studies, clinical trials were launched in 1942 that ushered in the modern era of chemotherapy. In 1948, methotrexate became available, which led Hertz and colleagues[2] to demonstrate cure of metastatic choriocarcinoma with this single agent. Shortly thereafter, 5-fluorouracil was synthesized. During the 1960s, investigation of certain medicinal plants resulted in the development of the vinca alkaloids and podophyllotoxin derivatives. Late in that decade, DeVita[3] showed that combinations of chemotherapeutic drugs produce better results than can be achieved with single-agent therapy. Since then, the incorporation of daunorubicin, doxorubicin, and cytosine arabinoside in the oncologic armamentarium has resulted in a significant impact in the curability of non-Hodgkin lymphomas and acute leukemias. Importantly, a quarter of century after the discovery of methotrexate's activity in choriocarcinoma, cisplatin was demonstrated to have equal specificity against germ cell tumors. Clinical trials have since produced a number of useful chemotherapeutic regimens.

This chapter reviews the pharmacology of antineoplastic drugs, with special focus on the cytotoxic agents employed in the treatment of hematologic malignancies. In addition, it provides an overview of their mechanisms of action as well as potential strategies designed to overcome drug resistance.

CELLULAR KINETICS AND TUMOR GROWTH

The key to cancer therapeutics lies in understanding the differential regulation of cell growth and proliferation between normal and neoplastic cells. Tumor growth is closely related to tumor cell kill with therapy, which in turn is a complex function of rate of cell division and cell loss. Initial studies conducted by Skipper[4] in L1210 tumor cells demonstrated two principles of tumor cell kinetics: (1) cell doubling time is tumor specific and forms a straight line on a semilog plot; and (2) drug-induced cell kill follows first-order kinetics, in that a fixed percentage of cells are killed, regardless of tumor burden. These principles had limited applicability because the L1210 mouse leukemia cells are all actively dividing in logarithmic phase of growth. Most neoplasms do not follow this pattern of growth. At any given time, only a portion of the cells in a tumor are actively dividing; this subset of cells is called the growth fraction. When a malignancy arises, most of the tumor cells are dividing, and the growth fraction is high. As the tumor grows, a larger proportion of the cells become inactive and assume a resting state. The decline in growth fraction may be due to restrictions of space, nutrient availability, and blood supply. This pattern of growth does not follow a classic exponential growth curve and is best described by the Gompertz equation. The growth fraction depends on the type of tumor with values ranging from <10% for some adenocarcinomas to >90% for some lymphomas.[5] This concept is crucial, as most chemotherapeutic agents are more effective against dividing cells than against resting cells.

A schematic presentation of the events that occur during the cell cycle is shown in Figure 61-1. In the past, classic autoradiographic techniques designed to study cytokinetics included stathmokinetic techniques of measuring mitotic index and radioactive thymidine incorporation. The latter technique permitted investigators to determine accurately the percentage of cells in S phase. A further refinement of this technique yielded a percentage of labeled mitoses curve, which determined the percentage of cells in M phase. Today, DNA and RNA flow cytometry has largely replaced these labor-intensive procedures. Flow cytometry evaluates changes in DNA and RNA content during the various phases of the cell cycle. One major limitation of the technique is that it is unable to distinguish normal from neoplastic cells. Meticulous technique and controls are required. Despite these disadvantages, flow cytometry is applicable to the study of solid tumors, cells in fluid suspension, leukemias, and paraffin-embedded specimens.[6,7]

Measurement of DNA is the primary goal of flow cytometry. The clinically useful indices measured include percentage of S-phase fraction and DNA ploidy. The percentage of S-phase fraction is defined as the percentage of cells having a DNA content of 2–4N. In most human tumors, at any point of time, approximately 2–25% of cells are in S phase. This correlates well with a growth fraction of 4–80%. Diploid DNA (2N) is found in cells in G_0–G_1 phase; tetraploid DNA (4N) is found in cells in G_2–M phase; aneuploid reflects abnormal DNA content (N) in cells in G_0–G_1 phase. The DNA index is a ratio of cellular DNA content of neoplastic cells in G_0–G_1 to normal diploid cells in G_0–G_1. DNA indices >1.1 or <0.9 are abnormal.[7,8]

Cytokinetic studies of human tumors have produced interesting clinical correlates. For example, in node-negative breast cancer, a high percentage S-phase fraction is predictive of a high relapse rate.[9] In childhood acute lymphocytic leukemia (ALL), multivariate analysis demonstrates that the presence of hyperdiploid blasts is predictive of an improved response to chemotherapy.[10] Proliferation rates or cell cycle time (Tc) become important and meaningful when applied to outcome measures of S-phase-specific drugs. In acute leukemia, for example, several interesting correlates arise. First, pretherapy proliferative rate (Tc) is an independent prognostic variable for induction remission duration in newly diagnosed cases of adult acute myeloid leukemia (AML).[11] Second, the extent of S-phase-specific cytotoxic therapy cell kill is a direct but complex function of the proliferative rate. The faster the initial proliferative rate, the larger the number of cells in S phase, and the larger the final fraction of cells killed. At the completion of therapy, the rate of relapse will depend to a large extent on the individual proliferative rates of the remaining leukemic cells untouched by therapy.[12] Finally, during chemotherapy there seems to be a direct correlation between extent of leukemic cell differentiation and slow proliferative rates.[13]

TUMOR HETEROGENEITY

Cancer has been shown to be a clonal disease (i.e., the cancer cells descend from a single progenitor cell). However, as cancers progress they become markedly heterogeneous. Within a single tumor this heterogeneity is expressed as variations in histopathology, cytogenetics, expression of surface antigens, growth rate, metastatic potential, and, more importantly, sensitivity to cytotoxic agents. The major factor responsible for this heterogeneity is spontaneous mutation. Tumors are also heterogeneous in their supply of nutrients and oxygen, factors that may further increase their genetic instability.[14,15] The overall growth of a tumor is dictated by the number of cell doublings, its growth fraction, and the death rate of the cancer cells. For example, in a given tumor (Fig. 61-2A) for which a constant mutation rate and a death rate of zero are assumed, the higher the number of cell doublings, the larger the tumor, the larger the number of mutations, and thus the higher the chance of having chemotherapy-resistant clones. If a constant mutation rate is assumed in a tumor with a high death rate (Fig. 61-2B), many more cell doublings and therefore many more mutations must occur for the tumor to reach the same size.[16] The latter situation applies to tumors that are slow growing, apparently because the rate of cell loss is high. Thus, by the time these slow-growing tumors are clinically detectable, they have already undergone multiple mutations and consist of a large number of cells that are resistant to virtually all available anti-

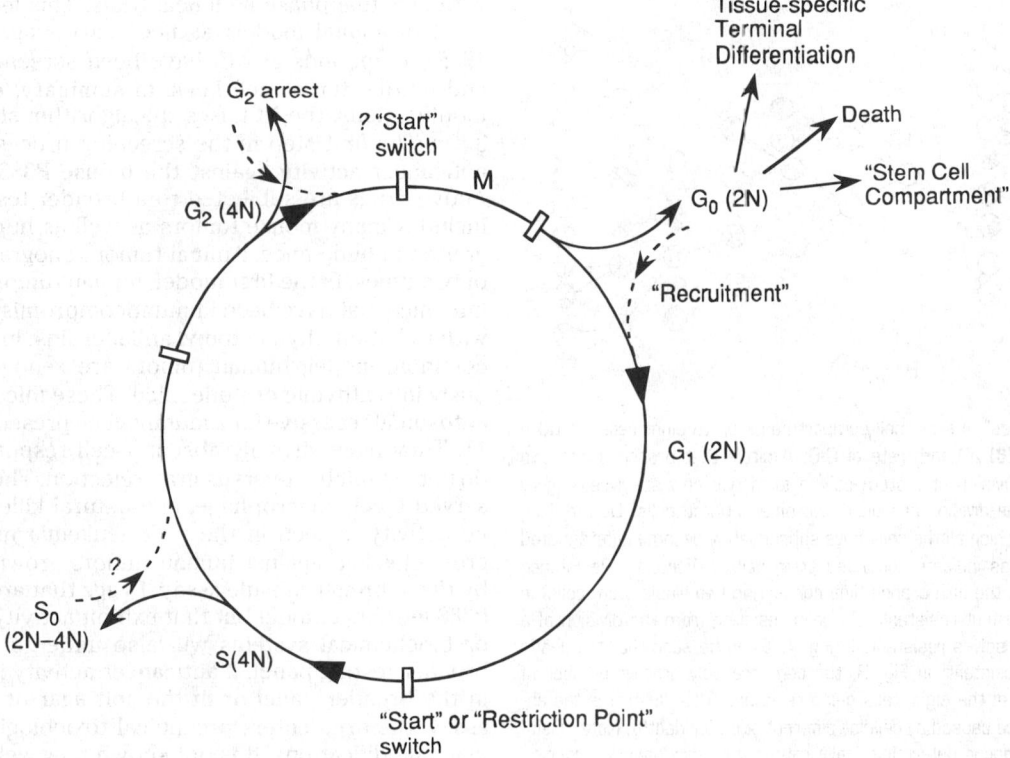

Fig. 61-1. Phases of the cell cycle. G_0 or gap time zero is the resting phase (nonproliferation of cells). There is no intention of entering into DNA synthesis. G_0 cells are small, possess low levels of RNA/protein, the Ki67 antigen is absent, and there is presumed diminution of mitochondrial activity. The cell cycle length is variable and the DNA content is diploid (2N). Cells may undergo terminal differentiation (e.g., neurons), enter the stem cell compartment, or die. Under appropriate external stimuli, G_0 cells may be recruited to enter G_1 phase, which signals a commitment to DNA synthesis. The point at which cells actively enter the S phase is variably known as "start" or "restriction point" and is thought to be regulated by a serine (threonine) kinase p34^{cdc2}. At this point, p34^{cdc2} is phosphorylated, and it interacts with newly synthesized cyclins during the S–G_2 phase to yield an inactive M-phase promoting factor complex (MFP). Cyclins are transient proteins that oscillate during the cell cycle. They are destroyed by cellular proteases at the end of M phase under the influence of cellular calcium concentrations. The pre-DNA synthetic phase or G_1 lasts 12 hours to few days. The S phase usually lasts 12–24 hours with DNA content increasing to 4N. Few cells may develop an intrinsic block to further replication of its DNA and enter S_0 phase. Subsequent events during this phase of cell cycle are unclear. In the G_2 phase (usually lasting 2–4 hours), cells are tetraploid. Rarely, cells enter into growth arrest and do not proceed to M phase (G_2 arrest phase). At a predetermined point, the inactive MFP complex undergoes dephosphorylation and subsequent activation that triggers entry into M phase. The released dephosphorylated p34^{cdc2} is then ready to enter another cycle with the help of as yet unidentified protein kinases. The cyclins are destroyed in G_1 and resynthesis occurs when the cell enters the S phase. In M phase, cells go through prophase, metaphase, anaphase, and telophase and detailed intracellular events have been well described. This phase usually lasts 1–2 hours. It is important to note that the entire duration of cell cycle (Tc) is quite variable, depending on the system being studied (i.e., in vivo, in vitro, normal versus neoplastic). Generally, Tc varies at 0.5–10 days in human cancers.

cancer agents. Consequently, current chemotherapy is seldom successful in patients with this type of condition.

An extension of the original Delbruck-Luria model of emergence of drug resistance, the mathematical model designed by Goldie and Coldman[16] permits the development of a better intuitive understanding of the events that occur during the treatment of cancer. This model substantiates the concept of dose intensity developed by Hryniuk and Bush[17] and also validates the importance of employing multiple cytotoxic drugs instead of single drugs to decrease the development of resistance. For example, the Goldie-Coldman model predicts that a single drug-sensitive clone is capable of being cured 90% of the time at cell volumes of 10^5. Hence, $<10^5$ cells should be completely cured by single agents. Larger tumors will not be cured. Stated differently, let us assume that a 1-cm tumor with 10^{10} cells has a spontaneous mutation rate toward drug resistance at 10^{-5}. This means that 1 cell out of every 10^5 cells will be drug resistant. In 10^{10} cells, 2 cells will be resistant. If the same drug resistance rate were to apply to another drug, the combination of two drugs would result in a spontaneous mutation rate toward resistance of $10^{-5} \times 10^{-5} = 10^{-10}$. Hence, only one cell would be resistant to this combination regimen. Eventually, enough agents may be added to completely nullify the effects of drug resistance, making intensive early combination chemotherapy the best defense. This hypothesis has also resulted in the use of alternating non-cross-resistant regimens. This approach has recently gained wide popularity. However, since most available chemotherapy regimens are at best only partially non-cross-resistant, such as MOPP (mechlorethamine, vincristine [Oncovin], procarbazine, and prednisone) alternating with ABVD (doxorubicin [Adriamycin], bleomycin, vinblastine, and dacarbazine), the therapeutic value of this strategy has not been properly tested.

DEVELOPMENT OF CHEMOTHERAPEUTIC AGENTS

Chemotherapeutic agents may be developed (1) by synthetic procedures using new biochemical and pharmacologic concepts and structure/activity relationships; (2) from natural

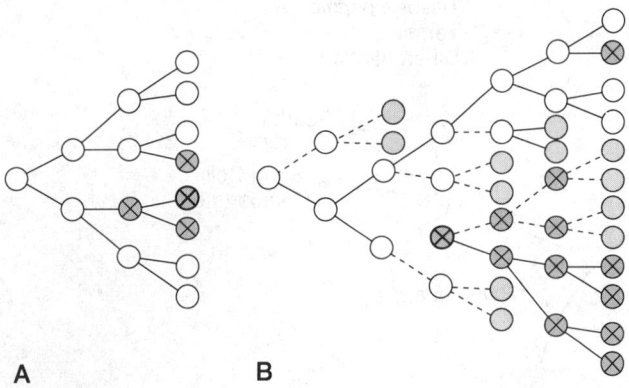

Fig. 61-2. "Growth trees" of stem cell compartments up to eight cells for **(A)** a death rate of 0, and **(B)** a death rate of 0.6. A circle that branches into two circles indicates the division of a stem cell to form two new stem cells; gray circles indicate that the division produced two differentiated cells. Dotted lines indicate ancestries in which all the cells have subsequently become differentiated (or died), and solid lines indicate continued stem cell proliferation. Resistance (pink circles) occurs at the fifth branch (line connecting two viable stem cells) in cells that are sensitive (not resistant). All cells resulting from the division of a resistant cell are themselves resistant. In Fig. A it can be seen that this leads to three cells being resistant; in Fig. B, the comparatively greater number of branches leads to five of the eight cells being resistant. This illustrates the enhancement of resistance caused by cellular differentiation (or death). Note: resistance is assumed to occur deterministically rather than randomly in order to simplify illustration, but it would not be expected to do so in reality. (Modified from Goldie and Coldman,[16] with permission.)

sources (e.g., plant extracts, microbial fermentation, and marine organisms); and (3) by examining new synthetic compounds made for other purposes. Since only a small fraction of the large number of compounds screened become clinically useful, the National Cancer Institute (NCI) has developed a decision analysis program to include initial screening, animal toxicity studies, drug formulation, and finally, clinical phase trials.

Screening for Antitumor Activity

The concept of screening agents for antitumor activity is based on the rationale that an appropriate bioassay may reliably indicate activity against human cancers. Since the mid-1940s, the NCI made major efforts toward drug discovery and development. In 1955, murine leukemia models P388 and L1210 were made available to test potentially new compounds.[18] During the mid- to late 1970s, the NCI developed the Drug Information System, which catalogued the structure and activity of all tested compounds. The generalization of efficacy was limited because compounds were initially tested only in leukemia models with high growth fractions. In order to circumvent this problem, a broader testing panel was instituted. This included a program of Rational Drug Screening (1975) with the availability of new rodent models (including transplantable murine tumors such as melanoma, lung, colon, and breast). Later, athymic or nude mice were used to screen compounds against transplantable human tumors or xenografts (e.g., lung, breast, colon). This resulted in a two-tier testing program, with the P388/L1210 murine leukemia model representing stage I and solid tumor animal models stage II screen. The limitations of this approach included high overall cost and the significantly poor correlation of preclinical tumor-specific screen activity

with eventual phase II clinical trials. This led to the abandonment of animal models as necessary stage II screens; since 1985, compounds at NCI have been screened against human and murine tumor cell lines. In summary, despite individual modifications, the NCI uses the algorithm shown in Figure 61-3.[18,19] The first step in the screening process is evaluation of anticancer activity against the mouse P388 leukemia model. Active drugs are subjected to a broader testing panel, which includes many mouse tumors as well as human tumors xenografted in nude mice. Animal tumor xenografts are essentially of two types. In the first model, human tumors are xenografted into mice that have been immunocompromised after treatment with radiation, thymectomy, and steroids. In the second, more common, model, human tumors are xenografted subcutaneously into athymic or nude mice. These mice are homozygous autosomal recessive for a mutant gene present on chromosome 11. They have virtually absent T-cell response and therefore do not exhibit host-versus-graft rejection. They do possess preserved B-cell, macrophage, and natural killer cell activity.[20] If no activity is seen in the P388 leukemia model, the drug is cross-checked against human tumors grown in soft agar and by the subrenal capsule assay. Drugs that are not active in the P388 leukemia model but that exhibit activity in other biologic or biochemical systems will also undergo evaluation in the broader testing panel. If anticancer activity is observed either in the broader panel or in the soft agar or subrenal capsule assay, the drug enters preclinical toxicologic testing. Despite many modifications, it is not known how well this current system identifies potentially active antineoplastic agents.

Animal Toxicity Studies

Once compounds have passed at least in vivo drug screens, toxicologic studies are performed in animals. Generally, two or more species are tested. Although there is no perfect correlation between doses toxic to animals and those toxic to humans, lethal doses seem to correlate well when averaged over two or more species. The common measures, LD_{50} and LD_{10} signify the dose that is lethal to 50% and 10% of animals tested, respectively. The NCI currently uses severe reversible toxicity or the maximum tolerated dose (MTD) as its end point. Concomitantly, pharmacokinetic measurements are performed in different animal species with the goal of eventually formulating a dosing schedule for human trials. Generally, the initial dose used in human phase I trials is calculated as a small fraction of the smallest dose that will cause reversible toxicity or as a fraction of LD_{10}.[18,19]

Clinical Trials

After extensive toxicologic and formulation studies, the new drug usually enters clinical trials in humans, divided into four phases. Phase I trials are designed to determine the toxicity profile, the MTD, and pharmacologic data; the determination of anticancer activity is a secondary goal. Patients with refractory cancers who are not bedridden and who are able to carry out the activities of daily living for most of the day are candidates for phase I trials. These patients must have normal hepatic, renal, and bone marrow function. They should not be receiving concomitant chemotherapy or radiotherapy. The initial dose employed is usually 10% of the lethal dose (LD_{10}) found in rodents during the preclinical studies. This dose is progressively escalated, generally according to a modified Fibonacci scale (Table 61-1). At least three patients are usually enrolled, and

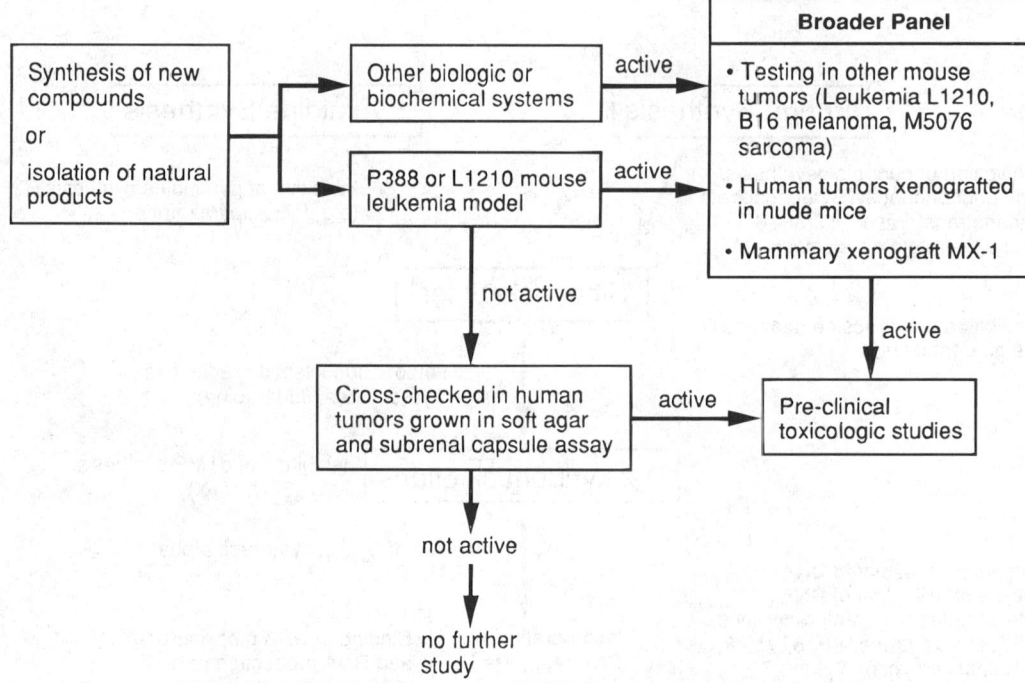

Fig. 61-3. Algorithm used for drug screening at the NCI.

toxicity is evaluated at each dose level. When a predefined fraction of patients experience overt but reversible toxicity, that particular dose is defined as the MTD. Therefore, each schedule of dosing has its own MTD; once the MTD and toxicity profile are determined, the drug enters phase II studies. Generally, the initial dose for phase II studies is 10–25% less than the MTD for that particular schedule. Phase II studies are designed primarily to determine the efficacy of the new compound in different types of cancer, generally the 7–10 most common ones. A secondary aim is to achieve a cleaner definition of human toxicity and dosing. Eligibility differs from the phase I studies in that patients accrued into phase II trials have more stringent guidelines concerning prior chemotherapy, entry performance status, and evidence for measurable disease. An important consideration in designing phase II trials is to accrue enough patients to accept or reject the null hypothesis with confidence. Statistical evaluation depends not only on the number of patients but also on the level of activity of the drug. For example, in lymphomas, assessing activity at <50% is of little value, since known single agents produce responses of >50%. Therefore, the new drug would be of interest only if it were to show response rates of ≥50%. Response is strictly defined as complete response (CR), partial response (PR), or progressive disease (PD). CR is defined as a complete absence of disease evaluated ≥4 weeks after treatment. PR is defined

as ≥50% reduction of the largest evaluable tumor mass measured in its two greatest diameters. PD is defined as the appearance of new lesions after treatment and/or a ≥25% increase of the largest evaluable tumor mass measured in its two greatest diameters. Phase III trials generally compare the efficacy of the new drug in a randomized fashion with the existing "standard therapy." Because differences in treatment efficacy between the randomized groups are small, large patient numbers are generally required through cooperative groups. In phase IV trials, usually conducted after the drug has been marketed, the drug is combined with other treatment modalities (e.g., radiation and/or surgery) and compared in a randomized study with the standard therapy.[19,21]

PHARMACOLOGY OF CHEMOTHERAPEUTIC AGENTS

Cytotoxic agents can be divided into phase-specific and phase-nonspecific, according to their predominant effect on the cell cycle.

1. *Phase-nonspecific agents* are effective in any phase of the cell cycle. Agents that fall into this category usually have a linear dose-response curve (i.e., the greater the dose administered, the greater the fraction of cell kill). They are divided into two subgroups:
   a. *Cycle-specific agents* kill cells that are proceeding through the cell cycle independent of whether the cell is in G_1, G_2, S, or M phase (e.g., alkylating agents, cisplatin)
   b. *Cycle-nonspecific agents* kill nondividing cells (e.g., steroids and antitumor antibiotics, except bleomycin)
2. *Phase-specific agents* are effective only if present during a certain phase of the cell cycle. Within a certain dose range agents in this category show no increase in cell kill with further increase in dose. If the drug is maintained over a period of time, however, more cells will enter the specific lethal phase of the cycle and be killed. Examples include L-asparaginase (G_1 phase), antimetabolites (S phase), and vinca alkaloids (M phase)

Table 61-1. Modified Fibonacci Dose Escalation Scheme Used in Phase I Trials

Drug Dose (mg/m²)	Percentage of Increment above Prior Dose Level
n	(Initial dose level)
2n	100
3.3n	65
5n	51
7n	40
9n	28
12n	33
16n	33

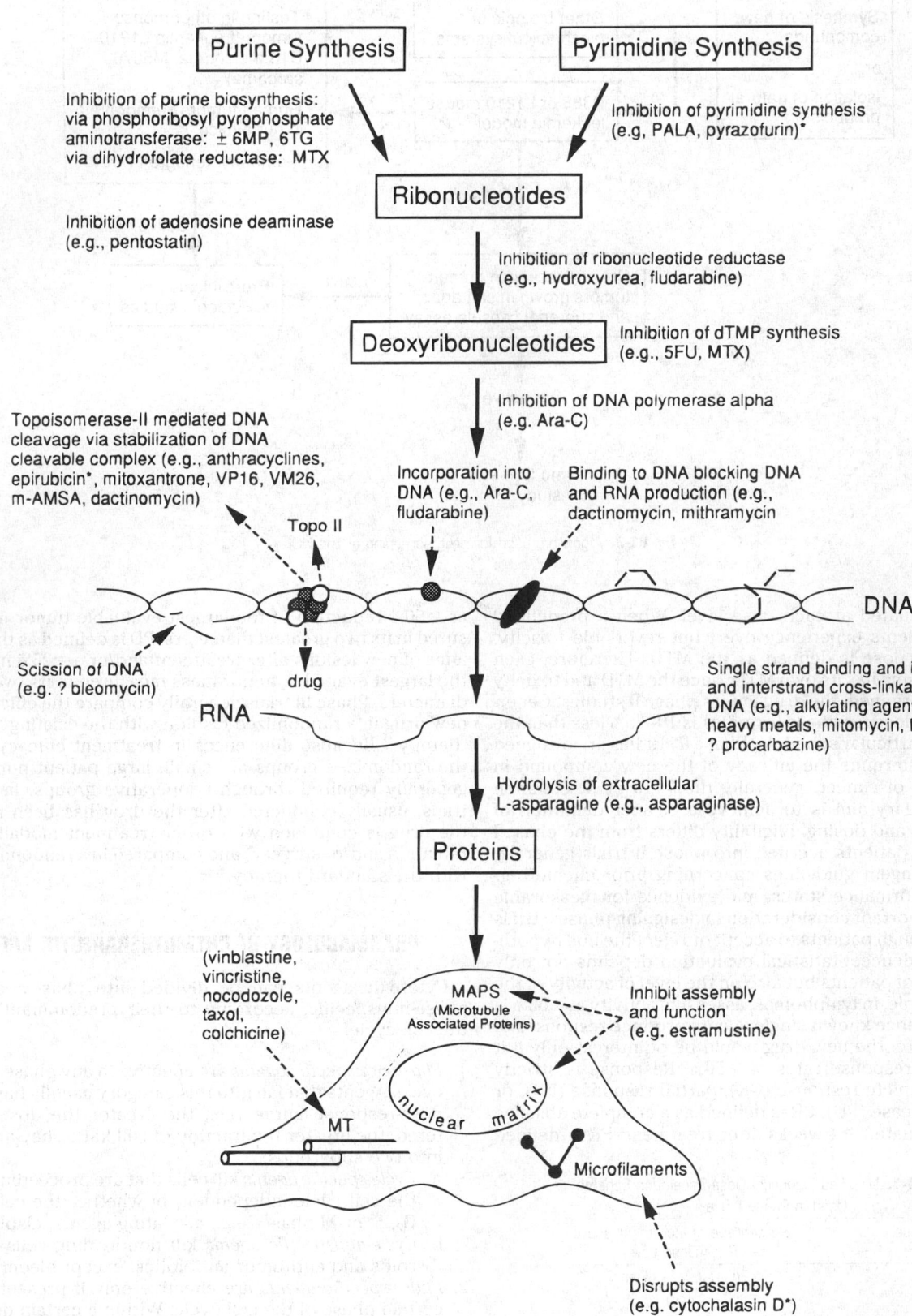

Fig. 61-4. Overview of sites and mechanism of action of the most useful chemotherapeutic agents.

Chemotherapeutic agents are not completely specific and affect normal as well as neoplastic cells. This effect is most pronounced with rapidly proliferating cells, such as the mucosa of the gastrointestinal tract and the bone marrow. This limits dose escalation and usually determines the MTD. Cytotoxic agents have been classically divided into alkylating agents, plant alkaloids, antitumor antibiotics, antimetabolites, and a miscellaneous group. The current number is >40 standard (i.e., commercially available) chemotherapeutic agents. The pharmacology and cellular mechanisms of those agents used in the treatment of hematologic malignancies are schematically presented in Figure 61-4.

Alkylating Agents

Alkylating agents contain alkyl groups that bond covalently with nucleophilic substances of the DNA and/or proteins associated with the DNA. On the basis of their chemical structure, the alkylating agents are divided into the five groups shown in Table 61-2.

The cytotoxic as well as the mutagenic effects of the alkylating agents are directly related to the alkylation and disruption of DNA. Figure 61-5 shows the various mechanisms by which mechlorethamine (nitrogen mustard) can alkylate the DNA. While mechlorethamine illustrates the effects of the alkylating agents on the DNA, the same basic mechanisms apply to the other alkylating agents. N-7 in guanine is particularly suscepti-

Table 61-2. Alkylating Agents

Nitrogen mustards
  Mechlorethamine
  Cyclophosphamide
  Ifosfamide
  Chlorambucil
  Melphalan
Ethylenimines
  Thiotepa
  Hexamethylmelamine
Alkylsulfonates
  Busulfan
Nitrosoureas
  Carmustine (BCNU)
  Lomustine (CCNU)
  Semustine (methyl/CCNU)
  Chlorozotocin
  Streptozocin
Triazines
  Dacarbazine (DTIC)
  Procarbazine
Others
  Mitomicin C

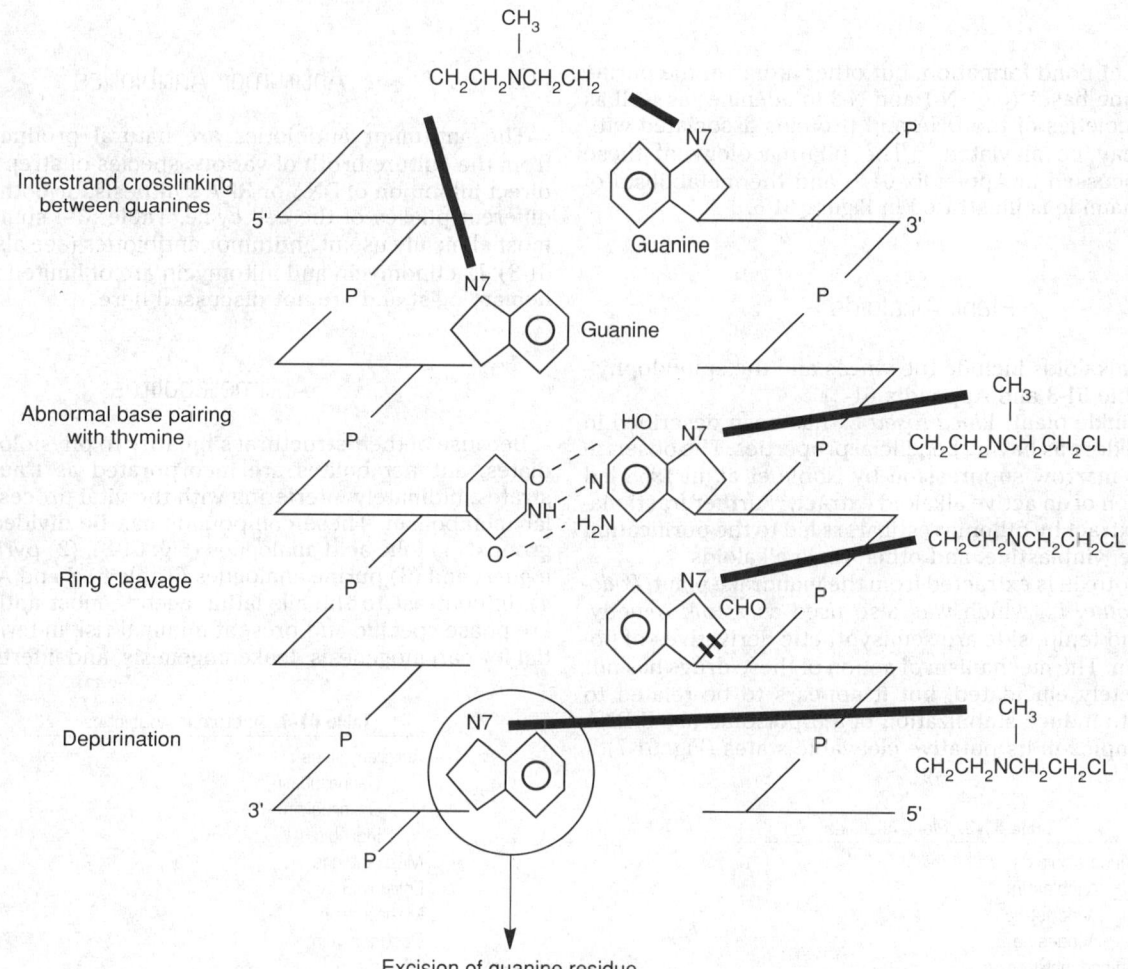

Fig. 61-5. Mechanism of action of alkylating agents, illustrated by mechlorethamine.

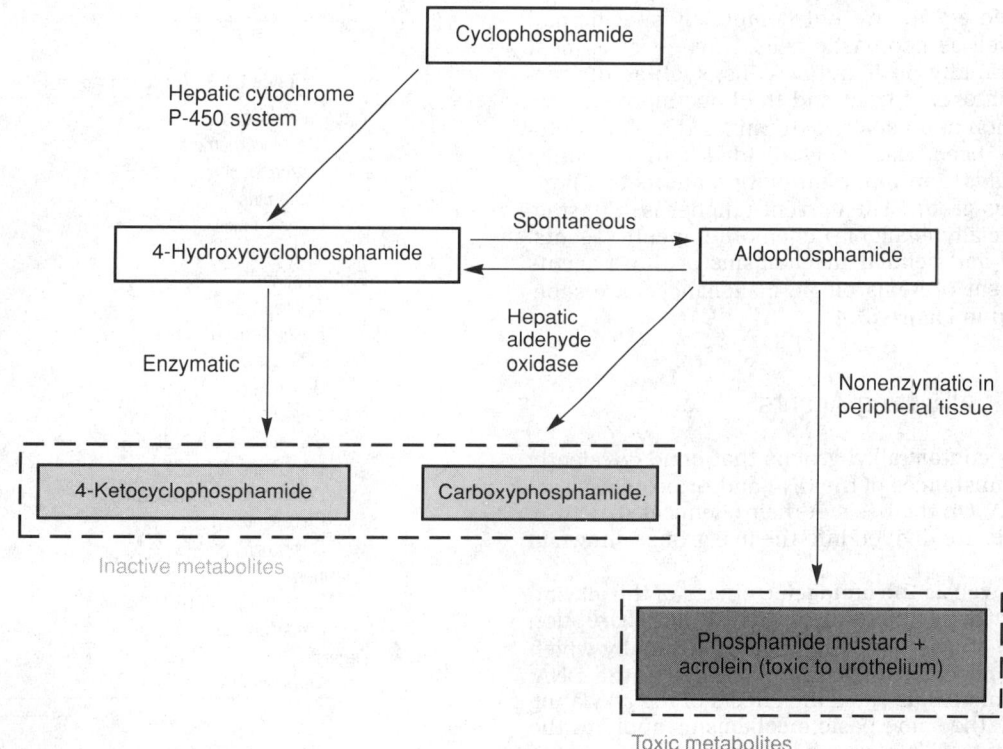

Fig. 61-6. Metabolism of cyclophosphamide.

ble to covalent bond formation, but other atoms in the purine and pyrimidine bases (e.g., N-1 and N-3 in adenine) as well as phosphate moieties of the DNA and proteins associated with DNA also may be alkylated.[22] The pharmacology of these agents is discussed in Appendix 61-1, and the metabolism of cyclophosphamide is illustrated in Figure 61-6.

Plant Alkaloids

The plant alkaloids include the vincas and the epipodophyllotoxins (Table 61-3 and Appendix 61-2).

The periwinkle plant, *Vinca rosea* L., has been described in medicinal folklore as having beneficial properties. The observation of bone marrow suppression by Noble et al. in 1958 led to the isolation of an active alkaloid extract.[1] Further fractionation of this extract by other investigators led to the purification of vincristine, vinblastine, and other vinca alkaloids.

Podophyllotoxin is extracted from the mandrake plant, *Podophyllum peltatum* L., which was also used as a folk remedy. Etoposide and teniposide are semisynthetic derivatives of podophyllotoxin. The mechanism of action of these drugs has not been completely elucidated, but it appears to be related to their ability to induce stabilization of a topoisomerase II/DNA cleavage complex in its putative cleavable states (Fig. 61-7).

Table 61-3. Plant Alkaloids

Vinca alkaloids
  Vinblastine
  Vincristine
  Vindesine
Epipodophyllotoxin
  Etoposide (VP-16)
  Teniposide (VM-26)

Antitumor Antibiotics

The antitumor antibiotics are natural products obtained from the culture broth of various species of streptomyces. By direct inhibition of DNA or RNA synthesis, or both, they affect different phases of the cell cycle. Table 61-4 summarizes the most clinically useful antitumor antibiotics (see also Appendix 61-3). Dactinomycin and mitomycin are of limited value to the hematologist and are not discussed here.

Antimetabolites

Because of their structural similarity to physiologic intermediates, antimetabolites are incorporated as fraudulent substrates, ultimately interfering with the vital processes of cellular metabolism. These compounds can be divided into three groups: (1) folic acid analogues (Fig. 61-8), (2) pyrimidine analogues, and (3) purine analogues (Table 61-5 and Appendix 61-4). In contrast to the alkylating agents, most antimetabolites are phase specific and present minimal risk in terms of potential for carcinogenesis, leukemogenesis, and infertility. Fluoro-

Table 61-4. Antitumor Antibiotics

Anthracyclines
  Daunorubicin
  Doxorubicin
  Idarubicin
Mitoxantrone
Epirubicin
Mithramycin
Dactinomycin
Plicamycin
Mitomycin
Bleomycin

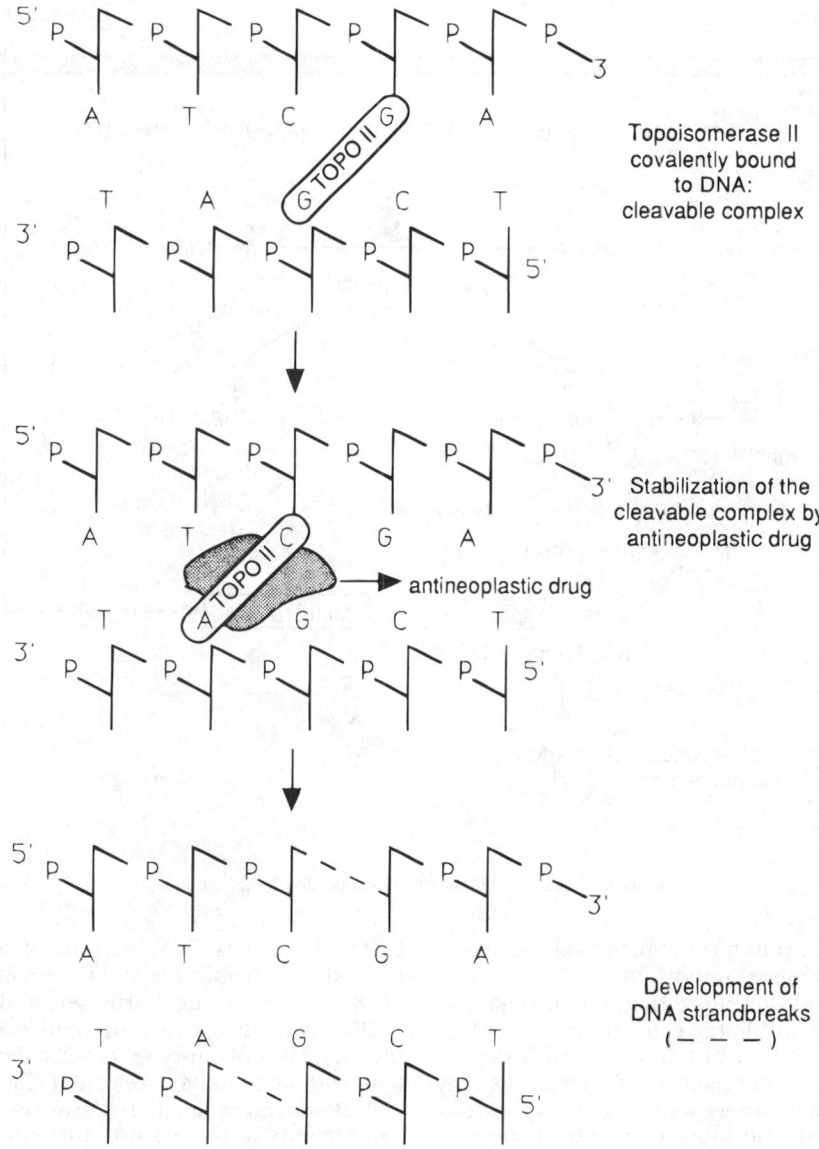

Fig. 61-7. Topoisomerase II-mediated DNA cleavage.

uracil and floxuridine are of limited value to the hematologist and are not discussed here.

Miscellaneous Agents

The agents included in the miscellaneous category are summarized in Table 61-6 and Appendix 61-5. Of these, only the heavy metals, hydroxyurea, procarbazine, L-asparaginase, amsacrine, and gallium nitrate, and the glucocorticoids are currently of clinical relevance to the hematologist.

MULTIDRUG RESISTANCE IN CANCER

The use of chemotherapy as a modality for cancer treatment has been hampered by the development of cellular resistance. Although many advances in drug therapy were made in the past decades, most patients still die of recurrence and disseminated disease. To a large extent, the cancer cells adapt to chemotherapeutic agents or de novo express resistance to these agents. Although drug resistance may be due to a variety of factors, the current discussion focuses only on the biochemical cellular

changes that enable cells to resist cytotoxic drug kill. Concepts of optimal tumor oxygenation and vascular hypertension as potential barriers of cytotoxic chemotherapy are less applicable to hematologic malignancies. Detailed reviews of these topics are available.[23,24]

In vivo drug resistance is difficult to study in patients; however, in vitro cell culture techniques have enabled investigators to understand the molecular details of drug resistance. In vitro, resistance is usually defined as the degree of growth resistance of a particular cell line in reference to its parent cell line. By contrast, clinical resistance to cytotoxic chemotherapy may be defined as lack of initial response to chemotherapy (drug-resistant clones) or initial response followed by progression after chemotherapy (tumor cell adaptation or selection). This biologic explanation is expressed in the form of the Goldie-Coldman hypothesis, suggesting that drug-resistant clones are selected by spontaneous mutation. Over the years, this rationale has been used in part to justify combination chemotherapy, dose intensification, and scheduling. Multidrug resistance (MDR) has many causes, broadly classified as resistance due to altered cell kinetics, intrinsic cellular factors, and host factors. Table 61-7 lists factors that may adversely influence the efficacy of chemotherapeutic agents and result in clinical resis-

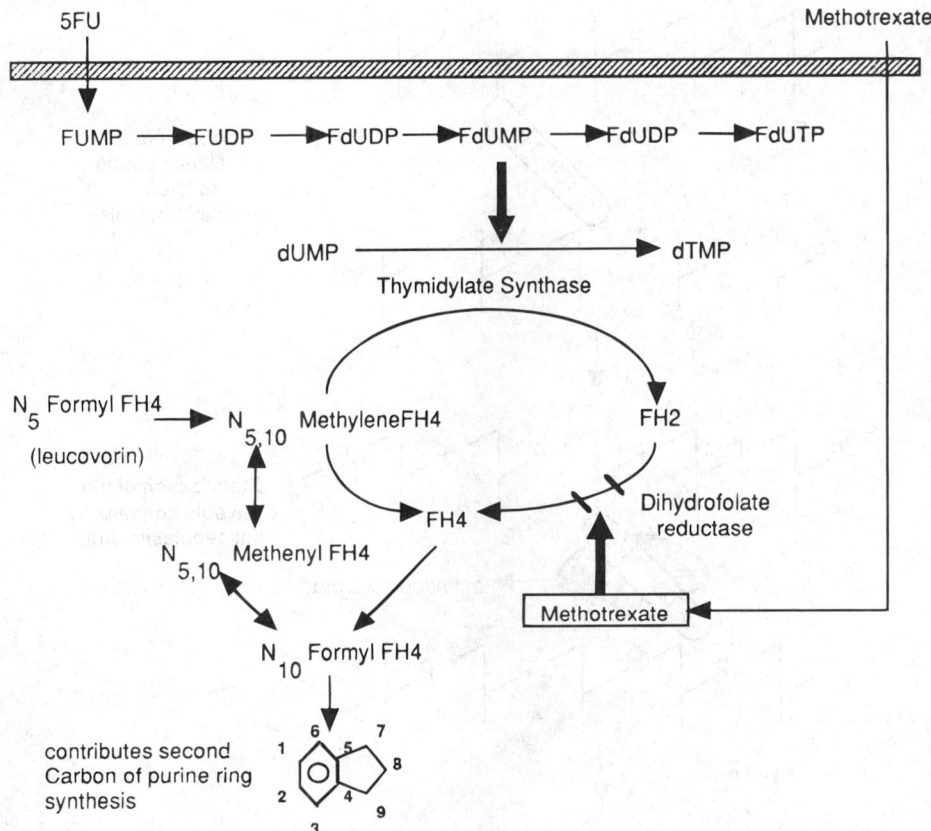

Fig. 61-8. Sites of action of methotrexate and 5-fluorouracil.

tance, of which intrinsic or acquired resistance to chemotherapeutic drugs is probably the most important.

MDR implies the likelihood that more than one mechanism is operative in vivo, not only within the same tumor but within the same cancer cell as well. In a broad sense, MDR can be defined as resistance to dissimilar agents.[25] Cancer cells may develop resistance to the chemotherapeutic agents by various mechanisms; an overview of the most common of these is shown in Figure 61-9. In most cases, these mechanisms have been characterized primarily in cell lines, and their clinical relevance has yet to be defined. Each of the mechanisms for MDR is discussed.

P-Glycoprotein System

Cancer cells selected in vitro by single cytotoxic agents for resistance are frequently cross-resistant to structurally dissimilar agents, including the vinca alkaloids and the podophyllo-

toxin derivatives. This pattern of drug resistance has been termed pleiotropic resistance, or MDR.[26] Early evidence for MDR came from single drug-selected cell lines and, in the late 1960s, from drug-resistant mouse leukemia models. Subsequently, MDR phenotype was also demonstrated for daunorubicin- and dactinomycin-resistant Chinese hamster lung cancer cells. Reduced radiolabeled drug uptake was observed in most experiments of this nature; this suggested decreased plasma membrane permeability as a mechanism of resistance.[27] In 1973, Dano[28] postulated that his Erhlich ascites tumor cells actively extruded daunorubicin, making these cells resistant. In 1976, Juliano and Ling[29] reported a pleiotropically resistant cell line derived from Chinese hamster ovary cells that accumulated less colchicine than its drug-sensitive parent. Believing changes in cell permeability to be responsible for decreased drug accumulation, their group investigated the cell membranes of these drug-resistant cells and identified a highly amplified 170-kd phosphoglycoprotein.[29] The existence of a 170–190-kd P-glycoprotein was also confirmed in vinblastine-resistant human leukemia cell lines. Subsequent work demonstrated that this phosphoglycoprotein, termed P-glycoprotein, actually functioned as an ATP-dependent drug efflux pump ca-

Table 61-5. Antimetabolites

Folic acid analogues
    Methotrexate
Pyrimidine analogues
    Cytarabine (ara-C)
    Fludarabine
    Azacytidine[a]
    Fluorouracil (5-FU)
    Floxuridine (FUDR)
Purine analogues
    Mercaptopurine (6-MP)
    Thioguanine (6-TG)
    Pentostatin
    2-Chlorodeoxyadenosine (CdA)

Table 61-6. Miscellaneous Agents

Heavy metals
    Cisplatin
    Carboplatin
Hydroxyurea
Procarbazine
Asparaginase
Amsacrine
Gallium nitrate
Hormones and antihormones

Table 61-7. Factors that May Adversely Influence the Efficacy of Chemotherapeutic Agents

Host factors
   Failure of the drug to undergo activation
   Alteration of drug pharmacokinetics such that a given dose results in altered distribution of metabolism (e.g., increased catabolism)
   Strategic location of the tumor, resulting in poor access of the drug to the tumor site (e.g., testis, central nervous system)
Tumor factors
   Intrinsic or acquired chemotherapy drug resistance
   Alteration of blood flow to the tumor, resulting in an inadequate dose reaching the tumor
   Changes in the tumor environment, reducing the effectiveness of the drug (e.g., low oxygen pressure, low pH)
   Presence of tumor cells predominantly in G_0 phase (kinetic resistance)

pable of extruding plant alkaloids and antitumor antibiotics from the cancer cells, rather than decreasing drug uptake.[26]

Genetics

Examination of the chromosomes of highly resistant cell lines often reveals the presence of many amplified sequences of DNA (gene-amplification-associated cytogenetic abnormalities). These may exist either as small extrachromosomal circles, termed minutes or double minutes (DM), or integrated into the chromosome as a homogeneously staining region (HSR) or abnormally banding (ABR) regions of metaphase chromosomes. These regions are known to arise when gene amplifi-

cation occurs and contain many copies of the amplified gene. The isolation and sequencing of these amplified regions provided evidence that the MDR phenotype could be ascribed to specific DNA sequences encoding the P-glycoprotein. Specific probe in situ hybridization to metaphase chromosomes of highly resistant Chinese hamster cell lines indicates that HSR and ABR are sites of resistance gene amplification. Most often, amplification of the MDR-1 gene appears to be the basis for increased P-glycoprotein expression in highly resistant cell lines. Gene amplification is not observed, however, in some P-glycoprotein-positive cell lines selected for low levels of resistance. Thus, it appears that overexpression of P-glycoprotein is not always dependent on gene amplification and may also be affected at levels such as transcription or translation.[26,27] In hamsters, three P-glycoprotein genes have been mapped to chromosome 1q26. Each amplicon contains 4–5 co-amplified genes in addition to the P-glycoprotein genes. Whether any one or all genes co-amplified confer or assist in confering the MDR phenotype is unknown. One closely juxtaposed gene class, the 22-kd cytoplasmic calcium-binding protein sorcin, has also been detected in P-glycoprotein-positive cells. However, overexpression of this protein is not sufficient, nor is it necessary, for acquisition of the MDR phenotype.[30] The in vitro demonstration that transfection of the MDR-1 gene into sensitive cell lines confers expression of both the P-glycoprotein and the MDR phenotype represents the most important evidence that the presence of the MDR-1 gene is a sufficient and necessary condition for expression of the MDR phenotype.[31]

P-glycoprotein, also known as PGY-1, is the product of the

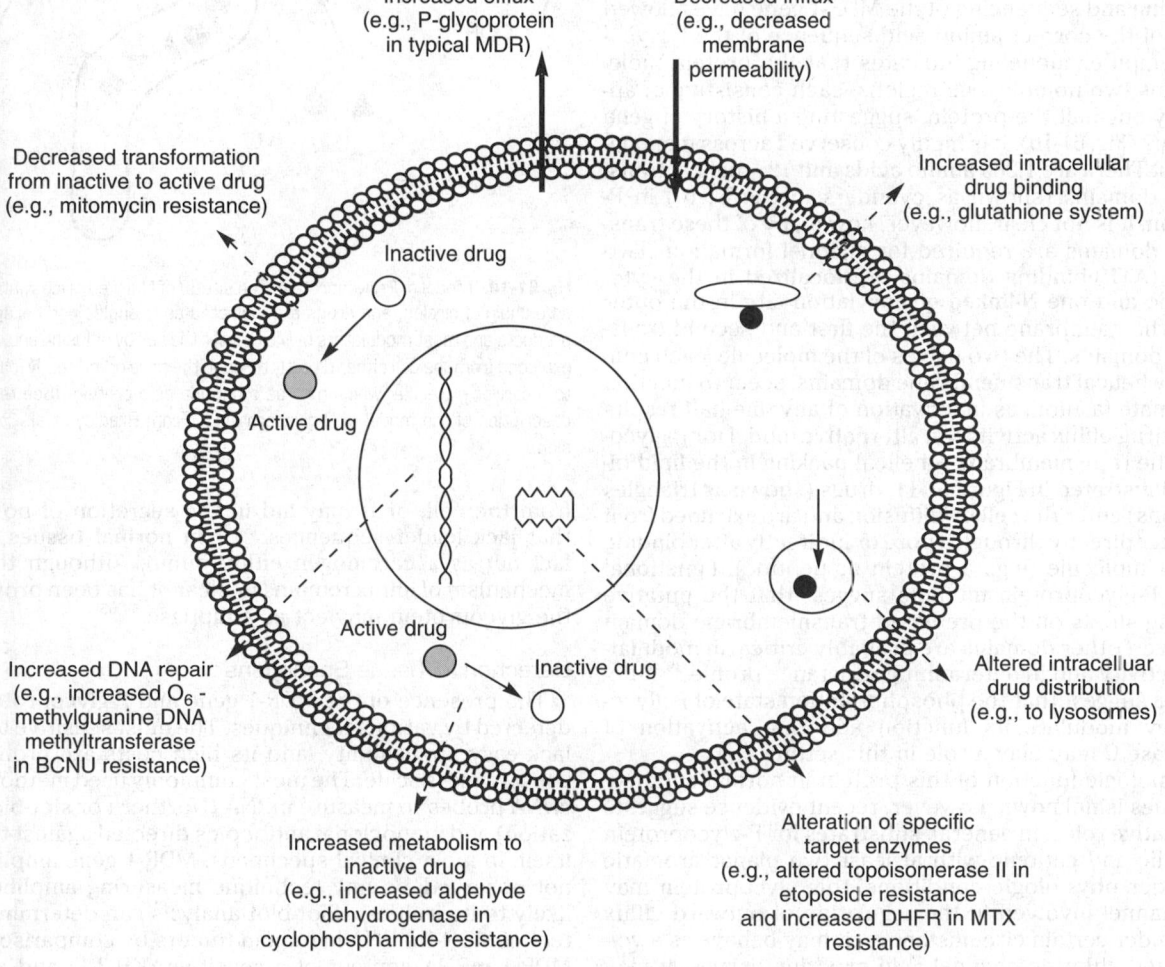

Fig. 61-9. Overview of potential sites for drug resistance at the cellular level.

MDR-1 gene (a member of the MDR multigene family),[32] which in humans is located on chromosome 7q21.1.[33] At this point, little is known about the molecular controls of MDR-1 gene expression; however, there is evidence for alternative splicing of MDR-1 mRNA, different topologic forms of the translational products, and extensive post-translational modification. It was recently shown that certain mutants of cellular oncogenes like p53 and *ras* may upregulate the expression of MDR-1.[34] Furthermore, at least one other homologous MDR gene, termed MDR-2 (also known as MDR-3), is also located on chromosome 7q21.1 and is separated from the MDR-1 gene by 34 kb.[35] Another gene related to the MDR multigene family has been identified on chromosome 16p13.1. Although this gene encodes an ATP-binding transmembrane transport protein, it does not appear to play a role in cytotoxic drug efflux.[36]

Recent evidence suggests that the MDR-2 gene product does not produce cellular resistance to known cytotoxic agents; however, this gene may be important in certain B-cell prolymphocytic leukemias, as it is seen to be highly expressed before initiation of therapy. Moreover, the mammalian MDR genes show striking homology with other prokaryotic and eukaryotic transport protein genes (see Table 61-13). To date, ≥30 ATP-binding proteins have been identified in eukaryotes that share striking sequence homology with P-glycoprotein. In certain cases, such as the adenylcyclase transport protein, despite minimal sequence homology, both proteins share structural similarities. The former protein seems to be involved in exporting cAMP from cells.[27]

Structure and Function

The cloning and sequencing of the MDR-1 gene have allowed prediction of the correct amino acid sequence of the P-glycoprotein. Computer modeling indicates that the protein molecule contains two homologous regions, each consisting of approximately one-half the protein, suggesting a history of gene duplication[26] (Fig. 61-10). It is highly conserved across mammalian species. There are 1,280 amino acids and 12 γ-helical transmembrane domains (shown as cylinders in Fig. 61-10) in P-glycoprotein. It is not clear, however, how many of these transmembrane domains are required for channel formation. Two nucleotide (ATP)-binding domains are localized in the cytoplasmic side and one N-linked glycosylation site in the outer portion of the membrane between the first and second transmembrane domains. The two halves of the molecule, each containing six γ-helical transmembrane domains, seem to function in a coordinate fashion, as inactivation of any one half results in a loss of drug-efflux activity. An alternative model for P-glycoprotein is the transmembrane α-helical packing in the lipid bilayer.[37] As illustrated in Figure 61-11, drugs (shown as triangles and hexagons) enter the cell by diffusion and are extruded from the cell either directly through a pore or indirectly after binding to a carrier molecule (e.g., a protein or peptide). Functional studies on P-glycoprotein mutants suggest that the putative drug-binding site is on the predicted transmembrane domain 11.[38] However, other domains are probably critical in modulating efflux activity and in determining resistance profile.[39,40] Recent studies suggest that the phosphorylation state of P-glycoprotein may modulate its function and that activation of protein kinase C may play a role in this setting.[26,41]

The physiologic function of this protein in normal and neoplastic tissues is unknown; however, recent evidence suggests several putative roles. In general, substrates for P-glycoprotein are lipophilic and cationic with at least two planar aromatic rings.[42] Under physiologic conditions, this glycoprotein may act as a channel involved in the regulation of outward efflux of ATP.[43] Under certain circumstances, it may behave as a volume-regulated chloride channel.[44] In exocrine tissues, it may serve as a channel that actively extrudes toxic metabolites

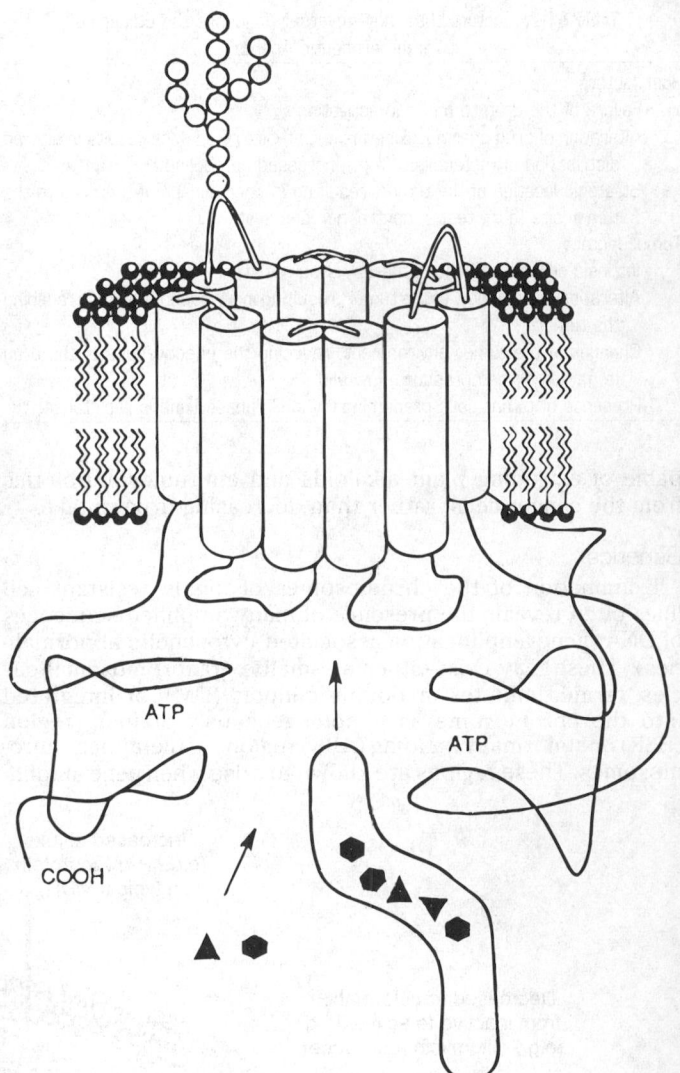

Fig. 61-10. Model of P-glycoprotein. The site(s) of N-linked glycosylation are shown as a chain of circles, and drugs are indicated as triangles and hexagons. Natural products and most modulators of MDR enter the cell by diffusion and are vectorially extruded from the cell either directly through the pore or indirectly following binding to a carrier molecule, which may be a peptide or a protein. (See text for further description of the model of P-glycoprotein.) (From Bradley et al.,[26] with permission.)

from the cell, or it may aid in the secretion of polypeptides that lack leader sequences.[45–53] In normal tissues, it may in fact act as a carcinogen efflux pump. Although the precise mechanism of efflux remains unclear, it has been proposed that the glycoprotein may act as a flippase.[54,55]

Detection in Tissue Specimens

The presence of the MDR-1 gene and P-glycoprotein can be detected by various techniques. The most sensitive techniques lack easy applicability, and its high costs are prohibitive for use on a mass scale. The most commonly used methods include cDNA probes to measure mRNA (Northern or slot-blot hybridization) and monoclonal antibodies directed against the protein itself. In most clinical specimens, MDR-1 gene amplification is not observed, so any technique measuring amplified DNA is likely to be fruitless. Slot-blot analysis can determine the content of MDR-1 mRNA in human tumors by comparison with the MDR-1 mRNA content of a sensitive (KB-3-1) and a resistant (KB-8-5) human cell line.[56] In addition to the slot-blot tech-

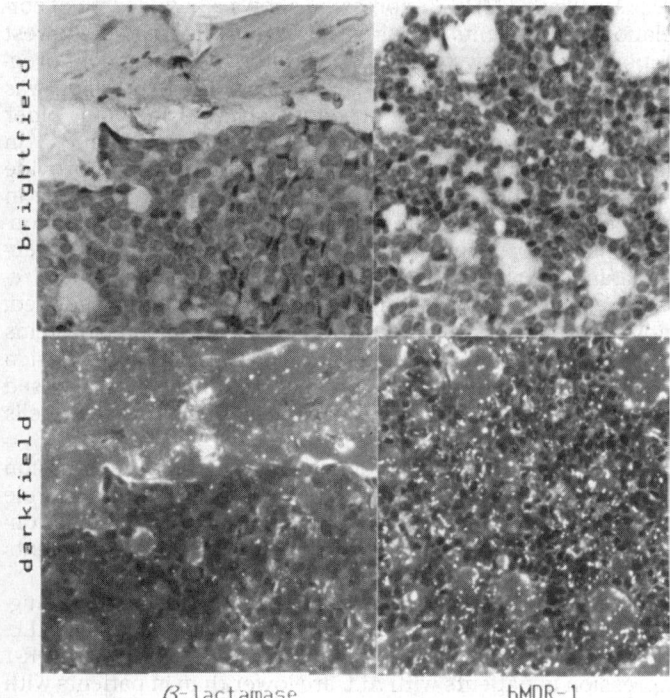

Fig. 61-11. Detection of the MDR-1 mRNA by in situ hybridization in a breast cancer specimen. The bright spots shown in the autoradiograph (dark-field) indicate sites at which hybridization occurred. β-Lactamase represents the negative control. (Courtesy of Dr. Barry M. Kacinski, Department of Therapeutic Radiology, Yale University School of Medicine.)

nique, in situ hybridization with autoradiography can be used to quantitate the MDR-1 gene.[57] Figure 61-11 presents an autoradiograph of an MDR-1-positive breast cancer specimen.

Slot-blot analysis of MDR-1 RNA levels is a relatively simple and easily reproducible technique. It is limited, however, because it only measures total MDR-1 mRNA in a tumor specimen. This is also the limiting factor when using polymerase chain reaction (PCR) or the measurement of P-glycoprotein expression by Western blot analysis. By contrast, in situ hybridization may permit determination of the MDR phenotype in individual tumor cells. With these techniques, benign tissue can be distinguished from the malignant tumor within the same surgical specimen. In addition, the heterogeneity of MDR expression within a tumor can be demonstrated. While in situ hybridization is probably more sensitive than immunohistochemical staining, it is a much more laborious technique.

The use of monoclonal antibodies against P-glycoprotein in conjunction with a peroxidase stain provides another way of assessing the expression of the MDR phenotype.[58] This rapid and easy technique is useful when good controls are available in the laboratory. In hematologic malignancies, the direct measurement of cell-surface glycoprotein by immunofluorescence provides reproducible results with good specificity. In tissues in which there is poor correlation between MDR-1 mRNA and cell glycoprotein levels, it is prudent to stain directly for the presence of the glycoprotein. However, none of these techniques has been standardized to the extent that direct comparison can be made between levels in different tissues or laboratories. In fact, the extent of MDR-1 glycoprotein expression cannot be entirely differentiated in tissue specimens containing normal and neoplastic cells. Many monoclonal antibodies are available for the detection of epitopes of P-glycoprotein, including JSB-1, C-219, MRK-16, HYB-241, HYB-612, C-494, UIC-2, and 4E-3. Functional measurement of the P-glycoprotein using rhodamine-123 efflux or organotechnetium labels is becoming

increasingly universal and provides a dynamic assessment of drug resistance.[59,60]

Distribution in Normal Human Tissue

Table 61-8 summarizes the results of these studies in normal tissues,[58,61-77] showing cell- and organ-specific distribution of the various MDR gene products. For example, in the liver, muscle, kidney, and placenta, MDR-2 is the commonly expressed gene.[66,67] Note that in the adrenal gland, P-glycoprotein is diffusely distributed over the surface of both cortical and medullary cells, while in other tissues it is localized in a highly polarized fashion consistent with its proposed role in drug transport and excretion of toxic natural products. P-Glycoprotein and/or increased levels of MDR-1 RNA have not been demonstrated in cells of the stomach, lung, cerebral cortex, cerebellum, spinal cord, ovary, spleen, cardiac muscle, or prostate. Recent data on MDR-1 expression in hematopoietic tissues demonstrate that immature hematopoietic elements contain high levels of P-glycoprotein; however, with differentiation, these levels diminish, suggesting differential regulation of MDR-1 in hematopoietic tissues. High levels of expression of MDR-1 may be found in the mature hematopoietic compartment consisting of CD8[+] T cells, activated monocytes, and natural killer cells.[64,65]

Distribution in Hematologic Malignancies

Determinations of the frequency of the MDR phenotype in many hematologic malignancies are summarized in Table 61-9. Although there is an increasing body of data in this field, rigorous serial evaluation for the MDR phenotype in a group of patients at diagnosis and then at relapse from chemotherapy-induced remissions is lacking for most tumors.

In AML, accumulating evidence demonstrates acquired resistance by P-glycoprotein after initial exposure to natural products. In particular, some but not all studies have shown P-glycoprotein-mediated anthracycline efflux from leukemic blasts, which may explain resistance to anthracyclines in some AML specimens.[77,90-92] In about 20% of patients with de novo AML, MDR-reversing agents have increased cellular retention of daunorubicin.[90-92] This correlates with the observed frequency of MDR-1 mRNA or P-glycoprotein expressed in 15–30% of patients with de novo AML (Table 61-9). Retrospective studies suggest that P-glycoprotein may be more highly expressed at relapse, although this needs to be confirmed by larger prospective studies.[91,92]

MDR phenotype may be important, especially in the subgroup of patients likely to have shorter disease-free survival

Table 61-8. Localization of P-Glycoprotein in Normal Human Tissues Detected by Immunoperoxidase Staining Using Monoclonal Antibodies

Tissue[a]	Localization of P-Glycoprotein
Liver[61,66]	Biliary canalicular surface of hepatocytes
Jejunum and colon[61]	Apical surface of columnar epithelial cells
Kidney[61,66]	Brush border of proximal tubules
Muscle[67,71]	Myocytes
Pancreas[61]	Apical surface of small ductules
Adrenal[61]	Diffusely on the surface of cells in medulla and cortex
Placenta[62,66]	Trophoblasts
Uterus[72]	Endometrial tissue and epithelia
Fetal tissues[69]	Differential expression in various organs
Central nervous system[45]	Endothelial cells of capillaries
Testis[45]	Endothelial cells of the capillaries
Skin[45]	Endothelial cells of the capillaries
Blood[64,65,70]	CD34[+] cells, myeloid and B lymphocytes

[a] In reference 45, two monoclonal antibodies (HYB-241 and C-219) were used. In references 61 and 62, only the monoclonal antibody MRK-16 was used.

Table 61-9. Frequency of the MDR Phenotype in Various Hematologic Malignancies from Untreated and Chemotherapy-Treated Patients

	No. of Tumors Positive/Total[a]			
	Untreated at		Chemotherapy Treated or	
Type of Malignancy[a]	Diagnosis	(%)	Relapsed	(%)
Acute leukemias				
AML (adult)[56]	3/24	(13)	4/5	(80)
AML (adult)[73]	0/11	(0)	0/14	(0)
AML (adult)[75]	5/24	(21)	4/7	(57)
AML (adult)[76]	9/38	(25)	9/17	(53)
AML (adult)[77]	1/7	(14)	8/10	(80)
AML (adult)[78]	18/67	(27)	7/26	(27)
AML (adult)[79]	1/12	(8)	6/8	(75)
AML (adult)[80]	2/8	(25)	5/8	(62)
AML (adult)[81]	1/6	(17)	6/10	(60)
ALL (adult)[56]	2/15	(13)	1/1	(100)
ALL (adult)[73]	0/4	(0)	0/5	(0)
ALL (adult)[77]	4/8	(50)	1/1	(100)
ALL (adult)[79]	2/20	(10)	7/12	(58)
ALL (childhood)[56]	1/9	(11)	3/20	(15)
ALL (childhood)[82]	47/175	(27)	10/25	(40)
ALL (childhood)[83]	1/9	(11)	3/20	(15)
ALL (childhood)[84]	0/28	(0)	0/14	(0)
T-cell (adult)[85]	8/20	(40)	6/6	(100
Chronic leukemias				
Chronic phase CML[56]	0/3	(0)	Not done	
Blast crisis CML[56]	3/3	(100)	2/3	(66)
B-CLL[86]	4/7	(57)	14/27	(52)
B-CLL[77]	17/17	(100)	—	
B-CLL[89]	34/42	(81)	—	
NHL[56]	4/18	(22)	3/5	(60)
NHL[74,87]	1/42	(2)	7/11	(64)
Multiple myeloma[88]	3/47	(6)	21/49	(43)

Abbreviation: NHL, non-Hodgkin lymphoma.

[a] In reference 56, MDR-1 mRNA was measured by slot-blot analysis. In this series, a sample was considered positive when the MDR-1 mRNA content was higher than in the KB-3-1-sensitive cell line. In reference 73, P-glycoprotein was detected by immunoperoxidase using the MRK-16 monoclonal antibody. In references 74 and 88, P-glycoprotein was detected by immunoperoxidase, using either C-219 or JSB-1 monoclonal antibody. In reference 76, MDR-1 mRNA was measured by slot-blot; reference 77 used the RNAse protection assay. In reference 79, immunocytochemistry was used to detect P-glycoprotein. In reference 82, rt-PCR was employed. Reference 83 used the sensitive RNAse protection assay, and reference 84 used immunocytochemistry. References 74 and 87 (the same investigators) report the use of immunocytochemistry to detect P-glycoprotein. In reference 89, rhodamine-123 assay for P-glycoprotein function and PCR for MDR-1 and MDR-3 was performed.

or in those who respond poorly to induction chemotherapy. The latter category includes elderly patients, AML with unfavorable cytogenetics, and secondary and relapsed AML. In most but not all studies, ≥20% of leukemic cells are MDR-1[+] and that its expression is an independent negative prognostic factor.[47,92–95] Conflicting reports on outcomes in patients with MDR-1[+] AML are attributable to the varied techniques of measuring MDR-1 gene expression and/or products; furthermore, the probes used in most situations were unable to distinguish between MDR-1 and MDR-2 mRNA transcripts and/or glycoprotein. In addition, none of the studies looked at the functional status of the P-glycoprotein. However, studies carefully performed to distinguish MDR-1 transcripts in leukemic cells accurately, using PCR coupled with flow cytometric assays, suggest that in AML, MDR-1 is associated with treatment failure.[96] In patients with de novo AML-, MDR-1 expression is not a significantly independent prognostic factor; however, it is associated with the presence of CD34[+] cells.[92–97] In the subgroup of patients with poor risk or relapsed AML, again the presence of

CD34[+] cells and MDR-1 expression shows a high degree of correlation.[92–97] Patients who were MDR-1[+] CD34[+] had the lowest response rates; however, MDR-1 was not an independent prognostic factor by multivariate analysis. MDR-1 expression was associated with other poor prognostic factors, including older age, dysplastic bone marrow, and high S-phase fraction.[93–97] In summary, although such correlative structural studies provide evidence for MDR-1 as a predictor of treatment outcome in patients with AML, it is far from clear whether MDR-1 functionally confers most drug resistance in relapsed or refractory leukemia. In fact, growing data on many other mechanisms of resistance include topoisomerase defects, glutathione-mediated, and more recently, the description of other transport proteins mediating drug efflux.[36] The data thus far justify careful design of clinical trials using MDR modulators for newly diagnosed leukemic patients in the hopes of suppressing MDR tumor cells from regrowth.

Patients with blast-phase CML have a high MDR expression rate, and it is likely that P-glycoprotein plays an important role in mediating resistance to natural products.[56,98] Currently ongoing trials are assessing the efficacy of MDR-reversing agents (cyclosporine) in blast-phase CML.[92]

Once again, there are too few studies to derive any meaningful conclusions regarding patients with newly diagnosed ALL. Several investigators have noted that the levels of MDR-1 expression in patients with ALL are lower than in patients with AML[56,91,92,99] (Table 61-9). In principle, given the high complete remissions to induction chemotherapy it is likely that P-glycoprotein is probably important only after exposure to natural products. However, at relapse, the original drugs used for induction remission are usually effective and therefore MDR expression may not be significantly different from that at diagnosis. In fact, in a summary of clinical studies in childhood ALL, it is noted that there is little acquisition of the MDR phenotype at relapse[56,82–84] (Table 61-9). These studies used a variety of methods to detect P-glycoprotein; however, one study using rt-PCR assay for MDR expression revealed that 40% of patients were MDR-1[+] at relapse (N = 25), compared with 27% at diagnosis (N = 175).[82] In adult ALL, MDR expression patterns may be more significant. Musto et al.[79] studied MDR expression by immunocytochemistry in 20 patients with adult ALL; 10% of cases at diagnosis were MDR-1[+], and 58% of the 12 patients that relapsed were MDR-1[+]. Although preliminary, a recent large study in patients with de novo ALL concluded that MDR-1 expression may confer a significant negative prognostic feature with respect to complete remission rates and risk of relapse; however, further confirmation of this finding is clearly required.[99] Once again, this study employed two monoclonal antibodies, JSB1 (MDR-1 specific) and C219 (IgG2A mouse monoclonal) to detect P-glycoprotein in cells from marrow aspirates, but the glycoprotein was not functionally assessed.[99]

In patients with T-cell ALL, some but not all studies demonstrate a high frequency of MDR expression.[77,85,99] At relapse, most if not all patients in these studies showed MDR overexpression. These studies are not confirmatory; larger prospective evaluations using both PCR and immunocytochemistry are awaited.

Few studies have been performed in patients with chronic lymphocytic leukemia (CLL) and chronic myeloid leukemia (CML) in chronic phase.[56,77,86,89,93,94] At least three studies show moderate MDR-1 mRNA expression both in untreated and in treated CLL patients.[77,86,89] However, the data on how MDR expression is regulated in treated and relapsed CLL are inconclusive. Herweijer et al.[77] used an RNAse protection assay to document MDR-1 mRNA in all their patients with CLL. There was no correlation between MDR-1 expression and prior treatment. In the same cohort of patients, MDR-3 (or MDR-2) expression was seen in all patients; on average, its expression was higher in treated than in untreated patients. They concluded that alternative splice variants of MDR may explain drug resistance in some patients.[77] Ludescher et al.[89] used PCR and dual fluorescence by flow cytometry to detect rhodamine-123 efflux from cells in patients with treated and untreated CLL. Their findings suggested that P-glycoprotein overexpression in B-CLL is intrinsic and its expression increased after exposure to MDR drugs. The expression of P-glycoprotein was not associated with aggressive disease potential or with the stage of disease.[89] In CML, MDR expression is usually limited to blast cells apparent on transformation. In a small study of three patients with chronic-phase CML, Goldstein et al.[56] studied MDR-1 mRNA expression and concluded that none of these patients had detectable levels of mRNA. Unfortunately, larger studies are lacking; however, it seems likely that MDR plays an important role only in blast crisis.

By contrast, refractory lymphomas and myelomas frequently appear to be MDR-1[+].[56,73,74,87] The clinical course of response to treatment in both diseases parallels the augmented expression of P-glycoprotein at relapse after initial treatment. In malignant lymphoma, at least two recent studies show augmented expression of P-glycoprotein at relapse—one study used immunocytochemistry and the other study used RNA slot-blot to detect MDR expression[56,74] (Table 61-9). In multiple myeloma, MDR expression is probably an acquired phenomenon, related to past exposure to natural products. Using immunocytochemistry and flow cytometry, Epstein et al.[100] demonstrated that almost all patients who failed VAD (vincristine, [Adriamycin], dexamethasone) treatment had detectable P-glycoprotein in their myeloma cells. A more recent study from the University of Arizona demonstrated that <5% of newly diagnosed or melphalan-treated patients with myeloma had P-glycoprotein; however, the introduction of either vincristine and/or Adriamycin-based regimens produced an overall MDR expression rate of 75%.[88]

Of the solid tumors (Table 61-10), pancreas, hepatoma, colon and renal cancer, carcinoid, and neoplasms of the adrenal gland show the highest expression of MDR-1 mRNA in untreated patients, but data on chemotherapy-treated patients with solid tumors other than neuroblastoma are still very limited.[56] Untreated tumors with low levels of MDR-1 mRNA levels include non-neuroendocrine-derived lung cancer, esophagus, head and neck, stomach, melanoma, breast, and ovary. Rates of P-glycoprotein expression increase with relapse, especially in breast cancer (10% at diagnosis to 50% at relapse), neuroblastoma (10% at diagnosis to 30% at relapse), and ovarian cancer (16% at diagnosis to 33% at relapse).[101] In summary, these studies suggest that there may be a correlation between MDR-1 expression and clinical drug resistance; however, these studies do not prove that MDR-1 expression is associated with, or causally affects, treatment outcome or survival. Two studies provide exceptions to the above rule. One, conducted by Chan et al.,[102] retrospectively analyzed 30 cases of childhood rhabdomyosarcoma and undifferentiated sarcoma for P-glycoprotein expression by immunohistochemistry. Nine patients had P-glycoprotein positive tumors, and all relapsed after initial chemotherapy, whereas of the 20 patients with P-glycoprotein-negative tumors, only 1 patient relapsed. Similar results have been observed with neuroblastoma.[103] In this tumor, P-glycoprotein expression before treatment predicts response to chemotherapy. Additionally, patients with P-glycoprotein positive tumors have poorer disease-free-survival and overall survival.[103]

Overcoming the MDR Phenotype

Extensive laboratory studies have identified many drugs (Table 61-11) capable of overcoming the MDR phenotype.[104–125] These drugs block the increased efflux of the cytotoxic agents from the resistant cells, which decreases the 50% inhibitory

Table 61-10. Distribution of MDR-1 mRNA Levels Measured by Slot-Blot Analysis in Various Solid Tumors Obtained from Untreated and Chemotherapy-Treated Patients

Cancer Type	No. MDR-1[+a]/Total			
	Untreated	(%)	Chemotherapy Treated	(%)
Hepatoma	12/12	(100)	Not done	
Colon cancer	35/41	(85)	Not done	
Renal cancer	40/50	(80)	Not done	
Carcinoid	7/9	(77)	Not done	
Adrenocortical cancer	7/9	(77)	Not done	
Pheochromocytoma	15/20	(75)	1/1	(100)
Pancreatic islet cell	2/4	(50)	Not done	
Neuroblastoma	17/34	(50)	16/16	(100)
Lung cancer	7/19	(36)	Not done	
Breast cancer	9/57	(16)	2/2	(100)
Bladder cancer	1/16	(16)	Not done	
Prostate cancer	0/3	(0)	Not done	
Thyroid cancer	0/4	(0)	Not done	
Wilms tumor	0/20	(0)	Not done	
Sarcomas	0/11	(0)	Not done	
Thymoma	0/1	(0)	Not done	
Esophageal cancer	0/14	(0)	Not done	
Head and neck cancer	0/14	(0)	Not done	
Gastric cancer	0/2	(0)	Not done	
Ovarian cancer	0/16	(0)	Not done	
Melanoma	0/3	(0)	Not done	

[a] A sample was considered positive when the MDR-1 mRNA content was higher than that in the KB-3-1-sensitive cell line.

(Data from Goldstein et al.[56])

Table 61-11. Agents Capable of Overcoming the MDR Phenotype (Typical MDR)

Agent
Cefoperazone[101]
Erythromycin[101]
Monoclonal antibodies—MRK-16, UIC-2[101]
Reserpine[104]
SDB-Ethylenediamine[104]
Chloroquine[104]
Atropine[104]
Amphotericin[105]
Amiodarone[106,107]
Ceftriaxone[108]
Cyclosporine and derivatives[109–112]
Diltiazem[113,114]
Dipyridamole[115]
Megestrol acetate[101,119]
Nifedipine and related derivatives[101,116]
Phenothiazines and derivatives[118]
Progesterone[119]
Quinidine[120]
Verapamil and derivatives[101,121,124]
Tamoxifen and toremifine[122,123]
FK506[125]
Rapamycin[125]
Miscellaneous (liposomal taxol, tumor necrosis factor, retinoids, oligomers)[101,117]

concentration of the resistant cell lines to a level approaching the IC_{50} of the sensitive parental line. The mechanisms by which these drugs block the efflux of the cytotoxic agents is not completely understood. Studies suggest that various agents, including quinidine, Cyclosporin A and its analogues, reserpine, and calcium-channel blockers (e.g., verapamil, nifedipine, and diltiazem), compete with the cytotoxic agents at the P-glycoprotein level.[104,123,124] However, other drugs, including chloroquine, progesterone, and phenothiazines, may overcome resistance by another mechanism or may interact with the P-glycoprotein at a different site.[104,123] In general, failures in complete reversal of MDR phenotype may relate to the following reasons, including inadequate levels of chemosensitizing agents, MDR-1 gene mutations, increased P-glycoprotein levels in progressing tumor tissue, and existence of alternative MDR mechanisms.

Investigators have initiated clinical trials combining a sensitizing agent with one or more cytotoxic natural products. Dalton et al.[126] reported on the efficacy of verapamil in overcoming resistance in patients who progressed on VAD chemotherapy. Of eight patients studied, seven had multiple myeloma, and one had diffuse large cell lymphoma. Except for one patient who failed the VMCP/VBAP regimen (vincristine, melphalan, cyclophosphamide, doxorubicin [Adriamycin], bischloronitrosourea [BCNU], prednisone), all patients showed unequivocal evidence of progression on VAD alone before the addition of verapamil. Verapamil was given by continuous infusion starting 12 hours before, and continuing 24 hours after, VAD infusion. Of six patients whose tumor cells were positive for P-glycoprotein, three responded, one with a complete remission of 6 months duration and two with partial responses of 4 and 5 months' duration.

This strategy has been extended to 18 patients with refractory lymphomas.[74,87] All patients received verapamil by continuous infusion along with a CVAD regimen consisting of cyclophosphamide 600 mg/m^2 on day 1 only and vincristine 0.4 mg/day, doxorubicin 10 mg/m^2/day, and dexamethasone 40 mg/day on days 1–4. All drug-resistant patients selected had high MDR-1 expression. The complete remission rate was 28% (5 patients) and another 44% (8 patients) had partial response. However, the side effects were significant, comprising mainly hypotension, heart block, arrhythmias, and edema requiring intensive care admission. Although preliminary, these results provide the first clinical evidence that the presence of P-glycoprotein in patients with refractory myeloma and lymphomas is of clinical importance and can be overcome in some cases by a sensitizing agent such as verapamil. This is usually achieved at a high cost of side effects.

The clinical relevance of the MDR phenotype in solid tumors such as renal, ovarian, and colon cancer and in other hematologic malignancies has yet to be determined. Various groups of investigators are now trying to find agents that are more effective and less toxic than verapamil. More recently, several investigators have shown that there is a correlation between MDR-1 expression with treatment failure and shorter remission rates. The total number of patients in each study is small and prohibits important subgroup analysis.[102,127,128]

Recently, MDR-1 phenotype-reversing agents have been extended to patients with AML. In a study by Nooter et al.[81] cyclosporine was more effective than verapamil in increasing in vitro intracellular retention of daunorubicin in patients with AML. In phase I/II studies, Cyclosporin A in serum concentrations of 1,000–2,000 ng/ml have been administered with daunorubicin to patients with poor-risk AML. Of the 42 cases studied, 70% had MDR-1 expression before treatment. These patients were given sequential high-dose cytosine arabinoside and daunorubicin, followed by Cyclosporin A infusion. The overall response rate was 69% with reversible moderate toxicity. Of particular note was a reversal or down-regulation of MDR-1 mRNA transcripts in seven patients with relapsing disease.[129] Cyclosporin A has been postulated to be capable of reversing or eliminating MDR-1$^+$ leukemic cells, paving a path for the expression of non-MDR multidrug resistance mechanisms.[129,130] These studies remain preliminary; the most important assessment of the role of MDR-1 in AML will be assays for biologic and functional presence of P-glycoprotein.

The problem of using chemosensitizers in the clinical setting is limited by its inherent toxicity, not by enhanced chemotherapy toxicity. In studies using S-verapamil in high doses, cardiac toxicity was dose limiting.[81] Other phase I studies, using tamoxifen and trifluoperazine, found neurotoxicity to be dose limiting.[131,132] In phase I/II studies using Cyclosporine A, severe neutropenia has limited dose escalation. Hyperbilirubinemia has been observed and is thought to result from inhibition of the P-glycoprotein in biliary canaliculi. Despite these side effects, serum levels of ≤4,800 ng/ml have been achieved with moderate toxicity. It is also possible that Cyclosporin A decreases the clearance of certain chemotherapeutic agents such as etoposide and doxorubicin.[133–135] A 50% reduction of etoposide dose, when used concomitantly with Cyclosporin A in a patient with normal liver and renal function has been advocated.[135]

In order to increase the therapeutic index of MDR-reversing agents, several approaches are ongoing. Stereoisomers of drugs such as verapamil are equally effective in reversing MDR; however, the R-isomer is far less cardiotoxic than the S-isomer.[135,136] Rational drug design may produce less toxic drugs with greater efficacy. For example, preclinical assessment of an analogue of Cyclosporin D, PSC 833, is more potent than Cyclosporin A in modulating MDR. PSC 833 is considerably less immunosuppressive and nephrotoxic.[137] Finally, an MDR-1 transgenic mouse model has been developed that may be used to test the efficacy of newly developed drugs.[138]

Atypical Multidrug Resistance

DNA topology is crucial in influencing DNA transcription and replication. The cellular regulation of DNA topology is largely achieved by topoisomerases. Two major topoisomerases have been identified. Topoisomerase I induces transient single-strand breaks in DNA; however, its precise role in DNA replication and recombination is unknown. Topoisomerase II induces transient double-strand knicks and catalyzes unknotting of DNA and decatenation of interposed DNA molecules. This enzyme directly influences DNA replication, repair, and recombination by preserving DNA topology through chromosome assembly and chromatin matrix attachment. Unlike topoisomerase I, topoisomerase II is tightly regulated throughout the cell cycle and is profoundly up-regulated during S phase.[139] Drugs that bind specifically to topoisomerases I and II inhibit further DNA replication by blocking DNA religation, eventually resulting in DNA cleavage.[139–141] Topoisomerase-related mechanisms of tumor drug resistance have only recently been described and may sometimes be associated with the coexistence of enhanced MDR-1 gene expression, resulting in decreased intracellular drug accumulation.[139,142] True resistance to topoisomerases usually results from low levels of cellular enzyme (decreased target concentration) or altered cellular enzyme (aberrant target). In 1987, Danks et al.[143] described a human leukemic cell line, resistant to teniposide (VM-26), that expressed a different form of MDR. This cell line, CEM/VM-1, was as resistant to epipodophyllotoxins and anthracyclines as the "typical" MDR cells, but it was completely sensitive to the vinca alkaloids. Unlike typical MDR cells, the CEM/VM-1 cells did not express the MDR-1 gene and had about the same steady-state levels of drug as the sensitive parent line. In addition, the drug-resistant phenotype could not be reversed by verapamil. Danks et al.[144] demonstrated that resistance to the CEM/VM-1 cell line was due to an alteration in both catalytic (unknotting) and DNA cleavage activity of topoisomerase II. This type of MDR was called *at*-MDR (altered topoisomerase).[145,146] *at*-MDR is characterized by absence of associated MDR-1 gene expression, sensitivity to vinca alkaloids, and cross-resistance to drugs that interfere with its activity.[139,144–146] This must be differentiated from cell lines that exhibit resistance to multiple toposiomerase II-specific agents as well as to multiple natural products (e.g., vincristine). These cell lines usually overexpress P-glycoprotein.[139,142] Pure *at*-MDR is seen with several well-characterized resistant cell lines in which the topoisomerase II alteration includes decreased activity, content, and point mutation in its gene.[139,147,148] Depletion of nuclear matrix topoisomerase II also results in a form of *at*-MDR; in other cases decreased activity of this enzyme has also been described.[139,149] Further work has revealed that the type of topoisomerase II alteration determines cross-resistance spectra. For example, amsacrine-induced topoisomerase II changes show cross-resistance to anthracycline and antibiotic intercalators, but not to epipodophyllotoxins.[150] Besides structural and functional alteration of the enzyme, absolute levels of topoisomerase II may determine drug resistance. In tumors that contain a high level of quiescent cells with low levels of topoisomerase II, drug insensitivity may be common. With the recent development of biochemical assays for the detection of *at*-MDR phenotype, clinical studies are being conducted in a prospective manner to determine its importance. Clinically useful topoisomerase inhibitors include doxorubicin, daunorubicin, etoposide, teniposide, amsacrine, mitoxantrone, and actinomycin D.

Topoisomerase I-mediated drug resistance is due primarily to changes in concentration or activity of target enzyme. In tumor cell lines mechanisms underlying resistance specifically include deletion of the topoisomerase I gene, decreased topoisomerase concentration or mutant topoisomerases.[139,151,152] All these cell lines are selected with camptothecin or its derivatives; clinical studies are ongoing to determine both the natural

occurrence, as well as the induced occurrence of camptothecin resistance in vivo.

Glutathione System

In the models of chemical carcinogenesis, several important biochemical and biophysical changes have been described that predominantly affect drug-conjugating and drug-metabolizing enzymes. Most situations show a down-regulation of the former and an up-regulation of the latter set of enzymes. Glutathione S-transferases are a family of drug-metabolizing enzymes (π, μ, α, θ) that have been evaluated the most and are able to bind covalently and noncovalently to toxins and to detoxify organic peroxides to less-reactive alcohols. At least 12 isoenzymes have been described.[153] These sets of enzymes convert hydrophobic compounds to glutathione (GSH)-conjugated inactive products. GSH, a tripeptide thiol, accounts for most of the intracellular nonprotein sulfhydryl content of most cell types. It plays an important role either directly or indirectly in many cellular functions, including detoxification of xenobiotics, amino acid transport, synthesis of DNA precursors, protection from free radical damage, and possibly DNA repair (Fig. 61-12).

Many lines of evidence suggest that GSH plays a vital role in protecting cancer cells from the cytotoxic effects of a wide variety of chemotherapeutic agents and of radiation therapy. Ozols et al.[154] demonstrated that the emergence of resistance to melphalan in ovarian cancer patients was positively correlated with an elevation in tumor cell GSH concentration. Furthermore, when these tumor cells were depleted of GSH by buthionine sulfoximine, a specific inhibitor of γ-glutamylcysteine synthetase, sensitivity to melphalan was restored. These in vitro findings have been corroborated by animal studies, which demonstrated an increased survival in nude mice bearing a transplantable human ovarian carcinoma following treatment with melphalan plus BSO as compared with those treated

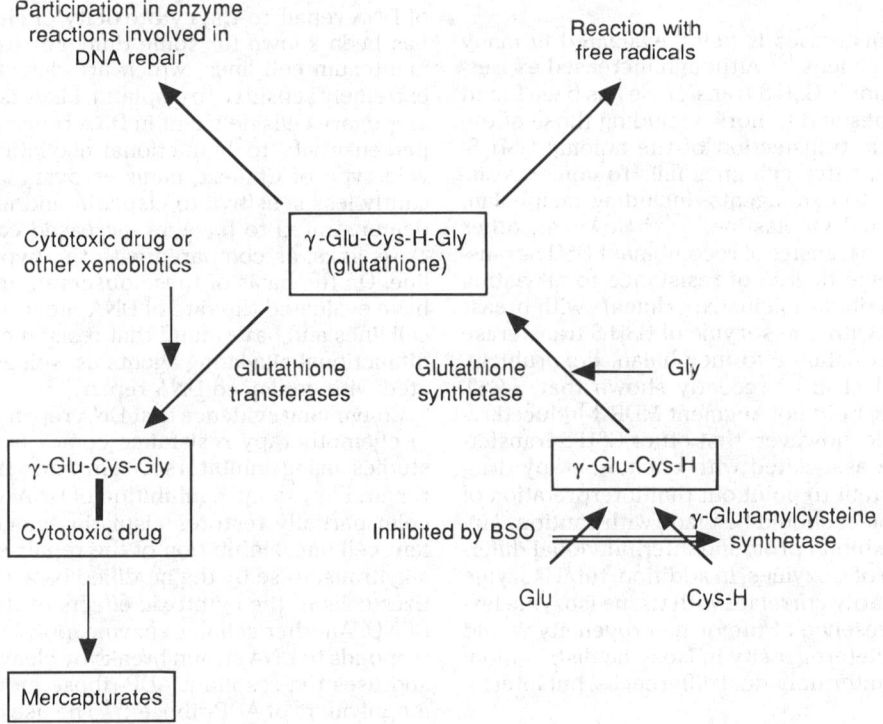

Fig. 61-12. Glutathione system.

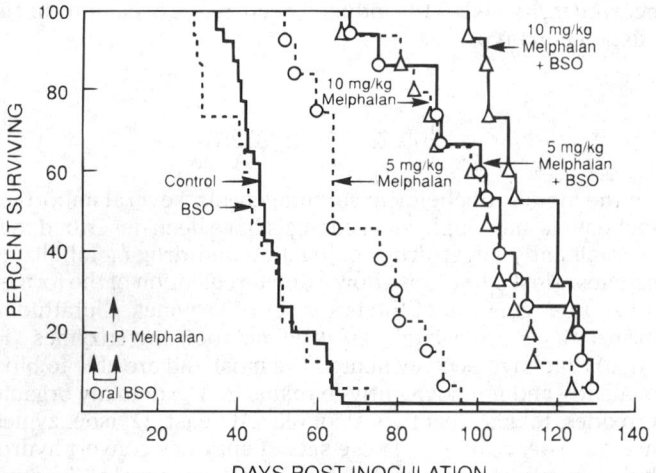

Fig. 61-13. Prolongation of survival of nude mice bearing intraperitoneal ovarian carcinoma (OVCAR-3) cells by L-BSO in combination with melphalan versus melphalan alone. Survivals are shown for untreated controls (—); L-BSO controls (----); melphalan-treated animals (5 mg/kg, —O—; 10 mg/g, —△—); and animals treated with melphalan while receiving oral L-BSO (5 mg/kg, —O—; 10 mg/kg, —△—) are shown above. Percentage of survival was calculated as $(C_T/15) \times 100$, where C_T represents animals surviving at the given day in the appropriate treatment or control group. (From Ozols et al.,[154] with permission.)

with melphalan alone (Fig. 61-13). Similar results have been found by other investigators.[155] Furthermore, pretreatment of cells with L-BSO (which depletes cellular GSH) results in an aerobic radiation response and greater lethality. In fact, it has been shown that ascites bearing mice injected with L-BSO have a profound decrease in the rate of tumor growth. It is conceivable that GSH-dependent drug detoxification of anthracyclines may also confer added drug resistance, although further proof is awaited. The mechanism(s) by which GSH protects cells are still poorly understood, although it appears that GSH is involved in direct scavenging of free radicals and in the repair of DNA damage.[156]

The role of GSH S-transferases is being evaluated in many cell lines and tumor specimens.[157] Although increased expression of the isoenzyme anionic GSH S-transferase has been found in some resistant cell lines and tumors, including those of the lung and head and neck, transfection of the anionic GSH S-transferase gene into sensitive cell lines fails to confer resistance to a number of cytotoxic agents, including melphalan, cisplatin, doxorubicin, and vinblastine.[157,158] However, other experiments using in vitro transfer of recombinant GSH S-transferase genes suggest some degree of resistance to alkylating agents, cisplatinum, and doxorubicin. Experiments with breast cancer cells transfected with a π-isozyme of GSH S-transferase (π-GST) did not show resistance to melphalan, doxorubicin, or cisplatin.[159] Fairchild et al.[158] recently shown that π-GST cotransfection with MDR-1 did not augment MDR-1-induced resistance. It is conceivable, however, that other GSH-S-transferase isoenzymes may be associated with chemotherapy drug resistance.[159] It is important to point out that interpretation of most studies on this subject should be made with caution. Any given tissue specimen exhibits profound interindividual differences in the distribution of isozymes. In addition, total isozyme activity does not necessarily correlate with tissue isozyme levels. Furthermore, the presence of tumor heterogeneity would also lead one to expect heterogeneity in isozyme distribution. Thus, not only are there interindividual differences, but intertumor variation as well.

Despite these inherent problems, few studies have shown the role of GSH S-transferase in clinical drug resistance. Schis-

selbauer et al.[160] showed that a twofold increase in GSH S-transferase was associated with clinical drug resistance in CLL cells obtained from patients clinically resistant to nitrogen mustards. In comparison with untreated CLL patients, clinically resistant patients had increased GSH S-transferase in the face of a preserved isozyme profile or development of a novel enzyme selected by chemotherapy. Lewis et al.[161] found that the α-isozyme of GSH S-transferase may be more directly involved with nitrogen mustard resistance. In cell lines resistant to nitrogen mustard, these investigators found increased α-isozyme protein levels and amplification of the α-isozyme gene.[161] Additional studies are needed to help clarify the role played by these enzymes in clinical drug resistance.

Conventional antineoplastic agents detoxified by the GSH S-transferase pathway include the nitrogen mustards (chlorambucil, melphalan), cyclophosphamide, nitrosurea (BCNU), and mitoxantrone. Clinical trials using BSO for GSH depletion and ethacrynic acid for GSH S-transferase inactivation are under way in an effort to enhance anthracycline and alkylating agent cytotoxicity.

Increased DNA Repair

DNA repair may be defined as a succession of cellular processes associated with restoration of the normal nucleotide sequence and stereochemistry of DNA following damage. DNA repair is a complex phenomenon involving many enzymes in the following sequence: (1) recognition of the DNA damage before incision, (2) incision of the damaged DNA strand at or near the site of the defect, (3) excision of the defective site and localized degradation of the affected strand, (4) repair replication to replace the excised region with a corresponding stretch of normal nucleotides, and (5) ligation to join the repair to the contiguous parental DNA strand.[162]

Since DNA is the principal cytotoxic target for alkylating and intercalating agents and heavy metals such as cisplatin, it is not surprising that tumor cells may acquire drug resistance due to altered DNA responses to these agents. The importance of DNA repair to the cytotoxicity of chemotherapeutic agents has been known for some time. For example, xeroderma pigmentosum cell lines, which are defective in DNA repair, are extremely sensitive to cisplatin. Likewise, mutant Chinese hamster ovary cells deficient in DNA repair have demonstrated hypersensitivity to bifunctional alkylating agents, whereas the wild type of Chinese hamster ovary cells, which are significantly less sensitive to cisplatin and mitomycin C, have been demonstrated to have an increased capacity to remove DNA cross-links, as compared with the hypersensitive mutant cell line. On the basis of these observations, several investigators have evaluated the rate of DNA repair in a number of resistant cell lines and have found that resistance to cisplatin and other bifunctional alkylating agents as well as to radiation is associated with enhanced DNA repair.[163]

Convincing evidence that DNA repair plays an important role in chemotherapy resistance comes from in vitro and in vivo studies using inhibitors of enzymes that participate in DNA repair. For example, inhibition of DNA α-polymerase by aphidicolin partially restores cisplatin sensitivity in cisplatin-resistant cell lines. Inhibition of the repair enzyme O_6-alkylguanine alkyltransferase by the modified base O_6-methylguanine sensitizes cells to the cytotoxic effects of the nitrosoureas such as BCNU. Another cellular enzyme, poly(ADP-ribose)polymerase, responds to DNA strand breaks by cleaving its substrate, NAD^+ and uses the resultant ADP-ribose moieties to synthesize homopolymers of ADP-ribose.[164] The use of agents such as 3-aminobenzamide, which inhibits poly(ADP-ribose) polymerase, results in accumulation of DNA strand breaks and potentiates the tumoricidal effect of some cytotoxic agents such as bleomycin and cisplatin.[165]

Inhibition studies of other enzymes that participate in DNA repair include inhibition of topoisomerases I and II by camptothecin and etoposide, respectively; inhibition of DNA ligase I and II by β-lapachone; inhibition of terminal transferase by dideoxyadenosine; interference in the pyridine nucleotide metabolism by tiazofurin; and modulation of the cell cycle by methylxanthines. An example of a methylxanthine is caffeine, which short-circuits the cell cycle and prevents damaged cells from arresting in G_2 and repairing their DNA.[164]

It is important to emphasize that many of these modulating agents are usually incapable of completely reversing the resistant phenotype, which indicates that other concomitant mechanisms may also be operative. In fact, many other distinct mechanisms have been described to account for resistance to cisplatin and other cytotoxic agents.[166] Ultimately, clinical trials will be required to assess the clinical value of these modulating agents in affecting DNA repair.

Metallothionein System

Metallothioneins are cytoplasmic low-molecular-weight cysteine-rich proteins. They are present in a wide variety of eukaryotes and participate extensively in Zn^{2+} and Cu^{2+} homeostasis and heavy metal detoxification. In addition, indirect evidence demonstrates that the abundant nucleophilic sulfhydryl groups in MTs can interact with many nucleophilic toxins, play a role in controlling intracellular redox potential, and act as scavengers of oxygen radicals generated during the metabolism of xenobiotics. The transcription of the MT gene is regulated by many factors, including metals and environmental stimuli such as epinephrine, glucocorticoids, thermal injury, cytokines, cyclic nucleotides, and phorbol esters.[167] There seems to be some tissue specificity to MT induction. In the kidneys, for example, MTs are specifically induced by certain heavy metals.[168] Additionally, there are at least two major MT isoforms: MT I and MT II. The subtype of each isoform has been difficult to isolate and characterize, since the epitopes on each of these proteins are highly conserved. Antisera raised against these epitopes are cross-reactive. MT mRNA may be detected in tissue by Northern analysis. For each MT isoform protein, specific oligonucleotides have been synthesized for the non-translated 5′ and 3′ regions.[168]

The potential role of MTs in chemotherapy drug resistance has been demonstrated by several investigators who have looked at cisplatin resistance.[169–173] Kelley et al.[169] demonstrated that cell lines selected for resistance to cadmium (a potent inducer of MTs) showed marked cross-resistance to chlorambucil, an ester of chlorambucil and prednisolone, estramustine, and cisplatin and also to radiation. Kelley et al.[169] also demonstrated that human carcinoma cell lines transfected with bovine papillomavirus expression vectors containing DNA-encoding human MT IIA were resistant to cisplatin, melphalan, and chlorambucil, but not to 5-fluorouracil or vincristine. Other workers have also provided indirect evidence for a possible association between elevated MT and cisplatin resistance[170–173]; however, a comprehensive study looking at MT overexpression at the gene and protein level in relationship to drug exposure is lacking. The important findings of Kelley et al.[169] have yet to be confirmed. Schilder et al.[172] described similar cell lines with overexpressed MT that did not have cisplatin cross-resistance. The differences in findings between the two studies using the same cell lines cannot be fully explained. Farnworth et al.[171] studied MT levels in cisplatin-resistant L1210 cell lines. These workers were unable to correlate levels or inducibility of MT with resistance to cisplatin; they con-

cluded that cisplatin resistance is not causally associated with MT expression.

Since MTs are thiols, it is theoretically possible that it has a role as a free radical scavenger. Thornalley and Vasak[174] showed a concentration-dependent removal of superoxide anions by MTs. More recent studies were unable to show this effect.[175,176] Clinically, the induction of MT seems to play a role in doxorubicin toxicity. Sato et al.[177] and Naganuma et al.[178] demonstrated that in mice, pretreatment induction of MT with bismuth subnitrate (BSN) significantly decreased cardiac and bone marrow toxicity. The levels of MT in these two tissues correlated with degree of BSN protection against doxorubicin toxicity. BSN-pretreated mice had equivalent levels of doxorubicin antitumor activity as compared with controls. Naganuma and colleagues hypothesized that BSN may preferentially induce MT in normal tissues, yielding a protective effect against doxorubicin. It was further postulated that this protective effect may result from MT-related free radical scavenging or inhibition.[177,178] Similar data have been shown for X-irradiated tissue[179]; however, it is still premature to conclude that MTs have a clinically significant role in preventing free radical-mediated damage.

Finally, resistance to alkylating agents may in part be associated with MT overexpression. Whether this is mediated by direct regulation or as a cofactor in the DNA repair mechanism after alkylation is unknown. Data reported by Endersen et al.[180] and by Kelley et al.[169] indicate that MT overexpression protects cells from directly repairing damaged DNA and not from free radical scavenging. Follow-up studies with Chinese hamster ovary cells selected for various DNA repair deficiencies suggest that MT overexpression is necessary but not sufficient to protect cells from alkylating DNA damage.[181,182] In conclusion, the potential role of MT in MDR remains unclear.

Decreased Influx of Cytotoxic Agents

Most drugs enter cells by facilitated diffusion that is receptor mediated. Phenotypic alterations in the receptor protein or changes in membrane protein concentration lead to decreased intracellular accumulation of the drug. This phenomenon, as opposed to increased efflux, has been demonstrated in many cell lines as a component of MDR or as the predominant mechanism of resistance to cisplatin and other cytotoxic agents.[183–185] In methotrexate and nitrogen mustard drug resistance models, a variety of membrane transport protein alterations have been documented. The importance of decreased drug uptake as a form of MDR, however, has not been well characterized. In 1988, Ferguson et al.[186] described a human KB cell line that was resistant to etoposide by at least two mechanisms: reduced levels of topoisomerase II and decreased drug uptake. Of note, the cell line was also cross-resistant to vincristine and methotrexate, apparently also attributable to decreased uptake. Thus, decreased drug uptake, probably due to alterations in membrane permeability, may also lead to MDR.

Growth Factors and Oncogenes in Multidrug Resistance

A very controversial emerging field involves growth factors and oncogenes. With the recent isolation of several oncogenes responsible in part for metastatic potential, investigators have tried to relate this to the development of MDR. Metastatic cells at the primary site probably exhibit clonal dominance over nonmetastatic tumor cells, which appears to be due to escape from the normal suppressive effects of certain growth factors like transforming growth factor-β and fibroblast growth factor. These metastatic cells may be more drug resistant than their counterpart nonmetastatic tumor cells; however, this remains speculative. In fact, cell lines selected for MDR in vitro against several chemotherapeutic agents tend to be less aggressive in vivo as measured by tumorigenicity assays. This is contrary to what one would expect, possibly reflecting the hazards of generalizing from in vitro studies.[187]

SUMMARY

Although the term MDR is generally used as a synonym for the P-glycoprotein-associated MDR, many other mechanisms may be involved, including atypical MDR, increased DNA repair, increased GSH, decreased drug influx, and possibly increased metallothionein content. It is very likely that additional mechanisms exist. Furthermore, MDR may be due to combinations of different mechanisms in the same cancer cell, a condition termed multifactorial resistance.

Distinct mechanisms of resistance have been found to be specific for certain cytotoxic agents. These include increased dehydrofolate reductase due to gene amplification in methotrexate resistance, increased aldehyde dehydrogenase in cyclophosphamide resistance, and deficiency in deoxycytidine kinase in cytosine arabinoside resistance. Unlike those causing MDR, these mechanisms do not result in resistance to other dissimilar cytotoxic agents.

It is important to emphasize that most of the mechanisms that lead to drug resistance have been characterized chiefly in cell lines. The clinical relevance of each of these mechanisms has yet to be defined.

FUTURE THERAPEUTIC IMPLICATIONS OF CANCER BIOLOGY

The basis for future curative therapeutics will depend largely on our fundamental understanding of cancer cell biology. Most likely no single magic bullet will be discovered; however, several target systems involved in unregulated growth may be modulated in vivo. As shown in Table 61-12, potential new targets are being actively sought with promising initial results in animal tumor models. It is premature to make conclusions on the basis of our current successes; however, at least two new

Table 61-12. Potential New Targets to Aim for Future Chemotherapy

Target	Potential Inhibitor(s)
Immune system	Vaccines,[a] adoptive immunotherapy[a]
Cell-cycle regulatory genes/protein	Cyclin/p34[cdc2] antisense oligonucleotides
Oncogenes	Antisense oligonucleotides, tumor suppressor gene products
DNA topoisomerases	Camptothecin analogues[a]
Signal transduction proteins	Suramin,[a] ether lipid analogues, Staurosporine, SH2 peptide inhibitors
Growth factor receptors	Suramin,[a] pentosanpolysulfate, monoclonal antibodies[a]
Other unique cell antigens	Monoclonal antibodies[a]
Microtubules	Taxol, taxotere[a]
Mitochondria	Diarylsulfonylureas
Cell adhesion molecules	Suramin,[a] P-selectin inhibitors
Metalloproteinases	TIMP-2
P-Glycoprotein	Cyclosporines,[a] tamoxifen, calcium channel blockers[a]
Angiogenic inhibitors	Collagenase inhibitors, penicillamine, gold, interferons[a]

[a] Currently in clinical trials.

Table 61-13. P-Glycoprotein Homology with Other Transport Proteins

E. coli Malk transporter
E. coli Hly-B α-hemolysin exporter
S. typhimurium Opp D,F oligopeptide transporter
Human CFTR
Bovine adenylylcyclase transporter
Bacterial Ars A,B,C arsenate transporter
D. melanogaster white, brown pigment
P. falciparum pfMDR gene product
S. cervisiae STE6 a-factor pheromone exporter

Abbreviation: CFTR, cystic fibrosis transmembrane conductance regulator.

classes of drugs, camptothecins (e.g., CPT-11) and taxanes have done remarkably well in early clinical trials. CPT-11 has shown significant activity in refractory lung, colon, and ovarian cancer.[188] Taxol has shown a 30% partial response rate in patients with refractory ovarian cancer and also has significant efficacy in advanced breast cancer.[189]

Given our current limitations with cytotoxic chemotherapy, several alternative modalities of treatment are being tested. Cytokines have allowed unimaginable chemotherapy dose escalations that would otherwise be intolerable. In the future, cytokines such as interleukin-3 or interleukin-6 may be used in protecting individual marrow elements (e.g., platelets). Apart from our moderate success using biologic response modifiers in both solid and hematologic malignancies, monoclonal antibodies will be useful in both the diagnosis and management of certain malignancies. Hybridoma technology, in particular CDR grafting, has enabled us to develop less antigenic monoclonal antibodies (humanized mouse antibodies); more recently, repertoire cloning has enabled us to create purely human monoclonal antibodies. The latter should be least antigenic and best tolerated by the patient. In cancer imaging or radioimmunodetection, radionuclides such as ^{131}I are tagged onto either bivalent F(ab')$_2$ or monovalent F(ab') and F(ab) fragments specific to a target antigen on cancer cells. Intravenous administration followed by tomographic imaging provides excellent detection capabilities of minute amounts of tumor undetected by conventional means.[190] This could be used in conjunction with immunotherapy. Other uses of monoclonal antibodies are as anti-idiotypic vaccines (e.g., melanoma, colorectal cancer) and conjugated drugs or toxins (e.g., conjugated cytotoxic drugs, tagged *Pseudomonas* exotoxin).[190]

Targeting intracellular signal transduction events for rational drug design is a new and exciting field. For example, growth factor receptors contain unique binding sites that, when occupied, engage in receptor autophosphorylation. These autophosphorylated domains along with neighboring amino acids cluster into recognition domains called *src* homology-2 (SH2), which in turn serve a crucial function in downstream protein-protein interactions. The SH2 domains are attractive sites for inhibition because small peptides of up to five amino acids may bind SH2 with high affinity in vitro.[191] We are far from constructing such mimetics, but it is hoped that further understanding of the biophysical properties of such domains will enhance development of cell-specific targets.

Probably the most significant advance of the decade has been the introduction of gene therapy. Early detection of genetic mutations in premalignant lesions has paved the way for gene therapy in the primary prevention of cancer. Several oncogenes have been identified as overexpressed or deleted in malignancies. Externally altering the expression of these oncogene products has proved to be useful in retarding cancer growth in animal tumor models. For example, antisense technology has recently been used to reverse k-*ras* expression in non-small cell lung cancer. A further step has been the recent approval for a human gene therapy protocol that will test whether antisense k-*ras* and wild-type p53 constructs are capable of retarding non-small cell lung cancer. Several other human gene therapy experiments have been approved for the treatment of various types of cancers[192,193] (also Kulver K, personal communication). In a similar vein, modulation of MDR gene products (P-glycoprotein) remains an important area of investigation (Table 61-13). Insertion of the MDR-1 gene into normal bone marrow hematopoietic stem cells may allow for extreme chemotherapy dose escalations.[194] Another example is the modulation of programmed cell death or apoptosis in indolent or slowly growing neoplasms. Follicular lymphomas carry a characteristic chromosomal translocation t(14;18) that involves the *bcl*-2 oncogene. The latter normally aides in apoptosis, but its altered expression causes an inhibition of programmed cell death. This results in persistent follicular lymphoma. Genetic alteration of *bcl*-2 may help us provide better treatment of these neoplasms.[194] Finally, designs of gene therapy protocols are limited by efficient gene transfer/delivery in vivo and the transient nature of inserted gene expression.[195] It is likely that, in cancer, gene therapy will be used in conjunction with existing cytokines and chemotherapy to achieve the best possible results.

REFERENCES

1. Marshall EK Jr: Historical perspectives in chemotherapy. p. 1. In Goldin A, Hawking IF (eds): Advances in Chemotherapy. Vol. 1. Academic Press, San Diego, 1964
2. Hertz R, Lewis J Jr, Lipsett M: Five years experience with chemotherapy of metastatic choriocarcinoma and related trophoblastic tumors in women. Am J Obstet Gynecol 82:631, 1961
3. DeVita VT: The evolution of therapeutic research in cancer. N Engl J Med 298:907, 1978
4. Skipper HE: Historic milestones in cancer biology: a few that are important to cancer treatment (revisited). Semin Oncol 6:506, 1979
5. Tubiana M: Tumor cell proliferation kinetics and tumor growth rate. Acta Oncol 2:113, 1989
6. Steel GG: Autoradiographic analysis of the cell cycle: Howard and Pelc to the present day. Int J Radiat Biol 49:227, 1986
7. Dressler LG, Bartow SA: DNA flow cytometry in solid tumors: practical aspects and clinical applications. Semin Diagn Pathol 6:55, 1989
8. Merkel DE, McGuire WL: Ploidy, proliferative activity and prognosis. Cancer 65:1194, 1990
9. Clark GM, Dressler LG, Owens MA et al: Prediction of relapse or survival in patients with node-negative breast cancer by DNA flow cytometry. N Engl J Med 320:627, 1989
10. Look AT, Robertson PK, Williams DL, et al: Prognostic importance of blast cell DNA content in childhood acute lymphoblastic leukemia. Blood 65:1079, 1985
11. Raza A, Preisler HD, Day R et al: Direct relationship between remission duration in acute myeloid leukemia and cell cycle kinetics. A leukemia Intergroup Study. Blood 76:2191, 1990
12. Preisler HD, Raza A, Larson R et al: Some reasons for the lack of progress in the treatment of acute myelogenous leukemia. Leuk Res 15:773, 1991
13. Raza A, Preisler HD, Lampkin B et al: Clinical and prognostic significance of in vivo differentiation in acute myelogenous leukemia. Am J Hematol 42:147, 1993
14. Heppner GH: Tumor heterogeneity. Cancer Res 44:2259, 1984
15. Schnipper LE: Clinical implications of tumor-cell heterogeneity. N Engl J Med 314:1423, 1986
16. Goldie JH, Coldman AJ: Quantitative model for multiple levels of drug resistance in tumors. Cancer Treat Rep 67:923, 1983
17. Hryniuk W, Bush H: The importance of dose intensity in chemotherapy of metastatic breast cancer. J Clin Oncol 2:1281, 1984
18. Boyd MR: Status of the NCI preclinical antitumor drug discovery screen. Principles and Practice of Oncology (PPO) Updates 3:1, 1989
19. Grever MR, Schepartz SA, Chabner BA: The National Cancer Institute: Cancer Drug Discovery and Development Program. Semin Oncol 19:622, 1992
20. Rygaard J, Povisen CO: Athymic (nude) mice. p. 51. In Foster HL, Small JD, Fox JG (eds): The Mouse in Biochemical Research. Vol VI. Academic Press, San Diego, 1982
21. Wittes RE, Leventhal BG (eds): Research Methods in Clinical Oncology. Raven Press, New York, 1988

22. Price CC: Chemistry of alkylation. p. 1. In Sartorelli AC, Johns DG (eds): Antineoplastic and Immunosuppressive Agents. Part II. Handbuch der Experimentellen Pharmakologie. Vol. 38. Springer-Verlag, Berlin, 1975
23. Vaupel P, Jain RK (eds): Tumor Blood Supply and Metabolic Microenvironment. Fischer, Stuttgart, 1991, p. 1
24. Boucher Y, Baxter LT, Jain RK: Interstitial pressure gradients in tissue-isolated and subcutaneous tumors: implications for therapy. Cancer Res 50:4478, 1990
25. Gerlach JH, Kartner N, Bell DR, Ling V: Multidrug resistance. Cancer Surv 5:25, 1986
26. Bradley G, Juranka PF, Ling V: Mechanisms of multidrug resistance. Biochim Biophys Acta 948:87, 1988
27. Biedler JL: Genetic aspects of multidrug resistance. Cancer 70:1799, 1992
28. Dano K: Active outward transport of daunomycin in resistant Ehrlich ascites tumor cells. Biochim Biophys Acta 323:466, 1973
29. Juliano RL, Ling V: A surface glycoprotein modulating drug permeability in Chinese hamster ovary cell mutants. Biochim Biophys Acta 455:152, 1976
30. Hamada H, Okochi E, Oh-hara T, Tsuruo T: Purification of the M_r 22,000 calcium-binding protein (Sorcin) associated with multidrug resistance and its detection with monoclonal antibodies. Cancer Res 48:3173, 1988
31. Pastan I, Gottesman MM, Ueda K et al: A retrovirus carrying an MDR1 cDNA confers multidrug resistance and polarized expression of P-glycoprotein in MDCK cells. Proc Natl Acad Sci USA 85:4486, 1988
32. Riordan JR, Ling V: Genetic and biochemical characterization of multidrug resistance. Pharmacol Ther 28:51, 1985
33. Trent JM, Witkowski CM: Clarification of the chromosomal assignment of the human P-glycoprotein/MDR-1 gene: possible coincidence with the cystic fibrosis and c-met oncogene. Cancer Genet Cytogenet 26:187, 1987
34. Chin KV, Ueda K, Pastan I, Gottesman MM: Modulation of activity of the promoter of the human MDR1 gene by Ras and p53. Science 255:459, 1992
35. NG WF, Sarangi F, Sastawny RL et al: Identification of members of the P-glycoprotein multigene family. Mol Cell Biol 9:1224, 1989
36. Cole SPC, Bhardwaj G, Gerlach JN et al: Overexpression of a transporter gene in a multidrug resistant human lung cancer cell line. Science 258:1650, 1993
37. Georges E, Tsuruo T, Ling V: Topology of P-glycoprotein as determined by epitope mapping of MRK-16 monoclonal antibody. J Biol Chem 268:1792, 1993
38. Kajiji S, Talbot F, Grizzuti K et al: Functional analysis of P-glycoprotein mutants identifies predicted transmembrane domain 11 as a putative drug binding site. Biochemistry 32:4185, 1993
39. Loo TW, Clarke DM: Functional consequences of proline mutations in the predicted transmembrane domain of P-glycoprotein. J Biol Chem 268:3143, 1993
40. Devine SE, Ling V, Melera PW: Amino acid substitutions in the sixth transmembrane domain of P-glycoprotein alter multidrug resistance. Proc Natl Acad Sci USA 89:4564, 1992
41. Chambers TC, Pohl J, Raynor RL, Kuo JF: Identification of specific sites in human P-glycoprotein phosphorylated by protein kinase C. J Biol Chem 268:4592, 1993
42. Dellinger M, Pressman BC, Calderon-Higginson C et al: Structural requirements of simple organic cations for recognition by multi-drug resistant cells. Cancer Res 52:6385, 1992
43. Abraham E, Prat AG, Gerweck L et al: The multidrug resistance (mdr1) gene product functions as an ATP channel. Proc Natl Acad Sci USA 90:312, 1993
44. Valverde MA, Diaz M, Sepulveda FV et al: Volume-regulated chloride channels associated with the human multidrug-resistance P-glycoprotein. Nature 355:830, 1992
45. Cordon CC, O'Brien JP, Casals D et al: Multidrug-resistance gene (P-glycoprotein) is expressed by endothelial cells at the blood-brain barrier sites. Proc Natl Acad Sci USA 86:695, 1989
46. Muesch A, Hartman E, Rohde K et al: A novel pathway for secretory proteins? Trends Biochem Sci 2:86, 1990
47. Arceci RJ: Clinical significance of P-glycoprotein in multidrug-resistance malignancies. Blood 81:2215, 1993
48. Chambers TC, Raynor RL, Kuo JF: Multidrug resistant human KB carcinoma cells are highly resistant to the protein phosphatase inhibitors okadaic acid and calyculin A. Analysis of potential mechanisms involved in toxin resistance. Int J Cancer 53:323, 1993
49. Delannoy IA, Silverman M: The MDR-1 gene product, P-glycoprotein, mediates the transport of the cardiac glycoside, digoxin. Biochem Biophys Res Commun 189:551, 1992
50. Ueda K, Okamura N, Hirai M et al: Human P-glycoprotein transports cortisol, aldosterone and dexamethasone, but not progesterone. J Biol Chem 267:24248, 1992
51. Becker KF, Allmeier H, Hollt V: New mechanisms of hormone secretion:

MDR-like gene products as extrusion pumps for hormones? Horm Metab Res 24:210, 1992

52. Gill DR, Hyde SC, Higgins CF et al: Separation of drug transport and chloride channel function of the human multidrug resistance P-glycoprotein. Cell 71: 23, 1992

53. Sharma RC, Inoue S, Roitelman J et al: Peptide transport by the multidrug resistance pump. J Biol Chem 267:5731, 1992

54. Higgins CF, Gottesman MM: Is the multidrug transporter a flippase? Trends Biochem Sci 17:18, 1992

55. Smit JJM, Schinkel AH, OudeElferink RPJ et al: Homozygous Disruption of the murine mdr2 P-glycoprotein gene leads to a complete absence of phospholipid from bile and to liver disease. Cell 75:451, 1993

56. Goldstein LJ, Galski H, Fojo A et al: Expression of a multidrug resistance gene in human cancers. J Natl Cancer Inst 81:116, 1989

57. Kacinski B, Yee LD, Carter D: Quantitation of tumor cell expression of the P-glycoprotein (mdr1) gene in human breast carcinoma clinical specimens. Cancer Bull 41:44, 1989

58. Dalton WS, Grogan TM, Rybski JA et al: Immunohistochemical detection and quantitation of P-glycoprotein in multiple drug-resistant myeloma cells: association with level of drug resistance and drug accumulation. Blood 73: 747, 1989

59. Ludescher C, Thaler J, Drach D et al: Detection of activity of P-glycoprotein in human tumor samples using rhodamine 123. Br J Haematol 82:161, 1992

60. Piwnica-Worms D, Chiu ML, Budding M et al: Functional imaging of multidrug resistant P-glycoprotein with an organotechnetium complex. Cancer Res 53:977, 1993

61. Thiebaut F, Tsuruo T, Hamada H et al: Cellular localization of the multidrug-resistance gene product P-glycoprotein in normal human tissues. Proc Natl Acad Sci USA 84:7735, 1987

62. Sugawara I, Kataoka I, Morishita Y et al: Tissue distribution of P-glycoprotein encoded by a multidrug-resistant gene as revealed by a monoclonal antibody, MRK-16. Cancer Res 48:1926, 1988

63. Hitchins RN, Harman DH, Davey RA, Bell DR: Identification of a multidrug resistance associated antigen (P-glycoprotein) in normal human tissues. Eur J Cancer Clin Oncol 24:449, 1988

64. Chaudhary PM, Roninson IB: Expression and activity of P-glycoprotein, a multidrug efflux pump, in human hematopoietic stem cells. Cell 66:85, 1991

65. Drach D, Shourong Z, Johannes D et al: Subpopulations of normal peripheral blood and bone marrow cells express a functional multidrug resistant phenotype. Blood 80:2729, 1992

66. Buschman E, Arceci RJ, Croop JM et al: MDR-2 encodes P-glycoprotein expressed in the bile canalicular membrane as determined by isoform specific antibodies. J Biol Chem 267:18093, 1992

67. Chin JE, Soffir R, Noonan KE et al: Structure and expression of the human mdr (P-glycoprotein) gene family. Mol Cell Biol 9:3808, 1989

68. Yamamoto T, Iwasaki T, Watanabe Y et al: Expression of multidrug resistance P-glycoprotein on peripheral blood mononuclear cells of patients with granular lymphocyte proliferative disorders. Blood 81:1342, 1993

69. VanKalken C, Giaccone G, Van der Valk P et al: Multidrug resistance gene (P-glycoprotein) expression in the human fetus. Am J Pathol 141:1063, 1992

70. Hegewisch-Becker S, Fliegner M et al: P-glycoprotein expression in normal and reactive bone marrows. Br J Cancer 67:430, 1993

71. Garberoglio C, Dudas M, Casper ES et al: Expression of P-glycoprotein in normal muscle cells and myogenic tumors. Arch Pathol Lab Med 116:1055, 1992

72. Schneider J, Efferth T, Centeno MM et al: High rate of expression of multidrug resistance-associated P-glycoprotein in human endometrial carcinoma and normal endometrial tissue. Eur J Cancer 29A:554, 1993

73. Ito Y, Tanimoto M, Kumazawa T et al: Increased P-glycoprotein expression and multidrug-resistant gene (mdr1) amplification are infrequently found in fresh acute leukemia cells. Cancer 63:1534, 1989

74. Miller TP, Grogan TM, Spier CM, Salmon SE: High-dose verapamil infusion added to chemotherapy reverses drug resistance in lymphoma patients in relapse. Proc Am Soc Clin Oncol 8:252, 1989

75. List AF, Glinsmann-Gibson B: Multidrug resistance and its pharmacologic modulation in acute myeloid leukemia. p. 178. In Foster JG, Rhodes JE (eds): Accomplishments in Cancer Research. JB Lippincott, Philadelphia, 1992

76. Sato H, Preisler H, Day R et al: mdr1 transcript levels as an indication of resistant disease in acute myelogenous leukemia. Br J Haematol 75:340, 1990

77. Herweijer H, Sonneveld P, Boas F et al: Expression of MDR1 and MDR3 multidrug resistant genes in human acute and chronic leukemias in association with stimulation of drug accumulation by cyclosporine. J Natl Cancer Inst 82:1133, 1990

78. Zhou DC, Marie JP, Suberville AM et al: Relevance of mdr1 gene expression in acute myeloid leukemia and comparison of different diagnostic methods. Leukemia 6:879, 1992

79. Musto P, Melillo L, Lombardi G et al: High risk of early relapse for leukemic patients with presence of multidrug resistance associated with P-glycoprotein positive cells in complete remission. Br J Haematol 77:50, 1991

80. Homes J, Jacobs A, Carter G et al: Multidrug resistance in hematopoietic cell lines, myelodysplastic syndromes and acute myeloblastic leukemia. Br J Haematol 72:40, 1989

81. Nooter K, Sonneveld P, Oostrum R et al: Overexpression of the mdr 1 gene in blast cells from patients with acute myelocytic leukemia is associated with decreased anthracycline accumulation that can be restored by cyclosporine. Int J Cancer 45:263, 1990

82. Ivy SP, Smith JK, Speciale A et al: Detection of mdr1 gene expression using polymerase chain reaction (PCR) in childhood acute lymphoblastic leukemia (ALL) at diagnosis. Proc Am Assoc Cancer Res 33:473A, 1992

83. Rothenberg ML, Mickley LA, Cole DE et al: Expression of the mdr1/P-170 gene in patients with acute lymphoblastic leukemia. Blood 74:1388, 1989

84. Pieters R, Hongo T, Loonen AH et al: Different types of non-P-glycoprotein mediated multiple drug resistance in children with relapsed acute lymphoblastic leukemia. Br J Cancer 65:691, 1992

85. Kuwazuru Y, Hanada S, Furukawa T et al: Expression of P-glycoprotein in adult T-cell leukemia cells. Blood 76:2065, 1990

86. Holmes JA, Jacobs A, Carter G et al: Is the mdr1 gene relevant in chronic lymphocytic leukemia? Leukemia 4:216, 1990

87. Miller TP, Grogan TM, Dalton WS et al: P-glycoprotein expression in malignant lymphoma and reversal of clinical drug resistance with chemotherapy plus high dose verapamil. J Clin Oncol 9:17, 1991

88. Grogan TM, Spier CM, Salmon SE et al: P-glycoprotein expression in human plasma cell myeloma: correlation with prior chemotherapy. Blood 81:490, 1993

89. Ludescher C, Hilbe W, Eisterer W et al: Activity of P-glycoprotein in B-cell chronic lymphocytic leukemia determined by flow cytometric assay. J Natl Cancer Inst 85:1751, 1993

90. Rischin D, Ling V: Multidrug resistance in leukemia. Cancer Treat Res 64: 269, 1993

91. List AF, Spier CM: Multidrug resistance in acute leukemia: a conserved physiologic function. Leuk Lymphoma 8:9, 1992

92. List AF: Multidrug resistance: clinical relevance in acute leukemia. Oncology 7:23, 1993

93. Campos L, Guyotat D, Archimbaud E et al: Clinical significance of multidrug-resistance P-glycoprotein expression on acute nonlymphoblastic leukemia cells at diagnosis. Blood 79:473, 1992

94. Marie JP, Zittoun R, Sikic BI: Multidrug resistance (mdr1) gene expression in adult acute leukemias: correlations with treatment outcome and in vitro drug sensitivity. Blood 78:586, 1991

95. Pirker R, Wallner J, Geissler K et al: MDR1 gene expression and treatment outcome in acute myeloidleukemia. J Natl Cancer Inst 83:708, 1991

96. Willman CL, Kopecky K, Griffith B et al: Multiparameter analysis of the expression of the multidrug resistance genes mdr1 and mdr2 (mdr3) in de novo AML by polymerase chain reaction in multicolor flow cytometry: identification of a biological subset of CD34+, mdr1+ AML cases. Blood, suppl 1. 78:172A, 1991

97. Willman CL, Kopecky KJ, Chen IM et al: Biologic parameters that predict response in de nove acute myeloid leukemia: CD34, but not multidrug-resistance gene expression, is associated with decreased complete remission (CR) rate and CD34 patients more frequently achieve CR with high-dose cytosine arabinoside. Proc Am Soc Clin Oncol 11:264a, 1992

98. Carulli G, Petrini M, Marini A et al: P-glycoprotein in acute nonlymphoblastic leukemia and in the blastic crisis of myeloid leukemia. N Engl J Med 319: 797, 1988

99. Goagsuen JE, Dossot JM, Fardel O et al: Expression of the multidrug-resistance associated P-glycoprotein (P-170) in 59 cases of de novo acute lymphoblastic leukemia prognostic implications. Blood 81:2394, 1993

100. Epstein J, Xiao H, Oba BK: P-glycoprotein expression in plasma cell myeloma is associated with resistance to VAD. Blood 74:913, 1989

101. Lum BL, Gosland MP, Kaubisch S, Sikic BI: Molecular targets in oncology: implications of the multidrug resistance gene. Pharmacotherapy 13:88, 1993

102. Chan HSL, Thorner PS, Haddad G, Ling V: Immunohistochemical detection of P-glycoprotein: prognostic correlation in soft tissue sarcoma of childhood. J Clin Oncol 8:689, 1990

103. Chan HSL, Haddad G, Thorner PS et al: P-glycoprotein expression as a predictor of the outcome of therapy for neuroblastoma. N Engl J Med 325:1608, 1991

104. Akiyama SI, Cornwell MM, Kuwano M et al: Most drugs that reverse multidrug resistance also inhibit photoaffinity labeling of P-glycoprotein by a vinblastine analog. Mol Pharmacol 33:144, 1988

105. Krishan A, Sauerteig A, Gordon K: Effect of amphotericin on adriamycin transport in P388 cells. Cancer Res 45:4097, 1985

106. Chauffert B, Martin M, Hammann A et al: Amiodarone-induced enhancement of doxorubicin and 4'-deoxydoxorubicin cytotoxicity to rat colon cancer cells in vitro and in vivo. Cancer Res 46:825, 1986

107. Chauffert B, Rey D, Coudert B et al: Amiodarone is more efficient than verapamil in reversing resistance to anthracyclines in tumor cells. Br J Cancer 56:119, 1987

108. Gosland MP, Lum BL, Sikic BI: Modulation of multidrug resistance by cephalosporin antibiotics: structure-activity relationships with human P-glycoprotein. Proc Am Assoc Cancer Res 30:567, 1989

109. Slater LM, Sweet P, Stupecky M et al: Cyclosporin A corrects daunorubicin resistance in Ehrlich ascites carcinoma. Br J Cancer 54:235, 1986

110. Twentyman PR: A possible role for cyclosporins in cancer chemotherapy. Anticancer Res 8:985, 1988

111. Hait WN, Stein JM, Koletsky AJ et al: Modulation of doxorubicin (DOX) resistance by cyclosporin-A (CsA) and a non-immunosuppressive homolog. Proc Am Assoc Cancer Res 28:298, 1987

112. Safa AR, Choe MM, Morrow M, Manley SA: Cyclosporin A and its nonimmunosuppressive analogs reverse vinca alkaloid resistance by interacting with P-glycoprotein. Proc Am Assoc Cancer Res 30:498, 1989

113. Klohs WD, Steinkampf RW, Havlick MJ, Jackson RC: Resistance to anthrapyrazoles and anthracyclines in multidrug-resistant P-388 murine leukemia cells: reversal by calcium channel blockers and calmodulin antagonists. Cancer Res 46:4352, 1986

114. Yalowich JC, Ross WE: Potentiation of etoposide-induced DNA damage by calcium antagonists in L1210 cells in vitro. Cancer Res 44:3360, 1984

115. Shalinsky DR, Howell SB: Synergistic enhancement of the cytotoxicity of vinblastine (VBL) and colchicine (COL) by dipyridamole (DPM) in drug-resistant KB carcinoma cells. Proc Am Assoc Cancer Res 30:2097, 1989

116. Tsuruo T, Iida H, Tsukagoshi S, Sakurai Y: Increased accumulation of vincristine and Adriamycin in drug-resistant tumor cells following incubation with calcium antagonists and calmodulin inhibitors. Cancer Res 42:4730, 1982

117. Corrias MV, Tonini GP: An oligomer complementary to the 5' end region of MDR1 gene decreases resistance to doxorubicin of human adenocarcinoma-resistant cells. Anticancer Res 12:1431, 1992

118. Ford JM, Prozialeck WC, Hait W: Structural features determining activity of phenothiazines and related drugs for inhibition of cell growth and reversal of multidrug resistance. Mol Pharmacol 35:105, 1989

119. Yang CPH, DePinho SG, Greenberger LM et al: Progesterone interacts with P-glycoprotein in multidrug-resistant cells and in the endometrium of gravid uterus. J Biol Chem 264:782, 1989

120. Tsuruo T, Iida H, Kitatani Y et al: Effects of quinidine and related compounds on cytotoxicity and cellular accumulation of vincristine and adriamycin in drug-resistant tumor cells. Cancer Res 44:4303, 1984

121. Willigham MC, Cornwell MM, Cardarell CO et al: Single cell analysis of daunorubicin uptake and efflux in multidrug-resistant and -sensitive KB cells: effects of verapamil and other drugs. Cancer Res 46:5941, 1986

122. Ramu A, Glaubiger D, Fuks Z: Reversal of acquired resistance to doxorubicin P388 murine leukemia cells by tamoxifen and other triparanol analogues. Cancer Res 44:4392, 1984

123. Kesse D: Interactions among membrane transport systems: anthracyclines, calcium antagonists and anti-estrogens. Biochem Pharmacol 35:2825, 1986

124. Naito M, Tsuruo T: Competitive inhibition by verapamil of ATP-dependent high affinity vincristine binding to the plasma membrane of multidrug resistance K 562 cells without calcium ion involvement. Cancer Res 49:1452, 1989

125. Arceci RJ, Stieglitz K, Bierer BE: Immunosuppressants FK506 and rapamycin function as reversal agents of the multidrug resistance phenotype. Blood 80:1528, 1992

126. Dalton WS, Grogan TM, Meltzer PS et al: Drug-resistance in multiple myeloma and non-Hodgkin's lymphoma: detection of P-glycoprotein and potential circumvention by addition of verapamil to chemotherapy. J Clin Oncol 7:415, 1989

127. Schneider J, Bak M, Efferth T et al: P-glycoprotein expression in treated and untreated human breast cancer. Br J Cancer 60:815, 1989

128. Niehans GA, Jaazcz W, Brunetto V et al: Immunohistochemical identification of P-glycoprotein in previously untreated, diffuse large cell and immunoblastic lymphomas. Cancer Res 52:3768, 1992

129. List AF, Spier C, Green J et al: Biochemical modulation of anthracycline resistance (MDR) in acute Leukemia with cyclosporin-A. Proc Am Soc Clin Oncol 11:264a, 1992

130. Slater L, Sweet P, Stupecky M, Gupta S: Cyclosporin-A reverses vincristine and daunorubicin resistance in acute lymphatic leukemia in vitro. J Clin Invest 77:1405, 1986

131. Trump D, Rogers M, Fine R et al: Phase I trial of high dose tamoxifen and five day infusion of vinblastine as an approach to reverse multidrug resistance. Proc Am Assoc Cancer Res 31:205, 1990

132. Miller RL, Bukowski RM, Budd GT et al: Clinical modulation of doxorubicin resistance by the calmodulin inhibitor trifluoperazine: A phase I trial. J Clin Oncol 6:880, 1988

133. Yahanda AM, Adler KM, Fisher GA et al: A phase I trial of etoposide with cyclosporine as a modulator of multidrug resistance. J Clin Oncol 10:1624, 1992

134. List AF, Spier C, Greer J et al: Biochemical modulation of anthracycline resistance (MDR) in acute leukemia with cyclosporine A. Proc Am Assoc Cancer Res 11:264, 1992

135. Jones BL, Dalton W, Fisher GA, Sikic BI: Reversal of multidrug resistance to cancer chemotherapy. Cancer 72:3484, 1993

136. Kellhauer E, Emling F, Raschack M et al: The use of R-verapamil (R-VPM) is superior to racemic VPM in breaking multidrug resistance (MDR) of malignant cells. Proc Am Assoc Cancer Res 30:503, 1989

137. Twentyman PR, Bleehan NM: Resistance modification by PSC-833, a novel nonimmunosuppressive cyclosporine A. Eur J Cancer 27:1639, 1991

138. Mickisch GH, Pastan I, Gottesman MM: Multidrug resistant transgenic mice as anivel pharmacologic tool. Bioassays 13:381, 1991

139. Fernandes DJ, Catapano CV, Townsend AJ: Topoisomerase related mechanisms of drug resistance. p. 479. In Teicher BA (ed): Drug Resistance in Oncology. Marcel Dekker, New York, 1993

140. Hertzberg RP, Busby RW, Caranfa MJ et al: Irreversible trapping of the DNA-topoisomerase I covalent complex: affinity labelling of the camptothecin binding site. J Biol Chem 265:19287, 1990

141. Liu LF: DNA topoisomerase poisons as antitumor drugs. Annu Rev Biochem 58:351, 1989

142. Long BH, Wang L, Lorico A et al: Mechanisms of resistance to etoposide and teniposide in acquired resistant human colon and lung carcinoma cells. Cancer Res 51:5275, 1991

143. Danks MK, Yalowich JC, Beck WT: Atypical multiple drug resistance in a human leukemic cell line selected for resistance to teniposide (VM-26). Cancer Res 47:1297, 1987

144. Danks MK, Schmidt CA, Cirtain MC et al: Altered catalytic activity of and DNA cleavage by DNA topoisomerase II from human leukemic cells selected for resistance to VM-26. Biochemistry 27:8861, 1988

145. Harker WG, Slade DL, Dalton WS et al: Multidrug resistance in mitoxantrone-selected HL-60 leukemia cells in the absence of P-glycoprotein overexpression. Cancer Res 49:4542, 1989

146. Takano H, Kohno K, Ono M et al: Increased phosphorylation of DNA topoisomerase II in etoposide-resistant mutants of human cancer KB cells. Cancer Res 51:3951, 1991

147. Takano H, Kohno K, Ono M et al: Increased phosphorylation of DNA topoisomerase II in etoposide-resistant mutants of human cancer KB cells. Cancer Res 51:3951, 1991

148. Hinds M, Deisseroth K, Mayes J et al: Identification of a point mutation in the topoisomerase II gene from a human leukemia cell line containing an amsacrine-resistant form of topoisomerase II. Cancer Res 51:4729, 1991

149. Fernandes DJ, Catapano CV: Nuclear matrix targets for anticancer agents. Cancer Cells 3:134, 1991

150. Zhang H, D'Arpa P, Liu LF: A model for tumor cell killing by topoisomerase poisons. Cancer Cells 2:23, 1990

151. Eng WK, McCabe FL, Tan KB et al: Development of stable camptothecin-resistant tumor cell subline of P388 leukemia with reduced topoisomerase content. Mol Pharmacol 38:471, 1990

152. Sugimoto Y, Tsukahara S, Oh-hara T et al: Decreased expression of DNA topoisomerase I in camptothecin-resistant tumor cell lines as determined by a monoclonal antibody. Cancer Res 50:6925, 1990

153. Meister A: Glutathione metabolism and its selective modification. J Biol Chem 263:17205, 1988

154. Ozols RF, Louie KG, Plowman J et al: Enhanced melphalan cytotoxicity in human ovarian cancer in vitro and in tumor-bearing nude mice by buthionine sulfoximine depletion by glutathione. Biochem Pharmacol 36:147, 1987

155. Friedman HS, Colvin OM, Griffith OW et al: Increased melphalan activity in intracranial human medulloblastoma and glioma xenografts following buthionine sulfoximine-mediated glutathione depletion. J Natl Cancer Inst 81:524, 1989

156. Lai GM, Ozols RF, Young RC, Hamilton TC: Effect of glutathione on DNA repair in cisplatin-resistant human ovarian cancer cell lines. J Natl Cancer Inst 81:535, 1989

157. Moscow JA, Fairchild CR, Madden MJ et al: Expression of anionic glutathione-S-transferase and P-glycoprotein genes in human tissues and tumors. Cancer Res 49:1422, 1989

158. Fairchild CR, Moscow JA, Cowan KH: Effect of GST-Pi expression on the pattern of the P-glycoprotein. Proc Am Assoc Cancer Res 30:2100, 1989

159. Singh SV, Nair S, Ahmad H et al: Glutathione S-transferase isoenzymes in doxorubicin sensitive and resistant cells. Proc Am Assoc Cancer Res 30:2096, 1989

160. Schisselbauer JC, Silber R, Papadopoulos E et al: Characterization of glutathione S-transferase expression in lymphocytes from chronic lymphocytic leukemia patients. Cancer Res 50:3562, 1990

161. Lewis AD, Hayes JD, Wolf CR: Glutathione and glutathione dependant enzymes in ovarian adenocarcinoma cell lines derived from a patient before and after the onset of drug resistance: intrinsic differences and cell cycle effects. Carcinogenesis 9:1283, 1988

162. Bohr VA, Phillips DW, Hanawalt PC: Heterogeneous DNA damage and repair in the mammalian genome. Cancer Res 47:6426, 1987

163. Fox M, Roberts JJ: Drug resistance and DNA repair. Cancer Metast Rev 6: 261, 1987

164. Berger NA, Berger SJ, Gerson SL: DNA-repair, ADP-ribosylation and pyridine nucleotide metabolism as targets for cancer chemotherapy. Anticancer Drug Des 2:203, 1987

165. Chen G, Pan Q: Potentiation of the antitumor activity of cisplatin in mice by 3-aminobenzamide and nicotinamide. Cancer Chemother Pharmacol 22: 303, 1988

166. DeGraeff A, Slebos RJC, Rodenhuis S: Resistance to cisplatin and analogues: mechanisms and potential clinical applications. Cancer Chemother Pharmacol 22:325, 1988

167. Seguin C, Felber BK, Carter AD, Hamer DH: Competition for cellular factors that activate metallothionein gene transcription. Nature 312:781, 1984

168. Jahroudi N, Foster R, Price-Haughey J et al: Cell-type specific and differential regulation of the human metallothionien genes. J Biol Chem 265:6506, 1990

169. Kelley SL, Basu A, Teicher BA et al: Overexpression of metallothionein confers resistance to anticancer drugs. Science 241:1813, 1988

170. Basu A, Lazo JS: A hypothesis regarding the protective role of metallothioneins against the toxicity of DNA interactive anticancer drugs. Toxicol Lett 50:123, 1990

171. Farnworth P, Hillcott B, Roos I: Metallothionein like proteins and cell resistance to cis-dichlorodiammenplatinum (II) in L1210 cells. Cancer Chemother Pharmacol 25:411, 1990

172. Schilder RJ, Hall L, Monks A et al: Metallothionein gene expression and resistance to cisplatin in human ovarian cancer. Int J Cancer 45:416, 1990

173. Hall KS, Endersen L, Huitfeldt HE: Induction of in vitro resistance to 4′-epidoxorubicin and cis-diamminedichloroplatinum in hepatoma cells. Anticancer Res 11:817, 1991

174. Thornalley P, Vasak M: Possible role for metallothionein in protection against radiation induced oxidative stress. Kinetics and mechanism of its reaction with superoxide and hydroxyl radicals. Biochim Biophys Acta 827: 36, 1985

175. Kaina B, Lohrer H, Karin M, Herrlich P: Overexpressed human metallothionein IIA gene protects Chinese hamster ovary cells from killing by alkylating agents. Carcinogenesis 10:2279, 1989

176. Lohrer H, Robson T: Overexpression of metallothionein in CE-10 cells and its effect on cell killing by ionizing radiation and alkylating agents. Carcinogenesis 10:2279, 1989

177. Sato M, Naganuma A, Imura N: Involvement of cardiac metallothionein in prevention of Adriamycin induced lipid peroxidation in the heart. Toxicology 53:231, 1988

178. Naganuma A, Sato M, Imura N: Specific reduction of side effects of adriamycin by induction of metallothionein in mice. Jpn J Cancer Res 79:406, 1988

179. Sato M, Imura N, Naganuma A et al: Prevention of adverse effects of X-ray irradiation after metallothionein induction by bismuth subnitrate in mice. Eur J Cancer Clin Oncol 25:1727, 1989

180. Endersen L, Bakka A, Rugstad HE: Increased resistance to chlorambucil in cultured cells with high concentration of cytoplasmic metallothionein. Cancer Res 43:2918, 1983

181. Lohrer H, Robson T, Grindley H et al: Differential effects on cell killing in metallothionein overexpressing CHO mutant cell lines. Carcinogenesis 11: 1937, 1990

182. Saijo N, Lazo JS: Metallothionein in drug resistance. p. 347. In Teicher BA (ed): Drug Resistance in Oncology. Marcel Dekker, New York, 1993

183. Fry DW, Jackson RC: Membrane transport alterations as a mechanism of resistance to anticancer agents. Cancer Surv 5:47, 1986

184. Waud WR: Differential uptake of cis-diamminedichloroplatinum (II) by sensitive and resistant murine L1210 leukemia cells. Cancer Res 47:6549, 1987

185. Andrews PA, Velury S, Mann SC, Howell SB: Cis-diamminedichloroplatinum (II) accumulation in sensitive and resistant human ovarian carcinoma cells. Cancer Res 48:68, 1988

186. Ferguson PJ, Fisher MH, Stephenson J et al: Combined modalities of resistance in etoposide-resistant human KB cell lines. Cancer Res 48:5956, 1988

187. Kerbel RS, MacDougall JR: Possible contribution of growth factors to the evolution of metastasis and de novo resistance in cancer. p. 583. In Teicher BA (ed): Drug Resistance in Oncology. Marcel Dekker, New York, 1993

188. Burris HA, Rothenberg ML, Kuhn JG et al: Clinical trials with the Topoisomerase I inhibitors. Semin Oncol 19:663, 1992

189. Rowinsky EK, Onetto N, Canetta RM, Arbuck SG: Taxol: the first of the taxanes, an important new class of antitumor agents. Semin Oncol 19:646, 1992

190. Goldenberg DM: Monoclonal antibodies in cancer detection and therapy. Am J Med 94:297, 1993

191. Brugge JS: New Intracellular targets for therapeutic drug design. Science 260:918, 1993

192. Anderson WF: Human gene therapy. Science 256:808, 1992

193. Miller AD: Human gene therapy comes of age. Nature 357:455, 1992

194. Chabner BA: Biological basis for cancer treatment. Ann Intern Med 118:633, 1993

195. Mulligan RC: The basic science of gene therapy. Science 260:926, 1993

196. Colvin M: The alkylating agents. p. 276. In Chabner BA (ed): Pharmacologic Principles of Cancer Chemotherapy. WB Saunders, Philadelphia, 1982

197. Balis FM: Pharmacokinetic drug interactions of commonly used anticancer drugs. Clin Pharmacokinet 11:223, 1986

198. Connors TA: Alkylating agents. Can Chem Biol Resp Mod 13:31, 1992

199. Webberley MJ, Murray JA: Life-threatening acute hyponatremia induced by low dose cyclophosphamide and indomethacin. Postgrad Med J 65:950, 1989

200. Nomoto K, Eto M, Yanaga K et al: Interference with cyclophosphamide-induced skin allograft tolerance by cyclosporin A. J Immunol 149:2668, 1992

201. Zalupski M, Baker LH: Ifosfamide. J Natl Cancer Inst 80:556, 1988

202. Hall G, Lind MJ, Huang M et al: Intravenous infusions of ifosfamide/mesna and perturbation of warfarin anticoagulant control. Postgrad Med J 66:860, 1990

203. Loehrer PJ, Einhorn LH, Williams SD: VP-16 plus ifosfamide plus cisplatin as salvage therapy in refractory germ cell cancer. J Clin Oncol 4:528, 1986

204. Cabanillas F, Hagemeister FB, Bodey GP et al: IMVP-16: an effective regimen for patients with lymphomas who have relapsed after initial combination chemotherapy. Blood 6:693, 1982

205. Morgenstern GR, Powles R, Robinson B et al: Cyclosporine interaction with ketoconazole and melphalan, letter. Lancet 2:1342, 1982

206. Lejeune FJ, Lienard D, Leyvraz S et al: Regional therapy of melanoma, review. Eur J Cancer 29A:606, 1993

207. Alberts DS, Chang SY, Chen HSG et al: Pharmacokinetics and metabolism of chlorambucil in man: a preliminary report. Cancer Treat Rev 6:9, 1979

208. Warwick GP: The mechanism of action of alkylating agents. Cancer Res 23: 1315, 1963

209. Kyle RA: A syndrome resembling adrenocortical insufficiency associated with long-term busulfan (myleran) therapy. Blood 18:497, 1961

210. Heard BE, Cooke RA: Busulfan lung. Thorax 23:187, 1968

211. Fitzsimmons WE, Ghalie R, Kaiser H: Anticonvulsants and busulfan, letter. Ann Intern Med 112:552, 1990

212. Levin VA, Hoffman W, Weinkam RJ: Pharmacokinetics of BCNU in man: a preliminary study of 20 patients. Cancer Treat Rep 62:1305, 1978

213. Ginsberg S, Comis R: The pulmonary toxicity of antineoplastic agents. Semin Oncol 9:34, 1982

214. Sponzo RW, DeVita VT, Oliverio VT: Physiologic disposition of 1-(2-chloroethyl)-3-cyclohexyl-1-nitrosourea (CCNU) and 1-(2-chloroethyl)-3-(4-methyl cyclohexyl)-1-nitrosourea (McCCNU) in man. Cancer 31:1154, 1973

215. Adolphe AB, Glasofer ED, Troetel WM et al: Fate of streptozotocin (NSC-85998) in patients with advanced cancer. Cancer Chemother Rep 59:547, 1975

216. Loo TL, Householder CE, Gerulath AH et al: Mechanism of action and pharmacology studies of DTIC (NSC-45399). Cancer Treat Rep 60:149, 1976

217. Merello M, Esteguy M, Perazzo F, Leiguarda R: Impaired levodopa response in Parkinson's disease during melanoma therapy. Clin Neuropharmacol 15: 69, 1992

218. Jackson DV, Castle MC, Bender RA: Biliary excretion of vincristine. Clin Pharmacol Ther 24:101, 1978

219. Owellen RJ, Hartke CA, Hains FO: Pharmacokinetics and metabolism of vinblastine in humans. Cancer Res 37:2597, 1977

220. Dorr RT, Fritz WL: Drug interactions. p. 75. In Pinedo I (ed): Cancer Chemotherapy Handbook. Elsevier Science, New York, 1980

221. Ozols RF, Hogan WM, Ostchega Y et al: MVP (mitomycin, vinblastine, and progesterone): a second line regimen in ovarian cancer with high incidence of pulmonary toxicity. Cancer Treat Rep 67:721, 1983

222. Echizen H, Ishizaki T: A possible drug interaction between cyclophosphamide and digoxin, letter. BMJ 291:1172, 1985

223. Ganapathi R, Hercbergs A, Grabowski D, Ford J: Selective enhancement of vincristine cytotoxicity in multi-drug resistant tumor cells by dilantin (phenytoin). Cancer Res 53:3262, 1993

224. Ross W, Rowe T, Glisson B et al: Role of topoisomerase II in mediating epipodophyllotoxin-induced DNA cleavage. Cancer Res 44:5857, 1984

225. Vogelsang NJ, Raghavan D, Kennedy BJ: VP-16-213 (etoposide): the mandrake root from Issyk-Kul. Am J Med 72:136, 1982

226. O'Dwyer PJ, Alonso MT, Leyland-Jones B, Marsoni S: Teniposide: a review of 12 years of experience. Cancer Treat Rep 68:1455, 1984

227. D'Incalci M, Garattini S: Podophylotoxin derivatives. Can Chem Biol Resp Mod 13:75, 1992

228. Ehninger G, Proksch B, Wanner T et al: Intracellular cytosine arabinoside triphosphate formation in leukemic blast cells is inhibited by etoposide and teniposide. Leukemia 6:582, 1992

229. Howell S: Comparison of the synergistic potentiation of etoposide, doxorubicin and vinblastine cytotoxicity by dipyridamoles. Cancer Res 49:3178, 1989

230. Wampler GL, Carter WH, Campbell ED et al: Exploration of methods for demonstrating therapeutic synergism utilizing a time-interval between the interacting drugs methotrexate and teniposide. Proc Am Assoc Cancer Res 24:268, 1983

231. Baker DK, Relling MV, Pui CH et al: Increased teniposide clearance with concomitant anticonvulsant therapy. J Clin Onc 10:311, 1992

232. Keller RP, Altermatt HJ, Donatsch P et al: Pharmacologic interactions between the resistance-modifying cyclosporine SDZ PSC 833 and etoposide (VP 16-213) enhance in vivo cytostatic activity and toxicity. Int J Cancer 51:433, 1992

233. Sehested M, Jensen PB, Sorensen BS et al: Antagonistic effect of the cardioprotector (+)-1,2-bis (3,5-dioxopiperazinyl-1-yl) propane (ICRF-187) on DNA breaks and cytotoxicity induced by the topoisomerase II directed drugs daunorubicin and etoposide (VP-16). Biochem Pharm 46:389, 1993

234. Yamazaki H, Dilworth A, Myers CE, Sinha BK: Suramin inhibits DNA damage in human prostate cancer cells treated with topoisomerase inhibitors in vitro. Prostate 23:25, 1993

235. Rivera GK, Evans WE: Clinical trials of teniposide (VM-26) in childhood acute lymphocytic leukemia. Semin Oncol 19:51, 1992

236. Sonneveld P: Teniposide in lymphomas and leukemias. Semin Oncol 19:59, 1992

237. Gass GD, Vincent M, Corringham R et al: Teniposide (VM-26) and carboplatin as initial therapy for small cell lung cancer. Semin Oncol 19:69, 1992

238. Pigram WJ, Fuller W, Amilton LDH: Stereochemistry of intercalation: interaction of daunorubicin with DNA. Nature 235:17, 1972

239. Wang JC: Recent studies of DNA topoisomerases. Biochim Biophys Acta 909:1, 1987

240. Myers C: Anthracyclines. p. 416. In Chabner BA (ed): Pharmacologic Principles of Cancer Treatment. WB Saunders, Philadelphia, 1982

241. Sadzuka Y, Mochizuki E, Takino Y: Caffeine modulates the antitumor activity and toxic side effects of Adriamycin. Jap J Cancer Res 84:348, 1993

242. Smith DB, Margison JM, Lucas SB et al: Clinical pharmacology of oral and intravenous 4-demethoxydaunorubicin. Cancer Chemother Pharmacol 19:138, 1987

243. Shenkenberg TD, Von Hoff DD: Mitoxantrone: a new anticancer drug with significant clinical activity. Ann Intern Med 105:67, 1986

244. Johnson SA, Prentice AG, Phillips MJ: A randomized trial of daunorubicin/cytosine (2 + 5) and mitoxantrone/cytosine in the treatment of acute myeloid leukemia. In the Fourth European Conference of Clinical Oncology in Cancer Nursing (ECCO-4). November 1–4, 1987, Madrid, Proceedings of the Federation of European Cancer Societies 1987, p. 173

245. Glaubiger D, Ramu A: Antitumor antibiotics. p. 402. In Chabner BA (ed): Pharmacologic Principles of Cancer Treatment. WB Saunders, Philadelphia, 1982

246. Koller CA, Miller DM: Preliminary observations on the therapy of the myeloid blast phase of chronic granulocytic leukemia with plicamycin and hydroxyurea. N Engl J Med 315:1433, 1986

247. Sikic BI, Rozencweig M, Carter SK (eds): Bleomycin Chemotherapy. Academic Press, San Diego, 1985

248. Bjornsson TD, Huang AT, Roth P et al: Effects of high-dose cancer chemotherapy on the absorption of digoxin in two different formulations. Clin Pharmacol Ther 39:25, 1986

249. Finchman RW, Schottelius DD: Decreased phenytoin levels in antineoplastic therapy. Ther Drug Monit 1:277, 1979

250. McAuliffe MS, Hartshorn EA: Anesthetic drug interactions, review. CRNA 3:44, 1992

251. O'Dwyer PJ, Wittes RE (eds): Development of folates and folic acid antagonists in cancer chemotherapy. Natl Cancer Inst Monog 5, 1:1, 1987

252. Lafforgue P, Monjanel-Mouterde S, Durand A et al: Is there an interaction between low doses of corticosteroids and methotrexate in patients with rheumatoid arthritis? A pharmacokinetic study in 33 patients. J Rheumatol 20:263, 1993

253. Thyss A, Milano G, Renee N et al: Severe interactions between methotrexate and macrolide-like antibiotic, letter. J Natl Cancer Inst 85:582, 1993

254. Dean R, Nachman J, Lorenzana AN: Possible mehtotrexate-mezlocillin interaction, letter. Am J Pediatr Hematol Oncol 14:88, 1992

255. Preisler H, Royer G (eds): Cytosar-U sterile powder: therapeutic biological effects. Semin Oncol, suppl. 1 14:1–275, 1987

256. Kemena A, Gandhi V, Shewach DS et al: Inhibition of fludarabine metabolism by arabinosylcytosine during therapy. Cancer Chemother Pharmacol 31:193, 1992

257. Brockman RW, Schabel FM Jr, Montgomery JA: Biologic activity of 9-beta-D-arabinofuranosyl-2-fluoroadenine, a metabolically stable analog of 9-beta-D-arabinofuranosyladenine. Biochem Pharmacol 26:2193, 1977

258. Avramis VI, Plunkett W: 2-Fluoro-ATP: a toxic metabolite of 9-beta-D-arabinosyl-2-fluoroadenine. Biochem Biophys Res Commun 113:35, 1983

259. Hutton JJ, Von Hoff D, Kuhn J et al: Phase I clinical investigation of 9-beta-D-arabinofuranosyl-2-fluoradenine-5″-monophosphate (NSC 312887), a new purine antimetabolite. Cancer Res 44:4183, 1984

260. Hersh MR, Kuhn JG, Phillips JL et al: Pharmacokinetic study of fludarabine phosphate (NSC 312887). Cancer Chemother Pharmacol 17:277, 1986

261. Malspeis L, De Souza JJV, Staubus AE et al: Pharmacokinetics of 2-F-Ara-AMP in man during a phase I clinical trial. Invest New Drugs 2:116, 1984

262. Spriggs DR, Stopa E, Mayer RJ et al: Fludarabine phosphate (NSC 312887) infusions for the treatment of acute leukemia: phase I and neuropathological study. Cancer Res 46:5953, 1986

263. Chun HG, Leyland-Jones BR, Caryk SM, Hoth DF: Central nervous system toxicity of fludarabine phosphate. Cancer Treat Rep 70:1225, 1986

264. Hurst PG, Habib MP, Garewal H et al: Pulmonary toxicity associated with fludarabine monophosphate. Invest New Drugs 5:207, 1987

265. Wijermans PW, Gerrits WB, Haak HL: Severe immunodeficiency in patients treated with fludarabine monophosphate. Eur J Hematol 50:292, 1993

266. Saven A, Piro LA: The newer purine analogues. Significant therapeutic advance in the management of lymphoid malignancies. Cancer 72:3470, 1993

267. Estey E, Plunkett W, Gandhi V et al: Fludarabine and arabinosylcytosine therapy of refractory and relapsed acute myelogenous leukemia. Leuk Lymphoma 9:343, 1993

268. Robertson LE, Keating MJ: Fludarabine phosphate in the treatment of chronic lymphocytic leukemia: biology, clinical impact, and future directions, review. Can Treat Res 64:105, 1993

269. Feldman EJ, Keating MJ: Fludarabine in the treatment of lymphoproliferative malignancies. Cancer Invest 11:314, 1993

270. Redman JR, Canabillas F, Velasquez WS et al: Phase II trial of fludarabine phosphate in lymphoma: an effective new agent in low-grade lymphoma. J Clin Oncol 10:790, 1992

271. Dimopoulos MA, O'Brien S, Kantarjian H et al: Fludarabine therapy in Waldenström's macroglobulinemia. Am J Med 95:49, 1993

272. VonHoff DD, Dahlberg S, Hartstock RJ, Eyre HJ: Activity of fludarabine monophosphate in patients with advanced mycosis fungoides: a Southwest Oncology Group study. J Natl Cancer Inst 82:1353, 1990

273. Glover AB, Leyland-Jones BR: Biochemistry of azacytidine: a review. Cancer Treat Rep 71:959, 1987

274. Glover AB, Leyland-Jones BR: Azacytidine: 10 years later. Cancer Treat Rep 71:737, 1987

275. McCormack JJ, Johns DG: Purine antimetabolites. p. 213. In Chabner BA (ed): Pharmacologic Principles of Cancer Treatment. WB Saunders, Philadelphia, 1982

276. O'Dwyer PJ, Marsoni S, Alonso MT et al: 2′-deoxycoformycin: summary and future directions. Cancer Treat Symp 2:1, 1984

277. Airhart MJ, Robbins CM, Knudsen TB et al: Occurrence of embryotoxicity in mouse embryo's following in utero exposure to 2′-deoxycoformycin (pentostatin). Teratology 47:17, 1993

278. McEvoy GK (ed): AHFS Drug Information-American Hospital Formulary Service. American Society of Hospital Pharmacy, 1993

279. Piro LD, Carrera CJ, Carson DA, Beutler E: Lasting remissions in hairy cell leukemia induced by a single infusion of 2-chlorodeoxyadenosine. N Engl J Med 322:1117, 1990

280. Seto S, Carrera CJ, Kubata M et al: Mechanism of deoxyadenine and 2-chlorodeoxyadenosine toxicity in nondividing human lymphocytes. Clin Invest 75:377, 1985

281. Loehrer PJ, Einhorn LH: Cisplatin. Ann Intern Med 100:704, 1984

282. Bennett WM, Pastore L. Houghton DC: Fatal pulmonary toxicity in cisplatin-induced acute renal failure. Cancer Treat Rep 64:921, 1980

283. Haim N, Kedar A, Robinson E: Methotrexate-related deaths in patients previously treated with cis-diamminedichloride platinum. Cancer Chemother Pharmacol 13:223, 1984

284. Koeller JM, Trump DL, Tutsch KD et al: Phase I clinical trial and pharmacokinetics of carboplatin (NSC 241240) by single monthly 30-minute infusion. Cancer 57:222, 1986

285. Egorin MJ, Van Echo DA, Tipping SJ et al: Pharmacokinetics and dosage

reduction of cis-diammine (1,1-cyclobutanedicarboxylato)platinum in patients with impaired renal function. Cancer Res 44:5432, 1984

286. Shea TC, Flaherty M, Elias A et al: A phase I clinical and pharmacokinetic study of carboplatin and autologous bone marrow support. J Clin Oncol 7: 651, 1989

287. Donehower RC: Hydroxyurea. p. 269. In Chabner BA (ed): Pharmacologic Principles of Cancer Treatment. WB Saunders, Philadelphia, 1982

288. Schilsky RL, Ratain MJ, Vokes EE et al: Laboratory and clinical studies of biochemical modulation by hydroxyurea, review. Sem Oncol 19:84, 1992

289. Weinkam RJ, Shiba D: Procarbazine. p. 340. In Chabner BA (ed): Pharmacologic Principles of Cancer Treatment. WB Saunders, Philadelphia, 1982

290. Liu YP, Chabner BA: Enzyme therapy: L-asparaginase. p. 435. In Chabner BA (ed): Pharmacologic Principles of Cancer Treatment. WB Saunders, Philadelphia, 1982

291. Issell BF: Amsacrine (AMSA). Cancer Treat Rev 7:73, 1980

292. Marshall B, Ralph RK: A reassessment of the mechanism of action of 4′-[(9-acridinyl)amino]methanesulphon-m-anisidide. Eur J Clin Oncol 15:553, 1982

293. Nelson EM, Tewey KM, Liu LF: Mechanism of antitumor drug action: poisoning of mammalian topoisomerase II on DNA by m-AMSA. Proc Natl Acad Sci USA 81:1361, 1984

294. Van Echo DA, Chiuten DF, Gormley PE et al: Phase I clinical and pharmacological study of 4′-(9-acridinylamino)methanesulfon-m-anisidide using an intermittent biweekly schedule. Cancer Res 39:3881, 1979

295. Kano Y, Sakamoto S, Kasahara T et al: Effects of amsacrine in combination with other anticancer agents in human acute lymphoblastic leukemic cells in culture. Leuk Res 15:1059, 1991

296. Van Hoff DD, Howser D, Gormley P et al: Phase I study of methanesulfonamide,N-,4-(9-acridinyl-amino)-3-methoxy-phenyl-(m-AMSA) using a single dose schedule. Cancer Treat Rep 62:1421, 1978

297. Louie AC, Issell BF: Amsacrine (AMSA)—a clinical review. J Clin Oncol 3: 562, 1985

298. Foster BJ, Clagett-Carr K, Hoth D, Leyland-Jones B: Gallium nitrate: the second metal with clinical activity. Cancer Treat Rep 70:1311, 1986

299. Warrell RP Jr, Israel R, Frisone M et al: Gallium nitrate for acute treatment of cancer-related hypercalcemia: a randomized double-blind comparison with calcitonin. Ann Intern Med 108:669, 1988

300. Alnemri ES, Litwack G: Glucocorticoid-induced lymphocytolysis is not mediated by an induced endonuclease. J Biol Chem 264:4104, 1989

301. Lippman ME, Eil C: Steroid therapy of cancer. p. 132. In Chabner BA (ed): Pharmacologic Principles of Cancer Treatment. WB Saunders, Philadelphia, 1982

Appendix 61-1

Clinical Pharmacology of Alkylating Agents

Mechlorethamine (Mustargen)

Chemistry: Mechlorethamine, also called nitrogen mustard, is a water- and alcohol-soluble analogue of sulfur mustard gas.

Absorption, Fate, and Excretion: The parent compound is highly reactive and has a biologic half-life of approximately 15 minutes. The principal route of degradation is spontaneous hydrolysis, but some enzymatic demethylation also occurs.[196]

Preparation and Administration: Mechlorethamine is supplied in vials of 10 mg with 100 mg of sodium chloride and is reconstituted with 10 ml sterile water to yield a 1-mg/ml solution, ideally prepared immediately before use. However, the manufacturer considers the drug expired 1 hour after reconstitution. The drug is injected over a few minutes through a tubing as a freely running intravenous infusion. For topical application (e.g., in mycosis fungoides), 10 mg of drug is dissolved in 60 ml of tap water. Alternatively, a 10 mg% ointment has been used by dissolving the drug in 95% ethyl alcohol and petrolatum (Aquaphor). Mechlorethamine is a powerful vesicant. In the event of extravasation, vigorous irrigation followed by 0.25% sodium thiosulfate injection at the site of extravasation should be attempted. Ice packs may be placed for 6–12 hours to minimize the local reaction.

Toxic Effects: Myelosuppression is the dose-limiting systemic side effect. This worsens with each additive cycle. Severe nausea and vomiting, infertility, alopecia, and pain at the site of injection, which can sometimes spread to involve the venous system (tracking) are also common. Occasionally, a macular papular rash is observed, but this does not appear to be allergic in nature and does not contraindicate continua-tion of therapy. Infrequent adverse effects include alopecia, anorexia, weakness, and diarrhea. The drug has also been shown to induce chromosomal abnormalities and may contribute to the development of secondary leukemias, as seen in patients treated with this agent as part of the MOPP regimen.

Potential Drug Interactions: None has been reported.

Therapeutic Indications in Hematology: Mechlorethamine is incorporated in many chemotherapy combinations used in the treatment of Hodgkin disease (MOPP and MOPP/ABV [Adriamycin, bleomycin, and vinblastine] hybrid) and in some non-Hodgkin lymphomas (etoposide, methotrexate, doxirubicin [Adriamycin], cyclophosphamide, Leucovorin [PROMACE]/MOPP).

Cyclophosphamide (Cytoxan)

Chemistry: Cyclophosphamide is a cyclic phosphamide ester of mechlorethamine.

Absorption, Fate, and Excretion: The drug is relatively well absorbed orally, with approximately 75% oral bioavailability. The parent compound is not active. The drug is metabolized by the hepatic cytochrome P-450 system, which ultimately generates at least two active compounds: phosphoramide mustard and acrolein. The latter appears to be responsible for cyclophosphamide's bladder toxicities. The plasma half-life of cyclophosphamide varies from 4 to 6.5 hours. Approximately 15% of the drug is excreted unchanged in the urine. Dose reduction should be considered in patients with severe renal failure.[196]

Preparation and Administration: Cyclophosphamide is supplied as 25- and 50-mg tablets and as a powder for parenteral administration in 100-, 200-, and 500-mg and 1- and 2-g vials. It is dissolved by adding 5 ml of preservative-free sterile water for every 100 mg of drug. Cyclophosphamide is chemically stable for 24 hours at room temperature and for 6 days, if refrigerated.

Toxic Effects: Marrow suppression is the major side effect. The myeloid series is primarily affected, although thrombocytopenia also occurs at high doses, and alopecia is common. Nausea and vomiting can be severe and are usually delayed, occurring 6–8 hours after administration. Hemorrhagic cystitis occurs in ≤10% of patients receiving nontransplant doses and is apparently due to the formation of the urotoxin acrolein (Fig. 61-6). Because of this potential side effect, patients should be well hydrated. Mesna disulfide (sodium 2-mercaptoethanesulfonate disulfide) has also been used to ameliorate cyclophosphamide-induced bladder toxicity. Other potential toxic effects include stomatitis, skin and nail hyperpigmentation, interstitial pulmonary fibrosis, and the syndrome of inappropriate secretion of antidiuretic hormone. After bone marrow transplant doses, hemorrhagic cystitis is common, and cardiac toxicity (cardiomyopathy) may be seen. Late sequelae include bladder fibrosis, more common with daily (oral) therapy, bladder cancer, leukemogenesis, and infertility.

Potential Drug Interactions: Allopurinol has been reported to increase the half-life of cyclophosphamide, but this interaction was not been confirmed in a randomized study in which patients received allopurinol during either three or six cycles of chemotherapy. In animal studies, conflicting results were reported when the P-450 enzyme inducer phenobarbital was given with cyclophosphamide. Most investigators, however, have observed a reduction in the amounts of active metabolites. Conversely, when cimetidine (but not ranitidine) was administered in leukemia-bearing mice before treatment with cyclophosphamide, a significant prolongation of their survival and higher plasma concentrations of alkylating metabolites were observed. Although one should remain alert for these potential drug interactions, none has been demonstrated in humans. Cyclophosphamide reduces serum pseudocholinesterase levels, which may prolong the neuromuscular blocking effects if given simultaneously. Caution must be exercised when administering high doses of these two drugs to critically ill patients.[197,198] Life-threatening hyponatremia may develop when used in conjunction with indomethacin, although the precise incidence is unknown.[199] In mouse transplant models, Cyclosporin A may interfere with cyclophosphamide-induced skin allograft tolerance.[200]

Therapeutic Indications in Hematology: Cyclophosphamide is a key drug in the treatment of lymphomas and myeloma. It is incorporated in many chemotherapy regimens, including CHOP, MACOP-B, PROMACE/CYTABOM, CVP, and VMCP. In addition, cyclophosphamide is the drug most commonly used in preparatory regimens for bone marrow transplantation.

Ifosfamide (Ifex)

Chemistry: Ifosfamide is an oxazaphosphine nitrogen mustard that differs from cyclophosphamide by the placement of chloroethyl groups.

Absorption, Fate, and Excretion: As in the case of cyclophosphamide, the parent compound is inactive and is metabolized by the cytochrome P-450 system in the liver. The metabolism of ifosfamide is influenced by the dose and schedule of administration. When administered as a single bolus, 60%

is eliminated into the urine, 53% as unchanged inactive drug. When administered daily for 5 consecutive days, 56% is excreted into the urine, 15% as the inactive parent compound. The half-life is 7 hours when administered daily for 5 consecutive days and 15 hours when given as a single bolus dose.

Preparation and Administration: The drug is provided in 1-g vials and should be reconstituted in sterile water or bacteriostatic water to a final concentration of 50 mg/ml. Ifosfamide can be diluted further in 5% dextrose, normal saline, or Ringer's solution for injection to achieve concentrations of 0.6–20 mg/ml. The solution should be infused over ≥30 minutes. To prevent hemorrhagic cystitis, patients must receive mesna disulfide for protection against urotoxicity and must be kept well hydrated (≥2 L/day). Mesna is a thiol compound that is rapidly oxidized to dimesna in vivo. Both mesna and dimesna are filtered by the glomeruli, reabsorbed in the proximal tubule, and finally secreted back into the tubular lumen of the kidney. In the tubules, approximately one-third of the filtered dimesna is readily converted back to mesna, the free sulfhydryl group of which reacts with the urotoxic metabolite acrolein produced by both ifosfamide and cyclophosphamide (Fig. 61-6). This reaction creates a nontoxic acrolein/mesna thioether that is safely eliminated in the urine. Mesna has also been shown to inhibit the degradation of ifosfamide or cyclophosphamide to acrolein.

Mesna has been given in combination with ifosfamide in different doses and schedules. One recommended schedule employs intravenous bolus injection in a dosage equal to 20% of the ifosfamide dose (on a milligram-to-milligram basis) at the time of ifosfamide administration and 4 and 8 hours after each dose of ifosfamide. Mesna has also been given by continuous infusion, with excellent results. The two agents may be mixed together in the same intravenous solution; however, mesna is not compatible with cisplatin.

Toxic Effects: With the use of mesna to protect against urotoxicity, myelosuppression, especially leukopenia and to a lesser extent thrombocytopenia, is the dose-limiting side effect. Renal tubular acidosis can occur. Central nervous system effects, observed in approximately 10% of patients treated, include somnolence, confusion, depressive psychosis, and hallucinations. Less commonly, dizziness, disorientation, and cranial nerve dysfunction occur. Nausea and vomiting are common. Low serum albumin and elevated serum creatinine may enhance central nervous system toxicity. As with cyclophosphamide, such side effects as alopecia, leukemogenesis, and infertility also occur.[201]

Potential Drug Interactions: Since ifosfamide is also metabolized by the P-450 system, one should remain alert for the same type of potential drug interactions that have been reported with cyclophosphamide. A recent report advises close monitoring of warfarin anticoagulant control in patients receiving ifosfamide/mesna.[202]

Therapeutic Indications in Hematology: Ifosfamide was recently approved for treatment of patients with refractory testicular cancer.[203] In hematologic malignancies its major indication is in the treatment of refractory lymphomas (IMVP-16 regimen).[204]

Melphalan (Melphalan)

Chemistry: Melphalan is synthesized from nitrogen mustard and phenylalanine.

Absorption, Fate, and Excretion: The oral bioavailability of melphalan is quite variable, 20–50% of the drug being excreted in the stool. Some patients show virtually no oral absorption. This fact is particularly pertinent in the treatment of myeloma patients, in whom a lack of response to melphalan may be due simply to poor oral absorption. Melphalan has a half-life of approximately 2 hours. It is extensively metabolized, with only about 10–15% of an administered dose excreted unchanged in the urine.[196]

Preparation and Administration: Melphalan is commercially available in 2-mg tablets and in intravenous formulation.

Toxic Effects: The dose-limiting toxicity is myelosuppression, manifested by leukopenia and thrombocytopenia and generally occurring 2–3 weeks after therapy. Recovery may take ≤6 weeks, however, in patients who have been heavily pretreated with chemotherapy drugs or radiotherapy, or both. Nausea, vomiting, and alopecia are uncommon side effects and are usually mild. Occasionally, amenorrhea and azoospermia, pulmonary fibrosis, dermatitis, and secondary malignancies (e.g., leukemia) occur, especially in patients receiving the drug over the long term. At cumulative doses of <600 mg, the incidence of second hematologic malignancy is probably <2%. Higher doses used in transplant patients result in gastrointestinal toxicity that is dose limiting. At these doses, the syndrome of inappropriate secretion of antidiuretic hormone, pneumonitis, and hepatic veno-occlusive disease have been observed.

Potential Drug Interactions: Administration of high-dose intravenous melphalan with cyclosporine increases the risk of cyclosporine nephrotoxicity.[205]

Therapeutic Indications: The major use of melphalan is for the treatment of multiple myeloma, either as a single agent or in combination with other alkylating agents and prednisone (e.g., the *M*P and V*M*CP regimens [CP, cyclophosphamide]). The intravenous formulation has been approved for isolated limb perfusion in melanoma.[206]

Chlorambucil (Chlorambucil)

Chemistry: Chlorambucil is an aromatic derivative of mechlorethamine.

Absorption, Fate, and Excretion: Chlorambucil is well absorbed after oral administration. It is extensively metabolized in the liver to its major metabolite, phenylacetic acid mustard (PAAM), which also has bifunctional alkylating activity. The half-lives of chlorambucil and PAAM are 1.5 and 2.5 hours, respectively; <1% of either chlorambucil or PAAM is excreted in the urine.[207]

Preparation and Administration: Chlorambucil is commercially available as 2-mg tablets.

Toxic Effects: Treatment is usually well tolerated, with myelosuppression the dose-limiting toxic effect. Patients on a daily oral schedule should have biweekly CBCs. Nausea and vomiting are uncommon, but mild alopecia and skin rashes occasionally occur. As with the other alkylating agents, azoospermia (especially above cummulative dose of 400 mg), amenorrhea, and secondary leukemia are potential risks of prolonged therapy. Rare cases of pulmonary fibrosis have also been reported.

Potential Drug Interactions: None has been reported.

Therapeutic Indications in Hematology: The major uses are in the treatment of Waldenström's macroglobulinemia, low-grade lymphomas, CLL, and Hodgkin disease.

Busulfan (Myleran)

Chemistry: Busulfan is an alkylsulfonate not chemically related to mechlorethamine.

Absorption, Fate, and Excretion: Busulfan is well absorbed after oral administration. When given by the intravenous route, >90% is cleared from the plasma after 3 minutes. The drug is extensively metabolized to inactive compounds, which are excreted renally. The major metabolite is methanesulfonic acid, although >10 other not fully identified metabolites exist. Virtually no intact busulfan is found in the urine.[208] The biologic half-life of busulfan is approximately 2.5 hours.

Preparation and Administration: The drug is commercially available as 2-mg tablets.

Toxic Effects: Although at low doses, the major effect of busulfan is on the granulocytic series, at high doses all three hematologic series are affected. As compared with the other alkylating agents, its nadir of myelosuppression may be relatively late, in a range of 11–30 days. Hematologic recovery is also prolonged and may take ≤54 days. A relatively common side effect is an addisonian-like syndrome characterized by skin hyperpigmentation and weakness but without abnormalities in adrenal function.[209] Cumulative pulmonary toxicity has been well described and consists of a mixed alveolar and interstitial pneumonitis.[210] As with the other alkylating agents, infertility and leukemogenesis can occur. Nausea and vomiting are rare.

Potential Drug Interactions: A metabolic interaction may take place between busulfan and various anticonvulsant medications; however, further description of the specific effects are awaited.[211]

Therapeutic Indications in Hematology: Busulfan is used mainly in the treatment of CML. More recently, high-dose busulfan has been incorporated into preparatory regimens for bone marrow transplantation.

Carmustine (BCNU)

Chemistry: Carmustine, also called BCNU (bischloronitrosourea), decomposes spontaneously into a chloroethyl hydroxide that can alkylate the DNA, and into an isocyanate molecule, which may produce carbamoylation of proteins.[212]

Absorption, Fate, and Excretion: Intravenously administered carmustine is rapidly metabolized, with a half-life of 70 minutes. Approximately 30–80% of metabolites are eliminated in the urine within 24 hours. The drug and/or its metabolites readily cross the blood-brain barrier, resulting in cerebrospinal fluid concentrations within the range of 15–70% of plasma levels.[212]

Preparation and Administration: Carmustine is commercially available in 100-mg vials as a white lyophilized powder. The drug is reconstituted with 3 ml of absolute alcohol provided by the manufacturer and 27 ml of sterile water and can be further diluted with normal saline or 5% dextrose in water. It should be used immediately after reconstitution and can be infused over 1–2 hours. Carmustine is chemically stable for 3 hours at room temperature and for 24 hours when refrigerated.

Toxic Effects: Myelosuppression is the dose-limiting toxic effect and tends to increase with successive cycles of therapy. Leukopenia and thrombocytopenia are characteristically delayed and reach their maximum between the third and sixth weeks after drug administration. Nausea and vomiting can be severe. Abnormal liver function tests may be found in ≤25% of patients, but the abnormalities are usually mild and reversible. Two rare but serious toxic effects include cumulative pulmonary fibrosis and progressive renal damage, which are dose related. Patients who receive >1,100 mg/m² are at increased risk of pulmonary fibrosis. Carmustine is not a vesicant, but rapid infusion often produces a burning pain at the injection site.

Potential Drug Interactins: Cimetidine may enhance the myelosuppressive effect of carmustine. Carmustine may decrease the pharmacologic effects of phenytoin. In rats with intracerebrally implanted tumors, pretreatment with phenobarbital eliminated the antitumor activity of carmustine. The reduction in carmustine antitumor activity correlated with increased carmustine metabolism, which is apparently the result of hepatic microsomal enzyme induction.[213]

Therapeutic Indications in Hematology: Carmustine in combination with other cytotoxic agents may be used in the initial treatment of Hodgkin disease (BCVPP regimen) and multiple myeloma (VBAP regimen).

Lomustine (CCNU)

Chemistry: Lomustine, also called CCNU, is a nitrosourea derivative with choloroethyl and cyclohexyl side chains.

Absorption, Fate, and Excretion: The drug is rapidly absorbed from the gastrointestinal tract and is rapidly and completely metabolized. Its active metabolites have prolonged plasma half-lives, within a range of 16–48 hours. Approximately 50% of an administered dose is detectable (as metabolites) in the urine within 24 hours, and 75% is detectable within 4 days. Active metabolites cross the blood-brain barrier and can be detected in significant concentrations in the cerebrospinal fluid.[214]

Preparation and Administration: The drug is commercially available in 10-, 40-, and 100-mg capsules.

Toxic Effects: The toxicity profile of lomustine is similar to that of carmustine. Since lomustine can produce vomiting, and the drug is given orally, special attention should be directed to emesis control. If the patient vomits soon after ingestion, the vomitus should be inspected for the presence of intact capsules. The drug should be given again if capsules are identified with certainty.

Potential Drug Interactions: These are probably similar to those of carmustine.

Therapeutic Indications in Hematology: Lomustine is occasionally used as second-line treatment for patients with Hodgkin disease and non-Hodgkin lymphoma.

Streptozocin (Zanosar)

Chemistry: Streptozocin is a naturally occurring nitrosourea derived from *Streptomyces acromogenes*. The drug is a glucosamine-1-methyl-nitrosourea, which, unlike the other nitrosoureas, does not have a chloroethyl side chain.

Absorption, Fate, and Excretion: After intravenous administration, the drug is rapidly metabolized, with no intact drug detectable in the plasma after 3 hours. Its half-life is 40 hours. Within the first 24 hours after administration, approximately 10% of the parent compound is excreted in the urine.[215]

Preparation and Administration: The drug is commercially available in 1-g vials and is reconstituted with either 9.5 ml of normal saline or 5% dextrose in water for injection to form a 100-mg/ml solution. Intravenous infusion of the drug over 30–45 minutes usually prevents discomfort at the injection site. Patients should be kept well hydrated to preclude renal tubular toxicity.

Toxic Effects: Although nausea and vomiting have been considered by some investigators to be the limiting toxic effects, in most phase I trials nephrotoxicity was the principal dose-limiting effect. Nausea and vomiting are severe and require aggressive antiemetic support. Streptozocin may also aggravate duodenal ulcers. Renal toxicity frequently occurs and includes mild proteinuria, glycosuria, hypophosphatemia, renal tubular acidosis, and occasionally irreversible azotemia. Although the myelosuppressive effect of streptozocin is mild, it can potentiate the bone marrow suppression of other cytotoxic drugs. Slight increases in hepatic enzymes can also occur. Occasionally, patients (primarily those with insulinomas) may experience transient alterations in glucose metabolism.

Potential Drug Interactions: Streptozocin can potentiate the hyperglycemic effect of glucocorticosteroids. Phenytoin therapy decreases the cytotoxic effect of streptozocin on the pancreatic β cells, leading to potential interference with its therapeutic effect in patients with pancreatic islet cell tumors. Streptozocin is a potent renal toxin, and every effort should be made to avoid concomitant administration of other nephrotoxins.

Therapeutic Indications in Hematology: Streptozocin has been used in the initial treatment of both Hodgkin disease and less commonly in non-Hodgkin lymphomas.

Dacarbazine (DTIC-Dome)

Chemistry: Dacarbazine is also called DTIC [5-(3,3-dimethyl-1-triazeno)imidazole-4-carboxamide]. After undergoing metabolic activation by microsomal enzymes in the liver, it acts primarily as an alkylating agent.[216]

Absorption, Fate, and Excretion: After intravenous administration, the drug is extensively metabolized. Activated dacarbazine has an elimination half-life of 5–7 hours. Approximately 40–50% of the parent drug is found in the urine within the first 24 hours after administration.[216]

Preparation and Administration: Dacarbazine is commercially available in 100- and 200-mg vials, which must be protected from light and stored at 2–8°C. The drug is reconstituted with normal saline or sterile water to produce a 10-mg/ml solution. It can be administered as a slow intravenous push or by infusion over ≥15–30 minutes.

Toxic Effects: Myelosuppression, primarily represented by leukopenia, is the dose-limiting toxic effect. Use of the drug leads to considerable problems with emesis and requires aggressive antiemetic support. A flu-like syndrome, consisting of fever, malaise, and myalgias, may occur. Direct sunlight during the first 2 days after drug administration may result in facial flushing, facial paresthesias, and light-headedness. Hepatotoxicity and diarrhea have also been reported. Pain along the injection site can occur if the drug is rapidly infused but can usually be lessened by prolonging the infusion rate.

Potential Drug Interactions: Dacarbazine activation may be enhanced by phenytoin or phenobarbital, although the clinical significance of this potential interaction remains uncertain. There may be a potential as yet poorly characterized drug interaction with levodopa, whereby the response to levodopa is diminished.[217]

Therapeutic Indications in Hematology: Dacarbazine is used primarily in the treatment of Hodgkin disease as part of the ABVD (doxorubicin [Adriamycin], bleomycin, vinblastine, and dacarbazine) regimen.

Clinical Pharmacology of Plant Alkaloids

Vincristine (Oncovin) and Vinblastine (Velban)

Chemistry and Mechanism of Action: Both vincristine and vinblastine are asymmetric dimeric compounds that bind to the protein tubulin, resulting in metaphase arrest. They are M phase specific.

Absorption, Fate, and Excretion: After intravenous injection, both drugs are rapidly distributed to the body tissues, especially the red blood cells and platelets. Their elimination follows a triphasic pattern—the distribution and elimination half-lives of vincristine are 0.85, 7.4, and 164 minutes,[218] and those of vinblastine are 3.5 minutes, 53 minutes, and 19–27 hours.[219] Both vinca alkaloids are primarily eliminated through the liver into the bile and feces, making patients with obstructive liver disease more susceptible to toxic effects.

Preparation and Administration: Vincristine is commercially available in 1-, 2-, and 5-mg vials. Each milliliter contains 1 mg vincristine sulfate, 100 mg mannitol, 1.3 mg methylparaben, and 0.2 mg propylparaben. Vincristine is a powerful vesicant that should be administered only intravenously into a freely running infusion of normal saline or dextrose solution. If the drug is given by continuous infusion it must be infused through a central intravenous line. In case of extravasation, the manufacturer recommends infiltrating the area with 1–2 ml of hyaluronidase, 150 U/ml, and then applying warm compresses for 72 hours to facilitate dispersion of the drug.

Vinblastine is commercially available as a lyophilized powder and a 1-mg/ml solution in 10-mg vials. The lyophilized drug is reconstituted by adding sodium chloride for injection (which may be preserved with either phenols or benzyl alcohol) to the 10-mg vial. Administration of vinblastine should follow the same guidelines described for vincristine.

Toxic Effects: Vincristine's dose-limiting toxic effect is neurotoxicity, which appears to be related to its relative polarity. Peripheral neurotoxicity is usually manifested by sensory impairment, decreased deep tendon reflexes, and paresthesias. Less commonly, severe painful dysesthesias, ataxia, foot drop, and cranial nerve palsy (e.g., affecting the extraocular and laryngeal muscles) can occur. Autonomic neurotoxicities include constipation, abdominal cramps, and ileus, which may be prevented by use of mild laxatives. Alopecia occurs frequently, but myelosuppressive effects are minimal. Rare side effects include inappropriate secretion of antidiuretic hormone and ischemic cardiac toxicity.

Vinblastine's dose-limiting toxic effect is myelosuppression, with leukopenia more pronounced than thrombocytopenia. Anemia is uncommon. Neurotoxicity can also occur but is significantly less common than with vincristine. Vinblastine is also a vesicant.

Potential Drug Interactions: Both vinca alkaloids have been reported to increase the accumulation of methotrexate and etoposide in tumor cells.[220] Acute shortness of breath and bronchospasm can occur when vincristine or vinblastine is given in conjunction with mitomycin C.[221] Since asparaginase may impair the hepatic clearance of vincristine, it is preferable to give the latter 12–24 hours prior to L-asparaginase administration. Vincristine may decrease the absorption and plasma levels of orally administered drugs such as digoxin.[222] Dilantin may increase the cytotoxicity of vincristine in multidrug-resistant tumor cells; however, this remains to be demonstrated in the clinic.[223]

Therapeutic Indications in Hematology: The vinca alkaloids are among the most important drugs in the treatment of hematologic malignancies. They have a broad spectrum of activity and are often incorporated into many chemotherapy regimens used in the treatment of ALL, Hodgkin disease, non-Hodgkin lymphomas, CLL, and multiple myeloma.

Etoposide (Vepesid) and Teniposide (Vehem, Vumon)

Chemistry and Mechanism of Action: Both etoposide (VP-16) and teniposide (VM-26) are semisynthetic derivatives of podophyllotoxin. The mechanism of action of these drugs has not yet been completely elucidated, but it appears to be related to their ability to induce stabilization of a topoisomerase II/DNA cleavable complex in its putative cleavable state. Another proposed mechanism involves metabolic activation of the drugs, with formation of highly reactive species that produce DNA damage. Unlike podophyllotoxin and the vinca alkaloids, neither etoposide nor teniposide causes mitotic arrest by binding to microtubules.[224]

Absorption, Fate, and Excretion: Etoposide has an oral bioavailability of 25–75%. Its half-life is within a range of 3–12 hours, with approximately 30–40% excreted in the urine, two-thirds as unchanged drug.[225] There is no accumulation with consecutive daily administration, but cytotoxicity has strict schedule dependancy. Clinical studies suggest that in patients with plasma creatinine >130 μmol/L, the etoposide dose should be reduced by ≥25%.

Teniposide has a multiphasic pattern of clearance from plasma with a half-life of 20–39 hours. Unlike those of etoposide, metabolites of teniposide account for ≥80% of the drug excreted in the urine.[226] Like etoposide, there is significant interpatient and intrapatient variation in clinical pharmacokinetics. Teniposide has greater cellular uptake and retention, albumin binding, and plasma half-life than that of etoposide. Although the potency in inhibiting the catalytic domain of topoisomerase II is equivalent for both drugs, teniposide has greater cytotoxicity than etoposide due to its increased cellular retention. There are currently no formal recommendations for dose modification in patients with renal insufficiency.

Preparation and Administration: Etoposide is commercially available as 50-mg capsules and in vials of 50 and 100 mg at a concentration of 20 mg/ml. When the drug is diluted with normal saline or 5% dextrose in water to a concentrations of 0.2 or 0.4 mg/ml, it is stable for 96 or 48 hours, respectively. Etoposide must be administered slowly over ≥30 minutes to prevent hypotension.

Teniposide is supplied by Bristol-Myers Oncology Division in 50-mg vials for intravenous use only. The intravenous solution maybe taken orally but is unpalatable. Additives in the vial include benzyl alcohol 0.15 mg, N,N-dimethylacetamidine 0.3 g, polyethoxylated castor oil 2.5 g, maleic acid to pH 5.1, and absolute alcohol 5 ml. Currently, no oral preparation is available in the market; however, for investigational purposes each 50-mg vial may be dissolved in 50–100 mg of syrup or juice. A single oral dose of 60 mg/m² is advised to achieve optimal absorption, which may be repeated at 6-hour intervals. As with etoposide, rapid infusion can produce hypotension.

Toxic Effects: Myelosuppression, especially leukopenia, is the dose-limiting toxic effect of both etoposide and teniposide. Nausea and vomiting are usually mild and easily prevented with antiemetics. Rapid infusion of etoposide (over >30 minutes) may cause hypotension. Anaphylactoid reactions (e.g., bronchospasm) occur in ≤2% of patients and may be related to the cremaphor vehicle. Alopecia occurs in approximately 20% of patients treated with etoposide. This side effect is more common with teniposide. When the drug is given in bone marrow transplantation doses, mucositis and diarrhea are prominent and may be dose limiting.

Potential Drug Interactions: Theoretically, any drug that increases the S-phase fraction will increase the cytotoxicity of epipodophyllotoxins and other topoisomerase inhibitors. Conversely, drugs that inhibit DNA synthesis antagonize the effect of etoposide and teniposide (e.g 5-fluoro-2'-deoxyuridine given before etoposide in some human cancer cell lines decreases cytotoxicity of the latter). However, teniposide activity in B16 melanoma cells is reported to be potentiated by lonidamine, which impairs mitochondrial ATP metabolism in cells. Although such drug interactions may exist, there is no general clinical rule for its final effect; therefore, its clinical significance remains unknown.[227] In hematology, etoposide and teniposide may inhibit intracellular ara-CTP formation, leading to reduced cytosine arabinoside cytotoxicity.[228] Potentiation of teniposide activity has been seen

with methotrexate and dipyridamoles.[229,230] There is at least a twofold increase in the clearance of teniposide with concomitant administration of phenobarbital or phenytoin.[231] Cyclosporine and other MDR antagonists (PSC 833) potentiates the cytotoxic effects of etoposide.[232] ICRF-187, a cardioprotector against anthracycline-mediated cardiomyopathy, antagonizes the cytotoxicity of daunorubicin and VP-16.[233] More recently, it has been demonstrated that suramin (an investigational agent with activity in prostate cancer) inhibits the cytotoxicity of topoisomerase inhibitors by preventing drug-induced DNA damage.[234]

Therapeutic Indications: Etoposide is employed in the treatment of non-Hodgkin lymphomas (PROMACE-CYTABOM regimen), and as second-line treatment for Hodgkin disease. It is also incorporated in the preparatory regimens for bone marrow transplantation of refractory lymphomas (CBV) and acute leukemia. Teniposide has been approved as a front-line agent in combination chemotherapy for childhood ALL.[235] Combination chemotherapy with teniposide has been used successfully in some cases of refractory adult ALL and acute monocytic leukemia, but duration of remission is not significantly different fron that with other standard salvage regimens. In non-Hodgkin lymphoma, teniposide has shown comparable activity to vincristine. Teniposide has also been used in the investigational setting in bone marrow transplant-conditioning regimens for leukemia and lymphoma.[236] Teniposide combination chemotherapy compares favorably with etoposide combination chemotherapy as first-line treatment against small cell lung cancer and provides effective palliation against brain metastases.[237] In other tumors, like gliomas, bladder and ovarian, teniposide remains investigational.

Appendix 61-3

Clinical Pharmacology of Antitumor Antibiotics

Daunorubicin

Chemistry and Mechanism of Action: Daunorubicin is an anthracycline in which the sugar daunosamine is linked to the tetracycline ring. The drug inhibits DNA synthesis and DNA-dependent RNA synthesis by intercalating between base pairs of the DNA helix.[238] Daunorubicin also induces stabilization of the topoisomerase II cleavable complex. The most important mechanism related to cell kill remains debatable, however.[239]

Absorption, Fate, and Excretion: After intravenous injection, daunorubicin undergoes rapid tissue uptake and concentration. It is rapidly metabolized in the liver, where approximately 25% of the drug concentrates and has a half-life of 25–50 hours. The principal metabolite is daunorubicinol, which also displays antineoplastic activity. Biliary excretion accounts for approximately 75% of the drug and metabolite

elimination. Approximately 23% of combined drug and metabolites is eliminated in the urine within 5 days after injection. Patients with significant hepatic dysfunction should receive an attenuated dose of daunorubicin.

Preparation and Administration: Daunorubicin is supplied with 100 mg of mannitol in 20-mg vials, from which it is reconstituted with 4 ml of sterile water for injection. The vials should be protected from sunlight. Daunorubicin is a powerful vesicant that should be administered into the tubing of a freely flowing intravenous infusion of either 5% dextrose in water or normal saline. In the event of extravasation, as much infiltrated drug as possible should be aspirated from the tissue, and cold compresses should be maintained on the site for several hours. Despite these measures, skin grafting may be necessary. Daunorubicin is not physically compatible with heparin, and the two drugs should not be co-administered in the same intravenous tubing. Patients should be informed that daunorubicin may impart a red color to their urine for ≤72 hours after administration.

Toxic Effects: Myelosuppression, predominantly leukopenia, is the dose-limiting toxic effect. Mucositis, nausea and vomiting, and alopecia are common; facial flushing, conjunctivitis, and lacrimation may occur in rare cases. Erythematous streaking near the site of injection occurs as a benign local allergic reaction and should not be confused with extravasation. The drug can produce a severe local reaction (e.g., pneumonitis, esophagitis) in previously irradiated areas, even when both therapies are not administered concomitantly (radiation recall).

Cardiotoxicity is a unique characteristic of the anthracycline antibiotics and can be acute or chronic. In the acute form, abnormal electrocardiographic changes such as ST-T wave elevations and arrhythmias may be seen. A transient reduction in the ejection fraction can also occur acutely and is often associated with pericarditis (pericarditis/myocarditis syndrome). The chronic form of anthracycline cardiotoxicity is related to the cumulative dose and occurs in >20% of patients at total doses of >550 mg/m². It is clinically characterized by congestive heart failure, usually refractory to medical therapy. Cardiac irradiation or administration of cyclophosphamide or other related antibiotics may increase the risk of cardiotoxicity. The cardiotoxic effects appear to be related to the formation of free radicals and can be prevented by the concurrent use of the ethylenediaminetetraacetate analogue ICRF-187 (also called ADR-529).

Potential Drug Interactions: Daunorubicin is not physically compatible with heparin or dexamethasone. The drug interactions described for doxorubicin (see below) probably occur with daunorubicin as well.

Therapeutic Indications in Hematology: Daunorubicin is used in combination with other drugs in the treatment of AML and ALL.

Doxorubicin (Adriamycin)

Chemistry and Mechanism of Action: Doxorubicin is also an anthracycline glycoside antibiotic. It differs from daunorubicin at C-8, where a hydroxyacetyl group replaces an acetyl group; because of this, doxorubicin is also called hydroxyldaunorubicin. Its mechanism of action is similar to that of daunorubicin.

Absorption, Fate, and Excretion: Doxorubicin has a triphasic plasma clearance with a half-life of approximately 30 hours. The drug is extensively metabolized in the liver to yield an active metabolite (doxorubicinol) and a number of inactive metabolites (aglycones). Within 7 days, ≥50% of an injected dose is excreted in the bile, but only 5–10% of the drug is excreted in the urine. Penetration into the cerebrospinal fluid is poor.[240]

Preparation and Administration: Doxorubicin is commercially available in 10-, 20-, 50-, 150-, and 200-mg vials. The lyophilized powder is reconstituted with either normal saline or sterile water for injection to yield a 2-mg/ml solution. The reconstituted solution must be protected from sunlight. The drug should be injected slowly into the tubing of a freely running intravenous infusion of normal saline or 5% dextrose in water. Erythematous streaking along the vein is often an indication that the administration rate is too rapid. The drug is a powerful vesicant, and in case of extravasation the measures described above for daunorubicin should be followed.

Toxic Effects: The toxic effects are similar to those of daunorubicin. It is important to emphasize that weekly low-dose regimens or administration by continuous infusion decreases the risk of cardiotoxicity with doxorubicin. Caffiene may potentiate the in vivo antitumor activity of doxorubicin without increasing its toxicity profile.[241]

Potential Drug Interactions: When used in combination with other drugs as treatment for leukemia or lymphoma, doxorubicin may decrease the oral bioavailability of digoxin. It is not physically compatible with heparin or 5-fluorouracil.[220] Barbiturates may increase the plasma clearance of doxorubicin and decrease its cytotoxic effect. In rats, cyclophosphamide pretreatment significantly decreases doxorubicin clearance.[197] Doxorubicin is compatible with vincristine; the two drugs can be administered together in the same intravenous solution.

Therapeutic Indications in Hematology: Doxorubicin is one of the most important drugs in the treatment of hematologic malignancies. It is used in the treatment of Hodgkin disease (ABVD regimen), non-Hodgkin lymphomas (CHOP, PROMACE/CYTABOM, MACOP-B, and M-BACOD), CLL (CHOP), and multiple myeloma (VBAP, VAD).

Idarubicin (Idamycin)

Chemistry and Mechanism of Action: Idarubicin, also called 4′-demethoxydaunorubicin (4-DMDR), is an analogue of daunorubicin in which the methoxy group from the aglycone has been replaced with hydrogen. The drug binds to DNA with a marked inhibitory effect on DNA polymerases and is more active than daunorubicin in inhibiting RNA synthesis.

Absorption, Fate, and Excretion: After its intravenous injection, idarubicin follows a triphasic pattern of elimination, with a half-life of 23 hours. The oral bioavailability of the drug is approximately 25%. Idarubicinol is the major metabolite and is as cytotoxic as idarubicin. The prolonged retention of idarubicinol in the plasma may explain the higher potency of idarubicin in vivo. Biliary and urinary excretion of the unchanged drug and its metabolites account for about 25% of an intravenous dose in 5 days.[242]

Preparation and Administration: Idarubicin is supplied by Adria Laboratories in 5- and 10-mg vials from which it is reconstituted with sterile water or normal saline to obtain a 1-mg/ml solution. The drug should be infused over 10–15 minutes through the tubing of a freely running intravenous infusion. Extravasation precautions should be instituted during administration. The oral formulation remains investigational.

Toxic Effects: The side effects of idarubicin are similar to those of daunorubicin and doxorubicin but are of lesser intensity at equally myelosuppressive doses.

Potential Drug Interactions: None has been reported.

Therapeutic Indications in Hematology: Idarubicin in combination with cytosine arabinoside is equivalent, if not superior to combination chemotherapy with daunorubicin in the treatment of adult AML and myelodysplastic syndrome. Idarubicin has been approved for use in combination therapy for adult AML.

Mitoxantrone (Novantrone)

Chemistry and Mechanism of Action: Mitoxantrone is a synthetic anthracenedione. Although its mechanism of action has not been fully elucidated, it is a DNA-reactive agent and, like the anthracyclines, it stabilizes topoisomerase II cleavable complex. The drug has a cytocidal effect on both proliferating and nonproliferating cells.[243]

Absorption, Fate, and Excretion: Mitoxantrone is excreted via the renal and hepatobiliary systems, but the hepatobiliary elimination accounts for approximately 30% of active drug elimination and appears to be of greater importance. The half-life is quite variable, within a range of 17–250 hours. Patients with severe hepatic dysfunction have been shown to eliminate the drug more slowly.

Preparation and Administration: Mitoxantrone is commercially available as a 2-mg/ml solution in 10-, 12.5-, and 15-ml vials (20, 25, and 30 mg per vial, respectively). The drug is further diluted in normal saline or 5% dextrose in water for injection and is administered over ≥15–30 minutes into the tubing of a freely running intravenous infusion. As with the anthracyclines, erythema or streaking along the vein of infusion indicates that the drug is being infused too rapidly. Although mitoxantrone is not a vesicant, there have been rare reports of tissue necrosis following extravasation.

Toxic Effects: Myelosuppression, principally leukopenia, is the dose-limiting toxic effect. Thrombocytopenia is relatively mild. Nausea, vomiting, and alopecia are usually mild and occur in <30% of patients treated. Rarely, mucositis and elevation of liver enzymes occur. The drug imparts a blue color to the urine of patients treated. Like the anthracyclines, mitoxantrone is cardiotoxic, both congestive heart failure and arrhythmias having been documented. In a randomized trial in which patients were treated with either cytarabine plus daunorubicin or cytarabine plus mitoxantrone, approximately 5% of patients in each treatment group developed congestive heart failure.[244] Thus, caution should be used when the drug is given to patients with pre-existing heart disease or to whom prior anthracyclines have previously been administered.

Potential Drug Interaction: None has been reported.

Therapeutic Indications in Hematology: Mitoxantrone has recently been approved for induction therapy of AML in adults.

Plicamycin

Chemistry and Mechanism of Action: Plicamycin, also called mithramycin, forms complexes with DNA and inhibits DNA-directed synthesis of RNA. Plicamycin also inhibits the effect of parathyrin on osteoclasts. The hypocalcemic effect is independent of the antitumor effect.

Absorption, Fate, and Excretion: The pharmacology of plicamycin has been poorly described. Within 15 hours of intravenous administration, 40% is excreted in the urine. The elimination half-life has been estimated to be approximately 2 hours.[245]

Preparation and Administration: Plicamycin is commercially available as a lyophilized powder in 2.5-mg vials, from which it is reconstituted with 4.9 ml of sterile water for injection. This dose should be further diluted in 1 L of 5% dextrose in water or normal saline and infused over 4–6 hours.

Toxic Effects: When plicamycin is employed as an antitumor agent, its most common side effects include myelosuppression, elevated liver enzymes, increased serum creatinine and proteinuria, and coagulopathy due to decreased clotting factors II, V, VII, and X. The drug also causes nausea and vomiting, diarrhea, stomatitis, headache, and irritability. Cutaneous toxicity may occur in up to one-third of patients, manifested by progressive blushing of the face and thickening and coarsening of the skinfolds. The drug can produce severe local irritation if extravasation occurs.[245]

Potential Drug Interactions: None has been reported.

Therapeutic Indications in Hematology: Presently, plicamycin is primarily used to treat hypercalcemia of malignancy. Claims of antitumor activity in the blast phase of CML have been made[246] but have not been confirmed.

Bleomycin

Chemistry and Mechanism of Action: Bleomycin is a glycopeptide. Its antitumor effect correlates with its ability to cause scission of both double- and single-stranded DNA via activated oxygen formed by the iron/bleomycin complex. Bleomycin also affects DNA repair by inhibiting DNA ligase.[247]

Absorption, Fate, and Excretion: Bleomycin is rapidly distributed throughout the body and concentrates in the skin, lung, kidney, peritoneum, and lymph nodes. Its plasma half-life is 2–4 hours. Within 24 hours of injection, approximately 50% of an administered dose is excreted unchanged in the urine. Bleomycin elimination correlates well with creatinine clearance; accordingly, patients with renal failure should receive a reduced dose. In the tissues, bleomycin is inactivated by bleomycin hydrolase. Tissues lacking this enzyme, such as lung and skin, are more susceptible to the drug's toxic effects.[247]

Preparation and Administration: Bleomycin is commercially available in vials containing 15 U (approximately equivalent to 15 mg), from which it is reconstituted for injection with 3–5 ml of sterile water, normal saline, 5% dextrose in water, or bacteriostatic water. For intravenous infusion, the reconstituted solution can be further diluted with either normal saline or 5% dextrose in water and administered over ≥5 minutes. Bleomycin can also be administered by the subcutaneous, intravenous, intramuscular, intracavitary, and intraarterial routes. Because patients with lymphomas are at an increased risk of anaphylactoid reactions, which may not occur until 12 hours after administration, the first two doses should be intramuscular "test doses" of 1–2 mg. If no reactions occur, full doses may be given.

Toxic Effects: The most serious toxic effect is interstitial pneumonitis, which is dose related and occurs in approximately 10% of patients treated with cumulative doses of >350–400 U. The interstitial pneumonitis may evolve into life-threatening pulmonary fibrosis. Pulmonary toxicity is more common in patients >70 years, in those receiving a total dose of >400 U, and in those who received prior radiotherapy to the lung. It is important to emphasize, however, that the pulmonary toxicity is unpredictable; it has been reported in patients who had none of these risk factors and has occurred in a patient after administration of only 20 U. Some reports suggest that an increased concentration of inspired oxygen acts synergistically with bleomycin to produce pulmonary fibrosis. During critical illness and perioperatively, therefore, an attempt should be made to maintain the inspired oxygen concentration at ≤21%. The early phases of the pulmonary toxicity are clinically manifested by dyspnea and fine rales. Although corticosteroids are often employed in this setting, it is not clear that they are of benefit.

Mucocutaneous toxicity occurs in ≥50% of patients treated and is manifested by hyperpigmentation, pruritic erythema, mucositis, desquamation of the plantar surface skin of the hands and/or feet, ridging of the nails, and alopecia. The mucositis can be severe and is the acute dose-limiting toxic effect. Febrile reactions, which occur a few hours after bleomycin administration and may last 4–12 hours, are also common. Fever becomes less frequent with continued use of the drug and can usually be prevented by concurrent administration of glucocorticosteroids (e.g., 100 mg of hydrocortisone). Bleomycin has virtually no myelosuppressive effect. Anaphylactoid reactions are observed in approximately 1 percent (≤8% in some series) of patients with lymphomas treated with bleomycin.[247]

Potential Drug Interaction: Bleomycin, administered with other drugs for the treatment of lymphorrla, can decrease the oral bioavailability of digoxin and the pharmacologic effect of phenytoin and certain anesthetic drugs.[247–250]

Therapeutic Indications in Hematology: Bleomycin is often incorporated in the chemotherapy regimens of Hodgkin disease (ABVD and MOPP/ABV hybrid regimens) and non-Hodgkin lymphomas (MACOP-B, PROMACE/CYTABOM, M-BACOD, and CHOP-Bleo).

Appendix 61-4

Clinical Pharmacology of Antimetabolites

Methotrexate (Folex, Mexate)

Chemistry and Mechanism of Action: Methotrexate is a folic acid analogue, which contains ≥85% of 4-amino-10-methylfolic acid and small amounts of related compounds. It exerts its cytotoxic effect by inhibiting the enzyme dihydrofolate reductase and thereby depleting the intracellular pool of tetrahydrofolate, which functions as a carrier of one carbon group required for the synthesis of purine nucleotides and thymidilate. As shown in Figure 61-8, the blockade produced by methotrexate can be circumvented by providing an exogenously reduced folate such as folinic acid (leucovorin [N^5-formyltetrahydrofolate]).[251]

Absorption, Fate, and Excretion: Orally administered methotrexate is rapidly absorbed from the gastrointestinal tract and reaches peak levels in about 1 hour. Methotrexate is reportedly 100% bioavailable at oral doses of <30 mg/m^2. At higher doses gastrointestinal absorption is reduced. The half-life varies with the route of administration (9 hours after oral, 3 hours after intramuscular, and 27 hours after intravenous administration). Methotrexate is widely distributed, primarily to body water. Accordingly, it accumulates in third-space fluids such as pleural effusions and ascites, which may function as a reservoir, resulting in prolonged slow release of the drug and increased toxicity. Methotrexate is primarily (>90%) excreted unchanged in the urine, with renal elimination correlating well with creatinine clearance. High doses of the drug may reach therapeutic concentrations in the cerebrospinal fluid.[252]

Preparation and Administration: Methotrexate is commercially available in various dosage forms and strengths: (1) as 2.5-mg tablets for oral use; (2) as a preservative-free parenteral preparation in vials containing 20, 25, 50, 100, 200, 250, and 1,000 mg; (3) as a low-sodium sterile preparation in 100-mg vials; and (4) in vials of 2.5 and 25 mg/ml containing preservatives (benzyl alcohol and sodium chloride). The lyophilized form of the drug should be reconstituted with preservative-free sodium chloride or 5% dextrose in water to a final concentration of ≤25 mg/ml. For intrathecal injections, solutions containing 1–1.5 mg/ml should be prepared with pre-servative-free 0.9% sodium chloride as the diluent (e.g., 12 mg of methotrexate in 10 ml of diluent). When methotrexate is employed in intermediate or high doses, leucovorin must be used as a rescue agent. Depending on the regimen chosen, leucovorin is administered 12–24 hours following methotrexate. Adequate hydration and alkalinization of the urine are essential to prevent excessive toxicity. Patients with body fluid third-space compartments are poor candidates for high-dose methotrexate regimens. When high-dose (≥500 mg/m^2) regimens are used, the 24-hour methotrexate level must be monitored along with the 24-hour serum creatinine. If at 24 hours the methotrexate concentration is ≥5 × 10^{-7} M, leuco-vorin should be added according to the following schedule:

Methotrexate Level (M)	Dose of Leucovorin (mg/m^2 q6h × 8 doses)
≥5 × 10^{-7}	15
≥1 × 10^{-6}	100
≥2 × 10^{-6}	200

Methotrexate levels must be determined every 48 hours and leucovorin administered until the methotrexate level has fallen to <5 × 10^{-7}M.

Toxic Effects: The dose-limiting toxic effects are myelosuppression and mucositis. Leukopenia and thrombocytopenia usually occur 7–14 days after administration. Diarrhea occurs in some cases. When methotrexate is used in high doses, an acute and transient elevation of liver enzymes can occur. Conversely, when it is employed in low doses but for prolonged periods, chronic hepatic fibrosis is more common. Nephrotoxicity is uncommon with standard doses of methotrexate but may occur with high-dose regimens owing to precipitation of 7-hydroxymethotrexate in the renal tubules. Methotrexate may produce rashes, generally of the maculopapular type. An idiosyncratic nonrecurring acute pulmonary toxicity also has been reported. Unlike the uniformly dose-related pulmonary fibrosis observed with carmustine, busulfan, and bleomycin, methotrexate toxicity is a self-limited process characterized by cough, fever, and an interstitial infiltrate.

Several complications have been associated with the intrathecal administration of methotrexate. These include (1) chemical arachnoiditis; (2) a subacute onset of motor paralysis manifested by cranial nerve dysfunction, seizures, and coma; and more rarely, (3) a chronic demyelinating syndrome characterized by motor spasticity and dementia. Cranial irradiation increases the frequency of these side effects.

Potential Drug Interactions: Salicylates, sulfonamides, phenytoin, tetracycline, and p-aminobenzoic acid can displace methotrexate from its protein-binding sites and increase the concentration of free drug. However, the clinical significance of these protein-binding interactions is debatable. Prednisone may influence methotrexate pharmacokinetics.[252] Pyrimethamine uses the same carrier protein and will compete for the cellular uptake of methotrexate. Salicylates and probenecid may compete with methotrexate for renal tubular secretion and may prolong the drug's half-life. Methotrexate can augment the anticoagulant effect of warfarin. Nonsteroidal anti-inflammatory drugs may enhance methotrexate toxicity and should be discontinued ≥48–72 hours prior to treatment with moderate or high-dose methotrexate. Methotrexate interacts with many cytotoxic agents. For example, when administered prior to 5-fluorouracil, it increases cell kill due to increased intracellular accumulation of PRPP (phosphoribosylpyrophosphate), but when given after 5-fluorouracil, it decreases cell kill. When methotrexate is given prior to L-asparaginase, its cytotoxicity in normal tissues is decreased.[197,220] Certain macrolide antibiotics may potentiate the effect of methotrexate, but the mechanism remains to be clearly defined.[253,254]

Therapeutic Indication in Hematology: Methotrexate is employed in the treatment of ALL (especially in the maintenance phase) and non-Hodgkin lymphomas (MACOP-B, M-BACOD, PROMACE/CYTABOM).

Cytarabine (Cytosar-U)

Chemistry and Mechanism of Action: Cytarabine, also called cytosine arabinoside (ara-C), is one of several arabinose nucleosides. Cytarabine enters cells via carrier and is metabolized by salvage pathway enzymes to its active form, ara-CTP. This nucleotide interferes with the action of DNA polymerase α, but the primary cytotoxic action appears to result from incorporation of ara-C into DNA, leading to a marked slowing of the elongating chain and a defect in the ligation of fragments of newly synthesized DNA. Cytarabine is S phase specific.[255] In addition to its direct cytotoxic effect, ara-C induces terminal differentiation of leukemic cells, which in some cases is associated with decreased c-*myc* amplification.

Absorption, Fate, and Excretion: Following intravenous administration, ara-C follows a biphasic elimination with a terminal half-life within a range of 1–3 hours. The drug is rapidly and extensively metabolized by cytidine deaminase, which is widely distributed in the liver as well as other tissues of the body. Approximately 90% of the dose is eliminated through the kidneys as ara-U and other inactive metabolites. After 2 hours of continuous intravenous administration, the concentration of ara-C in the spinal fluid reaches approximately 50% of the simultaneous plasma levels.[255]

Preparation and Administration: Cytarabine is commercially available as freeze-dried powder in 100- and 500-mg and 1- and 2-g vials. For reconstitution, the manufacturers recommends adding 5, 10, 10, and 20 ml of diluent (0.9% benzyl alcohol in water) to the 100-mg, 500-mg, 1-g, and 2-g vials, respectively. The reconstituted solution may be further diluted with 5% dextrose water or normal saline to obtain a desired lower dose. ara-C can be administered by various routes, including intravenous, subcutaneous, and intrathecal. The diluent provided by the manufacturer contains preservatives and *should not* be administered intrathecally.

Toxic Effects: Myelosuppression is the dose-limiting toxic effect. Leukopenia and thrombocytopenia reach their nadir in 7–14 days. Gastrointestinal toxicity is common and includes nausea, vomiting, mucositis, and elevation of liver enzymes. Occasionally, a flu-like syndrome is seen. Alopecia occurs commonly in patients receiving high-dose therapy, less commonly when receiving "standard" or low-dose ara-C. When ara-C is used in high doses (2–3 g/m^2 per dose for 6–12 doses), unique side effects may occur, including diarrhea, conjunctivitis, and, most importantly, neurotoxicity. The conjunctivitis may be severe but can be minimized or prevented by prophylactic administration of an ophthalmic corticosteroid. The neurotoxicity is primarily manifested as a cerebellar dysfunction syndrome with or without a cerebral component. Although it is usually reversible, it may take months to resolve. Rare cases of pulmonary toxicity, peripheral neuropathy, and the syndrome of inappropriate secretion of antidiuretic hormone have been reported.[255] Intrathecally administered ara-C can cause adverse effects similar to those mentioned for methotrexate.

Potential Drug Interactions: ara-C enhances cytotoxicity induced by cyclophosphamide, VP-16, m-AMSA, BCNU, and cisplatin. The probable mechanism is inhibition of DNA strand repair by ara-C. Additionally, thymidine and hydroxyurea both lower cellular dCDP levels and enhance ara-C cytotoxicity. Cyclopentenyl cytosine inhibits CTP synthetase, lowers CTP levels, and enhances ara-C cytotoxicity. Methotrexate enhances ara-C toxicity by an unclear mechanism. ara-C inhibits fludarabine metabolism in leukemic blast cells in vivo.[256] Finally, certain biologic response modifiers such as interleukin-3 and colony-stimulating factor-granulocyte/macrophage are able to cycle more cells into S phase and therefore may increase the therapeutic efficacy of ara-C.

Therapeutic Indications in Hematology: ara-C is probably one of the most important drugs for induction therapy of AML. It is also useful as a second-line agent in the treatment of Hodgkin disease and non-Hodgkin lymphomas.

Fludarabine (Fludara)

Chemistry and Mechanism of Action: Fludarabine phosphate is the 2-fluoro-5'-phosphate derivative of the antileukemic agent 9-β-D-arabinofuranosyl adenine (ara-A). It inhibits ribonucleotide reductase, and the triphosphate form, fluoro-ara-ATP, through incorporation into DNA inhibits DNA polymerase and thereby subsequent inhibits DNA synthesis.[257,258]

Absorption, Fate, and Excretion: After intravenous injection, fludarabine is rapidly dephosphorylated in the plasma to 2-fluoro-ara-A and is detectable as fludarabine phosphate at low levels after 2–4 minutes. 2-Fluoro-ara-A, the putative anticancer moiety, has a half-life of about 10 hours and is primarily excreted in the urine.[258–260]

Preparation and Administration: Fludarabine is supplied in vials containing 50 mg of fludarabine as a white lyophilized powder, with sodium hydroxide to adjust pH. The drug is reconstituted with 2 ml of sterile water to yield a 25-mg/ml solution for injection. The reconstituted solution is chemically stable for ≥48 hours at room temperature when further diluted to yield a 0.04–1 mg/ml solution in normal saline or 5% dextrose in water.

Toxic Effects: The acute dose-limiting toxic effect of fludarabine is myelosuppression. Occasionally, nausea, vomiting, and hepatocellular toxicity occur. The most serious side effect, however, is an irreversible neurotoxicity syndrome characterized by cortical blindness, encephalopathy, and coma. Neuropathologic findings include a diffuse necrotizing leukoencephalopathy that is most severe in the occipital lobes, medullary pyramids, and posterior columns. The neurotoxicity syndrome has been described primarily in patients receiving fludarabine in high doses (>40 mg/m²/day for 5 days).[259,261-263] Interstitial pneumonitis and respiratory failure has also been reported.[264] Severe T-cell immunodeficiency is common; however, infection with *Pneumocystis carinii* and cytomegalovirus is uncommon.[265]

Potential Drug Interactions: Concomitant administration of fludarabine (10 mg/m²/day for 4 days every 28 days) and pentostatin (4 mg/m² every 2 weeks) *may* be associated with fatal pneumonitis. ara-C also decreases the metabolism of fludarabine to its active metabolite both in vivo and in vitro. Fludarabine may enhance the metabolic activation of ara-C in vivo; however, the clinical significance of these findings remain to be ascertained.[256,267]

Clinical Indications in Hematology: Fludarabine remains the most active drug in CLL to date.[268] Further uses include marked antitumor activity in low-grade lymphomas, especially follicular small cleaved.[269,270] Other uses include salvage treatment of refractory of Waldenström's macroglobulinemia and mycosis fungoides.[271,272]

Azacytidine (5-aza-C) and 5-Azacytosine Arabinosde (ara-AC)

Chemistry and Mechanism of Action: Azacytidine is an analogue of the pyrimidine nucleoside cytidine. Intracellular azacytidine undergoes phosphorylated to azacytidine triphosphate, which is incorporated into RNA and ultimately leads to inhibition of protein synthesis. Azacytidine is also incorporated, but to a lesser extent, into DNA.[273] ara-AC is a synthetic pyrimidine analogue that is activated by deoxycytidine kinase to a phosphorylated compound and incorporated into DNA.

Absorption, Fate, and Excretion: Azacytidine is rapidly deaminated by cytidine deaminase, which is found in the liver, granulocytes, and gastrointestinal epithelium. Azacytidine (the parent compound plus metabolites) has a plasma half-life of 3.5–6.4 hours. Approximately 20% of the drug is excreted into the urine unchanged. The drug does not penetrate the cerebrospinal fluid.[274]

Toxic Effects: The dose-limiting side effect is myelosuppression, especially leukopenia. Nausea and vomiting can be severe and require aggressive antiemetic prophylaxis, but these effects can be significantly reduced if azacytidine is administered by continuous infusion. Diarrhea is also a common adverse effect. Occasionally the drug may produce fever, which may be seen at ≤24 hours after drug administration. In rare cases, hepatotoxicity, hypophosphatemia, and neuromuscular side effects occur.[274]

Potential Drug Interactions: None has been reported.

Therapeutic Indications in Hematology: Azacytidine is primarily used for the induction treatment of refractory AML. ara-AC has greater clinical activity both in vivo and in vitro against many different solid tumors including testicular and breast neoplasms.

Mercaptopurine (Purinethol)

Chemistry and Mechanism of Action: Mercaptopurine (6-MP) is a purine analogue that affects the synthesis of DNA and RNA by inhibiting de novo purine synthesis. The drug is also a potent immunosuppressive agent.[275]

Absorption, Fate, and Excretion: The oral bioavailability of 6-MP is extremely variable, within a range of 5–37% (average 16%). It has been suggested that this is due to metabolism in the gastrointestinal mucosa and/or during the first pass through the liver. After a single oral dose, peak concentrations are reached within 2 hours, and the drug is not detectable in the serum after 8 hours. Intravenously administered 6-MP has a half-life of 0.3–0.9 hours. 6-MP is rapidly and extensively metabolized in the liver by the enzyme xanthine oxidase. The parent drug and its metabolites are excreted in the urine.[275]

Preparation and Administration: 6-MP is commercially supplied as 50-mg oral tablets. An intravenous formulation, 500-mg per vial, is investigational and is supplied by Burroughs-Wellcome.

Toxic Effects: The dose-limiting side effect is myelosuppression. This may take several weeks to occur, although recovery of blood counts is usually rapid after drug discontinuation. Mild nausea, vomiting, and occasionally mucositis and diarrhea are also seen. Hepatotoxicity occurs in 10–40% of adult patients and consists of intrahepatic cholestasis and a variable degree of hepatocellular necrosis. Close monitoring of liver function is recommended and if liver function tests are abnormal, the drug should be discontinued until recovery. Other less common side effects include fever, eosinophilia, and scaling rash. Patients on prolonged 6-MP therapy should be considered immunosuppressed.[275]

Potential Drug Interactions: Allopurinol, an inhibitor of xanthine oxidase, significantly increases 6-MP blood levels resulting from *oral* administration. No effect is observed when allopurinol is combined with the intravenous form of 6-MP. This differential effect is attributed to inhibition of first-pass metabolism of oral 6-MP by allopurinol. Patients on allopurinol should receive one-fourth of the usual oral 6-MP dose. 6-MP has been reported to both increase and decrease the anticoagulant effect of warfarin.[197]

Therapeutic Indications in Hematology: The use of 6-MP is restricted to the maintenance phase of ALL.

Thioguanine

Chemistry and Mechanism of Action: Thioguanine (6-TG) is an analogue of guanine in which a sulfydryl group replaces the hydroxyl group in position 6. The cytotoxic effect of 6-TG is associated with depletion of purine nucleotides and more importantly, with its incorporation into DNA as "false" nucleotides. The drug appears to be 5 phase specific.[275]

Absorption, Fate, and Excretion: The oral bioavailability of 6-TG is approximately 30%, with the peak concentration reached 2–4 hours after oral administration. 6-TG has a half-life of about 90 minutes after intravenous administration. The drug does not enter the central nervous system. It is completely excreted by the kidneys in the form of metabolites.[275]

Preparation and Administration: 6-TG is commercially available as 40-mg tablets, from which oral suspensions containing 40 mg/ml may be prepared. An intravenous formulation is under investigation.

Toxic Effects: The dose-limiting toxic effect is myelosuppression, primarily leukopenia and thrombocytopenia. Nausea, vomiting, diarrhea, and jaundice may occur but are uncommon.

Potential Drug Interactions: Unlike 6-MP, 6-TG does not interact with allopurinol.

Therapeutic Indications in Hematology: 6-TG is used in the treatment of AML, although its usefulness has been recently questioned.

Pentostatin (Pentostatin, Nipent)

Chemistry and Mechanism of Action: Pentostatin, also called 2'-deoxycoformycin, is an adenosine analogue whose cytotoxic effect is mediated by inhibition of adenosine deaminase. This results in larger quantities of dATP, which appear to be cytoxic. Although adenosine deaminase is found in virtually every tissue, it is most abundant in lymphoid tissue. The pentostatin is toxic to dividing as well as to nondividing cells.[266]

Absorption, Fate, and Excretion: After intravenous injection, the plasma clearance of pentostatin follows a biphasic pattern, with a half-life of approximately 3–10 hours. About 90% of an administered dose is recovered in the urine within 24 hours of administration. The total body clearance of pentostatin correlates well with the creatinine clearance.[266]

Preparation and Administration: Pentostatin is provided in vials containing 10 mg of the drug, 50 mg of mannitol, and sodium hydroxide to adjust the pH. The drug is given as an intravenous infusion over ≥10–30 minutes. The patients should be well hydrated both before and after pentostatin infusion.

Toxic Effects: Pentostatin causes myelosuppression, immunosuppression, nausea, vomiting, renal failure, keratoconjunctivitis, fever, and elevation of liver enzymes. When high doses are used, neurotoxic effects, including seizures and coma, can occur. At the doses presently used in the treatment of hairy cell leukemia, however, side effects are usually minor.[266–276] Mouse embryotoxicity (neural tube defects) following in utero exposure to pentostatin has been reported but no such correlation has been observed in humans.[2]

Potential Drug Interactions: See drug interactions for fludarabine. There may be some increased abnormalities in renal or hepatic function when used with allopurinol, although cause and effect is established with combined administration. Therefore, allopurinol should only be used in selected cases where profound tumor lysis expected.[278]

Therapeutic Indications in Hematology: Pentostatin is approved for the treatment of hairy cell leukemia and has also clinically demonstrated activity against B-cell prolymphocytic leukemia low-grade non-Hodgkin lymphoma, cutaneous T-cell lymphomas, and CLL.[266,279]

2-Chlorodeoxyadenosine (Leustatin, 2-CdA)

Chemistry and Mechanism of Action: CdA is an ADA-resistant purine analogue that is predominantly toxic to lymphocytes. It is phosphorylated intracellularly to chlorodeoxy ATP and inhibits DNA synthesis. It may also independently activate cellular apoptosis.

Preparation and Administration: This drug is usually supplied as a 0.1% solution (1 mg/ml) in sterile 0.9% sodium chloride. The dosing schedule is 0.1 mg/kg/day given as a continuous infusion for 7 days, which may be repeated every 5 weeks.

Toxic Effects: Moderately severe leukopenic fever develops in 40% of patients. Most patients have reversible myelosuppression and immunosuppression.

Potential Drug Interactions: None has been reported.

Therapeutic Indications in Hematology: CdA is most useful as a first-line agent for hairy cell leukemia and also for interferon resistant hairy cell leukemia. It has reported efficacy in lymphoid malignancies such as CLL, CTCL, T-cell CLL, CML, multiple myeloma, and possibly low-grade lymphomas. In these diseases, however, the precise role for institution of CdA is unknown and subject to further investigation.[266,280]

Appendix 61-5

Clinical Pharmacology of Miscellaneous Agents

Cisplatin (Platinol)

Chemistry and Mechanism of Action: Cisplatin [cisdiaminedichloroplatinum(II)] is an inorganic heavy metal coordination complex. It produces its cytotoxic effect by forming intrastrand and interstrand DNA cross-links. The drug also binds to nuclear and cytoplasmic proteins. Cisplatin is cell cycle nonspecific.[281]

Absorption, Fate, and Excretion: Following its intravenous injection, the drug concentrates in the liver, kidneys, and bowel. Approximately 25–45% of it is eliminated via the kidneys. Plasma levels of cisplatin decay in a biphasic manner with an initial half-life of 25–49 minutes and a terminal half-life of 58–73 hours.[281]

Preparation and Administration: Cisplatin is commercially available as a lyophilized powder, supplied in 10- and 50-mg vials also containing mannitol, sodium chloride, and hydrochloric acid and as an aqueous solution in 50- and 100-mg vials. Reconstitution of the powder for injection is achieved by adding sterile water to make a 1-mg/ml solution. The reconstituted solution should be further diluted in normal saline (usually 500 ml to 1 L) and administered over 1–3 hours. To prevent nephrotoxic effects, 25–50 g of mannitol is often added to the saline solution, and patients are aggressively hydrated before and after cisplatin infusion. Magnesium sulfate (12–24 mEq) is commonly added to the saline solution to preclude the development of hypomagnesemia.

Toxic Effects: Nephrotoxicity is the dose-limiting toxic effect. Cisplatin produces a dose-dependent impairment of renal tubular function, manifested by an increase in serum creatinine and by hypomagnesemia. The renal dysfunction is usually reversible, but repeated treatments may produce a permanent mild-to-moderate impairment of renal function. Nausea and vomiting are usually severe and require the use of aggressive antiemetic support. When doses >70 mg/m^2 are used, it is also important to protect against delayed nausea and vomiting by administering antiemetic agents (e.g., prochlorperazine plus dexamethasone) for ≥ 3 days following therapy. Myelosuppression is usually mild. High-frequency hearing loss, tinnitus, and frank deafness may occur. Peripheral neurotoxicity, characterized by paresthesias or sensory loss in a glove-and-stocking distribution or as muscular weakness, is relatively common in patients who receive total cumulative doses of >500 mg/m^2. The peripheral neuropathy may take many months to resolve, if it does at all. Vestibular toxicity and anaphylactic reactions may occur rarely.

Potential Drug Interactions: Aminoglycosides and amphotericin may enhance cisplatin nephrotoxicity. Caution should be exercised when cisplatin is administered with bleomycin[282] and methotrexate,[283] as cisplatin-induced renal damage may delay the excretion and thus increase the toxicity of these agents.

Therapeutic Indications in Hematology: Cisplatin is used in the treatment of refractory lymphomas, usually in combination with cytosine arabinoside and high-dose dexamethasone.

Carboplatin (Paraplatin)

Chemistry and Mechanism of Action: Carboplatin is a second-generation platinum (II) complex. Its mechanism of action is very similar to that of cisplatin.

Absorption, Fate, and Excretion: Carboplatin is primarily eliminated through the kidneys and has a half-life of approximately 1.5 hours. Following intravenous injection, approximately 60% of the total drug is excreted within 24 hours.[284]

Preparation and Administration: Carboplatin is commercially available as a lyophilized powder in 50- and 150-mg vials containing carboplatin and mannitol. It is reconstituted with sterile water to a final concentration of 10 mg/ml. For injection further dilution with 5% dextrose and water or normal saline to a concentration of 0.5 or 2 mg/ml, it is stable for ≥ 24 hours at room temperature. Carboplatin is often administered by intravenous injection over 15–30 minutes. Patients with reduced renal function (creatinine clearance of <60 ml/min) should have the dose of carboplatin decreased according to the formula described by Egorin et al.[285]
For previously untreated patients:

$$\text{Dosage (mg/m}^2\text{)} = (0.091) \left(\frac{\text{creatinine clearance}}{\text{body surface area}} \right)$$

$$\times \left[\frac{\text{pretreatment platelet count} - \text{platelet nadir desired}}{\text{pretreatment platelet count}} \right.$$

$$\left. \times\ 100 \right] + 86$$

For heavily pretreated patients:

$$\text{Dosage (mg/m}^2\text{)} = (0.091) \left(\frac{\text{creatinine clearance}}{\text{body surface area}} \right)$$

$$\times \left[\left(\frac{\text{pretreatment platelet count} - \text{platelet nadir desired}}{\text{pretreatment platelet count}} \right. \right.$$

$$\left. \left. \times\ 100 \right) - 17 \right] + 86$$

Toxic Effects: The dose-limiting toxic effect is myelosuppression, thrombocytopenia being more significant than leukopenia. Carboplatin leads to less emesis than cisplatin. Although nausea and vomiting are common, they can be easily controlled with antiemetics. At high doses such as those used for bone marrow transplantation, hepatotoxicity, renal dysfunction, and moderate to severe ototoxicity can occur.[286]

Potential Drug Interactions: None has been reported.

Clinical Indications in Hematology: Carboplatin has been recently approved for the treatment of ovarian cancer. High-dose carboplatin is presently under evaluation in acute leukemias and lymphomas.

Hydroxyurea ((Hydrea)

Chemistry and Mechanism of Action: Hydroxyurea affects DNA systhesis through inhibition of ribonucleotide reductase. The drug is S phase specific.[287]

Absorption, Fate, and Excretion: Hydroyurea is well absorbed by the oral route. It has a half-life of 1.7–5 hours, and approximately 30–40% is eliminated through the kidneys. It achieves peak serum levels in 2 hours and is undetectable in the blood by 6 hours. About 50% of an oral dose is metabolized in the liver and excreted as urea and as carbon dioxide. The drug penetrates well into the central nervous system.

Preparation and Administration: Hydroxyurea is commercially available as 500-mg capsules.

Toxic Effects: The dose-limiting toxic effect is leukopenia, which resolves rapidly on discontinuation of the drug. Self-limiting megaloblastic erythropoiesis is also common; at high doses, nausea, vomiting, and mucositis can occur.

Potential Drug Interactions: Hydroxyurea inhibits DNA repair and therefore, interacts synergistically with DNA damaging agents such as topoisomerase II inhibitors. It increases cytosine arabinoside cytotoxicity by enhancing ara-C uptake and phosphorylation to cytosine arabinoside triphosphate. It is capable of suppressing high levels of deoxyuridine monophosphate, reducing 5-fluorouracil resistance. Recently, it has been demonstrated to enhance amsacrine-induced DNA strand breaks leading to synergistic cytotoxicity.[288]

Therapeutic Indications in Hematology: Hydroxyurea is primarily used in the treatment of the chronic phase of CLL, polycythemia vera, primary thrombocytosis, and agnogenic myeloid metaplasia. It is also useful in the treatment of leukostasis.

Procarbazine

Chemistry and Mechanism of Action: Procarbazine is a substituted hydrazine derivative with a chemical structure similar to that of the monoamine oxidase inhibitors (MAOI). Accordingly, procarbazine exhibits weak MAOI effects. Procarbazine itself is inert and must undergo metabolic activation to generate cytotoxic reactants, the mode of action of which is not clear. They may inhibit transmethylation of methyl groups of methionine into tRNA or may also directly damage DNA. Hydrogen peroxide, formed during the auto-oxidation of procarbazine, may attack protein sulfhydryl groups contained in residual proteins tightly bound to DNA.[289]

Absorption, Fate, and Excretion: Procarbazine is rapidly and completely absorbed by the oral route, peak plasma levels occurring within 60 minutes. It penetrates well into the cerebrospinal fluid. The drug is readily metabolized in the liver and has a plasma half-life of 10 minutes after intravenous injection. The major sites of elimination are the kidneys, where approximately 70% of the drug is excreted as N-isopropylterephthalamic acid and <5% is excreted unchanged.[289]

Preparation and Administration: Procarbazine is commercially available as 50-mg capsules.

Toxic Effects: The usual dose-limiting toxic effect is myelosuppression. Occasionally nausea and vomiting may be dose limiting, although tolerance to those effects may develop during continued administration. Other less common side effects include paresthesias, headache, dizziness, depression, apprehension, insomnia, nightmares, hallucinations, drowsiness, ataxia, foot drop, decreased reflexes, tremors, coma, confusion, convulsions, skin rash, alopecia, myalgia, and arthralgia. Procarbazine may possibly be leukemogenic.

Potential Drug Interactions: Combination chemotherapy that includes procarbazine may result in a decrease in digoxin plasma levels. Because procarbazine is a weak MAOI, hypertensive reactions could theoretically occur following concurrent ingestion of sympathomimetics, levodopa, tricyclic antidepressants, or foods with high tyramine content (e.g., dark beer, yogurt, cheeses, and red wines). However, such reactions have not been reported. Concomitant use of narcotics or other strong sedatives may result in exaggerated depressant effects, leading to coma and possibly death. Procarbazine also interacts with alcohol causing a disulfiram-like reaction.[289]

Therapeutic Indications in Hematology: Procarbazine is often used in combination with other cytotoxic agents in the treatment of Hodgkin disease (MOPP and MOPP derivatives) and to a lesser extent in the treatment of non-Hodgkin lymphomas (PROMACE/MOPP).

Asparaginase

Chemistry and Mechanism of Action: Asparaginase contains the high-molecular-weight enzyme L-asparaginase amidohydrolase, type EC-2, derived from *Escherichia coli*. Asparaginase hydrolyzes serum asparagine to nonfunctional aspartic acid and ammonia, depriving tumor cells of a required amino acid; thus, tumor cell proliferation is blocked by the interruption of asparagine-dependent protein synthesis. The drug appears to be most active in the G_1 phase.[290]

Absorption, Fate, and Excretion: Asparaginase is not absorbed orally. Its plasma half-life varies from 8 to 30 hours and is not influenced by dosage, age, sex, surface area, or renal or hepatic function.[290]

Preparation and Administration: Asparaginase is commercially available in vials containing 10,000 IU of asparaginase in 80 mg of mannitol. For intravenous use, the drug should be reconstituted with 5 ml of either sterile water or sodium chloride for injection and injected in the tubing of a freely running infusion of either normal saline or 5% dextrose in water over ≥30 minutes. For intramuscular or subcutaneous use, each vial should be reconstituted with 2 ml of sodium chloride for injection to obtain a 5,000-U/ml solution. For dosages that exceed 2 ml, use of two injection sites is recommended. For both intravenous and intramuscular administration, the drug must be used within 8 hours of reconstitution, and only if it is clear. Because of the possibility of hypersensitivity reactions (particularly in patients with lymphomas), an intradermal skin test is recommended before initial administration of asparaginase or when ≥1 week has elapsed between doses. For this test, 2 IU should be injected intradermally and observed for a wheal or erythema for ≥1 hour. A negative skin test, however, does not preclude possible development of a hypersensitivity reaction. It is recommended that oxygen, epinephrine, and corticosteroids be available at the bedside during administration of the drug. For allergic patients, the *E. coli* form of asparaginase should be replaced by the asparaginase derived from *Erwinia carotovora*, provided by the National Cancer Institute as an investigational group C agent.

Toxic Effects: The toxicity of asparaginase is reported to be greater in adults than in children. Anorexia, nausea, or vomiting occurs in approximately one-third of patients. Most of the other side effects can be divided into two main groups, those related to hypersensitivity reactions to the foreign protein and those resulting from decreased protein synthesis. The hypersensitivity reaction is characterized by urticaria, laryngeal edema, bronchospasm, or hypotension and may occur with the initial dose of the drug, even if the skin test is negative. More commonly, however, allergic phenomena are observed after multiple courses of treatment. Adverse effects related to the inhibition of protein synthesis include hypoalbuminemia and decreases in serum fibrinogen, prothrombin, antithrombin III, and other coagulation factors, which may lead to both clotting and hemorrhagic complications; decreased serum insulin with hyperglycemia; and decreased serum lipoproteins. In ≤25% of patients cerebral dysfunction, characterized by confusion, stupor, and frank coma, can occur. Although the neurotoxic effects resemble those of ammonia toxicity, they are apparently due to low concentrations of either L-asparagine or L-glutamine in the brain. Acute pancreatitis, which may progress to severe hemorrhagic pancreatitis, may occur in ≤15% of patients. Elevation of liver enzymes and serum bilirubin is almost universal and is histologically represented by fatty metamorphosis. Liver toxicity, although usually not clinically significant, has resulted in occasional fatalities. Asparaginase can occasionally produce renal functional impairment with oliguric renal failure.[290]

Potential Drug Interactions: When asparaginase is administered *immediately before or concurrent* with methotrexate, it decreases the cytotoxic effect of the latter. When administered to patients with acute leukemia 9–10 days *before or shortly after* methotrexate, however, asparaginase appears to enhance the cytotoxic effect of methotrexate. Concurrent administration of asparaginase with vincristine may increase vincristine's neurotoxic effects, but this effect appears to be less pronounced when asparaginase is given after vincristine. The effects of asparaginase on liver function may potentially interfere with the activation or metabolism of other cytotoxic agents.[290]

Therapeutic Indications in Hematology: Asparaginase is used in combination therapy for remission induction of patients with ALL.

Amsacrine

Chemistry and Mechanism of Action: Amsacrine, or 4'-(9-acridinylamino)methanesulfon-*M*-anisidide) (AMSA) is a synthetic aminoacridine derivative. Although its mechanism of action has not been completely elucidated, the drug is capable of DNA intercalation and of stabilizing the topoisomerase II cleavable complex, leading to the formation of DNA strand breaks.[291–297]

Absorption, Fate, and Excretion: Following intravenous injection, the drug exhibits a biphasic distribution of both the total and free drug, the half-life of free drug with a range of 3–10 hours. Approximately 50% of the drug is eliminated in bile. Cumulative urinary excretion amounts to approximately one-third within 3 days of administration. Patients with liver disease, however, have a prolonged plasma elimination, and excrete about 50% of the drug through the kidneys.[293,296]

Preparation and Administration: Amsacrine is an investigational agent supplied by the National Cancer Institute as a group C drug or by the Warner–Lambert Company. It is provided in a dual pack containing two sterile liquids that must be combined prior to use. One vial contains 1.5 ml of a 50-

mg/ml solution of AMSA in anhydrous N,N-dimethylacetamide, and the other contains 13.5 ml of 0.0353 M L-lactic acid diluent. When these are combined, the resulting orange-red solution contains 5 mg/ml of AMSA. Because of the N,N-dimethylactetamide solvent, plastic syringes should not be used with the undiluted AMSA solution.

Toxic Effects: The dose-limiting toxic effect is myelosuppression, predominantly affecting granulocytes. Alopecia is common, and nausea, vomiting, and mucositis can occur. Cardiotoxicity, manifested as a decrease in ejection fraction, acute arrhythmias, or electrocardiographic changes, was reported in 2.3% of 3,200 patients in a 1985 review, but most of these patients had been heavily pretreated with anthracyclines. Hypokalemia seems to enhance amsacrine cardiotoxicity and if present should be corrected prior to administration of the drug. Other, less common, side effects include elevation of liver enzymes and neurotoxic effects such as seizures.[291-297]

Potential Drug Interactions: The reconstituted solution is physically incompatible with chloride-containing solutions. In cell lines, there is additive effect with bleomycin, CPT-11, cisplatin, daunorubicin, doxorubicin, etoposide, 6-mercaptopurine, 5-fluorouracil, homoharringtonine, mitomycin C, and vincristine.[296]

Theapeutic Indications in Hematology: Amsacrine is a group C investigational drug approved for the treatment of refractory AML, although it is being evaluated in combination with other cytotoxic agents in the initial treatment of this disease. As a group C drug, amsacrine must be administered as a single agent.

Gallium Nitrate

Chemistry and Mechanism of Action: Gallium nitrate is a group IIA metal salt, of which the mechanism of action is not completely understood. Its selective cytotoxic effects in humans are probably related to its predominant concentration in certain malignant tumors. Gallium nitrate binds to intracellular calcium and magnesium sites. Transferrin binding appears to be necessary to produce the cytotoxic effect.[298]

Absorption, Fate, and Metabolism: Gallium nitrate is primarily eliminated by renal excretion and follows a biphasic pharmacokinetic pattern. The reported half-life is within a range of 6–36 hours.[298,299]

Preparation and Administration: Gallium nitrate is an investigational agent supplied as a 25-mg/ml solution in 20-ml vials (500 mg per vial), which also contain trisodium citrate and sodium hydroxide to adjust the pH. Gallium nitrate can be administered by slow intravenous infusion, although in the treatment of hypercalcemia it is usually given by continuous infusion over 5–7 days.

Toxic Effects: When gallium nitrate is given as a single bolus injection, the dose-limiting toxicity is renal impairment. The renal toxicity is significantly minimized when the drug is given by continuous infusion. Other toxic effects include mild myelosuppression, hypocalcemia (when not desired), nausea, vomiting, diarrhea, and mucositis. Rarely, gallium nitrate can produce neurotoxic effects such as hearing loss, visual disturbances, paresthesias, and mental status changes.[298,299]

Potential Drug Interactions: None has been reported.

Clinical Indications in Hematology: Gallium nitrate has shown promising results in the treatment of hypercalcemia associated with malignancy, in prevention of bone loss in patients with multiple myeloma, and in the treatment of refractory lymphomas.[298,299]

Glucocorticoids

Chemistry and Mechanism of Action: Glucocorticoids are synthetic compounds derived from the natural adrenal hormone cortisol. Glucocorticoids, like other steroids, are thought to act by interfering with protein synthesis, but their precise mechanism of action is still not completely understood. Lymphocytes treated with glucocorticoids undergo apoptosis or programmed cell death mediated by glucocorticoid receptors.[300,301] An early cytostatic phase is marked by growth inhibition and cessation of proliferation due to inhibition of cellular uptake of glucose, amino acids, and nucleosides as well as inhibition of macromolecular synthesis. This is followed by a cytolytic phase characterized by chromatin condensation and internucleosomal DNA cleavage.

Absorption, Fate, and Excretion: Many synthetic glucocorticoids are available, the three most commonly used in hematology being prednisone, dexamethasone, and methylprednisolone. The glucocorticoids are well absorbed orally and are primarily metabolized in the liver. Unlike the other two glucocorticoids, the activity of prednisone is dependent on hepatic conversion to the 11-hydroxy form (prednisolone). The biologic half-lives of prednisone and methylprednisolone are approximately 12–36 hours, whereas dexamethasone has a biologic half-life of 36–72 hours. Plasma half-lives for all three drugs are within the range of 3–4 hours. Compared with cortisol, the relative anti-inflammatory potencies of dexamethasone, methylprednisolone, and prednisone are 25, 5, and 4, respectively, for equivalent doses.

Preparation and Administration: Prednisone is available only for oral administration, whereas methylprednisolone and dexamethasone are available in oral and parenteral dosage forms.

Toxic Effects: When glucocorticoids are used for <14 days, as is often done when they are employed in combination with other cytotoxic agents, the most common side effects include euphoria, insomnia, psychosis, hyperglycemia, hypokalemia, increased appetite, metabolic alkalosis, proximal muscular weakness, and fluid retention with edema formation and hypertension. When used on a chronic basis, glucocorticoids also may induce a "cushingoid" appearance, easy bruisability, peptic ulcers, osteoporosis, subcapsular cataracts, and increased susceptibility to infections related to impaired cellular immunity. Because of this, H_2 blockers, antifungal agents (e.g., ketoconazole), and/or sulfamethoxazole trimethoprim have been employed in certain glucocorticoid chemotherapy combinations.

Potential Drug Interactions: Glucocorticoids interact with a variety of drugs, including barbiturates, oral contraceptives, erythromycin, hydantoins, rifampin, isoniazid, and salicylates. Given the wide range of doses of glucocorticoids used, however, these interactions are of no major clinical relevance.

Clinical Indications in Hematology: Glucocorticoids have direct anticancer activity in many hematologic malignancies, including ALL and CLL, Hodgkin and non-Hodgkin lymphomas, and plasma cell neoplasms. Because of their efficacy and toxic profiles, which do not overlap with the toxic effects of the other cytotoxic agents, glucocorticoids are employed in many chemotherapy regimens. In addition, they are useful in the management of hypercalcemia secondary to myeloma and lymphomas and are of paramount importance in the treatment of autoimmune hematologic disorders.

Clinical Application of Cytokines and Biologic Response Modifiers

62

Michael S. Gordon and Lynn M. Schuchter

INTRODUCTION

Cytokines and biologic response modifiers (BRMs) represent a broad class of therapeutic agents that modify the host's response to cancer or cancer therapy. Table 62-1 summarizes the biologic therapies currently in clinical use or undergoing clinical evaluation. While many of the biologic agents evaluated to date have potent immune-modulating activity, it should be emphasized that the term biologic response modifier is not synonymous with immunotherapy. Many of these agents exhibit differentiating, antiproliferative, and/or cytotoxic activities against malignant cells independent of immunomodulatory effects. The considerable focus on cytokines and BRMs in the treatment of cancer patients over the past decade is the result of several factors. Advances in cellular and molecular biology have permitted the production of large amounts of purified recombinant proteins that were previously available only in scant quantities. In addition, significant progress has been made in understanding the regulation of the immune system and the molecular nature of an immunologic response to cell-surface antigens within the context of the MHC.

Cytokines represent a class of proteins that include lymphokines, interleukins (ILs), interferons (IFNs), and colony-stimulating factors (CSFs). The term interleukin was originally used to describe molecules that mediate signals between leukocytes. However, we now know that such proteins can be produced by other cell types. Therefore, a system for naming cytokines has been developed by the International Congress of Immunology. A cytokine is initially described based on biologic properties, but once the amino acid sequence is defined, an interleukin number is assigned. The system has some exceptions and inconsistencies; for historical reasons, some cytokines retain their original names (i.e., IFNs and CSFs). To date, 13 ILs have been identified.

Over the past 10 years, cytokine therapy has in many ways revolutionized the field of hematology and oncology. The use of CSFs and hematopoietic growth factors (HGFs) to support patients receiving chemotherapy has permitted the implementation of higher chemotherapy doses with a significant reduction in toxicity.[1] In addition, cytokine therapy has expanded treatment options for patients with various malignancies, particularly hematologic malignancies.

Table 62-1. Biologic Response Modifier Therapy

Interferons (α, β, γ) and interferon inducers (poly IC:LC)
Interleukins (IL-1, IL-2, IL-3, IL-4, IL-6, IL-11, IL-12)
Colony-stimulating factors (CSF-G, CSF-GM, CSF-M, EPO, SCF, PIXY321)
Tumor necrosis factor (TNF-α)
Lymphotoxin (TNF-β)
Monoclonal antibodies
Adoptive immunotherapy (TIL and LAK cells)
Transforming growth factor-β
Vaccines
Differentiating agents (retinoids)

When considering the use of cytokines during the treatment of malignancies, one must be aware of the increasing evidence that some cytokines are aberrantly expressed by hematologic malignancies and may participate pathogenetically through autocrine or paracrine regulatory loops in the expansion of the tumor.[2] IL-1β and tumor necrosis factor-α(TNF-α) have been found to be constitutively expressed by virtually all leukemias, both myeloid and lymphoid.[3,4] Receptors for TNF have been detected on the surface of hairy cell leukemia (HCL) and B-cell chronic lymphocytic leukemia (CLL) cells; in vitro studies have shown that TNF promotes survival and induces proliferation of these malignant cells.[5] The mRNA for TNF, IL-1, and IL-6 have been detected in some malignant lymphoid cell lines.[6] Contradictory data have been reported concerning the expression of other cytokines by CLL cells and the consequences of this cytokine production on stimulation of leukemia cell proliferation.[7] With the exception of acute myeloid leukemias (AMLs), cytokines have not been found to have an in vivo proliferative effect on malignant tumors.

General Principles of Therapy

Cytokines are low-molecular-weight glycoproteins that act primarily in a paracrine or autocrine fashion and are therefore short-range mediators. Each cytokine interacts with a specific cell-surface receptor and, through various signal transduction pathways, communicates to the nucleus to enhance or diminish transcription of a number of genes.[8] Ultimately, changes in protein synthesis lead to alterations in cellular proliferation, growth inhibition, enhanced cytotoxicity, production of secondary cytokines, and/or modulation of the biologic effects of other cytokines. Many of the cytokines have multiple and overlapping functions. The action of a cytokine may depend on the local concentration of the cytokine, target cell type, available effector cells, and presence of other signal molecules.

Several principles of cytokine therapy are distinct from those used during the administration of traditional chemotherapy. First, for most of the cytokines, a simple dose-response relationship does not exist. More is not necessarily better. Preclinical and clinical studies have demonstrated that the optimal immunomodulatory dose is not necessarily the maximum tolerated dose.[9] Too high a dose may abrogate the desired immunologic response due to the complexity of cytokine action. Second, treatment with chemotherapy, if effective, is associated with a prompt response. By contrast, the therapeutic response to cytokines may develop slowly and take months to document. In addition, cytokine therapy is associated with unique toxicities, including fever, rigors, flu-like symptoms, and, for many agents, a capillary leak syndrome at higher doses. The side effects occur acutely, are generally short-lived, and abate with discontinuation of therapy. Long-term chronic toxicities are rare.[10,11]

The cytokines approved by the Food and Drug Administration (FDA) for clinical use are still few in number and include CSF-granulocyte (G) and CSF-granulocyte/macrophage (GM) to accelerate recovery of granulocytopenia following myelosuppressive chemotherapy or bone marrow transplantation (BMT), respectively; erythropoietin (EPO), for the treatment of chemotherapy-associated anemia, human immunodeficiency virus (HIV)-associated anemia and the anemia associated with renal failure; IFN-α for the treatment of HCL, Kaposi sarcoma in patients with acquired immunodeficiency syndrome (AIDS) and for certain viral syndromes, IFN-β for the treatment of multiple sclerosis, IFN-γ for the treatment of chronic granulomatous disease, and IL-2 for the treatment of metastatic renal cell cancer.

This chapter covers each of the HGFs and BRMs currently in clinical use, or undergoing clinical evaluation. For a review of the biology of these agents, the reader should refer to Chapter 16. The term cytokine is used to refer to the HGFs and the ILs. By contrast, the term BRM refers to agents that have a primarily antitumor effect, including the IFNs, TNF, CSF-M, and monoclonal antibodies.

CYTOKINES/HEMATOPOIETIC GROWTH FACTORS

The HGFs are a family of glycoproteins primarily responsible for the proliferation, differentiation, and maturation of the hematopoietic system. Many of these agents have effects not only on blood-forming cells, but also on bone marrow stroma, stimulating the secondary release of cytokines, or enhancing the microenvironment to favor cellular growth. These factors can broadly be divided into early-acting and late-acting agents. The early-acting HGFs act primarily at the level of noncommitted progenitors, resulting in proliferation of these often pluripotential cells. The late-acting factors exert their effects at the level of committed progenitors. They are responsible for the differentiation of these more mature cells, as well as having effects on terminally differentiated effector cells. Table 62-2 classifies the known HGFs on the basis of their site of action. The potential clinical effects of HGFs are summarized in Table 62-3.

The clinical use of the HGFs has concentrated mainly on their ability to stimulate the production of increased numbers of peripheral blood cells. The use of HGFs in the treatment of various diseases, both malignant and nonmalignant, has been studied. HGFs have found their greatest potential application with their use following the administration of intensive chemotherapy with or without progenitor cell support. The primary concern regarding the use of HGFs in patients with cancer is whether cytokines can stimulate malignant cell growth. While in vitro studies have provided some evidence that some HGFs promote tumor cell growth, with the exception of AML, no malignancy has been shown in vivo to be stimulated by HGF therapy.[12] The following sections discuss the clinical development of the clinically applicable cytokines.

Table 62-2. Stratification of HGFs

Early-acting factor
    IL-1
    IL-3
    Stem cell factor
    PIXY321
    IL-6

Late-acting factor
    CSF-G
    CSF-GM
    EPO
    CSF-M
    IL-6
    IL-11

Table 62-3. Potential Clinical Effects of HGFs

Agent	Erythroid	Lineage Myeloid	Megakaryocyte
EPO	Yes	No	No
CSF-G	No	Yes[a]	No
CSF-GM	No	Yes	No
CSF-M	No	Yes[b]	No
PIXY321	Yes	Yes	Yes
SCF	Yes	Yes	Yes
IL-1	Yes	Yes	Yes
IL-3	Yes	Yes	Yes
IL-6	No	No	Yes
IL-11	No	Yes	Yes

[a] Specific for neutrophilic granulocytes.
[b] Specific for monocyte/macrophage.

Colony-Stimulating Factor-Granulocyte

CSF-G was the first of the myeloid growth factors to be approved by the FDA. Its primary use is in the postchemotherapy setting, reducing the depth and duration of chemotherapy-induced neutropenia. CSF-G was initially identified and purified by investigators at Memorial Sloan-Kettering Cancer Center during the mid-1980s.[13]

The biologic properties of CSF-G have been well studied, and it appears to be a lineage restricted HGF, having its principle effect on the neutrophilic granulocyte series.[14] It is present in serum during normal conditions and in disease states.[15] CSF-G is capable not only of reducing the time required for maturation of a committed progenitor pool, but of prolonging the life span of mature effector cells (neutrophilic granulocytes) in the circulation. In addition, CSF-G is an activator of neutrophil function and has been demonstrated to have the ability, both in vitro and in vivo, to prime neutrophils for the activation of the respiratory burst, enhance chemotaxis, and increase phagocytosis. These effects are seen not only on neutrophils of normal subjects, but also in those with hematologic disorders, such as the myelodysplastic syndromes, characterized by distinct abnormalities of polymorphonuclear leukocyte function.[16]

Clinical Applications

Phase I trials with CSF-G demonstrated minimal toxicity over a wide range of doses tested. Dose-related increases in peripheral blood neutrophils were observed, but effects on other nonmyeloid lineages were not evident. Increased bone marrow cellularity with enhanced numbers of committed bone marrow progenitors as well as mobilization of these cells into the circulation was observed following treatment. Side effects of CSF-G include bone pain (due to medullary expansion), elevation of certain serum enzymes (leukocyte alkaline phosphatase and lactate dehydrogenase), exacerbation of dermatologic conditions such as psoriasis, and with chronic therapy, splenomegaly, and hair loss.

After Chemotherapy

Following the recognition by Bodey et al.[17] that both the depth and duration of neutropenia correlate with the incidence of infection in myelosuppressed hosts, the need for an agent that could reduce this risk was evident. Because of its ability to promote increases in peripheral blood neutrophil numbers, CSF-G was judged to be an ideal agent to alter the incidence and severity of chemotherapy-induced myelosuppression. Initial studies performed in the postchemotherapy setting demonstrated significant benefit associated with CSF-G therapy. In a phase I trial reported by Gabrilove et al.,[18] treatment with CSF-

G resulted in a reduction in the severity of neutropenia as well as in the ability to deliver significantly more chemotherapy in a timely fashion. These investigators also noted a reduction in the incidence of mucositis following treatment with CSF-G. Bronchud et al.,[19] demonstrated that with the use of CSF-G, doxorubicin chemotherapy for women with breast and ovarian cancer could be intensified from doses of 75–mg/m^2 to doses of 150 mg/m^2 administered every 2 weeks. Morstyn et al.[20] studied the relationship between the time of CSF-G administration and the administration of chemotherapy. While a delay in the initiation of CSF-G therapy was associated with a deeper neutrophil nadir, the neutrophil recovery was essentially the same as seen in patients for whom CSF-G therapy was initiated 1 day after chemotherapy.

The greatest benefit from the administration of CSF-G occurs after the use of chemotherapy regimens commonly associated with a high risk of developing neutropenic fever (defined as fever occurring during prolonged, severe neutropenia). Neidhart et al.[1] demonstrated that repeated cycles of high-dose chemotherapy can be safely administered with the adjunctive use of CSF-G.[1] Recovery of granulocytes was found to be significantly faster in cycles containing CSF-G than in those without. The benefit of the administration of CSF-G after chemotherapy was tested in two large phase III trials conducted in the United States and Europe.[21,22] These trials compared the use of CSF-G versus placebo in patients with small cell lung cancer receiving chemotherapy composed of cyclophosphamide, doxorubicin, and etoposide. While these studies have been criticized for the use of overly intensive doses of chemotherapy, they clearly demonstrate that with adequate myelosuppression, a benefit for CSF-G can be identified. The study by Crawford et al.,[21] conducted in the United States, allowed crossover to the CSF-G arm for any patients who received placebo therapy and experienced a neutropenic fever during any course of therapy. For this reason, the maximum data derived from this study are from the first cycle of chemotherapy when all patient therapy was double-blinded. These data demonstrate that the use of CSF-G results in a reduction of the incidence of neutropenic fever by approximately 25–30% when the overall incidence of the event approaches 50–60%. In addition, the number of days of antibiotics required, as well as the number of days of hospitalization, were reduced by the administration of CSF-G. In the European study, which precluded patients from crossover, and therefore maintained the double-blind format, similar results were observed with regard to the incidence of neutropenic fever. No survival benefit for the patients treated on the CSF-G arm has been seen. While there is little doubt that CSF-G has the ability to reduce neutropenia following chemotherapy, it has become critical to determine which regimens are myelosuppressive enough to warrant the routine use of this agent. Pettengell et al.[23] performed a randomized trial of CSF-G versus placebo in lymphoma patients receiving VAPEC-B chemotherapy. While this study has been criticized, it demonstrates a reduction of febrile neutropenic episodes and increased dose intensity for patients receiving CSF-G. However, a survival benefit associated with CSF-G use has not yet been documented.

Most clinical studies have focused on the use of CSF-G to prevent episodes of neutropenic fever. The question of whether there is a clinical benefit to the administration of CSF-G once neutropenia has developed has recently been addressed. Two studies have been performed evaluating the use of CSF-G in patients with an established neutropenic fever.[24,25] In the largest study, 216 patients with solid tumors, lymphoma, or acute lymphocytic leukemia (ALL), were randomized on admission to receive either CSF-G or placebo by continuous subcutaneous infusion. While patients treated with CSF-G generally had fewer days of hospitalization, fewer days of neutropenia, and fewer febrile days, the true benefit appeared to be experienced by patients with solid tumors or those with clinically documented or culture-positive infections. Similar results were seen in the second study. While these two studies appear to define a subset of patients who may benefit from the use of CSF-G in this setting, they also demonstrate the lack of necessity for every patient to be treated in this manner.

While the use of CSF-G following high-dose chemotherapy for patients with solid tumors has been defined, its use in patients with hematologic malignancies has remained a focus for controversy. It is clear that myeloid growth factors can increase the fraction of leukemic cells in S phase in vivo, but whether this translates into a benefit or drawback for patients is unknown. Over the past several years, the use of myeloid growth factors in leukemia patients has been studied by various investigators. Ohno et al.[26] published their observations in patients with both myeloid and lymphoid leukemias treated with CSF-G following intensive induction chemotherapy. There appeared to be a reduction of chemotherapy-related toxicity in the patients treated on the CSF-G arm. No evidence of increased relapse rate or poorer outcome with CSF-G therapy was seen. The use of CSF-G following induction chemotherapy in elderly patients with myeloid malignancies has been studied. CSF-G resulted in an apparent reduction in therapy-related morbidity and mortality characterized by fewer severe infections compared with historical controls. No negative impact on remission induction was seen, however the effect on survival remains unknown. The use of myeloid growth factors in patients with ALL or AML is currently under intensive investigation in controlled randomized trials, which should determine the role of HGFs in patients with these diseases.

Following Autologous and Allogeneic Bone Marrow Transplantation

The use of CSF-G following high-dose chemotherapy with progenitor cell support has been shown to reduce the time to engraftment and recovery from neutropenia in patients receiving progenitors derived from either bone marrow or peripheral blood.[27] CSF-G as a single agent, however, does not appear to have an impact on the time for engraftment of either platelets or red cells. The most frequently studied doses of CSF-G in this setting are in a range of 5–10 µg/kg/day administered either by subcutaneous or intravenous bolus or continuous infusion. The benefits of CSF-G in this setting have been seen in patients with solid tumors as well as lymphomas. No large randomized trials have been performed to study the use of the myeloid growth factors in patients with AML undergoing autologous BMT. The theoretical risks associated with stimulating the proliferation of residual leukemia either in the graft, or in the patient, warrants significant consideration before initiation of this therapy.

Clinical data on the use of CSF-G following allogeneic BMT are limited. Several small series of patients have been reported, demonstrating reduced time to myeloid engraftment, and no increase in the incidence of acute graft-versus-host disease (GVHD). These studies, however, are preliminary and therefore cannot address the larger issue of risk of leukemic relapse in the AML or ALL patients treated. For this reason, it is prudent to consider the use of CSF-G in these patients as investigational.

CSF-G has long been known to have the ability to mobilize progenitor cells into the peripheral blood. The use of these mobilized peripheral blood progenitor cells (PBPC) after chemotherapy has resulted in rapid multilineage engraftment. CSF-G is administered for 7 days by either subcutaneous bolus or continuous subcutaneous infusion. This results in mobilization of significant numbers of (PBPC) which are then collected by leukopheresis on days 5–7.[28]

Bone Marrow Failure States

Negrin et al.[29,30] evaluated the use of CSF-G in patients with the myelodysplastic syndromes (MDSs). Serial dose escalation of CSF-G in patients with <20% blasts resulted in significant increases in white blood cell (WBC) counts and absolute neutrophil counts (ANC). In 18 patients with MDS treated for 6–8 weeks with subcutaneously administered CSF-G, 16 of the 18 patients demonstrated an increase in both leukocyte and granulocyte counts. There were no changes in platelet counts, while 3 of 12 red cell transfusion-dependent patients experienced a decrease in their transfusion requirement. All peripheral counts returned to pretreatment values after discontinuation of the agent. Eleven of the patients received chronic administration of CSF-G for ≤11 months, with persistence of the leukocyte effects. No patients experienced transformation of their MDS to AML while on CSF-G. Current studies are focusing on the combination of CSF-G and EPO in this patient population. An initial study performed by Negrin et al.[31] demonstrated that the combination of CSF-G with EPO therapy resulted in neutrophilic responses in all evaluable patients, and erythroid responses in 42% of those treated. Responding patients generally had a lower endogenous serum EPO level than that of nonresponders. Similar findings for CSF-G alone have been seen in patients with other bone marrow failure states such as aplastic anemia.

Patients with Primary or Secondary Neutropenia

The neutropenic states represent a category of diseases for which CSF-G has become the therapy of choice. Most adults presenting with mild to moderate neutropenia (for whom increased neutrophil margination and drug-induced neutropenia have been ruled out) are categorized as having idiopathic neutropenia. This disorder is characterized by a neutrophil count of <500 cells/μl and a slight increase in infectious complications. Cyclic neutropenia is characterized by cyclical hematopoiesis affecting multiple lineages. Neutrophil counts in these patients oscillate with a periodicity of 14–21 days, often dropping to levels of near zero. During these periods of neutropenia, patients are at increased risk of infectious complications. These patients often develop painful ulcerations of their mucosal surfaces. Finally, congenital forms of neutropenia, such as Kostmann or Schwachmann-Diamond syndrome, are associated with severe neutropenia and infectious complications that are usually manifested in the first year of life and can be life-threatening. The use of CSF-G in each of these states has been studied; therapy results in an increase the number of circulating neutrophils and reduction in the number of infectious complications.[32–35] CSF-G should be the initial line of therapy once the appropriate diagnostic workup has been completed.

Neutropenia that complicates hematologic diseases such as HCL or CLL has been shown to be responsive to CSF-G therapy.[36] Neutropenia of an autoimmune etiology such as occurs in Felty syndrome or that associated with systemic lupus erythematosus tends to respond less well to CSF-G, probably due to the presence of antineutrophil antibodies.

Infectious Disease

Whether CSF-G will be of benefit in patients suffering from severe infections not associated with neutropenia is the focus of a randomized trial in patients with pneumonia. It is likely that there are subsets of patients such as those with severe burns who may benefit from CSF-G therapy in this setting. The beneficial effect of CSF-G may be a result of its ability to enhance effector cell function and to reduce the mortality due to superinfection in these patients.

The use of CSF-G in patients with AIDS has been studied. CSF-G has been shown to reduce neutropenia related to retroviral therapy, permitting the administration of high doses of antiviral drugs.[37,38]

Colony-Stimulating Factor-Granulocyte/Macrophage

CSF-GM has been approved by the FDA for its use in patients undergoing high-dose chemotherapy and BMT. CSF-GM is a glycosylated molecule with a molecular weight of 14.5–32. It is encoded for by a gene on the short arm of chromosome 5.

Unlike CSF-G, CSF-GM has effects on multiple aspects of hematopoiesis. In vitro, is appears to act synergistically with other factors (e.g., IL-3) to stimulate the production of erythroid and multipotential colonies.[39] In vivo, CSF-GM stimulates the proliferation and maturation of multiple myeloid cells, including neutrophils and eosinophils. In addition, at higher doses, CSF-GM has potent monocyte/macrophage potentiating ability. Like CSF-G, CSF-GM can activate effector cells and enhance their function. CSF-GM primes neutrophils for the respiratory burst and enhances phagocytosis. Unlike CSF-G, CSF-GM reduces chemotaxis. CSF-GM is a locally active factor at the site of inflammation, inhibiting the ability of effector cells to migrate away from this site.

Clinical Applications

Phase I trials with CSF-GM demonstrated several important aspects of its use. Generally, toxicity of CSF-GM comprises of arthralgias, myalgias, fever, serositis (pleuropericarditis), and a first-dose effect. These side effects appear to be dose related and are seen to a much lesser degree in doses that are clinically practical. At doses of 5–10 μg/kg/day, CSF-GM appears to have a primarily myeloid effect, promoting increased production of neutrophils and eosinophils. At higher doses, macrophage production and activation become apparent, and it is possible that the toxicity related to CSF-GM is primarily associated with this monocyte/macrophage activation. Toxicity due to CSF-GM appears to be altered depending on the route of administration. Lieschke et al.[40] reported on the first-dose effect seen in their phase I clinical trial. This toxicity occurred much more frequently in patients treated with intravenous bolus than in those with subcutaneous therapy. The first-dose effect is characterized by a constellation of symptoms, including dyspnea, flushing, tachycardia, hypotension, and musculoskeletal pain. It typically occurs several hours after the first dose of CSF-GM in a given cycle and may occur with the first dose of each cycle that a patient receives. It is self-limiting, and patients need only be treated with supportive care. This phenomenon, which may be related to sequestration of neutrophils in the pulmonary microcirculation, appears to be more prevalent with the nonglycosylated bacterially derived formulation of CSF-GM as compared with the glycosylated yeast-derived agent.

After Chemotherapy

As with CSF-G, CSF-GM has been studied for its ability to reduce the depth and duration of neutropenia following the administration of chemotherapy. While chemotherapy-induced neutropenia is not the primary indication for this agent, several studies address its use in this clinical setting. In a randomized trial of lymphoma patients receiving COP-BLAM, CSF-GM reduced chemotherapy-induced neutropenia as well as days of fever and hospitalization.[41] Other randomized trials have been less impressive. Bunn et al.[42] demonstrated an inferior response rate to primary therapy in patients with limited-stage small cell lung cancer receiving CSF-GM treated with chemotherapy and radiotherapy. Patients treated with CSF-GM, while having a reduction in granulocytopenia, experienced more infections and febrile days as well as a greater degree of thrombocytopenia. The presence of fevers as a side effect of CSF-GM confounds the interpretation of randomized trials. For this reason, the ability of CSF-GM to have an impact on chemotherapy-induced neutropenia remains to be proved in a large-scale randomized trial.

After Autologous and Allogeneic Bone Marrow Transplantation

CSF-GM has been studied extensively in patients undergoing high-dose chemotherapy with autologous progenitor cell support. Nemunaitis et al.[43,44] reported on the use of this agent in patients undergoing autologous bone marrow transplantation for lymphoid malignancies. Therapy with CSF-GM following reinfusion of marrow resulted in a shorter time to myeloid recovery, fewer infections, and shorter hospitalizations. This effect on has been confirmed by other investigators in a similar patient populations.[45,46] Similar results have been seen in patients with solid tumors undergoing high-dose chemotherapy with autologous BMT.[47]

CSF-GM was evaluated for its effects in 37 patients with marrow graft failure following allogeneic (15 patients), autologous (21 patients), or syngeneic (1 patient) BMT.[48] CSF-GM was administered as a 2-hour infusion for 14–21 days at doses of 60–1,000 μg/m^2/day. Nine of 15 allogeneic BMTs, 11 of 21 autologous BMTs, and 1 syngeneic BMT responded with increases of granulocytes to $\geq$500 cells/μl. Most patients maintained their granulocyte counts at >500 cells/μl after discontinuation of CSF-GM. CSF-GM had no effect on platelet or red blood cell (RBC) counts. Fevers resolved in all responding patients. Toxicities were typical for CSF-GM and were composed primarily of constitutional complaints.

Similar to CSF-G, the use of CSF-GM in the allogeneic BMT setting is currently under study. Early results suggest that CSF-GM may be capable of reducing the time to myeloid engraftment without a significant impact on the development of GVHD.[49] Long-term follow-up will be required to determine whether the use of these myeloid agents will affect long-term disease-free survival.

Gianni et al.[50] were the first group to demonstrate that the use of CSF-GM after intensive chemotherapy resulted in the mobilization of PBPCs. Such grafts are highly effective following high-dose chemotherapy. Since that time, various investigators have used CSF-GM for this purpose.[51–53] Timing of pheresis has generally been on a schedule similar to that of CSF-G, although some physicians use CD34 counts as an indication of when to harvest.[54]

Bone Marrow Failure States

CSF-GM has been studied in a series of phase I and II trials in patients with MDS. In three studies, CSF-GM was administered intravenously over a variety of doses.[55–57] Of the 26 patients studied in this manner, 23 demonstrated increases in leukocyte and granulocyte counts. Only 3 displayed any evidence of effect on other hematopoietic lineages. Similar to the responses seen with CSF-G, peripheral blood counts returned to pretreatment values after cessation of the administration of CSF-GM. Thompson et al.[58] studied the effect of subcutaneously administered CSF-GM to 16 patients with MDS.[58] Of 13 patients treated at doses of $\geq$1.0 μg/kg/day, 11 demonstrated a significant increase in granulocytes that returned to pretreatment values after completion of therapy. Effects on other hematopoietic lineages were seen in only two patients. Progression to acute leukemia occurred in a total of seven patients and was directly related to the pretreatment bone marrow blast percentage. The preliminary results of a randomized trial demonstrate a twofold or gratr rise in granulocyte counts in 27 of 28 patients at a dose of 3.0 μg/kg/day.[59] No benefit on platelet counts or hemoglobin was detected, and only 1 patient on therapy progressed to acute leukemia.

The use of CSF-GM in patients with aplastic anemia has demonstrated its ability to improve peripheral blood neutrophils transiently but lacks a multilineage effect that had initially been sought.[55] In addition, similar to patients with MDS, responses in aplastic anemia patients are generally not durable, and counts quickly drop to pretreatment levels following cessation of therapy.

Patients with AIDS or HIV Infection

Patients with HIV infection or AIDS have received CSF-GM either to reduce neutropenia resulting from retroviral therapy or as a component of a treatment plan in those with Kaposi sarcoma.[60,61] Levine et al.[62] reported on a small randomized trial in which patients who were hematologically intolerant of zidovudine (AZT) received CSF-GM either before the AZT was restarted or with continued AZT therapy. CSF-GM was administered subcutaneously in a phase I fashion for each patient. All patients started at a dose of 1.0 μg/kg/day and underwent dose escalation every 2 weeks to 3, 5, and 10 μg/kg/day to maintain the ANC >1,000 cells/μl. All patients were able to continue AZT therapy without significant neutropenia, while CSF-GM was administered. No evidence of HIV proliferation (assayed by p24 antigen levels) was seen, and the regimen did not alter the ability to culture the virus from the peripheral blood mononuclear cells.

CSF-GM has not had demonstrable benefit in patients with primary neutropenic disorders. It has been studied with some success both alone and in combination with IL-3 in children with amegakaryocytic thrombocytopenia.[63]

Erythropoietin

EPO is a 34-kd glycoprotein produced principally by the proximal renal tubular cells whose primary function is the regulation of erythrocyte production. It is essentially lineage specific with regard to its effects on red blood cells, and the regulation of EPO production is under the control of a simple feedback mechanism. EPO production is increased in hypoxemic conditions, and suppressed during times of hyperoxemia.[64,65] Under normal conditions, the EPO level is maintained at approximately 10–20 U/L of plasma. This level can rise exponentially when anemia develops.

The gene for EPO was initially cloned by two separate groups. Depending on the expression vector used, one can obtain either a glycosylated (Chinese hamster ovary cells) or nonglycosylated (*Escherichia coli*) form of the drug. Because native EPO is glycosylated, the mammalian cell-derived product is nearer to the natural product than the latter.[66,67] In addition, the product derived from *E. coli* appears to have reduced in vivo activity, probably related to the lack of glycosylation.[68]

It was evident very early in the evaluation of the clinical value of EPO that it may have a significant impact on diseases associated with anemia. The availability of sensitive radioimmunoassays permitted identification of disorders of EPO deficiency.[69]

Anemia of Renal Failure

Among the patients who were initially designated for the study of EPO were those with chronic renal failure (CRF). The use of EPO in this patient population is one of the most important advances in the field of clinical hematology. As one would expect, patients with nonfunctioning kidneys fail to produce EPO in sufficient amounts to support RBC production. The theory that the anemia related to CRF was at least partially due to EPO deficiency was confirmed by investigators in the United States and United Kingdom.[70,71] Doses of 25–500 U/kg three times per week were administered intravenously and demonstrated a dose-dependent increase in hematocrits, while signifi-

WHICH PATIENTS SHOULD RECEIVE HGF THERAPY?

While it is clear that both CSF-G and CSF-GM can reduce the depth and duration of neutropenia following myelosuppressive therapy, not all patients receiving chemotherapy are candidates for the use of these agents. In general, the use of hematopoietic growth factors benefits those patients who are at a high risk of developing neutropenic febrile complications. Most standard regimens used in hematology/oncology do not promote sufficient neutropenia to warrant the routine use of these agents in cancer patients. Regimens associated with an incidence of febrile neutropenia of <30% probably will not be affected by the addition of HGFs. In light of this, many cooperative groups as well as the National Cancer Institute are developing guidelines for the routine use of HGFs in clinical medicine.

Patients at high risk of the development of febrile neutropenic complications will generally benefit from the use of HGFs. Such patients include, but are not limited to the following groups, and this list is meant to serve as a rough guide for the initiation of HGF therapy.

Patients with prior episode of febrile neutropenia in whom a dose reduction is not planned or patients with febrile neutropenia following dose reduction
Patients receiving intensive chemotherapy either front line or salvage with an increased incidence of febrile neutropenia complications (i.e., VIP salvage in germ cell tumors with 70% febrile neutropenia incidence)
Elderly or debilitated patients who in the judgment of the clinician will not tolerate a febrile neutropenia episode
Patients who are predisposed to severe myelosuppression (i.e., post-BMT or patients with bone marrow involvement)

For these patients, therapy with CSF-G or CSF-GM can be instituted after completion of chemotherapy.

GUIDELINES FOR THE USE OF CSFs

Therapy with both CSF-G and CSF-GM should be instituted approximately 24 hours after the last dose of chemotherapy. The use of CSF-G or CSF-GM concomitant with chemotherapy should still be considered investigational pending adequate data regarding toxicity of this approach.

Both CSF-G and CSF-GM can be administered by daily subcutaneous injection.
Both CSF-G and CSF-GM should be administered at a dosage of 5 μg/kg/day.
The last dose of CSF-G or CSF-GM should precede chemotherapy by ≥24 hours.
Since premature discontinuation of CSF-G or CSF-GM can result in a drop in absolute neutrophil count, therapy should be continued until the ANC is >10,000 cells/μl.
Monitor CBC and differential counts twice weekly while on therapy.

cantly reducing and even eliminating the need for RBC transfusion. In the large multicenter phase III trial reported by Eschbach et al.,[72] patients treated with EPO experienced increases in hematocrits from baseline values of 0.223–0.35. Those who were treated at initial dose of 300 U/kg three times per week achieved their target hematocrit within 6–8 weeks of therapy. Patients treated with a dose of 150 U/kg (same schedule) achieved their target hematocrit in approximately 10 weeks. The 333 patients enrolled in this study required 1,030 erythrocyte transfusions over the 6 months before study initiation. Within 2 months of EPO therapy, all patients were erythrocyte-transfusion independent and remained as such with continued EPO maintenance. The only significant toxicities related to EPO therapy were the development of iron deficiency (related to utilization), hypertension, and seizures. The hypertension related to EPO therapy is thought to be secondary to a reversal of the vasodilatory effects of anemia. In the large study by Eschbach et al.,[72] blood pressure increases were noted in 35% of patients previously hypertensive patients. In addition, 44% of the patients who were not hypertensive before EPO therapy experienced increases in blood pressure, with 32% requiring the institution of antihypertensive therapy. There is no specific etiology regarding the incidence of seizures, although the investigators note that the incidence is not significantly higher than that of an untreated group of CRF patients (EPO 5.4%, untreated 8%). The recommended starting dose of EPO for dialysis-requiring CRF patients is 50–100 U/kg body weight IV three times per week. A phase IV study by Nissenson et al.[73] evaluated the treatment practices for patients receiving EPO therapy for CRF. They found that in general, relatively low doses of EPO were being used with resultant marginal increases in hematocrit levels. This suggests that uniformity is lacking regarding the maintenance of patients with CRF on EPO. While EPO therapy has produced improvements in hematocrit levels in patients with CRF not requiring dialysis, the degree of anemia in these patients, hence the benefit from therapy is not great enough to warrant a universal recommendation for this group. Recent studies have suggested that the subcutaneous route of administration is more efficacious than the intravenous route due to the better pharmacokinetics and length of exposure.[74] Patients treated on this study were able to reduce their dose of EPO by 30–50% when the drug was administered subcutaneously compared with their intravenous EPO dose.

Patients with AIDS or HIV Infection

Because of the beneficial effects of EPO therapy in patients with CRF, EPO therapy has been evaluated in other diseases. Many patients infected with the HIV have leukopenia and lymphopenia. In addition, chronic illness can result in the development of anemia. Therapies developed to treat HIV and its related infections are associated with hematologic toxicity. Retroviral therapy, particularly AZT, is associated with the development of anemia, which in many patients is the dose-limiting toxicity.[75] Henry et al.[76] reported on four randomized placebo controlled trials evaluating the effect of EPO on the anemia of HIV infection and AZT therapy. In these studies patients with endogenous EPO levels of <500 U/L experienced a statistically significant increase in hematocrit and a reduction in RBC transfusion requirements compared with placebo-treated controls. This benefit was associated with an overall improved sense of well-being. Patients with endogenous EPO levels of >500 U/L obtained no benefit. No significant effect of EPO therapy on the incidence of opportunistic infections was found. EPO has subsequently been further studied and has been approved by the FDA for use in this patient population.

Cancer Patients Receiving Chemotherapy

A recent development regarding EPO is its use in patients with malignancies. The anemia that develops in these patients is very similar to that of the anemia of chronic disease (i.e., an anemia in the presence of increased circulating levels of EPO). Many cancer patients have elevated levels of circulating cytokines such as TNF, which are negative regulators of hematopoiesis. In addition, chemotherapy, particularly with platinum analogues is often associated with the development of progressive anemia.[77,78] Miller et al.[79] previously demonstrated that an impaired EPO response is at least partially responsible for the anemia of cancer and is worsened with subsequent chemotherapy. EPO administration has been studied in patients with malignancies in various settings. Initial phase I/II trials demonstrated benefit from EPO therapy in patients receiving cisplatin therapy.[80,81] Subsequent randomized trials have been performed studying EPO in patients receiving chemotherapy. They have demonstrated a reduction in the transfusion requirements, particularly in platinum-treated patients.[82,83] The use of EPO for the treatment of anemia in patients not receiving chemotherapy has also been studied. In both multiple myeloma and other malignancies with bone marrow infiltration, EPO therapy has resulted in increases in hematocrit levels and reduction in the need for RBC transfusions.[84,85] Similar to the anemia of malignancy, the etiology of the anemia associated with diseases such as rheumatoid arthritis is multifactorial. Because one component of the development of anemia in this patient population is a blunted EPO response, the use of EPO has become a therapeutic option in these patients.[86]

Bone Marrow Failure States

Primary bone marrow failure states are often associated with anemia, requiring frequent transfusions and therefore the risk of developing iron overload. Among these, the MDSs have been most aggressively studied with regard to the role of EPO therapy. Circulating EPO levels have been studied in patients with MDS. Jacobs and co-workers[87] found an inverse relationship between EPO level and degree of anemia. They noted, however, that among patients with the same hemoglobin concentrations, a wide variation existed in EPO levels. Many investigators have studied EPO therapy in patients with MDS. Overall, the results have been disappointing.[87–90] Responding patients tend to be those patients who have extremely low EPO levels (<100 U/L). Even at high doses of EPO, while responses can be seen, they are often not durable.[91–93] EPO alone[94] or with CSF-G[95] has been studied in patients with aplastic anemia with some improvement in RBC transfusion requirements noted.

Autologous Blood Donation

The use of EPO to prime for autologous RBC donation has been perceived as a major step toward reducing the risks associated with blood transfusions. While the actual risk of contracting a viral infection from a unit of RBC has dropped significantly with improved testing, it still remains a concern. The use of EPO preoperatively has been demonstrated to promote an increase in the number of autologous units of blood donated. In a randomized, placebo-controlled, double-blind trial reported by Goodnough et al.,[96] the mean number of units collected from the EPO-treated group (600 U/kg twice weekly) was 5.4 ± 0.2 compared with 4.1 ± 0.2 in the placebo arm. In addition, the preoperative hematocrits in the EPO-treated patients were 3.4% higher (38.6 versus 35.2) than those of the placebo-treated patients. In a second study, the administration of EPO preoperatively has been shown to increase the amount of blood donated by patients by about 40%.[97] Results of a randomized trial conducted by the Canadian Orthopedic Perioperative Erythropoietin Study Group demonstrated that patients who received EPO preoperatively had a statistically significantly lower incidence of requiring any blood transfusions or of having a hemoglobin level <8 g/dl following hip replacement surgery.[98] EPO therapy preoperatively reduces the need for RBC transfusions as well as providing a method for autologous red cell donation.

Anemia of Prematurity

The use of EPO for the treatment of the anemia of prematurity has been widely studied. In this disorder, EPO levels are low and are not appropriately elevated in response to the anemia. This disorder is usually self-limiting and resolves spontaneously after 1–2 months. A pilot study with EPO appeared to demonstrate promise for the treatment of this disorder.[99] In a randomized double-blind study, however, Shannon et al.[100] showed no significant benefit to EPO treatment. While treated patients experienced a more rapid rise in reticulocytes, untreated patients spontaneously recovered precluding a clinical benefit. This topic has been reviewed by Phipps et al,[101] who propose that higher doses of EPO may be necessary. Other investigational, and as yet unproven, roles for EPO, include the treatment of anemia after BMT.[102]

Stem Cell Factor

Stem cell factor (SCF) is the ligand for the proto-oncogene receptor c-kit.[103–106] Also known as the c-kit ligand or mast cell growth factor, SCF has the ability to stimulate the proliferation of cells that bear its receptor. Cells that bear the c-kit receptor are ubiquitous, with expression on most normal tissue, if not, all early cells. In particular, c-kit is present on the hematopoietic stem cell, and acts to stimulate the proliferation and, in concert with other HGFs, the differentiation of these early cells. The recombinant protein is 165 amino acids long and has a molecular weight of 38. SCF as a single agent appears to have only modest effects on the in vitro growth of hematopoietic progenitors (see Ch. 16). However, when combined with other agents, such as IL-1 or IL-3, or with more lineage-specific factors, such as CSF-G, CSF-GM, IL-6, and EPO, SCF has potent synergistic effects on the proliferative capacity of these cells.[107–110] While the receptor for SCF is present on malignant cells, no clear evidence shows that SCF actually stimulates the growth of tumor cells, with the exception of myeloid leukemia cells.[111,112]

SCF has been studied in several preclinical animal models. Of primary importance is the ability of SCF to stimulate the mobilization of hematopoietic progenitors into the peripheral blood. Initial studies by Andrews et al.[113] demonstrated that PBPCs mobilized by SCF at a dose of 200 μg/kg/day for 11 days have the ability to engraft and rescue lethally irradiated baboons. This was compared with nonprimed mononuclear cells that failed to engraft in control animals, resulting in their death. Subsequent work by the same investigator has demonstrated that a significantly lower dose of SCF is required (20 μg/kg/day) if CSF-G is co-administered to baboons before pheresis.[114] The apparent synergistic interaction between these two agents facilitates the collection of PBPCs in the future.

Clinical Applications

The initial phase I trials of SCF have been recently completed.[115,116] Two separate phase I trials were performed in patients with breast cancer and non-small cell lung cancer. In each of the studies, patients received a period of SCF administration before chemotherapy as part of the study of effects of SCFs on unperturbed hematopoiesis.

In each trial, doses of 10, 25, and 50 μg/kg/day were studied. SCF alone demonstrated a modest dose-related increase in peripheral blood neutrophils. Less substantial increases at the higher doses were seen in platelets and reticulocytes, suggesting a possible multilineage effect. At the doses studied, no significant increases in bone marrow cellularity were found. SCF, however, did have substantial effects on bone marrow hematopoietic elements. Immunohistochemical stains of bone marrow biopsies demonstrated significant increases in CD34 expression as well as for Ki-67 and proliferating cell nuclear antigen (PCNA), both of which are proliferation-associated antigens.[117] These results suggest that even at low doses, SCF has the ability to stimulate the proliferation of hematopoietic stem cells. This effect was further investigated by Tong et al.,[118] who performed flow cytometric phenotyping of bone marrow and demonstrated statistically significant increases in various subsets of CD34$^+$ cells, including CD34$^+$DR$^+$ and CD34$^+$DR$^-$CD15$^-$ cells, the latter is believed to include the human hematopoietic stem cell. Additional assays demonstrated significant increases in the number of both primitive (colony-forming cell-high proliferative potential [CFC-HPP], burst-forming unit-megakaryocyte [BFU-Mk], and long-term bone marrow culture-initiating cell [LTBMC-IC]), as well as committed (colony-forming unit [CFU]-GM, CFU-GEMM, BFU-erythroid [E], and CFU-Mk) progenitors following therapy with SCF. Studies evaluating the ability of SCF to mobilize progenitors into the peripheral blood demonstrated mild increases in the number of BFU-E and CFU-GM at the highest dose levels studied.[118,119]

Toxicities in these studies were composed primarily of allergic-like reactions. These were somewhat expected based on the preclinical data, as well as the knowledge that c-kit is present in high numbers on the surface of mast cells. Dose escalation was limited in each study by respiratory (throat tightness, laryngospasm) and/or cutaneous toxicity (urticaria) to ≤50 µg/kg/day. Treatment was delivered by subcutaneous injection daily for 14 days. The effects of SCF following chemotherapy have only been preliminarily reported in the lung cancer study.[120] While a trend toward earlier recovery of neutrophils and platelets was seen at the highest dose, it is unlikely that this agent will have a major impact on postchemotherapy recovery.

Further clinical trials investigating SCFs ability to mobilize progenitor cells into the peripheral blood for use following high-dose chemotherapy are ongoing. McNiece et al[121] reported the preliminary results of a phase I/II trial of CSF-G ± SCF to mobilize PBPCs Women with breast cancer preparing to undergo high-dose chemotherapy were treated with either CSF-G alone (10 µg/kg/ lay SC) for 7 days or CSF-G (10 µg/kg/day sc) and SCF (5 or 10 µg/kg/day SC) for 13 days. Leukapheresis was performed on days 5–7 (CSF-G alone) or 11–13 (SCF + CSF-G). The addition of SCF to CSF-G resulted in a dose-dependent increase in number of peripheral blood CD34$^+$ cells in the day 1 apheresis product (0.18 ± 0.11; 0.39 ± 0.2, and 0.75 ± 0.13 for SCF 0, 5, and 10 µg/kg/day, respectively). Additionally, these increases were maintained over the 3 days of apheresis for the SCF-containing arms, while the CSF-G alone arm experienced a 50% dropoff from day 1 values. Data regarding the engraftment of these progenitors following high-dose chemotherapy are not available.

The use of SCF to prime bone marrow in vivo before bone marrow harvest is another interesting potential use of this agent.[118] Unquestionably, the two other major areas of interest for this factor are its use in ex vivo expansion and in patients with bone marrow failure states. Ex vivo expansion of bone marrow could theoretically replace the need to harvest large numbers of PBPCs or bone marrow progenitor cells. Multiple studies of this technique have demonstrated substantial increases in progenitor cells affording the opportunity to generate in the laboratory transplantable quantities of progenitors from a small volume of bone marrow.[122] All these studies have demonstrated the importance of SCF as a component of the cytokine "cocktail" needed for maximal expansion. In addition, SCF has been shown to increase erythroid progenitor numbers in vitro from patients with various bone marrow failure syndromes.[123]

PIXY321

PIXY321 is a genetically engineered fusion protein that links the genes encoding IL-3 and CSF-GM by a flexible amino acid linker.[124] In vitro, PIXY321 appears to have equal, if not superior, effects on hematopoiesis compared with the combination of IL-3 and CSF-GM as individual agents.[124–126] Preclinical animal studies have demonstrated that PIXY321 has the ability to effect multilineage responses following the administration of chemotherapy.[127,128]

After Chemotherapy

Several phase I clinical trials with PIXY321 have been conducted. Vadhan-Raj et al[129] have studied effects of PIXY321 on normal hematopoiesis in patients with sarcoma. PIXY321 was administered subcutaneously in two divided doses (25–1000 µg/m^2/day) for 14 days. PIXY321 treatment was associated with modest increases in peripheral blood WBC count, neutrophils, and platelets. Bone marrow biopsy specimens demonstrated a significant increase in cellularity. In addition, treatment with PIXY321 resulted in increases in assayable committed progenitors, including CFU-GM, CFU-GEMM, and BFU-E, as well as the number of circulating CD34$^+$ cells.[130] This suggests that PIXY321 may have the capability of mobilizing peripheral blood progenitors. At the doses studied, toxicity in this study was comprised primarily of local erythema at the injection site.

The effect of PIXY321 on hematologic recovery after the administration of chemotherapy has been studied by a variety of investigators. As a part of their phase I trial in sarcoma patients, Vadhan-Raj et al.[129] examined the effects of PIXY321 following cyclophosphamide, doxorubicin, dacarbazine (CyADIC) chemotherapy. These investigators found that the administration of PIXY321 at doses of >500 µg/m^2/day resulted in a reduction in mean nadir neutrophil counts following chemotherapy cycles in which PIXY321 was administered compared with those without PIXY321 therapy (90 cells/µl versus 380 cells/µl). The duration of neutropenia was also reduced from 6.7 to 3.1 days by PIXY321. Mean nadir platelet counts were also improved with PIXY321 therapy at doses of >500 µg/m^2/day with a reduction in the development of cumulative thrombocytopenia after two cycles of chemotherapy. Small numbers of patients preclude statistical conclusions from being drawn, but comparison to historical controls treated with CSF-GM reportedly demonstrates trends toward reduced myelosuppression. Additional phase I trials have reported similar results in patients treated for ovarian, breast, gastrointestinal, and refractory malignancies.[131–134] The toxicity profile in these studies appears to be similar to that seen in the study conducted by Vadhan-Raj et al. It appears from the phase I trials, that PIXY321 in doses of ≥750 µg/m^2/day demonstrates effects similar to those predicted based on the activity of CSF-GM and IL-3 independently. The confirmation of these effects in larger studies, and eventually in randomized phase III trials will determine whether this agent can produce true multilineage effects.

After Autologous Bone Marrow Transplantation

The effects of PIXY321 following high-dose chemotherapy and BMT are currently being studied by investigators at the University of Nebraska. Patients with lymphoma undergoing high-dose chemotherapy with autologous BMT are being treated on a phase I trial of PIXY321 to determine its ability to speed engraftment and reduce the morbidity of this procedure. Initial results suggest that doses lower than those used in the chemotherapy models may be effective for speeding engraftment and reducing the duration of neutropenia and thrombocytopenia.[135] In this initial study, doses as low as 250 µg/m^2/day appeared to demonstrate some benefit. Toxicities in this patient population were similar to those seen in the chemotherapy model and included local injection site reactions and headaches. A comparison with historical controls receiving CSF-GM demonstrated that treatment with PIXY321 at doses of ≥ 250 µg/m^2/day resulted in neutrophil recovery to 500 cells/µl within 18–20 days compared with 19 days for historical CSF-GM-treated patients. Days to platelet independence and time to discharge were shorter with PIXY321 (range 16–21 days and 19–23 days, respectively) than with CSF-GM (26 and 27 days, respectively). A randomized phase III trial is planned to confirm the true benefit of this agent in the setting of high-dose chemotherapy.

Interleukin-1

Interleukin-1 consists of two forms: IL-1α and IL-1β that exert their effects via a common receptor. In vitro studies with both agents have demonstrated their ability to stimulate the proliferation of early hematopoietic progenitors and produce a multilineage effect. In addition, their administration in preclinical models results in enhanced hematopoietic recovery following both chemotherapy and radiotherapy-induced myelosuppression.[137-139]

Clinical Applications

Clinical studies have been performed with both IL-1α and IL-1β. The initial phase I trial with IL-1β by Crown et al.[140] demonstrated that a short infusion of IL-1β resulted in a dose-dependent increase in WBC counts (primarily neutrophils) within the first hours of administration. A delayed thrombopoietic effect of IL-1β was seen approximately 3–4 weeks after administration. Whether this increase in platelet count is a direct effect of IL-1β, or indirect through the induction of secondary cytokines, remains unanswered. The major toxic events encountered were composed primarily of constitutional symptoms at the lower doses; however, hypotension became the dose-limiting toxicity at a dose of 0.1 µg/kg/day. The administration of IL-1β following 5-fluorouracil chemotherapy in subsequent cycles of treatment demonstrated no significant impact on altering chemotherapy-induced leukopenia or thrombocytopenia at the dose levels studied.

IL-1α has been evaluated in various clinical trials as an antitumor agent. In a phase I trial performed by Smith et al.[141] doses of ≤ 0.3 µg/kg/day were administered by rapid intravenous infusion. Therapy was tolerated, but the principal side effect at these doses was hypotension requiring vasopressor support. Nonetheless, a dose-related increase in WBCs (primarily neutrophils) during therapy, as well as increments in platelet counts occurring 1–2 weeks after completion of therapy were seen.[141] Serum levels of IL-6, a factor with known thrombopoietic effects, were increased following treatment with IL-1, raising the question as to whether the thrombopoietic effects of IL-1 are actually mediated through the induction of IL-6. Regardless, because of the hematologic effects seen in this initial trial with IL-1α, a subsequent study was performed in which IL-1α was administered following intensive carboplatin chemotherapy in patients with advanced cancer.[142] In this study, 43 patients received carboplatin at a dose of 800 mg/m^2. Patients were treated with one of three doses of intravenous IL-1α, ranging from 0.03 to 0.3 µg/kg/day for 3 days. Various schedules of IL-1α administration were used. These patients were compared with a control group who received chemotherapy alone. Treatment with IL-1α resulted in significant blunting of the platelet and WBC nadirs after chemotherapy. The optimal schedule was the administration of IL-1α after the completion of chemotherapy, in an optimal dose of 0.1–0.3 µg/kg/day. Toxicity was significant, consisting of reversible hypotension (requiring intensive care unit monitoring and vasopressor support), supraventricular tachycardias, and capillary leak syndrome.

After High-Dose Chemotherapy and Progenitor Cell Support

IL-1β has been investigated regarding its potential to accelerate engraftment following high-dose chemotherapy and autologous progenitor cell support. An initial dose escalation study conducted by Vredenburgh et al.[143] examined the effect of 7 days of subcutaneously administered IL-1β following reinfusion of progenitor cells. Doses of IL-1β of 4–32 ng/kg/day were studied. Of 14 patients, 7 experienced local pain at the injection site; 1 patient, at the highest dose studied, had severe hypotension. No benefit regarding accelerated hematologic recovery was noted, although IL-1β treated patients were found to have greater numbers of bone marrow CFU-GM progenitors on day +21. Similar results and toxicities were seen by Nemunaitas et al.[144] when IL-1β was administered by short intravenous infusion.

Weisdorf et al.[145] studied IL-1α following high-dose chemotherapy and autologous BMT. Patients received IL-1α for 14 days after reinfusion of autologous progenitor cells at doses of 0.1–10 µg/m^2/day by 6-hour intravenous infusion. Dose-limiting toxicity was hypotension, seen at the 10-µg/m^2 dose level. Engraftment of neutrophils (ANC $>$500 cells/µl) occurred at a median of 24 days for historical controls, and patients receiving IL-1β at 0.1–1.0 µg/m^2/day compared with 13 days for patients treated with IL-1β at 3.0 µg/m^2/day. Similar trends for platelet engraftment were seen.

In a small study by Walsh et al.[146] IL-1α was administered intravenously in 5-day courses to four patients with severe refractory aplastic anemia. No significant changes occurred in peripheral blood counts or bone marrow morphology associated with the IL-1α therapy.

Although both IL-1α and IL-1β are both potentially capable of reducing the myelosuppressive effects of chemotherapy, neither appears to exert these effects at doses that have been well tolerated. Attempts at using agents such as indomethacin to reduce the hypotension of IL-1 have proved ineffective.[141] Additional studies evaluating other potential applications of IL-1 are ongoing and include studying the ability of IL-1 to mobilize progenitor cells into the peripheral blood for collection and use after high-dose chemotherapy. If the toxicity of IL-1 can be significantly reduced, further clinical investigation is warranted.

Interleukin-2

IL-2 is a 15-kd lymphokine, coded for by a single gene on chromosome 4 that possesses a much more restricted range of biologic activities than that of other cytokines, with effects on T cells, which produce it, as well as B cells and natural killer (NK) cells.[8,147] Although IL-2 is a growth factor for T cells, resting T cells do not express IL-2 receptors (IL-2R), which are rapidly expressed after T-cell activation. The activation of T cells begins with mitogen or antigen stimulation of specific receptors on the surface of resting T cells in conjunction with macrophages and/or macrophage-produced cytokines (IL-1 and IL-6), which induce the synthesis and secretion of IL-2.[8,148] IL-2 effects are mediated through interaction with specific high-affinity membrane receptors.[149,150] The IL-2R is composed of three IL-2R peptide chains; the α-chain (or Tac molecule), a 55-kd peptide; the β-chain, a 75-kd peptide; and the newly described γ-chain, a 64-kd protein.[151,152] When all three chains are present in close approximation, a high-affinity IL-2R is formed that has 1,000-fold greater binding affinity compared to cells that express only the 55-kd chain. As a result of interaction of IL-2 with its receptor, T cells are activated to proliferate, and specific effector cells that mediate helper, suppressor, and cytotoxic functions are generated. Thus the specificity, duration and magnitude of a T-cell response is in part regulated by IL-2. IL-2Rs have a fairly restricted pattern of expression (NK cells, T cells, activated B cells, activated macrophages, and on some cells of malignant lymphoproliferative disorders).[153] In addition, IL-2 stimulates a resting population of lymphocytes that, when activated, have cytotoxic activity against isolated tumor cells and tumor cell lines that is not restricted by the MHC.[154,155] These cells have been termed lymphokine activated killer (LAK) cells; although no single effector cell is responsible for LAK activity, cell-surface phenotyping studies suggest that LAK activity is primarily mediated by $CD3^-$, $CD56^+CD16^+$ NK cells.[156] A minor contribution is also derived from cytotoxic T cells. In addition, IL-2 activation of effector cells results in the release of secondary cytokines, including IL-1, TNF, IFN-γ, and CSF-GM, which further recruit and activate monocytes.[8,157] This secondary release of cytokines may account for the therapeutic activity of IL-2 and certainly contributes to the toxicity associated with treatment.

In addition to the expression of the IL-2R by activated T cells, a fully soluble form of this molecule has been described and referred to as soluble IL-2R (sIL-2R).[158] Low levels of sIL-2R have been detected in the sera of healthy individuals and markedly increased levels have been detected in patients with hematologic malignancies.[159] This has been most extensively evaluated in patients with human T-cell leukemia/lymphome virus-1 (HTLV-1)-associated T-cell leukemia.

Clinical Application

IL-2 has undergone extensive clinical evaluation, first as a single agent, then in combination with effector cells, including LAK cells and tumor-infiltrating lymphocytes and, more recently, in combination with other cytokines and chemotherapy. Early studies, based on extensive animal experiments, used IL-2 combined with ex-vivo IL-2-activated LAK cells.[160] The LAK cells were obtained by daily leukopheresis, which were then cultured in vitro with IL-2. Initial clinical studies, reported in 1986, revealed objective regressions in traditionally unresponsive tumors that generated considerable interest.[161] Since then, numerous studies have been performed to define both the optimal dose and schedule of IL-2 therapy, as well as the overall antitumor activity. Phase II studies have demonstrated activity of IL-2 with and without LAK cells against a few cancers, most notably melanoma and renal cell carcinoma.[162,163] Thus far, no randomized studies have convincingly demonstrated a clear advantage to the administration of LAK cells in conjunction with IL-2 therapy.[164]

The therapeutic potential of high-dose IL-2 has been limited by the significant toxicities associated with this therapy, which was not entirely predicted by the murine experiments. Most of the side effects are thought to be due to IL-2-mediated release of secondary cytokines, including IFN-γ, CSF-GM, and TNF-α, which are released from activated NK cells and IL-1, IL-6, TNF-α, and CSF-GM from activated monocytes.[8,165] Minimal toxicity is associated with LAK cell administration. The toxicities associated with IL-2 can be severe and are clearly dose related. One of the most problematic is the capillary leak syndrome, manifested as weight gain, peripheral edema, and pulmonary edema, complicated by hypotension, oliguria, and respiratory failure. All patients experience a reversible malaise and flu-like syndrome with fever, chills, and gastrointestinal symptoms. Other end-organ toxicities have included hepatic dysfunction manifested as elevated bilirubin due to intrahepatic cholestasis, endocrinologic abnormalities, most notably autoimmune thyroiditis, myocardial infarction and myocarditis, dermatologic complications, and neuropsychiatric effects

in patients treated with intensive regimens.[165] Hematologic toxicities include thrombocytopenia and anemia, requiring transfusion, transient neutropenia and lymphopenia, and rebound lymphocytosis following discontinuation of IL-2.[166] The lymphopenia occurs early in therapy and may be the result of margination. The mechanism of the pancytopenia is not clear but may be due to IL-2-induced IFN-γ production, a potent inhibitor of hematopoietic cell proliferation in vitro. Eosinophilia has been seen following prolonged IL-2 therapy. Virtually all the side effects are rapidly reversible with discontinuation of therapy.

Therapy for Hematologic Malignancies

To date, most of the antitumor responses to IL-2 have been reported in patients with melanoma and renal cell cancer. Early studies with high-dose IL-2 regimens (i.e., 1.5 mg/m^2) suggested activity against lymphoma. Therefore, several phase II studies of IL-2 have performed in patients with large cell and indolent lymphomas, summarized in Table 62-4. Responses have been disappointing at 10–50%.[160,167] Duggan et al.[168] recently reported a phase II study of recombinant IL-2 with or without IFN-β in patients with relapsed or refractory non-Hodgkin lymphoma. Although designed as an outpatient regimen, toxicity was severe and the response rate was only 17%.

A potentially more promising approach has been the incorporation of IL-2 into BMT regimens to augment immunologic recovery after BMT and, possibly, to stimulate graft-versus-leukemia activity.[169,170] Defective IL-2 production and defective T-cell proliferation have been reported following BMT.[171] Higuchi et al.[172] reported that IL-2-responsive LAK precursor cells are available in the peripheral circulation as early as 3 weeks after autologous BMT. Therefore, several studies have been conducted in which IL-2 is administered post-BMT (Table 62-4). Higuchi et al.[173] evaluated the safety and immunomodulatory effects of continuous intravenous infusion of IL-2 in 16 patients undergoing autologous BMT for acute leukemia, lymphoma, or multiple myeloma. IL-2 was administered 14–91 days after autologous BMT. Dose-limiting toxicity was hypotension and thrombocytopenia. At the highest doses of IL-2, increased percentages of peripheral blood mononuclear cells expressing CD16 and CD56 with augmented LAK and NK cytotoxicity were demonstrated. Soiffer et al.[174] reported the clinical and immunologic effect of continuous low-dose IL-2 after BMT, administered in the outpatient setting. Thirteen patients (7 autologous, 6 CD6 T-cell-depleted allogeneic BMT) received IL-2 for 90 days. Again, low-dose IL-2 resulted in significant immunologic changes, including a fivefold increase in NK cell number and enhanced in vitro cytotoxicity. The immunologic effects of rIL-2 treatment were similar in both autologous and allogeneic marrow recipients. Overall, treatment was well tolerated. In this limited study, there were no signs of GVHD. More recent data suggest that the timing and duration of IL-2 treatment post-BMT appear important factors in the immunologic response to IL-2 and the antitumor activity. Based on these pilot data, additional clinical studies are ongoing to further explore the use of IL-2 with or without LAK cells after autologous BMT to reduce the risk of relapse.

Future studies with IL-2 for the treatment of malignancies will include investigation of effector cells supported by IL-2 including tumor-infiltrating lymphocytes and effector cells transfected with cytokine genes.[175] Additional studies will focus on ways of ameliorating the toxicity associated with IL-2 treatment. Potential leads include the use of TNF inhibitors (e.g., pentoxifylline) and nitric oxide synthase inhibitors (e.g., N-monomethylarginine or ciprofloxacin)[176,177] and further evaluation of low-dose IL-2 regimens.[178]

Table 62-4. Clinical Trials of IL-2 in Hematologic Malignancies

Patient Population	Dose/Schedule IL-2	Toxicity	Results	Reference
CLL Lymphoma	3 MU/m² IV bolus 5 days/wk × 4 weeks	Fever, fatigue thrombocytopenia, hypotension, weight gain, myocardial infarction	3/9 PR in patients with lymphoma and CLL	167
Non-Hodgkin lymphoma	5 MU/m² IV TIW or 2.5 MU/m² IV TIW and IFN-β5 MU/m² TIW	Severe toxicity, 17 life-threatening, 3 therapy-related deaths	Response rate overall 17%, no difference with IFN-β	168
Autologous BMT for non-Hodgkin lymphoma	Dose escalation IL-2 30–134 days following engraftment 3–34 MU/m²/day × 5 days, CI	Decreased platelets during therapy, pericarditis, hypotension, acute respiratory distress	Dose-related increase CD56⁺ cells, increase NK and LAK activity; immunologic effects short-lived	170
Autologous BMT or allogeneic BMT for ALL, AML, CML	2 × 105 U/m²/day CI × 3 mo	Decreased platelets, fever, fatigue, nausea, weight gain, well tolerated	Increased NK cells and activity, minimal effects on T cells; no signs of GVHD	174
Autologous BMT for hematologic	Induction: 0.3–4.5 MU/m²/day, days 1–5 Maintenance: 0.3 MU/m²/day, days 1–21	Fever, nausea, low platelets, hypotension	Dose-related increase in CD16⁺, CD56⁺ cells, increased LAK and NK activity	173

TIW, three times per week; PR, partial response; CI, continuous infusion.

Interleukin-3

IL-3 is the first of the early-acting hematopoietic growth factors to be broadly studied in various clinical trials. IL-3 has its action on early uncommitted progenitor cells and has been shown to act synergistically with various other HGFs, such as CSF-GM, CSF-G, and EPO to support in vitro colony formation.[179,180] In vivo, IL-3 has been shown to increase WBCs, RBCs, and platelets in normal animals, and to enhance the hematologic recovery of all lineages following chemotherapy or radiotherapy. IL-3 has a molecular weight 14–28 and is encoded for by a gene on chromosome 5q23–q31.

Patients with Refractory Malignancy and After Chemotherapy

The multilineage effects of IL-3 in patients with malignancy and following chemotherapy are currently the focus of clinical investigation. As a single agent in patients with normal bone marrow, IL-3 results in a dose-dependent increase in neutrophil and platelet numbers over doses of 0.25–10 μg/kg/day.[181] Lindemann et al.[182] treated 30 patients with refractory malignancies. IL-3 was administered as a single intravenous bolus on day 1, followed by 14 days of subcutaneously administered IL-3 (days 2–15). Doses studied were in the range of 60–500 μg/m²/day. Dose-dependent increases in WBC and neutrophil counts were seen. Platelets were mildly increased (twofold). Interestingly, significant increases in circulating numbers of basophils and eosinophils were seen. Toxicities were primarily constitutional in nature and consisted of mild fever and headache that were clinically significant. Therefore, Bhatia et al.[183] added propranolol to the IL-3 therapy to ameliorate the headache associated with IL-3. Doses of 60–4,000 μg/kg were evaluated. Hematologic effects were similar to the previously noted trial. No grade III or greater toxicity (including headache) or antitumor activity was reported in either of these studies. The effects of IL-3 on bone marrow and PBPCs were reported by Ottmann et al.[184] These investigators studied the effect of IL-3 administered for 15 days in various patients with normal and abnormal hematopoiesis. Patients were treated with doses of 60–500 μg/m²/day SC. Significant increases in peripheral blood CFU-GM and CFU-GEMM over baseline values were seen after 7 days of therapy (100% and 72% increased respectively). These effects were not seen after the second week of therapy (25% and 28%, respectively). Peripheral blood BFU-E were reduced in nearly all patients with normal hematopoiesis. Cycling rates of progenitors in the bone marrow were increased with therapy, as was bone marrow cellularity. Again, dose-dependent

increases in peripheral blood WBC, neutrophil, and eosinophil counts were seen, with peak values at or about day 13 of treatment.

Several studies have been performed using IL-3 as a single agent after chemotherapy.[185–187] In phase I studies, IL-3 has tolerable side effects below doses of approximately 15 μg/kg/day. Above this level, headache has been the dose-limiting toxicity. Other toxicities seen at lower dose levels include constitutional symptoms, such as fever, malaise, fatigue, arthralgias, and myalgias. Overall these studies demonstrate that IL-3 does not appear to alter the degree of neutropenia or thrombocytopenia but may, at higher doses, hasten the recovery of these nadirs. At least in one study by Biesma et al.,[185] this effect appeared to be associated with a reduction of platelet transfusions. The impact of IL-3 as a single agent, however, appears to be minimal, since equivalent or greater neutrophil effects can be obtained with either CSF-G or CSF-GM, and dose escalation of IL-3 to doses that might affect platelet numbers appears to be limited due to toxicity.

Combinations of HGFs such as CSF-G or CSF-GM with IL-3 have been pursued. Preclinical data suggest that sequential, as opposed to simultaneous, administration of IL-3 with CSF-GM results in increased platelet production via enhanced megakaryocyte maturational effect.[188] Combination HGF therapy, including IL-3, in humans has been studied after chemotherapy. Brugger et al.[189] reported the clinical results of sequential treatment, with 5 days of IL-3 (days 1–5) and 10 days of CSF-GM (days 5–15) following intensive VIP chemotherapy. This combination and schedule resulted in neutrophil effects similar to those of CSF-GM alone with additional platelet effects seen only in those patients who were previously heavily pretreated. Other combination trials of IL-3 with CSF-G have been reported with similar results.[190–192]

After High-Dose Chemotherapy

The use of IL-3 after high-dose chemotherapy and autologous progenitor cell transplants has been investigated. Nemunaitis et al.[193] administered IL-3 as a 2-hour infusion following reinfusion of bone marrow. Doses of 1–10 μg/kg/day were studied; however, doses of >5 μg/kg/day were not well tolerated due to constitutional side effects. Compared to historical controls treated with CSF-GM, IL-3 appeared to produce neutrophil recovery at a rate similar to that of CSF-GM. Peters et al.[194] reported on an initial study of IL-3 administered by continuous intravenous infusion in women with breast cancer receiving high-dose chemotherapy and reinfusion of a purged bone marrow. Dose-limiting toxicity consisting of fluid retention and neurologic changes (parkinsonian-like syndrome) at doses of 500 μg/m^2/day. Engraftment in patents receiving IL-3 was more rapid than in historical controls who received purged BMT without cytokines. Combinations of IL-3 with later-acting factors have been studied in the autologous BMT setting. Fay et al.[195] studied sequential IL-3 and CSF-GM in patients undergoing autologous BMT for lymphoma. Patients received IL-3 at a dose of 2.5 μg/kg/day as a 2-hour intravenous infusion, or subcutaneously. This was followed by CSF-GM at 250 μg/m^2/day as a 2-hour infusion until hematologic recovery. Rapid engraftment was seen in the few patients treated with a median ANC recovery to >1,000 cells/μl in 12.5 days. In a similar study, Wolff et al.[196] studied simultaneous IL-3 and CSF-G following BMT. Again, a trend toward an improved hematologic recovery profile for the combination versus historical controls treated with CSF-G was seen. Of note, Gupton et al.[197] demonstrated that therapy with IL-3 after BMT results in an apparent suppression of endogenous level of other cytokines, such as IL-6, CSF-M, and CSF-GM. These data suggest that additional randomized studies to evaluate the benefit of combination cytokine therapy in BMT are required.

Because of its effects on early hematopoietic cells, IL-3 is a potential agent to prime the bone marrow progenitor cells or PBPCs before the collection of progenitor cells that will be used as a graft. The pre-clinical primate studies performed by Geissler et al.[198] have shown that combinations of IL-3 with later-acting factors may be the optimal means with which to mobilize PBPCs. Wheeler et al.[199] harvested and reinfused bone marrow progenitors collected following 7 days of 50, 250, or 500 μg/m^2/day of IL-3 therapy. No impact of IL-3 pretreatment on hematopoietic reconstitution was seen in patients who received infusions of these progenitor cells following high-dose chemotherapy.

The effect of IL-3 on the mobilization of PBPCs was studied by Bregni et al.[200] They treated women with breast cancer with high-dose cyclophosphamide, followed by continuous intravenous infusion of IL-3 at doses of 1–10 μg/kg/day. While IL-3 increased the number of CD34$^+$ cells in the peripheral blood during recovery compared with historical controls treated without cytokines, this increase was less than that seen with CSF-GM. D'Hondt et al.[201] studied combined cytokine therapy with IL-3 and CSF-G administered on three different schedules with the purpose of optimizing PBPC mobilization. No comment was made regarding which of the schedules was optimal. PBPC mobilized by IL-3-containing regimens appeared to engraft without delay.

Other

Because IL-3 results in the proliferation of early hematopoietic cells, its effect on the recruitment of leukemic blasts into S phase has been studied. Brach et al.[202] demonstrated in vitro that IL-3 increases the number of leukemic cells in S phase, which resulted in an enhanced cytotoxic effect following cytosine arabinoside therapy. The preliminary results of a clinical trial seeking to take advantage of this effect were reported by Andreef et al.[203] and demonstrate that the in vivo administration of IL-3 has the ability to increase the number of leukemic cells in S phase. This therapy was thought to contribute to an enhanced antileukemic effect.

The multilineage effects of IL-3 make it a potential agent to study alone and in combination with other cytokines in patients with pancytopenia. Ganser et al.[204] studied the effects of subcutaneously administered IL-3 in doses of 250–500 μg/m^2/day in nine patients with the myelodysplastic syndromes (six refractory anemia), three refractory anemia with excess blasts. Patients were treated for 15 days. Increases in leukocyte counts (consisting of neutrophils, eosinophils, basophils, lymphocytes, and monocytes) were seen in all patients. Increments

in platelet numbers occurred in two severely thrombocytopenic patients, while RBC transfusion requirements decreased in one other patient. Therapy was tolerated with acceptable constitutional symptoms. Only one patient experienced an increase in the number of blasts. Other trials with IL-3 in patients with MDS have demonstrated similar findings with some patients experiencing multilineage responses.[205–208]

While patients with MDS appear to obtain multilineage responses to IL-3, patients with aplastic anemia tend to have less significant hematologic responses. Ganser et al[209] treated nine patients with aplastic anemia with subcutaneous IL-3 administered for 15 days at doses of 250–500 μg/kg/day. A platelet response was seen in one patient, and transient leukocyte responses were seen in several others. Two patients were found to have significant increases in bone marrow cellularity without significant increases in peripheral blood counts. This suggests that while IL-3 is capable of stimulating increases in early bone marrow cells, additional factors may be required to produce maturation and peripheral mobilization of these cells. Kurzrock et al.[206] demonstrated similar findings in their phase I trial, which included eight patients with aplastic anemia, as did Gillio et al.[208] in their trial. Guinan et al.[210] studied the effects of escalating doses of IL-3 in five patients with amegakaryocytic thrombocytopenia. Increases in all three (platelet, erythroid, myeloid) lineages were seen. This prompted a trial of combination IL-3 and CSF-GM that, in the first patient treated, resulted in a significant multilineage response.

Other uses of IL-3 that have been explored include its use as a single agent in HIV-infected patients. In a phase I trial, Scadden et al.[211] reported on 11 HIV-positive patients who were treated with 14 days of subcutaneous IL-3. While no significant hematologic improvements were seen, treatment with IL-3 was not associated with increases in HIV replication as measured by HIV p24 antigen levels or quantitative virus cultures.

It is hoped that the continued investigation of IL-3, particularly in combination with other HGFs, will lead to improved therapy for various hematologic disorders.

Interleukin-4

IL-4 is a 20-kd glycoprotein cytokine produced by activated T cells, first described as a B-cell stimulatory factor.[8,212] More recent studies have demonstrated a broad range of regulatory activities. It may have clinical application in the immunotherapy of cancer as a potent stimulator of cytotoxic T cells. IL-4 induces T-cell proliferation and enhances cytotoxicity of T cells and granulocytes. It enhances the generation of antigen-specific T lymphocytes from tumor-infiltrating lymphocytes.[213–215] IL-4 enhances the growth of mast cells and stimulates macrophage antitumor cytotoxicity.[8] Eosinophilic proliferation, enhancement of IgE production, and Fc receptor expression on B cells are also mediated in part by IL-4.[216] Preclinical studies of IL-2 and IL-4 in combination results in inhibition of IL-2-induced LAK activity.[217,218] In addition, IL-4 inhibits cytokine production and certain effector functions in human monocytes.[219] IL-4 can antagonize some of the responses induced by IFN and TNF.[220,221] Therefore, IL-4 appears to play an important role in the down-regulation and resolution of an inflammatory response. IL-4 has also been shown to inhibit megakaryocyte colony formation strongly in a dose-dependent fashion and to suppress CFU-GM.[222] The high-affinity IL-4 receptor can be found on T cells, mast cells, macrophages, and hematopoietic progenitors, as well as fibroblasts, brains cells, and most epithelial cells. The IL-4 gene is found on human chromosome 5.

The effects of IL-4 on human lymphoid and plasma cell malignancies have been investigated. IL-4 inhibited the in vitro growth of most tumor specimens, with <10% of specimens studied demonstrating a proliferative response.[223] The addition of IL-4 to chronic myeloid leukemia (CML) cell cultures has resulted in divergent effects with suppression of CML CFU-GM in some patients and stimulation in other samples.[224] IL-4 has also been shown to inhibit the growth of Philadelphia-positive ALL cells in vitro.[225] Therefore, IL-4 may have potential clinical application in the treatment of lymphoid malignancies, which is the focus of ongoing phase II studies.

The results of clinical studies with IL-4 are limited. Atkins et al.[226] reported the results of a phase I trial of IL-4 in patients with refractory malignancies. The maximum tolerated dose for this schedule was 10 μg/kg/dose. Phenotypic analysis of peripheral blood mononuclear cells showed a decrease in the percentage of circulating $CD16^+CD14^+$ monocytes, suggesting that IL-4 was wither suppressing transforming growth factor-β-induced CD16 expression, or stimulating $CD16^+$ monocytes to migrate into tissue. No antitumor responses were seen. Toxicities included nasal congestion, diarrhea, nausea, headache, and capillary leak syndrome.

Interleukin-5

IL-5 is a lineage-specific cytokine primarily involved with regulation of eosinophils, both stimulating eosinophilic growth and activation.[227–229] Eosinophils are bone marrow-derived granulocytes capable of killing parasites and protozoa. The role of eosinophils as mediators of tumor cytotoxicity is much less well defined. IL-5 is released by activated T lymphocytes and possibly by certain tumors when eosinophilia is a clinical sequelae. The release of IL-5 may contribute to the eosinophilia observed in patients treated with IL-2. Clinical studies with IL-5 have not been initiated.

Interleukin-6

IL-6 is a 21–30-kd protein that was initially characterized and independently identified by multiple investigators. Investigators have identified this protein as B-cell-stimulating factor-2,[230] IFN-β2,[231] hepatocyte-stimulating factor,[232] hybridoma growth factor,[233] T-cell replacement factor,[234] and monocyte granulocyte inducer-2.[235] By international convention, all the above factors are now referred to as IL-6.

IL-6 expression and production is increased by various other cytokines, such as IL-1 and TNF, as well as in response to a large number of conditions, including chronic inflammation, autoimmune diseases, and sepsis.[236–239]

The hematopoietic effects of IL-6 have been well studied in vitro, where its primary effect is on megakaryocyte maturation. IL-6 is a potent megakaryocyte maturational factor that has demonstrated the ability to increase the number of megakaryocyte progenitors (CFU-Mk) in vitro.[240] Mei et al.[241] demonstrated that IL-6 bioactivity in long-term bone marrow cultures correlated directly with megakaryocyte size and ploidy. However, there was no correlation between IL-6 bioactivity and megakaryocyte number, suggesting that IL-6 acts not to increase megakaryocyte numbers, but rather to influence the maturation of these cells.

IL-6 also has been shown to have the ability to stimulate the generation of granulocyte, granulocyte/macrophage, and megakaryocyte progenitor colonies.[242] These effects, while seen with IL-6 alone, are significantly enhanced by the addition of other cytokines such as IL-3 or CSF-GM.[243,244] In addition, IL-6 appears to stimulate the proliferation of both murine and human stem cells, as demonstrated by increased thymidine incorporation after incubation with this factor. These data suggest that in addition to a lineage-specific effect on megakaryocytes, IL-6 may also be an early-acting factor with the ability to activate progenitor cells.[242,245–249]

Preclinical studies in both mice and nonhuman primates have demonstrated that treatment with IL-6 results in significant increases in peripheral blood platelet counts.[250–252] The effects of IL-6 on thrombopoiesis appear to be mediated by its effects on megakaryocyte maturation. This conclusion is based on the observations that IL-6 increases megakaryocyte ploidy and that the maximal elevation in platelet counts is delayed, occurring primarily after completion of IL-6 therapy. Unlike the effects of CSF-G and CSF-GM on neutrophils, IL-6 does not appear to function as a platelet-releasing factor. IL-6 therapy results in the induction of acute-phase proteins, including C-reactive protein, fibrinogen, and haptoglobin. Following chemotherapy or irradiation, IL-6 enhances the hematologic recovery, thereby reducing the duration of myelosuppression.

Clinical Applications

Initial clinical studies with IL-6 have been completed. The results are promising regarding the use of this agent to reduce thrombocytopenia after chemotherapy. In separate phase I trials, IL-6 was studied in patients receiving chemotherapy for sarcoma or advanced malignancies.[253,254] In the first study, patients were treated with IL-6 before the initiation of chemotherapy to study the effects of this agent on normal hematopoiesis. Patients received 10 days of IL-6 by daily subcutaneous injections at doses of 1.0–25.0 μg/kg/day. IL-6 therapy resulted in significant dose-dependent increases in platelet counts that peaked following completion of the IL-6 therapy. Toxicities of IL-6 included fevers, chills, malaise, fatigue, and a transient therapy-related anemia. This anemia characteristically developed early after the initiation of IL-6 therapy and rapidly resolved after completion of treatment. The precise etiology is unknown, but changes in plasma volume or sequestration in the spleen are most likely. Dose-related increases in C-reactive protein and fibrinogen were consistent with the known effects of IL-6 on acute-phase proteins; elevations in these parameters can serve as an indicator of IL-6 activity.

After administration of chemotherapy, at the lowest doses studied, IL-6 appears to reduce the duration of platelet nadirs. At higher doses (10 and 25 μg/kg/day), IL-6 appears to reduce depth of platelet nadir as well. As a single agent, IL-6 appears to have no effect on the depth or duration of neutropenia.

IL-6 was also studied in patients with myelodysplasia and thrombocytopenia. In a phase I trial, 22 patients with refractory anemia, refractory anemia with ringed sideroblasts, or chronic myelomonocytic leukemia with <5% bone marrow blasts were with doses of IL-6 ranging from 1.0–5.0 μg/kg/day.[255] Dose-limiting toxicity of malaise and fatigue was reached at 5.0 μg/kg/day, and the maximum tolerated dose in this population was 3.75 μg/kg/day. Of 22 patients, 5 had transient (3 patients) or lasting (2 patients) responses to IL-6 therapy. Only 1 patient demonstrated progression of MDS to acute leukemia.

In addition to its hematopoietic effects, IL-6 has potential antitumor activity. IL-6 is synergistic with IL-2 in the generation of cytotoxic T lymphocytes.[256] This action is possibly mediated by the ability of IL-6 to up-regulate the expression of the IL-2R on thymocytes.[257] Mulé et al.[258] demonstrated that IL-6 therapy results in the regression of established pulmonary metastases in mice that appears to be mediated via both $CD4^+$ and $CD8^+$ lymphocytes.

Clinical studies testing the antitumor effects of IL-6 are just beginning. Weber[259] treated 11 patients with advanced malignancies with daily subcutaneous injections of IL-6. Patients were treated on an every-other-week schedule for 3 weeks at doses of 3, 10, and 30 μg/kg/day. Dose-limiting toxicity of hepatotoxicity and cardiac arrhythmias precluded further dose-escalation by this route of administration. Other side effects included fevers, chills, and malaise. While there were no antitumor responses reported in this study, peripheral blood immunophenotyping did demonstrate an up-regulation in the expression of the low affinity IL-2R on CD3$^+$ cells, suggesting the activation of peripheral blood lymphocytes. Olencki et al[260] reported the preliminary results of a clinical trial using subcutaneously administered IL-6 to patients with refractory malignancies. Dose-limiting toxicity has not been reached at a dose of 25 µg/kg/day, nor had any antitumor effects been seen. Functional studies of peripheral blood mononuclear cells demonstrated no increase in LAK activity, induction of IL-2, or change in IL-2R-α.[260] While studies are continuing by both the subcutaneous and intravenous routes of administration, it is not likely that IL-6 as a single agent will prove to be an active antitumor agent. Future studies will include combinations of IL-6 with other cytokines such as IL-2. The use of antagonists or antibodies to IL-6 or its receptor may have clinical value in diseases such as multiple myeloma, in which IL-6 appears to be an autocrine growth factor.[261]

Interleukin-11

IL-11 is a 199-amino acid polypeptide that was initially cloned from an immortalized and IL-1-induced primate bone marrow stromal cell line, PU-34. The human gene was subsequently cloned from a fetal pulmonary fibroblast cell line.[262] IL-11 has similar effects to IL-6 and is capable of stimulating the proliferation of the IL-6-dependent plasmacytoma cell line, T1165. IL-11 has the ability in vitro to synergize with other early-acting hematopoietic factors, including IL-3. Studies performed by Yin and Yang[263] demonstrated that IL-11 most likely uses the same signal transduction pathway as IL-6 but appears to operate through an independent receptor. IL-11 results in enhanced recovery of platelets as well as neutrophils after both chemotherapy and lethal irradiation following the infusion of progenitor cell transplants.[264]

IL-11 has also been shown to inhibit adipogenesis.[265] Keller et al.[266] recently demonstrated that IL-11 has the ability to promote myelopoiesis in long-term bone marrow cultures. This effect may be mediated by the inhibition of adipogenesis and promotion of stromal cell and macrophage development by IL-11. These findings could be relevant for the treatment of various bone marrow failure states in which bone marrow microenvironmental defects could play a role in the pathogenesis of the disorders.

Clinical Applications

The phase I trial of IL-11 has been performed in women with locally advanced or metastatic breast cancer.[267,268] Patients received IL-11 at doses of 10–100 µg/kg/day. Therapy was administered initially by daily subcutaneous injection for 14 consecutive days during a 28-day prechemotherapy period. Following completion of the prechemotherapy portion of the study, all patients received IL-11 at their assigned dose level after each of four cycles of chemotherapy. Chemotherapy consisted of cyclophosphamide (1,500 mg/m^2/day) and doxorubicin (60 mg/m^2/day) given on day 1 of each 28-day cycle. IL-11 was administered for 12 consecutive days on days 3–14.

Toxicity of IL-11 was primarily comprised of reversible grade 2 fatigue, myalgias, and arthralgias and extremity edema seen in all patients treated at 75 µg/kg/day. One patient treated at 100 µg/kg/day after 4 days of therapy developed transient expressive aphasia with radiologic evidence of cerebral ischemia. In addition, a transient therapy-related anemia was seen at all doses studied. This anemia is similar in character to that described for IL-6. Based on blood volume studies (RBC mass and plasma volume), it was thought to be secondary to plasma volume expansion. IL-11 therapy was associated with a dose-related increase in mean peak platelet counts over baseline of

76%, 93%, 108%, 180% (for doses of 10, 25, 50, and 75 µg/kg/day, respectively). For all doses studied, maximum platelet counts occurred after the completion of IL-11 therapy. No effect was seen on the WBC count. Acute-phase proteins, including C-reactive protein, haptoglobin, and fibrinogen, were increased at all doses. Platelet aggregation studies performed pretreatment and after 14 days of IL-11 demonstrated no therapy-related changes.

Trephine bone marrow biopsies performed pretreatment and after 14 days of IL-11 demonstrated significant increases in megakaryocyte numbers following doses of $\geq$50 µg/kg/day.[269] In addition, immunohistochemical stains with PC10, an monoclonal antibody that recognizes the PCNA demonstrated an increase in the number of PCNA-positive cells (20.8 ± 7.8% to 40.2 ± 14.0%, P <0.001). Most of these cells were erythroblasts and myeloid precursors. Flow cytometric ploidy analysis of bone marrow megakaryocytes revealed a greater number of 32N and 64N bone marrow megakaryocytes following 14 days of IL-11. In addition, the proportion of PCNA-positive bone marrow karyocytes increased from 19.6 ± 13.4% to 37.6 ± 24.6% (P <0.001). Treatment with IL-11 had no significant effect on the numbers of committed or primitive assayable progenitors in bone marrow or peripheral blood.

IL-11 administered after chemotherapy was associated with a similar side effect profile. One additional patient with a history of hypertension developed an hemorrhagic cerebral infarct during cycle 1 of chemotherapy. Compared to patients at the 10-µg/kg/day dose level, patients treated at doses of $\geq$25 µg/kg/day experienced less thrombocytopenia. Nadir platelet counts in the first cycle of chemotherapy were 67, 159, and 136,000/µl for the 10-, 25-, and 50-µg/kg/day doses, respectively. In addition, cumulative thrombocytopenia appeared to be attenuated by IL-11 therapy. No effect of IL-11 on neutrophil nadirs was seen. A similar therapy-related anemia was seen during chemotherapy cycles. IL-11 appears to be an effective thrombopoietic agent at doses associated with minimal toxicity. Further studies with more intensive chemotherapy regimens as well as autologous BMT will be required to define its value and role in these settings.

Interleukin-12

Preliminary preclinical studies with IL-12 suggest that this cytokine may be a particularly useful immunostimulant. IL-12, also named natural killer stimulatory factor or cytotoxic lymphocyte maturation factor has a molecular weight of 70 with an unusual heterodimeric structure.[270,271] Biologic activities of IL-12 include stimulation of CD4$^+$ and CD8$^+$ subsets, activation of NK-mediated cytotoxicity and induction of IFN-γ production by resting and activated peripheral blood lymphocytes, T cells, and NK cells.[272,273,274,275] Phagocytic and B cells appear to be the predominant producers of IL-12.[276] IL-12 induces production of several cytokines, including CSF-GM, TNF, IL-8, and IFN-γ.[277] IL-12 also induces LAK cell generation and is synergistic with IL-2 in this effect.[278] Preclinical studies support a therapeutic potential of IL-12 as an activator of T-helper response and NK cytotoxicity. Additional studies have demonstrated that peripheral blood lymphocytes from patients with metastatic cancer or following allogeneic BMT are activated by IL-12.[279] Future clinical studies with IL-12 will focus the potent immuno-enhancing properties of this cytokine both alone and in combination with IL-2.[279,280]

Biologic Response Modifiers

The rationale for using BRMs for the treatment of malignancies is based primarily on preclinical data and indirect clinical evidence that suggest an important relationship between the

Table 62-5. Biologic Effects of BRM Relevant for Use as Anticancer Therapy

Biologic Effect	Example of Agent
Direct cytotoxic effect against cancer cells	IFN
Alteration of tumor vascular supply	TNF
Stimulation of host immune response to the tumor	IL-2
Direct regulator of cell growth and differentiation	Retinoic acid
Stimulation of hematopoiesis following chemotherapy	CSF-G

immune system and the neoplastic process. These clinical and histopathologic observations include favorable clinical prognosis associated with brisk lymphocytic infiltrate in solid tumors, increased risk of malignancies in the setting of immunodeficiency states or immunosuppression, rare spontaneous regression of metastasis after resection of primary tumor, and the presence of antitumor antibodies in sera and specific cytotoxic T lymphocytes in the peripheral blood of cancer patients. More recently, compelling preclinical animal data have further supported the use of BRM for the treatment of cancer.[160,281,282] Table 62-5 summarizes some of the biologic effects of these agents that may be relevant for their potential in cancer treatment.

Interferons

The IFNs are a family of glycoproteins that were initially discovered in 1957, named for their ability to "interfere" with viral replication.[11] It has since become clear that IFNs have pleotropic biologic effects, including immunostimulatory effects, direct antiproliferative effects, and antiviral properties.[8] IFNs represent a multigene family that can be divided into three types—α, β, and γ—based on their antigenicity, chemical properties, and amino acid sequences. IFN-α and -β are classified as type I IFN and have similar biologic effects and interact with identical receptors. Virtually every nucleated cell produces this protein in response to a variety of stimuli, including viruses, other pathogens, and double-stranded RNA. IFN-γ, referred to as type II IFN, has distinct biologic properties and binds to a unique cell-surface receptor. It is a potent activator of monocytes and macrophages, enhances NK cell cytotoxicity, and results in the up-regulation and expression of both class I and class II MHC antigens. In part, IFNs mediate their action by enhancing or inhibiting a series of IFN-inducible genes.[283] The biologic role for most of the proteins activated by IFN is not known, but two of the best characterized regulate protein translation.[8,283] Table 62-6 summarizes the biologic effects of IFN.

Both IFN-β and IFN-γ have a single gene, but ≥23 genes exist for IFN-α, all located on the short arm of chromosome 9. The IFN-β gene is also located on chromosome 9, and the gene for IFN-γ is located on chromosome 12.[8] Interestingly, some malignant hematopoietic cell lines have been demonstrated to have homozygous deletions of type I IFN genes on chromosome 9, suggesting that these genes may function as tumor suppressor genes; therefore, their loss may be associated with tumor progression.[284]

Clinical Application

The IFNs were the first of the cytokines to undergo extensive clinical evaluation, and most of the trials have used IFN-α. Initial clinical studies began in the 1970s with a partially purified IFN

Table 62-6. Biologic Effects of IFN

Induce expression of class I and II MHC antigens on normal and malignant cells
Stimulates secretion of other cytokines
Enhances cytotoxicity of NK cells, macrophages, neutrophils and T cells
Regulation of antibody production by B cells
Potent antiviral effects
Regulate cell growth and cell differentiation

product. Over the previous decade, numerous phase II studies of IFN-α have been completed, with antitumor activity primarily being directed against hematologic malignancies. IFN has reproducible antitumor activity against HCL, low-grade non-Hodgkin lymphoma, multiple myeloma, cutaneous T-cell lymphoma, and CML.[284–288] Limited studies have been conducted with IFN-γ, and results to date demonstrate little role for this cytokine as a therapeutic anticancer agent.[289,290]

IFN-α is administered at a wide range of recommended doses that vary depending on the clinical indication. Clearly, the toxicities associated with IFN are dose related. The most common side effects include fever, chills, fatigue, headache, myalgias, arthralgias, and a flu-like syndrome.[11] Patients generally develop a tolerance to the fever and chills after repetitive treatment. However, there is no tolerance to the other constitutional symptoms, which are usually dose limiting. Higher doses of IFN are associated with neurologic toxicity (depression, confusion, seizures); cardiac abnormalities (atrial arrhythmias), and laboratory abnormalities, including transaminase elevation, leukopenia, thrombocytopenia, and anemia. Bone marrow suppression must be monitored closely in patients with compromised marrow reserve due to underlying malignancy, concomitant drug administration (AZT), and/or chemotherapy.

The salient features of IFN therapy in hematologic malignancies are discussed below. More detailed information regarding IFN and specific hematologic malignancies can be found elsewhere in this text. In limited pilot studies, IFN-α has been used to treat patients with polycythemia vera,[291] agnogenic myeloid metaplasia,[292] and primary thrombocythemia[293,294] with activity in subsets of patients. Similar to the effects seen in CML, IFN-α has the ability to suppress hematopoiesis of affected lineages, thereby reducing peripheral blood counts. Clearly, IFN-α has potential clinical application for the treatment of myeloproliferative disorders.[295]

Chronic Myeloid Leukemia

IFN-α and IFN-γ have been evaluated in patients with CML. Initial studies in patients with chronic phase demonstrated activity as documented by a decrease in splenomegaly and improvement in peripheral counts. More importantly, in a significant proportion of patients there was a reduction or complete elimination in the number of Philadelphia chromosome-positive metaphases. Overall, complete "hematologic remission" occurs in approximately 75% of patients, with 30–50% demonstrating cytogenetic improvement.[296–298] In some patients, cytogenetic improvement has been observed without hematologic responses. However, even with complete hematologic and cytogenetic responses after treatment with IFN-α, the bcr-abl rearrangement sometimes persists as detected by polymerase chain reaction assay.[298] These data suggest that IFN may suppress the proliferation of Philadelphia-positive clones, but does not completely eradicate the Philadelphia-positive stem cells. Whether patients who are rendered bcr-abl negative have a prolonged survival is unclear but preliminary results are promising.[297,299] Several studies suggest that a cytogenetic response may be correlated with improved survival. Investigators have recently reported the results of a prospective trial in which patients with chronic phase CML were randomized to IFN-α2A or chemotherapy with hydroxyurea. Of the 322 patients who entered the trial, 29% of patients treated with IFN progressed to blast crisis versus 39% of patients in the chemotherapy arm. Overall, patients treated with IFN had a significantly greater number of major karyotypic responses, which was correlated with longer survival compared with those treated with chemotherapy.[300]

IFN is most effective when used to treat patients with early-stage CML with very little activity in accelerated phase and no benefit when used in blast crisis.[291] Many patients experienced significant side effects from IFN, as relatively high doses are required to induce responses. Most studies have administered IFN as a daily subcutaneous injection at a dose of 5 MU/m². Using lower doses and less frequent administration, as in the treatment of HCL, results in fewer hematologic and cytogenetic responses. Therapy is generally continued for ≥1 year if the patient demonstrates continued sensitivity to IFN.

IFN-γ has also been evaluated in patients with CML, but the available data suggest that IFN-α has greater activity in CML and the incidence of toxic events have been greater with IFN-γ.[290] Additional approaches currently being explored include combining IFN with chemotherapy and the use of maintenance IFN after allogeneic BMT for CML.

Hairy Cell Leukemia

HCL is extremely responsive to IFN-α therapy, with an overall response rate of 80–90% and a 5% complete response rate.[301,302] Recovery of the platelet count can occur within 2 weeks; reduction in splenic size and improvement in peripheral blood counts usually occurs within 2–3 months of therapy. IFN is generally administered in low doses (2–3 million U), three times a week. Responses to IFN have been reported in splenectomized and previously untreated patients.[301] Progression of HCL has been associated with the development of neutralizing anti-IFN antibodies.[303]

The precise mechanism of IFN activity against HCL is not entirely clear but probably includes direct antitumor effects, modification of oncogene expression, modulation of cytokine expression, and specific alterations in protein synthesis, which leads to partial differentiation of the malignant leukemia cells.[304] Interesting preclinical and clinical data suggest that TNF may act as an autocrine growth factor for some cases of B-CLL and HCL. Digel et al.[7] recently found increased circulating levels of soluble TNF-binding proteins (TNF-BP) in the sera of patients with B-CLL and HCL compared with human sera from healthy controls. Levels of TNF-BP have been reported to be decreased after effective therapy with IFN-α.[7,305] In addition, preclinical studies have shown that IFN-α can inhibit TNF-dependent hairy cell growth with decreases in TNF mRNA occurring after IFN treatment.[305]

Multiple Myeloma

Despite years of evaluation, the role of IFN in the treatment of multiple myeloma remains unclear. Early studies that explored the activity of IFN-α as a single agent resulted in response rates of only 20–25%, considerably less than that achieved with chemotherapy.[306–309] However, more recent studies have focused on the use of IFN as maintenance therapy after chemotherapy and in combination with chemotherapy at conventional doses or in the setting of autologousBMT. The results of randomized trials suggest improved response rates and prolonged remission time in patients receiving IFN.[310] In this trial, patients treated with standard cytotoxic chemotherapy to maximal response were randomly assigned to receive or not receive IFN-α. IFN-α was initially administered by subcutaneous injection three times a week at a dose of 10 MU/m²/day. The dose was subsequently reduced to 3 MU/m²/day due to therapy-related toxicity. One hundred one patients were entered into the study. According to the investigators, 66 of 101 patients relapsed at the time of the report. The median duration of response (from the time of randomization) was 26 months in the patients given IFN and 14 months in the untreated patients ($P = 0.0002$). Survival similarly favored the IFN-treated patients who had a median duration of survival of 52 months compared with 39 months in the untreated group ($P = 0.0526$). This survival advantage was more pronounced for the patients who experienced a substantial objective response to their induction chemotherapy.

Non-Hodgkin Lymphoma

IFN studies in patients with non-Hodgkin lymphoma have focused on single-agent activity, maintenance therapy after induction chemotherapy, and in combination with chemotherapy. For the most part, these studies have been limited to indolent or "favorable" lymphomas in which the overall response rate is approximately 25–40%.[287,311] Patients with intermediate-grade non-Hodgkin lymphoma tend to have fewer objective responses. IFN has also been studied in combination with cytotoxic chemotherapy in patients with low-grade lymphomas. The results of an Eastern Cooperative Oncology Group prospective randomized trial designed to evaluate the efficacy of IFN-α added to multidrug cytotoxic therapy (COPA [cyclophosphamide, vincristine, prednisone, doxorubicin]) were recently reported. Two hundred ninety-one patients with low-grade lymphoma were randomized. The regimens produced comparable objective response rates, but the addition of IFN resulted in the prolongation of time to treatment failure, duration of complete response, and overall survival.[312] Similarly, in patients with follicular lymphomas, the addition of IFN-α to m-CAVP (methotrexate, cyclophosphamide, doxorubicin, VM-26, and prednisone) demonstrated higher response rates than were achieved in those receiving chemotherapy alone.[313] By contrast, the preliminary results of a large prospective trial in which patients with follicular low-grade lymphoma were randomized to chemotherapy or chemotherapy and IFN-α suggest no difference in complete response rates and overall survival between the two groups.[314] The results of ongoing randomized trials should address whether the combination of IFN and chemotherapy impact favorably on response rates and disease-free or overall survival in patients with low-grade lymphoma.[315]

Tumor Necrosis Factor

TNF-α and lymphotoxin (TNF-β) are closely related cytokines that share a common receptor and have similar biologic effects, playing a central role in immunity and the inflammatory response.[8] Release of TNF-α and lymphotoxin is stimulated by endotoxin, and other cytokines, including IFN-γ, IL-1, and CSF-GM.[316] Monocytes/macrophages are the primary producers of TNF-α, and activated T cells are the primary sources of TNF-β. In humans, the genes for TNF-α and LT are closely linked on the short arm of chromosome 6.[317] Recently two distinct types of cellular TNF receptors have been identified by molecular cloning that are differentially expressed on various human cells, normal and malignant.[318]

Interest in the use of TNF for the treatment of human cancers stems from intriguing animal studies in which TNF resulted in dramatic regression and hemorrhagic necrosis of tumors.[9,319] In addition, the in vitro antitumor effects of TNF are very specific for malignant cells, with very few cytotoxic effects observed against normal cells.[320] The biologic effects of TNF include profound effects on immune effector cells, hematopoietic cells, inhibition of enzymes involved in adipocyte differentiation, and lipid metabolism and stimulation of both collagen production and collagenase activity.[321] TNF specifically induces a number of proteins in vascular endothelial cells closely linked to the hemostatic properties of TNF.[322–324] Neutrophil activity is greatly stimulated by TNF. However, TNF suppresses the colony growth of CFU-GM and CFU-E.[325] The inhibitory effects of TNF on hematopoietic progenitor cells depend on prolonged exposure and high concentrations. In addition, TNF activates macrophages and is an important inducer of acute-phase reactants.[8] TNF-α is identical to the protein associated with cachexia, hence the alternative name, cachetin.[321] Importantly, TNF also induces secretion of a number of cytokines, including CSF-GM, IL-1, IL-6, as well as other mediators of inflammation.[8]

The precise mechanism whereby TNF mediates its antitumor

activity is unclear, but evidence to date suggests that direct cytotoxicity against malignant cells is one important mechanism that may be due to free radical formation.[8] In vivo antitumor effects may also depend on procoagulant effects of TNF on tumor vasculature.[322,324]

TNF appears to act as a growth factor for some malignant cells. In vitro stimulatory effects of TNF have been reported in patients with HCL, B-CLL, and AML.[325] Interesting preclinical and clinical data suggest that TNF may act as an autocrine growth factor for some cases of B-CLL and HCL. Digel et al.[7] recently found increased circulating levels of soluble TNF-BP in the sera of patients with B-CLL and HCL compared to human sera from healthy controls.

Several studies suggest that TNF may play a role in the induction of coagulation disorders associated with sepsis. Van der Poll et al.[326] reported the effects of low-dose TNF on activation of the coagulation cascade. Normal subjects received a single dose of TNF that resulted in subclinical activation of the coagulation system measured by an increase in plasma levels of factor X activation peptide. In addition, marked elevation in plasma plasminogen activator activity has been demonstrated in patients treated with TNF. The release of TNF-α in the setting of gram-negative sepsis and in patients treated with high-dose IL-2 may be responsible for the hemodynamic consequences of sepsis, namely, fever, hypotension, and the capillary leak syndrome.[327]

Phase I and II studies with TNF have been completed; little single-agent activity has been demonstrated against hematologic malignancies or solid tumors.[328–330] However, in studies to date, only modest doses of TNF have been administered due to considerable toxicity, including fever and hypotension. Thus, therapeutically inadequate doses of TNF have been administered due to the significant toxicity associated with the systemic administration of TNF. Strategies designed to overcome this limitation have included the use of agents to reduce hypotension associated with TNF, such as nitric oxide inhibitors[176] and the use of effector cells (tumor-infiltrating lymphocytes) transfected with the gene for TNF, augmenting the local delivery of TNF to tumors and limiting systemic exposure.[331]

Colony-Stimulating Factor-Macrophage

CSF-M, or CSF-1, is a homodimer composed of two monomers of approximately 45 kd connected by a disulfide link. Produced primarily by monocytes, fibroblasts, and endothelial cells, it stimulates the proliferation, differentiation, and activation of the monocyte/macrophage lineage. The receptor for CSF-M is the product of the proto-oncogene c-*fms*. CSF-M is detectable in the serum at low levels in normal healthy adults.[332]

When administered to mice, CSF-M results in an initial increase in cycling rates of bone marrow and splenic committed progenitors. Further treatment with CSF-M (>2 doses) leads to a reduction in cycling rates.[333] The precise mechanism of this effect is unclear. CSF-M is a potent activator of monocyte/macrophage function.[334] The mechanism by which macrophages promote their antitumor activity may involve the elaboration of secondary cytokines such as IL-1 or TNF or the promotion of oxygen free radicals. Activation of monocytes/macrophages by CSF-M significantly enhances their antitumor effects and particularly their antibody-dependent cellular cytotoxicity (ADCC).[334]

Munn et al.[335] studied the effects of parenteral CSF-M on the ADCC of monocytes of nonhuman primates. CSF-M administered by continuous intravenous infusion or subcutaneous injection daily for 14 days at doses of 50–100 μg/kg/day resulted in significant increases in peripheral blood monocyte number. ADCC of monocytes from treated animals incubated for 3 days with CSF-M demonstrated significantly enhanced tumoricidal

activity against a melanoma cell line (SKMel-1) in the presence of the monoclonal antibody 3F8. CSF-M therapy was associated with a mild decrease in peripheral blood platelet counts. No other significant toxicity was noted.

Antitumor Agent

Several clinical studies in humans have been conducted with CSF-M. Bajorin et al.[336] reported the results of a phase I trial of continuous intravenous infusion CSF-M in patients with metastatic melanoma. Patients were treated with CSF-M at doses of 10–120 μg/kg/day for 7 days. Significant increases in circulating monocytes were seen at all dose levels. Monocytes from patients at doses of >50 μg/kg/day demonstrated enhanced antibody-dependent monocyte cytotoxicity against tumor target cells in vitro. Only one delayed antitumor response was seen. Toxicity included dose-related thrombocytopenia and a lowering of serum cholesterol. Additional studies of CSF-M as an antitumor agent have been carried out using different routes of administration and schedules.[337,338] None has demonstrated significant antitumor activity. Future studies will focus on the use of CSF-M with other biologic agents.[339]

After Chemotherapy

Since CSF-M is an agent that exerts a proliferative and maturational effect on hematopoietic cells, several trials have examined its ability to reduce the myelosuppressive effects of chemotherapy. Studies with recombinant human CSF-M in patients undergoing autologous BMT have demonstrated no significant effect on the rate of engraftment of platelets or neutrophils. In several studies, natural CSF-M, purified from human urine, has demonstrated a significantly more rapid engraftment of neutrophils in one randomized study[340] and a more rapid engraftment of platelets in another.[341] These two studies have been criticized for the possible contamination of the CSF-M with other hematopoietic factors that may be present in human urine and could have contributed to the effects seen.

Infectious Diseases

Because of its ability to prime and activate monocytes and macrophages, CSF-M is a potentially attractive agent for the use in diseases in which enhanced effector cell function may contribute to therapy. CSF-M has been shown to enhance antifungal activity of its target effector cells, making invasive fungal infections an ideal scenario in which to test its potential.[342] Nemunaitis et al.[343,344] treated 24 BMT patients with invasive fungal infections with CSF-M doses of 100–2,000 μg/m² day. CSF-M was administered as a 2-hour infusion for 7 days, after which patients were eligible for dose escalation to the next level. All patients had failed aggressive prior antifungal therapy but were maintained on the best available therapy at their maximum tolerated dose during CSF-M therapy. Overall, 6 patients had resolution of their infections. Only 1 out of 16 patients treated following an allogeneic BMT experienced worsening of GVHD. A randomized trial designed to define the true benefit of CSF-M as an antifungal adjunct is currently being conducted.

Osteopetrosis

Another particularly interesting area of research regarding CSF-M is in osteopetrosis. Osteopetrosis is a heterogeneous family of disorders characterized by the inability of osteoclasts to resorb bone. This results in failure of the remodeling of bone, and obliteration of the medullary cavity that leads to extramedullary hematopoiesis. Additional complications of this disease include blindness and deafness due to nerve compression by bone.[345] Since osteoclasts and macrophages are thought to be derived from a common hematopoietic precursor, CSF-M could possibly enhance osteoclast function or recruit new osteoclasts into bone with resultant normalization of bone resorption.[346,347] While Orchard et al.[348] demonstrated that serum levels of biologically active CSF-M are normal in patients with osteopetrosis, other investigators have shown absence of bioactive CSF-M in *op/op* mice (an animal osteopetrosis model).[349] For this reason, a phase I trial of intravenous CSF-M has been performed.[350] While doses of CSF-M were low (100–2,000 μg/m²/day), some clinical benefit defined as reduced bone density, eruption of new teeth, and improved bone architecture, was seen in several of the patients suggesting that more prolonged therapy, beginning at an earlier age may be of benefit.

Monoclonal Antibodies

The successful use of monoclonal antibodies as a therapeutic approach to the treatment of cancer depends on two principles, that cancer cells are immunologically distinct from normal cells and that recognition of these differences can result in an effective antitumor response through specific binding to target antigens expressed on tumor cells.[351] Ideally, one can identify tumor-specific antigens (i.e., an antigen expressed solely on the tumor cell but not on normal cells) as the target for a monoclonal antibody. Unfortunately, truly tumor-specific antigens are rare and limited to B-cell malignancies in which the variable region of the immunoglobulin molecule serves as a unique marker referred to as the idiotype determinant.[351] Similarly, the T-cell receptor expressed on malignant cells of T-cell leukemia and lymphoma provides a unique tumor-specific antigen.[352] Except for these examples, no truly tumor-specific antigens have been identified to date. Currently identified tumor antigens represent differentiation antigens and are therefore expressed on both malignant cells and normal cells, albeit the expression of these antigens may be at lower levels on nonmalignant cells.[351,352] In addition, the products of cellular oncogenes have been defined as cell-surface receptors (i.e., platelet-derived growth factor, epidermal growth factor) and represent potential targets for monoclonal antibodies.[353]

Recent advances in technology have allowed for the large-scale production of monoclonal antibodies with defined specificity. The variable region of the immunoglobulin determines the antigen-binding characteristics, and the constant region defines the effector properties. Strategies for using monoclonal antibodies include activation of immune effector cell function (activation of complement cascade or activation of ADCC; conjugating the monoclonal antibody to a toxin or radionuclide, thereby delivering cytotoxic molecules to tumor targets; or interfering with tumor cell growth through binding to growth factors or their receptors. Only one monoclonal antibody has been approved by the FDA for clinical use—the OKT3 murine monoclonal antibody, which is directed against the T-cell receptor complex. It was approved for the prevention of renal graft rejection.

Considerable obstacles to the therapeutic use of monoclonal antibodies have been identified and include the short half-life of administered antibody due to the presence of free circulating antigen and the development of neutralizing antibodies to the murine antibody (human antimouse antibody).[354,355] Tumor cells can escape the monoclonal antibody through the phenomenon of antigenic modulation, in which binding of the antibody to the antigen results in the transient disappearance of the antigen. In addition, only a proportion of the cancer cells express the relevant antigen due to antigenic heterogeneity, again limiting efficacy. Other barriers to this approach include poor affinity of the antibody to the tumor target antigen and impaired delivery of the antibody due to poor tumor vascularity and necrotic centers. The use of human monoclonal antibodies may overcome some of these obstacles, but the production of

human reagents remains technically difficult. Only a few human monoclonal antibodies have been clinically evaluated. Early results suggest that they are less immunogenic and have a longer half-life than murine antibodies.[356] The distinct problems associated with murine antibodies (immunogenicity) and human antibodies (limited availability) have led to the construct of so-called chimeric antibodies, which retain the murine antigen-binding sites of the murine antibody but closely resemble the constant region of the human immunoglobulin. Chimeric antibodies have been shown to be less immunogenic, with longer half-lives than murine antibodies.[357]

The clinical effectiveness of native (unconjugated or unmodified) monoclonal antibodies has been disappointing. That has led to the development of new strategies in which a cytotoxic molecule is conjugated to the antibody, thereby delivering a cytotoxic agent directly to tumor targets with reduced systemic exposure, hence toxicity. A wide range of cytotoxic agents have been identified, including chemotherapeutic agents, radioisotopes, and toxins modified to remove their normal tissue-binding domains. The resulting immunotoxin has the advantage of specificity of the attached antibody combined with the potency of the toxin or radionuclide. Some examples of toxins evaluated to date include ricin, *Pseudomonas* exotoxin A, and diphtheria toxin, which inhibit specific steps in protein synthesis.[358–361] Monoclonal antibodies directed against high-affinity cell-surface receptors that are rapidly internalized have been the most successful and include antibodies to growth factor receptors, the IL-2 receptor, as well many lymphoid differentiation antigens.[359,362] Similarly, chemotherapeutic agents, including doxorubicin, methotrexate, vinblastine, and melphalan, have been linked to monoclonal antibodies. However, obstacles such as limited drug delivery to tumor sites and significant technologic challenges remain, limiting the clinical evaluation of this approach.

Clinical Application

Numerous phase I and II studies of monoclonal antibodies have been completed in patients with solid tumors and hematologic malignancies.[351,363–366] Initial studies focused on the safety and pharmacology of unconjugated murine antibodies in patients with leukemia and lymphoma. The tumor-associated antigens identified were differentiation surface markers expressed by both malignant and normal lymphoid cells. Many studies have used a monoclonal antibody directed against CD5, an antigen expressed on normal and malignant T cells as well as B-cell CLL. Generally the side effects of unconjugated monoclonal antibodies have been mild and include fever, chills, urticaria, bronchospasm, and pain.[366] Rarely, patients have developed symptoms of anaphylaxis and serum sickness, which in all reported cases has been reversible. Overall the antitumor response has been limited, primarily in patients with cutaneous T-cell lymphoma. Details of these early studies have been extensively reviewed.[363,366]

An alternative strategy for testing immune intervention in patients with hematologic malignancies is to target the IL-2R.[367] Waldmann et al.[368] developed a murine monoclonal antibody, anti-Tac, that binds to IL-2R and prevents interaction of IL-2 with this subunit. The rational for this approach is that resting normal cells do not express the high-affinity IL-2R, whereas expression of this receptor is found on a proportion of lymphoid neoplasms, including HCL, large and mixed-cell lymphomas, T-cell and B-cell monocytic leukemias, T-cell lymphoma, and some Reed-Sternberg cells in Hodgkin disease. In addition, virtually all patients with HTLV-1 associated adult T-cell leukemia express the IL-2R. Therefore, initial clinical with the anti-Tac antibody have focused on patients with HTLV-1 T-cell leukemia. Preliminary results with 19 patients have shown that therapy is well tolerated. Seven patients had partial or complete remission, lasting 9 weeks to >3 years.[368] The elimination of clonal malignant cells was confirmed by molecular genetic analysis of HTLV-1 proviral integration and T-cell receptor rearrangements. The mechanism of action of anti-Tac is not clear, but it does not appear to be mediated by ADCC.

One very intriguing approach that is extremely labor intensive has involved the use of anti-idiotype monoclonal antibodies for the treatment of indolent lymphomas. Levy et al. generated monoclonal antibodies that recognize the specific idiotype of surface immunoglobulin on the patient's lymphoma cells. Initial clinical trials reported a 50–70% reduction in the tumor size with some patients obtaining complete responses.[365]

Monoclonal antibodies have also been extensively studied to deplete neoplastic cells from the bone marrow of patients with leukemia and lymphoma undergoing autologous BMT.[369,370] Early trials, which have focused on non-T-cell ALL and B-cell non-Hodgkin lymphoma, confirm the value of antibodies and complement for purging bone marrow with very little toxicity being documented against hematopoietic progenitor cells. Thus, hematologic engraftment has not been affected; however, relapse of leukemia and lymphoma remains a significant problem. Monoclonal antibodies have also been used to prevent GVHD in patients undergoing allogeneic transplants for hematologic malignancies.[371,372] However, the use of anti-T-cell monoclonal antibodies for the treatment of donor marrow to decrease GVHD has been associated with reduced frequency of bone marrow engraftment and a higher incidence of leukemia recurrence.[373]

One of the limitations of monoclonal antibody therapy has been the generation of human antimouse antibody.[355] Therefore, newer strategies involve the production of chimeric antibodies. One such antibody is CAMPATH-1H, a "humanized" IgG monoclonal antibody that recognizes lymphocytes and mediates cell lysis through ADCC. The six hypervariable regions from the heavy and light chain domains of the rodent antibody have been reshaped into a human IgG-1 framework. This antibody recognizes CDw52, which is an antigen abundantly expressed on T and B lymphocytes, but not on erythrocytes, platelets, or bone marrow stem cells, and infrequently expressed on granulocytes. Additional data suggest that the antigen is expressed on the lymphocytes from most patients with

non-Hodgkin lymphoma, CLL, and ALL. Initial clinical studies in patients with non-Hodgkin lymphoma and CLL appear promising.[374] In patients with CLL, nearly all patients with high circulating lymphocyte counts experienced a ≥50% reduction in peripheral blood lymphocyte counts. Approximately one-third of patients with measurable lymphadenopathy achieved a ≥25% reduction in nodal size. However, toxicities associated with treatment are substantial including transient neutropenia, thrombocytopenia, hypotension, fever, rigors, and gastrointestinal symptoms.

An alternative approach involves conjugating a radioisotope to a monoclonal antibody. Various radioisotopes have been selected and governed by energy of γ-rays, safety, half-life, and ease of linkage to a particular antibody. Most therapeutic trials with radioimmunoconjugates have used α-emitters such as ^{131}I; more recently, long-range β-emitters such as ^{90}Yt and ^{188}Rh have been evaluated.[375,376] Responses have been reported in patients with B-cell non-Hodgkin lymphoma treated with the ^{131}I-Lym-1 antibody (Lym-1 reacts with a variant HLA-DR molecule expressed on many B-cell tumors) and in cutaneous T-cell lymphoma in patients treated with the ^{131}I-T101 antibody.[377] Toxicities associated with therapy were predictable and were principally myelosuppression due to the radiation dose delivered. Numerous clinical studies in patients with Hodgkin lymphoma, non-Hodgkin lymphoma, and chronic leukemias have been completed and are summarized in recent reviews.[378] For the most part, the responses have been partial and short lived. More recently, Kaminski et al.[379] evaluated the effect of ^{131}I-labeled B-cell-specific anti-CD20 murine (anti-B1) monoclonal antibody in 10 patients with refractory B-cell lymphoma. Six of nine patients had significant tumor responses, four with complete responses, and two had partial responses. Therapy was associated with minimal toxicity. These results are promising, and ongoing clinical studies will address the potential of radioimmunotherapy as a treatment for lymphoma.

The clinical application of immunotoxins has focused on the treatment of hematologic malignancies and in the setting of BMT where they have been used to deplete the marrow of T cells and to prevent GVHD.[372,380,381] Early results are summarized in Table 62-7. Clinical trials with ricin-A-chain immunotoxins are under way in patients with ALL, CLL, and non-Hodgkin lymphoma. Overall, the results have been disappointing and,

Table 62-7. Clinical Studies of Immunotoxin in the Treatment of Hematologic Malignancies

Patient Population	Immunotoxin	Target	Toxicity	Results	Reference
IL-2R expressing hematologic malignancies	DAB$_{486}$ IL-2 (diphtheria)	IL-2 receptor	Nausea, rash, reversible increased creatinine, SGOT/SGPT	50% developed antibody to immunotoxin, few antitumor responses	382
Allogeneic BMT (T-cell depletion to decrease GVHD)	Anti-T-cell monoclonal antibody T101-ricin-A	CD5 receptor (T cell)	—	Depleted T cells by 97.5–100%, decrease severity GVHD	380
Allogeneic BMT (T-cell depletion to decrease GVHD)	Anti-CD3-ricin-A	CD3 receptor	—	3 log depletion of CD3+ T cells in bone marrow, GVHD prevented, graft failure in 2/8 patients	372
Autologous BMT for refractory T-ALL (bone marrow purging)	Anti-CD5-ricin-A	CD5 receptor	—	Marrow engraftment not affected, 5/7 patients relapsed	381
CLL (B cell)	Anti-CD5-ricin-A	CD5 receptor	—	No response, rapid clearance of immunotoxin	363
Acute or chronic GVHD	Anti-CD5-ricin-A	CD5 receptor	Capillary leak syndrome, renal insult	50% of patients developed antibody to immunotoxin, significant activity in both acute and chronic GVHD	356

in some circumstances, toxicity significant. The toxicity may be the result of nonspecific binding of free toxin or binding of the immunotoxin to nontumor tissues.

A newer strategy involves the use of chimeric toxins, in which bacterial toxin genes are fused with cytokines genes or their receptors. The first such construct for clinical use involves the gene for IL-2 fused to a gene for diphtheria or pseudomonas exotoxin.[362] These fused proteins recognize cells bearing the IL-2R, are subsequently internalized by receptor-mediated endocytosis, and result in cell lysis mediated by the toxin. Clinical studies are now underway in malignancies in which the malignant cells express the IL-2Rs, including HTLV-1-associated leukemia, T-cell leukemia and lymphoma, and non-Hodgkin lymphoma.[382]

REFERENCES

1. Neidhart J, Mangalik A, Kohler W et al: Granulocyte colony-stimulating factor stimulates recovery of granulocytes in patients receiving dose-intensive chemotherapy without bone marrow transplantation. J Clin Oncol 7:1685, 1989
2. Kurzrock R, Kantarjian H, Wetzler M et al: Ubiquitous expression of cytokines in diverse leukemias of lymphoid and myeloid lineage. Exp Hematol 21:80, 1993
3. Duncombe AS, Heslop HE, Turner M et al: Tumor necrosis factor mediates autocrine growth inhibition in a chronic leukemia. J Immunol 143:3828, 1989
4. Oster W, Cicco NA, Klein H et al: Participation of the cytokines interleukin-6, tumor necrosis factor-alpha, and interleukin-1 beta secreted by acute myelogenous leukemia blasts in autocrine and paracrine leukemia growth control. J Clin Invest 84:451, 1989
5. Heslop HE, Brenner MK, Ganeshaguru K et al: Possible mechanism of action of interferon alpha in chronic B-cell malignancies. Br J Haematol 79:14, 1991
6. Biondi A, Ross B, Bassan R et al: Constitutive expression of the interleukin-6 gene in chronic lymphocytic leukemia. Blood 73:1279, 1989
7. Digel W, Stefanic M, Shoniger W et al: Tumor necrosis factor induces proliferation of neoplastic B cells from chronic lymphocytic leukemia. Blood 73:1242, 1989
8. Balkwill FR: Cytokines in Cancer Therapy. Oxford University Press, New York, 1989
9. Maluish AE, Urba W, Longo DL et al: The determination of an immunologically active dose of interferon-gamma in patients with melanoma. J Clin Oncol 6:434, 1988
10. Siegel JP, Puri RK: Interleukin-2 toxicity. J Clin Oncol 9:694, 1991
11. Foon KA: Biological response modifiers: the new immunotherapy. Cancer Res 49:1621, 1989
12. Salmon S, Liu R: Effects of granulocyte-macrophage colony-stimulating factor on in vitro growth of human solid tumors. J Clin Oncol 7:1346, 1989
13. Souza L, Boone T, Gabrilove J et al: Recombinant human granulocyte colony-stimulating factor: effects on normal and leukemic myeloid cells. Science 232:61, 1991
14. Demetri G, Griffin J: Granulocyte colony-stimulating factor and its receptor. Blood 78:2791, 1991
15. Watari K, Asano S, Shirafuji N et al: Serum granulocyte colony-stimulating factor levels in healthy volunteers and patients with various disorders as estimated by enzyme immunoassay. Blood 73:117, 1989
16. Yuo A, Kitagawa S, Okabe T et al: Recombinant human granulocyte colony-stimulating factor repairs the abnormalities of neutrophils in patients with myelodysplastic syndromes and chronic myelogenous leukemia. Blood 70:404, 1987
17. Bodey G, Buckley M, Sathe Y, Freireich E: Quantitative relationships between circulating leukocytes and infection in patients with acute leukemia. Ann Intern Med 64:328, 1966
18. Gabrilove J, Jakubowski A, Scher H et al: Effect of granulocyte colony-stimulating factor on neutropenia and associated morbidity due to chemotherapy for transitional-cell carcinoma of the urothelium. N Engl J Med 318:1414, 1988
19. Bronchud M, Howell A, Crowther D et al: The use of granulocyte colony-stimulating factor to increase the intensity of treatment with doxorubicin in patients wth advanced breast and ovarian cancer. Br J Cancer 60:121, 1989
20. Morstyn G, Souza L, Keech J et al: Effect of granulocyte colony-stimulating factor on neutropenia induced by cytotoxic chemotherapy. Lancet 1:667, 1988
21. Crawford J, Ozer H, Stoller R et al: Reduction by granulocyte colony-stimulating factor of fever and neutropenia by chemotherapy in patients with small-cell lung cancer. N Engl J Med 325:164, 1991
22. Trillet-Lenoir V, Green J, Manegold C et al: Recombinant granulocyte colony-stimulating factor reduces the infectious complications of cytotoxic chemotherapy. Eur J Cancer 29A:319, 1993
23. Pettengell R, Gurney H, Radford J et al: A randomized trial of recombinant human granulocyte colony-stimulating factor to preserve dose intensity in non-Hodgkin's lymphoma. Proc ASCO 11:1083a, 1992
24. Maher D, Bishop J, Stuart-Harris R et al: Randomized, placebo-controlled trial of filgrastim in patients with febrile neutropenia. Proc ASCO 12:1498a, 1993
25. Mayordomo J, Rivera F, Diaz-Puente M et al: Decreasing morbidity and cost of treating febrile neutropenia by adding G-CSF and GM-CSF to standard antibiotic therapy: results of a randomized trial. Proc ASCO 12:1510a, 1993
26. Ohno R, Tomonaga M, Kobayashi T et al: Effect of granulocyte colony-stimulating factor after intensive induction therapy in relapsed or refractory acute leukemia. N Engl J Med 323:871, 1990
27. Sheridan W, Morstyn G, Wolf M et al: Granulocyte colony-stimulating factor and neutrophil recovery after high-dose chemotherapy and autologous bone marrow transplantation. Lancet 2:891, 1992
28. Sheridan W, Begley G, Juttner C et al: Effect of peripheral-blood progenitor cells mobilized by filgrastim on platelet recovery after high-dose chemotherapy. Lancet 339:640, 1992
29. Negrin RS, Haeuber DH, Nagler A et al: Treatment of myelodysplatic syndromes with recombinant human granulocyte colony-stimulating factor. Ann Intern Med 110:976, 1989
30. Negrin R, Haeuber D, Nagler A et al: Maintenance treatment of patients with myelodysplastic syndromes using recombinant human granulocyte colony-stimulating factor. Blood 76:36, 1990
31. Negrin R, Stein R, Vardiman J et al: Treatment of the anemia of myelodysplastic syndromes using recombinant human granulocyte colony-stimulating factor in combination with erythropoietin. Blood 82:737, 1993
32. Bonilla M, Gillio A, Ruggeiro M et al: Effects of recombinant granulocyte colony-stimulating factor on neutropenia in patients with congenital agranulocytosis. N Engl J Med 320:1574, 1989
33. Dale D, Bonilla M, Davis M et al: A randomized, controlled phase II trial of recombinant human granulocyte colony-stimulating factor for the treatment of severe chronic neutropenia. Blood 81:2496, 1993
34. Hammond IV, W, Price T, Souza L, Dale D: Treatment of cyclic neutropenia with granulocyte colony-stimulating factor. N Engl J Med 320:1306, 1989
35. Jakubowski A, Souza L, Kelly F et al: Effects of human granulocyte colony-stimulating factor in a patient with idiopathic neutropenia. N Engl J Med 320:38, 1989
36. Glasby J, Baldwin G, Robertson P et al: Therapy for neutropenia in hairy cell leukemia with recombinant human granulocyte colony-stimulating factor. Ann Intern Med 109:789, 1988
37. Miles S: The use of hematopoietic growth factors in HIV infection and AIDS-related malignancies. Cancer Invest 9:229, 1991
38. Miles S, Mitsuyasu R, Moreno J et al: Combined therapy with recombinant granulocyte colony-stimulating factor and erythropoietin decreases hematologic toxicity from zidovudine. Blood 77:2109, 1991
39. Sieff C, Emerson S, Donahue R, Nathan D: Human granulocyte-macrophage colony-stimulating factor: a multilineage hematopoietin. Science 230:1171, 1985
40. Lieschke G, Cebon J, Morstyn G: Characterization of the clinical effects after the first dose of bacterially synthesized recombinant human granulocyte-macrophage colony-stimulating factor. Blood 74:2634, 1989
41. Gerhartz H, Engelhard M, Meusers P et al: Randomized double-blind placebo-controlled phase III study of recombinant human granulocyte-macrophage colony-stimulating factor (rhGM-CSF) as adjunct to induction treatment of high-grade malignant non-Hodgkin's lymphomas. Blood 82:2329, 1993
42. Bunn P Jr, Crowley J, Hazuka M et al: The role of GM-CSF in limited stage SCLC: a randomized phase II study of the Southwest Oncology Group (SWOG). Proc ASCO 11:974a, 1992
43. Nemunaitis J, Singer J, Buckner C et al: Long-term follow-up of patients who received recombinant human granulocyte-macrophage colony-stimulating factor after autologous bone marrow transplantation for lymphoid malignancies. Bone Marrow Transplant 7:49, 1991
44. Nemunaitis J, Rabinowe S, Singer J et al: Recombinant granulocyte-macrophage colony-stimulating factor after autologous bone marrow transplantation for lymphoid cancer. N Engl J Med 324:1773, 1991
45. Gulati S, Bennett C: Granulocyte-macrophage colony-stimulating factor (GM-CSF) as adjuvant therapy in relapsed Hodgkin disease. Ann Intern Med 116:177, 1992
46. Gorin N, Coiffier B, Hayat M et al: Recombinant human granulocyte-macrophage colony-stimulating factor after high-dose chemotherapy and autologous bone marrow transplantation with unpurged and purged marrow in

non-Hodgkin's lymphoma: a double-blind placebo-controlled trial. Blood 80: 1149, 1992

47. Brandt JS, Peters WP, Atwater SK et al: Effect of recombinant human granulocyte-macrophage colony-stimulating factor on hematopoietic reconstitution after high-dose chemotherapy and autologous bone marrow transplantation. N Engl J Med 318:869, 1988

48. Nemunaitis J, Singer JW, Buckner CD et al: Use of recombinant human granulocyte-macrophage colony-stimulating factor in graft failure after bone marrow transplantation. Blood 76:245, 1990

49. De Witte T, Gratwohl A, Van Der Lely N et al: Recombinant human granulocyte-macrophage colony-stimulating factor accelerates neutrophil and monocyte recovery after allogeneic T-cell depleted bone marrow transplantation. Blood 79:1359, 1992

50. Gianni A, Siena S, Bregni M et al: Granulocyte-macrophage colony-stimulating factor to harvest circulating haematopoietic stem cells for autotransplantation. Lancet 2:580, 1989

51. Haas R, Hohaus S, Egrer G et al: Recombinant human granulocyte-macrophage colony-stimulating factor (rhGM-CSF) subsequent to chemotherapy improves collection of blood stem cells for autografting in patients not eligible for bone marrow harvest. Bone Marrow Transplant 9:459, 1992

52. Patrone F, Ballestrero A, Balleari E et al: High-dose cyclophosphamide followed by GM-CSF is a safe and effective procedure for the recruitment of trilineage circulating progenitor cells. Haematological 77:457, 1992

53. Peters W, Rosner G, Ross M et al: Comparative effects of granulocyte-macrophage colony-stimulating factor (GM-CSF) and granulocyte colony-stimulating factor (G-CSF) on priming peripheral blood progenitor cells for use with autologous bone marrow after high-dose chemotherapy. Blood 81:1709, 1993

54. Siena S, Bregni M, Brando B et al: Flow cytometry for clinical estimation of circulating hematopoietic progenitors for autologous transplantation in cancer patients. Blood 77:400, 1991

55. Antin J, Smith BR, Holmes W, Rosenthal DS: Phase I/II study of recombinant human granulocyte-macrophage colony-stimulating factor in aplastic anemia and myelodysplastic syndrome. Blood 72:705, 1988

56. Ganser A, Volkers B, Hoelzer D: Recombinant human granulocyte-macrophage colony-stimulating factor in patients with myelodysplastic syndromes—a phase I/II trial. Blood 73:31, 1989

57. Vadhan-Raj S, Keating M, Hittelman W et al: Effects of recombinant human granulocyte-macrophage colony-stimulating factor in patients with myelodysplastic syndromes. N Engl J Med 317:1545, 1987

58. Thompson J, Lee DJ, Kidd P et al: Subcutaneous granulocyte-macrophage colony-stimulating factor in patients with myelodysplastic syndrome: toxicity, pharmacokinetics, and hematological effects. J Clin Oncol 7:629, 1989

59. Schuster M, Thompson J, Larson R et al: Randomized trial of subcutaneous granulocyte-macrophage colony-stimulating factor (GM-CSF) versus observation in patients with myelodysplastic syndrome. Proc ASCO 9:793a, 1990

60. Krown S, Paredes J, Bundow D et al: Interferon-alpha, zidovudine, and granulocyte-macrophage colony-stimulating factor: a phase I AIDS Clinical Trials Group study in patients with Kaposi's sarcoma associated with AIDS. J Clin Oncol 10:1344, 1992

61. Groopman J, Mitsuyasu R, DeLeo M et al: Effect of recombinant human granulocyte-macrophage colony-stimulating factor on myelopoiesis in the acquired immunodeficiency syndrome. N Engl J Med 317:593, 1987

62. Levine J, Allan J, Tessitore J et al: Recombinant huma granulocyte-macrophage colony-stimulating factor ameliorates zidovudine-induced neutropenia in patients with acquired immunodeficiency syndrome (AIDS)/AIDS-related complex. Blood 78:3148, 1991

63. Guinan E, Nathan D, Lee Y et al: Phase I/II trial of recombinant human inerleukin-3 (IL-3) and granulocyte-macrophage colony-stimulating factor (GM-CSF) in patients with amegakaryocytic thrombocytopenia (AMT). Blood 78: 9a, 1991

64. Krantz S, Jacobson L: Erythropoietin and the Regulation of Erythropoiesis. University of Chicago Press, Chicago, 1970

65. Goldberg M, Dunning S, Bunn H: Regulation of the erythropoietin gene: evidence that the oxygen sensor is a heme protein. Science 242:1412, 1988

66. Browne J, Cohen A, Egrie J et al: Erythropoietin, gene cloning protein structure, and biologic properties. Cold Spring Harbor Symp Quant Biol 51:693, 1986

67. Miyake T, Kung C, Goldwasser E: Purification of human erythropoietin. J Biol Chem 252:5558, 1977

68. Dordal M, Wang F, Goldwasser E: The role of carbohydrate in erythropoietin action. Endocrinology 116:2293, 1985

69. Cohen R, Clemons G, Ebbe S: Correlation between bioassay and radioimmunoassay for erythropoietin in human serum and urine concentrates. Proc Soc Exp Biol Med 110:29, 1985

70. Eschbach J, Egrie J, Downing M et al: Correction of the anemia of end-stage renal disease with recombinant human erythropoietin: results of a combined phase I and II clinical trial. N Engl J Med 316:73, 1987

71. Winearls C, Oliver D, Pippard M et al: Effect of human erythropoietin derived from recombinant DNA on the anaemia of patients maintained by chronic haemodialysis. Lancet 2:1175, 1986

72. Eschbach J, Abdulhadi M, Browne J et al: Recombinant human erythropoietin in anemic patients with end-stage renal disease. Results of a phase III multicenter clinical trial. Ann Intern Med 111:992, 1989

73. Nissenson AR, the National Cooperative rHu Erythropoietin Study Group: National cooperative rHu erythropoietin study in patients with chronic renal failure: a phase IV multi-center study. Am J Kidney Dis 18:24, 1991

74. Horl W: Optimal route of administration of erythropoietin in chronic renal failure patients: intravenous versus subcutaneous. Acta Haematol 87:16, 1992

75. Richman D, Fischl M, Grieco M et al: The toxicity of azidothymidine (AZT) in the treatment of patients with AIDS and AIDS-related complex. A double-blind, placebo-controlled trial. N Engl J Med 317:192, 1987

76. Henry D, Beall G, Benson C et al: Recombinant human erythropoietin in the treatment of anemia associated with human immunodeficiency virus (HIV) infection and zidovudine therapy. Ann Intern Med 117:739, 1992

77. Rossof A, Slayton R, Perlia C: Preliminary clinical experience with cis-diamminedichloroplatinum(II) (NSC 119875, CACP). Cancer 30:1451, 1972

78. Von Hoff D, Schilsky R, Reichert C et al: Toxic effects of cis-dischlorodiammineplatinum(II) in man. Can Treat Rev 63:1527, 1979

79. Miller C, Jones R, Piantadosi S: Decreased erythropoietin response in patients with the anemia of cancer. N Engl J Med 322:1689, 1990

80. James R, Wilkinson P, Belli F et al: Recombinant human erythropoietin in patients with ovarian carcinoma and anemia secondary to cisplatin and carboplatin chemotherapy: preliminary results. Acta Haematol 87:12, 1992

81. Miller C, Platanias L, Milles S et al: Phase I-II trial of erythroipoietin in the treatment if cisplatin-associated anemia. J Natl Cancer Inst 84:98, 1992

82. Gamucci T, Thorel M, Frasca A et al: Antianemic activity of erythropoietin in cisplatin-treated patients: a randomized trial. Proc ASCO 11:1431a, 1992

83. Abels R, Larholt K, Krantz K, Bryant E: Recombinant human erythropoietin (r-HuEPO) for the treatment of the anemia of cancer. p. 121. In Murphy M Jr (ed): Blood Cell Growth Factors: Their Present and Future Use in Hematology and Oncology. Proceedings of the Beijing Symposium, AlphaMed Press, Dayton, OH, 1991

84. Oster W, Herrmann F, Gamm H et al: Erythropoietin for the treatment of anemia of malignancy associated with neoplastic bone marrow infiltration. J Clin Oncol 8:956, 1990

85. Ludwig H, Fritz E, Kotzmann H et al: Erythropoietin treatment of anemia associated with multiple myeloma. N Engl J Med 322:1693, 1990

86. Baer A, Dessypris E, Goldwasser E, Krantz S: Blunted erythropoietin response to anemia in rheumatoid arthritis. Br J Haematol 66:559, 1987

87. Bowen D, Culligan D, Jacobs A: The treatment of anemia in the myelodysplastic syndromes with recombinant human erythropoietin. Br J Haematol 77:419, 1991

88. Van Kamp H, Prinsze-Postema T, Kluin P et al: Effects of subcutaneously-administered human recombinant erythropoietin on erythropoiesis in patients with myelodysplasia. Blood 76:170a, 1990

89. Adamson J, Schuster M, Allen S, Haley N: Effectiveness of recombinant human erythropoietin therapy in myelodysplastic syndromes. Acta Haematol 87:20, 1992

90. Stein R, Abels R, Krantz S: Pharmacologic doses of recombinant human erythropoietin in the treatment of myelodysplastic syndromes. Blood 78: 1658, 1991

91. Stebler C, Tichelli A, Dazzi H et al: High-dose recombinant human erythropoietin for treatment of anemia in myelodysplastic syndromes and paroxysmal nocturnal hemoglobinuria: a pilot study. Exp Hematol 18:1204, 1990

92. Zeigler Z, Jones D, Rosenfeld C, Shadduck R: Treatment of myelodysplasia (MDS) with recombinant erythropoietin (rHuEPO). Blood 78:352a, 1991

93. Casadevall N, Belanger C, Goy A et al: High-dose recombinant human erythropoietin administered intravenously for the treatment of anemia in myelodysplastic syndromes. Acta Haematol 87:25, 1992

94. Bessho M, Jinnai I, Matsuda A et al: Improvement of anemia by recombinant erythropoetin in patients with myelodysplastic syndromes and apastic anemia. Int J Cell Clon 8:445, 1990

95. Beesho M, Toyoda A, Itoh Y et al: Trilineage recovery by combination therapy with recombinant human granulocyte colony-stimulating factor (rhG-CSF) and erythropoietin (rhEpo) in severe aplastic anemia. Br J Haematol 80:409, 1991

96. Goodnough L, Rudnick S, Price T: Increased preoperative collection of autologous blood with recombinant human erythropoietin therapy. N Engl J Med 321:1163, 1989

97. Maeda H, Hitomi Y, Hirata R: Erythropoietin and autologous blood donation. Lancet 2:284, 1989

98. Canadian Orthopedic Perioperative Erythropoietin Study Group: Effectiveness of perioperative recombinant human erythropoietin in elective hip replacement. Lancet 341:1227, 1993

99. Halperin D, Wacker P, Lacourt G et al: Effects of recombinant erythropoietin in infants with the anemia of prematurity: a pilot study. J Pediatr 1990;116: 779

100. Shannon K, Mentzer W, Abels R: Recombinant human erythropoietin in infants with anemia of prematurity: a pilot study. J Pediatr 118:949, 1991

101. Phipps R, Shannon K, Mentzer W: Potential for treatment of anemia of prematurity with recombinant human erythropoietin: preliminary results. Acta Haematol 87:28, 1992

102. Miller C, Jones R, Zahurak L et al: Imparined erythropoietin response to anemia after bone marrow transplantation. Blood 80:2677, 1992

103. Copeland N, Gilbert D, Cho B et al: Mast cell growth factor maps near the steel locus on mouse chromosome 10 and is deleted in a number of steel alleles. Cell 63:175, 1990

104. Williams DE, Eisenman J, Baird A et al: Identification of a ligand for the c-kit proto-oncogene. Cell 63:167, 1990

105. Zsebo K, Wypych J, McNiece I et al: Identification, purification, and biological characterization of hematopoietic stem cell factor from buffalo rat liver-conditioned medium. Cell 63:195, 1990

106. Zsebo K, Williams D, Geissler E et al: Stem cell factor is encoded at the Sl locus of the mouse and is the ligand for the c-kit tyrosine kinase receptor. Cell 63:213, 1990

107. Ulrich T, del Castillo J, Yi E et al: Hematologic effects of stem cell factor in vivo and in vitro in rodents. Blood 78:645, 1991

108. Srour E, Brandt J, Briddell R et al: Long-term generation and expansion of human primative hematopoietic progenitor cells in vitro. Blood 81:661, 1993

109. McNiece I, Langley K, Zsebo K: Recombinant human stem cell factor synergises with CSFs and EPO to stimulate colony formation of myeloid and erythroid cells. Blood 76:606a, 1990

110. Brandt J, Briddell R, Srour E et al: Role of c-kit ligand in the expansion of human hematopoietic progenitor cells. Blood 79:634, 1992

111. Strohmeyer T, Peter S, Hartmann M et al: Expression of the hst-1 and c-kit protooncogenes in human testicular germ cell tumors. Can Res 51:1811, 1991

112. Broudy VC, Smith FO, Lin N et al: Blasts from patients with acute myelogenous leukemia express functional receptors for stem cell factor. Blood 80:60, 1992

113. Andrews R, Bensinger W, Knitter G et al: The ligand for c-kit, stem cell factor, stimulates the circulation of cells that engraft lethally irradiated baboons. Blood 80:2715, 1992

114. Andrews R, Briddell R, Appelbaum F et al: Stem cell factor synergistically enhances the in vivo response to G-CSF for stimulating increased WBC and progenitor cells in blood of baboons. Exp Hematol 21:519, 1993

115. Demetri G, Costa J, Hayes D et al: A phase I trial of recombinant methionyl human stem cell factor in patients with advanced breast carcinoma pre- and post-chemotherapy with cyclophosphamide and doxorubicin. Proc ASCO 12:367a, 1993

116. Crawford J, Lau D, Erwin R et al: A phase I trial of recombinant methionyl human stem cell factor in patients with non-small cell lung cancer. Proc ASCO 12:338a, 1993

117. Orazi A, Gordon M, Neiman R et al: Bone marrow effects of recombinant methionyl human stem cell factor (SCF) in patients with normal hematopoiesis. Proc AACR 34:2777a, 1993

118. Tong J, Gordon M, Srour E et al: In vivo administration of recombinant methionyl human stem cell factor expands the number of human marrow hematopoietic stem cells. Blood 82:784, 1993

119. Demetri G, Gordon M, Hoffman R et al: Effects of recombinant methionyl human stem cell factor on hematopoietic progenitor cells in vivo: preliminary results of a phase I trial. Proc AACR 34:1295, 1993

120. Crawford J, Lau D, Erwin R et al: A phase I trial of recombinant methionyl human stem cell factor in patients with non-small cell lung cancer. Proc ASCO 12:338, 1993

121. McNiece I, Glasby J, LeMaistre F et al: Effects of recombinant methionyl human tem cell factor (rhSCF) and filgrastim (rhG-CSF) on mobilization of peripheral blood progenitor cells: preliminary laboratory results from a phase I/II study. Blood 82:325a, 1993

122. Haylock D, To L, Dowse T et al: Ex vivo expansion and maturation of peripheral blood CD34$^+$ cells into the myeloid lineage. Blood 80:1405, 1992

123. Alter B, Knobloch M, He L et al: Effect of stem cell factor on in vitro erythropoiesis in patients with bone marrow failure states. Blood 80:3000, 1992

124. Curtis B, Williams D, Broxmeyer H: Enhanced hematopoietic activity of a human GM-CSF/IL-3 fusion protein. Proc Natl Acad Sci 88:5809, 1991

125. Bruno E, Briddell R, Cooper R et al: Recombinant GM-CSF/IL-3 fusion protein: its effect on in vitro human megakaryocytopoiesis. Exp Hematol 20:494, 1992

126. Broxmeyer H, Benninger L, Cooper S, Vadhan-Raj S: Effects of treatment of patients with sarcoma with PIXY321 (a genetically engineered GM-CSF/IL-3 fusion protein) on proliferation kinetics of bone marrow and blood myeloid progenitor cells. Blood 80:87a, 1992

127. MacVittie T, Farese A, Patchen M, Williams DE: Hematologic effects of in vivo administration of recombinant GM-CSF/IL-3 fusion protein (PIXY 321) in normal primates. Exp Hematol 19:177a, 1991

128. Williams DE, Farese A, Dunn J et al: In vivo effects of a GM-CSF/IL-3 fusion protein (PIXY321) in sublethally irradiated monkeys. Exp Hematol 19:479a, 1991

129. Vadhan-Raj S, Papadoupoulos N, Burgess M et al: Optimization of dose and schedule of PIXY321 to attenuate chemotherapy-induced multilineage myelosuppression in patients with sarcoma. Proc ASCO 12:1640a, 1993

130. Broxmeyer HE, Benninger L, Cooper S, Vadhan-Raj S: Effects of treatment of patients with sarcoma with PIXY321 (a genetically engineered GM-CSF/IL-3 fusion protein) on proliferation kinetics of bone marrow and blood myeloid progenitor cells. Blood 80:339a, 1992

131. Runowicz C, Mandeli J, Speyer J et al: Phase I/II study of PIXY321 in combination with cyclophosphamide and carboplatin in the treatment of patients with ovarian cancer. Proc ASCO 12:825a, 1993

132. Raptis G, Gilewski T, Gabrilove JL et al: Evaluation of PIXY321 as a myeloprotective agent in patients with metastatic breast cancer receiving doxorubicin and thiotepa. Proc ASCO 12:235a, 1993

133. Taylor C, Modiano M, Garrison L et al: PIXY plus carboplatin and adriamycin in patients with advanced gastrointestinal malignancy. Proc ASCO 12:569a, 1993

134. Miller L, Smith II J, Urba W et al: A phase I study of an IL-3/GM-CSF fusion protein (PIXY321) and high-dose carboplatin in patients with advanced cancer. Proc ASCO 12:353a, 1993

135. Vose J, Anderson J, Bierman P et al: Initial trial of PIXY321 following high-dose chemotherapy and autologous bone marrow transplantation for lymphoid malignancy. Proc ASCO 12:1237a, 1993

136. Tiberghien P, Laithier V, Mabed M et al: Interleukin-1 administration before lethal irradiation and allogeneic bone marrow transplantation: early transient increase of peripheral granulocytes and successful engraftment with accelerated leukocyte, erythrocyte, and platelet recovery. Blood 81:1933, 1993

137. Moore MAS, Warren DJ: Synergy of interleukin-1 and granulocyte colony-stimulating factor: in vivo stimulation of stem-cell recovery and hematopoietic regeneration following 5-fluorouracil treatment of mice. Proc Natl Acad Sci USA 84:7134, 1987

138. Stork L, Barczuk L, Kissinger M, Robinson W: Interleukin-1 accelerates murine granulocyte recovery following treatment with cyclophosphamide. Blood 73:938, 1989

139. Neta R, Douches S, Oppenheim J: Interleukin-1 is a radioprotector. J Immunol 136:2483, 1986

140. Crown J, Kemeny N, Jakubowski A et al: Phase I-II trial of recombinant human interleukin-1B with and without 5-fluorouracil in patients with gastrointestinal cancer. Blood 78:1420, 1991

141. Smith II J, Urba W, Curti B et al: The toxic and hematologic effects of interleukin-1 alpha administered in a phase I trial to patients with advanced malignancies. J Clin Oncol 10:1141, 1992

142. Smith II J, Longo D, Alvord W et al: The effects of treatment with interleukin-1 alpha on platelet recovery after high-dose carboplatin. N Eng J Med 328:756, 1993

143. Vredenburgh J, Ross M, Kurtzberg J et al: Phase I trial of interleukin-1β (IL-1β) following high-dose chemotherapy and autologous bone marrow transplantation (ABMT). Blood 78:13a, 1991

144. Nemunaitis J, Buckner C, Press O et al: Phase I trial with interleukin-1β (IL-1β) in patients undergoing autologous bone marrow transplantation (ABMT) for acute myelogenous leukemia (AML). Blood 78:21a, 1991

145. Weisdorf D, Katsanis E, Verfaillie C et al: Interleukin-1 alpha after autologous transplantation for lymphoma/Hodgkin's disease: clinical and hematologic effects. Blood 80:1321a, 1992

146. Walsh C, Liu J, Anderson S et al: A trial of recombinant human interleukin-1 in patients with severe refractory aplastic anemia. Br J Haematol 80:106, 1992

147. Kasakura S, Lowenstein L: A factor stimulating DNA synthesis derived from the medium of leucocyte cultures. Nature 208:794, 1965

148. Nossal GJB: The basic components of the immune system. N Engl J Med 316:1320, 1987

149. Horak ID, Gress RE, Lucas PJ et al: T-lymphocyte interleukin 2-dependent

tyrosine protein kinase signal transduction involves the activation of p^{56lck}. Proc Natl Acad Sci USA 88:1996, 1991

150. Bazan JF: Unraveling the structure of IL-2. Science 257:410, 1992

151. Takeshita T, Asao H, Ohtani K et al: Cloning of the γ chain of the human IL-2 receptor. Science 257:379, 1992

152. Hatakeyama M, Tsudo M, Minamoto S et al: Interleukin-2 receptor β chain gene: generation of three receptor forms by cloned human α and β chain cDNA's. Science 244:551, 1989

153. Grimm EA, Mazumder A, Zhang HZ et al: The lymphokine activated killer cell phenomenon: lysis of NK resistant fresh solid tumor cells by IL-2 activated autologous human peripheral blood lymphocytes. J Exp Med 155:1823, 1982

154. Philips JH, Lanier LL: Dissection of the lymphokine activated killer phenomenon. Relative contribution of peripheral blood natural killer cells and T lymphocytes to cytolysis. J Exp Med 164:814, 1986

155. Lotze MT, Grimm EA, Mazumder A et al: Lysis of fresh and cultured autologous tumor by human lymphocytes cultures in T-cell growth factor. Cancer Res 41:4420, 1981

156. Gemlo BT, Palladino MA, Jaffe HS et al: Circulating cytokines in patients with metastatic cancer treated with recombinant Interleukin-2 and lymphokine-activated killer cells. Cancer Res 48:5864, 1988

157. Rubin LA, Nelson DL: The soluble interleukin-2 receptor: biology, function and clinical application. Ann Intern Med 113:619, 1990

158. Steis RG, Marcon L, Clark J et al: Serum soluble IL-2 receptor as a tumor marker in patients with hairy cell leukemia. Blood 71:1304, 1988

159. Rosenberg SA: Adoptive immunotherapy of cancer using lymphokine activated killer cells and recombinant interleukin-2. In DeVita VT, Hellman S, Rosenberg SA (eds): Important Advances in Oncology. JB Lippincott, Philadelphia, 1986

160. Rosenberg SA, Lotz MT, Muul LM et al: A progress report on the treatment of 157 patients with advanced cancer using lymphokine-activated killer cells and interleukin-2 or high dose interleukin-2 alone. N Engl J Med 316:889, 1987

161. Lotze MT, Chang AR, Seipp CA et al: High-dose recombinant interleukin 2 in the treatment of patients with disseminated cancer: responses, treatment-related morbidity, and histologic findings. JAMA 256:3117, 1986

162. West WH, Tauer KW, Yanelli JR et al: Constant-infusion recombinant interleukin-2 in adoptive immunotherapy of advanced cancer. N Engl J Med 316:898, 1987

163. Dutcher JP, Creekmore S, Weiss GR et al: A phase II study of interleukin-2 and lymphokine activated killer cells in patients with metastatic malignant melanoma. J Clin Oncol 7:477, 1989

164. McCabe MS, Stablein D, Hawkins MJ: The modified group C experience-phase III randomized trials of IL-2 vs. IL-2/LAK in advanced renal cell carcinoma and advanced melanoma. Proc ASCO 10:714a, 1991

165. Margolin KA, Rayner AA, Hawkins MJ et al: Interleukin-2 and lymphokine-activated killer cell therapy of solid tumors: analysis of toxicity and management guidelines. J Clin Oncol 7:486, 1989

166. Ettinghausen SE, Moore JG, White DE et al: Hematologic effects of immunotherapy with lymphokine-activated killer cells and recombinant interleukin-2 in cancer patients. Blood 69:1654, 1987

167. Allison MAK, Jones SE, McGuffey P: Phase II trial of outpatient interleukin-2 in malignant lymphoma, chronic lymphocytic leukemia, and selected solid tumors. J Clin Oncol 7:75, 1989

168. Duggan DB, Santarelli MR, Zamkoff K et al: A phase II study of recombinant interleukin-2 with or without recombinant interferon-β in non-Hodgkin's lymphoma. A study of the Cancer and Leukemia Group. J Immunother 12:115, 1992

169. Bosly A, Guillaume T, Brice P et al: Effects of escalating doses of recombinant human interleukin-2 in correcting functional T-cell defects following ABMT for lymphoma and solid tumors. Exp Hematol 20:968, 1992

170. Blaise D, Olive A, Stoppa et al: Hematologic and immunologic effects of systemic administration of recombinant IL-2 after autologous bone marrow transplant. Blood 76:1092, 1990

171. Armitage RJ, Goldstone AH, Richards JDM et al: Lymphocyte function after autologous bone marrow transplantation (BMT): a comparison with patients treated with allogeneic BMT and with chemotherapy. Br J Haematol 63:637, 1986

172. Higuchi CM, Thompson JA, Cox T et al: Lymphokine-activated killer function following autologous bone marrow transplantation for refractory hematological malignancies. Cancer Res 49:5509, 1989

173. Higuchi CM, Thompson JA, Petersen FB et al: Toxicity and immunomodulatory effects of interleukin-2 after autologous bone marrow transplantation for hematologic malignancies. Blood 77:2561, 1991

174. Soiffer RJ, Murray C, Cochran K et al: Clinical and immunologic effects of prolonged infusion of low-dose recombinant interleukin-2 after autologous

175. Rosenberg SA: The immunotherapy and gene therapy of cancer. J Clin Oncol 10:180, 1992

176. Kilbourn R, Owen-Schaub L, Griffith O et al: Interleukin-2 mediated hypotension in dogs is reversed by N^G-Methyl-L-Arginine (NMA), an inhibitor of nitric oxide formation. Proc AACR 33:1958, 1992

177. Thompson JA, Bianco J, Benyunesm et al: Pentoxifylline and ciprofloxacin reduce the toxicity of high dose continuous infusion IL-2 and LAK cell therapy. Proc ASCO 12:946a, 1993

178. Smith KA: Lowest dose interleukin-2 immunotherapy. Blood 81:1414, 1993

179. Lopez A, To L, Yang Y-C et al: Stimulation of proliferation, differentiation, and function of human cells by primate interleukin 3. Proc Natl Acad Sci USA 84:2761, 1987

180. Bot F, van Eijk L, Schipper P, Lowenberg B: Effects of human interleukin-3 on granulocytic colony-forming cells in human bone marrow. Blood 73:1157, 1989

181. D'Hondt V, Weynants P, Humblet Y et al: Dose-dependent interleukin-3 stimulation of thrombopoiesis and neutropoiesis in patients with small cell lung carcinoma before and after chemotherapy: a placebo controlled randomized phase Ib study. J Clin Oncol 11:2063, 1993

182. Lindemann A, Ganser A, Herrmann F et al: Biologic effects of recombinant human interleukin-3 in vivo. Blood 9:2120, 1991

183. Bhatia A, Olencki T, Murthy S et al: Phase IA/IB trial of rhIL-3 in patients with refractory malignancies: hematologic and immunologic effects. Blood 80:1632a, 1992

184. Ottmann O, Ganser A, Seipelt G et al: Effects of recombinant human interleukin-3 on human hematopoietic progenitor and precursor cells in vivo. Blood 76:1494, 1990

185. Biesma B, Willemse P, Mulder N et al: Effects of interleukin-3 after chemotherapy for advanced ovarian cancer. Blood 80:1141, 1992

186. Demetri G, Young D, Merica E et al: Clinical effects of interleukin-3 (IL-3) in patients with advanced sarcomas: a phase I/II trial. Blood 78:12a, 1991

187. Postmus P, Gietema J, Damsma O et al: Effects of recombinant human interleukin-3 in patients with relapsed small-cell cancer treated with chemotherapy: a dose-finding study. J Clin Oncol 10:1131, 1992

188. Stahl C, Winton E, Monroe M et al: Differential effects of sequential, simultaneous, and single agent interleukin-3 and granulocyte-macrophage colony-stimulating factor on megakaryocyte maturation and platelet response in primates. Blood 80:2479, 1992

189. Brugger W, Frisch J, Schulz G et al: Sequential administration of interleukin-3 and granulocyte-macrophage colony-stimulating factor following standard-dose combination chemotherapy with etoposide, ifosfamide, and cisplatin. J Clin Oncol 10:1452, 1992

190. Hovgaard D, Nissen N: Interleukin-3 as monotherapy and combinations of IL-3/GM-CSF and IL-3/G-CSF in non-Hodgkin's lymphoma. Proc ASCO 12:1268a, 1993

191. Bretti S, Kamthan A, Hicks F et al: Phase I study of sequential IL-3 and GM-CSF by continuous intravenous infusion. Proc ASCO 11:537a, 1992

192. Tepler I, Hamm J, Shulman L et al: Combination cytokine therapy with recombinant human interleukin-3 and granulocyte colony-stimulating factor after "ICE" chemotherapy for lung cancer: sequential and simultaneous schedules. Proc ASCO 12:1110a, 1993

193. Nemunaitis J, Buckner C, Appelbaum F et al: Phase I trial with recombinant human interleukin-3 in patients with lymphoid cancer undergoing autologous bone marrow transplantation. Blood 80:331a, 1992

194. Peters W, Hussein A, Kurtzberg J et al: Use of recombinant human interleukin-3 in patients with metastatic breast cancer receiving high-dose chemotherapy and chemo-immunologically purged bone marrow transplantation. Blood 78:640a, 1991

195. Fay J, Bernstein S, Herzig R et al: A phase I study of sequential rhIL-3 and rhGM-CSF following autologous bone marrow transplantation therapy for lymphoma. Blood 80:334a, 1992

196. Wolff S, Ahmed T, Schuster M et al: Simultaneous rhIL-3 and rhG-CSF post autologous bone marrow transplantation (ABMT) for lymphoma: a phase I study. Proc ASCO 12:1555a, 1993

197. Gupton C, Rabinowitz J, Petros W et al: Interleukin-3 therapy suppresses endogenous cytokine concentrations following high-dose chemotherapy and autologous bone marrow transplantation. Blood 80:332a, 1992

198. Geissler K, Valent P, Mayer P et al: Recombinant human interleukin-3 expands the pool of circulating hematopoietic progenitor cells in primates—synergism with recombinant human granulocyte/macrophage colony-stimulating factor. Blood 75:2305, 1990

199. Wheeler C, Guinan E, Sieff C et al: Interleukin-3 before marrow harvest and GM-CSF post-autotransplant in patients with relapsed lymphoma: no enhancement of hematopoietic recovery. Blood 80:330a, 1992

200. Bregni M, Siena S, Di Nicola M et al: Circulation of hematopoietic progenitors in the peripheral blood of breast cancer patients treated with high-dose cyclophosphamide and recombinant human interleukin-3. Proc ASCO 11: 1333a, 1992

201. D'Hondt V, Guillaume T, Humblet Y et al: Tolerance and therapeutic effectiveness of sequential or simultaneous administration of IL-3 and G-CSF in improving peripheral blood stem cells harvesting following multi-agent chemotherapy. Proc ASCO 12:1564a, 1993

202. Brach M, Klein H, Platzer E et al: Effect of interleukin-3 on cytosine arabinoside-mediated cytotoxicity of leukemic myeloblasts. Exp Hematol 18:748, 1990

203. Andreef M, Drach J, Tafuri A et al: Interleukin-3 before and during idarubicin/ara-C in acute myeloblastic leukemia: phase I clinical and laboratory study. Blood 80:435a, 1992

204. Ganser A, Seipelt G, Lindemann A et al: Effects of human recombinant interleukin-3 in patients with myelodysplastic syndromes. Blood 76:455, 1990

205. Nimer S, Paquette R, Ireland P et al: Interleukin-3 (IL-3) therapy for aplastic anemia and myelodysplastic syndromes. Blood 78:371a, 1991

206. Kurzrock R, Talpaz M, Estrov Z et al: Phase I study of recombinant human interleukin-3 in patients with bone marrow failure. J Clin Oncol 9:1241, 1991

207. Bernstein S, Gilliland D, Aster J et al: A randomized trial of two doses of recombinant human interleukin-3 in patients with myelodysplastic syndrome. Blood 80:1631a, 1992

208. Gillio A, Castro-Malaspina H, Gasparetto C et al: Human recombinant interleukin-3 treatment in patients with myelodysplastic syndrome and aplastic anemia. Blood 78:372a, 1991

209. Ganser A, Lindemann A, Seipelt G et al: Effects of recombinant human interleukin-3 in aplastic anemia. Blood 76:1287, 1990

210. Guinan E, Nathan D, Lee Y et al: Phase I/II trial of recombinant human interleukin-3 (IL-3) and granulocyte-macrophage colony-stimulating factor (GM-CSF) in patients with amegakaryocytic thrombocytopenia (AMT). Blood 78:9a, 1991

211. Scadden D, Levine J, Hammer S et al: Recombinant human interleukin-3 for cytopenia in AIDS: a phase I study. Blood 80:2050a, 1992

212. Paul WE, Ohara J: B-cell stimulatory factor-1/interleukin 4. Annu Rev Immunol 5:429, 1987

213. Spits H, Yssel H, Takebe Y et al: Recombinant interleukin 4 promotes the growth of human T cells. J Immunol 139:1142, 1987

214. Hu-Li J, Shevach EM, Mizuguchi et al: B-cell stimulatory factor-1 (interleukin-4) is a potent costimulant for normal resting T-lymphocytes. J Exp Med 165: 157, 1987

215. Howard M, Farrar J, Hilfiker M et al: Identification of a T-cell derived B-cell growth factor distinct from interleukin-2. J Exp Med 155:914, 1982

216. Claasen JL, Levine AD, Buckley RH: Recombinant human IL-4 induces IgE and IgG synthesis by normal and atopic donor mononuclear cells. J Immunol 144:2123, 1990

217. Kawakami Y, Rosenberg SA, Lotze MT: Interleukin-4 promotes the growth of tumor-infiltrating lymphocytes cytotoxic for human autologous melanoma. J Exp Med 168:2183, 1988

218. Ito K, Plastoucas CD, Balch CM: Autologous tumor-specific cytotoxic T lymphocytes in the infiltrate of human metastatic melanomas. Activation by interleukin 2 and autologous tumor cells, and involvement of the T-cell receptor. J Exp Med 168:1419, 1988

219. Te Velde AA, Huibens RJF, Heije K et al: Interleukin-4 (IL-4) inhibits secretion of IL-1β, TNF alpha, and IL-6 by human monocytes. Blood 76:1392, 1990

220. Larner AC, Petricoin EF, Nakagawa Y et al: IL-4 attenuates the transcriptional activation of both IFN-alpha and IFN-gamma-induced cellular gene expression in monocytes and monocytic cell lines. J Immuno 150:1944–50, 1993

221. Wong HL, Costa GL, Lotz MT, Wahl SM: Interleukin (IL) 4 differentially regulates monocyte IL-1 family gene expression and synthesis in vitro and in vivo. J Exp Med 177:7575, 1993

222. Sonada Y, Kuzuyama Y, Tanka S et al: Human Interleukin-4 inhibits proliferation of megakaryocyte progenitor cells in culture. Blood 81:624, 1993

223. Taylor CW, Grogan TM, Salmon SE: Effects of interleukin-4 on the in vitro growth of human lymphoid and plasma cell neoplasms. Blood 74:1114, 1990

224. Estrov Z, Markowitz AB, Jurzrock R et al: Suppression of chronic myelogenous leukemia colony growth by interleukin-4. Leukemia 7:214, 1993

225. Okabe M, Saiki I, Miyazaki T: Inhibitory anti-tumor effects of interleukin-4 on Philadelphia chromosome-positive acute lymphocytic leukemia and other hematopoietic malignancies. Leuk Lymphoma 8:57, 1992

226. Atkins MB, Vachino G, Tilg HJ et al: Phase I evaluation of thrice-daily intravenous bolus interleukin-4 in patients with refractory malignancy. J Clin Oncol 10:1802, 1992

227. Sanderson CJ, Warren DJ, Strath M: Identification of a lymphokine that stimulates eosinophillic differentiation in-vitro. J Exp Med 162:60, 1985

228. Yokota T, Coffman RL, Hagiwara H et al: Isolation and characterization of lymphokine cDNA clones encoding mouse and human IgA enhancing factor and eosinophil colony-stimulating factor activities: relationship to interleukin-5. Proc Natl Acad Sci USA 84:7388, 1987

229. Takatsu K, Kikuchi Y, Takahashi T et al: Interleukin 5, a T-cell derived B-cell differentiation factor also induces cytotoxic T lymphocytes. Proc Natl Acad Sci USA 84:4234, 1987

230. Hirano T, Yasukawa K, Harada H et al: Complementary DNA for a novel human interleukin (BSF-2) that induces B lymphocytes to produce immunoglobulin. Nature 324:73, 1986

231. Sehgal P, May L: Human interferon-B2. J Interferon Res 7:521, 1987

232. Gauldie J, Richards C, Harnish D et al: Interferon B2/B-cell stimulating factor 2 shares identity with monocyte-derived hepatocyte-stimulating factor and regulates the major acute phase protein response in liver cells. Proc Natl Acad Sci USA 84:7251, 1987

233. Nordan R, Pumphrey J, Rudikoff S: Purification and NH2-sequence of a plasmacytoma growth factor derived from the murine macrophage cell line P388D1. J Immunol 139:813, 1987

234. Kishimoto T, Ishizaka K: Regulation of antibody response in vitro. VII. Enhancing soluble factors for IgG and IgE antibody response. J Immunol 111: 1194, 1973

235. Shabo Y, Lotem J, Sachs L: Target cell specificity of hematopoietic regulatory proteins for different clones of myeloid leukemic cells: two regulators secreted by Krebs carcinoma cells. Int J Cancer 41:622, 1988

236. Tovey M, Gresser I, Blanchard B, Guymarho J: Expression of IL-6 in normal individuals and in patients with autoimmune disease. Ann NY Acad Sci 557: 363, 1989

237. Lemay L, Otterness I, Vander A, Kluger M: In vivo evidence that the rise in plasma IL-6 following injection of a fever-inducing dose of LPS is mediated by IL-1B. Cytokine 2:199, 1990

238. Sheron N, Lau J, Hofman J et al: Dose-dependent increase in plasma interleukin-6 after recombinant tumor necrosis factor infusion in humans. Clin Exp Immunol 82:427, 1990

239. Hack C, DeGroot E, Felt-Bersma J et al: Increased plasma levels if interleukin-6 in sepsis. Blood 74:1704, 1989

240. Bruno E, Hoffman R: Effect of interleukin 6 on in vitro human megakaryocytopoiesis: its interactions with other cytokines. Exp Hematol 17:1038, 1989

241. Mei R-L, Burstein S: Megakaryocytic maturation in murine long-term bone marrow culture: role of interleukin-6. Blood 78:1438, 1991

242. Suda T, Yamaguchi Y, Suda J et al: Effect of interleukin-6 on the differentiation and proliferation of murine and human hematopoietic progenitors. Exp Hematol 16:891, 1988

243. Wong G, Clark S, Ikebuchi K, Ogawa M: Stimulation of murine hemopoietic colony formation by human IL-6. J Immunol 140:3040, 1988

244. Koike K: Synergism of BSF-2/interleukin-6 and interleukin-3 on development of multipotential hemopoietic progenitors in serum-free culture. J Exp Med 168:879, 1988

245. Gardner J, Liechty K, Christensen R: Effects of interleukin-6 on fetal hematopoietic progenitors. Blood 75:2150, 1990

246. Koike K, Nakahata T, Kubo T et al: Interleukin-6 enhances murine megakaryocytopoiesis in serum-free culture. Blood 75:2286, 1990

247. Long M, Hutchinson R, Gragowski L et al: Synergistic regulation of human megakaryocyte development. J Clin Invest 82:1779, 1988

248. Migliaccio G, Migliaccio A, Adamson J: In vitro differentiation and proliferation of human hematopoietic progenitors: the effects of interleukins 1 and 6 are indirectly mediated by production of granulocyte-macrophage colony-stimulating factor and interleukin 3. Exp Hematol 19:3, 1991

249. Quesenberry P, McGrath H, Williams M et al: Multifactor stimulation of megakaryocytopoiesis: effects of interleukin 6. Exp Hematol 19:35, 1991

250. Hill R, Warren M, Levin J: Stimulation of thrombopoiesis in mice by human recombinant interleukin 6. J Clin Invest 85:1242, 1990

251. Asano S, Okano A, Ozawa K et al: In vivo effects of recombinant human interleukin-6 in primates: stimulated production of platelets. Blood 75:1602, 1990

252. Pojda Z, Tsuboi A: In vivo effects of human recombinant interleukin 6 on hemopoietic stem and progenitor cells and circulating blood cells in normal mice. Exp Hematol 18:1034, 1990

253. Samuels B, Bukowski R, Gordon M et al: Phase I study of rhIL-6 with chemotherapy in advanced sarcoma. Proc ASCO 12:948a, 1993

254. Chang A, Boros L, Asbury R et al: Effects of interleukin-6 in cancer patients treated with ifosfamide, carboplatin, and etoposide. Proc ASCO 12:936a, 1993

255. Gordon M, Nemunaitis J, Hoffman R et al: Phase I trial of subcutaneous recombinant human interleukin-6 in patients with myelodysplasia and thrombocytopenia. Blood 80:986a, 1992

256. Takai Y, Wong G, Clark S et al: B cell stimulatory factor-2 is involved in the differentiation of cytotoxic T lymphocytes. J Immunol 140:508, 1988

257. Le J, Fredrickson G, Reis L et al: Interleukin 2-dependent and interleukin 2-independent pathways of regulation of thymocyte function by interleukin-6. Proc Natl Acad Sci USA 85:8643, 1988

258. Mule J, McIntosh J, Jablons D et al: Cellular mechanisms of the antitumor activity of recombinant human IL-6 in mice. J Immunol 148:2622, 1992

259. Weber J: Interleukin-6: Multifunctional cytokine. In DeVita VT, Hellman S, Rosenberg SA (eds): Biologic Therapy of Cancer Updates. JB Lippincott, Philadelphia, 1993

260. Olencki T, Budd GT, Murthy S et al: Immunoregulatory and hematopoietic effects of interleukin-6 in cancer patients. Proc ASCO 12:950a, 1993

261. Klein B, Wijdenes J, Zhang X-G et al: Murine anti-interleukin-6 monoclonal antibody therapy for a patient with plasma cell leukemia. Blood 78:1198, 1991

262. Paul SR, Bennett F, Calvetti JA et al: Molecular cloning of a cDNA encoding interleukin 11, a stromal cell-derived lymphopoietic and hematopoietic cytokine. Proc Natl Acad Sci USA 87:7512, 1990

263. Yin T, Yang Y-C: Interleukin-11 induces protein tyrosine phosphorylation and TIS11, and JUNB early response gene expression in H-35 hepatoma cells. Blood 80:351a, 1992

264. Du XX, Neben T, Goldman S et al: Effects of recombinant human interleukin-11 on hematopoietic reconstitution in transplant mice: acceleration of recovery of peripheral blood neutrophils and platelets. Blood 81:27, 1993

265. Kawashima I, Ohsumi J, Mita-Honjo K et al: Molecular cloning of cDNA encoding adipogenesis inhibitory factor and identity with interleukin-11. FEBS Lett 283:199, 1991

266. Keller D, Du XX, Srour E et al: Interleukin-11 inhibits adipogenesis and stimulates myelopoiesis in human long-term marrow cultures. Blood 82:1428, 1993

267. Gordon MS, Sledge GW Jr, Battiato L et al: The in vivo effects of subcutaneously administered recombinant human interleukin-11 (NEUMEGA™ rhIL-11 growth factor; rhIL-11) in women with breast cancer. Blood 82:1976a, 1993

268. Gordon MS, Battiato L, Hoffman R et al: Subcutaneously administered recombinant human interleukin-11 (NEUMEGA™ rhIL-11 growth factor; rhIL-11) prevents thrombocytopenia following chemotherapy with cyclophosphamide and doxorubicin in women with breast cancer. Blood 82:1258a, 1993

269. Orazi A, Cooper R, Tong J et al: Recombinant human interleukin-11 (NEUMEGA™ rhIL-11 growth factor; rhIL-11) has profound effects on human hematopoiesis. Blood 82:1460, 1993

270. Schoenhaut D, Chua A, Wolitzky A et al: Cloning and expression of murine IL-12. J Immunol 148:3433, 1992

271. Wolf S, Temple P, Kobayashi M et al: Cloning of cDNA for natural-killer-cell stimulatory factor, a heterodimeric cytokine with multiple biologic effects on T-cells and natural-killer cells. J Immunol 146:3074, 1991

272. Robertson M, Soiffer R, Wolf S et al: Response of human natural killer (NK) cells to NK cell stimulatory factor (NKSF): cytolytic activity and proliferation of NK cells are differentially regulated by NKSF. J Exp Med 175:779, 1992

273. Lieberman M, Sigal R, Williams N II et al: Natural killer cell stimulatory factor (NKSF) augments natural killer cell and antibody-dependent tumoricidal response against colon carcinoma cell lines. J Surg Res 50:410, 1991

274. Bertagnolli M, Lin B-Y, Young D et al: IL-12 augments antigen-dependent proliferation of activated T lymphocytes. J Immunol 149:3778, 1992

275. Gately M, Desai B, Wolitzky A et al: Regulation of human lymphocyte proliferation by a heterodimeric cytokine, IL-12 (cytotoxic lymphocyte maturation factor). J Immunol 147:874, 1991

276. Kobayashi M, Fitz L, Ryan M et al: Identification and purification of natural killer stimulatory factor (NKSF), a cytokine with multiple biologic effects on human lymphocytes. J Exp Med 170:827, 1989

277. Li L, Young D, Wolf S et al: Recombinant human natural-killer cell stimulatory factor stimulates B-cell growth by inducing IFN-gamma in B-cells. J Cell Biochem S17B:112, 1993

278. Stern A, Podlaski F, Hulmes J et al: Purification to homogeneity and partial characterization of cytotoxic lymphocyte maturation factor from human B-lymphoblastoid cells. Proc Natl Acad Sci USA 87:6808, 1991

279. Soiffer R, Robertson M, Murray C et al: Interleukin-12 augments cytolytic activity of peripheral blood lymphocytes from patients with hematologic and solid malignancies. Blood 82:2790, 1993

280. Chehimi J, Starr S, Frank I et al: Natural killer (NK) stimulatory factor increases the cytotoxic activity of NK cells from both healthy donors and human immunodeficiency virus-infected patients. J Exp Med 175:789, 1992

281. Weber JS, Jay G, Tamaka K et al: Immunotherapy of a murine tumor with interleukin-2: an increased sensitivity after MHC class I gene transfection. J Exp Med 166:1716, 1987

282. Currie GA: Eighty years of immunotherapy: a review of immunological methods in the treatment of cancer. Int J Cancer 26:141, 1972

283. Kessler DS, Levy DE, Darnell JE Jr: Two interferon-induced nuclear factors bind a single promoter element in interferon-stimulated genes. Proc Natl Acad Sci USA 85:8521, 1988

284. Diaz MO, Ziemin S, LeBeau MM et al: Homozygous deletion of the a and b-interferon genes in human leukemia and derived cell lines. Proc Natl Acad Sci USA 85:8521, 1988

285. Quesada JR, Reuben J, Manning JT et al: α interferon for induction of remission in hairy cell leukemia. N Engl J Med 310:15, 1984

286. Leavitt RD, Ratanatharathorn V, Ozer H et al: α-2b Interferon in the treatment of Hodgkin's disease and non-Hodgkin's lymphoma. Semin Oncol 14:18, 1987

287. Horning SJ, Merigan TC, Krown SE et al: Human interferon α in malignant lymphoma and Hodgkin's disease. Cancer 56:1310, 1985

288. Talpaz M, Kantarjian HM, McCredie K et al: Hematologic remission and cytogenetic improvement induced by recombinant human interferon alpha in chronic myelogenous leukemia. N Engl J Med 314:1065, 1986

289. Silver RT, Benn F, Verma SA et al: Recombinant gamma-interferon has activity in chronic myeloid leukemia. J Clin Oncol 13:49, 1990

290. Kurzrock R, Talpaz M, Kantarjian H et al: Therapy of chronic myelogeneous leukemia with recombinant interferon-gamma. Blood 70:943, 1987

291. Silver R: Interferon in the treatment of myeloproliferative diseases. Semin Hematol 27:6, 1990

292. Gilvert HS: Persistence of remission of myeloid metaplasia after treatment with recombinant interferon alpha-2b, abstracted. Blood 72:200a, 1988

293. Giles FJ, Singer CRJ, Gray AG et al: Alpha-interferon therapy for essential thrombocythaemia. Lancet 2:70, 1988

294. Velu T, Delwiche F, Gangi D et al: Therapeutic effect of human recombinant interferon alpha-2a in essential thrombocythaemia. Oncology 42:10, 1985

295. Gisslinger H, Ludwig H, Linksech W et al: Long-term interferon therapy for thrombocytosis in myeloproliferative diseases. Lancet 1:634, 1989

296. Alimena G, Morra E, Lazzarino M et al: Interferon alpha-2b as therapy for Ph-positive chronic myelogenous leukemia: a study of 82 patients treated with intermittent or daily administration. Blood 72:642, 1988

297. Ozer H, Dear K, Testa J et al: Prolonged administration of subcutaneous α interferon induces major clinical and complete cytogenetic remissions in untreated Philadelphia chromosome positive (Ph+) chronic myelogenous leukemia (CML), abstracted. Proc Am Soc Clin Oncol 9:783, 1990

298. Lee MS, LeMaistre A, Kantarjian HM et al: Detection of two alternative bcr/abl mRNA junctions and minimal residual disease in Philadelphia positive chronic myelogenous leukemia by polymerase chain reaction. Blood 73:2165, 1989

299. Ozer H, George S, Pettenati M et al: Subcutaneous α-interferon (αIFN) in untreated chronic phase Philadelphia chromosome positive (Ph+) chronic myelogenous leukemia (CML): no evidence for significant improvement in response duration or survival (CALGB 8583). Blood, suppl. 1. 80:358a, 1992

300. Zuffa E, Italian Cooperative Study Group on Chronic Myeloid Leukemia: A prospective study of interferon alpha-2A versus chemotherapy in chronic myeloid leukemia (CML): karyotypic response and survival. ASCO Proc 12:980a, 1993

301. Golomb HM, Ratain MJ, Mick R et al: Interferon treatment for hairy cell leukemia: an update on a cohort of 69 patients treated from 1983–1986. Leukemia 6:1177, 1992

302. Quesada JR, Hersh EM, Manning JT et al: Treatment of hairy cell leukemia with recombinant α interferon. Blood 68:493, 1986

303. Steis RG, Smith JW, Urba WJ et al: Resistance to recombinant interferon alfa-2a and hairy-cell leukemia associated with neutralizing anti-interferon antibodies. N Engl J Med 22:1409, 1988

304. Vedantham S, Gamliel H, Golomb H et al: Mechanism of interferon action in hairy cell leukemia: a model of effective cancer biotherapy. Cancer Res 52:1056, 1992

305. Werner D, Porzsolt F, Schmid M et al: High levels of circulating soluble receptors for tumor necrosis factor in hairy cell leukemia and type B chronic lymphocytic leukemia. Am Soc Clinic Invest 89:1690, 1992

306. Wagstaff J, Loynds P, Scarffe JH: Phase II study of rDNA human α-2 interferon in multiple myeloma. Cancer Treat Rep 69:495, 1985

307. Costanzi JJ, Cooper MR, Scarffe JH et al: Phase II study of recombinant α-2 interferon in resistant multiple myeloma. J Clin Oncol 3:654, 1985

308. Salmon SE, Crowley J, for the Southwest Oncology Group (SWOG): Impact of glucocorticoids (GC) and interferon (IFN) on outcome in multiple myeloma. Proc Am Soc Clin Oncol 11:316, 1992

309. Quesada JR, Alexanian R, Hawkins M et al: Treatment of multiple myeloma with recombinant interferon. Blood 67:275, 1986

310. Mandelli F, Avvisati G, Amadori S et al: Maintenance treatment with recombinant interferon alfa-2b in patients with multiple myeloma responding to conventional induction chemotherapy. N Engl J Med 322:1430, 1990

311. Foon KA, Sherwin SA, Abrams PG: Treatment of advanced non-Hodgkin's

lymphoma with recombinant leukocyte A interferon. N Engl J Med 311:1148, 1984

312. Smalley RV, Andersen JW, Hawkins MJ et al: Interferon alfa combined with cytotoxic chemotherapy for patients with non-Hodgkin's lymphoma. N Engl J Med 327:1336, 1992

313. Solal-Celigny Ph, Lepage E, Brousse N et al: Alpha-interferon and chemotherapy in patients with high-tumor burden follicular lymphoma—preliminary results of the "groupe d'étude des lymphomes folliculaires." Proc ASCO 10: 955a, 1991

314. Price CGA, Rohatiner AZS, Steward W et al: Interferon-α_{2b} in the treatment of follicular lymphoma: preliminary results of a trial in progress. Ann Oncol, suppl. 2. 2:141, 1991

315. O'Connell, Colgan MJ, Oken JP et al: Clinical trial of recombinant leukocyte A interferon as initial therapy for favorable histology non-Hodgkin's lymphomas and chronic lymphocytic leukemia. An Eastern Cooperative Oncology Group pilot study. J Clin Oncol 4:128, 1986

316. Rosenblum MG, Donato NJ: Tumor necrosis factor alpha: a multifaceted peptide hormone. CRC Crit Rev Immunol 9:21, 1989

317. Aggarwal BB, Kohr WJ, Hass PE et al: Human tumor necrosis factor: production, purification and characterization. J Biol Chem 260:2345, 1985

318. Aggarwal BB, Eessalu TE, Hass PE: Characterization of receptors for human tumor necrosis factor and their regulation by γ-interferon. Nature 318:665, 1985

319. Frei E III, Spriggs D: Tumor Necrosis Factor: still a promising agent. J Clin Oncol 7:291, 1989

320. Sugarman BJ, Aggarwal BB, Hass PE et al: Recombinant tumor necrosis factor-alpha: Effects on proliferation of normal and transformed cells in vitro. Science 230:943, 1985

321. Beutler B, Cerami A: Cachectin and tumor necrosis factor as two sides of the same biological coin. Nature 320:584, 1986

322. Nawroth PP, Stern DM: Modulation of endothelial cell hemostatic properties by tumor necrosis factor. J Exp Med 163:740, 1986

323. Bevilacqua MP, Pober JS, Majeau GR et al: Recombinant tumor necrosis factor induces procoagulant activity in cultured human vascular endothelium: characterization and comparison with the actions of interleukin 1. Proc Natl Acad Sci USA 83:4533, 1986

324. Silverman P, Goldsmith GH, Spitzer TR et al: Effect of tumor necrosis factor on the human fibrinolytic system. J Clin Oncol 8:468, 1990

325. Beutler B, Cerami A: The biology of cachectin/TNF. A primary mediator of the host response. Annu Rev Immunol 7:625, 1989

326. Van Der Poll T, Buller HR, Ten Cate H et al: Activation of coagulation after administration of tumor necrosis factor to normal subjects. N Engl J Med 433:1622, 1990

327. Mier JW, Vachino G, van Der Meer JWM et al: Induction of circulating tumor necrosis factor (TNFα) as the mechanism for the febrile response to interleukin-2 (IL-2) in cancer patients. J Clin Immunol 8:426, 1988

328. Spriggs DR, Sherman ML, Michie H et al: Recombinant human tumor necrosis factor administered as a 24 hour intravenous infusion. A phase I and pharmacologic study. J Natl Cancer Inst 80:1039, 1988

329. Feinberg B, Kurzrock R, Talpaz M et al: A phase I trial of intravenously administered recombinant tumor necrosis factor alpha in cancer patients. J Clin Oncol 6:1328, 1988

330. Jakubowski AA, Casper ES, Gabrilove JL et al: Phase I trial of intramuscularly administered tumor necrosis factor in patients with advanced cancer. J Clin Oncol 7:298, 1989

331. Rosenberg SA, Aebersold P, Cornetta K et al: Gene transfer into humans: immunology of patients with advanced melanoma using tumor-infiltrating lymphocytes modified by retroviral gene transduction. N Engl J Med 323: 570, 1990

332. Bajorin D, Cheung N-K, Houghton A: Macrophage colony-stimulating factor: biological effects and potential applications for cancer therapy. Sem Hematol 28:42, 1991

333. Chikkappa G, Broxmeyer H, Cooper S et al: Effect in vivo of multiple injections of purified murine and recombinant human macrophage colony-stimulating factor to mice. Cancer Res 49:3558, 1989

334. Sanda M, Bolton E, Mule J, Rosenberg S: In vivo administration of recombinant macrophage colony-stimulating factor induces macrophage-mediated antibody-dependent cytotoxicity of tumor cells. J Immunother 12:132, 1992

335. Munn D, Garnick M, Cheung N-K: Effects of parenteral recombinant macrophage colony-stimulating factor on monocyte number, phenotype and antitumor cytotoxicity in non-human primates. Blood 75:2042, 1990

336. Bajorin D, Jakubowski A, Cody B et al: Recombinant macrophage colony-stimulating factor (rhM-CSF): a phase I trial in patients with metastatic melanoma. Proc ASCO 9:707a, 1990

337. Zamkoff KW, Hudson ES, Childs A et al: A phase I trial of human macrophage colony-stimulating factor by rapid intravenous infusion in patients with refractory malignancy. J Immunother 11:103, 1992

338. Sanda MG, Yang JC, Topalian SL et al: Intravenous administration of recombinant human macrophage colony-stimulating factor to patients with metastatic cancer: a phase I study. J Clin Oncol 10:1643, 1992

339. Weiner L, Li W, Catalano R et al: Phase I trial of recombinant macrophage-colony stimulating factor (M-CSF) and recombinant gamma-interferon: peripheral blood mononuclear cell phagocyte proliferation and differentiation. Proc ASCO 12:947a, 1993

340. Masaoka T, Shibata H, Ohno R et al: Double-blind test of human urinary macrophage colony-stimulating factor for allogeneic and syngeneic bone marrow transplantation: effectiveness of treatment and 2-year follow-up for relapse of leukemia. Br J Haematol 76:501, 1990

341. Khwaja A, Yong K, Jones H et al: The effect of macrophage colony-stimulating factor on haematopoietic recovery after autologous bone marrow transplantation. Br J Haematol 81:288, 1992

342. Hume D, Pavli P, Donahue R et al: The effect of human recombinant macrophage colony-stimulating factor (CSF-1) on the murine mononuclear phagocyte system in vivo. J Immunol 141:3405, 1988

343. Nemunaitis J, Meyers J, Buckner C et al: Phase I trial of recombinant human macrophage colony-stimulating factor in patients with invasive fungal infections. Blood 78:907, 1991

344. Nemunaitis J, Shannon-Dorcy K, Appelbaum FR et al: Long-term follow-up of patients with invasive fungal disease who received adjunctive therapy with recombinant human macrophage colony-stimulating factor. Blood 82: 1422, 1993

345. Sorell M, Kapoor N, Kirkpatrick D et al: Marrow transplantation for juvenile osteopetrosis. Am J Med 70:1280, 1981

346. MacDonald B, Mundy G, Clark S et al: Effects on human recombinant CSF-GM and highly purified CSF-1 on the formation of multi-nucleated cells with osteclast characteristics in long-term bone marrow cultures. J Bone Miner Res 1:227, 1986

347. Burger E, van der Meer J, van de Gevel J et al: In vitro formation of osteoclasts from long-term cultures of bone marrow mononuclear phagocytes. J Exp Med 156:1604, 1982

348. Orchard P, Dahl N, Aukerman L et al: Circulating macrophage colony-stimulating factor is not reduced in malignant osteopetrosis. Exp Hematol 20:103, 1992

349. Wiktor-Jedrzejczak W, Bartocci A, Ferrante AJ et al: Total absence of colony-stimulating factor-1 in the macrophage deficient osteopetrotic (op/op) mouse. Proc Natl Acad Sci USA 87:4828, 1990

350. Wang W, Morris S, Vilmer E et al: Treatment of osteopetrosis with macrophage colony-stimulating factor (M-CSF). Blood 80:988a, 1992

351. Freedman AS, Pedrazzini, Nadler LM et al: B-cell monoclonal antibodies and their use in clinical oncology. Cancer Invest 9:69, 1991

352. Miller RA, Oseroff AR, Stratte PT, Levy R: Monoclonal antibody therapeutic trials in seven patients with T-cell lymphoma. Blood 62:988, 1983

353. Masui H, Kawamoto T, Sato JD et al: Growth inhibition of human tumor cells in athymic mice by anti-epidermal growth factor receptor monoclonal antibodies. Cancer Res 44:1002, 1984

354. Shawler D, Bartholomew R, Smith L, Dillman R: Human immune response to multiple injections of murine monoclonal IgG. J Immunol 135:1530, 1985

355. Schroff RW, Foon KA, Beatty SM et al: Human anti-murine immunoglobulin responses in patients receiving monoclonal antibody therapy. Cancer Res 45:879, 1985

356. Byers VS, Baldwin RW: Therapeutic strategies with monoclonal antibodies and immunoconjugates. Immunology 65:329, 1988

357. Liu AY, Robinson RR, Hellstrom KE et al: Chimeric mouse-human IgG1 antibody that can mediate lysis of cancer cells. Proc Natl Acad Sci USA 84:3439, 1987

358. FitzGerald D, Pastan I: Targeted toxin therapy for the treatment of cancer. J Natl Cancer Inst 81:1455, 1989

359. Vitetta ES, Uhr JW: Immunotoxin. Annu Rev Immunol 3:197, 1985

360. Olsnes S, Sandvig K: How protein toxins enter and kill cells. p. 39. In Frankel AE (ed): Immunotoxins. Kluwer-Academic Boston, 1988

361. Hertler AA, Frankel AE: Immunotoxins: a clinical review of their use in the treatment of malignancies. J Clin Oncol 7:1932, 1989

362. Bacha P, Williams DP, Waters C et al: Interleukin-2 receptor-targeted cytotoxicity: interleukin-2 receptor-mediated action of a diphteria toxin-related interleukin-2 fusion protein. J Exp Med 167:612, 1988

363. Freedman AS, Pedrazzini A, Nadler LM: B-cell monoclonal antibodies and their use in clinical oncology. Cancer Invest 9:69, 1991

364. Miller RA, Maloney DG, Warnke R, Levy R: Treatment of B cell lymphoma with monoclonal anti-idiotype antibody. N Engl J Med 306:517, 1982

365. Houghton AN, Scheinberg DA: Monoclonal antibodies: potential applications to the treatment of cancer. Semin Oncol 13:165, 1986

366. Foon KA: Biological response modifiers: the new immunotherapy. Cancer Res 49:1621, 1989
367. Uchiyama T, Nelson DL, Fleischer et al: A monoclonal antibody (anti-Tac) reactive with activated and functionally mature T-cells. J Immunol 126:1398, 1981
368. Waldmann T, White J, Goldman C et al: The IL-2 receptor: a target for monoclonal antibody treatment of human T-cell lymphotropic virus-1 induced adult T-cell leukemia. Blood 82:1701, 1993
369. Jansen J, Falkenburg JHF, Stepan DE et al: Removal of neoplastic cells from autologous bone marrow grafts with monoclonal antibodies. Semin Hematol 21:164, 1984
370. Lowder JN, Meeker TC, Levy R: Monoclonal antibody therapy of lymphoid malignancy. p. 359. In Hoppe R (ed): Cancer Surveys: Advances and Prospects in Clinical, Epidemiological and Laboratory Oncology. Vol 4: Recent Advances in the Treatment and Research in Lymphoma and Hodgkin's Disease. Oxford University Press, Oxford, 1985
371. Martin PJ, Hansen JA, Torok-Storb B et al: Effects of treating marrow with CD3-specific immunotoxin for prevention of acute graft-versus-host disease. Bone Marrow Transplantation 3:437, 1988
372. Filipovich AH, Vallera DA, Youle RJ et al: Graft-versus-host disease prevention in allogeneic bone marrow transplantation from histocompatible siblings. Transplantation 44:62, 1987
373. Waldmann H, Polliak A, Hale G et al: Elimination of graft-versus-host disease by in vitro depletion of alloreactive lymphocytes with a monoclonal rat anti-human lymphocyte antibody (CAMPATH-1). Lancet 2:483, 1984
374. Hale G, Clark MR, Marcuss R et al: Remission induction in non-Hodgkin's lymphoma with relapsed human monoclonal antibody CAMPATH-1H. Lancet 2:1394, 1988
375. Badger C, Krohn K, Shulman H et al: Experimental radioimmunotherapy of murine lymphoma with ^{131}I-labeled anti-T-cell antibodies. Cancer Res 46:6223, 1986
376. Press O, Badger C, Eary J et al: Radioimmunotherapy of refractory human malignant B cell lymphomas. Blood, suppl. 1. 70:2481, 1988
377. DeNardo S, DeNardo G, O'Grady L et al: Pilot studies of radioimmunotherapy of B cell lymphoma and leukemia using I-131 Lym-1 monoclonal antibody. Antibody Immunoconjugates Radiopharm 1:17, 1988
378. Carrasquillo JA, Bunn PA Jr, Keenan AM et al: Radioimmunodetection of cutaneous T-cell lymphoma with ^{111}In-labeled T101 monoclonal antibody. N Engl J Med 315:673, 1985
379. Kaminski M, Zasadny Z, Francis IR et al: Radioimmunotherapy of B-cell lymphoma with ^{131}I antiB1 (anti-CD20) antibody. N Engl J Med 329:459, 1993
380. Fauser AA, Shustik C, Langleben A et al: T-cell depletion with ricin A-chain T101 in allogeneic bone marrow transplantation to prevent severe graft-versus-host disease. Clin Invest Med 11:40, 1988
381. Vallera DA: Immunotoxins for ex vivo bone marrow purging in human bone marrow transplantation. p. 515. In Frankel AE (ed): Immunotoxins. Kluwer-Academic, Boston, 1988
382. LeMaistre DF, Kuzel T, Foss F: DAB$_{389}$IL-2 is well tolerated at doses inducing response in IL-2 receptor expressing lymphomas. Blood 82:532a, 1993

Appendix 62-1

Approved Agents

Trade name: Proleukin

Generic name: Interleukin-2

Other names: Aldesleukin

FDA status: Approved

Current approved indications: Indicated for adult patients with metastatic renal cell cancer

Investigational uses: Melanoma, bone marrow transplantation, hematologic malignancies

Dosing: 600,000 IU/kg administered IV over 15 minutes, q8h, for two 5-day treatment cycles

Toxicity: Fever, chills, hypotension, capillary leak syndrome, oliguria, pulmonary edema, anemia, elevated liver function studies, atrial and ventricular cardiac arrhythmias

Trade name: Actimmune

Generic name: Interferon-γ1B

Other names: None

FDA status: Approved, limited indication

Current approved indications: Reducing the frequency and severity of serious infections associated with chronic granulomatous disease

Investigational uses: Anticancer agent, immunomodulator

Dosing: 50 µg^2 for patients whose body surface area is >0.5 m^2 and 1.5 µg/kg/dose for patients whose body surface area is ≤0.5 m^2; injections should be administered subcutaneously three times weekly

Toxicity: Flu-like or constitutional symptoms such as headache, fever, chills, myalgias

Trade name: Roferon-A, Intron-A, Alferon N

Generic name: Interferon-α$_{2a}$, interferon-α$_{2b}$, human leukocyte derived (interferon-α$_{n3}$)

Other names: None

FDA status: Approved

Current approved indications: Indicated for use in hairy cell leukemia and AIDS-related Kaposi sarcoma; Alferon N approved for refractory or recurrent external condylomata accuminata.

Investigational uses: Malignant melanoma, hematologic malignancies, carcinoid

Dosing: Hairy cell leukemia—induction dose is 3 million IU/day for 16–24 weeks, administered as a subcutaneous or intramuscular injection; recommended maintenance dose is 3 million IU, three times per week; dose reduction by one-half or withholding of individual doses may be needed when severe adverse reactions occur; use of doses >3 million IU is not recommended in hairy cell leukemia
Kaposi sarcoma—recommended induction dose is 36 million IU/day for 10–12 weeks, administered as an intramuscular or subcutaneous injection; recommended maintenance dose is 36 million IU, three times per week; dose reduction by one-

half or withholding of individual doses may be required when severe adverse reactions occur

Condylomata accuminata—recommended doses of Alferon N injection (interferon-α_{n3}) for treatment is 0.05 ml (250,000 IU) per wart; Alferon N injection should be administered twice weekly for $\leq$8 weeks

Toxicity: Flu-like syndrome, fever, fatigue, chills, arthralgia, anorexia, and headache

Trade name: Neupogen

Generic name: Filgrastim

Other names: CSF-G

FDA status: Approved

Current approved indications: Chemotherapy-induced neutropenia

Investigational uses: HIV infection, bone marrow failure, primary neutropenic disorders, peripheral blood progenitor cell mobilization

Dosing: 5 μg/kg/day by subcutaneous injection or intravenous infusion; Check CBC twice per week; discontinue Neupogen when absolute neutrophil count >10,000 cells/μl

Toxicity: Elevation of serum chemistries (lactate dehydrogenase, leukocyte alkaline phosphatase), hair thinning, and splenomegaly (with chronic use), exacerbation of pre-existing vasculitis, bone pain

Trade name: Leukine, Prokine
Leukomax (investigational)

Generic name: Sargramostim

Other names: CSF-GM

FDA status: Approved

Current approved indications: High-dose chemotherapy with autologous bone marrow transplantation

Investigational uses: Chemotherapy-induced myelosuppression, bone marrow failure states, HIV infection

Dosing: 5 μg/kg/day administered by subcutaneous injection or intravenous infusion, continue therapy until neutrophil count has recovered; decrease dose by 50% if absolute neutrophil count >20,000 cells/μl; check CBC twice per week

Toxicity: Fever, chills, arthralgias, myalgias, pericarditis, pleuritis, "first-dose" effect, bone pain, fatigue, malaise

Trade name: Procrit, Epogen

Generic name: Erythropoietin

Other names: Not applicable

FDA status: Approved

Current approved indications: Anemia associated with chronic renal failure, chemotherapy-induced anemia, and anemia associated with HIV infection

Investigational uses: Anemia of prematurity, bone marrow failure states

Dosing: Chronic renal failure—starting doses 5–100 U/kg three times per week; dose is usually administered by intravenous bolus to patients on dialysis; dose may be increased at intervals of 25 U/kg three times per week until target hematocrit level is reached (36%); maintenance dosing can be either at a lower dose, or increased interval of therapy

HIV—before initiating therapy, check endogenous erythropoietin level, since most patients with erythropoietin levels >500 mU/ml will not respond to erythropoietin therapy; recommended starting dose for patients with erythropoietin levels <500 mU/ml and AZT doses <4200 mg/wk is 100 U/kg three times per week for 8 weeks; dose can be increased by 50–100 U/kg three times per week every 4–8 weeks and response monitored; erythropoietin therapy should be held when the hematocrit is >40% and resumed at 25% dose reduction when the hematocrit is <36%

Toxicity: Iron deficiency, hypertension, seizures, thrombotic events, headache, allergic reaction

Appendix 62-2

Investigational Agents

Name: Interleukin-1

FDA status: Investigational

Current approved indications: None

Investigational uses: Chemotherapy-induced myelosuppression, bone marrow transplantation, bone marrow failure states, antitumor agent

Dosing: To be established

Toxicity: Hypotension, hypertension, fevers, chills, rigors

Name: Interleukin-3

FDA status: Investigational

Current approved indications: None

Investigational uses: Chemotherapy-induced myelosuppression, bone marrow failure states, HIV infection, bone marrow transplantation, peripheral blood progenitor cell mobilization

Dosing: 2.5–5 μg/kg/day administered by subcutaneous injection

Toxicity: Fever, chills, arthralgias, myalgias, pericarditis, pleuritis, fatigue, malaise, rash, thromboembolic phenomena

Name: Interleukin-6

Other names: Sigosix (mammalian derived)

FDA status: Investigational

Current approved indications: None

Investigational uses: Chemotherapy-induced thrombocytopenia, bone marrow failure states, bone marrow transplantation, antitumor agent

Dosing: To be defined based on further clinical studies

Toxicity: Fever, chills, arthralgias, myalgias, fatigue, malaise

Name: Interleukin-11

Other names: Neumega

FDA status: Investigational

Current approved indications: None

Investigational uses: Chemotherapy-induced thrombocytopenia, bone marrow transplantation

Dosing: Administered subcutaneously, dosage to be defined by further studies

Toxicity: Fatigue, arthralgias, myalgias, malaise, rhinorrhea

Name: PIXY321 (interleukin-3/CSF-GM fusion protein)

FDA status: Investigational

Current approved indications: None

Investigational uses: Chemotherapy-induced myelosuppression, bone marrow failure states, bone marrow transplantation, peripheral blood progenitor cell mobilization

Dosing: $500–750$ µg/m^2/day administered by subcutaneous injection

Toxicity: Fever, chills, arthralgias, myalgias, injection site reaction, bone pain, fatigue, malaise

Name: Colony-stimulating factor-macrophage (CSF-M)

FDA status: Investigational

Current approved indications: None

Investigational uses: Antitumor agent, hypercholesterolemia, antifungal adjunct, bone marrow transplantation, chemotherapy-induced myelosuppression

Dosing: Not established

Toxicity: Thrombocytopenia, hypocholesterolemia

Name: Stem cell factor

Other names: c-kit ligand, mast cell growth factor, steel factor

FDA status: Investigational

Current approved indications: None

Investigational uses: Peripheral blood progenitor cell mobilization, bone marrow failure states, bone marrow priming

Dosing: To be established; $5–20$ µg/kg/day, subcutaneous administration only

Toxicity: Allergic-like reactions, including urticaria, shortness of breath, laryngospasm (at doses ≥ 25 µg/kg/day)

Pathobiology of Human Acute Myeloid Leukemia

63

Steven J. Collins

INTRODUCTION

Acute myeloid leukemia (AML) describes a heterogeneous group of hematologic disorders characterized by a block in the terminal differentiation of particular hematopoietic cell lineages. Like normal hematopoietic stem cells, the leukemia cells retain the capability to divide and proliferate, resulting in self-renewal, but their capacity to differentiate terminally to morphologically and functionally mature hematopoietic cells is markedly compromised. This results in the progressive accumulation of relatively immature, poorly functioning cells that eventually inhibit the production and differentiation of cells within the normal hematopoietic compartments. This inhibition of normal marrow function that characterizes AML eventually results in severe bleeding, infections, and metabolic complications that, left untreated, invariably prove lethal.

The heterogeneity in the clinical presentation and pathophysiology of AML reflects both the different hematopoietic lineages that can be affected by this differentiation block, as well as the different developmental stages within a given hematopoietic lineage in which this differentiation block occurs. The terms acute nonlymphocytic leukemia, acute myeloid leukemia, and acute myelogenous leukemia are generally used interchangeably.[1] Thus, the broad term AML commonly includes disorders affecting differentiation within the granulocyte, monocyte/macrophage, erythroid, and megakaryocytic lineages (i.e., nonlymphoid, marrow-derived lineages). This heterogeneity is reflected in the different terms frequently used to describe AML, including acute granulocytic, promyelocytic, monocytic, myelomonocytic, erythroid, megakaryocytic, or undifferentiated leukemia.

CLONAL ORIGIN

Studies using X-chromosome inactivation cellular mosaicism have clearly demonstrated the clonal origin of AML and have given considerable insight into the nature of the hematopoietic stem cell that may be involved in various cases of AML. This approach is based on the observation that early in female embryogenesis one of the two X chromosomes in each somatic cell is inactivated so that all progeny of that cell have either an active paternally derived X (X^P) chromosome or an active maternally derived X (X^M). Thus, females who are heterozygous for the X-linked glucose-6-phosphate dehydrogenase (G6PD) gene exhibit two populations of somatic cells—one expressing the usual B allele and the other expressing a variant allele with altered electrophoretic mobility such as A. Normal tissues are composed of mixtures of such cells and exhibit both B- and A-type enzymes. By contrast, cells of clonal origin exhibit either B- or A-type enzyme, but not both. Studies of female patients with AML who are heterozygous at the G6PD locus indicate that virtually all cases of AML at clinical presentation are clonal.[2–4] A G6PD analysis of cells derived from different hematopoietic lineages within individual AML patients indicates that in some cases the disease is restricted to granulocyte/monocyte progenitors; in other cases, the leukemic progenitors are multipotent giving rise to cells of the granulocyte, erythroid, and megakaryocytic lineages.[2–4] Moreover, in some AML patients who have achieved remission after chemotherapy, the marrow appears to be morphologically normal but nevertheless expresses a single G6PD enzyme type indicating the presence of a "clonal remission."[5,6] These studies reflect heterogeneity in the cell of origin in different cases of AML. That is, in some patients the disease appears to be restricted to cells of the granulocyte/monocyte lineage, while in other cases the disease involves a multipotential stem cell, capable of differentiation along the erythroid and megakaryocytic in addition to the granulocyte/monocyte lineages (Fig. 63-1).

The presence of clonal remission in certain patients with AML[5,6] most likely reflects the multistep pathogenesis of this disease. The clonal remission marrow may represent "preleukemic" stem cells that have undergone an initial transformation event. The overt leukemia cells that responded to chemotherapy most likely represent a subclone of these cells that have acquired additional genetic abnormalities conferring an enhanced block to differentiation. This situation in AML is analogous to that in patients with Philadelphia chromosome-positive chronic myeloid leukemia (CML) who undergo aggressive chemotherapy after entering blast crisis phase. The blast crisis cells frequently harbor additional cytogenetic abnormalities compared with the chronic-phase CML cells. A remission in these patients generally involves restoring the marrow back to the chronic phase, which represents a cytogenetically abnormal (i.e., Philadelphia chromosome positive) clonal stage of the disease.[7]

The observation that AML cells are clonally derived suggests

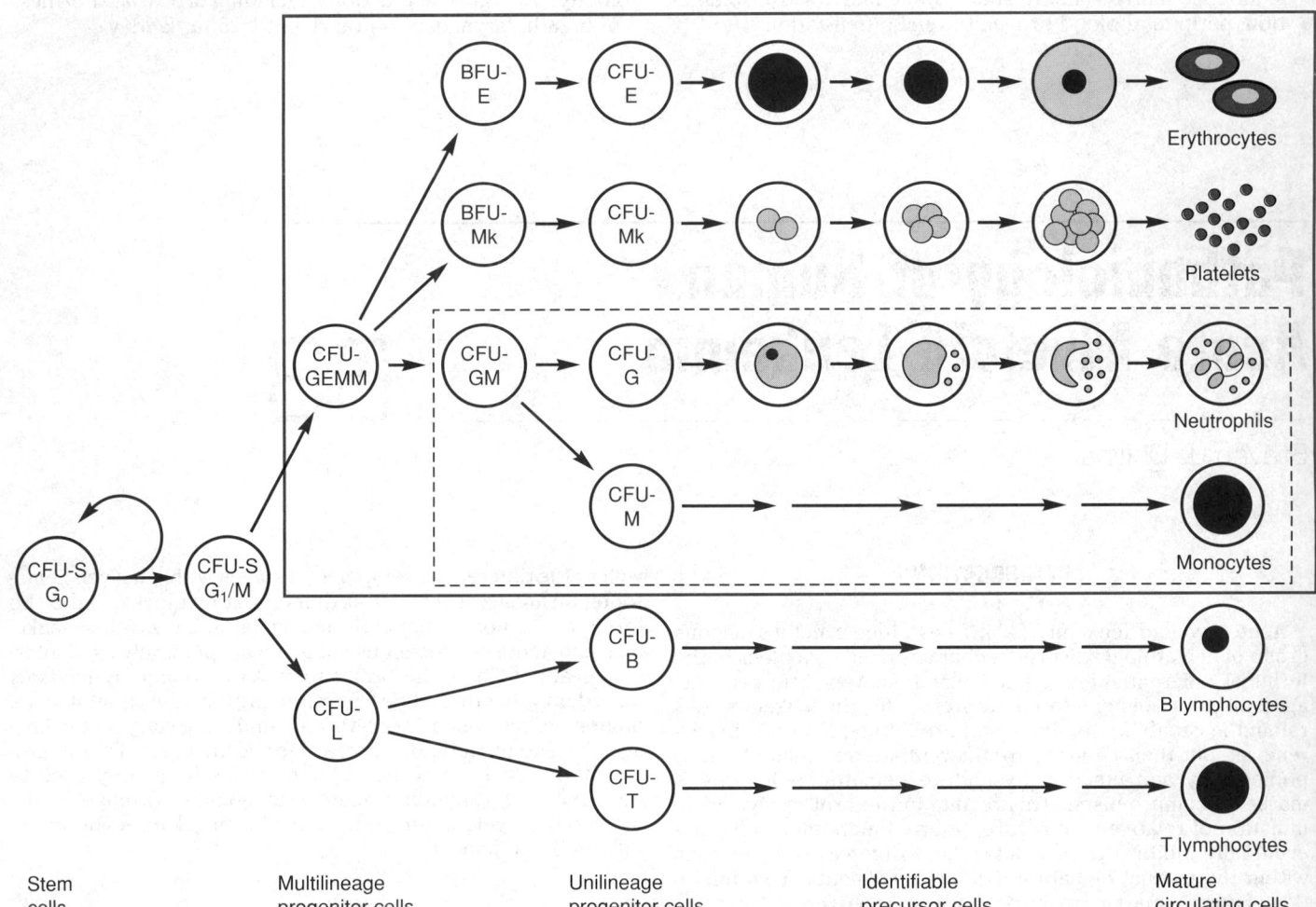

Stem cells   Multilineage progenitor cells   Unilineage progenitor cells   Identifiable precursor cells   Mature circulating cells

Fig. 63-1. Heterogeneity in the hematopoietic stem cell origin of AML. In some cases of AML, the disease appears restricted to stem cells committed to granulocyte/monocyte/macrophage differentiation (dotted box). In other cases of AML, the disease involves a pluripotential stem cell that is capable of differentiating to erythrocytes and megakaryocytes, in addition to granulocyte/monocyte/macrophages (red box).

that a rare event, such as genetic mutation(s), is critical to the development of AML. Moreover, the presence of a clonal remission in some cases of AML indicates that the pathogenesis of AML is a multistage phenomenon; that is, AML results not from a single mutation but from a series of mutations. This multistep development of AML is probably common to most human malignancies, best exemplified by the specific genetic events involving alterations in certain oncogenes and "tumor suppressor" genes that occur during the evolution of colon carcinoma from premalignant to overtly malignant stages.[8]

ETIOLOGY

Exposure to a number of different environmental insults, including radiation, hydrocarbons, and certain anticancer chemotherapeutic agents, has been associated with the development of AML. These agents have in common the potential to damage DNA. Such damage may lead to particular mutations or chromosome aberrations that are critical to the hematopoietic differentiation block that characterizes the development of AML.

An increased incidence of AML has been noted in atomic bomb survivors. This increased risk may be directly proportional to the estimated dose of γ-irradiation to which the individual was exposed.[9,10] Patients treated with certain chemotherapy drugs, particularly the radiomimetic agents, including alkylating agents and nitrosoureas, are at increased risk of the development of AML.[11-14] This risk is further increased in patients treated with a combination of radiotherapy and chemotherapy.[15] Exposure to chemicals, particularly benzene,[16] as well as other petroleum products,[17] is also associated with an increased risk of AML.

RNA tumor viruses (retroviruses) are leukemogenic in a number of different animal models, including mice, cats, and gibbon apes,[18,19] and provide important laboratory models for studying leukemogenesis. Moreover, the human retrovirus T-cell leukemia virus I is associated with the development of certain human lymphoid leukemias.[20] Nevertheless, despite extensive study, a clear role for the involvement of retroviruses in human AML has not been established.[21]

Families demonstrating an increased risk of the development of AML have been reported,[22] but such families appear to be extremely rare. Patients with Down syndrome (trisomy 21) have an increased incidence of the development of AML.[23] A predisposition to the development of AML as well as other types of malignancies is also noted in certain congenital disorders associated with DNA and chromosomal instability, including ataxia/telangiectasia, Bloom syndrome, and Fanconi's anemia.

Although these environmental and hereditary conditions clearly contribute to the development of certain cases of AML, it should be emphasized that the vast majority of patients presenting with de novo AML show no evidence of these risk factors, and the etiologic factors contributing to the development of the disease are unknown.

MULTISTEP PATHOGENESIS—FRIEND ERYTHROLEUKEMIA MODEL

A number of different experimental animal models correspond to different types of human leukemia. The erythroleukemias induced in susceptible mouse strains by the Friend leukemia virus[24] have been particularly well studied. In recent years considerable data have been obtained regarding the specific molecular events and mutations that occur in the different biologic stages of Friend virus-induced erythroleukemias[25] (Fig. 63-2). These genetic events provide important insights into the multiple stages that might occur in the pathogenesis of human AML.

The initial stage in Friend virus-induced disease occurs soon after the injection of susceptible adult mice with the FV-P variant of the Friend murine leukemia virus, which leads to a rapid polyclonal expansion of erythroid progenitors (burst-forming unit-erythroid and colony-forming unit-erythroid) within the spleen. While erythroid precursors from uninjected animals require erythropoietin (EPO) for growth, the erythroid precursors from the FV-P infected mice proliferate autonomously without the addition of EPO. These EPO-independent erythroid cells are not immortal and, when transplanted into susceptible mice, do not give rise to leukemia. However, some 4–6 weeks later, clones of cells that are indeed tumorigenic arise in the spleen of infected animals, giving rise to overt leukemia when transplanted into other mice. Thus, this initial polyclonal expansion of nontumorigenic erythroid precursors occurring soon after Friend virus injection appears to represent a distinct preleukemic stage of the leukemia from which later develops a clonal expansion of overt leukemia cells.

The molecular basis for this retrovirus-induced preleukemic expansion of the erythroid precursors has recently been determined. EPO is known to mediate the proliferation of erythroid precursors by binding to and activating its specific EPO receptor (EPO-R), a membrane-spanning glycoprotein found on the surface of erythroid precursors.[26] The activated EPO-R is involved in the signal transduction pathway to stimulate erythroid precursor proliferation. The Friend virus genome harbors an envelope glycoprotein (GP55) that when expressed in erythroid precursors binds to and activates the EPO-R.[27,28] Thus, by binding to EPO-R, the GP55 protein can stimulate erythroid proliferation in the absence of EPO. This most likely accounts for the enhanced polyclonal proliferation of preleukemic erythroid precursors noted relatively soon after injection of Friend virus.

Several weeks after this polyclonal erythroid expansion occurs, clonal subsets of these cells arise that exhibit characteristics of overt transplantable leukemia. The delayed development of these cells as well as their clonal nature suggest that rare leukemogenic mutation(s) has occurred. What specific genes are involved in such genetic events leading from the preleukemic to overtly leukemic phase of the Friend retrovirus-induced disease? Mutations of at least two different genes have been implicated in the progression of these erythroleukemias. First, in most of the overt Friend retrovirus-induced leukemias, proviral integration occurs in a region of the genome in close proximity to the Spi-1 gene.[29,30] This Friend provirus integration into the Spi-1 locus results in enhanced transcription of this gene, since mRNA transcripts of the Spi-1 gene are increased in these erythroleukemia cells. Such activation of endogenous cellular genes by proviral integration has been referred to as "promoter insertion" and has been noted in a number of different animal models of retrovirus-induced malignancies.[31,32] The Spi-1 gene is a member of the ets family of transcription factors and harbors a distinct DNA-binding domain and transcriptional activation domain.[30] Spi-1 presumably regulates the expression of specific target genes, and the activation of the Spi-1 transcription factor in Friend erythroleukemia may lead to the inappropriate expression of specific genes that are critical to leukemogenesis.

Another important genetic event in the progression of Friend erythroleukemia involves inactivation of the p53 gene. p53 is a tumor suppressor, or anti-oncogene, that when inactivated may play an important role in the development of malignancy.[33,34] Inactivation can occur through a number of different mechanisms, including point mutations, proviral integrations, intrachromosomal deletions, and complete chromosomal loss.[35] Inactivation of p53 appears to be one of the critical

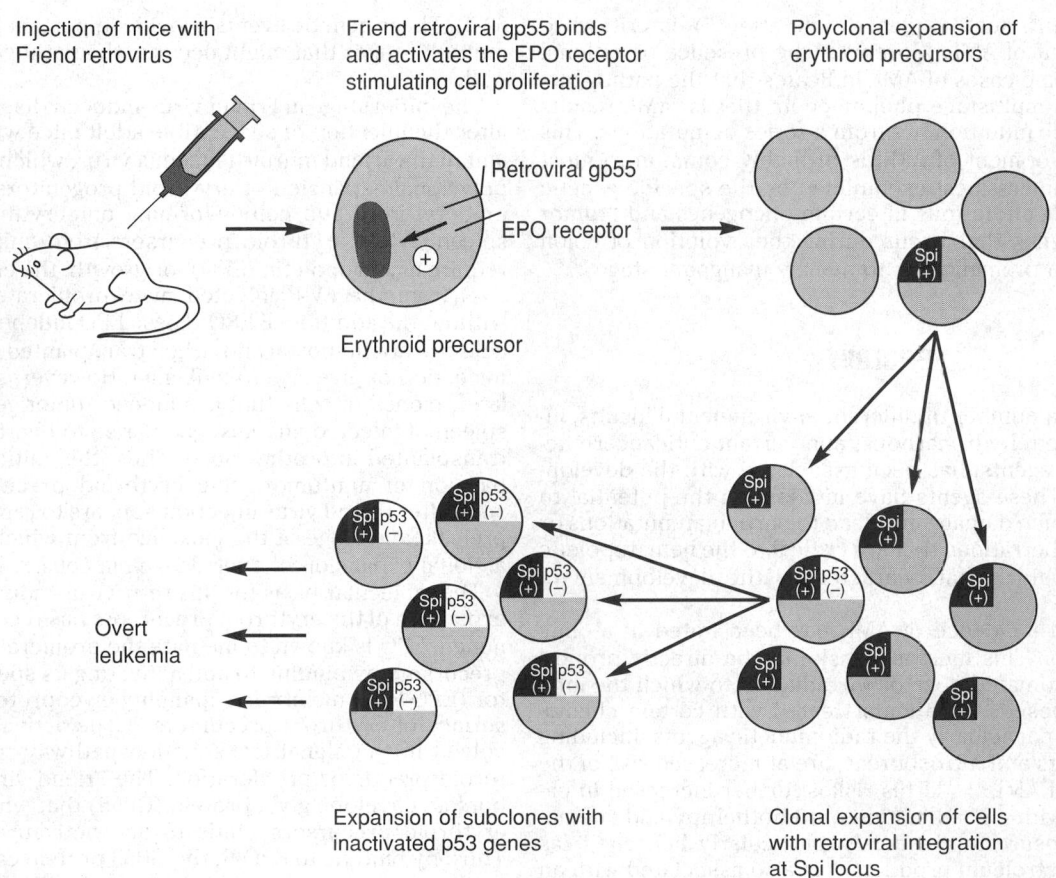

Injection of mice with Friend retrovirus

Friend retroviral gp55 binds and activates the EPO receptor stimulating cell proliferation

Polyclonal expansion of erythroid precursors

Retroviral gp55

EPO receptor

Erythroid precursor

Overt leukemia

Expansion of subclones with inactivated p53 genes

Clonal expansion of cells with retroviral integration at Spi locus

Fig. 63-2. Molecular events in the pathogenesis of Friend virus-induced erythroleukemia. Injection of the Friend retrovirus into susceptible mice results in retroviral infection of erythroid precursors. In these infected cells, the Friend virus glycoprotein GP55 binds to and activates the EPO-R, leading to the EPO-independent polyclonal proliferation of red cell precursors. Continued replication of the Friend virus within this expanding erythroid compartment results in multiple proviral integration events. A selective growth advantage occurs in clones in which retroviral integration activates transcription of the Spi-1 gene. Further proliferation occurs in subclones in which both p53 genes have been inactivated by retroviral integration or genetic mutation. Accumulation of these multiple genetic events leads to overt leukemia.

clonal events in the progression of Friend virus-induced erythroleukemia[35]; such p53 inactivation is frequently noted in human malignancies as well.[36]

What is the function of the normal p53 gene? p53 appears to be a transcription factor involved in mediating cell cycle arrest at G_1.[37] This G_1 arrest frequently occurs in cells subject to stress, including anoxia, exposure to X-irradiation, or administration of certain drugs. These agents may potentially damage DNA, and the G_1 arrest allows the enzymatic machinery of the cell sufficient time to recognize and repair this damage before DNA replication. Thus, p53 may serve as a brake on the cell cycle to arrest the growth of stressed cells temporarily to allow any DNA damage to be repaired prior to cell division[37–39] (Fig. 63-3). Malignant or premalignant cells in which p53 is inactivated have lost this brake mechanism on cell division; as a result, enhanced proliferation may ensue. Moreover, because of the inhibition of DNA repair associated with the loss of G_1 arrest, such cells harboring inactivated p53 genes may also be more susceptible to the accumulation of other DNA mutations or chromosomal abnormalities critical to tumor progression.[40]

The Friend virus-induced mouse erythroleukemia model thus involves at least three different genetic events to give rise to overt leukemia: (1) stimulation of the EPO-R by the viral GP55, resulting in the activation of this receptor in the absence of its normal ligand (EPO); (2) activation of the *Spi*-1 transcription factor resulting from viral integration at this locus; and (3) inactivation of the p53 tumor suppressor gene as a result of genetic mutations (Fig. 63-2). The pathobiology of the Friend

erythroleukemia model has several important parallels with human AML: (1) the development of human AML also appears to involve multiple genetic events that give rise to overt leukemia, (2) the activation or inappropriate expression of specific hematopoietic growth factors or growth factor receptors may also have a role in the pathogenesis of some cases of human AML, and (3) activation and/or inappropriate expression of specific transcription factors is also relatively common in human AML. Interestingly, in the Friend erythroleukemia model, this activation results from retrovirus promoter insertion at the *Spi*-1 locus, while in human AML, activation of transcription factors results from specific chromosome translocations. The genetic mutations and chromosome translocations that appear important in the pathogenesis of human AML are discussed below.

HEMATOPOIETIC GROWTH FACTORS

The development over the past 30 years of various in vitro clonogenic assays for normal hematopoietic cell precursors[41,42] has defined a number of different hematopoietic growth factors (HGFs) involved in regulating the proliferation and differentiation of normal hematopoietic cells (see Ch. 6). The more recent availability of recombinant HGFs and the molecular cloning of their corresponding receptors has markedly accelerated research into how these specific factors may control the growth and differentiation of both normal and leukemic

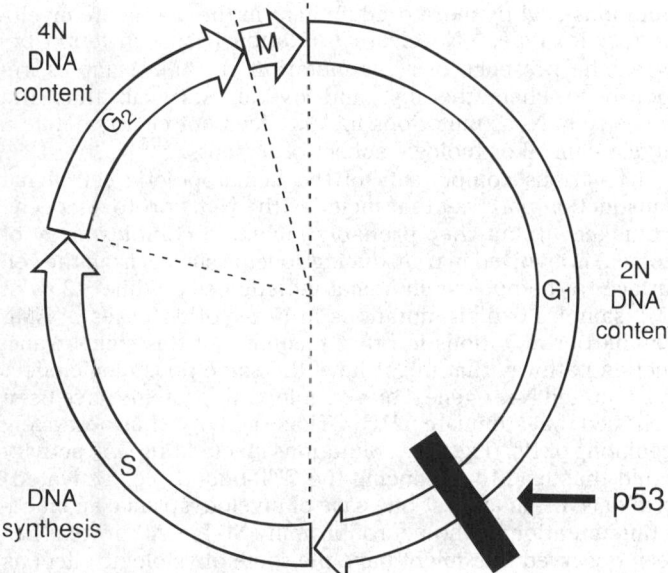

Fig. 63-3. The p53 gene product mediates G_1 cell cycle arrest. p53 is a transcription factor responsible for regulating the expression of genes involved in temporarily arresting the growth of stressed cells in the G_1 phase of the cell cycle. Cells subject to different forms of stress, including anoxia, ultraviolet irradiation, X-irradiation, or certain drugs, develop enhanced expression of p53. The resulting G_1 arrest delays the entry into S phase, allowing the enzymatic machinery of the stressed cells sufficient time to recognize and repair any DNA damage prior to further DNA replication and cell division.

blood cells.[43] There is clear evidence that most leukemic blasts demonstrate a proliferative or differentiative response to one or more of these HGFs. However, this response is a complex, mixed picture that varies markedly among individual AML patient samples. This complexity most likely reflects both the intricate network of HGF and cytokine ligand-receptor interaction that controls normal hematopoiesis and the marked heterogeneity in the developmental stage at which different patient AML cells are "frozen" in differentiation.

AML cells proliferate poorly in liquid suspension culture in vitro, and HGF independent myeloid leukemia cell lines are difficult to establish.[44] This poor in vitro proliferation most likely reflects the marked dependence of AML blasts on endogenous in vivo growth factors. Similarly, AML progenitor cells proliferate poorly in colony-forming assays in vitro, but colony formation is markedly enhanced with the addition of specific HGFs, including colony-stimulating factor-granulocyte, -macrophage, and -granulocyte/macrophage (CSF-G, CSF-M, CSF-GM), interleukin-3 (IL-3), and stem cell factor.[45-47] Different types of AML cells exhibit variation in their proliferative response to these various HGFs. Combinations of such factors generally enhance leukemic colony formation. In particular, stem cell factor can enhance by some 10–20-fold the proliferation of leukemic blasts induced by CSF-G, CSF-GM, and IL-3.[48,49]

The response of AML cells to HGFs is most likely mediated through specific growth factor receptors that are frequently expressed on the surface of AML cells.[43,50-52] Receptors for CSF-M, CSF-GM, CSF-G, EPO, IL-3, IL-4, IL-5, IL-6, and IL-7 have been demonstrated on the surface of different AML samples. Overexpression of these growth factor receptors might account for the enhanced proliferation of AML cells, but this has not been experimentally confirmed. The interaction of specific HGFs with their corresponding receptor presumably triggers a cascade of molecular events that leads to the stimulation of cell division. The molecular events involved in this hematopoietic cell signal transduction cascade following receptor activa-

tion are poorly understood but are currently the subject of intense investigation.

Since some AML cells produce specific HGFs and express the corresponding receptor, it is possible that an autocrine mechanism contributes to the continuous proliferation of AML cells.[53] In at least one case of AML, the leukemia cells produced CSF-GM, and the proliferation of these cells was inhibited by antibodies to CSF-GM, suggesting that an autocrine mechanism was at work.[54] Interestingly, it has been demonstrated that such an autocrine mechanism may occur intracellularly without requiring secretion of the synthesized ligand.[55] Production of mitogenic growth factors by AML cells may occur constitutively or in response to other cytokines, particularly IL-1,[56] and tumor necrosis factor-α.[57,58]

Particular mutations in HGF receptors may lead to their activation in the absence of specific ligands. A point mutation in the EPO-R extracellular domain leading to its constitutive activation has been observed in mouse erythroleukemias.[59] Point mutations at position 969 of the c-*fms* (CSF-1 receptor) gene have been noted in approximately 10% of AML samples.[60-62] This point mutation results in activation of the tyrosine kinase activity of the receptor, and c-*fms* constructs harboring this mutation exhibit transforming activity in mouse NIH3T3 transformation assays.[62] Other AML cells may harbor mutations within the genes coding for the critical enzymes involved in the signal transduction pathway triggered by the activated CSF-M receptor.

Thus, activation of surface membrane HGF receptors leading to the proliferation of AML cells may occur in a number of ways: (1) interaction with normal endogenous hematopoietic growth factors; (2) interaction with autocrine growth factors; and (3) by activation of mutations within the receptors themselves. However, this activation is only one of several events that lead to the development of AML. For example, mice reconstituted with bone marrow infected with retroviral vectors expressing CSF-GM or IL-3 will develop myeloproliferative syndromes, but not overt leukemia.[63-65] Infection of susceptible mice with Friend virus leads to activation of the EPO-Rs receptors, with subsequent polyclonal erythroid expansion, but not leukemia. Other genetic events appear to be critical to the development of full-blown AML, including point mutations and chromosomal translocations.

PROTO-ONCOGENE MUTATIONS

N-*ras* Point Mutations

Proto-oncogenes are normal cellular genes involved in critical cell functions related to cell growth and differentiation including growth factor receptor activation, signal transduction and gene transcription. Mutations within these proto-oncogenes have been described in a variety of different malignancies. In human AML, mutations within the N-*ras* gene are the most commonly described proto-oncogene mutation occurring in ≤25% of patient samples.

The *ras* proto-oncogene family includes Ha- Ki-, and N-*ras,* each of which codes for a 21-kd protein (p21^{ras}) that localizes to the inner plasma membrane. These proteins are structurally similar to and share the GTP binding and hydrolysis activity with the GTPase family of highly conserved proteins (G proteins) that are involved in signal transduction pathways from the extracellular environment to the cytoplasm.[66] Membrane receptor activation triggers a cascade of molecular events leading to the activation of p21^{ras}.[67] This "active" form of the p21^{ras} protein is the GTP-bound molecule, and the intrinsic GTPase activity of p21^{ras} returns it to its inactive form.[66,67] A cytoplasmic protein termed GAP (GTPase-activating protein) markedly accelerates this intrinsic GTPase activity, leading to down-

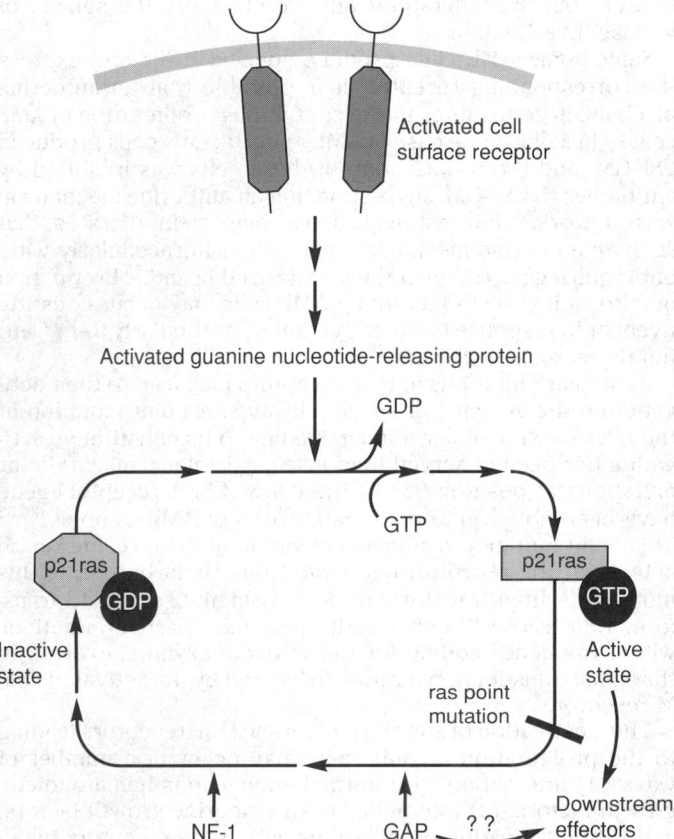

Fig. 63-4. *ras* point mutations enhance p21^ras activity. Activation of specific cell surface receptors results in a cascade of events leading to the active GTP-bound state of p21^ras. GTPase-activating proteins, including GAP and NF-1, normally down-regulate p21^ras activity by converting p21 from the GTP to the inactive GDP-bound state. p21^ras proteins harboring specific point mutations at codons 12, 13, or 61 are relatively resistant to this GAP-induced down-regulation and are therefore maintained in the active GTP-bound state. Mutations in the GAP or NF-1 genes that inactivate their p21^ras down-regulatory function will also result in enhanced p21^ras activity.

regulation of p21^ras (Fig. 63-4). N-*ras* genes cloned from AML cells can transform mouse NIH3T3 cells in vitro and this transformation is associated with point mutations within the N-*ras* genes that occur selectively at codons 12, 13, and 61.[68–71] These point mutations are all associated with decreased GTPase activity of N-ras, which leads to the accumulation of the activated GTP-bound N-ras product (Fig. 63-4).

Although point mutations in Ha-, Ki-, and N-*ras* have all been described in human malignancies, nearly 90% of the mutations within the *ras* family that occur in AML involve N-*ras,* with most of the others involving Ki-*ras*. Presumably the mutated N-*ras* gene deregulates a signal transduction pathway that is ordinarily involved in controlling the growth and differentiation of relatively immature myeloid precursors. It is unclear whether these N-*ras* mutations are a relatively early or a relatively late genetic event in the development of AML. In one patient exhibiting a clonal remission, a mutant N-*ras* allele was observed in the overt leukemia sample, but not in the remission cells, suggesting that the N-*ras* point mutation was a relatively late event in the development of the leukemia.[72] In other patient samples, however, N-*ras* mutations have been noted to be absent in patients relapsing after chemotherapy for AML, even though the initial leukemic cells exhibited an N-*ras* point mutation.[73]

N-*ras* mutations have been noted in all the different types of AML French-American-British (FAB) classifications, with such mutations slightly more predominant in the M4 (acute myelomonocytic) type.[74] No clear correlation has been found between the presence of N-*ras* mutations in AML samples, response to chemotherapy, and overall survival; thus the presence of N-*ras* mutations in AML does not clearly define a unique clinical or biologic subset of patients.[74,75]

The various components of the hematopoietic cell signal transduction pathway that includes the N-*ras* proto-oncogene are unknown, but they probably include a complex array of molecules involved in transducing specific signals from the cell surface to the nucleus in hematopoietic cells. While ≤25% of AML samples exhibit mutations in N-*ras*, other cases of AML may harbor mutations in other members of this signal transduction pathway that might have the same physiologic effect as a mutated N-*ras* gene. For example, GAP proteins have been identified that stimulate p21^ras GTPase activity, thus negatively regulating p21^ras (Fig. 63-4). Mutations inactivating GAP activity would thus lead to enhancing the GTP-bound (i.e., activated) form of N-*ras*. In at least one case of myelodysplasia, an inactivating mutation of the neurofibromin (NF-1) GAP protein has been observed that might have the same physiologic effect as an activating mutation within N-*ras* itself[76] (Fig. 63-4).

p53 Mutations

Mutations within the p53 tumor suppressor gene appear to be the most common genetic alteration that occurs in human malignancies. Inactivation of the p53 gene also appears to be a common, critical event in the development of Friend mouse erythroleukemias (Fig. 63-2). By contrast, mutations of p53 appear to be relatively infrequent in human AML, demonstrated in <20% of patient samples.[77,78] p53 is located on chromosome 17, and p53 mutations appear to be more common in patient samples displaying a loss of chromosome 17.[79] In addition, human myeloid leukemia cell lines established in continuous liquid suspension culture commonly harbor p53 allele point mutations and deletions.[80] No relationship between the presence of p53 mutations and the FAB AML classification has been described.

CHROMOSOMAL TRANSLOCATIONS

Chromosomal translocations involving the aberrant breakage and fusion of specific chromosomes are frequently noted in AML. In contrast with N-*ras* point mutations, there appears to be a marked correlation between the presence of specific chromosomal translocations and the FAB classification of AML. In recent years, a number of genes involved in these translocations have been cloned and sequenced. The relationship between the specific fusion genes that result from these translocations and the pathogenesis of the various types of AML is the subject of active laboratory investigation.

DNA sequence analysis indicates that most of the genes involved in these chromosome translocations in AML have the molecular structure of transcription factors.[81] Transcription factors belong to a number of discrete families and generally consist of modular structures, including a DNA-binding domain, a dimerization domain, and an activation domain. The DNA-binding domain is involved in sequence-specific recognition of DNA sequences in the regulatory region of target genes, and transcription factors generally bind to these regions as homodimers or heterodimers. The activation domain of specific transcription factors appears to interact with a complex of proteins, including RNA polymerase II, that bind near the transcriptional start site, and this interaction may be involved in tissue-specific enhancement or inhibition of target gene expression.[82]

The different chromosome translocations associated with

various forms of AML, and the specific genes involved in each of these translocations are described below.

t(15;17) PML/RAR-α

Acute promyelocytic leukemia (APL), classified as FAB M3, makes up approximately 10% of AML and is characterized by hypergranular promyelocytes populating the bone marrow. This subtype of AML is frequently associated with disseminated intravascular coagulation and is generally sensitive to conventional combination chemotherapy.[83] The cytogenetic hallmark of APL is the t(15;17), which occurs in approximately 80% of cases and is noted almost exclusively in APL.[84]

Molecular cloning of the chromosome breakpoint regions in APL have identified two genes that are involved in this translocation[85–89] (Fig. 63-5). Most of the breaks on chromosome 17 in the APL-specific t(15;17) occur in the first intron of the retinoic acid receptor-α (RAR-α) gene, a member of the steroid/thyroid hormone superfamily of nuclear transcription factors.[90] The RAR-α receptor is of particular interest, since the multiple diverse effects of retinoic acid (RA), one of the biologically active metabolites of vitamin A (retinol), are thought to be mediated through this and other closely related nuclear receptors. RAR-α exhibits a modular structure, including a discrete DNA-binding and hormone (ligand)-binding domain, as well as an NH_2-terminal activation domain. The RA receptors act as specific transcription factors by binding to specific cis-acting regulatory sequences in target genes, and this target gene expression may be modified by the interaction of RA with the RA receptor ligand-binding domain.[90]

As a result of the t(15;17), the NH_2-terminal "activation" domain of the RAR-α is replaced with the N-terminus of a gene on chromosome 15 termed promyelocytic leukemia (PML), resulting in a PML/RAR-α fusion gene[85–87] (Fig. 63-5). A DNA sequence analysis of PML indicates that it may also be a transcription factor with a zinc finger-like DNA-binding domain and a proline-rich activation domain.[85–87] Thus, the aberrant PML/RAR-α fusion gene that characterizes APL is a chimeric protein that consists of two specific transcription factors. PML is widely expressed in both hematopoietic and nonhematopoietic tissue, but the specific target genes that PML may ordinarily regulate are unknown. The reciprocal RAR-α/PML transcript is also expressed in APL cells and might also be involved in the pathogenesis of the disease[91] (Fig. 63-5).

The relationship of the generation of the aberrant PML/RAR-α fusion transcript and the pathogenesis of APL is unclear. Of particular interest is that RA induces APL cells to terminally differentiate to mature granulocytes both in vitro and in vivo.[92–97] Indeed, as a single agent, RA induces complete remissions in most patients with APL.[92–94] Molecular genetic studies indicate that it is the leukemic clone that differentiates to granulocytes in RA-treated patients. APL is generally the only subtype of AML that exhibits such a response to RA. These observations raise a curious paradox: the RA receptor most likely mediates the differentiative response to RA,[97] yet the subtype of AML that appears to be most sensitive to RA (i.e., APL) is the only known type of leukemia that harbors an aberrant RA receptor. One possible explanation of this paradox is that normal promyelocytes may be sensitive to differentiation induction by the relatively low concentrations of RA that are normally present in serum (10^{-8}–10^{-9} M), but in leukemic promyelocytes harboring the t(15;17), the aberrant PML/RAR-α gene inhibits normal RAR function such that considerably higher doses of RA (10^{-6} M) are required to induce differentiation. This hypothesis suggests that the aberrant PML/RAR gene product inhibits normal RAR activity. However, this inhibition has not been consistently demonstrated in RA receptor functional assays.[86,87]

The PML/RAR-α fusion gene is only present in the leukemia clone and this has been exploited to assess the presence of minimal residual disease in patients treated for APL. Specific oligonucleotide primers flanking the fusion point and complementary to the PML and RAR-α regions of the fusion transcript can be used in the polymerase chain reaction to detect this aberrant leukemia-specific fusion transcript.[98,99] (Fig. 63-5C). This approach is much more sensitive than morphologic, cytogenetic, or Southern blot analysis to detect residual promyelocytic leukemia cells and can detect one leukemia cell in 10^4–10^5 cells. Initial studies that employed this technique detected the presence of residual cells harboring the leukemia specific PML/RAR-α transcript in bone marrow that appeared to be in complete remission by morphologic criteria.[98,99]

t(8;21) ETO/AML1

Approximately 15–20% of AML samples harbor a specific reciprocal translocation involving chromosome 8 and 21.[100] Most of these t(8;21) leukemias are classified as FAB M2 (AML with maturation) and are frequently associated with cytoplasmic Auer rods, bone marrow eosinophilia and a relatively good response to chemotherapy.[101,102]

The specific genes involved in this translocation include the ETO gene on chromosome 8 and the AML1 gene on chromosome 21 resulting in an ETO/AML1 fusion transcript.[103–106] The DNA sequence of the AML1 gene indicates significant similarity between it and the *Drosophila* runt gene, which is involved in regulating expression of genes during *Drosophila* embryogenesis.[107] Thus it is likely that AML1 also codes for a transcription factor, but the target genes it is presumably regulating are unknown. The ETO gene on chromosome 8 has not been completely sequenced to date, and its function is unknown. The ETO gene is normally not expressed in hematopoietic cells, and its transcription appears to be activated as a result of the t(8;21) translocation.[104]

As with t(15;17)-positive APL cells, the presence of minimal residual disease can be detected with considerable sensitivity in remission bone marrow from patients with AML exhibiting the t(8;21) by using oligonucleotide primers flanking the fusion point of the ETO and AML1 genes in the polymerase chain reaction.[106]

t(6;9) dek/can

The t(6;9) is an uncommon translocation that occurs in AML and is associated with a relatively poor prognosis.[108,109] It usually involves the FAB M2 (AML with maturation) or FAB M4 (acute myelomonocytic leukemia) classification. Chromosomal breakpoints generally occur in a single intron within the *dek* gene on chromosome 6 and an intron within the *can* gene on chromosome 9.[110] As a result of this specific translocation, the 5′ sequences of the *dek* gene are fused with the 3′ sequences of the *can* gene resulting in the leukemia specific *dek/can* fusion transcript coding for the chimeric dek/can fusion protein.[111] DNA sequence analysis indicates that the *dek* gene encodes regions of highly acidic amino acids often noted in transcription factors. The *can* gene encodes regions consistent with dimerization and DNA-binding domains. This analysis together with the observation that the dek/can fusion protein is localized to the nucleus suggests that this aberrant fusion protein may also be functioning as a transcription factor.[111]

Interestingly, in an AML patient with a normal karyotype, the fusion of *can* with another gene on chromosome 9 termed *set* results in an aberrant *set/can* fusion transcript,[112] indicating that aberrant fusion genes can occur in AML in the absence of cytogenetically evident chromosomal translocations.

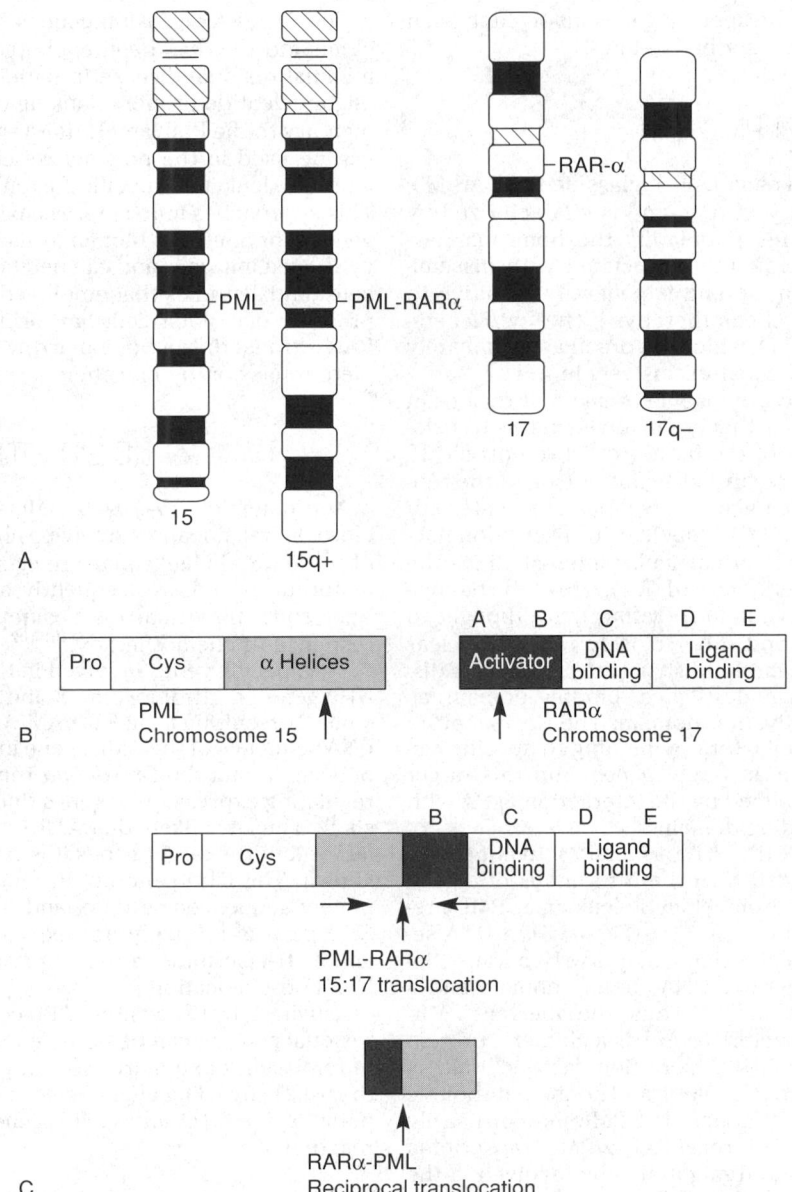

Fig. 63-5. Genes involved in the 15;17 chromosomal translocation characterizing APL. **(A)** The 15;17 reciprocal chromosomal translocation is noted in most cases of human APL with breaks occurring within the PML gene on chromosome 15 and the RAR-α gene on chromosome 17. **(B)** cDNA structures of the PML and RAR-α genes, with the vertical arrows indicating the corresponding fusion breakpoints leading to **(C)** the PML/RAR-α fusion gene. In the fusion PML/RAR-α gene, the NH₂-terminal activation domain of RAR-α is replaced with the PML NH₂-terminal sequences. Horizontal arrows indicate the approximate position of polymerase chain reaction oligonucleotide primers flanking the breakpoint that are used to detect the leukemia-specific PML/RAR-α fusion gene. The reciprocal RAR-α PML fusion cDNA is also expressed in most cases of APL.

5q-Deletions

Abnormalities involving the 5q chromosome have frequently been noted in AML. Although these abnormalities generally involve specific chromosomal deletions rather than chromosomal translocations, they are of sufficient interest to be discussed here. Deletions of 5q occur in approximately 15% of de novo AML and are particularly common in patients with AML evolving from myelodysplasia (MDS) and in patients with chemotherapy-related AML.[113,114] The amount of chromosome 5 deleted varies from patient to patient; some samples demonstrate a complete loss of chromosome 5, while others show that relatively small regions of 5 q are deleted. This chromosome region has been of particular interest to hematologists since a variety of different hematologic growth factors and

growth factor receptors, including CSF-1, CSF-GM, IL-3, IL-4, Il-5, EGR-1, and the CSF-1 receptor, map to this chromosome region.[115]

Comparison of the banded karyotypes of different patient samples indicates that the region of 5q that appears to be commonly deleted is 5q31.1.[114,115] Thus, a tumor suppressor gene, whose loss may be important in the evolution of MDS/AML, may map to this region. One such candidate tumor suppressor gene is the interferon regulatory factor-1 (IRF-1).[116] This gene maps to 5q31.1 and was noted to be consistently deleted in 13 cases of 5q⁻ MDS/AML.[117] The IRF-1 gene is a transcription factor involved in the activation of interferon (IFN)-α- and β- as well as other IFN-inducible genes.[116,117] The interferons are cytokines that can act as negative growth regulators. Thus, IRF-1 is a particularly attractive candidate for a tumor suppressor gene, since loss of its activity may lead to decreased IFN production with subsequent decreased inhibition of target cell growth. Indeed expression of IRF-1 inhibits the transformed phenotype of certain NIH3T3 cells, and thus inactivation of IRF-1 may contribute to the transformed phenotype in 5q⁻ AML cells.[118]

11q23 Chromosomal Translocations

Chromosomal translocations involving 11q23 have been observed in approximately 10–15% of acute lymphocytic leukemia (ALL) samples as well as 5–6% of AML patients. In AML, these translocations involve reciprocal events with a variety of other chromosome regions, including 9p22, 6q27, 1p21, 2p21, 10p11, 17q25, and 19p13.[119] The translocations involving 11q23 have been frequently observed in leukemia samples exhibiting both lymphoid and myeloid "biphenotypic" or "mixed lineage" markers. They have also been commonly noted in AML cells that evolve in children with ALL who have been treated with epipodophyllotoxins.[120]

The gene mapping to 11q23 involved in these chromosome translocations has been recently cloned and designated ALL-1.[121,122] A relatively large mRNA (15 kb) is transcribed from this locus, and DNA sequencing indicates that the ALL-1 gene exhibits marked homology to the *Drosophila trithorax* gene. This species harbors a DNA-binding zinc-finger domain and likely codes for a transcription factor that plays an important role in the embryonic development of *Drosophila*.[123] Presumably the ALL-1 gene also acts as a transcription factor to regulate the expression of specific target genes that might be involved in both lymphoid and myeloid differentiation.

The identification of the specific genes involved in the chromosomal translocations that characterize certain types of AML has provided not only a practical and sensitive polymerase chain reaction-based approach to the detection of minimal residual disease in patient samples but also important clues in identifying the particular transcription factors key to the regulation of normal hematopoiesis. Particularly intriguing in this regard is the relationship between specific chromosomal translocations and FAB subtypes of AML, as this may indicate the specific transcription factors that are involved in regulating the different stages of hematopoietic cell growth and differentiation. Future studies assessing the functional activity of the particular genes involved in these AML-specific translocations in both normal and leukemic cells should provide valuable insight into the specific gene regulatory mechanisms involved in both normal and malignant hematopoiesis.

REFERENCES

1. Stedman's Medical Dictionary. 21st Edition. p. 1044. Williams & Wilkins, Baltimore, 1966
2. Fialkow P, Singer J, Adamson J et al: Acute nonlymphocytic leukemia: expression in cells restricted to granulocytic differentiation. N Engl J Med 301:1, 1979
3. Fialkow P, Singer J, Adamson J et al: Acute nonlymphocytic leukemia: heterogeneity of stem cell origin. Blood 57:1068, 1981
4. Jacobson R, Temple M, Singer J et al: A clonal complete remission in a patient with acute nonlymphocytic leukemia originating in a multipotent stem cell. N Engl J Med 310:1513, 1984
5. Fialkow P, Singer J, Raskind R et al: Clonal development, stem-cell differentiation and clinical remissions in acute nonlymphocytic leukemia. N Engl J Med 317:468, 1987
6. Fialkow P, Janssen J, Bartram C: Clonal remissions in acute nonlymphocytic leukemia: evidence for a multistep pathogenesis of the malignancy. Blood 77:1415, 1990
7. Fialkow P, Jacobson R, Papayannopoulou T: Chronic myelocytic leukemia: clonal origin in a stem cell common to the granulocyte, erythroid, platelet and monocyte/macrophage. Am J Med 63:125, 1977
8. Fearon E, Vogelstein B: A genetic model for colorectal tumorigenesis. Cell 61:759, 1990

9. Bizzozero O, Johnson K, Ciocco A et al: Radiation-related leukemia in Hiroshima and Nagasaki. N Engl J Med 274:1095, 1966
10. Ishimaru T, Otake M, Ichimaru M: Dose response relationship of neutrons and gamma rays to leukemia incidence among atomic bomb survivors in Hiroshima and Nagasaki by type of leukemia 1950–1971. Radiat Res 77:377, 1979
11. Pedersen-Bjergaard J, Larsen S: Incidence of acute nonlymphocytic leukemia, preleukemia, and acute myeloproliferative syndrome up to 10 years after treatment of Hodgkin's disease. N Engl J Med 307:965, 1982
12. Greene M, Boice J, Greer B et al: Acute nonlymphocytic leukemia after therapy with alkylating agents for ovarian cancer: a study of five randomized clinical trials. N Engl J Med 307:1416, 1982
13. Reimer R, Hoover R, Fraumeni et al: Acute leukemia after alkylating agent therapy of ovarian cancer. N Engl J Med 297:177, 1977
14. Boice J, Greene M, Killen J et al: Leukemia and preleukemia after adjuvant treatment of gastrointestinal cancer with semustine (methyl-CCNU). N Engl J Med 309:1079, 1983
15. Coltman C, Dixon D: Second malignancies complicating Hodgkin's disease: a Southwest Oncology Group 10-year follow up. Cancer Treatm Rep 66:1023, 1982
16. Austin A, Delzell E, Cole P: Benzene and leukemia. A review of the literature and a risk assessment. Am J Epidemiol 127:419, 1988
17. Brandt L, Nilsson P, Mitelman F: Occupational exposure to petroleum products in men with acute nonlymphocytic leukemia. Br Med J 4:553, 1978
18. Hartley J, Wolford N, Old L, Rowe W: A new class of murine leukemia virus associated with development of spontaneous lymphomas. Proc Natl Acad Sci USA 74:789, 1977
19. Neil J, Hughes D, McFarlane R et al: Transduction and rearrangement of the *myc* gene by feline leukemia virus in naturally occurring T-cell leukemias. Nature 308:814, 1984
20. Poiesz B, Ruscetti F, Gazdar A et al: Detection and isolation of type-C retrovirus particles from fresh and cultured lymphocytes of a patient with cutaneous T-cell lymphoma. Proc Natl Acad Sci USA 77:7415, 1980
21. Gallo R, Ruscetti F, Collins S, Gallagher R: Human myeloid leukemia cells: studies on oncornaviral related information and in vitro growth and differentiation. p. 335. In Golde D, Cline M, Metcalf D, Fox D (eds): Hematopoietic Cell Differentiation. Vol. 10 Academic Press, Orlando, FL, 1979
22. Lee E, Schiffer C, Misawa S, Testa J: Clinical and cytogenetic features of familial erythroleukemia. Br J Haematol 65:313, 1987
23. Suton W, Welsh V: Acute leukemia and mongolism. J Pediatr 52:170, 1985
24. Friend C: Cell-free transmission in adult Swiss mice of a disease having the character of leukemia. J Exp Med 105:307, 1957
25. Ben-David Y, Bernstein A: Friend virus-induced erythroleukemia and the multistage nature of cancer. Cell 66:831, 1991
26. Krantz S: Erythropoietin. Blood 77:419, 1991
27. Li J, D'Andrea A, Lodish H, Baltimore D: Activation of cell growth by binding of Friend spleen focus-forming virus gp55 glycoprotein to the erythropoietin receptor. Nature 343:762, 1990
28. Ruscetti S, Janesch N, Chakraborti A et al: Friend spleen focus-forming virus induces factor independence in an erythropoietin-dependent erythroleukemia cell line. J Virol 64:1057, 1990
29. Moreau-Gachelin F, Ray D, de Both N: Spi-1 oncogene activation in Rauscher and Friend murine virus-induced acute erythroleukemias. Leukemia 4:20, 1990
30. Paul R, Schuetz S, Kozak S et al: The Spi-1 proviral integration site of Friend erytholeukemia encodes the ets-related transcription factor Pu.1. J Virol 65:464, 1991
31. Neel B, Hayward W, Robinson H et al: Avian leukosis virus-induced tumors have common proviral integration sites and synthesize discrete new RNAs: oncogenesis by promoter insertion. Cell 23:323, 1981
32. O'Donnell P, Fleissner E, Lonial H et al: Early clonality and high-frequency proviral integration into the c-myc locus in AKR leukemias. J Virol 55:500, 1985
33. Finlay C, Hinds P, Levine A: The p53 proto-oncogene can act as a suppressor of transformation. Cell 57:1083, 1989
34. Nigro J, Baker S, Preisinger A et al: Mutations in the p53 gene occur in diverse human tumour types. Nature 342:705, 1989
35. Levine A, Momand J, Finlay C: The p53 tumour suppressor gene. Nature 351:453, 1991
36. Chow V, Ben-David Y, Bernstein A et al: Multistage Friend erythroleukemia: independent origin of tumor clones with normal or rearranged p53 cellular oncogenes. J Virol 61:2777, 1987
37. Kern S, Kinzler K, Bruskin A et al: Identification of p53 as a sequence-specific DNA-binding protein. Science 252:1708, 1991
38. Vogelstein B, Kinzler K: p53 function and dysfunction. Cell 70:523, 1992
39. Kastan M, Zhan Q, El-Deiry W et al: A mammalian cell cycle checkpoint

pathway utilizing p53 and GADD45 is defective in ataxia-telangiectasia. Cell 71:587, 1992

40. Livingstone L, White A, Sprouse J et al: Altered cell cycle arrest and gene amplification potential accompany loss of wild-type p53. Cell 70:923, 1992

41. Pluznik D, Sachs L: The cloning of normal "mast cells" in tissue culture. J Cell Comp Physiol 66:319, 1965

42. Bradley T, Metcalf D: The growth of mouse bone marrow cells in vitro. Aust J Exp Biol Med Sci 44:287, 1966

43. Lowenberg B, Touw I: Hematopoietic growth factors and their receptors in acute leukemia. Blood 81:281, 1993

44. Collins S: The HL-60 promyelocytic leukemia cell line: proliferation, differentiation, and cellular oncogene expression. Blood 70:1233, 1987

45. Delwel R, Salem M, Dorssers L et al: Growth regulation of human acute myeloid leukemia: effects of five recombinant hematopoietic factors in a serum-free culture system. Blood 72:1944, 1988

46. Miyauchi J, Kelleher C, Yang Y-C et al: The effects of three recombinant growth factors, IL-3 GM-CSF and G-CSF on the blast cells of acute myeloblastic leukemia maintained in short term suspension culture. Blood 70:657, 1987

47. Vellenga E, Ostapovicz D, O'Rourke B, Griffin J: Effects of recombinant IL-3 GM-CSF and G-CSF on the proliferation of leukemic clonogenic cells in short-term and long-term cultures. Leukemia 1:584, 1987

48. Ikeda H, Kanakura Y, Tamaki T et al: Expression and functional role of the proto-oncogene c-kit in acute myeloblastic leukemia cells. Blood 78:2962, 1991

49. Kuriu A, Ikeda H, Kanakura Y et al: Proliferation of human myeloid leukemia cell line associated with the tyrosine-phosphorylation and activation of the proto-oncogene c-kit product. Blood 78:2834, 1991

50. Kelleher C, Wong G, Clark S et al: Binding of iodinated recombinant human GM-CSF to the blast cells of acute myeloblastic leukemia. Leukemia 2:211, 1988

51. Budel L, Touw I, Delwel R et al: Interleukin-3 and granulocyte-monocyte colony-stimulating factor receptors on human acute myelocytic leukemia cells and relationship to the proliferative response. Blood 74:565, 1989

52. Park L, Waldron P, Friend D et al: Interleukin-3, GM-CSF, and G-CSF receptor expression on cell lines and primary leukemia cells: receptor heterogeneity and relationship to growth factor responsiveness. Blood 74:56, 1989

53. Murohashi I, Tohda S, Suzuki T et al: Autocrine growth mechanisms of the progenitors of blast cells in acute myeloblastic leukemia. Blood 74:35, 1989

54. Young D, Griffin J: Autocrine secretion of GM-CSF in acute myeloblastic leukemia. Blood 68:1178, 1988

55. Dunbar C, Browder T, Abrams J, Nienhuis A: COOH-terminal-modified interleukin-3 is retained intracellularly and stimulates autocrine growth. Science 245:1493, 1989

56. Delwel R, Van Buitenen C, Salem M et al: Interleukin 1 stimulates proliferation of acute myeloblastic leukemia cells in induction of granulocyte-macrophage stimulating factor release. Blood 74:586, 1989

57. Hoang T, Levy B, Onetto N et al: Tumor necrosis factor alpha stimulates the growth of the clonogenic cells of acute myeloblastic leukemia in synergy with granulocyte/macrophage colony-stimulating factor. J Exp Med 170:15, 1989

58. Elbaz O, Budel L, Hoogerbrugge H et al: Tumour necrosis factor regulates the expression of GM-CSF and IL-3 receptors on human AML cells. Blood 77:989, 1991

59. Longmore G, Lodish H: An activating mutation in the murine erythropoietin receptor induces erythroleukemia in mice: a cytokine receptor superfamily oncogene. Cell 67:1089, 1991

60. Ridge S, Worwood M, Oscier D et al: FMS mutations in myelodysplastic leukemic and normal subjects. Proc Natl Acad Sci USA 87:1377, 1990

61. Roussel MM, Downing J, Sherr C: Transforming activities of human CSF-1 receptors with different point mutations at codon 301 in their extracellular domains. Oncogene 5:25, 1990

62. Tobal K, Pagliuca A, Bhatt B et al: Mutation of the human fms gene (M-CSF receptor) in myelodysplastic syndromes and acute myeloid leukemia. Leukemia 4:486, 1990

63. Chang J, Metcalf D, Lang R et al: Non neoplastic hematopoietic myeloproliferative syndrome induced by dysregulated multi-CSF (IL-3) expression. Blood 73:1487, 1989

64. Johnson G, Gonda T, Metcalf D et al: A lethal myeloproliferative syndrome in mice transplanted with bone marrow cells infected with a retrovirus expressing GM-CSF. EMBO J 8:441, 1988

65. Wong P, Chungf S, Dunbar C et al: Retrovirus mediated transfer and expression of the IL-3 gene in mouse hematopoietic cells results in a myeloproliferative disorder. Mol Cell Biol 9:797, 1989

66. McCormick F: Ras GTPase activating protein: signal transmitter and signal terminator. Cell 56:5, 1989

67. Egan S, Giddings B, Brooks M et al: Association of Sos Ras exchange protein with Grb2 is implicated in tyrosine kinase signal transduction and transformation. Nature 363:45, 1993

68. Bos J, Toksoz D, Marshall C et al: Amino-acid substitutions at codon 13 of the N-ras oncogene in human acute myeloid leukemia. Nature 315:726, 1985

69. Needleman S, Kraus M, Srivastava S et al: High frequency of N-ras activation in acute myelogenous leukemia. Blood 67:753, 1986

70. Bos J, Verlaan-deVries M, van der Eb A et al: Mutations in N-ras predominate in acute myeloid leukemia. Blood 69:1237, 1987

71. Farr C, Saiki R, Erlich H et al: Analysis of RAS gene mutations in acute myeloid leukemia by polymerase chain reaction and oligonucleotide probes. Proc Natl Acad Sci USA 85:1629, 1988

72. Bartram C, Ludwig W-D, Hiddemann W et al: Acute myeloid leukemia: analysis of Ras gene mutations and clonality defined by polymorphic-linked loci. Leukemia 3:247, 1989

73. Senn H, Jiricny J, Fopp M et al: Relapse cell population differs from acute onset clone as shown by absence of the initially activated N-ras oncogene in a patient with acute monocytic leukemia. Blood 72:931, 1988

74. Radich J, Kopecky K, Willman C et al: N-ras mutations in adult de novo acute myelogenous leukemia: prevalence and clinical significance. Blood 76:801, 1990

75. Radich J, Kopecky K, Appelbaum F et al: N-ras mutations in acute myelogenous leukemia: a review of the current literature and an update of the Southwest Oncology Group Experience. Leuk Lymphoma 6:325, 1992

76. Li Y, Bollag G, Clark R et al: Somatic mutations in the neurofibromatosis 1 gene in human tumors. Cell 69:275, 1992

77. Slingerland J, Minden M, Benchimol S: Mutations of the p53 gene in human acute myelogenous leukemia. Blood 77:1500, 1991

78. Fenaux P, Preudhomme C, Quiqandron I et al: Mutations of the p53 gene in acute myeloid leukemia. Br Haematol 80:178, 1992

79. Fenaux P, Jonveaux P, Quiquandon I et al: p53 gene mutations in acute myeloid leukemia with 17p monosomy. Blood 78:1652, 1991

80. Sugimoto K, Toyoshima H, Sakai R et al: Frequent mutations in the p53 gene in human myeloid leukemia cell lines. Blood 79:2378, 1992

81. Nichols J, Nimer S: Transcription factors, translocations and leukemia. Blood 80:2953, 1992

82. Sharp P: TATA-binding protein is a classless factor. Cell 68:819, 1992

83. Stone R, Mayer R: The unique aspects of acute promyelocytic leukemia. J Clin Oncol 8:1913, 1990

84. Rowley J, Golumb H, Dougherty C: 15/17 translocation, a consistent chromosomal change in acute promyelocytic leukemia. Lancet 1:549, 1977

85. Pandolfi P, Grignani F, Alcalay M et al: Structure and origin of the acute promyelocytic leukemia myl/RAR-alpha cDNA and characterization of its retinoid-binding and transactivation properties. Oncogene 6:1285, 1991

86. Kakizuka A, Miller WH, Umesono K et al: Chromosomal translocation t(15;17) in human acute promyelocytic leukemia fuses RAR-alpha with a novel putative transcription factor, PML. Cell 66:663, 1991

87. de The H, Lavau C, Marhcio A et al: The PML-RAR-alpha fusion mRNA generated by the t(15;17) translocation in acute promyelocytic leukemia encodes a functionally altered RAR. Cell 66:675, 1991

88. Alcalay M, Zangrilli D, Pandolfi P et al: Translocation breakpoint of acute promyelocytic leukemia lies within the retinoic acid receptor alpha locus. Proc Natl Acad Sci USA 88:1977, 1991

89. Chomienne C, Ballerini P, Balitrand N et al: The retinoic acid receptor alpha gene is rearranged in retinoic-acid sensitive promyelocytic leukemia. Leukemia 4:802, 1990

90. Evans R: The steroid and thyroid hormone receptor superfamily. Science 240:889, 1988

91. Chang K-S, Stass S, Chu D-T et al: Characterization of a fusion cDNA (RAR-alpha/myl) transcribed from the t(15;17) translocation breakpoint in acute promyelocytic leukemia. Mol Cell Biol 12:800, 1992

92. Huang M-E, Ye Y-C, Chen S-R et al: Use of all-trans retinoic acid in the treatment of acute promyelocytic leukemia. Blood 72:567, 1988

93. Castaigne S, Chomienne C, Daniel M et al: All-transretinoic acid as a differentiation therapy for acute promyelocytic leukemia. I. Clinical results. Blood 76:1704, 1990

94. Warrell R, Frankel S, Miller W et al: Differentiation therapy of acute promyelocytic leukemia with tretinoin (all-trans retinoic acid). N Engl J Med 324:1385, 1991

95. Breitman TR, Collins S, Keene B: Terminal differentiation of human promyelocytic leukemia cells in primary culture in response to retinoic acid. Blood 57:1000, 1981

96. Chomienne C, Ballerini P, Balitrand N et al: All-trans retinoic acid in acute promyelocytic leukemias. In vitro studies: structure-function relationship. Blood 76:1710, 1990

97. Collins S, Robertson K, Mueller L: Retinoic acid-induced granulocytic differ-

entiation of HL-60 myeloid leukemia cells is mediated directly through the retinoic acid receptor (RAR-alpha). Mol Cell Biol 10:2154, 1990

98. Biondi A, Rambaldi A, Pandolfi P et al: Molecular monitoring of the myl/ retinoic acid receptor-alpha fusion gene in acute promyelocytic leukemia by polymerase chain reaction. Blood 80:492, 1992

99. Miller W, Kakizuka A, Frankel S et al: Reverse transcription polymerase chain reaction for the rearranged retinoic acid receptor alpha clarifies diagnosis and detects minimal residual disease in acute promyelocytic leukemia. Proc. Natl Acad Sci USA 89:2694, 1992

100. Rowley J: Identification of a translocation with quinicrine fluorescence in a patient with acute leukemia. Ann Genet 16:109, 1973

101. Trujillo J, Cork A, Hart J et al: Clinical implications of aneuploic cytogenetic profiles in adult acute leukemia. Cancer 33:824, 1974

102. Swirsky D, Li Y, Matthews J: Translocation in acute granulocytic leukemia: cytological, cytochemical and clinical features. Br J Haematol 56:119, 1984

103. Gao J, Erickson P, Gardiner K et al: Isolation of a yeast artificial chromosome spanning the 8;21 translocation breakpoint t(8;21) (q22;q22.3) in acute myelogenous leukemia. Proc Natl Acad Sci USA 88:4882, 1991

104. Miyoshi H, Shimizu K, Maseki N et al: t(8;21) Breakpoints on chromosome 21 in acute myeloid leukemia are clustered within a limited region of a single gene, AML1. Proc Natl Acad Sci USA 88:10431, 1991

105. Erickson P, Gao J, Chang K et al: Identification of breakpoints in t(8;21) acute myelogenous leukemia and isolation of a fusion transcript, AML/ETO, with similarity to *Drosophila* segmentation gene, runt. Blood 80:1825, 1992

106. Chang K-S, Fan Y-H, Stass S et al: Expression of AML1-ETO fusion transcripts and detection of minimal residual disease in t(8;21)-positive acute myeloid leukemia. Oncogene 8:983, 1993

107. Duffy J, Gergen J: The Drosophila segmentation gene runt acts as a position-specific numerator element necessary for the uniform expression of the sex-determining gene Sex-lethal. Genes Dev 5:2176, 1991

108. Sandberg A, Morgan R, McCallister J et al: Acute myeloblastic leukemia with t(6;9) (p23;q34): a specific subgroup of AML? Cancer Genet Cytogenet 10: 139, 1983

109. Adriaansen H, Van Dongen J, Hooijkaas H et al: Translocation (6;9) may be associated with a specific TdT-positive immunological phenotype in ANLL. Leukemia 2:136, 1988

110. von Lindern M, Poustka A, Lerach H, Grosveld G: The (6;9) chromosome translocation, associated with a specific subtype of acute nonlymphocytic

leukemia, leads to aberrant transcription of a target gene on 9q34. Mol Cell Biol 10: 4016, 1990

111. von Lindern M, Fornerod M, van Baal S et al: The translocation (6;9) associated with a specific subtype of acute myeloid leukemia, results in the fusion of two genes, dek and can, and the expression of a chimeric, leukemia specific dek-can mRNA. Mol Cell Biol 12:1687, 1992

112. von Lindern M, van Baal S, Wiegant J et al: can, a putative oncogene associated with myeloid leukemogenesis, may be activated by fusion of its 3' half to different genes: characterization of the set gene. Mol Cell Biol 12:3346, 1992

113. Pedersen-Bjergaard J, Philip P, Larsen S et al: Chromosome aberrations and prognostic factors in therapy-related myelodysplasia and acute nonlymphocytic leukemia. Blood 76:1083, 1990

114. Pederson B, Jensen I: Clinical and prognostic implications of chromosome 5q deletions: 96 high resolution studied patients. Leukemia 5:566, 1991

115. LeBeau M, Lemons R, Espinosa R et al: IL-4 and IL-5 map to human chromosome 5 in a region encoding growth factors and receptors and are deleted in myeloid leukemias with a del(5q). Blood 73:647, 1989

116. Miyamoto M, Fujita T, Kimura Y et al: Regulated expression of a gene encoding a nuclear factor, IRF-1, that specifically binds to IFN-beta gene regulatory elements. Cell 54:903, 1988

117. Willman C, Sever C, Pallavicini M et al: Deletion of IRF-1, mapping to chromosome 5q31.1, in human leukemia and preleukemic myelodysplasia. Science 259:968, 1993

118. Harada H, Kitagawa M, Tanaka N et al: Anti-oncogenic and oncogenic potentials of interferon regulatory factors-1 and -2. Science 259:971, 1993

119. Heim S, Mitelman F: Cancer Cytogenetics. Alan R Liss, New York, 1987

120. Piu C-H, Ribeiro R, Hancock M et al: Acute myeloid leukemias in children treated with epipodophyllotoxins for acute lymphoblastic leukemia. N Engl J Med 325:1682, 1991

121. Tkachuk D, Kohler S. Cleary M: Involvement of a homolog of *Drosophila trithorax* by 11q23 chromosomal translocations in acute leukemias. Cell 71: 691, 1992

122. Gu Y, Nakamura T, Alder H et al: The t(4;11) chromosome translocation of human acute leukemias fuses the ALL-1 gene, related to *Drosophila trithorax* to the AF-4 gene. Cell 71:701:1992

123. Mazo A, Huang D-H, Mozer B, Dawid I: The trithorax complex in Drosophila encodes a protein with zinc-binding domains. Proc. Natl Acad Sci USA 87: 2112, 1990

Clinical Manifestations of Acute Myeloid Leukemia

64

Kenneth B. Miller

INTRODUCTION

Acute myeloid leukemia (AML) is not a single disease but rather a group of neoplastic disorders characterized by the proliferation and accumulation in the bone marrow and peripheral blood of immature hematopoietic cells. These malignant cells gradually replace and inhibit the growth and maturation of normal erythroid, myeloid, and megakaryocytic precursors. If untreated, AML is usually fatal within weeks to months after diagnosis.

The clinical evaluation and prognosis of, and therapy for, patients with AML has changed dramatically over the past two decades. The initial evaluation of a patient with acute leukemia

should be directed at defining the factors important in planning therapy and assessing the long-term prognosis. Molecular, cytogenetic, and immunologic studies have contributed to our understanding of the pathogenesis and prognosis of the acute leukemias. Knowledge of environmental or occupational exposures to known or suspected leukemogenic agents or a prior illnesses that predisposes an individual to develop AML must be considered in planning treatment and evaluating the response to therapy.

Velpeau in 1827 reported the first accurate description of a case of leukemia.[1] The patient was a 63-year-old florist who developed an illness characterized by fever, weakness, urinary stones, and massive hepatosplenomegaly. Velpeau reported that the blood of this patient was "like gruel." He found no infectious cause for this disorder and speculated that the elevated number of white corpuscles and the unique appearance of the blood may not have been the result of infection.

In 1845, Bennett,[2] a brilliant and controversial pathologist from Edinburgh, published a report of a series of patients who died with enlarged spleens and changes in the "color and consistency of their blood." While he also found no infectious etiology for the peculiar appearance of the blood, he attributed these changes to the presence of "purulent material" in the blood and introduced the term *leucocythemia.* Virchow, the noted German pathologist, reported a similar case.[3] Virchow, however, commented on the reversal of the normal ratio of pigmented, red to colorless, white cells, in this patient but did not attribute these changes to an infection. Unsure of the etiology of his finding, he was content simply to describe his observations and used the descriptive name *white blood.* Later, in a monograph entitled *Die Leukemia,* Virchow introduced the word *leukemia,* which he derived from the Greek meaning "white blood."[4]

The name and the interpretation of this new pathologic condition were acrimoniously debated by these two leading pathologists of the day. Virchow noted that the leukemias constituted not one disorder but a heterogeneous group of disorders, and he attempted to subdivide them into a splenic, probably myeloid, and a lymphatic type. In addition, he noted that some patients had a chronic or indolent course, while others presented with a rapidly progressive fatal illness. Virchow's and Bennett's observations and interpretations were remarkable, as neither had the tools to stain blood smears and little was known about the mechanisms of hematopoiesis or the fate, origin, or function of the various cellular elements.

Neumann[5] in the 1870s were the first to suggest that the colorless white cells were made in the bone marrow independently of red cells. Ehrlich in 1877 developed the first aniline-based stains that permitted the clear definition of cellular detail in air-dried films of blood. He was then able to accurately describe and differentiate the various types of normal and abnormal normal white blood cells (WBCs). Ebstein[6] in 1889 introduced the term *acute leukemia* to describe a rapidly fatal illness that failed to respond to available therapy. Neumann in 1899 first suggested that the WBCs were made in the bone marrow and not the spleen. This concept gave rise to the term *myeloid,* meaning "marrow derived." Naegeli[7] in 1900 described the myeloblast and divided the leukemias into a myelocytic and a lymphocytic type. Hirschfeld,[8] Di Guglielmo,[9] and Reschad and Schilling[10] described the granulocytic, erythroid, and monocytic leukemic variants, respectively.

The development of histochemical stains and cytogenetic, immunologic, molecular, and biochemical markers has helped to define further the lineage of the leukemic cell and to classify the leukemias. Effective therapy and advances in supportive care have resulted in dramatic changes in the approach to the patient with AML. The treatment and prognosis of patients with AML have changed from a disease that was formerly uniformly fatal to one that responds to chemotherapy and is potentially curable.

ETIOLOGY

AML accounts for approximately 1.2% of all cancer deaths in the United States, being responsible for an annual death rate of 2.2 per 100,000. The incidence increases with age and has remained remarkably steady since the late 1960s. In adults,

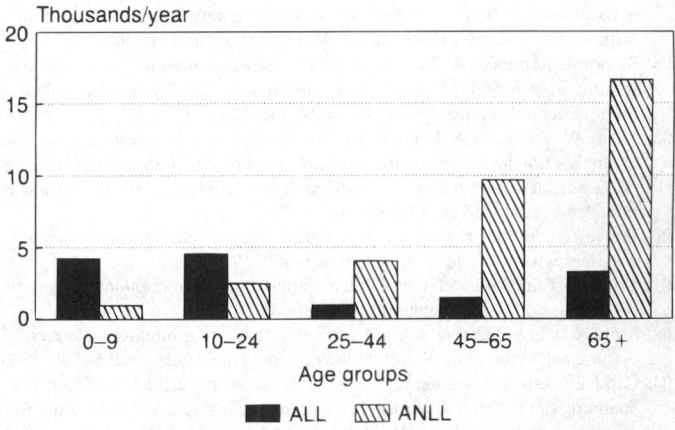

Fig. 64-1. Relative incidence of ALL versus AML (ANLL) in different age groups.

AML represents approximately 90% of all acute leukemias[11] (Fig. 64-1).

Genetic predisposition, drug and environmental exposure, and occupational factors have been implicated as possible leukemogenic agents in children and adults.[12] Current evidence suggests that leukemogenesis is a multistep process that requires the susceptibility of a hematopoietic progenitor cell to inductive agents at multiple stages. No one factor has been shown to cause leukemia in all exposed persons.

Evidence supporting a genetic predisposition for human leukemia has come from epidemiologic and family studies.[13] The incidence of AML is increased in eastern European Jews and decreased in Orientals.[13,14] Numerous reports of multiple cases of both acute lymphocytic leukemia (ALL) and AML occurring within the same family appear in the literature.[15] The concordance of each of the leukemia subtypes in families is also more common than could be expected on the basis of chance alone.[16-18] For all types, there is a threefold increase in leukemia incidence among first-degree relatives of patients with acute leukemia.[19]

Monozygotic twins show ≤25% concordance for childhood AML.[20,21] The clinical presentation of the AML in twins is atypical: the leukemia occurs at <2 years of age; it occurs in both twins in close succession, typically in the same year; and it is of the same morphologic and cytogenetic subtype.[22-24] The twin studies are compatible with a genetic or a nongenetic intrauterine postzygotic event that affects both twins simultaneously.[25-27] Moreover, no similar excess of leukemia has been observed in nonidentical twins of children with leukemia, and adult twin studies do not demonstrate such a high concordance for acute leukemia.[27,28] A possible explanation for these observations is that a single leukemogenic event occurring in utero leads to involvement of both twins, owing to the shared placental fetal circulation of monozygotic twins.[29]

The existence of a genetic predisposition for the development of AML is suggested by the increased leukemia incidence associated with a number of congenital disorders, including Down and Klinefelter syndromes.[30,31] In Down syndrome, the incidence of acute leukemia is 10 times that of the general population.[32-35] Moreover, families that have a Down syndrome child may have an overall higher incidence of acute leukemias in the genetically normal family members.[13,36] Parents of children with Down syndrome may also have an increased incidence of AML.[36-39] These reports of familial clustering of Down syndrome and leukemia have led to the speculations that a familial tendency to meiotic nondisjunction may be a risk factor for leukemia.[32] However, the familial association of Down syndrome and acute leukemia remains controversial.[40] In addition, the risk of childhood AML appears to increase with increasing maternal age, independent of the presence of Down syndrome.[41-43] Disorders associated with chromosomal instability and increased chromosome breakage, including Fanconi anemia, ataxia-telangiectasia, and Bloom syndrome, are associated with an increased incidence of AML.[44-46] The development of leukemia in these disorders appears to be a multistep process and not a single transforming event. The genetic disorders give rise to a cellular environment that results in chromosomal instability, a hypersensitivity to DNA damage, and an increased susceptibility to mutations.[47] Von Recklinghausen disease, congenital neurofibromatosis, is also associated with an increased incidence of childhood AML.[48]

Exposure to ionizing radiation and to a number of chemicals has been linked to the development of acute leukemia. The evidence linking radiation exposure and leukemia comes in part from the long-term follow-up of survivors of the atomic bomb explosions in Hiroshima and Nagasaki.[49-52] The latency time from exposure to the development of leukemia was 5–21 years, and the risk was related to age at exposure and to radiation dose.[49] The development of leukemia was predictable and dose related. In Hiroshima, there was a 30-fold increase in the incidence of both AML and chronic myeloid leukemia (CML). The highest rates were observed in persons <10 or >50 years at exposure. In utero exposure, however, was not associated with an increased risk of childhood leukemia.[50] In Nagasaki, where victims were exposed to a higher amount of γ-radiation, the incidence of AML was even greater.[51] All variants of AML, except the M3, acute promyelocytic leukemia (APL) subtype, were observed.[53]

Exposure to even moderate doses of radiotherapy appears to be associated with an increase risk of the development of AML. Workers at radium plants and military personnel who were exposed to ionizing radiation during nuclear test explosions have a higher-than-expected incidence of AML.[54,55] Patients who received low doses of radiation for benign disorders such as ankylosing spondylitis,[56,57] menorrhagia,[58] tinea capitis,[59] benign thymic enlargement,[60] and rheumatoid arthritis,[61] develop AML at a greater-than-expected rate. Exposure to thorotrast, a colloidal suspension of thorium dioxide used widely during the 1940s as a radiographic contrast medium, has been associated with an increased risk of AML, specifically the acute erythroleukemia subtype.[62,63] The principal thorium isotope is ^{232}Th which, on decay, exposes the individual to chronic low dose α-particles. The thorotrast-associated leukemia occurred 10–30 years after exposure.[62] The incidence of α-particle-induced AML after thorotrast exposure was related to the combined effects of the amount of thorotrast administered, the exposure time and the attained age of the individual.[62] Individuals living near high-intensity electrical wires have also been reported to have an increased incidence of acute leukemia, but this association remains controversial.[64,65] The incidence of AML is increased in workers with chronic magnetic and electrical field exposures; these include telegraph, telephone, and other communication equipment operators.[66,67] There appears to be an associated between the duration of electric field exposure and the risk of the subsequent development of AML.[68] Workers exposed to extremely low-frequency magnetic fields also have an increased incidence of AML.[69] Childhood leukemia had been linked to exposure to electromagnetic radiation associated with certain wiring configuration of a child's home.[70] These observations remain controversial; it is unclear from the reported case-control studies whether exposure to electromagnetic radiation generated from wiring and power lines is clinically or epidemiologically important.[71]

Chronic exposure to a number of chemicals has been associated with the development of acute leukemia.[72] Benzene is the best studied and has been the most widely used chemical leukemogenic agent.[72-75] Leather and rubber industry workers chronically exposed to benzene and to benzene derivatives have a significantly increased incidence of AML.[76] Case-control studies have found that truck drivers, filling station attendants, and painters have an increased incidence of AML, perhaps related to their chronic exposure to benzene and other hydrocarbons.[77,78] Persons exposed to embalming fluid, ethylene oxides, and herbicides also appear to be at increased risk of acute leukemia.[79-81] Workers exposed to organic solvents used in the processing of medical radiographs and the manufacturing of electrical wiring may have an increased incidence of AML.[82,83] Cigarette smokers and those chronically exposed to cigarette smoke appear to be at an increased risk of developing AML.[84-86] Heavy cigarette smoking is associated with the development of clonal, nonrandom, cytogenetic abnormalities.[87] Metabolites of benzene are found in the urine of chronic cigarette smokers.[88] Moreover, cigarette smoke contains measurable quantities of other known and suspected leukemogens and mutagens.[89,90]

An increased incidence of acute leukemia has been reported in patients who have received chemotherapy for a number of malignant and nonmalignant disorders. The nitrosoureas, the alkylating agents, and procarbazine appear to have the highest leukemogenic potential.[91-93] The development of AML after exposure to prior chemotherapy is usually preceded by a myelodysplastic syndrome.[94,95] All the commonly used alkylating agents, including cyclophosphamide, mechlorethamine, chlorambucil, busulfan, BCNU, and CCNU, have been associated with an increased risk of AML.[91] The combination of chemotherapy and radiotherapy further increases the risk of developing leukemia,[96] which is also proportional to the age of the patient and the cumulative dose of the administered alkylating agent. In Hodgkin disease, the cumulative risk of developing AML after treatment with alkylating agents increases steadily from 1 year after the start of treatment and reaches a peak of 13% at 7 years.[96,97] The post-treatment incidence of AML increases most markedly in the first 2 years and plateaus after 8–10 years[96,97]; this increase is related to the administration of a chemotherapy regimen that contains an alkylating agent. The incidence of AML in patients treated with the MOPP (mechlorethamine, vincristine [Oncovin] procarbazine, prednisone) regimen containing the alkylating agent mechlorethamine, is 3%, 4%, and 7% at 3, 5, and 7 years, respectively. This is in contrast to <1% incidence of treatment-related AML in patients treated with a nonalkylating containing regimen, or with radiotherapy alone.

An increased incidence of leukemia has been reported in patients receiving alkylating agents for small cell lung cancer,[98] ovarian cancer,[99] germ cell tumors,[100] breast cancer,[101] non-Hodgkin lymphoma,[102] chronic lymphocytic leukemia,[103] multiple myeloma,[104,105] polycythemia vera,[106] and other malignancies.[95] Patients with non-neoplastic disorders such as nephritis, rheumatoid arthritis, psoriasis, multiple sclerosis, systemic lupus erythematosus, and Wegener's granulomatosis who have received alkylating agents also have an increased incidence of AML.[107,108]

Therapy-related leukemias now represent 10–15% of all cases presenting with AML.[95] These treatment-related or so-called secondary leukemias are clinically and prognostically different from de novo AML. The secondary leukemias are frequently preceded by a variable period of anemia, neutropenia, or thrombocytopenia. Dysplastic changes can be found in all cell lines. Circulating platelets may be large, with abnormal granulation; neutrophils may be hypogranular or agranular with pseudo-Pelger-Huët nuclei; and the red cells may demonstrate coarse basophilic stippling with prominent anisocytosis. The bone marrow early in the course may demonstrate dysplastic changes characterized by megaloblastic erythroblasts, micromegakaryocytes, ringed sideroblasts, and an increased number of myeloblasts (5–25%) with abnormal maturation. These morphologic abnormalities may also be accompanied by functional defects. Platelet and neutrophil function may be markedly impaired, resulting in excess bleeding and recurrent infections despite an adequate number of circulating platelets and granulocytes. These findings in the peripheral blood and bone marrow may precede the development of overt AML by many months.[109] Clonal nonrandom cytogenetic abnormalities involving chromosomes 7, 5, and 8 occur in 50–90% of patients with therapy-related leukemia.[110,111] These leukemias are associated with an overall poor prognosis. Although some patients may attain a complete hematologic remission with intensive chemotherapy, these responses are usually of short duration.[110,112,113]

A clinically and cytogenetically distinct group of secondary leukemias has been reported in individuals who have received one of the topoisomerase II inhibitors. This group includes the epipodophyllotoxins, etoposide and teniposide, and the anthracyclines, daunomycin and doxorubicin. In contrast to alkylating agent-related AML, the topoisomerase II therapy-related leukemias typically lack a preceding myelodysplastic phase and are characterized by a shorter latency of onset.[114–116] Most reported patients have received combination therapy, including alkylating agents or radiotherapy, or both.[117,118] These topoisomerase II-related secondary leukemias are associated with chromosomal rearrangement involving chromosomes 11 and 21, characterized by a balanced translocation involving bands 11q23 and 21q22. Most patients developed morphologic M4 or M5 leukemias. The treatment outcome for these patients is much worse than for patients with de novo AML with these otherwise favorable cytogenetic abnormalities. In children with ALL, the incidence of secondary AML after exposure to one of the epipodophyllotoxins is approximately 5%.[117] However, in children treated for a T-cell ALL, the incidence of secondary AML approaches 19% after exposure to one of the topoisomerase II inhibitors.[117] Cytogenetic studies suggest that the second leukemogenic event occurs in a normal hematopoietic progenitor, and not in the initial leukemic clone. The outcome for these children with standard treatment remains poor. Topoisomerase II inhibitors have also been associated with the development of secondary acute promyelocytic leukemia, with the characteristic 15;17 translocation.[118] Whether the topoisomerase II inhibitors are leukemogenic by themselves or require the addition of other agents such as the prior or concomitant administration of alkylating agents or radiotherapy is unknown.

Drugs other than the cytotoxic agents reportedly associated with the development of acute leukemia include chloramphenicol,[119] phenylbutazone,[120] chloroquine,[121] methoxypsoralen,[122] and LSD.[123] The strength of such associations, however, remains unclear.

Certain acquired diseases are associated with transformation to AML. The myeloproliferative disorders, including polycythemia vera, primary thrombocythemia, and agnogenic myeloid metaplasia, are especially susceptible to such an event.[124–126] In polycythemia vera, the incidence of AML is approximately 1% for patients treated only with periodic phlebotomies; the addition of chemotherapy or radiotherapy significantly increases this incidence.[127–129] Moreover, the incidence of acute leukemia is related to the intensity and duration of alkylating agent therapy. The relative risk of AML was four times as great for those patients treated with daily continuous doses of an alkylating agent as for those treated by intermittent-pulse therapy.[128] A similar phenomenon has been observed in patients with multiple myeloma and Waldenström macroglobulinemia. Aplastic anemia is associated with the late development of acute leukemia.[130] In patients with aplastic anemia treated successfully with antithymocyte globulin, 26% developed AML or one of the myelodysplastic syndromes after 8 years. The risk of AML appears to be higher in patients with aplastic anemia after irradiation or chemical exposure.[130,131]

AML occurs in patients with paroxysmal nocturnal hemoglobinuria and appears to involve the same clone from which the abnormal erythrocytes are derived.[132] Multiple myeloma is associated with the development of AML.[133] The association between AML, multiple myeloma, and administration of multiple alkylating drugs is well documented, but AML can occur in patients with myeloma who have not received prior chemotherapy or radiotherapy.[134]

Primary nonseminomatous mediastinal germ cell tumors are associated with the development of AML.[135] The acute megakaryocytic leukemia (M7) subtype is a frequent type of AML after the occurrence of these germ cell tumors. This secondary leukemia appears associated with the primary disease and is unrelated to prior treatment of the germ cell neoplasm.

CLINICAL MANIFESTATIONS

The presenting signs and symptoms of AML are usually nonspecific and are related to the decreased production of normal hematopoietic cells and invasion of other organs by the leukemic cells. Patients usually complain of a brief virus-like illness characterized by fatigue and malaise or may present with a progressive skin infection after a minor abrasion. While anorexia is common, weight loss is unusual, generally reflecting the acute onset of the disease. Diffuse bone tenderness involving the long bones, ribs, and sternum is the initial clinical manifestation in 25% of patients. Joint pain and swelling, localized to the large joints, may antedate other symptoms by weeks. The bone pain, which can be severe, is caused by the expansion of the intramedullary space or direct involvement of the periosteum by the leukemic cells.

The findings on physical examination relate to the interference with normal hematopoiesis by the leukemic cells. Typically, all three cell lines are affected. Anemia results in pallor and the onset of cardiovascular symptoms. Thrombocytopenia produces hemostatic defects, which result in petechiae and ecchymosis. Oozing from the gums, epistaxis, and excess bleeding after dental procedures or minor trauma are common initial manifestations. Petechiae are most prominent in the lower extremities and may appear suddenly after minor physical activity or standing for prolonged periods. Splenomegaly occurs in ≤50% of patients with AML, but the splenic enlargement is usually modest and rarely extends >5 cm below the left costal margin. A very large spleen suggests that the leukemia has evolved from an underlying prior myeloproliferative disorder. Lymphadenopathy is rare in AML, in contrast to ALL, in which peripheral lymphadenopathy may be a prominent presenting finding. Involvement of the thymus or hilar nodes is very uncommon in AML. Skin involvement, leukemia cutis, occurs in about 10% of patients, usually presenting as violaceous, raised, nontender plaques or nodules,[136,137] which on biopsy are found to be infiltrated with myeloblasts (Plate 64-1). Skin involvement is more common with the monocytic subtypes, including the acute monocytic and myelomonocytic leukemias. Sweet syndrome, acute neutrophilic dermatosis, is a cutaneous paraneoplastic syndrome associated with AML.[138] It is characterized by tender red plaques and nodules, usually on the upper extremities, and may precede the diagnosis of AML by several months (Plate 64-2). The histologic finding in Sweet syndrome is a dense infiltrate composed primarily of mature neutrophils located predominantly in the mid- and upper dermis.[139] The pathogenesis of Sweet syndrome in AML is unknown. It has been postulated that leukemia-related growth substances or antigens may directly or indirectly stimulate epidermal or dermal cells.[140]

Chloromas, local collections of blasts, may present as isolated subcutaneous masses, hence the confusion with a primary or metastatic carcinoma.[137] Gingival hyperplasia due to leukemic infiltration is frequent in the monocytic leukemias (Plate 64-3). The patient may present initially to the dentist, complaining of painful gums, rapidly progressive gingival disease, and gum bleeding after dental brushing.

Central nervous system involvement in AML is an uncommon presenting finding, but 5–7% of all patients will have asymptomatic central nervous system involvement, as determined by positive cerebrospinal fluid cytology.[141] The finding of asymptomatic central nervous system disease does not alone appear to predict a poor prognosis.[142] Patients at highest risk of the development of central nervous system leukemia include those with a high circulating blast count, elevated lactate dehydrogenase (LDH) activity, and the presence of a monocytic leukemic subtype.[141,143] Of note is the very high frequency of central nervous system leukemia, ≤35%, in AML with increased eosinophils, the M4Eo variant, which is associated with an inversion of chromosome 16. Leptomeningeal leukemia and intracerebral myeloblastomas are common in this otherwise prognostically favorable subtype.[144] In the absence of signs of overt central nervous system involvement requiring therapy, it is preferable to defer a lumbar puncture until the peripheral blasts have been cleared with chemotherapy, to prevent the possibility of accidentally contaminating the spinal fluid with circulating leukemic cells.[145]

Most patients with leukemic involvement of the central nervous system are asymptomatic.[146] Some patients, however, present with meningeal signs and symptoms due to increased intracranial pressure. In these patients, a lumbar puncture is required, typically revealing an elevated opening pressure with an increased protein and a low glucose concentration in the cerebrospinal fluid. The cell count may be low, requiring a Millipore filter technique or cytocentrifuge preparation of the cerebrospinal fluid, to detect the presence of leukemic cells. Cranial nerve palsies secondary to leukemic infiltration of the nerve sheath are rare in AML. When they do occur, the fifth and seventh cranial nerves are most frequently involved.[147,148] Patients may present with a sudden onset of facial muscle weakness, rapidly progressing to paralysis. Optic nerve infiltration can result in papilledema and the sudden onset of unilateral blindness. Cranial nerve involvement can occur in the absence of overt central nervous system disease, therefore, the cerebrospinal fluid can be negative for leukemic cells in these cases.[146,148] A computed tomography (CT) or magnetic resonance imaging scan of the affected nerve root may demonstrate thickening of the nerve sheath, suggestive of leukemic involvement. To prevent permanent loss of cranial nerve function, the affected cranial nerve roots should be irradiated within 24 hours of the onset of symptoms. Patients presenting with neurologic findings and >50,000/mm³ circulating leukemic cells are at high risk of a major central nervous system event and require emergency intervention to rapidly lower the blast count.[149] The high number of circulating blasts increases the blood viscosity and is associated with small vessel leukoblastic emboli, resulting in leukostasis in the cerebral vessels (Fig. 64-2). The leukemic blasts can infiltrate the arteriolar endothelial walls and cause a secondary hemorrhage (Fig. 64-3). Suspected or developing central nervous system leukostasis requires emergency efforts to rapidly lower the blast count. Patients may complain of diffuse headaches and fatigue, which rapidly progress to confusion and coma. Leukostatic hemorrhage clinically resembles a major cerebrovascular accident. Despite most efforts to rapidly lower the WBC count and blood viscosity, the prognosis for patients with central nervous system leukostasis remains very poor.[150]

Metabolic and electrolyte derangements are common in patients with AML.[151] Hyperuricemia is the most frequent leukemia-related biochemical abnormality, resulting from increased turnover of the proliferating leukemic clone and subsequent purine catabolism. Hyperuricemia and hyperuricuria can de-

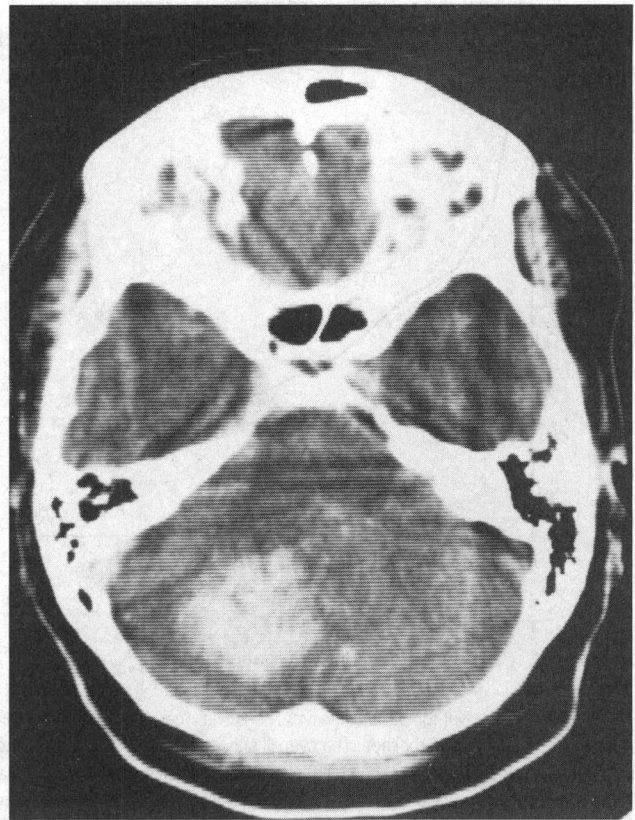

Fig. 64-2. Head CT scan of a patient with a presenting WBC count of 100,000/mm³ and a massive intracranial hemorrhage secondary to leukostasis.

velop before therapy is started. Typically, however, the uric acid level rises rapidly once therapy is initiated, owing to the release of intracellular nucleic acids by the lysis of large numbers of cells. Urate crystals can precipitate in the renal tubules and ureters, causing acute renal failure. To prevent the development of urate nephropathy, all patients should receive intravenous hydration and should be started on allopurinol before beginning chemotherapy. By inhibiting xanthine oxidase, allopurinol causes an increase in the urine xanthine and can produce xanthine crystalluria and calculi.[152] Therefore, it is important to maintain adequate hydration in addition to administering allopurinol both before and during induction chemotherapy. Rarely, leukemic cells produce an obstructive uropathy as a result of direct infiltration of the prostate gland.[153] Direct kidney involvement in AML, in contrast to ALL, is uncommon. Hyperkalemia may occur as a result of rapid cell breakdown,[154] but hypokalemia is more common.[155] The hypokalemia can be profound, requiring large doses of intravenous potassium. It is most pronounced in the myelomonocytic and monocytic leukemias, in which intracellular levels of the lysozyme, muramidase, which is toxic to renal tubular cells are high.[156–158] Ineffective myelopoiesis or destruction of the leukemic cells with therapy causes the release of large amounts of this enzyme, which produces a proximal renal tubular dysfunction and leads to renal potassium wasting. In most cases, however, muramidase-induced tubular damage is not the sole mechanism of the hypokalemia.[159] Attempts to correlate the elevated serum and urinary muramidase lysozyme level directly with the leukemic subtype and the development of hypokalemia and the renal tubular defect have produced conflicting results.[158,160] Antibiotics and chemotherapy-induced nephropathy, diarrhea, vomiting, and the development of hypomagnesemia all contribute to the development of potentially life-

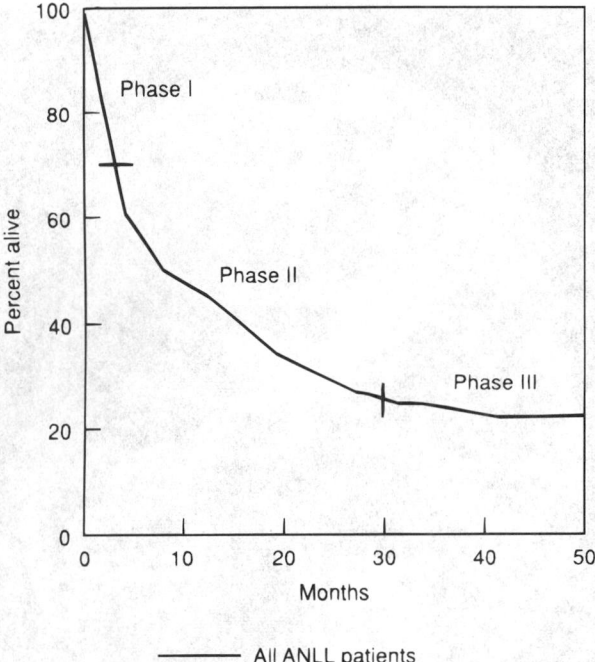

Fig. 64-3. Overall survival for patients with AML (ANLL) can be divided into three phases. Phase I is induction therapy. The overall survival during this phase reflects the complete remission rate and the ability of the patient to tolerate chemotherapy and prolonged neutropenia and thrombocytopenia. Most patients who fail to respond die of infections or hemorrhage. True resistant disease accounts for <15% of induction failures. The complete response rate is approximately 60–80%. Phase II is the first 2 years after attainment of complete remission. Most patients in complete remission will relapse and die of their leukemia in these first 2 years. While much of the attention in therapy for acute leukemia has focused on the first phase—surviving induction therapy and attaining complete remission—as this curve suggests, most patients fail after attaining complete remission. This reflects occult disease not recognized at the time of complete remission. In an effort to prolong this phase, multiple studies are addressing the use of post-induction consolidation and maintenance therapy. Treatment of minimal residual disease remains a controversial area of investigation. Phase III begins 2 years after complete remission is attained. Patients in remission for >2 years have a markedly increased chance of prolonged survival; 75–80% of patients in complete remission at 2 years will have a prolonged disease-free survival. However, the curve of this phase is not flat, and patients continue to relapse 3–10 years after attaining complete remission. The biologic factors responsible for these late relapses are unknown and may reflect one or more of the etiologic events in the development of AML.

threatening hypokalemia during and before induction therapy for AML.[160]

Hypercalcemia has been reported in association with AML.[161] The mechanism is unclear, but may be related to the release of parathyrin or parathyrin-like fragments produced by the leukemic cells.[162] In these instances, the blood calcium level parallels the activity of the disease. Hypocalcemia, presumably due to release by the leukemic cells of factors that result in accelerated bone formation, has been reported. The hypocalcemia can be profound, and patients can present with tetany and potentially fatal cardiac arrhythmias.[163] The hyperphosphatemia and hyperphosphaturia associated with underlying renal insufficiency can also contribute to the hypocalcemia.

The rapid lysis of leukemic cells can acutely precipitate a number of serious metabolic problems caused by the release of intracellular phosphate, potassium, and urate.[164] This so-called tumor lysis syndrome is characterized by the rapid development of hyperuricemia, hyperkalemia, hyperphospha-

temia, and hypocalcemia.[165] The consequences of tumor lysis syndrome are directly related to the metabolic abnormalities: the hyperuricemia produces a urate nephropathy and acute renal failure; the hyperkalemia is associated with potentially lethal cardiac arrhythmias; and the hyperphosphatemia causes a reciprocal depression of the serum calcium and progressive renal insufficiency, with further reduction of the excretion of potassium and phosphate. The hypocalcemia, a result of the hyperphosphatemia, can cause tetany, cardiac arrhythmias, and muscle cramps. The tumor lysis syndrome occurs in patients with a rapidly rising or very high blast count.[166–168] It is important to recognize those patients at risk of this syndrome and to address and correct metabolic and electrolyte abnormalities before starting therapy. Allopurinol and intravenous hydration should be started early, before beginning chemotherapy. Serum electrolytes, including potassium, calcium, phosphate, and uric acid, and renal function should be carefully monitored. Renal function can rapidly deteriorate, and patients should be monitored daily to correct developing electrolyte abnormalities. Dialysis may be required and should be considered early in the course to prevent the complications of rapidly rising serum potassium, phosphate, and uric acid.[169,170] In many patients, recovery of renal function after tumor lysis occurs early, and patients can be supported through the relatively brief period of renal insufficiency.[171,172] With careful attention to electrolytes and the use of intensive hydration, the tumor lysis syndrome remains a rare complication in the treatment of AML. In most patients with AML, the development of renal insufficiency is associated with acute tubular necrosis, sepsis, and the use of nephrotoxic drugs.[170] The use of nephrotoxic antibiotics and other medications is a frequent contributing factor for the development of renal failure during induction therapy. Many of the renal complications of AML and its treatment can be prevented with close attention to the medications given and the fluid status of the patient.[170]

Lactic acidosis has been associated with AML.[173] The etiology of this metabolic acidosis may result from anaerobic glycolysis by the leukemia cells. Lactic acidosis is usually associated with a very high blast count, extramedullary disease, and leukostasis. Lactic acidosis parallels the disease activity in these cases.[174]

Hypocholesteremia and a reduction in total low-density lipoproteins in the plasma are frequently noted in untreated patients with AML.[175] The mechanism of the reduced lipoproteins is unclear but may involve the leukemic cell's use of cholesterol for membrane synthesis. Alternatively, the leukemic cells may secrete growth factors associated with changes in the concentration of cholesterol.[176]

A spuriously low serum glucose level and arterial oxygen saturation can occur in the presence of high numbers of circulating blasts.[177] These spuriously low values reflect utilization by the leukemic blasts of the glucose and oxygen, typically reflecting a delay in processing the test sample. Spurious hyperkalemia may result from potassium release in vitro by lysed leukemic cells. Again, this phenomenon is more common in patients with a high blast count. If a spuriously elevated potassium is suspected, the serum electrolyte studies should be repeated with an anticoagulated blood sample to prevent the in vitro lysis of leukemic blasts.[178]

Ophthalmic problems occur in patients with AML.[179] All portions of the eye may be involved, including the optic nerve, choroid, and retina. Chloromas, a collection of blasts, can occur anywhere in the eye. Leukemia can involve the optic disc and optic nerve, resulting in the sudden onset of blurred vision, which can rapidly progress to total blindness.[180] This diagnosis should be suspected when the funduscopic examination reveals papilledema and disc pallor. Iritis may present with photophobia, excess lacrimation, and orbital pain. Ophthalmic involvement is very suggestive of meningeal leukemia.

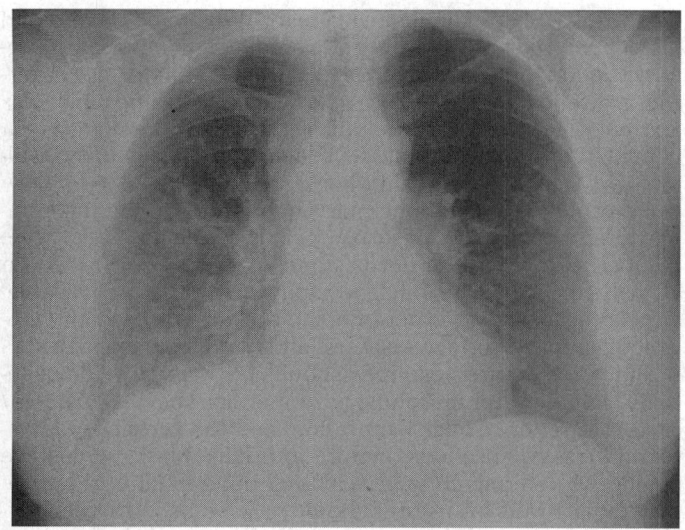

Fig. 64-4. Plumonary leukostasis in a patient with monoblastic leukemia and a presenting WBC count of 150,000/mm³.

Ophthalmic involvement can occur in all the leukemic subtypes and is associated with a higher relapse rate and shorter survival as compared to patients without eye involvement.[181]

Cardiorespiratory symptoms are common in patients with acute leukemia, pneumonias being the most common pulmonary problems. At presentation, gram-positive and gram-negative bacteria are the major pathogens. However, patients who have a history of prolonged neutropenia or abnormal neutrophil function or who are receiving broad-spectrum antibiotics are at an increased risk of pulmonary infection with fungi or other opportunistic organisms. Pulmonary leukostasis is a serious potential problem for patients who present with a blast count of >50,000/mm³.[182,183] In this setting, leukocyte thrombi and plugging of pulmonary microvascular channels lead to vascular rupture and infiltration of the lung parenchyma. Patients may note the sudden onset of shortness of breath and progressive dyspnea; on physical examination, they are tachypneic, with diffuse bilateral rales. The chest radiograph usually demonstrates a diffuse interstitial infiltrate (Fig. 64-4). Fever is common. Hypercapnia, hypoxemia, and progressive respiratory acidosis are signs of a very poor prognosis, despite intensive efforts to rapidly lower the blast count and institution of ventilatory support. Pulmonary leukostasis and the hyperleukocytosis syndrome are more common in patients with one of the monocytic subtypes and the microgranular variant of APL.[183]

Pulmonary hemorrhage and leukostasis may mimic the signs and symptoms of a bacterial or fungal pneumonia. Pulmonary hemorrhage may be diffuse, involving both lungs, or localized to a single segment or lobe. Patients typically complain of the sudden onset of shortness of breath. Hemoptysis may occur, and hypoxemia and hypercapnia are common. The presentation may be similar to other forms of noncardiogenic pulmonary edema.[184] The physical examination may indicate little by way of objective pulmonary findings, while the chest radiograph typically reveals an interstitial pattern in the area of the hemorrhage. The treatment of suspected pulmonary hemorrhage should be directed at correcting the underlying coagulopathy.

Cardiovascular abnormalities are usually due to derangements in metabolic, electrolyte, and pulmonary function. Leukemic infiltration of the heart or great vessels is rare, but there are reports of leukemic involvement of the conduction system, pericardium, and myocardium,[185] as well as involvement of the arterial endothelial wall with monoblasts and subsequent formation and rupture of an aortic aneurysm.[186] Chemotherapy-related toxicities produce most the cardiovascular problems in patients with AML. The cardiac toxicity of the anthracyclines is dose related; these agents act synergistically with other cardiotoxic agents. Cardiac function should be assessed before beginning therapy. The left and right ventricle ejection fractions should be measured in all patients who have received a known cardiotoxic drug or who have a prior history of cardiac disease, before they are given an anthracycline. A echocardiogram may be more helpful in assessing wall motion abnormalities than a ejection fraction. A pretherapy "baseline" ejection fraction, or echocardiogram is not, however, warranted for all patients before starting induction therapy. Unless the patient has a known or suspected cardiac disease that would alter the chemotherapy regimen, treatment need not be delayed pending the result of ejection fraction.

Gastrointestinal abnormalities are frequent in AML patients. Dysphagia is common and is usually due to oral or pharyngeal infections, mucosal involvement with leukemia, or chemotherapy-induced mucositis. Oral candidiasis is a common presenting finding that may involve the tongue or the soft or hard palate, or both. Esophageal candidiasis can produce substernal pain and a mid-epigastric burning sensation and dysphagia is common with oral and esophageal candidiasis. These symptoms may be severe, interfering with the patient's ability to eat and to take oral medication. A barium swallow is usually sufficient to confirm the diagnosis of Candida esophagitis. For patients who fail treatment, for atypical cases, or for cases in which the barium swallow is not diagnostic, an upper endoscopy is helpful. It is important to obtain a culture at endoscopy. The clinical appearance of the lesions may be deceiving, and mixed fungal and viral infections are common.[187,188] Candida infections can obscure an underlying herpes simplex virus (HSV) or cytomegalovirus infection, and HSV re-activation frequently occurs during therapy for AML. Viral lesions may be atypical, and superinfection with bacteria or fungi is common. Viral cultures for HSV should be obtained for all atypical lesions in and around the oral cavity. Serologic viral studies are usually not helpful, since most patients (>80%) will have had prior exposure to HSV and will have a positive serology. Patients with microbiologic documented or clinically suspected HSV infection should be treated with acyclovir while undergoing induction therapy. Gingival involvement can occur in any of the myeloid subtypes. Gingival hypertrophy is most frequent in the well-differentiated monocytic types. Small bowel involvement in AML is rare, but chloromas or granulocytic sarcomas can form in the small intestine, producing obstructive symptoms.[189,190]

In patients with leukemia, the anal and perirectal areas are important potential sources for infection, the first signs of which may be induration and tenderness in the perirectal area without other signs of inflammation or infection. Patients may initially complain only of pain on defecation and of diffuse anal tenderness. It is of the utmost importance to recognize and treat these potential sources of infection early. Perirectal abscesses are usually due to gram-negative bacteria and, in the setting of granulocytopenia, can rapidly progress to perirectal cellulitis and septicemia. While digital rectal examination is generally avoided in patients who are granulocytopenic, the perirectal area should be carefully and gently examined.

Patients should be instructed on the importance of perirectal hygiene. Constipation should be avoided in order to prevent small mucosal tears. Diarrhea and drugs or agents that cause diarrhea should be carefully monitored. The need for laxatives or agents that cause prolonged diarrhea should be avoided. The use of contrast agents that are cathartics must be critically evaluated before their use. Hemorrhoids must be closely followed and treated early. The perirectal and oral areas are important portals for infection; patients should be instructed on how to perform daily oral and perirectal care.

Typhlitis, a fulminant necrotizing colitis related to granulocytopenia and cytotoxic therapy, occurs in ≤10% of patients with leukemia who are undergoing intensive therapy.[191] This entity may present a diagnostic and therapeutic dilemma. Patients present with the sudden onset of abdominal pain, fever, and a distended and tense abdomen. Bowel sounds are decreased, and abdominal radiographs are nonspecific, usually revealing an incomplete small bowel obstruction, a questionable right lower quadrant mass, pneumatosis, or no appreciable abnormality. CT scanning frequently demonstrates an edematous right colon with spiculation of the pericolic fat and subcutaneous edema. The clinical presentation frequently mimics that of acute appendicitis. The diagnosis is usually made on clinical and CT scan findings in the febrile neutropenic patient who has recently received chemotherapy.

Treatment of typhlitis is controversial, and for many patients the prognosis is poor.[192,193] Medical management includes nasogastric suction with bowel rest, broad-spectrum antibiotics directed at bowel pathogens, intravenous fluid replacement, total parental nutrition, and transfusion support. Surgical intervention, usually a hemicolectomy, should be reserved for patients with localized peritoneal signs or clear evidence of perforation and for those who do not respond to medical therapy. Although patients with AML who are neutropenic and thrombocytopenic can tolerate an exploratory laparotomy, postoperative management of these patients is difficult. The morbidity and mortality of surgery must be carefully weighed against the risk of medical therapy in the individual patient. Most of these patients can be managed medically with intensive support, and only a few patients will require surgical intervention.

DIAGNOSIS

The diagnosis of acute leukemia is usually apparent after examining the patient and reviewing the peripheral smear. Most patients present with pancytopenia and circulating blast forms, which are apparent on the peripheral blood smear. The total WBC count may be within the range of $<1,000/mm^3$ to $>200,000/mm^3$, with most patients having a total WBC count of $5,000–30,000/mm^3$. The peripheral blood smear is usually sufficient to make the diagnosis of AML, but in the 10% of patients who present with only with a modest thrombocytopenia, low-grade anemia, and a normal WBC count without circulating immature cells, bone marrow aspiration is required to make the diagnosis. The bone marrow aspiration and biopsy should be performed when the necessary pretherapy studies can be obtained. While many patients and physicians feel compelled to start treatment for AML immediately, emergency therapy is not needed in most instances. Treatment can usually be delayed until the necessary clinical and laboratory evaluations are available. Patients may also need time to accept the diagnosis and address personal, financial, and family needs. As part of the initial evaluation, the psychological and emotional needs and concerns of patients and their families must be considered. Moreover, prior medical and dental problems and intercurrent illnesses need to be evaluated or treated before starting induction chemotherapy.

Even in the severely neutropenic and thrombocytopenic patient, a bone marrow biopsy and aspiration can be safely performed. Local bleeding or infection at the site of the procedure is very rare. The posterior iliac crest is the preferred site, unless the patient has received prior radiotherapy to the pelvis or has evidence of an active infection at the site. The sternum is an alternate site for performing a bone marrow aspirate. Marrow biopsies cannot be performed through the sternal route.

Bone marrow smears from the aspirate and touch preparations from the biopsy should be prepared at the bedside for best results. Slides should be made for Wright and Giemsa and histochemical stains. Cytogenetic studies are important prognostic indicators and should be performed at initial bone marrow aspiration and biopsy. Cell-surface markers and molecular and enzyme studies are helpful if there is a possibility of a lymphoid or a biphenotypic leukemia. The bone marrow aspirate provides for the qualitative assessment of bone marrow cell morphology. The bone marrow biopsy permits quantitative assessment of bone marrow cellularity,[194] megakaryocyte number, and reticulum fibrosis and should be performed on all patients. When insufficient aspirate material is available, circulating blasts in the peripheral blood may be used for cytogenetic studies, surface markers, and histochemical stains.

The bone marrow aspirate should be evaluated for cellularity, number and morphology of megakaryocytes, myeloid/erythroid ratio, cellular maturation, and the presence of dysplasia or asynchronous maturation. The blast percentage should be determined with ≥200-cell differential of the bone marrow aspirate. Iron stores should be assessed with the Prussian blue stain and the presence or absence of ringed sideroblasts specifically noted. Evaluation of the cellularity of a bone marrow aspirate is a qualitative assessment that may reflect the number of spicules obtained, slide preparation technique, and volume of diluting blood. Despite these limitations, a number of criteria have been adopted by cooperative groups to evaluate the cellularity of a bone marrow aspirate. Changes in cellularity during therapy are important for evaluating the response to chemotherapy.[195] Marrow aspirate cellularity is grouped into five broad categories from 0 to +4: aplastic, hypocellular, normal cellular, hypercellular, and intensely hypercellular.

The initial bone marrow in a patient with AML is typically hypercellular, with absent or decreased megakaryocytes. However, patients who develop secondary or treatment-related AML may have a normal cellular or hypocellular marrow. The bone marrow aspirate is usually replaced by leukemic cells, which constitute >30% of the marrow nucleated cells. Abnormalities of myeloid and erythroid maturation, with bizarre and asynchronous granulation of the myeloid precursors, are common. Auer bodies or rods, which are reddish rod-like filaments of aggregated lysosomes, may be present in the leukemic cells. These bodies, or rods, first described by Joseph Auer, are derived from incorporation of primary azurophilic granules into autophagic vacuoles. The term φ bodies has also been used to describe small spindle-shaped Auer bodies, and single cells containing multiple Auer bodies are sometimes referred to as faggot cells (from the term meaning "bundle of sticks"). Auer rods are faintly birefringent in polarized light. Ultrastructurally, they have a defined three-dimensional crystal structure with a characteristic 6–13-nm periodicity, which is different for each of the leukemic subtypes.[196] Auer rods have been considered virtually pathognomonic of AML. The French-American-British (FAB) Cooperative Group, however, does not place this degree of importance to the Auer rods and, in fact, includes the presence of Auer rods as part of the definition of one of the myelodysplastic syndrome, which it terms refractory anemia with excess blasts in transformation.[197,198] Auer rods should therefore not be considered unequivocal evidence of AML but as a manifestation of a malignant myeloid disorder with abnormal maturation. Auer rods are found in approximately 50% of newly diagnosed patients with AML and are found most frequently in the M1 and M2 subtypes.[199] The remission rate and duration of remission may be higher in patients in whom the leukemic cells demonstrate Auer rods.[199]

The diagnosis of acute leukemia is made when ≥30% of either total nucleated cells or nonerythroid cells in the bone marrow are blast forms. This includes type I and type II blasts. The determination of the number of blasts in the bone marrow is crucial, and the distinction between a blast and a promyelocyte can be difficult. The FAB Cooperative Group has recognized two types of myeloblasts.[200] The type I blast lacks granules and has uncondensed chromatin, a high nucleocytoplasmic ratio, and prominent nucleoli. The type II blasts are similar to the type I blasts except for the presence of a few azurophilic granules and a lower nucleocytoplasmic ratio. These type II blasts can be confused with promyelocytes. Myeloid precursors are classified as promyelocytes when they develop a eccentric nucleus, a defined clear Golgi zone, cytoplasmic granules, and a low nuclear/cytoplasmic ratio. The nucleus has nucleoli, and the cytoplasm remains basophilic. In a patient with acute leukemia, the most important initial morphologic evaluation is to distinguish between ALL, one of the myelodysplastic syndromes (MDSs), and AML. The prognosis and therapeutic strategies remain very different for adults with these disorders. In most cases, the morphologic evaluation and histochemical stains will define the appropriate lineage. It may, however, be difficult to differentiate between an MDS, refractory anemia with excess blasts in transformation, and AML. The MDSs are most frequently confused with the M6 variant, acute erythroleukemia, or a hypoplastic AML.[201] In cases in which the nucleated erythroid cells constitute >50% of all bone marrow nucleated marrow cells, the diagnosis may be difficult. In these cases, if the combined total of all blasts, type I and II, is <30%, the case is classified as a MDS.[198] If the nucleated red cells comprise <50% of bone marrow cells, the percentage of blasts is calculated as the percentage of all nucleated cells. In many cases, the difference between one of the MDSs and AML can present a difficult diagnostic problem. Cytogenetic studies may help define specific abnormalities associated with AML or MDS. In some cases, the morphologic distinction between an undifferentiated myeloid leukemia and a lymphocytic leukemia can be difficult. The AMLs with no or minimal differentiation, the monoblastic leukemias without differentiation, and some of the acute megakaryocytic leukemias can be difficult to differentiate from ALL on the basis of morphology or histochemical stains alone. In these instances, the use of monoclonal antibody markers for lineage-associated markers is important. When the blasts demonstrate <3% positivity with either myeloperoxidase or Sudan black stain, immunologic markers are needed to define the lineage of the leukemia. In most cases of acute leukemia, morphology and histochemistry are sufficient to assign the correct lineage. In approximately 15% of cases, however, the distinction between an immature AML variant and ALL cannot be made morphologically. The use of monoclonal antibodies that identify myeloid and lymphoid-associated antigens is very useful in these cases[202,203] (Table 64-1). A number of monoclonal antibodies have been generated that react with specific antigens expressed on the surface of normal and leukemic myeloid and lymphoid cells. To identify AML, the percentage of positive-reacting blasts should be >20% with one or more of the myeloid associated antigens: CD33 or CD14. The blasts should also be negative for the lymphoid-associated antigens, including the common ALL antigen, CD10 (CALLA), and CD19.[204,205] The determination of cellular terminal deoxynucleotidyltransferase (TdT) activity, in combination with

other markers of lymphoid differentiation, may be useful in selected cases.[206] However, TdT activity is not lineage specific and can be found in low levels in 15–50% of myeloblasts.[207]

In ALL, the immunologic markers are important in assigning cell lineage, in defining specific leukemic subsets, and in assessing prognosis. In AML, biochemical and immunologic markers have been less widely applied. The expression of these antigens corresponds to the normal stages of myeloid and monocytic differentiation. None of the available myeloid monoclonal antibodies identifies leukemia-specific determinants.

The monoclonal antibodies have been useful tools for defining the maturation and differentiation of normal myeloid and monocytic precursors.[208] However, leukemic cells frequently express markers of multiple levels of maturation and different lineages. Therefore, unlike morphologic classifications that attempt to place the predominant cell type within a specific defined group, surface marker studies have demonstrated that AML cells are antigenically and morphologically heterogeneous.[209,210] Surface markers have been most useful in distinguishing between AML and lymphoid leukemias and in defining hybrid or biphenotypic leukemias. Immunologic studies appear to define functionally and prognostically relevant subgroups unrelated to both morphology and histochemistry.[209] While a number of the individual antibodies correlate well with the morphologic classification, as in the expression of CD34 with M1 and M3 and of CD14 (MY4) in the M4 and M5 subtypes, overall the expression of surface antigens does not entirely agree with either morphology or histochemical staining.[209–212] The use of multiple monoclonal antibodies has identified certain phenotypic groups that may be clinically important, such as the association of the M2 subtype a t(8;21) cytogenetic abnormality and the expression of CD34 and the B-cell antigen CD19.[213] The use of monoclonal markers has demonstrated that most myeloid blast cells express differentiation markers asynchronously and that the unusual co-expression of normal differentiation antigens is common.[207] Moreover, myeloid blasts frequently express lymphoid-associated antigens. A meaningful proportion (20–40%) of myeloid blasts express lymphoid-associated antigens, most frequently CD2 and CD19. The CD2 antigen, known as the sheep erythrocyte receptor, which is found on mature T cells, is expressed on approximately 20% of myeloid leukemias. CD19, found on B cells, is frequently noted in association with the 8;21 translocation and is found in ≤34% of newly diagnosed myeloid leukemias.[213,214] The myeloid blasts cells frequently express both myeloid and lymphoid differentiation antigens. The prognostic significance of this phenotypic heterogeneity is unclear but is not associated with a uniformly adverse prognosis.[209–211,214] The use of surface markers in the diagnosis of AML is most appropriate for the evaluation of morphologically atypical or undifferentiated leukemias or suspected hybrid leukemias. The AML with minimal differentiation (M0) and the megakaryocytic leukemia (M7) require the use of monoclonal antibodies for diagnosis.[215] The use of surface marker analysis has demonstrated the phenotypic heterogeneity and mixed lineage heritage of many myeloid leukemias[216] (Table 64-2).

HISTOCHEMICAL STAINS USEFUL IN THE EVALUATION OF AML

The acute leukemias are classified according to the predominant neoplastic cell type. The FAB Cooperative Group in 1976 introduced a classification system for the AML subtypes[217] and periodically updates its recommendations and reviews diagnostic criteria. The recommendations of the FAB group have gained wide acceptance and are now used by most cooperative groups, cancer centers, and international workshops involved in clinical trials and studies of AML.

Table 64-1. Monoclonal Antibodies Commonly Used to Distinguish AML from ALL

AML	ALL
CD11 (anti Mo1)	CD10 (CALLA)
CD13 (MY7)	CD2 (T11, Leu 5)
CD14 (MY4)	CD4 (T4, Leu 3)
CD15	CD5 (Leu 1)
CD33 (MY 9)	CD3 (T8, Leu 2)
CD41 (platelet glycoprotein IIb/IIIa)	CD19 (anti B4)
	CD20 (anti B1)

Table 64-2. Immunophenotypic Markers in AML

AML Subtype	CD11	CD13	CD14	CD15	CD33	CD34	CD41	CD42b	HLA-DR	TdT	CD7
M0	−	+	−	−	+	+	−	−	−	+	±
M1	−	±	−	−	+	+	−	−	+	±	±
M2	+	+	±	+	+	−	−	−	+	−	−
M3	+	+	−	±	+	−	−	−	−	−	−
M4	+	+	+	+	+	−	−	−	+	−	−
M5	+	+	+	±	+	−	−	−	+	−	−
M6	−	−	−	−	−	−	−	−	−	−	−
M7	−	−	−	−	±	±	+	+	−	−	−

The FAB group has divided the myeloid leukemias into eight broad categories based on the morphology, cytochemical staining, and immunologic phenotype of the predominant cell type (Table 64-3 and Plates 64-4 through 64-14). While this classification system was initially proposed solely to define the subtypes of the acute leukemias morphologically, it has subsequently expanded to include ultrastructural morphology, cytochemistry, and immunologic markers. This classification system been shown to be both clinically and prognostically useful. The FAB criteria are based on a Wright-stained peripheral blood smear and on examination of the bone marrow aspirate or biopsy. Four basic histochemical stains are required, including periodic acid-Schiff (PAS) reagent, Sudan black, peroxidase, and esterase (specific and nonspecific).

PAS stains carbohydrates, including monosaccharides, polysaccharides, mucoproteins, and phosphorylated sugars. Myeloblasts are PAS negative, while most lymphoblasts are PAS positive with a distinctive pattern. PAS-positive lymphoblasts usually demonstrate several concentric rings of coarse granules or heavy "blocks" against a negative cytoplasmic background. Since not all lymphoblasts on a bone marrow sample stain with PAS, it is the pattern of the staining, rather than the number of positive cells, that suggests the diagnosis of ALL. Promyelocytes show a faint diffuse PAS-positive tinge, often with fine cytoplasmic granules, Auer rods are usually negative, and monoblasts stain variably with PAS. Immature monoblasts are usually PAS negative, while more differentiated monoblasts and monocytes may react, as do normal mature monocytes, with a diffuse reddish background superimposed on fine or coarse granules. Erythroblasts generally demonstrate strong PAS positivity, with a diffusely coarse granular reaction. Maturing erythrocytes may also show heavy PAS positivity, with concentric annular rings of moderately coarse cytoplasmic granules. Megakaryoblasts stain variably with PAS; the mature megakaryocyte is positive, but the megakaryoblast may be negative; therefore, the PAS stain is not a reliable marker for identification of this subtype. The PAS stain is most useful for differentiating a lymphoid from a nonlymphoid leukemia and is less helpful in defining the AML subtype.

Sudan black B is a lipophilic dye, which stains phospholipids and lipoprotein complexes. The Sudan black staining pattern is similar to the profile of the peroxidase reactivity, but the reaction is usually more strongly positive in myeloblasts and shows a different distribution from the peroxidase reaction in monocytes and monoblasts. Myeloblasts, promyelocytes, and myelomonoblasts are positive, while erythroid, megakaryocyte, and lymphoid precursors are negative. Myeloblasts are usually positive, with coarse heavy granules. Myeloblasts without azurophilic or specific granules on Wright stains may stain with Sudan black, and the myelomonocytic leukemias demonstrate both coarse and fine granules. Pure monoblasts are usually Sudan black negative. Auer rods stain prominently with Sudan black even when not apparent on the standard Wright preparation. In general, the Sudan black B stain represent a sensitive marker of myeloblasts and myelomonocytes. It is most helpful in differentiating immature cells that appear undifferentiated on smear, characterized by a negative peroxidase reaction.

The esterase stains are biochemically complex and are based on the reaction of a specific substrate with a cellular enzyme. This nomenclature is confusing and depends on the substrate used. In hematopoietic cells, nine esterase isoenzymes have been identified, all of which cleave the α-naphthylacetate or α-naphthylbutyrate substrate; this activity is referred to as nonspecific esterase activity. The substrate in the chloracetate esterase stains is the chloroacetate of α-naphthol or naphthol AS, which react with enzymes in the myeloid series at all stages of maturation; the reaction therefore is referred to as a specific esterase reaction.

The chloracetate esterase reaction gives sharply localized granular staining in the cytoplasm of nearly all granulocytes. The reactivity of this stain increases with cell maturity, and myeloblasts without granules are esterase negative. Thus, this reaction is less sensitive than the peroxidase or Sudan black stain for the diagnosis of AML without maturation (M1). The chloroacetate stain is intensively positive in promyelocytic leukemia (M3), but monoblasts, lymphoblasts, erythroblasts, megakaryocytes, eosinophils, basophils, and monocytes are chloroacetate esterase negative.

Table 64-3. Prognostic Factors in AML

Factor	Favorable	Unfavorable
Clinical		
Age	<40 years	>60 years
Leukemia	De novo	Secondary
WBC count	<10,000/Mm³	>100,000/mm³
DIC	Absent	Present
LDH	Normal	High
Serum albumin	Normal	Low
FAB type	M3, M4Eo	M0, M5a, M5b, M6, M7
Cytogenetics	t(15;17), inv16, t(8;21) normal	5q−, 7, +8
Auer rods	Present	Absent
In vitro		
Clonogenic assay	Normal growth	Autonomous growth
ara-C triphosphate retention	High	Low
Labeling index	High	Low
Bone marrow		
Fibrosis	Absent	Present
Cytoreduction	Rapid	Slow
Courses to complete remission	Single	Multiple
Pronormoblasts	Rare	Many
Eosinophils	Present	Absent

The nonspecific esterase stain has a markedly different spectrum of reactivity; the naphthylacetate and -butyrate reactions are largely confined to cells of the monocytic lineage, including monoblasts and monocytes. Monocytes contain two isoenzymes that react strongly with the nonspecific esterase substrate but are dramatically inhibited by addition of sodium fluoride. Therefore, a positive esterase activity inhibited by sodium fluoride is characteristic of monocytic differentiation. The two subclasses of the monocytic leukemias, the M5a undifferentiated and the M5b differentiated types, react with the nonspecific esterase stain. Neutrophil precursors and B lymphocytes are nonspecific esterase negative; other cells may show varying patterns of positivity not inhibited by sodium fluoride. Some T-cell lymphocytic leukemias may show a granular nonspecific esterase activity that is resistant to fluoride inhibition. The nonspecific esterase reaction aids in recognizing a monocytic component to the leukemia.

In the myeloid leukemias, the specific esterase stain is positive and the nonspecific esterase is negative. Auer rods are positive with the specific esterase. In myelomonocytic leukemia, ≥20% of the cells must show monocytic differentiation that is nonspecific esterase positive and inhibited by sodium fluoride. In this type of leukemia, both activities may be present in the same cell. In the pure monocytic leukemias, 80–100% of the blasts are nonspecific esterase positive and specific esterase negative. Therefore, the esterase stains are particularly useful in distinguishing an undifferentiated monocytic leukemia (M5b) from undifferentiated myeloid (M1, M0) or lymphoid leukemias.

SUBTYPES OF ACUTE MYELOID LEUKEMIA

The FAB group has defined eight subtypes of AML (Table 64-2 and Plates 64-4 through 64-14) on the basis of morphologic, immunologic, and cytochemical criteria. The FAB group's purpose was to subdivide the myeloid leukemias according to their predominant cell type and to define the leukemic cell's position in the maturation sequence of that specific lineage. The classification attempts to assign a single lineage to each leukemia, but this process is difficult at times because many cases demonstrate some admixture of cell lines and express features of multiple lineages. Some cases of AML cannot be classified according to the FAB criteria. These unclassifiable cases occur more frequently among patients with secondary leukemia and represent approximately 2–5% of all cases.[218,219] The FAB classification does not include hybrid or biphenotypic leukemias that cannot be identified on the basis of morphology or histochemistry alone. Moreover, the FAB group classification did not consider clinical characteristics, cytogenetic patterns, response to therapy, or prognosis in its formulation.[220] While other classification systems have been proposed, and despite its limitations, the FAB classification is used almost universally.[204,205,221] The classification system does try to take into account the heterogeneous nature of AML and recognizes that it is not a single disease but a group of disorders affecting the hematopoietic precursors in the bone marrow.

The FAB group defines four subsets of myeloid leukemia based on the percentage of maturing cells beyond the myeloblast stage. These range from the myeloid leukemia without morphologic evidence of maturation to the promyelocytic leukemia in which the dominant cell is a abnormal promyelocyte (M0, M1, M2, M3). The division between myeloblast groups, M0, M1, and M2 is somewhat arbitrary, and in many cases there is a spectrum of myeloid differentiation.

M0 Subtype (AML Without Differentiation or Maturation)

Myeloid leukemia without differentiation (M0) (Plate 64-4) constitutes 3% of all cases of AML. Morphologically, this group is most difficult to differentiate from the L2 variant of ALL. The blasts are very immature appearing and <3% of the blast cells are positive with myeloperoxidase, Sudan black B, or nonspecific esterase. Lymphoid markers are negative except for the enzyme TdT, which is expressed in about one-half of cases.[222] The bone marrow has >30% blasts. The blasts are identified as myeloid on the basis of either ultrastructural or immunologic markers. The blasts are usually large, with open chromatin and prominent single or multiple nucleoli. The nuclear/cytoplasmic ratio is variable, and cells may resemble lymphoblasts. Some evidence of trilineage dysplasia is frequently noted. Azurophilic granules and Auer rods are absent. Myeloperoxidase stain may be positive by ultrastructural cytochemistry or by the use of a monoclonal antibody.[223,224] The use of monoclonal antibodies to identify the myeloid lineage is essential in this subtype. The lymphoid markers characteristic of B- and T-lineage ALL, including CD10, CD19, CD24, CD3, and CD5, are negative. Rarely, the blasts can mark with the T-cell markers CD4 and CD7. CD4 is a marker of mature T cells expressed on some myeloid cells. The CD7 antigen is one of the early T-cell antigens and is usually expressed on immature T cells and prothymocytes. This subtype of AML can mark with CD7, usually in association TdT expression.[225,226] Myeloid-specific monoclonal antibodies are positive, including CD13 and CD33. Other myeloid antigens may be positive but are less helpful in establishing the diagnosis. M0 blasts may also resemble megakaryoblasts (M7) or undifferentiated monoblasts (M5a). The diagnosis of the M0 subtype cannot be made on the basis of morphology criteria alone and requires confirmation with monoclonal markers demonstrating myeloid antigens or ultrastructural cytochemistry.

M1 Subtype (AML Without Maturation)

The M1 subtype accounts for 15–20% of AML cases. Auer rods are rare or absent. The bone marrow is infiltrated with poorly differentiated blasts with rare azurophilic granules (Plate 64-5). If granules are absent, the myeloblasts resemble the lymphoblasts of the L2 variant of ALL, and cytochemical stains are necessary to distinguish these two leukemias. The peroxidase reaction is positive in >3% of blast cells, and the PAS stain is negative. The bone marrow contains <3% promyelocytes and <10% maturing granulocytes. Morphologically, the cells may appear pleomorphic, having irregular nuclei with an open chromatin. Some of the cells express the CD7, a antigen present on early T cells.[225,226]

M2 Subtype (AML with Maturation)

Myeloid leukemia with maturation (M2) (Plate 64-6) demonstrates clear evidence of maturation to and beyond the promyelocyte. It occurs in approximately 25–30% of all AML patients and represents the most common subtype in most reported series. Promyelocytes account for 3–20% of all myeloid cells. The myeloid series shows evidence of maturation, with occasional maturation to eosinophils and basophils. The bone marrow monocytic component represents <20% of nonerythroid cells. Auer rods are usually found, and the myeloblasts contain prominent azurophilic granules. Peroxidase and Sudan black stain are both strongly positive; chloracetate esterase (specific esterase) stain is positive, reflecting maturation beyond the myeloblast; and α-naphthylacetate and butyrate esterase (nonspecific esterase) stains are negative. On Wright-Giemsa stain, the blasts have a higher nuclear/cytoplasmic ratio than in the M1 variant, and the nuclear chromatin is condensed with less distinct nuclei.[227]

About one-half of patients in this subtype will have a translocation involving chromosomes 8 and 21 [t(8;21)].[228,229] About 25% of these patients will present with splenomegaly, and 20% will develop extramedullary disease during their course.[230] The marrow may have an increased number of eosinophil precursors, some of which may contain Auer rods. Some patients exhibit abnormal granulocytic maturation, with dysplastic granulocytes with a pseudo-Pelger-Huët abnormality. Histochemical staining with Sudan black and peroxidase demonstrates localized densely staining clumps, usually on one side of the nucleus or in a cleft of the nucleus, in contrast to the diffuse staining seen in patients without the 8;21 translocation. This variant has a high remission induction rate after standard chemotherapy. However, the remission duration is variable, with studies demonstrating a similar overall average remission duration for all AML patients.[229,231]

M3 Subtype (Acute Promyelocytic Leukemia)

Acute promyelocytic leukemia (APL) (M3) (Plate 64-7) is characterized by the presence of atypical promyelocytes in the bone marrow and peripheral blood. The M3 subtype accounts for 5–10% of all cases of AML. APL is distinguished from other subtypes of AML by its distinctive morphology, younger patient age at presentation, specific chromosomal abnormality, associated coagulopathy, and unique response to treatment with retinoic acid. APL has two morphologic variants: a hypergranular (M3) and an atypical microgranular (M3v) form.[232] These two variants differ in their clinical presentation, prognosis, and morphologic and histochemical appearance. The hypergranular form is the more common form of APL, representing 75% of cases. In this form, the cytoplasm of the promyelocyte typically demonstrates bright pink or dark purplish granules with abundant Auer rods. The promyelocytes are larger than nonmalignant promyelocytes with pleiomorphic nucleoli. The Sudan black and peroxidase stains are strongly positive; the PAS stain is usually negative but in some cases may show a diffuse positive tinge with fine cytoplasmic granules; the chloroacetate esterase stain is usually strongly positive; and the nonspecific esterase stain is negative. Promyelocytes account for ≥30% of the myeloid cells. Auer rods may be so numerous as to form Auer bundles.

Patients are typically younger, with a median age of 31 years, and present with a lower WBC count, most in the range of 3,000–15,000/mm^3. Most patients present with a WBC count of <5,000/mm^3. Approximately 25% of patients with APL present with the microgranular variant (M3v). The microgranular variant presents with a higher WBC count (50,000–200,000/mm^3) and morphologically atypical promyelocytes.[233–235]

Cytogenetic studies the M3 and M3v demonstrate the characteristic 15;17 translocation, a balanced translocation from the long arm of chromosome 17 to the long arm of chromosome 15 [t(15q+;17q−)]. This cytogenetic finding is present in 80–100% of patients with this variant.[236] The chromosome break point on chromosome 17 has been mapped to the site of the retinoic acid receptor-α (RAR-α).[237] The RAR is a member of a family of steroid hormone nuclear receptors that are important in the regulation and control of both normal and malignant cellular differentiation and proliferation.[238] In APL the cytogenetic translocation results in a fusion of the retinoic acid α-gene on chromosome 17 and in a region from chromosome 15 referred to as promyelocytic leukemia (PML).[239] The translocation encodes for a novel DNA-binding protein that results in

the expression of an abnormal mRNA transcript for the RAR-α and confers a unique therapeutic sensitivity to one of its ligands, all-trans-retinoic acid. Myeloid differentiation appears to be blocked by the abnormal PML-RAR-α fusion protein. This abnormal receptor is the target of all trans-retinoic acid treatment.[240] Treatment of patients with APL with all-trans-retinoic acid, a vitamin A derivative, results in differentiation of the leukemic cells, with approximately 85% of patients attaining a complete remission. Moreover, unlike standard induction therapy, treatment with oral all-trans-retinoic acid is not associated with bone marrow hypoplasia and the usual complications of cytotoxic chemotherapy. All-trans-retinoic acid induces leukemic cells to replicate and differentiate into cells capable of undergoing normal senescence and cell death.

Patients with APL often present with thrombocytopenia and evidence of disseminated intravascular coagulation (DIC), the latter attributed to the spontaneous or chemotherapy-associated release of a tissue factor with procoagulant activity present in the granules of the leukemic promyelocytes.[241,242] The bleeding disorder, however, cannot always be related solely to the development of DIC, and many patients show signs of primary fibrinolysis.[243,244] The promyelocytic leukemic cell has both strong procoagulant activity on its cell membrane and proteolytic activity in the cytoplasmic granules, a combination unique to the leukemic promyelocyte that may explain the severe coagulopathy seen in some patients.[245–247] Enhanced fibrinolysis is suggested by the increase in fibrin/fibrinogen degradation products, reduced α$_2$-antiplasmin levels, and normal antithrombin III and protein C levels present in all patients at diagnosis and up to initiation of therapy.[242,245] Plasma from patients with APL contains a plasminogen activator of tissue origin[245]—the mechanism of the coagulopathy remains unclear.[248] The treatment of the bleeding disorders in patients with APL is also controversial, with some groups using either heparin, antifibrinolytic therapy, or supportive therapy alone.[248–250] The role of either heparin or antifibrinolytic therapy during chemotherapy is unknown.[248]

The prognosis for patients of this subtype is usually favorable. The introduction of trans-retinoic acid with or without chemotherapy has changed the prognosis and management of this subtype. Patients are at high risk of life-threatening bleeding, including intracranial and pulmonary hemorrhage before and during induction therapy. Age, underlying renal function, pretreatment fibrinogen, and WBC count are important prognostic variables; younger age, lower WBC count, stable coagulation studies, and a normal fibrinogen level before starting therapy are all favorable indicators.[246,251]

The microgranular variant typically, presents with a very elevated WBC count, frequently >100,000/mm^3, and the cells have minimal rather than excessive cytoplasmic granulation.[235] Auer rods are rare. The nucleus is typically irregular, folded, or bilobed and resembles the nucleus of a monocytic precursor. Most cells are devoid of granules or contain a few fine dust-like azurophilic granules, often concentrated in one area of the cytoplasm. Histochemical stains reveal that the cells are peroxidase positive, Sudan black positive, and chloracetate esterase positive. Ultrastructural examination has demonstrated that most cells contain numerous "microgranules" (<250 nm), hence below the limit of resolution of light microscopy.[252] These patients have the typical 15;17 translocation of the "standard" hypergranular promyelocytic leukemia. The microgranular form can be confused morphologically with a monocytic leukemia. A few patients with M3v present with hyperbasophilic cytoplasm and cytoplasmic projections that may resemble megakaryoblasts.[235]

In the microgranular variant, the appearance of the blasts in the peripheral blood and bone marrow may be very different (Plate 64-8). In the bone marrow, many of the cells are frequently closer in appearance to that of the typical M3 hypergranular variant.[253] In questionable cases, cytochemical, ultrastructural, and cytogenetic studies may all be needed to confirm the diagnosis. The very high presenting blast count and the coagulopathy associated with this variant affect the outcome of remission induction. Leukostasis and fatal central nervous system and pulmonary hemorrhage are more common in this subtype.

M4 Subtype (Acute Myelomonocytic Leukemia)

In the M4 subtype (Plate 64-9), cells have characteristics of both AML and acute monocytic leukemia. Patients often present with extramedullary disease; gingival hypertrophy, leukemia cutis, and meningeal leukemia are more common in subtype than in the myeloid leukemias (M0–M3). Morphologically this subtype is similar to AML (M2), except that the proportion of promonocytes and monocytes is >20% in the bone marrow or peripheral blood, or both. This subtype represents 20–30% of all AML patients. Histochemical stains are helpful in identifying the monocytes in the peripheral blood and bone marrow. The bone marrow typically stains with the histochemical markers for both myelocytic and monocytic precursors, and the leukemic blasts stain positive with peroxidase, Sudan black, and chloroacetate esterase, as well as the nonspecific esterase that is inhibited by addition of sodium fluoride. Serum and urinary lysozyme levels, reflecting the monocytic component, are frequently elevated.

A variant of this subtype, called acute myelomonocytic leukemia with abnormal eosinophils (M4Eo) (Plate 64-10), is characterized by the presence myelomonocytic blasts and ≤30% of morphologically and histochemically abnormal eosinophils.[254] This variant represents approximately 5–10% of all patients with AML or about one-third of all patients with the M4 subtype. Patients with the M4Eo subtype often present with a high peripheral WBC count (30,000–100,000/mm^3) and organomegaly. The eosinophils have monocytic nuclei with abnormal, often basophilic, granules and lack the typical eosinophil crystals. The eosinophilic granules stain positive with PAS, Sudan black, chloroacetate esterase, and nonspecific esterase, typical of granulocytic but not of eosinophilic precursors. Presumably the hybrid morphologic and histochemical features of monocytes, eosinophils, and granulocytes in these cells result from abnormal differentiation of a primitive uncommitted leukemic cell before the divergence of the three cell lines. These cells also expresses the T-cell antigen, CD2. The myeloblasts are typically negative for other T-cell markers.[255] The peripheral blood typically contains myeloblasts and increased monocytes with abnormal-appearing eosinophils. Central nervous system involvement is very common in this variant. In one study, 35% of patients relapsed with leptomeningeal disease.[144]

The M4Eo variant has a unique karyotypic abnormality involving the long arm of chromosome 16. All patients have an inversion of chromosome 16 between the long and short arm or a balanced translocation between two homologous chromosomes 16. The cytogenetic feature in both translocations is the break in long arm of chromosome 16 at band q22.[256,257]

The overall complete response rate for patients with myelomonocytic leukemia is 50–65. However, patients with the M4Eo variant have a complete response rate of 70–80%, which is significantly higher than the standard M4 subtype.[258,259] The median duration of the remission and overall survival is also significantly prolonged in the M4Eo variant, as compared with that in other acute myelomonocytic leukemia cases.[259,260] It is therefore important to recognize patients with the M4Eo phenotype, as they appear to have a very responsive disease and may have a very favorable prognosis with currently available therapies.

M5 Subtype (Acute Monocytic Leukemia)

The acute monocytic subtype (Plates 64-11 and 64-12) represents 2–9% of all cases of AML.[261–263] The monocytic leukemias are divided into two variants, a poorly differentiated monoblastic leukemia (M5a) and a differentiated monocytic leukemia (M5b). The FAB criteria for the diagnosis of M5 (AMoL) require that ≥80% of the nonerythroid cells in the bone marrow be monoblasts, promonocytes, or monocytes. The blasts in the M5a variant (Plate 64-11) are poorly differentiated monoblasts, with rare granules and occasional cytoplasmic vacuoles. The undifferentiated monoblasts are large cells with plentiful cytoplasm that may contain vacuoles; they are usually basophilic. Auer rods are not usually seen. These cells may resemble lymphoblasts morphologically. The M5a subtype classification requires that >80% of the bone marrow monocytic component are monoblasts. The M5b variant (Plate 64-12) consists of more differentiated monocytes, which have the typical monocytic cerebriform nucleus. Nucleoli are not always present. The cytoplasm typically is grayish blue, and Auer rods are rare. Monoblasts comprise <80% of the monocytic component. The diagnosis of AMoL is confirmed by the positive nonspecific esterase reaction inhibited by sodium fluoride. The peroxidase, Sudan black, and chloroacetate esterase stains are usually negative in the blasts, but Sudan black can be positive in the more mature monocytic precursors. The PAS reaction is variable, while most of the monocytic leukemias are PAS negative; some will stain with coarse positive granules on a background of diffuse positivity.

There are meaningful clinical differences between the two monocytic leukemias.[264] Patients with the M5a variant are younger, present with a higher blast count in the peripheral blood and bone marrow, and have an overall poorer prognosis.[265] The M5b variant has a increased incidence of gingival hypertrophy and a higher percentage of circulating monocytes. The peripheral blood may show cells of the monocytic lineage that are more mature appearing and differentiated than found in the bone marrow. The diagnosis of this subtype is determined by the bone marrow findings.

Extramedullary disease involving the liver, spleen, and lymph nodes is more common in the monocytic leukemias than in other AMLs. An elevated WBC count is seen in most cases; ≤30% of patients present with a WBC count of >100,000/mm^3.[266,267] Laboratory evidence of DIC is common at presentation. Central nervous system involvement occurs in <22% of all patients.[267] However, prophylactic central nervous system therapy has not improved survival or prolonged remission.[266] Gingival hyperplasia and skin involvement are frequent prominent features of the monocytic leukemias and in many patients may be the presenting complaint.

The response of patients with the monocytic leukemias is variable. The complete remission rate is 50–70%, comparable to that in the other types of AML. However, the duration of the complete response and the overall survival are significantly shorter in this leukemic subtype.[267–269] This resistance to standard chemotherapy is also reflected in the increased relapse rate for patients with both variants of the monocytic leukemia after allogeneic bone marrow transplantation.[270]

M6 Subtype (Acute Erythroleukemia)

Acute erythroleukemia (Plate 64-13) represents 3–5% of all cases of AML. This subtype (M6) was initially described by Di Guglielmo and is still often referred to as the acute Di Guglielmo syndrome. The FAB criteria for erythroleukemia originally required that the abnormal erythropoietic cells be >50% of the nucleated bone marrow cells with ≥30% myeloblasts and promyelocytes present. However, the FAB group recently revised the criteria for this subtype to allow 30% of the nucleated cells to include type I or II blasts, but 50% of the total number of nucleated cells must still be erythroblasts. Type I blasts are defined as myeloblasts with prominent nucleoli and no cytoplasmic granules. By contrast, the type II blasts have primary azurophilic granules with a centrally placed nucleus, decreased nuclear/cytoplasmic ratio, and less conspicuous nucleoli. This classification recognizes the continuous spectrum of the mixed proportion of cells in this leukemic subtype and parallels the involvement of myeloid and monocytic precursors.

The erythroblasts are morphologically abnormal, with multilobed nuclei, multiple nuclei, nuclear fragments, and giant pronormoblasts with megaloblastic features. The PAS stain is usually positive, with a granular or diffuse cytoplasmic pattern. The intensity of the stain and the percentage of positive staining erythroblasts vary considerably in this subtype. Typically, the cells with the most abnormal cytologic appearance demonstrate the strongest PAS reaction. Because the PAS reaction is variable, a negative reaction should not exclude the diagnosis of erythroleukemia if the other morphologic features are present. Erythroblasts are Sudan black, peroxidase, and generally esterase negative. However, considering the usual involvement of the myeloid line, myeloblasts with Auer rods are often present. The granulocytic component demonstrates the typical positive cytochemical staining with Sudan black, peroxidase, and chloracetate esterase. Iron stains such as Prussian blue are useful in this subtype and may reveal prominent ringed sideroblasts. A monoclonal antibody that binds to glycophorin A on the cytoplasmic membrane appears to be specific for the erythroblast.[271]

Patients with erythroleukemia tend to be older at diagnosis, with a mean age of >50 years in most studies.[272,273] The presenting complaints are usually associated with the development of anemia. The peripheral smear may have only rare circulating blast forms. Hepatomegaly and splenomegaly occur in <25% of patients. Some patients present with peculiar rheumatic and immunologic findings, and up to one-third will complain of diffuse joint pain and abdominal, back, and chest pain.[274] Many patients will have a positive rheumatoid factor, increased polyclonal immunoglobulins, a positive antinuclear antibody test, and a positive Coombs test.[275] The erythroleukemias, frequently preceded by a myelodysplastic syndrome, represents 10–20% of the secondary leukemias and 3–5% of all de novo AML cases.[274] The preceding myelodysplastic or "erythremic myelosis" stage is characterized by progressive anemia, often associated with intense erythroid hyperplasia in the bone marrow. The peripheral blood may demonstrate prominent basophilic stippling, with abnormal red blood cells with rare circulating blast forms. The bone marrow frequently demonstrates dysplasia of all cell lines. Patients with this subtype generally respond to therapy poorly with a short remission duration.[276] The response to treatment may reflect the increased incidence of secondary leukemias and patients with a prior MDS with this subtype.

M7 Subtype (Acute Megakaryocytic Leukemia)

Acute megakaryocytic leukemia (M7) (Plate 64-14) is a recent addition to the FAB classification.[277] However, this not a not a new entity; previous cases have been described,[278] and many, if not all, of the previously reported cases of so-called acute myelofibrosis or malignant myelosclerosis probably represented acute megakaryocytic leukemia. Acute megakaryocytic leukemia represents 3–12% of all cases of AML, but its incidence may be much higher when cases are considered in patients in whom it represents a transformation from a prior myeloproliferative disorder.[279,280] The incidence of acute

megakaryocytic leukemia in patients with a prior myeloproliferative disorder, myelofibrosis, or CML is 24–51%.[281,282] Megakaryoblasts are morphologically heterogeneous and vary from small round cells, resembling cells found in the L2 variant of ALL or in an undifferentiated M0 or M1 leukemia, to large atypical megakaryocytes with or without cytoplasmic granules. Binuclear or multinuclear blasts with deeply basophilic cytoplasm, cytoplasmic projections, and vacuoles are common. Undifferentiated blasts may be surrounded by shed platelets and recognizable micromegakaryocytes. In the peripheral blood, megakaryocytic fragments are seen, along with large atypical cells with prominent cytoplasmic blebs representing megakaryoblasts. The bone marrow aspirate typically yields a dry tap, and the biopsy shows increased reticulin and fibrosis, the latter due to the stimulation of the normal fibroblasts in the bone marrow by the local secretion of platelet-derived growth factor by the leukemic cells.[283,284]

The megakaryoblast is Sudan black, peroxidase, and chloroacetate esterase negative. The nonspecific esterase reaction is difficult to interpret in this leukemic subtype. The α-naphthylacetate esterase reaction may be positive and is inhibited by the addition of fluoride, but the other nonspecific esterase stain, the α-naphthylbutyrate esterase, is usually negative. This differential staining distinguishes the megakaryoblast from the monocyte or monoblast. The PAS reaction is often but not universally positive. The FAB group recognized the difficulty of using routine morphology and cytochemistry to diagnose this subtype and included ultrastructural analysis and immunologic and cytogenetic criteria. In many cases, megakaryocytic features may not be recognized by light or electron microscopy, so the use of monoclonal antibodies to specific platelet glycoproteins is necessary to define this subtype.[285,286] Immunophenotyping with monoclonal antibodies to platelet glycoproteins IIb/IIIa (CD41a) or to factor VIII-related antigen may be needed to identify the megakaryoblasts. The ultrastructural platelet peroxidase reaction is technically difficult to perform and largely has been replaced by immunologic techniques. When flow cytometric techniques are used to determine the surface antigen profile of leukemic cells, platelets adherent to the leukemic cells may cause a false-positive result with antibodies to platelet glycoproteins.[287] Cytospin immunofluorescence techniques are important to distinguish adherent platelets versus a true positive cytoplasmic and membrane activity.

Cytogenetic abnormalities of chromosome 21 have been associated with the M7 subtype.[288,289] For the diagnosis of the M7 subtype, ≥30% of the blast cells must be megakaryoblasts, as defined by the use of one of the above methods.

The clinical and hematologic features of the M7 subtype are varied and reflect that, in many patients, the disease evolved from a prior myeloproliferative disorder. These patients frequently present with hepatomegaly and splenomegaly, an uncommon finding in patients with in patients with de novo acute megakaryocytic leukemia.[290] The presenting WBC count is usually low (<5,000/mm³) in 50% of cases, and the platelet count is normal or increased in more than one-third of cases. Anemia is usually present. The bone marrow aspirate is frequently a dry tap, and the bone marrow biopsy is fibrotic in >90% of patients. The response to conventional induction chemotherapy is generally poor, with a complete response rate of <40%. A complete remission is frequently associated with reversal of the bone marrow fibrosis.[291] The clinical course can be quite variable and atypical for an acute leukemia. Some patients whose disease has evolved from a pre-existing myeloproliferative disorder may have a slowly progressive indolent disease that extends over a number of months to years.[292]

Biphenotypic, Hybrid, and Bilineage Leukemias

The classification of AML is based on the predominant cell type and is an arbitrary system that does not reflect the biologic of the disease or the leukemogenic events. In many cases, it is impossible to define a single lineage or cell type of a leukemic cell either morphologically or histochemically or with the use of phenotypic markers. In an attempt to explain this phenomenon, a number of different terms have been described, including lineage infidelity, mixed-lineage leukemias, biphenotypic or bilineal leukemias, hybrid or biclonal leukemias, and lineage switches.[293-296] The confused and arbitrary terminology in this area reflects the heterogeneous nature of these disorders and the lack of specificity of available markers. Lineage infidelity refers to the expression of markers of more than one cell type by the same leukemic cell.[295] While many of the reported cases reflect the lack of specificity of the phenotypic markers, clear examples of blasts express markers of more than one lineage. The monoclonal antibodies used to characterize lymphoid or myeloid leukemias recognize hematopoietic differentiation antigens. These antigens, which are expressed on a number of epithelial cells and overlapping subsets of hematopoietic cells, have important roles in the biology of normal and malignant hematopoiesis.[297] Leukemic cells can demonstrate histochemical and phenotypic markers of both myeloid and lymphoid precursors.[297-299] This phenomenon may reflect a fundamental abnormality of gene expression specific to the malignant clone.[296,298] Alternatively, the leukemic cells may express markers of more than one lineage, reflecting the abnormal maturation of an earlier uncommitted stem cell.[300]

The use of specific monoclonal antibodies and other molecular probes has shown that leukemic cells can demonstrate characteristics of more than one hematopoietic lineage. By the standard FAB criteria, 10–25% of patients with AML may express markers of T-cell lineage.[209,211,296,297,301] These cells may contain Auer rods, stain with peroxidase and/or Sudan black, and react with monoclonal antibodies typical of both myeloid precursors and mature T cells.[302] A number of classification systems have attempted to address the biphenotypic leukemias, but none has been widely accepted.[205,302] Myeloblasts can react with B-lineage (CD19) and T-lineage (CD2 and CD7) markers.[209,225] These monoclonal antibodies are not lineage restricted and are usually found in the absence of other lymphoid markers. These cases do not represent evidence of biphenotypic leukemia but reflect the inappropriate expression of lymphoid antigens on immature myeloblasts.[225,299] While many of the monoclonal antibodies are considered lineage nonspecific, the two myeloid-associated monoclonals, CD13 and CD33, remain myeloid specific.

The term biclonal, or bilineage, leukemia is used to indicate a disorder that has two distinct leukemic cell populations—one that usually marks with myeloid markers and the other with lymphoid markers.[302,303] In these cases, the malignant transformation presumably occurred in a progenitor cell capable of differentiating into two distinct lines. This is in contrast to mixed-lineage, biphenotypic, or hybrid leukemias, in which the leukemic cell expresses characteristics of more than one lineage.[304] Bilineage leukemias can be suspected on morphologic grounds when two distinct population of blast cells are noted. However, immunologic markers are needed to define a bilineage leukemia. In this setting, two distinct population should be noted on immunophenotyping.

Lineage switch is the expression of markers of one lineage at diagnosis, but markers of a different phenotype or lineage at leukemic relapse.[303-306] This transformation, which usually occurs after a treatment interval of ≥1 year from initial diagnosis, may reflect the selection of a clone from a bilineage leukemia or modulation of antigens expressed on leukemic cells. This phenomenon has been frequently reported in leukemias of the T-cell subtype, in which relapse occurred as AML or acute myelomonocytic leukemia.[307]

Hybrid leukemias do not fit into a morphologically or histochemically defined group. Hybrid leukemias demonstrate malignant transformation of both lymphoid and myeloid cells.[308] The hybrid leukemias are morphologically heterogeneous and can present with undifferentiated or differentiated blasts. The undifferentiated myeloid leukemias present with agranular blasts with a high nuclear/cytoplasmic ratio, morphologically similar to those found in the lymphocytic leukemias.[309-311] Some of these undifferentiated leukemias express the CD34 antigen, a marker expressed by hematopoietic stem cells, and early progenitor cells. Some of these disorders may in fact represent true stem cell leukemias and generally have a poor prognosis.[312] More typically, the hybrid leukemias demonstrate commitment toward myeloid differentiation with morphologically identifiable myeloblasts. The myeloblasts may contain rare granules, but most of the blasts do not demonstrate evidence of maturation or reaction with standard histochemical stains that would indicate a myeloid phenotype. The blasts may, however, be peroxidase positive on electron microscopy or immunoelectron microscopy. The use of monoclonal antibodies against lymphoid and myeloid surface antigens is necessary to define these hybrid leukemias.

Clinically, the biphenotypic and hybrid leukemias present with the usual findings of AML. However, they may present with findings of myeloid and lymphoid leukemias, including prominent diffuse lymphadenopathy and a higher circulating blast count and platelet count.[313,314] Otherwise, the clinical presentations are indistinguishable from those of the other forms of AML.

Complete remission rates for the hybrid and biphenotypic leukemias are variable as is their clinical course. The undifferentiated and minimally differentiated hybrid leukemias do poorly with standard induction chemotherapy.[312] Myeloid leukemias that are TdT positive and that express T-lymphoid markers are a more heterogeneous population and show variable response to induction therapy, with some patients having a better prognosis than those with other AMLs.[209,313] Patients who fail standard AML treatment and who demonstrate lymphoid markers may respond to the addition of vincristine, prednisone, and L-asparaginase to their induction regimen.[299,312] The true incidence of hybrid and biphenotypic leukemias remains to be determined. Monoclonal antibodies to cell-surface markers are necessary to define these morphologically atypical leukemias. Their use should be part of the initial evaluation in selected patients who present with an atypical morphologic or clinical pattern.[209]

Current models of hematopoietic differentiation are based on the evidence that normal pluripotential precursors give rise to committed precursors of a single cell lineage and then undergo a series of discrete developmental steps.[309] The AMLs are believed to arise from a single clone that is arrested at a normal stage of differentiation. The currently used classification system is based on the premise that leukemic cells adhere morphologically and immunologically to a single lineage. These cases of biphenotypic leukemias, hybrid leukemias, lineage infidelity, mixed-lineage, or lineage-switch leukemias demonstrate the heterogeneity of these neoplastic disorders and support the concept that, in at least some acute leukemias, the transforming event occurs at the level of the pluripotential stem cell. Moreover, these data suggest that leukemic cells can differentiate, although aberrantly, and express differentiation markers.

PREDICTORS OF RESPONSE

A number of clinical characteristics have been defined that are important prognostic factors (Table 64-3). Age is the most consistent prognostic variable for induction therapy. While some single institution studies have treated elderly patients with intensive therapy, most patients who are >60 years of age tolerate intensive treatment poorly.[313–315] However, once an elderly patient attains a complete remission, subsequent survival, and remission duration are not age dependent.[313] Patients with secondary AML or a prior MDS or myeloproliferative disorder respond poorly to standard chemotherapy regimens.[316] Patients presenting with blast cell counts of >100,000/mm^3 and signs of leukostasis also respond poorly to induction therapy. The pretreatment serum albumin, serum LDH level and performance status are important predictors of response.[317] The lower the serum albumin, the less likely the patient will attain a complete remission and the higher the likelihood of having a fatal complication after treatment.[316] A poor performance status or elevated serum LDH is also associated with a lower complete response rate and shorter remission duration.

A number of in vitro studies have attempted to correlate leukemic progenitor cell growth characteristics, drug sensitivity, and drug metabolism, retention, and incorporation with outcome of therapy. In vitro growth characteristics may be predictive of the outcome of remission induction therapy and remission duration, but results from such studies remain conflicting.[318–321] The in vitro growth patterns and the presence of autonomous blast cell colony formation may be predictive of a response to treatment.[319,322] Additional in vitro studies that correlate with the probability of attaining a complete remission include the proliferative characteristics of leukemic cells including the percentage of cells in S phase, the cell cycle time, and the expression of the multidrug resistance gene.[323,324] Prospective studies are needed, however, before therapy can be altered on the basis of labeling indices or in vitro growth characteristics. The expression of multidrug resistance gene has been implicated as a predictor of a poor response to treatment.[319] These in vitro studies have failed to provide prognostic information for a change of therapy.

The major determinant of the outcome of remission induction therapy is the capacity of the patient to tolerate intensive therapy. Most patients who fail to attain a complete remission do so because of the complications of the therapy. Resistant disease accounts for approximately 20% of all induction failures. Most patients initially treated for AML die as a result of a complication of treatment, including infection or hemorrhage. Therefore, prior medical problems and performance status are important predictors of response. Underlying renal insufficiency and impaired cardiac or hepatic function limit the amount of chemotherapy that can be administered. Factors that predispose to serious infections decrease the likelihood that a patient will attain complete remission. Patients with diseases that impair their immune response or who are on medications that predispose to fungal or other opportunistic infections have increased infectious complications and a higher mortality rate during induction therapy. Infections account for >70% of deaths during the induction phase.[325] It remains unclear whether the introduction of hematopoietic growth factors will decrease the incidence of serious infections in patients receiving induction chemotherapy.[326]

In most studies, 55–65% of patients have attained complete remission with induction therapy, and 50–70% will relapse during the first 18–24 months (Fig. 64-3). Those factors that determine remission duration are still controversial and dependent in part on the type of postinduction chemotherapy employed.[327] Cytogenetic abnormalities can be demonstrated in the leukemic cells of most patients with AML. Recent studies on specific and nonspecific chromosomal abnormalities have defined favorable and unfavorable patterns[328]: cytogenetic abnormalities, including t(8;21) and inv(16), are associated with significantly longer remission and survival, while abnormalities of chromosomes 5, 7, and 11q are associated with a poor response to therapy and shorter overall survival. These and other studies have suggested that chromosomal abnormalities

constitute an important independent prognostic factor for remission duration but not for remission induction.[329] Other factors that are predictors of remission duration include the previously noted FAB subtypes, with M0, M4, M5, M6, and M7 having a poorer prognosis and M2, M3, and M4E having a better prognosis.[330–332] The absolute percentage of erythroblasts appears to correlate inversely with remission duration.[333] Auer rods and an increase in the bone marrow eosinophils may also be associated with longer remission and survival.[334] The in vivo sensitivity of the leukemic cell, as determined by the number of courses needed to attain a complete remission and the rate of cytoreduction in bone marrow cellularity, appears to be an independent predictor of remission duration. The morphologic appearance of the bone marrow biopsy at complete remission may also be an important predictor of remission duration. The presence of morphologic dysplasia involving more than one cell line is associated with a poor response to treatment.[335] The complete remission rate and the duration of the first remission is decreased in patients with trilineage dysplasia. All these factors are determined on the basis of retrospective studies. None of these variables has been critically analyzed in controlled prospective trials. No studies have demonstrated that modifying therapy on the basis of a specific constellation of prognostic factors will alter a patient's outcome or response to treatment.

REFERENCES

1. Virchow R: Weisses Blut and Wilztumoren. Med Z 16:9, 1847
2. Bennett JH: Two cases of hypertrophy of the spleen ard liver, in which death took place from suppuration of blood. Edinb Med Surg J 64:413, 1845
3. Virchow RE: Weisses Blut. Froiep Notizen 30:151, 1845
4. Virchow R: Die Leukemia. p. 190. In Virchow R (ed): Cesammelte Abhandlunge zur Wissenschaftlichen Medizin. Meidinger, Frankfurt, 1856
5. Neumann E: Ein Fall von Leukamie mit Erkrankung des Knochenmarkes. Arch Heilk 11:1, 1870
6. Ebstein W: Ueber die acute Leukamie und Pseudoleukamie. Dtsch Arch Klin Med 44:343, 1889
7. Naegeli O: Über richt Knochenmark und Myeloblasten. Dtsch Med Wochenschr 26:287, 1900
8. Hirschfeld H: Zur Kenntnis der histogenese der granulierten Knochenmark Zellen. Virchows Arch A Pathol Anat Histopathol 153:335, 1889
9. Di Guglielmo C: Un caso di eritroleucemia. Folia Med 13:380, 1917
10. Reschad H, Schilling V: Über eine neue Leukamie durch echte Uebergangs formen (splenozytenleukamie) und ihre Bedeutung für die Selbststandigkeit dieser Zellen. Munch Med Wochenschr 60:1981, 1913
11. Selvin S, Levin LI, Merrill DN, Winkelstein W: Selected epidemiologic observation of cell specific leukemia mortality in the United States 1969–1977. Am J Epidemiol 117:140, 1983
12. Sandler D: Epidemiology of acute myelogenous leukemia. Semin Oncol 14:359, 1987
13. Kessler IL, Lilienfeld AM: Perspectives in the epidemiology of leukemia. Adv Cancer Res 12:225, 1979
14. Linet MS: The leukemias: epidemiologic aspects. p. 1. In Lilienfeld AM (ed): Monographs in Epidemiology and Biostatistics. Oxford University Press, New York, 1985
15. Morse H, Hays T, Peakman D, et al: Acute nonlymphoblastic leukaemia in childhood. High incidence of clonal abnormalities and non-random changes. Cancer 44:164, 1979
16. Gunz FW, Fitzegerald PH, Crossen PE et al: Multiple cases of leukemia in a sibling. Blood 27:482, 1966
17. Crittenden LB: An interpretation of familial aggregation based on multiple genetic and environmental factors. Ann NY Acad Sci 91:764, 1978
18. Gunz FW, Gunz JP, Vincent PC et al: Thirteen cases of leukemia in a family. J Natl Cancer Inst 60:1243, 1978
19. Gunz FW, Veale AMO: Leukemia in close relatives—accident or predisposition? J Natl Cancer Inst 42:517, 1969
20. Pearson HA, Grello FW, Cone TE Jr: Leukemia in identical twins. N Engl J Med 268:1151, 1963
21. Anderson RC, Herrmann HW: Leukemia in twin children. JAMA 158:652, 1955
22. Hilton HB, Lewis IC, Trowell HR: C group trisomy in identical twins with acute leukemia. Blood 35:222, 1969
23. Joachim H: Acute leukemia in uniovular twins: review of genetic aspect of human leukemia. Cancer 15:539, 1962

24. Hartley SE, Sainsbury C: Acute leukemia and the same chromosome abnormality in monoygotic twins. Hum Genet 58:408, 1981
25. Crittenden LB: An interpretation of familial aggregation based on multiple genetic and environmental factors. Ann NY Acad Sci 91:764, 1978
26. MacMahon B, Levy MA: Prenatal origin of childhood leukaemia: evidence from twins. N Engl J Med 270:1082, 1964
27. Keith L, Brown E: Epidemiologic study of leukemia in twins (1928–1969). Acta Genet Med Gemmellol (Roma) 20:9, 1971
28. Kurita S: Familial leukemia. Acta Haematol Jpn 31:748, 1968
29. Clarkson BD, Boyse EA: Possible explanation of the high concordance of acute leukemia in monoygotic twins. Lancet 1:699, 1971
30. Miller OJ, Berg WR, Schmike RN et al: A family with XXXXY male, a leukaemic male, and two 21-trisomic mongoloid females. Lancet 2:78, 1961
31. Krivit W, Good RA: Simultaneous occurrence of mongolism and leukemia. Am J Dis Child 94:289, 1957
32. Fong C, Brodeur GM: Down's syndrome and leukemia: epidemiology, genetics, cytogenetics and mechanisms of leukemogenesis. Cancer Genet Cytogenet 28:55, 1987
33. Stiller CA, Wilson LMK: Down's syndrome and acute leukemia. Lancet 2:1343, 1981
34. Suton WN, Welsh VC: Acute leukemia and mongolism. J Pediatr 52:170, 1985
35. Rosner F, Lee SL: Down's syndrome and acute leukemia: myeloblastic or lymphoblastic? Am J Med 53:203, 1972
36. Holland WW, Doll R, Carter CO: The mortality from leukemia and other cancers among patients with Down's syndrome and among their parents. Br J Cancer 16:177, 1982
37. Gunz FW, Fitzgerald PH, Crossen PE et al: Multiple cases of leukemia in a sibship. Blood 27:482, 1966
38. Gunz FW, Gunz JP, Veale AMO et al: Familial leukaemia: a study of 909 families. Scand J Haematol 15:117, 1975
39. Gunz FW, Gunz JP, Vincent PC et al: Thirteen cases of leukemia in a family. J Natl Cancer Inst 60:1243, 1978
40. Eunpu DL, Mcdonald DM, Zackei EH: Trisomy 21: rate in second-degree relatives. Am J Med Genet 25:361, 1986
41. Shaw G, Lavey R, Jackson R, Austin D: Epidemiological studies, State of California, Department of Health Services Berkeley: association of childhood leukemia with maternal age, birth order, and paternal occupation. A case-control study. Am J Epidemiol 119:788, 1984
42. Stark CR, Mantel N: Effects of maternal age and birth order on the risk of mongolism and leukemia. J Natl Cancer Inst 37:687, 1966
43. Stark CR, Mantel N: Maternal age and birth order effects in childhood leukemia: age of child and type of leukemia. J Natl Cancer Inst 42:857, 1969
44. Sawitsky A, Bloom D, German JL: Chromosomal breakage and acute leukemia in congenital telangiectatic erythema and stunted growth. Ann Intern Med 65:489, 1966
45. Morrell D, Cromartie E, Swift M: Mortality and cancer incidence in 263 patients with ataxia-telangiectasia. J Natl Cancer Inst 77:89, 1986
46. Auerbach AD, Wolman SR: Susceptibility of Fanconi's anemia fibroblasts to chromosome change by carcinogens. Nature 261:494, 1976
47. Auerbach AD: Fanconi anemia and leukemia: tracking the genes. Leukemia 6:1, 1992
48. Bader JL, Miller RW: Neurofibromatosis and childhood leukemia. J Pediatr 92:925, 1978
49. Ichimaru M, Ishimaru T, Belsky JL: Incidence of leukemia in atomic bomb survivors belonging to a fixed cohort in Hiroshima and Nagasaki, 1950–71: radiation dose years after exposure, age at exposure, and type of leukemia. J Radiat Res (Tokyo) 1:262, 1978
50. Jablon S, Kato H: Childhood cancer in relation to prenatal exposure to atomic bomb radiation. Lancet 2:1000, 1970
51. Ishimaru T, Otake M, Ichimaru M: Dose response relationship of neutrons and gamma rays to leukemia incidence among atomic bomb survivors in Hiroshima and Nagasaki by type of leukemia 1950–1971. Radiat Res 77:377, 1979
52. Kato H, Schull WJ: Studies of the mortality of A-bomb survivors and mortality, 1950–1978. Part 1. Cancer mortality. Radiat Res 90:395, 1982
53. Ichimaru M, Tomognaga M, Amenomori T, Matsuo T: Atomic bomb and leukemia. J Radiat Res 32:162, 1991
54. Rowland RE: Dose and damage in long-term radium cases. In Medical Radionuclides Radiation Dose and Effect. AEC Symp Ser 20:369, 1970
55. Caldwell G, Kelley D, Health C: Leukemia among participants in military maneuvers at a nuclear bomb test: a preliminary report. JAMA 244:1575, 1980
56. Darby SC, Doll R, Smith PG: Long term mortality after a single treatment course with x-ray in patients treated for ankylosing spondylitis. Br J Cancer 55:179, 1987
57. Court-Brown WM, Doll R: Mortality from cancer and other causes after radiotherapy for ankylosing spondylitis. BMJ 2:1327, 1965
58. Smith P, Dall R: Late effects of x-irradiation in patients treated for metropathia haemorrhagica. Br J Radiol 49:224, 1976
59. Hempelmann LH, Hall WJ, Phillips M et al: Neoplasms in persons treated with x-rays in infancy: fourth survey in 20 years. J Natl Cancer Inst 55:519, 1975
60. Krivit E, Good RA: Simultaneous occurrence of mongolism and leukemia. Am J Dis Child 94:289, 1957
61. Urowitz MD, Rider WD: Myeloproliferative disorders in patients with rheumatoid arthritis treated with total body irradiation Am J Med, suppl. 78:1A, 5064, 1985
62. Andersson M, Carstensen B, Visfeldt J: Leukemia and other related hematological disorders among Danish patients exposed to thorotrast. Radiat Res 132:224, 1993
63. Janower ML, Miettinen OS, Flynn MJ: Effects of long-term thorotrast exposure. Radiology 103:13, 1972
64. Savik DA, Calle EE: Leukemia and occupational exposure to electromagnetic fields: review of epidemiologic surveys. J Occup Med 29:47, 1987
65. McDowall ME: Mortality of persons resident in the vicinity of electricity transmission facilities. Br J Cancer 53:271, 1986
66. Matonoski GM, Elliott EA, Breysse PN, Lynberg MC: Leukemia and telephone linemen. Am J Epidemiol 137:609, 1993
67. Juutilainen J, Laara E, Pukkala E: Incidence of leukemia and brain tumors in Finish workers exposed to ELF magnetic fields. Int Arch Occup Environ Health 62:289, 1990
68. Robinson CF, Lalich NR, Nurnet CA et al: Electromagnetic field exposure and leukemia mortality in the United States. J Occup Med 33:160, 1991
69. Sahl JD, Kelsh MA, Greenland S: Cohort and nested case-control studies of hematopoietic cancer among electric utility workers. Epidemiology 4:104, 1993
70. Pool R. Is there an EMF–cancer connection? Science 249:1096, 1990
71. Macklis RM. Magnetic healing, quackery, and the debate about the health effects of electromagnetic fields. Ann Intern Med 118:376, 1993
72. Adamson RH, Seiber SM: Chemically induced leukemia in humans. Environ Health Perspect 39:93, 1981
73. Askoy M, Erdern S: Follow-up study on the mortality and development of leukemia in 44 pancytopenic patients with chronic exposure to benzene. Blood 52:285, 1978
74. Nicholson WJ, Landrigan PJ: Quantitative assessment of lives lost due to delay in the regulation of occupational exposure to benzene. Environ Health Perspect 82:185, 1989
75. Bernard J: The epidemiology of leukemias (past, present and future). Nouv Rev Fr Hematol 31:103, 1989
76. Checkoway H, Wilcosky T, Wolf P et al: An evaluation of the association of leukemia and rubber industry solvent exposures. Am J Ind Med 5:239, 1984
77. Brandt L, Nilsson PG, Mitelman F: Occupational exposure to petroleum products in men with acute nonlymphocytic leukemia. BMJ 4:553, 1978
78. Williams RR, Stegens NK, Goldsmith JR: Associations of cancer site and type with occupation and industry from the Third Nation Cancer Survey interview. J Natl Cancer Inst 59:1147, 1977
79. Hogstedt C, Arlinger L, Gustavsson A: Epidemiologic support for ethylene oxide as a cancer-causing agent. JAMA 255:1575, 1986
80. Burkhart JA: Leukemia in hospital patients with occupational exposure to the sawmill industry. West J Med 137:440, 1982
81. Lynge E: A follow-up study of cancer incidence among workers in manufacture of phenoxy herbicides in Denmark. Br J Cancer 52:259, 1985
82. Flodin U, Anderson L, Anjou CG et al: A case-referral study on acute myeloid leukemia, background radiation and exposure to solvents and other agents. Scand J Work Environ Health 7:169, 1981
83. Jarvisalo J, Tola S, Korkala ML et al: A cancer-register based case study of occupations of patients with acute myeloid leukemia. Cancer 54:785, 1984
84. Brownson RC, Novotny TE, Perry MC: Cigarette smoking and adult leukemia. A meta-analysis. Arch Intern Med 153:469, 1993
85. Sandler DP, Evereson RB, Wilcox AJ et al: Cancer risks in adulthood from early life exposure to parent's smoking. Am J Public Health 75:487, 1985
86. Williams RR, Horm JW: Association of cancer sites with tobacco and alcohol consumption and socioeconomic status of patients: interview study from the Third National Cancer Suney. J Natl Cancer Inst 58:525, 1977
87. Crane MM, Keating MJ, Trujillo JM et al: Environmental exposure in cytogenetically defined subsets of acute nonlymphocytic leukemia. JAMA 262:634, 1989
88. Melikian AA, Prahalad AK, Hoffman D: Urinary trans,trans-muconic acid as an indicator of exposure to benzene in cigarette smokers. Cancer Epidemiol Biomarkers Prev 2:47, 1993
89. Greenberg RA, Haley NJ, Etzel RA et al: Measuring the exposure of infants

to tobacco smoke: nicotine and cotinine in urine and saliva. N Engl J Med 310:1075, 1984

90. DeMarini DM: Genotoxicity to tobacco smoke and tobacco smoke condensate. Mutat Res 114:59, 1983

91. Kyle R: Second malignancies associated with chemotherapeutic agents. Semin Oncol 9:133, 1982

92. Rieche K: Carcinogenicity of antineoplastic agents in man. Cancer Treat Rev 11:39, 1984

93. Pedersen-Bjergaard J, Phillip P: Balanced translocations involving chromosome bands 11q23 and 21q22 are highly characteristic of myelodysplasia and leukemia following therapy with cytostatic agents targeting at DNA-topoisomerase II. Blood 78:1147, 1991

94. Levine EG, Bloomfield CD: Leukemias and myelodysplastic syndromes secondary to drug, radiation and environmental exposure. Semin Oncol 19:47, 1992

95. Kantarjian HM, Keating MJ: Therapy-related leukemia and myelodysplastic syndrome. Semin Oncol 14:435, 1987

96. Cadman EC, Capizzi RL, Bertino JR: Acute nonlymphocytic leukemia. A delayed complication of Hodgkin's disease therapy: analysis of 109 cases. Cancer 40:1280, 1977

97. Pedersen-Bjergaard J, Larsen SO: Incidence of acute nonlymphocytic leukemia, preleukemia, and acute myeloproliferative syndrome up to 10 years after treatment of Hodgkin's disease. N Engl J Med 307:955, 1984

98. Markman M, Pavy M, Aheloff MP: Acute leukemia following intensive therapy for small cell carcinoma of the lung. Cancer 50:670, 1981

99. Reimer RR, Hoover R, Fraumeni JF et al: Acute leukemia after alkylating agent therapy of ovarian cancer. N Engl J Med 297:177, 1977

100. Redman JR, Vugrin P, Arlin ZA et al: Leukemia following treatment of germ cell tumors in men. J Clin Oncol 2:1080, 1984

101. Rosner F, Carey RW, Zarrabi MH: Breast cancer and acute leukemia. Report of 24 cases and review of the literature. Cancer 44:1070, 1979

102. Zarrabi MH, Rosner F, Bennett JM: Non-Hodgkin's lymphoma and acute myeloblastic leukemia. A report of 12 cases and review of the literature. Cancer 44:1070, 1979

103. Zarrabi MH, Grunwald HW, Rosner F: Chronic lymphocytic leukemia terminating in acute leukemia. Arch Intern Med 2:1513, 1977

104. Kempin S, Lee BJ III, Thaler HT et al: Combination chemotherapy of advanced chronic lymphocytic leukemia. The M-2 protocol (vincristine, BCNU, cyclophosphamide, melphalan and prednisone). Blood 60:1110, 1982

105. Bergsagel DE, Bailey AL, Langley GR et al: The chemotherapy of plasma cell myeloma and the incidence of acute leukemia. N Engl J Med 301:743, 1979

106. Berk PD, Goldberg AJ, Silverstein MN et al: Increased incidence of acute leukemia in polycythemia vera associated with chlorambucil therapy. N Engl J Med 304:441, 1981

107. Louis S, Schwartz RS: Immunodeficiency in the pathogenesis of lymphoma and leukemia. Semin Hematol 156:117, 1978

108. Hakulinen T, Isomaki H, Knekt P: Rheumatoid arthritis and cancer studies based on linking nation wide registries in Finland. Am J Med 78:29, 1985

109. Pedersen-Bjergaard J, Philip P, Larsen SO et al: Chromosme aberrations and prognostic factors in therapy-related myelodysplasia and acute nonlymphocytic leukemia. Blood 76:1083, 1990

110. Rubin CM, Arthur DC, Woods WG et al: Therapy-related myelodysplastic syndrome and acute myeloid leukemia in children: correlation between chromosmal abnormalities and prior therapy. Blood 78:2982, 1991

111. Heim S, Mitelman F: Cytogenetic analysis in the diagnosis of acute leukemia. Cancer 70:1701, 1992

112. Preisler H, Early A, Raza A et al: Therapy of secondary acute leukemia with cytarabine. N Engl J Med 308:21, 1983

113. Ratain MJ, Kaminer LS, Bitran JD et al: Acute nonlymphocytic leukemia following etoposide and cisplatin combination chemotherapy for advanced non small cell carcinoma of the lung. Blood 70:1412, 1987

114. Pui C-H, Behm FG, Raimondi SC et al: Secondary acute myeloid leukemia in children treated for acute lymphoid leukemia. N Engl J Med 321:136, 1989

115. Ratain MJ, Rowley JD: Therapy-related acute myeloid leukemia secondary to inhibitors of topoisomerase II: from bedside to the target genes. Ann Oncol 3:107, 1992

116. Sandoval C, Pui C-H, Bowman LC et al: Secondary acute myeloid leukemia in children previously treated with alkylating agents, intercalating topoisomerase II inhibitors, and irradiation. J Clin Oncol 11:1039, 1993

117. Albain KS, LeBeau MM, Ullirsch R et al: Implication of prior treatment with drug combinations including inhibitors of topoisomerase II in therapy-related monocytic leukemia with a 9;11 translocation. Genes Chromosome Cancer 2:53, 1990

118. Detourmignies L, Castigne S, Stoppa AM et al: Therapy related acute promyelocytic leukemia: a report on sixteen cases. J Clin Oncol 10:1430, 1992

119. Creger WP: Acute myeloid leukemia following seven years of aplastic anemia induced by chloramphenicol. Am J Med 43:762, 1967

120. Friedman GD: Phenylbutazone, musculoskeletal disease and leukemia. J Chron Dis 35:233, 1983

121. The International Agranuloqtosis and Aplastic Anemia Study: Risk of agranulocytosis and aplastic anemia: a first report of their relation to drug use with special reference to analgesics. JAMA 256:1749, 1986

122. Hansen NE: Development of acute leukemia in a patient treated with oral methoxypsoralen and long wave ultraviolet light. Scand J Haematol 22:57, 1979

123. Adamson RH, Seiber SM: Chemically induced leukemia in humans. Environ Health Perpect 39:93, 1981

124. Bloomfield CD, Brunnig RD: Acute leukemia as a temminal event in leukemic hematopoietic disorders. Semin Oncol 3:297, 1976

125. Sedlacek SM, Curtis JL, Weintraub J et al: Essential thrombocytemia and leukemic transformation. Medicine 65:353, 1986

126. van den Anker-Lugtenburg PJ, Sizoo W: Myelodysplastic syndrome and secondary acute leukemia after treatment of essential thrombocytemia with hydroxyurea. Am J Hematol 33:152, 1990

127. Najean Y, Deschamps A, Dresch C et al: Acute leukemias and myelodysplasia in polycythemia vera: a clinical study with long-term follow up. Cancer 61:89, 1988

128. Nand S, Messmore H, Fisher H et al: Leukemic transformation in polycythemia vera: analysis of risk factors. Am J Hematol 34:32, 1990

129. Berk PD, Goldberg JD, Donovan PB et al: Therapeutic recommendations in polycythemia vera based on polycythemia vera Study Group protocols. Semin Hematol 23:132, 1986

130. Tischelli A, Gratwohl A, Wursch A et al: Late complications in serve aplastic anemia. Br J Haematol 69:413, 1988

131. de Planque MM, Kluin-Nelemans HC, van Krieken HJM et al: Evolution of acquired severe aplastic anemia to myelodyspasia and subsequent leukeamia in adults. Br J Haematol 70:55, 1988

132. Devine DV, Gluck WL, Rosse WF, Weinberg JB: Acute myeloblastic leukemia in paroxymal nocturnal hemoglobinuria. J Clin Invest 79:314, 1987

133. Gonzales F, Trujillo J, Alexanian R: Acute leukemia in multiple myeloma. Ann Intern Med 86:440, 1977

134. Tursz T, Flandrin G, Brouet JC et al: Simultaneous occurrence of acute myeloblastic leukemia and multiple myeloma without previous chemotherapy. BMJ 2:642, 1974

135. Nichols CR, Roth B, Heerema N et al: Hematologic neoplasms associated with primary mediastinal germ cell tumors. N Engl J Med 322:1425, 1990

136. Shaikin BS, Frantz E, Lookingbill DP: Histologically proven leukemia cutis carries a poor prognosis in acute nonlymphocytic leukemia. Cutis 39:57, 1987

137. Geelhoed GW, Graff KS, Duttera MJ et al: Acute leukemia presenting as a breast mass. JAMA 223:1488, 1973

138. Cohen PR, Talpaz M, Kurzock R: Malignancy associated Sweet's syndrome: review of the world literature. J Clin Oncol 6:1887, 1988

139. Cohen PR: Acral erythema: a clinical review. Cutis 51:175, 1993

140. Cohen PR, Holder WR, Rapini RP: Concurrent Sweet's syndrome and erythema noduosum: case report, world literature review and mechanism of pathogenesis. J Rheumatol 19:814, 1992

141. Dekker AW, Elderson A, Punt K et al: Meningeal involvement in patients with acute nonlymphocytic leukemia. Cancer 56:2078, 1985

142. Meyer RJ, Ferreira PPC, Cuttner J et al: Central nervous system involvement at presentation in acute granulocytic leukemia. A prospective centrifuge study. Am J Med 68:691, 1980

143. Cassileth PA, Sylvester LS, Bennett JM, Begg CB: High peripheral blast count in adult acute myelogenous leukemia is a primary risk factor for CNS leukemia. J Clin Oncol 6:495, 1988

144. Holmes R, Keating MJ, Cork A: A unique pattern of central nervous system leukemia in acute myelomonocytic leukemia associated with inv(16) (pl3q22). Blood 65:1071, 1985

145. Armitage JO, Bums CP: Maintenance therapy of adult acute nonlymphoblastic leukemia: an argument against the need for central nervous system prophylaxis. Cancer 41:697, 1978

146. Law IP, Blom J: Adult central nervous system leukemia: incidence and clinicopathologic features. South Med J 69:1054, 1976

147. Tobelem G, Jacquillat C, Chastang C et al: Acute monoblastic leukemia: a clinical and biologic study of 74 cases. Blood 55:71, 1980

148. Brinch L, Evensen SA, Stavem P: Leukemia in the central nervous system. J Intern Med 224:173, 1988

149. Buchem MA, Velde J, Willemze R, Spaander PJ: Leucostasis an underestimated cause of death in leukemia. Blut 56:39, 1988

150. McKee LC Jr, Collins RD: Intravascular leucocyte thrombi and aggregates as a course of morbidity and mortality in leukemia. Medicine 52:463, 1974

151. O'Regan S, Carson S, Chesney RW et al: Electrolyte and acid base disturbances in the management of leukemia. Blood 49:345, 1977
152. Band PR, Silverberg DS, Hendenon JF et al: Xanthine nephropathy in a patient with lymphosarcoma treated with allopurinol. N Engl J Med 283:354, 1970
153. Frame R, Head D, Lee R et al: Granulocytic sarcoma of the prostate. Two cases causing urinary obstruction. Cancer 59:142, 1987
154. Fennelly JJ, Smyth H, Muldowney FP: Extreme hyperkalemia due to rapid lysis of leukaemic cells. Lancet 1:27, 1974
155. Mir MA, Brabin B, Tang CT et al: Hypokaemia in acute myeloid leukemia. Ann Intern Med 82:54, 1975
156. Ossemman EF, Lawlor DP: Serum and urinary Lysoyme (muramidase) in monocytic and monomyelocytic leukemia. J Exp Med 124:921, 1966
157. Muggia FM, Heinemmann HO, Farhangi M et al: Lysozymuria and renal tubular dysfunction in monocytic and myelomonocytic leukemia. Am J Med 47:351, 1969
158. Oberg G, Dahl R, Ellegaard J et al: Diagnostic and prognostic significance of serum measurements of lactoferrin, lysozyme and myeloperoxidase in acute myeloid leukemia (AML): recognition of a new variant, high lactoferrin AML. Eur J Haematol 38:148, 1987
159. Perry M, Bauer JH, Farhangi M: Hypokalemia in acute myelogenous leukemia. South Med J 76:958, 1983
160. Seymour JF: Induction of hypomagnesemia during amascrine treatment. Am J Hematol 42:262, 1993
161. Gewirtz AM, Stewart AF, Vignery A et al: Hypercalcemia complicating acute myelogenous leukemia: a syndrome of multiple aetiologies. Br J Haematol 54:133, 1983
162. Mundy GR, Luben RA, Raisz IG et al: Bone resorbing activity in supernatants from lymphoid cell lines. N Engl J Med 290:867, 1974
163. Schenkein DP, O'Niel W, Shapiro J et al: Accelerated bone formation causing profound hypocalcemia in acute leukemia. Ann Intern Med 105:375, 1986
164. Boles JM, Dutel JL, Briere J et al: Acute renal failure caused by extreme hyperphosphatemia after chemotherapy of an acute lymphoblastic leukemia. Cancer 53:2425, 1984
165. Cervantes F, Ribera JM, Granena A et al: Tumor lysis syndrome with hypocalcemia in chronic granulocytic leukemia. Acta Haematol 68:157, 1981
166. Warrell RP Jr, Coonley CJ, Gee TS: Homoharringtonine: an effective new drug for remission induction in refractory nonlymphoblastic leukemia. J Clin Oncol 3:617, 1985
167. Thomas MR, Robinson WA, Mughal TL, Glode LM: Tumor lysis syndrome following VP-16-213 in chronic myeloid leukemia in blast crisis. Am J Hematol 16:185, 1984
168. Lenov Y, Golik A, Kaufman S, Gilboa Y: Acute tumour lysis syndrome with extreme metabolic abnormalities. Clin Lab Haematol 9:85, 1987
169. Paciussi PA, Cuttner J, Holland JF: Sequential intermediate dose cytosine arabinoside and mitoxantrone for patients with relapsed and refractory acute myelocytic leukemia. Am J Hematol 35:22, 1990
170. Harris KP, Hattersley JM, Feehally J, Walls J: Acute renal failure associated with haemotological malignancies: a review of 10 years experience. Eur J Haematol 47:119, 1991
171. Schilsky RL: Renal and metabolic complications of cancer chemotherapy. Semin Oncol 9:75, 1982
172. O'Connor NT, Prientice HG, Hoffbrand AV: Prevention of urate nephropathy in the tumour lysis syndrome. Clin Lab Haematol 11:97, 1989
173. Wainer RA, Wiernik PH, Thompson WL: Metabolic and therapeutic studies of a patient with acute leukemia and severe lactic acidosis of prolonged duration. Am J Med 55:255, 1973
174. Ventura GL, Hester JP, Smith TL, Keating MJ: Acute myeloblastic leukemia with hyperleukocytosis: risk factor for early mortality in induction. Am J Med 69:34, 1988
175. Budd D, Ginserg H: Hypocholesterolemia and acute myelogenous leukemia. Cancer 58:1361, 1986
176. Nimer SD, Champlin RE, Golde DW: Serum cholesterol lowering activity of granulocyte-macrophage colony stimulating factor. JAMA 260:3297, 1988
177. Chillar RK, Belman MJ, Farbstein M: Explanation for apparent hypoxemia associated with extreme leukocytosis: leukocyte oxygen consumption. Blood 55:922, 1980
178. Salomon J: Spurious hypoglycemia and hyperkalemia in myelomonocytic leukemia. Am J Med Sci 267:359, 1974
179. Robb RM, Ervin LD, Sallan SE: An autopsy study of eye involvement in acute leukemia of childhood. Med Pediatr Oncol 6:171, 1979
180. Ridgway EW, Jaffe N, Wafton DS: Leukemic ophthalmopathy in children. Cancer 38:1744, 1976
181. Cavdar AO, Babacan E, Gozdasoglu S et al: High risk subgroup of acute myelomonocytic leukemia (AMML) with orbito-ocular granulocytic sarcoma (OOGS) in Turkish children. Retrospective analysis of clinical, hematological, ultrastructural and therapeutic findings of thirty-three OOGS. Acta Haematol 81:80, 1989
182. Lister TJ, Johnson JW, Cuttner J et al: Pulmonary leukostasis as the single worst prognostic factor in patients with acute myelocytic leukemia and hyperleukocytosis. Am J Med 70:43, 1985
183. Cuttner J, Conjalka MS, Reilly M et al: Association of monocytic leukemia in patients who present with extreme leukocytosis. Am J Med 69:555, 1980
184. Jehn U, Goldel N, Rienmuller R, Wilmanns W: Non-cardiogenic pulmonary edema complicating intermediate and high dose Ara C treatment for relapsed acute leukemia. Med Oncol Tumor Pharmacother 5:41, 1988
185. Wiernik PH, Sutherland JC, Stechmiller BK et al: Clinically significant cardiac infiltration in acute leukemia, lymphocytic lymphoma and plasma cell myeloma. Med Pediatr Oncol 2:75, 1976
186. Shifrin EG, Drenger B, Matzner Y et al: Ruptured inflammatory abdominal aortic aneurysm due to acute myelomonocytic leukemia. J Cardiovasc Surg 28:32, 1987
187. Greenberg MS, Friedman H, Cohen SG et al: A comparative study of herpes simplex infections in renal transplant and leukemic patients. J Infect Dis 156:280, 1987
188. Lam MT, Pszin GJ, Armstrong JA et al: Herpes simplex infection in acute myelogenous leukemia and other hematologic malignancies. A prospective study. Cancer 48:2168, 1981
189. Strauss DJ, Mertelsman R, Kozine B et al: The monocytic leukemia: multidisciplinary studies in 45 patients. Medicine 59:409, 1980
190. Brago EA, Marshall RB, Riberi AM et al: Preleukemic granulocytic sarcoma of the gastrointestinal tract. Am J Clin Pathol 68:616, 1977
191. Steinbert D, Gold J, Brodin A: Necrotizing enterocolitis in leukemia. Arch Intern Med 131:538, 1973
192. Kunkel JM, Rosenthal D: Management of ileocecal syndrome. Dis Colon Rectum 29:196, 1986
193. Keidan R, Fanning J, Gatenby RA, Weese JL: Recurrent typhlitis. Dis Colon Rectum 32:206, 1989
194. Miller KB, McKanna JA, Tischler AS et al: Computer assessment of bone marrow cellularity. Pathology 4:247, 1986
195. Miller KB, Grunwald H, Preisler H et al: A prognostic indicator for AML induction: the day 6 bone marrow aspirate and biopsy. Blood 60:156a, 1982
196. Peanon EC: Crystal structure of Auer rods in acute myeloblastic leukemia. Clin Pathol 39:569, 1986
197. Seigneurin D, Audhuy B: Auer rods in refractory anemia with excess of blasts: presence and significance. Am J Clin Pathol 80:359, 1983
198. Bennett JM, Catovsky D, Daniel MT et al: Proposals for the classification of the myelodysplastic syndromes. Br J Haematol 51:184, 1982
199. Ritter J, Vormoor J, Creutzig U, Schellong G: Prognostic significance of auer rods in acute myelogenous leukemia: results of the studies AML-BMF-78 and -83. Med Pediatr Oncol 17:202, 1989
200. Bennett JM, Catovsky D, Daniel MT et al: Proposed revised criteria for the classification of acute myeloid leukemia. A report of the French-American-British Cooperative Group. Ann Intern Med 103:620, 1985
201. Miller KB, Kim K, Morrison FS et al: The evaluation of low dose cytarabine in the treatment of myelodysplastic syndromes: a phase III intergroup study. Ann Hematol 65:162, 1992
202. Catovsky D, Matutes E, Buccheri V et al: A classification of acute leukemia for the 1990's. Ann Hematol 62:16, 1991
203. Ryan DH: Phenotypic heterogeneity of acute leukemia. Clin Chim Acta 206:9, 1992
204. Cheson BD, Cassileth PA, Head DR et al: Report of the national cancer institue sponsored workshop on definitions of diagnosis and response in acute myeloid leukemia. J Clin Oncol 8:813, 1990
205. Van den Berghe: Morphology, immunologic and cytogenetic (MIC) working classification of the acute myeloid leukaemias. Br J Haematol 68:487, 1988
206. Stark AN, MacKarill ID, Limbert HS et al: TdT expression in acute myeloid leukemia. Blut 56:33, 1988
207. Painetta E, Van Ness B, Bennett J: Lymphoid lineage associated features in acute myeloid leukemia: phenotypic and genotypic correlations. Br J Haematol 82:324, 1992
208. Foon K, Gale RP, Todd RF: Recent advances in the immunologic classification of leukemia. Semin Hematol 23:257, 1986
209. Ball ED, Davis RB, Griffin JD et al: Prognostic value of lymphocyte surface markers in acute myeloid leukemia. Blood 77:2242, 1991
210. Griffin JD, Davis R, Nelson DA et al: Use of surface marker analysis to predict outcome of adult acute myeloblastic leukemia. Blood 68:1232, 1986
211. Reading C, Estey EH, Huh YO et al: Expression of unusual immunophenotype combination in acute myelogenous leukemia. Blood 81:3083, 1993
212. Ispizu AU, Matute E, Villamor N et al: The value of detecting surface and cytoplasmic antigens in acute myeloid leukemia. Br J Haematol 81:178, 1992
213. Kita K, Nakase K, Minwa H: Phenotypical characteristics of acute myelocytic

leukemia associated with the t(8;21) (q22•2) chromosomal abnormality: frequent expression of immature B-cell antigen CD19 together with stem cell anmtigen CD34. Blood 80:470, 1992

214. Smith OF, Lampkin BC, Versteeg C et al: Expression of lymphoid-associated cell surface antigens by childhood acute myeloid leukemia cells lack prognostic significance. Blood 79:2415, 1992

215. Bennett JM, Catovsky D, Daniel MT et al: Proposal for the recognition of minimally differentiated acute myeloid leukemia (AML-MO). Br J Haematol 78:325, 1991

216. Hanson CA, Abaza M, Sheldon S: Acute biphenotypic leukemia: immunophenotypic and cytogenetic analysis. Br J Haematol 84:49, 1993

217. Bennett JM, Catovsky D, Daniel MT et al: Proposals for the classification of the acute leukemias. Br J Haematol 33:451, 1976

218. Fourth International Workshop on Chromosomes in Leukemia, 1982: Correlation between morphology and karyotype. Cancer Genet Cytogenet 11:275, 1984

219. Bennet JM, Moloney WC, Greene MH, Boyce JD: Acute myeloid leukemia and other myelopathic disorders following treatment with alkylating agents. Hematologic Pathol 1:99, 1987

220. Bloomfield CD, Burning RD: The revised French-American-British classification of acute myeloid leukemia: is new better? Ann Intern Med 103:614, 1985

221. Hayhoe FGJ: Classification of acute leukemias. Blood Rev 2:186, 1988

222. Parreira A, Pombo de Oliveira MS, Matutes E et al: Terminal deoxynucleotidyl transferase positive acute myeloid leukaemia: an association with immature myeloblastic leukaemia. Br J Haematol 69:219, 1988

223. Vainchenker W, Villeval JL, Tabilio E et al: Immunophenotype of leukemic blasts with small peroxidase-positive granules detected by electron microscopy. Leukemia 2:274, 1988

224. Matutes E, Pombo de Oliveira M, Foroni L et al: The role of ultrastructural cytochemistry and monoclonal antibodies in clarifying the nature of undifferentiated cells in acute leukaemia. Br J Haematol 69:205, 1988

225. Lo Coco F, De Rossi G, Pasqualetti D et al: CD7 positive acute myeloid leukaemia: a subtype associated with cell immaturity. Br J Haematol 73:480, 1989

226. Eto T, Akashi K, Harada M et al: Biological characteristics of CD7 positive acute myelogenous leukaemia. Br J Haematol 82:508, 1992

227. Flandrin G, Bemard J: Cytological classification of acute leukemias. A survey of 1400 cases. Blood Cells 1:7, 1975

228. A Prospective Study of Acute Nonlymphocytic Leukemia. Fourth International Workshop on Chromosomes in Leukemia, Chicago, Sept 2–7, 1982. Cancer Genet Cytogenet 11:49, 1984

229. Swirsky DM, Li YS, Matthews JG et al: 8;21 translocation in acute granulocytic leukemia: cytological, cytochemical and clinical features. Br J Haematol 56:199 1984

230. Trujillo JM, Cork A, Ahearn MJ et al: Hematologic and cytologic characterization of 8;21 translocation acute granulocytic leukemia. Blood 53:695, 1979

231. Schiffer CA, Lee EJ, Tomisasa T et al: Prognostic impact of cytogenetic abnormalities in patients with de novo AML. Blood 73:263, 1989

232. Warrell RP, De The H, Wang Z-Y, Degos L: Acute promyelocytic leukemia. N Engl J Med 329:177, 1993

233. Golomb HM, Rowley JD, Vardiman JW et al: Microgranular acute promyelocytic leukemia: a distinct clinical, ultrastructural and cytogenetic entity. Blood 55:253, 1980

234. Mckenna RW, Parkin J, Bloomfield CD et al: Acute promyelocytic leukaemia: a study of 39 cases with identification of a hyperbasophilic microgranular variant. Br J Haematol 50:201, 1982

235. Krause JR, Stolc V, Kaplan SS, Penchansky L: Microgranular promyelocytic leukemia: a multiparameter examination. Am J Hematol 30:158, 1989

236. Larson RA, Kondo K, Vardiman JW et al: Evidence for a 15;17 translocation in every patient with acute promyelocytic leukemia. Am J Med 76:827, 1984

237. Kakizuka A, Miller WH, Umesona K et al: Chromosomal translocation t(15;17) in human acute promyelocytic leukemia fuses RARα with a novel putative transcription factor, PML. Cell 66:663, 1991

238. Evans RM: The steroid and thyroid hormone receptor super family. Science 240:889, 1988

239. Warrell RP, Frankel SR, Miller WH et al: Differentiation therapy of acute promyelocytic leukemia with tretinoin (all-trans-retinoic acid). N Engl J Med 324:1385, 1991

240. Chomienne C, Ballerini P, Balitrand N et al: All-trans retinoic acid in acute promyelocytic leukemias. II. In vitro studies: structure-function relationship. Blood 76:1710, 1990

241. Andop K, Kuboh T, Takada M et al: Tissue factor activity in leukemia cells. Cancer 59:748, 1987

242. Avvisti G, ten Cate JW, Mandelli F: The coagulopathy in acute promyelocytic leukemia: DIC? p. 91. In Muzzbeth L (ed): Hemostasis and Cancer. CRC Press, Boca Raton, FL, 1987

243. Imaoka S, Ueda T, Shibata H et al: Fibrinolysis in patients with acute promyelocytic leukemia and disseminated intravascular coagulation during heparin therapy. Cancer 58:173, 1986

244. Sterrenberg L, Haak HL, Brommer EJP, Nieuwenhuizen W: Evidence of fibrinogen breakdown by leukocyte enyme in a patient with acute promyelocytic leukemia. Haemostasis 15:126, 1985

245. Wijemmans PW, Rebel VI, Ossenkoppele GJ et al: Combined procoagulant activity and proteolytic activity of acute promyelocytic leukemic cells: reversal of the bleeding disorder by cell differentiation. Blood 73:800, 1989

246. Guarini A, Gugliotta L, Catani L et al: Procoagulant cellular activity (PCA) in the classification of acute leukemia. Thromb Res 45:545, 1987

247. Bennett B, Booth NA, Croll A et al: The bleeding disorder in acute proymelocytic leukemia: fibrinolysis due to U-PA rather than defibrination. Br J Haematol 71:511, 1989

248. Tallman M, Kwaan HC: Reassessing the hemostatic disorders associated with acute promyelocytic leukemia. Blood 79:543, 1992

249. Goldberg MA, Ginsburg D, Mayer PJ et al: Is heparin administration necessary during induction chemotherapy for patients with acute promyelocytic leukemia? Blood 69:187, 1987

250. Hoyle CF, Swinky PM, Freedman L, Hayhoe FG: Beneficial effects of heparin in the management of patients with APL. Br J Haematol 68:283, 1988

251. Sanz MA, Jarque 1, Martin G et al: Acute promyelocytic leukemia. Therapy and prognostic factors. Cancer 61:7, 1988

252. Bennett JM, Catovsky D, Daniel MT et al: A variant form of hypergranular promyelocytic leukemia. Br J Haematol 44:109, 1978

253. Golomb HM, Rowley JD, Vardiman JW et al: "Microgranular" acute promyelocytic leukemia: a distinct clinical, ultrastructural and cytogenetic entity. Blood 55:253, 1980

254. Le Beau MM, Larson RA, Bitter MA et al: Association of an inversion of chromosome 16 with abnormal marrow eosinophils in acute myelomonocytic leukemia. A unique cytogenetic-clinicopathological association. N Engl J Med 309:630, 1983

255. Neri G, Daniel A, Hammond N: Chromosome 16 eosinophilia and leukemia. Cancer Genet Cytogenet 14:371, 1985

256. Adriaansen HJ, Boekhorst AW, Hagemeijer AM et al: Acute myeloid leukemia M4 with bone marrow eosinophilia (m4Eo) and inv(16) (p13q22) exhibits a specific immunophenotype with CD2 expression. Blood 81:3043, 1993

257. Larson RA, Williams SF, LeBeau MM et al: Acute myelomonocytic leukemia with abnormal eosinophils and inv(16) or t(16:16) has a favorable prognosis. Blood 68:1242, 1986

258. David P, Lacombe B, Brouset F: Acute nonlymphocytic leukemia with marrow eosinophilia and chromosome 16 abnormality: a report of 18 cases. Leukemia 3:740, 1989

259. Schiffer CA, Lee EJ, Tomiyasu T et al: Prognostic impact of cytogenetic abnormalities in patients with de novo acute nonlymphocytic leukemia. Blood 73:263, 1989

260. Haferlach T, Gassmann W, Loffler H et al: Clinical aspects of acute myeloid leukemias of the FAB types M3 and M4Eo. Ann Hematol 66:165, 1993

261. Peterson BA, Levine EG: Uncommon subtypes of acute nonlymphocytic leukemia. Clinical features and management of FAB M5, M7. Semin Oncol 14:425, 1987

262. Scott SS, Stark AN, Limbert HJ, Master PS: Diagnostic and prognostic factors in acute monocytic leukaemia: an analysis of 51 cases. Br J Haematol 69:247, 1988

263. Tobelem G, Jacquillat C, Chastang C et al: Acute monoblastic leukemia: a clinical and biologic study of 74 cases. Blood 55:71, 1980

264. Report of the Medical Research Council's Working Party on Leukemia in Adults: The relationship between morphology and other features of acute myeloid leukemia and their prognostic significance. Br J Haematol, suppl. 31:165, 1975

265. Weil M, Jacquillat C, Tobelem G: Therapy of acute monoblastic leukemia. Hamatol Bluttransfus 27:189, 1981

266. Rees JKH, Gray RG, Swirsky D et al: Principal results of the Medical Research Council's 8th acute myeloid leukemia trial Lancet 2:1236, 1986

267. Hug V, Keating M, McCredie K et al: Clinical course and response to treatment of patients with acute myelogenous leukemia presenting with high leukocyte count. Cancer 52:773, 1983

268. Hiddemann W, Martin WR, Sauerland CM et al: Definition of refractoriness against conventional chemotherapy in acute myeloid leukemia: a proposal based on the results of retreatment by thioguanine, cytosine arabinoside, and daunorubicin (TAD 9) in 150 patients after standardized first line therapy. Leukemia 4:184, 1990

269. Hoyle CF, Gray RG, Wheatley K et al: Prognostic importance of sudan black positivity: a study of bone marrow slides from 1386 patients with de novo acute myeloid leukemia. Br J Haematol 79:398, 1991

270. Bodtrom B, Brunning RD, McGlave P et al: Bone marrow transplantation for

acute nonlymphocytic leukemia in first remission. Analysis of prognostic factors. Blood 55:1191, 1985

271. Greaves MF, Sieff C, Edwards PAW: Monoclonal antiglycophorin as a probe for erythroleukemias. Blood 61:645, 1983

272. Stanley M, McKenna RW, Ellinger G et al: Classification of 358 cases of acute myeloid leukemia by FAB criteria analysis of clinical and morphologic features. p. 155. In Bloomfield CD (ed): Chronic and Acute Leukemias in Adults. Martinus Nijhoff, Hingham, MA, 1985

273. Atkinson J, Hrisinko MA, Weil SC: Erythroleukemia: a review of 15 cases meeting 1985 FAB criteria and survey of the literature. Blood 6:204, 1992

274. Cuneo A, VanOrshoven A, Michaux JL et al: Morphologic, immunologic and cytogenetic studies in erythroleukaemia: evidence for multilineage involvement and identification of two distinct cytogenetic-clinicopathological types. Br J Haematol 75:346, 1990

275. Roggli VL, Saleem A: Erythroleukemia: a study of 15 cases and literature review. Cancer 49:101, 1982

276. Hetzel P, Gee TS: A new observation in the clinical spectrums of erythroleukemia. Am J Med 64:765, 1978

277. Bennett JM, Catovsky D, Daniel MT et al: Criteria for the diagnosis of acute leukemia of megakaryocytic lineage. Ann Intern Med 103:460, 1985

278. Von Boros J, Korenyi A: Uber einen Fall von akuter megakaryoblasten Leukamie: zugleich einige Bemerkungen zum Problem der akuten Leukamie. Z Klin Med 17:118, 1931

279. Ruiz-Arguelles GJ, Marin-Lopez A, Lobato-Mendizaba E et al: Acute megakaryoblastic leukaemia: a prospective study of its identification and treatment. Br J Haematol 62:55, 1986

280. Polli N, O'Brien M, Tavares De Castro J et al: Characterization of blast cells in chronic granulocytic leukemia in transformation, acute myelofibrosis and undifferentiated leukemia. 1. Ultrastructural morphology and cytochemistry. Br J Haematol 59:277, 1984

281. Amberger DM, Saleem A, Kemp BL: Acute myelofibrosis—a leukemia of pluripotent stem cell. A report of three cases and review of the literature. Ann Clin Lab Sci 11/12:409, 1990

282. Smith RE, Chelmowski MK, Szabo EJ: Myelofibrosis: a review of clinical and pathologic features and treatment. Crit Rev Oncol Hematol 10:305, 1990

283. Ross R, Raines EW, Bowen-Pope DF: The biology of platelet derived growth factor. Cell 46:155, 1986

284. San Miguel JF, Gonzales M, Canizo MS et al: Leukemia with megakaryoblastic involvement: clinical hematologic and immunologic characteristics. Blood 72:402, 1988

285. San Miguel JF, Tavares De Castro J, Matutes E: Characterization of blast cells in chronic granulocytic leukemia in transformation, acute myelofibrosis and undifferentiated leukemia. II. Studies with monoclonal antibodies and terminal transferase. Br J Haematol 59:297, 1985

286. Choate JJ, Domenico DR, McGraw TP et al: Diagnosis of acute megakaryoblastic leukemia by flow cytometry and immunoalkaline phosphatase techniques. Utilization of new monoclonal antibodies. Am J Clin Pathol 89:247, 1988

287. Betz SA, Foucar K, Head DR et al: False-positive flow cytometric platelet glycoprotein IIb/IIIa expression in myeloid leukemias secondary to platelet adherence to blasts. Blood 79:2399, 1992

288. Chan WC, Brynes RK, Kim TH et al: Acute megakaryoblastic leukemia in early childhood. Blood 62:92, 1983

289. Berger R, Flanrin G, Bernheim A et al: Cytogenetic studies on 519 consecutive de novo acute nonlymphocytic leukemias. Cancer Genet Cytogenet 29: 9, 1987

290. Ruiz-Arguelles GJ, Lobato-Mendiazabal E, San Miguel JF et al: Long term treatment results for acute megakaryoblastic leukaemia patients a multicentre study. Br J Haematol 82:651, 1992

291. Mehta AB, Baughan ASJ, Catovsky D et al: Revenal of marrow fibrosis in acute megakaryoblastic leukaemia after remission-induction and consolidation chemotherapy followed by bone marrow transplantation. Br J Haematol 53:445, 1983

292. Jacobs P, Le Roux 1, Jacobs L: Megakaryoblastic transformation in myeloproliferative disorder. Cancer 54:297, 1984

293. Greaves MF, Chan LC, Furley AJW et al: Lineage promiscuity in hemopoietic difkrentiation and leukemia. Blood 67:1, 1986

294. Stass S, Mirro J, Melvin S et al: Lineage switch in acute leukemia. Blood 64: 701, 1984

295. Smith LJ, Curtis JE, Messner HA et al: Lineage infidelity in acute leukemia. Blood 61:1138, 1983

296. Hanson C, Abaza M, Sheldon M et al: Acute biphenotypic leukemia: immunophenotypic and cytogenetic analysis. Br J Haematol 84:49, 1993

297. Bordessoule D, Jones M, Glatter KC et al: Immunohistological patterns of myeloid antigens: tissue distribution of CD13, CD14, CD16, CD31, CD36, CD65, CD66 and CD67. Br J Haematol 83:370, 1993

298. Paietta E, Racevkis J, Bennett JM et al: Differential expression of terminal transferase (TdT) in acute lymphocytic leukaemia expressing myeloid antigens and TDT positive acute myeloid leukaemia as compared to myeloid antigen negative acute lymphocytic leukaemia. Br J Haematol 84:416, 1993

299. Pui CH, Raimondi SC, Head D et al: Characterization of childhood acute leukemia with multiple myeloid and lymphoid markers at diagnosis and at relapse. Blood 78:1327, 1991

300. Drexler HG, Thiel E, Ludwig WD: Review of the incidence and clinical relevance of myeloid antigen-positive acute lymphoblastic leukemia. Leukemia 5:637, 1991

301. Mirro J, Antoun GR, Zipf TF et al: The E-rosette-associated antigen of T cells can be identified on blasts from patients with acute myeloblastic leukemia. Blood 65:363, 1985

302. Cross AH, Goorha RM, Nuss R et al: Acute myeloid leukemia with lymphoid features: a distinct biologic and clinical entity. Blood 72:579, 1988

303. Childs CC, Hirsch-Ginsberg C, Walters RS et al: Myeloid surface antigenpositive acute lymphoblastic leukemia (My+ ALL): immunophenotypic, ultrastructural and molecular characteristics. Leukemia 3:777, 1989

304. Nosaka T, Ohno H, Doi S et al: Phenotypic conversion of T lymphoblastic lymphoma to acute biphenotypic leukemia composed of lymphoblasts and myeloblasts. J Clin Invest 81:1824, 1988

305. Thomas X, Campos L, Archimbaud E et al: Surface marker expression in acute myeloid leukaemia at first relapse. Br J Haematol 81:40, 1992

306. Pui CH, Behm FG, Raimondi SC et al: Secondary acute myeloid leukemia in children treated for acute lymphoid leukemia. N Engl J Med 321:136, 1989

307. Griffin JD: The use of monoclonal antibodies in the characterization of myeloid leukemia. Hematol Pathol 1:81, 1987

308. Gale RP, Ben Bassat I: Hybrid acute leukemia. Br J Haematol 65:261, 1987

309. Greaves MF: Differentiation linked leukogenesis. Science 234:697, 1986

310. Youness E, Trujillo JM, Ahern MJ et al: Acute unclassified leukemia. A clincopathologic study with diagnostic implications of electron microscopy. Am J Hematol 9:79, 1980

311. Vaugh WP, Civin Cl, Weisenburger DD et al: Acute leukemia expression with the normal human hematopoietic stem cell membrane glycoprotein, CD34. Leukemia 2:661, 1988

312. Lee EL, Pollak A, Leavitt RD et al: Minimally differentiated acute nonlymphocytic leukemia. A distinct entity. Blood 70:1400, 1987

313. Schachner J, Kantarjian H, Dalton WT et al: Cytogenetic association and prognostic significance of bone marrow blast cell terminal transferase in patients with acute myeloblastic leukemia. Leukemia 2:667, 1988

314. Mirro J, Zipf TF, Pui C-H et al: Acute mixed lineage leukemia: clinicopathologic correlations and prognostic significance. Blood 66:115, 1985

315. Stone RM, Mayer RJ: The approach to the elderly patient with acute myeloid leukemia. Hematol Oncol Clin North Am 7:64, 1993

316. Preisler HD, Raza A, Barcos M et al: High dose cytosine arabinoside as the initial treatment of poor risk patients with acute nonlymphocytic leukemia: a leukemia intergroup study. J Clinical Oncology 5:75, 1987

317. Willemze R, Jager U, Jehn U et al: Intermediate- and high-dose ara-C and m-AMSA for remission induction and consolidation treatment of patients with acute myeloid leukemia: an EORTC leukemia cooperative group phase II. Eur J Cancer Clin Oncol 24:1721, 1988

318. Nara N, Chen GJ, Murohashi I: The *in vitro* growth patterns and drug sensitivities of leukemic blast progenitors among the subtypes of acute myelocytic leukemia. Exp Hematol 20:904, 1992

319. Hunter AE, Rogers SY, Roberts IA et al: Autonomous growth of blast cells is associated with reduced survival in acute myeloblastic leukemia. Blood 82:899, 1993

320. Bowman G, Preisler HD, Vogler WR et al: The clonogenic assay as a reproducible in vitro system to study predictive parameter of treatment outcome in acute nonlymphocytic leukemia. Am J Hematol 15:227, 1983

321. Short T, Miller KB, Desforges JD: The predictive value of in vitro techniques in acute nonlymphocytic leukemia. Leuk Res 11:687, 1987

322. Lowenberg B, van Putten Win LJ, Touw IP et al: Autonomous proliferation of leukemic cells in vitro as a determinant of prognosis in adult acute myeloid leukemia. N Engl J Med 328:614, 1993

323. Raza A, Preisler HD, Day R et al: Direct relationship between remission duration in acute myeloid leukemia and cell cycle kinetics. A leukemia intergroup study. Blood 76:2191, 1990

324. Campos L, Guyotat D, Archimbaud E et al: Clinical significance of multidrug resistance P-glycoprotein expression on acute nonlymphoblastic leukemia cells at diagnosis. Blood 79:473, 1992

325. Hughes WT, Armstrong D, Bodey GP et al: Guidelines for the use of antimicrobial agents in neutropenic patients with unexplained fever. A statement by the Infectious Disease Society of America. J Infect Dis 161:381, 1991

326. Ohno R, Tomonaga M, Kobayashi T et al: Effect of granulocyte colony-stimu-

lating factor after intensive induction therapy in relapse or refractory acute leukemia. N Engl J Med 323:871, 1990

327. Zittoun R, Jehn U, Fiere D et al: Alternating versus repeated postremission treatment in adult acute myelogenous leukemia: a randomized phase-III study (AML6) of the EORTC leukemia cooperative group. Blood 73:896, 1989

328. Schiffer CA, Lee EJ, Romiyasu T et al: Prognostic impact of cytogenetic abnormalities in patients with de novo acute nonlymphocytic leukemia. Blood 73:263, 1989

329. Arthur DC, Berger R, Golomb HM et al: The clinical significance of karyotype in acute myelogenous leukemia. Cancer Genet Cytogenet 40:203, 1989

330. Lobato ME, Ruiz-Arguelles GJ, Gomez Almaguer D: Long term treatment and prognostic factors in adult acute myeloblastic leukemia. (Experience of the INNSZ group Puebla Monterrey Mexico.) Rev Invest Clin 43:215, 1991

331. Solary E, Casasnovas RO, Campos et al: Surface markers in adult acute myeloblastic leukemia: correlation of CD19+, CD23+ and CD14+/ DR—phenotypes with shorter survival. Groupe d'Etude Immunologique des Leucemies (Geil). Leukemia 6:393, 1992

332. Caldwell FJ, Burns CP, Dick FR et al: Minimally differentiated acute leukemia. Leuk Res 17:199, 1993

333. Kowal VA, Cotelingam J, Schumacher HR: The prognostic significance of proerythroblasts in acute erythroleukemia. Am J Clin Pathol 98:34, 1992

334. Ritter J, Vormoor J, Creutzig U, Schellong G: Prognostic significance of Auer rods in childhood acute myelogenous leukemia: results of the studies AML-BFM and -3. Med Pediatr Oncol 17:202, 1989

335. Nagai K, Matsuo T, Atogami S et al: Remission with morphological myelodys-plasia: implications for early relapse. Br J Haematol 81:33, 1992

Therapy for Acute Myeloid Leukemia

65

Elihu H. Estey, Hagop Kantarjian, and Michael J. Keating

INTRODUCTION

The goal of therapy in acute myeloid leukemia (AML) is to produce and maintain a complete remission (CR). As defined by a National Cancer Institute-sponsored workshop,[1] CR means circulating neutrophil and platelet counts >1,500/mm^3 and 100,000/mm^3 respectively, and a bone marrow consisting of <5% blasts and >20% cellularity and showing normal maturation of all lineages. Defined in this way, CRs are more durable than lesser degrees of hematologic response and are associated with longer survival.[2] Approximately 10–15% of patients with AML treated with chemotherapy are alive ≥5 years after diagnosis. In these patients, virtually the entire period after the initial month of treatment will have been spent in CR, establishing achievement and maintenance of CR as the key to potential cure of AML.

Treatment of AML is divided into remission induction and postremission phases. Postremission therapy consists of maintenance, consolidation, and intensification, or a combination of all three. Maintenance therapy is usually defined as therapy less myelosuppressive than that used to induce remission. Consolidation and intensification therapies generally approach or surpass the myelosuppressive toxicity of induction therapy. This chapter considers remission induction, maintenance, and consolidation/intensification separately.

REMISSION INDUCTION THERAPY

Remission induction therapy is based on the principle of combining drugs that are each active as single agents. The most active single agents are arabinosylcytosine (ara-C) and drugs that interact with the enzyme topoisomerase II, in particular the anthracyclines. A pyrimidine nucleoside analogue of cytosine, ara-C was first used to treat AML during the late 1960s.[3] To exert cytotoxicity, the drug must be converted to its

triphosphate, ara-CTP, by the enzyme deoxycytidine kinase.[4] It was originally postulated that ara-CTP competed with deoxycytidine triphosphate (dCTP) for DNA polymerase. More recent evidence suggests that ara-C is incorporated into DNA, serving to terminate growing DNA chains.[5] The drug's half-life is very short[6] (15 minutes), providing a rationale for the use of continuous, rather than intermittent, dosing schedules. The duration of the continuous infusion clearly affects response rate. For example, early studies of the Southwestern Oncology Group (SWOG) demonstrated that at similar total doses patients who received the drug over 5 days had higher CR rates than those of patients who received the drug over 2 days.[7] Used at 200 mg/m^2/day for 5 days by continuous infusion, ara-C produces CR rates of approximately 40%. The median remission duration is approximately 1 year, and about 10% of patients will be in initial remission 8–10 years after treatment.[8] At this dose, the drug's major toxicities are myelosuppression and gastrointestinal problems.

The initial anthracycline used in the treatment of AML was daunorubicin. Doses of 60 mg/m^2 for 3–7 days produce CR rates similar to those observed with single-agent ara-C.[9] The principal toxicities are also similar, with the exceptions of alopecia and a cardiomyopathy that can be prevented by limiting the total dose received. Anthracyclines are believed to stabilize a complex between DNA and the enzyme topoisomerase II. This complex is a normal intermediate in the topologic alternations of DNA induced by the enzyme.[10] The stabilized complex leads to cell death, by a mechanism that is poorly understood.

Daunorubicin was first combined with ara-C during the 1970s; a regimen consisting of daunorubicin (45–60 mg/m^2/ day) on days 1–3 and ara-C (100 mg/m^2/day by continuous infusion) on days 1–7 became standard therapy. This regimen, commonly known as 3 + 7, remains the most widely used regimen for treatment of newly diagnosed AML. Typically, a bone marrow aspirate is examined 2 weeks after 3 + 7 is begun. If blast cells are evident in this day 14 marrow, and the marrow is cellular, a second course of therapy is commenced. If the day 14 marrow has <5% blasts or is hypocellular, therapy is delayed and the marrow examined one or two times weekly. If an increased number of blasts is again apparent, a second course of therapy is begun. If CR is not obtained after this course, patients are usually offered alternative therapies. This is principally because the remissions attained after >2 courses of therapy are typically very short.[11]

In comparison to the approximately 40% CR rates seen following single-agent ara-C or daunorubicin, the 3 + 7 regimen typically produces CR rates of 50–70%.[12–15] Approximately one-half of patients who fail to enter CR will die during induction, chiefly of infection, especially fungal pneumonia, or hemorrhage, the latter especially if the diagnosis is acute promyelocytic leukemia (APL).[16] The other half will survive induction but be resistant to chemotherapy.[16] These patients are divided into those in whom therapy does not produce significant marrow cytoreduction and those in whom regrowth of leukemia follows a period of cytoreduction.[16,17] Despite the use of maintenance therapy, median remission durations remain only about 1–1.5 years, and only about 15–20% of patients achieving CR are still in CR 5–7 years later.[12–15] The likelihood of relapse begins to decrease after 2–3 years of remission and has decreased to such an extent after 5 years that patients in CR at this time can be considered potentially cured.[12–15,18] To improve CR rates and remission duration, various permutations of the basic 3 + 7 regimen have been investigated. These have included modification of the number of days of drug administration, choice of anthracycline, dose of ara-C, addition of other drugs, and, most recently, use of recombinant hematopoietic growth factors.

Number of Days of Drug Administration

In a randomized study[19] involving 385 patients, the Cancer and Acute Leukemia Group B (CALGB) demonstrated that the 3 + 7 regimen (daunorubicin 45 mg/m^2/day IV × 3 days + ara-C 100 mg/m^2/day × 7 days by continuous intravenous infusion) produced higher CR rates than daunorubicin and ara-C at the same doses, but given for 2 and 5 days, respectively (2 + 5). CR rates were 52% for 3 + 7 versus 30% for 2 + 5. CRs were obtained on average 9 days earlier with 3 + 7 than with 2 + 5. As a result, duration of myelosuppression and likelihood of fatal sepsis or hemorrhage were less. The same conclusion was reached from a trial conducted by the Medical Research Council of the United Kingdom[20] in which patients were randomly allocated to receive either 1 day of daunorubicin and 5 days of ara-C (1 + 5) or 3 and 10 days of the 2 drugs, respectively (3 + 10). Not only was the CR rate higher in patients given 3 + 10 but, due to the more rapid achievement of CR, red cell and platelet transfusion requirements were less with 3 + 10, as were the number of days spent on antibiotics and in hospital. The same was true if only patients who entered CR were considered.

While 5 days of ara-C and 1–2 days of daunorubicin appear inferior to 3 + 7 or 3 + 10, another CALGB study[21] suggests that there is little difference between the latter 2 regimens. Among 452 randomized patients CR rates were statistically the same (53%, 3 + 7 versus 57%, 3 + 10) as was median remission duration (1 year for either group) and percentage of long-term remissions (22% at 3 years in either group).

Choice of Anthracycline

Doxorubicin (Adriamycin), amsacrine, mitoxantrone, aclarubicin, and idarubicin have all been substituted for daunorubicin in the basic 3 + 7 regimen. In a randomized comparison, the CALGB[22] found CR rates following doxorubicin to be lower than following daunorubicin and that doxorubicin produced more severe gastrointestinal toxicity. By contrast, amsacrine,[23] mitoxantrone,[24] and aclarubicin[25] have been reported in randomized studies to produce higher CR rates and, in the case of amsacrine, longer survival, than achieved with daunorubicin. These studies await confirmation. Indeed another randomized study[26] using virtually the same doses of ara-C, daunorubicin, and amsacrine found identical CR rates and more toxicity in the amsacrine-treated group.

Idarubicin is the anthracycline that has received the most recent attention. Three large randomized studies have been conducted comparing standard-dose ara-C plus either daunorubicin or idarubicin (12–13 mg/m^2/day × 3 days) as induction therapy.[27–29] In each study, patients once in remission received two to three courses of the induction regimen at reduced total dose. Each study found idarubicin + ara-C to be superior to daunorubicin + ara-C. These studies are summarized in Table 65-1. Although the Berman et al.[27] study was limited to adults <60 years of age, older patients were eligible in the studies performed by Wiernik et al.[28] and Vogler et al.[29]; in both, CR rates were higher following idarubicin + ara-C in the older as well as the younger patients. Extramedullary toxicity was similar with both regimens, although duration of myelosuppression was greater in the idarubicin + ara-C arm in the studies conducted by Wiernik et al.[28] and Vogler et al.[29] These investigations appear to establish idarubicin, at the doses investigated, + ara-C as the standard induction regimen in newly diagnosed AML. Reasons for the superiority of idarubicin may include the activity of its metabolite, idarubicinol, or the relative inability of leukemia cells to pump out idarubicin, possibly because idarubicin is a comparatively poor substrate for the P170 glycoprotein involved in the transport of drugs such as anthracyclines and etoposide out of cells.

High-Dose ara-C

High-dose ara-C (HDAC) generally denotes daily doses of 2–6 g/m^2 and conventional-dose ara-C denotes daily doses of 100 or 200 mg/m^2, either of these 2 latter doses producing similar outcomes when given for 7 days in combination with daunorubicin.[30] Use of HDAC for remission induction in newly diagnosed patients stems from observations that patients in relapse after maintenance with conventional ara-C doses could again be induced into CR following doses of 3 g/m^2 bid IV for 6–12 doses.[31–34] Several toxicities also became apparent at these higher doses. These included cerebellar and cerebral dysfunction,[35] noncardiogeneic pulmonary edema,[36] pericardial effusion,[36] and conjunctivitis. The risk of nervous system toxicity increases sharply with age and decreasing renal function.[35] The effectiveness of HDAC was presumed a result of higher intracellular concentrations of ara-CTP. It was therefore of interest that Plunkett et al.[37] found that plasma ara-C concentrations of 7–10 μM, achieved at ara-C dose rates of approximately 0.5–1 g/m^2 over 2 hours, resulted in maximal intracellular accumulation of ara-CTP, presumably reflecting saturation of deoxycytidine kinase at higher ara-C concentrations. These observations suggested that ara-C dose rates of 0.5–1 g/m^2 over 2 hours (intermediate dose ara-C [IDAC]) might be as effective as HDAC and might produce less toxicity consequent to lower plasma ara-C concentrations. Results from studies in relapsed disease supported this hypothesis[38,39] and led to studies in newly diagnosed disease comparing anthracycline + conventional-dose ara-C to anthracycline + HDAC or anthracycline + IDAC.

Several nonrandomized studies have investigated HDAC-containing induction therapy. Phillips et al.[40] noted a 90% CR rate and a 27% probability of long-term (5–7 year) disease-free sur-

THERAPY FOR ACUTE MYELOID LEUKEMIA

Initial Assessment

The diagnosis of AML is made when the bone marrow contains >30% blasts of which >3% stain for myeloperoxidase. Acute monocytic leukemia can be peroxidase negative but will usually show positivity with butyrate or nonspecific esterase stains. Surface markers and electron microscopy may be useful in diagnosing erythroleukemia and megakaryocytic leukemia. When the initial marrow is obtained, specimens are sent for cytogenetics. HLA typing of the patient and family members is also done at diagnosis.

Once the diagnosis of AML is made, the need for emergency treatment should be assessed. Such treatment is required if the circulating blast count is >50,000/mm^3 or if the patient has APL, DIC, or organ dysfunction attributed to leukemic infiltration. Patients most likely to have leukemic infiltration are those with circulating blast counts of >10,000/mm^3. Patients with a temperature >101°F are begun on intravenous ceftazidime and vancomycin and prophylactically placed on fluconazole. Patients with platelet counts of <20,000/mm^3 receive platelet transfusions as described below.

Supportive Care

Patients are given 2–3 L of bicarbonate-containing intravenous fluid daily to prevent the development of tumor lysis syndrome and attendant hyperuricemia. Allopurinol is given only if the white blood cell (WBC) count is >10,000/mm^3. If the WBC count is >50,000/mm^3, leukapheresis is begun immediately, in conjunction with chemotherapy. By reducing tumor burden, pheresis may prevent development of tumor lysis syndrome. If renal function deteriorates or hyperphosphatemia or hyperkalemia ensues nonetheless, hemodialysis is instituted.

Patients who are afebrile (<101°F) at presentation are begun prophylactically on trimethoprim sulfamethoxazole, 1 double strength tablet bid, and fluconazole, 400 mg tid. If temperature >101°F develops unrelated to blood product administration, patients are begun on intravenous ceftazidime and vancomycin. If fever persists and cultures are unrevealing after 3 days, amphotericin B therapy is instituted. We use 1 mg/kg. There is no need for a test dose if appropriate premedication (meperidine, diphenhydramine, low-dose hydrocortisone) is used. If, despite the addition of amphotericin, there is evidence of progressive infection (development of pneumonia, persistently positive cultures) and persistent neutropenia, we begin administration of CSF-G and consider granulocyte transfusions from family donors if the donors can be treated with CSF-G to raise their granulocyte count.

Platelet transfusions are given routinely if the platelet count is <20,000. Exceptions may be made if the count has been below this level for weeks, if the patient is not bleeding, and if the patient does not have mucositis or DIC. If bleeding or DIC is present, platelet transfusions should be given if the platelet count is <50,000. If significant increments in platelet count are not obtained with pooled platelet concentrates, family members are used as donors. Transfusions of cryoprecipitate are given to maintain the fibrinogen level at >200 in patients with APL.

Remission Induction Therapy

We treat our patients with APL with all-trans-retinoic acid (ATRA) 45 mg/m^2 day until CR is achieved. Idarubicin (12 mg/m^2/day × 4 days) is begun 5 days after initiation of ATRA or sooner if leukocytosis >10,000 develops. If ATRA syndrome develops, we discontinue ATRA and administer dexamethasone (10 mg IV) bid for 3 days, followed by rapid taper. If the marrow shows persistent blasts, a second course of idarubicin is not begun until 5 weeks have elapsed after initial treatment, unless DIC ensues before then.

Patients with other types of AML are given idarubicin (12 mg/m^2/day on days 1–3) + high-dose ara-C (1.5 g/m^2/day on days 1–4 by continuous infusion or 2 g/m^2 over 4 hours once daily on days 1–4), if they are <age 60 and have a good performance status. Otherwise they receive idarubicin as above, plus conventional-dose ara-C (100 mg/m^2 day × 7 days by continuous infusion). A second course of therapy is not begun before day 21 of the first course, unless the circulating blast count rises before then. Patients not in remission after two courses are first considered for allo-BMT; if this is not feasible, they are offered investigational chemotherapy.

An alternative approach would be to assign patients to treatment on the basis of cytogenetic results, provided these are available within 3–4 days of presentation. With this approach, patients with abnormalities of chromosome 5 or 7, or both, would be immediately offered investigational therapies based on their low likelihood of achieving CR with conventional therapy or HDAC.

Postremission Therapy

By the time remission is achieved, pretreatment cytogenetic information should be available and used to plan therapy. Patients with inv(16) or t(8;21) are given HDAC (1.5 g/m^2 day × 2 days by continuous infusion) + idarubicin (8 mg/m^2/day on days 1 and 2) alternating with ara-C (100 mg/m^2/day on days 1–5) until they have been in CR for 6 months. For patients aged >60, the duration of each course of HDAC is decreased by 25%. Patients with t(15;17) (APL) receive one course of idarubicin (12 mg/m^2/day × 2 days), alternating with three courses of POMP until in CR for 1 year. Patients with other karyotypes are offered allo-BMT if <55 years of age, with an HLA-identical sibling donor. Otherwise, they are considered for investigational therapy.

Bone Marrow Transplantation

Aside from use in poor-prognosis patients in first remission, we recommend allo-BMT in first relapse if the patient is <55 years of age and has an HLA-matched sibling donor, or is <46 years old and has an HLA-identical unrelated donor.

Table 65-1. Randomized Comparisons of 3 + 7 Regimen Given with 3 Days of Either Daunorubicin or Idarubicin

		CR (%)		Median Months CR Duration		Median Months Survival	
Study	No. of Patients	3 + 7 Dauno	3 + 7 Ida	3 + 7 Dauno	3 + 7 Ida	3 + 7 Dauno	3 + 7 Ida
Berman et al.[27] (1991)	120	58	80[a]	Not given	Not given	13.5	19.7[a]
Wiernik et al.[28] (1992)	208	59	70	8.4	9.4[a]	8.7	12.9[a]
Vogler et al.[29] (1992)	230	55	69[a]	10.9	14.4	9.2	9.9

Abbreviations: Dauno, daunorubicin; Ida, idarubicin.
[a] $P < 0.05$ favoring idarubicin.

vival in a study involving 70 patients <age 60 who received HDAC bid for 12 doses + daunorubicin for both induction and intensification. Severe cerebellar toxicity occurred in 18% of cases. Using 12 doses of HDAC as a single agent in 43 patients, Curtis et al.[41] reported a higher CR rate than seen among 57 similarly aged patients given a 3 + 7 regimen using doxorubicin rather than daunorubicin (63% versus 37%, $P=0.01$).

Randomized studies, however, have not found higher CR rates following HDAC- or IDAC-containing induction therapy. Table 65-2 summarizes results from 3 such studies.[42–44] The SWOG[42] and UCLA[44] studies compared daunorubicin + ara-C at 200 mg/m² on days 1–7 versus either ara-C at 2 g/m² bid for 6 days (SWOG) or at 0.5 g/m² bid for 6 days (UCLA). The Australian Leukemia Study Group (ALSG) compared daunorubicin + etoposide with ara-C at 100 mg/m²/day × 7 or at 3 g/m² bid for 4 days.[43] While none of the studies found statistically significantly differences in CR rates among the regimens, all three studies found increased toxicity with the IDAC or HDAC regimens. This was most striking in the SWOG study,[42] in which both fatal toxicity and central nervous system toxicity were statistically greater ($P <0.001$) in the HDAC patients. Although neither the UCLA[44] nor the ALSG[43] study found an increased rate of toxic deaths or neurotoxicity in HDAC- or IDAC-treated patients, these patients had more gastrointestinal toxicity in both studies and more myelosuppression in the ALSG study.

Thus, direct comparisons to date indicate that IDAC or HDAC induction regimens have a lower therapeutic index than that found in conventional-dose regimens. However, as shown in Table 65-2, the ALSG study[43] suggests that the use of HDAC during induction may prolong remission duration.

Addition of Other Drugs to Daunorubicin + ara-C Induction

The purine analogue 6-thioguanine (6-TG) is frequently added to the basic 3 + 7 combination. This three-drug combination is known as TAD or DAT. However, a CALGB study[21] in which 668 patients were randomized to receive either daunorubicin + ara-C with or without 6-TG found no difference in CR rate, remission duration, or survival between the regimens.

Recent attention has focused on etoposide. Although etoposide, like the anthracyclines, stabilizes the DNA-topoisomerase II complex,[45] these drugs may have different binding sites on topoisomerase II.[46] Etoposide has activity in disease that has relapsed following anthracycline therapy.[47–49] These observations led the ALSG[50] to assign 264 newly diagnosed patients randomly to receive either the standard 3 + 7 regimen or the same regimen with the addition of etoposide (75 mg/m²/day on days 1–7). In remission, patients received the same regimen used for induction, but at a reduced dose. Remission rates were approximately the same in the two groups (56% versus 59%), but remission duration was significantly ($P=0.01$) longer in the etoposide-treated patients, with medians of 12 versus 18 months. This finding reflected the results in patients <55 years of age; these patients also showed evidence ($P = 0.03$) of a survival advantage for the etoposide-containing regimen with medians of 9 and 17 months, respectively. Diarrhea was more frequent during induction and myelosuppression during maintenance courses more pronounced in the etoposide-treated group. Further follow-up evaluation will be needed to determine whether these toxicities are counterbalanced by improvements in long-term survival.

Use of Hematopoietic Growth Factors During Induction

The availability of hematopoietic growth factors through the use of molecular cloning techniques[51] has focused attention on the potential use of these compounds in AML. Trials conducted to date have employed colony-stimulating factor-granulocyte/macrophage (CSF-GM) and colony-stimulating factor-granulocyte (CSF-G). These molecules have been used in two general ways. First, they have been administered after the completion of chemotherapy generally until return of the neutrophil count to >1,000/mm³. The objective has been to accelerate the recovery of functional neutrophils, decreasing the period of risk of fatal infection, and, accordingly, improving CR rate. Second, they have been administered either before or during chemotherapy, or both. Here the intent has been to enhance the sensitivity of the blasts to chemotherapy, possibly

Table 65-2. Randomized Trials Comparing High-Dose or Intermediate-Dose ara-C with Conventional-Dose ara-C

			CR Rate		Remission Duration	
Study	HDAC or IDAC Given During	No. of Patients	Conventional-Dose ara-C Regimen	HDAC or IDAC Regimen	Conventional-Dose ara-C Regimen	HDAC or IDAC Regimen
Weick et al.[42] (1992)	Induction and intensification	639	Age <50 (59%) Age 50–64 (54%)	Age <50 (54%) Age 50–64 (45%)	Not given	Not given
Bishop et al.[43] (1992)	Induction only	279	74%	70%	Median 12.7 mo	Median 36.9 mo[a]
Schiller et al.[44] (1992)	Induction only	101	71%	74%	Median 8.5 mo	Median 8.5 mo
Cassileth et al.[78] (1992)	Intensification only	170	NA	NA	16 ± 8% at 4 yr	27 ± 10% at 4 yr[b]
Mayer et al.[79] (1992)	Intensification only	596	NA	NA	22% projected at 3 yr	42% projected at 3 yr

Abbreviation: NA, not applicable.
[a] $P < 0.05$ favoring HDAC regimen.
[b] $P < 0.07$ favoring HDAC regimen.

Table 65-3. Comparisons of Chemotherapy with or without CSF-GM or CSF-G

Study	CSF	Given	No. of Patients	Statistically Significant ($P < 0.05$) Effect on		
				CR Rate	Infection Rate	RD
Estey et al.[54] (1990)	GM	After CHDAC induction	65	No	No	No
Büchner et al.[55] (1991)	GM	After TAD induction if no leukemia in marrow	92	No	No	No
Ohno et al.[56] (1990)	G	After MAE induction if no leukemia in marrow	61	No	Yes	No
Estey et al.[57] (1992)	GM	Before and during dauno rubicin + CHDAC induction	232	Lower with GM	Not given	No
Büchner et al.[58] (1993)	GM	Before, during, and after induction and consolidation with TAD/HAM	72	No	Not given	Currently longer with GM
Estey et al.[59] (1993)	G	Before, during, and after FA induction	197	No	No	Currently longer with G

Abbreviations: RD, remission duration; CHDAC, continuous-infusion high-dose ara-C; TAD, 6-thioguanine, ara-C, daunorubicin; MAE, mitoxantrone, ara-C, etoposide; HAM, high-dose ara-C, mitoxantrone; FA, fludarabine, ara-C.

by increasing the proportion of these cells in the S phase of the cell cycle.[52,53] Either approach entails the risk of stimulating growth of leukemia cells. The second approach has the additional potential to sensitize normal as well as leukemic progenitors to chemotherapy, resulting in prolonged myelosuppression.

Table 65-3 summarizes six trials[54–59] of CSF-GM and CSF-G in chemotherapy for newly diagnosed or relapsed AML. In five of these trials,[54–56,58,59] administration of growth factor either began after, or continued after, completion of chemotherapy. In none of these five was CSF-GM in doses of 120 μg/m^2/day[54] or 250 μg/m^2/day[55,58] or CSF-G in doses of 200 μg/m^2/day[56] or 400 μg/m^2/day[59] found to accelerate regrowth of leukemia compared with patients receiving the same chemotherapy without growth factor. Three[55,56,59] of the four studies[54–56,59] for which data were available noted that time to neutrophil recovery was accelerated by an average of about 1 week in patients receiving growth factor after completion of chemotherapy. However, none of the five studies demonstrated a statistically significant ($P < 0.05$) improvement in CR rate in patients receiving CSF-GM or CSF-G. Only the Ohno et al.[56] study reported a statistically significant decrease in the rate of documented infection. Further information on these issues will be forthcoming from trials being conducted by the CALGB and Eastern Cooperative Oncology Group (ECOG), in which patients >65 years of age are randomly assigned to receive CSF-GM or placebo after completion of chemotherapy.

Bettelheim et al.[60] were the first to report the administration of growth factor (CSF-GM 250 μg/m^2/day) 1–2 days before and/or during the standard 3 + 7 regimen, with the objective of sensitizing blasts. Although the CR rate of 83% (15 of 18) appeared encouraging, three subsequent studies have found either no improvement[58,61] or a decrease[57] in the CR rate in newly diagnosed[57,58] or relapsed[61] patients receiving CSF-GM for 1–7 days before and/or during anthracycline + ara-C with or without etoposide. Similarly, administration of CSF-G (400 μg/m^2/day) beginning 1 day before and continuing during fludarabine + ara-C chemotherapy did not significantly improve the CR rate compared to that demonstrated in previous patients receiving the same chemotherapy without CSF-G.[59] Both this study[59] and a randomized comparison[58] of CSF-GM or placebo given before, during, and after a regimen, including both TAD and high-dose ara-C + mitoxantrone, currently report a longer remission duration in patients given growth factor. However, follow-up time of patients in remission in these studies is short, averaging only a few months. Until further information is provided, administration of CSF-GM or CSF-G, either before, during, or after chemotherapy of AML, is not warranted, except as part of a formal clinical trial.

THERAPY IN REMISSION

Maintenance Therapy

Traditionally, once in remission after treatment with the 3 + 7 regimen, patients continued to receive similar chemotherapy at approximately monthly intervals for 3–5 years.[19] Such chemotherapy was less myelosuppressive than that used to induce remission. This is called maintenance therapy. The need for maintenance therapy in first remission has been addressed in several randomized trials. Table 65-4 summarizes representative trials. The ECOG[62] randomized patients attaining remission either to receive no further therapy or to receive each week for 2 years a regimen consisting of 6-TG on days 1–4 and ara-C 60 mg/m^2 SC on day 5. Remission duration was clearly superior among patients assigned to receive maintenance. The likelihood of achieving a second remission was the same in both groups, while survival was significantly ($P < 0.05$) longer in the maintenance group. A similar result was obtained in an ECOG study in patients in second remission.[66]

Although the ECOG study indicates a need for further therapy in patients who attain CR, it does not indicate how long maintenance therapy should be continued. As shown in Table 65-4, this question was addressed by trials conducted by the CALGB[21] and cooperative groups in Switzerland,[63] Italy,[64] and Germany,[65] in which patients were randomized to continue or discontinue maintenance after they had been in CR for 1–8 months. The data indicate that once patients have received 3–4 months of maintenance, further maintenance therapy is of no benefit. In addition to the randomized studies listed in Table 65-4, a British study[67] in which patients were to receive six courses of 3 + 7 type therapy indicated that patients who received only the first three cycles had remissions equivalent to those of patients who received all six cycles. UCLA investigators[68] also reported similar remission duration (median 14 months) in patients who received only two postremission courses and in previous patients who received 2.5 years of continued maintenance. After administering ara-C + 6-TG for 3 years to 86 patients, Dutcher et al.[69] reported that 55% of the patients were alive and in CR at 1 year and that 23% were alive and in CR at 5 years, results similar to those reported, after much shorter durations of therapy, by the Italian,[64] British,[67] and UCLA[68] investigators. In summary, data from both randomized and nonrandomized studies do not support the practice of administering more than two to four courses of maintenance therapy to patients with AML.

Consolidation/Intensification

Consolidation therapy is taken to mean therapy that is more myelosuppressive than maintenance therapy. The CALGB conducted an early randomized study assessing the value of con-

Table 65-4. Randomized Comparisons of Maintenance Versus No Maintenance in Patients in First Remission

Study	No. of Patients	Months in CR When Randomized	Months of Further Maintenance	Median Months' CR Duration Maintenance Versus No Maintenance Groups	Statistical Difference ($P < 0.05$)
ECOG (Cassileth et al., 1988)[62]	51	0	24	8 vs. 4	Yes
CALGB (Preisler et al., 1987)[21]	94	8	36	16.9 vs. 10.7	No
Swiss (Sauter et al., 1984)[63]	74	3–4	24	18 vs. 18	No
Italian (Mandelli et al., 1990)[64]	107	3–4	18	18 vs. 18	No
German (Büchner et al., 1985)[65]	145	1	36	13 vs. 8	Yes

solidation therapy.[70] Patients in CR were assigned to receive maintenance therapy (6-TG on days 1–4, ara-C 60 mg/m^2 on day 5 weekly) for 2 years with or without two preceding courses of "consolidation" (i.e., 2 days of daunorubicin, 5 days of ara-C at conventional doses). The results were similar in both groups, and the investigators concluded that "for consolidation therapy to provide substantial improvement in CR duration intensive regimens with non-cross-resistant drugs will be required." A similar conclusion had been drawn from a historically controlled M.D. Anderson trial,[71] that led to the concept of intensification therapy. Most studies of intensification therapy have included HDAC, which, because it produced CRs in disease relapsing after conventional dose ara-C, has been considered a potentially "non-cross-resistant" therapy.

At least four studies[72–75] employing HDAC as intensification have reported favorable results. Patients treated have been generally young, similar to patients who would be eligible to receive an allogeneic transplant. Disease-free survival rates noted 5 years after entering CR have been 35–50%, rivaling those achieved after allogeneic transplantation. It is unclear whether more than one course of intensification is required, as several studies[74,75] have reported no difference in outcome between patients who received one or two courses. It must be noted that HDAC intensification therapy entails substantial myelosuppressive toxicity that will prove fatal in approximately 5–15% of patients.[72,73,75,76] Toxicity often limits the number of courses of HDAC that can be given.[72,74,75] Furthermore nonrandomized trials are not unanimous in finding HDAC-based intensification beneficial.[77]

Because of uncertainties surrounding the efficacy of HDAC intensification, especially in view of the regimen's toxicity, both the ECOG[78] and CALGB[79] undertook randomized trials comparing intensification with HDAC to more traditional maintenance. In the ECOG study[78] (Table 65-2), patients achieving CR with a DAT regimen, who were not candidates for allogeneic marrow transplantation, received either one course of HDAC (3 g/m^2 bid × 6 days) + amsacrine or 2 years of weekly 6-TG (days 1–4) + ara-C (60 mg/m^2 on day 5). Probabilities of event-free survival 4 years after randomization were 27 ± 10% for the HDAC group versus 16 ± 8% for the maintenance group ($P = 0.07$). Considering only patients <60 years of age (most patients), these probabilities were 28 ± 11% versus 15 ± 9% ($P = 0.04$) in favor of HDAC intensification. Treatment-related deaths occurred in 0% of the maintenance but in 21% of the HDAC group. Of the 14 patients >60 years of age, 57% died during HDAC intensification versus 13% of younger patients. Hence the benefit of HDAC intensification in this study was limited to patients aged <60.

The CALGB study[79] reached the same conclusion. In this trial, patients achieving CR after a 3 + 7 regimen were randomized to receive four courses of either HDAC (3 g/m^2 bid every other day for six doses), ara-C (400 mg/m^2/day × 5 days by continuous intravenous infusion), or a more traditional ara-C maintenance regimen (100 mg/m^2/day × 5 days by continuous intravenous infusion). Probabilities of continued remission 3 years after randomization were 42%, 35%, and 22% for HDAC, ara-C 400 mg/m^2/day × 5 days, and ara-C 100 mg/m^2/day × 5

days, respectively ($P = 0.006$). Further analysis showed that HDAC and 400 mg/m^2/day were each better than 100 mg/m^2/day × 5 days in patients <40 years of age and that HDAC was superior to both of the two lower doses in patients aged 41–60. All three regimens were equivalent in older patients who had shorter remissions than achieved by the younger patients ($P <0.01$). Deaths in remission occurred in 1% of patients treated with 100 mg/m^2 × 5 days but in 5–6% of those treated with 400 mg/m^2 × 5 days, or HDAC. Hospitalizations due to fever and neutropenia were needed in 70% of the HDAC courses and in 59% of courses of 400 mg/m^2/day × 5 days, but in only 16% of courses of 100 mg/m^2 × 5 days. Central nervous system toxicity occurred in 12% of HDAC-treated patients.

A review of the data presented in Table 65-2 shows that the three large randomized cooperative group trials[43,78,79] for which remission duration are available all currently report statistically longer remissions in patients given HDAC for induction or for intensification in CR. This superiority is limited to patients <60 years of age. The HDAC regimens are clearly more toxic; longer follow-up evaluation is required before the value of those regimens, even in younger patients, can be fully established.

Non-Cross-resistant Drugs

The concept of using multiple drugs to avoid the development of therapeutic resistance has received considerable attention in oncology. A difficulty with this approach in AML is the shortage of active drugs that are not mutually cross-resistant. For example, although agents such as amsacrine or mitoxantrone can produce CR in patients who have relapsed after treatment with other topoisomerase II-reactive drugs, the remissions are usually short.[80,81] Furthermore, the probability of CR after relapse has a strong association with duration of first remission.[82–84] One possible non-cross-resistant regimen, POMP (6-mercaptopurine, vincristine [Oncovin], methotrexate, prednisone), was investigated by the SWOG.[85] The SWOG randomized patients who had been maintained in CR for 10 months with conventional-dose ara-C to continue to receive ara-C for an additional 3 months or to receive three cycles of POMP. With a median follow-up of 9 years, median survivals from time of randomization were 34 months in the POMP-treated group versus 19 months in the ara-C-treated group ($P = 0.03$). This result was similar to one reported earlier from a historically controlled M.D. Anderson study.[86] Although awaiting further confirmation, the data suggest that non-cross-resistant therapies can be found in AML.

Allogeneic Bone Marrow Transplantation

The use of allogeneic bone marrow transplantation (allo-BMT) was first investigated in patients in chemotherapy-resistant relapse.[87] Sustained remissions were observed in 10–20% of patients.[87] This led to trials of allo-BMT in first remission; the relative merits of chemotherapy versus allo-BMT in these

Table 65-5. Comparisons of Allogeneic Transplant Versus Chemotherapy in First Remission in Adults

Study	No. of Patients	Actuarial Rates[a]						Statistically Significant Differences ($P < 0.05$)
		Relapse		Disease-Free Survival		Survival		
		Chemo (%)	Trans (%)	Chemo (%)	Trans (%)	Chemo (%)	Trans (%)	
Cassileth et al.[78] (1992)	54 Trans 29 Chemo	Not given	Not given	30	42	43	42	None
Schiller et al.[88] (1992)	28 Trans 54 Chemo	60	32	38	48	53	45	Relapse rate
Reiffers et al.[89] (1989)	23 Trans 20 Chemo	82	22	16	66	Not given	Not given	Relapse rate, disease-free survival rate
Appelbaum et al.[90] (1988)	44 Trans 46 Chemo	Not given	Not given	20	40	30	40	None
Conde et al.[91] (1988)	14 Trans 25 Chemo	78	10	17	70	Not given	Not given	Relapse rate
Champlin et al.[92] (1985)	23 Trans 44 Chemo	70	40	Not given	Not given	27	40	Relapse rate

Abbreviations: Chemo, chemotherapy; Trans, transplant.

[a] At 5 years in studies by Schiller et al., Appelbaum et al., and Champlin et al.; at 4 years in study by Cassileth et al.; at 3 years in study by Conde et al.; at 2.5 years in study by Reiffers et al.

patients remains highly controversial. Table 65-5 summarizes six trials[78,88–92] formally comparing these two therapeutic modalities in patients in first remission. Patients <41–50 years old who had an HLA-matched sibling donor were to receive allo-BMT, while similarly aged,[78,88–91] or similarly aged and older,[92] patients without a donor received chemotherapy. Chemotherapy included HDAC in four studies,[78,88,89,91] and conventional-dose ara-C + anthracycline with or without POMP in the remaining two.[90,92] In each study, patients assigned to receive allo-BMT at time of CR, but who were not transplanted because of early relapse or intercurrent illness, were analyzed with the patients who were actually transplanted. As shown in Table 65-5, the relapse rate is invariably lower in transplanted patients. This probably results not only from the effects of the high-dose chemotherapy with or without total body radiation given as the "preparative regimen" but also from an immunologic graft-versus-leukemia effect. This effect is presumed to exist because of the inverse relationship between extent of graft-versus-host disease and relapse rate.[93,94]

Although allo-BMT clearly demonstrates a decreased relapse rate, Table 65-5 indicates that only one of the five studies in which disease-free survival (DFS) data are provided found a statistically significant difference favoring allo-BMT. Nonetheless, the invariable trend is for higher DFS rates among transplanted patients, raising the possibility that statistical differences might have been found had more patients been treated. Differences between allo-BMT and chemotherapy are least when survival becomes the end point. Indeed, the two most recent studies, each with median follow-up periods of 4 years since assignment to treatment, have reported no differences or a difference favoring chemotherapy. The discrepancies between the effect of transplant on relapse rates on the one hand and DFS and survival rate on the other reflect the toxicity of the allo-BMT procedure and perhaps a shorter survival after relapse in transplanted patients as well.

The DFS and survival data in Table 65-5 indicate that either allo-BMT or continued chemotherapy could currently be recommended for the patient achieving CR. Might some patients be better served by allo-BMT and others by chemotherapy? Currently, age is the characteristic that best identifies such patients.[87] Survival after allo-BMT is inversely related to age. The mortality rate following the procedure in patients >55–60 years old is such that benefit/risk considerations favor chemotherapy in these patients. The opposite is probably true in patients aged <20 years.[95] Data indicating that DFS in patients

transplanted only in second CR are influenced by length of first chemotherapy-maintained CR suggest that, aside from the extremes of age noted above, similar prognostic factors are operative for allo-BMT and chemotherapy.[96] However, Tallman et al.[97] retrospectively identified a group characterized not only by younger age, but also by female sex, need for more than one induction course to achieve CR, and presence of circulating blasts at diagnosis in whom survival is superior with allo-BMT than with chemotherapy. This finding awaits confirmation.

Autologous Marrow Transplantation

Only 30–45% of patients will have an HLA-matched sibling who can serve as a donor for allo-BMT. This has led to an increasing use of donors who, although HLA-matched, are not siblings.[98,99] Still, no donors will be available for many patients, or the wait to identify an unrelated donor may be unrealistically long (median 6.5 months).[99] As a result, interest in autologous bone marrow transplantation (auto-BMT) in first CR is likely to continue. In this procedure, high-dose chemotherapy with or without total body irradiation regimens similar to those used in allo-BMT are administered. Hematopoietic rescue from this therapy is accomplished by infusion of the patient's own marrow collected and stored previously. In auto-BMT, relapse could result not only from an inadequate preparative regimen, but also from the infusion of leukemia cells in the stored marrow. This possibility has led to use of techniques to purge the stored marrow of such cells. These include in vitro treatment of the stored marrow with either chemotherapeutic agents[100] or leukemia cell-specific monoclonal antibodies.[101]

Most reports with auto-BMT in first CR with or without purging have been from Europe. DFS probabilities of 40–60% have been reported.[102–106] Frequently patients appear to have been referred in CR to the auto-BMT center for the express purpose of undergoing the procedure. This raises the possibility of selection bias, that is, the referring physician may have sent a disproportionate number of patients considered likely to fare either particularly well or particularly poorly. The median time from first CR to auto-BMT in these studies is usually 3–6 months. Patients who relapse before this time are excluded from auto-BMT. Exclusion of these poor-prognosis patients could produce a misleadingly optimistic result.

Because of these uncertainties and reports of less favorable results with auto-BMT in first CR,[107] several trials directly com-

Table 65-6. Comparison of Allogeneic and Autologous Transplantation in First Remission

Study	No. of Patients	Relapse		Disease-Free Survival		Survival		Statistically Significant Differences $(P < 0.05)$
		Auto-BMT (%)	Allo-BMT (%)	Auto-BMT (%)	Allo-BMT (%)	Auto-BMT (%)	Allo-BMT (%)	
Cassileth et al.[108] (1993)	19 Allo 39 Auto	Not given	Not given	54	41	Not given	Not given	None
Löwenberg et al.[109] (1990)	21 Allo 32 Auto	60	34	35	51	37	66	Relapse and survival rates
Reiffers et al.[89] (1989)	20 Allo 15 Auto	59	22	41	61	Not given	Not given	Relapse and DFS rates
Amadori et al.[95] (1993)	22 Allo 35 Auto	78	45	21	51	Not given	Not given	Relapse and DFS rates

^{a} At 5 years in study by Amadori et al.; at 3 years in studies by Cassileth et al. and Löwenberg et al.; at 2.5 years in study by Reiffers et al.

paring auto-BMT with allo-BMT,[89,95,108,109] and less frequently with chemotherapy,[89,95] have been conducted. Adults aged <41–45 years with an HLA-sibling donor have been assigned to allo-BMT, while similarly aged patients without a donor have received auto-BMT or have been randomized to auto-BMT or chemotherapy. As shown in Table 65-6, two studies of adults[89,109] and one pediatric study[95] have found lower relapse rates and superior DFS or survival rates after allo-BMT. The autologous marrow was not subjected to purging. By contrast, an ECOG study[108] suggests that results following auto- and allo-BMT are similar. This latter study employed purging. Although the discrepancies between these studies may reflect the use of purging or differences between the preparative regimens, they may also reflect the exclusion from several analyses of patients who, although assigned to a transplant, were not transplanted, usually because of intercurrent illness. Such patients invariably did worse than the transplanted patients. Only two small studies directly comparing auto-BMT with chemotherapy in first CR have appeared.[89,95] In each relapse and DFS rates with the two modalities were similar. In summary, routine performance of auto-BMT in first CR does not appear to be warranted.

THERAPY FOR RELAPSED OR REFRACTORY AML

Relapse occurs in most of newly diagnosed patients who attain CR. The likelihood of a second CR is very strongly related to the duration of first CR.[82–84] Patients with first CR of >6 months in one study,[82] 10 months in a second study,[84] and 12 months in a third study[83] have CR rates of 60% with 3 + 7 or TAD regimens. The CR rate with the same therapy in patients with shorter first CR durations is only 20–30%. One large study[83] found a CR rate of 20% both in patients with initial CR duration <1 year and in those who fail to enter CR with initial induction therapy. There is no indication that HDAC improves the CR rate in these poor prognosis patients.[82,110,111] Median second CR duration averages 6–12 months (i.e., roughly one-half of first CR duration[82–84]) and seems to be directly proportional to first CR duration.[82] Importantly, approximately 5% of all patients in first relapse or refractory to initial induction therapy and 15% of all such patients achieving a second CR can be projected to be alive at 5 years.[83] In one study,[83] all such long-term survivors who had initial first CRs of <1 year, and most of those with longer first CRs, received an allo-BMT at relapse or in second CR. The only exceptions were patients with the prognostically favorable cytogenetic abnormalities pericentric inversion of chromosome 16 [inv(16)] or translocation between chromosomes 8 and 21 [t(8;21)], who received only chemotherapy at relapse and thereafter.

Given this information, it seems appropriate to perform allo-BMT in all patients in first relapse aged <55 if an HLA-compatible sibling donor is available. If a sibling donor is unavailable

and the patient is <45 years old, strong consideration should be given to the use of allo-BMT using an unrelated but matched donor. Allo-BMT should not be delayed until second CR.[112] Allo-BMT is also the procedure of choice for patients refractory to initial induction therapy. Forman et al.[113] reported a 50% probability of DFS at >2 years in these patients, although these results were largely confined to patients <30 years of age.

If an allo-BMT cannot be performed, patients with first CRs of >1 year should receive an induction regimen similar to that used initially. In CR, however, they can be offered investigational therapies. Patients with shorter first CRs or who are refractory to initial therapy should be offered investigational therapies at relapse if allo-BMT is not an option.

As with chemotherapy, the prognosis after relapse after allo-BMT is heavily dependent on duration of CR.[114] Recent data[115] suggest that remissions in some patients can be produced by CSF-G, which presumably stimulates the graft-versus-leukemia effect and is well tolerated. If this therapy is unsuccessful and the patient had a CR of >1 year after the previous allo-BMT, consideration should be given to a second allo-BMT.[116] Otherwise, the patient should be referred for investigational therapy.

PROGNOSTIC FACTORS

The discovery of prognostic factors is important because it permits more accurate comparison of results with different therapies. The striking effect of exclusion of patients with unfavorable prognostic characteristics on results of a single therapy is illustrated in a report from the Toronto Leukemia Study Group.[117] Berman et al.[118] noted the frequent exclusion of eligible patients from receiving an allo-BMT.

Prognostic factors in AML can be divided into those associated with death during chemotherapy and those associated with resistance to chemotherapy, manifested either by failure to enter CR despite surviving induction therapy or by a short CR duration. Characteristics predictive of early death are poor pretreatment performance status, age >60 years, low pretreatment serum albumin, and abnormal pretreatment hepatic and renal function.[119] Characteristics associated with sensitivity or resistance to chemotherapy are presented in Table 65-7. Probably the most well established are pretreatment leukemia cell cytogenetics.[120–123] Pericentric inversion of chromosome 16 [inv(16) associated with AML subtype M4EO[124]] or a translocation between chromosomes 8 and 21 [t(8;21) associated with M2[124]] or between chromosomes 15 and 17 [t(15;17) associated with M3, acute promyelocytic leukemia[124]], is predictive of high CR rates (>90%) or long CR durations (median 2 years), or both. Evidence suggests that the relatively long CR durations observed in patients with inv(16) or t(8;21) following anthracycline + conventional ara-C regimens can be prolonged significantly with HDAC-containing regimens.[125,126] Furthermore, the

Table 65-7. Characteristics Predicting Sensitivity of Leukemic Blasts to Chemotherapy

Characteristic	Effect	References
inv(16), t(8;21), t(15;17)	Favorable	120–123
−5, 5q−, −7, 7q−, +8, 11q−	Unfavorable	120–123
Antecedent hematologic disorder	Unfavorable	122,133,134
Secondary AML[a]	Unfavorable	128
CD34 expression	Unfavorable	135–139
	None	140–142
CD7 expression	Unfavorable	143–145
	None	141,146
CD19 expression	Unfavorable	139
	None	141,146
	Favorable	147
TdT expression	Unfavorable	137
	None	148
MDR expression	Unfavorable	149–151
	None	138,142
Short duration of first CR	Unfavorable	82–84
Persistent blasts in day 6 marrow	Unfavorable	152

Abbreviations: inv, inversion; t, translocation; −, loss; q−, deletion of long arm of chromosome.

[a] AML developing after chemotherapy or radiation therapy for another malignancy.

use of HDAC appears to eliminate the central nervous system relapses seen when patients with inv(16) were given conventional dose ara-C for maintenance.[126,127] By contrast, monosomies of chromosomes 5 or 7, deletions of the long arm (q) of these chromosomes or chromosome 11, and trisomy of chromosome 8 are associated with low CR rates (<50% for −5, 5q−, −7, 7q−, and +8) and short CR durations (median 6 months), regardless of whether therapy includes HDAC. The negative impact of secondary AML is largely due to its association with unfavorable cytogenetic abnormalities,[128] in particular, −5, −7, 7q−, and 5q− in patients previously treated with alkylating agents, and 11q− in patients treated with toposomerase II-reactive drugs.[129] For example, patients with APL and the t(15;17) do equally well, regardless of whether it develops de novo or as a secondary abnormality.[130] Similarly, the poor prognosis of patients with the rare AML subtypes M6 (erythroleukemia) and M7 (megakaryocytic leukemia) probably largely reflects the association of M6 and M7 with unfavorable cytogenetic abnormalities.[131,132] Factors suggesting the origin of the blasts from a primitive multipotential cell (CD34 expression), or from a myeloblast that has undergone genetic dysregulation, as evidenced by expression of lymphoid as well as myeloid cell-surface antigens, have been associated with therapeutic resistance. However, these findings have not been confirmed by other groups (Table 65-6).

The multidrug-resistant (MDR) phenotype, the hallmark of which is the presence of glycoprotein P170, has also been found to be correlated with resistance.[149–151] This protein promotes efflux of anthracyclines, although perhaps not idarubicin, and etoposide from blast cells.[149–151] However, because patients with unfavorable cytogenetic abnormalities do equally poorly, whether treated with or without drugs pumped by P170 glycoprotein,[126] the cytogenetic abnormality may be of primary, and MDR expression of secondary, importance.

It should be noted that currently known prognostic factors have been largely established in patients treated with 3 + 7 or TAD regimens. It is possible that some of these factors are therapy specific. Together with the very poor prognosis of patients with the cytogenetic abnormalities depicted in Table 65-6, this possibility suggests that allo-BMT or investigational

therapies might be considered in these patients either at diagnosis or at first CR.

INVESTIGATIONAL APPROACHES

Table 65-8 gives examples of therapies being actively investigated in poor-prognosis AML. The ultimate role, if any, of all these agents awaits further patient entry and correlation of results with these patients' prognostic factors. The topoisomerase I-reactive drug topotecan,[153] and the adenosine analogue 2 chlorodexoxydenosine,[154] have each produced CRs as single agents in relapsed disease and will soon be combined with known active agents. Fludarabine may potentiate the effects of ara-C.[111,155] Using cyclosporine together with HDAC and daunorubicin, List et al.[156] reported a CR rate of 67% in 15 patients, the great majority of whom had first remissions at <1 year or were refractory to initial therapy. The documented importance of the graft-versus-leukemia effect following allo-BMT[93] has led to attempts to reproduce graft-versus-leukemia effect without an allo-BMT, such as through the use of interleukin-2.[158]

Approaches to detect minimal residual disease in patients in CR by traditional hematologic criteria are also being investigated. These include cytogenetics,[159] fluorescence in situ hybridization (FISH), and the polymerase chain reaction (PCR). Whereas the usual cytogenetic techniques are limited to analysis of approximately 25 cells, FISH, and especially PCR, permit examination of cells at several more orders of magnitude to detect residual cytogenetic abnormalities. Miller et al.[160] reported that patients with APL who remained PCR positive for the t(15;17) are much more likely to relapse than are patients in whom the PCR reverted to negative. This type of information could eventually be useful in deciding when to change or discontinue therapy in patients in hematologic CR.

Acute Promyelocytic Leukemia

APL is distinguished clinically by a bleeding diathesis and morphologically by promyelocytes containing coarse, large granules and numerous Auer rods. A microgranular variant retains the bleeding diathesis, but the granules can be resolved only with electron microscopy.[161] Both types are characterized by a translocation between the long arms of chromosomes 15 and 17. The translocation breakpoint involves the retinoic acid receptor-α (RAR-α) gene on chromosome 17 and the *myl* gene on chromosome 15.[162] This RAR-α rearrangement can be identified by the PCR reaction in cases in which APL is diagnosed morphologically but in which the cytogenetics are normal.[163]

Risk factors for fatal hemorrhage in APL include high circulating blast and promyelocyte count,[164–166] low platelet count,[164–166] and, possibly, older age[164] and low hemoglobin.[164] The bleeding diathesis has been attributed to disseminated intravascular coagulation (DIC) or accelerated fibrinolysis,[167] leading to the use of heparin or antifibrinolytic agents. More important than these measures are prompt initiation of anthracycline-containing chemotherapy, or therapy with all-trans-retinoic acid (ATRA), together with frequent platelet,

Table 65-8. Investigational Therapies for AML

Class of Agent	Example	References
Topoisomerase I-reactive	Topotecan	153
Adenosine analogue	2-Chlorodeoxyadenosine	154
	Fludarabine	111,155
MDR reversing agent	Cyclosporine	156
Monoclonal antibody + toxin	Anti-CD33 + [131]I	157
Graft-versus-leukemia enhancing	Interleukin-2	158

Table 65-9. Outcome of Chemotherapy with or without Heparin or Antifibrinolytic Therapy for APL

Study	No. of Patients	Chemotherapy	No. on Heparin	No. on Antifibrinolytic Therapy	Fatal Hemorrhage During Induction (%)	CR (%)	Median Remission Duration
Kantarjian et al.[164] (1986)	60	Anthracycline + ara-C or HDAC	32	No	32	53	24 mo
Goldberg et al.[169] (1987)	27	Anthracycline + ara-C	2	No	15	74	Not given
Sanz et al.[170] (1988)	34	Daunorubicin	34	No	9	68	24 mo
Cunningham et al.[165] (1989)	57	ara-C + 6-TG or anthracycline + ara-C	57	No	14	72	25 mo
Rodeghiero et al.[166] (1990)	268	Daunorubicin or daunorubicin + ara-C	94	67	14	62	Not given
Avvisati et al.[171] (1990)	27	Idarubicin	4	17	4	81	Not given
Rotoli et al.[172] (1992)	90	Idarubicin	Not stated	Not stated	Not given	77	Not given

cryoprecipitate, and fresh frozen plasma transfusions. When ara-C + 6-TG was used to treat APL, 70% of patients died of hemorrhage.[165] This rate fell to 21% when single-agent daunorubicin was employed.[168] As shown in Table 65-9, rates of fatal hemorrhage in subsequent studies appear to be the same regardless of whether heparin was given. This was specifically noted in the study conducted by Rodeghiero et al.,[166] who also noted that the use of antifibrinolytic therapy failed to influence the rate of fatal hemorrhage. Thus there appears to be no reason for routine use of heparin in APL; more data are needed regarding antifibrolytic therapy, particularly given a possible association between ATRA and thrombosis.[173,174] As noted in Table 65-9, CR rates appear to be similar, regardless of whether anthracycline or anthracycline plus ara-C is given. The bone marrow in APL has been typically slow to clear of blasts[175,176] and, if blasts do persist, it is advisable to wait until ≥day 35 of the first course before beginning a second course, unless DIC reappears. As seen in Table 65-9, CR durations in APL are usually longer than in other types of AML. Two studies have cited the effectiveness of POMP in extending CR duration in APL.[177,178]

The use of ATRA in APL has received increasing attention. Several reports note CR rates of >90% in untreated patients or patients in first relapse.[179-182] The CR rate appears much lower after subsequent relapse.[182] DIC appears to reverse more rapidly with ATRA than with chemotherapy in newly diagnosed cases or in first relapse. A median of 5–6 weeks is required to achieve CR. By comparison, chemotherapy programs require about 1 week less to achieve CR. The effectiveness of ATRA is attributed to its ability to overcome the "differentiation block" responsible for APL.[183] This block results from the production of abnormal retinoic acid receptors consequent to the t(15;17). These receptors prevent physiologically occurring ATRA from differentiating promyelocytes to more mature myeloid cells. However, pharmacologic concentrations of ATRA induce the expression of normal retinoic acid receptors, which may then "outcompete" the abnormal receptors.[183] A problem with ATRA is the development of potentially fatal ATRA syndrome in 25% of patients.[184] This is characterized by fever, dyspnea, pleural and pericardial effusion, and hypotension. The syndrome is generally accompanied by leukocytosis, but only a few cases of ATRA-induced leukocytosis show the development of this syndrome. Treatment has included high-dose steroids[184]; some investigators initiate chemotherapy when leukocytosis develops.[185,186] Other toxicities of ATRA are erythema nodosum,[187] hyperhistaminemia,[188] and possibly thromboses,[173,174] which may produce pseudotumor cerebri.

Although effective in inducing CR, the use of ATRA alone in remission is ineffective in maintaining CR, with reported median remission durations of 5–6 months.[182] This may result from falling ATRA serum concentrations,[189] although it is unclear at what point concentrations fall relative to the loss of effectiveness of ATRA. To improve duration of remission, investigators either combine ATRA with chemotherapy during induction or administer chemotherapy when ATRA-induced CR is achieved, or attempt both approaches. Fenaux et al.[185,186] recently found that patients randomized to receive ATRA for induction with daunorubicin + ara-C added either in CR or when leukocytosis developed during induction had significantly lower ($P = 0.002$) relapse rates than those found in patients given chemotherapy alone for induction and maintenance. Substituting chemotherapy for ATRA once in CR may also maintain sensitivity to ATRA longer, as patients who relapse off ATRA are more likely to obtain subsequent CR following reinstitution of ATRA than are patients who relapse while being maintained on ATRA.[180]

Acute Myeloid Leukemia in the Elderly

The median age of AML patients has been estimated to be 64 years.[190] The age-specific incidence rate increases until ≥75 years of age,[190] in contrast with the linearly decreasing CR rate after age 25–30.[191] While patients <60 years old have average CR rates of 70%, the rate is 50% in older patients,[16,192] reflecting primarily an increased death rate during induction in older patients. This propensity partially reflects the association of older age with poor performance status, low serum albumin, and abnormal organ function.[119] Remission durations are also shorter in elderly patients, largely as a result of the association between older age, unfavorable cytogenetic abnormalities, and an antecedent hematologic disorder.[122,193]

The poor prognosis of elderly AML patients treated with standard chemotherapy led Löwenberg et al.[194] to randomly assign 60 otherwise healthy patients >65 years old to receive the 3 + 7 regimen or supportive care, the latter continuing until leukocytosis >50,000, symptomatic thrombopenia, organ infiltration, or clinical deterioration occurred, at which time ara-C was commenced. Supportive care-only strategy shortened survival and did not decrease the frequency of hospital admission. A similar strategy in 24 patients aged >50 who presented with low blast counts or low marrow cellularity resulted in a median survival of 9.3 months.[195] These data argue against a supportive care-only approach, unless the patient refuses therapy or is bedridden.

In an effort to reduce mortality during induction, investigators have administered attenuated doses of ara-C or daunorubicin, or both. Five randomized[19,20,196-198] and two nonrandomized[199,200] studies have compared this strategy to administration of usual doses in patients aged >60–70 years. The results, illustrated in Table 65-10, suggest that while dose reduction may decrease early death rate, at best it will produce an equivalent CR rate. Reflecting the relatively high early death rate, standard-dose chemotherapy does not improve, and may even decrease, overall survival. However, neither the reduced- nor the standard-dose approach produces encouraging sur-

Table 65-10. Comparisons of Standard-Dose with Attenuated-Dose Chemotherapy in Elderly Patients with Newly Diagnosed AML

Study	Induction Regimen	No. of Patients	Age of Patients	Early Deaths (%)	CR (%)	Median Remission Duration (mo)	Median Survival (mo)	Probability Survival at 2 yr (%)
Kahn et al.[196] (1984)	FDAT	20	>70	60[a]	25	Not given	1[a]	0
	ADAT	20	≥70	25[a]	30	Not given	5[a]	0
Tilly et al.[197] (1990)	4 + 7	46	>65	31[a]	52	13.8	12.8	20
	LDAC	41	>65	10[a]	32	8.3	8.8	25
Büchner et al.[198] (1992)	FDAT	218	≥60	18	54	11	Not given	Not given
	ADAT	104	≥60	26	42	9	Not given	Not given
Dutcher et al.[199] (1984)	3 + 7	35	≥60	31	51	12	Not given	Not given
	LDAC	13	≥60	18	24	3	Not given	Not given
Sebban et al.[200] (1988)	3 + 7	35	>60	29	48[a]	16	7	20
	LDAC	22	>60	9	23[a]	5	8	0
Rai et al.[19] (1981)	3 + 7	43	≥60	35[a]	42[a]	Not given	Not given	Not given
	2 + 5	62	≥60	68[a]	16[a]	Not given	Not given	Not given
Rees[20] (1989)	3 + 10	113	≥60	Not given	44	Not given	Not given	Not given
	1 + 5	115	≥60	Not given	39	Not given	Not given	Not given

Abbreviations: FDAT, full-dose daunorubicin, ara-C, 6-TG; ADAT, attenuated-dose daunorubicin, ara-C, 6TG; 4 + 7, 4 days anthracycline + 7 days ara-C; LDAC, low-dose ara-C; 3 + 7, 3 days anthracycline + 7 days ara-C; 2 + 5, 2 days anthracycline + 5 days ara-C; 3 + 10, 3 days anthracycline + 10 days ara-C; 1 + 5, 1 day anthracycline + 5 days ara-C.
[a] $P \leq 0.05$.

vival data, and ECOG[78] and CALGB[79] results argue against use of high-dose, rather than standard-dose, ara-C in elderly patients. Most newly diagnosed elderly patients should therefore be considered for investigational approaches in the setting of a formal clinical trial. Exceptions would be patients with favorable cytogenetic abnormalities who are <70 years of age with good performance status and normal organ function. Since the same prognostic factors operate in older as in younger patients,[201,202] at least some of these patients can expect durable remissions after chemotherapy.[198,202] Investigational approaches in the poorer-prognosis older patients should be directed at decreasing therapy-induced mortality or improving chemosensitivity of leukemia cells, or both. Examples of the former approach under active investigation include the administration of newer azoles, such as fluconazole or itraconzole, to prevent fungal infection[203]; white blood cell transfusions from family relatives given CSF-G to increase donor granulocyte count[204,205]; and administration of recombinant CSF-M in patients with disseminated candidiasis.[206] Example of strategies to overcome therapeutic resistance are provided in Table 65-8. The same investigational approaches taken to reduce mortality during induction or decrease resistance in elderly patients could be considered in younger high-risk patients, such as those with poor performance status or unfavorable cytogenetics.

REFERENCES

1. Cheson BD, Cassileth PA, Head DR et al: Report of the National Cancer Institute-sponsored workshop on definitions of diagnosis and response in acute myeloid leukemia. J Clin Oncol 8:813, 1990
2. Freireich EJ, Gehan EA, Sulman D et al: The effect of chemotherapy on acute leukemia in the human. J Chron Dis 14:593, 1961
3. Freireich EJ: Arabinosyl cytosine: a 20-year update. J Clin Oncol 5:523, 1987
4. Chu MY, Fischer GA: Comparative studies of leukemia cells sensitive and resistant to cytosine arabinoside. Biochem Pharmacol 14:333, 1965
5. Major P, Egan EM, Beardsley G et al: Lethality of human myeloblasts correlates with the incorporation of ara-C into DNA. Proc Natl Acad Sci USA 78:3235, 1981
6. Ho DHW, Frei E III: Clinical pharmacology of 1-beta-D-arabinofuranosylcytosine. Clin Pharmacol Ther 12:944, 1971
7. Southwest Oncology Group: Cytarabine for acute leukemia in adults. Arch Intern Med 133:251, 1974
8. Coltman CA, Freireich EJ, Pendleton O et al: Adult acute leukemia studies utilizing cytarabine: early Southwest Oncology Group trials. Med Pediatr Oncol, suppl. 1:173, 1982
9. Weil M, Glidewell OJ, Jacquillat C et al: Daunorubicin in the therapy of acute granulocytic leukemia. Cancer Res 33:921, 1973
10. Liu L: DNA topoisomerase poisons as antitumor drugs. Annu Rev Biochem 58:351, 1989
11. Keating MJ, Smith TL, Gehan EA et al: Factors related to length of complete remission in adult acute leukemia. Cancer 45:2017, 1980
12. Preisler HD, Anderson K, Rai K et al: The frequency of long-term remission in patients with acute myelogenous leukaemia treated with conventional maintenance chemotherapy: a study of 760 patients with a minimal follow-up time of 6 years. Br J Haematol 71:189, 1989
13. Bandini G, Zuffa E, Rosti G et al: Long-term outcome of adults with acute myelogenous leukaemia: results of a prospective, randomized study of chemotherapy with a minimal follow-up of 7 years. Br J Haematol 77:486, 1991
14. Keating MJ, McCredie KB, Bodey GP et al: Improved prospects for long-term survival in adults with acute myelogenous leukemia. JAMA 248:2481, 1982
15. Passe S, Mikè V, Mertelsmann R et al: Acute nonlymphoblastic leukemia prognostic factors in adults with long-term follow-up. Cancer 50:1462, 1982
16. Estey, Keating MJ, McCredie KB et al: Causes of initial remission induction failure in acute myelogenous leukemia. Blood 60:309, 1982
17. Preisler HD: Failure of remission induction in acute myelocytic leukemia. Med Pediatr Oncol 4:275, 1978
18. Whittaker JA, Reizenstein P, Callender ST et al: Long survival in acute myelogenous leukaemia: an international collaborative study. BMJ 282:692, 1981
19. Rai KR, Holland JF, Glidewell OJ et al: Treatment of acute myelocytic leukemia: a study by Cancer and Leukemia Group B. Blood 58:1203, 1981
20. Rees JKH: Chemotherapy of acute myeloid leukaemia in UK: past, present and future. Bone Marrow Transplant, suppl. 1. 4:110, 1989
21. Preisler H, Davis RB, Kirshner J et al and the Cancer and Leukemia Group B: Comparison of three remission induction regimens and two postinduction strategies for the treatment of acute nonlymphocytic leukemia: a Cancer and Leukemia Group B study. Blood 69:1441, 1987
22. Yates J, Glidewell O, Wiernik P et al: Cytosine arabinoside with daunorubicin or adriamycin for therapy of acute myelocytic leukemia: a CALGB study. Blood 60:454, 1982
23. Berman E, Arlin ZA, Gaynor J et al: Comparative trial of cytarabine and thioguanine in combination with amsacrine or daunorubicin in patients with untreated acute nonlymphocytic leukemia: results of the L-16M protocol. Leukemia 3:115, 1989
24. Arlin Z, Case DC, Moore J et al and the Lederle Cooperative Group: Randomized multicenter trial of cytosine arabinoside with mitoxantrone or daunorubicin in previously untreated adult patients with acute nonlymphocytic leukemia. Leukemia 4:177, 1990
25. Hansen OP, Pedersen-Bjergaard J, Ellegaard J et al for The Danish Society of Hematology Study Group on AML: Aclarubicin plus cytosine arabinoside versus daunorubicin plus cytosine arabinoside in previously untreated pa-

tients with acute myeloid leukemia: a Danish National Phase III Trial. Leukemia 5:510, 1991

26. Stein RS, Vogler R, Winton EF et al: Therapy of acute myelogenous leukemia in patients over the age of 50: a randomized Southeastern Cancer Study Group Trial. Leuk Res 14:895, 1990

27. Berman E, Heller G, Santorsa J et al: Results of a randomized trial comparing idarubicin and cytosine arabinoside with daunorubicin and cytosine arabinoside in adult patients with newly diagnosed acute myelogenous leukemia. Blood 77:1666, 1991

28. Wiernik PH, Banks PLC, Case DC et al: Cytarabine plus idarubicin or daunorubicin as induction and consolidation therapy for previously untreated adult patients with acute myeloid leukemia. Blood 79:313, 1992

29. Vogler WR, Velez-Garcia E, Weiner RS et al: A phase III trial comparing idarubicin and daunorubicin in combination with cytarabine in acute myelogenous leukemia: a Southeastern Cancer Study Group study. J Clin Oncol 10: 1103, 1992

30. Dilman RO, Davis RB, Green MR et al: A comparative study of two different doses of cytarabine for acute myeloid leukemia: a phase III trial of Cancer and Leukemia Group B. Blood 78:2520, 1991

31. Rudnick SA, Cadman EC, Capizzi RL et al: High dose cytosine arabinoside in refractory acute leukemia. Cancer 44:1189, 1979

32. Herzig RH, Wolff SN, Lazarus HM et al: High-dose cytosine arabinoside therapy for refractory leukemia. Blood 62:361, 1983

33. Kantarjian HM, Estey EH, Plunkett W et al: Phase I-II clinical and pharmacologic studies of high-dose cytosine arabinoside in refractory leukemia. Am J Med 81:387, 1986

34. Estey E, Plunkett W, Dixon D et al: Variables predicting response to high dose cytosine arabinoside therapy in patients with refractory acute leukemia. Leukemia 8:580, 1987

35. Baker WJ, Royer GL, Weiss RB: Cytarabine and neurologic toxicity. J Clin Oncol 9:679, 1991

36. Anderson B, Cogan B, Keating M et al: Subacute pulmonary failure complicating therapy with high-dose ara-C in acute leukemia. Cancer 56:2181, 1985

37. Plunkett W, Liliemark OJ, Adams TM et al: Saturation of 1-β-D-arabinosylcytosine 5'-triphosphate accumulation in leukemia cells during high-dose 1-β-D-arabinosylcytosine therapy. Cancer Res 47:3005, 1987

38. Estey EH, Plunkett W, Kantarjian H et al: Treatment of relapsed or refractory AML with intermediate-dose arabinosylcytosine: confirmation of the importance of ara-C triphosphate formation in mediating response to ara-C. Leuk Lymphoma, suppl. 10:115, 1993

39. Hiddemann W, Schleyer E, Uhrmeister C et al: High-dose versus intermediate-dose cytosine arabinoside in combination with mitoxantrone for the treatment of relapsed and refractory acute myeloid leukemia—preliminary clinical and pharmacological data of a randomized comparison. Cancer Treat Rev 17:279, 1990

40. Phillips GL, Reece DE, Shepherd JD et al: High-dose cytarabine and daunorubicin induction and post-remission chemotherapy for the treatment of acute myelogenous leukemia in adults. Blood 77:1429, 1991

41. Curtis JE, Messner HA, Minden MD et al: High-dose cytosine arabinoside in the treatment of acute myelogenous leukemia: contributions to outcome of clinical and laboratory attributes. J Clin Oncol 5:532, 1987

42. Weick J, Kopecky K, Appelbaum F et al for the Southwest Oncology Group: A randomized investigation of high-dose versus standard dose cytosine arabinoside with daunorubicin in patients with acute myelogenous leukemia, abstracted. Proc ASCO 11:261, 1992

43. Bishop JF, Young GA, Szer J et al for the Australian Leukemia Study Group: Randomized trial of high dose cytosine arabinoside (ARA-C) combination in induction in acute myeloid leukemia (AML), abstracted. Proc ASCO 11: 260, 1992

44. Schiller G, Gajewski J, Nimer S et al: A randomized study of intermediate versus conventional-dose cytarabine as intensive induction for acute myelogenous leukaemia. Br J Haematol 81:170, 1992

45. Ross WE, Rowe T, Yalowich J et al: Role of topoisomerase II in mediating epipodophyllotoxin-induced DNA cleavage. Cancer Res 44:5857, 1984

46. Estey EH, Silberman L, Beran M et al: The interaction between nuclear topoisomerase II activity from human leukemia cells, exogenous DNA, and 4'-(9-acridinylamino)methanesulfon-m-anisidide (m-AMSA) or 4-(4,6-0-ethylidene-β-D-glucopyranoside) (VP-16) indicates the sensitivity of the cells to the drugs. Biochem Biophys Res Commun 144:787, 1987

47. Smith IE, Clink HD, Gerken ME, McElwain TJ: VP-16-213 in acute myelogenous leukemia. Postgrad Med J 52:66, 1976

48. Bennett JM, Lymann GH, Cassileth PA et al: A phase II trail of VP-123 in adults with refractory acute myeloid leukemia. Am J Clin Oncol 7:471, 1984

49. Varini M, Cavilli F: Etoposide in the treatment of acute leukemia in adults. Cancer Treat Rev 9:59, 1982

50. Bishop JF, Lowenthal RM, Joshua D et al for the Australian Leukemia Study Group: Etoposide in acute nonlymphocytic leukemia. Blood 75:27, 1990

51. Lieschke GJ, Burgess AW: Granulocyte colony-stimulating factor and granulocyte-macrophage colony-stimulating factor. N Engl J Med 327:28, 99, 1992

52. Tafuri A, Andreeff M: Kinetic rationale for cytokine-induced recruitment of myeloblastic leukemia followed by cycle-specific chemotherapy in vitro. Leukemia 4:826, 1990

53. Koistinen P, Wang C, Curtis JE, McCulloch EA: Granulocyte-macrophage colony-stimulating factor and interleukin-3 protect leukemic blast cells from ara-C toxicity. Leukemia 5:789, 1991

54. Estey EH, Dixon D, Kantarjian HM et al: Treatment of poor-prognosis, newly diagnosed acute myeloid leukemia with ara-C and recombinant human granulocyte-macrophage colony-stimulating factor. Blood 75:1766, 1990

55. Büchner T, Hiddemann W, Koenigsmann M et al: Recombinant human granulocyte-macrophage colony-stimulating factor after chemotherapy in patients with acute myeloid leukemia at higher age or after relapse. Blood 78: 1190, 1991

56. Ohno R, Tomonaga M, Kobayashi T et al: Effect of granulocyte colony-stimulating factor after intensive induction therapy in relapsed or refractory acute leukemia. N Engl J Med 323:871, 1990

57. Estey E, Thall PF, Kantarjian H et al: Treatment of newly diagnosed acute myelogenous leukemia with granulocyte-macrophage colony-stimulating factor before and during continuous-infusion high-dose ara-C + daunorubicin: comparison to patients treated without GM-CSF. Blood 79:2246, 1992

58. Büchner TH, Hiddemann W, Rottmann R et al: Multiple course chemotherapy with or without GM-CSF priming and long-term administration for newly diagnosed AML, abstracted, (985). Proc ASCO 12:301, 1993

59. Estey E, Gandhi V, Keating M, Plunkett W: G-CSF potentiates clinical and pharmacokinetics response to fludarabine and ara-C in AML and MDS, abstracted (986). Proc ASCO 12:301, 1993

60. Bettelheim P, Valent P, Andreeff M et al: Recombinant human granulocyte-macrophage colony-stimulating factor in combination with standard induction chemotherapy in de novo acute myeloid leukemia. Blood 77:700, 1991

61. Archimbaud E, Fenaux P, Reiffers J et al: Granulocyte-macrophage colony-stimulating factor in association to timed-sequential chemotherapy with mitoxantrone, etoposide, and cytarabine for refractory acute myelogenous leukemia. Leukemia 7:372, 1993

62. Cassileth PA, Harrington DP, Hines JD et al: Maintenance chemotherapy prolongs remission duration in adult acute nonlymphocytic leukemia. J Clin Oncol 6:583, 1988

63. Sauter C, Fopp M, Imbach P et al: Acute myelogenous leukaemia: maintenance chemotherapy after early consolidation treatment does not prolong survival. Lancet 1:379, 1984

64. Mandelli F, Petti MC, Avvisati G et al for the Cooperative Group GIMEMA, Italy: Gimema experience in the treatment of adult acute myelogenous leukemia. p. 273. In Gale RP (ed): Acute Myelogenous Leukemia: Progress and Controversies. Wiley-Liss, New York, 1990

65. Büchner T, Urbanitz D, Hiddemann W et al: Intensified induction and consolidation with or without maintenance chemotherapy for acute myeloid leukemia (AML): two multicenter studies of the German AML Cooperative Group. J Clin Oncol 3:1583, 1985

66. Rowe JM, Oken MM, Cassileth PA et al: Clinical trials in adults with relapsed and refractory acute myelogenous leukemia: the ECOG and the University of Rochester Experience. Haematol Blood Transfus 34:392, 1992

67. Rohatiner AZS, Gregory WM, Bassan R et al: Short-term therapy for acute myelogenous leukemia. J Clin Oncol 6:218, 1988

68. Champlin R, Gale RP, Elashoff R et al: Prolonged survival in acute myelogenous leukemia without maintenance chemotherapy. Lancet 1:894, 1984

69. Dutcher JP, Wiernik PH, Markus S et al: Intensive maintenance therapy improves survival in adult acute nonlymphocytic leukemia: an eight-year follow-up. Leukemia 2:413, 1988

70. Cassileth PA, Begg CB, Bennett JM et al: A randomized study of the efficacy of consolidation therapy in adult acute nonlymphocytic leukemia. Blood 63:843, 1984

71. Bodey GP, Rodriguez V, McCredie KB, Freireich EJ: Early consolidation chemotherapy for adults with acute leukemia in remission. Med Pediatr Oncol 2:299, 1975

72. Wolff SN, Herzig RH, Fay JW et al: High-dose cytarabine and daunorubicin as consolidation therapy for acute myeloid leukemia in first remission: long-term follow-up and results. J Clin Oncol 7:1260, 1989

73. Champlin R, Gajewski J, Nimer S et al: Post-remission chemotherapy for adults with acute myelogenous leukemia: improved survival with high-dose cytarabine and daunorubicin consolidation treatment. J Clin Oncol 8:1199, 1990

74. Schiller G, Gajewski J, Territo M et al: Long-term outcome of high-dose

cytarabine-based consolidation chemotherapy for adults with acute myelogenous leukemia. Blood 80:2977, 1992

75. Harousseau JL, Milpied N, Briere J et al: Double intensive consolidation chemotherapy in adult acute myeloid leukemia. J Clin Oncol 9:1432, 1991

76. Cassileth PA, Begg CB, Silber R et al: Prolonged un-maintained remission after intensive consolidation therapy in adult acute nonlymphocytic leukemia. Cancer Treat Rep 71:137, 1987

77. Preisler HD, Raza A, Early A et al: Intensive remission consolidation therapy in the treatment of acute nonlymphocytic leukemia. J Clin Oncol 5:722, 1987

78. Cassileth PA, Lynch E, Hines JD et al: Varying intensity of post-remission therapy in acute myeloid leukemia. Blood 79:1924, 1992

79. Mayer RJ, Davis RB, Schiffer CA et al for the CALGB: Comparative evaluation of intensive post-remission therapy with different dose schedules of ara-C in adults with acute myeloid leukemia, abstracted. Proc ASCO 11:261, 1992

80. Estey EH, Keating MJ, McCredie KB et al: Phase II trial of mitoxantrone in refractory acute leukemia. Cancer Treat Rep 67:389, 1983

81. Legha SS, Keating MJ, McCredie KB et al: Evaluation of AMSA in previously treated patients with acute leukemia: results of therapy in 109 adults. Blood 60:484, 1982

82. Hiddemann W, Martin WR, Sauerland CM et al: Definition of refractoriness against conventional chemotherapy in acute myeloid leukemia: a proposal based on the results of retreatment by thioguanine, cytosine arabinoside, and daunorubicin (TAD 9) in 150 patients with relapse after standardized first line therapy. Leukemia 4:184, 1990

83. Keating MJ, Kantarjian H, Smith TL et al: Response to salvage therapy and survival after relapse in acute myelogenous leukemia. J Clin Oncol 7:1071, 1989

84. Angelov L, Brandwein JM, Baker MA et al: Results of therapy for acute myeloid leukemia in first relapse. Leuk Lymphoma 6:15, 1991

85. Morrison FS, Kopecky KJ, Head DR et al: Late intensification with POMP chemotherapy prolongs survival in acute myelogenous leukemia—results of a Southwest Oncology Group study of rubidazone versus adriamycin for remission induction, prophylactic intrathecal therapy, late intensification, and levamisole maintenance. Leukemia 6:708, 1992

86. Bodey GP, Freireich EJ, Gehan E et al: Late intensification therapy for acute leukemia in remission. JAMA 235:1021, 1976

87. Clift RA, Buckner CD, Thomas ED et al: The treatment of acute non-lymphoblastic leukemia by allogeneic marrow transplantation. Bone Marrow Transplant 2:243, 1987

88. Schiller GJ, Nimer SD, Territo MC et al: Bone marrow transplantation versus high-dose cytarabine-based consolidation chemotherapy for acute myelogenous leukemia in first remission. J Clin Oncol 10:41, 1992

89. Reiffers J, Gaspard MH, Maraninchi D et al: Comparison of allogeneic or autologous bone marrow transplantation and chemotherapy in patients with acute myeloid leukaemia in first remission: a prospective controlled trial. Br J Haematol 72:57, 1989

90. Appelbaum FR, Fisher LD, Thomas ED and the Seattle Marrow Transplant Team: Chemotherapy v marrow transplantation for adult with acute nonlymphocytic leukemia: a five-year follow-up. Blood 72:179, 1988

91. Conde E, Iriondo A, Rayon C et al: Allogeneic bone marrow transplantation versus intensification chemotherapy for acute myelogenous leukaemia in first remission: a prospective controlled trial. Br J Haematol 68:219, 1988

92. Champlin RE, Ho WG, Gale RP et al: Treatment of acute myelogenous leukemia, a prospective controlled trial of bone marrow transplantation versus consolidation chemotherapy. Ann Intern Med 102:285, 1985

93. Gale RP, Champlin RE: How does bone-marrow transplantation cure leukemia? Lancet 2:28, 1984

94. Maraninchi D, Blaise D, Rio B et al: Impact of T-cell depletion on outcome of allogeneic bone-marrow transplantation for standard-risk leukaemias. Lancet 2:175, 1987

95. Amadori S, Testi AM, Aricò M et al for the Associazione Italiana Ematologia ed Oncologia Pediatrica Cooperative Group: Prospective comparative study of bone marrow transplantation and postremission chemotherapy for childhood acute myelogenous leukemia. J Clin Oncol 11:1046, 1993

96. Butturini A, Gale RP: Chemotherapy versus transplantation in acute leukaemia. Br J Haematol 72:1, 1989

97. Tallman MS, Kopecky KJ, Amos D et al: Analysis of prognostic factors for the outcome of marrow transplantation or further chemotherapy for patients with acute nonlymphocytic leukemia in first remission. J Clin Oncol 7:326, 1989

98. Sonnenberg FA, Eckman MH, Pauker SG: Bone marrow donor registries: the relation between registry size and probability of finding complete and partial matches. Blood 74:2569, 1989

99. Kernan NA, Bartsch G, Ash RC et al: Analysis of 462 transplantations from unrelated donors facilitated by the national marrow donor program. N Engl J Med 328:593, 1993

100. Yeager AM, Kaizer H, Santos GW et al: Autologous bone marrow transplantation in patients with acute nonlymphocytic leukemia, using ex vivo marrow treatment with 4-hydroperoxycyclophosphamide. N Engl J Med 315:141, 1986

101. Ball ED, Mills LE, Coughlin CT: Autologous bone marrow transplantation in acute myelogenous leukemia: in vitro treatment with myeloid cell-specific monoclonal antibodies. Blood 68:1311, 1986

102. Gorin NC, Labopin M, Meloni G et al for the European Co-operative Group for Bone Marrow Transplantation (EBMT): Autologous bone marrow transplantation for acute myeloblastic leukemia in Europe: further evidence of the role of marrow purging by mafosfamide. Leukemia 5:896, 1991

103. Gorin NC, Aegerter P, Auvert B et al: Autologous bone marrow transplantation for acute myelocytic leukemia in first remission: a European survey of the role of marrow purging. Blood 75:1606, 1990

104. Beelen DW, Quabeck K, Graeven U et al: Acute toxicity and first clinical results of intensive postinduction therapy using a modified busulfan and cyclophosphamide regimen with autologous bone marrow rescue in first remission of acute myeloid leukemia. Blood 74:1507, 1989

105. Körbling M, Hunstein W, Fliedner TM et al: Disease-free survival after autologous bone marrow transplantation in patients with acute myelogenous leukemia. Blood 74:1898, 1989

106. McMillan AK, Goldstone AH, Linch DC et al: High-dose chemotherapy and autologous bone marrow transplantation in acute myeloid leukemia. Blood 76:480, 1990

107. Stewart P, Buckner CD, Bensinger W et al: Autologous marrow transplantation in patients with acute nonlymphocytic leukemia in first remission. Exp Hematol 13:267, 1985

108. Cassileth PA, Andersen J, Lazarus HM et al: Autologous bone marrow transplant in acute myeloid leukemia in first remission. J Clin Oncol 11:314, 1993

109. Löwenberg B, Verdonck LJ, Dekker AW et al: Autologous bone marrow transplantation in acute myeloid leukemia in first remission: results of a Dutch prospective study. J Clin Oncol 8:287, 1990

110. Estey E, Plunkett W, Dixon D et al: Variables predicting response to high dose cytosine arabinoside therapy in patients with refractory acute leukemia. Leukemia 1:580, 1987

111. Estey E, Plunkett W, Gandhi V et al: Fludarabine and arabinosylcytosine therapy of refractory and relapsed acute myelogenous leukemia. Leuk Lymphoma 9:343, 1993

112. Buckner CD, Sanders J, Appelbaum FR: Allogeneic marrow transplantation for acute non-lymphoblastic leukemia: first remission versus after first relapse. Bone Marrow Transplant, suppl. 1. 4:244, 1989

113. Forman SJ, Schmidt GM, Nademanee AP et al: Allogeneic bone marrow transplantation as therapy for primary induction failure of patients with acute leukemia. J Clin Oncol 9:1570, 1991

114. Mortimer J, Blinder MA, Schulman S et al: Relapse of acute leukemia after marrow transplantation: natural history and results of subsequent therapy. J Clin Oncol 7:50, 1989

115. Giralt S, Escudier S, Kantarjian H et al: Preliminary results of treatment with filgrastim for relapse of leukemia and myelodysplasia after allogeneic bone marrow transplantation. N Engl J Med 329:757, 1993

116. Barrett AJ, Locatelli F, Treleaven JG et al: Second transplants for leukaemic relapse after bone marrow transplantation: high early mortality but favorable effect of chronic GVHD on continued remission, a report by the EBMT Leukaemia Working Party. Br J Haematol 79:567, 1991

117. The Toronto Leukemia Study Group: Results of chemotherapy for unselected patients with acute myeloblastic leukaemia: effect of exclusions on interpretation of results. Lancet 1:786, 1986

118. Berman E, Little C, Gee T et al: Reasons that patients with acute myelogenous leukemia do not undergo allogeneic bone marrow transplantation. N Engl J Med 326:156, 1992

119. Estey EH, Smith TL, Keating MJ et al: Prediction of survival during induction therapy in patients with newly diagnosed acute myeloblastic leukemia. Leukemia 3:257, 1989

120. Arthur DC, Berger R, Golomb HM et al: The clinical significance of karyotype in acute myelogenous leukemia. Cancer Genet Cytogenet 40:203, 1989

121. Samuels BL, Larson RA, Le Beau MM et al: Specific chromosomal abnormalities in acute nonlymphocytic leukemia correlate with drug susceptibility in vivo. Leukemia 2:79, 1988

122. Keating MJ, Smith TL, Kantarjian H et al: Cytogenetic pattern in acute myelogenous leukemia: a major reproducible determinant of outcome. Leukemia 2:403, 1988

123. Schiffer CA, Lee EJ, Tomiyasu T et al: Prognostic impact of cytogenetic abnormalities in patients with de novo acute nonlymphocytic leukemia. Blood 73:263, 1989

124. Fourth International Workshop on Chromosomes in Leukemia, 1982: Corre-

lation between morphology and karyotype. Cancer Genet Cytogenet 11:275, 1984

125. Bloomfield C: Prognostic factors for selecting curative therapy for adult acute myeloid leukemia. Leukemia, suppl. 4. 6:65, 1992

126. Estey E, Kantarjian H, Freireich E et al: Long-term results in newly-diagnosed AML treated with continuous-infusion high-dose ara-C, abstracted. Blood, suppl. 1. 80:112a, 1992

127. Holmes R, Keating MJ, Cork A et al: A unique pattern of central nervous system leukemia in aucte myelomonocytic leukemia associated with inv(16) (p13q22). Blood 65:1071, 1985

128. Kantarjian H, Keating M, Walters R et al: Therapy-related leukemia and myelodysplastic syndrome: clinical cytogenetic, and prognostic features. J Clin Oncol 4:1738, 1986

129. Pedersen-Bjergaard J, Philip P: Balanced translocations involving chromosome bands 11q23 and 21q22 are highly characteristic of myelodysplasia and leukemia following therapy with cytostatic agents targeting at DNA-topoisomerase II. Blood 78:1147, 1991

130. Detourmignies L, Castaigne S, Stoppa AM et al: Therapy-related acute promyelocytic leukemia: a report on 16 cases. J Clin Oncol 10:1430, 1992

131. Olopade OI, Thangavelu M, Larson RA et al: Clinical, morphologic, and cytogenetic characteristics of 26 patients with acute erythroblastic leukemia. Blood 80:2873, 1992

132. Cuneo A, Mecucci C, Kerim S et al: Multipotent stem cell involvement in megakaryoblastic leukemia: cytologic and cytogenetic evidence in 15 patients. Blood 74:1781, 1989

133. Gajewski JL, Ho WG, Nimer SD et al: Efficacy of intensive chemotherapy for acute myelogenous leukemia associated with a preleukemic syndrome. J Clin Oncol 7:1637, 1989

134. Clarkson B, Berman E, Little C et al: Update on clinical trials of chemotherapy and bone marrow transplantation in acute myelogenous leukemia in adults at Memorial Sloan-Kettering Cancer Center 1966 to 1989. p. 239. In Gale RP (ed): Acute Myelogenous Leukemia: Progress and Controversies. Wiley-Liss, New York, 1990

135. Geller RB, Zahurak M, Hurwitz CA et al: Prognostic importance of immunophenotyping in adults with acute myelocytic leukaemia: the significance of the stem-cell glycoprotein CD34 (My10). Br J Haematol 76:340, 1990

136. Borowitz MJ, Gockerman JP, Moore JO et al: Clinicopathologic and cytogenic features of CD35 (My 10)-positive acute nonlymphocytic leukemia. Am J Clin Pathol 91:265, 1989

137. Lee EJ, Yang J, Leavitt RD et al: The significance of CD34 and TdT determinations in patients with untreated de novo acute myeloid leukemia. Leukemia 6:1203, 1992

138. Willman CL, Kopecky KJ, Weick J et al: Biologic parameters that predict treatment response in de novo acute myeloid leukemia: CD34, but not multidrug resistance gene expression, is associated with a decreased complete remission rate and CD34+ patients more frequently achieve CR with high dose cytosine arabinoside, aabstracted. Proc ASCO 11:262, 1992

139. Solary E, Casasnovas RO, Campos L et al and Groupe d'Etude Immunologique des Leucémies: Surface markers in adult acute myeloblastic leukemia: correlation of CD19+, CD34+ and CD14+/DR− phenotypes with shorter survival. Leukemia 6:393, 1992

140. Selleri C, Notaro R, Catalano L et al: Prognostic irrelevance of CD34 in acute myeloid leukaemia. Br J Haemat 82:479, 1992

141. Smith FO, Lampkin BC, Versteeg C et al: Expression of lymphoid-associated cell surface antigens by childhood acute myeloid leukemia cells lacks prognostic significance. Blood 79:2415, 1992

142. Ball ED, Lawrence D, Malnar M et al: Correlation of CD34 and multi-drug resistance P170 with FAB and cytogenetics but not prognosis in acute myeloid leukemia, abstracted. Blood, suppl. 1. 76:252a, 1990

143. Kita K, Miwa H, Nakase K et al (The Japan Cooperative Group of Leukemia/Lymphoma): Clinical importance of CD7 expression in acute myelocytic leukemia. Blood 81:2399, 1993

144. Urbano-Ispizua A, Matutes E, Villamor N et al: The value of detecting surface and cytoplasmic antigens in acute myeloid leukaemia. Br J Haematol 81: 178, 1992

145. Paietta E, Andersen J, Cassileth P et al: Prognostic implication of lymphoid-associated antigens in adult acute myeloid leukemia: an Eastern Cooperative Oncology Group (ECOG) Study, abstracted. Blood, suppl. 1. 80:256a, 1992

146. Kuerbitz SJ, Civin CI, Krischer JP et al: Expression of myeloid-associated and lymphoid-associated cell-surface antigens in acute myeloid leukemia of childhood: a Pediatric Oncology Group study. J Clin Oncol 10:1419, 1992

147. Ball ED, Davis RB, Griffin JD et al: Prognostic value of lymphocyte surface markers in acute myeloid leukemia. Blood 77:2242, 1991

148. Schachner J, Kantarjian H, Dalton W et al: Cytogenetic association and prog-

149. Campos L, Guyotat D, Archimbaud E et al: Clinical significance of multidrug resistance P-glycoprotein expression on acute nonlymphoblastic leukemia cells at diagnosis. Blood 79:473, 1992

150. Marie JP, Zittoun R, Sikic BI: Multidrug resistance (mdr 1) gene expression in adult acute leukemias: correlations with treatment outcome and in vitro drug sensitivity. Blood 78:586, 1991

151. Sato H, Preisler H, Day R et al: MDR$_1$ transcript levels as an indication of resistant disease in acute myelogenous leukaemia. Br J Haematol 75:340, 1990

152. Preisler H, Barcos M, Reese P et al: Recognition of drug resistance during remission induction therapy for acute nonlymphocytic leukemia: utility of day 6 bone marrow biopsy. Leuk Res 7:67, 1983

153. Kantarjian HM, Beran M, Ellis A et al: Phase I study of topotecan, a new topoisomerase I inhibitor, in patients with refractory or relapsed acute leukemia. Blood 81:1146, 1993

154. Santana VM, Mirro J, Kearns C et al: 2-Chlorodeoxyadenosine produces a high rate of complete hematologic remission in relapsed acute myeloid leukemia. J Clin Oncol 10:364, 1992

155. Gandhi V, Estey E, Keating MJ, Plunkett W: Fludarabine potentiates metabolism of cytarabine in patients with acute myelogenous leukemia during therapy. J Clin Oncol 11:116, 1993

156. List AF, Spier C, Greer J et al: Phase I/II trial of cyclosporine as a chemotherapy-resistance modifier in acute leukemia. J Clin Oncol 11:1652, 1993

157. Schwartz MA, Lovett DR, Redner A et al: Dose-escalation trial of M195 labeled with iodine 131 for cytoreduction and marrow ablation in relapsed or refractory myeloid leukemias. J Clin Oncol 11:294, 1993

158. Foa R, Meloni G, Tosti S et al: Treatment of acute myeloid leukaemia patients with recombinant interleukin 2: a pilot study. Br J Haematol 77:491, 1991

159. Freireich EJ, Cork A, Stass SA et al: Cytogenetics for detection of minimal residual disease in acute myeloblastic leukemia. Leukemia 6:500, 1992

160. Miller WH, Levine K, DeBlasio A et al: Detection of minimal residual disease in acute promyelocytic leukemia by a reverse transcription polymerase chain reaction assay for the PML/RAR-α fusion mRNA. Blood 82:1689, 1993

161. Golomb HM, Rowley JD, Vardiman JW et al: "Microgranular" acute promyelocytic leukemia: a distinct clinical, ultrastructural, and cytogenetic entity. Blood 55:253, 1980

162. de Thè H, Chomienne C, Lanotte M et al: The t(15;17) translocation of acute promyelocytic leukaemia fuses the retinoic acid receptor α gene to a novel transcribed locus. Nature 347:558, 1990

163. Biondi A, Rambaldi A, Alcalay M et al: RAR-α gene rearrangements as a genetic marker for diagnosis and monitoring in acute promyelocytic leukemia. Blood 77:1418, 1991

164. Kantarjian HM, Keating MJ, Walters RS et al: Acute promyelocytic leukemia M.D. Anderson Hospital experience. Am J Med 80:789, 1986

165. Cunningham I, Gee TS, Reich LM et al: Acute promyelocytic leukemia: treatment results during a decade at Memorial Hospital. Blood 73:1116, 1989

166. Rodeghiero F, Avvisati G, Castaman G et al: Early deaths and anti-hemorrhagic treatments in acute promyelocytic leukemia. A GIMEMA retrospective study in 268 consecutive patients. Blood 75:2112, 1990

167. Tallman MS, Kwaan HC: Reassessing the hemostatic disorder associated with acute promyelocytic leukemia. Blood 79:543, 1992

168. Bernard J, Weil M, Boiron M et al: Acute promyelocytic leukemia: results of treatment by daunorubicin. Blood 61:489, 1973

169. Goldberg MA, Ginsburg D, Mayer RJ et al: Is heparin administration necessary during induction chemotherapy for patients with acute promyelocytic leukemia? Blood 69:187, 1987

170. Sanz MA, Jarque I, Martín G et al: Acute promyelocytic leukemia: therapy results and prognostic factors. Cancer 61:7, 1988

171. Avvisati G, Mandelli F, Petti MC et al: Idarubicin (4-demethoxydaunorubicin) as single agent for remission induction of previously untreated acute promyelocytic leukemia: a pilot study of the Italian cooperative group GIMEMA. Eur J Haematol 44:257, 1990

172. Rotoli B for the GIMEMA Cooperative Group, Italy: The GIMEMA protocol LAP 0389 for the treatment of acute promyelocytic leukemia: preliminary results, abstracted (842). In Abstracts of the Twenty-fourth Congress of the International Society of Haematology, 1992

173. Runde V, Aul G, Heyll A, Schneider W: All-trans retinoic acid: not only a differentiating agent, but also an inducer of thromboembolic events in patients with M3 leukemia, letter. Blood 79:534, 1992

174. Escudier S, Kantarjian H, Estey E: Thrombosis in acute promyelocytic leukemia patients treated with all-trans retinoic acid, abstracted. Proc ASCO 12: 310, 1993

175. Kantarjian HM, Keating MJ, McCredie KB: A characteristic pattern of leu-

kemic cell differentiation without cytoreduction during remission induction in acute promyelocytic leukemia. J Clin Oncol 3:793, 1985

176. Stone RM, Maguire M, Goldberg MA et al: Complete remission in acute promyelocytic leukemia despite persistence of abnormal bone marrow promyelocytes during induction therapy: experience in 34 patients. Blood 71:690, 1988

177. Kantarjian HM, Keating MJ, Walters RS et al: Role of maintenance chemotherapy in acute promyelocytic leukemia. Cancer 59:1258, 1987

178. Ganem G, Fischer J, Marty M et al: Prognostic factors in acute promyelocytic leukemia: a retrospective study of 101 pts treated by DNR containing remission induction regimen, abstracted. Blood, suppl. 1. 62:171a, 1983

179. Huang M-E, Ye Y-C, Chen S-R et al: Use of all-trans retinoic acid in the treatment of acute promyelocytic leukemia. Blood 72:567, 1988

180. Chen Z-X, Xue Y-Q, Zhang R et al: A clinical and experimental study on all-trans retinoic acid-treated acute promyelocytic leukemia patients. Blood 78:1413, 1991

181. Warrell RP, Frankel SR, Miller WH et al: Differentiation therapy of acute promyelocytic leukemia with tretinoin (all-trans-retinoic acid). N Engl J Med 324:1385, 1991

182. Fenaux P, Castaigne S, Chomienne C et al: All trans retinoic acid treatment for patients with acute promyelocytic leukemia. Leukemia, suppl. 1. 6:64, 1992

183. Warrell RP, De Thé H, Wang Z-Y, Degos L: Acute promyelocytic leukemia. N Engl J Med 329:177, 1993

184. Frankel SR, Eardley A, Lauwers G et al: The "retinoic acid syndrome" in acute promyelocytic leukemia. Ann Intern Med 117:292, 1992

185. Fenaux P, Castaigne S, Dombret H et al: All-transretinoic acid followed by intensive chemotherapy gives a high complete remission rate and may prolong remissions in newly diagnosed acute promyelocytic leukemia: a pilot study on 26 cases. Blood 80:2176, 1992

186. Fenaux P, Robert MC, Castaigne S et al and the French, German, Spanish, Swiss APL groups: A multicenter trial comparing all trans retinoic acid plus chemotherapy (ATRA + CT) and CT alone in newly-diagnosed acute promyelocytic leukemia, abstracted. Proc ASCO 12:300, 1993

187. Hakimian D, Tallman MS, Zugerman C, Caro WA: Erythema nodosum associated with all-trans-retinoic acid in the treatment of acute promyelocytic leukemia. Leukemia 7:758, 1993

188. Koike T, Tatewaki W, Aoki A et al: Brief report: severe symptoms of hyperhistaminemia after the treatment of acute promyelocytic leukemia with tretinoin (all-trans-retinoic acid). N Engl J Med 327:385, 1992

189. Muindi J, Frankel SR, Miller WH et al: Continuous treatment with all-trans retinoic acid causes a progressive reduction in plasma drug concentrations: implications for relapse and retinoid "resistance" in patients with acute promyelocytic leukemia. Blood 79:299, 1992

190. Brincker H: Population-based age- and sex-specific incidence rates in the 4 main types of leukaemia. Scand J Haematol 29:241, 1982

191. Brincker H: Estimate of overall treatment results in acute non-lymphocytic leukemia based on age-specific rates of incidence and of complete remission. Cancer Treat Rep 69:5, 1985

192. Johnson PRE, Liu Yin JA: Acute myeloid leukaemia in the elderly: biology and treatment. Br J Haematol 83:1, 1993

193. Keating MJ, Cork A, Broach Y et al: Toward a clinically relevant cytogenetic classification of acute myelogenous leukemia. Leuk Res 11:119, 1987

194. Löwenberg B, Zittoun R, Kerkhofs H et al: On the value of intensive remission-induction chemotherapy in elderly patients of 65+ years with acute myeloid leukemia: a randomized phase III study of the European Organization for Research and Treatment of Cancer Leukemia Group. J Clin Oncol 7:1268, 1989

195. Van Slyck EJ, Rebuck JW, Waddell CC, Janakiraman N: Smoldering acute granulocytic leukemia, observations on its natural history and morphologic characteristics. Arch Intern Med 143:37, 1983

196. Kahn SB, Begg CB, Mazza JJ et al: Full dose versus attenuated dose daunorubicin, cytosine arabinoside, and 6-thioguanine in the treatment of acute nonlymphocytic leukemia in the elderly. J Clin Oncol 2:865, 1984

197. Tilly H, Castaigne S, Bordessoule D et al: Low-dose cytarabine versus intensive chemotherapy in the treatment of acute nonlymphocytic leukemia in the elderly. J Clin Oncol 8:272, 1990

198. Büchner TH, Hiddemann W, Maschmeyer G et al: AML in patients of 60+ years: full versus reduced dose induction. Randomized study by AMLCG, abstracted. Blood, suppl. 1. 80:209a, 1992

199. Dutcher JP, Strauman JJ, Wiernik PH: Treatment of acute nonlymphocytic leukemia in patients older than 60 years of age, abstracted. Blood, suppl. 1. 64:163a, 1984

200. Sebban C, Archimbaud E, Coiffier B et al: Treatment of acute myeloid leukemia in elderly patients. Cancer 61:227, 1988

201. Johnson PRE, Hunt LP, Liu Yin JA: Prognostic factors in elderly patients with acute myeloid leukaemia: development of a model to predict survival. Br J Haematol 85:300, 1993

202. Keating MJ, McCredie KB, Benjamin RS et al: Treatment of patients over 50 years of age with acute myelogenous leukemia with a combination of rubidazone and cytosine arabinoside, vincristine, and prednisone (ROAP). Blood 58:584, 1981

203. Winston DJ, Islam Z, Buell DN and Acute Leukemia Study Group: Fluconazole prophylaxis of fungal infections in acute leukemia patients: results of a placebo-controlled, double-blind, multicenter trial, abstracted (6). p. 99. In Programs and Abstracts of the Thirty-first Interscience Conference on Antimicrobial Agents and Chemotherapy, Chicago, 1991

204. Caspar CB, Seger RA, Burger J, Gmür J: Effective stimulation of donors for granulocyte transfusions with recombinant methionyl granulocyte colony-stimulating factor. Blood 11:2866, 1993

205. Bensinger WI, Price TH, Dale DC et al: The effects of daily recombinant human granulocyte colony-stimulating factor administration on normal granulocyte donors undergoing leukapheresis. Blood 81:1883, 1993

206. Nemunaitis J, Shannon-Dorcy K, Appelbaum FR et al: Long-term follow-up of patients with invasive fungal disease who received adjunctive therapy with recombinant human macrophage colony-stimulating factor. Blood 82:1422, 1993

Acute Myeloid Leukemia in Children

66

Lorrie F. Odom

CONGENITAL LEUKEMIA

Strictly defined, congenital leukemia is diagnosed between birth and 4 weeks of age. However, some reports extend this period to 6–12 months. Unless otherwise specified, information in this chapter refers to the strict definition of this disorder.

Criteria for diagnosis of congenital leukemia are the following: (1) proliferation of immature leukemic cells; (2) infiltration of these cells into nonhematopoietic tissues unrelated to extramedullary hematopoiesis; (3) absence of other disease processes such as congenital infections, hypoxia, and erythroblastosis fetalis that can cause a leukemoid or leukoerythroblastic reaction mimicking congenital leukemia; and (4) absence of constitutional chromosomal disorders that may be associated with "unstable" hematopoiesis such as trisomy 21.

Leukemia at this age is rare, with approximately 200 cases described. Congenital leukemia may be associated with Down syndrome,[1-3] Turner syndrome,[4] mosaic monosomy 7,[5] mosaic trisomy 9,[6] Klinefelter syndrome,[7] trisomy 13, or Bloom syndrome. Acute myeloid leukemia (AML) appears to occur more frequently at this young age than acute lymphocytic leukemia (ALL). AML ranges in various studies from 50% to 90% of congenital leukemia cases.[8-10] The variability in reported frequency of AML and ALL may be related to difficulty in determining blast cell type. Most infants with congenital AML have monocytoid leukemias, predominantly acute monocytic leukemia (AMoL) or M5 disease.

Newborn infants with Down syndrome or who are mosaic for trisomy 21 may present with a transient myeloproliferative disorder (TMD) that can be clinically indistinguishable from congenital leukemia.[11-13] The diagnosis of congenital leukemia therefore can be difficult and an important clinical problem.

Etiology and Pathogenesis

As is the case with other forms of leukemia, the etiology of congenital leukemia has not been elucidated. Congenital leukemia has not been reported in infants whose mothers had leukemia before or during pregnancy. There are no consistent relationships between fetal or extrauterine x-ray or other known potential toxic exposures and subsequent development of leukemia. The short latency time and lack of known carcinogenic exposures suggest that strong and perhaps unusual genetic mechanisms may be involved in the pathogenesis of this process. Genomic instability is suggested by studies in a few cases of congenital leukemia that show multiple immunoglobulin heavy chain hybridization bands using recombinant DNA technology.[14]

Breaks in 11q23 are seen in both congenital lymphoid and myeloid disease, leading to the speculation that rearrangements of a gene at 11q23 may affect a pluripotential progenitor cell or cause deregulation of a mechanism for differentiation shared by lymphoid and myeloid stem cells. It has previously been questioned whether one or more genes on band 11q23 are involved in these translocations. Recently, a single gene has been cloned that spans all 11q23 breakpoints. Several groups have cloned and sequenced the same gene; it has been called Htrx,[15] ALL-1,[16] HRX,[17] and MLL.[18] The increased frequency of 11q23 rearrangements in congenital leukemia may indicate that this gene region is subjected to different transcriptional control in fetal as compared with adult life or that this gene is particularly vulnerable to neoplastic rearrangement in fetal life.[19] Support for the hypothesis that MLL translocations may occur prenatally was demonstrated by Ford et al.,[20] in three pairs of identical twins who developed leukemia in infancy. The leukemia cells from each twin pair shared identical MLL rearrangements unique to each pair.

Transient megakaryoblastic proliferation appears to be particularly common in neonates with trisomy 21.[11,21-24] Although resembling congenital leukemia, in patients with trisomy 21 ineffective regulation of granulopoiesis, erythropoiesis, and thrombopoiesis is nearly always associated with complete clinical and hematologic recovery within weeks or months without antileukemic therapy. The syndrome is therefore called TMD. Controversy still exists over whether TMD is a manifestation of ineffective myelopoiesis or a spontaneous prolonged remission of true congenital leukemia. Although most affected children recover completely, there have been a few reports of development of acute leukemia in children with Down syndrome years after prior resolution of abnormal clinical and laboratory

findings consistent with TMD.[3,25] Karyotype analysis with banding may be helpful in distinguishing between acute leukemia and TMD. Clonal abnormalities detected with this syndrome should disappear with spontaneous remission and presumably recur with the evolution of acute leukemia. Hayashi et al.[11] found clonal cytogenetic abnormalities in the cells of 13 patients with Down syndrome and acute leukemia (DS-AL) but not in 15 neonates with Down syndrome and TMD (DS-TMD). The age range for DS-AL patients was 6–30 months and for the DS-TMD patients 0–34 days. The oldest DS-TMD patient had a spontaneous regression but developed AL at 18 months of age associated with clonal cytogenetic abnormalities. There are also reports of spontaneous disappearance of the 5q abnormality deletion and monosomy 7 clonal cytogenetic abnormalities in neonates with Down syndrome and apparent TMD.[12]

As discussed above, both TMD and leukemia have been associated with mosaic trisomy 21.[13] In all such patients trisomy was present in the abnormal hematologic cells. Nine phenotypically normal infants with TMD have been described. Mosaicism for trisomy 21 was present in eight of these infants, with the malignant cell line part of the trisomic clone in each instance. In four infants the trisomic karyotype appeared to be limited to the transient leukemic clone. The one patient who had apparent TMD not associated with trisomy 21 was initially reported by Lampkin et al.[26] in 1985 and continues to have no evidence of leukemia (Lampkin BC, personal communication, 1993).

Clinical Manifestations

The clinical manifestations of congenital leukemia differ in varying degrees from the typical findings in older infants and children. At least one-half of newborns with leukemia have nodular skin lesions (also called leukemia cutis). The baby is often described as looking like a "blueberry muffin"[27,28] (Fig. 66-1). These lesions are composed of nests of leukemic cells, may involve over half the body surface area, vary from a few millimeters to several centimeters in diameter, are firm, usually freely mobile, and the color of overlying skin ranges from blue-gray to brown-red.[29] Importantly, skin nodules may precede bone marrow and other organ manifestations of leukemia. Other signs and symptoms of congenital leukemia may include petechiae, purpura, hepatosplenomegaly, lethargy, pallor, and failure to thrive. Transient spontaneous remissions have occasionally been reported but are usually followed by reappearance of leukemia, frequently with more organ involvement and as a more clinically aggressive process.

Laboratory Evaluation

Laboratory findings are similar to those seen in older children with leukemia. Marked leukocytosis is common, with white blood cell (WBC) counts of 300,000–500,000/mm^3, and a preponderance of immature cells in the bone marrow and peripheral blood. Most congenital leukemias are classified as acute myeloid and most of these are of the monoblastic subtype (M5a in the French-American-British [FAB] system). Rarely, acute megakaryoblastic leukemia[30] and acute erythroleukemia[31] have been documented in neonates with congenital leukemia. The platelet peroxidase reaction and immunologic phenotyping of blast cells of patients with Down syndrome and infant leukemia have shown an especially high incidence of megakaryoblastic leukemia.[11,32,33]

Cytogenetic abnormalities appear to be more frequent in congenital leukemia than in other acute leukemias,[34] perhaps indirect evidence of the profound genetic damage necessary

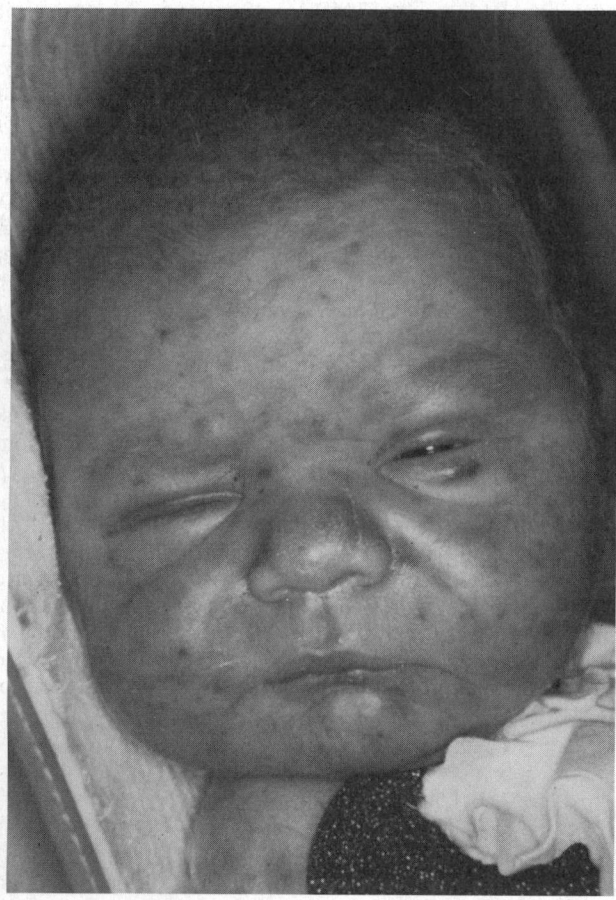

Fig. 66-1. The gray-blue lesions commonly seen in congenital leukemia. The child is often said to look like a "blueberry muffin" when these lesions appear.

to precipitate leukemia at such an early age. A parallel situation may be the presence of aberrations in most patients with leukemia secondary to mutagen exposure. In a review of cytogenetic findings in infant leukemia by Heim et al.,[34] selecting infants diagnosed ≤4 weeks of age, the following abnormalities were found: t(4;11)(q21 or 13;q22 or 23) in 4 of 6 infants with ALL; t(4;11;17)(q21;q23;q11) in 1 of 6 with ALL; 4 of 6 infants with AML had AMoL and variable cytogenetic abnormalities, including t(8;16)(p11;p13), t(x;10)(q28;q11), t(11;19)(q23;q13), and t(7;12)(q31;p12)+19. The predominance of t(4;11) in congenital ALL contrasts with the lower incidence of this translocation among pediatric ALL patients in general (about 70% compared with 10%). Translocations involving 11q23 are the single most common cytogenetic abnormality in congenital leukemia.[35]

Abnormalities of chromosome 10 within the region 10(p11-13) [e.g., del 10(p12)] have been reported frequently in congenital AMoL with cutaneous involvement. In one series, 4 of 10 cases had such chromosome 10 abnormalities.[28]

Additionally, there are two reported cases of infant ALL (newborn 2 months) who had t(x;6) rearrangements with breakpoints in bands q15-16 of chromosome 6 [t(x;6)(p22.1;q15) and t(x;5;6)(p11;q12;q16)]. These findings suggest that this chromosome 6 breakpoint may be another characteristic of congenital ALL.[36]

Studies incorporating recombinant DNA technology show an association between multiple immunoglobulin heavy chain hybridization bands in childhood leukemia and poor prognosis.[37] A study reported by Rechavi et al.[14] showed an abnormal immunoglobulin heavy chain J region multiband pattern to be a con-

sistent finding by Southern blot analysis in congenital leukemia. This possible association awaits further confirmation.

Differential Diagnosis

The differential diagnosis of congenital leukemia encompasses many disease processes. Severe neonatal hemolysis, bacterial infections, and hypoxemia can all cause a leukoerythroblastic peripheral blood smear. Other entities that can mimic congenital leukemia include ineffective granulopoiesis associated with trisomy 21, intrauterine viral disease (herpes simplex, rubella, cytomegalovirus, adenovirus), other congenital infections such as syphilis or toxoplasmosis, or proliferative processes such as neuroblastoma, Langerhans cell histiocytosis, and malignant histiocytosis.

Differentiating tests include TORCH (toxoplasmosis, other [viruses], rubella, cytomegalovirus, herpes [simplex viruses]) titers, cultures, Venereal Disease Research Laboratory (VDRL) determination, Coombs test, investigation of congenital defects such as intracerebral calcifications or chorioretinitis, serial bone marrow morphology, and cytogenetic studies. Importantly, all phenotypically normal infants with possible congenital leukemia should be evaluated for trisomy 21 mosaicism by obtaining bone marrow cytogenetic studies.

Congenital syphilis is characterized by a positive VDRL test without intramedullary blast cell proliferation. Intrauterine viral infections are usually associated with normal bone marrow morphology, although congenital defects, intracerebral calcifications, and chorioretinitis may be present. Positive serology for cytomegalovirus, rubella, or toxoplasmosis is helpful in making the diagnosis of intrauterine infection. Neuroblastoma in the neonate is diagnosed by biopsy of the primary tumor or skin nodule; the finding of elevated urinary catecholamine metabolites and/or the presence of marrow tumor invasion may provide supportive diagnostic information.

Newborns with trisomy 21 or who are mosaic for trisomy 21 may have transient clinical and hematologic features resembling those of congenital leukemia (TMD). This syndrome may be associated with a peripheral WBC count ≤400,000/mm^3; ≤95% monoblasts, myeloblasts, or erythroblasts peripherally; and thrombocytopenia.[1,11,38] Initial bone marrow findings may be even more confusing, showing erythroid or myeloid hyperplasia or sometimes ≤60% blasts with a reduction in normal hematopoietic elements.

Therapy and Prognosis

Because it can be difficult to distinguish infants clinically and biologically with true congenital leukemia from those with TMD, therapeutic alternatives must be carefully evaluated. It is believed by most observers that supportive care with close monitoring is the most judicious form of initial treatment. If clinical or hematologic deterioration becomes apparent during supportive therapy, chemotherapy may be instituted. In infants with Down syndrome, this option should be weighed even more heavily because of the strong correlation of trisomy 21 with TMD as well as increased chemotherapy-associated complications in this group.[39,40] These complications are related to both infections and direct toxicity, especially to mucous membranes (oral and gastrointestinal).

In addition to infants with trisomy 21, spontaneous remissions may occur in a small subset of newborns with AMoL and "monocytic leukemia cutis." The spontaneous remissions in infants with trisomy 21 are usually durable (i.e., permanent or lasting for years). In infants with AMoL, such remissions are usually transient. Of five reported neonates with congenital leukemia, skin nodules, and normal blast karyotype who underwent spontaneous remission, four had transient remissions.[26,30,41–43] Three of these infants had AML and the cell type was not reported for the other two infants.

Most patients with congenital leukemia die within a few days to months after diagnosis. Pierce[8] reported that 8 of 21 patients were dead within 2 weeks of presentation and the remainder died within 2 months. The disease is characterized by progressive signs of organ infiltration and hemorrhage. Patients frequently die as a consequence of cerebral hemorrhage or respiratory failure, often related to leukostasis.[44]

The treatment of congenital leukemia with chemotherapy has not been as successful as similar therapy in older children. Standard induction regimens of daunorubicin and cytosine arabinoside (ara-C) have yielded poor results. In 1984 Odom and Gordon[45] reported five infants and children with AMoL treated with an epipodophyllotoxin (VP-16 or VM-26). Four of the five children (including the three infants with congenital leukemia) were off therapy 11 months to 6 years at the time of the report and continue to be disease free. Other investigators have not had similar success with this regimen in older infants. There is an important need for further organized study of the neonatal leukemias, focusing on treatment as well as biologic and prognostic parameters.

Future Directions

The clinical and biologic significance of congenital leukemia far outweighs its incidence relative to other types of childhood cancer. Knowledge gained in better understanding this disease process will be relevant to oncogenesis in general.

Future efforts will be directed at improving outcome and the understanding of biologic mechanisms involved in its etiology, clinical presentation, sporadic occurrence of spontaneous remission or resolution, and response to therapy. Because of the rarity of this form of leukemia, cooperative therapeutic trials with concomitant biologic investigations are needed.

A few of the many biologic questions related to congenital leukemia that require further elucidation are the following: (1) the unusual genetic mechanisms involved in its pathogenesis; (2) the close association of 11q23 aberrations, specifically MLL gene translocations, with congenital leukemia; (3) verification of the preliminary finding of a high frequency of multiple immunoglobulin heavy chain rearrangements in congenital leukemia; (4) whether the multiple rearrangements represent multiclonal disease from the onset and whether this finding is a reflection of genomic instability that can lead to early acquisition of drug resistance; (5) the seemingly paradoxical role of an extra chromosome 21, which appears to be associated with self-limited TMD in infancy as well as an increased incidence of leukemia in childhood. Additional questions include (1) could suppression of an abnormal clone of hematopoietic cells be a normal mechanism exaggerated to the point of visibility in trisomy 21 cells; and (2) are some of these clones truly leukemic and suppressed for a variable period, possibly later re-expanding to a full-blown acute leukemia in a proportion of cases, thus accounting for the increased incidence of acute leukemia in children with Down syndrome?

The acquisition of a proliferative advantage by malignant hematopoietic cells in the highly specialized environment of fetal growth and differentiation is intriguing. Increased understanding of the unique aspects of congenital leukemia and the associations with chromosome 21 and 11q23 will perhaps help elucidate general mechanisms of oncogenesis and growth regulation.

PEDIATRIC ACUTE MYELOID LEUKEMIA

Childhood AML is increasingly recognized as a heterogeneous group of leukemias with varied clinical, morphologic, immunophenotypic, kinetic, cytogenetic, and molecular features,

and diverse responses to therapy. Currently, seven morphologic variants are officially recognized. Similarities in biologic behavior between respective subtypes in adult and pediatric populations appear to exist, with the notable exception of more frequent and extensive extramedullary involvement by the M5 subtype in infants and young children.

In the 1960s, AML was regarded as incurable and the average duration of remission for children with this disease was 3–6 months.[47] With more aggressive treatment, including intensive conventional chemotherapy or bone marrow transplantation in early first remission, attention to specific central nervous system treatment for certain subtypes, and aggressive supportive measures, 35–45% of children with AML now remain in long-term remission and appear to be cured of this disease. Greater understanding of the biologic, morphologic, kinetic, cytogenetic, and molecular distinctiveness of these leukemias will inevitably lead to more refined and specific treatment approaches and further improvements in outcome.

Epidemiology

AML represents approximately 25% of leukemias in children and adolescents.[48] Unlike ALL, AML is equally distributed among racial groups and its incidence remains stable from birth through age 10. Leukemia that has its onset within the first 4 weeks of life is most often AML.[8–10,44] There is increasing evidence that chemical exposures are linked to the development of some forms of AML. These exposures, including environmental carcinogens and certain chemotherapeutic agents, are discussed in more detail later.

Certain genetic diseases predispose to the development of AML in childhood. Acute leukemia is nearly 20 times more likely to occur in children with Down syndrome than in the general population. The cell type of leukemia in these children follows the usual distribution for this age group[1] with the exception that acute megakaryoblastic leukemia (AMeL) is more likely to occur in young children with Down syndrome.[49–51] As noted in Table 66-1, conditions associated with chromosomal instability and defective DNA repair, such as Fanconi anemia, Bloom syndrome, ataxia-telangiectasia, and incontinentia pigmenti are associated with an increased risk of AML.[52,53] Children with congenital disorders of myelopoiesis such as Kostmann syndrome and Diamond-Blackfan anemia are also predisposed to AML.[54] Additionally, there appears to be predisposition to the development of AML in children with Schwachman, Klinefelter, and Turner syndromes and von Recklinghausen's neurofibromatosis.[55–57]

There exists an apparent association between acute leukemia (frequently AML), brain tumors, and soft tissue tumors in family members, suggesting a "familial syndrome" of neoplastic diseases.[58–60] Meadows et al.[61] analyzing patterns of second malignant neoplasms in pediatric cancer patients and their siblings, described a "hereditary cancer syndrome" associating glioma, acute leukemia, and lymphoma. Farwell and Flannery[62] suggested an increased likelihood of childhood cancer, including leukemia, in siblings of children with brain tumors.

Biologic and Molecular Aspects

Investigations that further elucidate the molecular and cellular basis of hematopoiesis, such as in vitro bone marrow culture patterns, biochemical markers, cell-surface antigens, leukemia cell kinetics, nonrandom cytogenetic and molecular aberrations, and oncogene expression will lead to improved understanding of the biology of AML.

Molecular events associated with normal myeloid maturation and malignant transformation remain incompletely under-

Initial Evaluation

The workup of an infant with suspected congenital leukemia should first include a detailed history with particular attention to ruling out the possibility of congenitally acquired infection, blood type incompatibility, and the hereditary form of Down syndrome. A thorough physical examination should include inspection for stigmata of congenital infection, Down syndrome, and attention to the presence or absence of skin lesions, hepatosplenomegaly, adenopathy, extramedullary palpable tumor masses, and cranial nerve palsies.

Suggested initial laboratory studies consist of a CBC, reticulocyte count, platelet count, TORCH titers, appropriate cultures, VDRL and Coombs tests, chemistries (including electrolytes, calcium, phosphorus, lactate dehydrogenase, uric acid, urinalysis, and oximetry), coagulation profile (including prothrombin time, partial thromboplastin time, fibrinogen, and fibrin split products), chest radiograph, bone marrow aspirate with samples for cytogenetic analysis, cytochemical stains, and complete immunophenotyping, and cerebrospinal fluid assessment for chemistries and cytocentrifuge examination for morphology.

Because the administration of chemotherapy to the neonate is associated with so many potential toxicities, it is imperative that the diagnosis of acute leukemia be absolutely proven before the use of chemotherapy is considered. All other causes for the suspicious findings must be ruled out, such as infection, hemolysis, and hypoxemia. Additionally, trisomy 21 in the bone marrow cells must be ruled out because of the very high likelihood of spontaneous regression of the TMD associated with that cytogenetic abnormality.

Therapeutic Approach for Infants with Proven Congenital Acute Leukemia

Before the use of chemotherapy is contemplated, the infant should be stabilized with regard to renal, metabolic, and coagulation parameters. Depending on the type of leukemia, different approaches are indicated.

AMoL (FAB M5a) is one of the most common forms of congenital leukemia. It is usually associated with obvious skin nodules with purplish or reddish-brown discoloration of overlying skin. It also usually undergoes spontaneous temporary regression. Therefore, withholding treatment until the infant is absolutely stable is advisable, even if a few weeks elapse before treatment is initiated. If the leukemia does follow the typical course of regression, the use of single-agent systemic and intrathecal chemotherapy is often effective if initiated when the tumor burden is minimal. This leukemia usually responds rapidly to treatment with an epipodophyllotoxin such as etoposide or teniposide. Use of etoposide given three times weekly for the first 2 weeks during induction and then twice weekly for 15–18 months along with intermittent intrathecal ara-C may be curative in this setting. However, if treatment is not initiated until disease recurs, single-agent therapy is unlikely to be effective and cranial radiation may become necessary. Because of the very high likelihood of disease recurrence after an initial regression, beginning less aggressive treatment at the time of initial disease diagnosis or regression is recommended.

AML other than the FAB M5a subtype and ALL in the neonate usually behave aggressively and may become recalcitrant to multiagent chemotherapy. As above, it is important to stabilize the infant first before considering chemotherapy. Additionally, the potential of significant toxicity related to the use of chemotherapy at this age and the likelihood of poor outcome despite the use of appropriate chemotherapy must be explained to the family. Unfavorable outcome is especially likely if an 11q23 aberration other than t(9;11) is present in the leukemia cells. The pros and cons of initiating chemotherapy must be carefully weighed. A decision to give only supportive care and withhold chemotherapy can be appropriate in this situation as long as the family is fully informed. If a decision to initiate chemotherapy is made, supportive care becomes a major factor in the ongoing management of the infant.

Chemotherapeutic agents incorporated in the treatment are usually determined by the type of leukemia. Congenital leukemias frequently involve an 11q23 chromosomal aberration and as such probably involve a pluripotent progenitor cell in the leukemic clone. Thus the treatment of infant acute leukemia may optimally incorporate chemotherapy that is effective in both myeloid and lymphoid disease. Agents such as vincristine, prednisone, daunomycin, etoposide, 6-thioguanine, ara-C, and high-dose methotrexate are cautiously administered. Doses are determined by body weight rather than surface area. Careful attention must be given to possible vincristine-associated neuropathy such as hoarse cry or difficulty with swallowing or gag, to which infants are particularly predisposed.

Overt or subclinical meningeal leukemic involvement is common in this age group. Special attention must be given to treatment of the central nervous system with intrathecal medications and systemic chemotherapy that can penetrate that area such as high-dose methotrexate and ara-C. Every effort is made to postpone or ideally avoid cranial radiation (CRT) in this age group. If CRT does become necessary, giving it in "intermittent protracted" scheduling may be more protective in terms of later neuropsychological sequelae.[46] However, efficacy of this approach in infants remains to be proven.

As noted above, aggressive supportive care is needed when treating any infant with chemotherapy. Appropriate modifications of drug dosages for toxicity are made, with special attention to mucositis and vincristine-associated neuropathy. Central venous access with an indwelling double lumen catheter is necessary. All blood products are irradiated, leukocyte-depleted, and type and cytomegalovirus appropriate. Platelets are administered prophylactically to maintain a platelet count >20,000/mm³. Prophylactic trimethoprim-sulfamethoxazole (2.5 mg/kg every 12 hours × 4 consecutive doses each week) should provide adequate Pneumocystis protection without significant myelosuppression while mycostatin administration serves as prophylaxis for thrush. Infants with severe neutropenia (absolute granulocyte count <500/mm³) who become febrile (or hypothermic) are started promptly on empirical broad-spectrum antibiotic therapy after appropriate cultures are obtained, including blood cultures from each central catheter lumen. An initial choice of antimicrobial agents may include ceftazidime and vancomycin. If fever persists and anaerobic or candida infection is suspected, flagyl or fluconazole, respectively, should be promptly added to the regimen. It may become necessary to substitute amphotericin B for fluconazole if fever continues to persist. Intravenous antibiotics should be administered alternately through each catheter lumen.

Table 66-1. Genetic Diseases Predisposing to Childhood AML

Down syndrome

Fanconi anemia

Bloom syndrome

Ataxia-telangiectasia

Kostmann syndrome

Diamond-Blackfan anemia

Shwachman syndrome

Klinefelter syndrome

Turner syndrome

Neurofibromatosis

Incontinentia pigmenti

stood. The transforming event can theoretically occur in any cell along the pathway from a very potent stem cell to a committed progenitor cell. There is substantial evidence that the vast majority of myeloid leukemias are derived from a single cell. The demonstration that only one of two possible X-linked electrophoretically distinct glucose-6-phosphate dehydrogenase isoenzymes were present in leukemic blasts from females heterozygous for these enzymes provided the earliest evidence of clonal origin of AML.[63] Subsequently, restriction fragment length polymorphism analysis of a sex-linked lyonized gene, such as that for hypoxanthine guanosine phosphoribosyl transferase, demonstrated that progeny of AML leukemic cells express only one functional allele whereas normal cells randomly express one or the other.[64] Using enzyme and cytogenetic analyses, it became apparent that involvement of erythroid precursors and their progeny in the leukemic process is variable.[63–66] Presumably this variability is determined by whether the transforming event took place in a multipotent progenitor or a more committed granulocyte/macrophage progenitor. It was suggested by Keinanen et al.[67] that monosomy 7 and some trisomy 8 and FAB M2 leukemias involve erythroid precursors whereas other myeloid leukemias (e.g., subtype FAB M4) may more commonly be restricted to granulocytic/macrophage lineage. Occasional patients with AML continue to have clonal hematopoiesis when the bone marrow is morphologically and cytogenetically in remission.[64,68] The frequency of occurrence of hematopoiesis derived from the abnormal clone is controversial. A study of 17 female children with AML showed only one patient to have clonally derived granulocytes, suggesting that clonal remission is an infrequent event in this age group.[69] Importantly, this study included normal tissue controls.

Several proto-oncogenes appear to be overexpressed in AML cells, but their exact role in transformation remains to be elucidated.[70] Using a hybridization technique that permits detection of as few as five copies of mRNA per cell, Evinger-Hodges and associates[71–73] reported that expression levels of c-*myc* and c-*sis* are higher in hematopoietic cells obtained from leukemia patients than in normal hematopoietic cells. In a large proportion of remission marrows, a subpopulation of cells has been detected that expresses *myc* at very high levels.[73] Leukemic origin of this abnormal cell population is supported by double labeling experiments that show close correlation between gene overexpression and leukemic phenotype.[73] Moreover, there is a suggested correlation between overexpression of *myc* or *sis* in remission marrows of patients who relapse within 1 year.[74] Oncogene products may contribute to leukemogenesis as growth factors, growth factor receptors, or intracellular messengers. It is possible that aberrant expression of such oncogenes as *myc* and *sis* could contribute to the unregulated growth potential of myeloid leukemia cells.

An important finding at the molecular level has clinical relevance to the AML FAB M3 subtype, acute promyelocytic leuke-

mia (APL). In 1987, the gene encoding the retinoic acid receptor-α (RAR-α) was mapped to chromosome 17q21, the breakpoint in the nonrandom translocation associated with APL [t(15;17)(q22,q21)].[75] Subsequently, the breakpoint in this translocation was cloned and the RAR-α gene was found to be rearranged in the leukemic cells of all patients tested.[76] The breakpoints on chromosome 15 were found to cluster tightly in a region containing a gene that was named PML.[77,78] It is probable that this translocation generates a disease-specific fusion protein that presumably is involved in carcinogenesis.

Genetic Aspects

As techniques improve, karyotypically abnormal clones can be identified in an increasing proportion of children with AML at the time of diagnosis. The collaboration between oncologists and cytogeneticists has resulted in appropriate specimen collection and rapid processing, both of which affect the yield and quality of mitotic cells. Most laboratories use several culture systems for each sample, including direct preparations and short-term unstimulated cultures, and accurately analyze at least the 400 band level of chromosome condensation, allowing delineation of subtle chromosome abnormalities. The use of culture additives such as conditioned supernatant from giant cell tumor cultures also enhances the chromosome morphology of myeloid leukemia cells.

Nonrandom clonal aberrations are currently identified in leukemia cells from >80% of patients with AML.[79–83] During hematologic remission, the bone marrow karyotype usually returns to normal; at relapse, the initial cytogenetic abnormality, with or without additional aberrations, usually reappears.

Identifiable nonrandom chromosomal abnormalities are characteristic of specific morphologic and clinical subsets of AML and of leukemia arising after environmental exposures to possible carcinogens or prior treatment with certain chemotherapeutic agents[84–93] (Table 66-2). Six of seven infants who had been exposed to marijuana in utero had clonal abnormalities of the long or short arm of chromosome 11 (four) and/or trisomy 8 (three).[94]

Observations predominantly but not exclusively in adults show a correlation between environmental exposure to benzene and therapeutic exposure to leukemogenic agents such as cyclophosphamide, melphalan, and nitrogen mustard with the development of monosomy 5/5q− or monosomy 7/7q− myelodysplastic syndromes with a high risk of progression to overt AML.[95–100] More recently, AML following treatment with etoposide or teniposide has been reported, especially in pediatric patients initially treated for ALL.[90,93,101] This secondary leukemia is commonly associated with abnormalities in the 11q23 chromosomal region of the leukemic blasts (approximately 50% of the cases).[90,101]

Etiology and Pathogenesis

The etiology of AML is complex, appears to be multifactorial, and is far from completely understood. There is increasing evidence that environmental factors are linked to the development of some forms of AML. A large case control study from the Childrens Cancer Group[94] suggests a 10-fold increase in the risk of developing monocytoid leukemia in infants born to mothers who used marijuana while pregnant. The median age of these children at diagnosis was significantly younger than for children with other subtypes of AML. The risk for children <6 years of age of developing acute myelomonocytic leukemia (AMML) or AMoL was significantly elevated by direct exposure of the child to pesticides, maternal exposure to household pesticides during pregnancy, or by prolonged paternal or maternal

Table 66-2. AML Cytogenetic Abnormalities: Morphologic and Clinical Correlation

Primary Chromosome Abnormality[a]	Morphologic (FAB)[b]/Clinical Correlation	Prognosis
Structural rearrangements		
t(8;21)	M2; chloroma may be present	Good
t(15;17)	M3; severe bleeding common at onset; excellent initial response to all-trans retinoic acid[178]	Good[c]
t(9;11)	M5 in infants or young children	Good
t(A;11q23) (A = 6, 9, 10, or 17)	M5 or M4 (in infants, possible relationship to in utero marijuana exposure)[94]	Poor to intermediate
inv/del(16q22)	M4; usually with marrow eosinophilia; frequent meningeal involvement[230]	Good
t(9;22)	M1, rarely M2	Poor
t(6;9)	M2 or M4, often with basophilia	—
inv(3)	M1, rarely M2, M4, M7, with thrombocytosis	—
t(8;16)	M5b with erythrophagocytosis	—
t/del(12)	M2 with basophilia	—
Chromosome loss		
−5(5q−)	Myelodysplasia, preleukemia; exposure to leukemogenic agents	Poor
−7(7q−)	Myelodysplasia, preleukemia; exposure to leukemogenic agents	Poor
−Y	Myelodysplasia, preleukemia; M4	Poor
Chromosome gain		
+8	M1; M4 or M5 (in infants, possible relationship to in utero marijuana exposure)[94]	Intermediate
+4	M4, rarely M2	—

[a] Data from Second MIC Cooperative Study Group.[83]
[b] FAB morphologic classification (Data from Bennett et al.[74,136]).
[c] If fatal hemorrhage during induction can be avoided, prognosis is good.

occupational pesticide exposure.[102] Paternal exposure to solvents, plastics, petroleum products, or lead and maternal exposure to paints, pigments, metal dust, and sawdust were also significantly more often reported by case than control parents. Previous reports in smaller pediatric populations show an increased risk of childhood AML with parental exposure to pesticides[103]; maternal exposure to metal refining and processing, benzene, and gasoline[104]; and patient exposure to insecticides.[105]

Exposure to alkylating agents[106–108] and ionizing irradiation[109,110] are associated with development of AML in adults. Increased leukemia risk appears proportional to the total alkylating agent dose.[108] Such exposures are becoming increasingly pertinent to the development of AML in the pediatric population. Further elucidating this important relationship is the recently well-documented association of exposure to epipodophyllotoxins for treatment of primary pediatric cancers and subsequent development of secondary AML.[90–93,101,111–113] AML in this setting is typically monocytoid and has been most commonly reported after use of these topoisomerase II-reactive agents for treatment of pediatric ALL, especially but not exclusively T-cell ALL.[90,92,93,101,112] Secondary AML in the pediatric population has also been reported after exposure to epipodophyllotoxins for treatment of T-cell non-Hodgkin lymphoma[112] and other solid tumors.[91]

Lack of preceding myelodysplasia[90,101] and a relatively short median latency period, varying from 21 to 40.5 months from initial exposure to chemotherapy,[93,101,111,112] are characteristic of epipodophyllin-related AML. In addition to primary T-cell leukemia or lymphoma, factors that may be related to the likelihood of developing secondary epipodophyllin-related AML are schedule and total cumulative dose of these agents. Increased risk of secondary AML has been documented with twice-weekly or weekly administration of teniposide,[101] five daily doses of etoposide every 3 weeks,[114] and on days 1, 3, and 5 of an 8-week cycle.[115] The risk of acquiring secondary AML also appears to be potentiated by concomitant use of alkylating agents, methotrexate, mercaptopurine, cisplatin, ara-C, asparaginase, and/or irradiation.[113,116,117] It has been demonstrated in vitro that agents such as methotrexate and mercaptopurine can reduce purine nucleotide pools and increase epipodophyllotoxin-induced DNA alterations.[69]

The leukemic progenitor cell has a decreased capacity to differentiate in response to normal physiologic stimuli and gradually becomes a predominant cell. This process usually takes place in the bone marrow, but occasionally a chloroma originates in an extramedullary site[118] or the disease process begins in the skin, not uncommon in M5 disease in infants.[27] Leukemia may also proliferate in other reticuloendothelial tissues and extramedullary sites such as the central nervous system.

Suppression of normal hematopoiesis is caused by overcrowding normal marrow cells or production of inhibitory humoral factors such as acidic isoferritins, or both.[119,120] Certain characteristics of leukemic cells can be determined by in vitro culturing of bone marrow from patients with AML. Standard techniques for growing normal marrow progenitors result in the formation of leukemic blast colonies from approximately 30% of patients.[121] Alteration of culture conditions to include phytohemagglutinin-stimulated allogeneic leukocytes either in a feeder underlayer or mixed with leukemic cells yields growth of blast colonies, which are generally smaller than normal colonies, in 80–90% of patients.[121,122] Cell-surface phenotypes of these clonogenic leukemia cells often differ from the phenotypes of the marrow leukemic blasts.[123,124] The colony pattern generally reverts to normal after successful remission induction.[98]

Clinical Manifestations

Presenting manifestations of AML in childhood are protean. A comparison of common presenting features in children with AML and ALL is presented in Table 66-3. Symptoms related to bone marrow failure are prominent in both categories. Fever at diagnosis is less common in AML, perhaps because fever is less likely to be caused by the underlying disease process than in ALL. Bone and joint pain or inflammation are also less common presenting features of AML.

An association between certain clinical manifestations and FAB subtypes at diagnosis is recognized. Many of these clinical findings have important therapeutic implications (Table 66-4). Neurologic manifestations such as headaches and blurred vision are more common in AML than ALL at diagnosis, especially

Table 66-3. Comparison of Common Presenting Features in Childhood AML and ALL

Sign or Symptoms	Children (%)	
	AML[a]	ALL[b]
Fever	34	61
Pallor	25	55
Bleeding	33	48
Bone or joint pain	18	38
Anorexia, weight loss	22	33
Weakness, fatigue	19	30
Lymphadenopathy	14	15
Hepatosplenomegaly	70	68
Neurologic signs/symptoms	10	Rare
Swollen gingiva	8	—
Skin infiltrates	5	—

[a] Data from Choi and Simone.[259]
[b] Data from Miller.[260]

in association with central nervous system involvement or hyperleukocytosis with resultant hyperviscosity and sludging. Skin, gingival, or retinal infiltration at presentation is essentially unique to the monocytoid variants[125–127] (Plate 66-1). Skin involvement varies from discrete nodules 1–3 cm in diameter, usually with overlying violaceous discoloration, to a diffuse maculopapular rash with interposed discrete nodules (Plate 66-1). Leukemia cutis is most commonly a presenting manifestation of the M5a subtype in infants or neonates. Occasionally isolated skin involvement precedes disease in the bone marrow or other sites by weeks to months. Over one-half of children with AMoL are <2 years of age at diagnosis.[125,126,128]

The frequency of central nervous system involvement at diagnosis has been reported to be 14–52%.[129,130] Hyperleukocytosis,[131,132] age <2 years,[128,131] and/or AMoL[132,133] or AMML[132–134] are associated with a greater likelihood of central nervous system involvement at presentation. Such involvement may manifest as typical meningeal infiltration with leu-

Table 66-4. Presenting Manifestations of Specific Childhood AML Variants

Subtype	Frequently Associated Presenting Manifestations
M2 t(8;21) (AML with differentiation)	Chloroma: epidural, periorbital, perineural (occasional symptoms of nerve compression)
M3 (APL)	Spontaneous bleeding; central nervous system hemorrhage; DIC; secondary fibrinolysis
M4 (AMML)	Hyperleukocytosis and related complications: central nervous system symptoms and bleeding; renal tubular damage; hyperuricemia
	Extramedullary involvement: central nervous system, nodes, skin; DIC
M5 (AMoL)	Young age (<2 yr) and congenital
	Extramedullary disease: skin, gingiva, meninges, nodes, lungs, periosteum, tumor masses (epidural, sinus, mediastinal, rarely testicular)
	Hyperleukocytosis and associated leukostasis; DIC
M7 (AMeL)	Down syndrome
	Low WBC count and few circulating blasts; no organomegaly
	Bone marrow "dry," commonly with myelofibrosis

Abbreviation: DIC, disseminated intravascular coagulation.

kemic cells apparent in cytocentrifuge specimens of cerebrospinal fluid, cranial nerve palsies, or rarely, as a tumor mass.

Laboratory Evaluation

Seven morphologic variants of AML are presently described in the standardized FAB classification of AML[74,135,136] (Table 66-5). With explicit morphologic definition in the original classification of 1976[74] and the modifications in 1985,[135,136] concordance between institutional and review pathologists improved from 50% to 80% between 1983 and 1988.[137] A histologic analysis of 364 children with AML showed that the distribution of FAB subtypes was similar to that reported for adults.[137]

The M7 subtype, AMeL, was added to the original FAB classification in 1985.[135] Megakaryoblasts may be difficult to distinguish morphologically from lymphoblasts and FAB M1 AML. Histochemical staining properties of M7, M5, and L2 leukemias may be similar.[135,138,139] Confirmation of M7 leukemia usually requires ultrastructural evidence of platelet peroxidase positivity in the nuclear envelope and endoplasmic reticulum or the presence of platelet-specific cell-surface markers (factor VIII-related antigen or platelet glycoproteins IIb/IIIa).[11,136] Importantly, AMeL is often associated with abnormalities of chromosome 21,[11,139] Down syndrome,[11,140,141] myelofibrosis, and/or increased bone marrow reticulin.[142]

Antigen expression among the FAB subtypes of AML as detected by monoclonal antibodies is varied and may be helpful in diagnostic confirmation[143,144] (Table 66-5). M4 and M5 leukemia cells tend to express later antigens such as MY8, Mo1, and MY4; these antigens are generally not expressed by the M1–M3 variants. Additionally, there are a small number of patients with minimally differentiated AML, emerging as a clinically distinct subtype that responds poorly to chemotherapy.[145] The cells in this M0 category are myeloid by morphology, ultrastructure, and cell-surface markers and are defined by the presence of myeloperoxidase detectable only at the ultrastructural level.[145]

Leukemias with both lymphoid and nonlymphoid features also constitute a distinct clinical entity. Up to 30% of cells from children with AML may possess lymphoid-associated surface antigens.[146,147] The diagnosis of mixed lineage leukemia is also inferred when molecular studies demonstrate the presence of T-cell receptor or immunoglobulin gene rearrangements in cells from a patient with AML.[148] Mixed lineage leukemias may originate in a pluripotent progenitor, represent two distinct clonal populations of coexisting leukemias (biphenotypic), or in some cases represent aberrant gene expression as a result of the leukemogenic event.[129,146]

Critical analysis of laboratory data enables confirmation of a specific diagnosis and assessment of those parameters that may necessitate prompt institution of supportive measures. When AML is suspected, the diagnostic and ancillary evaluations should proceed simultaneously. In addition to an aspirate, a bone marrow biopsy is necessary to determine cellularity and "absolute leukemic infiltrate." Serial assessment of this parameter determines response to therapy and possibly the timing and composition of further treatment.

Routine histochemistries in addition to the Wright-Giemsa stain include peroxidase, Sudan black, nonspecific esterase, and periodic acid-Schiff. Because identification of the type of acute leukemia in one of five patients may be unclear by morphology and histochemistries,[149] the addition of ultrastructural analysis, immunophenotyping, cytogenetic studies, and molecular analysis can be important adjunctive diagnostic studies.

If the bone marrow evaluation is not diagnostic but accessible extramedullary disease is present (e.g., chloroma, skin or node infiltration), one of these areas should be biopsied. Ideally, this tumor tissue should be processed for all of the afore-

Table 66-5. Classification of AML According to FAB Subtype, Histochemistries, Antigen Expression, and Distribution in Childhood

FAB Class[74,135,136] and Subtype	Histochemistries			Antigen Expression[a]						Distribution[137] (%)
	MP	SB	NSE	Ia (HLA-DR)	MY9 (CD33)	MY7 (CD13)	MY8	Mo1 (CD11)	MY4 (CD14)	
M1: acute undifferentiated myeloid leukemia (AML without differentiation)	+	+ (>3% of blasts)	−	+	+	+	−	−	−	25
M2: acute differentiated myeloid leukemia (AML with differentiation)	+	+	−	+	+	+	−	−	−	27
M3: acute promyelocytic leukemia (APL)	+	+	−	−	+	+	−	−	−	9
M4: acute myelomonocytic leukemia (AMML)	+	+	+	+	+	+	+	+	+	21
M5a: acute monocytic leukemia (AMoL without differentiation)	−	−	+	+	+	−	+	+	+	11.5
M5b: acute differentiated monocytic leukemia (AMoL with differentiation)	−	−	+	+	+	−	+	+	+	
M6: acute erythroleukemia (AEL)	+	+ (Erythroid precursors PAS+)	−	−	+	+	−	−	−	3.5
M7: acute megakaryoblastic leukemia (AMeL)	−	−	+[b] (PAS diffusely +)	(Platelet-specific cell surface mrkers +: glycoproteins Ib, IIb/IIIa or factor VIII-related antigen)						3

Abbreviations: MP, myeloperoxidase; SB, Sudan black; NSE, nonspecific esterase (α-naphthylacetate or butyrate substrate); PAS, periodic acid-Schiff.

[a] Expression positive if antigen present on >50% of cells.

[b] Acetate-positive, butyrate-negative.

mentioned studies and cryopreserved. Histochemical stains of biopsy touch preparations may be of diagnostic importance. Examination of cerebrospinal fluid by the quantitative hemocytometer count and qualitatively using a cytocentrifuge preparation is important at diagnosis and serially during the course of therapy (Plate 66-2).

According to the revised FAB criteria,[136] the diagnosis of AML is confirmed when >30% abnormal blasts are present in the bone marrow. A marrow recovering from the effects of chemotherapy may have ≤15% myeloblasts, making interpretation difficult. Therefore, the Childrens Cancer Group adopted the following guidelines for categorization of bone marrow findings after treatment: M1, ≤5% blasts; M2A, 6–15% blasts; M2B, 16–39% blasts; M3, ≥40% blasts. In order to fulfill broad criteria for remission status with an M1 marrow aspirate, the bone marrow biopsy should show at least 1+ cellularity, and the platelet count should rise to >75,000/mm^3 and absolute neutrophil count to >750/mm^3 within 1 week. If peripheral counts show improvement despite M2a or even M2b marrow status, the bone marrow should be repeated weekly because the increased blasts may be normal regenerating cells.

Ancillary laboratory investigations are relevant to potential clinical complications secondary to the disease process. Early recognition of hypokalemia, hypophosphatemia, hyponatremia, and/or metabolic acidosis related to the toxic effect of lysozyme on the glomerulus and proximal renal tubule, is clinically important. The same rationale pertains to assessment of coagulation status.

Chemistries (uric acid, lytes, calcium, phosphorus, magnesium, BUN, creatinine) and clotting studies may change rapidly after the initiation of therapy, and therefore should be reassessed at least every 12 hours until stable. Imaging studies may localize possible extramedullary disease. An abdominal/pelvic sonogram enables noninvasive gross visualization of kidneys, liver, spleen, periaortic lymph nodes, and ovaries. If bulky extramedullary disease is identified at diagnosis, pertinent sequential imaging studies are warranted until resolution is apparent.

Differential Diagnosis

Misleading presenting clinical signs, symptoms, or hematologic findings, such as those mimicking juvenile rheumatoid arthritis or idiopathic thrombocytopenic purpura, not uncommon in ALL, are rare in children with AML. Clinical findings related to AML usually prompt appropriate diagnostic laboratory investigations.

An exception to the above generalization is leukemia cutis, which may precede by weeks to months other signs or symptoms of disease. This presentation usually occurs in the infant, neonate, or toddler and may initially be attributed to a bruise or insect bite (Plate 66-1A). If such a lesion does not disappear over the expected time course, biopsy of the lesion is the only means of establishing a diagnosis while disease remains localized.

Other diagnoses that occasionally may be difficult to distinguish based on peripheral blood and bone marrow findings are leukemoid reactions and preleukemia. In general, leukemoid reactions that are secondary to bacterial infections, acute hemolysis, granulomatous diseases, vasculitis, and metastatic tumor are associated with bone marrow aspirates that show evidence of myeloid hyperplasia with normal maturation. However, bacterial sepsis may cause a transient maturation arrest of the granulocyte precursors at the promyelocyte stage, which morphologically may be difficult to distinguish from leukemic promyelocytes except by cytogenetic and/or molecular studies. Signs and symptoms of bone marrow failure, and rarely myeloblastic infiltration in the skin, may be present in neonates with this syndrome.[44] A transient uncontrolled myeloproliferative syndrome, clinically indistinguishable from congenital leukemia, can be seen in neonates with classic or mosaic trisomy 21 or, extremely rarely, in phenotypically and chromosomally normal infants.[8,11,38,150,151] This myeloproliferative disorder in infants with either form of trisomy 21 and no other cytogenetic aberration in the marrow cells generally regresses spontaneously within a few weeks to months. Very rarely, AML may ensue[3] (see the section Congenital Leukemia).

In the absence of extramedullary involvement, the distinction between myelodysplasia, especially refractory anemia with excess blasts in transformation (RAEBIT), may be difficult. Similar karyotypic changes are present in children and adults with myelodysplasia.[152] There seems to be increased likelihood of progression to AML in patients with a detectable clonal cytogenetic abnormality.[95,153] The development of additional cytogenetic abnormalities[154] or extramedullary invasion, or both, can be helpful in making the distinction between AML and myelodysplasia. Some investigators contend that AML may be preceded by myelodysplasia more commonly than previously recognized. In one retrospective review of children with AML, six (17%) had clear evidence of preleukemia.[155]

Therapy

Therapy for the child with AML involves three important aspects: (1) acute management of potentially life-threatening metabolic and hematologic derangements, (2) treatment of the leukemia, and (3) ongoing supportive care.

Acute management guidelines are summarized in Table 66-6. When the WBC count at presentation is >150,000–200,000/mm^3, the patient is at risk of developing a "sludging" syndrome or leukostasis. Common symptoms of this problem are visual disturbance, mental status change, respiratory distress, and/or priapism. Complications of stasis in the pulmonary or cerebral vasculature are more likely to occur in children with AML than ALL.[156] Larger size of the myeloblast may contribute to an increased risk of sequestration, aggregation, and vascular damage.[157] Cytoreduction before initiation of primary therapy, using leukapheresis or exchange transfusion depending on the size of the child, may reduce the morbidity and mortality associated with hyperleukocytosis in children with AML.[158]

The M3, M4, and M5 variants commonly have evidence of disseminated intravascular coagulation (DIC) at diagnosis or shortly after therapy is initiated. Several reports suggest that

Table 66-6. Acute Management

Problem	Commonly Associated Subtypes	Intervention
Hyperleukocytosis (WBC count >150,000/mm^3 or symptoms of leukostasis)	M4, M5	Leukapheresis or exchange transfusion
Bleeding	M3, M4, M5	Transfusion of platelets, PRBCs, and FFP or fresh whole blood[a]
Disseminated intravascular coagulation	M3, M4, M5	Heparin[b], FFP, platelets
Thrombocytopenia and/or anemia	M1–M7	Platelet[c] and/or PRBC[d] transfusion when indicated
Fever and neutropenia (absolute neutrophil count <500/mm^3)	M1–M7	Prompt cultures and broad-spectrum intravenous antimicrobials (including early addition of antifungal coverage)
Lysozymuria	M2, M4	Replacement of Na, K, P, Ca, Mg, NaHCO$_3$, as indicated
Hyperuricemia	M4, M5	Hydration, alkalinization to urine pH 7, allopurinol; close monitoring of metabolic status

Abbreviations: PRBCs, packed red blood cells; FFP, fresh frozen plasma.

[a] Use leukocyte depleted and irradiated blood products that are cytomegavirus (CMV) negative until cytomegalovirus serostatus of patient is known; avoid transfusion with blood products from relatives; use single donor platelet product.

[b] Heparin may be used in a dose of 10–15 U/kg/hr continuous intravenous infusion.

[c] Platelet transfusion(s) indicated to maintain platelet count >30,000/mm^3 if one or more of the following present: (1) bleeding at any site, (2) WBC count >75,000/mm^3, (3) fever or infection, and (4) petechiae of face, palate, or conjunctivae.

[d] Transfusion of PRBC contraindicated if WBC count >75,000/mm^3 (to avoid increase in viscosity use leukapheresis or exchange transfusion to increase hemoglobin if necessary).

the use of heparin along with fresh frozen plasma and platelets is beneficial in preventing hemorrhagic episodes.[159-162] However, in the absence of concurrent controlled studies, the use of heparin remains controversial.[163]

Lysozyme is released from some variants of AML (particularly M4 and M5, occasionally M3), sometimes in massive quantities. Lysozyme is toxic to the renal glomerulus and proximal tubule, resulting in proteinuria, mild elevation of creatinine, and urinary loss of sodium, potassium, calcium, magnesium, phosphate, and bicarbonate.[164] Monitoring and replacement of these electrolytes, including phosphate, is therefore indicated. Acute respiratory and cardiac failure and hemolytic anemia have been described with severely depleted phosphate levels.[165,166]

Guidelines for supportive care during periods of very intensive chemotherapy are outlined in the box titled Supportive Care During Periods of Intensive Therapy. As chemotherapy becomes more aggressive, the thoroughness and intensity of supportive care measures must concomitantly increase. Attention to subtle changes in the host is of crucial importance during periods of highly intensive therapy.

Induction chemotherapy may be promptly instituted after stabilization of parameters outlined in Table 66-6. In general, chemotherapy is initiated in full dose in order to begin rapid cell lysis. However, when a high tumor burden is associated with AMoL, some investigators recommend gradual tumor lysis with cytostatic therapy such as hydroxyurea or low-dose ara-C.[167] This approach is suggested to minimize the occurrence of local DIC, a phenomenon that may be exacerbated when cell destruction is too rapid, perhaps contributing to pulmonary or central nervous system hemorrhage.

Most AML induction regimens are designed to achieve bone marrow aplasia or marked hypoplasia, an apparent requirement for successful remission induction for all subtypes except APL. Combination chemotherapy including ara-C, an antimetabolite, and an anthracycline, most commonly daunorubicin, has come to be the mainstay of induction therapy for AML.[168] Using variations of this combination, remission rates of 75–80% are achieved.[128,134,169-171] An induction regimen that also incorporated etoposide and 6-thioguanine (and additional dexamethasone for children with M5 disease), showed promising results in a single institution study.[132]

For patients with APL, the observation was made that remission could be achieved without a period of hypoplasia.[172] In addition, the finding that abnormal promyelocytes sometimes persisted after chemotherapy[173] suggested that some malignant cells may have been induced to undergo terminal differentiation. In 1980, Breitman et al.[174] reported that retinoic acid induced differentiation of the human promyelocytic cell line HL-60. Initial reports of clinical efficacy of 13-(cis)-retinoic acid[175-177] perhaps represented a publication bias.[178] In vitro studies show that all-(trans)-retinoic acid (ATRA) is at least one log more effective than 13-(cis)-retinoic acid in inducing differentiation of fresh human leukemic cells in culture.[179] In 1986, the first patients with APL were treated with ATRA in Shanghai; its efficacy was reported by Huang et al.[180] in 1987. By early 1993, approximately 1,500 patients with APL worldwide had been treated with ATRA. About 95% of patients with cytogenetic or molecular confirmation of APL achieved remission using ATRA within a median of 5–7 weeks.[178] However, the median duration of remission maintained by ATRA is about 3.5 months.[181] There appears to be no advantage to continuing treatment with ATRA in complete remission alone or in combination with chemotherapy and in fact there may be some disadvantage to its continued administration.[182] Currently, both pediatric and adult patients are eligible for a national intergroup phase III randomized study comparing the efficacy and toxicity of conventional chemotherapy versus ATRA for induction of remission in previously untreated APL.

SUPPORTIVE CARE DURING PERIODS OF INTENSIVE THERAPY

Double lumen central venous access device

Administration of daunomycin by continuous infusion (minimization of cardiotoxicity)

Transfusion of blood products:

    All products should be irradiated: 3,000 cGy

    Use *leukocyte-depleted* platelets or packed red blood cells (e.g., Pall filter)

    Avoid blood products from relatives unless family member bone marrow transplant is not an option

    Platelets: guidelines for transfusion as in Table 66-6; use apheresis single-donor products

    Packed red blood cells to maintain hemoglobin ≥12 g%

    WBCs: institute once or twice daily for gram-negative sepsis unresponsive to 48 hours of appropriate intravenous antibiotics

Low microbial diet (avoid fresh fruits/vegetables)

Maintain soft stools

Suppress menses in females

Prophylactic trimethoprim sulfamethoxazole, clotrimazole, or mycostatin, and good dental hygiene

Empirical addition of acyclovir for suspected herpetic gingivitis while awaiting culture results

Consider administration of CSF-G and/or intravenous immunoglobulins

Fever and neutropenia (see Table 66-6)*

    Consider empirical administration of fluconazole with broad-spectrum intravenous antibiotics; administer antimicrobials alternately through each central line lumen

    For persistent fever >3 days despite broad-spectrum antibiotics and negative fungal cultures:

        Workup for occult fungal disease with echocardiogram; computed tomography scan of sinuses; sonogram or computed tomography scan of abdomen to evaluate liver, spleen, kidneys; funduscopic examination of retinae

        Empirical addition of amphotericin

Exposure to varicella or zoster: if antibody titer is negative, administer zoster immunoglobulin intramuscularly within 96 hours of exposure

---

* If fever develops after a course of ara-C, a vancomycin-containing broad-spectrum antibiotic regimen should be immediately instituted after appropriate cultures to treat possible α-strep sepsis (potentially a fulminant infection in such a host).

Because AML in general is relatively resistant to chemotherapy, treatment intensity has gradually increased over the last few decades. Treatment strategies are usually based on certain theoretical concepts regarding cytoreduction. The Goldie-Coldman hypothesis predicts that the simultaneous use of many effective non-cross-resistant drugs prevents emergence of multiply resistant clones.[183,184] The administration of combination therapy in high doses but over an abbreviated period allows for more tolerable toxicity.[185] Another hypothesis suggests that timing of chemotherapy is crucial to the recruitment of resting or G0 cells into an actively dividing cell population that is more sensitive to certain classes of chemotherapeutic agents such as antimetabolites.[186,187]

Postremission treatment appears beneficial, but its optimum intensity and duration remain controversial. Bloomfield[188] clearly defined the three general categories of maintenance, consolidation, and intensification. Maintenance and consolidation regimens incorporate chemotherapy that results in either less or essentially the same myelosuppression as during induction. Intensification is defined as administration of induction agents at significantly higher doses or the use of non-cross-resistant alternate agents in myelosuppressive doses.

The efficacy of maintenance therapy, consolidation, and intensification is under investigation. Maintenance has been a traditional component of most chemotherapy regimens for childhood AML.[132,134,189,190] Multi-institution trials incorporating this traditional approach generally achieved survival plateaus of 30–40%. Table 66-7 summarizes data from reports of several pediatric trials, with variable periods of follow-up. Trials incorporating more intensive postremission therapy[133,171,191] do not yet show significant improvement in outcome. A recent Childrens Cancer Group trial that incorporated intensive induction and two different intervals of high-dose ara-C administration during intensification with or without maintenance chemotherapy showed no benefit from maintenance chemotherapy in patients who received aggressive intensification timing.[191] Actuarial 3-year disease-free survival from the end of consolidation was 62% in the 16 patients allocated to maintenance chemotherapy and 59% in the 27 patients who were allocated to not receive maintenance treatment (P = 0.49). Importantly, there was a 6% mortality rate among patients receiving the aggressive ara-C timing (marrow or stem cell "rescue" was not employed). Patients who received the less aggressive ara-C timing (every 28 as opposed to every 7 days) had an improved survival rate if maintenance therapy was administered (actuarial survival at 3 years was 65% of 17 patients receiving maintenance therapy versus 39% of 24 patients not receiving maintenance therapy).

Other more aggressive intensification regimens are also undergoing investigation, most are marrow ablative and subsequently rescued by allogeneic, syngeneic, or autologous bone marrow transplantation (BMT).[193–198] Whether purging of autologous marrow harvested in remission and stored in liquid nitrogen is necessary for optimum outcome is still controversial.[195–197] Meloni et al.[199] reported on an Italian survey of 93 children with AML from 15 centers who received autologous BMT in first or second remission. Although no definitive conclusions could be drawn from this review because of the heterogeneity of marrow procurement methods and conditioning regimens, this procedure appeared to be particularly effective in second complete remission (CR) (of 31 patients in second CR, 59% projected disease-free survival at 65 months as opposed to 39% projected disease-free survival at 66 months in 62 patients transplanted in first CR).[199] A recent report by Woods et al.[198] showed no difference between aggressively timed induction therapy followed by marrow ablation and BMT rescue with either allogeneic or 4-hydroperoxy-cyclophosphamide-purged autologous grafts for children with newly diagnosed AML or myelodysplasia. The actuarial disease-free survival rates at 3 years from the day of transplant were 55% and 51%, respectively.[198]

The role of BMT in early first remission in the treatment of AML remains to be clearly defined. In the future, pretreatment parameters may identify subgroups of patients for whom either BMT or continued conventional chemotherapy is most likely to be beneficial.[200] Several transplant studies have identified an adverse influence of M4 and M5 FAB subtypes on disease-free survival after early first remission allogeneic BMT.[201–203] By contrast, early primary BMT for children and young adults with myelodysplastic syndromes shows promising efficacy.[204]

The role of growth factors in the therapy of AML also remains to be more clearly elucidated. Mirro et al.[205] showed that in vitro response of blasts from pediatric patients with AML to growth factors such as colony-stimulating factor-granulocyte (CSF-G) or colony-stimulating factor-granulocyte/macrophage

Table 66-7. Outcome Associated with Childhood AML Treatment Regimens

Agents[a] (Duration, mo)		Patients (N) (age range)	CR (%)	EFS at 5 Years	Author (Yr)
(V, P, Ad, AC), AZA, MP, MTX (~16 mo)	(VAPA)	61 (0–18)	45 (74)	33%	Grier[133] (1987)
(D, AC, TG, VP, ±P); I-AC, CRT (26 mo)		23 (0–17 yrs)	22 (95)	39%	Odom[132] (1988)
(D, VP) (AC), V, P, TG, C; I-AC, CRT (26 mo)	(BFM-83)	182 (0–17 yr)	146 (80)	49% (an additional 5% of patients died before initiation of therapy)	Creutzig[257] (1990)
(D, HDAC, VP, AZA) (~9 mo)	(HI-C DAZE)	103 (0–18 yr)	82 (80)	30%	Grier[133] (1987)
(D, TG), (AC), HDAC, VP, AZA, P, V, MTX, MP, I-AC) (15 mo)	(POG8498)	145 (group II) (0–21 yr)	123 (85)	34% (at 3 yr)	Ravindranath[258] (1991)
(D, AC, VP, TG, P) HDAC, ASP, C, AZA; (I-AC) (26 mo or ~8 mo, with or without maintenance)	(CCG-213P)	194 (0–21 yr)	134 (69)	35% (at 3 yr)	Woods[192,198] (1990, 1993)

Abbreviations: EFS, event-free survival; V, vincristine; P, prednisone, (methyl)prednisolone, or dexamethasone; Ad, adriamycin; HDAC, high-dose cytosine arabinoside; ASP, asparaginase; AZA, 5-azacytidine; MP, 6-mercaptopurine; MTX, methotrexate; TG, thioguanine; C, cytoxan; I-AC, intrathecal ara-C; CRT, cranial radiation; D, daunomycin; VP, VP-16.

[a] Agents used in induction and continuation noted by parentheses ( ); agents used only in induction noted by brackets [ ].

(CSF-GM) was variable. There appeared to be no correlation of responsiveness with easily identifiable biologic features such as FAB classification or cytogenetic abnormalities. Using a [³H]thymidine incorporation assay, Mirro and colleagues[205] found that leukemic blasts from approximately 50% of children with AML were responsive to CSF-G, interleukin-3, and to a lesser extent, CSF-GM. Incorporation of growth factors into myeloablative chemotherapy trials for AML appears to have accelerated neutrophil recovery and reduced the incidence of documented infection without preferentially promoting the regrowth of leukemic cells.[205,206] However, additional controlled trials are needed to prove definitively that the relapse rate is not increased in this population of patients. CSF-GM has also been incorporated as an adjunct to chemotherapy in adults with AML to stimulate leukemic blasts into cell cycle, thereby making them more sensitive to cell cycle-specific killing.[207] There does not appear to be significant clinical efficacy using this approach. Moreover, the data of Mirro et al.[205] would suggest that this use of growth factors would be unpredictably successful in <50% of pediatric patients with AML.

For children who relapse after treatment with conventional chemotherapy, ≥25% may be salvaged with subsequent BMT in second remission or early relapse.[199,208,209] However, a study analyzing the outcome of relapse after allogeneic or syngeneic BMT for AML showed that time from BMT to relapse was the most important predictor of response to reinduction therapy.[210] Only 1–2% of patients with AML who relapsed after BMT achieved long-term survival.[210]

Certain subtypes of childhood AML may warrant a modified therapeutic approach based on observations of unique biologic behavior and response to specific chemotherapeutic agents. In several studies, children with the M5 variant, especially <2 years of age, had notably poor remission induction success[167,201] or poor remission duration, related particularly to extramedullary recurrence, commonly in the central nervous system.[133] Efficacy of rubidazone[125,126] and the epipodophyllotoxins[45,212–215] for patients with this subtype has been documented. Moreover, the M4 and M5 subtypes appear more sensitive to induction therapy with etoposide and ara-C, whereas the M1–M3 subtypes show better response to daunorubicin, ara-C, and 6-thioguanine.[191] In support of this clinical observation, in vitro susceptibility of myelomonocytic and monocytic leukemia cells to DNA damage from etoposide was fivefold greater than that demonstrated for cells of myelocytic origin.[191]

Treatment of the central nervous system remains a controversial issue. Several reports document the termination of remission in children with AML by central nervous system re-

lapse.[125,128,131,133,216,217] The incidence of this complication appears related to time at risk, diagnostic WBC count, and AML subtype. Reports for both pediatric and adult AML suggest that meningeal involvement is most frequent and clinically important for M4 and M5 subtypes.[125,128,132,218,219] Updated results of a German trial for childhood AML (BFM-87) are noteworthy in this regard. This trial was designed to prospectively determine whether cranial irradiation could be replaced by late intensification therapy with high-dose ara-C and etoposide in patients with a *low risk* of central nervous system relapse (i.e., no initial central nervous system disease and a WBC count ≤70,000/mm³ at diagnosis).[220] Intrathecal ara-C was administered initially and four times during consolidation to all patients. Analysis of this study after 2.5 years showed no increase in central nervous system relapse in nonirradiated patients compared with irradiated patients. However, subsequent actuarial analysis showed 78% of 29 irradiated patients surviving without relapse at 4 years versus 41% of 71 nonirradiated patients ($P = 0.007$).[220] Additionally, a slightly higher, although not statistically significant incidence, of central nervous system relapse was observed in nonirradiated patients. It is postulated from these results that residual blasts in the central nervous system, possibly at least partially resistant to the chemotherapy previously employed, may reseed the bone marrow and lead to marrow relapse. Whether more intensive and protracted systemic chemotherapy than incorporated in the BFM-87 trial can effectively replace the beneficial effect of cranial irradiation remains to be determined by long-term follow-up of future pediatric AML trials. On the other hand, for patients with AML and central nervous system involvement at diagnosis or at high risk of central nervous system relapse, several studies have shown that cranial irradiation decreases the incidence of central nervous system relapse.[126,132,134,221]

It is apparent that treatment of childhood AML is in a state of evolution. Therapy designed to address the unique aspects of M3, M5, and to a lesser extent M4 disease should be considered in the design of future approaches to the treatment of childhood AML. Relying more heavily on agents with known therapeutic efficacy in these subtypes, and treating known or potential central nervous system involvement in M4 and M5 subtypes appears warranted. Knowledge regarding the significance of varied clinical presentations, blast cell morphology, immunophenotype, karyotype, molecular aberrations, the presence of the multidrug resistance (MDR) gene, early marrow response, and down-regulation of specific proto-oncogenes, is rapidly accumulating. Based on preliminary observations, a theoretical approach to the treatment of newly diagnosed childhood AML is depicted in Figure 66-2. Aggressive suppor-

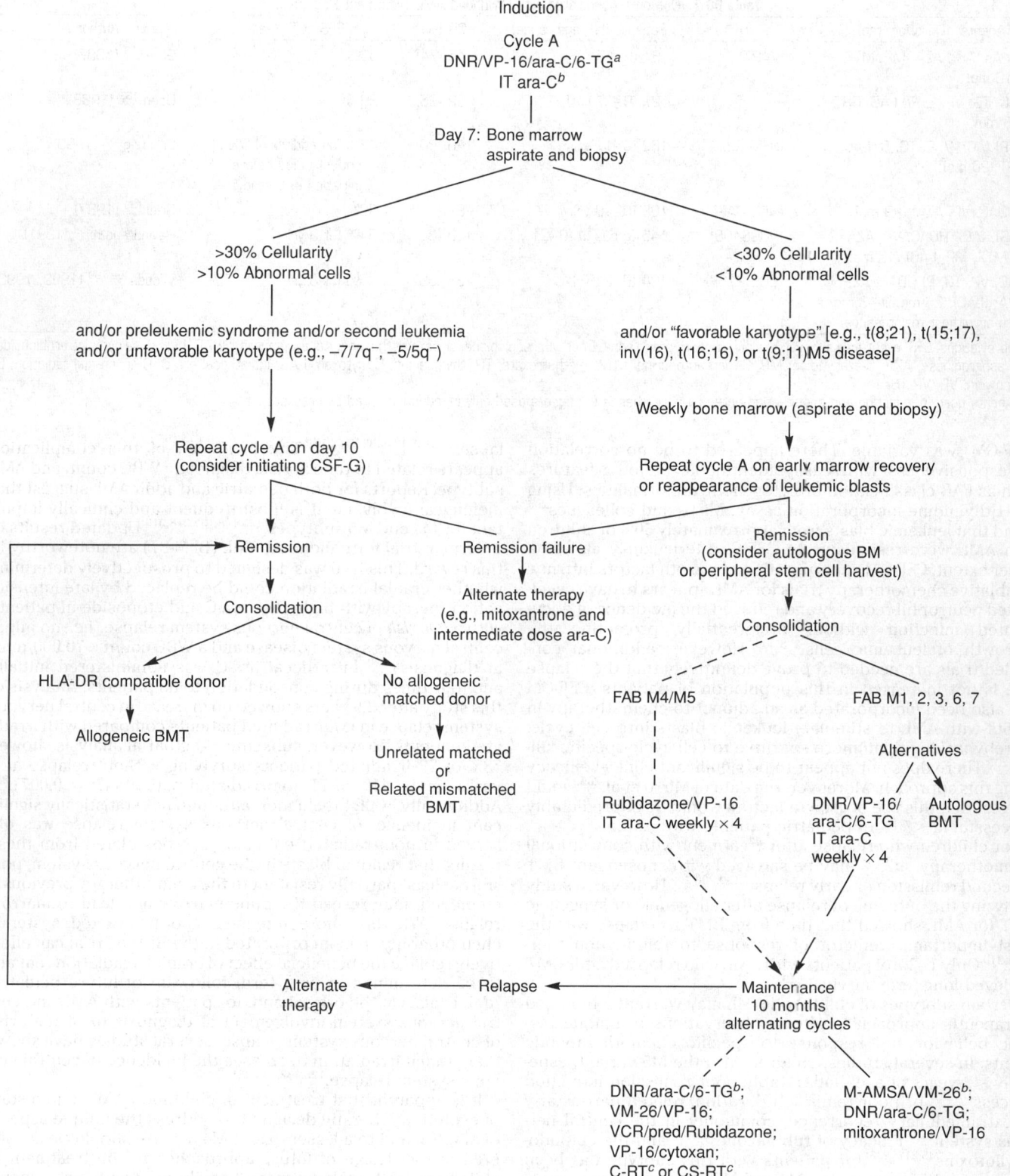

Induction

Cycle A
DNR/VP-16/ara-C/6-TG[a]
IT ara-C[b]

Day 7: Bone marrow
aspirate and biopsy

>30% Cellularity
>10% Abnormal cells

and/or preleukemic syndrome and/or second leukemia
and/or unfavorable karyotype (e.g., −7/7q⁻, −5/5q⁻)

<30% Cellularity
<10% Abnormal cells

and/or "favorable karyotype" [e.g., t(8;21), t(15;17),
inv(16), t(16;16), or t(9;11)M5 disease]

Repeat cycle A on day 10
(consider initiating CSF-G)

Weekly bone marrow (aspirate and biopsy)

Repeat cycle A on early marrow recovery
or reappearance of leukemic blasts

Remission

Remission failure

Remission
(consider autologous BM
or peripheral stem cell harvest)

Consolidation

Alternate therapy
(e.g., mitoxantrone and
intermediate dose ara-C)

Consolidation

HLA-DR compatible donor

Allogeneic BMT

No allogeneic
matched donor

Unrelated matched
or
Related mismatched
BMT

FAB M4/M5

Rubidazone/VP-16
IT ara-C weekly × 4

FAB M1, 2, 3, 6, 7

Alternatives

DNR/VP-16/
ara-C/6-TG
IT ara-C
weekly × 4

Autologous
BMT

Alternate
therapy

Relapse

Maintenance
10 months
alternating cycles

DNR/ara-C/6-TG[b];
VM-26/VP-16;
VCR/pred/Rubidazone;
VP-16/cytoxan;
C-RT[c] or CS-RT[c]

M-AMSA/VM-26[b];
DNR/ara-C/6-TG;
mitoxantrone/VP-16

[a]Patients with FAB M5 AML also receive Decadron × 4 days during each induction cycle; patients with FAB M3 subtype (APL) and identifiable t(15;17) or its molecular rearrangement should be treated with ATRA during induction or an investigational study incorporating that agent, followed by conventional chemotherapy.

[b]IT ara-C at beginning of each cycle of chemotherapy; C- or CS-RT for M4/M5 subtypes only; weekly IT ara-C × 4 during C-RT.

[c]C-RT, cranial radiation; CS-RT, craniospinal radiation and should be administered if >5 WBC/mm³ and leukemic blasts in diagnostic spinal fluid that do not clear after five twice weekly instillations of IT ara-C; if blasts appear or recur later, CS-RT should be administered.

Fig. 66-2. An approach to the therapy for childhood AML.

tive care during periods of intensive treatment is tantamount in importance to the intensity of cytoreductive therapy.

Prognosis

Using current treatment approaches, approximately 75–85% of children with newly diagnosed AML enter remission and 35–45% become long-term survivors. Children with Down syndrome appear to have a more favorable initial and long-term response to conventional AML therapy than children without Down syndrome. In a report from the Pediatric Oncology Group,[51] 100% of children with Down syndrome and AML survived event-free at 4 years compared with 28% ± 6.2% of children without Down syndrome. Of 12 children with Down syndrome in this series, 5 had the FAB M7 subtype, AMeL. This subtype in children with Down syndrome appears to have a particularly favorable response to regimens containing daunorubicin, ara-C, and etoposide.[49]

Diagnostic variables that appear to be associated with a poorer prognosis include the M4 and M5 morphologic subtypes, age <2 years particularly with the M5 subtype, and a WBC count ≥100,000/mm³.[128,133,169,222,223] Factors related to the adverse prognostic significance of the M5 subtype are early hemorrhage,[167] failure of initial response,[171] and/or termination of remission with bone marrow or extramedullary disease, especially in the central nervous system.[125–128] There is also an increased incidence of life-threatening hemorrhagic episodes during "cytoreductive" induction for the M3 subtype, particularly associated with a high diagnostic WBC count and serum lactate dehydrogenase.[161,162] This problem is minimized with vigilant coagulation support or with a differentiation approach to remission induction with ATRA as previously described.[161,162,178] However, the latter approach may be complicated by a clinically significant retinoic acid syndrome in about 25% of the patients. This syndrome is characterized by respiratory distress, pleural effusions and pulmonary infiltrates, elevated WBC count, fever, and weight gain.[224] Patients have died of progressive hypoxemia and multiorgan failure. Although the cause is not understood, the progression of the syndrome can be stopped in most patients by early treatment with a corticosteroid such as dexamethasone.[224] When remission is successfully achieved in patients with APL, remission duration reported for adolescents and adults appears to be superior to that of other AML subtypes.[162]

There have been several attempts to correlate patterns of in vitro colony growth at diagnosis with prognosis in AML.[154,225–227] In one study, cells from 12 of 50 children with acute leukemia grew in suspension culture containing CSFs for ≥12 weeks. Cells from 11 of these 12 patients had nonrandom chromosome abnormalities and 11 of the 12 subsequently died of disease.[228]

Initial clonal cytogenetic abnormalities have important prognostic implications, as noted in Table 66-2. A high CR rate is associated with trisomy 8, t(8;21), t(9;11), and structural abnormalities of chromosome 16.[85,229,230] CR rate for a group of 33 patients with t(8;21) <16 years of age was 90% with a 49% probability of 5-year survival.[231] One or more additional chromosome abnormalities, such as sex chromosome loss, trisomy 8, or 9q, are frequently associated with t(8;21). Prognostic significance of these additional abnormalities is yet to be determined.[231] Loss or deletion of chromosomes 7 and 5 is associated with a poor CR rate.[85] As noted previously, hemorrhagic episodes during cytoreductive induction are common for patients with t(15;17) disease (APL), but subsequent response to chemotherapy is good.[162]

Leukemic cell antigenic phenotype correlates with response to treatment in some studies. The presence of My4 and My7 antigens in adults is associated with a low CR rate and HLA-DR, My8, and MO1 with a decreased remission duration.[232] Adult patients with antigenically mature cells seem more likely to show a response to remission induction treatment and to survive long term.[233] The prognostic implications of these immunophenotype correlations in children require further investigation. A prospective study of 176 pediatric patients with AML treated according to Childrens Cancer Group Protocol 213 showed that the expression of both lymphoid and myeloid-associated cell-surface antigens lacked prognostic significance.[147]

Early leukemic cytoreduction as determined by bone marrow aspirate and biopsy 1 week after initiation of chemotherapy appears to be a promising prognostic indicator.[234,235] In 200 adult patients with AML, patients who ultimately failed induction had a median day 6 reduction in cellularity of 4% and reduction in blast count of 24% compared with 77% and 80% cellularity reductions, respectively, for those who responded to induction treatment.[235] Focal residual leukemia in day 6–10 marrow biopsies from adults with AML who received no further therapy correlated with early relapse; an early marrow free of leukemia correlated with improved remission duration.[234]

Additional parameters that show potential correlation with

AN APPROACH TO THE DIAGNOSIS OF AND THERAPY FOR CENTRAL NERVOUS SYSTEM LEUKEMIA IN CHILDHOOD AML

Definition: >5% leukemic blasts on cytocentrifuge preparation of atraumatic cerebrospinal fluid specimen.

Evaluation: Cerebrospinal fluid hemacytometer count and cytocentrifuge differential count; computed tomography or magnetic resonance imaging scan of head if neurologic examination is abnormal and/or for FAB M4 or M5 subtypes with overt or suspected central nervous system involvement.

Therapy:

1. Intrathecal ara-C twice weekly until blasts clear; intrathecal ara-C with commencement of each subsequent cycle of systemic chemotherapy.
2. For patients with central nervous system chloroma or retinal involvement, add local radiation; add craniospinal radiation (CSRT) if cerebrospinal fluid blasts have not cleared after five twice-weekly instillations of intrathecal ara-C.
3. For children >8 years of age with clearing of cerebrospinal fluid blasts after five doses of intrathecal ara-C: conventional cranial radiation (CRT) and four weekly instillations of intrathecal ara-C during early complete remission.
4. For children >8 years of age requiring more than five doses intrathecal ara-C to clear cerebrospinal fluid blasts: four weekly instillations of intrathecal ara-C in early CR and at beginning of each subsequent cycle of chemotherapy until definitive conventional CSRT is administered in later CR.
5. Total body radiation with BMT in early CR may substitute for CSRT or CRT in numbers 2, 3, or 4 above.
6. Central nervous system involvement that clears after (1) five or (2) more than five doses of intrathecal ara-C in children <8 years of age: intermittent protracted[46] (1) CRT or (2) CSRT, respectively; also consider early intermittent protracted CRT for children with FAB M5 subtype <2 years of age who have cytogenetic aberrations other than t(9;11) with normal cerebrospinal fluid at diagnosis.

response to treatment include cell kinetics,[236,237] down-regulation of proto-oncogene expression,[71,72,238] and expression of the MDR gene, MDR-1.[239,240] An initial myeloblastic labeling index >10% in children with AML appears to correlate with shorter remission duration.[236] In adult patients, an increase of ≥1.5-fold in the diagnostic leukemic cell labeling index by day 8 after a 3-day infusion of ara-C correlated with an improved CR rate when compared with an increase in the labeling index of <1.2-fold.[237] Elaborate kinetic studies demonstrate a marked variability in leukemic cell cycling time from 12 to 300 hours that does not appear to correlate with the FAB classification.[241,242] Patients whose leukemic cells are at the extremes of the cell cycle time show poor response to chemotherapy.[243] Demonstration of early down-regulation of the c-*myc* proto-oncogene appears to correlate with a favorable response to induction chemotherapy.[244]

MDR is related to the production of a 170-kd P-glycoprotein that functions as a transmembrane drug efflux pump and is encoded by the MDR-1 gene.[245] Cells expressing this protein exhibit reduced accumulation of different agents, including anthracyclines, vincristine, amsacrine, mitoxantrone, and etoposide.[246] MDR-1 expression in adult AML has been correlated with both treatment outcome and in vitro sensitivity of leukemic clonogenic cells.[240] Expression of MDR-1 at diagnosis has been shown to correlate with both decreased rate of CR[240] and with shorter remission duration.[247] Further investigations are needed to determine the importance and optimum application of this and the other in vitro prognostic parameters.

Future Directions

An important goal of future research will be to elucidate more clearly the carcinogenic exposures to parents or children (or both) that are associated with an increased risk of developing AML in childhood or adolescence. The ultimate goal will be to minimize or eliminate such exposures.

Increased sophistication in understanding the biologic heterogeneity of AML will undoubtedly lead to stratified treatment approaches. Improved outcome should result from decreasing unnecessary toxicity and increasing intensity of treatment as appropriate for specific biologic subtypes. These biologic variants should relate to behavior of the disease and response to treatment even more specifically than the FAB subclassification. In addition to present clinical parameters, more sophisticated cytogenetic and molecular studies, determination of proto-oncogene expression and early down-regulation, greater understanding of variations in cell cycle time, analysis of MDR gene expression, and determination of early histologic response to chemotherapy will contribute to a more precise definition of biologic subtypes and more specific and refined chemotherapy approaches.

Attention to extramedullary disease in children with M5, M4, or t(8;21) M2 subtypes will become increasingly important as control of bone marrow disease improves. With more specific delineation of biologic variants of childhood AML, patients within these FAB categories for whom extramedullary disease is likely to be a problem can be more readily identified. Alternative approaches to the treatment of young children and infants with central nervous system involvement will include more intensive use of intrathecal and high-dose systemic chemotherapy[248] in addition to new systemic agents with improved penetration of that sanctuary site and perhaps innovative dose-rate delivery of radiation.

The role of allogeneic or autologous BMT will be more clearly defined for specific subgroups of children with AML. For some patients, conventional chemotherapy with or even without intensification may be optimum, whereas for others early definitive BMT will be the therapeutic approach of choice. Autolo-

gous peripheral blood stem cell reconstitution potentially allows for faster hematopoietic recovery and lower infectious and hemorrhagic morbidity than autologous marrow reconstitution.[249] This approach will be explored in children and adolescents.

The chemotherapeutic armamentarium will increase with the development of new active agents or less toxic congeners of known agents as well as increasingly effective usage of agents in combination. Administration of a fludarabine infusion before ara-C to augment the rate of active metabolite (ara-CTP) synthesis in AML blasts is an example of the latter approach.[250] Additionally, administration of agents such as cyclosporine to overcome myeloblast resistance to certain chemotherapeutic agents, such as that related to the P-glycoprotein product of the MDR gene, is another possible approach.[251]

It is unlikely that carefully timed incorporation of one or more hematopoietic growth factors in early treatment will effectively enhance chemotherapy-induced cytoreduction of leukemic cells by recruitment and synchronization.[205,207] Cautious administration of certain growth factors such as CSF-G after heavily myelosuppressive chemotherapy does appear to safely and effectively hasten normal hematopoietic recovery, although additional studies to verify this outcome are warranted.[205,206] The use of interleukin-2 after autologous BMT to potentially simulate a graft-versus-leukemia-like effect is currently undergoing investigation in children.[199,252]

An area of exciting potential, based on the prototype of the efficacy of ATRA in APL, is the use of differentiating agents. In addition to retinoids, there are other compounds that have cytodifferentiating actions in model systems such as vitamin D_3, glucocorticoids, and sex steroids.[253,254] These agents in combination with each other, with biologic response modifiers such as the interferons, and/or with chemotherapy, represent promising advances in the future therapeutic armamentarium for AML.

Increasingly sophisticated methods for assessing minimal residual disease are on the horizon and may eventually prove useful in determining the need for early BMT. The detection of PML/RAR-(2) fusion transcripts, which show close correlation with clinical responsiveness to ATRA, is a prototype for this assessment.[255,256]

Progressive approaches to supportive care, such as earlier empirical administration of less toxic antifungal treatments, improved oral/gastrointestinal prophylaxis, new antiviral agents, and more selective treatment of graft-versus-host disease are on the horizon. In addition to improved supportive care measures, therapy tailored to a more specific biologic and functional classification to maximize the cytoreductive potential of the most effective agents should make possible steady improvement in the proportion of children with AML who become long-term survivors.

REFERENCES

1. Rosner F, Lee SL: Down's syndrome and acute leukemia: myeloblastic or lymphoblastic. Report of forty-three cases and review of the literature. Am J Med 53:203, 1972
2. Fong C, Brodeur GM: Down's syndrome and leukemia: epidemiology, genetics, cytogenetics, and mechanisms of leukemogenesis. Cancer Genet Cytogenet 28:55, 1987
3. Morgan R, Hecht F, Cleary ML et al: Leukemia with Down's syndrome: translocation between chromosomes 1 and 19 in acute myelomonocytic leukemia following transient congenital myeloproliferative syndrome. Blood 66:1466, 1985
4. Van Den Berghe H, Fryns J: Congenital leukemia with 46,xx,t(Bq Cq) cells. J Med Genet 9:468, 1978
5. MacDougall L, Brown J: C-monosomy myeloproliferative syndrome: a case of 7-monosomy. J Pediatr 88:596, 1976
6. Djernes BW, Soukup SW, Bove KE, Wong KY: Congenital leukemia associated with mosaic trisomy 9. J Pediatr 88:596, 1976

7. Gale GB, Toledano SR: Congenital acute lymphocytic leukemia in a newborn with Klinefelter syndrome. Pediatr Hematol Oncol 6:338, 1984

8. Pierce MI: Leukemia in the newborn infant. J Pediatr 54:691, 1959

9. Spier CM, Kjeldsberg CR, O'Brien R, Marty J: Pre-B cell acute lymphoblastic leukemia in the newborn. Blood 64:1064, 1984

10. Abe R, Ryan D, Cecalupo A: Cytogenetic findings in congenital leukemia: case report and review of the literature. Cancer Genet Cytogenet 9:139, 1983

11. Hayashi Y, Eguchi M, Sugita K et al: Cytogenetic findings and clinical features in acute leukemia and transient myeloproliferative disorders in Down's syndrome. Blood 72:15, 1988

12. Ghosh K: Transient abnormal myelopoiesis in Down's syndrome—are some of them truly leukaemic? Leukemia Res 16:545, 1992

13. Ridgway D, Benda G, Magenis E et al: Transient myeloproliferative disorder of the Down type in the normal newborn. Am J Dis Child 144:1117, 1990

14. Rechavi G, Brok-Simoni F, Katzir N et al: More than two immunoglobulin heavy chain J region genes in the majority of infant leukemia. Leukemia 2:347, 1988

15. Djabali M, Selleri L, Parry P et al: A trithorax-like gene is interrupted by chromosome 11q23 translocations in acute leukaemias. Nat Genet 2:113, 1992

16. Gu Y, Nakamura T, Alder H et al: The t(4;11) chromosome translocation of human acute leukemias fuses the ALL-1 gene, related to Drosophila trithorax, to the AF-4 gene. Cell 71:701, 1992

17. Tkachuk DC, Kohler S, Cleary ML: Involvement of a homolog of Drosophila trithorax by 11q23 chromosomal translocations in acute leukemias. Cell 71:691, 1992

18. Thirman MJ, Gill HJ, Burnett RC et al: Rearrangement of the MLL gene in acute lymphoblastic and acute myeloid leukemias with 11q23 chromosomal translocations. N Engl J Med 329:909, 1993

19. Cleary ML: A promiscuous oncogene in acute leukemia (editorial). N Engl J Med 329:958, 1993

20. Ford AM, Ridge SA, Cabrera MD et al: In utero rearrangements in the trithorax-related oncogene in infant leukaemias. Nature 363:358, 1993

21. Koike T, Aoki S, Maruyama S et al: Cell surface phenotyping of megakaryoblasts. Blood 69:957, 1987

22. Coulombel L, Derycke M, Villeval JL et al: Characterization of the blast cell population in two neonates with Down's syndrome and transient myeloproliferative disorder. Br J Haematol 66:69, 1987

23. Hayashi T, Hanada R, Yamamoto K et al: Transient megakaryoblastic proliferation in a newborn infant with Down's syndrome. Cancer Genet Cytogenet 28:373, 1987

24. Zipursky A, Peeters M, Poon A: Megakaryoblastic leukemia and Down's syndrome: a review. Prog Clin Biol Res 246:33, 1987

25. Lin HP, Menaka H, Lim KH, Yong HS: Congenital leukemoid reaction followed by fatal leukemia. Am J Dis Child 134:939, 1980

26. Lampkin BC, Bove KE, Peipon JJ et al: Spontaneous remission of presumed congenital acute nonlymphoblastic leukemia (ANLL) in a karyotypically normal neonate. Am J Pediatr Hematol Oncol 7:346, 1985

27. Reimann DL, Clemmons RL, Pillsbury WA: Congenital acute leukemia: skin nodules, a first sign. J Pediatr 46:415, 1958

28. Seo IS, McGuire WA, Heerema NA et al: Congenital monoblastic leukemia cutis. A case report with chromosomal abnormality: del (10p). Am J Pediatr Hematol Oncol 8:158, 1986

29. Francis J, Sybert V, Benjamin D: Congenital monocytic leukemia. Pediatr Dermatol 6:306, 1989

30. Jani Sait SN, Brecher ML, Green DM, Sandberg AA: Translocation t(1;22) in congenital acute megakaryocytic leukemia. Cancer Genet Cytogenet 34:277, 1988

31. Lasson U, Goos M: Congenital erythroleukemia—a case report. Blut 43:237, 1981

32. Suda T, Suda J, Miura Y et al: Clonal analysis of basophil differentiation in bone marrow cultures from a Down's syndrome patient with megakaryoblastic leukemia. Blood 66:1278, 1985

33. Eguchi M, Sakakibara H, Suda J et al: Ultrastructural and ultracytochemical differences between transient myeloproliferative disorder and megakaryoblastic leukemia in Down's syndrome. Br J Hematol 73:315, 1989

34. Heim S, Bekassy A, Garwicz S et al: New structural chromosomal rearrangements in congenital leukemia. Leukemia 1:16, 1987

35. Kaneko Y, Shikano T, Maseki N et al: Clinical characteristics of infant acute leukemia with or without 11q23 translocations. Leukemia 2:672, 1988

36. Carney L, Kinney J, Higgins R et al: X;6 translocation in a child with congenital acute lymphocytic leukemia. Cancer 69:799, 1992

37. Kitchingman GR, Mirro J, Stass S et al: Biologic and prognostic significance of the presence of more than two heavy chain genes in childhood acute lymphoblastic leukemia of B precursor cell origin. Blood 67:698, 1986

38. Okada H, Liu PI, Hoshino T et al: Down's syndrome associated with a myeloproliferative disorder. Am J Dis Child 124:107, 1972

39. Levitt GA, Stiller CA, Chessells JM: Prognosis of Down's syndrome with acute leukemia. Arch Dis Child 65:212, 1990

40. Peeters M, Poon A: Down syndrome and leukemia; unusual clinical aspects and unexpected methotrexate sensitivity. Eur J Pediatr 146:416, 1987

41. Van Eys J, Flexner JM: Transient spontaneous remission in a case of untreated congenital leukemia. Am J Dis Child 118:507, 1969

42. Lilleyman JS: Congenital monocytic leukemia. Clin Lab Hematol 2:243, 1980

43. Chu J-Y, O'Connor DM, Gale GB, Silberstein MJ: Congenital leukemia: two transient regressions without treatment in one patient. Pediatrics 71:277, 1983

44. Weinstein HJ: Congenital leukemia and the neonatal myeloproliferative disorders associated with Down's syndrome. Clin Hematol 7:147, 1978

45. Odom LF, Gordon EM: Acute monoblastic leukemia in infancy and early childhood: successful treatment with an epipodophyllotoxin. Blood 64:875, 1984

46. Kim TH, Ramsay NK, Steeves RA, Nesbit ME: Intermittent central nervous system irradiation and intrathecal chemotherapy for central nervous system leukemia in children. Int J Radiat Oncol Biol Phys 13:1451, 1987

47. Freedman MH, Finklestein JZ, Hammond GD, Karon M: The effect of chemotherapy on acute myelogenous leukemia in children. J Pediatr 78:526, 1971

48. Young JL, Miller RW: Incidence of malignant tumors in U.S. children. J Pediatr 96:254, 1975

49. Kojima S, Kato K, Matsuyama T et al: Favorable treatment outcome in children with acute myeloid leukemia and Down syndrome. Blood 81:3164, 1993

50. Kojima S, Matsuyama T, Sato T et al: Down's syndrome and acute leukemia in children. An analysis of phenotype by use of monoclonal antibodies and electron microscopic platelet peroxidase reaction. Blood 76:2348, 1990

51. Ravindranath Y, Abella E, Krischer JP et al: Acute myeloid leukemia (AML) in Down's syndrome is highly responsive to chemotherapy: experience on pediatric oncology group AML study 8498. Blood 80:2210, 1992

52. Pierre RV: Preleukemic states. Semin Hematol 11:73, 1974

53. Roberts WM, Jenkins JJ, Moorhead EL, Douglass EC: Incontinentia pigmenti, a chromosomal instability syndrome, is associated with childhood malignancy. Cancer 62:2370, 1988

54. Wasser JS, Yolken RH, Miller DR et al: Congenital hypoplastic anemia (Diamond-Blackfan syndrome) terminating in acute myelogenous leukemia. Blood 51:991, 1978

55. Woods WG, Roloff JS, Lukens JN et al: The occurrence of leukemia in patients with the Schwachman syndrome. J Pediatr 99:425, 1981

56. Reich SD, Wiernik PH: Von Recklinghausen neurofibromatosis and acute leukemia. Am J Dis Child 130:888, 1976

57. Blatt J, Jaffe R, Deutsch M, Adkins JC: Neurofibromatosis and childhood tumors. Cancer 57:1225, 1986

58. Li FP, Fraumeni JF: Soft-tissue sarcomas, breast cancer, and other neoplasms: a familial syndrome? Ann Intern Med 71:747, 1969

59. Lynch HT, Krush AJ, Harlan WL, Sharp EA: Association of soft tissue sarcoma, leukemia, and brain tumors in families affected with breast cancer. Am Surg 39:199, 1973

60. Bottomly RH, Trainer AL, Condit PT: Chromosome studies in a "cancer family." Cancer 28:519, 1971

61. Meadows AT, D'Angio GJ, Mike' et al: Patterns of second malignant neoplasms in children. Cancer 40:1903, 1977

62. Farwell J, Flannery JT: Cancer in relatives of children with central-nervous-system neoplasms. N Engl J Med 311:749, 1984

63. Fialkow PJ, Singer JW, Adamson JW et al: Acute nonlymphocytic leukemia: heterogeneity of stem cell origin. Blood 57:1068, 1981

64. Fearon ER, Burke PJ, Schiffer CA et al: Differentiation of leukemia cells to polymorphonuclear leukocytes in patients with acute nonlymphocytic leukemia. N Engl J Med 315:15, 1986

65. Fialkow PJ, Singer JW, Adamson JW et al: Acute nonlymphoblastic leukemia. Expression in cells restricted to granulocytic and monocytic differentiation. N Engl J Med 301:1, 1979

66. Grier HE, Weinstein HJ, Revesz T et al: Cytogenetic evidence for involvement of erythroid progenitors in a child with therapy linked myelodysplasia. Br J Haematol 64:513, 1986

67. Keinanen M, Griffin JD, Bloomfield CD et al: Clonal chromosomal abnormalities showing multiple-cell-lineage involvement in acute myeloid leukemia. N Engl J Med 318:1153, 1988

68. Jacobson RJ, Temple MJ, Singer JW et al: A clonal complete remission in a patient with acute nonlymphocytic leukemia originating in a multipotent stem cell. N Engl J Med 310:1513, 1984

69. Smith FO, Raskind WH, Waldron P et al: Clonal remission in childhood acute myeloid leukemia is an infrequent event. Leukemia 7:929, 1993

70. Rothberg PG, Erisman MD, Diehl RE et al: Structure and expression of the

oncogene c-myc in fresh tumor material from patients with hematopoietic malignancies. Mol Cell Biol 4:1096, 1984

71. Evinger-Hodges MJ, Dicke KA, Gutterman JU, Blick M: Proto-oncogene expression in human normal bone marrow. Leukemia 1:597, 1987

72. Evinger-Hodges MJ, Blick M, Bresser J, Dicke KA: Comparison of oncogene expression in human normal bone marrow and leukemia. Ann NY Acad Sci 511:284, 1987

73. Evinger-Hodges MJ, Bresser J, Brouwer R et al: Myc and sis expression in acute myelogenous leukemia. Leukemia 2:45, 1988

74. Bennett JM, Catovsky D, Daniel MT et al: Proposals for the classification of the acute leukaemias. French-American-British (FAB) cooperative group. Br J Haematol 33:451, 1976

75. Mattei MG, Petkovich M, Mattei JF et al: Mapping of the human retinoic acid receptor to the q21 band of chromosome 17. Hum Genet 80:186, 1988

76. Longo L, Pandolfi PO, Biondi A: Rearrangements and aberrant expression of the retinoic acid receptor α gene in acute promyelocytic leukemias. J Exp Med 172:1571, 1990

77. Lemmons R, Eilender D, Waldmann R: Cloning and characterization of the t(15;17) translocation breakpoint region in acute promyelocytic leukemia. Genes Chromosom Cancer 2:79, 1990

78. Kakizuka A, Miller WH Jr, Umesono K: Chromosomal translocation t(15;17) in human acute promyelocytic leukemia fuses RAR α with a novel putative transcription factor, PML. Cell 66:663, 1991

79. Rowley JD: Chromosome changes in acute leukemia. Br J Haematol 44:339, 1980

80. Yunis JJ: Recurrent chromosomal defects are found in most patients with acute nonlymphocytic leukemia. Cancer Genet Cytogenet 11:125, 1984

81. Kaneko Y, Rowley JD, Maurer HS et al: Chromosome pattern in childhood acute nonlymphocytic leukemia. (ANLL). Blood 60:389, 1982

82. Bitter MA, LeBeau MM, Rowley JD et al: Associations between morphology, karyotype, and clinical features in myeloid leukemias. Hum Pathol 18:211, 1987

83. Second MIC Cooperative Study Group (1988): Morphologic, immunologic, and cytogenetic (MIC) working classification of acute myeloid leukemias. Cancer Genet Cytogenet 30:1, 1988

84. Larson RA, Le Beau MM, Vardiman JW et al: The predictive value of initial cytogenetic studies in 148 adults with acute nonlymphocytic leukemia: a 12-year study (1970–1982). Cancer Genet Cytogenet 10:219, 1983

85. Fourth International Workshop on Chromosomes in Leukemia: A prospective study of acute nonlymphocytic leukemia. Cancer Genet Cytogenet 11:249, 1984

86. Yunis JJ, Brunning RD, Howe RB, Lobell M: High-resolution chromosomes as an independent prognostic indicator in adult acute nonlymphocytic leukemia. N Engl J Med 311:812, 1984

87. Le Beau MM, Larson RA, Bitter MA et al: Association of an inversion of chromosome 16 with abnormal marrow eosinophils in acute myelomonocytic leukemia: a unique cytogenetic-clinicopathological association. N Engl J Med 309:630, 1983

88. Brodeur GM, Williams DL, Kalwinsky DK et al: Cytogenetic features of acute nonlymphoblastic leukemia in 73 children and adolescents. Cancer Genet Cytogenet 8:93, 1983

89. Larson RA, Kondo K, Vardiman JW et al: Evidence for a 15;17 translocation in every patient with acute promyelocytic leukemia. Am J Med 76:827, 1984

90. Pui C-H, Behm F, Raimondi S. Secondary acute myeloid leukemia in children treated for acute lymphoid leukemia. N Engl J Med 321:136, 1989

91. Pui C, Hancock M, Raimondi S: Myeloid neoplasia in children treated for solid tumors. Lancet 336:417, 1990

92. Rubin CM, Arthur DC, Woods WG et al: Therapy-related myelodysplastic syndrome and acute myeloid leukemia in children: correlation between chromosomal abnormalities and prior therapy. Blood 78:2982, 1991

93. Winick NJ, McKenna RW, Shuster JJ et al: Secondary acute myeloid leukemia in children with acute lymphoblastic leukemia treated with etoposide. J Clin Oncol 11:209, 1993

94. Robison LL, Buckley JD, Daigle A et al: Maternal drug use and risk of childhood non-lymphoblastic leukemia among offspring. Cancer 63:1904, 1989

95. Nowell PC: Cytogenetics of preleukemia. Cancer Genet Cytogenet 5:265, 1982

96. Preisler HD, Lyman GH: Acute myelogenous leukemia subsequent to therapy for a different neoplasm: clinical features and response to therapy. Am J Hematol 3:209, 1977

97. Rinsky RA, Smith AB, Hornung R et al: Benzene and leukemia: an epidemiologic risk assessment. N Engl J Med 316:1044, 1987

98. Moore MA, Williams N, Metcalf D et al: In vitro colony formation by normal and leukemic human hematopoietic cells: characterization of the colony forming cells. J Natl Cancer Inst 50:603, 1973

99. Rowley JD, Golomb HM, Vardiman JW: Nonrandom chromosome abnormalities in acute leukemia and dysmyelopoietic syndromes in patients with previously treated malignant disease. Blood 58:759, 1981

100. Le Beau MM, Albain KS, Larson RA et al: Clinical and cytogenetic correlations in 63 patients with therapy-related myelodysplastic syndromes and acute nonlymphocytic leukemia: further evidence for characteristic abnormalities of chromosomes no. 5 and 7. J Clin Oncol 4:325, 1986

101. Pui C-H, Ribeiro R, Hancock M: Acute myeloid leukemia in children treated with epipodophyllotoxins for acute lymphoblastic leukemia. N Engl J Med 325:1682, 1991

102. Buckley JD, Robison LL, Swotinsky R et al: Occupational exposures of parents of children with acute nonlymphocytic leukemia. Cancer Res 49:4030, 1989

103. Lowengart RA, Peters JM, Cicioni C et al: Childhood leukemia and parent's occupational and home exposures. J Natl Cancer Inst 79:39, 1987

104. Shu XO, Gao YT, Brinton LA et al: A population-based case-control study of childhood leukemia in Shanghai. Cancer 62:635, 1988

105. Reeves JD, Driggers DA, Kiley VA: Household insecticide associated aplastic anemia and leukaemia in children. Lancet 2:300, 1981

106. Meadows AT, Baum E, Fossati-Bellani F et al: Second malignant neoplasms in children: an update from the Late Effects Study Group. J Clin Oncol 3:532, 1985

107. de Gramont A, Louvet C, Krulik M et al: Preleukemic changes in cases of nonlymphocytic leukemia secondary to cytotoxic therapy. Cancer 58:630, 1986

108. Tucker MA, Meadows AT, Boice JD et al: Leukemia after therapy with alkylating agents for childhood cancer. J Natl Cancer Inst 78:459, 1987

109. Archer VE. Occupational exposure to radiation as a cancer hazard. Cancer 39:1802, 1977

110. Matanoski GM, Seltser R, Sartwell PE et al: The current mortality rates of radiologists and other physician specialists: deaths from all causes and from cancer. Am J Epidemiol 101:188, 1975

111. Sandoval C, Head DR, Mirro J Jr et al: Translocation t(9;11)(p21q23) in pediatric de novo and secondary acute myeloblastic leukemia. Leukemia 6:513, 1992

112. Sugita K, Furukawa T, Tsuchida M et al: High frequency of etoposide (VP-16)-related secondary leukemia in children with non-Hodgkin's lymphoma. Am J Pediatr Hematol Oncol 15:99, 1993

113. Murphy S: Secondary acute myeloid leukemia following treatment with epipodophyllotoxins. J Clin Oncol 11:199, 1993

114. Pedersen-Bjergaard J, Daugaard G, Hansen SW: Increased risk of myelodysplasia and leukemia after etoposide, cisplatin, and bleomycin for germ-cell tumours. Lancet 338:359, 1991

115. Markman M, Pavy MD, Abeloff MD: Acute leukemia following intensive therapy for small-cell carcinoma of the lung. Cancer 50:672, 1982

116. Ratain MJ, Kaminer LS, Bitran JD: Acute nonlymphocytic leukemia following etoposide and cisplatin combination chemotherapy for advanced non-small-cell carcinoma of the lung. Blood 70:1412, 1987

117. Amylon MD, Carroll AJ, Link MP: Second malignancies in children treated with teniposide (VM-26) for T-cell lymphoid malignancy: a role for asparaginase? [a Pediatric Oncology Group (POG) study]. Blood, suppl. 1. 80:206a, 1992

118. Peterson L, Dehner LP, Brunning RD: Extramedullary masses as presenting features of acute monoblastic leukemia. Am J Clin Pathol 75:140, 1981

119. Broxmeyer HE, Grossbard E, Jacobsen N et al: Persistence of inhibitory activity against normal bone-marrow cells during remission of acute leukemia. N Engl J Med 301:346, 1979

120. Broxmeyer HE, Bognacki J, Dorner MH et al: The identification of leukemia-associated inhibitory activity as acidic isoferritins: a regulatory role for acidic isoferritins in the production of granulocytes and macrophages. J Exp Med 153:1426, 1981

121. Lampkin BC, Lange B, Bernstein I et al: Biologic characteristics and treatment of acute nonlymphocytic leukemia in children. Pediatr Clin North Am 4:743, 1988

122. Swart K, Lowenberg B: Feeder cell requirements for leukemia cell colony formation in cultures supplemented with phytohemagglutinin. Cancer Res 44:657, 1984

123. Lange B, Ferrero D, Pessano S et al: Surface phenotype of clonogenic cells in acute myeloid leukemia defined by monoclonal antibodies. Blood 64:693, 1984

124. Sabbath KD, Ball ED, Larcom P et al: Heterogeneity of clonogenic cells in acute myeloblastic leukemia. J Clin Invest 75:746, 1985

125. Tobelem G, Jacquillat C, Chastang C et al: Acute monoblastic leukemia: a clinical and biologic study of 74 cases. Blood 55:71, 1980

126. Janvier M, Tobelem G, Daniel MT et al: Acute monoblastic leukemia. Clinical, biological data and survival in 45 cases. Scand J Haematol 32:385, 1984

127. Darbyshire PJ, Smith JH, Oakhill A, Mott MG: Monocytic leukemia in infancy. A review of eight children. Cancer 56:1584, 1985

128. Weinstein HJ, Mayer RJ, Rosenthal DS et al: Chemotherapy for acute myelogenous leukemia in children and adults: VAPA update. Blood 62:315, 1983

129. Smith LJ, Curtis JE, Messner HA et al: Lineage infidelity in acute leukemia. Blood 61:1138, 1983

130. Walters TR: Special neurological complications due to acute non-lymphocytic leukemia. p. 41. In Pochedly C (ed): Leukemia and Lymphoma in the Nervous System. Charles C Thomas, Springfield, 1976

131. Pui C-H, Dahl GV, Kalwinsky KD et al: Central nervous system leukemia in children with acute nonlymphoblastic leukemia. Blood 66:1062, 1985

132. Odom LF, Morse H, Tubergen DG, Blake M: Long-term survival of children with acute non-lymphoblastic leukemia. Med Pediatr Oncol 16:248, 1988

133. Grier HE, Gelber RD, Camitta BM et al: Prognostic factors in childhood acute myelogenous leukemia. J Clin Oncol 5:1026, 1987

134. Creutzig U, Ritter J, Riehm H et al: Improved treatment results in childhood acute myelogenous leukemia: a report of the German cooperative study AML-BFM-78. Blood 65:298, 1985

135. Bennett JM, Catovsky D, Daniel MT et al: Criteria for the diagnosis of acute leukemia of megakaryocyte lineage (M7). A report of the French-American-British Cooperative Group. Ann Intern Med 103:460, 1985

136. Bennett JM, Catovsky D, Daniel MT et al: Proposed revised criteria for the classification of acute myeloid leukemia. Ann Intern Med 103:626, 1985

137. Argyle JC, Benjamin DR, Lampkin BC, Hammond D: Acute nonlymphocytic leukemias of childhood: inter-observer variability and problems in the use of the FAB classification. Cancer 63:295, 1989

138. Koike T: Megakaryoblastic leukemia: the characterization and identification of megakaryoblasts. Blood 64:683, 1984

139. Sariban E, Oliver C, Corash L et al: Acute megakaryoblastic leukemia in childhood. Cancer 54:1423, 1984

140. Cairney AE, McKenna R, Arthur DC et al: Acute megakaryoblastic leukemia in children. Br J Haematol 63:541, 1986

141. Lewis DS, Thompson M, Hudson E et al: Down's syndrome and acute megakaryoblastic leukemia. Case report and review of the literature. Acta Haematol 70:236, 1983

142. Chan WC, Byrnes RK, Kim TH et al: Acute megakaryoblastic leukemia in early childhood. Blood 62:92, 1983

143. Griffin JD, Ritz J, Nadler LM et al: Expression of myeloid differentiation antigens on normal and malignant myeloid cells. J Clin Invest 68:932, 1981

144. Ball ED, Fanger MW: The expression of myeloid-specific antigens on myeloid leukemia cells: correlations with leukemia subclasses and implications for normal myeloid differentiation. Blood 61:456, 1983

145. Lee EJ, Pollak A, Leavitt RD et al: Minimally differentiated acute nonlymphocytic leukemia: a distinct entity. Blood 70:1400, 1987

146. Mirro J, Zipf TF, Pui CH et al: Acute mixed lineage leukemia: clinicopathologic correlations and prognostic significance. Blood 66:1115, 1985

147. Smith FO, Lampkin BC, Versteeg C et al: Expression of lymphoid-associated cell surface antigens by childhood acute myeloid leukemia cells lacks prognostic significance. Blood 79:2415, 1992

148. Rovigatti U, Mirro J, Kitchingman G et al: Heavy chain immunoglobulin gene rearrangement in acute nonlymphocytic leukemia. Blood 63:1023, 1984

149. Chan LC, Pegram SM, Greaves MF: Contribution of immunophenotype to the classification and differential diagnosis of acute leukaemia. Lancet 1:475, 1985

150. Brodeur GM, Dahl GV, Williams DL et al: Transient leukemoid reaction and trisomy 21 mosaicism in a phenotypically normal newborn. Blood 55:691, 1980

151. Seibel NL, Sommer A, Miser J: Transient neonatal leukemoid reactions in mosaic trisomy 21. J Pediatr 104:251, 1984

152. Nowell P, Wilmoth D, Lange B: Cytogenetics of childhood preleukemia. Cancer Genet Cytogenet 10:261, 1983

153. Anderson RL, Bagby GC Jr: The prognostic value of chromosome studies in patients with the preleukemic syndrome (hemopoietic dysplasia). Leukemia Res 6:175, 1982

154. Moore MA, Spitzer G, Williams N et al: Agar culture studies in 127 cases of untreated acute leukemia: the prognostic value of reclassification of leukemia according to in vitro growth characteristics. Blood 44:1, 1974

155. Blank J, Lange B: Preleukemia in children. J Pediatr 98:565, 1981

156. Bunin NJ, Pui C-H: Differing complications of hyperleukocytosis in children with acute lymphoblastic or acute nonlymphoblastic leukemia. J Clin Oncol 3:1590, 1985

157. Litchman MA, Rowe JM: Hyperleukocytic leukemias: rheological, clinical and therapeutic considerations. Blood 60:279, 1982

158. Bunin NJ, Kunkel K, Callihan TR: Cytoreductive procedures in the early management in cases of leukemia and hyperleukocytosis in children. Med Pediatr Oncol 15:232, 1987

159. Gralnick HR, Bagley J, Abrell E: Heparin treatment for the hemorrhagic diathesis of acute promyelocytic leukemia. Am J Med 52:167, 1972

160. Drapkin RL, Gee TS, Dowlings MD et al: Prophylactic heparin therapy in acute promyelocytic leukemia. Cancer 41:2484, 1978

161. Cordonnier C, Vernant JP, Brun B et al: Acute promyelocytic leukemia in 57 previously untreated patients. Cancer 55:18, 1985

162. Cunningham I, Gee TS, Reich LJ et al: Acute promyelocytic leukemia: treatment results during a decade at Memorial Hospital. Blood 73:1116, 1989

163. Goldberg MA, Ginsburg D, Mayer RJ et al: Is heparin administration necessary during induction chemotherapy for patients with acute promyelocytic leukemia? Blood 69:187, 1987

164. Kobrinsky NL, Robison LL, Nesbit ME: Acute nonlymphocytic leukemia. Pediatr Clin North Am 27:345, 1980

165. Newman JH, Neff TA, Ziporin P: Acute respiratory failure associated with hypophosphatemia. N Engl J Med 296:1101, 1977

166. O'Connor LR, Wheeler WS, Bethune JE: Effect of hypophosphatemia on myocardial performance in man. N Engl J Med 297:901, 1977

167. Creutzig U, Ritter J, Budde M et al: Early deaths due to hemorrhage and leukostasis in childhood acute myelogenous leukemia. Cancer 60:3071, 1987

168. Steuber CP: Therapy in childhood non-lymphocytic leukemia (ANLL): evolution of current concepts of chemotherapy. Am J Pediatr Hematol Oncol 3:379, 1981

169. Chessells JM, O'Callaghan U, Hardisty RM: Acute myeloid leukaemia in childhood: clinical features and prognosis. Br J Haematol 53:555, 1986

170. Lampkin BC, Masterson M, Sambrano JE et al: Current chemotherapeutic treatment strategies in childhood acute nonlymphocytic leukemia. Semin Oncol 14:397, 1987

171. Amadori S, Ceci A, Comelli A et al: Treatment of acute myelogenous leukemia in children: results of the Italian Cooperative Study AIEOP/LAM 8204. J Clin Oncol 5:1356, 1987

172. Kantarjian HM, Keating MJ, McCredie KB et al: A characteristic pattern of leukemic cell differentiation without cytoreduction during remission induction in acute promyelocytic leukemia. J Clin Oncol 3:793, 1985

173. Stone RM, Magurie M, Goldberg MA et al: Complete remission in acute promyeleocytic leukemia despite persistence of abnormal bone marrow promyelocytes during induction therapy: experience in 34 patients. Blood 71:690, 1988

174. Breitman TR, Selonick SE, Collins SJ: Induction of differentiation of the human promyelocytic leukemia cell line (HL-60) by retinoic acid. Proc Natl Acad Sci USA 77:2936, 1980

175. Nilsson B: Probably in vivo induction of differentiation by retinoic acid of promyelocytes in acute promyelocytic leukaemia. Br J Haematol 57:365, 1984

176. Daenen S, Vellenga E, van Dobbenburgh OA, Halie MR: Retinoic acid as antileukemic therapy in a patient with acute promyelocytic leukemia and *Aspergillus* pneumonia. Blood 67:559, 1986

177. Fontana JA, Rogers JS II, Durham JP: The role of 13 cis-retinoic acid in the remission induction of a patient with acute promyelocytic leukemia. Cancer 57:209, 1986

178. Warrell RP Jr, De The' H, Wang Z, Degos L: Acute promyelocytic leukemia. N Engl J Med 329:177, 1993

179. Chomienne C, Ballerini P, Balitrand N: All-trans retinoic acid in acute promyelocytic leukemias. II. In vitro studies: structure-function relationship. Blood 76:1710, 1990

180. Huang ME, Ye YC, Chen SR: All-trans retinoic acid with or without low dose cytosine arabinoside in acute promyelocytic leukemia: report of 6 cases. Chin Med J (Engl) 100:949, 1987

181. Warrell RP Jr, Frankel SR, Miller WH Jr et al: All-trans retinoic acid for remission induction of acute promyelocytic leukemia: results of the New York study, abstracted. Blood, suppl. 80:360a, 1992

182. Chen ZX, Xue YQ, Zhang RI: A clinical and experimental study on all-trans retinoic acid-treated acute promyelocytic leukemia patients. Blood 78:1413, 1991

183. Goldie JH, Coldman AJ. Gudauskas GA: Rationale for the use of alternating non-cross-resistant chemotherapy. Cancer Treat Rep 66:439, 1982

184. Goldie JH, Coldman AJ: Quantitative model for multiple levels of drug resistance in clinical tumors. Cancer Treat Rep 67:923, 1983

185. Geyer JR, Pendergrass TW, Milstein JM, Bleyer WA: Eight drugs in one day chemotherapy in children with brain tumors: a critical toxicity appraisal. J Clin Oncol 6:996, 1988

186. Vaughan WP, Karp JE, Burke PJ: Long chemotherapy-free remissions after single-cycle timed sequential chemotherapy for acute myelocytic leukemia. Cancer 45:859, 1980

187. Vaughan WP, Karp JE, Burke PJ: Two-cycle timed sequential chemotherapy for adult acute non-lymphocytic leukemia. Blood 64:975, 1984

188. Bloomfield CD: Postremission therapy in acute myeloid leukemia. J Clin Oncol 3:1570, 1985

189. Baehner RL, Bernstein ID, Sather H et al: Contrasting benefits of two maintenance programs following identical induction in children with acute nonlymphocytic leukemia: a report from the Children's Cancer Study Group. Cancer Treat Rep 68:1269, 1984

190. Buckley JD, Chard RL, Baehner RL et al: Improvement in outcome for children with acute nonlymphocytic leukemia. Cancer 63:1457, 1989

191. Kalwinsky D, Mirro J, Schell M et al: Early intensification of chemotherapy for childhood acute nonlymphocytic leukemia: improved remission induction with a five-drug regimen including etoposide. J Clin Oncol 6:1134, 1988

192. Woods WG, Ruymann FB, Lampkin BC et al: The role of timing of high-dose cytosine arabinoside intensification and of maintenance therapy in the treatment of children with acute nonlymphocytic leukemia. Cancer 66:1106, 1990

193. Sanders JE, Donnall TE, Buckner CD et al: Marrow transplantation for children in first remission of acute nonlymphoblastic leukemia: an update. Blood 66:460, 1985

194. Johnson FL, Sanders JE, Ruggiero M et al: Bone marrow transplantation for the treatment of acute nonlymphoblastic leukemia in children aged less than 2 years. Blood 71:1277, 1988

195. Burnett AK, Tansey P, Watkins R et al: Transplantation of unpurged autologous bone marrow in acute myeloid leukaemia in first remission. Lancet 2:1068, 1984

196. Ball ED, Mills LE, Coughlin CT et al: Autologous bone marrow transplantation in acute myelogenous leukemia: in vitro treatment with myeloid cell-specific monoclonal antibodies. Blood 68:1311, 1986

197. Yeager AM, Kaizer H, Santos GW et al: Autologous bone marrow transplantation in patients with acute nonlymphocytic leukemia, using ex vivo marrow treatment with 4-hydroperoxycyclophosphamide. N Engl J Med 315:141, 1986

198. Woods WG, Kobrinsky N, Buckley J et al: Intensively timed induction therapy followed by autologous or allogeneic bone marrow transplantation for children with acute myeloid leukemia or myelodysplastic syndrome: a Children's Cancer Group pilot study. J Clin Oncol 11:1448, 1993

199. Meloni G, Vignetti M, Andrizzi C et al: ABMT for children AML: Italian experience. Bone Marrow Transplant 7:80, 1991

200. Tallman MS, Kopecky KJ, Amos D et al: Analysis of prognostic factors for the outcome of marrow transplantation or further chemotherapy for patients with acute nonlymphocytic leukemia in first remission. J Clin Oncol 7:326, 1989

201. Zwaan FE, Hermans J, Barrett AJ, Speck B: Bone marrow transplantation for acute nonlymphoblastic leukaemia: a survey of the European Group for Bone Marrow Transplantation (E.G.B.M.T.). Br J Haematol 56:645, 1984

202. Bostrum B, Brunning RD, McGlave P et al: Bone marrow transplantation for acute nonlymphocytic leukemia in first remission: analysis of prognostic factors. Blood 65:1191, 1985

203. Dicke KA: International Bone Marrow Transplant Registry (IBMTR): current status of bone marrow transplantation (BMT) for acute myelogenous leukemia (AML), abstracted. Proc ASCO 5:167, 1986

204. Appelbaum FR, Storb R, Ramberg RE et al: Treatment of preleukemic syndromes with marrow transplantation. Blood 69:92, 1987

205. Mirro J Jr, Hurwitz CA, Behm FG et al: Effects of recombinant human hematopoietic growth factors on leukemic blasts from children with acute myeloblastic or lymphoblastic leukemia. Leukemia 7:1026, 1993

206. Ohno R, Tomonaga M, Kobayashi T et al: Effect of granulocyte colony-stimulating factor after intensive induction therapy in relapsed or refractory acute leukemia. N Engl J Med 323:871, 1990

207. Taffuri A, Hegewisch S, Souze LM: Stimulation of leukemic blast cells in vitro by colony stimulating: evidence of recombinant and increased cell killing with cytosine arabinoside. Blood 72:329, 1988

208. Appelbaum FR, Clift RA, Buckner CD et al: Allogeneic marrow transplantation for acute nonlymphoblastic leukemia after first relapse. Blood 61:949, 1983

209. Thomas ED: Karnofsky Memorial Lecture. Marrow transplantation for malignant disease. J Clin Oncol 1:517, 1983

210. Mortimer J, Blinder MA, Schulman S et al: Relapse of acute leukemia after marrow transplantation: natural history and results of subsequent therapy. J Clin Oncol 7:50, 1989

211. Mathe G, Schwarzenberg L, Pouilart P et al: Two epipodophyllotoxin derivatives, VM-26 and VP16-213 in the treatment of leukemias, hematosarcomas, and lymphomas. Cancer 34:985, 1974

212. McKenna RW, Bloomfield CD, Dick F et al: Acute monoblastic leukemia: diagnosis and treatment of ten cases. Blood 46:481, 1975

213. Chard RL, Krivit LV, Bleyer WA et al: Phase II study of VP-16-213 in childhood malignant disease: a Children's Cancer Study Group report. Cancer Treat Rep 63:1755, 1979

214. Nishikawa A, Nakamura Y, Nobori U et al: Acute monocytic leukemia in children. Response to VP-16-213 as a single agent. Cancer 60:2146, 1987

215. Odom L, Lampkin B, Grem J et al: Successful induction of children with acute monoblastic leukemia (AMoL) of infancy and early childhood with epipodophyllotoxin, abstracted. Proc ASCO 7:183, 1988

216. Evans AE, Gilbert ES, Zandstra R: The increasing incidence of central nervous system leukemia in children. Cancer 26:404, 1970

217. Fleming I, Simone JV, Jackson R et al: Splenectomy and chemotherapy in acute myelocytic leukemia of childhood. Cancer 33:427, 1974

218. Meyer RJ, Ferreira PPC, Cuttner J et al: Central nervous system involvement at presentation in acute granulocytic leukemia. Am J Med 68:691, 1980

219. Haaxma-Reiche H, Daenen S, Witteveen RJW: Experiences with the Ommaya Reservoir for prophylaxis and treatment of the central nervous system in adult myelocytic leukemia. Blut 57:351, 1988

220. Creutzig U, Ritter J, Zimmermann M, Schellong G: Does cranial irradiation reduce the risk for bone marrow relapse in acute myelogenous leukemia? Unexpected results of the childhood acute myelogenous leukemia study BFM-87. J Clin Oncol 11:279, 1993

221. Vowels MR, White L, Hughes DO: Results of a pilot study for the treatment of childhood acute nonlymphoblastic leukemia. Cancer 55:2337, 1985

222. Odom LF, Lampkin BC, Tannous R et al: Acute monoblastic leukemia: a unique subtype. Leukemia Res 14:1, 1990

223. Lampkin B, Buckley J, Nesbit M et al: Biologic characteristics and outcome in infants with acute nonlymphocytic leukemia. (in press)

224. Frankel SR, Eardley A, Lauwers G et al: The "retinoic acid syndrome" in acute promyelocytic leukemia. Ann Intern Med 117:292, 1992

225. Spitzer D, Dicke KA, Gehan EA et al: A simplified in vitro classification for prognosis in adult acute leukemia: the application of in vitro results in remission-predictive models. Blood 48:795, 1976

226. Browman G, Goldberg J, Gottlieb AJ et al: The clonogenic assay as a reproducible in vitro system to study predictive parameters of treatment outcome in acute nonlymphoblastic leukemia. Am J Hematol 15:227, 1983

227. Nara N, McCulloch EA: The proliferation in suspension of the progenitors of the blast cells in acute myeloblastic leukemia. Blood 65:1484, 1985

228. Lange B, Valtieri M, Santoli D et al: Growth factor requirements of childhood acute leukemia: establishment of GM-CSF dependent cell lines. Blood 70:192, 1987

229. Woods WG, Nesbit ME, Buckley J et al: Correlation of chromosome abnormalities with patient characteristics, histologic subtype, and induction success in children with acute nonlymphocytic leukemia. J Clin Oncol 3:3, 1985

230. Kalwinsky D, Raimondi S, Schell M et al: Prognostic importance of cytogenetic subgroups in de novo pediatric acute nonlymphocytic leukemia. J Clin Oncol 8:1:75, 1990

231. Tanzer J, Fraysse J: Acute myelogenous leukemia with an 8;21 translocation. Cancer Genet Cytogenet 44:169, 1990

232. Griffin JD, Davis R, Nelson DA et al: Use of surface marker analysis to predict outcome of adult acute myeloblastic leukemia. Blood 68:1232, 1986

233. Vaughan WP, Strauss LC, Burke PJ: Surface marker phenotype (SMP) predicts response to therapy in acute non-lymphocytic leukemia (ANLL), abstracted. Proc ASCO 23:183, 1983

234. Cassileth PA, Gerson SL, Bonner H et al: Identification of early relapsing patients with adult acute nonlymphocytic leukemia by bone marrow biopsy after initial induction chemotherapy. J Clin Oncol 2:107, 1984

235. Preisler HD, Priore R, Azarnia N et al: Prediction of response of patients with acute nonlymphocytic leukaemia to remission induction therapy: use of clinical measurements. Br J Haematol 63:625, 1986

236. Dahl GV, Kalwinsky DK, Murphy S et al: Cytokinetically based induction chemotherapy and splenectomy for childhood acute nonlymphocytic leukemia. Blood 60:856, 1982

237. Karp JE, Donehower RC, Enterline JP et al: In vivo cell growth and pharmacologic determinants of clinical response in acute myelogenous leukemia. Blood 73:24, 1989

238. Gordon H: Oncogenes. Mayo Clin Proc 60:697, 1985

239. Sato H, Gottesman MM, Goldstein LJ et al: Expression of the multidrug resistance gene in myeloid leukemias. Leuk Res 14:11, 1990

240. Marie JP, Zittoun R, Sikic BI: Multidrug resistance (mdr1) gene expression in adult acute leukemias: correlations with treatment outcome and in vitro drug sensitivity. Blood 78:586, 1991

241. Raza A, Preisler HD: The use of BrdU and 3HTdr for double labeling of human leukemia cells. Biotechniques 2:262, 1984

242. Raza A, Ucar K, Preisler HD: Double labeling and in vitro versus in vivo incorporation of bromodeoxyuridine in patients with acute nonlymphocytic leukemia. Cytometry 6:633, 1985

243. Raza A, Mehdi I, Yasin Z et al: Cell cycle kinetics and drug sensitivity studies as determinants of response in AML. Int Soc Exp Hematol 1989

244. Venturelli D, Lange B, Narni F et al: Prognostic significance of short term effects of chemotherapy on myc and histone H3 m-RNA levels in acute leukemia patients. Proc Natl Acad Sci USA 85:3590, 1988

245. Kartner N, Riordan JP, Ling V: Cell surface P-glycoprotein associated with multidrug resistance in mammalian cell lines. Science 221:1285, 1983

246. Hamada H, Tsuruo T: Functional role for the 170-180 KDa glycoprotein in drug resistant tumor cells as revealed by monoclonal antibodies. Proc Natl Acad Sci USA 83:7785, 1986

247. Preisler HD, Gottesman M, Raza A et al: The clinical significance of expression of the multidrug resistance (MDR) gene in acute nonlymphocytic leukemia (ANLL), abstracted. Proc ASCO 8:201, 1989

248. Morra E, Lazzarino M, Brusamolino E et al: The role of systemic high-dose cytarabine in the treatment of central nervous system leukemia. Cancer 72: 439, 1993

249. Sanz MA, Rubia J, Sanz G et al: Busulfan plus cyclophosphamide followed by autologous blood stem-cell transplantation for patients with acute myeloblastic leukemia in first complete remission: a report from a single institution. J Clin Oncol 11:1661, 1993

250. Gandhi V, Estey E, Keating MJ, Plunkett W: Fludarabine potentiates metabolism of cytarabine in patients with acute myelogenous leukemia during therapy. J Clin Oncol 11:116, 1993

251. List AF, Spier C, Greer J et al: Phase I/II trial of cyclosporine as a chemotherapy-resistance modifier in acute leukemia. J Clin Oncol II:1652, 1993

252. Meloni G, Foa R, Tosti S et al: Autologous bone marrow transplantation followed by interleukin-2 in children with advanced leukemia: a pilot study. Leukemia 6:780, 1992

253. Kizaki M, Norman AW, Bishop JE et al: 1,24-Dihydroxyvitamin D3 receptor RNA: expression in hematopoietic cells. Blood 77:1238, 1991

254. Perlman K, Kutner A, Prahl J: 24-Homologated 1,25-dihydroxyvitamin D3 compounds: separation of calcium and cell differentiation activities. Biochemistry 29:190, 1990

255. Miller WH Jr, Kakizuka A, Frankel SR et al: Reverse transcription polymerase chain reaction for the rearranged retinoic acid receptor α clarifies diagnosis and detects minimal residual disease in acute promyelocytic leukemia. Proc Natl Acad Sci USA 89:2694, 1992

256. Biondi A, Rambaldi A, Pandolfi PP: Molecular monitoring of the myl/retinoic acid receptor-α fusion gene in acute promyelocytic leukemia by polymerase chain reaction. Blood 80:492, 1992

257. Creutzig U, Ritter J, Schellong G: Identification of two risk groups in childhood acute myelogenous leukemia after therapy intensification in study AML-BFM-83 as compared with study AML-BFM-78. Blood 75:1932, 1990

258. Ravindranath Y, Steuber CPS, Krischer J et al: High-dose cytarabine for intensification of early therapy of childhood acute myeloid leukemia: a Pediatric Oncology Group study. J Clin Oncol 9:572, 1991

259. Choi SI, Simone JV: Acute nonlymphocytic leukemia in 171 children. Med Pediatr Oncol 2:119, 1976

260. Miller DR: Acute lymphoblastic leukemia. Pediatr Clin North Am 27:269, 1980

Pathobiology of Acute Lymphocytic Leukemia

67

A. Thomas Look

INTRODUCTION

Normal lymphoid cell populations undergo diverse, clonal rearrangements of their immunoglobulin or T-cell receptor (TCR) genes, followed by highly regulated proliferation of the cells that successfully complete these genetic changes. This developmental process generates B cells and T cells with the specificities needed to support a fully competent immune system. When a lymphoid progenitor cell becomes genetically altered, the result can be dysregulated proliferation and clonal expansion eventually leading to acute lymphocytic leukemia (ALL). In most cases, the pathobiology of transformed lymphoid cells reflects the altered expression of genes whose products contribute to the normal phenotypes of B- and T-cell progenitors, but it may also involve the aberrant expression of otherwise quiescent genes.

Because leukemic lymphoid cells represent the clonal expansion of hematopoietic progenitors that are blocked in differentiation at discrete stages of development, they provide large uniform populations for molecular and functional analyses. Despite the disordered gene expression that accompanies malignant transformation, leukemic cells duplicate most of the features of normal lymphoid progenitors and thus can be studied profitably as normal surrogates, especially for rare cell types.[1] They also provide models for elucidating the regulatory cascades disrupted by specific genetic changes. For instance, molecular studies of chromosomal breakpoint regions in ALL cells have identified genes whose protein products are transcription factors that control the expression of developmentally important responder genes.[2,3] Indeed, most of the recent progress in understanding ALL pathobiology has come from the study of rearranged or mutated genes and their associated proteins.

CLONAL ORIGIN OF LEUKEMIC LYMPHOID CELLS

Human ALLs arise from a single progenitor cell that has undergone genetic damage leading to dysregulated growth and arrested differentiation. Evidence that each leukemic cell has descended from a single transformed progenitor comes from cytogenetic studies showing common numerical and structural chromosomal abnormalities within discrete leukemic cell populations. Cell lines with different karyotypes can be identified in about one-fourth of ALL cases,[4] but in most instances there are sufficient cytogenetic similarities to indicate that these lines arose from a common progenitor, diverging later as a result of the evolution of independent subclones. The unicellular development of leukemic cell populations is further demonstrated by uniform rearrangements of immunoglobulin or TCR genes, as compared with the heterogeneous pattern of rearrangements observed in populations of normal T and B lymphocytes.

The best evidence of clonality is provided by X-chromosome-linked genes that are inactivated during embryogenesis. This process occurs before somatically acquired transformation events and thus is independent of changes induced by differentiation and stem line evolution. In accord with the Lyon principle, one or the other of the X chromosomes is randomly inactivated early in the embryogenesis of females, in large part through DNA methylation, leading to a heterozygous pattern of inactivation of either the paternally or maternally derived X chromosome in all tissues, including the hematopoietic system. By contrast, in clonally derived cell populations, as found in the leukemias and other malignancies, every cell is characterized by inactivation of the same X chromosome. Thus, the unicellular development of a leukemic cell population can be demonstrated by detecting a single type of glucose-6-phosphate dehydrogenase—an enzyme encoded by a gene on the X chromosome—in the neoplastic cells of heterozygous female patients who express a double-enzyme pattern in their normal tissues.[5] By this method, a group of 19 girls and young women with B, pro-B, T, or undifferentiated ALL were found to have clonally derived leukemic cells.[6]

The methylation patterns of restriction fragment length polymorphisms (RFLPs) in X-linked genes, detected by Southern blot analysis, have been used to show that even rare ALL cases with two completely different cytogenetic stem lines probably arise by clonal evolution from a single transformed progenitor.[7] Immunoglobulin and TCR gene rearrangements and X-linked RFLPs were analyzed in five cases of ALL with two cytogenetically independent leukemic cell populations at diagnosis. Three female patients were found to be heterozygous for an X-linked RFLP with use of a probe from the phosphoglycerate kinase (PGK) gene, but only one parental allele was active in each case. Similarly, results of analysis in another case heterozygous for a hypoxanthine phosphoribosyl transferase (HPRT) BamHI RFLP revealed a single active parental allele. The most likely explanation is that these patients' leukemias developed clonally from transformed progenitors that were initially cytogenetically normal and that the two apparently unrelated abnormal karyotypes arose by clonal evolution. Thus, in patients with relapsed acute leukemia, a karyotype that differs entirely from the one at diagnosis may not represent a second leukemic transformation event, as is discussed in the section on acute myeloid leukemia (AML) developing after therapy for ALL.

LINEAGE-SPECIFIC FEATURES OF LEUKEMIC LYMPHOBLASTS

An important advance in the understanding of ALL pathobiology was the realization that malignant lymphoblasts share many of the features of normal lymphoid progenitors. Thus, ALL cells rearrange their immunoglobulin and TCR genes, and express components of antigen receptor molecules and other differentiation-linked cell-surface glycoproteins, in ways that correspond to developing normal B and T lymphocytes. In many cases, leukemic cells appear to represent the clonal expansion of a lymphoid progenitor that is blocked or "frozen" in an early stage of B- or T-cell differentiation.[1] With better understanding of the normal patterns of antigen-independent lymphoid cell development, however, it has become clear that leukemic lymphoblasts can show asynchronous gene expression with subtle variations in phenotype.[8,9] Hence, it should not be surprising that in some cases of ALL, the blast cell phenotypes differ from those of normal lymphocyte progenitors, presumably because of aberrant regulation of gene expression. Still, the general concept that leukemic cells should be classified according to their "normal" developmental stage remains an important one, providing a basis for the study of immuno-

phenotype-specific genetic changes and for the assignment of patients to risk-group-directed therapy.

B-Cell ALL

The diagnosis of B-cell leukemia depends on the detection of surface immunoglobulin on leukemic blasts. This rare phenotype accounts for only 2–3% of ALL cases, and the lymphoblasts generally have distinctive morphology, with deeply basophilic cytoplasm containing prominent vacuoles; this morphologic pattern is designated L3 in the French-American-British (FAB) system.[10] Prominent clinical features include concomitant extramedullary lymphomatous masses in the abdomen or head and neck, frequent involvement of the central nervous system and cranial nerves, and hyperuricemia with acute renal failure due to uric acid nephropathy. Most investigators believe that acute B-cell leukemia is a disseminated form of Burkitt lymphoma, as these conditions share common cytogenetic, molecular genetic, immunologic, cytologic, and clinical features.[11]

Acute B-cell leukemia does not respond well to chemotherapy traditionally used for childhood ALL. Better responses have been obtained with treatments designed for Burkitt lymphoma, which emphasize cyclophosphamide and the rapid rotation of antimetabolites in high dosages.[12] Thus, B-cell leukemia is the first form of ALL to be recognized as a distinct clinical entity based on immunophenotypic and cytogenetic features, and the first to be treated by separate protocols designed specifically for the leukemia's unique features.

Pro-B and Pre-B ALL

Approximately 80% of patients with ALL have lymphoblasts with phenotypes corresponding to those of B-cell progenitors. These cases can be identified on the basis of cell-surface expression of HLA-DR and at least one of the recognized B lineage-specific antigens: CD19, CD10 (neutral endopeptidase[13–15]), CD20, CD24, CD22, and CD21.[8] The lymphoblasts also express nuclear terminal deoxynucleotidyl transferase (TdT) at high levels, which can be detected by immunofluorescence assays applied to fixed cells.[16] A subset of cells co-express CD34, an antigen of unknown function whose normal expression is restricted to lymphoid and hematopoietic progenitors.[17,18] About one-fourth of the cases of B-progenitor ALL (20% overall) express cytoplasmic immunoglobulin μ heavy chain proteins and are designated pre-B-cell ALL[19,20]; the remainder do not express cytoplasmic immunoglobulin and are designated pro-B-cell ALL.[9] Pre-B cases were originally shown to have a worse long-term response to therapy than pro-B cases, an observation that was later attributed to the presence of a specific t(1;19) chromosomal translocation in about one-fourth of the pre-B cases.[21] The adverse effect of this cytogenetic feature appears to have been nullified by the development of effective chemotherapy.[22,23]

DNA rearrangement of immunoglobulin genes occurs before heavy chain gene expression in B-cell development, providing a genetic marker of B-lymphocyte ontogeny.[24,25] The variable region of immunoglobulin heavy chain genes is assembled from three classes of DNA segments on human chromosome 14, termed V_H (variable), D_H (diversity), and J_H (joining), which must recombine correctly during cell development to produce a functional protein. The initial attempt at rearrangement may be productive, resulting in immunoglobulin heavy chain synthesis, or it may be aberrant with no production of heavy chain molecules, in which case rearrangement of the other heavy chain allele is attempted. Similar rearrangements occur between the V and J regions of the κ and λ light chain genes on chromosomes 2 and 22, with attempts to rearrange the κ alleles occurring first, followed by recombination of λ alleles if these attempts are nonproductive. Rearrangement of each of these genes results in deletion of introns containing restriction endonuclease cleavage sites. This, in turn, causes changes in the sizes of restriction fragments bearing the rearranged gene under study, which can be detected by Southern blot analysis. Because lymphocytic leukemias are clonal, the DNA from each cell contains identical rearrangements apparent as discrete bands that differ from unrearranged germline bands.

The use of immunoglobulin heavy and light chain gene rearrangements to support an early B-lineage origin of most ALL blasts was pioneered by Korsmeyer and co-workers.[24,25] This work was extended to establish synchrony between immunoglobulin gene rearrangements and the expression of B lineage-restricted cell-surface antigens.[26] Immunoglobulin heavy chain gene rearrangements have also been documented in about 15% of cases of T-cell ALL[27-29] and a similar percentage of cases of AML.[30-32] Thus, caution must be exercised when assigning cell lineage on the basis of studies of immunoglobulin gene rearrangement.

T-Cell ALL

Leukemias of T-cell precursors are identified and classified according to the sequence of expression of T-cell-associated surface antigens during normal thymocyte ontogeny.[33,34] Thymocyte differentiation begins with the prothymocyte, which expresses CD7, TdT, and cytoplasmic T3 antigen. Next is the early thymocyte, which retains these markers and acquires CD5 and CD2, the receptor for sheep erythrocytes. Intermediate thymocytes co-express CD4 and CD8, as well as CD1. Mature thymocytes lose CD1 expression and produce functional TCRs, leading to expression of CD3 on the cell surface. Using a battery of monoclonal antibodies specific for these cell-surface glycoproteins, one can identify patterns of expression that correspond to equivalent stages of normal thymocyte development.[35-39] Leukemias with prothymocyte or early thymocyte phenotypes generally present as typical ALL, whereas those characterized by more mature thymocytes usually present with a localized thymic mass.[35,36,38] The clinical features most closely associated with T-cell ALL are high blood leukocyte counts, central nervous system involvement, and radiographic evidence of a thymic mass in about one-half of cases at presentation. Historically, patients with T-cell ALL have had an adverse prognosis in comparison with patients with pro-B ALL. With wider use of intensive chemotherapy, however, the outlook for patients with T-cell leukemia appears improved.[23,40-42]

The human antigen-specific TCR molecule is a heterodimer composed of disulfide-linked α and β polypeptide subunits, each encoded by gene families containing variable, joining, and constant sequence elements that rearrange at the DNA level to generate diversity, in a manner analogous to the immunoglobulin genes. Hence, rearrangement of the TCR β-chain genes can be used to establish clonality and lineage derivation within leukemias of T-cell progenitors.[43-45] Although TCR β-chain genes are generally in a germline configuration in B-lineage leukemic cells, about 10% of cases possess aberrant rearrangements.[46-48] Clonal rearrangements of the TCR γ- and δ-chain genes are even less restricted to the T-cell lineage, being observed in a significant number of pro-B ALL cases.[49,50]

Mixed-Lineage Leukemia

Acute mixed-lineage leukemias are defined by blast cells that co-express markers of both the lymphoid and myeloid lineages. Two distinct forms of these leukemias are recognized: those

with lymphoid morphology that co-express myeloid-associated antigen,[51-54] and those with myeloid morphology and reactivity to myeloperoxidase staining that co-express cell-surface antigens normally restricted to lymphoid cells.[55,56] The origin of mixed-lineage leukemias has not been established. One possibility is malignant transformation of pluripotent progenitor cells that retain the ability to differentiate in both the myeloid and lymphoid lineages; another is immortalization of rare progenitor cells that normally co-express features of both lineages; and a third is aberrant gene expression due to specific genetic alterations.[57]

Controversy exists over whether cases of lymphocytic leukemia with expression of one or more myeloid cell-surface antigens (e.g., CD13, CD33, or CD14) have an adverse prognosis. Sobol et al.[52] reported a lower complete remission rate and shorter survival in the one-third of adult ALL patients whose blasts expressed myeloid antigens. By contrast, Pui et al.[53] found that in the 16% of childhood ALL cases with expression of myeloid antigens, prognosis was no worse than in cases without this feature. The expression of T-lymphoid properties, such as cytoplasmic T3 and cell-surface CD2 and CD7, by predominantly myeloid leukemias appears to identify patients with a lower likelihood of complete remission with standard AML therapy but who respond well to induction agents commonly used in ALL therapy.[56]

GENETIC BASIS OF LYMPHOCYTIC LEUKEMIA

Multiple somatically acquired genetic abnormalities are responsible for the malignant transformation and disordered cell growth and differentiation seen in ALL. These include microscopically evident chromosomal rearrangements as well as lesions detectable only by molecular analysis of lymphoblast DNA (e.g., point mutations). The inability to define these changes in a precise, consistent manner and to relate them to the clinical course of the disease has hampered efforts to develop risk-specific therapy. It is worth noting that most children with leukemia have normal constitutional karyotypes, indicating that the genetic abnormalities in their leukemic cells are acquired somatically and thus are restricted to the malignant clone.

Transcriptional Control Genes

Chromosomal translocations are found in 50% of ALL cases[58,59] (Fig. 67-1). They can be broadly classified as recurring phenotype-specific, lineage-restricted abnormalities accounting for approximately half of the translocations in ALL, and as so-called random translocations, which have been identified in single cases only. As more "random" alterations have been characterized, the proportion affecting common breakpoints has increased, suggesting their involvement in oncogenic activation of specific genes.

Molecular studies of the breakpoints of specific chromosomal translocations of human leukemic cells have recently focused on transcription factor genes (Table 67-1), whose alteration apparently leads to the differentiation arrest and aberrant growth of leukemic lymphoid and myeloid progenitors.[2,3,60] Eventually, it may be possible to classify ALL according to the transcription factors involved in each subtype and their effects on normal cell growth and differentiation, but this development awaits a more complete understanding of the gene programs controlled by these proteins.

Conserved amino acid sequence motifs within the sequence-specific DNA binding domains of these nuclear trans-activating proteins allow them to be grouped into families, which in many cases appear to be involved in similar regulatory processes.

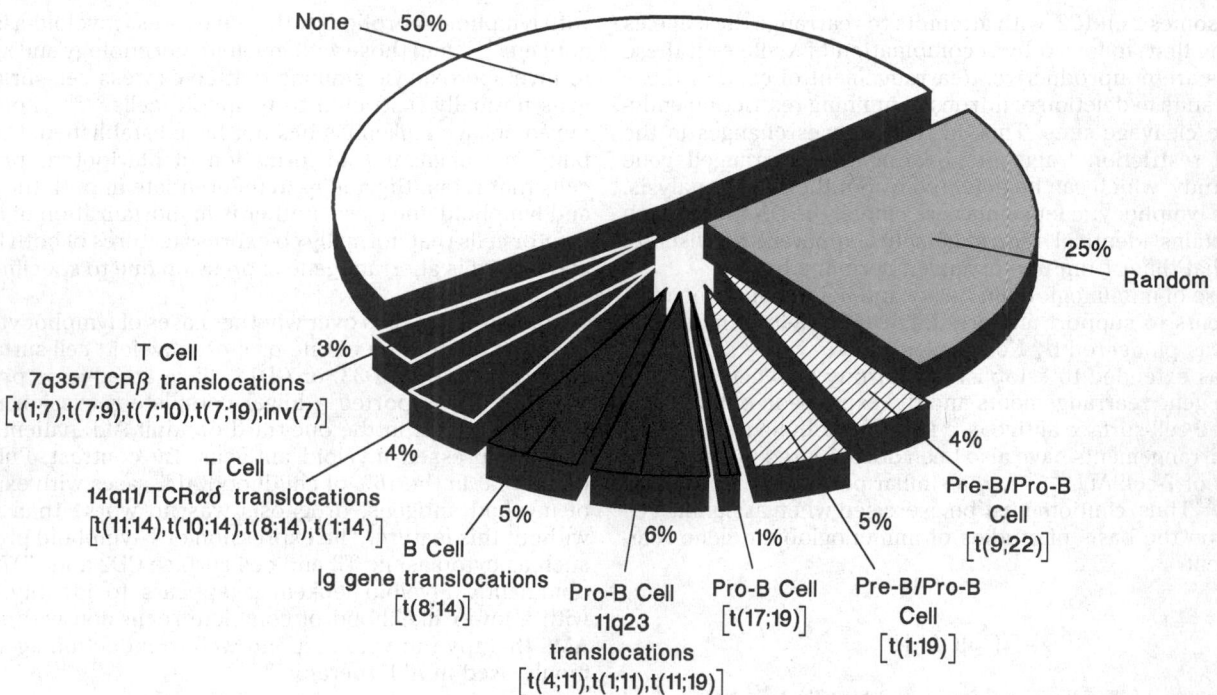

Fig. 67-1. Distribution of chromosomal translocations among the commonly recognized immunologic subtypes of ALL. One-half of the cases lack discernible rearrangements, and one-fourth have sporadic rearrangements that so far have only been observed in the leukemia cells from single patients.

Thus, the transcription factor genes in Table 67-1 are grouped according to shared structural features of their basic region-helix-loop-helix (bHLH), cysteine-rich (LIM), homeodomain (HOX), basic region-leucine zipper (bZip), A-T hook minor groove, or zinc-finger DNA-binding domains. Another important association is the lineage restriction of transcription factor genes affected by specific chromosomal translocations, suggesting that the proteins they encode may disrupt the differentiation programs of specific lymphoid progenitors. This interpretation implicates transcription factors as preferred targets

Table 67-1. Transcription Factors Genes Affected by Chromosomal Breakpoints in Human Acute Leukemias

Family[a]	Translocation	Affected Gene	Disease	References
Basic region-helix-loop-helix (bHLH) proteins	t(8;14)(q24;q32)	MYC	Burkitt lymphoma and B-cell ALL	62, 63, 293
	t(2;8)(p12;q24)	MYC		
	t(8;22)(q24;q11)	MYC		
	t(8;14)(q24;q11)	MYC	T-cell ALL	79–81
	t(7;19)(q35;p13)	LYL1	T-cell ALL	85
	t(1;14)(p32;q11)	TAL1/SCL/TCL5	T-cell ALL	82–84
	t(7;9)(q35;q34)	TAL2	T-cell ALL	84
Cysteine-rich (LIM) proteins	t(11;14)(p15;q11)	RHOMB1/TTG1	T-cell ALL	88, 89
	t(11;14)(p13;q11)	RHOMB2/TTG2	T-cell ALL	90, 91
	t(7;11)(q35;p13)	RHOMB2/TTG2	T-cell ALL	
Homeodomain (HOX) proteins	t(10;14)(q24;q11)	HOX11	T-cell ALL	94–97
	t(7;10)(q35;q24)	HOX11	T-cell ALL	
	t(1;19)(q23;p13)	E2A-PBX1	Pre-B-cell ALL	294, 295
Basic region-leucine zipper (bZip) proteins	t(17;19)(q22;p13)	E2A-HLF[b]	Pro-B-cell ALL	104, 105
Zinc-finger proteins	t(15;17)(q21;q11-22)	PML-RAR[b]	AML (promyelocytic)	270–274
	t(11;17)(q23;q21)	PLZF-RAR[b]	AML (promyelocytic)	296
	t(3;v)(q26;v)	EVI1	AML	297, 298
A-T hook minor groove binding proteins	t(4;11)(q21;q23)	HRX-FEL[b]/ALL1-AF4[b]/MLL-PBM1[b]	Pro-B-cell ALL	123, 125, 131
	t(9;11)(p21;q23)	HRX/ALL1/MLL[b]	AML (monocytic)	
	t(11;19)(q23;p13)	HRX-ENL[b]	ALL or AML	124
Others	t(8;21)(q22;q22)	AML1/ETO[b]	AML	299–302
	t(6;9)(p23;q34)	DEK-CAN[b]	AML	303

[a] Based on DNA-binding domain.
[b] Fusion gene.
(Modified from Rabbitts,[2] with permission.)

in leukemia induction. It also suggests that the normal developmental programs of progenitor cells of different lineages are controlled by different regulatory programs.

Rabbitts[2] has aptly described a key group of regulatory transcription factors as the products of "master genes." In his model, the nuclear proteins encoded by these genes act positively to up-regulate critical target genes or negatively to interfere with normal regulatory pathways. The net effect is disruption of gene regulatory cascades that control and coordinate the expression of large numbers of proteins required for completion of lymphoid cell differentiation programs.

Dysregulated Expression of Structurally Intact Transcription Factor Genes

One of the mechanisms by which chromosomal translocations can alter the expression of transcription factors in leukemic cells is dysregulated expression of structurally intact proteins. In this class of translocations, promoter/enhancer sequences from a gene expressed in progenitors of each lineage are rearranged adjacent to a gene encoding an oncogenic transcription factor, resulting in its untimely or lineage-inappropriate expression. The result is aberrant expression of a nuclear regulatory protein that controls the differentiation of hematopoietic progenitors within a given lineage.

Activation of MYC in B-Cell ALL

In B-cell acute leukemia and Burkitt lymphoma, translocation of one allele of the prototypic bHLH gene, *MYC,* on chromosome 8 into the vicinity of an immunoglobulin gene, either the heavy chain gene on chromosome 14q32 or the λ or κ light chain genes on chromosomes 2 and 22, leads to dysregulation of that allele.[61-69] In the predominant t(8;14) translocation, the involved *MYC* locus is translocated into the heavy chain gene on chromosome 14, adjacent to the coding sequences of the immunoglobulin constant region. The coding sequences of the immunoglobulin variable region generally are reciprocally translocated to the distal tip of chromosome 8. In variant translocations, the *MYC* gene remains on chromosome 8, and portions of the respective light chain genes are translocated to that chromosome downstream of the *MYC* locus.

The *MYC* proto-oncogene product acts in the nucleus and appears to be involved in the regulation of the transition of cells from a resting to a proliferative state.[70-75] These translocations are thought to disrupt the regulation of *MYC* expression in the involved B-cell progenitor through a complex array of molecular mechanisms, including removal of a portion of the promoter sequences from the coding region of the *MYC* gene, repositioning strong immunoglobulin gene enhancers close to the *MYC* gene on the rearranged chromosome, and dysregulating *MYC* expression by mutations that occur coincident with the translocation.[61-69] Dysregulation of *MYC* expression as a result of the translocation may contribute to malignant transformation or the high proliferative rate that is characteristic of these neoplasms. This hypothesis is supported by the induction of B-cell neoplasms in transgenic mice that carry the *MYC* oncogene driven by an immunoglobulin gene enhancer.[76,77] An activated *MYC* oncogene also induces malignant conversion when it is introduced into human Epstein-Barr virus-infected B lymphoblasts in vitro.[78]

bHLH, LIM, and HOX11 Genes in T-Cell ALL

In leukemias with a T-cell phenotype, chromosomal breakpoints consistently appear near enhancers included in the TCR β-chain locus on chromosome 7, band q34, or the αδ locus on chromosome 14, band q11. These enhancers, which are highly active in committed T-cell progenitors, cause dysregulated expression of one of a series of transcription factors located

at the breakpoint on the reciprocal chromosome involved in these phenotype-specific rearrangements (Table 67-1). Within the bHLH class of transcriptional regulators, chromosomal translocations affect the *MYC,*[79-81] *TAL1/SCL,*[82-84] and *LYL1*[85] genes in T-cell lymphoid malignancies. The bHLH domains of these proteins mediate dimerization and sequence-specific DNA binding to sequences located in the promoter/enhancer regions of target genes. Understanding of the normal roles of these proteins in the regulation of lymphoid and myeloid cell proliferation is still rudimentary, although studies of myogenic HLH proteins, of which MyoD is the prototype, have emphasized the potential of aberrant expression of such proteins to alter both lineage-specific differentiation and the control of cellular proliferation.[86,87]

Other genes whose expression can be altered by translocation into the proximity of one of the TCR loci include those encoding the cysteine-rich LIM proteins RHOMB1 and RHOMB2 (also called TTG1 and TTG2).[88-91] Both of these genes encode proteins that possess duplicated cysteine-rich LIM domains but lack homeobox DNA-binding domains as found in other transcription factors in this family. Thus, the LIM domain may function in protein-protein rather than protein-DNA interactions, and the rhombotin proteins could act as dominant negative suppressors through their ability to form complexes with other transcription factors.[2]

The rhombotin proteins are normally expressed at high levels in the central nervous system, in developmentally and segmentally regulated patterns.[89-92] They are normally minimally expressed or absent in T cells and their progenitors, implying that inappropriately high levels of expression resulting from chromosomal translocations may contribute to aberrant gene regulation in T-lymphoid leukemias. The *TTG1* gene has been experimentally introduced into developing thymocytes in transgenic mice under the control of the proximal *LCK* promoter, and shown to reproducibly induce thymic lymphomas within the first few months of life.[93] The tumor cells express high levels of the TTG1 transgene, and most have an unusual T-cell immunophenotype. Despite their CD8[+] and CD4[−] phenotype, the lymphoma cells lack the TCR for antigen, as indicated by the absence of the CD3 complex. The cells also express heat-stable antigen, detected by the J11d monoclonal antibody, indicating that a previously recognized rare subset of CD8[+] immature thymocytes are susceptible to transformation induced by inappropriate expression of the TTG1 protein.

The homeodomain protein HOX11, located on chromosome 10, band 24, is one of the more interesting proteins activated by translocation into the vicinity of the TCR loci.[94-97] Within the homeodomain transcription factor superfamily, *HOX11* is most closely related to *HLX,* a recently described murine gene homeobox gene expressed in specific hematopoietic cell lineages and during embryogenesis[98]; it also shows kinship to the *Antennapedia* homeobox genes of *Drosophila. HOX11* is normally expressed during embryogenesis in specific regions of the branchial arches and ectoderm of the pharyngeal pouches of the developing hindbrain in the mouse, but not by developing thymocytes or resting or activated T cells (Korsmeyer S, personal communication). Thus, *HOX11* conforms to the model of a gene whose expression is aberrantly activated by chromosomal translocation and whose product interferes with normal thymocyte development and predisposes these cells to neoplastic transformation.

Chimeric Transcription Factor Genes

Formation of chimeric proteins whose functional domains come from two normally separate genes represents a second mechanism of aberrant transcription factor activation. Thus, chromosomal translocations may produce a chimeric protein by fusing the DNA-binding, dimerization, and trans-effector regions of discrete genes, a process facilitated by the molecular structure of transcription factors.

E2A-PBX1 Fusion Genes in Pre-B ALL

A well-known example of a chimeric transcription factor with oncogenic potential is the *E2A-PBX1* rearrangement, which results from a t(1;19)(q23;p13) chromosomal translocation in human pre-B-cell ALL. This translocation breakpoint fuses the *E2A* gene on chromosome 19, which encodes a basic HLH transcription factor, to a homeobox gene *(PBX1)* on chromosome 1, leading to the expression of several forms of hybrid E2A-PBX1 oncoproteins (Fig. 67-2). In contrast to the products of other rearrangements affecting HLH genes, the hybrid proteins resulting from the t(1;19) retain only the N-terminal trans-activation domain of E2A. The bHLH domain is absent, replaced by the homeobox DNA-binding domain of PBX1. Thus, the target genes affected by this chimeric transcription factor are presumably recognized by the homeodomain of the PBX1 protein, which is not normally expressed by lymphoid or other hematopoietic cells. Although E2A-PBX1 proteins have been shown to have transforming potential in vitro[99] and in vivo[100,101] it is not clear whether the trans-activating domain of E2A plays an active role in this process or whether high levels of expression of truncated pbx1 proteins, driven by the *E2A* gene promoter, account for the transforming potential of the hybrid transcription factor.

Although the t(1;19) is found only in cytoplasmic immunoglobulin-positive pre-B-cell ALL in humans, recent studies by Kamps and Baltimore[100] have demonstrated the rapid induction of AML in lethally irradiated mice repopulated with bone marrow stem cells that had been infected with recombinant retroviruses containing *E2A-PBX1* genes. Using a different approach, Dedera and co-workers[101] reproducibly induced thymic lymphomas in transgenic mice that harbored *E2A-PBX1* genes in the germline. However, they observed lymphopenia in both B cells and T cells, suggesting induction of apoptotic cell death, which preceded malignant transformation in T cells expressing E2A-PBX1 proteins. Murine pre-B cells may be more susceptible to the programmed cell death effects of E2A-PBX1, which may be why pre-B-cell leukemias were not observed in either of the murine model systems. Because E2A-PBX1 is a potent transforming gene in murine T cells and myeloid cells, this explanation still leaves open the question of why the t(1;19) translocation is found only in human pre-B ALLs that express cytoplasmic but not surface immunoglobulin μ-chains.

Chimeric *E2A-PBX1* transcripts can be readily detected by using the reverse polymerase chain reaction (PCR) to amplify junctional sequences from leukemic cell RNA.[102,103] In our analysis of 17 cases with the t(1;19),[102] 10 of 11 pre-B cell cases expressing cytoplasmic immunoglobulin (cIg) heavy chains had typical *E2A-PBX1* chimeric transcripts with identical junctions. By contrast, none of the six cases of t(1;19)-positive, cIg⁻ ALL had evidence of detectable *E2A-PBX1* chimeric transcripts. These findings suggest that although the t(1;19) is cytogenetically indistinguishable in cIg⁺ and cIg⁻ ALLs, it does not produce E2A-PBX1 chimeras in the latter cases, presumably because it affects entirely different loci on chromosomes 1 and 19.

E2A-HLF Fusion Genes in Pro-B-Cell ALL

We and others recently identified a second fusion gene that combines *E2A* elements with those of a previously unidentified hepatic leukemia factor (HLF) gene,[104,105] which belongs to the bZip family of transcription factors (Fig. 67-3).[106] The hybrid E2A-HLF protein expressed by leukemic cells contains the E2A trans-activation domain linked to the basic region and leucine zipper domains of HLF. Within the superfamily of leucine zipper proteins, HLF is most closely related to an albumin gene promoter D-box binding protein (DBP),[107] and thyrotroph embryonic factor (TEF), which trans-activates the thyroid-stimulating hormone β-gene during anterior pituitary development.[108] HLF may regulate gene expression in hepatocytes and renal cells where it is normally expressed; its unscheduled expression as a chimeric protein in leukemic cells could alter normal regulatory circuits controlling early B-lymphocyte growth and differentiation.

HRX/MLL/ALL1 Fusion Genes in Leukemias with 11q23 Rearrangements

One of the most common chromosomal breakpoints involved by translocations in ALL and AML occurs on chromosome 11 in band q23. Cytogenetic studies have implicated ≥10 different chromosomal loci as partner chromosomes involved in 11q23 translocations, the most common of which is chromosome 4, band q21. In childhood ALL, approximately 4% of the cases overall and an even higher percentage of infant cases have 11q23 translocations, one-third of which involve chromosome 4; the remainder involve other diverse chromosomal regions.[109] The t(4;11)(q21;q23) translocation can occur in both children and adults with ALL,[110–112] and leukemic blasts from these patients have a B-cell precursor phenotype, with expression of HLA-DR antigens and rearranged immunoglobulin heavy chain genes.[113–116] Patients whose blast cells contain this translocation tend to have very high leukocyte counts at diagnosis (>100 × 10⁹/L) and an adverse prognosis when treated with combination chemotherapy.[23,110,117] Lymphoid leukemia cells with 11q23 rearrangements can be induced to express monocytic features in vitro, implying that the transformed progenitors may have the potential to differentiate in either the lymphoid or myeloid pathway.[115,116] Furthermore, translocations involving this chromosomal band occur as a t(9;11)(p22;q23), the most common single translocation in acute monocytic leukemia (AMoL; M5 subtype in the FAB classification).[118,119] 11q23 translocations of diverse types are found in a disproportionately high percentage of infants with both ALL and AMoL[120,121]; they also occur frequently in patients who develop myeloid leukemia after treatment for ALL.[122]

Cloning of a gene that is bisected at the breakpoint of translocations involving chromosome 11q23 has begun to reveal the significance of structural changes affecting this region.[123–130] Called *HRX, MLL,* or *ALL1* by the separate groups who have identified it, the gene encodes a large (430 kD) protein that shares sequence homology with the *Drosophila* trithorax protein, a regulator of homeotic gene function during the embryogenesis of this organism. The HRX/MLL/ALL1 protein has nuclear localization signals and other features, suggesting that it is a transcriptional regulatory protein, including both zinc-finger and A-T hook potential DNA-binding domains. Recent reports have indicated that the *HRX/MLL/ALL1* gene is rearranged within a defined breakpoint cluster region in several types of 11q23 translocations,[123–130] and potential fusion proteins have been identified for the t(4;11) and t(11;19) rearrangements.[123–125,131] Although both derivative chromosomes in these rearrangements are transcriptionally active and encode potential chimeric products, variant translocations occurring in rare leukemia cases implicate the fusion protein encoded by the der(11) chromosome. This protein contains N-terminal sequences from the *HRX/MLL/ALl1* gene, including the A-T hook potential DNA-binding domain, but sequences homologous to the zinc fingers of *Trithorax* are downstream of the break and are not included in the fusion protein. The genes encoded by the partner chromosomes in these two translocations, *AF4/PBM1/FEL* on chromosome 4 and *ENL* on chromosome 19, are serine- and proline-rich proteins with nuclear localization sequences, which contribute their C-terminal sequences to the

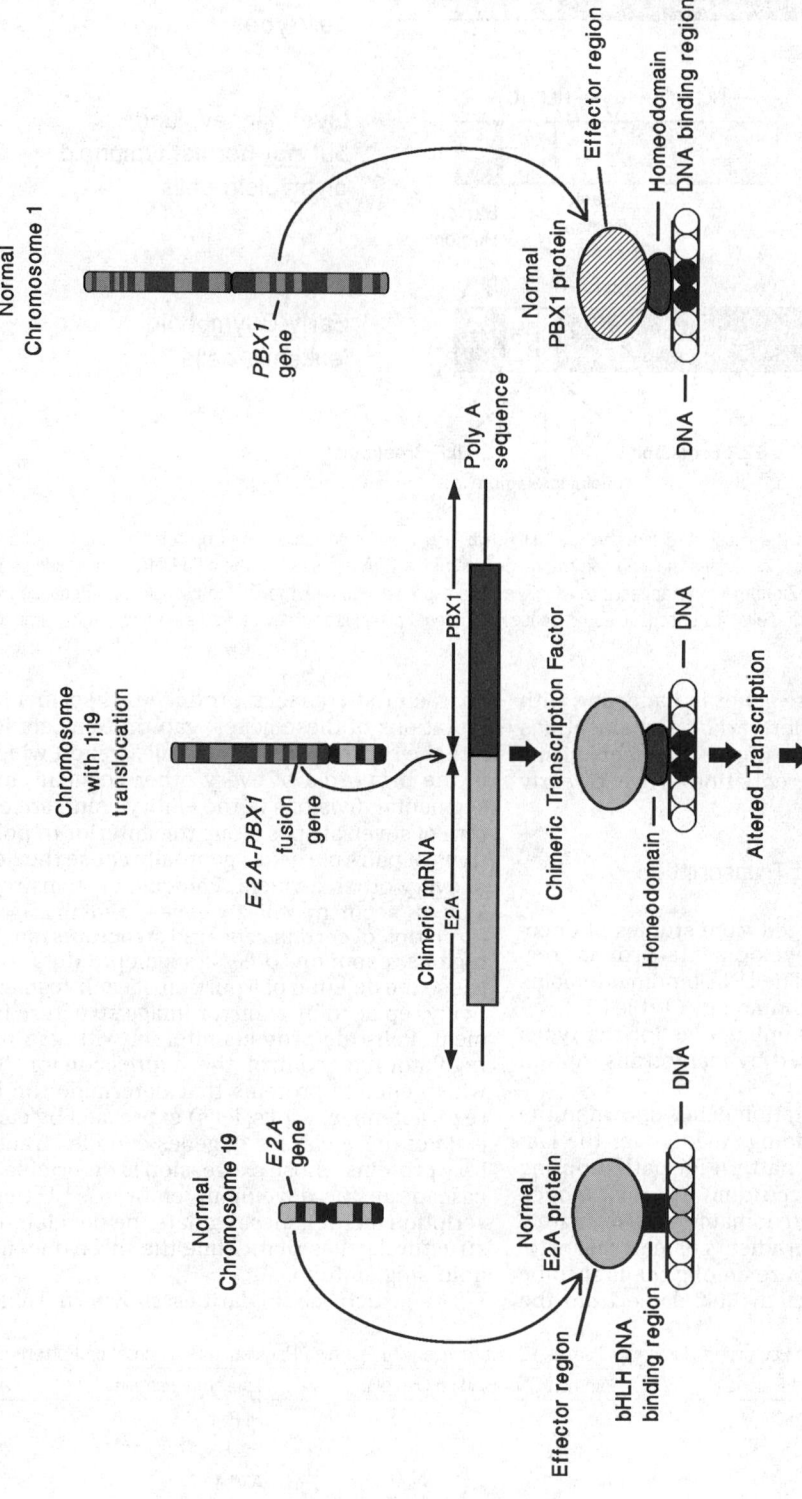

Fig. 67-2. Proposed role of the E2A-*PBX1* chimeric protein in ALL. Joining of the chromosome fragments produced by the t(1;19) translocation creates a fusion gene consisting of *E2A* and *PBX1* coding segments. The resulting protein binds to the DNA sequences normally recognized by the homeobox PBX1 protein; however, its effector (or trans-activator) region may interact with the transcription machinery in a manner analogous to that of the normal E2A protein. Consequently, transcription may be dysregulated and contribute to the development of ALL.

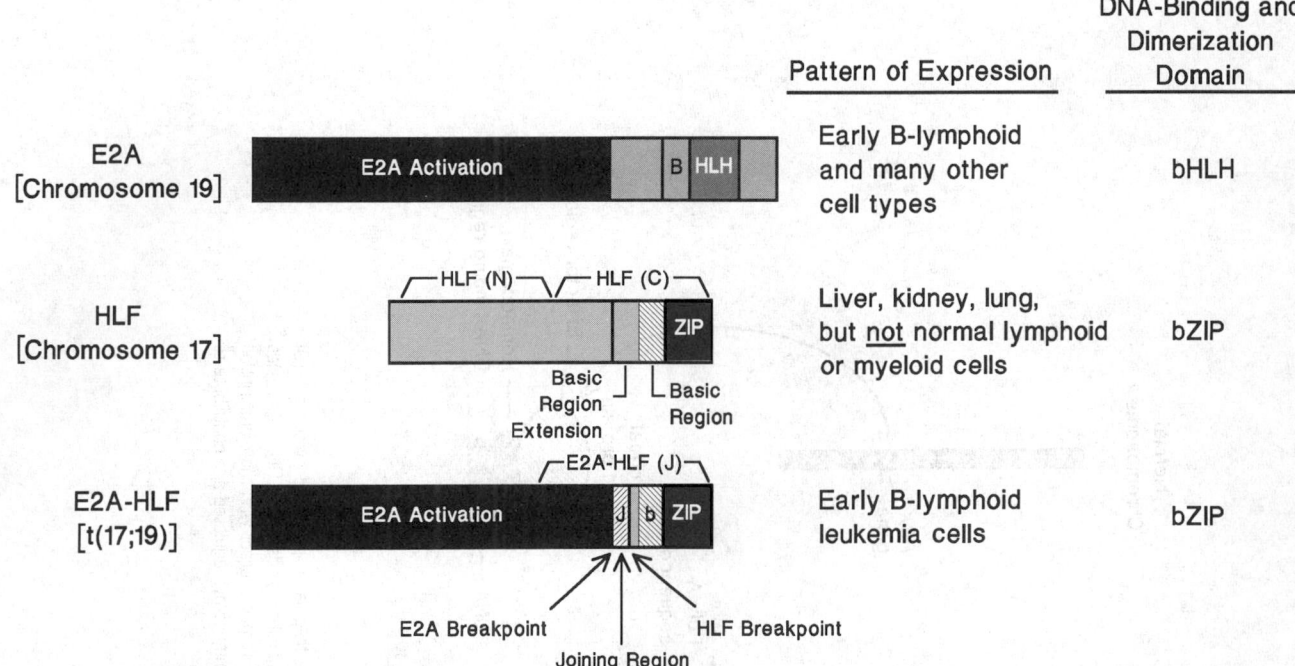

| | | Pattern of Expression | DNA-Binding and Dimerization Domain |

Fig. 67-3. Schematic diagram of the recently discovered E2A-HLF hybrid transcription factor. This protein, a result of the t(17;19) translocation in pro-B lymphoblasts, combines the trans-activation domain of the E2A protein with the bZip DNA-binding and dimerization domain of HLF, a protein of the bZip family that appears to regulate gene expression in hepatocytes and renal cells. Because HLF is not usually expressed in hematopoietic cells, its unscheduled presence in lymphoid progenitors may serve as an oncogenic stimulus. (From Inaba et al.,[304] with permission.)

respective fusion proteins. With these genes in hand, and with the cloning of genes involved in other variant translocations close behind, it will be possible to investigate the mechanisms underlying transformation and differentiation arrest of early lymphoid and myeloid stem cells.

Developmental Biology of Oncogenic Transcription Factors

A surprising connection has emerged from studies of oncogenic transcription factors and the developmental proteins regulating segmentation in *Drosophila*. The DNA-binding domains of these proteins often show striking homology (Table 67-2), an observation that carries important implications for the types of DNA sequence elements recognized by many transcription factors.

The classes of *Drosophila* segmentation genes shown in the first column of Table 67-2 reflect findings made over the last decade on the molecular control of pattern formation during *Drosophila* embryogenesis.[132,133] According to this model, "gap" proteins are expressed in broad domains, approximately three segments wide, in response to gradients of maternal cytoplasmic polarity proteins. *gap* genes are among the first to be transcribed in the embryo and earned their name from the

characteristic spaces produced in segmentation patterns by mutations of these genes. gap proteins act in concert to regulate the expression of "pair-rule" genes, which are transcribed in the primordia of every other segment and form repetitive segmental divisions in the embryo, and are expressed in a pattern of seven stripes along the anterior to posterior axis. Mutations of pair-rule genes generally cause the deletion of portions of every other segment. Pair-rule proteins regulate the expression of "segment polarity genes," which are responsible for the formation of certain repeated structures, such as the boundary regions, common to each segment. Mutations of these genes cause the deletion of a portion of each segment, which is repetitively replaced by a mirror-image structure from the same segment. Pair-rule proteins interact with gap proteins and other regulators to control the expression of "homeotic genes," which encode proteins that determine the unique structures (e.g., antennae, wings, legs) expressed by each segment. Thus, each of these classes of genes encodes transcriptional regulatory proteins whose expression is determined as a hierarchical cascade in the developing embryo.[134] Ultimately, these transcription factor genes regulate the developmental programs of structural genes that define the three-dimensional form of the unfolding embryo.

The structural similarities shown in Table 67-2 among the

Table 67-2. Oncogenic Transcription Factors in Human Leukemia—Convergence with Proteins Regulating Segmentation Pattern in *Drosophila*

Drosophila Protein	Morphogenetic Role	Common DNA-Binding Domain	Leukemia Protein	Activating Translocation
Giant	Gap	bZip	HLF	t(17;19)(q22;p13)
Krüppel	Gap	Zinc finger	PLZF	t(11;17)(q23;q21)
Runt	Pair-rule	Undefined	AML1	t(8;21)(q22;q22)
Antennapedia	Homeotic	Homeobox	HOX11	t(10;14)(q24;q11)
Extradenticle	Homeotic	Homeobox	PBX1	t(1;19)(q23;p13)
Trithorax	Homeotic gene regulator	A-T hook	HRX/ALL1/MLL	t(4;11)(q21;q23)
				t(9;11)(p21;q23)
				t(11;19)(q23;p13)

proteins regulating segmentation pattern in *Drosophila* and the oncogenic transcription factors activated by chromosomal translocation in acute leukemia suggest that these two classes of proteins may share functional properties as well. An obvious difference, however, is that the *Drosophila* proteins have been identified by the morphologic effects of recessive mutations that cause loss of function, whereas in ALL the proteins arise from dominant lesions that activate expression from one copy of the affected gene or genes, most of which are normally quiescent in lymphoid cells. The suggestion from this body of research is that the morphologic changes associated with lymphoid and myeloid cell differentiation are regulated by proteins analogous to those regulating the segmentation pattern during *Drosophila* embryogenesis. Hence, the proteins participating in leukemogenesis apparently interfere with a network of hematopoietic transcription factors leading to arrested cell development at stages corresponding to those of early lymphoid or myeloid progenitors. In this model, the oncogenic transcription factors inappropriately activate or suppress the expression of target genes involved in normal lymphohematopoietic cell development.

Tyrosine Kinase Genes: *BCR-ABL*

The 22q− chromosomal marker, originally identified in patients with chronic myeloid leukemia (CML), is also found in about 4% of childhood cases and 19% of adult cases of ALL.[111,135,136] This derivative chromosome generally arises from a reciprocal chromosomal translocation, t(9;22)(q34; q11), that cannot be distinguished at the cytogenetic level from the translocation found in CML, a hematopoietic stem cell disorder with unique clinical features.[137] The t(9;22) in ALL tends to be associated with a pro-B or pre-B phenotype, but it also appears in T-cell cases.[58] Patients with this rearrangement, termed the Philadelphia chromosome, have not responded well to standard treatment for ALL, often failing to achieve remission or relapsing soon after remission induction.[117,136,138,139] Chemotherapy with an intensive early phase, followed by allogeneic bone marrow transplantation in first remission, is warranted for ALL patients with Philadelphia chromosome-positive blast cells.

The t(9;22) breakpoints on the distal tip of the long arm of chromosome 9 are variable in CML and may occur over a distance of >100 kb within the *ABL* proto-oncogene, upstream of the tyrosine kinase domain.[140–142] By contrast, the CML breakpoints on chromosome 22 are confined to a 5.8-kb region of DNA known as the breakpoint cluster region.[143] This region of chromosome 22 is within a gene called *BCR*[143,144] that encodes a 160-kd phosphoprotein with undetermined function. As a result of the translocation, a *BCR-ABL* fusion gene is produced, consisting of 5′ (upstream) sequences from *BCR* and 3′ (downstream) sequences of *ABL*.[145–149] The 8.5-kb fusion transcript found in CML encodes a 210-kd hybrid protein,[150–153] which is activated as a tyrosine-specific protein kinase similar to the v-abl protein in assays that do not detect activity of the normal abl protein.[150–153]

Although the t(9;22) is identical by karyotyping in CML and ALL, molecular studies of the *BCR* and *ABL* proto-oncogenes, which are rearranged in both diseases, have revealed potentially important differences.[154–156] In ALL, the rearrangement produces a 6.5–7.0-kb fusion transcript and a 185–190-kd hybrid protein, which are distinct from the products of the rearranged *BCR-ABL* fusion gene in CML.[154–156] The breakpoints on chromosome 22 in ALL cases are not within the 5.8-kb region of *BCR* that contains the breakpoints in CML, but lie further upstream within the *BCR* gene.[157–159] The ALL fusion protein includes N-terminal BCR amino acids but lacks the internal residues found in the CML fusion proteins near the BCR-ABL junction.

N-terminal sequences of *ABL* are replaced in activated forms of the gene, with the Moloney virus *gag* gene in the case of v-*abl*[160–162] and with *BCR* in the 9;22 translocation of CML.[150–153] Both the v-*abl* and the *BCR-ABL* fusion genes can transform pre-B cells, but the *BCR-ABL* fusion gene is unable to transform fibroblasts unless it is also fused to the *gag* gene.[163] Thus, N-terminal alterations not only influence the ability of *ABL* to function as a lineage-specific transforming gene but also the tyrosine kinase activity of its protein product.

An attractive hypothesis is that, in CML, the *BCR-ABL* fusion gene affects a pluripotent hematopoietic stem cell, whereas in ALL it transforms a more committed lymphoid progenitor. The ability to manipulate molecular clones of both types of *BCR-ABL* hybrid genes should make it possible to assess the transforming effects of the respective protein products in lymphoid progenitor cells.

Chromosomal Deletion Syndromes and Tumor Suppressor Genes

Much recent attention has been focused on recessively acting oncogenes whose products normally suppress tumor formation in differentiating cells of a particular lineage. Loss of function of a tumor suppressor protein, occurring through deletion or mutational inactivation of both chromosomal loci of the gene that encodes it, leads to malignant transformation. Knudson[164] first proposed that inactivation of both alleles of a single locus is needed to initiate the development of retinoblastoma, basing his ideas on the observed frequencies of hereditary and sporadic forms of this disease.[164] The predicted retinoblastoma susceptibility locus, *RB1*, was localized to the long arm of chromosome 13 by cytogenetic and molecular genetic studies.[165,166] A candidate cDNA clone with properties predicted for the *RB1* gene was originally isolated by Friend and co-workers,[167] shown to encode a 110-kd nuclear phosphoprotein with DNA-binding properties.[168,169] Several lines of evidence suggest that the *RB1* gene encodes the bona fide retinoblastoma susceptibility locus: (1) the gene has been shown to be disrupted by constitutional chromosomal translocations in patients with the hereditary form of retinoblastoma[170]; (2) internal deletions within the *RB1* locus have been identified in retinoblastomas and osteosarcomas[168,171–173]; (3) replacement of the *RB1* gene appears to reverse the malignant phenotype in retinoblastoma cells[174]; and (4) the *RB1* product has been shown to bind the adenovirus E1A nuclear oncoprotein[175,176] and the SV40 large T antigen[177,178] in regions predicted by deletional analysis to be important for transformation of infected cells. Thus, these viral transforming proteins may deplete the *RB1* product by binding to it, thereby producing the same effect as the inactivation of both *RB1* alleles in human retinoblastoma.[176]

Allelic loss of defined regions of many different chromosomes has been linked to specific types of human tumors.[179,180] By analogy with the findings in retinoblastoma, a reasonable hypothesis is that each of these regions harbors a tumor suppressor gene whose product is uniquely involved in the inhibition of cell cycle progression and promotion of terminal differentiation of the normal cells that give rise to these different types of tumors. Additional tumor suppressor genes have also been identified at the molecular level. One is located on chromosome 11, band p13, in the region deleted in Wilms embryonic renal tumors,[181–184] and encodes a protein with properties of a transcriptional regulatory protein.[185] Another, on chromosome 17, band p13, encodes the p53 nuclear protein,[186–189] which is mutated or lost through chromosomal deletion in a wide variety of human tumors,[190] including colon cancer,[191,192] lung cancer,[193] breast cancer,[194] and osteosarcoma.[195] Recent reports document heritable cancer-associated changes of the p53 tumor suppressor gene in families with Li-Fraumeni syndrome—an unusual aggregation of sarcomas, brain tumors, leukemias, adrenocortical carcinomas, and premenopausal breast cancers.[196–199] Both inherited and sporadic p53 mutations are associated with lymphoid leukemias; although rarely found in T-cell and early B-progenitor ALL phenotypes, p53 mutations are commonly identified in Burkitt lymphoma and B-cell leukemia.[200,201]

Identification of recurring chromosome deletion syndromes in human ALL indicates that other tumor suppressor loci may be involved in this disease. These syndromes, which affect the long arm of chromosome 6, the short arm of chromosome 9, or the short arm of chromosome 12, can be found in leukemic cells from approximately 10% of patients with ALL, making them among the most frequent cytogenetic abnormalities in this disease. Functional deletion can result either from interstitial deletion of the involved chromosome arm or from derivative chromosomes that result from unbalanced chromosomal translocations. For each chromosome, the deleted regions overlap a single target region, which may contain key genes of the tumor suppressor type, whose loss could be an important step in leukemic transformation. From studies in other tumors,[166,167,181,182,184,202,203] one would predict that allelic loss of one copy of a tumor suppressor locus could occur through more subtle mechanisms, such as mitotic recombination or chromosomal loss and reduplication.

Deletions Involving the Long Arm of Chromosome 6

Deletions of the long arm of chromosome 6 are consistently found in about 10% of cases of ALL.[111,204–208] Interstitial deletions affecting bands 6q15-q24 have been reported most frequently; translocations with breakpoints within this region are also common. Band q21 of chromosome 6 seems to be involved in each of the abnormalities, suggesting that the target gene(s) resides in this region. It is clear from molecular studies that the *myb* gene, located on band 6q23-24, is distal to the target region and thus is retained by deleted chromosomes.[209] Deletions of chromosome 6q occur with equal frequency in pro-B, pre-B, and T-cell cases.

Deletions Involving the Short Arm of Chromosome 12

Deletions or translocations involving the short arm of chromosome 12 are also found in about 10% of ALL cases, with most clustered around band 12p12.[58,210] These cases generally have a pro-B or pre-B-cell phenotype, and blast cells usually express CD10/neutral endopeptidase and HLA-DR on the cell surface. Abnormalities of the short arm of chromosome 12 are rarely found in T-cell cases. Translocations involving chromosome 12p12 may be balanced or unbalanced and can involve multiple different donor chromosomes.[210] In the cases with unbalanced translocations, DNA sequences distal to the breakpoint are lost from the affected homologue and subsequently from the leukemia cell genome, so the result is similar to interstitial deletion. Among the only reciprocal translocations that have been seen in more than one case are t(7;12)(q11;p12) and t(12;13)(p13;q14). The unusual variation in donor chromosomes and breakpoints among the unbalanced translocations, as well as the frequency of deletions involving the 12p12 region, suggests that these lesions primarily inactivate one allele of a tumor suppressor gene in this chromosomal region.

Deletions Involving the Short Arm of Chromosome 9

Deletions affecting the short arm of chromosome 9 were first recognized as a nonrandom abnormality in ALL by Kowalczyk and Sandberg.[211] Initially, this deletion syndrome was thought to be specific for ALL patients with T-cell disease, bulky lymphadenopathy, splenomegaly, hyperleukocytosis, and a high risk of treatment failure. More recent evaluations of larger groups of children with ALL support the association of deletions of 9p with these high-risk features, but indicate that this abnormality can occur in patients with standard-risk pro-B ALL as well as those with T-cell ALL.[212,213] Molecular analysis has indicated homozygous deletion of the interferon-α and interferon-β_1 genes, which have been assigned to chromosome 9, bands p21-22, supporting the theory that this deletion may inactivate a tumor suppressor gene located within these chromosome bands.[214]

Deletions of Other Chromosomal Regions in ALL

In addition to 6q, 9p, and 12p, other regions are lost from the chromosomes of ALL blasts in a nonrandom fashion. Pui et al.[215] have documented selective loss of chromosomes 3, 7, 13, 16, and 17 in hypodiploid ALL cases with 30–40 chromosomes. Further study will be needed to define the frequency of loss of heterozygosity with probes localized to these chromosomes in cases with two normal-appearing homologues.

Mutated *RAS* Genes

Activation of cellular proto-oncogenes by point mutation is difficult to detect, because such lesions lack the cytogenetic abnormalities that signal other forms of transforming alterations. Genes of this type must be identified in experimental systems, so that investigators know in advance the type of activating point mutations that are likely to occur in human tumors. The prototypic genes of this class are genes of the *RAS* family, with mutations affecting defined amino acids of the corresponding proteins. Human tumor DNAs were initially found to contain activated homologues of either the *HRAS* or *KRAS* genes,[216–218] proto-oncogenes that had already been identified on the basis of their homology with viral oncogenes. Gene transfer methods identified an additional member of the *RAS* gene family, called *NRAS*,[219,220] that had not been previously observed as a component of a transforming retrovirus.

Proto-oncogenes of the *RAS* family—*HRAS*, *KRAS*, and *NRAS*—encode 21-kd proteins that are associated with the inner surface of the cytoplasmic membrane.[221] These proteins bind guanidine nucleotides and function as intermediates in signal transduction pathways that regulate the growth of cells. The *RAS* proto-oncogenes are activated to transforming oncogenes by somatic mutations that alter the amino acids specified by codons 12, 13, or 61.[222] Mutated *RAS* genes also bind guanine nucleotides, but have diminished capacity to hydrolyze GTP to GDP.[223–225] Transforming properties of activated RAS proteins may result from their inability to hydrolyze GTP, which could play an important role in modulating signal transduction.

The transforming potential of human *RAS* genes activated by point mutation has been documented in experimental systems. The *RAS* oncogenes will transform NIH-3T3 murine fibroblasts in vitro, and will collaborate with other oncogenes to transform primary cultures of embryo fibroblasts.[226–229] In addition, their role in mammalian tumorigenesis has been documented in carcinogen-induced animal tumor model systems.[230–232]

Activated *NRAS* genes appear to be preferentially involved in hematopoietic malignancies. They were detected in the myeloid cell lines HL-60, KG1, and Rc2A[233,234]; in fresh leukemic cell samples from patients with AML and CML[235–237]; and in lymphocytic leukemias with a T-cell immunophenotype.[238] In AML, *NRAS* gene mutations involving codon 13 or 61 were found in approximately 20% of cases, regardless of morphologic subtype.[235,239] Mutation of codon 12 of the *KRAS* gene was also observed in two of 37 cases studied.[239] In a study of lymphoblasts from children with ALL, 2 of 19 patients showed mutated *NRAS* genes, both involving codon 12.[240] Mutated *RAS* genes have also been documented in patients with preleukemic syndromes, indicating the potential involvement of activation of these genes in an early stage in the biogenesis of some leukemias.[241,242]

Gene Amplification

Gene amplification at the DNA level provides the cell a means to increase expression of critical genes whose products are ordinarily tightly controlled. Clinically important examples of proto-oncogene amplification have been documented in solid tumors of adults and children. The *NMYC* gene is amplified from 10–300-fold in tumor cells from about one-third of cases of childhood neuroblastoma; such amplification has been linked to an advanced stage of disease and a poor prognosis.[243–245] Members of the *MYC* gene family, including *NMYC*, *MYC*, or *LMYC*, are amplified in DNA extracted from cell lines of patients with small cell lung cancer, and are amplified more often in tumors from patients treated with chemotherapy.[246,247] The *HER2/NEU/ERBB2* proto-oncogene, a relative of the epidermal growth factor receptor gene, is amplified in approximately one-third of human breast cancers, and amplified levels are associated with shortened disease-free and overall survival.[248,249]

Gene amplification has been reported in isolated cases of human leukemia. The *MYC* gene has been shown to be amplified 8–32-fold in DNA from the HL-60 myeloid leukemia cell line, and in fresh leukemia cells from the same patient.[250,251] *MYB* has also been shown to be amplified in rare cases of AML,[252,253] and the *E2F-1* gene has recently been shown to be amplified and overexpressed in the HEL human erythroleukemia cell line.[254] The cytogenetic hallmarks of gene amplification—double-minute chromatin bodies and homogeneously staining regions—are rarely found in karyotypes of human leukemia cells, making it unlikely that consistently amplified cellular proto-oncogenes will be identified in this disease. Nonetheless, the detection of gene amplification in clinical samples holds promise for improving the staging of patients with certain types of solid tumors.[243–249]

Abnormalities of Leukemia Cell Ploidy

Karyotype Analysis

Secker-Walker and co-workers[255] first recognized that the chromosome number, or ploidy, of leukemic lymphoblasts was an important prognostic factor. Children with favorable responses to therapy have >50 chromosomes per leukemic cell,[117,139,256,257] whereas those with less favorable responses have fewer chromosomes (pseudodiploid, hypodiploid, and hyperdiploid 47–49 groups).[139,208,215,257] Analysis of leukemic cell karyotypes with >50 chromosomes has revealed other distinctive cytogenetic features, such as trisomies of specific chromosomes and a relatively low frequency of chromosomal translocations.[139] This subgroup comprises about 20% of children with ALL and is a subset of a larger group with pre-B or pro-B phenotypes, whose blasts express CD10/neutral endopeptidase.[258] Karyotypes from these patients generally have modal chromosome numbers in the range of 51–60 per leukemic cell, with a median of 55. These cases are cytogenetically distinct from those with 47–49 chromosomes, because trisomies of different chromosomes are found in the >50 group.[139,259] They also differ from tetraploid cases, which have four copies of each chromosome. Although the trisomies presumably result from nondisjunction, with unequal pairing of chromosomes in daughter cells after mitosis, the mechanisms underlying the preferential involvement of certain chromosomes and the clustering of the modal number at 51–60 chromosomes remain unknown.

DNA Flow Cytometry

Patients with hyperdiploid ALL can be identified rapidly by flow cytometric measurement of the DNA of leukemic blast cells.[258,260] With flow cytometry, nuclei stained with a DNA-specific dye are analyzed for the amount of DNA per cell, and the results are plotted as a frequency histogram. This DNA measurement is expressed as the ratio of the cellular DNA content of G_1/G_0-phase leukemic cells compared with that of normal diploid cells. As is described in detail in the next section, the speed, convenience, and uniformity of success of flow cytometric analysis of DNA ploidy has made this the technique of choice for detecting the favorable risk group in childhood ALL with >53 chromosomes or a DNA index >1.16 in the leukemic lymphoblasts.

IMPLICATIONS OF GENETIC FINDINGS FOR LEUKEMIA THERAPY

Detailed characterization of unique chimeric or dysregulated transcription factors in leukemic cells may well lead to new therapeutic approaches based on targeted drug development or antisense nucleotide technology, in which the goal would be to arrest cell growth or promote cell differentiation. Currently, however, gene-based clinical management strategies in acute leukemia focus on refinement of patient risk groups to permit more precise use of cytotoxic agents.

Childhood ALL—A Model for Gene-Based Risk Assessment

Chromosomal and molecular genetic abnormalities in the leukemic blasts of children with ALL are among the best predictors of response to currently available chemotherapy. Initially performed by time-consuming and labor-intensive cytogenetic methods, the classification of chromosomal abnormalities in leukemic lymphoblasts has been aided by flow cytometric techniques (to detect hyperdiploidy) and by a clinically applicable reverse PCR method (to detect translocations resulting in chimeric transcription factors or *BCR-ABL* rearrangements). Thus, at St. Jude Children's Research Hospital, leukemic blast cells from each new case of childhood ALL are examined for the ploidy of leukemic stem lines and for intermediate-risk (*E2A-PBX1*), high-risk (*HRX/ALL1/MLL*), or ultra-high-risk (*BCR-ABL*) fusion transcripts (Table 67-3). Flow cytometry and reverse PCR are complementary techniques offering the greatest likelihood of identifying clinically useful cytogenetic abnormalities in leukemic cells.

Our analysis of patients treated in St. Jude Total Therapy Study X revealed that a leukemic cell DNA index >1.16, corresponding to >53 chromosomes per leukemic cell by standard cytogenetic analysis, conferred the most favorable prognosis of any clinical or biologic feature analyzed.[260–262] These findings were particularly striking in a subset of patients treated with intravenous-intrathecal (IVIT) methotrexate in addition to prednisone, L-asparaginase, vincristine, and 6-mercaptopurine—a regimen characterized by modest acute toxicity and virtually none of the serious delayed effects associated with cranial irradiation and genotoxic drugs, such as cyclophosphamide, epipodophyllotoxins, and anthracyclines.

With this so-called IVIT therapy, 89% of the patients whose blasts had a DNA index >1.16 remained in continuous complete remission for 3 years, and 82% for 5 years. Therefore, one should be able to use this measurement of cellular DNA content to select a subgroup of children with ALL who might be spared the toxicity of highly aggressive treatment programs. To test this concept, we collaborated with other members of the Pedi-

Table 67-3. Clinical Risk Assignment in Childhood ALL by Genetic Characterization of Leukemic Lymphoblasts

Abnormality (Risk)	Method of Detection	Therapy
Hyperdiploidy (DNA index >1.16; >53 chromosomes per blast cell) (good risk)	DNA flow cytometry	Antimetabolite therapy emphasizing high-dose methotrexate
E2A-PBX1 fusion genes due to t(1;19) translocation (intermediate risk)	Reverse PCR to detect E2A-PBX1 fusion transcripts	Intensified chemotherapy based on alkylating agents and topoisomerase II inhibitors
HRX/ALL1/MLL fusion genes due to 11q23 translocations (high risk)	Reverse PCR to detect HRX/ALL1/MLL fusion transcripts	Experimental chemotherapy or bone marrow transplantation
BCR-ABL fusion genes due to t(9;22) (ultra-high risk)	Reverse PCR to detect BCR/ABL fusion transcripts	Bone marrow transplantation in first remission

atric Oncology Group to study 1,000 children who had received antimetabolite-based therapy similar to that in the St. Jude trial. Again, a DNA index of >1.16 was the most important prognostic feature, defining a good-risk subgroup with a 3-year relapse-free survival probability of 90%[263] (Fig. 67-4). These children were 12 times less likely to fail than were those with lower blast cell DNA indexes. We now recommend a risk-oriented protocol design in which children with a favorable DNA index are treated exclusively with antimetabolites, whereas others receive more intensive chemotherapy.

In the initial reports of chromosomal abnormalities and leukemia prognosis, virtually all translocations were thought to carry an increased risk of treatment failure in childhood ALL.[139] With improvements in therapy, however, several groups showed that the adverse prognostic influence of most chromosomal rearrangements is nullified by the greater cytoreductive effects of intensified chemotherapy.[23,264,265] Thus, one should be concerned primarily with the translocations listed in Table 67-3. Our approach has been to distinguish cases of t(1;19)-positive B-lineage ALL with E2A-PBX1 fusion transcripts from those without such transcripts, as the former have a poor prognosis on antimetabolite-based chemotherapy, whereas the latter respond well. The detection of E2A-PBX1 transcripts is particularly important, because patients whose lymphoblasts harbor this gene fusion respond well to more intensive chemo-

therapy regimens emphasizing rotational treatment with epipodophyllotoxins and other genotoxic drugs.[22,23] We have now extended this approach to detect fusion transcripts that result from the t(4;11) (Downing, J, personal communication), which have been variously termed HRX-FEL, ALL1-AF4, and MLL-PBM1.[123-125,131] The reverse PCR assay is particularly well-suited for this purpose, because a small amount of leukemic cell RNA can be used to prepare a universal first-strand cDNA with random primers, and the various fusion transcripts can be detected by PCR with specific oligonucleotide primers. In contrast to the t(1;19), 11q23 translocations and the Philadelphia chromosome [t(9;22)] confer a uniformly high risk of treatment failure, regardless of the chemotherapy program. Thus, cases with PCR evidence of BCR-ABL hybrid transcripts (a consequence of the 9;22 translocation), and possibly 11q23 translocations, should be considered for bone marrow transplantation in first remission.

Therapy Targeted to Oncogenic Transcription Factors

Elucidation of the leukemia-inducing pathways of aberrantly controlled transcription factors has provided a mechanistic underpinning for the positive responses of acute promyelo-

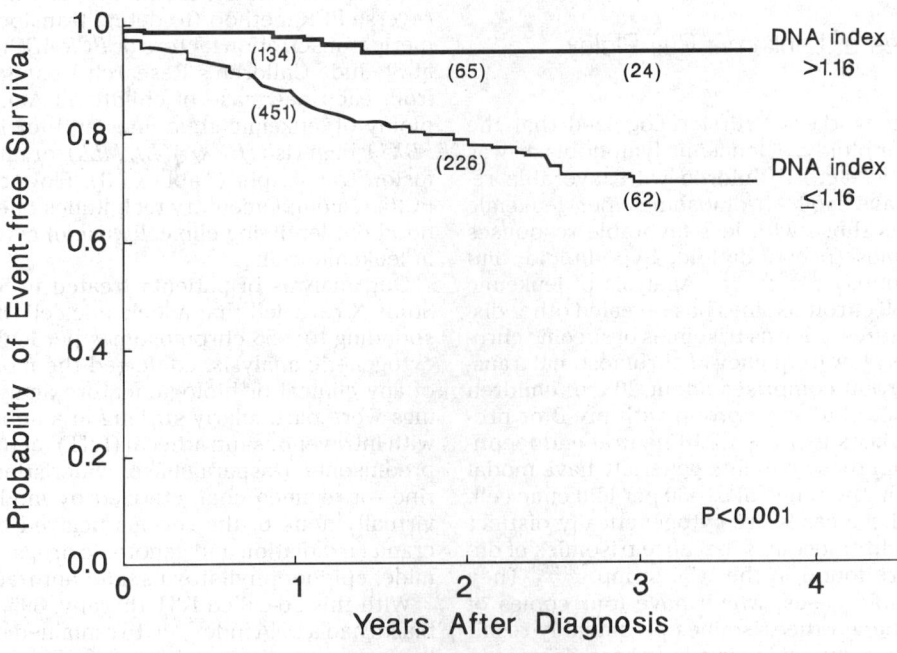

Fig. 67-4. Relation of chromosome number (ploidy) to treatment outcome in patients with B-cell precursor ALL. In this Pediatric Oncology Group clinical trial, patients were segregated according to a lymphoblast DNA index of ≤1.16 or >1.16 (equivalent to 53 chromosomes per leukemic cell). Treatment consisted essentially of antimetabolites and agents without known genotoxic effects. Event-free survival was significantly better for the hyperdiploid group, demonstrating the value of this cytogenetic measure in treatment planning.

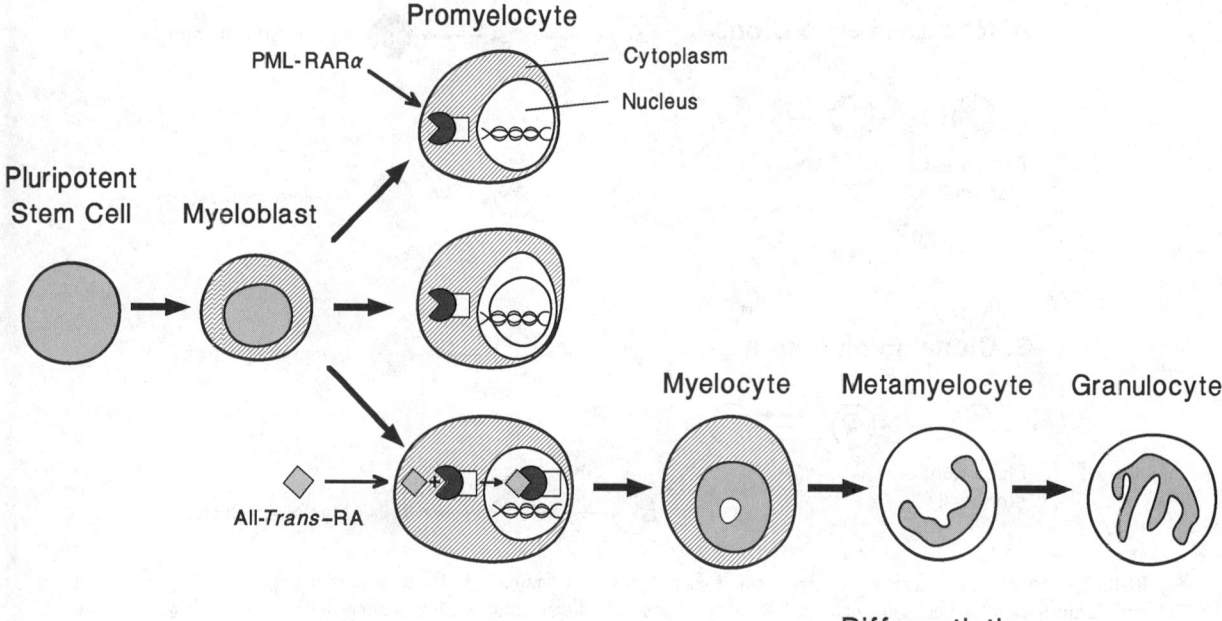

Fig. 67-5. All-trans-retinoic acid (RA) therapy for APL expressing PML-RARα fusion proteins. In patients with this form of AML, the t(15; 17) rearrangement produces a fusion protein, PML-RARα, whose ligand binding domain is specific for α-retinoic acid. As PML-RARα proteins accumulate in the cytoplasm of promyelocytes, they interfere with normal cell development, leading to leukemic conversion. By treating patients with pharmacologic doses of the retinoid compound, which binds to PML-RARα causing nuclear localization of the protein, it has been possible to induce leukemic promyelocytes to differentiate into mature cells with a finite life span. This advance illustrates the potential of transcription factor modulation as a mode of therapy for the human leukemias.

cytic leukemia (APL) patients to therapy with all-trans-retinoic acid.[266–269] The vast majority of leukemias with this morphologic feature have a t(15;17) that produces PML-RARα fusion proteins, whose DNA and ligand binding domains, encoded by the α-retinoic acid receptor gene on chromosome 17, are linked to amino acids encoded by the *PML* gene on chromosome 15.[270–274] PML-RARα fusion proteins are expressed in the cytoplasm and appear to interfere with normal myeloid cell development, leading to arrested differentiation in the promyelocyte stage, possibly through a dominant negative mechanism.[273–275] In response to pharmacologic doses of all-trans-retinoic acid, the fusion proteins are translocated into the nucleus, and the leukemic cells differentiate into mature myeloid cells with a limited life span[269] (Fig. 67-5). This therapy is specific for APL blasts that express PML-RARα fusion proteins; it is ineffective for other types of myeloid leukemia. Although resistance to all-trans-retinoic acid develops quickly, within 3–4 months on the average, this specific modulator of PML-RARα chimeric receptors has proved a useful adjunct to cytotoxic chemotherapy for inducing remissions in APL patients.

Whether knowledge of the mechanisms of action of other chimeric or dysregulated leukemogenic transcriptional control proteins will lead to improved therapy is difficult to answer. Unfortunately, most transcription factors do not contain convenient ligand binding domains, so the model provided by chimeric PML-RARα proteins in APL will be difficult to reproduce in leukemias with the activated transcription factor genes listed in Table 67-1. Nonetheless, new drugs may be found that interfere with the modulation of gene expression by specific transcription factors and lack many of the side effects of available cytotoxic agents. Other approaches, such as antisense strategies to block chimeric transcripts and gene therapy to introduce dominant negative inhibitors of protein-protein or protein-DNA interactions essential for transcription factor function, could yield novel therapies.

AML DEVELOPING AFTER THERAPY FOR ALL

In most cases of relapsed ALL, there are minor shifts in phenotypic markers and karyotypes, but these changes do not interfere with recognition of the original stem line. Thus, one is tempted to conclude that relapse uniformly signals the emergence of drug-resistant variants of the original malignant clone. Yet, the data supporting this interpretation are incomplete and do not reflect systematic multimarker analysis of leukemic cells at diagnosis and relapse. An emerging set of observations indicates that intensive chemotherapy can induce second lymphoid or myeloid malignancies.[276–278]

Clinical and Biologic Aspects

With wider use of genotoxic drugs in recent clinical trials, coupled with the improved ability to detect cell lineage-associated phenotypic markers, an apparent increase has been observed in the number of secondary AMLs developing in patients with ALL.[122,279] Because of the ominous prognosis of secondary AML, Pui et al.[122,280] sought to establish its cumulative risk during initial remission and the probable mechanisms of its pathogenesis in a cohort of 734 children with ALL who achieved complete remission in the Total Therapy X and XI studies at St. Jude Children's Research Hospital. Secondary AML was identified by standard morphologic and cytochemical criteria in 21 patients, representing 10% of all initial hematologic relapses during continuous complete remission. The median time from the diagnosis of ALL to the development of AML was 40 months (range 15–100 months). The cumulative probability (95% confidence interval) that AML would develop in any child during initial hematologic remission was 3.8% (2.3–6.1%) at 6 years from diagnosis.

A constellation of presenting features related to T-cell ALL was associated with the development of secondary AML. How-

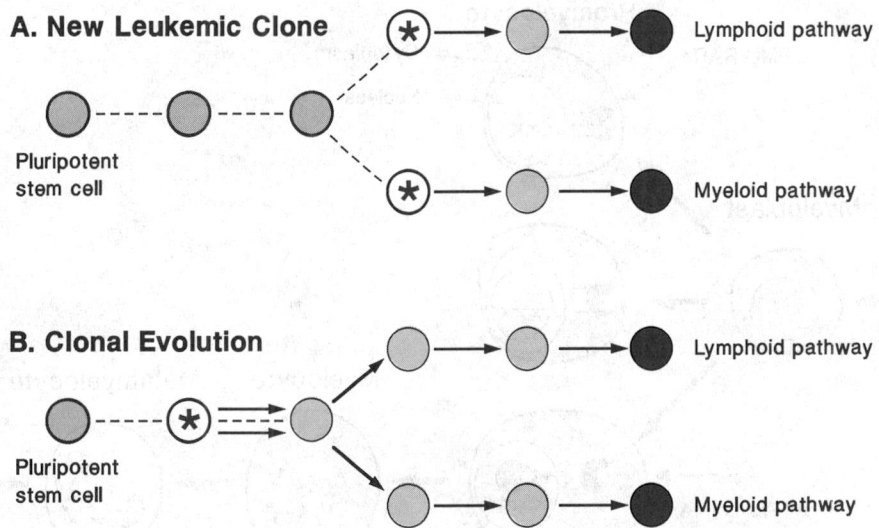

Fig. 67-6. Two hypotheses to account for the origin of secondary AML following ALL. **(A)** New leukemic clone and **(B)** clonal evolution. The transforming event is indicated by an asterisk, with subsequent differentiation leading to either a lymphoid or a myeloid leukemia.

ever, after adjustment for the competing effects of multiple covariates, only prolonged administration of epipodophyllotoxin therapy (teniposide with or without etoposide) retained statistical significance. The authors concluded that the risk of epipodophyllotoxin-related AML depends largely on the schedule of drug administration, irrespective of the total drug dosage or the initial features of the leukemic blasts.

None of the 21 cases had a loss of DNA from chromosome 5 or 7, a karyotypic change commonly observed in treatment-related AML developing in patients with Hodgkin disease or other solid tumors.[281–287] Blast cells from 16 patients had abnormalities of the 11q23 chromosomal region, which have been linked to malignant transformation of pluripotential stem cells. Importantly, the t(9;11)(p21;q23) associated with AML in 7 of the patients has been identified in patients who developed AML after treatment for solid tumors that included an epipodophyllotoxin.[288–290]

Attempts to reinduce and maintain complete remissions in patients with secondary AML included use of anthracycline antibiotics, cytarabine, and other agents commonly employed in therapy for AML. Two patients died before or shortly after reinduction therapy was begun. Of the 13 patients who attained a second complete remission, only 2 remain free of leukemia. Thus, bone marrow transplantation appears warranted for patients with this complication and a histocompatible donor.

Do Secondary AMLs Arise from an Independent Clone

The finding that ALL patients may develop AML as the primary cause of treatment failure raises questions about clonality in relation to the basic mechanisms of leukemogenesis. Of the 21 secondary AML cases reported by Pui et al.,[122,280] 18 were fully characterized cytogenetically both at the time of diagnosis and at relapse. In 9 of these cases, completely new karyotypic abnormalities were found in the AML clones with no evidence of retention of the abnormalities in ALL clones. A second piece of evidence is that sequential studies have shown clonal rearrangement of the immunoglobin heavy chain genes in three of the ALLs and germline bands in the AMLs that arose in the same patients at relapse. These results clearly support the concept that certain antileukemic agents can induce AML in otherwise normal hematopoietic progenitors. Nonetheless, one cannot rule out the possibility that some cases of secondary AML arise from extreme clonal evolution.

Figure 67-6 illustrates two pathways for the emergence of secondary AML. In the first, the initial transformation event affects a committed lymphoid progenitor and leads to the development of lymphoid leukemia. A second, completely independent transformation event occurs in a committed myeloid progenitor, leading to secondary AML. The second explanation involves a form of clonal evolution. Cytogenetic and immunoglobulin gene rearrangement studies have already ruled out certain types of lineage switching options, but it is still possible that the transformation event occurs in a stem cell that has not committed to differentiate in either the lymphoid or myeloid pathway. At diagnosis, differentiation of the transformed clone is directed through the lymphoid pathway leading to a lymphoid leukemia. According to this model, lymphoid phenotype-specific chromosomal translocations and immunoglobulin or TCR gene rearrangements occur as the transformed cell differentiates through the lymphoid lineage. At relapse, it is possible that the same transformed progenitor develops new secondary events, including an 11q23 breakpoint translocation, and differentiates along the myeloid lineage to yield a myeloid leukemia.

Whether these new leukemias represent unusual evolution of the original clone or induction of a second malignancy cannot be determined by standard phenotyping and cytogenetic analysis alone. Studies are needed to examine the clonality of relapsed AML, using methylation-sensitive X-chromosome-linked RFLPs[7,291,292] to detect X chromosome inactivation in female patients. This approach should provide direct evidence regarding the frequency of each mode of transformation.

Systematic analysis of the immunophenotype, karyotype, and immunoglobulin and TCR gene rearrangements in leukemic cells from ALL patients, both at diagnosis and relapse, should help to resolve key questions related to the biology of recurrent leukemia. Are the patterns of clonal evolution in patients who relapse on therapy similar to those of children relapsing off treatment? That is, do changes in phenotype reflect the development of drug-resistant variants within the leukemic clone? Does phenotypic shift correlate with the sensitivity of a patient's blast cells to a second course of chemotherapy? If different subclones are evident at diagnosis, which will be suppressed by chemotherapy and which will emerge at relapse?

FUTURE DIRECTIONS

Better treatment based on the molecular biology of ALL is clearly a priority for the future, and will likely take the form of targeted therapies described in the preceding section. More immediate applications of the emerging molecular information would include a redefinition of risk factors to emphasize somatically acquired genetic abnormalities that carry a defined risk of therapeutic failure. Currently, patients are assigned to treatment according to their initial clinical features and, in isolated instances, the biologic properties of their leukemic cells. We are now in a position to begin to view ALL as a group of heterogeneous diseases defined by discrete molecular lesions. Once these lesions are identified and characterized for larger numbers of patients, it should be possible to devise a new classification of ALL that will reflect prognosis with exquisite precision.

It will also be important to refine the current definition of complete remission by using molecular techniques to detect minimal residual disease. Although PCR will amplify DNA sequences unique to the malignant clone, such as chimeric gene transcripts, it can be difficult to quantify the numbers of residual leukemia cells, especially with RNA-based PCR assays. Fluorescence in situ hybridization with chromosome-specific probes and strategies to detect aberrant patterns of phenotypic markers can be used to augment results obtained with PCR. As additional probes are made available through molecular genetic research now under way, consistent recognition and monitoring of minimal residual leukemia should become an attainable goal.

ACKNOWLEDGMENTS

I would like to thank John Gilbert for editorial review and critical comments.

Supported in part by Cancer Center Support (CORE) grant CA-21765, Leukemia Program Project grant CA-20180, and by the American Lebanese Syrian Associated Charities (ALSAC).

REFERENCES

1. Greaves MF: Differentiation-linked leukemogenesis in lymphocytes. Science 234:697, 1986
2. Rabbits TH: Translocations, master genes, and differences between the origins of acute and chronic leukemias. Cell 67:641, 1991
3. Cleary ML: Oncogenic conversion of transcription factors by chromosomal translocations. Cell 66:619, 1991
4. Alimena G: Fourth International Workshop on Chromosomes in Leukemia, 1982. Karyotypic patterns in multiple clones. Cancer Genet Cytogenet 11:322, 1984
5. Raskind WR, Fialkow PJ: The use of cell markers in the study of human hematopoietic neoplasia. Adv Cancer Res 49:127, 1987
6. Dow LW, Martin P, Moohr J et al: Evidence for clonal development of childhood acute lymphoblastic leukemia. Blood 66:902, 1985
7. Pui C-H, Raskind WH, Kitchingman GR et al: Clonal analysis of childhood acute lymphoblastic leukemia with "cytogenetically independent" cell populations. J Clin Invest 83:1971, 1989
8. Hurwitz CA, Loken MR, Graham ML et al: Asynchronous antigen expression in B-lineage acute lymphoblastic leukemia. Blood 72:299, 1988
9. Crist WM, Grossi CE, Pullen J, Cooper MD: Immunologic markers in childhood acute lymphocytic leukemia. Semin Oncol 12:105, 1985
10. Bennett JM, Catovsky D, Daniel MT et al: Morphological classification of acute lymphoblastic leukaemia: concordance among observers and clinical correlations. Br J Haematol 47:553, 1981
11. Magrath IT, Ziegler JL: Bone marrow involvement in Burkitt's lymphoma and its relationship to acute B-cell leukemia. Leuk Res 4:33, 1979
12. Murphy SB, Bowman WP, Abomowitch M et al: Results of treatment of advanced-stage Burkitt's lymphoma and B-cell (SIg+) acute lymphoblastic leukemia with high-dose fractionated cyclophosphamide and coordinated high-dose methotrexate and cytarabine. J Clin Oncol 4:1732, 1986
13. Letarte M, Vera S, Tran R et al: Common acute lymphoblastic leukemia antigen is identical to neutral endopeptidase. J Exp Med 168:1247, 1988
14. Jongeneel CV, Quackenbush EJ, Ronco P et al: Common acute lymphoblastic leukemia antigen expressed on leukemia and melanoma cell lines has neutral endopeptidase activity. J Clin Invest 830:713, 1989
15. Shipp MA, Vijayaraghavan J, Schmidt EV et al: Common acute lymphoblastic leukemia antigen (CALLA) is active neutral endopeptidase 24.11 ("enkepha-

16. Bollum J: Terminal deoxynucleotidyl transferase as a hematopoietic cell marker. Blood 54:1203, 1979
17. Civin CI, Strauss LC, Brovall C et al: Antigenic analysis of hematopoiesis. III. Hematopoietic progenitor cell surface antigen defined by a monoclonal antibody raised against KG-1a cells. J Immunol 133:157, 1984
18. Borowitz MJ, Shuster JJ, Civin CI et al: Prognostic significance of CD34 expression in childhood B-precursor acute lymphocytic leukemia: a Pediatric Oncology Group study. J Clin Oncol 8:1389, 1990
19. Vogler LB, Crist WM, Bockman DE et al: Pre B-cell leukemia: a new phenotype of childhood lymphoblastic leukemia. N Engl J Med 298:872, 1978
20. Vogler LB, Crist WM, Sarrif AM et al: An analysis of clinical and laboratory features of acute lymphocytic leukemias with emphasis on 35 children with pre-B leukemia. Blood 58:135, 1981
21. Crist WM, Carroll AJ, Shuster JJ et al: The poor prognosis of children with pre-B acute lymphoblastic leukemia (ALL) is associated with the t(1;19)(q23;p13). Blood 74:1970, 1989
22. Raimondi SC, Behm FG, Roberson PK et al: Cytogenetics of pre-B-cell acute lymphoblastic leukemia with emphasis on prognostic implications of the t(1;19). J Clin Oncol 8:1380, 1990
23. Rivera GK, Raimondi SC, Hancock ML et al: Improved outcome in childhood acute lymphoblastic leukaemia with reinforced early treatment and rotational combination chemotherapy. Lancet 337:61, 1991
24. Korsmeyer SJ, Hieter PA, Ravetch JV et al: Developmental hierarchy of immunoglobulin gene rearrangements in human leukemic pre-B-cells. Proc Natl Acad Sci USA 78:7096, 1981
25. Korsmeyer SJ, Arnold A, Bakshi A et al: Immunoglobulin gene rearrangement and cell surface antigen expression in acute lymphocytic leukemias of T-cell and B-cell precursor origins. J Clin Invest 71:301, 1983
26. Nadler LM, Korsmeyer SJ, Anderson KC et al: B cell origin of non-T cell acute lymphoblastic leukemia. A model for discrete stages of neoplastic and normal pre-B cell differentiation. J Clin Invest 74:332, 1984
27. Kitchingman GR, Rovigatti U, Mauer AM et al: Rearrangement of immunoglobulin heavy chain genes in T-cell acute lymphoblastic leukemia. Blood 65:725, 1985
28. Ford AM, Molgaard HV, Greaves MF, Gould HJ: Immunoglobulin gene organization and expression in haemopoietic stem cell leukaemia. EMBO J 2:997, 1983
29. Ha K, Minden M, Hozumi N, Gelfand EW: Immunoglobulin mu-chain gene rearrangement in a patient with T-cell acute lymphoblastic leukemia. J Clin Invest 73:1232, 1984
30. Rovigatti U, Mirro J, Kitchingman G et al: Heavy chain immunoglobulin gene rearrangement in acute nonlymphocytic leukemia. Blood 63:1023, 1984
31. Ha K, Minden M, Hozumi N, Gelfand EW: Immunoglobulin gene rearrangement in acute myelogenous leukemia. Cancer Res 44:4658, 1984
32. Palumbo A, Minowada J, Erikson J et al: Lineage infidelity of a human myelogenous leukemia cell line. Blood 64:1059, 1984
33. Reinherz EL, Schlossman SF: The differentiation and function of human T lymphocytes. Cell 19:821, 1980
34. Reinherz EL, Schlossman SF: Current concepts in immunology: regulation of the immune response-inducer and suppressor T-lymphocyte subsets in human beings. N Engl J Med 303:370, 1980
35. Roper M, Crist WM, Metzgar R et al: Monoclonal antibody characterization of surface antigens in childhood T-cell lymphoid malignancies. Blood 61:830, 1983
36. Reinherz EL, Nadler LM, Sallan SE, Schlossman SF: Subset derivation of T-cell acute lymphoblastic leukemia in man. J Clin Invest 64:392, 1979
37. Nadler LM, Reinherz RL, Weinstein HJ et al: Heterogeneity of T-cell lymphoblastic malignancies. Blood 55:806, 1980
38. Bernard A, Boumsell L, Reinherz EL et al: Cell surface characterization of malignant T-cell from lymphoblastic lymphoma using monoclonal antibodies: Evidence for phenotypic differences between malignant T-cells from patients with acute lymphoblastic leukemia and lymphoblastic lymphoma. Blood 57:1105, 1981
39. Koziner B, Gebhard D, Denny T et al: Analysis of T-cell differentiation antigens in acute lymphatic leukemia using monoclonal antibodies. Blood 60:752, 1982
40. Clavel LA, Gelber RD, Cohen HJ et al: Four-agent induction and intensive asparaginase therapy for treatment of childhood acute lymphoblastic leukemia. N Engl J Med 315:657, 1986
41. Dahl GV, Rivera GK, Look AT et al: Teniposide (VM-26) plus cytarabine improves outcome in childhood acute lymphoblastic leukemia presenting with a very high leukocyte count greater than or equal to 100×10^9/L. J Clin Oncol 5:1015, 1987
42. Pullen DJ, Sullivan MP, Falletta JM et al: Modified LSA_2L_2 treatment in 53

children with E-rosette-positive T-cell leukemia: results and prognostic factors. Blood 60:1159, 1982

43. Waldmann TA, Davis MM, Bongioanni KF, Korsmeyer SJ: Rearrangements of genes for the antigen receptor on T-cell receptor in T-cell chronic lymphocytic leukemia and related disorders. N Engl J Med 313:776, 1985

44. Toyonaga B, Yanagi Y, Suciu-Foca N et al: Rearrangements of T-cell receptor gene YT35 in human DNA from thymic leukemia T-cell lines and functional T-cell clones. Nature 311:385, 1984

45. Waldmann TA: The arrangement of immunoglobulin and T-cell receptor genes in human lymphoproliferative disorders. Adv Immunol 40:247, 1987

46. Pelicci P-G, Knowles DM II, Dalla-Favera R: Lymphoid tumors displaying rearrangements of both immunoglobulin and T cell receptor genes. J Exp Med 162:1015, 1985

47. Tawa A, Hozumi N, Minden M et al: Rearrangement of T-cell receptor B-chain gene in non-T-cell, non-B-cell acute lymphoblastic leukemia of childhood. N Engl J Med 313:1033, 1985

48. O'Connor NTJ, Weatherall DJ, Feller AC et al: Rearrangement of the T cell-receptor B-chain gene in the diagnosis of lymphoproliferative disorders. Lancet 1:1295, 1985

49. Asou N, Matsuoka M, Hattori T et al: T-cell gamma gene rearrangements in hematologic neoplasms. Blood 69:968, 1987

50. Tkachuk DC, Griesser H, Takihara Y et al: Rearrangement of T-cell delta locus in lymphoproliferative disorders. Blood 72:353, 1988

51. Mirro J, Zipf TF, Pui C-H et al: Acute mixed lineage leukemia: clinicopathologic correlations and prognostic significance. Blood 66:1115, 1985

52. Sobol RE, Mick R, Royston I et al: Clinical importance of myeloid antigen expression of adult acute lymphoblastic leukemia. N Engl J Med 316:1111, 1987

53. Pui C-H, Behm FG, Singh B et al: Myeloid-associated antigen expression lacks prognostic value in childhood acute lymphoblastic leukemia treated with intensive multiagent chemotherapy. Blood 75:198, 1990

54. Smith LJ, Curtis JE, Messner HA et al: Lineage infidelity in acute leukemia. Blood 61:1138, 1983

55. Pui C-H, Dahl GV, Melvin S et al: Acute leukaemia with mixed lymphoid and myeloid phenotype. Br J Haematol 56:121, 1984

56. Cross AH, Goorha RM, Nuss R et al: Acute myeloid leukemia with T-lymphoid features: a distinct biologic and clinical entity. Blood 72:579, 1988

57. Greaves MF, Chan LC, Furley AJW et al: Lineage promiscuity in hemopoietic differentiation and leukemia. Blood 67:1, 1986

58. Williams DL, Look AT, Melvin SL et al: New chromosomal translocations correlate with specific immunophenotypes of childhood acute lymphoblastic leukemia. Cell 36:101, 1984

59. Pui C-H, Crist WM, Look AT: Biology and clinical significance of cytogenetic abnormalities in childhood acute lymphoblastic leukemia. Blood 76:1449, 1990

60. Solomon E, Borrow J, Goddard AD: Chromosome aberrations and cancer. Science 254:1153, 1991

61. Adams JM, Gerondakis S, Webb E et al: Cellular *myc* oncogene is altered by chromosome translocation to an immunoglobulin locus in murine plasmacytomas and is rearranged similarly in Burkitt lymphomas. Proc Natl Acad Sci USA 80:1982, 1983

62. Dalla-Favera R, Bregni M, Erikson J et al: Human c-myc onc gene is located on the region of chromosome 8 that is translocated in Burkitt lymphoma cells. Proc Natl Acad Sci USA 79:7824, 1982

63. Taub R, Kirsch I, Morton C et al: Translocation of the c-myc gene into the immunoglobulin heavy chain locus in human Burkitt lymphoma and murine plasmacytoma cells. Proc Natl Acad Sci USA 79:7837, 1982

64. Emanuel BS, Selden JR, Chaganti RSK et al: The 2p breakpoint of a 2;8 translocation in Burkitt lymphoma interrupts the V kappa locus. Proc Natl Acad Sci USA 81:2444, 1984

65. Erikson J, Nishikura K, ar-Rushdi A et al: Translocation of an immunoglobulin kappa locus to a region 3′ of an unrearranged c-myc oncogene enhances c-myc transcription. Proc Natl Acad Sci USA 80:7581, 1983

66. Hollis GF, Mitchell KF, Battey J et al: A variant translocation places the lambda immunoglobulin genes 3′ to the c-myc oncogene in Burkitt's lymphoma. Nature 307:752, 1984

67. Rappold GA, Hameister H, Cremer T et al: c-myc and immunoglobulin kappa light chain constant genes are on the 8q + chromosome of three Burkitt lymphoma lines with t(2;8) translocations. EMBO J 3:2951, 1984

68. Croce CM, Thierfelder W, Erikson J et al: Transcriptional activation of an unrearranged and untranslocated c-myc oncogene by translocation of a C lambda locus in Burkitt. Proc Natl Acad Sci USA 80:6922, 1983

69. Taub R, Kelly K, Battey J et al: A novel alteration in the structure of an activated c-myc gene in a variant t(2;8) Burkitt lymphoma. Cell 37:511, 1984

70. Abrams HD, Rohrschneider LR, Eisenman RN: Nuclear location of the putative transforming protein of avian myelocytomatosis virus. Cell 29:427, 1982

71. Blanchard JM, Piechaczyk M, Dani C et al: C-*myc* gene is transcribed at high rate in G_0-arrested fibroblasts and is post-transcriptionally regulated in response to growth factors. Nature 317:443, 1985

72. Donner P, Greiser-Wilke I, Moelling K: Nuclear localization and DNA binding of the transforming gene product of avian myelocytomatosis virus. Nature 296:262, 1982

73. Evans GI, Hancock DC: Studies on the interaction of the human c-*myc* protein with cell nuclei: p62 c-*myc* as a member of a discrete subset of nuclear proteins. Cell 43:253, 1985

74. Kelly K, Cochran BH, Stiles CD, Leder P: Cell-specific regulation of the c-*myc* gene by lymphocyte mitogens and platelet-derived growth factor. Cell 35:603, 1983

75. Armelin HA, Armelin MC, Kelly K: Functional role for c-*myc* in mitogenic response to platelet-derived growth factor. Nature 310:655, 1984

76. Adams JM, Harris AW, Pinkert CA et al: The c-*myc* oncogene driven by immunoglobulin enhancers induces lymphoid malignancy in transgenic mice. Nature 318:533, 1985

77. Langdon WY, Harris AW, Cory S, Adams JM: The c-*myc* oncogene perturbs B lymphocyte development in Emu-*myc* transgenic mice. Cell 47:11, 1986

78. Lombardi L, Newcomb EW, Dalla-Favera R: Pathogenesis of Burkitt lymphoma: expression of an activated c-*myc* oncogene causes the tumorigenic conversion of EBV-infected human B lymphoblasts. Cell 49:161, 1987

79. Finger LR, Harvey RC, Moore RC et al: A common mechanism of chromosomal translocation in T- and B-cell neoplasia. Science 234:982, 1986

80. McKeithan TW, Shima EA, Le Beau MM et al: Molecular cloning of the breakpoint junction of a human chromosomal 8;14 translocation involving the T-cell receptor alpha-chain gene and sequences on the 3′ side of MYC. Proc Natl Acad Sci USA 83:6636, 1986

81. Shima EA, Le Beau MM, McKeithan TW et al: Gene encoding the alpha chain of the T-cell receptor is moved immediately downstream of c-myc in a chromosomal 8;14 translocation in a cell line from a human T-cell leukemia. Proc Natl Acad Sci USA 83:3439, 1986

82. Begley CG, Aplan PD, Davey MP et al: Chromosomal translocation in a human leukemic stem-cell line disrupts the T-cell antigen receptor delta-chain diversity region and results in a previously unreported fusion transcript. Proc Natl Acad Sci USA 86:2031, 1989

83. Chen Q, Cheng JT, Tasi LH et al: The tal gene undergoes chromosome translocation in T cell leukemia and potentially encodes a helix-loop-helix protein. EMBO J 9:415, 1990

84. Xia Y, Brown L, Yang CY et al: TAL2, a helix-loop-helix gene activated by the (7;9)(q35;q34) translocation in human T-cell leukemia. Proc Natl Acad Sci USA 88:11416, 1991

85. Mellentin JD, Smith SD, Cleary ML: *lyl-l*, A novel gene altered by chromosomal translocation in T-cell leukemia, codes for a protein with a helix-loop-helix DNA binding motif. Cell 58:77, 1989

86. Lassar AB, Thayer MJ, Overell RW, Weintraub H: Transformation by activated ras or fos prevents myogenesis by inhibiting expression of MyoD1. Cell 58:659, 1989

87. Weintraub H, Tapscott SJ, Davis RL et al: Activation of muscle-specific genes in pigment, nerve, fat, liver, and fibroblast cell lines by forced expression of MyoD. Proc Natl Acad Sci USA 86:5434, 1989

88. McGuire EA, Hockett RD, Pollock KM et al: The t(11;14)(p15;q11) in a T-cell acute lymphoblastic leukemia cell line activates multiple transcripts, including *ttg-1*, a gene encoding a potential zinc finger protein. Mol Cell Biol 9:2124, 1989

89. Greenberg JM, Boehm T, Sofroniew MV et al: Segmental and developmental regulation of a presumptive T-cell oncogene in the central nervous system. Nature 344:158, 1990

90. Boehm T, Foroni L, Kaneko Y et al: The rhombotin family of cysteine-rich LIM-domain oncogenes: distinct members are involved in T-cell translocations to human chromosomes 11p15 and 11p13. Proc Natl Acad Sci USA 88:4367, 1991

91. Royer-Pokora B, Loos U, Ludwig WD: TTG-2, a new gene encoding a cysteine-rich protein with the LIM motif, is overexpressed in acute T-cell leukaemia with the t(11;14)(p13;q11). Oncogene 6:1887, 1991

92. Boehm T, Foroni L, Kennedy M, Rabbitts TH: The rhombotin gene belongs to a class of transcriptional regulators with a potential novel protein dimerization motif. Oncogene 5:1103, 1990

93. McGuire EA, Rintoul CE, Sclar GM, Korsmeyer SJ: Thymic overexpression of ttg-1 in transgenic mice results in T-cell acute lymphoblastic leukemia/lymphoma. Mol Cell Biol 12:4186, 1992

94. Hatano M, Roberts CW, Minden M et al: Deregulation of a homeobox gene, HOX11, by the t(10;14) in T cell leukemia. Science 253:79, 1991

95. Kennedy MA, Gonzalez-Sarmiento R, Kees UR et al: HOX11, a homeobox-containing T-cell oncogene on human chromosome 10q24. Proc Natl Acad Sci USA 88:8900, 1991

96. Lu M, Gong ZY, Shen WF, Ho AD: The tcl-3 proto-oncogene altered by chromosomal translocation in T-cell leukemia codes for a homeobox protein. EMBO J 10:2905, 1991
97. Dube ID, Kamel-Reid S, Yuan CC et al: A novel human homeobox gene lies at the chromosome 10 breakpoint in lymphoid neoplasias with chromosomal translocation t(10;14). Blood 78:2996, 1991
98. Allen JD, Lints T, Jenkins NA et al: Novel murine homeobox gene on chromosome 1 expressed in specific hematopoietic lineages and during embryogenesis. Genes Dev 5:509, 1991
99. Kamps MP, Look AT, Baltimore D: The human t(1;19) translocation in pre-B ALL produces multiple nuclear E2A-Pbx1 fusion proteins with differing transforming potentials. Genes Dev 5:358, 1991
100. Kamps MP, Baltimore D: E2A-Pbx1, the t(1;19) translocation protein of human pre-B-cell acute lymphocytic leukemia, causes acute myeloid leukemia in mice. Mol Cell Biol 13:351, 1993
101. Dedera DA, Waller EK, LeBrun DP et al: Chimeric homeobox gene E2A-PBX1 induces proliferation, apoptosis, and malignant lymphomas in transgenic mice. Cell 74:833, 1993
102. Privitera E, Kamps MP, Hayashi Y et al: Different molecular consequences of the 1;19 chromosomal translocation in childhood B-cell precursor acute lymphoblastic leukemia. Blood 79:1781, 1992
103. Hunger SP, Galili N, Carroll AJ et al: The t(1;19)(q23;p13) results in consistent fusion of E2A and PBX1 coding sequences in acute lymphoblastic leukemias. Blood 77:687, 1991
104. Inaba T, Roberts WM, Shapiro LH et al: Fusion of the leucine zipper gene HLF to the E2A gene in human acute B-lineage leukemia. Science 257:531, 1992
105. Hunger SP, Ohyashiki K, Toyama K, Cleary ML: HLF, a novel hepatic bZIP protein, shows altered DNA-binding properties following fusion to E2A in t(17;19) acute lymphoblastic leukemia. Genes Dev 6:1608, 1992
106. Vinson CR, Sigler PB, McKnight SL: Scissors-grip model for DNA recognition by a family of leucine zipper proteins. Science 246:911, 1989
107. Mueller CR, Maire P, Schibler U: DBP, a liver-enriched transcriptional activator, is expressed late in ontogeny and its tissue specificity is determined posttranscriptionally. Cell 61:279, 1990
108. Drolet DW, Scully KM, Simmons DM et al: TEF, a transcription factor expressed specifically in the anterior pituitary during embryogenesis, defines a new class of leucine zipper proteins. Genes Dev 5:1739, 1991
109. Mitelman F: Catalog of Chromosome Aberrations in Cancer. 4th Ed. Wiley-Liss, New York, 1988
110. Arthur DC, Bloomfield CD, Linquist LL, Nesbit ME Jr: Translocation 4;11 in acute lymphoblastic leukemia: clinical characteristics and prognostic significance. Blood 59:96, 1982
111. Chromosomal abnormalities and their clinical significance in acute lymphoblastic leukemia. Third International Workshop on Chromosomes in Leukemia. Cancer Res 43:868, 1983
112. Parkin JL, Arthur DC, Abramson CS et al: Acute leukemia associated with the t(4;11) chromosome rearrangement: ultrastructural and immunologic characteristics. Blood 60:1321, 1982
113. Crist WM, Cleary ML, Grossi CE et al: Acute leukemias associated with the 4;11 chromosome translocation have arranged immunoglobulin heavy chain genes. Blood 66:33, 1985
114. Mirro J, Kitchingman G, Willimas D et al: Clinical and laboratory characteristics of acute leukemia with the 4;11 translocation. Blood 67:689, 1986
115. Nagasaka M, Maeda S, Maeda H et al: Four cases of t(4;11) acute leukemia and its myelomonocytic nature in infants. Blood 61:1174, 1983
116. Stong RC, Korsmeyer SJ, Parkin JL et al: Human acute leukemia cell line with the t(4;11) chromosomal rearrangement exhibits B-lineage and monocytic characteristics. Blood 65:21, 1985
117. Bloomfield CD, Goldman AL, Berger AR et al: Chromosomal abnormalities identify high-risk and low-risk patients with acute lymphoblastic leukemia. Blood 67:415, 1986
118. Diaz MO, Le Beau MM, Pitha P, Rowley JD: Interferon and c-ets-1 genes in the translocation (9;11) (p22;q23) in human acute monocytic leukemia. Science 231:265, 1986
119. Fourth International Workshop on Chromosomes in Leukemia: A prospective study of acute nonlymphocytic leukemia. Cancer Genet Cytogenet 11:249, 1984
120. Abe R, Sandberg AA: Significance of abnormalities involving chromosomal segment 11q22-25 in acute leukemia. Cancer Genet Cytogenet 13:121, 1984
121. Pui C-H, Raimondi SC, Murphy SB et al: An analysis of leukemic cell chromosomal features in infants. Blood 69:1289, 1987
122. Pui C-H, Behm FG, Raimondi SC et al: Secondary acute myeloid leukemia in children treated for acute lymphoid leukemia. N Engl J Med 321:136, 1989
123. Morrissey J, Tkachuk DC, Milatovich A et al: A serine/proline-rich protein is fused to HRX in t(4;11) acute leukemias. Blood 81:1124, 1993
124. Tkachuk DC, Kohler S, Cleary ML: Involvement of a homolog of Drosophila trithorax by 11q23 chromosomal translocations in acute leukemias. Cell 71:691, 1992
125. Gu Y, Nakamura T, Alder H et al: The t(4;11) chromosome translocation of human acute leukemias fuses the ALL-1 gene, related to Drosophila trithorax, to the AF-4 gene. Cell 71:701, 1992
126. Rowley JD, Diaz MO, Espinosa R et al: Mapping chromosome band 11q23 in human acute leukemia with biotinylated probes: identification of 11q23 translocation breakpoints with a yeast artificial chromosome. Proc Natl Acad Sci USA 87:9358, 1990
127. Ziemin-van der Poel S, McCabe NR, Gill HJ et al: Identification of a gene, MLL, that spans the breakpoint in 11q23 translocations associated with human leukemias. Proc Natl Acad Sci USA 86:10735, 1991
128. Djabali M, Selleri L, Parry P et al: A trithorax-like gene is interrupted by chromosome 11q23 translocations in acute leukemias. Nature Genet 2:113, 1992
129. Mazo AM, Huang DH, Mozer BA, Dawid IB: The trithorax gene, a trans-acting regulator of the bithorax-complex in Drosophila, encodes a protein with zinc-binding domains. Proc Natl Acad Sci USA 87:2112, 1990
130. Gu Y, Cimino G, Alder H et al: The t(4;11)(q21;q23) chromosome translocations in acute leukemias involve the VDJ recombinase. Proc Natl Acad Sci USA 89:10464, 1992
131. Domer PH, Fakharzadeh SS, Chen CS et al: Acute mixed-lineage leukemia t(4;11)(q21;q23) generates an MLL-AF4 fusion product. Proc Natl Acad Sci USA 90:7884, 1993
132. Nusslein-Volhard C, Wieschaus E: Mutations affecting segment number and polarity in Drosophila. Nature 287:795, 1980
133. Nusslein-Volhard C, Frohnhofer HG, Lehmann R: Determination of antero-posterior polarity in Drosophila. Science 238:1675, 1987
134. Levine MS, Harding KW: Drosophila: the zygotic contribution. p 39. In Glover DM, Hames BD (eds): Genes and Embryos. IRL, New York, 1989
135. Rowley JD: Biological implications of consistent chromosome rearrangements in leukemia and lymphoma. Cancer Res 44:3159, 1984
136. Ribeiro RC, Abromowitch M, Raimondi SC et al: Clinical and biologic hallmarks of the Philadelphia chromosome in childhood acute lymphoblastic leukemia. Blood 70:948, 1987
137. Champlin RE, Golde DW: Chronic myelogenous leukemia: recent advances. Blood 65:1039, 1985
138. Jain K, Arlin Z, Mertelsmann R et al: Philadelphia chromosome and terminal transferase-positive acute leukemia: similarity of terminal phase of chronic myelogenous leukemia and de novo acute presentation. J Clin Oncol 1:669, 1983
139. Williams DL, Harber J, Murphy SB et al: Chromosomal translocation play a unique role in influencing prognosis in childhood acute lymphoblastic leukemia. Blood 68:205, 1986
140. Heisterkamp N, Stephenson JR, Groffen J et al: Localization of the c-abl oncogene adjacent to a translocation breakpoint in chronic myelocytic leukaemia. Nature 306:239, 1983
141. Leibowitz D, Schaefer-Rego K, Popenoe DW et al: Variable breakpoints on the Philadelphia chromosome in chronic myelogenous leukemia. Blood 66:243, 1985
142. Grosveld G, Verwoerd T, van Agthoven T et al: The chronic myelocytic cell line K562 contains a breakpoint in bcr and produces a chimeric bcr/c-abl transcript. Mol Cell Biol 6:607, 1986
143. Groffen J, Stephenson JR, Heisterkamp N et al: Philadelphia chromosomal breakpoints are clustered within a limited region, bcr, on chromosome 22. Cell 36:93, 1984
144. Heisterkamp N, Stam K, Groffen J et al: Structural organization of the bcr gene and its role in Ph[1] translocation. Nature 315:758, 1985
145. Gale RP, Canaani E: An 8-kilobase abl RNA transcript in chronic myelogenous leukemia. Proc Natl Acad Sci USA 81:5648, 1984
146. Collins SJ, Kubonishi I, Miyoshi I, Groudine MT: Altered transcription of the c-abl oncogene in K562 and other chronic myelogenous leukemia cells. Science 225:72, 1984
147. Stam K, Heisterkamp N, Grosveld G et al: Evidence of a new chimeric bcr/c-abl mRNA in patients with chronic myelocytic leukemia and the Philadelphia chromosome. N Engl J Med 313:1429, 1985
148. Canaani E, Gale RP, Steiner-Saltz D et al: Altered transcription of an oncogene in chronic myeloid leukemia. Lancet 1:593, 1984
149. Shtivelman E, Lifshitz B, Gale RP, Canaani E: Fused transcript of abl and bcr genes in chronic myelogenous leukemia. Nature 315:550, 1985
150. Kloetzer W, Kurzrock R, Smith L et al: The human cellular abl gene product in the chronic myelogenous leukemia cell line K562 has an associated tyrosine protein kinase activity. Virology 140:230, 1985
151. Konopka JB, Watanabe SM, Witte ON: An alteration of the human c-abl pro-

tein in K562 leukemia cells unmasks associated tyrosine kinase activity. Cell 37:1935, 1984

152. Konopka JB, Watanabe SM, Singer JW et al: Cell lines and clinical isolates derived from Ph1-positive chronic myelogenous leukemia patients express c-abl proteins with a common structural alteration. Proc Natl Acad Sci USA 82:1810, 1985

153. Naldini L, Stacchini A, Cirillo DM et al: Phosphotyrosine antibodies identify the p210 c-abl tyrosine kinase and proteins phosphorylated on tyrosine in human chronic myelogenous leukemia cells. Mol Cell Biol 6:1803, 1986

154. Chan LC, Karhi KK, Rayter SI et al: A novel abl protein expressed in Philadelphia chromosome-positive acute lymphoblastic leukaemia. Nature 325:635, 1987

155. Clark SS, McLaughlin J, Crist WM et al: Unique forms of the abl tyrosine kinase distinguish Ph¹-positive CML from Ph¹-positive ALL. Science 235:85, 1987

156. Kurzrock R, Shtalrid M, Romero P et al: A novel c-abl protein product in Philadelphia-positive acute lymphoblastic leukemia. Nature 325:631, 1987

157. Hermans A, Heisterkamp N, von Linden M et al: Unique fusion of bcr and c-abl genes in Philadelphia chromosome positive acute lymphoblastic leukemia. Cell 51:33, 1987

158. Walker LC, Ganesan TS, Dhut S et al: Novel chimaeric protein expressed in Philadelphia positive acute lymphoblastic leukemia. Nature 329:851, 1987

159. Fainstein E, Marcelle C, Rosener A et al: A new fused transcript in Philadelphia chromosome positive acute lymphocytic leukemia. Nature 330:386, 1987

160. Witte ON, Ponticelli A, Gifford A et al: Phosphorylation of the Abelson murine leukemia virus transforming protein. J Virol 39:870, 1981

161. Reynolds FH Jr, Oroszlan S, Stephenson JR: Abelson urine leukemia virus p120: identification and characterization of tyrosine phosphorylation sites. J Virol 44:1097, 1982

162. Srinivasan A, Dunn CY, Yuasa Y et al: Abelson murine leukemia virus: structural requirements for transforming gene function. Proc Natl Acad Sci USA 79:5508, 1982

163. Daley GQ, McLaughlin J, Witte ON, Baltimore D: The CML-specific P210 bcr/abl protein, unlike v-abl, does not transform NIH/3T3 fibroblasts. Science 237:532, 1987

164. Knudson AG Jr: Mutation and cancer: statistical study of retinoblastoma. Proc Natl Acad Sci USA 68:820, 1971

165. Yunis JJ, Ramsay N: Retinoblastoma and subband deletion of chromosome 13. Am J Dis Child 132:161, 1978

166. Cavenee WK, Dryja TP, Phillips RA et al: Expression of recessive alleles by chromosomal mechanisms in retinoblastoma. Nature 305:779, 1983

167. Friend SH, Bernards R, Rogelj S et al: A human DNA segment with properties of the gene that predisposes to retinoblastoma and osteosarcoma. Nature 323:643, 1986

168. Lee WH, Bookstein R, Hong F et al: Human retinoblastoma susceptibility gene: cloning, identification, and sequence. Science 235:1394, 1987

169. Lee WH, Shew FY, Hong FD et al: The retinoblastoma susceptibility gene encodes a nuclear phosphoprotein associated with DNA binding activity. Nature 329:642, 1987

170. Higgins MJ, Hansen MF, Cavenee WK, Lalande M: Molecular detection of chromosomal translocations that disrupt the putative retinoblastoma susceptibility locus. Mol Cell Biol 9:1, 1989

171. Friend SH, Horowitz JM, Gerber MR et al: Deletions of a DNA sequence in retinoblastomas and mesenchymal tumors: organization of the sequence and its encoded protein. Proc Natl Acad Sci USA 84:9059, 1987

172. Fung Y-KT, Murphree AL, T'ang A et al: Structural evidence for the authenticity of the human retinoblastoma gene. Science 236:1657, 1987

173. Bookstein R, Lee EY-H, To H et al: Human retinoblastoma susceptibility gene: genomic organization and analysis of heterozygous intragenic deletion mutants. Proc Natl Acad Sci USA 85:2210, 1988

174. Huang H-J, Yee JK, Shew JY et al: Suppression of the neoplastic phenotype by replacement of the RB gene in human cancer cells. Science 242:1563, 1988

175. Whyte P, Buchkovich KJ, Horowitz JM et al: Association between an oncogene and an anti-oncogene: the adenovirus E1A proteins bind to the retinoblastoma gene product. Nature 334:124, 1988

176. Whyte P, Williamson NM, Harlow E: Cellular targets for transformation by the adenovirus E1A protein. Cell 56:67, 1989

177. DeCapiro JA, Ludlow JW, Figge J et al: SV40 large tumor antigen forms a specific complex with the product of the retinoblastoma susceptibility gene. Cell 54:275, 1988

178. Ludlow JW, DeCaprio JA, Huang CH et al: SV40 large T antigen binds preferentially to an underphosphorylated member of the retinoblastoma susceptibility gene product family. Cell 56:57, 1989

179. Sager R: Tumor suppressor genes: the puzzle and the promise. Science 246:1406, 1989

180. Weinberg RA: Tumor suppressor genes. Science 254:1138, 1991

181. Orkin SH, Goldman DS, Sallan SE: Development of homozygosity for chromosome 11p markers in Wilms' tumour. Nature 309:172, 1984

182. Reeve AE, Housiaux PJ, Gardner RJM et al: Loss of a Harvey ras allele in sporadic Wilms' tumour. Nature 309:174, 1984

183. Riccardi VM, Hittner HM, Francke U et al: The aniridia-Wilms' tumor association: the critical role of chromosome b and 11p13. Cancer Genet Cytogenet 2:131, 1980

184. Koufos A, Hanse MF, Lampkin BC et al: Loss of alleles at loci on human chromosome 11 during genesis of Wilms' tumour. Nature 309:170, 1984

185. Haber DA, Buckler AJ: WT1: a novel tumor suppressor gene inactivated in Wilms' tumor. New Biol 4:97, 1992

186. Pennica D, Goeddel DV, Hayflick JS et al: The amino acid sequence of murine p53 determined from a cDNA clone. Virology 134:477, 1984

187. Matlashewski G, Lamb P, Pim D et al: Isolation and characterization of a human p53 cDNA clone: expression of the human p53 gene. EMBO J 3:3257, 1984

188. Zakut-Houri R, Bienz-Tadmor B, Givol D, Oren M: Human p53 cellular tumor antigen: cDNA sequence and expression in COS cells. EMBO J 4:1251, 1985

189. Benchimol S, Lamb P, Crawford LV et al: Transformation associated p53 protein is encoded by a gene on human chromosome 17. Somat Cell Mol Genet 11:505, 1985

190. Nigro JM, Baker SJ, Preisinger AC et al: Mutations in the p53 gene occur in diverse human tumour types. Nature 342:705, 1989

191. Baker SJ, Fearon ER, Nigro JM et al: Chromosome 17 deletions and p53 gene mutations in colorectal carcinomas. Science 244:217, 1989

192. Baker SJ, Markowitz S, Fearon ER et al: Suppression of human colorectal carcinoma cell growth by wild-type p53. Science 249:912, 1990

193. Iggo R, Gatter K, Bartek J et al: Increased expression of mutant forms of p53 oncogene in primary lung cancer. Lancet 335:675, 1990

194. Devilee P, van den Broek M, Kuipers-Dijkshoorn N et al: At least four different chromosomal regions are involved in loss of heterozygosity in human breast carcinoma. Genomics 5:554, 1989

195. Masuda H, Miller C, Koeffler HP et al: Rearrangement of the p53 gene in human osteogenic sarcomas. Proc Natl Acad Sci USA 84:7716, 1987

196. Li FP, Fraumeni JF Jr, Mulvihill JJ et al: A cancer family syndrome in twenty-four kindreds. Cancer Res 48:5358, 1988

197. Malkin D, Li FP, Strong LC et al: Germ line p53 mutations in a familial syndrome of breast cancer, sarcomas, and other neoplasms. Science 250:1233, 1990

198. Srivastava S, Zou Z, Pirollo K et al: Germ-line transmission of a mutated p53 gene in a cancer-prone family with Li-Fraumeni syndrome. Nature 348:747, 1990

199. Frebourg T, Friend SH: Cancer risks from germline p53 mutations. J Clin Invest 90:1637, 1992

200. Felix CA, Nau MM, Takahashi T et al: Herditary and acquired p53 gene mutations in childhood acute lymphoblastic leukemia. J Clin Invest 89:640, 1992

201. Gaidano G, Ballerini P, Gong JZ et al: p53 mutations in human lymphoid malignancies: association with Burkitt lymphoma and chronic lymphocytic leukemia. Proc Natl Acad Sci USA 88:5413, 1991

202. Murphree AL, Benedict WF: Retinoblastoma: clues to human carcinogenesis. Science 223:1028, 1984

203. Scrable H, Witte DP, Lampkin BC, Cavenee WK: Chromosomal localization of the human rhabdomyosarcoma locus by mitotic recombination mapping. Nature 329:645, 1987

204. Third International Workshop on Chromosomes in Leukemia. Cancer Genet Cytogenet 4:101, 1981

205. Oshimura M, Freeman AI, Sandberg AA: Chromosomes and causation of human cancer and leukemia. XXVI. Banding studies in acute lymphoblastic leukemia (ALL). Cancer Res 40:1161, 1977

206. Kaneko Y, Rowley JD, Variakojis D et al: Correlation of karyotype with clinical features in acute lymphoblastic leukemia. Cancer Res 42:2918, 1982

207. Kowalczyk JR, Grossi M, Sandberg AA: Cytogenetic findings in childhood acute lymphoblastic leukemia. Cancer Genet Cytogenet 15:47, 1985

208. Prigogina EL, Puchkova GP, Mayakova SA: Nonrandom chromosomal abnormalities in acute lymphoblastic leukemia of childhood. Cancer Genet Cytogenet 32:183, 1988

209. Ohyashiki K, Ohyashiki JH, Kinniburgh AJ et al: myb oncogene in human hematopoietic neoplasia with 6q-anomaly. Cancer Genet Cytogenet 33:83, 1989

210. Raimondi SC, Williams DL, Callihan T et al: Nonrandom involvement of the 12p12 breakpoint in chromosome abnormalities of childhood acute lymphoblasts leukemia. Blood 68:69, 1986

211. Kowalczyk J, Sandberg AA: A possible subgroup of ALL wth 9p−: short communication. Cancer Genet Cytogenet 9:383, 1983

212. Carroll AJ, Castleberry RP, Crist WM: Lack of association between abnormalities of the chromosome 9 short arm and either "lymphomatous" features or T cell phenotype in childhood acute lymphocytic leukemia. Blood 69:735, 1987

213. Murphy SB, Raimondi SC, Rivera GK et al: Nonrandom abnormalities of chromosome 9p in childhood acute lymphoblastic leukemia: association with high-risk clinical features. Blood 74:409, 1989

214. Diaz MO, Ziemin S, Le Beau MM et al: Homozygous deletion of the alpha and beta$_1$-interferon genes in human leukemia and derived cell lines. Proc Natl Acad Sci USA 85:5259, 1988

215. Pui C-H, Williams DL, Raimondi SC et al: Hypodiploidy is associated with a poor prognosis in childhood acute lymphoblastic leukemia. Blood 70:247, 1987

216. Der CJ, Krontiris TG, Cooper GM: Transforming genes of human bladder and lung carcinoma cell lines are homologous to the *ras* genes of Harvey and Kirsten sarcoma viruses. Proc Natl Acad Sci USA 79:3637, 1982

217. Parada LF, Tabin CJ, Shih C, Weinberg RA: Human EJ bladder carcinoma oncogene is homologue of Harvey sarcoma virus *ras* gene. Nature 297:474, 1982

218. Santos E, Tronick SR, Aaronson SA et al: T24 human bladder carcinoma oncogene is an activated form of the normal human homologue of BALB- and Harvey-MSV transforming genes. Nature 298:343, 1982

219. Shimizu K, Goldfarb M, Perucho M, Wigler M: Isolation and preliminary characterization of the transforming gene of a huma neuroblastoma cell line. Proc Natl Acad Sci USA 80:383, 1983

220. Shimizu K, Goldfarb M, Suard U et al: Three human transforming genes are related to the viral *ras* oncogenes. Proc Natl Acad Sci USA 80:2112, 1983

221. Ellis RW, Lowy DR, Scolnick EM: The Viral and Cellular p21 *ras* Gene Family. Raven Press, New York, 1982, p. 107

222. Barbacid M: Human oncogenes. p. 3. In DeVita VT Jr, Hellman S, Rosenberg SA (eds.): Important Advances in Oncology. JB Lippincott, Philadelphia, 1986

223. Gibbs JB, Sigal IS, Poe M, Scolnick EM: Intrinsic GPTase activity distinguishes normal and oncogenic *ras* p21 molecules. Proc Natl Acad Sci USA 81:5704, 1984

224. McGrath JP, Capon DJ, Goeddel DV, Levinson AD: Comparative biochemical properties of normal and activated human *ras* p21 protein. Nature 310:644, 1984

225. Sweet RW, Yokoyama S, Kamata T et al: The product of *ras* is a GTPase and the T24 oncogenic mutant is deficient in this activity. Nature 311:273, 1984

226. Land H, Parada LF, Weinberg RA: Cellular oncogenes and multistep carcinogenesis. Science 222:771, 1983

227. Land H, Parada LF, Weinberg RA: Tumorigenic conversion of primary embryo fibroblasts requires at least two cooperation oncogenes. Nature 304:596, 1983

228. Eliyahu D, Raz A, Gruss P et al: Participation of p53 cellular tumour antigen in transformation of normal embryonic cells. Nature 312:646, 1984

229. Parada LF, Land H, Weinberg RA et al: Cooperation between gene encoding p53 tumour antigen and *ras* in cellular transformation. Nature 312:649, 1984

230. Balmain A, Pragnell IB: Mouse skin carcinomas induced *in vivo* by chemical carcinogens have a transforming Harvey-*ras* oncogene. Nature 303:72, 1983

231. Sukumar S, Notario V, Martin-Zanca D, Barbacid M: Induction of mammary carcinomas in rats by nitro-methylurea involves malignant activation of H-*ras*-1 locus by single point mutations. Nature 306:658, 1983

232. Guerrero I, Calzada P, Mayer A, Pellicer A: A molecular approach to leukemogenesis: mouse lymphomas contain an activated c-*ras* oncogene. Proc Natl Acad Sci USA 81:202, 1984

233. Janssen JWG, Steenvoorden ACM, Collar JG, Nusse R: Oncogene activation in human myeloid leukemia. Cancer Res 45:3262, 1985

234. Murray MJ, Cunningham JM, Parada LF et al: The HL-60 transforming sequence: a *ras* oncogene coexisting with altered *myc* genes in hematopoietic tumors. Cell 33:749, 1983

235. Bos JL, Toksoz D, Marshall CJ et al: Amino-acid substitutions at codon 13 of the N-*ras* oncogene in human acute myeloid leukaemia. Nature 315:726, 1985

236. Gambke C, Signer E, Moroni C: Activation of N-*ras* gene in bone marrow cells from a patient with acute myeloblastic leukaemia. Nature 307:476, 1984

237. Hirai H, Tanaka S, Azuma M et al: Transforming genes in human leukemia cells. Blood 66:1371, 1985

238. Souyri M, Fleissner E: Identification by transfection of transforming sequences in DNA of human T-cell leukemias. Proc Natl Acad Sci USA 80:6676, 1983

239. Bos JL, Verlaan-de Vries M, van der Eb AJ et al: Mutations in N-*ras* predominate in acute myeloid leukemia. Blood 69:1237, 1987

240. Rodenhuis S, Bos JL, Slater RM et al: Absence of oncogene amplifications and occasional activation of N-*ras* in lymphoblastic leukemia of childhood. Blood 67:1698, 1986

241. Liu E, Hjelle B, Morgan R, Bishop JM: The role of mutant *ras* genes in preleukemic states. Blood, suppl. 1. 70:282a, 1987

242. Padua RA, Carter G, Hughes D et al: *RAS* mutations in myelodysplasia detected by amplification, oligonucleotide hybridization and transformation. Leukemia 2:503, 1988

243. Brodeur GM, Seeger RC, Schwab M et al: Amplification of N-myc in untreated human neuroblastomas correlates with advanced disease stage. Science 224:1121, 1984

244. Seeger RC, Brodeur GM, Sather H et al: Association of multiple copies of the N-*myc* oncogene with rapid progression of neuroblastomas. N Engl J Med 313:1111, 1985

245. Look AT, Hayes FA, Shuster JJ et al: Clinical relevance of tumor cell ploidy and N-myc gene amplification in childhood neuroblastoma: a Pediatric Oncology Group Study. J Clin Oncol 9:581, 1991

246. Johnson BE, Ihde DC, Makuch RW et al: *myc* family oncogene amplification in tumor cell lines established from small cell lung cancer patients and its relationship to clinical status and course. J Clin Invest 79:1629, 1987

247. Wong AJ, Ruppert JM, Eggleston J et al: Gene amplification of c-*myc* and N-*myc* in small cell carcinoma of the lung. Science 233:461, 1986

248. Slamon DJ, Clark GM, Wong SG et al: Human breast cancer: correlation of relapse and survival and amplification of the HER-2/neu oncogene. Science 235:177, 1987

249. Slamon DJ, Godolphin W, Jones LA et al: Studies of the HER-2/*neu* proto-oncogene in human breast and ovarian cancer. Science 244:707, 1989

250. Collins SJ, Groudine M: Amplification of endogenous *myc*-related DNA sequences in a human myeloid leukemia cell line. Nature 298:679, 1982

251. Dalla-Favera R, Wong-Staal F, Gallo RC: Onc gene amplification in promyelocytic leukemia cell line HL-60 and primary leukemic cells of the same patient. Nature 299:61, 1982

252. Barletta C, Pelicci PG, Kenyon LC et al: Relationship between the c-*myb* locus and the 6q-chromosomal aberration in leukemias and lymphomas. Science 235:1064, 1987

253. Pelicci PG, Lanfrancone L, Braithwaite MD et al: Amplification of the c-*myb* oncogene in a case of human acute myelogenous leukemia. Science 224:1117, 1984

254. Saito M, Helin K, Valentine MB et al: Amplification of the E2F-1 transcription factor gene in the HEL erythroleukemia cell line. Blood 1993 (submitted)

255. Secker-Walker LM, Lawler SD, Hardisty RM: Prognostic implications of chromosomal findings in acute lymphoblastic leukemia at diagnosis. BMJ 2:1529, 1978

256. Secker-Walker LM, Swansbury GJ, Hardisty RM et al: Cytogenetics of acute lymphoblastic leukemia in children as a factor in the prediction of long-term survival. Br J Haematol 52:389, 1982

257. Williams DL, Tsiatis A, Brodeur GM et al: Prognostic importance of chromosome number in 136 untreated children with acute lymphoblastic leukemia. Blood 60:864, 1982

258. Look AT, Melvin SL, Williams DL et al: Aneuploidy and percentage of S-phase cells determined by flow cytometry correlate with cell phenotype of childhood acute leukemia. Blood 60:959, 1982

259. Harris MB, Shuster JJ, Carroll A et al: Trisomy of leukemic cell chromosomes 4 and 10 identifies children with B-progenitor cell acute lymphoblastic leukemia with a very low risk of treatment failure: a Pediatric Oncology Group study. Blood 79:3316, 1992

260. Look AT, Roberson PK, Williams DL et al: Prognostic importance of blast cell DNA content in childhood acute lymphoblastic leukemia. Blood 4:33, 1979

261. Abromowitch M, Ochs J, Pui CH et al: High-dose methotrexate improves clinical outcome in children with acute lymphoblastic leukemia: St. Jude Total Therapy Study X. Med Pediatr Oncol 16:297, 1988

262. Look AT, Roberson PK, Murphy SB: Prognostic value of cellular DNA content in acute lymphoblastic leukemia of childhood. N Engl J Med 317:1666, 1987

263. Trueworthy R, Shuster J, Look T et al: Ploidy of lymphoblasts is the strongest predictor of treatment outcome in B-progenitor cell acute lymphoblastic leukemia of childhood: a Pediatric Oncology Group study. J Clin Oncol 10:606, 1992

264. Fletcher JA, Kimball VM, Lynch E et al: Prognostic implications of cytogenetic studies in an intensively treated group of children with acute lymphoblastic leukemia. Blood 74:2130, 1989

265. Rubin CM, Le Beau MM, Mick R et al: Impact of chromosomal translocations on prognosis in childhood acute lymphoblastic leukemia. J Clin Oncol 9:2183, 1991

266. Huang ME, Ye YC, Chen SR et al: Use of all-trans retinoic acid in the treatment of acute promyelocytic leukemia. Blood 72:567, 1988

267. Castaigne S, Chomienne C, Daniel MT et al: All-trans retinoic acid as a differentiation therapy for acute promyelocytic leukemia I. Clinical results. Blood 76:1704, 1990

268. Chen ZX, Xue YQ, Zhang R et al: A clinical and experimental study on all-trans retinoic acid-treated acute promyelocytic leukemia patients. Blood 78:1413, 1991

269. Warrell RP Jr, Frankel SR, Miller WH Jr et al: Differentiation therapy of acute promyelocytic leukemia with tretinoin (all-trans-retinoic acid). N Engl J Med 324:1385, 1991

270. de The H, Chomienne C, Lanotte M et al: The t(15;17) translocation of acute promyelocytic leukaemia fuses the retinoic acid receptor alpha gene to a novel transcribed locus. Nature 347:558, 1990

271. Borrow J, Goddard AD, Sheer D, Solomon E: Molecular analysis of acute promyelocytic leukemia breakpoint cluster region on chromosome 17. Science 249:1577, 1990

272. Longo L, Pandolfi PP, Biondi A et al: Rearrangements and aberrant expression of the retinoic acid receptor alpha gene in acute promyelocytic leukemias. J Exp Med 172:1571, 1990

273. de The H, Lavau C, Marchio A et al: The PML-RAR alpha fusion mRNA generated by the t(15;17) translocation in acute promyelocytic leukemia encodes a functionally altered RAR. Cell 66:675, 1991

274. Kakizuka A, Miller WH Jr, Umesono K et al: Chromosomal translocation t(15;17) in human acute promyelocytic leukemia fuses RAR alpha with a novel putative transcription factor, PML. Cell 66:663, 1991

275. Kastner P, Perez A, Lutz Y et al: Structure, localization and transcriptional properties of two classes of retinoic acid receptor alpha fusion proteins in acute promyelocytic leukemia (APL): structural similarities with a new family of oncoproteins. EMBO J 11:629, 1992

276. Stass S, Mirro J, Melvin S et al: Lineage switch in acute leukemia. Blood 64:701, 1984

277. Neame PB, Soamboonsrup P, Browman G et al: Simultaneous or sequential expression of lymphoid and myeloid phenotypes in acute leukemia. Blood 65:142, 1985

278. Pui C-H, Raimondi SC, Behm FG et al: Shifts in blast cell phenotype and karyotype at relapse of childhood lymphoblastic leukemia. Blood 68:1306, 1986

279. Gagnon GA, Childs CC, LeMaistre A et al: Molecular heterogeneity in acute leukemia lineage switch. Blood 74:2088, 1989

280. Pui CH, Ribeiro RC, Hancock ML et al: Acute myeloid leukemia in children treated with epipodophyllotoxins for acute lymphoblastic leukemia. N Engl J Med 325:1682, 1991

281. Fourth International Workshop on Chromosomes and Leukemia: a prospective study of acute nonlymphocytic leukemia. Cancer Genet Cytogenet 11:249, 1984

282. Pedersen-Bjergaad J, Larsen SO: Incidence of acute nonlymphocytic leukemia, preleukemia, and acute myeloproliferative syndrome up to 10 years after treatment of Hodgkin's disease. N Engl J Med 307:965, 1982

283. Aisenberg AC: Acute nonlymphocytic leukemia after treatment of Hodgkin's disease. Am J Med 75:449, 1983

284. Koletsky AJ, Bertino JR, Farber LR et al: Second neoplasms in patients with Hodgkin's disease following combined modality therapy—the Yale experience. J Clin Oncol 4:311, 1986

285. Blayney DW, Longo DL, Young RC et al: Decreasing risk of leukemia with prolonged follow-up after chemotherapy and radiotherapy for Hodgkin's disease. N Engl J Med 316:710, 1987

286. Tucker MA, Coleman CN, Cox RS et al: Risk of second cancers after treatment of Hodgkin's disease. N Engl J Med 318:76, 1988

287. van der Velden JW, van Putten WL, Guinee VF et al: Subsequent development of acute non-lymphocytic leukemia in patients treated for Hodgkin's disease. Int J Cancer 42:252, 1988

288. Ratain MJ, Kraminer LS, Bitran JD et al: Acute nonlymphocytic leukemia following etoposide and cisplatin combination chemotherapy for advanced non-small-cell carcinoma of the lung. Blood 70:1412, 1987

289. Weh HJ, Kabisch H, Landbeck G, Hossfeld DK: Translocation (q;11)(p21; q23) in a child with acute monoblastic leukemia following 2 1/2 years after successful chemotherapy for neuroblastoma. J Clin Oncol 4:1518, 1986

290. Pedersen-Bjergaard J, Philip P, Ravn V et al: Therapy-related acute non-lymphocytic leukemia of FAB type M4 or M5 with early onset and t(9;11)(p21;q23) or a normal karyotype: a separate entity? J Clin Oncol 6:395, 1988

291. Vogelstein B, Fearon ER, Hamilton SR et al: Clonal analysis using recombinant DNA probes from the X-chromosome. Cancer Res 47:4806, 1987

292. Fearon ER, Burke PJ, Schiffer CA et al: Differentiation of leukemia cells to polymorphonuclear leukocytes in patients with acute nonlymphocytic leukemia. N Engl J Med 315:15, 1986

293. Rappold GA, Hameister H, Cremer T et al: c-myc and immunoglobulin kappa light chain constant genes are on the 8q− chromosome of three Burkitt lymphoma lines with t(2;8) translocations. EMBO J 3:2951, 1984

294. Kamps MP, Murre C, Sun XH, Baltimore D: A new homeobox gene contributes the DNA binding domain of the t(1;19) translocation protein in pre-B ALL. Cell 60:547, 1990

295. Nourse J, Mellentin JD, Galili N et al: Chromosomal translocation t(1;19) results in synthesis of a homeobox fusion mRNA that codes for a potential chimeric transcription factor. Cell 60:535, 1990

296. Chen Z, Brand NJ, Chen A et al: Fusion between a novel Krüppel-like zinc finger gene and the retinoic acid receptor-α locus due to a variant t(11;17) translocation associated with acute promyelocytic leukaemia. EMBO J 12:1161, 1993

297. Morishita K, Parganas E, Bartholomew C et al: The human Evi-1 gene is located on chromosome 3q24-q28 but is not rearranged in three cases of acute nonlymphocytic leukemias containing t(3;5)(q25;q34) translocations. Oncogene Res 5:221, 1990

298. Morishita K, Parganas E, Willman CL et al: Activation of Evi-1 gene expression in human acute myelogenous leukemias by translocations spanning 300-400 kb on chromosome 3q26. Proc Natl Acad Sci USA 1992

299. Miyoshi H, Shimizu K, Kozu T et al: t(8;21) breakpoints on chromosome 21 in acute myeloid leukemia are clustered within a limited region of a single gene, AML1. Proc Natl Acad Sci USA 88:10431, 1991

300. Gao J, Erickson P, Gardiner K et al: Isolation of a yeast artificial chromosome spanning the 8;21 translocation breakpoint t(8;21)(q22;q22.3) in acute myelogenous leukemia. Proc Natl Acad Sci USA 88:4882, 1991

301. Erickson P, Gao J, Chang KS et al: Identification of breakpoints in t(8;21) acute myelogenous leukemia and isolation of a fusion transcript. AML1/ETO, with similarity to Drosophila segmentation gene, runt. Blood 80:1825, 1992

302. Shimizu K, Miyoshi H, Kozu T et al: Consistent disruption of the AML1 gene occurs within a single intron in the t(8;21) chromosomal translocation. Cancer Res 52:6945, 1992

303. von Lindern M, Poustka A, Lerach H, Grosveld G: The (6;9) chromosome translocation, associated with a specific subtype of acute nonlymphocytic leukemia, leads to aberrant transcription of a target gene on 9q34. Mol Cell Biol 10:4016, 1990

304. Inaba T, Shapiro LH, Funabiki T et al: DNA-binding specificity and trans-activating potential of the leukemia-associated E2A-hepatic leukemia factor fusion protein. Mol Cell Biol 14:3403, 1994

Clinical Manifestations of Acute Lymphocytic Leukemia in Children

68

Stacey Berg and David G. Poplack

INTRODUCTION

Prior to the institution of modern chemotherapy, acute lymphocytic leukemia (ALL) was a uniformly fatal disease, most patients surviving only 2–3 months. With current chemotherapy, most children with ALL have prolonged disease-free survival, and up to approximately 60% are considered cured. Although most adults also attain complete remission with chemotherapy, 3–5-year actuarial survivals range from only 20–35%.[1–3]

EPIDEMIOLOGY

Each year approximately 3,000 cases of ALL are diagnosed in the United States. Two-thirds of these cases occur in childhood, where ALL is the most common malignancy and the most frequent type of leukemia. In children, ALL is three times more frequent than acute myeloid leukemia (AML). By contrast, the nearly 1,000 cases of ALL diagnosed per year in adults account for <20% of the acute leukemias in this population.[4–6] In children, the peak incidence of ALL occurs at approximately 4 years of age. In adults, the greatest number of cases occur in those >65 years of age.

Some children are at particular risk of developing ALL. Children with certain chromosomal abnormalities, including Down syndrome,[7] Bloom syndrome,[8] Fanconi anemia,[9] and ataxia telangiectasia,[10] are all at higher risk than the general population for developing leukemia. In addition, siblings, especially twins, of children with leukemia are at greater risk of developing leukemia, although this risk may be only approximately twice that of the general population.[11,12] Some cases of childhood ALL may be related to hereditary or acquired mutations in the p53 gene.[13]

CLINICAL MANIFESTATIONS

Patients with ALL present most frequently with signs and symptoms of the uncontrolled growth of leukemic cells in bone marrow, lymphoid organs, and other sites of extramedullary spread. Bone marrow involvement results in varying in degrees of anemia, thrombocytopenia, and granulocytopenia, which may be manifested by pallor and fatigue, petechiae, purpura, or bleeding and fever. Liver, spleen, and nodal enlargement are present in most patients and are the most common sites of extramedullary disease spread. Both hepatosplenomegaly, which occurs in approximately two-thirds of patients, and lymphadenopathy, clinically detectable in more than one-half of presenting cases, are usually asymptomatic. Bone pain, however, is a common presenting feature, particularly in the young child with ALL whose first symptom may be the onset of a limp or refusal to walk.

Symptoms may be present from a few days to several weeks before the diagnosis of ALL is made, although in some cases a relevant clinical history may precede the diagnosis by several months. The nonspecific nature of the signs and symptoms of ALL occasionally leads to delay in diagnosis. In addition, because ALL may imitate a variety of disorders, there may be diagnostic confusion. For example, arthralgias arising from leukemic infiltration of the joints may be confused with juvenile rheumatoid arthritis or osteomyelitis. In rare cases, ALL has presented with unusual symptoms, such as aplastic anemia or even as hypereosinophilia[14,15] (Table 68-1).

Extramedullary Spread

ALL frequently involves organs other than bone marrow. Most patients have some extramedullary disease at diagnosis, and extramedullary relapse is a known complication of the disease. The incidence of occult extramedullary involvement in patients presumed to be in clinical remission is difficult to ascertain but has been estimated to be as high as 50%.[16–18] Actual organ dysfunction secondary to leukemic involvement is rare and is usually seen in patients with progressive end-stage disease. The occurrence of an extramedullary relapse is significant because it frequently heralds the development of bone marrow relapse. The most commonly affected extramedullary sites of disease include the central nervous system, testes, lymph nodes, liver, spleen, and kidney. Of these sites, the central nervous system and the testes have the greatest clinical significance.

Central Nervous System

Central nervous system involvement is relatively uncommon at diagnosis. Less than 5% of children and up to 15% of adults have evidence of central nervous system disease on initial evaluation.[19] Unless adequate central nervous system preventive therapy is administered, however, most patients will eventually develop central nervous system disease. This is presumed to be related, in part, to the blood-brain barrier, which effectively makes the central nervous system a "pharmacologic sanctuary" and prevents many systemically administered antileukemic agents from penetrating adequately into the central nervous system. For this reason, specific central nervous system treatment, in the form of intrathecal chemotherapy or cranial radiation, or both, is required to prevent the development

Table 68-1. Some Unusual Clinical Presentations of ALL

Aplastic anemia	Pericardial effusion[93]
Eosinophilia[90]	Hypoglycemia[94]
Isolated renal failure	Skin nodules[95]
Pulmonary nodules[91]	Cyclic neutropenia[96]
Bone marrow necrosis[92]	

(Adapted from Nesbit,[97] with permission.)

of central nervous system leukemia. Once present, central nervous system leukemia, although usually controllable in the short term, frequently recurs. The primary consequence of central nervous system leukemia is that it places patients at a high risk of subsequent bone marrow relapse. Therefore, the development of effective means of preventing central nervous system disease has become an important focus of clinical investigation, particularly (but not solely) in childhood ALL, in which the incidence of central nervous system disease has historically been higher than in adults.

Central nervous system leukemia is presumed to develop from hematogenous spread, through "seeding" of the meninges by circulating leukemic cells, or by direct extension from involved cranial bone marrow.[20-22] The meninges are the primary site of disease but, particularly in advanced disease, other sites within the brain parenchyma and spinal cord may be involved.[19] In patients with clinically overt central nervous system leukemia, signs and symptoms are usually caused by increased intracranial pressure and include headache, nausea and vomiting, lethargy or irritability, papilledema, and nuchal rigidity. Cranial nerves, most commonly in the 7th, 3rd, 4th, and 6th, may be involved and may on rare occasions be an isolated site of central nervous system relapse. The hypothalamic-obesity syndrome, in which infiltration of the hypothalamus produces hyperphagia and pathologic weight gain, is a rare complication of central nervous system leukemia. Because of its varied symptomatology, central nervous system leukemia must be considered as a possible diagnosis in any patient with ALL in whom neurologic signs and symptoms develop.

The diagnosis of central nervous system leukemia is made by evaluation of cerebrospinal fluid obtained by lumbar puncture. In symptomatic patients, the opening cerebrospinal fluid pressure is usually increased, the cerebrospinal fluid cell count is usually elevated, the cerebrospinal fluid protein is frequently elevated, and the cerebrospinal fluid glucose may or may not be decreased. Cerebrospinal fluid examination following concentration of cells by cytocentrifugation, reveals the presence of leukemic lymphoblasts. The heightened awareness of central nervous system leukemia has led to routine lumbar puncture surveillance of patients undergoing treatment. As a consequence, in many patients, the diagnosis of central nervous system leukemia is being made earlier in the course of the disease. In such cases, the cerebrospinal fluid opening pressure, cell count, protein and glucose may all be normal and only careful examination of a cytocentrifuged cerebrospinal fluid specimen may help identify leukemic lymphoblasts. Other techniques have been explored in an attempt to improve the ability to diagnose central nervous system leukemia in equivocal cases, including terminal deoxynucleotidyl transferase (TdT) determination and the use of monoclonal antibodies.

Testicular Leukemia

As the survival of patients with ALL has increased, so has the incidence of testicular involvement, particularly in children, in whom testicular leukemia has become a major site of disease recurrence. This complication occurs in approximately 10–15% of boys undergoing chemotherapy. The testes are also a site of late relapse in a substantial proportion of boys who had previously successfully completed a full chemotherapy regimen.[23,24] Although clinically evident testicular involvement is rare at initial diagnosis, occult testicular disease has been reported in ≤25% of newly diagnosed boys.[25] When clinically overt, testicular leukemia presents as a painless testicular enlargement that is usually unilateral. The diagnosis of testicular involvement is made using wedge biopsies, which should be done bilaterally because of the high incidence of contralateral testicular involvement.[26] Testicular leukemia is characterized by infiltration of leukemic cells into the interstitium; involve-

ment of the seminiferous tubules occurs in more advanced disease.[27] Although the testes were believed to be a leukemic sanctuary site, protected from systemic chemotherapy by a blood-testes barrier, animal studies suggest this is not the case.[28]

Testicular disease frequently occurs as an "isolated" clinical relapse in patients in bone marrow remission. The actual incidence of true isolated testicular disease, however, may be lower than previously believed. In one study, a high percentage of patients with testicular relapse who were presumed to be in bone marrow remission were found to have occult leukemia in other abdominal sites, including lymph nodes, liver, and spleen, when evaluated by exploratory laparotomy.[29] Thus, the frequent diagnosis of testicular involvement may simply reflect the relative ease with which recurrence can be clinically detected at this anatomic site. This point is underscored by the observation that the most successful treatment regimens for testicular recurrence employ both bilateral testicular radiation (usually ≥2,400 cGy) and intensive systemic reinduction and retreatment.[29-32]

As in the case of central nervous system leukemia, testicular recurrence is frequently followed by systemic relapse. This fact, and the observation that occult disease can be detected in ≤15% of boys who have "successfully" completed a full treatment course, led to the practice of performing routine testicular biopsies during maintenance treatment or immediately prior to its completion. Histopathologically, however, testicular biopsies are notoriously difficult to assess and are associated with a relatively high false-negative rate. This has caused investigators to question the wisdom of performing surveillance testicular biopsies, in view of their relative inability to predict eventual testicular relapse.[31-35]

Lymph Nodes

Nodal involvement is a characteristic feature of ALL and is often responsible for bringing the patient to medical attention. Leukemic involvement usually results in obliteration of the normal microscopic structure of the node. Typically, the lymphadenopathy is generalized, and enlarged nodes are painless and freely movable. Nodal enlargement is an indirect measure of tumor burden and has been associated with patient prognosis. The presence of massive lymphadenopathy or a large mediastinal mass, a particular feature of patients with T-cell ALL, has been associated with a poor prognosis.[36-38]

Liver and Spleen

Hepatosplenomegaly is common in newly diagnosed patients with ALL. As in the case of nodal enlargement, there is a correlation between the extent of hepatic and splenic enlargement and prognosis, with significant enlargement being linked to a poor outcome.[38,39] Pathologically, these organs show diffuse enlargement secondary to infiltration by leukemic lymphoblasts. In the spleen, the normal distinction between red and white pulp is lost. In the liver, leukemic infiltration of the portal areas is common. Even in cases associated with marked hepatomegaly, liver function abnormalities, if present, are usually mild.

Kidneys

Renal enlargement at diagnosis is common and represents diffuse infiltration by leukemic blast cells.[40,41] Preferential involvement of the cortex occurs. Renal dysfunction, in the absence of the development of uric acid nephropathy, is a rare phenomenon.

Table 68-2. Differential Diagnosis of ALL[a]

Nonmalignant disorders
    Aplastic Anemia
    Myelodysplastic syndrome (a)
    Myelofibrosis (a)
    Autoimmune diseases (e.g., systemic lupus erythematosus) (a)
    Infectious mononucleosis
    Juvenile rheumatoid arthritis (c)
    Idiopathic thrombocytopenia purpura (c)
    Leukemic reactions secondary to infection
Malignant disorders
    Other leukemias
    Hodgkin and non-Hodgkin lymphoma
    Bone marrow metastases from solid tumors (e.g., neuroblastoma) (c)
    Multiple myeloma (a)

[a] Where indicated, symbols denote disorders that are to be particularly considered in the differential diagnosis of children (c) or of adults (a).

DIFFERENTIAL DIAGNOSIS

In the differential diagnosis of ALL, the clinician must include a variety of malignant and nonmalignant disorders, some of which are listed in Table 68-2.

ALL must be distinguished from malignancies, including both Hodgkin and non-Hodgkin lymphomas and those solid tumors that may exhibit metastatic spread to bone marrow. For example, the morphologic appearance of neuroblastoma in the bone marrow may be difficult to differentiate from that of ALL, especially in the absence of pseudorosettes.

Infectious mononucleosis, idiopathic thrombocytopenic purpura, aplastic anemia, and infectious causes of lymphocytosis (e.g., pertussis) are other conditions that may mimic ALL.

Careful evaluation of a bone marrow aspirate using special strains as well as a panel of monoclonal antibodies will usually permit the clinician to make the definitive diagnosis of ALL (see below).

LABORATORY EVALUATION
Hematologic Findings

More than 90% of patients with ALL have clinically evident hematologic abnormalities at diagnosis, generally reflecting the degree to which normal marrow is replaced with leukemic cells. Anemia, usually normochromic and normocytic and characteristically accompanied by a low reticulocyte count, is present in approximately 80% of cases. In approximately 50% of patients, the initial leukocyte count is elevated; in ≤25% it is >50,000/ml at presentation. Patients with a profoundly elevated leukocyte count at diagnosis (>50,000/ml) have a particularly poor prognosis. Despite the elevation in leukocyte count at diagnosis, however, many patients present with severe neutropenia (<500 granulocytes/mm³) and are at significant risk of serious infection.[42] Thrombocytopenia is extremely common; more than three-fourths of patients present with platelet counts of <100,000/ml. Only approximately one-third of patients have a platelet count of <50,000/ml at diagnosis. Although petechiae and purpura are present in many patients, severe bleeding is unusual at initial presentation, even when the platelet count is <20,000/ml, unless fever, infection, or an accompanying coagulopathy (e.g., disseminated intravascular coagulation) is present as well.

Diagnostic examination of the peripheral blood smear will demonstrate the presence of leukemic lymphoblasts in most patients. Definitive diagnosis (see panel) requires examination of the bone marrow, which is usually hypercellular and infiltrated with leukemic lymphoblasts. Technically, the presence of >5% leukemic blasts cells confirms the diagnosis. Most institutions, however, require ≥25% blast cells before definitive diagnosis is rendered. More than three-fourths of patients have >50% lymphoblasts in their bone marrow at initial presentation.

Morphologic Classification

ALL cells manifest significant heterogeneity and have been subclassified on the basis of differences in their appearance under the light microscope. The most widely used system, developed by the French-American-British (FAB) Cooperative Working Group (Table 68-3) divides lymphoblasts into three categories. L1 lymphoblasts are small, with scanty cytoplasm and inconspicuous nucleoli (Plate 68-1A). L2 lymphoblasts are generally larger, although they may demonstrate considerable variation in size, and have more prominent nucleoli and abundant cytoplasm (Plate 68-1B). Lymphoblasts of the L3 type are large, manifest deep cytoplasmic basophilia and prominent cytoplasmic vacuolation, and are identical cytomorphologically to Burkitt lymphoma cells (Plate 68-1C). The L1 morphology is predominant in childhood ALL, occurring in approximately 85% of childhood cases. The L2 subtype is more common in adults.[43] Lymphoblasts of the L3 are characteristic of only 1–2% of ALL cases. Although there is no apparent correlation between the FAB L1 and L2 morphologic types and immunologic cell surface markers, cells of the L3 variety possess cell surface immunoglobulin and other characteristic B-cell markers.[44–46] The association between FAB classification and prognosis is discussed below.

Immunophenotyping

Immunophenotyping now plays a major role in the diagnosis of the acute leukemias. The use of monoclonal antibodies specific for various stages of B-cell, T-cell, and myeloid differentiation enables the clinician to determine more definitively that a leukemia is lymphoid in origin. In most cases, immunophenotyping also permits assignment of the relative stage in the process of B-cell or T-cell differentiation from which the leukemic clone is believed to have arisen. An example of the type of monoclonal antibody panel used in the immunophenotypic diagnosis of the acute leukemias is shown in Table 68-4. Approximately 80–85% of childhood ALL is believed to develop from the monoclonal proliferation of B-cell precursors. By contrast, only approximately 1–2% of cases manifest surface immunoglobulin and are classified as mature B-cell ALL. The remainder of cases are of T-cell origin. A variety of classification schemes have been developed that define both B-cell precursor ALL and T-cell ALL, according to their degree of differentiation or maturation. One prognostically useful system, devised by the Pediatric Oncology Group, separates childhood ALL into T-cell, B-cell, "early pre-B," and "pre-B" cell disease.[47,48] According to this classification system, approximately two-thirds of the cases of B-cell precursor ALL represent early pre-B ALL. These leukemias manifest early B-cell precursors antigens but no evidence of cytoplasmic immunoglobulin. The remaining one-third of B-cell precursor ALL cases are considered pre-B. These cases have demonstrable cytoplasmic immunoglobulin and represent leukemias derived from a more mature B-cell precursor. These B-cell precursor leukemias have different prognoses (see below).

The development of recombinant DNA technology permits identification of immunoglobulin gene and T-cell receptor gene rearrangement in leukemic cells. Although it is possible to relate the patterns of immunoglobulin gene rearrangement and T-cell receptor gene rearrangement to the stages of develop-

DIAGNOSTIC EVALUATION

The diagnostic evaluation of a patient with acute leukemia is a comprehensive process that includes a detailed history and complete physical examination, morphologic and laboratory assessment of peripheral blood and bone marrow, blood chemistries, comprehensive clotting studies (prothrombin time, partial thromboplastin time, thrombin time, and fibrinogen), a lumbar puncture and cerebrospinal fluid examination, and other studies necessary to ensure that the newly diagnosed patient will receive optimal supportive care.

History and Physical Examination

A detailed history is obtained to determine the nature of presenting symptoms and their duration. Specific attention is paid to signs and symptoms of anemia, thrombocytopenia, and neutropenia. Information is garnered regarding possible adverse environmental exposures (e.g., chemicals, radiation) and a detailed family history that includes the occurrence and nature of any malignancies among family members is obtained. On physical examination, signs that reflect leukemic marrow involvement and its sequelae are sought. The degree of pallor, evidence of bleeding (e.g., petechiae and/or purpura), and the presence of any signs of infection are noted. The degree of lymphadenopathy and hepatosplenomegaly is carefully assessed and documented. The pattern of lymph node enlargement provides helpful information. Generalized lymphadenopathy is more common than regional enlargement. In children, palpable small axillary, cervical and inguinal nodes are common, but enlargement of posterior auricular, epitrochlear, or supraclavicular nodes is abnormal. Careful examination of the optic fundi to rule out evidence of retinal hemorrhages secondary to thrombocytopenia or leukemic infiltration, or both, is important. The oropharynx is evaluated, including the gingivae, a common site of hypertrophy in patients with acute myelomonocytic or monocytic leukemia.

Hematologic Evaluation

A CBC will usually reveal evidence of varying degrees of anemia, thrombocytopenia, and anemia. These changes are also detectable on peripheral blood smear, which in most patients will display the presence of leukemic cells. Although examination of the peripheral smear may strongly suggest the diagnosis of leukemia, definitive diagnosis requires evaluation of a bone marrow aspirate. The posterior iliac crest is the preferred site for marrow aspiration. In cases in which aspiration does not yield sufficient material for evaluation, bone marrow biopsy is performed. Bone marrow biopsy also is helpful in assessment of the degree of marrow cellularity. Sternal marrows are rarely required and, because of the risk of retrosternal bleeding, the sternum is not an appropriate site for marrow biopsy. Once the diagnosis of leukemia is confirmed, definitive assignment of the type of leukemia is crucial if appropriate treatment is to be delivered. In the past, the distinction between ALL and AML was based solely on the morphologic assessment of a bone marrow specimen. Although this is the appropriate initial step in evaluating a bone marrow specimen, additional diagnos-

tic techniques must always be used. These include histopathologic evaluation with special cytochemical stains, biochemical assessment (i.e., TdT determination), comprehensive immunophenotyping, and cytogenetic analysis.

Special histochemical stains may be particularly helpful in delineating ALL from AML (see table) and should be performed routinely in the diagnostic evaluation of bone marrow aspirate specimens.[89] The myeloperoxidase stain defects myeloperoxidase in primary granules and is considered specific for cells of the myeloid lineage. Classically, an acute leukemia in which ≥3% of cells in the bone marrow are myeloperoxidase positive has been considered to be myeloid, although this definition is arbitrary and may cause confusion in cases of mixed lineage leukemia. Sudan black stain has sometimes been used as a substitute for myeloperoxidase, but because rare cases of ALL demonstrate Sudan black positivity, the myeloperoxidase stain is preferred. The periodic acid-Schiff (PAS) stain is positive in approximately 50% of cases of ALL and often shows a characteristic pattern of block positivity. The PAS reaction may be negative in ALL, however, and has been positive in rare cases of AML, limiting its diagnostic value. Naphthyl ASD chloroacetate esterase is an enzyme found in cells of neutrophilic lineage that may help define myeloid disease but is generally considered less sensitive than the myeloperoxidase stain. The α-naphthyl acetate esterase and α-naphthyl butyrate esterase stains are helpful particularly in defining monocytic lineage.

Analysis of TdT present in lymphoblasts of T- and B-cell precursor lineage, but not usually found in mature B-cell ALL or in AML, is also a helpful diagnostic procedure. Detailed immunophenotyping using a panel of monoclonal antibodies is undertaken in all newly diagnosed cases of acute leukemia. The use of a sufficiently comprehensive monoclonal antibody panel capable of detecting the major lymphoid (both B- and T-cell), myeloid, and platelet-related antigens permits a definitive lineage assignment in most cases of acute leukemia. Molecular phenotyping provides useful information regarding the status of the immunoglobulin or T-cell receptor gene rearrangement in lymphoid leukemic cells. However, because immunoglobulin gene rearrangement has been observed in T-cell ALL and T-cell receptor gene rearrangement in B-cell precursor ALL, molecular phenotyping cannot be used to distinguish definitively between immunologic subtypes of ALL.

Cytogenetic analysis, including evaluation of both chromosomal number and structure, is routinely performed and may reveal characteristic chromosomal abnormalities (e.g., t8;14, t4;11).

When this overall diagnostic strategy is used, it is rare to encounter a leukemia that defies classification.

Lumbar Puncture

Lumbar puncture is performed in all newly diagnosed patients to rule out central nervous system leukemia. In patients with marked thrombocytopenia, platelet transfusions are given to ensure that the platelet count is optimal ($>40,000/mm^3$) prior to performing the lumbar puncture. In addition to measurement of cerebrospinal fluid opening pressure, the cerebrospinal fluid cell count, protein, and glucose are determined. Examination of a cytocentrifuged specimen of cerebrospinal fluid is always performed, as this technique increases diagnostic sensitivity.

Other Diagnostic and Laboratory Studies

A chest radiograph is routinely obtained in newly diagnosed patients. When significant mediastinal enlargement is detected, computed tomography can help define its extent more accurately. Patients presenting with significant bone pain undergo radiologic examination of the involved site. All newly diagnosed patients have a comprehensive battery of blood chemistries performed, including uric acid, electrolytes, calcium, phosphorus, BUN, serum creatinine, and liver function tests (including lactate dehydrogenase).

Supportive Care

The blood type of all patients is determined and appropriate cross-matching instituted if transfusion is required. Platelets are administered prophylactically to maintain the platelet count >20,000/mm^3. Packed red cell transfusions are used to maintain a hemoglobin >8 g/dl. Where possible, HLA typing is performed. This information may be useful if the patient becomes refractory to random donor platelets and requires HLA-matched platelets. HLA typing of both patient and family also provides useful information regarding the possible bone marrow transplantation options. should this therapeutic approach be warranted.

All newly diagnosed patients receive allopurinol and vigorous hydration to prevent uric acid nephropathy and complications from tumor lysis. In patients with extremely high initial white blood cell counts (e.g., >100,000/ml), leukapheresis or, in very young patients, exchange transfusion is sometime necessary.

Newly diagnosed patients who are febrile receive an extensive evaluation to rule out infection. The febrile neutropenic patient is placed on broad-spectrum antibiotic coverage.

The diagnosis of leukemia places extraordinary stress on patient and family alike. Starting at the time of initial diagnosis, careful attention is given to evaluating the psychosocial profile of patient and family, so that appropriate psychosocial support for both can be instituted. Optimal psychosocial support requires a concerted, coordinated effort of physician, nurses, social workers, clergy, and other skilled health care personnel.

Morphologic, Cytochemical, and Biochemical Characteristics Helpful in Distinguishing ALL from AML[a]

Characteristic	ALL	AML
Nuclear/cytoplasmic ratio	High	Low
Nuclear chromatin	Clumped	Spongy
Nucleoli	0–2	2–5
Granules	–	+
Auer rods	–	±
Cytoplasm	Blue	Blue-gray
Cytochemical reaction		
Peroxidase	–	+
Sudan Black B	–	+
Periodic acid-Schiff	±	–
Naphthyl ASD chloracetate esterase	–	±
α-Napthyl acetate esterase	–	±
α-Naphthyl butyrate esterase	–	–
TdT	+[b]	–

[a] Table provides information on characteristics that may be useful in differentiating ALL from AML (see text for details). Wide variation in morphology is encountered in both disease categories. Diagnostic evaluation should include more refined classification of disease according to FAB subtype.

[b] TdT is usually negative in typical FAB L3 ALL.

ment of B-cell precursor and T-cell ALL, respectively, the occurrence of immunoglobulin gene rearrangement in some cases of T-cell ALL and the presence of T-cell receptor gene rearrangement in cases of B-cell precursor ALL undermines the value of molecular phenotyping to assign B-cell or T-cell lineage.[49–51]

Most cases of ALL express surface antigens and molecular markers that help identify them as derived from a specific lineage. However, cases of lineage infidelity, or biphenotypy, exist in which leukemia cells exhibit markers of more than one cell type on the same leukemic cell. Simultaneous expression of lymphoid and myeloid markers also occurs both in childhood and in adult ALL and is associated with a poor prognosis[45,52] (see below).

Other Laboratory Studies

At diagnosis, many patients with ALL have elevated serum uric acid levels, a by-product of the increased purine metabolism of leukemic cells. The degree of uric acid elevation reflects

Table 68-3. FAB Classification of Lymphocytic Leukemia

Cytologic Features	L1	L2	L3
Cell size	Small cells predominate	Large, heterogeneous in size	Large and homogeneous
Nuclear chromatin	Homogeneous in any one case	Variable; heterogeneous in any one case	Finely stippled and homogeneous
Nuclear shape	Regular; occasional clefting or indentation	Irregular; clefting and indentation common	Regular, oval to round
Nucleoli	Not visible, or small and inconspicuous	One or more present, often large	Prominent; one or more
Amount of cytoplasm	Scanty	Variable, often moderately abundant	Moderately abundant
Basophilia of cytoplasm	Slight or moderate, rarely intense	Variable, deep in some	Very deep
Cytoplasmic vacuolation	Variable	Variable	Often prominent

(From Bennett et al.,[98] with permission.)

Table 68-4. Monoclonal Antibodies Commonly Used to Immunophenotype Leukemia[a]

CD	Antibody	Predominant Reactivity
T Cell		
CD1	T6	Thymocytes
CD2	T1 1	Pan-T
CD3	T3	Pan-T
CD4	T4/Leu3	T-helper/inducer
CD5	T101/Leu1	Pan-T, B-CLL
CD7	Leu9	Pan-T
CD8	T8/Leu2	T cytotoxic/suppressor
CDw29	4B4	T4+/4B4+ = helper inducer
		T4+/2H4+ = suppressor inducer
B Cell		
CD19	B4	Pan-B
CD20	B1	Pan-B
CD21	B2	C3dR
CD24	BA1	Pan-B
	PCA-1	Plasma cells
Myeloid		
CD11c	LeuM5	Monocytes, hairy cell
CD13	My7	Pan-myeloid
CD14	LeuM3/MY4/MO2	Monocytes
CD15	LeuM1	Monocytes, granulocytes
CD33	My9	Pan-myeloid
Miscellaneous		
CD9	BA2	Hematopoietic Progenitor/leukemic blasts
CD10	CALLA/J5	ALL/Burkitt/follicular lymphoma
CD34	My10/HPCA-1	Hematopoietic progenitor cells/HTLV-infected cells
CD41a	Plt-1	Platelets/megakaryocytes
CD45	T-200/LCA	Pan-leukocyte
	T9	Transferrin Receptor/proliferating cells

[a] CD classification number, corresponding antibodies, and their predominant reactivity are listed.

(Data from Jane Trepel, Ph.D., Medicine Branch, National Cancer Institute.)

the extent of tumor burden, higher levels occurring in patients with high initial leukocyte counts, and pronounced lymphadenopathy and hepatosplenomegaly. Hyperuricemia must be corrected by vigorous use of hydration and administration of the xanthine oxidase inhibitor allopurinol in order to prevent uric acid nephropathy and renal failure.

Abnormalities in a number of lysosomal enzymes are also evident at diagnosis. Serum lactate dehydrogenase is frequently elevated. The degree of elevation appears to correlate with tumor burden and also with prognosis.[33,53] In addition, isoenzyme I, an acid hydrolase hexosaminidase, is frequently elevated in B-cell precursor ALL.[54]

A variety of metabolic abnormalities, including elevated serum levels of calcium, potassium, and phosphorus, may be observed in the newly diagnosed patient with ALL. These are more frequently encountered in those patients with a high leukocyte count and extensive tumor burden. Hypercalcemia may be due either to extensive infiltration of bone or to the ectopic release of a parathyrin-like substance by leukemic lymphoblasts.[40] Hyperphosphatemia may accompany the extensive destruction of tumor cells. It may occur either as a result of ineffective leukopoiesis or as a consequence of chemotherapy-induced tumor lysis.[55] Hyperkalemia also can occur as a result of extensive leukemic cell lysis. Spurious hyperkalemia, the result of the release of potassium from leukemic cells during the process of clotting in vitro, must be ruled out as a cause of high potassium levels.[56]

Other laboratory abnormalities are also occasionally present at diagnosis. Low serum immunoglobulin levels at diagnosis have been reported in ≤30% of children with ALL and have been associated with a poor prognosis.[57,58] Significant coagulation abnormalities are not a typical feature of ALL at diagnosis. Although disseminated intravascular coagulation may occur, it is infrequent. Clotting abnormalities are observed, however, in many patients who are under active treatment with L-asparaginase.[59]

PROGNOSIS

A number of clinical and laboratory features evident at diagnosis have prognostic value for predicting the remission duration of patients treated for ALL (Table 68-5). The identification of these prognostic factors has provided a means of stratifying patients into different risk groups and "tailoring" treatment accordingly. This approach has become an important feature of many current treatment protocols, particularly in children. In assessing the relative prognostic value of any feature, it is important to determine whether it functions as an independent prognostic determinant rather than a dependent one. Multivariate analysis is helpful in this regard.

The initial leukocyte count at diagnosis has proven to be an important prognostic factor in virtually all ALL studies. In general, the prognosis is inversely related to the leukocyte count. Those patients with initial leukocyte counts >50,000/ ml have a particularly poor prognosis.[60–62] The relationship between white count and prognosis appears to be linear and continuous.

Age at diagnosis also has prognostic importance. Patients who are very young (<2 years) and older patients (>10 years) tend to have a worse prognosis.[63–66] Among children, infants <12 months of age have the poorest prognosis; their disease has a number of unique biologic features, which in part may explain their relative resistance to therapy.[67] In adults, progressively older age is associated with lower rates of remission induction and shorter remission duration.[2,68]

Cytogenetic analysis also provides important prognostic information.[69–71] The association between chromosomal number and prognosis is well characterized. Patients with hyperdiploidy (>50 chromosomes) have a favorable prognosis, whereas those with hypoploidy and pseudodiploidy do not fare as well. Abnormalities in chromosome structures also conveys important prognostic information. A number of chromosomal translocations are associated with both a high rate of induction failure and early relapse, including the t(8;14) translocation associated with B-cell ALL, the t(9;22) found in Philadelphia chromosome positive ALL, and the t(4;11) translocation occurring most frequently in infants.[72]

There is also a relationship between sex and prognosis. Females have a more favorable outcome. This appears to be related to the impact of testicular relapse and to the higher incidence of T-cell disease in males.[61,65,73]

Immunophenotype also correlates with prognosis.[48,74,75] Patients with mature B-cell ALL have the worst prognosis. Conversely, the best prognosis appears to be for those patients with B-cell precursor ALL whose lymphoblasts do not show

Table 68-5. Factors Associated With Prognosis in ALL

Initial white blood cell count	Organomegaly and lymphadenopathy
Age at diagnosis	Hemoglobin level
Sex	Race
Cytogenetics	Platelet count
Immunophenotype	Serum immunoglobulins
FAB morphology	Rapidity of leukemic cytoreduction
Mediastinal mass	

evidence of cytoplasmic immunoglobulin (early pre-B ALL). Those cases of B-cell precursor ALL in which cytoplasmic immunoglobulin is present (known as pre-B ALL) have a poor outcome, as do patients with the T-cell phenotype.[47] Although earlier studies indicated that T-cell disease is associated with a poor prognosis, the prognostic influence of T-cell phenotype is less striking after adjustment for its association with high initial leukocyte count. The intensity of treatment appears to influence the degree to which T-cell phenotype influences prognosis. In some recent, more intensive, treatment protocols, the prognostic influence of T-cell phenotype has not been evident.[36,39,76–78]

The expression of myeloid markers on ALL cells appears to be associated with a poor prognosis, both in children and in adults with ALL.[45,52] There is also a relationship between morphologic subtype and prognosis. The FAB L3 subtype is associated with B-cell ALL and therefore conveys a poor prognosis. In many studies of childhood ALL, the L2 subtype has also been associated with a poor prognosis,[36,46,79,80] while the L1 subtype is associated with a more favorable outcome. This finding has not been universal, however, and may not be a helpful distinction in adult ALL.[1,81–83]

Race appears to be an important prognostic determinant. Blacks have a lower remission induction rate and a higher likelihood of experiencing bone marrow relapse.[81,84,85] The reasons for this poor outcome are related in part to the more frequent recurrence of very elevated initial leukocyte counts, mediastinal masses, and L2 morphology in blacks.[76,81,86]

Tumor burden can be assessed indirectly by evaluating the degree of hepatosplenomegaly and lymphadenopathy. In numerous studies, hepatomegaly, splenomegaly, and mediastinal mass have been demonstrated to have prognostic importance, although on multivariate analysis they are found to be closely dependent on the initial leukocyte count. Despite this, hepatomegaly and splenomegaly have been useful to some investigators in the prospective definition of risk groups. For example, the West German BFM (Berlin-Franfurt-Munich) study group uses a "risk factor" index, computed on the basis of initial leukocyte count and measurement of hepatosplenomegaly, to define different treatment groups for childhood ALL.[87]

In addition to the features noted above, a variety of other characteristics have been found to have prognostic value. In children, low serum immunoglobulins, particularly low IgM levels, are associated with poor event-free survival.[57,58,88]

Perhaps one of the most significant prognostic factors is the response to initial treatment, although, strictly speaking, it is not a presenting clinical or laboratory feature of patients with ALL. Nonetheless, patients who fail to achieve complete remission after completing an initial course of induction therapy have markedly reduced remission duration and survival. The rapidity of initial cytoreduction appears to be extremely important. For example, the presence of residual leukemia on day 14 of induction therapy has been associated with shorter event-free survival compared with patients whose day 14 marrow shows no evidence of residual disease.[36,62,76]

Current treatment regimens for childhood ALL use prognostic factors to define different risk groups, which are subsequently treated according to their relative risk of failure. At most centers, patients with poor risk features receive more intensive treatment, while those with good risk features receive treatment designed to be effective, yet minimize treatment-related adverse sequelae. Such treatment stratification has been applied primarily in children with ALL, a population in which patients with good risk features are more readily identified than in adults. The success of this strategy and the general principles of treatment for the patient with ALL are detailed in Chapter 69.

REFERENCES

1. Hoelzer D, Gale R: Acute lymphoblastic leukemia in adults: recent progress, future directions. Semin Hematol 24:27, 1987
2. Gaynor J, Chapman D, Little C et al: A cause-speciifc hazard rate analysis of prognostic factors among 199 adults with acute lymphoblastic leukemia: the Memorial Hospital Experience since 1969. J Clin Oncol 6:1014, 1988
3. Linker C, Levitt J, O'Donnell M et al: Improved results of treatment of adult acute lymphoblastic leukemia. Blood 69:1242, 1987
4. Pierce M, Borges W, Heyn R et al: Epidemiological factors and survival experience in 1770 children with acute leukemia treated by members of Children's Study Group A between 1957 and 1964. Cancer 23:1296, 1969
5. Committee on Leukemia and Working Party on Leukemia in Childhood: Duration of survival of children with acute leukemia. Br Med J 4:7, 1971
6. Tivey H: The natural history of untreated acute leukemia. Ann NY Acad Sci 60:322, 1954
7. Miller R: Down's syndrome, other malformations, and cancer among the sibs of leukemia children. N Engl J Med 268:393, 1963
8. Miller R: Relation between cancer and congenital defects: an epidemiologic evaluation. J Natl Cancer Inst 40:1079, 1968
9. Swift M: Fanconi's anemia in the genetics of neoplasia. Nature 230:370, 1971
10. Toledano S, Lange B: Ataxia-telangiectasia and acute lymphoblastic leukemia. Cancer 45:1675, 1980
11. Miller R: Persons with exceptionally high risk of leukemia. Part 1. Cancer Res 27:2420, 1967
12. Draper G, Heaf M, Wilson LK: Occurrence of childhood cancers among sibs and estimation of familial risks. J Med Genet 14:81, 1977
13. Felix C, Nau M, Takahashi T et al: Hereditary and acquired p53 gene mutations in childhood acute lymphoblastic leukemia. J Clin Invest 89:640, 1992
14. Melhorn D, Gross S, Newman A: Acute childhood leukemia presenting as aplastic anemia. The response to corticosteroids. J Pediatr 77:647, 1970
15. Nelken R, Stockman J: The hypereosinophilic syndrome in association with acute lymphoblastic leukemia. J Pediatr 89:771, 1976
16. Mathe G, Schwarzenberg L, Mery A et al: Extensive histological and cytological survey of patients with acute leukemia in "complete remission." Br Med J 1:640, 1966
17. Nies B, Bodey G, Thomas L et al: The persistence of extramedullary leukemic infiltrates during bone marrow remission of acute leukemia. Blood 26:133, 1965
18. Simone J, Holland E, Johnson W: Fatalities during remission of childhood leukemia. Blood 39:759, 1972
19. Bleyer WA: Central nervous system leukemia. Pediatr Clin North Am 35:789, 1988
20. Price R, Johnson W: The central nervous system and childhood leukemia. I. The arachnoid. Cancer 31:530, 1973
21. Thomas L, Chirigos M, Humphreys S, Golden A: Pathology of the spread of L1210 leukemia in the central nervous system of mice and effect of treatment with cytoxan. J Natl Cancer Inst 28:1355, 1962
22. Thomas L: Pathology of leukemia in the brain and meninges: postmortem studies of patients with acute leukemia and of mice given inoculations of L1210 leukemia. Cancer Res 25:1555, 1965
23. Baum E, Land V, Joo P et al: Cessation of chemotherapy during complete remission of childhood acute lymphoblastic leukemia. Proc Am Soc Clin Oncol 18:290, 1977
24. Stoffel T, Nesbit M, Livitt S: Extramedullary involvement of the testes in childhood. Cancer 35:1203, 1975
25. Kim T, Hargreaves H, Byrnes R et al: Pretreatment testicular biopsy in childhood acute lymphocytic leukemia. Lancet 2:652, 1981
26. Bowman W, Aur R, Hustu H, Rivera G: Isolated testicular relapse in acute lymphocytic leukemia of childhood: categories and influence on survival. J Clin Oncol 2:924, 1984
27. Kuo T, Tschang T, Chu J: Testicular relapse in childhood acute lymphocytic leukemia during bone marrow remission. Cancer 38:2604, 1976
28. Riccardi R, Vigersky R, Barnes S et al: Methotrexate levels in the interstitial space and seminiferous tubule of rat testis. Cancer Res 42:1617, 1982
29. Baum E, Heyn R, Nesbit M et al: Occult abdominal involvement with apparently isolated testicular relapse in children with acute lymphocytic leukemia. Am J Pediatr Hematol Oncol 6:3343, 1984
30. Brecher M, Weinberg V, Boyett J et al: Intermediate dose methotrexate in childhood acute lymphoblastic leukemia resulting in decreased incidence of testicular relapse. Cancer 58:1024, 1986
31. Haghbin M: Chemotherapy of acute lymphoblastic leukemia in children. Am J Hematol 1:201, 1976
32. Russo A, Schiliro G: The enigma of testicular leukemia: a critical review. Med Pediatr Oncol 14:300, 1986
33. Pui H, Parwaresch M, Kulenkampff C et al: Lysosomal acid esterase: activity and isoenzymes in separated normal human blood cells. Blood 55:891, 1985

34. Hudson M, Frankel L, Mullins J, Swanson D: Diagnostic value of surgical testicular biopsy after therapy for acute lymphocytic leukemia. J Pediatr 107:50, 1985

35. Kim T, Hargreaves H, Chan W et al: Sequential testicular biopsies in childhood acute lymphocytic leukemia. Cancer 57:1038, 1986

36. Hammond G, Sather H, Bleyer W, Coccia P: Stratification by prognostic factors in the design and analysis of clinical trials for acute lymphoblastic leukemia. Haematology and blood transfusion. p. 161. In Buchner T, Schellong G, Hiddemann W, Urbanitz D, Ritter J (eds): Acute Leukemias. Springer-Verlag, Berlin, 1987

37. Steinherz P, Siegel S, Bleyer A et al: Lymphomatous presentation of acute lymphoblastic leukemia. Proc Am Soc Clin Oncol 5:153, 1986

38. Reaman G, Poplack D, Wesley R et al: Prognostic factors for central nervous system (CNS) relapse in acute lymphoblastic leukemia (ALL) of childhood, abstracted (C-787). Proc Am Soc Clin Oncol 3:202, 1984

39. Steinherz P, Gaynon P, Miller D et al: Improved disease-free survival of children with acute lymphoblastic leukemia at high risk for early relapse with the New York regimen—a new intensive therapy protocol: a report from the Childrens Cancer Study Group. J Clin Oncol 4:744, 1986

40. Hann I, Lees F, Palmer M et al: Renal size as a prognostic factor in childhood acute lymphoblastic leukemia. Cancer 48:207, 1981

41. Kushner D, Weinstein H, Kirkpatrick J: The radiological diagnosis of leukemia and lymphoma in children. Semin Roentgenol 115:316, 1980

42. Bodey G, Buckley M, Sathe U: Quantitative relationships between circulating leukocytes and infections in patients with acute leukemia. Ann Intern Med 64:328, 1966

43. Brearly R, Johnson S, Lister T: Acute lymphoblastic leukemia in adults: clinicopathological correlations with the French-Amreican-British (FAB) Co-operative group classification. Eur J Cancer 15:909, 1979

44. First MIC Cooperative Study Group: Morphologic, immunologic, and cytogenetic (MIC) working classification of acute lymphoblastic leukemias. Report of the Workshop held in Leuven, Belgium, April 22–23, 1985. Cancer Genet Cytogenet 23:189, 1986

45. Sobol R, Mick R, Royston I et al: Clinical importance of myeloid antigen expression in adult acute lymphoblastic leukemia. N Engl J Med 316:1111, 1987

46. Miller D, Krailo M, Bleyer W et al: Prognostic implications of blast cell morphology in childhood acute lymphoblastic leukemia: a report from the Childrens Cancer Study Group. Cancer Treat Rep 69:1211, 1985

47. Crist W, Boyett J, Jackson J et al: Prognostic importance of the Pre-cell immunophenotype and other presenting features in B-lineage childhood acute lymphoblastic leukemia: a Pediatric Oncology Group Study. Blood 74:1252, 1989

48. Crist W, Grosse C, Pullen J, Cooper M: Immunologic markers in childhood acute lymphocytic leukemia. Semin Oncol 12:105, 1985

49. Felix C, Wright J, Poplack D et al: T cell receptor a-, b-, and g-genes in T cell and pre-B cell acute lymphoblastic leukemia. J Clin Invest 80:545, 1987

50. Kitchingman G, Rovigatti U, Mauer A et al: Rearrangement of immunoglobulin heavy chain genes in T cell acute lymphoblastic leukemia. Blood 65:725, 1985

51. Tawa A, Hozumi N, Minden M et al: Rearrangement of the T-cell receptor B-chain gene in non-T-cell, non-B-cell acute lymphoblastic leukemia of childhood. N Engl J Med 313:1033, 1985

52. Mirro J, Zipf T, Pui C et al: Acute mixed lineage leukemia: clinicopathologic correlations and prognostic significance. Blood 65:1115, 1985

53. Kornberg A, Polliack A: Serum lactic dehydrogenase (LDH) levels in acute leukemia: marked elevations in lymphoblastic leukemia. Blood 56:351, 1980

54. Ellis R, Rapson N, Patrick A, Greaves M: Expressions of hexosaminidase isoenzymes in childhood leukemia. N Engl J Med 298:476, 1978

55. Wiernik P: Acute leukemias. p. 1809. DeVita VJ, Hellman S, Rosenberg S (eds): Principles and Practice of Oncology. 3rd Ed. JB Lippincott, Philadelphia, 1989

56. Salomon J: Spurious hypoglycemia and hyperkalemia in myelomonocytic leukemia. Am J Med Sci 267:359, 1974

57. Leiken S, Miller D, Sather H et al: Immunologic evaluation in the prognosis of acute lymphoblastic leukemia. A report from Childrens Cancer Study Group. Blood 58:5601, 1981

58. Hann I, Morris-Jones P, Evans D et al: Low IgG or IgA: a further indicator of poor prognosis in childhood acute lymphoblastic leukaemia. Br J Cancer 41:317, 1980

59. Priest J, Ramsay N, Steinherz P et al: A syndrome of thrombosis and hemorrhage complicating L-asparaginase therapy for childhood acute lymphoblastic leukemia. J Pediatr 100:984, 1982

60. Mastrangelo R, Poplack D, Bleyer W et al: Report and recommendations of the Rome Workshop concerning poor-prognosis acute lymphoblastic leukemia in children: biologic bases for staging, stratification, and treatment. Med Pediatr Oncol 14:191, 1986

61. Robison L, Sather H, Coccia P et al: Assessment of the interrelationship of prognostic factors in childhood acute lymphoblastic leukemia. Am J Pediatr Hematol Oncol 2:3, 1980

62. Miller D: Prognostic factors in childhood acute lymphoblastic leukemia. J Pediatr 87:672, 1974

63. Sather H: Statistical evaluation of prognostic factors in ALL and treatment results. Med Pediatr Oncol 14:158, 1986

64. Zuelzer W, Flatz G: Acute childhood leukemia: a ten year study. Am J Dis Child 100:886, 1960

65. Hammond D, Sather H, Nesbit M et al: Analysis of prognostic factors in acute lymphoblastic leukemia. Med Pediatr Oncol 14:124, 1986

66. Crist W, Pullen J, Boyett J et al: Acute lymphoid leukemia in adolescents: clinical and biologic features predict a poor prognosis: a Pediatric Oncology Group Study. J Clin Oncol 6:34, 1988

67. Reaman G, Zeltzer P, Bleyer W et al: Acute lymphoblastic leukemia in infants less than one year of age: a cumulative experience of the Childrens Cancer Study Group. J Clin Oncol 3:1513, 1985

68. Marcus R, Catovsky D, Johnson S et al: Adult acute lymphoblastic leukemia: a study of prognostic features and response to treatment over a ten year period. Br J Cancer 53:175, 1986

69. Look AT: The cytogenetics of childhood leukemia: clinical and biologic implications. Pediatr Clin North Am 35:723, 1988

70. Bloomfield C, Goldman A, Alimena G et al: Chromosomal abnormalities identify high-risk and low-risk patients with acute lymphoblastic leukemia. Blood 67:415, 1986

71. Sandberg A: The chromosomes in human leukemia. Semin Hematol 23:201, 1986

72. Williams D, Raimondi S, Rivera G et al: Presence of clonal chromosome abnormalities in virtually all cases of acute lymphoblastic leukemia. N Engl J Med 10:640, 1985

73. Baumer J, Mott M: Sex and prognosis in childhood acute lymphoblastic leukemia. Lancet 2:128, 1978

74. Brouet J, Seligmann M: The immunological classification of acute lymphoblastic leukemias. Cancer 42:817, 1978

75. Foon K, Todd RI: Immunologic classification of leukemia and lymphoma. Blood 68:1, 1986

76. Kalwinsky D, Roberson P, Dahl G et al: Clinical relevance of lymphoblast biological features in children with acute lymphoblastic leukemia. J Clin Oncol 3:477, 1985

77. Henze G, Langermann H, Kaurmann U et al: Thymic involvement and initial white blood count in childhood acute lymphoblastic leukemia. Am J Pediatr Hematol Oncol 3:369, 1981

78. Riehm H, Gadner H, Henze G et al: The five therapy trials ALL-BFM 1970–1986: a synopsis of results. Proc Am Soc Clin Oncol 6:636, 1987

79. Lilleyman J, Hann I, Stevens R: The clinical significance of blast cell morphology in childhood lymphoblastic leukaemia. Med Pediatr Oncol 14:144, 1986

80. Chessells J, Hardisty R, Richards S: Long survival in childhood lymphoblastic leukaemia. Br J Cancer 55:315, 1987

81. Kalwinsky D, Rivera G, Dahl G et al: Variation by race in presenting clinical and biologic features of childhood acute lymphoblastic leukaemia: implications for treatment outcome. Leuk Res 9:817, 1985

82. van Eyes J, Pullen J, Head D et al: The French-American-British (FAB) classification of leukemia. The Pediatric Oncology Group experience with lymphocytic leukemia. Cancer 57:1046, 1986

83. Champlin R, Gale RP: Acute lymphoblastic leukemia: recent advances in biology and therapy. Blood 73:2051, 1989

84. Sklo M, Gordis L, Tonascia J, Kaplan E: The changing survivorship of white and black children with leukemia. Cancer 42:59, 1978

85. Walters T, Bushmore M, Simone J: Poor prognosis in Negro children with acute lymphoblastic leukemia. Cancer 29:210, 1972

86. Harousseau J, Tobelem G, Schaison G et al: High risk acute lymphocytic leukemia: a study of 141 cases with initial white blood counts over 100,000/cu. mm. Cancer 46:1996, 1980

87. Riehm H, Gadner H, Henze G et al: The Berlin childhood acute lymphoblastic leukemia therapy study, 1970–1976. Am J Pediatr Hematol Oncol 2:299, 1980

88. Khalifa A, Take H, Cejka J, Zuelzer W: Immunoglobulins in acute leukemia in children. J Pediatr 85:788, 1974

89. Dalton WJ, Stass SA: Morphologic and cytochemical approach to the diagnosis of acute leukemia. p. 27. In Stass SA (ed): Hematology. The Acute Leukemias: Biologic, Diagnostic, and Therapeutic Determinants. Marcel Dekker, New York, 1987

90. Troxell M, Mills G, Allen R: The hypereosinophilic syndrome in acute lymphocytic leukemia. Cancer 54:1058, 1984

91. Carbaton J, Monoz A, Modero L, Camarero C: Pulmonary leukemia in a child presenting with infiltrative and nodular lesions. Pediatr Radiol 14:431, 1984

92. Niebrugge D, Benjamin D: Bone marrow necrosis preceding acute lymphoblastic leukemia in childhood. Cancer 52:2162, 1983

93. Mancuso L, Marchi S, Giuliano P, Pitrolo F: Cardiac tamponade as first manifestation of acute lymphoblastic leukemia in a patient with echographic evidence of mediastinal lymph nodal enlargement. Am Heart J 110:1303, 1985

94. Canivet B, Squara P, Elbaze P et al: Consommation de glucose in vitro au cours des grandes hyperleucocytoses. Une cause d'hypoglycemia factice. Pathol Biol 30:843, 1982

95. Dunn N, McWilliams N, Mohanokumer T: Clinical and immunological correlates of leukemia cutis in childhood. Cancer 50:2049, 1982

96. Lensink D, Barton A, Applebaum F, Hammond, WD: Cyclic neutropenia as a premalignant manifestation of acute lymphoblastic leukemia. Am J Hematol 22:9, 1986

97. Nesbit ME: Clinical assessment and differential diagnosis of the child with suspected cancer. p. 83. In Pizzo PA, Poplack DG (eds): Principles and Practice of Pediatric Oncology. JB Lippincott, Philadelphia, 1988

98. Bennett JM, Catovsky D, Daniel MT et al: French-American-British (FAB) Co-operative Group: the morphological classification of acute lymphoblastic leukaemia—concordance among obesrvers and clinical correlations. Br J Haematol 47:553, 1981

Therapy for Acute Lymphocytic Leukemia in Children

69

Stephen E. Sallan and Harvey J. Cohen

INTRODUCTION

Advances in the treatment of childhood acute lymphocytic leukemia (ALL) have been the product of clinical trials and the prospective evaluation thereof (Fig. 69-1). Further advances in the treatment of this disease and attempts to limit toxicity from treatment require ongoing prospective studies. Thus, in the 1990s no child with newly diagnosed ALL should receive individualized treatment; rather every child with this diagnosis should be enrolled in a trial to ensure optimal treatment and subsequent advances for future generations of children with leukemia.

HISTORY AND PHILOSOPHY OF THERAPY

Before 1947, when the first complete remission in childhood ALL was attained by Farber and co-workers,[1] median duration of survival from the time of diagnosis was 2 months.[2] The development of a model for the scientific methodology of clinical therapeutic research in childhood ALL has been elegantly summarized in detail by Frei.[2] During the 1950s drugs such as 6-mercaptopurine, methotrexate, and corticosteroids were found to be active in leukemia-bearing mice[3] and subsequently in human leukemias.[4] The first controlled clinical trials were conducted by Frei and associates,[5] who ushered in the era of single-agent (and soon thereafter combination-agent) antileukemic chemotherapy trials[6] (Table 69-1).

Active drugs introduced in the 1960s and 1970s, such as the anthracyclines (doxorubicin and daunorubicin), asparaginase, and the epipodophyllotoxins (VP-16 and VM-26), usually underwent initial evaluation in patients whose leukemia had become resistant to the drugs listed in Table 69-1. Thus, their single-agent efficacy, as measured by the frequency of complete remissions (CRs), was underestimated because they were tested in patients with previously treated and potentially drug-resis-

tant disease. Nonetheless, these agents proved active. CR rates of 24–48% with doxorubicin[7] and 50–60% with asparaginase[8,9] were achieved.

Critical to those pioneering efforts was an understanding of the principles of the first-order cytokinetic effect of chemotherapeutic agents, and the need for clonal eradication. In the early 1960s, Skipper and associates[10] initiated a series of studies that addressed the quantitative biology of leukemia in mice and its perturbation by chemotherapy. The first-order cytokinetic effect of chemotherapy on tumor (leukemia) cells means that for a given treatment there is a constant fractional reduction of leukemia cells that is independent of the total leukemia burden. The cytokinetic model for antileukemic therapy is depicted in Figure 69-2.

From mouse leukemia models of Skipper et al.[10] it was shown that the time of death after treatment was a precise measure of the number of leukemia cells persisting at the end of treat-

Table 69-1. Chemotherapy of Childhood ALL: Historical Perspective

	Frequency of Complete Remission (%)
Single agents	
Prednisone	57
Vincristine	55
6-Mercaptopurine	27
Methotrexate	21
Cyclophosphamide	18
Combination agents	
Prednisone + vincristine	85
Prednisone + 6-mercaptopurine	81
Methotrexate + 6-mercaptopurine	45
Vincristine + prednisone + methotrexate + 6-mercaptopurine	94

(From Freireich and Frei,[6] with permission.)

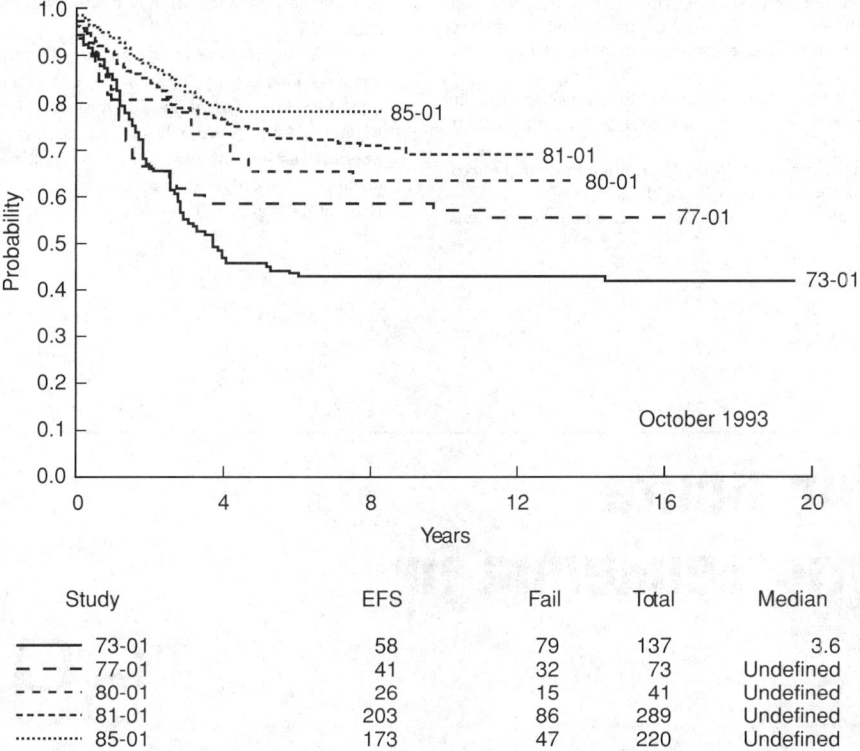

Study	EFS	Fail	Total	Median
——— 73-01	58	79	137	3.6
— — — 77-01	41	32	73	Undefined
– – – – 80-01	26	15	41	Undefined
- - - - - 81-01	203	86	289	Undefined
·········· 85-01	173	47	220	Undefined

Fig. 69-1. Event-free survival of children with ALL treated between 1973 and 1987 on Dana-Farber Cancer Institute/The Children's Hospital-based protocols. (Adapted from Sallan et al.,[13] with permission.)

ment.[11] They further demonstrated that having only one L1210 leukemic cell present was enough to cause the death of the animal. This observation led to the understanding of the need for clonal eradication. Moreover, their models provided important observations with respect to drug resistance, combination chemotherapy, and the cycling of chemotherapeutic agents. By the 1960s effective systemic chemotherapy and the development of improved supportive care with blood products and antibiotics resulted in an increased percentage of CRs and an increased duration of remissions. The ability to support a patient through prolonged myelosuppression has permitted clinical investigations that have demonstrated the importance of using maximal tolerable doses of drugs.[12,13]

In the 1960s the incidence of central nervous system leukemia as an initial site of relapse became progressively more common,[14,15] and the concept of the central nervous system as a "pharmacologic sanctuary" (i.e., an anatomic space that is poorly penetrated by systemically administered chemother-apeutic agents) emerged. Several avenues of approach to the problem of central nervous system leukemia and its treatment and prevention have been explored. These include intrathecal administration of drugs,[16] craniospinal irradiation,[17] cranial irradiation plus intrathecal drugs,[18] and high doses of systemically administered drugs that result in therapeutic concentrations in the cerebrospinal fluid.[19,20] The optimal delivery of central nervous system treatment remains controversial.

Current regimens for the treatment of ALL result in high proportions (>95%) of children achieving CR and favorable long-term outcome for most patients. This is true even though, with few exceptions, the drugs used for the treatment of ALL in the 1980s were all available by the late 1960s. Philosophically, treatment should be with curative (not palliative) intent—which means that all complications of the disease and its therapy need to be vigorously treated, and that the major effort should be directed at eradication of disease rather than relief of symptoms.

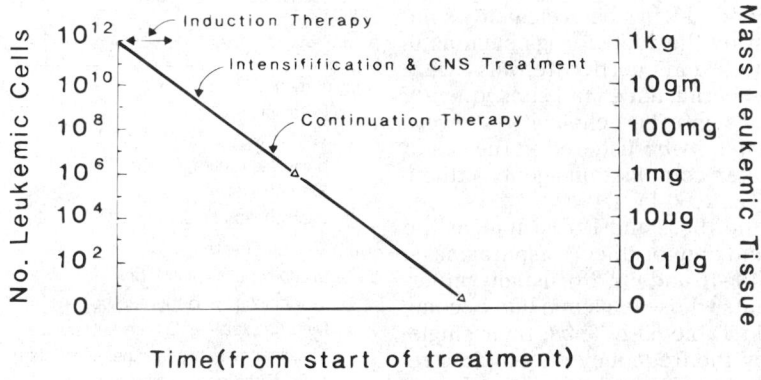

Fig. 69-2. A cytokinetic model for antileukemic therapy relating to hypothetical cell kill with components of treatment.

PRECHEMOTHERAPY SUPPORTIVE CARE

Immediately before beginning chemotherapy, patients should be treated intensively for any documented or presumed infection.[21] For a temperature >38.5°C, broad-spectrum intravenous antibiotic coverage should be given before obtaining laboratory confirmation of an infectious etiology. Chemotherapy should be started as soon as possible after diagnosis despite the need for antibiotics. Although newly diagnosed patients might not have severe neutropenia (granulocyte counts <500/mm^3), the usual state of marrow replacement with lymphoblasts and the anticipated marrow hypocellularity associated with antileukemic treatment make such antibiotic recommendations prudent. In the experience of one large referral center, 50% of newly diagnosed children with ALL had fever and neutropenia, although only 10% had blood culture documentation of bacterial sepsis.[22] Prophylaxis with trimethoprim sulfamethoxazole, usually from the time of complete remission, successfully prevents *Pneumocystis carinii* pneumonia.[23]

Thrombocytopenia, in association with neutropenia and anemia, is a common presenting feature of ALL[24]; however, active bleeding is a relatively unusual feature at the time of diagnosis. Despite this, most investigators recommend prophylactic platelet transfusions for patients with thrombocytopenia (platelet count <15,000/mm^3), as opposed to transfusions only for active bleeding. Any active hemorrhage, associated with a platelet count of <100,000/mm^3, should be treated with platelet transfusions. Similarly, symptomatic anemia should be treated by transfusion of packed red blood cells. Most investigators recommend prophylactic transfusions for a hematocrit <20–25 vol%. Stabilization of these two hematologic parameters should take no longer than 12–24 hours and should therefore not delay the start of antileukemic therapy.

Additional supportive care before institution of chemotherapy is directed at the burden of leukemic cells at the time of diagnosis, and the necessity for lysis and clearance thereof. Thus, intravenous hydration (usually with twice the maintenance volumes of fluids) and urinary alkalinization (pH ≥7.5) (usually with 0.25 N NaHCO$_3$) are important early components of supportive care. If urinary alkalinization is difficult, NaHCO$_3$-containing solutions can be increased to 0.5 N strength and acetazolamide can be added. Because the latter acts at the level of the renal tubule, care should be taken not to abruptly stop acetazolamide treatment at times of anticipated high urinary urate concentration. The purpose of the increased hydration and urinary alkalinization is to ensure that uric acid, a natural breakdown product of leukemic cell lysis, remains in solution for optimal excretion. In addition, administration of a xanthine oxidase inhibitor such as allopurinol should be started before institution of antileukemic drugs. Allopurinol prevents the formation of uric acid during cell lysis. For patients with white blood cell counts >200,000/mm^3, leukapheresis has been advocated to prevent hyperviscosity and lysis-related problems.[25]

CONCEPTUAL APPROACH TO THERAPY

Current concepts underlying therapy for newly diagnosed ALL include four components—induction, intensification, central nervous system treatment, and continuation. The induction component of therapy is designed to rapidly destroy measurable leukemic cells and minimize residual leukemic burden (i.e., the total number of leukemic cells in the body). The intensification component is designed to further reduce the total body leukemic cell burden and address issues of antileukemic drug resistance. Such treatment usually consists of higher doses of the same drugs used during induction, or of high doses of different drugs. When induction drugs are used again in the same doses, the treatment is known as reinduction therapy (also called consolidation therapy). The central nervous system treatment component is used to address the issue of pharmacologic sanctuary sites (i.e., areas of the body, such as the brain and spinal cord, that are not well penetrated by conventional doses of most antileukemic drugs). The continuation component is designed to eradicate the residual leukemic cell burden. In the past, this part of treatment was referred to as maintenance therapy. However, because the current concept is to eradicate all remaining leukemic cells, as opposed to maintaining a low tumor burden, the newer terminology is preferred.

Induction Therapy

As soon as the patient has been stabilized by the supportive measures discussed above, antileukemic chemotherapy is begun. The goal of remission induction therapy, which is provided during the first 3–4 weeks, is to rapidly induce a CR. Hematologic remission is defined as attainment of a normocellular bone marrow with ≤5% blasts, and peripheral blood without lymphoblasts, with a granulocyte count >500/mm^3, and with a platelet count >100,000/mm^3. CR is defined as achievement of the above criteria plus the absence of any demonstrable signs and symptoms of leukemia.

The percentage of children who can be induced into CR (the CR rate) is important because a CR must be induced before the next component of therapy is begun, and the achievement of CR is necessary to prolong survival. Because of the relative ease of inducing CRs in ALL, it is difficult to estimate the long-term outcome of treatment based only on the CR rate. In theory the rapidity and magnitude of the initial leukemic cell lysis might enhance the likelihood of preventing the emergence of leukemic clones, which develop drug resistance.[26] In one study, children were randomly assigned to receive identical therapy except for induction drugs; one group received vincristine and prednisone and the other received those two drugs plus an anthracycline. Although the CR rates for both groups exceeded 90%, there was long-term benefit for the more intensively treated group (event-free survival for the two groups at 16 years was 37% and 63%, respectively).[27] Thus, most investigative trials currently employ at least three drugs (e.g., vincristine, prednisone, and asparaginase)[28] and often use one or more additional drugs (e.g., an anthracycline; methotrexate).

CRs can be induced in approximately 95% of children with ALL. Although induction failures are uncommon, the current use of more intensive induction regimens might result in a slightly increased number of induction deaths. The reasons for the inability to induce rapid complete remissions, so-called induction failures, are generally equally divided between refractory disease and death from drug or disease toxicity. Successful treatment of refractory ALL has been reported with the use of drugs such as cytosine arabinoside (ara-C), etoposide, teniposide, and cyclophosphamide.[29,30]

Pharmacologic sanctuary sites, such as the central nervous system, should be treated during induction. Some commonly used systemic drugs such as glucocorticoids, asparaginase, and high-dose methotrexate affect central nervous system leukemic cells, but intrathecal agents such as ara-C and methotrexate are also recommended. Intrathecal ara-C has the advantage of having no additive myelosuppression because it is immediately inactivated by deaminases in the blood.

Although clinical CR is the goal of multidrug induction therapy, it must be recognized that "clinical" remissions are not *biologic* remissions (i.e., even after the induction of CR, leukemic cells remain in the marrow, undetected by light microscopy). Indirect evidence for this observation was derived from early clinical trials in which chemotherapy was stopped after induction of a clinical CR; all patients relapsed within 6 months.[31] Based on the principle of first-order cytokinetic killing of leukemic cells according to which a fixed proportion (≥99%, ≥99.9%, ≥99.99%) of cells are destroyed with any given dose of drugs, a fixed proportion (≥1%, ≥0.1%, ≥0.01%) of leukemic cells remains after each dose of therapy. It is the remaining tumor burden that necessitates postinduction treatment.

The use of multiagent chemotherapy during intensification and continuation phases of therapy is supported by the need to minimize the number of residual cells after each treatment. An alternative approach might be the use of very high doses of fewer drugs, such as methotrexate and ara-C (as long as post-treatment bone marrow recovery time is not increased). However, the latter approach is not as attractive because it less adequately addresses the issue of drug resistance.

An important area of investigation in leukemia pertains to the evaluation of microscopically and antigenically inapparent minimal residual disease. Immunologic and biochemical efforts to recognize residual leukemia have been relatively unsuccessful.[32,33] Most patients will have clonal abnormalities of their leukemic, but not of their normal, hematopoietic cells. Thus, cytogenetic complete remissions are also measurable, but even molecular genetic techniques have not been sensitive enough to assess small numbers of residual leukemic cells.[34] Current efforts to address minimal residual disease have focused on the use of polymerase chain reaction (PCR) techniques for the detection of extremely low numbers of cells.[35,36] Currently, the absence of detectable residual leukemia at the end of chemotherapy is insufficient to assure that the patient is cured.[37] In the future it is reasonable to expect that the duration and adequacy of treatment will in part be determined by the accurate assessment of minimal residual disease.

The Children's Cancer Group (CCG) and a Dana-Farber Cancer Institute (DFCI)-based leukemia therapy group have both attempted to assess the importance of early antileukemic responses.[38–41] In an era of relatively less intensive induction therapy it was shown that the time required to enter CR was predictive of subsequent outcome; shorter times of induction were associated with more favorable outcomes.[39] Subsequently the CCG assessed bone marrows on day 14 of treatment and found that early CRs were associated with better long-term results.[38] The use of PCR technology may aid in assessing whether the rate or degree of initial cell killing will be a predictive factor for long-term survival. Investigators in Germany have found that the clinical response to a 1-week course of steroids (plus intrathecal methotrexate) is one of the most sensitive predictors of subsequent event-free survival.[42]

The DFCI-based group also used the concept of an "investigational window" to assess early response to antileukemic agents after a 5-day exposure to the drugs in varying doses.[41,43,44] They found that high-dose methotrexate might be more effective than conventional-dose methotrexate,[41] and that although no dose response relationships were noted for asparaginase, there was a positive relationship between in vivo and in vitro leukemic cell killing.[43] In pharmacologic studies of different species of asparaginase (as well as the polyethylene glycol-modified *Escherichia coli* species) conducted in the context of an investigational window, it was shown that the half-life of asparaginase was dependent on the enzyme preparation used, but not affected by dose or repeated use. Also, patients who had a hypersensitivity reaction to one species had a decreased half-life with alternative preparations.[44]

Intensification Chemotherapy

The goals of intensification therapy are to reduce further the disease burden and to adjust the intensity of treatment based on the risk of subsequent relapse (i.e., to formulate risk-group-

specific therapy). Further reduction of the disease burden necessitates intensive cytoreductive treatment, which can be given at the time of CR because the bone marrow is relatively normocellular at the beginning of this phase of treatment.

Clinical trials conducted during the 1970s and early 1980s established groups of patients whose risk of subsequent relapse varied according to different characteristics. Current clinical trials approach individual groups of patients with different forms of therapy. For example, children with the least likelihood of relapse can be assessed to determine whether some of the more morbid components of therapy can be modified or eliminated. In contradistinction, individuals at a greater risk of relapse can be more intensively treated, and the potential higher risks of such intensified therapy can be limited to only these patients.

Because the treatment per se is the most important prognostic factor, one must be mindful of the potential misuse of pejorative terms such as good risk, average risk, or high risk patient groups. Philosophically, ALL is a high-risk disease inasmuch as 20–40% of affected children are unsuccessfully treated and die as a result of their disease.[45,46] Originally, the prognostic terms were retrospectively established in an era when there was one treatment for all children. As modern therapies based on the clinical and biologic heterogeneity of ALL have evolved, it is likely that terms such as low risk and high risk will no longer be valid, and risk factors or prognostic factors will be called therapy factors.

Therapy for the Central Nervous System

Central nervous system treatment is usually initiated during induction therapy, and definitive central nervous system treatment is usually begun immediately after induction of CR (to prevent seeding from the central nervous system to the periphery). This concept is based on data from the 1960s that demonstrated that most children who developed central nervous system leukemia, did so within the first year of therapy. However, at least some recent clinical trials delayed definitive central nervous system treatment for several months to permit more intensive systemic therapy.[47,48] There was no increase in central nervous system leukemia. The routine use of intrathecal therapy during and after induction might make the timing of definitive central nervous system treatment less critical.

Although the incidence of primary ("isolated") central nervous system relapse has been the hallmark for evaluating the efficacy of a central nervous system treatment regimen, any central nervous system involvement (whether "isolated" relapse or combined with relapse at another site) is probably the appropriate measure of efficacy of central nervous system treatment.[49,50] For example, in one clinical trial an otherwise highly successful treatment program that diminished central nervous system treatment for a group of "favorable risk" patients resulted in a high incidence (15%) of central nervous system leukemia, which in most instances was due to combined central nervous system and bone marrow involvement.[50,51]

Less well understood, but undoubtedly of importance, is the role of systemic therapy in the prevention of central nervous system leukemia. Penetration of the cerebrospinal fluid by drugs has been clearly demonstrated with the use of glucocorticoids[52] or very high doses of methotrexate or ara-C.[19,20] It has also been shown that systemically administered asparaginase, whose efficacy is a function of asparagine depletion, effectively lowers cerebrospinal fluid asparagine levels,[53] and lowers the number of lymphoblasts in the cerebrospinal fluid of children with central nervous system disease.

Another uncertainty in therapy pertains to the duration of central nervous system treatment. Whether treatment only during induction and postinduction sanctuary therapy is adequate or whether prolonged intermittent central nervous system treatment is more effective has not been adequately evaluated. However, trials with the lowest reported incidence of central nervous system leukemia used prolonged central nervous system treatment.[49,54-56]

Optimal central nervous system treatment should provide maximum antileukemic efficacy with minimum morbidity. It is important that efficacy be measured not only by the prevention of central nervous system leukemia, but by the effect of the entire therapy regimen on overall event-free survival. Equally important, the morbidity of the various treatment modalities must be clearly delineated.

Controversies surrounding the risk/benefit aspects of cranial irradiation are based on studies of ALL survivors who have brain damage, growth and neuroendocrinologic abnormalities, and an increased incidence of second malignant neoplasms.[57,58] Uncertainties about such morbidity have resulted in a wide range of treatment philosophies. For example, by the mid-1980s the proportion of children receiving cranial irradiation as a component of primary treatment varied from 0%[59] to 60%[56] among different national and international trials. Based on our own experience[49,56,60] and that of others,[61] we recommend cranial irradiation and intrathecal drugs (methotrexate and ara-C) for the 60% of children we place into a high-risk group.[56] Although other investigators have found that radiation can be successfully eliminated in the other 40% of patients,[62,63] we have recently observed that boys with standard risk leukemia who were treated without cranial irradiation had a very high incidence of central nervous system relapse.[64] Infants <1 year of age should not be irradiated because of the risk of excessive morbidity to the developing brain. The overall outcome for these patients is not as good as for older children with ALL, presumably because infants have a biologically different form of the disease.[65-67] The approach to the treatment of these children should include intensive chemotherapy designed to treat both systemic and central nervous system disease.

Bleyer and Poplack[68] have comprehensively summarized approaches to the treatment of central nervous system leukemia present at the time of diagnosis. For these children we recommend treatment with twice-weekly intrathecal ara-C until the cerebrospinal fluid no longer has detectable blasts. Thereafter, at the time of CR the central nervous system is treated with cranial irradiation and intrathecal drugs (usually methotrexate and ara-C).

Continuation Therapy

The ideal duration of intensive therapy remains unknown, as does the ideal duration of postintensification continuation therapy. Again, the inability to assess accurately minimal residual disease results in a necessary dependence on randomized clinical trials that assess the duration of treatment. It is difficult to use historical controls for such studies because so much of what was done early in therapy undoubtedly affected the later components of treatment, including the necessary length of treatment. In addition to presumably variable (and currently immeasurable) quantities of residual leukemic cells, there are also differences in the proliferative and growth potentials of the remaining leukemic cells. For example, clinical trials of rapidly proliferating, mature B-cell ALL have shown that short, intensive regimens (lasting only 2-3 months) have been quite effective.[69,70] On the other hand, slower-paced disease might benefit from a longer course of therapy. Drugs used during continuation therapy include methotrexate, 6-mercaptopurine, vincristine, and glucocorticoids (prednisone or dexamethasone).

LATE EFFECTS OF THERAPY

The treatment of children with ALL has resulted in prolonged, event-free survival for 60-70% of patients.[56] However, even for these successfully treated children, long-term effects of the disease and its treatment often result in organ toxicity of varying magnitude. Detailed analyses of the long-term complications of therapy have been thoroughly summarized by Green.[71] The consequences of treatment to the normal tissue are a function of the organ system involved and the type of therapy. The most common, and often most problematic, late effects involve the central nervous system,[72] but other problems include cataracts,[73] cardiac abnormalities,[74] hepatic toxicity,[75] abnormalities of gonadal function and reproduction,[76] and second malignant neoplasms.[57,58]

The magnitude of brain damage varies within the treatment population. For example, younger children (<5 years old) were more vulnerable than older children,[77,78] and in at least one set of reports, girls were more vulnerable than boys.[77,79]

Although most toxicity has been attributed to cranial irradiation, usually administered concomitantly with intrathecal drugs, including methotrexate, studies of children treated with intrathecal methotrexate and no irradiation have also shown that the use of methotrexate alone has been associated with central nervous system abnormalities.[80,81] The role of systemic and intrathecal chemotherapy in the causation of late central nervous system toxicity is difficult to assess, but in at least one study escalating doses of systemic methotrexate in children who had received cranial irradiation were associated with brain damage.[82] Low and low-average intelligence quotients have been frequent findings in survivors of ALL.[78,83] More detailed neuropsychological studies have demonstrated that learning disabilities are related to a slow speed of processing information, as well as to difficulty in dealing with complex or conceptually demanding material.[84] Increased dose intensity of methotrexate has been associated with lower intelligence quotients in girls, and higher doses of cranial irradiation (28 Gy) may be associated with impairment of verbal memory.[77] Microcephaly has also been reported as a late effect of central nervous system treatment and was found to be dependent on the radiation dose.[79]

In some studies, survivors of ALL are shorter than expected for their age,[85-88] but one study showed normal linear growth in children treated without cranial irradiation.[89] Young age and female sex are associated with greater growth failure.[87,88] Normal pubertal growth spurts, at least for girls, may not occur. Some instances of short stature have been associated with growth hormone deficiency,[90] although other investigations have failed to show impaired growth hormone secretion.[91] Short stature can sometimes be treated with growth hormone, but controversy surrounding possible additive cardiac toxicity of such therapy (especially in patients with anthracycline-induced cardiomyopathy),[92] as well as the possible risk of leukemic recurrence, necessitates that growth hormone be prescribed with great care.

Small, nonprogressive posterior subcapsular cataracts, which did not impair vision or require surgical treatment, have been reported in >50% of children treated for ALL.[73] Although the cataracts were thought to be related to the administration of steroids, the patients described had also received cranial irradiation (which included treatment of the posterior half of the globes and the optic nerves).

Echocardiographic abnormalities, particularly increased afterload and decreased contractility, are common late effects of prior anthracycline therapy.[74] The mechanism of this toxicity is impairment of myocardial growth. Patients treated with high doses of cyclophosphamide or ifosfamide, often in preparation for bone marrow transplantation (BMT), have also experienced cardiac toxicity.[93,94]

Late occurring hepatotoxicity is a relatively uncommon effect of ALL therapy.[75,76] Despite the large number of patients treated with regular doses of methotrexate, there have been few reports of fibrosis or other abnormalities.[75]

Ovarian and testicular function are relatively unaffected by most antileukemic therapy,[95] with the possible exception of programs that use alkylating agents (such as cyclophosphamide), high doses of ara-C,[96] or prophylactic gonadal irradiation. Several normal children have been born of patients successfully treated for childhood ALL.[97,98]

Second malignant neoplasms, especially malignant gliomas[57,58] and epipodophyllotoxin-treatment-related acute myeloid leukemia,[99,100] as well as carcinomas of the parotid and thyroid glands,[57,101] have been reported in survivors of ALL. Although cranial or craniospinal irradiation has been associated with many of these tumors, some second malignancies (especially brain tumors) might occur irrespective of central nervous system treatment.[102]

THERAPY FOR RELAPSED ALL

The recurrence of ALL is a life-threatening event. Factors that influence subsequent treatment include whether the recurrence is (1) in the bone marrow or at an extramedullary site, such as the central nervous system, testis, ovary, eye, or a combination of sites[103]; and (2) after a relatively short initial remission (<18–24 months) or after a longer first remission.[103–109] The latter factor is sometimes thought of as the distinction between recurrence during therapy and recurrence after cessation of therapy[103]; however, variable lengths of treatment programs make this criterion a less sensitive determinant of the outcome of subsequent therapy. Our observation has been that the time to relapse was more important than whether the relapse occurred while the patient was on or off therapy.[105]

Depending on the intensity of initial therapy, induction of second CRs can be expected in 50–90% of children, with conflicting data pertaining to whether some patients who were initially more intensively treated have a lower likelihood of second remission.[109,110] Second induction treatment usually consists of multiple drugs, most often combinations of vincristine, prednisone, asparaginase, and an anthracycline (with or without methotrexate, an epipodophyllotoxin, and ara-C). If the central nervous system has been involved as a site of relapse, intrathecal therapy with one or more drugs (methotrexate, ara-C, hydrocortisone, thiotepa) is usually recommended on a weekly or twice-weekly basis until the cerebrospinal fluid is clear. Thereafter, when the patient is in CR, subsequent central nervous system treatment ("reprophylaxis") is indicated.[111] Testicular relapses are usually treated with bilateral gonadal irradiation as well as with systemic chemotherapy.[112–114]

After a second complete remission has been attained, the options for subsequent treatment include BMT and chemotherapy. Most trials of the latter have been unsuccessful at producing long-term survival.[115,116] This is especially true for patients who relapse within 18 months of diagnosis and those with T-cell ALL.[109] However, the results of some chemotherapy trials have led to controversy pertaining to whether patients should receive chemotherapy or BMT. The most successful chemotherapy trials were achieved with patients whose initial CR was >18 months[103,106,109]; several other drug studies have resulted in the cure of few, if any, patients.[115,116] Clinical trials comparing BMT with chemotherapy have generally been complicated by variability of patient selection criteria and treatment.[117] One controlled study of children initially similarly treated and subsequently treated with BMT or chemotherapy (depending on the availability of an allogeneic donor), showed short-term equivalence between the two modalities,[118] although long-term follow-up demonstrated late relapses in the chemotherapy-treated but not the BMT-treated group.[119]

BMT—syngeneic, allogeneic, or autologous—has achieved varying degrees of success.[104,105,107–109,117,119–122] Allogeneic BMT for relapsed ALL has resulted in long-term survival for 25–50% of patients.[107–109,117,119,120,122] BMT in second remission has generally been more favorable than in third or subsequent remission, and the most common cause of failure is recurrence of leukemia.[120] Graft-versus-host disease is the other major complication of allogeneic BMT, but the concomitant phenomenon of graft-versus-leukemia sometimes counterbalances that adverse effect.[123] A very important prognostic factor in predicting the outcome of BMT for patients with relapsed ALL is the duration of their initial remission. In some studies better outcomes have been associated with initial remissions of >18–24 months.[107–109]

Results of autologous BMT for common ALL antigen-positive disease have been comparable to the experience with allogeneic BMT. The absence of graft-versus-host disease and the need for long-term immunosuppression, as well as the expanded donor pool, offer advantages for this form of treatment.[104,105,107]

Transplants from unrelated, computer-matched donors have been successful for some children with recurrent leukemia.[124] The major obstacle to the use of this source of grafts has been graft-versus-host disease.

Although some investigators argue for chemotherapeutic treatment of a bone marrow relapse that occurs ≥1 year after elective cessation of chemotherapy, we recommend BMT because we think that long-term event-free survival will be better in BMT-treated patients. Waiting for a second relapse before BMT may result in a decreased number of BMT candidates because of the difficulty of inducing third and subsequent CRs (especially in the era of more intensive initial ALL therapy).

Extramedullary relapses, usually central nervous system or testicular, are manifestations of systemic disease. Therefore, we recommend reinduction with systemic chemotherapy, intensification to the local site of disease (i.e., twice-weekly intrathecal drugs for central nervous system or bilateral testicular irradiation for testicular relapse), and BMT in second CR. Other investigators have reported treatment of central nervous system leukemia with craniospinal irradiation or cranial irradiation and intrathecal drugs.[125,126] However, the long-term efficacy of such treatments has not been good, and adverse central nervous system sequelae are common.[126–128] Alternative approaches to central nervous system relapse include treatment with systemically administered high doses of methotrexate or ara-C.[129–131] For isolated testicular relapses, systemic reinduction chemotherapy and testicular irradiation have been successful for 85% of patients with late occurring, and ≤50% for early occurring, testicular leukemia.[114]

FUTURE DIRECTIONS

Future approaches to the treatment of childhood ALL include redefinition of prognostic factors, so that only children at high risk of relapse are treated more intensively, and attempts to diminish long-term toxicity can be addressed in those patients who can be successfully treated with current therapies. Areas of investigation include the evaluation of more specific treatments (i.e., monoclonal antibodies linked to toxins), the use of hematopoietic growth factors to permit the administration of higher doses or more frequent dosing of chemotherapy and thus reduce infections and hemorrhagic toxicity, and the documentation of minimal residual disease. The possibility of developing patient-specific treatment regimens based on in vitro cytotoxicity assays also is a promising new approach to the improved treatment of this disease.[132]

THERAPEUTIC APPROACH TO CHILDHOOD ALL

The proper treatment of all children with newly diagnosed ALL must begin in a specialized pediatric hematology/oncology center and must subsequently be continued or closely supervised by experienced specialists. As soon as the diagnosis is confirmed and the patient stabilized with appropriate supportive care (hydration, blood products, antibiotics, and so forth), chemotherapy should be instituted. Such treatment should be part of a prospective clinical protocol to ensure that each of the children with this disease, who collectively form a rare human resource for one another, ultimately contributes to the development of more effective and less morbid treatment regimens.

Conceptually, early treatment should be with high doses of multiple drugs to ensure maximal leukemic cell kill and to address the issues of drug resistance. Although it is impossible to assess the importance of early intensive treatment on the basis of only the percentage of CRs or the time to induce a CR, long-term results support the use of intensive induction therapy. We use vincristine, prednisone, doxorubicin, methotrexate, and intrathecal ara-C. Each agent is individually cytotoxic to leukemic cells, and in combination the agents presumably are maximally cytotoxic. The dose-limiting aspect of induction therapy is the potentially additive side effects of the drugs; for example, doxorubicin and methotrexate both can result in damage to the gastrointestinal mucosa, and therefore the doses of each must be modified.

After obtaining a complete remission, attention is focused on central nervous system treatment and further reduction of the total (currently immeasurable) residual leukemic cells (the minimal residual leukemia). The treatment of the central nervous system should be maximally effective and minimally harmful, a balance that is difficult to attain (and controversial among clinical investigators). We treat all children with intensive systemic chemotherapy, including repeated doses of prednisone and high-dose asparaginase, which are also effective for central nervous system leukemia. Patients at higher risk of central nervous system relapse (white blood cell count >20,000/mm³, age 1–2 or >9 years, and T-cell ALL), who comprise 60% of all patients, are treated with cranial irradiation (18 Gy) and concurrently two-drug (methotrexate and ara-C) intrathecal therapy. Based on a high incidence of central nervous system leukemia in boys with standard risk disease, we give them cranial irradiation and concurrent intrathecal drugs. The remainder of the population is similarly treated except that no cranial irradiation is given. Intrathecal therapy is continued intermittently for 2 years.

Intensive systemic therapy with multiple drugs (including vincristine, dexamethasone, asparaginase, 6-mercaptopurine, and methotrexate or doxorubicin, depending on the risk group of the patient) is administered with central nervous system treatment for approximately 6 months. Thereafter continuation therapy (with vincristine, dexamethasone, 6-mercaptopurine, and methotrexate) is administered to complete a total of 2 years of treatment. Bone marrow transplantation in initial CR is recommended for the 3–4% of children with ALL who have lymphoblasts that express the Philadelphia chromosome [t(9;22)]. Children with mature B-cell ALL (surface immunoglobulin-positive) are treated on a separate protocol that features B-cell-specific drugs.

All current antileukemic therapy is leukemia-nonspecific, which means that all the drugs have acute toxicities and many of them also have long-term adverse effects. Thus, treatment programs must be balanced with regard to the risk/benefit ratio. The first goal must be eradication of the leukemic clone. When identical treatment is used, patients characterized as being at standard risk of relapse have a higher likelihood of successful outcome (cure) than those characterized as high-risk patients. Therefore, it is our practice to gradually diminish the potential toxicity in new therapy programs for the standard risk group, which always being mindful of the risk of more treatment failures. By contrast, as long as the high-risk group is inadequately treated (too many relapses), we believe that treatment of these patients, albeit associated with known acute and late toxicity, should be intensified. Despite that, efforts need to be made to modify both short- and long-term devastating toxicities (stroke, congestive heart failure, learning disorders, second malignant neoplasms) even in these high-risk patients, while at the same time attempting to increase their overall survival. Thus, we are searching for less toxic forms of asparaginase and less cardiotoxic ways of administering anthracyclines, and altering methods for the delivery of cranial irradiation. Hopefully, in the near future we will be able to use more specific antileukemic therapy, measure the number of residual leukemic cells, and base the intensity and duration of therapy on individual needs.

REFERENCES

1. Farber S, Diamond LK, Mercer RD et al: Temporary remissions in acute leukemia in children produced by folic acid antagonist, 4-aminopteroyl-glutamic acid (aminopterin). N Engl J Med 238:787, 1948
2. Frei E III: Acute leukemia in children. Model for the development of scientific methodology for clinical therapeutic research in cancer. Cancer 53:2013, 1984
3. Elion GB, Hitchings GH: Metabolic basis for the actions of analogs of purines and pyrimidines. Adv Chemother 2:91, 1965
4. Burchenal JH, Murphy ML, Ellison RB et al: Clinical evaluation of a new antimetabolite: 6-mercaptopurine in the treatment of leukemia and allied diseases. Blood 8:965, 1953
5. Frei E III, Holland JF, Schneiderman MA et al: A comparative study of two regimens of combination chemotherapy in acute leukemia. Blood 13:1126, 1958
6. Freireich EJ, Frei E III: Recent advances in acute leukemia. Prog Hematol 4:187, 1964
7. Blum RH, Carter SK: Adriamycin. A new anticancer drug with significant clinical activity. Ann Intern Med 80:249, 1974
8. Tallal L, Tan C, Oettgen H et al: E. coli L-asparaginase in the treatment of leukemia and solid tumors in 131 children. Cancer 25:306, 1969
9. Jaffe N, Traggis D, Das L et al: Comparison of daily and twice-weekly schedule of L-asparaginase in childhood leukemia. Pediatrics 49:590, 1972
10. Skipper HE, Schabel FM, Jay R et al: Experimental evaluation of potential antitumor agents: on the criteria and kinetics associated with curability of experimental leukemia. Cancer Chemother Rep 35:1, 1964
11. Frei E III, Freireich EJ: Progress and perspectives in the chemotherapy of acute leukemia. Adv Chemother 2:269, 1965
12. Pinkel D, Hernandez K, Borella L et al: Drug dosage and remission duration in childhood lymphocytic leukemia. Cancer 27:247, 1971
13. Sallan SE, Gelber RD, Kimball V et al: More is better! Update of Dana-Farber

Cancer Institute/Children's Hospital childhood acute lymphoblastic leukemia trials. Hematol Blood Transfus 33:459, 1990

14. Pinkel D: Five-year follow-up of "total therapy" of childhood lymphocytic leukemia. JAMA 216:648, 1971

15. Evans AE, Gilbert ES, Zandstra R: The increasing incidence of central nervous system leukemia in children (Children's Cancer Study Group A). Cancer 26:404, 1970

16. Haghbin M, Murphy ML, Tan CC et al: A long-term clinical follow-up of children with acute lymphoblastic leukemia treated with intensive chemotherapy regimens. Cancer 46:241, 1980

17. Aur RJA, Simone JV, Hustu HO et al: A comparative study of central nervous system irradiation and intensive chemotherapy early in remission of childhood acute lymphocytic leukemia. Cancer 29:381, 1972

18. Hustu HO, Aur RJA, Verzosa MS et al: Prevention of central nervous system leukemia by irradiation. Cancer 32:585, 1973

19. Wang JJ, Freeman AI, Sinks LF: Treatment of acute lymphocytic leukemia by high dose intravenous methotrexate. Cancer Res 36:1441, 1976

20. Early AP, Preisler HD, Slocum H et al: A pilot study of high-dose 1-βD-arabinofuranosylcytosine for acute leukemia and refractory lymphoma: clinical response and pharmacology. Cancer Res 42:1587, 1982

21. Pizzo PA: Infectious complications in the child with cancer. II. Management of specific infectious organisms. J Pediatr 98:513, 1981

22. Nakamura S, Gelber R, Blattner S et al: Infectious complications of intensive therapy for childhood acute lymphoblastic leukemia. Blood 74:366a, 1989

23. Hughes WT, Rivera GK, Schell MJ et al: Successful intermittent chemoprophylaxis for *Pneumocystis carinii* pneumonitis. N Engl J Med 316:1627, 1987

24. Dubansky AS, Boyett JM, Falletta J et al: Isolated thrombocytopenia in children with acute lymphoblastic leukemia: a rare event in a Pediatric Oncology Group Study. Pediatrics 84:1068, 1989

25. Bunin NJ, Pui C-H: Differing complications of hyperleukocytosis in children with acute lymphoblastic or acute nonlymphoblastic leukemia. J Clin Oncol 3:1590, 1985

26. Goldie JH, Coldman AJ, Gudauskas GA: Rationale for the use of alternating non-cross-resistant chemotherapy. Cancer Chemother Rep 66:439, 1982

27. Hitchcock-Bryan S, Gelber R, Cassady JR, Sallan SE: The impact of induction anthracycline on long-term failure-free survival in childhood acute lymphoblastic leukemia. Med Pediatr Oncol 14:211, 1986

28. Ortega JA, Nesbit ME Jr, Donaldson MH et al: L-asparaginase, vincristine and prednisone for induction of first remission in acute lymphocytic leukemia. Cancer Res 37:535, 1977

29. Rivera G, Dahl GV, Bowman WP et al: VM-26 and cytosine arabinoside combination chemotherapy for initial induction failures in childhood acute lymphocytic leukemia. Cancer 46:1727, 1980

30. Lay HN, Ekert H, Colebatch JH: Combination chemotherapy for children with acute lymphocytic leukemia who fail to respond to standard remission induction therapy. Cancer 36:1220, 1975

31. Freireich EJ, Gehan E, Frei E III et al: The effect of 6-mercaptopurine on the duration of steroid-induced remissions in acute leukemia: a model for evaluation of other potentially useful therapy. Blood 21:699, 1963

32. Hagenbeek A, Martens ACM: Detection of minimal residual leukemia utilizing monoclonal antibodies and fluorescence activated cell sorting (FACS). p. 45. In Lowenberg B, Hagenbeek A (eds): Minimal Residual Disease in Acute Leukemias. Martinus Nijhoff, The Hague, 1984

33. Smith RG, Kitchens RL: Phenotypic heterogeneity of TDT+ cells in the blood and bone marrow: implications for surveillance of residual leukemia. Blood 74:312, 1989

34. Zehnbauer BA, Pardoll DM, Burke PJ et al: Immunoglobulin gene rearrangements in remission bone marrow specimens from patients with acute lymphoblastic leukemia. Blood 67:835, 1986

35. Tycko B, Palmer JD, Link MP et al: Polymerase chain reaction amplification of rearranged receptor genes using junction-specific oligonucleotides: possible application for detection of minimal residual disease in acute lymphoblastic leukemia. Cancer Cells 7:47, 1989

36. Yamada M, Wasserman R, Lange B et al: Minimal residual disease in childhood B-lineage lymphoblastic leukemia. N Engl J Med 323:448, 1990

37. Ito Y, Wasserman R, Galili N et al: Molecular residual disease status at the end of chemotherapy fails to predict subsequent relapse in children with B-lineage acute lymphoblastic leukemia. J Clin Oncol 11:546, 1993

38. Miller DR, Coccia PF, Bleyer WA et al: Early response to induction therapy as a predictor of disease-free survival and late recurrence of childhood acute lymphoblastic leukemia: a report from the Children's Cancer Study Group. J Clin Oncol 7:1807, 1989

39. Sallan SE, Camitta BM, Cassady JR et al: Intermittent combination chemotherapy with Adriamycin for childhood acute lymphoblastic leukemia. Clinical results. Blood 51:425, 1978

40. Frei E III, Sallan SE: Acute lymphoblastic leukemia: treatment. Cancer 42:828, 1978

41. Niemeyer C, Gelber RD, Blattner SR et al: Importance of early intensive therapy in childhood ALL. Blood 70:234a, 1987

42. Riehm H, Reiter A, Schrappe M et al: Die corticosteroid-abhängige Dezimierung der Leukämiezellzahl im Blut als Prognosefaktor bei der akuten lymphoblastischen Leukämie im Kindesalter (Therapiestudie ALL-BFM 83). Klin Padiatr 199:151, 1986

43. Asselin BL, Ryan D, Frantz CN et al: *In vitro* and *in vivo* killing of acute lymphoblastic leukemia cells by L-asparaginase. Cancer Res 49:4363, 1989

44. Asselin BL, Whitin JC, Coppola DJ et al: Comparative pharmacokinetic studies of three L-asparaginase preparations. J Clin Oncol 11:1780, 1993

45. Niemeyer CM, Hitchcock-Bryan S, Sallan SE: Comparative analysis of treatment programs for childhood acute lymphoblastic leukemia. Semin Oncol 12:122, 1985

46. Niemeyer CM, Reiter A, Riehm H et al: Comparative results of two intensive treatment programs for childhood acute lymphoblastic leukemia: the Berlin-Frankfurt-Munster and Dana-Farber Cancer Institute protocols. Ann Oncol 2:745, 1991

47. Dahl GV, Rivera GK, Look AT et al: Teniposide plus cytarabine improves outcome in childhood acute lymphoblastic leukemia presenting with a leukocyte count >100 × 10⁹/L. J Clin Oncol 5:1015, 1987

48. Rivera GK, Raimondi SC, Hancock ML et al: Improved outcome in childhood acute lymphoblastic leukaemia with reinforced early treatment and rotational combination chemotherapy. Lancet 337:61, 1991

49. Gelber RD, Sallan SE, Cohen HJ et al: Central nervous system treatment in childhood acute lymphoblastic leukemia. Long-term follow-up of patients diagnosed between 1973–1985. Cancer 72:261, 1993

50. Schrappe M, Beck J, Brandeis WE et al: Die Behandlung der akuten lymphoblastischen Leukamie im Kindes- und Jugendalter: Ergebnisse der multizentrischen Therapiestudie ALL-BFM 81. Klin Padiatr 199:133, 1987

51. Riehm H, Gadner H, Henze G et al: Results and significance of six randomized trials in four consecutive ALL-BFM studies. Hematol Blood Transfus 33:439, 1990

52. Balis FM, Lester CM, Chrousos GP et al: Differences in cerebrospinal fluid penetration of corticosteroids: possible relationship to the prevention of meningeal leukemia. J Clin Oncol 5:202, 1987

53. Faller DV, Beardsley GP, Mikta T, Sallan SE: Prolonged asparagine (Asn) depletion after high dose asparaginase (HDA) therapy in childhood acute lymphoblastic leukemia. Proc Am Assoc Cancer Res 26:156, 1985

54. Sallan SE, Ritz J, Pesando J et al: Cell surface antigens: prognostic implications in childhood acute lymphoblastic leukemia. Blood 55:395, 1980

55. Sallan SE, Hitchcock-Bryan S, Gelber R et al: Influence of intensive asparaginase in the treatment of childhood non-T-cell acute lymphoblastic leukemia. Cancer Res 43:5601, 1983

56. Clavell LA, Gelber RD, Cohen HJ et al: Four-agent induction and intensive asparaginase therapy for treatment of childhood acute lymphoblastic leukemia. N Engl J Med 315:657, 1986

57. Ochs J, Mulhern RK: Late effects of antileukemic treatment. Pediatr Clin North Am 35:815, 1988

58. Rimm IJ, Li FP, Tarbell NJ et al: Brain tumors after cranial irradiation for childhood acute lymphoblastic leukemia. Cancer 59:1506, 1987

59. Morris M, Savitch J, Balis F et al: Altered central nervous system pharmacology of methotrexate in childhood leukemia: another sign of meningeal relapse. J Clin Oncol 3:19, 1985

60. Inati A, Sallan SE, Cassady JR et al: Efficacy and morbidity of central nervous system "prophylaxis" in childhood acute lymphoblastic leukemia: eight years' experience with cranial irradiation and intrathecal methotrexate. Blood 61:297, 1983

61. Abromowitch M, Ochs J, Pui C-H et al: Efficacy of high-dose methotrexate in childhood acute lymphocytic leukemia: analysis by contemporary risk classifications. Blood 71:866, 1988

62. Pullen J, Boyett J, Shuster J et al: Extended triple intrathecal chemotherapy trial for prevention of CNS relapse in good risk and poor risk patients with B-progenitor acute lymphoblastic leukemia: a Pediatric Oncology Group Study. J Clin Oncol 11:839, 1993

63. Tubergen DG, Gilchrist GS, O'Brien RT et al: Prevention of CNS disease in intermediate-risk acute lymphoblastic leukemia: Comparison of cranial radiation and intrathecal methotrexate and the importance of systemic therapy: a Children's Cancer Group Report. J Clin Oncol 11:520, 1993

64. Billett AL, Gelber RD, Tarbell NJ et al: Sex differences in the risk of central nervous system (CNS) relapse in childhood acute lymphoblastic leukemia, abstracted. Proc Am Soc Clin Oncol 12:316, 1993

65. Reaman GH, Steinherz PG, Gaynon PS et al: Improved survival of infants less than 1 year of age with acute lymphoblastic leukemia treated with intensive multiagent chemotherapy. Cancer Treat Rep 71:1033, 1987

66. Crist W, Pullen J, Boyett J et al: Clinical and biological features predict a poor prognosis in acute lymphoid leukemias in infants: a Pediatric Oncology Group Study. Blood 67:135, 1986

67. Chen C-S, Sorensen PHB, Domer PH et al: Molecular rearrangements on chromosome 11q23 predominate in infant acute lymphoblastic leukemia and are associated with specific biologic variables and poor outcome. Blood 81:2386, 1993

68. Bleyer WA, Poplack DG: Prophylaxis and treatment of leukemia in the central nervous system and other sanctuaries. Semin Oncol 12:131, 1985

69. Murphy SB, Bowman WP, Abromowitch M et al: Results of treatment of advanced-stage Burkitt's lymphoma and B-cell (SIg+) acute lymphoblastic leukemia with high dose fractionated cyclophosphamide and coordinated high-dose methotrexate and cytarabine. J Clin Oncol 4:1732, 1986

70. Patte C, Philip T, Rodary C et al: Improved survival rate in children with stage III and IV B cell non-Hodgkin's lymphoma and leukemia using multiagent chemotherapy: results of a study of 114 children from the French Pediatric Oncology Society. J Clin Oncol 4:1219, 1986

71. Green DM: Long-Term Complications of Therapy for Cancer in Childhood and Adolescence. Johns Hopkins University Press, Baltimore, 1989

72. Riccardi R, Brouwers P, DiChiro G, Poplack DG: Abnormal computed tomography brain scans in children with acute lymphoblastic leukemia: serial long-term follow-up. J Clin Oncol 3:12, 1985

73. Hoover DL, Smith LEH, Turner SJ et al: Ophthalmic evaluation of survivors of ALL. Ophthalmology 95:151, 1988

74. Lipshultz SE, Colan SD, Gelber RD et al: Late cardiac effects of doxorubicin therapy for acute lymphoblastic leukemia in childhood. N Engl J Med 324:808, 1991

75. Nesbit M, Krivit W, Heyn R et al: Acute and chronic effects of methotrexate on hepatic, pulmonary, and skeletal systems. Cancer 37:1048, 1976

76. Chessells JM: Childhood acute lymphoblastic leukaemia: the late effects of treatment. Br J Haematol 53:369, 1983

77. Waber DP, Tarbell NJ, Kahn CM et al: The relationship of sex and treatment modality to neuropsychologic outcome in childhood acute lymphoblastic leukemia. J Clin Oncol 10:810, 1992

78. Eiser C: Effects of chronic illness on intellectual development. Arch Dis Child 55:766, 1980

79. Waber DP, Urion DK, Tarbell NJ et al: Late effects of central nervous system treatment in long-term survivors of childhood acute lymphoblastic leukemia are sex dependent. Dev Med Child Neurol 32:164, 1990

80. Mulhern RK, Wasserman AL, Fairclough D, Ochs J: Memory function in disease-free survivors of childhood acute lymphocytic leukemia given CNS prophylaxis with or without 1800 cGy cranial irradiation. J Clin Oncol 6:315, 1988

81. Whitt JK, Wells RJ, Lauria MM et al: Cranial irradiation in childhood acute lymphocytic leukemia: neuropsychologic sequelae. Am J Dis Child 138:730, 1984

82. Aur RJA, Simone JV, Verzosa MS et al: Childhood acute lymphocytic leukemia: study VIII. Cancer 42:2123, 1978

83. Moss HA, Nannis ED, Poplack DG: The effects of prophylactic treatment of the central nervous system on the intellectual functioning of children with acute lymphocytic leukemia. Am J Med 71:47, 1981

84. Waber DP, Gioia G, Paccia J et al: Sex differences in cognitive processing in children treated with central nervous system prophylaxis for acute lymphoblastic leukemia (ALL). J Pediatr Psychol 15:105, 1990

85. Robison LL, Nesbit ME Jr, Sather HN et al: Height of children successfully treated for acute lymphoblastic leukemia: a report from the Late Effects Committee of the Children's Cancer Study Group. Med Pediatr Oncol 13:14, 1985

86. Clayton PE, Shalet SM, Morris-Jones PH, Price DA: Growth in children treated for acute lymphoblastic leukaemia. Lancet 1:460, 1988

87. Sklar C, Mertens A, Walter A et al: Final height after treatment for childhood acute lymphoblastic leukemia: comparison of no cranial irradiation with 1800 and 2400 centigrays of cranial irradiation. J Pediatr 123:59, 1993

88. Schell MJ, Ochs JJ, Schriock EA, Carter M: A method of predicting adult height and obesity in long-term survivors of childhood acute lymphoblastic leukemia. J Clin Oncol 10:128, 1992

89. Katz JA, Chambers B, Everhart C et al: Linear growth in children with acute lymphoblastic leukemia treated without cranial irradiation. J Pediatr 118:575, 1991

90. Voorhess ML, Brecher ML, Glicksman AS et al: Hypothalamic-pituitary function of children with acute lymphocytic leukemia after three forms of central nervous system prophylaxis. Cancer 57:1287, 1986

91. Swift PGF, Kearney PJ, Dalton RG et al: Growth and hormonal status of children treated for acute lymphoblastic leukemia. Arch Dis Child 53:890, 1978

92. Lipshultz SE, Colan SD, Sanders SP, Sallan SE: Cardiac mechanics after

93. growth hormone therapy in pediatric Adriamycin recipients. Pediatr Res 25:153a, 1989

93. Goldberg MA, Antin JH, Guinan EC, Rappeport JM: Cyclophosphamide cardiotoxicity: an analysis of dosing as a risk factor. Blood 68:1114, 1986

94. Quezado ZMN, Wilson WH, Cunnion RE et al: High dose ifosfamide is associated with severe, reversible cardiac dysfunction. Ann Intern Med 118:31, 1993

95. Blatt J, Poplack DG, Sherins RJ: Testicular function in boys after chemotherapy for acute lymphoblastic leukemia. N Engl J Med 304:1121, 1981

96. Lendon M, Palmer MK, Morris-Jones PH et al: Testicular histology after combination chemotherapy in childhood lymphoblastic leukaemia. Lancet 2:439, 1978

97. Moe PJ, Lethinen M, Wegelius R et al: Progeny of survivors of acute lymphocytic leukemia. Acta Paediatr Scand 68:301, 1979

98. Blatt J, Mulvihill JJ, Ziegler JL et al: Pregnancy outcome following cancer chemotherapy. Am J Med 69:828, 1980

99. Pui C-H, Behm FG, Raimondi SC et al: Secondary acute myeloid leukemia in children treated for acute lymphoid leukemia. N Engl J Med 321:136, 1989

100. Winick NJ, McKenna RW, Shuster J et al: Secondary acute myeloid leukemia in children with acute lymphoblastic leukemia treated with etoposide. J Clin Oncol 11:209, 1993

101. Tang TT, Holcenberg JS, Duck SC et al: Thyroid carcinoma following treatment for acute lymphoblastic leukemia. Cancer 46:1572, 1980

102. Tefft M, Vawter GF, Mitus A: Secondary primary neoplasms in children. AJR 103:800, 1968

103. Bleyer WA, Sather H, Hammond GD: Prognosis and treatment after relapse of acute lymphoblastic leukemia and non-Hodgkin's lymphoma: 1985. A report from the Children's Cancer Study Group. Cancer 58:590, 1986

104. Sallan SE, Niemeyer CN, Billett AL et al: Autologous bone marrow transplantation for acute lymphoblastic leukemia. J Clin Oncol 7:1594, 1989

105. Billett AL, Kornmehl E, Tarbell NJ et al: Autologous bone marrow transplantation after a long first remission for children with recurrent acute lymphoblastic leukemia. Blood 81:1651, 1993

106. Rivera GK, Buchanan G, Boyett JM et al: Intensive retreatment of childhood acute lymphoblastic leukemia in first bone marrow relapse. A Pediatric Oncology Group study. N Engl J Med 315:273, 1986

107. Kersey JH, Weisdorf D, Nesbit ME et al: Comparison of autologous and allogeneic bone marrow transplantation for treatment of high risk refractory acute lymphoblastic leukemia. N Engl J Med 317:461, 1987

108. Barrett AJ, Joshi R, Kendra JR et al: Prediction and prevention of relapse of acute lymphoblastic leukaemia after bone marrow transplantation. Br J Haematol 64:179, 1986

109. Henze G, Fengler R, Hartmann R et al: Six-year experience with a comprehensive approach to the treatment of recurrent childhood acute lymphoblastic leukemia (ALL-REZ 85). A relapse study of the BFM group. Blood 78:1166, 1991

110. Buchanan GR, Rivera GK, Boyett JM et al: Reinduction therapy in 297 children with acute lymphoblastic leukemia in first bone marrow relapse: a Pediatric Oncology Group study. Blood 72:1288, 1988

111. Rivera G, George SL, Bowman WP et al: Second central nervous system prophylaxis in children with acute lymphoblastic leukemia who relapse after elective cessation of therapy. J Clin Oncol 1:471, 1983

112. Nesbit ME Jr, Robison LL, Ortega JA et al: Testicular relapse in childhood acute lymphoblastic leukemia: association with pretreatment patient characteristics and treatment. A report for Children's Cancer Study Group. Cancer 45:2009, 1980

113. Bowman WP, Aur RJA, Hustu HO, Rivera G: Isolated testicular relapse in acute lymphocytic leukemia of childhood: categories and influence on survival. J Clin Oncol 2:924, 1984

114. Wofford MM, Smith SD, Shuster JJ et al: Treatment of occult or late overt testicular relapse in children with acute lymphoblastic leukemia: a Pediatric Oncology Group Study. J Clin Oncol 10:624, 1992

115. Butturini A, Gale RP: Chemotherapy versus transplantation in acute leukaemia. Br J Haematol 72:1, 1989

116. Johnson FL, Thomas ED, Clark BS et al: A comparison of marrow transplantation with chemotherapy for children with acute lymphoblastic leukemia in second or subsequent remission. N Engl J Med 305:846, 1981

117. Sanders JE, Thomas ED, Buckner CD, Doney K: Marrow transplantation for children with acute lymphoblastic leukemia in second remission. Blood 70:324, 1987

118. Chessells JM, Rogers DW, Leiper AD et al: Bone marrow transplantation has a limited role in prolonging second remission in childhood lymphoblastic leukaemia. Lancet 1:1239, 1986

119. Chessells JM: Allogeneic bone marrow transplantation in childhood leukemia: another form of intensive treatment. Leukemia 3:543, 1989

120. Brochstein JA, Kernan NA, Groshan S et al: Allogeneic bone marrow trans-

plantation after hyperfractionated total body irradiation and cyclophosphamide in children with acute leukemia. N Engl J Med 317:1618, 1987

121. Fefer A, Cheever MA, Greenberg PD: Identical-twin (syngeneic) marrow transplantation for hematologic cancers. J Natl Cancer Inst 76:1269, 1986

122. Dopfer R, Henze G, Bender-Gotze C et al: Allogeneic bone marrow transplantation for childhood acute lymphoblastic leukemia in second remission after intensive primary and relapse therapy according to the BFM- and CoALL-protocols: results of the German Cooperative Study. Blood 78:2780, 1991

123. Sullivan KM, Weiden PL, Storb R et al: Influence of acute and chronic graft-versus-host disease on relapse and survival after bone marrow transplantation from HLA-identical siblings as treatment of acute and chronic leukemia. Blood 73:1720, 1989

124. Kernan NA, Bartsch G, Ash RC et al: Analysis of 462 transplantations from unrelated donors facilitated by the national marrow donor program. N Engl J Med 328:593, 1993

125. Kun LE, Camitta BM, Mulhern RK et al: Treatment of meningeal relapse in childhood acute lymphoblastic leukemia. I. Results of craniospinal irradiation. J Clin Oncol 2:359, 1984

126. Mulhern RK, Ochs J, Fairclough D et al: Intellectual and academic achieve-

ment status after CNS relapse: a retrospective analysis of 40 children treated for acute lymphoblastic leukemia. J Clin Oncol 5:933, 1987

127. Behrendt H, van Leeuwen EF, Shuwirth C et al: The significance of an isolated central nervous system relapse, occurring as first relapse in children with acute lymphoblastic leukemia. Cancer 63:2066, 1989

128. Pinkerton CR, Chessells JM: Failed central nervous system prophylaxis in children with acute lymphoblastic leukaemia: treatment and outcome. Br J Haematol 57:553, 1984

129. Balis FM, Savitch JL, Bleyer WA et al: Remission induction of meningeal leukemia with high-dose intravenous methotrexate. J Clin Oncol 3:485, 1985

130. Morra E, Lazzarino M, Inverardi D et al: Systemic high-dose ara-C for the treatment of meningeal leukemia in adult acute lymphoblastic leukemia and non-Hodgkin's lymphoma. J Clin Oncol 4:1207, 1986

131. Amadori S, Papa G, Avvisati G et al: Sequential combination of systemic high-dose ara-C and asparaginase for the treatment of central nervous system leukemia and lymphoma. J Clin Oncol 2:98, 1984

132. Pieters R, Huismans DR, Loonen AH et al: Relation of cellular drug resistance to long-term clinical outcome in childhood acute lymphoblastic leukaemia. Lancet 338:399, 1991

Acute Lymphocytic Leukemia in Adults

70

Dieter Hoelzer

INTRODUCTION

Acute lymphocytic leukemia (ALL) is a malignant disease characterized by the accumulation of lymphoblasts. About two-thirds of the children and about one-third of the adults with the disorder can be cured with therapy presently available. Prognostic factors for leukemia-free survival in adults with ALL allow ALL patients at presentation to be stratified into low- and high-risk groups. This stratification is necessary for the recognition of patients who require bone marrow transplantation (BMT) as curative therapy during first or second remission.

The difference in outcome of treatment between children and adults is probably not due to the presence of a different disease in adults with more resistant blast cells, but rather a result of the higher frequency of ALL subtypes associated with adverse prognoses, such as Philadelphia (Ph) chromosome-positive ALL.[1] Furthermore, the lower tolerance of adults to hematologic and nonhematologic toxicity contributes to their poorer outcome, particularly in the ALL patients >50 years of age.

ETIOLOGY

The cause of ALL remains unknown. However, certain factors are related to its development.[2,3]

Genetic predisposition. In epidemiologic studies, patients with a rare congenital chromosomal abnormality have been shown to have an increased risk of the development of acute leukemias, including ALL. In children with leukemia there is

a 20-fold higher incidence of Down syndrome than would be expected. The leukemia in children with Down syndrome is usually acute myeloid leukemia (AML) but ALL is also increased in incidence. There is also an increased risk of ALL associated with inherited disorders such as Klinefelter syndrome, Fanconi anemia, Bloom syndrome, ataxia-telangiectasia, and neurofibromatosis. That genetic disposition is of importance in the pathobiology of ALL may also be inferred from reports of the simultaneous development of ALL in identical twins.[4-6] Such observations may also indicate that the disease is caused by an intrauterine event affecting both twins.[7]

Irradiation. The incidence of acute leukemias, mainly myeloid leukemias, but also ALL, was increased almost 20-fold in survivors of the atomic bomb explosions (>1 Gy exposure) in Japan,[8] with a peak incidence occurring 6–7 years after the radiation exposure. Induction of leukemia by emissions from nuclear power stations has also been raised as a possible environmental leukemogenic risk. An increased incidence of leukemia in children living near nuclear power stations has been observed in at least two reports. In one it could not be directly related to radioactive emission[9] and in the other it was shown to be related to the preconceptual radiation exposure of fathers working at the nuclear plant.[10] However, an increased incidence of leukemia was not found in children of Japanese men who survived the atomic bomb explosions, so some additional factor(s), such as radiation dosage rate or duration of exposure, must be involved in the pathobiology of acute leukemia in this setting.

Chemical. The risk of developing ALL may also be increased following exposure to chemical agents such as benzene[11] or other agents capable of producing bone marrow aplasia, including chemotherapeutic drugs. Because secondary therapy-related AMLs occur mostly after exposure to alkylating agents such as cyclophosphamide, epipodophyllotoxins, and rarely in anthracyclines[12,13] (all used extensively in the treatment of ALL), future treatment strategies might involve reduction of exposure of the patient to these drugs.

Viral. There is no direct evidence that a virus causes human ALL. There are, however, indirect findings in two lymphoid neoplasias, Burkitt lymphoma, and adult T-cell leukemia/lymphoma, which suggest involvement of a virus in the biogenesis of these disorders.

In Burkitt lymphoma, the Epstein-Barr virus, a DNA virus of the herpes family, has been implicated as a potential causative agent. Lymphoma cells containing Epstein-Barr virus genomic inserts have been identified. The pathogenesis of Burkitt lymphoma, however, is most likely a multistep process.

Human T-cell leukemia virus I (HTLV-I) has been shown to be the etiologic agent for adult T-cell leukemia/lymphoma.[14] Type C retroviral particles have been found in cells of patients with acute T-cell leukemia (ATL).[15,16] The etiologic association of HTLV-I with ATL is primarily based on seroepidemiologic evidence. The virus is endemic in a few areas of Japan and the Caribbean, where 98–99% of persons are infected with HTLV-I. Only few of those manifest ATL,[16,17] indicating that immunity to the virus may protect against the development of malignant disease.

CLASSIFICATION

Classification of the phenotype of the blast cells in acute leukemia requires morphologic and cytochemical evaluation, immunophenotyping, cytogenetic analysis, and molecular genetic analysis. Morphology remains the means by which acute leukemia is initially detected and is a major aid in distinguishing between ALL and AML. Cytochemical reactions provide additional information with which to distinguish between the two distinct acute leukemia entities. For more precise subclassification of ALL into B lineage or T lineage, one must employ immunologic techniques to detect lineage-specific antigens as well as surface or intracytoplasmic molecules. The presence of terminal deoxynucleotidyl transferase (TdT) activity in leukemic blasts can facilitate the diagnosis of ALL. Cytogenetic analysis is a prerequisite for diagnosis of ALL because it has strong prognostic value. Molecular genetic techniques for confirmation of diagnosis in particular subsets of ALL (e.g., *bcr-abl* positive ALL), as well as to evaluate the therapeutic efficacy by detection of minimal residual disease, are of increasing importance.

Morphology

The cytologic features of leukemic blast cells in ALL and their division into L1–L3 according to the French-American-British (FAB) classification are discussed in Chapter 68. As seen in Table 70-1 the L1 type ALL is most common form of childhood ALL, the L2 type is observed in about one-third of cases, and the L3 type is very rare. In adult ALL the L1 type is less common and L2 is the more frequent form of ALL. In a series of 471 adult patients with ALL/acute undifferentiated leukemia, type L1 was observed in 27%, L2 in 68%, and L3 in 5% of patients.[18]

Cell-Surface Marker Analysis

ALL is divided into subtypes by immunologic criteria based on the presence of specific receptors or antigens on the cell surface of leukemic blast cells. Within the B-lineage or T-lineage

Table 70-1. Classification of Childhood and Adult ALL

	Children (%)	Adults (%)
Morphology (FAB)		N = 471[18]
L1	60–90	27
L2	20–40	68
L3	1–2	5
Surface markers	N = 1756[20]	N = 946[20]
B-lineage		
Early pre-B-All	5	11
HLA-DR$^+$, TdT$^+$, CD19$^+$		
Common-ALL	65	51
HLA-DR$^+$, TdT$^+$, CD10$^+$, CD19$^+$		
Pre-B-ALL	15	10
HLA-DR$^+$, TdT$^+$, CD10$^\pm$, CD19$^+$, cytoplasmic immunoglobulin-positive		
B-ALL	3	4
HLA-DR$^+$, CD10$^\pm$, CD19$^+$, surface immunoglobulin-positive		
T-lineage		
Early T-ALL	1	7
TdT$^+$, cytoplasmic CD3$^+$, CD7$^+$		
T-ALL	11	17
TdT$^+$, cytoplasmic CD3$^+$, CD7$^+$, CD1a/2/3$^\pm$		

ALLs the subtypes are defined according to their stage of differentiation.[19,20] For more details of the immunologic classification of ALL, see Chapters 67 and 68.

The frequency of ALL subtypes in adult and childhood ALL is compared in Table 70-1. In the German multicenter trials for childhood and adult ALL, the phenotypic analysis of 1,756 children and 946 adults with ALL was analyzed prospectively. Of the adults, 76% had a B-precursor ALL compared with 88% of children, and 24% of adult patients had a T-ALL compared with 12% of children. Within the B and T lineages the more immature subtypes early-pre-B-ALL and pre-T-ALL occur more frequently in adults. Both these subtypes are frequently characterized by the expression of additional myeloid markers by the leukemic blasts cells, and have a poor prognosis.[20]

B-Lineage ALL

Early pre-B-ALL, also termed pre-pre-B-ALL or B-progenitor cell ALL, lacks B, T, and pre-B cell markers but expresses HLA-DR, TdT, CD19, and has rearranged immunoglobulin genes. It occurs in >10% of adults with ALL and 5% of childhood ALL (Table 70-1).

Common ALL is the major immunologic subtype in childhood as well as in adult ALL. It comprises >50% of cases of adult ALL. Common ALL is characterized by the presence of CD10 (formerly, CALLA) and a glycoprotein (gp100/CD10). Common ALL blast cells do not express markers that characterize relatively mature B cells such as cytoplasmic immunoglobulins or surface membrane immunoglobulins. The blast cells are positive for CD19 and TdT.

Pre-B-ALL is characterized by the expression of cytoplasmic immunoglobulin, which is absent in common ALL, but is identical to common ALL with respect to the expression of all other cell markers (Table 70-1). Only very rarely may CD10 be absent in this subtype. Pre-B-ALL comprises nearly 10% and 15% of adult and childhood ALL, respectively.

About 4% of adult and 3% of childhood ALL patients are categorized as having mature B-ALL. The blast cells express surface antigens of mature B cells, including surface membrane immunoglobulin. CD10 may be present and occasionally also cytoplasmic immunoglobulin.

T-Lineage ALL

Approximately 25% of adult ALL cases have blast cells with a T-cell phenotype. All cases express the T-cell antigen gp40 (CD7), and in addition they may, according to their position in the scheme of T-cell differentiation, express other T-cell antigens (e.g., the E rosette receptor [CD2] and/or the cortical thymocyte antigen T6 [CD1]). A minority of T-ALL blast cells may also express CD10 together with T-cell antigens. In most cases of T-ALL one or more of the T-cell receptor genes is rearranged. These properties make it possible to classify T-ALLs according to their stage of differentiation into early T-precursor-ALL (or pre-T-ALL), 7% and 1% of adult and childhood ALL, respectively, and more mature T-ALL, 17% and 11% of adult and childhood ALL, respectively.[21-23]

Mixed or hybrid leukemias are those in which blast cells express lymphoid as well as myeloid antigens; they may also be termed biphenotypic or bilineage leukemias. Biphenotypic leukemias are defined as those in which markers of lymphoid and myeloid lineages are co-expressed on the same leukemic cells. Bilineage leukemias are those with two populations of blast cells that have either lymphoid or myeloid antigens. The detection of leukemic cells that express both lymphoid and myeloid antigens is increasing, as might be expected with more detailed marker analysis, reaching 33% in adult ALL patients[24]; with more stringent criteria, the levels are 18% in adults compared with 6–8% in children.[19]

After careful phenotypic analysis only a small number of cases of ALL remain unclassified and as a result the truly undefinable acute leukemias comprise only 1.4% of 500 cases studied.[25]

CYTOGENETIC ANALYSIS

Cytogenetic abnormalities are the most important independent prognostic variables for predicting the outcome of adult ALL.[26] In two studies clonal chromosomal aberrations could be detected in about 50–70% of ALL patients.[27,28] Approximately 20% of cases had normal metaphases, whereas 10% of the karyotype cases were not analyzable for technical reasons. With careful attention to collection of the bone marrow cells, and their rapid transport and preservation, the success rate in analysis of ALL marrow can be increased, and the identification of clonal abnormalities can be achieved in >90% of cases.[29]

The major cytogenetic abnormalities[28] in ALL are clonal abnormalities, structural aberrations [t(4;11), t(9;22) or t(8;14)], and other abnormalities [14q+, 6q−]. If none of the structural aberrations are present, the abnormalities can be classified according to the modal chromosomal number (<46, 46 with other structural abnormalities, 47–50, >50)[28,30] (Table 70-2). The demonstration of chromosomal abnormalities in ALL is relevant for several reasons: the presence of such defects may

confirm the diagnosis if a karyotype specific for ALL is found; chromosomal abnormalities are closely correlated with clinical features, immunologic subtype, and morphologic class of ALL; and cytogenetic abnormalities are independent prognostic variables for predicting remission duration. Some current protocols for treatment of adult ALL are stratified according to the presence of the Ph chromosome.

A suggestion by the Morphological, Immunological, and Cytogenetic Study Group to correlate morphologic criteria, immunologic classification, and cytogenetic analysis was published in 1986.[31]

Genetic Aspects

Molecular analyses, detecting gene rearrangements in ALL by the polymerase chain reaction (PCR), Southern blot blast cell analysis, or fluorescent in situ hybridization with chromosome-specific DNA probes, are of increasing importance. This approach is not only useful in establishing the more exact diagnosis but is also helpful in defining the quality of remission achieved after chemotherapy and/or BMT. Using these methods, 1 in 10^5 or even 1 in 10^6 leukemic blast cells can be detected compared with morphology (1 in 10^2). Thus these molecular methods allow the detection of a few remaining leukemic cells in patients with clinically, morphologically, and immunologically defined complete remission (CR). The ability to detect minimal residual disease can now be used to judge the effectiveness of single treatment elements, the maintenance therapy, and may eventually allow individually tailored therapy.[32]

The Ph chromosome t(9;22)(q34q11) results from a translocation involving the breakpoint cluster region of the *bcr* gene and the *abl* gene. The *bcr-abl* gene rearrangement can be demonstrated by molecular techniques such as PCR or Southern blot analysis. PCR analysis of patients with ALL revealed an incidence of 20–30% Ph ALL in adults with ALL[33-36] compared with 3% of patients with childhood ALL. One-third of adult ALL patients with a Ph chromosome have m-bcr rearrangements (resulting in a 210-kd protein), similar to patients with chronic myeloid leukemia, whereas two-thirds have m-bcr rearrangements (resulting in a 190-kd protein). The outcome for patients with either variant is equally poor. It is noteworthy that very rarely patients are *bcr-abl*-positive without the cytogenetic demonstration of the Ph chromosome.

CLINICAL MANIFESTATIONS

Most adult patients initially present with clinical symptoms resulting from bone marrow failure. Physical findings such as pallor, tachycardia, weakness, and fatigue are due to anemia; petechiae or other hemorrhagic manifestations are attributable to thrombocytopenia; infectious complications are due to neutropenia. Clinical signs of leukemia related directly to infiltration of organs with leukemic blasts, such as lymphadenopathy, splenomegaly, and hepatomegaly, are present in most patients but are infrequently problems for which the patient first seeks medical advice.

Symptoms and clinical manifestations of patients with adult ALL were analyzed in 938 patients, 15–65 years of age, entering two consecutive German multicenter trials (Table 70-3). One-third had infection or fever at presentation, and one-third presented with hemorrhagic episodes. Weight loss was only occasionally observed. About one-half of the patients presented at diagnosis with lymphadenopathy, splenomegaly, and hepatomegaly, and hilar lymph node enlargement or a thymic mass (detected on chest radiographs or computed tomography scans in about 14% of patients). Most (85%) of patients with mediational masses had T-cell ALL. Massive thymic enlarge-

Table 70-2. Chromosomal Abnormalities in Adult ALL

	Frequency (%)
Numerical abnormalities[28,30]	
Normal	15–20
Hyperdiploid	30
>50 chromosomes	10–20
47–50 chromosomes	10
46 Abnormal (pseudodiploid)	30–50
Hypodiploid	5–8
Translocations[28,30]	
t(9;22)	17
t(4;11)	5
t(8;14)	6
t(1;19)	Rare

Table 70-3. Symptoms and Clinical Signs at Diagnosis of ALL in 938 Adult Patients

Sign or Symptom	Patients (%)
Symptoms	
Infections/fever	36
Hemorrhages	33
Physical findings	
Lymphadenopathy	57
Splenomegaly	56
Hepatomegaly	47
Mediastinal mass	14
Central nervous system involvement	7
Other organ involvement	9
Pleura	2.9
Bone	1.2
Pericardium	1.0
Retina	1.0
Skin	0.6
Tonsils	0.6
Lung	0.5
Kidney	0.4
Testis	0.3

Table 70-4. Laboratory Findings (Leukocyte Counts) at Time of Diagnosis of ALL in 938 Adult Patients

	Patients (%)
Total leukocytes ($\times 10^6$/L)	
<5,000	27
5,000–10,000	14
10,000–50,000	31
50,000–100,000	12
>100,000	16
Leukemic blast cells in peripheral blood	
Present	92
Not present	8
Leukemic blast cells in bone marrow	
<50%	3
51–90%	51
>90%	46
Bone marrow aspirable	84

ment can cause dyspnea, especially when associated with pleural effusions. Although 7% of ALL patients at presentation had central nervous system involvement (as demonstrated by leukemic blast cells in the cerebrospinal fluid) only 4% of these initially had central nervous system symptoms such as headache, vomiting, lethargy, nuchal rigidity, and cranial nerve or peripheral nerve dysfunction.

Virtually any organ can be infiltrated by ALL blast cells, and about one-tenth of the patients had such organ involvement (Table 70-3). Most often a pleural effusion was observed, and this occurred almost exclusively in those patients with mediastinal enlargement. Some of those patients also had a pericardial effusion. Bone or joint pain was rarely observed as compared with childhood ALL; bone lesions could be found in only 1.2% of cases. Initial involvement of the testis was very rare (<1%). Rarely, lymphoblastic infiltration was observed in the retina, skin, tonsils, lung, or kidney. Such organ infiltration can result in the typical clinical pattern associated with non-Hodgkin lymphoma (NHL). The distinction between NHL in leukemic phase and ALL is difficult or even impossible in this situation, and is usually based on an arbitrary decision made by determination of the extent of infiltration of bone marrow with leukemic blasts.

LABORATORY EVALUATION AND DIAGNOSIS

Evaluation of bone marrow and peripheral smears is essential for the diagnosis of ALL. The peripheral blood cell values at diagnosis in a cohort of 938 adult ALL patients 15–65 years old are shown in Tables 70-4 through 70-6.

The leukocyte count (Table 70-4) was elevated in 59%, 14% had normal counts, and 27% had leukopenia. However, in >90% of the patients, leukemic blast cells were seen in the blood smear. Thus, "aleukemic" leukemias account for only a small proportion of cases of adult ALL. With automated blood counting, the diagnosis may be missed in patients with normal or decreased white blood cell (WBC) counts and with low blast cell contents. For this reason the need for microscopic examination of blood smears in individuals suspected of having acute leukemia should be stressed. An elevated blood count >100,000 $\times 10^6$/L was observed in 16% of the patients, and occasionally WBC counts >500,000 $\times 10^6$/L have been observed. Neutrophils (Table 70-5) were <500 $\times 10^6$/L leading

to an increased risk of infection in only 23% of the patients. Thrombocytopenia <25,000 $\times 10^6$/L was seen in only 30% of patients, corresponding roughly with the symptoms of infection and bleeding present at diagnosis. Anemia at diagnosis is observed in most adult ALL patients.

Bone marrow aspiration and/or biopsy is mandatory for diagnosis of ALL. In <20% of patients, the bone marrow cannot be aspirated and a biopsy must be performed. Most patients have >50%, or even >90%, of blast cells in the bone marrow (Table 70-4). In <3% of cases, the blast cells constitute <50% of the nucleated marrow cells. In these rare cases an arbitrary distinction between ALL and NHL is made according to the degree of bone marrow infiltration with blast cells. ALL is diagnosed when >25–40% of the marrow cells are lymphoblasts, and NHL is diagnosed when <25% of the marrow cells are blasts.

Performance of lumbar puncture is obligatory before therapy to determine whether the central nervous system is involved. A lumbar puncture should be omitted only when there is a danger of bleeding due to a very low platelet count. When the leukocyte count in the spinal fluid is low, or the morphologic detection of blasts is inconclusive, demonstration of an immunologically defined clonal cell population often confirms a diagnosis of central nervous system involvement.

The most frequent metabolic abnormality, an increased serum uric acid level, was found in approximately one-half the patients; hypercalcemia was rare. Serum lactate dehydrogenase (LDH) may be elevated as a result of cell destruction in

Table 70-5. Peripheral Blood Counts at Time of Diagnosis of ALL in 938 Adult Patients

	Patients (%)
Neutrophils ($\times 10^6$/L)	
<500	23
500–1,000	14
1,000–1,500	9
>1,500	54
Platelets ($\times 10^6$/L)	
<25,000	30
25,000–50,000	22
50,000–150,000	33
>150,000	15
Hemoglobin (g/dl)	
<6	8
6–8	20
8–10	27
10–12	24
>12	21

Table 70-6. Coagulation Studies at Time of Diagnosis of ALL in 938 Adult Patients

	Patients (%)
Fibrinogen (mg/dl)	
<100	4
>100	96
Prothrombin time (%)	
<50	7
50–75	34
75–100	34
>100	25
Partial thromboplastin time (sec)	
<30	33
30–40	53
40–50	11
>50	3

patients with a large tumor mass, particularly in B-ALL. In a small proportion of patients (Table 70-6) the initial fibrinogen level was <100 mg/dl. Disseminated intravascular coagulation in ALL was rarely observed at diagnosis.

THERAPY

Initial Evaluation and Supportive Therapy

The initial evaluation of an adult with ALL should include a history and a careful physical examination. Speed in clinical evaluation and diagnosis is important in order to initiate supportive measures and to decide on appropriate therapy.

Treatment of initial complications and therapy to avoid complications expected during chemotherapy must be commenced immediately. Only in a few cases is the leukemic process so far advanced that immediate treatment of leukemia is necessary (e.g., in patients with symptoms due to a large mediastinal mass and pleural effusions or to a rapidly progressing B-cell ALL).

A few general measures should be initiated at once. Sufficient fluid intake to guarantee urine production of ≥100 ml/hr throughout induction therapy should be maintained to reduce the danger of uric acid formation. Parenteral fluid administration may be required when the patient's oral intake is inadequate due to nausea or difficulty in swallowing. Placement of a Hickman catheter or Portacath is advantageous when anticipating a long period of induction therapy or when part of the therapy will be carried out on an outpatient basis.

Patients should receive allopurinol to reduce the formation of uric acid and avoid the danger of urate nephropathy. Allopurinol should be given at a dose of 300 mg/day, which may be increased to 600 mg/day if high leukocyte counts or organomegaly persist. The dose of allopurinol should be reduced when 6-mercaptopurine is given due to pharmacologic interactions between there two agents. Allopurinol can cause skin rashes but rarely causes severe allergic reactions.

Approximately one-third of adult patients present with infection and bleeding. Because thrombocytopenia and granulocytopenia are aggravated by chemotherapy, the patient is at high risk of infectious and hemorrhagic complications during the induction period.

In general, platelet transfusions should be given in response to bleeding episodes and to prevent bleeding when platelet counts fall to <20,000 × 10⁶/L, especially during febrile periods. Most often 4–8 U/day of platelets are given until bleeding ceases. HLA-matched platelets are given to patients who become refractory to random donor platelets.[37] The incidence of fatal hemorrhage during induction therapy has been significantly lowered by these measures.

Infection Prophylaxis

Although improvements have been made in the diagnosis and treatment of infectious complications, infections remain the principal cause of morbidity and death during induction therapy. Careful physical examination, chest radiography, and cultures of blood, urine, sputum, and other sites of suspected infections are necessary. In patients with severe infections, empirical broad-spectrum antibiotics should be given immediately, even before the results of cultures are available.

Much attention has been paid to prophylactic measures to prevent infection. Such precautions include the regular use of mouthwash, careful disinfection of the anogenital region, and general body hygiene. Other routine procedures include reverse protective isolation or air filtration, if available. Simple measures that should always be carried out include the following: no live plants in the room, no humidifiers, no intramuscular or subcutaneous injections, no uncooked vegetables, no unpeeled fruits, and no visitors who have any kind of infection. Prophylactic medication includes agents with activity against bacterial and fungal infection. Gastrointestinal decontamination with nonabsorbable antibiotics is of some benefit. For patients who will receive intensive chemotherapy, with expected long-lasting granulocytopenia and high risk of infection, prophylactic antibiotic treatment should be started before initiation of chemotherapy. Particularly, prophylaxis with trimethoprim sulfamethoxazole has proven to be effective in preventing *Pneumocystis carinii* infection. In a study of children with ALL with a 23% incidence of *P. carinii* pneumonia (which proved fatal in 20% of the cases), the death rate was reduced to 0.7% by the introduction of this prophylactic measure.[37] Trimethoprim sulfamethoxazole in combination with prophylactic polymyxin B and amphotericin B prevented severe infection in 40% of the patients in a large, albeit uncontrolled, multicenter adult ALL trial.[38]

With more intensive chemotherapy and more prolonged periods of granulocytopenia, the incidence of fungal infections has markedly increased.[39] Morbidity due to *Candida* and *Aspergillus* infections in 5–20% of patients has been observed. Up to one-half of those fungal infections may be fatal, and are now the major complications in the treatment of acute leukemias.[40,41] The difficulty in managing fungal infections is not only due to the limited availability of effective drugs, but is also due to the lack of a speedy means of diagnosis. Because pulmonary mycoses, particularly with aspergillus, have a very unfavorable outcome, immediate diagnostic procedures with computed tomographic chest scans and bronchial-alveolar lavage are necessary. With early antifungal therapy, such as amphotericin B and 5-fluocytosine or new formulations of amphotericin B allowing application of higher dosages, the cure rates of systemic mycoses are expected to improve.[42] Prophylaxis of fungal infections with oral polyenes and the new triazoles, particularly fluconazole, for prevention of candida infections is effective. Aerosol administration of amphotericin B is also currently under investigation.[43]

Hemopoietic Growth Factors

The use of hemopoietic growth factors is a valuable component of supportive therapy during the treatment of ALL. Colony-stimulating factor-granulocyte (CSF-G) and colony-stimulating factor-granulocyte/macrophage (CSF-GM) have been used to accelerate recovery from neutropenia after chemotherapy, resulting in a reduction of risk from infectious complications. The use of growth factors also enhances marrow recovery, allowing closer adherence to the dose and schedule of chemotherapeutic regimens. In a randomized study in which CSF-G was given 2 days after the induction chemotherapy for AML/ALL, the neutrophil recovery time was shortened by about 1 week from 28 to 20 days, and infections were also

Table 70-7. Application of CSF-G and CSF-GM in Adult ALL

Author	N	Therapy	Schedule	Recovery of Neutrophils (days to >500/mm³) With	Recovery of Neutrophils (days to >500/mm³) Without	Days of Infection With	Days of Infection Without
CSF-G							
Ottmann et al.[48] (1993)	76	Induction weeks 5–8	During CT	8[a]	12[a]		
Scherrer et al.[47] (1993)	16	Induction weeks 1–4	During CT	17[a]	26[a]	No difference	
Kantarjian et al.[45] (1992)	28	Consolidation	Post-CT	14	18	2	4
Blaise et al.[46] (1992)	45	Autologous BMT	Post-BMT	10.5	13.5	8	22.5
		Allogeneic BMT	Post-BMT	15	17	11	19
CSF-GM							
Calderwood et al.[49] (1992)	36	Consolidation weeks 1–4	During CT	7.1	14.8	1.5	5.0

Abbreviation: CT, chemotherapy.
[a] Days to >1000/mm³.

significantly less frequent in the CSF-G treated group.[44] Another study confirmed the more rapid recovery of neutrophils in patients given CSF-G after chemotherapy.[45] When CSF-G was given after autologous or allogeneic BMT in patients with ALL, the time of recovery of neutrophils was shortened.[46] In ALL, particular interest has focused on using these growth factors during the period of chemotherapy administration. In contrast to other malignant diseases with short chemotherapy treatment cycles, the induction regimens for ALL often continue for several weeks, thereby inducing cytopenias during this treatment period. In one study in which patients received CSF-G together with induction therapy consisting of vincristine, prednisone, daunorubicin, L-asparaginase, cytarabine, cyclophosphamide, and 6-mercaptopurine, plus intrathecal therapy and central nervous system irradiation, the duration of the period of granulocytopenia was shortened by from 21.5 to 14.5 days in the group receiving CSF-G[47] (Table 70-7). In a larger randomized trial, when CSF-G was applied concomitantly with induction chemotherapy the time needed to administer the chemotherapy scheme and the total duration of neutropenia were shortened.[48] In another randomized study in which CSF-GM was given with a similar induction schedule for ALL,[49] the recovery of neutrophils could also be shortened by 1 week and the number of infectious episodes was reduced. Thus CSF-G and CSF-GM can reduce the duration of neutropenia, resulting in a shorter period of treatment and a lower rate of infectious complications. Whether this will result in an improvement in survival awaits longer follow-up.

Chemotherapy

Chemotherapy of ALL is generally divided into several phases beginning with remission induction, which is followed by a postremission or continuation therapy. The objective of induction chemotherapy is to achieve CR, that is, eradication of leukemia as determined by morphologic criteria. Whereas the induction phase is usually well defined, postremission therapy can be subdivided into consolidation, intensification, and maintenance phases and usually also a phase of central nervous system prophylaxis.

Remission Induction Therapy

Exact diagnosis and management of initial complications are the prerequisites for successful induction therapy. Patients with all immunologic subtypes of ALL except mature B-ALL are initially treated with a combination of chemotherapeutic agents that include vincristine and prednisone. For the patients with mature B-ALL, different regimens that initially include cyclophosphamide are recommended.

Cautious preinduction therapy is recommended for patients with a large leukemic cell burden and/or a high leukocyte count (>25,000 × 10⁶/L). Patients with extreme leukocytosis (>100,000 × 10⁶/L) have been treated initially with leukapheresis. However, patients with high leukocyte counts can also be managed with vincristine and prednisone (e.g., vincristine, 0.75 mg/m² on day 1 and prednisone, 30 mg/m² on days 1–7) in nearly all cases without complications. Thus, leukapheresis in adult ALL is not recommended except in rare instances, such as when leukemia occurs during pregnancy.[50] For mature B-ALL, initial treatment with cyclophosphamide (200 mg/m²) and prednisone (60 mg/m²) for 1 week usually results in lysis of large tumor masses.

Standard induction therapy for ALL in most studies consists of vincristine, prednisone, asparaginase, and an anthracycline. The combination of vincristine and prednisone alone produces CR rates of approximately 36–67% but a median remission duration of only 3–7 months. The addition of anthracyclines, daunorubicin or doxorubicin (Adriamycin), increases the CR rate to 72–92% (doxorubicin) or 72–89% (daunorubicin).[51] However, without use of an anthracycline higher CR rates can be obtained by adding moderate-dose methotrexate to vincristine (Oncovin), asparaginase, and dexamethasone therapy.[52] Asparaginase does not affect the CR rate but improves remission quality and if not used during induction therapy is often included as part of the consolidation treatment. The use of cyclophosphamide and cytosine arabinoside (ara-C) during induction therapy is a more recent strategy (Table 70-8). The use of these drugs may not raise the overall CR rate but possibly improves the remission quality. Cyclophosphamide ara-C therapy is particularly useful for treating special subgroups (e.g., T-ALL).

After induction therapy with vincristine, prednisone, and doxorubicin, some investigators have added high-dose ara-C (1–3 g/m² generally for 12 doses). The addition of high-dose ara-C has resulted in a median CR rate of 73%.[53] These results are not superior to conventional treatment. Whether the disease-free survival (DFS) for subgroups (e.g., T-ALL or B-ALL) will be improved with the implementation of this approach remains uncertain. It is also uncertain whether the potentially greater antileukemic effect of high-dose chemotherapy may be outweighed by the increased toxicity. That there are limits to the extent of intensification therapy during induction treatment in adult ALL is indicated by experience with simultaneous use of high-dose cyclophosphamide and vincristine[54] and the combination of doxorubicin, etoposide, and ara-C,[55] which led to considerable gastrointestinal toxicity.

Refractory ALL or Failure During Induction Therapy

Of adult ALL patients, 15–20% will not achieve CR after induction therapy, in contrast to <5% of children with ALL. About 10% of adult ALL patients die during the 8-week period in which the diagnosis is made and therapy is initiated. Mortality during induction is age-dependent, increasing with age from <3% in children to 20–30% in patients ≥60 years of age. The main

Table 70-8. Results of Chemotherapy in Adult ALL in Recent Large Studies[a]

Group	Year	No. of Patients	Median Age	Induction	Consolidation	Maintenance	CNS Treatment	CR (%)	MRD (mo)	DFS/CCR (%)	(yr)
SWOG Hussein et al.[123]	1989	168	28	V, P, Ad, C	M, AC, TG A, V, P, C	V, P, Ad, MP, M actD, C, BCNU	IT-M	68	23	30	7
GIMEMA 0183 Mandelli et al.[69]	1989	358	31	V, P, A, D	V, IDM, IDAC, P VM, AC	V, P, M, MP (A, Ac, VM, IDAC)	IT-M, IT-P	79	15	25	5
MDACC Kantarjian et al.[63]	1990	105	30	V, Ad, Dx, C	M, A, Ad, HDAC, V, P	IDM, D, MP, P, C, BCNU, VP	None	84	22	34	5
MSKCC Clarkson et al.[117]	1990	199	25	V, P, (D, A, Ad, C)	AC, TG, A, V, P, M, C, BCNU	actD, BCNU V, P, Ad, M, MP, C	IT-M	82	28	33	18
GATLA Lluesma-Gonalons et al.[124]	1991	145	29	V, P, D, A, C, AC, MP	Ad, V, Dx, A, AC, C, MP	MP, M, V, P	IT-M, IT-Dx	78	28	34	6
JALSG Tomonaga et al.[125]	1991	117	38	V, P, Ad, A, C	VP, Mi, and other	MP, M, A, and other	IT-M, IT-AC	81		30	4
Swedish ALL Smedmyr et al.[126]	1991	113	38	V, P, A, D, C	V, D, VP, AC, P	MP, M, V, P, (AC, C, Ad)	IT-M, IT-AC	77			
FGTALL Fiere et al.[127]	1991	467		V, P, AC/R, C	Ad, AC, A	MP, M, V, C, P, Ad, AC	IT-M, CI	76		39	4
CALGB 8011 Ellison et al.[60]	1991	277	33	V, P, A, D	(AC, D), M, MP	V, P, MP, M	IT-M, CI	64	21	29	9
CALGB 8513 Cuttner et al.[70]	1991	164	32	V, P, Mi/D HDM	V, P, D/Mi, HdM AC, MP, A	None	None	64	11	18	3
GMALL 01 Hoelzer et al.[62]	1992	368	25	V, P, A, D, C AC, M, MP	V, Dx, Ad AC, C, TG	MP, M	IT-M, CI	74	24	35	10
GMALL 02 Hoelzer et al.[62]	1992	562	28	V, P, A, D, C AC, M, MP	V, Dx, Ad AC, C, TG VM, AC	MP, M	IT-M, CI	75	27	40	7
EORTC Stryckmans et al.[128]	1992	106	27	V, P, Ad, (HDAC)	A, HDC, (M, TG, AC)	V, P, M, Ad, BCNU, C, MP, M	IT-M, CI	74	32	40	8
L + B + V Bassan et al.[82]	1992	212	27	V, P, Ad, A, (HDC/ HDAC)	V, P, Ad, A, (HDC/ HDAC)	MP, M, C	IT-M, IT-AC CI/HDAC	71	23	32	10
Total		3361	29[b]					74	23[b]	33%[b]	

Abbreviations: ( ), with or without; X/Y, either X or Y; CR, rate of complete remission; MRD, median remission duration; DFS, disease-free survival; CCR, continuous complete remission; V, vincristine; P, prednisone; A, asparaginase; D, daunorubicin; Ad, Adriamycin; C, cyclophosphamide; AC, cytosine arabinoside; MP, mercaptopurine; M, methotrexate; BCNU, carmustine; TG, thioguanine; Dx, dexamethasone; HDM, high-dose M; IDM, intermediate-dose M; HDAC, high-dose AC; IDAC, intermediate-dose AC; HDC, high-dose C; VM, teniposide; VP, etoposide; Mi, mitoxantrone; actD, actinomycin D; SWOG, Southwest Oncology Group; GIMEMA, Gruppo Italiano Malattie Ematologiche Maligne Adupo; MDACC, M. D. Anderson Cancer Center; MSKCC, Memorial Sloan-Kettering Cancer Center; GATLA, Argentine Group for Treatment of Acute Leukemia; JALSG, Japan Adult Leukemia Study Group; Swedish ALL, Swedish ALL Group; FGTALL, French Group for Treatment of Adult Acute Lymphoblastic Leukemia; CALGB, Cancer and Leukemia Group B; GMALL, German Multicenter Trials in Adult ALL; EORTC, European Organisation for Research and Treatment of Cancer, L + B + V, London (St. Bartholomew's Hospital) + Bergamo (Ospedale Riuniti) + Vicenza (Ospedale San Bartolo).
[a] >100 patients and follow-up of ≥3 years.
[b] Weighted mean.

cause of death in about two-thirds of the patients is infection, in part fungal infection. The remaining nonresponders may achieve a partial remission or may be refractory to standard treatment. The number of patients (10–15%) who are currently refractory to chemotherapy is steadily decreasing with the use of more intensive induction regimens. These, however, lead more frequently to aplasia or toxic death. This trend suggests that leukemic blast cells in adult ALL are no more resistant to chemotherapy than those in children. It also stresses the need for implementation of optimal supportive treatment to overcome hematologic and nonhematologic toxicity in older patients undergoing more aggressive induction therapy.

Table 70-9. Drugs Commonly Used for the Chemotherapy of Adult ALL

Induction
    V, P, D/Ida, A
    AC, C, M
Postinduction
    HDAC
    HDM
    m-AMSA/Mi
      VM/VP
    IdMP

Abbreviations: Ida, idarubicin; m-AMSA, m-amsacrine; for other abbreviations, see Table 70-8.

Continuation Therapy

Continuation or postremission therapy may consist of intensification, consolidation, and maintenance. Consolidation and intensification refer either to high-dose chemotherapy, to the use of multiple new agents, or to readministration of the induction regimen. These measures are aimed at eliminating clinically undetectable residual leukemia after induction chemotherapy and thereby preventing relapse as well as emergence of drug-resistant cells. Maintenance usually involves less intensive therapy. In most studies that involve repeated consolidation cycles given over the entire treatment period it is difficult to distinguish these various phases of therapy or to analyze critically the effect of each phase of treatment on outcome.

In adult ALL, consolidation and/or intensification therapy can prolong DFS (Table 70-8). Recent consolidation schedules (Table 70-9) include teniposide, etoposide, m-amsacrine, mitoxantrone, idarubicin and high-dose ara-C, intermediate- or high-dose methotrexate, or intermediate-dose 6-mercaptopurine. BMT should also be considered as a form of intensive postinduction therapy.

Data that illustrate the effect of postinduction therapy have resulted from nonrandomized trials, comparing induction and consolidation therapy but without maintenance therapy. There is evidence from these trials that consolidation therapy does improve outcome.[32,56] The advantage of a consolidation therapy has not, however, been demonstrated unequivocally in randomized trials. In earlier studies the results of treatment of patients who did not receive consolidation therapy were reported to be poor.[57,58] This was also true in an European Organization for the Research and Treatment of Cancer study where consolidation with asparaginase and cyclophosphamide was compared with asparaginase, cyclophosphamide + ara-C, methotrexate, and thioguanine with a median DFS of 24 versus 45 months, respectively.[59] However, the difficulty in assessing the efficacy of certain consolidation schemes is evident from a recent Cancer and Leukemia Group B study. Therapy consisting of two consolidation courses with "DA 7+3" (daunorubicin × 7 days + ara-C × 3 days) and "DA 5+2," in addition to 6-mercaptopurine and methotrexate, was not superior to therapy with 6-mercaptopurine and methotrexate alone.[60]

High-Dose Chemotherapy

High-dose chemotherapy has been used mainly to overcome drug resistance or to achieve therapeutic drug levels in the cerebrospinal fluid.

High-Dose ara-C

A great deal of experience with high-dose ara-C exists for the treatment of ALL.[51,53] It still remains uncertain what dose of ara-C is optional. In refractory or relapsed adult ALL, 4–12 doses of high-dose ara-C (1–3 g/m²) administered with various other chemotherapeutic drugs result in similar CR rates (50–60%) and similar remission durations (3–4 months).[53,61] It is unknown whether specific subgroups of ALL, especially those with very poor outcome such as Ph-positive ALL, may benefit from high-dose ara-C therapy, and if so, what the optimal dose is (lower [1 g/m²] or higher [3 g/m²]). In a few studies, improved outcomes for adult high-risk ALL patients treated with higher-dose ara-C have been reported.[62–64]

An additional argument for the use of higher-dose ara-C might be its effectiveness in treating central nervous system leukemia. There is evidence that in ALL and NHL higher levels of ara-C triphosphate can be reached with 3 g/m² compared with the lower dose of 1 g/m² ara-C; in addition, with the higher dose, the cerebrospinal fluid can be cleared of blast cells,[65] which may not be the case with use of the lower dose. Thus for high-risk adult ALL patients the higher-dose ara-C (3 g/m²) still seems to be justified despite a higher associated morbidity.

High-Dose Methotrexate

The use of high-dose methotrexate has been extensively studied for the treatment of childhood ALL. Intermediate doses (0.5 g/m²), high doses of 1, 2, 3, 5, or 8 g/m², and even doses of 33 g/m² have been used. In children with low-risk ALL, CR rates of 91–100% and DFS rates between 63% and 94% have been achieved with high-dose methotrexate.[53] High-dose methotrexate appears to be effective in preventing systemic and testicular relapses.[66]

The effect of high-dose methotrexate on central nervous system leukemia may account for the favorable results reported with its use. High-dose methotrexate at a dose of 6 g/m² resulted in an 80% CR rate in children with central nervous system relapse,[67] indicating that systemic high-dose methotrexate reaches cytotoxic levels in the cerebrospinal fluid.

There are ongoing studies to explore the efficacy of high-dose methotrexate as consolidation in therapy combinations with other chemotherapeutic agents during the treatment of de novo adult ALL.[55,62]

High-Dose Etoposide

High-dose etoposide is apparently effective for the treatment of ALL as part of a preparative regimen before allogeneic or autologous BMT. Only very limited data are available on the use of high-dose etoposide without BMT in adult ALL. In a study in which high-dose etoposide was administered in total doses of 1.8–4.8 g/m² together with cyclophosphamide to a total dose of 6 g/m² in 14 patients with resistant ALL, a CR rate of 28% was reported.[68]

Maintenance Therapy

The optimal duration and form of maintenance therapy in adult ALL is unknown. Because the aim of maintenance or continuation therapy is to eliminate minimal residual disease, the optimal form of maintenance therapy will not be identified until reliable methods for detection of minimal residual disease are available.

Maintenance therapy with mercaptopurine and methotrexate, together with repeated cycles of consolidation therapy, appears to be superior to mercaptopurine and methotrexate alone. However, there has been no study of adult ALL to assess this approach in patients who have received adequate induction and early consolidation therapy. In a large multicenter Italian study[69] patients were randomly assigned, after an intensive consolidation, to postconsolidation therapy with conventional maintenance therapy consisting of mercaptopurine and methotrexate and alternating treatment courses of different intensity. In this report there was no difference in the survival rate at 4 years between the different treatment groups, which may suggest that after adequate early consolidation therapy, the intensity of the maintenance therapy has no influence on survival. However, attempts to omit maintenance altogether after induction and consolidation therapy have resulted in inferior results.[34,70,71] The performance of prospective trials of maintenance schedules dependent on immunologic subtypes of ALL (e.g., longer for common ALL, shorter for T-ALL, and none for B-ALL) or on cytogenetic subgroups (e.g., Ph/bcr-abl-positive ALL chemotherapy maintenance versus interferon-α/interleukin-2) are needed.

Central Nervous System Leukemia

Central nervous system leukemia occurs in <10% of patients with adult ALL at diagnosis.[56] Risk factors often associated with development of central nervous system leukemia include an elevated WBC count[72]; T-ALL phenotype, where in a large series the incidence was 15%[73]; and L3 or Burkitt morphology, with 33% of patients having central nervous system involvement.[74] Treatment of central nervous system leukemia consists of intrathecal methotrexate alone or in combination with ara-C or prednisone, similar intraventricular therapy administered via an Ommaya reservoir, or cranial irradiation. When adult ALL patients with central nervous system leukemia at diagnosis are treated adequately, they do not have an inferior outcome with regard to disease-free survival or central nervous system relapse rate.[69,75,76]

Central Nervous System Prophylaxis

Adult ALL patients who do not receive specific prophylactic central nervous system treatment have a central nervous system relapse rate of 21–50%,[74,77] similar to that observed in children who do not receive central nervous system prophylaxis.[78] In earlier studies the standard central nervous system prophylaxis adopted from childhood ALL experience was cranial radiotherapy with 24 Gy and intrathecal methotrexate, which reduced the central nervous system relapse rate to about 10–15%.[74]

The modalities for central nervous system prophylaxis now comprise a wide range of methods. These include cranial irradiation; intrathecal administration of methotrexate or the triple combination of methotrexate, ara-C, and prednisone therapy via an intraventricular reservoir; or systemic high-dose chemotherapy with high-dose methotrexate or high-dose ara-C whereby sufficient cerebrospinal fluid levels can be reached.[65,78]

Prophylactic treatment of the central nervous system may result in acute or chronic neurotoxicity. Adverse effects include febrile reactions, arachnoiditis, leukoencephalopathy, and subclinical dysfunctions, including learning disabilities. These adverse reactions occur primarily in children and are often subclinical in adults.[79]

Because this neurotoxicity has been mainly related to cranial irradiation, it has prompted a search for alternative approaches. Chemotherapy in the form of intrathecal methotrexate, intraventricular methotrexate by Ommaya reservoir,[80] high-dose systemic methotrexate,[81] or high-dose systemic ara-C[65,82] has been used without cranial irradiation. These approaches have proven to be as effective in preventing central nervous system relapses as combined intrathecal methotrexate and cranial irradiation but are not superior and may even cause more neurotoxicity when used at high doses in older patients. Central nervous system leukemia relapse rates, however, should not be the only means of assessing the effectiveness of such therapy; DFS should also be considered.

Because the risk for central nervous system relapse is associated with other risk factors such as T-ALL, B-ALL, extreme leu-kocytosis, high leukemia cell proliferation rate, and high serum LDH levels,[74] future protocols for adult ALL will be required to test risk-adapted central nervous system prophylaxis.

Therapy for Relapsed and Resistant Leukemia

Use of single-agent high-dose methotrexate, high-dose ara-C, and probably the anthracycline derivatives mitoxantrone and rubidazone result in a second remission in ≤30% of patients, whereas other agents such as amsacrine, teniposide, and etoposide are effective in 10–15%.[56] By using either these or other drugs in combination, second remissions can be achieved in ≤50–60% of relapsed adult ALL patients. The most effective regimens appear to be (1) moderate- to high-dose methotrexate with L-asparaginase or folinic acid rescue; (2) the combination of teniposide and ara-C; and (3) high-dose ara-C in combination with amsacrine, an anthracycline, or other agents.[61] Median remission duration after treatment of refractory or relapsed ALL is usually <6 months and long-term DFS occurs in <5% of cases. Thus relapsed adult ALL patients are candidates for alternative forms of therapy such as BMT.

Allogeneic Bone Marrow Transplantation in Adult ALL

BMT is one of the postremission strategies for eradication of residual disease in ALL. An antileukemic effect is achieved by the use of total body irradiation and chemotherapeutic drugs administered as part of the preparative regimen. In addition, there is evidence for an antileukemic effect resulting from graft-versus-host disease and most probably a graft-versus-leukemia effect.

The outcome of allogeneic BMT for ALL depends on age and remission status of the patient.[83] The best results have been obtained with patients transplanted during the first remission. Survival for adult transplant recipients with ALL during first remission is 21–61% (Table 70-10). In second remission, DFS after allogeneic BMT is 15–45%. In more advanced cases allogeneic BMT will result in 10–15% long-term survivors. When comparing these results with those achieved by chemotherapy it is obvious that all patients in second remission should receive transplants, since the outcome after BMT is clearly superior to the 5% cure rate achieved with chemotherapy alone. The use of BMT during first remission of ALL remains more controversial. The DFS of ≤61% after BMT is superior to that obtained with chemotherapy alone; however, when these results are adjusted for age, risk factors, and time to BMT (thereby excluding early relapses), the differences between BMT and chemotherapy are smaller.[84] It therefore appears advisable that low-risk groups having a DFS of about 50% after chemotherapy should receive a BMT only after a second remission. For high-risk adult ALL patients, BMT in first remission results in a survival advantage as compared with chemotherapy alone. BMT in advanced, either refractory or relapsed ALL, result in 12–23% DFS at 3 years.

Prognostic factors for remission duration after chemother-

Table 70-10. Results of Chemotherapy and Allogeneic and Autologous BMT in Adult ALL

	Probability of Leukemia-Free Survival (%)	
	First Remission	Second Remission
Chemotherapy	35	5
Low-risk	50	
High-risk	25	
Allogeneic BMT	21–61	15–45
Autologous BMT	21–65	10–40

apy (i.e., age, WBC count, immunophenotype) are also predictive for the outcome after BMT.[85] An exception seems to be Ph-positive ALL, in which results with chemotherapy alone are very poor,[30,34,75] whereas results with allogeneic BMT are much more favorable, with a DFS of ≥40%.[86,87]

The conditioning regimens used for BMT in most studies have consisted of total body irradiation plus cyclophosphamide and other drugs. More recently, conditioning regimens without irradiation have also been used. These regimens appear to be a suitable alternative to radiation-based regimens.

Mismatched Bone Marrow Transplantation

Only one-third of potential BMT candidates with ALL will have an HLA-identical sibling donor. To extend the possibilities of allogeneic BMT by enlarging the number of bone marrow donors available, mismatched BMT from related or unrelated donors has been considered.[88] In a recent report[89] 31 patients were given mismatched BMT (3 unrelated, 28 related and genotypically identical for one haplotype but mismatched for up to three HLA antigens); 17 survive in remission but the mean follow-up of 16 months is too short to evaluate the therapeutic potential of this approach.

Autologous Bone Marrow Transplantation

Another attempt to overcome the limited availability of bone marrow donors is autologous BMT.[83] This form of BMT is associated with a risk of reinfusing residual leukemic cells and also of a higher relapse rate owing to the lack of a graft-versus-leukemia effect. For autologous BMT, bone marrow cells are harvested from patients during CR and are then cryopreserved. The patients then receive high-dose chemotherapy and/or radiation conditioning regimens equal or similar to those used for allogeneic BMT before infusion of the graft. The elimination of residual leukemic cells in the remission bone marrow, which is used as a graft, remains problematic.[90]

Several methods are currently in use to eliminate these leukemic cells in the graft. Monoclonal antibodies that are reactive to B- or T-lymphocyte differentiation antigens present on leukemic cells are used to purge marrow. Chemotherapeutic drugs such as 4-hydroperoxycyclophosphamide, mafosfamide, or etoposide have also been used for these purposes. At present it remains uncertain which of these methods is the most effective procedure in eliminating the minimal residual leukemic cells present in the graft. Some form of marrow purging seems necessary for autologous BMT therapy to be successful.

A large number of adults with ALL in second or later remission have been treated with autologous transplantation (overall results are shown in Table 70-10). In second remission the DFS rate at 3 years is 10–40%, a result somewhat inferior to that with allogeneic BMT, but clearly superior to that achieved with chemotherapy alone. DFS after autologous BMT in first remission in adults is 21–65%. This substantial range in outcome probably reflects selection of patients more than differences in the therapeutic approaches. These results are no better than those achieved with intensive chemotherapy alone in comparable risk groups. Thus the role of autologous BMT in the treatment of adult ALL remains uncertain. The value of autologous BMT during first remission needs to be evaluated in prospective trials.

Peripheral Blood Stem Cell Transplantation

A recent strategy for the treatment of adult ALL is to transplant autologous peripheral blood stem cells. In a study with 9 high-risk adult ALL patients, including those with the cytogenetic abnormalities t(4;11), t(9;22), or t(8;14), 5 of 9 patients

remain alive, and 1 is still leukemia-free post-transplant.[91] Similarly, in another study, 6 of 18 high-risk patients have not relapsed 2–15 months post-transplant.[92]

PROGNOSIS

Up to 80% of adult patients achieve a CR after induction chemotherapy. The major risk factor for attaining a CR is advanced age. Prognostic factors can be useful for estimating the duration of remission. Appreciation of the impact of such risk factors can result in the generation of risk-adapted treatment protocols for adult ALL, a strategy already well established for childhood ALL.

Age

Age is an important prognostic factor in ALL; its greatest impact is on remission duration and survival. There is a continuous decline in CR rate from 95% in children to 40–60% in patients >50–60 years of age.[1] Most trials demonstrate that increasing age is also associated with shorter remission duration and decreased survival. In almost all recent studies DFS in patients >50 or 60 years of age is inferior.[60,93–96] Patients <50 years of age are candidates for BMT.

The optimal treatment of elderly ALL patients remains unclear. Supportive treatment alone results in no cures and short survival. Moderate or intensive treatment has led to remission rates of 37–50% in patients 60 to >80 years of age but a survival time of only 3 months.[95,96] In four consecutive German multicenter studies the survival in CR for elderly ALL patients (50–65 years of age) could be improved from 19% to 32% at 6 years. Unexpectedly, elderly patients did not benefit from an intensive consolidation with high-dose ara-C (1 g/m^2) and mitoxantrone, but did benefit from a mild consolidation with teniposide and ara-C.[94] Elderly patients >50 years of age who have achieved a CR and good clinical condition are potential candidates for autologous BMT.

White Blood Cell Count

A high WBC count at presentation adversely influences the remission rate of patients with ALL as well as the remission duration.[60,69,75,76] Fewer long-term survivors are found among patients with a markedly elevated leukocyte count at diagnosis. The WBC elevations used to indicate a poor prognosis vary from a WBC count of $10,000 \times 10^6/L$ to one of $100,000 \times 10^6/L$ depending on the study cited. In recent studies the critical level of WBC elevation appears to be $25,000–35,000 \times 10^6/L$, a limit similar to that defined in childhood ALL.

Time to Response

The time required to achieve CR is inversely related to remission duration.[97] In four recent adult ALL studies the achievement of CR within 4 or 5 weeks[63,76,93,98] was associated with a significantly better long-term outcome, the DFS being 42–46% compared with 0–26% when additional therapy was required to achieve CR. In studies in which overall CR rates of 70–80% are obtained, the proportion of patients who require >4 weeks

Table 70-11. Outcome of Immunologic Subtypes in Adult ALL

Subtype	No. of Patients	CR rate (%)[a]	Probability of Continuous CR (%)[a]
T-ALL			
− ara-C/C	47	72	<10
+ ara-C/C	253	85	46
B-ALL			
"ALL" therapy	63	44	<10
"NHL" therapy	62	79	53
C-ALL	702	78	34

[a] Weighted mean values.

of treatment is ≤10%, and it is obvious that these patients have a poor prognosis.

Immunophenotype

T-ALL

T-ALL, which constitutes about 20–25% of adult ALL, was previously reported to have a very poor outcome (Table 70-11), particularly for patients with mediastinal mass, with a leukemia-free survival of <10%. With more innovative therapy, the CR rate of these patients has improved to about 80% and leukemia-free survival has increased to 45%.[99] The use of cyclophosphamide and ara-C during induction therapy is mainly responsible for this improvement in survival. The inclusion of ara-C and cyclophosphamide pulses during continuation therapy was selectively beneficial in childhood T-ALL.[100] Also, in adult ALL the combination of ara-C and cyclophosphamide with the usual chemotherapeutic drugs improved CR rate and DFS in T-ALL.[75,99] Improved CR rate and leukemia-free survival for T-ALL was also observed in a recent study in which cyclophosphamide was added to conventional induction therapy with vincristine, prednisone, daunorubicin, and asparaginase.[101] Although there are no randomized data available, it appears that cyclophosphamide and ara-C play a major role in the recently observed improved outcome of T-ALL patients (Table 70-11).

In patients with T-ALL and mediastinal mass, giving mediastinal irradiation after initial cell reduction by chemotherapy, either after complete disappearance of tumor or to a residual tumor, was shown to be of benefit in two German multicenter ALL trials.[99] The benefit of such additional mediastinal irradiation in T-ALL is not, however, yet confirmed in other trials.

In recent studies the latest relapses for T-ALL patients occur at approximately 3 years. The optimal duration of treatment for T-ALL patients is as yet undefined as is the value of conventional maintenance with 6-mercaptopurine and methotrexate, with or without reinforcement therapy.

B-ALL

There has been a significant change in the reported outcome of patients with B-ALL and Burkitt lymphomas after combination chemotherapy. In childhood B-ALL the outcome was significantly improved. CR rates of 81–96% and DFS rates of 76% have been achieved.[102] The drugs responsible for this improvement in care are high-dose cyclophosphamide, high-dose methotrexate (0.5–8 g/m^2), and high-dose ara-C, giving an 81% CR rate in the Pediatric Oncology Group study[103] and an 88% CR rate in the French Pediatric Oncology Society trial.[104] In the Berlin-Frankfurt-Münster protocols, CR rates of 92–96% were reported after the administration of higher doses of cyclophosphamide or ifosphamide and high-dose methotrexate (0.5–5 g/m^2), but without high-dose ara-C.[102] In addition to cyclophosphamide, high-dose methotrexate, or high-dose ara-C, the regimens contain the additional chemotherapeutic drugs doxoru-

bicin, ara-C, vincristine, prednisone, daunorubicin, and etoposide.

In earlier adult ALL trials, results of the treatment of patients with B-ALL were very poor with a weighted mean CR rate of 44%, a median remission duration of 11 months, and leukemia-free survival of <10% (Table 70-11). When the recent childhood B-ALL protocols were used to treat adult patients with B-ALL, results were substantially improved with CR rates of >80% and leukemia-free survival rates of 57% reported.[62,105]

Myeloid Antigen-Positive ALL

With the pursuit of a more detailed immunologic analysis of the phenotype of ALL blast cells, increasing numbers of patients with myeloid antigen-positive (My+) ALL have been reported.[24] These cases have been described as hybrid acute leukemia, biphenotypic leukemia, and acute mixed-lineage leukemia. A common property of these leukemias is that in addition to the markers specific for ALL, the myeloid markers CD13, CD14, CD33, and CDw65 are expressed by leukemia blast cells.[106] These leukemias were previously included in the subtype "null"-ALL.

Whether My+ ALL is associated with a poor prognosis is not clear. In childhood ALL there are some studies that report a significantly lower leukemia-free survival rate for My+ patients (38% and 39% compared with 75% and 78% for patients with leukemia blast cells that do not have myeloid markers).[107,108] Other studies, including those of the Berlin-Frankfurt-Münster group, have found no difference in CR rates or leukemia-free survival rates for My+ patients.[109] The few studies of adult My+ ALL have indicated that My+ ALL is associated with a poor outcome.[24,110,111] Larger patient numbers and longer follow-up are required before it can be definitely stated that, even with intensified treatment schedules, My+ ALL is associated with a poor prognosis.

Cytogenetics

Philadelphia Chromosome/bcr-abl-Positive ALL

Ph/bcr-abl-positive ALL is the subgroup of ALL having the worst prognosis in children as well as in adults. In 11 studies with a total of 213 patients, the weighted mean CR rate was 60%. The median duration of remission in all series is short (5–10 months), and the survival rate is from 0 to <20% at 3–5 years.[112,113] Ph-positive ALL comprises 2–5% of ALL cases in children to >44% of ALL patients >50 years of age.[112]

A new approach for the diagnosis of Ph-positive ALL is the detection of bcr-abl rearrangements by molecular analysis. Cytogenetic detection of the Ph chromosome remains the standard method but is tedious. In four adult ALL trials the incidence of Ph/bcr-abl-positive ALL ranged from 25% to 30% using molecular methods.[33–36]

In two German multicenter ALL trials, detection of the bcr-abl abnormality was of prognostic significance, since 15–23% of bcr-abl-positive patients survived at 3 years compared with 40–49% of the bcr-abl-negative group. Similarly in a Cancer and Leukemia Group B study, the median duration of remission was only 9.5 months for the bcr-abl-positive patients whereas the median duration of remission had not been reached for the bcr-abl-negative group.[36]

The successful treatment of Ph/bcr-abl-positive ALL patients remains problematic. With intensified induction regimens a >70% CR rate can be achieved. Thus the problem is not obtaining CR but maintaining remission. High-dose ara-C (3 g/m^2 × 6–8 days) with vincristine, doxorubicin, and dexamethasone,[63] or high-dose ara-C with mitoxantrone in the German ALL trials appear to be useful as consolidation therapy.

Biologic response modifiers have been used as a new form of maintenance treatment for Ph-positive ALL. There are reports indicating that interferon-α administered to patients in CR can maintain remission.[114,115] Studies evaluating a combination of interferon-α and interleukin-2 as maintenance therapy are ongoing.

The most promising approach at present for the treatment of Ph-positive ALL is BMT. After allogeneic BMT, 42% of 12 patients transplanted in first or second CR were reported to survive in one study.[87] A leukemia-free survival rate of 44% for 32 Ph-positive ALL patients transplanted in first CR has been reported by the International BMT Registry.[116] The role of autologous BMT in the treatment of Ph ALL has not been established.[35,117] Single long-term survivors have been reported after autologous BMT.[118] The difficulty with autologous BMT is the development of the means to purge Ph-positive bone marrow.[117] The detection of leukemia cells with the *bcr-abl* gene by semiquantitative PCR methods[119] may offer a method by which to monitor the effectiveness of such purging methods.

t(4;11), t(8;14)

Adult ALL patients with the cytogenetic translocation t(4;11) have a poor prognosis similar to those with t(9;22).[26,30] The presence of t(8;14) translocation has lost its adverse prognostic implications with the improved treatment results for patients with B-ALL and Burkitt lymphoma. With more intensive treatment regimens the outcome for patients with t(4;11), mostly the immunologic subtype pre-pre-B-ALL, has substantially improved (German multicenter ALL trials, unpublished results).

Sex

A tendency toward higher remission rates has been observed in women in most studies of adult ALL patients. Sex had no influence on remission duration in most series. When, however, a sex-related difference in long-term outcome was observed, survival was always inferior in men.[56] This trend is similar to that observed in children, in whom the inferior outcome of boys may partly be accounted for by the occurrence of testicular relapses. Reports of the incidence of testicular relapse in adults are rare; in three studies that included intensive therapy, testicular relapse was reported in ≤1% of cases.[72,76,120] Thus, the inferior outcome for adult men with ALL remains unexplained.

Other Risk Factors

Clinical features that were found to have an adverse influence on remission rate or duration include organ involvement at presentation, such as extensive lymphadenopathy, hepatomegaly, splenomegaly, central nervous system leukemia, or mediastinal involvement.[56] Other factors reported to have an adverse influence[56] include the morphology according to the FAB classification, degree of bone marrow involvement, the number of immature cells in the peripheral blood, low platelets at diagnosis, high serum LDH levels, elevated serum glutamic oxaloacetic transaminase levels, weight loss, and race.[121] The value of most of these variables as prognosticators has been proven in single studies only and, apart from LDH, are not used for treatment stratification.

Stratification into Risk Groups

Prognostic factors for predicting remission duration in adult ALL (Table 70-12) have been used to identify low- and high-risk patient groups. It is of interest that from recent adult ALL trials

Table 70-12. Adverse Prognostic Factors for Remission Duration in Adult ALL

Late achievement of complete remission (>4 or 5 wk)
High WBC count (>10,000->25,000->100,000/mm^{3a})
Advanced age (>50 years)
Immunologic subtypes
Mixed ALL or hybrid ALL (?)
Pre-T-ALL (?)
Chromosomal abnormalities
Ph-ALL [t(9;22)]
t(4;11)

^{a} Continuous variable.

employing intensive but different treatment regimens, consistent or similar prognostic factors have emerged,[75,76] including time to achieve CR, initial WBC count, age, immunologic subtype, and cytogenetic abnormalities (Table 70-12). In these studies low-risk patients can be identified and their probability of remaining in continuous CR beyond 5 years has been reported to be about 50% as compared with <25% for high-risk patients.[76,117] Thus, it no longer seems justified to consider all adult ALL patients as being in a poor-risk group. The stratification into risk groups forms a basis for selecting patients for different therapeutic strategies (e.g., BMT in first or second remission).

Relapse Time and Site

More than one-half of adult patients with ALL relapse after the completion of chemotherapy. The overall relapse rate is highest within the first 2 years after CR and lower thereafter. Relapse patterns seem to be dependent on the subtype of ALL: in common ALL nearly all relapses occur within 5–6 years, for T-ALL relapses occur within 3–4 years, and for B-ALL they occur within 1 year. This conclusion is limited because only a small number of reports of adult ALL treatment analyze the relapse pattern with regard to subtype.

Approximately 80% of all relapses occur in the bone marrow, with the remainder occurring in extramedullary sites, predominantly the central nervous system. Other extramedullary sites, such as lymph nodes, skin, or other organ sites, account for <3–5% of relapses in adult ALL. Testicular relapse has been estimated to occur in <1% of patients. This could be an underestimate of the incidence of testicular relapse because this event might not be as carefully and closely sought in adults as in children.[122] Relapses at other sites, such as the mediastinum, are rare, even in those patients with initial mediastinal involvement. Patients with an isolated extramedullary relapse are at high risk of subsequent marrow relapse and require local treatment followed by systemic reinduction therapy. Thus bone marrow relapse is the major concern in adult ALL. Methods to detect minimal residual disease are rapidly being developed and should be useful in monitoring the intensity and duration of therapy for individuals and in deciding whether alternative approaches such as BMT are necessary.

REFERENCES

1. Hoelzer D: Which factors influence the different outcome of therapy in adults and children with ALL. Bone Marrow Transplant, suppl. 1. 4:98, 1989
2. Cutler SJ, Young IL Jr (eds): National Cancer Institute: Third National Cancer Survey: Incidence Data. National Cancer Institute Monograph no. 41. U.S. Government Printing Office, Washington, DC, 1975, p. 102
3. McKinney PA, Alexander FE, Cartwright RA, Ricketts TJ: The Leukaemia Research Fund Data Collection Study: descriptive epidemiology of acute lymphoblastic leukaemia. Leukemia 3:880, 1989
4. Boggs DR, Wintrobe MM, Cartwright GE: The acute leukemias. Medicine 41: 163, 1962

5. Chaganti RSK, Miller DR, Meyers PA et al: Cytogenetic evidence of the intrauterine origin of acute leukemia in monozygotic twins. N Engl J Med 300: 1032, 1979

6. Hecht T, Henke M, Schempp W et al: Acute lymphoblastic leukemia in adult identical twins. Blut 56:261, 1988

7. Keith L, Brown E: Epidemiological study of leukemia in twins (1928–1969). Acta Genet Med Gemmellol (Roma) 20:9, 1971

8. Heath CW: Leukemogenesis and low-dose exposure to radiation and chemical agents. p. 23. In Yohn DS, Blakeslee JR (eds): Advances in Comparative Leukemia Research. North-Holland/Elsevier, Amsterdam, 1982

9. Haesman MA, Kemp JW, MacLaren A-M et al: Incidence of leukaemia in young persons in West of Scotland. Lancet 1:1188, 1984

10. Gardner MJ, Snee MP, Hall AJ et al: Results of case-control study of leukaemia and lymphoma among young people near Sellafield nuclear plant in West Cumbria. BMJ 300:423, 1990

11. Aksoy M, Erdem S, Dincol G: Types of leukemia in chronic benzene poisoning. A study in thirty-four patients. Acta Haematol 55:65, 1976

12. Pui C-H, Behm FG, Raimondi SC et al: Secondary acute myeloid leukemia in children treated for acute lymphoid leukemia. N Engl J Med 321:136, 1989

13. Pui C-H, Ribiero RC, Hancock MD et al: Acute myeloid leukemia in children treated with epipodophyllotoxins for acute lymphoblastic leukemia. N Engl J Med 325:1682, 1991

14. Manns A: Natural history of HTLV-1 infection: relation to leukemogenesis. Leukemia, suppl. 2. 7:75, 1993

15. Poiesz BJ, Ruscetti FW, Gadzar AF et al: Detection and isolation of type C retrovirus particles from fresh and cultured lymphocytes of a patient with cutaneous T-cell lymphoma. Proc Natl Acad Sci USA 77:7415, 1980

16. Hinuma Y, Nagata K, Hanaola M et al: Adult T-cell leukemia: antigen in an ATL cell line and detection of antibodies to the antigen in human sera. Proc Natl Acad USA 78:6476, 1981

17. Gallo RC, Kalyanaraman VS, Sarngadharan MG et al: Association of the human type C retrovirus with a subset of adult T-cell cancers. Cancer Res 43:3892, 1983

18. Löffler H, Kayser W, Schmitz N et al: Morphological and cytochemical classification of adult acute leukemias in two multicenter studies in the Federal Republic of Germany. Haematol Blood Transfus 30:21, 1987

19. Pui C-H, Behm FG, Crist WM: Clinical and biologic relevance of immunologic marker studies in childhood acute lymphoblastic leukemia. Blood 82:323, 1993

20. Ludwig W-D, Schwartz S, Martin M et al: Die immunzytologische Diagnose und Klassifizierung akuter Leukämien. Lab Med 17:465, 1993

21. Kersey J, Nesbit M, Halligren H et al: Evidence of origin of certain childhood acute lymphoblastic leukemias and lymphomas in thymus-derived lymphocytes. Cancer 36:1348, 1975

22. Reinherz EL, Kung PC, Goldstein G et al: Discrete stages of human intrathymic differentiation. Analysis of normal thymocytes and leukemic lymphoblasts of T-cell lineage. Proc Natl Acad Sci USA 77:1588, 1980

23. Thiel E, Kranz BR, Raghavachar A et al: Prethymic phenotype and genotype of pre-T (CD7+/ER−)-cell leukemia and its clinical significance within adult acute lymphoblastic leukemia. Blood 73:1247, 1989

24. Sobol RE, Mick R, Royston I et al: Clinical importance of myeloid antigen expression in adult acute lymphoblastic leukemia. N Engl J Med 316:1111, 1987

25. Janossy G, Coustan-Smith E, Campana D: The reliability of cytoplasmic CD3 and CD33 antigen expression in the immunodiagnosis of acute leukemia: a study of 500 cases. Leukemia 3:170, 1989

26. Bloomfield CD, Secker-Walker LM, Goldman AI et al: Six-year follow-up of the clinical significance of karyotype in acute lymphoblastic leukemia. Cancer Genet Cytogenet 40:171, 1989

27. Bloomfield CD, Rowley JD, Goldman AI et al (for the Third International Workshop on Chromosomes in Leukemia): Chromosomal abnormalities and their clinical significance in acute lymphoblastic leukemia. Cancer Res 43: 868, 1983

28. Bloomfield CD, Goldman AI, Alimena G et al: Chromosomal abnormalities identify high-risk and low-risk patients with acute lymphoblastic leukemia. Blood 67:415, 1986

29. Williams DL, Raimondi SC, Rivera G et al: Presence of clonal chromosome abnormalities in virtually all cases of acute lymphoblastic leukemia. N Engl J Med 313:640, 1985

30. Hagemeijer A, van der Plas DC: Clinical relevance of cytogenetics in acute leukemia. Haematol Blood Transfus 33:23, 1990

31. First MIC Cooperative Study Group: Morphologic, immunologic, and cytogenetic (MIC) working classification of acute lymphoblastic leukemias. Cancer Genet Cytogenet 23:189, 1986

32. Hoelzer D: Treatment of acute lymphoblastic leukemia. Semin Hematol 31: 1, 1994

33. Maurer J, Janssen JWG, Thiel E et al: Detection of chimeric BCR-ABL genes in acute lymphoblastic leukaemia by the polymerase chain reaction. Lancet 337:1055, 1991

34. Cassileth PA, Anderson JW, Hoagland HD et al: High-dose cytarabine therapy in adult acute lymphocytic leukemia. p. 197. In Gale RP, Hoelzer D (eds): Acute Lymphoblastic Leukemia. Wiley-Liss, New York, 1990

35. Gehly GB, Bryant EM, Lee AM et al: Chimeric BCR-abl messenger RNA as a marker for minimal residual disease in patients transplanted for Philadelphia chromosome-positive lymphoblastic leukemia. Blood 78:458, 1991

36. Westbrook CA, Hooberman AL, Spino C et al: Clinical significance of the BCR-ABL fusion gene in adult acute lymphoblastic leukemia: a Cancer and Leukemia Group B study (8762). Blood 80:2983, 1992

37. Schiffer CA, Wade JC: Supportive care issues in the use of blood products and treatment of infection. Semin Oncol 14:454, 1987

38. Hoelzer D, Thiel E, Löffler H et al: Intensified therapy in acute lymphoblastic and acute undifferentiated leukemia in adults. Blood 64:38, 1984

39. Walsh TJ, Pizzo PA: Fungal infections in granulocytopenic patients: current approaches to classification, diagnosis and treatment. p. 47. In Holmberg K, Meyer R (eds): Diagnosis and Therapy of Systemic Fungal Infections. Raven Press, New York, 1989

40. Bodey GP, Vartivarian S: Aspergillosis. Eur J Clin Microbiol Infect Dis 8:65, 1989

41. Meunier F: Fungal infections in the compromised host. p. 193. In Rubin RH, Young LS (eds): Clinical Approach to Infection in the Compromised Host. Plenum, New York, 1988

42. Ringden O, Meunier F, Tollemar J et al: Efficacy of amphotericin B encapsulated in liposomes (AmBisome) in the treatment of invasive fungal infections in immunocompromised patients. J Antimicrob Chemother, suppl. B. 28:73, 1991

43. Myers SE, Devine SM, Topper RL et al: A pilot study of prophylactic aerosolized amphotericin B in patients at risk for prolonged neutropenia. Leuk Lymphoma 8:229, 1992

44. Ohno R, Tomonaga M, Kobayashi T et al: Effect of granulocyte colony-stimulating factor after intensive therapy in relapsed or refractory acute leukemia. N Engl J Med 323:871, 1990

45. Kantarjian HM, Estey E, O'Brien S et al: Granulocyte-colony stimulating factor (G-CSF) supportive care following intensive chemotherapy consolidation in acute lymphocytic leukemia (ALL) in first remission. Blood, suppl. 1. 80:112a, 1992

46. Blaise D, Vernant JP, Fière D et al: A randomised, controlled, multicenter trial of recombinant human granulocyte colony stimulating factor (Filgrastim) in patients treated by bone marrow transplantation (BMT) with total body irradiation (TBI) for acute lymphoblastic leukemia (ALL) or lymphoblastic lymphoma (LL). Blood, suppl. 1. 80:248a, 1992

47. Scherrer R, Geissler K, Kyrle PA et al: Granulocyte colony-stimulating factor (G-CSF) as an adjunct to induction chemotherapy of adult acute lymphoblastic leukemia (ALL). Ann Hematol 66:283, 1993

48. Ottmann OG, Ganser A, Freund M et al: Simultaneous administration of granulocyte colony-stimulating factor (Filgrastim) and induction chemotherapy in adult acute lymphoblastic leukemia. Ann Hematol 67:161, 1993

49. Calderwood S, Rumeyer F, Freedman MH: GM-CSF in childhood acute lymphoblastic leukemia: randomized double blind trial during intensification phase. Blood, suppl. 1. 80:288a, 1992

50. Caligiuri MA, Mayer RJ: Pregnancy and leukemia. Semin Oncol 16:388, 1989

51. Stryckmans P, Debusscher L: Chemotherapy of adult acute lymphoblastic leukaemia. Baillières Clin Haematol 4:115, 1991

52. Wiernik PH, Dutcher JP, Paietta E et al: Long-term follow-up of treatment and potential cure of adult acute lymphocytic leukemia with MOAD: a nonanthracycline containing regimen. Leukemia 7:1236, 1993

53. Hoelzer D: High-dose chemotherapy in adult acute lymphoblastic leukemia. Semin Hematol, suppl. 4. 28:84, 1991

54. Berman E, Hudis C, Offit K et al: Therapy of adult acute lymphocytic leukemia (ALL). Haematologica, suppl. 4. 76:106, 1991

55. Elonen E, Almqvist A, Hänninen A et al: Intensive treatment of acute lymphatic leukaemia in adults: ALL86 protocol. Haematologica, suppl. 4. 76: 133, 1991

56. Hoelzer D, Gale RP: Acute lymphoblastic leukemia in adults: recent progress, future directions. Semin Hematol 24:27, 1987

57. Fière D, Extra JM, David B et al: Treatment of 218 adult acute lymphoblastic leukemias. Semin Oncol, suppl. 1. 14:64, 1987

58. Sackmann-Muriel F, Svarch E, Eppinger-Helft M et al: Evaluation of intensification and maintenance programs in the treatment of acute lymphoblastic leukemia. Cancer 42:1730, 1978

59. Stryckmans P, De Witte Th, Bitar N et al: Cytosine arabinoside for induction, salvage, and consolidation therapy of adult acute lymphoblastic leukemia. Semin Oncol 14:67, 1987

60. Ellison RR, Mick R, Cuttner J et al: The effects of postinduction intensification treatment with cytarabine and daunorubicin in adult acute lymphocytic

leukemia: a prospective randomized clinical trial by Cancer and Leukemia Group B. J Clin Oncol 9:2002, 1991

61. Freund M, Diedrich H, Ganser A et al: Treatment of relapsed or refractory adult lymphocytic leukemia. Cancer 69:709, 1992

62. Hoelzer D, Thiel E, Ludwig WD et al: The German multicenter trials for treatment of acute lymphoblastic leukemia in adults. Leukemia, suppl. 2. 6: 175, 1992

63. Kantarjian HM, Walters RS, Keating MJ et al: Results of the vincristine, doxorubicin, and dexamethasone regimen in adults with standard- and high-risk acute lymphocytic leukemia. J Clin Oncol 8:994, 1990

64. Rohatiner AZS, Bassan R, Battista R et al: High dose cytosine arabinoside in the initial treatment of adult with acute lymphoblastic leukaemia. Br J Cancer 62:454, 1990

65. Morra E, Lazzarino M, Inverdadi D et al: Systemic high-dose ara-C for the treatment of meningeal leukemia in adult acute lymphoblastic leukemia and non-Hodgkin's lymphoma. J Clin Oncol 4:1207, 1986

66. Freeman AI, Weinberg V, Brecher ML et al: Comparison of intermediate methotrexate with cranial irradiation for the post-induction treatment of acute lymphocytic leukemia in children. N Engl J Med 308:477, 1983

67. Balis FM, Savitch JL, Bleyer WA et al: Remission induction of meningeal leukemia with high-dose intravenous methotrexate. J Clin Oncol 3:485, 1985

68. Brown RA, Herzig RH, Wolff SN et al: High dose etoposide and cyclophosphamide without bone marrow transplantation for resistant hematologic malignancy. Blood 76:473, 1990

69. Mandelli F, Rotoli B, Aloe Spiriti MA et al: GIMEMA ALL 0183: a multicentric study on adult acute lymphoblastic leukaemia in Italy. Br J Haematol 71: 377, 1989

70. Cuttner J, Mick R, Budman DR et al: Phase III trial of brief intensive treatment of adult acute lymphocytic leukemia comparing daunorubicin and mitoxantrone: a CALGB study. Leukemia 5:425, 1991

71. Wernli M, Gratwohl A, von Fliedner V et al: Behandlung der akuten lymphatischen Leukämie beim Erwachsenen: Pilotversuch mit intensiver Frühtherapie und ohne Erhaltungsphase. Schweiz Med Wochenschr 121:194, 1991

72. Schauer P, Arlin ZA, Mertelsmann R et al: Treatment of acute lymphoblastic leukemia in adults: results of the L-10 and L-10 M protocols. J Clin Oncol 1:462, 1983

73. Ludwig W-D, Thiel E, Bartram CR et al: Clinical importance of T-ALL subclassification according to thymic or prethymic maturation stage. Haematol Blood Transfus 33:419, 1990

74. Kantarjian HM, Walters RS, Smith TL et al: Identification of risk groups for development of central nervous system leukemia in adults with acute lymphoblastic leukemia. Blood 72:1784, 1988

75. Clarkson B, Ellis S, Little C et al: Acute lymphoblastic leukemia in adults. Semin Oncol 12:160, 1985

76. Hoelzer D, Thiel E, Löffler H et al: Prognostic factors in a multicenter study for treatment of acute lymphoblastic leukemia in adults. Blood 71:123, 1988

77. Hoelzer D: Current status of ALL/AUL therapy in adults. Recent Results Cancer Res 93:182, 1984

78. Bleyer WA: Central nervous system leukemia. p. 733. In Henderson ES, Lister TA (eds): Leukemia. 5th Ed. W.B. Saunders, Philadelphia, 1990

79. Tucker J, Prior PF, Green CR et al: Minimal neuropsychological sequelae following prophylactic treatment of the central nervous system in adult leukaemia and lymphoma. Br J Cancer 60:775, 1989

80. Clarkson BD, Haghbin M, Murphy ML et al: Prevention of central nervous system leukaemia in acute lymphoblastic leukaemia with prophylactic chemotherapy alone. p. 36. In Whitehouse JMA, Kay HEM (eds): CNS Complications of Malignant Disease. Macmillan, London, 1979

81. Esterhay RJ, Wiernik PH, Grove WR et al: Moderate dose methotrexate, vincristine, asparaginase, and dexamethasone for treatment of adult acute lymphocytic leukemia. Blood 59:334, 1982

82. Bassan R, Battista R, Rohatiner AZS et al: Treatment of adult acute lymphoblastic leukaemia (ALL) over a 16 year period. Leukemia, suppl. 2. 6:186, 1992

83. Dicke KA, Hoelzer DF, Gorin NC et al: The role of bone marrow transplantation in adult acute lymphocytic leukemia. Ann Oncol, suppl. 1. 4:881, 1993

84. Horowitz MM, Messerer D, Hoelzer D et al: Chemotherapy compared with bone marrow transplantation for adults with acute lymphoblastic leukemia in first remission. Ann Intern Med 115:13, 1991

85. Barrett AJ, Horowitz MM, Gale RP et al: Marrow transplantation for acute lymphoblastic leukemia: factors affecting relapse and survival. Blood 74: 862, 1989

86. Forman SJ, O'Donnell MR, Nademanee AP et al: Bone marrow transplantation for patients with Philadelphia chromosome positive acute lymphoblastic leukemia. Blood 70:587, 1987

87. Blume KG, Schmidt GM, Chao NJ et al: Bone marrow transplantation for

acute lymphoblastic leukemia. p. 279. In Gale RP, Hoelzer D (eds): Acute Lymphoblastic Leukemia. Wiley-Liss, New York, 1990

88. Beatty PG: Results of allogeneic bone marrow transplantation with unrelated or mismatched donors. Semin Oncol, suppl. 3. 19:13, 1992

89. Henslee-Downey PJ, Fleming D, Kryscio R et al: Does mismatched bone marrow transplant (MMBMT) from related or unrelated donors offer successful salvage therapy for patients (pts) with relapsed acute lymphoblastic leukemia? Haematologica, suppl. 4. 76:69, 1991

90. Uckun FM, Kersey JH, Haake R et al: Pretransplantation burden of leukemic progenitor cells as a predictor of relapse after bone marrow transplantation for acute lymphoblastic leukemia. N Engl J Med 329:1296, 1993

91. Carella AM, Pollicardo N, Carlier P et al: "Normal" peripheral blood stem cells (PBSC) mobilization by myelosuppressive chemotherapy in very high-risk acute lymphoblastic leukemia (ALL) with cytogenetic translocations. Leuk Lymphoma, suppl. 2. 7:19, 1992

92. Henon PH: New developments in peripheral blood stem transplants. Leukemia, suppl. 1. 6:106, 1992

93. Gaynor J, Chapman D, Little C et al: A cause-specific hazard rate analysis of prognostic factors among 199 adults with acute lymphoblastic leukemia: the Memorial Hospital experience since 1969. J Clin Oncol 6:1014, 1988

94. Hoelzer D: Aggressive chemotherapy of ALL in elderly patients. Hematol Oncol, suppl. 1. 11:12, 1993

95. Delannoy A, Ferrant A, Bosly A et al: Acute lymphoblastic leukemia in the elderly. Eur J Haematol 45:90, 1990

96. Taylor PRA, Reid MM, Bown N et al: Acute lymphoblastic leukemia in patients aged 60 years and over: a population-based study of incidence and outcome. Blood 80:1813, 1992

97. Miller DR, Coccia PF, Bleyer WA et al: Early response to induction therapy as a predictor of disease-free survival and late recurrence of childhood acute lymphoblastic leukemia: a report from the Children's Cancer Study Group. J Clin Oncol 7:1807, 1989

98. Linker CA, Levitt LJ, O'Donnell M et al: Improved results of treatment of adult acute lymphoblastic leukemia. Blood 69:1242, 1987

99. Hoelzer D, Thiel E, Löffler H et al: Intensified chemotherapy and mediastinal irradiation in adult T-cell acute lymphoblastic leukemia. p. 221. In Gale RP, Hoelzer D (eds): Acute Lymphoblastic Leukemia. Wiley-Liss, New York, 1990

100. Lauer SJ, Pinkel D, Buchanan GR et al: Cytosine arabinoside/cyclophosphamide pulses during continuation therapy for childhood acute lymphoblastic leukemia. Cancer 60:2366, 1987

101. Schiffer CA, Larson RA, Bloomfield CD, for the CALGB: Cancer and Leukemia Group B (CALBG) studies in adult acute lymphocytic leukemia. Leukemia, suppl. 1. 6:171, 1992

102. Reiter A, Schrappe M, Ludwig W-D et al: Favorable outcome of B-cell acute lymphoblastic leukemia in childhood: a report of three consecutive studies of the BFM group. Blood 80:2471, 1992

103. Sullivan MP, Pullen DJ, Crist WM et al: Clinical and biological heterogeneity of childhood B cell acute lymphocytic leukemia: implications for clinical trials. Leukemia 4:6, 1990

104. Patte C, Philip T, Rodary C et al: High survival rate in advanced-stage B-cell lymphomas and leukemias without CNS involvement with a short intensive polychemotherapy: results from the French Pediatric Oncology Society of a randomized trial of 216 children. J Clin Oncol 9:123, 1991

105. Fenaux P, Lai JL, Miaux O et al: Burkitt cell acute leukaemia (L3 ALL) in adults: a report of 18 cases. Br J Haematol 71:371, 1989

106. Drexler HG, Thiel E, Ludwig WD: Review of the incidence and clinical relevance of myeloid antigen-positive acute lymphoblastic leukemia. Leukemia 5:637, 1991

107. Fink FM, Köller U, Mayer H et al: Prognostic significance of myeloid-associated antigen expression on blast cells in children with acute lymphoblastic leukemia (ALL). Onkologie, suppl. 2. 14:41, 1991

108. Wiersma SR, Ortega J, Sobel E, Weinberg KI: Clinical importance of myeloid antigen expression in acute lymphoblastic leukemia of childhood. N Engl J Med 324:800, 1991

109. Ludwig WD, Harbott J, Bartram CR et al: Maturational stage, cell biological features and clinical significance of myeloid antigen positive acute lymphoblastic leukemia (My+ ALL). Onkologie, suppl. 2. 14:100, 1991

110. Guyotat D, Campos L, Shi Z-H et al: Myeloid surface antigen expression in adult acute lymphoblastic leukemia. Leukemia 4:664, 1990

111. Urbano-Ispizua A, Matutes E, Villamor N et al: Clinical significance of the presence of myeloid associated antigens in acute lymphoblastic leukemia. Br J Haematol 75:202, 1990

112. Secker-Walker LM, Craig JM, Hawkins JM, Hoffbrand AV: Philadelphia positive acute lymphoblastic leukemia in adults: age distribution, BCR breakpoint and prognostic significance. Leukemia 5:196, 1991

113. Lestingi TM, Hooberman AL: Philadelphia chromosome positive acute lymphoblastic leukemia. Hematol Oncol Clin North Am 7:161, 1993

114. Haas OA, Mor W, Gadner H, Bartram CR: Treatment of Ph-positive acute lymphoblastic leukemia with α-interferon. Leukemia 2:555, 1988

115. Ohyashiki K, Ohyashiki JH, Tauchi T et al: Treatment of Philadelphia chromosome-positive acute lymphoblastic leukemia: a pilot study which raises important questions. Leukemia 5:611, 1991

116. Barrett AJ, Horowitz MM, Bortin MM, for the IBMTR: HLA-identical sibling bone marrow transplants for Ph'-chromosome positive acute lymphoblastic leukemia in first remission. Exp Haematol 19:569, 1991

117. Clarkson B, Gaynor J, Little C et al: Importance of long-term follow-up in evaluating treatment regimens for adults with acute lymphoblastic leukemia. Haematol Blood Transfus 33:397, 1990

118. Brennan C, Weisdorf D, Kersey J et al: Bone marrow transplantation (BMT) for Philadelphia chromosome-positive acute lymphoblastic leukemia (Ph' + ALL). Proc ASCO 10:222, 1991

119. Martin H, Hoelzer D, Atta J et al: Autologous bone marrow transplantation in Ph'-positive/BCR-ABL positive acute lymphoblastic leukemia. Blood, suppl. 1. 82:167a, 1993

120. Rodriguez C, Hart JS, Freireich EJ et al: POMP combination chemotherapy of adult leukemia. Cancer 32:69, 1973

121. Kalwinsky DK, Rivera G, Dahl GV et al: Variation by race in presenting clinical and biological features of childhood acute lymphoblastic leukemia: implications for treatment outcome. Leuk Res 9:817, 1985

122. Miller DR, Leikin SL, Albo VC et al: The prognostic value of testicular biopsy in childhood acute lymphoblastic leukemia: a report from the Children's Cancer Study Group. J Clin Oncol 8:57, 1990

123. Hussein KK, Dahlberg S, Head D et al: Treatment of acute lymphoblastic leukemia in adults with intensive induction, consolidation, and maintenance chemotherapy. Blood 73:57, 1989

124. Lluesma-Gonalons M, Pavlovsky S, Santarelli MT et al: Improved results of an intensified therapy in adult acute lymphocytic leukemia. Ann Oncol 2: 33, 1991

125. Tomonaga M, Omine M, Morishima Y et al: Individualized induction therapy followed by intensive consolidation and maintenance including asparaginase in adult ALL: JALSG-ALL87 study. Haematologica, suppl. 4. 76:68, 1991

126. Smedmyr B, Simonsson B, Björkholm M et al: Treatment of adult acute lymphoblastic and undifferentiated (ALL/AUL) leukemia, according to a national protocol, in Sweden. Haematologica, suppl. 4. 76:107, 1991

127. Fière D, Gisselbrecht C, Chauvin P et al: Adult acute lymphoblastic leukemia (ALL). First interim analysis of the evolution of 467 patients (French Multicentric Trial LALA 87). Haematologica, suppl. 4. 76:108, 1991

128. Stryckmans P, de Witte TH, Marie JP et al: Therapy of adult ALL: overview of 2 successive EORTC studies: (ALL-2 & ALL-3). Leukemia, suppl. 2. 6:199, 1992

Myelodysplastic Syndrome 71

Peter L. Greenberg

INTRODUCTION

Terminology describing the indolent myeloid clonal hemopathies has undergone an evolution from their initial description in 1953.[1] Numerous terms, including preleukemia (or hematopoietic dysplasia), refractory anemia with excess blasts (RAEB), subacute or smoldering myeloid leukemia, oligoleukemia, and myelodysplastic and dysmyelopoietic syndromes,[2–9] have been used to describe patients with refractory cytopenias whose marrows are characterized by morphologic evidence of dysplastic changes in at least two of the three hematopoietic cell lines and who have a propensity to undergo transformation into acute myeloid leukemia (AML). The term myelodysplastic syndrome (MDS) is currently used to describe this clinical entity. It should be recognized, however, that although the leukemic transition of these patients morphologically resembles de novo AML, the leukemic transformation developing after MDS is generally more resistant to standard induction chemotherapy. The poor prognosis of patients with this leukemic transformation is similar to the prognosis of leukemic transformations in patients with chronic myeloproliferative disorders (MPDs) (Fig. 71-1).

Heterogeneity of MDS patients has been recognized based on variations in marrow morphology and differing potential for survival and transformation to AML. To aid in categorizing patients with this disorder, the French-American-British (FAB) Morphology Cooperative Group formulated a set of categories based on marrow morphology, including the proportion of myeloblasts and degree of derangement of the hematopoietic cell lines.[10] This morphologic classification scheme subdivides patients into five subgroups: refractory anemia (RA), refractory anemia with ringed sideroblasts (RARS), RAEB, refractory anemia with excess blasts in transformation (RAEB-T), and chronic myelomonocytic leukemia (CMML) (Table 71-1). The first four entities are characterized by abnormal marrow myeloid cell differentiation patterns (dysplasia). RA and RARS patients have marrows that contain <5% blasts, associated with dysplasia of three hematopoietic cell lines; RAEB is characterized by 5–20% blasts in the marrow; and RAEB-T is characterized by 20–30% blasts in the marrow. By contrast, AML is considered to be present if the patient's marrow contains >30% blasts. This morphologic characterization has been helpful for assessing prognosis of these patients. However, due to evolution of these diseases into aggressive stages, an additional criterion necessary for categorizing individuals with MDS is the pace of the leukemic progression. This characteristic is important in distinguishing the patient with an indolent form of MDS from the patient with MDS with rapid evolution to frank AML. Therefore, stability of the patients' peripheral blood counts and marrow morphology for a period of 2–6 weeks aids in categorizing MDS patients. The inclusion of CMML in the category of MDS is problematic as this entity is predominantly a myeloproliferative rather than a myelodysplastic disorder and may (depending on marrow and blood findings) either be more akin to chronic myeloid leukemia (CML) with an excess of monocytes or RAEB with monocytosis.

Most patients with primary MDS develop this disorder de novo. However, an increasing number of patients who had previously been treated with chemotherapy or chemoradiotherapy for other malignancies or who had been extensively ex-

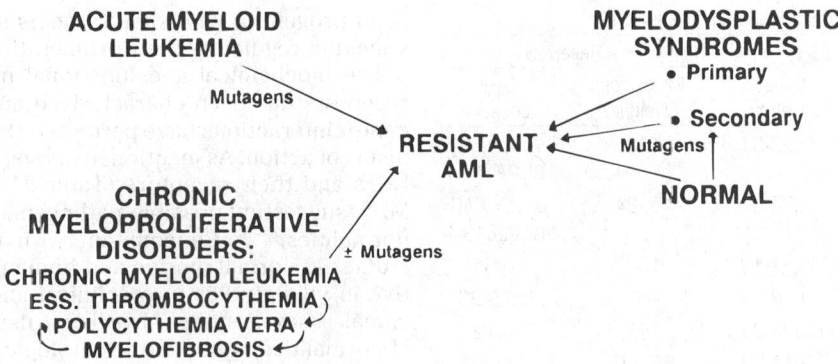

Fig. 71-1. Evolutionary transitions occurring in clonal myeloid hemopathies.

posed to a variety of marrow toxins develop a secondary form of MDS.[11] This secondary form of MDS generally has a more aggressive course than primary MDS.

Table 71-1. Myelodysplastic Syndrome Subtypes: FAB Cooperative Group Criteria

	Bone Marrow Blasts (%)	Peripheral Blood Blasts (%)	Auer Rods	Monocytes >1 × 10⁹/L	Ring Sideroblasts >15% of Nucleated Marrow Cells
RA	<5	≤1	−	−	−
RARS	<5	≤1	−	−	+
RAEB	5–20	<5	−	−	±
CMML	≤20	<5	−	+	±
RAEB-T	21–30 or	≥5 or	±	±	±

PATHOGENESIS

MDS provides a clinical model for evaluating the evolution of a relatively benign clonal myeloid hemopathy into a frankly malignant neoplasm, AML. Biologic data, particularly marrow cytogenetics, in vitro myeloid colony formation, and clonal analysis using restriction fragment length polymorphisms (RFLP), indicate that biologically the marrow cells of MDS patients are derived from a malignant clone of marrow stem cells.[12–14] These experimental approaches have been used to improve our understanding of mechanisms underlying MDS.

Cells derived from hematopoietic stem cells—neutrophils, monocytes, erythrocytes, and platelets—are clonally derived in MDS. Evidence for this breadth of hematopoietic cell involvement has been obtained using karyotypic markers[15–21] and by RFLP analysis using X-linked inactivation assays.[15,18–20,22–25] In some studies, combined cytogenetic and X-linked inactivation studies have been performed,[19,20] and results have been concordant in identifying the clonal derivation of the hematopoietic cells. With these techniques, the clonal origin of lymphoid cells of MDS patients has also been examined. Lymphoid cells appear to be part of the abnormal clone in some but not all cases, as clonal T cells[16,18,21,22,25] and both clonal[21] and polyclonal B cells[23] have been demonstrated in MDS.

Cytogenetic Abnormalities

Cytogenetic abnormalities occur in the marrow cells of patients with de novo MDS in approximately 40–60% of cases at diagnosis, whereas >80% of cases with secondary MDS have abnormal karyotypes.[26] Single or complex chromosomal abnormalities may be present initially and evolutionary changes may occur during the course of the disorder. These genetic derange-

ments reflect the multistep process believed to underlie the evolution of MDS. Generally, the more aggressive stage of the disorder, in terms of rapidity of clinical course and high number of marrow blasts is characterized by more complex abnormal karyotypes. Major karyotypic aberrations, including many structural changes, rings, and dicentrics, are usually seen in RAEB and RAEB-T, but only sporadically in RA.

Both structural and numeric changes may be found in MDS. Compared with AML, MDS is often associated with chromosomal deletions as a primary karyotypic anomaly. Deletions leading to gene loss suggest that a recessive mechanism is acting during the process of leukemic transformation.[27] With regard to specific associations between chromosome markers and the FAB morphologic subgroups, apart from the 5q− abnormality that is observed most often in RA, most other aberrations are distributed throughout all MDS subgroups. The 5q− abnormality associated with other abnormalities is unusual in CMML. Monosomy 7 is virtually absent in RA patients. The most frequently occurring clonal chromosomal abnormalities in MDS involve chromosomes 5, 7, 8, 11, 12, and 20.[26,28,29] The incidence of chromosomal anomalies in secondary MDS is higher and more complex, with the most common single abnormality being monosomy 7, followed by 5q−, trisomy 8, monosomy 5, and 20q−.

Chromosomal abnormalities identify areas of the genome that are susceptible to damage or that may be important in the pathogenesis of disease. The frequent occurrence of the 5q− chromosome abnormality implicates the involvement of one or more genes residing on chromosome 5q in the development and maintenance of abnormal hematopoiesis. Within the critical regions involved in the deleted region in the 5q abnormality cluster several genes coding for hematopoietic growth factors (HGFs) occur (Table 71-2). In addition, other genes such as *EGR-1*, which encodes the GTPase-activating protein for p21RAS, are also present in this chromosomal region.[30] Recently, the interferon (IFN) regulatory factor-1 gene was found to be deleted in the 5q− syndrome.[31] This gene, when activated, decreases cell proliferation. Loss of IRF-1 as well as the loss of genes encoding HGFs have possible implications for the pathobiology of abnormal cell proliferation occurring in the 5q− syndrome. Other as yet unidentified tumor suppressor genes may also be deleted in 5q− chromosomes.

A detailed analysis of chromosome aberrations in MDS reveals similarities between those abnormalities and those observed in other myeloid clonal hemopathies, such as AML and MPDs.[26] These observations suggest that a continuum exists between differing FAB subgroups of MDS and that similar genetic events at the level of the stem cell may result in a variety of clinical conditions, including MDS, AML, and MPD.

Secondary MDS is associated with karyotypic abnormalities in >80% of cases. As in primary MDS, recurrent aberrations frequently involve chromosomes 5 and 7 with partial or total

Table 71-2. Human HGFs and Receptors

			Receptor	
Factor	Molecular Weight	Gene Location	Molecular Weight	Gene Location
IL-3	15–30	5q23-31	140	α: X,Y-PAR[a]
				β: 22q13.1
CSF-GM	18–30	5q23-31	45, 84	α: X,Y-PAR[a]
				β: 22q13.1
CSF-G	20	17q11-12	150	1p35
CSF-M	70–90	1p13-21	160	5q23-33
c-kit ligand[b]	40	12q22-24	145	4q12
EPO	39	7q11-22	55–60	19p
IL-1	17	2q13-21	68, 80	2q12
IL-6	21	7p21	80	1q21
IFN-α	17–25	9	110, 130	21
IFN-β	17–25	9	110, 130	21
IFN-γ	17–25	9	54	6

Abbreviations: IL, interleukin; CSF, colony-stimulating factor; G, granulocyte; M, macrophage; EPO, erythropoietin; IFN, interferon.
[a] Pseudoautosomal region of the X,Y chromosome.
[b] Stem cell factor, mast cell growth factor.

monosomy, although with a differing incidence[12,26,32] (Table 71-3). Loss of material from the long arm of chromosome 5 and 7 may also be due to unbalanced translocations typically observed in secondary MDS/AML.[12,26,32–35] MDS or AML may arise as a secondary disorder independent of the type of preceding malignancy or treatment, suggesting biologic relatedness between secondary MDS and AML. Accordingly, both are characterized by the same chromosomal aberrations and a very short survival. In addition to deletions of chromosome 5 and 7, other commonly involved regions in secondary MDS and AML have been identified. Regions on chromosome 3p14-21, 6p23, 12p11-p12, 17p11-p12, 19q13, and 21q21-22[26,36] frequently undergo structural rearrangements such as deletions and translocations. The pathogenetic implications of these abnormalities have not been clarified to date.

Hematopoietic Regulatory Interactions

MDS marrow hematopoietic precursors are characterized by an uncoupling of their proliferative and differentiative abilities, leading to ineffective hematopoiesis. The lesion underlying this defect resides predominantly at the level of the hematopoietic stem cell, and phenotypic expression of such aberrant cells is clonal in nature. Use of in vitro assays for hematopoietic progenitor cells is a means of analysis of the hematopoietic

Table 71-3. Karyotypic Abnormalities in Primary and Therapy-Related MDSs

	Patients (%)		
Characteristic	Primary MDS (n = 371)	Therapy-Related MDS (n = 65)	P Value
Karyotype			
Normal	43	12	<0.01
Chromosome 5 or 7 abnormalities	23	55	<0.01
Trisomy 8	27	11	0.29
t(8;21), inversion 16	1	2	NS
Other abnormalities	14	5	0.04
Insufficient metaphases	10	12	NS
Missing	2	3	NS

Abbreviation: NS, not significant.
(Modified from Kantarjian et al.,[11] with permission.)

stem/progenitor cell compartments and the humoral HGFs involved in regulating their proliferation and differentiation.

The biochemical and functional nature of HGFs and their receptors has been characterized and assessment of HGF-receptor interactions have permitted the analysis of their mechanisms of action. As mentioned above, chromosomes coding for HGFs and their receptors (Table 71-2) are often deranged in MDS, suggesting possible pathogenetic relevance of these abnormalities.[37–43] Concomitant with in vitro marrow culture studies in normal murine and human marrow, and corroborative in vivo studies in preclinical and clinical settings, these clonal assay systems have been used to analyze regulatory abnormalities in human hematologic disorders.

Hematopoiesis

Despite the more indolent nature of MDS than AML, many parameters of in vitro myelopoiesis evident in AML are also present in MDS. These biologic parameters have been useful for evaluating pathogenetic mechanisms and prognosis in MDS patients.[37,44] The cloning efficiency of each of the marrow hematopoietic progenitor cells colony-forming unit-granulocyte/erythroid/macrophage/megakaryocyte (CFU-GEMM) burst-forming unit-erythroid (BFU-E), CFU-E, CFU-granulocyte/microphage (GM), CFU-megakaryocyte (Mk) is quite low or absent in most MDS patients as well as AML patients.[37,44–48] Also similar to leukemic patients, an increased proportion of CFU-GM are of light buoyant density, and abortive myeloid cluster formation and defective cellular maturation is observed.[37]

In MDS, in vitro hematopoietic regulatory derangements have been shown by use of the clonogenic assays. Decreased responsiveness of hematopoietic precursors to proliferative and differentiative and inhibitory HGFs, as well as diminished production of certain HGFs has been documented[37] (Table 71-4). These findings suggest that the ineffective hematopoiesis existing in MDS may be related to such biologic abnormalities. In MDS, colony-stimulating factor (CSF)-GM and interleukin (IL)-3 have greater myeloid proliferative effects in vitro than CSF-G, whereas CSF-G has greater myeloid differentiative effects.[49] This is particularly evident in RAEB/RAEB-T patients and those patients with normal cytogenetics. These in vitro studies have provided a biologic rationale for differentiation induction therapy used in an attempt to counter the relative uncoupling of proliferative and differentiative signals existing in MDS. Such marrow myeloid clonogenic assays also provide prognostic information and, as such, complement evaluation of marrow morphology and cytogenetics regarding analysis of disease progression in these patients.

In vitro studies and preclinical data indicate that a critical lesion underlying leukemia and MDS relates to an uncoupling of proliferation and differentiation at the level of the hematopoietic stem cell.[50,51] Induction of differentiation in vitro diminishes the ability of leukemic stem cells to self-generate and reduces in vivo leukemogenicity in murine models.[52–54] Studies with these murine models have demonstrated increased survival of animals with leukemia after in vivo treatment with inducers of myeloid differentiation, such as myeloid differentiation factors (CSF-G, MGI-2) and vitamin D.[51–56] Other studies have also demonstrated monocyte/macrophage differentiation of hematopoietic colonies cloned from human normal, leukemic, and MDS marrow after in vitro exposure to retinoids and vitamin D.[48,54,57,58] The in vitro myeloid differentiative and proliferative responses of normal and MDS cells to pharmacologic levels of CSF-G and CSF-GM[49] are consistent with the high proportion of in vivo neutrophil responses to the therapeutic use of these agents in MDS. Increased numbers of marrow CFU-GM after treatment with CSF-GM have been demonstrated in the responding patients.[59]

Table 71-4. Growth Factor Regulation of Hematopoiesis

	HGF Production			HGF Responsiveness		
	Proliferative	Differentiative	Inhibitory	Proliferative	Differentiative	Inhibitory
Normal	+ +	+ +	+ +	+ +	+ +	+ +
AML	+ +	±	+ + + +	+ + + +	−	−
CML	+ + +	+ +	+ + + +	+ + + +	+ +	−
MDS	+ +	+	+ +	+	+	+

In MDS, suboptimal responses of MDS erythroid progenitor cells to erythropoietin (EPO) have been reported.[48,60,61] Analysis of the relationship between EPO levels in MDS and the size of the patients' erythroid progenitor pool indicates that the anemia in MDS cannot be attributed to an abnormality in the capacity of EPO to induce the generation of CFU-E, but is influenced by the size of the BFU-E population. A contraction of the size of the BFU-E pool in MDS results in insufficient influx of EPO-responsive cells.[60] CSF-G markedly augments the in vitro EPO responsiveness of BFU-E in normal and MDS marrow.[61]

Hematopoietic growth factor production has also been analyzed in MDS. Marrow cells and peripheral blood T cells from MDS patients produce decreased amounts of CSF-GM, IL-3, CSF-M, and IL-6.[62] Production of CSF-G is predominantly stimulated by microbe-stimulated monocytes.[63] Decreased levels of monocyte-derived CSF-G has been demonstrated in MDS patients. This abnormality is difficult to interpret because most of these patients are elderly, and decreased monocyte CSF-G production was also absent from elderly control subjects.[63] Thus, the defective production of a variety of HGFs, in addition to decreased precursor cell responsiveness to some of these factors, may contribute to ineffective granulopoiesis observed in MDS (Table 71-4). The effects of IL-1 and IL-6 in combination with CSF-GM on in vitro colony formation by MDS myeloid progenitor cells indicates that neither IL-1 nor IL-6 alone possess colony-stimulating activity. These factors do not alter the stimulatory effects of CSF-GM when promoting colony formation by normal myeloid progenitor cells.[64] However, in most MDS cases, an enhancing effect of IL-6 or IL-1 in combination with CSF-GM was observed. Other studies indicate that the actions of IL-1 and IL-6 on hematopoiesis are mainly indirect and are mediated by enhancing the production of CSF-GM, CSF-G, and/or IL-3 by accessory cells.[65]

Transforming growth factor-β is inhibitory for early normal and leukemic stem cells in vitro.[66–70] IFN-α, -β, and -γ are also inhibitory against both normal and leukemic hematopoietic precursors.[71,72] By contrast, inhibitory factors leukemia-associated activity (LIA, acidic H-isoferritin) and prostaglandin E have been shown to have less inhibitory activity for MDS and AML hematopoietic precursors than for normal cells.[73–77] Similarly, macrophage inflammatory protein (MIP)-1α is inhibitory for normal early stem cells,[78–82] but with lesser effects on leukemic precursors. Thus, the selective functional nature of these inhibitors may permit a growth advantage of leukemic over normal cells. Further, tumor necrosis factor-α (TNF-α) generation is increased in MDS and AML and, in addition to its ability to increase CSF production, may be inhibitory to hematopoietic precursors.[83,84] These findings suggest that in addition to defective responsiveness of hematopoietic precursors to stimulatory cytokines, cytokine-mediated inhibition of hematopoiesis may play a role in the abnormal hematopoiesis that characterizes MDS (Table 71-4).

Immunologic cell dysfunction has also been demonstrated in MDS patients. In these individuals, T cells, natural killer cells, and B cells all appear to be diminished in numbers and to have defective function. Quantitative deficiencies of the T-helper cell population and abnormalities of the mitogenic response of T cells have been recognized.[85–88] These abnormalities may also contribute to the decreased HGF production in MDS.

Oncogenes

Conversion of normal cells into preleukemic and ultimately leukemic cells is a multistep process requiring the accumulation of genetic lesions. To evaluate the role of genetic derangements in MDS the incidence of alterations of a variety of oncogenes in this disorder has been determined. The *fms* gene encodes the CSF-1 receptor (CSF-M receptor).[89] Mutations of *fms* have been observed in 12–18% of MDS patients,[90] with the highest incidence occurring in the CMML subgroup, consistent with the observation that CSF-M is a monocytic growth factor.

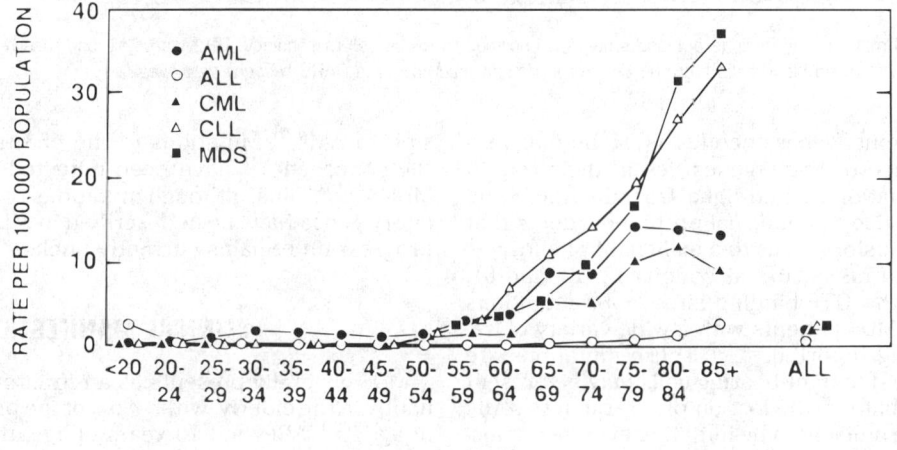

Fig. 71-2. Age-specific incidence of MDS in comparison with acute and chronic leukemias. (Data extrapolated from references 102 and 104.)

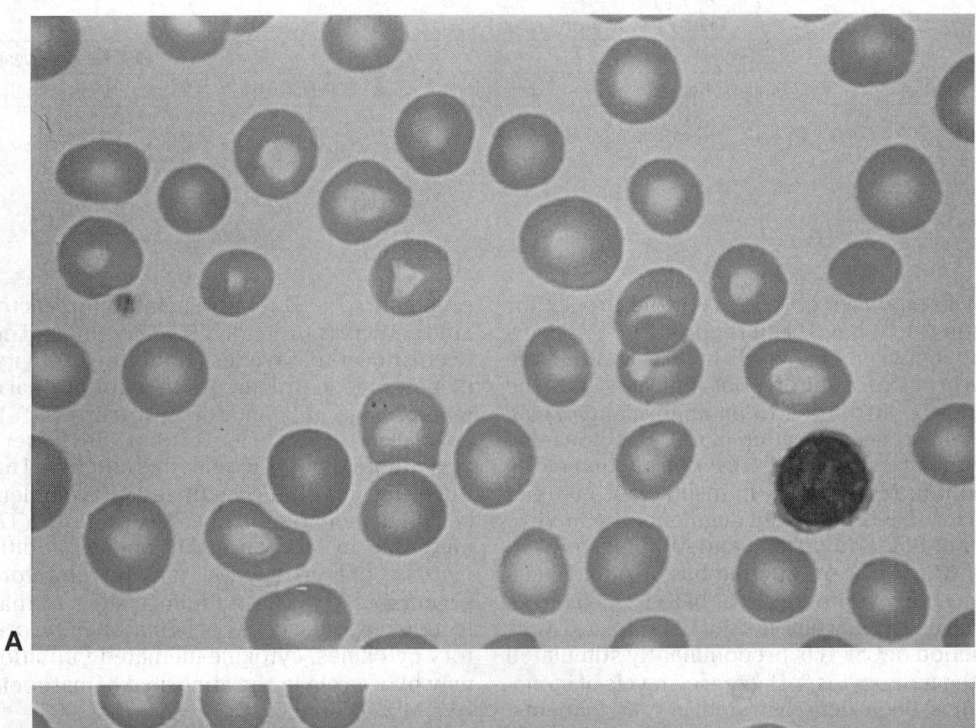

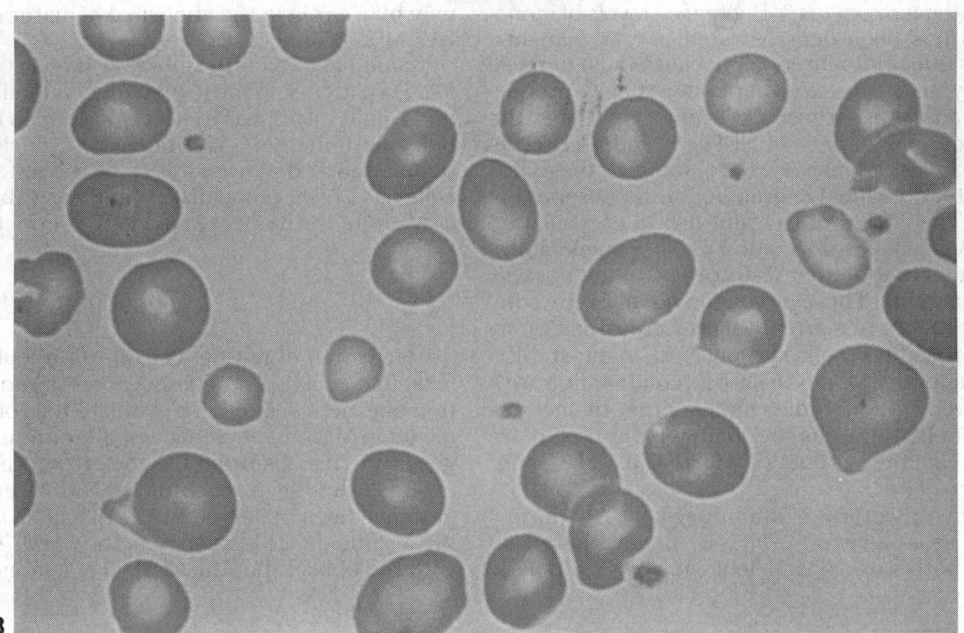

Fig. 71-3. MDS morphology: Peripheral blood smears. Abnormal red blood cell morphology. **(A)** Macrocytic and macro-ovalocytic cells in RA. **(B)** Dimorphic red blood cells (normocytic/microcytic and macrocytic) in RARS. *(Figure continues.)*

The *ras* family of proto-oncogenes encodes a GTP-binding protein.[91,92] The importance of these genes lies in their role in mitogenic and differentiation-related signal transduction.[93] Mutations of *ras* may give rise to abnormal protein products that have the capacity to transform cells to a malignant phenotype. Mutational activation of *ras* occurs at codons 12, 13, and 61, which correspond to the GTP-binding sites.[94] *ras* mutations have been detected in MDS patients with a wide variety of frequencies (3–33%) being reported.[95–100] These mutations are somatically acquired and mutant-bearing cells may be present as minor populations that may be lost on progression to AML, indicating that they are unlikely to be initiating events in transformation. The incidence of *ras* mutations varies between FAB types, with the highest occurrence being in CMML patients. In some studies, *ras* mutations have been reported to be associated with poor prognosis either in terms of survival or progression to AML.[91] Mutations of the p53 tumor suppressor gene (anti-oncogene)[27] have been detected at a low frequency in MDS.[5–8,101] Thus, although mutations of these cell growth regulatory genes have been described in MDS, their role in disease progression remains currently unclear.

CLINICAL MANIFESTATIONS

MDS generally presents as a refractory cytopenia, predominantly in the elderly, with >80% of the patients being >60 years of age.[102,103] Beyond 70 years of age, the incidence of MDS is approximately 22–45 per 10^5 population,[102,103] indicating that MDS is as prevalent as the other most common hematologic malignancies of the aged (i.e., chronic lymphocytic leukemia and multiple myeloma)[102–104] (Fig. 71-2).

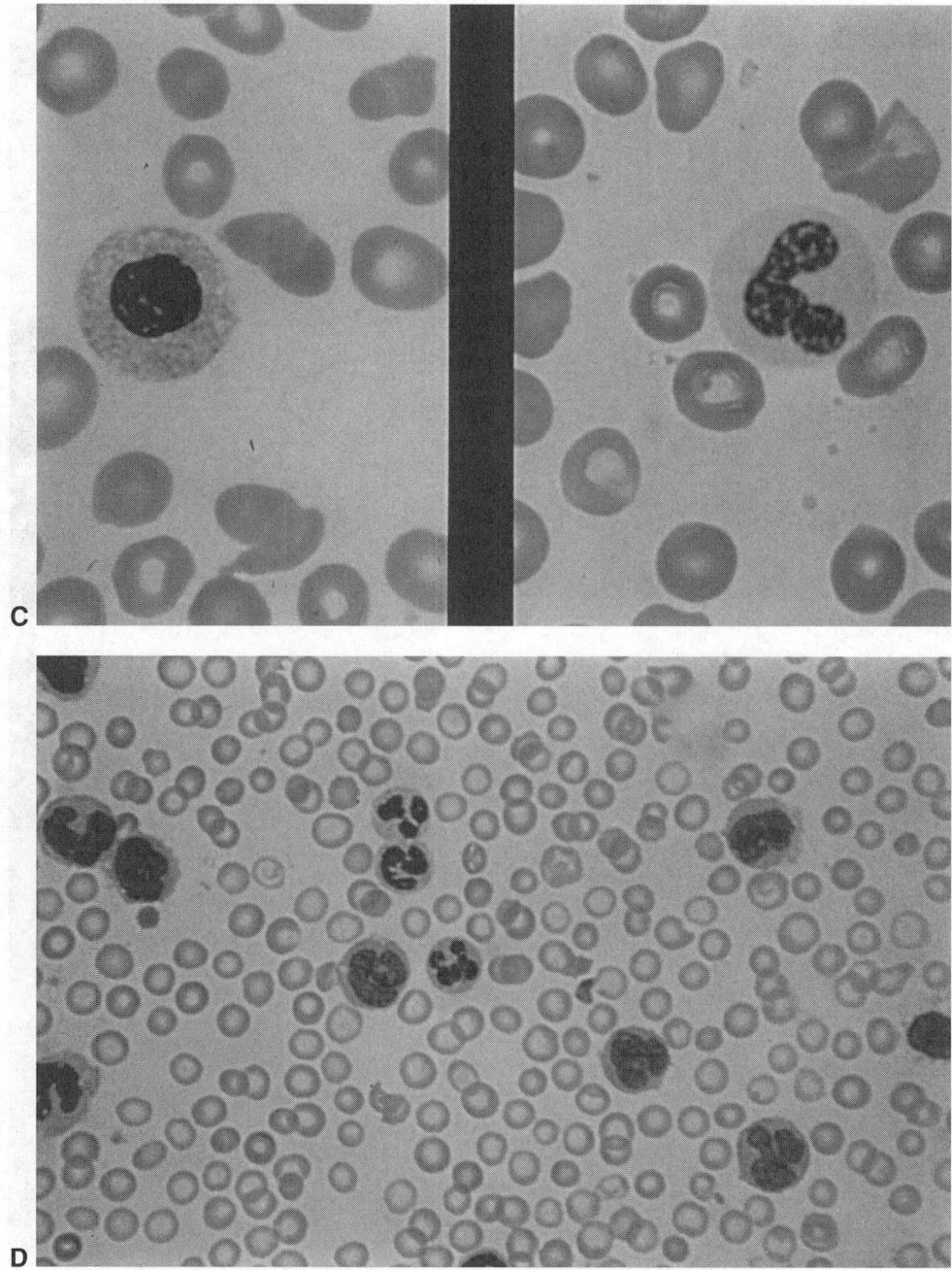

Fig. 71-3 *(Continued)*. **(C)** Dysplastic neutrophils showing hyposegmentation and hypogranularity. **(D)** Monocytes in CMML. (Wright stain × 1000.) (Courtesy of Dr. James W. Vardiman, University of Chicago Hospitals.)

Blood and Bone Marrow

Anemia/Fatigue

Nearly all MDS patients are anemic, with a substantial proportion having associated fatigue. The anemia is usually macrocytic with a low reticulocyte response. In this elderly patient population, it is necessary to exclude vitamin B_{12} or folate deficiency as a cause of the macrocytic anemia. The anemia of MDS is usually due to ineffective erythropoiesis. In addition, these patients may have findings consistent with abnormal iron metabolism,[105] disordered globin chain synthesis,[106] decreased levels of red cell enzymes,[107] raised levels of fetal hemoglobin,[108] hemoglobin H inclusions,[109,110] abnormal red cell antigens,[111] or a positive Ham test.[112] Low levels of pyruvate kinase may occur,[107] with associated hemolysis. Together with the requirement for long-term red cell transfusions, the abnor-

malities in iron metabolism may lead to hemochromatosis with subsequent organ (hepatic, pancreatic islet cell, testicular, and cardiac) dysfunction.

Morphologic evidence of dyserythropoiesis in MDS includes ringed sideroblasts, multinuclear fragments, bizarre nuclear shapes, internuclear bridging, mitosis, abnormal dense chromatin or fine chromatin with asynchronous cytoplasm, and abnormal cytoplasmic features (intense basophilia, Howell-Jolly bodies). The red blood cells (RBCs) may be characterized by anisocytosis, poikilocytosis, nucleated forms, and acanthocytosis (Fig. 71-3). Erythroid precursors appear with megaloblastoid changes (Figs. 71-4A and 71-5A). Because of the macrocytosis in these patients, vitamin B_{12} and folic acid deficiency must be excluded. The occurrence of five or more siderotic granules is considered pathologic and when these granules comprise more than one-third of the nuclear rim, the

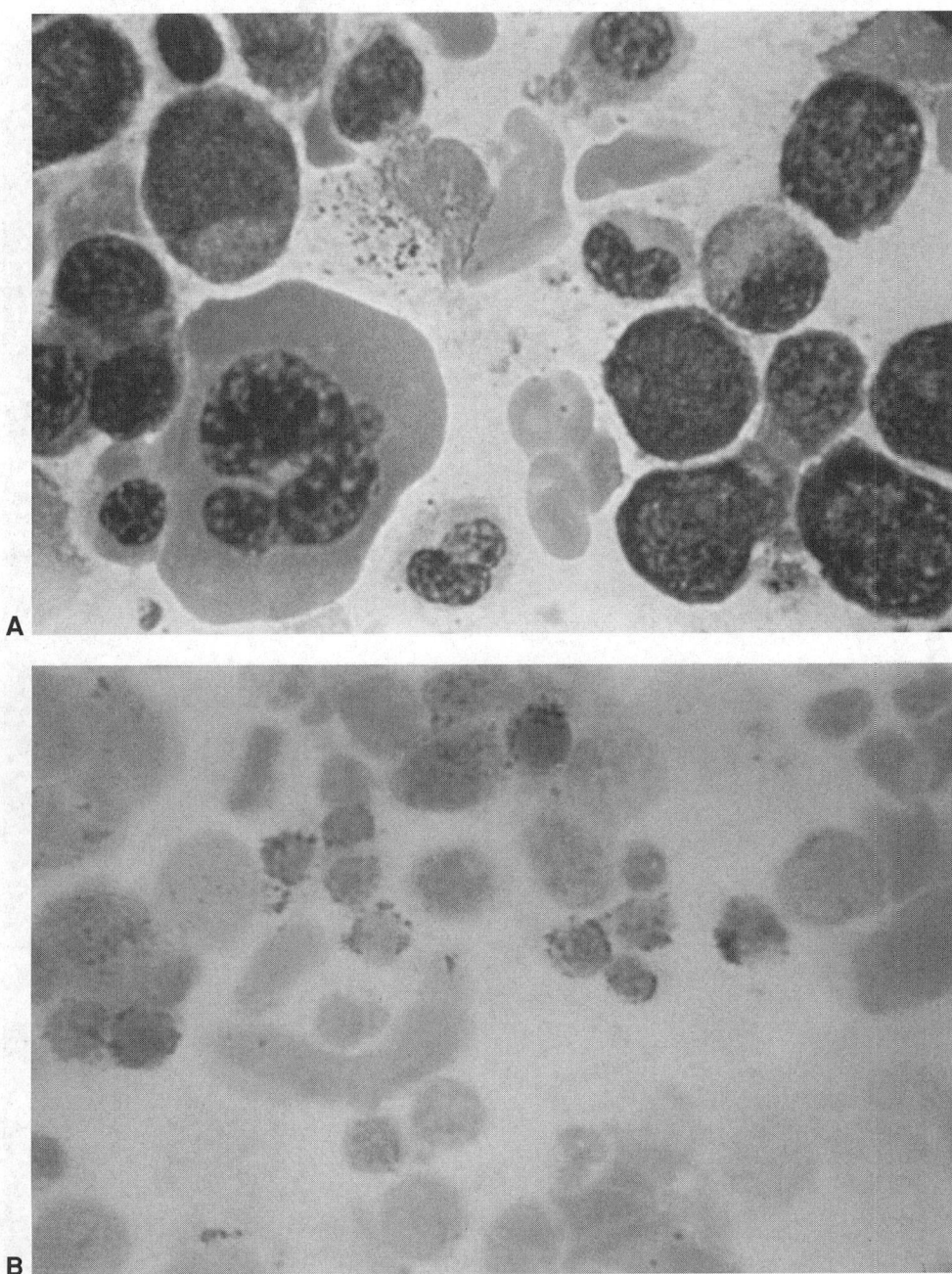

Fig. 71-4. MDS morphology: Bone marrow aspirates. **(A)** Megablastoid dyserythropoiesis. **(B)** Ringed sideroblasts in RARS (Prussian blue stain). *(Figure continues.)*

term ringed sideroblast has been used[113] (Fig. 71-4B). The disruption of mitochondria by these siderotic granules and observed changes in heme synthesis relate to the ineffective erythropoiesis, premature erythroid destruction, and RA in this disorder. Very rarely, the sideroblastic anemia will respond to pyridoxine. RA is differentiated from RARS by the presence of >15% ringed sideroblasts. If erythroid precursors account for >50% of bone marrow cells with >30% of the myeloid cells being blasts, the diagnosis of erythroleukemia is made (M6 variant of AML).

Neutropenia/Infections

A substantial proportion (about 60%) of MDS patients are neutropenic and are also often unable to mount an appropriate inflammatory response to infection. This defect is likely is due to the poor myeloid marrow responsiveness to and decreased production of HGFs. Qualitative abnormalities occur in MDS neutrophils, which are derived from the abnormal clone.[15–21] In addition, because HGFs play important roles in modulating mature neutrophil and monocyte cell functions, decreased production of the HGFs contributes to the phagocyte abnormalities noted in these patients.

Morphologic abnormalities of granulocytes are common in MDS and are present in both the peripheral blood and bone marrow. The most common abnormalities are hypogranulation, which may be associated with a negative peroxidase reaction, low levels of leukocyte alkaline phosphatase, and hyposegmentation of the polymorphonuclear leukocytes with abnormal chromatin condensation (Pelger-Huët-like anomaly) (Figs. 71-3C and 71-4C). Occasionally, the chromatin appears excessively clumped, leading to an appearance of nuclear frag-

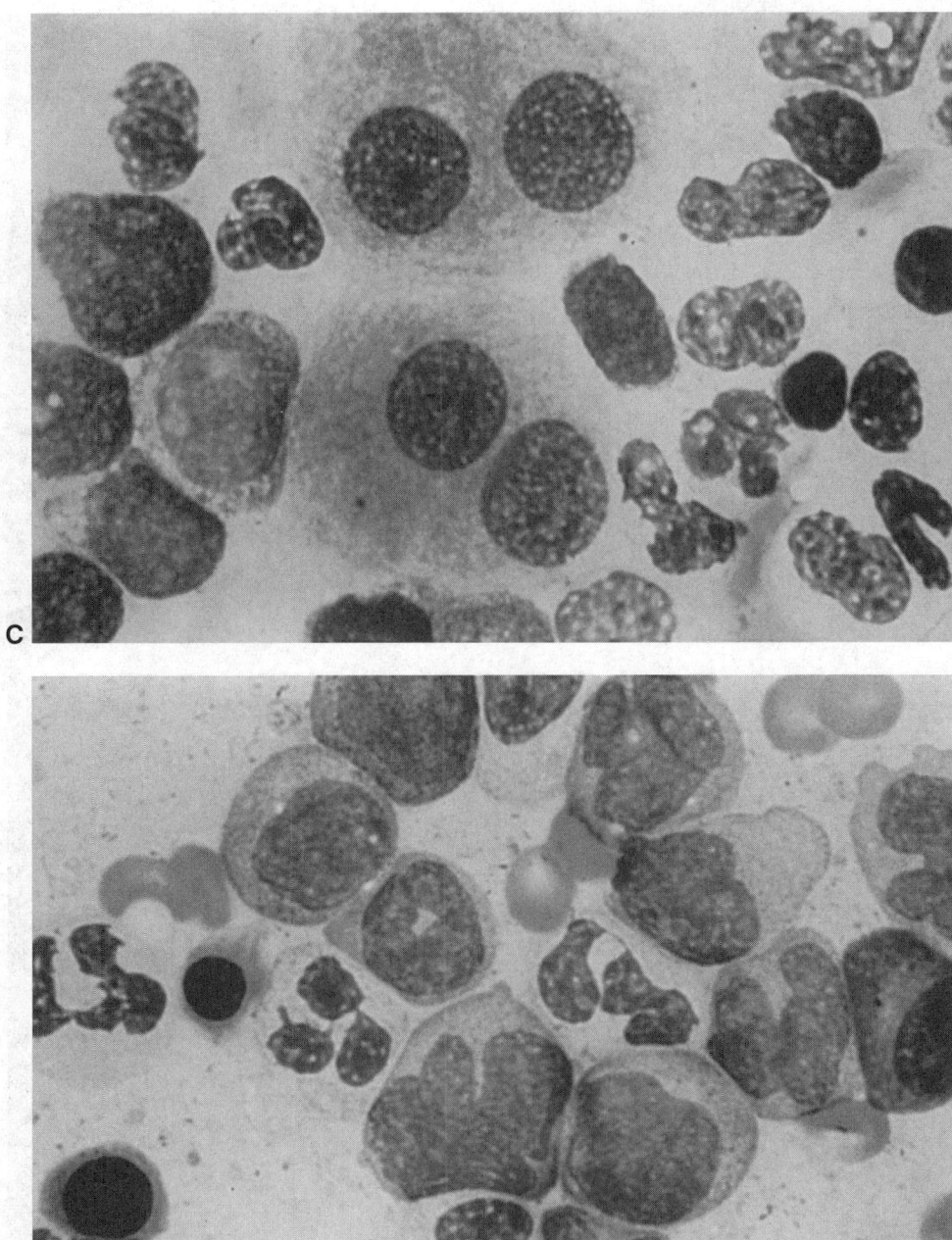

Fig. 71-4 *(Continued)*. **(C)** Dysgranulopoiesis with increased blasts, hypogranular neutrophils, and hypolobated megakaryocytes in RAEB. **(D)** Abnormal monocytes and neutrophils in CMML. (Wright stain × 1000.) (Courtesy of Dr. James W. Vardiman, University of Chicago Hospitals.)

mentation associated with a loss of segmentation. A critical finding of dysplasia within the marrow is that of nuclear-cytoplasmic asynchrony in abnormal early myeloid cells (type III blasts or abnormal promyelocytes), showing granular cytoplasm, reticulated nucleus possessing a nucleolus, and a prominent perinuclear Golgi zone. The proportion of type I marrow myeloblasts determines the subtype of MDS (Table 71-1) and is a major reflection of the differentiative abnormality present.

Infections are common in MDS. Approximately 10% of patients present with evidence of infection[12]; in 21% it is the major cause of death.[114,115] Most infections in MDS are bacterial, usually with host organisms, and are associated with neutropenia. Defective adhesion, phagocytosis, and bacterial killing are commonly found.[116–118] The migration of qualitatively abnormal granulocytes into sites of infection often leads to poorly resolving abscesses, which may be occult.[119] In MDS, blood monocytes are derived from the abnormal clone, and in CMML proliferate in a poorly controlled manner. Certain monocyte functions are impaired, including decreased phagocytosis.[120,121] Furthermore, natural killer cells in MDS are reduced in number and are functionally immature, leading to an impaired ability to produce interferon.[122–123]

Thrombocytopenia/Bleeding

Thrombocytopenia is common (approximately 60%) in MDS and occasionally becomes severe. In about 5% of cases it is the only cytopenia detected.[102] Giant and agranular platelets are often seen and platelet function may be abnormal, including prolonged bleeding times (even without thrombocytopenia)

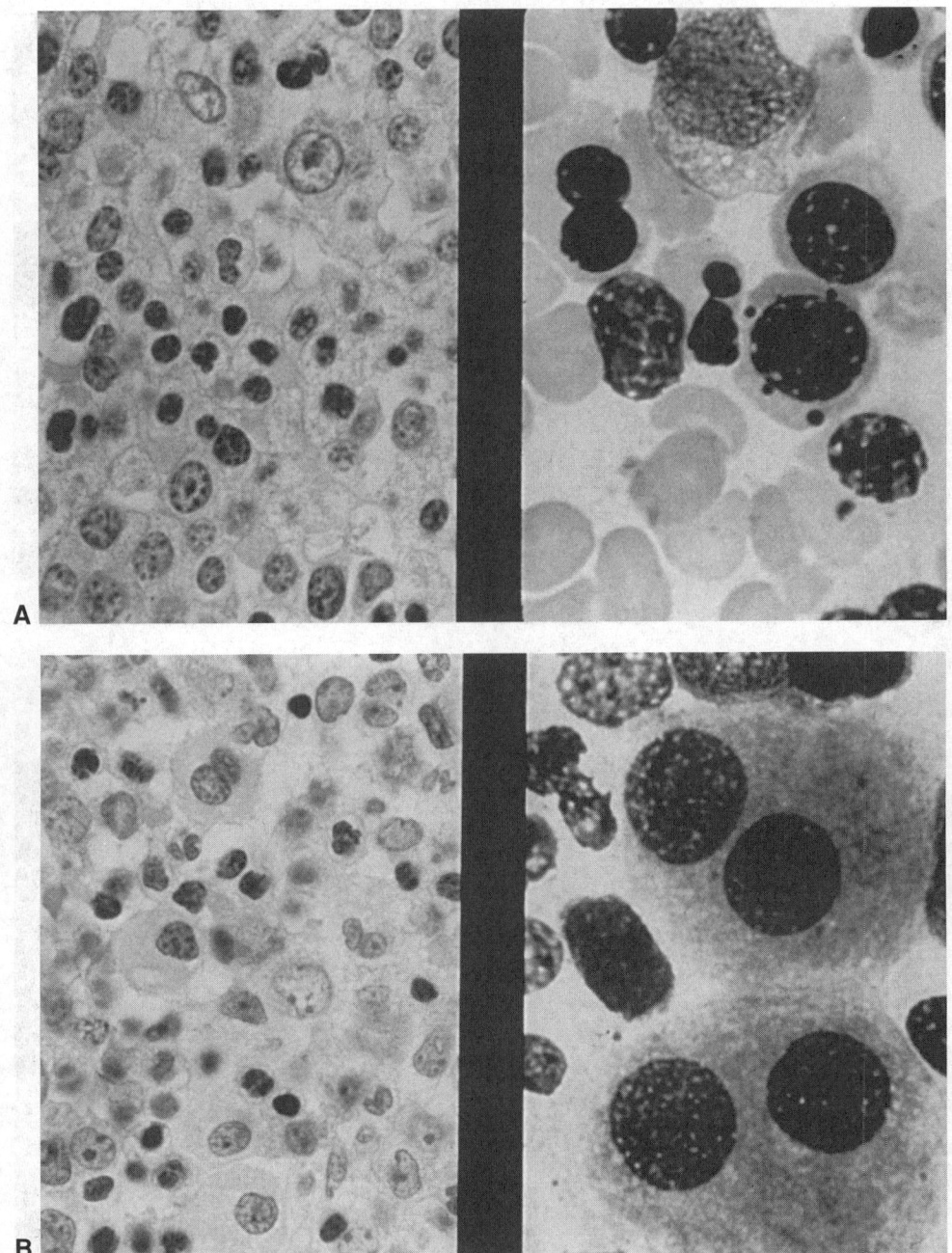

Fig. 71-5. MDS morphology: Bone marrow biopsies and aspirates. **(A)** Dyserythropoiesis in RA. **(B)** Dysmegakaryopoiesis in RAEB. *(Figure continues.)*

and reduced platelet aggregation.[124] Progressive thrombocytopenia is often a harbinger of disease evolution. The risk of hemorrhage during surgery or after trauma is increased because of defective platelet function. Thus, bleeding in these circumstances may occur at relatively normal platelet counts, and platelet transfusions should be administered in these conditions. Splenomegaly occurs in about 10% of MDS patients and may contribute, by sequestration of platelets, to the thrombocytopenia.

Common morphologic abnormalities of megakaryocytes in MDS occur and include micromegakaryocytes, mononuclear megakaryocytes, multiple small nuclei separated by strands of nuclear material, dysmorphic nuclear features, and hypogranularity (Figs. 71-4C, 71-5B, and 71-5D). The 5q− syndrome is frequently associated with morphologic abnormalities of mega-

karyocytes, which are usually small, with single eccentric round nuclei.

Clinical Variants

Rheumatic and immunologic processes occur, albeit uncommonly, in association with MDS. These features include cutaneous vasculitis, peripheral neuropathy, and lupus-like syndromes.[125] A subgroup of MDS patients have acute seronegative inflammatory arthritis temporally related to the discovery of cytopenia.[126] Episodes of oligoarthritis or polyarthritis may occur along with systemic features, including fever, pleuritis, pericarditis, and hemolytic anemia. The arthritis and systemic features often respond to corticosteroid therapy.

The association of MDS and lymphoid tumors, particularly

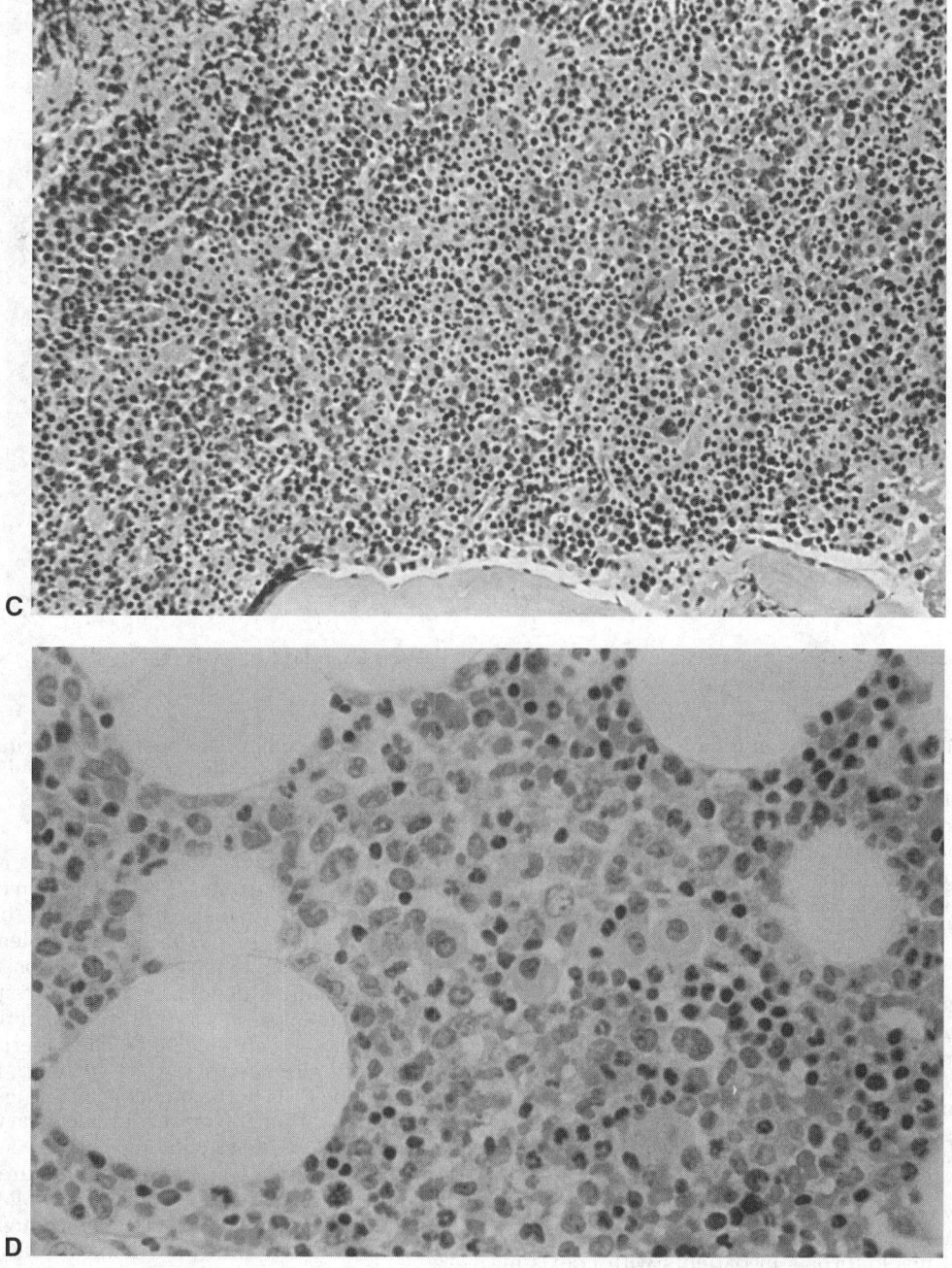

Fig. 71-5 *(Continued)*. **(C)** RARS with erythroid hyperplasia. (H&E × 200). **(D)** Myeloid hyperplasia with increased immature forms and abnormal megakaryocytes in RAEB. (× 400.) *(Figure continues.)*

B-cell neoplasias, has been reported. Chronic lymphocytic leukemia, hairy cell leukemia, lymphocytic lymphoma, multiple myeloma, large granular lymphocytic leukemia, and T-helper-cell lymphoma have all been diagnosed simultaneously with MDS.[127] The mechanism whereby this association occurs is unknown, but its presence suggests involvement of a common hematolymphoid stem cell as the inciting event. Following alkylating agent chemotherapy, secondary MDS may develop in some patients and contribute to problematic cytopenias.

The 5q− syndrome is an MDS variant, usually seen in RA, which demonstrates characteristic morphologic features (i.e., macrocytic anemia, normal or high platelet counts, nonlobulated micromegakaryocytes, and hypoplastic erythroid cells). When the 5q− defect is the sole karyotypic abnormality, evolution to acute leukemia is uncommon.[128-131] Superimposed cyto-

genetic lesions, however, are associated with a poorer prognosis.

Overlap Syndromes

Hypocellular MDS

Although most patients with MDS have hypercellular or normocellular bone marrows, a small subgroup of MDS patients (<15%) have marrow hypoplasia at the time of diagnosis.[132,133] Differentiation of these patients from either aplastic anemia or hypoplastic AML may be difficult. When marrow cellularity is low, recognition of hematopoietic dysplasia by examination of either the aspirate or biopsy may be problematic. Most hypocellular MDS cases fit into the categories of RA and RAEB.[133-135] CMML, which classically is characterized by a hypercellular bone marrow, has not been reported to have a hypocellular

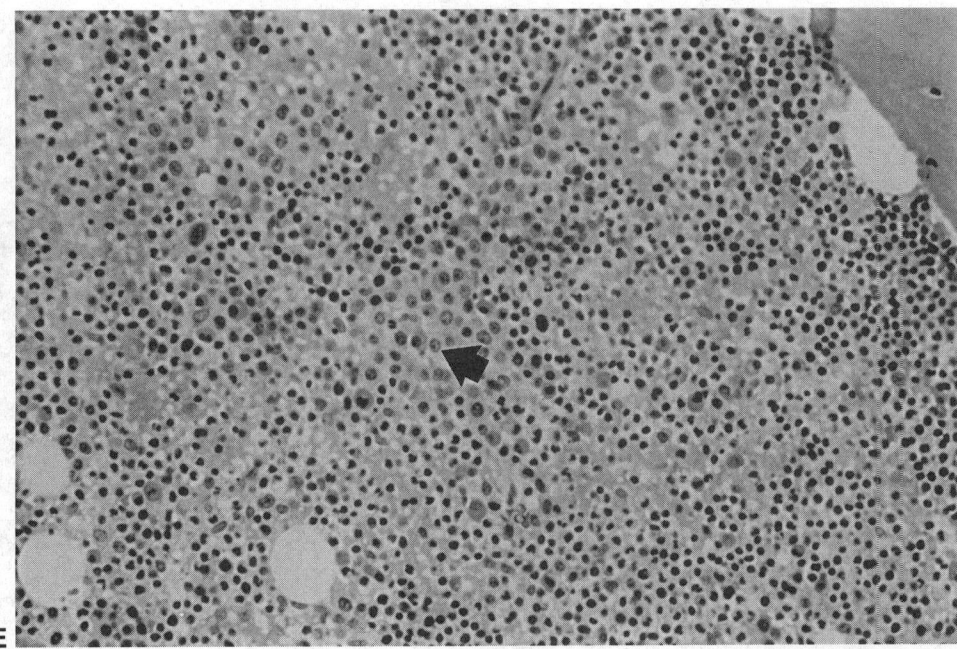

Fig. 71-5 *(Continued).* **(E)** Atypical localization of immature myeloid precursors (ALIP) (arrow). (× 250.) (Courtesy of Dr. James W. Vardiman, University of Chicago Hospitals.)

variant. A potentially useful means of identifying hypocellular MDS is the finding of an associated clonal cytogenetic abnormality characteristic for MDS (e.g., -5, -7, $5q-$, $7q-$, $+8$).[136-138] In a recent large series of patients with aplastic anemia, clonal chromosomal abnormalities were present in only 4% of individuals, but such clonal chromosomal abnormalities were frequently seen in MDS and AML.[136]

MDS with Fibrosis

Myelofibrosis refers to the generalized increase in the number and thickness of reticulin fibers detected by use of a silver stain of a bone marrow biopsy specimen.[139] Mild-to-moderate myelofibrosis has been reported in ≤50% of MDS, with marked fibrosis occurring in <15% of cases.[140-142] Myelofibrosis occurs in all FAB subclassifications of MDS.[140-142] The incidence of myelofibrosis in therapy-related MDS is greater than that in primary MDS.[143,144] Marked fibrosis has been reported to occur in ≤50% of therapy-related MDS, with mild fibrosis occurring in ≤85% of such cases.[143,144]

The syndrome of myelofibrosis in patients with coexisting MDS is characterized by the abrupt onset of pancytopenia without organomegaly, but with substantial red blood cell anisopoikilocytosis, a hypercellular bone marrow with myelofibrosis, trilineage dysplasia, atypical megakaryocyte proliferation with hypolobated forms, and increased numbers of marrow blasts.[142,143] Occasionally a leukoerythroblastic peripheral blood picture is evident. The clinical course is generally rapidly progressive.[145]

Distinguishing between this entity and MPDs may be difficult. Other diagnostic entities that should be excluded before the diagnosis of MDS with myelofibrosis include primary myelofibrosis; the accelerated phase of chronic myelocytic leukemia; post-polycythemia vera myelofibrosis with myeloid metaplasia; AML, especially acute megakaryoblastic leukemia (AML M7); AML with trilineage dysplasia; and acute myelofibrosis.[146] A period of myelodysplasia may herald transformation in ≤50% of patients who develop acute leukemia as a terminal episode in polycythemia vera.[147,148] In most cases, this event is related to previous cytotoxic therapy, and therefore resembles other therapy-related myelodysplastic disorders, although a myelo-

dysplastic phase has also been reported in polycythemia vera patients treated by phlebotomy alone.[147,148]

Chronic Myelomonocytic Leukemia

Some patients have a disorder from the outset with features of both MDS and chronic MPD. Included in this group are those who exhibit leukocytosis, hypercellular bone marrows with variable amounts of dysplasia, and splenomegaly. Some of these patients (i.e., those with monocytosis) may have CMML. Although CMML is defined as a myelodysplastic disorder by the FAB group, it serves as a prototype of those disorders that straddle MDS and chronic MPD. The criteria for CMML include a peripheral monocytosis $>1 \times 10^3/mm^3$; increased numbers of monocytic cells in the bone marrow (Figs. 71-3D and 71-4D); dysplasia in either the erythroid, megakaryocytic, or granulocytic series; <5% circulating blasts; and <30% marrow blasts[10,149] (Table 71-1). Pericardial, pleural, synovial, and ascitic effusions have been reported in CMML.[150] These serous effusions appear to be associated with high peripheral monocyte counts. CMML was placed in the MDS category primarily because of the dysplasia occurring in some patients, and because cytopenias of one or more peripheral-blood elements are not uncommon.[149] However, the nosologic position of CMML as a subtype of MDS is not accepted by all investigators, since features associated with MPD predominate in a substantial portion of the patients.[151] These latter features include marked monocytosis or neutrophilic leukocytosis in nearly 50% of patients, the finding of tissue infiltration by monocytes, splenomegaly in 50%, and hepatomegaly in ≤20% of patients.[151-153] In addition, the cloning efficiency of myeloid progenitor cells in CMML resembles that of chronic MPD, with increased numbers of colonies and clusters, rather than the pattern of MDS, in which progenitor cells form few colonies in short-term cultures.[149] Therefore, CMML may be considered as a disorder that encompasses features of both chronic MPD and MDS.

Atypical CML

Another disorder, Philadelphia (Ph) chromosome-negative CML, in some cases, has features of MDS as well as those of an MPD.[154] These features include dysplastic granulocytes; a low percentage of basophils; a sum of promyelocytes, myelocytes, and metamyelocytes >10%; and, often, monocytosis and thrombocytopenia.[146] In a retrospective study of cases previously diagnosed as Ph chromosome-negative CML, 60% of the patients had significant dysplasia, and 30–40% of the cases met the criteria for CMML.[146] Subsequent studies, however, demonstrated that, in some cases of Ph chromosome-negative CML, the breakpoint cluster region gene *(bcr)* on chromosome 22 was rearranged as in Ph-positive CML, despite the absence of a cytogenetically detectable Ph chromosome.[155,156] Patients lacking the Ph chromosome t(9;22) but possessing the *bcr* rearrangement have morphologic and clinical features indistinguishable from Ph chromosome-positive CML.[157] The remaining patients (i.e., those possessing some features of CML but lacking the Ph chromosome and *bcr* rearrangement) are a heterogeneous population that includes patients with features of both MDS and chronic MPD. Some, but not all, of these patients have findings that fulfill the criteria for CMML. Thus, many of these patients defy placement into current classification schemes and have been termed atypical CML.

Secondary MDS

Secondary (i.e., therapy-related and toxic chemical-related) MDS is emerging as a significant clinical problem and may cause morbidity and mortality with or without progression to AML.[158–161] The increasing incidence of secondary MDS and AML reflects a number of factors, including a longer period of risk resulting from successful treatment of solid tumors, more intensive treatment regimens combining high-dose chemotherapy and irradiation, broader utilization of adjuvant chemoirradiation in solid tumor therapy, and environmental pollution and exposure to chemicals and carcinogens (particularly organic solvents)[160,161] in industrialized nations. Generally these patients have poorer prognoses than those with primary MDS.[158]

In secondary MDS, abnormal karyotypes are evident in almost all patients, the presence of multiple chromosome aberrations is the rule, and chromosomes 5 and 7 are most frequently (85%) involved (Table 71-3). Accumulating experience in therapy-related leukemia suggests that chemotherapeutic agents may have different leukemogenic potentials that are associated with differing pathophysiologic processes. The classic therapy-related leukemia involving chromosome 5 and 7 abnormalities, and implicating alkylating agents and irradiation, remains the most common form. Two additional forms of therapy-related leukemia have recently been described: one attributed to exposure to topoisomerase II-active chemotherapeutic agents and involving the chromosome 11q23 locus, and the other involving the chromosome 21q22 locus.[162–164]

THERAPY

A variety of treatment approaches have been used in MDS, with supportive care generally being the mainstay of therapy. Patients should be treated as needed with antibiotics for infection and with RBC and platelet transfusions for symptomatic anemia and thrombocytopenic bleeding. Long-term RBC transfusion support may lead to iron overload and hemochromatosis. When it is anticipated that patients will have prolonged transfusion requirements, regular desferrioxamine chelation treatment should be considered. As MDS is relatively indolent and predominates in the elderly, a therapeutic challenge has been to provide treatment modalities having adequate support for the patients' dominant cytopenias without causing excessive toxicity. These elderly patients frequently have concomitant medical illnesses that markedly limit therapeutic options. Patients with abnormal cytogenetics, leukemic-

like in vitro marrow myeloid progenitor cell colony growth patterns, and more deranged clinical and marrow morphologic features have poorer prognoses. These abnormalities generally correlate with the more advanced FAB classifications. Due to this variability of prognoses in subgroups of patients with MDS, stratification according to these risk categories is necessary in order to analyze the therapeutic efficacy of different treatments.

Chemotherapy

Chemotherapeutic options for this disease have ranged from intensive cytotoxic therapy to low-dose therapy with DNA synthesis inhibitors such as cytosine arabinoside or hydroxyurea. Intensive chemotherapy in these generally elderly individuals is often poorly tolerated. In addition, a high proportion of these patients have marrow cells expressing surface P-glycoprotein that is associated with the multidrug resistance (MDR) phenotype.[165] Thus, in addition to MDS patients showing poor marrow recovery after marrow hypoplasia induced by intensive therapy, difficulty often exists in eradicating their abnormal clonal cells. In secondary MDS, the increased frequency of MDR positivity, unfavorable cytogenetics, and treatment-related stromal damage contribute to their poorer therapeutic responses.[166,167]

In studies evaluating the use of intensive chemotherapy in MDS, variable complete remission (CR) rates have been reported (13–51%) but with a high proportion of significant morbidity and toxic deaths due to therapy.[168–172] Better results have been achieved with younger patients and those having favorable karyotypes. In addition to the severe toxicity of this treatment for these patients, the durations of these responses are generally short.

Numerous studies have evaluated the use of low-dose cytosine arabinoside (ara-C) to treat these patients, generally with 10–20% of these individuals achieving CR.[173–176] However, the durability of these responses is usually short and in a randomized trial evaluating low-dose ara-C versus supportive care alone, the CR rate was only 8% and no improvement in survival was noted.[177] In addition, marrow toxicity, particularly thrombocytopenia, provided attendant difficulties with such management of these patients. Organomegaly, skin lesions, and serous effusions in CMML may be responsive to low-dose oral chemotherapy.

Bone Marrow Transplantation

The use of allogeneic bone marrow transplantation (BMT) for MDS patients has been reported.[178–180] The median age of these individuals (i.e., 29–39 years) was much younger than that of most MDS patients (>65 years). In a recent large study, the probabilities of disease-free survival (DFS), relapse, and nonrelapse mortality at 4 years were 41%, 28%, and 43%, respectively.[178] Multivariate analysis indicated that younger age (<40 years old) and low marrow blast counts (<5%) had better prognoses (62% DFS). However, for older patients (>40 years old) and those with >5% blasts (i.e., RAEB, RAEB-T), the DFS was only 17% and 32%, respectively; 51% of patients with >5% blasts relapsed. For patients in this study with secondary MDS, only two of eight individuals remain alive and disease free. In seven MDS patients with associated myelofibrosis none survived after BMT.

In a study by the European BMT Group, the DFS after BMT of patients with RAEB and RAEB-T was somewhat better, approximately 50–74%.[179] In this study, however, age criteria were not given for the responding individuals. In another study, DFS of 40% was found for 15 MDS patients who underwent

BMT.[180] Of these patients, 9 (60%) died of BMT-related complications within the first 100 days. Three of nine RAEB or RAEB-T patients relapsed. Increased marrow blasts had a negative impact on outcome as only 2 of 10 patients in this group survived compared with 6 of 10 patients with less blasts pre-BMT. Taken together, these data suggest that matched sibling allogeneic BMT may be useful for a portion of relatively young patients with low-risk MDS. However, those with more advanced forms of MDS (RAEB, RAEB-T), particularly if they are elderly, require other forms of therapy.

Hormonal Therapy

Corticosteroids have been used in a small number of MDS patients with approximately 10% having transient responses.[181] These responses often correlated with in vitro marrow culture studies, which demonstrated T-cell-mediated inhibition of hematopoiesis.[181] Androgens have also been used to treat MDS patients. However survival data indicated that patients who received the androgens did no better than those being observed and supportively treated with supportive care.[182] A randomized trial using androgens versus low-dose ara-C or observation only revealed similar survival in these three groups.[183] Treatment with danazol has been used in some individuals with MDS who were believed to have immune-associated thrombocytopenia.[184] Some improvement in the degree of thrombocytopenia was observed, but the incidence of such responses was generally quite low, and clinically useful responses were rare.

Nonspecific Differentiation-Inducing Agents

The use of differentiation-inducing agents for treating MDS is based on a large body of in vitro marrow culture studies and preclinical data indicating that such drugs may diminish self-replication of abnormal cell clones concomitant with enhancing their differentiation.[49-56] A variety of differentiation-inducing agents have been used for treating MDS, including retinoic acid,[79,185,186] vitamin D,[187] and HGFs. Although trials using 13-cis retinoic acid were associated with an increase in neutrophils in 30–50% of MDS patients, a randomized trial demonstrated that survival was not improved.[186] Similar results, indicating a low response rate, were seen recently in a trial using all trans-retinoic acid.[188] The use of 1,25 dihydroxy-vitamin D_3 to treat MDS was found not to be beneficial.[187] 5-Azacytidine has been shown to enhance cellular differentiation. In a recent phase II trial for 5-azacytidine for MDS, however, it was not found to be superior to ara-C.[190]

Interferons

Because of its effect on enhancing monocytic differentiation of myeloid cells, IFN-γ has been used to treat MDS patients. In a study using high and low doses of IFN-γ, 30 MDS patients were treated, 18 of whom had RAEB and 10 of whom had RAEB-T.[191] The median survival of these patients was 12 months. Two patients had partial responses and 12 individuals underwent transformation to AML. No clear differences were demonstrated between patients receiving the high- or low-dose therapy. Clinical benefit with regard to numbers of infectious episodes or improvement in blood counts was not demonstrated and no complete responses were noted. In another study, none of 25 MDS patients had complete responses to IFN-γ although 3 patients had good responses.[192]

IFN-α has also been used to treat patients with MDS. In one study of 14 patients (3 RA, 9 RAEB, 2 CMML) myelosuppression

was noted in 11 individuals, 5 of whom evolved in AML.[193] No sustained improvement in blood counts occurred in these patients. In other studies, 3 of 10 "low-risk" MDS patients[194] and 2 of 8 "high-risk" patients had transient responses.[195] These data did not demonstrate efficacy for the use of IFN-γ or IFN-α in treating MDS.

Hematopoietic Growth Factors

HGFs have been demonstrated to play critical physiologic roles in the control of hematopoiesis in vivo.[196,197] Several of these growth factors, IL-3 and CSF-GM, have predominantly proliferative effects on early hematopoietic cell compartments, whereas CSF-G and CSF-M have major differentiative, as well as proliferative, effects on later more lineage-restricted precursor cells (i.e., for granulocytes and monocytes, respectively). Each hematopoietic cell lineage appears to be regulated by both proliferative and differentiative stimuli. These factors have been used to improve the cytopenias and natural history of MDS.

Colony-Stimulating Factor-Granulocyte/Macrophage

Five phase I/II therapeutic trials have been reported using short-term recombinant human CSF-GM therapy (generally treatment was administered for 7–14 days, with 1–5 courses of therapy) to treat primary MDS.[198-203] The combined data from these studies indicated that 38 of 45 patients treated with CSF-GM had improvements in neutrophil counts, 9 with associated increases in marrow myeloid maturation, 14 had increased reticulocyte counts with 3 of these individuals having decreased RBC transfusion requirements, and 8 had transient increases in platelets (Table 71-5). In 12 patients an increase in marrow and/or peripheral blood blasts was noted. Seven patients progressed to AML, particularly individuals with >15% marrow blasts (i.e., those with RAEB or RAEB-T).

A trial using CSF-GM to treat patients with secondary MDS (i.e., after prior cytotoxic chemotherapy for other malignancies) demonstrated neutrophil responses in 8 of 10 patients evaluated.[204] Several patients had transient improvements in platelet counts and three experienced resolution of active in-

Table 71-5. Effects of Recombinant Human CSF-GM and CSF-G in Phase I/II Clinical Trials of Patients with MDS

	198–202	208,209
Short-term treatment		
Duration	7–14 days × 1–5 courses daily, IV or SC	42–56 days daily SC
Daily dose	30–750 µg/m²	0.1–3 µg/kg
No. of patients	45	18
FAB subtypes		
RA/RAEB/RAEB-T/CMML	14/26/5	2/16/0
Responses		
Neutrophils	38 (84%)	16 (89%)
Reticulocytes	14	5
Platelets	8	1
Marrow maturation	9	16
Increased blasts	12	4
Progression to AML	7	5
Long-term treatment		
Duration	2–9 wks	6–28 months
Persistent neutrophil responses/patients	1/5 patients	10/11 patients

(From Greenberg,[203] with permission.)

fections. Transformation to AML occurred in four patients after 5–11 months of therapy and three other patients died of their underlying malignancy. The median survival of these patients (11 months) reflected the poor prognosis of this group of patients.

A recent multicenter phase III study[205] provided information regarding the use of CSF-GM in relatively low-risk MDS patients (i.e., RA, RAEB patients with <10% marrow blasts), for longer periods (i.e., periods ≤2 months). Eighty-two patients (50 RA, 32 RAEB) received either of two different fixed daily dose levels of CSF-GM. These low-risk MDS patients untreated would have been expected to generally have relatively good prognoses, with median survivals of several years and a low incidence of evolution to AML. Nearly all of the MDS patients treated with CSF-GM responded with increased neutrophil counts. However, only 35% of the patients completed 8 weeks of treatment and the drug was discontinued in the others due to progression of disease, local infiltrates, flu-like syndromes, hyperleukocytosis, or bone pain. In 25% of the patients, platelet counts decreased during CSF-GM administration to <50% of baseline values, whereas two patients had increases in platelets. Six patients had progressive disease, two of whom with RAEB developed acute leukemia; improvements in erythropoiesis were not observed. No differences in the rate or quality of hematologic responses were demonstrated between the two dose levels of CSF-GM used. The impact of CSF-GM on progression of disease could not be addressed because of the small number of patients and short duration of treatment. A preliminary report of another multi-institutional randomized trial of CSF-GM treatment for periods ≤6 months versus observation in 21 patients with MDS, with crossover occurring in patients with infections has resulted in similar results.[206] A decrease in infections in the CSF-GM group was reported. Severe toxicity requiring reduction or discontinuation of CSF-GM dose occurred in a substantial proportion of the patients. No improvements in the patients' platelet counts or hemoglobin levels were noted. Further patient accrual and follow-up is occurring to determine the impact of this therapy on transformation to AML. These studies demonstrated some of the potential difficulties and benefits of chronic administration of a predominantly proliferative myeloid growth factor, such as CSF-GM, in patients with MDS.

In another recent study,[207] low-risk (4 patients), high-risk (14 patients), and CMML (3 patients) subtypes of MDS were randomly assigned to receive either CSF-GM alone or CSF-GM plus low-dose ara-C for 2 weeks, repeated monthly for three cycles. Patients receiving CSF-GM alone generally had increases in leukocyte and neutrophil counts, with only one patient having an improvement in the numbers of platelets. In the group receiving both CSF-GM and low-dose ara-C, leukocytes also increased during administration of the combined treatment, whereas platelet counts significantly declined. In the four patients who received three courses of combined treatment, partial short-term responses occurred, with some decreased percentage of blasts observed. These transient improvements with combined CSF-GM and low-dose ara-C suggest that further studies using HGFs combined with low-dose cytotoxic chemotherapy are warranted in this clinical setting. It will be important to analyze long-term as well as short-term outcomes of these individuals, and determine which subtypes of patients may respond and the degree of supportive care needed during such therapy.

Colony-Stimulating Factor-Granulocyte

Treatment of 18 MDS patients (2 RA, 9 RAEB, 7 RAEB-T) has been reported, using daily subcutaneous injections of CSF-G, escalating dosage levels every 2 weeks 0.1–3.0 μg/kg/day for a 2-month period.[208,209] Sixteen patients, including those with severe neutropenia, had substantial elevations in both white blood cell (WBC) count and absolute neutrophil count (ANC). In 5 patients, a greater than twofold rise in reticulocyte counts occurred and 3 of 12 RBC transfusion-dependent patients had decreases in RBC transfusions. Improved marrow myeloid maturation was noted in 16 of 18 patients. No significant changes in other blood counts were found during treatment of 17 of 18 patients (Table 71-5). After discontinuing CSF-G treatment, peripheral WBC counts returned to baseline levels over 2–4 weeks.

Results of a short-term trial of 40 MDS patients (20 RA, 20 RAEB/RAEB-T) treated with CSF-G have recently been reported.[210] Twenty of 22 patients (7-day treatment) and 16 of 18 patients (14-day treatment) had substantial improvement in neutrophil levels associated with decrements in marrow blasts in 8 of 13 evaluated patients. Of 11 patients with infections before CSF-G therapy, 7 experienced resolution of infectious processes after CSF-G and antibiotics.

As a result of the clinical responsiveness and tolerance of MDS patients to short-term CSF-G treatment, prolonged maintenance therapy was administered, and 10 of the 11 patients studied had persistent improvements of their neutrophil counts for 6–28 months.[209] Marrow granulocytic maturation improved in seven of nine patients. Two of four RBC transfusion-dependent patients had decreases in their transfusion requirements. Platelet counts were generally not altered by this therapy. Neutrophil function (in vitro chemotaxis and phagocytosis), which was maintained or improved after 2 months of treatment, was further augmented in five patients after an additional 6 months of CSF-G therapy. A significant reduction in the risk of developing an infection was retrospectively demonstrated in responding patients who achieved an ANC >1,500/mm^3 after CSF-G treatment. Toxicity to CSF-G was minimal. Five of 18 patients treated with long-term CSF-G, 4 with RAEB-T, converted to AML after 6–16 months of the study. These data indicated that chronic CSF-G administration was well tolerated and effective for promoting persistent improvement in neutrophil counts and neutrophil function, marrow myeloid maturation, and possibly decreasing the incidence of bacterial infections and RBC transfusion requirements in MDS patients. A phase III multi-institutional randomized trial for patients with high-risk MDS (RAEB/RAEB-T), comparing long-term CSF-G administration to observation, is ongoing to attempt to determine the impact of CSF-G on the natural history of the disease.

Evidence of Clonal Responses

Cytogenetic evaluations and investigations analyzing RFLPs of X-linked genes were performed in several of these cytokine trials[24,209,211] to determine whether the HGFs lead to selective responses of normal versus abnormal clones in MDS. The general persistence of cytogenetic abnormalities and clonal hematopoiesis after treatment with CSF-GM and CSF-G suggested that these cytokines each induced differentiation of the abnormal clone in MDS. In one case, however, polyclonal hematopoiesis developed after CSF-GM treatment.[211] In most cases, however, CSF-GM or CSF-G did not preferentially stimulate normal marrow stem cells, nor had the ability to eradicate the cytogenetically abnormal clone by inducing terminal differentiation.

Interleukin-3

Two studies have reported the effects of short-term IL-3 therapy in 22 MDS patients.[212,213] These studies indicated modest improvements in neutrophils; however, they were not as prominent as those demonstrated with CSF-G or CSF-GM (Table 71-6). Furthermore, only limited responses occurred in the other hematopoietic cell lines. Similar results were found in a recent longer term study treating low-risk (RA/RARS) MDS patients for 3 months with IL-3.[214] Transient improvements in platelet

Table 71-6. Effects of Recombinant Human IL-3 Treatment in MDS

	Reference 212	Reference 213
Treatment duration	15 days × 1–3 courses	28 days
Daily dose	250–500 μg/m² SC	30–1000 μg/m² IV
No. of patients	9	13
FAB subtypes		
RA/RAEB-RAEB-T/ CMML	6/3/0	5/5/3
Responses		
Leukocytes	9	8
Neutrophils	7;3[a]	6;3[a]
Reticulocytes	3; ↓transfusions 1/9	1
Platelets	3[b]; ↓transfusions 2/4	2
↑Blasts	2 PB; 1 BM	1 BM
Progression to AML	1	0

Abbreviations: BM, bone marrow; PB, peripheral blood.
[a] Increased ANC from <1,000 to >1,000/mm³.
[b] Unsustained.
(From Greenberg,[203] with permission.)

counts occurred in 2 of 5 patients who initially had <50,000 platelets/mm³. These data indicate that IL-3 will require combination with other HGFs to achieve substantial improvement in the cytopenias of MDS.

Interleukin-6

Fifteen low-risk MDS patients and one with CMML were treated with IL-6 to attempt to improve their platelet counts.[215] Preliminary information indicates that platelet responses occurred in 5 of 16 patients, including 2 patients with <50,000 platelets/mm³. Moderate to severe toxicity with constitutional symptoms occurred without leukocyte improvement, and worsening anemia developed in a substantial portion of these patients. The durability of these platelet responses and long-term tolerance to this agent remain to be determined.

Erythropoietin

Serum EPO levels may be suboptimally elevated in MDS patients relative to the degree of anemia.[216] Thus, recombinant human EPO therapy has been used in an attempt to correct the hypoproliferative anemias associated with MDS. A number of published reports have detailed the responses of MDS patients to this form of treatment. Results of the initial seven studies using EPO in MDS[217–223] indicated that 14 of 75 (19%) patients responded to EPO (Table 71-7). Generally, the patients required relatively high doses of EPO (>200 U/kg/day). This limited in vivo responsiveness of MDS marrow cells to EPO is not totally unexpected because the defective erythroid progen-

itor cells in MDS have demonstrated in vitro to respond suboptimally to EPO alone.[37,60]

HGFs such as CSF-G synergized with EPO in promoting in vitro erythropoiesis, enhancing normal and MDS marrow BFU-E numbers or responsiveness to EPO in vitro.[61] Such studies suggest that CSF-G and EPO might produce more prominent in vivo erythroid responses. EPO is a relatively late-acting factor that acts predominantly on CFU-E and on a portion of the late BFU-E that generate CFU-E. Defective in vitro erythropoiesis has been demonstrated in MDS.[37] Two clinical studies describing effects of such combination therapy with CSF-G plus EPO to treat the anemia of MDS[224,225] have shown an enhanced number of hematologic responses. Therapy was initiated with CSF-G at 1 μg/kg/day SC and adjusted to either normalize or double the neutrophil count. EPO was then administered by daily subcutaneous dose of 100 U/kg and dose escalated to 150–300 U/kg every 4 weeks in one study or kept at 120 U/kg/day in the other study, while continuing the CSF-G. Ten of 24 patients (42%) in one study[224] and 8 of 21 (38%) in the other[225] demonstrated substantial erythroid responses, and all patients had neutrophil responses. Six and five patients in these studies, respectively, who had previously required RBC transfusion support, no longer required transfusions during the treatment period. Responses were more frequent in patients with less advanced pancytopenia, lower endogenous EPO levels,[224,225] and in those with responsive marrow BFU-E.[226] Patients with ringed sideroblasts, who respond poorly to EPO alone, showed a response rate of 60%. These findings suggest synergistic in vivo effects of CSF-G and EPO for the anemia of patients with MDS. The durability of these short-term responses and determination of which patients require both growth factors rather than EPO alone are currently under study.

PROGNOSIS

Marrow Histologic Features

The FAB morphologic classification has been useful for helping to determine prognoses in MDS. Although MDSs are heterogeneous disorders with an incidence of AML evolution varying between 10% and 50%,[10] there has been relative consistency of prognostic findings regarding survival and AML evolution in a number of large studies, using FAB subgroup morphologic criteria[150,227–232] (Table 71-8 and Fig. 71-6). Patients with RAEB and RAEB-T had relatively poor prognoses, with median survivals generally in the range of 5–12 months, in contrast to RA or RARS patients who had median survivals of about 3–6 years. The proportion of these individuals whose disease transformed to AML varied similarly: in the high-risk RAEB and RAEB-T patients this incidence was 40–50%, whereas in the low-risk group it was 5–15%. In a recent study evaluating time to disease evolution, 25% and 55% of patients with RAEB and

Table 71-7. Erythroid Responses to Recombinant Human EPO in MDS

MDS Subtype		EPO Dose (U/kg)	Responses/Patients (%)	Responder Serum EPO Levels (mU/ml)	References
RA/RARS	RAEB/RAEB-T				
4	4	200–400 IV 3×/wk	2/8 (25)	694, 919	216
2	0	50–500 IV 3×/wk	0/2	—	217
7	5	200–1,000 IV 3×/wk	5/12 (42)	360 (mean)	218
17	0	800–1,600 IV 2×/wk	4/17 (24)	16, 515, 589, 1,030	219
11	1	50–250 SC 3×/wk	0/12	—	220
10	4	80–640 SC 3×/wk	1/14 (7)	1,750	221
8	2	60–90 SC daily	2/10 (20)	49, 199	222
59	16		14/75 (19)		

(From Greenberg,[203] with permission.)

Table 71-8. MDS: Survival and Leukemic Evolution Related to Morphologic Subgroups[a]

	FAB Subgroups				
	RA	RARS	RAEB	RAEB-T	CMML
Median survival (mo)	43	73	12	5	20
Transformation to AML (%)	15	5	40	50	35
Proportion of patients (%)	25	15	35	15	10

[a] Meta-analysis of results from references 227–232.

RAEB-T, respectively, underwent transformation to AML at 1 year, and 35% and 65% at 2 years. By contrast, for patients with RA the incidence of transformation was 5% and 10% at 1 and 2 years, whereas none of the RARS patients underwent leukemic transformation within 2 years.

The prognosis of MDS patients with "overlap syndromes" has been evaluated. The major prognostic feature for survival of CMML patients (as for the other MDS subgroups) is the marrow blast percentage.[149,231,233,234] Median survival of CMML patients with <5% marrow blasts was 53 months, whereas for those with 5–20% blasts it was 16 months (similar to RAEB). Monocytosis greater than $2.6 \times 10^9/L$ and abnormal cytogenetics also correlated with poor survival. Controversy exists regarding whether the hypocellular subtype of MDS has prognostic significance, as these patients have been reported to either progress to AML less frequently and have a longer survival or to have similar clinical outcome as other MDS patients.[133–135] A tendency toward hypocellularity in therapy-related MDS has been reported, and these patients generally have short survival times.[80] MDS patients with myelofibrosis generally have shorter survivals than those for MDS patients without fibrosis.[145] According to FAB classification, the presence of Auer rods in myeloid cells implies the diagnosis of RAEB-T.[10] However, the adverse influence of Auer rods per se has not been demonstrated.

Mortality in MDS is related to the morphologic subtype and is due to a variety of causes, including evolution to AML and infectious or bleeding complications related to the individual patient's dominant cytopenias. Because most of these patients are elderly, concomitant nonhematologic diseases associated with an elderly patient population also substantially contribute to their eventual outcome. In RAEB and RAEB-T patients, AML is the cause of death in 20–55% of patients, whereas infection and hemorrhage due to marrow failure causes 36–50% of the deaths, and nonhematologic causes account for 10–20% of the deaths.[150,227–232] In RA and RARS, these figures are somewhat

reversed: AML caused death in 0–29% of the deaths, infection and hemorrhage caused 15–44% of the deaths, and nonhematologic causes accounted for 25–42% of the deaths.

As adjuncts to FAB morphologic categorization, other classification systems using clinical or cytogenetic features have also been used for prognostic assessment. In all of these systems, the proportion of type I marrow blast cells was the most useful clinical prognostic marker in MDS, and probably the most important factor accounting for the striking differences in survival and progression to AML observed among the FAB subtypes.[150,227–232] Survival was progressively shorter as the marrow blast count increased.[231,232] These studies have reported clear differences in survival for patients with <5% and ≥5% marrow blasts, with survival curves of patients with 10–20% and 20–30% marrow blasts being almost identical (Fig. 71-7). Significant differences have also been demonstrated for the risk of developing AML when the patients are characterized according to marrow blast counts (Fig. 71-7). The cumulative probability of evolving into AML for patients with >20% marrow blasts was 100% at 30 months, a finding emphasizing that the border between RAEB-T and AML is somewhat arbitrary.[231] These data suggest that an additional cut-off point of 10% in the percentage of marrow blasts (i.e., including RAEB and RAEB-T patients with >10% blasts) would add significant prognostic information to the current FAB criteria. A categorized scoring system for MDS patients based on clinical risk features, including marrow blast percentage, platelet count, and age, which segregated patients into high-, intermediate-, and low-risk groups (Table 71-9), has been prognostically quite useful regarding survival and appears to improve upon FAB categorization alone[231] (Fig. 71-8).

Studies analyzing plastic-embedded marrow biopsies have suggested that the presence of small clusters of blast cells in central marrow regions, rather than in paratrabecular areas, has prognostic significance. Such blast cell clusters are referred to as ALIP (abnormal localization of immature myeloid precursors)[229] (Fig. 71-5E). ALIP-positive cases were characterized by a significantly shorter survival in all subtypes of MDS, including those patients with <5% total blasts. ALIP-positive cases were somewhat more common in RAEB, RAEB-T, and CMML.

Marrow Cytogenetics

Approximately 40–60% of patients with primary MDS have abnormal marrow karyotypes by conventional karyotyping methods[229,235,236]; however, with more refined techniques,

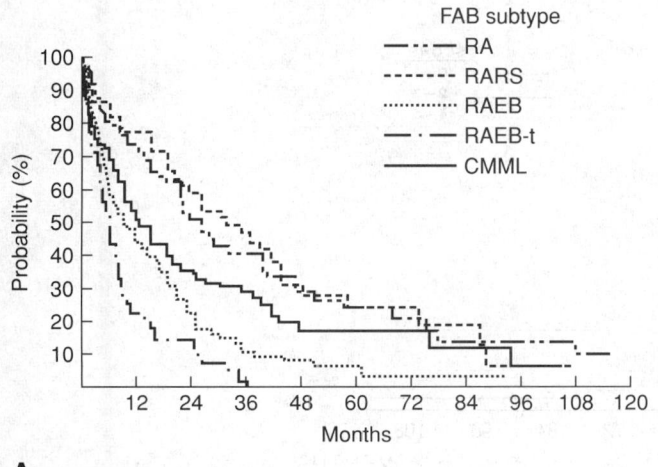

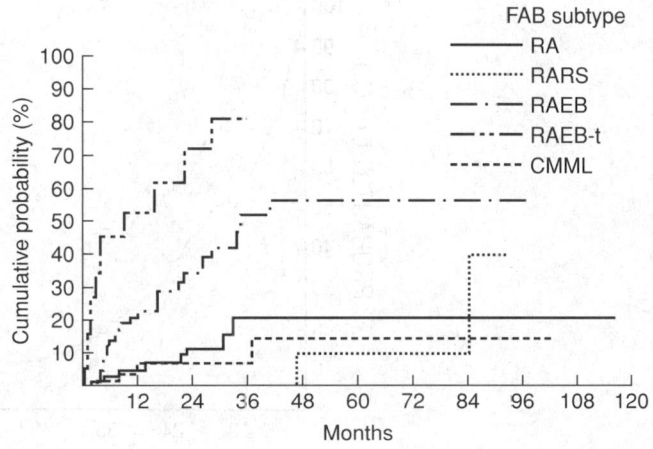

Fig. 71-6. (A) Survival and **(B)** AML evolution in MDS according to FAB morphologic subtypes. Analysis of 370 patients. (From Sanz et al.,[231] with permission.)

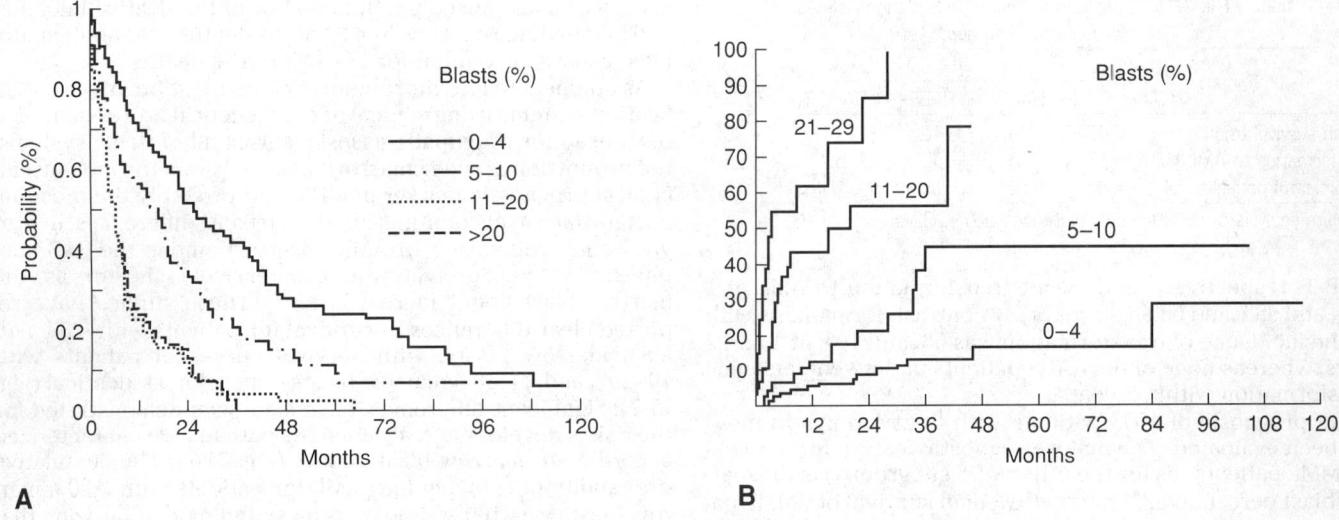

Fig. 71-7. (A) Survival and **(B)** AML evolution in MDS according to percentage of marrow blasts. Analysis of 370 patients. (From Sanz and Sanz,[233] with permission.)

chromosome abnormalities have been detected in ≤73% of cases.[237] Clinical correlative studies with multivariate analyses have established that marrow cytogenetics are an independent prognostic factor in MDS (Table 71-10), complementing analyses using clinical features of these patients. The highest incidence of abnormalities is concentrated in the poor prognostic subgroups of the FAB classification (RAEB and RAEB-T). In early studies, MDS cases with normal karyotypes had better prognoses than patients with abnormal chromosomes.[28,29] However, recent investigations, using more precisely defined abnormal karyotypes, have modified this conclusion. Current data indicate that patients with poor prognosis are those with marrow cell clones that have complex chromosome abnormalities[233,235–238] or who have a single chromosome abnormality involving −7 or 7q− or +8 (Fig. 71-9 and Table 71-10). Conversely, patients with the 5q− deletion [i.e., del(5) (q12q33)] as the sole abnormality have relatively longer survivals.[129,233,235,237] However, the 5q− abnormality combined with other karyotypic derangements is indicative of a poor prognosis. Survival was >2 years in cases with either normal chromosomes or 5q−, between 1 and 2 years in cases with trisomy 8, and <1 year in cases with either deletions of chromosome 7 or multiple abnormalities. The higher incidence of complex

chromosomal abnormalities in patients with secondary MDS partly explains their poor prognosis.[236] The acquisition of a chromosomally abnormal clone in MDS patients with a previously normal karyotype or additional karyotypic changes in a patient with previously abnormal clone is associated with progression to a more aggressive FAB subtype or AML evolution and early death.[166,239–241] However, karyotype stability does not preclude transformation to AML because most MDS patients do not acquire new chromosome abnormalities at the time overt AML develops.[240,242] A composite risk categorization for MDS patients comprised of clinical, morphologic, and cytogenetic features is presented in Table 71-11.

In Vitro Myeloid Clonogenic Assays

Patterns of in vitro marrow myeloid colony formation in MDS may be classified as leukemic and nonleukemic.[37] Leukemic-type growth is characterized by micro- or macrocluster formation with defective maturation or blasts within the aggregates, single persisting blasts, or very low cloning efficiency (<2 colonies per 10^5 marrow cells). Nonleukemic growth is marked by near normal colony formation, even if moderately decreased

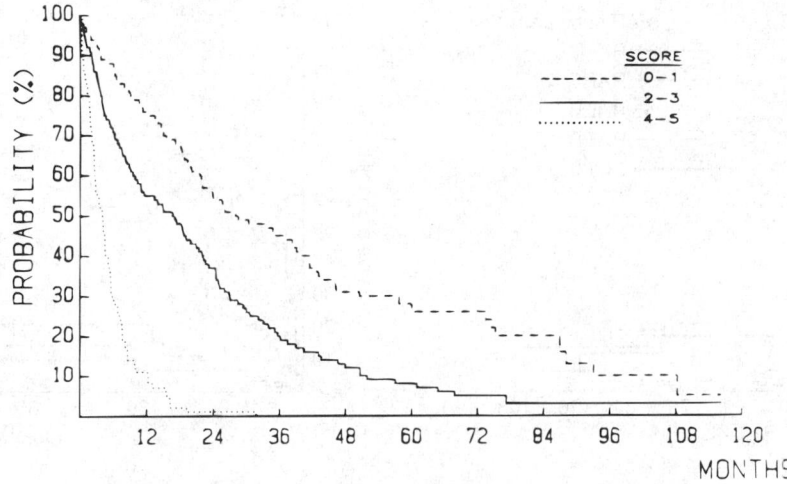

Fig. 71-8. Survival in MDS according to categorized clinical risk scores. Analysis of 370 patients. Risk: low 0–1, intermediate 2–3, high 4–5. See Table 71-9 for the clinical risk prognostic scoring system. (From Sanz et al.,[231] with permission.)

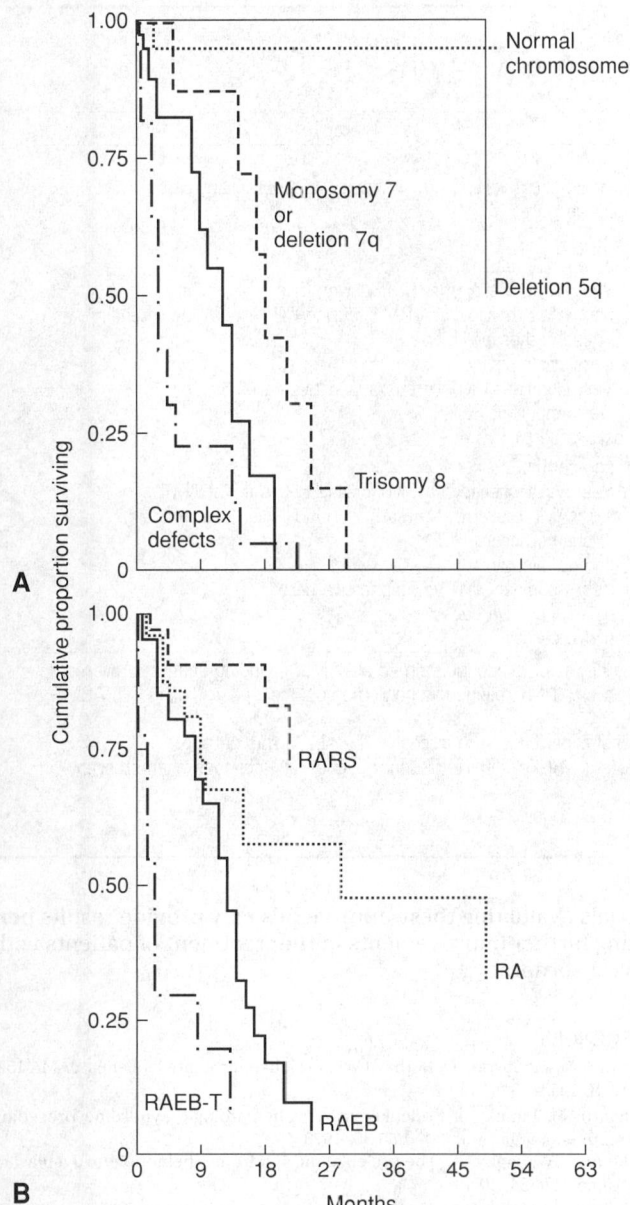

Fig. 71-9. Survival in myelodysplastic syndrome according to analysis of **(A)** refined cytogenetic abnormalities and **(B)** FAB morphologic subtypes. Analysis of 90 patients. (From Yunis et al.,[237] with permission.)

in frequency. As shown in Table 71-12, six studies involving 179 MDS patients with differing FAB morphologic subtypes demonstrated a correlation between clinical outcome and in vitro proliferative patterns.[37,44,243–248] When patients were stratified according to their in vitro myeloid growth patterns, subgroups of MDS patients with nonleukemic growth patterns

Table 71-9. Survival in MDS: Categorized Scoring System

Prognostic variable	Score Value		
	0	1	2
Marrow blasts (%)	<5	5–10	>10
Platelets (× 10^3/mm^3)	>100	51–100	<50
Age (yr)	≤60	>60	
Risk groups			Score
Low	A		0 or 1
Intermediate	B		2 or 3
High	C		4 or 5

(From Sanz et al.,[231] with permission.)

Table 71-10. Multivariate Analysis of Survival in Patients with Primary MDS

Characteristic	P Value	Unfavorable Values
Karyotype	<0.0001	Monosomy 7 or 7q− Trisomy 8 Complex abnormalities
Marrow blasts	0.004	Higher percentage
Age	0.01	Increased age
Platelets	0.02	Lower count

(From Sanz and Sanz,[233] with permission.)

had a 20–31% incidence of transformation to AML and a median survival of 20–47 months. By contrast, MDS patients with leukemic growth patterns had a 60–100% incidence of transformation and a 7–10 month median survival. MDS patients with single hematopoietic cell line defects, such as idiopathic sideroblastic anemia and idiopathic neutropenia, which are associated with a low propensity to leukemic evolution, had normal in vitro marrow myeloid progenitor cell growth parameters.[44] Patients who died without undergoing transformation generally did so as a result of infectious or bleeding complications. The decreased marrow granulopoiesis in vitro (low frequency of normal CFU-GM) may reflect the patients' marrows being less capable of responding to demand for new cells. Factors other than in vitro growth patterns contribute to transformation, as not all patients with abnormal clonal growth had poor prognoses. A correlation has been demonstrated between in vitro myeloid growth abnormalities, abnormal marrow cytogenetics, and poor prognoses.[37] The findings of decreasing CFU-GM incidence, a higher proportion of light density CFU-GM, and increased cluster/colony ratios provide functional evidence of clonal evolution and an indication of disease progression toward acute leukemia.

Such in vitro clonogenic assay permits the assay of blast cell progenitors from marrow and blood of patients with AML.[249] Whereas these colonies are generally not present in the marrow of normal individuals, most patients in a study of MDS demonstrated these circulating blast cell progenitors, some of which were in active phases of the cell counts cycle.[250] Further investigations correlating this in vitro feature with peripheral blast, clinical status, and subsequent course will be important to determine the significance of this finding.

Table 71-11. Prognostic Groups in MDS

Risk	Cytopenia	Marrow Blasts (%)	A_IP	Cytogenetics
Low	1	<5	−	Normal, 5q−
Intermediate	2	5–9	+	Simple, +8
High	3	≥10		Complex, −7

THERAPEUTIC DIRECTIONS

To determine the potential long-term effects of CSF-G and CSF-GM in MDS, competing hypotheses are being evaluated in phase III clinical trials, which are assessing the long-term effects of chronic CSF administration.[206,251] The theses being analyzed are differentiation induction, which potentially decreases self-replication of the abnormal clone,[50–54] versus enhanced survival/proliferation of the leukemic cells induced by these stimulatory factors.[37,252] This issue is particularly important to resolve because some leukemic cells are characterized by enhanced proliferative responses to HGFs in vitro.[253,254] Thus, concern exists about the safety of these agents regarding their potential for enhancing leukemic progression. Despite the demonstration of improvements in neutrophil levels and marrow morphology in a substantial proportion of MDS patients with

APPROACH TO THERAPY OF PATIENTS WITH MDS

	Therapy
Patients >60 years old[a]	
Excellent clinical condition	Supportive care[b] versus "low intensity" chemotherapy/HGFs
Poor clinical condition	Supportive Care[b]
Patients >50 and ≤60 years old[a]	
Excellent Clinical Condition	HLA compatible sibling
High-risk category[c]	Yes: rAML therapy → BMT during CR
	No: rAML therapy → ABMT$_p$ during CR versus "low intensity" chemotherapy/HGFs
Low/intermediate risk category[c]	HLA compatible sibling
	Yes: Consider BMT versus supportive care[b]
	No: Supportive care[b]
Poor clinical condition	Supportive care[b]
Patients ≤50 Years Old[a]	HLA compatible sibling
Good/excellent clinical condition	Yes: rAML therapy → BMT during CR vs initial BMT
	No: rAML therapy → ABMT$_p$ during CR vs. "low intensity" chemotherapy/HGFs
Low/intermediate risk category[c]	HLA compatible sibling
	Yes: Consider BMT vs. supportive care[b]
	No: Supportive care[b]
Poor clinical condition	Supportive care[b]

Abbreviations: CR, complete remission; rAML, resistant AML; rAML therapy, chemotherapeutic induction aimed at rAML, including agents to overcome multidrug resistance and HGFs such as CSF-G or CSF-GM to assist hemopoietic recovery; BMT, allogeneic bone marrow transplant during CR; ABMT$_p$, autologous purged bone marrow transplant during CR.

[a] Age guidelines are approximate and depend on patient's clinical condition and local experience with intensive therapy in this setting.

[b] Consider participation in experimental protocols with "low intensity" treatment (e.g., HGFs, differentiation induction ± low-dose chemotherapy) in addition to transfusion/antibiotic support.

[c] Risk category based on Sanz et al. [231] prognostic scores; high 4–5, intermediate 2–3, low 0–1.

these cytokines, results of ongoing randomized controlled studies are needed to determine whether the natural history of these disorders (survival, evolution to AML, or infectious complications) will be altered by treatment with the CSFs. Also, growth factors are needed that are able to augment platelet levels in order to modify a major cause of morbidity, thrombocytopenia. Until results of these trials are available, extended use of HGFs in MDS should still be considered experimental.

Given the generally advanced age of MDS patients, the relatively poor complete responses to most standard therapeutic modalities and the variability of prognoses of patients with these disorders, approaches to treatment of this patient population remain problematic. The standard of care remains to be symptomatic supportive therapy. However, subgroups of MDS patients (based on age, clinical condition, and risk category) could be considered for other forms of therapy. It should be understood, however, that at this time many of these treatment strategies remain experimental. Appropriately designed clinical trials evaluating these approaches may provide results permitting further improvements in the treatment of patients with these disorders.

REFERENCES

1. Block M, Jacobson LO, Bethard WF: Preleukemic acute leukemia. JAMA 152: 1018, 1953
2. Saarni M, Linman J: Preleukemia. The hematologic syndrome preceding acute leukemia. Am J Med 55:38, 1973
3. Linman JW, Bagby GC: The preleukemic syndrome (hemopoietic dysplasia). Cancer 42:854, 1978
4. Rheingold JJ, Kaufman R, Adelson E, Lear A: Smoldering acute leukemia. N Engl J Med 268:812, 1963
5. Knospe WH, Gregory SA: Smoldering acute-leukemia. Arch Intern Med 127: 910, 1971
6. Sexauer J, Kass L, Schnitzer B: Subacute myelomonocytic leukemia. Am J Med 57:853, 1974
7. Dreyfus B: Preleukemic states. II. Refractory anemia with excess of myeloblasts. Blood Cells 2:33, 1976
8. Dreyfus B, Rochant H, Sultan C et al: Les anemies refractaires avec exces de myeloblasts dans la moelle. Etude de 11 observations. Presse Med 787: 359, 1970
9. Izrael V, Jacquillat C, Chastaing G et al: Donnees nouvelles sur les leucemies oligoblastiques. A propos d'une analyse de 120 cas. Nouvelle Presse Med 4:947, 1975
10. Bennett JM, Catovsky D, Daniel T et al: FAB Cooperative Group. Proposal for the classification of the myelodysplastic syndromes. Br J Haematol 51: 189, 1982
11. Kantarjian HM, Estey EH, Keating MJ: Treatment of therapy-related leukemia and myelodysplastic syndromes. Hematol Oncol Clin North Am 7:81, 1993
12. LeBeau MM, Albain KS, Larson R et al: Clinical and cytogenetic correlations in 63 patients with therapy-related myelodysplastic syndromes and acute nonlymphocytic leukemia: further evidence for characteristic abnormalities of chromosomes no. 5 and 7. J Clin Oncol 4:325, 1986
13. Janssen JWG, Buschle M, Layton M et al: Clonal analysis of myelodysplastic syndromes: evidence of multipotent stem cell origin. Blood 73:248, 1989
14. Greenberg PL: In vitro culture techniques defining biologic abnormalities in the myelodysplastic syndromes and myeloproliferative disorders. Clin Haematol 15:973, 1986

Table 71-12. Prognosis of MDS: Utility of In Vitro Marrow Myeloid Clonogenic Culture Studies

Growth Patterns	Incidence (%)	Transformation to AML (%)	Median Survival (mo)
RAEB-T (n = 80)[243,244]		51 (45–60)[a]	9 (7–11)
Nonleukemic growth	33 (27–38)	31 (29–33)	20 (15–25)
Leukemic growth	68 (62–73)	60 (50–70)	7 (5–8)
RAEB (n = 17)[245,246]		41	41
Nonleukemic growth	70	29	21
Leukemic growth	30	100	10
RA (n = 82)[44,247,248]		39 (35–44)	24 (9–20)
Nonleukemic growth	54 (30–74)	20 (21–40)	47 (9–50)
Leukemic growth	46 (26–70)	60 (50–80)	8 (4–10)

[a] Mean values and ranges of means for cited studies.
(From Greenberg,[37] with permission.)

15. Gilliland DG, Blanchard KL, Levy J et al: Clonality in myeloproliferative disorders: analysis by means of the polymerase chain reaction. Proc Natl Acad Sci 88:6848, 1991
16. Kere J, Rutu T, de la Chappelle A: Monosomy 7 in granulocytes and monocytes in myelodysplastic syndrome. N Engl J Med 316:499, 1987
17. Grier HE, Weinstein HJ, Revesz R et al: Cytogenetic evidence for involvement of erythroid progenitors in a child with therapy linked myelodysplasia. Br J Haematol 64:513, 1986
18. Gerritsen WR, Donohue J, Bauman J et al: Clonal analysis of myelodysplastic syndrome: monosomy 7 is expressed in the myeloid lineage, but not in the lymphoid lineage as detected by fluorescent in situ hybridization. Blood 80:217, 1992
19. Abrahamson G, Boultwood J, Madden J et al: Clonality of cell populations in refractory anaemia using combined approach of gene loss and X-linked restriction fragment length polymorphism-methylation analysis. Br J Haematol 79:550, 1991
20. Kroef MJPL, Fibbe WE, Mout R et al: Myeloid but not lymphoid cells carry the 5q deletion: polymerase chain reaction analysis of loss of heterozygosity using mini-repeat sequences on highly purified cell fractions. Blood 81:1849, 1993
21. Anastasi J, Feng J, LeBeau MM et al: Cytogenetic clonality in myelodysplastic syndromes studied with fluorescence in-situ hybridization: lineage, response to growth factor therapy and clonal expansion. Blood 81:1580, 1993
22. Tsukamoto N, Morita K, Maehara T et al: Clonality in MDS: demonstration of pluripotent stem cell origin using X-linked restriction fragment length polymorphisms. Br J Haematol 83:589, 1993
23. van Kamp H, Fibbe WE, Jansen RPM et al: Clonal involvement of granulocytes and monocytes, but not of T and B lymphocytes and natural killer cells in patients with myelodysplasia: analysis by X-linked restriction fragment length polymorphisms and polymerase chain reaction of the phosphoglycerate kinase gene. Blood 80:1774, 1992
24. Janssen JWG, Buschle M, Layton M et al: Clonal analysis of myelodysplastic syndromes: evidence of multipotent stem cell origin. Blood 73:248, 1989
25. Culligan DJ, Cachai P, Whittaker J et al: Clonal lymphocytes are detectable in only some cases of MDS. Br J Haematol 81:346, 1992
26. Mecucci C, van den Berghe H: Cytogenetics. Hematol Oncol Clin North Am 6:522, 1992
27. Marshall C: Tumor suppressor genes. Cell 64:313, 1991
28. Pierre RV, Catovsky D, Mufti GJ et al: Clinical-cytogenetic correlations in myelodysplasia (preleukemia). Cancer Genet Cytogenet 40:149, 1989
29. Mufti G: Chromosomal deletions in the myelodysplastic syndromes. Leuk Res 15:35, 1992
30. Carter G, Ridge S, Padua R: Genetic lesions in preleukemia. Crit Rev Oncogen 3:339, 1992
31. Willman CL, Sever CE, Pallavicini MG et al: Deletion of IRF-1 mapping to chromosome 5q31.1, in human leukemia and preleukemic myelodysplasia. Science 259:968, 1993
32. Thangaveleu M, Bitter MA, Larson RA et al: del (5) t(5;7) (q 11.2;p 11.2): a new recurring abnormality in malignant myeloid disorders. Cancer Genet Cytogenet 37:1, 1989
33. van den Berghe H, Mecucci C, Delannoy A, van den Berghe H: Deletion of 5q by t(5;17) in therapy-related myelodysplastic syndrome. Cancer Genet Cytogenet 48:49, 1990
34. Bloomfield CD: Chromosome abnormalities in myelodysplastic syndromes. Scand J Haematol 36:82, 1986
35. Nowell P: Chromosome abnormalities in myelodysplastic syndrome. Sem Oncol 19:25, 1992
36. Pedersen-Bjergaard J, Philip P: Cytogenetic characteristics of therapy-related acute nonlymphocytic leukemia, preleukemia and acute myeloproliferative syndrome: correlation with clinical data for 61 consecutive cases. Br J Haematol 66:199, 1987
37. Greenberg P: In vitro culture studies in the myelodysplastic syndromes. Sem Oncol 19:34, 1992
38. Kremer E, Baker E, D'Andrea RJ et al: A cytokine receptor gene cluster in the X-Y pseudoautosomal region? Blood 82:22, 1993
39. Morris SW, Valentine MB, Shapiro DN et al: Reassignment of the human CSF1 gene to chromosome 1p12-p21. Blood 78:2013, 1991
40. Kluck PM, Wiegant J, Raap AK et al: Order of human hematopoietic growth factor and receptor genes on the long arm of chromosome 5, as determined by fluorescence in situ hybridization. Ann Hematol 66:15, 1993
41. Kluck PM, Wiegant J, Jansen RP et al: The human interleukin-6 receptor alpha chain gene is localized on chromosome 1 band q21. Hum Genet 90:542, 1993
42. Giebel LB, Strunk KM, Holmes SA, Spritz RA: Organization and nucleotide sequence of the human KIT (mast/stem cell growth factor receptor) proto-oncogene. Oncogene 7:2207, 1992
43. Sprintz RA, Droetto S, Fukushima Y: Deletion of the KIT and PDGFRA genes in a patients with piebaldism. Am J Med Genet 44:492, 1992
44. Greenberg PL, Mara B: The preleukemic syndrome: correlation of in vitro parameters of granulopoiesis with clinical features. Am J Med 66:951, 1979
45. Chiu DH, Clark BJ: Abnormal erythroid progenitor cells in human preleukemia. Blood 60:362, 1982
46. Juvonen E, Partanen S, Knuutila S et al: Megakaryocyte colony formation by bone marrow progenitors in myelodysplastic syndromes. Br J Haematol 64:331, 1985
47. Swanson G, Picozzi V, Morgan R et al: Response of hemopoietic precursors to 13-cis retinoic acid and 1,25 dihydroxyvitamin D₃ in the myelodysplastic syndromes. Blood 67:1154, 1986
48. Nagler A, Ginzton N, Bangs C et al: In vitro differentiative and proliferative effects of human recombinant colony-stimulating factors on marrow hemopoiesis in myelodysplastic syndromes. Leukemia 4:193, 1990
49. Nagler A, Binet C, Mackichan ML et al: Impact of marrow cytogenetics and morphology on in vitro hemopoiesis in the myelodysplastic syndromes: comparison between recombinant human granulocyte colony-stimulating factor and granulocyte-macrophage colony-stimulating factor. Blood 76:1299, 1990
50. Lotem J, Sachs L: Mechanisms that uncouple growth and differentiation in myeloid leukemia cells: restoration of requirement for normal growth-inducing protein without restoring induction of differentiation-inducing protein. Proc Natl Acad Sci USA 79:4347, 1982
51. Hozumi M: Fundamentals of chemotherapy of myeloid leukemia by induction of leukemia cell differentiation. Adv Cancer Res 38:121, 1983
52. Lotem J, Sachs L: In vivo inhibition of the development of myeloid leukemia by injection of macrophage and granulocyte-inducing protein. Int J Cancer 28:375, 1981
53. Honma Y, Hozumi H, Abe E et al: 1a, 25-dihydroxyvitamin D₃ prolong survival time of mice inoculated with myeloid leukemia cells. Proc Natl Acad Sci USA 80:201, 1983
54. Block A: Induced cell differentiation in cancer therapy. Cancer Treat Rep 68:199, 1984
55. Nicola N, Metcalf D: Binding to the differentiation-inductor, granulocyte-colony-stimulating factor, to responsive but not unresponsive leukemic cell lines. Proc Natl Acad Sci USA 81:3765, 1984
56. McCarthy DM, San Miguel JF, Freake HC et al: 1,25-dihydroxyvitamin D₃ inhibits proliferation of human promyelocytic leukaemic (HL-60) cells and induces monocyte-macrophage differentiation in HL-60 and normal human bone marrow. Leuk Res 7:51, 1983
57. Koeffler PH, Hirji K, Itri L: 1,25 dihydroxyvitamin D₃: in vivo and in vitro effects on human preleukemic and leukemic cells. Cancer Treat Rep 69:1399, 1985
58. Nienhuis AW, Bunn HF, Turner P et al: Expression of the human c-fms proto-oncogene in hematopoietic cells and its deletion in the 5q − syndrome. Cell 42:421, 1985
59. Nagler A, Ginzton N, Negrin RS et al: In vitro hemopoiesis in myelodysplastic syndrome patients treated with recombinant human granulocyte colony-stimulating factor, abstracted. Blood 72:128a, 1988
60. Merchav S, Nielsen OJ, Rosenbaum H et al: In vitro studies of erythropoietin-dependent regulation of erythropoiesis in myelodysplastic syndromes. Leukemia 4:771, 1990
61. Greenberg PL, Negrin RS, Ginzton N: G-CSF synergizes with erythropoietin for enhancing erythroid colony-formation in myelodysplastic syndromes. Blood, suppl. 1. 78:38a, 1991
62. Schipperus MR, Sonneveld P, Lindemans J et al: The combined effects of IL-3, GM-CSF and G-CSF on the in vitro growth of myelodysplastic myeloid progenitor cells. Leuk Res 14:1019, 1990
63. Greenberg PL, Mackichan ML, Negrin R: Production of granulocyte colony-stimulating factor by normal and myelodysplastic syndrome peripheral blood cells, abstracted. Blood suppl. 1. 76:146a, 1990
64. Migliaccio G, Migliaccio AR, Adamson JW: In vitro differentiation and proliferation of human hematopoietic progenitors: the effects of interleukins 1 and 6 are indirectly mediated by production of granulocyte-macrophage colony-stimulating factor and interleukin 3. Exp Hematol 19:3, 1991
65. Anderson RW, Volsky D, Greenberg B et al: Lymphocyte abnormalities in preleukemia. Decreased NK activity, anomalous immunoregulatory cell subsets and deficient EBV receptors. Leuk Res 7:389, 1983
66. Sporn MB, Roberts AB, Wakefield LM et al: Some recent advances in the chemistry and biology of transforming growth factor-beta. J Cell Biol 195:1039, 1987
67. Grotendorst GR, Smale G, Pencev D: Production of transforming growth factor beta by human peripheral blood monocytes and neutrophils. J Cell Physiol 140:396, 1989

68. Massague J: The TGF-beta family of growth and differentiation factors. Cell 49:437, 1987

69. Sing GK, Keller JR, Ellingsworth JR et al: Transforming growth factor beta selectively inhibits normal and leukemic human bone marrow cell growth in vitro. Blood 72:1504, 1988

70. Axelrad A: Some hemopoietic negative regulators. Exp Hematol 18:143, 1990

71. Greenberg PL, Mosny S: Cytotoxic effects of interferon in vitro on granulocytic progenitor cells. Cancer Res 37:1794, 1977

72. Broxmeyer HE, Lu L, Platzer E et al: Comparative analysis of the influence of human gamma, alpha, and beta interferons on human multipotential, erythroid and granulocyte-macrophage progenitor cells. J Immunol 131:1300, 1983

73. Pelus LM, Broxmeyer HE, Moore MAS: Regulation of human myelopoiesis by prostaglandin E and lactoferrin. Cell Tissue Kinet 14:515, 1981

74. Broxmeyer HE, Bognacki J, Dormer MH: Identification of leukemia-associated inhibitory activity as acidic isoferritins. A regulatory role for acidic isoferritins in the production of granulocytes and macrophages. J Exp Med 152:1426, 1981

75. Broxmeyer HE, Gentile P, Cooper S et al: Functional activities of acid isoferritins and lactoferrin in vitro and in vivo. Blood Cells 10:397, 1985

76. Olofsson T, Nilsson E, Olsson I: Characterization of the cells in myeloid leukemia that produce leukemia-associated inhibitor (LAI) and demonstration of LAI-producing cells in normal bone marrow. Leuk Res 48:387, 1984

77. Gold EJ, Canjalka M, Pelus LM et al: Marrow cytogenetic and cell-culture analyses of the myelodysplastic syndromes: insights to pathophysiology and prognosis. J Clin Oncol 1:627, 1983

78. Broxmeyer HE, Sherry B, Cooper S et al: Comparative analysis of the human macrophage inflammatory protein family of cytokines (chemokines) on proliferation of human myeloid progenitor cells. J Immunol 150:3448, 1993

79. Lord BI, Dexter TM, Clements JM et al: Macrophage-inflammatory protein protects multipotent hematopoietic cells from the cytotoxic effects of hydroxyurea in vivo. Blood 79:2605, 1992

80. Maze R, Sherry B, Kwon BS et al: Myelosuppressive effects in vivo of purified recombinant murine macrophage inflammatory protein 1α. J Immunol 149:1004, 1992

81. Dunlop DJ, Wright EG, Lorimore S et al: Demonstration of stem cell inhibition and myeloprotective effects of SCI/RHMIP-1α. Blood 79:2221, 1992

82. Lord B, Dexter M: Inhibitors of haematopoietic stem cell proliferation. Focus Growth Factors 3:1, 1992

83. Peetre C, Gullberg U, Nilsson E et al: Effects of recombinant tumor necrosis factor on proliferation and differentiation of leukemic and normal hemopoietic cells in vitro: relationship to cell surface receptor. J Clin Invest 78:1694, 1986

84. Murase T, Hotta T, Saito H et al: Effect of recombinant human tumor necrosis factor on the colony growth of human leukemia progenitor cells and normal hematopoietic progenitor cells. Blood 69:467, 1987

85. Bynoe AG, Scott CS, Ford P et al: Decreased T helper cells in the myelodysplastic syndromes. Br J Haematol 54:97, 1983

86. Knox SJ, Greenberg BR, Anderson RW et al: Studies of T-lymphocytes in preleukemic disorders and acute nonlymphocytic leukemia: in vitro radiosensitivity, mitogenic responsiveness, colony formation, and enumeration of lymphocytic subpopulations. Blood 61:449, 1983

87. Kerndrup G, Meyer K, Ellegaard J: Natural killer (NK)-cell activity and antibody-dependent cellular cytotoxicity (ADCC) in primary preleukemic syndrome. Leuk Res 8:239, 1984

88. Justesen J, Hokland P, Hokland M: The interferon/2-5A synthase system in primary preleukemia patients. Prog Clin Biol Res 202:349, 1985

89. Sherr CJ, Rettenmier CW, Sacca R et al: The *c-fms* proto-oncogene product is related to the receptor for the mononuclear phagocyte growth factor, CSF-1. Cell 41:665, 1985

90. Carter C, Ridge S, Padua R: Genetic lesions in preleukemia. Crit Rev Oncogen 3:339, 1992

91. Barbacid M: *ras* genes. Ann Rev Biochem 56:779, 1987

92. Downward J, Graves JD, Warne PH et al: Stimulation of p21^{ras} upon T-cell activation. Nature 346:719, 1990

93. Cantley LC, Auger KR, Carpenter C et al: Oncogenes and signal transduction. Cell 6:281, 1991

94. Bos JL: ras oncogenes in human cancer: a review. Cancer Res 49:4682, 1989

95. Janssen JWG, Steenvoorden ACM, Lyons J et al: *RAS* gene mutations in acute and chronic myelocytic leukemias, chronic myeloproliferative disorders and myelodysplastic syndromes. Proc Natl Acad Sci USA 84:9228, 1987

96. Lyons J, Janssen JWG, Bartram C et al: Mutation of Ki-*ras* and N-*ras* oncogenes in myelodysplastic syndromes. Blood 71:1707, 1988

97. Padua RA, Carter G, Hughes D et al: RAS mutations in myelodysplasia detected by amplification, oligonucleotide hybridization and transformation. Leukemia 2:203, 1988

98. Bar-Eli M, Ahuja H, Gonzales-Cadavid et al: Analysis of N-RAS exon-1 mutations in myelodysplastic syndromes by polymerase chain reaction and direct sequencing. Blood 73:281, 1989

99. Yunis JJ, Boot AJM, Mayer MG, Bos JL: Mechanisms of *ras* mutation in myelodysplastic syndrome. Oncogene 4:609, 1989

100. Paquette RL, Landaw EM, Pierre RV et al: N-*ras*-mutations are associated with poor prognosis and increased risk of leukemia in myelodysplastic syndrome. Blood 82:590, 1993

101. Jonveaux PH, Fenaux P, Quiquandon I et al: Mutations in the p53 gene in myelodysplastic syndromes. Oncogene 6:2243, 1991

102. Oscier D: Myelodysplastic syndromes. Ballieres Clin Haematol 1:389, 1987

103. Aul C, Gatterman N, Schneider W: Age-related incidence and other epidemiological aspects of myelodysplastic syndrome. Br J Haematol 82:385, 1992

104. Young JL, Pollack ES: The incidence of cancer in the United States. p.138. In Schottenfeld D, Fraumeni JF (eds): Cancer Epidemiology and Prevention. WB Saunders, Philadelphia, 1982

105. May SJ, Smith SA, Jacobs A et al: The myelodysplastic syndrome: analysis of laboratory characteristics in relation to the FAB classification. Br J Haematol 59:311, 1985

106. Chalevelakis G, Karaoulis S, Yalouris AG et al: Globin chain synthesis in myelodysplastic syndromes. J Clin Pathol 44:134, 1991

107. Lintula R: Red cell enzymes in myelodysplastic syndromes: a review. Scand J Haematol, suppl. 45. 36:56, 1986

108. Newman DR, Pierre RV, Linman JW: Studies on the diagnostic significance of haemoglobin F levels. Mayo Clin Proc 48:199, 1973

109. Annino L, Di Giovanni S, Tentori L Jr et al: Acquired haemoglobin H disease in a case of refractory anaemia with excess of blasts (RAEB) evolving into acute nonlymphoid leukemia. Acta Haematol 72:41, 1984

110. Higgs DR, Wood WG, Barton C, Weatherall DJ: Clinical features and molecular analysis of acquired hemoglobin H disease. Am J Med 75:181, 1983

111. Salmon A: Blood group changes in preleukaemic states. Blood Cells 2:211, 1976

112. Hauptman GM, Sondag D, Lang JM, Oberling F: False positive acidified serum lysis test in preleukaemic dyserythropoiesis. Acta Haematol 59:73, 1978

113. Galton DAG: The myelodysplastic syndromes. Scand J Hematol, suppl. 45. 36:16, 1986

114. Garcia S, Sanz MA, Amigo V et al: Prognostic factors in chronic myelodysplastic syndromes. Am J Hematol 27:163, 1988

115. Mufti GJ, Stevens JR, Oscier DG et al: Myelodysplastic syndromes: a scoring system with prognostic significance. Br J Haematol 59:311, 1985

116. Ruutu T: Granulocyte function in the myelodysplastic syndromes. Scand J Haematol, suppl. 45. 36:66, 1986

117. Boogaerts MA, Nelissen V, Roelant C, Goosens W: Blood neutrophil function in primary myelodysplastic syndromes. Br J Haematol 55:217, 1983

118. Martin S, Baldock SC, Ghoneim ATM, Child JA: Defective neutrophil function and microbicidal mechanisms in the myelodysplastic syndromes. J Clin Pathol 36:1120, 1983

119. Williamson PJ, Oscier DG, Mufti GJ, Hamblin TJ: Pyogenic abscesses in the myelodysplastic syndrome. Br Med J 299:375, 1990

120. Zwierzina H, Sepp N, Ringler E, Schmalzl R: Delayed maturation of skin window macrophages in myelodysplastic syndromes. J Clin Pathol 13:433, 1989

121. Clark RE, Hoy TG, Jacobs A: Granulocyte and monocyte surface membrane markers in the myelodysplastic syndromes. J Clin Pathol 38:301, 1985

122. Takagi S, Kitagawa S, Takeda A et al: Natural killer-interferon system in patients with preleukaemic states. Br J Haematol 58:71, 1984

123. Takaku S, Takaku F: Natural killer cell activity and preleukaemia. Lancet 2:1178, 1981

124. Rasi V, Lintula R: Platelet function in the myelodysplastic syndrome. Scand J Haematol 36:71, 1986

125. Castro M, Conn D, Su W et al: Rheumatic manifestations in myelodysplastic syndromes. J Rheumatol 18:721, 1991

126. George S, Newman E: Seronegative inflammatory arthritis in the myelodysplastic syndromes. Sem Auth Rheumatol 21:345, 1992

127. Hamblin T: Immunologic abnormalities in myelodysplastic syndromes. Hematol Oncol Clin North Am 6:571, 1992

128. van den Berghe H, Cassiman JJ, David G et al: Distinct haematological disorder with deletion of long arm of the 5 chromosome. Nature 251:437, 1974

129. van den Berghe H, Vermaelen K, Mecucci C et al: The 5q− anomaly. Cancer Genet Cytogenet 17:189, 1985

130. Riccardi A, Giordano M, Girino M, et al: Refractory cytopenias: clinical course according to bone marrow cytology and cellularity. Blut 54:153, 1987

131. Kokil G, Michaux JL, van den Berghe H et al: A new hematologic syndrome with a distinct karyotype: The 5q− chromosome. Blood 46:519, 1975

132. Coiffier B, Adeleine P, Viala JJ et al: Dysmyelopoietic syndromes: a search for prognostic factors in 193 patients. Cancer 52:83, 1983

133. Yoshida Y, Oguma S, Uchino H et al: Refractory myelodysplastic anaemias with hypocellular bone marrow. J Clin Pathol 41:763, 1988

134. Nand S, Godwin JE: Hypoplastic myelodysplastic syndrome. Cancer 62:958, 1988

135. Riccardi A, Giordana M, Girino M et al: Clinical course according to bone marrow cytology and cellularity. Blut 54:153, 1987

136. Appelbaum FR, Barrall J, Storb R et al: Clonal cytogenetic abnormalities in patients with otherwise typical aplastic anemia. Exp Hematol 15:1134, 1987

137. DePlanque MM, Bacigalup A, Wursch A et al: Long-term follow up of severe aplastic anaemia patients treated with antihymocyte globulin. Br J Haematol 73:121, 1989

138. Tichelli A, Gratwohl A, Wursch A: Late haematological complications in severe aplastic anaemia. Br J Haematol 69:413, 1988

139. Zsebo KM, Williams DA, Geissler EN et al: Stem cell factor is encoded at the *Sl* locus of the mouse and is the ligand for the *c-kit* tyrosine kinase receptor. Cell 63:213, 1990

140. Ohyashiki K, Ohyashiki JH, Iwabuchi A et al: Clinical and cytogenetic characteristics of myelodysplastic syndromes developing myelofibrosis. Cancer 68:178, 1991

141. Pagliuca A, Layton DM, Manoharan A et al: Myelofibrosis in primary myelodysplastic syndromes: a clinico-morphological study of 10 cases. Br J Haematol 71:499, 1989

142. Rios A, Canizo MC, Sanz MA et al: Bone marrow biopsy in myelodysplastic syndromes: morphological characteristics and contribution to the study of prognostic factors. Br J Haematol 75:26, 1990

143. Michels SD, McKenna RW, Arthur DC et al: Therapy-related acute myeloid leukemia and myelodysplastic syndrome: a clinical and morphologic study of 65 cases. Blood 65:1365, 1985

144. Vardiman JW, Le Beau MM, Albain K et al: Myelodysplasia: a comparison of therapy-related and primary forms. Ann Biol Clin (Paris) 43:369, 1985

145. Lambertenghi-Deliliers G, Orazi A, Luksch R et al: Myelodysplastic syndrome with increased marrow fibrosis: a distinct clinicopathological entity. Br J Haematol 78:161, 1991

146. Kampmeier P, Anastasi J, Vardiman JM: Issues in the pathology of myelodysplastic syndromes. Hematol Oncol Clin North Am 6:501, 1992

147. Najean Y, Deschamps A, Dresch C et al: Acute leukemia and myelodysplasia in polycythemia vera: a clinical study with long-term follow up. Cancer 61:89, 1988

148. Shamdas GJ, Spier CM, List AF: Myelodysplastic transformation of polycythemia vera: case report and review of the literature. Am J Hematol 37:45, 1991

149. Storniolo AM, Moloney WC, Rosenthal DS et al: Chronic myelomonocytic leukemia. Leukemia 4:766, 1990

150. Foucar K, Langdon RM, Armitage JO et al: Myelodysplastic syndromes: a clinical and pathologic analysis of 109 cases. Cancer 56:553, 1985

151. Tefferi A, Hoagland HC, Therneau TM et al: Chronic myelomonocytic leukemia: natural history and prognostic determinants. Mayo Clin Proc 64:1246, 1989

152. Fenaux P, Jouet JP, Zandecki M et al: Chronic and subacute myelomonocytic leukaemia in the adult: a report of 60 cases with special reference to prognostic factors. Br J Haematol 65:101, 1987

153. Solal-Celigny P, Desaint B, Herrera A et al: Chronic myelomonocytic leukemia according to FAB classification: analysis of 35 cases. Blood 63:634, 1984

154. Pugh WC, Pearson M, Vardiman JW et al: Philadelphia chromosome-negative chronic myelogenous leukaemia: a morphological reassessment. Br J Haematol 60:457, 1985

155. Fitzgerald PH, Beard MEJ, Morris CM et al: Ph-negative chronic myeloid leukaemia. Br J Haematol 66:311, 1987

156. Wiedemann LM, Karhi KK, Shivji MKK et al: The correlation of breakpoint cluster region rearrangement and p210 *phl/abl* expression with morphological analysis of Ph-negative chronic myeloid leukaemia and other myeloproliferative diseases. Blood 71:349, 1988

157. Frindel E, Masse A, Pradelles P et al: Correlation of endogenous acetyl-ser-asp-lys-pro plasma levels in mice and the kinetics of pluripotent hemopoietic stem cells entry into the cycle after cytosine arabinoside treatment. Leukemia 6:599, 1992

158. Kantarjian H, Keating M, Walters R et al: Therapy-related leukemia and myelodysplastic syndrome: clinical, cytogenetic, and prognostic features. J Clin Oncol 4:1743, 1986

159. Pedersen-Bjergaard J: Radiotherapy- and chemotherapy-induced myelodysplasia and acute myeloid leukemia. A review. Leuk Res 16:61, 1992

160. Farrow A, Jacobs A, West RR: Myelodysplasia, chemical exposure and other environmental factors. Leukemia 3:33, 1989

161. Brandt L: Exposure to organic solvents and risk of haematological malignancies. Leuk Res 16:67, 1992

162. Ratain MJ, Kaminer LS, Bitran JD et al: Acute nonlymphocytic leukemia following etoposide and cisplatin combination chemotherapy for advanced non-small-cell carcinoma of the lung. Blood 70:1412, 1987

163. Pedersen-Bjergaard J, Philip P, Larsen SO et al: Chromosome aberrations and prognostic factors in therapy-related myelodysplasia and acute non-lymphocytic leukemia. Blood 76:1083, 1990

164. Pedersen-Bjergaard J, Philip P: Balanced translocations involving chromosome bands 11q23 and 21q22 are highly characteristic of myelodysplasia and leukemia following therapy with cytostatic agents targeting at DNA-topoisomerase II. Blood 78:1147, 1991

165. Holmes J, Jacobs A, Carter G et al: Multidrug resistance in haemopoietic cell lines, myelodysplastic syndromes and acute myeloblastic leukemia. Br J Haematol 72:40, 1989

166. Horiike S, Taniwaki M, Misawa S, Abe T: Chromosome abnormalities and karyotypic evolution in 83 patients with myelodysplastic syndrome and predictive value for prognosis. Cancer 62:1129, 1988

167. List AF, Spier CM, Cline A et al: Expression of the multidrug resistance gene product (P-glycoprotein) in myelodysplasia is associated with a stem cell phenotype. Br J Haematol 78:28, 1991

168. Armitage JO, Dick FR, Needleman SW, Burns CP: Effect of chemotherapy for the dysmyelopoietic syndrome. Cancer Treat Rep 65:601, 1981

169. Preisler HD, Raza A, Barcos M et al: High-dose cytosine arabinoside in the treatment of preleukemic disorders. Am J Hematol 23:131, 1986

170. Mertelsmann R, Tzvi-Thaler H, To L et al: Morphological classification, response to therapy, and survival in 263 adult patients with acute non-lymphoblastic leukemia. Blood 56:773, 1980

171. Tricot G, Boogaerts MA, Verwilghen RL: Treatment of patients with myelodysplastic syndromes: a review. Scand J Haematol, suppl. 45:121, 1986

172. Fenaux P, Lai JL, Jouet JP et al: Aggressive chemotherapy in adult primary myelodysplastic syndromes. A report on 29 cases. Blut 57:297, 1988

173. Baccarani M, Tura S: Differentiation of myeloid leukaemic cells: new possibilities for therapy. Br J Haematol 42:485, 1979

174. Wisch JS, Griffin JD, Kufe DW: Response of preleukemic syndromes to continuous infusion of low-dose cytarabine. N Engl J Med 309:1599, 1983

175. Chesson BD, Jasperse DM, Simon R et al: A critical appraisal of low-dose cytosine arabinoside in patients with acute non-lymphocytic leukemia and myelodysplastic syndromes. J Clin Oncol 4:1857, 1986

176. Cheson BD, Simon R: Low-dose ara-C in acute nonlymphocytic leukemia and myelodysplastic syndromes: a review of 20 years' experience. Sem Oncol, suppl. 1. 14:126, 1987

177. Miller KB, Kim K, Morrison FS et al: Evaluation of low dose ara-C versus supportive care in the treatment of myelodysplastic syndromes, abstracted. Blood, suppl. 1. 72:215A, 1988

178. Anderson JE, Appelbaum FR, Fisher LD et al: Allogeneic bone marrow transplantation for 93 patients with myelodysplastic syndrome. Blood 82:677, 1993

179. DeWitte T, Zwaan F, Hermans J et al: Allogeneic bone marrow transplantation for secondary leukaemia and myelodysplastic syndrome. Br J Haematol 74:151, 1989

180. O'Donnell MR, Nadamanee AP, Snyder DS et al: Bone marrow transplantation for myelodysplastic and myeloproliferative syndromes. J Clin Oncol 5:1822, 1987

181. Bagby GC Jr, Gabourel JD, Linman JW: Glucocorticoid therapy in the preleukemia syndrome (hemopoietic dysplasia): identification of responsive patients using in-vitro techniques. Ann Intern Med 92:55, 1980

182. Najean Y, Pecking A: Refractory anaemia with excess of myeloblasts in the bone marrow: a clinical trial of androgens in 90 patients. Br J Haematol 37:25, 1977

183. Najean Y, Pecking A: Refractory anemia with excess of blast cells: prognostic factors and effects of treatment with androgens or cytosine arabinoside. Results of a prospective trial in 58 patients. Cancer 44:1976, 1979

184. Cines CB, Cassileth PA, Kiss JE: Danazol therapy in myelodysplasia. Ann Intern Med 103:58, 1985

185. Picozzi VJ Jr, Swanson GF, Morgan R et al: 13-cis-retinoic acid treatment for myelodysplastic syndromes. J Clin Oncol 4:589, 1986

186. Koeffler HP, Heitgan D, Mertelsmann R et al: Randomized study of 13 cis-retinoic acid vs placebo in the myelodysplastic disorders. Blood 71:703, 1988

187. Koeffler HP, Hirji K, Itri L: 1,25-dihydroxyvitamin D_3: in vivo and in vitro effects of human preleukemic and leukemic cells. Cancer Treat Rep 69:1399, 1985

188. Ohno R, Naoe T, Hirano M et al: Treatment of myelodysplastic syndromes with all-trans retinoic acid. Blood 81:1152, 1993

189. Itoh N, Yonehara S, Schreurs J et al: Cloning of an interleukin-3 receptor gene: a member of a distinct receptor gene family. Science 247:324, 1990

190. Silverman LR, Davis RB, Holland JF et al: 5-azacytidine as a low dose continu-

ous infusion is an effective therapy for patients with myelodysplastic syndromes. Proc Am Soc Clin Oncol 8:198, 1989

191. Maiolo AT, Cortelezzi A, Calori R, Polli EE, for the Italian Study Group: Recombinant gamma-interferon as first line therapy for high risk myelodysplastic syndromes. Leukemia 4:480, 1990

192. Ogawa M, Yoshida Y, Moriyama Y et al: A phase II clinical trial of recombinant interferon-gamma on myelodysplastic syndromes, abstracted. Blut 56: c21, 1988

193. Elias L, Hoffman R, Boswell S et al: A trial of recombinant α2 interferon in the myelodysplastic syndromes. Leukemia 1:105, 1987

194. Gisslinger H, Chott A, Linkesch W et al: Long-term α-interferon therapy in myelodysplastic syndromes. Leukemia 4:91, 1990

195. Galvani DW, Nethersell ABW, Cawley JC: α-Interferon in myelodysplasia: clinical observations and effects on NK cells. Leuk Res 12:257, 1988

196. Metcalf D: The molecular biology and functions of the granulocyte-macrophage colony-stimulating factors. Blood 67:257, 1986

197. Sieff CA: Hematopoietic growth factors. J Clin Invest 79:1549, 1987

198. Vadhan-Raj S, Keating M, LeMaistre A et al: Effects of recombinant human granulocyte-macrophage colony-stimulating factor in patients with myelodysplastic syndromes. N Engl J Med 317:1545, 1987

199. Antin JH, Smith BR, Holmes W et al: Phase I/II study of recombinant granulocyte-macrophage colony-stimulating factor in aplastic anemia and myelodysplastic syndrome. Blood 72:705, 1988

200. Ganser A, Volkers B, Greher J et al: Recombinant human granulocyte-macrophage colony-stimulating factor in patients with myelodysplastic syndromes—a Phase I/II trial. Blood 73:31, 1989

201. Herrmann F, Lindemann A, Klein H et al: Effect of recombinant granulocyte-macrophage colony-stimulating factor in patients with myelodysplastic syndrome with excess blasts. Leukemia 3:335, 1989

202. Thompson JA, Lee DJ, Kidd P et al: Subcutaneous granulocyte-macrophage colony-stimulating factor in patients with myelodysplastic syndrome: toxicity, pharmacokinetics, and hematological effects. J Clin Oncol 7:629, 1989

203. Greenberg PL: Treatment of myelodysplastic syndromes with hemopoietic growth factors. Semin Oncol 19:106, 1992

204. Gradishar W, Le Beau MM, O'Laughlin R et al: Clinical and cytogenetic responses to GM-CSF in therapy-related myelodysplastic syndrome. Blood 80: 2463, 1992

205. Willemze R, van der Lely N, Zwierzina H et al: A randomized phase I/II multicenter study of recombinant human GM-CSF therapy for patients with myelodysplastic syndromes and a relatively low risk of acute leukemia. Ann Hematol 464:173, 1992

206. Schuster MW, Thompson JA, Larson R et al: Randomized trial of subcutaneous granulocyte-macrophage colony-stimulating factor versus observation in patients with myelodysplastic syndrome or aplastic anemia. Proc Am Soc Clin Oncol A793, 1990

207. Economopoulos T, Papageorgiou E, Stathakis N et al: Treatment of myelodysplastic syndromes with human granulocyte-macrophage colony-stimulating factor (GM-CSF) or GM-CSF combined with low-dose cytosine arabinoside. Eur J Haematol 49:138, 1992

208. Negrin RS, Haeuber DH, Nagler A et al: Treatment of myelodysplastic syndromes with recombinant human granulocyte colony stimulating factor. Ann Intern Med 110:976, 1992

209. Negrin RS, Nagler A, Kobayashi Y et al: Maintenance treatment of patients with myelodysplastic syndromes using recombinant human granulocyte colony stimulating factor. Blood 78:36, 1992

210. Yoshida Y, Hirashima K, Asano S et al: A phase II trial of recombinant human granulocyte colony-stimulating factor in the myelodysplastic syndromes. Br J Haematol 78:378, 1991

211. Vadhan-Raj S, Broxmeyer HE, Spitzer G et al: Stimulation of nonclonal hematopoiesis and suppression of the neoplastic clone after treatment with recombinant human GM-CSF in a patient with therapy-related myelodysplastic syndrome. Blood 74:1491, 1989

212. Ganser A, Seipelt G, Lindemann A et al: Effects of recombinant human interleukin-3 in patients with myelodysplastic syndromes. Blood 6:455, 1990

213. Kurzrock R, Talpaz M, Estrov Z et al: Phase I study of recombinant human interleukin-3 in patients with bone marrow failure. J Clin Oncol 9:1241, 1991

214. Ganser A, Ottmann OG, Seipelt G et al: Effect of long-term treatment with recombinant human interleukin-3 in patients with myelodysplastic syndromes. Leukemia 7:696, 1993

215. Gordon MS, Nemunaitis J, Hoffman R et al: Phase I trial of subcutaneous recombinant human interleukin-6 in patents with myelodysplasia and thrombocytopenia. Blood, suppl. 1. 80:249a, 1992

216. Jacobs A, Janowska-Wieczorek A, Caro J et al: Circulating erythropoietin in patients with myelodysplastic syndromes. Br J Haematol 73:36, 1989

217. Bessho M, Jinnai I, Matsuda A: Improvement of anemia by recombinant erythropoietin in patients with myelodysplastic syndromes and aplastic anemia. Int J Cell Cloning 8:445, 1990

218. Stebler C, Tichelli A, Dazzi H et al: High-dose recombinant human erythropoietin for treatment of anemia in MDS and paroxysmal nocturnal hemoglobinuria: a pilot study. Exp Hematol 18:1204, 1990

219. Stein R, Abels R, Krantz S: Pharmacologic doses of recombinant human erythropoietin in the treatment of myelodysplastic syndromes. Blood 78: 1658, 1991

220. van Kamp H, Prinsze-Postema T, Kluin PM et al: Effect of subcutaneously administered human recombinant erythropoietin in patients with myelodysplasia. Br J Haematol 78:488, 1991

221. Hellstrom E, Birgegaård G, Lockner D et al: Treatment of myelodysplastic syndromes with recombinant human erythropoietin. Eur J Haematol 47:355, 1991

222. Schouten HC, Vellenga E, van Rhenen D et al: Recombinant human erythropoietin for patients with a myelodysplastic syndrome. Blood 76:317, 1990

223. Bowen D, Culligan D, Jacobs AJ: The treatment of anaemia in the myelodysplastic syndromes with recombinant human erythropoietin. Br J Haematol 77:419, 1991

224. Negrin RS, Stein R, Doherty K et al: Treatment of the anemias of MDS using recombinant human granulocyte colony-stimulating factor in combination with erythropoietin. Blood 82:737, 1993

225. Hellstrom-Lindberg E, Birgegard G, Carlsson M et al: A combination of G-CSF and erythropoietin may synergistically improve the anaemia in patients with myelodysplastic syndromes. Leuk Lymphoma 11:221, 1993

226. Greenberg PL, Negrin RS, Ginzton N: In vitro-in vivo correlations of erythroid responses to G-CSF plus erythropoietin in myelodysplastic syndromes. Exp Hematol 20:733a, 1992

227. Mufti GJ, Stevens JR, Oscier DG et al: Myelodysplastic syndromes: a scoring system with prognostic significance. Br J Haematol 59:425, 1985

228. Kerkhofs H, Hermans J, Haak HL et al: Utility of the FAB classification for myelodysplastic syndromes: investigation of prognostic factors in 237 cases. Br J Haematol 65:73, 1987

229. Tricot G, Vlietinck R, Boogaerts MA et al: Prognostic factors in the myelodysplastic syndromes: importance of initial data on peripheral blood counts, bone marrow cytology, trephine biopsy and chromosomal analysis. Br J Haematol 60:19, 1985

230. Vallespi T, Torrabadella M, Julia A et al: A study of 101 cases according to the FAB classification. Br J Haematol 61:83, 1985

231. Sanz GF, Sanz MA, Vallespi T et al: Two regression models and a scoring system for predicting survival and planning treatment in myelodysplastic syndromes: a multivariate analysis of prognostic factors in 370 patients. Blood 74:395, 1989

232. Coiffier B, Adeleine P, Viala JJ et al: Dysmyelopoietic syndromes. A search for prognostic factors in 193 patients. Cancer 52:83, 1983

233. Sanz GF, Sanz MA: Prognostic factors in myelodysplastic syndromes. Leuk Res 16:77, 1992

234. Fenaux P, Benscart R, Lai J: Prognostic factors in adult CMML. Analysis of 107 cases. J Clin Oncol 6:1417, 1990

235. Billstrom R, Thiede T, Hansen S et al: Bone marrow karyotype and prognosis in primary myelodysplastic syndromes. Eur J Haematol 41:341, 1988

236. Pedersen-Bjergaard J, Philip P, Larsen SO et al: Chromosome aberrations and prognostic factors in therapy-related myelodysplasia and acute nonlymphocytic leukemia. Blood 76:1083, 1990

237. Yunis JJ, Lobell M, Arnesen MA et al: Refined chromosome subgroups helps define prognostic subgroups in most patients with primary myelodysplastic syndrome and acute myelogenous leukaemia. Br J Haematol 68:189, 1988

238. Le Beau MM, Albain KS, Larson RA et al: Clinical and cytogenetic correlations in 63 patients with therapy-related myelodysplastic syndromes and acute nonlymphocytic leukemias: further incidence for characteristic abnormalities of chromosomes nos. 5 and 7. J Clin Oncol 4:325, 1986

239. Yunis JJ, Rydell RE, Oken MM et al: Refined chromosome analysis as an independent prognostic indicator in *de novo* myelodysplastic syndromes. Blood 67:1721, 1986

240. Tricot G, Boogaerts MA, De Wolf-Peeters C et al: The myelodysplastic syndromes: different evolution patterns based on sequential morphological and cytogenetic investigations. Br J Haematol 58:759, 1985

241. Geddes AD, Bowen DT, Jacobs A: Clonal karyotype abnormalities and clinical progression in the myelodysplastic syndrome. Br J Haematol 76:194, 1990

242. Benitez J, Carbonell F, Sanchez Fayos J. Heimpel H: Karyotypic evolution in patients with myelodysplastic syndromes. Cancer Genet Cytogenet 16: 157, 1985

243. Berthier R, Douady F, Metral J et al: In vitro granulopoiesis in oligoblastic leukemia: prognostic value, characterization and serial cloning of bone mar-

row colony and cluster forming cells in agar culture. Biomedicine 30:305, 1979

244. Greenberg PL, Bax I, Mara B et al: The myeloproliferative disorders: correlation between clinical evolution and alteration of granulopoiesis. Am J Med 61:878, 1976

245. Faille A, Dresch C, Poirer O et al: Prognostic value of in vitro bone marrow culture in refractory anaemia with excess of myeloblasts. Scand J Haematol 20:280, 1978

246. Milner GR, Testa NG, Geary CG et al: Bone marrow studies in refractory cytopenia and smoldering leukaemia. Br J Haematol 35:251, 1977

247. Spitzer G, Verma D, Dicke K et al: Subgroups of oligoleukemia as identified by in vitro agar culture. Leuk Res 3:29, 1979

248. Verma DS, Spitzer G, Dicke KA et al: In vitro agar culture patterns in preleukemia and their clinical significance. Leuk Res 3:41, 1979

249. Buick RN, Till JR, McCulloch EA: Colony assay for proliferating blast cells circulating in myeloblastic leukaemia. Lancet 1:862, 1977

250. Senn JS, Messner HA, Pinkerton PH: Peripheral blood blast cell progenitors in human preleukemia. Blood 59:106, 1982

251. Greenberg P, Taylor K, Larson R et al: Phase III randomized multicenter trial of recombinant human G-CSF in MDS. Blood, suppl. 1. 82:196a, 1993

252. Metcalf D: The roles of stem cell self-renewal and autocrine growth factor production in the biology of myeloid leukemia. Cancer Res 49:2305, 1989

253. Miyauchi J, Kelleher CA, Yang YC et al: The effects of three recombinant growth factors, IL3, GM-CSF and G-CSF, on the blast cells of acute myeloblastic leukemia maintained in short-term suspension culture. Blood 76:657, 1987

254. Vellenga E, Young DC, Wagner K et al: The effects of GM-CSF and G-CSF in promoting growth of clonogenic cells in acute myeloblastic leukemia. Blood 69:1771, 1987

Polycythemia Vera

72

Ronald Hoffman and H. Scott Boswell

INTRODUCTION

Polycythemia vera is a hematologic malignancy that leads to excessive proliferation of erythroid, myeloid, and megakaryocytic elements within the bone marrow. Vaquez[1] first described this clinical entity in 1892, noting the characteristic physical findings. At the turn of this century, Vaquez,[1] Cabot,[2] and finally Osler[3] associated the name polycythemia vera with this newly described clinical disorder. Polycythemia vera is a clonal, chronic, progressive myeloproliferative disorder, often of insidious onset, characterized by an absolute increase in red cell mass and usually leukocytosis, thrombocytosis, and splenomegaly.[4,5]

Recently, new insight into the pathogenesis of this disorder has been gained. Studies have been performed to investigate the response of hematopoietic progenitor cells derived from the malignant clone to hematopoietic regulatory factors.[6-8] In the absence of definitive evidence for changes in the number of receptors for the known hematopoietic growth factors, these progenitor cells are characterized by increased responsiveness to a variety of hematopoietic regulatory molecules. This heightened responsiveness probably arises from an undefined event that occurs at a receptor or postreceptor level.

Polycythemia vera differs from many other hematologic malignancies, in that prolonged survival is enjoyed by most patients if the excessive production of red blood cells and platelets can be controlled.[9] This prolonged survival, however, is punctuated by the development of other syndromes, such as myelofibrosis and acute leukemia[9-11] (Table 72-1). Frequently patients present asymptomatically to a physician only to find that they have either splenomegaly, isolated erythrocytosis, or thrombocytosis; left untreated, these patients will become symptomatic, owing to the consequences of the excessive production of red blood cells or platelets, or both. After a number of years, the erythrocytotic phase of the disease frequently becomes inactive, and the patient may no longer suffer from the sequelae of excessive red cell production. Subsequently, these patients can develop so-called spent-phase or postpolycythemic myeloid metaplasia, which is frequently indistinguishable from another myeloproliferative disorder, agnogenic myeloid metaplasia.[9-11] Finally, a significant proportion of these patients will eventually go on to develop acute myeloid leukemia.

The constantly changing clinical picture of this malignant hematologic disorder requires careful observation and treatment to deal with the numerous problems that can be encountered.

Table 72-1. Evolution of Polycythemia Vera

Stage	Clinical Findings
Asymptomatic	Splenomegaly
	Isolated erythrocytosis
	Isolated thrombocytosis
↓	
Erythrocytotic phase	Erythrocytosis
	Thrombocytosis
	Leukocytosis
	Splenomegaly
	Thrombosis
	Hemorrhage
	Pruritus
↓	
Inactive phase	No longer requires phlebotomy or chemotherapy
	? Iron deficient
↓	
Postpolycythemic myeloid metaplasia	Anemia
	Leukoerythroblastosis
	Thrombocytopenia or thrombocytosis
	Enlarging splenomegaly
	Systemic symptoms (fever, weight loss)
↓	
Acute myeloid leukemia	

EPIDEMIOLOGY AND PATHOGENESIS

Polycythemia vera is a rare disorder, with an annual incidence in Western Europe and the United States of approximately 5–17 cases per 1 million population per year.[12–14] Actual determination of its prevalence is a difficult process because of the need for an extensive diagnostic evaluation to differentiate this disorder from other causes of spurious or absolute erythrocytosis.[15] The prevalence of polycythemia vera has been stated by several investigators to be higher among American Jews and lower among black Americans.[12,16,17] The incidence of the disorder is greater among Ashkenazi Jews, who originate from eastern and central Europe, than among Arabs and Sephardic Jews.[18] Interestingly, extremely low occurrence rates have been reported from Japan, where the incidence was found to be two cases per million per year.[19] These findings suggest that important environmental or genetic factors might be involved in the biogenesis of this disorder. One notable exception to the low prevalence of polycythemia vera in Japan has been the higher incidence observed among populations exposed to atomic bomb explosions.[20] The possibility that radiation exposure is an etiologic factor in the generation of polycythemia vera was also raised by the observation in the United States of four cases of polycythemia vera 10–20 years after a nuclear explosion to which somewhat >3,000 military observers were exposed.[21]

An epidemiologic investigation focused on occupational exposure among petroleum refinery and chemical plant workers has revealed an increased incidence of polycythemia vera relative to the general population.[22] In this study, the increased incidence of polycythemia vera was linked to similar increases in the frequency of multiple myeloma and non-Hodgkin lymphoma, suggesting involvement of a putative environmental toxin that may have broad hematopoietic toxicity.[22]

The importance of genetic factors in the origin of this disease is further emphasized by several case reports of polycythemia vera within families.[23–26] A greater than expected prevalence has been reported in the parents of patients with this disorder.[27] In addition, one family of three sisters all having the disorder has been reported.[28] An additional report describes a father and son who were both exposed to organic solvents and in whom polycythemia vera subsequently developed.[29] These forms of familial polycythemia vera must be distinguished from a familial polycythemic illness characterized by isolated erythrocytosis inherited as an autosomal dominant.[30] None of the affected family members with this familial polycythemia has experienced health-related problems similar to those observed in patients with polycythemia vera. The reports of families in which multiple members have polycythemia vera raise the possibility that a genetic predisposition occurring in concert with several additional external insults might lead to the development of polycythemia vera. Slightly more males than females develop this disorder; the male/female ratio is approximately 1.2:1.[12] The average age at diagnosis is 60 years,[12] and the disease is extremely rare <30 years of age. In several large studies, 5% of patients with polycythemia vera were <40 years of age, 1% were <25 years old at diagnosis, and 0.1% were calculated to be <20 years old.[4,10,31] To date, <12 patients with polycythemia vera have been reported who presented with this disorder during childhood.[32]

BIOLOGIC AND MOLECULAR ASPECTS

Considerable speculation has centered on the pathobiology of the erythrocytosis that characterizes polycythemia vera.[33] London et al.[34] established that the expanded red cell mass of polycythemia vera was due to a two- to threefold increase in the production of red blood cells by a hyperplastic marrow and was not attributable to prolongation of the red cell life span. Granulocyte and platelet production are also increased in this disorder. This overly exuberant production of all cellular elements of the blood suggests that the basic defect resides at the level of the cell from which each of these cells originates, the pluripotent hematopoietic stem cell.

The hematopoietic growth factor erythropoietin (EPO) is considered to be the physiologic regulator of the later phases of erythropoiesis.[35] Alterations in its production are followed by adjustments in the rate of formation of red blood cells.[36] In humans, EPO production is controlled by the relative supply of oxygen to the kidney, the major site of erythropoietin formation.[35] Studies in animals have indicated that in response to anemia the liver may contribute 10–25% of the total EPO mRNA, whose production appears to be regulated by alterations in the rate of gene transcription.[37,38] EPO causes the differentiation and proliferation of a pool of erythroid progenitor cells, which eventually results in increased production of mature red blood cells.[35,39] These committed erythroid progenitor cells ultimately originate from a pluripotential hematopoietic stem cell also capable of producing myeloid and megakaryocytic elements.[35] The novel multipotential hematopoietin Steel locus factor, the ligand for c-kit, is also strongly implicated in the earliest steps of erythropoietic development from the pluripotential hematopoietic progenitor cell.[40] Interleukin-3 (IL-3) and colony-stimulating factor-granulocyte/macrophage may contribute to the early proliferative expansion of these multipotential progenitors.[41]

Alterations in EPO production can lead to the development of anemia and erythrocytosis.[36] An increased red cell mass, for instance, can be the result of EPO elaboration resulting from chronic hypoxia or can be the consequence of EPO secretion by a tumor or cyst, which is independent of physiologic control mechanisms.[42,43] By contrast, decreased production of EPO is an important component in the pathobiology of the anemia of chronic renal failure.[44] This deficiency was the initial focus for pharmaceutical development of EPO, an endeavor that has been highly successful.[44]

A large body of information has been obtained over the years addressing EPO physiology in patients with erythrocytosis.[42,43] A variety of assays for quantitation of levels of this hormone have been developed.[45–52] EPO concentrations in the past have been estimated by in vivo bioassays using posthypoxic polycythemic mice.[45–47] In these assays, patient plasma or urine preparations containing EPO are injected into animals, and the incorporation of radioactive iron into newly produced erythrocytes is monitored. The proportional increase in radioactive iron incorporation into red blood cells is then correlated with the EPO content of the particular specimen.[45–47] Basal levels of EPO excretion have been defined by using urine samples obtained from normal subjects.[45–47] Following phlebotomy of a healthy person, urinary EPO excretion increases, and an inverse logarithmic relationship between hematocrit and EPO excretion rate is observed.[36] Patients with secondary erythrocytosis due to chronic hypoxia have either normal or increased basal values, but all have increased values following reduction of hematocrit to normal levels by phlebotomy.[36] By contrast, urinary EPO excretion is invariably low in patients with polycythemia vera, which demonstrates that this disorder is not due to excessive EPO production.[36]

The use of in vivo assays to measure EPO levels has not been entirely satisfactory, however. Such bioassays are impractical when quantitating hormone levels in large numbers of samples, as their performance is expensive and if normal or low concentrations of EPO are present, a substantial sample volume must be concentrated.[35] In vitro bioassays that use bone marrow cells in culture have been developed but vary in their specificity.[49] Following the purification of EPO and its subsequent cloning, radioimmunoassay (RIA) and enzyme-linked immunosor-

Table 72-2. Serum EPO Levels Obtained by RIA in Patients with Erythrocytosis

Patient Diagnosis	Patients (n)	Hematocrit (%)	Erythropoietin (Mean ±SD) (mU/ml)
Polycythemia vera	26	54	17 ± 8
Secondary polycythemia	33	56	94 ± 101
Lung-associated disease	7	55	80 ± 99
Heart disease	13	58	151 ± 126
Kidney disease	6	55	55 ± 19
Cancer	3	56	39 ± 5
Unknown	4	53	35 ± 19
Normal donors	26	41	15 ± 4

(From Koeffler and Goldwasser,[43] with permission.)

bent assay (ELISA) techniques for this hormone have been developed and have now entered widespread clinical use.[50–52] The RIAs provide great promise for further defining the role of EPO in the biogenesis of erythrocytosis.

A study by Koeffler and Goldwasser[43] was among the first reports to distinguish serum EPO levels in primary polycythemia vera, in secondary erythrocytosis, and in normal adults for diagnostic purposes. These investigators measured serum concentrations of EPO in 59 patients with polycythemia, using such a RIA system. The mean EPO concentration was 17.5 ± 8.4 mU/ml in normal persons and 14.9 ± 4.2 mU/ml in 26 patients with polycythemia vera.[43] In 33 patients with secondary polycythemia, a significant elevation of serum EPO concentration was observed, with an average concentration of 94.3 ± 101.2 mU/ml (Table 72-2). Of the patients with polycythemia vera, 92% had concentrations of <30 mU/ml and 94% of those with secondary polycythemia had concentrations of >30 mU/ml.[43] It is important to emphasize that the average hematocrit value in polycythemia vera and in secondary polycythemia patients did not differ. This study indicates an overall correct classification of 93% of patients using an RIA for quantitation of serum EPO.[43] These observations have now been confirmed by other groups.[42,52–54]

Recently, investigators have used highly purified recombinant EPO as the reference standard for RIAs of the hormone levels in patient serum. These studies have reported that patients with polycythemia vera most frequently exhibit serum EPO levels below the 95% confidence intervals for the range in normal controls. In two studies, the subnormal serum EPO levels were maintained even after several phlebotomies had been performed to normalize the serum hemoglobin concentration in polycythemia vera patients.[55,56]

In 1951 Dameshek[5] postulated that chronic myeloid leukemia (CML), polycythemia vera, primary thrombocythemia, and agnogenic myeloid metaplasia with myelofibrosis were related disorders, which he called myeloproliferative syndromes. He concluded that these disorders resulted from a generalized hyperresponsiveness of marrow cells to myelostimulatory factors and speculated that these disorders were neoplastic in origin.[5]

Since the mid-1970s, a substantial amount of data has accumulated that conclusively demonstrates polycythemia vera to be the result of a neoplastic proliferation of hematopoietic cells as first proposed by Dameshek.[57,58] The cellular origin of the disorder was first established by the analysis of glucose-6-phosphate dehydrogenase (G6PD) isoenzymes in black women who were heterozygous for this X-linked gene (Fig. 72-1). This approach was based on the random irreversible inactivation of one X chromosome in each female somatic cell during embryogenesis. Inactivation of the same X chromosome occurs in the progeny of these cells.[59] A normal black female heterozygous for G6PD will therefore have approximately equal populations of marrow cells with a different G6PD isoenzyme.[59] The

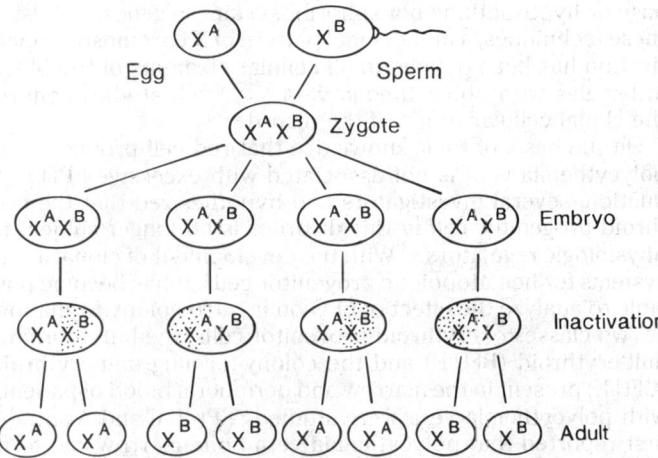

Fig. 72-1. Schematic presentation of X chromosome inactivation in an embryo heterozygous at the G6PD locus (Gd^b/Gd^a). In this diagram, the maternal X chromosome bears an A gene for G6PD(X^a) and the paternal X chromosome a B gene (X^b). During embryogenesis, one X chromosome in each somatic cell is randomly inactivated, so that one-half the somatic cells will have an active X^a and the other half an active X^b. Inactivation is fixed for a particular cell and its progeny. All progeny of an active X^a gene will express X^a. Female G6PD heterozygotes are mosaics, with some cells active X^a and others X^b. A tumor with clonal origin will consist entirely of either X^a or X^b cells and therefore will contain only G6PD type A or B but not both. Tumors with multicellular origin will contain both X^a and X^b cells and therefore both G6PD types. (From Fialkow,[261] with permission.)

G6PD isoenzymes can be readily distinguished by electrophoretic methods.

This approach was exploited by Adamson and co-workers[60] in an effort to determine the cellular origin of polycythemia vera. They presumed that cells composing a tumor that arises from a single cell in a G6PD heterozygote would express a single isoenzyme type, whereas a neoplasm originating from multiple cells would express both isoenzyme types.[59] These investigators found that circulating red cells, granulocytes, and platelets obtained from black females who were G6PD heterozygotes express the same isoenzyme, while skin and cultured marrow fibroblasts obtained from these same patients demonstrate both isoenzymes[60] (Table 72-3). They concluded that polycythemia vera represented a clonal proliferation of neoplastic hematopoietic stem cells and was not multicellular in origin or the consequence of excessive proliferation of normal hematopoietic stem cells.[60]

Using similar methods, Raskind et al.,[61] have demonstrated that the multipotential stem cell that is involved by the neoplastic process in polycythemia vera can also differentiate to B cells. The clonality of blood cell production in polycythemia vera has subsequently been confirmed by an alternative methodology; evaluation of X-linked restriction fragment length DNA analysis of polymorphisms of either the phosphoglycerate ki-

Table 72-3. Relative Amounts of G6PD Isoenzymes in Various Mesenchymal Tissues in Two Patients with Polycythemia Vera

Tissue	% A/% B Case 1	% A/% B Case 2
Skin	55:45	55:45
Lymphocytes	85:15[a]	55:45
Erythrocytes	100/0	100/0
Granulocytes	100/0	100/0
Platelets	100/0	100/0

[a] Contaminated with erythrocytes.
(From Adamson et al.,[57] with permission.)

nase or hypoxanthine phosphoribosyl kinase genes.[62,63] Using these techniques, a monoclonal pattern of X chromosome inactivation has been defined in all cellular elements of the blood in females with polycythemia vera.[62,63] Such studies confirm the clonal cellular origin of the disorder.

On the basis of their knowledge that red cell production in polycythemia vera is not associated with excessive EPO production, several investigators had hypothesized that the erythroid progenitor cell in this disorder is no longer subject to physiologic regulators.[33] With the development of clonal assay systems for hematopoietic progenitor cells, it has become possible to analyze the effect of EPO on in vitro colony formation.

Two classes of erythroid progenitor cells, the burst-forming unit-erythroid (BFU-E) and the colony-forming unit-erythroid (CFU-E) present in the marrow and peripheral blood of patients with polycythemia vera were studied.[64] Prchal and Axelrad[65] first reported that polycythemia vera bone marrow can form substantial numbers of erythroid colonies in vitro in the absence of exogenous EPO, whereas normal human bone marrow is incapable of forming such colonies without the addition of EPO. These erythroid colonies have been termed endogenous colonies.[65–67] When both polycythemia vera and normal bone marrow were subsequently assayed in the presence of EPO, polycythemia vera marrow was characterized by a higher cloning efficiency.[65–67] Several groups have reported that mixed colony formation was also enhanced in polycythemia vera.[68,69] Mixed colonies originate from multilineage progenitor cells. Their formation by polycythemia vera, but not by normal marrow, also occurs in vitro in the absence of exogenous EPO.[68,69] These observations suggest that the altered response to EPO in polycythemia vera is characteristic not only of erythroid progenitor cells but of more primitive hematopoietic progenitor cells as well. Cell cycle analysis of polycythemia vera colony-forming unit-multilineage (CFU-GEMM) BFU-E, CFU-E, and colony-forming unit-granulocyte/macrophage (CFU-GM) revealed another cell progenitor abnormality[68,70]; a higher proportion of polycythemia vera progenitor cells were in the synthetic phase of the cell cycle than was observed in normal subjects.[68,70]

Further insight into the cellular defect in polycythemia vera was provided by the studies of Prchal et al.[71] (Table 72-4). These workers cloned marrow cells from black female G6PD heterozygotes with polycythemia vera both in the presence and in the absence of exogenous EPO and demonstrated that the erythroid colonies that formed in the absence of exogenous EPO contained the same G6PD isoenzyme type as that expressed by peripheral blood elements.[71] Thus, the so-called endogenous colonies arose from the abnormal clone that was responsible for supplying red cells, granulocytes, and platelets to the peripheral blood. When exogenous EPO was added, increasing numbers of colonies were formed containing cellular elements expressing the other G6PD isoenzymes; presumably these colonies originated from cells not involved in the malignant process. Similarly, small numbers of granulocyte/macrophage colonies not originating from the polycythemia vera

clone were also observed in these assays. These data collectively indicate the existence of both malignant and nonmalignant populations of hematopoietic progenitor cells in polycythemia vera marrow. The relative frequency of the neoplastic clone in relationship to normal progenitor cells was further examined by Adamson and co-workers,[72] who, by monitoring the proportion of neoplastic erythroid clones and their numerical relationship to normal clones over a period of several years, showed disease progression to be associated with a significant decline in the frequency of normal colony-forming cells and increasing preponderance of the neoplastic clone.[72]

The clonal assay systems first used to obtain "endogenous erythroid colonies" used serum containing trace amounts of EPO.[66] This EPO contamination led to confusion about the responsiveness of the polycythemia vera cells to the actions of this hormone. Two conflicting hypotheses were entertained, one suggesting that proliferation of abnormal populations of erythroid progenitor cells is completely independent of EPO and the other consistent with hypersensitivity of polycythemia progenitors to EPO.[66,67] Using an anti-EPO antiserum to remove trace amounts of EPO present in serum, Zanjani et al.[66] concluded that erythroid progenitor cells from polycythemia vera patients do not proliferate in the absence of EPO but are, in fact, abnormally sensitive to the actions of this hormone. This increased responsiveness allowed these cells to form colonies in the presence of serum containing small amounts of EPO. By constructing EPO dose-response curves from polycythemia vera marrows and comparing them with those obtained from normal marrow cells, Eaves and Eaves[73] drew similar conclusions. Their studies showed that most polycythemia patients possess two distinct populations of erythroid progenitor cells: a normally EPO-responsive population and a population of cells similar in proliferative and maturational behavior in vitro but requiring little or no EPO.[73] These investigators suggested that because of the exquisite EPO sensitivity of the malignant clone, the proliferation of the normal progenitor cells in vivo was at a disadvantage.[73] The EPO dependence of polycythemia vera progenitor cells was further demonstrated by Casadevall and co-workers,[74] who used a serum-free culture system, which no longer was contaminated with EPO. They were unable to demonstrate endogenous erythroid colony formation by normal or polycythemia vera marrow and were able to show that polycythemia vera erythroid progenitor cells were exquisitely sensitive to EPO as compared with normal progenitors[66] (Fig. 72-2). These data collectively indicate that the abnormality in the erythroid progenitor cell in polycythemia vera is not only quantitative but also qualitative.

More recently, using semipurified populations of blood and bone marrow BFU-E, Krantz and colleagues[6,7] demonstrated that the increased responsiveness of these marrow progenitor populations extends to their response to IL-3 and CSF-GM. In fact, these studies have revealed a 38-fold increase in sensitivity to IL-3 compared to a 4.3-fold increase in response to EPO by cells from polycythemia vera patients. These studies also demonstrated that bone marrow fractions enriched for granulocyte/macrophage progenitors as well as megakaryocyte progenitors from the patients had a heightened responsiveness to IL-3 and CSF-GM. No differences in receptor numbers for EPO, IL-3, or CSF-GM were found, strongly supporting the possibility that quantitatively abnormal growth factor receptors or postreceptor events might account for this growth factor hyperresponsiveness. Other investigators have suggested a role for the c-*kit* receptor and its ligand, Steel locus factor, in the biogenesis of polycythemia vera.[75] There is in fact some precedence for growth factor receptor abnormalities leading to growth factor hypersensitivity. D'Andrea et al.[76] showed that truncation of the cytoplasmic domain of the EPO receptor increases the sensitivity to EPO of murine cell lines expressing this form of the EPO receptor. In addition, de la Chapelle et al.[77] performed genetic linkage studies in members of a family with a familial form of polycythemia characterized by in-

Table 72-4. G6PD Isoenzyme Analysis of Erythroid Colonies Cloned from Marrow Cells of G6PD Heterozygotes with Polycythemia Vera

Erythropoietin (U/ml)	Patient 1		Patient 2	
	Colonies[a]	A/B[b]	Colonies[a]	A/B[b]
0	15	19/0	36	27/0
0.25	32	21/1	75	12/0
1.0	47	28/3	115	22/1
5.0	68	26/10	156	44/2
10.0	—	—	161	30/8

[a] Colonies per 10^5 cells.
[b] Number of individual colonies analyzed of specific G6PD isoenzyme type per 10^5 cells.
(From Prchal et al.,[71] with permission.)

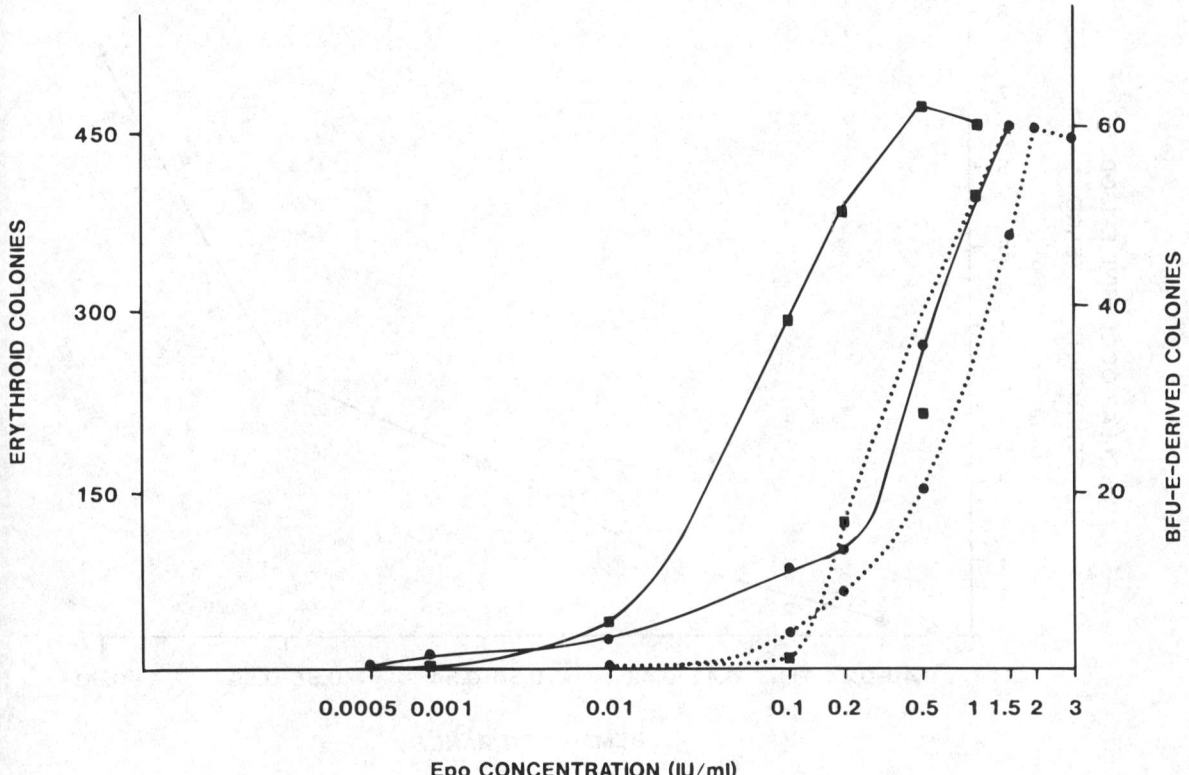

Fig. 72-2. Comparison of the EPO dose-response curves in serum-free cultures of colonies derived from CFU-Es (■) and BFU-Es (●) of marrow cells obtained from normal (dotted line) patients or individuals with polycythemia vera (solid line). (From Casadevall et al.,[74] with permission.)

creased sensitivity of erythroid progenitor cells to EPO; they presented data suggesting that a mutation in the EPO receptor is responsible for the disease phenotype. However, Correa et al.[77a] have recently presented data that questions the presence of EPO hypersensitivity of polycythemia vera hematopoietic progenitor cells. Their data indicates that the erythroid progenitor cell in polycythemia vera is hypersensitive to insulin-like growth factor-1 (IGF-1) and not EPO.[77a] Further investigation of the role of these two growth factors in the pathobiology of polycythemia vera is obviously warranted.

Cashman and co-workers[78] used long-term cultures of polycythemia vera bone marrow to further investigate the neoplastic proliferation of hematopoietic cells in such marrow. Polycythemia vera hematopoietic progenitor cells in the adherent layer of these long-term cultures proliferated continuously, unlike normal adherent progenitors, which were extremely quiescent. These investigators hypothesized that polycythemia vera progenitor cells were able to bypass or ignore negative regulatory signals derived from marrow adherent cells and that such signals were normally responsible for maintaining hematopoietic progenitor cells in a quiescent state.[78] Progenitor cells free of such inhibitory influences would be expected to be more sensitive to cytokines required for their further proliferation and differentiation, the precise situation observed in polycythemia vera with EPO or IGF-1. However, no conclusive studies linking the neoplastic hyperproliferation to abrogation of specific antiproliferative pathways in polycythemia vera clones has been achieved.

Certain clonal chromosomal abnormalities have been found in some polycythemia vera patients at diagnosis (see the section Laboratory Evaluation). Because these karyotypic abnormalities are not present in most patients, it remains unclear what role the putative products of these clonal chromosomal aberrations might play in the biogenesis of polycythemia vera. Some have conjectured that multiple etiologies of this disorder

might be possible due to the presence of different nonrandom karyotypic abnormalities in a number of cases. However, in one case of polycythemia vera characterized by the presence of trisomy 8, "endogenous erythroid colonies" derived from bone marrow cells assayed in vitro without the addition of exogenous EPO were analyzed by the technique of fluorescence in situ hybridization in order to determine the number of colonies containing cells with this cytogenetic abnormality. The bone marrow progenitors that presumably represent the malignant clone were found to produce not only colonies containing cells with trisomy 8, but also colonies with a normal complement of chromosome 8. This study strongly suggests that the acquisition of trisomy 8 occurs as a secondary event during the biogenesis of the malignant polycythemia vera clone.[77]

ETIOLOGY AND PATHOGENESIS

The most frequent cause of mortality in polycythemia vera patients is vascular thrombosis.[10,80,81] This increased thrombotic tendency is a direct consequence of the expanded red cell mass that characterizes this disorder.[82] Although the contributions of coexisting thrombocytosis and qualitative platelet abnormalities to this thrombotic tendency have remained uncertain, there is increasing evidence that abnormal platelet metabolism occurs in all polycythemia vera patients.

A markedly increased number of thrombotic events in polycythemia vera patients >70 years of age, particularly those with a history of prior thrombosis, has been reported.[81] The relationship between risk of thrombosis and age suggests that coexisting vascular disease is an important contributory factor in the development of thrombosis in polycythemia vera patients. This conclusion is probably correct but does not negate the increased incidence of thrombotic incidents also observed in younger patients with this disorder.[80] In a series of 58 polycy-

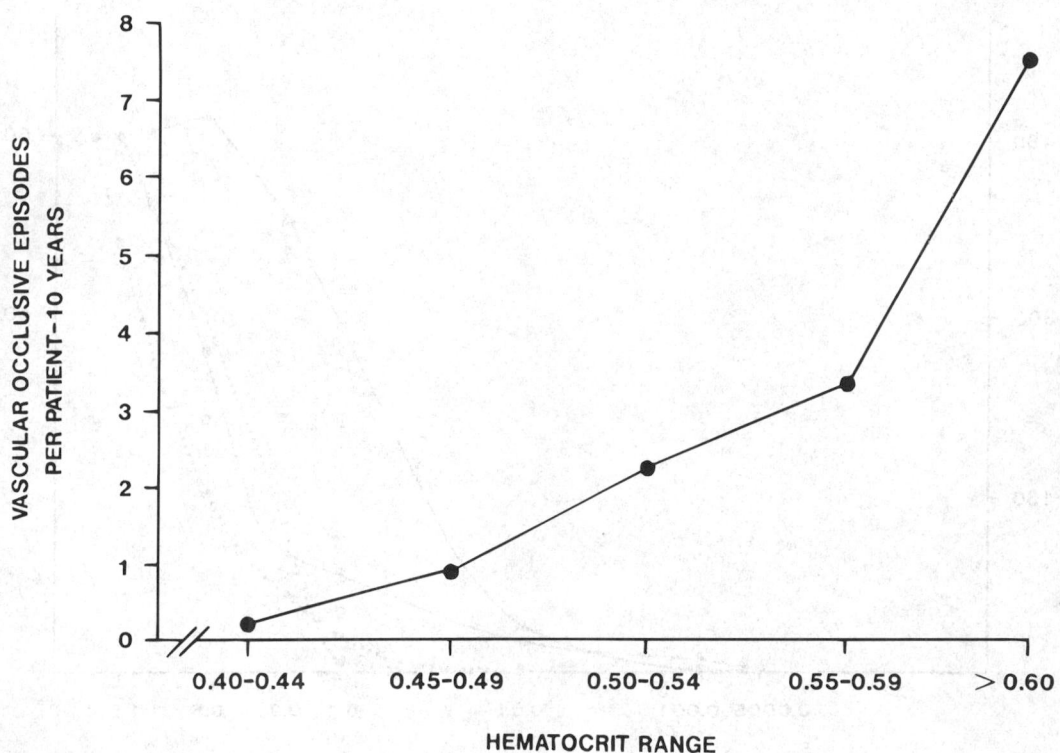

Fig. 72-3. Relationship of hematocrit to number of vascular occlusive episodes per 10 patient years in patients with polycythemia vera. (From Pearson and Wetherley-Mein,[82] with permission.)

themia vera patients diagnosed <40 years of age, a disturbingly high incidence of life-threatening thrombotic events was observed—in fact, 7 of the 10 patients in this series who died during the period of observation died from thrombotic events—4 from Budd-Chiari syndrome, 1 from a pulmonary embolism, and 2 from cerebral thrombosis.[80] Therefore, although a significant factor, pre-existing atherosclerotic disease is not the sole etiologic factor in the genesis of thrombosis in polycythemia vera. Some have suggested an important role for smoking as a secondary factor leading to the increased incidence of thrombotic events in this patient population.

In a retrospective analysis of the records of 69 polycythemia vera patients with a history of vascular thrombosis, Pearson and Wetherley-Mein[82] demonstrated a strong correlation between hematocrit level and development of thrombotic episodes, including many cerebrovascular occlusions (Fig. 72-3). The strength of this relationship has been questioned by others.[81] Thomas et al.[83] showed that cerebral blood flow is reduced in patients with polycythemia vera in whom the hematocrit is 53–62%. These abnormalities were observed even in patients with hematocrits at the lower levels of normal, 46–52%.[82] Reductions in cerebral blood flow were correctable with phlebotomy. Reduction of the hematocrit by relatively small amounts frequently led to substantial improvements in whole blood viscosity and cerebral blood flow.

A number of possible explanations have been suggested for the observed relationship between hematocrit and development of thrombotic events in polycythemia vera patients. Turrito and Weiss[84] presented evidence to indicate that platelet adhesion and thrombus formation on the vascular subendothelium are determined in part by the rate at which platelets are transported to the vascular surface. In a polycythemic condition in which increased numbers of red cells are present, a greater number of intercellular collisions between red cells and platelets occur. These collisions could lead to increased platelet movement in a direction perpendicular to blood flow. This facilitation of platelet transport to the vessel wall may be an important factor in the development of thrombosis.[84] An alternative explanation for the association between hematocrit level and risk of thrombosis is based on the knowledge that blood viscosity is particularly sensitive to hematocrit levels.[85,86] Increased hematocrits lead to increased blood viscosity, in turn leading to increased peripheral vascular resistance and an actual reduction in blood flow to a variety of organs, predisposing them to the development of thrombosis.[85,86]

Additional factors have been implicated in the development of thrombosis in polycythemia vera patients. Almost all patients with this disorder are iron deficient.[87] Decreased red cell deformability has been said to accompany iron deficiency, leading to increased blood viscosity and a decreased ability of red cells to pass through small-bore polycarbonate filters.[88,89] Such abnormalities have been shown by Tillman and Schröter[90] and Yip et al.[91] to be due to increased membrane stiffness rather than to reduced surface/volume ratio, as has been suggested by others. This increased membrane stiffness, however, might be counterbalanced by the effect of a reduced red blood cell size on the adherence of blood platelets to arteriolar subendothelium. Aarts et al.[92] have shown that red cell size is a major determinant of platelet adherence, with larger red blood cells leading to increased and smaller red cells to decreased platelet adherence. Whether the increased membrane stiffness associated with iron deficiency is counterbalanced by the decreased platelet adherence associated with smaller red blood cells is yet to be determined.

Study of patients with hemoglobinopathies due to abnormal oxygen binding who have secondary erythrocytosis provide further support to the belief that hematocrit elevations are not the sole cause of the thrombotic tendency in polycythemia vera. A survey of 200 patients with these types of hemoglobinopathies has not demonstrated a higher incidence of myocardial ischemia or any other form of thrombosis, even though the red cell mass is frequently as elevated as that in patients with polycythemia vera.[93]

Thrombocytosis and qualitative platelet abnormalities occur frequently and are likely important contributory factors to the development of thrombosis.[11,94,95] Dawson and Ogston[96] have implicated uncontrolled thrombocytosis as a cause of thrombosis in these patients, but this relationship has not been confirmed by Kessler et al.[81] or Berk et al.[94]

Polycythemia vera patients also are at an increased risk of the development of life-threatening hemorrhagic complications. Abnormalities in platelet function and number have been implicated as the cause of this hemorrhagic tendency.[10,11] Qualitative platelet abnormalities frequently found in these patients include platelet hypofunction as demonstrated by defective in vitro platelet aggregation, acquired storage pool disease, platelet membrane defects, increased platelet reactivity as demonstrated by enhanced platelet aggregation, increased plasma β-thromboglobulin levels, and shortened platelet survival.[97–102] Recently, increased plasma and urinary thromboxane production has been linked to increased platelet activation in these patients.[95] A low-dose aspirin regimen selective for inhibition of platelet cyclo-oxygenase was found to suppress increased thromboxane production in vivo.

Despite conflicting data, no clear clinical relationship between platelet number or function and the incidence of hemorrhage or thrombosis has been found.[97–102] Further evidence that the extent of thrombocytosis is not alone a determinant of the development of thrombosis or hemorrhage is provided by analysis of patients with secondary thrombocytosis who have been reported not to be at increased risk of the development of thrombosis.[103,104] However, selected patients with polycythemia vera have been afforded prompt resolution of vascular complications following institution of platelet antiaggregating agents or plateletpheresis.[105,106] What distinguishes the clinical course of these patients from that of others is unknown. These anecdotal reports, coupled with the knowledge of abnormal thromboxane metabolism of platelets in polycythemia vera, provide substance to the belief by many that platelets contribute to generation of the thrombotic and hemorrhagic tendencies observed in polycythemia vera.[10,11,97–102]

Although a variety of clinical assessments of platelet function have been used to identify patients who are potentially at a high risk of developing a life-threatening hemorrhagic or thrombotic event, the results of these studies to date have been very disappointing. One is left with the impression that the etiology of thrombosis and hemorrhage in polycythemia vera is multifactorial and that the available tools are inadequate to identify biochemically those patients at highest risk.

A major cause of morbidity and mortality in polycythemia vera results from the transition from the polycythemic phase of the disease to postpolycythemic myeloid metaplasia (PPMM) and to acute leukemia. PPMM is characterized by cytopenias, myelofibrosis, and extramedullary hematopoiesis.[107–109] In a variety of myeloproliferative disorders, the fibroblastic component of the bone marrow has been shown not to be directly involved in the malignant process but to be a reactive event to the neoplastic clone.[57] Several investigators have suggested that release of growth factors, particularly plateletderived growth factor from megakaryocytes or platelets, which are present in abundance in patients with myeloproliferative disorders, might be responsible for this fibroblastic proliferation.[110,111]

Whether the use of any particular therapeutic agents for treatment of polycythemia vera accelerates the development of the spent phase is unknown. Some have suggested that the use of radioactive phosphorus favors such a transition, yet others have not noted any relationship between the treatment modality used and more rapid progression to PPMM.[107,108,111–114] However, after treatment with alkylating agents or irradiation during the proliferative phase, patients with PPMM are more likely to transform to acute leukemia.[115]

This appears to be closely linked with acquisition of specific marrow clonal chromosomal abnormalities (see the section Therapy).

CLINICAL MANIFESTATIONS

The principal clinical manifestations of polycythemia vera are a direct consequence of the excessive proliferation of cellular elements of the various hematopoietic cellular lineages involved in the neoplastic process. With the current widespread use of laboratory screening tests during routine patient examinations, increasing numbers of persons are being diagnosed with polycythemia vera before the development of symptoms related to this neoplastic process. Symptomatic patients with polycythemia vera may present to a physician with a myriad of nonspecific complaints, including headache, weakness, pruritus, dizziness, excessive sweating, visual disturbances, paresthesias, joint symptoms, epigastric distress, and weight loss.[4,10] At diagnosis, in fact, one-third of patients have already lost 10% of their body weight, presumably secondary to the hypermetabolism associated with this disorder.[10] Arthropathies that are frequently observed in these patients are largely due to the clinical manifestations of gout. The hyperproliferative bone marrow state characteristic of polycythemia vera and the increased nucleoprotein degradation are contributing factors in the development of hyperuricemia.

The principal findings on physical examination of a patient with polycythemia vera include ruddy cyanosis, conjunctival plethora, hepatomegaly, splenomegaly, and hypertension.[4,10]

Untreated patients are at particularly high risk of both thrombotic and hemorrhagic events.[4,10,12] In several large series of patients with polycythemia vera, thrombosis was the cause of death in 30–40% of patients.[4,80–82] Patients may present with deep venous thrombosis in the lower extremities, pulmonary embolism, or cerebrovascular, coronary, and peripheral vascular occlusions. It is not unusual for patients with polycythemia vera to develop thromboses at unusual anatomic sites; in particular, thromboses are relatively frequent in the splenic, hepatic, portal, and mesenteric vessels.[4,10]

A particularly serious thrombotic event associated with polycythemia vera is Budd-Chiari syndrome,[80,116–118] due to hepatic venous or inferior vena caval thrombosis and obstruction. This syndrome is characterized by hepatosplenomegaly, ascites, edema of the peripheral extremities, jaundice, abdominal pain, and distension of superficial abdominal veins due to resultant portal hypertension.[117,118] Routine biochemical determinations of hepatocellular function and injury are frequently of little diagnostic value in patients with suspected Budd-Chiari syndrome.[117,118] Liver scans using ^{99}Tc-labeled sulfur colloid may provide important diagnostic information, a characteristic pattern being central accumulation of the tracer and an enlarged hypertrophic caudate lobe of the liver, with apparent diminished or even absent tracer accumulation over the right lobe.[118] Percutaneous liver biopsy specimens usually reveal intense congestion and cellular atrophy. Hepatic venous and inferior venal caval catheterization are key diagnostic procedures that indicate the sites of venous obstruction.[118]

Of patients with Budd-Chiari syndrome reported in the literature, 10% have had coexisting polycythemia vera.[117,118] Therefore, anyone who develops Budd-Chiari syndrome should be suspected of having polycythemia vera, and that diagnosis should be quickly excluded. The factors operational in the polycythemia vera patient that lead to the development of hepatic vein thrombosis are thought to be multiple. Splenomegaly causes increased portal blood flow and extramedullary hematopoiesis within the hepatic sinusoids, and frequently compromises hepatic blood flow. These processes are surely important contributory factors, in addition to the other previously discussed risk factors that are thought to lead to the development of thrombosis.

Neurologic abnormalities occur in almost 60–80% of untreated or poorly controlled polycythemia vera patients and include transient ischemic attacks, cerebral infarction, cerebral hemorrhage, fluctuating dementia, confusional states, and choreic syndromes.[119] In addition, complaints of dizziness, paresthesias, visual disturbances, tinnitus, and headache have been attributed to the increased blood viscosity[119] and reduced cerebral blood flow caused by erythrocytosis. The transient neurologic symptoms can also be the consequence of small infarcts in the region of the basal ganglia, which can be detected by computed tomography.[120] These small infarcts are known as lacunae and result from the occlusion of small penetrating arteries, which are particularly susceptible to thrombosis.[120] Cerebrovascular thrombosis occurs more often in polycythemia vera patients than in the general population.[120,121] Symptoms due to intermittent carotid or vertebral basilar insufficiency (or both) occur so frequently in polycythemia vera that Millikan et al.[122] suggest that every patient with focal cerebrovascular insufficiency be examined to rule out an underlying myeloproliferative disorder.

Cavernous sinus thrombosis is usually associated with a primary infectious etiology involving a focus in the face, throat, mouth, ear, or sinuses.[123] Aseptic cavernous sinus thrombosis is an extremely rare phenomenon that has been reported in patients with polycythemia vera.[124,125] These patients present with monocular blindness and the characteristic features of ipsilateral cavernous sinus thrombosis, and only retrospectively is the diagnosis of polycythemia vera made.[125] Therefore, patients found to have this symptom complex who have no known infectious predisposing causes should be carefully evaluated to rule out this diagnosis.

Thrombosis of large-caliber arteries is a relatively rare event in polycythemia vera patients, but there have been case reports of thromboses within the chambers of the heart leading to refractory congestive heart failure and acute aortic occlusion.[126,127] Such catastrophic thrombotic events in the heart or large vessels would suggest that cardiac catheterization be performed with some caution.[127]

Polycythemia vera frequently presents with symptoms due to peripheral vascular disease.[128–130] In these cases, patients may first be seen by surgeons or dermatologists.[128] Intense redness or cyanosis of digits with or without burning, classical erythromelalgia, digital ischemia with palpable pulses, or thrombophlebitis without other known cause may be the presenting symptoms.[128–132]

Erythromelalgia is characterized by burning pain in the digits, an objective sensation of increased temperature, and relief by cooling.[131–133] Polycythemia vera is the most common cause of erythromelalgia and is one of the few disorders in which digital ischemia with or without ulceration may exist in the presence of palpable pulses.[133] Other disorders that can lead to this abnormality include embolism, trauma, cutaneous infarction, neuritis, infection, and various types of arteritis.[128,134] Painful and ulcerating toes and fingers have been frequently observed to be a presenting symptom in patients with polycythemia vera.[128–130] The likelihood that arterial insufficiency is the cause of such ulceration is quite small in patients who have a palpable dorsalis pedis and posterior tibialis pulses; in this situation, the possibility of an underlying hematologic disorder such as polycythemia vera should be entertained. Foot pain at rest is a distressing but not widely recognized symptom of polycythemia vera. In patients with this complaint, peripheral pulses are of normal character and cutaneous circulation appears to be adequate.[128,130] The pain is most severe at night, is dull in nature, and occurs primarily in the feet or legs. These symptoms have been reported to be rapidly reversible after the institution of antiplatelet aggregation therapy. Therefore,

the cause of erythromelalgia appears to be closely linked to abnormal arachidonic acid metabolism that occurs within platelets in this disorder.[95]

Hemorrhagic complications are the cause of death in 5–10% of polycythemia vera patients.[10,12,97] The gastrointestinal tract is the most frequent site of hemorrhage. These patients have an increased incidence of peptic ulcer disease,[12] and esophageal varices due to portal hypertension occur frequently. Cerebral hemorrhage is a common cause of morbidity and mortality.[119] As many as 30–40% of patients with polycythemia vera experience some sort of hemorrhagic event,[10,135] which can be relatively trivial, such as epistaxis or gingival hemorrhage, or can be life-threatening, such as gastrointestinal hemorrhage or hematomas involving vital organs.[10] In large part this hemorrhagic tendency has been attributed to qualitative platelet abnormalities.[45] In one study of platelets from a patient with polycythemia vera and a bleeding diathesis, the coupling between the thromboxane A_2 receptor and intracellular signal transducers was found to be defective.[136]

Bleeding events frequently occur with the use of anti-inflammatory agents[137,138]; an association between the hemorrhage and the use of these platelet-paralyzing drugs has been made in almost one-third of such instances.[94,137,138] Spontaneous bleeding in patients with polycythemia vera is relatively rare,[96,135] although spontaneous retropharyngeal hematomas leading to acute upper airway obstruction or hematomas in the groin have been reported.[139]

The polycythemia vera patient who undergoes a surgical procedure is at a very high risk of the development of postoperative complications.[140–143] In one series of 62 major operations on 54 patients with polycythemia vera, postoperative complications occurred in 47%[142]; 52% of complications were due to hemorrhage, 18% to thrombosis, and 14% to hemorrhage and thrombosis.[142] The postoperative mortality in this patient population was 18%.[142] In another series of 15 patients, 5 suffered serious complications secondary to thrombosis and hemorrhage.[140] Data analysis of polycythemia vera patients undergoing surgery has shown the complication rate to be highest in those who had uncontrolled erythrocytosis before surgery. Patients whose disease was inadequately controlled had a 79% incidence of complications, while in those who enjoyed adequate hematologic control prior to surgery the rate of perioperative and postoperative complications was reduced to 28%.[142] In addition, duration of disease control was an important factor in decreasing surgical risk[142]; a prolonged period of effective disease control prior to surgery reduced the complication rate to 5%.[142] Complication rates following surgery can therefore be dramatically reduced by appropriate therapeutic interventions with normalization of blood counts. The chief deterrent to such an approach has been the failure by physicians to recognize the risk associated with polycythemia vera in the surgical setting.

Generalized pruritus occurs in approximately 50% of cases of polycythemia vera.[4,12,144] Water contact, such as during showers or bathing, induces attacks of intolerable pruritus.[145] There appears to be no clear relationship between the degree of the pruritus and severity of the disease,[146] and 20% of patients continue to experience itching despite reduction of their red blood cell masses to the normal range.[146] The degree of pruritus is so severe in some patients that they are unable to tolerate bathing at all and find it necessary to substitute gentle skin swabbing or simply not to bathe. The etiology of the pruritus in polycythemia vera remains uncertain. Several groups have attempted to implicate elevated blood and urine histamine levels in its pathobiology.[144,146] Steinman et al.[146] have presented data suggesting that water exposure in patients with polycythemia vera actually leads to elevated histamine levels, which would provide an explanation for the exacerbation of the pruritus frequently observed with water contact. Jackson et al.[147] have been able to establish a strong correlation be-

Table 72-5. Progression of Polycythemia Vera to PPMM in 29 Patients

	Male	Female
Number	15	14
Median age at onset of polycythemia vera	50	53
Median age at onset of postpolycythemia myeloid metaplasia	60	62

(From Silverstein,[107] with permission.

tween skin mast cell numbers and the severity of itching. However, the failure of the pruritus to respond to antihistamine therapy in many patients suggests that abnormally high histamine levels probably do not constitute the sole factor in its development.[148]

Iron deficiency has also been implicated as a factor contributing to pruritus in polycythemia vera patients who are almost invariably iron deficient.[149] Iron substitution therapy has resulted in symptomatic improvement,[149] but this approach is less than optimal because it frequently results in uncontrollable erythrocytosis.

A great deal of information suggests that patients suffer from serious nonhematologic symptoms secondary to iron deficiency.[150-152] Rector et al.[153] evaluated these sequelae in patients with polycythemia vera who were uniformly iron deficient and followed these patients for >25 years. Their data are unique in that they indicate that quantitative evaluation of symptoms fails to provide convincing evidence that undue fatigue occurs as a result of iron deficiency.[153] In fact, treadmill performance by six patients was equivalent to that observed among normal subjects.[153] None of the patients experienced dysphagia or the esophageal changes associated with chronic iron deficiency.[153] The one symptom that was observed to occur regularly, particularly in women, was picophagia, a pica consisting of compulsive ice eating.[153]

PPMM occurs in 5–15% of patients with polycythemia vera.[10,11,107-109] The transition to this stage of the disease occurs, on average, 10 years after initial diagnosis, but in individual cases it can occur after either shorter or longer intervals[107-109] (Table 72-5). PPMM is characterized by (1) increasing splenomegaly, (2) teardrop red blood cell morphology, (3) extensive bone marrow fibrosis, (4) a leukoerythroblastic blood picture, and (5) a normal or decreasing red blood cell mass. The patients may be entirely asymptomatic but often complain of fatigue, dizziness, weight loss, and anorexia[107-109] (Table 72-6). Splenomegaly can lead to abdominal pain due to repeated splenic infarcts and to early satiety due to mechanical obstruction of the upper gastrointestinal tract.

The anemia that characterizes the spent phase is primarily a result of splenic pooling, ineffective erythropoiesis, and extramedullary production of red blood cells with a shortened survival. Occasionally, the anemia is exacerbated by folate or iron deficiency.[107,109,154] Before assuming that a patient has entered the spent phase, it is prudent to assess bone marrow iron stores. Replacement therapy with iron may lead to the resurgence of erythropoiesis and prevent the faulty categorization of disease progression.

Bleeding abnormalities due to thrombocytopenia or qualita-

tive platelet abnormalities are especially common during this phase of the disease. Frequent instances of epistaxis or ecchymoses occur,[109] and gastrointestinal hemorrhage due to esophageal varices arising from portal hypertension is a recurrent problem.[102,104] Frequently patients suffer from generalized wasting characterized by progressive asthenia and weight loss. Severe hyperuricemia, leading to secondary gout or uric acid nephropathy, may also complicate the clinical course.

Patients with PPMM are at high risk of the development of acute leukemia.[87,107-109,115,155-159] Of those patients who enter the spent phase of polycythemia vera, 25–50% will eventually undergo leukemic transformation.[87,107-109,115,155-159] Approximately 70% of patients who enter the spent phase will be dead 3 years after this transition; however, the other 30% of these patients will have a much longer survival, averaging 6.5 years.[107,109,156]

The leukemic transformation of polycythemia vera has been extensively described.[115,147-160] The possibility that a relationship exists between the therapeutic modality used during the erythrocytotic phase and the frequency of development of acute leukemia has been a point of heated discussion.[161-166] Some of the controversy surrounding this question was formerly due to a lack of understanding of the basic origins of polycythemia vera. Clinical hematologists in the 1950s and 1960s frequently thought of polycythemia vera as a benign hematologic abnormality and believed that therapeutic interventions either with alkylating agents or radiotherapy were solely responsible for the development of acute leukemia. That concept has proved erroneous, and polycythemia vera, like the other myeloproliferative disorders, has been shown to be a clonal malignant hematologic disorder.[57,59] The evolution to acute leukemia can therefore be thought of as a natural consequence of this malignant disorder, which can be accentuated by the therapeutic interventions discussed above.

Further insight into relationships between acute leukemia and polycythemia vera has been best provided by the published results of the Polycythemia Vera Study Group (PVSG), which described a randomized trial comparing the use of phlebotomy, chlorambucil, and ^{32}P for the treatment of this disorder.[167] The incidence of acute leukemia was approximately 1.5% in patients treated with phlebotomy alone, 13.5% in patients treated with chlorambucil, and 10.2% in patients treated with ^{32}P.[81,168] The incidence of acute leukemia in the patients treated with phlebotomy alone is therefore much higher than that expected in a normal age-matched control group, again indicating that leukemia is a natural evolutionary event in the clinical course of an individual with polycythemia vera. The incidence of acute leukemia can be increased, however, by institution of therapy with either alkylating agents or ^{32}P.[115] Approximately 30–50% of patients with polycythemia vera who develop acute leukemia have previously entered the spent phase[115] (Table 72-7). By contrast, approximately 50% of pa-

Table 72-6. Symptoms of Patients with PPMM at Presentation

	Cases	%
Asymptomatic	9	31
Symptomatic	20	69
Anemia	10	50
Pressure	9	45
Bleeding	4	20

(From Silverstein,[107] with permission.)

Table 72-7. Incidence of Acute Leukemia in Three Study Arms of PVSG Randomized Trial According to Development of Myelofibrosis–Myeloid Metaplasia

Treatment Arm	Myelofibrosis–Myeloid Metaplasia	Cases	Acute Leukemia Cases	Acute Leukemia %
Phlebotomy	No	120	1	0.8
	Yes	14	1	7.1
Chlorambucil	No	127	14	11.0
	Yes	14	5	36.0
^{32}P	No	140	12	8.6
	Yes	16	4	25.0
Total	No	387	27	7.0
	Yes	44	10	23.0

(From Berk et al.,[168] with permission.)

tients progress directly from the erythrocytotic phase to acute leukemia.[115] The phenotype of the leukemia cells that characterize the leukemic phase is overwhelmingly myeloid.[115] Unusual cases of lymphoblastic transformation of polycythemia vera have, however, been reported, as have rare cases of biphenotypic leukemias.[169–172] Another adverse effect solely associated with the use of chlorambucil has been the development of large cell lymphoma in 3.5% of patients.[81]

Acute leukemia rarely develops before the eighth year following the diagnosis of polycythemia vera.[115,155–160] Its development can be abrupt, however. In some instances, a preleukemic phase characterized by refractory anemia with excess blasts has been described.[158] In fact, one-half of such cases of acute leukemia in one series were preceded by a myelodysplastic disorder.[158]

LABORATORY EVALUATION

Laboratory evaluation of the patient with polycythemia vera involves the careful utilization of a broad range of diagnostic studies. These studies must be employed in a rational manner, or the evaluation can become extremely costly. Since polycythemia vera is a panmyelosis, the overwhelming number of patients have elevated hematocrits, white blood cell counts, and platelet counts.[4] In order to document the absolute increase in red cell mass, the performance of a blood volume study with direct quantitation of both the red cell mass and plasma volume is mandatory.[173,174] This study will eliminate costly, unnecessary investigations, which are unfortunately often pursued in patients who have spurious polycythemia.[175]

Indirect calculations of the red cell mass from plasma volume measurements assume a normal body venous hematocrit ratio. Unfortunately, this ratio may be abnormal in patients with spurious polycythemia vera, and calculations derived from venous packed red cell volumes may overestimate the red cell mass.[175] Because polycythemia patients are most often iron deficient, at times it may be necessary to replenish iron stores before the extent of the red cell mass elevation can be appreciated.[166]

Leukocytosis is present in approximately two-thirds of cases, and thrombocytosis is observed in 50%.[4] Abnormalities of red blood cell, white blood cell, and platelet morphology are frequently observed. The morphologic red blood cell changes observed during the erythrocytotic phases are characteristic of iron deficiency and include microcytosis, hypochromia, and frequently polychromatophilia.[166] Some anisocytosis and poikilocytosis can be seen. Fetal hemoglobin levels and the number of red cells containing fetal hemoglobin, known as F cells, may be increased.[176] The white blood cells are characterized by normal morphology, although the preponderance of basophils, eosinophils, and immature myeloid forms is increased.[9] Platelet morphology is also quite striking in polycythemia vera. Frequently, megathrombocytes (platelets having the size of red blood cells) are seen on the peripheral blood smear. Patients frequently have platelet counts of $<1 \times 10^6/mm^3$, but it is not unusual to observe a patient with a platelet count higher than this value. The postpolycythemic myeloid metaplasia phase of the disease is characterized by a leukoerythroblastic blood picture, with the appearance in the peripheral blood of myelocytes, metamyelocytes, and, rarely, blasts and promyelocytes in addition to nucleated red blood cells in the peripheral blood.[107–109]

Platelet aggregation studies and bleeding times are frequently abnormal in patients with polycythemia vera, but many patients can have normal results.[97–102] Prothrombin time and partial thromboplastin time, as well as fibrinogen levels, are normal.[177,178] Tytgat et al.[177] have detected a shortened fibrinogen half-life in polycythemia vera patients and a significantly increased fractional catabolic rate of the plasma fibrinogen pool per day. Boughton and Dallinger[178] have confirmed these

findings. In addition, elevated platelet β-thromboglobulin and plasma β-thromboglobulin levels are observed. The constellation of findings is indicative of increased platelet turnover rates due to ongoing low-grade disseminated intravascular coagulopathy.

Abnormal multimeric forms of von Willebrand factor have been detected in 50% of patients and are thought to be due in part to a specific inhibitor of polymerization of this factor.[179] This abnormality has led to the diagnosis of acquired von Willebrand disease in a small number of patients.[179] The leukocyte alkaline phosphatase activity level is elevated in 70% of patients.[4] Serum B_{12} concentrations have been found to be elevated in 40% of patients, whereas serum B_{12}-binding proteins are elevated in 70% of cases.[4] Hyperuricemia occurs in the overwhelming number of patients, while elevated histamine levels are also frequently observed.[4,144] Bone marrow aspirates and biopsies obtained at the diagnosis of patients with polycythemia vera are hypercellular and display characteristic erythroid, granulocytic, and megakaryocytic hyperplasia.[87,114,180–183] This is not a uniform finding, as 13% of the pretreatment biopsies in one series demonstrated an initial marrow cellularity of <60%, which lies within the normal range.[87] The cellular elements are frequently morphologically normal. Iron stores are almost uniformly absent in pretreatment biopsy specimens.[87,183] Significant increases in bone marrow reticulin may be present in biopsies obtained early in the course; they also may develop during the erythrocytotic phase and be present for long periods before the onset of the spent phase.[87,114] The presence of increased reticulin at diagnosis is not predictive of imminent development of postpolycythemic myeloid metaplasia. In those patients who enter the spent phase of the disease, a moderate to marked increase in reticulin fiber is observed, either simultaneously with or within 1 year of this clinical transformation.[114]

Several investigators have attempted to use bone marrow biopsy morphology as a differential diagnostic tool to discriminate between polycythemia vera and secondary forms of erythrocytosis.[181,182] The marked hypercellularity and megakaryocytic hyperplasia that are the hallmarks of myeloproliferative disorders are useful parameters for distinguishing such individuals[182,183] (Fig. 72-4). It is imperative to use the bone marrow biopsy rather than aspirate specimens for this purpose.[87,114,180–183]

The pathologic appearance of the spleen in polycythemia vera depends on the stage of the disease at which that organ is examined.[184] Spleens from patients in the erythrocytotic phase of the disease are characterized by striking congestion with mature erythrocytes.[184] Small numbers of hematopoietic precursor cells are frequently present. By contrast, spleens examined during the PPMM phase are characterized by prominent numbers of foci of extramedullary hematopoiesis, with representation of all marrow precursor elements.[184]

The proliferative capacity of polycythemia vera hematopoietic progenitor cells from bone marrow has recently been shown to be a useful laboratory adjunctive study.[185–193] Lemoine et al.[191] prospectively used the formation of endogenous erythroid colonies as a diagnostic tool to confirm the diagnosis of polycythemia vera in the evaluation of a group of patients with isolated erythrocytosis (Table 72-8). In this study, the clinical course of those patients with marrow cells that formed endogenous colonies was very similar to that of patients who met standard criteria for the diagnosis of polycythemia vera.[191] Slightly >70% of these patients developed difficulties that eventually required treatment. Conversely, those patients whose marrow cells did not form colonies in the absence of erythropoietin enjoyed a benign clinical course not requiring therapeutic intervention.

Laboratory evaluation of patients with polycythemia vera has been further facilitated by the more widespread availability of quantitative assays of EPO.[35–56] More generalized use of well-

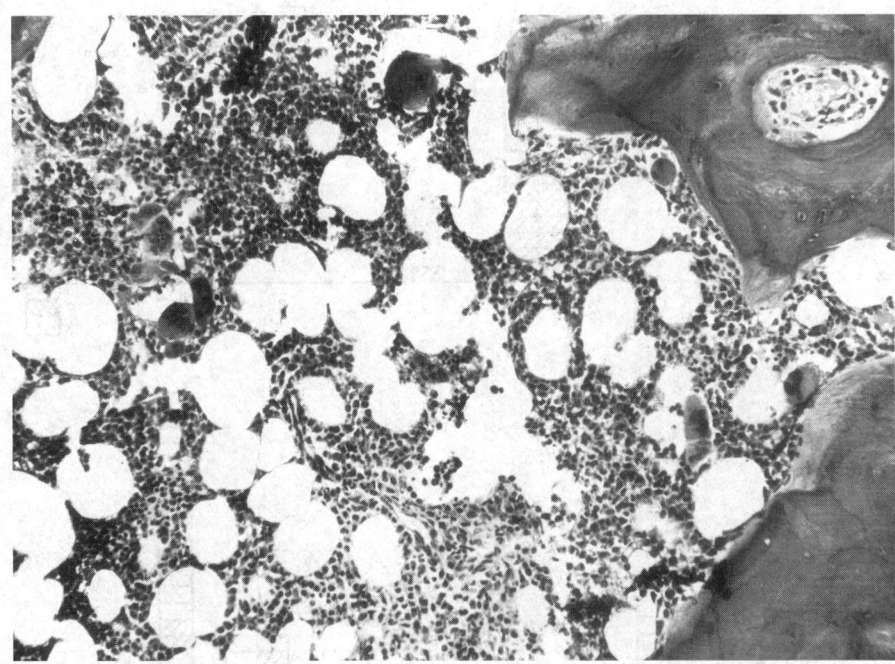

Fig. 72-4. Photomicrograph of bone marrow biopsy obtained from polycythemia vera patient in spent phase demonstrating hypercellularity and increased number of megakaryocytes. (× 160.)

defined clinical criteria, in conjunction with bone marrow histology, in vitro proliferative capacity of erythroid progenitor cells, and EPO levels might be useful in defining the appropriate roles of these newly available diagnostic tests in evaluating the patient with polycythemia vera.

The occurrence of nonrandom cytogenetic abnormalities in polycythemia vera is not unexpected, as this is a feature of most hematologic malignancies.[57,194–203] Such abnormalities have been observed, with no single characteristic chromosomal abnormality; abnormalities of chromosomes 1, 5, 7, 8, 9, 12, 13, and 20 have each been detected.[194–202] These cytogenetic abnormalities can be categorized according to the phase of disease (onset, erythrocytotic, or spent phase) in which they are most frequently observed.[194–202] Also, certain cytogenetic abnormalities are clearly a result of treatment-induced muta-

tion, associated with the use of ^{32}P or alkylating agents.[194–196] The frequency of detection of cytogenetic abnormalities in polycythemia vera is a cumulative function, with 15–20% at diagnosis; 35–55% following a number of years of treatment; and >80% in those patients in whom acute leukemia eventually develops.[194–196,201] Therefore, clonal progression from a normal to abnormal karyotype, especially acquisition of abnormalities involving chromosomes 5 and 7, is an important adverse prognostic parameter[194–196,201] (Fig. 72-5).

Trisomy of chromosomes 8 and 9 and deletion of the long arm of chromosome 20 (20q−) are most frequently observed at diagnosis.[194,195] In one study the single most common abnormality was 20q− (q11),[192] which is a recognized genomic constitutive fragile site subject to mutagenic insult in vitro.[194] High-resolution analysis of a subset of patients with myeloproliferative disorders and an apparent terminal deletion of this region (20 qter) has been reported by LeBeau et al.[205] Using in situ chromosomal hybridization, these investigators found that the 20q− (q11) deletion was actually an interstitial deletion, associated with conservation of the c-src proto-oncogene whose normal chromosomal location is (20q 13.2).[205] This finding suggests that src might be altered as a consequence of this chromosomal abnormality, to augment its function. Experimental verification of this hypothesis is not available. This observation, if correct, might provide an attractive potential functional correlation relevant to the observed growth advantage of the polycythemia vera marrow cells.

The observation of a single karyotypic abnormality of 8, 9, or 20q is not of prognostic importance.[194] Other abnormalities most often acquired with progression of the disease are 13q−, 12q−, and 1q−. These particular abnormalities do not necessarily herald transition to acute leukemia, but leukemia or myelofibrosis was observed in 8 of 12 patients with 1q− abnormality of one study.[194,195] Deletion of the long arm of chromosome 13 has been observed during the myelofibrotic phase of polycythemia vera, but this abnormality has been detected also during the erythrocytotic phase. It does not appear, therefore, that a chromosome 13q abnormality heralds disease transition.[196] PPMM occurring after the use of chemotherapy is often accom-

Table 72-8. Study of Diagnostic Utility of Marrow Erythroid Progenitor Cell Cultures in Patients Suspected of Polycythemia Vera Based on Standard Clinical Criteria

Diagnosis	Standard Criteria[a]	Endogenous Erythroid Colonies[b]
Group A[c]		
Polycythemia vera	46	43 (93%)
Secondary polycythemia	12	0
Unclassifiable polycythemia	29	18
Total	87	61 (70%)
Group B[c]		
Secondary polycythemia	5	0
Unclassifiable polycythemia	16	4 (25%)
Total	21	4 (20%)

[a] Standard criteria were criteria proposed by the PVSG and criteria routinely used for the diagnosis of causes of secondary polycythemia.[4]

[b] Endogenous erythroid colonies derived from bone marrow cells developing without exogenous EPO.

[c] Group A is defined to include male patients having a red cell mass of ≥36 ml/kg and female patients with a red cell mass of ≥32 ml/kg. Group B is defined as male patients having a red cell mass of 30–36 ml/kg and female patients with a red cell mass of 25–32 ml/kg.

(From Lemoine et al.,[191] with permission.)

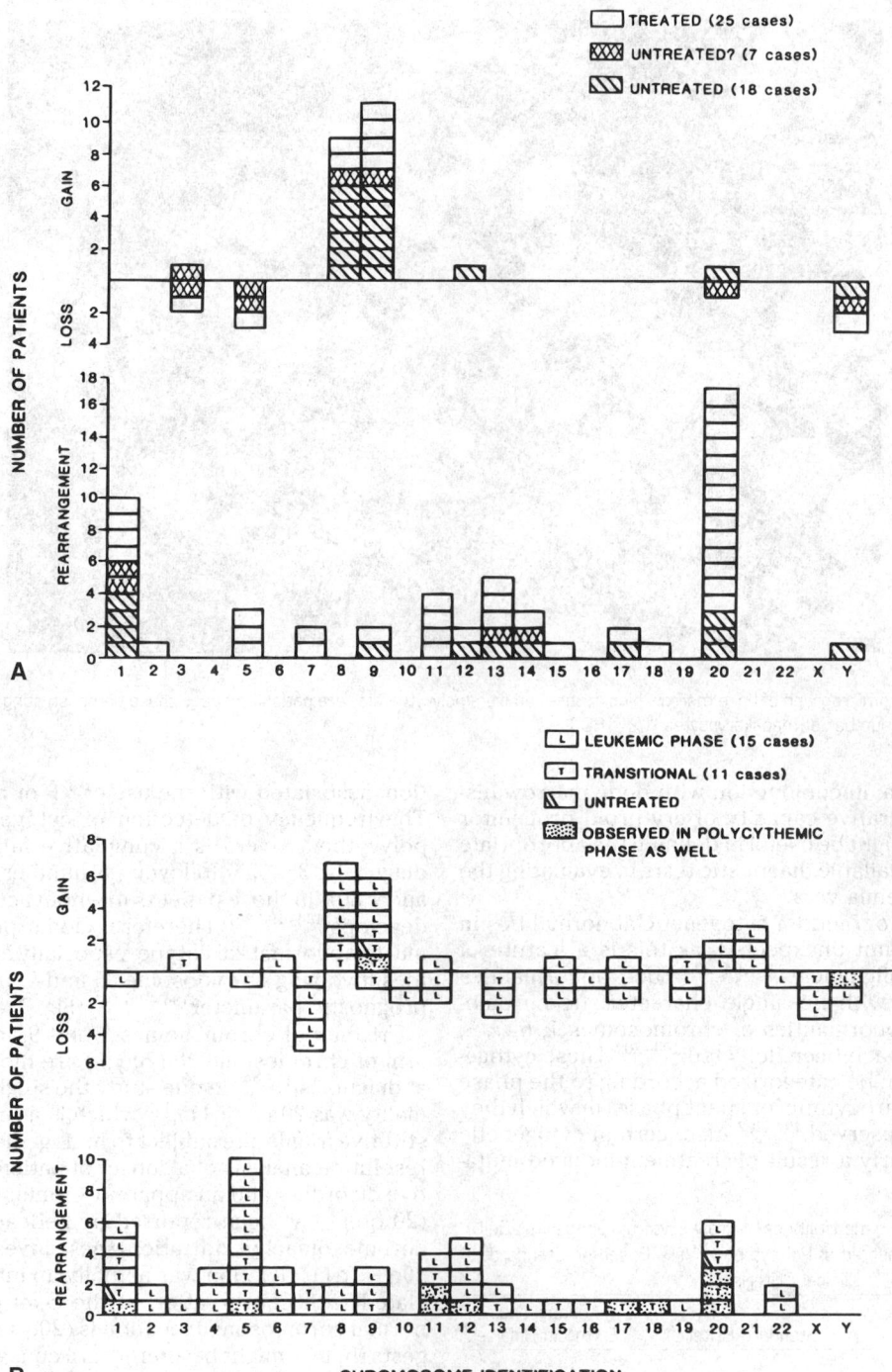

Fig. 72-5. (A) Histogram of clonal karyotypic abnormalities observed in 50 untreated and treated patients with polycythemia vera. Each box represents a clonal abnormality seen in a single patient. **(B)** Histogram of clonal karyotypic abnormalities seen in 26 polycythemia vera patients during a transitional or leukemic phase. In contrast to the pattern seen in the erythrocytotic phase, rearrangement of chromosome 5 and loss of chromosome 7 are quite common in the more advanced stages of polycythemia vera. (From Testa et al.,[197] with permission.)

panied by additional karyotypic abnormalities, with chromosomes 5 and 7 being most frequently involved.[196,197]

DIFFERENTIAL DIAGNOSIS

In the overwhelming number of patients, the establishment of the diagnosis of polycythemia vera is not difficult. Characteristically, the patient will present with erythrocytosis, leukocy-

tosis, and thrombocytosis.[4] The bone marrow biopsy shows hypercellularity with trilinear cellular hyperplasia.[180–184] A direct determination of red blood cell mass is necessary for documentation of the presence of absolute erythrocytosis and should be performed in every patient.[173,174] The presence of splenomegaly is an important finding on clinical examination, and adjunctive laboratory findings include normal arterial oxygen saturation, elevated leukocyte alkaline phosphatase activity, elevated serum vitamin B_{12}, and B_{12}-binding proteins.[4]

Table 72-9. Clinical and Laboratory Criteria for Diagnosis of Polycythemia Vera[a]

1. Elevated red blood cell mass of ≥36 ml/kg for male and ≥32 ml/kg for female patients

2. Normal arterial oxygen saturation (≥92%) in the presence of erythrocytosis as defined in criterion 1

3. Splenomegaly

4. Thrombocytosis (platelet count of ≥400,000/mm³) and leukocytosis (white blood cell count of ≥12,000/mm³)

5. Bone marrow hypercellularity associated with megakaryocytic hyperplasia and absent iron stores

6. Low serum EPO levels (<30 mU/ml) in the presence of an increased red blood cell mass as defined in criterion 1

7. Abnormal marrow proliferative capacity as manifested by formation of erythroid colonies in the absence of exogenous EPO

[a] The presence of four of these criteria indicates that the patient's hematologic disorder is polycythemia vera.

It is initially important to discriminate polycythemia vera from the large number of other causes of secondary erythrocytosis and spurious polycythemia. (This subject is discussed in greater detail in Ch. 37.) Two tests that are especially useful for this purpose are the ability of bone marrow cells to form erythroid colonies in the absence of exogenous EPO and quantitation of serum and urinary EPO levels by either RIA, ELISA, or in vivo biologic assay.[185–193] The availability of newly defined genetic markers employing DNA restriction fragment length polymorphisms to establish clonality of a bone marrow proliferative disorder may also expedite the diagnosis in affected females.[62,63] The impact of these new diagnostic tools in establishing the diagnosis of polycythemia vera in an individual patient is only now becoming apparent.

Clinical criteria for the diagnosis have been defined by the PVSG and have been successfully used to obtain a uniform patient population with polycythemia vera for evaluation of therapeutic modalities.[4,81,167] It is important, however, for the clinician to realize that some patients undoubtedly have a myeloproliferative disorder resembling polycythemia vera but do not fulfill all the clinical criteria of the PVSG.[191] The diagnostic criteria of the PVSG do not include measurement of bone marrow proliferative capacity or serum erythropoietin. More useful—and, it is hoped, more flexible—criteria for the diagnosis of polycythemia vera are suggested in Table 72-9. There will always be unusual cases showing clinical characteristics that cannot be pigeonholed in a particular diagnostic category. If asymptomatic, these patients should be followed carefully until the disorder evolves into a more recognizable entity. This would appear prudent in order to avoid unnecessary therapeutic interventions. If these patients have serious symptoms, the individual physician must make treatment decisions on the basis of the risk/benefit ratio for that patient.

A particularly difficult dilemma occurs when evaluating patients with isolated pure erythrocytosis. These patients have elevated red blood cell masses, normal white blood cell counts, normal platelet counts, no evidence of splenomegaly, and no evidence of any recognizable cause of secondary erythrocytosis. Russell and Conley[206] and Modan and Modan,[207] as well as Najean et al.,[208] believe that these cases represent a clinical entity distinct from polycythemia vera. By contrast, Pearson and Wetherley-Mein[209] have suggested that at least some of these cases can be reclassified as polycythemia vera at a later time in their clinical course. In the report of Najean et al., 7 of 51 such patients after prolonged follow-up developed a clinical picture similar to that of polycythemia vera or agnogenic myeloid metaplasia with myelofibrosis, or both.[208] The course of the other patients with primary pure erythrocytosis was also frequently complicated by thrombotic vascular episodes. These patients were treated with myelosuppressive therapy to avoid additional complications. Of these 51 patients, 5 eventually developed some form of acute myeloid leukemia.[208] On the basis of this information, a significant number of these patients appear to have a disorder that closely resembles polycythemia vera and should be accordingly treated. The familial form of polycythemia characterized by increased sensitivity of erythroid progenitor cells to EPO is clearly distinct from polycythemia vera. These patients are frequently asymptomatic and do not require therapeutic intervention.[30]

The ability of bone marrow cells to form endogenous erythroid colonies has also been used to analyze etiologic factors in the development of Budd-Chiari syndrome.[210] Valla et al.[210] studied the marrow proliferative capacity of 20 patients with this syndrome and observed endogenous erythroid colony formation in 16 cases. In 2 of these 16 patients, it was quite obvious that a myeloproliferative disorder was the underlying etiologic factor in the development of hepatic vein thrombosis. This abnormality in the other 14 patients suggests that the development of Budd-Chiari syndrome may represent, in some cases, a forme fruste of a myeloproliferative disorder.

Polycythemia vera must also be differentiated from the other myeloproliferative disorders, such as CML, primary thrombocythemia, and agnogenic myeloid metaplasia with myelofibrosis. Such classification has major prognostic implications on which important therapeutic decisions should be based. With the distinctive cytogenetic abnormalities and molecular genetic abnormalities that are unique to CML (Philadelphia chromosome, *bcr-abl* gene fusion), these two disorders should not be difficult to differentiate.[57,211] A less complex test, the leukocyte alkaline phosphatase activity, be used for this purpose. The leukocyte alkaline phosphatase score is elevated in polycythemia vera but is decreased in patients with CML.[4,57] In addition, the incidence of elevated red cell masses in patients with CML is low.

Patients with agnogenic myeloid metaplasia with myelofibrosis can present with abnormalities that are virtually indistinguishable from those of patients with PPMM.[107–109] The survival of patients with the latter disorder is much shorter than that of patients with the former condition.[107–109] A preceding history of polycythemia vera permits differentiation between these two situations. Primary thrombocythemia and polycythemia vera with marked thrombocytosis can easily be confused. When the red blood cell mass is used as a definitive diagnostic test, a distinction between primary thrombocythemia and erythrocytotic phase of polycythemia vera is usually readily apparent.[212] This measurement, however, can be normal or actually low in the patient with polycythemia vera who is iron deficient because of bleeding or excessive phlebotomy. To avoid this difficulty, Iland[213] has developed a logistic regression algorithm on the basis of clinical characteristics; this algorithm appears useful in differentiating primary thrombocythemia from polycythemia vera in cases in which either a red blood cell mass quantitation is unavailable or iron deficiency cannot be excluded.

THERAPY

Dramatic prolongation of survival over that expected from the natural history of untreated polycythemia vera has been achieved with several therapeutic strategies.[81,121,157,160] Historical evidence for an untreated median survival of approximately 18 months is derived from descriptive accounts.[10,167] Median survivals ranging >10 years in length are now commonplace with optimal management.[81,121,157,160,214] The choice of therapy however, remains an area of active debate.[161,164] Improvement of therapy might involve the use of newer biologic agents.[215–219]

GENERAL PRINCIPLES OF THERAPY

1. Etiology of erythrocytosis must be correctly categorized in order to be certain the patient has polycythemia vera. This will avoid inappropriate exposure of patients with nonmalignant disorders to radiation or chemotherapy.
2. Therapy should be individualized.
3. Initially blood volume should be reduced to normal as rapidly as possible. The speed of phlebotomy will depend on patient's general medical condition (250–500 ml every other day). Elderly patients with compromised cardiovascular or pulmonary systems should be more carefully phlebotomized (twice a week), or smaller volumes of blood should be removed.
4. Hematocrit should be maintained at 42–45%.
5. Excessive doses of chemotherapeutic agents should be avoided. Supplementary phlebotomy rather than potentially toxic doses of chemotherapeutic agents should be used in order to avoid excessive marrow and systemic toxicity.
6. Hyperuricemia is treated with allopurinol (100–300 mg/day).
7. Pruritus is treated with histamine (H_1 or H_2)-antagonists (cyproheptadine 4–16 mg/day; cimetidine 900 mg/day or ranitidine 300 mg/day). If unsuccessful, aspirin and myelosuppressive therapy should be tried, and if no response, PUVA plus psoralens or cholestyramine should be considered. Iron therapy can be considered but will probably have to be discontinued because of an unacceptable rise in the patient's red cell mass.
8. Elective surgery or dental procedures should be delayed until red cell mass and platelet counts have been normalized for ≥2 months. If emergency surgery is contemplated, phlebotomy and cytopheresis should be pursued.
9. Women and men who are contemplating having children should be treated by phlebotomy in order to avoid teratogenic effects of chemotherapy and radiotherapy. Such avoidance will also prevent deleterious effects on fertility. During pregnancy therapy is frequently not necessary; if it is, phlebotomy should be exclusively used.

A series of studies performed over a 17-year period (1967–1984) by the PVSG has answered several very important questions regarding the efficacy and associated complications of particular therapeutic modalities. These investigations, however, have not resulted in the identification of the single best therapy but rather have emphasized that treatment of an individual patient must be selected on the basis of age and comorbid disease status in order to minimize treatment-related complications.[81,114,115,167,168]

The PVSGs first randomized trial (01 trial) examined three treatment arms: (1) phlebotomy alone, to maintain the hematocrit at <45%; (2) intravenous ^{32}P, 2.3 mCi/m² repeated every 12 weeks if needed (maximum 5 mCi per dose), supplemented by phlebotomy to maintain the hematocrit at ≤45; and (3) myelosuppression with chlorambucil 10 mg/day PO for 6 weeks, then daily on alternate months, with necessary dose reductions and supplemental phlebotomy.[167] More than 400 patients were randomly assigned to this protocol. An early finding was the appearance during the first 5 years of a significant excess

of deaths from acute leukemia in the chlorambucil arm, with the rate >10% by the fifth year.[167] These patients had a reduced overall survival compared with those on the other treatment arms. As a result, the chlorambucil arm was discontinued, and patients were assigned randomly to one of the other two arms. Even though no statistical difference in overall survival between ^{32}P and phlebotomy alone was apparent through the first 10 years, the morbidity and mortality associated with each type of therapy were attributable to distinctly different causes.[81] Thrombosis as a cause of death was much more frequent in the phlebotomy-only group during the first 5–7 years of follow-up. Analysis of factors associated with thrombosis revealed that the performance of phlebotomy, the rate of phlebotomy, advancing age, and history of previous thrombosis were statistically significant factors predictive of this outcome.[81,114] By contrast, the use of ^{32}P led to a lower rate of thrombosis during the first 5 years, but the incidence of leukemias, lymphoma, and nonhematologic malignancies increased during the next 5 years to nearly 10%.[81] Following a comparable period of observation, the incidence of leukemia and lymphoma in the chlorambucil group had risen to >15%.[81,114] A statistically significant increase in skin and gastrointestinal cancers occurred in the [32]P- and chlorambucil-treated cohorts, as compared with the group treated with phlebotomy alone.[81]

Given the paradox of equal 10-year survivals, but demise due to distinct causes, in comparable populations of patients treated by phlebotomy alone or by phlebotomy plus ^{32}P, it seemed reasonable to pursue reduction of thrombotic risk in the phlebotomy-only group as a goal of greater ease of attainment. One study attempted reduction of the thrombotic risk by combination antiplatelet therapy. It appeared possible that qualitative antiplatelet therapy might reduce the frequency of thrombosis.[137] Therefore, a randomized trial was performed in which phlebotomy supplemented with the platelet antiaggregating agents aspirin and dipyridamole was compared with [32]P (PVSG trial 05). The outcome for the phlebotomy/aspirin/dipyridamole-treated group was disappointingly inferior to the ^{32}P results.[137] In fact, more thromboses occurred in the former than in the latter group, but surprisingly, there was also a significantly greater incidence of severe gastrointestinal hemorrhages.[137]

In light of more recent knowledge of the dose requirements for selective antiplatelet therapy with aspirin, it appears this study might have failed due to excessive aspirin dosages (900 mg/day) which appear to diminish vascular endothelial production of the platelet antiaggregatory factor, prostacyclin (PGI_2).[137,220]

It is interesting to compare the results of the PVSG with those of a randomized trial of ^{32}P versus busulfan for the treatment of polycythemia vera conducted by the European Organization for Research and Treatment of Cancer.[214] The two studies were comparable in size, design, and duration of follow-up. In the EORTC trial induction courses of busulfan 4–6 mg/day for 4–8 weeks were compared with ^{32}P treatment.[214] Patients treated with busulfan enjoyed a survival advantage over ^{32}P-treated patients.[214] This difference was due primarily to a threefold greater incidence of fatal thrombotic events in the ^{32}P group. Interestingly, the incidence of leukemia in both groups was very low (<2%), with an overall malignancy rate of <10% (involving mostly solid tumors).[214]

It is reasonable to conclude from this trial that busulfan is a myelosuppressive agent of relatively low leukemogenic potential when used on an intermittent schedule.[163,164,221,222] A retrospective study of patients in England treated with phlebotomy and intermittent busulfan supports these same conclusions.[163,164,221,222]

After the disappointing results experienced with the alkylating agent chlorambucil, the PVSG began a nonrandomized phase II investigation of hydroxyurea, an S-phase-specific ribonucleotide reductase inhibitor.[223,224] Of 53 patients with polycythemia vera who had never received other forms of myelosuppression, follow-up for a median period of 5 years did not indicate a higher incidence of leukemia than that reported previously in patients treated with phlebotomy alone.[223,224] Other investigators have reported similar findings.[225–227] Najean[228] recently reported an 11-year randomized trial comparing hydroxyurea and pipobroman (vercyte) for the treatment of polycythemia vera. Both therapies were comparable in terms of induction of remission, but pipobroman was less well tolerated during maintenance therapy because of gastrointestinal side effects. Low dosages of hydroxyurea were accompanied by inadequate suppression of platelets (range 400–900 $\times$ 106/μl). Progressive resistance to these therapies occurred in 5% of cases. There was no evidence of an increased incidence of leukemia in the hydroxyurea group.

Although longer follow-up of larger cohorts of patients treated with hydroxyurea will be required before the true significance of these findings are known, a prospective study of the consequences of continuous hydroxyurea therapy on acquisition of new cytogenetic abnormalities sheds additional light on the leukemogenic potential of hydroxyurea. This study indicates that the incidence of new karyotypic abnormalities is very low in a hydroxyurea-treated population. The incidence of cytogenetic abnormalities before and after treatment for this period was 9% and 15%, respectively.[229] This rate of increase is markedly lower than previously seen with ^{32}P or chlorambu-

cil. In addition, none of the acquired cytogenetic abnormalities involved the specific chromosomes (particularly 5 and 7) typical of treatment-related myelodysplastic disorders.

Some clinical investigators have suggested that a program of phlebotomy alone would be the most appropriate for younger patients, in whom the risk of cerebrovascular or cardiovascular thromboses might be predicted to be low.[11,81,166] In fact, analysis by Najean et al.[80] of a series of patients with polycythemia vera presenting <40 years of age indicated that such suppositions are erroneous. A striking incidence of serious thrombotic events was observed, with Budd-Chiari syndrome (hepatic vein thrombosis) and cerebrovascular accidents the leading causes of death.[80] These investigators recommended a program of myelosuppression for the treatment of these young patients. There was a low incidence of acute leukemia in this group of 58 patients, who were followed for ≤15 years (only one developed acute leukemia). This finding is surprising, as most patients received either ^{32}P, an alkylating agent, or hydroxyurea as supplemental therapy.[80]

It is well recognized that the platelets of patients with polycythemia vera are qualitatively abnormal.[97–102] The inability to attribute an increased thrombotic risk directly to quantitative increases in platelet numbers does not necessarily imply that reducing the number of dysfunctional platelets by myelosuppression is of no therapeutic importance. In addition, the failure of aspirin and dipyridamole therapy to reduce the rate of thrombosis in the overall population of polycythemia vera

ALGORITHM FOR MANAGEMENT OF PATIENTS WITH POLYCYTHEMIA VERA

Young patients (<40 years) or standard risk
    (>40 years)
        ↓

Phlebotomy alone to maintain hematocrit ≤ 45%
    ↓

Thrombosis or hemorrhage
Systemic symptoms
Severe pruritus refractory to histamine antagonists
Painful splenomegaly
    ↓

Myelosuppression
    Hydroxyurea: 30 mg/kg PO for 1 week, then 15–20 mg/kg
        Supplemental phlebotomy if hematocrit is >47%
or
    Busulfan: 4–6 mg/day PO for 4–8 weeks; stop when blood counts are normalized or platelet count is <300,000/mm³
        Supplemental phlebotomy if hematocrit is >47%
    When patient relapses, initiate therapy again at same dose
    ↓

Thrombocytosis with repeated thrombosis
    ↓

Anagrelide, interferon, or low-dose aspirin
    ↓

Painful splenomegaly or repeated thrombosis
    ↓
    [32]P

High-risk patients >40 years
Previous thrombosis
High rate of phlebotomy
Age >69 years
    ↓

Myelosuppression
    Hydroxyurea 30 mg/kg for 1 week, then 15 mg/kg
or
    Busulfan 4–6 mg/day PO for 4–8 weeks
    Stop when blood counts are normalized or platelet count is <300,000/mm³.
    Occasional supplemental phlebotomy if hematocrit is >47%; when patient relapses (phlebotomy more often than one every 2–3 months or patient is symptomatic), initiate therapy again at same dose
    ↓

No response
    ↓

[32]P: 2.3 mCi/m² IV every 12 weeks as needed (limit 5 mCi per dose)
Phlebotomize for hematocrit >47%
Increase dose by 25% if no response
    ↓

Persistent thrombosis and thrombocytosis
    ↓

    Anagrelide
    Low-dose aspirin
    Interferon

patients treated with phlebotomy (as in PSVG 05 trial) does not imply that selective qualitative antiplatelet therapy cannot be effective.[137] In fact, it has been suggested that high-dose aspirin is a therapeutic double-edged sword, that can promote platelet aggregation by blocking production of the antiaggregatory PGI_2 by the vascular endothelium.[220] PGI_2 is a potent inhibitor of platelet aggregation.[50] It has been proposed that very low dose aspirin (e.g., 40–80 mg) may be superior in inhibiting platelet aggregation and thromboxane synthesis while sparing vascular endothelial PGI_2 synthesis. In addition, Schaefer has suggested restricting the use of aspirin to patients with digital or cerebrovascular ischemia who have normal bleeding times and normal or spontaneous platelet aggregation.[97] Patients with a prior history of bleeding problems or with prolonged bleeding times and/or abnormal platelet aggregation studies are at a high risk of bleeding following use of aspirin.[97]

Silverstein et al.[230,231] have suggested the use of anagrelide, a selective inhibitor of platelet production, for the treatment of thrombocytosis in such patients. This agent appears to be nonleukemogenic and acts by impairing megakaryocyte maturation.[232] Its use leads to a selective reduction in platelet numbers, and it has been effective in patients refractory to hydroxyurea and interferon. In addition, a protocol for combination treatment with hydroxyurea and anagrelide has been developed. This regimen might be considered in certain clinical situations because of the inability of low-dose hydroxyurea maintenance therapy to control platelet counts.[228] Approximately 15–20% of patients treated with anagrelide discontinued the medication due to nonmyelosuppressive side effects. The spectrum of adverse effects involved neurologic (headaches and dizziness), cardiac (vasodilation, fluid retention, congestive heart failure, palpitations, and tachycardia), and gastrointestinal (nausea) toxicities. These toxicities reflect the novel mechanism of action of anagrelide as a cyclic nucleotide phosphodiesterase inhibitor. Anagrelide should be used with caution in patients with known or suspected cardiac disease.[230] This might include a large fraction of the elderly population with polycythemia vera.

Another potential approach to controlling the erythrocytosis and thrombocytosis in polycythemia vera involves use of an interferon-α.[215–217] Several small trials of interferon therapy in myeloproliferative disorders have been performed.[216,218,219] The patients treated have experienced reduction in red cell counts and platelet counts, but there is no information regarding possible beneficial effects in avoiding thrombotic complications.[216,218,219]

Symptomatic management of the polycythemia vera patient may be complicated by the occurrence of intractable pruritus.[4,144–149] Classically the pruritus occurs on exposure to sudden body cooling, especially after a warm bath,[4,144–149] and is experienced by as many as 40–60% of patients treated with phlebotomy.[26,145] The frequency of pruritus appears to be somewhat lower in patients treated with myelosuppressive agents.[233] This observation is related to the probable relationship between pruritus and degranulation of tissue mast cells and circulating basophils.[144,146,147] Some uncontrolled studies have attributed pruritus to hyperhistaminemia or severe iron deficiency, with relief associated with the use of histamine antagonists or ferrous sulfate.[149,233,234–239] Chanarin and Szur[234] have suggested empirical use of cholestyramine. The success rate of these treatment modalities remains low. Iron replacement is frequently not possible since it can lead to dangerous elevations of the red cell mass. In one study, myelosuppressive therapy in combination with aspirin resulted in relief from pruritus.[147] The association between pruritus and tissue infiltration by mast cells would appear to explain the response of occasional patients to photochemotherapy with psoralens and ultraviolet irradiation.[239] No uniformly successful treatment for

pruritus is available, and the clinician must resort to the empirical use of the above-mentioned modalities.

Budd-Chiari syndrome is a catastrophic illness, which can lead to significant morbidity and mortality in a patient with polycythemia vera.[116–118] Patients with myeloproliferative disorders are at a high risk of developing this syndrome,[116–118] and independently, use of oral contraceptive pills is a risk factor for its development, a number of cases of hepatic vein thrombosis having been reported in nonpolycythemic women taking oral contraceptives.[240–242] Although no data are available, one must be concerned about use of oral contraceptives in women with polycythemia vera.

The optimal approach to the problem of Budd-Chiari syndrome is obviously preventive and involves maintenance of normal blood values in the patient with polycythemia vera.[118] Once the Budd-Chiari syndrome develops, the prognosis without treatment is dismal. The goals of therapy are to prevent further propagation of thrombus, relieve the intense hepatic congestion, and manage the severe ascites that often plagues these patients.[118] If untreated, these patients often have a slowly progressive course, with deterioration and death within 3.5 years.[118] Spontaneous resolution of the hepatic vein occlusion rarely occurs. Diuretics may be of value in the treatment of the ascites but do not affect the long-term outcome.[118] Thrombolytic therapy may be expected to have some role in the treatment of patients with acute thrombosis.[124] Anticoagulant therapy may have a role in the prevention of further clot formation, but there has been no definitive evidence that such therapy promotes resolution of established thromboses.[118]

The clinical deterioration of patients with Budd-Chiari syndrome is due to damage to the hepatocytes from necrosis associated with marked elevation in sinusoidal pressure, coupled with ischemia from reduced hepatic arteriole perfusion.[118] The only rational therapeutic intervention therefore involves some sort of portal decompression to achieve effective reduction of sinusoidal pressure.[118] A variety of surgical procedures resulting in portasystemic decompression have been shown to be of value in patients with Budd-Chiari syndrome.[243–245] Liver transplantation is currently also a potential option for treatment of these patients.[246] The hematologic consequences of polycythemia must be aggressively treated in the post-transplant setting, since the hepatic vein occlusion may recur in the transplanted liver.[246] However, the frequent use following liver transplantation of 6-mercaptopurine, in addition to cyclosporine, for immunosuppression appears to contribute to control of excessive hematopoietic proliferation due to the underlying polycythemia vera.

The performance of any surgical procedures on patients with polycythemia vera is, as previously discussed, accompanied by excessively high morbidity and mortality.[140–143] Elective surgery should not be contemplated unless the patient's hematologic values have been normalized for several months.[142,143] The longer the hematologic control has been in effect, the lower the incidence of postoperative complications. If emergency surgery is required, the patient should be phlebotomized rapidly until a normal hematocrit is reached.[142,143] Following both emergency and elective surgery, the patient should be mobilized as soon as possible. Dental extractions can also result in excessive hemorrhage and should not be performed unless the patient is under strict hematologic control.[142,143]

Perhaps the most difficult and frustrating period encountered during the clinical course of a patient with polycythemia vera is the development of PPMM.[107–109] These patients are frequently symptomatic, owing to the sequelae of anemia, infection, bleeding, and splenic enlargement.[107–109] Because few of these patients have been treated in a uniform, controlled fashion, it is difficult to make strict therapeutic recommendations.

The anemia that characterizes the spent phase is usually multifactorial in origin. An important factor is splenic pooling of red cells and expansion of the plasma volume, which occurs as a consequence of splenomegaly.[247-249] It is therefore important in these patients to obtain red blood cell mass measurements and to quantitate the degree of anemia directly in order to detect those patients who have a low hematocrit but normal red cell mass. Folate or iron deficiency may be important in already anemic patients and should be corrected.[107-109,154] Almost 20% of patients with PPMM develop overt hemolytic anemia.[107-109] Some of these patients respond to prednisone therapy, but most require splenectomy. By far the most common cause of anemia is ineffective erythropoiesis,[250] and these patients often require transfusion therapy. Androgen therapy may be effective in stimulating effective hematopoiesis and diminishing transfusion requirements.[251] The possibility of iron overload syndrome secondary to ineffective erythropoiesis or transfusion therapy is a danger. In this situation, some consideration should be given to chronic iron chelation therapy.

Perhaps the most troubling aspects of the clinical course of these patients are the pressure symptoms secondary to splenic enlargement and repeated splenic infarcts.[107-109,252-254] Treatment must be directed toward decreasing the expansion of a rapidly enlarging spleen. Small doses of busulfan or hydroxyurea may result in the relief of such symptoms[107,109]; radiotherapy in small doses is also sometimes helpful. Unfortunately, its effect is frequently transient.[109,255] The chemotherapy or radiation dose must be carefully determined since overzealous use may lead to granulocytopenia and thrombocytopenia. Often, as a last resort, splenectomy is the only reasonable therapeutic maneuver. This procedure in far advanced disease is associated with an operative mortality of 25% and should be performed by only the most experienced of surgeons.[252-254] Surgical intervention should not be inappropriately delayed.[252-254] Splenectomy in such patients is frequently complicated by excessive hemorrhage and infected hematomas.[252-254]

Thrombocytopenia may lead to life-threatening hemorrhage in PPMM patients.[107-109] Its development is due to ineffective thrombopoiesis and/or platelet sequestration by an enlarged spleen and patients may respond to splenectomy.[252-254] Bleeding due to qualitative platelet abnormalities has been noted in these patients[109]; when it is severe, platelet transfusions are often required, although because of marked splenomegaly such transfusions frequently do not increase platelet numbers. The clinician therefore must follow the extent of hemorrhage as a means of determining the effectiveness of such transfusions. Disseminated intravascular coagulopathy occasionally complicates the PPMM and can lead to life-threatening hemorrhage.[252] After careful laboratory documentation, replacement therapy with fresh frozen plasma should be pursued; if that is unsuccessful, a course of low-dose heparin therapy is warranted. If bleeding increases with institution of heparin therapy, the heparin should be quickly discontinued.[233] Some mention should also be made of the use of biological response modifiers for the treatment of PPMM. A number of investigators have suggested that interferon might be useful in the treatment of agnogenic myeloid metaplasia and might be successful in reducing spleen size.[216-219] Experience with this drug for the treatment of PPMM has not been published, and its use is not without adverse effects. Interferon can suppress hematopoiesis and might be a particularly difficult agent to use in the management of patients who are already anemic and thrombocytopenic.[218]

Some information is available concerning the treatment of those patients who develop acute leukemia following polycythemia vera.[81,87,115] The overwhelming majority of such cases involve myeloid leukemias, but a small number of patients have a lymphoblastic phenotype.[115,169-171] The optimal treatment of such patients is unknown. In the elderly, the choice not to institute chemotherapy is a reasonable option, since results with treatment are so poor. In those patients with a lymphoid phenotype, a brief course of vincristine and prednisone with or without Adriamycin or daunomycin might be considered.[233] The PVSG has treated 13 patients, irrespective of phenotypic markers with vincristine and prednisone without a successful response.[115] This group treated the remaining nine patients with a combination including cytosine arabinoside and Adriamycin and were able to achieve a complete remission in one patient and a partial remission in another.[115] The survival for the 13 patients, however, was 32 days from the time of institution of chemotherapy.[115] Hoyle et al.,[256] however, have reported more favorable results with an induction regimen of daunomycin, cytosine arabinoside, and 6-thioguanine.

Rare prolonged remissions of acute leukemia following polycythemia vera have been reported in the literature.[257] Some investigators have suggested that the poor prognosis of these patients merits immediate treatment with high-dose cytosine arabinoside in combination with either daunomycin or Adriamycin.[258] Because these patients are frequently elderly, poor results with standard regimens have been reported, and an alternative approach using low-dose cytosine arabinoside might be considered.[158]

Polycythemia vera occurs infrequently during the childbearing years.[233] When it does, it has been reported to lead to an increased incidence of fetal wastage, with 30% of pregnancies in polycythemia vera patients terminating in spontaneous abortions.[259,260] In addition, pre-eclampsia occurs more frequently in these women.[259,260] Pregnancy in polycythemia vera patients is associated with a gradual normalization of blood values, and it is not unusual for a woman who has required extensive therapy for control of her disease to no longer require phlebotomies during pregnancy.[259,260] Delivery appears not to be complicated by excessive hemorrhage or by an increased risk of venous thrombosis.[233,259,260] However, one must be concerned about the possible occurrence of such events.

The normalization of the hematocrit during pregnancy in polycythemia vera has been associated with lowering of the red cell mass into the normal range in the few patients in whom these measurements have been performed.[233] Although some degree of hematocrit normalization can be explained by expansion of the plasma volume or by nutritional deficiencies that occur during pregnancy, it is unlikely that these factors can be solely responsible.[233] It seems more reasonable to assume that the high estrogen levels characteristic of pregnancy suppress erythropoiesis. In the few male patients with polycythemia vera who have been treated with estrogen, suppression of the red cell production has been noted.[233] After termination of the pregnancy, the patients' hematologic values slowly drift back to their previously elevated values coincidentally with the return to normal estrogen levels.[233] Because pregnancy is usually associated with spontaneous control of the polycythemic state, no specific therapy is required, except for careful observation. If needed, therapy should be limited to phlebotomy because of the mutagenic effects of chemotherapeutic agents.

PROGNOSIS

The prognosis of a patient with polycythemia vera is dependent on the nature and severity of the complications that occur during the clinical course of that particular patient's disorder.[10,11,81] In addition, an individual patient's prognosis depends on the duration of the erythrocytotic phase or the time for transition to PPMM or acute leukemia.[9,81,121,154] Survival is also influenced by whether appropriate treatment is instituted during the erythrocytotic phase of the illness. Patients who have uncontrolled erythrocytosis are at an extremely high risk of the development of thromboses.[81,82] The median survival from onset of symptoms may be as short as 1.5 years in untreated patients.[10,167] Determination of the optimal management of patients with polycythemia vera has been a difficult task, as the disease, when treated, is associated with a survival of 10–15 years. Studies of new potential therapeutic interventions therefore require prospective study with prolonged follow-up before meaningful results can be generated.[167]

The PVSG has shown quite conclusively that survival is significantly poorer for patients treated with chlorambucil than for those treated with either ^{32}P or phlebotomy.[81] On the basis of this study, chlorambucil is not a desirable choice.[81] In this particular study, at least, median survival from entry until death was 11.8 years for ^{32}P-treated patients, 8.9 years for chlorambucil-treated patients, and 13.9 years for the phlebotomy-treated group.[81]

Thrombosis occurred predominantly among the phlebotomy-treated patients, especially during the first 4 years of this study.[81] However, longer follow-up demonstrates a greater number of deaths due to both hematologic and nonhematologic malignancies in patients treated with either of the myelosuppressive regimens.[81,114] One is left with a serious dilemma in defining treatment for a particular patient. Those who are treated with phlebotomy alone for the first 5–7 years of their course appear to be at a very high risk of dying from thrombosis. However, with more prolonged follow-up after this 5–7-year period, patients treated with ^{32}P or one of the other alkylating agents would appear to be at a much higher risk of dying from a malignant disorder.[81,114]

Therefore, optimal management for a particular patient remains problematic. In a young patient, who potentially will have a more prolonged course lasting several decades, it would appear best to treat with phlebotomy alone. In many patients with serious hemorrhagic or thrombotic complications however, this may not be possible. This situation warrants the use of interferon-α, phlebotomy with supplemental use of anagrelide, intermittent use of busulfan, or the use of hydroxyurea. Although a great concern for potential leukemogenic activity of hydroxyurea has been registered, so far this fear has not been realized in >10 years of use. In elderly patients, who have a more limited survival because of their age, the use of either ^{32}P or another agent such as hydroxyurea might be optimal.

FUTURE DIRECTIONS

Future directions in the treatment of patients with polycythemia vera is highly dependent on obtaining a more comprehensive understanding of the pathophysiology of this clonal neoplastic disorder. Further definition of oncogenic alterations in intracellular signaling within these clonal malignant cells should permit the development of more specific therapies. Further definition of risk factors for the development of fatal thrombotic and hemorrhagic events will be important for the rational design of therapeutic interventions to prevent these complications. It will also be important to test whether sequential therapy in younger patients with polycythemia vera might be optimal.[81] This would include the use of hydroxyurea, or busulfan for the first 3–5 years in order to decrease the incidence of thrombotic events early in the clinical course and subsequently to treat with phlebotomy in order to decrease neoplastic deaths from prolonged administration of these agents.[81]

REFERENCES

1. Vaquez H: Sur une forme spéciale de cyanose s'accompagnant d'hyperglobule excessive et persistente. CR Soc Biol 44:384, 1892
2. Cabot RC: A case of chronic cyanosis without discoverable cause, ending in cerebral hemorrhage. Boston Med Surg J 141:574, 1899
3. Osler W: Chronic cyanosis with polycythemia and enlarged spleen: a new clinical entity. Am J Med Sci 126:187, 1903
4. Berlin N: Diagnosis and classification of the polycythemias. Semin Hematol 12:339, 1975
5. Dameshek W: Some speculations on the myeloproliferative syndromes. Blood 6:372, 1951
6. Dai CH, Krantz SB, Means RT Jr et al: Polycythemia vera blood burst-forming units-erythroid are hypersensitive to interleukin-3. J Clin Invest 87:391, 1991
7. Dai CH, Krantz SB, Dessypris EN et al: Polycythemia vera. II. hypersensitivity of bone marrow erythroid, granulocyte-macrophage, and megakaryocyte progenitor cells to interleukin-3 and granulocyte-macrophage colony-stimulating factor. Blood 80:891, 1992
8. de Wolf JI, Beentjes JA, Esselink MI, Smit JW et al: In polycythemia vera human interleukin 3 and granulocyte-macrophage colony-stimulating factor enhance erythroid colony growth in the absence of erythropoietin. Exp Hematol 17:981, 1989
9. Wasserman LR: Polycythemia vera—its course and treatment: relation to myeloid metaplasia and leukemia. Bull NY Acad Med 3:343, 1954
10. Chievitz E, Thiede T: Complications and causes of death in polycythemia vera. J Intern Med 172:513, 1962
11. Wasserman LR: The treatment of polycythemia vera. Semin Hematol 13:57, 1976
12. Modan B: An epidemiological study of polycythemia vera. Blood 26:657, 1965
13. Silverstein MN, Lanier AP: Polycythemia vera, 1935–1969: an epidemiologic survey in Rochester, Minnesota. Mayo Clin Proc 46:751, 1971
14. Prochazka AV, Markowe HLG: The epidemiology of polycythaemia rubra vera in England and Wales 1968–1982. Br J Cancer 53:59, 1986
15. Dougan LE, Mathews MVL, Armstrong BK: The effect of diagnostic review on the incidence of lymphatic and haematopoietic neoplasms in western Australia. Cancer 48:866, 1987
16. Damon A, Holub DA: Host factors in polycythemia vera. Ann Intern Med 49:43, 1958
17. Wasi P, Block M: Polycythemia vera in a Negro woman. Arch Intern Med 107:260, 1961
18. Chaiter Y, Brenner B, Aghai E, Tatarsky I: High incidence of myeloproliferative disorders in Ashkenazi Jews in northern Israel. Leuk Lymphoma 7:251, 1992
19. Kurita S: Epidemiological studies of polycythemia vera in Japan. Acta Haematol 37:793, 1974
20. The Committee for the Compilation of Materials on Damage Caused by the Atomic Bombs in Hiroshima and Nagasaki. p. 200. In Ishikara R, Swain DL (transl): The Physical, Medical and Social Effects of the Atomic Bombings. Basic Books, New York, 1981
21. Caldwell GG, Kelly DB, Heath CW, Zack M: Polycythemia vera among participants of a nuclear weapons test. JAMA 252:662, 1984
22. Marsh GM, Enterline PE, McCraw D: Mortality patterns among petroleum refinery and chemical plant workers. Am J Ind Med 19:29, 1991
23. Lawrence JH, Goetsch AT: Familial occurrence of polycythemia and leukemia. West J Med 73:361, 1950
24. Friedland ML, Wittels EG, Robinson RJ: Polycythemia vera in identical twins. Am J Hematol 10:101, 1981
25. Erf LA: Radioactive phosphorus in the treatment of primary polycythemia (vera). Prog Hematol 1:153, 1956
26. Levin WC, Houston EW, Ritzman SE: Polycythemia vera with Ph[1] chromosomes in two brothers. Blood 30:503, 1967
27. Brubaker LH, Wasserman LR, Goldberg JD et al: Increased prevalence of polycythemia vera in parents of patients on Polycythemia Vera Study Group protocols. Am J Hematol 16:367, 1984
28. Manoharan A, Garson OM: Familial polycythaemia vera: a study of 3 sisters. Scand J Haematol 17:10, 1976
29. Ratnoff OD, Gress RE: The familial occurrence of polycythemia vera: report of a father and son with consideration of the probable role of exposure to organic solvents including tetrachloroethylene. Blood 56:233, 1980
30. Emanuel PD, Eaves CJ, Broudy VC et al: Familial and congenital polycythemia in three unrelated families. Blood 79:3019, 1992
31. Osgood EE: Polycythemia vera: age relationship and survival. Blood 26:293, 1965
32. Danish EH, Rasch CA, Harris JW: Polycythemia vera in childhood: case report and review of the literature. Am J Hematol 9:421, 1980
33. Gurney CW: Polycythemia vera and some possible pathogenetic mechanisms. Annu Rev Med 16:169, 1965
34. London IM, Shemin D, West R, Rittenberg D: Heme synthesis and red blood cell dynamics in normal humans and in subjects with polycythemia vera, sickle cell anemia and pernicious anemia. J Biol Chem 179:463, 1943
35. Zanjani ED, Ascensao JL: Erythropoietin. Transfusion 29:46, 1989

36. Adamson JW: The erythropoietin/hematocrit relationship in normal and polycythemic man: implications of marrow regulation. Blood 32:597, 1968

37. Goldberg MA, Gaut CC, Bunn HF: Erythropoietin mRNA levels are governed by both the rate of gene transcription and posttranscriptional events. Blood 77:271, 1991

38. Fandrey J, Bunn HF: In vivo and in vitro regulation of erythropoietin mRNA: measurement by competitive polymerase chain reaction. Blood 81:617, 1993

39. Erslev A: Erythropoietin coming of age. N Engl J Med 316:101, 1987

40. Williams DE, de Vries P, Namen AE et al: The Steel factor. Dev Biol 151:368, 1992

41. Brandt J, Briddell RA, Srour EF et al: Role of c-kit ligand in the expansion of human hematopoietic progenitor cells. Blood 79:634, 1992

42. Erslev A, Caro J: Erythrocytosis classified according to erythropoietin titers. Am J Med 76:57, 1984

43. Koeffler HP, Goldwasser E: Erythropoietin radioimmunoassay in evaluating patients with polycythemia. Ann Intern Med 94:44, 1981

44. Eschbach JW, Egric JC, Downing MR et al: Correction of the anemia of end stage renal disease with recombinant human erythropoietin. N Engl J Med 31:673, 1987

45. Camiscoli JF, Weintraub AH, Gordon AS: Comparative assay of erythropoietin standards. Ann NY Acad Sci 149:40, 1968

46. Limman JW, Pierre RV: Studies on the erythropoietin effects of hyperbaric hyperoxia. Ann NY Acad Sci 149:25, 1968

47. Cotes PM, Bangham DR: Bio-assay of erythropoietin in mice made polycythaemic by exposure to air in reduced pressure. Nature 191:1065, 1961

48. Garcia JF, Ebbe SN, Hollander L et al: Radioimmunoassay of erythropoietin: circulating levels in normal and polycythemic human beings. J Lab Clin Med 99:624, 1982

49. Krystal G: A simple microassay for erythropoietin based on ^{3}H-thymidine incorporation into spleen cells from phenylhydrazine treated mice. Exp Hematol 11:649, 1983

50. Sherwood JB, Goldwasser E: A radioimmunoassay for erythropoietin. Blood 54:889, 1979

51. Cotes PM: Immunoreactive erythropoietin in serum. I. Evidence for the validity of the assay method and physiological relevance of estimate. Br J Haematol 50:427, 1982

52. Wognum AW, Lansdorp PM, Eaves AC, Krystal G: An enzyme-linked immunosorbent assay for erythropoietin using monoclonal antibodies, tetrameric immune complexes, and substrate amplification. Blood 74:622, 1989

53. Cotes PM, Dore CJ, Lin Yin JA et al: Determination of serum immunoreactive erythropoietin in the investigation of erythrocytosis. N Engl J Med 315:283, 1986

54. Birgegård G, Miller O, Caro J, Erslev A: Serum erythropoietin levels by radioimmunoassay in polycythaemia. Scand J Haematol 29:161, 1982

55. Birgegård G, Wide L: Serum erythropoietin in the diagnosis of polycythaemia and after phlebotomy treatment. Br J Haematol 81:603, 1992

56. Schlageter M-H, Toubert M-E, Podgorniak M-P, Najean Y: Radioimmunoassay of erythropoietin: analytical performance and clinical use in hematology. Clin Chem 36:1731, 1990

57. Adamson JW, Fialkow PJ: The pathogenesis of myeloproliferative syndromes. Br J Haematol 38:299, 1978

58. Adamson JW: Analysis of haemopoiesis: the use of cell markers and in vitro culture techniques in studies of clonal haemopathies in man. Clin Haematol 13:484, 1984

59. Fialkow PJ: The origin and development of human tumors studied with cell markers. N Engl J Med 291:26, 1974

60. Adamson JW, Fialkow PJ, Murphy S et al: Polycythemia vera stem-cell and probable clonal origin of the disease. N Engl J Med 295:913, 1976

61. Raskind WH, Jacobson R, Murphy S et al: Evidence for the involvement of B lymphoid cells in polycythemia vera and essential thrombocythemia. J Clin Invest 75:1388, 1985

62. Gilliland DG, Blanchard KL, Levy J et al: Clonality in myeloproliferative disorders: analysis by means of the polymerase chain reaction. Proc Natl Acad Sci USA 88:6848, 1991

63. Lucas GS, Padua RA, Masters GS et al: The application of X chromosome gene probes to the diagnosis of myeloproliferative disease. Br J Haematol 72:530, 1989

64. Gregory CJ, Eaves AC: Human marrow cells capable of erythropoietic differentiation in vitro. Definition of three erythroid colony responses. Blood 49:855, 1977

65. Prchal JF, Axelrad AA: Bone marrow responses in polycythemia vera. N Engl J Med 290:1382, 1974

66. Zanjani ED, Lutton JD, Hoffman R, Wasserman LR: Erythroid colony formation by polycythemia vera bone marrow in vitro: dependence on erythropoietin. J Clin Invest 59:841, 1977

67. Golde DW, Bersch N, Cline MJ: Polycythemia vera: hormonal modulation of erythropoiesis in vitro. Blood 49:399, 1977

68. Fauser AA, Messner HA: Pluripotent hemopoietic progenitors (CFU-GEMM) in polycythemia vera: analysis of erythropoietin requirement and proliferative activity. Blood 58:1224, 1981

69. Ash RC, Detrick RA, Zanjani ED: In vitro studies of human pluripotent hematopoietic progenitors in polycythemia vera. J Clin Invest 69:1112, 1982

70. Singer JW, Fialkow PJ, Adamson JW et al: Polycythemia vera: increased expression of normal committed granulocytic stem cells in vitro after exposure of marrow to tritiated thymidine. J Clin Invest 64:1320, 1979

71. Prchal JF, Adamson JW, Murphy S et al: Polycythemia vera: the in vitro response of normal and abnormal stem cell lines to erythropoietin. J Clin Invest 61:1044, 1978

72. Adamson JW, Singer JW, Catalano P et al: Polycythemia vera: further in vitro studies of hematopoietic regulation. J Clin Invest 66:1363, 1980

73. Eaves CJ, Eaves AC: Erythropoietin (Ep) dose-response curves for three classes of erythroid progenitors in normal human marrow and in patients with polycythemia vera. Blood 52:1196, 1978

74. Casadevall N, Vainchenker W, Lacombe C et al: Erythroid progenitors in polycythemia vera: demonstration of their hypersensitivity to erythropoietin in serum free cultures. Blood 59:447, 1982

75. Ratajczak MZ, Luger SM, DeRiel K et al: Role of the KIT protooncogene in normal and malignant human hematopoiesis. Proc Natl Acad Sci USA 89:1710, 1992

76. D'Andrea AD, Yoshimura A, Youssoufian H et al: The cytoplasmic region of the erythropoietin receptor contains nonoverlapping positive and negative growth-regulatory domains. Mol Cell Biol 11:1980, 1991

77. De La Chapelle A, Sistonen P, Lehväshaiho H et al: Familial erythrocytosis genetically linked to erythropoietin receptor gene. Lancet 341:82, 1993

77a. Correa PN, Eskinazi D, Axelrad A: Circulating erythroid progenitors in polycythemia vera are hypersensitive to insulin-like growth factor 1 in vitro: studies in an improved serum-free medium. Blood 83:99, 1994

78. Cashman JD, Eaves CJ, Eaves AC: Unregulated proliferation of primitive neoplastic progenitors in long term polycythemia vera marrow cultures. J Clin Invest 81:87, 1988

79. Kanfer E, Price CM, Colman SM, Barrett AJ: Erythropoietin-independent colony growth in polycythaemia vera is not restricted to progenitor cells with trisomy of chromosome 8. Br J Haematol 82:773, 1992

80. Najean Y, Mugnier P, Dresch C, Didier Rain J: Polycythemia vera in young people: an analysis of 58 cases diagnosed before 40 years. Br J Haematol 67:285, 1987

81. Berk PD, Goldberg JN, Donovan PB et al: Therapeutic recommendations in polycythemia vera based on Polycythemia Vera Study Group protocols. Semin Hematol 23:132, 1986

82. Pearson TC, Wetherley-Mein G: Vascular occlusive episodes and venous haematocrit in primary proliferative polycythemia. Lancet 2:1219, 1978

83. Thomas DJ, Marshall J, Ross Russell RW et al: Cerebral blood flow in polycythemia. Lancet 2:161, 1977

84. Turitto VT, Weiss HJ: Red blood cells: their dual role in thrombus formation. Science 207:541, 1989

85. Lowes GDO, Forbes CD: Blood rheology and thrombosis. Clin Haematol 10:343, 1981

86. Pearson TC, Humphrey PRD, Thomas DJ, Wetherley-Mein G: Haematocrit, blood viscosity, cerebral blood flow and vascular occlusion. In Lowe GDO, Barbenel JC, Forbes CD (eds): Clinical Aspects of Blood Viscosity and Cell Deformability. Springer-Verlag, Berlin, 1981

87. Ellis JT, Silver RT, Colman M, Geller SA: The bone marrow in polycythemia vera. Semin Hematol 12:433, 1975

88. Hutton RD: The effect of iron deficiency on whole blood viscosity in polycythaemic patients. Br J Haematol 43:191, 1971

89. Card RT: Metabolic abnormalities of erythrocytes in severe iron deficiency. Blood 37:725, 1971

90. Tillman W, Schröter W: Deformability of erythrocytes in iron deficiency anemia. Blut 40:179, 1980

91. Yip R, Mohandas N, Clark MR et al: Red cell membrane stiffness in iron deficiency. Blood 62:99, 1983

92. Aarts PAM, Bolhuis PA, Sakariassen KS et al: Red blood cell size is important for adherence of blood platelets to artery subendothelium. Blood 62:214, 1983

93. Bunn HF, Forget BG: Hemogloginopathy due to abnormal oxygen binding. p. 611. In Bunn HF, Forget BG (eds): Hemoglobin: Molecular, Genetic and Clinical Aspects. WB Saunders, Philadelphia, 1986

94. Kessler CM, Klein HG, Havlik RJ: Uncontolled thrombocytosis in chronic myeloproliferative disorders. Br J Haematol 50:157, 1982

95. Landolfi R, Ciabattoni G, Patrignani P et al: Increased thromboxane biosynthesis in patients with polycythemia vera: evidence for aspirin-suppressible platelet activation in vivo. Blood 80:1965, 1992

96. Dawson AA, Ogston D: The influence of the platelet count on the incidence

of thrombotic and haemorrhagic complications in polycythemia vera. Postgrad Med J 46:76, 1970

97. Schafer AI: Bleeding and thrombosis in myeloproliferative disorders. Blood 64:1, 1984

98. Murphy S, Davis JL, Walsh PN, Gardner FH: Template bleeding time and clinical hemorrhage in myeloproliferative disorders. Arch Intern Med 138:1251, 1978

99. Phadke K, Dean S, Pitney WR: Platelet dysfunction in myeloproliferative syndrome. Am J Hematol 10:57, 1981

100. Baker RT, Monohoran A: Platelet function in myeloproliferative disorders: characterization and sequential studies show multiple platelet abnormalities, and change with time. Eur J Haematol 40:267, 1988

101. Murphy S: Thrombocytosis and thrombocythemia. Clin Haematol 12:89, 1983

102. Berger S, Aledort IM, Gilbert HS et al: Abnormalities of platelet function in patients with polycythemia vera. Cancer Res 33:2683, 1973

103. Coon WW, Penner J, Clagett GP: Deep venous thrombosis and post splenectomy thrombocytosis. Arch Surg 113:429, 1978

104. Starksen NF, Day AT, Gazzaniga AB: Does splenectomy result in a higher incidence of limb deep venous thrombosis? Am J Surg 135:202, 1978

105. Singh AK, Wetherly-Mein G: Microvascular occlusive lesions in primary thrombocythemia. Br J Haematol 36:553, 1977

106. Orlin JB, Berkman EM: Improvement of platelet function following plateletpheresis in patients with myeloproliferative diseases. Transfusion 20:540, 1980

107. Silverstein MH: Postpolycythemia myeloid metaplasia. Arch Intern Med 134:113, 1974

108. Najean Y, Arrago JP, Rain JD, Dresch C: The spent phase of polycythemia vera: hypersplenism in the absence of myelofibrosis. Br J Haematol 56:163, 1984

109. Silverstein MN: The evolution into and treatment of late stage polycythemia vera. Semin Hematol 3:79, 1976

110. Castro-Malaspina H, Rabellino EM, Yen A et al: Human megakaryocytic stimulation of proliferation of bone marrow fibroblasts. Blood 57:781, 1981

111. Pettit JE, Lewis SM, Goolden AWG: Polycythemia vera transformation to myelofibrosis and subsequent reversal. Scand J Haematol 20:63, 1978

112. Pettit JE, Lewis SM, Nicholas AW: Transitional myeloproliferative disorder. Br J Haematol 43:167, 1979

113. Perkins J, Israels MCG, Wilkinson JF: Polycythemia vera: clinical studies on a series of 127 patients managed without radiation therapy. Q J Med 33:499, 1965

114. Ellis JT, Peterson P, Gellar SA, Rappaport H: Studies of bone marrow in polycythemia vera and the evolution of myelofibrosis and second hematologic malignancies. Semin Hematol 23:144, 1986

115. Landaw SA: Acute leukemia in polycythemia vera. Semin Hematol 23:156, 1986

116. Noble JA: Hepatic vein thrombosis complicating polycythemia vera: successful treatment with a portacaval shunt. Arch Intern Med 120:105, 1967

117. Parker RGF: Occlusion of the hepatic veins in man. Medicine 38:369, 1954

118. Mitchell MC, Boitnott JK, Kaufman S et al: Budd-Chiari syndrome: etiology, diagnosis and management. Medicine 61:199, 1982

119. Silverstein A, Gilbert H, Wasserman LR: Neurologic complications of polycythemia. Ann Intern Med 57:909, 1962

120. Pearch JMS, Chandrasekera CP, Ladusans EJ: Lacunar infarcts in polycythemia with raised packed cell volumes. Br Med J 287:935, 1983

121. Lawrence JH, Berlin NI, Huff RL: The nature and treatment of polycythemia: studies on 263 patients. Medicine 32:323, 1953

122. Millikan CH, Sickert RG, Whisnant JP: Intermittent carotid and vertebral-basilar insufficiency associated with polycythemia. Neurology 10:188, 1960

123. Clune JP: Septic thrombosis within the cavernous chamber: review of the literature with recent advances in diagnosis and treatment. Am J Ophthalmol 56:33, 1963

124. Boniuk M: The ocular manifestations of ophthalmic vein and aseptic cavernous thrombosis. Trans Am Acad Ophthalmol Otolaryngol 76:1519, 1972

125. Melamed E, Rachmilewitz EA, Reches A, Lavy S: Aseptic cavernous sinus thrombosis after internal carotid arterial occlusion in polycythemia vera. J Neurol Neurosurg Psychiatry 39:320, 1976

126. Ali M, Fayemi AP, Malcolm D, Braun EV: Intraventricular thrombosis in polycythemia vera: a cause of intractable cardiac failure. Am Heart J 100:520, 1980

127. Zinn P, Applegate RJ, Walsh RA: Acute total aortic occlusion during cardiac catheterization associated with polycythemia vera. Cathet Cardiovasc Diagn 14:108, 1988

128. Edwards EA, Cooley MH: Peripheral vascular symptoms as the initial manifestation of polycythemia vera. JAMA 214:1463, 1970

129. Salem HH, Van der Weyden MB, Koutts J, Firkin BG: Leg pain and platelet aggregates in thrombocythemic myeloproliferative disease. JAMA 244:1122, 1980

130. Fagrell B, Mellstedt H: Polycythemia vera as a cause of ischemic digital neurosis. Acta Chir Scand 144:129, 1978

131. Kurzrock R, Cohen PR: Erythromelalgia and myeloproliferative disorders. Arch Intern Med 149:105, 1989

132. Kurzrock R, Cohen PR: Erythromelalgia: review of clinical characteristics and pathophysiology. Am J Med 91:416, 1991

133. Babb RR, Alarcon-Segovia D, Fairbairn JF: Erythromelalgia: review of 51 cases. Circulation 29:136, 1964

134. Berdel WE, Theiss W, Fink U, Rastetler J: Peripheral arterial occlusion and amaurosis fugax as the first manifestation of polycythemia vera. Blut 48:177, 1984

135. Askeir A: Spontaneous bleeding in polycythemia vera. Med J Aust 21:456, 1980

136. Ushikubi F, Ishibashi T, Narumiya S, Okuma M: Analysis of the defective signal transduction mechanism through the platelet thromboxane A_2 receptor in a patient with polycythemia vera. Thromb Haematol 67:144, 1992

137. Tartaglia AP, Goldberg TD, Berk PD, Wasserman LR: Adverse effects of anti-aggregating platelet therapy in the treatment of polycythemia vera. Semin Hematol 23:172, 1986

138. Barbui S, Buelli M, Cortellazzo S et al: Aspirin and risk of bleeding in patients with thrombocythemia. Am J Med 83:255, 1987

139. Mackenzie JW, Jellieve JA: Acute upper airway obstruction: spontaneous retropharyngeal hematoma in a patient with polycythemia rubra vera. Anesthesiology 41:57, 1986

140. Rigby PG, Leavell BS, Polycythemia vera: a review of fifty cases with emphasis on the risk of surgery. Arch Intern Med 5:622, 1960

141. Fitts WT, Erde A, Peskin GW, Frost JW: Surgical complications of polycythemia vera. Ann Surg 152:548, 1960

142. Wasserman LR, Gilbert HS: Surgery in polycythemia vera. N Engl J Med 23:1226, 1963

143. Wasserman LR, Gilbert HS: Surgical bleeding in polycythemia vera. Ann NY Acad Sci 115:122, 1964

144. Gilbert HS, Warner RRP, Wasserman LR: A study of histamine in myeloproliferative disease. Blood 28:795, 1966

145. Klein H: Polycythemia: Theory and Management. Charles C Thomas, Springfield, IL, 1973, p. 90

146. Steinman HK, Kabza-Black H, Lotti TM et al: Polycythemia rubra vera and water induced pruritus: blood histamine levels and cutaneous fibrinolytic activity before and after water challenge. Br J Dermatol 116:329, 1987

147. Jackson N, Burt D, Crocker J, Boughten B: Skin mast cells in polycythemia vera: relationship to the pathogenesis and treatment of pruritus. Br J Dermatol 116:21, 1987

148. Denman ST: A review of pruritus. J Am Acad Dermatol 14:375, 1986

149. Salem HH, Van Der Weyden MB, Young IF, Wiley DS: Pruritus and severe iron deficiency in polycythaemia. BMJ 285:91, 1982

150. Dallman PR: Manifestations of iron deficiency. Semin Hematol 19:19, 1982

151. Dallman PR, Beutler E, Finch CH: Effects of iron deficiency exclusive of anemia. Br J Haematol 40:179, 1978

152. Jacobs A: The non-haematological effects of iron deficiency. Clin Sci 53:105, 1977

153. Rector WG Jr, Fortuin NJ, Conley CL: Nonhematologic effects of chronic iron deficiency: a study of patients with polycythemia vera treated solely with venesections. Medicine 61:382, 1982

154. Hoffbrand AV, Chanarin I, Kremenchuzky S et al: Megaloblastic anemia in myelosclerosis. Q J Med 37:493, 1968

155. Lawrence JH, Winchell HS, Donall WG: Leukemia in polycythemia vera: relationship to splenic myeloid metaplasia and therapeutic radiation dose. Ann Intern Med 70:763, 1964

156. Szur L, Lewis SM: The haematological complications of polycythemia and treatment with radioactive phosphorus. Br J Radiol 39:122, 1966

157. Tubiana M, Flamant R, Attie E, Hayatt M: A study of hematological complications occurring in patients with polycythemia vera treated with [32]P. Blood 32:536, 1968

158. Najean Y, Deschamps A, Dresch C et al: Acute leukemia and myelodysplasia in polycythemia vera: a clinical study with long-term follow up. Cancer 61:89, 1988

159. Modan B: Inter-relationship between polycythemia vera, leukemia and myeloid metaplasia. Clin Haematol 4:427, 1975

160. Modan B, Lilienfeld AM: Polycythemia vera and leukemia—the role of radiation—study of 1,122 patients. Medicine 44:305, 1965

161. Dameshek W: The case for phlebotomy in polycythemia vera. Blood 32:488, 1968

162. Osgood EE: The case for ^{32}P in treatment of polycythemia vera. Blood 32:492, 1968

163. Brodsky I: Speculations on the treatment and pathophysiology of polycythemia vera and chronic myelogenous leukemia. Cancer Invest 4:281, 1986
164. Brodsky I: Busulphan treatment of polycythemia vera. Br J Haematol 56:1, 1982
165. Gilbert HS: Problems relating to control of polycythemia vera: the use of alkylating agents. Blood 32:500, 1968
166. Conley CL: Polycythemia vera: diagnosis and treatment. Hosp Pract 21:181, 1987
167. Wasserman LR: The management of polycythemia vera. Br J Haematol 21:371, 1971
168. Berk PD, Goldberg JD, Silverstein M et al: Increased incidence of acute leukemia in polycythemia vera associated with chlorambucil. N Engl J Med 304:441, 1981
169. Hoffman R, Estren S, Kopel S et al: Lymphoblastic-like transformation of polycythemia vera. Ann Intern Med 89:71, 1978
170. Braich TA, Grogan TM, Hicks MJ, Greenberg BR: Terminal lymphoblastic transformation in polycythemia vera. Am J Med 80:304, 1986
171. Hann HWL, Festa RS, Rosenstock JG, Cifuentes E: Polycythemia vera in a child with acute lymphocytic leukemia. Cancer 43:1862, 1974
172. Anastasi J, Pettenot MJ, LeBeau MM et al: Acute lymphoblastic leukemia in a patient with long standing polycythemia vera: cytogenetic analysis reveals two distinct abnormal clones. Am J Hematol 29:33, 1988
173. Zhang B, Lewis SM: Use of radionuclides in vivo. J Clin Pathol 40:508, 1987
174. International Committee for Standardization in Haematology: Recommended methods for measurement of red cell and plasma volume. J Nucl Med 21:793, 1980
175. Balcerzak SP, Bromberg PA: Secondary polycythemia. Semin Hematol 12:353, 1975
176. Hoffman R, Papyannopoulou T, Landaw S et al: Fetal hemoglobin in polycythemia vera: cellular distribution in 50 unselected patients. Blood 53:1148, 1979
177. Tytgat GN, Collen D, Vermylen J: Metabolism and distribution of fibrinogen. II. Fibrinogen turnover in polycythemia, thrombocytosis, hemophilia, congenital afibrinogenemia and during streptokinase therapy. Br J Haematol 22:70, 1972
178. Boughton BJ, Dallinger KJ: ^{125}I fibrinogen turnover in polycythemia: the effect of phlebotomy. Br J Haematol 53:97, 1983
179. Mohri H: Acquired von Willebrand disease in patients with polycythemia rubra vera. Am J Hematol 26:135, 1987
180. Kurnick JE, Ward HP, Block MH: Bone marrow sections in the differential diagnosis of polycythemia. Arch Pathol Lab Med 94:489, 1972
181. Luce NP, Young G: Marrow cellularity in the diagnosis of polycythemia. J Clin Pathol 36:180, 1983
182. Ellis JT, Petersen P: The bone marrow in polycythemia vera. Pathol Annu 1:383, 1979
183. Wolf BC, Neiman RS: The bone marrow in myeloproliferative and dysmyelopoietic syndromes. Hematol Oncol Clin North Am 2:669, 1988
184. Wolf BC, Bank PM, Mann RB, Neiman RS: Splenic hematopoiesis in polycythemia vera: a morphologic and immunohistologic study. Am J Clin Pathol 89:69, 1988
185. Lutton JD, Levere RD: Endogenous erythroid colony formation by peripheral blood mononuclear cells from patients with myelofibrosis and polycythemia vera. Acta Haematol 62:94, 1979
186. Lacombe C, Casadevall N, Varet B: Polycythemia vera: in vitro studies of circulating erythroid progenitors. Br J Haematol 44:189, 1980
187. Clement S, Eberlin A, Najean Y, Chedville A: Two different in vitro growth patterns for erythroid precursors in 18 patients with pure erythrocytosis. Scand J Haematol 29:319, 1982
188. Yuen E, Gibson J, Rickard KA, Kronenberg H: An analysis of peripheral blood burst forming units-erythroid in the polycythaemic states. Scand J Haematol 31:293, 1983
189. Partanen S: Spontaneous erythroid colony formation in erythrocytosis. J Intern Med 214:159, 1983
190. Mladenovic J, Adamson JW: Characteristics of circulatory erythroid colony forming cells in normal and polycythemic man. Br J Haematol 51:377, 1982
191. Lemoine F, Najman A, Baillou C et al: A prospective study of the value of bone marrow erythroid progenitor cultures in polycythemia. Blood 63:996, 1986
192. Reid CDL, Kirk A: Endogenous erythroid clones (EEC) in polycythemia and their relationship to diagnosis and the response to treatment. Br J Haematol 68:395, 1988
193. Weinberg RS, Worsley A, Gilbert HS et al: Comparison of erythroid progenitor cell growth in vitro in polycythemia vera and chronic myelogenous leukemia: only polycythemia vera has endogenous colonies. Leuk Res 13:331, 1989
194. Rege-Cambrin G, Mecucci C, Tricot G et al: A chromosomal profile of polycythemia vera. Cancer Genet Cytogenet 25:233, 1987
195. Swolin B, Weinfeld A, Westin J: A prospective long-term cytogenetic study in polycythemia in relationship to treatment and clinical course. Blood 72:386, 1988
196. Groupe Français de Cytogénétique Hématologique: Cytogenetics of acutely transformed chronic myeloproliferative syndromes without a Philadelphia chromosome. Cancer Genet Cytogenet 32:157, 1988
197. Testa JR, Kanofsky JR, Rowley JA et al: Karyotypic patterns and their clinical significance in polycythemia vera. Am J Hematol 11:29, 1981
198. Wurster-Hill D, Whang-Peng J, McIntyre OR et al: Cytogenetic studies in polycythemia vera. Semin Hematol 13:13, 1976
199. Swolin B, Weinfeld A, Westin J: Trisomy 1q in polycythemia vera and its relation to disease transition. Am J Hematol 22:155, 1986
200. Johnson DD, DeWald GW, Pierre RV et al: Deletions of chromosome 13 in malignant hematologic disorders. Cancer Genet Cytogenet 18:235, 1985
201. Diez-Martin JL, Graham DL, Petitt RM, Dewald GW: Chromosome studies in 104 patients with polycythemia vera. Mayo Clin Proc 66:287, 1991
202. Aatola M, Armstrong E, Teerenhovi L, Borgström GH: Clinical significance of the del(20q) chromosome in hematologic disorders. Cancer Genet Cytogenet 62:75, 1992
203. Mertens F, Johansson B, Heim S et al: Karyotypic patterns in chronic myeloproliferative disorders: report on 74 cases and review of the literature. Leukemia 5:214, 1991
204. Yunis JJ, Soreng AL, Bowe AE: Fragile sites are targets of diverse mutagens and carcinogens. Oncogene 1:59, 1987
205. LeBeau MM, Westbrook CA, Diaz MO, Rowley JD: C-Src is consistently conserved in the chromosomal deletion (20q) observed in myeloid disorders. Proc Natl Acad Sci USA 82:6692, 1985
206. Russell PR, Conley CL: Benign polycythemia Gaisbock's syndrome. Arch Intern Med 114:734, 1964
207. Modan B, Modan M: Benign erythrocytosis. Br J Haematol 14:375, 1968
208. Najean Y, Tribeil F, Dresch C: Pure erythrocytosis: reappraisal of a study of 51 cases. Am J Hematol 10:124, 1981
209. Pearson TC, Wetherley-Mein G: The course and complications of idiopathic erythrocytosis. Clin Lab Haematol 11:189, 1979
210. Valla D, Casadevall N, Lacombe C et al: Primary myeloproliferative disorder and hepatic vein thrombosis: a prospective study of erythroid colony formation in vitro in 20 patients with Budd-Chiari syndrome. Ann Intern Med 103:324, 1985
211. Kurzrock R, Gutterman JU, Talpaz M: The molecular genetics of Philadelphia chromosome positive leukemias. N Engl J Med 319:990, 1988
212. Iland HJ, Lazlo J, Peterson P et al: Essential thrombocythemia: clinical and laboratory characteristics at presentation. Trans Assoc Am Physicians 96:165, 1983
213. Iland HJ, Lazlo J, Case DC Jr et al: Differentiation between essential thrombocythemia and polycythemia vera with marked thrombocytosis. Am J Hematol 25:191, 1981
214. Haanen C, Mathe G, Hayat M (European Organization for Research and Treatment of Cancer, Leukemia/Hematosarcoma Cooperative Group): Treatment of polycythemia vera by radiophosphorus or busulphan: a randomized trial. Br J Cancer 44:75, 1981
215. Broxmeyer HE, Lu L, Platzer E et al: Comparative analysis of the influences of human gamma, alpha and beta interferons on human multipotential (CFU-GEMM), erythroid (BFU-E) and granulocyte-macrophage (CFU-GM) progenitor cells. J Immunol 131:1300, 1983
216. Silver RT: Recombinant interferon-alpha for treatment of polycythemia vera. Lancet 1:403, 1988
217. Lazzarino M, Vitale A, Morra E: Interferon alpha-2b as treatment for Philadelphia-negative chronic myeloproliferative disorders with excessive thrombocytosis. Br J Haematol 72:173, 1989
218. Talpaz M, Kurzrock R, Kantargian H et al: Recombinant interferon-alpha therapy of Philadelphia chromosome-negative myeloproliferative disorders with thrombocytosis. Am J Med 86:554, 1989
219. Ludwig H, Linkesch W, Gisslinger H et al: Interferon-alpha corrects thrombocytosis in patients with myeloproliferative disorders. Cancer Immunol Immunother 25:266, 1988
220. Hirsh J, Dalen JE, Fuster V et al: Aspirin and other platelet-active drugs. The relationship between dose, effectiveness, and side effects. Chest 102:327S, 1992
221. Messinezy M, Pearson TC, Prochazka A, Wetherly-Mein G: Treatment of primary proliferative polycythemia by venesection and low-dose busulphan: retrospective study from one centre. Br J Haematol 61:657, 1985
222. Zittoun R, EORTC Leukemia and Haematosarcoma Cooperative Group: Busulfan versus ^{32}P in polycythemia vera. Drugs Exp Clin Res 12:283, 1986

223. Donovan PB, Kaplan ME, Goldberg JD et al: Treatment of polycythemia vera with hydroxyurea. Am J Hematol 17:329, 1984

224. Kaplan ME, Mack K, Goldberg JD et al: Long-term management of polycythemia vera with hydroxyurea: a progress report. Semin Hematol 23:167, 1986

225. West W: Hydroxyurea in the treatment of polycythemia vera: a prospective study of 100 patients over a 20-year period. South Med J 80:323, 1987

226. Sharon R, Tatersky I, Ben-Arieh Y: Treatment of polycythemia vera with hydroxyurea. Cancer 57:718, 1986

227. Lofvenbey E, Wahlin A: Management of polycythemia vera, essential thrombocythemia and myelofibrosis with hydroxyurea. Eur J Haematol 41:375, 1988

228. Najean Y: Treatment of polycythemia vera with hydroxyurea or pipobroman. Efficacy and toxicity analysed from a protocol of 96 patients under 65 years of age. Le Groupe d'Etude des Polyglobulies. Presse Med 21:1753, 1992

229. Löfvenberg E, Nordenson I, Wahlin A: Cytogenetic abnormalities and leukemic transformation in hydroxyurea-treated patients with Philadelphia chromosome negative chronic myeloproliferative disease. Cancer Genet Cytogenet 49:57, 1990

230. Silverstein MN et al: Anagreline, a therapy for thrombocythemic states: experience in 577 patients. Am J Med 92:69, 1992

231. Silverstein MN, Pettit RM, Solberg LA et al: Anagrelide: a new drug for treating thrombocytosis. N Engl J Med 318:1292, 1988

232. Solberg LA Jr, Gles KJ, Tarach J et al: the effects of anagrelide on human megakaryocytopoiesis. Nouv Rev Fr Hematol 31:238, 1989

233. Hoffman R, Wasserman LR: Natural history and management of polycythemia vera. Adv Intern Med 24:255, 1979

234. Chanarin I, Szur L: Relief of intractable pruritis in polycythemia rubra vera with cholestyramine. Br J Haematol 29:669, 1975

235. Easton P, Galbraith PR: Cimetidine treatment of pruritus in polycythemia vera. N Engl J Med 299:1134, 1979

236. Hess CE: Cimetidine for the treatment of pruritus. N Engl J Med 300:370, 1979

237. Weick JK, Donovan PB, Najean Y et al: The use of cimetidine for the treatment of pruritus in polycythemia vera. Arch Intern Med 142:241, 1982

238. Fitzsimons EJ, Dugg JH, McAllister EJ: Pruritus of polycythemia vera: a place for pizotifen. Br Med J 283:277, 1981

239. Swerlide RA: Photochemotherapy treatment of pruritus associated with polycythemia vera. J Am Acad Dermatol 13:675, 1985

240. Ecker JA, McKittrick JE, Failing RM: Thrombosis of the hepatic veins: "the Budd-Chiari syndrome." A possible link between oral contraceptives and thrombosis formation. Am J Gastroenterol 45:429, 1966

241. Hoympa AM Jr, Schiff L, Helfman EL: Budd-Chiari syndrome in women taking oral contraceptives. Am J Med 50:137, 1971

242. Lewis JH, Tice HL, Zimmerman HJ: Budd-Chairi syndrome associated with oral contraceptive steroids: review of treatment of 47 cases. Dig Dis Sci 28:673, 1983

243. Langer B, Store RM, Colapinto RF et al: Clinical speculation of Budd-Chiari syndrome and its surgical management. Am J Surg 129:137, 1975

244. Prandi P, Rueff B, Benhamou JP: Side to side portacaval shunt in the treatment of Budd-Chiari syndrome. Gastroenterology 68:138, 1975

245. Nishikawa M, Miyoshi S, Imai Y et al: Treatment of the Budd-Chiari syndrome in polycythemia vera by repeated percutaneous transluminal angioplasty of a hepatic vein stenosis. Postgrad Med J 58:511, 1982

246. Maddry WC, Van Thiel DH: Liver transplantation: an overview. Hepatology 8:948, 1988

247. Huber H, Lewis SM, Szur L: The influence of anemia, polycythemia and splenomegaly on the relationship between venous haematocrit and red cell volume. Br J Haematol 10:567, 1967

248. Bowdler AJ: Plasma volume and splenomegaly in polycythemia vera. Br J Haematol 22:231, 1972

249. Zhang B, Lewis SM: The splenomegaly of myeloproliferative disorders: effects on blood volume and red blood count. Eur J Haematol 42:250, 1989

250. Najean Y, Caccione R, Cast-Malaspina H, Dresch C: Erythrokinetic studies in myelofibrosis. Their significance for prognosis. Br J Haematol 40:205, 1978

251. Besa EC, Nowell PC, Geller NC, Gardner FH: Analysis of the androgen response of 23 patients with agnogenic myeloid metaplasia: the value of chromosomal studies in predicting response and survival. Cancer 49:308, 1982

252. Silverstein MH, Remine WH: Splenectomy in myeloid metaplasia. Blood 53:515, 1979

253. Brennon B, Hagler A, Tatarsky I, Hashmonai M: Splenectomy in agnogenic myeloid metaplasia and post-polycythemia myeloid metaplasia. Arch Intern Med 148:250, 1988

254. Bennbasset J, Penchas S, Ligumski M: Splenectomy in patients with agnogenic myeloid metaplasia: an analysis of 321 published cases. Br J Haematol 42:207, 1979

255. Wagner I, McKeough PG, Desforges J: Splenic irradiation in the treatment of patients with chronic myelogenous leukemia or myelofibrosis with myeloid metaplasia. Cancer 58:1204, 1986

256. Hoyle CF, De Bastos M, Barzilai D, Wheatley K: AML associated with previous cytotoxic therapy, MDS or myeloproliferative disorders: results from the MRC's 9th AML trial. Br J Haematol 72:45, 1989

257. Hazani A, Tatarsky T, Burzila: Prolonged remission of leukemia associated with polycythemia vera. Cancer 40:1297, 1977

258. Preisler H, Early A, Raza A et al: Therapy of secondary acute nonlymphocytic leukemia with cytarabine. N Engl J Med 308:21, 1983

259. Harris RE, Conrad FG: Polycythemia in the childbearing age. Arch Intern Med 120:697, 1967

260. Hochman A, Stein JA: Polycythemia and pregnancy. Obstet Gynecol 18:230, 1961

261. Fialkow PJ: Clonal origin of human tumors. Annu Rev Med 30:135, 1979

Chronic Myeloid Leukemia

73

Timothy P. Hughes and John M. Goldman

INTRODUCTION

Several forms of leukemia have been included under the generic term chronic myeloid leukemia (CML). The commonest form, sometimes designated chronic granulocytic leukemia (CGI),[1] is the main focus of this chapter and further use of the term CML will refer to this specific entity. Other forms of CML are discussed at the end of the chapter.

In about 90% of patients with CML, the classic Philadelphia (Ph) chromosome is present in myeloid cells. The most common presenting features of CML are anemia, bleeding, and splenomegaly; however, increasingly the diagnosis is being made after a routine blood test taken for unrelated reasons. The disease is biphasic, with an initial (chronic) phase lasting on average 3 years and a terminal (blast) phase, which is refractory to treatment and has a median duration of 2–4 months.

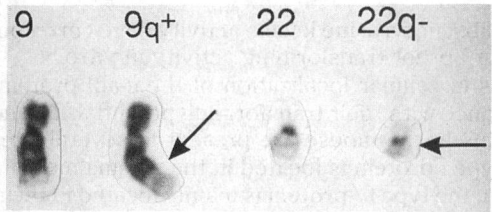

Fig. 73-1. Partial karyotype showing the standard Ph translocation (9;22)(q34; q11). Arrows show the rearranged chromosomal regions. (Courtesy of J. Bungey.)

EPIDEMIOLOGY AND ETIOLOGY

CML accounts for about 20% of all leukemias, with an annual incidence of 1 per 100,000 population; this incidence appears to be constant worldwide.[2] There is a slight male predominance (male/female ratio 1.4:1). The disease is seen in all age groups, with a peak incidence in the fifth and sixth decades of life. Lack of concordance of CML in monozygotic twins suggests that CML is an acquired disorder, but in most cases there are no known predisposing factors. The incidence of CML was significantly increased in survivors of the atomic bomb explosions at Hiroshima and Nagasaki who were exposed to high levels of radiation[3,4] and in a group of patients given radiotherapy for ankylosing spondylitis,[5] but for most patients radiation plays no definite role in causation. There is as yet no evidence that toxic chemicals or viruses are risk factors for CML.

GENETIC ASPECTS

Philadelphia Chromosome

A distinctive chromosomal deletion, later designated the Ph chromosome (Fig. 73-1) was first described in 1960, when the presence of a minute chromosome in leukemic cells of patients with CML was reported.[6] This G group chromosome (later designated chromosome 22) had extensive deletions from its long arm. In 1973 newly available banding techniques were used to establish that the Ph chromosome almost always coexisted with a gain of material on the long arm of one of the number 9 chromosomes.[7] Subsequently it became clear that the breakpoints on the two chromosomes occurred consistently within the same bands in different patients. Thus a translocation between the long arms of chromosomes 9 and 22 [t(9;22)(q34; q11)] was recognized, generating two derivative chromosomes 9q + and 22q − (Fig. 73-2).

Variant Ph Translocations

The classic t(9;22) translocation is present in about 90% of cases of CML, and variant forms of the Ph translocation are present in about 5% of cases.[8,9] Three major cytogenetic variants have been described:

1. Simple translocations involving the distal part of chromosome 22 and another chromosome without apparent involvement of chromosome 9.
2. Complex translocations involving chromosomes 9 and 22 and a third chromosome, which is the recipient of the deleted part of 22q −, while chromosome 9 is the recipient of the deleted part of the third chromosome.
3. Simple or complex translocations involving chromosome 22 that obscure the typical Ph translocation, resulting in a so-called masked Ph chromosome.[10]

The mechanisms by which variant translocations arise are unclear. In some cases there is evidence for secondary occurrence of a variant translocation (e.g., when standard and variant translocations are observed simultaneously in different metaphases or sequentially[11,12] or when a proximal breakpoint on 9q + is demonstrated by translocation of part of 9q together with the 22q distal segment).[13] In most cases, however, there is no evidence for sequential events, and a rearrangement involving multiple simultaneous breaks is the most probable explanation.[14]

Cytogenetic Evolution in Chronic Phase

During the chronic phase of CML, karyotypic abnormalities in addition to the Ph chromosome are seen in 10–20% of patients and are in general associated with a worse prognosis independent of all other disease characteristics.[15] Loss of the Y chromosome is an exception—it appears to be a favorable feature during the chronic phase.[16] These cases most often involve duplication of Ph, isochromosome (17q), and trisomy 8. These changes are characterized by their stability—they do not usually predominate and may be transient.[14]

Cytogenetic Evolution in Acute Phase

In 80% of patients who have progressed to the acute phase, random and nonrandom chromosomal abnormalities are seen in addition to the Ph chromosome; in the remaining 20% of cases no additional chromosomal changes are seen.[17] Duplication of the Ph chromosome, trisomy 8, trisomy 19, and isochro-

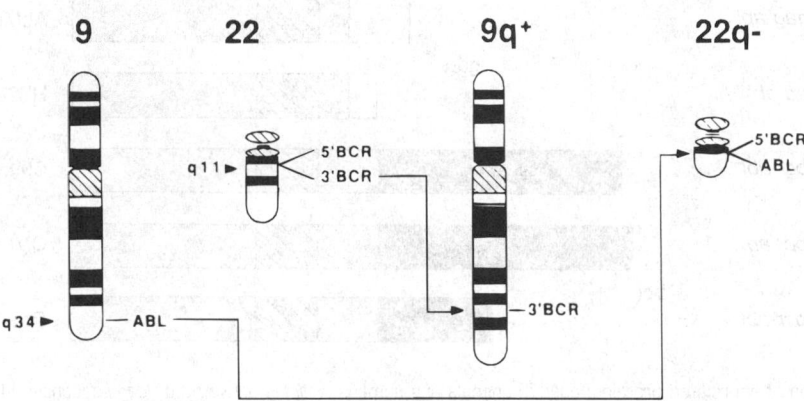

Fig. 73-2. Scheme of the t(9;22) showing the regional localization of the *abl* and *bcr* genes. Note that the 5' portion of *bcr* remains on 22q − whereas the 3' portion of *bcr* moves to 9q +.

Table 73-1. Major Discoveries in CML

1845:	First description of what was later called "splenic leukemia"
1960:	Discovery of Ph chromosome, later designated 22q−
1973:	Recognition of translocation t(9;22)(q34;q11)
1982:	Finding that *abl* translocates to 22q−
1984:	Description of BCR on chromosome 22
	Discovery of P210 protein with tyrosine kinase activity
1989:	CML-like syndrome induced in mice transfected with a *bcr/abl* construct

mosome 17q (iso-17q) replacing a normal chromosome 17 are the four most frequently observed.[18] Diagnosis of the acute phase based on chromosomal changes alone is unreliable, but sequential studies showing expansion and increase in complexity of the karyotype almost always indicate actual or impending transformation to the acute phase.[19] The isochromosome (17q) is also highly characteristic of impending transformation and is virtually never found as a stable abnormality in chronic phase disease.

BIOLOGIC AND MOLECULAR ASPECTS

Molecular Aspects

The cytogenetic characterization of CML that took place in the 1960s and early 1970s has been followed by a series of discoveries at the molecular level (Table 73-1) that have shown that the Ph translocation results in formation of a fusion gene, which encodes a leukemia-specific protein. It now seems likely that this protein, called P210, may induce normal hematopoietic cells to undergo transformation to the chronic phase CML phenotype.[20,21]

The discovery of the human *abl* oncogene resulted from studies of the Abelson murine leukemia virus (A-MuLV) (Fig. 73-3). A-MuLV was isolated from a thymectomized mouse inoculated with Moloney murine leukemia virus (M-MuLV),[22] which developed an acute B-cell leukemia. The virus isolated from this mouse differed from the M-MuLV virus in that it could transform lymphoid cells in vitro.[23] Molecular cloning and DNA sequencing confirmed that A-MuLV arose from recombination between M-MuLV and the normal mouse c-*abl* gene (designated v-*abl* in the virus). A-MuLV produces a fusion protein, encoded by M-MuLV gag polyprotein sequences joined to v-*abl* sequences (called P160$^{gag/v-abl}$), which has tyrosine kinase activity. The transforming activity of the virus seems closely related to this tyrosine kinase activity, as mutants of A-MuLV with re-

duced or absent tyrosine kinase activity have correspondingly reduced or absent transforming activity in vitro.[24]

Changes in cellular localization of the c-abl proteins occur in accordance with their transforming potential. The normal c-abl proteins in the mouse are present in several sites in the cell; the type I protein is located in the plasma membrane and cytoplasm; the type IV protein is mainly located in the nucleus. The viral transforming protein P160$^{gag/v-abl}$ is predominantly cytoplasmic or membrane-associated. Deletion of a small N-terminal regulatory region of the mouse abl type IV protein sufficient to activate its transforming potential changes the distribution of this protein from the nucleus to the cytoplasm.[25]

The human genome contains on the long arm of chromosome 9 a "cellular" gene highly homologous to the v-*abl* oncogene.[26] This human *abl* proto-oncogene (Fig. 73-3) is a large gene, in which v-*abl* homologous sequences are dispersed over nine exons.[27] Upstream of this v-*abl* homologous region two exons, 1a and 1b, act as alternative first exons for two mRNAs of 6 and 7 kb, respectively.[28] At the DNA level exons 1a and 1b are located approximately 18 and 200 kb upstream of exon 2 (the first common exon), respectively.[29] It appears that when transcription begins at exon 1b, exon 1a is spliced out and fusion of exon 1b to exon 2 occurs,[30] so that two mRNA species are formed that correspond closely to the two most abundant murine abl mRNAs, called type I and type IV. These two mRNA species are translated into proteins that differ by 19 amino acids at the amino termini. Both proteins are called P145 and have intrinsic tyrosine kinase activity. The human mRNA corresponding to the murine type IV species encodes an acceptor site for myristylation, which allows this P145 to localize to the cell membrane. Whether these two abl proteins subserve different cellular functions is not known.

The actual breakpoint appears to be distributed over an area >200 kb between exon 1b and exon 2, as determined in a number of patients with Ph-positive CML.[26,31]

The exchange of chromosomal material between the long arms of chromosomes 9 and 22 in Ph-positive cells results in the bulk of the *abl* gene translocating to the 22q− chromosome.[32–34] Furthermore, most cases of variant Ph translocation have also shown translocation of *abl* to the 22q− chromosome.[31]

The breakpoint on the Ph chromosome has been localized in many patients and (in contrast to the extensive region of possible breakpoints on chromosome 9) is confined to a very small region (5.8 kb),[35] which has been designated the major breakpoint cluster region (M-BCR).[36] M-BCR includes five exons

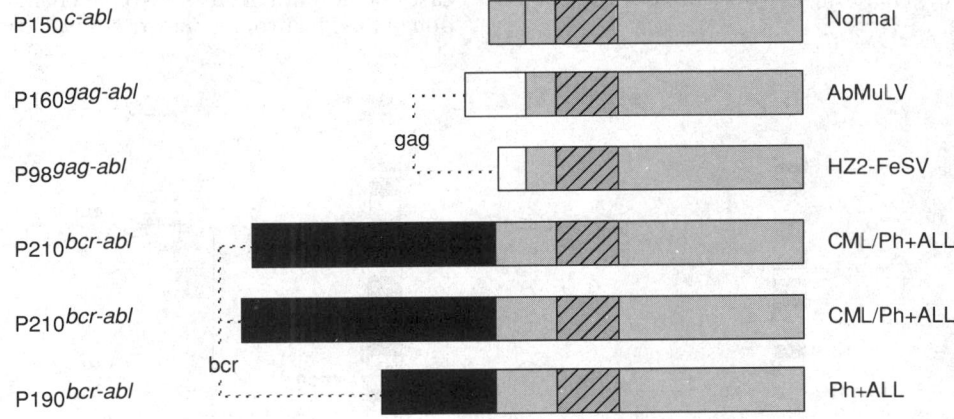

Fig. 73-3. Comparison of abl-related proteins found in animals and humans. v-*abl* is activated by *gag* sequences in the Abelson mutant of Moloney murine leukemia virus (A-MuLV) and the Hardy-Zuckerman feline sarcoma virus (HZ2-FeSV). The juxtapositioning of different sequences of the *bcr* gene is associated with activation of the human *abl* gene. The "TINT" areas show the tyrosine kinase domain common to all *abl* sequences. (From Gale and Goldman,[36] with permission.)

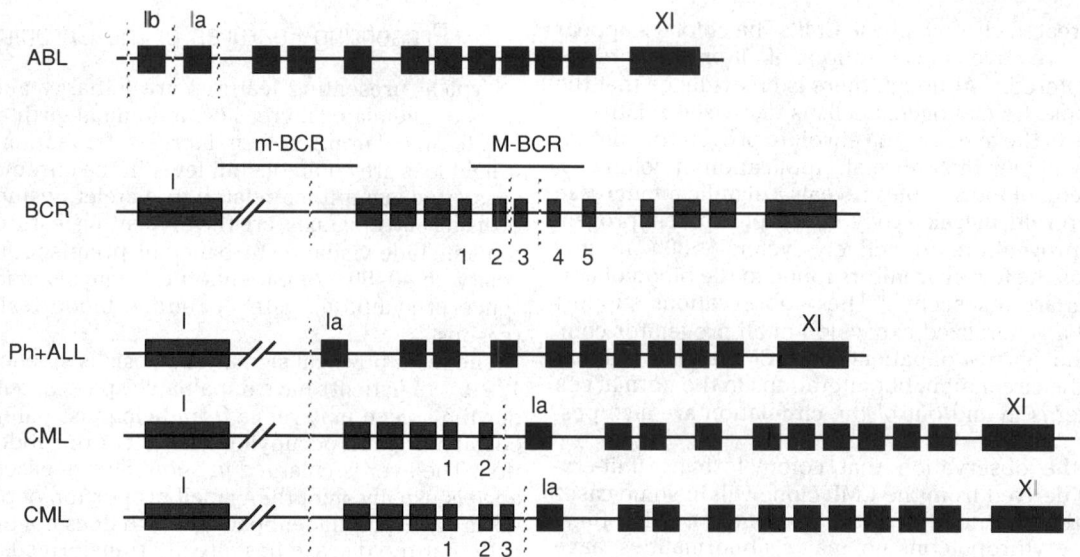

Fig. 73-4. Molecular events in CML and related disorders. The genomic structure of the *abl* and *bcr* genes are indicated with exons represented schematically as black or red boxes. The possible positions for breakpoints in the *abl* and *bcr* genes are shown as dashed vertical lines. The major and minor breakpoint cluster regions are designated M-BCR and m-BCR, respectively. Rearrangements seen in Ph-positive ALL and two alternative translocations seen in CML are shown. (From Gale and Goldman,[36] with permission.)

(Fig. 73-4) and forms part of a larger gene referred to as the *bcr* gene. The *bcr* coding region spans ≥100 kb and contains >20 exons. Two bcr proteins of 130 and 160 kd are encoded and are widely expressed in normal tissues. There also appear to be three *bcr*-related genes on chromosome 22 at band q11, which may be pseudogenes.[37]

The Ph translocation results in the fusion of the *bcr* and *abl* genes in a head-to-tail fashion. The *bcr* gene loses a 3' section, which is replaced by 3' *abl* sequences from chromosome 9. The chimeric *bcr/abl* gene transcribes an mRNA of approximately 8.5 kb[38] with 5' *bcr* and 3' *abl* sequences. Although the hybrid *bcr/abl* gene produced will vary from patient to patient depending on the location of the intronic breakpoints, the chimeric mRNA formed after processing is in almost all cases one of two possible types with either the second or the third exon in the M-BCR region of the *bcr* gene linked to the second *abl* exon. These mRNAs are referred to as b2a2 and b3a2, respectively. They can be characterized by reverse transcription to cDNA and subsequent use of the polymerase chain reaction (PCR) with selected primers. Thus, the only difference between the two possible mRNAs produced is the inclusion or exclusion of the b3 exon, which is 75 bases long.

An abnormal protein of 210 kd, isolated from Ph-positive cells,[39] was shown to bind to antisera specific for the N-terminal segment of the bcr protein as well as to v-abl antisera; this protein must therefore be a bcr/abl fusion protein, P210. It has greatly enhanced tyrosine kinase activity relative to P145, the normal abl product.[40] It can form a complex with the GRB-2/SOS proteins thought to act as exchange factors for activating P21[ras],[41] so it may act by inducing inappropriate mitosis in a target cell.

As to the question of whether P210 directly induces CML, it should be noted that the viral transforming protein P160[gag/v-abl] has enhanced tyrosine kinase activity and altered subcellular localization as compared with the normal mouse c-abl protein (type IV). Both changes appear to be central to the ability of the P160[gag/v-abl] protein to transform cells in vitro.

Similar alterations of function between the normal human abl proteins and P210 may underlie transformation of a normal cell (or possibly a preleukemic cell) to the CML phenotype. An important approach to the study of the function of the bcr/abl fusion protein involves attempts to transform cells in vitro or to produce a disease simulating CML in animals by transfection with bcr/abl or related constructs. A disease resembling CML has been observed in mice transplanted with hematopoietic stem cells containing a bcr/abl construct and the experimental leukemia so produced can be transplanted to secondary recipients.[42,43]

Even though most patients whose disease has transformed have nonrandom cytogenetic changes, consistent molecular changes likely to be pathogenetically involved in transformation have not been identified. Most patients with phenotypically lymphoid blast cells have clonal rearrangement of immunoglobulin genes, and some also have rearrangement of T-cell receptor (TCR) genes.[44,45] A minority of patients with myeloid transformation have deletions or point mutations involving the p53 tumor suppressor gene[46,47] and rare changes in the retinoblastoma (Rb) gene are reported. ras mutations occur very occasionally and are probably not pathogenetically relevant.[48,49]

Cellular Aspects

Extensive data, including studies of the presence of the Ph chromosome, expression of polymorphic genetic loci, and analysis of X chromosome-linked restriction fragment length polymorphisms, indicate that malignant transformation in CML occurs in a pluripotent hematopoietic stem cell.[50,51] This cell can differentiate along erythroid, megakaryoblastic, monocytic, eosinophilic, and basophilic pathways. At least some B lymphocytes[52] and probably in some cases a minority of T lymphocytes also appear to derive from the Ph-positive clone. Despite the pluripotent origin of the leukemia, only the myeloid, monocytic, and megakaryocytic lineages are significantly increased in the bone marrow. The cause of this selective expansion is unknown.

During the chronic phase the leukemic cells mature normally and have a near normal life span. The patient is dependent on these leukemic cells for vital hematopoietic functions. Granulocyte and erythroid functions are generally normal, although platelet function is mildly impaired in some cases.

Standard in vitro colony assays to detect hematopoietic progenitors have not revealed any important differences between normal marrow and marrow taken from patients with newly diagnosed or treated chronic phase CML. The colonies appear normal, and the relative concentrations of all progenitors are not markedly altered.[53] Although there is no evidence that the number of neoplastic clonogenic cells is increased relative to other cell types in the marrow, the absolute progenitor content is considerably higher than normal. Application of colony assays to peripheral blood samples reveals a significant increase in myeloid, erythroid, megakaryocytic, and pluripotent progenitors.[54] These progenitors are actively cycling (>30% are in S phase), whereas the few progenitors found in the blood of normal individuals are quiescent.[54] These observations support the concept of a generalized expansion of all progenitor compartments in the marrow of patients with CML and a resultant spillover into the circulation, but alterations in the normal cell migration patterns in and out of the circulation are also possible.

Except for the observation that colony-forming unit-erythroid (CFU-E) derived from the CML clone will in some cases proliferate in the absence (or in the presence of suboptimal quantities) of erythropoietin, no major abnormalities have been identified in the growth factor requirements of Ph-positive cells. Autonomous or autocrine growth of Ph-positive cells has not been found, and altered growth factor responsiveness has not been demonstrated.[55]

If marrow from newly diagnosed CML patients is cultured in vitro for several weeks, the Ph-positive cells will sometimes die at an early stage and a population of predominantly Ph-negative cells will survive.[56] This provides further evidence that Ph-negative cells are present in CML marrow despite frequent failure to detect them by cytogenetic means. The therapeutic potential of autografting with marrow cultured in vitro is discussed below.

CLINICAL MANIFESTATIONS

In most cases CML is a biphasic or triphasic disease. The initial chronic phase may last several years without change, but ultimately it either changes abruptly to an acute phase or, more commonly, evolves slowly into a phase of "acceleration," which later progresses to the acute phase. The acute phase is usually defined by the observation of >30% blasts or blasts plus promyelocytes in the blood or marrow,[57] but criteria for defining the accelerated phase are imprecise.[58] A reasonable classification has been proposed by the International Bone Marrow Transplant Registry (Table 73-2).

Table 73-2. Criteria Established by the International Bone Marrow Transplant Registry for Classifying the Phases of CML

Chronic phase
    No significant symptoms *(after treatment)*
    None of the features of accelerated phase or blastic phase
Accelerated phase
    WBC count difficult to control with conventional use of busulfan or hydroxyurea in terms of doses required or shortening of intervals between courses
    Rapid doubling of WBC count (<5 days)
    ≥10% blasts in blood or marrow
    ≥20% blasts plus promyelocytes in blood or marrow
    ≥20% basophils plus eosinophils in blood
    Anemia or thrombocytopenia unresponsive to busulfan or hydroxyurea
    Persisent thrombocytosis
    Additional chromosome changes (evolving new clone)
    Increasing splenomegaly
    Development of chloromas or myelofibrosis
Blastic phase
    ≥30% blasts plus promyelocytes in the blood or bone marrow

(Data from International Bone Marrow Transplant Registry.)

Presenting Features of the Chronic Phase

Typical presenting features are lethargy and other symptoms of anemia or increasing abdominal girth and discomfort due to an enlarging spleen. Increased sweating and moderate weight loss are common, but fever in the chronic phase is rare. Less often, symptoms related to platelet dysfunction, such as bruising and epistaxis, are the presenting features. Rarer symptoms include visual disturbance or priapism due to hyperviscosity. In 40–50% of patients the diagnosis is made in the absence of symptoms after a routine blood test for unrelated reasons.

The main physical sign at diagnosis is splenomegaly. About 10–15% of patients have impalpable spleens, but in the remainder the spleen may range from being just palpable below the costal margin to occupying the bulk of the abdomen on palpation. The liver is enlarged in about 50% of cases, but its lower edge is usually smooth. A small proportion of patients at diagnosis have lymphadenopathy, which does not necessarily indicate that the disease has already transformed.

Clinical Features of the Acute Phase

The patient may or may not have symptoms when the disease begins to accelerate.[59] Fever and night sweats may occur and the spleen may enlarge. Often the only change will be seen on examination of the peripheral blood and bone marrow, as discussed below. With appropriate treatment a patient may remain in the accelerated phase for many months, but eventually the disease will progress to a blastic phase.

Blast phase is commonly associated with the onset of symptoms, including fever, sweats, weight loss, and/or bone pain, which may be generalized or localized, and pain over the splenic area, which may be pleuritic. The patient may have a bleeding tendency or have symptoms related to anemia. Rarely, patients have generalized lymphadenopathy or multiple subcutaneous nodules. Symptoms of hyperviscosity due to intracerebral or intrapulmonary leukostasis are sometimes present. Very rarely, patients may present in blastic transformation with symptoms of disease in the central nervous system, including features of raised intracranial pressure or focal neurologic signs.

PROGNOSIS

Chronic phase CML is a "benign" disease, which with modern management is compatible with a period of survival in good health. By contrast, the outlook for a patient who has entered the acute phase is very poor, with a median survival of <3 months. Thus, survival duration in CML is essentially determined by the time taken to transformation. This may occur so early that the patient first presents in acute phase or it may take >10 years, but it usually occurs between 2 and 6 years after diagnosis. (The various phases of CML are defined in Table 73-2). A survival curve for a large series of patients with chronic phase disease at diagnosis[15] (Fig. 73-5) shows a low annual death rate within the first 2 years, which increases to 25% by the third year and remains fairly constant in subsequent years. Transformation appears to occur randomly; for an individual patient the risk of transformation and death can be specified but the actual time when it will occur cannot be predicted. There is no evidence that conventional antileukemic therapy changes the risk of transformation, so survival is determined principally by the intrinsic biology of the disease.[60]

Several groups have constructed models that use a series of parameters to classify patients with CML into low-risk, intermediate-risk, and high-risk groups.[15,61–64] The International CGL

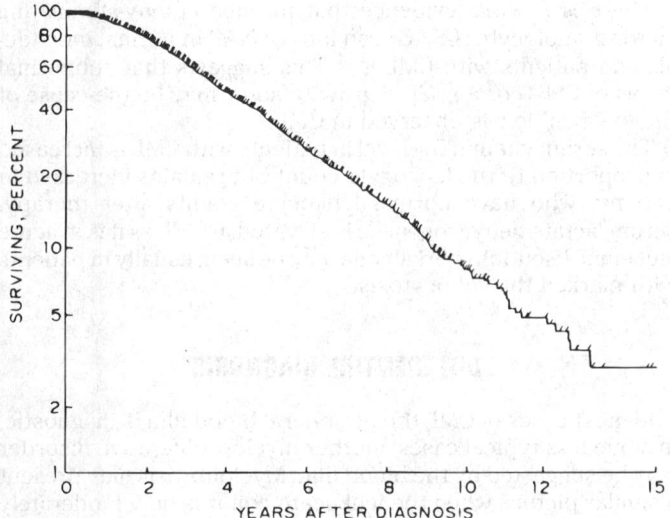

Fig. 73-5. Actuarial survival curve for 1,635 patients with Ph-positive, nonblastic CML registered in the International CGL Prognosis Study. The semilogarithmic plot becomes linear during the third year, indicating a constant risk of death thereafter. Diagonal ticks indicate surviving patients. (From Sokal et al.,[15] with permission.)

Prognosis Study Group[15] reported 678 cases of nonblastic Ph-positive CML, which were followed for ≥4 years from diagnosis to identify features with prognostic significance when analyzed by multivariate regression analysis. Age, spleen size, platelet count, and percentage of blasts at diagnosis had an unequivocal association with survival, and a Cox model[65] was generated with these four variables (Fig. 73-6). This model was tested in a 1988 prospective study[66] and successfully classified patients into three groups with significantly different outcomes. The proportion of patients surviving ≥2 years from diagnosis in the high-, intermediate-, and low-risk groups was 70%, 80%, and 93%, respectively. This classification may be useful when decisions are being made about the timing of an allogeneic bone marrow transplantation (BMT).

In practice, prognosis in individual patients may be assessed most reliably on the basis of response to initial treatment. Patients who have a relatively low requirement for treatment with busulfan or patients who respond rapidly to interferon-α (IFN-α) may fare particularly well.[67]

Several reports have suggested that the position of the breakpoint within the M-BCR on chromosome 22 may influence the prognosis.[68,69] Survival of patients with more downstream (or 3′) breakpoints was inferior to survival of patients with more upstream (or 5′) breakpoints. In one study, patients who expressed the chimeric mRNA that includes M-BCR exon 3 appeared to have a significantly worse prognosis than the remainder who expressed the same chimeric message without exon 3. In other studies, there was no correlation at the DNA level between position of the breakpoint and survival[70,71] and the prognostic value of this type of analysis now seems to be limited.

LABORATORY EVALUATION

Peripheral Blood

The leukocyte count is usually between 100 and 300 × 10⁹/ L at diagnosis but, rarely, may be 500–1,000 × 10⁹/L. Thrombocytosis is seen in about 30% of patients, and in some cases the disease may resemble essential thrombocythemia. Anemia is almost always a feature of untreated CML if the leukocyte count is >150 × 10⁹/L. It is usually normochromic and normocytic. The major causes for anemia appear to be decreased erythropoiesis and shortened red cell survival related to splenomegaly. Rarely, erythrocytosis may be seen, and the disease may resemble polycythemia rubra vera. The blood film usually reveals several diagnostic features (Table 73-3 and Fig. 73-7). There is a leukocytosis, which shows a full spectrum of immature and mature myeloid cells with "peaks" of myelocytes and mature neutrophils. The myeloid series appears normal in morphology. Blast cells may constitute ≤12% of the differential, their percentage rising in parallel with the total leukocyte count. Monocytes may be increased in absolute numbers but are usually <3% of the leukocytes.[72] Basophilia and eosino-

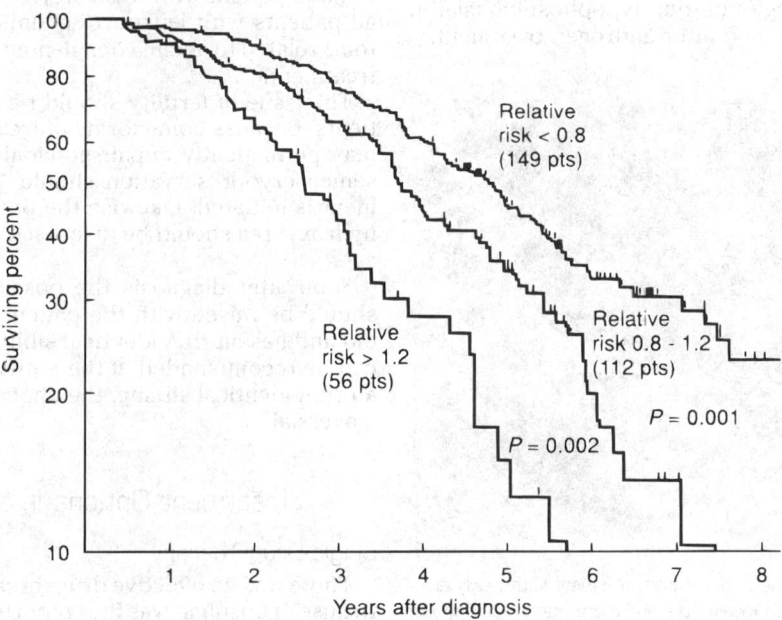

Fig. 73-6. Survival of 317 patients divided into high-, intermediate-, and low-risk groups according to relative risk calculated from the hazard ratio formula. (From Sokal,[60] with permission.)

Table 73-3. Hematologic Features of CML

Mean platelet count above the upper limit of the normal range

Differential count showing two large peaks involving neutrophils and myelocytes; the mean myelocyte percentage increasing with increasing total leukocyte count

Absolute basophilia present in all cases

Low percentage of monocytes, which decreased further with increasing leukocyte count; however, absolute monocyte counts were often 1×10^9/L

Dysplastic features in the granulocytic series were minimal or absent and found in <10% of cases

(Data from Spiers et al.[220])

philia are usually seen. Occasional nucleated red cells may appear in the blood.

Bone Marrow

The marrow aspirate frequently does not show any fragments but instead shows a dense population of myeloid cells. The mean myeloid/erythroid ratio is 25:1 (normal range 2:1 to 5:1). Mitotic figures are usually increased. Megakaryocytes are usually increased and often dysplastic, with low numbers of nuclei and relatively sparse cytoplasm.[72] Features of dysplasia in other lineages are not usually prominent. Cells that resemble Gaucher cells may be present, as well as sea-blue histiocytes.

The trephine usually shows marked hypercellularity with loss of fat spaces. Reticulin staining may be mildly increased. In some cases marked fibrosis is evident.

Other Investigations

Elevation in plasma and urinary uric acid occurs in untreated CML but rarely causes problems in the chronic phase. Neutrophil alkaline phosphatase (NAP) is usually markedly decreased in CML when measured by histochemical and biochemical techniques. This can be a useful diagnostic test, as the NAP score is usually elevated in other myeloproliferative disorders and also in reactive causes of leukocytosis (stress, infection, and so forth). The enzyme activity may also be reduced in paroxysmal nocturnal hemoglobinuria, hypophosphatasia, in some cases of myelofibrosis, and after androgen treatment.

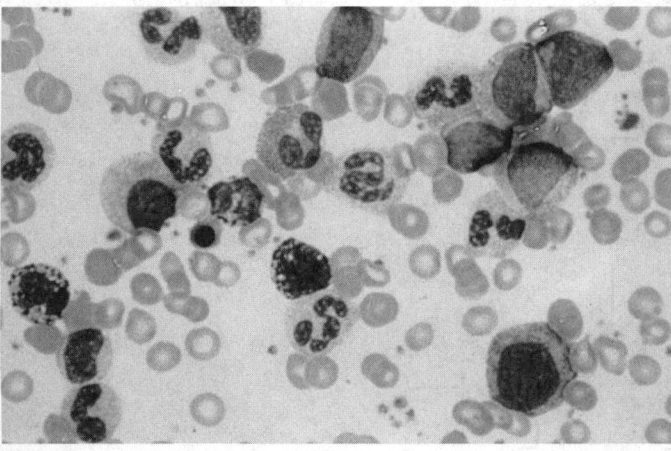

Fig. 73-7. Photomicrograph of peripheral blood from a patient with newly diagnosed CML, showing leukocytosis with myelocytes and more mature cells in the granulocyte series. Three basophils, one eosinophil, and a nucleated red blood cell are present. There is thrombocytosis with platelet anisocytosis. (Courtesy of D. Swirsky.)

There is in vitro evidence that purified colony-stimulating factor-granulocyte (CSF-G) can induce NAP in normal individuals and patients with CML.[73,74] This suggests that subnormal levels of CSF-G or a related growth factor may be the cause of the low NAP levels observed in CML.

The serum vitamin B_{12} level in patients with CML is increased in proportion to the leukocyte count but remains increased in patients who have normal leukocyte counts after therapy. Serum lactate dehydrogenase is elevated in CML as it is in acute leukemia. Pseudohyperkalemia may be seen, usually in patients with marked thrombocytosis.

DIFFERENTIAL DIAGNOSIS

In most cases of CML the peripheral blood film is diagnostic. In some less typical cases another myeloproliferative disorder may be suggested by the blood film. Myelofibrosis may present a similar picture when the leukocyte count is only moderately elevated, and teardrop poikilocytes are seen. Marrow fibrosis is usually more marked in myelofibrosis. The finding of a low NAP and the presence of the Ph chromosome in myeloid cells can help to differentiate CML from other myeloproliferative disorders.

A mildly elevated leukocyte count with immature myeloid cells and nucleated red blood cells on the blood film (leukoerythroblastic reaction) can occur in patients with shock, hemolysis, hemorrhage, metastatic carcinoma, myeloma, or chronic inflammation. This can usually be differentiated from CML by examination of the marrow.

THERAPY
Initial Management

Once the diagnosis of CML has been confirmed, the nature of the disease should be explained to the patient and the overall therapeutic strategy discussed. The initial objective of treatment should be to alleviate symptoms or delay their onset, which can usually be achieved by maintaining the leukocyte count $<100 \times 10^9$/L, but treatment is not urgent in the asymptomatic patient with a leukocyte count $<200 \times 10^9$/L. Almost all patients with leukocyte counts $>200 \times 10^9$/L have symptoms related to anemia or splenomegaly and require immediate treatment.

The issue of fertility should be discussed with younger patients. Because some forms of treatment (e.g., busulfan, BMT) may permanently impair gonadal function, the possibility of semen cryopreservation should be considered before treatment is initiated. Likewise the probable teratogenic effects of hydroxyurea should be discussed with women of childbearing age.

Soon after diagnosis the possibility of treatment by BMT should be raised with the patient. If the patient is <50 years old and has an HLA-identical sibling donor, an allogeneic BMT can be recommended. If the patient is older or does not have an HLA-identical sibling, the choice of initial treatment is controversial.

Treatment Options in the Chronic Phase

Single-Drug Therapy

There was no effective drug therapy for CML until 1953, when the use of busulfan was first reported[75] (Table 73-4). The capacity of busulfan to control CML for longer periods than radiotherapy was demonstrated in results of a randomized controlled trial published 15 years later.[76] It is conventional to

Table 73-4. Landmarks in the Treatment of CML

1860:	Introduction of Fowler's solution (potassium arsenite)
1902:	Radium therapy for chronic leukemias
1930:	Splenic irradiation
1952:	Busulfan
1966:	Hydroxyurea
1979:	Syngeneic transplants in chronic phase
1981:	Allografting with HLA-identical siblings
1983:	IFN-α
1985:	Unrelated donor transplants

start treatment with busulfan at a dosage of 4–6 mg/day and to monitor the leukocyte count on a weekly basis. The rate of fall of the leukocyte count differs in different patients, but usually the drug is discontinued or the dosage reduced very substantially when the leukocyte count has fallen to 30 or 20 × 10^9/L, because the leukocyte count will continue to fall for 2–4 weeks after stopping the drug.[77] Thereafter some clinicians continue treatment at a dose level (1–3 mg/day) intended to maintain the leukocyte count in the normal range, whereas others prefer to await the rise of the leukocyte count and then to initiate another course of treatment lasting 2–6 weeks. Another method of giving busulfan involves use of large single doses (50 or 100 mg) administered on a single occasion at intervals of ≥4 weeks.[78] This last method is particularly useful for patients whose ability to comply with daily dosage is in doubt.

Busulfan can cause a variety of toxic effects.[79,80] It damages the gonads in both sexes; males develop aspermia, and menstruation in females ceases after 3–6 months of treatment.[79,81] These effects are seldom reversible. Occasional patients (perhaps 1 in 100) are hypersensitive to the drug and develop pancytopenia and marrow aplasia after treatment with standard doses; such patients may die or may recover if supportive care can be maintained for weeks or months. Their hematopoiesis may then be exclusively or mainly Ph-negative.[75,82,83] A similar clinical picture can be achieved by "overdosing" other patients (i.e., if busulfan treatment is continued at full dosage for weeks or months after the leukocyte has been restored to normal). Occasionally patients treated for some years develop a pulmonary syndrome characterized by cough, fever, pulmonary infiltrates, and respiratory failure; this has been termed busulfan lung[80,84,85] and could be due to cytomegalovirus (CMV) infection in some cases. Other rare complications include a wasting syndrome resembling Addison disease[80] and cataract formation.[86]

Hydroxyurea, first reported in 1966 for use in CML,[87] is a cycle-specific inhibitor of DNA synthesis, which is now commonly used as the agent of first choice for disease control. Although it produces less smooth control of the leukocyte count than does busulfan, it is far less toxic.[88,89] It does not produce prolonged or irreversible marrow aplasia and indeed the leukocyte count begins to rise within days of stopping or reducing therapy. It is usual to start treatment for the high count patient with 2.0 g/day and to reduce dosage to 1.5 or 1.0 g/day once the leukocyte count has reached normal levels. With hydroxyurea, unlike busulfan, treatment must be maintained indefinitely and effectively. The aim is to titrate the leukocyte level against the hydroxyurea dosage. The usual maintenance level is between 1.0 and 1.5 g/day, but counts can be controlled in some patients at much lower drug levels.

Most patients experience no toxic effects of hydroxyurea even if treatment is maintained for many years. Most do, however, develop macrocytosis and megaloblastic features in the marrow. Very rarely patients develop allergic features, including rashes or aphthous-type ulcers in the mouth. Doses of ≥2.0 g/day may cause gastrointestinal disturbances, including nausea, vomiting, or diarrhea. The drug may damage the fetus if

administered during the first trimester of pregnancy. Partly because of its relative lack of toxicity, there has been an increased tendency in Western countries during the last decade to use hydroxyurea in preference to busulfan for treating the newly diagnosed CML patient. One recent report showed significantly superior survival for hydroxyurea compared with busulfan,[90] but this needs confirmation.

Combination Therapy

Regimens using busulfan in combination with 6-mercaptopurine or 6-thioguanine have been compared with use of busulfan alone. Although disease control is achieved more rapidly with combination therapy, there is no evidence of a survival advantage.

Intensive Therapy

Aggressive combination chemotherapy has been used in the hope that genuine remission could be induced. Considerable suppression of the Ph-positive clone can be achieved in some cases, and in rare instances the Ph-positive clone temporarily disappears.[91] However, none of the regimens used so far has been curative or has improved survival.[92]

Interferons

The use of IFN-α in CML has been evaluated since the early 1980s by several groups.[93–95] The consensus appears to be that IFN-α will produce good hematologic control in about 70% of patients in the chronic phase whether they have had previous therapy or not, although previous therapy may make the disease slightly more resistant. Control generally takes ≥3 months to achieve. It is also clear that IFN-α does not prevent transformation to the acute phase. Some patients will develop resistance to therapy, which may be related to the development of anti-IFN-α neutralizing antibodies. Patients whose leukocyte counts are restored to normal may have some degree of Ph-negative hematopoiesis and this may be prolonged; thus, 20–40% of patients may achieve complete disappearance or major reduction in the proportion of Ph-positive metaphases in the marrow. Very occasional patients have no evidence of residual leukemia even when blood or marrow is tested by the very sensitive PCR,[96–98] but in most patients the Ph negativity is partial and transient.

The Houston group has recently updated its initial experience with use of IFN-α.[99] Patients who obtain major or complete chromosomal responses survived significantly longer than those who did not and the survival for all IFN-α-treated patients was >6 years. The preliminary Houston experience provided the stimulus for design of a number of multicenter studies intended to prove (or disprove) a clinical benefit from treatment with IFN-α. The results to date are conflicting. A recent analysis of the Italian multicenter study showed that the median survival for IFN-α-treated patients was significantly longer than for those treated with hydroxyurea and also confirmed the Houston data, showing that patients who obtained chromosomal responses lived longer than those who did not. However, preliminary reports from the United Kingdom and German multicenter studies have not revealed any survival advantage for IFN-α-treated patients.[90] Moreover, a recent report from the U.S. study group Cancer and Acute Leukemia Group B failed to demonstrate any survival advantage for chromosome responders among patients treated with IFN-α.[100] Thus, one must for the present conclude that IFN-α may prolong survival for some patients and this benefit may be more pronounced in patients with "low-grade" disease or in those who obtain some reduction in the degree of Ph-positive hematopoiesis. The case, however, is not yet proved.

The major disadvantages of IFN-α therapy are its high cost

and the frequency of unpleasant side effects. Most patients will experience an influenzalike syndrome, with lethargy, fever, chills, myalgia, and bone pain; less common side effects include diarrhea, abnormal liver function, and impotence. Side effects are generally dose-related but tend to diminish with time if the patient persists with therapy. Little is known about the mechanism of action of IFN-α. In vitro studies suggest that the main effect is to suppress proliferation of hematopoietic cells,[101] but the basis for the selectivity is unknown.

IFN-γ also suppresses the proliferation of hematopoietic progenitor cells. The use of IFN-γ alone or in combination with IFN-α has not yielded superior results.[102]

Autologous Bone Marrow Transplantation

Studies performed in the 1970s showed that patients in the acute phase treated with high-dose chemotherapy or chemoradiotherapy followed by autografting with hematopoietic stem cells collected from the blood or marrow at diagnosis and cryopreserved during the chronic phase derived short-term benefit from the procedure.[103] Of great interest is the recent observation that some patients treated with chemoradiotherapy and autografting while still in the chronic phase may achieve partial or complete Ph negativity. It is possible that the onset of transformation has been delayed in many of these patients.[104]

The probability of achieving complete Ph negativity may be increased if the harvested marrow or blood-derived stem cells could be treated in vitro in a manner that favored the survival of Ph-negative stem cells, for example, with cytotoxic drugs or biologic response modifiers (such as IFN or interleukin-2). Autologous bone marrow that has been held in culture for 10 days has been given after high-dose chemotherapy to a small number of selected patients and has resulted in successful engraftment and predominant Ph-negative hematopoiesis in the short term.[105] Of equal interest is the recent observation that stem cells can be collected from the peripheral blood in the recovery phase after combination chemotherapy, stored in liquid nitrogen, and then used to reconstitute hematopoiesis after high-dose chemotherapy[106]; such hematopoiesis may also be predominantly Ph negative.

Splenectomy

There are now very few indications for splenectomy in the management of CML. It was at one time thought possible that removal of the spleen might delay the onset of transformation. A randomized trial conducted by the British Medical Research Council reported no effect on duration of chronic phase or survival.[107] Furthermore, no special group could be identified that would benefit from splenectomy nor was there evidence that splenectomy improved the quality of life, particularly in the terminal phase. Nevertheless some indications for splenectomy remain. It may be appropriate for massive splenomegaly that is causing discomfort. It may decrease the platelet and red cell transfusion requirement of some patients in acute phase[108] and improve their response to chemotherapy.

Management of Acute Phase CML

Accelerated Phase

The management of a patient in the accelerated phase must be individualized. For example, the patient with increasing splenomegaly may benefit from splenectomy or splenic irradiation; splenectomy may be particularly valuable for the patient with splenomegaly and thrombocytopenia and/or anemia. A rising leukocyte or platelet count resistant to busulfan or to hydroxyurea may be held in check for a period by switching to another drug or to a combination of two cytotoxic drugs,

such as busulfan plus 6-thioguanine or hydroxyurea plus 6-thioguanine. If the platelet count is $>1,000 \times 10^9$/L, it may be expedient to treat the patient with antiplatelet drugs. A low-grade fever may also be a manifestation of acceleration and may respond to a change in schedule of cytotoxic drugs.

If the transformation from chronic phase to acute phase occurs over weeks or months, a change in treatment may be indicated because of a rise in leukocyte or platelet count on the current therapy or the onset of new symptoms. Hydroxyurea will often be effective in reducing the leukocyte count and controlling symptoms if the patient is not already receiving it. For patients already receiving hydroxyurea a higher dose may be effective in the short term.

Once the patient has entered the blast phase of disease, survival is often a matter of weeks if no treatment is given. The options at this stage are supportive care alone or chemotherapy, which will often alleviate symptoms and prolong survival for weeks or months. If chemotherapy is to be used, the initial choice of therapy will be dictated by the type of transformation. The blast cell lineage should be determined by morphology, cytochemistry, and cell-surface markers. Most (60%) cell lineages are myeloid, including the rarely predominantly involved megakaryoblastic, basophilic, or erythroid cell lineages. Lymphoblastic characteristics are seen in 25–30%, 4% are biphenotypic with both lymphoid and myeloid markers, and the remainder are undifferentiated.[109,110]

Lymphoblastic Transformation

Lymphoblastic transformations respond in 60% of cases to regimens that include vincristine and prednisolone.[111] Response rates may be higher in patients whose blasts are both terminal deoxynucleotidyl transferase (TdT)- and CD10-positive.[112] The median duration of survival is still very short, however, around 4–6 months. The combination of continuous infusions of vincristine and Adriamycin with dexamethasone (VAD) was reported to provide a median remission duration of 10 months.[113]

In those patients with lymphoid transformation who have been successfully restored to a second chronic phase, the best approach to further treatment is probably use of a maintenance protocol similar to the regimen used in adult acute lymphocytic leukemia (ALL).[114] This typically involves 6-mercaptopurine and intermittent methotrexate, with reinductions using an anthracycline, vincristine, and steroid combination. It would also be wise to include some form of neuroprophylaxis, such as intrathecal methotrexate with or without cranial irradiation.

Myeloid Transformation

Patients with myeloid transformation do not usually respond to vincristine and steroid combinations. Results of chemotherapy have universally been poor, with <20% of patients achieving complete remission (defined as <5% blasts in the marrow aspirate). A few patients will revert to the chronic phase for short periods. Even for patients who do respond the median survival is only 6 months; patients who have no response have a median survival of 2 months.[115]

The usual regimen would be similar to those currently used in acute myeloid leukemia, with an anthracycline as well as cytosine arabinoside at standard or high doses. The combination of mithramycin and hydroxyurea has been tried with some success. Koller and Miller[116] used this combination in six patients with myeloid blast crisis; all patients responded and in four cases control was maintained for 5–19 months without significant toxicity and with improvement in clinical symptoms. The value of using these two drugs in combination has not been confirmed by others.

Management of Specific Problems

Thrombocytosis

Marked thrombocytosis, with a platelet count >1,000 × 10⁹/L, is found at diagnosis in 8% of patients, occurring more frequently in females. Splenectomy will often lead to marked sustained thrombocytosis. Thrombocytosis that develops later in the chronic phase often heralds acceleration of the disease. It is rarely associated with thrombosis or hemorrhage[117] and does not usually require specific therapy.

Attempts to reduce the platelet count toward normal with hydroxyurea or busulfan often lead to excessive depression of the leukocyte count. Therapy with IFN-α or -γ, however, can often control thrombocytosis without excessive leukocyte depression.[102,118]

Extramedullary Disease

Disease in sites other than the bone marrow, spleen, or liver is usually associated with transformation of the disease to the acute phase. Lymph nodes, bones, skin, and subcutaneous tissues are all recognized sites of disease. If the lesion is isolated, radiotherapy will often be effective, but evidence of blastic transformation should be sought.

Hyperviscosity

Hyperviscosity is a relatively rare complication of CML. In the second Medical Research Council CML trial, it occurred in 1% of patients, and the total leukocyte count was >300 × 10⁹/L in all but one case. Treatment is usually aimed at reducing the leukocyte count as rapidly as possible by urgent leukapheresis and chemotherapy. High-dose hydroxyurea is a safe and effective treatment at doses of ≤4 g/day. If anemia is also present, blood transfusion should be delayed until the leukocytosis is under control.

Priapism

Priapism is sometimes a presenting feature of CML[119,120] and is often associated with a high leukocyte and platelet count. The patient may give a history of previous transient episodes of sustained erection. Treatment is difficult; direct aspiration of the pooled blood may relieve congestion, but sexual potency may still be lost. Leukapheresis is seldom effective, and thrombolytic therapy has not been successful. Surgical intervention is a last resort, but sexual potency will usually be destroyed.

Tumor Lysis Syndrome

Tumor lysis syndrome is a rare complication of chemotherapy during the blast phase of CML.[120,121] The usual clinical findings are hypocalcemia, hyperphosphatemia, hyperkalemia, hyperuricemia, and renal failure. Acidosis and shock are often present. The syndrome can usually but not always be prevented by adequate hydration during therapy and treatment with allopurinol for ≥24 hours before chemotherapy. Once the syndrome is evident, the patient should be closely monitored with close attention to hydration, and any metabolic abnormalities should be reversed.

CML Presenting During Pregnancy

Occasionally one of the blood tests performed in the prenatal clinic reveals that a pregnant woman also has asymptomatic CML. Because there is no evidence that pregnancy affects the course of CML adversely, the pregnancy should not automatically be terminated. If the decision is taken to proceed with the pregnancy, the CML can usually be managed in the first and second trimester by repeated leukapheresis.[128,129] Busul-

fan and hydroxyurea may both be teratogenic but interestingly administration of IFN-α seems not to be harmful to the fetus.[130,131]

Bone Marrow Transplantation

Since about 1980 a large number of patients with CML have been treated with high-dose chemotherapy or chemoradiotherapy followed by transplantation of marrow from HLA-identical siblings.[122–125] The early studies were performed mainly on patients already in the acute phase. Most patients died either of BMT-related causes or of recurrent leukemia, but a small number became long-term leukemia-free survivors. This encouraged various investigators to offer BMT to patients with HLA-identical sibling donors while they were still in the chronic phase.

Timing of Transplantation

It is now very clear that the treatment of choice for younger patients with CML who have an HLA-identical sibling donor is a transplant while in the chronic phase (Fig. 73-8), but the optimal timing within the chronic phase remains controversial. For patients receiving BMT in the chronic phase the BMT-related mortality within the first 2 years after the procedure is approximately 20%. This means that if one could accurately define a cohort of patients likely to live 4 or 5 years without BMT, it might be reasonable for these patients to delay the procedure for 2 or 3 years. Segel et al.[126] have constructed a computer program that attempts to balance in individual patients the risk of transformation against the risk of BMT-related mortality and to predict the optimal time after diagnosis for the BMT to be performed. However, doubt is cast on this approach by data reported by a Seattle team, who found an inverse correlation between the interval from diagnosis to BMT and the probability of survival after BMT in the chronic phase.[123] A recent analysis performed by the International Bone Marrow Transplant Registry (IBMTR) confirmed this trend.[127] This observation could not be explained on the basis of an increased probability of relapse after BMT in patients with more "evolved" chronic phase disease, since relapse was not a major cause of death in these patients. It is possible that prolonged treatment with

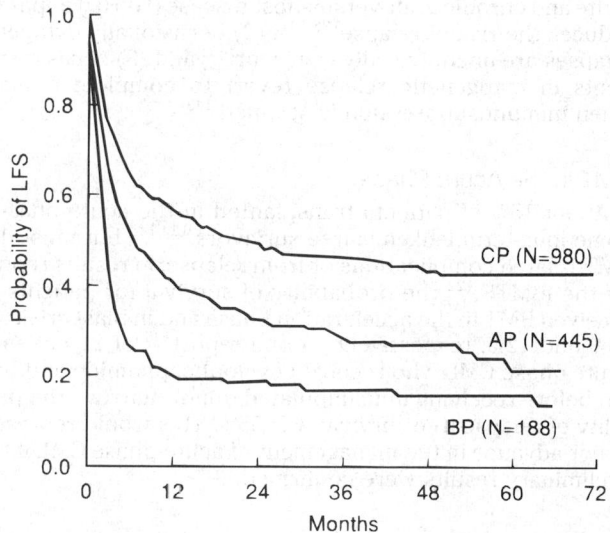

Fig. 73-8. Actuarial probability of leukemia-free survival (LFS) after allogeneic BMT from HLA-identical sibling donors for patients with CML, according to the disease status at the time of transplantation. The data presented here were obtained from the Statistical Center of the International Bone Marrow Transplant Registry.

cytotoxic drugs, especially busulfan, might reduce the probability of survival post-BMT.

Conditioning Regimens

The initial attempts to perform BMT in patients with CML in the acute phase[132] used cyclophosphamide (usually 60 mg/kg for 2 days) followed by total body irradiation (TBI), usually 10 Gy. Similar protocols were adopted[133–137] to treat patients in the chronic phase. Thus, for example, the Seattle group has in general used cyclophosphamide and TBI, either single dose or fractionated,[97,103] whereas the protocol used at the Hammersmith Hospital (London) has been cyclophosphamide followed by fractionated TBI (2 Gy fractions twice daily for five or six doses).[124,135] At the Memorial Sloan Kettering Cancer Center in New York the standard protocol is cyclophosphamide with hyperfractionated TBI (120 cGy three times daily to a total dose of 1,320 or 1,440 cGy).[138]

There is no clear evidence that radiotherapy forms an essential component of conditioning for patients undergoing allogeneic transplantation for CML. The Baltimore group has accumulated extensive experience with the use of busulfan (4 mg/kg/day for 4 days) followed by cyclophosphamide (50 mg/kg/day for 4 days).[139,140] Although this combination may be unduly toxic for patients who have already received substantial doses of busulfan before BMT, it is certainly an effective conditioning schedule for patients with acute leukemia, and success with its use in CML casts doubt on the necessity for including TBI in the conditioning regimen.

Importance of Graft-Versus-Leukemia Effects

Most patients with chronic-phase CML who are given conventional chemoradiotherapy followed by unmanipulated donor marrow will probably never relapse.[123,125] By contrast most patients who are treated with similar chemoradiotherapy regimens but receive donor marrow cells depleted in vitro of lymphoid cells do relapse within 2 or 3 years of BMT.[125] These data suggest that chemoradiotherapy alone rarely, if ever, eradicates the leukemic clone and that the lymphoid cells present in the donor marrow must exert an important antileukemic influence, which has been designated a graft-versus-leukemia effect. Further evidence for the role of such an effect comes from the following related observations: (1) the occurrence of acute and chronic graft-versus-host disease (GVHD) apparently reduces the risk of relapse[125,141]; (2) occasionally cytogenetic relapses are unequivocally transient[142]; and (3) occasional patients in cytogenetic relapse revert to complete remission when immunosuppression is stopped.[143]

BMT in the Acute Phase

About 15% of patients transplanted in the acute phase become long-term leukemia-free survivors,[124,144] but most die of BMT-related complications or from relapse. In results reported by the IBMTR,[122] the probability of survival for patients who received BMT in the acceleration phase and in blast crisis were 35% and 12%, respectively. In one report[145] of 21 patients in acute-phase CML who received cyclophosphamide and busulfan before receiving unmanipulated donor marrow, the probability of relapse-free survival was 55%. This would represent a major advance in the management of acute-phase CML if these preliminary results were confirmed.

BMT in Chronic Phase

A number of individual centers have now reported the results of BMT performed for CML in the chronic phase using HLA-identical sibling donors.[123,124,146–149] The results of BMT worldwide have been reported at intervals by the

IBMTR,[122,125,150] although many of the patients in the individual reports are included in the IBMTR analyses. In summary, the probabilities of survival and relapse at 4 years are about 55% and 19%, respectively.[125] It should be noted, however, that this IBMTR analysis included some patients who had received T-cell-depleted bone marrow grafts. If these are excluded from the analysis, the probability of relapse is 9%, and the probability of leukemia-free survival is 47%. These results agree relatively well with those of the large series reported independently from Seattle, in which the actuarial probabilities of survival and of relapse were 49% and 20%, respectively.[123] It should be noted that the term relapse for the purposes of these figures includes hematologic or clinical relapses but excludes cytogenetic-only relapse (see below).

The status of residual leukemia can be monitored after BMT by use of PCR to identify small numbers of *bcr-abl* transcripts. Peripheral blood and marrow serve this purpose equally well. It is not unusual for patients to show PCR positivity for 6–9 months after BMT but most have become negative by 1 year.[151–153] Persisting or recurrent PCR positivity beyond 1 year suggests that a patient may be at increased risk of relapse. Among 10-year survivors most are PCR negative but occasional patients are positive in blood or marrow without other evidence of relapse.[154]

Donor Selection

To minimize the risk of serious GVHD, donors for BMT have hitherto been mainly syngeneic or genotypically HLA-identical siblings. In western Europe and North America, however, the average size of families indicates that only about one-third of patients who would otherwise be eligible for BMT have HLA-identical siblings.[155] For BMT to make a greater impact on the management of CML, the donor pool must be extended by using partially matched family donors or matched unrelated donors.

Partially Matched Family Donors

Although the role of histocompatibility in transplantation has been well defined in laboratory animals,[156,157] there were until recently few clinical data available to assess the extent of HLA incompatibility permissible in human BMT. This made it difficult to predict the risk of graft failure or of GVHD. BMT using related donors mismatched for two or more HLA-A, -B, or -DR loci are associated with poorer results.[158,159] If, however, the degree of mismatch involves only a single HLA-A, -B, or -DR antigen, such partially mismatched family donor BMTs can apparently be as successful as those using fully matched siblings in "good risk" patients.[159] There has been some success with T-cell-depleted BMT from partially matched family donors for patients with leukemia, which have resulted in good engraftment and a reduced incidence of GVHD.[160] Despite this extension of the donor pool, most patients otherwise eligible for BMT still lack a suitable family member donor. For this reason the possibility of extending the donor pool further by using HLA-matched unrelated volunteer donors has been investigated.

Unrelated Donors

A number of registers holding data on individuals who have volunteered to donate bone marrow have now been established in various countries. In the United Kingdom the Anthony Nolan Research Centre has data on 300,000 persons typed for HLA-A and -B, of whom about 100,000 have also been DR-typed. Other registries in Europe and North America have a total of >1 million HLA-A- and -B-typed donors. The relationship between the size of the donor panel and the chance of finding a donor for an individual patient was examined by Bradley et al.[161] Their calculations took into account the known linkage disequilibrium between A, B, and DR genes in the donor population and assumed that only one of eight A-, B-, and DR-matched donors would be unreactive in mixed lymphocyte reaction (MLR) with the prospective recipient. With a donor pool size of 1,400,000, approximately the size of all current registries combined, one or more donors matched for A, B, and DR antigens and negative in MLR could be found for 59% of patients. Furthermore, if a transplant center were prepared to make use of an unrelated donor mismatched for one class I antigen, then suitable donors could be found for 82% of patients. In practice, the complexity of the HLA region makes it difficult to identify a suitably matched unrelated donor for a given patient. In contrast to HLA-identical sibling donor/recipient pairs, initial serologic screening of unrelated donor/recipient pairs only ensures limited phenotypic identity rather than genotypic identity for the whole HLA region. Additional matching procedures using the MLR, complement-typing,[162] DNA restriction fragment length polymorphism,[163] and DNA typing with PCR using sequence-specific primers (SCR-SSP), may be of value in predicting the outcome of BMT.

In a recent analysis of the combined results of unrelated donor BMTs for CML from four centers the projected 1,000-day survival was 55% for chronic-phase patients and 22% for those in the acute phase. For patients who received BMTs during the chronic phase, results appeared to be comparable whether the donor was fully HLA-matched or mismatched for one HLA locus.[164] Viral infections may be a particular problem.[165]

Management of the Spleen at BMT

The spleen of a patient in the chronic phase should be relatively small; if it is not, the classification as chronic phase is suspect. Nonetheless there was at one time some suspicion that relapse might be more likely in patients who retained even normal-size spleens than in those subjected to splenectomy before BMT.[166] This led investigators at some centers to recommend routine splenectomy or additional splenic irradiation before BMT.[124,137,147] No clear-cut benefit from splenectomy or splenic irradiation has been demonstrated.[167,168] The European Bone Marrow Transplant Group is currently assessing the value of additional splenic irradiation in a randomized multicenter study.[169] There is no clear benefit to be derived from splenectomy or splenic irradiation before BMT.

Drug Therapy to Prevent GVHD

Most attempts to prevent GVHD have involved use of immunosuppressive therapy. Methotrexate was initially used by the Seattle group, starting within 24 hours of BMT and continuing for approximately 3 months,[170] but GVHD remained a serious problem affecting 25–60% of patients. More recently, cyclosporine has been used for prophylaxis of GVHD. Although initial uncontrolled studies suggested that it was more effective than methotrexate,[171] a controlled study in CML patients found no difference in incidence of GVHD between patients given methotrexate and those given cyclosporin.[172] Because of the generally disappointing results, several attempts at combination therapy have been tried. No significant benefit was observed from combining methotrexate with antithymocyte globulin when compared with methotrexate alone.[132] The Minneapolis group, however, reported a significant reduction in the incidence of GVHD, albeit without significant improvement in survival, in patients given methotrexate combined with corticosteroids and antithymocyte globulin as compared with patients given methotrexate alone.[173] More recently, cyclosporine combined with "short methotrexate" has resulted in a significantly

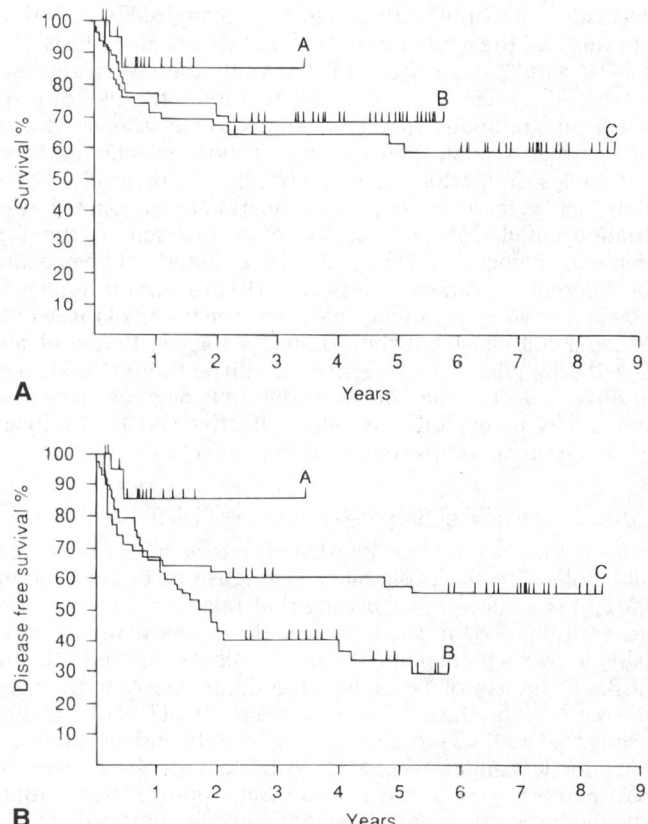

Fig. 73-9. Actuarial probability of **(A)** survival and **(B)** leukemia-free survival for patients who received transplants in the chronic phase of CML at the Hammersmith Hospital, London, according to the GVHD prophylaxis used. Group A (n = 17) received unmanipulated donor marrow with cyclosporine and methotrexate; group B (n = 51) received T-cell-depleted donor marrow; group C (n = 43) received unmanipulated donor marrow with cyclosporine only. Vertical marks indicate surviving patients.

lower incidence of GVHD and better survival than can be achieved by using either agent alone[144,174] (Fig. 73-9).

T-Cell Depletion of the Donor Marrow

Various methods of depleting donor marrow of T cells have been used. The most common and convenient technique is to incubate donor marrow in vitro with anti-T-lymphocyte monoclonal antibodies and complement to induce T-cell lysis. The Royal Free Hospital group in London used antibodies with CD6 and CD8 specificities,[175] and the University of California at Los Angeles group used a CD2 antibody.[176] Much experience worldwide has been accumulated with the use of Campath-1, an IgM monoclonal antibody active against incompletely defined antigens on T and B lymphocytes and on some monocytes, which fixes human complement in vitro.[177–181] Other techniques for the elimination of T cells include soybean lectin agglutination in conjunction with E-rosette formation and counterflow elutriation.[138,182] In general, these different methods reduce the number of residual T cells in the marrow to <1% of the pretreatment levels.

The use of T-cell-depleted donor marrow is associated with a lower incidence and severity of GVHD but a higher risk of graft failure.[181] The graft failure may be due to survival in the host of chemotherapy-resistant, radioresistant, immunologically competent cells, which in the absence of T cells of donor origin are capable of mediating graft rejection.[183] In patients with CML the major problem associated with the use of T-cell-depleted bone marrow is a substantial increase in the risk of relapse, which applies to patients receiving BMTs in both the chronic and the acute phase (Fig. 73-9). Recent analysis of the IBMTR data[184] has suggested that while the risk of relapse is increased by all T-cell depletion methods, the use of broad-spectrum antibodies (such as Campath-1) is associated with a higher relative risk than the use of more specific anti-T-cell antibodies. Somewhat surprisingly, physical methods of depletion such as lectin soybean agglutination and counterflow elutriation entailed the lowest risk of relapse among the T-cell depletion categories. These differences could not be explained by differences in effectiveness of GVHD prevention, as all methods appeared to be equally effective. The cause of these differences is not clear, but these findings suggest that equivalent GVHD prophylaxis can be achieved with methods that abrogate graft-versus-leukemia effects to different degrees. This could potentially be exploited to allow effective GVHD prophylaxis while retaining graft-versus-leukemia effects.

Other Factors Affecting the Outcome of BMT

In view of the relatively long list of factors that could theoretically influence the probability of relapse or of survival after BMT, it is somewhat surprising that relatively few have been generally agreed on. These include the degree of histocompatibility between patient and donor, the disease status at the time of BMT, the use of T-cell-depleted donor marrow, the age of the patient, and the incidence and severity of GVHD post-BMT.

It is a general observation that morbidity and mortality after BMT for leukemia are related to the age of the patient, and CML in this regard is no exception. Data reported by the IBMTR and by the Seattle group show that mortality post-BMT is lower in patients <20 years old than in older patients.[123,125] It is not clear, however, whether this age-related risk is a continuous or a dichotomized variable. In some reports patients in the age ranges of 20–30, 30–40, and 40–50 fare equally well. In the Seattle study, older age was related to a greater frequency and severity of GVHD and to an increasing interval from diagnosis to BMT, but age was found to have no additional effect on mortality after adjustment for these two factors.[124]

Acute or chronic GVHD is one of the principal causes of death in patients who receive BMTs in the chronic phase.[123] It may lead directly to death or may contribute indirectly to death from other causes such as infection or interstitial pneumonitis. The survival of patients in chronic phase who develop grades II–IV acute GVHD is significantly worse than that of patients who do not.[126] Conversely, in an IBMTR analysis of 405 CML patients who received allografts in the chronic phase, the probability of relapse was 24% in those who did not develop chronic GVHD versus only 12% in those who did,[125] with $P < 0.004$.

Relapse of Leukemia

The recognition of relapse after transplant for CML is not always straightforward. In some cases the clinical, hematologic, and cytogenetic features of the relapse are obvious; such cases we have designated hematologic relapse. In other cases the only evidence for relapse is the finding of Ph-positive metaphases in a minority of marrow cells after BMT; these we have called cytogenetic relapses.[142] In other cases, there is no hematologic or cytogenetic evidence of relapse but the PCR is persistently positive or positive with increasing numbers of *bcr-abl* transcripts; these cases we have called molecular relapses.[152,154] Most intriguing are the cases reported in which relapse has occurred in cells apparently of donor origin.

Cytogenetic Relapse

In all large series in which cytogenetic analysis of the marrow was carried out at regular intervals, a small number of cases have been seen in which a low proportion of the Ph-positive metaphases was identified within 1 or 2 years of BMT without progression to hematologic relapse.[125,142,185–187] The clinical significance of these transient cytogenetic relapses is unclear. It may be that the cytogenetic analysis has revealed evidence of a leukemic clone that is small and doomed to extinction. Alternatively, the Ph-positive metaphases may be derived from lymphoid cells that have no capacity to maintain hematopoiesis. If, however, the T-cell component of the graft is important in suppressing leukemia post-BMT, it is possible that these transient cytogenetic relapses are a manifestation of the temporary failure of this putative graft-versus-leukemia effect. In other cases the finding of Ph-positive marrow metaphases persists for months or years or proceeds to overt hematologic relapse.[142,143]

Relapse in Cells of Donor Origin

Two cases have been reported in which relapse after BMT occurred in cells that appeared to be of donor origin.[188,189] Both patients received BMT from HLA-identical siblings of the opposite sex, and in both cases blast cells at relapse had the sex chromosome pattern of the donor. It may be of significance that both patients received their BMTs in the second chronic phase after treatment for lymphoid transformation and both relapsed directly to a second blastic phase without an obvious preceding chronic phase.

There are in theory many mechanisms by which relapse after BMT could occur in cells of donor origin.[190,191] For example, a powerful microenvironmental influence could exist, which caused the original leukemia in the host and later induced leukemia in the donor cells. Alternatively, the appearance of relapse in donor cells might be artifactual if exchange of sex chromosomes had taken place between the host's leukemic cells and normal cells of donor origin. Perhaps the most likely interpretation is transfer or transfection of a "transforming" sequence of DNA from residual leukemic cells of host origin to the donor cells.

Hematologic Relapse

Relapse is usually recognized within 2 years of BMT but may occasionally occur at intervals ≤6 years after BMT.[126,154] The first indication of relapse is frequently the finding in the peripheral blood of abnormalities suggestive of CML (e.g., basophilia or the presence of myelocytes) in the absence of leukocytosis. Examination of the marrow trephine at this stage may show a degree of cellularity in excess of what would normally be expected within 1 or 2 years of BMT.[192] Cytogenetic analysis will then reveal the Ph chromosome in most metaphases.[187,193] Despite evidence of hematologic relapse, some of these patients remain well, with stable or only slowly rising leukocyte count, and do not require treatment for many months or years.[193]

Management of Hematologic Relapse. Several groups have reported encouraging results using IFN-α after BMT: hematologic control in most cases treated, partial Ph negativity in a minority, and complete cytogenetic and hematologic remission in a few cases.[194–196] A second BMT carries a high chance of transplant-related mortality. In several studies[197–199] the probability of survival was strongly related to the interval between transplants. In view of the high risk of a second BMT performed soon after the first and the relatively low risk of early transformation after hematologic relapse, it is probably reasonable to delay a second BMT for ≥24 months from the first in patients who received the first BMT during the chronic phase and who then relapse to chronic phase.

Of great interest has been the recent demonstration that patients in hematologic relapse after BMT can be treated by transfusion of leukocytes collected from their original donor without the use of cytotoxic drugs.[200-203] Most patients so treated are restored to complete remission with normal marrow cytogenetics (consistent with donor origin) and negative PCR results. The response usually occurs within 4–12 weeks and is then durable but some patients do not respond. Some patients develop GVHD and this can on occasion be fatal. Others in whom leukemia cell numbers diminished have become pancytopenic and aplastic but this state can usually be reversed by transfusion of marrow cells from the original donor.

This efficacy of leukocyte transfusions in this situation is further evidence of a graft-versus-leukemia effect, but the nature of the effector cells is not known. Because of the relatively high success rate for this technique, it should probably be attempted before submitting a patient formally to a second transplant procedure. It is not clear whether a patient who receives leukocyte transfusions for treatment of relapse should or should not also receive GVHD prophylaxis.

Future Directions

The major obstacles to improving survival after BMT remain graft-versus-host disease and interstitial pneumonitis. Improved post-BMT immunosuppressive therapy with regimens such as cyclosporine plus methotrexate may reduce the morbidity and mortality of acute GVHD,[174] but it is still a major and not infrequently lethal complication. Attempts to prevent it with T-cell depletion have been associated with a significantly increased risk of relapse. It remains to be seen whether any of the modifications to the technique of T-cell depletion now under study will reduce the risk of relapse while retaining its benefits. The incidence of CMV pneumonitis has been reduced in CMV-seronegative recipients with the use of CMV-negative blood products,[204] and there is some evidence that early (or prophylactic) use of ganciclovir may benefit some patients.

DISEASES CLOSELY RELATED TO CHRONIC MYELOID LEUKEMIA

Ph-Negative Chronic Myeloid Leukemia

In series reported before 1980 as many as 10–15% of patients with CML were Ph-negative.[205,206] With the establishment of well-defined clinical and morphologic criteria for CML, many of these Ph-negative cases have been reclassified. There remain about 5% of patients with CML who are Ph-negative.[207] At the molecular level many of these patients have evidence of the same DNA rearrangement as Ph-positive patients, with formation of a *bcr/abl* chimeric gene, presumably by a different mechanism.[208-211] This group is generally impossible to separate clinically and hematologically from those with Ph-positive CML. Those patients who lack cytogenetic and molecular evidence of *bcr/abl* formation tend to have subtle atypical hematologic features, namely, dysgranulopoiesis, elevated monocyte counts, and low basophil counts.[72,212]

Juvenile Chronic Myeloid Leukemia

Juvenile CML is a rare disorder seen in young children.[213,214] The child presents with sweats, fever, weight loss, or a variety of septic lesions. The spleen and liver are markedly enlarged, lymphadenopathy is prominent, and rashes may also be seen. The degree of leukocytosis is variable, but the blood film cannot usually be confused with that of Ph-positive CML. Immature granulocytes and blasts are present but myelocytes are not prominent, and eosinophilia and basophilia are lacking. Monocytes are often increased, platelets are often mildly decreased, and the NAP score is normal or raised. The karyotype is usually

normal. These patients respond poorly to cytotoxic drugs, although some can have partial responses that last months or years. An allogeneic BMT is the treatment of choice if a suitable donor can be identified.

Eosinophilic Leukemia

Eosinophilic leukemia is a very rare and poorly defined entity, which may present with a variety of symptoms, including sweats, weight loss, nonspecific rashes, and cardiac abnormalities.[215] Splenomegaly may be a feature. The cardiac lesions include various dysrhythmias and disturbance of valvular function, probably due to the direct toxic action of eosinophil cationic proteins and other enzymes on the endomyocardium. The blood film shows marked eosinophilia, and some eosinophils have cytoplasmic areas of vacuolation and degranulation. A few immature eosinophils and blasts may be present. Various cytogenetic abnormalities have been described, including trisomy for C group chromosomes and an isochromosome 17. The finding of a Ph chromosome suggests that the diagnosis is not eosinophilic leukemia but rather eosinophilic blastic transformation of CML. Eosinophilic leukemia must be distinguished from other causes of eosinophilia (including the hypereosinophilic syndrome). In these cases eosinophilia may be marked but immature cells are usually absent.

Eosinophilic leukemia may remain under control for several years but eventually enters a blastic and terminal phase.

Chronic Neutrophilic Leukemia

Chronic neutrophilic leukemia is a rare disorder in which the patient has marked neutrophilia without an increase in basophils, eosinophils, or less mature granulocytes.[216] There are usually no associated symptoms and signs, although some patients have mild splenomegaly. The marrow usually shows myeloid hyperplasia and is cytogenetically normal.[217] It is often difficult to exclude reactive causes of neutrophilia such as occult infection or malignancy. When other causes of neutrophilia have been excluded, the diagnosis of chronic neutrophilic leukemia can be made. In the absence of symptoms treatment is not usually required.

Chronic Myelomonocytic Leukemia

Chronic myelomonocytic leukemia (CMML) is classified as a myelodysplastic disorder.[218] It is diagnosed mainly in older men, who may present with weight loss or symptoms of anemia. The spleen is often moderately enlarged, and the blood film reveals marked monocytosis and neutrophilia. Features of myelodysplasia are usually present in the blood or bone marrow, such as hypogranular neutrophils, Pelger-Huët forms of granulocytes, dyserythropoiesis with ringed sideroblasts, and micromegakaryocytes. Serum lysozyme levels are greatly elevated and hypokalemia is sometimes seen. The marrow is usually hypercellular, with increased immature and mature monocytes. The Ph chromosome is not seen. The disease is usually indolent for many years, requiring supportive measures only, but in many patients it will eventually transform to acute leukemia that responds poorly to conventional therapy for acute myeloid leukemia.

Ph-Positive Acute Lymphocytic Leukemia

About 20% of adults and 2–3% of children who present with ALL have blast cells with a Ph chromosome indistinguishable on cytogenetic grounds from that found in patients with Ph-positive CML. In general these patients do not have clinical or hematologic features suggestive of CML. The prognosis for this group is significantly worse than for those with Ph-negative ALL. Studies at the molecular level show that 20–30% of the patients have chromosome breakpoints within the M-BCR region, while the others have breakpoints located upstream of M-BCR in the first intron of the bcr gene. The latter patients have a relatively smaller bcr/abl mRNA (7.0 kb) and a smaller 190-kd hybrid protein (P190).[219]

Most of those patients who achieve complete remission have normal hematopoiesis and no evidence of the Ph chromosome. Some patients will recover from chemotherapy to reveal the picture of chronic-phase CML with Ph-positivity and are presumed to have been in CML blast crisis.

REFERENCES

1. Galton DAG: The chronic myeloid leukemia. p. 877. In Hardisty RM, Weatherall DJ (eds): Blood and its Disorders. Blackwell Scientific Publications, Oxford, 1982
2. Gunz FW: The epidemiology and genetics of the chronic leukaemias. Clin Haematol 6:3, 1977
3. Lange R, Moloney W, Yamawaki T: Leukemia in atomic bomb survivors. 1. General observations. Blood 9:574, 1954
4. Heyssel R, Brill B, Woodbury L: Leukemia in Hiroshima atomic bomb survivors. Blood 15:313, 1960
5. Court Brown W, Abbatt J: Mortality from cancer and other causes after radiotherapy for ankylosing spondylitis. BMJ 2:1327, 1965
6. Nowell PC, Hungerford DA: A minute chromosome in human chronic granulocytic leukemia. Science 132:1497, 1960
7. Rowley JD: A new consistent chromosomal abnormality in chronic myelogenous leukaemia identified by quinacrine fluorescence and Giemsa banding. Nature 243:290, 1973
8. Sandberg AA: The cytogenetics of chronic myelocytic leukemia (CML): chronic phase and blast crisis. Cancer Genet Cytogenet 1:217, 1980
9. De Braekeleer D: Variant Philadelphia translocations in chronic myeloid leukemia. Cytogenet Cell Genet 44:215, 1987
10. Hagemeijer A, deKlein A, Godde-Salz E et al: Translocation of c-abl to "masked" Ph in chronic myeloid leukemia. Cancer Genet Cytogenet 18:95, 1985
11. Pederson B: Coexistence of cells with unmasked and masked Ph in a case of chronic myeloid leukemia in blast phase. Cancer Genet Cytogenet 12:129, 1984
12. Ohyashiki K, Ohyashiki JH, Otaki K et al: Four cases with complex Philadelphia translocations, including one with appearance de novo of a "masked" Ph. Cancer Genet Cytogenet 24:281, 1987
13. Hagemeijer A, Bartram CR, Smit EME et al: Is the chromosomal region 9q34 always involved in variants of the Ph¹ translocation? Cancer Genet Cytogenet 13:1, 1984
14. Hagemeijer A: Chromosome abnormalities in CML. Baillieres Clin Haematol 4:963, 1987
15. Sokal JE, Cox EB, Baccarani M et al: Prognostic discrimination in 'good risk' chronic granulocytic leukemia. Blood 63:789, 1984
16. Sakurai M, Sandberg AA: The chromosomes and causation of human cancer and leukemia. XVIII. The missing Y in acute myeloblastic leukemia (AML) and Ph1-positive chronic myelocytic leukemia (CML). Cancer 38:762, 1976
17. Lawler SD: The cytogenetics of chronic granulocytic leukaemia. Clin Haematol 6:55, 1977
18. Bernstein R: Cytogenetics of chronic myelogenous leukemia. Semin Hematol 25:20, 1988
19. Watmore AE, Potter AM, Sokal RJ et al: Value of cytogenetic studies in prediction of acute phase of CML. Cancer Genet Cytogenet 14:293, 1985
20. Kurzrock R, Gutterman JU, Talpaz M: The molecular genetics of Philadelphia chromosome-positive leukemias. N Engl J Med 319:990, 1988
21. Gale RP, Goldman JM, Grosveld G, Goldman JM: Chronic myelogenous leukemia: biology and therapy. (Meeting Report). Leukemia 7:653, 1993
22. Abelson HT, Rabstein LS: Lymphosarcoma: virus induced thymic-independent disease in mice. Cancer Res 30:2213, 1970
23. Baltimore D, Rosenberg N, Witte O: Transformation of immature lymphoid cells by Abelson murine leukemia virus. Immunol Rev 48:3, 1979
24. Witte ON, Goff SP, Rosenberg N, Baltimore D: A transformation defective mutant of Abelson murine leukemia virus protein lacks protein kinase activity. Proc Natl Acad Sci USA 77:4993, 1980
25. Van Etten RA, Jackson P, Baltimore D: The mouse type IV c-abl gene product

is a nuclear protein, and activation of transforming ability is associated with cytoplasmic localisation. Cell 58:669, 1989
26. Heisterkamp N, Groffen J, Stephenson JR: The human v-abl cellular homologue. J Mol Appl Genet 2:57, 1983
27. Groffen J, Heisterkamp N, Grosveld F et al: Isolation of human oncogene sequences (v-fes homolog) from a cosmid library. Science 216:1136, 1982
28. Bernards A, Rubin CM, Westbrook CA et al: The first intron in the human c-abl gene is at least 200 kilobases long and is a target for translocation in chronic myelogenous leukemia. Mol Cell Biol 7:3231, 1987
29. Westbrook C, Rubin C, Carrino J et al: Long-range mapping of the Philadelphia chromosome by pulse-field gel electrophoresis. Blood 71:697, 1988
30. Schtivelman E, Lifshitz B, Gale RP et al: Alternative splicing of RNAs transcribed from the human ABL gene and from the bcr-abl gene. Cell 42:277, 1986
31. Groffen J, Heisterkamp N: The BCR/ABL hybrid gene. Ballieres Clin Haematol 4:983, 1987
32. Heisterkamp N, Groffen J, Stephenson JR et al: Chromosomal localisation of human cellular homologues of two viral oncogenes. Nature 299:747, 1982
33. De Klein A, Geurts van Kessel A, Grosfeld G et al: A cellular oncogene is translocated to the Philadelphia chromosome in chronic myelocytic leukaemia. Nature 300:765, 1982
34. Bartram CR, de Klein A, Hagenmeijer A: Translocation of c-abl oncogene correlates with the presence of a Philadelphia chromosome in chronic myelocytic leukaemia. Nature 306:277, 1983
35. Groffen J, Stephenson JR, Heisterkamp N et al: Philadelphia chromosomal breakpoints are clustered within a limited region, bcr, on chromosome 22. Cell 36:93, 1984
36. Gale RP, Goldman JM: Workshop letter: rapid progress in chronic myelogenous leukemia. Leukemia 2:321, 1988
37. Croce CM, Huebner K, Isobe M et al: Mapping of 4 distinct BCR-related loci to chromosome region 22q11: order of BCR loci relative to chronic myelogenous leukemia and acute lymphoblastic leukemia. Proc Natl Acad Sci USA 84:7174, 1987
38. Collins SJ, Groudine MT: Rearrangement and amplification of c-abl sequences in the human chronic myelogenous leukemia cell line K562. Proc Natl Acad Sci USA 80:4813, 1983
39. Konopka JB, Watanabe SN, Witte ON: An alteration of the human c-abl protein in K562 leukemia cells unmasks associated tyrosine kinase activity. Cell 37:1035, 1984
40. Ben-Neriah Y, Daley GQ, Mes-Masson AM et al: The chronic myelogenous leukemia specific p210 protein is the product of the bcr/abl hybrid gene. Science 223:212, 1986
41. Pendergast AM, Quilliam LA, Cripe LD et al: BCR-ABL-induced oncogenesis is mediated by direct interaction with the SH2 domain of the GRB-2 adaptor protein. Cell 75:175, 1993
42. Daley GQ, Van Etten RA, Baltimore D: Induction of chronic myelogenous leukemia in mice by the P210^bcr/abl gene of the Philadelphia chromosome. Science 247:824, 1990
43. Daley GQ, van Etten RA, Baltimore D: Blast crisis in a murine model of chronic myelogenous leukemia. Proc Natl Acad Sci USA 88:11335, 1991
44. Bakhshi A, Minowada J, Arnold A et al: Lymphoid blast crisis of chronic myelogenous leukemia represent stages in the development of B-cell precursors. N Engl J Med 309:826, 1983
45. Uike N, Takeichi N, Kimura N et al: Dual rearrangement of immunoglobulin and T cell receptor genes in blast crisis of CML. Eur J Haematol 42:460, 1989
46. Ahuja H, Bar-Eli M, Advani SH et al: Alterations in the P53 gene and the clonal evolution of the blast crisis of chronic myelocytic leukemia. Proc Natl Acad Sci USA 86:6783, 1989
47. Kelman Z, Prokocimer M, Peller S et al: Rearrangements in the p53 gene in Philadelphia chromosome positive myelogenous leukemia. Blood 74:2318, 1989
48. Liu E, Hjelle B, Bishop JM et al: Transforming genes in chronic myelogenous leukemia. Proc Natl Acad Sci USA 85:1952, 1988
49. Collins SJ, Howard M, Andrews DF et al: Rare occurrence of N-ras point mutations in Philadelphia chromosome positive chronic myeloid leukemia. Blood 73:1028, 1989
50. Fialkow PJ, Jacobson RJ, Papayannopoulou T: Chronic myelocytic leukemia: clonal origin in a stem cell common to the granulocyte, erythrocyte, platelet and monocyte/macrophage. Am J Med 63:125, 1977
51. Yoffe G, Chinault AC, Talpaz M et al: Clonal nature of Philadelphia chromosome positive and negative chronic myelogenous leukemia by DNA hybridization analysis. Exp Hematol 15:725, 1987
52. Martin PJ, Najfeld V, Fialkow PJ: B-lymphoid cell involvement in chronic myelogenous leukemia: implications for the pathogenesis of the disease. Cancer Genet Cytogenet 6:359, 1982
53. Eaves AC, Henkelman DH, Eaves CJ: Abnormal erythropoiesis in the myelo-

proliferative disorders: an analysis of underlying cellular and humoral mechanisms. Exp Hematol, suppl 8. 8:235, 1980

54. Eaves CJ, Eaves AC: Cell culture studies in CML. Baillieres Clin Haematol 4: 931, 1987
55. Metcalf D: Hemopoietic colonies. Recent Res Cancer Res 61:1, 1977
56. Coulombel L, Kalousek DK, Eaves CJ et al: Long term marrow culture reveals chromosomally normal hemopoietic progenitor cells in patients with Philadelphia-positive chronic myelogenous leukemia. N Engl J Med 308:1493, 1983
57. Karanas A, Silver RT: Characteristics of the terminal phase of chronic granulocytic leukemia. Blood 32:445, 1968
58. Kantarjian HM, Dixon D, Keating MJ et al: Characteristics of accelerated disease in chronic myelogenous leukemia. Cancer 61:1441, 1988
59. Kantarjian HM, Keating MJ, Talpaz M et al: Chronic myelogenous leukemia in blast crisis. Am J Med 83:445, 1987
60. Sokal JE: Prognosis in chronic myeloid leukaemia: biology of the disease vs. treatment. Baillieres Clin Haematol 4:907, 1987
61. Tura S, Baccarani M, Corbelli G et al: Staging of chronic myeloid leukaemia. Br J Haematol 47:105, 1981
62. Cervantes F, Rozman C: A multivariate analysis of prognostic factors in chronic myeloid leukemia. Blood 60:1298, 1982
63. Kantarjian HM, Smith TL, McCredie KB et al: Chronic myelogenous leukemia: a multivariate analysis of the associations of patient characteristics and therapy with survival. Blood 66:1326, 1985
64. Kantarjian H, Keating M, Smith T et al: Proposal for a simple synthesis prognostic staging system in chronic myelogenous leukemia. Am J Med 88: 1, 1990
65. Cox DR: Regression models and life tables. J R Stat Soc [B] 34:187, 1972
66. Italian Cooperative Study Group on Chronic Myeloid Leukaemia: Prospective confirmation of a prognostic classification for Ph-positive chronic myeloid leukaemia. Br J Haematol 69:463, 1988
67. Wareham NJ, Johnson SA, Goldman JM: Relationship of the duration of chronic phase in the chronic granulocytic leukaemia to the need for treatment during the first year after diagnosis. Cancer Chemother Pharmacol 8: 205, 1982
68. Schaefer-Rego K, Dudek H, Popenoe D et al: CML patients in blast crisis have breakpoints localised to a specific region of the BCR. Blood 70:448, 1987
69. Mills KI, Mackenzie ED, Birnie GD: The site of the breakpoint within the bcr is a prognostic factor in Philadelphia-positive CML patients. Blood 72:1237, 1988
70. Dyck JA, Bosco JJ: Clinical stage of chronic granulocytic leukaemia and BCR breakpoint location in south-east Asian patients. Br J Haematol 72:64, 1989
71. Jaubert J, Martiat P, Dowding C et al: The position of the M-BCR breakpoint does not predict the duration of chronic phase or survival in chronic myeloid leukaemia. Br J Haematol 74:30, 1990
72. Shepherd PA, Ganesan TS, Galton DAG: Haematological classification of the chronic myeloid leukaemias. Baillieres Clin Haematol 4:887, 1987
73. Yuo A, Kitagawa S, Okabe T et al: Recombinant human granulocyte colony-stimulating factor repairs the abnormalities of neutrophils in patients with myelodysplastic syndromes and chronic myelogenous leukaemia. Blood 70: 404, 1987
74. Chikkappa G, Wang GJ, Santella D et al: Granulocyte colony-stimulating factor (G-CSF) induces synthesis of alkaline phosphatase in neutrophilic granulocytes of chronic myelogenous leukemia patients. Leuk Res 12:491, 1988
75. Galton DAG: Myleran in chronic myeloid leukaemia. Results of treatment. Lancet 1:208, 1953
76. Medical Research Council: Chronic granulocytic leukemia: comparison of radiotherapy and busulphan therapy. BMJ 1:201, 1968
77. Galton DAG: Treatment of the chronic leukaemias. Br Med Bull 15:79, 1959
78. Vicariot M, Goldman JM, Catovsky D, Galton DAG: Treatment of chronic granulocytic leukaemia with repeated single doses of busulphan. Eur J Cancer 15:559, 1979
79. Galton DAG: Busulphan (1,4 dimethanesulphonyloxybutane): summary of clinical results. Ann NY Acad Sci 68:967, 1958
80. Kyle RA, Schwartz RS, Oliner HL, Dameshek W: A syndrome resembling adrenal cortical insufficiency associated with long term busulfan (myleran) therapy. Blood 18:497, 1961
81. Kenis Y, Dustin P, Henry JA, Tagnon HJ: Action du myleran dans 22 cas de leucemie myeloide chronique. Rev Fr Etudes Clin Biol 1:435, 1956
82. Djaldetti M, Padeh B, Pinkhas J, Devries A: Prolonged remission in chronic myeloid leukemia after one course of busulfan. Blood 27:103, 1966
83. Finney R, McDonald GA, Baikie AG, Douglas AS: Chronic granulocytic leukaemia with Ph[1] cells in bone marrow and 10 year remission after busulphan hypoplasia. Br J Haematol 23:283, 1972

84. Oliner HL, Schwartz RS, Rubio F, Dameshek W: Interstitial pulmonary fibrosis following busulfan therapy. Am J Med 31:134, 1961
85. Podoll LN, Winkler SS: Busulfan lung. Report of two cases and review of the literature. Am J Roentgenol Radium Ther Nucl Med 120:151, 1974
86. Podos SM, Canellos GP: Lens changes in chronic granulocytic leukemia: possible relationship to chemotherapy. Am J Ophthalmol 68:500, 1969
87. Kennedy BJ, Yarbro KW: Metabolic and therapeutic effects of hydroxyurea in chronic myeloid leukemia. JAMA 195:1038, 1966
88. Kennedy BJ: Hydroxyurea in chronic myelogenous leukemia. Ann Intern Med 70:1084, 1969
89. Bolin R, Robinson W, Sutherland J, Hamman R: Busulfan versus hydroxyurea in long term therapy of chronic myelogenous leukemia. Cancer 50:1683, 1982
90. Hehlmann R, Heimpel H, Hasford J et al: Randomized comparison of busulfan and hydroxyurea in chronic myelogenous leukemia: prolongation of survival by hydroxyurea. Blood 82:398, 1993
91. Cunningham I, Gee T, Dowling M et al: Results of treatment of Ph' + chronic myelogenous leukemia with an intensive treatment regimen (L-5 protocol). Blood 53:375, 1979
92. Clarkson B: Chronic myelogenous leukemia: is aggressive treatment indicated? J Clin Oncol 3:135, 1985
93. Talpaz M, Kantarjian HM, McCredie KB et al: Clinical investigation of human alpha interferon in chronic myelogenous leukemia. Blood 69:1280, 1987
94. Niederle N, Kloke O, May D et al: Treatment of chronic myelogenous leukemia with recombinant interferon alpha-2b. Invest New Drugs 5:19, 1987
95. Alimena G, Morra E, Lazzarino M et al: Interferon alpha-2b as therapy for Ph-positive chronic myelogenous leukemia: a study of 82 patients treated with intermittent or daily administration. Blood 72:642, 1988
96. Dhingra K, Kurzrock R, Kantarjian H et al: Polymerase chain reaction (PCR) for minimal residual disease in 20 CML patients in complete cytogenetic remission induced by interferon therapy. Blood, suppl. 1. 74:235a, 1989
97. Lee M-S, Kantarjian H, Talpaz M et al: Detection of minimal residual disease by polymerase chain reaction in Philadelphia chromosome-positive chronic myelogenous leukemia following interferon therapy. Blood 79:1920, 1992
98. Malinge M-C, Mahon FX, Delfau MH et al: Quantitative determination of the hybrid Bcr-Abl RNA in patients with chronic myelogenous leukaemia under interferon therapy. Br J Haematol 82:701, 1992
99. Talpaz M, Kantarjian H, Kurzrock R et al: Interferon alpha produces sustained cytogenetic responses in chronic myelogenous leukemia Philadelphia chromosome-positive patients. Ann Intern Med 114:532, 1991
100. Ozer H, George SL, Schiffer CA et al: Prolonged subcutaneous administration of recombinant α2b interferon in patients with previously untreated Philadelphia chromosome-positive myelogenous leukemia: effect on remission duration and survival: Cancer and Leukemia Group B Study 8583. Blood 82: 2975, 1993.
101. Opalka B, Wandl U, Koppe J et al: Molecular and in vitro stem cell analysis on patients (PTS) with chronic myelogenous leukemia (CML) under therapy with recombinant interferon alpha (IFN alfa-2B). Proc Am Assoc Cancer Res 28:206, 1987
102. Kurzrock R, Talpaz M, Kantarjian H et al: Therapy of chronic myelogenous leukemia with recombinant interferon gamma. Blood 70:943, 1987
103. Haines ME, Goldman JM, Worsley AM et al: Chemotherapy and autografting for patients with chronic granulocytic leukemia in transformation: probable prolongation of life for some patients. Br J Haematol 58:711, 1984
104. Brito-Babapulle F, Bowcock SJ, Marcus RE et al: Autografting for patients with chronic myeloid leukaemia in chronic phase: peripheral blood stem cells may have a finite capacity for maintaining haemopoiesis. Br J Haematol 73:76, 1989
105. Barnett MJ, Eaves CJ, Phillips GL: Successful autografting in chronic myeloid leukaemia after maintenance of marrow in culture. Bone Marrow Transplant 4:345, 1989
106. Carella A, Gaozza E, Raffo MR et al: Therapy of acute phase chronic myelogenous leukemia with intensive chemotherapy, blood cell autograft and cyclosporine A. Leukemia 5:517, 1991
107. Medical Research Council: Randomised trial of splenectomy in Ph positive chronic granulocytic leukaemia including an analysis of prognostic features. Br J Haematol 54:415, 1983
108. Gomez GA, Sokal JE, Mittelman A, Aungst CW: Splenectomy for palliation of chronic myeloid leukemia. Am J Med 61:14, 1976
109. Griffen JD, Todd RF, Ritz J et al: Differentiation patterns in the blastic phase of chronic myeloid leukemia. Blood 61:85, 1983
110. Bettelheim P, Lutz D, Majdic O et al: Cell lineage heterogeneity in blast crisis of chronic myeloid leukaemia. Br J Haematol 59:395, 1985
111. Marks SM, McCaffrey R, Rosenthal DS et al: Blastic transformation in chronic myelogenous leukemia: experience with 50 patients. Med Pediatr Oncol 4: 159, 1978
112. Janossy G, Woodruff RK, Pippard MJ et al: Relation of 'lymphoid' phenotype

and response to chemotherapy incorporating vincristine-prednisolone in the acute phase of Ph' positive leukemia. Cancer 43:426, 1979

113. Walters RS, Kantarjian HM, Keating MJ et al: Therapy of lymphoid and undifferentiated chronic myelogenous leukemia in blast crisis with continuous vincristine and adriamycin infusions plus high dose decadron. Cancer 60: 1708, 1987

114. Nathwani A, Goldman JM: The management of chronic myeloid leukemia in lymphoid blast crisis. Haematologica 78:162, 1993

115. Coleman M, Silver R, Pajak T et al: Combination chemotherapy for terminal phase chronic myelocytic leukemia. Blood 55:29, 1980

116. Koller CA, Miller DM: Preliminary observations in the therapy of myeloid blast phase of chronic granulocytic leukemia with plicamycin and hydroxyurea. N Engl J Med 315:1433, 1986

117. Mason JE, DeVita VT, Cannelos GP: Thrombocytosis in chronic granulocytic leukemia. Incidence and clinical significance. Blood 44:483, 1974

118. Talpaz M, Mavligit G, Keating M et al: Human leukocyte interferon to control thrombocytosis in chronic myelogenous leukemia. Ann Med Intern 99:789, 1983

119. Suri R, Goldman JM, Catovsky D et al: Priapism complicating chronic granulocytic leukemia. Am J Hematol 9:295, 1980

120. Goldman JM, Baughan ASJ: Chronic granulocytic leukemia: treatment. p. 239. In Goldman JM, Priesler HD (eds): Butterworth International Medical Reviews. Vol. 8. Leukemias. Butterworth, London, 1984

121. Thomas MR, Robinson WA, Mughal TI et al: Tumour lysis syndrome following VP 16-213 in chronic myeloid leukemia in blast crisis. Am J Hematol 16: 185, 1984

122. Speck B, Bortin MM, Champlin R et al: Allogeneic marrow transplantation for chronic myelogenous leukaemia. Lancet 1:665, 1984

123. Thomas ED, Clift RA, Fefer A et al: Marrow transplantation for the treatment of chronic myelogenous leukemia. Ann Intern Med 104:155, 1986

124. Goldman JM, Apperley JF, Jones L et al: Bone marrow transplantation for patients with chronic myeloid leukemia. N Engl J Med 314:202, 1986

125. Goldman JM, Gale RP, Horowitz MM et al: Bone marrow transplantation for chronic myelogenous leukemia in chronic phase: increased risk of relapse associated with T-cell depletion. Ann Intern Med 108:806, 1988

126. Segel GB, Simon W, Lichtman MA: Variables influencing the timing of marrow transplantation in patients with chronic myelogenous leukemia. Blood 68:1055, 1986

127. Goldman JM, Szydlo R, Horowitz MM et al: Choice of pretransplant treatment and timing of transplants for chronic myelogenous leukemia in chronic phase. Blood 82:2235, 1993

128. Lowenthal RM, Buskard NA, Goldman JM et al: Intensive leukapheresis as initial therapy of chronic granulocytic leukemia. Blood 46:835, 1975

129. Arthur CK, Mijovic A, Dannie E et al: Management of chronic myeloid leukaemia in pregnancy. J Obstet Gynaecol 11:396, 1991

130. Baer MR, Ozer H, Foon FA: Interferon-α therapy during pregnancy in chronic myelogenous leukaemia and hairy cell leukaemia. Br J Haematol 81:167, 1992

131. Delmer A, Rio B, Bauduer F et al: Pregnancy during myelosuppressive treatment for chronic myelogenous leukaemia, letter. Br J Haematol 82:781, 1992

132. Doney K, Buckner CD, Thomas ED et al: Allogeneic bone marrow transplantation for chronic granulocytic leukaemia. Exp Hematol 9:966, 1981

133. Curtis JE, Messner HA: Bone marrow transplantation for leukemia and aplastic anemia: management of ABO incompatibility. Can Med Assoc J 126:649, 1982

134. Clift RA, Thomas ED, Buckner CD et al: Treatment of chronic granulocytic leukemia in chronic phase by bone marrow transplantation. Lancet 2:621, 1982

135. Goldman JM, Baughan ASJ, McCarthy DM et al: Marrow transplantation for patients in chronic phase of chronic granulocytic leukaemia. Lancet 2:623, 1982

136. Champlin R, Ho W, Arenson E, Gale RP: Allogeneic bone marrow transplantation for chronic myelogenous leukemia. Blood 60:1038, 1982

137. Speck B, Gratwohl A, Nissen C et al: Allogeneic bone marrow transplantation for chronic granulocytic leukemia. Blut 45:237, 1982

138. Cunningham I, Castro-Malaspina H, Flomenberg N et al: Improved results of bone marrow transplantation (BMT) for chronic myeloid leukemia using marrow depleted of T cells by soy bean lectin agglutination and E-rosette depletion. p. 359. In Gale RP, Champlin RE (eds): Progress in Bone Marrow Transplantation. Alan R Liss, New York, 1987

139. Santos GW, Tutschka PJ, Brookmeyer R et al: Marrow transplantation for acute nonlymphocytic leukemia after treatment with busulfan and cyclophosphamide. N Engl J Med 309:1347, 1985

140. Tutschka PJ, Copelan EA: Bone marrow transplantation following a new busulfan and cyclophosphamide regimen—results after three years of observation. Exp Hematol 15:601, 1987

141. Marmont AM, Horowitz MM, Gale RP et al: T-cell depletion of HLA-identical transplants in leukemia. Blood 78:2120, 1991

142. Arthur CK, Apperley JF, Guo AP et al: Cytogenetic events after bone marrow transplantation for chronic myeloid leukemia in chronic phase. Blood 71: 1179, 1988

143. Zaccaria A, Rosti G: Karyotypic conversion by BMT. p. 44. In Proceedings of the Tenth Congress of the International Society of Haematology, 1989

144. Thomas ED, Clift RA: Indications for marrow transplantation in chronic myelogenous leukemia. Blood 73:861, 1989

145. Copelan EA, Grever MR, Kapoor N, Tutschka PJ: Marrow transplantation following busulfan and cyclophosphamide for chronic myelogenous leukemia in accelerated or blastic phase. Br J Haematol 71:487, 1989

146. Armitage JO, Klassen LW, Patil SR et al: Marrow transplantation for stable phase chronic granulocytic leukemia. Exp Hematol 12:717, 1984

147. Lehn P, Devergie A, Benbunan M et al: Bone marrow transplantation for chronic granulocytic leukemia. J Natl Cancer Inst 314:202, 1986

148. Bacigalupo A, Frassoni F, van Lint MT et al: Bone marrow transplantation for chronic granulocytic leukemia. Cancer 58:2307, 1986

149. McGlave PB, Scott E, Ramsay N et al: Unrelated donor bone marrow transplantation therapy for chronic myelogenous leukemia. Blood 70:877, 1987

150. Goldman JM, Bortin MM, Champlin RE et al: Bone marrow transplantation for chronic myelogenous leukaemia, letter. Lancet 2:1925, 1985

151. Cross NCP, Hughes TP, Mackinnon S et al: Minimal residual disease after allogeneic bone marrow transplantation for chronic myeloid leukaemia in chronic phase: correlations with probability of relapse. Br J Haematol 84: 67, 1993

152. Cross NCP, Feng L, Chase A et al: Competitive PCR to estimate the number of BCR-ABL transcripts in chronic myeloid leukemia patients after bone marrow transplantation. Blood 82:1929, 1993

153. Lion T, Henn T, Gaiger A et al: Early detection of relapse after bone marrow transplantation in patients with chronic myelogenous leukaemia. Lancet 341:275, 1993

154. van Rhee F, Pisula A, Goldman JM: Long term survivors after bone marrow transplantation for chronic myeloid leukaemia, abstracted. Exp Hematol 8: 1019, 1993

155. Black D: Report on the Working Group on Bone Marrow Transplantation. HM Stationery Office, London, 1982

156. Simonsen M: Graft versus host reactions: their natural history, and applicability as tools of research. Prog Allergy 6:349, 1962

157. Storb R, Weiden PL, Graham TC et al: Marrow grafts between DLA-identical and homozygous unrelated dogs: evidence for an additional locus involved in graft versus host disease. Transplantation 24:165, 1977

158. Powles RL, Morgenstern GR, Kay HEM et al: Mismatched family donors for bone marrow transplantation as treatment for acute leukaemia. Lancet 1: 612, 1983

159. Beatty PG, Clift RA, Michelson EM et al: Marrow transplantation from related donors other than HLA-identical siblings. N Engl J Med 313:765, 1985

160. Ash RC, Casper J, Serwint MS et al: Extending the application of allogeneic marrow transplantation for leukemic patients who lack matched sibling donors, utilizing partially matched donors in concert with T-cell depletion for GVHD prophylaxis. p. 365. In Gale RP, Champlin R (eds): Progress in Bone Marrow Transplantation. Alan R Liss, New York, 1987

161. Bradley BA, Gilks WR, Gore SM, Klouda PT: How many HLA typed volunteer donors for marrow transplantation are needed to provide an effective service? Bone Marrow Transplant, suppl. 1. 2:79, 1987

162. Awdeh ZL, Alper CA, Eynon E et al: Unrelated individuals matched for MHC extended haplotypes and HLA-identical siblings show comparable responses in mixed lymphocyte culture. Lancet 2:853, 1986

163. Bidwell JL, Jarrold EA: HLA-DR allogenotyping using exon specific cDNA probes and application of rapid minigel methods. Mol Immunol 23:1111, 1986

164. Beatty PG, Ash R, Hows JM, McGlave PB: The use of unrelated bone marrow donors in the treatment of patients with chronic myelogenous leukemia: experience of four marrow transplant centers. Bone Marrow Transplant 4: 287, 1989

165. Marks DI, Cullis JO, Ward KN et al: Allogeneic bone marrow transplantation for chronic myeloid leukemia using sibling and volunteer unrelated donors: a comparison of complications in the first two years. Ann Intern Med 119: 207, 1993

166. Gluckman E, Devergie A, Bernheim A, Berger R: Splenectomy and bone marrow transplantation in chronic granulocytic leukaemia, letter. Lancet 2:1392, 1982

167. Baughan ASJ, Worsley AM, McCarthy DM et al: Haematological reconstitution and severity of graft-versus-host disease after bone marrow transplantation for chronic granulocytic leukaemia: the influence of previous splenectomy. Br J Haematol 56:445, 1984

168. Gratwohl A, Goldman JM, Gluckman E, Zwaan F: Effect of splenectomy before bone marrow transplantation on survival in chronic granulocytic leukaemia. Lancet 2:1290, 1985
169. Gratwohl A, Hermans J, Biezen A et al: No advantage for patients who receive splenic irradiation before bone marrow transplantation for chronic myeloid leukaemia: results of a prospective randomized study. Bone Marrow Transplant 10:147, 1992
170. Storb R, Epstein RB, Graham TC et al: Methotrexate regimens for control of graft-versus-host disease in dogs with allogeneic marrow grafts. Transplantation 9:240, 1970
171. Powles RL, Clink HM, Spence D et al: Cyclosporin A to prevent graft-versus-host disease in man after allogeneic bone marrow transplantation. Lancet 1:327, 1980
172. Storb R, Deeg HJ, Thomas ED et al: Preliminary results of prospective randomized trials comparing methotrexate and cyclosporine for prophylaxis of graft-vs-host disease after HLA identical marrow transplantations. Transplant Proc 15:2620, 1983
173. Ramsay NK, Kersey JH, Robison LL et al: A randomized study of the prevention of acute graft-versus-host disease. N Engl J Med 306:392, 1982
174. Storb R, Deeg HJ, Whitehead J et al: Methotrexate and cyclosporine compared with cyclosporine alone for prophylaxis of acute graft versus host disease after marrow transplantation for leukemia. N Engl J Med 314:729, 1986
175. Prentice HG, Blacklock HA, Janossy G et al: Depletion of T-lymphocytes in donor marrow prevents significant graft-versus-host disease in matched allogeneic leukaemic marrow transplant recipients. Lancet 1:472, 1984
176. Mitsuyasu RT, Champlin RE, Gale RP et al: Treatment of donor bone marrow with monoclonal anti-T-cell antibody and complement for the prevention of graft-versus-host disease: a prospective randomized double blind trial. Ann Intern Med 105:20, 1986
177. Apperley J, Jones L, Hale G et al: Bone marrow transplantation for patients with chronic myeloid leukaemia: T-cell depletion with Campath 1 reduces the incidence of graft-versus-host disease but may increase the risk of leukaemic relapse. Bone Marrow Transplant 1:53, 1986
178. Apperley JF, Mauro F, Goldman JM et al: Bone marrow transplantation for chronic myeloid leukaemia in chronic phase: importance of a graft-versus-leukaemia effect. Br J Haematol 69:239, 1988
179. Heit W, Bunjes D, Wiesneth M et al: Ex vivo T-cell depletion with the monoclonal antibody Campath-1 plus human complement effectively prevents acute graft-versus-host disease in allogeneic bone marrow transplantation. Br J Haematol 64:479, 1986
180. Papa G, Arcese W, Mauro FR et al: Standard conditioning regimen and T-cell depleted donor marrow for transplantation in chronic myeloid leukemia. Leuk Res 10:1469, 1986
181. Hale G, Cobbold S, Waldmann H: T-cell depletion with Campath-1 in allogeneic bone marrow transplantation. Transplantation 45:753, 1988
182. De Witte T, Hoogenhout J, De Pauw B et al: Depletion of donor lymphocytes by counterflow centrifugation successfully prevents graft-versus-host disease in matched allogeneic marrow transplantation. Blood 67:1302, 1986
183. Butturini A, Seeger RC, Gale RP: Recipient immune competent T lymphocytes can survive intensive conditioning for bone marrow transplantation. Blood 68:954, 1986
184. Marmont AM, Horowitz MM, Gale RP et al: T-cell depletion of HLA-identical transplants in leukemia. Blood 78:2120, 1991
185. Apperley JF, Rassool F, Parreira S et al: Philadelphia positive metaphases in the marrow after bone marrow transplantation for chronic granulocytic leukemia. Am J Hematol 22:199, 1986
186. Sessarego M, Frassoni F, van Lint MT et al: Competition between Ph positive and Ph negative cell populations after bone marrow transplantation for chronic granulocytic leukemia. p. 243. In Proceedings of the Fourth International Symposium on Therapy of Acute Leukemias, Rome, 1987
187. Zaccaria A, Rosti G, Sessarego M et al: Relapse after allogeneic bone marrow transplantation for Philadelphia chromosome positive chronic myeloid leukaemia: cytogenetic analysis of 24 patients. Bone Marrow Transplant 3:413, 1988
188. Marmont A, Frassoni F, Bacigalupo A et al: Recurrence of Ph[1] positive leukemia after marrow transplantation for chronic granulocytic leukaemia. N Engl J Med 310:903, 1984
189. Smith JL, Heerema NA, Provisor AJ: Leukaemic transformation of engrafted bone marrow cells. Br J Haematol 60:415, 1985
190. Fialkow PJ, Thomas ED, Bryant JI, Neiman P: Leukaemic transformation of engrafted human marrow cells in vivo. Lancet 1:251, 1971
191. Leukaemic transfection in vitro?, editorial. Lancet 1:1001, 1984
192. Lampert IA, Piaza-Biza P, Thompson I et al: Reduced marrow cellularity at varying intervals after allogeneic bone marrow transplantation for chronic myeloid leukaemia. Bone Marrow Transplant, suppl. 1. 2:111, 1987
193. Hughes TP, Economou K, Mackinnon S et al: Slow evolution of chronic myeloid leukaemia relapsing after BMT with T-cell depleted donor marrow. Br J Haematol 73:462, 1989
194. Arcese W, Mauro FR, Alimena G et al: Interferon therapy for Ph+ CML patients relapsed after T cell depleted BMT. Bone Marrow Transplant, suppl. 1. 3:185, 1988
195. Borgies P, Ferrant A, Delannoy A et al: Interferon alpha induced and maintained complete remission in chronic granulocytic leukaemia in relapse after bone marrow transplantation. Bone Marrow Transplant 4:127, 1988
196. Newland AC, Jones L, Mir M et al: Alpha 2 interferon in chronic myeloid leukaemia following relapse post-allogeneic transplant. Br J Haematol 66:141, 1987
197. Sanders JE, Buckner CD, Clift RA et al: Second marrow transplants in patients with leukemia who relapse after allogeneic marrow transplantation. Bone Marrow Transplant 3:11, 1988
198. Atkinson K, Biggs J, Concannon A et al: Second marrow transplants for recurrence of haematological malignancy. Bone Marrow Transplant 1:159, 1986
199. Champlin RE, Ho WG, Lenarsky C et al: Successful second bone marrow transplants for treatment of acute myelogenous leukemia or acute lymphoblastic leukemia. Transplant Proc 17:496, 1985
200. Kolb HJ, Mittermuller J, Clemm CH et al: Donor leukocyte transfusions for treatment of recurrent chronic myelogenous leukemia in marrow transplant patients. Blood 76:2462, 1990
201. Cullis JO, Jiang YZ, Schwarer AP et al: Donor leukocyte infusions in the treatment of chronic myeloid leukemia in relapse following allogeneic bone marrow transplantation, letter. Blood 79:1379, 1992
202. Drobyski WR, Keever CA, Roth MS et al: Salvage immunotherapy using donor leukocyte infusions as treatment for relapsed chronic myelogenous leukemia after allogeneic bone marrow transplantation: efficacy and toxicity of a defined T-cell dose. Blood 82:2310, 1993
203. Van Rhee F, Lin F, Cullis JO et al: Relapse of chronic myeloid leukemia after allogeneic bone marrow transplant: the case for giving donor leukocyte transfusions before the onset of hematologic relapse. (submitted)
204. Bowden RA, Sayers M, Flournoy N et al: Cytomegalovirus immune globulin and seronegative blood products to prevent primary cytomegalovirus infection after bone marrow transplantation. N Engl J Med 314:1006, 1986
205. Ezdinli EZ, Sokal JE, Crosswhite L et al: Philadelphia chromosome-positive and -negative chronic myelocytic leukemia. Ann Intern Med 72:175, 1970
206. Canellos GP, Whang-Peng J, DaVita VT: Chronic granulocytic leukemia without the Philadelphia chromosome. Am J Clin Pathol 65:467, 1976
207. First International Workshop on Chromosomes in Leukaemia: Chromosomes in Ph[1] positive chronic granulocytic leukaemia. Br J Haematol 39:305, 1978
208. Ganesan TS, Rassool F, Guo A-P et al: Rearrangement of the BCR gene in Philadelphia chromosome negative chronic myeloid leukemia. Blood 68:957, 1986
209. Kurzrock R, Blick MB, Talpaz M et al: Rearrangement of the breakpoint cluster region in Philadelphia-negative chronic myelogenous leukemia. Ann Intern Med 105:673, 1986
210. Dreazen O, Klisak I, Rassool F et al: Do oncogenes determine clinical features in chronic myeloid leukaemia? Lancet 1:1402, 1987
211. Van der Plas DC, Hermans ABC, Soekarman D et al: Cytogenetic and molecular analysis in Philadelphia negative CML. Blood 73:1038, 1989
212. Wiedemann LM, Karhi KK, Shivji M et al: The correlation of breakpoint cluster region rearrangement and P210 Ph1/abl expression with morphological analysis of Ph-negative chronic myeloid leukemia and other myeloproliferative diseases. Blood 71:349, 1988
213. Weatherall DJ, Brown MJ: Juvenile chronic myeloid leukaemia. Lancet 1:526, 1970
214. Smith KL, Johnson W: Classification of chronic myelocytic leukemia in children. Cancer 34:670, 1974
215. Faud AS, Harley JB, Roberts WC et al: The idiopathic hypereosinophilia syndrome: clinical, pathophysiologic and therapeutic considerations. Ann Intern Med 92:78, 1982
216. You W, Weisbrot IM: Chronic neutrophilic leukemia: report of 2 cases and a review of the literature. Am J Clin Pathol 72:233, 1979
217. Tanzer J, Harel P, Boiron M et al: Cytochemical and cytogenetic findings in a case of neutrophilic leukemia of mature cell type. Lancet 1:387, 1964
218. Bennett JM, Catovsky D, Daniel MT et al: Proposals for the classification of the myelodysplastic syndromes. Br J Haematol 51:189, 1982
219. Walker LC, Ganesan TS, Dhut S et al: Novel chimeric protein expressed in Philadelphia positive acute lymphoblastic leukemia. Nature 329:851, 1987
220. Spiers ASD, Bain BJ, Turner JE: The peripheral blood in chronic granulocytic leukaemia: study of 50 untreated Philadelphia positive cases. Scand J Haematol 18:25, 1977

Agnogenic Myeloid Metaplasia

74

Ronald Hoffman and Murray N. Silverstein

INTRODUCTION

Agnogenic myeloid metaplasia (AMM) is a chronic, malignant hematologic disorder characterized by splenomegaly, a leukoerythroblastic blood picture, teardrop poikilocytosis, varying degrees of marrow fibrosis, and extramedullary hematopoiesis.[1-10] This disorder was first described in 1879 by Heuck,[11] who reported the presence of marrow fibrosis and extramedullary hematopoiesis in the liver and spleen of two patients. AMM has also been referred to by a variety of other terms, including myelofibrosis, myelosclerosis, idiopathic myeloid metaplasia, and osteosclerosis.[6] Fibrosis of the bone marrow is not unique to AMM and may accompany many other disorders[9,10] (Table 74-1). In AMM, the marrow fibrosis is thought to be a response to a clonal proliferation of hematopoietic stem cells. This syndrome frequently leads to progressive marrow failure,[12] but whether the marrow failure is a consequence of the excessive marrow fibrosis or of the underlying hematologic malignancy remains unknown. Dameshek[13] in 1951 included AMM among the myeloproliferative disorders. This hypothesis was largely based on clinical observations of patients with polycythemia vera, chronic myeloid leukemia (CML), and primary thrombocythemia who developed marrow fibrosis and a clinical picture resembling AMM. In addition, Dameshek[13] noted that each of these myeloproliferative disorders frequently terminates in a leukemic phase.

EPIDEMIOLOGY

No epidemiologic studies are available to estimate the actual incidence of AMM. From an examination of the number of cases encountered at a variety of medical centers, one can arrive at some estimate of the frequency of the disorder. The Mayo Clinic cared for 137 patients with AMM from 1960–1965; 110 patients were seen at the Johns Hopkins Hospital over an 18-year period; 100 cases were observed at the Ohio State University over a 16-year period; and 65 patients were seen from 1968–1980 at Barnes Hospital in St. Louis.[1,5,6,8,14]

In Japan AMM is considered a rare disorder, with only 84 cases per 100,000 at autopsy.[15,16] This figure was obtained by monitoring autopsy protocols from all Japanese medical schools, universities, general hospitals, and research institutes over a 10-year period.[15] The autopsy incidence of myelofibrosis among survivors who were ≤10,000 m from the hypocenter of the atomic bomb explosion at Hiroshima was 18 times the incidence reported from the remainder of Japan.[17] These patients became symptomatic an average of 6 years after the bomb blast.[17] Such data indicate a strong link between excessive radiation exposure and development of AMM, which is further substantiated by the high incidence of myelofibrosis in patients who have received the contrast material Thorotrast (which contains ^{232}Th, a radioactive element with a half-life of 1.41×10^{10} years).[18] Thorotrast is taken up and retained indefinitely by cells of the reticuloendothelial system, which results in continuous irradiation of the liver, spleen, lymph nodes, and bone marrow. Chronic exposure to several industrial solvents, including benzene and toluene, has also been associated with development of AMM.[19-21] AMM has been reported as a complication of chronic benzene poisoning since the chemical was first used in the leather and shoe industry during the 1930s and 1940s.[19]

The average age at diagnosis of AMM is approximately 60 years, most patients being diagnosed at 50–69 years of age.[1-8] In several series, males have been reported to be affected more frequently than females, but others have failed to confirm this male predominance.[1-8] Rarely, AMM has been reported in the pediatric age group.[22] No evidence of genetic transmission exists.

BIOLOGIC AND MOLECULAR ASPECTS

Ward and Block[7] originally proposed that AMM represents a response of an intrinsically normal stem cell to an unidentified stimulus, while Dameshek[13] conjectured that the abnormal fibroblastic proliferation in AMM is not an integral part of the primary disorder.

These conflicting hypotheses were tested in studies using a variety of genetic markers to define the cellular origin of AMM. Jacobson et al[12] demonstrated in a black female AMM patient

Table 74-1. Conditions Associated With Myelofibrosis

Nonmalignant conditions
    Infections: tuberculosis, histoplasmosis
    Renal osteodystrophy
    Vitamin D deficiency
    Hypoparathyroidism
    Hyperparathyroidism
    Gray platelet syndrome
    Systemic lupus erythematosus
    Scleroderma
    Radiation exposure
    Osteopetrosis
    Paget disease
    Benzene exposure
    Thorotrast exposure
    Gaucher disease
Malignant disorders
    Agnogenic myeloid metaplasia
    Other chronic myeloproliferative disorders: polycythemia vera, chronic myeloid leukemia, primary thrombocythemia
    Acute myelofibrosis
    Acute myeloid leukemia
    Acute lymphocytic leukemia
    Hairy cell leukemia
    Hodgkin disease
    Acute myelodysplasia with myelofibrosis
    Multiple myeloma
    Systemic mastocytosis
    Non-Hodgkin lymphoma
    Carcinoma: breast, lung, prostate, stomach

who was heterozygous for glucose-6-phosphate dehydrogenase (G6PD) that circulating hematopoietic cells were derived from a common hematopoietic stem cell and that the bone marrow fibroblasts were nonclonal in origin. Using X-chromosome gene probes, Lucas et al.[23] have confirmed the clonal origin of hematopoiesis in AMM. Furthermore, using a similar molecular biologic approach Anger et al.[24] reported that in each of three cases of AMM suitable for clonal analysis a clear-cut monoclonal X-inactivation pattern was observed. Furthermore, Greenberg et al.[25] studied the cytogenetic composition of bone marrow fibroblasts of an AMM patient who had a clonal cytogenetic abnormality in unstimulated peripheral blood cells, which, however, was absent in the marrow fibroblasts.

The fully developed fibrosis of the bone arrow in AMM is frequently preceded by a hypercellular phase of variable duration. Because characteristic blood cell findings of the cellular phase of AMM do not exist, the diagnosis depends on the demonstration of atypical megakaryocytes and an increase of fibers within marrow biopsies and the exclusion of other myeloproliferative disorders. Kriepe et al.[26] have used an analysis of X-linked restriction length polymorphisms of blood cells of patients at various stages of AMM, to demonstrate clonality of hematopoiesis not only in advanced stages of AMM but also in the cellular phase. In addition, an N-ras mutation present in hematopoietic cells in an AMM patient indicated that T and B cells were also involved in the malignant process perhaps providing some explanation for the immunologic abnormalities in AMM.[27] These studies indicate that AMM is a clonal hematologic malignancy and that the marrow fibrosis represents a secondary non-neoplastic reaction of marrow stromal cells.[23–28] If myelofibrosis is truly an epiphenomenon of the neoplastic hematopoietic cell proliferation it may be expected to disappear if this cell population is eradicated. Reversal of myelofibrosis has, in fact, been observed following allogeneic bone marrow transplantation and following long-term administration of chemotherapy.[29–31] Such findings indicate that the bone marrow fibrosis in AMM is not irreversible and is clearly a consequence of the neoplastic cellular proliferation.

The concept that the primary defect in AMM resides in hematopoietic stem cells or progenitor cells is further supported by the observations of a number of investigators concerning the number of uinlineage and multilineage hematopoietic progenitor cells present in the blood of AMM patients.[32–37] Circulating assayable progenitor cells are increased from 9- to 20-fold above that present in normal peripheral blood.[32–37] Patients with secondary myelofibrosis have a much smaller (threefold) increase in circulating assayable progenitor cells.[33] Secondary myelofibrosis is thought to result from insults to the marrow microvascular system rather than from an intrinsic hematopoietic cell defect.[9,10] Erythroid and megakaryocyte colony formation has been observed to occur in the absence of added exogenous cytokines in AMM, a finding common to other myeloproliferative disorders.[32–38] The hypothesis that marrow fibrosis in AMM is a secondary process is further supported by the work of Castro-Malaspina et al.,[39] Wang,[40] and Hirata et al.[41] These groups have each found that fibroblasts derived from marrow explants obtained from AMM patients displayed the same physical and proliferative characteristics as normal marrow fibroblasts. Both AMM and normal marrow fibroblasts exhibited anchorage and serum dependence, contact inhibition of growth, and similar production of hematopoietic colon-stimulating activities. These data suggest that marrow fibroblasts and their precursor cells in AMM patients do not differ from those in normal subjects.

One of the characteristic features of AMM is reversion of hematopoiesis to a fetal distribution.[7] Hematopoietic tissue is present not only in the marrow cavity but also in extramedullary sites such as the spleen and liver (myeloid metaplasia). Gilbert et al.[42] recently studied the role of colony-stimulating

factor-macrophage (CSF-M) in myeloproliferative disorders.[42] Using a radioimmunoassay, they found that serum CSF-M levels were increased in patients with polycythemia vera, primary thrombocythemia,and AMM.[42] The highest levels of CSF-M were detected in those patients with extensive extramedullary hematopoiesis. Serum CSF-M concentrations were positively correlated with spleen size and peripheral bone marrow expansion. These authors have suggested that CSF-M might alter the distribution of active hematopoietic tissue by directly stimulating macrophage proliferation or macrophage cytokine production. CSF-M could also act by direct synergism with other hematopoietic growth factors that alter the homing behavior of AMM pluripotent hematopoietic stem cells.[42]

Groopman[43] first hypothesized that growth factors released from neoplastic hematopoietic cells in AMM were capable of stimulating marrow fibroblast proliferation and suggested that the megakaryocyte was the primary source of such proliferation factors. Castro-Malaspina et al.[44] subsequently showed that megakaryocyte-enriched marrow cell homogenates and platelet homogenates induced DNA synthesis by human marrow fibroblasts. This group hypothesized that ineffective megakaryocytopoiesis in AMM results in liberation of excessive amounts of such growth factors, leading to marrow fibroblast expansion and collagen synthesis.[44] Platelet-derived growth factor (PDGF), transforming growth factor (TGF-β), and epidermal growth factor (EGF), each of which is contained within platelet and megakaryocyte α-granules, have been shown to stimulate marrow fibroblast proliferation.[45–47] In fact, TGF-β enhances type I and type III procollagen and fibronectin synthesis by marrow fibroblasts.[46] Kimura et al.[48] have presented data to suggest that myeloproliferative disease fibroblasts are more sensitive to human serum mitogens than normal marrow fibroblasts. The PDGF content of platelets from AMM patients is known to be decreased, indicating that a release or leakage of such growth factors by marrow megakaryocytes may occur.[47] Burstein et al.[49] were unable to detect any connection between marrow fibrosis and plasma levels or platelet content of platelet factor 4, another α-granule constituent. Their studies indicated that if α-granule constituents were important in the development of marrow fibrosis, their release or leakage would likely occur within the marrow cavity. Such local effects could result in fibrosis without leading to increased concentrations of α-granule constituents in the general circulation.[49]

Martyré et al.[50] have further examined the possibility that platelet α-granule constituents may account for marrow fibrosis in AMM. In these studies, AMM platelet PDGF and TGF-β levels were found to be 2–3.5- and 1.5–3-fold greater respectively in AMM than in normal controls while EGF levels in AMM were similar to that of control platelets.[50] The role of PDGF and TGF-β in the biogenesis of AMM is likely not restricted merely to promoting fibroblastic proliferation but is due to the effect of these two growth factors on synthesis, secretion, and degradation of extracellular matrix components.[45,46]

TGF-β enhances fibronectin and collagens type I, III, IV as well as chondroitin/dermatan sulphate and proteoglycan gene expression.[57,58] TGF-β decreases the synthesis of various collagenase-like enzymes that degrade extracellular matrices, while at the same time stimulating the synthesis of protease inhibitors such as plasminogen activator inhibitor I.[59] The net effect of these complex interactions is the accumulation of extracellular matrix, which likely contributes to further progression of fibrosis.[60]

In AMM, characteristic changes of the marrow vascular architecture have also been observed.[52] These alterations consist of increased quantities of collagen type IV deposits associated with endothelial cell proliferation. Moreover, sinusoidal hyperplasia and hypervascularity resulting in increased blood flow occurs.[52] The excessively dilated marrow sinusoids in AMM contain prominent intraluminal foci of hematopoiesis.[52,53] Thiele et al.[51] pursued a morphometric analysis of marrow vascular structures and collagen type IV deposits in AMM. In comparison to normal controls and patients with polycythemia vera, a significant increase in the number of marrow sinusoids as well as subendothelial collagen type IV in AMM was observed. Furthermore, evolution of the fibro-osteosclerotic changes in AMM was accompanied by a striking accumulation of collagen IV and a marked luminal expansion and irregularity. Thiele et al.[51] have hypothesized that neovascularization of the bone marrow stroma in AMM is likely mediated by megakaryocyte α-granule constituents. TGF-β for instance has a profound effect on angiogenesis.[54,55] The evolution of the fibro-osclerotic process in AMM appears to be a coordinated process closely related to the vascular proliferation and to also be modulated by growth factors present within abnormal megakaryocytes.

ETIOLOGY AND PATHOGENESIS

The etiology of AMM remains unknown. In experimental systems the exposure of a variety of animal models to chemical agents, industrial solvents, hormones, viruses, immunologic stimuli, and ionizing radiation have led to the development of AMM.[6] A model of AMM has been established in the rabbit,[61–67] in which saponin administered intravenously induces extramedullary hematopoiesis and myelofibrosis over a period of weeks.[62] Interestingly, mice and rats fail to respond to the same doses of saponin.[61] Hoshi and Weiss[61] have provided ultrastructural evidence to suggest that saponin causes damage to the endothelium of marrow vascular cells, rendering them incompetent. A series of hemorrhagic events appears to occur, leading to release of normoblasts into the peripheral blood, marrow hypoplasia, fibrosis, and regeneration.[61] This effect is accompanied by the appearance of increased numbers of hematopoietic progenitor cells in the blood and spleen and a simultaneous depletion of such cells in the marrow.[61] Such marrow vascular injury may be a common link leading to the development of myelofibrosis.

Progress has recently been made in defining the nature of the connective tissue matrix present in normal marrow and in patients with AMM.[10] Reticulin fibrosis of the marrow represents an exaggeration of the fibrous pattern of normal marrow. By contrast, collagen fibrosis occurs in primary and secondary AMM and results in the disruption and obliteration of the sinusoidal architecture of the bone marrow. Bone marrow reticulin has been shown to be composed of types I and III collagen and fibronectin.[64–66] Charron et al.[67] documented a constant increase in marrow collagen content during the course of AMM. The increment in collagen was highest in those patients in whom the disease was of longest duration.[67] As compared with collagen extracts from normal individuals, AMM extracts showed a moderate increase in neutral soluble collagen and a larger increase in polymeric collagen.[67] Charron et al.[67] also noted changes in the pattern of marrow collagen deposition during the course of AMM. Early in the course there is a higher percentage of newly synthesized fibers, while later on more polymeric collagen is present, presumably owing to progressive cross-linking and insolubilization. Both Charron et al.[67] and Gay et al.[65] claim that type III collagen preferentially increases in the early stages of the disease but that it is subsequently replaced by type I collagen. Serum procollagen NH$_2$-terminal peptide III (PC III), which is cleared extracellularly during collagen biosynthesis, is increased in most AMM patients.[52–54] This finding supports the concept that type III collagen synthesis is increased in AMM.[68–70] Some investigators have suggested that PC III levels do not reflect the extent of marrow fibrosis in AMM,[68,69] yet PC III elevation in a longitudinal study of patients with AMM was found to be a sensitive

marker of disease activity.[71,72] PC III levels were observed to fall in patients responding to chemotherapy and to rise 1–2 weeks prior to elevations in white cell and blast cell counts in patients unresponsive to chemotherapy.[72] Bone marrow fibrosis appears to depend not only on the accumulation of collagen but also on the establishment of an equilibrium between collagen production and destruction. PC III levels would therefore be expected to reflect collagen synthesis more adequately than total marrow collagen content.

CLINICAL MANIFESTATIONS

Table 74-2 lists the symptoms of patients with AMM at presentation.[6,8] Approximately 20% of patients are entirely asymptomatic and come to medical attention because of an enlarged spleen detected during routine physical examination or because of an abnormal peripheral blood smear. The most common symptoms in AMM are due to the consequences of anemia, which leads to complaints of weakness, fatigue, dyspnea on exertion, and palpitations. With enlargement of the spleen, various syndromes characterized by abdominal discomfort may emerge.[73] Pressure of the spleen on the stomach may lead to delayed gastric emptying and early satiety.[73] Patients may merely complain of a dull, heavy sensation in the left upper quadrant. Splenic infarction may produce pain of extreme severity, simulating an acute abdominal emergency. Severe diarrhea in patients with AMM may be particularly disabling; since studies of gut flora and motility have been unrevealing, it appears that the pressure of the spleen on the colon or small bowel may be responsible for this symptom. Rarely, the development of AMM can be preceded by the appearance of multiple cutaneous edematous plaques and modules characteristic of Sweet syndrome, a reactive cutaneous process to a number of hematologic malignancies.[74]

Bleeding problems may complicate the clinical course of AMM patients. Bleeding may be trivial, as manifested by petechiae and ecchymoses, or may be life-threatening as a result of uncontrollable esophageal bleeding.[1–8] It may be secondary to thrombocytopenia or to poor platelet aggregation.[1–8] Bleeding may be only initially encountered during a surgical proce-

Table 74-2. Summary of Symptoms and Physical Findings of Patients with AMM Detected at Diagnosis

Symptom or Finding	Incidence (%)		
	Varki et al.[8]	Silverstein[6]	Visani et al.[182]
Asymptomatic	21	30	16
Fatigue	71	58	47
Fever	5	10	5
Symptoms due to enlarged spleen	11	23	48
Bleeding	20	17	5
Gout/renal stones	13	6	NR
Weight loss	39	15	7
Night sweats	21	6	NR
Pallor	NR	60	NR
Petechiae/ecchymoses	20	15	NR
Splenomegaly	89	90	99
Hepatomegaly	64	70	39
Peripheral edema	13	NR	NR
Evidence of portal hypertension	2	6	2
Lymphadenopathy	2	10	1
Jaundice	0	4	NR

Abbreviation: NR, not reported.

dure such as splenectomy; in this case, the bleeding diathesis may be secondary to "inapparent disseminated intravascular coagulation" (DIC) and has the potential for catastrophic consequences.[6]

In addition to the above three major modes of clinical presentation of AMM, occurrence of isolated sites of ectopic myeloid metaplasia has been reported, particularly in the pulmonary, gastrointestinal, central nervous, and genitourinary systems.[1-8,14] such patients present with cough and "large lung tumors," headache, or paralysis secondary to "brain tumors or spinal cord tumors," "urinary tumors present in either the bladder or kidney," small bowel obstruction, or intractable ascites secondary to ectopic implants of hematopoietic tissue in the gut or peritoneum.[1-8,14,56,75-82]

Myeloid metaplasia of the renal pelvis, ureters, and bladder as well as renal parenchymal infiltration have been observed. In addition, expansion of hematopoietic tissue at the urethral meatus may be confused with a urethral caruncle.[79] Such strategically localized sites of extramurally hematopoiesis may lead to renal failure or obstruction of both kidneys and bladder dysfunction.[79] Ascites occurring in a patient with AMM may result from peritoneal or mesenteric implants of extramedullary hematopoietic tissue and/or from portal hypertension.[80,81] If the ascites is secondary to peritoneal implants the fluid is always exudative and sterile and frequently contains myeloid, erythroid, and megakaryocytic elements.[81] Such cytologic studies should routinely be performed on ascitic or pleural fluid obtained from patients with AMM.

Nonspecific systems are not infrequent in AMM and include fever, night sweats, anorexia, and weight loss.[5] Table 74-2 lists the prominent physical findings in patients with AMM.[5,8] Splenomegaly serves as the hallmark of the disease. Its extent may vary, but massive splenomegaly, with the organ occupying the entire left side of the abdomen and extending into the pelvis, may occur in 35% of patients. Hepatomegaly occurs in almost 70% of cases,[1-8] and lymphadenopathy is observed in 10–20%, but the degree of nodal enlargement is frequently only moderate.[5,8] Other important physical findings include pallor, peripheral edema, jaundice, and bony tenderness. Acute monarticular inflammation due to secondary gout is seen in 6% of patients.[5] Peritoneal implants of extramedullary tissue may lead to development of ascites.[80,81] Portal hypertension may occur and is due to massive increases in hepatic blood flow and intrahepatic obstruction.[3,5-7,73,82,83]

Clinical features of portal hypertension, such as ascites or esophageal varices, are known to occur in 9–18% of patients with AMM.[80-83] Occasionally, cirrhosis or evidence of thrombosis of the portal or hepatic veins has been reported.[82,83] The liver histologic findings in AMM have previously been considered normal or to be characterized by minimal portal fibrosis, which has led to the view that the splenomegaly in AMM may be due to increase hepatic blood flow with resultant portal hypertension. Wanless et al, however, analyzed a large autopsy series of patients with AMM and found frequent thromboses in small or medium-size portal veins as well as extrahepatic portal veins in patients with portal hypertension.[80,82]

LABORATORY EVALUATION

Careful examination of the peripheral blood smear (Fig. 74-1) and bone marrow (Fig. 74-2) permits ready diagnosis of AMM. The presence of a leukoerythroblastic blood picture with teardrop poikilocytosis strongly suggests this diagnosis. A leukoerythroblastic blood picture characterized by the presence of nucleated red blood cells and immature myeloid elements is seen in 96% of cases.[1-8] Megathrombocytes and megakaryocytic fragments are a constant finding. The teardrop erythrocytes have been noted to decrease in number following sple-

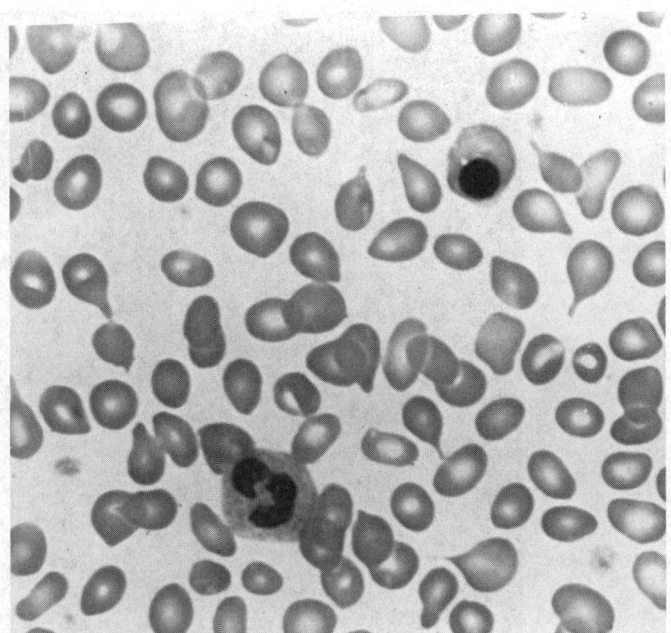

Fig. 74-1. Peripheral blood smear showing normoblasts and teardrop poikilocytes in AMM. (Wright stain, × 700.)

nectomy or institution of chemotherapy,[84,85] which has led some to suggest that splenic fibrosis may lead to development of these red cell changes.[83,84] In approximately 60% of patients, hemoglobin levels drop to <10 g/dl.[1-8] The degree of anemia is difficult to estimate by hemoglobin or hematocrit determinations, since individuals with large spleens often have expanded plasma volumes. Such alterations in hemodynamics may lead to apparent anemia, which is largely dilutional in nature. Of patients with decreased red cell masses, 95% have normochromic normocytic red cell indices.[86] The anemia is due to both ineffective red cell production and shortened red cell survival.[87-90] Ineffective red cell production in AMM can be demonstrated by ferrokinetic studies, which are characterized by increased iron turnover but decreased incorporation of radioactive iron into circulating red cells.[87-90] Silverstein[6] found ineffective iron incorporation into red cells to occur in 90% of patients with AMM. Fifteen percent of patients have major hemolytic episodes during their clinical course.[6]

The cause of the hemolytic anemia is usually multifactorial, with contributions from hypersplenism, a defect in red cells resembling that in paroxysmal nocturnal hemoglobinuria, and antierythrocyte autoantibodies.[87-93] In one series, 55% of patients with AMM had a positive acid hemolysis or sucrose hemolysis test, or both, and 10% had decreased haptoglobin levels and hemosiderinuria, suggestive of intravascular hemolysis.[92,93] Hypochromic microcytic anemia due to blood loss may develop in 5% of AMM patients. The etiology of the blood loss may be leaking esophageal varices, duodenal ulceration, gastritis, or intravascular hemolysis. Occasionally, a patient with AMM may develop an occult malignancy or a site of extramedullary hematopoiesis within the gastrointestinal tract, which may serve as a bleeding source.[94] Macrocytic anemia may complicate AMM.[95] Folic acid absorption is normal in these patients, but the folic acid deficiency is probably due to increased utilization.[95]

Leukopenia can occur in 13–25% of patients, while leukocytosis is seen in one-third.[1-8] In one series,[8] the mean white count was 16,600/mm[3]. Occasional blast cells and granulocytes with the pseudo-Pelger-Huët anomaly are frequent findings.[6] The leukocyte alkaline phosphatase score was studied in 78 patients by Silverstein and Elveback[96] and was high in 41 patients

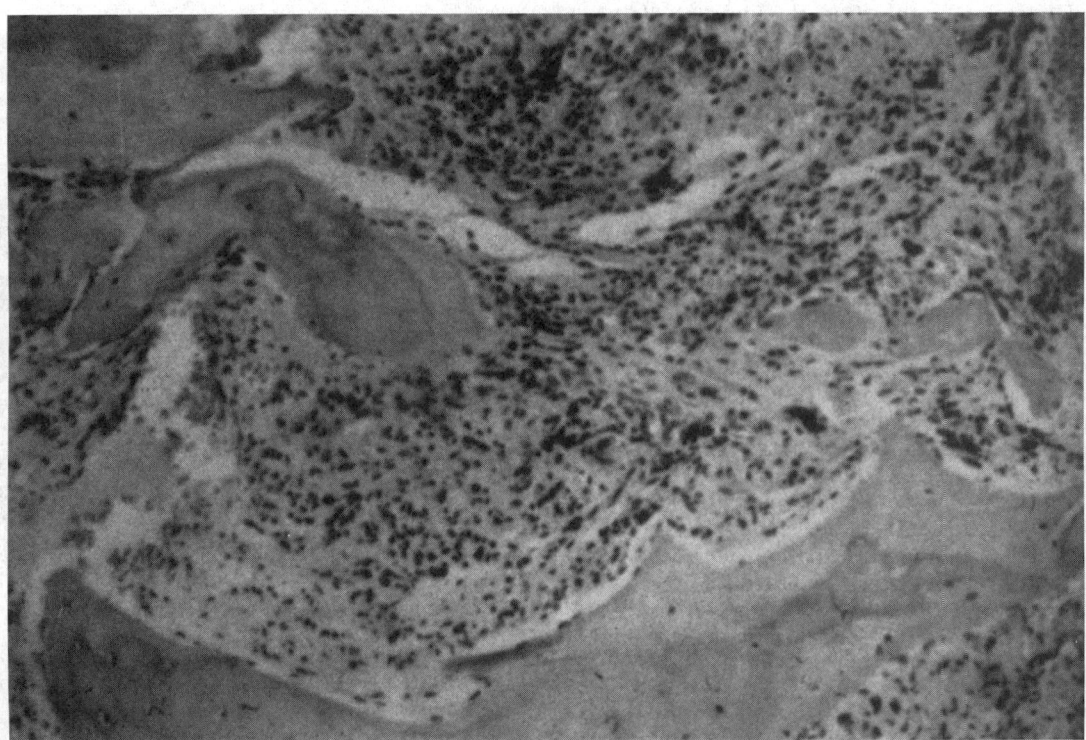

Fig. 74-2. Marrow section from a patient with diffuse myelofibrosis and osteosclerosis. (H&E, × 135). (From Silverstein,[6] with permission.)

(>100), normal in 17 patients (30–100), and low in 20 patients (<30). Such a distribution of leukocyte alkaline phosphatase scores has been reported by others.[8]

In the Mayo Clinic series of 169 patients, platelet counts of <100,000/mm³ were observed in 31% of patients, while platelet counts of >800,000 were observed in 12%.[6] Defective platelet aggregation is common, and platelets frequently do not respond to either collagen or epinephrine.[6,97,98] Didisheim and Bunting[97] reported that 5 of 10 patients with AMM had prolonged bleeding times. A variety of qualitative platelet anomalies documented by abnormal in vitro aggregation patterns has been documented in AMM.[97] In 15% of patients, abnormalities suggestive of ongoing DIC are found, including decreased platelet numbers, decreased levels of coagulation factors V and VIII, an increased fibrin-split products.[6] Usually, when DIC occurs in AMM, it produces no symptoms and unfortunately may only become clinically apparent following surgical intervention. Approximately 75% of patients with AMM have increased prothrombin times due to isolated deficiencies in factor V or to the presence of circulating anticoagulants.[6] Associated liver dysfunction may also be a contributory factor to prolongation of the prothrombin time. Additional laboratory abnormalities are quite frequent. In one series lactic acid levels were elevated in 95% of patients, bilirubin levels in 40%, uric acid in 60%, and alkaline phosphate and serum glutamic oxaloacetic transaminase levels in 50%.[8] Patients with AMM have been noted to have decreased levels of total cholesterol.[99–100] The ratio of high-density lipoprotein cholesterol to low-density lipoprotein cholesterol has been shown to be diminished.[99]

Ferrokinetic and red cell survival studies may be useful in defining sites of extramedullary hematopoiesis and determining the cause of anemia in AMM.[6,87–90] Furthermore, the presence of erythroid hyperplasia, intense hemolysis, increased plasma volume, and significant ineffective erythropoiesis appears to define a subpopulation of patients with an especially poor prognosis.[6]

A variety of immunologic abnormalities have been reported in AMM, including the presence of positive antinuclear antibodies, elevated rheumatoid factor titers, direct Coombs test positivity, lupus-type circulating anticoagulants, hypocomplementemia, marrow lymphoid nodules, and increased circulating immune complexes.[101–105] In one series of 50 patients with AMM, increased quantities of circulating immune complexes were detected[101] and found to be associated with increased disease activity as manifested by increased transfusion requirements, bone pain, and fever.[101] Some investigators have suggested that abnormalities of the complement system may be important in disease progression of AMM,[104] while others have hypothesized that low levels of C3 may predispose these patients to develop serious bacterial infections.[101] A remarkably high incidence of monoclonal gammopathies has been reported in AMM, with such benign gammopathies occurring in 8–10% of patients in some series.[104,105] Ten cases of the simultaneous occurrence of a plasma cell dyscrasia and AMM have been reported.[6,105–107]

Successful bone marrow aspiration is unusual, being accomplished in only 6 of 48 cases in one series, with the tap completely dry in 50% of cases.[8] A bone marrow biopsy is necessary in all cases to assess the amount of residual hematopoietic cellular tissue and the degree of marrow fibrosis. Table 74-3 summarizes the appearance of bone marrow biopsies in the series of Varki et al.[8] Salgado et al.[108] recently suggested that some caution should be taken in using repeated bone marrow biopsies specimens to diagnose AMM. They reported two cases in which a marrow biopsy was performed at the site of a previous bone injury during the healing process as primary callus formation was occurring. Intense myelofibrosis with new bone formation was noted. They suggest that marrow biopsies performed at the site of previous biopsies or aspirates may potentially lead to an erroneous diagnosis of AMM and recommend that marrow biopsies intended for diagnosis of AMM be performed at a site previously spared.[108] Most marrow biopsies in AMM are hypercellular and were remarkable for increased numbers of megakaryocytes (Table 74-3). Bone marrow fibrosis

Table 74-3. Bone Marrow Biopsy Findings at Diagnosis of Patients with AMM[a]

Findings	Incidence (%)
Percentage of hematopoietic cells	
0–25	6
26–50	10
51–75	31
76–100	52
Pattern of cellularity	
Diffuse	71
Patchy	29
Megakaryocytes	
Increased	90
Decreased	4
Normal	6
Granulocytes	
Increased	70
Immaturity	8
Percentage of fibrosis/collagen (H&E stain)	
0–10	79
11–25	15
26–50	2
51–100	4
Reticulin fibrosis (Gomori stain)[b]	
1 +	12
2 +	21
3 +	46
4 +	21
Osteosclerosis	54

Abbreviation: H&E, hematoxylin and eosin.
[a] Based on a total of 48 biopsies.
[b] Based on a scale of 1 + to 4 +.
(From Varki et al.,[8] with permission.)

and osteosclerosis were seen in 67% and 54% of cases, respectively.[8] Wolf and Neiman[53] have reported three characteristic morphologic features: (1) patchiness of the hematopoietic cellularity and the reticulin fibrosis, some microscopic fields being cellular and others depleted of hematopoietic cells and the amount of reticulin varying from field to field; (2) increased numbers of megakaryocytes, which often appeared in clusters and displayed dysplastic features with bizarre nuclear configurations; and (3) distended marrow sinusoids frequently containing intravascular hematopoiesis. In Wolf and Neiman's series, morphologic evidence of progression of fibrosis was present in only 1 of 21 cases in which sequential biopsies were obtained.[53] In addition, no connection was observed between bone marrow cellularity and fibrosis and splenic size.[53] By contrast, Lohmann and Beckman[109] observed progressive fibrosis in 18 of 20 patients who did not have maximal myelofibrosis at the time of the initial biopsy. Thiele et al.[110] presented data to indicate an early hyperplastic subtype of AMM with no or minimal medullary reticulin and another phase with conspicuous fibrosis and osteosclerotic changes of the marrow. They concluded based on a careful histomorphometric evaluation of the bone marrow that there was a progressive fibro-osteosclerotic process during the evolution of the disease that was paralleled by an increase in small megakaryocytes with irregular perimeters and megakaryocytes with naked nuclei.[110] Cervantes et al.[111] also observed an unexpectedly high incidence of bone marrow lymphoid nodules in AMM, which they believe favors an immunologic component to this disorder.

Morphologic examination of the spleen reveals foci of extramedullary hematopoiesis in the sinusoids of the red pulp, where megakaryocytes, myeloid elements, and nucleated erythroid elements are seen.[53] Follicular atrophy in the white pulp frequently occurs.[53] Pathologic examination of the liver reveals hematopoietic cellular elements within the sinusoids. Sinusoi-

dal dilation is a frequent finding, as well as prominent intraheptocytic and Kupffer cell hemosiderin deposition. A marked increase in the hepatic reticulin network has also been observed.[53,83]

Clinical features of portal hypertension such as ascites or esophageal varices are known to occur in 9–18% of patients with agnogenic myeloid metaplasia.[79–83] The liver histologic findings have usually been considered normal or to be characterized by minimal portal fibrosis, which has led to the view that the splenomegaly in AMM may be due to increase hepatic blood flow with resultant portal hypertension. Wanless et al.,[82] however, analyzed a large series of patients with polycythemia vera and AMM at autopsy. In those patients with portal hypertension, thrombotic lesions in small or medium-size portal veins as well as extrahepatic portal veins were observed. In addition, nodular regenerative liver hyperplasia occurred in 14.6% of cases and correlated closely with the presence of portal vein lesions. They have concluded that thrombosis is the most likely cause of portal venous obliteration and portal hypertension in AMM and that clinically significant thrombosis confined to small intrahepatic veins or large hepatic veins should be considered in any patient with AMM. In this autopsy series portal and hepatic venous disease occurred even in the absence of signs of portal hypertension. Such a finding is consistent with subclinical thrombosis with recanalization occurring fairly commonly in this patient group.[82]

Approximately 50–60% of patients with AMM have karyotypic abnormalities at diagnosis.[112–116] It is important to perform cytogenetic analysis on this patient population in order to discriminate AMM from CML. Detection of a Philadelphia chromosome and/or a *bcr/abl* fusion gene indicates that the myelofibrosis is secondary to CML.[117,118] Chromosomal abnormalities in AMM have been reported to involve chromosomes 1, 2, 5–13, 15, 17, 18,20, and 21 and the Y chromosome.[112–116] There appears to be a pronounced increase in observed abnormalities in the C group chromosomes, but no abnormality specific to AMM has been identified. The most common abnormalities include trisomies 8, 1q, 9, 21, and 13q.[112–116] Partial or complete losses of chromosomes, particularly chromosomes 5 and 7, appear to be associated with the use of chemotherapeutic agents for treatment of AMM.[117] Recently an association between erythroid hypoplasia in AMM and a defect on chromosome 11 has been reported.[119] It is not unusual for a leukemic transformation of AMM to precede additional cytogenetic abnormalities; a finding consistent with a multistep process leading to a leukemic transformation.[120]

On radiographic examination the characteristic features of AMM are a diffuse increase in bone density and increased prominence of the bony trabeculae. This increased bone density may be patchy and can produce a mottled appearance. In 25–66% of patients with AMM, such abnormalities have been reported.[6]

Magnetic resonance imaging (MRI) is a promising noninvasive means of evaluating the bone marrow status of patients with AMM. MRI can portray the conversion or reconversion of fatty to cellular marrow.[121,122] Fibrotic marrow is easily distinguished from cellular marrow by its strikingly low signal intensity with all pulse signals.[120] Kaplan et al.[121] reported that marrow patterns in the proximal femurs of AMM patients correlates with the clinical severity of the disease and that MRI of the proximal femurs may be useful in both staging and evaluating the progression of the disease process. Careful clinical prospective studies correlating marrow MRI and the clinical course of AMM patients are required to define the appropriate role of MRI in the evaluation and progression of this disorder.[122]

DIFFERENTIAL DIAGNOSIS

A patient with hepatosplenomegaly, peripheral cytopenias, teardrop poikilocytosis, and leukoerythroblastosis and marrow fibrosis likely suffers from AMM. It must be appreciated, however, that a number of other disorders besides AMM may lead to this clinical picture[9,10] (Table 74-1). Secondary myelofibrosis frequently occurs in patients with lymphoma or metastatic carcinoma of the stomach, prostate, lung, and breast.[9,10,123–126] Successful treatment of Hodgkin disease or breast cancer has resulted in reversal of such marrow fibrosis.[123–126] One should be extremely careful of making the diagnosis of AMM in a patient who has a previous history of a primary neoplasm. The demonstration of carcinoma cells in the marrow establishes that metastatic carcinoma is the cause of the marrow fibrosis. Careful breast examination and mammography are indicated in all women suspected of having AMM, in order to rule out the possibility of metastatic breast cancer. The finding of blastic or lytic bone lesions in patients with myelofibrosis suggests the presence of an underlying carcinoma.

Disseminated tuberculosis and histoplasmosis have also been associated with the development of secondary myelofibrosis.[6,127] Caseating or noncaseating granulomas observed on bone marrow biopsy suggests the presence of these infectious disorders. Identification of the causative organisms by culture techniques should be pursued.

A number of other primary hematologic disorders can also be accompanied by marrow fibrosis. A variant myelodysplastic syndrome with myelofibrosis has been described by Pagliuca et al.[128] These patients frequently present with cytopenias and have cellular dysplastic abnormalities indistinguishable from those of other patients with myelodysplasia. Their marrows, however, are characterized by the presence of marrow fibrosis and a striking megakaryocytic hyperplasia, with a predominance of small hypolobulated forms, in some cases surrounding fibrosis. Reticulocytopenia is characteristic of these patients as well as teardrop red blood cells and a leukoerythroblastic blood picture.[127,128] Unlike patients with AMM, patients with myelodysplasia and marrow fibrosis do not have hepatic or splenic enlargement extending beyond 3 cm below the costal margin.[129,130] The overall survival of patients with this variant of myelodysplasia has been reported to be 30 months, with death resulting from the effects of cytopenias or transformation to acute leukemia.[128] Two additional studies have, however, indicated that the presence of myelofibrosis in patients with myelodysplasia is associated with a particularly short survival (9.6 months) as compared with patients with myelodysplasia without fibrosis (17.4 months).[129,130]

Hairy cell leukemia can also be confused with AMM.[8] In one study, 5 of 61 patients who had originally been diagnosed as having AMM were shown retrospectively to have had hairy cell leukemia.[8] Hairy cell leukemia can present as pancytopenia with splenomegaly and is associated with a dry marrow tap. In one series, marrow reticulin content was increased in 26 of 29 patients with hairy cell leukemia.[131] The presence of hairy mononuclear cells possessing tartrate-resistant acid phosphatase in the peripheral blood or marrow should facilitate differentiation of AMM from hairy cell leukemia. This exercise is important because of the different modalities of treatment that can be successfully employed for hairy cell leukemia.[131]

Myelofibrosis can occur in patients with other myeloproliferative disorders, especially polycythemia vera and CML and rarely primary thrombocytopenia.[132] In the latter, progressive marrow fibrosis may herald the onset of accelerated disease or blast crisis.[132] Myelofibrosis in CML occurs in two distinct patterns, one in which patients present with CML and significant associated marrow fibrosis, and a second in which the myelofibrosis develops late in the course of the CML.[118] The myelofibrosis in this latter group appears at a mean of 36 months after the diagnosis of CML is associated with a mean survival of 4.9 months from the detection of myelofibrosis, and therefore represents an ominous prognostic sign.[118]

Postpolycythemic myeloid metaplasia occurs in 5–15% of patients with polycythemia vera.[133,134] This transition occurs, on the average, 10 years after the initial diagnosis of polycythemia vera is made, but in individual cases it may appear after either shorter or longer intervals.[132–134] AMM is clinically indistinguishable from postpolycythemic myeloid metaplasia except for the previous history of erythrocytosis in the latter group. Of patients with postpolycythemic myeloid metaplasia, 25–50% will develop leukemia, and 70% will be dead within 3 years of this transition.[132–134] Postpolycythemic myeloid metaplasia represents a transitional myeloproliferative syndrome with relatively grave prognostic implications. Myelofibrosis has also reported following primary thrombocythemia.[135]

Acute myelofibrosis represents a clinical entity distinct from AMM.[136–139] Patients characteristically present with pancytopenia, fever, absence of clinically significant splenomegaly, minimal or absent teardrop poikilocytosis, and fibrotic bone marrow.[134–137] The bone marrow is characterized by the appearance of immature myeloid elements, and the blast cells frequently express megakaryocytic phenotypic properties.[136–139] Although the number of circulating blast cells is frequently low, these cells have been reported to range from 13% to 55% of the total number of leukocytes.[136–139] Survival ranges from 1 to 9 months following diagnosis. Most clinicians consider acute myelofibrosis to be a form of acute megakaryoblastic leukemia. Its distinction from AMM is vital, since aggressive chemotherapy and possibly bone marrow transplantation are the treatments of choice for acute myelofibrosis.

THERAPY

AMM remains an incurable disease. The optimal forms of treatment have to date not been defined. A conservative approach to management is generally accepted, asymptomatic patients being observed and therapeutic intervention being reserved for those patients with symptoms. An alternative approach proposed by Pegrum et al.[140] provides for the institution of single-agent chemotherapy early in the course of the disease. Chemotherapeutic regimens used have included busulfan (2–4 mg/day), 6-thioguanine (20–40 mg/day), and a combination of chlorambucil (15 mg/day) and prednisone (30 mg/day), administered intermittently for a course of 3–4 weeks with a 2-week rest interval between courses.[1–8,27,103,140–147] Such an approach is associated with reduction in spleen size, and some authors have claimed reversal of marrow fibrosis with reduction in the amount of teardrop red cells, poikilocytosis, and leukoerythroblastosis.[27,85,86,140–147]

Hydroxyurea appears to be a particularly useful agent for the treatment of AMM. Its use has been reported to be associated with significantly reduced platelet production and a reduction of megakaryocytic abnormalities as well as a significant reduction of myelofibrosis.[145,146] Some investigators have hypothesized that hydroxyurea-induced suppression of megakaryocytopoiesis, causes a reduction in platelet PDGF levels resulting in reduced fibroblast proliferation and deposition of reticulin.[145] Manoharan et al.[145] have shown that moderate doses (20–30 mg/kg) of hydroxyurea given twice or three times weekly are effective and safe in AMM patients requiring treatment. Furthermore, Chang and Gross[146] reported three patients with AMM who responded to daily busulfan therapy with the achievement of hematologic remission and reversal of myelofibrosis and myeloid metaplasia. Not only did hematologic parameters, including the hemoglobin and hematocrit levels, improve, but a reduction of teardrop erythrocytes and lessening of leukoerythroblastosis was noted as well as reversal of myeloid metaplasia and marrow fibrosis. Most importantly the quality of life of these individuals improved.[147] Judicious use of busulfan is recommended in this setting, however, because of its potential for producing delayed marrow suppression.[149] The long-term effects of such early chemotherapeutic intervention on prognosis and frequency of leukemic transformation of AMM remains unknown. Selection of such an "aggressive" therapeutic approach at present appears unwarranted, but this strategy clearly merits further investigation. A randomized clinical trial comparing early use of chemotherapy with a supportive approach is needed to clarify the merit of these two different strategies. The remainder of the discussion of AMM treatment is devoted to measures for the care of symptomatic patients.

Therapy is indicated for patients with the following conditions: (1) symptoms attributable to anemia, (2) pressure symptoms related to splenomegaly, (3) bleeding problems or life-threatening thrombocytopenia, (4) significant hyperuricemia, and (5) portal hypertension and life-threatening gastrointestinal bleeding.[6] Hyperuricemia should be aggressively treated in all patients with AMM. Hydration and chronic administration of allopurinol (300 mg/day) are suggested.[6]

Anemia is a common problem in patients with AMM. It is usually multifactorial in origin, contributing factors being folate deficiency, iron deficiency, ineffective erythropoiesis, and hemolysis.[87-96] Kinetic studies and red cell survival studies using radioisotopes can be helpful in defining the etiology of the anemia. It is also important to directly measure the patient's red cell mass to be assured that the low hemoglobin level is not merely dilutional in origin.[87-90] Transfusion therapy with packed red cells is clearly indicated in these patients who are symptomatic from their anemia. Patients with documented nutritional deficiencies should receive either folate or iron supplementation, or both. Chronic transfusion therapy will frequently be required; one should try to attain a hemoglobin level at which symptoms resolve. Since AMM is a chronic disease, long-term transfusion therapy potentially may lead to the development of the iron overload syndrome. Serious consideration should be given to early institution of iron chelation therapy.

The remainder of approaches to the anemic patient deal with therapeutic interventions designed to avoid or diminish the number of transfusions administered. Ineffective erythropoiesis in AMM may be treated with anabolic steroids.[1-8,148-151] Gardner and Nathan[148] have recommended that all patients with AMM and anemia should receive a trial of androgens. A number of preparations have been suggested, including testosterone enanthate (600 mg/wk IM), stanozolol (12 mg/day PO), nandrolone (3 mg/kg/wk IM), fluoxymesterone (10 mg tid PO), and oxymethalone (50 mg qid PO). It is unknown whether any of these preparations is superior to the others, but a good response, as defined by a decrease or total avoidance of transfusion therapy, occurs in about 50% of patients. A course of 3–6 months of androgen therapy is indicated in order to identify responsive patients,[148] but the development of hepatic dysfunction or virilizing side effects may limit long-term androgen administration. Besa et al.[151] have indicated that patients with associated chromosomal abnormalities are less likely to respond to androgen therapy. Rojer et al.[152] have also reported successful treatment with pyridoxine (250 mg/day PO) of 40% of patients with anemia and AMM. Confirmatory reports of such excellent responses have not been published to date. Some preliminary success with the use of recombinant human erythropoietin to treat the anemia of AMM has been reported.[153]

Corticosteroids (e.g., prednisone 1 mg/kg/day PO) have been successfully employed for treatment of the hemolytic anemia associated with AMM.[1-8] Bouroncle and Doan[1] reported favorable results in approximately 25% of patients, while Silverstein[6]

reported a 2-g increase in hemoglobin in 29% of men and 52% of women. Folate should be simultaneously administered to all such patients. Bouroncle and Doan[1] reported even more encouraging results with simultaneous administration of busulfan and corticosteroids, with clinical responses lasting 6–12 months. Once patients have reached a peak response, tapering of prednisone should be initiated to determine an acceptable maintenance dose. Frequently the hemolytic process recurs following such tapering. Appropriate patients should be referred for splenectomy at that time.

Pressure symptoms secondary to splenic enlargement can be treated initially with cytotoxic chemotherapy. Busulfan, chlorambucil and prednisone, 6-thioguanine, radioactive phosphorus, and hydroxyurea (15–20 mg/kg three times a week) have been used for this purpose.[1-8,27,101,140-147] In the Mayo Clinic series a significant reduction in spleen size with relief of pressure symptoms occurred in 70% of patients receiving chemotherapy.[6] Responses are unfortunately short-lived, lasting a median of only 4.5 months.[6] Only 16% of these patients with long-term maintenance therapy enjoyed sustained relief of symptoms.[6] Hematologic toxicity was not infrequent and often necessitated cessation of therapy.

Splenic irradiation has also been frequently used for treatment of the painful big spleen syndrome.[6,7,154-157] Irradiation in fractions of 0.15–1 Gy administered either daily or by an intermittent fractionation schedule (two or three times per week) to a total dose per treatment course of 2.5–6.5 Gy may be effective.[6,7,151-157] Responses are transient, lasting an average of 3.5 months, and hemotopoietic toxicity is frequently significant. Wagner et al.[156] have recommended for this purpose simultaneous treatment with splenic irradiation and oral hydroxyurea and have obtained some promising preliminary results. Silverstein[6] has reported that splenic irradiation is especially useful for treatment of splenic pain of sudden onset and also for treatment of ascites due to implants of hematopoietic tissue. Radiation therapy should be considered as a temporary measure to be employed in patients who are too ill to tolerate splenectomy or chemotherapy.

Radiotherapy offers a viable treatment option and at times may be the therapy of choice for the treatment of peritoneal or pleural implants leading to ascites or pleural efficiency and extramedullary hematopoiesis in vital organs leading to organ dysfunction.[158] Because of the inherent sensitivity of myeloid tissue to irradiation and profound marrow suppression that may occur following irradiation, therapy is usually initiated at low doses (20–25 cGy/day) with modification of the dose as the clinical situation dictates.[158]

Parmeggiani et al.[159] reported the use of interferon-α (IFN-α) for the treatment of painful splenomegaly in AMM.[159] Splenic pain and pressure symptoms disappeared with a decrease in splenic size, but peripheral blood counts deteriorated. Gilbert has, however, reported a similar reduction in spleen size with maintenance IFN-α therapy but without hematologic compromise.[160] Barosi et al.[161] have suggested that IFN-α might be useful in treating thrombocytosis that follows splenectomy in AMM patients. Several investigators have noted, however, that although IFN-α has cytoreductive activity in AMM, its use is often limited by debilitating toxic effects such as severe flu-like symptoms and worsening of anemia. These investigators believe that the use of IFN-α has limited applicability.[162] Martyré et al.[163] also reported that IFN-γ administration results in the reduction of PDGF and TGF-β levels present within AMM platelets. These investigators have suggested that such an approach might lead to a cessation or slowing of the marrow fibrosis but this hypothesis has not been proven to date.[163] The appropriate role of the IFNs in the treatment of AMM is at present uncertain and requires further investigation.

The role of splenectomy in the management of AMM remains a controversial issue.[164-173] Splenectomy is indicated in pa-

THERAPY FOR AGNOGENIC MYELOID METAPLASIA

The treatment of AMM is dependent on the major manifestations of the disease in the individual patient. One must consider treatment of anemia patients, patients with symptoms due to splenomegaly, those with bleeding abnormalities, those with portal hypertension, and those with ascites, bone pain, or symptoms due to hypermetabolism.

Blood volume studies should be performed in anemic patients. Those who have normal red cell masses and marked increases in plasma volume have a dilutional form of anemia requiring no treatment. Treatment for ineffective erythropoiesis includes use of androgens, the androgen of choice being oxymethalone in doses of 50 mg qid. In those patients who do not respond to androgens, a trial of erythropoietin therapy is merited, yet should be considered important therapy. Those patients who demonstrate a shortened red cell survival, benefit from addition of prednisone at a dose of 60 mg/day. In patients with iron deficiency anemia, every attempt should be made to determine the underlying etiology of blood loss. If a patient develops esophageal varices or peptic ulcer disease, these lesions must be specifically treated. Occasional patients may develop an underlying occult gastrointestinal carcinoma. When the cause of iron deficiency has been determined, iron therapy (ferrous sulfate 300 mg/day for ≥ 3 months) should be added.

In those patients with symptoms due to splenomegaly, treatment will depend on the severity and nature of these difficulties. Various measures to reduce the size of the spleen have been used to alleviate uncontrollable splenic pain; these measures may include the use of radiotherapy or of chemotherapy in the form of busulfan or hydroxyurea. Approximately two-thirds of patients treated with these agents will have some reduction of spleen size, but on discontinuation of chemotherapy, rapid enlargement of the spleen usually occurs.

Individuals with acute splenic infarction who do not respond to administration of analgesics may gain pain relief from local irradiation over the spleen at doses of 0.25–0.50 Gy/day for 4–5 days. Those with huge, painful spleens in whom splenectomy is too risky a procedure may benefit from a cautious trial of radiotherapy. Our overall experience indicates that patients with symptoms due to a profoundly enlarged spleen are best treated by splenectomy.

Whenever a patient is considered a candidate for splenectomy, an extensive preoperative evaluation must be pursued. A patient must be considered an acceptable surgical risk in terms of cardiac, hepatic, renal, and metabolic function. All patients must have an extensive preoperative evaluation of the coagulation system, which should include assays for coagulation factors V and VIII, fibrin-split products, and platelet function. Patients with qualitative platelet abnormalities remain candidates for splenectomy, but successful surgical intervention may require use of adrenal steroids preoperatively and platelet transfusion at the time of surgery. In patients with "inapparent DIC," surgery is definitely contraindicated. The operation itself must be considered a major procedure. Only a senior staff surgeon who has performed this type of surgery many times should attempt such an operation.

In treating patients with myelofibrosis, one must appreciate that bleeding may be multifactorial in origin. Invariably, patients with myelofibrosis will have qualitative platelet abnormalities. In addition, thrombocytopenia and apparent DIC may lead to a hemorrhagic diathesis. In those patients who have qualitatively abnormal platelet function, platelet transfusions are suggested for serious bleeding or when preparing a patient for surgery. Patients with thrombocytopenia secondary to marrow failure and hypersplenism can often be managed by administering androgenic or adrenal steroids, or both. In those patients with life-threatening thrombocytopenia who do not respond to steroids, splenectomy should be seriously considered. Patients with inapparent DIC require no treatment. In those patients who develop DIC seondary to infection or other identifiable etiologies, treatment is best directed toward controlling the underlying etiology of the coagulopathy and initiating replacement therapy with platelets and fresh frozen plasma.

Portal hypertension may complicate myelofibrosis in 6–8% of patients. Careful assessment of patients with this potentially catastrophic problem is mandatory. Portal hypertension in AMM may be secondary to increased blood flow from the spleen to the liver (i.e., forward-flow portal hypertension) or secondary to an intrahepatic block due to postnecrotic cirrhosis or intrahepatic extramedullary hematopoiesis. The treatment of portal hypertension is surgical. Our experience suggests that this complication is secondary to forward-flow portal hypertension in 70% of patients and results from an intrahepatic block in the other 30%. At surgery, forward-flow portal hypertension can be demonstrated by a marked increase in hepatic blood flow and collapse of varices following clamping of splenic vessels. In this situation splenectomy will produce beneficial effects. If portal hypertension is secondary to intrahepatic obstruction, our group has favored a splenorenal shunt as the decompressive procedure of choice. Our data indicate limited survival in patients treated medically with variceal bleeding but prolonged survival in patients treated surgically.

Patients with ascites, bone pain, or hypermetabolism present unique problems. If the ascites is due to portal hypertension, management should be directed toward relieving the hypertension. Development of ascites in AMM may also, however, be due to seeding of the peritoneal cavity with extramedullary hematopoiesis. In all patients with myelofibrosis who develop ascites, paracentesis should be performed and careful study of the ascitic fluid pursued. If megakaryocytes are found in the samples of ascitic fluid, the ascites is likely due to peritoneal implants of myeloid tissue. These implants are treated by abdominal radiation. We have found that administration of fractional doses of radiation at 0.25 Gy/day with rotation into the four quadrants of the abdomen is extremely effective. Radiation therapy to a total dose 5–10 Gy may be very rewarding.

Patients with myelofibrosis who develop severe bone pain have an extremely guarded prognosis. Our experience suggests that this complication represents leukemic transformation in evolution. In these patients, biopsies at sites of pain may reveal pure populations of leukemic blasts. The pain appears to be the result of invasion of the periosteum by blast cells. Bone pain is best treated with local radiation for several days.

Symptoms due to hypermetabolism such as weight loss, sweating, and asthenia are not unusual. Such patients may benefit from low-dose adrenal steroids or hydroxyurea.

Table 74-4. Indications for and Responses to Splenectomy in Patients with AMM

	Combined Series	
Indication	No. of Patients	No. of Responders
Painful splenomegaly	40	38
Refractory thrombocytopenia	13	6
Refractory hemolytic anemia	19	11
Portal hypertension	11	9

(Data from Silverstein and Remine[167] and Brenner et al.[171])

tients with hemolysis, thrombocytopenia, or painful splenomegaly refractory to other therapeutic modalities.[6] Crosby[164] and Mulder et al.[165] have suggested that splenectomy be performed in every patient with AMM immediately after the diagnosis is made. However, Benbassat et al.[166] reviewed the role of splenectomy in AMM by evaluating 321 published AMM splenectomy cases and concluded that this procedure should be considered only in selected individuals for specific indications. Table 74-4 shows the combined results from two representative published series of splenectomized patients. These series indicate that for specific indications splenectomy is an excellent therapeutic choice.[167,171] It is important to note, however, that 10 of the 72 patients in these series died postoperatively and that significant postoperative morbidity due to septicemia and hemorrhage was present.[167,171] Benbassat et al.[166] further explored the risks and benefits of splenectomy by reviewing and performing a formal decision analysis of 15 reports in the literature dealing with splenectomy in AMM that were published after 1970. They determined that the operative mortality was 13.4% and early morbidity due to atelectasis, hemorrhage, thromboembolism, and subphrenic infections was 45.5%.[168] However, anemia was improved in 70% of patients, painful splenomegaly in 97% of patients, thrombocytopenia in 56% of patients and portal hypertension in 83% of individuals.[168] Splenectomy however was not demonstrated to alter survival but was recognized to improve the quality of life. In one series, an extraordinarily high incidence of leukemic transformation was noted following splenectomy.[172] Whether this was a function of the absence of the spleen or more likely the consequence of the natural history of the disease is unknown. Splenectomy should be considered for symptomatic patients after they have been informed of the operative mortality and chances of palliation.[168] Ferrokinetic measures of total erythropoiesis and of plasma volume previously claimed to be useful guides for the choice of splenectomy have little value for predicting outcome.[172,173] The clinician should not agonize over the decision of whether or not to splenectomize a patient with AMM. Splenectomy often results in improved quality of life due to resolution of cytopenias or relief from painful splenomegaly.[167–172] It is important to be aware that compensatory hepatic myeloid metaplasia may accelerate following splenectomy, leading to rapid enlargement of the liver.[8,169,170] This complication can, however, frequently be treated with chemotherapy.[169] Occasionally, however, massive myeloid metaplasia and sinusoidal dilation can occur following splenectomy resulting in liver failure and death.[169,170]

McCarthy et al.[174] first suggested that 1,25-vitamin D_3 may have a role in control of bone marrow collagen synthesis in AMM. This hypothesis was based on the known reversal of the myelofibrosis of rickets with vitamin D_3 therapy.[174] Although some investigators have reported hematologic improvement in 50% of AMM patients treated with 1,25-vitamin D_3, others have not confirmed these results.[174–178]

Excessive bleeding in patients with AMM can be due to either thrombocytopenia, qualitative platelet defects, or DIC.[6] Based on his clinical observations, Silverstein[6,167] has suggested that

splenectomy is contraindicated in patients with DIC. Actively bleeding patients with consumption coagulopathy should receive platelet and plasma replacement therapy. Low-dose heparinization has resulted in improvement in occasional patients.[6] Platelet transfusions are suggested in bleeding patients who are thrombocytopenic or are known to have qualitative platelet abnormalities.

Bone marrow transplantation is a potentially useful therapeutic tool in young patients with AMM who have an appropriate donor available.[25,26,179] Successful transplantation is associated with gradual resolution of marrow fibrosis and normalization of hematopoiesis.[26,179] Allogeneic bone marrow transplantation offers the best chance for cure and should be seriously considered in all patients <40 years of age. However, the feasibility of successful bone marrow transplantation remains questionable, since Rajantie et al.[179] have reported that severe marrow fibrosis can adversely affect post-transplantation hematopoietic reconstitution. According to the International Bone Marrow Transplantation Registry, a total of 13 patients with AMM have been reported to the Registry, with 8 patients surviving 4–71 months after allogeneic transplantation.[180]

PROGNOSIS

The median overall survival from the time of diagnosis of AMM varies from series to series but is approximately 5 years[1–8] (Fig. 74-3). Individual survival has been reported to range from 1 year to >30 years.[1–8] Silverstein was able to define specific prognostic indicators based upon observations made at diagnosis. Patients who were asymptomatic (Fig. 74-4), not anemic (Fig. 74-5), and not thrombocytopenic (Fig. 74-6), and who did not have a massively enlarged liver (Fig. 74-7) appeared to enjoy a survival advantage.[6] Varki et al.[8] found that the presence of unexplained fever, night sweats, weight loss, anemia, and thrombocytopenia identified patients with a particularly short survival, but that the size of the spleen or liver, overall marrow cellularity, relative number of megakaryocytes, degree of marrow fibrosis, degree of collagen formation, and degree of reticulin fibrosis were of no use in predicting survival. Using a multivariate analysis, Barosi et al.[181] developed a set of prognostic factors that appear to be useful in identifying patients with an extremely poor or extremely good prognosis.

Furthermore, Visani and co-workers[182] analyzed the prognostic significance of 11 different variables in AMM patients and showed that the percentage of peripheral white blood cells that are blasts, promyelocytes, and myelocytes at the time of initial diagnosis correlated closely with survival. In addition,

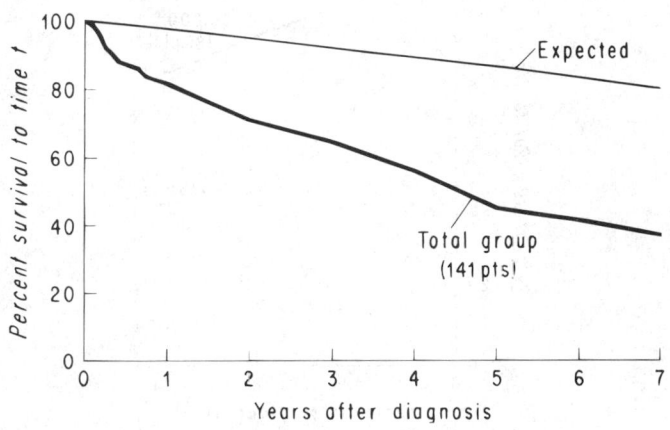

Fig. 74-3. Overall survival from time of diagnosis of 141 patients with AMM. (From Silverstein,[6] with permission.)

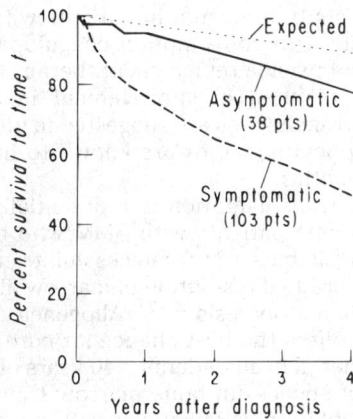

Fig. 74-4. Suvivorship of patients with AMM asymptomatic at diagnosis compared with those who were symptomatic. (From Silverstein,[6] with permission.)

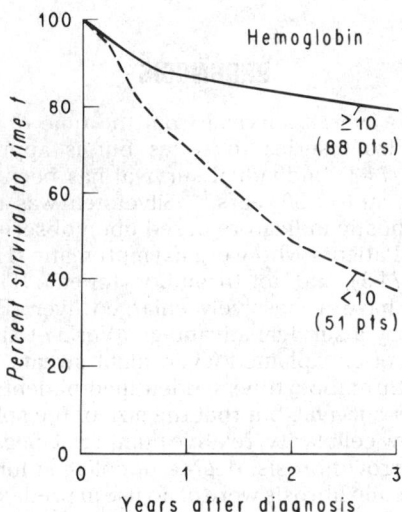

Fig. 74-5. Survivorship of patients with AMM based on hemoglobin level at time of diagnosis. (From Silverstein,[6] with permission.)

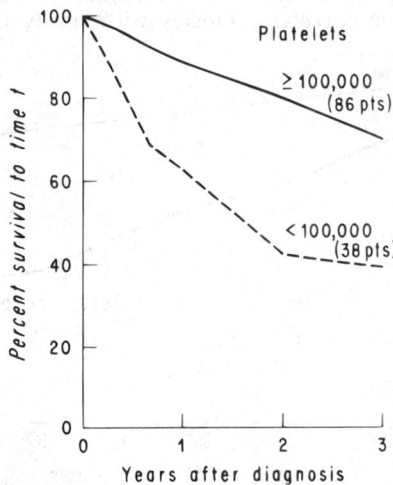

Fig. 74-6. Survivorship of patients with AMM based on platelet count at diagnosis. (From Silverstein,[6] with permission.)

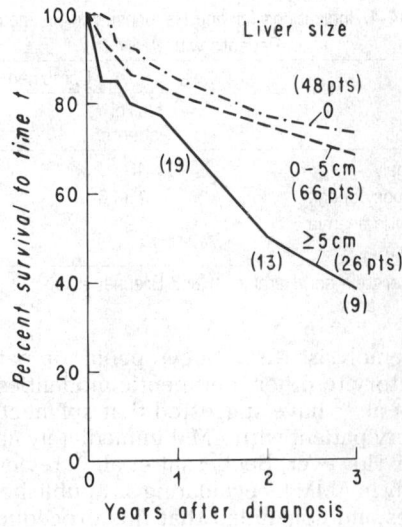

Fig. 74-7. Survivorship of patients with AMM based on liver size at diagnosis. (From Silverstein,[6] with permission.)

hemoglobin levels, white blood cell (WBC) counts, and delay from first symptoms to diagnosis gave significant additional prognostic information. Using simple hematologic parameters at diagnosis this group was able to divide AMM patients into three groups with significantly different survivals: (1) good-risk patients (median survival 81 months) with hemoglobin (Hb) >10 g/dl and percentage of WBC precursors <10%); (2) intermediate-risk patients (median survival 39 months) with Hb <10 g/dl and percentage of WBC precursors <10%; and (3) high-risk group (median survival 31 months) with >10% WBC precursors independent of the Hb level. The risk of leukemic conversion in patients with group III was twice that observed in either group I or II.[182] Hasselbalch and Jensen[183] have also found that a Hb level <10 g/dl to be an adverse prognostic factor, while patients with osteomyelosclerosis to have a significantly better prognosis. Identification of the prognosis of an individual patient may be useful in defining high-risk patients in whom experimental forms of therapy might be indicated. The causes of death in one series of 53 cases of AMM were as follows: cardiac (infarction or failure) 33%, hemorrhage 26%, acute leukemia 22%, infection 13%, carcinoma 4%, and mesenteric thrombosis 2%.[184] The incidence of acute leukemia as a terminal event ranges from 5 to 22% of patients depending on the series cited.[1–8,184–192] Approximately one-half of the patients who develop acute leukemia have received previous treatment with alkylating agents or radiotherapy, suggesting that the evolution into acute leukemia might be part of the natural history of AMM.[181,186–192] Immunologic and morphologic phenotypic characterization of the blasts comprising these leukemias reveals that a typical myeloid phenotype is most commonly detected; other cell lineages, such as megakaryocytic, erythroid, and even lymphoid, may also be involved, leading to the existence of both mixed myeloid and hybrid transformations.[192] Megakaryoblastic transformation have been detected in one-third of cases in one series, an incidence clearly higher than that found in de novo acute myeloid leukemia.[192] Survival in these blast transformations is limited, a phenomena that is probably due to patient age and the aggressive biology of these leukemias. Successful leukemia induction of these patients is a rare event.

FUTURE DIRECTIONS

Rapid strides have been made in understanding the biosynthesis of collagen in myelofibrosis. As myelofibrosis progresses, parallel insolubilization of collagen occurs, leading to progressive fibrosis. Conversion of soluble to insoluble collagen requires monoamine oxidase oxidation of lysine to lysylaldehydes, which then cross-link collagen, resulting in insoluble collagen formation. Monoamine oxidase inhibitors (e.g., penicillamine) prevent the formation of lysylaldehydes. At the Mayo Clinic, of 18 patients with asymptomatic myelofibrosis who were treated with penicillamine, 12 remained stable over a 3-year period, 4 suffered deterioration in their clinical course during treatment, and in 2 penicillamine toxicity required cessation of the drug (Silverstein MN, unpublished observations, 1991). Since about 80% of patients with asymptomatic myelofibrosis will remain so over a 5-year period of observation, it did not appear in this preliminary study that penicillamine was of any value in altering the natural history of this disorder.

Colchicine is able to disrupt microtubule formation and leads to decreased rates of procollagen secretion. Recently, 18 patients were treated with 0.625 mg colchicine bid. These patients have not been on study long enough to assess the value of this form of treatment (Silverstein MN, unpublished observations, 1991).

If it is indeed true that PDGF and TGF-β play a major role in promoting fibroblastic proliferation in patients with AMM, agents capable of neutralizing the biologic functions of such growth factors may be of potential clinical use. This hypothesis was recently tested in a clinical trial of suramin, an antiparasitic agent that inhibits TGF-β. In a phase II trial suramin was administered in a 24-hour continuous infusion at dose levels of 280–350 mg/m^2 for 5–10 days every 5 weeks.[194] No biologic evidence or clinical evidence of suramin activity in AMM was observed. Instead progressive splenomegaly and severe pancytopenia was observed in all patients. Further exploration of the use of biologic response modifiers or drugs that might alter the fibrotic process in AMM will likely be pursued in the future.[194]

Rozman et al.[195] recently analyzed survival data for each of the chronic nonleukemic myeloproliferative disorders. In this study the survival of patients with polycythemia vera and essential thrombocythemia receiving modern therapy did not differ from that of a control population while the survival of patients with AMM was strikingly reduced with respect to a control population. This information emphasizes the need for new therapeutic approaches for the treatment of AMM.

REFERENCES

1. Bouroncle BA, Doan CA: Myelofibrosis: clinical hematologic and pathologic study of 110 patients. Am J Med Sci 243:697, 1962
2. Linman JW, Bethel FH: Agnogenic myeloid metaplasia. Am J Med 22:107, 1957
3. Pitcock JA, Reinhard EJ, Justus BW, Mendelson RS: A clinical and pathological study of 70 cases of myelofibrosis. Ann Intern Med 57:73, 1962
4. Rosenthal DS, Molony WC: Myeloid metaplasia: a study of 98 cases. Postgrad Med 45:136, 1964
5. Silverstein MN, Gomes MN, ReMine WH, Elveback LR: Agnogenic myeloid metaplasia. Natural history and treatment. Arch Intern Med 120:545, 1967
6. Silverstein MN: Agnogenic Myeloid Metaplasia. Publishing Sciences Group, Acton, MA, 1975
7. Ward HP, Block MH: The natural history of agnogenic myeloid metaplasia. Medicine (Baltimore) 50:357,1971
8. Varki A, Lottenberg R, Griffin R, Reinhard E: The syndrome of idiopathic myelofibrosis: clinicopathologic review with emphasis on the prognostic variables predicting survival. Medicine (Baltimore) 62:353, 1983
9. Myelofibrosis, editorial. Lancet 1:127, 1980
10. McCarthy DM: Fibrosis of the bone marrow: contents and causes. Br J Haematol 59:1, 1985
11. Heuck G: Zwei Fälle von Leukämie mit eigenthümlichem Blut-resp Knochenmarksebefund. Virchows Arch A Pathol Anat Histopathol 78:475, 1879
12. Jacbobson RJ, Salo A, Fialkow PJ: Agnogenic myeloid metaplasia: a clonal proliferation of hematopoietic stem cells with a secondary myelofibrosis. Blood 51:189, 1978
13. Dameshek W: Some speculations on the myeloproliferative syndromes. Blood 6:372, 1951
14. Glen RH, Haese WH, McIntyre PA: Myeloid metaplasia with myelofibrosis. The clinical spectrum of extramedullary hematopoiesis and tumor formation. Johns Hopkins Med J 132:253, 1973
15. Sawada K: Statistical studies on autopsy cases in Japan excluding malignant tumors from 1946 to 1955 inclusive as compared with eastern and western parts of Japan. Med J Osaka Univ 11:1075, 1959
16. Mitaji T, Yuk H, Oda T et al: The incidence of malignant tumors in autopsy cases of Japan during the ten years from 1946 to 1955 inclusive. Gann 48:523, 1957
17. Anderson RE, Hoshino T, Yamamoto T: Myelofibrosis with myeloid metaplasia in survivors of the atomic bomb in Hiroshima. Ann Intern Med 60:1, 1964
18. Johnson SAN, Bateman CJT, Beard MEJ et al: Long term hematological complications of thorotrast. Q J Med 182:259, 1977
19. Rawson R, Parker F Jr, Jackson H Jr: Industrial solvents as possible etiologic agents in myeloid metaplasia. Science 93:541, 1941
20. Hu H: Benzene associated myelofibrosis. Ann Intern Med 106:171, 1987
21. Bosch X, Campistal JM, Montolia J et al: Toluene-associated myelofibrosis. Blut 58:219, 1989
22. Tobin MS, Tan C, Argano SA: Myelofibrosis in the pediatric age group. NY State J Med 69:1080, 1969
23. Lucas GS, Padua RA, Masters GS et al: The application of X chromosome gene probes to the diagnosis of myeloproliferative disease. Br J Haematol 72:530, 1989
24. Anger B, Janssen JWG, Schrezenmeier H et al: Clonal analysis of chronic myeloproliferative disorders using X-linked DNA polymorphisms. Leukemia 4:258, 1990
25. Greenberg BR, Woo L, Veomett IC: Cytogenetics of bone marrow fibroblastic cells in idiopathic chronic myelofibrosis. Br J Haematol 66:487, 1987
26. Kreipe H, Jaquet K, Felgner J et al: Clonal granulocytes and bone marrow cells in the cellular phase of agnogenic myeloid metaplasia. Blood 78:1814, 1991
27. Buschle M, Janssen JWG, Drexler H et al: Evidence for pluripotent stem cell origin of idoipatihc myelofibrosis: clonal analysis of a case characterised by a N-ras gene mutation. Leukaemia 2:658, 1988
28. Wang JC, Lang H-D, Lichter S et al: Cytogenetic studies of bone marrow fibroblasts cultured from patients with myelofibrosis and myeloid metaplasia. Br J Haematol 80:184, 1992
29. Reversible myelofibrosis, editorial. Lancet 1:497, 1985
30. Dokal I, Jones L, Deenmamode M et al: Allogeneic bone marrow transplantation for primary myelofibrosis. Br J Haematol 71:158, 1989
31. Manoharan A, Pitney WR: Chemotherapy resolves symptoms and reverses marrow fibrosis in myelofibrosis. Scand J Haematol 33:453, 1984
32. Chevenick PA: Increase in circulating stem cells in patients with myelofibrosis. Blood 41:67, 1973
33. Wang JC, Cheung CP, Fakhiuddin A et al: Circulating granulocyte and macrophage progenitor cells in primary and secondary myelofibrosis. Br J Haematol 54:301, 1983
34. Hibbin JA, Njoku OS, Matutes E et al: Myeloid progenitor cells in the circulation of patients with myelofibrosis and other myeloproliferative disorders. Br J Haematol 57:495, 1984
35. Carlo-Stella C, Cazzola M, Gasner A et al: Effects of recombinant α and γ interferons on in vitro growth of circulating hematopoietic progenitor cells (CFU-GEMM, CFU-MK, BFU-E and CFU-GM) from patients with myelofibrosis with myeloid metaplasia. Blood 70:1014, 1987
36. Juvonen E: Megakaryocyte colony formation in chronic myeloid leukemia and myelofibrosis. Leuk Res 12:751, 1988
37. Han ZC, Briere J, Nedellec G et al: Characteristics of circulating megakaryocyte progenitors (CFU-MK) in patients with primary myelofibrosis. Eur J Haematol 40:130, 1988
38. Adamson JW, Failkow PJ: The pathogenesis of myeloproliferative syndromes, annotation. Br J Haematol 38:299, 1978
39. Castro-Malaspina H, Gay RE, Jhanwar SC: Characteristics of bone marrow fibroblast colony forming cells (CFU-F) and their progress in patients with myeloproliferative disorders. Blood 59:1046, 1982
40. Wang JC: Myelopoietic effect of bone marrow fibroblasts cultured from patients with myelofibrosis. Am J Hematol 27:235, 1988
41. Hirata J, Takahira H, Kaneko S et al: Bone marrow stromal cells in myeloproliferative disorders. Acta Haematol 82:35, 1989
42. Gilbert HS, Prolaran V, Stanley ER: Increased circulating CSF-1 (M-CSF) in myeloproliferative disease: association with myeloid metaplasia and peripheral bone marrow extension. Blood 74:1231, 1989
43. Groopman JE: The pathogenesis of myelofibrosis in myeloproliferative disorders. Ann Intern Med 92:857, 1980
44. Castro-Malaspina H, Rabellino EM, Yen A et al: Human megakaryocyte stimulation of proliferation of bone marrow fibroblasts. Blood 57:781, 1981
45. Kimura A, Katoh O, Kuramoto A: Effect of platelet derived growth factor,

epidermal growth factor and transforming growth factor-B on the growth of human marrow fibroblasts. Br J Haematol 69:9, 1988

46. Kimura A, Katoh O, Hyodo H, Kuramoto A: Transforming growth factor-B regulates growth as well as collagen and fibronectin synthesis of human marrow fibroblasts. Br J Haematol 72:486, 1989

47. Katoh O, Kimura A, Kuramoto A: Platelet derived growth factor is decreased in patients with myeloproliferative disorders. Am J Hematol 27:276, 1988

48. Kimura A, Katoh O, Kuramoto A: Marrow fibroblasts from patients with myeloproliferative disorders showed increased sensitivity to human serum mitogens. Br J Haematol 69:153, 1989

49. Burstein SA, Malpass TW, Yee E: Platelet factor 4 excretion in myeloproliferative disease: implications for the etiology of myelofibrosis. Br J Haematol 51:383, 1989

50. Martyré M-C, Magdelenat H, Bryckaert M-C et al: Increased intraplatelet levels of platelet-derived growth factor and transforming growth factor-β in patients with myelofibrosis with myeloid metaplasia. Br J Haematol 77: 80, 1991

51. Thiele J, Rompcik V, Wagner S, Fischer R: Vascular architecture and collagen type IV in primary myelofibrosis and polycythaemia vera: an immunomorphometric study on trephine biopsies of the bone marrow. Br J Haematol 80:227, 1992

52. Charbord P: Increased vascularity of bone marrow in myelofibrosis. Br J Haematol 62:595, 1986

53. Wolf BC, Neiman RS: Myelofibrosis with myeloid metaplasia: pathophysiologic implications between bone marrow changes and progression of splenomegaly. Blood 65:803, 1985

54. Roberts AB, Heine UI, Flanders KC, Sporn MB: Transforming growth factor-β: major role in regulation of extracellular matrix. Ann NY Acad Sci 580:225, 1990

55. Folkman J, Klagsbrun M: Angiogenic factors. Science 235:442, 1987

56. Reilly JT: Pathogenesis of idiopathic myelofibrosis: role of growth factors. J Clin Pathol 45:461, 1992

57. Varga J, Rosenbloom J, Jimenez SA: Transforming growth factor-β (TGF-β) causes a persistent increase in steady-state amounts of type I and type III collagen and fibronectin mRNAs in normal human dermal fibroblasts. Biochem J 247:597, 1987

58. Nakamura T, Okuda S, Miller D et al: Transforming growth factor-β (TGF-β) regulates production of extracellular matrix (ECM) components by glomerular epithelial cells. Kidney Int 37:221, 1990

59. Overall CM, Wrana JL, Sodek J: Independent regulation of collagenase, 72 Kda-progelatinase, and metalloendoproteinase inhibitor (TIMP) expression in human fibroblasts by transforming growth factor-B. J Biol Chem 264:1860, 1989

60. Terui T, Niitsu Y, Mahara K et al: The production of transforming growth factor-β in acute megakaryoblastic leukemia and its possible implications in myelofibrosis. Blood 75:1540, 1990

61. Hoshi H, Weiss L: Rabbit bone marrow after administration of saponin. Lab Invest 37:67, 1978

62. Argano SAP, Tobin MS, Spain DM: Experimental induction of myelofibrosis with myeloid metaplasia. Blood 33:851, 1989

63. Wang JC, Tobin MS: Mechanism of extramedullary hematopoiesis in rabbits with saponin-induced myelofibrosis and myeloid metaplasia. Br J Haematol 51:271, 1987

64. Bentley SA, Alabaster O, Foidart JM: Collagen heterogeneity in normal human bone marrow. Br J Haematol 48:287, 1981

65. Gay S, Gay R, Prchal JT: Immunohistological studies of bone marrow collagen. p. 291. In Berk PD, Castro-Malaspina H (eds): Myelofibrosis and the Biology of Connective Tissue. Alan R Liss, New York, 1984

66. Zuckerman KS, Wicha MS: Extracellular matrix production by the adherent cells of long term bone marrow cultures. Blood 61:540, 1983

67. Charron D, Robert L, Couty MC, Biner JL: Biochemical and histological analysis of bone marrow collagen in myelofibrosis. Br J Hematol 41:151, 1979

68. Hochweiss S, Fruchtman S, Hahn EG et al: Increased serum procollagen II amino terminal peptide in myelofibrosis. Am J Hematol 15:343, 1983

69. Barosi G, Costa LN, Liberato G et al: Serum procollagen III peptide level correlates with the disease activity in myelofibrosis with myeloid metaplasia. Br J Haematol 72:16, 1989

70. Arrago JP, Poirer O, Chomienne C et al: Type III amino terminal peptide of procollagen in some haematological malignancies. Scand J Haematol 36: 288, 1986

71. Hasselbalch H, Junker P, Hørslev-Petersen K et al: Procollagen type III aminoterminal peptide in serum in idiopathic myelofibrosis and allied conditions: relation to disease activity and effect of chemotherapy. Am J Hematol 33:18, 1990

72. Hasselbalch H, Junker P, Lisse I et al: Circulating hyaluronan in the myelofi-

brosis/osteomyelosclerosis syndrome and other myeloproliferative disorders. Am J Hematol 36:1, 1991

73. Silverstein MN, Wollaeger EE, Baggenstoss AH: Gastrointestinal and abdominal manifestations of agnogenic myeloid metaplasia. Arch Intern Med 131: 532, 1973

74. Su WPD, Alegre VA, White WL: Myelofibrosis discovered after diagnosis of Sweet's syndrome. Int J Dermatol 29:201, 1990

75. Landolfi R, Colosimo C Jr, De Candia E et al: Meningeal hematopoiesis causing exophthalmus and hemiparesis in myelofibrosis: effect of radiotherapy. Cancer 62:2346, 1988

76. Periera A, Bruguera M, Cervantes F, Rozman C: Liver involvement at diagnosis of primary myelofibrosis: a clinicopathological study of twenty-two cases. Eur J Haematol 40:355, 1988

77. Lara JF, Rosen PP: Extramedullary hematopoiesis in a bronchial carcinoid tumor. Arch Pathol Lab Med 114:1283, 1990

78. Fedeli G, Certo M, Cannizzaro O et al: Extramedullary hematopoiesis involving the esophagus in myelofibrosis. Am J Gastroenterol 85:1512, 1990

79. Oesterling JE, Keating JP, Leroy AJ et al: Idiopathic myelofibrosis with myeloid metaplasia involving the renal pelves, ureters and bladder. J Urol 147: 1360, 1992

80. Gorshein D, Brauer MJ: Ascites in myeloid metaplasia due to ectopic peritoneal implantation. Cancer 23:1408, 1969

81. Lioté F, Yeni P, Teillet-Thiebaud F et al: Ascites revealing peritoneal and hepatic extramedullary hematopoiesis with peliosis in agnogenic myeloid metaplasia: case report and review of the literature. Am J Med 90:111, 1991

82. Wanless IR, Peterson P, Das A et al: Heptic vascular disease and portal hypertension in polycythemia vera and agnogenic myeloid metaplasia: a clinicopathological study of 145 patients examined at autopsy. Hepatology 12:1166, 1990

83. Tsao M-S: Hepatic sinusoidal fibrosis in agnogenic myeloid metaplasia. Am J Clin Pathol 91:302, 1989

84. DiBella NJ, Silverstein MN, Hoagland HC: Effect of splenectomy on teardrop-shaped erythrocytes in agnogenic myeloid metaplasia. Arch Intern Med 137: 308, 1977

85. Manoharan A, Hargrave M, Gordon S: Effect of chemotherapy on teardrop poikilocytes and other peripheral blood findings in myelofibrosis. Pathology 20:7, 1988

86. Christensen BE: Red cell kinetics. Clin Haematol 4:393, 1975

87. Najean Y, Cacchione R, Castro-Malaspina H, Dresch C: Erythrokinetic studies in myelofibrosis: their significance for prognosis. Br J Haematol 40:205, 1978

88. Barosi G, Cazzola M, Frassoni F et al: Erythropoiesis in myelofibrosis with myeloid metaplasia: recognition of different classes of patients by erythrokinetics. Br J Haematol 48:263, 1981

89. Njoku OS, Lewis SM, Catovsky D, Gordon-Smith EC: Anemia in myelofibrosis: its value in prognosis. Br J Haematol 54:79, 1983

90. Beguin Y, Fillet G, Bury J, Fairon Y: Ferrokinetic study of splenic erythropoiesis: relationships among clinical diagnosis, myelofibrosis, splenectomy and extramedullary erythropoiesis. Am J Hematol 52:123, 1989

91. Khumbanonda M, Horowitz HI, Eyster ME: Coomb's positive hemolytic anemia in myelofibrosis with myeloid metaplasia. Am J Med Sci 258:89, 1969

92. Lewis SM, Pettit JE, Tattersall Pepys MB: Myelosclerosis and paroxysmal nocturnal haemoglobinuria. Scand J Haematol 8:451, 1971

93. Kuo CY, Van Voolen A, Morrison AN: Primary and secondary myelofibrosis: its relationship to "PNH-like defect." Blood 40:875, 1972

94. Schreibman P, Brenner B, Jacobs R et al: Small intestinal myeloid metaplasia. JAMA 259:2580, 1988

95. Forshaw J, Harwood L, Weatherall DJ: Folic acid deficiency and megaloblastic erythropoiesis. Br Med J 1:671, 1964

96. Silverstein MN, Elveback LR: Leukocyte alkaline phosphatase in agnogenic myeloid metaplasia. Am J Clin Pathol 61:307, 1974

97. Didsheim P, Bunting D: Abnormal platelet function in myelofibrosis. Am J Clin Pathol 45:566, 1966

98. Balduini CL, Bertolino G, Gamba G et al: Platelet aggregation in platelet rich plasma and whole blood in 18 patients affected by idiopathic myelofibrosis. Eur J Haematol 41:267, 1988

99. Leglise D, Abgrall JF, DesFontaine B et al: Lipoprotein composition in agnogenic myeloid metaplasia. Biomed Pharmacother 39:135, 1985

100. Gilbert HS, Ginsberg H, Fagerstrom R, Brown WV: Characterization of hypocholesterolemia in myeloproliferative disease: relation to disease manifestation and activity. Am J Med 71:595, 1981

101. Gordon BR, Colman M, Kohen P, Day NK: Immunologic abnormalities in myelofibrosis with activation of the complement system. Blood 58:904, 1981

102. Bernhardt B, Valletta M: Lupus anticoagulant in myelofibrosis. Am J Med Sci 272;229, 1976

103. Lewis CM, Pegrum GD: Immune complexes in myelofibrosis: a possible guide to management. Br J Haematol 39:233, 1978
104. Caligaris Cappio F, Vigliani R et al: Idiopathic myelofibrosis: a possible role for immune-complexes in the pathogenesis of bone marrow fibrosis. Br J Haematol 49:17, 1981
105. Rondeau E, Solal-Celigny P, Dhermy S et al: Immune disorders in agnogenic myeloid metaplasia: relations to myelofibrosis. Br J Haematol 53:467, 1983
106. Duhrsen U, Uppenkamp M, Meusers P et al: Frequent association of idiopathic myelofibrosis with plasma cell dyscrasias. Blut 56:97, 1988
107. Humphrey CA, Morris TC: The intimate relationships of myelofibrosis and myeloma: effect of therapy. Br J Haematol 73:269, 1989
108. Salgado C, Feliu E, Blade J et al: A second bone marrow biopsy as a cause of a false diagnosis of myelofibrosis. Br J Haematol 80:407, 1992
109. Lohmann TP, Beckman EN: Progressive myelofibrosis in agnogenic myeloid metaplasia. Arch Pathol Lab Med 107:593,1983
110. Thiele J, Hoeppner B, Zankovich R, Fischer R: Histomorphometry of bone marrow biopsies in primary osteomyelofibrosis/sclerosis (agnogenic myeloid metaplasia)—correlations between clinical and morphological features. Virchows Arch A Pathol Anat Histopathol 415:191, 1989
111. Cervantes F, Pereira A, Marti JM et al: Bone marrow lymphoid nodules in myeloproliferative disorders: association with non myelosclreotic phases of idiopathic myelofibrosis and immunological significance. Br J Haematol 70:279, 1988
112. Miller JB, Testa JR, Lindgren V, Rowley JD: The pattern and clinical significance of karyotypic abnormalities in patients with idiopathic and post polycythemic myelofibrosis. Cancer 55:582, 1985
113. Whang-Peng J, Lee E, Knutson T et al: Cytogenetic studies in patients with myelofibrosis and myeloid metaplasia. Leuk Res 2:41, 1978
114. Castoldi G, Cuneo A, Tomas P, Ferrari L: Chromosome abnormalities in myelofibrosis. Acta Haematol, suppl 1. 78:104, 1987
115. Lawler SD, Swansberg GJ: Cytogenetic studies in myelofibrosis and related conditions. p. 167. In Lewis SM (ed): Myelofibrosis Pathophysiology and Clinical Management. Marcel Dekker, New York, 1985
116. Dewald GW, Pierre RV: Cytogenetic studies in neoplastic hematologic diseases. p. 231. In Fairbanks VF (ed): Current Hematology and Oncology. Vol. 6. Year Book Medical, Chicago, 1988
117. Clough V, Geary CG, Hashimi K et al: Myelofibrosis in chronic granulocytic leukemia. Br J Haematol 42:515, 1979
118. Gralnick HR, Harbor J, Vogel C: Myelofibrosis in chronic granulocytic leukemia. Blood 37:152, 1971
119. Patton WN, Bunce CM, Larkin S, Brown G: Defective erythropoiesis in primary myelofibrosis associated with a chromosome 11 abnormality. Br J Cancer 64:128, 1991
120. Kerim S, Rege-Cambrin G, Scaravaglio P et al: Trisomy 8 and an unbalanced t(5;17) (q11;p11) characterize two karyotypically independent clones in a case of idiopathic myelofibrosis evolving to acute nonlymphoid leukemia. Cancer Genet Cytogenet 52:63, 1991
121. Kaplan KR, Mitchell DG, Steiner RM et al: Polycythemia vera and myelofibrosis: correlation of MR imaging, clinical, and laboratory findings. Radiology 183:329, 1992
122. Jones RJ: The role of bone marrow imaging. Radiology 183:321, 1992
123. Kiely JM, Silverstein MN: Metastatic carcinoma simulating agnogenic myeloid metaplasia and myelofibrosis. Cancer 24:1041, 1969
124. Kiang DT, McKenna RW, Keneddy BJ: Reversal of myelofibrosis in advanced breast cancer. Am J Med 64:173, 1978
125. Viola MV, Kovi J, Nukhopahyay M: Reversal of myelofibrosis in Hodgkin's disease. JAMA 223:1145, 1973
126. Myers CE, Chabner BA, DeVita VT et al: Bone marrow involvement in Hodgkin's disease: pathology and response to MOPP chemotherapy. Blood 44:197, 1974
127. Crail HW, Alt HL, Nadler WH: Myelofibrosis associated with tuberculosis—a report of four cases. Blood 3:1426, 1948
128. Pagliuca A, Layton DM, Manoharan A et al: Myelofibrosis in primary myelodysplastic syndromes: a clinico-morphological study of 10 cases. Br J Haematol 71:499, 1989
129. Maschek H, Georgii A, Kaloutsi V et al: Myelofibrosis in primary myelodysplastic syndromes: a retrospective study of 352 patients. Eur J Haematol 48:208, 1992
130. Ohyashiki K, Sasao I, Ohyashiki JH et al: Clinical and cytogenetic characteristics of myelodysplastic syndromes developing myelofibrosis. Cancer 68:178, 1991
131. Golomb HM, Catovsky D, Golde DW: Hairy cell leukemia: a clinical review of 71 cases. Ann Intern Med 89:677, 1978
132. Silverstein MN: Postpolycythemia myeloid metaplasia. Arch Intern Med 134:113, 1974
133. Najean Y, Arrago JP, Rain JD, Dresch C: The spent phase of polycythemia vera: hypersplenism in the absence of myelofibrosis. Br J Haematol 56:163, 1984
134. Silverstein MN: The evolution into and treatment of late stage polycythemia vera. Semin Hematol 3:79, 1976
135. Llberato NL, Barosi G, Costa A et al: Myelofibrosis with myeloid metaplasia following essential thrombocythaemia. Acta Haematol 82:150, 1989
136. Kergsman KL, VanSlyck EJ: Acute myelofibrosis: an accelerated variant of agnogenic myeloid metaplasia. Ann Intern Med 74:232, 1971
137. Bearman RM, Pangalis GA, Rappaport H: Acute malignant myelosclerosis. Cancer 43:279, 1979
138. Sultan C, Sigaux F, Imbert M, Reyes F: Acute myelodysplasia wiht myelofibrosis: a report of eight cases. Br J Haematol 49:11, 1981
139. Ottolander GJD, Velde JT, Brederoo P et al: Megakaryoblastic leukemia (acute myelofibrosis): a report of three cases. Br J Haematol 42:9, 1979
140. Perum GD, Foadi M, Boots M, Clarke M: How should we manage myelofibrosis? J Coll Physicians Lond 15:17, 1981
141. Manoharan A: Myelofibrosis: prognostic factors and treatment, annotation. Br J Haematol 69:295, 1988
142. Manoharan A, Chen CF, Wilson LS et al: Ultrasonic characterization of splenic tissue in myelofibrosis: further evidence for reversal of fibrosis with chemotherapy. Eur J Haematol 40:149, 1988
143. Löfvenberg E, Wahlin A, Roos G, Öst Å: Reversal of myelofibrosis by hydroxyurea. Eur J Haematol 44:33, 1990
144. Hasselbalch H, Lisse I: A sequential histological study of bone marrow fibrosis in idiopathic myelofibrosis. Eur J Haematol 46:285, 1991
145. Löfvenberg E, Wahlin A: Management of polycythaemia vera, essential thrombocythaemia and myelofibrosis with hydroxyurea. Eur J Haematol 41:375, 1988
146. Manoharan A: Management of myelofibrosis with intermittent hydroxyurea. Br J Haematol 77:252, 1991
147. Chang JC, Gross HM: Case report: remission of chronic idiopathic myelofibrosis to busulfan treatment. Am J Med Sci 295:472, 1988
148. Gardner FH, Nathan DG: Androgens and erythropoiesis. III. Further evaluation of testosterone treatment of myelofibrosis. N Engl J Med 274:420, 1966
149. Gardner FH, Pringle JC Jr. Androgens and erythropoiesis. II: treatment of myeloid metaplasia. N Engl J Med 264:104, 1961
150. Silver RT, Jenkins DE, Engle RL Jr: Use of testosterone and busulfan in the treatment of myelofibrosis with myeloid metaplasia. Blood 23:341, 1964
151. Besa EC, Nowell PC, Geller NL, Gardner FH: Analysis of the androgen response of 23 patients with agnogenic myeloid metaplasia. The value of chromosomal studies in predicting response and survival. Cancer 49:308, 1982
152. Rojer RA, Mulder NH, Nieweg HO: Response to pyridoxine hydrochloride in refractory anemia due to myelofibrosis. Am J Med 65:655, 1978
153. Petti MC, Aloe Spiriti MA, Latagliata R et al: A new approach with rHuEPO in the treatment of myelodysplastic syndromes (MDS) and idiopathic myelofibrosis (IMF), abstracted. Blood, suppl 1. 78:92a, 1991
154. Parmentier C, Charbord P, Tibl M, Tubiana M: Splenic irradiation in myelofibrosis. Clinical findings and ferrokinetics. Int J Radiat Oncol Biol Phys 2:1075, 1975
155. Koeffler HP, Cline MJ, Golde DW: Splenic irradiation in myelofibrosis: effect on circulating myeloid progenitor cells. Br J Haematol 43:69, 1979
156. Wagner H Jr, McKeough PG, Desforges J, Madoc-Jones H: Splenic irradiation in the treatment of patients with chronic myelogenous leukemia or myelofibrosis with myeloid metaplasia. Effects of daily and intermittent fractionation with or without concomitant hydroxyurea. Cancer 58:1204, 1986
157. Szur L, Pettit JC: The effect of radiation on splenic function in myelosclerosis: studies with ^{52}Fe and ^{99m}Tc. Br J Radiol 46:295, 1973
158. Leinweber C, Order SE, Calkins AR: Whole-abdominal irradiation for the management of gastrointestinal and abdominal manifestations of agnogenic myeloid metaplasia. Cancer 68:1251, 1991
159. Parmeggiani L, Ferrant A, Rodhain J et al: Alpha interferon in the treatment of symptomatic myelofibrosis with myeloid metaplasia. Eur J Haematol 39:228, 1987
160. Gilbert HS: Persistence of remission of myeloid metaplasia after treatment with recombinant interferon alpha 2B. Blood, suppl. 1. 72:711, 1987
161. Barosi G, Liberato LN, Costa A, Ascari E: Cytoreductive effect of recombinant alpha interferon in patients with myelofibrosis with myeloid metaplasia. Blut 58:271, 1989
162. Lawlor E: Myeloid antigen expression in childhood acute lymphoblastic leukaemia. Br J Haematol 80:566, 1992
163. Martyré M-C, Magdelenat H, Calvo F: Interferon-γ in vivo reverses the increased platelet levels of platelet-derived growth factor and transforming growth factor-β in patients with myelofibrosis with myeloid metaplasia. Br J Haematol 77:431, 1991
164. Crosby WH: Splenectomy in hematologic disorders. N Engl J Med 286:1533, 1972

165. Mulder H, Steinberg J, Haanen C: Clinical course and survival after elective splenectomy in 19 patients wih primary myelofibrosis. Br J Haematol 35: 419, 1977

166. Benbassat J, Penchas S, Ligumski M: Splenectomy in patients with agnogenic myeloid metaplasia: an analysis of 321 published cases. Br J Haematol 42: 207, 1979

167. Silverstein MN, Remine WH: Splenectomy in myeloid metaplasia. Blood 53: 515, 1979

168. Benbassat J, Gilon D, Penchas S: The choice betewen splenectomy and medical treatment in patients with advanced agnogenic myeloid metaplasia. Am J Hematol 33:128, 1990

169. Towel BL, Levine SP: Massive hepatomegaly following splenectomy for myeloid metaplasia. Am J Med 82:371, 1987

170. Löpez-Guillermo A, Cervantes F, Bruguera M et al: Liver dysfunction following splenectomy in idiopathic myelofibrosis: a study of 10 patients. Acta Haematol 85:184, 1991

171. Brenner B, Nagler A, Tatarsky I, Hashmonai M: Splenectomy in agnogenic myeloid metaplasia and postpolycythemic myeloid metaplasia. Arch Intern Med 108:2501, 1988

172. Barosi G, Ambrosetti A, Buratti A et al: Splenectomy for patients with myelofibrosis and myeloid metaplasia: pretreatment variables and outcome prediction. Leukemia 7:200, 1993

173. Milner JR, Geary CG, Wadswoth LD et al: Erythrokinetic studies as a guide to the value of splenectomy in primary myeloid metaplasia. Br J Haematol 25:467, 1973

174. McCarthy DM, Hibbin JA, Goldman JM: A role for 1,25 dihydroxyvitamin D_3 in control of bone marrow collagen deposition. Lancet 1:78, 1984

175. Coopenberg AA, Singer OP: Reversible myelofibrosis in vitamin D deficiency rickets. Can Med Assoc J 94:392, 1966

176. Duncombe AS, Pearson TC, Nunan TO et al: 1,25-Dihydroxy vitamin D_3 $(1,25(OH)_2D_3)$ in the treatment of idiopathic myelofibrosis. Br J Haematol 66:579, 1987

177. Petrini M, Cecconi N, Azzara A et al: 1,25-Dihydroxy-vitamin D_3 $(1,25(OH)_2$ vit $D_3)$ in the treatment of idiopathic myelofibrosis. Br J Haematol 64:624, 1986

178. Richard C, Mazzora F, Iriondo A et al: The usefulness of 1,25-dihydroxy-vitamin D_3 $(1,25(OH)_2$ vit $D_3)$ in the treatment of idiopathic myelofibrosis. Br J Haematol 62:399, 1986

179. Rajantie J, Sale GE, Deeg HJ et al: Adverse effect of severe marrow fibrosis on hematologic recovery after chemotherapy and allogeneic bone marrow transplantation. Blood 67:1693, 1986

180. Creemers GJ, Löwenberg B, Hagenbeek A: Allogeneic bone marrow transplantation for primary myelofibrosis. Br J Haematol 82:772, 1992

181. Barosi G, Berzuini C, Liberato LN et al: A prognostic classification of myelofibrosis with myeloid metaplasia. Br J Haematol 70:397, 1988

182. Visani G, Finelli C, Castelli U et al: Myelofibrosis with myeloid metaplasia: clinical and haematological parameters predicting survival in a series of 133 patients. Br J Haematol 75:4, 1990

183. Hasselbalch H, Jensen BA: Prognostic factors in idiopathic myelofibrosis: a simple scoring system with prognostic significance. Eur J Haematol 44: 172, 1990

184. Silverstein MN, Linman JW: Causes of death in agnogenic myeloid metaplasia. Mayo Clin Proc 44:36, 1969

185. Silverstein MN, Brown AL, Linman JW: Idiopathic myeloid metaplasia: its evolution into acute leukemia. Arch Intern Med 132:709, 1973

186. Bentley SA, Murray KH, Lewis SM, Roberts PD: Erythroid hypoplasia in myelofibrosis: a feature associated with blastic transformation. Br J Haematol 36:41, 1977

187. Jara S, Migud A, Miguel A et al: Idiopathic myelofibrosis terminating in erythroleukemia. Am J Hematol 32:70, 1989

188. Choate JJ, Domenico DR, McGraw TD et al: Diagnosis of acute megakaryoblastic leukemia by flow cytometry and immunoalkaline phosphatase techniques. Am J Clin Pathol 89:247, 1988

189. Polliack A, Prokocimer M, Matzner Y: Lymphoblastic leukemia transformation (lymphoblastic crisis) in myelofibrosis and myeloid metaplasia. Am J Hematol 9:211, 1989

190. Hasselbalch H: Idoipathic myelofibrosis: a clinical study of 80 patients. Am J Hematol 29:174, 1988

191. Garcia S, Miguel A, Zinares M et al: Idiopathic myelofibrosis terminating in erythroleukemia. Am J Hematol 32:70, 1989

192. Hernandez JM, Miguel S, Gonzalez M et al: Development of acute leukemia after idiopathic myelofibrosis. J Clin Patohl 45:427, 1992

193. Hoyle CF, deBastos M, Wheatley K et al: AML associated with previous cytotoxic therapy, MDS or myeloproliferative disorders: results from the MRC's 9th AML trial. Br J Haematol 72:45, 1989

194. Tefferi A, Silverstein MN, Plumhoff EA. Petitt RM: Suramin therapy in agnogenic myeloid metaplasia, abstracted. Blood, suppl 1. 80:461a, 1992

195. Rozman C, Girallt M, Felia E et al: Life expectancy of patients with chronic nonleukemic myeloproliferative disorders. Cancer 67:2658, 1991

Primary Thrombocythemia

75

Ronald Hoffman, Murray N. Silverstein, and Robert Hromas

INTRODUCTION

Primary thrombocythemia is a chronic myeloproliferative disorder characterized by a sustained proliferation of megakaryocytes, which leads to increased numbers of circulating platelets.[1-16] In addition to platelet counts in excess of 600,000/mm³, this disorder is characterized by profound marrow megakaryocyte hyperplasia, splenomegaly, and a clinical course punctuated by hemorrhagic or thrombotic episodes or both.[1-16]

Primary thrombocythemia was first reported in 1934 by Epstein and Goedel,[17] who described a patient with an elevated platelet count who suffered from repeated hemorrhagic episodes.[17] This disease entity has been referred to by a variety of names, including essential thrombocythemia, idiopathic thrombocythemia, essential thrombophilia, and essential thrombocytosis.[1-16]

Originally, many clinical investigators questioned whether primary thrombocythemia represents a distinct clinical entity. However, extensive descriptions of larger series of patients have provided information to overcome this initial skepticism.[1-18] Dameshek[19] in 1951 speculated that primary thrombocythemia may represent one of the myeloproliferative disorders. Subsequent laboratory investigations have confirmed this concept and clearly demonstrated that the disorder is a clonal hematologic malignancy.[20-24]

EPIDEMIOLOGY

The true incidence of primary thrombocythemia is unknown, since extensive epidemiologic studies are not available. While many investigators have indicated that this disorder is very rare, information from several institutions suggests that it occurs considerably more frequently than originally appreciated.[1-16] Thus, 94 cases of newly diagnosed primary thrombocythemia were identified from 1961–1982 at the Saint Louis Hospital in France, while 61 patients with this disorder were discovered from 1974 through 1987 at the Medizinische Poliklinik in Munich.[13,14] Similarly, 63 primary thrombocythemia patients were diagnosed over a 10-year period at the University of Padua in Italy.[25] Data from the Mayo Clinic in fact have led to estimates of a frequency rate of 10 new primary polycythemia patients per year per million in the population diagnosed each year (Silverstein MN, unpublished observations, 1991). Primary thrombocythemia and polycythemia vera appear to have approximately a 1:4 relative incidence.[7]

The disorder appears to affect primarily middle-aged people, with an average age at diagnosis of 50–60 years.[1-16] In most series, there appears to be no sexual predilection; however, in the report from the Saint Louis Hospital in France, there was a female prevalence, with a 1.76:1 female/male ratio.[7,12-16] This discrepancy might be due to an equal frequency in older patients of both sexes but to a second peak frequency at around 30 years of age for women.[13] This predisposition of young women to develop primary thrombocythemia has been reported previously.[26]

Genetic transmission of the disorder is unusual, although two families with multiple members having primary thrombocythemia have been described.[27,28] In one of these families, thrombocythemia occurred in five members of three successive generations, ranging in age from 2 to 62 years.[27] Several cases have been reported in patients in the pediatric age group, but this is an extremely unusual finding.[29,30] The disorder occurs more frequently in young adults, however, with 13 of 94 patients in one series <20 years of age.[13]

ETIOLOGY

The mechanisms leading to thrombocytosis in primary thrombocythemia are poorly understood. Patients with primary thrombocythemia have normal or near-normal platelet survival.[31,32] The best evidence indicates that the thrombocytosis is due to increased platelet production by megakaryocytes. Effective platelet production is increased as much as 10-fold and is associated with an increase in megakaryocyte clustering, volume, nuclear lobe number, and nuclear ploidy.[31-35]

Analysis of circulating blood cells of females with primary thrombocythemia who were heterozygotes for isoenzymes of glucose-6-phosphate dehydrogenase has revealed that platelets, erythrocytes, and neutrophils express a single isoenzyme type.[20-23] In addition, Raskind et al.[23] have presented data to indicate that B cells are also involved in this neoplastic process. Such findings indicate that primary thrombocythemia is a clonal hematopoietic disorder originating at the level of the pluripotential hematopoietic stem cell. The clonal origin of primary thrombocythemia has been subsequently confirmed using restriction fragment length polymorphisms of X chromosome genes.[36]

However, in this disorder, such clonal analyses often detect a significant proportion of nonclonally derived leukocytes in addition to the clonally derived population of leukocytes. It is possible that small numbers of normal hematopoietic stem cells persist to account for this admixture of nonclonal populations. In one patient, Anger et al.[36] determined that although the total leukocyte fraction was clonally derived, the T-lymphocyte population was nonclonal in origin. Other studies mentioned above, however, have indicated a common origin of granulocytes, platelets, and B lymphocytes in this disorder.[23] These studies raise the possibility that the malignant transformation leading to primary thrombocythemia may occur at different stages of the hematopoietic cellular hierarchy.[37] Such a model would predict that in some cases a primitive stem cell would be the site of the initial oncogenic event, while in others this event might occur in a more differentiated progenitor cell. Data supporting such a hypothesis were recently supplied in an analysis of two sisters with primary thrombocythemia.[37] In one sister, granulocytes, monocytes, and T lymphocytes were clonally derived; in the other sister, the granulocytes fraction was monoclonal, but the T lymphocytes were polyclonal in origin. This study confirms the heterogeneity of the affected hematopoietic cell at which primary thrombocythemia might originate.

The biologic behavior of megakaryocyte progenitor cells present either in the marrow or in the peripheral blood of patients with primary thrombocythemia has been extensively studied.[39-44] In each of these studies, the use of serum-containing culture systems has led to the detection of increased numbers of assayable progenitors. In addition, colonies were noted to appear in the absence of exogenous cytokines.[39-44] A subpopulation of colony-forming unit-megakaryocyte (CFU-MK) assayed from patients with primary thrombocythemia was also shown to remain responsive to addition of cytokines.[39-44]

However, recent studies using serum-free assay systems have found that megakaryocyte colony formation is entirely dependent on the addition of cytokines.[45] This indicates that the proliferation of CFU-MKs is not autonomous, but rather is cytokine dependent.[46] The formation of "endogenous" megakaryocyte colonies in serum-containing systems is probably attributable to small amounts of cytokines in the serum.[39-44] In addition, megakaryocyte progenitors from primary thrombocythemia are less responsive to growth inhibitors such as transforming growth factor (TGF-β).[47] There is also evidence to suggest that the spontaneous formation of megakaryocyte progenitors may be due to a lack of platelet factor 4.[48] Both TGF-β and platelet factor 4 are α-granule constituents, which are known to inhibit megakaryocyte colony formation.[49] Interestingly, the presence of "endogenous" megakaryocyte colony formation in marrow cells obtained from primary thrombocythemic patients is associated with an increased risk of thrombohemorrhagic complications.[50]

Erythroid progenitor cells in primary thrombocythemia can also proliferate in response to the small amount of cytokines present in serum alone. Erythroid colony formation in the absence of exogenous erythropoietin is a hallmark of the proliferative defect that characterizes polycythemia vera.[51,52] Burst-forming unit-erythroid assayed from both marrow and peripheral blood from patients with primary thrombocythemia form erythroid colonies in the absence of exogenous erythropoietin.[53-56] Such an abnormality in these nonpolycythemic patients probably indicates an underlying defect shared by progenitor cells in many myeloproliferative disorders.[53-56]

Careful study of one woman with primary thrombocythemia, who entered a spontaneous clinical remission while pregnant, has indicated the existence of normal hematopoietic progenitor cells in the marrow of this patient.[24] This information suggests the coexistence of normal and neoplastic hematopoietic progenitor cells in primary thrombocythemia.[24] This hypothesis is further corroborated by the finding, in some patients, of polyclonal granulocytes, indicating a normal stem cell population alongside the thrombocythemic stem cell clone.[37,38] Thus, during active phases of the disease the neoplastic cells apparently predominate over normal progenitor cell populations.

There appears to be a rare variant of primary thrombocythemia, in which the clonal expansion of platelets is associated with systemic mastocytosis.[57] Affected patients have the pathologic evidence of systemic mastocytosis but rarely have symptoms of systemic mastocytosis, in contrast to the finding of systemic mastocytosis alone. The pathogenetic significance of this association is poorly understood.

PATHOBIOLOGY

Most clinical sequelae of primary thrombocythemia are related to hemorrhagic and thrombotic episodes, which frequently punctuate the clinical course of individual patients.[1–16] Such thrombohemorrhagic complications occur most often in older patients.[10,58,59] Hoagland and Silverstein[26] have described a subset of young patients who are remarkably free of such complications. Such age-related differences in the frequency of these events have been attributed to the coexistence of vascular disease among older patients.[59] This is controversial, however, as other studies have described younger patients with significant vascular thrombosis.[13,60,61] Microvascular thrombosis causing digital or central nervous system ischemia leads to a variety of clinical syndromes closely associated with primary thrombocythemia.[9,58–71]

Past studies have concluded that the degree of elevation of the platelet count in primary thrombocythemia is an important determinant of the frequency of thrombotic and hemorrhagic events.[1,4,5] These conclusions were, however, based on observations of a limited number of patients. More recently, four different studies have failed to find a relationship between frequency of thrombotic complications and platelet numbers.[13,14,58,72] The relationship between frequency of bleeding episodes and platelet counts is also cloudy. In two studies, patients with extreme thrombocytosis (above $1 \times 10^6/mm^3$) were reported to have a much higher incidence of hemorrhagic events, although such a relationship was not confirmed in a third study.[13,59,72]

Platelets in patients with primary thrombocythemia have been known for a considerable time to be qualitatively abnormal.[4,7,8,73–77] Numerous investigators have attempted to characterize these qualitative abnormalities in the hope of further defining the thrombohemorrhagic tendencies of such patients.[4,7,8,59,73–77] While both increased and decreased platelet reactivity have been identified, these findings have not been definitively associated with thrombohemorrhagic complications.[4,7,8,59,73–77] A variety of individual functional platelet abnormalities have been demonstrated by the liberation of β-thromboglobulin, an α-granule constituent.[84,85] A defect in the metabolism of arachidonic acid by lipoxygenase has been identified, as have decreased numbers of platelet receptors for prostaglandin D_2 and adrenergic receptors for epinephrine.[79,82] Platelets from patients with thrombotic episodes have been found to have increased generation of thromboxane B_2 and increased affinity for fibrinogen.[86,87] Observed elevations in β-thromboglobulin and serum thromboxane B_2 in primary thrombocythemia patients are suggestive of the presence of enhanced in vivo platelet activation and possibly thrombin generation. These same abnormalities are not detected in patients with secondary thrombocythemia and may provide some explanation for the thrombosis associated with primary thrombocythemia. Platelets from patients who have hemorrhagic tendencies often have acquired von Willebrand defects.[88]

Many platelet structural abnormalities have also been reported in primary thrombocythemia, including a decrease in the number of dense bodies and α-granules.[89,90] Although each of these abnormalities indicates the presence of qualitatively abnormal platelets, their contribution to the development of thrombohemorrhagic events remains unknown, as does their molecular basis. It is possible that these abnormalities reflect either the formation of defective platelets from malignant hematopoietic progenitor cells or the activation of platelets in the circulation. The correction of several of these biochemical abnormalities following allogeneic bone marrow transplantation from normal donors suggests that the platelet abnormalities result from the neoplastic process involving the hematopoietic progenitor cell pool.[59]

CLINICAL MANIFESTATIONS

The presenting symptoms of patients with primary thrombocythemia are quite variable. Many patients (12–67%) reach medical attention fortuitously, owing to the extreme degree of thrombocytosis detected when obtaining a routine blood cell count.[1–16] After thrombocytosis has been detected, 13–37% of patients relate symptoms due to hemorrhagic events, while 22–84% of patients report thromboembolic complications.[1–16] Table 75-1 lists the symptoms at diagnosis from one large series of patients.[14] The thrombotic events primarily involved the microvasculature, with thrombosis of large vessels occurring less frequently. Neurologic complications are common;[1–16,62–65] Table 75-2 lists representative neurologic complaints,[62] of which headache was the most common, with paresthesias of the extremities a close second. There was an extremely high incidence of transient ischemic attacks involving both the anterior and posterior cerebral circulation.

Microvascular occlusions involving the toes and fingers are frequent.[63–68] Such events can lead to digital pain, enhanced by warmth; distal extremity gangrene (Fig. 75-1); and classic erythromelalgia.[9,63–68] The term *erythromelalgia* refers to a syndrome of redness and burning pain in the extremities.[63,64] The

Table 75-1. Symptoms at Diagnosis of Primary Thrombocythemia

Symptoms	Patients N[a]	%
Thromboembolic complications	51	84
Microcirculation	41	67
Peripheral (tips of fingers and/or toes)	32	53
Gangrene	16	26
Acrocyanosis	16	26
Paresthesias	15	25
Cold tip feeling	5	8
Cerebral	17	28
Dizziness	15	25
Acoustic phenomena	4	7
Disorientation	2	3
Transient ischemic attack	2	3
Epilepsy	1	2
Apoplectic insult	1	2
Organic psychosyndrome	1	2
Large vessels	31	51
Arteries	29	48
Lower extremities	18	30
Coronary arteries	11	18
Carotid arteries	3	5
Renal arteries	6	10
Mesenteric arteries	2	3
Subclavian artery	1	2
Veins	4	7
Portal vein	3	5
Splenic vein	3	5
Leg and pelvic veins	2	3
Hemorrhages	8	13
Gastrointestinal	2	3
Urogenital	2	3
Epistaxis	2	3
Postoperative	2	3
No symptoms	7	12

[a] Total number of patients: 61.
(From Hehlmann et al.,[14] with permission.)

Table 75-2. Frequency of Neurologic Complaints Associated with Primary Thrombocythemia

Manifestations	Patients[a] (N)
Headache	13
Paresthesias	10
Posterior cerebral circulatory ischemia	9
Anterior cerebral circulatory ischemia	6
Visual disturbances	6
Epileptic seizures	2

[a] Total number of patients: 33.
(From Jabaily et al.,[62] with permission.)

relief of such pain for several days after a single dose of aspirin is diagnostic or erythromelalgia.[63] The specific microvascular syndrome of erythromelalgia is readily explained by platelet-mediated arteriolar inflammation and occlusive thrombosis leading to acrocyanosis and even gangrene.[69,70] Skin biopsies from affected sites reveal arteriolar lesions without involvement of venules, capillaries, or nerves.[63] The arteriolar endothelial cells are swollen and the vessel walls thickened by cellular swelling and deposition of intracellular material.[63] In contrast to atherosclerotic circulatory obstruction, arterial pulses in patients with erythromelalgia remain normal.[63,64] Some evidence has been obtained indicating that platelet consumption is increased in these patients.[91] This shortened platelet survival can be normalized by administration of aspirin, but not coumarin.[91] Platelet activation in vivo in the microcirculation likely leads to microthrombi formation and results in obstruction of small vessels.

Although thrombosis of the microvasculature is generally more frequent, thrombosis of large veins and arteries in patients with primary thrombocythemia still occurs commonly.[13,14] In one series, 51% of patients had symptoms related to large vessel thrombosis, mostly in the arteries of the legs (30%), the coronary arteries (18%), and the renal arteries (10%).[14] Involvement of the carotid, mesenteric, and subclavian arteries is not unusual. In the same series, 7% of patients suffered from venous thrombosis involving either the splenic vein, hepatic veins, or veins of the legs and pelvis.[14] Unexplained thrombosis of the hepatic veins leads to Budd-Chiari syndrome, while thrombosis of the renal vein can result in the development of the nephrotic syndrome.[92] Priapism is a rare complication of primary thrombocythemia, presumably caused by platelet sludging in the corpus cavernosum.[93] In addition, myocardial ischemia or infarction, or both, associated with normal coronary angiograms has been reported in pa-

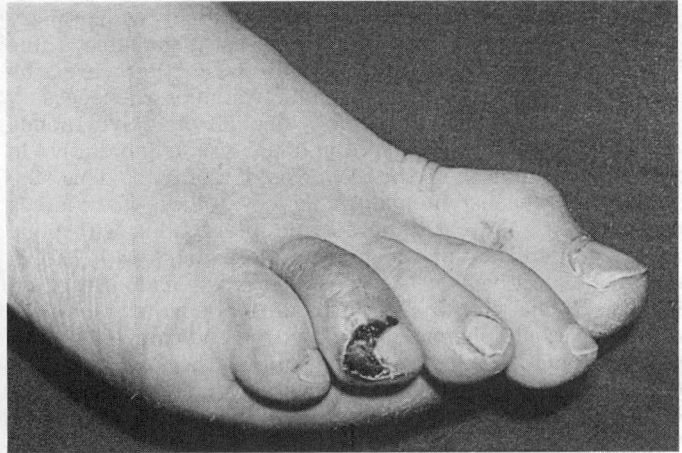

Fig. 75-1. Gangrene of the toe in a patient with primary thrombocythemia.

tients with primary thrombocythemia, as has a high incidence of anginal symptoms.[94,95] Reisner et al.[96] recently reported a high incidence of aortic and mitral valvular lesions in patients with myeloproliferative disorders, including primary thrombocythemia. These valvular lesions resemble previous descriptions of nonbacterial thrombotic endocarditis and may be the origin of the peripheral arterial emboli observed in these patients. In addition, acute renal failure was observed after thrombosis of renal arteries and veins in one patient with primary thrombocythemia.[97]

Hemorrhagic problems plague many patients with primary thrombocythemia;[1-14] the primary site of bleeding is the gastrointestinal tract.[5,59] At least 40% of patients with primary thrombocythemia may have duodenal arcade thrombosis with sloughing of duodenal mucosa, simulating a duodenal ulcer.[5] Other sites of bleeding may be the skin, eyes, urinary tract, gums, tooth sockets (following extraction), joints or brain.[1-14] Bleeding most often is not severe but occasionally may require red cell transfusion support.[1,8,13] The postoperative period appears to be an extremely precarious time, with a high incidence of bleeding episodes following surgical insult.[98]

In one large study in which 97 primary thrombocythemia patients were followed for an average of 7 years, the incidence of thrombohemorrhagic complications was significant, although these were rarely life-threatening.[99] Of the 97 patients, 26 had some type of hemorrhage, mostly of gastrointestinal or mucosal origin; 33 of the 97 patients had some form of thrombosis, mainly in the peripheral arteries. Risk factors for atherosclerotic disease, especially cigarette smoking, increased the risk of thrombosis.[99,100] Of the patients with thrombohemorrhagic events, 11 were shared between the groups, having at least one incident of both types of complication.

It is important to emphasize that individual patients can suffer from both thrombotic and hemorrhagic episodes and that patients are not necessarily consistent "bleeders" or "clotters."[59] Constitutional symptoms, such as weight loss, sweating, low-grade fever, and pruritus, can occur in 20–30% of patients.[10]

Physical examination is relatively unremarkable in most cases. Most patients are not severely ill at diagnosis, a median Karnofsky score of 90% being reported in one series.[10,12] Splenomegaly is detectable in 40–50% of patients, and approximately 20% have hepatomegaly.[10,12] During the course of the disorder, further increase in degree of hepatosplenomegaly does not appear to occur.[10,12]

Although splenomegaly is the more common finding in primary thrombocythemia, splenic atrophy due to silent autoinfarction of the spleen may lead to an acquired form of hyposplenism.[6,7,101] The appearance of Howell-Jolly bodies and target erythrocytes in the peripheral blood smear suggests the occurrence of splenic autoinfarction.[5]

LABORATORY EVALUATION

The hallmark of primary thrombocythemia is a sustained and unexplained elevation of the platelet count. The level of thrombocytosis required for the diagnosis is arbitrarily determined; the range is 450,000–1,000,000/mm^3, depending on the series cited.[1-16] Table 75-3 shows the laboratory findings reported in one large series of patients with this disorder.[13] These findings might be considered representative, as only patients with platelet counts of >600,000/mm^3 were evaluated, and relatively rigorous diagnostic criteria were used. Accompanying leukocytosis was a common finding in this series, as in others reported in the literature.[1-16] Occasional immature myeloid precursor cells (myelocytes or metamyelocytes) and nucleated red blood cells can be seen in the peripheral blood of 25% of patients.[10,12] In one series, mild eosinophilia (>400/mm^3) and

Table 75-3. Laboratory Findings Associated with Primary Thrombocythemia

Findings	Patients N	%
Hemoglobin level		
>16 g/100 ml	6	6
12–16 g/dl	64	68
<12 g/dl	23	24
Leukocytosis		
<8 × 10⁹/L	23	24
8–12 × 10⁹/L	41	44
12–20 × 10⁹/L	22	22
20–29 × 10⁹/L	8	8
Platelet count		
<1 × 10¹²/L	37	38
1–1.5 × 10¹²/L	37	39
>1.5 × 10¹²/L	20	22
Reticulum fibrosis	38/70	54
Normal cytogenetics	49/51	99
Platelet aggregation		
Normal	4/64	6
Decreased		
After ADP	19/64	30
After collagen	6/64	9
After ADP & collagen	35/64	55

(From Bellucci et al.,[13] with permission.)

basophilia (>100/mm³) were present in more than one-third of patients.[10,12]

The most common morphologic abnormalities are variations in red cell size and shape and the presence of megathrombocytes.[1–16] The mean leukocyte alkaline phosphatase activity in one series was 79, with levels below 20 in only three patients.[10,12] Table 75-4 summarizes the bone marrow biopsy findings.[10,12] In this careful study performed by the Polycythemia Vera Study Group, marrow cellularity was increased in almost 90% of patients. In two-thirds of patients, marked megakaryocytic hyperplasia, morphologically bizarre megakaryocytes with nuclear pleomorphism, and clustering of megakaryocytes were frequently present.[10,12,35] Reticulin content was increased in 25% of patients, but collagen fibrosis was not evident.[10,12] In 70–80% of patients, iron stores were present in the marrow, albeit at reduced levels.[14,102] Almost all patients have normal serum ferritin levels.[102] Cervantes et al.[102] have suggested that the absence of iron stores in ≤30% of patients may merely be an epiphenomenon of a chronic myeloproliferative syndrome, and not truly reflective of an iron deficiency state. Bleeding times are prolonged in 10–20% of patients.[13,74] Platelet aggregation studies are frequently abnormal, most often demonstrating impaired aggregation in response to epinephrine or ADP, but not to collagen.[13,73,74,77] Spontaneous platelet aggregation has been reported to occur frequently in such patients, but this has not been a universal finding.[13,75]

About 25% of patients with primary thrombocythemia have been reported to have elevated uric acid levels at diagno-

Table 75-4. Bone Marrow Biopsy Findings in Primary Thrombocythemia

Parameter	Normal	Slightly Increased	Moderately Increased	Markedly Increased
Cellularity	4	7	22	4
Megakaryocyte number	0	3	10	24
Erythroid elements	6	12	15	4
Myeloid elements	7	11	17	2
Reticulin content	29	7	1	0

(From Iland et al.,[10] with permission.)

sis.[10,12,14] The average value of the serum potassium at diagnosis is usually within the normal range, although 23% of patients have been reported to have pseudohyperkalemia.[14,103] Pseudohypoxemia has also been observed in primary thrombocythemia patients with extreme degrees of thrombocytosis.[104] The serum B_{12} level can be increased in 25% of cases.[10,12,13]

The marrow karyotypes are characteristically normal.[10–14,105] The absence of the Philadelphia chromosome rules out the diagnosis of chronic myeloid leukemia (CML).[106,107] Aneuploidy is seen in the minority of cases. In fact, analysis of 170 cases of primary thrombocytosis revealed a definite chromosomal abnormality in only 5.3% of cases. Marker chromosomal abnormalities, such as 1q⁻, 20q⁻, 21q⁻, or 1q⁺, have been reported, but no consistent chromosomal abnormality has been identified.[10–14,105–112]

DIFFERENTIAL DIAGNOSIS

Primary thrombocythemia must be distinguished from reactive or secondary forms of thrombocytosis and from other myeloproliferative disorders, such as polycythemia vera, agnogenic myeloid metaplasia, and CML, which are also characterized by thrombocytosis.[1–14] Patients with myelodysplastic syndromes can also present with a moderate or marked degree of thrombocytosis; this is especially true of patients with the 5q⁻ syndrome and of patients with idiopathic acquired sideroblastic anemia.[113,114] The causes of secondary or reactive forms of thrombocytosis are numerous. They include acute or chronic infections, rheumatoid arthritis, ankylosing spondylitis, chronic inflammatory bowel disease, iron deficiency anemia, nonhematologic malignancies, and sickle cell anemia.[97,115] Thrombocytosis also occurs frequently postoperatively, especially following splenectomy.[97,115,116] The cause of thrombocytosis was evaluated in a study of inpatients at the Mayo Clinic.[116a] It was found that 512 of 279,000 patients who had Coulter counter examinations in 1979 had platelet counts of >800,000/mm³. In one-third of the patients, thrombocytosis was due to a myeloproliferative disorder, either primary thrombocythemia, CML, or polycythemia vera. Interestingly, one-third of patients developed thrombocytosis postoperatively; these were primarily patients who had recently been splenectomized, but others were recovering from orthopaedic surgical procedures or organ transplants. The final one-third of patients developed thrombocytosis following either an infection, a sterile inflammatory process such as inflammatory bowel disease, or a neoplastic process primarily involving the lung and gastrointestinal tract.[116a]

A number of investigators have constructed lists of diagnostic criteria useful in identifying individual patients with primary thrombocythemia.[10,13,14,117,118] No such list is infallible. Table 75-5 lists useful diagnostic criteria, but these criteria are arbitrary. Red cell mass and plasma volume studies are necessary to differentiate primary thrombocythemia from polycythemia vera.[118,119] Bone marrow karyotypic analysis is imperative in every patient to exclude the diagnosis of CML.[106,107] This step is necessary because the natural history of these disorders is very different, and early therapeutic intervention with bone marrow transplantation for appropriate patients with CML is potentially curative.[106,107] In one series, six women presented with the clinical picture of primary thrombocythemia *without* anemia, marked splenomegaly, or extreme leukocytosis characteristic of CML.[107] Each of these patients was shown to have a Philadelphia chromosome on karyotypic analysis, and five of the six entered the accelerated phase or blast crisis within 5–7 years of diagnosis.[107]

A highly instructive case was reported in 1988 by Morris et al.[106] The patient was a 23-year-old woman who presented with

Table 75-5. Criteria for Diagnosis of Primary Thrombocythemia[a]

1. Platelet count >600,000/mm³ on two different occasions, separated by a 1-month interval

2. Absence of identifiable cause of thrombocytosis, such as infections, inflammatory disorders, or nonhematologic malignant disorders

3. Normal red cell mass (males <36 ml/kg; females <32 ml/kg)

4. Absence of significant fibrosis of the marrow (>⅓ cross-sectional area of the bone marrow biopsy).

5. Absence of the Philadelphia chromosome and the fusion *bcr/abl* gene

6. Presence of splenomegaly

7. Bone marrow hypercellularity, as appreciated by a bone marrow biopsy (marrow should be remarkable for megakaryocytic hyperplasia with aggregates of megakaryocytes being present)

8. Absence of iron deficiency, as documented by the presence of stainable marrow iron and/or normal serum ferritin

9. In females, demonstration of clonal hematopoiesis by means of restriction fragment length polymorphism analysis of genes present on the X chromosome

10. Presence of abnormal marrow hematopoietic progenitor cells, as determined by the formation of endogenous erythroid and/or megakaryocytic colonies

11. Abnormal platelet aggregation studies in response to epinephrine and ADP at a time when the patient is not taking any drug that might impair platelet function

[a] Patients who meet criteria 1–5 and ≥3 of criteria 6–11 should be considered to have primary thrombocythemia.

a syndrome indistinguishable from primary thrombocythemia.[106] Although no Philadelphia chromosome was detected, the patient did develop blast crisis after 4 years of follow-up. By Southern blot analysis, she was shown to have the *bcr/abl* fusion gene, suggesting that she actually suffered from CML and not from primary thrombocythemia.[107] This case emphasizes the importance of molecular studies when evaluating patients suspected of having primary thrombocythemia.[107]

Differentiation between reactive thrombocytosis or secondary thrombocytosis and primary thrombocythemia may be a difficult task. Some clinicians have considered the degree of thrombocytosis useful for this purpose.[8] Platelet counts of >1 × 10⁶/mm³ are not unusual in patients with secondary thrombocytosis.[115] Platelet aggregation in response to a variety of stimuli (e.g., ADP, epinephrine, and collagen) has also been suggested as a means of differentiating secondary thrombocytosis from primary thrombocythemia.[74,76,115] A number of investigators have concluded that detection of severe abnormalities of platelet aggregation, particularly in response to several agonists, is very suggestive of primary thrombocythemia, while the detection of only minimal defects or none at all suggests that some other underlying disease process is responsible for the thrombocytosis.[13,74,76,119]

The presence of clonal hematopoiesis quickly establishes the diagnosis of primary thrombocythemia.[20–22] Such studies may be particularly useful in young females with thrombocytosis.[26] Probes derived from the hypoxanthine phosphoribosyl transferase gene and phosphoglycerate kinase gene can be used for clonal analysis of blood cell production in >50% of American females.[121] In such patients, analysis of restriction fragment length polymorphism can be used to establish a pattern of clonal hematopoiesis, which is indicative of a hematologic malignancy and establishes the diagnosis of primary thrombocythemia in a young female with thrombocytosis.[24]

A number of diagnostic tests, including platelet volume analysis, splenic volume estimates, and assays of bone marrow progenitor cells (erythroid or megakaryocyte), have been suggested as useful means of differentiating reactive thrombocytosis from primary thrombocythemia.[38–46,122,123] Insufficient numbers of patients as well as a lack of long-term follow-up make it impossible to assess the clinical value of such tests.

At times it is impossible to define the cause of an individual patient's thrombocytosis. In an asymptomatic patient, the resolution of this problem is easy, since one should simply provide follow-up and determine whether the degree of thrombocytosis increases. If additional clues to the cause of the thrombocytosis are subsequently revealed, a diagnosis will become apparent. In a patient with thrombohemorrhagic difficulties, one must make a presumptive diagnosis of the cause of the thrombocytosis and then, after weighing the benefits versus the risks of various treatment plans, determine whether reduction of platelet numbers or simple observation is indicated. Some reassurance is provided by the report of Schilling, who followed >102 patients, each with platelet counts of >1 × 10⁶/mm³, for 18 months. None of the patients with reactive thrombocytosis developed a cerebrovascular accident, thrombophlebitis, or peripheral arterial thrombosis.[72,115] These findings are consistent with the conclusions of Buss et al.[72] that thrombohemorrhagic complications are rare in patients with secondary thrombocytosis.

THERAPY

The treatment of patients with primary thrombocythemia is controversial and largely problematic.[15] Handling of primary thrombocythemia patients with life-threatening hemorrhagic or thrombotic episodes is more straightforward and is best approached by plateletpheresis in combination with institution of myelosuppressive therapy.[124–126] Rapid plateletpheresis using continuous or discontinuous flow centrifugation devices has proved effective in preventing additional morbidity in patients with primary thrombocythemia.[124–126] In this situation, immediate physical removal of large numbers of platelets is preferred. Since chemotherapeutic agents generally require 18–20 days before platelet counts can be reduced to normal levels, Taft et al.[126] have recommended reducing the platelet count to 500,000/mm³ by each plateletpheresis and suggest that achievement of such a goal requires the passage of two blood volumes over a 3–4-hour period.

Such a therapeutic approach has been employed to treat acutely ill patients with problems such as cerebrovascular accidents, myocardial infarction, transient ischemic attacks, or life-threatening gastrointestinal hemorrhage.[124–126] Long-term plateletpheresis has proved an ineffective means of controlling thrombocythemia, presumably owing to the rapid rate of production of platelets.[127] Therefore, most clinicians begin by administering a chemotherapeutic agent that has a rapid onset of action, such as hydroxyurea, simultaneously with the institution of plateletpheresis.[126] If plateletpheresis is not an available therapeutic option, administration of nitrogen mustard (0.4 mg/kg) is usually effective in lowering the platelet count within several days.[128]

In those patients found to have chronic primary thrombocythemia and who are clearly symptomatic, little controversy exists as to the need for lowering the platelet count. The large number of thrombotic complications that occur in primary thrombocythemic patients who smoke, point to the urgent need for these patients to stop smoking immediately.[100] Since a relationship between degree of platelet count elevation and risk of thrombosis or hemorrhage is at best tenuous, the level of platelet count reduction necessary to reduce subsequent morbidity or mortality is unknown.[13,58,59,72] Most investigators try to normalize the platelet count or to reach a platelet count at which the patient's symptoms resolve. Groups of patients have been successfully treated with a variety of chemotherapeutic agents, including busulfan, melphalan, chlorambucil, pi-

PERSONAL APPROACH TO THERAPY FOR PRIMARY THROMBOCYTHEMIA

The optimal therapy for primary thrombocythemia, and even the need for therapy at all, remains an area of active debate. Studies can be found to support completely different approaches. The guidelines presented here are derived from the overall thrust of the literature and personal experience. It must be stated that individual cases may often require unique approaches. There are precepts that apply to all patients, however. One is that all patients with primary thrombocythemia should stop smoking to minimize the thrombotic risk factors associated with athersoclerotic disease. Another is to avoid the indiscriminant use of nonsteroidal anti-inflammatory drugs, which can lead to an increased risk of hemorrhage. Such agents are particularly common in the elderly age group in which primary thrombocythemia is common.

Therapy should only be initiated when a diagnosis is firmly established. Our first choice for therapy has been hydroxyurea, starting at 1 g/day and then adjusted to achieve normal platelet counts (1.5–$4.5 \times 10^5/mm^3$) without leukopenia. In those patients who either do not tolerate hyrdroxyurea or fail to respond, we then proceed to anegrelide. This is started at 0.5 mg qid and increased by 0.5 mg/day every 5–7 days, if platelet counts do not begin to decrease. The usual dose, however, is 2–2.5 mg/day. There are patients who do not tolerate either hydroxyurea or anegrelide, mostly because of significant gastrointestinal distress or headaches. In this patient group, interferon-α started at 3 million units three times per week subcutaneously is one possibility. Another is busulphan at 4 mg/day for 2-week courses every time the platelet count rises above the normal range.

In general, we do not routinely treat patients <40 years of age, unless they have already have had thrombohemorrhagic symptoms or have significant risk factors for atherosclerotic disease. We have had no complications in young otherwise healthy untreated patients despite prolonged platelet counts of $>2.0 \times 10^6/mm^3$.

However, in certain situations, in young, risk-free patients, treatment is instituted. Surgery can increase the risk of thrombosis, and many anti-inflammatory agents can increase the risk of bleeding. If these circumstances arise, the platelet count should be lowered to the normal range.

In pregnant patients with primary polycythemia, our tendency has been to intervene as little as possible. Weekly plateletpheresis and 300 mg/day of aspirin are the first possibilities for treatment should it be needed. Both hydroxyurea and busulphan have been successfully used to treat myeloproliferative disorders during pregnancy, but they are probably teratogenic during the first trimester. If such agents are needed, they should be instituted after the first trimester. The risk of leukemia is unknown, but not something to be ignored. Little information is available on the risks of anegrelide or interferon during pregnancy.

In a patient with primary thrombocythemia and a serious acute hemorrhage, the site of bleeding should be immediately determined, and any antiplatelet aggregating agents stopped. Although the platelet count may be high, these platelets are qualitatively abnormal, leading to defective hemostasis. In this situation, the transfusion of normal platelets is suggested. In those patients with persistent hemorrhage, immediate reduction of the platelet count can be achieved by plateletpheresis. Hydroxyurea at 2–4 g/day for 3–5 days should be administered beginning immediately, then reduced to 1 g/day. Any patient receiving hydroxyurea should be monitered for granulocytopenia or thrombocytopenia, or both. Reduction of platelet counts is usually observed within 3–5 days of hydroxyurea treatment.

By contrast, patients with acute arterial thrombosis require immediate institution of platelet antiaggregating agents. Aspirin at a dose of 300 mg/day is suggested. Patients with erythromelalgia will have a rapid cessation of symptoms. In addition, the platelet count should be lowered with either a combination of apheresis and hydroxyurea or with hydroxyurea alone, depending on the severity of the event. In patients with severe thrombosis, such as myocardial or cerebral infarction, heparin anticoagulation can also be instituted, unless there is a medical contraindication. Since anticoagulation increases the risk of concurrent hemorrhage, the choice for anticoagulation should be made on an individual basis, after the risks and benefits have been weighed.

---

pobroman, thiotepa, radioactive phosphorus, hydroxyurea, nitrogen mustard, uracil mustard, and CCNU (lomustine).[1,6,8,12,128-136] Many of these agents have been used to treat a variety of myeloproliferative disorders and solid tumors, and their use has been associated with an increased risk of leukemia.[137,138] Phase III studies comparing the efficacy of such agents for the treatment of primary thrombocythemia have not been completed.

One exception is a study of a small group of patients whose response to either melphalan or radioactive phosphorus during the first year of therapy was compared. The only conclusion that could be drawn from this study was that time to response as defined by platelet count reduction was considerably shorter for patients receiving melphalan than for those receiving radioactive phosphorus.[132] Hydroxyurea (15 mg/kg for the first week, followed by a maintenance dose adjusted to maintain an acceptable platelet count but avoiding leukopenia) is the drug of choice.[112] Hydroxyurea is quite efficient in lowering the platelet count; its leukemogenic effect has been said to be

less than that associated with other chemotherapeutic agents.[12,135] Intermittent use of busulfan (4 mg/day, until the platelet count falls to 400,000/mm³, followed by a series of 2-week courses when the platelet count rises to >400,000/mm³) has proved a relatively nontoxic and effective regimen.[129] These conclusions were based on a lengthy examination of the course of 37 patients.[129]

Biologic response modifiers have also recently been employed to treat the thrombocytosis associated with myeloproliferative disorders.[139-141] A report of 26 patients with primary thrombocythemia treated with interferon-α (IFN-α) has appeared.[139] Slightly more than 60% of these patients achieved a complete hematologic response following such therapy. After achievement of a complete remission, maintenance therapy at a lower dose of IFN alone or in combination with pipobroman was successful in maintaining an acceptable platelet count.[141] Toxicity was not minimal, however, since 28% of patients did not tolerate dose escalation.[139] Two smaller trials have reported higher response rates using IFN-α, with a combined total of 14 of 16 patients achieving a significant lowering of platelet counts.[141-143] These responses were quite durable, ≤4 years. None of the responding patients suffered a thrombohemorrhagic event. Still, the future role of IFN-α as compared to other therapy remains to be defined by prospective randomized trials investigating the relative rates of thrombohemorrhagic events.

The use of platelet antiaggregating agents remains an extremely controversial area. Patients with primary thrombocythemia have an increased predisposition to hemorrhage, which is likely potentiated by the use of drugs that affect platelet function.[1-16,58,59] Transient ischemic attacks and erythromelalgia associated with primary thrombocythemia have been reported to respond rapidly to aspirin alone, to aspirin and dipyridamole in combination, or to indomethacin alone.[62-67] In erythromelalgia, symptoms disappear for 2–4 days after administration of a single 500-mg dose of aspirin.[63] Although these agents surely have a role in the treatment of these specific complications, their use should be pursued with extreme caution because of the increased risk of hemorrhage. Kessler et al.[58] have, in fact, determined that 32% of bleeding episodes in patients with extreme thrombocytosis and myeloproliferative disorders occurred concurrently with the use of anti-inflammatory agents. By contrast, Hehlmann et al.[14] have reported the treatment of 46 patients with primary thrombocythemia with 250 mg/day of aspirin without any bleeding complications.

Of great interest has been the development of a new drug, anagrelide, for the treatment of primary thrombocythemia.[144] Anagrelide is a member of the imidazo(2,1-b)quinazolin-2-one series of compounds. During studies in humans, it was noted that anagrelide in small doses produced profound thrombocythemia. The drug acts primarily by inhibiting megakaryocyte maturation and platelet release;[144] it does not appear to affect DNA synthesis. A major new study of 577 patients treated with anagrelide has confirmed its usefulness.[145] Anagrelide in low doses was effective in lowering the platelet count in 93% of patients. Most importantly, it was effective despite resistance to previous therapy. Few patients developed resistance to anagrelide, but 16% eventually had to discontinue the drug at some time because of intolerable side effects, especially headaches, nausea, and fluid retention, which sometimes resulted in frank congestive heart failure. Anagrelide has also been successfully used to treat children with primary thrombocythemia.[146] This new agent appears to be extremely promising for the treatment of primary thrombocythemia.

A challenging therapeutic dilemma is whether any treatment is indicated in patients with primary thrombocythemia in whom the platelet count elevation is initially detected fortuitously and who remain largely asymptomatic. Such a decision is particularly important, as the use of most chemotherapeutic agents is associated with an increased risk of the development of leukemia, and the use of platelet antiaggregating agents is not without risk.[58,59,137,138] The need for such treatment can be questioned, since in several studies a relationship between frequency of thrombotic episodes and degree of platelet elevation has not been established.[13,58,72] One should not lapse into false security in deferring therapy, however, since the course of primary thrombocythemia is characterized by infrequent but dangerous thromboembolic complications, and patients may function normally for long periods of time without experiencing a life-threatening event.[1-14] Still, it would seem reasonable to withhold therapy in younger, asymptomatic patients until the development of a clinically significant thrombotic or hemorrhagic event. The elderly patient with other significant risk factors for cardiovascular complications is probably best served by immediate institution of therapy.

Table 75-6. Causes of Death in Primary Thrombocythemia

Cause of Death	Patients (N)
Sudden cardiac death or myocardial infarction	7
Acute leukemia	2
Infarction of mesenteric artery	1
Pulmonary embolism	1
Renal insufficiency	1
Stroke	1
Unknown	1

(From Hehlmann et al.,[14] with permission.)

PROGNOSIS

The probability that a patient with primary thrombocythemia will survive 10 years is within the range of 64–80%. Complications continue to arise after the diagnosis. Obstetric problems are frequent—in one series, six spontaneous abortions, two premature deliveries, and one abruptio placentae were noted in 3 of 22 young women with primary polycythemia. Only two pregnancies resulted in full-term deliveries.[13] In another study, however, mild intervention with low-dose aspirin and occasional plateletpheresis resulted in eight normal deliveries in nine pregnancies among six patients.[147]

Table 75-6 presents the causes of death in one series of 61 patients with primary thrombocythemia.[14] Death predominantly ensued from thrombotic complications.[14] Transformation to acute myeloid leukemia has been reported with increasing frequency in patients with primary thrombocythemia and is an important cause of mortality.[1-14,27,131,148-152] The blast cell phenotype that characterizes this transformation can be either myeloid, myelomonoblastic, megakaryocytic, or of mixed lineage.[148-152] Only one patient to date has been reported who developed acute leukemia who had not been previously treated with chemotherapeutic agents.[149] Whether this patient truly suffered from primary thrombocythemia is debatable, since appropriate cytogenetic and molecular studies were not performed to exclude the diagnosis of CML.[149] With these reservations in mind, several investigators have concluded that the transformation of primary thrombocythemia into acute leukemia is a rare event, which can be accelerated by the administration of chemotherapeutic agents.[13,14,151]

It is sobering to note that two patients with primary thrombocythemia who developed acute leukemia were treated solely with hydroxyurea.[14] The report of these patients suggests that the use of hydroxyurea might not be as safe as previously suggested.[12,135] The acute leukemia, that occurs following primary thrombocythemia is difficult to treat.[27] Transformation of primary thrombocythemia to a clinical stage that resembles agnogenic myeloid metaplasia with or without myelofibrosis has been sporadically reported but is at best a rare event.[6,7,9] In one retrospective study of 94 patients, no patient developed clinically significant myelofibrosis or myeloid metaplasia.[13] Singh and Wetherley-Mein[9] have, however, reported two patients with primary thrombocythemia who developed myelofibrosis 3 and 5 years after presentation and who died 8 and 9 years, respectively, after this transition occurred. The exact incidence of such transitions remains unknown.

An actuarial study of survival of 247 patients with primary thrombocythemia followed for a median of 27 months found no statistically significant survival difference as compared to the normal population.[153] Several other studies have also concluded that the life expectancy of patients with primary thrombocythemia is that of a matched population without primary thrombocythemia.[13,14]

FUTURE DIRECTIONS

Primary thrombocythemia is now firmly established as a clonal hematologic malignancy with its own distinct clinical manifestations and associated complications. Better means of identifying patients at risk of fatal thrombotic or hemorrhagic complications are necessary to bring about the optimal care of such patients. The relationship between risk of thrombo-hemorrhagic phenomena and platelet numbers and function must be better defined. Platelet antiaggregating agents should be judiciously used only in patients with a high risk of thrombosis.

Multi-institutional comparisons of the efficacy of such promising agents as IFN and anagrelide with chemotherapeutic agents such as hydroxyurea or busulfan, for the initial treatment of primary thrombocythemia, must be completed before decisions on appropriate drug therapy can be made. These studies should include enrollment of large numbers of patients, who will require follow-up for long periods, before meaningful conclusions can be drawn. The effects of IFN and anagrelide use on patient survival, as well as the frequency of hemorrhagic and thrombotic events and the development of leukemia, must be determined. Only after completion of such studies can these agents be regarded as optimal therapeutic tools for the treatment of primary thrombocythemia.

REFERENCES

1. Gunz FW: Hemorrhagic thrombocythemia: a critical review. Blood 15:706, 1960
2. Ozer FL, Traux WE, Miesch DC, Levin WC: Primary hemorrhagic thrombocythemia. Am J Med 28:807, 1960
3. Frick PG: Primary thrombocythemia, clinical, hematological and chromosomal studies of 13 patients. Helv Chir Acta 35:20, 1989
4. Hardisty RM, Wolf HH: Haemorrhagic thrombocythemia: a clinical and laboratory study. Br J Haematol 1:390, 1955
5. Silverstein MN: Primary or hemorrhagic thrombocythemia. Arch Intern Med 122:18, 1968
6. Jameshidi K, Ansari A, Windschitl HE, Swaim WR: Primary thrombocythemia. Geriatrics 28:121, 1973
7. Lewis SM, Szur L, Hoffbrand AV: Thrombocythemia. Clin Haematol 1:339, 1978
8. Murphy S: Thrombocytosis and thrombocythemia. Clin Haematol 12:89, 1983
9. Singh AK, Wetherley-Mein G: Microvascular occlusive lesions in primary thrombocythemia. Br J Haematol 36:553, 1977
10. Iland HJ, Laszlo J, Peterson P et al: Essential thrombocythemia: clinical and laboratory characteristics at presentation. Trans Assoc Am Physicians 96: 165, 1983
11. Preston EE: Primary thrombocythemia. Lancet 1:1021, 1982
12. Murphy S, Iland H, Rosenthal D, Laszlo J: Essential thrombocythemia: an interim report from the Polycythemia Vera Study Group. Semin Hematol 23:177, 1986
13. Bellucci S, Janvier M, Tobelem G et al: Essential thrombocythemias: clinical, evolutionary and biological data. Cancer 58:2440, 1986
14. Hehlmann R, Jahn M, Baumann B, Kopcke W: Essential thrombocythemia: clinical characteristics and course of 61 cases. Cancer 61:2487, 1988
15. Pearson TC: Primary thrombocythemia: diagnosis and management. Br J Haematol 78:145, 1991
16. Schafer AI: Essential thrombocythemia. Prog Hemost Thromb 10:69, 1991
17. Epstein E, Goedel A: Hamorrhagische Thrombozythämie bei vascularer Schrumpfmilz. Virchows Arch A Pathol Anat Histophathol 293:233, 1934
18. McCabe WR, Bird RM, McLaughlin RA: Case reports: is primary hemorrhagic thrombocythemia a clinical myth? Ann Intern Med 43:1982, 1955
19. Dameshek W: Some speculations on the myeloproliferative syndromes. Blood 6:372, 1951
20. Fialkow PJ, Faguet GB, Jacobsen RJ et al: Evidence that essential thrombocythemia is a clonal disorder with origin in a multipotent stem cell. Blood 58: 916, 1981
21. Gaetani GF, Ferraris AM, Galiano S et al: Primary thrombocythemia: clonal origin of platelets, erythrocytes and granulocytes in a $Gd^B/Gd^{mediterranean}$ subject. Blood 59:76, 1982
22. Singal U, Prasad AS, Halton DM, Bishop C: Essential thrombocythemia: A clonal disorder of hematopoietic stem cell. Am J Hematol 14:193, 1983
23. Raskind WH, Jacobson R, Murphy S et al: Evidence for the involvement of B lymphoid cells in polycythemia vera and essential thrombocythemia. J Clin Invest 75:1388, 1985
24. Turhan AG, Humphries RK, Cashman JD: Transient suppression of hemopoi-
25. Randi ML, Fabris F, Vio C, Giorlami A: Familial thrombocythemia and or thrombocytosis: apparently a rare disorder. Acta Haematol 78:63, 1987
26. Hoagland HC, Silverstein MN: Primary thrombocythemia in the young patient. Mayo Clin Proc 53:578, 1978
27. Fickers M, Speck B: Thrombocythemia: familial occurrence and transition into blastic crisis. Acta Haematol 51:251, 1974
28. Eyster ME, Saletan SL, Rabellino EM: Familial essential thrombocythemia. Am J Med 80:497, 1986
29. Linch DC, Hutton R, Cowan D et al: Primary thrombocythemia in childhood. Scand J Haematol 28:72, 1982
30. Sceats DJ, Baitlon D: Primary thrombocythemia in a child. Clin Pediatr 19: 298, 1980
31. Harker LA, Finch CA: Thrombokinetics in man. J Clin Invest 48:963, 1969
32. Branehog I, Ridell B, Swolin B, Weinfeld A: Megakaryocyte quantifications in relation to thrombokinetics in primary thrombocythemia and allied diseases. Scand J Haematol 15:21, 1975
33. Mazur EM, Lindquist DL, de Alarcon PA, Cohen JL: Evaluation of bone marrow megakaryocyte ploidy distributions in individuals with normal and abnormal platelet counts. J Lab Clin Med 111:194, 1988
34. Tomer A, Friese P, Conklin R et al: Flow cytometric analysis of megakaryocytes from patients with abnormal platelet counts. Blood 74:594, 1989
35. Buss DH, O'Connor ML, Woodruff RD et al: Bone marrow and peripheral blood findings in patients with extreme thrombocytosis. Arch Pathol Lab Med 115:475, 1991
36. Anger B, Janssen JWG, Schrezenmeier H et al: Clonal analysis of chronic myeloproliferative disorders using X-linked DNA polymorphisms. Leukemia 4:258, 1990
37. Turhan AG, Cashman JD, Eaves CJ et al: Variable expression of features of normal and neoplastic stem cells in patients with thrombocytosis. Br J Haematol 82:50, 1992
38. Janssen JWG, Anger BR, Drexler HG et al: Essential thrombocythemia in two sisters originating from different stem cell levels. Blood 75:1633, 1990
39. Gewirtz AM, Bruno E, Elwell J, Hoffman R: In vitro studies of megakaryocytopoiesis in thrombocytic disorders of man. Blood 61:384, 1983
40. Kamatsu N, Suda T, Sakata Y: Megakaryocytopoiesis in vitro of patients with essential thrombocythemia: effect of plasma and serum on megakaryocytic colony formation. Br J Haematol 64:241, 1986
41. Juvoken E, Partenen S, Ruutu T: Colony formation by megakaryocytic progenitors in essential thrombocythemia. Br J Haematol 66:161, 1987
42. Kimura H, Ishibashi T, Sato T et al: Megakaryocytic colony formation (CFU-Meg) in essential thrombocythemia. Quantitative and qualitative abnormalities of bone marrow CFU-Meg. Am J Hematol 24:23, 1987
43. Mazur EM, Cohen JL, Bogart L: Growth characteristics of circulating hematopoietic progenitor cells from patients with essential thrombocythemia. Blood 71:1544, 1988
44. Han ZC, Briere J, Abgrall JF et al: Characteristics of megakaryocytic colony formation in normal individuals and in primary thrombocythemia. Studies using an optimal cloning system. Exp Hematol 17:46, 1989
45. Bruno E, Briddell R, Hoffman R: Effect of recombinant and purified hematopoietic growth factors in human megakaryocyte colony formation. Exp Hematol 16:371, 1988
46. Van Besien K, Bruno E, Hoffman R: Cytokine requirements for in vitro megakaryocyte colony formation in myeloproliferative disorders. Blood, suppl 1. 74:250a, 1989
47. Zauli G, Visani G, Catani L et al: Reduced responsiveness of bone marrow megakaryocyte progenitors to platelet-derived transforming growth factor beta-1, produced in normal amount, in patients with essential thrombocythemia. Br J Haematol 83:14, 1993
48. Abgrall J-F, Berthou C, Cauvin J-M et al: Spontaneous in vitro megakaryocyte colony formation in primary thrombocythemia: relation to platelet factor 4 plasma level and beta-thromboglobulin/platelet factor 4 ratio. Acta Haematol 87:118, 1992
49. Gordon MS, Hoffman R: Growth factors affecting human thrombocytopoiesis: potential agents for the treatment of thrombocytosis. Blood 80:302, 1992
50. Juvonen E, Ikkala E, Oksanen K, Ruutu T: Megakaryocyte and erythroid colony formation in essential thrombocythemia and reactive thrombocytosis: diagnostic value and correlation to complications. Br J Haematol 83:192, 1993
51. Prchal JF, Axelrad AA: Bone marrow response in polycythemia vera. N Engl J Med 290:1382, 1985
52. Zanjani ED, Lutton JD, Hoffman R, Wasserman LR: Erythroid colony formation by polycythemia vera bone marrow in vitro. J Clin Invest 59:841, 1977
53. Reid CD, Chanarin I, Lewis J: Formes frustes in myeloproliferative disorders.

esis associated with pregnancy in a patient with a myeloproliferative disorder. J Clin Invest 81:1999, 1988

Identification by growth of an endogenous erythroid clone in vitro in patients with arterial vascular disease. Lancet 1:14, 1982

54. Eridani S, Batten E, Sawyer B: Erythroid colony formation in primary thrombocythemia: evidence of hypersensitivity to erythropoietin. Br J Haematol 55:157, 1983

55. Eridani S, Dudley JM, Sawyer BM, Pearson TC: Erythropoietic colonies in a serum-free system: results in primary proliferative polycythaemia and thrombocythemia. Br J Haematol 67:387, 1987

56. Partanen S, Ruutu T, Vopio P: Haemopoietic progenitors in essential thrombocythemia. Scand J Haematol 30:130, 1983

57. LeTourneau A, Gaulard P, Agay MFD et al: Primary thrombocythemia associated with systemic mastocytosis: a report of five cases. Br J Haematol 79: 84, 1991

58. Kessler CM, Klein HG, Havlik RJ: Uncontrolled thrombocytosis in chronic myeloproliferative disorders. Br J Haematol 50:157, 1982

59. Schafer AI: Bleeding and thrombosis in myeloproliferative disorders. Blood 64:1, 1984

60. Mitus AJ, Barbui T, Shulman LN et al: Hemostatic complications in young patients with essential thrombocythemia. Am J Med 88:371, 1990

61. Randi ML, Fabris F, Girolami A: Thrombocytosis in young people: evaluation of 57 cases diagnosed before the age of 40. Blut 60:233, 1990

62. Jabaily J, Iland HJ, Laszlo J et al: Neurologic manifestations of essential thrombocythemia. Ann Intern Med 99:513, 1983

63. Michiels JJ, Abels J, Stekette J et al: Erythromelalgia caused by platelet-mediated arteriolar inflammation and thrombosis. Ann Intern Med 102:466, 1985

64. Kurzrock R, Cohen P: Erythromelalgia and myeloproliferative disorders. Arch Intern Med 149:105, 1989

65. Preston FE, Martin JF, Stewart RM, Davies-Jones GAB: Thrombocytosis, circulating platelet aggregates and neurological dysfunction. Br Med J 2:1561, 1979

66. Preston FE, Emmanuel IG, Winfield DA, Malia RG: Essential thrombocythemia and peripheral gangrene. Br Med J 3:548, 1974

67. Salem HH, Van Der Weyden MB, Kouts J, Firkin BG: Leg pain and platelet aggregates in thrombocythemia myeloproliferative disease. JAMA 244:1122, 1980

68. McDonald E, Marino C, Raftery T, Levine M: Gangrene of the fingers secondary to myeloproliferative disease. Postgrad Med 90:115, 1991

69. Michiels JJ, Tenkate FWJ, Vuzevski VD, Abels J: Histopathology of erythromelalgia in thrombocythemia. Histopathology 8:669, 1984

70. Michiels JJ, Tenkate FWJ: Erythromelalgia in thrombocythemia of various myeloproliferative disorders. Am J Hematol 39:131, 1992

71. Hussain S, Schwartz JM, Friedman SA, Chua SN: Arterial thrombosis in essential thrombocythemia. Am Heart J 96:31, 1978

72. Buss DH, Stuart JJ, Lipscomb GE: The incidence of thrombotic and hemorrhagic disorders in association with extreme thrombocytosis. An analysis of 129 cases. Am J Hematol 20:36, 1985

73. Spaet TH, Lejnieks I, Gaynor E, Goldstein ML: Defective platelets in essential thrombocythemia. Arch Intern Med 124:135, 1969

74. Ginsburg AD: Platelet function in patients with high platelet counts. Ann Intern Med 82:506, 1975

75. Wu KKY: Platelet hyperaggregability and thrombosis in patients with thrombocythemia. Ann Intern Med 88:7, 1978

76. Zucker S, Mielke CH: Classification of thrombocytosis based on platelet function tests: correlation with hemorrhagic and thrombotic complications. J Lab Clin Med 80:385, 1972

77. Weinfeld A, Branehog I, Kutti J: Platelets in the myeloproliferative syndrome. Clin Hematol 4:373, 1975

78. Cooper B, Schafer AI, Puchalsky D, Handin RI: Platelet resistance to prostaglandin D_2 in patients with myeloproliferative disorders. Blood 52:618, 1978

79. Kaywin P, McDonough M, Inset PA, Shattil SJ: Platelet function in essential thrombocythemia: decreased epinephrine responsiveness associated with platelet adrenergic receptors. N Engl J Med 299:505, 1978

80. Bolin RB, Okumura T, Jamieson GA: Changes in distribution of platelet membrane glycoproteins in patients with myeloproliferative disorders. Am J Hematol 3:63, 1977

81. Okuma M, Uchino H: Altered arachidonate metabolism by platelets in patients with myeloproliferative disorders. Blood 54:12, 1979

82. Schafer AI: Deficiency of platelet lipoxygenase activity in myeloproliferative disorders. N Engl J Med 306:381, 1981

83. Moore A, Nachman RL: Platelet Fc receptor: increased expression in myeloproliferative disorders. J Clin Invest 67:1064, 1981

84. Boughton BJ, Allington MJ, King A: Platelet and plasma B thromboglobulin in myeloproliferative syndromes and secondary thrombocytosis. Br J Haematol 40:125, 1978

85. Cortelazzo S, Viero P, Barbui T: Platelet activation in myeloproliferative disorders. Thromb Haemost 45:211, 1981

86. Zahavi J, Zahavi M, Firsteter E et al: An abnormal pattern of multiple platelet function abnormalities and increased thromboxane generation in patients with primary thrombocytosis and thrombotic complications. Eur J Haematol 47:326, 1991

87. Landolfi R, DeCristofaro R, Castagnola M et al: Increased platelet-fibrinogen affinity in patients with myeloproliferative disorders. Blood 71:978, 1988

88. Fabris F, Casoneti A, Del-Ben MG et al: Abnormalities of Von Willebrand factor in myeloproliferative disease: a relationship with bleeding diathesis. Br J Haematol 63:75, 1986

89. Pareti FI, Gugliotta L, Mannucci L et al: Biochemical and metabolic aspects of platelet dysfunction in chronic myeloproliferative disorders. Scand J Haematol 25:214, 1982

90. Carnobe C, Sie P, Nouvel C et al: Platelets in myeloproliferative disorders: serotonin uptake and storage correlates with mepacrine labelled dense bodies and with platelet dense bodies. Scand J Haematol 25:289, 1980

91. Michiels JJ, Lindemans J, Van Vliet HHDM, Abels J: Survival kinetics of platelets and fibrinogen in thrombocythemia related to erythromelalgia. Br J Haematol 50:691, 1982

92. Valle D, Casadevall N, Lacombe C et al: Primary myeloproliferative disorders and hepatic vein thrombosis: a prospective study of erythroid colony formation in vitro in 20 patients with Budd Chiari syndrome. Ann Intern Med 103: 320, 1985

93. Welford C, Spie SM, Green D: Priapism in primary thrombocythemia. Arch Intern Med 141:807, 1981

94. Barr I, Cohen P, Berken A, Lown B: Thrombocythemia and myocardial ischemia with normal coronary angiogram. Arch Intern Med 134:528, 1974

95. Virmani R, Popousky MA, Roberts WC: Thrombocytosis, coronary thrombosis and acute myocardial infarction. Am J Med 67:498, 1979

96. Reisner SA, Rinkivich D, Markiewicz W et al: Cardiac involvement in myeloproliferative disorders. Am J Cardiol 93:498, 1993

97. Nicolau IB, Zurita JMC, Gusman AB et al: Essential thrombocytosis with acute renal failure due to bilateral thrombosis of the renal arteries and veins. Nephron 32:73, 1982

98. Ravich RBM, Gunz FW, Reis CS, Thompson IL: The dangers of surgery in uncontrolled haemorrhagic thrombocytosis. Med J Aust 1:704, 1970

99. Randi ML, Stocco F, Rossi C et al: Thrombosis and hemostasis in thrombocytosis: evaluation of a large cohort of patients (357 cases). J Med 22:213, 1991

100. Watson KV, Key N: Vascular complications of essential thrombocythemia: a link to cardiovascular risk factors. Br J Haematol 83:198, 1993

101. Marsh GW, Lewis SM, Szur L: The use of ^{51}Cr-labelled heat damaged red cells to study splenic function. Br J Haematol 12:167, 1966

102. Cervantes F, Marti JM, Guillermo AL et al: Iron stores in essential thrombocythemia. Blut 58:291, 1989

103. Hartmann RC, Auditore JV, Jackson DP: Studies on thrombocytosis in hyperkalemia due to release of potassium from platelets during coagulation. J Clin Invest 37:699, 1958

104. Hess CE, Nichols AB, Suratt PM: Pseudohypoxemia secondary to leukemia and thrombocytosis. Med Intell 301:361, 1979

105. Third International Workshop on Chromosomes in Leukemia 1980: Report on essential thrombocythemia. Cancer Genet Cytogenet 4:138, 1981

106. Morris CM, Fitzgerald PH, Hollings PE et al: Essential thrombocythemia and the Philadelphia chromosome. Br J Haematol 70:13, 1988

107. Stoll DB, Peterson P, Exten R et al: Clinical presentation and natural history of patients with essential thrombocythemia and the Philadelphia chromosome. Am J Hematol 27:77, 1988

108. Knuutila S, Ruutu T, Partanen S, Vuopio P: Chromosome 1q$^+$ in erythroid and granulocyte-monocyte precursors in a patient with essential thrombocythemia. Cancer Genet Cytogenet 9:245, 1983

109. Petet P, Vanden Berghe H: A chromosomal abnormality (21q$^-$) in primary thrombocytosis. Hum Genet 50:105, 1979

110. Zaccaria A, Baccurani M, Gugliotta L et al: 21q$^-$ in primary thrombocythemia. Haematologia (Budap) 63:337, 1978

111. Woodliff HJ, Onesti P, Dougan L: Karyotypes in thrombocythemia. Lancet 1:114, 1967

112. Zaccaria A, Tura S: A chromosomal abnormality in primary thrombocythemia. N Engl J Med 298:1422, 1978

113. Swolin B, Weinfeld A, Ridell B et al: On the 5q$^-$ deletion, clinical and cytogenetic observations in ten patients and review of the literature. Blood 58: 986, 1981

114. Kushner JP, Lee GR, Wintrobe MM, Cartwright GE: Idiopathic refractory sideroblastic anemia: clinical and laboratory investigation of 17 patients and review of the literature. Medicine 50:139, 1971

115. Schilling RF: Platelet millionaires. Lancet 2:372, 1980

116. Boxer MA, Braun J, Ellman L: Thromboembolic risk of post splenectomy thrombocytosis. Arch Surg 113:808, 1978.

116a.Jones MJ, Pierre RV: The causes of extreme thrombocytosis. Am J Clin Pathol 76:349, 1981

117. Dudley JM, Messinerzy M, Eridani S et al: Primary thrombocythemia: diagnostic criteria and a simple scoring system for positive diagnosis. Br J Haematol 71:331, 1989

118. Iland HJ, Laszlo J, Case DC Jr: Differentiation between essential thrombocythemia and polycythemia vera with marked thrombocytosis. Am J Hematol 25:191, 1987

119. Waweru F, Lewis SM: Blood volume, erythrokinetics and spleen function in thrombocythemia. Acta Haematol 73:219, 1985

120. Fabris F, Randi M, Shrojavacca R et al: The possible value of platelet aggregation in patients with increased platelet numbers. Blut 43:279, 1981

121. Vogelstein B, Fearson ER, Hamilton SR et al: Clonal analysis using recombinant DNA probes for the X chromosome. Cancer Res 47:4806, 1987

122. Vander Lelie J, von dem Borne AEGR: Platelet volume analyses for differential diagnosis of thrombocytosis. J Clin Pathol 39:129, 1986

123. Messinezy M, Chapman R, Dudley JM et al: Use of splenic volume estimation to distinguish primary thrombocythaemias from reactive thrombocytosis. Eur J Haematol 40:339, 1988

124. Greenberg BR, Watson-Williams EJ: Successful control of life-threatening thrombocytosis with a blood processor. Transfusion 15:620, 1975

125. Panlilio AL, Reiss RF: Therapeutic plateletpheresis in thrombocythemia. Transfusion 19:147, 1979

126. Taft EG, Babcock RB, Scharfman WB, Tartaglia AP: Plateletpheresis in the management of thrombocytosis. Blood 50:927, 1977

127. Goldfinger D, Kurz L, Lowe C et al: Failure of long term plateletpheresis to control primary thrombocytosis. Transfusion 18:382, 1978

128. Hoagland HC, Perry MC: Thrombocythemia (thrombocytosis). JAMA 235:2330, 1976

129. Van de Pette EW, Prochazka AV, Pearson TC et al: Primary thrombocythemia treated with busulphan. Br J Haematol 62:229, 1986

130. Shamasunder HK, Gregory SA, Knopse WH: Uracil mustard for the treatment of thrombocytosis. JAMA 244:1454, 1980

131. Brusamolino E, Canevari A, Salvaneschi L et al: Efficacy of pipobroman in essential thrombocythemia. A study of 24 patients. Cancer Treat Rep 68:1339, 1984

132. Murphy S, Rosenthal DS, Weinfeld A et al: Essential thrombocythemia: response during first year of therapy with melphalan and radioactive phosphorus: a Polycythemia Vera Study Group report. Cancer Treat Rep 66:1495, 1982

133. Case DC Jr: Therapy of essential thrombocythemia with thiotepa and chlorambucil. Blood 63:51, 1984

134. Bensinger TA, Logue GL, Rendler RW: Hemorrhagic thrombocythemia: control of postsplenectomy thrombocytosis with melphalan. Blood 36:61, 1970

135. Lofunberg E, Wahlin A: Management of polycythaemia vera, essential thrombocythemia and myelofibrosis with hydroxyurea. Eur J Haematol 41:375, 1988

136. Leoni F, Grossi A, Ferrini PR: 1-(2-Chloroethyl)-cyclohexyl-nitrosourea induced remission in essential thrombocythemia. Acta Haematol 69:180, 1983

137. Sieber SM, Adamson RH: Toxicity of antineoplastic agents in man: chromosomal aberrations, antifertility effects, congenital malformations and carcinogenic potential. Adv Cancer Res 22:57, 1975

138. Berk PD, Goldberg JD, Silverstein MN et al: Increased incidence of acute leukemia in polycythemia vera associated with chlorambucil therapy. N Engl J Med 304:441, 1981

139. Lazzarino M, Vitale A, Morra E et al: Interferon alpha 2b as treatment for Philadelphia-negative myeloproliferative disorders with excessive thrombocytosis. Br J Haematol 72:173, 1989

140. Gugliotta L, Macchi S, Catani L et al: Recombinant alpha 2a interferon (alpha IFN) in the treatment of essential thrombocythemia: preliminary report. Haematologia (Budap) 72:277, 1987

141. Giles FJ, Singer CRJ, Gray AG et al: Alpha interferon for essential thrombocythemia. Lancet 2:70, 1988

142. Talpaz M, Kurzock R, Kantarzian H et al: Recombinant interferon-alpha therapy of Philadelphia chromosome negative myeloproliferative disorders with thrombocytosis. Am J Med 86:554, 1989

143. Middlehoff G, Boll I: A long term clinical trial of interferon-alpha therapy in essential thrombocythemia. Ann Hematol 64:207, 1992

144. Silverstein MN, Petitt RM, Solberg LA Jr: Anagrelide: a new drug for treating thrombocytosis. N Engl J Med 318:1292, 1988

145. Silverstein MN, the Anegrelide Study Group: Anagrelide, a therapy for thrombocythemic states: experience in 577 patients. Am J Med 92:69, 1992

146. Chintagumpala MM, Steuber P, Mahoney DH et al: Essential thrombocythemia in a child: management with anegrelide. Am J Pediatr Hematol Oncol 13:52, 1991

147. Beard J, Hillmen P, Anderson CC et al: Primary thrombocythemia in pregnancy. Br J Haematol 77:371, 1991

148. Frei-Lahr D, Barton JC, Hoffman R et al: Blastic transformation of essential thrombocythemia: dual expression of myelomonoblastic/megakaryoblastic phenotypes. Blood 63:866, 1984

149. Geller SA, Shapiro E: Acute leukemia as a natural sequel to primary thrombocythemia. Am J Clin Pathol 77:353, 1982

150. Toh BT, Gregory SA, Knopse WH: Acute leukemia following treatment of polycythemia vera and essential thrombocythemia with uracil mustard. Am J Hematol 28:58, 1988

151. Sedlacek SM, Curtis JL, Weintraub J, Levin J: Essential thrombocythemia and leukemic transformation. Medicine 65:353, 1986

152. Reiffers J, Dachary D, David B: Megakaryoblastic transformation of primary thrombocythemia. Acta Haematol 73:228, 1985

153. Rozman C, Giralt M, Feliu E et al: Life expectancy of patients with chronic non-leukemic myeloproliferative disorders. Cancer 67:2658, 1991

Myelodysplastic Syndromes and Myeloproliferative Syndromes in Children

76

Cindy L. Schwartz

INTRODUCTION

Myelodysplastic syndromes (MDS) and myeloproliferative syndromes (MPS) are clonal disorders observed only rarely during the childhood years. Unlike acute leukemia, in which abnormalities of both proliferation and differentiation are apparent at diagnosis, MDS and MPS are characterized by abnormalities of differentiation and proliferation, respectively. The propensity of patients with these disorders eventually to develop acute leukemia, with abnormalities of both proliferation and differentiation, suggests that an MPS or MDS represents an initial step in the process of leukemogenesis.

MYELODYSPLASTIC SYNDROMES

MDSs are characterized by ineffective hematopoiesis (peripheral cytopenias with a hypercellular bone marrow) and morphologic evidence of abnormal differentiation in at least one, and often multiple, cell lines. The likelihood that a patient with an MDS will develop acute myeloid leukemia (AML) accounts for the commonly used terms *preleukemia* and *smouldering leukemia*. Although MDSs occur most often in adults, 6 of 37 children with AML had an MDS prior to diagnosis. Thus, MDSs may precede AML in children as often as in adults.[1]

Five types of MDS are described in the 1982 French-American-British classification.[2] Children, however, usually present with refractory anemia with an excess of blasts (RAEB) or with RAEB in transformation (RAEBt). Although the other forms of MDS seen in adults may progress at a variable rate to AML, the two forms seen in childhood, RAEB and RAEBt, progress rapidly to AML. The main features of RAEB and RAEBt are anemia and an excessive number of blasts in the marrow. MDSs and AML have similar abnormalities of differentiation, but the proliferative abnormality is less apparent in MDSs.

Biologic and Molecular Aspects

Cells of multiple hematopoietic lineage are involved in MDSs, and chromosomal abnormalities have been noted in 50–60% of such patients.[3] Deletions of chromosome 5 or 7 are often found in adults, particularly those treated with cytotoxic therapies or exposed to toxins (petroleum solvents, pesticides, or industrial materials).[4,5,6] Trisomy 8 also occurs frequently in adults. Complex chromosomal aberrations in MDSs have been associated with rapid progression to AML and poor prognosis. In one review, 7 of 16 children in whom chromosome studies were performed had detectable chromosomal abnormalities.[7] Children with an MDS and monosomy 7 often appear to have features of an MPS initially. However, at the time of their leukemic conversion, they may be clinically indistinguishable from patients with an MDS only.

Assays of hematopoietic progenitor cells, performed in vitro with marrow cells from patients with RAEB and RAEBt, are characterized by increased numbers of abortive clusters of myeloid cells exhibiting defective maturation similar to that found in AML.[8] Hematopoietic colonies cloned from MDS colony-forming unit-granulocyte/macrophage (CFU-GM) and burst-forming unit-erythroid (BFU-E) are often morphologically normal, but decreased in numbers.[8,9] The proliferative abnormality of acute leukemia results in expansion of an abnormal clone at the expense of normal cells. In the MDSs, normal and abnormal cells may coexist for a prolonged period.[10] The abnormal hematopoiesis of MDSs may reflect the growth pattern of the abnormal clone itself or its effect on normal progenitors, perhaps mediated by inhibitors of hematopoiesis. Leukemic proliferation in a patient with an MDS may result from a karyotypic change in the original clone or from a subclone of malignant cells, which slowly predominates.

Clinical Manifestations

In contrast to adults, who are often asymptomatic initially, most children with an MDS are symptomatic. Fever, pallor, hemorrhage, and infection are most frequently seen.[1,11] Except in children with monosomy 7, hepatosplenomegaly is not common.[7,12] Macrocytic anemia and pancytopenia are classically found in adults with an MDS. Children, however, may present with a normocytic normochromic anemia,[1] with macrocytosis and ovalocytosis appearing later, followed by poikilocytosis and anisocytosis. Nucleated red blood cells (RBCs) and a low reticulocyte count may be seen. White blood cell (WBC) changes, including Pelger-Hüet abnormalities, hypersegmentation, and hypogranularity, may be subtle. Peripheral blasts may be seen with a normal marrow examination and hypogranular platelets are noted.

The marrow of patients with an MDS is often hypercellular, which is indicative of ineffective hematopoiesis. Megaloblastoid changes of erythroid and myeloid precursors are common. Decreased numbers of megakaryocytes have been reported in children,[1,13] although megakaryocytes are often increased in adults. Auer rods were present in 12 of 21 children in one study.[1]

Vitamin B_{12} levels were increased in six children tested in one study.[1] In another study, three of nine children had decreased leukocyte alkaline phosphatase activity.[8] Other neutrophil abnormalities noted in adults include decreased myeloperoxidase activity, defective chemotaxis, and phagocytosis, and diminished bactericidal activity.[14] RBC abnormalities include decreased RBC enzymatic activity, abnormal iron metabolism, increased fetal hemoglobin levels, and abnormal expression of RBC antigens.[13,15,16]

Differential Diagnosis

MDS is characterized by the presence of anemia with or without other cytopenias and a hypercellular dyserythropoietic marrow. The high likelihood of leukemic transformation in children with classic presentations of MDS, justifies the use of the term *preleukemia*. Two forms of preleukemia occur commonly in children: pre-AML and pre-acute lymphocytic leukemia (pre-ALL) (Table 76-1). As in the acute leukemias, the age frequency of pre-AML is approximately constant throughout the childhood period, while pre-ALL appears most often in children aged 1–6 years. Symptoms and peripheral blood findings may be similar, but the marrow findings usually differ, marrow hypoplasia being more common in pre-ALL. Although ineffective erythropoiesis and myelopoiesis may occur in either, ineffec-

Table 76-1. Preleukemia in Childhood

	Pre-AML	Pre-ALL
Patient population		
Sex	M > F	F > M
Age	All	1–6
Signs and symptoms		
Pallor	+	+
Fever/infection	+	+
Bleeding/bruising	+	+
Hepatosplenomegaly	+	+
Peripheral blood		
Anemia	+ +	+ +
Granulocytopenia	+	+ +
Thrombocytopenia	+	+
Morphology	Macrocytosis	Normal
	Ovalocytosis	
	Pelger-Hüet WBCs	
	Hypogranular WBCs	
	Hypogranular platelets	
Marrow		
Hypoplasia (all cell lines)	–	+
Erythroid hyperplasia	+ +	–
Myeloid hyperplasia	+	–
Megakaryocyte hyperplasia	+	–
Abnormal maturation	+	–
Chromosomes		
Detectable abnormality	+	–

Symbols: + +, >75%; +, 30–75%; +/–, 15–30%; –, <15%.

tive megakaryopoiesis is unique to pre-AML. The morphology of marrow precursor cells is abnormal in pre-AML and normal in pre-ALL, while karyotypic abnormalities are common in pre-AML and rare in pre-ALL.[11]

A review of 760 pediatric marrow samples identified seven children with hematopoietic dysplasia,[17] of whom one died of hemorrhage and four, including two with family histories of childhood leukemia, developed AML. One child suffered from Shwachman syndrome, which has a known association with hematopoietic dysplasia and progression to AML.[18] Six of the seven children had constitutional abnormalities, including skin abnormalities (five), short stature (four), unusual facies (four), mental retardation (three), and endocrinopathy (two). One otherwise normal child had a hydrocele. The incidence of leukemia is also increased in other constitutional disorders with hematologic manifestations, including Kostmann's agranulocytosis, Down syndrome, Bloom syndrome, Diamond-Blackfan syndrome, and Fanconi's anemia.[13,19]

Therapy and Prognosis

MDS of childhood is rapidly progressive; children rarely die of unrelated causes. Of 26 children with MDS, 23 developed overt leukemia, and 3 died in a preleukemic state.[7] The median preleukemic phase in children is short, lasting 12 months. The rapidity of disease progression necessitates consideration of therapeutic options beyond supportive care.

One approach uses maturational therapies, which attempt to cause differentiation of abnormal cells into normally functional cells. Agents used include low-dose cytosine arabinoside (which may actually exert its effect via cytotoxic clonal suppression), retinoic acid, and vitamin D_3. In general, these therapies have been disappointing. Hematopoiesis improved temporarily (3–27 months) in one-half of patients treated with low-dose cytosine arabinoside, but hospitalizations increased and survival was unchanged.[20,21] Retinoic acid was found to enhance in vitro CFU-GM and BFU-E cloning efficiency. The granulocyte count improved in some patients, but transfusion requirements were unchanged.[22] Although modification of the preleukemic disorder by induction of normal cellular maturation would be ideal, the means of doing so are currently inadequate. However, a recent phase II clinical trial of hexamethylene bisacetamide (a potent inducer of differentiation in vitro) in 41 patients with MDS resulted in 3 complete responses and 6 partial responses.[23]

A second approach is to employ chemotherapeutic regimens similar to those used for AML. Treatment with aggressive chemotherapy has been relatively unsuccessful in adult MDS patients, since periods of bone marrow aplasia are prolonged and responses limited.[24] Better remission rates have been noted in younger patients.[25,26] Of 11 children with MDS treated with intensive chemotherapy, 6 achieved complete remission, and 2 of these remained in complete remission at 48 and 69 months (i.e., 18% survived for >2 years).[12] Allogeneic bone marrow transplantation (BMT) from an HLA-matched sibling has resulted in long-term survival of 40–80% of patients[27–29] and is the preferred therapy, when feasible. Long-term survival with nonrelated allogeneic BMT has not yet been documented.[30]

The use of biologic response modifiers such as colony-stimulating factor-granulocyte/macrophage (CSF-GM) and the interferons (IFNs) are being studied in patients with MDS in the hope of affecting the control mechanisms that regulate hematopoiesis.[31–37] Phase I/II studies of these agents have shown definitive improvement in neutrophil counts in most patients, with occasional improvement in platelet counts and hemoglobin levels. Such studies are now in their infancy, and their role in the treatment of MDS remains unclear.

MYELOPROLIFERATIVE SYNDROMES

Classic MPSs, including adult-type chronic myeloid leukemia (ACML), polycythemia vera (PV), essential thrombocythemia (ET), and agnogenic myeloid metaplasia with myelofibrosis (AMMM), are disorders that were initially thought to be "pure" proliferations of granulocytes, RBCs, platelets, and fibroblasts, respectively. In 1951 they were grouped as MPSs by Dameshek, who noted that, to variable degrees, stimulation of all hematopoietic cell lineages occurs frequently in these disorders.[38] These syndromes are now known to be clonal disorders, with aberrant regulatory control of hematopoietic precursors causing excessive proliferation.[39–41]

Classic MPSs most frequently occur in adults, but MPSs unique to childhood also exist. Such syndromes include juvenile CML (JCML), the MPS of monosomy 7 in childhood, familial CML, the transient MPS of infants with trisomy 21, and childhood forms of myelofibrosis. Study of the biology of these syndromes gives clues to the pathogenesis of leukemia. Biologic and clinical features of MPSs in children are discussed.

Disorders Characterized by Leukocytosis

Table 76-2 lists the salient characteristics of ACML, JCML, familial CML, and the MPS of monosomy 7.

Adult Chronic Myeloid Leukemias

Biologic and Molecular Aspects

ACML is characterized primarily by granulocytosis, often in association with thrombocytosis, marrow hyperplasia, and fibrosis. A reciprocal translocation, with breakpoints involving the *bcr* oncogene of chromosome 22 and the *abl* oncogene of chromosome 9, results in the abnormal Philadelphia chromosome, which encodes for chimeric *bcr/abl* mRNA.[42,43] Two common molecular rearrangements between the *bcr* and *abl* genes occur in adults (*mbcr* exons 2 or 3 are joined to *abl* exon II. Most children have the *mbcr* exon 2 joined to *abl* exon II.[43] The translocated chromosome 9 is usually of paternal origin, while the translocated chromosome 22 is the maternal origin.[44] The c-abl/bcr protein product is an abnormal tyrosine kinase, which may bring about the proliferative state by functioning as an abnormal growth factor or receptor.[45] Occasional patients have variant translocations that may result in the formation of a similar abnormal protein.

Clinical Manifestations

ACML accounts for 1–3% of childhood leukemia and is the most common form of CML in children.[46–48] It occurs primarily in the older child. Generalized malaise, weakness, weight loss, fever, pallor, and hepatosplenomegaly are frequently the presenting findings. Hyperleukocytosis has been found to be a more prominent feature in patients <20 years of age (median presenting WBC count 360,000/mm³) as compared with older patients (137,000/mm³),[49] resulting in an increased incidence of central nervous system, retinal, and pulmonary dysfunction. Arthritis and priapism may occur.

In addition to leukocytosis with a WBC count of >100,000/mm³ and the appearance of some immature myeloid elements, such abnormalities as thrombocytosis, erythrocytosis, eosinophilia, and basophilia may be seen. The bone marrow shows myeloid hyperplasia but normal maturation. Other abnormalities include increased vitamin B_{12} levels and decreased leukocyte alkaline phosphatase levels.

The course of ACML is variable, but ultimately blast crisis

Table 76-2. Chronic Myeloid Leukemia in Childhood

	ACML	JCML	MPS of Monosomy 7	Familial CML
Patient population				
Sex	M = F	M > F	M > F	M = F
Age	>5	<2	<2	<2
Neurofibromatous	−	+	−	−
Signs and symptoms				
Fever/infection	+	+	+ +	+
Bleeding/bruising	−	+	+	+
Splenomegaly	+ +	+ +	+ +	+ +
Lymphadenopathy	−	+	+	+
Rash	−	+	+	−
Central nervous system symptoms	+	−	−	−
Philadelphia chromosome	+ +	−	−	−
Hematology				
Anemia	+ +	+ +	+ +	+ +
Leukocytes	+ +	+ +	+ +	+ +
Leukocytosis	+	−	−	+/−
Monocytosis	−	+ +	+ +	+
Thrombocytopenia	+	−	−	−
Thrombocytosis	+	−	−	−
Fetal hemoglobin	−	+ +	+/−	+/−
Leukocyte alkaline phosphatase	+ +	+ +	+/−	+ +
Course of disease				
Blast crisis	+ +	+/−	+ +	+
Type	AML (ALL)	Peripheral erythroblasts	AML	AML
Survival	3 yr	<9 mo	1–6 yr	<2 yr or recovery

Symbols: + +, >75%; +, 30–75%; +/−, 15–30%; −, <15%.

intervenes (0–10 years, median 2–3 years),[47,50,51] at which time a florid leukemic picture develops. Such a transformation may be heralded by increased fatigue, pallor, and splenomegaly. Although the blast crisis is generally of myeloid origin, lymphoid blast crisis does occur. Responses to standard therapeutic agents are usually brief.

Therapy

The traditional therapy of ACML has been palliative, employing agents such as busulfan and hydroxyurea to lower the granulocyte count and prevent complications. More intensive chemotherapy rarely eradicates the abnormal clone, never for more than a short time. Recombinant IFN-α induces hematologic and cytogenetic remissions in CML in adults[52,53] and in children.[54] However, the *bcr/abl* rearrangement can still be detected in such patients if a sensitive assay is used.[55,56] Combination regimens (e.g., IFN-α and low-dose cytoarabine) may show improved response rates.[57] Allogeneic BMT has been used and is currently the only known curative approach.[58] Transplantation is most successful when performed during the chronic phase of the disease. Although patients may remain clinically well during the chronic phase, it is not possible to predict when blast crisis will intervene. Thus, early BMT is recommended for children with HLA-matched siblings. For those without such donors, transplantation using other closely matched family members and unrelated individuals as donors is being evaluated, but long-term results are not available.[58]

Juvenile Chronic Myeloid Leukemia

Biologic and Molecular Aspects

ACML and JCML are very different disorders, both biologically and clinically. Peripheral blood and marrow monocytosis is more characteristic of JCML. In patients with ACML, BFU-E growth is exuberant, and colony-forming unit-granulocyte (CFU-G) predominate. The blood and marrow of patients with JCML produce large numbers of assayable colony-forming unit-macrophages (CFU-Ms).[59,60] Defects in JCML considered by Estrov et al[60] to be hallmarks of the disease include (1) CFU-M growth in the absence of added growth factors and (2) inhibition of normal hematopoietic colony formation, presumably due to elaboration of a monokine by the abnormal cells.[61] These clinical and laboratory findings have led to the suggestion that JCML is most closely related to myelomonocytic leukemia. Enhanced BFU-E-derived colony formation, fetal hematopoiesis, and terminal erythroblastosis suggest that a pluripotent stem cell may be involved, at least in some JCML patients.[61]

Bagby and co-workers[62] recently examined the etiology of the spontaneous myeloid colony growth that characterizes JCML. Such spontaneous colony growth was virtually eliminated after depletion of marrow auxiliary cells.[62] This group then showed that monocytes in JCML released interleukin-1, which then induced the release of high levels of colony-stimulating activity by other cells. Interleukin-1-dependent, paracrine-stimulated granulopoiesis appears therefore to be a unique feature of JCML.[62] Emanuel et al.[63] have also suggested that the defects likely responsible for the exuberant myelomonocytic proliferation in JCML is selective hypersensitivity of hematopoietic progenitor cells to CSF-GM. These workers were unable to demonstrate any differences in CSF-GM receptor number or affinity to account for this observation and suggest that enhanced signal transduction after normal CSF-GM binding is an explanation for the observed selective CSF-GM hypersensitivity.[64,65]

The Philadelphia chromosome has not been detected in patients with JCML, although 18% of patients have other chromosomal abnormalities.[66] Monosomy 7 has been reported in a number of patients with a clinical syndrome very much like that of JCML.[67,68] The course of that disorder appears different, and these patients are probably best categorized as having a distinct MPS. However, the similarity of the disorders has resulted in a tendency to group these patients together, perhaps accounting in part for the conflicting clinical and biologic information reported.

Clinical Manifestations

Children with JCML are younger than those with ACML. Most are <2 years of age, and 95% are <4 years old.[47,50,69] At presentation, malaise, bleeding, and fever are common. Occasional patients present with cough, tachypnea, and wheezing, with an interstitial pulmonary pattern observed on chest radiography. Leukemic pulmonary infiltrates have been reported.[55] Physical examination reveals splenomegaly, pallor, hepatomegaly, and lymphadenopathy. A facial eczematoid rash may occur, particularly in patients with neurofibromatosis (which has been associated with JCML).[47,59,70–74] Biopsy reveals a leukemic infiltrate in the dermal layer. The rash may precede the diagnosis of JCML by 1 year.

Laboratory findings include thrombocytopenia, anemia, and an elevated leukocyte count (usually <100,000/mm^3) with a prominent monocytosis. Occasional blasts may be noted in the peripheral blood, but myeloid cells in all stages of development are noted. The bone marrow shows myeloid and erythroid hyperplasia with myeloid/erythroid ratios (M/E) of 2:1–5:1 (lower than in ACML).[50] Dysplastic features are not present. Other laboratory features include increased fetal hemoglobin levels and glucose-6-phosphate dehydrogenase activity levels, and decreased I antigen, carbonic anhydrase activity, and hemoglobin A$_2$, all of which are consistent with an increased number of fetal RBC. Leukocyte alkaline phosphatase activity is decreased.

JCML is associated with an acute deteriorating course, with death from bone marrow failure occurring within 9 months. Increasing myeloid blasts appear, and thrombocytopenia with progressive splenomegaly occurs terminally. An increase in pronormoblasts without evidence of leukemic marrow infiltration has been noted in some patients.[47,50] In patients with JCML in association with neurofibromatosis, deletion of the whole or part of certain chromosomes (e.g., 6, 7) may be an important step in the evolution of JCML into the accelerated or blast phase. Erythroid progenitor cells remain responsive to erythropoietin, even at this terminal erythroblastic period.[74]

Two patients have been reported with classic features of JCML who remitted spontaneously. They were found to have serologic evidence of persistent Epstein-Barr virus (EBV) infection.[73] Serologic tests should be performed to rule out an EBV infection before chemotherapy is administered. Monsomy 7 has also been noted in patients with persistent EBV infection.[75] Further biologic studies will be necessary to understand the relationship of monosomy 7 and EBV to JCML-like disorders. The association of neurofibromatosis, monosomy 7, and JCML suggests a multistep mechanism of oncogenesis.[76,77]

Therapy

Early reports suggested that agents active in ACML (e.g., busulfan) were ineffective in JCML, while 6-mercaptopurine was efficacious, although not curative.[47,48] In 1987, an intensive chemotherapeutic regimen used for the treatment of acute myelomonocytic leukemia was reported to induce complete remissions in all four children to whom it was administered.[78] However, all except one child had continued inhibition of normal hematopoietic colony formation and autonomous CFU-M-derived colony formation when marrow cells were assayed in vitro. Only the patient with normal in vitro hematopoiesis was still in remission after >32 months.[79] Recently, Emanuel et al[63] reported transient responses to cis-retinoic acid therapy in JCML.

As in myelomonocytic leukemia, more intensive regimens may be necessary to improve survival rates. Allogeneic BMT has resulted in survival of 6 of 14 children with JCML for >0.5 to >11.5 years.[80]

Myeloproliferative Disease of Monosomy 7

Biologic and Molecular Aspects

In patients with AML, monosomy 7 suggests involvement by the leukemic process of a pluripotent hematopoietic stem cell.[81] Monosomy 7 has also occurred in some patients who have been reported as having JCML involving a multilineage progenitor.[61] Since the natural history of those with monosomy 7 differs from that of other JCML patients, the MPS of monosomy 7 is considered here as a distinct disorder.

Clinical Manifestations

Patients have been reported with monosomy 7 (or a missing C chromosome in earlier studies) and with a clinical presentation similar to JCML.[67,68,75,82,83] Both syndromes present in children <2 years of age. Pallor, lymphadenopathy, hepatosplenomegaly, infection, facial rash, and petechial bleeding are frequently present. The hematologic picture is characterized by leukocytosis with a monocytosis, anemia, and thrombocytopenia. However leukocyte alkaline phosphatase activity is reduced in JCML, and hemoglobin F levels, which are increased in JCML, are variable in patients with monosomy 7. It is important to distinguish these two disorders because of their different natural histories. The course of JCML is brief, with most patients dying within 9 months. Patients with monosomy 7 often present initially with repeated bacterial infections and develop AML after a latent period of 3–6 years. Those patients with monosomy 7 who are diagnosed while their disorder is evolving to AML may appear clinically identical to patients with RAEBt or chronic myelomonocytic leukemia and may be classified as such.

Therapy

Patients with the MPS of monosomy 7 eventually develop AML. Chemotherapy has not proved effective. Allogeneic BMT remains the only means of curing such patients.

Familial Chronic Myeloid Leukemia

In 1965 Randall et al.[83] reported a large kindred of nine cousins afflicted with an MPS characterized by early onset (age 5 months to 4 years), hepatosplenomegaly, anemia, thrombocytopenia, and leukocytosis (with a monocytosis documented in some). The marrow, liver, and spleen of these patients showed marked granulocytic and slight erythroid hyperplasia. Leukocyte alkaline phosphatase levels were low in all patients tested as well as in parents and grandparents. Three of these patients died of complications, while six eventually improved (<14 years from diagnosis). Other sibling groups with JCML-like illnesses have been reported,[84,85] particularly in association with monosomy 7 (or a missing C chromosome).[86,87] Cerebellar ataxia was also noted in two families described with monosomy 7-associated JCML.[86,87] It is unclear whether these reported cases arise as a result of an undetected constitutive abnormality or as a result of an exogenous exposure. The genetic predisposition is not limited to chromosome 7.[89] Thus, a multistep mechanism involving another constitutive gene as well as loss of chromosome 7 may result in leukemia.[90] Potential marrow donors for transplantation should be examined for chromosomal abnormalities in addition to other hematologic abnormalities similar to that of their sibling.

Myeloproliferative Syndrome Associated with Trisomy 21

Newborns with trisomy 21 may present with an MPS that appears morphologically identical to AML. The WBC count may be as high as 400,000/mm^3, with peripheral myeloblasts accounting for ≤95% of the WBCs. Anemia, thrombocytopenia, hepatosplenomegaly, and skin infiltrates may be seen.[91] Spontaneous remission occurs within a few months in some of these patients, but others have a persistent leukemia. It is unclear whether the transient cases are clonal leukemic disorders or are due to nonclonal abnormalities of hematopoietic regulation, although three female neonates with Down syndrome and transient MDS have recently been shown to have clonal disorders by analysis of methylation patterns of the X chromosome by restriction fragment length polymorphism.[92]

A recent study reported 15 neonates with transient MPS, all with trisomy 21 as the only abnormality.[93] None of the initial leukemias persisted, although 1 patient later developed true leukemia at 18 months of age. At that time, trisomy 8 and another marker chromosome were present. Some patients have been reported to have chromosomal abnormalities other than trisomy 21, which were no longer detectable as the MPS resolved.[94,95] These findings are suggestive of a clonal leukemic or preleukemic disorder that remits, possibly as regulatory influences allow the normal trisomic hematopoietic cells to gain dominance over the abnormal clone. In one infant with a transient MPS, an extra chromosome C was noted in 6% of his cells.[96] This abnormal clone persisted as a minor cell line until 26 months of age, at which time leukemia appeared, and the extra chromosome was present in 93% of the cells. The extra C chromosome may have caused genetic instability, predisposing the cells to leukemic transformation. Alternatively, the clone may have been at truly leukemic line that was suppressed initially but that then expanded. Transient MPS with trisomy 21 in blast cells has occasionally been noted in phenotypically normal infants,[97] suggesting an increased proliferative potential in cells with trisomy 21.

CFU-GM assays have been performed in an attempt to determine whether the transient disorder can be differentiated from persistent leukemia.[98-101] In several children with the transient form, the CFU-GM cloning efficiency was normal. In one patient, abortive myeloid clusters were observed, a finding common in AML. This patient had a persistent leukemia. The numbers of patients who have been studied with such in vitro techniques are too few to permit routine use of hematopoietic colony assays to predict outcome. Children with this disorder should receive supportive care as long as possible to determine whether the abnormality is transient or whether the patient has a true leukemic process.

Disorders Associated with Myelofibrosis

Some characteristics of the three myelofibrosis-associated myeloproliferative disorders are listed in Table 76-3.

Agnogenic Myeloid Metaplasia with Myelofibrosis

AMMM is characterized by myelofibrosis, myeloid metaplasia (splenomegaly), and a leukoerythroblastic blood picture. AMMM is virtually unheard of in children; there is only one

Table 76-3. Myelofibrosis

	AMMM	AMF	C-AMF
Patient population			
Age	Adult	Adult	<4
Trisomy 21	−	−	+
Hepatosplenomegaly	+	−	+
Leukoerythroblastosis	+	−	+
Marrow fibrosis	+ +	+ +	+ +
Survival	10 yr (median)	<1 yr	>1 yr

Abbreviations and symbols: AMMM, agnogenic myeloid metaplasia with myelofibrosis; AMF, acute myelofibrosis in adults; C-AMF, child acute myelofibrosis; + +, >75%; +, 30–75%; +/−, 15–30%; −, <15%.

published case in which the child clearly fits the criteria for AMMM.[102]

Acute Myelofibrosis

Acute myelofibrosis (AMF) in adults presents as a rapidly fatal disorder with nonspecific symptoms of fatigue and weight loss. Splenomegaly is absent. The peripheral smear shows pancytopenia with morphologically normal cells, but the marrow shows bizarre megakaryocytes with fibrosis.[103] Unclassifiable blast cells may be present. Electron microscopic examination and platelet peroxidase assays reveal features of megakaryoblasts, suggesting that this may be a variant of acute megakaryocytic leukemia. Classic AMF is rare in childhood.[103] However, a number of children have been reported with a similar syndrome characterized by myelofibrosis, unclassifiable blast cells, and bizarre megakaryocytes.[104-110] Unlike adults with this disorder, children commonly have splenomegaly, and a leukoerythroblastic blood smear may be seen. These children are acutely ill and survival is brief. This childhood form of AMF (C-AMF) occurs most commonly in toddlers (<3 years old) with trisomy 21 (Table 76-3). Trisomy 21 is also known to be associated with acute megakaryocytic leukemia. Although marrow infiltration with leukemic blasts is less prominent, C-AMF overlaps with childhood acute megakaryocytic leukemia in clinical symptomology, marrow findings, and the population at risk.[111] Children with C-AMF treated with chemotherapeutic regimens used for AML have had prolonged remissions,[89] as did a child who received an allogeneic BMT.[104]

Congenital Myelofibrosis

Two siblings were found to have myelofibrosis and myeloid metaplasia at the ages of 7 and 8 weeks.[112] No evidence of a clonal disorder was present. A constitutional abnormality may have caused abnormal regulation of marrow fibroblast function or megakaryocytic proliferation.

Disorders Characterized by Erythrocytosis or Thrombocytosis

Polycythemia Vera

Biologic and Molecular Aspects

PV is a clonal disorder resulting in an increase in RBC mass. An increased proliferative response to erythropoietin has been noted for the colony-forming unit-erythroid (CFU-E) and the BFU-E of patients with PV,[113-115] allowing them to establish dominance over normal hematopoietic progenitor cells.

Clinical Manifestations

PV is rarely seen in children, with only 0.1% of patients <20 years of age.[116] Fewer than 20 children have been reported, and not all have clearly been documented to have PV.[117-123]

During the proliferative phase, hyperplasia of all marrow elements is present, leading to varying degrees of thrombocytosis and leukocytosis. Splenomegaly is common. When making the diagnosis of PV, one must exclude causes of relative, or spurious, polycythemia and secondary polycythemia. Erythrocytosis may cause plethora, cardiac symptoms (dyspnea and hypertension), and symptoms of disturbed cerebral circulation (dizziness and paresthesias). Thrombosis and hemorrhage are due to the combination of abnormal platelet function and thrombocytosis. Granulocytic proliferation is associated with increased histamine turnover, causing gastrointestinal symptoms and pruritus. Hyperuricemia and hypermetabolic symptoms of weakness and weight loss are common. During this phase, thrombohemorrhagic events are of greatest concern.

Table 76-4. Causes of Thrombocytosis in Children

I:	Infection/immune disorder
S:	Surgery/splenic dysfunction
T:	Trauma/thrombosis
O:	Oncologic (lymphoma, neuroblastoma, acute megakaryocytic leukemia)
P:	Pharmacologic (epinephrine, exogenous or endogenous steroids, Vinca alkaloids, leucovorin)
U:	Unclassifiable diseases (histiocytosis, sarcoid, Caffey disease)
P:	Proliferative disorders (ET, PV, ACML)
A:	Anemia (iron/vitamin E deficiency, hemolytic megaloblastic)
BLEED:	Hemmorrhage

(Data from Addiego et al.,[136] and Schwartz and Cohen.[140])

In children, serious complications have been noted, including hypersplenism, splenic infarction, hypertension, strokes, and hemorrhage.[118]

Some patients progress to the "stable phase," during which time blood counts normalize without therapy. Eventually they enter the "spent" phase of postpolycythemic myeloid metaplasia (PPMM), characterized by extensive marrow fibrosis, hepatosplenomegaly, and peripheral cytopenias.[124] Leukemia most often arises in patients with PPMM.

Therapy

Therapeutic modalities used during the proliferative phase in an attempt to decrease the incidence of thrombohemorrhagic phenomena include phlebotomy, ^{32}P, chlorambucil, and hydroxyurea.[125,126] In children, phlebotomy is recommended, since chlorambucil and ^{32}P increase the incidence of leukemia and other malignancies.[125] If the phlebotomy requirement is excessive or if thrombotic events have occurred, use of hydroxyurea, a nonalkylating myelosuppressive agent, which may be less mutagenic than chlorambucil, has been recommended.[125,126] More recently, IFN-α has been shown to decrease the need for phlebotomy.[127]

Essential Thrombocythemia

Clinical Manifestations

ET is a clonal disorder that causes thrombocytosis (Table 76-4). ET is rarely reported in children,[128,129] although a recent study claimed that 13 of 94 patients (14%) with ET were <20 years of age.[130] Approximately one-third of young patients present with thrombohemorrhagic events, including transient cerebral ischemia, peripheral vascular ischemia, deep vein thrombosis, and priapism.[130] Pruritus, splenomegaly, and hepatomegaly may occur but are less severe and less frequent in ET than in PV. Laboratory abnormalities related to the hyperproliferative hematopoietic state include elevations in granulocyte count, leukocyte alkaline phosphatase activity, vitamin B_{12}, uric acid, and cholesterol levels.[130,131] Platelet aggregation is abnormal,[128,130,132] and platelet clumps may be seen on the peripheral blood smear, with megakaryocytic hyperplasia in the marrow.

The course of ET in children is relatively benign. Of 10 children described in the literature, 1 died of leukemia after ^{32}P treatment,[129,133] and 1 developed idiopathic myelofibrosis.[134] Among adults, 80% survive >100 months, with 5 of 95 treated patients experiencing a leukemic conversion.[130] Children appear to have a more benign course than that of adults,[135,136] perhaps because they are more tolerant of thrombocytosis regardless of etiology.

Therapy

Asymptomatic children need not be treated. Treatment with hydroxyurea should be considered for those who have had thrombohemorrhagic episodes. IFN-α has been used successfully to control thrombocytosis in ET.[137] Another potentially useful agent for the treatment of thrombocytosis in ET is anagrelide.[138,139]

SUMMARY

Myeloproliferative disorders of childhood include those classic for adults (e.g., CML, PV, AMMM, and ET), as well as some unique to childhood. The increased risk of leukemic conversion in these MPSs and in the MDSs suggests that an abnormality of proliferation or differentiation may be the first in a two-step process of leukemogenesis.[140] Understanding the biologic processes involved may help improve our ability to treat these patients appropriately.[140]

REFERENCES

1. Blank J, Lange B: Preleukemia in children. J Pediatr 98:565, 1981
2. Bennett JM, Catovsky D, Daniel MT et al: Proposals for the classification of the myelodysplastic syndromes. Br J Haematol 51:189, 1982
3. Nowell PC: Cytogenetics of preleukemia. Cancer Genet Cytogenet 5:265, 1982
4. Golumb HM, Alimena G, Rowley JC et al: Correlation of occupation and karyotype in adults with acute nonlymphocytic leukemia. Blood 60:404, 1982
5. Rowley JD, Golomb HM, Vardiman JW: Nonrandom chromosome abnormalities in acute leukemia and dysmyelopoietic syndromes in patients with previously treated malignant disease. Blood 58:759, 1981
6. Toyama K, Ohyashiki K, Yoshida Y et al: Clinical implications of chromosomal abnormalities in 401 patients with myelodysplastic syndromes: a mutlicentric study in Japan. Leukemia 7:499, 1993
7. Wegelius R: Preleukaemic states in children. Scand J Haematol 36:133, 1986
8. Ruutu T, Partanen S, Lintula R et al: Erythroid and granulocyte-macrophage colony formation in myelodysplastic syndromes. Scand J Haematol 32:395, 1984
9. Chui DH, Clark BJ: Abnormal erythroid progenitor cells in human preleukemia. Blood 60:362, 1982
10. Streuli RA, Testa JR, Vardiman JW et al: Dysmyelopoietic syndrome: sequential clinical and cytogenetic studies. Blood 55:636, 1980
11. Saarinen UM, Wegelius R: Preleukemic syndrome in children. Am J Pediatr Hematol Oncol 6:127, 1984
12. Creutzig U, Cantu-Rajnoldi A, Ritter J et al: Myelodysplastic syndromes in childhood. Am J Pediatr Hematol Oncol 9:324, 1987
13. Linman JW, Bagby GC: The preleukemic syndrome (hemopoietic dysplasia). Cancer 42:854, 1978
14. Ruutu P, Ruutu T, Vuopio P et al: Function of neutrophils in preleukemia. Scand J Haematol 18:317, 1977
15. Dreyfus B, Sultan C, Rochant H et al: Anomalies of blood group antigens and erythrocyte enzymes in two types of chronic refractory anemia. Br J Haematol 16:303, 1969
16. Valentine WN, Konrad PN, Paglia DE: Dyserythropoiesis, refractory anemia, and "preleukemia": metabolic features of the erythrocytes. Blood 41:857, 1973
17. Kobrinsky NL, Nesbit ME, Ramsay NKC et al: Hematopoietic dysplasia and marrow hypocellularity in children: a preleukemic condition. J Pediatr 100:907, 1982
18. Woods WG, Roloff JS, Lukens JN et al: The occurrence of leukemia in patients with the Shwachman syndrome. J Pediatr 99:425, 1981
19. Kleihauer E: The preleukemic syndromes (hematopoietic dysplasia) in childhood. Eur J Pediatr 133:5, 1980
20. Griffin JD, Spriggs D, Wisch JS et al: Treatment of preleukemia syndromes with continuous intravenous infusion of low-dose cytosine arabinoside. J Clin Oncol 3:982, 1985
21. Koeffler HP: Myelodysplastic syndromes (preleukemia). Semin Hematol 22:284, 1986
22. Picozzi VJ, Swanson GF, Morgan R et al: 13-cis-Retinoic acid treatment for myelodysplastic syndromes. J Clin Oncol 4:589, 1986
23. Andreeff M, Stone J, Michaeli J et al: Hexamethylene bisacetamide in myelodysplastic syndrome and acute myelogenous leukemia: a phase II clinical trial with a differentiation-inducing agent. Blood 80:2604, 1992
24. Murray C, Cooper B, Kitchens LW: Remission of acute myelogenous leukemia in elderly patients with prior refractory dysmelopoietic anemia. Cancer 52:967, 1983
25. Armitage JO, Dick FR, Needleman SW, Burns CP: Effect of chemotherapy for the dysmyelopoietic syndrome. Cancer Treat Rep 65:601, 1981

26. Tricot G, Bogaerts MA: The role of aggressive chemotherapy in the treatment of the myelodysplastic syndromes. Br J Haematol 63:477, 1986
27. Deeg HJ: Marrow transplantation in preleukemia. J Natl Cancer Inst 76:1329, 1986
28. O'Donnell MR, Nademanee AP, Snyder DS et al: Bone marrow transplantation for myelodysplastic and myeloproliferative syndromes. J Clin Oncol 5:1822, 1987
29. Guinan EC, Tarbell NJ, Tantravahi R, Weinstein HJ: Bone marrow transplantation for children with myelodysplastic syndromes. Blood 73:619, 1989
30. Bunin NJ, Casper JT, Chitambar J et al: Partially matched bone marrow transplantation (BMT) using T-cell depletion in patients with myelodysplastic syndromes (MDS). Proc Am Soc Clin Oncol 7:175, 1988
31. Francis GE, Guimaraes JETE, Berney JJ et al: Synergistic interaction between differentiation inducers and DNA synthesis inhibitors: a new approach to differentiation induction in myelodysplasia and acute myeloid leukemia. Leuk Res 9:573, 1985
32. Antin JH, Smith BR, Holmes W, Rosenthal DS: Phase I/II study of recombinant human granulocyte-macrophage colony-stimulating factor in aplastic anemia and myelodysplastic syndrome. Blood 72:705, 1988
33. Blok WL, Lowenberg B, Sizoo W, den Hoed D: Disappearance of trisomy 8 after alpha-2 interferon in a patient with myelodysplastic syndrome. N Engl J Med 318:787, 1988
34. Galvani DW, Cawley JC, Nethersell A, Bottomley JM: Alpha-interferon in myelodysplasia. Br J Haematol 66:145, 1987
35. Ganser A, Seipelt G, Lindemann A, Ottman O et al: Effects of recombinant human interleukin-3 in patients with myelodysplastic syndromes. Blood 76:455, 1990
36. Gradishar W, LeBeau M, O'Laughlin R et al: Clinical and cytogenetic responses to granulocyte-macrophage colony-stimulating factor in therapy-related myelodysplasia. Blood 80:2463, 1992
37. Vadhan-Raj S, Keating M, LeMaistre A et al: Effects of recombinant human granulocyte-macrophage colony-stimulating factor in patients with myelodysplastic syndromes. N Engl J Med 317:1545, 1987
38. Dameshek W: Some speculations on the myeloproliferative syndromes, editorial. Blood 6:372, 1951
39. Adamson JW, Failkow PJ, Murphy S et al: Polycythemia vera: stem-cell and probable clonal origin of the disease. N Engl J Med 295:913, 1976
40. Fialkow RJ, Faguet GB, Jacobsen PJ et al: Evidence that essential thrombocythemia is a clonal disorder with origin in a multipotent stem cell. Blood 58:916, 1981
41. Jacobsen RJ, Salo A, Filkow PJ: Agnogenic myeloid metaplasia: a clonal proliferation of hematopoietic stem cells with secondary myelofibrosis. Blood 51:189, 1978
42. Stam K, Heisterkamp N, Grosveld G et al: Evidence of a new chimeric bcr/c-abl mRNA in patients with chronic myelocytic leukemia and the Philadelphia chromosome. N Engl J Med 313:1429, 1985
43. Shtivelman E, Lifshitz B, Gale RB, Canaani E: Fused transcript of abl and bcr genes in chronic myelogenous leukemia. Nature 315:550, 1985
44. Haas OA, Argyriou-Tirita A, Lion T: Parental origin of chromosomes involved in the translocation t(9;22). Nature 359:414, 1992
45. Konopka JB, Watanabe SM, Witte ON: An alteration of the human c-abl protein in K562 leukemia cells unmasking associated tyrosine kinase activity. Cell 37:1035, 1984
46. Cooke JV: Chronic myelogenous leukemia in children. J Pediatr 42:537, 1953
47. Hardisty RM, Speed DE, Till M: Granulocytic leukaemia in childhood. Br J Haematol 10:551, 1964
48. Reisman LE, Trujillo JM: Chronic granulocytic leukemia of childhood. J Pediatr 62:710, 1963
49. Rowe JM, Lichtman MA: Hyperleukocytosis and leukostasis: common features of childhood chronic myelogenous leukemia. Blood 63:1230, 1984
50. Smith KL, Johnson W: Classification of chronic myelocytic leukemia in children. Cancer 34:670, 1974
51. Galton DAG: Chemotherapy of chronic myelocytic leukemia. Semin Hematol 6:323, 1969
52. Talpaz M, Kantarjian HM, McCredie K et al: Hematologic remission and cytogenetic improvement induced by recombinant human interferon alpha in chronic myelogenous leukemia. N Engl J Med 314:1065, 1986
53. Talpaz M, Kantarjian HM, McCredie MB et al: Clinical investigation of human alpha interferon in chronic myelogenous leukemia. Blood 69:1280, 1987
54. Dow LW, Raimondi SC, Culbert SJ et al: Response to alpha-interferon in children with Philadelphia chromosome-positive chronic myelocytic leukemia. Cancer Clin Trials 1678, 1991
55. Opatka B, Wandl UB, Becher R et al: Minimal residual disease in patients with chronic myelogenous leukemia undergoing long-term treatment with recombinant interferon alpha-2b alone or in combination with interferon. Blood 78:2188, 1991
56. Malinge MC, Mahon FX, Delfau MG et al: Quantitative determination of the hybrid Bcr-Abl RNA in patients with chronic myelogenous leukemia under interferon therapy. Br J Haematol 82:701, 1992
57. Kantarjian HM, Keating MJ, Estey EH et al: Treatment of advanced stages of Philadelphia chromosome-positive chronic myelogenous leukemia with interferon-alpha and low-dose cytarabine. J of Clin Oncol 10:772, 1992
58. Thomas ED, Clift RA: Indications for marrow transplantation in chronic myelogenous leukemia. Blood 73:861, 1989
59. Altman AJ, Baehner RL: In vitro colony-forming characteristics of chronic granulocytic leukemia in childhood. J Pediatr 86:221, 1975
60. Estrov Z, Grunberger T, Chan HSL, Freedman MH: Juvenile chronic myelogenous leukemia: characterization of the disease using cell cultures. Blood 67:1382, 1986
61. Inoue S, Shibata T, Ravindranath Y, Gohle N: Clonal origin of erythroid cells in juvenile chronic myelogenous leukemia. Blood 68:975, 1987
62. Bagby GC Jr, Dinarello CA, Neerhout RC et al: Interleukin-1 dependent paracrine granulopoiesis in chronic granulocytic leukemia of the juvenile type. J Clin Invest 82:1430, 1989
63. Emanuel PN, Bates LJ, Castleberry RP et al: Selective hypersensitivity to granulocyte-macrophage colony-stimulating factor by juvenile chronic myeloid leukemia hematopoietic progenitors. Blood 77:925, 1991
64. Castleberry RP, Emanuel PN, Gaultieri R et al: Preliminary experiences with 13-cis retinoic acid in the treatment of juvenile chronic myelogenous leukemia (JCML). Blood, suppl 1. 78:17a, 1991
65. Emanuel PN, Peiper SC, Worth CA et al: Fluorescence-labelled cytokine analysis of GM-CSF receptors in juvenile chronic myelogenous leukemia. Blood, suppl 1. 78:12a, 1991
66. Brodeur GM, Dow LW, Williams DL: Cytogenetic features of juvenile chronic myelogenous leukemia. Blood 53:812, 1979
67. Sieff CA, Chessellis JM, Harvey BAM et al: Monosomy 7 in childhood: a myeloproliferative disorder. Am J Hematol 49:235, 1981
68. Gyger M, Bonny Y, Forest L: Childhood monosomy 7 syndrome. Am J Hematol 13:329, 1982
69. Castro-Malaspina H, Schaison G, Passe S et al: Subacute and chronic myelomonocytic leukemia in children (juvenile CML). Cancer 54:675, 1984
70. Mays JA, Neerhoust RC, Bagby GC, Koler RD: Juvenile chronic granulocytic leukemia. Am J Dis Child 134:654, 1980
71. Clark RD, Hutter JJ: Familial neurofibromatosis and juvenile chronic myelogenous leukemia. Hum Genet 60:230, 1982
72. Heskel NS, White CR, Fryberger S et al: Aleukemic leukemia cutis: juvenile chronic granulocytic leukemia presenting with figurate cutaneous lesions. J Am Acad Dermatol 9:423, 1983
73. Herrod HG, Dow LW, Sullivan JL: Persistent Epstein-Barr virus infection mimicking juvenile chronic myelogenous leukemia: immunologic and hematologic studies. Blood 61:1098, 1983
74. Hoffman R, Zanjani ED: Erythropoietin dependent erythropoiesis during the erythroblastic phase of juvenile chronic granulocytic leukaemia. Br J Haematol 38:511, 1978
75. Stollmann B, Fonatsch C, Havers W: Persistent Epstein-Barr virus infection associated with monosomy 7 or chromosome 3 abnormality in childhood myeloproliferative disorders. Br J Haematol 60:183, 1985
76. Kaneko Y, Maseki N, Sakarai M et al: Chromosome pattern in juvenile chronic myelogenous leukemia, myelodysplastic syndrome and acute leukemia associated with neurofibromatosis. Leukemia 3:36, 1989
77. Shannon KM, Watterson J, Johnson P et al: Monosomy 7 myeloproliferative disease in children with neurofibromatosis. Type 1: epidemiology and molecular analysis. Blood 79:1311, 1992
78. Chan HSL, Estrov Z, Weitzman SS, Freedman MH: The value of intensive combination chemotherapy for juvenile chronic myelogenous leukemia. J Clin Oncol 5:1960, 1987
79. Freedman MH, Estrov Z, Chan HSL: Juvenile chronic myelogenous leukemia. Am J Pediatr Hematol Oncol 10:261, 1988
80. Sanders JE, Buckner CD, Thomas ED et al: Allogeneic marrow transplantation for children with juvenile chronic myelogenous leukemia. Blood 71:1144, 1988
81. Sheer LC, Drysdale HC, Bevan D, Greaves MF: Monosomy 7 and multipotential stem cell transformation. Br J Haematol 61:531, 1985
82. Humbert JR, Hathaway WE, Robinson A et al: Preleukemia in children with a missing bone marrow C chromosome and a myeloproliferative disorder. Br J Haematol 21:705, 1971
83. Randall DL, Reiquam WC, Githens JH, Robinson A: Familial myeloproliferative disease. Am J Dis Child 110:479, 1965
84. Holton CP, Johnson WW: Chronic myelocytic leukemia in infant siblings. J Pediatr 72:377, 1968
85. Luddy RE, Champion LAA, Schwartz AD: A fatal myeloproliferative syn-

drome in a family with thrombocytopenia and platelet dysfunction. Cancer 41:1959, 1978

86. Li FP, Hecht F, Kaiser-McCaw B et al: Ataxia-pancytopenia: syndrome of cerebellar ataxia, hypoplastic anemia, monosomy 7, and acute myelogenous leukemia. Cancer Genet Cytogenet 4:189, 1981

87. Carroll WL, Morgan R, Glader BE: Childhood bone marrow monosomy 7 syndrome: a familial disorder? J Pediatr 107:578, 1985

88. Daghistani D, Curless R, Toledano SR, Ayyar DR: Ataxia-pancytopenia and monosomy 7 syndrome. J Pediatr 115:108, 1989

89. Shannon KM, Turhan AG, Chang SSY et al: Familial bone marrow monosomy 7. J Clin Invest 84:984, 1989

90. Gilchrist DM, Friedman JM, Rogers PCJ, Creighton SP: Myelodysplasia and leukemia syndrome with monosomy 7: a genetic perspective. Am J Med Genet 35:437, 1990

91. Weinstein HJ: Congenital leukemia and the neonatal myeloproliferative disorders associated with Down's syndrome. Clin Haematol 7:147, 1978

92. Kurahesi H, Hara J, Yumura-Yagi K et al: Monoclonal nature of transient abnormal myelopoesis in Down's syndrome. Blood 77:1161, 1991

93. Hayashi Y, Eguchi M, Sugita K et al: Cytogenetics findings and clinical features in acute leukemia and transient myeloproliferative disorder in Down's syndrome. Blood 72:15, 1988

94. Lazarus KH, Heerema NA, Palmer CG et al: The myeloproliferative reaction in a child with Down's syndrome: cytological and chromosomal evidence for a transient leukemia. Am J Hematol 11:417, 1981

95. Morgan R, Hecht F, Cleary ML et al: Leukemia with Down's syndrome: translocation between chromosomes 1 and 19 in acute myelomonocytic leukemia following transient congenital myeloproliferative syndrome. Blood 66:1466, 1985

96. Honda F, Punnett HH, Charney E et al: Serial cytogenetic and hematologic studies on mongol with trisomy-21 and acute congenital leukemia. J Pediatr 65:880, 1964

97. Broder GM, Dahl GU, William DC et al: Transient leukemoid reaction and trisomy 21 mosaicism in a phenotypically normal newborn. Blood 55:691, 1980

98. Barak Y, Mogilner BM, Karov Y et al: transient acute leukemia in a newborn with Down's syndrome. Acta Paediatr Scand 71:699, 1982

99. DeAlarcon PA, Goldberg J, Allen J: Leukemia in trisomy 21: progressive or transient? Pediatr Res 16:202A, 1982

100. Denegri JF, Rogers PCJ, Chan KW et al: In vitro cell growth in neonates with Down's syndrome and transient myeloproliferative disorders. Blood 58:6756, 1981

101. Inoue S, Ottenbreit MJ, Ravindrath Y et al: Leukemoid reaction in Down's syndrome in vitro maturation of circulating stem cells. Pediatr Res 15:579, 1981

102. Boxer LA, Camitta BM, Berenberg W et al: Myelofibrosis-myeloid metaplasia in childhood. Pediatrics 55:861, 1975

103. Lewis SM, Szur L: Malignant myelosclerosis. Br Med J 2:472, 1963

104. Brovall C, Mitchell M, Saral R et al: Acute myelofibrosis in a child. J Pediatr 103:91, 1983

105. Evans DIK: Acute myelofibrosis in children with Down's syndrome. Arch Dis Child 50:458, 1975

106. Hillman F, Forrester RM: Myelofibrosis simulating acute leukemia in a female infant with Down's syndrome. Ir J Med Sci 1:167, 1968

107. Okada H, Liu PI, Hoskino T et al: Down's syndrome associated with a myeloproliferative disorder. Am J Dis Child 124:107, 1972

108. Rosenberg HS, Taylor FM: The myeloproliferative syndrome in children. J Pediatr 52:407, 1958

109. Ueda K, Kawaguchi Y, Kodama M et al: Primary myelofibrosis with myeloid metaplasia and cytogenetically abnormal clones in 2 children with Down's syndrome. Scand J Haematol 27:152, 1981

110. Wood EE, Andrews CT: Subacute myelosclerosis. Lancet 2:739, 1949

111. Cairney AEL, McKenna R, Arthur DC et al: Acute megakaryoblastic leukemia in children. Br J Haematol 63:541, 1986

112. Sieff CA, Malleson P: Familial myelofibrosis. Arch Dis Child 55:888, 1980

113. Fauser AA, Messner HA: Pluripotent hematopoietic progenitors (CFU-GEMM) in polycythemia vera: analysis of erythropoietin requirement and proliferative activity. Blood 58:1224, 1981

114. Golde DW, Cline MJ: Erthropoietin responsiveness in polycythemia vera. Br J Haematol 29:567, 1975

115. Zanjani ED, Lutton JD, Hoffman R et al: Erythroid colony formation by polycythemia vera bone marrow in vitro. J Clin Invest 59:841, 1977

116. Berlin NI: Diagnosis and classification of the polycythemias. Semin Hematol 12:339, 1975

117. Aggeler PM, Pollycove M, Hoag S et al: Polycythemia vera in childhood. Studies of iron kinetics with Fe^{59} and blood clotting factors. Blood 17:345, 1961

118. Danish EH, Rasch CA, Harris JW: Polycythemia vera in childhood: case report and review of the literature. Am J Hematol 9:421, 1980

119. Dykstra OH, Halbertsma T: Polycythemia vera in childhood. Am J Dis Child 60:907, 1940

120. Hann HWL, Festa RS, Rosenstock JS et al: Polycythemia vera in a child with acute lymphocytic leukemia. Cancer 43:1962, 1979

121. Heilmann E, Klein CE, Beck JD: Primary polycythemia in childhood and adolescence. Folia Haematol (Leipz) 110:935, 1983

122. Marlow AA, Fairbanks VF: Polycythemia vera in an eleven-year-old girl. N Engl J Med 263:950, 1960

123. Natelson EA, Lynch EC, Britton HA et al: Polycythemia vera in childhood. Am J Dis Child 122:241, 1971

124. Silverstein MN: Postpolycythemia myeloid metaplasia. Arch Intern Med 134:113, 1974

125. Berk PD, Goldberg JC, Donovan PB et al: Therapeutic recommendations in polycythemia vera based on polycythemia vera study group protocols. Semin Hematol 23:132, 1986

126. Kaplan ME, Mack K, Goldberg JD et al: Long term management of polycythemia vera with hydroxyurea in a progress report. Semin Hematol 23:167, 1986

127. Silver RT: A new treatment for polycythemia vera: recombinant interferon alpha. Blood 76:664, 1990

128. Linch DC, Hutton R, Cowan D et al: Primary thrombocythemia in childhood. Scand J Haematol 28:72, 1982

129. Sceats DJ, Baitlon D: Primary thrombocythemia in a child. Clin Pediatr 19:298, 1980

130. Bellucci S, Janvier M, Tobelem G et al: Essential thrombocythemias. Cancer 58:2440, 1986

131. Murphy S, Iland H, Rosenthal D et al: Essential thrombocytopenia: an interim report from the polycythemia vera study group. Semin Hematol 23:177, 1986

132. Kaplan ME, Mack K, Goldberg JD et al: Platelet function in essential thrombocythemia. N Engl J Med 299:505, 1978

133. Ozer FL, Truax WE, Miesch DC et al: Primary hemorrhagic thrombocythemia. Am J Med 28:807, 1960

134. Amato D, Freedman MH: Editorial correspondence. Eleven-year follow-up of "primary thrombocythemia" in a child. J Pediatr 107:650, 1985

135. Hoagland HC, Silverstein MN: Primary thrombocythemia in the young patient. Mayo Clin Proc 53:578, 1978

136. Addiego JE, Mentzer WB, Dallman PR: Thrombocytosis in infants and children. J Pediatr 805, 1974

137. Giles FJ, Singer CRJ, Gray AG et al: Alpha-interferon therapy for essential thrombocythemia. Lancet 2:70, 1988

138. Silverstein MN, Petitt RM, Solberg LA et al: Anagrelide: a new drug for treating thrombocytosis. N Engl J Med 318:1292, 1988

139. Chintagumpala MM, Steuber P, Mahoney D et al: Essential thrombocythemia in a child: management with anagrelide. Am J Pediatr Hematol Oncol 13:52, 1991

140. Schwartz CL, Cohen HJ: Preleukemia syndromes and other syndromes predisposing to leukemia. Pediatr Clin North Am 85:853, 1988

Pathobiology of Lymphoproliferative Disease

77

Nancy Berliner and Brian R. Smith

LYMPHOCYTE DEVELOPMENT AND MALIGNANT TRANSFORMATION

The development of the normal lymphocyte immune repertoire depends on an orderly series of preprogrammed genetic maturational events that transform a differentiating totipotent hematopoietic stem cell into functional B and T lymphocytes. In the case of B cells, this maturation process occurs in the bone marrow (the human equivalent of the bursa of Fabricius), while T cells undergo the development of antigen specificity, tolerance, and immune competence under the predominant influence of the thymus.[1-7] In contrast to B- and T-cell development, the precise cell of origin and early events in maturation of the natural killer (NK) lymphocyte system remain a relative mystery.[8] Nevertheless, the different stages in normal development for B, T, and NK cells can be recognized by characteristic genetic changes and by the expression of particular cellular proteins (both intracellular and surface membrane), which in turn give rise to the particular functional attributes of the cell at each stage of differentiation. This orderly sequence of maturation events is illustrated in Figure 77-1.

In line with the remarkable diversity of response to non-self-antigens that is characteristic of the immune system, lymphocyte ontogeny differs from models of maturation in other tissues (including myeloid and erythroid maturation) in that this developmental process must give rise not only to different maturational states of the same cell but also to a large number of different clonal lymphocyte populations (as many as 10^{11}), each characterized by a different, highly specific, antigen receptor. In the case of B lymphocytes the surface antigen receptor is an immunoglobulin molecule, while for T cells the antigen receptor is a heterodimeric structure, either an $\alpha\beta$ T-cell receptor ($\alpha\beta$ TCR) or a $\gamma\delta$ TCR. The generation of this incredible diversity depends on an as yet incompletely understood molecular process.[9] Subsequent encounter with, and binding of, antigen to immunoglobulin or TCR triggers additional alterations in the structure and function of only those cells preprogrammed to recognize that specific antigen. Such triggering leads to further recognizable morphologic, structural, and functional changes in the cell, some of which are depicted in Figure 77-1. The encounter with antigen often occurs in anatomic sites removed from the original early developmental process in thymus and marrow, specifically in the peripheral lymphoid system, including lymph nodes, spleen, and other specialized microenvironments such as the mucosal-associated lymphoid tissue (MALT) and skin-associated lymphoid tissue (SALT).[10] It is also important to recognize that a variety of drugs, for example, cyclosporine, that are commonly used in marrow transplantation and in the treatment of lymphoproliferative disease, can have profound effects on normal (as well as abnormal) lymphocyte development.[11]

Any B- or T-lymphocyte population can be described in two ways: (1) with respect to the particular clone to which it belongs (defined by the clone's unique antigen receptor molecule that remains constant throughout development and throughout clonal expansion in response to antigen), and (2) with respect to the cell's maturational stage, defined by rapidly changing morphology, expression of structural genes and proteins,[12] antigen receptor genes and proteins,[13] growth factor and growth factor receptors,[14] and "homing" or adhesive structures.[15] While clonal analysis at the genomic or protein level provides a completely unique marker for all progeny of a particular progenitor cell, maturational changes define both the microenvironment most favorable for the cell's survival and the functional attributes of the cell. Neoplastic transformation of the immune system involves the poorly controlled growth of a single clone of cells (with either higher proliferative potential than normal or with greater longevity or both), while reactive proliferations involve multiple different clones proliferating in a self-limited fashion. In the case of B and T lymphocytes, this monoclonality of malignancy can always be determined by an examination of antigen receptor gene rearrangement (immunoglobulin or TCR), or, in the case of B cells, by whether or not surface immunoglobulin light chain is exclusively κ or λ for the entire population in question (implying a single progenitor cell of origin). Immunoglobulin and TCR antigen receptors provide a completely characteristic "tumor marker" shared by no normal cell. This property of malignant B and T cells, unique among cancers, makes it possible to follow truly "minimal residual disease" via very sensitive fluorescence- and molecular amplification-based assays and, moreover, serves as a totally cancer-specific target structure for highly precise therapies.[16-21]

For purposes of classification, it is often convenient to consider malignant transformation of cells of these lineages as representing a maturation arrest at a specific point in the normal ontogenic process,[22-25] outlined in Figure 77-1. Within broad boundaries, such nosology does in fact tend to group diseases of similar clinical behavior, proliferative potential, preferential sites of involvement, and functional concomitants such as cytokine production leading to characteristic clinical complications, natural history, and response to therapy. Thus correlation of marker characteristics of malignant lymphocytes with those of normal cells can aid in the diagnosis and prognosis of lymphoproliferative disease and also provide clues to the pathogenesis of these disorders.

Ontogeny of B-Lymphocyte-Derived Malignancies

In normal ontogeny, the earliest proto-B and -T cells (lymphoid stem cells) acquire the machinery to carry out immunoglobulin and TCR gene rearrangement but have not yet successfully rearranged these genes. Such cells are characterized by the intranuclear expression of the enzyme terminal deoxynucleotidyl transferase ([TdT] responsible for addition of nucleotides to joining regions of the genes), germline configuration of immunoglobulin and TCR genes, and surface expression of the stem cell antigen CD34.[26] The first definable stage of B-cell maturation occurs as the cell begins the process of producing immunoglobulin. The genetic heavy chain locus is rearranged but protein is not yet expressed in the cell and the light chain loci have not undergone alteration. At this early pre-B stage, two other characteristic proteins appear, both rel-

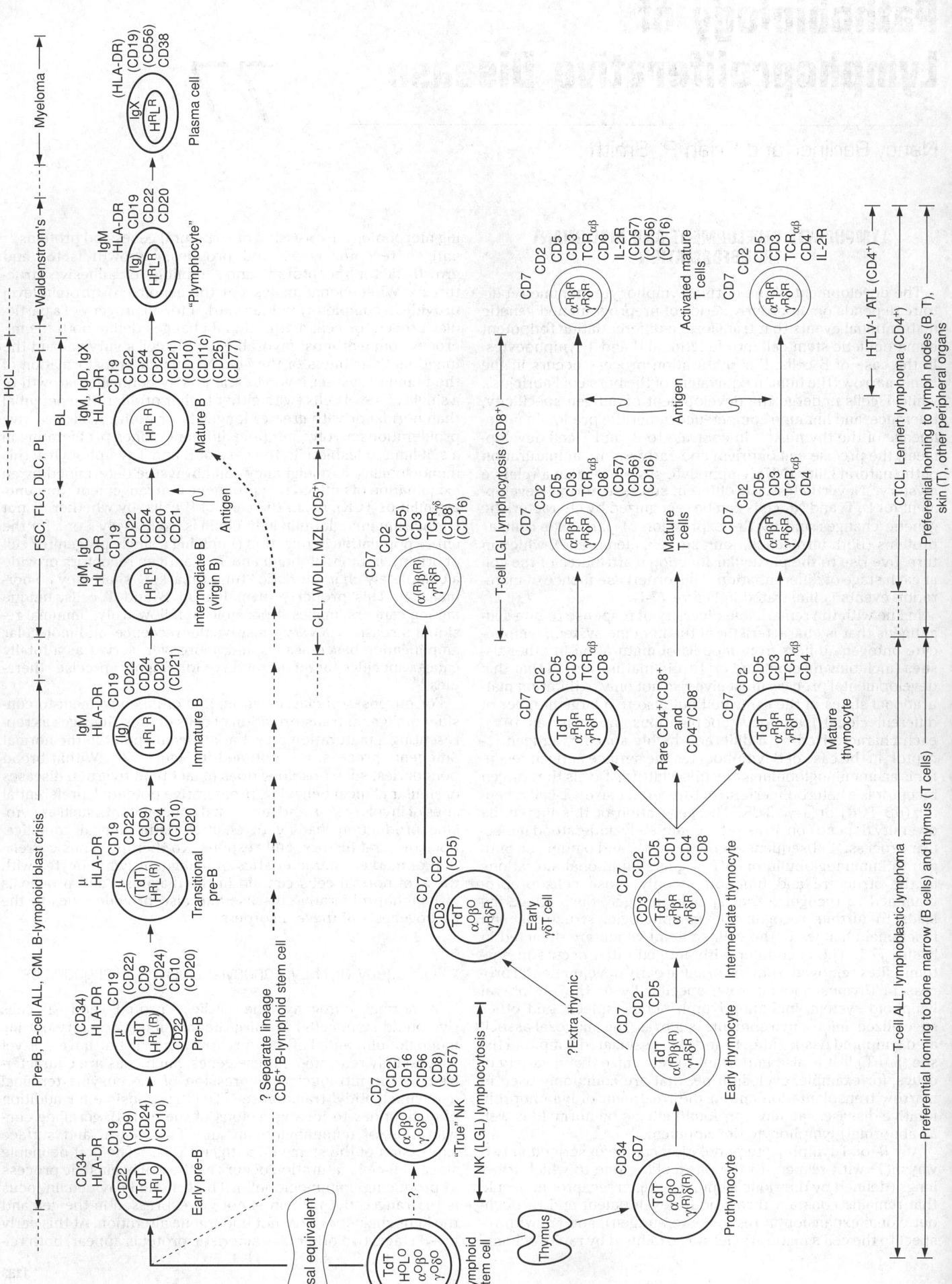

atively lineage specific and both retained throughout subsequent differentiation: CD19[27,28] and CD22. While the former is fully expressed on the surface of the cell, CD22 is found only in the cytoplasm at this particular stage of development. Differentiation obviously represents a continuum of changes in constituent gene expression and protein production so the number of "stages" in B-cell development that can be defined is nearly infinitely variable. Figure 77-1 uses a parsimonious approach based on stages that appear to have relevance to clinical correlation of B-cell malignancies. Thus the early pre-B cell stage depicted here includes both cells expressing and not expressing CD10[29] (the non-lineage specific common acute lymphocytic leukemia antigen [CALLA]), also known as neutral enkephalinase. CD10⁻ pre-B cells are sometimes referred to as pro-B cells (or, unfortunately, early early pre-B), while CD10⁺ cells are variably called, in different nomenclature schemes, early pre-B or pre-pre-B. When malignant transformation of this B-cell stage occurs, it seems easier to avoid these terminology problems by referring to CD10⁺ and CD10⁻ early pre-B cell acute lymphocytic leukemia (ALL).

CD10 remains on the membrane of the pre-B cell through subsequent light chain rearrangement, is then lost on further maturation, only to reappear again when mature B cells enter the lymph node germinal center at later stages of postantigenic stimulation differentiation. Within the hematopoietic system, the CD10 antigen is expressed only on normal and abnormal early pre-B and pre-B cells, on the more mature neoplastic cells of Burkitt lymphoma and the follicular non-Hodgkin lymphomas (NHLs), and on granulocytes. Coupled with CD19, it therefore serves as an excellent marker of B-cell lineage for the leukemias and lymphomas and is also a potential therapeutic target molecule for bone marrow purging protocols.[30] It is important to emphasize, however, that CD10⁺ precursor B cells are a normal constituent of marrow and may be increased in frequency after chemotherapy or stem cell transplantation. Therefore the presence of such immunophenotypically identified cells in specimens from patients with ALL does not necessarily imply relapse; only the presence of such cells with the patient's characteristic immunoglobulin gene rearrangement indicates recurrence of disease.[31]

After rearrangement of the heavy chain at the level of the genome, cytoplasmic μ-protein is expressed, with retention of the surface and intranuclear enzyme characteristics noted above. This defines the pre-B cell stage of development, sometimes also referred to as late pre-B. For physiologic reasons that are not yet fully understood, μ heavy chain can be expressed on the surface of the developing B cell in the absence of κ or λ light chain. In that case, the heavy chain is accompanied by another molecule known as surrogate light chain.[32] This phenomenon defines an additional stage in differentiation known as the transitional B cell, whose malignant transforma-

tion has been recently recognized as defining a clinically unique type of ALL requiring differential therapeutic intervention.[33]

A number of empirically determined clinical associations with particular leukemic immunophenotypes have been described, related to prognosis, patient age, and even geographic distribution of B-cell-derived leukemias.[33] As the function of particular markers of differentiation is elucidated, it is likely that these associations will be at least partly explicable from a physiologic standpoint.

The immunoglobulin light chain genetic locus is next rearranged, first with an attempt to obtain a productive κ-rearrangement and, if that fails, a productive λ-rearrangement. Surface expression of a complete IgM molecule defines the first stage in B-cell (as opposed to pre-B cell) development. It should be remembered that throughout this process of generating a particular B-cell clone's unique antigen receptor, the immune system requires each such clone to produce one and only one antibody with one and only one unique specificity. The same specificity is expressed as a cell membrane receptor on the B-cell clone awaiting its antigenic ligand and, once that antigen has been encountered, as a secreted antibody product. Because two chromosomes carrying heavy chain genes and four chromosomes carrying light chain genes can undergo rearrangement, the immune system requires the ability to carry out allelic exclusion. This term refers to the empirically described but mechanistically still uncertain process by which, after productive rearrangement of one chromosome's heavy chain locus, the other chromosome is forbidden to rearrange, and similarly, once a productive light chain rearrangement is obtained all other chromosomes carrying light chain genes are deactivated. The practical diagnostic consequence of this process is that each B-cell clone expresses one and only one type of light chain, either κ or λ, but never both, allowing the distinction between reactive versus neoplastic B-cell proliferations, the former including cells of both κ- and λ-phenotype while the latter are restricted to a single light chain.[34]

Between the time of light chain rearrangement and the expression of intact surface immunoglobulin, another lineage-specific B-cell marker, CD20, appears on the cell surface and remains throughout mature B-cell development. Although the variable, or antigen-binding, portions of the immunoglobulin heavy and light chains are now fixed and uniquely define a given B-cell clone, the constant, or complement-binding regions of the heavy chain can be switched, so that surface and secreted immunoglobulin can be of the μ, δ, α, γ, or ε heavy chain subclass. Several different immunoglobulin constant region classes may be simultaneously expressed on the cell surface. Note, however, that the variable region of each of these molecules will be identical and that the light chain portion of

Fig. 77-1. Lymphoproliferative diseases as they relate to normal lymphoid development. This schema of lymphoid differentiation should be regarded as an evolving working hypothesis. Similarly, the association of a particular stage in normal development with a particular clinical category of lymphoproliferative disease is an approximation. Many of these disorders have a particular cell type that is the easily identifiable portion of the malignant clone, but the true malignant "stem cell" is actually at a much more primitive maturational state. This is partly indicated by the use of dashed lines. Parentheses around a marker indicate that the protein is variably expressed at that stage of differentiation or is present on a subset of cells. μ refers to μ immunoglobulin heavy chain without accompanying κ or λ light chain. When this molecule is expressed on the surface of the B cell without light chain, it is instead accompanied by surrogate light chain. H°, germline immunoglobulin heavy chain; Hᴿ, rearranged immunoglobulin heavy chain; Lᴳ/ᴿ, germline or rearranged immunoglobulin light chain; Ig, immunoglobulin; TCR, T-cell receptor; α°, germline TCR α-gene; FSC, follicular small cell lymphoma; FLC, follicular large cell lymphoma; DLC, diffuse large cell lymphoma; PL, prolymphocytic leukemia; HCL, hairy cell leukemia; BL, Burkitt lymphoma; LGL, large granular lymphocyte; CTCL, cutaneous T-cell lymphoma; ATL, adult T-cell leukemia/lymphoma; LL, lymphoblastic lymphoma; αᴿ, rearranged TCR α gene (similar designations for TCR β-, γ-, δ-genes); IgX, IgG or IgA; MZL, mantle zone lymphoma; WDLL, well-differentiated lymphocytic lymphoma.

the intact molecule will always be the same, κ or λ, but never both.

The B cell first expresses IgM alone on the surface (immature B), which is followed by simultaneous expression of IgM and IgD (intermediate B or virgin B). At this point the cell has still not encountered antigen. The progenitor cell of chronic lymphocytic leukemia (CLL) appears to represent this stage of differentiation. However, CLL cells are not derived from the major B-cell subset, the so-called CD5⁻ B cell, but rather from the CD5⁺ B lineage.[35] CD5 is a surface membrane glycoprotein of 67,000 relative molecular weight, originally described as a pan-T marker but subsequently recognized on a subset of normal murine and human B lymphocytes.[36-42] In the mouse, CD5⁺ B cells represent a distinct lymphocyte subset that originates from a different progenitor than CD5⁻ B cells[43]; whether human B cells have a similar pattern of development remains controversial.[44-47] As noted below, this difference in B-subset lineage origin may help to account for some of the autoimmune clinical characteristics of CLL,[48,49] since normal CD5⁺ B cells, in addition to providing help to CD5⁻ B cells for antibody production, also themselves produce IgM rheumatoid factor and other "natural" autodirected antibodies[50-53] and are found in increased frequency in autoimmune disorders[54,55] and after marrow transplantation.[56]

Binding of antigen ligand to the membrane-bound immunoglobulin surface antigen receptor of a B-cell clone results in activation of the B cell. A number of intracellular events follow activation, all designed to accomplish two purposes: (1) further terminal differentiation of some members of the clone to antibody-secreting plasma cells, and (2) conversion of some progeny of the clone to memory B cells. At the molecular level, this process first involves immunoglobulin heavy chain class switching (from IgM and IgD to additional expression of γ, α, or ε heavy chains already expressed to produce IgG, IgA, or IgE, respectively). In normal physiology, then, the secondary antibody classes, IgG, IgE, and IgA (symbolized by IgX in Fig. 77-1), do not appear on the surface of virgin B cells but only on B cells previously stimulated by their appropriate antigen. Usually, a given cell expresses only one of these secondary classes on its surface, along with IgM ± IgD.

Most (85%) of the NHLs encountered in the United States are derived from B cells, most frequently B cells at mature stages of differentiation. The clinical characteristics of all these lymphomas demonstrate a wide range. While the follicular (nodular) lymphomas have a "low-grade" clinical behavior, acting as though their primary pathophysiology involves the persistence of long-lived cells rather than the vigorous proliferation of highly activated B cells, the diffuse large cell and immunoblastic B-cell lymphomas have an intermediate to high-grade pattern of growth and spread, corresponding to a high turnover rate and short cell cycle time.[57] Similarly, although most B-cell lymphomas that infiltrate the spleen are found in the white pulp (where normal lymphocytes traffic), the malignant cells of hairy cell leukemia (HCL) are found in the red pulp, intimately adhered to the high endothelial venule. The different clinical scenarios manifest by the non-Hodgkin lymphomas can be partly explained on the basis of two additional cellular characteristics: (1) activation of the cells manifested by the production of growth factors and cytokines by the cells themselves and by the appearance on the cell surface of growth factor receptors and "activation antigens" (e.g., interleukin-2 receptor [CD25], the receptor for the Fc portion of the IgE molecule [FcεR II, CD23], and the "Burkitt lymphoma associated antigen" [CD77]); and (2) "homing" or "adhesion" structures present on the surface membrane of these cells. For example, the neoplastic cells in HCL express high quantities of the β₂ integrin CD11c/CD18, which serves as a cellular adhesion receptor.[58] Similarly, although CLL cells and the malignant cells of patients

with well-differentiated small lymphocytic lymphoma (WDLL) originate from a similar normal B-cell counterpart (CD5⁺ B cell), in the latter case the cells express significantly increased quantities of another β₂ integrin, CD11a/CD18. The expression of these integrins has been postulated to explain the relatively exclusive lymph node homing of WDLL cells as compared to the more promiscuous homing behavior of CLL cells.[59]

These subset, activation, and adhesion characteristics of the various mature B-cell-derived lymphoproliferative disorders can also be used for the purposes of differential diagnosis. A summary of these characteristics useful in the diagnosis of lymphocytosis is presented in Table 77-1.

Once fully committed to antibody secretion, mature B cells become plasma cells, which are morphologically easily recognizable, passing through an intermediate stage whose cells are sometimes referred to as plymphocytes or plasmacytoid lymphocytes. At the molecular level, this involves a switch to the production of secretory immunoglobulin rather than cytoplasmic immunoglobulin. Malignant transformation of these stages of B-cell differentiation result in Waldenström's macroglobulinemia and multiple myeloma.[60] The traditional view of normal B-cell differentiation has held that plasma cells lose many of the usual B-cell surface markers (CD19, CD20) while expressing distinctly high amounts of the CD38 antigen. Recently, however, some investigators have suggested that normal plasma cells retain CD19, while myeloma cells lose this marker and may also acquire other surface markers associated with adhesion in the neural system and normally present on NK cells, specifically CD56.[61]

Ontogeny of T-Lymphocyte-Derived Malignances

Normal differentiation of the T lymphocyte involves a series of steps that parallel that of the B cell (Fig. 77-1). At least four genes (α, βα, γ, δ) demonstrate recombination events in order to produce a productive TCR. Current evidence supports the notion that a temporal sequence is followed in the rearrangements of these four genes during development but that ultimately any given T-cell clone expresses either an αβ or a γδ heterodimer, but not both, on its surface as its antigen receptor.[16,62-64] γδ T cells may undergo some of their differentiation in extrathymic locations, including the MALT and SALT, where they specifically home.[65]

In fetal development, the earliest identifiable proto-T cells express the CD7 marker on their cell membrane along with CD34. CD7 has been identified not only on thymocytes and T cells but also on a very small subset of normal myeloid precursors and on the blast cells of about 15% of cases of acute myeloid leukemia.[33] Thus it is not a lineage-specific molecule. The next developmental stage of the T cell is recognized in the thymus and is identified by the expression of CD2 and CD5 molecules on the cell membrane (early thymocyte, early cortical or stage I thymocyte). The γ and δ TCR genes are usually rearranged by this stage (regardless of whether the cell is destined to be an αβ or γδ T cell)[66,67] but are not expressed as protein. Progression to the next stage of T-cell development in the thymus (referred to as intermediate thymocyte in Fig. 77-1 but also variably referred to as common or inner cortical thymocyte or stage II) involves the rearrangement of αβ TCR genes for future αβ T cells and the production of cytoplasmic CD3. These cells are also dual positive for both CD4 and CD8 and express CD1. The final thymic stage involves generation of an intact TCR on the cell surface accompanied by the CD3 complex (mature thymocyte or stage III medullary thymocyte), along with commitment to either the CD4⁺/CD8⁻ or CD4⁻/CD8⁺ lineage for most of these cells. T cells then pass into the peripheral circulation. The identification of the two different TCR structures has allowed a more precise definition of the mature

Table 77-1. Evaluation of Lymphocytosis

	Cell Type	Maturation	T/B Subset	Activation	Adhesion
Chronic lymphocytic leukemia	Monoclonal B	Low density, IgM ± IgD CD19⁺ CD20⁺ CD22⁺ CD10⁻	CD5⁺	CD25± CD23⁺	CD11c⁻ CD21⁺
Prolymphocytic leukemia	Monoclonal B	High density, IgM + IgD CD19⁺ CD20⁺ CD22⁺ CD10⁻	CD5⁻	CD25⁻ CD23⁻	CD11c⁻ CD21⁺
Hairy cell leukemia	Monoclonal B	High density IgM + IgD + IgX CD19⁺ CD20⁺ CD22⁺ CD10⁻	CD5⁻	CD25⁺⁺	CD11c⁺⁺ CD21⁻
Follicular lymphoma (lymphosarcoma cell leukemia)	Monoclonal B	High density IgM + IgG CD19⁺ CD20⁺ CD22⁺ CD10±	CD5⁻	CD25± CD23⁺	CD11c⁻ CD21±
Burkitt lymphoma	Monoclonal B	High density, IgM + IgG CD19⁺ CD20⁺ CD22⁺ CD10⁺	CD5⁻	CD25± CD77⁺	CD11c⁻
Lymphoblastic lymphoma	Monoclonal T	TdT⁺ CD7⁺ Cytoplasmic CD3⁺ CD1± CD2± CD5±	Thymocyte CD4± CD8±	CD25±	—
Cutaneous T-cell lymphoma	Monoclonal T	CD3 + CD2 + CD5 + CD7±	CD4⁺ CD8⁻	CD25±	—
HTLV-1-associated adult T-cell leukemia/lymphoma	Monoclonal T	CD3⁺ CD2⁺ CD5⁺	CD4⁺ CD8⁻	CD25⁺⁺	—
Large granular T lymphocytosis	Monoclonal T	CD3⁺ CD2⁺ CD5±	CD8⁺ CD4⁻ CD57⁺	CD25±	CD16⁺ CD56⁺

Normal blood is approximately 75% T (CD3⁺), 15% NK (CD3⁻, CD16, and/or CD56⁺), and 10% B (CD19⁺, SIg⁺). Mature T cells express CD7, CD5, CD2, and either CD4 or CD8 (with approximately twice as many CD4⁺ cells as CD8⁺ cells). Mature B cells express CD19, CD20, IgM ± IgD ± IgG or IgA, and CD22. Approximately 15% of normal peripheral B cells are CD5⁺; the rest are CD5⁻. Normal mature B cells only rarely express CD10, but malignant B cells in ALL, Burkitt lymphoma, and the follicular (nodular) lymphomas express CD10. In normals, <10% of T cells and <5% of B cells express activation markers, including interleukin-2 receptor (CD25). Normal expression of homing and adhesion molecules is still being investigated, but only rare normal B cells express CD11c, and <10% of T cells express an Fc_γ receptor (CD16). The table represents the surface phenotype of the *majority* of cases of each disease, but many exceptions also exist.

blood T lymphocytes into both the very common cells (αβTCR⁺ CD4⁺/CD8⁻ and αβTCR+ CD8⁺/CD4⁻) and into four rarer phenotypes, namely αβTCR⁺ CD4⁺/CD8⁺, αβ TCR-positive CD4⁻/CD8⁻, γδ TCR⁺ CD4⁻/CD8⁻, γδTCR⁺ CD8⁺/CD4⁻. Again analogous to B-cell differentiation, these cells are activated on encounter with antigen, or, more precisely, class I MHC plus exogenous antigen for CD8⁺ mature T cells and class II MHC plus endogenous antigen for CD4⁺ T cells.

One important subset of the peripheral T-cell population is also readily defined both morphologically and by surface marker analysis, that is, the large granular lymphocyte (LGL) subset. This population of CD3⁺/CD8⁺ T cells usually expresses the CD57 antigen, often along with CD16 (an Fcγ receptor) and/or CD56 (an adhesion molecule).[68,69] Most of these cells will express the αβ TCR, while a smaller subpopulation are γδ TCR-positive. Two nosologic facts must be noted. First, these T-

LGLs are sometimes referred to as Tγ cells. The Tγ refers to the presence of an Fcγ receptor on the surface of the cells and not to the heterodimeric composition of their TCR. The vast majority of Tγ cells bear an αβ TCR. Second, morphologically identified LGLs contain both T-derived cells that are CD3⁺ and TCR⁺ and NK-derived cells, which are TCR⁻ CD3⁻, and have no rearrangement of their TCR genes (see below).

T-cell-derived ALL represents transformation of cells at the early thymocyte stages of T differentiation (Fig. 77-1 and Table 77-1); diffuse lymphoblastic lymphomas are similarly thymocyte in origin, usually at the intermediate thymocyte stage. T-ALL may be derived from either αβ TCR or γδ TCR T cells.[70] The preponderance of evidence now suggests that the exact stage of normal differentiation corresponding to the T-ALL (early, intermediate, or mature) has little influence on overall prognosis, clinical behavior, or therapeutic results,[33] although selected immunophenotype characteristics are reported by some to be associated with specific patterns of radiation resistance.[71] This is in contrast to several of the diseases of mature T cells. Cutaneous T-cell lymphomas are almost always derived from mature CD4⁺ T cells.[72] The dermatotropic nature of these diseases has been attributed in part to the normal behavior of CD4⁺ T cells, which includes migration through skin. Human T-cell leukemia/lymphoma virus-1 (HTLV-1)-associated adult T-cell leukemia/lymphoma is also virtually always CD4⁺ T-cell derived because of the tropism of the virus for that mature T-cell subset.[73] In addition, this neoplasm acts clinically as a highly proliferative T-cell malignancy. The molecular etiology of this activation and proliferation is now partly understood.[74] HTLV-1 is one of a class of retroviruses that contain potent trans-activating transcriptional regulating genes, in particular the *tax* gene. The tax protein results in trans-activation of the interleukin-2 receptor gene in the host T cell as well as activation of a variety of cytokines, including interleukin-2 itself and colony-stimulating factor-granulocyte/macrophage. Thus the virus establishes an autocrine stimulation of the infected cell. However, because most patients who have been infected with HTLV-1 never develop lymphoma and the disease state is usually associated with additional genetic events, the *tax* gene must not be acting alone in pathogenesis (see below).

While follicular lymphomas (characterized by their morphologic similarity to normal B-cell-containing germinal centers) are virtually always of B-cell origin, the diffuse large cell NHLs are derived from T-cell progenitors in 15–25% of cases (either αβ TCR T cells, or, much less commonly, γδ TCR T cells[75]), including many cases of angioimmunoblastic lymphadenopathy[76] and Lennert lymphoma.[77] There is a distinct lack of consistency in marker expression in these disorders and the malignant cells frequently lose common mature T-cell markers.[78] Although some studies demonstrate subgroups of patients in which immunophenotyping can be associated with prognostic patterns, most data suggest poor correlation of phenotype with clinical course.[79,80] An exception is T-cell prolymphocytic leukemia, which is clinically distinguishable from its B-cell cousin.[81]

One unique lymphoproliferative syndrome is derived from CD8⁺ LGL progenitors. This disorder, known by a host of names, including lymphoproliferative disease of large granular lymphocytes and Tγ lymphocytosis, is characterized by clonal proliferations of CD3⁺ T-cell LGLs in most cases and by proliferation of CD3⁻ NK-derived LGL progenitors in a minority of cases.[68,69,82] Characteristics include an association with cytopenias (especially anemia and neutropenia) that occur on a noninfiltrative basis and an association with rheumatoid arthritis. This entity is discussed in more detail below.

Ontogeny of Natural Killer Cell-Derived Malignancies

In normal blood, approximately 75% of the lymphocytes are CD3⁺ T cells (roughly 50% CD4⁺ and 25% CD8⁺) and about 10% B lymphocytes. The remaining 15% of cells might be said to suffer from semantic excess, having been described in the past from the surface marker point of view as null cells, non-B, non-T cells, or Fc receptor-rich cells.[83] The former two terms led to marked confusion with similar terms used historically to describe the cells of patients with ALL of immature type, which we now know to be predominantly of early pre-B and pre-B cell origin. Because the vast majority of these non-T, non-B cells demonstrate the in vitro function known as natural killing, they are commonly, and perhaps best, referred to as NK cells. Natural killing refers to the ability of some lymphocytes to spontaneously lyse particular target cell lines (virally infected or of tumor origin) to which the cell has not been previously sensi-

tized. The target structure being recognized by these cytolytic cells remains uncertain.[84] Most cells showing this function are TCR⁻ NK cells. It is important to note, however, that this function can also be displayed by some subsets of "true" T lymphocytes (defined as cells expressing a functional surface TCR), especially after lymphokine stimulation (lymphokine-activated killer cells).

Recognizing these problems, most authors consider a surface phenotypic designation of NK cells as CD3⁻ (and therefore TCR⁻) cells that express one or more other molecules associated with this population, most commonly CD16 or CD56. These cells do not show TCR gene rearrangements by molecular analysis. Most of these cells also express CD2 (and thus have previously been erroneously termed T cells on the basis of sheep erythrocyte rosetting) and CD7 but not CD5. The place of such cells in the normal ontogeny of the lymphocyte immune system and their relationship to T cells are incompletely defined[83] (Fig. 77-1).

Neoplastic transformation of NK cells appears to be a relatively unusual event. Most NK malignancies present as NK large granular lymphocytoses associated with cytopenias[68,85] (see below), although it should be again emphasized that most LGL syndromes are derived from CD3⁺ T cells rather than CD3⁻ NK cells. It is often technically impossible to demonstrate clonality in the CD3⁻ NK lymphocytosis patients and the chronic indolent course of some individuals may represent a reactive process rather than neoplastic transformation.[86] Some patients with true NK cell large granular lymphocytosis have an extremely aggressive disease course.[68]

Controversy exists as to the cell of origin of angiocentric lymphoproliferative disorders of the respiratory system, including lymphomatoid granulomatosis and lethal midline granuloma. Some evidence suggests an NK cell origin to these particular malignant proliferations of lymphocytes.[87,88] Other proliferations of NK cells have been associated with neuropathy,[89] and, very rarely, more aggressive ALL-like tumor variants.[90,91]

MONOCLONAL, OLIGOCLONAL, AND POLYCLONAL LYMPHOPROLIFERATION

Immunoglobulin and TCR Gene Rearrangements in the Diagnosis of Lymphoproliferative Disease

The carefully ordered sequence of events involved in immunoglobulin gene rearrangement defines the progressive stages of B-lymphocyte development outlined in Figure 77-1[92–94]: heavy chain rearrangement, surrogate light chain production, light chain rearrangement, allelic exclusion, heavy chain class switching, and switching from membrane-bound to secreted immunoglobulin.[95] Because the process of malignant transformation usually involves a single progenitor cell and gives rise to a tumor cell population that is arrested at a particular stage of differentiation, it results in a proliferation of cells manifesting an identical (clonal) pattern of DNA rearrangement. Examination of the state of immunoglobulin gene DNA consequently offers a sensitive means of establishing the clonality and lymphoid origin of malignant and nonmalignant B cells. Such studies also provide a powerful marker of alterations in the tumor cell population that can be used to follow the natural history of B-cell lymphoproliferative disease.[96–98]

As noted earlier, similar molecular events have been shown to occur in the TCR loci in the course of normal and malignant T-cell ontogeny. The most common TCR is expressed as a heterodimer of α- and β-chains, each of which undergoes V-D-J rearrangement comparable with that undergone by the immunoglobulin heavy chain genes. The exact timing of these rearrangement events in the ontogeny of the T cell is less well

Table 77-2. Use of Immunoglobulin and TCR Gene Rearrangements in the Diagnosis and Treatment of Lymphoproliferative Disease

Establishing lymphoid origin of poorly defined lymphoproliferative lesions with confusing histology or absent lymphoid surface markers

Defining clonality in monoclonal, biclonal, oligoclonal, or polyclonal disorders of indeterminate neoplastic potential

Determining extent of disease in patients with established lymphoproliferative disorders

Monitoring disease activity in patients undergoing treatment for lymphoproliferative malignancy

understood than the sequence of events in the immunoglobulin gene loci, although it is known that β-chain rearrangement precedes α-chain rearrangement. Rearrangement of the α-chain genes has proved technically difficult to study, because of their large size and possible more limited repertoire; hence, the α-genes are usually not used as a marker of T lineage or clonality. The TCR β-chain genes, however, have proved most useful as a marker of T-cell clonality in lymphoproliferative disease but less valuable as a clue to the degree of maturation of the T cell[99,100] (Table 70-1). Note, also, that for T cells there is no comparable surface protein clonality test analogous to light chain expression used in the assessment of clonality for B-cell-derived disorders.

In summary, the analysis of immunoglobulin and TCR gene rearrangement is a powerful means of establishing the clonality and stage of differentiation of a neoplastic lymphoid cell population. As outlined in Table 77-2, these studies have been used (1) to establish the lymphoid origin of tumors that lack definitive markers; (2) to resolve the question of clonality in poorly defined lymphoproliferative syndromes; and (3) to follow the natural history of lymphoid tumors and document their response to treatment.

Clonal Derangements in Lymphoproliferative Disease

Studies of immunoglobulin and TCR gene rearrangements have provided insight into derangements of the normal processes of lymphoid differentiation that occur in lymphoproliferative malignancies. These include (1) lineage infidelity, the occurrence of genetic events in one cell type that are usually limited to a different lymphocyte subtype (e.g., TCR rearrangements in B cells); (2) the production of structurally abnormal immunoglobulins; and (3) clonal evolution, that is, cellular alteration in an established clone that changes the natural history of a particular patient (e.g., Richter syndrome).[101] An additional derangement of normal maturation, that of chromosomal translocation, is thought to play a primary role in the pathogenesis of malignant transformation. It probably represents an error in the process of somatic rearrangement that is a part of the normal genetic program of the developing lymphocyte.

Lineage Infidelity

Southern blot analysis is a highly sensitive technique to establish lymphoid clonality, being capable of identifying single clones that represent ≥1% of the total cell population being studied. For this reason, it has come to be viewed as a standard for the study of lymphoid origin and clonality. It is important to keep in mind, however, that cells displaying immunoglobulin heavy chain rearrangement may occasionally also show rearrangements of TCR α-, β-, γ-, or δ-chains as well. Similarly, some T-cell clones contain rearrangements of the immunoglobulin heavy chain locus. This finding is characteristic of very immature cells; ≤40% of pre-B cell ALLs have been found to have TCR rearrangements. Such lineage infidelity has also been ob-

served in normal lymphocytes, and may therefore represent an aspect of normal immune physiology that is not yet completely understood.[102,103]

In general, concurrent immunoglobulin and TCR gene rearrangements may be considered at least to confirm a lymphoid origin for the cells in question, although a rare myeloid leukemia has been reported to demonstrate immunoglobulin heavy chain rearrangement, as well as TCR α- and β-chain rearrangement.[104] In contrast to immunoglobulin heavy chain and TCR rearrangement, immunoglobulin light chain rearrangement has been considered a definitive marker of B-cell lineage, although a single case has been reported in which κ-chain gene rearrangement was seen in a lymphoma of T-cell phenotype.[105]

Abnormal Immunoglobulin Gene Structure in Heavy Chain Disease

In most lymphoid malignancies, antigen receptor genes, mRNA, and protein are of normal structure. Heavy chain disease, however, is associated with surface expression and secretion of the immunoglobulin heavy chain in the absence of associated light chains; such expression is totally aberrant in the normal ontogeny of the B lymphocyte.[106] Isolated heavy chains are usually expressed only in the cytoplasm of developing B cells; the normal transitional B-cell stage allows the expression of normally structured μ heavy chain on the cell surface but only in association with surrogate light chain. Examination of the heavy chains expressed in the malignant cells of heavy chain disease has revealed that they are of aberrant size, usually lack a variable region, and contain a variety of molecular defects. Among these defects are deletion of a splice donor site leading to elimination of the V-D-J portion of the heavy chain, abnormal rearrangements that delete portions of the variable region, and abnormal heavy chain class switching, which results in deletion of part of the heavy chain gene.[107,108] Although the cells show DNA rearrangement of the light chain loci, they rarely express light chains; when light chains are produced, they are not associated with heavy chains and are detected only as Bence Jones proteins.[107] In the face of such nonproductive gene rearrangements, the factors that allow these cells to continue to differentiate to plasma cells are unknown.

Biclonality and Clonal Evolution

A neoplasm is usually defined as a clonal disorder arising from a single transformed cell. The availability of a sensitive means of confirming or disproving monoclonality in lymphoid cells has allowed this question to be assessed in a more rigorous manner. The results have been surprisingly complex, and have brought into question the validity of the concept that malignancy arises from a single transformed cell. The development of polyclonal malignant lymphoid expansions in immunocompromised patients, especially in association with Epstein-Barr virus (EBV), has recently been recognized. That entity should probably be distinguished from the emergence of biclonal or oligoclonal malignancy in the setting of lymphoid malignancy arising in the previously immunocompetent host.

The first observation of apparent biclonality of lymphoid tumors was documented by Sklar et al.[109] in studies of anti-idiotypic antibodies directed against typical B-cell lymphomas. Lymphoma populations were separated either by reactivity or nonreactivity with specific anti-idiotypic antibody, or by sorting with two independent anti-idiotypic antibodies. The two populations were then subjected to Southern blot analysis, which revealed distinct immunoglobulin gene rearrangements in the two different populations, suggesting independent clonal origins for the two subsets of tumor cells.[109]

Subsequent studies by the same group analyzed multiple

tumor specimens obtained over time from seven patients with lymphoma; they concentrated on samples in which the histology of the tumor varied between biopsies. The results showed three different patterns of clonality: (1) physically and temporally separate samples that shared identical rearrangements, suggesting multiple tumors arising from the same clone; (2) samples that exhibited clonally distinct monoclonal populations, suggesting true bi- or oligoclonal proliferations arising from independent cells; and (3) samples that shared some rearranged bands, but not others; this suggested that multiple tumors arose from the same clonal population, and that further genetic events had occurred to distinguish these subpopulations (clonal evolution).[110]

The major question surrounding these and similar studies is whether such variable populations of tumor cells represent independent stochastic events giving rise to totally distinct tumor cell populations, or represent evolution of a single clone to give rise to apparently dissimilar clones with a common progenitor cell. In the latter case, the finding of independent rearrangements of the immunoglobulin genes in different node samples could be explained by a clonal population that arose from an early progenitor cell in a stage before the rearrangement of the immunoglobulin genes. Such an explanation would imply a capacity for further differentiation after the initial oncogenic event, with subsequent gene rearrangement giving rise to multiple subclones with different DNA rearrangements.

Several lines of evidence support this explanation. First, within a given tumor, the DNA rearrangements were identical, suggesting clonal proliferation in each focus of the tumor. Second, the appearance of the involved nodes in the patients studied by Sklar et al. was nearly simultaneous; that two independent chance events should occur concurrently giving rise to two independent tumors seems unlikely. Finally, and most convincingly, a further study by the same group was made on a series of five apparently biclonal follicular lymphomas carrying the t(14;18) translocation. Despite the apparent indication of dissimilar clones in immunoglobulin gene rearrangement studies, studies of the t(14;18) translocation using a chromosome 18 probe for the translocation breakpoint revealed identical DNA rearrangements in four out of five tumors. The fifth tumor was apparently dissimilar by this analysis; however, cloning of the translocation breakpoint revealed sequence identity of the chromosomal crossover point in the two subclones. Furthermore, sequence analysis of the immunoglobulin gene rearrangements in the two subclones suggested that divergence of the two subclones had actually occurred after the rearrangement of the immunoglobulin genes, and that the differences in rearrangements detectable by Southern analysis reflected subsequent somatic rearrangements.[111] The results of this elegant study strongly suggest that at least the majority of apparently biclonal lymphomas arise from a common precursor cell, with any divergence of subclones being due to subsequent somatic mutation.

These studies have important practical clinical implications as well as adding to our understanding of the pathogenesis of lymphoproliferative disease. If the ultimate cell of origin for some lymphomas is an immunoglobulin uncommitted cell, then treatment with immunotargeting reagents that depend on surface immunoglobulin expression or on surface proteins expressed simultaneously with surface immunoglobulins will fail regardless of whether such reagents are used in vivo or as ex vivo purging drugs for autologous transplantation.

Biclonal M components have also been reported in monoclonal gammopathy of undetermined significance (MGUS), in lymphoma, and in multiple myeloma.[112–115] Although no molecular analysis of such cases has been performed, a similar sequence of events can probably be implicated in the explanation of this apparent biclonality.

Monoclonal and Oligoclonal Lymphoproliferations of Unknown Significance

The development of clinically applicable serum protein electrophoresis and immunoelectrophoresis led to the recognition by Kyle[116] and others[117] that small monoclonal components could be detected in the serum of many normal individuals who did not demonstrate any other signs or symptoms of lymphoproliferative disease. The incidence of these MGUSs increases significantly with age. There is a constant risk of overt lymphoproliferative disease developing in these individuals, increasing over time, but even after 20 years of observation most will be without obvious malignant disease. More sensitive screening techniques, such as immunofixation electrophoresis, further demonstrate an even larger number of patients with monoclonal and oligoclonal gammopathies. These occur particularly in patients with infections,[118–122] hypersensitivity reactions,[123] human immunodeficiency virus,[124,125] solid tumors,[126] HTLV-1 associated neuropathy,[127] and in immunosuppressed patients,[128] especially in patients after marrow[129] and solid organ transplantation.[130] Detection of oligoclonal γ-globulin production in these settings is also not predictive of overt lymphoproliferative disease.

The introduction of sensitive immunofluorescence techniques for detecting monoclonal and oligoclonal B cells (as opposed to their antibody product) similarly demonstrated that particular patient groups had a significant likelihood of having circulating oligoclonal B cells, for example, patients with rheumatoid arthritis.[131] Again, although these patient groups are at increased risk of lymphoproliferative disorders, the vast majority of patients who show small populations of monoclonal and oligoclonal B cells in the periphery never develop overt lymphoma.

There are also a number of diseases characterized by lymphocytic infiltration into nonlymphoid tissues that behave benignly over long periods. These include ocular/conjunctival pseudolymphoma[132] and salivary gland benign lymphoepithelial lesions.[133,134] Although many of these were originally thought to represent reactive, polyclonal processes, molecular gene rearrangement studies have shown them to involve mono- and oligoclonal B cells in many circumstances. Cases that are clearly monoclonal in origin do not necessarily have a different natural history from those that are polyclonal.[135] Moreover, in some cases, the B cells of the lesion are not only monoclonal but also demonstrate overexpression of oncogenes that have been associated with malignantly acting disorders, including bcl-2 and bcl-1[136–138] (see below).

Similarly, other lymphoid disorders that behave benignly can be shown to include mono- or oligoclonal T lymphocytes. These include ataxia-telangiectasia[139,140] and lymphomatoid papulosis.[141] Several studies have demonstrated the coexistence of oligoclonal T-cell expansions in patients with monoclonal B-cell disorders,[142–145] the existence of oligoclonal T-cell populations in the immunocompromised patient with concomitant herpes virus infections,[146] and also the presence of benign-behaving oligoclonal B-lymphocyte populations coexistent with monoclonal B-cell lymphoproliferative disease.[147] Furthermore, two otherwise healthy individuals have been identified who have approximately 5–20% of their circulating lymphocytes consisting of monoclonal T cells of the rare but normal TCRαβ[+] CD4[−]/CD8[−] phenotype[148,149] and an additional group of normal individuals with apparent oligoclonal TCRαβ CD4[+]/CD8[+] cells have also been described.[150]

These observations suggest that it is a relatively common occurrence to develop small mono- or oligoclonal lymphocyte populations, either in response to infection or inflammation, or as a consequence of the aging process. The reasons for this phenomenon are uncertain but it may simply represent a more

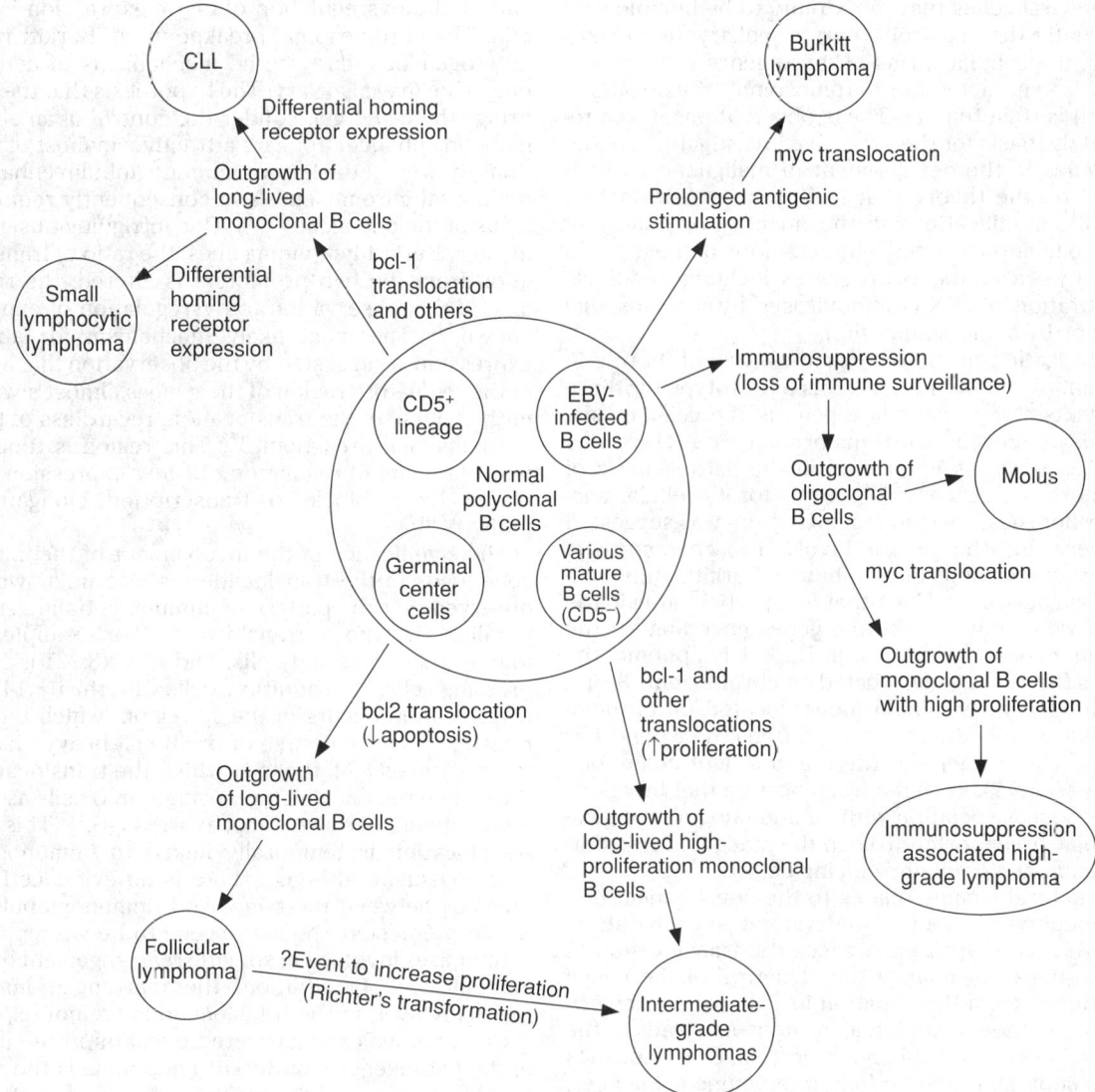

Fig. 77-2. The pathogenesis of B-cell lymphoma is incompletely understood. A progression of polyclonal to oligoclonal to monoclonal proliferations may occur in the setting of immunosuppression. If no other genetic event occurs, the result may be monoclonal or oligoclonal lymphoproliferations of unknown significance (MOLUS), including monoclonal gammopathies of unknown significance. If *myc* translocation to immunoglobulin gene sites occurs then a highly proliferative tumor results. By contrast, if *bcl-2* translocation to these loci occurs then a long-lived (apoptosis-resistant) B-cell malignancy results. The clinical behavior of different B-cell malignancies may also depend on both the particular B-cell subset that is transformed (CD5+ versus CD5−) and the concomitant expression of homing (adhesion) surface proteins, such as the β_2 integrin, CD11a/CD18.

extreme version of the normal immune response, which generates a progressively more restrictive antigen receptor repertoire over time.[151–153] Other possibilities include chronic stimulation of a limited repertoire of normal antigen receptor positive cells by superantigen[154] or primary stochastic dysregulation of one lymphocyte lineage resulting in further perturbations in others.[155] In any case, it is clear that further genetic alteration must occur in order for these incompletely regulated B or T lymphocytes to undergo true malignant transformation. Indeed, a large body of data suggest that several events must occur before such cells become neoplastic. The relative frequency of these events suggest that it might be useful to expand the venerable MGUS concept to a larger group, including both B and T cells at various stages of maturation. In Figure 77-2, this is referred to as monoclonal and oligoclonal lymphoproliferations of unknown significance (MOLUS) in order to reflect this expanded understanding of the condition.

MOLECULAR PATHOGENESIS OF LYMPHOID NEOPLASIA

The recent dramatic increase in our understanding of the process of malignant transformation has relied heavily on insights provided by the study of lymphoid neoplasia. The application of molecular techniques to the study of lymphoproliferative disease has allowed the integration of newly evolving concepts of the role of oncogenes in the origins of malignancy with older previously recognized concepts of cancer cytogenetics and viral carcinogenesis.

Chromosomal Translocation and c-*myc* in Burkitt Lymphoma

Current concepts of malignant transformation have evolved from two observations linking tumor virology to more general concepts of oncogenesis. First, the transforming capability of certain RNA tumor viruses was found to be attributable to oncogenes, single viral genes that were found to be homologous to, and apparently derived from, normal eukaryotic cellular genes. Second, the cellular forms of these genes were shown to be involved in characteristic chromosomal translocations associated with certain tumors. These observations, taken together, formed the basis for the extensive investigations of the role of oncogenes in the development of malignancy, which are predicated on the theory that malignant transformation involves specific modifications in the quantity or quality of expression of cellular oncogenes. The activation of these genes may occur by any of a number of processes, including modification by incorporation into RNA tumor viruses, by chromosomal translocation, or by somatic mutation.

The characterization of the oncogene c-*myc* and its role in the development of lymphoma serves as a prototype for these evolving concepts.[156-158] The c-*myc* gene is the cellular analogue of the v-*myc* oncogene, the transforming gene of the avian retrovirus MC29, which is implicated in the pathogenesis of numerous tumors in chickens.[159,160] A role for its cellular analogue in the pathogenesis of mammalian tumors was suggested by the discovery that the gene is involved in characteristic chromosomal translocations in both human Burkitt lymphoma and murine plasmacytomas. The other loci participating in the translocations were shown to be the genes encoding for the immunoglobulin genes.[161-164] Thus, in Burkitt lymphoma, the t(8;14) involves the c-*myc* gene, located on chromosome 8, and the immunoglobulin heavy chain locus, located on chromosome 14. Similarly, the variant translocations, t(2;8) and t(8;22), involve the c-*myc* gene and the κ and λ light chain loci, respectively. It seems likely that a translocation that brings an oncogene into close association with an immunoglobulin gene locus should play an important role in the malignant transformation of an immunoglobulin-producing cell.

How this structural change relates to the development of a transformed phenotype is not well understood. Intensive study has yielded evidence that in most cases the translocation of the c-*myc* gene does not change the structure of the c-myc protein. This differs from the situation in CML, where the *bcr-abl* translocation in the Philadelphia chromosome leads to the production of an aberrant c-abl fusion protein. c-*myc* consists of three exons separated by two long intervening sequences. The first exon contains two transcription initiation sites that are both used in the production of c-*myc* mRNA. However, the exon contains no initiation codon and has multiple termination codons in all three reading frames; hence, although it is transcribed, it cannot be translated into protein. Despite the inability to translate the first exon, its sequence is highly conserved in mouse and humans, suggesting that it serves an important regulatory function.[165]

Several observations support the hypothesis that translocation usually results in alterations in the regulatory regions of the gene, and that the tumorogenic action of c-*myc* arises from a quantitative rather than a qualitative abnormality in the level of the gene's expression. First, almost all the translocations that have been mapped have revealed chromosomal breakpoints lying upstream from the exons that encode for protein, which suggests that the protein structure is intact although portions of the regulatory sequences may be altered.[164] Second, studies in mouse erythroleukemia cells have shown that introduction of a normal c-*myc* gene under the control of a strong constitutive promoter will block induction of a mature phenotype in those cells.[166-169] Finally, studies in transgenic mice have shown that introduction of the normal c-*myc* structural gene as a transgene under the control of an inducible promoter results in tumorogenesis in the tissues in which that promoter may be activated.[170] All these studies suggest that the c-*myc* gene exerts its primary tumorigenic effect by changes in the level of expression of its normal gene product.

The mechanism by which chromosomal translocation causes the dysregulation of c-*myc* expression is also not certain. The chromosomal breakpoints in Burkitt lymphoma are heterogeneous, and so the mechanisms of activation of the oncogene may also vary. The hypothesis that the translocation brings the c-*myc* gene under the control of an active immunoglobulin enhancer appears attractive; in most of the translocations, however, the known immunoglobulin enhancer is on the reciprocal chromosome and consequently removed from the locus of the oncogene.[165,171] One intriguing observation is that in many Burkitt lymphoma lines, the ratio of transcription initiation from the two promoters is altered; the relationship, if any, of this observation to dysregulation of expression is unknown.[172] The most likely mechanism for aberrant c-*myc* expression is suggested by the observation that a small portion of the regulatory region of the gene is almost always disrupted in the course of the translocation, regardless of the site of the chromosomal breakpoint.[173] This region is thought to be an important site of regulation of c-*myc* expression, which is mediated by a block to transcription elongation of c-*myc* mRNA.[174,175]

The significance of the involvement of the immunoglobulin gene locus in the translocation is also unknown. It has been observed that the pattern of immunoglobulin gene expression parallels the site of translocation. For example, the t(2;8) is found in κ-expressing cells, and the t(8;22) is found in λ-expressing cells.[176] In addition, cells with the t(8;14) in which the translocation occurs in the J$_H$ region, which undergoes rearrangement in the course of pre-B cell heavy chain rearrangement, express IgM; those in which the translocation occurs in the switch region, which rearranges in B cells as they undergo heavy chain class switching, express IgG.[177] This suggests that translocation is temporally linked to immunoglobulin gene rearrangement, although there is no evidence for shared sequences between the c-*myc* and immunoglobulin genes that would predispose the c-*myc* gene to be susceptible to the recombinases involved in somatic rearrangement of the immunoglobulin loci. In addition, the rearranged immunoglobulin genes involved in the translocations are not expressed.

One final major unanswered question in the understanding of the pathogenesis of Burkitt lymphoma is the role of EBV in the development of the malignancy. There is strong evidence for the hypothesis that cooperation between two or more oncogenes is necessary for the development of the malignant phenotype.[178] In this regard, it is possible that EBV infection represents a preliminary oncogenic event, perhaps resulting in the immortalization of B lymphocytes, which then proliferate and subsequently acquire the c-*myc* mutation, which allows the development of the fully transformed phenotype. The strong epidemiologic relationship between EBV and endemic Burkitt lymphoma would then be primarily a reflection of the high rate of EBV infection in those areas. In support of this hypothesis, EBV-infected lymphoblastoid cell lines have been shown to develop full malignant potential upon introduction of a constitutively expressed c-*myc* gene.[179]

In summary, the translocation event between the c-*myc* oncogene and the immunoglobulin locus in Burkitt lymphoma is thought to result in dysregulation in the expression of the normal c-*myc* protein. Overexpression of the c-*myc* has been shown in many systems to result in abnormal growth of cells or in a block to their phenotypic maturation, although the specific function of the c-myc protein and therefore the basis of this tumorigenic effect are unknown. Consequently, the translocation event presumably has an important role in the pathogenesis of this malignancy and its particular highly proliferative clinical phenotype. However, much remains to be elucidated about the specific mechanism underlying the translocation event itself as well as the specific functions of the c-myc protein that allow it to induce a transformed phenotype.

14;18 Translocation in Follicular Lymphoma

The most common chromosomal translocation in NHL is t(14;18), seen in association with a small cleaved cell histology (nodular, diffuse, and mixed poorly differentiated lymphoma).[180] It has been found in ≤60% of follicular lymphomas in some series.[181] This translocation was found to include the immunoglobulin heavy chain locus in a manner similar to Burkitt lymphoma; this allowed identification of the chromosomal breakpoint and consequently the reciprocal locus of the translocation. The other gene involved in the translocation was cloned and called c-*bcl*2 (B-cell leukemia/lymphoma).[182–184] Hence, this gene was not found by homology to a known retroviral oncogene, but rather by its involvement in the chromosomal translocation in lymphoma.

The c-*bcl*2 DNA is transcribed in cells carrying the t(14;18) translocation, as well as in other hematopoietic cell lines.[185,186] In cells with t(14;18), the mRNA is part of a chimeric message with IgH; the normal c-*bcl*-2 gene is not expressed in these cells.[187] The fusion of the c-*bcl*-2 gene occurs in the 3′ untranslated region of the gene; consequently, as with c-*myc*, the protein product of the c-*bcl*-2 gene in these cells is normal, despite the aberrant size of the mRNA. The gene, by virtue of its involvement in the translocation and in the context of its preferential expression in cells carrying the translocation, is presumed to be an oncogene; as discussed below, it has been shown to be involved in apoptosis, but its specific function is unknown. There is some evidence for its increased expression in lymphocytes stimulated with mitogens.[188] The location of the reciprocal portion of the translocation mimics the situation in Burkitt lymphoma, with most cases occurring in the J_H region and some in the switch region, again suggesting a temporal relationship between normal immunoglobulin gene rearrangement and the translocation event.[186]

The analysis of the t(14;18) translocation illustrates the interplay between cancer cytogenetics and developing concepts of oncogenesis. The experiments that led to the discovery of the presence of the cellular analogue of a retroviral oncogene at the t(8;14) breakpoint in Burkitt lymphoma have now been extended to further studies that allow identification of previously unknown oncogenes through the analysis of similar chromosomal translocations.

Other Chromosomal Translocations in Lymphoproliferative Disease

Chromosome analysis of NHLs has revealed cytogenetic abnormalities in nearly all cases.[189] The most common translocations and the histology of the malignancies in which they are most common are listed in Table 77-3. The more common of these abnormalities are thought to be associated with the concomitant activation of a cellular oncogene. Some of these oncogenes have, like c-*myc*, been identified by homology to their known retroviral analogues. Others, like c-*bcl*-2, have been presumptively identified because of their association with characteristic chromosomal translocations; the malignant potential of these genes remains to be defined by further study. Future endeavors must be aimed at characterizing the further events that directly link these genetic mishaps to development of the malignant phenotype.

Detection of Other Activated Oncogenes in Lymphoid Malignancy

The study of chromosomal translocations has been an especially fruitful approach to the analysis of oncogenes in lymphoproliferative malignancy, because of the high frequency of

Table 77-3. Characteristic Chromosomal Translocations in Lymphoid Malignancy

Karyotypic Change	Tumor Histology	Involved Genes
t(8;14)(q24;q32)	Burkitt lymphoma (80%); ALL (5%); B-cell ALL (100%)	c-*myc*, IgH
t(2;8)(p12;q24)	Burkitt lymphoma (10%)	IgK, c-*myc*
t(8;22)(q24;p11)	Burkitt lymphoma (10%)	c-*myc*, IgL
t(14;18)(q32;p21)	Small cleaved cell (50–80%)	Ig, c-*bcl*-2
t(11;14)(q13;q32)	CLL, PDL, DHL	c-*bcl*-1, immunoglobulin
t(9;22)(q34;q11)	ALL (10–15%)	c-*abl*, bcr
t(4;11)(q21;q23)	ALL (5%)	?, c-*ets*-1
t(11;14)(p13;q11)	T-cell lymphoma	c-*tcl*-1, αTCR
t(8;14)(q24;q13)	T-cell lymphoma	c-*myc*, αTCR

Abbreviations: PDL, poorly differentiated lymphocytic lymphoma; DHL, diffuse histocytic lymphoma.

chromosomal abnormalities in those tumors. Two other approaches to the analysis of potential oncogenes involved in the pathogenesis of malignancy have been applied to the study of lymphoproliferative malignancy.

The first of these approaches, use of DNA-mediated gene transfer by transfection into stable cell lines, was originally used by Weinberg[190] in the landmark experiments identifying the point mutation in the c-H-*ras* gene as the origin of the malignant phenotype in the human EJ bladder carcinoma.[190] Genomic DNA derived from tumors is transfected into NIH-3T3 cells, which display a characteristic and easily scorable transformed phenotype on transfection with 10–15% of human tumors. It is especially sensitive in detecting transforming genes of the *ras* family.[190,191]

This approach has been used in the study of lymphoproliferative disease with limited results. An activated c-N-*ras* gene has been detected by this assay in the HL60 cell line, which also contains amplified c-*myc* sequences[192]; it is presumed that in these cells, the *ras* gene mutation represents the second transforming event in the development of the fully transformed phenotype. On the basis of such studies two other genes, *B-lym* and *T-lym*, were proposed as oncogenes, which are activated in B- and T-cell lymphomas, respectively.[193,194] Subsequent study has not confirmed the validity of these results, either by the demonstration of homology to known oncogenes, or by detection of mRNA encoding these genes in normal cells. The *B-lym* gene was subsequently shown to be a portion of murine repeated sequences.[195] In summary, this approach has not definitively implicated any novel oncogenes involved in the pathogenesis of lymphoid malignancy, although it may occasionally demonstrate the contribution of activated *ras* genes in sporadic cases.

Another approach to the detection of oncogenes active in malignancy is measurement of levels of expression of known oncogenes in RNA derived from tumors. This approach, too, is fraught with difficulty. The expression of many of the cellular oncogenes is cell-cycle specific, and levels of expression may reflect the rate of cellular proliferation rather than any pathogenetic mechanism underlying the transformation process itself. In many instances, as in the case of the c-*myc* gene, it is probably the timing rather than the absolute level of mRNA expression that reflects the significant disruption of normal gene regulation. In this regard, the level of c-*myc* mRNA expression in most Burkitt lymphoma lines studied is highly variable, and frequently not elevated.[172] Finally, many genes, such as the *ras* genes, are activated by somatic mutation rather than by regulatory defects; in such cases the level of mRNA expression in the tumors is irrelevant to the transforming potential of the oncogene product. Consequently, such studies are probably of limited value in the analysis of oncogene activation in malignancy.

APOPTOSIS AND THE ROLE OF ONCOGENES IN LYMPHOID MALIGNANCY

Recent studies on the control of apoptosis, or programmed cell death, have provided new insights into the potential role of activated oncogenes in the pathogenesis of lymphoma. Apoptosis was originally understood as a process by which normal growth and differentiation are regulated during embryogenesis; it is now clear that many adult tissues continue this dynamic process as part of the normal program of cell turnover and renewal.[196-198] Apoptosis is characterized by a specific morphologic phenotype, and is associated with a specific pattern of DNA fragmentation.[196-198] Apoptosis is energy dependent, and requires the activity of the Na^+/H^+ transporter.[199] In some studies, its occurrence has been shown to require protein synthesis, and is postulated to depend on the synthesis of specific endonucleases that result in the DNA fragmentation.[200,201] In others, the suppression of apoptosis is shown to depend on the transcription of genes that are hypothesized to block the action of these endonucleases.[202]

Hematopoietic cells, which are constantly undergoing cycles of differentiation and maturation, are especially dependent on this program of growth control. It has long been known that the growth and survival of hematopoietic progenitor cells depends on the presence of specific growth factors. It has now become clear that although some of these factors act directly to promote growth, other factors function to preserve the viability of the differentiating hematopoietic cell by suppressing apoptosis.[203-206] One recent study has shown that transfection of interleukin-3 dependent hematopoietic precursor cells with a constitutively expressed c-bcl-2 gene delays apoptosis induced by interleukin-3 deprivation, and surprisingly, actually allows multilineage differentiation in the absence of lineage-inducing growth factors; these results support the notion that the primary function of growth factors is to prevent apoptotic death.[207]

There is increasing evidence that the promotion of cellular survival and the induction of cell growth are closely related, but separable, activities that can be differentially regulated. This separation of growth-promoting activity from factors influencing programmed cell death has been demonstrated experimentally in in vitro studies of growth-factor-independent leukemic cell lines. Treatment of these cells with maturation-promoting factors has shown that phenotypic maturation is preceded by induction of growth-factor dependence. Withdrawal of the growth factor can then induce apoptosis without the induction of a mature phenotype.[208] Consequently, one may postulate that one mechanism for the development of malignant transformation could involve the uncoupling of the process of growth from the regulatory process of programmed cell death, resulting in uncontrolled growth of the transformed cell population.

Study of the interaction of growth factors and oncogenes in lymphoma has suggested that such modulations of the program of apoptosis may indeed have a crucial role in the pathogenesis of that malignancy. Studies of the c-myc and c-bcl-2 oncogenes serve as a paradigm for this theory of oncogenesis. The c-myc gene displays differential effects on apoptosis and cellular growth. Deregulated expression of c-myc has been associated with increased growth and inhibition of maturation; however, when tumor cells expressing high levels of c-myc are induced with promoters of differentiation, they undergo enhanced apoptosis.[209] When cells exhibiting this phenotype also express high levels of bcl-2, however, the increased apoptosis is abrogated, and the growth-promoting and differentiation-inhibiting effects of c-myc continue without the associated enhancement of programmed cell death. Similar interactions have been observed with a deregulated c-myc gene in association with a mutant p53 gene.[210] These observations fit well with the hypothesis that interaction of multiple oncogenes is necessary for the development of malignancy.

These studies have important implications for therapy of lymphoma as well. Many cancer chemotherapeutic drugs have been shown to act by inducing apoptosis in sensitive tumor cells.[211-213] This effect can be enhanced by deprivation of growth factors or cytokines that naturally protect the tumor cells from apoptosis. For example, myeloma cells from patients with high-level expression of IL-6 have been shown to be more resistant to chemotherapy[214,215]; they have also been shown to undergo increased apoptosis in response to antibodies directed against IL-6.[216] This suggests that in tumors dependent on growth factors, these factors may mediate resistance to therapy by blocking apoptosis, but may also provide a target for therapy. Alternatively, in apparently growth-factor-independent tumors, growth factors may give maturation signals that will induce susceptibility to apoptosis on therapy. Further analysis of the complex interaction of oncogene expression with the closely intertwined processes of growth, differentiation, and apoptosis, should provide further insights into the origins of lymphoma, and reveal potential innovative strategies for antilymphoma therapy.

ROLE OF VIRUSES IN THE PATHOGENESIS OF LYMPHOPROLIFERATIVE DISEASE

Epstein-Barr Virus

EBV is a herpesvirus that selectively infects B lymphocytes and pharyngeal epithelial cells. It is the only herpesvirus that is known to be lymphotropic, and infects B cells via the C3d complement receptor (CRII, CD21). The virus was first identified by its presence in cultured Burkitt lymphoma cells,[217] and has been implicated in a wide range of lymphoproliferative lesions on the basis of epidemiologic, serologic, and molecular studies.[218,219] The mechanism of its role in neoplastic disorders, however, remains obscure.[220]

Infection of B cells with EBV results in expression of viral antigens, polyclonal activation, induction of immunoglobulin secretion, and subsequent continuous infection and "immortalization" of a subset of the cells. The continuously infected cells express nuclear antigen (EBNA), and carry multiple copies of the EBV genome.[220] Continuously infected cells are immortalized in that they will grow continuously in culture, but they do not have the characteristics of malignant cells (i.e., they do not cause tumors in nude mice and will not grow in soft agar).[221] It is consequently believed that a further transforming event (such as one of the cytogenetic alterations described for Burkitt lymphoma) is necessary for the acquisition of a malignant phenotype.

EBV infections occur worldwide. The vast majority of primary infections are asymptomatic, especially in areas where exposure and infection occur in early childhood.[222] The primary effect of the virus is to cause lymphocytic proliferation of infected cells. Consequently, the symptomatic disease associated with later primary infections, as well as the rare later manifestations of malignancy, are related to the host response to the virus-induced proliferation. The spectrum of manifestations of EBV-related disease is a reflection of the host's ability to control and suppress the infected B-cell clones. The range

Table 77-4. Lymphoproliferative Syndromes Associated with EBV

Infectious mononucleosis
Disease associated with X-linked lymphoproliferative disease and other congenital
   immunodeficiency syndromes
      Overwhelming lymphoproliferative syndrome (fatal infectious mononucleosis)
      Malignant lymphoma
      Hypogammaglobulinemia
Burkitt lymphoma
Polyclonal lymphoma in patients with acquired immunodeficiency or post-trans-
   plant immunodeficiency

of lymphoproliferative manifestations of EBV infections is outlined in Table 77-4.

Infectious Mononucleosis Syndrome

Primary EBV infection is responsible for 80–90% of cases of infectious mononucleosis syndrome (IM). The remaining cases are caused by other agents, primarily cytomegalovirus. IM is characterized by lymphadenopathy, fever, pharyngitis, and hepatosplenomegaly. It is associated with exuberant proliferation of $CD8^+$ T cells, which are the characteristic atypical lymphocytes seen in the peripheral blood of affected patients. Heterophil antibodies appear in most patients during the acute infection, and convalescence is associated with the development of multiple antibodies to viral antigens; IgG antibodies to viral capsid antigen (VCA) and to EBNA persist lifelong.[223–225] The symptoms of IM presumably result both from the primary proliferation of infected B cells, and the exaggerated T-cell response. Control of the disease is probably related to cytotoxic T-cell activity and to the development of neutralizing antibody. Long-term suppression of latent virus is thought to be primarily dependent on the activity of suppressor/cytotoxic T cells, because reactivation of the virus is seen primarily in people with acquired defects in T-cell immunity.

Overwhelming Primary Infection in Congenital Immunodeficiency Syndromes

The lethal manifestations of EBV fall into two broad categories: overwhelming primary infection, and later development of malignancy. Fatal primary EBV infection has been described as the hallmark of the X-linked lymphoproliferative syndrome (XLP), a disease associated with a poorly defined immunodeficiency that leads to inability to control primary IM. Over 50% of patients with XLP die of overwhelming IM; the remainder die of malignant B-cell lymphoma or of the complications of acquired hypogammaglobulinemia. Death occurs by age 10 in 80–90% of affected persons.[226,227] Other immunodeficiency syndromes, most notably ataxia-telangiectasia and Wiskott-Aldrich syndrome, have been associated with fatal IM.[228] The pathogenesis of these fatal disorders is thought to be uncontrolled proliferation of infected lymphocytes in the face of an inadequate host immune response; however, there is also evidence that some of the manifestations of fatal infection in XLP are related to hyperactivity of $CD8^+$ T cells.[227]

Burkitt Lymphoma

The role of EBV in the development of Burkitt lymphoma is not well understood. The high rate of early EBV infection in Africa, where 95% of infections occur by age 2, makes epidemiologic distinctions difficult. In a prospective study of a large group of children, elevated VCA antibody titers were predictive of increased risk of development of Burkitt lymphoma.[229] In addition, EBV genome is detectable in all African Burkitt lymphoma cells. This is in contrast to sporadic (North American) Burkitt lymphoma, in which EBV DNA is frequently not detected in the tumor.[230] The low overall frequency of Burkitt lymphoma in the uniformly infected population, as well as a long latency period from the time of initial infection to the appearance of lymphoma, suggests that EBV infection is only a predisposing factor in the development of the lymphoma. It has been proposed that malaria may be a second predisposing factor by causing antigenic stimulation and lymphoid hyperplasia.[231,232] A complex interaction of these multiple factors has been proposed: (1) initial EBV infection selects a subset of B cells with the potential for uncontrolled proliferation, but this initial hyperproliferation is suppressed by antibody and T-cell responses; (2) the persistent antigenic challenge of endemic malaria may depress the effectiveness of the immunologic suppression of the persistent EBV-positive clones, allowing them to proliferate; (3) recurrent proliferation of the immortalized clones predisposes to the eventual development of the clonal cytogenetic abnormality that causes oncogene activation and development of the malignant phenotype.

Lymphoma in Patients with Acquired Immunodeficiency

Acquired immunodeficiency, resulting either from immunosuppressive regimens for organ transplant recipients or from the acquired immunodeficiency syndrome, is associated with an increased incidence of lymphoma. The direct role of EBV in the development of these tumors remains to be established.[233–236] However, there is again substantial evidence for the role of EBV-induced lymphoproliferation as the substrate for the development of malignancy in this setting. EBV reactivation is seen in these patients as evidenced by rising anti-VCA titers, and EBV genomes have been detected in some tumors. In addition, some transplant patients have manifested polyclonal, EBV-positive lymphoproliferations that have regressed on reduction of immunosuppression.[237–243]

Human T-Cell Leukemia/Lymphoma Virus

HTLV-I has been implicated as the etiologic agent in the development of adult T-cell leukemia/lymphoma (ATLL). The virus has a structure similar to that of an oncogenic retrovirus, but has no homology with any known oncogenes. It integrates randomly into DNA, and therefore does not activate cellular oncogenes by insertional mutagenesis. Hence, the mechanism by which it transforms cells remains uncertain.[244] Infection with HTLV-1 gives rise to immortalized $CD4^+$ T cells that are nontumorigenic in nude mice.

Infection with HTLV-1 is not widespread. The virus has limited means of spread, and is transmitted primarily by means of body fluids, namely semen, blood, and breast milk; it can also be transmitted transplacentally.[245,246]

The relationship of HTLV-1 infection to the development of ATLL is reminiscent of the role of EBV in the development of Burkitt lymphoma. ATLL develops as a late complication of latent infection with HTLV-1 in <2% of patients infected with the virus,[247] which suggests that the virus is necessary but insufficient to lead to the development of a fully malignant phenotype. The necessary complementary factors for the development of ATLL after HTLV-1 infection are unknown.

The lymphoproliferative disease associated with HTLV-1 infection falls within a spectrum ranging from subclinical disease to acute, fulminant T-cell lymphoma.[248,249] Chronic disease manifests itself as intermittent fever, rash, and adenopathy in association with chronic mild proliferation of abnormal lymphocytes. The chronic form of the disease may persist for many years, and the factors responsible for the progression to acute leukemia/lymphoma are unknown. Progression to ATLL is marked by prominent skin infiltration, leukemic involvement with abnormal lymphocytes, hepatosplenomegaly, adenopathy, and frequent hypercalcemia. Response to therapy in the acute phase of HTLV-1-related leukemia/lymphoma is poor, with survival ranging from 2 weeks to about 1 year.[250]

CELL BIOLOGY AND NATURAL HISTORY OF LYMPHOPROLIFERATIVE DISEASE

The lymphoproliferative disorders are clinically distinguishable by widely variant natural histories. CLL and WDLL are slow-growing disorders with relatively well-behaved neoplastic cells, that is, the cells tend to remain in those locations normally populated by B lymphocytes: the white pulp of spleen, blood, and nodes. Both diseases behave clinically as though their major pathophysiology involves the accumulation of long-lived but relatively slow-growing cells rather than the expansion of cells demonstrating a burst of proliferative activity. Even though both disorders appear to arise from a similar stage of B-cell maturation, CLL cells traffic widely in the blood whereas WDLL cells tend to remain highly localized in the peripheral lymphoid organs. In contrast to both disorders, diffuse large cell lymphoma often invades extranodal sites and shows a high mitotic index. Some lymphoproliferative disorders such as HCL show a very characteristic pattern of cell homing that includes common B-cell sites (the bone marrow) but also sites that normal B cells do not occupy (e.g., the red rather than the white pulp of spleen). Furthermore, it is clear that the condition we call "complete clinical remission" in the indolent lymphoproliferative disorders such as the follicular small cell lymphomas involves the continuing, easily measurable presence of small numbers of monoclonal cells derived from the original malignant clone.[251,252] During clinical relapse, these same cells, previously quiescent, proliferate vigorously.[253]

These differing patterns of growth and migration, and the movement into and out of clinical remission, must be the result of many interactive processes, including (1) lineage and clonality of the malignant cell population and corresponding stage of differentiation, (2) molecular alteration at the DNA, RNA, and protein level resulting in relative immortalization and/or uncontrolled proliferation (loss of lymphocyte homeostasis[254]), (3) specific homing patterns of lymphocytes to particular tissues, and (4) modification of the tumor's growth by the immune system. The first two aspects of the genesis of lymphoma have been discussed; in this section the last two aspects are reviewed. Figure 77-2 provides a hypothetical working framework in which to consider the factors involved both in the genesis of lymphoma and in the particular clinical behavior of different lymphomas.

Normal and Malignant Lymphocyte Homing

The lymphoid immune system is by no means static. Lymphocytes have an extensive recirculation pattern[255,256] into and out of peripheral lymphoid organs (nodes and spleen). The site of entry of lymphocytes into these organs is usually at the histologically recognizable postcapillary (high-endothelial) venule, a structure that also appears to be the primary site of lymphocyte migration into sites of inflammation. In recent years, the molecular components responsible for lymphocyte homing have begun to be elucidated.[257] These include the selectin and β₁, β₂, and β₃ integrin families of adhesion molecules as well as other structures such as CD54 (ICAM-1), CD58 (LFA-3), and CD44.[258-263]

The selectin family of adhesion molecules consists of three members: (1) E-selectin (ELAM-1), inducible by cytokines such as IL-1 and tumor necrosis factor on the surface of endothelial cells and providing an adhesive structure for granulocytes; (2) L-selectin (Leu8, Mel14, LECAM-1), expressed on most leuko-

cytes and known to support rolling of granulocytes along blood vessel walls; (3) P-selectin (CD62, GMP140), inducible on both platelets and endothelium and known to mediate platelet binding to granulocytes and monocytes.[264,265] Both E-selectin and L-selectin are involved in lymphocyte migration. E-selectin is important for homing of subsets of T cells to skin (SALT). L-selectin appears responsible for several lymphocyte subsets homing to the high endothelial venule.[257] The counter-ligands for these receptors remain incompletely described, but at least include sialated Lewis^X carbohydrate moieties and probably sulfatides.[266-268]

The β₂ integrin family[269] consists of (1) CD11a/CD18 (LFA-1), present on virtually all leukocytes, which binds counter-ligands ICAM-1 and ICAM-2, and is responsible for a variety of cell-cell adhesive processes, including neutrophil diapedesis; (2) CD11b/CD18 (Mac-1, CR3), present on NK cells and other lymphocyte subsets as well as granulocytes and monocytes, which binds a variety of ligands, including complement components and bacterial components (C3bi, lipopolysaccharide), coagulation system components (fibrinogen, factor X), and also shares with CD11a/CD18 important phagocyte diapedesis activities via ICAM-1; (3) CD11c/CD18 (p150,95), present on phagocytes and some activated B cells and cytolytic T cells, which shares some functional similarity to CD11b/CD18.[270] The β₁ integrin family (including VLA-4) is also involved in immunocyte adhesion.[271,272] Integrin molecules serve both adhesive and signal transduction functions.[273] The movement of neutrophils along vessel walls appears to be mediated by selectin moieties in the "rolling" phase and integrin molecules during directed diapedesis.[274] Rapid modulation of these moieties is similarly important for lymphocyte trafficking.[275]

CD44 has been identified by a number of investigators working in somewhat disparate fields over time but it has recently become apparent that the Hermes antigens, HUTCH1, B-cell p80, red cell blood group In(Lu)-related p80, extracellular matrix receptor-III, phagocytic glycoprotein-1, and F10-44-2 all represent the same molecule, which is widely distributed on hematopoietic and epithelial cells.[276,277] Evidence is emerging to suggest that this molecule is involved in lymphocyte-high endothelial venule interactions[278-280] and also that its expression could be involved in metastatic behavior of human epithelial tumors.[281]

The differential expression of these adhesion molecules on neoplastic lymphocytes has been described in several studies.[282-287] As noted earlier, CD11c is strongly expressed by hairy cell leukemia cells and has been postulated to help explain their peculiar anatomic preferences; its expression on the malignant cells of some patients with CLL has also been associated with a distinctive clinical course.[288,289] Other investigators have postulated that differential expression of CD11a/CD18 may help explain the different patterns of organ involvement of CLL versus WDLL.[59] Increased expression of CD44 in large cell lymphoma has been reported to correlate with advanced stage disease.[286,290] Similarly, using a biologic assay of lymphocyte-endothelial cell adherence, a correlation of enhanced adhesion with advanced stage disease has been observed in CLL.[291] Some investigators have also found that lymphomas with gastrointestinal tropism tend to lack L-selectin, whereas those with a nodal predilection express this molecule.[155,292,293] HTLV-1 adult T-cell leukemia cells are thought to home to endothelium via E-selectin and VCAM-1[244]. Expression of sialated Lewis^X determinants (counter-ligands for the selectins) may also affect malignant lymphocyte homing.[294]

At the present time it is impossible to fully predict clinical homing behavior of the lymphoproliferative diseases solely on the basis of quantitative expression of these known families of adhesion molecules. Undoubtedly, conformational changes in these receptors as well as the complex interaction of different classes of receptor, along with the likely contribution of as yet undiscovered adhesive structures, will all be important in the eventual elucidation of the pathobiology behind the natural history of these neoplasms.

Immune Surveillance of Lymphoproliferative Disease

The Ehrlich-Thomas-Burnet hypothesis of the immune surveillance of cancer[295] predicts that immunosuppressed individuals should have a higher incidence of neoplasia. The tumor most frequently associated with immunosuppression is lymphoma, and therefore it would seem likely that lymphoproliferative disease might provide an excellent model for the study of immune regulation of cancers.[296] Although a clear understanding of immune surveillance remains elusive,[297,298] clinical data clearly demonstrate the regression of even large cell lymphomas that develop during immunosuppressive treatment on the removal of the extraneous immunosuppressive agents.[299,300] Improved understanding of cell-cell adhesion has begun to shed more light on this process.[301,302]

With respect to adhesive interactions necessary for the action of cytolytic T cells against tumor targets,[303] much work has been carried out on the CD11/CD18 series of integrin molecules, and on the interactions of CD2 with LFA-3. In immune reactions, antigen-independent adhesion is thought to be an early crucial step in engaging cytolytic T cells with appropriate targets. This antigen-independent adhesion is mediated by two pathways, the CD11a-CD54 path and CD2-CD58 ligand-counterligand interaction. The importance of the former pathway is emphasized by the fact that congenital inability to express the CD11/CD18 molecules on the cell surface results in a fatal immunodeficiency syndrome.[304] CD11a-CD54 (and CD2-CD58) adhesion may therefore be crucially important for immune surveillance of tumors. Indeed, it has been shown that the characteristic rosette formation of T cells around the Reed-Sternberg cells of Hodgkin disease is mediated largely by these interactions.[305] Moreover, Burkitt lymphoma cells characteristically express very low levels of CD11a, CD54, and CD58 but acquire these molecules gradually during prolonged passage in tissue culture. As predicted, early passages of these cells are frequently resistant to EBV-specific cytolytic T cells, while they become more susceptible as the expression of the adhesion molecules increases.[306,307]

IMMUNE CYTOPENIAS IN LYMPHOPROLIFERATIVE DISEASE

Cytopenia in Lymphoproliferative Disorders of Large Granular Lymphocytes

The Tγ lymphocytosis syndrome, also termed T-suppressor leukemia, large granular lymphocyte leukemia, and T-cell lymphocytosis with cytopenia, is characterized by a proliferation of large granular lymphocytes in association with prominent cytopenias, most commonly neutropenia.[308–310] Neutropenia is found in >80% of these patients, and may be cyclic.[311] Anemia is also common, often with a marrow consistent with pure red cell aplasia. Coombs-positive hemolytic anemia has been described in one patient.[310] There is strong association of the syndrome with rheumatoid arthritis, and patients often have positive tests for antinuclear antibodies and rheumatoid factor, as well as polyclonal hypergammaglobulinemia. Many of these patients have been initially diagnosed as having Felty syndrome.[312]

The natural history of the LGL syndrome is variable. In many cases, the patients have a benign clinical course that rarely requires cytotoxic therapy.[313] However, some series have reported complications requiring therapy, usually recurrent infections, in up to two-thirds of patients.[314] The relatively indolent course of the disease, as well as its strong association with autoimmune disease, led to considerable controversy as to whether the syndrome represents a T-cell neoplasm or a benign disorder of immune regulation. This question has been largely resolved by studies that have revealed monoclonal rearrangements of the TCR in most cases.[102,315–317]

Although the cell population involved in this disorder is heterogeneous, the proliferating lymphocytes usually have a characteristic phenotype, most expressing CD2, CD3, and CD8. A striking abnormal feature of the cells is the absence of the T-cell marker CD5.[318–322] Functional analysis of the cells has given variable results. Cells from nearly all patients studied exhibit antibody-dependent cytotoxicity, which is consistent with the nearly uniform presence of Fc receptors for γ-globulin. Less than one-half of the cells studied have revealed spontaneous NK activity. In nearly all cases, responses to T-cell mitogens are poor, although up to one-half show suppressor activity as demonstrated by inhibition of pokeweed mitogen-induced immunoglobulin production by B lymphocytes.[321] The cases of large granular lymphocytosis derived from CD3− NK cells are also rather heterogeneous with respect to precise immunophenotype and measurements of in vitro cell function.

The suppressor/cytolytic phenotype of the proliferating large granular lymphocytes has led many investigators to attempt to relate the cytopenias associated with the syndrome to the functional activity of the cells involved. Suppression of erythroid progenitors, namely colony-forming unit-erythroid (CFU-E) and burst-forming unit-erythroid (BFU-E), has been seen in most cases studied that have been associated with pure red cell aplasia.[323,324] By contrast, suppression of myeloproliferation by the large granular lymphocytes has been more difficult to demonstrate. Normal CD3+/CD8+ T cells and CD3− NK cells coexist with myelopoietic stem cells.[325] In the LGL syndromes, one report has suggested limited evidence for active suppression of hematopoietic progenitor cells by this population of lymphocytes.[326] In the absence of proof of direct suppression of myeloid precursors by the proliferating lymphoid population, evidence has been sought for antibody-mediated neutropenia or for inhibition by soluble lymphokines. Antineutrophil antibodies have been found in many of these patients, but the functional significance of these in the etiology of neutropenia has not been proved. No direct evidence for lymphokine-mediated bone marrow suppression has been elucidated; however, some large granular lymphocytes from these patients have been shown to produce interferon, which is known to inhibit CFU-granulocyte/macrophage and BFU-E growth.[327]

The treatments for severe neutropenia in this syndrome have been based on the assumed immunologic basis of the neutropenia, namely splenectomy and cytotoxic agents. These interventions have proved of little efficacy in the treatment of neutropenia, although cytotoxic agents usually easily control adenopathy and other lymphomatous aspects of the disease.[328,329] Surprisingly, patients often respond to treatment with CSF-G, further compounding the confusion regarding the pathogenesis of neutropenia in this syndrome.[330,331] In summary, although the surface phenotype and functional profile of the proliferating large granular lymphocytes in Tγ lymphocytosis suggest that they are potentially active in suppressing hematopoiesis, direct evidence for their role in the pathogenesis of the cytopenias or their involvement in the other autoimmune manifestations of the syndrome remains to be elucidated.

Cytopenia in Chronic Lymphocytic Leukemia

Autoimmune hemolytic anemia and immune thrombocytopenia are common complications of CLL. The pathogenesis of these immune complications remains unclear. For the most part, these antibodies do not arise from the malignant clone, but instead arise from "bystander" lymphocytes.[332–334]

Recent attempts to understand the basis for the autoimmune manifestations of CLL have focused on the identity of the CD5$^+$ B cells as a lineage associated with autoantibody production.[40] CD5$^+$B cells are the predominant B lymphocytes found in the fetal spleen and peripheral blood. In addition, they comprise ≤10–25% of B lymphocytes in normal adults. These cells produce polyspecific antibodies, including autoreactive antibodies; it has also been hypothesized that they may play a significant role in the primary immune response to pathogens. CD5$^+$ B cells are increased in patients with rheumatoid arthritis.[334] This finding, in the context of the autoreactivity demonstrated by many of the antibodies produced by CD5$^+$ B cells, has led to the hypothesis that this subset of B cells is involved in autoimmune disease. However, their role is poorly understood, since they produce polyreactive antibodies quite different from the characteristic high-affinity antibodies found in rheumatoid arthritis.[335]

CLL is postulated to result from a clonal expansion of a cell from the normal subpopulation of CD5$^+$ B cells. In support of this is the observation that CD5$^+$ B cells in CLL patients can be stimulated with mitogens to produce autoantibodies.[336] There is also evidence that CLL may arise from a more global defect in immune regulation, since independent clones of autoantibody-producing cells can be isolated from mice with severe combined immunodeficiency engrafted with peripheral blood lymphocytes from CLL patients.[337]

One might therefore postulate that the autoimmune phenomena associated with CLL could be attributed to antibodies produced by other nonmalignant, but inadequately regulated, B cells. This would not explain the restriction of the autoimmune phenomena to the hematopoietic system, nor that only 20% of patients with CLL experience autoimmune hemolytic anemia or thrombocytopenia. In summary, the relationship of the significant clinical observations of autoimmune phenomena to the basic biology of CLL remains obscure.

REFERENCES

1. Uckon FM: Regulation of human B-cell ontogeny. Blood 76:1908, 1990
2. Blackman M, Kappler J, Marrack P: The role of the T cell receptor in positive and negative selection of developing T cells. Science 243:1335, 1990
3. von Boehmer H: Developmental biology of T cells in T cell-receptor transgenic mice. Ann Rev Immunol 8:531, 1990
4. Boyd RL, Hugo P: Towards an integrated view of thymopoiesis. Immunol Today 12:71, 1991
5. Clevers HC, Owen MJ: Towards a molecular understanding of T-cell differentiation. Immunol Today 12:86, 1991
6. Cooper MD: B lymphocytes. Normal development and function. N Engl J Med 317:1452, 1987
7. Smith BR: Regulation of hematopoiesis. Yale J Med Biol 63:371, 1990
8. Lanier LL, Spits H, Phillips JH: The developmental relationship between NK cells. Immunol Today 13:392, 1992
9. Oettinger MA, Schatz DG, Gorka C, Baltimore D: RAG-1 and RAG-2 adjacent genes that synergistically activate V(D)J recombination. Science 248:1517, 1990
10. Bos JD, Kapsenberg ML: The skin immune system: progress in cutaneous biology. Immunol Today 14:75, 1993
11. Jenkins MK, Schwartz RH, Pardoll DM: Effects of cyclosporine A on T cell development and clonal deletion. Science 241:1655, 1988
12. Clark EA, Ledbetter JA: Structure, function, and genetics of human B cell associated surface molecules. Adv Cancer Res 52:81, 1989
13. Korsmeyer SJ, Hieter PA, Ravetch JV et al: Developmental hierarchy of immunoglobulin gene rearrangements in human leukemic pre-B-cells. Proc Natl Acad Sci USA 78:7096, 1981

14. Kishimoto T, Hirano T: Molecular regulation of B lymphocyte response. Ann Rev Immunol 6:485, 1988
15. Butcher EC: Cellular and molecular mechanisms that direct leukocyte traffic. Am J Pathol 136:3, 1990
16. Griesser H, Tkachuk D, Reis MD, Mak TW: Gene rearrangements and translocations in lymphoproliferative diseases. Blood 73:1402, 1989
17. Smith BR: Qualitative versus quantitative immunophenotyping. Ann NY Acad Sci 677:152, 1993
18. Smith BR: Integrating flow cytometry into the hematology laboratory: a curmudgeon's view. Ann NY Acad Sci 677:326, 1993
19. Antin JH, Bierer BE, Smith BR et al: Depletion of bone marrow T lymphocytes with an anti-CD5 monoclonal immunotoxin (ST1-immunotoxin): effective prophylaxis for graft versus host disease. In Gross S, Gee AP, Worthington-White DA (eds): Bone Marrow Purging and Processing. Prog Clin Biol Res 333:207, 1993
20. Kwak LW, Campbell MJ, Czerwinski DK et al: Induction of immune responses in patients with B-cell lymphoma against the surface-immunoglobulin idiotype expressed by their tumors. N Engl J Med 327:1209, 1992
21. Miller RA, Hart S, Samoszuk M et al: Shared idiotypes expressed by human B-cell lymphomas. N Engl J Med 321:851, 1989
22. Uckun FM, Ledbetter JA: Immunobiologic differences between normal and leukemic human B-cell precursors. Proc Natl Acad Sci USA 85:8603, 1988
23. Foon KA, Todd RF: Immunologic classification of leukemia and lymphoma. Blood 68:1, 1986
24. Freedman AS, Nadler LM: Immunological markers in non-Hodgkin's lymphoma. Hematol Oncol Clin North Am 5:871, 1991
25. Kadin ME, Said J: T-cell lymphomas and leukemias of post-thymic differentiation. Clin Lab Med 8:135, 1988
26. Molgaard HV, Spurr NK, Greaves MF: The hematopoietic stem cell antigen, CD34, is encoded by a gene located on chromosome 1. Leukemia 3:773, 1989
27. Carter RH, Fearon DT: CD19: lowering the threshold for antigen receptor stimulation of B lymphocytes. Science 256:105, 1992
28. Bradbury LE, Goldmacher VS, Tedder TF: The CD19 signal transduction complex of B lymphocytes. J Immunol 151:2915, 1993
29. LeBien TW, McCormack RT: The common acute lymphoblastic leukemia antigen (CD10)—emancipation from a functional enigma. Blood 73:625, 1989
30. Grossbard ML, Press OW, Appelbaum FR et al: Monoclonal antibody based therapies of leukemia and lymphoma. Blood 80:863, 1992
31. Leitenberg D, Rappeport JM, Smith BR: Precursor B cell bone marrow reconstitution following marrow transplant. Am J Clin Pathol 1994 (in press)
32. Melchers F, Karasuyama H, Haasner D et al: The surrogate light chain in B-cell development. Immunol Today 14:60, 1993
33. Pui C-H, Behm FG, Crist WM: Clinical and biologic relevance of immunologic marker studies in childhood acute lymphoblastic leukemia. Blood 82:343, 1993
34. Smith BR, Ault KA: Circulating monoclonal B lymphocytes in non-Hodgkin's lymphoma. p. 142. In Hickey RC (ed): 1985 Yearbook of Cancer. Year Book Medical Publishers, Chicago, 1985
35. Dighiero G, Travade P, Chevret S et al: B-cell chronic lymphocytic leukemia: present status and future directions. Blood 78:1901, 1991
36. Van de Velde H, von Hoegen I, Luo W et al: The B-cell surface protein CD72/Lyb-2 is the ligand for CD5. Nature 351:662, 1991
37. Hayakawa K, Hardy RR: Normal, autoimmune, and malignant CD5 + cells: the Ly-1 B lineage? Ann Rev Immunol 6:197, 1988
38. Kipps TJ: The CD5 B cell. Adv Immunol 47:117, 1989
39. Herzenberg LA, Herzenberg LA: Toward a layered immune system. Cell 59:953, 1989
40. Kantor AB: The development and repertoire of B-1 cells (CD5 B cells). Immunol Today 12:389, 1991
41. Gadol N, Ault KA: Phenotypic and functional characterization of human Leu1 (CD5) B cells. Immunol Rev 93:23, 1986
42. Casali P, Notkins AL: CD5 + B lymphocytes, polyreactive antibodies and the B cell repertoire. Immunol Today 10:364, 1989
43. Hayakawa K, Hardy RR, Herzenberg LA: Progenitors for Ly-1 B cells are distinct from progenitors for other B cells. J Exp Med 151:1554, 1985
44. Antin JH, Ault KA, Rappeport JM, Smith BR: B lymphocyte reconstitution after human bone marrow transplantation: the Leu-1 antigen defines a functionally distinct population of B lymphocytes. J Clin Invest 80:325, 1987
45. Werner-Favre C, Vischer TL, Wohlwend D, Zubler RH: Cell surface CD5 is a marker for activated human B cells. Eur J Immunol 19:1209, 1989
46. Freedman AS, Freeman G, Whitman J et al: Expression and regulation of CD5 on in vitro activated human B cells. Eur J Immunol 19:849, 1989
47. Hayakawa K, Hardy RR, Herzenberg LA, Herzenberg LA: Progenitors for Ly-1 B cells are distinct from progenitors for other B cells. J Exp Med 161:1554, 1985
48. Sthoeger ZM, Wakai M, Tse DB et al: Production of autoantibodies by CD5–

expressing B lymphocytes from patients with chronic lymphocytic leukemia. J Exp Med 169:255, 1989

49. Kipps TJ, Carson DA: Autoantibodies in chronic lymphocytic leukemia and related systemic autoimmune diseases. Blood 81:2475, 1993

50. Casali P, Burastero SE, Nakamura M et al: Human lymphocytes making rheumatoid factor and antibody to ssDNA belong to the Leu-1+ B-cell subset. Science 236:77, 1987

51. Hardy RR, Hayakawa K, Shimizu M et al: Rheumatoid factor secretion from human Leu-1+ B cells. Science 236:81, 1987

52. Inghirami G, Foitl DR, Sabichi A et al: Autoantibody-associated cross-reactive idiotype-bearing human B lymphocytes: distribution and characterization, including Ig V_H gene and CD5 antigen expression. Blood 78:1503, 1991

53. Hardy RR, Hayakawa K, Shimizu M et al: Rheumatoid factor secretion from human Leu-1 + B cells. Science 236:81, 1987

54. Suzuki N, Sakane T, Engleman EG: Anti-DNA antibody production by CD5 and CD5− by cells of patients with systemic lupus erythematosus. J Clin Invest 85:238, 1990

55. Kasaian MT, Ikematsu H, Casali P: Identification and analysis of a novel human surface CD5− B lymphocyte subset producing natural antibodies. J Immunol 148:2690, 1992

56. Ault KA, Antin JH, Ginsburg D et al: Phenotype of recovering lymphoid cell populations following marrow transplantation. J Exp Med 161:1483, 1985

57. Longo DL: What's the deal with follicular lymphomas? J Clin Oncol 11:202, 1993

58. Chang KL, Stroup R, Weiss LM: Hairy cell leukemia. Anat Pathol 34:719, 1992

59. Freedman AS, Nadler LM: Immunological markers in non-Hodgkin's lymphoma. Hematol Oncol Clin North Am 5:871, 1991

60. Smith BR, Robert NJ, Ault KA: In Waldenström's macroglobulinemia the quantity of detectable circulating monoclonal B lymphocytes correlates with clinical course. Blood 61:911, 1983

61. Harada H, Kawano MM, Huang N et al: Phenotypic difference of normal plasma cells form mature myeloma cells. Blood 81:2658, 1993

62. Yamada M, Hudson S, Tournay O et al: Detection of minimal disease in hematopoietic malignancies of the B-cell lineage by using third-complementarity-determining region (CDR-III)-specific probes. Proc Natl Acad Sci USA 86:5123, 1989

63. Winoto A, Baltimore D: Separate lineages of T cells expressing the alpha beta and gamma delta receptors. Nature 338:430, 1989

64. de Villartay JP, Hockett RD, Coran D et al: Deletion of the human T-cell receptor delta-gene by a site-specific recombination. Nature 335:170, 1988

65. Itohara S, Farr AG, Lafaille JJ et al: Homing of a γδ thymocyte subset with homogeneous T-cell receptors to mucosal epithelia. Nature 343:754, 1990

66. Malissen M, Trucy J, Jouvin-Marche E et al: Regulation of TCR α and β gene allelic exclusion during T-cell development. Immunol Today 13:315, 1992

67. Foroni L, Laffan M, Boehm T et al: Rearrangement of the T-cell receptor δ genes in human t-cell leukemias. Blood 73:559, 1989

68. Loughran TP Jr: Clonal diseases of large granular lymphocytes. Blood 82: 1, 1993

69. de Totero D, Tazzari PL, DiSanto JP et al: Heterogeneous immunophenotype of granular lymphocyte expansions: differential expression of the CD8α and CD8β chains. Blood 80:1765, 1992

70. Maziarz RT, Arceci RJ, Bernstein SC et al: A γδ T cell leukemia bearing a novel variant t (8;14) (q24;q11) translocation demonstrates in vitro lymphocyte activated killing. Blood 79:1523, 1992

71. Uckun FM, Ramsay NKC, Waddick KG et al: In vitro and in vivo radiation resistance associated with CD3 surface antigen expression in T-lineage acute lymphoblastic leukemia. Blood 78:2945, 1991

72. Strair RK, Towle M, Heald P, Smith BR: Retroviral mediated transfer and expression of exogenous genes in primary lymphoid cells: assaying for a viral transactivator activity in normal and malignant cells. Blood 76:1201, 1990

73. Yodoi J, Uchiyama T: Disease associated with HTLV-I virus, IL-2 receptor dysregulation and redox regulation. Immunol Today 14:405, 1992

74. Hollsberg P, Hafler DA: Pathogenesis of diseases induced by human lymphotropic virus type I infection. N Engl J Med 328:1173, 1993

75. Burg G, Dummer R, Wilhelm M et al: A subcutaneous delta-positive t-cell lymphoma that produces interferon gamma. N Engl J Med 325:1078, 1991

76. Anagnostopoulos I, Hummel M, Finn T et al: Heterogeneous Epstein-Barr virus infection patterns in peripheral T-cell lymphoma of angioimmunoblastic lymphadenopathy type. Blood 80:1804, 1992

77. Feller AC, Griesser GH, Mak TW, Lennert K: Lymphoepithelioid lymphoma (Lennert's lymphoma) is a monoclonal proliferation of helper/inducer T cells. Blood 68:663, 1986

78. Gaulard P, Bourquelot P, Kanavaros P et al: Expression of the α/β and γ/δ T-cell receptors in 57 cases of peripheral T-cell lymphomas. Identification of a subset of γ/δ T-cell lymphomas. Am J Pathol 137:617, 1990

79. Kwak LW, Wilson M, Weiss LM et al: Similar outcome of treatment of B-cell and T-cell diffuse large-cell lymphomas: the Stanford experience. J Clin Oncol 9:1426, 1991

80. Armitage JC, Vose JM, Weisenburger D et al: Clinical significance of immunophenotype in diffuse aggressive non-Hodgkin's lymphoma. J Clin Oncol 7: 1783, 1989

81. Brunning RD: T-prolymphocytic leukemia. Blood 78:3111, 1991

82. Ault KA, Smith BR, Holmberg LA: Proliferation of Tγ cells with natural killer activity in patients with neutropenia, letter. N Engl J Med 303:881, 1980

83. Robertson MJ, Ritz J: Biology and clinical relevance of human natural killer cells. Blood 76:2421, 1990

84. Bridges KB, Smith BR: Discordance of transferrin receptor expression and susceptibility to lysis by natural killer cells. J Clin Invest 76:913, 1985

85. Zambello R, Trentin L, Ciccone E et al: Phenotypic diversity of natural killer (NK) populations in patients with NK-type lymphoproliferative disease of granular lymphocytes. Blood 81:2381, 1993

86. Nash R, McSweeney P, Zambello R et al: Clonal studies of CD3− lymphoproliferative disease of granular lymphocytes. Blood 81:2363, 1993

87. Kanavaros P, Lescs M-C, Briere J et al: Nasal T-cell lymphoma: a clinicopathologic entity associated with peculiar phenotype and with Epstein-Barr virus. Blood 81:2688, 1993

88. Peiper SC: Angiocentric lymphoproliferative disorders of the respiratory system: incrimination of Epstein-Barr virus in pathogenesis. Blood 82:687, 1993

89. Leitenberg D, Rinder H, Goldstein JM et al: Natural killer cell lymphocytosis in patients with chronic inflammatory demyelinating polyneuropathy. Blood, suppl. 1. 80:53a, 1992

90. Pirruccello SJ, Bicak MS, Gordon BG et al: Acute lymphoblastic leukemia of NK-cell lineage: responses to IL-2. Leuk Res 13:735, 1989

91. Sheridan W, Winton EF, Chan WC et al: Leukemia of non-T lineage natural killer cells. Blood 72:1701, 1988

92. Leder P: The genetics of antibody diversity. Sci Am 246:102, 1982

93. Tonegawa S: Somatic generation of antibody diversity. Nature 302:575, 1983

94. Brack C, Hirama M, Lehard-Schuller R et al: A complete immunoglobulin gene is created by somatic recombination. Cell 15:1, 1978

95. Noesel CJM, van Lier RAW: Architecture of the human B-cell antigen receptors. Blood 82:363, 1993

96. Korsmeyer SJ: Antigen receptor genes as molecular markers of lymphoid neoplasms. J Clin Invest 79:1291, 1987

97. Korsmeyer SJ: B-lymphoid neoplasms: immunoglobulin genes as molecular determinants of clonality, lineage, differentiation, and translocation. Adv Intern Med 33:1, 1988

98. Horning SJ, Galili N, Cleary M, Sklar J: Detection of non-Hodgkin's lymphoma in the peripheral blood by analysis of antigen receptor gene rearrangements: results of a prospective study. Blood 75:1139, 1990

99. Flug E, Pelicci PG, Bonetti F et al: T cell receptor gene rearrangements as markers of lineage and clonality in T cell neoplasms. Proc Natl Acad Sci USA 82:3460, 1985

100. Minden MD, Mak TW: The structure of the T cell antigen receptor genes in normal and malignant T cells. Blood 68:327, 1986

101. Foon KA, Thiruvengadam R, Saven A et al: Genetic relatedness of lymphoid malignancies. Ann Intern Med 119:63, 1993

102. Waldmann TA, Davis MM, Bongiovanni KF et al: Rearrangements of genes for the antigen receptor on T cells as markers of lineage and clonality in human lymphoid neoplasms. N Engl J Med 313:776, 1985

103. Felix CA, Wright JJ, Poplack DG et al: T cell receptor α, β, and genes in T cell and pre B cell acute lymphoblastic leukemia. J Clin Invest 80:545, 1987

104. Oster W, Konig K, Ludwig WD et al: Incidence of lineage promiscuity in acute myeloblastic leukemia: diagnostic implications of immunoglobulin and T-cell receptor gene rearrangement analysis and immunological phenotyping. Cancer Res 12:887, 1988

105. Ha-Kawa K, Hara J, Keiko Y et al: Kappa-chain gene rearrangement in an apparent T-lineage lymphoma. J Clin Invest 78:1439, 1986

106. Cogne M, Silvain C, Khamlichi AA, Preud'homme JL: Structurally abnormal immunoglobulins in human immunoproliferative disorders. Blood 79:2181, 1992

107. Bakhshi A, Guglielmi P, Siebenlist U et al: A DNA insertion/deletion necessitates an aberrant RNA splice accounting for a mu heavy chain disease protein. Proc Natl Acad Sci USA 83:2689, 1986

108. Alexander A, Steinmetz M, Barritault D: Gamma heavy chain disease in man: cDNA sequence supports partial gene deletion model. Proc Natl Acad Sci USA 79:3260, 1982

109. Sklar J, Cleary M, Thielemans K et al: Biclonal B-cell lymphoma. N Engl J Med 311:20, 1984

110. Siegelman MH, Cleary ML, Warnke R, Sklar J: Frequent biclonality and Ig

gene alterations among B cell lymphomas that show multiple histologic forms. J Exp Med 161:850, 1985

111. Cleary ML, Galili N, Trela M et al: Single cell origin of bigenotypic and biphenotypic B cell proliferations in human follicular lymphomas. J Exp Med 167: 582, 1988

112. Kyle RA, Robinson RA, Katzmann JA: The clinical aspects of biclonal gammopathies: review of 57 cases. Am J Med 71:999, 1981

113. Fine JM, Gorin NC, Gendre JP et al: Simultaneous occurrence of clinical manifestations of myeloma and Waldenstrom's macroglobulinemia with monoclonal IgG lambda and IgM kappa in a single patient. J Intern Med 209: 229, 1981

114. Weinstein S, Jain A, Bhagavan NV, Scottolini AG: Biclonal IgA and IgM gammopathy in lymphocytic lymphoma. Clin Chem 30:1710, 1984

115. Guarner J, Austin GE, Nassar VH et al: Biclonal gammopathy (IgG κ and IgG λ) in a patient with non-Hodgkin's lymphoma. Arch Pathol Lab Med 110: 445, 1986

116. Kyle RA: "Benign" monoclonal gammopathy—after 20 to 35 years follow-up. Mayo Clin Proc 68:26, 1993

117. Radl J: Monoclonal B-cell proliferative disorders and aging. Ann NY Acad Sci 621:418, 1991

118. Keshgegian AA: Oligoclonal banding in sera of hospitalized patients. Clin Chem 38:169, 1992

119. Harrison HH: The "ladder light chain" or pseudo-oligoclonal pattern in urinary immunofixation electrophoresis (IFE) studies: a distinctive IFE pattern and an explanatory hypothesis relating it to free polyclonal light chains. Clin Chem 37:1559, 1991

120. Papadopoulos NM, Tsianos EV, Costello R: Oligoclonal immunoglobulins in serum of patients with chronic viral hepatitis. J Clin Lab Anal 4:180, 1990

121. Probert CS, Roland JM, Simpson KR, Fairham SA: Dramatic oligoclonal paraproteinemia following a pneumococcal septicaemia. Postgrad Med J 67:295, 1991

122. Tsianos EV, DiBisceglie AM, Papadopoulos NM et al: Oligoclonal immunoglobulin bands in serum in association with chronic viral hepatitis. Am J Gastroenterol 85:1005, 1990

123. Del Carpio J, Espinoza LR, Lauter S, Osterland CK: Transient monoclonal proteins in drug hypersensitivity reactions. Am J Med 66:1051, 1979

124. Amadori A, Gallo P, Zamarchi R et al: IgG oligoclonal bands in sera of HIV-1 infected patients are mainly directed against HIV-1 determinants. AIDS Res Hum Retroviruses 6:581, 1990

125. Sinclair D, Galloway E, McKenzie S et al: Oligoclonal immunoglobulins in HIV infection. Clin Chem 35:1669, 1989

126. Yoshino I, Yano T, Yoshikai Y et al: Oligoclonal T lymphocytes infiltrating human lung cancer tissues. Int J Cancer 47:654, 1991

127. Link H, Cruz M, Gessain A et al: Chronic progressive myelopathy associated with HTLV-I: oligoclonal IgG and anti-HTLV-I IgG antibodies in cerebrospinal fluid and serum. Neurology 39:1566, 1989

128. Tissot JD, Schneider P, Pelet B et al: Mono-oligoclonal production of immunoglobulin in a child with the Wiskott-Aldrich syndrome. Br J Haematol 75: 436, 1990

129. Mitus AJ, Stein RS, Rappeport JM et al: Monoclonal and oligoclonal gammopathy after bone marrow transplantation. Blood 74:2764, 1989

130. Myara I, Quenum G, Storogenko M et al: Monoclonal and oligoclonal gammopathies in heart-transplant recipients. Clin Chem 37:1334, 1991

131. Fox DA, Smith BR: Evidence for oligoclonal B cell expansion in the peripheral blood of patients with rheumatoid arthritis. Ann Rheum Dis 45:991, 1986

132. Medeiros LJ, Harris NL: Lymphoid infiltrate of the orbit and conjunctiva. A morphologic and immunophenotypic study of 99 cases. Am J Surg Pathol 8:83, 1984

133. Falzon M, Isaacson PG: The natural history of benign lymphoepithelial lesion of the salivary gland in which there is a monoclonal population of B cells. A report of two cases. Am J Surg Pathol 15:59, 1991

134. Fishleder A, Tubbs R, Hesse B, Levine H: Uniform detection of immunoglobulin-gene rearrangement in benign lymphoepithelial lesions. N Engl J Med 316:1118, 1987

135. Knowles DM, Jakobiec FA: Cell marker analysis of extranodal lymphoid infiltrates: to what extent does the determination of mono or polyclonality resolve the diagnostic dilemma of malignant lymphoma vs pseudolymphoma in an extranodal site? Semin Diagn Pathol 2:163, 1985

136. Knowles DM, Athan E, Ubriaco A et al: Extranodal noncutaneous lymphoid hyperplasias represent a continuous spectrum of B-cell neoplasia: demonstration by molecular genetic analysis. Blood 73:1635, 1989

137. Korsmeyer SJ: Bcl-2 initiates a new category of oncogenes: regulators of cell death. Blood 80:879, 1992

138. Raffeld M, Jaffe ES: bcl-1, t(11;14) and mantle cell-derived lymphomas. Blood 78:259, 1991

139. Stern MH, Theodorou I, Aurias A et al: T-cell nonmalignant clonal prolifera-

tion in ataxia telangiectasia: a cytological, immunological, and molecular characterization. Blood 73:1285, 1989

140. Peterson RD, Funkhouser JD: Speculations on ataxia-telangiectasia: defective regulation of the immunoglobulin gene superfamily. Immunol Today 10:313, 1989

141. Weiss LM, Wood GS, Trela M et al: Clonal T-cell populations in lymphomatoid papulosis. N Engl J Med 315:475, 1986

142. Wen T, Mellstedt H, Jondal M: Presence of clonal T cell populations in chronic B lymphocytic leukemia and smoldering myeloma. J Exp Med 171: 659, 1990

143. Janson CH, Grunewald J, Osterborg A et al: Predominant T cell receptor V gene usage in patients with abnormal clones of B cells. Blood 77:1776, 1991

144. Balk SP, Ebert EC, Blumenthal RL et al: Oligoclonal expansion and CD1 recognition by human intestinal intraepithelial lymphocytes. Science 253:1411, 1991

145. Strickler JG, Movahed LA, Gajl-Peczalska KJ et al: Oligoclonal T cell receptor gene rearrangements in blood lymphocytes of patients with acute Epstein-Barr virus-induced infectious mononucleosis. J Clin Invest 86:1358, 1990

146. Leitenberg D, Chapin-Robertson K, Rappeport J, Smith BR: Large granular lymphocytosis and oligoclonal expression of the T cell receptor beta chain. Blood, suppl. 1. 78:176a, 1992

147. Dean M, Pappas H, Norton JD: Immunoglobulin heavy chain gene fingerprinting reveals widespread oligoclonality in B-lineage acute lymphoblastic leukaemia. Leukemia 5:832, 1991

148. Kusunoki Y, Hirai Y, Kyoizumi S, Akiyama M: Evidence for in vivo clonal proliferation of unique population of blood CD4-/CD8- T cells bearing T-cell receptor α and β chains in two normal men. Blood 79:2964, 1992

149. Ishikawa T, Imura A, Tanaka K et al: E-selectin and vascular cell adhesion molecule-1 mediate adult T-cell leukemia cell adhesion to endothelial cells. Blood 82:1590, 1993

150. Sala P, Tonutti E, Feruglio C et al: Persistent expansions of CD4+ CD8+ peripheral blood T cells. Blood 82:1546, 1993

151. French DL, Laskov R, Scharff MD: The role of somatic hypermutation in the generation of antibody diversity. Science 244:1152, 1989

152. Moebius U, Manns M, Hess G et al: T cell receptor gene rearrangements of T lymphocytes infiltrating the liver in chronic active hepatitis B and primary biliary cirrhosis (PBC): oligoclonality of PBC-derived T cell clones. Eur J Immunol 20:889, 1990

153. Davies TF, Martin A, Concepcion ES et al: Evidence of limited variability of antigen receptors on intrathyroidal T cells in autoimmune thyroid disease. N Engl J Med 325:238, 1991

154. Palliard X, West SG, Lafferty JA et al: Evidence for the effects of superantigen in rheumatoid arthritis. Science 253:325, 1991

155. Kunkel HG, Muller-Eberhard HJ, Fudenberg HH, Tomasi TB: Gamma globulin complexes in rheumatoid arthritis and certain other conditions. J Clin Invest 40:117, 1961

156. Leder P, Battey J, Lenoir G et al: Translocation among antibody genes in human cancer. Science 222:765, 1983

157. Chevenix-Trench G: The molecular genetics of human non-Hodgkin's lymphoma. Cancer Genet Cytogenet 22:191. 1987

158. Showe LC, Croce CM: The role of chromosomal translocations in B- and T-cell neoplasia. Ann Rev Immunol 5:253, 1987

159. Graf T, Beug H: Avian leukemia viruses: interaction with their target cells in vivo and in vitro. Biochem Biophys Acta 516:269, 1978

160. Shieness DK, Hughes SH, Varmus HE et al: The vertebrate homolog of the putative transforming gene of avian myelomatosis virus: characteristics of the DNA locus and its RNA transcript. Virology 28:600, 1978

161. Ohno S, Babonits MM, Wiener F et al: Nonrandom chromosome changes involving the Ig gene-carrying chromosomes 12 and 6 in pristane-induced mouse plasmacytoma. Cell 18:1001, 1979

162. Taub R, Kirsch I, Morton C et al: Translocation of the c-myc gene into the immunoglobulin heavy chain locus in human Burkitt lymphoma and murine plasmacytoma cells. Proc Natl Acad Sci USA 79:7841, 1982

163. Adams JM, Gerondakis S, Webb E et al: Cellular myc oncogene is altered by chromosome translocation to an immunoglobulin locus in murine plasmacytomas and is rearranged similarly in human Burkitt lymphomas. Proc Natl Acad Sci USA 80:1982, 1983

164. Hamlyn PH, Rabbits TH: Translocation joins c-myc and immunoglobulin gamma 1 genes in a Burkitt lymphoma revealing a third exon in the c-myc oncogene. Nature 304:135, 1983

165. Battey J, Moulding C, Taub R et al: The human c-myc oncogene: structural consequences of translocation into the IgH locus in Burkitt lymphoma. Cell 34:779, 1983

166. Coppola JA, Cole MD: Constitutive c-myc oncogene expression blocks mouse erythroleukemia cell differentiation but not commitment. Nature 320: 760, 1986

167. Dmitrovsky E, Kuehl WM, Hollis EF et al: Expression of a transfected human c-myc oncogene inhibits differentiation of a mouse erythroleukemia cell line. Nature 322:748, 1986

168. Prochownick EV, Kukowska J: Deregulated expression of c-myc by murine erythroleukemia cells prevents differentiation. Nature 322:848, 1986

169. Lachman HM, Cheng G, Skoultchi AI: Transfection of mouse erythroleukemia cells with myc sequences changes the rate of induced commitment to differentiation. Proc Natl Acad Sci USA 83:6480, 1986

170. Stewart TA, Pattengale PK, Leder P: Spontaneous mammary adenocarcinomas in transgenic mice that carry and express MTV/myc fusion genes. Cell 38:627, 1984

171. Moulding C, Rappoport A, Goldman P et al: Structural analysis of both products of a reciprocal translocation between c-myc and immunoglobulin loci in Burkitt lymphoma. Nucleic Acid Res 13:2141, 1985

172. Taub R, Moulding C, Battey J et al: Activation and somatic mutation of the translocated c-myc gene in Burkitt lymphoma cells. Cell 36:339, 1984

173. Cesarman E, Dalla-Favera R, Bentley DI, Groudine M: Mutations in the first exon are associated with altered transcription of c-myc in Burkitt lymphoma. Science 238:1272, 1987

174. Bentley DL, Groudine M: A block to elongation is largely responsible for decreased transcription of c-myc in differentiated HL60 cells. Nature 321:702, 1986

175. Bentley DL, Groudine M: Sequence requirements for premature termination of transcription of the human c-myc gene. Cell 53:245, 1988

176. Lenoir G, Preud'homme JL, Bernheim A, Berger R: Correlation between immunoglobulin light chain expression and variant translocation in Burkitt's lymphoma. Nature 298:474, 1982

177. Pelicci PG, Knowles DM II, Magrath I, Dalla-Favera R: Chromosomal breakpoints and structural rearrangements of the c-myc locus differ in endemic and sporadic forms of Burkitt lymphoma. Proc Natl Acad Sci USA 83:2984, 1986

178. Land H, Parada LF, Weinberg RA: Tumorigenic conversion of primary embryo fibroblasts requires at least two cooperating oncogenes. Nature 302:596, 1983

179. Lombardi L, Newcomb E, Dalla-Favera: Pathogenesis of Burkitt lymphoma: expression of an activated c-myc oncogene causes tumorigenic conversion of EBV-infected human B lymphoblasts. Cell 49:161, 1987

180. Rowley JD: Chromosome studies in the non-Hodgkin's lymphomas: the role of the 14;18 translocation. J Clin Oncol 6:919, 1988

181. Kaneko Y, Rowley JD, Variakojis D et al: Prognostic implications of karyotype and morphology in patients with non-Hodgkin's lymphoma. Int J Cancer 32:683, 1983

182. Tsujimoto Y, Finger LR, Yunis J et al: Cloning of the chromosome breakpoint of neoplastic B cells with the t(14;18) translocation. Science 226:1097, 1984

183. Bakshi A, Jensen JP, Goldman P et al: Cloning the chromosomal breakpoint of t(14;18) human lymphomas: clustering around J_H on chromosome 14 and near a transcriptional unity on 18. Cell 41:899, 1985

184. Cleary ML, Sklar J: Nucleotide sequence of a t(14;18) chromosomal breakpoint in follicular lymphoma and demonstration of a breakpoint cluster region near a transcriptionally active locus on chromosome 18. Proc Natl Acad Sci USA 82:7439, 1985

185. Tsujimoto Y, Cossman J, Jaffe E, Croce CM: Involvement of the bcl-2 gene in human follicular lymphoma. Science 228:1440, 1985

186. Tsujimoto Y, Croce CM: Analysis of the structure, transcripts, and protein products of bcl-2, the gene involved in human follicular lymphoma. Proc Natl Acad Sci USA 83:5214, 1986

187. Cleary ML, Smith SD, Sklar J: CLoning and structural analysis of cDNAs for bcl-2 and a hybrid bcl-2/ immunoglobulin transcript resulting from the t(14;18) translocation. Cell 47:19, 1986

188. Reed JC, Tsujimoto Y, Alpers JD et al: Regulation of bcl-2 proto-oncogene expression during normal human lymphocyte proliferation. Science 236:1295, 1987

189. Le Beau MM, Rowley JD: Chromosomal abnormalities in leukemia and lymphoma: clinical and biological significance. Adv Hum Genet 15:1, 1986

190. Weinberg RA: Oncogenes of spontaneous and chemically induced tumors. Adv Cancer Res 36:149, 1982

191. Cooper GM: Cellular transforming genes. Science 218:801, 1982

192. Murray MJ, Cunningham JM, Parada LF et al: The HL60 transforming sequence: a ras oncogene coexisting with altered myc genes in hematopoietic tumors. Cell 33:749, 1983

193. Goubin G, Goldman DS, Luce J et al: Molecular cloning and nucleotide sequence of a transforming gene detected by transfection of chicken B-cell lymphoma DNA. Nature 302:114, 1983

194. Lane M, Sainten A, Doherty KM, Cooper GM: Isolation and characterization of a stage-specific transforming gene, Tlym-1, from T-cell lymphomas. Proc Natl Acad Sci 81:2227, 1984

195. Rogers J: Relationship of Blym genes to repeated sequences. Nature 320:579, 1986

196. Sachs L, Lotem J: Control of programmed cell death in normal and leukemic cells: new implications for therapy. Blood 83:15, 1993

197. Williams GT, Smith CA: Molecular regulation of apoptosis: genetic controls on cell death. Cell 74:777, 1993

198. Waring P, Kos FJ, Mullbacher A: Apoptosis or programmed cell death. Med Res Rev 11:219, 1991

199. Cook N, Lord BI, Cragoe E, Dexter TM: Identification of a common signal associated with cellular proliferation stimulated by four haemopoietic growth factors in a highly enriched population of granulocyte/macrophage colony-forming cells. EMBO J 8:2967, 1989

200. Arends MJ, Morris RG, Wyllie AH: Apoptosis: the role of the endonuclease. Am J Pathol 136:593, 1990

201. Wyllie AH: Glucocorticoid-induced thymocyte apoptosis is associated with endogenous endonuclease activation. Nature 284:555, 1980

202. Deng G, Podacek ER: Suppression of apoptosis in a cytotoxic T-cell line by interleukin 2-mediated gene transcription and deregulated expression of the protooncogene bcl-2. Proc Natl Acad Sci USA 90:2189, 1993

203. Williams GT, Smith CA, Spooncer E et al: Haemopoietic colony stimulating factors promote cell survival by suppressing apoptosis. Nature 343:76, 1990

204. Sachs L: Control of normal cell differentiation and the phenotypic reversion of malignancy in myeloid leukemia. Nature 274:535, 1978

205. Martin SJ, Bradley JG, Cotter TG: HL-60 cells induced to differentiate towards neutrophils subsequently die via apoptosis. Clin Exp Immunol 79:448, 1990

206. Mangan DF, Wahl SM: Differential regulation of human monocyte programmed cell death (apoptosis) by chemotactic factors and proinflammatory cytokines. J Immunol 147:3408, 1991

207. Fairbairn LJ, Cowling GJ, Reipert BM, Dexter TM: Suppression of apoptosis allows differentiation and development of a multipotent hemopoietic cell line in the absence of added growth factors. Cell 74:823, 1993

208. Lotem J, Cragoe EJ Jr. Sachs L: Rescue from programmed cell death in leukemic and normal myeloid cells. Blood 78:953, 1991

209. Askew DS, Ashmun RA, Simmons BC, Cleveland JL: Constitutive c-myc expression in an IL-3-dependent myeloid cell line suppresses cell cycle arrest and accelerates apoptosis. Oncogene 6:1915, 1991

210. Lotem J, Sachs L: Regulation by bcl-2, c-myc, and p53 of susceptibility to induction of apoptosis by heat shock and cancer chemotherapy compounds in differentiation competent and defective myeloid leukemic cells. Cell Growth Differ 4:41, 1993

211. Gunji H, Kharbanda S, Kufe D: Induction of internucleosomal DNA fragmentation in human myeloid leukemia cells by 1-B-D-arabinofuranosylcytosine. Cancer Res 51:741, 1991

212. Barry MA, Behnke CA, Eastman A: Activation of programmed cell death (apoptosis) by cisplatin, other anticancer drugs, toxins, and hyperthermia. Biochem Pharmacol 40:2353, 1990

213. Walker PR, Smith C, Youdale T et al: Topoisomerase reactive drugs induce apoptosis in thymocytes. Cancer Res 51:1078, 1991

214. Kawano M, Hirano T, Matsuda T et al: Autocrine generation and requirement of BSF-2/IL-6 for human multiple myeloma. Nature 332:83, 1988

215. Bataille R, Jourdan M, Zhang X-G, Klein B: Serum levels of interleukin 6, a potent myeloma cell growth factor, as a reflection of disease severity in plasma cell dyscrasias. J Clin Invest 84:2008, 1989

216. Klein B, Wijdenes J, Ahang X-G et al: Murine anti-interleukin 6 monoclonal antibody therapy for a patient with plasma cell leukemia. Blood 78:1198, 1991

217. Epstein MA, Henle G, Achong BG, Barr YM: Morphological and biological studies on a virus in cultured lymphoblasts from Burkitt's lymphoma. J Exp Med 121:761, 1965

218. Schnipper LE: The Epstein-Barr virus and human lymphoproliferative disorders. Prog Hematol 12:275, 1981

219. Bird AG, Britton S: The relationship between Epstein-Barr virus and lymphoma. Semin Hematol 19:285, 1982

220. Straus SE, Cohen JI, Tosato G, Meier J: NIH Conference: Epstein-Barr virus infections: biology, pathogenesis, and management. Ann Intern Med 118:45, 1993

221. Nilsson K, Giovanella GJ, Shehlin JS et al: Tumorigenicity of human hematopoietic cell lines in athymic nude mice. Int J Cancer 19:337, 1977

222. Tischendorf P, Shraneck GJ, Balatas RC et al: Development and persistence of immunity to Epstein-Barr virus in man. J Infect Dis 122:401, 1970

223. Epstein MA, Achong BGF: Pathogenesis of infectious mononucleosis. Lancet 1:1270, 1977

224. Henle G, Henle W, Horwitz CA: Epstein-Barr virus specific diagnostic tests in infectious mononucleosis. Hum Pathol 5:551, 1974

225. Hewetson JF, Rocchi G, Henle W, Henle G: Neutralizing antibodies to Epstein-

Barr virus in healthy populations and patients with infectious mononucleosis. J Infect Dis 128:283, 1973

226. Purtilo DT, Strobach RS, Okano M, Davis JR: Biology of disease: Epstein-Barr virus-associated lymphoproliferative disorders. Lab Invest 67:5, 1992

227. Strauss SE: Acute progressive Epstein-Barr virus infections. Ann Rev Med 43:437, 1992

228. Gatti RA, Good RA: Occurrence of malignancy in immunodeficiency diseases: a literature review. Cancer 28:89, 1971

229. De The G, Gaser A, Day NE et al: Epidemiological evidence for a causal relationship between Epstein-Barr virus and Burkitt's lymphoma from Ugandan prospective study. Nature 274:756, 1970

230. Andersson M, Klein G, Ziegler JL et al: Association of Epstein-Barr viral genomes with American Burkitt lymphoma. Nature 260:357, 1976

231. O'Conor GT: Persistent immunologic stimulation as a factor in oncogenesis, with special reference to Burkitt's tumor. Am J Med 48:279, 1970

232. Burkitt DP: Etiology of Burkitt's lymphoma: an alternative hypothesis to a vectoral virus. J Natl Cancer Inst 42:19, 1969

233. Shibata D, Weiss LM, Hernandez AM et al: Epstein-Barr virus-associated non-Hodgkin's lymphoma in patients infected with the human immunodeficiency virus. Blood 81:2102, 1993

234. Ballerini P, Gaidano G, Gong JZ et al: Multiple genetic lesions in acquired immunodeficiency syndrome-related non-Hodgkin's lymphoma. Blood 81:166, 1993

235. Levine AM: Acquired immunodeficiency syndrome-related lymphoma. Blood 80:8, 1990

236. Niedobitek G, Herbst H, Young LS et al: Patterns of Epstein-Barr virus infection in non-neoplastic lymphoid tissue. Blood 79:2520, 1992

237. Klein G: Lymphoma development in mice and humans: diversity of initiation is followed by convergent cytogenetic evolution. Proc Natl Acad Sci USA 76:2442, 1979

238. Henle W, Henle G: Epstein-Barr virus serology in immunologically compromised individuals. Cancer Res 41:4222, 1981

239. Hanto D, Sakamoto K, Purtilo DT et al: The Epstein-Barr virus in the pathogenesis of posttransplant lymphoproliferative disorders. Surgery 90:204, 1981

240. Serraino D, Salamina G, Franceschi S et al: The epidemiology of AIDS-associated non-Hodgkins lymphoma in the World-Health-Organization European region. Br J Cancer 66:912, 1992

241. Reynolds P, Saunders LD, Layefsky ME, Lemp GF: The spectrum of acquired immunodeficiency syndrome (AIDS)-associated malignancies in San Francisco, 1980–1987. Am J Epidemiol 137:19, 1992

242. Starzl TE, Porter KA, Iwatsuki S et al: Reversibility of lymphomas and lymphoproliferative lesions developing under cyclosporin-steroid therapy. Lancet 1:583, 1984

243. Antin JH, Bierer BE, Smith BR et al: Selective depletion of bone marrow T-lymphocytes with anti-CD5 monoclonal antibodies: effective prophylaxis for graft-versus-host disease in patients with hematologic malignancies. Blood 78:2139, 1991

244. Ambinder RF: Human lymphotropic viruses associated with lymphoid malignancy: Epstein-Barr and HTLV-1. Hematol Oncol Clin North Am 4:821, 1990

245. Okochi K, Sato H: Transmission of human T-cell leukemia virus (HTLV I) by blood transfusion: demonstration of proviral DNA in recipients' blood lymphocytes. Int J Cancer 37:395, 1986

246. Hino S, Yamaguchi K, Ikada S et al: Mother-to-child transmission of human T cell leukemia virus type I. Jpn J Cancer Res 76:474, 1985

247. Wachsman W, Golde DW, Chen ISY: HTLV and human leukemia: perspectives 1986. Semin Hematol 23:245, 1986

248. Ratner L, Griffiths RC, Marselle L et al: A lymphoproliferative disorder caused by human T-lymphotropic virus type I: demonstration of a continuum between acute and chronic adult T-cell leukemia/lymphoma. Am J Med 83:953, 1987

249. Ratner L, Poisez BJ: Leukemias associated with human T-cell lymphotropic virus type I in a nonendemic region. Medicine 67:401, 1988

250. Neely SM: Adult T-cell leukemia/lymphoma. West J Med 150:5578, 1989

251. Smith BR, Weinberg DS, Robert NJ et al: Circulating monoclonal B lymphocytes in non-Hodgkin's lymphoma. N Engl J Med 331:1476, 1984

252. Berliner N, Ault KA, Martin P, Weinberg DS: Detection of clonal excess in lymphoproliferative disease by kappa/lambda analysis: correlation with immunoglobulin gene DNA rearrangement. Blood 67:80, 1986

253. Stetler-Stevenson M, Raffeled M, Cohen P, Cossman J: Detection of occult follicular lymphoma by specific DNA amplification. Blood 72:1822, 1988

254. Freitas AA, Rocha BB: Lymphocyte lifespans: homeostasis, selection and competition. Immunol Today 25, 1993

255. Berg EL, Goldstein LA, Jutila MA et al: Homing receptors and vascular addressins: cell adhesion molecules that direct lymphocyte traffic. Immunol Rev 108:5, 1989

256. Stoolman LM: Adhesion molecules controlling lymphocyte migration. Cell 56:907, 1989

257. Yednock TA, Rosen SD: Lymphocyte homing. Adv Immunol 44:313, 1989

258. Pardi R, Inverardi L, Bender JR: Regulatory mechanisms in leukocyte adhesion: flexible receptors for sophisticated travelers. Immunol Today 13:224, 1992

259. Albelda SM, Buck CA: Integrins and other cell adhesion molecules. FASEB J 4:2868, 1990

260. Haynes BF, Telen MJ, Hale LP, Denning SM: CD44—a molecule involved in leukocyte adherence and T-cell activation. Immunol Today 10:423, 1989

261. Murakami S, Miyake K, Kincade PW, Hodes RJ: Functional role of CD44 (pgp-1) on activated B cells. Immunol Res 10:15, 1991

262. Moller G (ed): Adhesion molecules. Immunol Rev 114:5, 1990

263. Lasky LA: Lectin cell adhesion molecules (LEC-CAMs): a new family of cell adhesion proteins involved with inflammation. J Cell Biochem 45:139, 1991

264. Rinder HM, Bonan J, Rinder CS et al: Activated and unactivated platelet adhesion to monocytes and neutrophils. Blood 78:1760, 1991

265. Rinder HM, Bonan J, Rinder CS et al: Dynamics of leukocyte-platelet adhesion in whole blood. Blood 78:1730, 1991

266. Mebius RE, Watson SR: L- and E-selectin can recognize the same naturally occurring ligands on high endothelial venules. J Immunol 151:3252, 1993

267. Polley MJ, Phillips ML, Wayner E et al: CD62 and endothelial cell-leukocyte adhesion molecule 1 (ELAM-1) recognize the same carbohydrate ligand, sialyl-Lewis X. Proc Natl Acad Sci USA 88:6224, 1991

268. Lasky LA, Singer M, Dowbenko D et al: An endothelial ligand for L-selectin is a novel mucin-like molecule. Cell 69:927, 1992

269. Springer TA: Adhesion receptors in the immune system. Nature 346:425, 1990

270. Postigo AA, Corbi AL, Sanchez-Madrid F, de Landazuri MO: Regulated expression and function of CD11c/CD18 integrin on human B lymphocytes. Relation between attachment to fibrinogen and triggering of proliferation through CD11c/CD18. J Exp Med 174:1313, 1991

271. Carter WG, Wayner EA, Bouchard TS, Kaur P: The role of integrins α2β1 and α3β1 in cell-cell and cell-substrate adhesion of human epidermal cells. J Cell Biol 110:1387, 1990

272. Hynes RO: Integrins: versatility, modulation, and signalling in cell adhesion. Cell 69:11, 1992

273. Juliano RL, Haskill S: Signal transduction from the extracellular matrix. J Cell Biol 120:577, 1993

274. Lawrence MB, Springer TA: Leukocytes roll on a selectin at physiologic flow rates: distinction from and prerequisite for adhesion through integrins. Cell 65:859, 1991

275. Kishimoto TK, Jutila MA, Butcher EC: Identification of a human peripheral lymph node homing receptor a rapidly down-regulated adhesion molecule. Proc Natl Acad Sci USA 87:2244, 1990

276. Gallatin WM, Wayner EA, Hoffman PA et al: Structural homology between lymphocyte receptors for high endothelium and class III extracellular matrix receptor. Proc Natl Acad Sci USA 86:4654, 1989

277. Haynes BF, Telen MJ, Hale LP, Denning SM: CD44-A molecule involved in leukocyte adherence and T cell activation. Immunol Today 10:423, 1989

278. Picker LJ, Nakache M, Butcher EC: Monoclonal antibodies to human lymphocyte homing receptors define a novel class of adhesion molecules on diverse cell types. J Cell Biol 109:927, 1989

279. Jalkanen S, Bargatze RF, de los Toyos J, Butcher EC: Lymphocyte recognition of high endothelium: antibodies to distinct epitopes of an 85-95-kD glycoprotein antigen differentially inhibit lymphocyte binding to lymph node, mucosal, or synovial endothelial cells. J Cell Biol 105:983, 1987

280. Kishimoto TK, Jutila MA, Berg EL, Butcher EC: Neutrophil Mac-1 and MEL-14 adhesion proteins inversely regulated by chemotactic factors. Science 245:1238, 1989

281. Stamenkovic I, Amiot M, Pesando JM, Seed B: A lymphocyte molecule implicated in lymph node homing is a member of the cartilage link protein family. Cell 56:1057, 1989

282. DeRossi G, Zarcone D, Mauro F et al: Adhesion molecule expression on B-cell chronic lymphocytic leukemia cells: malignant cell phenotypes define distinct disease subsets. Blood 81:2679, 1993

283. Maio M, Pinto A, Carbone A et al: Differential expression of CD54/intercellular adhesion molecule in myeloid leukemias and in lymphoproliferative disorders. Blood 76:783, 1990

284. Horst E, Mejjer CJLM, Radaskiewicz T et al: Adhesion molecules in the prognosis of diffuse large-cell lymphoma: expression of a lymphocyte homing receptor (CD44), LFA-1(CD11a/18), and ICAM-1 (CD54). Leukemia 8:595, 1990

285. Michie SA, Garcia CF, Strickler JG et al: Expression of the Leu8 antigen by B-cell lymphomas. Am J Pathol 88:486, 1987

286. Pals ST, Horst E, Ossekoppele GJ et al: Expression of lymphocyte homing receptor as a mechanism of dissemination in non-Hodgkin lymphoma. Blood 73:885, 1989
287. Picker LJ, Medeiros LJ, Weiss LM et al: Expression of lymphocyte homing receptor antigen in non-Hodgkin's lymphoma. Am J Pathol 130:496, 1988
288. Hanson CA, Gribbin TE, Schnitzer B et al: CD11C (LeuM5) expression characterizes a B-cell chronic lymphoproliferative disorder with features of both chronic lymphocytic leukemia and hairy cell leukemia. Blood 76:2360, 1990
289. Wormsley SB, Baird SM, Gadol H et al: Characteristics of CD11c+ CD5+ chronic B-cell leukemias and the identification of novel peripheral blood B-cell subsets with chronic lymphoid leukemia immunophenotype. Blood 76:123, 1990
290. Jalkanen S, Joensuu H, Klemi P: Prognostic value of lymphocyte homing receptor and S phase fraction in non-Hodgkin's lymphoma. Blood 75:1549, 1990
291. Stauder R, Hamader S, Fasching B et al: Adhesion to high endothelial venules: a model for dissemination mechanisms in non-Hodgkin's lymphoma. Blood 82:262, 1993
292. Moller P, Eichelmann A, Mechtersheimer G, Koretz K: Expression of β1-integrins, H-CAM (CD44) and Lecam-1 in primary gastro-intestinal B-cell lymphomas as compared to the adhesion receptor profile of the gut-associated lymphoid system, tonsil and peripheral lymph node. Int J Cancer 49:846, 1991
293. Pals ST, Meijer CJ, Radaskiewicz T: Expression of the human peripheral lymph node homing receptor (LECAM-1) in nodal and gastrointestinal non-Hodgkin's lymphomas. Leukemia 5:628, 1991
294. Ohmori K, Takada A, Yoneda T et al: Differentiation-dependent expression of sialyl state-specific embryonic antigen-1 and l-antigens on human lymphoid cells and its implications for carbohydrate-mediated adhesion to vascular endothelium. Blood 81:101, 1993
295. Burnet FM: The concept of immunological surveillance. Prog Exp Tumor Res 13:1, 1970
296. Nalesnik MA, Jaffe R, Starzl TE: The pathology of posttransplant lymphoproliferative disorders occurring in the setting of cyclosporine A-prednisone immunosuppression. Am J Pathol 133:173, 1988
297. Ritz J: The role of natural killer cells in immune surveillance. N Engl J Med 320:1748, 1989
298. Macklis RM, Mauch PM, Burakoff SJ, Smith BR: Lymphoid irradiation results in long term increases in natural killer cells in patients treated for Hodgkin's disease. Cancer 69:778, 1992
299. Kamel OW, van de Rijn M, Weiss LM et al: Brief report: reversible lymphomas associated with Epstein-Barr virus occurring during methotrexate therapy for rheumatoid arthritis and dermatomyositis. N Engl J Med 328:1317, 1993
300. Starzl TE, Nalesnik MA, Porter KA et al: Reversibility of lymphomas and lymphoproliferative lesions developing under cyclosporin-steroid therapy. Lancet 1:583, 1984
301. Larson RS, Corbi AL, Berman L, Springer T: Primary structure of the leukocyte function-associated molecule-1 alpha subunit: an integrin with an embedded domain defining a protein superfamily. J Cell Biol 108:703, 1989
302. Ginsberg MH, Loftus JC, Plow EF: Cytoadhesins, integrins, and platelets. Thromb Haemost 59:1, 1988
303. Mentzer SJ, Smith BR, Barbosa JA et al: CTL adhesion and antigen recognition are discrete steps in the human CTL-target cell interaction. J Immunol 138:1325, 1987
304. Fischer A, Lisowska-Grospierre B, Anderson DC, Springer TA: Leukocyte adhesion deficiency: molecular basis and functional consequences. Immunodefic Rev 1:39, 1988
305. Sanders ME, Makgoba MW, Sussman EH et al: Molecular pathways of adhesion in spontaneous rosetting of T-lymphocytes to the Hodgkin's cell line L428. Cancer Res 48:37, 1988
306. Gregory CD, Murray RJ, Edwards CF, Rickinson AB: Downregulation of cell adhesion molecules LFA-3 and ICAM-1 in Epstein-Barr virus-positive Burkitt's lymphoma underlies tumor cell escape from virus-specific T cell surveillance. J Exp Med 167:1811, 1988
307. Makgoba MW, Sanders ME, Shaw S: The CD2-LFA3 and LFA1-ICAM pathways: relevance to T cell recognition. Immunol Today 10:417, 1989
308. Broder S, Poplack D, Whang-Peng J et al: Characterization of a suppressor-cell leukemia. N Engl J Med 298:66, 1978
309. Bom-van Noorloos AA, Pegels HG, van Oers RHJ et al: Proliferation of T cells with killer-cell activity in two patients with neutropenia and recurrent infections. N Engl J Med 302:933, 1980
310. Loughran TP: Clonal diseases of large granular lymphocytes. Blood 82:1, 1993
311. Loughran TP, Hammond WP: Adult onset cyclic neutropenia is a benign neoplasm associated with clonal proliferation of large granular lymphocytes. J Exp Med 164:2089, 1986
312. Linch DC, Newland AC, Turnbull AL et al: Unusual T cell proliferations and neutropenia in rheumatoid arthritis: comparison with classical Felty's syndrome. Scand J Haematol 33:342, 1984
313. Newland AC, Catovsky D, Linch D et al: Chronic T cell lymphocytosis: a review of 21 cases. Br J Haematol 58:433, 1984
314. Pandolfi F, Loughran TP, Starkebaum G et al: Clinical course and prognosis of the lymphoproliferative disease of large granular lymphocytes. A multicenter study. Cancer 65:341, 1990
315. Aisenberg AC, Krontiris TG, Mak TW, Wilkes BM: Rearrangement of the gene for the beta chain of the T-cell receptor in T-cell chronic lymphocytic leukemia and related disorders. N Engl J Med 313:529, 1985
316. Bertness V, Kirsh I, Hollis G et al: T cell receptor gene rearrangements as clinical markers of human T-cell lymphomas. N Engl J Med 313:534, 1985
317. Berliner N, Duby AD, Linch DC et al: T cell receptor gene rearrangements define a monoclonal T cell proliferation in patients with T cell lymphocytosis and cytopenia. Blood 67:914, 1986
318. Miedema F, Melief CJM: Immunobiology of the expanded T cells in T-cell leukemia and T-gamma lymphocytosis. Leuk Res 10:469, 1986
319. Linch DC, Cawley JC, Worman CP et al: Abnormalities of T- cell subsets in patients with neutropenia and an excess of lymphocytes in the bone marrow. Br J Haematol 48:137, 1981
320. Rumke JC, Miedema F, ten Berge IJM et al: Functional properties of T cells in patients with chronic Tγ lymphocytosis and chronic T cell neoplasia. J Immunol 129:419, 1982
321. Bierer BE, Nishimura Y, Burakoff SJ, Smith BR: Phenotypic and functional characterization of human cytolytic T cells lacking expression of CD5. J Clin Invest 81:1390, 1988
322. Bierer BE, Burakoff SJ, Smith BR: A large proportion of T lymphocytes lack CD5 expression following bone marrow transplantation. Blood 73:1359, 1989
323. Grillot-Courvalin C, Vinci G, Tsapsi A et al: The syndrome of T8 hyperlymphocytosis: variation in phenotype and cytotoxic activities of granular cells and evaluation of their role in associated neutropenia. Blood 69:1204, 1987
324. Nagasawa T, Abe T, Nakagawa T: Pure red cell aplasia and hypogammaglobulinemia associated with Tr-cell chronic lymphocytic leukemia. Blood 57:1025, 1981
325. Niemeyer CM, Sieff CA, Smith BR et al: Hematopoiesis *in vitro* co-exists with natural killer lymphocytes. Blood 74:2376, 1989
326. Lipton JM, Nadler LM, Canellos GP et al: Evidence for genetic restriction in the suppression of erythropoiesis by a unique subset of T lymphocytes in man. J Am Soc Clin Invest 72:694, 1983
327. Standen GR, Masters G, Pill R et al: Production of hemopoietic growth factors and γ interferon by large granular lymphocytes from patients with T lymphocytosis. Int J Cell Cloning 5:302, 1987
328. Loughran TP, Starkebaum G, Clark E et al: Evaluation of splenectomy in large granular lymphocyte leukemia. Br J Haematol 67:135, 1987
329. Lang DF, Rosenfeld CS, Diamond HS et al: Successful treatment of Tγ-lymphoproliferative disease with human-recombinant granulocyte colony stimulating factor. Am J Hematol 40:66, 1992
330. Kaneko T, Ogawa Y, Hirata Y et al: Agranulocytosis associated with granular lymphocyte leukaemia: improvement of peripheral blood granulocyte count with human recombinant granulocyte colony-stimulating factor (G-CSF). Br J Haematol 74:121, 1990
331. Cooper DL, Henderson-Bakas M, Berliner N: Lymphoproliferative disorder of granular lymphocytes (LPGL) associated with severe neutropenia: response to granulocyte colony-stimulating factor. Cancer 72:1607, 1993
332. Kipps TJ, Carson DA: Autoantibodies in chronic lymphocytic leukemia and related systemic autoimmune diseases. Blood 81:2475, 1993
333. Borche L, Lim A, Binet J, Dighiero G: Evidence that chronic lymphocytic leukemia B lymphocytes are frequently committed to production of natural autoantibodies. Blood 76:562, 1990
334. Plater-Zyberk C, Maini RN, Lam K et al: A rheumatoid arthritis B cell subset expresses a phenotype similar to that in chronic lymphocytic leukemia. Arthritis Rheum 31:642, 1988
335. Casali P, Notkins AL: CD5+ B lymphocytes, polyreactive antibodies, and the human B-cell repertoire. Immunol Today 10:364, 1989
336. Stoeger ZM, Wakai M, Tse DB et al: Production of autoantibodies by CD5-expressing B lymphocytes from patients with chronic lymphocytic leukemia. J Exp Med 169:255, 1989
337. Mosier DE, Gulizia RJ, Baird SM, Wilson DB: Transfer of a functional human immune system to mice with severe combined immunodeficiency. Nature 335:256, 1989

Pathology and Histogenesis of Hodgkin Disease

78

Marshall E. Kadin

INTRODUCTION

The nature of the Reed-Sternberg (RS) cell and the cellular origin of Hodgkin disease (HD) have been an enigma for more than 150 years. Some authorities have doubted that HD represents a malignant process, in part because of its variable clinical behavior and multiple histologies. Recent progress in immunology and in cell culture studies has helped identify the RS cell as a part of the malignant cell population. The remaining cell types, which comprise the bulk of the HD lesion, appear to represent a combination of RS cell precursors, host inflammatory cells, and cells recruited to the site in response to cytokines liberated by RS cells. Somehow the mixture of these cell types and stromal elements determines the natural history of HD, thereby influencing the treatment and prognosis of the disease. This chapter re-evaluates the morphologic hallmarks of HD in light of new knowledge about the RS cell and its cellular immunology. Immunopathologic methods for the more accurate diagnosis of HD are emphasized. Recent information regarding the role of Epstein-Barr virus (EBV) in HD are presented. Finally, cytogenetic abnormalities and non-Hodgkin lymphomas associated with HD are discussed within the context of the histogenesis of HD.

HISTOPATHOLOGY

The histopathology of HD is more complex and variable than that of the non-Hodgkin lymphomas (NHL). To simplify the histopathologic interpretation of HD and make it clinically relevant, Lukes et al.[1] formulated a histopathologic classification of HD based on six different types: (1) lymphocytic and/or histiocytic (L&H), nodular; (2) L&H, diffuse; (3) nodular sclerosis; (4) mixed cellularity; (5) diffuse fibrosis; and (6) reticular (cellular) types. At the Rye conference on HD,[2] the nodular and diffuse subtypes of L&H were included under a single heading of lymphocyte predominance type; the diffuse fibrosis and reticular types were combined under the heading of lymphocyte depletion. In 1989 Wright[3] argued that clinicopathologic correlations since the late 1960s justify a return to the subtypes of HD proposed originally by Lukes and co-workers.

A definite relationship among histologic types, clinical stages, and survival has been demonstrated.[1] Nodular sclerosis is associated with a good prognosis and a marked propensity to involve the mediastinum and is often limited to stage I or II disease. Lymphocyte predominance has an excellent prognosis and is commonly restricted to localized stage I disease in the neck or inguinal areas. Lymphocyte depletion has a poor prognosis and usually presents with advanced stage III or IV disease and a high frequency of bone marrow and abdominal lymph node disease. Mixed cellularity has an intermediate prognosis, commonly presenting with abdominal disease and relatively infrequently being associated with mediastinal disease.

These relationships were confirmed and extended in a study of 719 patients with HD who underwent staging laparotomy with splenectomy between April 1969 and December 1986 at the Harvard Joint Center for Radiation. Mauch et al.[4] showed that the mediastinum and left and right sides of the neck are the most common sites involved in patients with nodular sclerosis or mixed cellularity types, each site being involved in 60% of cases. By contrast, the mediastinum was involved in only 8% of patients with lymphocyte predominance. Nodular sclerosis and mixed cellularity appeared to spread by contiguity, whereas lymphocyte predominance was limited to one site of involvement in approximately 50% of patients and was least likely to spread in a contiguous fashion.

Histologic Types

Nodular Sclerosis

In most series nodular sclerosis is the most frequent type of HD[1,4–6] (Plate 78-1). It comprises interconnecting dense bands of collagen, which circumscribe abnormal lymphoid nodules. As a result, the cut surface of lymph nodes show tan nodules of lymphoid tissue bulging out from gray-white connective tissue. This gross appearance should lead to a high suspicion of nodular sclerosing HD, which can sometimes be confirmed in the surgical suite by demonstrating RS variants in touch imprints of the lymph node. In permanent tissue sections stained with hematoxylin and eosin, eosinophilic collagen bands of varying width surround blue lymphoid nodules, a pattern that can be recognized with the naked eye by holding the slide up to the light. The collagen is birefringent in polarized light, which may aid in its recognition and quantitation. It appears to emanate from a thickened capsule or from the adventitia of blood vessels, or both.[1,5] Microscopically, there are large spaces around the RS variants, called lacunar cells. The lacunar artifact, best seen in formalin-fixed tissue, results from retraction of cytoplasm of the RS cells from surrounding tissues (Plate 78-1). The lacunar cells appear distinctive by virtue of pale, sometimes, transparent, cytoplasm and relatively small nuclei and nucleoli when compared with diagnostic RS cells. The nucleoli may be basophilic, in contrast to the eosinophilic nucleoli of RS cells. Lacunar cells may have one, two, or many nuclear lobes. Usually only an occasional lacunar cell will closely resemble an RS cell.

The amount of collagen sclerosis may vary considerably from marked (visible to the naked eye) to minimal, in which case the diagnosis is suspected mainly from the presence of distinctive lacunar cells. This latter type, with minimal or absent sclerosis, has been referred to as the cellular phase of nodular sclerosis.[5,7] The frequent finding of typical sclerotic lesions elsewhere in the same patient seemed to justify recognition of the cellular phase as part of the spectrum of nodular sclerosis.[5] This concept was supported by the study conducted by Strum and Rappaport,[8] who observed progression from the cellular phase to advanced sclerosis in serial biopsies from five of seven patients. Colby et al.[6] found that patients with the cellular phase of nodular sclerosis had some clinical features and an overall survival similar to those of patients with mixed cellularity HD, but relapse-free survival similar to that of nodular sclerosis patients. Recognizing that sampling sometimes demonstrates lymph node involvement in the cellular phase without collagen bands, Lukes[7] recommends that for reproducibility, the diagnosis of nodular sclerosis should be made only when the two criteria of collagen band formation and lacunar cells are met.

Colby et al.[6] described a fibroblastic variant of nodular sclerosis. They found the number of fibroblasts to be prognostically more significant than the number of lymphocytes; numerous fibroblasts correlated with a shorter relapse-free survival. This grading system is not in widespread use. Dorfman[9] has indicated that mediastinal biopsies from patients with the fibroblastic variant of nodular sclerosis may be misinterpreted as malignant fibrous histiocytoma.

In 1986 Strickler et al.[10] described a syncytial variant of nodular sclerosis, in which cohesive clusters or sheets of RS cells are found (Plate 78-2). Syncytial foci may be found anywhere in the node but often occur in interfollicular areas and in the trabecular sinuses of the lymph node. The atypical HD giant cells surround zones of necrosis and may be associated with numerous granulocytes. This histologic picture may be mistaken for metastatic carcinoma, malignant melanoma, thymoma, and large cell NHL.[10] The distinction of nodular sclerosing HD can be confirmed by immunophenotypic studies, as described later in this chapter.

The British National Lymphoma Investigation (BNLI) recognized that within the spectrum of nodular sclerosis there is wide variation in the relative numbers of pleomorphic HD giant cells and small lymphocytes.[11] The BNLI subclassified nodular sclerosis into grades I and II; grade II shows areas of lymphocyte depletion or numerous pleomorphic HD giant cells. Grade II, which accounts for 20–30% of all cases of nodular sclerosis, has a significantly worse prognosis than that of grade I. The prognostic significance of this grading of nodular sclerosis has been confirmed in a multivariate analysis.[12] Patients with nodular sclerosis grade I who relapse have a more successful salvage and longer period of survival than do patients with grade II nodular sclerosis.[13] Histologic subclassification of nodular sclerosis therefore appears to be clinically relevant and important in planning therapy. Unfortunately, there are nearly 207 interobserver disagreements in the subclassification of nodular sclerosis grades I and II.[14]

Nodular sclerosis occurs most often in females, a predilection that is present across all age groups. The prognostic advantage of nodular sclerosing HD is largely restricted to patients in clinical stages I and II. There is no survival advantage in stages III and IV, with the possible exception of patients with stage IV disease on the basis of contiguous spread to the lung or anterior chest wall.[15]

Lymphocyte Predominance

Lymphocyte predominance occurs in both diffuse and nodular forms[1] (Plate 78-3). The cut surface of the lymph node has a diffuse or faintly nodular fish flesh appearance. Both nodular and diffuse types consist primarily of small lymphocytes and of benign epithelioid histiocytes. Other cellular elements, such as eosinophils and plasma cells, are rare or absent. Necrosis and fibrosis are also negligible, and diagnostic RS cells are rare (Plate 78-3). There are, however, distinctive variants of RS cells, which have large folded, twisted, or multilobated nuclei and relatively small nucleoli (Plate 78-4). These variants of RS cells have become known as L&H cells or, because they resemble popcorn, as "popcorn cells." L&H/popcorn variants are sufficiently distinctive that some authorities will rely on their appearance to make a diagnosis of HD with lymphocyte predominance (LPHD) in the absence of diagnostic RS cells.

Because of the rarity of diagnostic RS cells, the diffuse form of LPHD can be mistaken for well-differentiated lymphocytic lymphoma or chronic lymphocytic leukemia.[7] When histiocytes predominate, the differential diagnosis includes lymphoepithelioid lymphoma (Lennert lymphoma) and granulomatous inflammation. Lennert lymphoma can be distinguished by a spectrum of atypical lymphoid cells and clustering of histiocytes. Granulomatous inflammation is often accompanied by necrosis not found in LPHD. In nodular LPHD, epithelioid histiocytes may be numerous within the nodules or surrounding them in a wreath-like arrangement. The diagnosis of LPHD is made when there are L&H/popcorn variants of RS cells.

Nodular LPHD is often found in association with progressively transformed germinal centers[16–19] (Plate 78-5), which occur in follicular hyperplasia when secondary follicles become large and the border between the germinal center and lymphocytes of the mantle zone becomes indistinct. In progressively transformed germinal centers, the small lymphocytes of the mantle zone appear to infiltrate and gradually overrun the germinal centers. Progressively transformed germinal centers may precede, follow, or coexist with nodular LPHD, but the condition is not sufficient for a diagnosis of LPHD.[18,19] It is essential that the diagnosis of nodular LPHD not be made unless diagnostic RS cells or their L&H/popcorn variants, or both, are found within some of the lymphoid nodules.

Regula et al.[20] emphasized clinical differences between the nodular and diffuse subtypes of LPHD. Patients with the diffuse form tend to have a course similar to that of the mixed cellularity and nodular sclerosing types of HD. By contrast, patients with nodular LPHD have significantly more relapses, independent of stage or treatment and occurring continuously for many years after initial therapy. Trudel et al.[21] noted differences in the clinical presentations of diffuse and nodular LPHD: nodular LPHD usually involves a single anatomic site, whereas the diffuse form often presents with more extensive disease.

Nodular LPHD sometimes progresses to lymphocyte depletion HD, or more likely, to large cell NHL.[16,22–24] Miettenen et al.[22] reported that 5 of 51 patients with nodular LPHD developed large cell NHL 4–11 years after the diagnosis of nodular LPHD and that only 1 of these patients had received radiotherapy. Hansmann et al.[23] observed the simultaneous presence of (n = 11) or subsequent transition into (n = 3) a large B-cell lymphoma in 14 nodular LPHD cases. Retrospective follow-up of these secondary large cell lymphomas in patients with nodular LPHD revealed a longer survival time than that of primary B-type large cell lymphomas and other secondary large cell lymphomas. Sundeen et al.[24] described seven cases of nodular LPHD in which mononuclear (L&H) RS cell variants occurred in large confluent sheets resembling large cell lymphoma. These findings were interpreted as histologic progression of nodular LPHD, with uncertain biologic significance. Six of these patients were in complete remission following radiation or chemotherapy, suggesting a good prognosis for large cell lymphomas occurring in patients with LPHD.

Lymphocyte Depletion

Lymphocyte depletion HD includes two major types: diffuse fibrosis and reticular[1] (Plate 78-6). Both types are characterized by a depletion of lymphocytes, and focal necrosis is common. The diffuse fibrosis type is characterized by amorphous proteinaceous material or disorderly fibrils without mature birefringent collagen, or both, whereas the reticular type shows numerous diagnostic RS cells (Plate 78-6) or RS cell variants of the pleomorphic and sarcomatous types. When the pleomorphic variants predominate, the process may be mistaken for a poorly differentiated nonlymphoid neoplasm. A morphologic distinction between the reticular type of lymphocyte depletion HD and anaplastic large cell lymphoma (ALCL) of the Ki-1+ (CD30+) type is difficult and will be aided by application of immunologic techniques.

Neiman et al.[25] noted that 13 patients with lymphocyte depletion had a distinctive clinicopatholoic syndrome of rapidly fatal disease with fever, pancytopenia, lymphocytopenia, and abnormal hepatic function, often without peripheral lymphadenopathy. In patients with the diffuse fibrosis type, the diagnosis was commonly made by bone marrow examination, at laparotomy, or at autopsy. Patients with the reticular type more often had peripheral lymphadenopathy. Lymphocyte depletion HD is predominantly subdiaphragmatic, with extensive involvement of liver, spleen, retroperitoneal lymph nodes, and multiple bone marrow sites, often accompanied by bone marrow hypoplasia and pancytopenia. Thus, multiple bone marrow biopsies and liver biopsies can frequently establish the diagnosis of lymphocyte depletion HD.

Bearman et al.[26] found no clinical or survival differences between reticular and diffuse types of lymphocyte depletion HD. However, Greer et al.[27] reported that patients with diffuse fibrosis more often had bone marrow involvement and less frequently had peripheral lymphadenopathy than patients with the reticular type. Among patients who received chemotherapy, median survival was longer for patients with diffuse fibrosis.

Kant et al.[28] found that of 39 patients treated for lymphocyte depletion HD at the National Cancer Institute between 1964 and 1976, 10 actually had large cell NHL and 13 had nodular sclerosing HD. Only 3 of 10 patients with NHL had complete remissions, and their median survival was only 7 months. Complete remissions were attained by 67% and 85% of patients with lymphocyte depletion and nodular sclerosing HD, respectively, and the median survival had not been reached in either group with a median follow-up of 14 years. These results suggest that more accurate diagnosis and classification of HD is needed not only for proper care of individual patients but also for accurate analysis of new treatment protocols.

Mixed Cellularity

Mixed cellularity is the second most common histologic type of HD and shows a relatively high frequency of abdominal involvement.[4,29] Reactive histiocytes, eosinophils, neutrophils, plasma cells, and small lymphocytes are numerous, and small foci of necrosis are common. Among the benign cellular elements are numerous diagnostic RS cells (Plate 78-7). In diffusely involved lymph nodes, the architecture is usually obliterated, and the capsular and subcapsular sinuses are compressed. In focally involved lymph nodes the sinuses may remain patent.

Mixed cellularity HD comprises a heterogeneous histologic group representing the center of a spectrum of lesions whose appearance ranges from that of lymphocyte predominance on one extreme to that of lymphocyte depletion on the other. Lukes[7] intended mixed cellularity also to serve as a catch-all classification for those lesions that lack typical features of the remaining types. For example, HD in which lymph nodes are focally or partially involved and lack characteristics of nodular sclerosis are included in the mixed cellularity type.

Reed-Sternberg Cells

Diagnostic RS cells have two or more nuclear lobes and huge, inclusion-like nucleoli (Plate 78-8). The classic RS cell has a symmetric mirror image nucleus. Other RS cells have multiple separate nuclei or an elongated and often twisted nucleus, which, when cut in thin tissue sections, simulates a multinucleated cell. Some RS cells are truely multinucleated. RS cell nucleoli are of relatively uniform density and eosinophilic to amphophilic in staining quality. Nuclear chromatin is condensed to the nuclear membrane, resulting in a clear halo around the nucleolus. The cytoplasm is variable in appearance but is generally abundant and eosinophilic to amphophilic in staining quality.

RS variants are associated with the different histologic types of HD (Table 78-1) and Plates 78-1, 78-4, and 78-6. The L&H/popcorn variant is characteristic of the lymphocyte predominance type, the lacunar variant is typical of nodular sclerosis, and the pleomorphic or sarcomatous variant is found in lymphocyte depletion.

In general, the number of diagnostic RS cells is inversely proportional to the number of small lymphocytes; hence, diagnostic RS cells are rare in lymphocyte predominance, frequent in lymphocyte depletion, and easily found in mixed cellularity types. In nodular sclerosis, the number of diagnostic RS cells is quite variable and may be low. This is rarely a problem for diagnosis, since lacunar variants in a background of collagen sclerosis are virtually diagnostic of nodular sclerosis HD.

Diagnostic Problems

Because of wide variation in the character and frequency of RS cells, HD may sometimes be confused with benign lymphadenopathies, with NHL, and even with epithelial and soft tissue malignancies.[6,30,31] Lukes et al.[30] reported cells indistinguishable from RS cells in infectious mononucleosis. Strum and Rappaport[31] expanded the list of conditions containing RS-like cells to include rubeola, myositis, thymoma, anticonvulsant-induced lymphadenopathy, carcinomas of the lung and breast, malignant melanoma, malignant fibroxanthoma, and various hematopoietic neoplasms. Colby et al.[6] added angioimmunoblastic lymphadenopathy, toxoplasmosis, and malignant histiocytosis to the list of disorders mimicking HD.

Coppleson et al.[32] found a high degree of inter- and intraobserver disagreement in the histologic classification of HD. These investigators recommended the use of a panel of pathologists for the reproducible classification of HD.

In an expert hematopathology panel review of initial diagnostic material from a Southwest Oncology Group trial of advanced HD, Miller et al.[33] found that 13% of 287 cases had been misdiagnosed as HD. The most common error was to confuse other malignant lymphomas with HD (14 of 21 patients), particularly in the case of large cell lymphomas with pleomorphic features

Table 78-1. Summary of Morphology and Phenotype of Reed-Sternberg Cells in Different Histologic Types of Hodgkin Disease

Histologic Type	Reed-Sternberg Cell Variant	Appearance
Mixed cellularity	Classic	Binucleate/multinucleated with hugh inclusion-like eosinophilic nucleoli
Nodular sclerosis	Lacunar cell	Pale retracted cytoplasm; one to many nuclei; small, sometimes basophilic nucleoli
Lymphocyte predominance	"Popcorn" cell	Wrinkled, twisted nucleus, small nucleoli
Lymphocyte depletion	Sarcomatous	Pleomorphic hyperchromatic nuclei, nucleoli often indistinct

Histologic Type	Pattern	Phenotype
Mixed cellularity	Interfollicular or diffuse	B or T/null; CD30$^+$, CD15$^+$
Nodular sclerosis	Inter- or intrafollicular with sclerosis	B or T/null; CD30$^+$, CD15$^+$
Lymphocyte predominance	Intrafollicular	B; CD30$^\pm$, CD 45$^+$; EMA$^+$, CD15$^-$
Lymphocyte depletion	Diffuse fibrosis	Unknown, CD30$^+$, CD15$^+$

(From American Society of Hematology Education Program, 1988, with permission.)

and RS-like cells. Lennert lymphoma and angioimmunoblastic lymphadenopathy were also confused with HD. Mixed cellularity and lymphocyte depletion HD were the types most frequently diagnosed incorrectly (14 of 21), and nodular sclerosis was least frequently mistaken for other disorders (2 of 21). One of the two patients mistakenly diagnosed as having nodular sclerosing HD actually had a sclerosing carcinoma; the other had a dermatopathic lymphadenopathy with multinucleate cells, which on review were found not to be RS cells. Atypical clinical presentations, particularly unusual extranodal sites of disease, characterized the group most often incorrectly diagnosed as HD. Overdiagnosis of HD is particularly common in elderly patients.[34]

Should We Continue to Subclassify HD

Advances in treatment have diminished the earlier prognostic significance of the histologic subtypes of HD, and the question has been raised: Should we bother subclassifying HD?[35] For now, the answer seems to be yes. Histologic classification continues to identify subcategories at greater or lesser risk of relapse. It also helps to predict the most likely sites and extent of disease and in so doing influences decisions about staging and therapy. Correlations of HD histology with new biologic markers should provide new insights into the etiology and pathophysiology of HD.

Pathologic Staging

Improved therapy protocols have placed greater emphasis on more accurate staging of HD. Staging considerations include recognition of early or focal involvement of abdominal lymph nodes, distinction of HD from nondiagnostic granulomas, and recognition of HD in the spleen and at extranodal sites, usually the liver and bone marrow.[36] In addition, HD may present at unusual extranodal sites such as the skin in patients with acquired immunodeficiency syndrome (AIDS), and at various sites, including body fluids, in patients who relapse from HD.

Clinically occult lymph node involvement is most often found in splenic hilar and celiac lymph nodes.[5,29] Early microscopic involvement of abdominal lymph nodes typically occurs in the interfollicular areas (Fig. 78-1), where it resembles the pattern described as interfollicular HD, sometimes encountered in initial biopsy specimens.[37] At least one diagnostic RS cell or variant thereof should be found before a staging lymph node is considered to be involved by HD. Occasionally, prominent immunoblasts in a perifollicular location may cause confusion with HD.

Splenic involvement almost always is apparent on gross inspection of the spleen sliced at thin (3–4-mm) intervals. The number of splenic nodules should be noted, since patients with ≥5 nodules may have a more unfavorable prognosis.[38] Splenic lesions begin in the white pulp and appear as more prominent than usual Malpighian corpuscles. Microscopically, the lesions of HD are first evident near the central artery in the periarterial lymphatic sheath[39] (Plate 78-9). Usually inflammatory cells are increased; patients with nodular sclerosis are commonly found to have bands of collagen.

Liver involvement histologically begins in the portal areas, where increased numbers of small lymphocytes, inflammatory cells, and occasional, often infrequent, HD giant cells are present. It is generally accepted that once the diagnosis of HD has been established, a mononuclear variant of the RS cell with a huge nucleolus is sufficient to confirm HD in the liver and other extranodal sites.[7]

Liver involvement almost never occurs in the absence of splenic HD, except in patients with AIDS who develop HD.[40] Liver function tests are poor predictors of hepatic involvement. The frequency of positive liver biopsies is doubled by performing laparotomy or peritoneoscopy after negative percutaneous biopsy.[41]

Bone marrow involvement occurs in no more than 10% of untreated patients with HD.[42] It is almost always detected in the biopsy and only rarely in the aspirate. This result is most likely due to the focal nature of bone marrow involvement and the increase in reticulum fibers in areas of HD. Bone marrow involvement is probably never recognized as isolated RS cells. Consequently, it can usually be detected at low and medium microscopic magnifications as nodular aggregates of inflammatory cells and/or fibrosis (Plate 78-10). RS cells or their variants may be confirmed at medium and high power (Plate 78-11). They must be distinguished from megakaryocytes, which lack large inclusion-like nucleoli.

In a patient with HD, bone marrow fibrosis is presumptive evidence of marrow involvement by HD. Further sections of the biopsy should be made until RS cells or their variants can

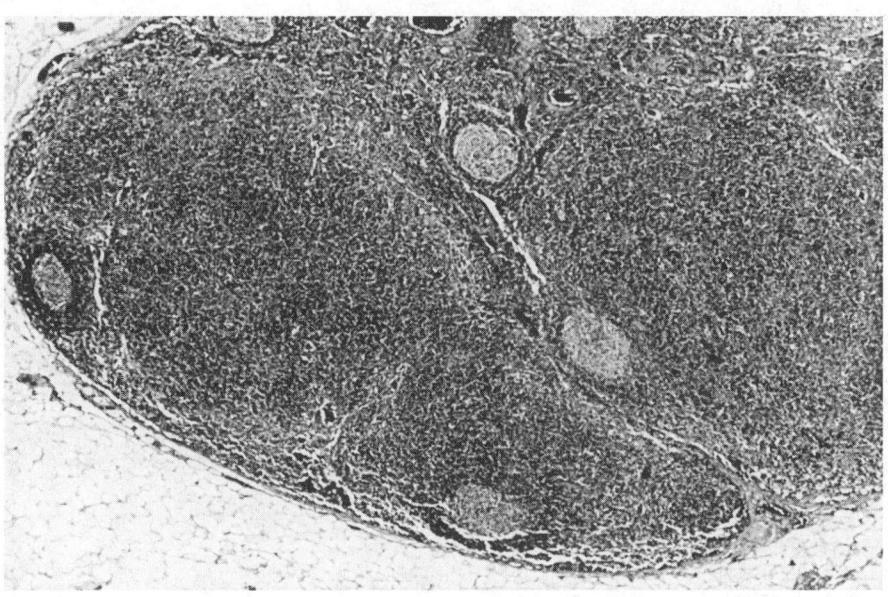

Fig. 78-1. Splenic hilar lymph node: interfollicular Hodgkin disease.

be found. Bone marrow fibrosis is usually not related to previous treatment, which more often causes bone marrow hypoplasia.

Isolated sarcoid-like granulomas may occur in any of the staging sites and should not be considered evidence of HD unless accompanied by RS cells.[43] These granulomas most often occur in a perivascular location (Plate 78-12). In one study, they were found to be associated with a more favorable prognosis and are thought to represent a host immune response to HD.[44] Isolated granulomas in HD seldom contain areas of necrosis but probably should be stained for acid-fast bacilli and fungus to exclude opportunistic infection, which can occur with higher incidence in immunocompromised patients with HD than in the normal population.

IMMUNOPATHOLOGY

The diagnosis and staging of HD is facilitated by the use of immunologic markers that define a characteristic profile of RS cells (Table 78-1 and 78-2; Plates 78-13 to 78-15). RS cells and their variants have the phenotype of activated lymphoid cells expressing antigens Ki-1 (CD30), Leu-M1 (CD15), HLA-DR, Tac (CD25), and T9 (transferrin receptor).[45–48] Other useful markers of RS cells include receptors for peanut agglutinin (PNA),[48,49] intermediate filaments of vimentin, certain myeloid antigens (CD13, My8)[50,51] and epithelial membrane antigen,[52] LN1, and LN2.[53] Polyclonal cytoplasmic immunoglobulin (IgG-κ and IG-λ) is a nearly constant feature of RS cells.[54,55] Monotypic immunoglobulin light chains have been found in RS cells in lymphocyte predominance.[56]

Using special immunohistochemical techniques, T- and/or B-cell antigens are detected on the surface and/or in the cytoplasm of RS cells in 50–100% of cases of HD.[46,47,57–62] Particularly useful for detection of B-cell related antigens on RS cell are antibodies BLA.36[61] and Fun-1.[62] Other B- and T-cell lineage-specific antigens are variably, and often weakly, expressed on RS cells in paraffin-embedded tissues, whereas CD30 and CD15 antigens can be detected in most cases of HD in formalin-fixed paraffin-embedded tissues.[48,51,52,63] Staining for Lewis X antigen may be more sensitive than staining for Leu-M1 in paraffin sections.[64] Bauhinia purpurea is another paraffin section marker with high sensitivity (97%) for RS cells in paraffin sections.[65] It also produces dense cytoplasmic staining of macrophage-histiocytes but shows less cross-reactivity than Ber-H2 or LN2 with NHL of T- or B-cell origin.

It should be appreciated that some investigators have found an inconsistency of immunophenotype of RS cells in simultaneous and consecutive specimens from the same patients.[66] Major immunophenotypic differences were related to cell lineage-specific antigens. Minor differences involved mainly CD15 and LN2 (CD74) antigens.[66]

Immunologic Distinction of Hodgkin Disease from Non-Hodgkin Lymphoma

It is important to distinguish HD from NHL for proper patient management and therapy. Immunologic markers can be used to facilitate this distinction. Leukocyte common antigen (LCA [CD45]) is absent in most cases of HD,[47,51] a feature that, together with other markers, helps distinguish HD from NHL, which is generally CD45[+] (Table 78-2). Among the lymphomas most easily confused with HD are CD30[+] ALCL,[45,67,68] post-thymic or peripheral T-cell lymphoma (PTCL),[69] mediastinal large B-cell lymphoma with sclerosis,[70,71] and T-cell-rich B-cell lymphoma.[72]

Anaplastic Large Cell Lymhoma

CD30[+] ALCL, resembles interfollicular HD because of the focal involvement of lymph nodes and the presence of occasional RS cells (Plate 78-16). However, CD30[+] ALCL has several features usually not found in HD, including infiltration of subcapsular lymph node sinuses and the appearance of monomorphous sheets of tumor cells. Clinically, CD30[+] ALCL involves extranodal sites, such as the skin, soft tissue, gastrointestinal tract, lung, and bone more often (>40%) than does HD (<10%). The peak age incidence of CD30[+] ALCL is in the second decade with a second peak after age 50,[73] whereas HD has a first peak age incidence in the third decade and a second peak after age 50.[74] Patients with CD30[+] ALCL often present with advanced-stage (III or IV) disease and respond to chemotherapy regimens used for diffuse large cell NHL.[73,75] Some cases of CD30[+] ALCL confined to the skin are controlled with local excision and radiation.[76] Antibody BNH9, which detects red blood cell H and Y antigens, can help distinguish CD30[+] ALCL from HD, since antibody BNH9 reacts with tumor cells in most CD30[+] ALCL, but only infrequently with RS cells in HD.[77] Simi-

Table 78-2. Comparison of Hodgkin Disease with Non-Hodgkin Lymphomas Resembling Hodgkin Disease

Disease	Histology	Principal Sites of Disease	Tumor Cell Immunophenotype
Hodgkin disease	RS cells a constant feature; sinus infiltration usually absent, sheets of cells can surround areas of necrosis in syncytial variant	Peripheral lymph node, mediastinum, spleen, para-aortic lymph node	CD30[+], CD45[−], CD15[+], B 50%, T 20%, N 30%
Anaplastic large cell lymphoma	RS cells rare, sinus infiltration, usually sheets of tumor cells with pleomorphic or histiocyte-like appearance	Peripheral lymph node, extranodal sites (skin, gastrointestinal tract, soft tissue, lung, pleura, bone)	CD30[+], CD45[+], CD15[−], BNH9[+], T 75%, B 15%, N 10%
Post-thymic or peripheral T-cell lymphoma	Some cases have numerous large cells, which are similar to or indistinguishable from RS cells; a spectrum of medium and small atypical cells is also found	Generalized lymphadenopathy, spleen, skin	CD30[−], CD45[+], CD15[±], B[−], T[+]
Mediastinal large B-cell lymphoma with sclerosis	RS cells rare or absent; large immunoblast-like cells, no lacunar cells, bands of collagen surround individual and small groups of cells	Mediastinum (thymus) and adjacent intrathoracic structures, late spread to kidneys, adrenal, liver	CD30[−], CD45[+], CD15[−], B[+], T[−]
T-cell-rich B-cell lymphoma	RS-like cells dispersed in a diffuse, small lymphocyte-rich background; mostly older patients (>50 years) with advanced-stage (III or IV) disease, splenomegaly common, poor response to HD treatment regimens	—	CD30[−], CD15[−], EMA[+], B[+]

(From American Society of Hematology Education Program, 1988, with permission.)

larly, epithelial membrane antigen (EMA) is expressed by tumor cells in 75% of CD30⁺ ALCL but is usually not expressed by RS cells in HD other than the nodular lymphocyte predominance subtype.[52]

Post-thymic or Peripheral T-cell Lymphoma

PTCLs, first described by Waldron et al,[69] comprise a spectrum of small and medium-sized atypical lymphoid cells as well as larger immunoblasts, including RS-like cells. The presence of RS cells in a background of inflammatory cells, especially eosinophils, closely resembles mixed cellularity HD (Plate 78-17). Mixed cellularity HD with a high content of epithelioid histiocytes is a newly recognized entity that is easily confused with PTCL.[78] The indistinct borders between PTCL and mixed cellularity HD have been further detailed by Tosi et al.[79] Fortunately, an immunologic distinction can be made in most instances because PTCLs usually are CD30⁻ and CD45⁺ and always express T-cell antigens on the tumor cells. Clinically, PTCLs have more generalized adenopathy than occurs with HD and a higher frequency of pulmonary, pleural, and cutaneous involvement. Most patients with PTCL are middle-aged or elderly, hence are older than most HD patients.

Mediastinal Large B-Cell Lymphoma with Sclerosis

Mediastinal large B-cell lymphoma is a disease that contains large cleaved and noncleaved cells and occasional RS-like cells in a background of sclerosis[70] (Plate 78-18). This entity is curable with full-dose CHOP chemotherapy and consolidation radiation.[71] It affects mainly, but not exclusively, young female patients and therefore can be easily mistaken for nodular sclerosing HD, which also has a preference for young females and mediastinal disease. Both diseases have a strong tendency to involve adjacent intrathoracic structures, but mediastinal large B-cell lymphoma also spreads to the liver, kidneys, and adrenals, rather than to periaortic lymph nodes and spleen, as does nodular sclerosing HD. Although both disorders are characterized by sclerosis, the sclerosis in mediastinal large B-cell lymphoma more often surrounds individual and small groups of tumor cells, in contrast to the coarse circumferential bands of collagen that surround lymphoid nodules in nodular sclerosing HD. Nevertheless, in small mediastinal biopsies, the distinction between the two conditions can at times be difficult but can be made with immunologic markers, as mediastinal large B-cell lymphoma always expresses B-cell antigens and is CD30⁻, CD15⁻, and CD45⁺.

T-cell-Rich B-cell Lymphoma

T-cell-rich B-cell lymphoma contains RS-like cells in a background of small lymphocytes. These cases represent about 4–5% of erroneous diagnoses of HD, being most often confused with diffuse lymphocyte predominance HD.[72] Immunologic distinction from HD is possible because the RS-like cells have a different phenotype than RS cells in HD (Table 78-2). This distinction is important because T-cell-rich B-cell lymphomas are poorly responsive to HD treatment regimens.

Soluble Cellular Antigens and Antigen Receptors in Staging and Prognosis

Elevated levels of soluble interleukin (IL)-2 receptor (CD25) have been detected in the serum of patients with lymphoproliferative disorders.[80] In HD, Pizzolo et al.[81] found that serum values of CD25 correlate with severity of disease and are significantly higher in patients with B symptoms. Low CD25 levels (<1,000 U/ml) are predictive of an excellent prognosis.[82] In addition, patients with high serum CD8 levels (>750 U/ml) have

a poor outcome.[82,83] Pui et al.[83] measured this surface antigen of suppressor/cytotoxic T cells in the serum of 90 children with untreated HD. CD8 levels retained prognostic value in a multivariate analysis when compared to other potentially useful parameters of HD.

CD30 appears to be a marker specific for the neoplastic component and not for the reactive cells in HD. Accordingly, elevated serum CD30 was detected only in patients with active HD and was never found in control sera or in the sera of patients in remission from HD.[82,84] Detectable levels of soluble CD30 were observed more often in patients with advanced stages (III and IV) and with B symptoms, and was detected overall in only 22% of HD patients. Thus, Serum CD30 is a more specific, but less sensitive, marker than CD25 or CD8. Serum CD30 appears to be of particular value for follow-up evaluation of HD patients in remission.

HISTOGENESIS

Nature of the Malignant Cell

In HD, unlike most other human tumors, the nature of the malignant cell remains controversial. In vitro studies indicate that the RS cell, widely regarded as representing the malignant cell in HD, is an end-stage nonproliferating cell,[85,86] and that the most proliferative or clonogenic cell is a small, less conspicuous mononuclear cell.[87] Much of the recent information about the nature of the malignant cell in HD has come from the study of cell lines established in most instances from clinically advanced HD.[88–94] Overall, 13 HD cell lines have been extensively characterized.[94] These cell lines exhibit three features indicative of the malignant cells of HD: (1) they share the same cytochemical and immunlogic staining characteristics as RS cells from fresh tissue biopsies, (2) the cell lines are monoclonal with constant marker chromosomes, and (3) the cultured cells are cytogenetically malignant, with aneuploidy and structural and numerical chromosome abnormalities. The phenotype of the HD cell lines is often not concordant with that of normal hematopoietic cells; some cell lines have features most consistent with a mixed cell lineage.[94] A similar conclusion has resulted from the study conducted by Trumper et al.,[95] who employed the polymerase chain reaction to amplify genes expressed by single RS cells isolated from lymph nodes at diagnosis of HD. These investigators found that single RS cells often co-express genes characteristic of several hematopoietic lineages (monocytes and lymphocytes) and concluded that RS cells resemble activated hematopoietic cells.

Monoclonal antibodies (CD30, Ber-H2, HeFi, HRS-1, and HRS-2) raised against HD cell lines react with RS and mononuclear HD giant cells in fresh tissue sections of HD.[96–98] These antibodies react with two molecules: a 120-kd membrane-associated glycolylated phosphoprotein (CD30/120), and a 57-kd nonglycosylated phosphoprotein (CD30/57), which is found only intracellularly. Both molecules are phosphorylated at serine residues.[99,100] The CD30/57 antigen, but not CD30/120, is a protein kinase capable of autophosphorylation that can also phosphorylate histones.[101] The 120-kd antigen develops from an intracellular precursor of 90 kd by N- and O-glycosidic glycoslyation.[102,103] It can be shed from the cell surface as a soluble CD30 antigen of approximately 90 kd.[99,104] cDNAs encoding the CD30 antigen have been cloned from expression libraries of the human HUT-102 cell line using monoclonal antibodies CD30 and Ber-H2. When expressed in COS-1 cells, the extracellular domain of the CD30 antigen proved homologous to members of the nerve growth factor/tumor necrosis factor (TNF) receptor superfamily.[105] The CD30 gene was mapped to the short arm of chromosome 1 in the region Ip36.[106]

The ligand for CD30 also has been expression-cloned, and

the C-terminal domain was found to show significant homology to TNF-α, TNF-β, and the CD40 ligand.[107] A recombinant human CD30 ligand enhanced proliferation of the HD line HDLM-2 and CD3-activated T cells, while the same ligand induced apoptosis of the Karpas 299 cell line derived from a CD30$^+$ ALCL. The gene for the CD30 ligand was localized to the proximal region of human chromosome 4.[107]

The CD30 antigen is expressed preferentially, if not exclusively, on activated lymphocytes, supporting the hypothesis that RS cells are derived from activated lymphocytes.[45] The normal counterparts of CD30$^+$ cells are found around, between, and at the inner margin of germinal centers.[45,96] CD30$^+$ cells have the appearance of mononuclear immunoblasts with large nucleoli in some inflammatory conditions, such as lymphadenopathy of toxoplasmosis.[96]

Stein et al.[45] and Froese et al.[103] have shown that CD30 can be induced, together with the IL-2 receptor (CD25), on normal B and T cells by exposure to phytohemagglutinin, human T-leukemia viruses, EBV, or *Staphylococcus aureus*.[45,103] CD30 antigen expression appears to represent a late event in lymphocyte activation.[45,108]

There is disagreement about the expression of CD30 antigen on monocyte/macrophages.[109] Stein et al.[110] suggested that apparent CD30 expression may be due to the binding of the CD30 antibody to high-affinity FC γ receptors, which may be induced by interferon (IFN)-γ. Pfreundschuh et al.[98] also detected epitopes of the CD30 antigen on activated monocytes and in some myelomonocytic leukemias. In this respect, it is interesting to note that RS cells in tissue sections express antigens associated with late granulocytic differentiation.[50,51] HD cell line L428KS expresses antigens found mainly on monocytes and immature myeloid cells.[89]

Some studies[111–113] have shown similarities between RS cells and interdigitating reticulum cells, which are antigen-presenting cells in interfollicular regions of lymph nodes. The L428 cell line has been shown to be capable of antigen presentation.[114] RS cells express antigens shared with activated interdigitating reticulum cells,[112] and both cell types have similar reactivities with CD15 antibody and PNA.[48] However, interdigitating reticulum cells in lymph nodes do not appear to react with CD30 antibodies.[45,63]

A recent study by Delsol et al.[115] purports to show a relation of RS cells to follicular dendritic reticulum cells (FDRC), as originally proposed by Curran and Jones.[116] The study of Delsol cites as support for this hypothesis the intimate association of RS cells with the lymph node FDRC network, expression of CD21 antigen by FDRC and RS cells, expression of IgG Fc receptors, and the presence of polyclonal IgG and IgE within the cytoplasm of both FDRC and RS cells.[55,117]

Lymphocyte-associated antigens have been detected on RS cells in 50–100% of HD cases.[45–47,57–62,118] In an immunocytochemical study of lymph node cytospins from 20 cases of HD, Falini et al.[46] found that a variable percentage of typical RS and mononuclear HD giant cells in eight cases expressed cytoplasmic or surface staining, or both, for T-cell antigens CD3, CD4, CD5, and CD6. In one case each of nodular sclerosis and mixed cellularity, the neoplastic cells weakly expressed B-cell antigens CD19 and CD22 but not T-cell or macrophage-associated antigens. Using a sensitive immunocytochemical technique and paraformaldehyde-lysine-periodated (PLP) fixed frozen tissues, Kadin et al.[118] and Agnarsson and Kadin[47] found that RS cells expressed either T-cell- or B-cell-specific antigens and sometimes co-expressed both, in 55% of nodular sclerosis and 80% of mixed cellularity HD cases. Expression of B-cell antigens was found on L&H RS cell variants in four of five cases of LPHD.[47] Similarly, Pinkus and Said[59] showed that virtually all cases of nodular LPHD express a B-cell immunophenotype. Schmid et al.[60] detected one or more B-cell antigens (CD19, CD20, CD22, CDw75, MB2) on RS cells in 87%, including all types

of HD. They also found reactivity of RS cells, mainly cytoplasmic, for T-cell markers CD3 and Bf1 in 14.5% of HD cases. Zuckerberg et al.[119] demonstrated co-expression of B-cell antigen CD20 and granulocyte-associated antigen CD15 by RS cells in 3 of 20 cases of nodular sclerosis and mixed cellularity HD. These investigators correlated the variable expression of these antigens in the remaining cases with the relative proportion of granulocytes in cellular background of HD. Imam et al.[61] and Nozawa et al.[62] detected B-cell-associated antigens on RS cells in virtually all cases of HD. In contrast to these findings, which support a B-cell origin for RS cells of HD, Ruprai et al.[120] Lauritzen et al.,[121] and Weiss et al.[122] were unable to detect immunoglobulin light-chain mRNA in RS cells. Moreover, Kuzu et al.[123] detected the immunoglobulin-associated heterodimer (mb-1 and B29) in six of seven cases of LPHD but could not find this heterodimer in nonlymphocyte predominance subtypes of HD. Their results confirm previous studies that suggest that LPHD is of B-cell origin but did not provide support for the hypothesis that nonlymphocyte predominance subtypes also have a B-cell origin.

Timens and co-workers[124] and Poppema and colleagues[16,17,125] have provided evidence that nodular LPHD is a germinal center lymphoma. Nodular LPHD is confined to follicles that predominantly contain B cells. A smaller population of T lymphocytes in these follicles belongs to a Leu 7$^+$ subpopulation of CD4 cells, which are present in normal germinal centers. This population, not found in other types of HD, is greatly increased ($\leq$30%) in nodular LPHD.[125] The L&H/popcorn variants of RS cells found in nodular LPHD express B-cell antigens and in some cases have membrane or cytoplasmic immunoglobulin, or both.[124] This immunoglobulin may show light-chain restriction.[56] These L&H variants also differ from other types of RS cells in their frequent expression of CD45 and EMA but inconstant expression of CD30 and CD15 antigens.[52]

Gene Rearrangement Studies

A lymphoid origin for the neoplastic cells in HD is supported by immunoglobulin and T-cell receptor (TCR) gene rearrangement studies.[126–130] Weiss et al.[126] found that tumors rich in RS cells often had rearranged bands of immunoglobulin genes. Brinker et al.[127] found rearrangements of immunoglobulin heavy- and light-chain genes in tissues from 5 of 11 patients, particularly in late stages of the disease, when lymphocyte depletion had occurred. Sundeen et al.[128] detected immunoglobulin gene rearrangements in three of five cases in which RS cells were enriched by cell separation techniques to >1%. These investigators found no rearrangements in lymphocyte fractions or unseparated cells prepared from the same tissues. Griesser et al.[129] found either immunoglobulin or TCR gene rearrangements in most of 22 cases of HD. Rearrangements of immunoglobulin heavy-chain gene were found in only two cases, both of lymphocyte depletion type. TCR-β chain gene rearrangements were found in three cases of HD, including one case each of mixed cellularity, nodular sclerosis, and lymphocyte predominance types. Most HD cases of any histologic type had rearrangements of TCR-γ chain genes, usually without TCR-β or immunoglobulin gene rearrangement.[129] Interestingly, similar results (TCR-γ chain gene rearrangements only) were also encountered in many cases of CD30$^+$ ALCL.[130,131] Among cases of HD and CD30$^+$ ALCL with only TCR-γ gene rearrangements were cases in which the tumor cells expressed a histiocytic phenotype. In these cases especially, it was concluded that a histiocytic derivation for RS cells could not be excluded.

It has been suggested from gene rearrangement studies that RS cells may represent polyclonal T-cell populations.[132] In three cases of lymphocyte depletion HD estimated to contain >25% RS-cell variants, Knowles et al.[132] found no immunoglobu-

Color Plates

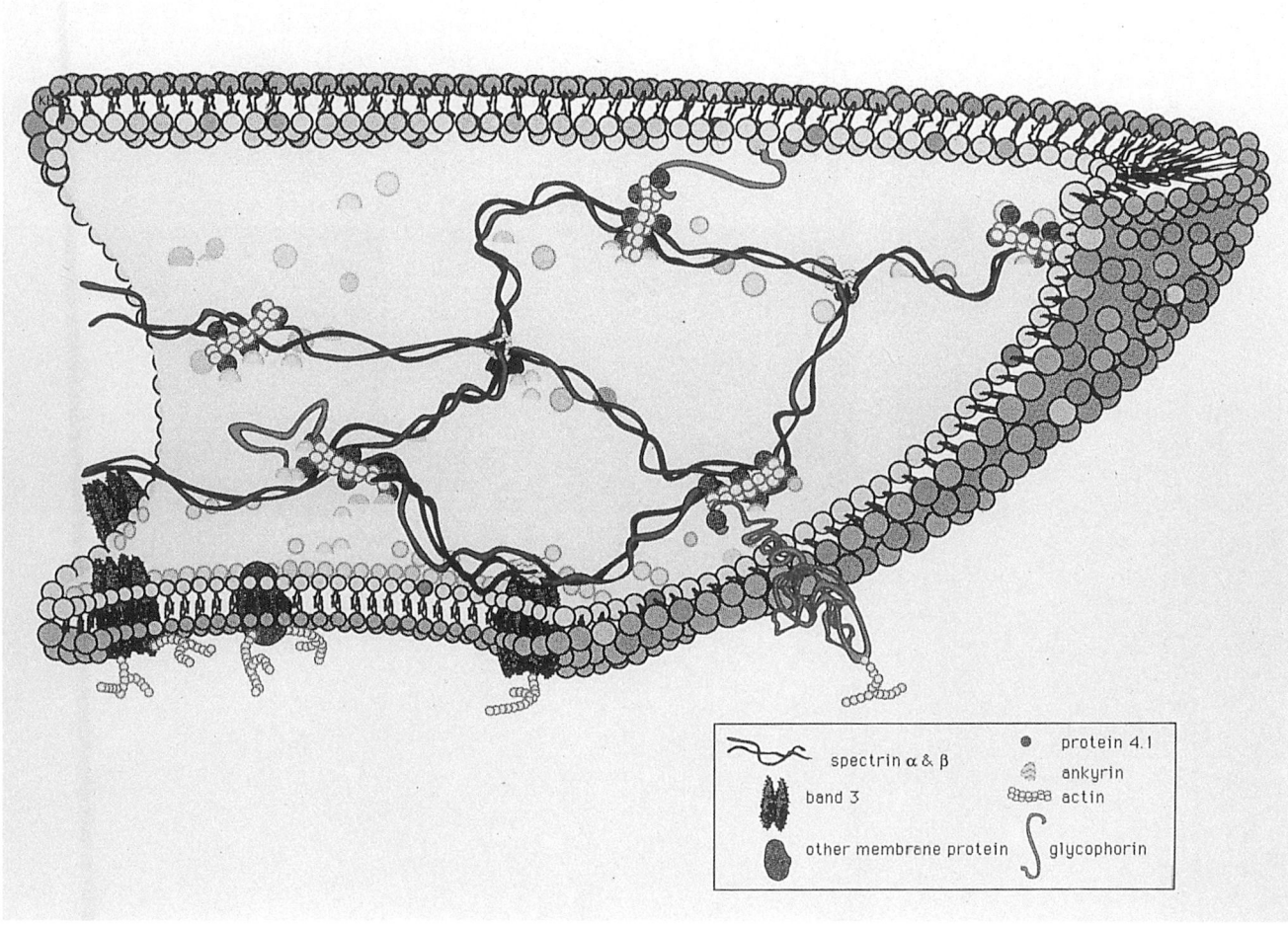

Plate 4-1.

Plate 4-1. Arrangement of integral and peripheral membrane proteins in the red cell. Note the asymmetric distribution of lipid, the anastomosing lattice formed by spectrin-spectrin and spectrin-actin junctions.

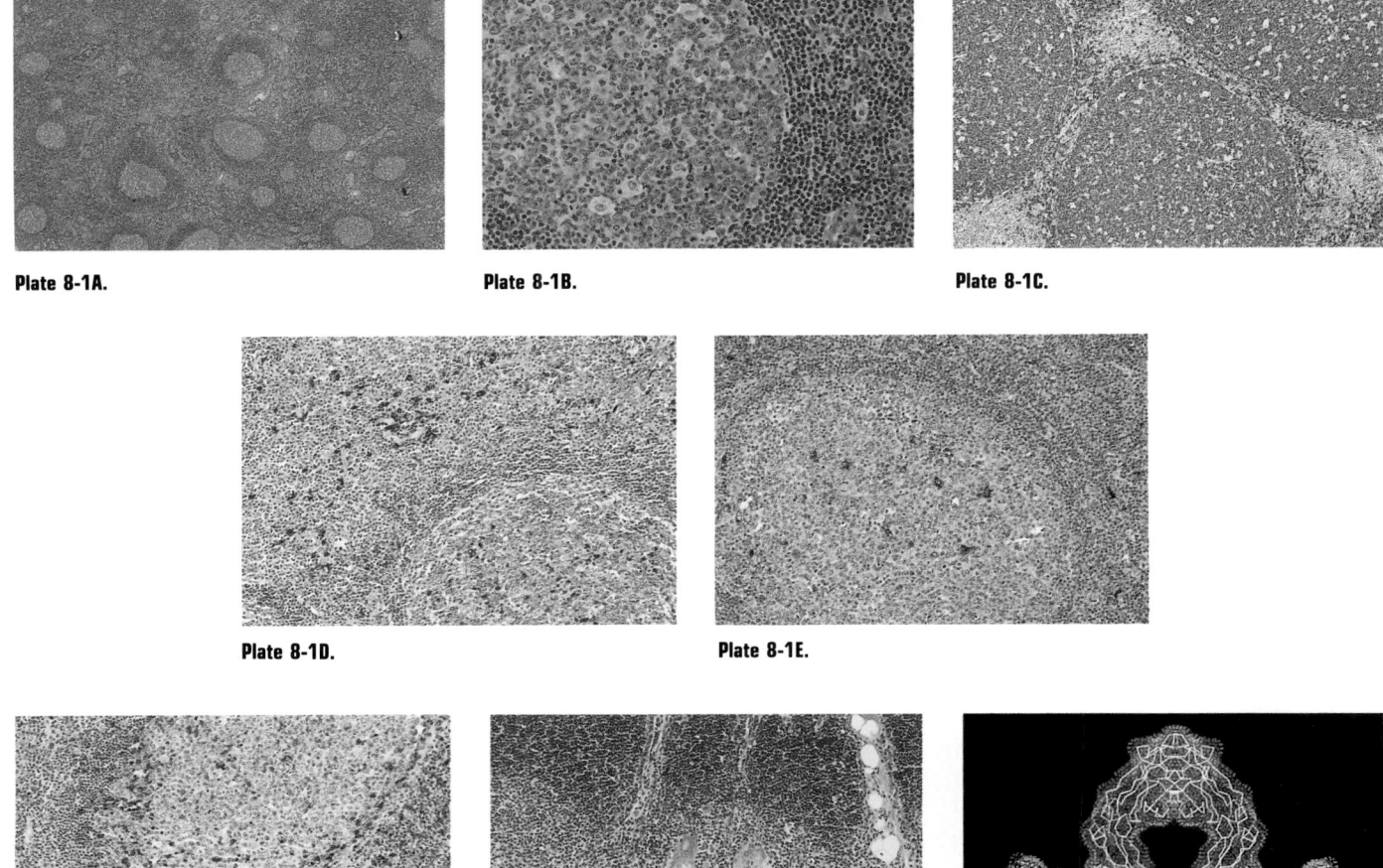

Plate 8-1A. **Plate 8-1B.** **Plate 8-1C.**

Plate 8-1D. **Plate 8-1E.**

Plate 8-1F. **Plate 8-1G.** **Plate 9-1.**

Plate 8-1. **(A)** Lymph node. Several lymphatic follicles with well-developed germinal centers are visible. (H&E × 200.) **(B)** Lymph node. Lymphatic follicle with prominent germinal center pushing away the follicular mantle. (H&E × 350.) **(C)** Lymph node. B cells are stained (brown color) with a peroxidase-labeled monoclonal antibody against CD20, a pan-B-cell marker. (× 250.) **(D)** Lymph node. B cells are stained (brown color) with a peroxidase-labeled monoclonal antibody against κ light chains. (× 300.) **(E)** Lymph node. Stain for lysozyme. Macrophages containing the enzyme are scattered throughout the germinal center and mantle zone. (× 300.) **(F)** Lymph node. T cells stained (brown color) by a peroxidase-labeled monoclonal antibody (UCHL-1) against the pan-T-cell antigen CD45RO. (× 300.) **(G)** Thymus. Thymic lobule with densely packed cellular cortex and less cellular medulla in which large, pale Hassal's corpuscles are visible. (H&E × 250.)

Plate 9-1. α-Carbon backbone and overall surface shape of the intact Dob IgG structure. The antigen combining sites are located at the ends of the two horizontal Fab arms formed by the association of the light chains (α-carbon backbone as red lines and surface as light blue dots) and heavy chains (α-carbon backbone as yellow lines and surface as blue dots). On the basis of amino acid sequence studies, Dob has a substantial deletion in the hinge region, and this probably limits its segmental flexibility. The molecular surface represents the area accessible to a probe sphere the size of a water molecule (1.4-Å radius). In this representation the surface of the IgG is composed of convex regions, formed by the solvent-accessible van der Waals' surface of individual atoms and concave regions. Small gaps and crevices inaccessible to the probe sphere are smoothed over. (From Getzoff et al.,[4] with permission.)

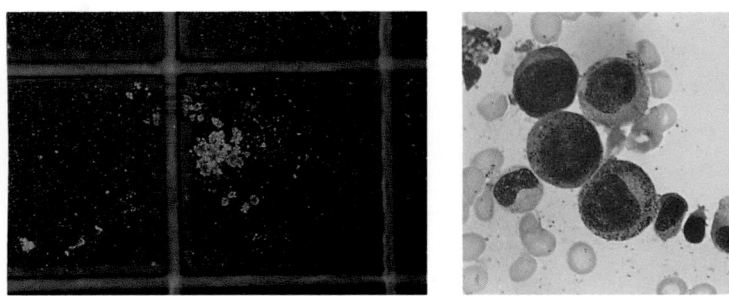

Plate 14-1.

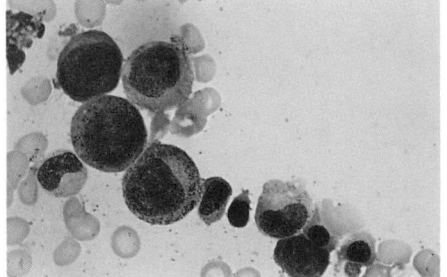

Plate 14-2.

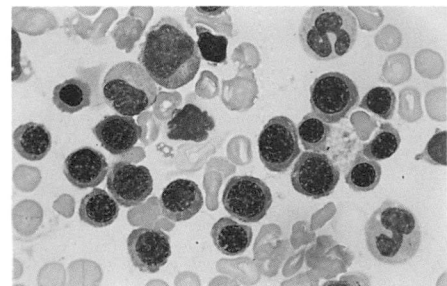

Plate 14-3.

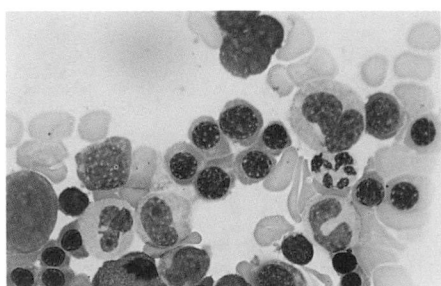

Plate 14-4.

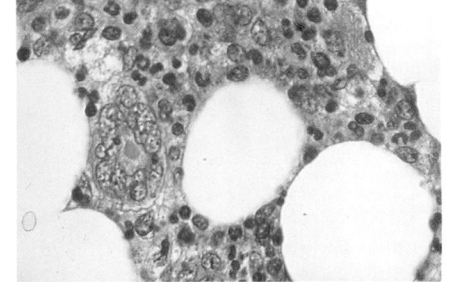

Plate 23-1A.

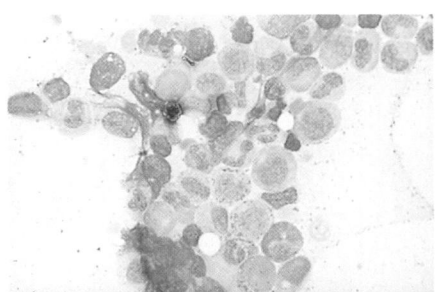

Plate 23-1B.

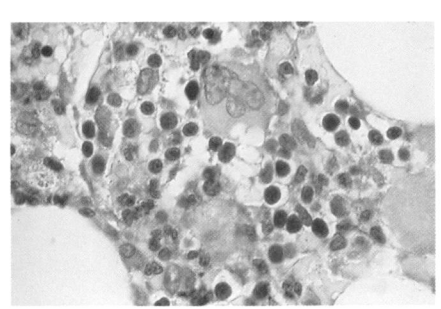

Plate 23-1C.

Plate 14-1. Colony-forming unit-mixed erythroid, myeloid, megakaryocyte (CFU-Mix). (See also Fig. 14-3.)

Plate 14-2. Proerythroblast (upper left corner), promyelocyte (middle) and myelocyte (below, right), and metamyelocyte (lower right).

Plate 14-3. Erythrocyte maturation. Basophilic (four in middle, middle right), polychromatic (three middle right) and orthochromatic erythroblast (upper left).

Plate 14-4. Cluster of polychromatophilic erythroblasts.

Plate 23-1. Bone marrow in PRCA. **(A)** Particle section showing normal cellularity with periodic acid-Schiff (PAS)-positive granulocyte precursors and megakaryocytes, but no erythroblasts. **(B)** Wright stain of particle smear showing absence of erythroblasts and predominance of granulocyte precursor cells and lymphocytes. **(C)** Particle section, after treatment and remission of PRCA, demonstrating marked increase in PAS-negative mature erythroblasts.

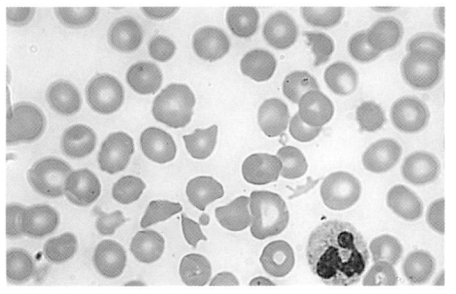

Plate 48-1.

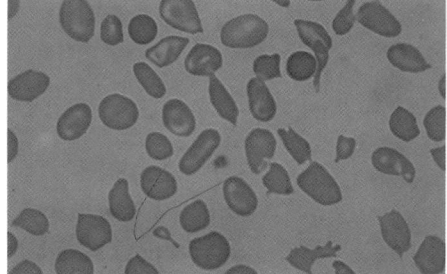

Plate 48-2.

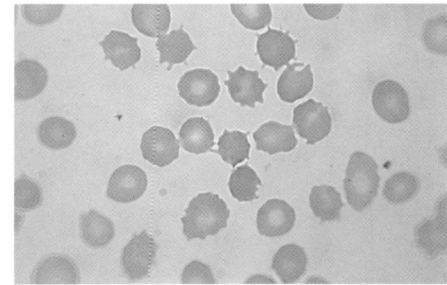

Plate 48-3.

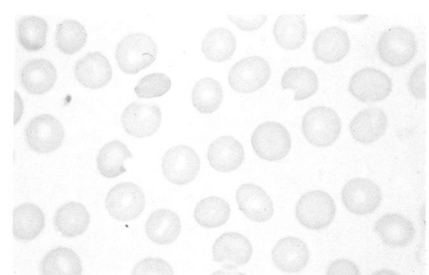

Plate 48-4.

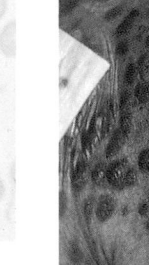

Plate 64-1.

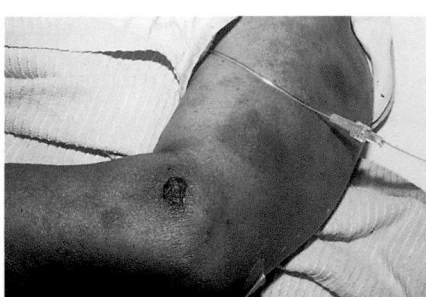

Plate 64-2.

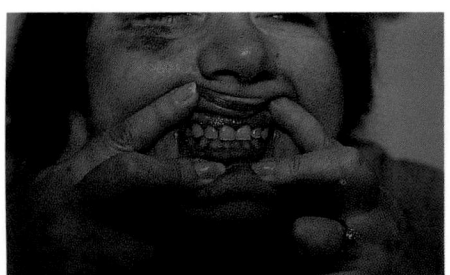

Plate 64-3.

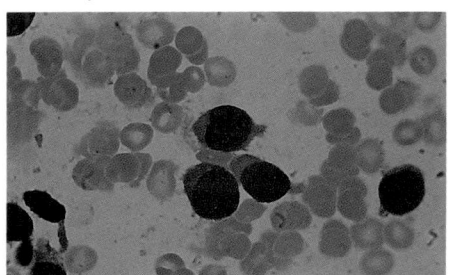

Plate 64-4.

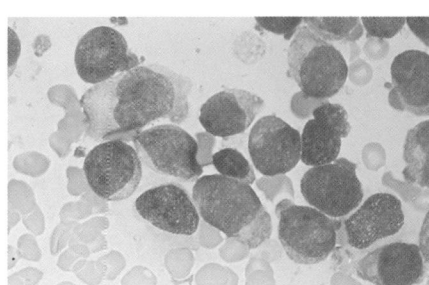

Plate 64-5.

Plate 48-1. Fragmentation hemolysis. Note the irregular, distorted forms and small fragments.

Plate 48-2. Peripheral smear from a patient with β-thalassemia intermedia shows the extensive tailed forms that largely disappear following splenectomy. Similar observations have been made on tailed RBCs in patients with agnogenic myeloid metaplasia and myelofibrosis.

Plate 48-3. Peripheral smear from a patient with severe alcoholic liver disease. Note the acanthocytes, spur cells, and transitional forms. Macrocytes are also present.

Plate 48-4. Bite cells from a patient with oxidative hemolysis. Note the thin veil of membrane across a clear zone, giving the appearance of a "blister."

Plate 64-1. Leukemia cutis in a patient with monoblastic leukemia.

Plate 64-2. Sweet syndrome in a patient with AML. Tender, pseudovescicular, erythematous plaques of Sweet syndrome. (From Cohen,[139] with permission.)

Plate 64-3. Gingival infiltration in a patient with myelomonocytic leukemia.

Plate 64-4–Plate 64-14. French-American-British Cooperative Group classification of acute myeloid leukemia.

Plate 64-4. M0: Acute myeloid leukemia.

Plate 64-5. M1: Acute myeloid leukemia. Cells demonstrate no evidence of maturation or differentiation. The blasts often have large irregular nuclei with varying amounts of eccentrically placed cytoplasm. There is no definite granulation, and Auer rods are absent.

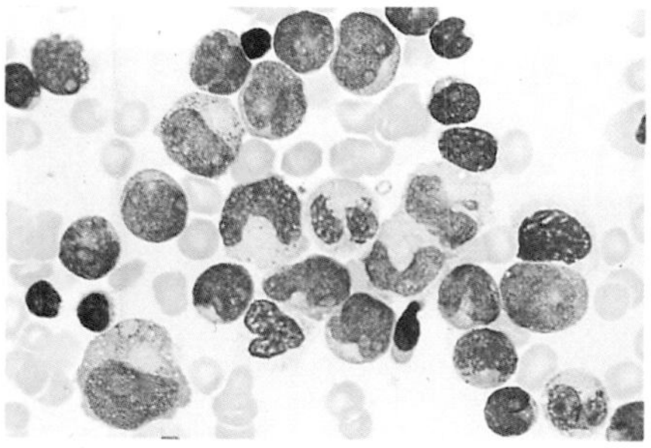

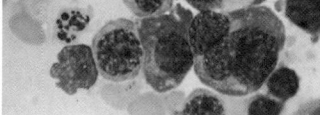**Plate 64-6.**	**Plate 64-7.**	**Plate 64-8.**
Plate 64-9.	**Plate 64-10.**	**Plate 64-11.**
Plate 64-12.	**Plate 64-13.**	**Plate 64-14.**

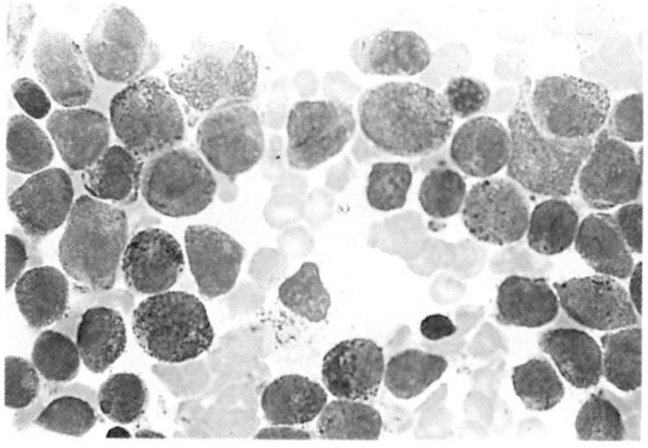

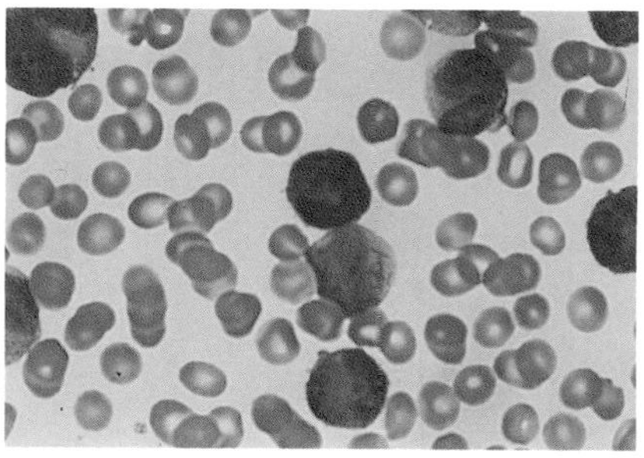

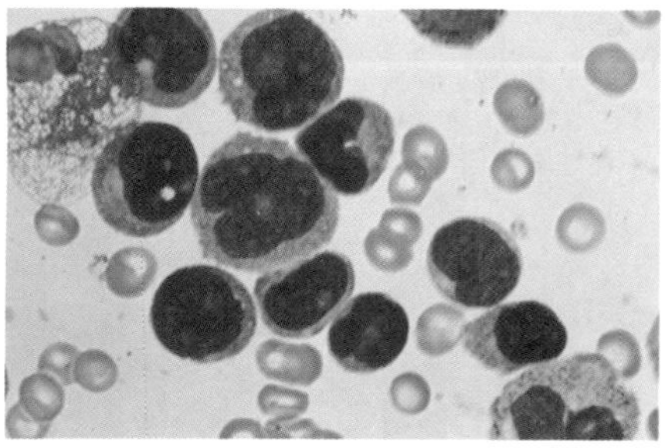

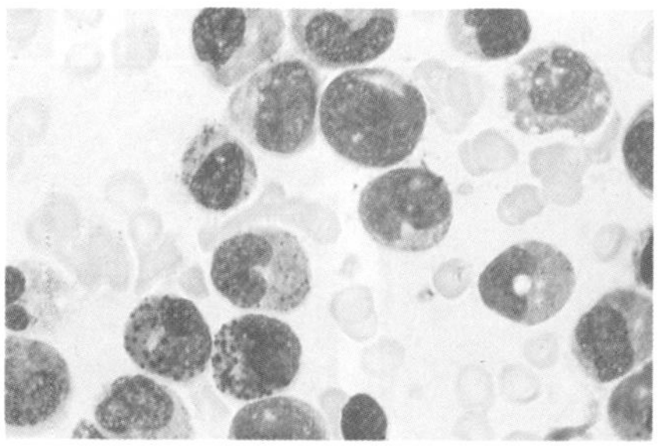

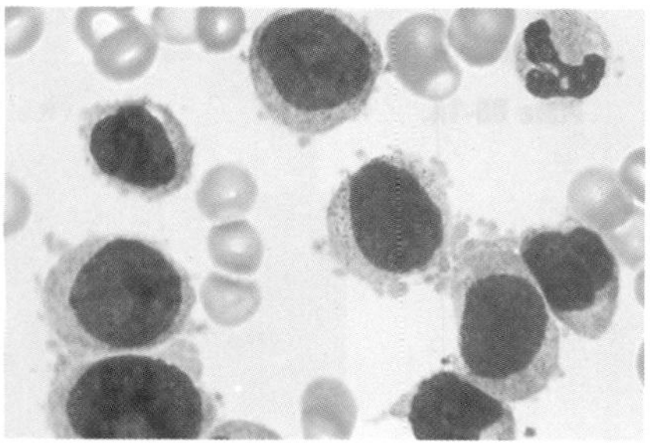

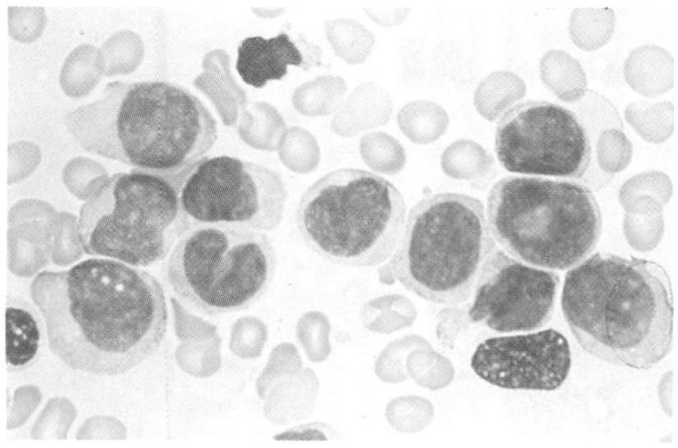

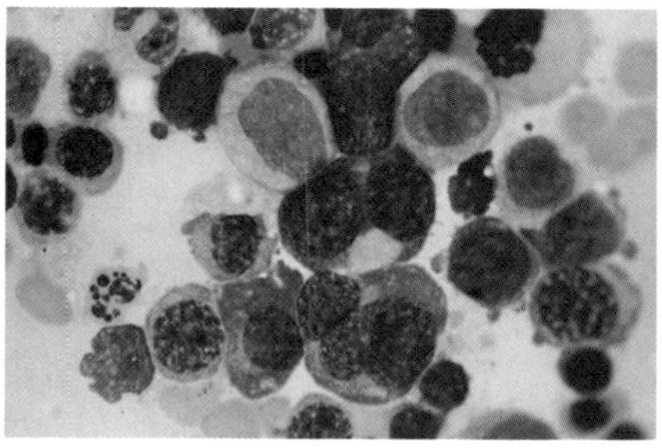

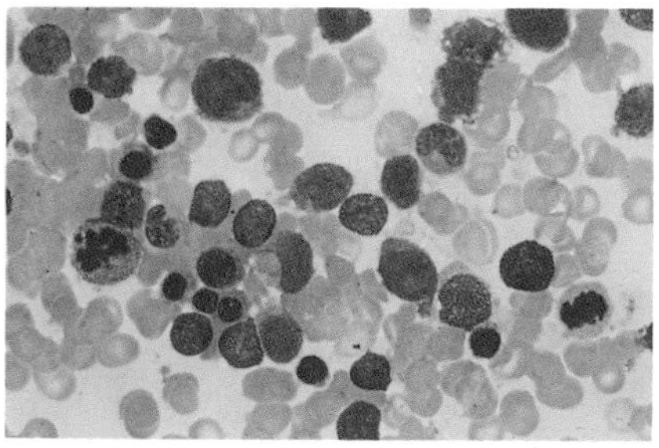

Plate 64-6. M2: Myeloblastic leukemia with differentiation. The leukemic cells demonstrate maturation through the promyelocytic stage. Azurophilic granules are seen with occasional Auer rods. (Courtesy of Guido J.K. Tricot, M.D., Ph.D.)

Plate 64-7. M3: Acute promyelocytic leukemia. The leukemic cells contain multiple abnormal, coarse azurophilic granules, and Auer rods are prominent. (Courtesy of Guido J.K. Tricot, M.D., Ph.D.)

Plate 64-8. M3v.

Plate 64-9. M4: Acute myelomonocytic leukemia. Both myeloid and monocytic elements are found, and myeloblasts differentiate through the promyelocyte stage. Monocytes and monoblasts make up <20% of the total number of nucleated cells. Monoblasts demonstrate a pale cytoplasm, with occasional vacuoles and granules with folded or rounded nuclei.

Plate 64-10. M4Eo: Acute myelomonocytic leukemia with eosinophils. Similar to the M4 variant but with increased eosinophils; eosinophils are atypical in appearance, with prominent basophilic granules.

Plate 64-11. M5a: Acute monocytic leukemia, undifferentiated. The predominant cell is an undifferentiated monoblast. The cytoplasm is pale, with occasional vacuoles. The nuclei are round and lack the usual folded monocytoid appearance.

Plate 64-12. M5b: Acute monocytic leukemia, differentiated. Most of the cells are mature-looking monocytes with centrally placed folded nuclei. Rare monoblasts are found. (Courtesy of Dr. Lorrie F. Odom.)

Plate 64-13. M6: Erythroleukemia. Abnormal erythroid precursors with megaloblastic features are prominent. All stages of the erythroid series are found, typically with many bizarre and dysplastic features. Typical myeloblasts are also noted. (Courtesy of the Blood and Bone Marrow Cell Recognition and Interpretation audiovisual seminars. American Society of Clinical Pathologists, Chicago, 1987.)

Plate 64-14. M7: Acute megakaryocytic leukemia. Increased marrow fibrosis is frequent. Note the cytoplasmic budding, which is typical of megakaryocytic leukemias.

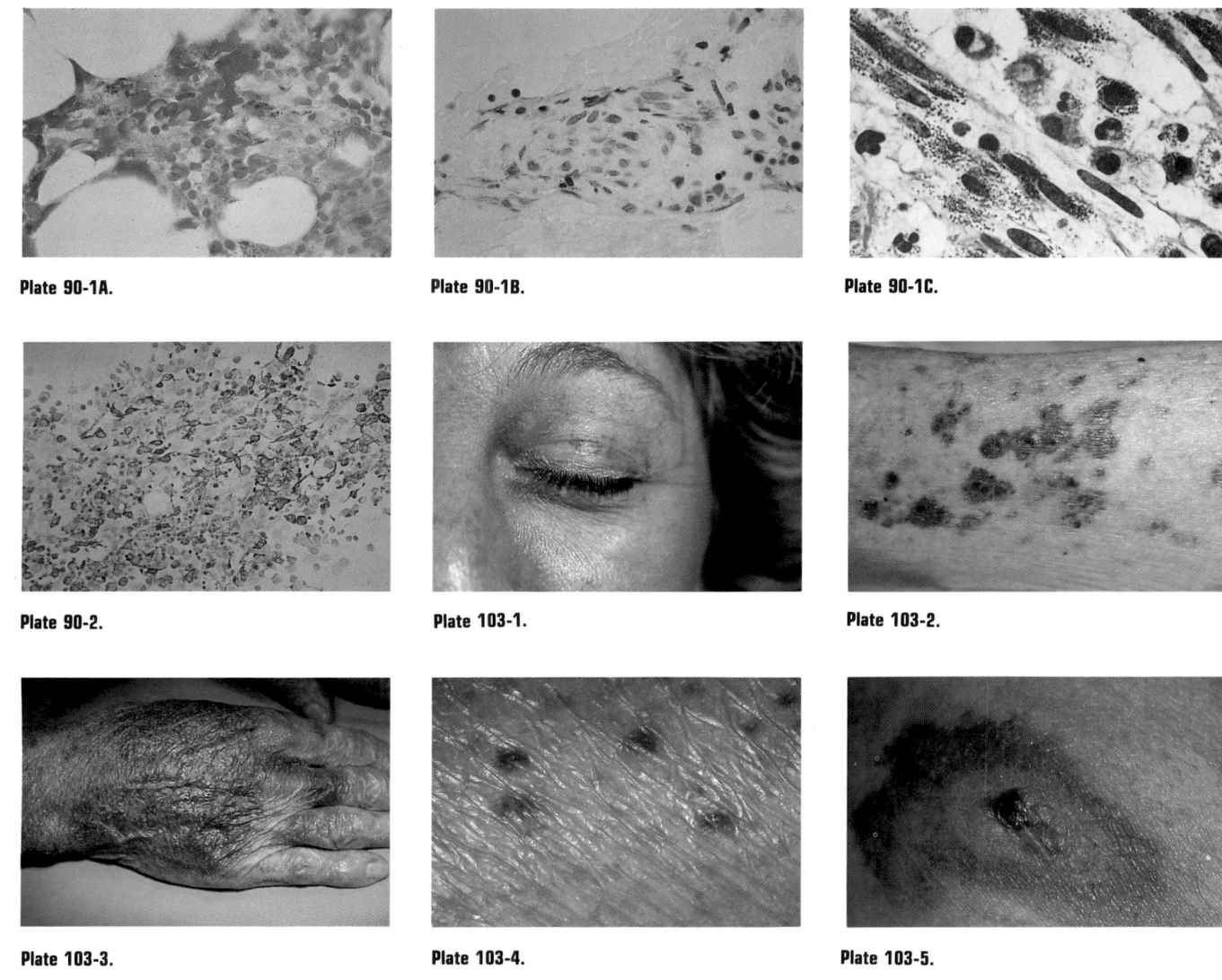

Plate 90-1A. **Plate 90-1B.** **Plate 90-1C.**

Plate 90-2. **Plate 103-1.** **Plate 103-2.**

Plate 103-3. **Plate 103-4.** **Plate 103-5.**

Plate 90-1. (A) High power (× 156) Geimsa stain of a mast cell lesion in a plastic embedded bone marrow. **(B)** High power (× 250) toluidine blue stain of a mast cell lesion in a plastic embedded bone marrow. Note that on Geimsa stains, mast cell granules stain dark blue, whereas eosinophils stain bright orange. (From Parker RI: Hematologic aspects of mastocytosis. 1. Bone marrow pathology in adult and pediatric systemic mast cell disease. J Invest Dermatol 96:47S, 1991, with permission.) **(C)** Giemsa plastic embedded bone marrow biopsy demonstrating metachromatic granules in mast cells. (× 1,000.) (From Travis WD, Li C-Y, Bergstralh EJ et al: Systemic mast cell disease: analysis of 58 cases and literature review. Medicine 67:345, 1988, with permission.)

Plate 90-2. Low power (× 20) of toluidine blue stain of mast cells in bone marrow aspirate smear. (From Parker RI: Hematologic aspects of mastocytosis. 1. Bone marrow pathology in adult and pediatric systemic mast cell disease. J Invest Dermatol 96:47S, 1991, with permission.)

Plate 103-1. Valsalva petechiae.

Plate 103-2. Stasis purpura (palpable).

Plate 103-3. Senile purpura.

Plate 103-4. Scurvy.

Plate 103-5. Ecthyma gangrenosum.

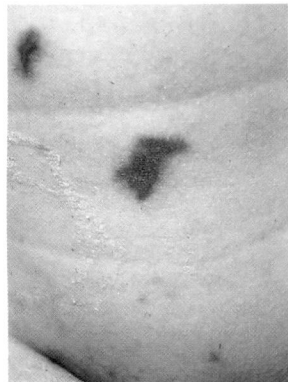

Plate 103-6.

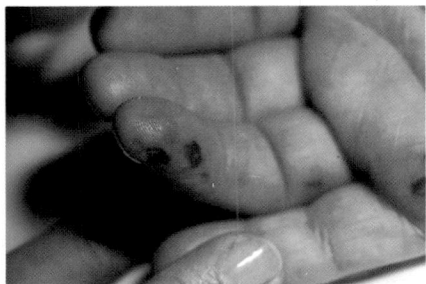

Plate 103-7.

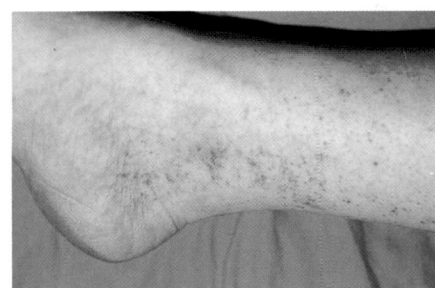

Plate 103-8.

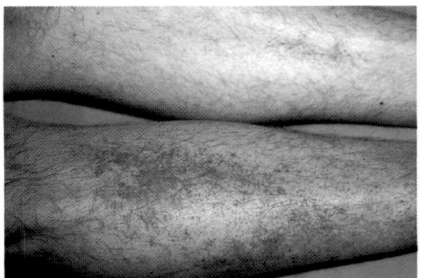

Plate 103-9.

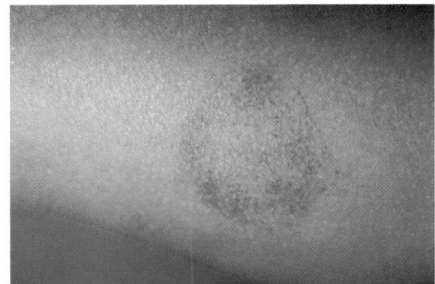

Plate 103-10.

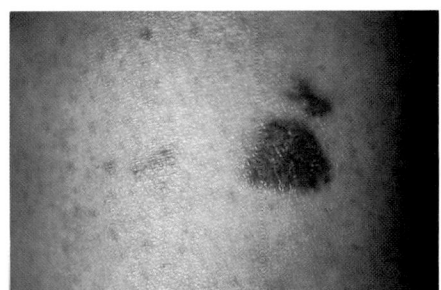

Plate 103-11.

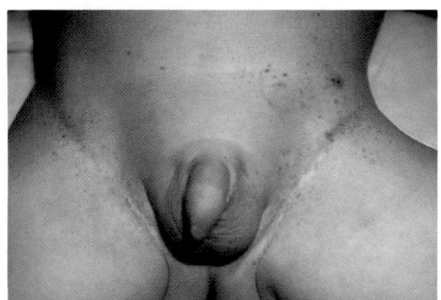

Plate 103-12.

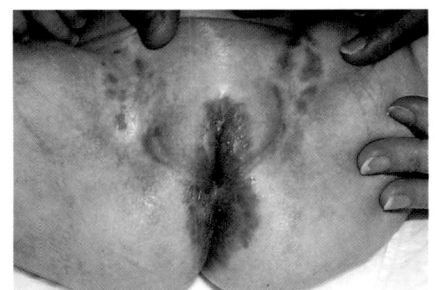

Plate 103-13.

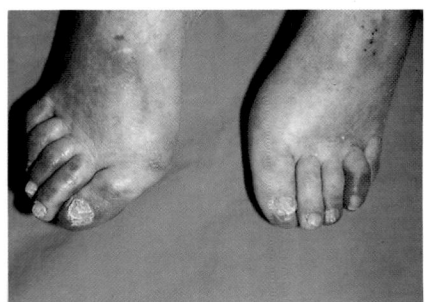

Plate 103-14.

Plate 103-6. Meningococcemia.

Plate 103-7. Acute bacterial endocarditis.

Plate 103-8. Rocky Mountain spotted fever.

Plate 103-9. Schamberg's pigmented purpuric eruption.

Plate 103-10. Majocchi's pigmented purpuric eruption.

Plate 103-11. Lichen aureus.

Plate 103-12. Letterer-Siwe disease.

Plate 103-13. Histiocytosis X.

Plate 103-14. Disseminated intravascular coagulation.

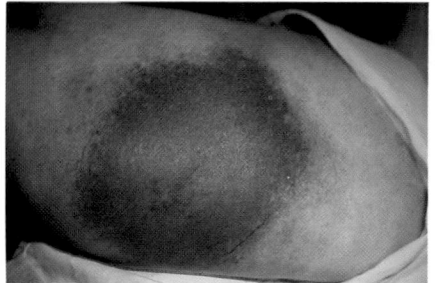

Plate 103-15.

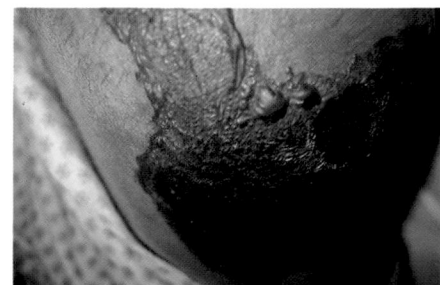

Plate 103-16.

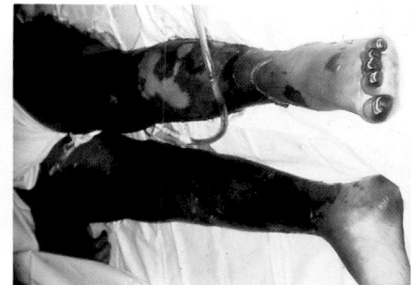

Plate 103-17.

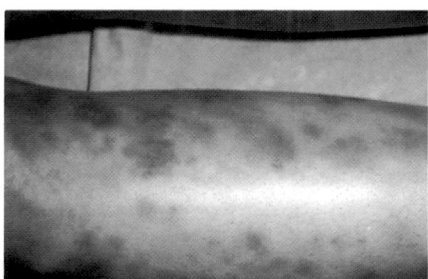

Plate 103-18.

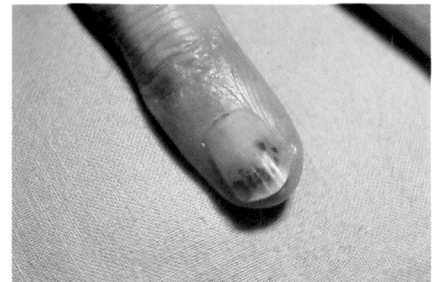

Plate 103-19.

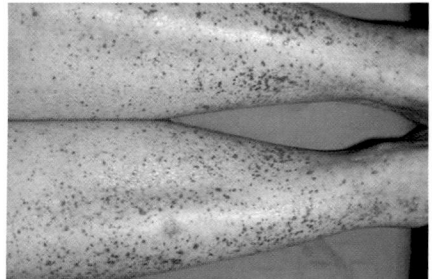

Plate 103-20.

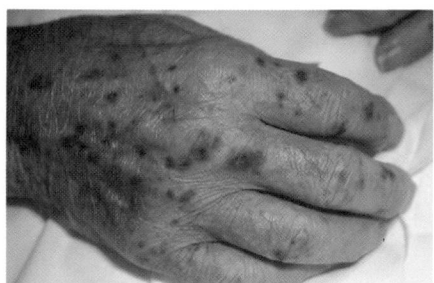

Plate 103-21.

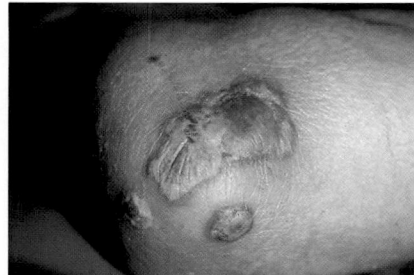

Plate 103-22.

Plate 103-15. Coumarin necrosis.

Plate 103-16. Coumarin necrosis.

Plate 103-17. Purpura fulminans status post herpes zoster.

Plate 103-18. Psychogenic purpura.

Plate 103-19. Subungual hemorrhage due to cryoglobulins.

Plate 103-20. Hyperglobulinemic purpura.

Plate 103-21. Rheumatoid vasculitis.

Plate 103-22. Wegener's granulomatosis.

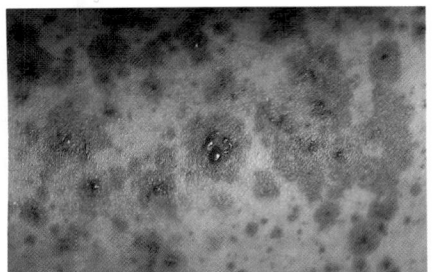

Plate 103-23.

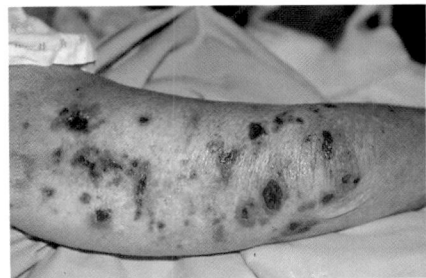

Plate 103-24.

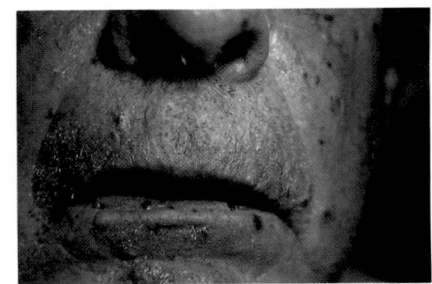

Plate 103-25.

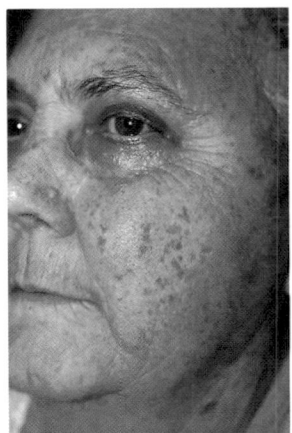

Plate 103-26.

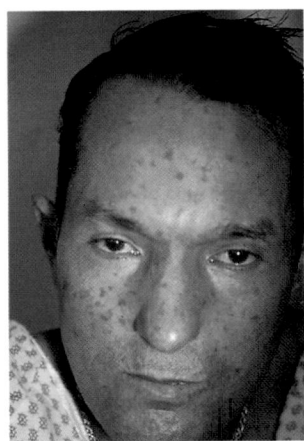

Plate 103-27.

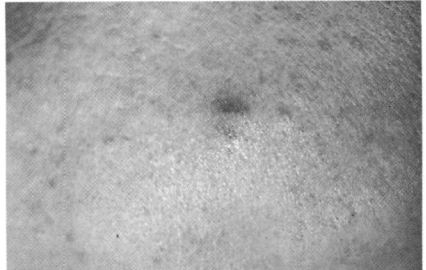

Plate 103-28.

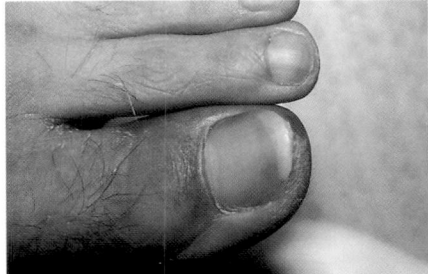

Plate 103-29.

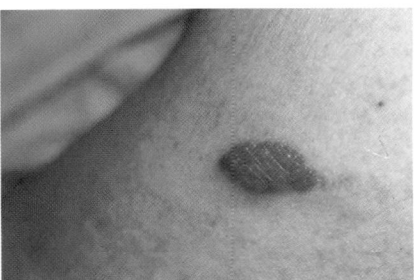

Plate 103-30.

Plate 103-23. Henoch-Schönlein purpura.

Plate 103-24. Leukocytoclastic vasculitis.

Plate 103-25. Hereditary hemorrhagic telangiectasia.

Plate 103-26. Telangiesctatic Mats.

Plate 103-27. CREST.

Plate 103-28. Kaposi sarcoma (AIDS).

Plate 103-29. Kaposi sarcoma (AIDS).

Plate 103-30. Kaposi sarcoma (AIDS).

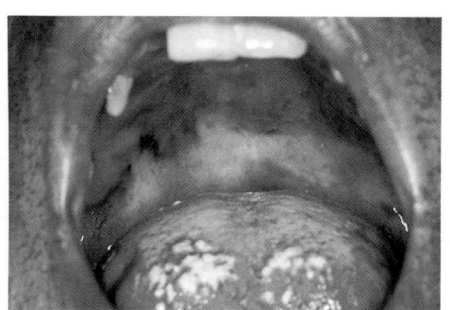

Plate 103-31.

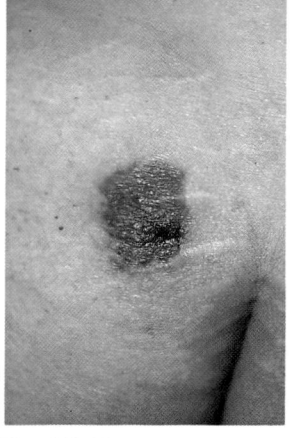

Plate 103-32.

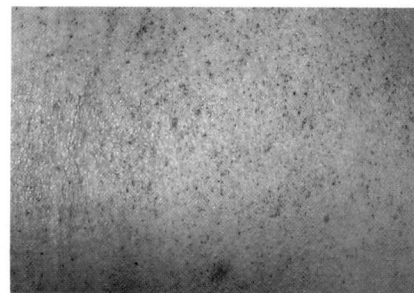

Plate 103-33.

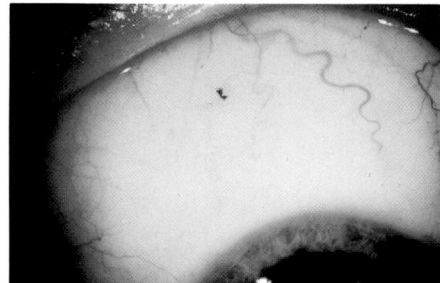

Plate 103-34.

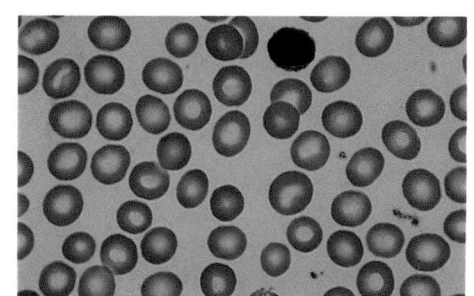

Plate 156-1A.

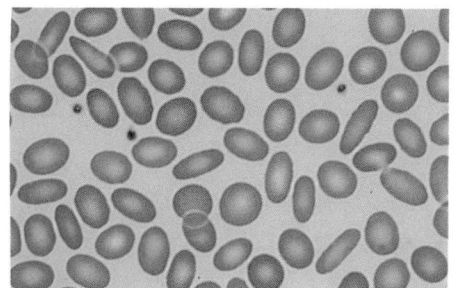

Plate 156-1B.

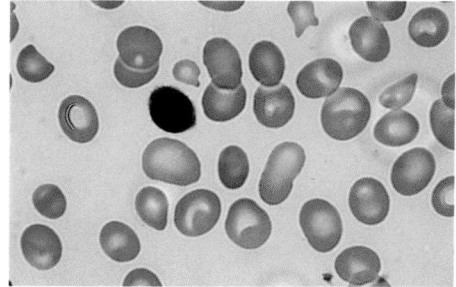

Plate 156-1C.

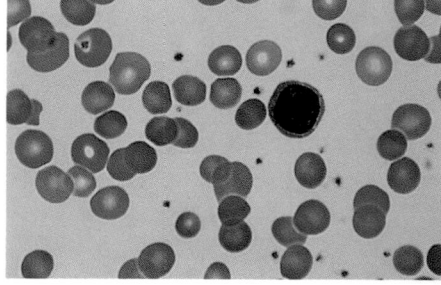

Plate 156-1D.

Plate 103-31. Kaposi sarcoma (AIDS).

Plate 103-32. Angiosarcoma.

Plate 103-33. Fabry disease.

Plate 103-34. Fabry disease.

Plate 156-1. Red cell morphology. **(A)** Discocytes (normocytic, normochromic). **(B)** Elliptocytes and ovalocytes. **(C)** Megalocytes (oval macrocytes). **(D)** Spherocytes. *(Plate 156-1 continues.)*

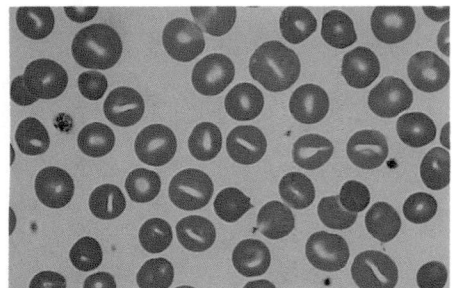

Plate 156-1E.

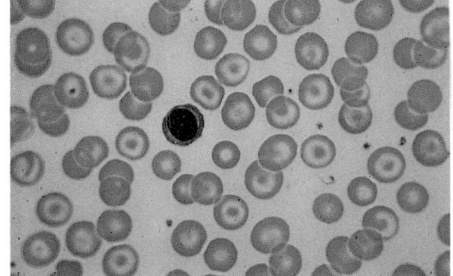

Plate 156-1F.

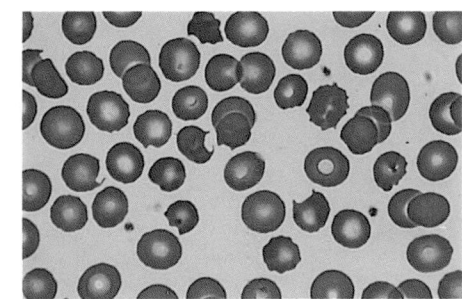

Plate 156-1G.

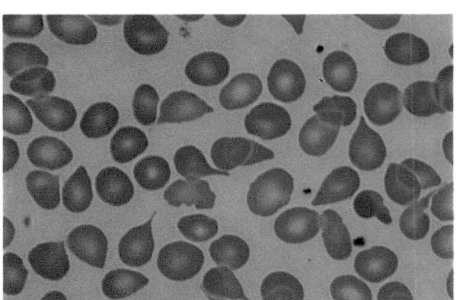

Plate 156-1H.

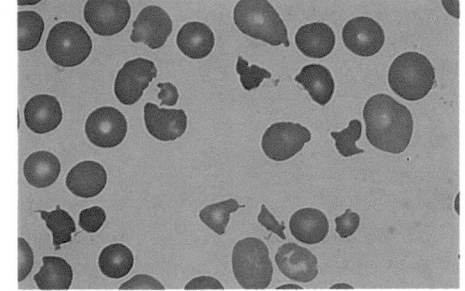

Plate 156-1I.

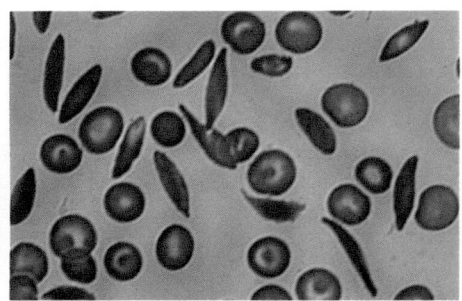

Plate 156-1J.

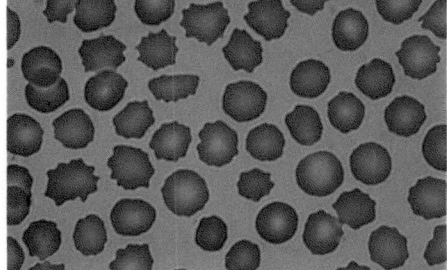

Plate 156-1K.

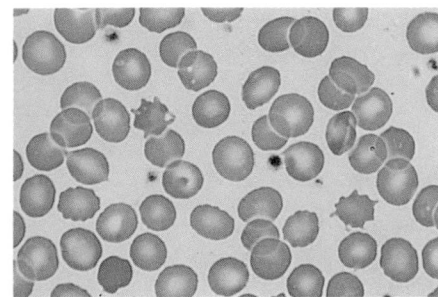

Plate 156-1L.

Plate 156-1 *(Continued).* **(E)** Stomatocytes. **(F)** Codocytes (target). **(G)** Keratocytes (helmet or bitten). **(H)** Dacrocytes (teardrops). **(I)** Schistocytes (fragments). **(J)** Drepanocytes (sickle). **(K)** Echinocytes (crenated or spiculated). **(L)** Acanthocytes (burr, spur, pyknocyte, or spiculated cell).

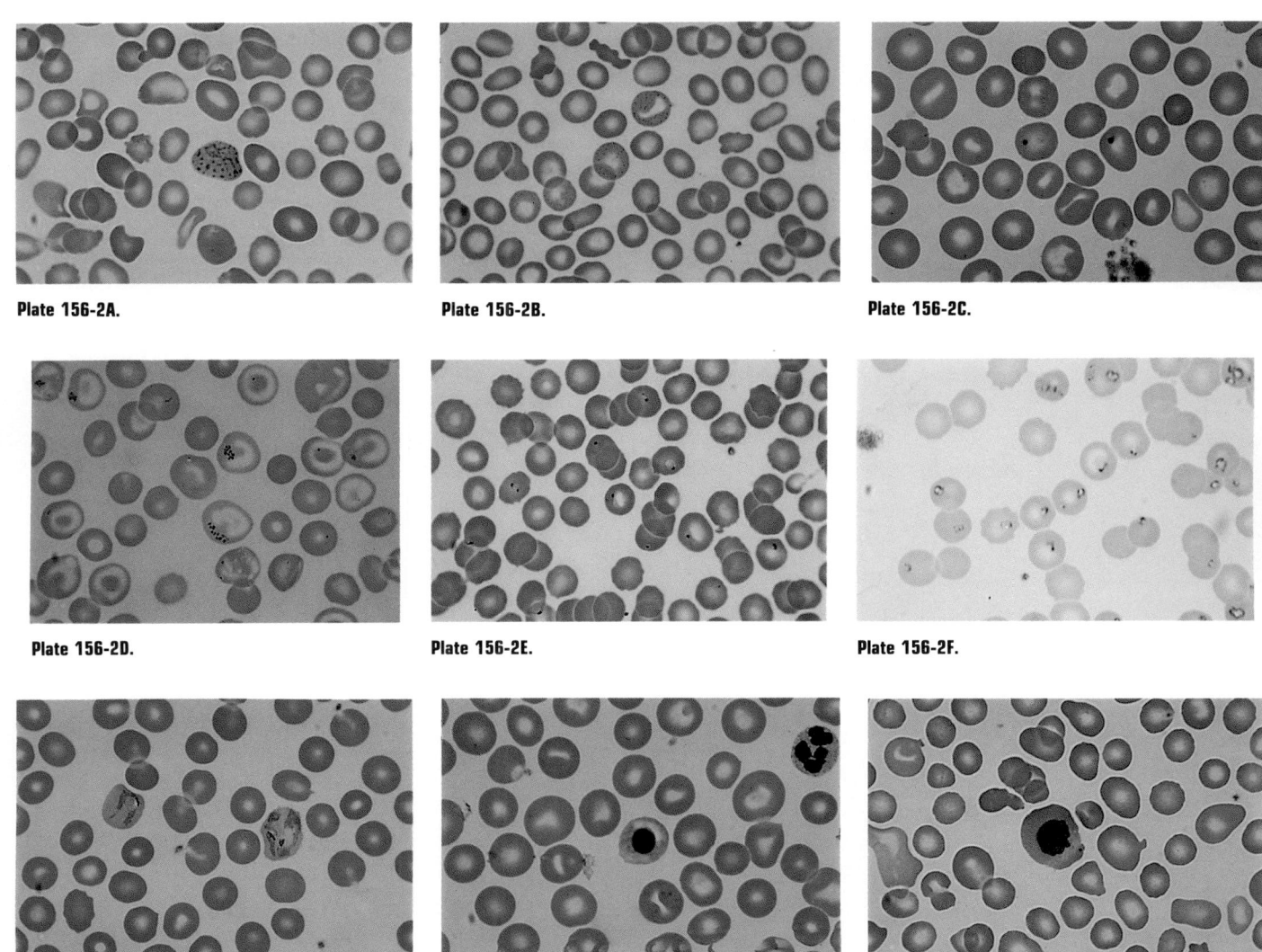

Plate 156-2A.

Plate 156-2B.

Plate 156-2C.

Plate 156-2D.

Plate 156-2E.

Plate 156-2F.

Plate 156-2G.

Plate 156-2H.

Plate 156-2I.

Plate 156-2. Red cell inclusions. **(A)** Coarse basophilic stippling. **(B)** Fine basophilic stippling. **(C)** Howell Jolly body. **(D)** Siderotic granules. **(E)** Falciparum malaria ring forms. **(F)** Babesia parasites. **(G)** Vivax malaria gametes. **(H)** Erythroblast, late form. **(I)** Megaloblast, late form.

Plate 156-3A.

Plate 156-3B.

Plate 156-3C.

Plate 156-4A.

Plate 156-4B.

Plate 156-4C.

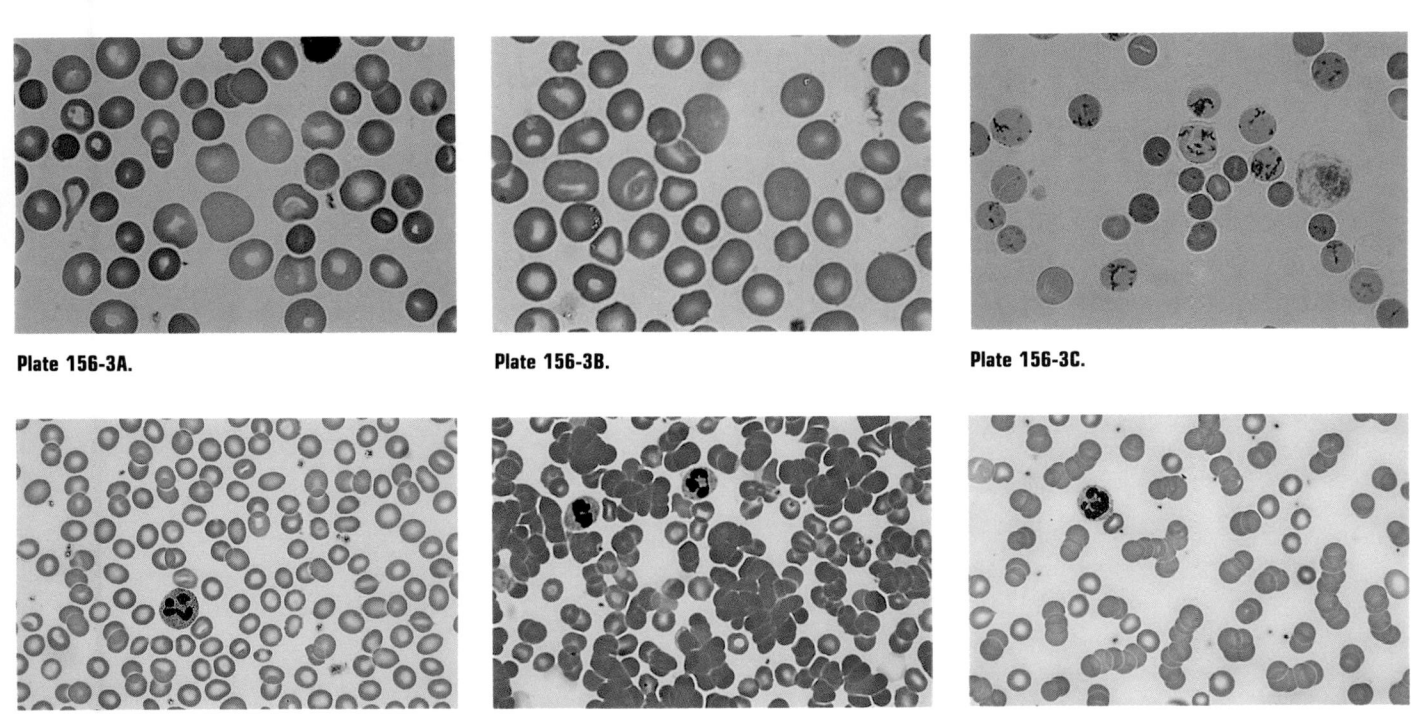

Plate 156-3. Polychromatophilic RBCs and reticulocytes. **(A)** Polychromatophilic RBCs (Wright stain). **(B)** Bone marrow reticulocytes (shift or stress reticulocytes, Wright stain). **(C)** Reticulocytes (new methylene blue stain).

Plate 156-4. Red cell distribution. **(A)** Normal red cell distribution. **(B)** RBC agglutination. **(C)** Rouleaux formation.

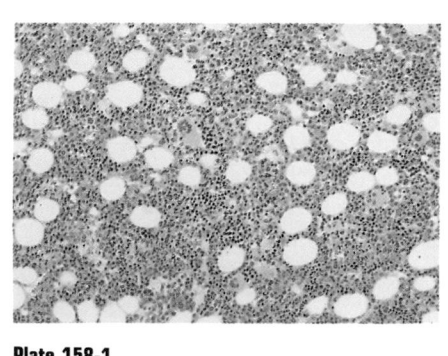

Plate 158-1.

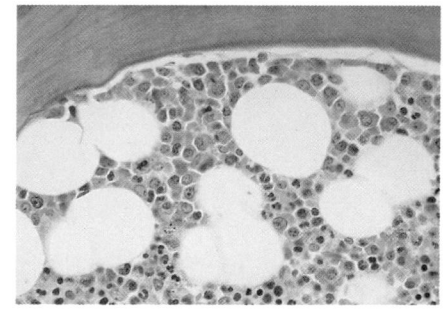

Plate 158-2.

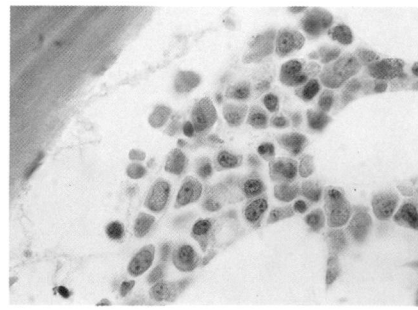

Plate 158-3.

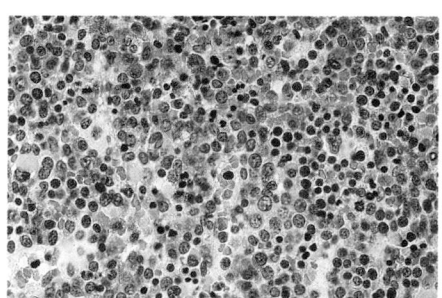

Plate 158-4.

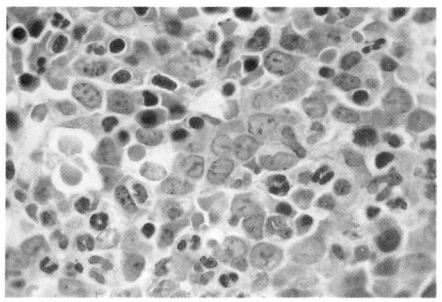

Plate 158-5.

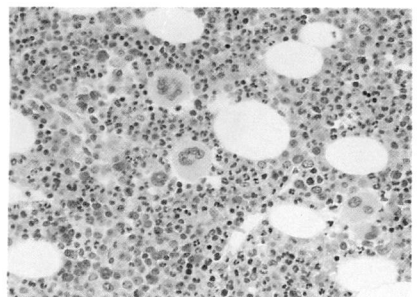

Plate 158-6.

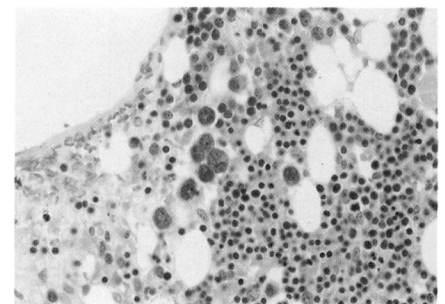

Plate 158-7.

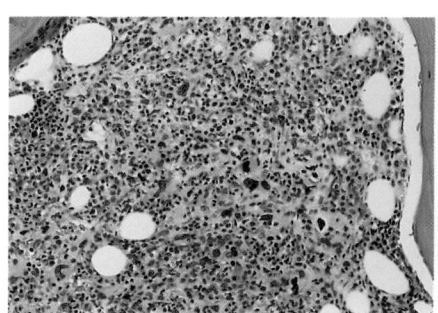

Plate 158-8.

Plate 158-1. Clusters of red cell precursors (dark, round nuclei) are evident in this bone marrow biopsy, even at low magnification. M/E ratio is 2:1 to 3:1; cellularity is 60–70%. (H&E × 40.)

Plate 158-2. Immature myelocytic precursors next to the bone. (H&E × 200.)

Plate 158-3. Cytologic detail of immature myelocytic precursors in a bone marrow biopsy. (H&E × 400.)

Plate 158-4. Mature and immature erythrocytic elements. Normoblasts have dark, round nuclei; less mature precursors have delicate chromatin, tiny nucleoli, and distinct nuclear membranes. (H&E × 200.)

Plate 158-5. Megaloblastic anemia. Marked left shift in erythrocytic maturation and erythrocytic hyperplasia may resemble acute leukemia. (H&E × 400.)

Plate 158-6. Mature megakaryocytes in a normal bone marrow biopsy. (H&E × 100.)

Plate 158-7. Immature megakaryocytes have dark, hypolobated nuclei and are smaller than the mature elements. (H&E × 200.)

Plate 158-8. Clusters of dark-staining abnormal megakaryocytes in a biopsy specimen from a patient with a myeloproliferative disorder. (H&E × 100.)

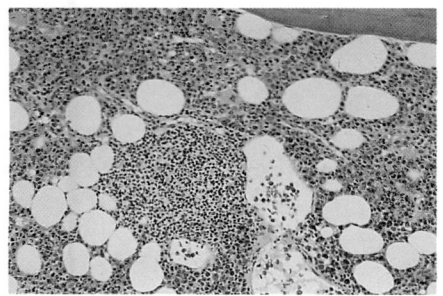

Plate 158-9.

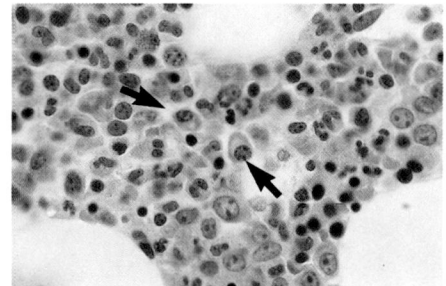

Plate 158-10.

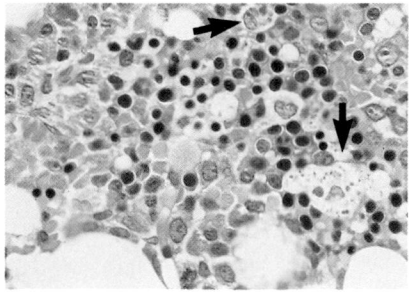

Plate 158-11.

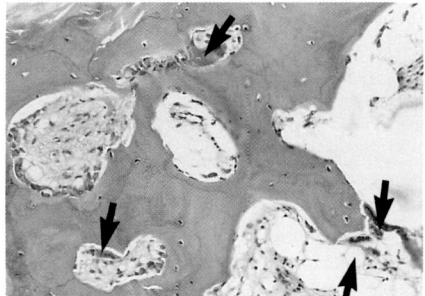

Plate 158-12.

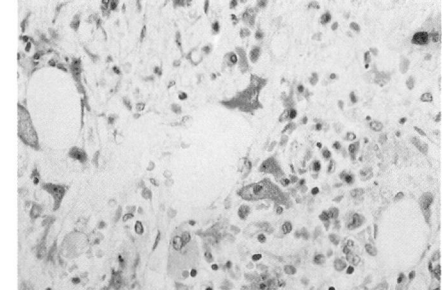

Plate 158-13.

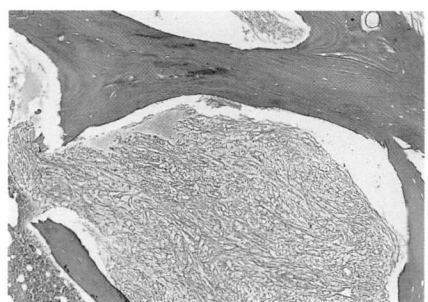

Plate 158-14.

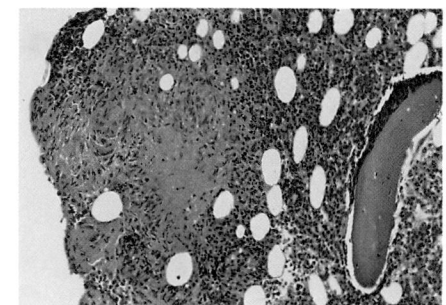

Plate 158-15.

Plate 158-9. Lymphoid aggregate in a bone marrow biopsy. (H&E × 100.)

Plate 158-10. Plasma cells (arrows) have eccentric nuclei, paranuclear clear zones, and "clockface" chromatin. (H&E × 400.)

Plate 158-11. Macrophages (arrows) containing cellular debris and brown hemosiderin pigment. (H&E × 400.)

Plate 158-12. Paget disease of bone. Plump osteoblasts line spaces within this bone, numerous osteoclastic giant cells are present (arrows), and cement lines are disordered (compare Plate 158-2) (H&E × 25.)

Plate 158-13. Macrophages containing storage iron. (Prussian blue × 200.)

Plate 158-14. Increased reticulin in a biopsy specimen from a patient with "myelofibrosis." (Reticulin × 40.)

Plate 158-15. Granuloma in a bone marrow biopsy. (H&E × 25.)

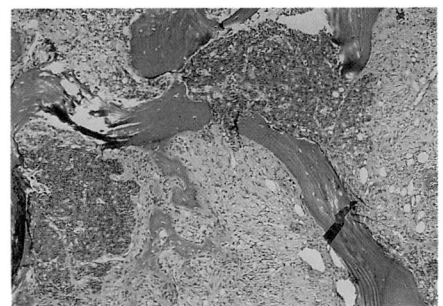

Plate 158-16.

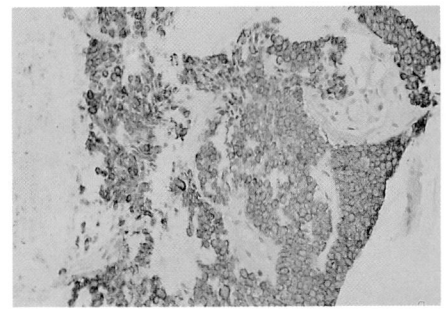

Plate 158-17.

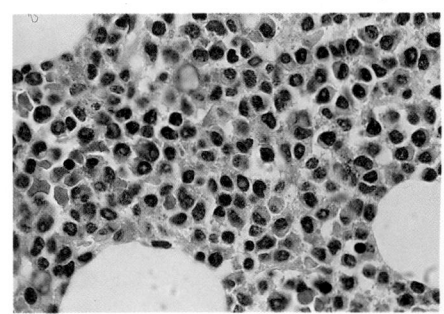

Plate 158-18.

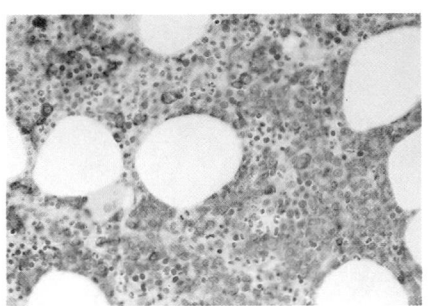

Plate 158-19.

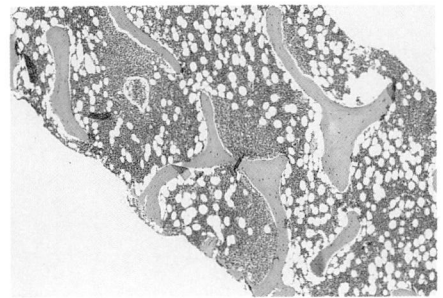

Plate 158-20.

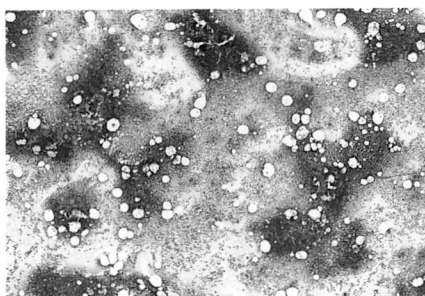

Plate 158-21.

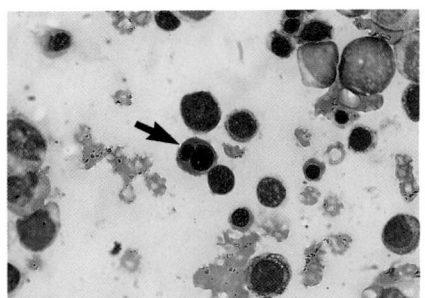

Plate 158-22.

Plate 158-16. Metastatic carcinoma in a bone marrow biopsy. Note the fibrotic (pink-staining) reaction to it. (H&E × 25.)

Plate 158-17. Metastatic carcinoma in a bone marrow biopsy specimen stained for cytokeratins. (Immunoperoxidase × 25.)

Plate 158-18. Multiple myeloma. Some of the plasma cells exhibit prominent red nucleoli. (H&E × 400.)

Plate 158-19. Multiple myeloma stained with an antibody to κ immunoglobulin light chain shows numerous positive cells. A stain for λ light chain was negative. (Immunoperoxidase × 200.)

Plate 158-20. Low grade non-Hodgkin lymphoma in a bone marrow biopsy exhibits a paratrabecular pattern. (H&E × 25.)

Plate 158-21. Bone marrow aspirate smear showing numerous particles. (Wright-Giemsa × 40.)

Plate 158-22. Binucleated red cell precursor (arrow) in an aspirate smear shows dyssynchronous maturation. Myelodysplastic syndrome. (Wright-Giemsa × 1,000.)

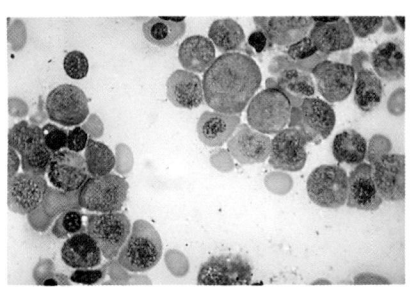

Plate 158-23.

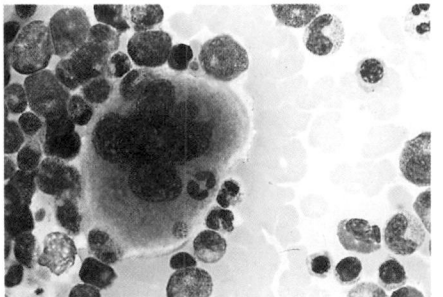

Plate 158-24.

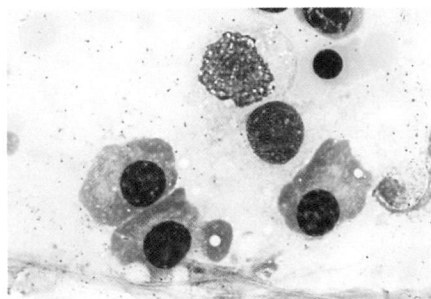

Plate 158-25.

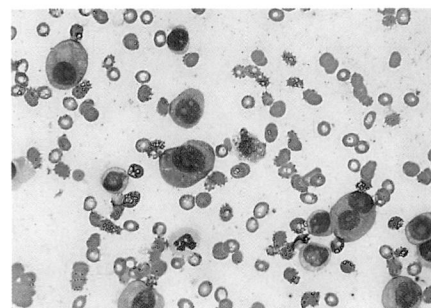

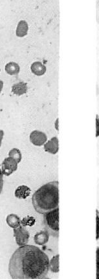

Plate 158-26.

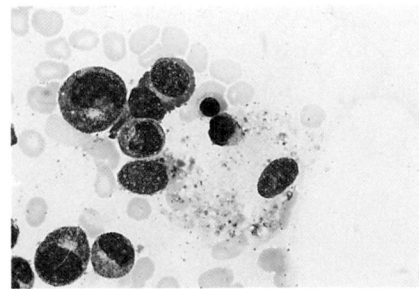

Plate 158-27.

Plate 158-23. Megaloblastic maturation, aspirate smear. These red cell precursors exhibit a moderate degree of nuclear/cytoplasmic dyssynchrony (nuclei are larger and have less condensed chromatin than is typical for this degree of cytoplasmic development). (Wright-Giemsa × 1,000.)

Plate 158-24. Megakaryocyte in an aspirate smear with an intact neutrophil in its cytoplasm (emperipolesis). (Wright-Giemsa × 1,000.)

Plate 158-25. Plasma cells in an aspirate smear. (Wright-Giemsa × 1,000.)

Plate 158-26. Multiple myeloma, bone marrow aspirate smear. Note the central nuclei and prominent nucleoli in some of the cells. (Wright-Giemsa × 1,000.)

Plate 158-27. Macrophage in an aspirate smear containing cytoplasmic debris and a degenerated cell. (Wright-Giemsa × 1,000.)

lin or TCR-β gene rearrangements. Instead, in Southern blots, they detected a markedly diminished *Eco*RI 12.0-kb band, which is characteristic of polyclonal T-cell populations.[132] Polyclonal T cells have also been found in some skin lesions of lymphomatoid papulosis, which contain RS-like cells and may closely resemble HD.[133]

Cytokines

It has been hypothesized that the different histologic types of HD, and perhaps systemic symptoms, are a consequence of cytokines secreted by the malignant RS cells.[45] IL-1 and colony-stimulating factor-granulocyte have been demonstrated in culture supernates of HD cell lines.[134,135] Eosinophilia may occur in response to IL-5 secreted by RS cells.[136] Nodular sclerosis may be explained by the stimulation of collagen synthesis by transforming growth factor-β secreted by RS cells,[137,138] and/or by eosinophils.[139] IL-6, which stimulates growth of B cells and plasma cells, was found in cell cultures and tissue sections of HD but did not correlate with the intensity or number of RS cells stained or degree of plasma cell infiltration.[140] IL-9, which stimulates T cell proliferation, appears to be uniquely associated with RS cells and tumor cells in CD30+ ALCL.[141] Kretschmer et al.[142] demonstrated synthesis of both TNF-α and TNF-β (lymphotoxin) by HD cell lines, and TNF-α protein and mRNA directly in HD tissue specimens. Sappino et al.[143] demonstrated high levels of lymphotoxin mRNA in Northern blots of tissue extracts from lymphocyte predominance HD. TNF-α and lymphotoxin have a broad range of biologic activities, which include neutrophil and eosinophil recruitment[144] macrophage activation,[145] stimulation of fibroblast growth,[146] and endothelial cell/leukocyte interactions,[147] each of which can contribute to the pathologic features and symptoms of HD. IFN-γ mRNA and protein are produced by the HD cell line SUP-HD1 derived from a patient with nodular sclerosing HD.[148] IFN-γ causes fever and chills, which are symptoms of HD. IFN-γ also induces lymphocyte proliferation, activation of phagocytes, recruitment of monocytes and T lymphocytes, and formation of multinucleated giant cells, which may account for some histologic features of HD.[149]

The cytokine hypothesis does not appear to provide an adequate explanation of the influence of environmental factors and patient age on the relative frequency of the different types of HD. For example, lymphocyte predominance and nodular sclerosis are more common in children from developed countries, whereas the less favorable mixed cellularity and lymphocyte depletion types are relatively more common among older patients and among children from underdeveloped countries.[150–152] These observations suggest that nutrition and host immune factors may also contribute significantly to the histopathology of HD.

Epstein-Barr Virus

EBV genomes have recently been demonstrated in RS cells in approximately one-half of HD cases.[153–156] Using a combined approach of slot blot, Southern blot, and in situ hybridization, Weis et al.[153,154] and Anagnostopoulos et al.[155] have demonstrated monclonality of EBV infected cells and localization of EBV nucleic acid to RS cells and their variants. EBV nuclear antigen had previously been demonstrated by immunoperoxidase staining of RS cells in a single case of mixed cellularity HD following a chronic EBV infection.[156] EBV appears to be associated particularly with mixed cellularity histology, less often with nodular sclerosis, and only occasionally with cases of lymphocyte predominance.[157] EBV is associated mainly with HD in children and older patients, and only rarely with HD in young adults.[158,159] These observations are consistent with the hypothesis proposed originally by MacMahon[74] that HD is a heterogeneous disorder comprising at least three subgroups with different etiologies.

RS cells commonly express the EBV gene product, latent membrane protein (LMP),[160] which can confer a growth advantage on these cells.[161] LMP up-regulates expression of bcl-2, which prevents cell death and thereby could help to maintain the viability of HD/RS cells.[162] At the same time, LMP is recognized by cytotoxic T cells, which may limit the growth of EBV infected cells.[163] A defect in T-cell immunosurveillance may contribute to the increased frequency of advanced HD in patients with AIDS.[40] Moreover, since there is some evidence for a genetic defect in immunity,[164] HD could result from the inability of certain immunodeficient individuals to control an EBV infection that in others of normal immunocompetence would go unnoticed or produce only a benign syndrome of infectious mononucleosis.

The finding of EBV in HD does not help identify conclusively the nature of the RS cell. Although EBV commonly infects B cells through the C3d receptor, the range of host cell types infected by EBV has been expanded to include T lymphocytes and epithelial and endothelial cells.[165] A T-cell phenotype was demonstrated in one of the HD cases in which Anagnostopolous et al.[156] detected EBV. EBV also has been detected in NHL, not only in Burkitt lymphomas and B-cell lymphomas of patients with immunodeficiency, but more recently in lymphomas with an activated helper T-cell phenotype.[166] EBV was noted with surprisingly high frequency in PTCL both in Europe[167] and Taiwan.[168] High titers of EBV antibodies have also been reported in children suffering from sinus histiocytosis with massive lymphadenopathy, a disorder of tissue histiocytes.[169,170]

CYTOGENETICS

Chromosome analyses of fresh HD tissue have usually revealed two populations of cells, one having a diploid modal chromosome number that is thought to represent the nonmalignant small lymphocyte population, and the other having a pseudodiploid or often hypotetraploid number that appears to represent the malignant cells. Seif and Spriggs[171] were the first to demonstrate marker chromosomes as evidence of a clone of malignant aneuploid cells in HD. Subsequent studies confirm that HD cells are usually aneuploid and frequently clonally related.[172] Cytogenetic markers are consistent with a lymphocytic origin of HD.[173] The most common breakpoints found by Cabanillas et al.[173–176] were at 11q23, 14q32, 6q11–q21, and 8q22–q24, which are also common breakpoints in B- and T-cell lymphomas. Moreover, the 11q23 breakpoint is also seen in a type of childhood B-cell acute lymphocytic leukemia characterized by the presence of aberrant myeloid and monocytic antigens,[174] a possible similarity to HD. Tilly et al.[175] found that some of the chromosome regions involved in HD are shared with NHL of either B-cell (e.g., 14q32, 8q24, 6q, and 11q21-q23) or T-cell origin (e.g., 4q28, 7q31-q35, 3q27) and demonstrated that significant differences occurred more often between HD and diffuse B-cell NHL than between HD and T-cell NHL. Schouten et al.[170] found recurrent breakpoints at 4q32-q34, 6q24, 12q13, 12q23-q24 and 13p11-q13: three patients had two or more clones, and one had subclones. In HD cell lines, Fonatsch et al.[177] found nonrandom marker chromosome abnormalities that are frequently associated with proto-oncogenes and other genes. Among the frequently involved sites are 1p21-p22, associated with N-*ras*, B-*lym*, and L-*myc*; 7q11.2-q36, associated with *met* and TCR-β chain gene; 11q21-q23, associated with c-*ets*1, CD3γ, δ, and ε chains; 14q32, associated with immunoglobulin heavy-chain gene; 15p12, associated with the nucleolus organizing region; and 21q21-q22, associated with c-*ets*2.

Rearrangement of *bcl*-2 can occur as a result of translocations involving chromosomes 14 and 18.[178] Rearrangements of the *bcl*-2 gene have been detected in ≤40% of HD cases and it has been suggested that these rearrangements may be involved in the pathogenesis of HD.[179] To determine whether the presence of translocations between chromosomes 14 and 18 explain the observed *bcl*-2 rearrangements in HD, Poppema et al.[180] performed cytogenetics and *bcl*-2 gene rearrangement analyses on biopsy specimens from 28 consecutive untreated patients with HD. Although 11 patients had chromosome abnormalities in the chromosome 14q region, and 6 of these had involvement of the 14q32 region that comprises the gene encoding for immunoglobulin heavy chain, only 1 patient had a t(14;18) translocation, whereas almost 40% of these 28 patients showed *bcl*-2 rearrangements by a PCR method. Thus, although most cases of HD contain a clonal population with an abnormal karyotype, comprising RS cells, and the 14q32 region is frequently involved, a t(14;18) is extremely infrequent in HD.

ASSOCIATION OF HODGKIN DISEASE WITH NON-HODGKIN LYMPHOMAS

HD can follow, coexist with, or precede a variety of lymphocytic malignancies.[181-184] This interrelationship has stimulated the hypothesis that both HD and NHL can be derived from a common stem cell. Validation of this hypothesis would support a lymphoid origin for RS cells. Among the lymphocytic malignancies repeatedly associated with HD are chronic lymphocytic leukemia, follicular lymphoma, diffuse large cell or immunoblastic lymphoma, and mycosis fungoides. The most common association between HD and NHL is that of nodular LPHD and large cell lymphoma. Meittenen et al.[22] described 5 cases of diffuse large cell lymphoma in 51 patients, occurring 4–11 years after the diagnosis of non-LPHD. Sundeen et al.[182] described 7 cases of localized large cell lymphoma that was coexistent with nodular non-LPHD. Momose et al.[183] described 13 cases of chronic lymphocytic leukemia/small lymphocytic lymphoma in which RS cells were present. The RS cells in 12 of 13 cases contained EBV RNA, but the surrounding neoplastic lymphocytes were negative for EBV RNA. In each of these cases the NHL was of B-cell phenotype. More than 20 cases of HD associated with mycosis fungoides, a T-cell malignancy, have been reported. In one such case, molecular genetic and immunophenotypic studies indicated that the RS cells and mycosis fungoides cells were derived from a common T-cell clone.[184] Together, these studies of HD and NHL in the same individual support the hypothesis that the RS cell of HD is often has a lymphocytic origin.

SUMMARY

HD has clearly been shown to be a malignant disorder in which the proportion of RS cells and their variants in affected tissues correspond to the clinical grade of malignancy. RS cells have a distinctive immunologic profile, which is characteristic of activated lymphocytes. A T-lymphocyte origin is suggested for some cases of nodular sclerosis and mixed cellularity HD. A B-lymphocyte origin is likely for some cases of nodular sclerosis and mixed cellularity types and for all the RS-cell variants in nodular lymphocyte predominance, which in many cases seems to arise in progressively transformed germinal centers. The diffuse lymphocyte predominance type is histogenetically and clinically more closely related to mixed cellularity and nodular sclerosis than to the nodular lymphocyte predominance type. Many cases formerly classified as lymphocyte depletion

HD actually represent variants of peripheral T-cell lymphoma or lymphocyte-depleted nodular sclerosis HD. True cases of lymphocyte depletion are rare and have a poor prognosis.

HD can be distinguished immunophenotypically from morphologically similar peripheral T-cell lymphomas, mediastinal B-cell lymphoma with sclerosis, CD30+ ALCLs, and T-cell-rich B-cell lymphomas, which have a different natural history and prognosis. Recent evidence implicates EBV in the pathogenesis of HD, especially mixed cellularity subtype, pediatric and older patients. EBV transformation could confer a growth advantage on HD/RS cells, whereas inadequate recognition of EBV antigens in genetically predisposed individuals or patients with acquired immunodeficiency could contribute to the development and progression of HD. Recurrent chromosomal abnormalities and frequent associations of HD with NHL are both consistent with a lymphocytic origin for the malignant cell in HD.

REFERENCES

1. Lukes RJ, Butler JJ, Hicks EB: Natural history of Hodgkin's disease as related to its pathologic picture. Cancer 19:317, 1966
2. Lukes RJ, Craver LF, Hall TC et al: Report of the nomenclature committee. Part 1. Cancer Res 26:1311, 1966
3. Wright DH: Hodgkin's disease: anything new? Recent Results Cancer Res 117:3, 1989
4. Mauch PM, Kalish LA, Kadin ME et al: Patterns of presentation of Hodgkin's disease. Implications for etiology and pathogenesis. Cancer 71:2062, 1993
5. Kadin ME, Glatstein E, Dorfman RF: Clinicopathologic studies of 117 untreated patients subjected to laparotomy for the staging of Hodgkin's disease. Cancer 27:1277, 1971
6. Colby TV, Hoppe RT, Warnke RA: Hodgkin's disease: a clinicopathologic study of 659 cases. Cancer 49:1948, 1981
7. Lukes RJ: Criteria for involvement of lymph node, bone marrow, spleen and liver in Hodgkin's disease. Cancer Res 31:1755, 1971
8. Strum SB, Rappaport H: Interrelations of the histologic types of Hodgkin's disease. Arch Pathol 10:470, 1971
9. Dorfman RF: The enigma of Hodgkin's disease: current concepts based on morphologic, clinical and immunologic observations. p. 167. In Hanaoka M, Kadin ME, Watanabe S et al (eds): Lymphoid Malignancy: Immunology and Cytogenetics. Field & Wood, Philadelphia, 1989
10. Strickler JG, Michie SA, Warnke RA, Dorfman RF: The "syncytial variant" of nodular sclerosing Hodgkin's disease. Am J Surg Pathol 10:470, 1986
11. Haybittle JL, Hayhoe FGJ, Easterling MJ et al: Review of British National Lymphoma Investigation studies of Hodgkin's disease and development of a prognostic index. Lancet 1:967, 1985
12. Wijlhuizen TJ, Vrints LW, Jairam R et al: Grades of nodular sclerosis (NSI-NSII) in Hodgkin's disease. Are they of independent prognostic value? Cancer 63:1150, 1989
13. Ferry JA, Linggood RM, Convery KM et al: Hodgkin disease, nodular sclerosis type. Implications of histologic subclassification. Cancer 71:457, 1993
14. Geogii A, Fischer R, Hubner K et al: Classification of Hodgkin's disease biopsies by a panel of four histopathologists. Report of 1,140 patients from the German national trial. Leukemia Lymphoma 9:365, 1993
15. Berard CW, Thomas LB, Axtell LM et al: The relationship of histopathologic subtype to clinical stage of Hodgkin's disease at diagnosis. Cancer Res 31:1776, 1971
16. Poppema S, Kaiserling E, Lennert K: Nodular paragranuloma with lymphocyte predominance nodular type (nodular paragranuloma) and progressively transformed germinal centers—a cytohistological study. Histopathology 3:295, 1979
17. Poppema S, Kaiserling E, Lennert K: Nodular paragranuloma and progressively transformed germinal centers. Virchows Arch B Cell Pathol 31:211, 1979
18. Burns BF, Colby TV, Dorfman RF: Differential diagnostic features of nodular L&H Hodgkin's disease, including progressively transformed germinal centers. Am J Surg Pathol 8:725, 1984
19. Osborne BM, Butler JJ: Clinical implications of progressive transformation of germinal centers. Am J Surg Pathol 8:725, 1984
20. Regula DP Jr, Hoppe RT, Weiss LM: Nodular and diffuse types of lymphocyte predominance Hodgkin' disease. N Engl J Med 318:214, 1988
21. Trudel MA, Krikorian JG, Neiman RS: Lymphocyte predominance Hodgkin's disease: a clinicopathologic reassessment. Cancer 59:99, 1987
22. Miettenen M, Fransilla KO, Saxen E: Hodgkin's disease lymphocyte predomi-

nance nodular. Increased risk for subsequent non-Hodgkin's lymphomas. Cancer 51:2293, 1983

23. Hansmann ML, Stein H, Fellbaum C et al: Nodular paragranuloma can transform into high-grade malignant lymphoma of B type. Hum Pathol 20:1169, 1989

24. Sundeen JT, Cossman J, Jaffe ES: Lymphocyte predominant Hodgkin's disease nodular subtype with coexistent "large cell lymphoma." Histological progression or composite malignancy? Am J Surg Pathol 12:599, 1988

25. Neiman RS, Rosen PJ, Lukes RJ: Lymphocyte depletion Hodgkin's disease. A clinicopathologic entity. N Engl J Med 288:751, 1973

26. Bearman RM, Pangalis GA, Rappaport H: Hodgkin's disease, lymphocyte depletion type: a clinicopathologic study of 39 patients. Cancer 41:293, 1978

27. Greer JP, Kinney MC, Cousar JB et al: Lymphocyte depleted Hodgkin's disease. Clinicopathologic review of 25 patients. Am J Med 81:208, 1986

28. Kant JA, Hubbard SM, Longo DL et al: The pathologic and clinical heterogeneity of lymphocyte depleted Hodgkin's disease. J Clin Oncol 4:284, 1986

29. Aisenberg AC, Qazi R: Abdominal involvement at the onset of Hodgkin's disease. Am J Med 57:870, 1974

30. Lukes RJ, Tindle BH, Parker JW: Reed-Sternberg-like cells in infectious mononucleosis. Lancet 2:1003, 1969

31. Strum SB, Rappaport H: Observation of cells resembling Reed-Sternberg cells in conditions other than Hodgkin's disease. Cancer 26:176, 1970

32. Coppleson LW, Factor RM, Strum SB et al: Observer disagreement in the classification and histology of Hodgkin's disease. J Natl Cancer Inst 45:731, 1970

33. Miller TP, Byrne GE, Jones SE: Mistaken clinical and pathologic diagnoses of Hodgkin's disease; a Southwest Oncology Group study. Cancer Treat Rep 66:645, 1982

34. Glaser SL, Swartz WG: Time trends in Hodgkin's disease incidence. The role of diagnostic accuracy. Cancer 66:2196, 1990

35. Rosen PJ: Should we bother subclassifying Hodgkin's disease? J Clin Oncol 4:275, 1986

36. Dorfman RF, Colby TV: The pathologist's role in management of patients with Hodgkin's disease. Cancer Treat Rep 66:675, 1982

37. Doggett RS, Colby TV, Dorfman RF: Interfollicular Hodgkin's disease. Am J Surg Pathol 7:145, 1983

38. Hoppe RT, Roenberg SA, Kaplan HS, Cox RS: Prognostic factors in pathologic stage IIIA Hodgkin's disease. Cancer 46:1240, 1980

39. Yam LT, Li CY: Histogenesis of splenic lesions in Hodgkin's disease. Am J Clin Pathol 66:976, 1976

40. Schoeppel SA, Hoppe RT, Dorfman RF et al: Hodgkin's disease in homosexual men with generalized lymphadenopathy. Ann Intern Med 102:68, 1985

41. Bagley CM, Roth JA, Thomas LB, De Vita VT: Liver biopsy in Hodgkin's disease. Clinicopathologic correlations in 127 patients. Ann Intern Med 76:219, 1972

42. Bartl R, Frisch B, Burkhardt R et al: Assessment of bone marrow histology in Hodgkin's disease: correlation with clinical factors. Br J Haematol 51:345, 1982

43. Kadin ME, Donaldson SS, Dorfman RF: Isolated granulomas in Hodgkin's disease. N Engl J Med 283:859, 1971

44. Sacks EL, Donaldson Gordon J, Dorfman RF: Epithelioid granulomas associated with Hodgkin's disease. Cancer 41:562, 1978

45. Stein H, Mason DY, Gerdes J et al: The expression of the Hodgkin's disease associated antigen Ki-1 in reactive and neoplastic lymphoid tissue: evidence that Reed-Sternberg cells and histiocytic malignancies are derived from activated lymphoid cells. Blood 66:848, 1985

46. Falini B, Stein H, Pileri S et al: Expression of lymphoid-associated antigens on Hodgkin's and Reed-Sternberg cells of Hodgkin's disease: an immunocytochemical study on lymph node cytospins using monoclonal antibodies. Histopathology 11:1229, 1987

47. Agnarsson BA, Kadin ME: The immunophenotype of Reed-Sternberg cells. A study of 50 cases of Hodgkin's disease using fixed frozen tissues. Cancer 63:2083, 1989

48. Hsu SM, Jaffe ES: Leu-M1 and peanut agglutinin stain the neoplastic cells of Hodgkin's disease. Am J Clin Pathol 82:29, 1984

49. Ree HJ, Kadin ME: Macrophage-histiocytes in Hodgkin's disease. The relation of peanut-agglutinin-binding macrophage-histiocytes to clinicopathologic presentation and course of disease. Cancer 56:333, 1985

50. Stein H, Uchanska-Ziegler B, Gerdes J et al: Hodgkin and Sternberg-Reed cells contain antigens specific to late cells of granulopoiesis. Int J Cancer 29:283, 1982

51. Dorfman RF, Gatter KC, Pulford KAF, Mason DY: An evaluation of the utility of anti-granulocyte and anti-leukocyte monoclonal antibodies in the diagnosis of Hodgkin's disease. Am J Pathol 123:508, 1986

52. Chittal SM, Caveriviere P, Schwarting R et al: Monoclonal antibodies in the

53. Sherrod AE, Felder B, Levy N et al: Immunohistologic identification of phenotypic antigens associated with Hodgkin and Reed-Sternberg cells. A paraffin section study. Cancer 57:2135, 1986

54. Taylor CR: An immunohistological study of follicular lymphoma, reticulum cell sarcoma and Hodgkin's disease. Eur J Cancer Clin Oncol 12:61, 1976

55. Landaas TO, Godal T, Halvorsen TB: Characterization of immunoglobulins in Hodgkin cells. Int J Cancer 20:717, 1977

56. Schmid C, Sargent C, Isaacson PG: L and H cells of nodular lymphocyte predominance Hodgkin's disease show immunoglobulin light-chain restriction. Am J Pathol 139:1281, 1991

57. Dallenbach FE, Stein H: Expression of T-cell receptor B chain in Reed-Sternberg cells. Lancet 2:828, 1989

58. Casey TT, Olson SJ, Cousar JB, Collins RD: Immunophenotype of Reed-Sternberg cells: a study of 19 cases of Hodgkin's disease in plastic-embedded sections. Blood 74:2624, 1989

59. Pinkus GS, Said JW: Hodgkin's disease, lymphocyte predominance type, nodular—further evidence for a B cell derivation. L&H variants of Reed-Sternberg cells express L26, a pan B cell marker. Am J Pathol 133:211, 1988

60. Schmid C, Pan L, Diss T, Isaacson PG: Expression of B-cell antigens by Hodgkin's and Reed-Sternberg cells. Am J Pathol 139:701, 1991

61. Imam A, Stathopoulos E, Holland SL et al: Characterization of a cell surface molecule expressed on B-lymphocytes and Hodgkin's cells. Cancer Res 50:1650, 1990

62. Nozawa Y, Wachi E, Tominaga K et al: A novel monoclonal antibody (Fun-1) identifies an activation antigen in cells of the B-cell lineage and Reed-Sternberg cells. J Pathol 169:309, 1993

63. Schwarting R, Gerdes J, Durkop H et al: Ber-H2: a new anti-Ki-1 (CD30) monoclonal antibody directed against a formol-resistant epitope. Blood 74:1678, 1989

64. Ree HJ, Teplitz C, Khan A: The Lewis X antigen. A new paraffin section marker for Reed-Sternberg cells. Cancer 67:138, 1991

65. Sarker AB, Akagi T, Jeon HJ et al: Bauhinia purpurea—a new paraffin section marker for Reed-Sternberg cells of Hodgkin's disease. A comparison with Leu-M1 (CD15), LN2 (CD74), peanut agglutinin, and Ber-H2 (CD30). Am J Pathol 141:19, 1992

66. Chu W-S, Abbondanzo SL, Frizzera G: Inconsistency of the immunophenotype of Reed-Sternberg cells in simultaneous and consecutive specimens from the same patients. A paraffin section evaluation in 56 patients. Am J Pathol 141:11, 1992

67. Kadin ME, Sako D, Berliner N et al: Childhood Ki-1 lymphoma presenting with skin lesions and peripheral lymphadenopathy. Blood 68:1042, 1986

68. Agnarsson BA, Kadin ME: Ki-1 positive large cell lymphoma. A morphologic and immunologic study of 19 cases. Am J Surg Pathol 12:264, 1988

69. Waldron JA, Leech JH, Click AD et al: Malignant lymphoma of peripheral T-lymphocyte origin. Immunologic, pathologic, and clinical features in six patients. Cancer 40:1604, 1977

70. Addis BJ, Isaacson PG: Large cell lymphoma of mediastinum: a B-cell tumour of probable thymic origin. Histopathology 10:379, 1986

71. Jacobson JO, Aisenberg AC, Lamarre L et al: Mediastinal large cell lymphoma. An uncommon subset of adult lymphoma curable with combined modality therapy. Cancer 62:1893, 1988

72. Chittal SM, Brousset P, Voight J-J, Delsol G: Large B-cell lymphoma rich in T-cells and simulating Hodgkin's disease. Histopathology 19:211, 1991

73. Greer JP, Kinney MC, Collins RD et al: Clinical features of 31 patients with Ki-1 anaplastic large-cell lymphoma. J Clin Oncol 9:539, 1991

74. MacMahon B: Epidemiology of Hodgkin's disease. Cancer Res 26:1189, 1966

75. Shulman LN, Frisard B, Antin JH et al: Primary Ki-1 anaplastic large-cell lymphoma in adults: clinical characteristics and therapeutic outcome. J Clin Oncol 11:937, 1993

76. Kaudewitz P, Stein H, Dallenbach F et al: Primary and secondary cutaneous Ki-1+ (CD30+) anaplastic large cell lymphomas. Morphologic, immunohistologic, and clinical characteristics. Am J Pathol 135:359, 1989

77. Delsol G, Blancher A, Al Saati T et al: Antibody BNH9 detects red blood cell related antigens on anaplastic large cell (CD30+) lymphomas. Br J Cancer 64:321, 1991

78. Patsouris E, Noel H, Lennert K: Cytohistologic and immunohistochemical findings in Hodgkin's disease, mixed cellularity type, with a high content of epithelioid cells. Am J Surg Pathol 13:1014, 1988

79. Tosi P, Leoncini L, Del Vecchio MT et al: Phenotypic overlaps between pleomorphic malignant T-cell lymphomas and mixed-cellularity Hodgkin's disease. Int J Cancer 52:202, 1992

80. Wagner D, Kiwanuka J, Edwards BK et al: Soluble interleukin-2 receptor levels in patients with undifferentiated and lymphoblastic lymphomas: correlation with survival. J Clin Oncol 5:1262, 1987

81. Pizzolo G, Chilosi M, Vinate F et al: Soluble interleukin-2 receptors in the serum of patients with Hodgkin's disease. Br J Cancer 55:427, 1987

82. Gause A, Jung W, Schmits R et al: Soluble CD8, CD25 and CD30 antigens as prognostic markers in patients with untreated Hodgkin's lymphoma. Ann Oncol, suppl 4. 3:S49, 1992

83. Pui CH, Ip SH, Thompson E et al: Increased serum CD8 antigen in childhood Hodgkin's disease relates to advanced stage and poor treatment outcome. Blood 73:209, 1989

84. Pizzolo G, Vinante F, Chilosi M et al: Serum levels of soluble CD30 molecule (Ki-1 antigen) in Hodgkin's disease: relationship with disease activity. Br J Haematol 75:282, 1990

85. Peckham MJ, Cooper EH: Proliferative characteristics of the various classes of cells in Hodgkin's disease. Cancer 24:135, 1969

86. Hsu SM, Zhao X, Chakroborty S et al: Reed-Sternberg cells in Hodgkin's cell lines HDLM, L-428, and KM-H2 are not actively replicating: Lack of bromo-deoxyuridine uptake by multinuclear cells in culture. Blood 71:1382, 1988

87. Newcom SR, Kadin ME, Phillips C: L-428 Reed-Sternberg cells and mononuclear Hodgkin's cells arise from a single cloned mononuclear cell. Int J Cell Cloning 6:417, 1988

88. Schaadt M, Diehl V, Stein H et al: Two neoplastic cell lines with unique features derived from Hodgkin's disease. Int J Cancer 26:723, 1980

89. Diehl V, Kirchner HH, Burrichter H et al: Characteristics of Hodgkin's disease cell lines. Cancer Treat Rep 66:615, 1982

90. Drexler HG, Gaedicke G, Lok MS et al: Hodgkin's disease derived cell lines HDLM-2 and L-428: comparison of morphology, immunological and isoenzyme profiles. Leuk Res 10:487, 1986

91. Jones DB, Scott CS, Wright DH et al: Phenotype analysis of an established cell line derived from a patient with Hodgkin's disease (HD). Hematol Oncol 3:133, 1985

92. Kamesaki H, Fukahara S, Tatsumi E et al: Cytochemical, immunologic, chromosomal, and molecular genetic analysis of a novel cell line derived from Hodgkin's disease. Blood 68:285, 1986

93. Poppema S, De Jong B, Atmosoerodjo J et al: Morphologic, immunologic, enzymehistochemical and chromosomal analysis of a cell line derived from Hodgkin's disease. Evidence for a B-cell origin of Reed-Sternberg cells. Cancer 55:683, 1985

94. Drexler HG: Recent results on the biology of Hodgkin and Reed-Sternberg cells. II. Continuous cell lines. Leukemia Lymphoma 9:1, 1993

95. Trumper LH, Brady G, Bagg A et al: Single-cell analysis of Hodgkin and Reed-Sternberg cells: molecular heterogeneity of gene expression and p53 mutations. Blood 81:3097, 1993

96. Schwab U, Stein H, Gerdes J et al: Production of a monoclonal antibody specific for Hodgkin and Sternberg-Reed cells of Hodgkin's disease and a subset of normal lymphoid cells. Nature 299:65, 1982

97. Hecht TT, Longo DL, Cossman J et al: Production and characterization of a monoclonal antibody that binds Reed-Sternberg cells. J Immunol 134:4231, 1985

98. Pfreundschuh M, Mommertz E, Meissner M et al: Hodgkin and Reed-Sternberg cell associated monoclonal antibodies HRS-1 and HRS-2 react with activated cells of lymphoid and monocytoid origin. Anticancer Res 8:217, 1988

99. Hansen H, Lemke H, Bredfeldt G et al: The Hodgkin-associated Ki-1 antigen exists in an intracellular and a membrane-bound form. Biol Chem Hoppe Seyler 370:409, 1989

100. Rohde D, Hansen H, Hafner M et al: Cellular localizations and processing of the two molecular forms of the Hodgkin-associated Ki-1 (CD30) antigen. The protein kinase Ki-1/57 occurs in the nucleus. Am J Pathol 140:473, 1992

101. Hansen H, Bredfeldt G, Havsteen B, Lemke H: Protein kinase activity of the intracellular but not of the membrane-associated form of the Ki-1 (CD30) antigen. Res Immunol 141:13, 1990

102. Nawrocki JF, Kirsten ES, Fisher RI: Biochemical and structural properties of a Hodgkin's disease-related membrane protein. J Immunol 141:672, 1988

103. Froese P, Lemke H, Gerdes J et al: Biochemical characterization and biosynthesis of the Ki-1 antigen in Hodgkin-derived and virus-transformed human B and T lymphoid cell lines. J Immunol 139:2081, 1987

104. Josimovic-Alasevic O, Durkop H, Schwarting R et al: Ki-1 (CD30) antigen is released by Ki-1 positive tumor cells in vitro and in vivo. I. Partial characterization of soluble Ki-1 antigen and detection of the antigen in cell culture supernatants and in serum by an enzyme-linked immunosorbent assay. Eur J Immunol 19:157, 1989

105. Durkop H, Latza U, Hummel M et al: Molecular cloning and expression of a new member of the nerve growth factor receptor family that is characteristic for Hodgkin's disease. Cell 68:421, 1992

106. Fonatsch C, Latza U, Durkop H et al: Assignment of the human CD30 (Ki-1) gene to 1p36. Genomics 14:825, 1992

107. Smith CA, Gruss H-J, Davis T et al: CD30 antigen, a marker for Hodgkin's lymphoma, is a receptor whose ligand defines an emerging family of cytokines with homology to TNF. Cell 73:1349, 1993

108. Chadburn A, Inghirami G, Knowles DM: Kinetics and temporal expression of T-cell activation-associated antigens CD15 (LeuM1), CD30 (Ki-1), EMA, and CD11c (Leu M5) by benign activated T-cells. Hematol Pathol 6:193, 1992

109. Andreesen R, Bruger W, Lohr GW, Bross KJ: Human macrophages express the Hodgkin's cell-associated antigen Ki-1 (CD30). Am J Pathol 134:187, 1989

110. Stein H, Schwarting R, Dallenbach F, Dienemann D: Immunology of Hodgkin and Reed-Sternberg cells. Recent Results Cancer Res 117:14, 1989

111. Hsu SM, Hsu PL, Lo SS, Wu KK: Expression of prostaglandin H synthetase (cyclooxygenase) in Hodgkin's mononuclear and Reed-Sternberg cells. Functional resemblance between H-RS cells and histiocytes or interdigitating reticulum cells. Am J Pathol 133:5, 1988

112. Hsu SM, Zhao X: The H-RS-like cells in infectious mononucleosis are transformed interdigitating reticulum cells. Am J Pathol 127:403, 1987

113. Kadin ME: Possible origin of the Reed-Sternberg cell from an interdigitating reticulum cell. Cancer Treat Rep 66:601, 1982

114. Fisher RI, Cossman J, Diehl V, Volkman DJ: Antigen presentation by Hodgkin's disease cells. J Immunol 135:3568, 1985

115. Delsol G, Meggetto F, Brouseset P et al: Relation of follicular dendritic reticulum cells to Reed-Sternberg cells of Hodgkin's disease with emphasis on the expression of CD21 antigen. Am J Pathol 142:1729, 1993

116. Curran RC, Jones EL: Dendritic cells and B lymphocytes in Hodgkin's disease. Lancet 2:349, 1977

117. Somozuk M: IgE in Reed-Sternberg cells of Hodgkin's disease with eosinophilia. Blood 79:1518, 1992

118. Kadin ME, Maramoto L, Said JW: Expression of T-cell antigens on Reed-Sternberg cells in a subset of patients with nodular sclerosis and mixed cellularity Hodgkin's disease. Am J Pathol 130:345, 1988

119. Zukerberg LR, Collins AB, Ferry JA, Harris NL: Coexpression of CD15 and CD20 by Reed-Sternberg cells in Hodgkin's disease. Am J Pathol 139:475, 1991

120. Ruprai AK, Pringle JH, Angel CA et al: Localization of immunoglobulin light chain mRNA expression in Hodgkin's disease by in situ hybridization. J Pathol 164:37, 1991

121. Lauritzen AF, Pluzek K-J, Kristensen LE, Nielsen HW: Detection of immunoglobulin light chain mRNA in nodular sclerosing Hodgkin's disease by in situ hybridization with biotinylated oligonucleotide probes compared with immunohistochemical staining with poly- and monoconal antibodies. Histopathology 21:353, 1992

122. Momose H, Chen YY, Ben-Ezra J, Weiss LM: Nodular lymphocyte-predominant Hodgkin's disease: study of immunoglobulin light chain protein and mRNA expression. Hum Pathol 23:1115, 1992

123. Kuzu I, Delsol G, Hones M et al: Expression of the Ig-associated heterodimer (mb-1 and B29) in Hodgkin's disease. Histopathology 22:141, 1993

124. Timens W, Visser L, Poppema S: Nodular lymphocyte predominance type of Hodgkin's disease is a germinal center lymphoma. Lab Invest 54:457, 1986

125. Poppema S: The nature of the lymphocytes surrounding Reed-Sternberg cells in nodular lymphocyte predominance and in other types of Hodgkin's disease. Am J Pathol 135:351, 1989

126. Weiss LM, Strickler JG, Hu E et al: Immunoglobulin gene rearrangements in Hodgkin's disease. Hum Pathol 17:1009, 1986

127. Brinker MGL, Poppema S, Buys CHCM et al: Clonal immunoglobulin gene rearrangements in tissues involved by Hodgkin's disease. Blood 70:186, 1987

128. Sundeen J, Lipford E, Uppenkamp M et al: Rearranged antigen receptor genes in Hodgkin's disease. Blood 70:96, 1987

129. Griesser H, Feller AC, Mak T, Lennert K: Clonal rearrangements of T-cell receptor and immunoglobulin genes and immunophenotypic antigen expression in different subclasses of Hodgkin's disease. Int J Cancer 40:157, 1987

130. Griesser H, Feller AC, Lennert K et al: The structure of the T-cell gamma chain gene in lymphoproliferative disorders and lymphoma cell lines. Blood 68:592, 1986

131. O'Connor NTJ, Stein H, Gatter KC et al: Genotypic analysis of large cell lymphomas which express the Ki-1 antigen. Histopathology 11:733, 1987

132. Knowles DM, Neri A, Pellici PG et al: Immunoglobulin and T-cell receptor beta chain gene rearrangement analysis of Hodgkin's disease: implications for lineage determination and differential diagnosis. Proc Natl Acad Sci USA 83:7942, 1986

133. Kadin ME, Vonderheid EC, Sako D et al: Clonal composition of T cells in lymphomatoid papulosis. Am J Pathol 126:13, 1987

134. Kortmann C, Burrichter H, Monner D et al: Interleukin-1-like activity constitutively generated by Hodgkin derived cell lines. I. Measurement in a human lymphocyte co-stimulator assay. Immunobiology 166:318, 1984

135. Burrichter H, Heit W, Schaadt M et al: Production of colony stimulating factors by Hodgkin's disease cell lines. Int J Cancer 31:269, 1983

136. Samoszuk M, Nansen LI: Interleukin-5 mRNA detected in Reed-Sternberg cells of Hodgkin's disease with eosinophilia. Blood 75:13, 1990
137. Kadin ME, Agnarsson BA, Ellingsworth LR, Newcom SR: Immunohistochemical evidence of a role for transforming growth factor-beta in the pathogenesis of nodular sclerosing Hodgkin's disease. Am J Pathol 136:1209, 1990
138. Hsu S-M, Lin J, Xie S-S et al: Abundant expression of transforming growth factor-B1 and -B2 by Hodgkin's Reed-Sternberg cells and by reactive T lymphocytes in Hodgkin's disease. Hum Pathol 24:249, 1993
139. Kadin ME, Butmarc J, Elovic A, Wong D: Eosinophils are the major source of transforming growth factor-B1 in nodular sclerosing Hodgkin's disease. Am J Pathol 142:11, 1993
140. Hsu S-M, Xie S-S, Hsu P-L, Waldron JA: Interleukin-6, but not interleukin-4, is expressed by Reed-Sternberg cells in Hodgkin's disease with or without histologic features of Castleman's disease. Am J Pathol 141:129, 1992
141. Merz H, Houssiau FA, Orscheschek K et al: Interleukin-9 expression in human malignant lymphomas: unique association with Hodgkin's disease and large cell anaplastic lymphoma. Blood 78:1311, 1991
142. Kretschmer C, Homes DB, Morrison K et al: Tumor necrosis factor alpha and lymphotoxin production in Hodgkin's disease. Am J Pathol 137:341, 1990
143. Sappino A-P, Seelentag W, Pelte M-F et al: Tumor necrosis factor/cachectin and lymphtoxin gene expression in lymph nodes from lymphoma patients. Blood 75:958, 1990
144. Perussia B, Kobayashi M, Rossi ME et al: Immune interferon enhances functional properties of human granulocytes: role of Fc receptor and effect of lymphotoxin tumor necrosis factor, and granulocyte-macrophage colony stimulating factor. J Immunol 138:765, 1987
145. Chang RJ, Lee SH: Effects of interferon-gamma and tumor necrosis factor-alpha on the expression of an Ia antigen on a murine macrophage cell line. J Immunol 138:2853, 1987
146. Sugarman RJ, Aggarwal BB, Hass PE et al: Recombinant human tumor necrosis factor-alpha: effects on proliferation of normal and transformed cells in vitro. Science 230:043, 1985
147. Pober JS, Lapierre LA, Stolpen AH et al: Activation of cultured human endothelial cells by recombinant lymphotoxin: comparison with tumor necrosis factor and interleukin-1 species. J Immunol 138:3319, 1987
148. Naumovski L, Utz PJ, Bergstrom SK et al: SUP-HD1: a new Hodgkin's disease derived cell line with lymphoid features produces interferon-gamma. Blood 74:2733, 1989
149. Murray JW: Interferon-gamma, the activated macrophage, and host defense against microbial challenge. Ann Intern Med 108:595, 1988
150. Strum SB, Rappaport H: Hodgkin's disease in the first decade of life. Pediatrics 46:748, 1970
151. Azzam SA: High incidence of Hodgkin's disease in children in Lebanon. Cancer Res 26:1202, 1966
152. Burn C, Davies JNP, Dodge OG, Nias BC: Hodgkin's disease in English and African children. J Natl Cancer Inst 46:37, 1971
153. Weiss LM, Strickler JG, Warnke RA et al: Epstein-Barr DNA in tissues of Hodgkin's disease. Am J Pathol 129:86, 1987
154. Weiss LM, Movahed, Warnke RA, Sklar J: Detection of Epstein-Barr viral genomes in Reed-Sternberg cells of Hodgkin's disease. N Engl J Med 320:502, 1989
155. Anagnostopoulos I, Herbst H, Niedobitek G, Stein H: Demonstration of monoclonal EBV genomes in Hodgkin's disease and Ki-1 positive anaplastic large cell lymphoma by combined Southern blot and in situ hybridization. Blood 74:810, 1989
156. Poppema S, van Imhoff G, Torensma R, Smit J: Lymphadenopathy morphologically consistent with Hodgkin's disease associated with Epstein-Barr virus infection. Am J Clin Pathol 84:385, 1985
157. Herbst H, Pallesen G, Weiss LM et al: Hodgkin's disease and Epstein-Barr virus. Ann Oncol, suppl. 3. 3:S27, 1992
158. Jarrett RF: Viral involvement in Hodgkin's disease. Int J Cell Cloning 10:315, 1992
159. Armstrong AA, Alexander FE, Paes RP et al: Association of Epstein-Barr virus with pediatric Hodgkin's disease. Am J Pathol 142:1683, 1993
160. Pallesen G, Hamilton-Dutoit MR, Young LS: Expression of Epstein-Barr virus latent gene products in tumor cells of Hodgkin's disease. Lancet 337:320, 1991
161. Wang D, Liebowitz D, Kieff E: An EBV membrane protein expressed in immortalized lymphocytes transforms established rodent cells. Cell 43:831, 1985
162. Henderson SM, Rowe D, Croom-Carter F et al: Induction of bcl-2 expression by Epstein-Barr virus latent membrane protein protects infected B cells from programmed cell death. Cell 65:1107, 1991
163. Murray RJ, Wang D, Young LS et al: Epstein-Barr virus-specific cytotoxic T-cell recognition of transfectants expressing the virus-encoded latent membrane protein LMP. J Virol 62:3747, 1988
164. Merk K, Bjokholm M, Tullgren O et al: Immune deficiency in family members of patients with Hodgkin's disease. Cancer 66:1938, 1990
165. Raab-Traub N, Flynn K: The structure of the termini of the Epstein-Barr virus as a marker of clonal cellular proliferation. Cell 47:883, 1986
166. Jones JF, Shurin S, Abramowsky C et al: T-cell lymphomas containing Epstein-Barr viral DNA in patients with chronic Epstein-Barr virus infections. N Engl J Med 318:733, 1988
167. Hamilton-Dutoit SJ, Pallesen G: A survey of Epstein-Barr virus gene expression in sporadic non-Hodgkin's lymphomas. Detection of Epstein-Barr virus in a subset of peripheral T-cell lymphomas. Am J Pathol 140:1315, 1992
168. Su I-J, Hsieh HC, Line KH et al: Spectrum of peripheral T-cell lymphomas containing Epstein-Barr viral DNA: a clinicopathologic and molecular analysis. Blood 77:799, 1991
169. Rosai J, Dorfman RF: Sinus histiocytosis with massive lymphadeonopathy: a pseudolymphomatous benign disorder. Analysis of 34 cases. Cancer 30:1174, 1972
170. Lober M, Rawlings W. Newell GR, Reed RJ: Sinus histiocytosis with massive lymphadenopathy. Report of a case associated with elevated EBV antibody titers. Cancer 32:421. 1973
171. Seif GSF, Spriggs AI: Chromosome changes in Hodgkin's disease. J Natl Cancer Inst 39:557, 1967
172. Boecker WR, Hossfeld DK, Gallmeier WM, Schmidt CG: Clonal growth of Hodgkin cells. Nature 258:235, 1975
173. Cabanillas F, Pathak S, Trujillo J et al: Cytogenetic features of Hodgkin's disease suggest possible origin from a lymphocyte. Blood 71:1625, 1988
174. Strong RS, Korsmeyer SJ, Parkin JL et al: Human acute leukemia cell line with the t(4:11) chromosomal rearrangement exhibits B lineage and monocytic characteristics. Blood 65:21, 1985
175. Tilly H, Bastard C, Delastre T et al: Cytogenetic studies in untreated Hodgkin's disease. Blood 77:1298, 1991
176. Schouten HC, Sanger WG, Duggan M et al: Chromosomal abnormalities in Hodgkin's disease. Blood 73:2149, 1989
177. Fonatsch C, Gradl G, Rademacher J: Genetics of Hodgkin's lymphoma. Recent Results Cancer Res 117:35, 1989
178. Stetler-Stevenson M, Crush-Stanton S, Cossman J: Involvement of bcl-2 gene in Hodgkin's disease. J Natl Cancer Inst 82:855, 1990
179. Weiss LM, Warnke A, Sklar J et al: Molecular analysis of the t(14;18) chromosomal translocation in malignant lymphomas. N Engl J Med 317:1185, 1987
180. Poppema S, Kaleta J, Hepperle B: Chromosomal abnormalities in patients with Hodgkin's disease: evidence for frequent involvement of the 14q region but infrequent bcl-2 gene rearrangement in Reed-Sternberg cells. J Natl Cancer Inst 84:1789, 1992
181. Jaffe ES, Zarate-Osorno A, Medeiros J: Interrelationship of Hodgkin's disease and non-Hodgkin's lymphomas—lessons learned from composite and sequential malignancies. Semin Diagn Pathol 9:297, 1992
182. Sundeen JT, Cossman J, Jaffe ES: Lymphocyte predominant Hodgkin's disease nodular subtype with coexistent "large cell lymphoma." Histological progression or composite malignancy? Am J Surg Pathol 12:599, 1988
183. Momose H, Jaffe ES, Sung SS et al: Chronic lymphocytic leukemia/small lymphocytic lymphoma with Reed-Sternberg-like cells and possible transformation to Hodgkin's disease. Mediation by Epstein-Barr virus. Am J Surg Pathol 16:859, 1992
184. Davis TH, Morton CC, Miller-Cassman R et al: Hodgkin's disease, lymphomatoid papulosis, and cutaneous T-cell lymphoma derived from a common T-cell clone. N Engl J Med 326:1115, 1992

Hodgkin Disease: Clinical Manifestations, Staging, and Therapy

79

John H. Glick and Carol S. Portlock

INTRODUCTION

Hodgkin disease (HD) is a unique malignancy of uncertain etiology and cell type that has become a prototype for curable neoplasms. Although the disease may involve the entire lymphoid system, the pattern of presentation and spread is usually predictable and initially localized, lending itself to the successful use of extended field radiotherapy. Since the first description of this disorder by Thomas Hodgkin in 1832, there has been much conjecture as to its nature and, in fact, whether it represents a true malignancy at all.

INCIDENCE AND EPIDEMIOLOGY

In the United States, HD is annually diagnosed in approximately 7 persons per 100,000. The median age of diagnosis is 26–31 years. A bimodal pattern of age distribution frequency for HD has been characteristically seen in the United States, with one peak at 20–29 years, followed by a trough at 40–59 years and a second peak at ≥60 years. It is now recognized that the second bimodal frequency peak was the result of pathologic misclassification.[1] The most recent SEER data (the National Cancer Institute's Surveillance, Epidemiology, and End Results Program) indicate that these cases were largely aggressive non-Hodgkin lymphomas (NHL), rather than HD, mixed cellularity or lymphocyte depletion subtypes, as often reported. The nodular sclerosis (NS) subtype is the most common diagnosis overall, with >75% of cases occurring at <40 years of age and without a second peak thereafter. The other histologic subtypes, lymphocyte predominance (LP), mixed cellularity (MC), and lymphocyte depletion (LD), occur with low but gradually increasing frequency in all age groups.[2]

The incidence of HD is approximately 1.4-fold greater in males. A male predominance has been noted in children <10 years old and again >50 years of age. Between the ages of 10 and 40 years, the ratio is reversed, with females predominating. This corresponds to the peak incidence of NSHD, which is more frequent in females. HD is primarily a malignancy of the white population in the United States, with whites accounting for more than 90% of all cases. In addition, the incidence is associated with small family size and a high standard of living in childhood, as well as a high level of maternal school education.[3,4] Other possible risk factors include human immunodeficiency virus (HIV)[5] infection, Epstein-Barr virus (EBV)[6] infection, genetic predisposition,[7] environmental exposure to herbicides, and certain occupations (woodworking, livestock, and meat processing).

EBV appears to be associated with HD (see Ch. 78). Many studies have documented an increased risk of HD among those with a history of infectious mononucleosis. Moreover, the proportion of patients with HD who have elevated antibody titers to EBV viral capsid antigen is significantly greater than expected.[8,9] Recent reports have also documented the presence of EBV genome in the Reed-Sternberg cell.[10] Its detection appears dependent on the sensitivity of the molecular techniques employed and the histology of the neoplasm (MCHD > NSHD; LPHD undetectable), among other factors. Additional epidemiologic and laboratory study will be necessary, however, before the role of EBV or other possible infectious etiologies can be further clarified.

CLINICAL MANIFESTATIONS

HD usually presents with supradiaphragmatic lymph node involvement and only later with generalized lymphatic and extralymphatic disease. Regional disease presenting below the diaphragm is distinctly unusual (<10% of all cases).[11] Lymph node involvement above the diaphragm frequently includes the anterior mediastinum and may become very large (>10 cm) without causing major symptoms. Complaints of dry nonproductive cough, substernal discomfort, and decreased exercise tolerance are common in this situation. Enlarged lymph nodes in the supraclavicular, cervical, and/or axillary regions are typically noted. Occasionally infraclavicular, submandibular, or even preauricular disease may be present. Waldeyer's ring adenopathy is distinctly unusual and suggests a NHL. Lymph nodes are characteristically firm and rubbery and are often bulky. Local inflammation or erythema is uncommon, although lymphadenopathy will occasionally wax and wane spontaneously or appear to respond partially to antibiotic therapy.

Mauch et al.[12] recently performed a detailed analysis of the initial sites of anatomic involvement, histopathologic findings, and clinical features in 719 patients with HD who underwent staging laparotomy and splenectomy. Table 79-1 presents the initial sites of involvement above the diaphragm, with the mediastinum, left side of neck, and right side of neck each present at diagnosis in >50% of patients with NSHD and MCHD. One of these sites of involvement was present in 92% of their patient population. The spleen was involved in 27% of patients (documented by splenectomy), while upper and lower abdominal nodes were found in 14% and 11% of patients, respectively. A strong association between splenic involvement and upper and lower abdominal disease was found. Only 5% of patients without splenic involvement had abdominal lymph node involvement. By contrast, 61% of patients with splenic involvement had abdominal lymph node disease.[12]

Bulky lymph node disease may result in certain regional complications. For example, tracheal or bronchial compression by massive mediastinal disease can result in complaints of cough or shortness of breath, often made worse in a supine rather than an upright position; obstructive pneumonia may also develop with hilar nodal compression. Extension of mediastinal and hilar adenopathy into adjacent lung, pericardium, chest wall, and pleura may be identified on chest radiograph and by computed tomography (CT) scanning. Pericardial and pleural

Table 79-1. Presenting Sites of Involvement Above the Diaphragm in Descending Order of Prevalence[a]

Site of Involvement[a]	Patients (N)	Prevalence (%)
Mediastinum	425	59
Left side of neck	414	58
Right side of neck	398	55
Left axilla	104	14
Right axilla	92	13
Left hilum	86	12
Right hilum	80	11
Upper neck	36	5
Infraclavicular	21	3
Epitrochlear	13	2
Cardiac	5	1

[a] Categories are not mutually exclusive because more than one site could be involved in a given patient.
(From Mauch et al.,[12] with permission.)

fluid collections are usually asymptomatic, and cytologic examination rarely reveals Reed-Sternberg cells. Chest wall extension may be so great that adjacent sternal or rib destruction occurs, and palpable parasternal disease may be appreciated on physical examination.

In spite of bulky intrathoracic disease presentations, it is rare for patients with HD to have superior vena cava syndrome, upper-extremity venous thrombosis, or phrenic nerve or recurrent laryngeal nerve entrapment. These clinical manifestations are more likely found in patients with NHLs.

Bulky intra-abdominal lymph node involvement is less common in HD and, when identified, is often associated with regional presentations (inguinal and iliac nodes) below the diaphragm. Ureteral obstruction, lower-extremity lymphedema, and venous thrombosis are rare complications and again suggest a NHL. Moreover, lymph node involvement rarely occurs in the mesentery or as isolated retroperitoneal adenopathy.

The spleen is often an occult site of HD spread (see the section Staging). Massive splenomegaly is rare, as are such complications as splenic infarct or hypersplenism. In addition, clinical and radiologic evidence of splenomegaly does not always indicate disease involvement.

Extranodal spread of HD may occur by two separate means: (1) direct extension from a nodal mass (e.g., hilar adenopathy extending into lung parenchyma) and (2) hematogenous dissemination (e.g., bone marrow disease). Regional extranodal extension usually occurs in the presence of local bulky adenopathy. For example, in the lung this may lead to a confusing picture of obstructive pneumonia and infiltrative pulmonary HD. Along the lumbosacral spine, the epidural cord or nerve root may be compressed in addition to direct invasion of one or more vertebral bodies.

Hematogenous spread may be manifested by such findings as multiple pulmonary nodules or diffuse infiltrative disease of the liver and/or bone marrow. Extranodal sites that are rarely involved with HD include skin, the gastrointestinal tract, and the central nervous system. Although recognized more often in patients with the acquired immunodeficiency syndrome and HD,[13] these extranodal disease sites suggest a NHL. The presence of disseminated extranodal disease is generally accompanied by generalized lymphadenopathy and splenic involvement. Since all such presentations are uncommon, it is important to document these extranodal sites pathologically, which usually requires a cutting-needle or open biopsy, since aspiration cytology is rarely if ever positive. Clinical judgment must be used in assessing the risk versus benefit of performing an extranodal site biopsy. For example, in a patient with multi-

ple pulmonary nodules and mediastinal and hilar adenopathy, lung biopsy is rarely indicated.

HD may have associated systemic symptoms such as unexplained fever of $\geq 101°F$, drenching night sweats, and/or weight loss of $>10\%$ body weight during the previous 6 months. Such "B" symptoms (see Table 79-3) correlate with disease stage, increasing in frequency with extent and bulk, and also correlate with overall prognosis. Other systemic manifestations of HD without known prognostic significance include generalized pruritus (often severe and difficult to treat symptomatically without control of the HD) and alcohol-induced lymph node pain after ingestion of alcoholic beverages. These systemic complaints may be the first indication of active HD, but more often they are elicited after the diagnosis has been established.

Patients with HD will often be anergic to skin test antigens at first diagnosis. Hyporesponsiveness increases with increasing disease stage. In addition, T-cell number, T-cell helper (CD4)/suppressor (CD8) ratio, and T-cell in vitro response to antigen may be altered. Although cell-mediated immunity may be mildly abnormal, patients with HD rarely develop opportunistic infections prior to treatment. An exception, however, is the increased frequency of herpes zoster, seen in previously untreated as well as treated patients.[14]

B-cell function appears to be normal in HD at diagnosis. Pneumococcal vaccination, for example, results in normal antibody response as long as subsequent treatment is delayed 10–14 days. Splenectomy does not interfere with an adequate antibody rise. By contrast, overwhelming bacterial sepsis with encapsulated organisms is still a potential risk among patients with HD after splenectomy or irradiation to the spleen.[15,16]

STAGING

Clinical and Pathologic Staging

Once a diagnosis has been established with an adequate biopsy and hematopathologic interpretation, systematic clinical staging should be initiated (Table 79-2). During a complete history and physical examination, the presence of systemic symptoms and the extent of lymphatic nodal involvement can be

Table 79-2. Clinical Staging Evaluation

1. Detailed history for unexplained fever, weight loss, night sweats, and pruritus
2. Physical examination to document all areas of lymphadenopathy; size of liver and spleen; bony tenderness; neurologic evaluation
3. Laboratory studies
   a. CBC, differential and platelet count, erythrocyte sedimentation rate
   b. Serum alkaline phosphatase, lactate dehydrogenase
   c. Renal function, including uric acid
   d. Liver function tests
4. Radiologic studies
   a. Chest radiograph
   b. Bipedal lymphogram
   c. Computed tomography of the chest and whole abdomen, including the pelvis
   d. Gallium scan
   e. Bone scan/bone radiographs obtained when areas of bone pain or tenderness are present
5. Biopsy studies
   a. Diagnostic biopsy of lymph node: review with experienced hematopathologist
   b. Bone marrow biopsy
   c. Biopsy of suspicious disseminated extranodal sites (i.e., pulmonary or liver lesions), if clinically indicated
6. Under special circumstances
   a. Magnetic resonance imaging
   b. Ultrasound

assessed. A chest radiograph will define the bulk of intrathoracic adenopathy and the possible presence of pulmonary extension, postobstructive pneumonia, or rarely, disseminated lung disease. CT scanning of the chest, abdomen, and pelvis will identify enlarged lymph nodes and their relationship to normal anatomic structures (e.g., pericardium, chest wall, kidney). Possible extranodal involvement (e.g., lung, liver, bone) may also be imaged. Although hepatosplenomegaly may be identified, its presence does not necessarily confirm disease involvement since nonspecific enlargement of these organs may occur. The lymphogram complements the abdominal and pelvic CT scan, since it may identify abnormal lymph nodes of borderline size, as well as identifying intranodal architecture. The lymphogram is more sensitive in detecting para-aortic disease (85–98% rate of true-positive results as compared with 40–65 for CT).[17,18] However, the lymphogram is not accurate above L2–L3 and is therefore unable to assess celiac axis, porta hepatis, or mesenteric (rare in HD) adenopathy; CT scanning is more accurate in assessing these nodal areas. Thus, both abdominal CT scanning and a bipedal lymphogram are recommended as part of the initial staging procedures. Although uncommon at diagnosis, bone marrow involvement should be excluded before regional therapy is initiated. Percutaneous bone marrow biopsies are indicated as part of routine clinical staging. They are more likely to be positive in patients with B symptoms, clinical stage III or IV disease, or MCHD or LDHD and in patients with leukopenia or thrombocytopenia. Routine laboratory blood work may reveal leukocytosis, often with eosinophilia, a mild thrombocytosis, and/or anemia with a reactive bone marrow picture. The alkaline phosphatase may be elevated nonspecifically or in association with bone and/or bone marrow or liver involvement. Elevation of lactate dehydrogenase is an indication of bulky disease and appears to have prognostic significance at high levels.

Other staging studies that are often used include gallium scanning and magnetic resonance imaging (MRI). Gallium scanning is most useful in the anterior mediastinum and chest when evaluating treatment outcome of bulky disease.[19] If initial and post-treatment studies indicate gallium avidity with a persistent mediastinal mass, the possibility of residual HD mandates biopsy confirmation. The gallium scan is less useful in the abdomen because of bowel uptake, although CT studies may improve the yield. MRI of the bone marrow in relapsed HD may be a particularly useful method of detecting occult disease.[20] Although MRI may provide excellent imaging of nodal and extranodal sites, its superiority to CT scanning has not been proved or shown to be cost effective.

The Ann Arbor staging classification[21] for HD (Table 79-3 presents the Cotswolds modification[22] of the Ann Arbor staging system) recognizes both a clinical and a pathologic stage. Staging designations are determined according to the number of lymph node regions (not sites) involved and whether there is disease on one or both sides of the diaphragm. Systemic or B symptoms include fever, night sweats, and weight loss. The E lesion is defined as a direct extranodal extension of lymph node disease that potentially can be encompassed in a radiation portal, such as hilar node extension into lung parenchyma.

Clinical staging includes the initial biopsy site and all other abnormalities detected by noninvasive methods, including physical examination and radiologic studies. Pathologic staging requires biopsy confirmation of potentially abnormal sites (e.g., liver or bone); if disease involvement appears to be limited to the lymph nodes, full staging laparotomy and splenectomy may be necessary. This latter procedure requires biopsy of para-aortic, celiac, porta hepatis, and other suspicious lymph nodes, and splenectomy (with placement of clips on the splenic pedicle), liver wedge and needle biopsies, and bone marrow biopsy (if not done prior to laparotomy). Pneumococcal vaccine is routinely administered prior to surgery.

Table 79-3. Cotswolds Staging Classification of Hodgkin Disease

Classification	Description
Stage I	Involvement of a single lymph node region or lymphoid structure
Stage II	Involvement of two or more lymph node regions on the same side of the diaphragm (the mediastinum is considered as a single site, whereas hilar lymph nodes are considered bilaterally); number of anatomic sites should be indicated by a subscript (e.g., stage II$_3$)
Stage III	Involvement of lymph node regions or structures on both sides of the diaphragm
III$_1$	With or without involvement of the spleen, splenic, hilar, celiac, or portal nodes
III$_2$	With involvement of para-aortic, iliac, and mesenteric nodes
Stage IV	Involvement of one or more extranodal sites in addition to a site for which the designation E has been used (see below)

Designations applicable to any disease stage

A	No symptoms
B	Fever (temperature, >38°C), drenching night sweats, unexplained loss of >10% body weight within the preceding 6 months
X	Bulky disease (a widening of the mediastinum by more than one-third or the presence of a nodal mass with a maximal dimension of >10 cm)
E	Involvement of a single extranodal site that is contiguous or proximal to the known nodal site
CS	Clinical stage
PS	Pathologic stage (as determined by laparotomy)

(Adapted from Lister and Crowther,[22] with permission.)

Although staging laparotomy has been widely applied in HD, its indications have decreased in recent years. Successful treatment of many clinically staged patients has become feasible with the use of combination chemotherapy. Moreover, very favorable subsets of patients with early-stage HD may be identified in whom the risk of intra-abdominal disease is <5–10% and in whom primary irradiation may be considered without laparotomy confirmation.

Following complete clinical and pathologic staging, the distribution of patients with HD is as shown in Table 79-4.[23] Prognostic factors not reflected in the Ann Arbor stage but that may influence treatment decisions and outcome include bulk of disease, number of nodal regions involved, distribution of intra-abdominal stage III adenopathy, and extent of splenic involvement.

In 1989, an international multidisciplinary committee[24] recommended further modifications in the Ann Arbor staging classification to reflect changes in clinical staging criteria, the in-

Table 79-4. Clinical Characteristics of Patients Treated for Hodgkin Disease at Stanford (1968–1988) According to Histologic Subtype

	Lymphocyte Predominance	Nodular Sclerosis	Mixed Cellularity	Lymphocyte Depletion
No.	78	1,301	282	13
Percentage	5%	78%	17%	1%
Age range	4–65	2–82	4–81	11–65
Median age	31	26	30	42.5
Stage				
I	42%	6%	13%	0
II	38%	51%	26%	8%
III	19%	31%	46%	38%
IV	0	12%	15%	54%
B symptoms	3%	33%	30%	62%

(Data from Hoppe.[23])

Table 79-5. Cotswolds Meeting Recommendations for Clinical Imaging Criteria

1. Lymph node involvement
   CT size criteria of >1.5 cm for a positive study
2. Spleen involvement
   Requires unequivocally palpable spleen or equivocally palpable spleen plus radiologic enlargement or splenic defects
3. Liver involvement
   Multiple focal defects confirmed by two imaging modalities
4. Definition of bulky dimension
   ≥10 cm in largest dimension
   Mediastinal mass greater than one-third of the internal transverse diameter of the thorax at T5-T6[e]

[a] Although the Cotswolds definition of a bulky mediastinal mass uses the internal transverse diameter of the thorax at T5-T6, most investigators define a large mediastinal mass as greater than one-third of the maximal intrathoracic diameter. (From Lister et al.,[24] with permission.)

creased use of new diagnostic tests such as CT scanning, newly recognized prognostic factors, and their impact on therapeutic decisions. Table 79-5 summarizes the Cotswolds Staging Classification recommendations for clinical imaging criteria.[22,24] This staging system acknowledges the value of CT and other imaging modalities in defining disease extent. However, it was again emphasized that biopsy confirmation is required if treatment recommendations might be altered by an equivocal study. This new staging system also clarified issues of disease distribution and bulk. In regional disease, the number of involved sites is denoted by a subscript (e.g., stage II_3). For stage III presentations, anatomic extent of intra-abdominal adenopathy is defined and denoted by subscript, with stage III_1 assigned to patients with spleen or splenic hilar, celiac, or portal node involvement; and stage III_2 to those with para-aortic, iliac, inguinal, or mesenteric involvement. Bulky disease is defined by maximum dimension (>10 cm) or by at least one-third mass/thorax ratio, designated by the subscript X. In the setting of bulky intrathoracic disease, contiguous spread to adjacent extranodal tissues is clearly distinguished from disseminated extranodal involvement (e.g., multiple pulmonary nodules). This common clinical stage II presentation would be designated with the subscript X for bulky or E for extranodal extension of lymph node disease into adjacent tissues (e.g., chest wall, pericardium, and sternum) and with a numerical subscript for the number of nodal sites involved above the diaphragm.

Staging Laparotomy

The Ann Arbor and Cotswolds staging systems are based on both clinical and pathologic staging. The extent to which disease is pathologically confirmed depends on the suspected sites involved and whether that information would influence treatment decisions. Most HD patients have involvement limited to lymph node areas. Therefore, suspected stage IV sites should be pathologically confirmed (e.g., liver lesions) if these sites are not unequivocally involved by disease (e.g., multiple obvious lung nodules or a positive radiographic bone scan with blastic involvement).

Moreover, the anatomic distribution of lymph node involvement in HD is not random. Supradiaphragmatic disease with or without intra-abdominal involvement is the rule, and regional disease limited to subdiaphragmatic sites is uncommon. During the 1960s, the extent of intra-abdominal involvement was recognized to be underestimated in many cases, since the disease status of the spleen could not be reliably assessed by clinical means alone. Staging laparotomy was introduced to more adequately evaluate the suspected clinical findings. The primary purpose behind the decision to perform a staging la-

poratomy is to determine whether radiation alone can be used for treatment.

Surprisingly, the accuracy of clinical abdominal disease assessment is often poor in spite of CT and lymphogram imaging.[11,25] More than 40% of clinical stage IIIA patients may be downstaged (negative laparotomy findings), and the extent of inaccuracy rises to 68% for patients <40 years of age with LPHD or NSHD. Likewise, for clinical stage I and II, staging laparotomy yields evidence of intra-abdominal disease in approximately one-third of patients. Those factors most likely to be associated with upstaging include male sex, presence of B symptoms, and two or more sites of disease involvement above the diaphragm.

Of equal importance, however, is the observation that certain subgroups have a very low likelihood of change in stage with laparotomy. Those with clinical stage IA disease that presents in the mediastinum have virtually no risk of intra-abdominal involvement. Females with clinical stage IA at other supradiaphragmatic sites have a 6% risk, whereas males with similar clinical characteristics are at an equally low risk only if they have LPHD or interfollicular HD. Other histologic subtypes are associated with positive laparotomy findings in up to one-third of clinical stage IA males.[25]

For clinical stage II patients, female sex confers a significantly lower risk of intra-abdominal disease (22% versus 36%) than for males. Moreover, a favorable subset (females with fewer than three disease sites ≤26 years of age) has been identified by the Stanford group[11]; laparotomy is positive in <10% of this subset. Such laparotomy data make it possible to identify subsets of patients in whom there is good correspondence between clinical and pathologic staging; these are summarized in Table 79-6.

For patients with favorable clinical stage I and II presentations, a correspondence of ≥90% with pathologic staging suggests that primary irradiation without staging laparotomy may be considered. This approach would be valid if other treatment parameters were satisfactory for primary irradiation (i.e., no bulk disease at any site). Similarly, for patients with clinical stage IIIB and IVB, correspondence is ≥80–90%, suggesting that few if any of these patients would be downstaged with complete staging laparotomy evaluation. In this situation, combination chemotherapy with or without irradiation would be the primary treatment approach chosen.

For all other clinical presentations of clinical stages I and II as well as clinical stage IIIA, full pathologic staging must be seriously considered if primary irradiation alone is to be used. In these situations, the correspondence is low enough (≤80%) that many patients may be inaccurately staged and treated if the clinical stage is not pathologically confirmed. Similarly, for rare patients with clinical stage IVA, correspondence may be low as a result of inaccurate extranodal disease assessment. With downstaging, a rare patient might then become a candidate for primary irradiation.

A high level of correspondence is not the only factor to be considered in treatment planning. Additional parameters that

Table 79-6. Correspondence of Clinical and Pathologic Staging

Correspondence	
≥90%	1. CS IA, females
	2. CS IA, males with LPHD or interfollicular HD
	3. CS I, mediastinum only
	4. CS II, females with ≤3 disease sites, and age ≤26 years
	5. CS IIIB, with MCHD or LDHD, and age >40 years
≥80%	1. CS IIIB
	2. CS IVB

Abbreviations: CS, clinical stage; LP, lymphocyte predominance; HD, Hodgkin disease; MC, mixed cellularity; LD, lymphocyte depletion.
(Data from Leibenhaut et al.[11] and Mauch et al.[25])

often exclude patients from primary irradiation include bulky disease[26] (best treated with combined chemotherapy and irradiation), clinical stage III$_2$A presentations,[27] and the extent of splenic involvement assessed pathologically.[28] The Stanford group defines extensive splenic disease as five or more nodules. Regardless of the intra-abdominal adenopathy pattern (III$_1$ or III$_2$), patients with extensive splenic involvement have a poor outcome with primary irradiation and require combination chemotherapy. Approximately 90% of patients will appear to have stage I or II disease on the basis of the initial physical examination and chest radiograph. One-third of these patients will be shown to have more advanced stage III or IV disease as assessed by lymphogram or CT scanning, or both. Another 20–33% of patients with early stage disease will be placed in a higher stage after laporatomy and splenectomy. After all staging procedures are completed, 40–50% of patients will be found to have stages I and II, while 50–60% will be noted as stage III and IV.[29] Patients with NSHD or LPHD are more likely to have stage I or II disease.

In summary, the concept of clinical and pathologic staging in HD remains a valid tool in selecting curative treatment strategies. By keeping in mind the likelihood of clinical and pathologic stage correlations, an accurate definition of subsets of patients may be possible for cases in which abdominal exploration would add little information to the treatment plan. However, if disease involvement is equivocal, if an extranodal site appears to be involved without direct extension, or if clinical/pathologic correlation is known to be low, biopsy or staging laparotomy, or both, must be considered.

THERAPY

The prognosis for patients with all stages of HD has improved dramatically since 1960 as a result of advances in precise staging, knowledge of important prognostic factors, the development of supervoltage radiotherapy, and the use of effective combination chemotherapy. The improved results achieved with modern therapy after accurate clinical and pathologic staging are possible only with experienced teams of pathologists, surgeons, radiotherapists, hematologists, and oncologists working closely together. This approach can produce the excellent cure rates now possible, while minimizing acute and long-term morbidity from treatment. It should be emphasized that the goal of treatment is to obtain the highest overall possible cure rate for all patients. Thus, freedom from first or even second relapse must be considered in the evaluation of both disease-free and overall survival when the results of past and current trials are analyzed. For example, an early-stage patient who has relapsed after radiation therapy alone may be cured with chemotherapy administered at relapse. The challenge for physicians caring for patients with all stages of HD is to weigh carefully the toxicity/benefit ratio for each treatment regimen and to design a treatment strategy that maximizes the overall survival rate.

Radiotherapy for Early-Stage Disease

The long-term survival of patients with early-stage HD is >85% in multiple studies using various staging techniques and treatment modalities.[30–38] Definitive radiotherapy has long been considered standard treatment for the vast majority of patients with stage I–II HD because of the excellent long-term survival with minimal complications. The results of radiotherapy for laparotomy-stage I and II patients are dependent on close attention to important technical considerations for radiotherapy, including total radiation dose per field; size, shape, and number of treatment fields and careful definition of in-

volved sites; use of appropriate voltage devices (e.g., linear accelerators); treatment simulation with individually shaped blocks for careful protection of normal tissues, such as the lungs and heart; equal doses from anterior and posterior fields; and use of cone-down fields and careful matching techniques with appropriate cord blocks.[31,39–43]

Kaplan[43] provided the critical data to indicate that radiotherapy of HD follows a dose-response curve. Permanent eradication of any given known site of involvement is achieved in the vast majority of cases with doses of 3,600–4,400 cGy delivered at a dose rate of 1,000 cGy/wk. Prophylactic radiation to a total dose of 3,000–3,600 cGy is delivered to apparently uninvolved areas treated for subclinical disease. Use of a linear accelerator in the 4–8-MeV range provides the advantage of precise beam margins with reduced lateral scatter, increased depth-dose, and improved skin tolerance.[42] It is important to define carefully the extent of disease and fields to be treated, using appropriate treatment simulators. Proper technique also includes the use of carefully shaped lead blocks to protect such vital structures as the lungs, heart, and spinal cord; frequent port films; and dose verification using precise dosimetry.

Current radiotherapy practice continues to emphasize the treatment of multiple lymph node chains within a few very large, carefully shaped fields. Figure 79-1 illustrates the radiation fields most frequently delivered in clinical practice. The mantle field treats the cervical, supraclavicular, infraclavicular, axillary, hilar, and mediastinal lymph nodes to the level of the diaphragm in one contiguous treatment volume. Prophylactic whole lung irradiation to a dose of 1,500–1,650 cGy in 150-cGy fractions is administered by some radiotherapists when the ipsilateral hilum is involved with HD.[40,42] Although this technique decreases relapse in the treated fields for patients with hilar disease, the routine use of whole-lung irradiation remains controversial. The para-aortic field covers the splenic pedicle, the spleen (if not removed at laparotomy), and the celiac and para-aortic lymph nodes from the diaphragm to the level of the aortic bifurcation. The mantle (M) and para-aortic fields are frequently referred to as extended-field (EF) or subtotal nodal (or lymphoid) irradiation (STNI). The radiotherapy approach known as total nodal irradiation (TNI) or total lymphoid irradiation, involves treating the mantle, para-aortic, and pelvic fields. As is discussed below, inclusion of pelvic irradiation, as part of TNI is rapidly disappearing. In addition, pelvic irradiation affects large amounts of bone marrow and therefore may subsequently preclude the use of full-dose chemotherapy. Pelvic radiotherapy also may increase the risk of infertility.

Delivering radiotherapy to apparently uninvolved lymph node regions has long been advocated because of the orderliness and contiguity of spread for patients who present with early stage disease.[13,44–45] This approach is based on the knowledge of sites of relapse of HD when treated only with involved field radiotherapy, the limitations of our diagnostic techniques to discover minute or microscopic foci of subclinical disease, and the advantage of avoiding overlapping fields. In the initial Stanford trials,[33] patients with stage I and IIA disease were randomly assigned to involved field (IF) irradiation, EF irradiation, or TNI. A highly significant difference in disease-free survival was observed in favor of either EF irradiation or TNI, although overall survival was similar (80% at 15 years). The studies from the Joint Center for Radiation Therapy (JCRT) in laparotomy stage I–IIA HD have been reviewed by Mauch et al.[30] At a median follow-up of 9 years, review of the 315 patients treated with mantle and para-aortic irradiation (M + PA) revealed a freedom from relapse of 82% and an overall survival of 90%. These results are illustrated in Figure 79-2. More than 80% of patients treated with mantle and para-aortic irradiation have been continuously relapse free and therefore have not required the use of salvage chemotherapy. Pelvic recurrences were noted in only 3% of cases, indicating that it is reasonable to omit the

SUMMARY OF INITIAL THERAPY RECOMMENDATIONS BY STAGE OF HODGKIN DISEASE

The recommended therapy for a patient with HD must be indivdualized. Advances in histopathologic classification, precise staging procedures, and selection of appropriate aggressive therapy have led to continuous improvement in both failure-free survival and overall survival. Any treatment recommendations must be viewed with the understanding that the management of HD is dynamic, constantly undergoing change and refinement. The goal is to provide each patient with the best probability of cure and the least possibility of long-term toxicity.

For most patients with pathologic stage I or IIA, mantle and para-aortic radiotherapy remains the treatment of choice for supradiaphragmatic presentations. However, younger laporatomy-staged patients with stage I or IIA disease of NS or LP histology who do not have mediastinal involvement can be treated with mantle radiotherapy alone, as can stage IA patients with these histologic subtypes and a small mediastinal mass. For favorable subsets of clinically staged IA and selected IIA patients, staging laparotomy and splenectomy are not required. These patients can be treated with either a mantle field, or mantle, para-aortic, and splenic fields, depending on their clinical prognostic factors. For early-stage asymptomatic patients with large mediastinal masses in whom definitive radiotherapy alone is not thought to be an acceptable option, owing to the location and size of the mediastinal disease, involvement of contiguous extranodal sites, or the potential morbidity from treating large volumes of normal tissues, a combined modality approach is appropriate. In the subgroup of patients who will receive initial combined modality therapy, staging laparotomy is not indicated, and treatment is initiated with one of the currently accepted regimens for advanced-stage disease. In this situation chemotherapy is given to maximal tumor response, which is then followed by limited-field radiotherapy.

Laparotomy-staged patients with stage I–IIB disease can be treated effectively with mantle and para-aortic radiotherapy alone, provided that they do not have both fever and weight loss and/or bulky mediastinal mass. This approach spares these patients the additional morbidity of initial combined modality therapy. The presence of a large mediastinal mass in a patient with early-stage HD and B symptoms is associated with a significantly greater risk of relapse. These patients should be treated with combined modality therapy.

Patients with subdiaphragmatic pathologic stage IA disease are generally treated with inverted Y radiotherapy, including the splenic pedicle. In patients with pathologic stage IIA and IIsA with limited splenic involvement, total nodal radiotherapy, and combined modality therapy appear to be of comparable efficacy. In patients with subdiaphragmatic clinical stage IIB disease, management

with primary chemotherapy or with combined modality therapy appears to be equally effective.

Although combined modality therapy is an attractive alternative for the management of early- and intermediate-stage disease, any potential disease-free survival advantage must be balanced by the potential risk of late complications, particularly second neoplasms or potential cardiac and pulmonary toxicity (with ABVD) and must be translated into an overall survival benefit before general acceptance.

The treatment of pathologic stage IIIA HD remains controversial. In laparotomy-staged patients with III$_1$A disease who have minimal splenic involvement, mantle and para-aortic radiotherapy, and total nodal irradiation are equally effective. However, for most patients with stage IIIA disease, combined modality therapy or chemotherapy alone should be used. Patients to be treated in this manner should meet one or more of the following criteria: extensive splenic involvement (more than four splenic nodules); pathologic stage III$_2$A disease; unequivocal clinical evidence of disease below the diaphragm on lymphogram and/or CT scan; and clinical stage IIIA disease with large mediastinal masses. From the limited data available, it would appear that chemotherapy alone using any one of the accepted combinations for advanced disease is as effective as combined modality therapy for most patients with extensive stage IIIA disease. Although the results with combined modality therapy for IIIB and IV disease are excellent in terms of freedom from progression and overall survival, they do not appear significantly different from the results obtained with chemotherapy alone. Thus, for the vast majority of patients with stage IIIB or IV disease, chemotherapy alone is recommended as initial treatment.

For many years, MOPP remained the standard of care for the treatment of patients with stage IIIB or IV disease. However, data from recent randomized trials indicate that alternating monthly MOPP/ABVD or the MOPP/ABV hybrid regimen result in improved failure-free and overall survival. The use of ABVD alone is intriguing because of its apparent reduced long-term toxicity, but the data with ABVD are still preliminary. Administration of radiotherapy to all sites of pretreatment involvement once a complete remission has been obtained with chemotherapy for advanced disease does not result in improved failure-free or overall survival and cannot be recommended. Limited-field irradiation to initial sites of bulky disease may be used in selected clinical situations.

The treatment of HD remains one of the great triumphs of cancer therapy since the middle 1960s. The overall 5-year survival rate for all patients has increased to ≥75% today. Thus, a treatment strategy for each patient should be designed to provide the highest probability of overall cure, while limiting late toxicities when possible.

---

pelvic field from the radiotherapy port. Other investigators using comparable staging and radiotherapy techniques have reported similar results, which are summarized in Table 79-7.

In the JCRT series, mediastinal size was the only factor that significantly predicted freedom from relapse.[30] Patients with large mediastinal masses were significantly less likely to have freedom from relapse than were those with less or no mediastinal involvement (53% versus 83%, respectively). However, the survival of these two groups of patients was not significantly

different. The approach to patients with large mediastinal masses is discussed in a subsequent section.

Gospodarowicz et al.[36] reported the long-term results of treating 521 clinically staged I and II patients with radiation alone at the Princess Margaret Hospital (Table 79-7). The overall actuarial survival for all irradiated patients was 78% at 10 years and 63% at 20 years, while the cause-specific survival was 87% and 83%, respectively. The use of mantle radiotherapy rather than IF radiotherapy was associated with a significant

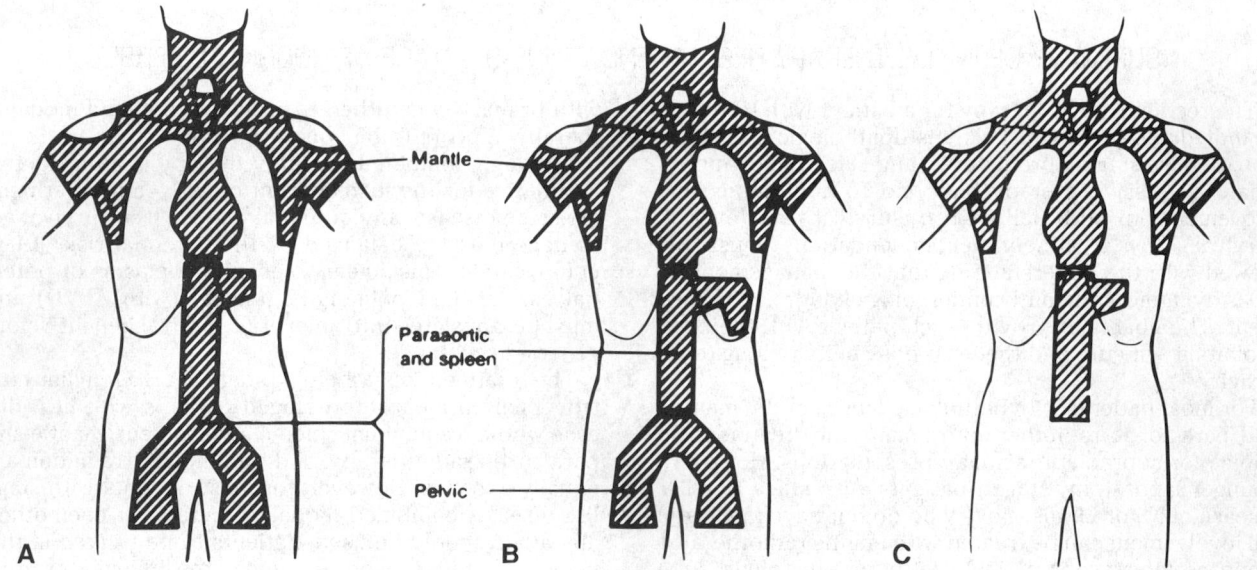

Fig. 79-1. Radiotherapy fields commonly used for Hodgkin disease. Total nodal irradiation consists of **(A)** a mantle and an inverted Y or **(B)** three fields. **(C)** Subtotal nodal irradiation after splenectomy consists of a mantle and para-aortic fields. (From Rosenberg,[39] with permission.)

improvement in the 10-year relapse-free survival (RFS) (M = 66%, IF = 51%) and in the 10-year actuarial survival (M = 80%, IF = 59%). There was further improvement in the 10-year RFS with the use of EF radiotherapy (76%), but this effect was not statistically significant when EF was compared with mantle radiotherapy alone in a multivariate analysis adjusting for other prognostic features. In a "low-risk" or very favorable cohort of patients (defined as clinical stage I and IIA, <50 years of age,

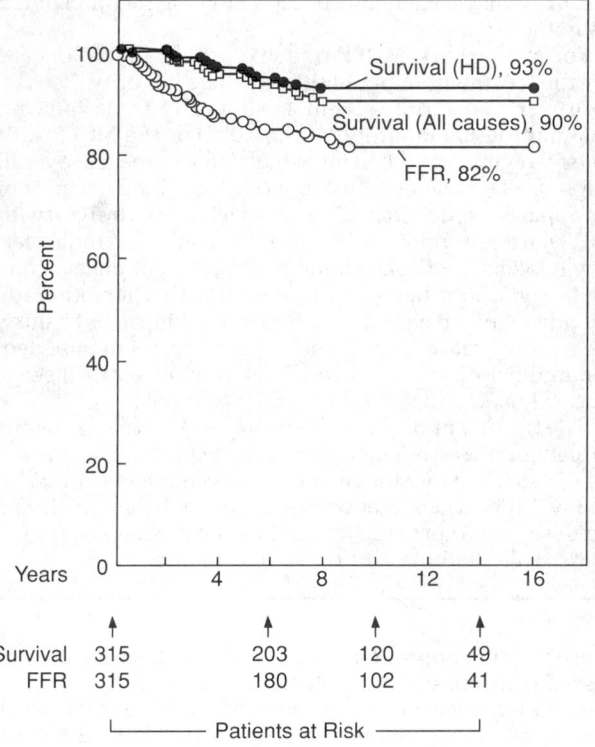

Fig. 79-2. Actuarial freedom from relapse (FFR) and survival for stage IA and IIA patients treated initially with mantle and para-aortic irradiation. Actuarial survival curves are shown censored for unrelated deaths (marked HD) and for survival, including deaths from all causes. (From Mauch et al.,[30] with permission.)

with LP or NS histology, erythrocyte sedimentation rate (ESR) <40, no large mediastinal mass, and no E lesion), the 10-year survival was 91%, with an RFS of 77%. The 10-year RFS for patients in this favorable subgroup was 80% for mantle radiotherapy, compared with 87% for EF radiotherapy (not statistically significant). The overall conclusions reached by Gospodarowicz et al.[36] were that the role of laparotomy and splenectomy in defining a favorable group of patients for treatment with radiotherapy alone may be offset by patient selection, using multiple clinical prognostic factors and by employing EF radiotherapy.

An alternative approach to the staging and treatment of early stage HD has been proposed by Cosset et al.,[35] reporting for the European Organization for the Research and Treatment of Cancer (EORTC). In the EORTC H2 trial, NSHD patients were randomized to either staging laparotomy and splenectomy followed by mantle and para-aortic radiotherapy, or to STNI and spleen radiotherapy (Table 79-7). At 12 years, RFS was 68% for STNI alone and 76% for laparotomy–STNI. Overall survival was virtually identical. In the subsequent H5 trial, a favorable prognostic group was defined with all the following characteristics: no B symptoms, age <40 years, ESR <70; LP or NS histology; and either clinical stage I or II without mediastinal involvement. All patients in this favorable group first underwent laparotomy and splenectomy. If negative, patients were randomly assigned to mantle irradiation alone or to mantle plus para-aortic radiotherapy. There was no difference in either RFS or overall survival between the two arms (Table 79-7). Therefore, in patients with all these initial favorable prognostic factors and with no infradiaphragmatic extension (i.e., negative laparotomy), the addition of para-aortic irradiation did not yield any benefit. The EORTC H6 trial then addressed the need for laparotomy in the favorable subgroup: patients in the first arm of the study underwent laparotomy with treatment adapted to the pathology findings; if the laparotomy was negative, mantle radiotherapy was given (plus para-aortic field for MC or LD histology); if the laparotomy was positive, combined modality treatment was administered. Patients in the second arm of the study without laparotomy directly received mantle, para-aortic, and spleen radiotherapy (STNI + spleen). In this trial, the end point was survival and not RFS. At 5 years, RFS was significantly lower in the STNI group than in the laparotomy (plus adapted treatment) patients, as expected. However, because of the effi-

Table 79-7. Comparison of Different Treatment Strategies for Stages I–II

Investigators	Stage	Follow-up	Comment	Treatment	FFP/RFS (%)	Survival (%)
Rosenberg and Kaplan[33]	I, IIA	15 yr	All patients	IF	32	79
				STNI/TNI	80	80
Mauch et al.[30]	I, IIA	14 yr	All patients	M + PA	82	90
			SMM	M + PA	86	93
			LMM	M + PA	53	88
			NS/LP	M + PA	88	97
			MC/LD	M + PA	80	84
Gospodarowicz et al.[36]	I, II	10 yr	All patients	M	66	80
				M + PA	76	NA
	I, II	10 yr	Very favorable[a]	M	80	88
				M + PA	87	97
Cosset et al.[35]	I, II	12 yr	All patients	M + PA (lap)	76	79
				M + PA + spleen (no lap)	68	77
	I, II	9	Favorable[b]	M	69	94
				M + PA	70	91
	I, II	5	Favorable[b]	M (lap negative)	89	90
				M + PA + spleen (no lap)	79	94
Horning et al.[65]	I, IIA	10 yr	All patients	M + PA	80	90
				IF + MOPP	82	84
Horning et al.[66]	I, II	10 yr	All patients	IF + VBM	97	100
Rosenberg[37]				STLI	70	91
Cosset et al.[35]	I, II	9 yr	Unfavorable[b]	TNI	66	73
				CMT (MOPP-M RT-MOPP)	83	88
Crnkovich et al.[48]	I, IIB	10 yr	All patients	M + PA/TNI	70	90
				CMT	80	85
Fuller et al.[46]	I, II	4 yr	Favorable[c]	M	79	92
			Unfavorable[c]	MOPP × 2 + IF RT	78	100
Pavlovsky et al.[69]	I, II	7 yr	Favorable[d]	CVPP	77	92
				CVPP + RT	70	91
			Unfavorable[d]	CVPP	34	66
				CVPP + RT	75	84
Longo et al.[70]	I, II		Excluding LMM	M + PA	67	85
				MOPP	82	90
Biti et al.[71]	I, II		All patients	M + PA	76	93
				MOPP	70	56

Abbreviations: M, mantle radiotherapy; PA, para-aortic radiotherapy; STNI, subtotal nodal irradiation; TNI, total nodal irradiation; lap, staging laparotomy and splenectomy; CMT, combined modality therapy; RT, radiotherapy; IF, involved field radiotherapy; MOPP, nitrogen mustard, vincristine, procarbazine, prednisone; CVPP, cyclophosphamide, vinblastine, procarbazine, prednisone; RFS, relapse-free survival; FFP, freedom from progression; ESR, erythrocyte sedimentation rate; SMM, small mediastinal mass; LMM, large mediastinal mass; NS, nodular sclerosis; LP, lymphocyte predominance; MC, mixed cellularity; LD, lymphocyte depletion; NA, results not available; VBM, vinblastine, bleomycin, methotrexate.

[a] Very favorable: clinical Stage IA or IIA with age <50, or lymphocyte predominance, ESR < 40, no LMM, and no E lesion.

[b] Favorable: age <40, ESR <70, NS or LP histology, clinical stage IA or clinical stage IIA without mediastinal involvement. Unfavorable: one or more of the following: age ≥40, ESR ≥70, MC or LD histology, clinical stage II with mediastinal involvement.

[c] Favorable: asymptomatic, mediastinal mass <7.5-cm diameter, negative hila. Unfavorable: not meeting all favorable criteria.

[d] Favorable: age ≤45, <3 sites of disease, nonbulky disease. Unfavorable: not meeting all favorable criteria.

cacy of salvage chemotherapy, 5-year overall survival was similar[35] (Table 79-7). Based on these studies, the EORTC decided to give up staging laparotomy for supradiaphragmatic disease and subsequently used clinical staging. On the basis of their data, they also defined a small cohort of patients who could be safely treated with a mantle field alone without laparotomy. This subgroup is very restrictively defined and only includes female NSHD or LPHD patients with clinical stage I, <40 years of age, without B symptoms, with an ESR of <50, and without bulky mediastinal involvement.[35]

Similar results were reported by Fuller et al.[46] for the M.D. Anderson group in a small number of prognostically favorable patients, who had supradiaphragmatic disease with either no mediastinal disease or limited mediastinal disease without hilar involvement and no B symptoms. These patients were treated with mantle radiotherapy alone. The British National Lymphoma Investigational Trials[47] also confirmed the equal effectiveness of more limited radiotherapy fields (i.e., mantle) for favorable subsets of stage I–IIA patients.

Thus, laparotomy-staged patients with pathologic stage I–IIA supradiaphragmatic disease of the NS or LP histology who do not have mediastinal involvement can be treated with mantle radiotherapy alone. Stage I patients with these histologies and a small mediastinal mass may also be treated with a mantle field. However, for stage I–IIA patients not meeting these criteria, mantle and para-aortic fields should be used; in clinically staged patients (i.e., no laparotomy), a splenic field should be also irradiated. Thus, for most patients with pathologic stage I–IIA, mantle and para-aortic radiotherapy remains the treatment of choice. For most clinically staged I–IIA patients with large mediastinal masses, combined modality therapy should be used as initial treatment.

The presence of constitutional or B symptoms has long been recognized as an important prognostic factor in HD. This observation is based primarily on data from patients with advanced disease, since patients with early-stage disease rarely present with B symptoms. This has led to different treatment recommendations for surgically staged patients with supradiaphragmatic stage I–IIB disease. Although several investigators have recommended the routine use of combined modality therapy for these patients,[30,47–50] this approach remains controversial. In one of the few randomized trials for this subset of patients, the Stanford investigators treated stage IB–IIB patients with either TNI alone or TNI followed by six cycles of adjuvant MOPP (mechlorethamine, vincristine [Oncovin], procarbazine, prednisone) chemotherapy.[33] This small controlled trial showed no difference in either freedom from progression or overall survival, with 78% of all patients surviving >10 years from initial treatment.

Crnkovich et al.[48] reviewed the treatment records of 180 patients with pathologic stage IB–IIB HD treated at Stanford and the JCRT. In this retrospective review, the two most important disease characteristics predictive of relapse were the number and type of B symptoms and the presence of a large mediastinal mass. Patients with both fever and weight loss had a 7-year freedom from relapse of 48% and an overall survival of only 57%. The poor prognosis in this subset was apparent for treatment either with radiation alone or with combined modality therapy. The presence of night sweats alone had no adverse effect on outcome. Among patients treated with radiation alone, there was similar freedom from relapse and overall survival irrespective of whether pelvic irradiation was included in the initial treatment fields. Although combined modality therapy improved the 7-year freedom from relapse when compared with radiotherapy alone (86% versus 74%, $P = 0.02$), overall survival in the two treatment groups was virtually identical (88% and 89%, respectively). It was concluded that the presence of B symptoms is not necessarily a poor prognostic factor in patients with pathologically staged IA–IIB HD, since their overall survival approached that of surgically staged IA–IIA patients.[48] Thus, many patients pathologically staged as having IB–IIB disease can be treated effectively with mantle and para-aortic radiotherapy alone, provided that they do not have both fever and weight loss and/or a large mediastinal mass. This approach spares the patient the additional morbidity of initial combined modality therapy. The presence of a large mediastinal mass in a patient with early-stage HD and B symptoms is associated with a significantly greater risk of relapse, and these patients should received combined modality therapy.

Radiation and Combined Modality Therapy for Large Mediastinal Masses

It is now well recognized that a subgroup of stage I and II patients with large mediastinal masses have a significantly greater risk of relapse than that of patients with little or no mediastinal disease when treated with radiotherapy alone.[26,30,51,52] The most commonly accepted definition of a large mediastinal mass is a mass greater than one-third of the maximal intrathoracic diameter. However, this measurement alone is not a sufficient criterion for selecting which patients should be treated by definitive irradiation alone rather than by combined modality therapy. Other important selection criteria that should be considered in the evaluation of patients with a large mediastinal mass include (1) location of the mass: wide versus long, anterior and superior mediastinum versus mid-mediastinum; (2) involvement of multiple E sites; and (3) estimated volume of normal tissue that would need treatment with shrinking radiation fields. Treatment of all patients with a large medi-

astinal mass with initial radiotherapy alone results in a RFS of approximately 50%. However, in 1990 Hoppe reported a Stanford study[52] of a small series of selected patients with bulky mediastinal disease, who were carefully staged with CT scans to determine tumor volume, and then were laparotomy-staged (some patients were irradiated before surgery). These patients were treated with aggressive mantle radiation, which often included prophylactic treatment to the lungs. This treatment resulted in a 7-year freedom from relapse in 80% of patients and an overall survival of 100%. Careful monitoring of the tumor response during radiotherapy and the use of a shrinking field technique helped the Stanford group keep complications to a minimum. However, radiotherapy alone is inappropriate for most patients with early-stage HD who present with large mediastinal masses. Treatment with initial radiotherapy in these patients often requires extensive irradiation of the heart and lungs in order to include the large mediastinal mass in the radiotherapy port, which causes significant subsequent morbidity.

Although it must be recognized that patients with early-stage HD and large mediastinal masses treated with initial combined modality therapy achieve significantly better freedom from relapse at 10 years (83%) than do those treated by radiotherapy alone (49%), overall survival is virtually identical (82–83%).[30] Despite the similarity in overall survival, most investigators concur that a 50% risk of relapse is too high, and therefore recommend combined modality therapy as the initial approach. Patients treated with radiotherapy alone tend to relapse in the initially irradiated field, as well as in adjacent untreated lymph nodes, while extranodal relapses are seen primarily in the lung.

For patients with large mediastinal masses in whom definitive radiation therapy alone is not considered an acceptable option, owing to the location and size of the mediastinal disease, involvement of contiguous extranodal sites, or the potential morbidity of treating large volumes of normal tissues, a combined modality approach is recommended. In the subgroup of patients who will receive initial combined modality therapy, staging laporatomy is not indicated, and treatment is initiated with one of the currently accepted regimens for advanced disease, such as MOPP/ABVD (Adriamycin, bleomycin, vinblastine, dacarbazine), the MOPP/ABV hybrid, or ABVD alone (Table 79-8). Chemotherapy is given to maximal tumor

Table 79-8. MOPP/ABV(D) Chemotherapy Regimens

MOPP/ABVD[a]
  Month 1
    Nitrogen mustard 6 mg/m² IV, days 1, 8
    Vincristine (Oncovin) 1.4 mg/m² IV, days 1, 8 (max = 2 mg/dose)
    Procarbazine 100 mg/m² PO, days 1–14
    Prednisone 40 mg/m², days 1–14
  Month 2
    Doxorubicin (Adriamycin) 25 mg/m² IV, days 1, 15
    Bleomycin 10 U/m² IV, days 1, 15
    Vinblastine 6 mg/m² IV, days 1, 15
    Dacarbazine 375 mg/m² IV, days 1, 15
      Alternate one cycle of monthly MOPP with one cycle of monthly ABVD

MOPP/ABV hybrid[b]
    Nitrogen mustard 6 mg/m² IV, day 1
    Vincristine (Oncovin) 1.4 mg/m² (max = 2 mg/dose)
    Procarbazine 100 mg/m² PO, days 1–7
    Prednisone 40 mg/m² PO, days 1–14
    Doxorubicin (Adriamycin) 35 mg/m² IV, day 8
    Vinblastine 6 mg/m² IV, day 8
    Bleomycin 10 U/m² IV, day 8
      Repeat every 28 days

[a] Data from Bonadonna.[97]
[b] Data from Klimo and Connors.[102]

response, as judged by chest radiographs and CT scans, after which two additional cycles of consolidation chemotherapy are given. Once maximal benefit from chemotherapy has been obtained, limited radiation therapy (generally to the mediastinum alone or a mantle field) is used. With this combined modality approach, approximately 83% of patients will remain disease free beyond 5 years.[30] The medical and psychological advantage to this approach with its high rate of RFS cannot be underestimated. However, it must be emphasized that the initial treatment of early-stage HD in patients with a large mediastinal mass must be individualized, in view of the potential increase in long-term morbidity after combined modality therapy as compared with radiotherapy alone. The goal is to achieve the highest rate of cure with the least long-term morbidity. One unresolved question is whether patients with stage III and IV disease who have large mediastinal masses at presentation and in whom initial chemotherapy is the treatment of choice should receive consolidation radiotherapy to the mediastinum to decrease the risk of relapse in this one particular site.[53]

It is also important to recognize that most patients with large mediastinal masses treated either with radiation therapy or with radiation plus chemotherapy will have a residual mediastinal abnormality after treatment. Jochelson et al.[54] noted that mediastinal abnormalities were common at the end of radiation or combined modality therapy for HD and that these abnormalities in themselves did not indicate persistent active disease or an increased risk of relapse. Persistent radiologic abnormalities may continue to improve in up to one-half of patients for >1 year after therapy. Biopsy or further treatment is not recommended if these radiographic abnormalities are stable for months after the end of radiotherapy or after two additional cycles of chemotherapy. The use of high-dose gallium scanning in this situation may be particularly helpful, especially if the gallium scan is positive before treatment and reverts to normal following the completion of radiotherapy or combined modality treatment.[55] In young patients (<25 years old), a regenerating thymus during the 6 months after treatment may present as an enlarging anterior mediastinal mass.[29] This can be a diagnostic problem, as this mass may be gallium positive.

Radiation and Combined Modality Therapy for Subdiaphragmatic Early-Stage Disease

HD below the diaphragm is a relatively rare clinical presentation, occurring in <5% of patients. Patients with early-stage subdiaphragmatic presentation tend to be older men with MC pathology.[11,56-57] Overall freedom from relapse and survival are similar to those of patients with supradiaphragmatic presentations, if compared stage for stage.[56-58] However, relapses tend to occur later in subdiaphragmatic presentations.

Lymphography, CT scanning, and staging laporatomy are integral parts of the management of patients with subdiaphragmatic HD disease. Clinically staged I–IIA patients with negative para-aortic nodes on lymphangiogram have only a 10% incidence of splenic involvement at laporatomy, as compared with a 52% incidence of splenic involvement when the para-aortic nodes are positive.[11,56] Thus, for patients with clinical stage I–IIA presentations below the diaphragm, staging laparotomy is indicated with treatment based on the pathologic findings.

The M.D. Anderson group[59] treated 60 patients with infradiaphragmatic presentations. In 22 patients with inguinal/femoral or pelvic disease who were treated with irradiation alone, the 10-year freedom from progression and overall survival were 86% and 90%, respectively. In this retrospective analysis, the small numbers of patients with abdominal disease who were treated with radiotherapy plus MOPP fared better than did similar patients treated with radiotherapy alone.

Patients with subdiaphragmatic pathologic stage IA are gen-

erally treated with inverted Y radiotherapy that includes the splenic pedicle. In patients with pathologic stage IIA and II$_S$A with limited splenic involvement, TNI (including the mediastinum) and combined modality therapy appear to be of comparable efficacy on the basis of limited data.[11,56,59] Patients who received TNI were less likely to relapse above the diaphragm than were patients who did not receive supradiaphragmatic radiation. In these patients, the degree of upper abdominal nodal involvement as well as the extent of splenic involvement helps determine the choice of treatment. For example, in pathologic stage II$_S$A patients with extensive histologic involvement of the spleen, either chemotherapy alone or combined modality therapy is a reasonable option. In patients with subdiaphragmatic clinical stage IIB disease, laparotomy should be omitted, since the risk of splenic disease is extremely high (89%), and management with primary chemotherapy or combined modality therapy is the treatment of choice.

Complications of Radiotherapy

Complications of radiotherapy are related to the technique employed, dosage administered, and irradiated volume.[39] Mantle and para-aortic radiotherapy or TNI is technically difficult and potentially hazardous. The complications of radiation are also directly related to the skill and experience of the radiotherapist. The acute side effects of radiotherapy include transient nausea and vomiting, dysphagia, and marrow suppression. These side effects subside shortly after radiotherapy is completed. Temporary alopecia may be expected in the occipital regions on either side of the mantle field. Late potential side effects of radiation include elevation of thyroid-stimulating hormone in 25–50% and clinical hypothyroidism in 10–20% of patients[60,61]; symptomatic radiation pneumonitis in <5%; transient myelitis (generally manifested as electric-like shocks in limbs on neck flexion, known as Lhermitte sign); and rarely, radiation pericarditis or chronic restrictive fibrosis. Peristent myelosuppression is also a rare late complication. Radiation-induced decrease in bone growth has been noted in children. The evidence suggesting that radiotherapy accelerates coronary artery disease is controversial.[62-64] No significant increase in cardiac-related deaths in HD was noted in one large epidemiologic study.[64] However, the Stanford group reported a 3.2 increased relative risk of death, primarily from late fatal myocardial infarction, in patients treated with radiotherapy.[63] The incidence of second neoplasms following radiotherapy alone or combined modality therapy is discussed in a separate section.

Combined Modality Therapy or Chemotherapy Alone for Early- and Intermediate-Stage Disease

Combinations of radiotherapy and chemotherapy in the treatment of early-stage HD have been used since about 1970, with the goal of increasing the cure rate. It is reasonable to assume that chemotherapy, effective in curing most patients with advanced disease, should be even more effective for subclinical disease that might be present after radiotherapy. Relapses after radiotherapy frequently do so in areas of extranodal disease, while relapses after chemotherapy most frequently occur in sites of pretreatment involvement, including bulky lymph node areas.

Randomized trials conducted at Stanford[33,37] in pathologic stage I–IIA HD demonstrated that adjuvant chemotherapy could replace prophylactic irradiation of areas of occult subclinical disease (Table 79-7). IF radiotherapy followed by MOPP or PAV (phenylalanine mustard, Alkeran, vinblastine) chemotherapy achieved freedom from relapse and overall survival results comparable to those of TNI or STNI.[33,37,65] In a more recent small study from Stanford,[37,66] asymptomatic patients with pathologic stage I and II HD were randomly assigned to involved field radiotherapy plus VBM (vinblastine, bleomycin, methotrexate) chemotherapy versus STNI. Again, there was no difference in either freedom from relapse or overall survival. The VBM combination was empirically developed because of its presumed lower long-term morbidity (i.e., less effect on fertility and lower risk of leukemia). Although less toxic than either adjuvant MOPP or PAV, the VBM combination is untested in large numbers of patients with advanced HD. Greater patient numbers and longer follow-up are needed before it can be concluded that adjuvant VBM chemotherapy plus IF irradiation are an effective alternative to standard radiotherapy with either mantle or mantle and para-aortic fields for favorable presentations of early-stage HD.

Cosset et al.[35] reported the updated EORTC results in clinical stage I–II patients classified as having any one or more of the following unfavorable prognostic factors: B symptoms, age ≥40 years, ESR ≥70, MC or LD histology, and/or clinical stage II with mediastinal involvement. In these patients, laparotomy was not performed. Patients were randomly assigned to either TNI or three cycles of MOPP, followed by mantle radiotherapy and a further three cycles of MOPP (Table 79-7). There was a significant difference in freedom from relapse at 9 years in favor of combined modality treatment (83% versus 66%), but overall survival showed only a borderline advantage for the combined modality patients (Table 79-7). In patients <40 years of age, no difference in long-term survival could be detected between the two forms of treatment.

A second EORTC trial in this unfavorable cohort randomized patients to MOPP for three cycles, mantle radiotherapy, MOPP for three cycles; or to ABVD for three cycles, mantle radiotherapy, ABVD for three cycles. At 5 years, RFS was significantly lower in the MOPP group (79%) than in the ABVD group (89%), but no difference in overall survival was noted (virtually identical at 89%).[35] The M.D. Anderson group[46,67] reported similar results with combined modality therapy using two cycles of MOPP and IF radiotherapy. The obvious conclusion can be drawn that staging laparotomy is unnecessary if combined modality treatment is to be used as initial therapy.

The demonstration of significant activity of MOPP chemotherapy in early-stage disease led to a National Cancer Institute (NCI) pilot study in patients with pathologic stages IB–II and IIIA randomly selected for treatment with EF radiotherapy followed by six cycles of MOPP, as compared with MOPP therapy alone.[68] The small number of patients in each stage precludes definitive conclusions from this study. However, to date, there are no significant differences in either disease-free survival, freedom from relapse, or overall survival among these two groups.

Pavlovsky et al.[69] reported the results of a randomized trial of CVPP (cyclophosphamide, vinblastine, procarbazine, prednisone) chemotherapy for six monthly cycles versus the same chemotherapy plus IF radiotherapy (3,000 cGy) in 277 patients with clinical stage I–II HD (Table 79-7). One or more of the following factors were considered prognostically unfavorable: age >45 years, more than two lymph node areas involved, or bulky disease. In the favorable group without any of these adverse prognostic factors, disease-free survival (77% versus 70%) or overall survival (92% versus 91%) were similar at 7 years for CVPP versus radiotherapy plus CVPP. These results do not represent any advantage over those obtained in comparable series of patients treated with mantle and para-aortic radiotherapy alone. Among patients in the unfavorable prognostic subgroup reported on by Pavlovsky et al.[69] those treated with radiotherapy plus CVPP had a longer disease-free survival (75% versus 34%) and overall survival (84% versus 66%) than experienced by those patients treated with CVPP alone. How-

ever, the results with CVPP chemotherapy alone in this subgroup appear distinctly inferior to those reported in a small series of early stage patients treated with MOPP at the NCI.[70]

Longo et al.[70] recently reported the updated results of a randomized trial of MOPP chemotherapy alone versus mantle and para-aortic radiotherapy in 106 patients with surgically staged IA, IB, IIA, IIB, and III₁A disease (Table 79-7). With a median follow-up of 7.5 years, 96% of MOPP-treated patients achieved complete remission, with 7 (13%) relapses. Of the radiotherapy-treated patients, 96% achieved a complete response, but 17 (35%) relapsed. However, the radiotherapy arm of the study contained more patients with large mediastinal masses than did the chemotherapy arm. Four MOPP-treated patients (7%) and 10 radiotherapy-treated patients (20%) have died. Although the curves of complete response duration significantly favor MOPP, overall survival is not significantly different.[70] When patients with either large mediastinal masses or stage III₁A are excluded from the analysis, there are no significant differences in either disease-free survival (67% for radiation versus 82% for MOPP) or overall survival (85% for radiation versus 90% for MOPP). Patients treated with MOPP had significantly more hospital admissions, episodes of febrile neutropenia, and documented infections and received more blood transfusions. The results from this study do not permit one to conclude that MOPP chemotherapy can be safely substituted for mantle and para-aortic radiotherapy for early-stage HD.

Biti et al.[71] recently updated the results of a small randomized trial comparing MOPP alone with mantle and para-aortic radiotherapy for 89 patients with pathologic stage I–IIA disease (Table 79-7). Complete remission was obtained in all radiotherapy patients compared with 40 of 44 (91%) of the MOPP patients. With a median follow-up of 8 years, overall survival was significantly higher in the radiation therapy group (93%) as compared to 56 percent in the MOPP group ($P < 0.001$), whereas freedom from progression and disease-free survival were similar. Relapsing patients had a much higher salvage rate in the radiotherapy group, reflected in the significantly improved overall survival. True recurrences (in sites of initial presentation) were significantly more frequent in the chemotherapy patients than in those treated with radiotherapy, who relapsed mainly in previously uninvolved sites. In addition, early relapses (within 1 year from the end of treatment) were also more frequent in the chemotherapy group.[72] These data suggest that curative radiotherapy may achieve better local control of HD than does MOPP chemotherapy. Treatment-related complications were more severe in the chemotherapy group.

The treatment of pathologic stage IIIA HD remains controversial. Table 79-9 summarizes the treatment results with either radiotherapy alone (generally mantle or para-aortic irradiation or TNI), combined modality therapy, or chemotherapy alone. The use of combined radiation therapy and chemotherapy is associated with both a lower risk of relapse and improved survival for most patients with stage IIIA disease, as compared with radiation therapy alone.[73,76] However, subsets of stage IIIA disease have been identified that can be treated with either mantle and para-aortic radiotherapy or with TNI alone.[77] Patients with pathologic stage III₁A disease (pathologic involvement of the spleen and/or upper abdominal nodes) and minimal splenic involvement (less than five splenic nodules) can be spared the initial toxicity of combined modality therapy or chemotherapy alone. For this subgroup of patients, mantle and para-aortic irradiation or TNI appears equally effective as an initial treatment, with chemotherapy reserved for those patients who relapse. With this approach, approximately one-third of patients with stage IIIA disease can be spared initial chemotherapy. It must be emphasized that significant differences in freedom from first relapse that favor initial combined modality therapy or chemotherapy alone do not argue for the

Table 79-9. Stage IIIA Hodgkin Disease: Treatment Results

Investigators	Stage	Treatment	FFR (%)	Survival (%)
Stein et al.[73]	III$_1$[a]	XRT	60	76
		CMT	92	88
	III$_2$[b]	XRT	20	41
		CMT	84	84
Mauch et al.[74]	III$_1$	XRT	53	73
		CMT	92	97
	III$_2$	XRT	15	44
		CMT	73	66
Hoppe et al.[76]	III$_1$	XRT	59	91
		CMT	93	89
	III$_2$	XRT	63	83
		CMT	77	90
Mauch et al.[74]	Minimal splenic	XRT	62	100
	involvment[c]	CMT	92	92
	Extensive splenic	XRT	35	58
	involvement[d]	CMT	81	77
Hoppe et al.[76]	Minimal splenic	XRT	80	80
	involvement[e]	CMT	80	85
	Extensive splenic	XRT	30	70
	involvement[d]	CMT	85	85
Henkelmann et al.[79]	III$_1$	MOPP × 2 + STLI/TNI	84	86
Lister et al.[81]	All IIIA	TNI	60	83
		MVPP	85	90
Crowther et al.[82]	All IIIA	MVPP	82	87
		MVPP + XRT	72	84
Santoro et al.[83]	All IIIA	MOPP × 3, XRT, MOPP × 3	65	NS
		ABVD × 3, XRT, ABVD × 3	92	NS

Abbreviations: XRT, radiotherapy (either mantle and para-aortic or TNI); TNI, total nodal irradiation; STLI, subtotal lymphoid irradiation; CMT, combined modality therapy (generally extended field radiotherapy + MOPP); MVPP, nitrogen mustard, vinblastine, procarbazine, prednisone; MOPP, nitrogen mustard, vincristine, procarbazine, prednisone; ABVD, Adriamycin, bleomycin, vinblastine, decarbazine; NS, not stated; FFR, freedom from relapse.

[a] III$_1$, pathologic involvement of any of the following sites: spleen; splenic hilar, celiac, porta hepatis nodes.

[b] III$_2$, pathologic involvement of para-aortic nodes, iliac, or inguinal nodes with or without involvement of the spleen and upper abdominal nodes.

[c] Minimal splenic Involvement: <5 splenic nodules.

[d] Extensive splenic involvement: ≥5 splenic nodules.

use of these modalities unless significant overall survival differences are seen as well.

However, for most patients with stage IIIA disease, combined modality therapy or chemotherapy alone should be used.[29,74,78–79] Patients to be treated in this manner should meet one or more of the following criteria: extensive splenic involvement (more than four splenic nodules); pathologic stage III$_2$A disease; unequivocal evidence of disease below the diaphragm on lymphangiogram and/or CT scan (i.e., clinical stage III$_2$A disease); clinical stage IIIA with large mediastinal masses. When combined modality therapy is used, these patients appear to have improved freedom from relapse and improved overall survival as compared with similar patients treated with TNI alone with chemotherapy reserved for relapse.

Therefore, the most important question pertaining to the treatment of most stage IIIA patients today is whether combined modality therapy is superior to chemotherapy alone. Investigators from the NCI reported a 94% 10-year disease-free survival in a small number of stage IIIA–IVA patients treated with MOPP alone.[80] Lister et al.[81] reported a 10-year freedom

from relapse rate of 85% with MVPP (mechlorethamine, vinblastine, procarbazine, prednisone) chemotherapy alone, as compared with 60% with TNI. However, there were no significant differences in overall survival between these two modalities. Crowther et al.[82] compared MVPP chemotherapy alone with the same chemotherapy regimen plus radiotherapy. There were no significant differences in either disease-free survival or overall survival between these two arms. Thus, it appears that chemotherapy alone is as effective as combined modality therapy for patients with stage IIIA disease who do not fit into the minimal risk group that may be treated with mantle and para-aortic irradiation alone. In view of the higher anticipated complication rate using combined modality therapy, it would appear that chemotherapy alone, using any one of the accepted combinations for advanced disease, is as effective as combined modality therapy for most patients with stage IIIA disease. The minimal risk subgroup of pathologically staged patients with limited splenic involvement and NS/LP histology can be treated with mantle and para-aortic radiation therapy alone; chemotherapy in this subgroup should be reserved for those who relapse. In a small randomized study from Milan of 63 stage IIIA patients treated with three cycles of either MOPP or ABVD followed by extensive irradiation and then in some cases by three additional cycles of the same chemotherapy, the 7-year results indicated both improved complete response rates and freedom from progression with ABVD.[83] Moreover, it was reported that irreversible gonadal dysfunction as well acute leukemia occurred only in patients subjected to MOPP, while cardiopulmonary studies failed to document a significant laboratory difference between the two treatment arms. However, the MOPP and ABVD groups compared in this Milan study did not receive comparable treatment, with only 40% of the MOPP group receiving the planned three postradiotherapy chemotherapy cycles, compared with 80% of the ABVD group.[83,84] However, if confirmed, these results would suggest that ABVD as part of a combined modality therapy program is at least as effective as MOPP, with decreased morbidity.

Patients with clinical or pathologic stage IIIB disease are generally treated with combination chemotherapy alone, as described in subsequent sections. However, selected small series suggest a role for combined modality in these patients. Mauch et al.[74] treated 43 stage IIIB patients with combined modality therapy (IF radiotherapy plus MOPP). At 12 years they observed excellent freedom from relapse (79%) and overall survival (76%). Rosenberg and Kaplan,[33] reporting for the Stanford group, performed a series of prospective trials in pathologic stage IIIB disease, in which, again, small numbers of patients were treated with each combined modality therapy regimen. TNI plus MOPP resulted in only a 51% freedom from progression rate and 52% overall survival at 10 years. The Stanford investigators then proceeded to use two courses of initial chemotherapy, followed by TNI, followed by four cycles of the same chemotherapy (split-course technique). In this series of 42 patients, freedom from relapse of 82% and overall survival of approximately 72% at 8 years were observed.[33] Henkelmann et al.[79] treated 26 patients with pathologic stage III$_1$B disease with two cycles of MOPP and TNI. They reported 78% freedom from progression and 91% overall survival at 10 years. In the randomized study conducted by Santoro et al.,[83] a total of only 28 patients were treated with three cycles of either MOPP or ABVD, followed by EF radiotherapy, and then by three cycles of the same drug regimen. In this series, 78% of IIIB patients achieved complete remission with MOPP, as compared with 94% with ABVD. Freedom from progression also favored the ABVD patients (92% at 7 years), as compared with MOPP (65%).

Although the results with combined modality therapy for stage IIIB disease are impressive in terms of their freedom from progression and overall survival, they do not appear to be significantly different from what can be obtained with today's chemotherapy regimens employing seven or eight drugs (MOPP/ABVD or the MOPP/ABV hybrid regimen). Thus, for the vast majority of patients with stage IIIB disease, chemotherapy alone is recommended as initial treatment.

Chemotherapy of Advanced Disease

Since the late 1960s, a dramatic improvement has been observed in the prognosis of patients with advanced HD resulting from the development of curative combination chemotherapy. Until recently, MOPP represented the standard against which all alternative chemotherapy or combined modality regimens were judged. The landmark studies of DeVita et al.[80,85] at the NCI demonstrated that >50% of patients with advanced HD are cured with chemotherapy alone. A recent update of the NCI data has been reported by Longo et al.[86] who reanalyzed 188 of the original NCI patients after a median of 14 years of follow-up. A complete remission rate of 84% was reported; also, 66% of the complete responders had remained disease-free for >10 years. Thus, 54% of patients were continuously free of disease, and 48% were alive between 9 and 21 years from the end of treatment. It is important to note that 19% of the complete responders died of intercurrent illnesses while free of HD.

The major factors adversely affecting complete response rate in the NCI MOPP trials were B symptoms, male sex, advanced-stage disease, and lower than projected rate of vincristine administration.[86] The most important factors predicting duration of complete response were B symptoms, age, rapidity of complete response (patients requiring five cycles or less had significantly longer remissions), number of extranodal sites of disease, and liver or pleural involvement. Maintenance chemotherapy after achieving complete remission had no influence on either disease-free or overall survival. The following are among the major considerations in the administration of MOPP at the NCI that have been emphasized by DeVita et al.,[42]: (1) MOPP is given for a minimum of six cycles or to complete remission plus two cycles; (2) dose intensity is emphasized, with administration of drugs on schedule using a sliding scale for dose adjustment; (3) vincristine is administered at 1.4 mg/m^2; (4) arbitrary dose modifications to circumvent manageable toxic effects such as nausea and vomiting are not allowed; (5) actual body weight is used in calculation of body surface area; (6) drugs are not arbitrarily omitted from the combination; and (7) rounding of drug doses to fit either procarbazine capsule size or reduction of intravenous drug doses to arbitrarily conform to a certain size of vial is not allowed.

The importance of administering full doses of MOPP in a timely fashion has been stressed by DeVita et al.,[42,85] as well as by Carde et al.,[87] and failure to do so may account for the disparate MOPP results reported in the literature by other authors. The NCI investigators concluded that the dose intensity of vincristine (but not of any of the other drugs) together with B symptoms predicted a significantly higher complete remission rate.[42,85] Although the NCI group administered vincristine at 1.4 mg/m^2, virtually all other trials limit the dose of vincristine to 2.0 mg. Thus, the optimal dose of vincristine remains an open question, but it is unlikely to be the subject of a prospective trial. Carde et al.[87] concluded that the geometric mean of nitrogen mustard, vincristine, and procarbazine were significantly associated with attainment of complete remission. In a report by van Rijswijk et al.,[88] the total dose of nitrogen mustard was significantly associated with complete remission and overall survival. However, Pillai et al.,[89] from M.D. Anderson Hospital, found no influence of dose or dose intensity on the complete remission rate of stage IV patients treated with MOPP. All the above studies were retrospective analyses, and there is no controlled trial that prospectively tests the concept of dose intensity in HD. Moreover, dose intensity of MOPP may

now be an outdated research issue, since current chemotherapy programs use seven or more drugs, with improved results.

In the NCI MOPP trials, most patients required six cycles of chemotherapy, but approximately 20–25% of patients required two or more additional cycles. Restaging studies were generally performed after the fourth cycle, and if they were negative, two more cycles were administered. However, if continued tumor response was observed between cycles 4 and 6, two additional cycles of chemotherapy were administered followed by repeat staging studies.[29] Thus, it is current practice to administer six to eight cycles of chemotherapy, using the general guideline of treating to clinical or pathologic complete response plus two additional cycles. In the case of a stable residual mass that is unchanged by radiography or CT scan after two or more additional cycles of chemotherapy, the patient is classified as a clinical complete responder and chemotherapy is stopped. Further evidence for complete response in this situation is gained if the tumor mass went from gallium scan-positive before chemotherapy to gallium scan-negative after chemotherapy. These same principles apply to the duration of therapy for the newer seven and eight drug combinations described later in this section.

The NCI MOPP trials and subsequent studies over the next decade continued to use the end points of complete response, disease-free survival, and overall survival as measures of efficacy. However, determination of complete response may be difficult and ambiguous in the setting of advanced HD. This is particularly true in bulky disease, where a residual mass on radiography is frequently observed after six to eight cycles of combination chemotherapy. Disease-free survival refers only to patients who achieve a complete remission and does not reflect the outcome of the whole population of patients treated. Moreover, some investigators censor out patients who die from causes other than HD from their disease-free survival curves, artificially improving their results. Therefore, the most accurate and definitive end point for determining the effectiveness of any chemotherapy regimen is failure-free survival, also referred to as freedom from progression. Failure-free survival is defined for the entire group of patients treated and therefore counts as an event the following parameters: progressive disease, relapse from complete or partial remission, and death from any cause. Overall survival remains the most important end point and reflects not only the effectiveness of the primary chemotherapy regimen but also the efficacy of any secondary or salvage treatments.

Although MOPP revolutionized the treatment of advanced HD, there is ample opportunity for improvement in these results, since ≥15–30% of patients do not achieve initial complete remission, and 30–40% of complete responders eventually relapse. While multiple studies with MOPP confirmed its efficacy in the treatment of advanced HD, numerous investigators attempted to design alternative combinations aimed at improving the therapeutic index of MOPP by reducing toxicity and attempting to improve the cure rate. These trials are described in detail in several reviews,[29,42,90] and selected alternative chemotherapy regimens are listed in Table 79-10. For example, the BCVPP regimen adds BCNU, while substituting cyclophosphamide for nitrogen mustard and vinblastine for vincristine. In a prospective controlled trial conducted by the Eastern Cooperative Oncology Group (ECOG), Bakemeier et al.[91] compared BCVPP directly with MOPP. Although the complete response rates were virtually identical, the duration of complete response and the overall survival of the complete responders were significantly longer with BCVPP. Moreover, despite inclusion of the additional myelosuppressive agent BCNU, there were no significant differences in hematologic toxicity. Both severe and life-threatening neurotoxicity and gastrointestinal toxicity were significantly reduced on the BCVPP arm. Report-

Table 79-10. Chemotherapy Regimens for Advanced Hodgkin Disease

MOPP (NCI)
Nitrogen mustard 6 mg/m² IV, days 1, 8
Vincristine (Oncovin) 1.4 mg/m² IV, days 1, 8
Procarbazine 100 mg/m² PO, days 1–14
Prednisone 40 mg/m² PO, days 1–14

MVPP
Nitrogen mustard 6 mg/m² IV, days 1, 8
Vinblastine 10 mg days 1, 8, 15
Procarbazine 100 mg/m², days 1–15
Prednisone 40 mg PO, days 1–15

LOPP (BNLI)
Chlorambucil 10 mg/day PO, days 1–10
Vincristine (Oncovin) 1.4 mg/m² IV, days 1, 8 (max 2 mg/dose)
Procarbazine 100 mg/m² PO, days 1–10
Prednisone 25 mg/m² PO, days 1–14

CVPP
Cyclophosphamide 300 mg/m² IV, days 1, 8
Vinblastine 10 mg IV, days 1, 8, 15
Procarbazine 100 mg/m² PO, days 1–14
Prednisone 40 mg/m² PO, days 1–14

BCVPP
BCNU 100 mg/m² IV, day 1
Cyclophosphamide 600 mg/m² IV, day 1
Vinblastine 5 mg/m² IV, day 1
Procarbazine 100 mg/m² PO, days 1–10
Prednisone 60 mg/m² PO, days 1–10

ChlVPP
Chlorambucil 6 mg/m² PO, days 1–14 (max 10 mg/day)
Vinblastine 6 mg/m² IV, days 1–8 (max 10 mg/dose)
Procarbazine 100 mg/m² PO days 1–14 (max 150 mg/day)
Prednisone 40 mg/m² PO, days 1–4

ABVD
Doxorubicin (Adriamycin) 25 mg/m² IV, days 1, 15
Bleomycin 10 U/m² IV, days 1, 15
Vinblastine 6 mg/m² IV, days 1, 15
Dacarbazine 375 mg/m² IV, days 1, 15

CEP
CCNU 80 mg/m² PO, day 1
Etoposide (VP-16) 100 mg/m², days 1–5
Prednimustine 60 mg/m², days 1–5

EVA
Etoposide (VP-16) 100 mg/m²/day IV, days 1–3
Vinblastine 6 mg/m³ IV day 1
Doxorubicin (Adriamycin) 50 mg/m² IV, day 1

CBV
Cyclophosphamide 1.5 g/m²/day, IV, days 1–4
Carmustine (BCNU) 300 mg/m² IV, day 1
Etoposide (VP-16) 125 mg/m² IV bid × 6 doses, days 1–3

High-dose CBV
Cyclophosphamide 1.8 g/m²/day IV, days 1–4
Carmustine (BCNU) 600 mg/m² IV, day 1
Etoposide (VP-16) 400 mg/m² IV bid × 6 doses, days 1–3

---

ing for the Southeast Oncology Group, Gams et al.[92] achieved similar results with BCVPP.

Several other alternatives to MOPP that are considered useful under specific circumstances emerged during the mid- to late 1970s. The MVPP combination substitutes vinblastine for vincristine (Oncovin) and has been used for patients who cannot tolerate the neurotoxicity of vincristine.[93] The LOPP regimen substitutes chlorambucil (Leukeran) for nitrogen mustard. A controlled trial compared LOPP with MOPP and achieved equivalent results with less toxicity for LOPP.[94] However, the results with both arms are inferior to other reports. The ChlVPP protocol[95,96] substitutes chlorambucil for mustard

and vinblastine for vincristine. Nausea, vomiting, and neurotoxicity are substantially reduced with ChlVPP, which makes it a valuable regimen, particularly for elderly patients. Selby et al.[95] updated the British experience with ChlVPP in 229 previously untreated patients, 85% of whom entered complete remission. The disease-free survival of complete responders was 71% at 10 years, and the 10-year overall survival for all patients was 65%. Acute toxicity was mild, and the 10-year actuarial risk of leukemia was 2.7%. Reporting for four research groups that pooled their data on the use of ChlVPP, Anderson et al.[96] observed an 89% and 72% complete response rate in stage IIIA and IIIB/IV patients, respectively. Failure-free survival and overall survival at 5 years were 67% and 78%, respectively, for the stage IIIA patients. For the IIIB/IV group, 5-year failure-free survival was 51%, and 5-year overall survival was 63%. Patients aged ≥50 years with all stages of disease did especially poorly on ChlVPP therapy, making this less toxic regimen much less useful in the older age population.[96] Although the BCVPP, MVPP, and ChlVPP regimens are attractive alternatives to MOPP, these combinations are generally no longer recommended as initial therapy, because more recent trials have demonstrated the superiority of seven- or eight-drug combinations (e.g., MOPP/ABVD), or ABVD alone, as described below. However, if MOPP is administered strictly according to NCI guidelines, this regimen remains an option for selected patients, who might not be able to tolerate Adriamycin and bleomycin, for example.

The identification of the ABVD regimen as an active non-cross-resistant combination in relapsed HD led to the investigation of this new and important regimen in the previously untreated patient. In the original comparison of MOPP and ABVD as initial treatment,[97] the complete response rate with MOPP was 63%, as compared with 72% with ABVD. In addition, disease-free and overall survival were similar. Bonadonna et al.[98] then proceeded with a controlled randomized trial in which 88 patients with stage IV HD previously untreated by chemotherapy were treated in a 12-month cycle with either MOPP alone or MOPP alternating every month with ABVD (Table 79-11). Although the complete remission rate with MOPP/ABVD was 89% compared with 74% with MOPP, this difference was not statistically significant, undoubtedly because of the small number of patients entered onto this trial. The 8-year actuarial results also indicated that MOPP/ABVD was superior to MOPP in terms of freedom from progression (64% vs 36%, respectively) as well as disease-free survival of the complete responders (73% vs 45%). Tumor mortality (only deaths from HD included) was also significantly reduced on the MOPP/ABVD arm. However, the overall survival (including deaths from all causes) at 8 years is 76% on MOPP/ABVD versus 62% on MOPP. This difference is not statistically significant, but again this may be due to the small sample size in this study. Favorable prognostic factors in this trial include the fact that 28% of patients relapsed after radiotherapy alone and 30% were asymptomatic. Although this study has been criticized for the lower-than-expected freedom from progression and disease-free survival in the MOPP alone arm, it is interesting to note that there are no differences in the overall survival rate between MOPP results seen in this study and the MOPP results from the NCI. However, a larger patient population and confirmatory clinical trials were clearly required before the apparent superiority of MOPP/ABVD could be accepted.

Two confirmatory trials have now been completed, and the results have been reported (Table 79-11). Canellos et al.[99] recently described the 5-year results of the Cancer and Acute Leukemia Group B (CALGB) controlled trial comparing MOPP, ABVD, and MOPP/ABVD in 361 eligible patients with HD stage III₂A–IVB. Patients received a minimum of six cycles of treatment with either MOPP or ABVD, which included two additional cycles after complete remission was obtained; MOPP/ABVD pa-

Table 79-11. Chemotherapy for Advanced Hodgkin Disease

Group	Regimen	N[a]	CR (%)	FFS (%)	OS (%)	Median Follow-Up (yr)
NCI–US[86]	MOPP	188	84	(55)	48	14
Milan[98]	MOPP	43	74	36	64	8
	vs MOPP/ABVD	45	89	65[b]	84[b]	
ECOG[100]	BCVPP ± RT	130	69	47	63	6
	vs MOPP/ABVD	98	80[b]	59[b]	73[b]	
CALGB[99]	MOPP	123	67	50	66	5
	vs ABVD	115	82[b]	61[b]	73	
	vs MOPP/ABVD	123	83[b]	65[b]	75	
Intergroup[105]	MOPP → ABVD	315	75	59	78	4.3
	vs MOPP/ABV hybrid	327	84[b]	69[b]	84[b]	
NCI Canada[106]	MOPP/ABVD ± RT	141	82	70	84	4
	vs MOPP/ABV hybrid ± RT	146	85	75	84	
Milan[107]	MOPP/ABVD	(150)	89	64	79	4
	vs MOPP/ABVD hybrid	(150)	88	69	79	

Abbreviations: N, number of eligible patients; CR, complete response rate; FFS, failure-free survival for all eligible patients entered in study; OS, overall survival for all patients; RT, radiotherapy. See Tables 79-9 and 79-10 for definitions and doses of the chemotherapy regimens.

[a] Numbers shown in parentheses had to be estimated from the original report.

[b] $P \leq 0.05$ for the comparison of the experimental arm compared with the MOPP-type regimen.

(Data from Connors.[104])

tients received 6 cycles of each combination for a total of 12 cycles. While this study has been criticized for the reduced doses of MOPP administered, doses were adjusted on the basis of observed toxicity and were not arbitrarily reduced. The complete response rate for MOPP/ABVD was 83%, compared with 67% for MOPP. However, the complete response rate for ABVD of 82% was similar to that with MOPP/ABVD. With a median follow-up of >4 years, these data have been reported in terms of 5-year actuarial results. Failure-free survival reported with MOPP/ABVD (65%) was significantly improved as compared with MOPP (50%) but was similar to that obtained with ABVD alone (61%). The overall 5-year survival for the treatment groups was similar and was not statistically significant: MOPP 66%, ABVD 73%, and MOPP/ABVD 75%. To date there is no advantage of MOPP/ABVD over ABVD alone. However, it would be premature to accept ABVD alone as an acceptable alternative for the initial treatment of advanced HD on the basis of this study alone, since a relatively small number of patients were treated with only ABVD. The ABVD regimen is theoretically attractive because of its relative lack of gonadal toxicity and induction of acute leukemia. The short follow-up and lack of long-term toxicity data also indicate that the ABVD regimen deserves further investigation. However, on the question of MOPP/ABVD versus MOPP, the CALGB trial clearly shows the superiority of MOPP/ABVD.

The ECOG compared the MOPP/ABVD regimen with BCVPP alone and with BCVPP followed by low-dose consolidation radiotherapy administered to sites of pretreatment involvement in patients achieving a complete response.[100] In this protocol, each of the three chemotherapy regimens was administered for a minimum of eight cycles (or to complete response plus two cycles). Since there were no differences in complete response rate, failure-free survival, or overall survival at 6 years between the two BCVPP arms, they have been combined and compared directly with MOPP/ABVD. The complete response rate on MOPP/ABVD of 80% was significantly better than the 69% complete response rate on the combined BCVPP arms. Although there are no significant differences in complete response duration, both failure-free survival and overall survival were significantly improved on MOPP/ABVD. At 6 years, the failure-free survival on MOPP/ABVD was 59% versus 47% on the combined BCVPP arms. At 6 years, 73% of the MOPP/ABVD patients were alive, compared with 63% of those receiving either of the BCVPP regimens. Importantly, the MOPP/ABVD data from ECOG[100] are virtually identical to those reported by

CALGB[99] and by Bonadonna et al[98] All three of these prospectively randomized trials provide strong evidence of the superiority of MOPP/ABVD over MOPP.

The MOPP/ABVD regimen was based on clinical empiricism (i.e., the therapeutic limitations of MOPP and the apparent effectiveness of ABVD as salvage therapy in MOPP-refractory patients) and preceded the mathematical model proposed by Goldie and Coldman.[101] The Goldie-Coldman hypothesis predicts that the efficacy of treatment will be enhanced by the earliest introduction of the most rapid alternation of all active single agents in a chemotherapy regimen to decrease drug resistance. Klimo and Connors[102–104] reported the updated results of a MOPP/ABV hybrid regimen (Tables 79-8 and 79-11) designed to test the Goldie-Coldman hypothesis prospectively. In this regimen, decarbazine is omitted, the Adriamycin dose is increased, prednisone is administered for 14 days, and MOPP is given on day 1, while ABV is given on day 8. Treatment is administered for a minimum of six courses of therapy, with patients in complete remission at that time receiving two additional courses. In patients who have a partial response limited to a single nodal area, local radiotherapy is administered, while for more extensive residual disease further MOPP/ABV is given. In the original report, of the 76 evaluable patients, 97.5% achieved complete remission, 84% on chemotherapy alone and 13% with IF radiotherapy. In Connors and Klimo's 1988 report,[103] only seven patients (9.5%) relapsed, most of these patients being males with large mediastinal masses and B symptoms. Actuarial RFS of the 74 complete responders was 94% with a median follow-up of almost 4 years; overall survival for all patients was 79%. The toxicity of this regimen was acceptable, with only one death from toxic effects and <10% of patients requiring hospitalization for a suspected or proven systemic infection. The impressive results from this regimen are the best reported to date by a single institution in the treatment of advanced HD. However, 40% of patients in this study were asymptomatic, 17% had stage II disease, and the very high complete response rate includes patients who received radiotherapy for residual disease. Nonetheless, the results with the MOPP/ABV hybrid regimen, if confirmed, represented a potential increase in the cure rate for advanced HD. In addition, it remained to be determined whether the MOPP/ABV hybrid was equivalent or superior to alternating monthly MOPP/ABVD.

Three confirmatory trials have now been reported (Table 79-11). The Intergroup trial led by ECOG compared the MOPP/ABV hybrid regimen to sequential MOPP followed by ABVD, in which MOPP alone is administered to the point of complete remission or stable partial response followed by three cycles of ABVD in consolidation.[105] No radiotherapy was administered in either arm of the Intergroup trial. The complete response rate on the MOPP/ABV hybrid was 84%, compared with 75% on the sequential regimen ($P < 0.01$) (Glick JH, personal communication). The 5-year failure-free survival of 69% on the hybrid program was also superior to the 59% 5-year FFS on the sequential arm ($P = 0.002$). Moreover, the 5-year overall survival of 84% on the MOPP/ABV hybrid was significantly better than the 78% overall survival on the sequential MOPP followed by ABVD ($P < 0.02$). In the poor prognostic subgroup of patients who were either >40 years old and/or who had stage IV disease, the MOPP/ABV hybrid also achieved significantly improved 5-year failure-free and overall survival. There was no difference in the incidence of severe or very severe leukopenia between the two arms, while significantly more patients on the sequential MOPP/ABV arm had thrombocytopenia. Infectious and pulmonary complications were greater on the hybrid arm, while there was no difference in neurotoxicity. Thus, the Intergroup trial provides definitive evidence for the superiority of MOPP/ABV hybrid over MOPP, even when MOPP is augmented by ABVD given as late consolidation to complete responders.

The NCI of Canada compared the MOPP/ABV hybrid regimen with Bonadonna's alternating monthly MOPP/ABVD, with radiotherapy administered in both arms to selected patients with residual nodal disease. The complete response rates were similar: 85% on the hybrid and 82% on MOPP/ABVD.[104,106] At 4 years, the FFS for both regimens is not different (Table 79-11). This important trial demonstrates the equivalence of the MOPP/ABV hybrid regimen and alternating monthly MOPP/ABVD. In an earlier report from the NCI of Milan, Viviani et al.[107] also compared alternating half-cycles of MOPP and ABVD with their original MOPP/ABVD program and found no significant differences between these two eight-drug regimens.

Thus, the results from the randomized prospective controlled trials of CALGB,[99] ECOG,[100] Intergroup,[105] and NCI of Milan[98,107] all confirm the superiority of MOPP/ABV ± D (decarbazine) over MOPP or MOPP-type chemotherapy alone. The preliminary results from the recent NCI of Canada and Milan trials show that the MOPP/ABV hybrid and alternating monthly MOPP/ABVD regimens appear equivalent. It remains to be determined whether ABVD alone as initial therapy is equivalent to either of these seven- or eight-drug chemotherapy combinations. This question will be answered by the current Intergroup trial, which compares ABVD to the MOPP/ABV hybrid program.

Since it is well known that most relapses following chemotherapy for advanced HD occur in nodal sites, other investigators have evaluated the additive role of low-dose radiotherapy administered following chemotherapy to sites of pretreatment involvement. Prosnitz et al.[108] updated their combined modality results for 102 previously untreated patients with stage IIIB–IV disease and for 82 patients who relapsed after initial treatment with radiotherapy. During the initial years of their studies, induction chemotherapy with MVVPP (mechlorethamine, vincristine, vinblastine, procarbazine, prednisone) for 6 months was followed by low-dose radiotherapy (1,500–2,500 cGy) to all disease sites present prior to chemotherapy. Subsequently, induction chemotherapy for poor-risk advanced-stage patients was changed to MOPP/ABVD and ultimately to a randomization between MVVPP and MOPP. The results of the three induction chemotherapy regimens were similar. The overall complete response rate was 82%, with a 5-year RFS of 70%. However, the 15-year actuarial overall survival of all treated patients was 54%, which is not significantly different from that reported by the NCI for MOPP alone. Of the 184 patients, 17 died of causes other than HD, 11 with secondary malignancies.[108]

ECOG attempted to reproduce the results reported by Prosnitz et al. in two separate controlled studies, reported by Glick et al.[100,109,110] In the first of these trials, sequential bleomycin-MOPP (Bleo-MOPP) followed by ABVD was compared with the same induction chemotherapy with Bleo-MOPP followed by low-dose radiotherapy administered according to the technique used by Prosnitz et al. The overall complete response rate in both arms was identical (75%), but the 8-year freedom from progression on the sequential Bleo-MOPP/ABVD arm was 62%, compared with 44% on the Bleo-MOPP/radiotherapy arm.[110] This difference is statistically significant. In addition, the 8-year overall survival rate of 78% for all patients on the sequential Bleo-MOPP/ABVD arm was significantly better than that achieved on the radiotherapy arm (65%). These results were not known at the time a second ECOG study was initiated in 1981. The Prosnitz radiotherapy technique was again used in an ECOG protocol in which alternating monthly MOPP/ABVD was compared with BCVPP alone or followed by low-dose radiotherapy. Again, no differences in complete response rates, disease-free survival, or overall survival were noted in the two BCVPP arms.[100] Thus, two large-scale randomized trials have failed to confirm any benefit for administration of low-dose radiotherapy to sites of pretreatment involvement once a complete remission has been obtained with chemotherapy. Straus and associates[111] also reported no advantage to adding low-dose radiotherapy to involved sites to a regimen of either MOPP/ABVD or MOPP/ABVD/CAD (CCNU, phenylalanine mustard, vindesine). Although this trial was not randomized, the authors concluded that disease-free and overall survival were similar to those reported for MOPP alone.

Thus, MOPP or its variants can no longer be considered standard initial therapy for advanced HD. Outside the context of a clinical trial, either MOPP/ABVD or the MOPP/ABV hybrid regimen should be used as first-line therapy for advanced HD. The use of ABVD alone is intriguing because of its apparently reduced long-term toxicity, but the data with ABVD are preliminary. The current Intergroup trial comparing ABVD alone with the MOPP/ABV hybrid will ultimately determine the role of ABVD as initial therapy.

Salvage Therapy for Advanced Disease

The choice of salvage therapy for HD relapsing after initial treatment is one of the most difficult challenges and must be individualized to the clinical circumstances of the relapse. Four broad categories of treatment failures after initial therapy have been identified: (1) patients with early-stage disease relapsing from primary radiotherapy; (2) patients whose initial complete response to front-line chemotherapy lasted >1 year; (3) patients whose initial complete response to chemotherapy lasted <1 year; and (4) patients who fail to achieve a complete remission with initial chemotherapy. The treatment of choice for the first category is one of the accepted chemotherapy regimens used as initial treatment for stage III or IV disease. Thus, ABVD, MOPP/ABVD or the MOPP/ABV hybrid regimen should be used in full doses with the realistic expectation of achieving complete response rates, failure-free survival, and overall survival as good as, or better than, that achieved with initial chemotherapy for stage IIIB and IV disease. Although the risk of significant myelosuppression is recognized under these circumstances, salvage chemotherapy results in the cure of ≥50% of patients who relapse after radiotherapy alone.[42,112] As the risk of secondary leukemia will approach 10% at 10 years in patients receiving MOPP salvage regimens, ABVD may represent an attractive alternative. However, patients relapsing after receiving mantle radiotherapy may experience an increased risk of cardiac or pulmonary toxicity when ABVD is used alone as a salvage treatment. Therefore, close cardiac and pulmonary monitoring is warranted.

Even for patients whose initial complete response to chemotherapy lasted >1 year, retreatment with the same or a crossover regimen (e.g., MOPP treated patients receiving MOPP a second time or crossing over to ABVD at relapse) will result in a durable remission in only one-third or less of cases.[113–119] The NCI recently updated their experience using retreatment with MOPP in patients with recurrent HD who had previously achieved complete remission with the same initial chemotherapy.[113] Among patients with long initial remissions (>1 year), RFS at 10 years was 45%, but the development of second neoplasms and other treatment-related mortality reduced the overall survival to 24%. Among patients with a short (<1-year) initial remission, only 11% survived >10 years. The recently published follow-up results from the Milan group on long-term salvage therapy with ABVD are similar to the NCI data.[114] Those patients whose initial response to chemotherapy lasted <1 year or who fail to achieve a complete response with initial chemotherapy represent a very poor risk group. Although complete response rates ranging from 13–72% have been reported with a variety of standard dose salvage regimens, prolonged disease-free survival is achieved in significantly <20% of patients.[113–119]

High-dose combination chemotherapy with autologous bone marrow or peripheral stem cell transplantation (ASCT), or both, has become the standard salvage approach for most patients relapsing after initial chemotherapy. This recommendation is based on (1) high rates of durable complete remission with ASCT regimens; (2) low rates of morbidity and mortality in selected patients with the availability of growth factors to hasten nadir myelosuppression recovery; and (3) poor outcomes in most patients treated with standard-dose salvage chemotherapy regimens.

ASCT in relapsed or refractory HD has several technical components that can influence outcome. These include timing of the intervention (second or later relapse); type of stem cell rescue product (bone marrow or peripheral blood stem cells, or rarely allogeneic bone marrow); type of cytoreductive induction chemotherapy prior to ASCT to demonstrate chemoresponsive disease (e.g., MOPP or ABVD-like regimens, or ifosfamide/cisplatin-based regimens); type of preparative regimen (e.g., CBV [cyclophosphamide, BCNU, VP-16]; BEAM [BCNU, VP-16, cytosine arabinoside, melphalan]; or VP-16, melphalan); the use of consolidative irradiation; and the use of growth factors and other supportive care measures.

The compiled results of ASCT reveal complete response rates of 34–80% with median progression-free survivals for all patients of 12–24 months.[120,121] Prognostic factors include performance status, number of prior chemotherapy regimens, disease sites, and remission status at ASCT. Using CBV with autologous bone marrow, Jagannath et al.[122] reported an overall complete response rate of 47% with an additional 10% achieving complete remission after local radiotherapy to sites of residual disease. With a minimum follow-up of 2 years and a median follow-up of nearly 3 years, 23 patients (38%) were alive and free of disease. Patients with no adverse risk factors and/or those given intensification treatment with CBV and ASCT while their HD was still responding to conventional chemotherapy achieved a complete remission rate of 63%, with ≥77% of these patients projected to be alive at 3 years. This regimen of CBV chemotherapy produced severe myelosuppression; also reported were four treatment-related deaths (7%). Other investigators have used different intensive preparative chemotherapy regimens with or without IF radiotherapy and have also reported prolonged disease-free survival in relapsed disease.[123–128]

Armitage et al.[125] and Kessinger et al.[126] have reported the results of the Nebraska ASCT experience and identified the number of prior chemotherapy regimens (two or fewer versus three or more) and the absence of bone marrow disease as important prognostic variables in predicting significantly im-

proved survival. Complete remission rates (82%, 58%, 45%) and disease-free survival at 4 years (44%, 33%, 21%) significantly favored patients who had failed one (17 patients), two (24 patients), or three or more (29 patients) chemotherapy regimens, respectively.[125] This same group has recently reported their results of ASCT in 84 patients in first relapse of HD.[128] Complete remission was achieved in 63% with an overall failure-free survival of 43% at 4 years. The 4-year failure-free survival was 35% for patients relapsing at <18 months after initial diagnosis compared to 57% for those with a relapse of >18 months after diagnosis. An early death was reported in 4% of patients. It was concluded that ASCT should be considered in any patient relapsing after initial chemotherapy, regardless of the remission duration.

However, the Milan group has reported their experience with standard combination chemotherapy (CEP [CCNU, VP-16, prednimustine]) or retreatment with the initial regimen in 27 patients relapsing at >12 months after initial chemotherapy complete remission.[129,130] Second complete remission was achieved in 85% and, at 5 years, the freedom from progression was 46%, with overall survival of 61%. These results appear to compare favorably with that of ASCT in second remission and further challenge the question of ASCT timing. A new salvage chemotherapy regimen of EVA (VP-16, vinblastine, and doxorubicin) has also shown significant activity in recurrent HD, but the follow-up evaluation is short.[131] Thirty-five patients who were refractory (10 patients) or in relapse (25 patients) following MOPP as the only prior therapy were treated. The complete response rate was 41% and the 2-year FFS was 38%; 2-year overall survival was 47%.

Thus, the treatment of choice for patients failing to achieve complete remission with initial chemotherapy alone or relapsing after a short initial complete remission is high-dose chemotherapy (e.g., CBV) plus ASCT. Since CBV plus ASCT appears to be more effective in a setting of low-volume chemotherapy-responsive disease, it would appear that the optimal approach to these subgroups of patients would be to use a conventional-dose chemotherapy regimen to maximum clinical response (with or without involved field radiotherapy to the sites of residual disease) before employing CBV or another preparative regimen and ASCT. With this approach, a significant survival advantage and a realistic increase in the long-term cure rate may be expected. It remains to be determined whether high-dose chemotherapy plus ASCT should be used as consolidative therapy in patients whose initial complete response to chemotherapy lasted >1 year and who have then relapsed but achieved a second complete remission. This is because prospective comparative trials of ASCT in second remission versus standard combination chemotherapy have not been performed, retrospective series of standard chemotherapy demonstrate durable remissions in up to one-third of patients, and newer standard dose regimens appear to have even greater remission durability (e.g., CEP and EVA).

Although salvage chemotherapy with non-cross-resistant regimens, combined modality therapy, or high-dose chemotherapy with ASCT is generally recommended for relapse from a chemotherapy-induced complete remission, extended-field radiotherapy alone may be curative in a small subset of this population. Several retrospective and selected series have been reported,[132,133] from which it has been concluded that comprehensive salvage radiotherapy is of benefit for patients who have long disease-free intervals after initial chemotherapy and who have relapsed only in nodal sites without systemic dissemination of their disease. High-dose extended-field radiotherapy in this situation generally included the areas of nodal recurrence as well as covering adjacent nodal sites in the same manner as would be used in treating patients with early-stage HD. Therefore, most patients received either mantle and para-aortic radiotherapy or TNI. All patients in these trials had relapsed or had failed to obtain a complete remission after combination chemotherapy. The 5-year disease-free survival in these three series ranged from 25% to 48%, and the 5-year overall survival ranged from 30% to 70%.[131-133] These results are not significantly different from those obtained with salvage chemotherapy alone in patients who had had a complete remission of >1 year with initial chemotherapy. However, for selected patients with nodal disease at recurrence, who have had prolonged initial remission with chemotherapy and for whom either salvage chemotherapy with a non-cross-resistant regimen or high-dose cytoreductive chemotherapy plus ASCT is not an option, extended-field radiotherapy alone may be curative.

Complications of Chemotherapy

A major complication of combination chemotherapy is bone marrow suppression, with increased risk of infection and, rarely, hemorrhage. Peripheral blood counts are monitored carefully during chemotherapy, and drug doses are adjusted according to the degree of myelosuppression. As a cautionary note, drug dose reductions made simply for the purpose of decreasing subjective toxicity are inappropriate. Significant myelosuppression is seen with all the chemotherapy regimens commonly used for advanced disease or as part of combined modality programs.

Treatment-induced sterility, more commonly seen in males, is a frequent and permanent side effect of chemotherapy. This is of particular importance because long-term survival is observed in most patients treated for advanced disease with combination chemotherapy. Irreversible sterility in males after treatment with MOPP and MOPP-like regimens has been reported in a high percentage of patients, regardless of age, whereas drug-induced ovarian failure among females resulting in premature menopause is much more common in older patients.[134,135] The ABVD combination produces significantly less infertility than does MOPP.[83]

The incidence of congestive heart failure does not appear to be significantly increased with ABVD, but the dose of Adriamycin is frequently limited to ≤ 300 mg/m^2. Patients treated with ABVD and mantle radiotherapy have a significantly higher incidence of post-irradiation paramediastinal fibrosis; persistent dyspnea on exertion has been observed in a small number of these patients at ≤ 3 years after completion of therapy.[83] Significant nausea and vomiting occur with MOPP and with the MOPP-like and ABVD regimens. These drug programs often produce serious psychological problems that require effective counseling as well as antiemetic agents. Mild to moderate peripheral neuropathy is commonly seen with vincristine, but paresthesias are not an indication to reduce drug doses. Aseptic necrosis of the femoral heads and rarely, the humeral heads, is an unusual late complication related to corticosteroid therapy.[39]

Second Primary Neoplasms

Patients cured of HD are at an increased risk of the development of second primary cancers. The most widely reported neoplasm is acute myeloid leukemia, generally thought to result from combination chemotherapy or from treatment with both chemotherapy and radiation. An increased risk of solid tumors, usually attributed to irradiation, is emerging as a significant problem, as patients cured of HD are being followed for longer times.[37]

Tester et al.[136] reviewed the NCI experience in 473 previously untreated patients, among whom 34 subsequent second malignant neoplasms were observed. At 10 years of follow-up, these investigators reported no increased risk of the development of leukemia in patients treated with radiotherapy alone. The estimated risk of leukemia following MOPP chemotherapy alone was 2%, and that following initial planned combined radiotherapy and MOPP chemotherapy was 6%, increasing to 9% in patients treated initially with radiotherapy who received MOPP chemotherapy at relapse. The 10-year estimated risk of solid tumors was 7% overall, with all treatment groups having similar risks. In contrast to other reports,[137] a greater risk of leukemia in patients who began treatment for HD at ≥ 40 years of age was not found. No case of acute leukemia occurred at >11 years after treatment. Actuarial analysis showed a peak onset of leukemia-related complications between 3 and 9 years after first treatment.[136]

Valagussa et al.,[138] reporting for the Milan group, retrospectively reviewed the records of 1,329 patients, in whom a total of 68 new cancers were documented. None of the 19 cases of acute myeloid leukemia reported was observed in patients treated with radiotherapy alone. The 12-year estimate of leukemia development by treatment was 1.4% for chemotherapy alone, 10.2% for radiotherapy plus MOPP, 0% for radiation plus ABVD, and 4.8% for radiation plus other drug regimens. The incidence of leukemia was particularly high in patients who received salvage MOPP after relapse from radiotherapy. Valagussa and co-workers[138] also noted a positive association between increasing age and the risk of second malignancies, especially leukemia, which had been reported initially by the Southwest Oncology Group.[137] The overall risk of NHL in the Milan series was only 1.3%, and that of solid tumors, excluding basal cell carcinomas, was 6.7%. The failure to document an increased risk of leukemia in patients treated with ABVD chemotherapy alone or with radiotherapy plus ABVD is an important observation, since it appears that ABVD is more effective than MOPP in its ability to achieve long-term disease-free survival as initial chemotherapy for advanced disease.[99]

In a case-controlled study of 163 cases of leukemia following treatment for HD, Kaldor et al.[139] observed that the use of chemotherapy alone to treat HD was associated with a relative risk of leukemia of 9.0, as compared with the use of radiation alone; patients treated with both modalities had a relative risk of 7.7. After treatment with more than six cycles of combination chemotherapy including nitrogen mustard and procarbazine, the risk of leukemia was 14 times as high as after radiotherapy alone. The use of radiotherapy in combination with chemotherapy did not increase the risk of leukemia above that produced by the use of chemotherapy alone. The peak in leukemia risk came approximately 5 years after the start of chemotherapy, and a large excess risk as compared with other treatment modalities persisted for ≥ 8 years after its discontinuance. Patients who had undergone splenectomy had at least twice the leukemia risk of patients who had not undergone this surgical procedure. Interestingly, Tura et al.[140] have confirmed the observation that splenectomy, in addition to exposure to MOPP chemotherapy, increases the risk of secondary leukemia. In their study of 503 patients treated with MOPP plus irradiation, only 1 of 145 without splenectomy developed leukemia as compared to 21 of 358 splenectomized patients (5.9%). Moreover, an increasing number of MOPP cycles correlated with increasing risk of secondary leukemia, as reported by other groups.

A review by Tucker et al.[141] of the Stanford series of 1,507 patients treated since 1968 indicated that 83 second cancers occurred >1 year after diagnosis. The mean 15-year actuarial risk was 18% for all second cancers, of which 13% were solid tumors. The risk of leukemia appeared to reach a plateau level of 3.3% at 10 years, whereas NHL continued to increase to 16% by the end of the follow-up period. Although these investigators noted that there was no increased risk of leukemia after radiotherapy alone, the risk of leukemia was significantly higher after either adjuvant chemotherapy or chemotherapy alone. The risk of a second solid tumor did not vary significantly according to treatment category, but the data did suggest that the risk of solid tumors after therapy for HD continues to increase with time. The Stanford group has recently updated this data base, examining the risk of breast cancer in a cohort of 885 women with a mean follow-up of 10 years.[142] The overall relative risk (RR) of breast cancer was 4.1, and age at irradiation was a significant prognostic factor. For girls treated before age 15, RR was 136; at 15–24 years, RR was 19; at 24–29 years, RR was 7; and interestingly, at >30 years, RR was not elevated (0.7). Length of follow-up was also correlated with RR: <15 years, RR was 2.0; ≥15 years, RR was 13.6. This finding explains the lack of significant breast cancer risk observed in the earlier Stanford analysis by Tucker et al.[141] Most breast cancers occurred within, or adjacent to, prior irradiation portals. Yahalom et al.[143] from Memorial Sloan-Kettering also confirmed the increased risk of breast cancer in patients irradiated for HD. In this series, patients in whom breast cancer developed were more likely to be younger (median age 43 years) and to have bilateral disease, and involvement of the medial half of the breast was more frequent. The median interval from the treatment of HD to the diagnosis of breast cancer was 15 years.

Van Leeuwen et al.[144] assessed the risk of second cancers in 744 patients admitted to the Netherlands Cancer Institute from 1966 to 1983. Among the 69 second cancers observed were lung cancer (14 cases), leukemia (16 cases), myelodysplastic syndrome (6 cases), and NHL (9 cases). The overall relative risk of the development of lung cancer was 4.9%. Excess lung cancer risk was noted only in treatment regimens including radiotherapy, and all lung cancers arose in irradiation fields. Kaldor et al.[145] reported the results of a collaborative group of population-based cancer registries and major treatment centers using a case-control study. Patients treated with chemotherapy had about twice the risk of the development of lung cancer than that of patients treated with radiotherapy alone or both modalities. Among patients treated with radiation alone, the increased risk was related to estimated radiation dose to the lung. There was also a strong association between cigarette smoking in this population and the risk of lung cancer.

It is evident from these studies and others in the literature that treated HD patients have an increased risk of second neoplasms. The incidence of leukemia appears lowest in patients treated with radiotherapy alone, while the development of solid tumors increases significantly over time in these patients. The risk of leukemia is seen in patients treated with chemotherapy alone using a MOPP-like regimen, with initial combined modality therapy using adjuvant MOPP, and with salvage alkylating agent-based chemotherapy following radiotherapy relapse. The peak risk of leukemia occurs at 5–8 years after initiation of chemotherapy, and no cases of leukemia have been observed at >10 years after the end of treatment. The risks of the development of solid tumors or acute leukemia must be taken into consideration in planning the initial treatment for an individual patient. Any predicted improvement in disease-free survival from initial therapy must be balanced against the significant risk of a second neoplasm at a later date. The risks and benefits of the initial treatment approach should be discussed with each patient and a treatment strategy designed to maximize the cure rate while minimizing long-term complications such as second neoplasms.

REFERENCES

1. Glaser S, Swartz W: Time trends in Hodgkin's disease incidence: the role of diagnostic accuracy. Cancer 66:2196, 1990
2. Davis S, Dahlberg S, Myers MH et al: Hodgkin's disease in the United States: a comparison of patient characteristics and survival in the centralized cancer patient data system and surveillance. Epidemiology and end results program. J Natl Cancer Inst 78:471, 1987
3. Gutensohn N, Cole P: Childhood social environment and Hodgkin's disease. N Engl J Med 304:135, 1981
4. Gutensohn NM: Social class and age at diagnosis of Hodgkin's disease. Cancer Treat Rep 66:689, 1982
5. Hessol N, Mitchell HK, Liu J et al: Increased incidence of Hodgkin's disease in homosexual men with HIV infection. Ann Intern Med 117:309, 1992
6. Klein G: Epstein-Barr virus-carrying cells in Hodgkin's disease. Blood 80:299, 1992
7. Lynch HT, Marcus JN, Lynch JF: Genetics of Hodgkin's and non-Hodgkin's lymphoma: a review. Cancer Invest 10:247, 1992
8. Johansson B, Klein G, Henle W, Henle G: Epstein-Barr virus (EBV)-associated antibody patterns and malignant lymphoma and leukemia. I. Hodgkin's disease. Int J Cancer 6:450, 1970
9. Mueller N, Evans A, Harris NL, et al: Hodgkin's disease and Epstein Barr virus: altered antibody pattern before diagnosis. N Engl J Med 320:689, 1989
10. Herbst H, Steinbrecher E, Niedobitek G et al: Distribution and phenotype of Epstein-Barr virus-harboring cells in Hodgkin's disease. Blood 80:484, 1992
11. Leibenhaut MH, Hoppe RT, Varghese A, Rosenberg SA: Subdiaphragmatic Hodgkin's disease: laparatomy and treatment results in 49 patients. J Clin Oncol 5:1050, 1987
12. Mauch P, Kalish L, Kadin M et al: Patterns of presentation of Hodgkin's disease: implications for etiology and pathogenesis. Cancer 71:2062, 1993
13. Knowles DM, Chamulak GA, Subar M et al: Lymphoid neoplasia associated with the acquired immunodeficiency syndrome (AIDS): the New York University Medical Center experience with 105 patients (1981–1986). Ann Intern Med 108:744, 1988
14. Fisher RI: Implications of persistent T-cell abnormalities for the etiology of Hodgkin's disease. Cancer Treat Rep 66:681, 1982
15. Donaldson SS, Vosti KL, Berberich FR et al: Response to pneumococcal vaccine among children with Hodgkin's disease. Rev Infect Dis 3:S133, 1981
16. Hays DM, Ternberg JL, Chen TT et al: Complications related to 234 staging laparotomies performed in the intergroup Hodgkin's disease in childhood study. Surgery 96:471, 1984
17. Mansfield CM, Fabian C, Joses S et al: Comparison of lymphangiography and computed tomography scanning in evaluating abdominal disease in stages III and IV Hodgkin's disease. Cancer 66:2295, 1990
18. Castellino RA, Hoppe RT, Blank N et al: Computed tomography, lymphography and staging laparotomy: correlations in initial staging of Hodgkin's disease. AJR 143:37, 1984
19. Front D, Ben-Haim S, Israel O et al: Lymphoma: predictive value of Ga-67 scintigraphy after treatment. Radiology 182:359, 1992
20. Hoane BR, Shields A, Porter B, Shulman H: Detection of lymphomatous bone marrow involvement with magnetic resonance imaging. Blood 78:728, 1991
21. Carbone P, Kaplan HS, Mushoff K et al: Report of the committee on Hodgkin's disease staging classification. Cancer Res 31:1860, 1971
22. Lister R, Crowther D: Staging for Hodgkin's disease. Semin Oncol 17:696, 1990
23. Hoppe RT: The contemporary management of Hodgkin's disease. Radiology 169:297, 1988
24. Lister TA, Crowther D, Sutcliffe SB et al: Report of a committee convened to discuss the evaluation and staging of patients with Hodgkin's disease: Cotswolds meeting. J Clin Oncol 7:1630, 1989
25. Mauch P, Larson D, Osteen R et al: Prognostic factors for possible surgical staging in patients with Hodgkin's disease. J Clin Oncol 8:257, 1990
26. Mauch P, Goodman R, Hellman S: The significance of mediastinal involvement in early stage Hodgkin's disease. Cancer 42:1039, 1978
27. Desser RK, Golomb HM, Ultmann JE et al: Prognostic classification of Hodgkin's disease in pathologic stage III, based on anatomic considerations. Blood 49:883, 1977
28. Hoppe RT, Rosenberg SA, Kaplan HS, Cox RS: Prognostic factors in pathologic stage IIIA Hodgkin's disease. Cancer 46:1240, 1980
29. Urba W, Longo D: Hodgkin's disease. N Engl J Med 326:678, 1992
30. Mauch P, Tarbell N, Weinstein H et al: Stage IA and IIA supradiaphragmatic Hodgkin's disease: prognostic factors in surgically staged patients treated with mantle and paraaortic irradiation. J Clin Oncol 6:1576, 1988
31. Kaplan HS: Hodgkin's Disease. 2nd Ed. Harvard University Press, Cambridge, MA, 1980
32. Hoppe RT, Coleman CN, Cox RS: The management of stage I–II Hodgkin's disease with irradiation alone or combined modality therapy: the Stanford experience. Blood 59:455, 1982
33. Rosenberg SA, Kaplan HS: The evolution and summary results of the Stanford randomized clinical trials of the management of Hodgkin's disease: 1962–1984. Int J Radiat Oncol Biol Phys 11:5, 1985
34. Tubiana M, Henry-Amar M, Van Der Werf-Messing B et al: A multivariate analysis of prognostic factors in early stage Hodgkin's disease. Int J Radiat Oncol Biol Phys 11:23, 1985

35. Cosset J, Henry-Amar M, Meerwaldt J et al: The EORTC trials for limited stage Hodgkin's disease. Eur J Cancer 28A:1847, 1992

36. Gospodarowicz M, Sutcliffe S, Bergsagel D et al: Radiation therapy in clinical stage I and II Hodgkin's disease. Eur J Cancer 28A:1841, 1992

37. Rosenberg S: The treatment of Hodgkin's disease. Ann Oncol 5:17, 1994

38. Ganesan T, Wrigley P, Murray P et al: Radiotherapy for stage I Hodgkin's disease: 20 years' experience at St. Bartholomew's Hospital. Br J Cancer 62:314, 1990

39. Rosenberg SA: Hodgkin's disease. p. 401. In Calabresi P, Schein P (eds): Medical Oncology. McGraw-Hill, New York, 1993

40. Carmel RJ, Kaplan HS: Mantle irradiation in Hodgkin's disease. An analysis of technique, tumor irradiation and complications. Cancer 37:2812, 1976

41. Lutz WR, Larsen RD: Technique to match mantle and para-aortic fields. Int J Radiat Oncol Biol Phys, suppl 2. 5:159, 1979

42. DeVita V Jr, Hellman S, Jaffe: Hodgkin's disease. p. 1819. In DeVita V Jr, Hellman S, Rosenberg S (eds): Cancer: Principles and Practice of Oncology. 4th Ed. JB Lippincott, Philadelphia, 1993

43. Kaplan HS: Evidence for a tumoricidal dose level in the radiotherapy of Hodgkin's disease. Cancer Res 26:1221, 1966

44. Kaplan HS: On the natural history, treatment and prognosis of Hodgkin's disease. p. 215. In Harvey Lectures 1968–1969. Academic Press, San Diego, 1970

45. Rosenberg SA, Kaplan HS: Evidence for an orderly progression in the spread of Hodgkin's disease. Cancer Res 26:1225, 1966

46. Fuller LM, Hagemeister FB, North LB et al: The adjuvant role of two cycles of MOPP and low-dose lung irradiation in stage IA through IIB Hodgkin's disease: preliminary results. Int J Radiat Oncol Biol Phys 14:683, 1987

47. Haybittle JL, Easterling MJ, Bennett MH et al: Review of British National Lymphoma Investigation studies of Hodgkin's disease and development of prognostic index. Lancet 1:967, 1985

48. Crnkovich MJ, Leopold K, Hoppe RT, Mauch PM: Stage I to IIB Hodgkin's disease: the combined experience at Stanford University and the Joint Center for Radiation Therapy. J Clin Oncol 5:1041, 1987

49. Crnkovich MJ, Hoppe RT, Rosenberg SA: Stage IIB Hodgkin's disease: the Stanford experience. J Clin Oncol 4:472, 1985

50. Anderson H, Deakin DP, Wagstaff J et al: A randomized study of adjuvant chemotherapy after mantle radiotherapy in supradiaphragmatic Hodgkin's disease PS IA–IIIB: a report from the Manchester lymphoma group. Br J Cancer 49:695, 1984

51. Mauch P, Hellman S: Supradiaphragmatic Hodgkin's disease: is there a role for MOPP chemotherapy in patients with bulky mediastinal disease? Int J Radiat Oncol Biol Phys 6:947, 1980

52. Hoppe RT, Behar RA: Radiation therapy in the management of bulky mediastinal Hodgkin's. Cancer 66:75, 1990

53. Longo D, Russo A, Duffey P et al: Treatment of advanced stage massive mediastinal Hodgkin's disease: the case for combined modality treatment. J Clin Oncol 9:227, 1991

54. Jochelson M, Mauch P, Balikian J et al: The significance of the residual mediastinal mass in treated Hodgkin's disease. J Clin Oncol 3:637, 1985

55. Tumeh SS, Rosenthal DS, Kaplan WD et al: Lymphoma: evaluation with Ga-67 SPECT. Radiology 164:111, 1987

56. Krikorian JG, Portlock CS, Mauch PM: Hodgkin's disease presenting below the diaphragm: a review. J Clin Oncol 4:1551, 1986

57. Mason M, Law M, Ashley S et al: Infradiaphragmatic Hodgkin's disease. Eur J Cancer, 28A:1851, 1992

58. Specht L, Nissen NI: Hodgkin's disease stages I and II with infradiaphragmatic presentation: a rare and prognostically unfavorable combination. Eur J Haematol 40:396, 1988

59. Givens S, Fuller L, Hagemeister F, Gehan E: Treatment of lower torso stages I and II Hodgkin's disease with radiation with or without adjuvant mechlorethamine, vincristine, procarbazine, and prednisone. Cancer 66:69, 1990

60. Morgan GW, Freeman AP, Mclean RG et al: Late cardiac, thyroid, and pulmonary sequelae of mantle radiotherapy for Hodgkin's disease. Int J Radiat Oncol Biol Phys 11:1925, 1985

61. Schimpff SC, Diggs CH, Wiswell JG et al: Radiation-related thyroid dysfunction: implications for the treatment of Hodgkin's disease. Ann Intern Med 92:91, 1980

62. Stewart JR, Fajardo LF: Radiation-induced heart disease: an update. Prog Cardiovasc Dis 27:173, 1984

63. Hancock SL, Hoppe RT, Horning SJ, Rosenberg SA: Intercurrent death after Hodgkin's disease therapy in radiotherapy and adjuvant MOPP trials. Ann Intern Med 109:183, 1988

64. Annest LS, Anderson RP, Li W et al: Coronary artery disease following mediastinal radiation therapy. J Thorac Cardiovasc Surg 85:257, 1983

65. Horning SJ, Hoppe RT, Rosenberg SA: The Stanford Hodgkin's disease trials:

1967–1984. p. 633. In Jones SE, Salmon SE (eds): Adjuvant Therapy of Cancer. Vol. 4. Grune & Stratton, Orlando, FL, 1984

66. Horning SJ, Hoppe RT, Hancock SL, Rosenberg SA: Vinblastine, bleomycin, and methotrexate: an effective adjuvant in favorable Hodgkin's disease. J Clin Oncol 6:1822, 1988

67. Hagemeister FB, Fuller LM, Sullivan JA et al: Treatment of patients with stages I and II nonmediastinal Hodgkin's disease. Cancer 50:2307, 1982

68. O'Dwyer PJ, Wiernik PH, Stewart MB et al: Treatment of early stage Hodgkin's disease: a randomized trial of radiotherapy plus chemotherapy versus chemotherapy alone. p. 329. In Cavalli F, Bonadonna G, Rozensweig N (eds): Malignant Lymphomas in Hodgkin's Disease: Experimental and Therapeutic Advances. Martinus Nijhoff, Boston, 1985

69. Pavlovsky S, Maschio M, Santarelli MT et al: Randomized trial of chemotherapy versus chemotherapy plus radiotherapy for stage I–II Hodgkin's disease. J Natl Cancer Inst 80:1466, 1988

70. Longo D, Glatstein E, Duffey P et al: Radiation therapy versus combination chemotherapy in the treatment of early-stage Hodgkin's disease: seven year results of a prospective randomized trial. J Clin Oncol 9:906, 1991

71. Biti G, Cimino C, Cartoni S et al: Extended-field radiotherapy is superior to MOPP chemotherapy for the treatment of pathologic stage I–IIA Hodgkin's disease: eight-year update of an Italian prospective randomized study. J Clin Oncol 10:378, 1992

72. Cimino G: Chemotherapy alone for the treatment of early-stage Hodgkin's disease. Eur J Cancer 26:1115, 1990

73. Stein RS, Golomb HM, Diggs CH et al: Anatomic substages of stage III-A Hodgkin's disease. Ann Intern Med 92:159, 1980

74. Mauch P, Goffman T, Rosenthal S et al: Stage III Hodgkin's disease: improved survival with combined modality therapy as compared with radiation therapy alone. J Clin Oncol 3:1166, 1985

75. Glick J: The treatment of stage IIIA Hodgkin's disease: what is the role of combined modality therapy? Int J Radiat Oncol Biol Phys 4:781, 1978

76. Hoppe RT, Cox RS, Rosenberg SA et al: Prognostic factors in pathologic stage III Hodgkin's disease. Cancer Treat Rep 66:743, 1982

77. Powlis WD, Mauch P, Goffman T: Treatment of patients with minimal stage IIIA Hodgkin's disease. Int J Radiat Oncol Biol Phys 13:1437, 1987

78. Prosnitz LR: Therapy of IIIA Hodgkin's disease. J Radiat Oncol Biol Phys 13:1595, 1987

79. Henkelmann GC, Hagemeister FB, Fuller LM: Two cycles of MOPP and radiotherapy for stage III₁A and stage III₁B Hodgkin's disease. J Clin Oncol 6:1293, 1988

80. DeVita VT, Serpick AA, Carbone PP: Combination chemotherapy in the treatment of advanced Hodgkin's disease. Ann Intern Med 73:891, 1970

81. Lister TA, Dorreen MS, Faux M et al: The treatment of stage IIIA Hodgkin's disease. J Clin Oncol 1:745, 1983

82. Crowther D, Wagstaff J, Deakin D et al: A randomized study comparing chemotherapy alone with chemotherapy followed by radiotherapy in patients with pathologically staged IIIA Hodgkin's disease. J Clin Oncol 2:892, 1984

83. Santoro A, Bonadonna G, Valagussa P et al: Long-term results of combined chemotherapy-radiotherapy approach in Hodgkin's disease: superiority of ABVD plus radiotherapy versus MOPP plus radiotherapy. J Clin Oncol 5:27, 1987

84. Rosenberg SA: ABVD versus MOPP: which is better? J Clin Oncol 5:7, 1987

85. DeVita VT, Hubbard SM, Longo DL: The chemotherapy of lymphomas: looking back, moving forward. Richard and Linda Rosenthal Foundation Award Lecture. Cancer Res 47:5810, 1987

86. Longo DL, Young RC, Wesley M et al: Twenty years of MOPP chemotherapy for Hodgkin's disease. J Clin Oncol 4:1295, 1986

87. Carde P, MacKintosh R, Rosenberg SA: A dose and time response analysis of the treatment of Hodgkin's disease with MOPP therapy. J Clin Oncol 1:146, 1983

88. Van Rijswijk R, Haanen C, Dekker AW et al: Dose intensity of MOPP chemotherapy and survival in Hodgkin's disease. J Clin Oncol 7:1776, 1989

89. Pillai GN, Hagemeister FB, Velasquez WS et al: Prognostic factors for stage IV Hodgkin's disease treated with MOPP, with or without bleomycin. Cancer 55:691, 1985

90. Glick JH: Chemotherapy of Hodgkin's and non-Hodgkin's lymphoma. p. 343. In Bennett JM (ed): Lymphomas. Vol. 1. Martinus Nijhoff, The Hague, 1981

91. Bakemeier RF, Anderson JR, Costello W et al: BCVPP chemotherapy for advanced Hodgkin's disease: evidence for greater duration of complete remission, greater survival and less toxicity than with a MOPP regimen. Ann Intern Med 101:447, 1984

92. Gams RA, Durant JR, Bartolucci AA: Chemotherapy for advanced Hodgkin's disease: conclusions from the Southeast Cancer Study Group. Cancer Treat Rep 66:899, 1982

93. Sutcliffe SB, Wrigley PFM, Peto J et al: MVPP chemotherapy regimen for advanced Hodgkin's disease. Br Med J 1:670, 1978

94. Hancock B, Hudson G, Hudson B et al: British National Lymphoma Investigation randomized study of MOPP (mustine, oncovin, procarbazine, prednisolone) against LOPP (Leukeran substituted for mustine) in advanced Hodgkin's disease: long term results. Br J Cancer 63:579, 1991

95. Selby P, Patel P, Milan S, et al: ChIVPP combination chemotherapy for Hodgkin's disease: long term results. Br J Cancer, 62:279, 1990

96. The International ChIVPP Treatment Group: ChIVPP therapy for Hodgkin's disease: experience of 960 patients abstracted. In Proceedings of the Fifth International Conference on Malignant Lymphoma, Lugano, Switzerland, 1993

97. Bonadonna G: Chemotherapy strategies to improve the control of Hodgkin's disease. Rosenthal Award Lecture. Cancer Res 42:4309, 1982

98. Bonadonna G, Valagussa P, Santoro A: Alternating non-cross resistant combination chemotherapy with ABVD or MOPP in stage IV Hodgkin's disease: a report of eight year results. Ann Intern Med 104:739, 1986

99. Canellos G, Anderson JR, Propert KJ et al: Chemotherapy of advanced Hodgkin's disease with MOPP, ABVD, or MOPP alternating with ABVD. N Engl J Med 327:1478, 1992

100. Glick J, Tsiatis A, Chen A et al: Improved survival with MOPP-ABVD compared to BCVPP ± radiotherapy for advanced Hodgkin's disease: 6-year ECOG results, abstracted. Blood 76:351, 1990

101. Goldie JH, Coldman AJ, Gudauskas GA: Rationale for the use of alternating non-cross-resistant chemotherapy. Cancer Treat Rep 66:439, 1982

102. Klimo P, Connors JM: MOPP/ABV hybrid program: combination chemotherapy based on early introduction of seven effective drugs for advanced Hodgkin's disease. J Clin Oncol 3:1174, 1985

103. Klimo P, Connors JM: An update on the Vancouver experience in the management of advanced Hodgkin's disease treated with the MOPP/ABV hybrid program. Semin Hematol, suppl 2.25:34, 1988

104. Connors JM: Is cyclical chemotherapy better than standard four drug chemotherapy for Hodgkin's disease? Yes. PPO Updates 7:1, 1933

105. Glick J, Tsiatis A, Schilsky R et al: A randomized phase III trial of MOPP/ABV hybrid vs. sequential MOPP-ABVD in advanced Hodgkin's disease: preliminary results of the Intergroup trial: ECOG, CALGB, SWOG. Proc Am Soc Clin Oncol 10:271, 1991

106. Connors JH, Klimo P, Adams G et al: MOPP/ABV hybrid versus alternating MOPP/ABVD for advanced Hodgkin's disease, abstracted. Proc Am Soc Clin Oncol 11:317, 1992

107. Viviani S, Bonadonna G, Santoro A et al: Alternating vs hybrid administration of MOPP-ABVD in Hodgkin's disease. Proc Am Soc Clin Oncol 9:254, 1990

108. Prosnitz LR, Farber LR, Kapp DS et al: Combined modality therapy for advanced Hodgkin's disease: 15-year follow-up data. J Clin Oncol 6:603, 1988

109. Glick JH, Tsiatis A: MOPP/ABVD chemotherapy for advanced Hodgkin's disease. Ann Intern Med 104:876, 1986

110. Glick JH, Tsiatis A, Rubin P, Bennett J: Improved survival with sequential Bleo-MOPP followed by ABVD for advanced Hodgkin's disease, abstracted. Blood 70:245, 1987

111. Strauss DJ, Myers J, Lee BJ et al: Treatment of advanced Hodgkin's disease with chemotherapy and irradiation. Am J Med 76:270, 1984

112. Portlock CS, Rosenberg SA, Glatstein E et al: Impact of salvage treatment on initial relapses in patients with Hodgkin's disease stages I to II. Blood 51:825, 1978

113. Longo D, Duffey P, Young R et al: Conventional-dose salvage combination chemotherapy in patients relapsing with Hodgkin's disease after combination chemotherapy: the low probability for cure. J Clin Oncol 10:210, 1992

114. Viviani S, Santoro A, Negretti E et al: Hodgkin's disease: results in patients relapsing more than 12 months after first complete remission. Ann Oncol 1:123, 1990

115. Santoro A, Bonfante V, Bonadonna G: Salvage chemotherapy with ABVD in MOPP-resistant Hodgkin's disease. Ann Intern Med 96:139, 1982

116. Tannir N, Hagemeister F, Valasquez W et al: Long-term followup with ABDIC salvage chemotherapy of MOPP-resistant Hodgkin's disease. J Clin Oncol 1:432, 1983

117. Piga A, Ambrosetti A, Todeschini et al: Doxorubicin, bleomycin, vinblastine and dacarbazine (ABVD) salvage of mechlorethamine, vincristine, prednisone, and procarbazine (MOPP)-resistant advanced Hodgkin's disease. Cancer Treat Rep 58:947, 1984

118. Harker GW, Kushlan P, Rosenberg SA: Combination chemotherapy for advanced Hodgkin's disease after failure of MOPP: ABVD and B-CAVe. Ann Intern Med 10:440, 1984

119. Hagemeister FBN, Tannir N, McLaughlin P et al: MIME chemotherapy (methyl-GAG, ifosamide, methotrexate, etoposide) as treatment for recurrent Hodgkin's disease. J Clin Oncol 5:556, 1987

120. Desch CE, Lasala MR, Smith TL, Hillner BE: The optimal timing of autologous bone marrow transplantation in Hodgkin's disease patients after a chemotherapy relapse. J Clin Oncol 10:200, 1993

121. Vose J, Armitage J: Bone marrow transplantation for Hodgkin's disease and lymphoma. Annu Rev Med 44:255, 1993

122. Jagannath S, Armitage JO, Dicke KA et al: Prognostic factors for response and survival after high-dose cyclophosphamide, carmustine, and etoposide with autologous bone marrow transplantation for relapsed Hodgkin's disease. J Clin Oncol 7:179, 1989

123. Reece D, Barnett M, Connors J et al: Intensive chemotherapy with cyclophosphamide, BCNU and etoposide followed by autologous bone marrow transplantation for relapsed Hodgkin's disease. J Clin Oncol 9:1871, 1991

124. Chopra R, Linch DC, Mc Millan AK et al: Mini-BEAM followed by BEAM and ABMT for very poor risk Hodgkin's disease. Br J Haematol 81:197, 1992

125. Armitage J, Bierman P, Vose J et al: Autologous bone marrow transplantation for patients with relapsed Hodgkin's disease. Am J Med 91:605, 1991

126. Kessinger A, Bierman PJ, Vose JM, Armitage JO: High dose cyclophosphamide, carmustine, and etoposide followed by autologous peripheral stem cell transplantation for patients with relapsed Hodgkin's disease. Blood 77:2322, 1991

127. Crump M, Smith AM, Brandwein J et al: High-dose etoposide and melphalan, and autologous bone marrow transplantation for patients with advanced Hodgkin's disease: importance of disease status at transplant. J Clin Oncol 11:704, 1993

128. Bierman P, Anderson J, Vose J et al: High-dose chemotherapy with autologous hematopoietic rescue for Hodgkin's disease following first relapse after chemotherapy. Proc Am Soc Clin Oncol 12:366, 1993

129. Santoro A, Viviani SS, Valagussa P et al: CCNU, etoposide, prednimustine (CEP) in refractory Hodgkin's disease. Semin Oncol 13:23, 1986

130. Bonfante V, Santoro A, Devizzi L et al: Outcome of patients with Hodgkin's disease relapsing after alternating MOPP/ABVD. Proc Am Soc Clin Oncol 12:364, 1993

131. Canellos G, Anderson J, Peterson B et al: EVA, etoposide, vinblastine, doxorubicin (Adriamycin): an effective regimen for the treatment of Hodgkin's disease in relapse following MOPP. Proc Am Soc Clin Oncol 10:273, 1991

132. Roach M III, Kapp DS, Rosenberg SA, Hoppe RT: Radiotherapy with curative intent: an option in selected patients relapsing after chemotherapy for advanced Hodgkin's disease. J Clin Oncol 5:550, 1987

133. Mauch P, Tarbell N, Skarin A et al: Wide-field radiation therapy alone or with chemotherapy for Hodgkin's disease in relapse from combination chemotherapy. J Clin Oncol 5:544, 1987

134. Sherins R, DeVita V: Effects of drug treatment for lymphoma on male reproductive capacity. Ann Intern Med 79:216, 1973

135. Horning S, Hoppe R, Kaplan H et al: Female reproductive potential after treatment for Hodgkin's disease. N Engl J Med 304:1377, 1981

136. Tester WJ, Kinsella TJ, Waller B et al: Second malignant neoplasms complicating Hodgkin's disease: the National Cancer Institute experience. J Clin Oncol 2:762, 1984

137. Coltman CA, Dixon DO: Second malignancies complicating Hodgkin's disease: a Southwest Oncology Group 10-year followup. Cancer Treat Rep 66:1023, 1982

138. Valagussa P, Santoro A, Fossati-Bellani F et al: Second acute leukemia and other malignancies following treatment for Hodgkin's disease. J Clin Oncol 4:830, 1986

139. Kaldor JM, Day NE, Clarke EA et al: Leukemia following Hodgkin's disease. N Engl J Med 322:7, 1990

140. Tura S, Fiacchini M, Zinzani PL et al: Splenectomy and the increasing risk of secondary acute leukemia in Hodgkin' disease. J Clin Oncol 11:925, 1993

141. Tucker MA, Coleman CN, Cox RS et al: Risk of second cancers after treatment for Hodgkin's disease. N Engl J Med 76, 1988

142. Hancock SL, Tucker MA, Hoppe RT: Breast cancer after treatment of Hodgkin's disease. J Natl Cancer Inst 85:25, 1993

143. Yahalom J, Petrek JA, Biddinger PW et al: Breast cancer in patients irradiated for Hodgkin's disease: a clinical and pathological analysis of 45 events in 37 patients. J Clin Oncol 10:1674, 1992

144. Van Leeuwen FE, Somers R, Taal BG et al: Increased risk of lung cancer, non-Hodgkin's lymphoma, and leukemia following Hodgkin's disease. J Clin Oncol 7:1046, 1989

145. Kaldor JM, Day NE, Bell J et al: Lung cancer following Hodgkin's disease: a case-control study. Int J Cancer 52:677, 1992

Non-Hodgkin Lymphomas: Pathologic Features and Clinical Correlations

80

Glauco Frizzera

INTRODUCTION

Until recently the term pathology of lymphomas has referred to the anatomic and histopathologic manifestations of lymphoproliferative disorders. Today the term includes a wealth of additional information provided by new techniques, which have immeasurably deepened our understanding of the biology of lymphopoiesis. These include the study of lymphoid cell-surface phenotypes with polyclonal and monoclonal antibodies, the analysis of associated chromosomal abnormalities, and the molecular genetic study of antigen receptor genes of B and T cells. Although the histologic diagnosis still remains the gold standard on which clinical management is based, the modern study of lymphomas requires the combined input of each of these approaches. It is important that the hematologist-oncologist be familiar not only with the theoretical aspects of these new techniques but also with their practical use.[1] Before discussing the specific types of non-Hodgkin lymphoma (NHL), the contributions of each of these techniques to the study of NHL are reviewed.

TECHNIQUES

Histopathology

Histopathology allows (1) the diagnosis of NHL by exclusion of non-neoplastic lymphoproliferation and nonhematopoietic malignancy, and (2) the correct classification of the type of NHL. Both goals are best approached by determining first the pattern of growth and second the cytologic features of the neoplastic population. The pattern is defined on the basis of the relationship between the neoplastic proliferation and the normal architecture of the lymphoid tissue and thus may be more difficult to evaluate in extranodal lesions. Four patterns of lymphoid proliferation are seen in NHLs, each of which suggests a different set of NHLs and requires distinction from specific reactive processes. These patterns include the nodular, paracortical, sinusal, and diffuse types.

A nodular pattern (i.e., the organization of the neoplastic infiltrate in discrete, rounded areas) is characteristic of follicular lymphomas (Fig. 80-1A). Thus the term nodular is often replaced by the term follicular, which, however, also carries a histogenetic connotation (i.e., composed of follicular center cells). A nodular pattern may also be observed characteristically in small lymphocytic lymphomas with prominent proliferation centers[2] (Fig. 80-1B), in mantle cell lymphoma,[3] and in monocytoid B-cell lymphoma.[4] Differentiation of a follicular lymphoma from benign reactive hyperplasia may be exceedingly difficult[5,6] and may not be possible without the use of immunophenotypic or -genotypic techniques.

A paracortical (or interfollicular) pattern (Fig. 80-1C) is produced by both T- and B-cell proliferations that spare the follicles. The presence of such a pattern effectively rules out the diagnosis of a follicular center cell neoplasm. This pattern is associated not only with NHL but also with a large number of other lymphoproliferative disorders, including Hodgkin disease, leukemias, viral and drug-induced lymphadenopathies, and some atypical lymphoproliferative processes.[7]

A sinusal pattern is found in monocytoid B-cell lymphoma,[4] some large cell lymphomas, especially of the Ki-1+ large cell type,[8] but also in leukemias, metastatic nonhematopoietic malignancies, and Langerhans cell histiocytosis.[7] A diffuse pattern is defined simply by the lack of nodularity; this may result from an initially paracortical or sinusal infiltration or from the confluence of the nodules of a follicular lymphoma.

Classification Systems

All classifications of NHLs rely on the distinction of cytologic types of neoplastic cells, based on nuclear and cytoplasmic characteristics, as well as on the proposed relationship of these types with "normal counterparts" in the lymphoid tissue. The cytologic categories recognized by the four most commonly used classifications and their incidence in each are listed in Tables 80-1 through 80-4.

The Rappaport classification[9] was introduced in 1956 as an alternative to the old subdivision into lymphosarcoma, reticulum cell sarcoma, and giant follicular lymphoma,[10] which was not easily reproducible and did not correlate well with clinical characteristics or outcome.[11] This classification scheme, recently modified with the inclusion of the lymphoblastic type[12] (Table 80-1), has been largely superseded, as rapid developments in immunology have allowed a combined morphologic-immunophenotypic definition of lymphoma. Such a combined approach is reflected in both the Kiel and the Lukes-Collins proposals.

The Kiel scheme,[13] a modification of Lennert's original classification,[14] gives prime importance to cytologic distinctions regardless of pattern of proliferation. The suffix -cytic is used to describe mature cellular elements and -blastic is used to identify more primitive cells. A recent update[15] (Table 80-2) has introduced two separate lists of categories for B- and T-cell lymphomas, both of which are subdivided into low- and high-grade tumors.

The Lukes-Collins classification[15,17] (Table 80-3), subdivides NHLs into B- and T-cell tumors and also provides for tumors of histiocytes and for those composed of morphologically primitive cells, the lineage of which cannot be determined by immunologic methods (U cells). As in the Kiel scheme, pattern of growth is not used as a parameter of classification.

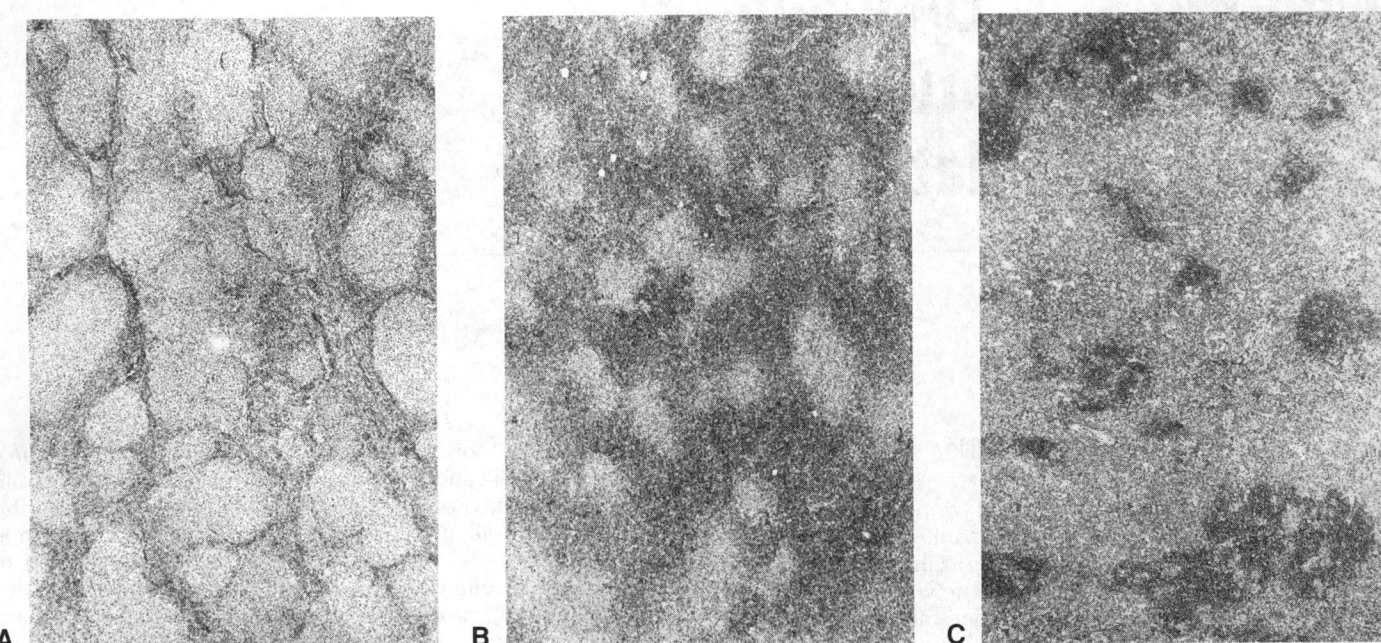

Fig. 80-1. Growth patterns of NHLs in lymph nodes. **(A)** Nodular pattern in a follicular lymphoma. **(B)** Nodular pattern in a small lymphocytic lymphoma with prominent proliferation centers. **(C)** Paracortical pattern in a T-zone lymphoma. (H&E × 30.)

The Working Formulation[12] (Table 80-4) is the result of an international multi-institutional clinicopathologic study sponsored by the National Cancer Institute. It was proposed in 1982 to serve as a common basis for comparison of data obtained from clinicopathologic studies of NHLs. It is closely related to the Rappaport scheme, but incorporates many terms used by Lukes and Collins. Recognition is given to the relationship of some cell types (cleaved and noncleaved cells) to germinal centers, and a designation of pattern (follicular or diffuse) is required. The diffuse large cell tumors are divided in two main types, follicular center cell and immunoblastic. The Working Formulation has been criticized for excluding immunophenotypic considerations and appears inadequate for classifying newly recognized histotypes, especially small B-cell neoplasms and the T-cell lymphomas. Nevertheless, its primary categories represent clinicopathologic entities well recognized by clinicians and widely referred to in the international literature. Therefore this system is used throughout this chapter, although additional new entities are described separately where appropriate.

Immunophenotyping

Evaluation of antigen expression by neoplastic cells has become an integral part of the pathologic workup of NHLs. Immunophenotyping may be performed by immunofluorescent or immunoenzymatic analysis of cell suspensions and/or frozen sections.[18] Only a more limited phenotypic evaluation can be obtained by using paraffin sections,[19–22] because most antigens do not resist the process of routine tissue embedding. However, the list of antibodies reactive in paraffin-embedded material continues to grow, expanding our diagnostic capabilities.[22] The variety of antigenic cell-surface determinants of lymphocytes and the monoclonal antibodies that identify them have been the focus of four international workshops,[23–26] which have resulted in a classification of antibodies (and their antigens) into 78 CDs.[27] The monoclonal antibodies most frequently used in the study of NHLs[18,28–30] (Table 80-5) may be grouped into five broad categories.

Panleukocyte Monoclonal Antibodies

Leukocyte common antigen (LCA) is a family of glycoproteins (five different isoforms) that are expressed exclusively on hematopoietic cells, except red blood cells and platelets,[20,31,32] and are clustered as CD45. Some antibodies to LCA, such as T29/33 (CD45) or PD7/26 (CD45RB), have panleukocyte reactivity: they are therefore most useful in the differential diagnosis of NHL versus a poorly differentiated nonhematopoietic malignancy,[33,34] but do not discriminate between lymphoid and myeloid malignancies. Other CD45 antibodies are restricted preferentially—but not exclusively—to B cells (CD45RA, such as 4KB5 or MB1) or T cells (CD45RO, such as UCHL-1).

Table 80-1. Rappaport Classification of NHLs

Lymphoma Type	Incidence (%)
Nodular lymphomas	
Well-differentiated lymphocytic	0.5
Poorly differentiated lymphocytic	18.6
Mixed, lymphocytic and histiocytic	8.0
Histiocytic	1.7
Diffuse lymphomas	
Well-differentiated lymphocytic	3.7
With plasmacytoid features	0.3
Poorly differentiated lymphocytic	9.4
Lymphoblastic	
Convoluted	5.4
Nonconvoluted	3.0
Mixed, lymphocytic and histiocytic	4.4
Histiocytic	28.4
Undifferentiated	1.1
Burkitt type	1.1

Based on unpublished data from the Working Formulation study.[12] The list does not include the miscellaneous category (unclassified, composite, etc.), which accounts for 14.4% of cases.

Table 80-2. Updated Kiel Classification of NHLs[a]

B Cell	%	T Cell	%
Low grade		Low grade	
Lymphocytic		Lymphocytic	
Chronic lymphocytic leukemia	17.3	Chronic lymphocytic leukemia	0.25
Prolymphocytic leukemia	0.05	Prolymphocytic leukemia	
Hairy cell leukemia	1.0	Small, cerebriform cell (mycosis fungoides/Sézary syndrome)	0.8
Lymphoplasmacytoid/cytic (LP immunocytoma)	17.8	Lymphoepithelioid (Lennert lymphoma)	
Plasmacytic	0.8	Angioimmunoblastic (AILD, LgX)	
Centroblastic/centrocytic	22.8		
Follicular ± diffuse		T zone	1.3
Diffuse		Pleomorphic, small cell (HTLV-1 ±)	
Centrocytic	10.0		
High grade		High grade	
Centroblastic	5.5	Pleomorphic, medium and large cell (HTLV-1 ±)	
Immunoblastic	8.0	Immunoblastic (HTLV-1 ±)	0.5
Large cell anaplastic (Ki-1[+])		Large cell anaplastic (Ki-1[+])	
Burkitt lymphoma	2.1		
Lymphoblastic		Lymphoblastic	5.8
Rare types		Rare types	

Abbreviations: AILD, angioimmunoblastic lymphadenopathy; LgX, lymphogranulomatosis X; HTLV-1, human T-cell leukemia virus-1.
[a] Percentages are those provided for the categories included in the 1981 version[243] and do not include lymphomas phenotypically null (6.0%).
(Modified from Stansfeld et al.,[15] with permission.)

Pan-B-Cell and Pan-T-Cell Antibodies

Pan-B-cell and pan-T-cell antibodies detect antigens restricted to either cell lineage.[35,36] The CD19, CD20, CD22, and CD24 antigens are expressed by B cells at most stages of differentiation, except the terminal plasma cell stage.[35] The CD2, CD3, and CD7 antigens, as well as the T-cell receptor (TCR) β-chain detected by the βF-1 monoclonal antibody,[37] span T-cell ontogeny. CD5, another pan-T antigen, is also expressed by a minor population of normal B cells and by some B-cell malignancies.[38] The antibodies in this category help identify the cell lineage of a lymphoid proliferation in frozen section specimens, and some, such as polyclonal CD3[39] or L26 (CD20),[40] also in paraffin sections. In addition, because they are consistently expressed by normal B or T cells, their absence constitutes an "abnormal" phenotype and is strong, but indirect, evidence for the neoplastic—rather than reactive—nature of a lymphoproliferation.[41] Direct evidence is only provided, for B-cell proliferations, by the light chain restriction (either κ or λ) of their surface and/or cytoplasmic immunoglobulins[42] (Fig. 80-2).

Table 80-3. Lukes-Collins Classification of NHLs

Type	%
B cell	
Small lymphocyte (B)	7.7
Plasmacytoid lymphocyte	7.7
Follicular center cell	41.2
Small cleaved	23.4
Large cleaved	6.4
Small noncleaved	7.7
Large noncleaved	3.7
Immunoblastic sarcoma (B)	3.0
Hairy cell leukemia	4.0
T-cell	
Small lymphocyte (T)	1.7
Convoluted lymphocyte	11.0
Cerebriform lymphocyte (Sézary-mycosis fungoides)	2.0
Immunoblastic sarcoma (T)	5.0
Lymphoepithelioid cell	1.3
Histiocyte	0.3
U cell	15.1

(From Lukes et al.,[16] with permission.)

T-Cell and B-Cell Subset Antibodies

T-cell subset antibodies can be used to identify in frozen sections the helper/inducer or cytotoxic/suppressor subsets of T cells. Preponderance of one subset cannot be taken as evidence of neoplasia, since great variations in such ratios can

Table 80-4. Working Formulation of NHLs for Clinical Use

Type	%
Low grade	
Malignant lymphoma, small lymphocytic	3.6
Consistent with chronic lymphocytic leukemia	
Plasmacytoid	
Malignant lymphoma follicular, predominantly small cleaved cell	22.5
Malignant lymphoma, follicular, mixed small cleaved and large cell	7.7
Intermediate grade	
Malignant lymphoma, follicular, predominantly large cell	3.8
Malignant lymphoma, diffuse, small cleaved cell	6.9
Malignant lymphoma, diffuse, mixed small and large cell	6.7
Malignant lymphoma, diffuse, large cell	19.7
Cleaved cell	
Noncleaved cell	
High-grade	
Malignant lymphoma, large cell, immunoblastic	7.9
Plasmacytoid	
Clear cell	
Polymorphous	
Epithelioid cell component	
Malignant lymphoma, lymphoblastic	4.2
Convoluted	
Nonconvoluted	
Malignant lymphoma, small noncleaved cell	5.0
Burkitt	
Miscellaneous	12.0
Composite	
Mycosis fungoides	
Histiocytic	
Extramedullary plasmacytoma	
Unclassifiable	

(From the Non-Hodgkin Lymphoma Pathologic Classification Project,[12] with permission.)

Table 80-5. Monoclonal Antibodies Most Frequently Used in the Study of NHL

Category	CD	Common Names	Reactivity
Panleukocyte	CD45	LCA, T29/33, PD7/26	Leukocytes (leukocyte common antigen)
Pan T	CD2	T11, OKT11, Leu-5, 9.6	Pan T (E-rosette receptor)
	CD3	T3, OKT3, Leu-4, UCHT1	Pan-T (T-receptor associated)
	CD5	OKT1, Leu-1, T101	Pan-T, rare B
	CD7	Leu-9, Tu14, 3A1	Pan-T
T subsets	CD4	T4, OKT4, Leu-3	T-helper/inducer, macrophages, monocytes
	CD8	T8, OKT8, Leu-2	T-cytotoxic/suppressor
Pan B	CD19	B4, Leu-12	Pan-B, B progenitors
	CD20	B1, Leu-16	Pan-peripheral B
	CD22	Leu-14, To15, SHCL1	Pan-B, B progenitors
	CD24	BA1	Pan-B, B progenitors, granulocytes, IDRCs
Activation	CD23	Tu1, blast 2	Restricted B, DRC
	CD25	TAC, anti-IL-2R	Activated T, B, and macrophages (IL-2R)
	CD30	Ki-1, Ber-H2	Reed-Sternberg cells, activated B and T
Other	CD10	J5, BA3, VilA1	Pre-B, Pre-T (CD10)
	—	HLA-DR (Ia-like)	B, activated T
	—	TdT	B and T precursors
	—	Ki-67	Proliferating cells

Abbreviations: DRC, dendritic reticulum cells; IL-2R, interleukin-2 receptor; IDRC, interdigitating dendritic cells; TdT, terminal deoxynucleotidyl transferase.

be seen in reactive processes. Lack of both markers or their co-expression on lymphoid proliferations outside the thymus is, however, suggestive of a neoplastic process.[41] CD1, being expressed only by immature T cells, is useful in separating thymic from post-thymic neoplasms.[28] Antibodies have re-cently become available that recognize the $\alpha\beta$ or the $\gamma\delta$ subset of T cells.[37,43] Within B-cell lymphomas, CD5 is restricted to tumors of small lymphocytic and mantle cell type and CD10 is characteristic of those of follicular center cell origin.[44]

Antibodies to Activation and Proliferation Antigens

A wide range of antigens are expressed by lymphoid cells during activation or proliferation[45]: among them are CD23, CD25 (interleukin-2 receptor), CD30 (Ki-1 antigen), the transferrin receptor (CD71),[46] and the nuclear antigen detected by Ki-67. Such a nuclear antigen, present in all phases of the cell cycle except G_0, is widely considered the best marker of cell proliferation.[47] Monoclonal antibodies in this general category have been applied to the study of NHLs for the definition of subtypes[48] or for correlations with clinical characteristics and survival.[49–53]

Other Antibodies

Several monoclonal antibodies are used to detect the HLA-DR locus, which is normally expressed by B cells at the earliest stages of development and by monocytes/macrophages, but by T cells only when activated.[54] Abnormal expression of this and other products of the major histocompatibility complex (HLA-DP and DQ) has been used as a possible predictor of clinical outcome.[55–57] Antibodies to CD10 (formerly, common ALL antigen [CALLA]) and terminal deoxynucleotidyl transferase (TdT) are most frequently used to classify acute leukemias.[18] However, since these antigens are also expressed by some lymphomas, such antibodies may also be useful in the definition of NHL types.[58,59] Recent studies have investigated the expression by NHLs of adhesion molecules,[60] such as lymphocyte function-associated antigen-1 (LFA-1),[61] lymphocyte homing receptor antigens,[61,62] and integrins,[63] in correlation with clinical outcome and dissemination patterns.[64–67]

Other Techniques

Throughout this chapter sporadic mention is made of data provided by other pathologic techniques less routinely employed in the study of NHLs. Lectin histochemistry investigates

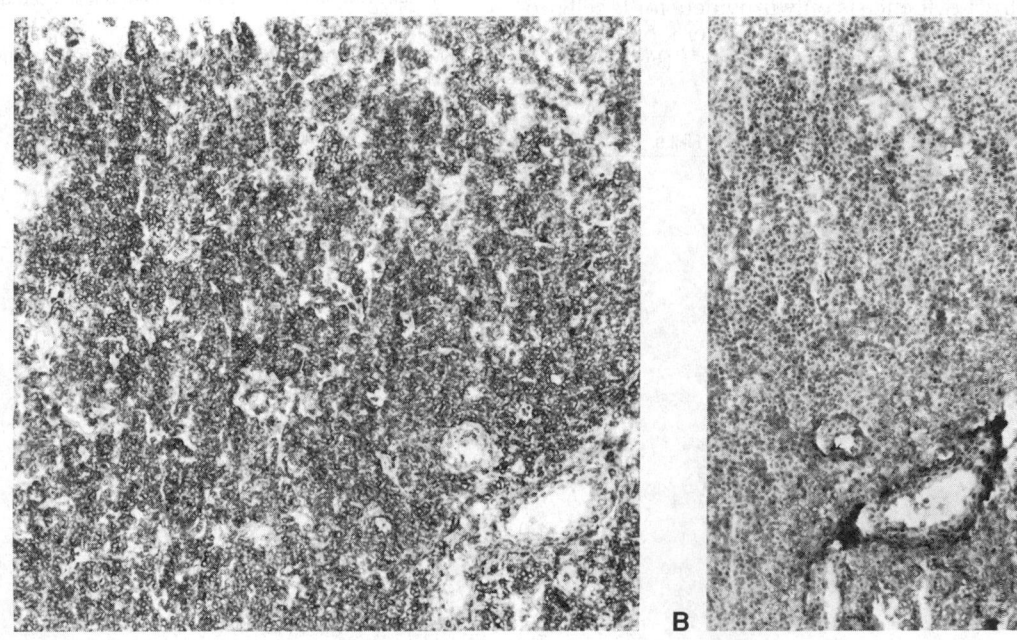

Fig. 80-2. The expression of **(A)** λ but not **(B)** κ surface immunoglobulin light chains by the neoplastic cells (on serial sections of the same area) indicates the monoclonality of this small lymphocytic lymphoma. (Immunoperoxidase-stained frozen section × 75.)

the expression of surface markers of carbohydrate nature (or lectin receptors) that bind plant proteins, called lectins,[68] which then can be detected by using antilectin antibodies. Lectin receptors, most frequently those for peanut agglutinin and concanavalin A, have been used to define subtypes of NHLs.[69-71] Enzyme histochemistry and cytochemistry are today rarely used to identify different lymphoid populations.[72,73] However, enzymatic markers still play a role in the identification of the rare true histiocytic/reticulum cell malignancies.[74,75] In addition to Ki-67 labeling, other techniques, such as autoradiography, quantitation of cellular tritiated thymidine incorporation by scintillation counting, and more recently flow cytometry,[76] have been used to study parameters of cell proliferation, including DNA synthesis, DNA content (aneuploidy), and fraction of cells in S phase. Many studies[76] have attempted, with mixed results, to establish correlations of these parameters with histologic type and patient prognosis.

Molecular Pathology and Cytogenetics

Antigen receptor gene analysis and cytogenetics (see Chs. 10 and 59) provide unique markers with which to establish clonality of a lymphoid proliferation. Thus, they have a definitive role in distinguishing polyclonal (reactive, hyperplastic) from clonal proliferations; in following the evolution of clonal populations within atypical lymphoproliferations[77-79]; and in investigating the natural history of a neoplasia during clinical remission (minimal residual disease) or progression.[80]

Genomic analysis of NHLs, in addition, provides specific markers with which to determine the B- or T-cell nature of lymphoid proliferations in which the neoplastic cells are admixed with an abundant population of reactive cells (e.g., the so-called T-cell-rich B-cell lymphomas),[81,82] or of proliferations in which no B- or T-cell surface markers are expressed (the so-called null lymphomas).[83,84] Cytogenetic analysis, although not helpful in the determination of cell lineage, has recognized strong correlations between specific chromosomal abnormalities and histopathologic types.[85,86] These correlations, in addition to providing invaluable clues to the pathogenesis of these neoplasias, have a role in the classification of NHLs and may help identify subtypes with different clinical characteristics and outcome. They are specifically discussed for each of the NHL categories.

NON-HODGKIN LYMPHOMAS

The discussion of the specific types of NHLs largely follows the histopathologic categories established by the Working Formulation, even though reference is often made to similarities or discordances with the subtypes defined by other classification schemes. Because some types of small cell lymphomas and most types of T-cell lymphomas are poorly represented by the Working Formulation categories, it was deemed necessary to add to the discussion of the NHLs two specific sections to discuss them. For each category of lymphoma the same order is followed: a concise summary of the defining pathologic characteristics; the histopathologic, immunophenotypic, genotypic, and chromosomal features in detail; and a discussion of those features that correlate with clinical characteristics and thus, provide information useful for clinical management and prognosis.

Small Lymphocytic Lymphoma

Pathologic Definition

In the Working Formulation, the term small lymphocytic lymphoma (SLL) describes a lymphoid tumor mass composed of small lymphocytes with a round regular nucleus and compact

chromatin structure; the cytoplasm is inconspicuous or may show plasmacytoid features. Patients with such a tumor may have chronic lymphocytic leukemia (CLL), a serum monoclonal gammopathy (see Ch. 87), or a lymphoma not associated with either peripheral lymphocytosis or monoclonal gammopathy. This histologic category thus corresponds roughly to the lymphocytic lymphoma and lymphoplasmacytic immunocytoma of the Kiel classification and to the small B lymphocytic and plasmacytoid lymphocytic lymphomas of Lukes and Collins. The vast majority of these tumors have a B-cell phenotype. They are commonly associated with trisomy 12 and chromosomal breaks at 11q and 14q.

Histopathology

SLL is characterized by a diffuse pattern of growth. However, vague nodular areas are frequently present (pseudofollicular proliferation centers)[14,87,88] (Fig. 80-1A), which are composed of a spectrum of transformed lymphocytes with a prominent central nucleolus and pale cytoplasm, the largest corresponding to Lennert's paraimmunoblasts.[2] Mitoses are seen mostly in these foci and are rare elsewhere. Occasionally, residual germinal centers may be found.[2] The neoplastic cells have a round, regular nucleus with compact chromatin and inconspicuous cytoplasm (Fig. 80-3A). In about 25% of cases, cells with the nucleus of a small lymphocyte and the cytoplasm of a plasma cell (so-called plasmacytoid lymphocytes) and/or bona fide plasma cells may be present.[87] Periodic acid-Schiff (PAS)-positive material representing immunoglobulins of the IgM or IgA class may also be observed as intracytoplasmic and/or intranuclear (Dutcher's body) spherules.[2]

Immunophenotyping

In the Western world, <5% of CLLs[89] and only rare nonleukemic SLLs[88,90] have a T-cell phenotype. All other SLLs are B cell in type[18,88,90-95] (Table 80-6); they express monotypic immunoglobulins (Fig. 80-2), most frequently IgM, with or without IgD, HLA-DR, and B-cell differentiation antigens. In addition, they characteristically manifest the pan-T antigen CD5,[96] and, strongly associated with it, CD43, also detectable in paraffin sections[41,97,98]; they also manifest the activation antigen CD23,[44,97] and inconsistently CD11c, a marker of hairy cell leukemia.[97] The cells of SLL express often cross-reactive idiotypes, suggesting little diversification of the immunoglobulin variable genes from the germline,[99] and almost always the adherence molecule LFA-1 (CD11a), which is absent in CLL cells.[65] The latter finding may account for the different distribution (lymph nodes versus systemic) of the two malignancies.[65] The SLLs with lymphoplasmacytoid features are obviously distinguished by the presence of easily detectable cytoplasmic immunoglobulins; whether other differences exist is somewhat controversial.[88,90,91,94-96,100,101] The normal cellular equivalent of SLL is thought to be the CD5+ autoantibody-producing B-cell subset,[102] which is normally found in small numbers at the edge of germinal centers in lymph nodes of adults[103] but represents a major population of primary follicles of fetal spleen and lymph nodes.

Cytogenetics

SLLs frequently have abnormalities of chromosomes 11, 12, and 14.[104] The most common abnormalities are trisomy 12 and breaks at 11q, 14q22-q24, or 14q32, which occur primarily as part of a t(11;14)(q13;q32) translocation.[104-109] Also, deletions at 6q23 appear strongly associated with SLLs.[110] In one study,[111] no differences were found in the cytogenetic pattern between CLL and tumors with plasmacytoid features. However, a new t(9;14)(p13;q32) appears to be strongly associated with the latter.[112]

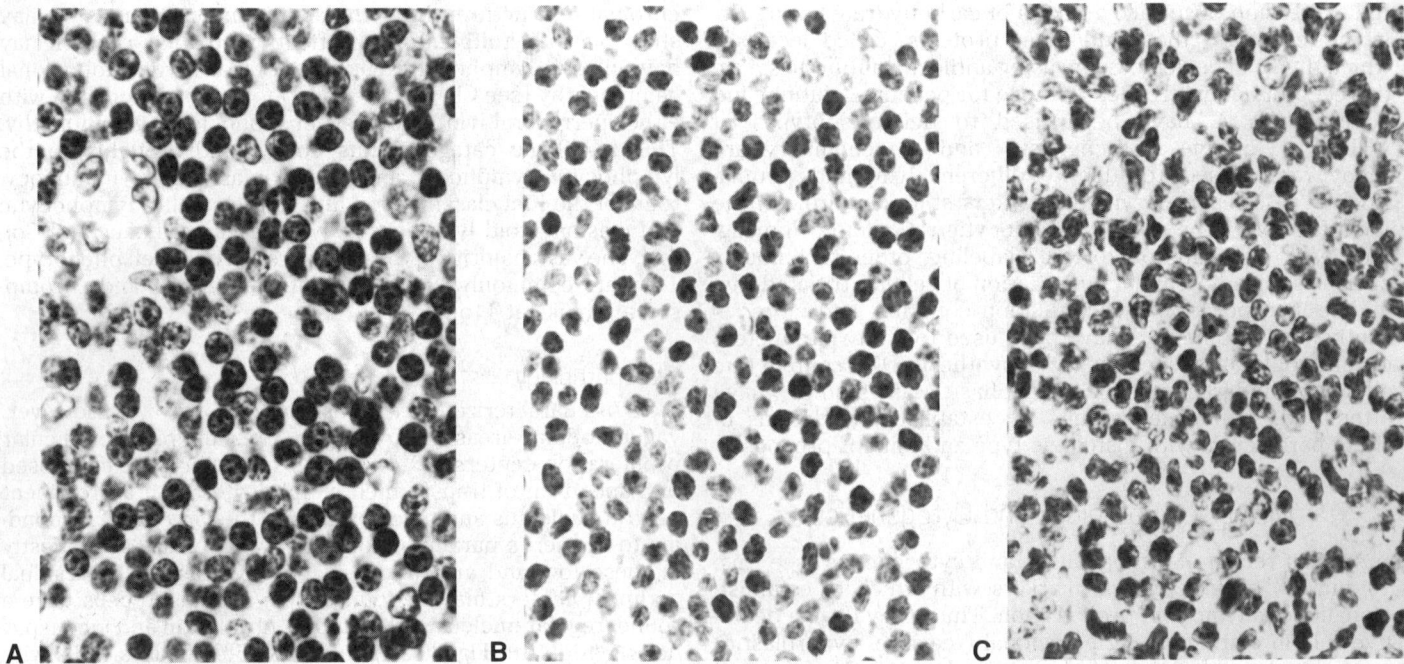

Fig. 80-3. Comparison of **(A)** the regularly round dark nuclei of the small lymphocytic type (Rappaport's well-differentiated lymphocytic); **(B)** the round but slightly irregular nuclei of the intermediately differentiated lymphocytic (mantle cell) type; and **(C)** the angulated and cleaved nuclei of the small cleaved cell (Rappaport's poorly differentiated lymphocytic) lymphoma. (All H&E × 900.)

Clinical Correlations

The term SLL encompasses three clinical entities: CLL, Waldenström's macroglobulinemia, and lymphoma without peripheral lymphocytosis or paraproteinemia.[87,113,114] This last entity has been characterized as differing from CLL by its lower incidence of generalized lymphadenopathy and/or hepatomegaly (47% versus 70% in CLL), bone marrow involvement (68% versus 93%), and hypogammaglobulinemia (5% versus 43%).[87] About one-quarter of patients with SLL present with stage I–II disease[115] and 15%[87] to 18.5%[115] will progress to CLL. The median survival for nonleukemic SLL, reported to be similar to that for CLL,[87] was longer in a more recent and larger series (84 versus 50 months; $P < 0.008$).[114]

Histopathologically no feature in a tumor of small lymphocytes can distinguish a leukemic from a nonleukemic form. Plasmacytoid lymphocytes and/or plasma cells and PAS-positive material are commonly, but not necessarily, associated with paraproteinemia.[87,116] Conversely, SLL with a serum monoclonal gammopathy may lack either of the above histologic features.[87] Therefore, there is not a complete correspondence between SLL with plasmacytoid features, which is a histopathologic category, and Waldenström's macroglobulinemia, which

is an entity defined by biochemical and clinical criteria, and the two terms should not be used interchangeably. Whether patients with lymphoplasmacytoid tumors differ with regard to clinical findings or survival from those with CLL/SLL[94,100] or whether they do not[87,111,114] remains controversial. A paraimmunoblastic variant of SLL, characterized by cells of medium to large size, all with prominent nucleoli, appears to have a more aggressive clinical course.[117] Cases characterized by circulating villous lymphocytes are associated with prominent, possibly primary, involvement of the spleen: they have pathologic and clinical features intermediate between those of SLL and those of hairy cell leukemia.[118] As for phenotypic features, expression of CD5 and IgD are said to be characteristic of SLL tumors associated with lymphocytosis but to be absent[94] or less common[88,100] in the nonleukemic forms. Cytogenetic analysis appears to contribute prognostic information. Shorter overall and therapy-free survivals have been reported for patients with trisomy 12[111,119] and for those with complex karyotypes,[111] and 14q+ has been associated with features of progressive disease and shorter median survival.[120] However, no correlation between any chromosome group and survival was found in another study.[121]

Table 80-6. Selected Immunohistologic Findings in B-Cell NHLs

Histologic Type	No. of Patients	Immunoglobulins[a]			Pan-B Antigens[a]				Activation Antigens[a]		Other Antigens[a]		References
		κ/λ	M/G	D	CD19	CD20	CD22	CD24	HLA-DR	CD25	CD5	CD10	
Small lymphocytic	141	1.6	4.2	40	95	82	88	96	97	34	70	4	88, 90–95
Follicular	201	1.1	1.2	25	93	97	98	67	96.5	41	4	79	91, 92, 95, 143, 149, 208, 209, 212
Diffuse, large cell	198	2.4	1.5	9	84	91.5	90	49	82	48	6	33	92, 208, 285, 287, 288
Small noncleaved cell, Burkitt type	43	1.6[b]	20[b]	18.5[b]	100	93	100	86	98	0	0	94.5	91, 92, 208, 287, 352

[a] Numbers represent percent positive among cases tested.
[b] Values do not include Garcia et al.[287] series.

Transformation of Small Lymphocytic Lymphoma (Richter Syndrome)

During the course of their disease, patients with SLL may develop a lymphoid malignancy of higher grade, which most frequently is a large cell lymphoma (Richter syndrome) or a prolymphocytoid transformation[122] and rarely a plasmacytoid blast crisis[123] or a lymphoblastic malignancy.[2,124] The incidence of Richter syndrome has been calculated to be 3–10% in CLL[125] and 6% in macroglobulinemia.[126] The large cell component may form nodal or extranodal tumor masses and is usually associated with evidence of SLL in the same or different tissues.[126,127] Cytologically it may manifest as a predominantly paraimmunoblastic tumor, a plasmacytoid immunoblastic sarcoma, or a mixed small and large cell NHL.[125–128] The large cell lymphomas of Richter syndrome that have been studied immunologically are B-cell neoplasms and mostly represent a progression of the original clone, as shown by the expression of the same immunoglobulins[128] or idiotypes,[129] or by the finding of identical immunoglobulin gene rearrangements[130–133] or the same cytogenetic abnormalities.[133] The interpretation of findings reported in favor of a different clonal origin for the SLL and Richter large cell lymphoma in some cases[134–136] has been disputed.[133]

Clinically, Richter syndrome develops 2–4 years[125–127] after the diagnosis of an otherwise typical SLL. In 15% of cases the two diseases are diagnosed concurrently. Richter syndrome is manifested by unexplained fever, weight loss, rapidly growing lymphadenopathy, and/or extranodal tumor mass; the large cell tumor is in most cases widely disseminated.[126,127] The median survival from the diagnosis of Richter syndrome is 4 months.[125,126] "Hodgkin disease variant of Richter syndrome" is an inappropriate term recently used[137] to describe a much less ominous event (i.e., the later development of a neoplasm morphologically, phenotypically, and clinically classic of Hodgkin disease in a patient with CLL). Such a combination, also described simultaneously in the same patient,[138] has been interpreted as the final in a series of steps starting with the emergence of a Reed-Sternberg cell phenotype from the neoplastic B cells.[139]

Other Small B-Cell Lymphomas

Mantle Cell Lymphoma

Mantle cell lymphoma (MCL) has been recently proposed by an international group[140] to replace the analogous terms of intermediately differentiated lymphocytic,[141] centrocytic of the Kiel classification,[2,142,143] and mantle zone lymphoma.[144] This neoplasm has no counterpart in the Working Formulation but deserves recognition as a specific clinicopathologic entity.[140,145,146] Cytologically it is characterized by small lymphocytes with somewhat open chromatin pattern and slightly irregular nuclei, which were considered "intermediate" between those of SLL and those of small cleaved cells (Fig. 80-3). Essential to the definition are also numerous mitoses and the lack of proliferation centers characteristic of SLL.[146,147] The neoplastic cells may grow in a diffuse pattern or form large lymphoid nodules (follicular variant) that may contain a more or less defined residual reactive germinal center.[3] Unusually one may observe a "blastic variant"[147] or a large cell variant.[2]

The immunophenotype of MCL cells is quite characteristic: in addition to surface immunoglobulins and B-cell-associated antigens, they express in most cases CD5, CD43, Leu8, and CD6[44,90,91,95,144,147–150]; they may[44,147] or may not express CD10 and lack CD23, this last being the most useful differential fea-

---

DIFFUSE SMALL CELL LYMPHOMAS

The categories described—SL, MCL, MoBCL, and MALT-type lymphomas—can be best understood as part of a histopathologic and immunophenotypic spectrum of diffuse small B-cell lymphomas that also includes the small cleaved cell (Rappaport's poorly differentiated lymphocytic) lymphoma. In this context, one may recognize affinities and differences among four distinct biologic families of neoplasms.

The follicular center cell neoplasms (centroblastic/centrocytic of the Kiel classification) are characterized by small cells with angulated and cleaved nuclei, associated with large noncleaved cells (centroblasts), and by the CD5−, CD10+, CD23±, CD43−, Leu8− phenotype. Mantle cell lymphomas are composed of small cells, with less irregular nuclei, unassociated with centroblasts, and manifesting a CD5+, CD10±, CD23−, CD43+, Leu8+ phenotype. SLLs, in addition to the predominant cells with round nuclei, most often show proliferation centers, and their phenotype is CD5+, CD10−, CD23+, CD43+, Leu8+. Finally, the family of marginal cell lymphomas, including MoBCL, MALT-type neoplasms, and splenic marginal cell lymphoma, is characterized especially by monocytoid B-cell cytology and the CD5−, CD10−, CD23±, CD43±, Leu8+ phenotype.

---

ture with SLL.[44] These cells are associated with a loose meshwork of dendritic reticulum cells (DRCs), as seen in the mantle zone of reactive follicles.[2,144,149,150] On the basis of these histopathologic and immunophenotypic characteristics, it is now generally accepted that MCL cells are the neoplastic counterpart of the cells of the mantle zone. MCL is strongly associated with the t(11;14)(q13;q32),[151–154] with rearrangements of a large DNA region on 11q13, named *bcl*-1 locus,[155–158] and with overexpression of a *bcl*-1-linked oncogene, named PRAD (parathyroid adenomatosis)-1.[158] This oncogene, which encodes for a protein involved in the regulation of the cell cycle (a cyclin),[159] is thought therefore to have an essential role in MCL lymphomagenesis.

The clinical presentation of MCL does not appear to differ substantially from that of SLL, in that both present at a median age in the late sixties, predominantly in males, without symptoms, with generalized lymphadenopathy, and mostly (78%) in stage III or IV.[141,146,147,160,161] A leukemic presentation is distinctly uncommon,[162] but bone marrow is commonly involved (63–93%).[161] Extranodal disease can be observed in 5–30% of cases,[161] mostly in the gastrointestinal tract, where MCL often presents as multiple lymphomatous polyposis.[163] Similar to other low-grade lymphomas, the survival curve of patients with MCL demonstrates a continuous slope, without plateau. Median survival for MCL varies from 36[44] to 56 months.[147] However, the follicular variant is associated with a longer survival (88 months)[164] than the diffuse form (46.5 months).[146] Trends for a worse prognosis are recorded for cases with the "blastic" cytology,[44,147,160] a higher proliferative rate,[147,164] or, within the follicular variant, for those with more abundant large cells.[164]

Monocytoid B-Cell Lymphoma/Mucosa-Associated Lymphoid Tissue-Type Lymphoma

Monocytoid B-cell lymphoma (MoBCL)[165,166] is characterized by small lymphocytes with bland ovoid nuclei and relatively abundant pale cytoplasm, which are indistinguishable from hairy cells.[166] In involved lymph nodes the neoplastic cells have a sinusal, perifollicular/interfollicular, or diffuse distribution[167]; in the spleen, they involve the marginal zone or the red pulp, or both[168]; and in the liver, mostly the sinusoids.[166] Phenotypically, they express surface and often cytoplasmic immunoglobulins, predominantly μ and κ[169]; B-cell-associated antigens; some macrophage-associated antigens, such as CD32,[170] KiM-1P,[167] and CD11c[165,171]; and, inconstantly, other, unusual antigens, such as muscle-specific actin and EMA.[172] Unlike SLLs, they never express CD5[165,167] and only rarely CD43[170,172]; and, unlike follicular center cell lymphomas, do not express CD10.[167] MoBCL is thought to be the neoplastic counterpart of so-called monocytoid B cells, a cell type that is prominent in toxoplasmosis and acquired immunodeficiency syndrome (AIDS)-related lymphadenopathies.[173,174] Clinically, patients with these tumors seem to differ in several respects from those with SLL: they are often female, at least in some studies[170,175]; many have associated Sjögren syndrome or rheumatoid arthritis[166,170,175]; often manifest extranodal involvement, in addition to or subsequent to their predominantly adenopathic disease[169,170,176]; only few have splenomegaly,[169,170] bone marrow involvement, or leukemic evolution[168]; and their disease is most often localized (62–67%).[166,169] Like SLLs, MoBCLs have an indolent course, the survival curve showing a continuous slope.[166,169,170]

There is now a general agreement that MoBCL is the nodal equivalent of the low-grade lymphoma of the mucosa-associated lymphoid tissue (MALT).[44,167,169,170,176] This tumor was originally described as arising in the MALT of the gastrointestinal tract,[177] from a specific B-cell type involved in a characteristic traffic pattern that leads back to the viscus: this pattern was reflected in the distribution and localized nature of the MALT tumor. This is characterized by cells of variable morphology (from regular or slightly irregular small lymphocytes, to "centrocyte-like" forms, or monocytoid B cells), often arranged around reactive follicles and consistently forming pockets of infiltration within the epithelia ("lymphoepithelial lesions").[178] Tumors with the same morphology and homing pattern have been later described in glandular organs, such as thyroid,[179] salivary glands,[180] and breast,[181] as well as in the lung,[182] skin, and other sites.[181] These MALT-type tumors are thought to arise from an "acquired MALT," which develops in response to local agents via an autoimmune mechanism.[183]

The overlap of MoBCL and MALT-type tumors is demonstrated by their frequent coexistence in the same patient[167,169,170,175,176] and by their similarities. These include one neoplastic cell type in common (i.e., the monocytoid B cell)[167]; the same perifollicular distribution and tendency to the "colonization" of the reactive germinal centers[176]; the common plasmacytic differentiation[176,184] and possible progression to a large cell lymphoma[167,176,185]; and, equally important, the same phenotypic features. Both tumor types, in fact, express consistently surface and/or cytoplasmic immunoglobulins, B-cell antigens, and Leu8, and inconstantly CD23 and CD43, and characteristically lack CD5 and CD10.[44] Another overlap is apparent between these neoplasms and the marginal cell lymphoma recently described in the spleen,[186,187] suggesting a unique category of tumors, all arising from the marginal cell. This cell type, well recognized in the splenic marginal zone,[188] is also found in sinusal and parafollicular position in the lymph node.[189]

Follicular Center Cell Lymphomas

Pathologic Definition

Follicular center cell lymphomas (FCCLs) are composed of cells that are morphologically and immunophenotypically similar to the lymphocytes of the normal germinal centers and are similarly associated with a characteristic microenvironment of DRCs and T-helper cells. Their growth pattern may be follicular (nodular), follicular and diffuse, or diffuse. Thus, they include the Working Formulation categories identified as follicular lymphomas (FLs), but also diffuse small cleaved cell lymphomas, and a portion of the tumors classified as diffuse, mixed, or large cell. They correspond to the Kiel centroblastic/centrocytic and centroblastic categories. FCCLs are characteristically associated with the (14;18) chromosomal translocation, which alters the expression of the bcl-2 oncogene.

Histopathology

In their follicular form of growth, FCCLs are composed of closely arranged nodules (Fig. 80-1A). Such nodules are most often round and uniform in size and have either infiltrative ill-defined or expansile sharply defined borders. A diffuse pattern results from the progressive coalescence of the nodules. The follicular center cells (FCCs)[2,17] include small cells with angulated and cleaved nuclear contours (small cleaved cells, centrocytes) (Fig. 80-3C); larger cells, with similar but larger nuclei and abundant, pale-staining cytoplasm (large cleaved cells); and medium-size and large cells, with round to oval nuclei, two or more prominent peripheral nucleoli, and a well-defined basophilic rim of cytoplasm (small and large noncleaved or "transformed" cells, centroblasts). Various subdivisions of FLs by cell composition have been described: by the estimated percentage of large cells (<20%, 20–50%, and >50%)[190]; by the actual average count of such cells at high dry magnification (<5, 5–15, and >15)[191]; or according to different cutoff points depending on the type of "transformed" cells present.[192] However, the rate of agreement among pathologists applying these subdivisions when examining the same material is low.[193] FCCLs with either follicular or diffuse patterns are often associated with two very characteristic types of sclerosis: one features short, interconnected collagenous trabeculae, and the other forms thick parallel bands of collagen, as in nodular sclerosis Hodgkin disease. Abundant PAS-positive proteinaceous material may be seen in the nodules,[194] as well as plasmacytoid differentiation[195] or cytoplasmic vacuoles of immunoglobulins[196] in the neoplastic cells (signet ring cells).

The histopathology of FCCLs may show differences in the same specimen, or at different sites or in consecutive biopsies of the same patient. When an FL is associated with a diffuse large cell or Burkitt-like tumor in the same specimen, the term composite lymphoma is used.[5,197] Divergent or discordant histologies are seen in 51% of FL patients in whom multiple simultaneous biopsies from different sites are examined.[198] One-third of the discordances involve only the cytologic subtype, while in the remaining two-thirds nodular and diffuse patterns are observed at different sites.[198,199] Finally, histologic changes may be seen in sequential biopsies: in three studies, two-thirds of the tumors retained a nodular pattern (and a low-grade category), while the other one-third converted to a diffuse pattern (and a higher category of malignancy).[200–202] The progression of FLs to a malignancy of higher grade can take several forms: most frequently a diffuse large cell type,[203] uncommonly a Burkitt-like lymphoma,[204] an acute lymphocytic leukemia (ALL),[205] or a "secondary" Ki-1+ anaplastic large cell lymphoma.[206]

Immunophenotyping

FCCLs are B-cell neoplasias[207] as defined by the expression of monoclonal surface immunoglobulins, usually without IgD and/or B lineage differentiation antigens (Table 80-6). The incidence of immunoglobulin-negative cases varies from 0[91,92,95,149,208] to 6–9%.[143,209–211] FCCLs virtually always express HLA-DR and, variably, other activation antigens.[92,208,212] In contrast to SLL, they rarely express CD5 (4%), CD23, CD43, or Leu8,[41,44,98,149,213] and instead quite frequently express CD10 (79%). In

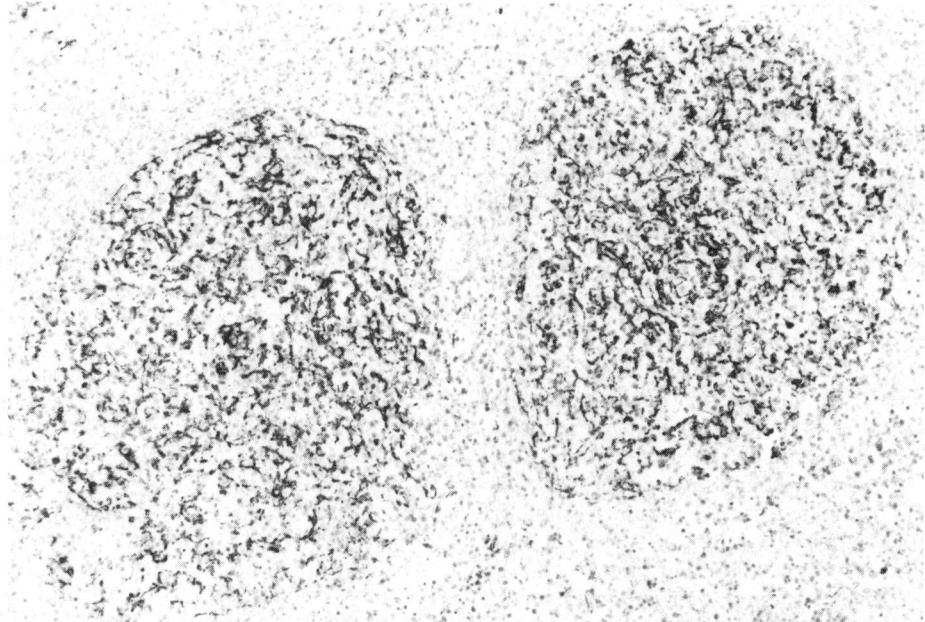

Fig. 80-4. The stairing for dendritic reticulum cells with the monoclonal antibody DRC shows the fine network of DRC projections in the nodules of a follicular lymphoma. (Immunoperoxidase-stained frozen section × 75.)

contrast to hyperplastic germinal centers, FL cells express MT2 in 47%[214] to >90%[215,216] of cases and the *bcl-2* product in 85%[217] to 88%.[215,216] of cases and the *bcl-2* product in 85%[217] to 88%.[218,219] In addition to the DRC network[92,143] (Fig. 80-4), the microenvironment of these tumors includes T cells, especially the CD4+ subset,[210,220,221] and natural killer (NK) cells.[92,222] This general phenotypic pattern is similar in all cytologic types of FLs[143] and in both the follicular and the diffuse forms of FCCL.[41,95,208,212] Differences in immunoglobulin or idiotype expression may be observed with time in tumors from the same patient.[223,224] However, these phenotypic changes (as well as genomic changes of the immunoglobulin genes) do not represent biclonality but mutations within clones arising from one progenitor cell.[225] With respect to both histologic and immunologic features, FLs are clearly the counterparts of normal germinal centers.[2,17] They have been thought to originate either from the neoplastic transformation of one of the cell types that compose the germinal centers of lymph nodes[17] or from the transformation of bone marrow pre-B cells that later home to the lymph nodes. The latter hypothesis might better explain the systemic nature of this disease.[226]

Cytogenetics and Molecular Genetics

Over 80% of FLs are associated with the t(14;18)(q32;q21) translocation,[105,227] which may also be observed in the diffuse forms of FCCLs[104,108,228] and rarely in non-FCC lymphomas.[108,228] This translocation results in an altered expression of the *bcl-2* gene, located at the 18q21 band.[229,230] The bcl-2 product is a protein that, by blocking apoptosis (programmed cell death), prolongs the survival of the cells and thus increases the probability of other genetic mistakes and tumor development.[231] Other translocations, however, have been reported in FLs, such as t(8;14)(q24;q32)[232] or the variant t(2;18)(p11;q21), which appears to involve another gene—FVT (follicular variant translocation)-1—close to the *bcl-2* locus.[233] Additional diverse chromosomal abnormalities, such as partial del6q and trisomies 7 and 12, are common,[104,108] especially with increasing histologic grade.[228,234] Progression of FLs to diffuse large cell lymphomas is associated strongly with p53 mutations,[235,236] less commonly with *myc* rearrangements.[237]

Clinical Correlations

FL constitutes a distinct clinicopathologic entity.[12,238] It is a disease of adults, very rarely observed in children,[239] which presents mostly at nodal rather than extranodal sites, usually without B symptoms[240,241] and with extensive dissemination (stages III–IV). Despite such widespread involvement, the prognosis is generally good. FLs may be controlled by therapy but are rarely cured.[242]

The clinical relevance of histopathologic features, such as pattern (nodular or diffuse), degree of nodularity, and cytologic composition, is still being debated. The following are among the findings to date. (1) The pattern appears to have no important prognostic significance in comparison with cytologic composition in studies based on the Kiel[243,244] classification. However, in the Working Formulation project, the pattern has been shown to be as strong an independent prognostic variable as cytologic type ($P < 0.00001$).[12] More favorable survival with the follicular than with the diffuse pattern has also been proved within cytologic categories.[12,245,246] (2) In most studies the distinction of different degrees of nodularity has provided no additional prognostic information in FL as a whole[244,245,247] or within its cytologic subtypes.[190,245,246,248–250] Degree of nodularity was an independent prognostic factor, however, in follicular, small cleaved, and mixed cell subtypes in two studies,[251,252] and in advanced stage large cell FLs in another.[253] (3) Most studies seem to agree that the differences in overall survival between the three cytologic types of FL are not statistically significant[192,241,254]; paired comparisons show a significant difference between the two extremes of the spectrum, the small cleaved and the large cell types,[241,245,248,254] but not between the mixed and the large cell types.[248,254–256] Whether the mixed cell variant is clinically different from the small cleaved cell type remains controversial. From some studies, it appears that the mixed cell type is clinically more aggressive,[216] has a significantly poorer survival,[245,255] and is associated with a longer remission duration after chemotherapy[257,258] than the small cleaved cell type and that it may even be curable with conventional chemotherapy.[257] In other studies, however, no differences were detected when comparing the two types as to rate of clinical remissions,[258,259] duration of remission,[241] or survival.[247,248,254,256,258,259]

As to the clinical significance of multiple histologies in FL, it has been shown that patients in whom biopsies obtained at the same time demonstrate nodular and diffuse patterns at different sites have complete remission rates and median survival times intermediate between those of patients showing only a nodular or only a diffuse pattern.[198] Progression with time from a follicular to a diffuse pattern is associated with a worsening prognosis: the survival from time of rebiopsy was 11 months in one series[201] and 8.5 months in another,[202] which is considerably shorter than that of patients with persistent nodular pattern on repeat biopsies.

In a few studies phenotypic characteristics appear to be correlated with clinical features and prognosis. The expression of the IgD and/or the receptor for C′3 has identified a subset of FL of small cleaved cell type with an indolent course and excellent prognosis.[260] LFA-1 was found to be less frequently expressed in recurrences of FL of small cleaved cell type than in the initial tumors, which suggests a role for this adherence molecule in the immunologic control of the neoplasia.[64] Similarly, the host cell infiltrates in FLs that underwent spontaneous regression were found to be significantly more abundant and to contain more CD4[+] cells than FLs in patients with progressive disease.[261] S-phase fraction, an index of cellular proliferation, when >5%, was associated with decreased survival of FLs in one study.[262] Cytogenetic studies suggest that chromosomal alterations in addition to t(14;18) may portend increased aggressiveness of FLs.[234] A low number of normal metaphases, breaks in chromosome 17,[263] and 10q23-25 abnormalities[264] have all been shown to correlate with a shorter survival.

Diffuse Mixed Cell Lymphomas

In the Working Formulation, as in the Rappaport classification, diffuse mixed cell lymphoma is a poorly defined category because its distinction from diffuse lymphomas composed of small cells and those composed of large cells is problematic,[265,266] and because this form of NHL is heterogeneous. From a morphologic viewpoint, in fact, diffuse mixed cell lymphoma[12] includes tumors composed of FCCs, tumors cytologically consistent with a T-cell phenotype,[267] and the Kiel polymorphic lymphoplasmacytoid lymphomas.[2] Commonly, SLLs with a high percentage of large transformed cells are also classified as diffuse mixed cell lymphomas.[266] From an immunophenotypic and genotypic viewpoint, the mixed cell category contains both B- and T-cell lymphomas.[268] In most B-cell mixed lymphoma, the small cells are predominantly reactive T cells,[268,269] suggesting that, perhaps, a diagnosis of T-cell-rich large B-cell lymphoma would be more appropriate.[269]

The diffuse mixed cell type, as a group, is considered by clinicians to constitute an aggressive lymphoma.[270–274] There appear to be no relevant differences in clinical characteristics or survival between this type of NHL and "undifferentiated" or diffuse large cell lymphomas.[12,241,274] Two studies have addressed the issue of whether clinical differences exist among the morphologic subtypes contained within the mixed cell category. In one, mixed cell tumors of the small lymphocytic, FCC, and immunoblastic types all had similar clinical features; however, those of the immunoblastic type responded less favorably to therapy than those of small lymphocytic type.[266] In a larger study the survival of patients with the FCC type was better than the survival of those with T-cell morphology, but it was not significantly prolonged by aggressive chemotherapy directed to achievement of complete remission, as was the case with T-cell tumor patients.[275]

Diffuse Large Cell Lymphomas

Pathologic Definition

The term diffuse large cell lymphoma (DLCL), which corresponds to Rappaport's diffuse histiocytic lymphoma, includes two categories of the Working Formulation: the neoplasms composed of large FCCs and those composed of immunoblasts of presumed B- or T-cell origin (Table 80-4). These two categories largely coincide with the diffuse large cleaved or noncleaved cell lymphoma and the immunoblastic sarcomas of the Lukes-Collins scheme and with the centroblastic diffuse and the immunoblastic categories of the Kiel system. The immunophenotype of DLCLs is heterogeneous: 79% are B-cell, 16% T-cell, and 5% non-T, non-B. Some tumors with this last phenotype may be of true histiocytic type. There are no cytogenetic abnormalities specific to either the DLCLs as a group or to the histologic subtypes of the group.

Histopathology

The morphologic heterogeneity of DLCLs remains a major obstacle to the accurate categorization of these tumors. Those of FCC type, the large noncleaved (centroblastic)[2] and the large cleaved cell type (Fig. 80-5A & B) have already been described. The immunoblastic lymphoma category of the Working Formulation[12] includes four morphologic subtypes, three of which (clear cell, polymorphous, and with an epithelioid component) are presumed to be of T-cell type (see the section Peripheral T-Cell Lymphomas) (Fig. 80-5C), while the one with plasmacytoid features is presumed to be of B-cell origin (Fig. 80-6) and consists of large cells with abundant intensely basophilic cytoplasm and nuclei with coarse chromatin and prominent central nucleoli. These cells are admixed with a variable proportion of smaller cells showing plasmacytic differentiation. In addition, a multilobated cell type of DLCL has been described, composed of large cells with very complex nuclear hypersegmentation.[276] It may have a T-cell phenotype (and thus reasonably belongs to the immunoblastic, clear cell category) or may be composed of B cells, which are of FCC derivation (and thus is best classified with the diffuse large cleaved cell lymphomas).[276–278] The same heterogeneity has been demonstrated for the immunoblastic clear cell lymphomas,[279] exemplifying the difficulty of predicting the immunologic phenotype of DLCLs from their cytologic characteristics.[280,281] Discordancies between a large cell type in the lymph node and a small cleaved or mixed cell lymphoma in the bone marrow of the same patient are quite common (52–77%).[282–284]

Immunophenotyping

Based on the presence or absence of cell-surface and cytoplasmic immunoglobulins and the expression of B- and T-cell-restricted antigens, 79% of DLCLs are found to be of B-cell origin and 16% of T-cell origin, and only 5% remain unclassifiable.[285,286] Exceptional cases of DLCL have been shown to express both T- and B-cell markers.[286] The phenotypic characterization of the DLCLs of T-cell type is discussed in the section Peripheral T-Cell Lymphomas. In a collation of data from frozen section phenotypic studies of B-cell DLCLs (Table 80-6), 73% were shown to express surface and/or cytoplasmic immunoglobulins, and the remaining 27% were immunoglobulin-negative.[92,208,285,287,288] Both lower (17%)[289] and higher (>60%)[206] incidences of immunoglobulin-negative DLCL are reported in more recent series. B-cell restricted markers CD19, CD20, and CD22 are expressed consistently, while activation antigens are variably expressed by B-DLCLs, HLA-DR being the most frequent and CD23 especially uncommon (0–25%).[206,289] Only minor phenotypic differences seem to exist between FCC

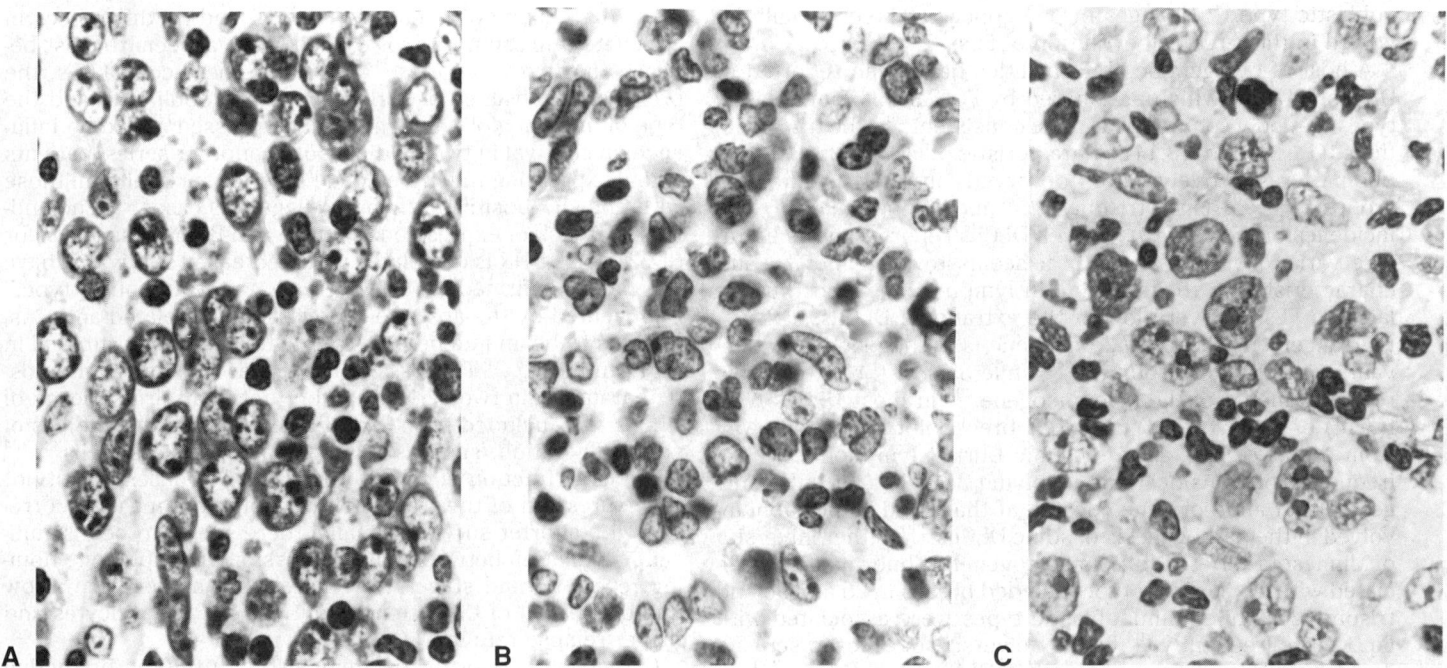

Fig. 80-5. Different cytologic types of diffuse large cell lymphomas. **(A)** Large noncleaved FCC; **(B)** large cleaved FCC; and **(C)** immunoblastic clear cell. (All H&E × 900.)

and B-cell immunoblastic types[92,206,208,288,290]: the former more frequently express CD10, while the latter more frequently express cytoplasmic immunoglobulins, and 14.5% of the former, but none of the latter, express CD21.[206] The presence of CD10 or CD5 suggests that at least a one-third of DLCLs are related to FLs and a small minority to small lymphocytic tumors. That most B-cell DLCLs infrequently express either immature B-cell markers (IgD and CD21) or plasma cell antigens has suggested that they are the neoplastic counterparts of normal B cells at midstages of differentiation.[291]

Genotyping and Cytogenetics

By DNA hybridization techniques the great majority of B-cell DLCLs (and of the "null" DLCLs)[292] demonstrate rearrangements of the immunoglobulin genes (in the absence of rearrangements of the Tβ subunit of the TCR gene), proving their B-cell lineage. However, approximately 9% of B-DLCLs show no evidence of immunoglobulin gene rearrangement and 18% show rearrangement only of the immunoglobulin heavy chain gene.[293] Mutations or allelic losses of the p53 tumor suppressor gene on 17p13.1 are common in DLCL, especially in the immu-

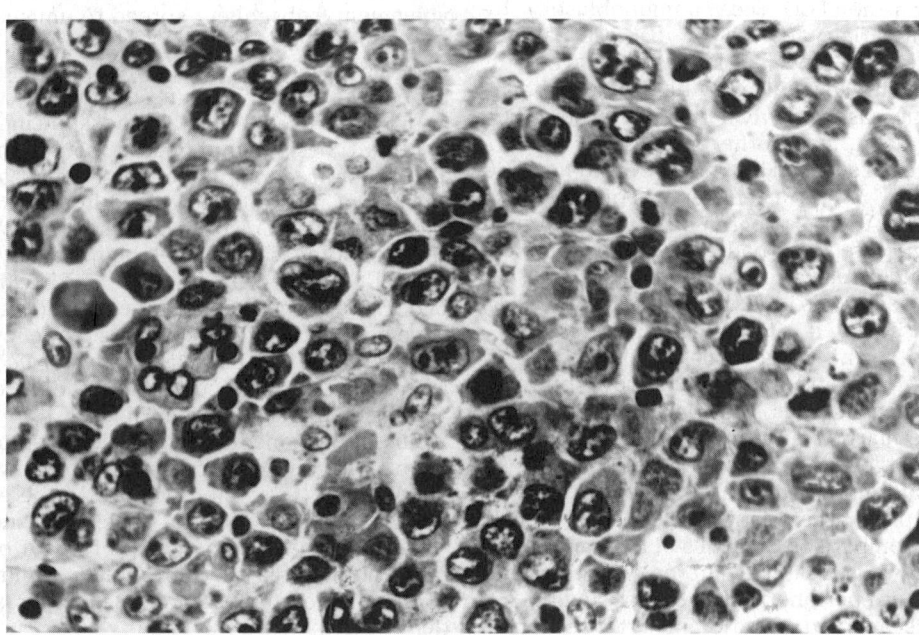

Fig. 80-6. Varying degrees of plasmacytoid differentiation are seen in this plasmacytoid immunoblastic lymphoma. (H&E × 450.)

noblastic type.[294] Changes of p53 appear to be especially involved in the large cell evolution of FLs.[235,236]

A host of cytogenetic abnormalities have been reported in DLCLs, most of which are shared by FCC and immunoblastic types, but only some appear to be consistent.[295] The translocations t(14;18) and t(8;14), characteristic of FL and Burkitt lymphoma, respectively, are observed in both histologic groups,[104,105,108] as are trisomy 12[108] and deletion of 6q.[106] The incidence of the t(14;18) in B-cell DLCLs reported in the literature varies from 12% to 40%; it seems to be higher in, and characteristic of, those arising in lymph nodes, and thus related to FLs, but very low in the extranodal DLCLs.[296] Thus, rearrangement of the bcl-2 oncogene is pathogenetically relevant in the former group,[296,297] while 35% of the latter show rearrangements of the myc oncogene.[296] In most DLCLs with t(8;14) or other t(8q24), the 8q24 breakpoint is located away from the myc gene, as in endemic Burkitt lymphoma.[298] The frequency of translocations involving 3q27 has recently suggested that another gene, located at that band, is possibly involved in the pathogenesis of some DLCLs.[299] In the University of Minnesota series, additional cytogenetic abnormalities associated with DLCL of FCC type included breaks in 2q and 9q and trisomy 21, while immunoblastic types were associated with 6q21 more frequently.[104] In the University of Chicago series a 3q+ chromosome was seen only in DLCLs of FCC type.[300]

Clinical Correlations

DLCLs represent a distinct clinical entity characterized by a wide patient age range, relatively frequent presentation in extranodal sites, and a tendency to present as localized disease but also to have rapid dissemination.[12] Bone marrow is involved in only one-quarter of patients at presentation[282-284] and a leukemic phase is very uncommon.[301] The once dismal prognosis has been dramatically improved by newer chemotherapy regimens, which have led to sustained complete remissions in 73–84% of cases.[302] Several clinical factors of prognostic importance have been identified,[272,303-308] but the influence of pathologic parameters on prognosis is controversial.

In the Working Formulation and other pioneering studies looking at the clinical significance of histologic type, the DLCLs of FCC morphology seemed to have a better overall and disease-free survival than non-FCC (i.e., immunoblastic) tumors.[12,309,310] In a multivariate analysis of 75 DLCL patients treated with CHOP chemotherapy, the large noncleaved FCC variant was associated with a significantly higher rate of complete remission and increased survival than all other DLCL types.[311] On the other hand, many other studies have shown no significant differences in survival between FCC and non-FCC variants of DLCLs.[241,306,308,312-314] Recent reports of the results of the COP-BLAM[315] and MACOP-B programs[316] have confirmed that these two histologic categories had comparable complete remission rates[315,316] and disease-free and overall survivals.[316] The presence of marked sclerosis in DLCL or a divergent histology at another site is associated with an increased risk of late relapses.[317] For patients with discordant histology (i.e., in whom the node shows DLCL and the bone marrow shows involvement with small cleaved cells), the prognosis is similar to those with negative marrow and much better than those with marrow showing large cell lymphoma.[282-284]

Many studies have attempted to establish correlations between immunophenotypic characteristics of DLCLs and clinical features or prognosis. Comparison of DLCLs of B- versus T-cell lineage has revealed only some clinical differences (the former more often presenting with peripheral adenopathy and the latter with extranodal disease and hepatic and retroperitoneal involvement)[318] and, in two studies from the same group, a shorter disease-free survival for T-cell tumors.[319,320] However,

these data have not been confirmed[321] and no differences in complete remission rate, or overall survival seem to exist between the two categories.[318,319,321] For the B-cell DLCLs, the presence or absence of surface immunoglobulins,[289] and the type of immunoglobulin light chain expressed[322] had no influence on survival in two studies, but in another series, patients with κ-expressing tumors enjoyed a better survival than those with non-κ (λ-positive or κ- and λ-negative) cases.[286] The findings that lack of expression of single pan-B antigens (CD20 or CD22) or HLA-DR is correlated with decreased survival[286] have not been confirmed.[289] However, an "aberrant phenotype," represented by the absence of several B-cell-related antigens, appears to be an independent predictor of shorter survival in both studies.[286,289] The loss of HLA-DR was also a poor prognostic parameter in two series,[56,320] but not in a third series[323] of DLCLs that included both B- and T-cell types. Some indices of cell proliferation, such as high numbers of Ki-67+ cells[320,324] and a large fraction of cells in the S and G_2 phases,[325] but not the expression of the transferrin receptor,[52] appear to correlate with shorter survival. Finally, there seems to be a significant correlation between high expression of lymphocyte homing receptors and stage III–IV disease[326] and between a low number (<6%) of CD8+ tumor infiltrating T lymphocytes and higher relapse rate in DLCL.[327]

Cytogenetic abnormalities may also be useful in predicting clinical outcome in DLCLs. Patients with karyotypes containing a break in 2p have been shown to survive longer than those without this abnormality[263]; in another study, a dup3p or trisomy 3 had a positive influence while dup2p or trisomy 2 adversely affected survival.[328] The patients with DLCL that show rearrangements of bcl-2 have a shorter disease-free survival than those without such rearrangements, a behavior reminiscent of the FLs to which they are related.[329]

Variants of Large Cell Lymphomas

Two variants of DLCLs have recently received much attention. One, the mediastinal large (clear) cell lymphoma with sclerosis (MLCL), represents a distinct clinicopathologic entity.[330-336] It has a predilection for women of young age, with medians/means from 25 to 36 years. The presentation is mostly localized to the mediastinum and thoracic cavity, without superficial node, bone marrow, or central nervous system involvement; subsequent spread to unusual sites (kidney, adrenals, thyroid) is common.[330,331,334,336] The contrasting literature data regarding response to therapy and prognosis of MLCL are probably accounted for not only by the variety of therapeutic approaches used, but by the possible inclusion in some series of other types of lymphomas arising in the mediastinum.[335,336] The most frequent histology is that of large cleaved/noncleaved or multilobated cells, often with clear cytoplasm and associated with fine trabecular sclerosis,[330-333,335] and the classic phenotype is immunoglobulin-negative, B-antigen-positive, HLA-DR+, CD30−, CD45+.[206,332,333,335] The frequent expression of CD11c[335] and the specific adhesion molecule profile of MLCL[337] have been thought to explain its tendency to remain localized. The lack of CD10 expression and of bcl-2 rearrangements[338] argues against an FCC origin. Instead the expression of plasma-cell-associated antigens, as in MoBCL,[339] and the lack of CD21, as in the intramedullary thymic B lymphocytes[340] and their neoplastic counterpart,[341] suggest that MLCL arises from thymic B cells[331,335,336] and belongs to the ever-expanding family of tumors of MoBCL/MALT type.[339] As such, it should be separated from mediastinal DLCL of nodal origin, most of which have immunoblastic morphology, immunoglobulin-positive CD21+ phenotype, and occur in older and mostly male patients.[335,336]

A second variant of DLCL, the T-cell-rich large B-cell lymphoma (TBL), is heterogeneous in its histology and is not a distinct clinical entity.[81,342–345] The classic cases feature a predominance of small reactive T lymphocytes intermixed with sparse large neoplastic B cells and, often, increased vascularity and Reed-Sternberg-like cells.[81,343,345] Therefore, histopathologically they may closely mimic T-cell lymphomas and Hodgkin disease, from which at times they can be distinguished only by detecting immunoglobulin gene rearrangements.[343,345,346] Although this distinction is clinically relevant, that of TBL from the other DLCLs is not. In fact, several studies[342–345] have demonstrated that there are no distinctive clinical characteristics to TBL, except perhaps a high frequency of splenomegaly,[344] and that, despite the striking T-cell component, the clinical outcome is not different from that of the usual DLCL in patients adequately treated.

Small Noncleaved Cell Lymphoma

Pathologic Definition

Small noncleaved cell lymphomas (SNCLs) are composed of lymphoid cells of intermediate size, with prominent basophilic cytoplasm and nuclei with prominent nucleoli. The growth pattern is primarily diffuse. The category of SNCL in the Working Formulation includes Burkitt lymphomas (BLs) and tumors that in the Rappaport classification were referred to as undifferentiated non-Burkitt type. The SNCL category corresponds to the Lukes-Collins SNCL and to the B-cell lymphoblastic lymphomas in the Kiel system. These tumors are of B-cell phenotype and are probably histogenetically related to FCCs. They are associated with three characteristic chromosomal translocations—t(8;14), t(2;8), and t(8;22)—which lead to the dysregulation of the c-*myc* oncogene.

Histopathology

The morphologic criteria for the diagnosis of BL[347] (Fig. 80-7A) include a monotonous proliferation of cells of intermediate size (10–25 μm in diameter), with round to oval nuclei, coarsely reticulated chromatin, and two to five prominent peripheral nucleoli. The cytoplasm is relatively abundant, sharply deline-

ated, and, owing to the abundance of RNA, strongly basophilic and pyroninophilic. When lymph node imprints or bone marrow smears are examined, the cytoplasm is noted to contain small vacuoles of neutral lipids, stainable with oil red O. This cell proliferation is consistently associated with a high number of mitoses and a prominent diffuse "starry sky" pattern, produced by scattered macrophages containing nuclear debris. The pattern of growth is diffuse. However, in approximately 20% of cases one finds follicular structures representing involved germinal centers.[348] This morphologic description applies to the two forms of BL, namely, the African or endemic form, which is nearly always (95%) associated with Epstein-Barr virus (EBV) infection, and the sporadic form, which occurs worldwide at a much lower incidence and is less commonly (20%) associated with EBV.[349]

A tumor very similar to BL that is included in the undifferentiated category of the Rappaport classification,[12] has been referred to as non-Burkitt or pleomorphic type (Fig. 80-7B). As compared with BL it is distinguished by greater variability in nuclear size and shape, a single central nucleolus, and a less abundant and paler cytoplasm.[350] By conventional histopathology the differentiation between these two types is somewhat subjective, as shown by the poor rate of agreement among pathologists and the poor reproducibility by the same pathologists.[351] However, significant dissimilarities between the Burkitt and the non-Burkitt types have been recognized by ultrastructural morphometric analysis,[352] and, more important, at the molecular level.[353] In some cases it may be difficult to separate SNCLs, especially the non-Burkitt variant, from DLCLs.[350,352,354] In fact, morphometric analysis of nuclear area and irregularity has demonstrated a continuum between the two types rather than a clear-cut distinction,[355] and transition from an SNCL morphology to a plasmacytoid immunoblastic one can be obtained in vitro by the addition of phorbol ester.[356]

Immunophenotyping

BL in both its endemic and sporadic form is a monoclonal B-cell tumor.[348] Immunophenotypic characterization based on studies of cultured BL cell lines has shown marked heterogene-

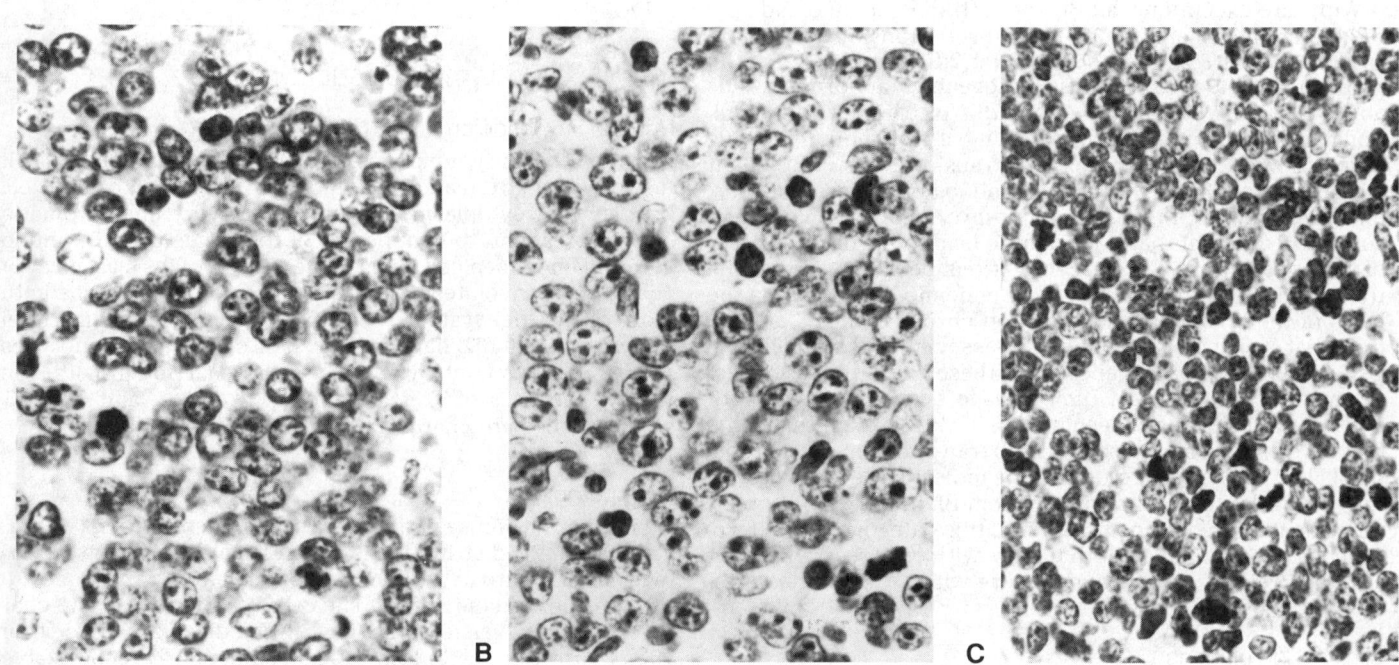

Fig. 80-7. Comparison of the cellular characteristics of **(A)** a Burkitt lymphoma; **(B)** a small noncleaved cell lymphoma of non-Burkitt (pleomorphic) type; and **(C)** a lymphoblastic lymphoma. (All H&E × 900.)

ity, which, however, appears to be generated during in vitro passages.[357–360] By contrast, studies of fresh tumor cells and frozen sections have revealed a rather consistent phenotype (Table 80-6), including surface κ- or λ-chains in proportions similar to those observed in normal B cells, surface IgM in striking predominance over IgG (20:1 ratio), and IgD in 18.5% of the cases.[91,92,208,352] These findings are in contrast with those of Garcia et al.,[287] which indicated an excess of lymphomas expressing λ-chains and IgD. BL cells express pan-B cell antigens, HLA-DR and CD10,[361] but not CD21 or, characteristically, activation antigens such as CD25 or CD35. The reactivity with the OKT9 (CD71) monoclonal antibody in most cases[52] and the high percentage of cells positive with Ki-67[287,352] are in keeping with the high proliferative rate of this tumor. EBV-related BLs have an identical phenotype to EBV-negative BLs, but express EB nuclear antigen (EBNA)-1, one of the proteins associated with the EBV latent cycle.[359,360] The lack of expression of other EBNA proteins and latent membrane protein (LMP) (which are responsible for the cytotoxic T-cell response) in the EBV-related BLs and the low expression of adhesion molecules, such as LFA-1 and -3 (which facilitate interaction with the T cells) in both EBV-positive and -negative BL-cell lines[362] may help the tumor escape the host immunosurveillance.

The considerable evidence indicating that BLs are related to FCCs, perhaps to "primary B blasts,"[363] includes the involvement of germinal centers[348] and the association with DRCs in some cases[91,92,287]; the expression of CD10[364] and the BL-associated antigen (BLA)[365,366]; and the absence of vimentin; all of which are frequent features of normal FCCs and FLs.[364,366,367] Finally, a small cell population obtained from normal tonsils and characterized, like BL cells, by co-expression of CD10 and BLA and lack of activation antigens, was found to be localized in the germinal centers.[368] Dissenting voices remain, however, as to the FCC derivation of BL.[92,369] Some phenotypic differences have been noted between Burkitt and non-Burkitt types,[92,352] which may suggest that non-Burkitt lymphomas are, in general, composed of cells more mature than those of BLs.[352] Also, exceptional cases of lymphomas, histologically identical to the non-Burkitt type, have expressed a T-cell phenotype.[370]

Cytogenetics and Molecular Biology

With rare exceptions, all BLs of both the endemic and sporadic variants manifest one of three translocations: t(8; 14)(q24;q32), t(8;22)(q24;q11), and t(2;8)(p11-p13;q24). The respective incidence of these cytogenetic abnormalities is about 80%, 15%, and 5%.[371] About 70% of patients have additional chromosomal abnormalities, most frequently involving chromosome 1. The chromosomal translocations in BL result in the juxtaposition of one of the immunoglobulin gene regions, on chromosome 2, 14, or 22, to the c-*myc* oncogene on chromosome 8,[372] an event that is thought to lead to the dysregulation of the oncogene.[373] More recently it has been shown that the t(8;14) translocation found in most endemic BLs differs on the basis of the breakpoint positions on chromosomes 8 and 14, from that seen in sporadic and AIDS-associated BLs, which suggests a different pathogenesis for these two groups of neoplasms.[374,375] Non-Burkitt tumors have been associated with the same translocations seen in BLs,[104,105,108] except that some of them have also shown the t(14;18) translocation characteristic of FLs.[108] In a recent study, at the molecular level, however, the non-Burkitt category differed from BL in that no *myc* rearrangements were found; in addition, this category was heterogeneous, as it contained both tumors with *bcl*-2 rearrangement and thus related to FLs, and tumors without that rearrangement.[353]

Clinical Correlations

BL in its endemic, African form is a well-characterized clinicopathologic entity.[376] Less certain is the clinical characterization of the sporadic form of BL, because of its controversial relation-

ships with the non-Burkitt variant. In a series of pediatric patients the distinction between BL and non-Burkitt lymphoma has been shown to be poorly reproducible histopathologically and irrelevant clinically.[354] In other studies, including children and adult patients, either the two groups have been dealt with together as SNCLs or "undifferentiated" lymphomas[12,377–379] or they have been compared with each other and found to be clinically distinct.[350,352,380,381] It is difficult, however, to draw firm conclusions from such comparisons since the criteria to separate the two groups may not be the same in all studies, as indicated by the wide spectrum of median ages at presentation given for the two types in different series: from 6.5 years[352] to 31 years[380] for BL and from 24.5 years[379] to 67 years[382] for non-Burkitt lymphoma.

With this caveat in mind, many similarities and some differences between the clinical presentation and course of the two groups have been defined. The similarities in clinical presentation include distribution by stage (with patients presenting mostly with Ann Arbor stage IV or equally distributed between low and high NCI-Pediatric Branch stages) and the incidence of B symptoms and bone and bone marrow involvement. BLs, however, tend to present with primary extranodal and intra-abdominal sites of disease, especially in the gastrointestinal tract, while non-Burkitt lymphomas tend to present more frequently with peripheral lymphadenopathy. These data seem to agree with those of the already mentioned molecular study, in which tumors with Burkitt histology (and *myc* rearrangement) were all extranodal in presentation, while those of non-Burkitt type (without *myc* rearrangement) often had nodal presentation.[353] Complete remission rates have been similar in the two groups in most studies.[350,379,380] Similarly, relapse rates,[350] disease-free survival,[378,379,383] median survival,[350,380,383] and projected survival rates[379] have not been significantly different. However, in two studies, patients with BL had higher complete remission rates (67% versus 25%),[352] better survival rates (42% versus 11%),[350] and longer median survival (63 versus 3 months)[352] than patients with non-Burkitt lymphoma. With new high-dose chemotherapy regimens, both Burkitt[384] and non-Burkitt lymphomas[385] have a high (57–85%) complete response rate and 50–60% rates of disease-free survival.

Lymphoblastic Lymphoma

Pathologic Definition

Lymphoblastic lymphomas (LBLs) are characterized by a diffuse growth pattern and are composed of medium to large cells having scant cytoplasm and nuclei with very fine chromatin. They correspond to lymphomas of the convoluted T lymphocyte and undefined cell types of the Lukes-Collins classification and to the convoluted cell and unclassified lymphoblastic tumors of the Kiel system. Most LBLs have an immature T-cell phenotype, but 16% have pre-B cell or other rare phenotypes. Almost all LBLs contain TdT. Chromosomal abnormalities involving the sites of TCR αδ (14q11), β (7q34), and γ (7p15) subunit genes are characteristic.

Histopathology

LBLs have a diffuse pattern of growth; when germinal centers are spared, the distribution is paracortical. At low power, very high mitotic activity, a starry-sky pattern, and infiltration of the capsule are common.[386] The cells of LBLs have quite characteristic cytologic features (Fig. 80-7C): they vary in size from 10 to 14 μm, their cytoplasm is scanty and poorly recognizable, the nuclei have a very fine, dusty chromatin pattern, and the nucleoli are inconspicuous. Nuclear contours may be irregular and convoluted or rounded (nonconvoluted).[386] Smaller cells,

Table 80-7. Selected Immunohistologic Findings in T-Cell NHLs

| Histologic Type | No. of Patients | Pan-T Antigens[a] | | | | Subset Antigens[b] | | | | | Activation Antigens[a] | | References |
		CD2	CD3	CD5	CD7	CD4+/CD8-	CD4-/CD8+	CD4-/CD8-	CD4+/CD8+	Other	HLA-DR	CD25	
Lymphoblastic	60	83	92.5	78	81	13	0	31	8	48[c]	43	4	208, 395, 398
PTCLs in general	123	81	76	71	66	64	12	16	8	0	77	44	208, 446, 450, 460, 463
Lymphoepithelioid	18	100	94	83	50	100	0	0	0	0	82		461, 470–472
AILD-like	48					48	6	0	0	46[d]			461, 473–476
Large anaplastic[e]	52	67	37	39	22	61	9	28	2	0	96	84	448, 477–481
Pleomorphic/immunoblastic	23	90	100	83	0	91	4.5	0	4.5	0	83	95	461, 482

[a] Numbers represent percentage of positive among cases tested.
[b] Numbers represent percentage with phenotype based on number tested: sum of subsets = 100%.
[c] CD1+.
[d] No predominance of either CD4- or CD8+ cells.
[e] Data refer only to the large anaplastic cell Ki-1+ lymphoma of T-cell phenotype.

with a more compact chromatin pattern, or prolymphocytes, may also be observed.[386] Rare LBLs feature a somewhat different cell type characterized by larger size and more obvious cytoplasm and/or relatively prominent nucleoli; this has been referred to as the "atypical lymphoblastic"[387,388] or "large cell" variant[389] and may be difficult to distinguish from Burkitt, large cell, or mixed cell lymphomas.[390,391] On immunochemical or biochemical assays, LBL cells demonstrate the presence of the nuclear enzyme TdT, which is thought to contribute to the generation of diversity of the antigen receptors in B and T precursor cells.[392] TdT activity is the most consistent marker of LBLs,[58,393–395] being absent[396,397] in only about 4% of the total reported cases. About 80% of LBLs have focal acid phosphatase reactivity.[2]

Immunophenotyping

The vast majority of LBLs (i.e., 84% of 110 cases)[92,393,395,397,398] have a T-cell phenotype (Table 80-7). There is, however, a marked degree of immunophenotypic heterogeneity within this category: two-thirds of the phenotypes can be correlated with the classic stages of normal T-cell development in the thymus,[399] but one-third of them do not conform to any normal pattern of T-cell development.[394,395,400] The distribution of T-cell LBLs among the normal thymic phenotypes (i.e., immature, common, mature) varies in different series; overall, values of 15%, 57%, and 28%, respectively, are obtained.[390,398,400,401] Thus most (common and mature thymocyte phenotype) express CD7, cytoplasmic or surface CD3, CD2, and CD5 and many express CD1 with both CD4 and CD8. A minority express CD7 only, with or without the hematopoietic precursor cell marker CD34[402] (prothymocyte), or CD7 with CD2 and CD5 (immature thymocyte). Similar disparate conclusions have been reached about the distribution of T-cell ALLs among the same thymic phenotypes: the values from several series[390,398,400,401] are 34%, 42%, and 24%, respectively, which are not significantly different from those obtained for T-LBL, confirming the close relationship between the two diseases. T-cell LBLs may also express HLA-DR (43%) and CD10 (25%),[393–395,398,400] as do B-cell tumors, but rarely express CD25. A few of them also manifest antigens associated with NK cells, such as CD57 or CD16.[395,403] Only 60% of T-cell LBLs co-express with CD3 the β-chain of the TCR.[404–406] Among the other 40%, some cases represent a phenotypic aberrancy of LBLs of Tαβ type[404]; others, however, co-express δ-chains and represent LBLs of Tγδ type.[407–409]

As mentioned, 16% of tumors with the morphology typical of LBLs are non-T in phenotype; most of them show pre-B features and rare ones manifest surface immunoglobulin[395,410] or co-expression of B- and T-cell markers[398] or of T-cell and myeloid markers.[411] The pre-B-cell tumors are clearly heterogeneous.[412] Some have been shown to contain cytoplasmic IgM only[391,393,412–416]; others, by virtue of the presence of HLA-DR, CD10, and early B-cell antigens, have a pre-pre B or precursor B-cell phenotype.[92,391,393,395,397,398,412,417–420] Most of the non-T-cell tumors are composed of convoluted cells[391,393,413–415,418] rather than nonconvoluted cells.[2,417]

Immunogenotyping and Cytogenetics

Most T-cell LBLs demonstrate rearrangements of the TCR genes.[394,421–423] There is a general but not consistent correlation between the degree of immunophenotypic differentiation and the postulated order of rearrangement of the TCR genes in ontogeny[424,425]: tumors with immature phenotypes are most often associated with rearranged γ- or δ-chain genes and germline α- and β-chain genes, while the rearrangements of the latter chains are more common in tumors with mature phenotype.[421–423] A small number of T-LBLs expressing prothymocyte phenotype have shown no rearrangements of the TCR genes or only rearrangements of the δ-chain gene.[394,421,423] All these molecular data do not confirm the purported strong correlation found in one study between T-LBL and immunohistochemical expression of β-chain (87%), as opposed to the expression of γδ chains in T-ALL (67%).[409]

The most common chromosomal abnormalities in T-cell LBLs are those involving 14q11-13; they include inv(14)(q11;q32)[104] and deletions[426] and translocations involving chromosomes 9,[426] 10,[427] and 11.[108,426] Others involve 7q34[428] and 7p15.[429] These are the sites at which the TCR α-, β-, and γ-subunit genes are located, which suggests that, in analogy with B-cell lymphomas, juxtaposition of receptor gene regions to oncogenes may play an essential role in the neoplastic transformation of T cells.[430] In a large study of T-cell lymphoblastic malignancies,[388] such translocations were found in T-cell LBLs and T-cell ALLs with similar frequency (47% and 36%, respectively). However, other translocations, such as t(9;17)(q34;q23), occurred only in LBLs, perhaps indicating the existence of subsets of LBLs that are distinct from T-cell ALL.[443]

Clinical Correlations

LBL was originally characterized as a rapidly fatal malignancy of children and adolescents, mostly males, which presents with a mediastinal mass and has a tendency to involve bone marrow and peripheral blood. Supradiaphragmatic lymphadenopathy and involvement of the central nervous system and gonads are also common and most patients have disseminated disease at presentation.[431] LBLs with similar clinical features also occur in older age groups.[432–434] The prognosis in all age groups has recently dramatically improved: with new intensive chemotherapies, as used for ALL,[435] the disease-free survival has reached 58%[436] or 65%[437] in children, and 56% in adults.[438] The clinical features of T-LBL may overlap those of T-cell ALL, to the point that at times the two diseases can only be distinguished by the extent of bone marrow involvement at presentation.[431,439,440] However, most cases of T-LBL are distinguished from T-ALL by having minimal or no involvement of peripheral blood and bone marrow, and normal hemoglobin values and cell blood counts, and by lacking organomegaly.[386]

Prognostic parameters in LBL are mostly of clinical nature.[435] The histopathologic distinction between convoluted and non-convoluted types is not clinically significant.[386] Unusual cytologic appearances, with tumoral and peripheral eosinophilia, have been associated with subsequent development of a myeloid malignancy.[441] Within the T-cell LBLs, the immunophenotypic subdivision into thymocyte of early, mid, and late stages does not appear to recognize significant clinical differences.[390,401] However, the group of patients with midstage LBLs had no generalized lymphadenopathy or initial bone marrow involvement in one study,[400] and those with mature-stage LBLs were less likely to have a mediastinal mass ($P = 0.02$) in another.[390] In the small group of T-LBLs that expressed NK cell-associated antigens, most patients were female and the clinical course was more aggressive.[403] In two large series the overall survival and disease-free survival were similar for all phenotypic subgroups of T-cell LBLs,[390,401] which suggests that phenotype need not be included in the stratification of patients for clinical trials.[390]

The smaller subgroup of non-T-cell LBLs has a clinical pattern somewhat different from that of T-cell LBLs. The median age of onset calculated from all reports of patients with the pre-B phenotype is 6 years, which is below the median age for LBLs in general (27 years in males and 50 years in females)[432] and in fact differs from that for all childhood LBLs (11.5 years)[442] and for childhood LBLs of T-cell phenotype (8.5 years).[401] This LBL subgroup is also distinguished by an unusually high incidence of cutaneous (about 43%) and osteolytic bone lesions (about 26%) and by the absence of a mediastinal mass, but the incidence of bone marrow involvement at presentation (about 33%) is similar to that found in LBLs in general.[432,442] There appear to be no significant differences in response to therapy as compared with the usual T-cell LBLs. In a series of LBLs treated with similar intensive chemotherapy protocols, the survival curves of T-cell and null LBLs were not statistically different.[397]

Subdivision of patients with T-cell LBLs (and T-cell ALL) according to cytogenetic abnormalities does not correlate with survival differences.[388] However, in our study, all patients with the t(9;17) translocation, who presented with a mediastinal mass and no bone marrow involvement, had a rapidly progressive disease and died without developing a leukemic phase.[443] This translocation may therefore identify a special subset of patients with a poor prognosis.

Peripheral T-Cell Lymphomas

The T-cell malignancies are traditionally divided according to the stages of normal T-cell ontogeny into two main categories: those corresponding to the early stages of T-cell differentiation in the bone marrow and thymus and those related to mature T cells.[444,445] The former category (prethymic and thymic) includes lymphoblastic lymphoma/leukemia. The latter (post-thymic) includes T-cell chronic lymphocytic/prolymphocytic leukemia and mycosis fungoides/Sézary syndrome, as well as a variety of T-cell NHLs, usually referred to as peripheral T-cell lymphomas (PTCLs).[267] In this section PTCLs are discussed as a group, unified by their phenotypic characteristics. Distinct subtypes are mentioned later.

Pathologic Definition

The PTCLs comprise a heterogenous group of diffuse NHLs with a mature or post-thymic phenotype, other than T-cell chronic lymphocytic/prolymphocytic leukemia and mycosis fungoides/Sézary syndrome. Histologically, PTCLs manifest various combinations of features, including increased vascularity, a pleomorphic cellular composition, cells with irregular nuclear contours and often optically clear cytoplasm, and a component of eosinophils and epithelioid macrophages. They are composed of mature T cells, most often of the helper/inducer subset, which characteristically often fail to express normal pan-T antigens and manifest activation antigens. Rearrangements of the TCR genes are demonstrated in most cases. PTCLs are associated with several karyotypic abnormalities, most frequently breaks in 14q11 and trisomy 3.

Histopathology

Despite a variable histopathologic picture, a composite of common pathologic features provides the basis for making a tentative diagnosis of PTCL[267,276,444–447]; such a diagnosis needs to be confirmed by immunophenotypic analysis. The growth pattern is diffuse or exclusively paracortical, as observed most characteristically in the T-zone lymphoma variant[2,445] (Fig. 80-1C). In other cases the neoplastic cells may preferentially involve the sinuses, a feature especially common in the so-called Ki-1 lymphomas.[448,449] Cytologically some PTCLs are composed of a monotonous population of distinctly atypical cells, such as in the pleomorphic (small, medium-size, and large cell) subtypes (Fig. 80-8B), in which the cells have very complex nuclear invaginations; in the immunoblastic cell type, characterized by large round to oval nuclei with prominent nucleoli and basophilic or pale cytoplasm; and in the anaplastic large cell type, in which the nuclei may have round contours or very prominent multilobulation and nucleoli.[445] However, usually PTCL cells cover a spectrum of sizes, including Reed-Sternberg-like giant cells, and have nuclear shapes varying from round to very irregular.[267] The cytoplasm of the neoplastic cells is pale in appearance and often characteristically optically clear.[445] Increased numbers of high-endothelial venules and reactive cells, such as plasma cells, eosinophils, and epithelioid macrophages, are common in the lymphoepithelioid, angioimmunoblastic lymphadenopathy (AILD)-like variants (Fig. 80-8A) and T-zone variants but are uncommon in the pleomorphic or immunoblastic cell types.[78,445,450,451] Such reactive components are thought to result from the action of lymphokines produced by the neoplastic T cells.[452,453] In the so-called angiocentric immunoproliferative lesions,[444,454] the wall of small arteries and veins is extensively infiltrated and destroyed by neoplastic cells. A histologic picture quite close to Hodgkin disease has been reported in both human T-cell leukemia/lymphoma virus (HTLV)-1-negative[447,451] and HTLV-1-positive[455] lymphomas.

The variety of PTCLs encompasses several categories of the Rappaport classification and the Working Formulation. In a compilation of studies that have used such classifications,[446,456–458] 12% were classified as small cell, 39% as mixed cell, 45% as large cell, and 4% could not be classified. Only in a few instances have T-cell tumors shown the morphology of SNCLs.[280,281,370] However, attempts to fit the PTCLs into the categories provided by the Working Formulation do not do justice to the extraordinary morphologic heterogeneity of these tumors. This has prompted the development of several detailed classifications of PTCLs,[444,445,459] one of which[445] has become part of the updated Kiel scheme[15] (Table 80-2) and has been extensively used in pathologic and clinical studies of PTCLs.

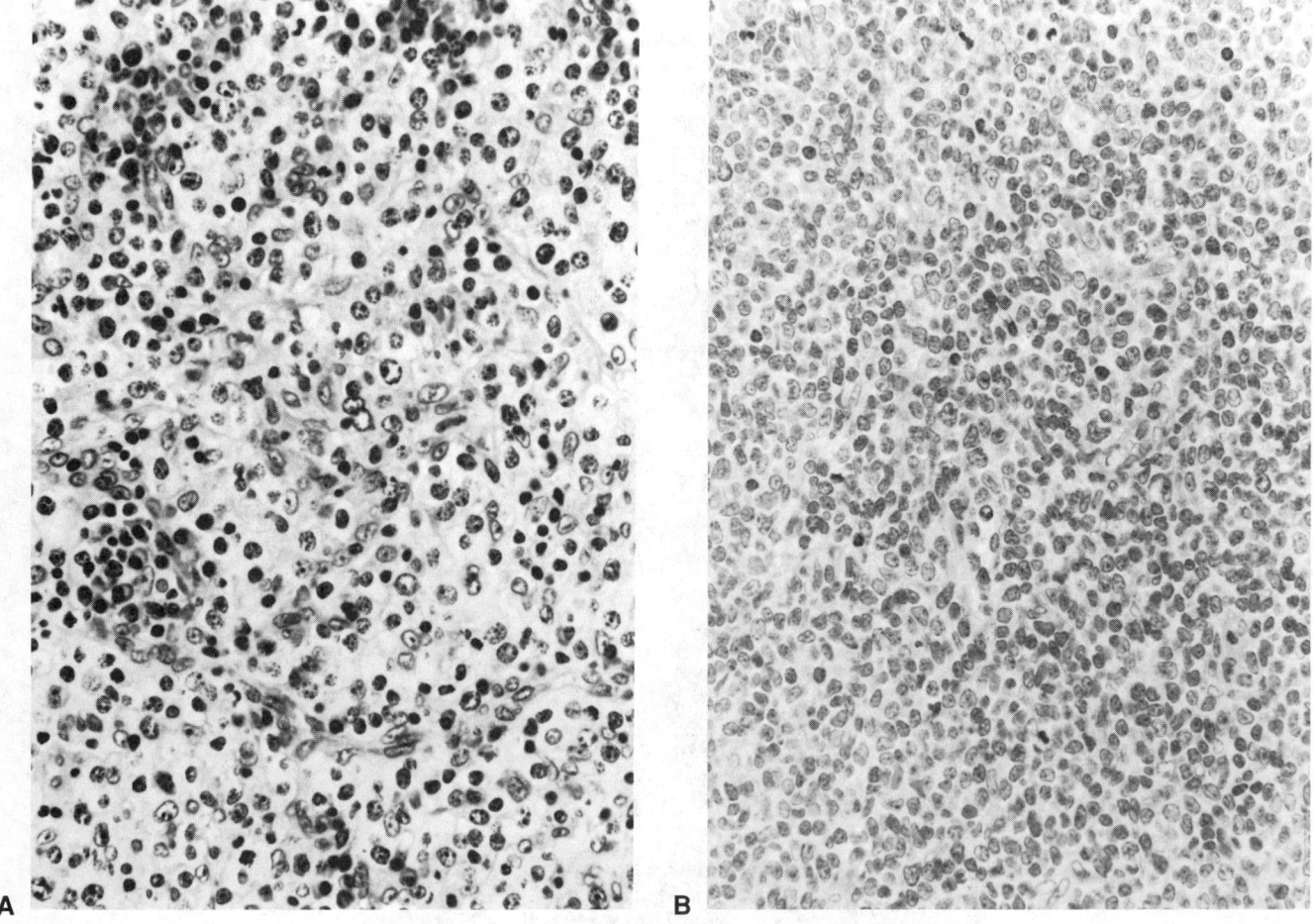

Fig. 80-8. (A) In an angioimmunoblastic lymphadenopathy (AILD)-like lymphoma, the mildly atypical neoplastic infiltrate, rich in clear cells, is associated with increased vascularity and plasma cells ("reactive" features). **(B)** These features are absent in a medium-sized pleomorphic cell lymphoma, which shows instead a monotonous proliferation of distinctly atypical neoplastic cells. (Both H&E × 300.)

Immunophenotyping

The usual definition of PTCLs includes expression of one or more of the normal pan-T antigens (CD2, CD3, CD5, CD7) in the absence both of the immature T-cell antigen CD1 and of B-cell antigens.[446,450,457,460,461] Within these limits, however, a marked phenotypic heterogeneity is observed. The phenotypes of most PTCLs, from 64% to 86%,[462] have been referred to as "abnormal," "novel," or "unusual," because they do not conform to those of the normal mature T cells. The most common abnormality (Table 80-7) is loss of expression of pan-T antigens present on normal T cells[208,446,450,460,463] (Fig. 80-9); this loss therefore provides very useful information in differentiating reactive from malignant T-cell lesions.[41] Loss of pan-T antigens in some studies is said to be characteristic of high-grade, but not of low-grade, lymphomas.[464,465] A second characteristic feature of PTCLs is the abnormal predominance of one T-cell subset (helper/inducer or cytotoxic/suppressor) over the other. In U.S. series,[446,450,460,463] and similarly in Europe[457] and Japan,[461] the large majority of these neoplasms (64%) manifest a CD4+/CD8− phenotype, whereas 12% are CD4−/CD8+. Interestingly, CD4−/CD8− and CD4+/CD8+ tumors can also be observed (16% and 8%, respectively).[462] In exception to the immunophenotypic definition given above, rare tumors with PTCL morphology express CD1.[462] A final immunophenotypic characteristic of PTCLs is the frequent expression of activation markers, such as HLA-DR,[208,446,450,460,461] transferrin receptor,[460] CD38,[208,463] interleukin-2 receptor (CD25),[460,461] and CD11c (Leu M5).[466] A few PTCLs have been found to express NK cell markers, such

as CD16 or CD76.[467–469] Table 80-7 summarizes selected immunophenotypic data available on distinct subtypes of PTCLs,[448,461,470–482] suggesting that some differences do exist among them, which may be both useful in diagnosis and indicative of a different biology.

In recent years, monoclonal antibodies have become available that detect the αβ or γδ chains of the TCR in frozen sections[41,404,407,483–485]; in good agreement with genotypic data,[486] it has been shown that 70% of PTCLs express the αβ chain (βF-1-positive), 10% the γδ chain (TCRδ-1-positive), and around 20% are "receptor-silent" (βF-1 and TCRδ-1-negative).[483] This last category may include neoplastic phenotypic aberrancies, disorders of immature thymocytes or of a third (non-αβ, non-γδ) T-cell subset, or NK-cell lymphomas.[483] All three categories showed loss of pan-T antigens and a variety of T-subset phenotypes, except that all γδ PTCLs were of CD4−/CD8− type.[483] Of these monoclonal antibodies only βF-1 is reactive in paraffin sections; its yield in diagnosing a PTCL in this material is, however, lower (37–67%)[487,488] than with the three classic antibodies—UCHL-1, CD3, and MT-1.[489] More recently, restricted usage of the TCR variable region families has been used in the diagnosis of T-cell malignancy[490–493]; this was detected in ≤33% of cases, the percentage growing with the increase in the number of clonotypic antibodies used. Neither this finding, which can occur also in several reactive conditions,[492] or any of the immunophenotypic markers mentioned above is by itself direct proof of the clonality of a T-cell malignancy. This can only be provided by the demonstration of rearrangements of the TCR genes.

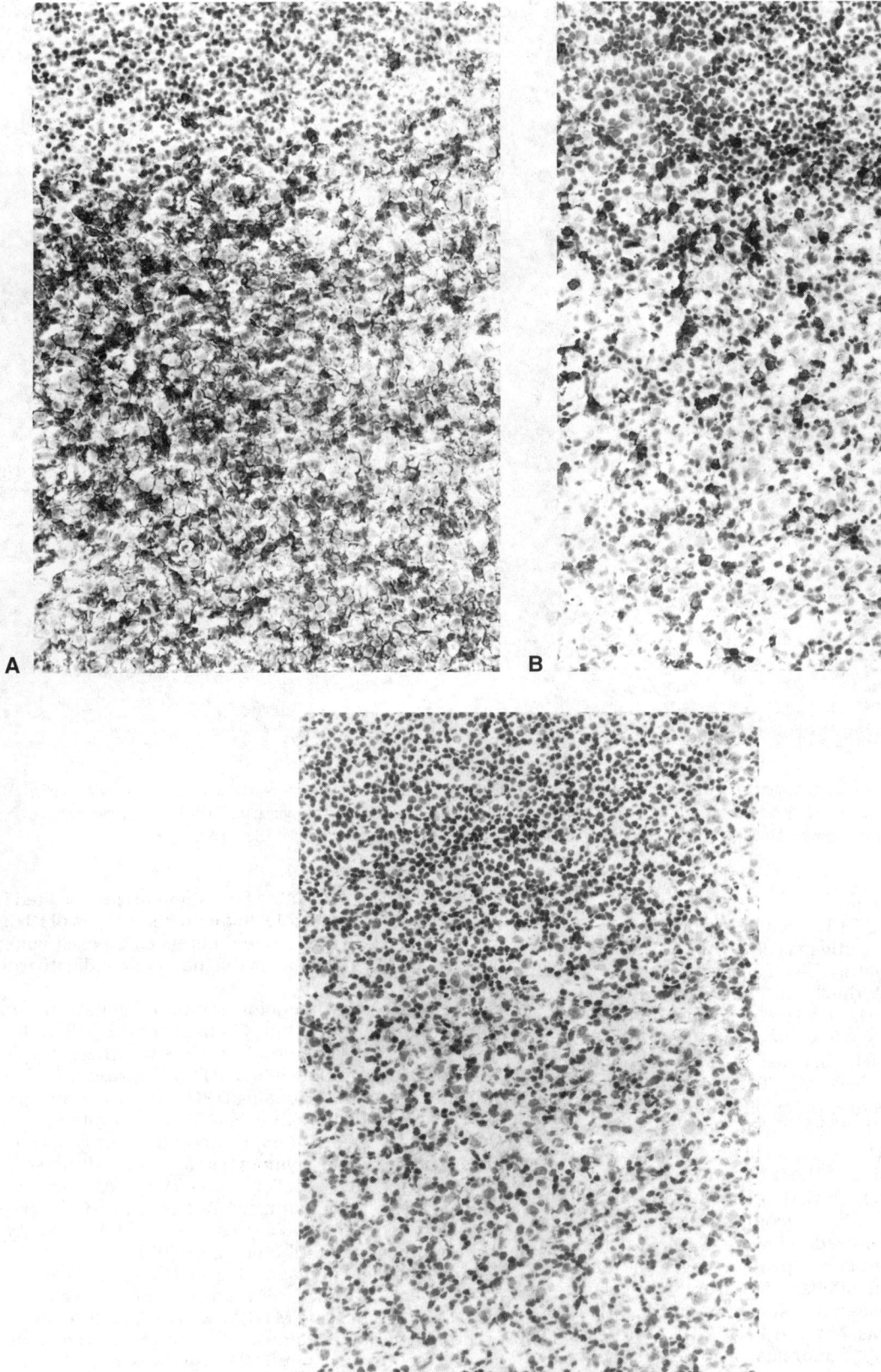

Fig. 80-9. Characteristic phenotype of a peripheral T-cell lymphoma. In serial sections of the same area, the neoplastic cells are **(A)** stained for OKT4 (CD4), but **(B)** negative for OKT8 (CD8) (a few reactive positive cells are seen) and **(C)** negative for OKT11 (CD2). (All immunoperoxidase-stained frozen sections × 150.)

Genotyping and Cytogenetics

The vast majority of PTCLs exhibit clonal rearrangements of the TCR β-chain gene and of the γ-chain gene.[483,484,486,494–496] A variable proportion of them in addition rearrange[497] or, more commonly, delete the δ-chain gene.[486,498,499] In contrast to the above data, 22% of PTCLs in one study showed germline configuration of the β-, γ-, and δ-genes.[486] Bigenotypic patterns may be observed in PTCLs that feature Tβ and immunoglobulin heavy[500] and, exceptionally, light chain[501] rearrangements. Molecular hybridization techniques have also demonstrated the presence of the EBV genome in 20% and 47% of PTCLs in Taiwan[502] and Europe,[503] respectively. The association with EBV is particularly strong (42–72%) for the angiocentric lymphoproliferative lesions,[504,505] especially those developing in the facial midline and nasal cavities.[506,507]

A host of chromosomal abnormalities have been reported in PTCLs, the most common of which are those involving the chromosome region 14q(11-13), where genes encoding for the α- and δ-chains of the TCR are located.[108,426,508] Other abnormalities include trisomy 3,[108] breaks in 1p,[108] trisomy 19,[509] and breaks in 6p21.[510,511] In a 1988 study,[78] a characteristic pattern of disease, which includes many normal mitotic cells, unrelated clonal and/or nonclonal cytogenetic abnormalities, and trisomies 3 and 5, was found to be associated with AILD-lesions and lymphomas (lymphoepithelioid and T-zone) with similar histologic "reactive" features, but was rare in a group of pleomorphic, immunoblastic, and anaplastic large cell types. Several studies have documented the strong association of breaks at 5q35, usually with t(2;5), in the Ki-1[+] anaplastic large cell or other large T-cell lymphoma.[478,512–515]

Clinical Correlations

The variability of the clinical descriptions of PTCLs in different studies has been discussed.[447,456,458,465] A survey of the three largest clinical series in the Western literature[456–458] indicates a wide range of age (4–97 years) but a similar median age of onset (56–57 years). Male/female ratio varies from 1.1 to 1.9 and the incidence of B symptoms from 27% to 60%.[456,457] The disease at presentation is in most cases nodal and disseminated (stage III–IV) (68–76%); however, it may involve extranodal sites, such as the skin (13–49%), the liver (7–22%), the bone marrow (10–35%), and the lung and/or pleura (11–15%).[456–458] Primary T-cell lymphomas are characteristic of the sinonasal areas and rhynopharynx (rather than the oropharynx, where B-cell lymphomas predominate),[516] especially in Asians[506,517]; they are instead uncommon in the intestine, where they usually occur in association with celiac disease.[518] Peripheral eosinophilia and hypogammaglobulinemia were reported in 8% and 16%, respectively, in one series.[457] Hypergammaglobulinemia is more frequent (29–52%) in other series.[465,517,519] The outcome appears to vary widely with median survivals of 17, 29, and 59 months being reported.[456–458] The clinical picture of PTCLs in Japan,[520] China,[521] and Taiwan[451,517] is similar in all respects.

Whether PTCLs are specifically different from the most common B-cell lymphomas is a contentious matter. This has already been discussed relative to the DLCLs. Other studies have compared histologically heterogeneous groups of B- and T-cell lymphomas. In some such studies no differences in clinical characteristics were found between PTCLs and B-cell tumors.[281,456,522] However, in two other series, PTCLs had a higher incidence of B symptoms and skin involvement,[517,521] and of bulky disease, and involvement of liver, spleen, bone marrow, and nasal cavities.[521] Complete remission rates and disease-free and overall survival are the same in the two phenotypic categories in most series.[281,456,517,521,522] However, differences have been reported in other studies: a worse overall survival for PTCLs than for B-cell lymphomas[457,517] and, only

in the subset of stage IV patients, a lower complete remission rate and shorter survival for those with T-cell tumors.[522]

Within the PTCLs, histopathologic classifications in most studies do not correlate significantly with clinical characteristics,[456] complete remission rates,[458,523] or survival.[447,456–458, 519,523] Even the clinical relevance of the simpler subdivision of PTCLs into low and high grade is uncertain. In a Japanese study using the Kiel classification, there were no differences in survival among low-grade PTCLs (lymphoepithelioid, T-zone, and AILD types), but their prognosis was significantly better than that of the high-grade neoplasms (pleomorphic and immunoblastic types).[524] Survival curves for the same two groups were instead no different in two other studies[519,525] or the differences were of borderline significance in another.[447] However, clinicopathologic correlations have been established for some cytologic types. The pleomorphic (or immunoblastic) cell type is strongly associated with adult T-cell leukemia/lymphoma (ATL), and thus with a grave prognosis.[445,451,461,482,526] In one study,[458] the incidence of bone marrow involvement was significantly higher in the small cell type (68%) than in either the mixed cell (33%) or the large cell (24%) type. Only a few immunophenotypic characteristics have been found to have prognostic value in the PTCLs. The CD4[+] phenotype, when compared with the CD8[+]/CD4[+]/CD8[+], was associated with both a higher complete remission rate and a longer survival.[457] Among non-B DLCLs (T cell or of ambiguous lineage) those that were Ki-1[+] had better overall survival than those that were Ki-1[−].[527]

Subtypes of Peripheral T-Cell Lymphomas

Although there are contradictory data about the prognostic discriminating power of the Kiel classification of PTCLs,[447,519, 524,525] some of its categories appear to have distinct characteristics. These and other recently reported disorders that fit well the definition of PTCLs are described below.

Angioimmunoblastic Lymphadenopathy-like Lymphoma and Other Low-Grade PTCLs

Lesions with morphologic features similar to AILD include a spectrum of lymphoproliferative disorders, from purely reactive to bona fide malignancies.[79] The unfortunate tendency of some groups[524,528,529] to lump all of them together as lymphomas makes it difficult to understand their biology and impossible to define with certainty the clinical characteristics, evolution, and outcome of the bona fide angioblastic lymphadenopathy-like lymphoma (AILL).

Its histopathologic distinction from AILD is difficult and is mostly based on the presence of clusters of clear cells in AILL (Fig. 80-8A), but not in AILD.[445,473,474,476] The immunophenotypic features are not different from those seen in PTCLs: often, however, there is no appreciable preponderance of either T-cell subset (Table 80-7). In addition to the proliferating T cells,[474,530] there is a consistent polyclonal population of small B cells and plasma cells,[474,476] as well as an abundant component of follicular DRCs.[530] A review of the molecular genetic studies of AILD-like lesions[79] showed that 73% manifested clonal populations at presentation; the clonal rearrangements involved the TCR β-gene in 81% of these cases, both the immunoglobulin heavy chain gene and one light chain gene in 7%, and the TCR β and the immunoglobulin heavy or light chain genes in 12%. The EBV genome can be detected in the vast majority of the AILD-like lesions.[531,532] Their characteristic cytogenetic pattern has already been mentioned. Sequential cytogenetic studies in our patients[78] have shown that some of the clonal or nonclonal abnormalities did not progress, some actually disappeared, and others became predominant in subsequent specimens. These findings, which parallel those obtained by DNA analysis,[77] support the concept that lesions with morphologic features of AILD are variable expressions of an unstable lymphoproliferative state characterized by the coexistence of a normal mitotic population and emerging, often multiple, unrelated clones. "Expanding clones would be susceptible to genetic errors during the repeating cell division process"; these errors might "produce malignant transformation and selective proliferation of the malignant clone."[77] Clinically, AILD-like lesions are characterized by a mostly acute presentation with prominent constitutional symptoms, generalized lymphadenopathy, hepatosplenomegaly, and frequently skin rashes; anemia and hypergammaglobulinemia are quite common.[524,528,533] Complete remission rates with chemotherapy are around 60%,[528,529] median survival varies from 13[524] or 15[529] to 18 months[528] and survival rates from 20%[528] to 40%[529] at 3 years.

It has often been noted that there is a great overlap in the histologic features of AILD-like, lymphoepithelioid, and T-zone lymphomas,[78,445,451,524,525] as all share in common a mild degree of cytologic atypia and are associated with "reactive" characteristics (prominent vascularity and inflammatory cell component); thus the reproducibility of these diagnoses among pathologists is poor.[534] In addition, these three types share a similar immunophenotypic and genotypic pattern,[464,465,535] the same chromosomal changes,[78] the rarity of an association with HTLV-1,[445,451,461,482,524] and, in at least one study, the same survival.[524] Thus, they may conceivably be different forms of one disorder characterized by a hyperplastic (hyperreactive) background in which clonal T-cell population(s) arise and may or not develop into full-blown clinical malignancy.[78]

High-Grade PTCLs (Pleomorphic or Immunoblastic)

High-grade PTCLs manifest characteristics in strong contrast with those of low-grade PTCLs. The histology is one of a monotonous population of markedly atypical cells with little or no associated "reactive" features[78,445,450,451] (Fig. 80-8B). Immunophenotypically, they show a prominent loss of pan-T antigens,[464,465] especially CD7,[461,482] and consistent expression of activation markers, especially CD25[461,482] (Table 80-7). Their cytogenetic pattern is one of multiple clonal abnormalities rather than single cell or nonclonal changes.[78] Finally, they are often associated with HTLV-1[445,451,461,482] and their survival is significantly worse than for the low-grade PTCLs in one study.[524] There is a strong correlation between these histologic types and ATL.[445,451,461,482,526]

ATL has emerged as a distinct clinicopathologic entity, observed mainly in southwestern Japan and the West Indies, but also in the southeastern United States and other areas, and is causally related to the HTLV-1 retrovirus.[536] Apart from cases referred to as of smoldering, chronic, or lymphomatous type,[537] most patients present acutely or subacutely, with disseminated disease characterized by lymphadenopathy, hepatosplenomegaly, skin and lytic bone lesions, a leukemic blood picture, and hypercalcemia. The circulating atypical cells have characteristic very complex, multilobulated nuclei.[445,538] Both changes in the immunophenotypic profiles of activation[539] and mutations of the p53 gene[540,541] have been associated with progression to the acute phase. Remissions with chemotherapy are short-lived, and median survival varies from 6.2 months for the acute form to 24 months and longer for the chronic and smoldering types.[537]

Ki-1+ Lymphoma

The Ki-1 (CD30) antibody, raised against a Hodgkin disease–derived cell line,[542] identifies an activation marker on Reed-Sternberg cells, activated B- and T-lymphoid cells,[448] and the cells of a variety of NHLs.[543] This widespread reactivity compounds any discussion of Ki-1+ (CD30+) lymphoma (KL), as this term may cover primary neoplasms and tumors that developed from other NHLs, mycosis fungoides, or Hodgkin disease; tumors of a specific cell type—the anaplastic large cell of the Kiel classification—and of several other cell types[544]; neoplasms in which the totality of the cells express the marker and others in which such reactivity is focal; and neoplasms of T-cell, B-cell, non-B non-T, biphenotypic B- and T-cell, and, rarely, histiocytic lineages. These different components of KL are often not clearly identified or treated together in literature reports. As much as possible, the following discussion is limited to primary neoplasms, composed of large cells, the totality or vast majority of which express Ki-1 (or its analogue, Ber-H2, also reactive in formalin-fixed material).[545]

The most characteristic histologic type—the anaplastic large cell—features cells of very large size, with abundant cytoplasm, and bizarre nuclei, often with a horseshoe, donut, or wreath shape.[445] Other CD30+ cell types include "Hodgkin related,"[206] giant cell rich,[206] lymphohistiocytic,[546] monomorphic,[547,548] as well as other large cell types[549] and even a small cell variant.[550] The neoplastic cells tend to grow in cohesive masses and within the sinuses.[8] The immunophenotypic findings vary widely in different series.[551] In the original study, 58% of KLs typed as T cell, 15.5% as B cell, and 7% were null on frozen sections,[448] but the figures for the three phenotypes vary, respectively, from 32%[477] to 80%,[552] from 0%[552] to 29%,[206] and from 18%[481] to 41%.[545] A small proportion of cases express both B- and T-cell antigens and rare examples manifest histiocytic markers.[553,554] A similar variability is obtained in immunophenotypic studies done on paraffin sections.[21,548,549] CD45 (LCA) is expressed in 50–100% of cases in frozen sections and 33–86% in paraffin sections.[551] The frequent lack of expression of LCA and the characteristic epithelial membrane antigen (EMA) positivity (55–89% on frozen and 20–92% in paraffin sections) may lead to a misdiagnosis of carcinoma.[548,555] The expression of CD15 (LeuM-1) by as many as 50% of cases in frozen and 27% in paraffin sections is one of the many overlapping features with Hodgkin disease.[551] Characteristics of the T-cell subset of anaplastic large cell lymphoma (Table 80-7) include the frequent loss of pan-T and T-subset antigens, and consistent expression of activation antigens and EMA.[448,477,479,480]

The immunogenotypic pattern of anaplastic large cell lymphoma is unusual in several regards. First, although most cases demonstrate rearrangements of TCR genes, immunoglobulin genes, or both sets of genes, in approximately one-third of the cases neither set of genes is rearranged.[481,556] Second, there is frequently a discrepancy between the lineage determination obtained by immunophenotyping and that obtained by molecular techniques.[481] Third, a dissociation is often observed between the immature (TCR- and immunoglobulin-negative) genotype and the expression of late activation markers.[206] The latter phenomenon has been attributed to a superimposed infection with EBV, a powerful inducer of an activated phenotype.[206] EBV-DNA was found by polymerase chain reaction in 32%[557] to 47%[558] of CD30+ anaplastic large cell lymphomas and by in situ hybridization in the neoplastic cells of 43%[558] to 82%[557] of the EBV-DNA-positive cases. In addition, however, 74% of non-anaplastic cell KLs were also EBV-positive and 67% of them demonstrated EBV in the neoplastic cells with the same techniques, strongly suggesting a causal correlation between the presence of EBV and the expression of CD30.[558] Many, but not all[559,560] KLs, whether of anaplastic cell type or not,[512,514,559] have translocations involving 5q35; all cases with this abnormality are of T-cell or undeterminate, but not B-cell, lineage.[559]

Somewhat different clinical characterization of KLs are gleaned from general series, reports limited to cutaneous disease or pediatric series. Three large studies—for a total of 88 patients—include all primary KLs of the anaplastic large cell type.[547,548,560] These show a bimodal age distribution, with a peak in young adults and another in older age; median age varies from 35[560] to 50[548] years. The presentation is with lymphadenopathy in the vast majority of patients but extranodal presentation is common (25%)[548]; this is limited to the skin in 10–13% of all cases.[548,560] Roughly equal proportions of patients present with localized or disseminated disease[548,560] and B symptoms occur in 42%.[560] Bone marrow involvement is reported in 3%[560] to 30%[548] of patients, mostly in the older age groups.[548] Relapses are frequent.[560] The overall survival rate in one series was 60%,[547] the median overall survival in another was 13 months,[548] and the median disease-free survival in the third was 16 months.[360] Three factors seem to be predictive of good prognosis: younger age,[547,548,560] localized stages of disease,[548,560] and presentation in the skin.[448,547,548] Patients <30 (or 40) years of age have better overall survival,[548,560] but not disease-free survival,[560] than those who are older. Patients with stage I–II disease have both better overall[548,560] and disease-free survival[560] than those in stage III–IV. Which histologic features influence prognosis is unclear. The largest subgroup of CD30[+] anaplastic large cell lymphoma, that of T- or null cell type, does better than CD30[+] nonanaplastic large cell type of all lineages[549] and better than all other CD30[−] non-B nonanaplastic large cell type[527] or CD30[−] PTCLs of all other types together.[561] Thus, it appears that it is the anaplastic large cell morphology that confers a better prognosis rather than the CD30 reactivity.

The primary cutaneous CD30[+] large cell lymphomas might be somewhat different. Those of anaplastic large cell type are all[562–565] or almost all[566] of T-cell type; show no bimodal age distribution, the median age varying between 49[563] and 67[566] years; and mostly have localized disease, presenting with solitary nodules or with several lesions in a circumscribed area. Recurrences in the skin, as well as spontaneous regressions, are quite common and only 15%[562] to 25%[563] of patients later develop involvement of nodes or other extracutaneous sites. From 58%[563] to 80%[566] or 85%[562] of patients have long survivals (median 66 months)[563] and only a minority, from 8%[562,566] to 25%,[563] die of their lymphoma. However, two studies contend that these features are characteristic of all primary cutaneous CD30[+] large T-cell lymphomas, there being no differences in clinical presentation, course, or survival between those of anaplastic and those of nonanaplastic large cell type.[564,565] CD30[−] large T-cell lymphomas primary in the skin, in contrast, tend to have more often (81%) multiple cutaneous sites of involvement, a shorter survival (median 17 months versus 52 months in CD30[+] cases), and a higher mortality rate, even among patients with initially localized disease.[564,565]

Studies of KLs in children and adolescents[449,480,567] confirm the favorable influence of young age on prognosis obtained from general studies.[548,560] These tumors are characteristically of anaplastic large cell type and of T-cell lineage. They present at a median age of 11–13 years with lymphadenopathies, frequent skin involvement (26–100%), and high-stage disease (67–77%). However, there is a high complete remission rate (67–100%) with aggressive chemotherapy; continuous complete remission rates are variable, from 33%[449] to 67%[480] and 74%.[567]

Other Variants

Angiocentric lymphoproliferative disorders (ACLPDs)[568] include a wide morphologic spectrum of lesions, from polymorphic with little atypia and necrosis (grade I) to increasingly monomorphic, atypical, and necrotic (grades II and III), all centered on, and destructive of, blood vessels.[454] This definition, recently proposed, partially overlaps the multiple histologies covered by terms such as lethal midline granuloma,[506] lymphomatoid granulomatosis,[569] or polymorphic reticulosis.[570] ACLPDs characteristically present at extranodal sites, especially nose and nasal cavities,[454,571,572] lung,[454,505] and skin.[573] They express a T-cell phenotype, often with a mixture of both subsets and little loss of pan-T markers.[454,571] Many also express surface markers, such as CD16, CD56 (N-CAM), or CD57,[468,469] as well as cytoplasmic azurophilic granules,[468] that are characteristic of cells with NK activity. TCR rearrangement is rarely demonstrated[574] and the EBV genome, of type A or B in equal proportion,[575] is found in a high number of cases.[502,504,505] These lesions are clinically aggressive; data on their responsiveness to cytotoxic therapy are conflicting[454,468,469] and it is unclear at the present time whether aggressiveness is related to the histologic grade,[454] the expression of the NK marker CD56,[468,469] or the association with EBV.[502]

Several other types of PTCLs have been reported that may represent distinct clinicopathologic entities. PTCL associated with hemophagocytic syndrome is an aggressive lymphoma presenting with prominent hepatosplenomegaly, little or no lymphadenopathy, and profound cytopenia.[576] Also associated with hemophagocytic syndrome, but localized to the subcutaneous tissues, is a panniculitis-like T-cell lymphoma.[577] The existence of a T γδ hepatosplenic lymphoma, characterized by sinusoidal involvement of spleen, liver, and bone marrow,[467] has already been mentioned. Massive hepatosplenomegaly without significant lymphadenopathy, and aggressive clinical course characterize rare lymphoproliferative disorders, both leukemic and lymphoma-like in presentation, which have their counterpart in a rare S-100-positive T-cell subset. They manifest predilection for sinusoidal involvement, express NK cell markers, and are of αβ subtype.[578]

REFERENCES

1. Weiss LM, Dorfman RF, Warnke RA: Lymph node workup. Adv Pathol 1:111, 1988
2. Lennert K, Feller AC: Histopathology of Non-Hodgkin's Lymphomas (based on the updated Kiel classification). Springer-Verlag, Berlin, 1992
3. Weisenburger DD, Chan WC: Lymphomas of follicles. Mantle cell and follicle center cell lymphomas. Am J Clin Pathol 99:409, 1993
4. Shin SS, Sheibani K: Monocytoid B-cell lymphoma. Am J Clin Pathol 99:421, 1993
5. Rappaport H: Tumors of the hematopoietic system. In Atlas of Tumor Pathology. Sect. III, Fascicle 8. Armed Forces Institute of Pathology, Washington, 1966
6. Nathwani BN, Winberg CD, Diamond LW et al: Morphologic criteria for the differentiation of follicular lymphoma from florid reactive follicular hyperplasia: a study of 80 cases. Cancer 48:1794, 1981
7. Krishnan J, Danon AD, Frizzera G: Reactive lymphadenopathies and atypical lymphoproliferative disorders. Am J Clin Pathol 99:385, 1993
8. Kinney MC, Glick AD, Stein H, Collins RD: Comparison of anaplastic large cell Ki-1 lymphomas and microvillous lymphomas in their immunologic and ultrastructural features. Am J Surg Pathol 14:1047, 1990
9. Rappaport H, Winter WJ, Hicks EB: Follicular lymphoma. A re-evaluation of its position in the scheme of malignant lymphoma, based on a survey of 253 cases. Cancer 9:792, 1956
10. Custer RP, Bernhard WG: The interrelationship of Hodgkin's disease and other lymphatic tumors. Am J Med Sci 216:625, 1948
11. Rosenberg SA, Diamond HD, Jaslowitz B, Craver LF: Lymphosarcoma: a review of 1,269 cases. Medicine 40:31, 1961
12. The Non-Hodgkin's Lymphoma Pathologic Classification Project: National Cancer Institute sponsored study of classifications of non-Hodgkin's lymphomas. Summary and description of a working formulation for clinical usage. Cancer 49:2112, 1982
13. Gerard-Marchant R, Hamlin I, Lennert K et al: Classification of non-Hodgkin's lymphomas. Lancet 2:406, 1974
14. Lennert K, Stein H, Kaiserling E: Cytological and functional criteria for the classification of malignant lymphomata. Br J Cancer, suppl. II. 31:29, 1975
15. Stansfeld AG, Diebold J, Noel H et al: Updated Kiel classification for lymphomas. Lancet 1:292, 1988
16. Lukes RJ, Taylor CR, Phil D et al: A morphologic and immunologic surface marker study of 299 cases of non-Hodgkin lymphomas and related leukemias. Am J Pathol 90:461, 1978
17. Lukes RJ, Collins RD: Immunologic characterization of human malignant lymphomas. Cancer 34:1488, 1974
18. Freedman AS, Nadler LM: Immunologic markers in non-Hodgkin's lymphoma. Hematol Oncol Clin North Am 5:871, 1991

19. Strickler JG, Weiss LM, Copenhaver CM et al: Monoclonal antibodies reactive in routinely processed tissue sections of malignant lymphoma, with emphasis on T-cell lymphomas. Hum Pathol 18:808, 1987

20. Norton AJ, Isaacson PG: Lymphoma phenotyping in formalin-fixed and paraffin wax-embedded tissues. I. Range of antibodies and staining patterns. Histopathology 14:437, 1989

21. Norton AJ, Isaacson PG: Lymphoma phenotyping in formalin-fixed and paraffin wax-embedded tissues. II. Profiles of reactivity in the various tumour types. Histopathology 14:557, 1989

22. Perkins SL, Kjeldsberg CR: Immunophenotyping of lymphomas and leukemias in paraffin-embedded tissues. Am J Clin Pathol 99:362, 1993

23. Bernard A, Boumsell L, Dausset J et al (eds): Leukocyte Typing: Human Leukocyte Differentiation Antigens Selected by Monoclonal Antibodies. Springer Verlag, New York, 1984

24. Reinherz EL, Haynes BF, Nadler LM, Bernstein ID (eds): Leukocyte Typing II. Springer Verlag, New York, 1986

25. McMichael AJ, Beverley PCL, Cobbold S et al (eds): Leukocyte Typing. III. White Cell Differentiation Antigens. Oxford University Press, Oxford, 1987

26. Knapp W, Doerken B, Gilks WR et al (eds): Leukocyte Typing. IV. White Cell Differentiation Antigens. Oxford University Press, Oxford, 1992

27. Knapp W, Doerken B, Rieber P et al: CD antigens 1989. Blood 74:1448, 1989

28. Jaffe ES: The role of immunophenotypic markers in the classification of non-Hodgkin's lymphomas. Semin Oncol 17:11, 1990

29. Pileri S, Falini B, Sabattini E et al: Immunohistochemistry of malignant lymphomas. Advantages and limitations of the new monoclonal antibodies working in paraffin sections. Haematologica (Pavia) 76:226, 1991

30. Knowles DM, Chadburn A, Inghirami G: Immunophenotypic markers useful in the diagnosis of hematopoietic neoplasms. p. 73. In Knowles DM (ed): Neoplastic Hematopathology. Williams & Wilkins, Baltimore, 1992

31. Cobbold S, Hale G, Waldmann H: Non-lineage, LFA-1 family, and leucocyte common antigens: new and previously defined clusters. p. 788. In McMichael AJ (ed): Leucocyte Typing. III. White Cell Differentiation Antigens. Oxford University Press, Oxford, 1987

32. Thomas ML, Lefrancois L: Differential expression of the leukocyte-common antigen family. Immunol Today 9:320, 1988

33. Gatter KC, Alcock C, Heryet A, Mason DY: Clinical importance of analysing malignant tumours of uncertain origin with immunohistological techniques. Lancet 1:1302, 1985

34. Kurtin PJ, Pinkus GS: Leukocyte common antigen. A diagnostic discriminant between hematopoietic and nonhematopoietic neoplasms in paraffin sections using monoclonal antibodies: correlation with immunologic studies and ultrastructural localization. Hum Pathol 16:353, 1985

35. Ling NR, MacLennan IGM, Mason DY: B-cell and plasma cell antigens: new and previously defined clusters. p. 302. In McMichael AJ (ed): Leucocyte Typing. III. White Cell Differentiation Antigens. Oxford University Press, Oxford, 1987

36. McMichael AJ, Gotch FM: T-cell antigens: new and previously defined clusters. p. 31. In McMichael AJ (ed): Leucocyte Typing. III. White Cel Differentiation Antigens. Oxford University Press, Oxford, 1987

37. Brenner MB, McLean J, Scheft H et al: Characterization and expression of the human β T cell receptor by using a framework monoclonal antibody. J Immunol 138:1502, 1987

38. Lydyard PM, Youinou PY, Cooke A: CD5-positive B cells in rheumatoid arthritis and chronic lymphocytic leukemia. Immunol Today 8:37, 1987

39. Mason DY, Cordell J, Brown M et al: Detection of T cells in paraffin wax embedded tissue using antibodies against a peptide sequence from the CD3 antigen. J Clin Pathol 42:1194, 1989

40. Mason DY, Comans-Bitter WM, Cordell JL et al: Antibody L26 recognizes an intracellular epitope on the B-cell-associated CD20 antigen. Am J Pathol 136:1215, 1990

41. Picker LJ, Weiss LM, Medeiros LJ et al: Immunophenotypic criteria for the diagnosis of non-Hodgkin's lymphoma. Am J Pathol 128:181, 1987

42. Levy R, Warnke R, Dorfman RF, Haimovich J: The monoclonality of human B-cell lymphomas. J Exp Med 145:1014, 1977

43. Band H, Hochstenbach F, McLean J et al: Immunohistochemical proof that a novel rearranging gene encodes the T cell receptor δ subunit. Science 238:682, 1987

44. Zukerberg LR, Medeiros LJ, Ferry JA, Harris NL: Diffuse low-grade B-cell lymphomas. Four clinically distinct subtypes defined by a combination of morphologic and immunophenotypic features. Am J Clin Pathol 100:373, 1993

45. Beverley PCL: Activation antigens: new and previously defined clusters. p. 516. In McMichael AJ (ed): Leucocyte Typing. III. White Cell Differentiation Antigens. Oxford University Press, Oxford 1987

46. Schwarting R, Stein H: Cluster report: CD71 p. 455. In Knapp W, Doerken B,
Gilks WR et al (eds): Leukocyte Typing. IV. White Cell Differentiation Antigens. Oxford University Press, Oxford, 1992

47. Brown DC, Gatter KC: Monoclonal antibody Ki-67: its use in histopathology. Histopathology 17:489, 1990

48. Salter DM, Krajewski AS, Cunningham S: Activation and differentiation antigen expression in B-cell non-Hodgkin's lymphoma. J Pathol 154:209, 1988

49. Hall PA, Richards MA, Gregory WM et al: The prognostic value of Ki67 immunostaining in non-Hodgkin's lymphoma. J Pathol 154:223, 1988

50. Holte H, Davies CD, Kvaloy S et al: The activation-associated antigen 4F2 predicts patient survival in low-grade B-cell lymphomas. Int J Cancer 39:590, 1987

51. Kvaloy S, Langholm R, Kaalhus O et al: Transferrin receptor and B-lymphoblast antigen. Their relationship to DNA synthesis, histology and survival in B-cell lymphomas. Int J Cancer 33:173, 1984

52. Medeiros LJ, Picker LJ, Horning SJ, Warnke RA: Transferrin receptor expression by non-Hodgkin's lymphomas. Correlation with morphologic grade and survival. Cancer 61:1844, 1988

53. Sheibani K, Winberg CD, van de Velde S et al: Distribution of lymphocytes with interleukin-2 receptors (TAC antigens) in reactive lymphoproliferative processes, Hodgkin's disease, and non-Hodgkin's lymphomas. Am J Pathol 127:27, 1987

54. Glimcher LH, Kara CJ: Sequences and factors: a guide to MHC class-II transcription. Annu Rev Immunol 10:13, 1992

55. Momburg F, Herrmann B, Moldenhauer G, Möller P: B-cell lymphomas of high-grade malignancy frequently lack HLA-DR, -DP and -DQ antigens and associated invariant chain. Int J Cancer 40:598, 1987

56. Miller TP, Lippman SM, Spier CM et al: HLA-DR (Ia) immune phenotype predicts outcome for patients with diffuse large cell lymphoma. J Clin Invest 82:370, 1988

57. Grogan TM, Miller TP: New biologic markers in non-Hodgkin's lymphomas. Hematol Oncol Clin North Am 5:925, 1991

58. Braziel RM, Keneklis T, Donlon JA et al: Terminal deoxynucleotidyl transferase in non-Hodgkin's lymphoma. Am J Clin Pathol 80:655, 1983

59. LeBien TW, McCormack RT: The common acute lymphoblastic leukemia antigen (CD10)—emancipation from a functional enigma. Blood 73:625, 1989

60. Freedman AS: Expression and function of adhesion receptors on normal B cells and B cell non-Hodgkin's lymphomas. Semin Hematol 30:318, 1993

61. Horst E, Meijer CJLM, Radaszkiewicz T et al: Adhesion molecules in the prognosis of diffuse large-cell lymphoma: expression of a lymphocyte homing receptor (CD44), LFA-1(CD11a/18), and ICAM-1 (CD54). Leukemia 4:595, 1990

62. Picker LJ, Butcher EC: Physiological and molecular mechanisms of lymphocyte homing. Annu Rev Immunol 10:561, 1992

63. Hynes RO: Integrins: versatility, modulation, and signaling in cell adhesion. Cell 69:11, 1992

64. Medeiros LJ, Weiss LM, Picker LJ et al: Expression of LFA-1 in non-Hodgkin's lymphoma. Cancer 63:255, 1989

65. Inghirami G, Wieczorek R, Zhu B-Y et al: Differential expression of LFA-1 molecules in non-Hodgkin's lymphoma and lymphoid leukemia. Blood 72:1431, 1988

66. Picker LJ, Medeiros LJ, Weiss LM et al: Expression of lymphocyte homing receptor antigen in non-Hodgkin's lymphoma. Am J Pathol 130:496, 1988

67. Baldini L, Cro L, Calori R et al: Differential expression of very late activation antigen-3 (VLA-3)/VLA-4 in B-cell non-Hodgkin lymphoma and B-cell chronic lymphocytic leukemia. Blood 79:2688, 1992

68. Damjanov I: Lectin cytochemistry and histochemistry. Lab Invest 57:5, 1987

69. Ree HJ, Hsu S-M; Lectin histochemistry of malignant tumors. I. Peanut agglutinin (PNA) receptors in follicular lymphoma and follicular hyperplasia: an immunohistochemical study. Cancer 51:1631, 1983

70. Strauchen JA: Lectin receptors as markers of lymphoid cells. I. Demonstration in tissue section by peroxidase technique. Am J Pathol 116:297, 1984

71. Ree HJ, Raine L, Crowley JP: Lectin binding patterns in diffuse large cell lymphoma. Cancer 52:2089, 1983

72. Ho AD, Doerken B, Ma DDF et al: Purine degradative enzymes and immunological phenotypes in chronic B-lymphocytic leukemia: indications that leukaemic immunocytoma is a separate entity. Br J Haematol 62:545, 1986

73. Khalaf MR, Aqel NM, Hayhoe FGJ: Histochemistry of dipeptidyl aminopeptidase (DAP) II and IV in reactive lymphoid tissues and malignant lymphoma. J Clin Pathol 40:480, 1987

74. Turner RR, Colby TV, Wood GS et al: Histiocyte malignancies. Morphologic, immunologic, and enzymatic heterogeneity. Am J Surg Pathol 8:485, 1984

75. Roholl PJM, Kleyne J, Pijpers HW, Van Unnik JAM: Comparative immunohistochemical investigations of markers for malignant histiocytes. Hum Pathol 16:763, 1985

76. Braylan RC: Flow-cytometric DNA analysis in the diagnosis and prognosis of lymphoma. Am J Clin Pathol 99:374, 1993

77. Lipford EH, Smith HR, Pittaluga S et al: Clonality of angioimmunoblastic lymphadenopathy and implications for its evolution to malignant lymphoma. J Clin Invest 79:637, 1987

78. Kaneko Y, Maseki N, Sakurai M et al: Characteristic karyotypic pattern in T-cell lymphoproliferative disorders with reactive "angioimmunoblastic lymphadenopathy with dysproteinemia-type" features. Blood 72:413, 1988

79. Frizzera G: Atypical lymphoproliferative disorders. p. 459. In Knowles DM (ed): Neoplastic Hematopathology. Williams & Wilkins, Baltimore, 1992

80. Korsmeyer SJ: Antigen receptor genes as molecular markers of lymphoid neoplasms. J Clin Invest 79:1291, 1987

81. Ramsay AD, Smith WJ, Isaacson PG: T-cell-rich B-cell lymphoma. Am J Surg Pathol 12:433, 1988

82. Lardelli P, Swaby RF, Medeiros LJ et al: Determination of lineage and clonality in diffuse lymphomas using the polymerase chain reaction technique. Hum Pathol 22:685, 1991

83. Knowles DM II, Dodson L, Burke JS et al: SIg−E− ("null-cell") non-Hodgkin's lymphomas. Multiparametric determination of their B- or T-cell lineage. Am J Pathol 120:356, 1985

84. Davis RE, Warnke RA, Dorfman RF et al: Utility of molecular genetic analysis for the diagnosis of neoplasia in morphologically and immunophenotypically equivocal hematolymphoid lesions. Cancer 67:2890, 1991

85. Le Beau MM: Chromosomal abnormalities in non-Hodgkin's lymphomas. Semin Oncol 17:20, 1990

86. Offit K, Chaganti RSK: Chromosomal aberrations in non-Hodgkin's lymphoma. Biologic and clinical correlations. Hematol Oncol Clin North Am 5:853, 1991

87. Pangalis GA, Nathwani BN, Rappaport H: Malignant lymphoma, well differentiated lymphocytic. Its relationship with chronic lymphocytic leukemia and macroglobulinemia of Waldenström. Cancer 39:999, 1977

88. Medeiros LJ, Strickler JG, Picker LJ et al: "Well-differentiated" lymphocytic neoplasms. Immunologic findings correlated with clinical presentation and morphologic features. Am J Pathol 129:523, 1987

89. Dighiero G, Travade P, Chevret S et al: B-cell chronic lymphocytic leukemia: present status and future directions. Blood 78:1901, 1991

90. Spier CM, Grogan TM, Fielder K et al: Immunophenotypes in "well-differentiated" lymphoproliferative disorders, with emphasis on small lymphocytic lymphoma. Hum Pathol 17:1126, 1986

91. van der Valk P, Jansen J, Daha MR, Meijer CJLM: Characterization of B-cell non-Hodgkin's lymphomas. A study using a panel of monoclonal and heterologous antibodies. Virchows Arch A Pathol Anat Histopathol 401:289, 1983

92. Stein H, Lennert K, Feller AC. Mason DY: Immunohistological analysis of human lymphoma: correlation of histological and immunological categories. Adv Cancer Res 42:67, 1984

93. Swerdlow SH, Murray LJ, Habeshaw JA, Stansfeld AG: Lymphocytic lymphoma/B-chronic lymphocytic leukaemia. An immunohistopathological study of peripheral B lymphocyte neoplasia. Br J Cancer 50:587, 1984

94. Harris NL, Bhan AK: B-cell neoplasms of the lymphocytic, lymphoplasmacytoid, and plasma cell types: immunohistologic analysis and clinical correlation. Hum Pathol 16:829, 1985

95. Weisenburger DD, Linder J, Daley DT, Armitage JO: Intermediate lymphocytic lymphoma: an immunohistologic study with comparison to other lymphocytic lymphomas. Hum Pathol 18:781, 1987

96. Sundeen JT, Longo DL, Jaffe ES: CD5 expression in B-cell small lymphocytic malignancies. Correlations with clinical presentation and sites of disease. Am J Surg Pathol 16:130, 1992

97. Hollema H, Visser L, Poppema S: Small lymphocytic lymphomas with predominant splenomegaly: a comparison of immunophenotypes with cases of predominant lymphadenopathy. Mod Pathol 4:712, 1991

98. Treasure J, Lane A, Jones DB, Wright DH: CD43 expression in B cell lymphoma. J Clin Pathol 45:1018, 1992

99. Kipps TJ, Robbins BA, Tefferi A et al: CD5-positive B-cell malignancies frequently express cross-reactive idiotypes associated with IgM autoantibodies. Am J Pathol 136:809, 1990

100. Hall PA, D'Ardenne AJ, Richards MA, Stansfeld AG: Lymphoplasmacytoid lymphoma: an immunohistological study. J Pathol 153:213, 1987

101. Gordon J, Mellstedt H, Aman P et al: Phenotypes in chronic B-lymphocytic leukemia probed by monoclonal antibodies and immunoglobulin secretion studies: identification of stages of maturation arrest and the relation to clinical findings. Blood 62:910, 1983

102. Kipps TJ: The CD5 B cell. Adv Immunol 47:117, 1989

103. Gobbi M, Caligaris-Cappio F, Janossy G: Normal equivalent cells of B cell malignancies: analysis with monoclonal antibodies. Br J Haematol 54:393, 1983

104. Levine EG, Arthur DC, Frizzera G et al: There are differences in cytogenetic abnormalities among histologic subtypes of the non-Hodgkin's lymphomas. Blood 66:1414, 1985

105. Yunis JJ, Oken MM, Kaplan ME et al: Distinctive chromosomal abnormalities in histologic subtypes of non-Hodgkin's lymphoma. N Engl J Med 307:1231, 1982

106. Koduru PRK, Filippa DA, Richardson ME et al: Cytogenetic and histologic correlations in malignant lymphoma. Blood 69:97, 1987

107. Speaks SL, Sanger WG. Linder J et al: Chromosomal abnormalities in indolent lymphoma. Cancer Genet Cytogenet 27:335, 1987

108. Fifth International Workshop on Chromosomes in Leukemia-Lymphoma: Correlation of chromosome abnormalities with histologic and immunologic characteristics in non-Hodgkin's lymphoma and adult T-cell leukemia-lymphoma. Blood 70:1554, 1987

109. Tilly H, Bastard C, Halkin E et al: Del(14)(q22) in diffuse B-cell lymphocytic lymphoma. Am J Clin Pathol 89:109, 1988

110. Offit K, Parsa NZ, Gaidano G et al: 6q deletions define clinicopathologic subsets of non-Hodgkin's lymphoma. Blood 82:2157, 1993

111. Juliusson G, Robert K-H, Oest A et al: Prognostic information from cytogenetic analysis in chronic B-lymphocytic leukemia and leukemic immunocytoma. Blood 65:134, 1985

112. Offit K, Parsa NZ, Filippa D et al: t(9;14)(p13;q32) denotes a subset of low-grade non-Hodgkin's lymphoma with plasmacytoid differentiation. Blood 80:2594, 1992

113. Pangalis GA, Boussiatis VA, Kittas K: Malignant disorders of small lymphocytes. Small lymphocytic lymphoma, lymphoplasmacytic lymphoma, and chronic lymphocytic leukemia: their clinical and laboratory relationship. Am J Clin Pathol 99:402, 1993

114. Ben-Ezra J, Burke JS, Swartz WG et al: Small lymphocytic lymphoma: a clinicopathologic analysis of 268 cases. Blood 73:579, 1989

115. Morrison WH, Hoppe RT, Weiss LM et al: Small lymphocytic lymphoma. J Clin Oncol 7:598, 1989

116. Levine AM, Lichtenstein A, Gresik MV et al: Clinical and immunologic spectrum of plasmacytoid lymphocytic lymphoma without serum monoclonal IgM. Br J Haematol 46:225, 1980

117. Pugh WC, Manning JT, Butler JJ: Paraimmunoblastic variant of small lymphocytic lymphoma/leukemia. Am J Surg Pathol 12:907, 1988

118. Melo JV, Hegde U, Parreira A et al: Splenic B cell lymphoma with circulating villous lymphocytes: differential diagnosis of B cell leukaemias with large spleens. J Clin Pathol 40:642, 1987

119. Robert K-H, Gahrton G, Friberg K et al: Extra chromosome 12 and prognosis in chronic lymphocytic leukemia. Scand J Haematol 28:163, 1982

120. Pittman S, Catovsky D: Prognostic significance of chromosome abnormalities in chronic lymphocytic leukaemia. Br J Haematol 58:649, 1984

121. Bird ML, Ueshima Y. Rowley JD et al: Chromosome abnormalities in B cell chronic lymphocytic leukemia and their clinical correlations. Leukemia 3:182, 1989

122. Enno A, Catovsky D, O'Brien M et al: 'Prolymphocytoid' transformation of chronic lymphocytic leukaemia. Br J Haematol 41:9, 1979

123. Paietta E, Tudoriu CD, Goldstein M et al: Plasmacytoid blast crisis in B-cell chronic lymphocytic leukemia: effect of estradiol on growth and differentiation in vitro. Leuk Res 9:19, 1985

124. Torelli UL, Torelli GM, Emilia G et al: Simultaneously increased expression of the c-myc and μ chain genes in the acute blastic transformation of a chronic lymphocytic leukaemia. Br J Haematol 65:165, 1987

125. Trump DL, Mann RB, Phelps R et al: Richter's syndrome. Diffuse histiocytic lymphoma in patients with chronic lymphocytic leukemia. A report of five cases and review of the literature. Am J Med 68:539, 1980

126. Harousseau JL, Flandrin G, Tricot G et al: Malignant lymphoma supervening in chronic lymphocytic leukemia and related disorders. Richter's syndrome: a study of 25 cases. Cancer 48:1302, 1981

127. Foucar K, Rydell RE: Richter's syndrome in chronic lymphocytic leukemia. Cancer 46:118, 1980

128. Chan WC, Dekmezian R: Phenotypic changes in large cell transformation of small cell lymphoid malignancies. Cancer 57:1971, 1986

129. Bertoli LF, Kubagawa H, Borzillo GV et al: Analysis with antiidiotype antibody of a patient with chronic lymphocytic leukemia and a large cell lymphoma (Richter's syndrome). Blood 70:45, 1987

130. Sun T, Susin M, Desner M et al: The clonal origin of two cell populations in Richter's syndrome. Hum Pathol 21:722, 1990

131. Miyamura K, Osada H, Yamauchi T et al: Single clonal origin of neoplastic B-cells with different immunoglobulin light chains in a patient with Richter's syndrome. Cancer 66:140, 1990

132. Schots R, Dehou M-F, Jochmans K et al: Southern blot analysis in a case of Richter's syndrome. Evidence for a postrearrangement heavy chain gene deletion associated with the altered phenotype. Am J Clin Pathol 95:571, 1991

133. Nakamine H, Masih AS, Sanger WG et al: Richter's syndrome with different immunoglobulin light chain types. Molecular and cytogenetic features indicate a common clonal origin. Am J Clin Pathol 97:656, 1992

134. van Dongen JJM, Hooijkaas H, Michiels JJ et al: Richter's syndrome with different immunoglobulin light chains and different heavy chain gene rearrangements. Blood 64:571, 1984

135. McDonnell JM, Beschorner WE, Staal SP et al: Richter's syndrome with two different B-cell clones. Cancer 58:2031, 1986

136. Ostrowski M, Minden M, Wang C, Bailey D: Immunophenotypic and gene probe analysis of a case of Richter's syndrome. Am J Clin Pathol 91:215, 1989

137. Brecher M, Banks PM: Hodgkin's disease variant of Richter's syndrome. Report of eight cases. Am J Clin Pathol 93:333, 1990

138. Williams J, Schned A, Cotelingam JD, Jaffe ES: Chronic lymphocytic leukemia with coexistent Hodgkin's disease. Implications for the origin of the Reed-Sternberg cells. Am J Surg Pathol 15:33, 1991

139. Tsang WYW, Chan JKC, Ng CS: The nature of Reed-Sternberg-like cells in chronic lymphocytic leukemia. Am J Clin Pathol 99:317, 1993

140. Banks PM, Chan J, Cleary ML et al: Mantle cell lymphoma. A proposal for unification of morphologic, immunologic, and molecular data. Am J Surg Pathol 16:637, 1992

141. Weisenburger DD, Nathwani BN, Diamond LW et al: Malignant lymphoma, intermediate lymphocytic type: a clinicopathologic study of 42 cases. Cancer 48:1415, 1981

142. Swerdlow SH, Habeshaw JA, Murray LJ et al: Centrocytic lymphoma: a distinct clinicopathologic and immunologic entity. A multiparameter study of 18 cases at diagnosis and relapse. Am J Pathol 113:181, 1983

143. Harris NL, Nadler LM, Bhan AK: Immunohistologic characterization of two malignant lymphomas of germinal center type (centroblastic/centrocytic and centrocytic) with monoclonal antibodies. Follicular and diffuse lymphomas of small-cleaved-cell type are related but distinct entities. Am J Pathol 117:262, 1984

144. van den Oord JJ, de Wolf-Peeters C, Pulford KAF et al: Mantle zone lymphoma. Immuno- and enzymehistochemical studies on the cell of origin. Am J Surg Pathol 10:780, 1986

145. Raffeld M, Jaffe ES: bcl-1, t(11;14), and mantle cell-derived lymphomas. Blood 78:259, 1991

146. Perry DA, Bast MA, Armitage JO, Weisenburger DD: Diffuse intermediate lymphocytic lymphoma. A clinicopathologic study and comparison with small lymphocytic lymphoma and diffuse small cleaved cell lymphoma. Cancer 66:1995, 1990

147. Lardelli P, Bookman MA, Sundeen J et al: Lymphocytic lymphoma of intermediate differentiation. Morphologic and immunophenotypic spectrum and clinical correlations. Am J Surg Pathol 14:752, 1990

148. Cossman J, Neckers LM, Hsu S-M et al: Low-grade lymphomas. Expression of developmentally regulated B-cell antigens. Am J Pathol 115:117, 1984

149. Hollema H, Poppema S: Immunophenotypes of malignant lymphoma centroblastic-centrocytic and malignant lymphoma centrocytic: an immunohistologic study indicating a derivation from different stages of B cell differentiation. Hum Pathol 19:1053, 1988

150. Strickler JG, Medeiros LJ, Copenhaver CM et al: Intermediate lymphocytic lymphoma: an immunophenotypic study with comparison to small lymphocytic lymphoma and diffuse small cleaved cell lymphoma. Hum Pathol 19:550, 1988

151. Weisenburger DD, Sanger WG, Armitage JO, Purtilo DT: Intermediate lymphocytic lymphoma: immunophenotypic and cytogenetic findings. Blood 69:1617, 1987

152. Leroux D, Le Marc'hadour F, Gressin R et al: Non-Hodgkin's lymphomas with t(11;14)(q13;q32): a subset of mantle zone/intermediate lymphocytic lymphoma? Br J Haematol 77:346, 1991

153. Frizzera G, Sakurai M, Notohara K, Konishi H: t(11;14)(q13;q32) in B-cell lymphomas (intermediately differentiated lymphocytic and follicular). A report of four cases. Am J Clin Pathol 95:684, 1991

154. Vandenberghe E, de Wolf Peeters C, Wlodarska I et al: Chromosome 11q rearrangements in B non Hodgkin's lymphoma. Br J Haematol 81:212, 1992

155. Medeiros LJ, van Krieken JH, Jaffe ES, Raffeld M: Association of bcl-1 rearrangement with lymphocytic lymphoma of intermediate differentiation. Blood 76:2086, 1990

156. Williams ME, Meeker TC, Swerdlow SH: Rearrangement of the chromosome 11 bcl-1 locus in centrocytic lymphoma: analysis with multiple breakpoint probes. Blood 78:493, 1991

157. Athan E, Foitl DR, Knowles DM: Bcl-1 rearrangement. Frequency and clinical significance among B-cell chronic lymphocytic leukemias and non-Hodgkin's lymphomas. Am J Pathol 138:591, 1991

158. Rimokh R, Berger F, Delsol G et al: Rearrangement and overexpression of the bcl-1/PRAD-1 gene in intermediate lymphocytic lymphomas and in t(11q13)-bearing leukemias. Blood 81:3063, 1993

159. Motokura T, Bloom T, Kim HG et al: A novel cyclin encoded by a bcl-1 linked candidate oncogene. Nature 350:512, 1991

160. Bookman MA, Lardelli P, Jaffe ES et al: Lymphocytic lymphoma of intermediate differentiation: morphologic, immunophenotypic, and prognostic factors. J Natl Cancer Inst 82:742, 1990

161. Shivdasani RA, Hess JL, Skarin AT, Pinkus GS: Intermediate lymphocytic lymphoma: clinical and pathologic features of a recently characterized subtype of non-Hodgkin's lymphoma. J Clin Oncol 11:802, 1993

162. Oliveira MSP, Jaffe ES, Catovsky D: Leukaemic phase of mantle zone (intermediate) lymphoma: its characterisation in 11 cases. J Clin Pathol 42:962, 1989

163. O'Briain DS, Kennedy MJ, Daley PA et al: Multiple lymphomatous polyposis of the gastrointestinal tract. A clinicopathologically distinctive form of non-Hodgkin's lymphoma of B-cell centrocytic type. Am J Surg Pathol 13:691, 1989

164. Duggan MJ, Weisenburger DD, Ye YL et al: Mantle zone lymphoma. A clinicopathologic study of 22 cases. Cancer 66:552, 1990

165. Sheibani K, Sohn CC, Burke JS et al: Monocytoid B-cell neoplasm. A novel B-cell neoplasm. Am J Pathol 124:310, 1986

166. Sheibani K, Burke JS, Swartz WG et al: Monocytoid B-cell lymphoma. Clinicopathologic study of 21 cases of a unique type of low-grade lymphoma. Cancer 62:1531, 1988

167. Nizze H, Cogliatti SB, von Schilling C et al: Monocytoid B-cell lymphoma: morphological variants and relationship to low grade B-cell lymphoma of the mucosa-associated lymphoid tissue. Histopathology 18:403, 1991

168. Traweek ST, Sheibani K: Monocytoid B-cell lymphoma. The biologic and clinical implications of peripheral blood involvement. Am J Clin Pathol 97:591, 1992

169. Cogliatti SB, Lennert K, Hansmann M-L, Zwingers TL: Monocytoid B cell lymphoma: clinical and prognostic features of 21 patients. J Clin Pathol 43:619, 1990

170. Ngan B-Y, Warnke RA, Wilson M et al: Monocytoid B-cell lymphoma: a study of 36 cases. Hum Pathol 22:4090, 1991

171. Traweek ST, Sheibani K, Winberg CD et al: Monocytoid B-cell lymphoma: its evolution and relationship to other low grade B-cell neoplasms. Blood 73:573, 1989

172. Stroup R, Sheibani K: Antigenic phenotypes of hairy cell leukemia and monocytoid B-cell lymphoma: an immunohistochemical evaluation of 66 cases. Hum Pathol 23:172, 1992

173. Sheibani K, Fritz RM, Winberg CD et al: "Monocytoid" cells in reactive follicular hyperplasia with and without multifocal histiocytic reactions: an immunohistochemical study of 21 cases including suspected cases of toxoplasmic lymphadenitis. Am J Clin Pathol 81:453, 1984

174. Sohn CC, Sheibani K, Winberg CD, Rappaport H: Monocytoid B lymphocytes: their relation to the patterns of the acquired immunodeficiency syndrome (AIDS) and AIDS-related lymphadenopathy. Hum Pathol 16:979, 1985

175. Shin SS, Sheibani K, Fishleder A et al: Monocytoid B-cell lymphoma in patients with Sjoegren's syndrome: a clinicopathologic study of 13 patients. Hum Pathol 22:422, 1991

176. Ortiz-Hidalgo C, Wright DH: The morphological spectrum of monocytoid B-cell lymphoma and its relationship to lymphomas of mucosa-associated lymphoid tissue. Histopathology 21:555, 1992

177. Isaacson PG, Spencer J: Malignant lymphoma of mucosa-associated lymphoid tissue. Histopathology 11:445, 1987

178. Isaacson PG: Lymphomas of mucosa-associated lymphoid tissue (MALT). Histopathology 16:617, 1990

179. Hyjek E, Isaacson PG: Primary B cell lymphoma of the thyroid and its relationship to Hashimoto's thyroiditis. Hum Pathol 19:1315, 1988

180. Hyjek E, Smith WJ, Isaacson PG: Primary B-cell lymphoma of salivary glands and its relationship to myoepithelial sialadenitis. Hum Pathol 19:766, 1988

181. Pelstring RJ, Essel JH, Kurtin PJ et al: Diversity of organ site involvement among malignant lymphomas of mucosa-associated tissues. Am J Clin Pathol 96:738, 1991

182. Li G, Hansmann M-L, Zwingers T, Lennert K: Primary lymphomas of the lung: morphological, immunohistochemical and clinical features. Histopathology 16:519, 1990

183. Isaacson PG, Spencer J: Malignant lymphoma and autoimmune disease. Histopathology 22:509, 1993

184. Davis GG, York JC, Glick AD et al: Plasmacytic differentiation in parafollicular (monocytoid) B-cell lymphoma. A study of 12 cases. Am J Surg Pathol 16:1066, 1992

185. Chan JK, Ng CS, Isaacson PG: Relationship between high-grade lymphoma and low grade B-cell mucosa-associated lymphoid tissue lymphoma (MALToma) of the stomach. Am J Pathol 136:1153, 1990

186. Schmid C, Kirkham N, Diss T, Isaacson PG: Splenic marginal zone cell lymphoma. Am J Surg Pathol 16:455, 1992
187. Fend F, Kraus-Huonder B, Müller-Hermelink, Feller AC: Monocytoid B-cell lymphoma: its relationship to and possible cellular origin from marginal zone cells. Hum Pathol 24:336, 1993
188. MacLellan ICM, Gray D, Kumararatne DS et al: The lymphocytes of splenic marginal zones: a distinct B-cell lineage. Immunol Today 3:305, 1982
189. van Krieken JHJM, von Schilling C. Kluin PhM, Lennert K: Splenic marginal zone lymphocytes and related cells in the lymph node: a morphologic and immunohistochemical study. Hum Pathol 20:320, 1989
190. Warnke RA, Kim H, Fuks Z, Dorfman RF: The coexistence of nodular and diffuse patterns in nodular non-Hodgkin's lymphomas. Significance and clinicopathologic correlation. Cancer 40:1229, 1977
191. Mann RB, Berard CW: Criteria for the cytologic subclassification of follicular lymphomas: a proposed alternative method. Hematol Oncol 1:187, 1983
192. Nathwani BN, Metter GE, Miller TP et al: What should be the morphologic criteria for the subdivision of follicular lymphomas? Blood 68:837, 1986
193. Metter GE, Nathwani BN, Burke JS et al: Morphological subclassification of follicular lymphoma: variability of diagnoses among hematopathologists, a collaborative study between the Repository Center and Pathology Panel for Lymphoma Clinical Studies. J Clin Oncol 3:25, 1985
194. Chittal SM, Caverivière P, Voigt J-J et al: Follicular lymphoma with abundant PAS-positive extracellular material. Immunohistochemical and ultrastructural observations. Am J Surg Pathol 11:618, 1987
195. Frizzera G, Anaya JS, Banks PM: Neoplastic plasma cells in follicular lymphomas: clinical and pathologic findings in six cases. Virchows Arch A Pathol Anat Histopathol 409:149, 1986
196. Silberman S, Fresco R, Steinecker PH: Signet ring cell lymphoma. A report of a case and review of the literature. Am J Clin Pathol 81:358, 1984
197. Kim H, Hendrickson MR, Dorfman RF: Composite lymphoma. Cancer 40:959, 1977
198. Fisher RI, Jones RB, DeVita VT Jr et al: Natural history of malignant lymphomas with divergent histologies at staging evaluation. Cancer 47:2022, 1981
199. Mead GM, Kushlan P, O'Neil M et al: Clinical aspects of non-Hodgkin's lymphomas presenting with discordant histologic subtypes. Cancer 52:1496, 1983
200. Ostrow SS, Diggs CH, Sutherland JC et al: Nodular poorly differentiated lymphocytic lymphoma: changes in histology and survival. Cancer Treat Rep 65:929, 1981
201. Hubbard SM, Chabner BA, DeVita VT Jr et al: Histologic progression in non-Hodgkin's lymphoma. Blood 59:258, 1982
202. Acker B, Hoppe RT, Colby TV et al: Histologic conversion in the non-Hodgkin's lymphomas. J Clin Oncol 1:11, 1983
203. Ersboll J, Schultz HB, Pedersen BJ, Nissen NI: Follicular low grade non-Hodgkin's lymphoma: long-term outcome with or without tumor progression. Eur J Haematol 42:155, 1989
204. Mintzer DM, Andreeff M, Filippa DA et al: Progression of nodular poorly differentiated lymphocytic lymphoma to Burkitt's-like lymphoma. Blood 64:415, 1984
205. De Jong D, Voetdijk MH, Beverstock GC et al: Activation of the c-myc oncogene in a precursor-B cell blast crisis of follicular lymphoma, presenting as a composite lymphoma. N Engl J Med 318:1373, 1988
206. Stein H, Dallenbach F: Diffuse large cell lymphomas of B and T cell type. p. 675. In Knowles DM (ed): Neoplastic Hematopathology. Williams & Wilkins, Baltimore, 1992
207. Warnke R, Levy R: Immunopathology of follicular lymphomas. A model of B-lymphocyte homing. N Engl J Med 298:481, 1978
208. Schuurman H-J, van Baarlen J, Huppes W et al: Immunophenotyping of non-Hodgkin's lymphoma. Lack of correlation between immunophenotype and cell morphology. Am J Pathol 129:140, 1987
209. Borowitz MJ, Bousvaros A, Brynes RK et al: Monoclonal antibody phenotyping of B-cell non-Hodgkin's lymphomas. The Southeastern Cancer Study Group experience. Am J Pathol 121:514, 1985
210. Swerdlow SH, Murray LJ, Habeshaw JA, Stansfeld AG: B- and T-cell subsets in follicular centroblastic/centrocytic (cleaved follicular center cell) lymphoma: an immunohistologic analysis of 26 lymph nodes and three spleens. Hum Pathol 16:339, 1985
211. Molenaar WM, van den Berg M, Halie MR, Poppema S: The heterogeneity of follicular center cell lymphomas. I. Cytohistologic, immunologic and enzymehistochemical aspects. Cancer 52:2269, 1983
212. Garcia CF, Warnke RA, Weiss LM: Follicular large cell lymphoma. An immunophenotype study. Am J Pathol 123:425, 1986
213. Michie SA, Garcia CF, Strickler JG et al: Expression of the Leu-8 antigen by B cell lymphomas. Am J Clin Pathol 88:486, 1987
214. Norton AJ, Rivas C, Isaacson PG: A comparison between monoclonal anti-

body MT2 and immunoglobulin staining in the differential diagnosis of follicular proliferations in routinely fixed wax-embedded biopsies. Am J Pathol 134:63, 1989
215. Chilosi M, Mombello A, Menestrina F et al: Immunohistochemical differentiation of follicular lymphoma from florid reactive follicular hyperplasia with monoclonal antibodies reactive on paraffin sections. Cancer 65:1562, 1990
216. Browne G, Tobin B, Carney DN, Dervan PA: Aberrant MT2 positivity distinguishes follicular lymphoma from reactive follicular hyperplasia in B5- and formalin-fixed paraffin sections. Am J Clin Pathol 96:90, 1991
217. Gaulard P, d'Agay M-F, Peuchmaur M et al: Expression of the bcl-2 gene product in follicular lymphoma. Am J Pathol 140:1089, 1992
218. Ngan BY, Chen-Levy Z, Weiss LM et al: Expression in non-Hodgkin's lymphoma of the bcl-2 protein associated with the t(14;18) chromosomal translocation. N Engl J Med 318:1638, 1988
219. Zutter M, Hockenbery D, Silverman GA, Korsmeyer SJ: Immunolocalization of the bcl-2 protein within hematopoietic neoplasms. Blood 78:1062, 1991
220. Dvoretsky P, Wood GS, Levy R, Warnke RA: T-lymphocyte subsets in follicular lymphomas compared with those in non-neoplastic lymph nodes and tonsils. Hum Pathol 13:618, 1982
221. Harris NL, Bhan AK: Distribution of T-cell subsets in follicular and diffuse lymphomas of B-cell type. Am J Pathol 113:172, 1983
222. Miller ML, Tubbs RR, Fishleder AJ et al: Immunoregulatory Leu-7+ and T8+ lymphocytes in B-cell follicular lymphomas. Hum Pathol 15:810, 1984
223. Raffeld ML, Neckers L, Longo DL, Cossman J: Spontaneous alteration of idiotype in a monoclonal B cell lymphoma: escape from detection by anti-idiotype. N Engl J Med 312:1653, 1985
224. Ngan B, Warnke RA, Cleary ML: Variability of immunoglobulin expression in follicular lymphoma. An immunohistologic and molecular genetic study. Am J Pathol 135:1139, 1989
225. Cleary ML, Gallili N, Trela M et al: Single cell origin of bigenotypic and biphenotypic B cell proliferations in human follicular lymphomas. J Exp Med 167:582, 1988
226. Bertoli LF, Kubagawa H, Borzillo GV et al: Bone marrow origin of a B-cell lymphoma. Blood 72:94, 1988
227. Bloomfield CD, Arthur DC, Frizzera G et al: Nonrandom chromosome abnormalities in lymphoma. Cancer Res 43:2975, 1983
228. Richardson ME, Quanguang C, Filippa DA et al: Intermediate- to high-grade histology of lymphomas carrying t(14;18) is associated with additional nonrandom chromosome changes. Blood 70:444, 1987
229. Cleary ML, Smith SD, Sklar J: Cloning and structural analysis of cDNAs for bcl-2 and a hybrid bcl-2/immunoglobulin transcript resulting from the t(14;18) translocation. Cell 47:19, 1986
230. Graninger WB, Seto M, Boutain B et al: Expression of bcl-2 and bcl-2-Ig fusion transcripts in normal and neoplastic cells. J Clin Invest 80:1512, 1987
231. McDonnell TJ, Korsmeyer SJ: Progression from lymphoid hyperplasia to high-grade malignant lymphoma in mice transgenic for the t(14;18). Nature 349:254, 1991
232. Ladanyi M, Offit K, Parsa NZ et al: Follicular lymphoma with t(8;14)(q24;q32): a distinct clinical and molecular subset of t(8;14)-bearing lymphomas. Blood 79:2124, 1992
233. Rimokh R, Gadoux M, Bertheas M-F et al: FVT-1, a novel human transcription unit affected by variant translocation t(2;18)(p11;q21) of follicular lymphoma. Blood 81:136, 1993
234. Yunis JJ, Frizzera G, Oken MM et al: Multiple recurrent genomic defects in follicular lymphoma. A possible model for cancer. N Engl J Med 316:79, 1987
235. Sander CA, Yano T, Clark HM et al: p53 mutation is associated with progression in follicular lymphomas. Blood 82:1994, 1993
236. Lo Coco F, Gaidano G, Louie DC et al: p53 mutations are associated with histologic transformation of follicular lymphoma. Blood 82:2289, 1993
237. Yano T, Jaffe ES, Longo DL, Raffeld M: MYC rearrangements in histologically progressed follicular lymphomas. Blood 80:758, 1992
238. Jones SE: Follicular lymphoma. Do no harm. Cancer Treat Rep 70:1055, 1986
239. Frizzera G, Murphy SB: Follicular (nodular) lymphoma in childhood: a rare clinical-pathological entity. Report of eight cases from four cancer centers. Cancer 44:2218, 1979
240. Anderson T, Chabner BA, Young RC et al: Malignant lymphoma. I. The histology and staging of 473 patients at the National Cancer Institute. Cancer 50:2699, 1982
241. Simon R, Durrleman S, Hoppe RT et al: The non-Hodgkin lympoma pathologic classification project. Longterm follow-up of 1153 patients with non-Hodgkin lymphomas. Ann Intern Med 109:939, 1988
242. Horning SJ: Natural history of and therapy for the indolent non-Hodgkin's lymphomas. Semin Oncol 20:75, 1993
243. Lennert K: Histopathology of Non-Hodgkin's Lymphomas (Based on the Kiel Classification). Springer-Verlag, Berlin, 1981
244. Brittinger G, Bartels H, Common H et al: Clinical and prognostic relevance of

the Kiel classification of non-Hodgkin lymphomas. Results of a prospective multicenter study by the Kiel lymphoma study group. Hematol Oncol 2:269, 1984

245. Anderson T, DeVita VT Jr, Simon RM et al: Malignant lymphoma. II. Prognostic factors and response to treatment of 473 patients at the National Cancer Institute. Cancer 50:2708, 1982

246. Glick JH, McFadden E, Costello W et al: Nodular histiocytic lymphoma: factors influencing prognosis and implications for aggressive chemotherapy. Cancer 49:840, 1982

247. Rudders RA, Kaddis M, DeLellis RA, Casey H Jr: Nodular non-Hodgkin's lymphoma (NHL). Factors influencing prognosis and indications for aggressive treatment. Cancer 43:1643, 1979

248. Colby TV, Hoppe RT, Burke JS: Nodular lymphoma: clinicopathologic correlations of parafollicular small lymphocytes and degree of nodularity. Cancer 45:2364, 1980

249. Kantarjian HM, McLaughlin P, Fuller LM et al: Follicular large cell lymphoma: analysis and prognostic factors in 62 patients. J Clin Oncol 2:811, 1984

250. Horning SJ, Weiss LM, Nevitt JB, Warnke RA: Clinical and pathologic features of follicular large cell (nodular histiocytic) lymphoma. Cancer 59:1470, 1987

251. Ezdinli EZ, Costello WG, Kucuk O, Berard CW: Effect of the degree of nodularity on the survival of patients with nodular lymphomas. J Clin Oncol 5: 413, 1987

252. Hu E, Weiss LM, Hoppe RT, Horning SJ: Follicular and diffuse mixed small-cleaved and large-cell lymphoma. A clinicopathologic study. J Clin Oncol 3:1183, 1985

253. Anderson JR, Vose JM, Bierman PJ et al: Clinical features and prognosis of follicular large-cell lymphoma: a report from the Nebraska Lymphoma Study Group. J Clin Oncol 11:218, 1993

254. Flippin T, McLaughlin P, Conrad FG et al: Stage III nodular lymphomas. Preliminary results of a combined chemotherapy/radiotherapy program. Cancer 51:987, 1983

255. Osborne CK, Norton L, Young RC et al: Nodular histiocytic lymphoma: an aggressive nodular lymphoma with potential for prolonged disease-free survival. Blood 56:98, 1980

256. Glick JH, Barnes JM, Ezdinli EZ et al: Nodular mixed lymphoma: results of a randomized trial failing to confirm prolonged disease-free survival with COPP chemotherapy. Blood 58:920, 1981

257. Longo DL, Young RC, Hubbard SM et al: Prolonged initial remission in patients with nodular mixed lymphoma. Ann Intern Med 100:651, 1984

258. Gallagher CJ, Gregory WM, Jones AE et al: Follicular lymphoma: prognostic factors for response and survival. J Clin Oncol 4:1470, 1986

259. Romaguera JE, McLaughlin P, North L et al: Multivariate analysis of prognostic factors in stage IV follicular low-grade lymphoma: a risk model. J Clin Oncol 9:762, 1991

260. Rudders RA, Ahl ET Jr, DeLellis RA et al: Surface marker identification of small cleaved follicular center cell lymphomas with a highly favorable prognosis. Cancer Res 42:349, 1982

261. Strickler JG, Copenhaver CM, Rojas VA et al: Comparison of "host cell infiltrates" in patients with follicular lymphoma with and without spontaneous regression. Am J Clin Pathol 90:257, 1988

262. Macartney JC, Camplejohn RS, Morris R et al: DNA flow cytometry of follicular non-Hodgkin's lymphoma. J Clin Pathol 44:215, 1991

263. Levine EG, Arthur DC, Frizzera G et al: Cytogenetic abnormalities predict clinical outcome in non-Hodgkin's lymphoma. Ann Intern Med 108:14, 1988

264. Speaks S, Harrington DS, Sanger W et al: Chromosome 10q23-25 abnormalities in follicular non-Hodgkin's lymphoma patients with t(14;18)(q32;q21): evidence defining a subgroup of patients with an aggressive clinical course. Lab Invest 60:90A, 1989

265. Nathwani BN, Kim H, Rappaport H et al: Non-Hodgkin's lymphoma: a clinicopathological study comparing two classifications. Cancer 41:303, 1978

266. Foucar K, Armitage JO, Dick FR: Malignant lymphoma, diffuse mixed small and large cell. A clinicopathologic study of 47 cases. Cancer 51:2090, 1983

267. Waldron JA, Leech JH, Glick AD et al: Malignant lymphoma of peripheral T-lymphocyte origin. Immunologic, pathologic, and clinical features in six patients. Cancer 40:1604, 1977

268. Medeiros LJ, Lardelli P, Stetler-Stevenson MA et al: Genotypic analysis of diffuse, mixed cell lymphomas. Comparison with morphologic and immunophenotypic findings. Am J Clin Pathol 95:547, 1991

269. Katzin WE, Linden MD, Fishleder AJ, Tubbs RR: Immunophenotypic and genotypic characterization of diffuse mixed non-Hodgkin's lymphomas. Am J Pathol 135:615, 1989

270. Gams RA, Rainey M, Dandy M et al: Phase III study of BCOP v CHOP in unfavorable categories of malignant lymphoma: a Southeastern cancer study group trial. J Clin Oncol 3:1188, 1985

271. Vose JM, Armitage JO, Weisenburger DD et al: The importance of age in

272. Coiffier B, Lepage E: Prognosis of aggressive lymphomas: a study of five prognostic models with patients included in the LNH-84 regimen. Blood 74: 558, 1989

survival of patients treated with chemotherapy for aggressive non-Hodgkin's lymphoma. J Clin Oncol 6:1838, 1988

273. Gordon LI, Harrington D, Andersen J et al: Comparison of a second-generation combination chemotherapeutic regimen (m-BACOD) with a standard regimen (CHOP) for advanced diffuse non-Hodgkin's lymphoma. N Engl J Med 327:1342, 1992

274. Tondini C, Zanini M, Lombardi F et al: Combined modality treatment with primary CHOP chemotherapy followed by locoregional irradiation in stage I or II histologically aggressive non-Hodgkin's lymphomas. J Clin Oncol 11: 720, 1993

275. Nathwani BN, Metter GE, Gams RA et al: Malignant lymphoma, mixed cell type, diffuse. Blood 62:200, 1983

276. Pinkus GS, Said JW, Hargreaves H: Malignant lymphoma, T-cell type. A distinct morphologic variant with large multilobated nuclei, with a report of four cases. Am J Clin Pathol 72:540, 1979

277. O'Hara CJ, Said JW, Pinkus GS: Non-Hodgkin's lymphoma, multilobated B-cell type: report of nine cases with immunohistochemical and immuno-ultrastructural evidence for a follicular center cell derivation. Hum Pathol 17:593, 1986

278. Baroni CD, Pescarmona E, Calogero A et al: B- and T-cell non-Hodgkin lymphomas with large multilobated cells: morphological, phenotypic and clinical heterogeneity. Histopathology 11:1121, 1987

279. Nakamine H, Mashi AS, Strobach RS et al: Immunoblastic lymphoma with abundant clear cytoplasm. A comparative study of B- and T-cell types. Am J Clin Pathol 96:177, 1991

280. Jaffe ES, Strauchen JA, Berard CW: Predictability of immunologic phenotype by morphologic criteria in diffuse aggressive non-Hodgkin's lymphomas. Am J Clin Pathol 77:46, 1982

281. Cossman J, Jaffe ES, Fisher RI: Immunologic phenotypes of diffuse, aggressive, non-Hodgkin's lymphomas. Correlation with clinical features. Cancer 54:1310, 1984

282. Fisher DE, Jacobson JO, Ault KA, Harris NL: Diffuse large cell lymphoma with discordant bone marrow histology. Clinical features and biological implications. Cancer 64:1879, 1989

283. Conlan MG, Bast M, Armitage JO et al: Bone marrow involvement by non-Hodgkin's lymphoma: the clinical significance of morphologic discordance between the lymph node and bone marrow. J Clin Oncol 8:1163, 1990

284. Robertson LE, Redman JR, Butler JJ et al: Discordant bone marrow involvement in diffuse large cell lymphoma: a distinct clinical-pathologic entity associated with a continuous risk of relapse. J Clin Oncol 9:236, 1991

285. Doggett RS, Wood GS, Horning S et al: The immunologic characterization of 95 nodal and extranodal diffuse large cell lymphomas in 89 patients. Am J Pathol 115:245, 1984

286. Spier CM, Grogan TM, Lippman SM et al: The aberrancy of immunophenotype and immunoglobulin status as indicators of prognosis in B cell diffuse large cell lymphoma. Am J Pathol 133:118, 1988

287. Garcia CF, Weiss LM, Warnke RA: Small noncleaved cell lymphoma: an immunophenotypic study of 18 cases and comparison with large cell lymphoma. Hum Pathol 17:454, 1986

288. Strickler JG, Audeh MW, Copenhaver CM, Warnke RA: Immunophenotypic differences between plasmacytoma/multiple myeloma and immunoblastic lymphoma. Cancer 61:1782, 1988

289. Nakamine H, Bagin RG, Vose JM et al: Prognostic significance of clinical and pathologic features in diffuse large B-cell lymphoma. Cancer 71:3130, 1993

290. van der Valk P, van den Besselaar-Dingjan G, Daha MR, Meijer CJLM: Analysis of large-cell lymphomas using monoclonal and heterologous antibodies. J Clin Pathol 36:44, 1983

291. Freedman AS, Boyd AW, Anderson KC et al: Immunologic heterogeneity of diffuse large cell lymphoma. Blood 65:630, 1985

292. Cleary ML, Trela MJ, Weiss LM et al: Most null large cell lymphomas are B lineage neoplasms. Lab Invest 53:521, 1985

293. Kneba M, Bergholz M, Bolz I et al: Heterogeneity of immunoglobulin gene rearrangements in B-cell lymphomas. Int J Cancer 45:609, 1990

294. Nakamura H, Said JW, Miller CW, Koeffler HP: Mutation and protein expression of p53 in acquired immunodeficiency syndrome-related lymphomas. Blood 82:920, 1993

295. Cabanillas F, Pathak S, Trujillo J et al: Frequent non-random chromosome abnormalities in 27 patients with untreated large cell lymphoma and immunoblastic lymphoma. Cancer Res 48:5557, 1988

296. Raghoebier S, Kramer MHH, van Krieken JHJM et al: Essential differences in oncogene involvement between primary nodal and extranodal large cell lymphoma. Blood 78:2680, 1991

297. Villuendas R, Piris MA, Orradre JL et al: Different bcl-2 protein expression

in high grade B-cell lymphomas derived from lymph node or mucosa-associated lymphoid tissue. Am J Pathol 139:989, 1991

298. Ladanyi M, Offit K, Jhanwar SC et al: MYC rearrangement and translocations involving band 8q24 in diffuse large cell lymphomas. Blood 77:1057, 1991

299. Bastard C, Tilly H, Lenormand B et al: Translocations involving band 3q27 and Ig gene regions in non-Hodgkin's lymphoma. Blood 79:2527, 1992

300. Kaneko Y, Rowley JD, Variakojis D et al: Prognostic implications of karyotype and morphology in patients with non-Hodgkin's lymphoma. Int J Cancer 32:683, 1983

301. Bain B, Matutes E, Robinson D et al: Leukaemia as a manifestation of large cell lymphoma. Br J Haematol 77:301, 1991

302. DeVita VT Jr, Molloy-Hubbard S, Young RC, Longo DL: The role of chemotherapy in diffuse aggressive lymphomas. Semin Hematol 25:2, 1988

303. Jagannath S, Velasquez WS, Tucker SL et al: Tumor burden assessment and its implications for a prognostic model in advanced diffuse large-cell lymphoma. J Clin Oncol 4:859, 1986

304. Shipp MA, Harrington DP, Klatt MM et al: Identification of major prognostic subgroups of patients with large-cell lymphoma treated with m-BACOD or M-BACOD. Ann Intern Med 104:757, 1986

305. Dixon DO, Neilan B, Jones SE et al: Effect of age on therapeutic outcome in advanced diffuse histiocytic lymphoma: the Southwest Oncology Group experience. J Clin Oncol 4:295, 1986

306. Hoskins PJ, Ng V, Spinelli JJ et al: Prognostic variables in patients with diffuse large-cell lymphoma treated with MACOP-B. J Clin Oncol 9:220, 1991

307. Velasquez WS, Fuller LM, Jagannath S et al: Stages I and II diffuse large cell lymphomas: prognostic factors and long-term results with CHOP-Bleo and radiotherapy. Blood 77:942, 1991

308. Vitolo U, Bertini M, Brusamolino E et al: MACOP-B treatment in diffuse large-cell lymphoma: identification of prognostic groups in an Italian multicenter study. J Clin Oncol 10:219, 1992

309. Warnke RA, Strauchen JA, Burke JS et al: Morphologic types of diffuse large-cell lymphoma. Cancer 50:690, 1982

310. Newcomer LN, Nerenberg MI, Cadman EC et al: The usefulness of the Lukes-Collins classification in identifying subsets of diffuse histiocytic lymphoma responsive to chemotherapy. Cancer 50:439, 1982

311. Armitage JO, Dick FR, Corder MP et al: Predicting therapeutic outcome in patients with diffuse histiocytic lymphoma treated with cyclophosphamide, Adriamycin, vincristine and prednisone (CHOP). Cancer 50:1695, 1982

312. Bloomfield CD, Gajl-Peczalska KJ, Frizzera G, LeBien TW: The clinical utility of cell surface markers in malignant lymphoma. p. 263. In Ford RJ, Fuller LM, Hagemeister FB (eds): University of Texas M.D. Anderson Clinical Conference on Cancer, Proceedings. Vol. 27. Raven Press, New York, 1984

313. Nathwani BN, Dixon DO, Jones SE et al: The clinical significance of the morphological subdivision of diffuse "histiocytic" lymphoma: a study of 162 patients treated by the Southwest Oncology Group. Blood 60:1068, 1982

314. Kwak LW, Wilson M, Weiss LM et al: Clinical significance of morphologic subdivision in diffuse large cell lymphoma. Cancer 68:1988, 1991

315. Coleman M, Armitage JO, Gaynor M et al: The COP-BLAM programs: evolving chemotherapy concepts in large cell lymphoma. Semin Hematol 25:23, 1988

316. Connors JM, Klimo P: MACOP-B chemotherapy for malignant lymphomas and related conditions: 1987 update and additional observations. Semin Hematol 25:41, 1988

317. Cabanillas F, Velasquez WS, Hagemeister FB et al: Clinical, biologic and histologic features of late relapses in diffuse large cell lymphoma. Blood 79:1024, 1992

318. Levine AM, Taylor CR, Schneider DR et al: Immunoblastic sarcoma of T-cell versus B-cell origin. I. Clinical features. Blood 58:52, 1981

319. Lippman SM, Miller TP, Spier CM et al: The prognostic significance of the immunotype in diffuse large-cell lymphoma: a comparative study of the T-cell and B-cell phenotype. Blood 72:436, 1988

320. Slymen DJ, Miller TP, Lippman SM et al: Immunobiologic factors predictive of clinical outcome in diffuse large-cell lymphoma. J Clin Oncol 8:986, 1990

321. Kwak LW, Wilson M, Weiss LM et al: Similar outcome of treatment of B-cell and T-cell diffuse large cell lymphomas: the Stanford experience. J Clin Oncol 9:1426, 1991

322. Horning SJ, Doggett RS, Warnke RA et al: Clinical relevance of immunologic phenotype in diffuse large cell lymphoma. Blood 63:1209, 1984

323. O'Keane JC, Mack C, Lynch E et al: Prognostic correlation of HLA-DR expression in large cell lymphoma as determined by LN3 staining. An Eastern Cooperative Oncology Group (ECOG) study. Cancer 66:1147, 1990

324. Grogan TM, Lippman SM, Spier CM et al: Independent prognostic significance of a nuclear proliferation antigen in diffuse large cell lymphomas as determined by the monoclonal antibody Ki-67. Blood 71:1157, 1988

325. Bauer KD, Merkel DE, Winter JN et al: Prognostic implications of ploidy and proliferative activity in diffuse large cell lymphomas. Cancer Res 46:3173, 1986

326. Pals ST, Horst E, Ossekoppele GJ et al: Expression of lymphocyte homing receptor as a mechanism of dissemination in non-Hodgkin's lymphoma. Blood 73:885, 1989

327. Lippman SM, Spier CM, Miller TP et al: Tumor-infiltrating T-lymphocytes in B-cell diffuse large cell lymphoma related to disease course. Mod Pathol 3: 361, 1990

328. Yunis JJ, Mayer MG, Arnesen MA et al: bcl-2 and other genomic alterations in the prognosis of large-cell lymphoma. N Engl J Med 320:1047, 1989

329. Offit K, Koduru PRK, Hollis R et al: 18q21 rearrangement in diffuse large cell lymphoma: incidence and clinical significance. Br J Haematol 72:178, 1989

330. Perrone T, Frizzera G, Rosai J: Mediastinal diffuse large-cell lymphoma with sclerosis. A clinicopathologic study of 60 cases. Am J Surg Pathol 10:176, 1986

331. Addis BJ, Isaacson PG: Large cell lymphoma of the mediastinum: a B-cell tumour of probably thymic origin. Histopathology 10:379, 1986

332. Moeller P, Moldenhauer G, Momburg F et al: Mediastinal lymphoma of clear cell type is a tumor corresponding to terminal steps of B cell differentiation. Blood 69:1087, 1987

333. Lamarre L, Jacobson JO, Aisenberg AC, Harris NL: Primary large cell lymphoma of the mediastinum. A histologic and immunophenotypic study of 29 cases. Am J Surg Pathol 13:730, 1989

334. Todeschini G, Ambrosetti A, Meneghini V et al: Mediastinal large B-cell lymphoma with sclerosis: a clinical study of 21 patients. J Clin Oncol 8:804, 1990

335. Al-Sharabati M, Chittal S, Duga-Neulat I et al: Primary anterior mediastinal B-cell lymphoma. A clinicopathologic and immunohistochemical study of 16 cases. Cancer 67:2579, 1991

336. Lavabre-Bertrand T, Donadio D, Fegueux N et al: A study of 15 cases of primary mediastinal lymphoma of B-cell type. Cancer 69:2561, 1992

337. Eichelmann A, Koretz K, Mechtersheimer G, Moeller P: Adhesion receptor profile of thymic B-cell lymphoma. Am J Pathol 141:729, 1992

338. Scarpa A, Borgato L, Chilosi M et al: Evidence of c-myc gene abnormalities in mediastinal large B-cell lymphoma of young adult age. Blood 78:780, 1991

339. Moeller P, Matthaei-Maurer DU, Hofmann WJ et al: Immunophenotypic similarities of mediastinal clear-cell lymphoma and sinusoidal (monocytoid) B cells. Int J Cancer 43:10, 1989

340. Isaacson PG, Norton AJ, Addis B: The human thymus contains a novel population of B lymphocytes. Lancet 2:1488, 1987

341. Isaacson PG, Chan JKC, Tang C, Addis BJ: Low grade B-cell lymphoma of mucosa-associated lymphoid tissue arising in the thymus. A thymic lymphoma mimicking myoepithelial sialadenitis. Am J Surg Pathol 14:342, 1990

342. Ng CS, Chan JKC, Hui PK, Lau WH: Large B-cell lymphomas with a high content of reactive T cells. Hum Pathol 20:1145, 1989

343. Macon WR, Williams ME, Greer JP et al: T-cell-rich B-cell lymphomas. A clinicopathologic study of 19 cases. Am J Surg Pathol 16:351, 1992

344. Rodriguez J, Pugh WC, Cabanillas F: T-cell-rich B-cell lymphoma. Blood 82: 1586, 1993

345. Krishnan J, Wallberg K, Frizzera G: T cell rich large B cell lymphoma: a study of 30 cases, supporting its histologic heterogeneity and lack of clinical distinctiveness. Am J Surg Pathol 18:455, 1994

346. Osborne BM, Butler JJ, Pugh WC: The value of immunophenotyping on paraffin sections in the identification of T-cell rich B-cell large-cell lymphomas: lineage confirmed by J$_H$ rearrangement. Am J Surg Pathol 14:933, 1990

347. Berard C, O'Conor GT, Thomas LB, Torloni H: Histopathological definition of Burkitt's tumour. Bull WHO 40:601, 1969

348. Mann RB, Jaffe ES, Braylan RC et al: Non-endemic Burkitt's lymphoma. A B-cell tumor related to germinal centers. N Engl J Med 295:685, 1976

349. Magrath IT, Jain V, Jaffe ES: Small noncleaved cell lymphoma. p. 749. In Knowles DM (ed): Neoplastic Hematopathology. Williams & Wilkins, Baltimore, 1992

350. Miliauskas JR, Berard CW, Young RC et al: Undifferentiated non-Hodgkin's lymphomas (Burkitt's and non-Burkitt's types). The relevance of making this histologic distinction. Cancer 50:2115, 1982

351. Wilson JF, Jenkin RDT, Anderson JR et al: Studies on the pathology of non-Hodgkin's lymphoma of childhood. 1. The role of routine histopathology as a prognostic factor: a report from the Childrens Cancer Study Group. Cancer 53:1695, 1984

352. Payne CM, Grogan TM, Cromey DW et al: An ultrastructural, morphometric and immunophenotypic evaluation of Burkitt's and Burkitt's-like lymphomas. Lab Invest 57:200, 1987

353. Yano T, van Krieken JHJM, Magrath IT et al: Histogenetic correlations between subcategories of small noncleaved cell lymphomas. Blood 79:1282, 1992

354. Kelly DR, Nathwani BN, Griffith RC et al: A morphologic study of childhood

lymphoma of the undifferentiated type. The Pediatric Oncology Group experience. Cancer 59:1132, 1987

355. Sigaux F, Berger R, Bernheim A et al: Malignant lymphomas with band 8q24 chromosome abnormality: a morphologic continuum extending from Burkitt's to immunoblastic lymphoma. Br J Haematol 57:393, 1984

356. Benjamin D, Magrath IT, Triche T et al: Induction of plasmacytoid differentiation by phorbol ester in B cell lymphoma cell lines bearing 8;14 translocations. Proc Natl Acad Sci USA 81:3547, 1984

357. Preud'homme JL, Dellagi K, Guglielmi P et al: Immunologic markers of Burkitt's lymphoma cells. IARC Sci Publ 60:47, 1985

358. Rooney CM, Gregory CD, Rowe M et al: Endemic Burkitt's lymphoma: phenotypic analysis of tumor biopsy cells and of derived tumor cell lines. J Natl Cancer Inst 77:681, 1986

359. Rowe M, Rowe DT, Gregory CD et al: Differences in B cell growth phenotype reflect novel patterns of Epstein-Barr virus latent gene expression in Burkitt's lymphoma cells. EMBO J 6:2743, 1987

360. Gregory CD, Rowe M, Rickinson AB: Different Epstein-Barr virus-B cell interactions in phenotypically distinct clones of a Burkitt's lymphoma cell line. J Gen Virol 71:1481, 1990

361. Gajl-Peczalska KJ, Bloomfield CD, Frizzera G et al: Diversity of phenotypes of non-Hodgkin's malignant lymphoma. p. 63. In Vitetta ES (ed): B and T Cell Tumors. Academic Press, San Diego, 1982

362. Billaud M, Rousset F, Calender A et al: Low expression of lymphocyte function-associated antigen (LFA)-1 and LFA-3 adhesion molecules is a common trait in Burkitt's lymphoma associated with and not associated with Epstein-Barr Virus. Blood 75:1827, 1990

363. MacLennan IC, Liu YL, Ling NR: B cell proliferation in follicles, germinal centre formation and the site of neoplastic transformation in Burkitt's lymphoma. Curr Top Microbiol Immunol 141:138, 1988

364. Hoffman-Fezer G, Knapp W, Thierfelder S: Anatomic distribution of CALL antigen expressing cells in normal lymphatic tissue and lymphomas. Leuk Res 6:761, 1982

365. Wiel J, Fellous M, Tursz T: Monoclonal antibody against a Burkitt lymphoma-associated antigen. Proc Natl Acad Sci USA 78:6485, 1981

366. Murray LJ, Habeshaw JA, Wiels J, Greaves MF: Expression of Burkitt lymphoma-associated antigen (defined by the monoclonal antibody 38.13) on both normal and malignant germinal center B cells. Int J Cancer 36:561, 1985

367. Moeller P, Momburg F, Hofmann WJ, Matthaei-Maurer DU: Lack of vimentin occurring during the intrafollicular stages of B cell development characterizes follicular center cell lymphomas. Blood 71:1033, 1988

368. Gregory CD, Tursz T, Edward CF et al: Identification of a subset of normal B cells with a Burkitt's lymphoma (BL)-like phenotype. J Immunol 139:313, 1987

369. Pallesen G, Zeuthen J: Distribution of the Burkitt's lymphoma-associated antigen (BLA) in normal human tissue and malignant lymphoma as defined by immunohistological staining with monoclonal antibody 38.13. J Cancer Res Clin Oncol 113:78, 1987

370. Oliver JD, Grogan TM, Payne CM et al: Burkitt's-like lymphoma of T-cell type. Mod Pathol 1:15, 1988

371. Berger R, Bernheim A: Cytogenetics of Burkitt's lymphoma-leukemia: a review. IARC Sci Publ 60:65, 1985

372. Croce CM, Nowell PC: Molecular basis of human B cell neoplasia. Blood 65:1, 1985

373. Klein G, Klein E: *Myc*/Ig juxtaposition by chromosomal translocations: some new insights, puzzles and paradoxes. Immunol Today 6:208, 1985

374. Lanfrancone L, Pelicci P-G, Dalla-Favera R: Structure and expression of translocated c-*myc* oncogenes: specific differences in endemic, sporadic and AIDS-associated forms of Burkitt's lymphomas. Curr Top Microbiol Immunol 132:257, 1986

375. Neri A, Barriga F, Knowles DM et al: Different regions of the immunoglobulin heavy chain locus are involved in chromosomal translocations in distinct pathogenetic forms of Burkitt lymphoma. Proc Natl Acad Sci USA 85:2748, 1988

376. Nkrumah FK, Olweny CLM: Clinical features of Burkitt's lymphoma: the African experience. IARC Sci Publ 60:87, 1985

377. Skarin AT, Canellos GP, Rosenthal DS et al: Improved prognosis of diffuse histiocytic and undifferentiated lymphoma by use of high dose methotrexate alternating with standard agents (M-BACOD). J Clin Oncol 1:91, 1983

378. Magrath IT, Janus C, Edwards BK et al: An effective therapy for both undifferentiated (including Burkitt's) lymphomas and lymphoblastic lymphomas in children and young adults. Blood 63:1102, 1984

379. Bernstein JI, Coleman CN, Strickler JG et al: Combined modality therapy for adults with small noncleaved cell lymphoma (Burkitt's and non-Burkitt's types). J Clin Oncol 4:847, 1986

380. Levine AM, Pavlova Z, Pockros AW et al: Small noncleaved follicular center cell (FCC) lymphoma: Burkitt and non-Burkitt variants in the United States. Cancer 52:1073, 1983

381. Oviatt DL, Cousar JB, Flexner JM et al: Malignant lymphoma of follicular center cell origin in humans. IV. Small transformed (noncleaved) cell lymphoma of the non-Burkitt's type. Cancer 52:1196, 1983

382. Grogan TM, Warnke RA, Kaplan HS: A comparative study of Burkitt's and non-Burkitt's "undifferentiated" malignant lymphoma: immunologic, cytochemical, ultrastructural, cytologic, histopathologic, clinical and cell culture features. Cancer 49:1817, 1982

383. Lopez TM, Hagemeister FB, McLaughlin P et al: Small noncleaved cell lymphoma in adults: superior results for stages I–III disease. J Clin Oncol 8:615, 1990

384. Straus DJ, Wong GY, Liu J et al: Small non-cleaved-cell lymphoma (undifferentiated lymphoma, Burkitt's type) in American adults: results with treatment designed for acute lymphoblastic leukemia. Am J Med 90:328, 1991

385. McMaster ML, Greer JP, Greco FA et al: Effective treatment of small-noncleaved-cell lymphoma with high-intensity, brief-duration chemotherapy. J Clin Oncol 9:941, 1991

386. Nathwani BN, Kim H, Rappaport H: Malignant lymphoma, lymphoblastic. Cancer 38:964, 1976

387. Kjeldsberg CR, Wilson JF, Berard CW: Non-Hodgkin's lymphoma in children. Hum Pathol 14:612, 1983

388. Kaneko Y, Frizzera G, Shikano T et al: Chromosomal and immunophenotypic patterns in T cell acute lymphoblastic leukemia (T ALL) and lymphoblastic lymphoma (LBL). Leukemia 3:886, 1989

389. Griffith RC, Kelly DR, Nathwani BN et al: A morphologic study of childhood lymphoma of the lymphoblastic type. The Pediatric Oncology Group experience. Cancer 59:1126, 1987

390. Crist WM, Shuster JJ, Falletta J et al: Clinical features and outcome in childhood T-cell leukemia-lymphoma according to stage of thymocyte differentiation: a Pediatric Oncology Group study. Blood 72:1891, 1988

391. Schwob VS, Weiner L, Hudes G, Ratech H: Extranodal non-T-cell lymphoblastic lymphoma in adults. A report of two cases. Am J Clin Pathol 90:602, 1988

392. Greenberg JM, Kersey JH: Terminal deoxynucleotidyl transferase expression can precede T cell receptor β chain and γ chain rearrangement in T cell acute lymphoblastic leukemia. Blood 69:356, 1987

393. Cossman J, Chused TM, Fisher RI et al: Diversity of immunological phenotypes of lymphoblastic lymphoma. Cancer Res 43:4486, 1983

394. Pittaluga S, Raffeld M, Lipford EH, Cossman J: 3A1 (CD7) expression precedes Tβ gene rearrangements in precursor T (lymphoblastic) neoplasms. Blood 68:134, 1986

395. Sheibani K, Nathwani BN, Winberg CD et al: Antigenically defined subgroups of lymphoblastic lymphoma. Relationship to clinical presentation and biologic behavior. Cancer 60:183, 1987

396. Vezzoni P, Giardini R, Lucchini R: Specificity of terminal deoxynucleotidyl transferase in non-Hodgkin's lymphoma, letter. Am J Clin Pathol 82:128, 1984

397. Slater DE, Mertelsmann R, Koziner B et al: Lymphoblastic lymphoma in adults. J Clin Oncol 4:57, 1986

398. Weiss LM, Bindl FM, Picozzi VJ et al: Lymphoblastic lymphoma: an immunophenotype study of 26 cases with comparison to T cell acute lymphoblastic leukemia. Blood 67:474, 1986

399. Reinherz EL, Kung PC, Goldstein G et al: Discrete stages of human intrathymic differentiation: analysis of normal thymocytes and leukemic lymphoblasts of T-cell lineage. Proc Natl Acad Sci USA 77:1588, 1980

400. Bernard A, Boumsell L, Reinherz E et al: Cell surface characterization of malignant T cells from lymphoblastic lymphoma using monoclonal antibodies: evidence for phenotypic differences between malignant T cells from patients with acute lymphoblastic leukemia and lymphoblastic lymphoma. Blood 57:1105, 1981

401. Roper M, Crist WM, Metzgar R et al: Monoclonal antibody characterization of surface antigens in childhood T-cell lymphoid malignancies. Blood 61:830, 1983

402. Quintanilla-Martinez L, Zukerberg LR, Harris NL: Prethymic adult lymphoblastic lymphoma. A clinicopathologic and immunohistochemical analysis. Am J Surg Pathol 16:1075, 1992

403. Sheibani K, Winberg CD, Burke JS et al: Lymphoblastic lymphoma expressing natural killer cell-associated antigens: a clinicopathologic study of six cases. Leuk Res 11:371, 1987

404. Picker LJ, Brenner MB, Weiss LM et al: Discordant expression of CD3 and T-cell receptor beta-chain antigens in T-lineage lymphomas. Am J Pathol 129:434, 1987

405. Ng CS, Chan JKC, Hui PK et al: Application of a T cell receptor antibody βF1 for immunophenotypic analysis of malignant lymphomas. Am J Pathol 132:365, 1988

406. Chan WC, Borowitz MJ, Hammani A et al: T cell receptor antibodies in the

immunohistochemical studies of normal and malignant lymphoid cells. Cancer 62:2118, 1988

407. Picker LJ, Brenner MB, Michie S, Warnke RA: Expression of the T cell receptor delta chain in benign and malignant T lineage lymphoproliferations. Am J Pathol 132:401, 1988

408. Falini B, Flenghi L, Fagioli M et al: T-lymphoblastic lymphomas expressing the non-disulfide-linked form of the T-cell receptor γ/δ: characterization with monoclonal antibodies and genotypic analysis. Blood 74:2501, 1989

409. Gouttefangeas C, Bensussan A, Boumsell L: Study of the CD-associated T-cell receptors reveals further differences between T-cell lymphoblastic lymphoma and leukemia. Blood 75:931, 1990

410. Stroup R, Sheibani K, Misset J-L et al: Surface immunoglobulin-positive lymphoblastic lymphoma. A report of three cases. Cancer 65:2559, 1990

411. Childs CC, Chrystal GS, Strauchen JA: Biphenotypic lymphoblastic lymphoma. An unusual tumor with lymphocytic and granulocytic differentiation. Cancer 57:1019, 1986

412. Gruemayer ER, Ladenstein RL, Slavc I et al: B-cell differentiation pattern of cutaneous lymphomas in infancy and childhood. Cancer 61:303, 1988

413. Link MP, Roper M, Dorfman RF et al: Cutaneous lymphoblastic lymphoma with pre-B markers. Blood 61:838, 1983

414. Smith RG: Parosteal lymphoblastic lymphoma. A human counterpart of Abelson virus-induced lymphosarcoma of mice. Cancer 54:471, 1984

415. Kamps WA, Poppema S: Pre-B-cell non-Hodgkin's lymphoma in childhood. Report of a case and review of the literature. Am J Clin Pathol 90:103, 1988

416. Sander CA, Medeiros LJ, Abruzzo LV et al: Lymphoblastic lymphoma in cutaneous sites: a clinico-pathologic analysis of six cases. J Am Acad Dermatol 25:1023, 1991

417. Bernard A, Murphy SB, Melvin S et al: Non-T, non-B lymphomas are rare in childhood and associated with cutaneous tumor. Blood 59:549, 1982

418. Borowitz MJ, Croker BP, Metzgar RS: Lymphoblastic lymphoma with the phenotype of common acute lymphoblastic leukemia. Am J Clin Pathol 79:387, 1983

419. Grogan TM, Spier CM, Wirt DP et al: Immunologic complexity of lymphoblastic lymphoma. Diagn Clin Immunol 4:81, 1986

420. Sander CA, Jaffe ES, Gebhardt FC et al: Mediastinal lymphoblastic lymphoma with an immature B-cell immunophenotype. Am J Surg Pathol 16:300, 1992

421. Pittaluga S, Uppenkamp M, Cossman J: Development of T3/T cell receptor gene expression in human pre-T neoplasms. Blood 69:1062, 1987

422. de Villartay J-P, Pullman AB. Andrade R et al: γ/δ lineage relationship within a consecutive series of human precursor T-cell neoplasms. Blood 74:2508, 1989

423. Kimura N, Takihara Y, Akiyoshi T et al: Rearrangement of the T cell receptor δ chain gene as a marker of lineage and clonality in T-cell lymphoproliferative disorders. Cancer Res 49:4488, 1989

424. Pardoll DM, Fowlkes BJ, Bluestone JA et al: Differential expression of two distinct T-cell receptors during thymocyte development. Nature 326:79, 1987

425. de Villartay J-P, Hockett R, Coran D et al: Deletion of the human T-cell receptor δ-gene by a site-specific recombination. Nature 335:170, 1988

426. Clare N, Boldt D, Messerschmidt G et al: Lymphocyte malignancy and chromosome 14: structural aberrations involving band q11. Blood 67:704, 1986

427. Dube ID, Raimondi SC, Pi D, Kalousek DK: A new translocation, t(10;14)(q24; q11), in T cell neoplasia. Blood 67:1181, 1986

428. Smith SD, Morgan R, Gemmell R et al: Clinical and biologic characterization of T-cell neoplasias with rearrangements of chromosome 7 band q34. Blood 71:395, 1988

429. Kaneko Y, Maseki N, Homma C et al: Chromosome translocations involving band 7q35 or 7p15 in childhood T-cell leukemia/lymphoma. Blood 72:534, 1988

430. Croce CM: Role of chromosome translocations in human neoplasia. Cell 49:155, 1987

431. Murphy S: Childhood non-Hodgkin's lymphoma. N Engl J Med 299:1446, 1978

432. Nathwani BN, Diamond LW, Winberg CD et al: Lymphoblastic lymphoma: a clinicopathologic study of 95 patients. Cancer 48:2347, 1981

433. Baldit C, Trojani M, Eghbali H et al: Lymphoblastic lymphoma with convoluted nuclei: a report of 19 cases. Oncology 41:252, 1984

434. Salloum E, Henry-Amar M, Caillou B et al: Lymphoblastic lymphoma in adults: a clinico-pathologic study of 34 cases treated at the Institut Gustave Roussy. Cancer Clin Oncol 24:1609, 1988

435. Picozzi VJ Jr, Coleman CN: Lymphoblastic lymphoma. Semin Oncol 17:96, 1990

436. Hvizdala EV, Berard C, Callihan T et al: Lymphoblastic lymphoma in children. A randomized trial comparing LSA₂-L₂ with A-COP+ therapeutic regimen: a Pediatric Oncology Group study. J Clin Oncol 6:26, 1988

437. Eden OB, Hann I, Imeson J et al: Treatment of advanced stage T cell lympho-

438. Coleman CN, Picozzi VJ, Cox RS et al: Treatment of lymphoblastic lymphoma in adults. J Clin Oncol 4:1628, 1986

439. Weinstein HJ, Cassady JR, Levey R: Long-term results of the APO protocol (vincristine, doxorubicin [Adriamycin], and prednisone) for treatment of mediastinal lymphoblastic lymphoma. J Clin Oncol 1:537, 1983

440. Morel P, Lepage E, Brice P et al: Prognosis and treatment of lymphoblastic lymphoma in adults: a report on 80 patients. J Clin Oncol 10:1078, 1992

441. Abruzzo LV, Jaffe ES, Cotelingam JD et al: T-cell lymphoblastic lymphoma with eosinophilia associated with subsequent myeloid malignancy. Am J Surg Pathol 16:236, 1992

442. Dahl GV, Rivera G, Pui C-H et al: A novel treatment of childhood lymphoblastic non-Hodgkin's lymphoma: early and intermittent use of teniposide plus cytarabine. Blood 66:1110, 1985

443. Kaneko Y, Frizzera G, Maseki N et al: A novel translocation, t(9;17)(q34; q23), in aggressive childhood lymphoblastic lymphoma. Leukemia 2:745, 1988

444. Jaffe ES: Pathologic and clinical spectrum of post-thymic T-cell malignancies. Cancer Invest 2:413, 1984

445. Suchi T, Lennert K, Tu L-Y et al: Histopathology and immunohistochemistry of peripheral T cell lymphomas: a proposal for their classification. J Clin Pathol 40:995, 1987

446. Grogan TM, Fielder K. Rangel C et al: Peripheral T-cell lymphoma: aggressive disease with heterogeneous immunotypes. Am J Clin Pathol 83:279, 1985

447. Pinkus GS, O'Hara CJ, Said JW: Peripheral/post-thymic T-cell lymphomas: a spectrum of disease. Clinical, pathologic, and immunologic features of 78 cases. Cancer 65:971, 1990

448. Stein H, Mason DY, Gerdes J et al: The expression of the Hodgkin's disease associated antigen Ki-1 in reactive and neoplastic lymphoid tissue: evidence that Reed-Sternberg cells and histiocytic malignancies are derived from activated lymphoid cells. Blood 66:848, 1985

449. Kadin ME, Sako D, Berliner N et al: Childhood Ki-1 lymphoma presenting with skin lesions and peripheral lymphadenopathy. Blood 68:1042, 1986

450. Weiss LM, Crabtree GS, Rouse RV, Warnke RA: Morphologic and immunologic characterization of 50 peripheral T-cell lymphomas. Am J Pathol 118:316, 1985

451. Su I-H, Wang C-H, Cheng A-L et al: Characterization of the spectrum of post-thymic T-cell malignancies in Taiwan. A clinicopathologic study of HTLV-1-positive and HTLV-1-negative cases. Cancer 61:2060, 1988

452. Jaffe ES, Costa J, Fauci AS et al: Malignant lymphoma and erythrophagocytosis simulating malignant histiocytosis. Am J Med 75:741, 1983

453. O'Shea JJ, Jaffe ES, Lane HC et al: Peripheral T cell lymphoma presenting as hypereosinophilia with vasculitis. Clinical, pathologic, and immunologic features. Am J Med 82:539, 1987

454. Lipford EH, Margolick JB, Longo DL et al: Angiocentric immunoproliferative lesions: a clinicopathologic spectrum of post-thymic T-cell proliferations. Blood 72:1674, 1988

455. Ohshima K, Kikuchi M, Yoshida T et al: Lymph nodes in incipient adult T-cell leukemia-lymphoma with Hodgkin's disease-like histologic features. Cancer 67:1622, 1991

456. Horning SJ, Weiss LM, Crabtree GS, Warnke RA: Clinical and phenotypic diversity of T cell lymphomas. Blood 67:1578, 1986

457. Coiffier B, Berger F, Bryon P-A, Magaud J-P: T-cell lymphomas: immunologic, histologic, clinical, and therapeutic analysis of 63 cases. J Clin Oncol 6:1584, 1988

458. Armitage JO, Greer JP, Levine AM et al: Peripheral T-cell lymphoma. Cancer 63:158, 1989

459. Stansfeld AG: Peripheral T-cell lymphomas. p. 300. In Stansfeld AG (ed): Lymph Node Biopsy Interpretation. Churchill Livingstone, Edinburgh, 1985

460. Borowitz MJ, Reichert TA, Brynes RK et al: The phenotypic diversity of peripheral T-cell lymphomas: the Southeastern Cancer Study Group experience. Hum Pathol 17:567, 1986

461. Doi S, Nasu K, Arita Y et al: Immunohistochemical analysis of peripheral T-cell lymphoma in Japanese patients. Am J Clin Pathol 91:152, 1989

462. Hastrup N, Ralfkiaer E, Pallesen G: Aberrant phenotypes in peripheral T cell lymphomas. J Clin Pathol 42:398, 1989

463. Wieczorek R. Burke JS, Knowles DM II: Leu-M1 antigen expression in T-cell neoplasia. Am J Pathol 121:374, 1985

464. Hollema H, Poppema S: T-lymphoblastic and peripheral T-cell lymphomas in the northern part of the Netherlands. An immunologic study of 29 cases. Cancer 64:1620, 1989

465. Chott A, Augustin I, Wrba F et al: Peripheral T-cell lymphomas: a clinicopathologic study of 75 cases. Hum Pathol 21:1117, 1990

466. Chadburn A, Inghirami G, Knowles DM: Hairy cell leukemia-associated anti-

gen LeuM5 (CD11c) is preferentially expressed by benign activated and neoplastic CD8 T cells. Am J Pathol 136:29, 1990

467. Farcet J-P, Gaulard P, Marolleau J-P et al: Hepatosplenic T-cell lymphoma: sinusal/sinusoidal localization of malignant cells expressing the T-cell receptor γδ. Blood 75:2213, 1990

468. Wong KF, Chan JKC, Ng CS et al: CD56 (NKH1)-positive hematolymphoid malignancies: an aggressive neoplasm featuring frequent cutaneous/mucosal involvement, cytoplasmic azurophilic granules and angiocentricity. Hum Pathol 23:798, 1992

469. Kern WF, Spier CM, Hanneman EH et al: Neural cell adhesion molecule-positive peripheral T-cell lymphoma: a rare variant with a propensity for unusual sites of involvement. Blood 79:2432, 1992

470. Feller AC, Griesser GH, Mak TW, Lennert K: Lymphoepithelioid lymphoma (Lennert's lymphoma) is a monoclonal proliferation of helper/inducer T cells. Blood 68:663, 1986

471. O'Connor NTJ, Feller AC, Wainscoat JS et al: T-cell origin of Lennert's lymphoma. Br J Haematol 64:521, 1986

472. Spier C, Lippman SM, Miller TP, Grogan TM: Lennert's lymphoma. A clinicopathologic study with emphasis on phenotype and its relationship to survival. Cancer 61:517, 1988

473. Weiss LM, Strickler JG, Dorfman RF et al: Clonal T-cell populations in angioimmunoblastic lymphadenopathy and angioimmunoblastic lymphadenopathy-like lymphoma. Am J Pathol 122:392, 1986

474. Namikawa R, Suchi T, Ueda R et al: Phenotyping of proliferating lymphocytes in angioimmunoblastic lymphadenopathy and related lesions by the double immunoenzymatic staining technique. Am J Pathol 127:279, 1987

475. Ohno T, Kita K, Miwa K, Shirakawa S: Immunophenotypical and molecular genetical examination of angioimmunoblastic lymphadenopathy. Nippon Ketsueki Gakkai Zasshi 50:1657, 1987

476. Jaffe ES: Angioimmunoblastic lymphadenopathy: morphologic features. p. 577. In Steinberg AD (moderator): Angioimmunoblastic lymphadenopathy with dysproteinemia. Ann Intern Med 108:575, 1988

477. Delsol G, Al Saati T, Gatter KC et al: Coexpression of epithelial membrane antigen (EMA), Ki-1, and interleukin-2 receptor by anaplastic large cell lymphomas. Diagnostic value in so-called malignant histiocytosis. Am J Pathol 130:59, 1988

478. Fischer P, Nacheva E, Mason DY et al: A Ki-1 (CD30)-positive human cell line (Karpas 299) established from a high-grade non-Hodgkin's lymphoma, showing a 2;5 translocation and rearrangement of the T-cell receptor β-chain gene. Blood 72:234, 1988

479. Fujimoto J, Hata J, Ishii E et al: Ki-1 lymphomas in childhood: immunohistochemical analysis and the significance of epithelial membrane antigen (EMA) as a new marker. Virchows Arch A Pathol Anat Histopathol 412:307, 1988

480. Schnitzer B, Roth MS, Hyder DM, Ginsburg D: Ki-1 lymphomas in children. Cancer 61:1213, 1988

481. Herbst H, Tippelmann G, Anagnostopoulos J et al: Immunoglobulin and T-cell receptor gene rearrangements in Hodgkin's disease and Ki-1-positive anaplastic large cell lymphoma: dissociation between phenotype and genotype. Leuk Res 13:103, 1989

482. Lennert K, Kikuchi M, Sato E et al: HTLV-positive and -negative T-cell lymphomas. Morphological and immunohistochemical differences between European and HTLV-positive Japanese T-cell lymphomas. Int J Cancer 35:65, 1985

483. Gaulard P, Bourquelot P, Kanavaros P et al: Expression of the alpha/beta and gamma/delta T-cell receptors in 57 cases of peripheral T-cell lymphomas. Identification of a subset of γ/δ T-cell lymphomas. Am J Pathol 137:617, 1990

484. Kasai K, Kameya T, Ono M et al: Relationships among expression, transcription and rearrangement of T-cell receptor β gene in T-cell lymphomas. Virchows Arch A Pathol Anat Histopathol 417:57, 1990

485. Mori N, Oka K, Yoda Y et al: T-cell receptor expression in the T-cell malignancies. Am J Clin Pathol 93:495, 1990

486. van Krieken JHJM, Elwood L, Andrade RE et al: Rearrangement of the T-cell receptor delta chain gene in T-cell lymphomas with a mature phenotype. Am J Pathol 139:161, 1991

487. Cabecadas JM, Isaacson PG: Phenotyping of T-cell lymphomas in paraffin sections—which antibodies? Histopathology 19:419, 1991

488. Said JW, Shintaku IP, Parekh K, Pinkus GS: Specific phenotyping of T cell proliferations in formalin-fixed paraffin-embedded tissues. Use of antibodies to the T cell receptor βF1. Am J Clin Pathol 93:382, 1990

489. Kurtin PJ, Roche PC: Immunoperoxidase staining of non-Hodgkin's lymphomas for T-cell lineage associated antigens in paraffin sections. Comparison of the performance characteristics of four commercially available antibody preparations. Am J Surg Pathol 17:898, 1993

490. Clark DM, Boylston AW, Hall PA, Carrel S: Antibodies to T cell antigen recep-

tor beta chain families detect monoclonal T cell proliferation. Lancet 2:835, 1986

491. O'Grady J, Krajewski AS, Ramage EF: Demonstration of clonality in T-cell lymphoma using an anti-T-cell receptor variable region antibody panel. Histopathology 17:553, 1990

492. Poppema S, Hepperle B: Restricted V gene usage in T-cell lymphomas as detected by anti-T-cell receptor variable region reagents. Am J Pathol 138:1479, 1991

493. Smith JL, Lane AC, Hodges E et al: T-cell receptor variable (V) gene usage by lymphoid populations in T-cell lymphoma. J Pathol 166:109, 1992

494. Griesser H, Feller A, Lennert K et al: The structure of the T cell gamma chain gene in lymphoproliferative disorders and lymphoma cell lines. Blood 68:592, 1986

495. Weiss LM, Picker LJ, Grogan TM et al: Absence of clonal beta and gamma T-cell receptor gene rearrangements in a subset of peripheral T-cell lymphomas. Am J Pathol 130:436, 1988

496. Knowles DM: Immunophenotypic and antigen receptor gene rearrangement analysis in T cell neoplasia. Am J Pathol 134:761, 1989

497. Tkachuk DC, Griesser H, Takihara Y et al: Rearrangement of T-cell δ locus in lymphoproliferative disorders. Blood 72:353, 1988

498. Asou N, Hattori T, Matsuoka M et al: Rearrangements of T-cell antigen receptor δ chain gene in hematologic neoplasms. Blood 74:2707, 1989

499. Dyer MJS: T-cell receptor delta-alpha rearrangements in lymphoid neoplasms. Blood 74:1073, 1989

500. Pelicci PG, Knowles DM, Dalla-Favera R: Lymphoid tumors displaying rearrangements of both immunoglobulin and T cell receptor genes. J Exp Med 162:1015, 1985

501. Sheibani K, Wu A, Ben-Ezra J et al: Rearrangement of κ-chain and T-cell receptor β-chain genes in malignant lymphomas of "T-cell" phenotype. Am J Pathol 129:201, 1987

502. Su I-J, Hsieh H-C, Lin K-H et al: Aggressive peripheral T-cell lymphomas containing Epstein-Barr viral DNA: a clinicopathologic and molecular analysis. Blood 77:799, 1991

503. Korbjuhn P, Anagnostopoulos I, Hummel M et al: Frequent latent Epstein-Barr virus infection of neoplastic T cells and bystander B cells in human immunodeficiency virus-negative European peripheral pleomorphic T-cell lymphomas. Blood 82:217, 1993

504. Medeiros LJ, Jaffe ES, Chen Y-Y, Weiss LM: Localization of Epstein-Barr viral genomes in angiocentric immunoproliferative lesions. Am J Surg Pathol 16:439, 1992

505. Katzenstein A-LA, Peiper SC: Detection of Epstein-Barr virus genomes in lymphomatoid granulomatosis: analysis of 29 cases by the polymerase chain reaction technique. Mod Pathol 3:435, 1990

506. Harabuchi Y, Yamanaka N, Kataura A et al: Epstein-Barr virus in nasal T-cell lymphomas in patients with lethal midline granuloma. Lancet 335:128, 1990

507. Weiss LM, Gaffey MJ, Chen Y-Y, Frierson HF: Frequency of Epstein-Barr viral DNA in "western" sinonasal and Waldeyer's ring non-Hodgkin's lymphomas. Am J Surg Pathol 16:156, 1992

508. Maseki N, Kaneko Y, Sakurai M et al: Chromosome abnormalities in malignant lymphoma in patients from Saitama. Cancer Res 47:6767, 1987

509. Levine EG, Arthur DC, Gajl-Peczalska KJ et al: Correlations between immunological phenotype and karyotype in malignant lymphoma. Cancer Res 46:6481, 1986

510. Mecucci C, Michaux J-L, Tricot G et al: Rearrangements of the short arm of chromosome no. 6 in T-cell lymphomas. Leuk Res 9:1139, 1985

511. Maseki N, Kaneko Y, Sakurai M: Interstitial deletion of the short arm of chromosome 6 as a new cytogenetic marker of T-cell lymphoma. Jpn J Cancer Res 77:334, 1986

512. Kaneko Y, Frizzera G, Edamura S et al: A novel translocation, t(2;5)(p23;q35), in childhood phagocytic large T-cell lymphoma mimicking malignant histiocytosis. Blood 73:806, 1989

513. Bitter MA, Franklin WA, Larson RA et al: Morphology in Ki-1 (CD30)-positive non-Hodgkin's lymphoma is correlated with clinical features and the presence of a unique chromosomal abnormality, t(2,5),(p23;q35). Am J Surg Pathol 14:305, 1990

514. Mason DY, Bastard C, Rimokh R et al: CD30-positive large cell lymphomas ('Ki-1 lymphoma') are associated with a chromosomal translocation involving 5q35. Br J Haematol 74:161, 1990

515. Gordon BG, Weisenburger DD, Warkentin PI et al: Peripheral T-cell lymphoma in childhood and adolescence: a clinicopathologic study of 22 patients. Cancer 71:257, 1993

516. Chan JKC, Ng CS, Lo STH: Immunohistological characterization of malignant lymphomas of the Waldeyer's ring other than the nasopharynx. Histopathology 11:885, 1987

517. Cheng A-L, Chen Y-C, Wang C-H et al: Direct comparisons of peripheral

T-cell lymphoma with diffuse B-cell lymphoma of comparable histological grades. Should peripheral T-cell lymphoma be considered separately? J Clin Oncol 7:725, 1989

518. Chott A, Dragosics B, Radaszkiewicz T: Peripheral T-cell lymphomas of the intestine. Am J Pathol 141:1361, 1992

519. Montalban C, Obeso G, Gallego A et al: Peripheral T-cell lymphoma: a clinico-pathological study of 41 cases and evaluation of the prognostic significance of the updated Kiel classification. Histopathology 22:303, 1993

520. The T- and B-cell Malignancy Study Group: Statistical analyses of clinico-pathological, virological and epidemiological data on lymphoid malignancies with special reference to adult T-cell leukemia/lymphoma: a report of the second nationwide study of Japan. Jpn J Clin Oncol 15:517, 1985

521. Liang R, Chiu E, Chan T-K et al: Direct comparison of peripheral T-cell lymphomas with their B-cell counterparts. Acta Haematol 85:179, 1991

522. Armitage JO, Vose JM, Linder J et al: Clinical significance of immunopheno-type in diffuse aggressive non-Hodgkin's lymphoma. J Clin Oncol 7:1783, 1989

523. Liang R, Todd D, Chan TK et al: Peripheral T cell lymphoma. J Clin Oncol 5:750, 1987

524. Nakamura S, Suchi T: A clinicopathologic study of node-based, low-grade, peripheral T-cell lymphoma. Angioimmunoblastic lymphoma, T-zone lymphoma, and lymphoepithelioid lymphoma. Cancer 67:2565, 1991

525. Noorduyn LA, van der Valk P, van Heerde P et al: Stage is a better prognostic indicator than morphologic subtype in primary noncutaneous T-cell lymphoma. Am J Clin Pathol 93:49, 1990

526. Chadburn A, Athan E, Wieczorek R, Knowles DM: Detection and characterization of human T-cell lymphotropic virus type I (HTLV-I) associated T-cell neoplasms in an HTLV-1 nonendemic region by polymerase chain reaction. Blood 77:2419, 1991

527. Offit K, Ladanyi M, Gangi MD et al: Ki-1 antigen expression defines a favorable clinical subset of non-B cell non-Hodgkin's lymphoma. Leukemia 4:625, 1990

528. Tobinai K, Minato K, Ohtsu T et al: Clinicopathologic, immunophenotypic, and immunogenotypic analyses of immunoblastic lymphadenopathy-like-T-cell lymphoma. Blood 72:1000, 1988

529. Siegert W, Agthe A, Griesser H et al: Treatment of angiommunoblastic lymphadenopathy (AILD)-type T-cell lymphoma using prednisone with or without the COPBLAM/IMVP-16 regimen. A multicenter study. Ann Intern Med 117:364, 1992

530. Feller A, Griesser H, Schilling CV et al: Clonal gene rearrangement patterns correlate with immunophenotype and clinical parameters in patients with angioimmunoblastic lymphadenopathy. Am J Pathol 133:549, 1988

531. Weiss LM, Jaffe ES, Liu X-F et al: Detection and localization of Epstein-Barr viral genomes in angioimmunoblastic lymphadenopathy and angioimmuno-blastic lymphadenopathy-like lymphoma. Blood 79:1789, 1992

532. Anagnostopoulos I, Hummel M, Finn T et al: Heterogeneous Epstein-Barr virus infection patterns in peripheral T-cell lymphoma of angioimmunoblas-tic lymphadenopathy type. Blood 80:1804, 1992

533. Knecht H: Angioimmunoblastic lymphadenopathy: ten years' experience and state of current knowledge. Semin Hematol 26:208, 1989

534. Hastrup N, Hamilton-Dutoit S, Ralfkiaer E, Pallesen G: Peripheral T-cell lymphomas: an evaluation of reproducibility of the updated Kiel classification. Histopathology 18:99, 1991

535. Takagi N, Nakamura S, Ueda R et al: A phenotypic and genotypic study of three node-based, low grade peripheral T-cell lymphomas: angioimmuno-blastic lymphoma, T-zone lymphoma, and lymphoepithelioid lymphoma. Cancer 69:2571, 1992

536. Kim JH, Durack DT: Manifestations of human T-lymphotropic virus type I infection. Am J Med 84:919, 1988

537. Shimoyama M et al: Diagnostic criteria and classification of clinical subtypes of adult T-cell leukaemia-lymphoma. A report from the Lymphoma Study Group (1984–87). Br J Haematol 79:428, 1991

538. Jaffe ES, Robert-Guroff M, Blattner WA et al: The pathologic spectrum of adult T-cell leukemia/lymphoma in the United States. Am J Surg Pathol 8: 263, 1984

539. Shirono K, Hattori T, Hata H et al: Profiles of expression of activated cell antigens on peripheral blood and lymph node cells from different clinical stages of adult T-cell leukemia. Blood 73:1664, 1989

540. Cesarman E, Chadburn A, Inghirami G et al: Structural and functional analysis of oncogenes and tumor suppressor genes in adult T-cell leukemia/lymphoma shows frequent p53 mutations. Blood 80:3205, 1992

541. Sakashita A, Hattori T, Miller CW et al: Mutations of the p53 gene in adult T-cell leukemia. Blood 79:477, 1992

542. Schwab U, Stein H, Gerdes J et al: Production of a monoclonal antibody specific for Hodgkin and Sternberg-Reed cells of Hodgkin's disease and a subset of normal lymphoid cells. Nature 299:65, 1982

543. Pallesen G: The diagnostic significance of the CD30 (Ki-1) antigen. Histopathology 16:409, 1990

544. Piris M, Brown DC, Gatter KC, Mason DY: CD30 expression in non-Hodgkin's lymphoma. Histopathology 17:211, 1990

545. Schwarting R, Gerdes J, Duerkop H et al: BerH2: a new anti-Ki-1 (CD30) monoclonal antibody directed at a formol-resistant epitope. Blood 74:1678, 1989

546. Pileri S, Falini B, Delsol G et al: Lymphohistiocytic T-cell lymphoma (anaplastic large cell lymphoma CD30 + /Ki-1 + with a high content of reactive histiocytes). Histopathology 16:383, 1990

547. Chan JKC, Ng CS, Hui PK et al: Anaplastic large cell Ki-1 lymphoma. Delineation of two morphological types. Histopathology 15:11, 1989

548. Chott A, Kaserer K, Augustin I et al: Ki-1 positive large cell lymphoma. A clinicopathologic study of 41 cases. Am J Surg Pathol 14:439, 1990

549. Penny RJ, Blaustein JC, Longtime JA, Pinkus GS: Ki-1-positive large cell lymphomas, a heterogeneous group of neoplasms. Morphologic, immunopheno-typic, genotypic, and clinical features of 24 cases. Cancer 68:362, 1991

550. Kinney MC, Collins RD, Greer JP et al: A small-cell-predominant variant of primary Ki-1 (CD30)+ T-cell lymphoma. Am J Surg Pathol 17:859, 1993

551. Frizzera G: The distinction of Hodgkin's disease from anaplastic large cell lymphoma. Semin Diagn Pathol 9:291, 1992

552. Nakamura S, Takagi N, Kojima M et al: Clinicopathologic study of large cell anaplastic lymphoma (Ki-1-positive large cell lymphoma) among the Japanese. Cancer 68:118, 1991

553. Carbone A, Gloghini A, De Re V et al: Histopathologic, immunophenotypic, and genotypic analysis of Ki-1 anaplastic large cell lymphomas that express histiocyte-associated antigens. Cancer 66:2547, 1990

554. Nezelof C, Barbey S, Gogusev J, Terrier-Lacombe M-J: Malignant histiocytosis in childhood: a distinctive CD30-positive clinicopathological entity associated with a chromosomal translocation involving 5q35. Semin Diagn Pathol 9:75, 1992

555. Falini B, Pileri S, Stein H et al: Variable expression of leukocyte-common (CD45) antigen in CD30 (Ki1)-positive anaplastic large-cell lymphoma. Implications for the differential diagnosis between lymphoid and nonlymphoid malignancies. Hum Pathol 21:624, 1990

556. O'Connor NTJ, Stein H, Gatter KC et al: Genotypic analysis of large cell lymphomas which express the Ki-1 antigen. Histopathology 11:733, 1987

557. Herbst H, Dallenbach F, Hummel M et al: Epstein-Barr virus DNA and latent gene products in Ki-1 (CD30)-positive anaplastic large cell lymphomas. Blood 78:2666, 1991

558. Kanavaros P, Jiwa NM, de Bruin PC et al: High incidence of EBV genome in CD30-positive non-Hodgkin's lymphomas. J Pathol 168:307, 1992

559. Ebrahim SAD, Ladanyi M, Desai SB et al: Immunohistochemical, molecular and cytogenetic analysis of a consecutive series of 20 peripheral T-cell lymphomas and lymphomas of uncertain lineage, including 12 Ki-1 positive lymphomas. Genes Chromosomes Cancer 2:27, 1990

560. Greer JP, Kinney MC, Collins RD et al: Clinical features of 31 patients with Ki-1 anaplastic large-cell lymphoma. J Clin Oncol 9:539, 1991

561. de Bruin PC, Noorduyn AL, van der Valk P et al: Noncutaneous T-cell lymphomas. Recognition of lymphoma type (large cell anaplastic) with a relatively favorable prognosis. Cancer 71:2604, 1993

562. Kaudewitz P, Stein H, Dallenbach F et al: Primary and secondary cutaneous Ki-1 + (CD30 +) anaplastic large cell lymphomas. Morphologic, immunohis-tologic, and clinical characteristics. Am J Pathol 135:359, 1989

563. Banerjee SS, Heald M, Harris M et al: Twelve cases of Ki-1 positive anaplastic large cell lymphoma of skin. J Clin Pathol 44:119, 1991

564. Belijaards RC, Meijer CJLM, Scheffer E et al: Prognostic significance of CD30 (Ki-1/Ber-H2) expression in primary cutaneous large-cell lymphomas of T-cell origin. A clinicopathologic and immunohistochemical study in 20 patients. Am J Pathol 135:1169, 1989

565. Belijaards RC, Kaudewitz P, Berti E et al: Primary cutaneous CD30-positive large cell lymphoma: definition of a new type of cutaneous lymphoma with a favorable prognosis. A European multicenter study of 47 patients. Cancer 71:2097, 1993

566. Krishnan J, Tomaszewski M-M, Kao GF: Primary cutaneous CD30-positive anaplastic large cell lymphoma. Report of 27 cases. J Cutaneous Pathol 20: 193, 1993

567. Heitger A, Gadner H, Bucsky P et al: Das grosszellige anaplastische Lymphom im Kindesalter. Klinische Erfahrungen bei einer histologisch neu definierten Entitaet. Klin Paediatr 201:237, 1989

568. Peiper SC: Angiocentric lymphoproliferative disorders of the respiratory system: incrimination of Epstein-Barr virus in pathogenesis. Blood 82:687, 1993

569. Liebow AA, Carrington CB, Friedman PJ: Lymphomatoid granulomatosis. Hum Pathol 3:457, 1972

570. DeRemee RA, Weiland LH, McDonald TJ: Polymorphic reticulosis, lymphomatoid granulomatosis. Two diseases or one? Mayo Clin Proc 53:634, 1978

571. Chott A, Rappersberger K, Schlossarek W, Radaszkiewicz T: Peripheral T cell lymphoma presenting primarily as lethal midline granuloma. Hum Pathol 19:1093, 1988

572. Lippman SM, Grogan TM, Spier CM et al: Lethal midline granuloma with a novel T-cell phenotype as found in peripheral T-cell lymphoma. Cancer 59: 936, 1987

573. Chan JKC, Ng CS, Ngan KC et al: Angiocentric T-cell lymphoma of the skin. An aggressive lymphoma distinct from mycosis fungoides. Am J Surg Pathol 12:861, 1988

574. Medeiros LJ, Peiper SC, Elwood L et al: Angiocentric immunoproliferative lesions: a molecular analysis of eight cases. Hum Pathol 22:1150, 1991

575. Borisch B, Hennig I, Laeng RH et al: Association of the subtype 2 of the Epstein-Barr virus with T-cell non-Hodgkin's lymphoma of the midline granuloma type. Blood 82:858, 1993

576. Falini B, Pileri S, De Solas I et al: Peripheral T-cell lymphoma associated with hemophagocytic syndrome. Blood 75:434, 1990

577. Gonzalez CL, Medeiros J, Braziel RM, Jaffe ES: T-cell lymphoma involving subcutaneous tissue. A clinicopathologic entity commonly associated with hemophagocytic syndrome. Am J Surg Pathol 15:17, 1991

578. Hanson CA, Bockenstedt PL, Schnitzer B et al: S100-positive, T-cell chronic lymphoproliferative disease: an aggressive disorder of an uncommon T-cell subset. Blood 78:1803, 1991

Clinical Manifestations and Staging of and Therapy for Non-Hodgkin Lymphomas

81

Philip J. Bierman, Julie M. Vose, and James O. Armitage

INTRODUCTION

In 1993 an estimated 43,000 new cases of non-Hodgkin lymphoma (NHL) were diagnosed in the United States.[1] It is estimated that these will account for 20,500 deaths. Although these cases account for <5% of all newly diagnosed cancers, they are among the five leading causes of cancer mortality in young men and women and may therefore have a disproportionate social and economic impact. The study of lymphomas has advanced our understanding of the function of the immune system, particularly in terms of lymphocyte development. Exciting discoveries have allowed new insights into the origins of these malignancies. Finally, with the introduction of combination chemotherapy >20 years ago,[2,3] it has become clear that these malignancies are curable. NHLs have thus become a proving ground for new chemotherapeutic agents. New chemotherapy dosing and administration schedules have validated previously described concepts of cell kinetics and have improved on early treatment results and allowed successful treatment even of patients with advanced or relapsed disease.

Because the goal in treating lymphomas is most often cure rather than palliation, a meticulous approach to diagnosis and staging is mandatory. The diagnosis of lymphoma is among the hardest for a pathologist to make. Fortunately, advances in immunophenotyping, cytogenetics, and molecular biology can provide help in situations in which diagnosis was previously impossible.[4] Since an accurate diagnosis may determine prognosis as well as therapy, any uncertainty should lead to review by a consulting pathologist or to a repeat biopsy if required. New drugs are currently under evaluation, along with other promising modalities, including biologic response modifiers, radioimmunoconjugates, and bone marrow transplantation (BMT). In addition, the use of hematopoietic growth factors as a means of increasing dose intensity is under active exploration. These, hopefully, will build on our past successes and improve our treatment results.

EPIDEMIOLOGY AND ETIOLOGY

The prevalence of NHLs shows wide geographic variations throughout the world. There is as much as an 8–10-fold range of occurrence, with the maximum rate reported in the Western developed countries.[5] The incidence rises steadily with age, especially beyond age 40.[6,7] However unlike Hodgkin disease, no peak in incidence of NHL exists for young adults. Males are affected more often than females, the ratio being 1.5:1.0, and in the United States the incidence is approximately twice as great among whites as among blacks. The differences in gender and racial incidence may reflect occupational risks that are experienced preferentially by the more frequently affected groups. The incidence of NHL has been steadily rising, not only in the United States but also worldwide.[6,7] Over the past 20 years, the incidence rates for NHL have increased 3–4% each year. This rate of increase is greater than for any other cancers except melanoma and lung cancer in woman. Although the reason for the increase in incidence is not completely understood, it is partly related to an increase in acquired immunodeficiency syndrome (AIDS)-associated lymphomas. This is supported by Surveillance Epidemiology and End Results (SEER) data that show the largest increase in NHL incidence is in San Francisco. As utilization of standardized reporting and classification methods for NHL increases, perhaps more information regarding true differences in the incidence of NHL will be obtained.

No common etiologic agent can be associated with all cases of NHL. However, a number of genetic, immunologic, and environmental factors have been associated with some cases. Several families have now been described with an unusually large number of lymphoproliferative diseases among their members.[8] A family history of NHL or other lymphoproliferative disorder is associated with a markedly increased risk of NHL. One category of familial NHL involves sibling pairs, with mostly young males affected. Many of these patients have had extranodal lymphoma at diagnosis. Another category of familial NHL affects adult siblings, and a third category has included families with adult NHL occurring in more than one generation. When such a familial incidence is noted, the entire family should be screened for an underlying immunodeficiency syndrome.

Although many families with an increased incidence of lymphoproliferative diseases do not have an underlying immunodeficiency syndrome, there are several immunologic disorders that do predispose to an increased incidence of lymphomas. Rare immunologic or inherited disorders that are associated with an increased incidence of NHL include ataxia-telangiectasia, Wiskott-Aldrich syndrome, common variable immunodeficiency syndrome, Bruton-type agammaglobulinemia, and Chédiak-Higashi syndrome.[9,10] Of particular interest is the X-linked lymphoproliferative syndrome, a rare condition, described in 1976 by Purtilo,[11] in which families exhibit impaired cellular immunity to the Epstein-Barr virus (EBV) in an X-linked recessive pattern. The affected male members of these families have uncontrolled EBV infections expressed as fatal infectious mononucleosis, NHL, or acquired agammaglobulinemia.[12,13]

Many cases of NHL are related to iatrogenic causes. The frequency of NHL is high in patients who have been treated for Hodgkin disease.[14] Iatrogenic immunodeficiency also leads to an increased risk of developing NHL. This risk applies to patients who are receiving immunosuppressive agents to prevent transplant rejection or for treatment of other conditions. The incidence of NHL in recipients of renal allografts has been approximately 40–100 times greater than expected. These lymphomas occur within 2–3 years of transplant on average, but may occur within a matter of months. The central nervous system is a frequent site of involvement, and other extranodal sites of presentation are common.[15–17] The allograft itself is a frequent site of microscopic or macroscopic disease. These tumors display a wide spectrum of histologic appearance and may be monoclonal or polyclonal proliferations of B lymphocytes.[18] The use of the monoclonal antibody OKT3 has been associated with an increased risk of lymphomas after cardiac transplantation.[19] An increased risk of lymphoproliferative syndromes after allogeneic BMT has been described as well.[20,21] There seems to be a correlation with HLA-mismatched and T-cell-depleted transplants, presumably as a result of increased immunosuppression. Lymphoma risk in persons receiving immunotherapy for other clinical conditions appears to be less pronounced.[22]

It is now clear that many, if not all, lymphomas that occur in the setting of acquired or congenital immunodeficiency are caused by EBV.[17,23,24] This virus, which infects B cells, is normally suppressed by T-cell-mediated immune mechanisms. When T-cell deficiencies, either congenital or acquired, occur, EBV-infected B cells can proliferate unchecked. Initially a polyclonal proliferation takes place; however, one clone eventually can escape immune surveillance to become autonomous. Various cytogenetic abnormalities have been associated with this second step in differentiation to a monoclonal proliferation.[25]

A wide range of disorders with impaired immunity have also been associated with an increased risk of lymphoma. Rheumatoid arthritis,[26] Sjögren-Larsson syndrome,[27] Hashimoto thyroiditis,[28] systemic lupus erythematosus,[26] and celiac sprue[29] have all been associated with this increase in incidence of lymphomas. The patients with celiac sprue often present with primary gastrointestinal lymphoma, the distal ileum being the most frequent site of involvement.[30]

Environmental factors may play a part in the induction of lymphomas. A small but significant increase in NHL incidence has been demonstrated in patients receiving radiation for ankylosing spondylitis,[31] as well as in Japanese atomic bomb survivors who had been exposed to >100 cGy.[32] Several surveys of cancer risk in relationship to occupational associations have suggested that some occupations may be associated with NHL.[33–35] These include vinyl chloride workers, anesthesiologists, rubber production workers, leather workers, and road transport workers. These exposures, however, are related to only a small percentage of lymphomas. An increase in the incidence of lymphoma among farmers has been noted in several epidemiologic studies. Use of the herbicide 2,4-D has been associated with a two- to eightfold increase in NHL. Risk of NHL can be directly correlated with duration of herbicide exposure. Exposure to hair dye has also been linked to the development of NHL.[34] It has been estimated that hair dye may account for as much as 20% of NHL in women.

Several lymphomas have now been associated with a viral agent; however, such an association has not been clearly delineated for most types of lymphoma.[36] In humans there is a strong association between EBV and Burkitt lymphoma in Africa, but the association is not as strong for Burkitt lymphoma cases diagnosed in the United States.[37] Another lymphoproliferative syndrome that has been associated with a viral agent is adult T-cell leukemia/lymphoma, which is endemic in southwestern Japan, the Caribbean, and also the southeastern United States.[38,39] The virus isolated from this type of lymphoproliferative disorder is a type C RNA retrovirus—the human T-cell leukemia/lymphoma virus-1 (HTLV-1).[40] Other viruses associated with lymphomas include HTLV-3 (human immunodeficiency virus-1 [HIV-1] the causative agent of AIDS,[41] and HTLV-4 (HIV-2), which is a similar retrovirus isolated from West African patients with AIDS.[42] A recently discovered agent, HTLV-5, may be associated with certain subtypes of cutaneous T-cell lymphoma, although questions remain regarding its actual role.[43]

Both host and environmental factors seem to be important in the etiology of NHLs. Host factors, including genetic predisposition and underlying immunodeficiency syndromes, may set the stage for the development of lymphoproliferative syndromes. Environmental agents such as chemicals, immunosuppressive drugs, radiation, or viruses may also predispose to lymphoma development. Further analysis of this complex group of diseases may uncover how these factors may interact to initiate lymphoproliferative disorders.

The large number of classification systems for NHLs has led to considerable confusion for both pathologists and practicing physicians when attempts were made to correlate diagnoses from one classification system to another.[44–58] The various classification systems are discussed in detail in Chapter 80. In order to relieve the confusion in terminology that resulted from these different systems of classification, an international multi-institutional study was undertaken in an attempt to assess the clinical applicability and reproducibility of the six major classification systems for NHL.[59] Pathologic material from 1,175 newly diagnosed patients seen at four institutions between July 1, 1971 and December 31, 1975 was reviewed and classified by six expert pathologists, each a proponent of one of the major classification systems. Six other hematopathologists were selected to review the same slides, and they also independently reviewed and classified all the cases according to all six systems of classification. The results of the analysis led to the development of a working formulation of the NHLs for clinical purposes, which is described in Chapter 80. It was concluded that all six classification symptoms were valuable and comparable in reproducibility and clinical correlations. The working formulation also confirmed the significance of follicular architecture independent of cell type. Ten major cell types were identified, along with a miscellaneous category, and subtypes were described that allowed comparisons between one system and another.

CLINICAL MANIFESTATIONS

Low-Grade Histologies

The subset of NHL with low-grade histology consists of the small lymphocytic, follicular small cleaved cell, and follicular mixed categories in the working formulation.[59] Because of their

Table 81-1. Characteristics of the Major Histologic Subtypes of the NHLs[a]

| Histologic Subtype[59] | Cases (%) | Distribution by Stage (%) | | | | Symptom Status (%) | Bone Marrow Involvement (%) | Median Survival (yr) | Cure with Aggressive Chemotherapy Possible |
		I	II	III	IV				
Small lymphocytic	4	3	8	8	81	20	71	5.8	No
Follicular small cleaved	22	8	10	16	66	20	51	7.2	No/rare
Follicular mixed	8	15	12	28	46	20	30	5.1	Uncertain
Follicular large cell	4	15	12	15	58	27	34	3.0	Probable
Diffuse small cleaved	7	9	19	12	60	18	32	3.4	Probable
Diffuse mixed	7	19	26	13	42	21	14	2.7	Yes
Diffuse large cell	20	16	30	10	44	28	10	1.5	Yes
Immunoblastic	8	23	29	16	33	32	12	1.3	Yes
Lymphoblastic	4	7	20	2	72	27	50	2.0	Yes
Small noncleaved	5	13	21	9	57	14	14	0.8	Yes

[a] A miscellaneous group comprises the remaining 12% of NHLs and are not included in this table. This category includes composite NHL, mycosis fungoides, histiocyte lymphoma, extramedullary plasmacytoma, and unclassifiable NHLs.

natural history and response to therapy they have often been referred to as "good prognosis" or "favorable prognosis" lymphomas. These histologies make up 23–43% of newly diagnosed NHLs[60–64] (Table 81-1). Although not uncommon in the third and fourth decades, these lymphomas occur most commonly in middle-aged patients and the elderly, with a median age at diagnosis of 50–60 years.[60–64] Bone marrow involvement is commonly seen at presentation, and ≥50–80% of patients will present with stage III or IV disease.[62,65–67] With few exceptions these lymphomas are composed of B lymphocytes.[68] By using flow cytometric κ-λ analysis or Southern analysis, circulating monoclonal B lymphocytes have been detected in ≤78% of these patients.[69,70] Numerous primary and secondary cytogenetic abnormalities have been described in patients with low-grade histologies. The specific abnormality, t(14;18) (q32; q21) has been seen in most patients with follicular lymphomas.[71–75] This cytogenetic abnormality is associated with deregulation of the bcl-2 proto-oncogene. This results in overexpression of the bcl-2 protein, which is known to inhibit programmed cell death.[76]

Although median survivals >7–8 years are reported from several series,[77–82] the low-grade lymphomas should be considered fatal malignancies. The median survival of a group of 83 patients with low-grade lymphoma who were managed initially with observation alone was 11 years.[80] With time, these lymphomas often transform into a more aggressive histologic pattern; when patients have a repeat biopsy during the course of their disease, 28–44% may show evidence of such a transformation.[61,80,83–86] Rates of such histologic transformation have been >70% when patients with residual disease are examined at autopsy.[87,88] These transformed lymphomas may be quite aggressive and poorly responsive to chemotherapy.[61,82]

Intermediate-Grade Lymphomas

Intermediate-grade lymphomas considered in the working formulation include follicular large cell, diffuse small cleaved, diffuse mixed, and diffuse large cell. Since clinically there is very little distinction between tumors labeled diffuse large cell and those classified as immunoblastic, that category is also included in this discussion. As can be seen in Table 81-1, intermediate grade tumors make up approximately 50% of NHLs. The most common are the diffuse large cell lymphomas.

Follicular large cell lymphomas are closely related to the other follicular lymphomas. They are the least common of the follicular lymphomas, making up 4% of the cases on which the working formulation was based. Like all other subtypes of follicular lymphoma, these tumors tend to be widely disseminated at diagnosis, and a minority of patients have systemic symptoms. Follicular large cell lymphomas can be identified by a variety

of criteria, of which perhaps the most useful is that of Mann and Berard,[89] who proposed that a distinction between follicular mixed and follicular large cell lymphoma should be made when there are >15 large cells per high-power field. The criteria for separating follicular mixed and follicular large cell NHL are not the same among the various classification systems, and the distinctions are difficult to reproduce among pathologists. This makes it difficult to interpret clinical trials involving patients with follicular large cell lymphoma. Follicular large cell lymphomas are of B-cell origin, but it must be remembered that reactive T cells can infiltrate the tumor and cause confusion in immunophenotyping.[90] The most common chromosomal abnormality seen in follicular large cell lymphoma is the t(14;18) (q32;q21) translocation that is characteristic of other follicular lymphomas. With the usual cytogenetic methods, this translocation is found in approximately 50% of follicular large cell lymphoma cases. It can be accompanied by a variety of other cytogenetic abnormalities.[91]

Follicular large cell lymphoma seems to have a more aggressive natural history than the other follicular lymphomas, particularly in patients with advanced-stage disease.[92–94] This tumor is more likely to progress quickly when patients are observed without therapy. The greater number of large cells in the tumor has led to some enthusiasm for the treatment of these patients with aggressive chemotherapy regimens in hopes of cure, although the percentage of large cells may not have prognostic influence.[86] Whether this tumor can be cured in a significant number of patients with aggressive chemotherapy regimens remains a point of controversy.

Diffuse small cleaved cell NHL is the diffuse counterpart of follicular small cleaved cell lymphoma.[95] This tumor has been diagnosed less commonly in the United States over the last several years. As outlined in Table 81-1, patients with diffuse small cleaved cell lymphoma generally have disseminated disease without systemic symptoms. This tumor usually represents a B-cell neoplasm, although occasional patients with peripheral T-cell lymphoma will be classified in this subcategory. The natural history of tumors in this category varies considerably. When patients with true lymphoblastic lymphoma are carefully excluded, the typical course of patients with this lymphoma subtype is usually one of response to therapy with frequent relapses. It is unclear whether these lymphomas are curable with standard chemotherapy, although the working formulation study[59] suggested that some proportion of these patients can be cured. However, many oncologists in the United States would believe that patients with small cleaved cell lymphoma should be managed similarly regardless of the degree of follicularity in the tumor. We favor a more aggressive approach and treat these patients initially much as we treat those with large cell lymphoma.

Diffuse mixed lymphoma is one of the most varied subtypes included in the working formulation. These tumors have a distribution similar to that of large cell lymphomas with respect to the percentage of patients with localized and with disseminated disease at diagnosis. Most patients will not have systemic symptoms at diagnosis. With the exception of lymphoblastic lymphoma, diffuse mixed lymphomas represent the subgroup with the highest proportion of T-cell lymphomas. These lymphomas are generally post-thymic or peripheral T-cell lymphomas. No single chromosomal abnormality is characteristic. It is important to note that peripheral T-cell lymphoma of the diffuse mixed cell type can easily be misdiagnosed as mixed-cellularity Hodgkin disease.

We have found the clinical course of patients with diffuse mixed lymphoma to be so similar to that of patients with large cell lymphomas that there is no useful distinction with regard to staging and therapy. Patients with diffuse mixed lymphoma have complete responses to therapy, and the proportion of long-term survivors is approximately the same as with diffuse large cell or immunoblastic lymphoma.

Diffuse large cell and immunoblastic lymphomas are aggressive neoplasms. These tumors present in a localized (i.e., stage I) manner approximately 20% of the time, and disease is confined to one side of the diaphragm (i.e., stage I or II) approximately 50% of the time. Disseminated extranodal disease (i.e., stage IV) is seen least frequently in these types of lymphomas. Approximately one in three patients have systemic symptoms. These tumors can have either a B- or a T-cell immunophenotype; in the United States approximately 80–90% of the patients will have B-cell lymphomas and the remainder will have the peripheral T-cell immunophenotype.[96,97] The cytogenetic abnormality t(14;18) (q32;q21) is the one most frequently seen in these subtypes, although a wide number of other cytogenetic abnormalities have been described.[74,98] The significance of the particular pattern of cytogenetic abnormalities remains uncertain, but it has been proposed that the pattern might have prognostic significance. For example, patients with abnormalities involving chromosome 17 or 7 have poor survival,[98–100] and patients with abnormalities involving chromosome 2 have improved survival.[98]

Patients with diffuse large cell or immunoblastic lymphoma have aggressive disease, which progress rapidly without therapy. However, with therapy these subtypes of lymphoma are curable in a significant proportion of patients. Most of those who present with localized disease are curable, and even patients with widely disseminated, symptomatic disease can be cured in a significant proportion of cases. This particular subtype of lymphoma can occasionally be misdiagnosed as an undifferentiated carcinoma. When patients present with undifferentiated malignant neoplasms, the diagnosis of large cell lymphoma should be considered because of the considerable therapeutic implications.[101]

High-Grade Lymphomas

The working formulation for NHL clinical usage divides the high-grade NHLs into three major categories: malignant lymphoma-large cell immunoblastic, malignant lymphoma-lymphoblastic, and malignant lymphoma-small noncleaved cell.[59] These high-grade lymphomas behave in a clinically aggressive manner if left untreated; however, with modern therapy long-term disease-free survival is possible. Overall, these lymphomas represent approximately 12–18% of all NHLs. Most cases of high-grade NHLs present in young patients and almost half of childhood NHL falls into this category. Other histologies in the working formulation that manifest aggressive biologic characteristics, such as advanced-stage peripheral T-cell lymphoma, may also be considered in this high-grade category and are discussed here.

The category of malignant lymphoma-large cell immunoblastic lymphoma would be considered diffuse "histiocytic" lymphoma in the Rappaport scheme, and thus diffuse histiocytic lymphoma was subclassified in the working formulation into large cell and large cell immunoblastic categories. Because of a small but significant difference in survival and certain morphologic distinctions, these cases were separated from the diffuse large cell type in the working formulation.[59] However, the studies, although showing survival trends in the same direction, failed to demonstrate a statistical difference in survival.[102] Furthermore, because the large cell and large cell immunoblastic categories share many clinical features, the intermediate- and high-grade categories of the working formulation have been controversial. Because of the clinical similarities most oncologists would evaluate and treat immunoblastic NHL in a manner similar to that used for diffuse large cell NHL, which has been considered under the intermediate-grade lymphomas.

Lymphoblastic NHL was originally included in the diffuse, poorly differentiated lymphocytic lymphomas of the Rappaport classification; however, on clinical and pathologic grounds it is clearly a distinct entity.[103] In 1975 Barcos and Lukes[104] used the term *convoluted lymphocytic lymphoma* to describe this clinical subgroup, seen predominantly in young males who present with a large mediastinal mass and progress rapidly to disseminated lymphoma. Nathwani et al.[105] subsequently recognized both convoluted and nonconvoluted cell types in these lymphomas and classified them as lymphoblastic lymphoma. This lymphoma shares many of the features of T-cell acute lymphocytic leukemia (T-ALL) and may be a close variant. In contrast to T-ALL, lymphoblastic NHL occurs in a slightly older age group with a peak incidence in the second decade of life, and males outnumber females in approximately a 2:1 ratio.[106]

Most patients (approximately 50–75%) present with a mediastinal mass, and emergent symptoms related to superior vena cava syndrome or tracheal obstruction often are initially present.[107] Although the disease occasionally appears to be localized at diagnosis, it evolves rapidly and is characterized by disseminated systemic involvement. Bone marrow involvement is present at diagnosis in approximately 30% of cases; however, as the disease progresses, ≤80% of patients eventually develop bone marrow and peripheral blood involvement.[108] Because of this clinical overlap, the boundaries between T-ALL and lymphoblastic lymphoma can be indistinct. The frequently used St. Jude Children's Hospital staging system for childhood NHL includes patients in the lymphoblastic lymphoma category if they have <25% blasts in their bone marrow.[109] However, other systems use a 10% lymphoblast cutoff.[110] In addition to the marrow and blood, central nervous system involvement is also detected in approximately one-third of patients at some time during the clinical course.

The small noncleaved lymphomas (SNCLs) of the working formulation were designated as undifferentiated lymphomas in the Rappaport classification. Within this subgroup a histologic distinction between Burkitt and non-Burkitt lymphoma can be made based on the degree of cellular pleomorphism and the proportion of cells with a single large nucleolus. However, the importance of this distinction clinically remains controversial. "Endemic" regions of the world, which include Africa and New Guinea,[111] have a relatively high incidence of SNCL—5–10 cases per 100,000 children, with few cases in the adult population. These cases are associated with significantly elevated antibody titers to a variety of EBV antigens, and 80–90% of the tumors contain multiple copies of the EBV DNA genome.[112,113] The "sporadic" regions for SNCL include most of the United States and Europe. The incidence is lower in the sporadic regions, with two to three cases per million children, which account for approximately 1–2% of NHLs in all age groups.[114] The association with EBV is not as clear in the sporadic as in the endemic cases of SNCL. Most Burkitt lymphomas (75%) have a chromosomal translocation identified as a t(8;14), with another 20% having a t(8;22) and 8% having a t(8;2).[99,115] The common features of these translocations are involvement of the c-*myc* oncogene located on chromosome 8 and juxtaposition of the protein coding region of this gene with sequences from one of the immunoglobulin gene loci. Chromosome 14 contains the immunoglobulin heavy chain locus, while chromosomes 2 and 22 contain the immunoglobulin κ and λ light chain loci, respectively.

The clinical features of endemic and sporadic cases of SNCL are somewhat different. The African endemic SNCL most often presents as large extranodal tumors affecting the bones of the jaws and abdominal viscera. Occasionally patients can present with isolated tumors of the thyroid, skin, breasts, testes, or long bones. Retroperitoneal or extradural tumors can cause paraplegia, either by vascular compromise or by direct spinal cord invasion. Involvement of the central nervous system is an unusual presenting feature, but it becomes increasingly common after relapse and may be manifested by cranial nerve palsies. The mean age of African patients with SNCL is 7 years, with a 2:1 male/female ratio. Patients with sporadic SNCL present most of the time with intra-abdominal tumors, arising apparently from Peyer's patches in the ileocecal region or from the mesenteric lymph nodes. Patients often have bowel obstruction or perforation as an initial clinical presentation. The remainder of the sporadic cases present as tumors involving the ovaries, kidneys, retroperitoneum, or peripheral lymph nodes or as diffuse bone marrow involvement. The mean age in the sporadic cases is slightly older, 11 years, with the same male/female ratio.

The final category that we would classify as high-grade lymphoma on the basis of clinical parameters consists of peripheral T-cell lymphomas, including those of advanced stage or with large tumor burden. Although not all previous studies have found peripheral T-cell lymphoma to be an important prognostic characteristic,[97,116,117] several recent studies of uniformly treated patients have found this to be the case.[95,96,118]

STAGING

One of the important concepts in managing patients with malignant disease is the concept of staging. This implies an evaluation of patients that classifies them into one of multiple categories to allow therapeutic decisions and/or accurate determination of the prognosis. Because lymphoma patients have illnesses that sometimes can be cured and in most other cases can be palliated with a variety of different chemotherapeutic and radiotherapeutic approaches, staging these patients is the most important initial responsibility of the physician after the diagnosis has been firmly determined. The importance, as the initial step, of confirming the histologic diagnosis by having an expert hematopathologist review the slides cannot be too strongly emphasized.

Staging is often considered to be based on determination of the sites of involvement by disease. However, there are other staging systems that can be used. For chronic lymphocytic leukemia the Rai system divides patients into groups based on the sites of involvement and the extent of marrow failure.[119] A popular staging system for multiple myeloma depends on sites of involvement, hypercalcemia, extent of protein abnormalities, and signs of marrow failure.[120] The most popular staging system for patients with lymphoma, often referred to as the Ann Arbor staging system,[121] was originally developed for patients with Hodgkin disease, and not those with NHL. The differences between these disorders make application of the Ann Arbor system to NHL patients not always simple. However, it remains the most popular system in use for patients with most types of NHL.

Table 81-2. Evaluation and Staging of Patients with NHL

Confirmation of histologic diagnosis
Careful history and physical examination
Routine studies (e.g., hemogram, chemistry profile, chest radiograph)
Bone marrow biopsy
Imaging studies to look for occult sites of involvement (e.g., CT scan, gallium scan, lymphangiogram, abdominal ultrasound)
Other tests as indicated by results of above (e.g., biopsy of suspicious area)

The Ann Arbor system assigns patients to stage I (disease confined to one lymph node site), stage II (disease confined to lymphatic tissue in more than one site but on only one side of the diaphragm), stage III (disease confined to lymphatic tissue or spleen but on both sides of the diaphragm), or stage IV (bone marrow involvement, liver involvement, or any other site of extranodal disease with widespread lymphoma). When patients present with localized extranodal disease (e.g., a disease originating in and confined to the stomach), they are designated as having stage IE disease, and patients with localized extranodal disease and regional lymph node involvement would be designated as having stage IIE. Some physicians would designate widespread lymphatic disease and one localized site of extranodal involvement other than the liver or bone marrow as stage IIIE, whereas others would classify such patients as having stage IV. Patients are further subdivided in the Ann Arbor classification depending on whether they have the systemic symptoms of fever (i.e., >38°C with no other cause), weight loss (i.e., >10% body weight in 6 months), or drenching night sweats. When the Ann Arbor classification is applied to patients with Hodgkin disease, there is a distinction made between clinical staging (examination, laboratory, and imaging studies) and pathologic staging (including the results of staging laparotomy). Because staging laparotomies are rarely done in NHL patients, this distinction is less useful for NHL.

Table 81-2 presents one approach to the staging of NHL patients. It cannot be stated too firmly that the first step is to confirm the histologic diagnosis by having the slides reviewed by an experienced hematopathologist. This should be followed by a careful history and physical examination to identify potential sites of involvement and the presence or absence of systemic symptoms. Findings from the history and physical examination may direct further biopsies to document a high stage. A variety of standard laboratory studies, including a hemogram, chemistry profile, chest radiograph, and bone marrow biopsy, should be performed on all patients. The first three tests also aid in identifying possible areas for documentation of advanced disease, and a positive bone marrow biopsy is especially important in that it would always make the patient stage IV. A wide variety of imaging studies beyond the use of the chest radiograph have been used with NHL. These include the computed tomography (CT) scan, gallium scan, lymphangiogram, ultrasound scan, and magnetic resonance imaging (MRI). Of the multiple other imaging studies available, radionuclide bone scans can sometimes be helpful. The most important reason for the more complex imaging studies in patients being staged for lymphoma is the possible detection of occult intra-abdominal disease. Staging laparotomies will be done only rarely in these patients, and physical examination, laboratory studies, and routine radiographic studies have limited value in identifying intra-abdominal adenopathy or organ involvement. Perhaps the most important advance in this regard was the development of the CT scan, which is fairly simple to use and has a high accuracy in identifying sites of lymphoma involvement.[122] CT scans are particularly useful in identifying high periaortic, mesenteric, and splenic hilar nodes, which are not seen by lymphangiography.[123]

Although performed with decreasing frequency, lymphangiography has been the standard test for identification of involvement of periaortic lymph nodes by Hodgkin disease or NHL. This procedure has a high accuracy,[124] but it has been replaced by CT scans to a significant degree. Ultrasonography provides a comparatively easy and noninvasive imaging approach, which can be used to study a number of sites of the body in addition to the abdomen.[125] It is worth remembering that ultrasound can be used to confirm or refute the suspicion of possible superficial adenopathy,[126] and endoscopic ultrasonography might extend the usefulness of this technique.[127] MRI offers a new approach to the imaging of patients with lymphoma; in addition to identifying usual sites of disease, MRI scans might be helpful in detecting bone marrow involvement without bone marrow biopsies.[128] In addition, MRI may prove to be a useful way to evaluate residual masses on CT scans after treatment.[129]

Of the radionuclide imaging techniques, gallium scans probably have the most utility in NHL patients. However, it must be remembered that this test is much more useful in patients with aggressive NHL than in those with indolent lymphomas, whose tumors are less likely to take up gallium.[130] When combined with single-photon emission computed tomography, gallium scans become especially useful.[131] Gallium scanning can be especially useful in re-evaluating patients after therapy, particularly those with residual, potentially fibrotic masses. This is true because gallium scanning reflects the metabolic activity of the tumor rather than anatomic findings. However, this technique is not perfect in that both false-positive and false-negative scans can occur.[132,133] The other radionuclide study that is often used in NHL patients is the bone scan. Although not recommended for routine use, this is a sensitive technique that can be used to identify bone marrow involvement in patients in whom it is suspected.[134]

A more subtle reason for careful staging of the lymphoma patient before therapy is to allow accurate determination of the response at the completion of therapy. This is often referred to as restaging. In general, all studies that gave abnormal results before therapy should be repeated at the completion of therapy. This will allow the accurate determination of a complete response. As noted above, some patients (particularly those with bulky mediastinal or retroperitoneal disease) are likely to have residual imaging abnormalities reflecting persistent fibrotic masses. In general, patients with stable, residual masses in sites of bulky disease, particularly if the mass has gone from gallium-positive to gallium-negative, should be followed without further therapy and treated as complete responders.[135] A new staging system for Hodgkin disease has been proposed in which patients with residual masses of uncertain significance are given the classification CR[u] to denote a complete remission of uncertain significance.[136] This designation is gaining usage for patients with NHL.

PROGNOSIS

A wide variety of factors have been determined to predict outcome in some groups of NHL patients, the most widely used prognostic factor being histologic subtype.[59,62] Although it should be remembered that the various histologic subtypes do not carry sharply different prognoses (e.g., some patients with follicular small cleaved cell lymphoma will have a poorer survival than patients with diffuse large cell lymphoma), this is still an important factor on which to base therapeutic decisions. Some other prognostic factors might be especially important only when histologic subtype is taken into account, and some would apply to all different subtypes of lymphomas. Prognostic factors can be divided into those related primarily to the patient (e.g., age, concomitant illnesses) and those related to the tumor itself (e.g., immunologic subtype, cytogenetic abnormalities). Of the patient-related prognostic variables, perhaps the most consistent is the poor outcome found with advanced age.[137–139] The apparent lack of importance of age in some series of patients with aggressive NHL is probably because few patients >60–65 years of age (at which point there seems to be a significant drop-off in favorable outcome) were actually treated.[140,141] The general health of patients as reflected in their performance status is an important factor in survival for many malignancies and seems to be important also in NHL patients.[142] Obviously, the existence of serious concomitant illnesses such as lung or heart disease might greatly limit the drugs that can be used and thus alter the physician's ability to treat the patient effectively. Patients who have failed previous chemotherapy regimens have a poor outlook with second-line therapy,[143] as do patients who have undergone progression from a low-grade to a more aggressive histology.[61,82–84,144]

Tumor-related variables such as bulkiness[142,145–150] or high growth fraction[151–154] are associated with a poor prognosis. The significance of stage in treatment outcome presumably is a reflection of both these variables.[148,155] Similarly, the adverse prognosis associated with an elevated serum lactate dehydrogenase (LDH) level reflects bulky tumor and/or particularly rapid growth.[145,146,148,150,156,157] More recently, the serum level of β_2-microglobulin has been identified as a prognostic factor not only in multiple myeloma but also in NHL.[158]

The influence of T-cell versus B-cell phenotype is controversial. Some reports have shown no difference in outcome related to phenotype.[97,159–161] However, a number of other investigations have noted a significantly poorer outcome in patients with a T-cell phenotype.[95,96,118,162] Certain cytogenetic abnormalities have also been associated with a poor outcome.[74,98,163] In addition, specific sites of tumor involvement, especially the bone marrow,[147,150,155] but also other sites such as the gastrointestinal tract,[147] have been identified as significant adverse prognostic factors. Several studies have shown that the rate of response of the tumor to initial therapy is highly predictive of outcome, with more rapidly responding patients having better outlooks.[164–166] This presumably is a direct reflection of the sensitivity of the tumor to the treatment being administered.

Recently, results from the International non-Hodgkin's Lymphoma Prognostic Factors Project[167] have been published. This study analyzed results of >3,000 patients with aggressive NHL in North America and Europe. An International Index was developed based on age, tumor stage, the number of extranodal sites of disease, performance status, and serum LDH. The influence of age (≤60 versus >60 years) was highly predictive, with elderly patients having significantly poorer outcomes. Therefore, an Age-Adjusted International Index was developed (Table 81-3) for patients ≤60 of age. This index was based on three variables: stage, serum LDH, and performance status. These models were more accurate than the Ann Arbor stage[121] in predicting survival, and these indexes are likely to be widely used in the future.

Table 81-4 outlines the other prognostic factors discussed above. It should be remembered that prognostic factors are useful for transmitting to patients some idea of their chances for successful therapy; they might also be useful in identifying

Table 81-3. Age-Adjusted International Prognostic Index for Aggressive NHL

Risk Factors (N)	Risk Group	5-yr Projected Survival (%)
0	Low	83
1	Low intermediate	69
2	High intermediate	46
3	High	32

Risk factor: (1) stage (I or II versus III or IV); (2) serum LDH (≤1 × normal versus >1 × normal); (3) performance status (0 or 1 versus 2–4).

(Modified from The International Non-Hodgkin's Lymphoma Prognostic Factors Project,[167] with permission.)

Table 81-4. Important Prognostic Factors in the Treatment of Patients with NHL[a]

Histologic subtype
Age
Other serious illnesses
Failed previous therapy
Histologic progression
Tumor bulk
Stage
Systemic symptoms
Performance status
Serum LDH
Serum β_2-microglobulin
Specific sites of involvement (e.g., bone marrow, gastrointestinal tract)
Immunophenotype
Cytogenetic abnormalities
Rate of tumor response

[a] See text for references.

patients who should receive one or another treatment. For example, patients with a particularly poor prognosis with primary therapy might be candidates for an alternate treatment such as BMT as part of the primary therapy.

THERAPY

Low-Grade Non-Hodgkin Lymphomas

No aspect of the optimal management of NHL patients is more controversial than that of patients with low-grade histologic subtypes. Although highly responsive to chemotherapy and radiation, most groups of patients with advanced disease have failed to show definite evidence of a plateau in their survival curves and have exhibited a continuous pattern of relapse.[81,86,168,169]

Interpretation of treatment results in these patients is difficult and should be undertaken with caution. Few studies are prospective or randomized, and many if not all are plagued by difficulties in classification. Small lymphocytic lymphomas, for example, are considered to be solid tumor counterparts of chronic lymphocytic leukemia.[170] A decision on whether to include those patients in lymphoma or chronic lymphocytic leukemia trials is often arbitrary. Other difficulties are seen when attempts are made to distinguish follicular mixed from diffuse mixed lymphomas or follicular mixed from follicular large cell histologies.

Follicular large cell lymphomas, although classified as belonging to an intermediate grade, are often grouped with low-grade histologies.[61,79,86,171,172] Since these lymphomas may respond differently to therapy, their inclusion in series containing low-grade histologies may influence results, and literature must be interpreted in this light.[61,172–174] How newer imaging technologies have influenced staging in more recent patient series is unknown, but their use certainly makes comparisons with older studies more difficult.

Localized Low-Grade Lymphomas

Although the treatment of patients with advanced low-grade lymphomas remains controversial, cure is sometimes possible with true stage I or minimal stage II. Table 81-5 shows treatment results for patients with localized low-grade lymphomas treated with radiation alone or in combination with chemotherapy.[171,172,175–180] A variety of radiation doses and treatment fields have been employed, but most series report 5-year disease-free survivals >50%. Differences in results may be accounted for in several ways.

Laparotomy has been used in staging some patients, generally those who would be more likely to have clinically occult disease outside the radiation ports, which may account for the superior disease-free survival (DFS) reported for laparotomy-staged patients in some series. Also, some series have reported superior DFS in patients treated with more extensive radiation fields. Despite a trend for improved DFS with more aggressive staging or more extensive radiation fields, it has been difficult to translate these findings into improved overall survival. Relapses have almost always occurred outside of radiation ports, however, which supports the concept that failure is often a result of inadequate treatment.

The question of whether adjuvant chemotherapy adds anything to the effectiveness of radiation alone is still unsettled. With few exceptions, the addition of chemotherapy has not been studied in a prospective randomized fashion. Furthermore, the length and type of chemotherapy employed has varied widely from study to study. Again, improvement in DFS has been reported with the addition of chemotherapy, but improvement in overall survival of patients with localized low-grade lymphomas is difficult to prove.

It seems that radiation alone can cure patients with low-grade NHL when disease is truly localized and all areas of disease are treated. The role of adjuvant chemotherapy and more extensive radiation is less clear, but improvements in DFS may indeed be translated into overall survival differences when these patients are followed long enough. We do not perform staging laparotomies. Patients are treated with three cycles of

Table 81-5. Radiotherapy for Localized Low-Grade NHLs

Reference	Patients (N)	Radiation Fields	Adjuvant Chemotherapy (N)	Results	Comments
171	57	IF	Yes (9)	FSC: 49% RFS, 5 yr FM: 44% RFS, 5 yr	5 patients with FSC received chemotherapy alone
172	124	IF, EF, or TLI	Yes (2)	54% RFS, 10 yr	Includes FLC
175	23	IF or EF	Yes (?)	55% RFS, 5 yr	Includes FLC
176	26	IF, EF, STNI, or TNI	No	83% RFS, 5 yr	Includes FLC
177	26	IF or EF	Yes, randomized (15)	54.6% RFS, 5 yr radiation alone 63.0% RFS, 5 yr radiation + chemotherapy	Includes FLC Includes FLC
178	190	IF	No	53% RFS, 12 yr	Includes FLC
179	25	IF or TLI	Yes, randomized (?)	55% CCR, median F/U 118 mo	
180	39	IF or EF	Yes (18)	28/39 CCR, median F/U 5 yr	

Abbreviations: IF, involved field radiation; EF, extended field radiation; STNI, subtotal nodal irradiation; TNI, total nodal irradiation; TLI, total lymphoid irradiation; RFS, relapse-free survival; CCR, continuous complete remission; FSC, follicular small cleaved; FM, follicular mixed; F/U, follow-up; FLC, follicular large cell.

Table 81-6. Initial Observation for Low-Grade Lymphomas

Reference	Patients (N)	Survival (%)	Median Time to Institution of Therapy	Comments
80	83	73 (10 yr)	3 yr	23% spontaneous regression
81	59	56 (5 yr)	20% still on watch and wait; median follow-up 88 months	Includes some intermediate histologies
170	16	66 (5 yr)	5.9 yr	Small lymphocytic histology
185	31	81 (3 yr)	Not reached	—
186	41	83 (4 yr)	56% still on watch and wait; median duration 24 months	Includes some intermediate histologies

combination chemotherapy, followed by 4,000 cGy of involved-field radiation.

Advanced Low-Grade Lymphomas

The treatment of advanced-stage low-grade lymphomas has been the subject of considerable debate, primarily centering around the question of curability of these patients and whether any therapy at all is indicated for asymptomatic patients.[168,181–183] Traditionally therapy for this group of patients has relied on three approaches: (1) watch and wait; (2) moderate therapy with limited chemotherapy or radiotherapy; and (3) aggressive chemotherapy and radiotherapy. The choice of therapy is more often based on the philosophy of the treating physician than on objective data.

Watch and Wait

In the light of studies showing a continuous relapse rate for aggressively treated patients with advanced low-grade lymphomas, many physicians choose to defer initial treatment in asymptomatic patients and adopt a conservative watch and wait approach. The long natural history of this disease and that patients are often elderly with coexisting medical problems make this approach attractive in many situations. There may be several potential benefits from withholding therapy initially in asymptomatic patients.[184] (1) It may be months or years after the initial diagnosis before therapy is required, and patients would almost certainly have a better quality of life without therapy during this time. (2) Withholding initial therapy will theoretically limit exposure to chemotherapeutic agents and, it is hoped, prevent resistance at a time when those drugs are truly needed. (3) Spontaneous regression of disease may occur, eliminating the need for treatment.[80] (4) Finally, it has been suggested that if those lymphomas transform into a more aggressive histology, treatment at that time might offer an improved chance of success.

The watch and wait approach has several potential disadvantages, however. Patients must be monitored closely to prevent insidious complications such as ureteral obstruction due to enlarging retroperitoneal adenopathy. It has also been suggested that waiting until the disease progresses and bulky adenopathy and systemic symptoms develop may make treatment at that time more difficult. Finally, many patients are unable to accept the option of letting their disease progress without therapy and insist on some form of treatment.

The natural history of patients managed with initial observation[80,81,170,185,186] is shown in Table 81-6. Overall survival in general is >5 years. Histologic transformation was seen in 6–15% of patients, while spontaneous remissions were seen in ≤23% of patients.[80] When patients were randomly assigned to the watch and wait approach versus aggressive chemotherapy and radiation, overall survival was not changed (83% versus 84%), while DFS was significantly influenced (0% versus 51%).[186] In another trial, which was nonrandomized, overall survival was significantly better in patients initially managed with a watch and wait approach.[81]

It is not certain whether aggressive initial therapy will influence overall survival. If patients are thought not to be candidates for such therapy and are asymptomatic and reliable, then an initial period of observation without treatment is acceptable. Factors associated with adverse prognosis in low-grade lymphoma patients have included advanced stage,[82,86,187] age,[82,187] and the presence of systemic symptoms.[61,81,86,170] The presence or absence of these factors may be helpful in deciding which patients can be initially managed with observation.

Moderate Therapy

Nonaggressive therapy has been used as initial therapy for some patients and as palliative therapy later in the course of disease in others. This approach has generally relied on single-agent alkylator therapy with chlorambucil or cyclophosphamide; combination chemotherapy with regimens such as CVP (cyclophosphamide, vincristine, prednisone); or radiotherapy. Single-agent alkylator therapy in patients with advanced disease has generally achieved response rates of 50–80%.[188–192] Cyclophosphamide may be given at a dose of 50–150 mg/day PO, or chlorambucil may be given at a dose of 0.1–0.2 mg/kg/day. Alternatively, chlorambucil may be given in pulses of 0.4–0.6 mg/kg every 2 weeks. Although this treatment is highly effective in controlling disease, patients are not cured and exhibit a continuous pattern of relapse.

CVP has been employed in several trials, and similar response rates of 80–90% have been observed.[190,193,194] Again, however, a continuous relapse pattern has been observed, and there is little evidence of cure in any of these patients. Trials comparing moderate with aggressive therapy have failed to show a survival advantage for patients treated aggressively.[77,168,182,186,190,194]

Radiation may also be extremely useful in managing patients with low-grade lymphomas,[195] who often develop localized problems related to painful adenopathy, cord compression, or ureteral obstruction. Those symptoms can be effectively palliated with local radiotherapy without resorting to systemic chemotherapy.

Aggressive Chemotherapy

Despite the success of modern chemotherapy regimens for intermediate- and high-grade lymphomas, these regimens have been used relatively infrequently for low-grade histologies.[77,78,169,174,186,187,196–199] Table 81-7 reviews several studies in which low-grade lymphomas have been treated with somewhat more aggressive chemotherapy regimens. High complete remission rates have been observed in some series. Differences in reported remission rates may relate to various criteria for defining remission, and to differences in restaging intensity. Some studies appear to show a plateau in DFS, which may indicate cures, but late relapses are still seen, again bringing into question whether any of these patients are actually cured. Most studies show a continuous pattern of relapse, however. Although improved relapse-free survival is seen with aggressive therapy, it remains to be proven whether any difference in overall survival will be seen.

Two prospective randomized studies have shown higher rates of remission duration and overall survival when patients were treated with interferon in addition to intensive chemo-

NEBRASKA APPROACH TO THE INITIAL MANAGEMENT OF LOW-GRADE LYMPHOMAS

Patients are first staged after diagnosis of a low-grade lymphoma. Our staging procedures include a history and physical examination, CBC, chemistry screen, chest radiograph, abdominal and pelvic CT scans, and a bone marrow biopsy. A chest CT is performed on patients with an abnormal chest radiograph. We do not use lymphangiography or perform a laparotomy on patients with clinically localized disease. If patients have localized disease (stage I or minimal stage II) they receive three cycles of CNOP[a] followed by 4,000 cGy involved-field radiation.

We explain the various treatment approaches to patients who present with advanced-stage disease. Younger patients (generally <60 years of age) with good performance status are generally offered aggressive therapy with CNOP with the goal of attaining a complete remission. Older patients, those with poor performance status or other medical problems, and patients who do not wish aggressive therapy are managed initially by a watch and wait approach. Palliative radiation or single-agent chemotherapy is used for symptomatic progression. Patients who achieve only a partial remission with initial anthracycline-based therapy are offered peripheral blood stem cell transplantation. Transplantation is also offered to patients who relapse.

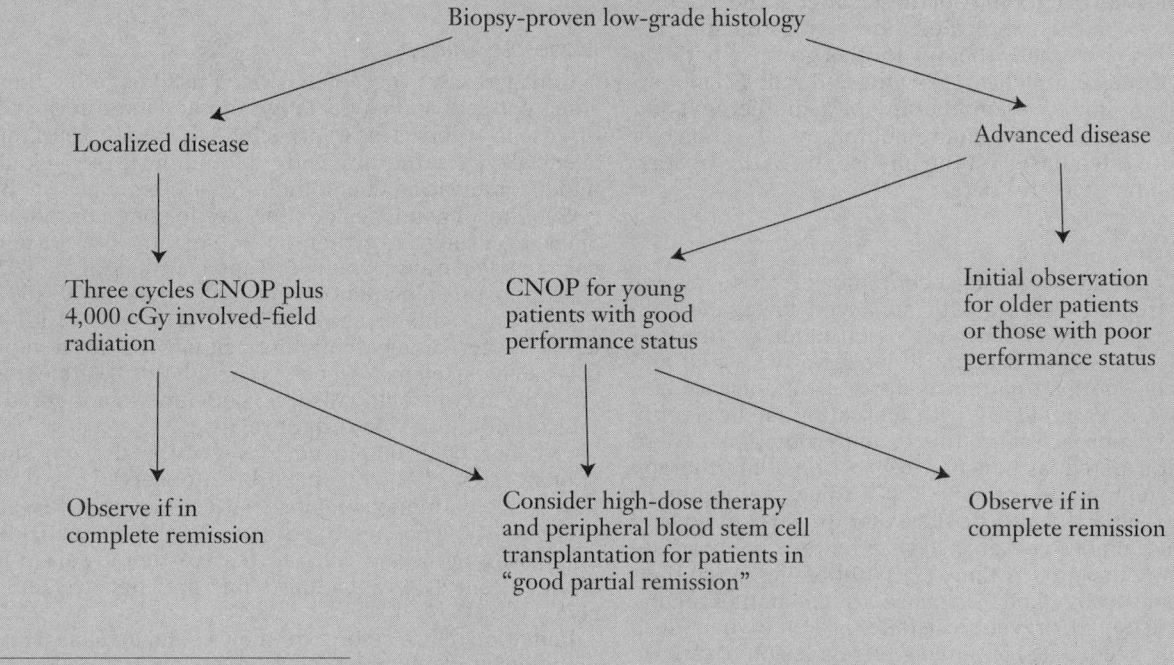

Biopsy-proven low-grade histology

Localized disease → Three cycles CNOP plus 4,000 cGy involved-field radiation → Observe if in complete remission

Advanced disease → CNOP for young patients with good performance status → Consider high-dose therapy and peripheral blood stem cell transplantation for patients in "good partial remission"

Advanced disease → Initial observation for older patients or those with poor performance status → Observe if in complete remission

---

[a] CNOP is identical to CHOP except mitoxantrone (12 mg/m^2 IV) is substituted for cyclophosphamide.

---

therapy.[198,199] Two purine analogues, fludarabine and 2-chlorodeoxyadenosine, have recently been introduced.[200-202] These new agents have shown high response rates in previously treated low-grade NHL. It is still unclear whether these drugs will become useful as initial therapy or in combination with other chemotherapy agents.

Aggressive Radiotherapy

Total body irradiation and total lymphoid irradiation have been used to treat patients with stage III and IV low-grade lymphomas.[203-205] Complete remission rates of 100% have been observed, along with 5-year DFS rates >60%. Although this approach is less often used than others, results are comparable with those of other forms of therapy.

Intermediate-Grade Lymphomas

For the purpose of this discussion intermediate-grade lymphomas include the follicular large cell, diffuse small cleaved, diffuse mixed, diffuse large cell, and immunoblastic histologic subtypes. The immunoblastic subtype is included in the intermediate category because of the lack of difference in response of diffuse large cell and immunoblastic lymphomas to modern, intensive chemotherapy regimens. Similarly, most investigators have not found a difference in outcome between diffuse mixed and diffuse large cell lymphoma. These three histologic subtypes are considered together.

Diffuse aggressive lymphomas are among the minority of neoplasms that can be cured by combination chemotherapy or, when localized, by radiotherapy. The treatment of these tumors has been one of the success stories of modern oncology. DeVita et al.[2] demonstrated that 37% of patients diagnosed as having diffuse histiocytic lymphoma could be cured with regimens previously demonstrated to be curative in patients with Hodgkin disease. A much smaller series of patients diagnosed with reticulum cell sarcoma had been reported 1 year earlier and seemed to demonstrate curability.[206] With the subsequent addition of doxorubicin and more recently etoposide, a large number of new regimens have been developed. The treatment of patients with localized and disseminated disease is considered in detail below.

Table 81-7. Aggressive Chemotherapy for Advanced Low-Grade Lymphomas

Reference	Patients (N)	Therapy	CR (%)	Follow-up	Comments
77	27	COPP	78	57% 5 yr PFS	Some received BCVP maintenance
	53	BCVP	64	26% 5 yr PFS	
78	74	CHOF-Bleo + IF	81	52% 5 yr RFS	Includes FLC, 78 mo median follow-up
174	64	C-MCPP	72	20/64 CCR	Median follow-up 7 yr
		CVP			
		TBI or TNI			
		MOPP			
		C-MOPP + TBI			
		BACOP			
		ProMACE-MOPP			
186	43	ProMACE-MOPP + TNI	78	25/43 CCR	4-yr median follow-up, includes intermediate histologies
	18	COFP	61	3/18 CCR	Median follow-up 3 yr
	14	BCVP	50	?	
197	18	M-BACOD	56	4/18 CCR	Median follow-up 58 mo, includes FLC
169	415	CHOP	64	6.9 yr median survival	Some received levamisole maintenance or
		CHOP + levamisole			chemotherapy maintenance
		CHOP + levamisole + BCG			
187	148	CHOP or CVP	69		Some received chemotherapy maintenance
		± IF or TBI			
		± BCG			
198	249	COPA	51		Improved outcome in interferon patients; includes some
		± Interferon			patients with intermediate histologies
199	242	CHVP	17		Improved outcome in interferon patients
		± Interferon			

Abbreviations: CR, complete remission; CCR, continuous complete response; PFS, progression-free survival; RFS, relapse-free survival; FLC, follicular large cell; COPP, cyclophosphamide, vincristine, procarbazine, prednisone; BCVP, BCNU, cyclophosphamide, vincristine, prednisone; M-BACOD, methotrexate, bleomycin, doxorubicin, cyclophosphamide, vincristine, prednisone; C-MOPP, cyclophosphamide, vincristine, procarbazine, prednisone; MOPP, nitrogen mustard, vincristine, procarbazine, prednisone; BACOP, bleomycin, doxorubicin, cyclophosphamide, vincristine, prednisone; ProMACE, prednisone, methotrexate, doxorubicin, cyclophosphamide, etoposide; CHOP/COPA, cyclophosphamide, doxorubicin, vincristine, prednisone; CHOP-Bleo, CHOP + bleomycin; CHVP, cyclophosphamide, doxorubicin, teniposide, prednisone; TBI, total body irradiation; TNI, total nodal irradiation; IF, involved field radiation.

Localized Diffuse Mixed, Diffuse Large Cell, and Immunoblastic Lymphoma

As might be expected, patients with localized minimal disease have a much better outlook than patients with more extensive disease. Patients with an especially good outlook and for whom less chemotherapy can be used are those with nonbulky (i.e., masses <10 cm) stage I or IE disease without systemic symptoms and occasional patients with stage II or IIE disease in whom the two sites of involvement are immediately adjacent and nonbulky and who are also without systemic symptoms. In such patients radiotherapy can be curative; however, the chances for cure with radiotherapy will be directly dependent on the thoroughness of the staging evaluation.[207] That is, patients who have undergone very aggressive staging procedures, including staging laparotomy, and are still found to have localized disease will have a significantly higher cure rate than patients who have undergone less aggressive staging. Because staging laparotomies are not often used in patients with aggressive NHLs, radiotherapy alone is not the preferred therapy for localized disease except in unusual situations, such as frail elderly patients, or those who refuse chemotherapy.

In patients treated initially with radiotherapy, a number of studies have demonstrated that following the radiotherapy with a course of chemotherapy reduces the frequency of relapse.[208–211] More recently, the opposite sequence of events has been studied (i.e., patients treated initially with an abbreviated course of chemotherapy followed by radiotherapy). When initial doxorubicin-based combination chemotherapy has been used, the long-term DFS rate has been very high.[212–215] Patients treated with an aggressive combination chemotherapy regimen for an abbreviated duration (e.g., three or four cycles rather than six) and then with involved-field radiotherapy have consistently showed a >80% DFS rate. A "full course" of chemo-

therapy alone is probably as effective as chemotherapy plus radiotherapy for patients with localized lymphomas.[213,216] This approach may be useful for patients who might have undesirable side effects from chemotherapy (e.g., dry mouth after radiation to the salivary glands).

Patients with certain sites of apparently localized, extranodal lymphoma should receive special attention. Those who present with lymphoma in the stomach or distal gastrointestinal tract are especially likely to have occult disease in Waldeyer's ring, and those who present with disease in Waldeyer's ring are likely to have disease more distally in the gastrointestinal tract. With either situation, a careful evaluation at the site of possible occult involvement is necessary before treating the patient for localized disease. Patients with testicular lymphoma should have the entire scrotal contents included in any radiation field to avoid the possibility of local relapse. Those with sinus or epidural lymphoma are at a high risk of central nervous system relapse and should be considered for prophylactic therapy to the central nervous system despite otherwise apparently localized disease. Patients who have radiotherapy to the thyroid are at high risk of eventually developing hypothyroidism and need to be followed expectantly.

Disseminated Disease

Several chemotherapy regimens can cure some patients with widely disseminated intermediate-grade NHL. However, certain principles must be followed in administering these drugs for them to be effective. The first principle is that the goal of therapy should be attainment of a complete remission as quickly as possible, as only patients who achieve a complete remission have any chance for cure with initial chemotherapy. The one possible exception to this rule is the patient who presents with bulky mediastinal or retroperitoneal disease with residual fi-

Table 81-8. Therapeutic Results for Diffuse Large Cell and Immunoblastic NHLs

Reference	Regimen[a]	CR Rate (%)	Relapse-Free Survival (%)	Overall Survival (%)
137	CAP-BOP	65	49	42 (3 yr)
148	LNH-84	75	70	67 (3 yr)
220	CHOP	53	60	30 (7 yr)
221	COP-BLAM	73	55	
222	MACOP-B	86	67	65 (6.5 yr)
223	m-BACOD	61	76	60 (5 yr)
224	ProMACE/Cyta-BOM	80	—	80 (2 yr)

[a] CHOP

	Days				
	1	5	10	15	22
Cyclophosphamide 750 mg/m^2 IV	X				Repeat cycle
Adriamycin 50 mg/m^2 IV	X				
Vincristine 1.4 mg/m^2 IV	X				
Prednisone 100 mg PO	X X X X X				

COP-BLAM

	Days				
	1	5	10	14	21
Cyclophosphamide 400 mg/m^2 IV	X				
Vincristine 1.4 mg/m^2 IV	X				
Prednisone 40 mg/m^2 PO × 10 days	X X X X X X X X X X				Repeat cycle
Bleomycin 15 U IV				X	
Doxorubicin 40 mg/m^2 IV	X				
Procarbazine 100 mg/m^2 PO × 10 days	X X X X X X X X X X				

MACOP-B

	Week of Therapy											
	1	2	3	4	5	6	7	8	9	10	11	12
Methotrexate 400 mg/m^2 IV		X				X				X		
Doxorubicin 50 mg/m^2 IV	X		X		X		X		X		X	
Cyclophosphamide 350 mg/m^2 IV	X		X		X		X		X		X	
Vincristine 1.4 mg/m^2 IV			X		X		X		X		X	X
Bleomycin 10 U/m^2 IV			X					X				X
Prednisone 75 mg PO	Daily dose tapered over the last 15 days											
Co-trimoxazole 2 tablets PO	Twice daily throughout											
Ketoconazole 200 mg PO	Once daily throughout											
Folinic acid 15 mg PO every 6 hr for 6 days, starting 24 hr after methotrexate												

m-BACOD

	Days									
	1	2	3	4	5	6	7	8	15	21
Methotrexate 200 mg/m^2 IV								X	X	Repeat cycle
Bleomycin 4 U/m^2 IV	X									
Doxorubicin 45 mg/m^2 IV	X									
Cyclophosphamide 600 mg/m^2 IV	X									
Vincristine 1 mg/m^2 IV	X									
Dexamethasone 6 mg/m^2 PO × 5 days	X X X X X									
Folinic acid 10 mg/m^2 PO every 6 hr for 8 doses, starting 24 hr after methotrexate										

(Table continues)

brotic masses.[135] Such patients can be identified by the existence of a mass that shrinks quickly early in therapy but thereafter remains stable in size. A gallium scan that goes from positive to negative can also be helpful in this determination.

Because salvage therapy is only marginally effective in these patients,[217] it is vital that patients be optimally managed initially and that a cure be achieved with the initial chemotherapy regimen if this is possible. This requires chemotherapy administered at full doses. Dose reduction for arbitrary reasons are never a favor to the patient. In studies in which reduced chemotherapy doses have been administered to patients with NHL, response rates have been significantly lower.[218]

It is not necessary to administer more than a few treatment cycles past the documentation of complete remission.[219] It is likely that prolonged therapy will increase treatment-related toxicity without increasing the chance for cure. New aggressive chemotherapy regimens reduce the treatment time to as few as 10–12 weeks in rapidly responding patients.

A summary of the results of several aggressive chemother-apy regimens with proven curative potential in aggressive NHL[137,148,220–224] is presented in Table 81-8. As can be seen, the complete remission rate varies from 53% to 86%, and the relapse-free survival for complete responders varies from 49% to 76%. Overall survival tends to be better in patients with shorter follow-up but averages approximately 60–75% at 3 years. The chances for cure can be obtained by multiplying the complete response rate by the relapse-free survival rate (i.e., the proportion of complete responders who do not relapse). This suggests that the cure rate for reported regimens might vary from approximately 30% with CHOP to approximately 60% with some newer regimens. However, it should be remembered that the CHOP regimen has the longest follow-up. In addition, it is difficult to compare the results of various trials due to differences in prognostic factors for patients in the trials. This has led to a prospective randomized trial comparing CHOP, m-BACOD, ProMACE-CytaBOM, and MACOP-B[225] (see Table 81-7 for definitions). No significant differences in response rates, time to treatment failure, or survival were noted

Table 81-8. *(Continued)*

ProMACE/Cyta-BOM	Days			
	1	8	9	14
Cyclophosphamide 650 mg/m² IV push	X			
Doxorubicin 25 mg/m² IV push	X			
Etoposide (VP-16) 120 mg/m² IV	X			
Prednisone 60 mg/m² PO × 14 days	X X X X X X X	X	X X X X X	X
Cytarabine 300 mg/m² IV push		X		Repeat cycle
Bleomycin 5 U/m² IV push		X		every 28 days
Vincristine 1.4 mg/m² IV push		X		
Methotrexate 120 mg/m² IV push		X		
Folinic acid 25 mg/m² PO every 6 hr × 6 doses			X	

LNH-84	Induction (wk)			Consolidation (wk)							Final Intensification (wk)		
	0	2	4	8	10	12	14	16	17	19	21	27	31
Cyclophosphamide 1,200 mg/m² IV	X	X	X									X	X
Doxorubicin 75 mg/m² IV	X	X	X										
Vindesine 2 mg/m² IV days 1,5	X	X	X										
Bleomycin 10 mg days 1,5	X	X	X									X	X
Prednisone 60 mg/m² IV × 5 days	X	X	X										X
Methotrexate 15 mg intrathecal	X	X	X										
Cytarabine 100 mg/m²/day SC × 4 days										X	X	X	X
Methotrexate 3 g/m² IV + leucovorin rescue 25 mg PO every 6 hr × 12 doses				X	X								
Etoposide 300 mg/m²						X	X						
Ifosfamide 1,500 mg/m²						X	X						
L-asparaginase 50,000 U/m² IM								X	X				
Teniposide 60 mg/m² IV												X	X

CAP-BOP	Schedule Days			
	1	7	15	21
Cyclophosphamide 650 mg/m² IV	X			
Doxorubicin 50 mg/m² IV	X			
Procarbazine 100 mg/m² PO × 7 days	X X X X	X X X		Repeat cycle
Bleomycin 10 U/m² SC			X	
Vincristine 1.4 mg/m² IV			X	
Prednisone 100 mg PO × 7 days			X X X X	X X X

among the various regimens. Several additional trials have failed to demonstrate the superiority of any particular chemotherapy regimen for NHL.[226] Many physicians are now using CHOP because of its ease of administration. The details of the administration of these, and other, regimens are presented in Table 81-8. Each regimen has proven curative potential in patients with diffuse large cell or other aggressive NHLs, and at present there is no basis for choosing one regimen over another.

It is important to remember that the treatment of aggressive lymphomas with chemotherapy is fraught with risks. Almost all treatment trials have resulted in treatment-related deaths. Clinical factors that appear to predispose patients to increased risk of morbidity and mortality include older age and poor performance status. Familiarity with the regimen being used is important. Treatment-related mortality declines with increased experience in administering a particular chemotherapy regimen.[227] For this reason it is a logical plan for each oncologist to choose one regimen that has been proven to be active in aggressive NHLs and to use that regimen exclusively. It is hoped that advances in supportive care, such as hematopoietic growth factors, will lead to improved treatment results for NHL. Growth factors can allow increases in dose intensity for NHL patients and can decrease neutropenia and infection.[228,229] However, it is unknown whether this will result in improved remission rates or survival.

At our institution, once the patient has been carefully evaluated to determine the extent of disease, treatment is initiated. We use combination chemotherapy consisting of cyclophosphamide, mitoxantrone, vincristine, and prednisone (CNOP). This regimen may be less toxic than CHOP and has equivalent results.[230,231] Patients who achieve complete remission are followed closely in the first year but at decreasing intervals over the next several years. We do not routinely restage patients unless clinically indicated.

High-Grade Lymphomas

The treatment of lymphoblastic lymphoma with conventional chemotherapy regimens used for NHL has demonstrated excellent initial response rates in most trials. However, most patients relapse and eventually die of progressive disease that is unresponsive to salvage chemotherapy. In 1971 Aur et al.[232] reported encouraging results using an intensified chemotherapy program with induction maintenance and central nervous system prophylaxis for localized NHL in children, a heterogeneous group with a large proportion of cases of lymphoblastic disease. Additional studies in children evaluated the type of regimens used in ALL for treatment of lymphoblastic lymphoma. The LSA₂-L₂ protocol (used for ALL) was subsequently shown to be significantly more effective therapy than COMP (cyclophosphamide, vincristine, methotrexate, and prednisone) therapy for lymphoblastic lymphoma in children (76% 2-year failure-free survival for the LSA₂-L₂ protocol versus 26% for the COMP protocol).[233] Similarly, Weinstein et al.[110] reported a 69% 5-year actuarial survival for 21 patients, aged 2.5–22 years, with mediastinal lymphoblastic lymphoma treated with the APO (doxirubicin [Adriamycin], prednisone, vincristine) protocol.

Treatment of lymphoblastic lymphoma in adults is less well documented in the literature than the treatment of children

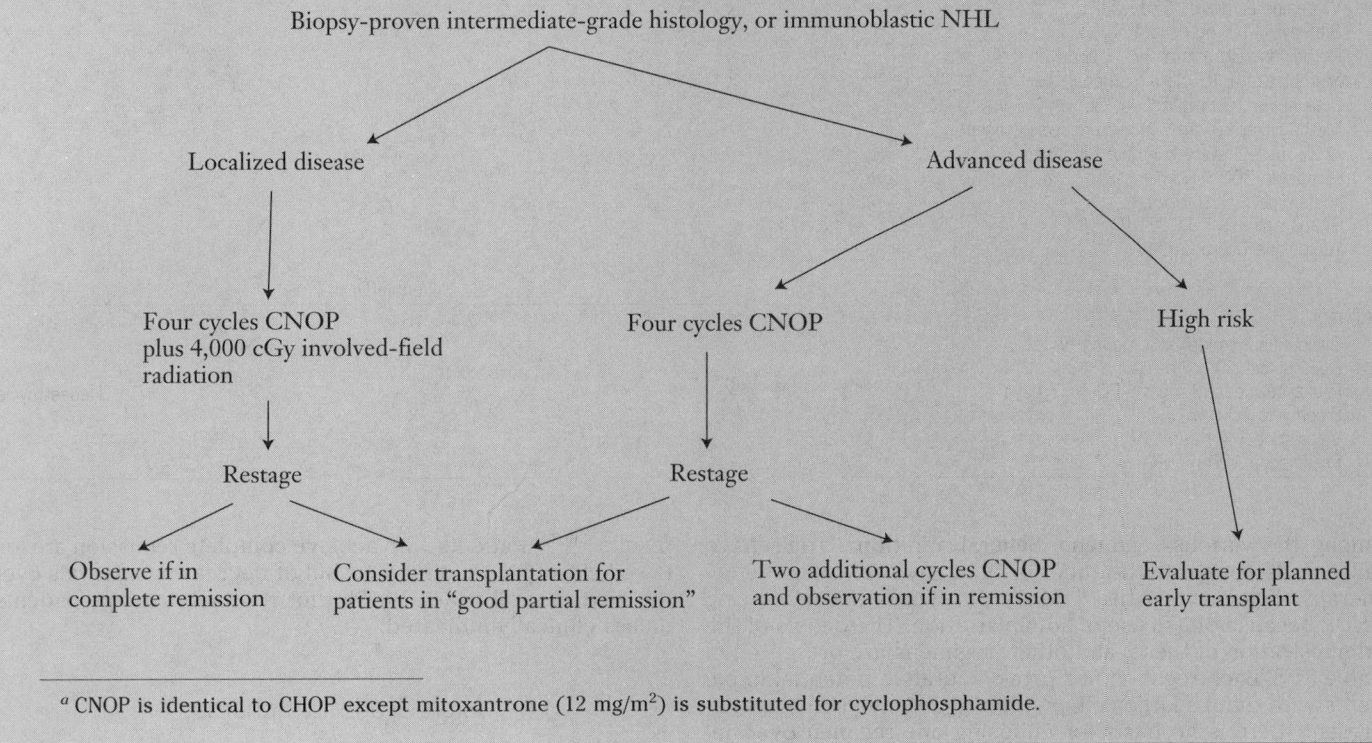

NEBRASKA APPROACH TO THE INITIAL MANAGEMENT OF INTERMEDIATE-GRADE LYMPHOMAS

Patients with intermediate-grade and immunoblastic lymphomas are staged in the same manner as for low-grade histologic subtypes. If patients have nonbulky, localized disease (stage I or minimal stage II), they receive four cycles of CNOP[a] followed by 4,000 cGy involved-field radiation. Patients with more advanced disease are eligible for planned early autologous transplantation if they have diffuse mixed, diffuse large cell, or immunoblastic histology and an age-adjusted International Prognostic Index[167] of 2 or 3. Patients with stage IV peripheral T-cell lymphomas and those with stage IV follicular large cell lymphomas are also eligible for early transplant.

Other patients receive four cycles of CNOP followed by restaging. Those in complete remission are given two more cycles of therapy, followed by observation. Patients not in remission are evaluated for transplantation. If patients are not eligible for transplantation, they receive two additional cycles of CNOP, followed by restaging. If in remission after six cycles of CNOP, they receive two more cycles of CNOP (total eight) followed by observation. Patients not in remission receive second-line chemotherapy regimens.

Biopsy-proven intermediate-grade histology, or immunoblastic NHL

Localized disease → Four cycles CNOP plus 4,000 cGy involved-field radiation → Restage → Observe if in complete remission / Consider transplantation for patients in "good partial remission"

Advanced disease → Four cycles CNOP → Restage → Consider transplantation for patients in "good partial remission" / Two additional cycles CNOP and observation if in remission

High risk → Evaluate for planned early transplant

---

[a] CNOP is identical to CHOP except mitoxantrone (12 mg/m^2) is substituted for cyclophosphamide.

---

with this disease. Pediatric results have led to treatment principles in adults that use regimens similar to those used in ALL. Coleman et al.[234] reported a trial involving the treatment of 13 patients with mediastinal lymphoblastic lymphoma with an intensive chemotherapy protocol using central nervous system prophylaxis and achieved a complete response rate of 100%, with a 3-year actuarial DFS rate of 56%. In a study by Levine et al.,[108] 15 patients were treated with a modified LSA$_2$-L$_2$ protocol for adult lymphoblastic lymphoma. In this evaluation 73% of the patients achieved a complete response rate and the actuarial survival rate at 5 years for all patients was 40%. In a later trial by Coleman et al.,[235] it was possible to divide patients into good and poor prognostic groups based on the presence of marrow or central nervous system disease and a serum LDH level of >300 IU/ml. The good prognosis patients had a 5-year freedom from relapse rate of 94%, whereas the poor prognosis patients had a 5-year freedom from relapse rate of 19%. However, one other study, by Slater et al.,[236] failed to find any difference in survival based on bone marrow involvement. Results from a number of institutions (Table 81-9) have confirmed the poor results of treatment of lymphoblastic lymphoma in adults.

The poor results of treatment for adult lymphoblastic lymphoma have led to evaluation of the use of high-dose therapy with allogeneic or autologous BMT for hematopoietic reconstitution. One such trial from the City of Hope National Medical Center evaluated five patients with lymphoblastic lymphoma and one with diffuse undifferentiated lymphoma who were treated with high-dose cyclophosphamide and total body irradiation, with allogeneic BMT in first complete remission.[240] Four of the patients were alive in complete remission at 8, 14, 21, and 47 months post-transplant. One patient died of recurrent lymphoma 17 months post-transplant, and one died of graft-versus-host disease without evidence of lymphoma at autopsy. These encouraging results demonstrated that allogeneic BMT could produce durable remission in patients with high-grade lymphomas who present with bone marrow, central nervous system, and/or skin involvement. Subsequent studies have demonstrated that BMT in first complete remission may improve the outcome of adult lymphoblastic lymphoma patients.[241,242] It is unclear whether selection bias influenced these results, and randomized trials will be needed to determine the role of early BMT in lymphoblastic lymphoma.

As in lymphoblastic lymphoma, most therapeutic trials for

Table 81-9. Therapy Results for High-Grade NHL in Adults

Type	Reference	Regimen	CR Rate (%)	Disease-Free Survival (%)
Lymphoblastic	108	Induction: cyclophosphamide, doxorubicin, vincristine, prednisone, cytarabine, thioguanine, asparaginase, lomustine	73	35 (5 yr)
		Maintenance: thioguanine, methotrexate, cyclophosphamide, hydroxyurea, doxorubicin, lomustine, cytarabine, vincristine		
	235	Induction: cyclophosphamide, doxorubicin, vincristine, prednisone, asparaginase	95	56 (3 yr)
		Maintenance: methotrexate, mercaptopurine		
		Variable		
		Variable		
	236	Variable	78	45 (5 yr)
	237	Variable	74	30 (3 yr)
	238	Variable	53	—
	239	Variable	82	38 (2½ yr)
Small non-cleaved cell	248	Cyclophosphamide, doxorubicin, vincristine, prednisone, methotrexate	77	71 (1 yr)
	249	Variable	80	60 (5 yr)
	250	Cyclophosphamide, etoposide, vincristine, bleomycin, doxorubicin, methotrexate, prednisone	85	60 (5 yr)

the treatment of SNCL have been carried out in the pediatric population, with few trials on adults available for analysis. In some initial African Burkitt lymphoma cases, long-term DFS with single-agent cyclophosphamide therapy has been reported. Several multiagent chemotherapy regimens combined with central nervous system prophylaxis have now been shown to achieve high remission rates and long-term DFS. Most of these protocols vary in their complexity and content but include cyclophosphamide combined with various other cytotoxic agents, including methotrexate, doxorubicin, cytarabine, and/or vincristine. The importance of central nervous system prophylaxis has now been documented in several trials, with decreased central nervous system relapse rates in the prophylactically treated patients. Protocols that were designed for lymphoblastic lymphoma or ALL (i.e., LSA$_2$-L$_2$ protocol) are clearly inferior to the specific SNCL protocols. This was confirmed in a Children's Cancer Study Group trial, in which children with SNCL had a much better prognosis when treated with COMP as compared with those children treated with LSA$_2$-L$_2$.[233] Most trials report 50–75% overall survival rates in childhood SNCL with modern multiagent chemotherapy.[243–247] The differences in survival characteristics between trials can often be accounted for by differences in the patient populations. Trials containing older patients or more patients with central nervous system disease or bone marrow involvement would generate poorer survival characteristics. Patients with limited disease, such as resectable abdominal disease, have an excellent prognosis and may require a shorter treatment time or less intensive chemotherapy.

The therapy for SNCL in adults is less well defined. One study from Stanford reported 18 adult patients with SNCL who were treated with cyclophosphamide, doxorubicin, vincristine, prednisone, and systemic and intrathecal methotrexate. These investigators also used radiotherapy to treat unresectable masses of >10 cm when possible.[248] The patients with prognostic signs, including unresected tumor bulk >10 cm, pretreatment LDH >500 IU/L (normal ≤200 IU/L), or involvement of the central nervous system or bone marrow, had significantly worse results than patients without these features, their relapse-free survival rate being 28.6% versus 100%. Treatment results of small noncleaved-cell NHL in adults are shown in Table 81-9.

These results have pointed out that for children and adults who present with these poor prognostic signs, more intensive therapy is needed to expect a higher percentage of curability. The BACT (carmustine, cytarabine, cyclophosphamide, 6-thioguanine) massive chemotherapy regimen followed by autologous bone marrow rescue for the treatment of relapsed or resistant Burkitt lymphoma was first reported by Appelbaum et al.[251] in 1978. In the original report 14 patients were treated

with this therapy, of whom three were alive at 9+, 19+, and 29+ months post-transplant. With improvement in the front-line treatment for Burkitt lymphoma, the indications for autologous BMT in Burkitt lymphoma have changed so that its use in poor prognosis, relapsed, or resistant patients is recommended at present. A 5-year experience in autologous BMT for Burkitt lymphoma was reported in 1986 by Philip et al.,[252] who performed BMT in 28 patients with Burkitt lymphoma using the BACT protocol or the BEAM (carmustine, etoposide, cytarabine, melphalan) protocol as high-dose chemotherapy. The overall DFS at the time of their report was 46%, with a median observation time post-transplant of 22 months. These excellent results were also achieved in the poor prognosis patients, with 5 of 10 long-term survivors having previous central nervous system disease. With conventional chemotherapy these results would have been difficult to achieve. Occult tumor cells are a potential problem when using autologous marrow for BMT in this setting. Explosive bone marrow relapse following autologous BMT for Burkitt lymphoma was reported in this trial as well as in other published trials. Also, it had previously been shown that Burkitt lymphoma cells can grow in a liquid culture system from cytologically and histologically normal marrow.[253] The role of marrow purging in this clinical setting is undergoing intensive evaluation. Alternatively, allogeneic marrow grafting may be useful in this clinical setting when a donor is available. Further clinical trials are ongoing to identify the patient population for whom high-dose therapy and BMT are appropriate.

The high-grade NHLs have distinct biologic properties that make timely evaluation and treatment important. Modern chemotherapeutic regimens and improvement with salvage treatments such as high-dose chemotherapy and autologous or allogeneic BMT have greatly improved the outlook for patients with these lymphomas. It is hoped that new trials will improve the survival of this difficult patient population.

Salvage Therapy

Despite the progress observed with first-line chemotherapy regimens for NHL, ≥30–50% of patients will not achieve remission. These patients have a poor prognosis, and almost all will die of progressive lymphoma without effective second-line (salvage) therapy.

Conventional Chemotherapy

Table 81-10 shows the results from several recent salvage chemotherapy regimens for NHL.[254–259] Although relatively high complete response rates are noted, <10% of patients with relapsed or refractory NHL will achieve long-term DFS. Numerous other regimens have been employed for relapsed or refrac-

NEBRASKA APPROACH TO THE INITIAL MANAGEMENT OF HIGH-GRADE LYMPHOMAS

Lymphoblastic NHL is Treated with the Following Regimen[a,b]

Agent	Pre	Induction				Central Nervous System Prophylaxis				Consolidation				Maintenance
		1	2	3	4	5	6	7	8	9	10	11	12–21	22–52
Cyclophosphamide 1.0 gm/m² IV	X	X			X					X				
Doxorubicin 50 mg/mn² IV	X	X			X					X	Repeat weeks 9–12 × 3			
Vincristine 2.0 mg IV	X	X	X		X	X	X			X				
Prednisone 40 mg/m² PO		←daily→		taper			5 days							
L-asparaginase 6,000 U/m² IM or IV (max 10,000 U)		5 doses												
Methotrexate 12 mg IT	X			X		←5 doses→								
Whole brain XRT 2,400 cGy in 12 fractions						←XRT→								
Methotrexate 30 mg/m² PO														Weekly
Mercaptopurine 75 mg/m² PO														Daily

[a] Patients are evaluated for autologous or allogeneic BMT at the end of consolidation.

[b] patients with small noncleaved histology are treated like advanced-stage intermediate-histology patients. Those with bulky disease, bone marrow involvement, central nervous system involvement, or high LDH are evaluated for autologous or allogeneic BMT in first complete remission or at best response.

tory lymphomas using both available and investigational agents.[217] Other treatment strategies such as infusional chemotherapy,[260,261] and chronic administration of oral etoposide have also been tried.[262] Similar response rates are seen, but only rare patients appear to be cured of their disease. The poor results are due to primary drug resistance following failure of front-line therapy and to the inability of patients to tolerate full doses of chemotherapy salvage regimens.

Marrow Transplantation

For the reasons cited above, high-dose therapy with BMT is now being used with increasing frequency to treat patients with relapsed or refractory NHL.[263] This technique allows delivery of radiation or chemotherapy in higher than normal doses, thereby taking advantage of the steep dose-response curves exhibited by these agents against lymphomas.[264–266] This dose escalation makes it possible to overcome drug resistance without regard for what might otherwise be lethal bone marrow toxicity, since patients can subsequently be rescued with syngeneic, allogeneic, or autologous marrow.

Syngeneic and allogeneic transplants for NHL have been performed relatively infrequently compared with autologous transplants.[267–274] It is clear, however, that a substantial proportion of patients can be cured with this technique and that results are superior when patients undergo BMT in a state of minimal disease. No significant differences in overall survival

Table 81-10. Salvage Chemotherapy Regimens for NHL

Reference	Drugs	Patients (N)	CR (%)	PR (%)	Follow-up
254	Etoposide Methylprednisolone Cytarabine Cisplatin	24	(CR + PR = 69%)		—
255	Dexamethasone Cytarabine Cisplatin	90	28 (31)	22 (24)	20, CCR median follow-up 11 mo
256	Ifosfamide Methotrexate Etoposide	52	19 (37)	13 (25)	10, CCR 12 mo median projected RFS for CR patients
257,258	Methyl-GAG Ifosfamide Methotrexate Etoposide	208	49 (24)	75 (36)	Approximately 25% of CR patients in CCR
259	Dexamethasone Ifosfamide Cisplatin Etoposide	22	6 (22)	11 (50)	—

Abbreviations: CR, complete response; CCR, continuous complete response; PR, partial response; RFS, relapse-free survival; TTR, time to relapse.

Table 81-11. Autologous BMT in NHL

Reference	Patients (N)	Histologies	Therapy	CR (%)	CCR
276	100	Intermediate and high grade	Variable	57 (57)	19 (21–75 mo)
277	50	Intermediate and high grade	Variable	15 (30)	6 (19–45 mo)
278	46	Low, intermediate, and high grade	Variable	—	25 (8–104 mo)
279	68	Intermediate and high grade	Cyclophosphamide and TBI	37 (54)	15 (37–109 mo)
280	70	Low, intermediate, and high grade	Variable	51 (73)	16 (12–78 mo)
281	44	Low, intermediate, and high grade	Cyclophosphamide, etoposide, and TBI	—	25 (14–84 mo)

Abbreviations: CR, complete remission; CCR, continuous complete remission; TBI, total body irradiation.

have been observed between syngeneic, allogeneic, and autologous BMT for NHL,[272–274] except that allogeneic BMT results may be better for patients with lymphoblastic lymphoma.[274] Allogeneic BMT eliminates the risk of infusing malignant cells back with the marrow. In addition, allogeneic BMT has the advantage of a possible graft-versus-lymphoma effect similar to the graft-versus-leukemia effect that has been observed after allogeneic BMT for leukemia.[275] Studies do show a lower relapse rate for allogeneic marrow recipients, compared with autologous marrow recipients.[273,274] This suggests that a graft-versus-lymphoma effect exists; however, the effect is offset by higher transplant-related mortality with allogeneic BMT. Autologous BMT eliminates the need to find a matched donor, can be more safely performed in older patients, and eliminates the problems of graft-versus-host disease found in allogeneic BMT. Although there is a theoretical risk of infusing malignant cells with autologous BMT, this technique, rather than allogeneic BMT, is the one most often used.

Table 81-11 shows the results of several large studies of autologous BMT for NHL.[276–281] Approximately 20–40% of patients experience prolonged DFS with this procedure and appear cured. Although mortality rates have averaged 15–20%, the safety of BMT has improved due to advances in supportive care such as hematopoietic growth factors. Retrospective evidence suggests that results of BMT are better than those of conventional salvage chemotherapy,[282] and prospective trials are under way to test this hypothesis.[283] Patients who receive transplants after relapse but whose tumors still respond to conventional chemotherapy (sensitive relapse) have superior results compared with those whose tumors do not respond to conventional chemotherapy (resistant relapse).[276–281] Current studies are attempting to define patients who might benefit from earlier BMT. Patients who fail to enter complete remission, or who respond slowly to initial chemotherapy, have a very poor prognosis. Several studies have shown that these patients may have an improved outcome if they are transplanted in first partial remission.[277,278,281] In addition recent evidence suggests that patients with poor prognostic features may have improved survival if transplanted in first complete remission.[284,285] There is now increasing use of autologous peripheral stem cells instead of autologous bone marrow for hematopoietic recovery after high-dose therapy. This technique allows patients to undergo BMT if their marrow contains malignant cells or if their marrow cannot be harvested (e.g., after radiation to the pelvis). Autologous peripheral stem cell transplantation has been used for relapsed NHL, and results are at least as good as those of BMT.[286] Most autologous transplants for NHL have been performed in patients with intermediate- and high-grade histologies. Comparatively few transplants have been performed for low-grade lymphomas. The results of these transplants show that complete remissions can be obtained, but these patients will need prolonged follow-up to determine whether this modality can effect a cure.[287–289]

Other Approaches

Several studies have examined the use of recombinant interferon for NHL.[290–292] Responses have been seen at various dosages and seem to occur in approximately 50% of patients with low-grade NHL and those with cutaneous T-cell lymphoma, even among heavily pretreated patients. Few responses have been noted with intermediate- and high-grade lymphomas. Recent evidence suggests that results of therapy for NHL may be improved by adding interferon to conventional chemotherapy regimens.[198,199]

Finally, the use of monoclonal antibodies is being investigated in NHL. Such antibodies might be used in various ways. Anti-idiotype antibodies can be developed that are directed against the unique variable region of the immunoglobulin molecule on the lymphoma cell surface. Such antibodies are primarily directly cytotoxic or impair the tumor cell proliferation. Responses were seen in 9 of 15 patients treated with this approach in one study.[293] In addition, it may be possible to use immunoglobulin idiotype as an antigen to form lymphoma vaccines.[294] Monoclonal antibodies might also be used to deliver toxins, radioactive isotopes, or chemotherapeutic agents specifically to tumor cells. Anti-B-cell antibodies labeled with ^{131}I have shown activity in refractory NHL.[295–297] Antibodies conjugated to various plant toxins are being investigated for activity in patients with relapsed NHL.[298–299]

REFERENCES

1. Boring CC, Squires TS, Tong T: Cancer Statistics, 1993. CA Cancer J Clin 43: 7, 1993
2. DeVita VT, Chabner B, Hubbard SP et al: Advanced diffuse histiocytic lymphoma, a potentially curable disease. Lancet 1:248, 1975
3. McKelvey EM, Gottlieb JA, Wilson HE et al: Hydroxyldaunomycin (Adriamycin) combination chemotherapy in malignant lymphoma. Cancer 38:1484, 1976
4. Isaacson PG: Recent advances in the biology of lymphomas. Eur J Cancer 27:795, 1991
5. Cancer Facts and Figures 1984. American Cancer Society, New York, 1983, p.8
6. Devesa SS, Fears T: Non-Hodgkin's lymphoma time trends: United States and international data. Cancer Res, suppl. 52:5432s, 1992
7. Weisenburger DD: An epidemic of non-Hodgkin's lymphoma: comments on time trends, possible etiologies, and the role of pathology. Mod Pathol 5: 481, 1992
8. Linet MS, Pottern LM: Familial aggregation of hematopoietic malignancies and risk of non-Hodgkin's lymphoma. Cancer Res, suppl. 52:5468s, 1992
9. Heath CW Jr: Heredity factors in leukemia and lymphoma. p. 233. In Lynch HT (ed): Cancer Genetics. Charles C Thomas, Springfield, IL, 1976
10. Tan C, Etcubanas E, Liberman P et al: Chediak-Higashi syndrome in a child with Hodgkin's disease. Am J Dis Child 121:135, 1971
11. Purtilo DT: Hypothesis: pathogenesis and phenotypes of an X-linked recessive lymphoproliferative syndrome. Lancet 2:882, 1976
12. Purtilo DT, Yang JPS, Cassell CK et al: X-linked recessive progressive combined variable immunodeficiency (Duncan's disease). Lancet 1:935, 1975
13. Purtilo DT: Opportunistic non-Hodgkin's lymphoma in X-linked recessive immunodeficiency and lymphoproliferative syndrome. Semin Oncol 4:335, 1977
14. Rodriguez MA, Fuller LM, Zimmerman O et al: Hodgkin's disease: study of treatment intensities and incidences of second malignancies. Ann Oncol 4: 125, 1993
15. Penn I: Cancers following cyclosporine therapy. Transplantation 43:32, 1987
16. Penn I: The changing pattern of posttransplant malignancies. Transplant Proc 23:1101, 1991
17. Swinnen LJ: Post-transplantation lymphoproliferative disorder. Leuk Lymphoma 6:289, 1992

18. Nalesnik MA, Jaffe R, Starzl TE et al: The pathology of posttransplant lymphoproliferative disorders occurring in the setting of cyclosporine A-prednisone immunosuppression. Am J Pathol 133:173, 1988

19. Swinnen LJ, Costanzo-Nordin MR, Fisher SG et al: Increased incidence of lymphoproliferative disorder after immunosuppression with the monoclonal antibody OKT3 in cardiac-transplant recipients. N Engl J Med 323:1723, 1990

20. Witherspoon RP, Fisher LD, Schoch G et al: Secondary cancers after bone marrow transplantation for leukemia or aplastic anemia. N Engl J Med 321:784, 1989

21. Lyttelton MPA, Browett PJ, Brenner MK et al: Prolonged remission of Epstein-Barr virus associated lymphoma secondary to T cell-depleted bone marrow transplantation. Bone Marrow Transplant 3:641, 1988

22. Kinlen LJ, Shiel AGR, Pets J et al: A collaborative study of cancer patients who have received immunosuppressive therapy. BMJ 2:1461, 1979

23. List AF, Greco FA, Vogler LB: Lymphoproliferative disease in immunocompromised hosts: the role of Epstein-Barr virus. J Clin Oncol 5:1673, 1987

24. Young L, Alfieri C, Hennessy K et al: Expression of Epstein-Barr virus transformation-associated genes in tissues of patients with EBV lymphoproliferative disease. N Engl J Med 321:1080, 1989

25. Docker J, Nalesnik M: Molecular genetic analysis of lymphoid tumors arising after organ transplantation. Am J Pathol 135:977, 1989

26. Louie S, Schwartz RS: Immunodeficiency and the pathogenesis of lymphoma and leukemia. Semin Hematol 15:117, 1978

27. Kassan SS, Thomas TL, Montsopoulos HM et al: Increased risk of lymphoma in sicca syndrome. Ann Intern Med 87:888, 1978

28. Burke JS, Butler JJ, Fuller LM: Malignant lymphomas of the thyroid. Cancer 39:1587, 1977

29. Swinson GM, Slavin G, Coles EC et al: Coeliac disease and malignancy. Lancet 2:111, 1983

30. Heath CW Jr: Epidemiology of gastrointestinal lymphomas. p. 147. In Correa P, Haenszel W (eds): Epidemiology of Cancer of the Digestive Tract. Martinus Nijhoff, The Hague, 1982

31. Court Brown WM, Doll R: Mortality from cancer and other causes after radiotherapy for ankylosing spondylitis. BJM 2:181, 1958

32. Beebe GN, Kato H, Land C: Studies of mortality of A-bomb survivors. 6. Mortality and radiation dose, 1950–1974. Radiat Res 75:138, 1978

33. Zahm SH, Blair A: Pesticides and non-Hodgkin's lymphoma. Cancer Research, suppl. 52:5485s, 1992

34. Pearce N, Bethwaite P: Increasing incidence of non-Hodgkin's lymphoma: occupational and environmental factors. Cancer Res, suppl. 52:5496s, 1992

35. Weisenburger DD: Human health effects of agrichemical use. Hum Pathol 24:572, 1993

36. Mueller NE, Mohar A, Evans A: Viruses other than HIV and non-Hodgkin's lymphoma. Cancer Res, suppl. 52:5479s, 1992

37. Reedman BM, Klein G: Cellular location of Epstein-Barr virus (EBV) associated complement fixing antigen in producer and non-producer lymphoblastoid cell lines. Int J Cancer 11:499, 1973

38. Robert-Guroff M, Nakao Y, Notake K et al: Natural antibodies to human retrovirus HTLV in a cluster of Japanese patients with adult T-cell leukemia. Science 215:975, 1982

39. Blayney DW, Blattner WA, Robert-Guroff M et al: The human T-cell leukemia/lymphoma virus (HTLV) in the Southwestern United States. JAMA 250:1048, 1983

40. Blayney DW, Jaffe ES, Blattner WA et al: The human T-cell leukemia/lymphoma virus associated with American T-cell leukemia/lymphoma. Blood 62:401, 1983

41. Gallo RC, Salahuddin SZ, Popovic M et al: Frequent detection and isolation of cytopathic retroviruses (HTLV-III) from patients with AIDS and at risk for AIDS. Science 224:500, 1984

42. Clavel F, Guetard D, Brun-Vezinet F et al: Isolation of a new human retrovirus from West African patients with AIDS. Science 233:343, 1986

43. Manzari V, Gismondi A, Barillari G et al: HTLV-V: a new human retrovirus in Tac-negative T-cell lymphoma/leukemia. Science 238:1581, 1987

44. Rappaport H: Tumors of the hematopoietic system. In Atlas of Tumor Pathology, Sect. 3, Fascicle 8. U.S. Armed Forces Institute of Pathology, Washington, DC, 1966

45. Rappaport H, Winter WJ, Gicks EB: Follicular lymphoma: a re-evaluation of its position in the scheme of malignant lymphoma based on a survey of 253 cases. Cancer 9:792, 1956

46. Brown TC, Peters MV, Bergsagel DE, Reid J: A retrospective analysis of the clinical results in relation to the Rappaport histologic classification. Br J Cancer 31:174, 1975

47. Lukes RJ, Collins RD: New observations on follicular lymphoma. p. 209. In Akazaki K, Rappaport H, Berard CW et al (eds): Malignant Diseases of the Hematopoietic System. Gann Monograph on Cancer Research No. 15, University of Tokyo Press, Tokyo, 1973

48. Lukes RJ, Collins RD: A functional approach to the classification of malignant lymphoma. Recent Results Cancer Res 46:18, 1974

49. Jaffe ES, Ethan MS, Frank MM et al: Nodular lymphoma—evidence for origin from follicular B lymphocytes. N Engl J Med 290:813, 1974

50. Lukes RJ, Collins RD: Lukes-Collins classification and its significance. Cancer Treat Rep 61:971, 1977

51. Dorfman RF: Classification of non-Hodgkin's lymphoma. Lancet 1:1295, 1978

52. Dorfman RF: The non-Hodgkin's lymphomas. p. 262. In The Reticuloendothelial System. International Academy of Pathology Monograph No. 16. Williams & Wilkins, Baltimore, 1975

53. Bennett MG, Farrer-Brown G, Henry K et al: Classification of non-Hodgkin's lymphomas. Lancet 2:405, 1975

54. Henry K, Bennett MH, Farrer-Brown G: Morphologic classification of non-Hodgkin's lymphomas. p. 38. In Mathe C, Seligmann M, Tubiana M (eds): Recent Results in Cancer Research. Springer-Verlag, Berlin, 1978

55. Gerard-Marchant R, Hamlin I, Lennert K et al: Classification of non-Hodgkin's lymphomas. Lancet 2:406, 1974

56. Lennert K, Mohri N, Stein H et al: The histopathology of malignant lymphoma. Br J Haematol, suppl. 31:193, 1975

57. Mathe G, Rappaport H, O'Connor GT et al: Histological and cytological typing of neoplastic diseases of hematopoietic and lymphoid tissues. In WHO International Histological Classification of Tumours, No. 14. World Health Organization, Geneva, 1976

58. Lukes RJ, Collins RD: Immunologic characterization of human malignant lymphomas. Cancer 34:1488, 1974

59. Summary and description of a working formulation for clinical usage. The non-Hodgkin's lymphoma pathologic classification project. NCI-sponsored study of classifications of Non-Hodgkin's lymphomas. Cancer 49:2112, 1982

60. Straus DJ, Filippa DA, Lieberman PH et al: A retrospective clinical and pathologic analysis of 499 cases diagnosed between 1958 and 1969. Cancer 51:101, 1983

61. Gallagher CJ, Gregory WM, Jones AE et al: Follicular lymphoma: prognostic factors for response and survival. J Clin Oncol 4:1470, 1986

62. Simon R, Durrleman S, Hoppe RT et al: The non-Hodgkin lymphoma pathologic classification project: long-term follow-up of 1153 patients with non-Hodgkin lymphomas. Ann Intern Med 109:939, 1988

63. Anderson T, Chabner BA, Young RC et al: Malignant lymphoma: the histology and staging of 473 patients at the National Cancer Institute. Cancer 50:2699, 1982

64. Jones SE, Fuks Z, Bull M et al: Non-Hodgkin's lymphomas IV. Clinicopathologic correlation in 405 cases. Cancer 31:806, 1973

65. Rosenberg SA: Bone marrow involvement in the non-Hodgkin's lymphomata. Br J Cancer 31:261, 1975

66. Stein RS, Ultmann JE, Byrne GE et al: Bone marrow involvement in non-Hodgkin's lymphoma: implications for staging and therapy. Cancer 37:629, 1976

67. Chabner BA, Johnson RE, Young RC et al: Sequential nonsurgical and surgical staging of non-Hodgkin's lymphoma. Ann Intern Med 85:149, 1976

68. Rudders RA, DeLellis RA, Ernest T et al: Adult non-Hodgkin's lymphoma: correlation of cell surface marker phenotype with prognosis, the New Working Formulation, and the Rappaport and Lukes-Collins histomorphologic schemes. Cancer 52:2289, 1983

69. Smith BR, Weinberg DS, Robert NJ et al: Circulating monoclonal B lymphocytes in non-Hodgkin's lymphoma. N Engl J Med 311:1476, 1984

70. Hu E, Trela M, Thompson J et al: Detection of B-cell lymphoma in peripheral blood by DNA hybridisation. Lancet 2:1092, 1985

71. Levine EG, Arthur DC, Frizzera G et al: Cytogenetic abnormalities predict clinical outcome in non-Hodgkin lymphoma. Ann Intern Med 108:14, 1988

72. Armitage JO, Sanger DD, Weisenberger DD et al: Correlation of secondary cytogenetic abnormalities with histologic appearance in non-Hodgkin's lymphoma bearing t(14;18) (q32;q21). J Natl Cancer Inst 80:576, 1988

73. Ngan BY, Chen-Levy Z, Weiss LM et al: Expression in non-Hodgkin's lymphoma of the bcl-2 protein associated with the t(14:18) chromosomal translocation. N Engl J Med 318:1638, 1988

74. Offit K, Wong G, Filippa DA et al: Cytogenetic analysis of 434 consecutively ascertained specimens of non-Hodgkin's lymphoma: clinical correlations. Blood 77:1508, 1991

75. Kluin PM, van Krieken JHJM et al: The molecular biology of B-cell lymphoma: clinicopathologic implications. Ann Hematol 62:95, 1991

76. Hockenbery D, Nunez, Milliman C et al: Bcl-2 is an inner mitochondrial membrane protein that blocks programmed cell death. Nature 348:334, 1990

77. Exdinli EZ, Anderson JR, Melvin F et al: Moderate versus aggressive chemotherapy of nodular lymphocytic poorly differentiated lymphoma. J Clin Oncol 3:769, 1985

78. McLaughlin P, Fuller LM, Velasquez WS et al: Stage III follicular lymphoma: durable remissions with a combined chemotherapy-radiotherapy regimen. J Clin Oncol 5:867, 1987

79. Kalter S, Holmes L, Cabanillas F: Long-term results of treatment of patients with follicular lymphomas. Hematol Oncol 5:127, 1987

80. Horning SJ, Rosenberg SA: The natural history of initially untreated low-grade non-Hodgkin's lymphomas. N Engl J Med 311:1471, 1984

81. O'Brien M, Easterbrook P, Powell J et al: The natural history of low grade non-Hodgkin's lymphoma and the impact of a no initial treatment policy on survival. Q J Med 80:651, 1991

82. Leonard RCF, Hayward RL, Prescott RJ et al: The identification of discrete prognostic groups in low grade non-Hodgkin's lymphoma. Ann Oncol 2:655, 1991

83. Hubbard SM, Chabner BA, DeVita VT et al: Histologic progression in non-Hodgkin's lymphoma. Blood 59:258, 1982

84. Acker B, Hoppe RT, Colby TV et al: Histologic conversion in the non-Hodgkin's lymphomas. J Clin Oncol 1:11, 1983

85. Ersboll J, Schultz HB, Pedersen-Bjergaard J et al: Follicular low-grade non-Hodgkin's lymphoma: long-term outcome with or without tumor progression. Eur H Haematol 42:155, 1989

86. Bastion Y, Berger F, Bryon P-A et al: Follicular lymphomas: assessment of prognostic factors in 127 patients followed for 10 years. Ann Oncol 2:123, 1991

87. Risdall R, Hoppe RT, Warnke R: Non-Hodgkin's lymphoma: a study of evolution of the disease based upon 92 autopsied cases. Cancer 44:529, 1979

88. Garvin AJ, Simon RM, Osborne CK et al: An autopsy study of histologic progression in non-Hodgkin's lymphomas: 192 cases from the National Cancer Institute. Cancer 52:393, 1983

89. Mann RB, Berard CW: Criteria for the cytologic subclassification of follicular lymphomas: a proposed alternative method. Hematol Oncol 1:187, 1983

90. Ree HJ, Leone LA: Prognostic significance of parafollicular small lymphocytes in follicular lymphoma. Cancer 41:1500, 1978

91. Levine AM, Arthur EG, Frizzera G et al: There are differences in cytogenetic abnormalities among histologic subtypes of the non-Hodgkin's lymphomas. Blood 66:1414, 1985

92. Kantarjian HM, McLaughlin P, Fuller LM et al: Follicular large cell lymphoma: analysis and prognostic factors in 62 patients. J Clin Oncol 2:811, 1984

93. Stewart ML, Felman IE, Nichols PW et al: Large noncleaved follicular center cell lymphoma: clinical features in 53 patients. Cancer 57:288, 1986

94. Anderson JR, Vose JM, Bierman PJ et al: Clinical features and prognosis of follicular large-cell lymphoma: a report from the Nebraska lymphoma study group. J Clin Oncol 11:218, 1993

95. Leith CP, Spier CM, Grogan TM et al: Diffuse small cleaved-cell lymphoma: a heterogeneous disease with distinct immunobiologic subsets. J Clin Oncol 10:1259, 1992

96. Armitage JO, Vose JM, Linder J et al: Clinical significance of immunophenotype in diffuse aggressive non-Hodgkin's lymphoma. J Clin Oncol 7:1783, 1989

97. Cheng A-L, Chen Y-C, Wang C-H et al: Direct comparisons of peripheral T-cell lymphoma with diffuse B-cell lymphoma of comparable histological grades—should peripheral T-cell lymphoma be considered separately? J Clin Oncol 7:725, 1989

98. Levine EG, Arthur DC, Frizzera G et al: Cytogenetic abnormalities predict clinical outcome in non-Hodgkin lymphoma. Ann Intern Med 108:14, 1988

99. Le Beau MM: Chromosomal abnormalities in non-Hodgkin's lymphomas. Semin Oncol 17:20, 1990

100. Cabanillas F, Pathak S, Grant G et al: Refractoriness to chemotherapy and poor survival related to abnormalities of chromosomes 17 and 7 in lymphoma. Am J Med 87:167, 1989

101. Horning SJ, Carrier EK, Rouse RV et al: Lymphomas presenting as histologically unclassified neoplasms: characteristics and response to treatment. J Clin Oncol 7:1281, 1989

102. Fisher RI, Hubbard SM, DeVita VT et al: Factors predicting long-term survival in diffuse mixed, histiocytic, or undifferentiated lymphoma. Blood 58:45, 1981

103. Picozzi VJ, Coleman CN: Lymphoblastic lymphoma. Semin Oncol 17:96, 1990

104. Barcos MP, Lukes RJ: Malignant lymphoma of convoluted lymphocytes—a new entity of possible T-cell type. p. 147. In Sinks LF, Godden JO (eds): Conflicts in Childhood Cancer. An Evaluation of Current Management. Vol. 4. Alan R Liss, New York, 1975

105. Nathwani BN, Kim H, Rappaport H: Malignant lymphoma, lymphoblastic. Cancer 38:964, 1976

106. Rosen PJ, Feinstein DI, Pattengale PK et al: Convoluted lymphocytic lymphomas in adults: a clinicopathologic entity. Ann Intern Med 89:319, 1978

107. Streuli RA, Laneko Y, Variakojis D et al: Lymphoblastic lymphoma in adults. Cancer 47:2510, 1981

108. Levine AM, Forman SJ, Meyer PR et al: Successful therapy of convoluted T-lymphoblastic lymphoma in adults. Blood 61:92, 1983

109. Murphy SB: Childhood non-Hodgkin's lymphoma. N Engl J Med 299:1446, 1978

110. Weinstein MJ, Cassidy JR, Levey R: Long term results of the APO protocol (vincristine, doxorubicin [Adriamycin] and prednisone) for treatment of mediastinal lymphoblastic lymphoma. J Clin Oncol 1:537, 1983

111. Burkitt D: A sarcoma involving the jaws in African children. Br J Surg 46:218, 1958

112. Henle G, Henle W, Clifford P et al: Antibodies to Epstein-Barr virus in Burkitt's lymphoma and control groups. J Natl Cancer Inst 43:1147, 1969

113. Lindahl T, Klein G, Reedman BM et al: Relationship between Epstein-Barr virus (EBV) DNA and the EBV-determined nuclear antigen (EBNA) in Burkitt's lymphoma biopsies and other lymphoproliferative malignancies. Int J Cancer 13:764, 1974

114. Magrath IT: Burkitt's lymphoma: clinical aspects and treatment. p. 103. In Molander DW (ed): Diseases of the Lymphatic System: Diagnosis and Therapy. Springer-Verlag, New York, 1983

115. Magrath IT: Biology and treatment of small non-cleaved cell lymphoma. Oncology 3:41, 1989

116. Horning SJ, Weiss CL, Crabtree CG et al: Clinical and phenotypic diversity of T-cell lymphomas. Blood 67:1578, 1986

117. Simoyama M, Ota K, Kikuchi M et al: Major prognostic factors of adult patients with advanced T-cell lymphoma/leukemia. J Clin Oncol 6:1088, 1988

118. Coiffier B, Berger F, Byron P-A et al: T-cell lymphomas: immunologic, histologic, clinical, and therapeutic analysis of 63 cases. J Clin Oncol 6:1584, 1988

119. Rai KR, Sawitsky A. Cronkite EP et al: Clinical staging of chronic lymphocytic leukemia. Blood 46:219, 1975

120. Durie BGM, Salmon SE: A clinical staging system for multiple myeloma: correlation of measured myeloma cell mass with presenting clinical features, response to treatment and survival. Cancer 36:842, 1975

121. Carbone PP, Kaplan HS, Musshoff K et al: Report of the Committee on Hodgkin's disease staging classification. Cancer Res 31:1860, 1971

122. Jones SE, Tobias DA, Waldman RF: Computed tomographic scanning in patients with lymphoma. Cancer 41:480, 1978

123. Breiman RS, Castellino RA, Harell GS et al: CT-pathologic correlations in Hodgkin's disease and non-Hodgkin's lymphoma. Radiology 126:159, 1978

124. Castellino RA, Dunnick NR, Goffinet DR et al: Predictive value of lymphography for subdiaphragmatic disease encountered at staging laparotomy in newly diagnosed Hodgkin's disease and non-Hodgkin's lymphoma. J Clin Oncol 1:532, 1983

125. Jackson FI, Lalani Z: Ultrasound and the diagnosis of lymphoma: a review. J Clin Ultrasound 17:145, 1989

126. Bruneton JN, Normand F, Balu-Maestro C et al: Lymphomatous superficial lymph node: US detection. Radiology 165:233, 1987

127. Tiot L, Jager H, Tigtgat NJ: Endoscopic ultrasonography of non-Hodgkin's lymphoma of the stomach. Gastroenterology 91:401, 1986

128. Richards MA, Webb JAW, Jewell SE et al: Low field strength magnetic resonance imaging of bone marrow in patients with malignant lymphoma. Br J Cancer 57:412, 1988

129. Hill M, Cunningham D, MacVicar D et al: Role of magnetic resonance imaging in predicting relapse in residual masses after treatment of lymphoma. J Clin Oncol 11:2273, 1993

130. Anderson KC, Leonard RCF, Canellos GP et al: High-dose gallium imaging in lymphomas. Am J Med 75:327, 1983

131. Tumeh SS, Rosenthal DS, Kaplan WD et al: Lymphoma: evaluation with GA-67 SPECT. Radiology 164:111, 1987

132. Longo DL, Schilsky RL, Blei L et al: Gallium-67 scanning: limited usefulness in staging patient with non-Hodgkin's lymphoma. Am J Med 68:695, 1980

133. Peylan-Ramu N, Haddy TB, Jones E et al: High frequency of benign mediastinal uptake of gallium-67 after completion of chemotherapy in children with high-grade non-Hodgkin's lymphoma. J Clin Oncol 7:1800, 1989

134. Anderson KC, Kaplan WD, Leonard RCF et al: Role of Tc methylene diphosphonate bone imaging in the management of lymphoma. Cancer Treat Rep 69:1347, 1985

135. Surbone A, Longo DL, DeVita VT et al: Residual abdominal masses in aggressive non-Hodgkin's lymphoma after combination chemotherapy: significance in management. J Clin Oncol 6:1832, 1988

136. Lister TA, Crowther D, Sutcliffe SB et al: Report of a committee convened to discuss the evaluation and staging of patients with Hodgkin's disease: Cotswolds meeting. J Clin Oncol 7:1630, 1989

137. Vose JM, Armitage JO, Weisenberger DD et al: The importance of age in survival of patients treated with chemotherapy for aggressive non-Hodgkin's lymphoma. J Clin Oncol 6:1838, 1988

138. Solal-Celigny P, Chastang C, Herrera A et al: Age as the main prognostic factor in adult aggressive non-Hodgkin's lymphoma. Am J Med 83:1075, 1987

139. Tirelli U, Zagonel V, Serraino D et al: Non-Hodgkin's lymphomas in 137 patients aged 70 years or older: a retrospective European organization for research and treatment of cancer lymphoma group study. J Clin Oncol 6: 1708, 1988

140. Klimo P, Connors JM: MACOP-B chemotherapy for the treatment of diffuse large cell lymphoma. Ann Intern Med 102:596, 1985

141. Skarin AT, Canillas GP, Rosenthal DS et al: Improved prognosis of diffuse histiocytic in differentiated lymphoma by use of high-dose methotrexate alternating with standard agents (M-BACOD). J Clin Oncol 1:91, 1983

142. Shipp MA, Harrington DP, Klatt MM et al: Identification of major prognostic subgroups of patients with large-cell lymphoma treated with M-BACOD or m-BACOD. Ann Intern Med 104:757, 1986

143. Armitage JO, Cheson BD: Interpretation of clinical trials in diffuse large-cell lymphoma. J Clin Oncol 6:1335, 1988

144. Armitage JO, Dick FR, Corder MP: Diffuse histiocytic lymphoma after histologic conversion: a poor prognostic variant. Cancer Treat Rep 65:413, 1981

145. Danieu L, Wong G, Koziner B et al: Predictive model for prognosis in advanced diffuse histiocytic lymphoma. Cancer Res 46:5372, 1986

146. Jagannath S, Valasquez WS, Tucker SL et al: Tumor burden assessment and its implication for a prognostic model in advanced diffuse large-cell lymphoma. J Clin Oncol 4:859, 1986

147. Fisher RI, DeVita VT, Johnson BL et al: Prognostic factors for advanced diffuse histiocytic lymphoma following treatment with combination chemotherapy. Am J Med 63:177, 1977

148. Coiffier B, Gisselbrecht C, Vose JM et al: Prognostic factors in aggressive malignant lymphomas: description and validation of a prognostic index that could identify patients requiring a more intensive therapy. J Clin Oncol 9: 211, 1991

149. Hoskins PJ, Ng V, Spinelli JJ et al: Prognostic variables in patients with diffuse large-cell lymphoma treated with MACOP-B. J Clin Oncol 9:220, 1991

150. Vitolo U, Bertini M, Brusamolino E et al: MACOP-B treatment in diffuse large-cell lymphoma: identification of prognostic groups in an Italian multicenter study. J Clin Oncol 10:219, 1992

151. Bauer KD, Merkel DE, Winter JN et al: Prognostic implications of ploidy and proliferative activity in diffuse large cell lymphomas. Cancer Res 46:3173, 1986

152. Woolridge TN, Grierson HL, Weisenberger DD et al: Association of DNA content and proliferative activity with clinical outcome in patients with diffuse mixed cell and large cell non-Hodgkin's lymphoma. Cancer Res 48: 6608, 1988

153. Christensson B, Lindemalm C, Johansson B et al: Flow cytometric DNA analysis: a prognostic tool in non-Hodgkin lymphoma. Leuk Res 13:307, 1989

154. Grogan TM, Lippman SM, Spier CM et al: Independent prognostic significance of a nuclear proliferation antigen in diffuse large cell lymphomas as determined by the monoclonal antibody Ki-67. Blood 71:1157, 1988

155. Todd MB, Portlock CS, Farber LR et al: Prognostic indicators in diffuse large-cell (histiocytic) lymphoma. Int J Radiat Oncol Biol Phys 12:593, 1986

156. Ferraris AA, Giuntini P, Gaetani GF: Serum lactic dehydrogenase as a prognostic tool for non-Hodgkin's lymphomas. Blood 54:928, 1979

157. Fasola G, Fanin R, Gherlinzoni F et al: Serum LDH concentration in non-Hodgkin's lymphomas. Relationship to histologic type, tumor mass, and presentation features. Acta Haematol 72:231, 1984

158. Swan F Jr, Velasquez WS, Tucker S et al: A new serologic staging system for large-cell lymphomas based on initial beta 2-microglobulin and lactate dehydrogenase levels. J Clin Oncol 7:1518, 1989

159. Horning SJ, Weiss LM, Crabtree GS et al: Clinical and phenotypic diversity of T-cell lymphomas. Blood 67:1578, 1986

160. Levine AM, Taylor CR, Schneider DR et al: Immunoblastic sarcoma of T-cell versus B-cell origin. I. Clinical features. Blood 58:52, 1981

161. Cossman J, Jaffe ES, Fisher RI: Immunologic phenotypes of diffuse aggressive non-Hodgkins lymphomas. Cancer 54:1310, 1984

162. Lippman SM, Miller TP, Spier CM et al: The prognostic significance of immunophenotype in diffuse large cell lymphoma: a comparative study of the T-cell and B-cell phenotype. Blood 72:436, 1988

163. Cabanillas F, Pathak S, Grant G et al: Refractoriness to chemotherapy and poor survival related to abnormalities of chromosomes 17 and 7 in lymphoma. Am J Med 87:167, 1989

164. Guglielmi C, Amadori S, Ruco LP et al: Combination chemotherapy for the treatment of diffuse aggressive lymphomas: F-MACHOP update. Semin Oncol 14:104, 1987

165. Armitage JO, Weisenberger DD, Hutchins M et al: Chemotherapy for diffuse large-cell lymphoma—rapidly responding patients have more durable remissions. J Clin Oncol 4:160, 1986

166. Coiffer B, Bryon PA, French M et al: Intensive chemotherapy in aggressive lymphomas: updated results of LNH-80 protocol and prognostic factors affecting response and survival. Blood 70:1394, 1987

167. The International Non-Hodgkin's Lymphoma Prognostic Factors Project: A predictive model for aggressive non-Hodgkin's lymphoma. N Engl J Med 329:987, 1993

168. Editorial: Durable remissions in stage III follicular lymphoma: interpret with caution. J Clin Oncol 6:838, 1987

169. Dana BW, Dahlberg S, Nathwani BN et al: Malignant lymphomas treated with doxorubicin-based chemotherapy or chemoimmunotherapy. J Clin Oncol 11:644, 1993

170. Morrison WH, Hoppe RT, Weiss LM et al: Small lymphocytic lymphoma. J Clin Oncol 7:598, 1989

171. McLaughlin P, Fuller LM, Velasquez WS et al: Stage I-II follicular lymphoma: treatment results for 76 patients. Cancer 58:1596, 1986

172. Paryani SB, Hoppe RT, Cox RS et al: Analysis of non-Hodgkin's lymphomas with nodular and favorable histologies, stages I and II. Cancer 52:2300, 1983

173. Osborne CK, Norton L, Young RC et al: Nodular histiocytic lymphoma: an aggressive nodular lymphoma with potential for prolonged disease-free survival. Blood 56:98, 1980

174. Longo DL, Young RC, Hubbard SM et al: Prolonged initial remission in patients with nodular mixed lymphoma. Ann Intern Med 100:651, 1984

175. Reddy S, Saxena VS, Pellettiere EV et al: Early nodal and extra-nodal non-Hodgkin's lymphomas. Cancer 40:98, 1977

176. Chen MG, Prosnitz LR, Gonzalez-Serva A et al: Results of radiotherapy in control of stage I and II non-Hodgkin's lymphoma. Cancer 43:1245, 1979

177. Monfardini S, Banfi A, Bonadonna G et al: Improved five year survival after combined radiotherapy-chemotherapy for stage I-II non-Hodgkin's lymphoma. Int Radiat Oncol Biol Phys 6:125, 1980

178. Gospodarowicz MK, Bush RS, Brown TC et al: Prognostic factors in nodular lymphomas: a multivariate analysis based on the Princess Margaret Hospital experience. Int J Radiat Oncol Biol Phys 10:489, 1984

179. Gomez GA, Barcos M, Krishnamsetty RM et al: Treatment of early—stages I and II—nodular, poorly differentiated lymphocytic lymphoma. Am J Clin Oncol 9:40, 1986

180. Richards MA, Gregory WM, Hall PA et al: Management of localized non-Hodgkin's lymphoma: the experience at St. Bartholomew's Hospital 1972–1985. Hematol Oncol 7:1, 1989

181. Cheson BD, Wittes RE, Friedman MA: Low-grade non-Hodgkin's lymphomas revisited. Cancer Treat Rep 70:1051, 1986

182. Jones SE: Follicular lymphoma—do no harm. Cancer Treat Rep 70:1055, 1986

183. Wright DH: The natural history of low grade non-Hodgkin's lymphoma and the impact of a no initial treatment policy on survival. Q J Med 80:631, 1991

184. Portlock CS: Deferral of initial therapy for advanced indolent lymphomas. Cancer Treat Rep 66:417, 1982

185. Mead GM, Macbeth FR, Ryall RDH et al: A report on a prospective trial of no initial therapy in patients with asymptomatic favourable prognosis non-Hodgkin's lymphoma. Hematol Oncol 2:179, 1984

186. Young RC, Longo DL, Glatstein E et al: The treatment of indolent lymphomas: watchful waiting. V. Aggressive combined modality treatment. Semin Hematol 25:11, 1988

187. Soubeyran P, Eghbali H, Bonichon F et al: Low-grade follicular lymphomas: analysis of prognosis in a series of 281 patients. Eur J Cancer 27:1606, 1991

188. Jones SE, Rosenberg SA, Kaplan HS et al: Non-Hodgkin's lymphomas: II. Single agent chemotherapy. Cancer 30:31, 1972

189. Pasmantier MW, Coleman M, Silver RT: Chemotherapy of the non-Hodgkin's lymphomas. Med Clin North Am 60:1043, 1976

190. Hoppe TE, Kushlan P, Kaplan HS et al: The treatment of advanced stage favorable histology non-Hodgkin's lymphoma: a preliminary report of a randomized trial comparing single agent chemotherapy, combination chemotherapy, and whole body irradiation. Blood 58:592, 1981

191. Cadman E, Drislane F, Waldron JA et al: High dose chlorambucil: effective therapy for rapid remission in nodular lymphocytic poorly differentiated lymphoma. Cancer 50:1037, 1982

192. Kennedy BJ, Bloomfield CD, Kiang DT et al: Combination versus successive single agent chemotherapy in lymphocytic lymphoma. Cancer 41:23, 1978

193. Canellos GP, Lister TA, Skarin AT: Chemotherapy of the non-Hodgkin's lymphomas. Cancer 42:932, 1978

194. Rosenberg SA: The low-grade non-Hodgkin's lymphomas: challenges and opportunities. J Clin Oncol 3:299, 1985

195. Hoppe RT: The role of radiation therapy in the management of the non-Hodgkin's lymphomas. Cancer 55:2176, 1985

196. Glick JH, Barnes JM, Ezdinli EZ et al: Nodular mixed lymphoma: results of a randomized trial failing to confirm prolonged disease-free survival with COPP chemotherapy. Blood 58:920, 1981

197. Anderson KC, Skarin AT, Rosenthal DS et al: Combination chemotherapy for advanced non-Hodgkin's lymphomas other than diffuse histiocytic or undifferentiated histologies. Cancer Treat Rep 68:1343, 1984

198. Smalley RV, Andersen JW, Hawkins MJ et al: Interferon ALFA combined with cytotoxic chemotherapy for patients with non-Hodgkin's lymphoma. N Engl J Med 327:1336, 1992

199. Solal-Celigny P, Lepage E, Brousse N et al: Recombinant interferon ALFA-2b combined with a regimen containing doxorubicin in patients with advanced follicular lymphoma. N Engl J Med 329:1608, 1993

200. Hochster HS, Kim K, Green MD et al: Activity of fludarabine in previously treated non-Hodgkin's low-grade lymphoma: results of an Eastern Cooperative Oncology Group study. J Clin Oncol 10:28, 1992

201. Kay AC, Saven A, Carrera CJ et al: 2-chlorodeoxyadenosine treatment of low-grade lymphomas. J Clin Oncol 10:371, 1992

202. Redman JR, Cabanillas F, Velasquez WS et al: Phase II trial of fludarabine phosphate in lymphoma: an effective new agent in low-grade lymphoma. J Clin Oncol 10:790, 1992

203. Mendenhall Price N, Noyes WD, Million RR: Total body irradiation for stage II-IV non-Hodgkin's lymphoma: ten-year follow-up. J Clin Oncol 7:67, 1989

204. Paryani SB, Hoppe RT, Cox RS et al: The role of radiation therapy in the management of stage III follicular lymphomas. J Clin Oncol 2:841, 1984

205. Cox JD, Komaki R, Lun LE et al: Stage III nodular lymphoreticular tumors (non-Hodgkin's lymphoma): results of central lymphatic irradiation. Cancer 47:2247, 1981

206. Levitt M, Marsh JC, DeConti R et al: Combination sequential chemotherapy in advanced reticulum cell sarcoma. Cancer 29:630, 1972

207. Sweet DL, Kinzie J, Gaeke ME et al: Survival of patients with localized diffuse histiocytic lymphoma. Blood 58:1218, 1981

208. Jones SE, Rosenberg SA, Kaplan HS et al: Non-Hodgkin's lymphomas II. Single agent chemotherapy. Cancer 30:31, 1972

209. Landberg TG, Hakansson LG, Moller TR et al: CVP-remission-maintenance in stage I or II non-Hodgkin's lymphomas: preliminary results of a randomized study. Cancer 44:831, 1979

210. Nisson NI, Ersboll J, Hansen HS et al: A randomized study of radiotherapy versus radiotherapy plus chemotherapy in stage I-II non-Hodgkin's lymphomas. Cancer 52:1, 1983

211. Carde P, Burges JMV, van Glabbekem M et al: Combined radiotherapy-chemotherapy for early stage non-Hodgkin's lymphoma: the 1975–1980 EDRTC controlled lymphoma trial. Radiother Oncol 2:301, 1984

212. Longo DL, Glastsein E, Suffey PL et al: Treatment of localized aggressive lymphomas with combination chemotherapy followed by involved-field radiation therapy. J Clin Oncol 7:1295, 1989

213. Jones SE, Miller TP, Connors JM: Long term follow up and analysis for prognostic factors for patients with limited-stage diffuse large-cell lymphoma treated with initial chemotherapy with or without adjuvant radiotherapy. J Clin Oncol 7:1186, 1989

214. Tondini C, Zanini M, Lombardi F et al: Combined modality treatment with primary CHOP chemotherapy followed by locoregional irradiation in stage I or II histologically aggressive non-Hodgkin's lymphomas. J Clin Oncol 11:720, 1993

215. Connors JM, Klimo P, Fairey RN et al: Brief chemotherapy and involved field radiation therapy for limited-stage, histologically aggressive lymphoma. Ann Intern Med 107:25, 1987

216. Miller TP, Jones SE: Initial chemotherapy for clinically localized lymphomas of unfavorable histology. Blood 62:413, 1983

217. Armitage JO, Vose JM, Bierman PJ: Salvage therapy for patients with non-Hodgkin's lymphoma. J Natl Cancer Inst Monogr 10:39, 1990

218. Dana BW, Dahlberg S, Miller TP et al: m-BACOD treatment for intermediate- and high-grade malignant lymphomas: a Southwest Oncology Group phase II trial. J Clin Oncol 8:1155, 1990

219. Coleman M: Chemotherapy for large-cell lymphoma: optimism and caution. Ann Intern Med 103:140, 1985

220. Coltman CA Jr, Dahlberg S, Jones SE et al: CHOP is curative in thirty percent of patients with large cell lymphoma: a twelve-year southwest oncology group follow-up. p. 71. In Skarin AT (ed): Update on Treatment for Diffuse Large Cell Lymphoma. John Wiley & Sons, New York, 1986

221. Laurence J, Coleman M, Allen SL et al: Combination chemotherapy of advanced diffuse histiocytic lymphoma with the six-drug COP-BLAM regimen. Ann Intern Med 97:190, 1982

222. Connors JM, Klimo P: MACOP-B chemotherapy for malignant lymphomas and related conditions: 1987 update and additional observations. Semin Hematol, suppl. 25:41, 1988

223. Shipp MA, Yeap BY, Harrington DP et al: The m-BACOD combination chemotherapy regimen in large-cell lymphoma: analysis of the completed trial and comparison with the M-BACOD regimen. J Clin Oncol 8:84, 1990

224. Fisher RI, DeVita BT, Hubbard SM et al: Randomized trial of ProMACE vs. ProMACE-CytaBOM in previously untreated advanced stage, diffuse aggressive lymphomas. Proc Am Soc Clin Oncol 3:242(a), 1984

225. Fisher RI, Gaynor ER, Dahlberg S et al: Comparison of a standard regimen (CHOP) with three intensive chemotherapy regimens for advanced non-Hodgkin's lymphoma. N Engl J Med 328:1002, 1993

226. Armitage JO: Treatment of non-Hodgkin's lymphoma. N Engl J Med 328:1023, 1993

227. Browne MJ, Hubbard SM, Longo DL et al: Excess prevalence of *Pneumocystis carinii* pneumonia in patients treated for lymphoma with combination chemotherapy. Ann Intern Med 104:338, 1986

228. Gerhartz HH, Englehard M, Meusers P et al: Randomized, double-blind, placebo-controlled, phase III study of recombinant human granulocyte-macrophage colony-stimulating factor as adjunct to induction treatment of high-grade malignant non-Hodgkin's lymphomas. Blood 82:2329, 1993

229. Pettengell R, Gurney H, Radford JA et al: Granulocyte colony-stimulating factor to prevent dose-limiting neutropenia in non-Hodgkin's lymphoma: a randomized controlled trial. Blood 80:1430, 1992

230. Brusamolino E, Bertini M, Guidi S et al: CHOP versus CNOP (N = mitoxantrone) in non-Hodgkin's lymphoma: an interim report comparing efficacy and toxicity. Haematologica 73:217, 1988

231. Pavlovsky S, Santarelli MT, Erazo A et al: Results of a randomized study of previously-untreated intermediate and high grade lymphoma using CHOP versus CNOP. Ann Oncol 3:205, 1992

232. Aur RJA, Hustu HO, Simone JV et al: Therapy of localized and regional lymphosarcoma of childhood. Cancer 27:1328, 1971

233. Anderson JR, Wilson JF, Jenkin DT et al: Childhood non-Hodgkin's lymphoma: the results of a randomized therapeutic trial comparing a 4-drug regimen (COMP) with a 10-drug regimen (LSA$_2$-L$_2$). N Engl J Med 308:559, 1983

234. Coleman CN, Cohen JR, Burke JS et al: Lymphoblastic lymphoma in adults: results of a pilot protocol. Blood 57:679, 1981

235. Coleman CN, Picozzi VJ, Cox RS et al: Treatment of lymphoblastic lymphoma in adults. J Clin Oncol 4:1628, 1986

236. Slater DE, Mertelsmann R, Koziner B et al: Lymphoblastic lymphoma in adults. J Clin Oncol 4:57, 1986

237. Salloum E, Henry-Amar M, Caillou B et al: Lymphoblastic lymphoma in adults: a clinicopathological study of 34 cases treated at the Institute Gustave-Roussy. Eur J Cancer Clin Oncol 24:1609, 1988

238. Voakes JB, Jones SE, McKelvey EM: The chemotherapy of lymphoblastic lymphoma. Blood 57:186, 1981

239. Morel P, Lepage E, Brice P et al: Prognosis and treatment of lymphoblastic lymphoma in adults: a report on 80 patients. J Clin Oncol 10:1078, 1992

240. Nademanee AP, Forman SJ, Schmidt GM et al: Allogeneic bone marrow transplantation for high risk non-Hodgkin's lymphoma during first complete remission. Blut 55:11, 1987

241. Verdonck LF, Dekker AW, de Gast GC et al: Autologous bone marrow transplantation for adult poor-risk lymphoblastic lymphoma in first remission. J Clin Oncol 10:644, 1992

242. Satini G, Congiu AM, Coser P et al: Autologous bone marrow transplantation for adult advanced stage lymphoblastic lymphoma in 1st CR. A study of the NHL CSG. Leukemia, suppl. 1. 5:42, 1991

243. Magrath IT, Janus C, Edwards BK et al: An effective therapy for both undifferentiated (including Burkitt's) lymphomas and lymphoblastic lymphomas in children and young adults. Blood 63:1102, 1984

244. Sullivan MP, Ramirez I: Curability of Burkitt's lymphoma with high-dose cyclophosphamide—high-dose methotrexate therapy and intrathecal chemoprophylaxis. J Clin Oncol 3:627, 1985

245. Murphy SB, Husto HO: A randomized trial of combined modality therapy of childhood non-Hodgkin's lymphoma. Cancer 45:630, 1980

246. Ziegler JL: Burkitt's lymphoma. N Engl J Med 305:735, 1981

247. Magrath IT, Lee YJ, Anderson T et al: Prognostic factors in Burkitt's lymphoma: importance of total tumor burden. Cancer 45:1507, 1980

248. Bernstein JI, Coleman N, Strickler JG et al: Combined modality therapy for adults with small non-cleaved cell lymphoma (Burkitt's and non-Burkitt's type). J Clin Oncol 4:847, 1986

249. Lopez TM, Hagenmeister FB, McLaughlin P et al: Small noncleaved cell lymphoma in adults: superior results for stages I-II disease. J Clin Oncol 8:615, 1990

250. McMaster ML, Greer JP, Greco FA et al: Effective treatment of small-non-cleaved-cell lymphoma with high-density, brief-duration chemotherapy. J Clin Oncol 9:941, 1991

251. Appelbaum FR, Deisseroth AB, Graw RG et al: Prolonged complete remission following high dose chemotherapy of Burkitt's lymphoma in relapse. Cancer 41:1059, 1978

252. Philip T, Biron P, Philip I et al: Massive therapy and autologous bone marrow transplantation in pediatric and young adults Burkitt's lymphoma (30 courses on 28 patients: a 5 year experience). Eur J Cancer Clin Oncol 22:1015, 1986

253. Philip I, Philip T, Favrot M et al: Establishment of lymphomatous cell lines

from bone marrow samples from patients with Burkitt's lymphoma. J Natl Cancer Inst 73:835, 1984

254. Cabanillas F, Velasquez WS, McLaughlin P et al: Results of recent salvage chemotherapy regimens for lymphoma and Hodgkin's disease. Semin Hematol 25:47, 1988

255. Velasquez WS, Cabanillas F, Salvador P et al: Effective salvage therapy for lymphoma with cisplatin in combination with high-dose Ara-C and dexamethasone (DHAP). Blood 71:117, 1988

256. Cabanillas F, Hagemeister FB, Bodey GP et al: IMVP-16: an effective regimen for patients with lymphoma who have relapsed after initial combination chemotherapy. Blood 60:693, 1982

257. Cabanillas F, Hagemeister FB, McLaughlin P et al: Results of MIME salvage regimen for recurrent or refractory lymphoma. J Clin Oncol 5:407, 1987

258. Cabanillas F: Experience with salvage regimens at M.D. Anderson Hospital. Ann Oncol, suppl. 1. 2:31, 1991

259. Goss PE, Shepherd FA, Scott JG et al: Dexamethasone/ifosfamide/cisplatin/etoposide (DICE) as therapy for patients with advanced refractory non-Hodgkin's lymphoma: preliminary report of phase II study. Ann Oncol, suppl. 1. 2:43, 1991

260. Jackson DV Jr, Paschold EH, Spurr CL et al: Treatment of advanced non-Hodgkin's lymphoma with vincristine infusion. Cancer 53:2601, 1984

261. Hollister D Jr, Silver RT, Gordon B et al: Continuous infusion vincristine and bleomycin with high dose methotrexate for resistant non-Hodgkin's lymphoma. Cancer 50:1690, 1982

262. Hainsworth JD: Chronic administration of etoposide in the treatment of non-Hodgkin's lymphoma. Leuk Lymphoma, suppl. 10:65, 1993

263. Gorin NC, Gale RP, Armitage JO: Autologous bone marrow transplants: different indications in Europe and North America. Lancet 2:317, 1989

264. Frei E III, Canellos GP: Dose: a critical factor in cancer chemotherapy. Am J Med 69:585, 1980

265. Gehan EA: Dose-response relationship in clinical oncology. Cancer 54:1204, 1984

266. Odaimi M, Ajani J: High-dose chemotherapy: concepts and strategies. Am J Clin Oncol 10:123, 1987

267. Ernst P, Maraninchi D, Jacobsen N et al: Marrow transplantation for non-Hodgkin's lymphoma: a multi-centre study from the European Co-operative Bone Marrow Transplant Group. Bone Marrow Transplant 1:81, 1986

268. Phillips GL, Herzig RH, Lazarus HM et al: High-dose chemotherapy, fractionated total-body irradiation, and allogeneic marrow transplantation for malignant lymphoma. J Clin Oncol 4:480, 1986

269. Appelbaum FR, Thomas ED, Buckner CD et al: Treatment of non-Hodgkin's lymphoma with chemoradiotherapy and allogeneic marrow transplantation. Hematol Oncol 1:149, 1983

270. O'Leary M, Ramsay NKC, Nesbit ME Jr et al: Bone marrow transplantation for non-Hodgkin's lymphoma in children and young adults. Am J Med 74:497, 1983

271. Appelbaum FR, Fefer A, Cheever MA et al: Treatment of non-Hodgkin's lymphoma with marrow transplantation in identical twins. Blood 58:509, 1981

272. Appelbaum FR, Sullivan KM, Buckner CD et al: Treatment of malignant lymphoma in 100 patients with chemotherapy, total body irradiation, and marrow transplantation. J Clin Oncol 5:1340, 1987

273. Jones RJ, Ambinder RF, Piantadosi S et al: Evidence of a graft-versus-host-lymphoma effect associated with allogeneic bone marrow transplantation. Blood 77:649, 1991

274. Chopra R, Goldstone AH, Pearce R et al: Autologous versus allogeneic bone marrow transplantation for non-Hodgkin's lymphoma: a case-controlled analysis of the European Bone Marrow Transplant Goup Registry data. J Clin Oncol 10:1690, 1992

275. Butturini A, Bortin MM, Gale RP: Graft-versus-leukemia following bone marrow transplantation. Bone Marrow Transplant 2:244, 1987

276. Philip T, Armitage JO, Spitzer G et al: High-dose therapy and autologous bone marrow transplantation after failure of conventional chemotherapy in adults with intermediate-grade or high-grade non-Hodgkin's lymphoma. N Engl J Med 316:1493, 1987

277. Gribben JG, Goldstone AH, Linch DC et al: Effectiveness of high-dose combination chemotherapy and autologous bone marrow transplantation for patients with non-Hodgkin's lymphomas who are still responsive to conventional-dose therapy. J Clin Oncol 7:1621, 1989

278. Colombat P, Gorin N-C, Lemonnier M-P et al: The role of autologous bone marrow transplantation in 46 adult patients with non-Hodgkin's lymphomas. J Clin Oncol 8:630, 1990

279. Phillips GL, Fay JW, Herzig RH et al: The treatment of progressive non-Hodgkin's lymphoma with intensive chemoradiotherapy and autologous marrow transplantation. Blood 75:831, 1990

280. Weisdorf DJ, Haake R, Miller WJ et al: Autologous bone marrow transplantation for progressive non-Hodgkin's lymphoma: clinical impact of immunophenotype and in vitro purging. Bone Marrow Transplant 8:135, 1991

281. Gulati S, Yahalom J, Acaba L et al: Treatment of patients with relapsed and resistant non-Hodgkin's lymphoma using total body irradiation, etoposide, and cyclophosphamide and autologous bone marrow transplantation. J Clin Oncol 10:936, 1992

282. Bosly A, Coiffier B, Gisselbrecht C et al: Bone marrow transplantation prolongs survival after relapse in aggressive-lymphoma patients treated with the LNH-84 regimen. J Clin Oncol 10:1615, 1992

283. Philip T, Chauvin F, Armitare J et al: PARMA international protocol: pilot study of DHAP followed by involved-field radiotherapy and BEAC with autologous bone marrow transplantation. Blood 77:1587, 1991

284. Nademanee A, Schmidt GM, O'Donnell MR et al: High-dose chemoradiotherapy followed by autologous bone marrow transplantation as consolidation therapy during first complete remission in adult patients with poor-risk aggressive lymphoma: a pilot study. Blood 80:1130, 1992

285. Freedman AS, Takvorian T, Neuberg D et al: Autologous bone marrow transplantation in poor-prognosis intermediate-grade and high-grade B-cell non-Hodgkin's lymphoma in first remission: a pilot study. J Clin Oncol 11:931, 1993

286. Vose JM, Anderson JR, Kessinger A et al: High-dose chemotherapy and autologous hematopoietic stem-cell transplantation for aggressive non-Hodgkin's lymphoma. J Clin Oncol 11:1846, 1993

287. Freedman AS, Ritz J, Neuberg D et al: Autologous bone marrow transplantation in 69 patients with a history of low-grade B-cell non-Hodgkin's lymphoma. Blood 77:2524, 1991

288. Rohatiner AZ, Price CG, Arnott S et al: Myeloablative therapy with autologous bone marrow transplantation as consolidation of remission in patients with follicular lymphoma. Ann Oncol, suppl. 2:147, 1991

289. Bierman P, Vose J, Armitage J et al: High-dose therapy followed by autologous hematopoietic rescue for follicular low grade non-Hodgkin's lymphoma (NHL). Proc ASCO 11:1074, 1992

290. Foon KA, Sherwin SA, Abrams PG et al: Treatment of advanced non-Hodgkin's lymphoma with recombinant leukocyte A interferon. N Engl J Med 311:1148, 1984

291. O'Connell MJ, Colgan JP, Oken RE et al: Clinical trial of recombinant leukocyte A interferon as initial therapy for favorable histology non-Hodgkin's lymphomas and chronic lymphocytic leukemia. An Eastern Cooperative Oncology Group Pilot Study. J Clin Oncol 4:128, 1986

292. Bunn PA Jr, Ihde DC, Foon KA: The role of recombinant interferon alpha-2a in the therapy of cutaneous T-cell lymphomas. Cancer, suppl. 57:1689, 1986

293. Brown SL, Miller RA, Levy R: Antiidiotype antibody therapy of B-cell lymphoma. Semin Oncol 16:199, 1989

294. Kwak LK, Campbell MJ, Czerwinski DK et al: Induction of immune responses in patients with B-cell lymphoma against the surface-immunoglobulin idiotype expressed by their tumors. N Engl J Med 327:1209, 1992

295. Press OW, Eary JF, Appelbaum FR et al: Radiolabeled-antibody therapy of B-cell lymphoma with autologous bone marrow support. N Engl J Med 329:1219, 1993

296. Kaminski MS, Zasadny KR, Francis IR et al: Radioimmunotherapy of B-cell lymphoma with [^{131}I]ANTI-B1 (ANTI-CD20) antibody. N Engl J Med 329:459, 1993

297. Czuczman MS, Straus DJ, Divgi CR et al: Phase I dose-escalation trial of iodine 131-labeled monoclonal antibody OKB7 in patients with non-Hodgkin's lymphoma. J Clin Oncol 11:2021, 1993

298. Grossbard ML, Lambert JM, Goldmacher VS et al: Anti-B4-blocked ricin: a phase I trial of 7-day continuous infusion in patients with B-cell neoplasms. J Clin Oncol 11:726, 1993

299. Amlot PL, Stone MJ, Cunningham D et al: A phase I study of an anti-CD22-deglycosylated ricin A chain immunotoxin in the treatment of B-cell lymphomas resistant to conventional therapy. Blood 82:2624, 1993

Childhood Lymphomas

82

Sharon B. Murphy

INTRODUCTION

The lymphomas occurring among children and adolescents, just as among adults, may be either Hodgkin disease (HD) or non-Hodgkin lymphomas (NHLs). There are major differences between childhood NHL and lymphomas that occur in adults. The dissimilarities in classification, staging, and end results of childhood lymphomas from patterns in adults have been reviewed elsewhere.[1] Important differences in cellular origins and natural history also exist. In childhood, practically all NHLs are diffuse, high-grade malignancies, and one virtually never sees intermediate or low-grade lymphomas. Characterization of the T- or B-cell nature of childhood lymphomas, furthermore, confirms a state of tumor cell differentiation very different from most lymphomas occurring in adult years, as the tumors of childhood are generally less functionally differentiated, more closely resembling lymphoid stem cells or early precursors. Optimal strategies for therapy and outcomes of treatment for children with NHL also differ markedly from those for adults.

By contrast, there is no compelling evidence to suggest that HD in children and adolescents differs materially from the disease in adults, except for the confounding impact of growth and pubertal development on treatment options and for the longer lifelong period of risk of adverse late consequences of treatment. In view of the recognized bone growth abnormalities known to accompany high-dose extended field radiotherapy, a combined modality approach using low-dose irradiation and combination chemotherapy is favored for the treatment of HD in children and adolescents. In other respects, the manifestations, staging, and treatment of HD in childhood are similar to those in adults and are presented in Chapter 79.

EPIDEMIOLOGY

The peak frequency of childhood NHL is in the middle childhood years, the median age being 9–10 years in most reported series. NHL occurs very rarely in children <3 years old at diagnosis.[2,3] In childhood NHL, a marked male predominance is present, with a male/female ratio of 3:1. The explanation for this unequal gender distribution remains obscure, although the sex-linked recessive lymphoproliferative syndrome reported by Purtilo[4] may provide a clue.

Infection by the Epstein-Barr virus (EBV), a polyclonal B-cell activator, has been implicated in the pathogenesis, not only of those lymphomas associated with the X-linked lymphoproliferative syndrome, but also of those associated with congenital immunodeficiency or the acquired immunodeficiency syndrome (AIDS) associated with infection by the human immunodeficiency virus (HIV).[5-7] At-risk populations mainly include the ever-increasing number of children perinatally infected with HIV, which parallels the increase in the number of women in their childbearing years who are HIV-infected. Also at risk are HIV-infected children and adolescents whose disease was transfusion transmitted (e.g., hemophiliacs) and adolescents engaged in high-risk behavior (e.g., unsafe sex, intravenous drug use). Estimates of the risk of lymphoma developing in a child with AIDS vary and appear to be influenced not only by the degree of immunosuppression, as reflected by the CD4+-cell count, but also by competing causes of mortality. If the adult experience with AIDS-related lymphoma is a model, one can predict that the risk of developing NHL in children with AIDS is roughly 5%.

CLASSIFICATION

In childhood, the histologic pattern of NHL is limited essentially to one of three diffuse high-grade types[8-11] (Table 82-1), with only a small proportion (about 5%) of cases of any histology other than lymphoblastic, small noncleaved cell (also termed undifferentiated, Burkitt or non-Burkitt pleomorphic), or large cell, usually immunoblastic. The working formulation for classification of NHL developed by the Non-Hodgkin's Lymphoma Pathologic Classification Project[12] has very limited applicability to children. One virtually never encounters well-differentiated lymphocytic tumors of intermediate or low-grade type, and follicular or nodular lymphomas of germinal center cell origin, while common in adults, are extremely rare in children. Frizzera and Murphy[13] were able to compile only eight bona fide cases of nodular lymphoma in children <15 years old from a total of 318 cases of childhood lymphomas seen over a span of two decades at four cancer centers. All the cases in children were of the mixed or histiocytic nodular type, with nodular tumors of poorly differentiated lymphocytic type notably absent. Furthermore, Winberg et al.[14] found only 12 cases of nodular lymphomas in children and adolescents <20 years old from a total of 1,760 cases of nodular lymphomas.

Among the high-grade lymphomas common in children and adolescents, some confusion and considerable controversy exist about the relevance of the morphologic distinctions between Burkitt and non-Burkitt types of small noncleaved cell (SNC) NHL. Recent studies have conclusively demonstrated that the morphologic distinctions, including nuclear and cell size and shape and prominence of nucleoli, are subtle, unreproducible, and of no demonstrable clinical significance.[10,15] Age at presentation, primary sites, extent of disease, and survival do not differ between the Burkitt and non-Burkitt subtypes of SNC lymphomas.[10,15] Furthermore, all SNC cell lymphomas that have been well studied are of B-cell origin, displaying monoclonal surface immunoglobulin (SIg) and carrying characteristic nonrandom chromosomal translocations [t(8;14), t(8;22), and t(2;8)], the common features of which juxtapose the c-myc oncogene on chromosome 8 with one of the genes coding for sequences from one of the immunoglobulin heavy- or light-chain loci.

The lymphoblastic lymphomas seen in childhood and ado-

Table 82-1. Distribution of Major Histologic Types of NHL in Children and Adolescents

	St. Jude Children's Research Hospital[8]	Pediatric Oncology Group[9-11]
No. of cases	338	227
Lymphoblastic	28%	47%
Large cell, diffuse	26%	32%
Small noncleaved cell, Burkitt and non-Burkitt	39%	21%
Other	7%	—

lescence are primarily T-cell-derived and are composed of cells cytologically indistinguishable from those seen in acute lymphocytic leukemia (ALL) (i.e., small, round, blue cells with scanty cytoplasm and indistinct nucleoli). Lymphoblastic lymphomas and leukemias of T-cell origin are composed of cells that resemble cells at the early, middle, or late stages of maturational differentiation.[16-17] While T-cell lymphoblastic leukemias are more often characterized by relatively less differentiated cells than are T-cell lymphoblastic lymphomas, there is considerable overlap. T-cell leukemias are equally distributed through the early, middle, and late stages of thymic differentiation, while the lymphomas tend to occur in the middle and late stages. These diseases might best be described as a continuum, with reported differences in response to treatment of lymphoblastic leukemias and lymphomas more a reflection of "stage" or tumor burden than of real biologic differences in the composition of malignant cells.

An interesting minor subgroup of cases, accounting for ≤5% of all childhood NHLs, has been described, which morphologically appear lymphoblastic and express the immunophenotype of common ALL (HLA-DR[+], CALLA[+] [CD10[+]]).[19,20] Fewer than 10% of cases of childhood NHL express neither T-cell antigens nor SIg[19]; these non-T, non-B cases predominantly involve young children presenting with cutaneous lymphoblastic lymphoma, often localized to the scalp, without evidence of bone marrow involvement. The blast cells comprising these cutaneous lymphomas express cytoplasmic IgM heavy chains characteristic of pre-B cells.[20] This entity of pre-B cutaneous lymphoblastic lymphoma thus represents a unique clinicopathologic entity that occurs in young children. Thus, while most childhood cases of lymphoblastic lymphoma are T-cell-derived, cases of localized lymphoblastic lymphomas presenting in sites outside the thymus often represent proliferations of B-precursor cells of the common ALL or pre-B phenotype in extramedullary sites.

Unlike the lymphoblastic lymphomas, which are usually T-cell in origin, the immunophenotype of the large cell lymphomas is quite variable.[21-23] In adult series, most of these lymphomas appear to be of B-cell origin, as demonstrated by either the expression of SIg or the presence of more primitive B-cell developmental antigens. About 15% of adult large cell lymphomas are of T-cell origin, and the immunophenotype is generally that of a more mature post-thymic peripheral T cell. Few indeed (<5%) appear to be true histiocytic neoplasms. In contrast to the large cell lymphomas prevalent among adults, which are mainly B-cell derived and of follicular center cell origin, most childhood large cell lymphomas are immunoblastic, and T-cell lineage is equally common as B.[8,22] Many pediatric large cell lymphomas express neither T- nor B-lineage markers.[23]

A subtype of childhood large cell NHL that has been reported to involve skin and lymph nodes preferentially is often referred to by its characteristic expression of the antigen Ki-1 (CD30), an antigen originally identified by a monoclonal antibody raised against a HD-derived cell line that reacts with Reed-Sternberg cells. Kadin et al.[24] initially described six pediatric cases of a clinicopathologic syndrome of skin and subcutaneous lesions (which may regress) in association with peripheral lymphadenopathy, a syndrome that may be confused with malignant histiocytosis, regressing atypical histiocytosis, lymphomatoid papulosis (when confined to skin) or HD. Histologically, the tumor cells are large, pleomorphic, and often anaplastic, and immunologic studies have shown that the tumor cells in some cases resemble activated T cells in that they are positive for Ia (HLA-DR) and Tac (interleukin-2 [IL-2] receptor), and Southern blot analysis confirms clonal rearrangements of the T-cell receptor β-chain. Schnitzer et al.[25] reported three pediatric cases of CD30[+] large cell lymphomas involving lymph nodes that lacked the reportedly characteristic skin involvement but expressed CD30 and T-cell markers. Subsequent reports of CD30[+]

large cell lymphomas underscore the difficulty in diagnosis and the phenotypic and clinical heterogeneity.[26,27]

A recent review of seven reported pediatric series of CD30[+] anaplastic large cell lymphomas (ALCL) concludes that the entity is relatively uncommon, accounting for roughly 8–12% of all pediatric NHL.[27] Survival of pediatric ALCL cases treated with modern therapy is reasonably good, in the range of 75–85%, despite presentation with advanced stage disseminated disease in most cases.[27]

CLINICAL MANIFESTATIONS

The clinical presentation of childhood NHL may be extremely varied, depending on the dominant anatomic site(s) involved and the extent of disease. Virtually any lymphatic tissue of the body may be involved, including lymph nodes, spleen, Peyer's patches, tonsils, and thymus. Extranodal extralymphatic disease is seen frequently. Disseminated NHL that is noncontiguous, particularly disease involving the central nervous system and bone marrow, also occurs. In some cases, it is impossible to specify exactly the primary site of the tumor owing to its extensive, apparently multifocal, distribution from the onset.

Painless peripheral lymph node enlargement, usually cervical, is the most common clinical presentation. Cervical lymphadenopathy may be solitary or a reflection of regional disease in association with a tumor either of the head and neck or of the mediastinum. NHL of the head and neck may primarily involve the sinuses, jaws, orbit, nasopharynx, tonsils, or adenoids and is often initially misdiagnosed as a comparatively trivial pediatric complaint, such as tonsillitis with peritonsillar abscess, serous otitis, or a dental problem. Mediastinal tumors are usually associated with upper torso adenopathy. Massive mediastinal tumors can frequently lead to stridor, dyspnea, a brassy cough, and venous engorgement and edema of the upper half of the body. Such a constellation of symptoms and findings constitutes a medical emergency and is an indication for immediate therapy to relieve the respiratory embarrassment.

Abdominal NHL in children is typically associated with a palpable mass and abdominal pain, characteristically intermittent, colicky, and in the periumbilical region or right lower quadrant.[28] Vomiting, weight loss, and ascites may be present as well. Tumors localized to the gastrointestinal tract generally involve the distal ileum, cecum, and mesenteric nodes and often lead to intussusception. Retroperitoneal and renal involvement is more common than is appreciated clinically.

The distribution of primary sites of tumor reported in large series of pediatric NHL cases[8,29] is shown in Table 82-2. Roughly one-third of patients present with intra-abdominal tumors, one-

Table 82-2. Distribution of Primary Sites of Tumor in Children and Adolescents with NHL

	St. Jude Children's Research Hospital[8]	The Hospital for Sick Children
No. of cases	338	102
Intra-abdominal	31%	40%
Mediastinal	26%	23%
Head and neck	29%[a]	11%[b]
Nodal	7%[c]	21%
Other[d]	7%	6%

[a] Includes Waldeyer's ring and/or cervical lymph nodes.

[b] Includes only Waldeyer's ring.

[c] Includes cases with primary nodal disease arising outside the head/neck region.

[d] Includes a variety of less common locations, including bone, skin, epidural space, thyroid.

Table 82-3. Relationship Between Histology, Immunophenotype, and Clinical Manifestations of Childhood NHL

Histology	Immunophenotype	Clinical Features
Lymphoblastic	T-cell (immature thymocyte)	Anterior mediastinal mass
	B precursor (pre-B) cell	Cutaneous tumor ± lymph node
Small noncleaved cell, so-called undifferentiated, Burkitt and non-Burkitt pleomorphic type	B (SIg$^+$) cell	Abdominal tumor ± ascites, Waldeyer's ring jaw, orbit
Large cell, immunoblastic anaplastic, polymorphous	B, T, or non-T, non-B	Mediastinum, lymph nodes, bone, skin, and other sites

quarter with mediastinal disease, and 30–35% with disease involving cervical lymph nodes or Waldeyer's ring, or both; the remainder of cases present with tumor in other sites.

The relationship between the primary location of tumor and the histology is strong,[8–11] as certain histologies correlate with certain sites, as shown in Table 82-3. For example, lymphoblastic disease typically presents within the chest, involving the mediastinum, usually in association with upper torso nodal disease, and seldom in other locations. By contrast, diffuse SNC tumors virtually never involve the mediastinum or peripheral nodes, but typically arise in the abdomen or Waldeyer's ring. Large cell lymphomas occur at all sites and predominate in other less common locations. Tumors of the head and neck may be of any histology. The usual interval of symptoms prior to the diagnosis of childhood NHL is brief, 4–6 weeks. Some children are desperately ill, developing rapidly progressive widespread disease within 1–2 weeks of their first symptoms.

LABORATORY FINDINGS

In the usual case of childhood NHL, the laboratory findings are frequently entirely normal, with the possible exception of an elevation in the serum levels of lactate dehydrogenase (LDH) and uric acid. Both levels are elevated because of the often high rate of cell proliferation and spontaneous tumor cell lysis and necrosis.

Peripheral blood findings are unremarkable in the absence of bone marrow involvement by tumor. A typical leukemic blood and bone marrow picture is found when tumor cells disseminate to replace normal marrow elements.

Since lymphomas (especially of B-cell origin) may occur as the first manifestation of AIDS, it is necessary to maintain a high index of suspicion and screen suspect cases for infection with HIV, for immunodeficiency (T_4 and T_8 cell counts, quantitative immunoglobulins), and for co-infections (e.g., with EBV or cytomegalovirus).

DIAGNOSIS AND DIFFERENTIAL DIAGNOSIS

The diagnosis of NHL in a child rests on demonstrating the typical histopathologic picture in an adequate biopsy specimen, usually obtained at surgery. Prompt and adequate tissue diagnosis is mandatory. The practice of repetitive fruitless trials of antibiotic therapy for progressive painless enlargement of peripheral lymph nodes must be avoided, although close observation of the response to antibiotic therapy for 10–14 days is reasonable if blood counts are normal and the

results of cultures, skin testing, and serology fail to identify an etiology for adenopathy. On occasion, lymphadenopathy simulating lymphoma may occur as a result of infectious mononucleosis, toxoplasmosis, histoplasmosis, or even juvenile rheumatoid arthritis. Patients presenting with a mediastinal mass without enlarged accessible cervical or supraclavicular nodes may require a limited thoracotomy or mediastinotomy for diagnosis, although one must recognize the additional risk of anesthesia. Children presenting with abdominal pain, a palpable abdominal mass, and/or symptoms suggestive of intussuception usually require laparotomy for tissue diagnosis. In such cases, in which the primary is gastrointestinal and localized to the ileocecal region, the preferred surgical approach is complete resection, usually by some variation of a right-sided hemicolectomy and removal of the distal ileum, cecum, appendix, and ascending colon with the associated mesentery and proximal mesenteric lymph nodes, followed by performance of an ileocolonic re-anastomosis. The importance of complete resection of localized gastrointestinal lymphoma whenever feasible, has been clearly shown by Fleming et al.,[28] who reported 100% survival for 24 such patients with localized gastrointestinal tumors who received modern treatment.

Under special circumstances, provided the clinical presentation is otherwise classic, the diagnosis of NHL may be established by cytologic examination and phenotyping of malignant cells aspirated from either pleural effusions, ascites, the marrow cavity, or spinal fluid. NHL may be difficult to distinguish from other lymphomas, leukemias, or histiocytic disorders. Expert hematopathologic consultation is required. Further immunologic and molecular phenotypic analysis can be extraordinarily useful, not only in distinguishing lymphoid tumors from other small round cell tumors of childhood, such as rhabdomyosarcoma, Ewing sarcoma, and neuroblastoma, but also in precisely classifying the nature and lineage of the lymphoid tumor. The addition of special immunologic, cytogenetic, and molecular studies to routine light microscopy is desirable in all cases (see Ch. 80).

STAGING

An expeditious investigation should be carried out in the child newly diagnosed with NHL to determine the anatomic extent of disease and the degree of organ impairment or biochemical disturbance present. The procedures recommended for a staging workup for childhood lymphomas are listed in Table 82-4.

A variety of radiographic and imaging techniques may be useful to demonstrate areas of tumor involvement. These studies include excretory urography, barium studies of the gastrointestinal tact, lateral soft tissue views of the nasopharynx, Panorex views of the mandible and maxilla, lymphangiography, ultrasound, myelography, bone scanning, whole-body gallium

Table 82-4. Recommended Staging Workup for Pediatric NHL

Required investigations
    Complete physical examination
    Complete blood counts
    Serum chemistries, particularly lactate dehydrogenase and uric acid
    Chest radiograph
    Computed tomographic scanning
    Radionuclide bone scanning
    Bone marrow examination
    Cerebrospinal fluid examination
Optional or contingent
    Gallium 67 scanning
    Cytologic examination of any effusions present
    Serologic studies for human immunodeficiency virus infection

scanning, and whole-body computed tomography (CT).[30,31] Disease is seldom demonstrated by such investigations unless it is already clinically suspected. An exception is the occasional otherwise occult finding of nephromegaly or hydronephrosis and hydroureter due to retroperitoneal or pelvic disease.

Given the range and variety of imaging modalities available nowadays, one can readily select from the menu of options the adequate minimum necessary to determine the initial extent of disease and to follow the response to therapy. Generally, plain films, barium studies, and contrast urography are now seldom performed. Lymphangiography is considerably less useful in childhood NHL than in HD, and the procedure should not be performed routinely in staging childhood NHL.

The effectiveness of CT for the accurate delineation of tumor extent, for treatment planning, and for monitoring response in lymphoma patients has been established.[32] The technique is particularly useful for imaging tumors in the head and neck, mediastinum, and/or abdominal and pelvic viscera. The roles of magnetic resonance imaging (MRI) and single photon emission computed tomographic (SPECT) scanning have not been clearly defined as yet. Unquestionably, these newer imaging modalities will increase the expense of a staging workup, with only scant likelihood of actually influencing therapeutic decision making. Since all children and adolescents with NHL require chemotherapy and the role of radiation therapy is extraordinarily limited, an excessive search for and definition of the anatomic limits of detectable disease is probably unwarranted.

Laparotomy and splenectomy for staging childhood NHL are not indicated, although as noted above (see the section Diagnosis and Differential Diagnosis), many children with abdominal lymphomas undergo exploratory laparotomy for diagnosis, biopsy, relief of intestinal obstruction, and partial or complete excision of abdominal tumor. For children with tumor localized to the gastrointestinal tract, in whom grossly complete excision of the tumor is possible, the staging designation is favorable (i.e., stage II), regardless of the status of mesenteric nodes. When only biopsy or incomplete surgical excision of abdominal lymphoma is possible, the stage of disease is upgraded and the prognosis is less favorable.[28]

Examination of the cerebrospinal fluid is essential to staging, although the initial examination can be deferred to coincide with the initiation of prophylactic intrathecal therapy at the onset of systemic treatment in order to spare the child an additional lumbar puncture. It is mandatory to review not only the number of cells present in the wet preparation of cerebrospinal fluid, but also their morphology on a Wright-stained cytocentrifuged cerebrospinal fluid specimen in order to assess adequately the presence or absence of initial leptomeningeal lymphoma. On occasion, focal neurologic deficits or cranial nerve palsies, or both, may signify involvement of the central nervous system in the absence of either detectable lymphoma cells in the lumbar cerebrospinal fluid or abnormalities on brain CT or MRI.

Examination of the bone marrow can generally be adequately achieved by percutaneous aspiration. Seldom will a bone marrow biopsy demonstrate disease that is not already apparent from inspection of a marrow smear.

At completion of the initial workup, a staging designation is assigned. The Ann Arbor staging system, developed for use in HD is not applicable to pediatric NHL. Alternative staging systems have been developed for pediatric NHL, which assist in determining prognosis, in selecting risk-adapted therapy, and in uniform reporting of end results.

One of the most widely used systems, the so-called Murphy staging or St. Jude system,[1] is outlined in Table 82-5. This clinical staging scheme is applicable to all histologic types of pediatric NHL and has the advantages of recognizing the major site(s) of tumor involvement for assignment of stage. It also

Table 82-5. Clinical Staging Classification for Childhood NHL

Stage	Criteria for Extent of Disease
I	Single tumor (extranodal) or single anatomic area (nodal), with the exclusion of mediastinum or abdomen
II	Single tumor (extranodal) with regional node involvement Two or more nodal areas on the same side of the diaphragm Two single (extranodal) tumors with or without regional node involvement on the same side of the diaphragm Primary gastrointestinal tract tumor, usually in the ileocecal area, with or without involvement of associated mesenteric nodes only, grossly completely resected
III	Two single tumors (extranodal) on opposite sides of the diaphragm Two or more nodal areas above and below the diaphragm All the primary intrathoracic tumors (mediastinal, pleural, thymic) All extensive primary intra-abdominal disease, unresectable; all paraspinal or epidural tumors, regardless of other tumor site(s)
IV	Any of the above with initial central nervous system and/or bone marrow involvement

(From Murphy,[1] with permission.)

reflects the prognostic advantage of complete surgical resection of abdominal disease (i.e., stage II) and in this regard resembles staging systems originally devised for African Burkitt lymphoma and modified for use at the National Cancer Institute.[33] A favorable prognosis is associated with localized regional disease (i.e., stage I or II), excluding the mediastinum. Furthermore, the system recognizes the grave prognosis (i.e, stage IV) associated with initial involvement of the marrow of the central nervous system, or both. The prognostic usefulness of this system has been extensively validated.[8,28,34–40]

Roughly 30–40% of pediatric NHL cases present with localized disease in favorable sites (i.e., stage I or II), while the remaining 60–70% of cases have more advanced disease.[8] Approximately 15% of patients present with tumors, normal blood counts, and <25% replacement of marrow elements by tumor (i.e., stage IV bone marrow-positive [BM+]).

THERAPY

General Stage- and Histology-Specific Strategy

In view of the diversity of histologies and immunophenotypes, each with variable natural histories, and the differences in stage or extent of disease at presentation, optimum management of lymphoma requires a risk-adapted, stage- and histology-specific approach.[8,34,40] The importance of adopting a histology-specific approach to therapy in advanced stages (III and IV) has been demonstrated convincingly by investigators of the Children's Cancer Study Group, who showed that the outcome of treatment is influenced by both the histologic subtype of disease and the therapeutic regimen followed. Thus, a 10-drug program (modified LSA$_2$-L$_2$) was more effective than a four-drug regimen (COMP) in patients with disseminated lymphoblastic disease (the 2-year failure-free survival rate was 76% versus 26%, respectively, $P = 0.0002$), whereas the four-drug program was more effective than the 10-drug program in patients with disseminated nonlymphoblastic disease (57% versus 28%, respectively, $P = 0.008$).[41] The need for further subclassification of diffuse advanced-stage nonlymphoblastic lymphomas into SNC cell (Burkitt and non-Burkitt pleomorphic) types and large cell tumors is based on distinct differences in natural history.[10,11,22] Large cell lymphomas are a histologically distinct, yet heterogeneous, group. When members of the Pediatric Oncology Group treated all nonlymphoblastic lymphomas with a uniform treatment plan consisting of multiple drugs (ACOP+) and radiation, large cell histology proved

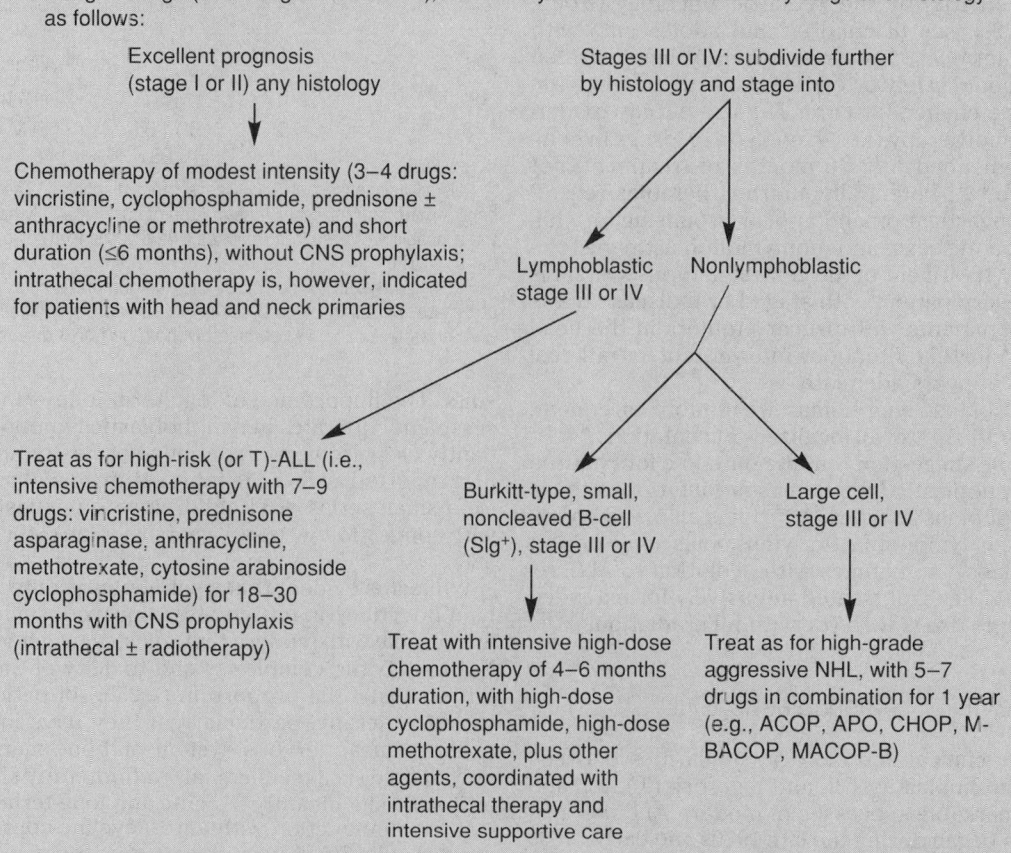

A STRATEGY FOR MANAGEMENT OF CHILDHOOD NHL

1. Establish diagnosis and classification by means of routine and special studies: tissue histopathology, immunophenotyping, cytogenetics, molecular diagnostics

2. Perform an expeditious staging evaluation (see Table 82-4)

3. Stabilize renal and metabolic status and anticipate risk of tumor lysis syndrome:
   Hydrate, alkalinize, begin allopurinol
   Check BUN, creatinine, uric acid, LDH, K^+, PO_4, Ca^{2+}, and urinary output

4. Assign a stage (according to Table 82-5), and stratify for treatment selection by stage and histology as follows:

Excellent prognosis (stage I or II) any histology

Stages III or IV: subdivide further by histology and stage into

Chemotherapy of modest intensity (3–4 drugs: vincristine, cyclophosphamide, prednisone ± anthracycline or methotrexate) and short duration (≤6 months), without CNS prophylaxis; intrathecal chemotherapy is, however, indicated for patients with head and neck primaries

Lymphoblastic stage III or IV

Nonlymphoblastic

Treat as for high-risk (or T)-ALL (i.e., intensive chemotherapy with 7–9 drugs: vincristine, prednisone asparaginase, anthracycline, methotrexate, cytosine arabinoside cyclophosphamide) for 18–30 months with CNS prophylaxis (intrathecal ± radiotherapy)

Burkitt-type, small, noncleaved B-cell (SIg^+), stage III or IV

Large cell, stage III or IV

Treat with intensive high-dose chemotherapy of 4–6 months duration, with high-dose cyclophosphamide, high-dose methotrexate, plus other agents, coordinated with intrathecal therapy and intensive supportive care

Treat as for high-grade aggressive NHL, with 5–7 drugs in combination for 1 year (e.g., ACOP, APO, CHOP, M-BACOP, MACOP-B)

1. No involved field radiotherapy should be used up front for any patient, regardless of histology or stage, but may be considered for biopsy-proven disease resistant to chemotherapy

2. High-dose ablative chemotherapy and autologous marrow re-infusion may be useful for refractory or relapsed NHL

---

to be an important favorable prognostic factor in patients with stage III and IV diseases (4-year event-free survival 67% for large cell cases versus 17% for SNC cases).[42] Although some approaches are reportedly effective for treatment of both lymphoblastic and nonlymphoblastic lymphomas, most major centers and all national pediatric cooperative clinical trials groups have adopted distinctly different strategies for different histologic types of childhood lymphomas.[35] Therapies effective for advanced-stage cases are clearly curative in the vast majority with less advanced disease.[35,37,41,42] Optimum therapy, however, requires proper consideration of the risk–benefit ratio of modern intensive therapies. Most patients treated are presently potentially curable, even those with advanced-stage disease. The 2-year event-free survival in 154 consecutive cases of children and adolescents with NHL who were seen and treated at St. Jude Children's Research Hospital from 1978–1986 was 77% ± 4%.[8] It is therefore imperative to adopt a risk-adapted strategy for management aimed at maximizing the chance for cure while minimizing the adverse acute and long-term consequences of treatment for children with lymphomas, most of whom will otherwise be at risk of potentially avoidable and unwanted late effects throughout their lives.

Stage I or II Localized Disease

The excellent outcome for children who present with localized disease in favorable areas (i.e., stage I or II) according to the staging classification shown in Table 82-5 is demonstrated by the series of end results presented in Table 82-6, demonstrating a cure rate of 84–90%.[36,43,45,46]

The trend in recent studies has been to eliminate radiotherapy and to lessen both the intensity and the duration of therapy for these children.[43,44] The use of involved field radiotherapy to encompass areas of localized disease dates back to the prechemotherapy era and has traditionally been considered part

Table 82-6. Results of Treatment of Localized (Stage I and II) NHL

No.	Event-Free Survival[a] (%)	Source
28	85.7	St. Jude Children's Research Hospital[36]
27	85–95	BFM Group[40]
73	84	Children's Cancer Study Group[45]
129	87	Pediatric Oncology Group[43]

[a] Usually assessed 2–3 years after diagnosis and roughly equivalent to cure rate, since the probability of late relapses is low.[46]

Table 82-7. Results of Treatment of Nonlocalized (Stage III and IV) Lymphoblastic NHL

No.	Event-Free Survival[a] (%)	Treatment	Source
124	64	LSA$_2$-L$_2$	Children's Cancer Study Group[46]
37	57	LSA$_2$-L$_2$	Pediatric Oncology Group[37]
15 (stage III)	93	LSA$_2$-L$_2$	Pediatric Oncology Group[49]
11 (stage IV)	12	LSA$_2$-L$_2$	Pediatric Oncology Group[49]
24	73	Total therapy	St. Jude Children's Research Hospital[50]
21	58	APO	Dana Farber[52]
84	75	LMT-81[b]	Institute Gustave Roussy[48]
178	75[c]	BFM-81, -83, -86	BFM Group[53,62]

[a] Usually assessed at 2–3 years after diagnosis. The percentages may be approximate but not precise estimates of cure rate in lymphoblastic lymphomas, the probability of even late relapses, (4–5 years from diagnosis) off therapy may be 10–15%.
[b] LSA$_2$-L$_2$ therapy, modified by the addition of 10 courses of high-dose methothrexate. Series includes 8 cases with stage I or II disease.
[c] Series includes 11% of cases with stage I or II disease.

of conventional management for lymphoma.[27,29,32,33,35] In a prospective randomized trial by the Pediatric Oncology Group, which included 129 cases of children and adolescents with stage I and II NHL, Link et al.,[43] however, recently demonstrated that radiotherapy could safely be omitted from treatment without jeopardizing the chance for cure. The use of only moderately intensive chemotherapy (i.e., 4, not 8 or 10, drugs in combination) is recommended[43,44]; ≤6 months of treatment, not longer, is adequate.[43,44] Potentially shorter therapies (e.g., 9 weeks) are under investigation and appear promising for children with localized disease and nonlymphoblastic histologies.[47] Prophylactic treatment of the central nervous system is not indicated for every patient with stage I or II disease but is reserved for those patients with primary tumors in the head and neck region.[43] In this situation, intermittent intrathecal chemoprophylaxis appears adequate.[43]

Localized lymphoblastic lymphomas are notably infrequent, accounting for only 10–15% of all localized presentations.[8,43–45] There has been some suggestion that the outcome for children with localized lymphoblastic lymphomas are inferior to those typical for nonlymphoblastic types.[43–45,47] It is also well appreciated that localized lymphoblastic lymphomas may exhibit late patterns of relapse, sometimes with evolution to ALL, regardless of treatment, even if treated intensively for extended periods with multiple drugs with (or without) radiation.[48,49]

Stage III–IV Lymphoblastic NHL

Because of many clinical and biologic similarities between advanced-stage lymphoblastic NHL and high-risk (T) ALL and because of the remarkable successes of modern ALL therapy, many investigators began during the late 1970s and early 1980s to apply intensive multiple-drug leukemia protocols and prophylactic treatment of the central nervous system (with or without involved field radiotherapy) to the treatment of lymphoblastic NHL.[41,48–53] This strategy of intensified chemotherapy with 7–10 agents over 2–3 years has led to impressive gains in disease-free survival, now in the ranges of 60–75% in published series of advanced-stage pediatric lymphoblastic lymphomas (Table 82-7).

One of the earliest reports of remarkable improvement in survival with intensive treatment was by Wollner et al.,[51] who in 1976 reported 76% overall disease-free survival (25 + months median follow-up) in a group of 43 children (all stages and histologies) treated with the 10-drug LSA$_2$-L$_2$ regimen (cyclophosphamide, prednisone, vincristine, daunomycin, methotrexate, cytosine arabinoside, thioguanine, L-asparaginase, BCNU, and hydroxyurea) for 2–3 years.[51] This reported success prompted many investigators and cooperative study groups to attempt to reproduce these results. Variable rates of success have resulted (Table 82-7). Careful review of all the data, both published and unpublished, from large numbers of cases of stage III and IV NHL treated with LSA$_2$-L$_2$ therapy and followed for 6–7 years suggests that overall cure rates of only about 60–75% are to be expected with LSA$_2$-L$_2$ type treatment, and modifications of LSA$_2$-L$_2$ or alternate approaches (e.g., strategies of the BFM group for the treatment of ALL[40] or Adriamycin, Vincristine [Oncovin], and prednisone) yield similar end re-

sults. The importance of long-term follow-up for adequate assessment cure rates in lymphoblastic lymphomas is also abundantly clear from the experience of Boston investigators, who first reported an 86% life-table estimate of disease-free survival for a small series of 11 children with mediastinal lymphomas; with longer follow-up (6 years median), this estimate fell to 58%.[52]

While it is evident that treatment and outcome for advanced lymphocytic NHL has greatly improved, such that most cases are curable with modern therapies, management is not optimal. Not only is the complexity and toxicity of therapy significant, but a substantial proportion (≥25%) of patients still may fail modern therapy, particularly if they have initial involvement of the central nervous system or bone marrow, or both. Involved field (i.e., mediastinal) radiotherapy should be avoided, as it adds significantly to acute and long-term morbidity (especially in conjunction with anthracycline-containing regimens); good results have been reported without it,[35,48,50] and a randomized prospective trial failed to demonstrate its benefit.[34] Rather than reliance on radiotherapy, better disease control is more apt to result from improved schedules of combination intravenous and intrathecal chemotherapy.

Stage III and IV Small Noncleaved Cell Lymphoma

Optimal management of advanced stage III and IV SNC, Burkitt-type lymphomas is based on intensive combination chemotherapy with high doses of both cyclophosphamide and methotrexate (at a minimum), together with intensive intrathecal chemotherapy plus other agents, including vincristine, high-dose cytosine arabinoside, ifosfamide, VP-16 (etoposide), and anthracyclines.[28,31,43–45]

On the basis of pioneering studies of African Burkitt patients, Ziegler applied high-dose cyclophosphamide-containing protocols to the treatment of nonendemic American Burkitt lymphoma patients and reported cures in 41% of advanced-stage patients.[56] Adopting a similar approach but escalating the dosage of methotrexate, Sullivan and Ramirez[55] reported survival of 75% of a group of 24 children (all stages) with Burkitt lymphoma. Murphy and colleagues[38] developed a regimen (Total B) using a novel fractionation scheme of high-dose cyclophosphamide (300 mg/m^2 bid for six doses) with coordinated in-

Table 82-8. Results of Treatment for Advanced SNC (Burkitt) Lymphomas

No.	Event-Free Survival (%)	Treatment	Source
37	41	74-0, 75-6	National Cancer Institute[56]
30 (stage III) 9 (stage IV)	57	77-04	National Cancer Institute[35]
72 (stage III) 48 (stage IV/B-ALL)	73 48	LMB-81	French Pediatric Oncology Society[54]
167 (stage III) 34 (stage IV/B-ALL)	80 68	LMB-84	French Pediatric Oncology Society[57]
105 (stage III) 22 (stage IV) 54 (B-ALL)	87 85 87	LMB-89	French Pediatric Oncology Society[58]
17 (stage III) 12 (stage IV/B-ALL)	81 20	Total B	St. Jude Children's Research Hospital[38]
52 (stage III)	76	Total B	Pediatric Oncology Group[59]
34 (stage IV) 47 (B-ALL)	75 60	Modified Total B[a]	Pediatric Oncology Group[60]
22 (B-ALL)	43	BFM-81	BFM Group[62]
24 (B-ALL)	50	BFM-83	
41 (B-ALL)	78	BFM-86	
94[b]	74	BFM-90	BFM Group[61]
18	90	Regimen II A-B	Instituto Nazional Tumori, Milan[63]
20	75%	HI C-COM	Boston[64]

[a] Modified by the substitution of high doses of cytarabine (3 g/m^2) for moderate doses by infusion.

[b] Includes patients with bone marrow involvement (n = 51) and/or central nervous system disease (n = 17) and those cases with unresectable abdominal disease and initial lactate dehydrogenase ≥500 U/L.

trathecal and intravenous methotrexate and cytosine arabinoside, which yielded improved results, producing cures of 14 of 17 (81%) stage III cases. These results were subsequently confirmed by the Pediatric Oncology Group in a large randomized trial (#8616) enrolling 126 stage III patients,[59] in which 76% of 52 children treated with Total B therapy[38] were disease-free at 2 years, compared to 62% treated with the regimen used by Sullivan et al.[55] Other pediatric groups from France, Germany, and Italy, have reported high cure rates for Burkitt lymphoma (80–90%), with intensive polychemotherapy regimens incorporating additional agents and higher drug dosages.[57,58,61,62]

Results of modern treatments of stage III and IV small noncleaved B (SIg$^+$) cell NHL and ALL (with >25% or complete replacement of marrow by blasts) are summarized in Table 82-8. The results demonstrate that even extensive disease is now curable in 80% or more of cases by aggressive chemotherapy, and that even patients with initially high tumor burdens (>500 IU serum LDH at diagnosis) or those presenting with initial involvement of the central nervous system or bone marrow, are curable with reported regimens. The acute toxicity from all reported regimens is severe, often life-threatening, requiring intensive supportive care.

It is clear that the duration of treatment for advanced stage SNC tumors need not be prolonged. Relatively short (2–4 months) intensive programs are able to eradicate disease in most patients, even in the presence of central nervous system or bone marrow involvement, or both.[57,63,64]

Stage III and IV Large Cell Lymphomas

Published data regarding the results of treatment of large cell lymphomas in children and adolescents are limited but demonstrate curability of most cases. Weinstein et al.[65] re-

ported a relapse-free survival rate of 86% for 16 patients with disseminated disease (stages III and IV) treated with the APO protocol (Adriamycin, vincristine [Oncovin], and prednisone) for 2 years with prophylactic cranial irradiation and regional radiotherapy. Santana and co-workers[66] reported 55% disease-free survival among 13 children and adolescents with advanced-stage (III and IV) large cell lymphomas treated for 12 weeks with MACOP-B (methotrexate, vincristine, bleomycin, cyclophosphamide, Adriamycin, and prednisone) without radiotherapy.

Five-year estimates for disease-free survival for 42 children and adolescents with disseminated large cell lymphoma treated by investigators of the Children's Cancer Study Group with the four-drug COMP regimen (cyclophosphamide, vincristine, methotrexate, and prednisone) plus radiation are 52%, compared to 43% for 18 treated with LSA$_2$-L$_2$ therapy.[46] Hvizadala et al.[42] reported 67% 4-year disease-free survival for 22 patients with stage III–IV large cell NHL treated with the ACOP+ regimen (Adriamycin, cyclophosphamide, vincristine, prednisone, methotrexate, mercaptopurine) plus radiation.

SALVAGE TREATMENT

Patients with relapsed or refractory NHL constitute a group with a particularly poor outlook, who may be considered for investigational therapies and/or myeloablative treatments supported by allogeneic or autologous bone marrow transplantation.[48,49] Post-transplant relapse or death from acute complications, however, still occurs in most pediatric (or adult) recipients of either allogeneic or autologous transplants for NHL. Clearly, improvement in conditioning regimens and refinements in transplantation techniques are needed.

SUPPORTIVE CARE

Meticulous attention to all aspects of supportive care is necessary to ensure success in end results of the intensive treatments necessary for patients with stage III or IV NHL. Supportive measures necessary at the onset of treatment routinely include initiation of allopurinol (100–300 mg/m^2/day) and measures to promote alkaline diuresis to prevent uric acid nephropathy and massive tumor cell lysis syndrome. Ensuring central venous access, usually by placement of a Hickman/Broviac catheter or totally implantable port, greatly facilitates management. Transfusions of irradiated packed red blood cells and platelets are needed for symptomatic anemia and bleeding. Administration of appropriate broad-spectrum antibiotics and/or antifungals is necessary for neutropenia, fever, and presumed or documented infection. Administration of recombinant human hematopoietic growth factors, such as colony-stimulating factor-granulocyte or colony-stimulating factor-granulocyte/macrophage, at intervals following high-dose chemotherapy will significantly shorten the duration of several neutropenia and reduce the frequency of febrile and septic episodes. The prophylactic use of trimethoprim-sulfamethoxazole is indicated to prevent *Pneumocystis carinii* pneumonitis. Total parenteral nutrition must be considered for patients who are in a catabolic state due to the effects of tumor and/or in whom the effects of intensive treatment and complications interfere with normal nutritional intake.

PROGNOSTIC FACTORS

The most important determinants of outcome in children and adolescents are the initial body burden of tumor and the adequacy of the primary treatment.[8] The initial tumor mass is reflected by stage or other serum markers, such as LDH, which accumulate as a consequence of tumor cell numbers. The adverse impact of either tumor bulk, advanced stage, or initially highly elevated levels of serum LDH (i.e., >1,000 IU) has been repeatedly demonstrated.[8,35,69] The serum level of soluble IL-2 receptors was reported by Pui et al.[70] to correlate with disease stage and serum LDH levels and to predict treatment failure in childhood NHL. The adverse impact of the presence of initial involvement of the bone marrow or central nervous system is well recognized but no longer constitutes an absolute obstacle to cure, provided therapies are appropriately intensified. The independent prognostic significance of immunophenotype, chromosomal alterations, or molecular genetic rearrangements in tumor tissues from children with NHL requires further study. As treatments have improved to the point where 8 of 10 children with lymphomas are cured, the impact of prognostic factors diminishes or vanishes.

FUTURE DIRECTIONS

Current problems remaining in the treatment of childhood NHL include relapse, undesirable side effects of therapy, and cost (financial and emotional), as well as the complexity of modern therapies. Clearly, the improved cure rates in advanced stages are the result of intensive therapy and vigorous supportive treatments, generally achievable only at centers with experienced teams capable of caring for myelosuppressed and immunocompromised patients. Aside form the acute toxicity typical of treatments necessary for children with advanced-stage disease, long-term adverse consequences of treatment in survivors, including sterility and second malignancies, are likewise cause for concern.

One would hope that future therapies could be developed that would be more rational, less empirical, and less toxic, relying more on strategies for growth control and regulation of gene expression and of cell proliferation than on cytotoxic or ablative treatments. The goal of future investigations must be a complete genetic and biochemical understanding of the molecular events that lead to NHL in children. Complete biochemical understanding may ultimately lead to identification of either unique or exaggerated metabolic steps in lymphoma cells, which may be amenable to specific manipulation. If either deregulated or mutated cellular proto-oncogenes, or both, are assumed to be the proximate causes of NHL, the proto-oncogenes or their growth factor products, or both, will be the likely targets for the next generation of anticancer therapy.

REFERENCES

1. Murphy SB: Classification, staging, and end results of treatment of childhood non-Hodgkin's lymphomas: dissimilarities from lymphomas in adults. Semin Oncol 7:332, 1980
2. Young JL, Miller RW: Incidence of malignant tumors in U.S. children. J Pediatr 85:254, 1975
3. Hutchison RE, Pui C-H, Murphy SB, Berard CW: Non-Hodgkin's lymphoma in children younger than 3 years. Cancer 62:1371, 1988
4. Purtilo DT: Opportunistic non-Hodgkin's lymphoma in X-linked recessive immunodeficiency and lymphoproliferative syndromes. Semin Oncol 4:335, 1977
5. Patton DF, Sixbey JW, Murphy SB: Epstein-Barr virus in human immunodeficiency virus-related Burkitt lymphoma. J Pediatr 113:951, 1988
6. McClain KL, Rosenblatt H: Pediatric HIV infection and AIDS: clinical expression of malignancy. Semin Pediatr Infect Dis 1:124, 1990
7. Aricò M, Caselli D, D'Argenio P et al: Malignancies in children with human immunodeficiency virus type 1 infection. Cancer 68:2473, 1991
8. Murphy SB, Fairclough DL, Hutchinson RE, Berard CW: Non-Hodgkin's lymphomas of childhood: an analysis of the histology, staging, and response to treatment of 338 cases at a single institution. J Clin Oncol 7:186, 1989
9. Griffith RC, Kelly DR, Nathwani BN et al: A morphologic study of childhood lymphoma of the lymphoblastic type: the Pediatric Oncology Group experience. Cancer 59:1126, 1987
10. Kelly DR, Nathwani BN, Griffith RC et al: A morphologic study of childhood lymphoma of the undifferentiated type: the Pediatric Oncology Group experience. Cancer 59:1132, 1987
11. Nathwani BN, Griffith RC, Kelly DR et al: A morphologic study of childhood lymphoma of the diffuse "histiocytic" type: the Pediatric Oncology Group experience. Cancer 59:1138, 1987
12. Report to the Writing Committee: National Cancer Institute sponsored study of classifications of non-Hodgkin's lymphomas: summary and description of a working formulation for clinical usage. The Non-Hodgkin's Lymphoma Pathologic Classification Project. Cancer 49:2112, 1982
13. Frizzera G, Murphy SB: Follicular (nodular) lymphoma in childhood: a rare clinical pathologic entity. Report of eight cases from four cancer centers. Cancer 44:2218, 1979
14. Winberg CD, Nathwani BN, Bearman RM et al: Follicular (nodular) lymphoma during the first two decades of life: a clinicopathologic study of 12 patients. Cancer 48:2223, 1981
15. Hutchison RE, Murphy SB, Fairclough DL et al: Diffuse small noncleaved-cell lymphoma in children, Burkitt's versus non-Burkitt's types: results from the Pediatric Oncology Group and St. Jude Children's Research Hospital. Cancer 64:23, 1989
16. Reinherz EL, Nadler LM, Sallan SE, Schlossman SF: Subset derivation of T-cell acute lymphoblastic leukemia in man. J Clin Invest 64:392, 1979
17. Roper M, Crist WM, Metzgar R et al: Monoclonal antibody characterization of surface antigens in childhood T-cell lymphoid malignancies. Blood 61:830, 1983
18. Bernard A, Boumsell L, Reinherz EL et al: Cell surface characterization of malignant T-cells from lymphoblastic lymphoma using monoclonal antibodies. Blood 57:1105, 1981
19. Bernard A, Murphy S, Melvin S et al: Non-T, non-B lymphomas are rare in childhood and associated with cutaneous tumor. Blood 59:549, 1982
20. Link M, Roper M, Dorfman R et al: Cutaneous lymphoblastic lymphoma with pre-B markers. Blood 61:838, 1983
21. Doggett RS, Wood GS, Horning S et al: The immunologic characterization of 95 nodal and extranodal diffuse large cell lymphomas in 89 patients. Am J Pathol 115:245, 1984
22. Hutchison RE, Fairclough DL, Holt H et al: Clinical significance of histology and immunophenotype in childhood diffuse large cell lymphoma. Am J Clin Pathol 95:787, 1991
23. Hutchison RE, Berard CW, Shuster JJ et al: Immunophenotype influences survival in pediatric large cell lymphoma. A Pediatric Oncology Group Study, abstracted (83). In Proceedings of the Fifth International Conference on Malignant Lymphomas, Lugano, 1993
24. Kadin ME, Sako D, Berliner N et al: Childhood Ki-1 lymphoma presenting with skin lesions and peripheral lymphadenopathy. Blood 68:1042, 1986
25. Schnitzer B, Roth MS, Hyder DM, Ginsburg D: Ki-1 lymphomas in children. Cancer 61:1213, 1988
26. Kadin ME. Ki-1-positive anaplastic large-cell lymphoma: a clinicopathologic entity? J Clin Oncol 9:533, 1991
27. Murphy SB: Pediatric lymphomas: recent advances and commentary on Ki-1 + anaplastic large cell lymphomas of childhood. Ann Oncol, suppl. 5:S31, 1994
28. Fleming ID, Turk PS, Murphy SB et al: Surgical implications of primary gastrointestinal lymphoma of childhood. Arch Surg 125:252, 1990
29. Jenkin RDT: The management of malignant lymphoma in childhood. p. 341. In Deeley TJ (ed): Modern Radiotherapy—Malignant Disease in Children. Butterworths, London, 1974
30. Castellino RA, Bellani FF, Gasparini M et al: Radiographic findings in previously untreated children with non-Hodgkin's lymphoma. Radiology 117:657, 1975
31. Martin DJ, Ash JM: Diagnostic radiology in non-Hodgkin's lymphoma. Semin Oncol 4:297, 1977
32. Pilepich MV, Rene JB, Munzenrider JE, Carter BL: Contribution of computed tomography to the treatment of lymphomas. AJR 131:69, 1978
33. Magrath I: Malignant non-Hodgkin's lymphomas. p. 554. In Pizzo PA, Poplack DG (eds): Principles and Practice of Pediatric Oncology. 2nd Ed. JB Lippincott, Philadelphia, 1993
34. Murphy SB, Hustu HO: A randomized trial of combined modality therapy of childhood non-Hodgkin's lymphoma. Cancer 45:630, 1980
35. Magrath IT, Janus C, Edwards BK et al: An effective therapy for both undifferentiated (including Burkitt's) lymphomas and lymphoblastic lymphomas in children and young adults. Blood 63:1102, 1984
36. Murphy SB, Hustu HO, Rivera G, Berard CW: End results of treating children with localized non-Hodgkin's lymphoma with a combined modality approach of lessened intensity. J Clin Oncol 1:326, 1983
37. Sullivan MP, Boyett J, Pullen J et al: Pediatric Oncology Group experience

with modified LSA$_2$-L$_2$ therapy in 107 children with non-Hodgkin's lymphoma (Burkitt's lymphoma excluded). Cancer 55:323, 1985

38. Murphy SB, Bowman WP, Abromowitch M et al: Results of treatment of advanced-stage Burkitt's lymphoma and B cell (SIg+) acute lymphoblastic leukemia with high-dose fractionated cyclophosphamide and coordinated high-dose methotrexate and cytarabine. J Clin Oncol 4:1732, 1986

39. Murphy SB: Strategies for management of childhood non-Hodgkin's lymphomas based upon stage and immunopathologic subtype: rationale and current results. p. 627. In Cavalli F, Bonadonna G, Rozencweig M (eds): Malignant Lymphomas and Hodgkin's Disease: Experimental and Therapeutic Advances. Martinus Nijhoff, Boston, 1985

40. Mueller-Weihrich S, Henze G, Odenwald E, Riehm H: BFM trials for childhood non-Hodgkin's lymphomas. p. 633. In Cavalli F, Bonadonna G, Rozencweig M (eds): Malignant Lymphomas and Hodgkin's Disease: Experimental and Therapeutic Advances. Martinus Nijhoff, Boston, 1985

41. Anderson JR, Wilson JF, Jenkin DT et al: Childhood non-Hodgkin's lymphoma: the results of a randomized therapeutic trial comparing a 4-drug regimen (COMP) with a 10-drug regimen (LSA$_2$-L$_2$). N Engl J Med 308:559, 1983

42. Hvizdala EV, Berard C, Callihan T et al: Non-lymphoblastic lymphoma in children: histology and stage related response to therapy: a Pediatric Oncology Group study. J Clin Oncol 9:1189, 1991

43. Link M, Donaldson SS, Berard CW et al: A randomized trial demonstrates that involved field radiotherapy can safely be omitted from treatment of localized non-Hodgkin's lymphoma childhood: a Pediatric Oncology Group study. N Engl J Med 322:1169, 1990

44. Meadows AT, Sposto R, Jenkin RDT et al: Similar efficacy of six and eighteen months of therapy with four drugs (COMP) for localized non-Hodgkin's lymphoma of children: a report from the Children's Cancer Study Group. J Clin Oncol 7:92, 1989

45. Jenkin RDT, Anderson JR, Chilcote RR et al: The treatment of localized non-Hodgkin's lymphoma in children: a report from the Children's Cancer Study Group. J Clin Oncol 2:88, 1984

46. Anderson JR, Jenkin DT, Wilson JF, Kjeldsberg CR: Long-term follow-up of patients treated with COMP or LSA$_2$L$_2$ therapy for childhood non-Hodgkin's lymphoma: a report of CCG-551 from the Children's Cancer Group. J Clin Oncol 11:1024, 1993

47. Link MP, Shuster JJ, Berard CW, Murphy SB: Nine weeks of chemotherapy without radiotherapy is sufficient treatment for most children with localized non-Hodgkin's lymphoma (NHL). Proc Am Soc Clin Oncol 12:384, 1993

48. Patte C, Kalifa C, Flamant F, Hartmann O: Results of the LMT81 protocol, a modified LSA$_2$L$_2$ protocol with high dose methotrexate, on 84 children with non-B-cell (lymphoblastic) lymphoma. Med Pediatr Oncol 20:105, 1992

49. Hvizdala EV, Berard C, Callihan T et al: Lymphoblastic lymphoma in children—a randomized trial comparing LSA$_2$L$_2$ with the A-COP+ therapeutic regimen: a Pediatric Oncology Group study. J Clin Oncol 6:26, 1988

50. Dahl GV, Rivera G, Pui C-H et al: A novel treatment of childhood lymphoblastic non-Hodgkin's lymphoma: early and intermittent use of teniposide plus cytarabine. Blood 66:1110, 1985

51. Wollner N, Burchenal JH, Lieberman PH et al: Non-Hodgkin's lymphoma in children: a comparative study of two modalities of therapy. Cancer 37:123, 1976

52. Weinstein HJ, Cassady JR, Levey R: Long-term results of the APO protocol (vincristine, doxorubicin, Adriamycin, and prednisone) for treatment of mediastinal lymphoblastic lymphoma. J Clin Oncol 1:537, 1983

53. Schrappe M, Reiter A, Gadner H et al: Childhood non-Hodgkin's lymphoma of the non-B-cell type (NB-NHL): treatment results of three BFM trials, abstracted (80). In Proceedings of the Fifth International Conference on Malignant Lymphoma, Lugano, 1993

54. Patte C, Philip T, Rodary C et al: Improved survival rate in children with stage III and IV B-cell non-Hodgkin's lymphoma and leukemia using multi-agent chemotherapy: results of a study of 114 children from the French Pediatric Oncology Society. J Clin Oncol 4:1219, 1986

55. Sullivan MP, Ramirez I: Curability of Burkitt's lymphoma with high-dose cyclophosphamide-high-dose methotrexate therapy and intrathecal chemophylaxis. J Clin Oncol 3:627, 1985

56. Ziegler JL: Treatment results of 54 American patients with Burkitt's lymphoma are similar to the African experience. N Engl J Med 297:75, 1977

57. Patte C, Philip T, Rodary C: High survival rate in advanced-stage B-cell lymphomas and leukemias without CNS involvement with a short intensive polychemotherapy: results from the French Pediatric Oncology Society of a randomized trial of 216 children. J Clin Oncol 9:123, 1991

58. Patte C, Leverger G, Michon J: High survival rate of childhood B-cell lymphoma and leukemia (ALL). As a result of the LMB 89 protocol of the SFOP (French Pediatric Oncology Society). In Proceedings of the Fifth International Conference on Malignant Lymphoma, Lugano, 1993

59. Brecher M, Murphy SB, Bowman P et al: Results of Pediatric Oncology Group (POG 8616): a randomized trial of two forms of therapy for stage III diffuse, small non-cleaved cell lymphoma in children. Proc ASCO 11:340, 1992

60. Bowman WP, Shuster J, Cook B et al: Improved survival for children with B cell (SIg+) Acute Lymphoblastic Leukemia (B-ALL) and stage IV small non-cleaved cell lymphoma (SNCCL). Proc ASCO 11:277, 1992

61. Reiter A, Henzler D, Schrappe M: B-Cell neoplasia in childhood: risk group stratification, treatment strategy and preliminary results of trial NHL-BFM 90. In Proceedings of the Fifth International Conference on Malignant Lymphoma, Lugano, 1993

62. Reiter A, Schrappe M, Ludwig WD, Lampert F: Favorable outcome of B-cell acute lymphoblastic leukemia in childhood: a report of three consecutive studies of the BFM group. Blood 80:2471, 1992

63. Gasparini M, Rottoli L, Massimino M, Gianni MC: Curability of advanced Burkitt's lymphoma in children by intensive short-term chemotherapy. Eur J Cancer 29A:692, 1993

64. Schwenn M, Blattner SR, Lynch E, Weinstein HJ: HiC-COM: a 2-month intensive chemotherapy regimen for children with stage III and IV Burkitt's lymphoma and B-cell acute lymphoblastic leukemia. J Clin Oncol 9:133, 1991

65. Weinstein HJ, Lack EE, Cassady JR: APO therapy for malignant lymphoma of large cell "histiocytic" type of childhood: analysis of treatment results for 29 patients. Blood 64:422, 1984

66. Santana VM, Abromowitch M, Sandlund JT et al: MACOP-B treatment in children and adolescents with advanced diffuse large cell non-Hodgkin's lymphoma. Leukemia 7:187, 1993

67. Philip T, Pinkerton R, Hartmann O et al: The role of massive therapy with autologous bone marrow transplantation in Burkitt's lymphoma. Baillieres Clin Haematol 15:205, 1984

68. Hartmann O, Pein F, Beaujean F et al: High-dose polychemotherapy with autologous bone marrow transplantation in children with relapsed lymphomas. J Clin Oncol 2:979, 1984

69. Magrath I, Lee YJ, Anderson T et al: Prognostic factors in Burkitt's lymphoma: importance of total tumor burden. Cancer 45:1507, 1980

70. Pui C-H, Ip SH, Kung P et al: High serum interleukin-2 receptor levels are related to advanced disease and a poor outcome in childhood non-Hodgkin's lymphoma. Blood 70:624, 1987

Chronic Lymphocytic Leukemia

83

Kanti R. Rai and Dilip V. Patel

INTRODUCTION

Chronic lymphocytic leukemia (CLL) as a distinct clinical entity was first identified in 1903 by Turk,[1] who gave us not only criteria for its diagnosis but also the features that distinguish it from lymphomas. In 1924 Minot and Isaacs[2] presented a detailed clinical description of CLL. Although several physicians studied this disease in the ensuing decades, it was not until 1966–1967 that the pathophysiology of CLL was fully explained. Galton[3] and Dameshek[4] independently but virtually simultaneously suggested that the main characteristic of CLL is a progressive accumulation of functionally incompetent, long-lived lymphocytes.

EPIDEMIOLOGY

CLL is the most common form of leukemia in the Western Hemisphere, accounting for about 25–30% of all leukemias. Approximately 10,000 new cases are diagnosed every year in the United States.[5] Characteristically, CLL is a disease of advancing age, the incidence being >20 per 100,000 persons >60 years of age.[6] However, the disease is being diagnosed in increasing frequency among younger age groups and is no longer considered unusual even in patients 35 years of age. The median age at diagnosis is 55 years. The incidence of CLL is higher among men, with the male/female ratio being nearly 2:1. CLL is rarely seen in Japan, China, and other Asian countries. The reason for this wide disparity in incidence of CLL in different parts of the world remains unknown. More than 95% of patients have a B-cell phenotype; T-cell CLL is a rare disease, accounting for only 2–5% of all cases. Unless otherwise specified, most descriptions of CLL pertain to B-cell disease.

GENETIC ASPECTS

CLL is an acquired disorder. There is one report in the literature of CLL occurring in twin sisters who were monozygous, but not identical. Immunoglobulin gene rearrangements in the CLL cells of these twins were found to differ from each other.[7] Relatives of CLL patients have an increased frequency of CLL, other B-cell malignancies, and autoimmune disorders.[8–11] The risk of developing CLL among first-degree relatives of patients with CLL is higher than expected. Consanguinity and chromosomal abnormalities have been proposed as possible explanations. No HLA haplotype has been found to be consistently associated with CLL.[12]

ETIOLOGY AND ONCOGENESIS

The etiology of B-CLL remains unknown. No causal relationship has been found with exposure to radiation, chemicals, and alkylating agents. Human T-cell leukemia/lymphoma virus 1 (HTLV-1) is known to cause adult T-cell leukemia. Although retroviruses and DNA viruses such as HTLV-1 and Epstein-Barr virus (EBV) are not considered to be etiologic agents for CLL, Mann et al.[13] have observed two patients with B-CLL who were HTLV-1 seropositive, but the virus was not present in the cellular genome.

In CLL there is a progressive accumulation of the leukemic lymphocytes, with no increase in their rate of proliferation. Lymphocytes in CLL are known to be long-lived. The early observations of Galton[3] and Dameshek[4] suggested that CLL lymphocytes are long-lived because they are functionally incompetent. The still unfolding story of the proto-oncogene bcl-2, however, indicates that at least in some cases of CLL the explanation for lymphocyte longevity may be the inhibition of programmed cell death (apoptosis). It was observed, initially in follicular lymphoma, that there is an association between the rearrangement of bcl-2 and t(14;18) chromosomal translocation. bcl-2 is known to interfere with apoptosis.

Early studies in CLL showed that only about 10% of patients had rearrangement of bcl-2.[14,15] However, subsequent studies have revealed that there are alternative mechanisms that result in accumulation of high levels of bcl-2 protein in CLL cells, which are independent of bcl-2 rearrangements.[16] One possible mechanism is DNA-hypomethylation. Hanada et al.[16] demonstrated DNA hypomethylation in a relatively selected region of the bcl-2 gene in 20 of 20 CLL cases studied. These data favor the explanation that an overexpression of bcl-2 protein, with its known ability to interfere with apoptosis, results in the long life of CLL lymphocytes.

GROWTH AND DIFFERENTIATION

Leukemic cells in CLL are known to be "arrested" in the G_0 phase of the cell cycle with a relatively rare cell in the peripheral blood showing evidence of being in the active proliferative cycle.[17,18] CLL cells, arrested in the late stages of B-cell differentiation, reveal certain characteristics in vitro that may explain at least some aspects of the pathophysiology of this disease. When cultured[19] without cytokines and mitogens, in vitro, CLL cells die rapidly by apoptosis. It has been demonstrated that CLL cells lose bcl-2 protein during culture.[20] Addition of interleukin (IL)-4[21] or interferon (IFN)-γ[22] to the cultures inhibits the cell death by apoptosis, an observation correlated with a simultaneous increased expression of bcl-2 protein in IL-4-treated B-CLL cells.[21] When CLL cells are cultured in the presence of B-cell mitogens or the phorbol ester TPA (12-0-tetradecanoylphorbol-13-acetate), they are capable of plasmacytoid differentiation, suggesting that these cells are not "frozen" at an intermediate stage in the B-cell differentiation pathway. The process of stimulation of differentiation of CLL cells, however, is complex and requires all the co-stimulatory factors necessary for normal B cells undergoing differentiation in vitro, including various cytokine producing non-neoplastic T cells.[23]

CHROMOSOMAL ABNORMALITIES

CLL lymphocytes are resting cells in G_0 and in vitro have no spontaneous mitoses. Until the recent introduction of B-cell mitogens, cytogenetic studies were not possible in CLL be-

1308

cause metaphases were only rarely inducible. In the past decade, however, several laboratories have been successful in performing cytogenetic studies in CLL following the availability of a battery of B-cell mitogens, including lipopolysaccharide, TPA, cytochalasin B, pokeweed mitogen, and EBV supernate, which induce readable metaphases in a large proportion of cases. Juliusson and Gahrton[24] in an update on the cytogenetic data pooled by the International Working Party on Chromosomes in CLL and from additional data from the published literature, have provided a detailed status report on this subject. In this collected series[24] of G-banded metaphase analysis of 1,244 cases of CLL, clonal chromosomal abnormalities were seen in 43% (533 cases), and trisomy 12 was the most frequently observed abnormality, occuring in about 15% of all patients studied and about one-third of all cases with clonal abnormalities. Structural abnormalities involving the long arm of chromosome 13 accounted for 20% of cases with clonal abnormalities, and other, less frequently occurring structural abnormalities involved the long arms of chromosomes 6 and 14.[24]

Although structural abnormalities of the long arm of chromosome 13 involved different breakpoints, most consisted of deletion of band 13q14, the site of retinoblastoma (Rb) suppressor gene. The Rb gene product, however, is normally expressed in patients with 13q14 deletion,[25,26] perhaps because the other allele has a normal Rb gene.

Structural abnormalities involving chromosome 14 is of particular interest because this chromosome is the site for the genes for immunoglobulin heavy chain at band q32 at the distal end of the long arm. Clonal abnormalities in B-cell malignancies sometimes involve 14q32, including t(11;14) (q13;q32), which juxtaposes the bcl-1 gene[27,28] and the immunoglobulin heavy chain gene.

Among the cases with chromosomal abnormalities, more than one-half are constituted by single abnormalities and complex abnormalities are seen in 10–15%.[24]

Fluorescence in situ hybridization (FISH) with a chromosome 12-specific α-centromeric probe has enabled a study of numerical abnormalities of this chromosome in interphase cells in CLL, thereby overcoming the problem of inconsistency in inducing mitoses by banding techniques that require readable metaphases.[29] Using the FISH technique, Que et al.[30] noted trisomy 12 in 21 of 183 (11.5%) cases of CLL, whereas the conventional cytogenetic techniques could detect trisomy 12 in only 15 of these 21 cases. It is likely that further studies with the FISH technique will be useful in establishing the exact incidence of trisomy 12 in CLL without the need to depend on obtaining adequate metaphase preparations. However, the need to identify chromosomal abnormalities other than trisomy 12 requires that both conventional cytogenetics and FISH are necessary. At this time, cytogentic studies are not performed in the routine clinical management of CLL—they remain in the research domain.

IMMUNOPHENOTYPIC PROFILE OF LYMPHOCYTES

B-Cells

The normal T-cell/B-cell ratio is reversed in CLL. In B-CLL, the B cells usually account for nearly 90% of all lymphocytes. There is a characteristic immunophenotypic profile of B-cells as shown in Table 83-1.[31–33] CLL B-cells express low surface density of immunoglobulins, usually IgM or IgM with IgD, which are monoclonal as revealed by expression of only one light chain, either κ or λ. These cells form rosettes with mouse erythrocytes. Intracytoplasmic immunoglobulins may be detectable in a few cases. Some B cells have receptors for Fc fragments, for IgG, and for complement (C3d). By using a wide range of monoclonal antibodies, it has been established that B cells of

Table 83-1. Immunophenotypic Pattern of B-CLL Cells

Surface immunoglobulin (sIg):
    Usually IgM or IgM and IgD of low intensity (infrequently, the amount of sIg may be so low that the cell is read as sIg negative)
Mouse-erythrocytes rosetting
One or more of the following B-cell markers
    CD19 (B4), CD20 (B1), CD24 (BA1), CD21 (C3dR), CD23 (activation marker)
Ia
CD5 (pan-T, Leu-1)
Heterogeneous with respect to
    CD11c (β₂ integrin)
    Surface adhesion molecules CD54, CD58, L-selectin, and CD25 (IL-2 receptor)

B-CLL stain positively with one pan-T-cell antibody Leu-1 (CD5),[34–36] while simultaneously also staining with at least one of the B-cell monoclonal antibodies B1 (CD20), B4 (CD19), and BA1 (CD24). These cells express HLA-DR, the MHC class II antigen. There is considerable degree of heterogeneity in the expression of CD25 (IL-2 receptor), CD23 (activation marker, low-affinity FcE receptor), and CD11c (β₂ integrin) and surface adhesion molecules CD54, CD58, and L-selectin.[31,32,37] The overall interpretation of this phenotypic expression is that CLL cells are relatively mature cells that are arrested at an intermediate stage in the pathway of B-cell differentiation.

The CD5 positivity of B cells in CLL has become a subject of active investigation. A very small subset of normal B lymphocytes is known to be CD5+.[34] It is not clear whether this normal CD5+ B-cell subpopulation is the one that proliferates and accumulates in CLL.[38] Normal CD5+ B cells express activation markers and >10% of these cells may be in active proliferative cycle, whereas only <1% of CD5+ B cells in CLL are in active cycle[38] (Table 83-1). Investigations in this area, however, do not provide clear evidence that CD5+ B cells constitute a separate B-cell lineage.[39]

T Cells and Natural Killer Cells

The absolute number of T cells in B-CLL may be normal, decreased, or increased according to the total lymphocyte count and percentage of T cells. There is usually a reversal of the normal T-helper (CD4)/T-suppressor (CD8) cell ratio.[40–42] The population of large granular lymphocytes (natural killer [NK] cells) is usually decreased.[38,41–44] The published work on the functional status of T cells and NK cells in CLL is contradictory and difficult to interpret.[39,45]

Autoimmune Complications

Autoimmune complications are known to occur frequently in CLL.[46] It has been suggested that CD5+ B cells may play an important role in the production of IgM autoantibodies. An increase in the number of CD5+ B cells has been reported in rheumatoid arthritis and other autoimmune diseases.[47] Autoimmune phenomena in CLL are often directed against hematopoietic cells. A positive direct antiglobulin test has been reported in ≤35% of CLL cases. Autoimmune hemolytic anemia may occur in 10–25% of cases at some time during the course of the disease.[39] In most cases the autoantibodies against erythrocytes are warm reactive and polyclonal[48] with or without red-cell-associated C₃b or C₃d. Immune thrombocytopenia occurs in about 2% of CLL cases. Pure red cell aplasia and autoantibodies against neutrophils are observed less frequently.

Table 83-2. Factors Contributing to Immunodeficiency in CLL

Reduced serum immunoglobulin
Reduced percentage of CD4+ cells, increased percentage of CD8+ cells (worsening with disease prognosis)
Reduced response to antigens and mitogens

(Modified from Foa,[45] with permission.)

Abnormalities in γ-Globulin Levels

Hypogammaglobulinemia is not an unusual feature of CLL. The levels of serum IgG, IgA, and IgM may all be markedly decreased or just one or two of the immunoglobulin classes may be involved. The pathogenesis of this complication is poorly understood but regulatory abnormalities of helper T, suppressor T, NK, and antibody-dependent cellular cytotoxicity (ADCC) cells may play a role. NK cells from CLL patients with hypogammaglobulinemia were found to cause a decrease in immunoglobulin secretion by normal B cells.[49] It is also possible that a decrease in or inhibition of normal B cells (CD5−) results in hypogammaglobulinemia.[39] CLL patients tend to have defective specific antibody response to infection and to immunization.[50] Infections with encapsulated organisms as well as with gram-negative bacteria are recognized as the most frequent cause of morbidity and mortality in CLL.[50,51]

A monoclonal serum immunoglobulin spike (usually IgM) has been observed in 5% of cases with CLL. However, Deegan et al.,[52] using high-resolution agarose gel electrophoresis and immunofixation, observed a small amount of monoclonal protein in the serum and urine of 60% of CLL patients.[52]

A summary of the presently recognized factors that may play a role in the heterogeneous immunologic abnormalities in CLL is shown in Table 83-2. There are additional factors (such as reduced NK, ADCC, and lymphokine-activated killer cell activity, increased levels of soluble IL-2 receptors, and reduced IL-2 availability), but their role is far from clearly proven. The available data strongly suggest that the abnormalities of the T- and cytotoxic cell compartments represent a secondary event occurring during the course of CLL.[45]

CLINICAL MANIFESTATIONS

Criteria for Diagnosis of CLL

The National Cancer Institute-sponsored Working Group (NCI-WG) on CLL was charged with the task of developing guidelines for protocol studies in this disease and in that context it recommended the following three diagnostic requirements[53]:

1. An absolute lymphocytosis in the blood, with a count of ≥5 × 10^9/L, and cells morphologically mature in appearance, sustained over at least a 4-week period.
2. ≥30% lymphocytes in a normocellular or hypercellular bone marrow.
3. A monoclonal B-cell phenotype expressed by the preponderant population of blood lymphocytes with low levels of surface immunoglobulins and simultaneously showing CD5 positivity (a pan-T-cell marker).

The requirement that the lymphocytosis should be sustained over a period of time is included in these diagnostic criteria in order to exclude those conditions (such as infectious mononucleosis, pertussis, toxoplasmosis, and cytomegalovirus infection) in which lymphocytosis is transient. In our view, if a bone marrow lymphocytosis also is required for the diagnosis of CLL, it is not necessary to prove that blood lymphocytosis is of a sustained nature because none of the conditions with transient lymphocytosis are associated with bone marrow involvement.

The International Workshop on CLL (IWCLL)[54] proposed somewhat similar diagnostic criteria, but it requires ≥10 × 10^9/L lymphocytes in the blood for the diagnosis to be made if facilities to obtain phenotyping are not available. IWCLL recommended that a diagnosis of CLL can be made in a patient with <10 × 10^9/L lymphocytes in the peripheral blood, provided phenotyping is performed and reveals the pattern characteristic of CLL as described above.

The FAB Cooperative Group[55] states that when >10% cells in the blood are large (or prolymphocytes) in appearance, the diagnosis of mixed cell type CLL should be considered. In our experience, clearly identifiable forms of prolymphocytic leukemia are a consistent clinical identity. The importance of occasional prolymphocyte appearing cells in the peripheral blood of a case of CLL is controversial.

Symptoms

The usual complaints of CLL patients are weakness, easy fatigue, night sweats, fever without infections, weight loss, frequent bacterial and viral infections, increased bleeding tendencies, and exaggerated responses to mosquito or other insect bites. These are symptoms often associated with malignancy and immunodeficiency. Symptoms may be entirely absent, or only some or all may be present in varying severity.

Findings on Physical Examination

The most frequently noted abnormal finding on physical examination is lymphadenopathy. Only a single node-bearing area may be involved, or lymph nodes may be palpably enlarged in the cervical, axillary, and inguinofemoral areas. These nodes may be small (e.g., about 1 cm in diameter) or massively enlarged. The enlarged lymph nodes in CLL are almost always nontender, nonpainful, discrete, firm, and easily movable on palpation. Enlargement of spleen and liver when present may range from barely palpable to ≤15 or 20 cm below the respective costal margin. In addition, infiltration by CLL cells may be manifested in virtually all other parts of the body, including the meninges and skin.

Laboratory Evaluation

Absolute lymphocytosis in blood, with mature-appearing cells, is one of the two major presenting features of CLL (Plate 83-1). The blood lymphocyte count may range from 5 to 500 × 10^9/L, but in most cases it is >20 × 10^9/L. Similarly, the differential count of bone marrow aspirate smear may reveal lymphocytes accounting for as little as 30% of all nucleated cells or as much as 99%; in the latter, the marrow is totally replaced by monotonously similar appearing lymphocytes. The overall cellularity of bone marrow is normal or increased; a hypocellular marrow is not a typical finding in CLL unless it is the result of cytotoxic therapy. Depending on the extent of lymphocytic infiltration, myeloid and erythroid precursors and megakaryocytes may be decreased or normal. Pure red cell aplasia,[56–58] however, may also occur in CLL. Bone marrow biopsy examination has become virtually routine whenever an aspiration procedure is performed in CLL. Biopsy specimens are characteristically infiltrated with lymphocytes, but the patterns of such infiltration may be diffuse, nodular, or interstitial[59–64] (Plates 83-2 to 83-4).

Lymphocytes in the blood and the marrow appear morphologically mature. However, it is now well recognized that func-

Table 83-3. Markers Useful in Distinguishing Chronic Lymphoid Leukemias

Marker	CLL	Prolymphocytic Leukemia	Hairy Cell Leukemia	Leukemic Phase of Follicular Non-Hodgkin Lymphoma	Plasma Cell Tumors	T-CLL	Sézary Syndrome
Surface immunoglobulin	Weak	Strong	Strong	Strong	Negative	Negative	Negative
Cytoplasmic immunoglobulin	−	±	±	−	+ +	−	−
Mouse red cell rosetting	+ +	−	±	±	−	−	−
Sheep red cell rosetting	−	−	−	−	−	+ +	+ +
CD2	−	−	−	−	−	+ +	+ +
CD3	−	−	−	−	−	+ +	+ +
CD4	−	−	−	−	−	+	+ +
CD5	+ +	±	−	−	−	+ +	+ +
CD7	−	−	−	−	−	+ +	−
CD8	−	−	−	−	−	+	−
CD19/20/24	+ +	+ +	+ +	+ +	−	−	−
Anticlass II MHC antigens	+ +	+ +	+ +	+ +	−	−	−
CD22	±	+ +	+ +	+	−	−	−
CD10	−	±	−	+	±	−	−
CD25	−	−	+ +	−	−	−	−
CD38	−	−	±	±	+ +	−	−

Symbols: +, incidence at which a marker is positive in >40% of cells in a particular leukemia; + +, 80–100%; ±, 10–40%; −, 0–9% of cases. (Modified from Bennett et al.,[55] with permission.)

tionally they are not mature inasmuch as they are arrested at an intermediate level of differentiation.[65] Lymphocytes in CLL are usually small, with the nucleus filling almost the entire cell, and the nuclear chromatin is dense and clumped and without any discernible nucleolus (Plate 83-1). Occasionally the CLL lymphocyte may be a large cell with round or somewhat notched nucleus, there may be an indistinct nucleolus, and the cytoplasm may be abundant and slightly basophilic or orthochromatic. Several morphologic variants of CLL have been described in the literature (e.g., prolymphocytic leukemia and Sézary cell leukemia).[55] Preparation of blood films may cause severe morphologic deformities of CLL lymphocytes, recognized as "smudge" cells (Plate No. 83-5).

Although CLL is characterized by leukocytosis, the proportion of neutrophils is always reduced, but to a varying degree—from as low as 1% to as high as 40%. Thus the absolute neutrophil count may be normal, extremely low, or extremely high, depending on total leukocyte count and percentage of neutrophils.

About 30% of all CLL patients may have somewhat decreased hemoglobin values or platelet counts, but these values are significantly decreased in only 15% of cases (hemoglobin <110 g/L, platelets <100 × 10⁹/L) at the time of initial diagnosis. Autoimmune complications, including Coombs-positive hemolytic anemia, immune thrombocytopenia, and hypogammaglobulinemia, are discussed above.

There is no characteristic abnormality of blood chemistry profile in CLL, but hypercalcemia and abnormal liver and kidney function tests may be encountered.

Differential Diagnosis

The differential diagnosis of CLL includes the entire spectrum of chronic lymphoproliferative disorders. Malignant lymphoma in leukemic phase may sometimes be indistinguishable from CLL, and the most helpful findings in such situations are phenotypic profiles of lymphocytes. Whereas the fluorescence intensity of surface immunoglobulins on B lymphocytes is bright in lymphomas, it is very faint in CLL; only B lymphocytes of CLL form rosettes with mouse erythrocytes and carry the T-cell marker denoted by CD5. T-cell CLL and morphologic variants of CLL (prolymphocytic leukemia, Sézary syndrome, hairy

cell leukemia, and so forth) are distinguished by their respective characteristic phenotypic and microscopic appearances.[55] The phenotypic characteristics useful in differentiating these various disorders are summarized in Table 83-3.

Prognosis

Just as the initial extent of disease is variable in CLL, the prognosis and clinical course also are extremely variable. Some patients have a rapid downhill course and die within 2–3 years after diagnosis, whereas others have a very benign, indolent course and live for 10 or 20 years without major problems from CLL. About one-half of CLL patients have a disease course somewhere in between the two extremes. Boggs et al.[66] studied several prognostic factors and concluded that the extent of disease at initial diagnosis correlates inversely with survival.

Clinical Staging System of Rai

Building on the work of Dameshek,[4] Boggs et al.,[66] and of Hansen,[67] my colleagues and I[68] were able to devise a clinical staging system in which patients with minimum evidence of disease (those merely satisfying the minimum diagnostic criteria) were considered to be in the earliest stage of disease, whereas those demonstrating significant compromise of bone marrow function (as an index of high leukemic cell burden) were considered to be in advanced stages. This staging system is detailed in Table 83-4.

Table 83-4. Rai Clinical Staging Systems

Level of Risk	Stage	Description
Low[a]	0	Lymphocytosis only (in blood and marrow)
	I	Lymphocytosis plus enlarged nodes
Intermediate[a]		
	II	Lymphocytosis plus enlarged spleen and/or liver with or without enlargement of nodes
	III	Lymphocytosis plus anemia (hemoglobin <110 g/L) with or without enlarged nodes, spleen, liver
High[a]		
	IV	Lymphocytosis plus thrombocytopenia (platelets <100 × 10⁹/L) with or without anemia and/or enlarged nodes, spleen, liver

[a] Modified Rai system.

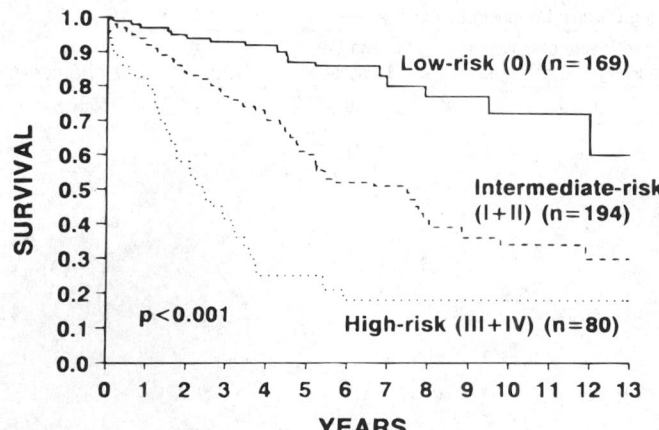

Fig. 83-1. Survival according to the modified Rai staging criteria in 443 patients with CLL followed at the Postgraduate School of Hematology, Barcelona, Spain. (From Montserrat and Rozman,[70] with permission.)

The definition of lymphocytosis in our original description consisted of a 15×10^9/L or higher absolute lymphocyte count in blood and $\geq 40\%$ of lymphocytes in the marrow differential count of all nucleated cells. However, following the recommendations of the NCI-WG[53] and the IWCLL[54] detailed above, we suggest that these thresholds be modified to $\geq 5 \times 10^9$/L and $>30\%$ in blood and marrow, respectively. The presence of palpably enlarged lymph nodes was found to be of prognostic value (stage I), but it did not seem to make much difference whether adenopathy was bulky or minimal or whether it involved a single node-bearing region or was generalized. Median survival correlated inversely with the clinical stage: stage 0, 12+ years; stage I, 8.5 years; stage II, 6 years; stage III, 1.5 years; and stage IV, 1.5 years.[68]

Modified Rai System

Although several investigators confirmed the validity of the staging system of Rai et al. as a reliable predictor of survival time in CLL, many workers found that having as many as five stages in the system made it difficult to plan prospective therapeutic trials. We had, however, acknowledged in our original proposal[68] in 1975 that in the actuarial survival curves, there were indeed only three, not five, distinct patterns: (1) stage 0, (2) stages I and II combined, and (3) stages III and IV combined.[68] Therefore, a formal modification[69] of the staging system was published in 1987, which assigns stage 0 to the low-risk group, stages I and II combined to the intermediate-risk group, and stages III and IV combined to the high-risk group (Table 83-4). The survival curves according to the modified Rai system in a large series of CLL patients followed in the Hematology Clinic of the University of Barcelona in Spain[70] are shown in Figure 83-1. These curves are statistically significantly different from each other and demonstrate that the low-risk group patients have the best outlook for survival. The NCI-WG recommends[53] using the modified Rai staging system for prospective therapeutic trials.

Staging System of Binet and Colleagues

The only other staging system that has found wide acceptance in clinical practice is the one devised by Binet et al.[71] This system is similar to the Rai system in concept. Stage C consists of all patients who have anemia (hemoglobin <100 g/L) and/or thrombocytopenia (platelets $<100 \times 10^9$/L). All other (non-C) patients are divided into A or B stages depending on the number of lymphoid-bearing areas palpably enlarged, two or less for A and more than three for B (there are five of

these areas: the cervical, axillary, and inguinofemoral nodes; spleen; and liver). This three-stage system is an excellent predictor of survival and is useful in planning therapeutic trials. Binet et al. have observed that the survival times of stage A patients do not differ from those of age- and sex-matched normal members of the French population. Inasmuch as stage A patients include those who have splenomegaly with one area of lymphadenopathy (or two areas of adenopathy without splenomegaly), it is somewhat surprising that the life expectancy of such patients is equal to that of the nonleukemic normal French population. Conceptually, in our opinion, the stage 0 subgroup of Binet's A should have a better prognosis than all other (non-stage-0) patients in stage A. In actual practice, both the Rai and the Binet systems are used in clinical management and in therapeutic protocols.

Other Staging Systems

The IWCLL recommends the use of an integrated Binet and Rai system in which each Binet stage (A, B, or C) is subclassified according to the corresponding Rai stage.[54] However, clinicians use either of the two systems without the recommended integration.

Jaksic and Vitale's[72] total tumor mass estimation yields a score indicating the size of the spleen and the largest palpable lymph node, while also including a factor related to the blood lymphocyte count. Other systems proposed include those of Mandelli et al.,[73] Lee et al.,[74] Baccarini et al.,[75] Skinnider et al.,[76] and Paolino et al.[77] Each of these systems has certain advantages and helps a physician in individual cases but none has found wide usage, perhaps because the Rai and Binet methods are simple to apply and succeed in segregating large populations of CLL patients into distinct groups of survival outlook.

Additional Prognostic Features

Numerous clinical, hematologic, and laboratory abnormalities, as well as immunophenotypic and cytogenetic characteristics have been reported to be indicative of adverse prognosis in CLL. Some of these are listed in Table 83-5. Perhaps only a

Table 83-5. Factors Associated with a Poor Prognosis

Clinical
    Lymphadenopathy
    Splenomegaly
    Hepatomegaly
    "Bulky" disease
    Poor performance status
Hematologic
    Anemia
    Thrombocytopenia
    Large and atypical lymphocytes in blood
    Diffuse bone marrow histopathologic pattern
Laboratory abnormalities
    Increased serum lactate dehydrogenase level
    Hypoalbuminemia
    Increased serum calcium level
Cytogenetic abnormalities
    Complex and multiple cytogenetic abnormalities (e.g., 14q32, 12+, others)
Immunologic
    Hypogammaglobulinemia
    Immunophenotype (different abnormalities related to poor prognosis [e.g., $SmIg^{+++}$, $CD5^-$, $CD23^-$])
    Increased serum-soluble CD25 receptors
    Increased serum-soluble CD23 receptors
Kinetic parameters
    Rapid doubling time
Others
    Poor response to therapy

(Adapted from Montserrat and Rozman,[70] with permission.)

few of these features have a consistent impact on prognosis and are described below.

Lymphocyte Doubling Time

Although the lymphocyte count acts as a continuous variable as a prognosis indicator, we have not found a threshold (such as a cut-off level of 40–50 × 10^9/L) count consistently reliable. However, the rate of increase of the absolute lymphocyte count in the blood of CLL patients not receiving cytotoxic therapy has proven to be a reliable indicator of disease activity. A serial plotting of blood lymphocyte counts provides a measure of this activity and either by extrapolation or by actual observation it can be determined whether the blood lymphocyte count doubles slowly (≥12 months) or rapidly (<12 months); the latter is associated with a worse prognosis.[78–80]

Bone marrow histopathology: The pattern of lymphocytic infiltration in the bone marrow biopsy specimens (Plates 83-2 to 83-4) can be classified as either diffuse or nondiffuse. The nondiffuse pattern may be nodular, interstitial, or mixed nodular and interstitial. Patients with diffuse infiltration have a worse prognosis than those with nondiffuse. The diffuse pattern is seen most frequently in advanced clinical stage CLL, while a nondiffuse infiltration is the more likely pattern in early stages of CLL.[59,62,63,81]

Immunophenotypic Features

A large, prospective study of flow-cytometric immunophenotyping in Denmark provides the most systematic analysis of prognostic value of these findings.[82] There were 503 CD5$^+$ and 37 CD5$^-$ cases. The survival of CD5$^-$ patients was on the borderline of being significantly shorter than that of CD5$^+$ patients. Most CD5$^-$ patients had malignant lymphocytes with strong sIgM fluorescence, and were FMC7$^+$ and CD23$^-$, indicating that CD5$^-$ cases represent an atypical variant of CLL.[82] Among the CD5$^+$ cases, by Cox multiple regression analysis a few features emerged with independent prognostic importance: higher age, low CD23 expression and high sIgM fluorescence intensity, and advanced clinical stage were all associated with worse prognosis. CD20, CD21, and CD22 expression did not have prognostic importance.[82]

Cytogenetics

A clonal chromosomal abnormality indicates a poorer prognosis as compared with a normal karyotype.[24] Although trisomy 12 as a single chromosomal abnormality is an adverse prognostic sign in CLL, multiple chromosomal abnormalities are associated with a worse prognosis. Patients with 13q abnormalities do not have as bad a prognosis as those with 12+ or 14q+.[24]

Prediction of Clinical Course in Patients with Early Stages

Neither the Rai nor the Binet system of clinical staging can reliably predict the clinical course of patients in the nonadvanced stages (0, I, and II for the Rai and A and B for the Binet) of CLL. It is widely recognized that there is a group of patients in these stages whose disease course remains indolent for prolonged periods (several years) and another group with a relatively progressive and active course. Several prognostic factors have been tested by numerous investigators since about the 1970s. These include a blood lymphocyte count above or below a certain threshold[75,83,84]; lymphocyte morphology and size[79,85]; serum levels of several enzymes (e.g., lactate dehydrogenase[86] and deoxythymidine kinase[87]); serum β-microglobulin levels[88]; phenotype of blood lymphocytes[82,89]; and chromosomal abnormalities.[24] The value of these criteria for predicting the clinical course of CLL has not been universally accepted.

Table 83-6. Definition of Smoldering CLL

Patients in Binet's stage A
Nondiffuse lymphocytic infiltration in bone marrow biopsy
Lymphocyte doubling time >12 months
Blood lymphocyte count ≤30 × 10^9/L
Hemoglobin ≥13 g/dl

(From Montserrat and Rozman,[70] with permission.)

Patients with early stages of CLL whose blood lymphocyte doubling time is long (>12 months) and whose bone marrow biopsy shows a nondiffuse pattern of lymphocytic infiltration tend to have an indolent course of the disease. The Spanish group[90] retrospectively tested certain criteria associated with nonprogressive (or stable) CLL among patients in Binet's A stage, which they call "smoldering CLL." They noted that (in addition to the two criteria mentioned above), a relatively low (≤30 × 10^9/L) absolute lymphocyte count and a relatively high (≥13 g/dL) hemoglobin (Table 83-6) characterize the category of smoldering CLL. The patients with smoldering CLL were found to have life expectancies no different than those of an age- and sex-matched control population and a significantly lower risk of disease progression compared with the other Binet's stage A patients not meeting the criteria of smoldering CLL (and were deemed to have "active" CLL)[70] (Table 83-7). The French Cooperative Group[91] on CLL recommended similar criteria associated with smoldering CLL in early stages of the disease. Thus, it seems that we are approaching a successful resolution of the problem of predicting disease activity in the nonadvanced stages of CLL.

CLL in the Younger Age Group

CLL is a disease of the elderly; the median age at diagnosis is 55 years. However, with the easy availability of routine blood counts in today's society, CLL is being diagnosed in increasing frequency both at earlier stages of the disease as well as in younger age groups. About 12% of patients are <50 years of age at diagnosis. Although nearly two-thirds of younger age CLL patients are >40 years of age, a recent Mayo Clinic report shows 18 years as the lower end of the age range.[80] With the advent of newer and more aggressive therapies in CLL, several studies have been conducted to determine whether younger age CLL patients have different outcomes than those in the more typical, older age groups. These studies show that there are no differences in the presenting features, treatment response rates, and median durations of response between the younger and the older age groups.[92–96] The Mayo Clinic study was confined to the prognostic features of nonadvanced stages of CLL in the younger patients and it showed that the survival curves for stages 0 and I were virtually superimposable with a median duration of 140 months and was significantly longer

Table 83-7. Disease Activity in Smoldering Versus Active CLL

	Smoldering CLL[a] (%)	"Active" CLL (Nonsmoldering)[b] (%)	
Risk of progression			
at 3 yr	8	57	
95% CI	6–16	42–72	
at 5 yr	13	57	
95% CI	3–24	42–72	$P < 0.001$
Surviving at 10 yr	78	43	
95% CI	56–99	22–64	$P < 0.05$

Abbreviation: CI, confidence interval.
[a] 38 patients.
[b] 161 patients.
(Data from Montserrat and Rozman.[70])

than the medium duration of 60 months for stage II patients. On multivariate analysis of several factors, only clinical stage (0 and I versus II) and lymphocyte doubling time (>12 versus ≤12 months) emerged as prognostically useful among younger age CLL patients in the nonadvanced stages.[80] These observations are helpful in planning long-term therapeutic options for these patients who do not find it particularly reassuring to be informed when they are 40 years of age that their median life expectancy is 10 or 12 years. The same prognosis may not have a grim impact on a 70-year-old person. Therefore, although it is helpful to know that there are no unique prognostic factors for the younger CLL patients, the ability of the physician as well as the patient to weigh the risks and benefits of various treatment options is greatly influenced by the patient's age.

THERAPY

Period of Observation Without Cytotoxic Therapy

It is prudent to withhold cytotoxic therapy after the initial diagnosis of CLL has been established.[97] A vast majority of patients can withstand a period without such therapy. As the clinical course is highly variable in this disease, the physician can use the therapy-free few weeks to observe whether the disease is stable or progressive in an individual patient on the basis of the following criteria:

1. The rate of increase of blood lymphocyte count is charted to determine whether the projected doubling time is long (>12 months) or short (≤12 months).
2. The clinical stage is clearly established.
3. The pattern of lymphocytic infiltration in bone marrow biopsy specimen is noted.
4. The presence or absence of constitutional symptoms is noted.
   The therapy-free period may be extended indefinitely for those patients whose disease appears to be indolent; such patients may need to return to the clinic less frequently (e.g., at 3-month intervals). A minority of patients have an aggressive course of CLL and require institution of some therapy within 2–4 weeks from the time of initial diagnosis.

Indications for Therapeutic Intervention

A decision to start antileukemia therapy is made in the presence of any of the following indications[97]:

1. Disease-related progressive symptoms (e.g., weight loss without trying, fever without overt infection, night sweats, weakness, or easy fatigability).
2. Progressively worsening anemia or thrombocytopenia.
3. Autoimmune (Coombs-positive) hemolytic anemia or autoimmune thrombocytopenic purpura.
4. "Bulky" lymphadenopathy that is getting progressively worse poses risk to the patient from pressure on underlying tissues, or causes significant cosmetic problems.
5. Massive splenomegaly that is worsening progressively or results in hypersplenism.
6. Progressive hyperlymphocytosis. It is not possible to set a rigid upper threshold for the blood lymphocyte count that must be met before starting therapy, but it is our current practice not to allow this count to be >150 × 10⁹/L. Hyperviscosity syndrome associated with hyperlymphocytosis in CLL can be catastrophic.[98,99] As noted earlier, the rate of increase of blood lymphocyte count is of equal importance; thus a short doubling time (≤12 months, actual or by extrapolation) is an indication for therapeutic intervention.
7. Increased susceptibility to bacterial infections.[50,51] This may

result from marked hypogammaglobulinemia, in which case intravenous high-dose γ-globulin therapy has a proven protective effect.[100] Severe neutropenia or agranulocytosis may occur in CLL, and may play a major role in the development of bacterial sepsis.[51]

Choices of Therapeutic Modalities

Alkylating Agents

Chlorambucil and cyclosphosphamide are the most frequently used initial drugs of choice. Chlorambucil is administered orally and is readily absorbed from the gastrointestinal tract. There are two methods of treatment with this drug: small-dose continuous therapy (0.07 mg/kg/day with adjustments as needed by monitoring blood counts at weekly or biweekly intervals) or large-dose bolus intermittent therapy (0.7 mg/kg at intervals of 3 or 4 weeks).[101] Both methods are approximately equally effective, markedly reducing the size of previously enlarged lymph nodes or spleen, but patient compliance is perhaps better with intermittent therapy. The premise[102,103] that the intermittent method may enable recovery of normal hematopoietic elements in the marrow before regrowth of leukemic cells between two successive doses and thus be superior to daily continuous administration of chlorambucil was not conclusively proven to be the case in a randomized trial sponsored by the Cancer and Leukemia Group B (CALGB).[101] Our own preference is for intermittent chlorambucil, but both methods are commonly used by physicians caring for CLL patients. The dose-limiting toxicity is bone marrow suppression, which is reversible if it is recognized promptly by frequent blood counts. Nausea, vomiting, mucositis, and so forth, are not major problems with chlorambucil.

The second most frequently used alkylating agent in CLL is cyclophosphamide, which may be given orally or intravenously. This drug, like chlorambucil, is also given either on a daily basis (50–150 mg/day PO) or intermittently (1,000–1,200 mg every 2–4 weeks PO). The intravenous dose is the same as the intermittent oral dose. Cyclophosphamide is equal to chlorambucil in its effectiveness in control of CLL, but some patients who are starting to show refractoriness to the latter respond to the former. Besides bone marrow suppression, chemical cystitis is a major side effect of cyclophosphamide, but is avoidable in most cases by ensuring adequate hydration and advising the patients to urinate frequently after each intermittently administered dose. The incidence of nausea is somewhat greater than with chlorambucil. Both drugs are effective as first-line single-agent therapy in CLL. Other alkylating agents (e.g., melphalan or nitrogen mustard) may also be effective, but they are associated with considerable toxicities and are rarely used in CLL.

Fludarabine monophosphate is a fluorinated analogue of adenine that is resistant to deamination by the enzyme adenosine deaminase. This drug has proved an effective therapy for CLL patients who are resistant to alkylating agents.[104] Fludarabine is given intravenously at a dose of 25 mg/m²/day for 5 consecutive days every month. Usually four to six treatments at monthly intervals are required to achieve the maximally achievable benefits from this drug. Although fludarabine does not cause nausea, vomiting, and hair loss, prolonged use may result in cumulative myelotoxicity and infectious complications. Precautions against tumor lysis syndrome during the initial phase of therapy with fludarabine are advised. Addition of prednisone does not increase response rates of fludarabine, but may increase the risk of opportunistic infections.[105,106]

Other Chemotherapeutic Drugs

Alkylating agents and fludarabine are the only cytotoxic drugs used as single agents in CLL, but vincristine, doxorubicin, nitrosoureas, and others are administered as part of several combination chemotherapy protocols. Even though vincristine has been administered frequently in CLL (being a part of several treatment schedules tested in lymphomas and used when a CLL patient is refractory to single-agent therapy), there is no clear evidence that this drug is indeed useful in the treatment of CLL. Considering the potential of significant peripheral neuropathy associated with vincristine therapy in CLL patients, who usually are elderly, we recommend either reduced dosage or avoidance of this drug when using a combination chemotherapy schedule that includes it.

Glucocorticosteroids

Glucocorticosteroids (e.g., prednisone) are frequently used in CLL either as single agents in the management of autoimmune hemolytic anemia and thrombocytopenia or as part of combination chemotherapy protocols in other cases. Prednisone has significant lymphocytolytic effect; it causes marked reduction in previously enlarged nodes and spleen, and after an initial phase of causing a further increase in blood lymphocytosis, eventually results in significant decrease when therapy is continued for several days or a few weeks. Side effects of prednisone use (especially in elderly CLL patients) that should be kept in mind are increased blood sugar levels, worsening of pre-existing osteoporosis, psychiatric reactions ranging from euphoria to severe depression, and increased susceptibility to infections, particularly reactivation of old healed tuberculous lesions. Prednisone is given orally on an intermittent schedule of 40–80 mg/day for 5–7 days every month. In some patients with persistent chronic hemolysis, a lower dosage maintenance schedule (e.g., 5–15 mg/day or twice a week) may be necessary.

Androgens or Anabolic Steroids

Androgens or anabolic steroids[107] have been used in CLL patients with marked anemia (considered to be due to leukemic infiltration of bone marrow or erythroid hypoplasia) to stimulate erythropoiesis. These agents are not uniformly effective but in some patients have been very beneficial; therefore, in selected situations, their use is justifiable. Side effects include hepatic toxicity, hirsutism, and prostatism. There have been reports of diethylstilbestrol causing significant reduction in blood lymphocyte counts when used in those patients with prostate cancer who happened also to have CLL,[108] but these results have not been confirmed in any controlled trials in CLL.

Radiotherapy

The most frequently used form of radiotherapy is splenic irradiation,[109,110] which in selected patients results in prompt reduction in the size of an enlarged spleen, accompanied by evidence of partial control of overall disease. This treatment is particularly beneficial in patients with marked splenomegaly who are not responsive to chemotherapy. Irradiation of large, bulky lymphoid masses localized in one region, nonresponsive to chemotherapy, is also an effective method of treatment. Experimental therapies, including extracorporeal irradiation of blood,[111] mediastinal irradiation,[112–114] total body irradiation,[109,115,116] and administration of radioactive isotopes,[117] have proved to be either too toxic or ineffective. A consultation with a radiation oncologist experienced in treating CLL and other hematologic malignancies is recommended in deciding whether radiotherapy is advisable.

Splenectomy

Splenectomy[118–123] is an effective treatment for CLL in specific clinical situations. Patients with extensive splenomegaly unresponsive to chemotherapy and with significant anemia or thrombocytopenia attributed to hypersplenism (some of these patients are not considered for splenic irradiation because of fear of worsening anemia or thrombocytopenia, and some of them may have failed radiotherapy) and patients whose response to steroid therapy is inadequate in the presence of autoimmune anemia are among those considered to be candidates for splenectomy. Beneficial response to splenectomy may last from a few months to several years. Pneumococcal vaccine should be administered before surgery.

Leukapheresis

Leukapheresis[124,125] has a very limited role in the long-term management of CLL. When the blood leukocyte count is >500 $\times 10^9$/L either at diagnosis or during the course of the disease, catastrophic complications of hyperviscosity and thromboembolic phenomena may be avoided by resorting to intensive leukapheresis (using one of the automatic cell-separating machines) while simultaneously providing adequate hydration and initiating cytotoxic chemotherapy. Leukapheresis as the sole therapeutic measure is of no benefit because the reduction in blood lymphocyte count so achieved is very transient.

Criteria for Evaluating Response

The NCI-WG[53] and the IWCLL[54] have separately proposed a series of criteria to objectively assess complete or partial remission in CLL. To qualify for complete remission a patient must have no adenopathy, no hepatosplenomegaly, no constitutional symptoms, normal hemogram (hemoglobin >110 g/L, platelets >100 $\times 10^9$/L, absolute lymphocytes <4 $\times 10^9$/L, and absolute neutrophils >1.5 $\times 10^9$/L), and the bone marrow must contain <30% lymphocytes. To qualify for partial remission, IWCLL criteria require an improvement in clinical stage (e.g., from Binet's C to B or A or from Binet's B to A). The NCI-WG recommends a similar approach (i.e., improvement in clinical stage), but in addition defines partial remission by a >50% reduction in the previously enlarged nodes, spleen, or liver, together with a >50% improvement of peripheral blood values over baseline (when they do not approach the levels described for complete remission).

Therapy Based on Clinical Stage

Low-risk (stage 0) patients should not be started on cytotoxic therapy unless significant constitutional symptoms develop or there is evidence of an active clinical course as described above.

Intermediate-risk (stage I and II) patients should also be observed without antileukemia therapy until there is evidence of an active clinical course as described above or of any of the indications for therapeutic intervention also as enumerated above. In randomized studies CALGB[126] and the French Cooperative Group[127] assigned early-stage patients to chlorambucil therapy or observation alone. Both these studies showed that early treatment with chlorambucil did not improve survival, although it did correlate with a somewhat slower progression to the more advanced stages. If treatment is indicated, chlorambucil as a single agent is the appropriate first-line therapy. The therapeutic end point is unclear; we do not know whether pushing treatment to try to achieve a complete remission is necessarily beneficial for the patient. The current practice, however, is to at least try to eliminate whatever indication required initiation of therapy in the first instance, and if possible, to maximize the best achievable level of response without subjecting the patient to undue toxicity.

High-risk (stages III and IV) patients have a uniformly poor

APPROACH TO THERAPY FOR CLL

We use the following diagnostic criteria for CLL: an absolute lymphocytosis in blood, with mature-appearing lymphocytes; lymphocytosis in the marrow, which is hypercellular or at least normocellular; and a monoclonal B-cell phenotype of the preponderant population of blood lymphocytes with low levels of surface immunoglobulins and simultaneously expressing CD5 positivity. The threshold for the absolute lymphocyte count in the blood is 5×10^9/L and the threshold for the proportion of lymphocytes among all nucleated cells in the marrow is 30%.

We begin treatment if a patient in the low- or intermediate-risk category shows a rapid rate of increase in blood lymphocyte count (doubling time, actual or projected, of ≤12 months) on several weeks of observation without cytotoxic therapy and, in addition, the marrow biopsy shows diffuse lymphocytic infiltration. We initiate therapy in all high-risk category patients. More specifically, we use the seven indications listed in the text; if any of these is present, we initiate therapy.

If, for any reason, the patient is not going to be placed on a research protocol for front-line therapy, in routine clinical management we continue to use chlorambucil for low- and intermediate-risk (stages 0, I, or II) CLL. We recommend an intermittent schedule in which 40 mg/m² total dose, taken orally in 1 day or divided over 2 days, is repeated every 4 weeks. In high-risk (stages III or IV) patients, we add prednisone (60 mg/day PO) for 5 days at each 4-week chlorambucil therapy. All patients starting this therapy for the first time also take allopurinol (300 mg/day PO) for 1 week with each cycle of therapy with chlorambucil. If there is no evidence of hyperuricemia, we do not continue with allopurinol after 2–3 months. When prednisone is prescribed, we monitor blood sugar levels to ensure that complications from hyperglycemia do not occur.

All patients have a weekly monitoring of blood counts and serum chemistries for the first 8 weeks. By then, each patient's nadir counts and rate of recovery are well established, as is also the dosage of chlorambucil (which needs to be adjusted upward or downward depending on the response in blood counts). Thereafter, patients return for an examination every 3–4 weeks.

As soon as we recognize that chlorambucil is not optimally effective we switch to the second-line drugs. Fludarabine is our drug of choice for all patients who show inadequate degree of response to chlorambucil or who start to show evidence of recurrent disease after having had a response to initial chlorambucil. Fludarabine dosage is 25 mg/m²/day IV for 5 days each month. We do not use prednisone with fludarabine because with this combination a patient has an increased risk of developing opportunistic infections. A maximally achievable beneficial response is usually attained after four to six cycles of fludarabine, when this therapy is stopped.

Patients who do not respond to fludarabine or relapse after an initial response are offered 2-chlorodeoxyadenosine (2cdA). 2cdA offers some hope for response, particularly in patients who have previously not been heavily treated with fludarabine and other drugs. In our experience combination chemotherapy schedules such as COP, CHOP, M-2 are not very effective.

For CLL patients <50 years of age, we consult with the bone marrow transplantation service. Allogeneic marrow transplantation is recommended if an HLA-matched sibling donor is available; otherwise autologous marrow transplantation is considered.

We use prednisone for patients with autoimmune anemia/thrombocytopenia. If prednisone does not produce satisfactory results, we add a 2–3-month trial of intravenous γ-globulin therapy, which consists of 200 mg/kg/day over a 3-hour period for 5 days initially (loading dose), followed by only one dose every 3 weeks. If there is a satisfactory response, we continue with prednisone plus intravenous γ-globulin therapy for 6–12 months. If the results are inadequate, we consider splenectomy.

With respect to pure red cell aplasia in CLL, if there is a true reticulocytopenia with severe anemia in Coombs-negative patients or if the marrow shows markedly decreased or absent erythroid precursors, we recommend Cyclosporin A at a dose of 600–1,000 mg/day PO; tapered to 400–600 mg/day after 2 weeks. Close monitoring of serum BUN, creatinine, and liver enzymes is necessary to adjust the dosage and to prevent undue toxicity. If a beneficial response is likely to occur, it will become evident within 2 weeks, by an increase in either reticulocytes or hemoglobin.

The patients to whom we give intravenous γ-globulin are primarily CLL patients who have had pneumonia or any other major documented bacterial infection, especially if their baseline serum IgG level is <6.0 g/L. We start intravenous γ-globulin without waiting for a second episode of infection. We give 200 mg/kg over a 3-hour period every 3 weeks for 6 months. Following that, we reduce the frequency of infusion to every 6 or 8 weeks (especially if the initial therapy has protected the patient from recurrence of bacterial infections).

We treat infections in CLL very vigorously. We obtain multiple blood, urine, and sputum cultures if indicated, and consult with colleagues in infectious diseases for their recommendation of empirically selected antibiotics. We discontinue or taper prednisone therapy. We actively look for tuberculosis and for infections caused by *Pneumocystis carinii* and other opportunistic organisms.

By way of supportive care we give packed cell transfusions to all anemic patients who are symptomatic from anemia and have not responded to prednisone. If the hematocrit is ≤24%, we tend to give transfusions to maintain it at >28%. If a patient's base-line serum erythropoietin level is low or within normal range we initiate a 4-week therapeutic trial with recombinant erythropoietin injections subcutaneously. This therapy is continued only if the initial trial reveals some improvement in anemia. We do not use prophylactic oral antibiotics, and we do not have a set policy concerning the use of pneumococcal vaccine or influenza vaccine.

We are very sensitive to patients' psychosocial needs and to their ability to cope with the stress of a terminal disease. We enlist the help of a psychiatrist specializing in oncology and of a social worker who has experience in oncology. We spend a considerable amount of our own time talking to the patients and their families—reassuring them, answering their questions, and helping them to anticipate problems rather than to have the problems descend on them without adequate preparation or warning.

prognosis and should be started on cytotoxic therapy. A large trial by CALGB[101] revealed that if at least a partial (complete if possible) remission is achieved after chlorambucil and prednisone therapy, there is a significant improvement in survival as compared with survival in those patients who failed to achieve such a response. This was the first study that defined the therapeutic end point in advanced CLL (i.e., a partial or complete remission). The French Cooperative Group[128] demonstrated a significantly better survival of advanced stage patients after treatment with COP (cyclosphosphamide, vincristine [Oncovin], prednisone) together with low-dose doxorubicin (CHOP) as compared with patients who received COP without doxorubicin.[128] The results of this study, however, have not been confirmed by subsequent trials, nor has there been any evidence that a somewhat higher response rate with CHOP provides a survival advantage over COP, or chlorambucil and prednisone therapy.[129–133]

Second-Line Therapy

Fludarabine

Fludarabine has proven to be an extremely effective drug for CLL patients who have failed prior therapy with an alkylating agent.[104–106] A large proportion of such patients obtain objective responses and responding patients have an improved survival.

Combination Chemotherapy

Other multiagent combination chemotherapies (e.g., POACH, [COP plus cytosine arabinoside and doxorubicin],[134] devised at the M.D. Anderson Hospital in Houston, Texas) or the M-2 protocol[135] (COP plus melphalan and carmustine, developed for treatment of multiple myeloma at the Memorial Sloan-Kettering Cancer Center in New York) also have some promise in the management of advanced stages of CLL but the results are not uniformly consistent.

Special Therapeutic Issues

High-Dose Intravenous Immunoglobulin

As mentioned earlier, significant hypogammaglobulinemia is frequently observed in CLL, rendering these patients highly vulnerable to bacterial infections. With the availability of purified immunoglobulins for intravenous administration, it is now possible to treat those CLL patients who are at increased risk of infections. In a multi-institutional, placebo-controlled randomized trial,[100] it was observed that replacement therapy with intravenous γ-globulin provides a significant protection from major bacterial infections in CLL patients who would otherwise be at risk. The γ-globulin dose in this study was 400 mg/kg body weight every 3 weeks for 1 year. Although such therapy appears rather expensive, when one considers the potential costs of treating bacterial pneumonia in a hospital inpatient setting, the cost of such preventive measures becomes justifiable in certain selected patients who are at high risk of infections. We have been using a lower dosage (200 mg/kg body weight) of intravenous immunoglobulin, which appears to provide protection from infections at significantly reduced costs. A multicenter trial comparing a high dose (500 mg/kg/mo) with a lower dose (250 mg/kg/mo) has been conducted and the preliminary results show that both dosages are equally effective in preventing bacterial infections in the at-risk patients with CLL.[136] Thus, if the patients are selected for their previous history of major bacterial infections and/or severe hypogammaglobulinemia and the dosage of intravenous immunoglobulin is lowered, the overall cost of such a preventive measure

would not remain as big an issue as was previously considered.[137] This therapy is well tolerated and can be given at the patient's home or in outpatient clinics.

Interferon-α

Although initial results[138] with IFN-α in advanced stages of CLL were very disappointing, subsequently performed studies suggest that this agent may benefit patients in early stages of the disease, or when the tumor burden is relatively low.[139–142] The clinical benefits from a combination of IFN-α and chlorambucil and prednisone are being studied.[143] The mechanism of action of IFN-α in CLL is not understood. In vitro, it causes differentiation of CLL cells,[144] and there are also data to suggest that it inhibits apoptosis of CLL cells. However, there is no evidence of direct cytotoxicity from IFN-α; it may interfere with cellular interactions necessary for the survival and growth of CLL cells, or alternatively, it may inhibit the proliferation of the small fraction of clonogenic CLL progenitors.[145] Until more data from some of the recently completed trials become available, IFN-α should be considered an experimental agent in the treatment of CLL.

Pure Red Cell Aplasia

Pure red cell aplasia is a relatively rare cause of anemia in CLL. Some studies suggest that suppressor cytotoxic T cells exert inhibitory effects on erythroid progenitor cells in the bone marrow.[56–58] Therefore, an immunosuppressive agent such as Cyclosporin A has been proposed for therapy of pure red cell aplasia with the objective of attacking the erythropoiesis-inhibiting effect of suppressor T cells.[56] Since the first report of Chikkappa et al.[146] of successful treatment of pure red cell aplasia in CLL with Cyclosporin A, others[147,148] have confirmed these results in a small number of patients. This therapy is well tolerated, the only reported side effect being mild and reversible renal toxicity. A reticulocyte response is noted within 2 weeks of therapy and is soon followed by an increase in hemoglobin levels. We have observed[147] that not only hemoglobin but also platelet counts increased in a CLL patient who had significant, refractory anemia and thrombocytopenia before Cyclosporin A therapy.

Late Complications and Terminal Events

The quality of life and performance status of CLL patients gradually deteriorate with progression of the disease, and a refractoriness to all cytotoxic therapies becomes increasingly evident. Marked degree of persistent anemia is not unusual in the last phases of this disease and the patients require frequent and regular transfusions of packed red cells. Recombinant human erythropoietin may be effective in some patients with anemia. Although platelet transfusions are not routinely recommended in patients with profound degrees of thrombocytopenia who have no evidence of any bleeding, such transfusions are necessary in the presence of bleeding.

Infections

Infections from bacterial, viral, and fungal agents are the most important cause of morbidity and mortality in CLL.[50,51] There are several factors that contribute to the increased incidence of infections in CLL, but advanced stages or long duration of the disease, hypogammaglobulinemia and neutropenia (from CLL or from myelosuppression effects of chemotherapy) are the most significant. The new nucleoside analogues, which have found increasing usage in the therapy of CLL, are known to cause marked lymphopenia, especially of the T-helper-cell populations.[104–106] This in turn renders the patients vulnerable to infections with opportunistic organisms. Therapy is directed at identification of the causative organisms and use of the appropriate antibiotics after consultation with an infectious diseases specialist. Judicious use of granulocyte-stimulating factor is helpful in septic patients with chemotherapy-induced neutropenia. Prophylactic use of high-dose intravenous immunoglobulin has been discussed above. Prophylactic use of antibiotics in neutropenic or hypogammaglobulinemic patients is not recommended.

Richter Syndrome

About 1–10% of patients with CLL develop a large cell lymphoma. It is known as Richter syndrome because it was Richter who first described this association.[149] In a retrospective review of 1,374 CLL patients seen at the M.D. Anderson Cancer Center during a 20-year period between 1972 and 1992, 2.8% were reported to have developed Richter transformation.[150] Richter syndrome is often characterized by sudden clinical deterioration, development of systemic symptoms, and usually a rapid increase in the size of a lymphoid mass at one site. Less frequently, a monoclonal gammopathy or lytic bone lesions are observed. The histology of lymphoma is either of diffuse large cell type or its immunoblastic variant.[150] One of our patients developed a lymphoma of Burkitt type pathology. Immunoglobulin gene rearrangements and light chain isotype analyses in the study at the M.D. Anderson Cancer Center suggest that CLL and Richter syndrome had a common origin, indicating that a bona fide transformation occurred in the CLL cells.[150] The published literature, however, supports both theories[151,152]: some studies show that lymphoma cells and CLL cells have identical features, while other studies show that lymphoma cells arise de novo with characteristics distinct from those of CLL cells. There have been separate reports of two cases extensively studied with molecular markers, one conclusively proving a common origin and another equally conclusively revealing that CLL cells and lymphoma cells were clonally distinct.[151,152] These reports prove that diffuse large cell lymphoma may occur both ways: a transformation of the original clone of CLL cells as well as a development of a new or second malignancy. It is customary to treat patients with Richter transformation with chemotherapeutic agents known to be effective in treating de novo diffuse large cell lymphoma. Therapy has so far proven to be uniformly unsuccessful and the overall survival of patients is approximately 6 months after Richter transformation.

Prolymphocytoid Transformation

In addition to Richter transformation, prolymphocytoid transformation may occur terminally in about 10% of cases with CLL. The morphology of blood lymphocytes changes into that of a large cell with convoluted nucleus, immature-appearing nuclear chromatin, and one or two large nucleoli. Therapy of this complication also is unsatisfactory. Besides the drugs commonly used in therapy of CLL, antilymphoma agents have also been tried but the success rate has been low. Acute leukemia and multiple myeloma are extremely rare late events in CLL.

CLL patients are known to have a higher incidence of developing a second malignancy (such as cancer of the gastrointestinal tract, lung, or any other organ) than the general population. Patients with CLL also have a high risk of developing skin cancers.

Paraneoplastic Pemphigus—An Autoimmune Complication

Anhalt et al.[153] have suggested that the term paraneoplastic pemphigus, which is clinically distinct from pemphigus vulgaris and pemphigus foliaceus, be applied to the painful, persistent, and treatment-resistant erosions of the oral mucosa, vermilion borders of the lips, and conjunctivitis that appear in patients with various types of cancers, including CLL. These acantholytic mucocutaneous lesions are characterized by autoantibodies that are pathogenic after passive transfer.

FUTURE DIRECTIONS

Although chlorambucil and cyclosphosphamide have been the mainstays of chemotherapy in CLL over the last 20–30 years and both drugs induce a high rate of partial remissions, it is also recognized that no treatment available to date has resulted in improvement of the natural history of this disease. The overall median survival time has remained at about 6 years.

Fludarabine

As mentioned earlier, fludarabine[104–106] has proven to be an extremely effective agent for those patients who have failed therapy with an alkylating agent. The potential role of fludarabine as front-line therapy for CLL is under active investigation in a large multi-institutional study in which patients are randomized to receive fludarabine or chlorambucil, or a combination of these two drugs. In this NCI-sponsored study led by Cancer and Leukemia Group B, NCI-Canada's Clinical Trials Group, South West Oncology Group, and Eastern Cooperative Oncology are participating. A single institution-based experience in a relatively small number of patients demonstrated a complete remission rate of 33% among previously untreated patients with active CLL.[104] It will be very important to determine whether the patients achieving complete remission with fludarabine have a prolonged survival—either equal to or better than the survival rate for stage 0 (low-risk group) patients.

2-Chlorodeoxyadenosine

2-Chlorodeoxyadenosine (2-CdA) is also a purine analogue like fludarabine, and is resistant to the action of adenosine deaminase. This drug has proven to be extremely effective in inducing lasting remissions in hairy cell leukemia. 2-CdA has been used in a relatively small number of CLL patients, mostly previously treated and refractory to alkylating agents.[154,155] The preliminary results are very encouraging and controlled clinical trials in previously untreated CLL are being planned; the results of such studies will have an impact on the future therapies of this disease. 2-CdA is given by a 2-hour intravenous infusion at a dose of 0.12–0.14 mg/kg/day for 5 days every month. Most patients obtain maximally attainable response after 4–6 months of therapy. Myelosuppression and immunosuppression are the major toxicities of 2-CdA.

Pentostatin

Pentostatin (deoxycoformycin) has a chemical structure somewhat similar to that of 2-Cda and is a potent inhibitor of adenosine deaminase. This drug also seems to offer benefit[156,157] to previously treated CLL patients, but it is used less often in CLL than fludarabine or 2-CdA.

Bone Marrow Transplantation as Therapy

With the recognition that CLL is being diagnosed today in increasing numbers in patients in the 35–50 age group, even a relatively long survival outlook of 6–10 years is not satisfactory for people this young. Simultaneously, we are developing an increasing level of expertise in performing bone marrow transplantation and in managing the various complications of this therapy in several other types of human malignancies. In the United States[158] and in Europe,[159] results of small trials have been reported that reveal that bone marrow transplantation is a feasible approach in properly selected groups of CLL patients. An allogeneic bone marrow transplantation is preferred if a sibling is available as an HLA-compatible donor. In the absence of a compatible donor, autologously harvested marrow (after intensive chemotherapy-induced maximal reduction of leukemic cell mass in the patient's bone marrow) is reinfused following myeloablation with massive doses of chemotherapy. The preliminary results are encouraging and in the next few years we expect to learn more about this interesting and promising therapy.[158,159]

Monoclonal Antibodies

Immunotherapy with monoclonal antibodies either alone or conjugated with toxins or radioisotopes are becoming very attractive treatment measures[160] because of their potential of killing only the targeted tumor cells and sparing the normal hematopoietic cells. However, so far these approaches in CLL have been in early experimental stages; most published reports demonstrate that such therapies are feasible.

Anti-B4 (CD19) blocked ricin,[161,162] an immunoconjugate, has shown some activity in phase I studies but there was an associated risk of development of antibodies to the murine monoclonal antibody being used. CAMPATH-1H monoclonal antibody was developed by "humanization" of rodent variable immunoglobulin regions with human immunoglobulin gene sequences that present fewer xenogenic-peptide sequences and are thus less immunogenic.[163] Our own limited experience with CAMPATH-1H has been extremely promising[164] and we are continuing these studies on a larger number of patients.

T-CELL CLL

The T-cell variant of CLL, a rare form accounting for only 2–5% of all CLL cases, is briefly reviewed here. The diagnosis is suspected when confirmation of a lymphocytosis in blood and bone marrow is accompanied by phenotype analysis of blood lymphocytes revealing a preponderance of T cells.[165] Within this rare group of diseases there is considerable heterogeneity with respect to clinical features, clinical course, and phenotypic markers.[165] The most benign end of the spectrum consists of large granular lymphocytic leukemia associated with neutropenia, a T8 +, T4 −, T3 + phenotype (suppressor T lymphocytes), multiple autoantibodies (rheumatoid factor, antinuclear antibodies), splenomegaly, and absence of lymphadenopathy. Cytogenetic, immunologic, and functional studies indicate that this disease results from a clonal proliferation of immature NK cells.[166] The clinical course is variable but in most cases is rather indolent. Treatment is generally based on corticosteroids with the addition of alkylating agents if there is evidence of disease progression. The T4 CLL variant[167,168] usually affects patients <40 years of age and is associated with hyperlymphocytosis and marked generalized lymphadenopathy, frequently involving the skin and central nervous system. The lymphocyte morphology reveals small, mature-appearing cells with a notched nucleus that lacks a nucleolus and without cytoplasmic granules. The phenotype is T3 +, T4 +, and T8 −. The clinical course is aggressive, the response to the usual cytotoxic therapy is inadequate, and overall survival is <2 years. Sézary syndrome is the leukemic manifestation of cutaneous T-cell lymphoma. The lymphocyte phenotype is CD4⁺, CD2⁺, CD3⁺, and CD5⁺. Treatment is directed to the underlying lymphoma. Adult T-cell leukemia, which is seen in certain areas of Japan, the Caribbean, and in the southeastern United States, is an HTLV-1 associated disease and bears little relation to CLL.

ACKNOWLEDGMENT

This work was made possible with grant support from Helena Rubinstein Foundation, Leon Lowenstein Foundation, Inc., Joel Finkelstein Foundation, Ruth and H. Bert Mack Family Fund, United Leukemia Fund, Inc., National Leukemia Association, and Wayne Goldsmith Leukemia Fund.

REFERENCES

1. Turk W: Ein System der Lymphomatosen. Wien Klin Wochenschr 16:1073, 1903
2. Minot GP, Isaacs R: Lymphatic leukemia. Age, incidence, duration and benefit derived from irradiation. Boston Med Surg J 191:1, 1924
3. Galton DAG: The pathogenesis of chronic lymphocytic leukemia. Can Med Assoc J 94:1005, 1966
4. Dameshek W: Chronic lymphocytic leukemia—an accumulative disease of immunologically incompetent lymphocytes. Blood 29:566, 1967
5. Bloomfield CD, Foon KA, Levine EG: Leukemia. p. 459. In Calabresi P, Schein PS (eds): Medical Oncology: Basic Principles and Clinical Management of Cancer. 2nd Ed. McGraw-Hill, New York, 1993
6. Linet MS, Blattner WA: The epidemiology of chronic lymphocytic leukemia. p. 11. In Polliack A, Catovsky D (eds): Chronic Lymphocytic Leukemia. Harwood Academic Publishers, Chur, Switzerland, 1988
7. Brok-Simoni F, Rechavi G, Katzir N et al: Chronic lymphocytic leukemia in twin sisters: monozygous but not identical. Lancet 1:329, 1987
8. Conley CL, Misiti J, Laster AJ: Genetic factors predisposing to chronic lymphocytic leukemia and to auto-immune disease. Medicine 5:323, 1980
9. Cuttner J: Increased incidence of hematological malignancies in first-degree relatives of patients with chronic lymphocytic leukemia. Cancer Invest 10:103, 1992
10. Cartwright RA, Bernard SM, Bird CC et al: Chronic lymphocytic leukaemia: case control epidemiological study in Yorkshire. Br J Cancer 56:59, 1987
11. Blattner WA, Dean JH, Fraumeni JF: Familial lymphoproliferative malignancy: clinical and laboratory follow-up. Ann Intern Med 90:943, 1979
12. Jones HP, Whittaker JA: Chronic lymphatic leukemia: an investigation of HLA antigen frequencies and white cell differential counts in patients, relatives, and controls. Leuk Res 15:543, 1991
13. Mann DL, LeSane F, Boumpas D et al: HTLV-I infection and chronic lymphocytic leukemia. Nouv Rev Fr Hematol 30:267, 1988
14. Adachi M, Tefferi A, Greipp PR et al: Preferential linkage of bcl-2 to immunoglobulin light-chain gene in chronic lymphocytic leukemia. J Exp Med 171:559, 1990
15. Raghobier S, van Krieken JHJM, Kluin-Nelemans JC et al: Oncogene rearrangements in chronic lymphocytic leukemia. Blood 77:1560, 1991
16. Hanada M, Delia D, Aiello A et al: Bcl-2 gene hypomethylation and high-level expression in B-cell chronic lymphocytic leukemia. Blood 82:1820, 1993
17. Dighiero G, Travade P, Chevret S et al: B-cell chronic lymphocytic leukemia: present status and future directions. Blood 78:1901, 1991
18. Gordone I, Matutes E, Catovsky D: Monoclonal antibody Ki-67 identifies B and T cells in cycle in chronic lymphocytic leukemia: correlation with disease activity. Leukemia 6:902, 1992
19. Collins RJ, Verschuer LA, Harmon BV et al: Spontaneous programmed cell death (apoptosis) of B-chronic lymphocytic leukaemia cells following their culture in vitro. Br J Haematol 71:343, 1989
20. Panayiotidis P, Ganeshguru K, Jabbar SAB, Hoffbrand AV: Interleukin-4 inhibits apoptotic cell death and loss of the bcl-2 protein in B-chronic lymphocytic leukaemia cells in vitro. Br J Haematol 85:439, 1993
21. Danescu M, Rubio-Trujillo M, Biron G et al: Interleukin-4 protects chronic lymphocytic leukemic B cells from death by apoptosis and upregulates bcl-2 expression. J Exp Med 176:1319, 1992
22. Buschle M, Campana D, Carding SR et al: Interferon gamma inhibits apoptotic cell death in B chronic lymphocytic leukemia. J Exp Med 177:213, 1993
23. Nilsson K: The control of growth and differentiation in chronic lymphocytic leukemia (B-CLL) cells. p. 33. In Cheson BD (ed): Chronic Lymphocytic Leukemia: Scientific Advances and Clinical Developments. Marcel Dekker, New York, 1993
24. Juliusson G, Gahrton G: Cytogenetics in CLL and related disorders. Baillieres Clin Haematol 6:821, 1993
25. Kay NE, Peterson LC, Ranheim E: Molecular and protein analysis of the

retinoblastoma (13q 12-14) locus in a subset of B-CLL patients with a retinoblastoma locus abnormality. Blood, suppl. 1. 78:385, 1991

26. Liu Y, Szekely L, Grander D et al: Chronic lymphocytic leukemia cells with allelic deletions at 13q14 commonly have one intact RB-1 gene. Evidence for a role of an adjacent locus. Proc Natl Acad Sci USA 90:8697, 1993

27. Tsujimoto Y, Yunis J, Onorato-Showe L et al: Molecular cloning of the chromosomal breakpoint of B-cell lymphomas and leukemias with the t(11;14) chromosome translocation. Science 224:1403, 1984

28. Meeker TC, Grimaldi JC, O'Rourke R et al: An additional breakpoint region in the bcl-1 locus associated with the t(11;14) (q13;q32) translocation of B-lymphocytic malignancy. Blood 74:1801, 1989

29. Anastasi J, LeBeau MM, Vardiman JW et al: Detection of trisomy 12 in chronic lymphocytic leukemia by fluorescence in situ hybridization to interphase cells: a simple and sensitive method. Blood 79:1796, 1992

30. Que TH, Garcia Marco J, Ellis J et al: Trisomy 12 in chronic lymphocytic leukemia detected by fluorescence in situ hybridization: analysis by stage, immunophenotype and morphology. Blood 82:571, 1993

31. Freedman AS, Nadler LM: Immunologic markers in B-cell chronic lymphocytic leukemia. p. 1. In Cheson BD (ed): Chronic Lymphocytic Leukemia: Scientific Advances and Clinical Developments. Marcel Dekker, New York, 1993

32. Litz CE, Brunning RD: Chronic lymphoproliferative disorders: classification and diagnosis. Baillieres Clin Haematol 6:767, 1993

33. Kurec AS, Threatte GA, Gottlieb AJ et al: Immunophenotypic subclassification of chronic lymphocytic leukemia (CLL). Br J Haematol 81:45, 1992

34. Caligaris-Cappio F, Gobbi M, Bofill M, Janossy G: Infrequent normal B lymphocytes express features of B-chronic lymphocytic leukemia. J Exp Med 155:623, 1982

35. Gadol N, Ault KA: Phenotypic and functional characterization of human Leu-1 (CD5) B cells. Immunol Rev 93:23, 1986

36. Foon KA, Todd RF III: Immunologic classification of leukemia and lymphoma. Blood 68:1, 1986

37. DeRossi G, Zarcone D, Mauro F et al: Adhesion molecule expression on B-cell chronic lymphocytic leukemia cells: malignant cell phenotypes define distinct disease subsets. Blood 81:2879, 1993

38. Riva M, Schena M, Bergui L et al: Comparative analysis of normal and malignant CD5⁻ B lymphocytes. Nouv Rev Fr Hematol 30:289, 1988

39. Dighiero G: Biology of the neoplastic lymphocytic in B-CLL. Baillieres Clin Haematol 6:807, 1993

40. Kay NE: Abnormal T-cell subpopulation function in CLL: excessive suppressor (T) and deficient helper (T) activity with respect to B-cell proliferation. Blood 57:418, 1981

41. Platsoucas CD, Galinski M, Kempin S et al: Abnormal T lymphocyte subpopulations in patients with B cell chronic lymphocytic leukemia: an analysis by monoclonal antibody. J Immunol 129:2305, 1982

42. Kay NE, Johnson JD, Stanek R et al: T-cell subpopulations in chronic lymphocytic leukemia: abnormalities in distribution and in vitro receptor maturations. Blood 54:540, 1979

43. Zeigler HW, Kay NE, Zarling JM: Deficiency of natural killer cell activity in patients with chronic lymphocytic leukemia. Int J Cancer 27:321, 1981

44. Bofill M, Janossy G, Janossa M et al: Human B cell development. II. Subpopulations in the human fetus. J Immunol 134:1531, 1985

45. Foa R: Pathogenesis of the immunodeficiency in B-cell chronic lymphocytic leukemia. p. 147. In Cheson BD (ed): Chronic Lymphocytic Leukemia: Scientific Advances and Clinical Developments. Marcel Dekker, New York, 1993

46. Foon KA, Rai KR, Gale RP: Chronic lymphocytic leukemia: new insights into biology and therapy. Ann Intern Med 113:525, 1990

47. Hardy RR, Hayakawa K, Shimizu M et al: Rheumatoid factor secretion from human Leu-1+ B-cells. Science 236:81, 1987

48. Hamblin TJ, Oscier DJ, Young BJ: Autoimmunity in chronic lymphocytic leukemia. J Clin Pathol 39:713, 1986

49. Kay NE, Perri RT: Evidence that large granular lymphocytes from B-CLL patients with hypogammaglobulinemia down-regulate B-cell immunoglobulin synthesis. Blood 73:1016, 1989

50. Chapel H, Bunch C: Mechanisms of infections in chronic lymphocytic leukemia. Semin Hematol 24:291, 1987

51. Kantoyiannis DP, Anaissie EJ, Bodey GP: Infection in chronic lymphocytic leukemia: a reappraisal. p. 399. In Cheson BD (ed): Chronic Lymphocytic Leukemia: Scientific Advances and Clinical Developments. Marcel Dekker, New York, 1993

52. Deegan MJ, Abraham JP, Sawdyk M, Van Slyck EJ: High incidence of monoclonal proteins in the serum and urine of chronic lymphocytic leukemia patients. Blood 64:1207, 1984

53. Cheson BD, Bennett JM, Rai KR et al: Guidelines for clinical protocols for chronic lymphocytic leukemia (CLL). Recommendations of the NCI-Sponsored Working Group. Am J Hematol 29:152, 1988

54. Binet JL, Catovsky D, Dighiero G et al: Chronic lymphocytic leukemia: recommendations for diagnosis, staging and response criteria. International Workshop on CLL. Ann Intern Med 110:236, 1989

55. Bennett JM, Catovsky D, Daniel MT et al: The French American British (FAB) Cooperative Group proposals for the classification of chronic (mature) B and T lymphoid leukemia. J Clin Pathol 42:567, 1989

56. Chikkappa G, Pasquale D, Phillips PG et al: Cyclosporin-A for the treatment of pure red cell aplasia in a patient with chronic lymphocytic leukemia. Am J Hematol 26:179, 1987

57. Mangan KF, Chikkappa G, Farley PC: T gamma cells suppress growth of erythroid colony-forming units in vitro in the pure red cell aplasia of B-cell chronic lymphocytic leukemia. J Clin Invest 70:1148, 1982

58. Mangan KF, D'Alessandro L: Hypoplastic anemia in B-cell chronic lymphocytic leukemia: evolution of T cell-mediated suppression of erythropoiesis in early-stage and late-stage disease. Blood 66:533, 1985

59. Geisler C, Ralfkiaer E, Hansen MM et al: The bone marrow histology pattern has independent prognostic value in chronic lymphocytic leukemia. Br J Haematol 62:47, 1986

60. Han T, Barcos M, Emrich L et al: Bone marrow infiltration patterns and their prognostic significance in chronic lymphocytic leukemia: correlations with clinical, immunologic, phenotypic, and cytogenetic data. J Clin Oncol 6:562, 1984

61. Hernandez-Nieto L, Montserrat-Costa E, Muncunill J et al: Bone marrow patterns and clinical staging in chronic lymphocytic leukemia, letter. Lancet 1:1269, 1977

62. Lipshutz MD, Mir R, Rai KR et al: Bone marrow biopsy and clinical staging in chronic lymphocytic leukemia. Cancer 46:1422, 1980

63. Montserrat E, Rozman C, Spanish Cooperative Group for CLL: Bone marrow biopsy in chronic lymphocytic leukemia: a study of 208 cases. Haematologia 16:73, 1983

64. Rozman C, Montserrat JM, Rodriquez-Fernandez R et al: Bone marrow histologic pattern—the best single prognostic parameter in chronic lymphocytic leukemia: a multivariate survival analysis of 329 cases. Blood 64:642, 1984

65. Preud'homme JL, Seligmann M: Surface-bound immunoglobulins as a cell marker in human lymphoproliferative diseases. Blood 40:777, 1972

66. Boggs DR, Sofferman SA, Wintrobe MM et al: Factors influencing the duration of survival of patients with chronic lymphocytic leukemia. Am J Med 40:243, 1966

67. Hansen MM: Chronic lymphocytic leukemia. Clinical studies based on 189 cases followed for a long time. Scand J Haematol, suppl. 18:1, 1973

68. Rai KR, Sawitsky A, Cronkite EP et al: Clinical staging of chronic lymphocytic leukemia. Blood 46:219, 1975

69. Rai KR: A critical analysis of staging in CLL. p. 253. In Gale RP, Rai KR (eds): Chronic Lymphocytic Leukemia Recent Progress and Future Directions. UCLA Symposia on Molecular and Cellular Biology, New Series. Vol. 59. Alan R Liss, New York, 1987

70. Montserrat E, Rozman C: Chronic lymphocytic leukaemia: prognostic factors and natural history. Baillieres Clin Haematol 6:849, 1993

71. Binet JL, Auquier A, Dighiero G et al: A new prognostic classification of chronic lymphocytic derived from a multivariate survival analysis. Cancer 48:198, 1981

72. Jaksic B, Vitale B: Total tumor mass score (TTM): a new parameter in chronic lymphocytic leukaemia. Br J Haematol 49:405, 1981

73. Mandelli F, DeRossi G, Mancini P et al: Prognosis in chronic lymphocytic leukemia: a retrospective multicentric study from the GIMEMA group. J Clin Oncol 5:398, 1987

74. Lee JS, Dixon DO, Kantarjian HM et al: Prognosis of chronic lymphocytic leukemia: a multivariate regression analysis of 325 untreated patients. Blood 69:929, 1987

75. Baccarini M, Cavo M, Gobbi M et al: Staging of chronic lymphocytic leukemia. Blood 59:1191, 1982

76. Skinnider LF, Tan L, Schmidt J, Armitage G: Chronic lymphocytic leukemia. A review of 745 cases and assessment of clinical staging. Cancer 50:2951, 1982

77. Paolino W, Infelise V, Levis A et al: Adenosplenomegaly and prognosis in uncomplicated and complicated chronic lymphocytic leukemia. A study of 362 cases. Cancer 54:339, 1984

78. Molica S, Alberti A: Prognostic value of the lymphocyte doubling time in chronic lymphocytic leukemia: analysis of its prognostic significance. Br J Haematol 62:567, 1986

79. Vallespi T, Montserrat E, Sanz M: Chronic lymphocytic leukaemia: prognostic value of lymphocyte morphological subtypes. A multivariate analysis of 146 patients. Br J Haematol 77:478, 1991

80. Dhodapkar M, Tefferi A, Su J, Phyliky RL: Prognostic features and survival in young adults with early/intermediate chronic lymphocytic leukemia (B-CLL): a single institution study. Leukemia 7:1232, 1993

81. Pangalis GA, Roussou PA, Kittas C et al: B-chronic lymphocytic leukemia. Prognostic implications of bone marrow histology in 120 patients. Experience from a single hematology unit. Cancer 59:767, 1987

82. Geisler CH, Larsen JK, Hansen NE et al: Prognostic importance of flow cytometric immunophenotyping of 540 consecutive patients with B-cell chronic lymphocytic leukemia. Blood 78:1795, 1991

83. Rozman C, Montserrat E, Feliu E et al: Prognosis of chronic lymphocytic leukemia: a multivariate survival analysis of 150 cases. Blood 59:1001, 1982

84. Phillips EA, Kempin S, Passe S et al: Prognostic factors in chronic lymphocytic leukaemia and their implications for therapy. Clin Haematol 6:203, 1977

85. Peterson LC, Bloomfield CD, Sundberg RD et al: Morphology of chronic lymphocytic leukemia and its relationship to survival. Am J Med 59:316, 1975

86. Han T, Emrich LJ, Ozer H et al: Clinical significance of lactate dehydrogenase in chronic lymphocytic leukemia. NY State J Med 85:685, 1985

87. Kallander CFR, Simonsson B, Hagberg H, Gronowitz JS: Serum deoxythymidine kinase gives prognostic information in chronic lymphocytic leukemia. Cancer 54:2450, 1984

88. Montserrat E, Marques-Pereira JP, Rozman C et al: Serum beta-2-microglobulin in chronic lymphocytic leukaemia. Clin Lab Haematol 4:323, 1982

89. Orfao A, Gonzalez M, San Miguel JF et al: B-cell chronic lymphocytic leukemia: prognostic values of the immunophenotype and clinico-hematologic features. Am J Hematol 31:26, 1989

90. Montserrat E, Vinolas N, Reverter JC, Rozman C: Natural history of chronic lymphocytic leukemia: on the progression and prognosis of early clinical stages. Nouv Rev Fr Hematol 30:359, 1988

91. French Cooperative Group on Chronic Lymphocytic Leukaemia: Natural history of Stage A chronic lymphocytic leukaemia untreated patients. Br J Haematol 76:45, 1990

92. DeRossi G, Mandelli F, Covelli A et al: Chronic lymphocytic leukemia in younger adults: a retrospective study of 133 cases. Hematol Oncol 7:127, 1989

93. Montserrat E, Gomis F, Vallespi T et al: Presenting features and prognosis of chronic lymphocytic leukemia in younger adults. Blood 78:1545, 1991

94. Pangalis GA, Reverter JC, Bussiotis VA, Montserrat E: Chronic lymphocytic leukemia in younger adults: preliminary results of a study based on 454 patients—IWCLL Working Group. Leuk Lymphoma, suppl. 5:175, 1991

95. Bennett JM, Raphael B, Oken MA, Silber R: The prognosis and therapy of chronic lymphocytic leukemia under age 50 years. Nouv Rev Fr Hematol 30:411, 1988

96. Cheson BD: Chronic lymphocytic leukemia: staging and prognostic factors. p. 253. In Cheson BD (ed): Chronic Lymphocytic Leukemia: Scientific Advances and Clinical Developments. Marcel Dekker, New York, 1993

97. Rai KR: An outline of clinical management of chronic lymphocytic leukemia. p. 241. In Cheson BD (ed): Chronic Lymphocytic Leukemia: Scientific Advances and Clinical Developments. Marcel Dekker, New York, 1993

98. Lichtman MA, Rowe JM: Hyperleukocytic leukemia: rheological, clinical and therapeutic considerations. Blood 60:279, 1982

99. Baer MR, Stein RS, Dessypris EN: Chronic lymphocytic leukemia with hyperleukocytosis. The hyperviscosity syndrome. Cancer 56:2865, 1985

100. Cooperative Group for the Study of Immunoglobulin in Chronic Lymphocytic Leukemia: Intravenous immunoglobulin for the prevention of infection in chronic lymphocytic leukemia. A randomized, controlled clinical trial. N Engl J Med 319:902, 1988

101. Sawitsky A, Rai KR, Glidewell O et al: Comparison of daily versus intermittent chlorambucil and prednisone therapy in the treatment of patients with chronic lymphocytic leukemia. Blood 50:1049, 1977

102. Huguley CM Jr: Treatment of chronic lymphocytic leukemia. Cancer Treat Rev 4:261, 1977

103. Knospe WH, Loeb V Jr, Huguley CM Jr: Biweekly chlorambucil treatment of chronic lymphocytic leukemia. Cancer 3:555, 1974

104. Keating MJ: Chemotherapy of chronic lymphocytic leukemia. p. 297. In Cheson BD (ed): Chronic Lymphocytic Leukemia: Scientific Advances and Clinical Developments. Marcel Dekker, New York, 1993

105. Robertson LE, Huh YO, Butler JJ et al: Response assessment in chronic lymphocytic leukemia after fludarabine plus prednisone: clinical pathologic, immunophenotypic and molecular analysis. Blood 80:29, 1992

106. O'Brien S, Kantarjian H, Beran M et al: Results of fludarabine and prednisone therapy in 264 patients with chronic lymphocytic leukemia with multivariate analysis-derived prognostic model for response to treatment. Blood 32:695, 1993

107. Presant CA, Safidar SH: Oxymethalone in myelofibrosis and chronic lymphocytic leukemia. Arch Intern Med 132:175, 1973

108. Narasimhan P, Amaral L: Lymphopenic response of patients presenting with chronic lymphocytic leukemia associated with carcinoma of the prostate

109. Kempin S, Shank B: Radiation in chronic lymphocytic leukemia. p. 337. In Gale RP, Rai KR (eds): Chronic Lymphocytic Leukemia: Recent Progress and Future Directions. UCLA Symposia on Molecular and Cellular Biology, New Series. Vol. 59. Alan R Liss, New York, 1987

110. Roncardin M, Arcicasa M, Trovo MG et al: Splenic irradiation in chronic lymphocytic leukemia. A 10-year experience at a single institution. Cancer 60:2624, 1987

111. Chanana AD, Cronkite EP, Rai KR: The role of extracorporeal irradiation of blood in the treatment of leukemia. Int J Radiat Oncol Biol Phys 1:539, 1976

112. Richards F, Spurr CL, Ferree C et al: Thymic irradiation. An approach to chronic lymphocytic leukemia. Am J Med 57:862, 1974

113. Richards F, Spurr CL, Ferree C et al: The control of chronic lymphocytic leukemia with mediastinal irradiation. Am J Med 64:947, 1978

114. Sawitsky A, Rai KR, Aral I et al: Mediastinal irradiation for chronic lymphocytic leukemia. Am J Med 71:892, 1976

115. Johnson RE: Treatment of chronic lymphocytic leukemia by total body irradiation alone and combined with chemotherapy. Int J Radiat Oncol Biol Phys 5:159, 1979

116. Bennett JM, Raphael B, Moore D et al: Comparison of chlorambucil and prednisone vs. total body irradiation and chlorambucil, prednisone vs. cytoxan, vincristine, prednisone for the therapy of active chronic lymphocytic leukemia. p. 317. In Gale RP, Rai KR (eds): Chronic Lymphocytic Leukemia: Recent Progress and Future Directions. UCLA Symposia on Molecular and Cellular Biology, New Series. Vol. 59. Alan R Liss, New York, 1987

117. Osgood EE: Titrated, regularly spaced radioactive phosphorous of spray roentgen therapy of leukemias. Arch Intern Med 87:329, 1951

118. Depero JR, Mouvenaeghel G, Gastaut JA et al: Splenectomy for hypersplenism in chronic lymphocytic leukemia and malignant non-Hodgkin's lymphoma. Br J Surg 77:443, 1990

119. Ferrant A, Michaux JL, Sokal G: Splenectomy in advanced chronic lymphocytic leukemia. Cancer 58:2130, 1986

120. Merl SA, Theodarakis ME, Goldberg J, Gottlieb AJ: Splenectomy for thrombocytopenia in chronic lymphocytic leukemia. Am J Hematol 15:253, 1983

121. Pegourie B, Sotto J-J, Holland D et al: Splenectomy during chronic lymphocytic leukemia. Cancer 59:1626, 1987

122. Neal TF Jr, Tefferi A, Witzig T: Splenectomy in advanced chronic lymphocytic leukemia: a single institution experience with 50 patients. Am J Med 93:435, 1992

123. Majumdar G, Singh AK: Role of splenectomy in chronic lymphocytic leukemia with massive splenomegaly and cytopenia. Leuk Lymphoma 7:131, 1992

124. Goldfinger D, Capostagno V, Lowe C et al: Use of long-term leukapheresis in the treatment of chronic lymphocytic leukemia. Transfusion 20:450, 1980

125. Marti GE, Folks T, Longo DL, Klein H: Therapeutic cytopheresis in chronic lymphocytic leukemia. J Clin Apheresis 1:243, 1983

126. Shustik C, Mick R, Silver R et al: Treatment of early chronic lymphocytic leukemia: intermittent chlorambucil vs. observation. Hematol Oncol 6:7, 1988

127. French Cooperative Group on Chronic Lymphocytic Leukemia: Effects of chlorambucil and therapeutic abstention in initial forms of chronic lymphocytic leukemia (stage A): results of a randomized clinical trial in 612 patients. Blood 75:1414, 1990

128. French Cooperative Group on CLL: Long-term results of the CHOP regimen in stage C chronic lymphocytic leukemia. Br J Haematol 73:334, 1989

129. Jaksic B, Brugiatelli M, for the IGCI (Vienna) CLL Study Group: High dose chlorambucil for the treatment of advanced B-chronic lymphocytic leukemia: results of two multicentric randomized trials. Blood, suppl. 1. 76:284, 1990

130. Bennett JM: The use of CHOP in the treatment of chronic lymphocytic leukemia. Br J Haematol 74:546, 1990

131. Hansen MM, Andersen E, Birgens H et al: CHOP versus chlorambucil plus prednisone in chronic lymphocytic leukemia. Leuk Lymphoma, suppl. 5:97, 1991

132. Spanish Cooperative Group on CLL: Treatment of chronic lymphocytic leukemia: a preliminary report of Spanish (PETHEMA) trials. Leuk Lymphoma, suppl. 5:89, 1991

133. Kimby E, Mellstedt H: Chlorambucil/prednisone versus CHOP in symptomatic chronic lymphocytic leukemia of B-cell type. A randomized trial. Leuk Lymphoma, suppl. 5:93:1991

134. Keating MJ, Scouros M, Murphy M et al: Multiple agent chemotherapy (POACH) in previously treated and untreated patients with chronic lymphocytic leukemia. Leukemia 2:157, 1988

135. Kempin S, Lee BJ, Thaler HT et al: Combination chemotherapy of advanced phosphamide, melphalan and prednisone. Blood 60:110, 1982

Pangalis GA, Roussou PA, Kittas C et al: B-chronic lymphocytic leukemia. — to diethylstilbestrol: correlation of response to the in vitro synthesis of RNA by patient lymphocytes and its relationship to transcortin. Am J Hematol 8: 569, 1980

136. Dicato M, Chapel H, Gamm H et al: Use of intravenous immunoglobulin in chronic lymphocytic leukemia. A brief review. Cancer, suppl. 1. 68:1437, 1991

137. Weeks JC, Tierney MR, Weinstein MC: Cost effectiveness of prophylactic intravenous immunoglobulin in chronic lymphocytic leukemia. N Engl J Med 325:81, 1991

138. Foon KA, Bottino GC, Abrams PG et al: Phase II trials of recombinant leukocyte A interferon in patients with advanced chronic lymphocytic leukemia. Am J Med 78:216, 1985

139. Boussiotis VA, Pangalis GA: Interferon alpha-2b therapy in untreated early stage B chronic lymphocytic leukaemia patients: one year follow-up. Br J Haematol, suppl. 1. 79:30, 1991

140. Montserrat E, Villamor N, Urbano Ispizua A et al: Alpha-interferon in chronic lymphocytic leukemia. Eur J Cancer, suppl. 27:74, 1991

141. Ferrara F, Rametta C, Mele G et al: Recombinant interferon alfa-2A as a maintenance treatment for patients with advanced stage chronic lymphocytic leukemia responding to chemotherapy. Am J Hematol 41:45, 1992

142. Ziegler-Heitbrock HWL, Schlag R, Flieger R, Thiel E: Favorable response of early stage B-CLL patients to treatment with IFN-alpha-2. Blood 73:1426, 1989

143. Molica S: Combined use of alpha-2b interferon, chlorambucil, and prednisone in the treatment of previously B-chronic lymphocytic leukemia patients. Am J Hematol 43:334, 1993

144. Ostlund L, Einhorn S, Robert KH et al: Chronic B lymphocytic leukemia cells proliferate and differentiate following exposure to interferon in vitro. Blood 67:152, 1986

145. Panayiotidis P, Ganeshguru K, Jabbar SAB, Hoffbrand AV: Alpha-interferon protects B-chronic lymphocytic leukaemia cells from apoptotic cell death in vitro. Br J Haematol 86:169, 1994

146. Chikkappa G, Pasquale D, Mangan K et al: Successful treatment of pure red cell aplasia in a patient with chronic lymphocytic leukemia with cyclosporine-A. Blood, suppl. 1. 68:1069, 1986

147. Rai KR, Jagthambal K, Siegal FP et al: Cyclosporine in treatment of refractory anemia and thrombocytopenia of chronic lymphocytic leukemia. Blood 70: 141a, 1987

148. Tura S, Finelli C, Bandini G et al: Cyclosporin A in the treatment of CLL, associated PRCA and bone marrow hypoplasia. Nouv Rev Fr Hematol 30: 479, 1988

149. Richter MN: Generalized reticular cell sarcoma of lymph nodes associated with lymphatic leukemia. Am J Pathol 4:285, 1928

150. Robertson LE, Pugh W, O'Brien S et al: Richter's syndrome: a report on 39 patients. J Clin Oncol 11:1985, 1993

151. Cherepakhin V, Baird SM, Meisenholder GW, Kipps TJ: Common clonal origin of chronic lymphocytic leukemia and high grade lymphoma of Richter's syndrome. Blood 82:3141, 1993

152. Kruger A, Sadullah S, Chapman R et al: Use of retinoblastoma gene probe to investigate clonality in Richter's syndrome. Leukemia 7:1891, 1993

153. Anhalt GJ, Kim SC, Stanley JR et al: Paraneoplastic pemphigus: an autoimmune mucocutaneous disease associated with neoplasia. N Engl J Med 323: 1729, 1990

154. Saven A, Carrera CJ, Carson DA et al: 2-chlorodeoxyadenosine treatment of refractory chronic lymphocytic leukemia. Leuk Lymphoma, suppl. 5:133, 1991

155. Juliusson G, Lilliemark J: High complete remission rate from 2-chloro-2'-deoxyadenosine in previously treated patients with B-cell chronic lymphocytic leukemia: response predicted by rapid decrease in blood lymphocyte count. J Clin Oncol 11:679, 1993

156. Grever MR, Leiby JM, Kraut EH et al: Low dose deoxycoformycin in lymphoid malignancy. J Clin Oncol 3:1196, 1985

157. Dillman RO, Mick R, McIntyre OR et al: Pentostatin in chronic lymphocytic leukemia: a phase II trial of Cancer and Leukemia Group B. J Clin Oncol 7: 433, 1989

158. Rabinowe SN, Soiffer RJ, Gribben JG et al: Autologous and allogeneic bone marrow transplantation for poor prognosis patients with B-cell chronic lymphocytic leukemia. Blood 82:1366, 1993

159. Michallet M, Corront B, Hollard D et al: Allogeneic bone marrow transplantation in chronic lymphocytic leukemia: 17 cases. Report from EBMTG. Bone Marrow Transplant 7:275, 1991

160. Vallera DA: Immunotoxins: will their clinical promise be fulfilled? Blood 83: 309, 1994

161. Grossbard ML, Press OW, Applebaum FR et al: Monoclonal antibody-based therapies of leukemia and lymphoma. Blood 80:863, 1992

162. Grossbard ML, Nadler LM: Immunotoxin therapy of malignancy. p. 111. In DeVita VT Jr, Hellman S, Rosenberg SA (eds): Important Advances in Oncology. JB Lippincott, Philadelphia, 1992

163. Dyer MJS, Hale G, Hayhoe FGJ, Waldmann H: Effects of CAMPATH-1H antibodies in vivo in patients with lymphoid malignancies: influence of antibody isotype. Blood 73:1431, 1989

164. Janson D, Nissel-Horowitz S, Sattler M, Rai KR: Complete and partial response (CR, PR) in treatment of advanced refractory B-cell chronic lymphcytic leukemia (B-CLL) using CAMPATH-1H. Blood, suppl. 1. 82:139a, 1993

165. Catovsky D: Diagnosis and treatment of CLL variants. p. 369. In Cheson BD (ed): Chronic Lymphocytic Leukemia: Scientific Advances and Clinical Developments. Marcel Dekker, New York, 1993

166. Loughran TP, Kadin ME, Starkebaum G et al: Leukemia of large granular lymphocytes: association with clonal chromosomal abnormalities and autoimmune neutropenia, thrombocytopenia and hemolytic anemia. Ann Intern Med 102:169, 1985

167. Knowles DM, Halper JP: Human T-cell malignancies: correlative clinical histopathologic, immunologic and cytochemical analysis of 23 cases. Am J Pathol 106:187, 1982

168. Pandolfi JC, DeRossi G, Semenzato G et al: Immunologic evaluation of T-chronic lymphocytic leukemia cells: correlations among phenotype, functional activities and morphology. Blood 59:688, 1982

Hairy Cell Leukemia

84

Alan Saven and Lawrence D. Piro

INTRODUCTION

Hairy cell leukemia (HCL), or leukemic reticuloendotheliosis, is a rare chronic lymphoproliferative disorder first described in the literature as a distinct clinicopathologic entity in 1958 by Bouroncle et al.[1] The disease is characterized by circulating B lymphocytes that display prominent cytoplasmic projections and have a characteristic pattern of infiltration in the bone marrow and spleen. Because of this characteristic pattern, the original name of leukemic reticuloendotheliosis was replaced in 1966 by the more descriptive name, hairy cell leukemia.[2] Patients tend to be elderly, often presenting with pancytopenia, splenomegaly, or recurrent infections. In recent years, interferon (IFN)-α, 2'-deoxycoformycin (dCF), and 2-chlorodeoxyadenosine (2-CdA) have been shown to be capable of regularly inducing remissions in HCL. These clinical advances have revolutionized the treatment and prognosis for patients with this disease.

EPIDEMIOLOGY

HCL is said to compromise approximately 2% of adult leukemias in the United States. Approximately 600 new patients are diagnosed each year. Several familial cases have been reported, but whether these result from common genetic or environmental factors is unclear.[3] HCL is predominantly a disease of middle-aged men with a median age at presentation of 52 years. There is a 4:1 male predominance, with Ashkenazi Jewish males being more frequently afflicted. Some geographic variation in incidence exists but has not resulted in meaningful insights except that the incidence in Japan is extremely low.[4]

ETIOLOGY AND PATHOGENESIS

No clear etiology of HCL has been documented. Previous exposure to ionizing radiation and organic chemicals in the workplace is higher among some HCL patients than controls.[5,6] A possible association of human T-cell leukemia virus (HTLV)-II infection with the T-cell variant of HCL has been described[7]; however, this has never been corroborated. In fact, there is little data even to support the existence of a T-cell variant of this disease.

BIOLOGY AND PATHOLOGY

Hairy cells are named for their characteristic cytoplasmic projections, which may be seen as fine wisps, pseudopods, or microvilli in blood smears viewed by light, phase contrast, and electron microscopy. The normal function and site of action of the cell from which HCL arises are unknown, although the malignant cell is known to be a B lymphocyte.[8] Hairy cells are mononuclear cells with eccentrically or centrally placed nuclei. They have a variety of morphologic appearances based on differences in cell size and nuclear shape.[9] Nuclear configurations may be round, ovoid, reniform, convoluted, and indented. Round and ovoid cells tend to be smallest in size with a mean diameter of 7 μm. Convoluted nuclear types average 9 μm in diameter and the indented types average 11 μm in diameter.

Small nucleoli may be present, which are more prominent in the larger indented forms. Most nuclear forms share a fine reticular chromatin, except for the round variety. which is more clumped. Cytoplasm is variable in amount but consistent in quality, and blue-gray in color with varying amounts of ruffled cell borders exhibiting thin cytoplasmic projections. The cytoplasm may rarely contain granules or broad-shaped inclusions that correspond to the ribosomal lamellar complex[10] (Fig. 84-1).

Most patients present with pancytopenia.[9,11–13] Leukopenia is marked by severe monocytopenia. Bone marrow aspirate smears typically lack spicules because of marrow reticulin fibrosis, but occasional cases will show typical hairy cells on aspirated material or on touch preparations of the core biopsy. The hairy cell morphology in bone marrow aspirate smears is similar to that found in the peripheral blood, except for slightly coarser reticular chromatin staining. Marrow biopsy sections usually show involvement by hairy cells, but because of patchy HCL involvement repeat biopsy may occasionally be necessary.[9,11–13] At low magnification power the pattern of HCL infiltration is characteristic. There is diffuse or focal infiltration by monotonous round, oval, or spindle-shaped nuclei separated by abundant amounts of pale cytoplasm in a fine fibrillar network that separates individual cells, a pattern often called "fried-egg" appearance. Nuclei have fine or vesicular chromatin with variably sized nucleoli. Admixed are varying numbers of small lymphocytes, plasma cells, mast cells, extravasated erythrocytes, and fibroblasts. At higher magnification, the nuclear morphology appears more heterogeneous, with round, ovoid, convoluted, and indented forms usually apparent. Round or ovoid cells tend to predominate. The cytoplasm is pale and a delicate network of fibrils extending around individual hairy cells can often be seen, especially with the periodic acid-Schiff stain. HCL infiltration may produce dilated sinuses with extravasated red blood cells similar to the red cell lakes typically seen in the spleen. Rarely, hairy cells may have a peritrabecular distribution. The most difficult pattern of HCL involvement to recognize is that of a hypocellular marrow with sparse infiltration by hairy cells within residual hematopoietic tissue and when hairy cell infiltrates merge with normal surrounding hematopoietic tissue without sharp boundaries delineated. There are typically small clusters of immature erythro-

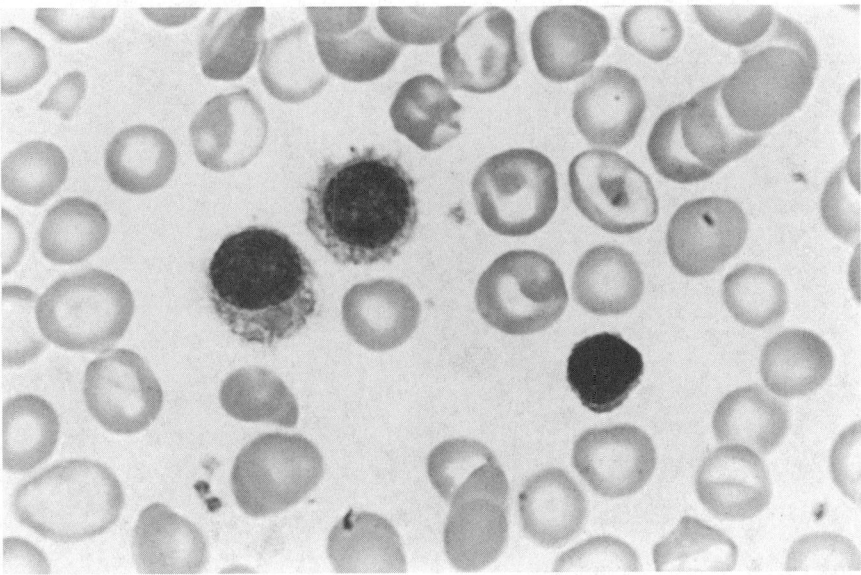

Fig. 84-1. Peripheral blood smear. Two hairy cells and one normal lymphocyte. Note the abundant frayed cytoplasm, and the round to oval nucleus with reticular chromatin. (× 1,600.)

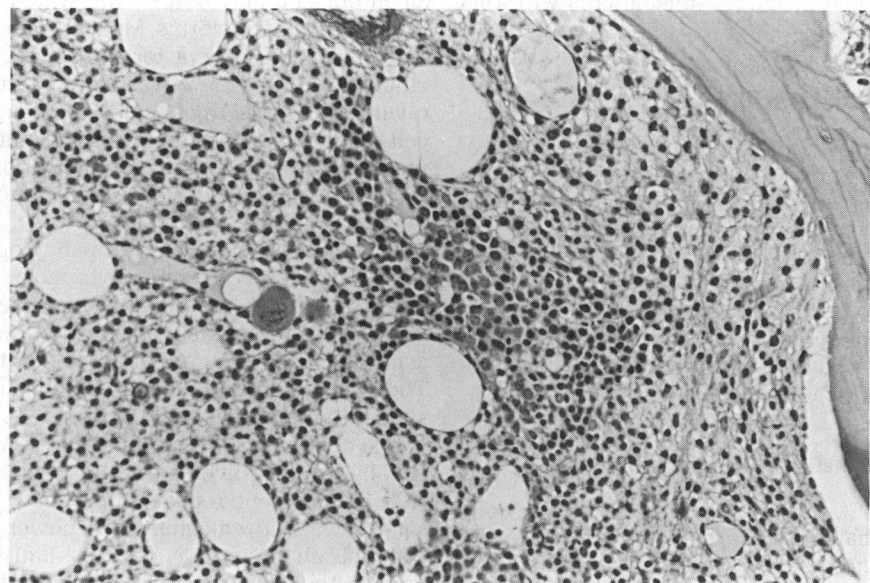

Fig. 84-2. Bone marrow biopsy. Note the central island of erythroblasts and the peripheral monotonous mononuclear cell infiltrate with abundant cytoplasm separating the cells.

blasts and granulocytic precursors are usually markedly diminished (Fig. 84-2).

The spleen is typically moderately enlarged with a median weight of 1,300 g.[14] The cut surface reveals a beefy-red homogeneous surface. Microscopically, hairy cells populate the red pulp, and eventually the white pulp atrophies and is replaced. Early HCL involvement is seen as focal infiltration of trabeculae and subendothelial infiltrates within trabecular veins.[15] A characteristic but not pathognomonic finding is red cell lakes, which are blood-filled spaces lined by hairy cells that have disrupted the normal sinus architecture.[16] Exceptional cases of HCL may involve only the spleen.[17]

Liver involvement is both sinusoidal and portal.[18] Lymph node involvement is marked by sinusoidal and interstitial involvement.[19] Hairy cell infiltrates of bone may extend from the medullary cavity to produce cortical osteolytic lesions.[20]

Cytochemical evaluation is important for diagnostic confirmation of these morphologic observations. Hairy cells demonstrate strong cytoplasmic positivity for tartrate-resistant acid phosphatase (TRAP) staining. Isoenzyme 5 acid phosphatases is unlike other acid phosphatases because of its resistance to tartrate.[21,22] Smears should be evaluated for adequate cellularity and morphology. When evaluating the stain, individual hairy cells exhibit a range of staining from weak to strongly positive, with typical cells showing moderate positivity. However, for the diagnosis, at least two cells with >40 granules or with numerous granules that obscure the nucleus, is required. When strongly positive TRAP-staining cells with morphology suggestive of hairy cells are found, the finding is highly specific for HCL. TRAP staining of peripheral blood buffy-coat smears will yield a positive result in approximately 90% of cases.[21] Moderate to weak staining is described in other diseases, some

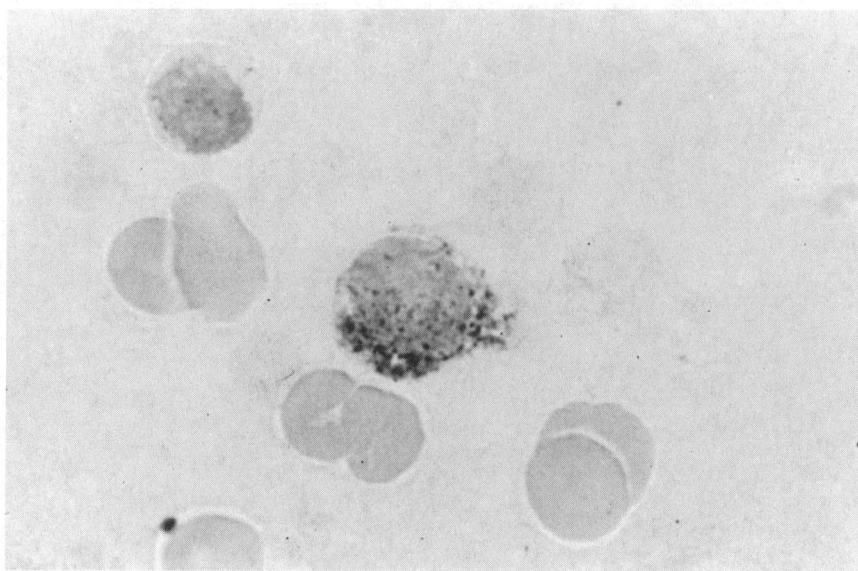

Fig. 84-3. TRAP-stained buffy coat smear. Note the TRAP-positive hairy cell with abundant cytoplasmic granules in contrast to the TRAP-negative small lymphocyte. (× 4,000.)

of which may be confused with HCL. Granulocytes and platelets both contain acid phosphatases that are not resistant to tartrate and should be TRAP-stain-negative (Fig. 84-3).

Electron microscopy may aid in the diagnosis when hairy cells with numerous circumferential cytoplasmic projections, appearing as ridges or villi, are visualized.[23] Electron microscopic studies of related disorders usually reveal fewer and blunter microvilli that also do not exhibit a circumferential pattern.[24,25] Under electron microscopy, ribosomal lamella complexes appear as membranous structures composed of concentric rings of lamellae lined by ribosomes.[21] Ribosomal lamella complexes may also be seen in approximately one-half the HCL cases, but these too have been described in other lymphoproliferative disorders.[26]

IMMUNOPHENOTYPIC ANALYSIS

Hairy cells have a mature B-cell phenotype and typically express single or multiple immunoglobulin heavy chains with monotypic light chains.[8,27–31] Hairy cells express receptors for the Fc portions of IgG and IgM,[32–35] but do not express the complement receptor.[32,36] Hairy cells form rosettes with mouse erythrocytes.[37] Hairy cells express the pan B-cell antigens CD19, CD20, and CD22; they do not express CD21, an antigen lost in the later stages of B-cell ontogeny. They also commonly express PCA-1, an early plasma cell antigen.

HCL has a characteristic phenotype as assessed by staining with a panel of monoclonal antibodies.[38] This pattern is best visualized by a combination of the pan B-cell markers with CD11c, CD25, and Bly-7.[39] CD11c gives a very strong pattern of staining, with a relative intensity virtually always greater than that seen in chronic lymphocytic leukemia and other chronic lymphoproliferative disorders.[40] This intensity is 30-fold higher than that seen in a typical case of chronic lymphocytic leukemia.

HCL was the first B-cell lymphoproliferative disorder recognized to express the interleukin-2 (IL-2) receptor CD25. Again, chronic lymphocytic leukemia and other B-cell chronic lymphoproliferative disorders may be positive for CD25, but the intensity of staining by HCL is six-fold greater. Serum levels of soluble IL-2 receptors are high in patients with HCL and correlates with disease activity.[41]

Monoclonal antibody Bly-7 has high sensitivity and specificity for HCL. This antibody recognizes an antigen that is associated with the subunit of the B7 integrin molecule, which may play a role in lymphocyte homing and adhesion.[42]

The B-cell antibody CD22 shows significantly higher intensity of staining in hairy cells than either normal B cells or leukemic cells from other B-cell chronic lymphoproliferative disorders. CD22 was found to stain 50 times more intensely in HCL cells than chronic lymphocytic leukemia, which only weakly expresses CD22.[38]

Subsets of hairy cells may be defined immunologically by weak expression of CD5 (in approximately 4% of cases) and by CD10 (formerly CALLA) (in 26% of cases).[38]

In 161 patients studied, circulating hairy cells could be identified by immunophenotypic features in 92% of cases, even when representing <1% of circulating lymphocytes. This is an advancement over morphologic examination of the peripheral blood, which reveals hairy cells in approximately 80% of cases.[38]

Immunohistochemistry on bone marrow biopsy sections may also be supportive of the diagnosis of HCL. The hairy cells stain with L26 (CD20) and DBA.44.[43] Staining with L26 is membranous and accentuates the ruffled abundant cytoplasm. DBA.44, an undefined antigen, stains a subpopulation of hairy cells, but in both a cytoplasmic granular and membranous pattern. DBA.44 also stains approximately 30% of all low-grade lymphomas.

Table 84-1. Clinical Manifestations of HCL

Splenomegaly (90%)
Circulating hairy cells (90%)
Pancytopenia (70%)
Hepatomegaly (35%)
Lymphadenopathy (25%)
Osteolytic lesions, autoimmune disease, vasculitis
Bone marrow findings
Dry tap; reticular fibrosis
Diffusely infiltrating mononuclear cells separated by clear cytoplasms giving bone marrow a "fried egg" appearance

CLINICAL MANIFESTATIONS

Patients usually present with symptoms related to their hematologic abnormalities (Table 84-1). About 25% of patients present with fatigue and weakness, 25% with infection, and 25% with the incidental finding of splenomegaly or an abnormal blood count.[44] In a series of 102 patients, at presentation 86 had anemia, 84 thrombocytopenia, and 78 neutropenia.[45] Splenomegaly was present in 93 patients. Bleeding and infectious complications tend to occur with increasing frequency as the disease progresses. Hepatomegaly occurs in 20% of patients. Peripheral adenopathy is rarely found clinically (<10% of patients have peripheral lymph nodes >2 cm); however, with the use of computed tomographic scans in the initial evaluation, internal lymphadenopathy is now recognized in up to one-third of patients. Although HCL is classically associated with leukopenia, almost 20% of patients may present in a leukemic phase[46] and 10% of patients may present without circulating hairy cells demonstrable on light microscopy. Other laboratory findings include abnormal liver function tests in 19% of patients, azotemia in 27%, and hypergammaglobulinemia in 18%, which may rarely be monoclonal. Hypogammaglobulinemia is uncommon.

Patients with HCL are susceptible to gram-positive and gram-negative bacterial infections as well as atypical mycobacterial disease, particularly *Mycobacterium kansasii*. The incidence of infection does not correlate with prior splenectomy or previous systemic therapy, but with the severity of neutropenia and monocytopenia. Nonpyogenic infections with *Aspergillus, Histoplasma, Cryptococcus,* and *Pneumocystis carinii* occur with greater frequency among HCL patients.

HCL has also been associated with other immunologic disorders, including leukocytoclastic vasculitis and polyarthritis nodosa. Rarely there may be cutaneous manifestations of the disease.[47,48] Skeletal involvement with HCL has also been reported.[20,49] This may be manifested as diffuse osteoporosis or more commonly as lytic lesions involving the axial skeleton, particularly the femoral heads. These patients tend to have higher tumor burdens with hypercellular marrows heavily infiltrated by HCL. Patients with chylous and serous ascites, and even pleural effusions, have also been reported.[50,51]

LABORATORY EVALUATION

As discussed, at the time of diagnosis many patients have pancytopenia and therefore evaluation of the blood smear is usually the first laboratory test to be performed. When anemia is present it can be severe, usually associated with a normal mean corpuscular volume and mild anisocytosis and poikilocytosis. If the bone marrow is heavily infiltrated, occasional nucleated red cells may also be observed. Most patients have leukopenia and granulocytopenia, although in about 20% of cases leukocytosis is observed. Patients with HCL usually demonstrate monocytopenia, and in >80% of cases thrombocytopenia is present.[44,46] Rarely, a qualitative platelet defect in ag-

Table 84-2. Differential Diagnosis of HCL

Hairy cell leukemia variant
Chronic lymphocytic leukemia
Prolymphocytic leukemia
Splenic lymphoma with circulating villous lymphocytes
Low-grade non-Hodgkin lymphoma
    Small-cleaved lymphoma
    Small cell lymphocytic lymphoma
    Marginal zone lymphoma of the spleen
    Monocytoid B-cell lymphoma

gregation has been reported that may improve with effective therapy.[52–54]

In approximately 90% of cases, circulating hairy cells are present, are of the classic appearance described earlier, and demonstrate TRAP positivity. Other laboratory parameters that have been reported in HCL include increased alkaline phosphatase levels,[55] and elevated immunoglobulin levels sometimes associated with a monoclonal immunoglobulin spike.[44,46] Blood chemistries are usually normal except as mentioned and for occasionally low serum cholesterol measurements.

The diagnosis of HCL is confirmed by bone marrow aspirate and biopsy where the characteristic appearance previously described is found. Aspiration of the marrow is unsuccessful due to "dry tap" in most patients. Occasionally HCL is not suspected until after splenectomy is performed for diagnostic evaluation. When this occurs the diagnosis is made by observing the classic red pulp involvement of the spleen already discussed.

In difficult cases, diagnosis may be confirmed with immunophenotypic analysis and electron microscopy as detailed in previous sections. Soluble IL-2 receptor levels are characteristically quite elevated in HCL and may provide additional supportive data in making a diagnosis.

DIFFERENTIAL DIAGNOSIS

The differential diagnosis of HCL includes hairy cell leukemia variant as well as the other low-grade B-cell lymphoproliferative disorders, such as chronic lymphocytic leukemia, splenic lymphoma with circulating villous lymphocytes, marginal zone lymphoma of the spleen, and monocytoid B-cell lymphoma (Tables 84-2 and 84-3). Splenic lymphoma with circulating villous lymphocytes typically has more basophilic cytoplasm than HCL, and has a lymphocyte-like nucleus.[24] Cytoplasmic projections may be present but are usually polar and not obvious in most of the circulating lymphocytes. Circulating plasmacytoid cells are frequently noted. Immunophenotyping reveals a monoclonal B-cell population lacking strong CD11c positivity, and without Bly-7 positivity. TRAP staining is negative or very weak. Again, the bone marrow is usually aspiratable and typically minimally involved. The lymphocytes appear as small round lymphocytes with plasmacytoid features and peripheral monocytopenia is typically lacking. Sections of spleen are diagnostic, with predominant involvement of the white pulp.

Other splenic lymphomas, including marginal zone lymphoma and monocytoid B-cell lymphoma involving the spleen, are less well characterized immunophenotypically.[56] Although their morphologic features may approximate hairy cells, they are generally TRAP-stain-negative. Extremely strong staining for CD11c and Bly-7 probably excludes these disease entities. Splenic morphology could be helpful in distinguishing these entities early in the disease course. When a patient presents with pancytopenia without splenic enlargement, a hypoplastic bone marrow due to aplastic anemia may be difficult to differentiate from a patchy infiltrate of hairy cells without performing special studies. The most significant single criterion of differentiation is the appearance of hairy cells in the bone marrow biopsy section, as this is usually the most accessible source of diagnostic material.[11] If the diagnosis cannot be established on the bone marrow biopsy, a diagnostic splenectomy may be required. It is important to recognize that the HCL appearance in the bone marrow may be simulated by an artifactual distortion of cytoplasmic clearing around the nuclei of lymphocytic lymphomas or surrounding granulocytic cells.

Finally, HCL must be differentiated from mast cell disease. Both the cytologic appearance and pattern of involvement of mast cell disease may mimic HCL, especially infiltrates composed of spindle-shaped cells. Mast cells contain metachromatic granules when stained with Giemsa and the granules are also positive for chloroacetate esterase.[57] Immunohistochemistry will show reactivity with KPI (CDBP), a marker of macrophages, and lack of reactivity with L26 (CD20).

VARIANTS OF HAIRY CELL LEUKEMIA

Hairy cell leukemia variant (HCL-V)[25] is a hybrid clinical entity between prolymphocytic leukemia and HCL with the nucleus resembling that of a prolymphocyte and the cytoplasm that of a hairy cell. Patients tend to have massive splenomegaly and a profound leukocytosis. These cells are usually TRAP-negative or weakly positive. Immunophenotypic analysis is similar to HCL, but HCL-V is usually CD25⁻ and Bly-7⁻. Distinction from HCL is based on nuclear morphology, leukemic pre-

Table 84-3. Differential Laboratory and Pathologic Features

Peripheral Blood	HCL	HCL-V	SLVL	MBCL/MRZL
Morphology				
Nuclear shape	Ovoid, reniform	Round	Round	Irregular
Chromatin	Reticular, ± nucleolus	Coarse with central nucleolus	Coarse, ± nucleolus	Coarse
Cytoplasm	Blue-gray, abundant	Blue-gray, abundant	Basophilic, scant to moderate	Pale, abundant
Monocytopenia	+	−	−	−
TRAP staining	+ + +	±	±	±
Aspiratable bone marrow	−	+	+	+
Predominant splenic involvement	Red pulp	Red pulp	White pulp	White pulp
Immunophenotype				
CD22	+ + +	+ +	+ +	+ +
CD11c	+ + +	+ +	+	±
CD25	+ +	−	±	±
Bly-7	+ +	±	−	NA

Abbreviations: HCL-V, hairy cell leukemia-variant; SLVL, splenic lymphoma with villous lymphocytes; MBCL, monocytoid B-cell lymphoma; MRZL, marginal zone lymphoma; NA, not available.

sentation, lack of monocytopenia, and appearance of the cells in the bone marrow biopsy as small round cytoplasmic lymphocytes. Unlike HCL, the bone marrow is typically aspiratable. A blastic variant of HCL has been described in which patients have massive splenomegaly, peripheral lymphadenopathy, and pancytopenia.[58] These cells stain positively with TRAP and negatively with myeloperoxidase.

THERAPY

Indications

Ten percent of patients, usually elderly males with moderate splenomegaly, will never require therapy (Table 84-4). Standard hematologic indications for the initiation of therapy in HCL include significant anemia (hemoglobin <8–10 g/dl), thrombocytopenia (platelet count <50–100 × 10^9/L), or neutropenia (absolute neutrophil count <0.5–1.0 × 10^9/L). Given the current availability of agents capable of achieving durable complete remissions together with the attendant risks of blood product support, in some cases it may be prudent to initiate therapy earlier than outlined by these rigid criteria, especially in those patients who have never been previously transfused with blood products. Less common indications for the initiation of therapy include leukocytosis with a high proportion of hairy cells, repeated life-threatening infections, symptomatic splenomegaly, bulky or painful lymphadenopathy, vasculitis, and bony involvement.

Splenectomy

Splenectomy was the first standard treatment modality employed in the treatment of HCL because it rapidly corrects peripheral cytopenias in most patients.[59,60] Thrombocytopenia reverses in 75% of patients and usually within a few days of splenectomy. Splenic size alone is not always predictive of response to splenectomy.[14] Patients with only patchy involvement of the marrow by HCL are reported to respond more favorably to splenectomy irrespective of their splenic size. Splenic red blood cell pooling is much greater in HCL than in other lymphoproliferative disorders with comparable splenomegaly, which likely accounts for the lack of a consistent correlation between splenic weight and response to splenectomy.[61] Given the availability of effective systemic agents in the treatment of HCL and since 50% of splenectomized patients require systemic therapy at a median of 8.3 months,[62] splenectomy is less commonly employed as primary treatment. Splenectomy is now usually reserved for those patients with active infection, active thrombocytopenic bleeding, or who fail systemic therapies.

Table 84-4. Common Indications for Therapy

Standard hematologic indications
  Hemoglobin <8–10 g/dl
  Platelets <50–100 × 10^9/L
  Absolute neutrophil count <0.5–1.0 × 10^9/L
Less common indications
  Leukocytosis with high proportion of hairy cells
  Severe or recurrent infections
  Symptomatic splenomegaly
  Bulky lymphadenopathy
  Vasculitis
  Bony involvement

Chlorambucil, Hormonal Therapy, and Radiotherapy

Chronic low-dose chlorambucil (4 mg/day PO for 6 months) induces a significant number of peripheral hematologic responses, but the absolute neutrophil count does not regularly increase, making this treatment of limited value.[63] Isolated reports document the salutatory effects of protracted androgen administration (oxymetholone)[64] and lithium to patients with HCL,[65] but these treatments are largely of historical interest. Lytic bone lesions may be successfully managed with low-dose irradiation.[20]

Interferon

IFN-α was the first systemic therapy to partially eradicate hairy cells from the bone marrow. The first report of the successful use of partially purified α (leukocyte) human IFN was in 1984.[66] In 1986 the use of recombinant IFN-α$_{2b}$ (Intron A; Schering Corporation, Kenilworth, NJ), at 2 million U/m^2 for 12 months, was reported in 64 HCL patients.[67] Of those 64 patients, 3 patients (5%) achieved a complete response and 45 patients (70%) a partial response. The same multicenter study was updated in 1987 with 128 patients accrued,[68] in 1988 with 193 patients,[69] and in 1990 with 195 patients.[69] The updated response rates were comparable to those previously reported. Studies have indicated that 12 months of therapy is optimal and that more protracted therapy does not substantially improve response rates or diminish relapse rates, but does increase toxicity.[70,71] After the discontinuation of IFN therapy, the median time to treatment failure is 18–25 months.[72] IFN reinstitution at relapse achieves a 77% response rate.[73] Recombinant IFN-α$_{2a}$ (Roferon; Hoffmann-La Roche, Nutley, NJ), which differs from IFN-α$_{2b}$ only in the amino acid residue at position 23 (α$_{2a}$ has a cysteine residue and α$_{2b}$ has an arginine residue), achieved similar response rates when administered to 30 patients with HCL.[74] Splenomegaly does not adversely affect response rates to IFN therapy.

When the results of five large studies are combined, the overall response rate is 65%, of which 10% are complete and 55% partial (Table 84-5). These results should be interpreted cautiously given the different methods, indications, and types of IFN administered.

A flu-like syndrome consisting of fever, myalgia, and malaise is the most common adverse effect. Tachyphylaxis often develops and acetaminophen may ameliorate these symptoms. Macular-papular rashes and gastrointestinal complaints occur in about 50% of patients. Rarely, central and peripheral nervous system complaints, hepatitis, alopecia, small joint arthritis, and decreased libido have been documented.

The mechanisms by which IFN induces remissions in HCL are poorly understood. IFN does stimulate natural killer cell activity, which is known to be suppressed in HCL.[75,76] IFN-α is also known to have a growth-inhibitory effect on lymphoma cell lines and to stimulate differentiation of leukemic cell lines.[77,78]

The standard dose recommendation for IFN therapy is 2 mil-

Table 84-5. Studies of IFN-α Therapy for HCL

Reference	Patients (N)	Response (%) Complete	Partial	Minor	None
107	30	9	17	4	0
108	14	1	12	0	1
109	25	7	6	12	0
110	195	7	152	10	26
89	152	16	42	0	94
Total	416	40 (10%)	229 (55%)	26 (6%)	121 (29%)

lion U/m^2 administered subcutaneously three times per week for 12 months.

Colony-Stimulating Factor-Granulocyte

Colony-stimulating factor-granulocyte (CSF-G) abrogates the early myelosuppressive effects of IFN[79] and reverses neutropenia in some HCL patients. The role of CSF-G in the management of HCL will likely be principally adjunctive to systemic therapy. It does have a role in the initial treatment of actively infected HCL patients. A single patient with HCL has been reported to have developed acute neutrophilic dermatosis (Sweet syndrome) after the administration of CSF-G.[79]

Purine Analogues

In 1972, Giblett and colleagues[80] made the seminal observation that 30% of children with severe combined immunodeficiency syndrome were deficient in the purine catabolic enzyme adenosine deaminase. Cohen et al.[81] established the relationship between the intracellular accumulation of deoxyadenosine triphosphate and lymphocytotoxicity. This then provided the rationale for the development of agents that mimic this experiment of nature either by the irreversible binding to adenosine deaminase (dCF) or by resisting deamination in the purine salvage pathway (2-CdA). 2-CdA, a chlorine-substituted purine deoxynucleoside, was found to be the most potent among a panel of substituted purine analogues screened for in vitro toxicity toward a L1210 murine leukemia.[82] dCF and 2-CdA have been demonstrated to have major activity in a variety of indolent lymphoid malignancies, but their action is most profound in the treatment of HCL.

2'-Deoxycoformycin

dCF, a natural product isolated from the cultured broth of *Streptomyces antibioticus,* is a tight-binding inhibitor of adenosine deaminase. In 1983, dCF was first shown to have activity in a single patient with HCL.[83] The successful administration of low-dose dCF (5 mg/m^2 for 2–3 days then weekly for 15–16 doses) was reported in 1984.[84]

Although dCF was introduced into clinical trials at about the same time as IFN, the published trials are fewer with less patients accrued. The Eastern Cooperative Oncology Group treated patients with dCF administered at 5 mg/m^2 for 2 days every other week until complete remission was achieved.[85] Of 27 evaluable patients with HCL, 16 (59%) achieved a complete remission, 10 (37%) a partial response, and 1 patient did not respond. These results were later updated with 50 patients accrued: 32 patients (64%) achieved a complete remission and 10 patients (20%) a partial remission.[86] dCF has also been evaluated by the European Organization for Research and Treatment of Cancer as salvage therapy for HCL patients resistant to or failing IFN-α therapy.[87] Of 33 evaluable patients, 11 patients (33%) achieved a complete remission and 15 patients a partial response, with an overall median response duration of 12 months. The National Cancer Institute made dCF available on a group C protocol for hairy cell leukemia patients failing IFN-α.[88] Of 208 patients accrued, 78 patients were evaluable. Of these 78 patients, 29 (37%) achieved a complete remission and 2 patients (6%) a partial remission. Responses were more likely in patients who were intolerant of or who had progressed after an initial response to IFN-α than in IFN-α refractory patients.

Preliminary results are available from the large Intergroup study comparing IFN with dCF in previously treated patients with HCL. Of 150 patients randomized to dCF, 103 (69%) had a complete remission and 9 (6%) a partial remission.[89] Of 103 patients who had a complete response, 4 relapsed at 13–37 months, and 2 patients died of infection. Of 152 patients ran-

Table 84-6. Studies of Purine Analogues of HCL

Reference	Patients (N)	Response (%)		
		Complete	Partial	None
dCF				
86	50	32	10	8
111	23	20	1	2
87	33	11	15	7
90	8	2	4	2
89	150	103	9	38
Total	264	168 (64%)	39 (15%)	57 (21%)
2-CdA				
95	144	123	17	3
100	46	36	5	5
99	16	12	0	4
102	11	9	2	0
98	9	7	2	0
101	8	6	2	0
Total	234	193 (82%)	28 (12%)	12 (5%)
Fludarabine				
104	3	0	2 (67%)	1 (33%)

domized to IFN-α, 16 (11%) had a complete remission and 42 (28%) had a partial remission. Of the 16 patients who had a complete response, 8 relapsed at 10–19 months, and there were no treatment-related deaths. The authors concluded that dCF was a more active agent than IFN-α in HCL but final interpretation of the analysis will require long-term survival information.

dCF therapy may be complicated by fever, nausea, vomiting, photosensitivity, and keratoconjunctivitis.[84,90] Severe myelosuppression may occur soon after the initiation of dCF therapy, especially in those patients with pre-existing marrow compromise.[86,91] Patients with reasonable pretreatment hematologic parameters tend to have less myelosuppression after dCF administration. Serious infections, including disseminated herpes zoster, *Escherichia coli, Haemophilus influenzae,* and pneumococcal infections have been documented early after the administration of dCF.[90] It is recommended that in patients with active infection, a poor performance status or impaired renal function dCF is best avoided.[85] dCF is potently immunosuppressive.[92] During dCF therapy and for ≥14 months after its administration, CD4 and CD8 lymphocytes may decrease to levels <200 cells/mm^3. In a separate study, even low doses of dCF resulted in a similar magnitude of immunosuppression.[93] Despite the severity of immunosuppression, there has been no significant increased incidence of either late infections or secondary malignancies.

When the results of five studies are combined, the overall response rate is 79%, of which 64% are complete and 15% are partial (Table 84-6). The recommended dose of dCF for patients with HCL is 4 mg/m^2 body surface area every other week for 3–6 months until maximum response is obtained.

2-Chlorodeoxyadenosine

In 1990, the first 12 HCL patients treated with a single 7-day course of 2-CdA at 0.1 mg/kg/day by continuous intravenous infusion were reported.[94] Since that report, >400 patients with HCL have been treated at Scripps Clinic and Research Foundation. Data on the first 144 patients who have been followed for a median of 14 months are available.[95] Of these 144 patients, 69 were untreated, 27 had undergone splenectomy and 26 had received IFN only, and 22 patients had undergone splenectomy and received interferon. One hundred twenty-three patients (85%) obtained complete responses, 17 (12%) partial responses, 3 (2%) did not respond, and 1 patient died of a cardiovascular event and was therefore unevaluable. Responses were independent of previous therapy and disease duration.

Table 84-7. Characteristics of IFN-α dCF and 2-CdA in Therapy for HCL

	IFN-α	dCF	2-CdA
Food and Drug Administration status	Approved	Approved	Approved
Synthesis	Recombinant technology	Complex	Simple
Route of administration	Subcutaneous	Intravenous bolus	Intravenous infusion
Recommended dose	2 million U/m² 3 ×/wk	4 mg/m² every other wk	0.1 mg/kg/day for 1 wk
Duration of treatment	12 mo	3–6 months	1 wk
Responses	65% overall, 10% complete	79% overall, 64% complete	94% overall, 84% complete
Major toxicities	Influenza-like syndrome, early infections	Nausea, early infections, immunosuppression	Culture-negative fever, immunosuppression

Five patients resistant (three patients) or intolerant (two patients) to dCF were also treated.[96] Of these five patients, four obtained complete responses with a median follow-up duration of ≥11 months. Three of the four complete responders remain in unmaintained remission, while the fourth patient has developed progressive splenic enlargement with stable hematologic parameters. Two of the five patients experienced culture-negative neutropenic fever associated with treatment. Thus, 2-CdA induced complete responses in a small number of patients with HCL resistant to dCF, suggesting a possible lack of cross-resistance between these two nucleosides. 2-CdA was not prohibitively toxic in patients intolerant to dCF.

Fever was the principal toxicity, occurring in 63 (43%) of the patients treated. The attainment of fever was related to the disappearance of hairy cells and appeared most marked in patients with the greatest pretreatment HCL burden, manifested principally as splenomegaly. Documented infections, unrelated to a peripherally inserted central catheter device, were uncommon, occurring in only four patients. Given the rarity of infection and the frequency of fever, it has been postulated that these febrile episodes are likely cytokine mediated. Like dCF, 2-CdA is also immunosuppressive. Some studies have shown a tendency toward restoration of T-cell subsets in most patients between 12 and 18 months after 2-CdA administration,[97,97a] whereas others have shown CD4⁺ lymphocytopenia beyond 2 years.[97b] Long-term follow-up, however, has shown no evidence of increased late infections or secondary malignancies.

Thus far, four patients have relapsed at a median of 36 months, typically with normal peripheral blood counts and 5–10% marrow medullary space infiltration. Three patients with primary refractoriness to 2-CdA therapy failed to respond to retreatment with a second course of 2-CdA administered at a median of 9 months after the first treatment. Other single-institution studies have documented similar response rates and toxicities after the administration of a single course of 2-CdA to patients with HCL.[98–102] More recently, it was shown that some patients in apparent complete remission after 2-CdA therapy have minimal residual disease by immunohistochemical staining done on serial marrow biopsy specimens.[102a]

When the results of six studies are combined, the overall response rate is 94%, of which 82% are complete and 12% are partial (Table 84-6). Given the complete and long-lasting remissions and the favorable toxicity profile that follow a single 7-day course of 2-CdA administered at 0.1 mg/kg/day by continuous intravenous infusion, 2-CdA is emerging as the treatment of choice for patients with HCL. 2-CdA is approved by the Food and Drug Administration for patients with untreated and treated active HCL, defined by the presence of cytopenias.

Fludarabine

Fludarabine does appear to have some activity in HCL but has only been evaluated in small numbers of patients and results have been less dramatic than with the other nucleoside analogues discussed.[103,104]

Considerations

The treatment indications and management for patients with HCL are currently in evolution. Splenectomy, the first standard treatment employed, is now less commonly used given the ability of systemic agents to induce pathologic complete responses. The three systemic agents, IFN-α, dCF, and 2-CdA, all have substantial activity in the treatment of HCL (Table 84-7). Although treatment with IFN-α is associated with high overall response rates, complete responses are distinctly uncommon; therefore, this agent alone is unlikely to have curative potential. dCF and 2-CdA both induce durable responses that are commonly complete responses. 2-CdA is emerging as the treatment of choice for this disease because the durable complete responses are achieved after only a brief exposure to therapy and because of its favorable toxicity spectrum. The bioavailability of 2-CdA administered subcutaneously and orally is 100% and 50%, respectively.[105] These routes of drug delivery remain to be tested in large numbers of patients with HCL, but if successful, would further simplify 2-CdA therapy and further reduce costs.[106]

Because HCL is an indolent disease, protracted follow-up will be necessary to determine relapse rates and whether some patients are indeed cured. Before the introduction of effective systemic therapy in this disease, the median survival for patients was only 53 months.[46] The development of the nucleoside analogues for the treatment of lymphoid malignancies, which serves as a model for rational drug design, has dramatically changed the therapeutic approach to HCL, and seems destined to alter survival in this disease.

FUTURE DIRECTIONS

Ongoing research in this disease is aimed at long-term follow-up of the spectacular responses achieved with modern drug therapy to determine whether this is a curable malignancy. Efforts are directed at establishing the cellular and biochemical reasons why hairy cells are so sensitive to these agents in hopes of influencing treatment similarly in other disease states and favorably effecting drug development for cancer in general.

REFERENCES

1. Bouroncle BA, Wiseman BK, Doan CA: Leukemic reticuloendotheliosis. Blood 13:609, 1958
2. Schrek R, Donnelly WJ: "Hairy" cells in blood in lymphoreticular neoplastic disease and "flagellated" cells of normal lymph nodes. Blood 27:199, 1966
3. Wylis RF, Greene MH, Palretke M et al: Hairy cell leukemia in three siblings: an apparent HLA-linked disease. Cancer 49:538, 1982
4. Katayama I, Mochino T, Honwa T, Falcada M: Hairy cell leukemia: a comparative study of Japanese and non-Japanese patients. Semin Oncol, suppl. 2: 486, 1984
5. Oleske D, Golomb HM, Farber MD, Levy PS: A case-control inquiry into the etiology of hairy cell leukemia. Am J Epidemiol 121:675, 1985

6. Stewart DJ, Keating MJ: Radiation exposure as a possible etiologic factor in hairy cell leukemia. Cancer 46:1577, 1980

7. Wachsman W, Golde DW, Chen IS: Hairy cell leukemia and human T cell leukemia virus. Semin Oncol 11:446, 1984

8. Korsmeyer SJ, Greene WC, Cossman J et al: Rearrangement and expression of immunoglobulin genes and expression of Tac antigen in hairy cell leukemia. Proc Natl Acad Sci USA 80:4522, 1983

9. Bartl R, Frisch B, Hill W et al: Bone marrow histology in hairy cell leukemia. Am J Clin Pathol 79:531, 1983

10. Katayama I: Bone marrow in hairy cell leukemia. Hematol Oncol Clin North Am 2:585, 1988

11. Burke JS: The value of the bone-marrow biopsy in the diagnosis of hairy cell leukemia. Am J Clin Pathol 70:876, 1978

12. Naeim F, Jacobs AD: Bone marrow changes in patients with hairy cell leukemia treated by recombinant alpha-2 interferon. Hum Pathol 16:1200, 1985

13. Ratain MJ, Golomb HM, Bardawil RG et al: Durability of responses to interferon alfa-2b in advanced hairy cell leukemia. Blood 69:872, 1987

14. Golomb HM, Vardiman JW: Response to splenectomy in 65 patients with hairy cell leukemia: an evaluation of spleen weight and bone marrow involvement. Blood 61:349, 1983

15. Burke JS, Sheibani K, Winberg CD, Rappaport H: Recognition of hairy cell leukemia in a spleen of normal weight: the contribution of immunologic studies. Am J Clin Pathol 87:276, 1987

16. Nanba K, Soban EJ, Bowling MC, Berard CW: Splenic pseudosinuses and hepatic angiomatous lesions: distinctive features of hairy cell leukemia. Am J Clin Pathol 67:415, 1977

17. Ng JP, Hogg RB, Cumming RL et al: Primary splenic hairy cell leukemia: a case report and review of the literature. Eur J Haematol 39:349, 1987

18. Roquet ML, Zafrani ES, Farcet JP et al: Histopathological lesions of the liver in hairy cell leukemia: a report of 14 cases. Hepatology 5:496, 1985

19. Vardiman JW, Golomb HM: Autopsy findings in hairy cell leukemia. Semin Oncol 11:370, 1984

20. Lembersky BC, Ratain MJ, Golomb HM: Skeletal complications in hairy cell leukemia: diagnosis and therapy. J Clin Oncol 6:1280, 1988

21. Yam LT, Janckila AJ, Li C-Y, Lam WKW: Cytochemistry of tartrate-resistant acid phosphatase: fifteen years' experience. Leukemia 1:285, 1987

22. Li CY, Yam LT, Lam KW: Studies of acid phosphatase isoenzymes in human leukocytes: demonstration of isoenzyme specificity. J Histochem Cytochem 18:901, 1970

23. Katayama I, Li CY, Yam LT: Ultrastructural characteristics of the "hairy cells" of leukemic reticuloendotheliosis. Am J Pathol 361:370, 1972

24. Melo JV, Robinson DSF, Gregory C, Catovsky D: Splenic B cell lymphoma with "villous" lymphocytes in the peripheral blood: a disorder distinct from hairy cell leukemia. Leukemia 1:294, 1987

25. Catovsky D, O'Brien M, Melo JV et al: Hairy cell leukemia variant: an intermediate disease between hairy cell leukemia and B prolymphocytic leukemia. Semin Oncol 11:362, 1984

26. Brunning RD, Parkin J: Ribosome-lamella complexes in neoplastic hematopoietic cells. Am J Pathol 79:565, 1975

27. Hsu S, Yang K, Jaffe ES: Hairy cell leukemia: a B cell neoplasm with a unique antigenic phenotype. Am J Clin Pathol 80:421, 1983

28. Melo JV, San Miguel JF, Moss VE, Catovsky D: The membrane phenotype of hairy cell leukemia: a study with monoclonal antibodies. Semin Oncol 11:381, 1984

29. Anderson KC, Boyd AW, Fisher DC et al: Hairy cell leukemia: a tumor of pre-plasma cells. Blood 65:620, 1985

30. Falini B, Pulford K, Erber WN et al: Use of a panel of monoclonal antibodies for the diagnosis of hairy cell leukemia: an immunocytochemical study of 36 cases. Histopathology 10:671, 1986

31. Falini B, Schwarting R, Erber W et al: The differential diagnosis of hairy cell leukemia with a panel of monoclonal antibodies. Am J Clin Pathol 83:289, 1985

32. Jansen J, Schmit HRE, van Zwet TL et al: Cell markers in hairy cell leukemia studied in cells from 51 patients. Blood 59:52, 1982

33. Fu SM, Winchester RJ, Rai KR, Kunkel HG: Hairy cell leukemia: proliferation of a cell with phagocytic and B-lymphocyte properties. Scand J Immunol 3:847, 1974

34. Jaffe ES, Shevach EM, Frank MM, Green I: Leukemic reticuloendotheliosis: presence of a receptor for cytophilic antibody. Am J Med 57:108, 1974

35. Burns GF, Cawley JC, Worman CP et al: The distribution of a receptor for (μFCR) on haemic cells. Am J Hematol 6:243, 1979

36. Burns GF, Cawley JC, Barker CR, Hazhoe FGJ: Absence of a receptor for C3 on the hairy cells of leukemia reticuloendotheliosis. Clin Exp Immunol 29:442, 1977

37. Catovsky D, Cherchi M, Okos A et al: Mouse red-cell rosettes in B-lymphoproliferative disorders. Br J Haematol 33:173, 1976

38. Robbins BA, Ellison DJ, Spinosa JC et al: Diagnostic application of two-color flow cytometry in 161 cases of hairy cell leukemia. Blood 82:1277, 1993

39. Visser L, Shaw A, Slupsky J et al: Monoclonal antibodies reactive with hairy cell leukemia. Blood 74:320, 1989

40. Hanson CA, Gribbin TE, Schnitzer B et al: CD11c (LEU-M5) expression characterizes a B-cell chronic lymphoproliferative disorder with features of both chronic lymphocytic leukemia and hairy cell leukemia. Blood 76:2360, 1990

41. Steis RG, Marcon L, Clark J et al: Serum soluble IL-2 receptor as a tumor marker in patients with hairy cell leukemia. Blood 77:1304, 1988

42. Micklem KJ, Dong Y, Willis A et al: HML-1 antigen on mucosa-associated T cells, activated cells, and hairy leukemic cells is a new integrin containing the β7 subunit. Am J Pathol 139:1297, 1991

43. Hounieu H, Chittal SM, al Saati T et al: Hairy cell leukemia. Diagnosis of bone marrow involvement in paraffin-embedded sections with monoclonal antibody DBA.44. Am J Clin Pathol 98:26, 1992

44. Flandrin G, Sigaux F, Sebahoun G et al: Hairy cell leukemia: clinical presentation and follow-up of 211 patients. Semin Oncol 11:458, 1984

45. Turner A, Kjeldsberg CR: Hairy cell leukemia: a review. Medicine 57:477, 1978

46. Golomb HM, Catovsky D, Golde DW: Hairy cell leukemia: a clinical review of 71 cases. Ann Intern Med 89:677, 1978

47. Dorsey JK, Penick GD: The association of hairy cell leukemia with unusual immunologic disorders. Arch Intern Med 142:902, 1982

48. Elkon KB, Hughes GRV, Catovsky D et al: Hairy-cell leukemia with polyarteritis nodosa. Lancet 2:280, 1979

49. Quesada JR, Keating MJ, Libshitz HI, Llamas L: Bone involvement in hairy cell leukemia. Am J Med 74:228, 1983

50. Davies GE, Wiernik PH: Hairy cell leukemia with chylous ascites. JAMA 238:1541, 1977

51. Krause JR, Dekker A: Hairy cell leukemia (leukemic reticuloendotheliosis) in serous effusions. Acta Cytol 22:80, 1978

52. Levine PH, Katayama I: The platelet in leukemic reticuloendotheliosis. Functional and morphological evidence of a qualitative disorder. Cancer 36:1353, 1975

53. Rosove MH, Naeim F, Harwig S, Sighelboim J: Severe platelet dysfunction in hairy cell leukemia with improvement after splenectomy. Blood 55:903, 1980

54. Depuy E, Sigaux F, Brychaert MC et al: Platelet acquired defect in PDGF and B-thromboglobulin content in hairy cell leukemia: improvement after interferon therapy. Br J Haematol 65:107, 1987

55. Aiba M, Raffa PP, Katayama I: Significance of leukocyte alkaline phosphatase in hairy cell leukemia. Am J Clin Pathol 74:297, 1980

56. Sheibani K, Burke JS, Swartz WG et al: Monocytoid B-cell lymphoma: clinicopathologic study of 21 cases of a unique type of low-grade lymphoma. Cancer 62:1531, 1988

57. Burke JS, Rappaport H: The differential diagnosis of hairy cell leukemia in bone marrow and spleen. Semin Oncol 11:334, 1984

58. Diez-Martin JL, Li CY, Banks PM: Blastic variant of hairy cell leukemia. Am J Clin Pathol 87:576, 1987

59. Mintz U, Golomb HM: Splenectomy as initial therapy in twenty-six patients with leukemic reticuloendotheliosis (hairy cell leukemia). Cancer Res 39:2366, 1979

60. Jansen J, Hermans J: Splenectomy in hairy cell leukemia: a retrospective multicenter analysis. Cancer 47:2066, 1981

61. Lewis SM, Catovsky D, Hows JM, Ardalan B: Splenic red cell pooling in hairy cell leukemia. Br J Haematol 35:351, 1977

62. Golde DW: Therapy of hairy-cell leukemia. N Engl J Med 307:495, 1982

63. Golomb HM: Progress report on chlorambucil therapy in postsplenectomy patients with progressive hairy cell leukemia. Blood 57:464, 1981

64. Lusch CJ, Ramsey HE, Katayama I: Leukemic reticuloendotheliosis: report of a case with peripheral blood remission on androgen therapy. Cancer 41:1964, 1978

65. Blum SF: Lithium in hairy cell leukemia. N Engl J Med 303:464, 1983

66. Quesada JR, Reuben J, Manning JT et al: Alpha-interferon for induction of remission in hairy cell leukemia. N Engl J Med 310:15, 1984

67. Golomb HM, Jacobs A, Fefer A et al: Alpha-2 interferon therapy of hairy cell leukemia: a multicenter study of 64 patients. J Clin Oncol 4:900, 1986

68. Golomb HM, Fefer A, Golde DW et al: Sequential evaluation of alpha-2b interferon treatment in 128 patients with hairy cell leukemia. Semin Oncol, suppl. 2. 14:13, 1987

69. Golomb HM, Fefer A, Golde DW et al: Report of a multi-institutional study of 193 patients with hairy cell leukemia treated with interferon alfa-2b. Semin Oncol suppl. 5. 15:7, 1988

70. Golomb HM, Ratain MJ, Fefer A et al: Randomized study of the duration of treatment with interferon alfa-2b in patients with hairy cell leukemia. J Natl Cancer Inst 80:369, 1988

71. Berman E, Heller G, Kempin S et al: Incidence of response and long-term follow-up in patients with hairy cell leukemia with recombinant alpha-2a. Blood 75:839, 1990
72. Ratain MJ, Golomb HM, Vardiman JW et al: Relapse after interferon alpha-2b therapy for hairy-cell leukemia: analysis of diagnostic variables. J Clin Oncol 6:1714, 1988
73. Ratain MJ, Golomb HM, Vardiman JW et al: Interferon alpha-2b therapy for hairy cell leukemia in 69 patients. A 6-year update, abstracted. Blood 74:76, 1989
74. Quesada JR, Hersh EM, Manning J et al: Treatment of hairy cell leukemia with recombinant alpha-interferon. Blood 68:493, 1986
75. Ruco LP, Procapio A, Maccallini V et al: Severe deficiency of natural killer activity in the peripheral blood of patients with hairy cell leukemia. Blood 61:1132, 1983
76. Lee SH, Kelley S, Chin H, Stebbing N: Stimulation of natural killer cell activity and inhibition of proliferation of various leukemic cells by purified human leukocyte interferon subtypes. Cancer Res 42:1312, 1982
77. Lieberman D, Voloch Z, Aviv H et al: Effects of interferon on hemoglobin synthesis and leukemia virus production in Friend cells. Mol Biol Rep 1:447, 1974
78. Taylor-Papadimitriou J: Effects of interferons on cell growth and function. p. 13. In Gresser I (ed): Interferon 1980. Vol. 2. Academic Press, San Diego, 1980
79. Glaspy JA, Baldwin GC, Robertson PA et al: Therapy for neutropenia in hairy cell leukemia with recombinant human granulocyte colony-stimulating factor. Ann Intern Med 109:789, 1988
80. Giblett ER, Anderson JE, Cohen F et al: Adenosine deaminase deficiency in two patients with severely impaired cellular immunity. Lancet 2:1067, 1972
81. Cohen A, Hirshhorn R, Horowitz SD et al: Deoxyadenosine triphosphate as a potentially toxic metabolite in adenosine deaminase deficiency. Proc Natl Acad Sci USA 75:472, 1978
82. Carson DA, Wasson DB, Kaye J et al: Deoxycytidine kinase-mediated toxicity of deoxyadenosine analogs towards malignant human lymphoblasts *in vitro* and toward murine L1210 leukemia *in vivo*. Proc Natl Acad Sci USA 77:6865, 1980
83. Spiers ASD, Parekh SJ: Pentostatin (2'-deoxycoformycin, DCF) is active in hairy cell leukemia (HCL), abstracted. Blood 62:208, 1983
84. Spiers ASD, Parekh SJ, Bishop MB: Hairy-cell leukemia: induction of complete remission with pentostatin (2'-deoxycoformycin). J Clin Oncol 2:1336, 1984
85. Spiers ASD, Moore D, Cassileth PA et al: Remissions in hairy cell leukemia with pentostatin (2'deoxycoformycin). N Engl J Med 316:825, 1987
86. Cassileth PA, Cheuvant B, Spiers ASD et al: Pentostatin induces durable remissions in hairy cell leukemia. J Clin Oncol 9:243, 1991
87. Ho AD, Thaler J, Stryckmans P et al: Pentostatin in resistant chronic lymphocytic leukemia. A phase II trial of the European organization for research and treatment of cancer. Proc Am Soc Clin Oncol 9:206, 1990
88. Sorensen JM, Chun HG, Vena D et al: Pentostatin (DCF) therapy for hairy cell leukemia (HCL): update of a Group C protocol of 208 patients (pts) who have failed interferon-alpha (IFNa), abstracted. Proc Am Soc Clin Oncol 10:232, 1991
89. Grever M, Kopecky K, Head D et al: A randomized comparison of deoxycoformycin (DCF) versus alpha-2a interferon (IFN) in previously untreated patients with hairy cell leukemia (HCL): an NCI-sponsored Intergroup Study (SWOG, ECOG, CALGB, NCIC, CTG), abstracted. Proc Am Soc Clin Oncol 11:868, 1992
90. Johnston JB, Glazer RI, Pugh L, Israels LG: The treatment of hairy-cell leukemia with 2'-deoxycoformycin. Br J Haematol 63:525, 1986
91. Ho AD, Thaler J, Stryckmans P et al: Pentostatin in refractory chronic lymphocytic leukemia: a phase II trial of the European Organization for Research and Treatment of Cancer. J Natl Cancer Inst 82:1416, 1990
92. Urba WJ, Baseler MW, Kopp WC et al: Deoxycoformycin-induced immunosuppression in patients with hairy cell leukemia. Blood 73:38, 1989
93. Kraut EH, Neff JC, Bouroncle BA et al: Immunosuppressive effects of pentostatin. J Clin Oncol 8:848, 1990
94. Piro LD, Carrera CJ, Carson DA, Beutler E: Lasting remissions in hairy-cell leukemia induced by a single infusion of 2-chlorodeoxyadenosine. N Engl J Med 322:1117, 1990
95. Piro LD, Saven A, Ellison D et al: Prolonged complete remissions following 2-chlorodeoxyadenosine (2-CdA) in hairy cell leukemia (HCL), abstracted. Proc Am Soc Clin Oncol 11:846, 1992
96. Saven A, Piro LD: Complete remissions in hairy cell leukemia with 2-chlorodeoxyadenosine after failure with 2'-deoxycoformycin. Ann Intern Med 119:278, 1993
97. Carrera CJ, Piro LD, Saven A et al: Restoration of lymphocyte subsets following 2-chlorodeoxyadenosine remission induction in hairy cell leukemia, abstracted. Blood, suppl. 1. 76:260a, 1990
97a. Juliusson G, Lenkei R, Liliemark J: Flow cytometry of blood and bone marrow cells from patients with hairy cell leukemia: phenotype of hairy cells and lymphocyte subsets after treatment with 2-chlorodeoxyadenosine. Blood 83:3672, 1994
97b. Seymour JF, Kurzrock R, Freireich EJ, Estey EH: 2-Chlorodeoxyadenosine induces durable remissions and prolonged suppression of CD4+ lymphocyte counts in patients with hairy cell leukemia. Blood 83:2906, 1994
98. Tallman MS, Hakimian D, Variakojis D et al: A single cycle of 2-chlorodeoxyadenosine results in complete remission in the majority of patients with hairy cell leukemia. Blood 9:2203, 1992
99. Juliusson G, Liliemark J: Rapid recovery from cytopenia in hairy cell leukemia after treatment with 2-chloro-2'-deoxyadenosine (CdA): relation to opportunistic infections. Blood 79:888, 1992
100. Estey EM, Kurzrock R, Kantarjian HM et al: Treatment of hairy cell leukemia with 2-chlorodeoxyadenosine (2-CdA). Blood 79:882, 1992
101. Lauria F, Benfenati D. Zinzani PL et al: 2-Chlorodeoxyadenosine in the treatment of hairy cell leukemia patients relapsed after α-interferon, abstracted. Blood, suppl. 1. 78:34a, 1991
102. Hoffman M, Rai K, Sawitsky A, Janson D: 2-chlorodeoxyadenosine (2-CdA) in hairy cell leukemia. Blood, suppl. 1. 78:454a, 1991
102a. Hakimian D, Tallman MS, Kiley C, Peterson LA: Detection of minimal residual disease by immunostaining of bone marrow biopsies after 2-chlorodeoxyadenosine for hairy cell leukemia. Blood 82:1798, 1993
103. Kantarjian HM, Redman J, Keating MJ: Fludarabine phosphate therapy in other lymphoid malignancies. Semin Oncol, suppl. 8. 17:66, 1990
104. Kantarjian HM, Schachner J, Keating MJ: Fludarabine therapy in hairy cell leukemia. Cancer 67:1291, 1991
105. Liliemark J, Albertioni F, Hassan M et al: On the bioavailability of oral and subcutaneous 2-chloro-2'-deoxyadenosine in humans: alternative routes of administration. J Clin Oncol 10:1514, 1992
106. Juliusson G, Liliemark J, Hippe E et al: Subcutaneous injections of 2-chloro-2'-deoxyadenosine (CDA) as treatment for symptomatic hairy cell leukemia (HCL), abstracted. Blood 80:1427, 1992
107. Quesada JR, Gutterman J, Hersh EM: Treatment of hairy cell leukemia with alpha interferons. Cancer 57:1678, 1986
108. Foon KA, Maluish AE, Abrams PG et al: Recombinant leukocyte A interferon therapy for advanced hairy cell leukemia. Therapeutic and immunologic results. Am J Med 80:351, 1986
109. Rai K, Mick R, Ozer H et al: Alpha-interferon therapy in untreated active hairy cell leukemia: a Cancer and Leukemia Group B (CALGB) study. Proc Am Soc Clin Oncol 6:159, 1987
110. Golomb H, Fefer A, Golde D et al: Update of a multi-institutional study of 195 patients (pts) with hairy cell leukemia (HCL) treated with interferon alfa-2b (IFN), abstracted. Proc Am Soc Clin Oncol 6:215, 1990
111. Kraut EH, Bouroncle BA, Grever MR: Pentostatin in the treatment of advanced hairy cell leukemia. J Clin Oncol 7:168, 1989

Cutaneous T-Cell Lymphomas

85

Peter W. Heald and Richard L. Edelson

INTRODUCTION

A distinctive feature of cutaneous T-cell lymphoma (CTCL) is the tropism of this mesenchymal tumor for the epidermis, which is of ectodermal origin. It is now known that this so-called epidermotropism exhibited by the malignant T cells is an amplification of a physiologic interaction between T cells and skin. The distribution of the immune repertoire and the functional coordination of spatially distinct compartments of the immune system is critically dependent on a closely regulated system of lymphocyte homing. This system directs naive T lymphocytes to the organized lymphoid microenvironment of secondary lymphoid tissues such as lymph nodes or Peyer's patches in which they can be specifically activated by their specific foreign antigen in conjunction with appropriate accessory cells. Memory/effector T cells (CD45RO$^+$), generated in secondary lymphoid tissues in response to stimulation by antigen, migrate efficiently to such sites where they "patrol" for the return of their particular antigen. Different subsets of memory/effector T cells exist, each with different tissue-selective homing properties.[1]

One such site receiving a distinct subset of memory T cells in response to inflammatory stimuli is the skin. The malignant cells of CTCL have been shown to have the distinctive characteristics of the cutaneous T cells.[2] Because common lymphocyte antigen (CLA) expression is not a feature of T-cell lymphomas in extracutaneous sites,[3] these observations suggest that the variants of CTCL that have appeared under such colorful names of mycosis fungoides, Pagetoid reticulosis, and Sézary syndrome, can not be unified by the concept that they are malignancies of cutaneous T cells. CTCLs are diseases characterized by cutaneous infiltrates of malignant clonally expanded T cells admixed with an inflammatory infiltrate.

BIOLOGIC AND MOLECULAR ASPECTS

The region-specific organization of the T-cell network has been recognized with skin- and mucosal-associated lymphoid tissues. The concept of T cells dedicated to patrolling cutaneous sites of inflammation (cutaneous T cells) has provided a basis for understanding region-specific lymphomas. In the spectrum of CTCLs, the epidermotropic stage biopsies demonstrate CLA expression, whereas the nonepidermotropic tumor stage is not associated with this expression. However, there are accessory molecules that assist in the adherence of cutaneous T cells to skin components. Intercellular adhesion molecule 1 (ICAM-1) and class II MHC protein molecules can be demonstrated in lesional but not in nonlesional keratinocytes in CTCL.[4] Class II MHC protein binds to the CD4 antigen of helper T cells, and ICAM-1 binds to lymphocytes that bear lymphocyte function-associated molecule 1 (LFA-1).

Keratinocytes constitutively produce immunologically active cytokines, many of which are membrane-associated and thus can provide an instant reserve when keratinocytes are activated or damaged. The first keratinocyte-derived cytokine identified was termed epidermal-derived T-cell activating factor (ETAF). Subsequently ETAF has been shown to include a family of cytokines including interleukin (IL)-1, colony-stimulating factor-granulocyte/macrophage (CSF-GM), and IL-6, -7, and -8. These factors activate T cells in proximity to the epidermis. In addition, several ETAFs stimulate T-cell growth and maturation. Of all the cytokines produced by keratinocytes, IL-7 has the greatest capacity to drive CTCL cell proliferation.[5] The importance of this in the pathogenesis of cutaneous lymphomas is also suggested by the cutaneous lymphomas that appear in IL-7 transgenic mice.[6] Thus, T-cell surface proteins that mediate adhesion and cytokine interaction play an important role in the pathophysiology of CTCL. A representative biopsy of a CTCL lesion demonstrating the influx of lymphocytes into the skin is shown in Figure 85-1.

ETIOLOGY AND PATHOGENESIS

Since the cells exhibit a marker that signifies they have encountered specific antigen, and malignant cells are apparently moving into and out of an activated stage that is triggered by T-cell receptor activation, it appears that they are continuing to encounter antigen in the host during the course and development of the lymphoma. This suggests that antigen-specific stimulation of the malignant cells is a real possibility in the pathogenesis of CTCL.[7]

One feature of CTCL cells is that when they are stimulated, they produce a cytokine profile consistent with that of a T-helper-2 type cell (T_{H2}). The dichotomy of T_{H1} and T_{H2} T cells was initially discovered in mice but the human analogues have been identified. The T_{H2} cells produce IL-4, IL-5, and IL-6 and they are inhibited by interferon (IFN)-γ. The T_{H2} cells appear most critical to driving antibody and eosinophil-mediated responses. T_{H1} cells produce IL-2 and IFN-γ and are more involved in directing the cytotoxic cell responses. Peripheral blood cells from leukemic CTCL patients, and resting and stimulated cells made cytokines of the T_{H2} type that is inhibited by IFN-γ.[8] This pattern of cytokine expression is consistent with the findings of hypergammaglobulinemias and of eosinophilia in CTCL patients. But this pattern is also intertwined with one of the crucial pathogenic steps in CTCL. When T_{H2} cells are stimulated they inhibit T_{H1} cells. Since CTCL cells appear to be stimulated in the course of the disease, they suppress T_{H1} cells in function; eventually this leads to the virtual depletion of normal T cells.[9] Since the patient's cell-mediated antitumor immunity resides within this depleted population of T cells, CTCL facilitates its own progression by dismantling the immune system.

The progression of the disease is associated not only with the disease-induced immunosuppression but also with transformation of the CTCL cells.[10] Transformation is associated with distinct morphologic features, such as nucleolar prominence, paler cytoplasm, and substantial failure of expression of markers associated with more mature cells.[11]

CLINICAL MANIFESTATIONS

The different surface phenotypes of the CTCL cells, the variable degrees of epidermotropism, varying rates of cellular replication, and differing degrees of host antitumor responses all cause the clinical expression of CTCL to vary greatly. This clinical diversity is reflected in the varied names and eponyms ap-

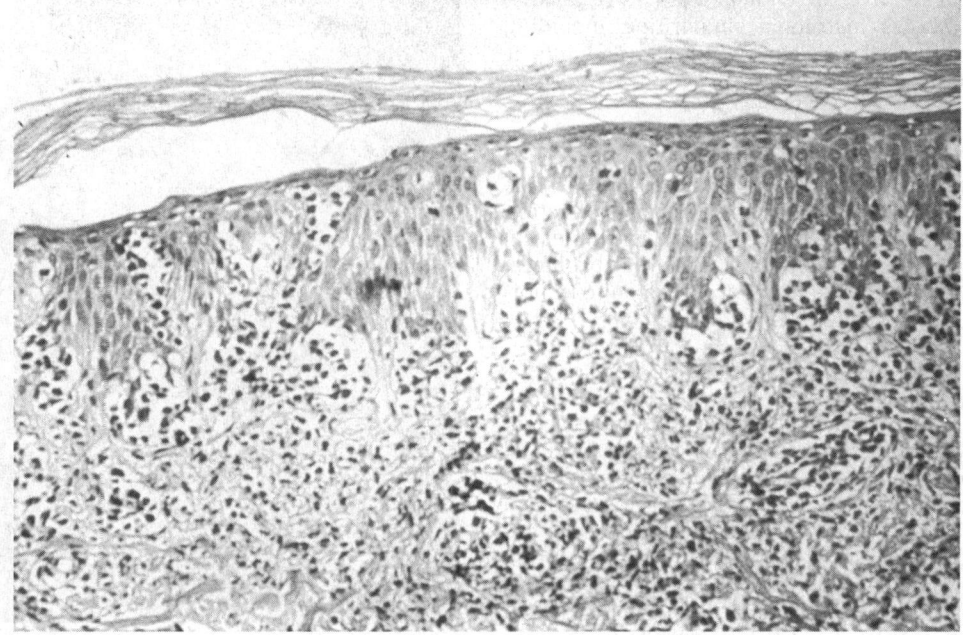

Fig. 85-1. Biopsy of classic CTCL shows the epidermotropism and dermal infiltrate of malignant cells.

plied to these conditions. The term cutaneous T-cell lymphoma was proposed as the unifying term at a 1979 international symposium, sponsored by the National Cancer Institute.[12] A partial list of recognized syndromes is given in Table 85-1. The common features in all these conditions are clonal T-cell proliferation in the skin (as defined by Southern blot analysis) and the sequential or concomitant presence in patients with CTCL of these conditions in any variety of patterns.

Premalignant Stages

The premalignant stages are typically nonspecific and are often misdiagnosed for many years as eczema or psoriasis. In several retrospective studies the latent period from onset of

Table 85-1. Classification of Lymphomas of Cutaneous T Cells

Premalignant conditions
    Large plaque parapsoriasis
    Poikiloderma vasculare atrophicans
    Jessner's infiltrate
    Alopecia mucinosa
Epidermotropic (mycosis fungoides variants)
    Clinicopathologic syndromes
        Woringer-Kolopp disease
        Mycosis fungoides
        Granulomatous slack skin
        Follicular mucinosis
    Erythrodermic CTCL and Sézary syndrome
    Tumor-stage mycosis fungoides
    Immunophenotypic entities
        $CD8^+$ CTCL
        $\gamma\delta^+$ CTCL
Lymphomatoid papulosis
$HTLV-1^+$ CTCL
$CD30^+$ (Ki-1) lymphoma
    Primary
    Secondary
$CD30^-$ lymphoma
    Angiotropic large cell lymphoma

the skin lesions to definitive diagnosis of CTCL was 4–10 years, with a mean of 6.1 years.[13] The eruptions are characteristically transitory but invariably reappear in either previously affected or unaffected sites. Classically a number of putative distinct clinical entities are included with the premalignant eruptions. Histologically the premalignant stages can often be nondescript, although several of those to be discussed have distinctive features. The premalignant stages include large plaque parapsoriasis, poikiloderma atrophicans vasculare, Jessner's infiltrate, alopecia mucinosa, and lymphomatoid papulosis.

Large Plaque Parapsoriasis

Large plaque parapsoriasis is characterized by erythematous, atrophic lesions, usually >6 cm, with a predilection for the trunk and buttocks. These lesions occur commonly in conjunction with other lesions of CTCL. Parapsoriasis defies easy definition, but when CTCL is at this stage, the histologic picture may be nonspecific, with only a banal upper dermal infiltrate. Examination of multiple biopsy specimens, however, may reveal changes indicative of the correct diagnosis. Scattered, atypical mononuclear cells may be present in the infiltrate; infiltration of the epidermis by mononuclear cells without evident spongiosis is suggestive of early CTCL. Immunotyping shows large plaque parapsoriasis to be identical to plaque-stage CTCL,[14] and these lesions are best considered as an early stage of malignant disease. As perhaps the most classic of the premalignant lesions, large plaque parapsoriasis can persist for years before showing any malignant decompensation.[15]

Poikiloderma Atrophicans Vasculare

Poikiloderma atrophicans vasculare has three clinical components: (1) reticulate hypo- and hyperpigmentation, (2) telangiectasia, and (3) atrophy of the skin. The age of onset is usually between 40 and 60 years, but no age group is exempt, and poikiloderma atrophicans vasculare has been recognized in the newborn. Typically, the eruption resolves on exposure to sunlight in the summer but recurs in the winter. Progression to overt CTCL is usually associated with induration of the skin and the development of papules and plaques. The greatest difficulty arises in distinguishing this from cutaneous lupus erythematosus, which may also have the clinical features of poikilo-derma. Skin biopsy shows histologic similarities, including basal layer vacuolization and deposits of immunoreactants at the basement membrane.[16]

Jessner's Infiltrate

The lymphocytic infiltrate of Jessner typically produces nod-ules and plaques, often solitary, with a dense dermal collection of cells. As shown in Figure 85-2, this clinically resembles tu-mor- or nodular-stage CTCL. This is a disease of T-cell prolifera-tion.[17,18] In addition, there are reports of progression to tumor-stage CTCL, although this is unusual.

Alopecia Mucinosa

Alopecia mucinosa, also termed follicular mucinosis, is an inflammatory disorder characterized by the accumulation of acid mucopolysaccharides in sebaceous glands and outer root sheaths of hair follicles in conjunction with a periappendageal T-cell infiltrate (Fig. 85-3). At the early stages, all lesions are centered on follicles, and hair loss is an early sign. The eruption evolves to indurated papules and plaques, which may be iso-lated or multiple. In 15% of patients with alopecia mucinosa, CTCL is also present, and these patients generally have more widely disseminated skin lesions. There is an adolescent and childhood form of alopecia mucinosa, which appears to be more benign. CTCL may be present before development of alo-pecia mucinosa or may be diagnosed for the first time on histo-logic examination of a biopsy specimen of the latter lesions.[19]

Lymphomatoid Papulosis

Lymphomatoid papulosis was clinically described as rhythmic paradoxical eruption. The "paradox" referred to the histology giving the disease a malignant appearance but the clinical outcome was benign in most cases. The age of onset is between 8 and 60 years, with a median age of 37.5 years. Lymphomatoid papulosis usually has a benign clinical course lasting from 6 months to 20 years. Lesions tend to appear in groups, and individual lesions resolve within 3–4 weeks. Typi-cally, lesions start as red-brown papules, which develop a scale or crust over the surface, or even central necrosis as seen in Figure 85-4. The lesions resolve, leaving residual pigmented areas or superficial atrophic scars. Patients with lympho-

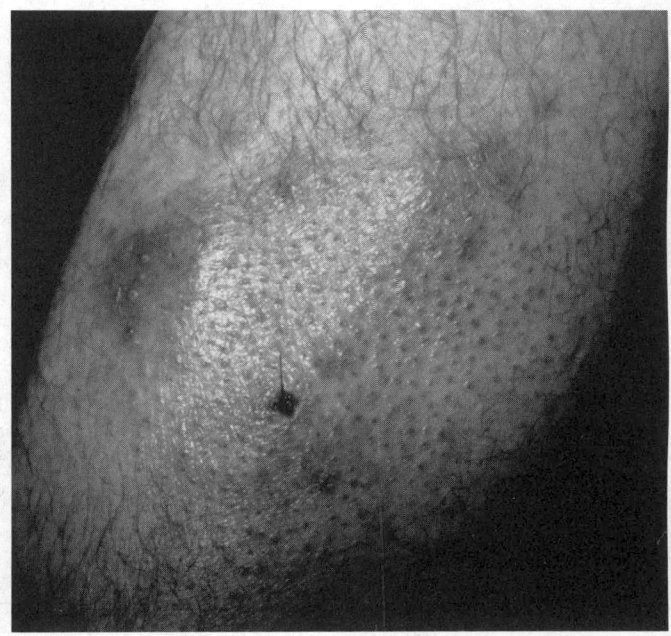

Fig. 85-3. Alopecia mucinosa produces follicular lesions that coalesce to form plaques.

matoid papulosis may subsequently develop CTCL, which is the most common lymphoma associated with lymphomatoid papulosis.[20,21] Clonality studies have demonstrated distinct clones in lymphomatoid papulosis lesions, which appear in the context of an already established clone of CTCL.[22]

The main histologic differential diagnosis of lymphomatoid papulosis is epidermotropic CTCL of the mycosis fungoides type and Hodgkin disease. The epidermis shows patchy para-keratosis, acanthosis, spongiosis, and occasional exocytosis of mononuclear cells into the epidermis. Central ulceration of the epidermis may also be present. The dermis shows a perivascu-lar lymphohistiocytic infiltrate, with extravasation of red blood cells. Bizarre pleomorphic and hyperchromatic cells present within this infiltrate resemble the Reed-Sternberg cell of Hodg-kin disease, with which they also share the surface marker Ki-1 (CD30). Mitotic figure may be prominent. The histology is thus strongly suggestive of a malignant condition. The clinical course of the disease, however, is unpredictable inasmuch as the patient may eventually succumb to malignant lymphoma or may simply have periodic skin discomfort. Treatment of lymphomatoid papulosis is controversial, but in patients with large numbers of lesions and frequent bouts, an approach such as that outlined in the section Therapy can lead to improve-ment and potentially provide a secure future for these patients.

Woringer-Kolopp Disease

Woringer-Kolopp disease (pagetoid reticulosis) is a solitary skin lesion of long duration and slow growth, which histologi-cally shows large numbers of abnormal mononuclear cells infil-trating the epidermis and an underlying reactive mixed dermal infiltrate.[23] The original description was of a solitary lesion on the arm of a 13-year-old boy with the distinctive histology char-acteristic of this disease. Pagetoid reticulosis represents an indolent, and particularly epidermotropic, form of CTCL. This has been difficult to establish by surface marker characteriza-tion because the abnormal cells in these lesions show very low intensity staining with any of the classic T-cell markers. The advent of molecular biologic techniques has led to the clear demonstration that this is a CTCL.[24]

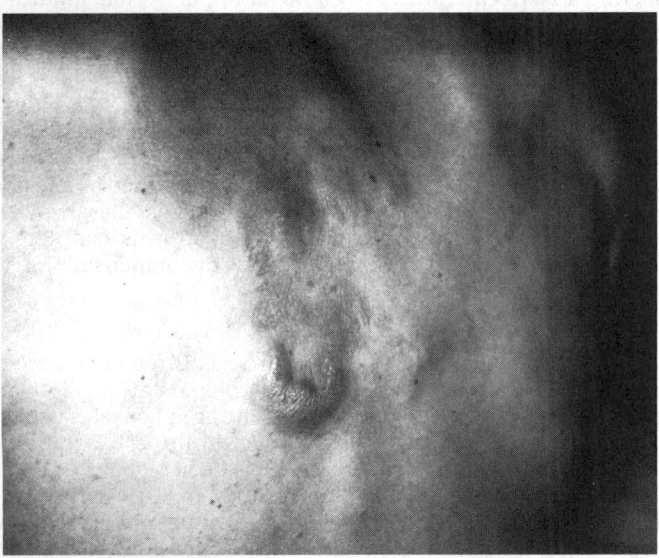

Fig. 85-2. Nodular lesions of Jessner's infiltrate.

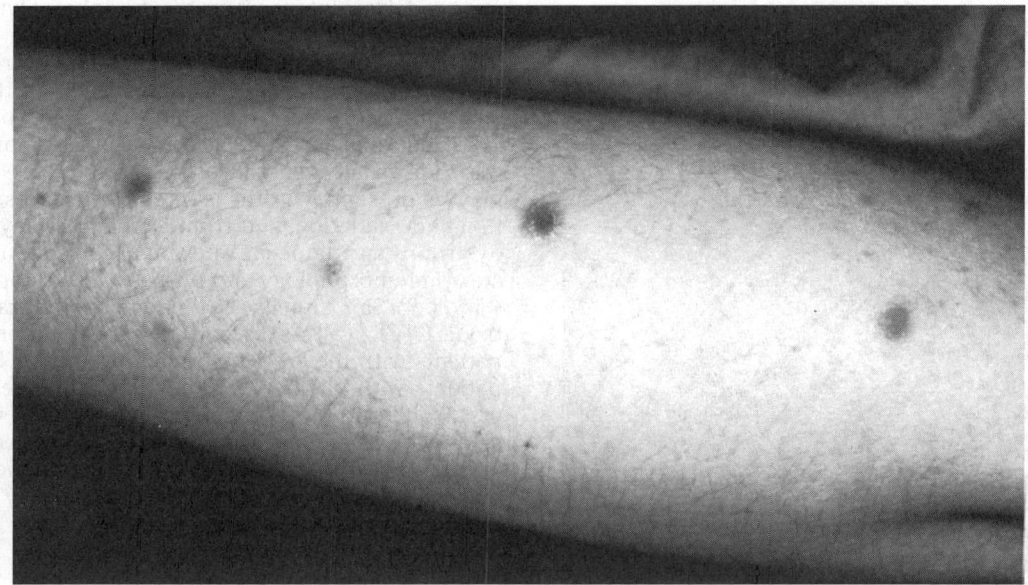

Fig. 85-4. Lesions of lymphomatoid papulosis appear in crops and consist of ulcerated papules that scar.

Diagnosis is made on clinicopathologic criteria. The long duration, slow growth, and solitary nature of the disease are characteristics of this CTCL variant. The histology of Woringer-Kolopp disease is diagnostic but should be distinguished from that of pagetoid melanoma and Paget disease. The striking histologic feature of this disorder is the infiltration of the epidermis by large atypical mononuclear cells. The nuclei are hyperchromatic and are of variable shape, ranging from oval to deeply indented. The staining of the cytoplasm of these cells is pale, which gives the appearance of a halo, similar to those seen in the epidermis, and a variable reactive infiltrate is present.

Plaque-Stage Mycosis Fungoides

Plaque-stage CTCL, the type usually referred to as mycosis fungoides,[25,26] is characterized by sharply demarcated plaques that are usually discoid in shape. Coalescence of adjacent lesions with central resolution of larger lesions can give a "geographic" appearance (Fig. 85-5). In each patient the lesions tend to be of uniform color, ranging from an erythematous to a violaceous hue. Occasionally the plaques are scaly, simulating psoriasis, or are associated with papules, vesicles, and crusts. Pruritus may be a prominent feature. More rarely, bullae or pustules may be present. A verrucous form, predominantly affecting the palms, soles, and body creases, has also been described. Because of the potential confusion of these presentations with nonmalignant cutaneous disorders, skin biopsy at an early stage is advisable.

Cytologically the cells may be either the same size as or considerably larger than normal small lymphocytes. The cells often possess scant cytoplasm, and the nuclei are hyperchromatic and irregular in shape. The tissue pattern is that of a polymorphous infiltrate, present in a band-like pattern in the upper dermis, which is composed of histiocytes, eosinophils, normal lymphoid cells, plasma cells, and a variable number of CTCL cells. The epidermis is generally infiltrated either by individual cells or by small groups of mononuclear cells surrounded by halo-like clear spaces, the Pautrier microabscesses.

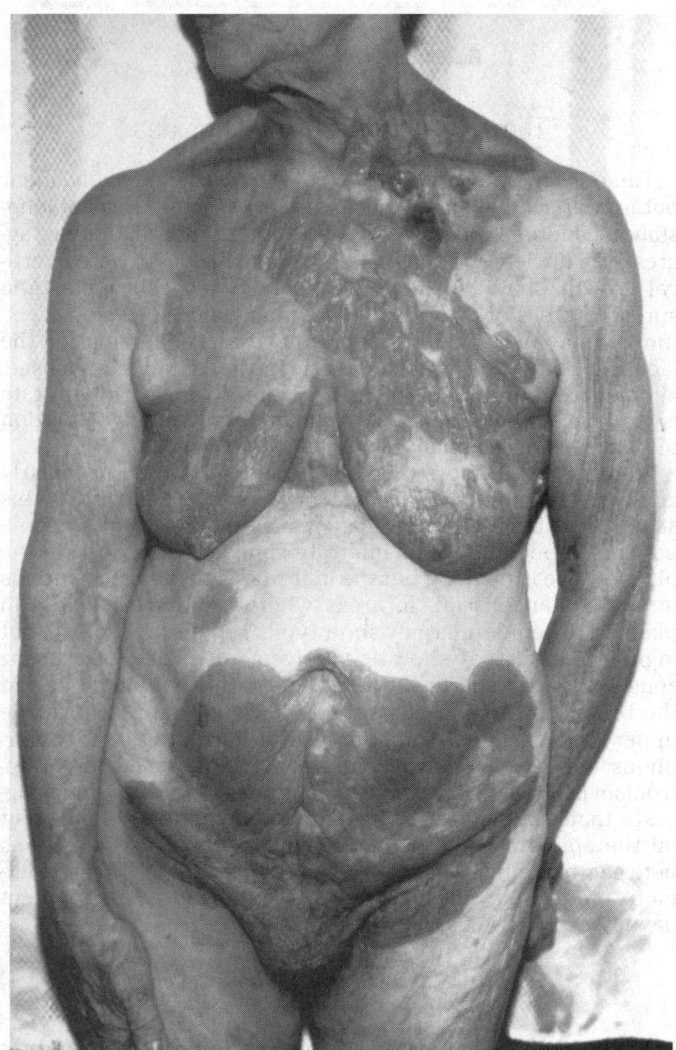

Fig. 85-5. Plaque lesion of CTCL.

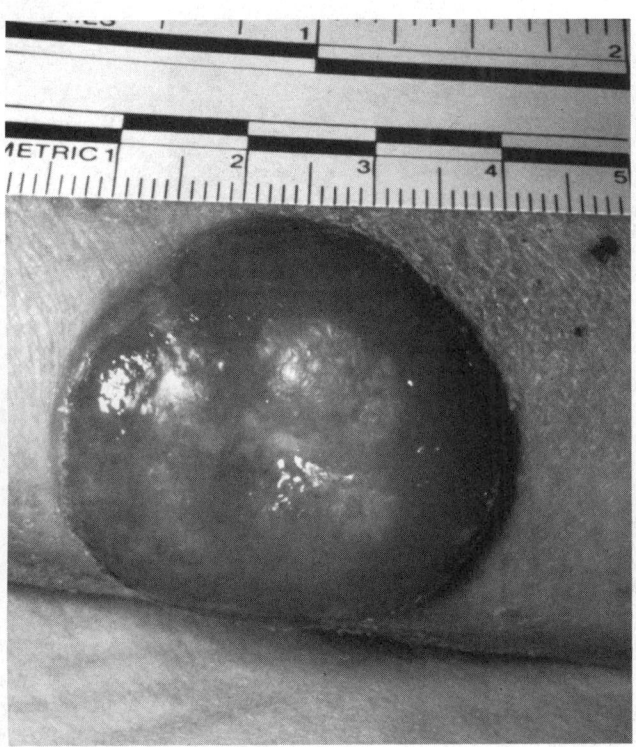

Fig. 85-6. Tumor stage of CTCL.

Tumor-Stage Mycosis Fungoides

Tumors generally arise at sites of previous skin involvement but may arise in clinically normal skin. Origin in areas of long-standing indolent plaques suggests local evolution of more aggressive subclones of malignant cells with an associated vertical growth phase. De novo occurrence suggests metastatic spread by cells of an already quite malignant T-cell clone. The tumors may occur anywhere but have a predilection for the face and body folds (i.e., the axillae, groin, antecubital fossae, and neck and in women the inframammary area). Growth rate is variable, and ulceration may occur. Spontaneous resolution of tumors is occasionally observed.

Patients with tumors (Fig. 85-6) tend to have a particularly aggressive form of the disease and a poor prognosis. At this stage, two histologic appearances may be observed. In some patients, a polymorphous infiltrate similar to that seen in the plaque stage is present, but the infiltrate is denser and extends into subcutaneous fat. In areas where tumors originated in plaques, the epidermis may show typical epidermotropism, but in other areas it may show no involvement, even when a grenz zone (an area of sparing between infiltrating lymphocytes and the basement membrane of the epidermis) is present in the upper dermis. In other patients, the infiltrate is monomorphous, composed almost exclusively of tumor cells. Epidermotropism is not a prominent feature in these tumors, which suggests that less mature malignant T cells are less dependent on the epidermal microenvironment for growth. Transitions between these histologic variants and evolution from epidermotropic to nonepidermotropic variants in the same patient have been observed.

Sézary Syndrome (Erythroderma)

The clinical variant of CTCL known as Sézary syndrome was first described in 1892 by Besnier and Hallopeau.[27] Sézary and Bouvrain[28] described patients with generalized exfoliating erythroderma, intense pruritus, peripheral lymphadenopathy, and abnormal hyperchromatic mononuclear cells in the skin and peripheral blood. Erythroderma may start de novo, follow a premalignant eruption, or appear after established plaque-stage disease. After a variable time some patients with the erythrodermic form of CTCL develop tumors. The erythroderma is usually generalized, but isolated areas of normal skin may be present. Pruritus is often intense, resulting in excoriation and exudation, and trophic changes may occur, with nail dystrophy and alopecia. The abnormal mononuclear cells have a distinct morphology and possess cerebriform-shaped nuclei (Fig. 85-7). Similar cells are found in the infiltrates of epidermotropic CTCL in all stages, and they are also found in the blood of patients with the erythrodermic form of CTCL and occasional patients with plaque- or tumor-stage disease. Thus, the term erythrodermic CTCL encompasses patients with widespread skin involvement and varying stages of leukemic disease. Sézary syndrome is best used as the term for patients with marked leukemia and large numbers of cytologically atypical cells in the peripheral circulation.

Granulomatous Slack Skin

Granulomatous changes are not infrequently encountered in the histology of CTCL. At the extreme end of this spectrum, however, is a distinctive syndrome called granulomatous slack skin. Patients with this condition develop large regions of slack skin accompanied by fibrotic bands (Fig. 85-8). In many respects this disease is a variant of tumor-stage CTCL. The histology shows malignant cells palisading around zones of necrobiotic degenerated connective tissue (Fig. 85-9). In addition, there may be circulating cells bearing the BE2 marker. After the demonstration that this disorder is a cutaneous T-cell lymphoma, its recognition as a subset of CTCL has increased.[29]

Adult T-Cell Lymphoma

The clustering of aggressive cutaneous T-cell lymphomas in southern Japan led to its recognition as the entity adult T-cell lymphoma (ATL).[30] A characteristic finding is a very high level of IL-2 receptor (Tac) expression by lymphocytes infiltrating the peripheral blood and skin. After its clinical discovery, human T-cell leukemia/lymphoma virus 1 (HTLV-1), a retrovirus, was isolated and identified as the causative agent of this condition.[31]

ATL provides a paradigm for understanding cutaneous lymphomas.[32] There are several stages of the disease, many of which are clinically and histologically indistinguishable from mycosis fungoides and Sézary-type CTCLs. Also, like these CTCLs, ATL is increasing in incidence worldwide. Epidemic foci are in southern Japan and the Caribbean and there have been >200 cases in the United States and Europe to date. Epidemiologic studies suggest that transmission occurs by several routes. The virus appears to be transmitted from mothers to children by breast-feeding, after which a latent infection is established. Once the disease has become active in a patient, it can be transmitted sexually. Cases of male to female transmission have been clearly demonstrated, along with transmission by blood products in a manner similar to the transmission of hepatitis B and human immunodeficiency virus infection.

The initial stage is that of the carrier state, which is characterized by positive HTLV-1 antibody but no circulating abnormal cells and no detectable proviral integration into the host genome. This stage then appears to be rather quiet until after the age of 40, when disease expression is most common. Factors that may play a role in subsequent exacerbation and expression of the disease have been postulated to be infectious

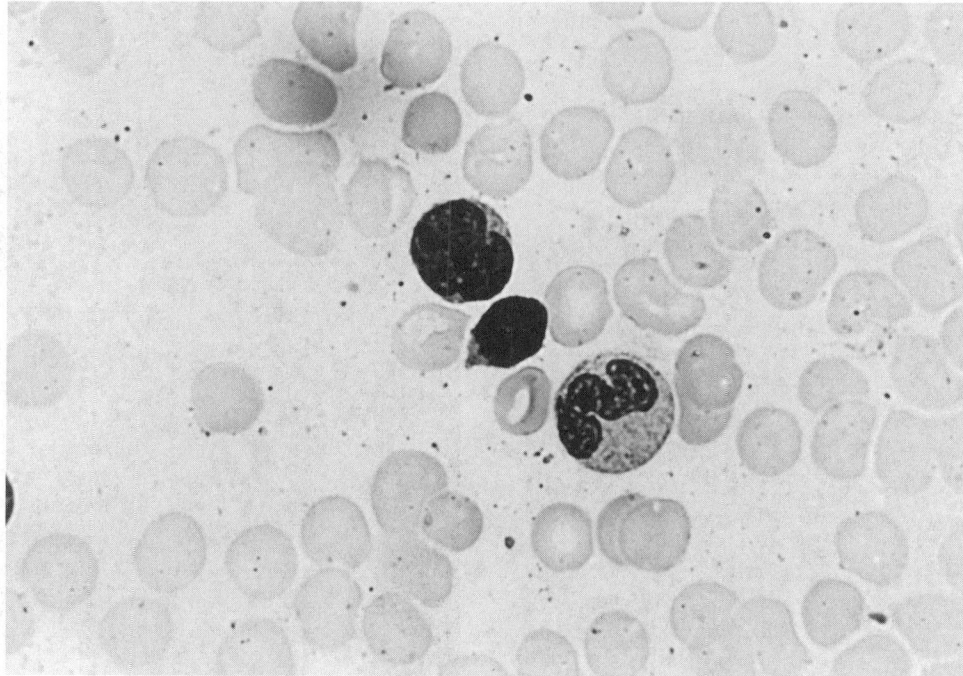

Fig. 85-7. Sézary cells: abnormal cells in peripheral blood with characteristic cerebriform, large, and clefted nuclei with fine chromatin and scanty cytoplasm. (Courtesy of Carol Bradford, M.T., Indiana University School of Medicine, Indianapolis, IN.)

in nature; the role of such factors would be similar to the mechanism by which infections exacerbate immunodeficiency retroviral disease. ATL initially becomes manifest as the *smoldering* state, characterized clinically by patch- and plaque-stage skin infiltration with malignant-appearing cells that bear high levels of IL-2 receptor and low levels of circulating abnormal cells (Fig. 85-10). As the disease subsequently progresses through the *chronic* and then the *acute* or *lymphoma* stage, it is characterized by increasing numbers of Tac-positive cells, immunodeficiency, hypercalcemia, and pulmonary compromise.

CD8⁺ Cutaneous Lymphoma

The discovery of CD8⁺ cutaneous lymphoma is testimony to the usefulness of immunoperoxidase typing of lymphoma infiltrates at the time of presentation. The antibody to CD8

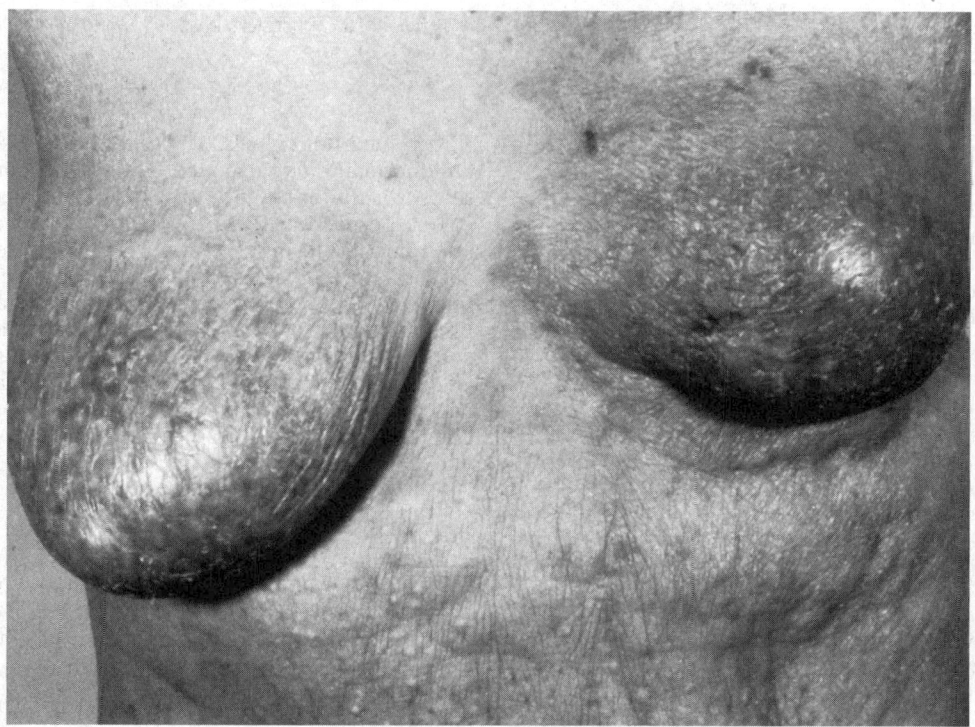

Fig. 85-8. Lesions of granulomatous slack skin produce atrophy and dermal and subcutic destruction.

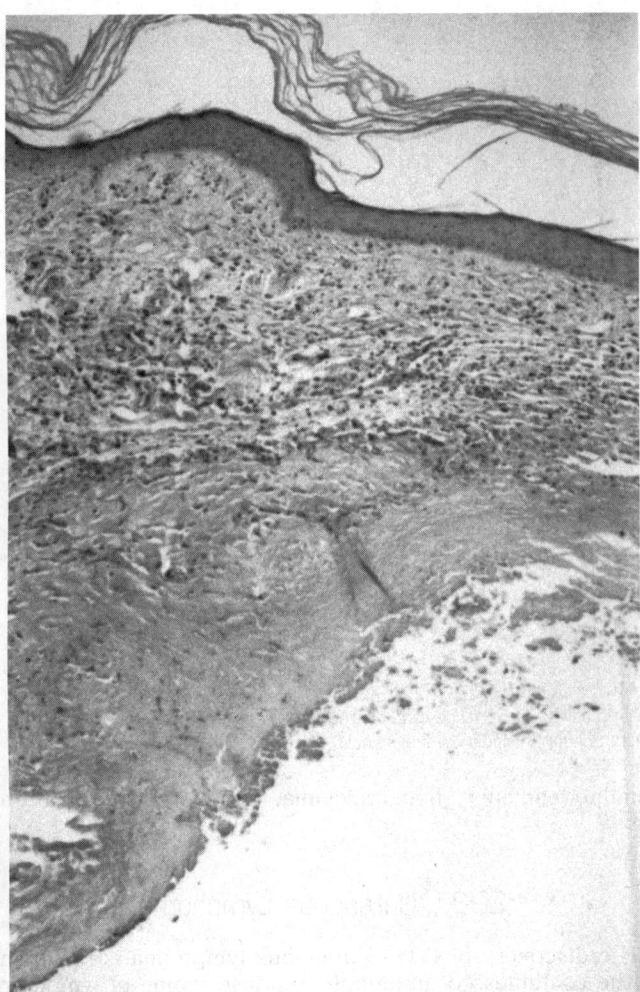

Fig. 85-9. Biopsy of granulomatous slack skin shows broad zones of tissue necrosis surrounded by malignant cells. Biopsy may facilitate the detection of involvement of these organs.

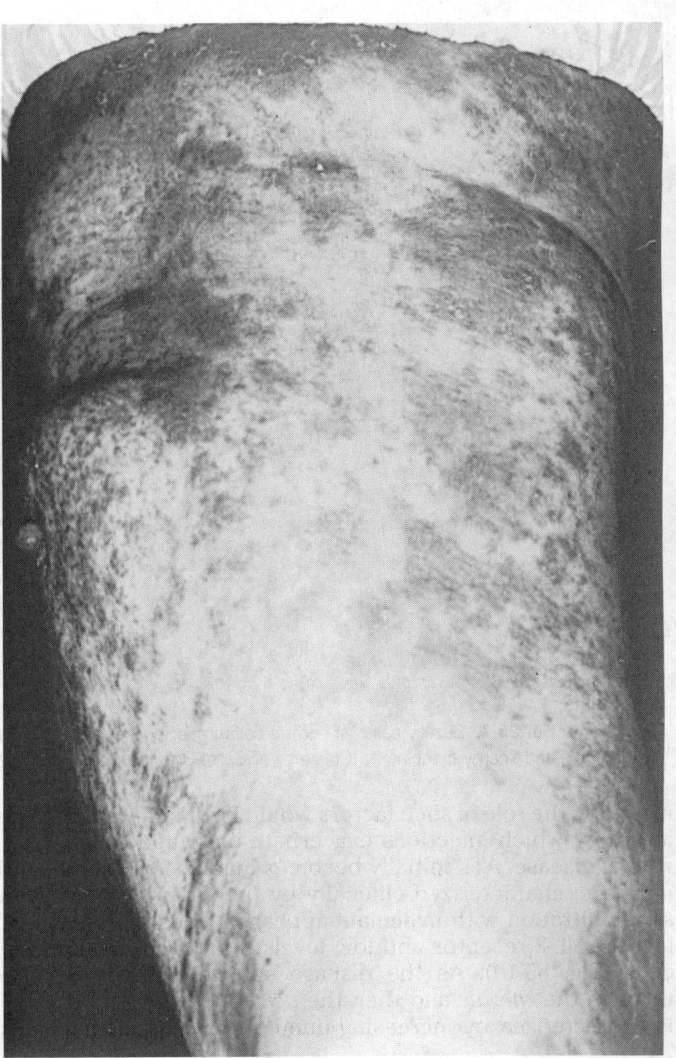

Fig. 85-10. Skin lesions in adult T-cell lymphoma/leukemia syndrome.

defines a population of cells that behave in functional assays as cells that suppress antibody production or cells that become cytotoxic T cells. There appear to be two clinical syndromes recognized to date. The first is a chronic disease with epidermotropism of cells that express CD8, CD2, and do not express CD7. The more common aggressive, angiodestructive subtype presents with a noduo-ulcerative disease (Fig. 85-11) characterized by epidermotropic cells expressing CD8 and CD7 and not expressing CD2. This aggressive subtype has been resistant to therapy.[33,34]

γδ T-Cell Lymphoma

CTCLs of "double negative" (CD3$^+$, CD4$^-$, CD8$^-$) T cells bear the γδ T-cell receptor complex. γδ cells have not been routinely demonstrated in normal human skin. The mouse analogues to these cells are abundantly present in murine skin. Their immunologic repertoire of "double negative" cells appear to include the ability to lyse target cells with natural killer (NK)-cell-like cytotoxicity.

Several cases have presented with pronounced epidermal necrosis in conjunction with γδ tumor cell epidermotropic infiltrates, suggesting that the malignant cells were participating in the keratinocyte lysis.[35] A lipotropic γδ lymphoma variant has also been described. In this syndrome, lymphocytic infiltrates of the fat produced tumid nodules.[36]

Ki-1 Lymphoma

Ki-1 lymphoma (CD30$^+$ lymphoma) occurs frequently in childhood and adolescence. The typical clinical appearance is that of a tumor-stage lesion with central ulceration (Fig. 85-12). A perplexing feature of this condition is a tendency to spontaneous resolution, along with a tendency to progress to aggressive malignant lymphoma. Its histology at an early stage mimics that of lymphomatoid papulosis. In addition to this lymphoma, which is a tumor of T-cell origin, Ki-1 is expressed in some cases of classic CTCL, lymphomatoid papulosis, and Hodgkin disease.[37] Despite the unpredictable course of this condition, aggressive radiotherapy, with or without follow-up chemotherapy, is recommended.

Extracutaneous Involvement with CTCL

Any organ may be involved in disseminated CTCL. At autopsy the most frequent sites of extracutaneous involvement are lymph nodes (75%), lungs (60%), liver (53%), and spleen (60%).[38] Despite the high incidence of extracutaneous CTCL found at autopsy, clinically apparent extracutaneous disease, other than that involving peripheral lymph nodes and blood, is uncommon.

As with other lymphomas, extracutaneous involvement is more common as the stage or extent of CTCL increases. Most

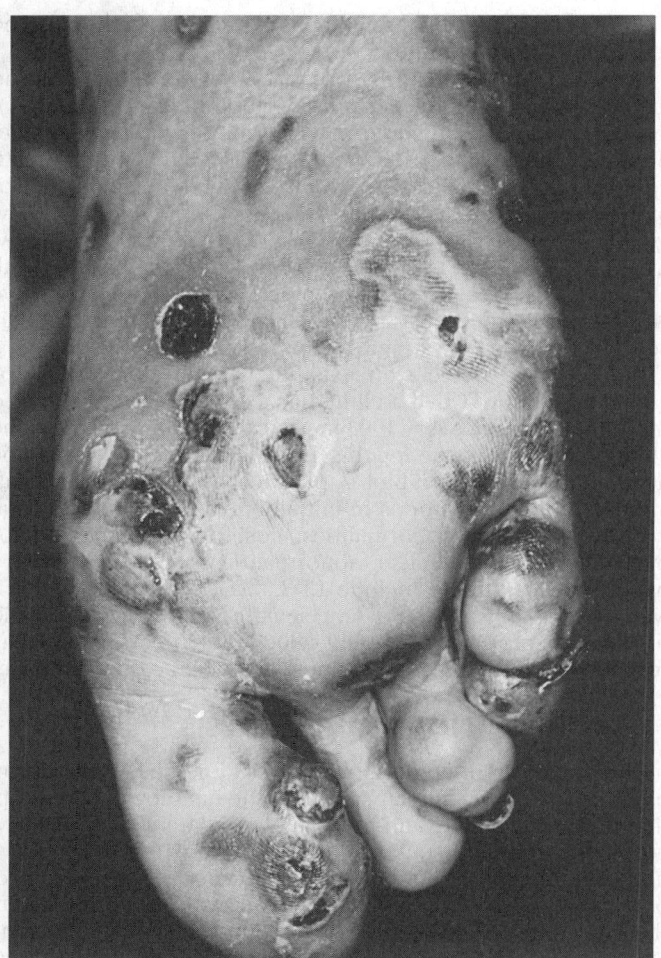

Fig. 85-11. Ulcerations of the plantar surface in a patient with CD8+ CTCL.

patients with generalized plaques and skin tumors have microscopic evidence of extracutaneous disease, most often affecting the peripheral blood and lymph nodes. Patients with the erythrodermic variant of CTCL invariably have microscopically demonstrable systemic disease.

When present, node involvement can be detected as lymphadenopathy as judged by computed tomography (CT) criteria. This technology is useful for measuring peripheral nodes and for detecting pelvic, abdominal, and thoracic node disease. Lymph node histology in CTCL is a controversial topic. Unlike the lymph nodes in B-cell lymphomas, lymph nodes in CTCL are rarely effaced by the lymphoma cells, but foci of abnormal cells are present in most enlarged "dermatopathic" nodes. Even this nonspecific node histology can be shown to represent nodal involvement by Southern blot analysis. Lymph node histology affects staging, but the prognostic importance of the newer molecular methods needs to be studied.

Pulmonary involvement in CTCL is usually asymptomatic and is rarely recognized ante mortem. Mediastinal or hilar adenopathy, parenchymal nodules, and pleural effusions may be evident on chest radiography or chest CT, but diagnosis necessitates biopsy of the lesion.[39] Pulmonary involvement is best treated with whole lung irradiation.[40]

Occult splenic and hepatic infiltrations are common (34% and 16%, respectively), but liver and spleen involvement is usually only diagnosed postmortem.[41] Liver-spleen scans, CT, and liver biopsies can be used to document lymphomatous involvement. Antitumor immunity is mediated by T cells, and there is an appreciable incidence of second malignancies in the CTCL population.[42,43] These malignancies may be of the lung, prostate, or bladder. Undoubtedly chemotherapy and radiation may be contributing factors. The clinical strategy is to pursue any abnormal symptom or laboratory finding with the knowledge that these patients are at risk of malignancy. Cutaneous malignancies occurring in CTCL patients can be due to multiple contributing factors. Nitrogen mustard, electron beam, and psoralens plus ultraviolet A (PUVA) therapy all put patients at increased risk of skin cancer, particularly squamous cell carcinoma. Nitrogen mustard has a unique predilection for in-

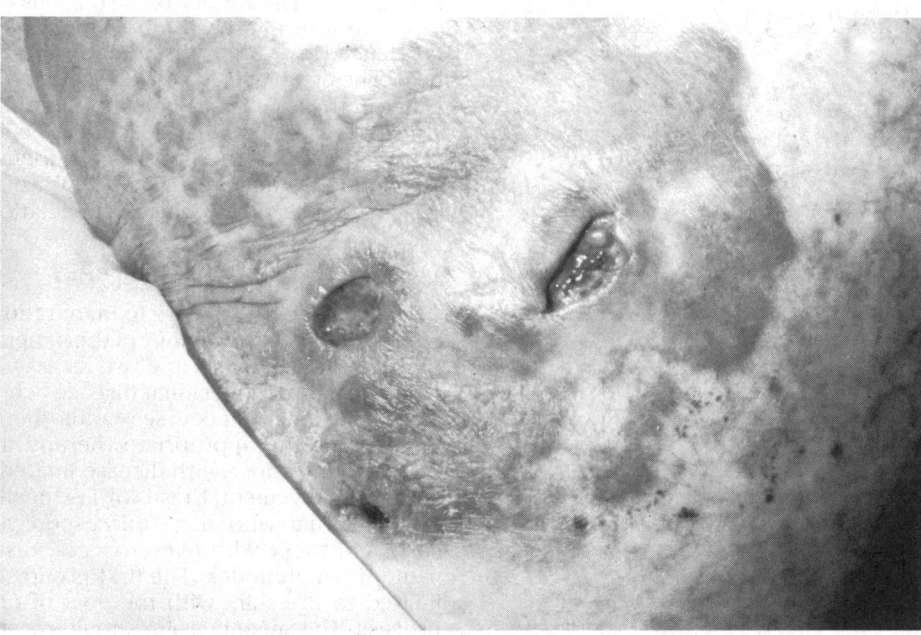

Fig. 85-12. Lesions of Ki-1 lymphoma tend to ulcerate.

ducing scrotal carcinomas, which is reminiscent of the observation of this condition in chimney sweeps. The role of retinoids in the chemical prevention of cutaneous carcinomas may lead to a greater use of retinoid therapy as an adjunct to the mutagenic first-line regimens of nitrogen mustard, PUVA, and electron beam radiation.

As with many other pruritic skin eruptions and lymphomas, eosinophilia may be associated with CTCL. Some of the severe pruritis associated with CTCL may be a systemic effect of lymphoma, similar to the severe pruritus of Hodgkin disease.

LABORATORY EVALUATION

Cutaneous T cells exhibit distinctive characteristics, in the skin and circulation, which have been described by cell-surface analysis and molecular biologic techniques. Cutaneous lymphocyte surface proteins that are expressed by CTCLs are listed in Table 85-2. Many of the surface proteins provide valuable insights for staging and follow-up of the disease. The antigens most frequently used are CD3, which transduces the signal from antigen receptor to cell activation; CD4, which binds MHC class II antigens; CD8, which binds MHC class I; CD25, the IL-2 receptor that increases with activation; CD30; UCHL1 (CD45RO), which is present on memory T-cells; and CLA, the cutaneous lymphocyte antigen discussed previously.

Immunochemical methods for studying cell-surface markers include immunoperoxidase staining of fixed tissue and flow cytometric analysis of cell suspensions. The surface proteins just described should be tested for on samples of skin, blood, and lymph node. These immunochemical techniques have shown that at early stages of the disease the predominant cell type is CD3$^+$/CD4$^+$ (Fig. 85-13). In addition to these standard markers, malignant lymphocytes that infiltrate the skin in CTCL have been shown to express activation markers.[7,44] The most diagnostic immunophenotypic cutaneous finding is the presence of >90% of CD4$^+$ cells. As this percentage decreases, so does the specificity of this finding.[45] The skin biopsy immunoperoxidase allows for the complete typing of the cutaneous

infiltrate and the proper assignment of the name of the subtype (e.g., $\gamma\delta$, Ki-1) of lymphoma.

In 1939, the state of the art of CTCL cell detection was the nuclear atypia seen on peripheral blood smear[28] (Fig. 85-7). Peripheral blood examination by light microscopy has tremendous variability and it has been demonstrated to underestimate the tumor burden when compared with more reproducible laboratory assessments of peripheral blood.[7] Flow cytometric analysis of peripheral blood lymphocytes is now widely available and this methodology is easily applied to evaluation of CTCL patients.[46] The most sensitive yet expensive and laborious method for studying the peripheral blood is Southern blotting for T-cell receptor gene rearrangements.[47] This technique detects an expanded T-cell clone blood or lymph node. In CTCL, if a clone has expanded, even if only to the extent that 1 of every 100 lymphocytes belongs to the same clone, the unique gene for this T-cell antigen receptor will be detected by a Southern blot. A practical approach for evaluating the peripheral blood is to initially review the CBC for total lymphocyte count abnormalities, eosinophil count, and for overt lymphocyte nuclear abnormalities. A flow cytometry panel should initially include CD3, CD4, CD8, and CD45RO, which are readily available. Any elevation of the CD4/CD8 ratio or elevation of CD45RO% would select out patients where gene rearrangement studies could confirm leukemic stage disease.

DIFFERENTIAL DIAGNOSIS

The diagnosis of epidermotropic CTCL is based on clinicopathologic criteria. In many patients the histology of the eruption is not distinctive, and there may be a latent period of several years from the onset of the eruption to the definitive histologic diagnosis. Early diagnostic criteria have been proposed for "patch" stage CTCL based on histology of the lesion; these include the presence of mononuclear cells infiltrating an epidermis that is devoid of spongiosis.[48] In many cases, however, the clinical diagnosis of CTCL cannot be confirmed histologically.

The characteristic morphology of the leukemic cell in the Sézary syndrome is also seen in the infiltrate of plaque-stage lesions and is now accepted to be characteristic of epidermotropic CTCL. The surface of the nucleus ranges from mild indentation to gross cerebriform shape. The nuclear chromatin is condensed in a patchy distribution, and nucleoli may be prominent. The cytoplasm is typically sparse[49] (Fig. 85-7). The significance of these cells has been brought into question by several studies in which similar cells have been described in benign skin disorders.[50] Whether the cells found in lichen planus, discoid lupus erythematosus, and psoriasis are the same as CTCL malignant cells is a matter of speculation.

THERAPY

The goals of therapy are to match the modality of treatment appropriately to the biology of the patient's disease. The exceptions to the approach of CTCL as a systemic disease are the unique cases of unilesional disease, which can often be cured by a single localized course of radiotherapy.[51] It is most useful in choosing the appropriate therapy to divide patients into three groups: those with disease limited to the skin but <10% surface involvement; those with extensive plaques, tumors, or erythroderma who have microscopically disseminated disease; and those with overt visceral disease, including effacement of lymph nodes. The first group should receive therapy limited to the skin, with the goal of eradicating the disease process. The second group should receive ablative therapy to the skin along with secondary systemic therapy. The third group requires palliative skin therapy and systemic therapy aimed at prolongation of an otherwise very limited life span.

In the more common plaque and patch stage of the disease,

Table 85-2. Cell-Surface Markers Involved in the Pathogenesis of CTCLs

Marker	Positive Cells	Description
CD2	T cells	Binds to LFA-3
CD3	T cells	Transduces the activation signal from TCR
CD4	Helper T cells Monocyte/ macrophages	Binds to class II MHC
CD8	Suppressor T cells	Binds to class 1 MHC
CD25	Activated T cells	IL-2 receptor (Tac), induced by HTLV-1
CD30	Activated T cells	Ki-1 marker, found in Hodgkin disease and lymphomatoid papulosis
CD45	Leukocyte common antigen	Isoforms of CD45 appear with T-cell activation
CD45RO (UCHL1)	Memory cells	Irreversibly formed after T-cell activation
CLA	Skin-associated lymphocytes	Homing receptor that binds endothelial leukocyte adhesion molecule-1
BE2	CTCL cells	Heat-shock protein found on CTCL cells
LFA-1	Lymphocytes	Binds ICAM-1, which can be found on keratinocytes
T-cell receptor	T cells	Two varieties: $\alpha\beta$ and $\gamma\delta$; these are proteins that bind specific antigens
V-β	T cells	Variable region-specific antibodies (~45 different regions)

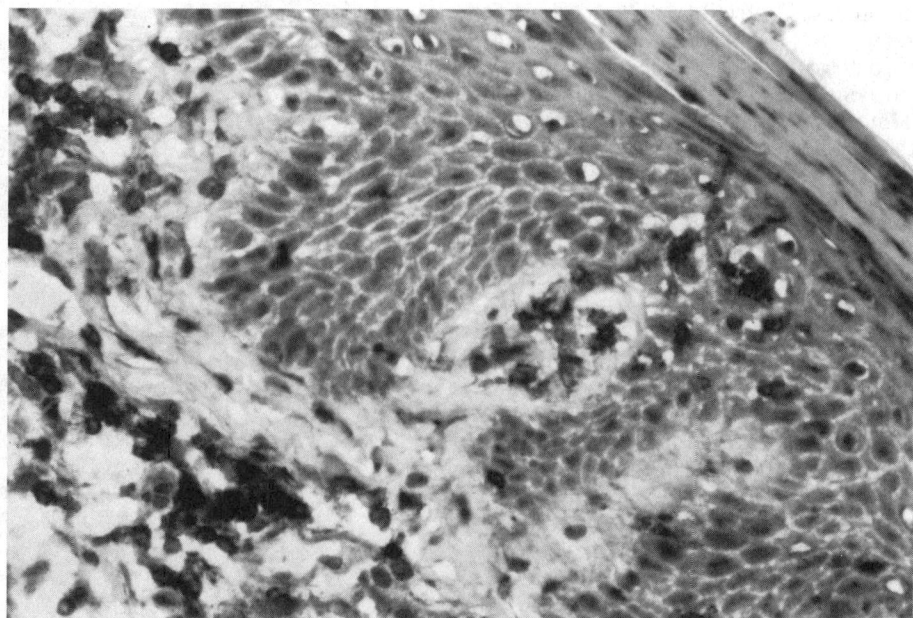

Fig. 85-13. Immunoperoxidase stain for CD3 shows epidermotropic cells.

the most successful regimens are those consisting of skin-directed therapy. Three methods of skin-directed therapy are available: (1) topical chemotherapy with mechlorethamine (nitrogen mustard) or carmustine (BCNU); (2) whole body electron beam irradiation; and (3) photochemotherapy with oral 8-methoxypsoralen and ultraviolet A light.

Topical chemotherapy with mechlorethamine has been successfully used in the treatment of limited cutaneous CTCL. The longest follow-up studies of any skin-directed therapy have been of patients treated with nitrogen mustard. A complete remission occurred in a majority, with a median survival of 8 years. Response rates were better in patients with early stage disease, and there were several apparent cures.[52] The major disadvantage of topical mechlorethamine is cutaneous hypersensitivity, which develops in ≤40% of patients treated in this manner. An alternative to the aqueous solutions of this agent, which must be prepared by the patient each night before total body application, is the use of an ointment-based compound.[53] For those who have become sensitive, there are topical or intravenous desensitization regimens. The best results are obtained if the entire skin is treated, not just the perilesional and lesional areas.

Topical carmustine therapy for limited plaque-stage CTCL may be as efficacious as topical nitrogen mustard, but it differs from the latter in having a topical and systemic effect. Patients with limited plaques undergo an intensive course of topical therapy, during which they may experience irritant but not allergic reactions. In addition, systemic absorption leads to bone marrow suppression. Once the treatment course is completed, most patients achieve a remission during which no further treatment is needed, although retreatment is always possible.[54]

Because electrons penetrate only to the upper dermis, electron beam therapy may be used without systemic effect. Whole body electron beam irradiation brings about complete remission in 84% of patients, whose median survival time is 9 years.[55] The relapse rate is highest in the later stages of CTCL (i.e., in those patients with tumors, lymphadenopathy, and visceral involvement). The total radiation dose is important; a dose of 36 Gy leads to higher complete remission rates and longer disease-free survival than do lower doses.[56] The major disadvantages are that this type of therapy is expensive, requires a

specialized center, and takes ≤3 months to complete. Local side effects include alopecia, atrophy of sweat glands and skin generally, radiodermatitis, and edema. Side effects, both short- and long-term, can be markedly diminished by dividing the dose so as to give ≤1 Gy per treatment. Follow-up treatment to prolong remission is currently under study, and the effects of nitrogen mustard,[57] cyclic doxorubicin and cyclophosphamide,[56] and photopheresis[58] have been documented.

Photochemotherapy with ultraviolet A light and 8-methoxypsoralen provides complete remission in most patients[59]; however, maintenance therapy is needed.[60] The response rate is better in early stage disease and decreases in patients with tumors or generalized erythroderma. The treatment is continual for years, and this aspect discourages some patients. Thus, patients on this therapy continue after remission is achieved with weekly and then biweekly treatments, which are further progressively tapered to a frequency as low as bimonthly. Long-term side effects include atrophy and dryness of the skin. Psoriasis patients treated by photochemotherapy have a 2–3% incidence of cutaneous epitheliomas, particularly those who have undergone previous x-ray irradiation of the skin or who sunburn easily.

Orthovoltage radiotherapy is ideal for all deep lesions such as tumors and for refractory plaques. Spot radiotherapy of this type is usually considered to be palliative and a component of a multiple-regimen approach.

Erythrodermic disease can often result in making patients cutaneous cripples. Palliative relief can be provided for patients with elevated leukocyte counts with the use of leukapheresis.[61] The treatment of choice for erythrodermic CTCL is photopheresis, in which a leukapheresis sample is obtained and treated with ultraviolet A light to activate 8-methoxypsoralen, which has been added to the leukapheresis sample. The photoinactivated cells are then reinfused. Patients are treated on a monthly basis, and >75% achieve improvement, many going into complete remission.[62,63] In view of the low toxicity of this therapy, it is currently being explored as an adjunct to the previously described cytoreductive treatments. Laboratory studies indicate that extracorporeal alteration of the pathogenic T cells provokes immunologic responses to them in a clonally limited way.[64] This observation is supported by the long-term remissions in responsive CTCL patients.

Of the immunomodulating agents tried to date, the best results have been achieved with IFN-α. Most patients treated with an average of 9 million U/day for 10 weeks achieved responses, and several experienced complete remissions in all stages of the disease.[65] The treatment can then be extended using an intermittent treatment schedule. The side effects are dose-related and extremely common. All patients develop flu-like fevers, myalgias, fatigue, and anorexia; central nervous system and marrow suppressive complications, which may necessitate cessation of treatment, are less frequent. Although the response to IFN-α is often incomplete, this therapy has been shown to be a useful adjunct to both PUVA treatment[66] and photopheresis.[67]

Systemic single-agent chemotherapy with mechlorethamine, cyclophosphamide, methotrexate, bleomycin, and doxorubicin and combination chemotherapy have been used in the treatment of CTCL. The response rates vary between 60% and 85%. Complete remission is seen in only 20–25% of patients, and this is associated with a high relapse rate.[68-70] There have been no reports of long-term disease-free survival after either single-agent or combination chemotherapy in patients with histologic evidence of extracutaneous CTCL. Prospective trials of various combinations of chemotherapeutic agents in advanced CTCL are under way at several centers. Three regimens have shown an impact on extensive disease when used in conjunction with radiotherapy: the previously mentioned doxorubicin and cyclophosphamide regimen[56]; alternating cycles of vincristine, doxorubicin, and bleomycin with cyclophosphamide, methotrexate, and prednisone; and monthly cycles of cyclophosphamide, vincristine, procarbazine, and prednisone.[71,72] However, currently the role of chemotherapy appears to remain a palliative one in patients with extensive CTCL. Newer, less toxic agents such as fludarabine are now being tested both alone and in conjunction with IFN. Initial results are encouraging.[73]

PROGNOSIS

The approach to the patient with CTCL should be to establish the diagnosis, determine the extent of disease, and embark on a therapeutic course with some awareness of the prognosis of the individual patient. The only parameter of CTCL that has been shown to have significant prognostic value is the extent of disease (extent and type of skin involvement). For this reason a modified TNM classification system was adopted by the Mycosis Fungoides Cooperative Study Group in 1975 and further modified by the Cutaneous T Cell Lymphoma Workshop (Table 85-3). Staging of the disease on the basis of this classification may allow for more rational treatment of patients with CTCL and for more organized assessment of different treatment modalities. Despite therapeutic intervention, surveys have not shown an appreciable increase in survival of CTCL patients.[74] In general, the median survival with early stage disease is ≥8 years, which decreases to <3 years with the development of tumor nodules or erythroderma.[74,75]

Skin Lesions

Lesion morphology is typically varied, and this creates the need to perform multiple biopsies. Often plaques can have tumor histology and plaque lesions can mimic tumors. Immunophenotyping is necessary to assign the diagnosis of T-cell lymphoma. In addition to biopsies, whole body photography is a useful adjunct in skin staging. The prognosis for patients with CTCL worsens with the extent of cutaneous involvement.[41] Patients with limited plaque lesions (<10% of body surface area) have a better prognosis than patients with generalized plaque lesions (T2, >10% of body surface). Prognosis is poorer in patients with tumors (T3) than in those with plaque lesions and is poorer still in those with erythroderma (T4).[41,75] Differences in prognosis in these groups may be related to the in-

Table 85-3. TNM Classification of CTCL

Classification	Description
T: skin[a]	
T0	Clinically and/or histopathologically suspicious lesions
T1	Limited plaques, papules, or eczematoid patches covering ≥10% of the skin surface
T2	Generalized plaques, papules, or erythematous patches covering ≥10% of the skin surface
T3	Tumors, one or more
T4	Generalized erythroderma
N: lymph nodes[b]	
N0	No clinically or palpably abnormal peripheral lymph nodes, pathology negative for CTCL
N1	Clinically abnormal peripheral lymph nodes, pathology negative for CTCL
N2	No clinically abnormal peripheral lymph nodes, pathology positive for CTCL
N3	Clinically abnormal peripheral lymph nodes, pathology positive for CTCL
B: peripheral blood	
B0	Atypical circulating cells not present or <5%
B1	Atypical circulating cells present in ≥5% of total blood lymphocytes; record total white blood cell count and total lymphocyte counts and number of atypical cells per 100 lymphocytes
M: visceral organs	
M0	No involvement of visceral organs
M1	Visceral involvement (must have confirmation of pathology and organ involved should be specified)

[a] Pathology of T1 to T4 is diagnostic of a CTCL. When characteristics of more than one T classification exist, both are recorded and the highest is used for staging (e.g., T4).[3]

[b] The number of sites of abnormal nodes is recorded, for example, cervical (left + right), axillary (left + right), axillary (left + right), inguinal (left + right), epitrochlear, submandibular, submaxillary, and so forth.

creased incidence of extracutaneous involvement with progressive stages of skin disease. The unique clinical syndrome of unilesional CTCL has a particularly good prognosis with frequent cures.[51]

Lymph Nodes

The incidence of lymphadenopathy increases with the stage of cutaneous involvement. Lymphadenopathy, whether dermatopathic lymphadenopathy (N1) or infiltration by CTCL (N2, N3), indicates a poor prognosis. In practice, enlarged nodes are biopsied at initial staging and whenever they appear. Flow cytometry, immunophenotyping, and Southern blot analysis are recommended for appropriate analysis of node samples. Because the Southern blot technique can even detect lymphoma in dermatopathic nodes, its impact on prognosis is unknown. In conjunction with imaging procedures for visceral disease, radiologic studies provide periodic assessments of thoracic, abdominal, and pelvic nodes.

Peripheral Blood

Circulating CTCL cells can be detected by light microscopy in about 20% of all patients with tumors and in almost all patients with the erythrodermic form of this disorder.[5] The presence of >5% circulating malignant cells in CTCL (B1) indicates a poor prognosis. However, the technology previously discussed that has improved the ability to detect CTCL cells has not been available for long-term follow-up at this point.

Visceral Involvement

Visceral involvement is clinically apparent only late in the course of CTCL. This type of involvement (M1) carries the poorest prognosis, with median survival only 6–8 months. Initial and periodic CT scans in conjunction with the physical examination are the best monitors of this stage of the disease.

The brain, peripheral nervous system, and leptomeninges are involved in about 10% of patients.[41] Symptoms depend on the site of involvement and the occurrence of secondary intracerebral hemorrhage. Involvement may simulate progressive multifocal leukoencephalopathy, myelopathy, or peripheral neuropathy or may present as space-occupying lesions. The appearance of any focal neurologic deficit should be investigated with a CT scan of the brain in conjunction with cerebrospinal fluid cytology. Leptomeningeal involvement can often be diagnosed by cytology alone. Care must be taken in the evaluation of results, since circulating cells are more common than neurologic involvement and can contaminate cerebrospinal fluid samples.

Paraneoplastic Phenomena

Additional clinical findings in CTCL are created by the variety of paraneoplastic phenomena that appear as a result of helper T-cell functions. Cutaneous infections that are dependent on T cells for their control are more common. In fact, disseminated herpetic eruptions are favored not only by the disruption in the T-cell compartment but also by the diffusely involved skin in some patients. Helper T cells are required for antibody production by B cells. Immunoglobulin abnormalities in CTCL include monoclonal gammopathies and polyclonal hypergammaglobulinemia.

FUTURE DIRECTIONS

Lymphomas of cutaneous T cells represent a pathologic exaggeration of physiologic interactions. As the molecular controls of T_{H1}-T_{H2} lymphocyte interactions, activated T-cell regulation, and antitumor immunity unfold, these advances will find clinical application in the syndromes discussed.

REFERENCES

1. Picker LJ, Bacher EC: Physiological and molecular mechanisms of lymphocyte homing. Ann Rev Immunol 10:561, 1992
2. Heald P, Yan SL, Edelson RL et al: Skin selective lymphocyte homing mechanisms in the pathogenesis of leukemic cutaneous T-cell lymphoma. J Invest Dermatol 101:222, 1993
3. Picker LJ, Michie SA, Rott LS, Butcher EC: A unique phenotype of skin-associated lymphocytes in humans. Am J Pathol 136:1053, 1990
4. Nickoloff BJ: Role of interferon gamma in cutaneous trafficking of lymphocytes with emphasis on molecular and cellular adhesion events. Arch Dermatol 124:1835, 1988
5. Dalloul A, Laroche L, Bagot M et al: Interleukin-7 is a growth factor for Sézary cells. J Clin Invest 90:1054, 1992
6. Rich BE, Campos-Torres J, Tepper RI et al: Cutaneous lymphoproliferation and lymphomas in interleukin 7 transgenic mice. J Exp Med 177:305, 1993
7. Heald P, Edelson R: The immunobiology of cutaneous T-cell lymphoma. J Natl Cancer Inst 83:400, 1991
8. Vowels BR, Cassin M, Vonderheid EC, Rook AH: Aberrant cytokine production by Sézary syndrome patients: cytokine secretion pattern resembles murine Th2 cells. J Invest Dermatol 99:90, 1992
9. Heald P, Yan SL, Edelson RL: Profound deficiency in normal circulating T cells in erythrodermic cutaneous T cell lymphoma. Arch Dermatol 130:198, 1994
10. Cerroni L, Rieger E, Hodl S, Kerl H: Clinicopathologic and immunologic features associated with transformation of mycosis fungoides to large-cell lymphomas. Am J Surg Pathol 16:543, 1992
11. Salhany KE, Cousar JB, Greer JP et al: Transformation of cutaneous T cell lymphoma to large cell lymphoma. Am J Pathol 132:265, 1988
12. Lamberg SI, Bunn PA: Proceeding of the workshop on cutaneous T cell lymphomas (mycosis fungoides and Sezary syndrome). Cancer Treat Rep 63:561, 1979
13. Carney DN, Bunn PA: Manifestations of cutaneous T cell lymphoma. J Dermatol Surg Oncol 6:369, 1980
14. Lindae ML, Abel EA, Hoppe RT, Wood GA: Poikilodermatous mycosis fungoides and atrophic large plaque parapsoriasis exhibit similar abnormalities of T-cell antigen expression. Arch Dermatol 124:366, 1988
15. Lambert WC, Everett MA: The nosology of parapsoriasis. J Am Acad Dermatol 5:373, 1981
16. Watsky MS, Lynnfield YL: Poikiloderma vasculare atrophicans. Cutis 17:938, 1976
17. Willenzer R, Dijkstra A, Meijr CJ: Lymphocytic infiltrate of the skin (Jessner): a T-cell lymphoproliferative disease. J Invest Dermatol 110:523, 1984
18. Von Hinen YT, Bergroth V, Johansson E et al: A long term clinicopathologic survey of patients with Jessner's lymphocytic infiltrate of the skin. J Invest Dermatol 110:523, 1984
19. Gibson LE, Muller S: Follicular mucinosis: clinical and histopathologic study. J Am Acad Dermatol 20:441, 1989
20. Black MM, Wilson-Jones E: Lymphomatoid pityriasis lichenoides: a variant with histological features simulating a lymphoma. Br J Dermatol 86:329, 1972
21. Thomsen K, Wantzin GL: Lymphomatoid papulosis. A follow up study of thirty patients. J Am Acad Dermatol 17:632, 1988
22. Weiss LM, Wood GA, Trela M et al: Clonal T-cell populations in lymphomatoid papulosis. Evidence of a lymphoproliferative origin for a clinically benign disease. N Engl J Med 315:475, 1986
23. Braun-Falco O, Schmoeckel C, Burg G et al: Pagetoid reticulosis: a further case report with a review of the literature. Acta Dermatol Venereal (Stockh), suppl. 85. 59:11, 1979
24. Wood GS, Weiss LM, Hu CH et al: T cell antigen deficiencies and clonal rearrangement of T-cell receptor genes in pagetoid reticulosis (Woringer-Kolopp disease). N Engl J Med 318:164, 1988
25. Alibert J: Monographie des dermatoses. Vol. 2. p. 413. G Bailliere, Paris, 1835
26. Bazin E: Leçons sur le Traitement des Maladies Chroniques en General Affection de la Peau, en Particulier par l'Emploi Compare des Eaux Minerales de l'Hydrotherapie et des Moyens Pharmaceutiques. Adrien Delahaye, Paris, 1870, p. 425
27. Besnier E, Hallopeau H: On the erythrodermia of mycosis fungoides. J Cutan Genitourin Dis 10:453, 1892
28. Sézary A, Bouvrain Y: Erythrodermie avec presence de cellules monstreuses dans le derme et le sang circulant. Bull Soc Fr Dermatol Syphil 45:254, 1938
29. LeBoit P, Beckstead JH, Bond B et al: Granulomatous slack skin: clonal rearrangement of the T-cell receptor beta gene is evidence for the lymphoproliferative nature of a cutaneous elastolytic disorder. J Invest Dermatol 89:183, 1987
30. Takatsuki K, Uchiyama T, Sagawa K, Yodoi J: Adult T cell leukaemia in Japan. p. 73. In Seno S, Takaku F, Irino S (eds): Topics in Haematology. Excerpta Medica, Amsterdam, 1977
31. Poiesz BJ, Ruscetti FW, Gazdar AF et al: Detection and isolation of type C retrovirus particles from fresh and cultured lymphocytes of a patient with cutaneous T cell lymphoma. Proc Natl Acad Sci USA 77:7415, 1980
32. Yamaguchi K, Kiyokawa T, Nakada K et al: Polyclonal integration of HTLV-I proviral DNA in lymphocytes from HTLV-I seropositive individuals: an intermediate state between the healthy carrier state and smoldering ATL. Br J Hematol 68:169, 1988
33. Fujiwara Y, Abe Y, Kuyama M et al: CD8+ cutaneous T-cell lymphoma with pagetoid epidermotropism and angiocentric and angiodestructive infiltration. Arch Dermatol 126:801, 1990
34. Agnarsson BA, Vonderheid EC, Kadin ME: Cutaneous T cell lymphoma with suppressor/cytotoxic (CD8) phenotype: identification of rapidly progressive and chronic subtypes. J Am Acad Dermatol 22:569, 1990
35. Heald P, Buckley P, Kacinski B et al: Correlations of unique clinical, immunotypic, and histologic findings in cutaneous gamma/delta T-cell lymphoma. J Am Acad Dermatol 26:865, 1992
36. Burg G, Dummer R, Wilhelm M et al: A subcutaneous delta positive T-cell lymphoma that produces interferon gamma. N Engl J Med 325:1078, 1991
37. Agnarsson BA, Kadin ME: Ki-1 positive large cell lymphoma. A morphologic and immunologic study of nineteen cases. Am J Surg Pathol 12:264, 1988
38. Bunn PA, Huberman MS, Whang-Peng J et al: Prospective staging evaluation of patients with cutaneous T cell lymphomas. Ann Intern Med 93:223, 1980
39. Stokar LM: Clinical manifestations of intrathoracic cutaneous T cell lymphoma. Cancer 56:2694, 1985
40. Patel DJ, Greim ML, Vijaykumar S, Greim SG: Treatment of pulmonary mycosis fungoides with whole lung radiation therapy. J Surg Oncol 38:118, 1988

41. Epstein EH Jr, Levin DL, Croft JD Jr et al: Mycosis fungoides. Survival, prognostic features, response to therapy and autopsy findings. Medicine 51:61, 1972

42. Kantor AF, Curtis RE, Vonderheid EC et al: Risk of second malignancy after cutaneous T-cell lymphoma. Cancer 63:1612, 1989

43. Olsen EA, Delzell E, Jegasothy BV: Second malignancies in cutaneous T-cell lymphoma. J Am Acad Dermatol 10:197, 1984

44. Heald P, Berger C, Yamamura T et al: BE-2 antigen: appearance during T cell activation and increase with stimulation and growth of T cells. J Invest Dermatol 94:452, 1990

45. Vonderheid EC, Tan E, Sobel EL et al: Clinical implications of immunologic phenotyping in cutaneous T cell lymphoma. J Am Acad Dermatol 17:40, 1987

46. Yan SL, Heald PW: Flow cytometry in the evaluation of dermatology patients. Clin Dermatol 9:31, 1991

47. Weiss LM, Hu E, Wood GS et al: Clonal rearrangements of T-cell receptor genes in mycosis fungoides and dermatopathic lymphadenopathy. N Engl J Med 313:539, 1985

48. Sanchez JL, Ackerman AB: The patch stage of mycosis fungoides: criteria for histologic diagnosis. Am J Dermatopathol 1:5, 1979

49. Lutzner MA, Hobbs JW, Horvath P: Ultra-structure of abnormal cells in Sezary syndrome. Mycosis fungoides and parapsoriasis en plaque. Arch Dermatol 103:375, 1971

50. Flaxman BA, Zelazny G, Van Scott EJ: Nonspecificity of characteristic cells in mycosis fungoides. Arch Dermatol 104:141, 1971

51. Oliver GF, Winkelmann RK: Unilesional mycosis fungoides: a distinct entity. J Am Acad Dermatol 20:63, 1989

52. Vonderheid EC, Tan ET, Cantor AF et al: Long term efficacy, curative potential, and carcinogenicity of topical mechlorethamine chemotherapy and cutaneous T-cell lymphoma. J Am Acad Dermatol 20:416, 1989

53. Price NM, Hoppe RT, Deneau G: Ointment based mechlorethamine treatment for mycosis fungoides. Cancer 52:2214, 1983

54. Zackheim HS, Epstein EH, Crain WR: Topical carmustine (BCNU) for cutaneous T cell lymphoma: a 15-year experience in 143 patients. J Am Acad Dermatol 22:802, 1990

55. Hoppe RT, Cox RS, Fuks Z et al: Electron-beam therapy for mycosis fungoides: the Stanford University experience. Cancer Treat Rep 63:691, 1979

56. Braverman IM, Yager NB, Chen M et al: Combined total body electron beam irradiation and chemotherapy for mycosis fungoides. J Am Acad Dermatol 17:40, 1987

57. Hamminga MD, Noorkijk EM, Van Vloten WA: Treatment of mycosis fungoides. Total skin electron beam irradiation vs topical mechlorethamine therapy. Arch Dermatol 118:150, 1982

58. Heald PW, Perez MI, Edelson RL: The use and efficacy of photopheresis in the treatment of cutaneous T cell lymphoma. Yale J Biol Med 62:629, 1989

59. Gilchrest BA: Methoxsalen photochemotherapy for mycosis fungoides. Cancer Treat Rep 63:663, 1979

60. Honigsmann H, Brenner W, Rauschmeier W et al: Photochemotherapy for cutaneous T cell lymphoma. J Am Acad Dermatol 10:238, 1984

61. Edelson R, Facktor M, Andrews A et al: Successful management of the Sézary syndrome: mobilization and removal of extravascular neoplastic T cells by leukapheresis. N Engl J Med 291:293, 1974

62. Edelson RL, Berger CL, Gasparro FP et al: Treatment of cutaneous T cell lymphoma by extracorporeal photochemotherapy. N Engl J Med 316:297, 1987

63. Heald PW, Rook A, Perez M et al: Treatment of erythrodermic cutaneous T-cell lymphoma patients with photopheresis. J Am Acad Dermatol 7:427, 1992

64. Heald PW, LaRoche L, Knobler R: Photoinactivated lymphocyte therapy for cutaneous T-cell lymphoma. Dermatol Clin 12:443, 1994

65. Olsen EA, Rosen ST, Vollmer RT et al: Interferon alfa-2a in the treatment of cutaneous T-cell lymphoma. J Am Acad Dermatol 20:395, 1989

66. Mostow EN, Neckel SL, Oberhelman L et al: Complete remissions in psoralen and ultraviolet A (PUVA) refractory mycosis fungoides type cutaneous T-cell lymphoma with combined interferon alfa and PUVA. Arch Dermatol 129:747, 1993

67. Rook A, Prystowsky M, Cassin M et al. Combined therapy for Sézary syndrome with extracorporeal photochemotherapy and low dose interferon alfa therapy. Arch Dermatol 127:1535, 1991

68. Van Scott EJ, Grekin DA, Kalmansory JD et al: Frequent low doses of intravenous mechlorethamine for late-stage mycosis fungoides lymphoma. Cancer 36:1613, 1975

69. Levi JA, Diggs CH, Wiernik PH: Adriamycin therapy in advanced mycosis fungoides. Cancer 39:1967, 1977

70. Wright JC, Gumport SL, Golomb FM: Remissions produced with the use of methotrexate in patients with mycosis fungoides. Cancer Chemother Rep 9:11, 1960

71. Hallahan DE, Griem ML, Griem SF et al: Combined modality therapy for tumor stage mycosis fungoides: results of a 10 year follow-up. J Clin Oncol 6:1177, 1988

72. Winkler CF, Sausville EA, Ihde DC et al: Combined modality treatment of cutaneous T cell lymphomas. Results of a 6 year follow-up. J Clin Oncol 4:1094, 1986

73. Von Hoff DD, Dahlberg S, Hartstock RJ et al: Activity of fludarabine monophosphate in patients with advanced mycosis fungoides: a Southwest Oncology Group study. J Natl Cancer Inst 82:1353, 1990

74. Weinstock MA, Horm JW: Mycosis fungoides in the United States. Increasing incidence and descriptive epidemiology. JAMA 260:42, 1988

75. Sauseville EA, Eddy JL, Makuch RW et al: Histopathologic staging at initial diagnosis of mycosis fungoides and the Sezary syndrome. Definition of three distinctive prognostic groups. Ann Intern Med 109:372, 1988

AIDS-Associated Lymphomas

86

David T. Scadden and Jerome E. Groopman

INTRODUCTION

Immunologic dysfunction leads to an increased incidence of non-Hodgkin lymphoma (NHL) in a number of different clinical settings, ranging from congenital immunodeficiency states such as Wiskott-Aldrich syndrome to autoimmune processes such as Sicca syndrome[1-10] (Table 86-1). Immunodeficiency induced by infection with the human immunodeficiency virus (HIV) is now strongly associated with NHL and is emerging as an important cause of high-grade NHL worldwide.[11-18] The pathophysiologic basis for this association of immune abnormalities and immune neoplasia are unknown, but several mechanisms are suggested by associated phenomena.

The incidence of lymphoma after organ transplantation cor-

Table 86-1. Magnitude of Relative Risk of Lymphoma[a]

High (RR >15)	Intermediate (RR >2)	Low (RR ≤2)
Multiple transplants	Sibling transplant	Splenectomy
Cadaver transplant	Mild sicca syndrome	Sarcoidosis
Severe sicca syndrome	Nontropical sprue	Hyperimmunization
Wiskott-Aldrich syndrome	Crohn disease	Asthma
Ataxia-telangiectasia	Short-term HIV infection	Hansen disease
Long-term HIV infection	Rheumatoid arthritis	Cytotoxic drug prescription
		Systemic lupus erythematosus

Abbreviation: RR, relative risk.

[a] Risk of lymphoma in patients with the condition relative to a risk of 1.0 to comparable individuals without the condition.

(From Hoover,[1] with permission.)

relates with the type of organ transplanted (Table 86-2) and is probably related to the intensity of associated immunosuppressive therapy.[3,19–21] During bone marrow transplantation, purging the donor marrow of T cells reduces graft-versus-host disease, but dramatically enhances the incidence of post-transplant lymphoproliferation[9,22,23] (Table 86-2). The depth of immunosuppression appears to be directly associated with the likelihood of developing lymphoma; however, the increased incidence of lymphoma observed in HLA-mismatched bone marrow transplantation and in autoimmune diseases suggests that immune activation also plays a contributory role.

Specific mechanisms that may lead to the emergence of malignancy in the setting of disordered immunity include an inadequate or inappropriate host response to transforming infectious pathogens.[3,24–26] The immune deficit after organ transplantation has been clearly shown to permit an Epstein-Barr virus (EBV)-driven lymphoproliferative condition that often behaves like frank lymphoma.[24–28] Similarly, a lack of immunologic response to a transformed cell and deficient tumor surveillance may facilitate the neoplastic outgrowth.[29] This may be particularly important in the setting where interactions between immune cells may be perturbed, leading to exuberant proliferation of a subset of cells. An expanded pool of proliferating cells, perhaps induced by aberrantly regulated production of cytokines, may provide the background for a transforming event. The possibility that each of these mechanisms may be playing a role in immunodysfunctional states in general and acquired immunodeficiency syndrome (AIDS) in particular, may only be indirectly inferred from several lines of evidence that are discussed in more detail below.

Although many types of immunologic abnormalities lead to lymphoid malignancy, they may not do so via a common path. Particular features of the immune abnormality may predispose

Table 86-2. Lymphoproliferative Disease Post-Transplantation

Transplant Type	Incidence[a] (%)
Renal	1.0
Heart	1.8
Liver	2.2
Heart and lung	5.0
Bone marrow (BM)	<1
T-depleted BM	12
Mismatched, T-depleted BM	24

[a] It should be noted that these numbers were reported using aggressive immunosuppressive regimens that have generally been modified substantially, likely decreasing the incidence of lymphoproliferative disease.

(Data from references 3, 9, and 19–23.)

to particular neoplastic manifestations. For example, the lymphoproliferative disease that occurs in the organ transplant patient is virtually uniformly associated with EBV and may be reversible with withdrawal of immunosuppressive drugs.[24,27] By contrast, the immunodeficiency of HIV disease results in lymphomas that are EBV associated in only a portion of cases (estimated at 33–66%)[30–35] and there is an apparently unique occurrence of polyclonal EBV-negative tumors in AIDS.[36] The frequency of rearrangements of c-*myc* in HIV-related tumors is also substantially higher (30–80%) than after organ transplants.[30,31,35–39] In addition, the small non-cleaved cell (SNCC) or Burkitt lymphoma is seen in approximately 20% of AIDS lymphomas, whereas it is extremely uncommon in other immunodysfunction-associated lymphomas.[12] These differing manifestations of malignancy in different settings of immunologic abnormalities may provide clues as to how immune perturbation results in malignancy, an issue with clear implications beyond the specific disorders in question.

EPIDEMIOLOGY

The increased frequency of NHL in HIV infection was first detected in 1984 and became a criterion for an AIDS-defining illness in 1987.[40–48] As treatments or prophylaxes for other complications of HIV disease have become more effective, NHL has become increasingly problematic.[12,16] NHL may occur at any time during the course of HIV disease and is the AIDS-defining event in approximately 4% of U.S. patients as reported to the Centers for Disease Control.[49] However, the frequency of NHL appears to increase with increasing immunosuppression and the development of primary central nervous system NHL is clearly associated with very advanced immunodeficiency.

All risk groups for HIV are susceptible to NHL with the degree of risk appearing to vary based on the type of exposure that led to HIV infection[12,15,17,18,50,51] (Table 86-3). The degree of variation may indicate important biologic differences among the risk groups such as exposure to co-infectious agents predisposing to malignancy. However, the data may also reflect differences in the quality of medical care or surveillance among different HIV infected subpopulations. The relatively slight differences in incidence of lymphoma among risk groups contrasts sharply with the other major neoplastic complication of HIV disease, Kaposi sarcoma, in which a striking association with particular sexual practices supports the hypothesis that a second sexually transmitted pathogen is required for tumor development.

The incidence of NHL in an HIV-infected population has been estimated to vary between 3% and 12% over a 2-year period of observation in patients with symptomatic HIV disease.[52–54] Moore et al.[52] reported an incidence of 3.2% at 24 months in >1,000 patients who had a diagnosis of AIDS based on clinical conditions other than lymphoma. Pluda et al.[54] reported a higher incidence of 8% per year with a cumulative incidence

Table 86-3. Relative Risk of Lymphoma by HIV Transmission Group

HIV Transmission Group	+Relative Risk (95% CI)
Hemophiliac or clotting disorder	1.66 +
Homosexual or bisexual men	1.13
Transfusion recipient	1.0
Children infected perinatally	0.90
Heterosexual contact, except those born in the Caribbean or Africa	0.77
Intravenous drug user	0.6 +
Heterosexual contact, born in the Caribbean or Africa	0.4 +

(From Beral et al.,[12] with permission.)

of 12% over 24 months of observation in 55 patients who had entered an anti-retroviral therapy study with a mean entry CD4 count of 71 cells/mm³. The latter study included postmortem diagnoses whereas the former did not, accounting for some of the differences in the estimate of risk.

NHL has been increasing in incidence steadily over the past two decades in the U.S. population, with a particularly striking increase in incidence in U.S. males. National Cancer Institute (NCI) statistics indicate approximately a 60% increase in the interval from 1976 to 1990.[55] The contribution of the HIV epidemic to this trend has not been fully documented to date, but estimates of the number of infected individuals in the United States suggest that AIDS lymphoma will accelerate the increase in NHL and may already constitute 8–27% of all NHL.[11]

PATHOPHYSIOLOGY

Neoplasia may be more common in the immunodeficient host on the basis of a number of different mechanisms: (1) opportunistic infection with a transforming infectious agent, (2) inadequate tumor surveillance, or (3) unregulated proliferation of cells responding to disordered production of growth factors. A critical point in AIDS lymphomas is that HIV itself is not transforming and is not detectable in the malignant cells (with the rare exception of some cases of T-cell lymphoma).[56] In general, there is no AIDS virus in AIDS lymphoma cells. NHL develops as an opportunistic neoplasm when HIV causes the immune system to falter in much the same manner as opportunistic infections occur with progressive immunodeficiency.[57,58]

The role of a second infectious agent inducing disordered cell growth in HIV disease is most apparent in development of cervical neoplasia in HIV-seropositive women with papillomavirus infection.[59–64] Similarly, squamous cell neoplasia of the anus seen in homosexual men, is associated with papillomavirus infection and hypothesized to be directly related to the transforming capacity of subtypes of the virus.[65,66] Although a specific infectious agent has not been confirmed in AIDS-associated Kaposi sarcoma, epidemiologic evidence supports the concept that a sexually transmitted agent is a critical cofactor in development of that tumor.[67] In AIDS lymphoma, there is a clear association between EBV and primary central nervous system lymphoma and to a lesser extent with systemic lymphomas.[32–34,57,68] EBV infection may precede the development of NHL in HIV-infected individuals and has been suggested as a risk factor for the progression of lymphadenopathy to lymphoma.[69,70] Large cell or immunoblastic histology tumors have been reported to contain EBV in ≤77%, whereas the small noncleaved or Burkitt-like tumors are associated with EBV in approximately 20–34%.[34,71] In addition, in the small number of T-cell lymphomas reported in AIDS patients, oral T-cell lymphomas have been shown to contain the EBV genome.[72]

The pattern of EBV gene expression in AIDS NHL tumors has been variably reported. Some investigators suggested that EBV gene expression in AIDS was similar to that of EBV transformed cells of similar histologic type in patients without HIV disease. Immunoblastic histology NHL resembled lymphoblastoid cells and the pattern of EBV gene expression in small non-cleaved or Burkitt histology mimicked that seen in classic Burkitt lymphoma.[33,34,71,73–75] In tissue obtained from patients with immunoblastic lymphoma or the lymphoproliferative disease after transplantation, a range of EBV latency genes are expressed, including Epstein-Barr nuclear antigens (EBNA)-2 through EBNA-5 and latent membrane protein (LMP)-1 and -2.[76–78] In Burkitt lymphoma only EBNA-1 is usually detectable.[76,79,80] Recently, it has been reported that AIDS tumors are unlike these other settings and uniquely express a combination of EBNA-1 and LMP-1.[35]

In vitro studies have confirmed the capacity for EBV LMP-1 to transform B lymphocytes and for LMP-2 to interact with growth regulatory intracellular tyrosine kinases.[81–83] How the limited EBV latent gene expression seen in Burkitt lymphoma cells may contribute to the development of malignancy remains undefined. However, other EBV products may be relevant such as those that contribute to immune recognition[84] or cell growth.[85,86] The EBV gene product, BCRF-1, mimics interleukin-10 (IL-10) in molecular and biologic structure.[85–88] BCRF-1 or IL-10 may enhance the proliferation of tumor cells and have other immunologic effects discussed below that may contribute to the emergence of malignant cells.[89] The pathogenic role of these EBV gene products in the development of AIDS lymphomas is likely to be similar to that in other settings, but precise mechanisms are not well understood at present.

The response of HIV-infected patients to immunogenic stimuli deteriorates over time, both as measured by laboratory tests and as evidenced by their clinical course.[90,91] Although some of the functional immunologic deficit is clearly attributable to the decline in number of the CD4⁺ subset of T lymphocytes, a range of functional defects has also been documented in T cells and cells of monocytic or granulocytic origin. Interactions between cells are also perturbed, thought to be partially attributable to disordered regulation of cytokine production.[92] In particular, the production of cytokines that may enhance the proliferation of B cells, such as IL-6 or IL-10, has been reported to be abnormal.[89,93–95] IL-10 (or the EBV product BCRF-1) may be of particular interest because it inhibits interferon-γ and IL-2 elaboration by a subset of helper T cells (T_{H1} cells), thereby potentially impairing the immunologic response.[86–88] It may be postulated that AIDS NHL cells are producing and responding to the growth-inducing signal, IL-10, and that this autocrine loop additionally inhibits an immunologic response that may be mounted against a transformed cell. Alternatively, it may be that the overexuberant growth of otherwise normal B cells (evident in the lymphadenopathy seen in most HIV-infected patients during the course of their disease) simply provides a larger denominator for causally independent, transforming events. There are reports of polyclonal EBV-negative tumors in AIDS NHL, which indirectly support this concept.[36]

Regulation of the B cell in HIV disease is abnormal on several levels, including an increased incidence of spontaneously activated B cells in the peripheral blood and the high levels of serum γ-globulin found in virtually all HIV-infected individuals.[96,97] The mechanism for this perturbation has been postulated to be due to a portion of the HIV envelope inducing T-cell-mediated B-cell effects.[98,99] The nature of the hypergammaglobulinemia has been characterized as oligoclonal often with HIV specificity.[100–105] Multiple myeloma (sporadically seen in HIV-infected patients, but apparently without increased frequency)[106] has been reported to develop from HIV-specific plasma cell clones.[107] The chronic stimulation of HIV-specific B cells by ongoing virus production[91,108] may provide the mitogenic background for mutagenesis, resulting in malignancy.

A number of genetic alterations in AIDS lymphomas have been characterized. Rearrangements of the c-*myc* proto-oncogene with the immunoglobulin locus, well characterized in Burkitt lymphoma, are the most prevalent genetic mutations reported.[31,36,37,39,67,109–111] The most common form of c-*myc* rearrangement resembles the abnormality associated with sporadic Burkitt lymphoma, rather than epidemic Burkitt lymphoma.[37,112–116] That is, c-*myc* is most often mutated and rearranged with the immunoglobulin heavy chain switch region. The presence of this rearrangement in the switch region suggests that the transforming event is occurring in a more mature B cell, which is undergoing the transition between heavy chain isotypes.

The frequency of c-*myc* rearrangement has been estimated at between 23% and 79%.[30,31,35–37,39] It is controversial whether specific histologic types of AIDS NHL are more commonly linked with c-*myc* alterations.[36,39] However, it is apparent that c-*myc* activation and EBV infection are not necessarily associ-

Table 86-4. Histology, Extranodal Sites, and Stage of Lymphoma in AIDS

	No. of Patients	Histology			Extranodal Sites				Stage	
		SNCC	IBS/ALC	LC	Gastrointestinal	Liver	Central Nervous System	Marrow	I, II	III, IV
Levine et al.	27	10	13	—	6	1	8	5	7	20
Kalter et al.	14	7	1	5	2	2	8	4	1	13
Gill et al.	22	16	6	—	5	5	3	7	1	21
Knowles et al.	89	36	25	25	14	14	19	19	27	57
Ziegler et al.	90	32	24	17	8	8	38	30	38	52
Bermudez et al.	31	8	6	10	6	6	8	10	1	30
Lowenthal et al.	43	16	8	16	11	6	11	13	9	26
Kaplan et al.	84	29	36	17	7	22	10	26	14	69
Kaplan et al.	30	7	16	3	?	?	?	7	12	14
Levine et al.	42	17	14	4	5	11	6	6	11	24
Remick et al.	18	0	7	10	5	?	?	?	5	13
Raphael et al.	113	41	33	35	18	3	22	17	—	—
Total (%)	603	219 (36)	189 (31)	142 (24)	87 (15)	78 (13)	133 (23)	144 (25)	126 (27)	339 (73)

Abbreviations: SNCC, small non-cleaved cell; IBS, immunoblastic; ALC, anaplastic large cell; LC, large cell.

ated in the AIDS lymphomas.[36,39] Each may be present independent of the other. It has been documented that c-*myc* rearrangement may precede EBV infection, further supporting the notion that there is no necessary causal linkage between EBV infection and c-*myc* mutation.[110]

A number of other oncogenic mutations have been surveyed and occur with lesser frequency than that of c-*myc*. Notably the tumor suppressor gene p53 has been found to be mutated in 14% of immunoblastic histology tumors regardless of their association with HIV disease.[117] Other investigators have reported an exclusive association of p53 inactivation and Burkitt-like tumors that is always present in conjunction with c-*myc* mutation.[39] Mutation of *ras* has been reported in approximately 15% of AIDS NHL.[39] The *bcr* rearrangement (11;14) linked to lower grade lymphomas is not associated with AIDS lymphomas.

CLINICAL MANIFESTATIONS

AIDS lymphomas are generally histologically intermediate or high-grade B-cell tumors (Table 86-4), proliferate rapidly, and are clinically very aggressive. However, rare cases of T-cell malignancies have been reported, including a range of histologies from large granular lymphoproliferative disease, large cell or anaplastic T-cell lymphoma, Sézary syndrome, and angiocentric T-cell lymphoproliferation.[56,72,118–127] Virus infection with human T-cell leukemia/lymphoma virus (HTLV)-1, EBV, or HIV has been implicated directly in at least some of these T-cell tumors.[56,72,127] One report documented EBV in the malignant cells from oral T-cell lymphomas.[72] In another case the site of HIV-1 integration appeared to serve as a genetic trigger to transformation.[56] These latter events appear to be extremely rare and are probably selected against by the deleterious effects of HIV on the survival of HIV-1-infected T cells.

Although controversial, it does appear that Hodgkin disease occurs with increased frequency in HIV disease (a fivefold increase in one study)[128,129] and has an aggressive clinical course. It has been reported that the mixed cellularity histologic subtype is particularly common in HIV-seropositive patients and that the clinical stage is often more advanced.[73,129–135] Stage III and IV at presentation occurred in 82% of HIV-seropositive patients compared with one-half that incidence in seronegative controls in one retrospective review.[131] As in AIDS-related NHL, extranodal disease and bone marrow involvement are more commonly present (67% and 48%, respectively).[131] Staging and treatment strategies are generally the same as for other Hodgkin patients with several caveats detailed below for the NHL patients. Treatment responses appear to occur with approximately equivalent frequency compared with the HIV-seronegative Hodgkin disease, but survival is limited by the other complications of HIV disease. Hodgkin disease has not been included as a criterion for the diagnosis of AIDS in an HIV-infected individual.

The most common histologic types of lymphoma in AIDS are SNCC (36%) and immunoblastic (32%) (Table 86-4), both considered high-grade lymphomas by the Working Formulation.[136] The expected frequency of these histologies in NHL outside the setting of immunodeficiency is only 10–15%.[37] Large cell histology, categorized as intermediate grade (although often clinically very aggressive), accounts for approximately 22% of AIDS lymphomas. Low-grade B-cell malignancies are a distinct minority in AIDS and it is not clear whether they are increased in frequency or have a different clinical behavior as compared with these disorders in the population at large.

Typical of high-grade B-cell malignancies, AIDS lymphomas often involve sites outside the confines of the lymph node (Table 86-5). Extranodal disease has been estimated to occur in ≤95% of patients with AIDS lymphoma and is often the site of diagnosis.[37,45,130,135–149] Exclusively extranodal disease has been reported in ≤56% of patients.[149] Approximately 15–20% of patients will present with disease restricted to the central nervous system. Patients with primary central nervous system lymphoma constitute a relatively unique subset of AIDS lymphoma patients and are discussed separately below.

The extent of involvement at the time of diagnosis is often stage II–IV (Ann Arbor classification) (Table 86-4). Although approximately 15–25% of patients will present with stage I or II disease, these patients often have extranodal disease and will generally relapse at remote sites if treated with local therapy alone. Sites of involvement vary somewhat with the histologic subtype. For example, immunoblastic B-cell tumors often involve the gastrointestinal tract and are the rule for mass le-

Table 86-5. NHL in Immunosuppression

	Organ Transplantation (%)	AIDS (%)
EBV genome	~100	38–68
SNCC histology	~1	36
myc translocation	No	23–79
Polyclonal phase	Yes	?

Table 86-6. AIDS Lymphoma: Clinical Subtypes

	Primary Central Nervous System	Systemic
Mean CD4/mm^3	~50	~180
Prior AIDS	73%	37%
Immunoblastic histology	100%	~30%
EBV genome	100%	38–68%
Median survival	2–5 mo	4–7 mo

(Data from references 31–33.)

sions in brain parenchyma. SNCC tumors are the histology most commonly involving the bone marrow.[37,149] The most common extranodal sites of involvement are the bone marrow (25%), central nervous system (23%), gastrointestinal tract (22%), and liver.[37,45,135–149] However, virtually any anatomic site may be involved in AIDS lymphoma. Clinicians caring for AIDS patients need to maintain a high level of suspicion for lymphoma with unusual presentations.

Many of the features of AIDS lymphomas are similar to those of comparable histology tumors in settings outside that of HIV infection. However, one study has indicated that specific features may distinguish the HIV-seropositive from HIV-negative high-grade lymphomas.[37,151] By molecular analysis, EBV is much more common in AIDS (33–67% versus 5%) as is c-*myc* rearrangement (23–79% versus 14%). HIV-positive and HIV-negative high-grade NHL both have a high frequency of extranodal disease, but there may be more frequent involvement of the central nervous system in AIDS and unusual sites of disease such as oral mucosa and rectum.[37] "B" symptoms such as night sweats, fevers, and weight loss may also be somewhat more prominent in the HIV-infected population.[37]

Some aspects of AIDS lymphomas resemble the lymphomas of other immunodeficiencies, but they can clearly not be equated (Table 86-5). The lymphomas of organ transplant, for example, lack the SNCC histology lymphoma that accounts for approximately 36% of AIDS lymphomas. In addition, the polyclonal lymphoproliferative tumors that occur in the setting of the organ transplant patient have been reported, but appear to be less common in patients with AIDS lymphoma.[31,36] Unlike the situation of the polyclonal tumors after organ transplantation, the same investigators have found no detectable EBV genome in a majority of the AIDS polyclonal lymphomas. The bases for these striking differences between AIDS-associated and other immunodeficiency lymphomas are unknown and suggest fundamental differences in pathophysiology.

PRIMARY CENTRAL NERVOUS SYSTEM LYMPHOMA

Where AIDS lymphomas and lymphomas associated with other immunodeficiency states overlap is in the high incidence of primary central nervous system lymphoma.[150] Lymphoma that presents as parenchymal mass lesions in the brain without systemic disease accounts for approximately 15–20% of all AIDS lymphomas. The epidemiology of primary central nervous system AIDS lymphoma is different from that of systemic AIDS lymphoma in that it tends to occur in the setting of more advanced immunosuppression. One study comparing primary central nervous system lymphoma with systemic lymphoma in AIDS found average CD4 cell counts of 30/mm^3 and 188/mm^3, respectively.[32] Other features that characterize the primary central nervous system AIDS lymphomas are the high frequency of large cell or immunoblastic histology and the virtual uniformity of detectable EBV gene expression[31,33] (Table 86-6).

In evaluating a patient with a central nervous system mass lesion and HIV disease, lymphoma must be considered along with abscess (toxoplasma or other infection) or progressive multifocal leukoencephalopathy (PML).[152–154] Among these,

toxoplasmosis is often the most difficult to distinguish from lymphoma by radiographic criteria.[153] Several radiologic characteristics have been reported to occur more often in AIDS lymphoma than in toxoplasma brain abscess, including large size (>2 mm), central location, lack of multifocality,[139,155] and, perhaps most definitive, central nervous system lymphoma, but not toxoplasmosis, may cross the midline. Definitive diagnosis requires a brain biopsy. However, many clinicians now obtain serologic samples for toxoplasma antibody and cryptococcal antigen; blood cultures for bacteria, fungus, and mycobacteria; and employ a therapeutic trial of 7–14 days of antitoxoplasma therapy (sulfadiazine or clindamycin and pyrimethamine). Oral antitoxoplasma therapy has been documented to induce a response in 65% of patients with toxoplasma encephalitis by day 14.[156] For patients who worsen after day 5 or fail to improve after 14 days, biopsy is recommended. Symptoms that may herald the occurrence of central nervous system lymphoma may be very vague (including personality changes) and a high level of suspicion should be maintained in patients with severely depressed CD4$^+$ cell counts.[139,155,157]

Treatment of primary central nervous system lymphoma in AIDS has generally been restricted to radiotherapy and steroids, although efforts to evaluate the role of systemic chemotherapy are ongoing. Responses to radiotherapy occur with high frequency (60–79%), but no randomized trials have been performed to evaluate whether there is a beneficial effect on survival.[158,159] The advanced stage of immunosuppression in these patients often limits their prognosis, which is estimated as 2–5 months. With improved therapies for the infectious complications of AIDS, some investigators have advocated testing more aggressive NHL treatment regimens and, where feasible, enrollment of patients in clinical trials is strongly encouraged. Defining better treatment strategies is clearly necessary in this devastating complication of AIDS. If no trial is available, the approach at our center is based on the underlying health status of the patient and active involvement of patient and family in the decision-making process. Patients with prior AIDS complications that significantly compromise their quality of life often prefer steroids alone or pain medications only.

SYSTEMIC LYMPHOMA

Staging

Staging evaluation of patients with systemic NHL should proceed along the usual grounds for evaluation of any patient with NHL. There are several considerations that require special attention, however. The first is the possibility of coincident infectious complications that may account for symptoms otherwise possibly attributable to tumor. Extensive microbiologic evaluation should be performed in any patient with fever or night sweats, but particularly in those with a CD4$^+$ count of <200 cells/mm^3 or a prior history of AIDS. Evaluation should include bacterial, fungal, and mycobacterial cultures; serologic tests for cryptococcus and toxoplasma; and evaluation for cytomegalovirus infection. Consideration should also be given to possible *Pneumocystis carinii* infection.

Special attention to the central nervous system should be included in the pretreatment evaluation of a patient with AIDS lymphoma because of the high frequency of involvement and the implications for therapy. There may be meningeal involvement without parenchymal mass lesions in patients with concurrent systemic lymphoma and, therefore, an imaging study and sampling of the cerebrospinal fluid are typically performed at our institution. At present, the sensitivity of detecting occult central nervous system lymphoma by cerebrospinal fluid analysis is poor; however, using markers for EBV has been suggested as a possible future tool in assessing these patients.[160]

Therapy

A number of different chemotherapeutic regimens have been tested in AIDS lymphomas, but to date no large-scale phase III comparative trials have been reported and no consensus has emerged.[137,140,142,144–148,161–163] In evaluating the efficacy of these regimens, it is important to keep in mind the progress that has been made in the care of AIDS patients and the contribution to outlook that is a consequence of better treatment and prevention of opportunistic infections. For example, early trials evaluating standard or intensive dose chemotherapy regimens were complicated by high rates of treatment-related morbidity and death. These trials set in motion efforts in the United States to find less toxic chemotherapy regimens. The result has been the development of the "modified" M-BACOD regimen[137] and a recently described oral chemotherapy regimen[146] (Table 86-7). However, other investigators (particularly in Europe) have continued to be concerned with the high-grade nature of the tumor and have pursued aggressive chemotherapy protocols such as LNH-84.[164]

Several general conclusions may be drawn from the therapeutic trials to date. The first is that most patients have chemosensitive tumors: responses have been recorded in ≤76%[164] and complete responses in ≤67%.[145] These data are similar to non-AIDS patients with aggressive lymphomas. The second is that responders do appear to achieve a survival benefit from the therapy with mean survivals of 6–20 months in patients with a complete response compared with 4–7 months for patients without a complete response.[137,142,145,146,164] Although this appears to support a self-evident maxim that patients who do better, do better, the underlying life-threatening HIV disease in these patients previously caused many to question the value of treating AIDS malignancies. The data do support the value of using antilymphoma therapy with curative intent at least in a subgroup of AIDS patients. Finally, there is a consensus that patients with advanced HIV disease do poorly. At present, there are no trials that have defined specific therapies for specific stages of HIV disease. However, such trials are anticipated and it is our practice to use palliative intent in selecting a treatment for patients with poor performance status prior to the NHL diagnosis or those with ongoing opportunistic infections.

Issues not systematically studied in clinical trials, but where a consensus has emerged, include the use of prophylaxis against *P. carinii* pneumonia regardless of the entry CD4$^+$ T-cell count. For patients who do not have lymphoma, this practice is generally reserved for those with CD4 counts of <200 cells/mm^3. Patients undergoing NHL therapy will have alterations in T-cell numbers and probably T-cell dysfunction due to drug treatment. Which specific PCP prophylaxis is optimal in this setting has not been defined. Also, patients with HIV appear to have unusual sensitivity to the myelotoxic effects of drugs and respond to the hematopoietic growth factors often used to mitigate cytopenia.[145,165–170] Only one randomized trial evaluating the effects of a growth factor (colony-stimulating factor-granulocyte/macrophage [CSF-GM]) in AIDS lymphoma has been reported to date.[145] Kaplan and colleagues[145] documented a significant benefit for those AIDS lymphoma patients randomized to receive CSF-GM with their CHOP chemotherapy as quantitated by days of neutropenia, fever and neutropenia, and adequacy of chemotherapy drug delivery.

More controversy revolves around the use of prophylactic intrathecal antitumor therapy. No randomized trial has been conducted. However, central nervous system relapse has been documented in ≤67% (8 of 12) of patients treated with systemic chemotherapy without intrathecal prophylaxis.[140] A subsequent study by the same investigators using intrathecal cytosine arabinoside (ara-C) in combination with systemic chemotherapy observed no central nervous system relapses in 35 patients.[137] Currently, it is the practice in chemotherapy trials sponsored by the AIDS Clinical Trials Group (ACTG) of the U.S. National Institute of Allergy and Infectious Diseases to include prophylactic central nervous system treatment. At our center we typically include four weekly doses of intrathecally administered ara-C (50 mg) when initiating chemotherapy for patients with systemic AIDS lymphoma.

Also controversial is the concurrent use of specific antiretroviral drugs in conjunction with chemotherapy. It is often impossible to continue zidovudine (AZT) during chemotherapy due to the myelosuppressive effects of AZT. Recent data suggest that it may be possible to give nonmyelosuppressive antiretroviral drugs such as dideoxycytidine (ddC) in conjunction with chemotherapy.[171] ddC is associated with neuropathy and pancreatitis, but no increase in those toxicities associated with concurrent chemotherapy has been shown to date. However, whether antiretroviral therapy provides additional clinical benefit remains unknown. Indirect data suggest that chemotherapy itself may provide antiviral effects.[145] This issue will require a randomized trial to be adequately addressed.

Finally, it remains unclear which chemotherapy regimen provides the optimal outcome for patients with AIDS lymphoma. The encouraging results of the preliminary trial using modified (approximately 60% dose) M-BACOD suggest that less chemotherapy may be given without sacrificing response rates.[137] This trial has provided the rationale for comparing the lower dose with standard dose M-BACOD (plus hematopoietic growth factor) in a randomized, multicentered trial under the auspices of the ACTG. This trial is approaching completion. Interpretation of its results will be complicated by the recent Southwest Oncology Group (SWOG) data comparing chemotherapy regimens in the non-HIV-infected population with NHL that demonstrated the superiority of CHOP.[172] If reduced dose M-BACOD appears equivalent in response rate, response durability, and survival to standard dose M-BACOD, the issue of modified dose CHOP will certainly be raised. At present, there do not appear to be significant clinical differences in the responses to treatment of the AIDS lymphomas compared with NHL in the non-AIDS population to suggest that different treatment principles apply. Although intensive chemotherapy protocols appear to

Table 86-7. Commonly Used Therapy Regimens for Systemic AIDS Lymphoma

CHOP	Cyclophosphamide	750 mg/m^2 (each cycle 21–28 days)
	Doxorubicin	50 mg/m^2
	Vincristine	1.4 mg/m^2
	Prednisone	100 mg × 5 days
Modified M-BACOD	Bleomycin	4 U/m^2 day 1 (each cycle 21–28 days)
	Cyclophosphamide	300 mg/m^2 day 1
	Doxorubicin	25 mg/m^2 day 1
	Vincristine	1.4 mg/m^2 day 1
	Dexamethasone	3 mg/m^2 days 1–5
	Methotrexate	200 mg/m^2 day 15 (with leukovorin rescue)
M-BACOD	Bleomycin	4 U/m^2 day 1 (each cycle 21–28 days)
	Cyclophosphamide	600 mg/m^2 day 1
	Doxorubicin	45 mg/m^2 day 1
	Vincristine	1 mg/m^2 day 1
	Dexamethasone	6 mg/m^2 days 1–5
	Methotrexate	200 mg/m^2 day 8, 15 (with leukovorin rescue)
"ORAL"	CCNU	100 mg/m^2 day 1 (cycles 1, 3, 5; each cycle 6 wk)
	Etoposide	200 mg/m^2 days 1–3
	Cyclophosphamide	100 mg/m^2 days 22–31
	Procarbazine	100 mg/m^2 days 22–31

now be more manageable in AIDS patients (likely due to better care and prevention of infections),[164] rationale for their use has been challenged by the SWOG data.

Prognosis

Prognostic factors have been evaluated in a number of studies.[32,135,140,143,144,164,173,174] By far the most significant issue in the long-term outlook for these patients is the status of their immune system. If patients have depressed CD4 counts (<100 cells/mm^3), a prior AIDS-defining illness, or a poor performance status the overall outlook is poor. Both the ability to tolerate therapy and the rate of opportunistic infections limit the prognosis for these patients. Other prognostic factors that are specific for the lymphoma have not been uniformly associated with outcome in all series. In particular, some studies have found bone marrow involvement,[32] immunoblastic histology,[164] tumor stage,[32,146] or EBV-negative tumors[174] to be significant negative indicators of prognosis; lactate dehydrogenase or tumor bulk has not correlated with outcome. Future studies will be needed to more clearly define whether the recently described criteria for determining high risk among patients with high-grade lymphomas will be applicable to AIDS patients.[175]

Overall median survival estimates for patients with AIDS lymphoma are 4–7 months.[32,45,135,141,143,144,145,164] However, mean survival times of 11.5–24 months have been reported for patients without high-risk factors.[32,164]

FUTURE DIRECTIONS

The ability to treat AIDS patients safely with multiagent chemotherapy and provide benefit to a responding subset has been one of the successes in AIDS oncology. However, the fraction of treatment refractory lymphomas (approximately one-third) and the number of patients that relapse (≤50% in some series) remains dauntingly high.[45,129,135,141–143] Because dose intensified chemotherapy schemas have been complicated in AIDS and do not appear to improve outcomes in the non-AIDS population, other approaches are in the process of development. Specifically, studies piloting the use of monoclonal antibody based therapeutics or novel chemotherapeutics are under way.[176] Immunologic manipulation is a direction of ongoing research that is supported by the possibility of cytotoxic T-cell therapies in humans.[177] These efforts may have a particularly appealing rationale in the setting of the EBV-positive AIDS tumors because of the foreign antigens they present.[29,84,178,179] Rare cases of spontaneous regression of NHL in AIDS are suggestive of an immunoresponsive tumor.[180] The current lack of an adequate salvage therapy for this disease argues for the further pursuit of these efforts. The use of bone marrow transplantation outside the setting of HIV has encouraged efforts to attempt this in AIDS lymphoma. However, the clinical data have suggested very poor outcomes, probably due to the added immunodeficiency implicit in the transplant process.

In addition to controversial treatment issues, a number of pathophysiologic questions that may be important in the adequate treatment of this disease remain outstanding. For example, the frequency of SNCC (Burkitt-like) histology is unique to the HIV immunosuppressed patient among immunosuppressed individuals. Does this point to a novel mechanism of disease or perhaps a novel infectious cofactor?[181,182] With other lymphomas reportedly responding to anti-infective therapy (e.g., mucosal-associated lymphoid tissue lymphomas improving with anti-*Helicobacter* therapy),[183] is a therapeutic opportunity possible with better understanding of potential infectious factors in AIDS? How critical a role does EBV play in AIDS lymphoma and would better control of this virus prevent the development of lymphoma? Is immune response to the malignant cells impaired by cytokines or cytokine-like viral products and can that cytokine milieu be altered for therapeutic advantage? Is manipulating the immune system with biologic response modifiers a possible potent supplement to chemotherapy? Many issues remain unresolved and many potential benefits to the non-HIV-infected population stand to be gained by understanding better the interplay of the HIV-impaired immune system and the development of lymphoma.

REFERENCES

1. Hoover RN: Lymphoma risks in populations with altered immunity—a search for mechanism. Cancer, suppl. 52:5477, 1992
2. Waldmann TA, Misiti J, Nelson DL, et al: Ataxia-telangiectasia: a multisystem hereditary disease with immunodeficiency, impaired organ maturation, x-ray hypersensitivity, and a high incidence of neoplasia. Ann Intern Med 99: 367, 1983
3. Penn I: Tumors arising in organ transplant recipients. Adv Cancer Res 28: 31, 1978
4. Cotelingam JD, Witebsky FG, Hsu SM et al: Malignant lymphoma in patients with Wiskott-Aldrich syndrome. Cancer Invest 3:515, 1985
5. Purtilo DT: Immune deficiency predisposing to Epstein-Barr virus-induced lymphoproliferative diseases. The X-linked lymphoproliferative syndrome as a model. Adv Cancer Res 34:279, 1981
6. Frizzera G, Rosai F, Dehner LP et al: Lymphoreticular disorders in primary immunodeficiency: new findings based on an updated histologic classification of 35 cases. Cancer 46:692, 1980
7. Grierson H, Purtilo DT: Epstein Barr virus infections in males with the x-linked lymphoproliferative syndrome. Ann Intern Med 106:538, 1987
8. Zulman J, Jaffe R, Talal N: Evidence that the malignant lymphoma of Sjögren's syndrome is a monoclonal B cell neoplasm. N Engl J Med 299:1215, 1978
9. Swinnen LJ, Costanzo-Nordin MR, Fisher SG et al: Increased incidence of lymphoproliferative disorders after immunosuppression with the monoclonal antibody OKT3 in cardiac transplant recipients. N Engl J Med 323: 1723, 1990
10. Lenoir GM, Delecluse H-J: Lymphoma and immunocompromised hosts. p. 173. In Revillard JP, Wierzbicki N (ed): Immune disorders and opportunistic infections. Foundation Franco-Allemande, Suresnes, 1989
11. Gail MH, Pluda JM, Rabkin CS et al: Projections of the incidence of non-Hodgkin's lymphoma related to acquired immunodeficiency syndrome. J Natl Cancer Inst 83:695, 1991
12. Beral V, Peterman T, Berkelman R et al: AIDS-associated non-Hodgkin's lymphoma. Lancet 337:805, 1991
13. Biggar RJ, Rabbin CS: The epidemiology of acquired immunodeficiency-related lymphomas. Curr Opin Oncol 4:883, 1992
14. Italian Cooperative Group for AIDS-Related Tumors: Malignant lymphomas in patients with or at risk for AIDS in Italy. J Natl Cancer Inst 80:855, 1988
15. Monfardini S, Vaccher E, Foa R, et al: for the Italian Cooperative Group on AIDS-related Tumors (GICAT): AIDS associated non-Hodgkin's lymphoma in Italy: intravenous drug users versus homosexual men. Ann Oncol 1:208, 1990
16. Reynolds P, Saunders LD, Layefsky ME, Lemp GF: The spectrum of acquired immunodeficiency syndrome (AIDS)-associated malignancies in San Francisco, 1980–1987. Am J Epidemiol 137:19, 1993
17. Arico et al: Malignancies in children with HIV type 1 infection. Cancer 68: 2473, 1991
18. Epstein LG, DiCarlo FJ Jr, Joshi VV et al: Primary lymphoma of the CNS in children with AIDS. Pediatrics 82:355, 1988
19. Israel P: Cancers complication organ transplantation. N Engl J Med 323: 1767, 1990
20. Nalesnik MA, Makowka L, Starzl TE: The diagnosis and treatment of post-transplant lymphoproliferative disorders. Curr Prob Surg 25:367, 1988
21. Hoover R, Fraumeni JF Jr: Risk of cancer in renal transplant recipients. Lancet 2:55, 1973
22. Shapiro RS, McClain K, Frizzera G et al: Epstein-Barr virus associated B cell lymphoproliferative disorders following bone marrow transplantation. Blood 71:1234, 1988
23. Witherspoon RP, Fisher LD, Schoch G et al: Secondary cancers after bone marrow transplant for leukemia or aplastic anemia. N Engl J Med 321:784, 1989
24. Hanto DW, Frizzera G, Gajl-Peczalska KJ et al: Epstein-Barr virus-induced B-cell lymphoma after renal transplantation: acyclovir therapy and transition from polyclonal to monoclonal B-cell proliferation. N Engl J Med 306:913, 1982

25. Hochberg FH, Miller G, Schooley RT et al: Central-nervous-system lymphoma related to Epstein-Barr virus. N Engl J Med 309:745, 1983

26. Shearer WT, Ritz J, Finegold MJ et al: Epstein-Barr virus associated B-cell proliferations of diverse clonal origins after bone marrow transplantation in a 12-year-old patient with severe combined immunodeficiency. N Engl J Med 312:1151, 1985

27. Starzl TE, Nalesnik MA, Porter KA et al: Reversibility of lymphomas and lymphoproliferative lesions developing under cyclosporin-steroid therapy. Lancet 1:583, 1984

28. Straus SE, Clhen JI, Tosato G, Meier J: Epstein-Barr virus infections: biology, pathogenesis, and management. Ann Intern Med 118:45, 1993

29. Rowe M, Young LS, Crocker J et al: Epstein-Barr virus (EBV)-associated lymphoproliferative disease in the SCID mouse model: implications for the pathogenesis of EBV-positive lymphomas in man. J Exp Med 173:147, 1991

30. Subar M, Neri A, Inghirami G et al: Frequent *c-myc* oncogene activation and infrequent presence of Epstein-Barr virus genome in AIDS-associated-lymphoma. Blood 72:667, 1988

31. Meeker TC, Shiramizu B, Kaplan L et al: Evidence for molecular subtypes of HIV-associated lymphoma: division into peripheral monoclonal, polyclonal and central nervous system lymphoma. AIDS 5:669, 1991

32. Levine AM, Sullivan-Halley J, Pike MC et al: HIV-related lymphoma: prognostic factors predictive of survival. Cancer 68:2466, 1991

33. MacMahon EME, Glass JD, Hayward SD et al: Epstein Barr virus in AIDS-related primary central nervous system lymphoma. Lancet 338:969, 1991

34. Hamilton-Dutoit SJ, Pallesen G, Franzmann MB et al: AIDS-related lymphoma: histopathology, immunophenotype and association with Epstein-Barr virus as demonstrated by in situ nucleic acid hybridisation. Am J Pathol 138:149, 1991

35. Shibata D, Weiss LM, Hernandez AM et al: Epstein-Barr virus-associated non-Hodgkin's lymphoma in patients infected with the human immunodeficiency virus. Blood 81:2102, 1993

36. Shirmizu B, Herndier B, Meeker T et al: Molecular and immunophenotypic characterization of AIDS-associated, Epstein-Barr virus-negative, polyclonal lymphoma. J Clin Oncol 10:383, 1992

37. Levine AM: Acquired immunodeficiency syndrome-related lymphoma. Blood 80:8, 1992

38. Pellicci P-G, Knowls DM, Arlin ZA et al: Multiple monoclonal B-cell expansions and *c-myc* oncogene rearrangements in acquired immune deficiency syndrome-related lymphoproliferative disorders. J Exp Med 164:2049, 1986

39. Ballerini P, Gaidano G, Gong JZ et al: Multiple genetic lesions in acquired immunodeficiency syndrome-related non-Hodgkin's lymphoma. Blood 81:166, 1993

40. Centers for Disease Control: Revision of the CDC sureveillance case definition for acquired immunodeficiency syndrome for national reporting—United States. MMWR 36:1, 1987

41. Harnly ME, Swan SH, Holly EA et al: Temporal trends in the incidence of non-Hodgkin's lymphoma and selected malignancies in a population with a high incidence of acquired immunodeficiency syndrome (AIDS). Am J Epidemiol 128:261, 1988

42. Ioachim HL, Cooper MC, Hellman GC: Lymphomas in men at high risk for acquired immune deficiency syndrome (AIDS). Cancer 56:2831, 1985

43. Levine AM, Gill PS, Meyer PR et al: Retrovirus and malignant lymphoma in homosexual men. JAMA 254:1921, 1985

44. Levine AM, Meyer PR, Bergandy MK et al: Development of B cell lymphoma in homosexual men: clinical and immunologic findings. Ann Intern Med 100:7, 1984

45. Ziegler JL, Beckstead JA, Volberding PA et al: Non-Hodgkin's lymphoma in 90 homosexual men: relation to generalized lymphadenopathy and the acquired immunodeficiency syndrome. N Engl J Med 311:565, 1984

46. Ross R, Dworsky R, Paganini-Hill A et al: Non-Hodgkin's lymphomas in never married men in Los Angeles. Br J Cancer 52:785, 1985

47. Levine AM, Burkes RL, Walker M et al: Development of B cell lymphoma in two monogamous homosexual men. Arch Intern Med 145:479, 1985

48. Kalter SP, Riggs SA, Cabanillas F et al: Aggressive non-Hodgkin's lymphoma in immunocompromised homosexual males. Blood 66:655, 1985

49. Statistics from the Center for Disease Control. AIDS 6:1992

50. Ragni MV, Belle SH, Jaffe RA et al: Acquired immunodeficiency syndrome-associated non-Hodgkin's lymphomas and other malignancies in patients with hemophilia. Blood 81:1889, 1993

51. Rabkin CS, Hilgartner MW, Hedberg KW et al: Incidence of lymphomas and other cancers in HIV-infected and HIV-uninfected patients with hemophilia. JAMA 267:1090, 1992

52. Moore RD, Kessler H, Richman DD et al: Non-Hodgkin's lymphoma in patients with advanced HIV infection treated with zidovudine. JAMA 265:2208, 1991

53. Pluda JM, Venzon DJ, Tosato G et al: Parameters affecting the development of non-Hodgkin's lymphoma in patients with severe human immunodeficiency virus infection receiving antiretroviral therapy. J Clin Oncol 11:1099, 1993

54. Pluda JM, Yarchoan R, Jaffe ES et al: Development on non-Hodgkin's lymphoma in a cohort of patients with severe human immunodeficiency virus (HIV) infection on long-term antiretroviral therapy. Ann Intern Med 113:276, 1990

55. Devesa SS, Fears T: Non-Hodgkin's lymphoma time trends: United States and international data. Cancer 52:5432s, 1992

56. Herndier BG, Chiramizu BT, Jewett NE et al: Acquired immunodeficiency syndrome-associated T-cell lymphoma: evidence for human immunodeficiency virus type 1-associated T-cell transformation. Blood 79:1768, 1992

57. Broder S: Factors in the development of AIDS-related lymphomas. Leukemia 3:6S, 1992

58. Ioachim HL: Lymphoma: an opportunistic neoplasia of AIDS. Leukemia 3:30S, 1992

59. Schafer A, Friedman W, Mielke M et al: The increased frequency of cervical dysplasia: neoplasia in women infected with HIV is related to degree of immunosuppression. Am J Obstet Gynecol 164:593, 1991

60. Schrager LK, Friedland GH, Maude D et al: Cervical and vaginal squamous cell abnormalities in women infected with HIV. J AIDS 2:570, 1989

61. Vermund SH, Kelley KF, Klein RS et al: High risk of human papillomavirus infection and cervical squamous intraepithelial lesions among women with symptomatic HIV infection. Am J Obstet Gynecol 165:392, 1991

62. Laga M, Icenogle JP, Marsella R et al: Genital papillomavirus infection and cervical dysplasia: opportunistic complications of HIV infection. Int J Cancer 50:45, 1992

63. Feingold AR, Vermund SH, Burk RD et al: Cervical cytologic abnormalities and papillomavirus in women infected with HIV. J AIDS 3:896, 1990

64. Maiman M, Fruchter RG, Serur E et al: HIV infection and cervical neoplasia. Gynecol Oncol 38:377, 1990

65. Palefsky JM, Gonzales J, Greenblatt RM et al: Anal intraepithelial neoplasia and anal papillomavirus infection among homosexual males with group IV HIV disease. JAMA 263:2911, 1990

66. Kiviat N, Rompalo A. Bowden R et al: Anal human papilloma-virus infection among human immunodeficiency virus-seropositive and -seronegative men. J Infect Dis 162:358, 1990

67. Beral V, Bull D, Darby S et al: Risk of Kaposi's sarcoma and sexual practices associated with faecal contact in homosexual or bisexual men with AIDS. Lancet 339:632, 1992

68. Knowles DM, Inghirami G, Ubriaco A et al: Molecular genetic analysis of three AIDS-associated neoplasms of uncertain lineage demonstrates their B-cell derivation and the possible pathogenetic role of the Epstein-Barr virus. Blood 73:792, 1989

69. Shibata D, Weiss LM, Nathwani BN et al: Epstein Barr virus in benign lymph node biopsies from individuals infected with the human immunodeficiency virus is associated with concurrent or subsequent development of non-Hodgkin's lymphoma. Blood 77:1527, 1991

70. Neri A, Barriga F, Inghirami G et al: Epstein-Barr virus infection precedes clonal expansion in Burkitt's and acquired immunodeficiency syndrome-associated lymphomas. Blood 77:1092, 1991

71. Hamilton-Dutoit S, Pallesen G, Karkov J et al: Identification of EBV-DNA in tumor cells of AIDS-related lymphomas by in situ hybridization. Lancet 1:554, 1989

72. Thomas JA, Cotter F, Hanby AM et al: Epstein-Barr virus-related oral T-cell lymphoma associated with human immunodeficiency virus immunosuppression. Blood 81:3350, 1993

73. Carbone A, Tirelli U, Vaccher E et al: A clinicopathologic study of lymphoid neoplasms associated with human immunodeficiency virus infection in Italy. Cancer 68:842, 1991

74. Haluska F, Russo G, Kant J et al: Molecular resemblance of an AIDS-associated lymphoma and endemic Burkitt lymphomas: implications for their pathogenesis. Proc Natl Acad Sci 86:8907, 1989

75. Borisch-Chappuis B, Nezelof C, Muller H, Muller Hermeling HK: Different Epstein-Barr virus expression in lymphomas from immunocompromised and immunocompetent patients. Am J Pathol 136:751, 1990

76. Young LS, Alfieri C, Hennessy K et al: Expression of Epstein-Barr virus transformation-associated genes in tissues of patients with EBV lymphoproliferative disease. N Engl J Med 321:1080, 1989

77. Thomas JA, Hotchin NA, Allday MJ et al: Immunohistology of Epstein-Barr virus-associated antigens in B cell disorders from immunocompromised individuals. Transplantation 49:944, 1990

78. Kieff E, and Liebowitz D: Epstein-Barr virus and its replication. p. 1889. In Fields B, Knipe D (eds): Virology. Raven Press. New York, 1990

79. Sample J, Brooks L, Sample C et al: Restricted Epstein-Barr virus protein

expression in Burkitt lymphoma is due to a deferent Epstein-Barr nuclear antigen 1 transductional initiation site. Proc Natl Acad Sci USA 88:6343, 1991

80. Rowe M, Rowe DT, Gregory CD et al: Differences in B-cell growth phenotype reflect novel patterns of Epstein-Barr virus latent gene expression in Burkitt's lymphoma cells. EMBO J 6:2743, 1987

81. Gregory CD, Dive C, Henderson S et al: Activation of Epstein-Barr virus latent genes protects human B cells from death by apoptosis. Nature 349:612, 1991

82. Klein G: Viral latecy and transformation: the strategy of Epstein-Barr virus. Cell 58:5, 1989

83. Burkhardt AL, Bolen JB, Kieff E, Longnecker R: An Epstein-Barr virus transformation-associated membrane protein interacts with *src* family tyrosine kinases. J Virol 66:5161, 1992

84. List AF, Spier CM, Miller TP, Grogan TM: Deficient tumor-infiltrating T-lymphocyte response in malignant lymphoma: relationship to HLA expression and host immunocompetence. Leukemia 7:398, 1993

85. Hsu D-H, Malefyt RD, Fiorentino DF et al: Expression of interleukin-10 activity by Epstein-Barr virus protein BCRF1. Science 250:830, 1990

86. Moore KW, Vieira P, Fiorentino DF et al: Homology of cytokine synthesis inhibitory factor (IL-10) to the Epstein-Barr virus gene BCRF1. Science 248:1230, 1990

87. Howard M, O'Garra A: Biological properties of interleukin 10. Immunol Today 13:198, 1992

88. Moore KW, O'Garra A, Dewaal Malefyt R et al: Interleukin-10. Ann Rev Immun 11:165, 1993

89. Benjamin D, Knobloch J, Dayton MA: Human B-cell interleukin-10: B-cell lines derived from patients with acquired immunodeficiency syndrome and Burkitt's lymphoma constitutively secrete large quantities of interleukin-10. Blood 80:1289, 1992

90. Pantaleo G, Graziosi C, Fauci AS: The immunopathogenesis of human immunodeficiency virus infection. N Engl J Med 328:327, 1993

91. Fauci AS: Immunopathogenic mechanisms in human immunodeficiency virus (HIV) infection. Ann Intern Med 114:678, 1991

92. Amadori A, Chieco-Bianchi L: B-cell activation and HIV-1 infection: deeds and misdeeds. Immunol Today 11:374, 1990

93. Breen EC, Rezai AR, Nakajima K et al: Infection with HIV is associated with elevated IL-6 during human immunodeficiency virus infection. J Immunol 144:480, 1990

94. Boue F, Wallon C, Goujard C et al: HIV induces IL-6 production by human B lymphocytes. J Immunol 148:3761, 1992

95. Emilie D, Coumbaras J, Raphael M et al: Interleukin-6 production in high-grade B lymphomas: correlation with the presence of malignant immunoblasts in acquired immunodeficiency syndrome and in human immunodeficiency virus-seronegative patients. Blood 80:498, 1992

96. Lane HC, Masur H, Edgar KC et al: Abnormalities of B-cell activation and immunoregulation in patients with the acquired immunodeficiency syndrome. N Engl J Med 309:453, 1983

97. Yarchoan R, Redfield RR, Broder S: Mechanisms of B cell activation in patients with acquired immunodeficiency syndrome and related disorders. Contribution of antibody producing B cells, or Epstein-Barr infected B cells, and of immunoglobulin production induced by human T cell lymphotropic virus, type III/lymphadenopathy associated virus. J Clin Invest 78:439, 1986

98. Chirmule N, Kalyanaraman VS, Saxinger C et al: Localization of B-cell stimulatory activity of HIV-1 to the carboxyl terminus of gp41. AIDS Res Hum Retroviruses 6:299, 1990

99. Rieckmann P, Poli G, Fox CH et al: Recombinant $_{gp}$120 specifically enhances tumor necrosis factor-alpha production and Ig secretion in B lymphocytes from HIV-infected individuals but not from seronegative donors. J Immunol 147:2922, 1991

100. Sala PG, Mazzolini S, Tonutti E, Bramezza M: Monoclonal immunoglobulins in HTLV-III-positive sera. Clin Chem 32:574, 1986

101. Papadopoulos NM, Lane HC, Costello HC et al: Oligoclonal immunoglobulins in patient with the acquired immunodeficiency syndrome. Clin Immunol Immunopathol 35:43, 1985

102. Crapper RM, Deam DR, Mackay IR: Paraproteins in homosexual men with HIV infection: lack of association with abnormal clinical or immunologic findings. Am J Clin Pathol 88:348, 1987

103. Heriot K, Harrquist AE, Tomar RH: Paraproteinemia in patients with acquired immunodeficiency syndrome (AIDS) or lymphadenopathy syndrome (LAS). Clin Chem 31:1224, 1985

104. Ng VL, Hwang KM, Reyes GR et al: High titer anti-HIV antibody reactivity associated with a paraprotein spike in a homosexual male with AIDS related complex. Blood 71:1397, 1988

105. Shirai A, Cosentino M, Leitman-Klinman SF, Klinman DM: Human immunodeficiency virus infection induces both polyclonal and virus-specific B cell activation. B Cell Act Hum Immun Virus 89:561, 1992

106. Vandermolen LA, Fehir KM, Rice L: Multiple myeloma in a homosexual man with chronic lymphadenopathy. Arch Intern Med 145:745, 1985

107. Konrad RJ, Kricka LJ, Goodman DB et al: Brief report: myeloma-associated paraprotein directed against the HIV-1 p24 antigen in an HIV-1-seropositive patient. N Engl J Med 328:1817, 1993

108. Freedman AR, Scadden DT: Viral activity in early HIV disease. Curr Opin Hematol 16:19, 1994

109. Groopman JE, Sullivan JL, Mulder C et al: Pathogenesis of B cell lymphoma in a patient with AIDS. Blood 67:612, 1986

110. Roncella S, Dicelle PF, Cutrona G et al: Cytogenetic rearrangement of c-myc oncogene occurs prior to infection with Epstein-Barr virus in the monoclonal malignant B cells from an AIDS patient. Leukem Lymphoma 9:157, 1993

111. Karp JE, Broder S: The pathogenesis of AIDS lymphomas: a foundation for addressing the challenges of therapy and prevention. Leukem Lymphoma 8:167, 1992

112. Chaganti RSK, Jhanwar SC, Koziner B et al: Specific translocations characterize Burkitt's like lymphoma of homosexual men with the acquired immunodeficiency syndrome. Blood 61:1269, 1983

113. Peterson JM, Tubbs RR, Savage RA et al: Small noncleaved B cell Burkitt-like lymphoma with chromosome t(8;14) translocation and Epstein Barr virus nuclear associated antigen in a homosexual man with acquired immunodeficiency syndrome. Am J Med 78:141, 1985

114. Pellici P-G, Knowles DM, Magrath I, Dalla-Favera: Chromosomal breakpoints and structural alterations of the *c-myc* locus differ in endemic and sporadic forms of Burkitt's lymphoma. Proc Natl Acad Sci USA 83:2984, 1986

115. Neri A, Barriga F, Knowles DM et al: Different regions of the immunoglobulin heavy chain locus are involved in chromosomal translocations indistinct pathogenetic forms of Burkitt's lymphoma. Proc Natl Acad Sci USA 85:2748, 1988

116. Haluska FG, Russo G, Kant J et al: Molecular resemblance of an AIDS-associated lymphoma and endemic Burkitt lymphomas: implications for their pathogenesis. Proc Natl Acad Sci USA 86:8907, 1989

117. Nakamura H, Said JW, Miller CW, Koeffler HP: Mutation and protein expression of p53 in acquired immunodeficiency syndrome-related lymphomas. Blood 82:920, 1993

118. Goldstein J, Becker N, Delrowe J, Davis L: Cutaneous T cell lymphoma in a patient infected with HIV, type 1. Cancer 66:1130, 1990

119. Crane GA, Variakojis D, Rosen ST et al: Cutaneous T cell lymphoma in patients with human immunodeficiency virus infection. Arch Dermatol 127:989, 1991

120. Ruff P, Bagg A, Papadopoulos K: Precursor T cell lymphoma associated with human immunodeficiency virus (HIV) type 1: first reported case. Cancer 64:39, 1989

121. Presant CA, Gala K, Wiseman C et al: Human immunodeficiency virus associated T cell lymphoblastic lymphoma in AIDS. Cancer 60:1459, 1987

122. Shibata D, Brynes R, Rabinowitz A et al: HTLV-1 associated adult T cell leukemia lymphoma in a patient infected with HIV-1. Ann Intern Med 111:871, 1989

123. Sternlieb J, Mintzer D, Kwa D, Gluckman S: Peripheral T cell lymphoma in a patient with the acquired immunodeficiency syndrome. Am J Med 85:445, 1988

124. Gonzalez-Clemente JM, Ribera JM, Campo E et al: Ki-1 positive anaplastic large cell lymphoma of T-cell origin in an HIV infected patient. AIDS 5:751, 1991

125. Ciobanu N, Andreef M, Safai B et al: Lymphoblastic neoplasia in a homosexual patient with Kaposi's sarcoma. Ann Intern Med 98:151, 1983

126. Gold JE, Ghali V, Gold S et al: Angiocentric immunoproliferative lesion/T-cell non-Hodgkin's lymphoma and the acquired immunodeficiency syndrome: a case report and review of the literature. Cancer 66:2407, 1990

127. Harper ME, Kaplan MH, Marselle BA et al: Concomitant infection with HTLV-I and HTLV-III in a patient with T8 lymphoproliferative disease. N Engl J Med 315:1073, 1986

128. Hessol NA, Katz MH, Liu JY et al: Increased incidence of Hodgkin disease in homosexual men with HIV infection. Ann Intern Med 117:309, 1992

129. Kaplan LD: AIDS-associated lymphomas. Infect Dis Clin North Am 2:525, 1988

130. Ioachim HL, Dorsett B, Cronin W et al: Acquired immunodeficiency syndrome associated lymphomas: clinical pathological, immunologic and viral characteristics of 111 cases. Hum Pathol 22:659, 1991

131. Ames ED, Conjalka MS, Goldberg AF et al: Hodgkin's disease and AIDS. Hematol Oncol Clin North Am 5:343, 1991

132. Schoeppel SL, Hoppe RT, Dorfman RF et al: Hodgkin's disease in homosexual men with generalized lymphadenopathy. Ann Intern Med 102:68, 1985

133. Monfardini S, Tirelli U, Vaccher E et al: Hodgkin's disease in 63 intravenous drug users with human immunodeficiency virus. Ann Oncol, suppl.:201, 1991

134. Tirelli A, Serraino D, Carbone A: Hodgkin disease and AIDS. Ann Intern Med 118:313, 1993

135. Lowenthal DA, Straus DJ, Campbell SW et al: AIDS-related lymphoid neoplasia: the Memorial Hospital experience. Cancer 61:2325, 1988

136. Non-Hodgkin's Lymphoma Pathologic Classification Project: National Cancer Institute sponsored study of classifications of non-Hodgkin's lymphomas: summary and description of a working formulation for clinical usage. Cancer 49:2112, 1982

137. Levine AM, Wernz JC, Kaplan L et al: Low-dose chemotherapy with central nervous system prophylaxis and zidovudine maintenance in AIDS-related lymphoma. A prospective multiinstitutional trial. JAMA 266:84, 1991

138. Kalter SP, Riggs SA, Cabanillas F et al: Aggressive non-Hodgkin's lymphomas in immunocompromised homosexual males. Blood 66:655, 1985

139. Gill PS, Levine AM, Meyer PR et al: Primary central nervous system lymphoma in homosexual men: clinical, immunologic and pathologic features. Am J Med 78:742, 1985

140. Gill PS, Levine AM, Krailo ML et al: AIDS related malignant lymphoma: results of prospective treatment trials. J Clin Oncol 5:1322, 1987

141. Knowles DM, Chamulak GA, Subar M et al: Lymphoid neoplasia associated with the acquired immunodeficiency syndrome (AIDS): the New York University experience. Ann Intern Med 108:744, 1988

142. Bermudez MA, Grant KM, Rodvien R, Mendes F: Non-Hodgkin's lymphoma in a population with or at risk for acquired immunodeficiency syndrome: indications for intensive chemotherapy. Am J Med 86:71, 1989

143. Kaplan LD, Abrams DI, Feigal E et al: AIDS-associated non-Hodgkin's lymphoma in San Francisco. JAMA 261:719, 1989

144. Kaplan MH, Susin M, Pahwa SG et al: Neoplastic complications of HTLV-III infection. Lymphomas and solid tumors. Am J Med 82:389, 1987

145. Kaplan LD, Kahn JO, Crowe S et al: Clinical and virologic effects of recombinant human granulocyte-macrophage colony-stimulating factor in patients receiving chemotherapy for human immunodeficiency virus-associated non-Hodgkin's lymphoma: results of a randomized trial. J Clin Oncol 9:929, 1991

146. Remick SC, McSharry JJ, Wolf BC et al: Novel oral combination chemotherapy in the treatment of intermediate and high-grade AIDS-related non-Hodgkin's lymphoma. J Clin Oncol 1993

147. Freter CD: Acquired immunodeficiency syndrome associated lymphoma. NCI Monographs 10:45, 1990

148. Von Gunten CF, Von Roenn JH: Clinical aspects of human immunodeficiency virus-related lymphoma. Curr Opin Oncol 4:894, 1992

149. Raphael J, Gentihomme O, Tulliez M et al: Histopathologic features of high grade non-Hodgkin's lymphomas in acquired immunodeficiency syndrome. Arch Pathol Lab Med 115:15, 1991

150. Remick SC, Diamond C, Migliozzi JA et al: Primary central nervous system lymphoma in patients with and without the acquired immune deficiency syndrome. A retrospective analysis and review of the literature. Medicine 69:345, 1990

151. Levine AM, Shibata D, Weiss LM et al: Molecular characteristics of intermediate/high (I/H) grade lymphomas (NHL) arising in HIV-positive vs. HIV-negative PTS: preliminary data from a population (POP) based study in the county of Los Angeles. Blood 80:1028, 1992

152. Bishburg E, Eng RHK, Slim J et al: Brain lesions in patients with acquired immunodeficiency syndrome. Arch Intern Med 149:941, 1989

153. Ciricillo SF, Rosenblum ML: Use of CT and MR imaging to distinguish intracranial lesions and to define the need for biopsy in AIDS patients. J Neurosurg 73:720, 1990

154. Goldstein JD, Dickson DW, Moser FG et al: Primary central nervous system lymphoma in acquired immunodeficiency syndrome: A clinical and pathologic study with results of treatment with radiation. Cancer 67:2756, 1991

155. Gill PS, Graham RA, Boswell W et al: A comparison of imaging, clinical and pathologic aspects of space-occupying lesions within the brain in patients with acquired immunodeficiency syndrome. Am J Phys Imaging 1:134, 1986

156. Luft BJ, Hafner R, Korzun AH et al: Toxoplasmic encephalitis in patients with the acquired immunodeficiency syndrome. N Engl J Med 329:995, 1993

157. So YT, Beckstead JH, Davis RL: Primary central nervous system lymphoma in acquired immune deficiency syndrome: a clinical and pathological study. Ann Neurol 20:566, 1986

158. Baumgartner JE, Rachlin JR, Beckstead JH et al: Primary central nervous system lymphomas: natural history and response to radiation therapy in 55 patients with acquired immunodeficiency syndrome. J Neurosurg 73:206, 1990

159. Formenti SC, Gill PS, Lean E et al: Primary central nervous system lymphoma in AIDS: results of radiation therapy. Cancer 63:937, 1989

160. Cinque P, Brytting M, Vago J et al: Epstein-Barr virus DNA in cerebrospinal fluid from patients with AIDS-related primary lymphoma of the central nervous system. Lancet 342:398, 1993

161. Karp JE, Broder S: Acquired immunodeficiency syndrome and non-Hodgkin's lymphomas. Cancer Res 51:4743, 1991

162. Walsh C, Wernz JC, Levine A et al: Phase I trial of m-BACOD and granulocyte macrophage colony stimulating factor in HIV-associated non-Hodgkin's lymphoma. J AIDS 6:265, 1993

163. Taillan B, Garnier G, Ferrari E et al: MACOP-B chemotherapy for the treatment of high-grade lymphomas in patients with HIV-1 infection. Acta Hematol 89:10, 1993

164. Gisselbrecht C, Lepage E, Tirelli U et al: Human immunodeficiency virus-related lymphoma treatment with intensive combination chemotherapy. ASCO Proc 12:1227, 1993

165. Groopman JE, Mitsuyasu RT, Deleo MJ et al: Effect of recombinant human granulocyte-macrophage colony-stimulating factor on myelopoiesis in the acquired immunodeficiency syndrome. N Engl J Med 317:593, 1987

166. Scadden DT, Bering HA, Levine JD et al: Granulocyte-macrophage colony-stimulation factor mitigates the neutropenia of combined interferon alfa and zidovudine treatment of acquired immune deficiency syndrome-associated Kaposi's sarcoma. J Clin Oncol 9:802, 1991

167. Hardy WD: Combined ganciclovir and recombinant granulocyte-macrophage colony-stimulation factor in the treatment of cytomegalovirus retinitis in AIDS patients. J AIDS 4:S22, 1991

168. Levine JD, Allan JD, Tessitore JH: Granulocyte-macrophage colony stimulating factor ameliorates the neutropenia induced by azidothymidine in AIDS/ARC patients. Proc Am Soc Clin Oncol 8:1, 1989

169. Miles SA, Mitsuyasu RT, Moreno J et al: Combined therapy with recombinant G-CSF and EPO decreased hematologic toxicity from zidovudine. Blood 77:2109, 1991

170. Krown SE, Paredes J, Bundow D et al: Interferon-α, zidovudine and granulocyte-macrophage colony-stimulating factor: a phase I trial in patients with Kaposi's sarcoma associated with the acquired immunodeficiency syndrome (AIDS). Ann Intern Med 112:812, 1990

171. Levine AM, Katz-Willson E, Espina B et al: Low dose m-BACOD with concomitant dideoxycytidine (ddC) in AIDS related lymphoma, abstracted. Blood 80:1301, 1992

172. Fisher RI, Gaynor ER, Dahlberg S et al: Comparison of a standard regimen (CHOP) with three intensive chemotherapy regimens for advanced non-Hodgkin's lymphoma. N Engl J Med 328:1002, 1993

173. Taillan B, Garnier G, Schneider S et al: Human immunodeficiency virus-related lymphoma: prognostic factors predictive of survival, letter. Cancer 71:2881, 1993

174. Kaplan L, Shiramizu B, Kahn J et al: Molecular predictors of survival in HIV-associated non-Hodgkin's lymphoma. Presented at the Seventh International Conference on AIDS. AIDS 1991

175. Shipp MA, Harrington DP, Anderson JR et al: A predictive model for aggressive non-Hodgkin's lymphoma. N Engl J Med 329:987, 1993

176. Scadden DT, Doweiko J, Schenkein D et al: A phase I/II trial of combined immunoconjugate and chemotherapy for AIDS-related lymphoma. Blood, suppl. 1. 82:386A, 1993

177. Riddell SR, Greenberg PD, Overell RW et al: Phase I study of cellular adoptive immunotherapy using genetically modified CD8− HIV-specific T cells for HIV seropositive patients undergoing allogeneic bone marrow transplant. Human Gene Ther 3:319, 1992

178. Murray RJ, Kurilla MG, Brooks JM et al: Identification of target antigens for the human cytotoxic T cell response to Epstein-Barr virus (EBV): implications for the immune control of EBV-positive malignancies. J Exp Med 176:157, 1992

179. Feichtinger H, Kaaya E, Putkonen P et al: Malignant lymphoma associated with human AIDS and with SIV-induced immunodeficiency in macaques. AIDS Res Hum Retroviruses 8:339, 1992

180. Karnad AB, Jaffar A, Lands RH: Spontaneous regression of acquired immune deficiency syndrome-related, high-grade, extranodal non-Hodgkin's lymphoma. Cancer 69:1856, 1992

181. Ford RJ, Goodacre A, Bohannon B, Donehower L: Identification of human retrovirus(es) in lymphoma cells from AIDS patients. AIDS Res Hum Retroviruses 6:142, 1990

182. Bohannon RC, Donehower LA: Isolation of a type D retrovirus from B-cell lymphomas of a patient with AIDS. J Virol 65:5663, 1991

183. Wotherspoon AC, Doglioni C, Diss TC, et al: Regression of primary low-grade B-cell gastric lymphoma of mucosa-associated lymphoid tissue type after eradication of *Helicobacter pylori*. Lancet 342:575, 1993

Multiple Myeloma and Other Plasma Cell Disorders

87

Robert A. Kyle

INTRODUCTION

The plasma cell proliferative disorders, or monoclonal gammopathies, are a group of diseases characterized by the proliferation of plasma cells (Table 87-1). Each monoclonal protein (M protein, paraprotein) is produced by a single clone of plasma cells and consists of one class of immunoglobulin heavy chains (γ in IgG, α in IgA, μ in IgM, δ in IgD, and ϵ in IgE) and one type of light chain (κ or λ) (see Chs. 8 and 9). Although M proteins in multiple myeloma and macroglobulinemia have a normal structure, the heavy chains found in heavy chain diseases have significant deletions of amino acids and are therefore abnormal. On electrophoresis, an M protein is seen as a narrow peak ("church spire") or as a localized band (Fig. 87-1).

In contrast to M proteins, polyclonal immunoglobulins consist of one or more heavy chain classes and of both light chain types. The electrophoretic pattern of a polyclonal increase in immunoglobulins is a broad-based peak or band, usually of γ-mobility (Fig. 87-2). The differential diagnosis of polyclonal gammopathies includes connective tissue (autoimmune) disorders, chronic liver disease (especially chronic active hepatitis), chronic infections, and lymphoproliferative diseases, as well as apparently normal persons.

The differentiation of a monoclonal from a polyclonal increase in immunoglobulins is essential because the former is associated with a neoplastic or potentially neoplastic process, whereas the latter is due to an inflammatory or a reactive process.

RECOGNITION OF MONOCLONAL PROTEINS

Analysis of Serum for M Proteins

Analysis of the serum and urine for M proteins requires a dependable screening method to detect the presence of an M protein. Electrophoresis on a cellulose acetate membrane is satisfactory for screening but may not detect small M proteins. High-resolution agarose gel electrophoresis is more sensitive than electrophoresis using cellulose acetate membranes.[1] Immunoelectrophoresis or immunofixation,[2] or both, should be used to confirm the presence of an M protein and to identify the heavy chain class and the light chain type.

Serum protein electrophoresis should be performed when a plasma cell proliferative process is suspected. Indications for serum protein electrophoresis are listed in Table 87-2. The presence of an M protein is suggestive of monoclonal gammopathy of undetermined significance (MGUS), multiple myeloma, Waldenström's macroglobulinemia or other lymphoproliferative conditions, or primary systemic amyloidosis.

Hypogammaglobulinemia (γ-globulin <0.6 g/dl) should be confirmed by quantitative determination of immunoglobulin levels. This abnormality is observed in about 10% of patients

Table 87-1. Classification of Plasma Cell Proliferative Disorders

Monoclonal gammopathies of undetermined significance
  Benign (IgG, IgA, IgD, IgM, and, rarely, free light chains)
  Associated neoplasms or other diseases not known to produce monoclonal proteins
  Biclonal gammopathies
  Idiopathic Bence Jones proteinuria
Malignant monoclonal gammopathies
  Multiple myeloma (IgG, IgA, IgD, IgE, and light chain)
    Smoldering multiple myeloma
    Plasma cell leukemia
    Nonsecretory myeloma
    IgD myeloma
    Osteosclerotic myeloma (polyneuropathy, organomegaly, endocrinopathy, M protein, and skin changes [POEMS])
  Plasmacytoma
    Solitary plasmacytoma of bone
    Extramedullary plasmacytoma
Malignant lymphoproliferative diseases
  Waldenström's macroglobulinemia (primary macroglobulinemia) (IgM)
  Malignant lymphoma
Heavy-chain diseases (HCD)
  γ-HCD
  α-HCD
  μ-HCD
Other
  Cryoglobulinemia
  Pyroglobulinemia
Primary amyloidosis (see Ch. 88)

(From Kyle,[245] with permission.)

with multiple myeloma and in approximately 25% of patients with primary systemic amyloidosis and is often associated with a monoclonal light chain in the urine (Bence Jones proteinuria).

An M protein may be present even when the total protein level, β- or γ-globulin concentrations, and quantitative immunoglobulin values are all within normal limits. The cellulose acetate strip must be carefully inspected because a small M protein may be present and not detected on the densitometer tracing. Even with careful inspection, a small M protein may be concealed within the β or γ components and be missed. Furthermore, a monoclonal light chain (Bence Jones proteinemia) is rarely visible on the cellulose acetate tracing. A localized band or peak is often not seen in the heavy chain diseases. Therefore, either immunoelectrophoresis or immunofixation is necessary for the identification of an M protein and should be performed when a narrow peak or band is found in the cellulose acetate tracing or when myeloma or a related plasma cell proliferative disorder is suspected (Fig. 87-3). Immunofixation is particularly helpful when an M protein is suspected and only bowing of a single heavy or light chain arc is found on immunoelectrophoresis, when a small M protein is present in

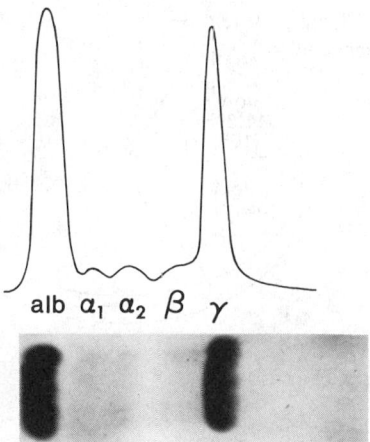

Fig. 87-1. (Top) Monoclonal pattern of serum protein from densitometer tracing after electrophoresis of serum on cellulose acetate (anode on left): tall, narrow-based peak of γ-mobility. **(Bottom)** Monoclonal pattern from electrophoresis of serum on cellulose acetate (anode on left): dense localized band representing monoclonal protein in γ-area. (From Kyle and Greipp,[243] with permission.)

Table 87-2. Indications for Serum Protein Electrophoresis

Diagnosis or suspected diagnosis of multiple myeloma, macroglobulinemia, or amyloidosis

Symptoms
    Weakness or fatigue
    Back pain
    Recurrent infections

Laboratory indications
    Anemia
    Elevated erythrocyte sedimentation rate
    Immunoglobulin deficiency
    Hypercalcemia
    Bence Jones proteinuria
    Renal insufficiency

Radiologic indications
    Osteoporosis
    Osteolytic lesions or fracture

Syndromes
    Peripheral neuropathy
    Carpal tunnel syndrome
    Refractory congestive heart failure
    Nephrotic syndrome
    Orthostatic hypotension
    Malabsorption

(From Kyle and Greipp,[173] with permission.)

a polyclonal increase in immunoglobulins, or when the second component of a biclonal gammopathy is not recognized.

The κ/λ ratio obtained from nephelometry may be helpful in the detection of the light chain type of large monoclonal gammopathies,[3] but small M proteins will have a normal ratio and will not be recognized. This is especially true with a small monoclonal IgG κ-protein.

Immunoelectrophoresis must be used to examine the sera of all patients with an apparently free monoclonal κ- or λ-light chain for the presence of an IgD or IgE heavy chain. Ouchterlony immunodiffusion can be used to screen for IgD and IgE.

Quantitation of immunoglobulins is more useful than immunoelectrophoresis or immunofixation for the demonstration of hypogammaglobulinemia. Rate nephelometry is the preferred method for quantitation of immunoglobulins because it is not affected by the molecular size of the antigen. For example, polymers of IgA or aggregates of IgG will produce spuriously low levels for IgA and IgG, respectively, with radial immunodiffusion because diffusion is less than with the 7S IgA standard. Low-molecular-weight 7S IgM produces a spuriously elevated level because its rate of diffusion is greater than that of the 19S IgM standard. Thus, radial immunodiffusion is not recommended.

Frequently, the nephelometry value for IgM and occasionally IgG or IgA is much higher than the value obtained with a densitometer tracing of serum protein electrophoresis.[4] Both nephelometry and densitometer tracing values are reproducible. Consequently, one must use either electrophoresis or nephelometry throughout the course of a patient's illness rather than alternating the techniques.

Analysis of Urine for M Proteins

The recognition of Bence Jones protein depends on the demonstration of a monoclonal light chain by immunoelectrophoresis or immunofixation. Dipsticks are used in many laboratories to screen for protein, but they are often insensitive to Bence Jones protein and should not be used. Sulfosalicylic acid or Exton's reagent is preferable because it detects both albumin

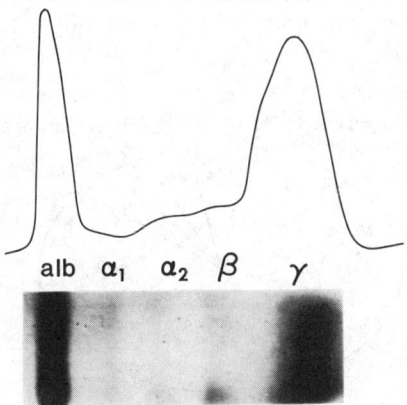

Fig. 87-2. (Top) Polyclonal pattern of serum protein from densitometer tracing after electrophoresis on cellulose acetate (anode on left): broad-based peak of γ-mobility. **(Bottom)** Polyclonal pattern from electrophoresis of serum on cellulose acetate (anode on left): γ-band is broad. (From Kyle and Greipp,[243] with permission.)

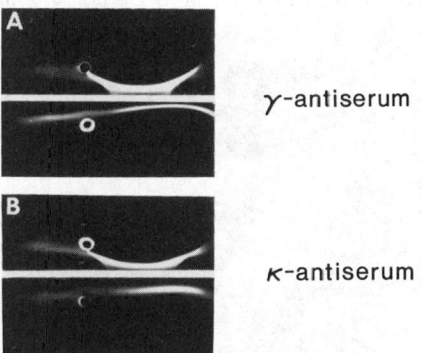

Fig. 87-3. Immunoelectrophoretic pattern of serum. **(A top)** Antiserum to IgG (γ) shows a thickened arc. **(B top)** Antiserum to κ-chains shows a thickened arc similar to the IgG arc. **(A & B bottom)** Antiserum to γ- and to κ-chains shows a faint normal arc. Patient's serum contains a monoclonal IgG κ-protein. (From Kyle and Greipp,[243] with permission.)

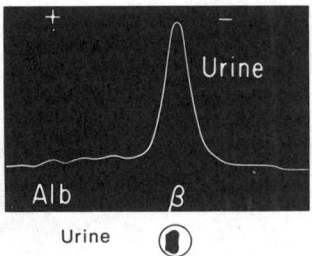

Fig. 87-4. Urinary monoclonal protein. **(Top)** Densitometer tracing showing a tall, narrow-based peak of β-mobility. **(Bottom)** Cellulose acetate electrophoretic pattern showing a dense band of β-mobility. This is consistent with a monoclonal urine protein (Bence Jones protein). (From Kyle and Greipp,[243] with permission.)

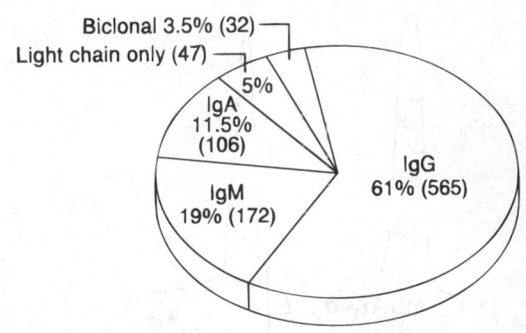

Fig. 87-6. Distribution of monoclonal serum proteins in 922 cases seen at the Mayo Clinic during 1992.

and globulin. The heat test for Bence Jones protein is not satisfactory because both false-positive and false-negative results occur.

An aliquot from a 24-hour collection of urine must be concentrated 150–200-fold, followed by electrophoresis, immunoelectrophoresis, and immunofixation in all cases of multiple myeloma, Waldenström's macroglobulinemia, amyloidosis, MGUS, and heavy chain diseases or on suspicion of these entities. The amount of M protein is calculated from the size of the spike on the densitometer tracing and the total 24-hour urine protein content. This M protein value correlates directly with the size of the patient's plasma cell burden.

A urinary M protein produces a dense band on the cellulose strip or a tall, narrow peak on the densitometer tracing (Fig. 87-4). Immunofixation of an M protein is characterized by a localized band with monospecific antisera. Occasionally, two discrete globulin bands may be seen. These may represent a monoclonal light chain plus a monoclonal immunoglobulin fragment from the serum (Fig. 87-5) or monomers and dimers of the monoclonal light chain. Although more sensitive than immunoelectrophoresis, immunofixation is technically more difficult.[5] Particular care must be taken to obtain the appropriate dilution because an M protein can be overdiagnosed or underdiagnosed when immunofixation is used. Immunofixation is most helpful when a monoclonal light chain occurs in the presence of a polyclonal increase in light chains such as in the nephrotic syndrome.

Incidence of Monoclonal Gammopathies

Monoclonal gammopathies are currently being found in clinical practice with greater frequency. Of 922 new cases of serum M protein recognized at the Mayo Clinic in 1992 (Fig. 87-6),

8.5% showed Bence Jones proteinemia or biclonal gammopathy—two entities that are often overlooked on a serum protein electrophoretic pattern. Each is recognized only if immunoelectrophoresis or immunofixation is performed. The clinical diagnoses associated with the detection of a monoclonal gammopathy are shown in Figure 87-7. Unexpectedly, multiple myeloma was found in only 18% of patients, and MGUS was found most frequently.

MONOCLONAL GAMMOPATHY OF UNDETERMINED SIGNIFICANCE

The term MGUS denotes the presence of an M protein in patients without multiple myeloma, macroglobulinemia, amyloidosis, or other related diseases. The term benign monoclonal gammopathy (BMG) is misleading because it is not known at the time of recognition of the M protein whether this protein will remain stable and benign, represents an early form of multiple myeloma, or will develop into symptomatic multiple myeloma, primary systemic amyloidosis, macroglobulinemia, or another malignant lymphoproliferative disease.

MGUS is characterized by a serum M protein concentration of <3 g/dl; <5% plasma cells in the bone marrow; little or no M protein in the urine; absence of lytic bone lesions, anemia, hypercalcemia, and renal insufficiency; and, most importantly, stability of the M protein and failure of additional abnormalities to develop during long periods of observation.

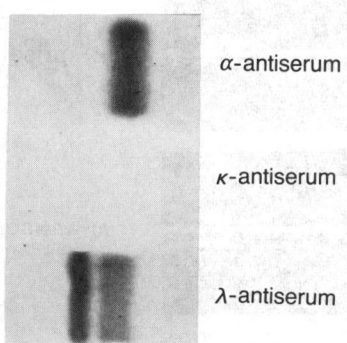

Fig. 87-5. Immunofixation of urine. **(Top)** Narrow, localized band with IgA (α) antiserum. **(Middle)** No reaction with κ-antiserum. **(Bottom)** Two discrete bands with λ-antiserum. This patient has a monoclonal λ-protein plus an IgA λ-fragment. (From Kyle and Garton,[244] with permission.)

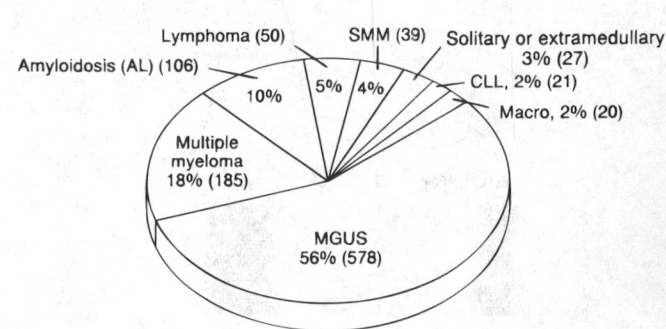

Fig. 87-7. Diagnoses in 1,026 cases of monoclonal gammopathy seen at the Mayo Clinic during 1992. CLL, chronic lymphocytic leukemia; SMM, smoldering multiple myeloma; Macro, macroglobulinemia; MGUS, monoclonal gammopathy of undetermined significance.

Epidemiology

Approximately 3% of persons >70 years of age in Sweden,[6] France,[7] and the United States[8] have a monoclonal gammopathy without evidence of myeloma, macroglobulinemia, or amyloidosis. Among patients ≥50 years of age who were residents of a small Minnesota community with a cluster of myeloma, 1.25% had an M protein,[8] and 1.7% of adults ≥50 years of age in Finistère, France, had an M protein.[7] The incidence increases with advancing age. Using agarose gel electrophoresis, Crawford et al.[9] found M proteins in 10% (11 of 111) of patients >80 years in a population of ambulatory residents of a retirement home. The incidence of monoclonal gammopathies in blacks is greater than that in the whites.[10,11]

More sensitive techniques such as high-resolution electrophoresis[12] and immunoisoelectric focusing[13] will detect a higher incidence of M proteins.

Biologic and Molecular Aspects

T cells have an important role in normal B-cell differentiation. Patients with multiple myeloma have reduced percentages of CD4 cells (helper T cells) and increased percentages of CD8 cells (suppressor T cells), and an increase in CD8 cells has been reported in MGUS.[14] T cells also have an important role in the development of M proteins; thus, infusion of corticosteroid-resistant T cells into BALB/c nude mice decreased the incidence of M proteins from 49% at 9 months to 20% at 15 months of age, while the incidence of M proteins in the control group increased from 40% at 9 months to 68% at 12 months.[15] These changes suggest that T-cell deficiency has a role in the development of MGUS.

Although benign monoclonal gammopathy spontaneously develops in aging C57BL mice, multiple myeloma does not.[16] By contrast, in humans with benign monoclonal gammopathy or MGUS, multiple myeloma or related disorders often occur.[17] Cytogenetic abnormalities probably do occur in patients with MGUS, but they have not been detected because of the low proliferative activity and the small number of plasma cells.

Clinical Presentation and Laboratory Evaluation

Because patients with MGUS have no symptoms or physical findings, the M protein is found only by electrophoresis and either immunoelectrophoresis or immunofixation. The clinical and laboratory features may best be described by analysis of a series of 241 patients seen at the Mayo Clinic before January 1, 1971. These patients all had a monoclonal gammopathy but no evidence of multiple myeloma, macroglobulinemia, amyloidosis, lymphoma, or related diseases. Their median age was 64 years, with only 4% <40 years old and 33% ≥70 years old; 58% were men. None of the findings, which included anemia, leukopenia, leukocytosis, thrombocytopenia, thrombocytosis, renal insufficiency, and hypoalbuminemia, could be directly attributed to MGUS.

The concentration of the M protein ranged from 0.3 to 3.2 g/dl, with a median of 1.7 g/dl. Immunoelectrophoresis revealed IgG in 73%, IgA in 11%, and IgM in 14% of patients; 86% of the IgG gammopathies were IgG$_1$. The light chain type was κ in 62% and λ in 38%. Five patients (2.1%) had a biclonal gammopathy and nine had a urinary monoclonal light chain. The uninvolved or background immunoglobulins were reduced in 52 (29%) of 181 patients in whom they were tested. The number of bone marrow plasma cells ranged from 1 to 10% (median, 3%).

Table 87-3. Course During First 22 Years (Median) of Follow-up in a Series of 241 Patients with "Benign" Monoclonal Gammopathy

		Patients	
Group	Status	N	%
1	No significant increase of serum or urinary M protein (benign)	46	19
2	Increase of M protein to >3 g/dl	23	10
3	Died of unrelated cause	113	47
4	Developed myeloma, macroglobulinemia, amyloidosis, or related diseases	59	24
		241	100

Follow-up Evaluation

The 241 patients were followed for a median of 22 years (range, 20–35 years). The number of patients whose M protein had remained stable and who could be classified as having BMG had decreased to 46 (19%) (Table 87-3). Six of these patients were found to have a monoclonal light chain in the urine. The hemoglobin level, amount of the serum M protein, and number of plasma cells in the bone marrow at diagnosis of the stable (benign) group did not differ substantially from those of the total group.

Twenty-three (10%) had an increase in M protein to >3 g/dl but did not require chemotherapy. Eight also had a small amount of monoclonal light chain in their urine. The median interval from the recognition of the M protein before reaching 3 g/dl was 9 years (range, 0–21 years). Five patients are still alive and must be followed because symptomatic multiple myeloma, macroglobulinemia, or amyloidosis is likely to develop.

As expected in an older population, 113 patients (47%) have died; the median interval from recognition of the M protein to death was 7 years. Cardiac disease was the most frequent cause of death, followed in frequency by cerebrovascular disease and non-plasma cell malignancy.

Multiple myeloma, macroglobulinemia, amyloidosis, or a malignant lymphoproliferative process developed in 59 (24%) of the 241 patients during follow-up (actuarial rate, 17% at 10 years and 33% at 20 years). Of these 59 patients, 39 (66%) had well-documented multiple myeloma. The median duration of survival after diagnosis of multiple myeloma was 34 months. The interval from the recognition of the M protein to the diagnosis of multiple myeloma ranged from 2 to 29 years (median, 10 years); this finding indicates that patients with an apparently benign monoclonal gammopathy must be followed indefinitely (Table 87-4). The mode of development of multiple myeloma was variable in that some patients remained stable for many years, with multiple myeloma then gradually or suddenly developing, whereas a few others had a steady increase in M protein until multiple myeloma was diagnosed 5–29 years later.

Waldenström's macroglobulinemia developed in seven patients at a median interval of 8.5 years after recognition of the M

Table 87-4. Interval Between Recognition of Monoclonal Protein and Diagnosis of Serious Disease in 59 Patients with MGUS

			Interval to Diagnosis[a]	
	N	%	Median (yr)	Range (yr)
Multiple myeloma	39	66	10	2–29
Macroglobulinemia	7	12	8.5	4–20
Amyloidosis	8	14	9	6–19
Lymphoproliferative	5	8	10.5	6–22
	59	100		

[a]Actuarial rate was 17% at 10 years and 33% at 20 years.

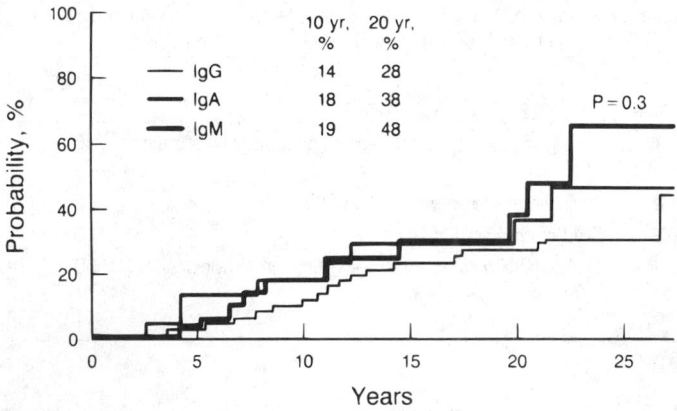

Fig. 87-8. Rate of development of lymphoplasmacytic disease in 241 patients with a serum monoclonal protein, stratified by immunoglobulin class. (From Kyle,[17] with permission.)

protein, and primary systemic amyloidosis developed in eight patients 6–16.5 years (median, 8 years) after recognition of the M protein. In five patients, a malignant lymphoproliferative process developed 9–22 years (median, 10.5 years) after detection of the M protein. In one patient with systemic lupus erythematosus and biclonal gammopathy, an aggressive diffuse undifferentiated malignant lymphoma developed 7 years later; in another patient, an immunoblastic lymphoma developed 22 years after recognition of an IgM λ-protein. Chronic lymphocytic leukemia (CLL) developed in one patient after 56 months of observation. Of the patients with IgG or IgA monoclonal gammopathy, 23% developed multiple myeloma or related disorders or had an M protein level of >3 g/dl during follow-up, as did 37% of those with an IgM monoclonal gammopathy. The rate of development of serious disease did not differ whether the monoclonal gammopathy was IgG, IgA, or IgM (Fig. 87-8).

The medical records of 430 patients in whom a serum IgM monoclonal gammopathy had been identified during 1956–1978 at the Mayo Clinic were reviewed and their gammopathies classified[18] (Table 87-5). Follow-up evaluation showed that 40 (17%) of the 242 patients with an IgM MGUS developed a malignant lymphoid disease; of these 40 patients, 22 had Waldenström's macroglobulinemia, 9 had a malignant lymphoproliferative process requiring chemotherapy, 6 had lymphoma, 2 developed amyloidosis, and 1 had CLL. The median duration from the recognition of the IgM protein until the diagnosis of lymphoid disease was >4 years (range 0.4–22 years). Patients with Waldenström's macroglobulinemia and lymphoproliferative disease differed mainly in the serum M protein concentration. Survival was virtually the same for both groups. Consequently, no rationale exists for differentiating patients with symptomatic lymphoproliferative disease requiring chemo-

Table 87-5. Classification of the IgM Monoclonal Gammopathies of 430 Patients

| | Patients | |
Classification	N	%
MGUS	242	56
Waldenström's macroglobulinemia	71	17
Lymphoma	28	7
CLL	21	5
Primary amyloidosis	6	1
Lymphoproliferative disease	62	14
	430	100

(From Kyle and Garton,[18] with permission.)

therapy and a modest M protein value from those with Waldenström's macroglobulinemia characterized by an M spike of >3 g/dl.

A 20-year follow-up study of 67 Swedish patients with an M protein revealed that 11% had progression of BMG.[19] In a series of 113 patients with MGUS, 8 developed multiple myeloma and 2 had amyloidosis during a follow-up of 1–17 years. The actuarial risk of myeloma or amyloidosis developing at 8 years was 30%.[20]

In a series of 191 patients with MGUS, the actuarial risk of the development of a malignant monoclonal gammopathy was 4.5% at 5 years, 15% at 10 years, and 26% at 15 years.[21] In another series of 128 patients, the actuarial probability of malignant transformation at 5 and 10 years was 8.5% and 19.2%, respectively.[22]

Differential Diagnosis of MGUS from Multiple Myeloma and Macroglobulinemia

Differentiation of the patient with BMG from one in whom myeloma or macroglobulinemia eventually develops is very difficult when the M protein is first recognized. The extent of the serum M protein is of some help; an M-protein concentration of ≥3 g/dl generally indicates overt multiple myeloma or macroglobulinemia, but some exceptions, such as smoldering multiple myeloma (SMM), exist. Levels of immunoglobulins not associated with the M protein (normal polyclonal or background immunoglobulins) may help because most patients with multiple myeloma have a reduction in normal polyclonal immunoglobulins, but a reduction may also occur in those with BMG.[23]

The presence of a monoclonal light chain (Bence Jones proteinuria) with the M protein is suggestive of a neoplastic process. However, 40% of a group of patients with apparent BMG had a small amount of monoclonal light chain in their urine.[24] The condition of many patients with a small amount of monoclonal light chain in their urine and an M protein in their serum has remained stable for many years.

The presence of >10% plasma cells in the bone marrow is suggestive of multiple myeloma, although some patients with a greater degree of plasmacytosis have remained stable for long periods. The bone marrow plasma cells in multiple myeloma are often atypical, but it is difficult to differentiate benign from malignant plasma cells on the basis of morphologic appearance. The presence of osteolytic lesions is strongly suggestive of multiple myeloma, but metastatic carcinoma may produce lytic lesions as well as plasmacytosis and may be associated with an unrelated serum M protein.

The plasma cell labeling index may be useful in differentiating patients with MGUS or SMM from those with multiple myeloma. A monoclonal antibody (BU-1) reactive with 5-bromo-2-deoxyuridine recognizes cells that synthesize DNA. The BU-1 monoclonal antibody does not require denaturation; consequently, fluorescein-conjugated immunoglobulin antisera (κ and λ) identify monoclonal plasma cells and plasmacytoid lymphocytes. The labeling index can be performed in 4–5 hours and is a practical aid in therapeutic decisions.[25] The plasma cell labeling index can also be performed on peripheral blood and correlates with the bone marrow labeling index.[26] An elevated plasma cell-labeling index strongly suggests that the patient has, or will soon have, symptomatic multiple myeloma, but it must be emphasized that at least one-third of patients with overt symptomatic multiple myeloma have a normal plasma cell labeling index.

Monoclonal plasma cells are found in the peripheral blood of 60% of patients who have active multiple myeloma and in >90% of those with relapsed or refractory myeloma. Patients with MGUS or SMM have few or no circulating plasma cells.[27]

With the use of consensus oligonucleotide primers to amplify the third complementary determining region of rearranged immunoglobulin heavy chain alleles by polymerase chain reaction, circulating malignant cells were identified in 13 of 14 previously untreated patients with multiple myeloma.[28]

Elevated levels of β_2-microglobulin, the presence of J chains, elevated plasma cell acid phosphatase levels, reduced numbers of CD4[+] T cells, increased numbers of monoclonal idiotype peripheral blood lymphocytes, or increased numbers of immunoglobulin-secreting cells in peripheral blood will not reliably differentiate multiple myeloma from MGUS. It has been suggested that expression of p170, the absence of CD56 expression, and a low proliferation rate with use of KI67 are characteristic of MGUS and help differentiate it from multiple myeloma.[29]

No single technique exists that differentiates benign from malignant plasma cell proliferative disease. The most dependable means is serial measurement of the M protein level in the serum and urine and periodic re-evaluation of clinical and laboratory features to determine whether multiple myeloma, systemic amyloidosis, macroglobulinemia, or other malignant lymphoplasma cell proliferative disease has developed.

If the serum M-protein level is <2 g/dl, electrophoresis should be repeated 6 months later, and if the concentration is stable, the study should be repeated annually thereafter. Bone marrow examination and a metastatic bone survey are unnecessary unless other features suggest multiple myeloma or related disorders. If the M-protein level is ≥2.0 g/dl, and myeloma or related disorders is not evident, electrophoresis should be repeated in 3–4 months. If the M-protein level is stable, electrophoresis should be repeated in 6 months; if no progression is noted, it should be performed annually thereafter. If the M-protein level increases by >0.5 g/dl, immunoelectrophoresis of a 24-hour urine specimen should be performed and hemoglobin, calcium, and creatinine levels determined. If abnormalities are found, bone marrow and radiographic examinations are indicated. If an M protein (Bence Jones proteinuria) is present in the urine, the patient should be followed more closely.

Follow-up evaluation may also involve quantitation of the immunoglobulin level. However, the quantitative immunoglobulin value may be as much as 2,000 mg/dl greater than that indicated by the densitometer tracing. Therefore, the M-protein level should be monitored either by a densitometer tracing of the electrophoretic pattern or by quantitation of immunoglobulins; however, the method selected for the measurement should not be changed.

Association of MGUS with Other Diseases

Although MGUS frequently exists without other abnormalities, certain diseases are associated with it, as would be expected in an older population. The association of two diseases depends on the frequency with which each occurs independently. There may be an apparent association because of a difference in the referral practice or in other selected patient groups. Valid epidemiologic and statistical methods must be used in evaluating these associations. Appropriate control populations are essential.

For example, the association of monoclonal gammopathy and hyperparathyroidism has been reported.[30] In an effort to clarify this relationship, we reviewed our cases of surgically proven parathyroid adenoma in which serum protein electrophoresis had been done within the 6 months preceding parathyroidectomy. Among 911 patients who met these criteria and who were >50 years old, 9 (1%) were shown by immunoelectrophoresis to have MGUS.[31] This prevalence of MGUS is similar to the 1.25–1.7% found in studies of three normal populations.[6–8] Thus, the association of hyperparathyroidism with MGUS appears to be due to chance alone.

The incidence of monoclonal gammopathies in patients with diffuse lymphomas is increased but in those with nodular lymphoma or Hodgkin disease it is not. In 1,150 patients with lymphoma, Alexanian[32] found M proteins in 29 (4.5%) of 640 patients with diffuse lymphoproliferative disease (chronic lymphocytic leukemia, lymphocytic lymphoma, and reticulum cell sarcoma) but in none of the 292 patients with nodular lymphoma.

M proteins have been found in the sera of patients with leukemia. We have described 100 patients with CLL and an M protein in the serum or urine.[33] IgG accounted for 51% and IgM for 21%. The M-protein level was modest, with a median concentration of 1 g/dl. There were no major differences between CLL patients who had an IgG and those who had an IgM M protein. Monoclonal gammopathies have been recognized in hairy cell leukemia, adult T-cell leukemia, chronic myeloid leukemia, and acute myelomonocytic leukemia, but data are inadequate to determine whether the incidence of M protein is greater than in a normal population.[34]

Rheumatoid arthritis[35] and seronegative erosive arthritis[36] have been reported with monoclonal gammopathies. Systemic lupus erythematosus, polymyalgia rheumatica, polymyositis, discoid lupus erythematosus, and psoriatic arthritis have all also been reported, but the relationship is questionable.

In a series of 279 patients with a clinically recognized sensorimotor peripheral neuropathy of unknown cause, Kelly et al.[37] reported 16 (6%) with MGUS. The incidence would be greater if the diagnosis were based on only electrophysiologic evidence of neuropathy. Latov et al.[38] demonstrated that a small monoclonal IgM λ-protein in a patient with peripheral neuropathy was directed against peripheral nerve myelin. This protein was subsequently identified as a specific glycoprotein component of myelin and referred to as myelin-associated glycoprotein. Reviews of neurologic disorders associated with monoclonal gammopathies have been published.[39,40]

Monoclonal gammopathies may be associated with lichen myxedematosus, scleredema, pyoderma gangrenosum, necrobiotic xanthogranuloma, Sézary syndrome, mycosis fungoides, diffuse plane xanthomatosis, Gaucher disease, acquired von Willebrand disease, myelodysplastic syndrome, acquired deficiency of Cl esterase inhibitor, periodic systemic capillary leak syndrome, acquired immunodeficiency syndrome, renal, bone marrow, and liver transplants, and a wide variety of other conditions.[34]

M Proteins with Antibody Activity

In some patients with MGUS, myeloma, or macroglobulinemia, the monoclonal immunoglobulin has exhibited unusual specificities to dextran, antistreptolysin O, antinuclear activity, riboflavin, von Willebrand factor, thyroglobulin, insulin, double-stranded DNA, apolipoprotein, thyroxine, cephalin, lactate dehydrogenase, anti-human immunodeficiency virus, actin, and antibiotic agents. After an infection, transient M proteins with antibody activity have been recognized. A comprehensive review of M proteins with antibody activity in plasma cell dyscrasias has been published.[41]

The binding of calcium by an M protein produces hypercalcemia without symptomatic or pathologic consequences; the situation must be recognized to prevent treatment of such patients for hypercalcemia.[42] Copper-binding M protein has been reported.[43] Binding of an M protein to phosphate produces a spurious hyperphosphatemia and should be recognized.

Biclonal Gammopathy

The clinical findings of biclonal gammopathies, detected in 3–4% of all patients with monoclonal gammopathy, are similar to those seen in monoclonal gammopathies.[44] About two-thirds of the patients have a biclonal gammopathy of undetermined significance, while the remainder have multiple myeloma, amyloidosis, macroglobulinemia, or other lymphoproliferative disease. More than 12 cases of triclonal gammopathy have been reported.[45]

Idiopathic Bence Jones Proteinuria

Although a recognized feature of multiple myeloma, primary amyloidosis, macroglobulinemia, or other lymphoproliferative disease, Bence Jones proteinuria may exist without evidence of malignant plasma cell proliferation. Some patients have excreted large amounts of Bence Jones protein in the urine and have remained asymptomatic for several years. In most of these patients, multiple myeloma or amyloidosis will eventually develop, but this may not occur for as long as 20 years.[46]

MULTIPLE MYELOMA

Multiple myeloma (plasma cell myeloma, myelomatosis, or Kahler disease) is characterized by the neoplastic proliferation of a single clone of plasma cells engaged in the production of a monoclonal immunoglobulin. Although multiple myeloma was described in 1844 by Solly and subsequently in 1850 by Macintyre, it was rarely recognized until 1889, in the famous case report of Dr. Loos by Kahler.[47]

Epidemiology

Multiple myeloma accounts for approximately 1% of all types of malignant disease and for slightly >10% of hematologic malignancies. Although two- to fivefold increases in the incidence of multiple myeloma have been reported in the United States, England, and Wales, the rates in Malmö, Sweden, have increased only slightly.[48] Data from Olmsted County, Minnesota, indicated a rate of 3 per 100,000 for 1945–1954 and a similar rate during the following two decades.[49] During 1978–1990, the annual incidence of multiple myeloma in Olmsted County was 4 per 100,000.[50] In Denmark during 1943–1962, the incidence of multiple myeloma increased nearly threefold but has since remained virtually stable.[51] The incidence of multiple myeloma probably has not changed significantly; the apparent increase in rates is probably related to increased availability and use of medical facilities, as well as improved diagnostic techniques.

Multiple myeloma has a peak incidence during the seventh decade of life. Only 3% of patients are <40 years of age. Although multiple myeloma has been well documented in a child,[52] the diagnosis of myeloma in persons <30 years of age is to be accepted only after critical evaluation of all data. The incidence in blacks is twice that in whites and is slightly more frequent in men than in women. Multiple myeloma occurs in all races and in all geographic areas, but the incidence is lower in Asian populations.

Biologic and Molecular Aspects

Cytogenetic studies in multiple myeloma have been hindered because of the low proliferative activity of plasma cells. Flow cytometric analysis has led to the demonstration of an aneuploid myeloma cell population in approximately 80% of patients, with hyperdiploidy the most common.[53] Aneuploidy was detected in the bone marrow of 54% of 25 patients with multiple myeloma and in only one case of benign monoclonal gammopathy.[54] Structural changes of chromosomes 1, 11, and 14, as well as monosomies and trisomies, have been reported.[55–57]

Approximately one-half of patients with myeloma have an abnormal karyotype, with trisomies 3, 5, 9, and 15 and monosomies 13 and 16 the most frequent abnormalities. More cytogenetic abnormalities would likely be found if the karyotype of plasma cells could be more easily studied.[58] Translocations have also been observed in myeloma and include t(8;14) (q24; q32) and t(11;14) (q13;q32), with the t(8;14) abnormality occurring only in patients with IgA monoclonal gammopathies—findings suggestive of a pathogenetic relationship.[56] Interestingly, 8q24 and 11q13 are the sites of the c-*myc* and *bcl*-1 proto-oncogenes, respectively, and 14q32 is the locus of the immunoglobulin heavy chain gene. Loss of restriction sites in a region 44 base pairs upstream from the 3' border of the first c-*myc* exon was found in 8 of 13 patients with multiple myeloma.[59] In one series, 4 of 70 patients with myeloma had a *bcl*-1 rearrangement.[60]

In another series, elevated levels of c-myc mRNA were found in 9 of 37 patients with myeloma.[61] Most of the 37 patients had distinct rearrangements of the immunoglobulin heavy and light chain genes, and 2 of the 9 with increased c-myc mRNA also had evidence of c-*myc* rearrangement. In still another report, 17 (74%) of 23 patients with active myeloma had higher fluorescence of H-ras p21 protein in aneuploid tumor cells than did patients with marrows in remission.[62] Elevated levels of c-myc mRNA and c-*myc* rearrangement[61] and higher fluorescence of H-ras p21 protein in aneuploid tumor cells have been seen in multiple myeloma[62]; *ras* gene mutations were reported in 47% of 30 cases of multiple myeloma. Two-thirds of the patients with *ras* gene mutations had fulminating disease.[63] Although increased expression of *bcl*-2 protein has been reported,[64] rearrangement of *bcl*-2 was not found in 16 patients with multiple myeloma.[65] Point mutations of the p53 gene were found in three recent reports.[63,66,67] Both *ras* and p53 mutations were found in patients with aggressive multiple myeloma. The biology of myeloma has been reviewed.[68]

Plasma cells express cytoplasmic immunoglobulin, CD38, and plasma cell antigen-1, and a minority express CD10, HLA-DR, and CD20. Most myeloma cells are positive for N-CAM (CD56), whereas patients with plasma cell leukemia or normal plasma cells express little or no CD56.[69] The nature of the clonogenic cell in multiple myeloma is unknown.[70] The presence of multiple hematopoietic surface antigens on malignant plasma cells suggests its origin from a pluripotent stem cell.[71] It is likely that plasma cell precursors of myeloma circulate in peripheral blood. These circulating clonogenic premyeloma cells may home to the bone marrow by means of adhesion molecules and find an appropriate microenvironment (cytokine network, including stromal cells) in which to differentiate and proliferate.[72]

Several growth factors are involved in the differentiation and growth of normal B cells. Overproduction of interleukin (IL)-1 and tumor necrosis factor, which have bone-resorbing activity, has been found in patients with multiple myeloma.[73,74] Resting B cells enter DNA synthesis following stimulation with IL-4, proliferate with IL-5, and differentiate into plasma cells with IL-6 stimulation.[73,75–77] Kawano et al.[78] showed that myeloma cells produce IL-6 and express IL-6 receptors. Elevated IL-6 levels in most patients with progressive terminal multiple myeloma and in those with plasma cell leukemia support the concept that this cytokine is an important factor in the progression of multiple myeloma.[79] The elevated levels also support the use of anti-IL-6 therapy in patients with aggressive plasma cell diseases that are resistant to chemotherapy.[80] The role of IL-6 in multiple myeloma was recently reviewed.[81,82]

Etiology

The cause of multiple myeloma is unknown, although radiation may be a factor in some cases. In atomic bomb survivors aged 20–59 years who had received >50 cGy,[83] 5 multiple myeloma cases were found, versus 1.8 expected, 20 years after exposure. Radiation workers at the Sellafield plant in England had an excessive death rate from multiple myeloma, with 7 cases observed versus 4.2 expected.[84] In a long-term follow-up study of 14,106 patients with ankylosing spondylitis who were given a single course of radiotherapy, the incidence of multiple myeloma was increased, with 8 cases observed versus 4.7 expected.[85]

Direct evidence that chemicals cause myeloma in humans is sparse, even though reports have linked multiple myeloma with benzene[86] and asbestos.[87] An increased risk of multiple myeloma has been recognized in farmers exposed to herbicides and insecticides.[88] Case control studies have reported an excess risk of multiple myeloma in workers in the food processing or agricultural industry in England and Wales.[89] Excess risk of multiple myeloma also has been noted in grain workers, rubber workers, cosmetologists, furniture workers, and persons exposed to pesticides and carbon monoxide. The number of cases is small, however, and more data are necessary.

Repeated antigenic stimulation of the reticuloendothelial system could contribute to the development of multiple myeloma. However, a case control study revealed that patients with multiple myeloma actually had fewer immune-stimulating conditions, such as chronic infections, connective tissue diseases, allergies, cholecystitis, or diverticulitis, than did the control population.[90]

Genetic Aspects

The likelihood of a genetic factor in some patients is supported by well-documented reports of familial clusters of two or more first-degree relatives (siblings or parents and children) with multiple myeloma.[91] A genetic factor is also supported by a report of multiple myeloma in monozygotic twins[92] and by its reported presence in two brothers, both of whom had an IgG κ-monoclonal protein and the same genotype.[93] However, in a study of 439 patients with multiple myeloma and 1,317 matched controls, only 3 patients and 4 controls reported multiple myeloma in their families.[94]

Clinical Manifestations and Laboratory Evaluation

Bone pain, typically in the back or chest and less often in the extremities, is present at diagnosis in more than two-thirds of patients. The pain is aggravated by movement, and the patient is usually comfortable at rest. The patient's height may be reduced by several inches because of vertebral collapse. Weakness and fatigue are common and are often associated with anemia. Fever from the disease itself is rare; most patients with multiple myeloma and fever have an infection. Abnormal bleeding, most often epistaxis or purpura, may be a prominent feature. Symptoms from an acute infection, renal insufficiency, hypercalcemia, or amyloidosis may be the initial manifestation.

Pallor is the most frequent physical finding. The liver is palpable in about 20% of patients and the spleen in 5%. Extramedullary plasmacytomas are not common and are usually seen late in the course of the disease as large, vascular, subcutaneous masses with a purplish hue.

Anemia is present at diagnosis in about two-thirds of multiple myeloma patients. The erythrocyte sedimentation rate is typically increased but is normal in 10% of patients. A serum protein electrophoretic pattern shows a spike or localized band in about 80% of patients; approximately 10% have hypogammaglobulinemia, and 10% have a normal-appearing pattern. Immunoelectrophoresis and immunofixation of the serum reveal an M protein in slightly >90% of patients. The serum creatinine level is elevated in one-half of patients, approximately one-fifth

having a level of ≥2 mg/dl at diagnosis. Immunoelectrophoresis or immunofixation reveals a urinary M protein in 80% of patients, with a κ/λ ratio of 2:1, and an M protein is found in the serum or urine of 99% during the course of the disease.

A bone marrow aspirate and biopsy usually contain >10% plasma cells in these cases. The finding of large homogeneous nodules or infiltrates of plasma cells in the bone marrow sections is the most reliable morphologic criterion for the diagnosis, but such nodules or infiltrates are not always present.[95]

Renal Involvement

The two major causes of renal insufficiency are "myeloma kidney" and hypercalcemia. Myeloma kidney is characterized by the presence of large, waxy, laminated casts in the distal and collecting tubules. These casts are composed mainly of precipitated monoclonal light chains and are surrounded by multinucleated syncytial epithelial cells (giant cells). Dilation and atrophy of the renal tubules develop, and eventually the entire nephron becomes nonfunctional. Interstitial fibrosis and nephrocalcinosis may occur.[96]

The extent of cast formation correlates directly with the amount of free urinary light chains and with the severity of renal insufficiency. The actual mechanism of nephrotoxicity from Bence Jones proteinuria is unknown, and the role of the isoelectric point of Bence Jones protein is controversial. While λ-light chains are believed to be more nephrotoxic than κ-light chains, the type of Bence Jones protein probably has no significant effect.

Hypercalcemia, present in nearly 25% of patients initially, is one of the most frequent causes of renal insufficiency. The use of nonsteroidal anti-inflammatory agents also may promote the development of renal failure. Acute renal failure may in some instances be due to antibiotics such as aminoglycosides but is rarely caused by radiographic contrast medium, particularly if dehydration is avoided.[97] Hyperuricemia may contribute to the development of renal insufficiency. Amyloidosis occurs in 10–15% of patients with multiple myeloma and may produce renal insufficiency or nephrotic syndrome, or both.

Acquired Fanconi syndrome, characterized by dysfunction of the proximal renal tubules and resulting in glycosuria, phosphaturia, and aminoaciduria, occurs infrequently. The plasma cells and renal tubular cells of these patients often have crystalline cytoplasmic inclusions.[98]

Monoclonal light chains may be deposited in the renal glomerulus and produce renal insufficiency or the nephrotic syndrome.[99,100] This is commonly called light chain deposition disease. Typically, nodular glomerulosclerosis is present, and electron microscopy reveals finely granular, electron-dense deposits. Most deposits consist of κ-light chains.

Neurologic Involvement

Radiculopathy is the single most frequent neurologic complication and is usually thoracic or lumbosacral. Root pain results from compression of the nerve by the vertebral lesion or by the collapsed bone itself. Compression of the spinal cord, most often produced by myeloma arising in the marrow cavity of the vertebra and extending into the extradural space, has been found in ≤10% of patients with multiple myeloma. The usual manifestations are back pain with radicular features, weakness or paralysis of the lower extremities, and bowel or bladder incontinence.

Peripheral neuropathy is uncommon in multiple myeloma. When present, it almost always results from the associated development of amyloidosis. Intracranial plasmacytomas usually represent extensions of myelomatous lesions of the skull. Infrequently, leptomeningeal infiltration by myeloma cells may occur.[101,102]

Other Systemic Involvement

Hepatomegaly from plasma cell infiltration is uncommon. Ascites due to peritoneal involvement is rare and is usually a preterminal event. Myeloma may involve the stomach and may present as an infiltrative process or as an ulceration of a plasmacytoma.[103] Plasmacytomas of the ribs are common and present either as expanding bony lesions or as soft tissue masses. Pleural effusion is uncommon, and involvement of the pericardium is very rare.

Skeletal involvement occurs in three-fourths of patients initially and is manifested as lytic lesions or generalized osteoporosis, or both. Pathologic fractures often occur. ^{99m}Tc bone scans are inferior to conventional radiographs for the detection of myelomatous lesions. Computed tomography (CT)[104] and magnetic resonance imaging (MRI)[105] are more sensitive and may be helpful when skeletal pain is atypical and radiographs show no abnormalities. Foci of presumed tumor were seen in 65% of patients with T_2-weighted MRI scans.[106]

The incidence of infection is increased in multiple myeloma. *Diplococcus pneumoniae* and *Staphylococcus aureus* have been the most frequent pathogens; more recently, gram-negative organisms have accounted for more than one-half of all infections.[107] Impaired antibody response, deficient normal immunoglobulins, impaired serum opsonic activity, and neutrophil dysfunction all may contribute to the increased incidence of infections. The propensity to infection is further increased by neutropenia and chemotherapeutic depression of the immune response. Herpes zoster is common.

Bleeding episodes occur frequently in myeloma patients.[108] The etiology of this hemorrhagic tendency is multifactorial and may occur from impairment of platelet function, thrombocytopenia, abnormalities in fibrinogen function, and the presence of an acquired von Willebrand disease. Hypercoagulability and a tendency to thrombosis have also been observed.[108]

Differential Diagnosis

Bone pain, anemia, and renal insufficiency constitute a triad that is strongly suggestive of multiple myeloma. Minimal criteria for the diagnosis of multiple myeloma are a bone marrow with >10% plasma cells or a plasmacytoma plus one of the following: (1) M protein in the serum (usually at a level >3 g/dl); (2) M protein in the urine; and (3) lytic bone lesions. These findings must not be related to metastatic carcinoma, connective tissue diseases, chronic infection, or lymphoma. Patients with multiple myeloma must be differentiated from those with MGUS and SMM. The differentiation of multiple myeloma from MGUS has been discussed in this chapter.

Therapy

The patient's symptoms, physical findings, and all laboratory data must be considered before therapy is begun. If there are doubts about whether to begin chemotherapy, treatment

---

APPROACH TO THERAPY FOR MULTIPLE MYELOMA

Therapy should be delayed until the patient is symptomatic or has significant laboratory or radiographic abnormalities indicating an imminent complication. Patients with MGUS or SMM should not be treated. If there is a question in the physician's mind concerning treatment or no treatment, it is generally better to delay therapy and to re-evaluate the situation in 2–3 months. Indications for therapy are an increasing M protein in the serum or urine; the development of anemia, hypercalcemia, or renal insufficiency; or the presence of lytic bone lesions or extramedullary diseases.

Chemotherapy with either single or multiple alkylating agents leaves much to be desired. We recommend that newly diagnosed patients be considered for a prospective randomized trial. We use the current Eastern Cooperative Oncology Group (ECOG) study, in which patients are randomly assigned to following regimens: (1) VBMCP (vincristine, BCNU (carmustine), melphalan, cyclophosphamide, prednisone); (2) VBMCP plus alternating courses of IFN-α_2; or (3) VBMCP with substitution of high-dose cyclophosphamide for VBMCP in cycles 3 and 5. Therapy is continued for 2 years. More importantly, bone marrow and peripheral blood samples are obtained at intervals for plasma cell labeling index determination, ploidy studies, β_2-microglobulin and C-reactive protein determinations, evaluation of morphology and of T- and B-cell subsets, and gene rearrangement studies.

If the patient does not choose to enter a protocol study, the advantages and disadvantages of melphalan and prednisone versus a combination of alkylating agents (VBMCP) are discussed. If the patient has aggressive disease, we suggest VBMCP. Chemotherapy with either single or multiple alkylating agents is continued until the patient reaches a plateau state in which the M protein in the serum and urine is decreased to a stable level and

there is no other evidence of progressive disease. The role of IFN-α_2 in maintenance therapy is discussed with the patient. If IFN-α_2 is used for maintenance, the dosage must be altered so that side effects do not interfere with the quality of the plateau state. In the event of relapse, treatment with the original chemotherapeutic regimen is resumed, and approximately 80% of patients will respond.

If the relapse occurs during chemotherapy, we recommend VBAP (vincristine, BCNU [carmustine], doxorubicin [Adriamycin], prednisone) or a new phase II agent. If no response occurs, VAD (vincristine, Adriamycin, dexamethasone) or dexamethasone alone is advised. If the patient has pancytopenia or prefers not to take VAD or dexamethasone, we use methylprednisolone in a dosage of 2 g IV three times weekly for a minimum of 4 weeks. If a response occurs, administration of methylprednisolone is reduced to once or twice weekly.

We have developed a protocol with peripheral stem cell bone marrow transplantation for patients with previously untreated multiple myeloma ≤65 years of age. After approval by the third-party carrier, the patient is treated with three courses of VAD and given colony-stimulating factor-granulocyte/macrophage, followed by collection of autologous peripheral blood stem cells. The patient is then treated with conventional chemotherapy to the plateau state and followed with or without IFN-α_2 maintenance. At the time of progression of disease, the patient is given high-dose melphalan and total body irradiation, followed by infusion of the peripheral blood stem cells. Allogeneic bone marrow transplantation is considered for patients <50 years who have an HLA-matched sibling. A national prospective study comparing autologous stem cell transplantation and chemotherapy is being planned.

should be withheld and the patient re-evaluated in 2 or 3 months. There is no evidence that early treatment of multiple myeloma is advantageous. A prospective study in which 50 patients with asymptomatic stage I multiple myeloma were randomized to receive melphalan and prednisone or deferred therapy until disease progression showed no difference in response rate, response duration, or survival.[109]

Therapy in multiple myeloma has been attempted for more than a century. The second recorded patient, Thomas Alexander McBean, had obtained relief of pain by removal of 1 lb of blood and application of leeches. At relapse, a combination of steel and quinine produced another pain-free period of approximately 6 months.[47] Urethane has been used for the treatment of myeloma, and an occasional patient has had an objective response. However, a prospective randomized study comparing the use of urethane with that of Coca Cola syrup found no difference in median survival.[110] These historical vignettes emphasize the need for a rational approach to the treatment of multiple myeloma in which newer modalities are compared with conventional therapy in a randomized manner.

Chemotherapy is the preferred initial treatment for overt symptomatic multiple myeloma. Palliative radiation, in a dose of 2,000–3,000 cGy, should be limited to patients with disabling pain who have a well-defined focal process that has not responded to chemotherapy. In most cases, analgesics plus chemotherapy suffice to control the pain. Many patients will respond to acetaminophen with codeine, but if this is not sufficient, methadone in a dosage of 5–10 mg PO qid is usually adequate. Morphine sulfate may be necessary in some patients. This approach is preferred to local radiation because the pain associated with myeloma frequently recurs at another site, and local radiation does not benefit the patient with systemic disease. Although radiotherapy may be repeated, its use is ultimately limited by the development of leukopenia or thrombocytopenia as a result of reduction in the bone marrow reserve of many patients.

A major controversy in chemotherapy is whether to use melphalan and prednisone or a combination of alkylating agents. Oral administration of melphalan (L-phenylalanine mustard [Alkeran]) and prednisone is a standard form of therapy and produces objective response in 50–60% of patients. Melphalan may be given (0.15 mg/kg/day PO for 7 days; amounting to 8–10 mg/day for an average-size person), along with prednisone (20 mg tid) for the same period; the dose of melphalan should be calculated on the basis of the patient's ideal body weight. This dosage should be repeated every 6 weeks. Leukocyte and platelet counts must be determined at 3-week intervals after the start of therapy, and the melphalan dose should be altered until midcycle cytopenia occurs.

Many combinations of chemotherapeutic agents have been used because of the obvious shortcomings of melphalan and prednisone. The best known combination, the M2 protocol, includes melphalan, cyclophosphamide, BCNU (carmustine), vincristine, and prednisone. This regimen produced objective responses in 78% of 81 previously untreated patients and a median survival of 38 months.[111] The ABCM (doxorubicin [Adriamycin], BCNU [carmustine], cyclophosphamide, melphalan) regimen increased both the proportion of patients reaching the plateau phase and the survival in comparison with melphalan alone.[112] A meta-analysis of 18 published prospective trials comparing multiple alkylating agents demonstrated no difference in overall survival.[113] Patients with good-risk prognostic factors seemed to fare better when treated with melphalan and prednisone, whereas those with poor prognostic variables did better with combination chemotherapy. The controversy regarding melphalan/prednisone versus combination alkylating agents has not been resolved. Newer agents with greater specificity must be found before chemotherapy for multiple myeloma can be significantly improved.

The ideal duration of chemotherapy is unknown. Cessation of chemotherapy usually results in relapse, but continued chemotherapy may lead to the development of a myelodysplastic syndrome or acute leukemia. A randomized trial found no difference in survival between patients receiving continuing melphalan and prednisone and those receiving no maintenance therapy.[114] Chemotherapy should be continued until the patient reaches a plateau state, defined as a stable M-protein value in the serum and urine and no evidence of progression of myeloma.

Since the first report suggesting the possible role of alkylating agents in the development of acute leukemia and multiple myeloma,[115] many cases have been recognized.[116,117] The (British) Medical Research Council's first two trials demonstrated the development of myelodysplasia or acute leukemia in 12 of 648 patients with myeloma. The 5-year actuarial prevalence was 3% and the 8-year prevalence 10%.[118] The peak incidence of acute leukemia occurs 3.5–5 years after initiation of therapy; thus, patients who die within the first 2 years after the diagnosis of myeloma are not included in the "at-risk" group for leukemia. In one series, the actuarial risk of the development of acute leukemia within 50 months was 19.6%.[119]

The duration of melphalan therapy may have some role in the incidence of myelodysplastic syndrome and acute myeloid leukemia; however, a 1987 study found the most important risk factor to be the total amount of melphalan given during the most recent 3-year period.[118] Multiple myeloma and acute leukemia have been recognized simultaneously or within a few months of each other in several cases in which patients have not received radiation or chemotherapy. This simultaneous occurrence is probably fortuitous.[116] The occurrence of second malignancies after chemotherapy was recently reviewed.[120]

Interferon-α_2 (IFN-α_2) prolonged the remission of patients with multiple myeloma in a randomized study of 101 patients who had achieved an objective response or stable disease after chemotherapy with single or multiple alkylating agents and who then received either IFN-α_2 or no maintenance treatment. However, the survival rate was not significantly different in the two groups.[121] Similar results have been reported from Sweden[122] and from the Southwest Oncology Group.[123]

IFN-α_2 may be used in conjunction with alkylating agents in an effort to improve response and survival. A combination of alternating cycles of VBMCP (vincristine, BCNU [carmustine], melphalan, cyclophosphamide, prednisone) and IFN-α_2 produced an objective response in 80% of 54 previously untreated patients with multiple myeloma. Complete response, defined as disappearance of an M protein and normalization of the bone marrow, occurred in 30%. The median duration of survival was 42 months, and the estimated 5-year survival rate was 42%.[124] Österborg et al[125] reported a response rate of 68% for patients given melphalan, prednisone, and natural IFN-α (Finnferon alpha) and of 42% in a trial of 335 previously untreated patients with multiple myeloma who were given only melphalan/prednisone. Surprisingly, 85% of IgA myelomas and 71% of Bence Jones myelomas responded to the melphalan/IFN regimen compared with 48% and 27%, respectively, in the melphalan/prednisone regimen ($P = 0.001$). However, another study showed that a combination of IFN-α_2 with melphalan and prednisone did not provide any survival advantage as compared with only melphalan and prednisone.[126]

Refractory Multiple Myeloma

Cure rarely, if ever, occurs in multiple myeloma; thus, almost all patients who respond to chemotherapy will eventually have relapse if they do not die of another disease. In addition, approximately one-third of patients treated initially with chemotherapy will not achieve an objective response. The highest response rates reported for patients with multiple myeloma resistant to alkylating agents have been achieved with VAD (vincristine plus doxorubicin [Adriamycin] by continuous infusion for 4 days plus dexamethasone [40 mg/day] on days 1–4, 9–12, and 17–20 of each 28-day cycle). Actually, the use of dexamethasone usually must be reduced to days 1–4 for even-numbered cycles because of toxicity. Most of the activity of VAD is from dexamethasone.[127]

If the patient has pancytopenia or elects not to take VAD because of the need for an indwelling catheter and steroid toxicity, methylprednisolone is an alternative. When given at a dosage of 2 g IV 3 times weekly for a minimum of 4 weeks, methylprednisolone produced objective response in 25% of patients refractory to alkylating agents. If a response occurs, administration of methylprednisolone is reduced to once or twice weekly. The median duration of survival in patients who responded was 70 weeks.[128] There are fewer side effects from methylprednisolone than from dexamethasone. VBAP—a regimen consisting of a combination of vincristine (2 mg), carmustine (BCNU; 30 mg), and doxorubicin (Adriamycin; 30 mg) on day 1 and prednisone (60 mg/day) for 5 days, with the entire regimen repeated every 3–4 weeks—has produced some benefit in 30–40% of patients. The use of IFN has been disappointing in the treatment of patients with multiple myeloma refractory to alkylating agents.[129]

Bone Marrow Transplantation

Bone marrow transplantation is an alternative therapy for multiple myeloma. Syngeneic transplantation from an identical twin donor has been performed in eight patients. Two patients were alive and in complete remission at 24 and 34 months, and another one was alive without evidence of disease except for an M protein at 9 years.[130]

Allogeneic Bone Marrow Transplantation

Allogeneic bone marrow transplantation has been performed for multiple myeloma for several years. The major advantage is that the graft contains no tumor cells that can subsequently lead to a relapse. A graft-versus-tumor effect may also be operative. Unfortunately, the early mortality rate is 15–25% within 6 months. Furthermore, graft-versus-host disease is troublesome and relapse of multiple myeloma common. In addition, only 18% of our patients are <50 years old, and approximately one-third have a suitable HLA-matched sibling donor. Thus, only 5–10% of patients with multiple myeloma are eligible for an allogeneic bone marrow transplantation.

The European Bone Marrow Transplant Registry published the results of a heterogeneous population of 90 myeloma patients with allogeneic transplantation from 26 different European centers. The complete response rate was 43% and the actuarial survival rate 40% at 76 months. Only 12% (11 of 90) were in complete remission 24–68 months after transplantation.[131] In another report, of 20 patients who received high-dose busulfan and cyclophosphamide followed by bone marrow transplantation from HLA-identical donors, a complete response was obtained in 12 of 15 evaluable patients. Of the 20 patients, 8 were still alive, but 10 died of complications related to transplantation and 2 died of progressive multiple myeloma. Seven of the eight living patients were in complete remission 6–42 months after transplantation.[132]

Autologous Bone Marrow Transplantation

Autologous bone marrow transplantation is applicable for more patients because the age limit is higher (approximately 65 years) and a matched donor is unnecessary. Transplantation has two major limitations: (1) eradication of the malignant clone and (2) the removal of myeloma cells and their precursors from the bone marrow or peripheral blood. The transplant-related mortality rate is <10%.

Cunningham et al.[133] described 50 previously untreated patients with myeloma treated with vincristine, doxorubicin (Adriamycin), and methylprednisolone followed by melphalan (200 mg/m² IV) and an autologous bone marrow transplantation. The overall survival rate was 3.5 years. In a series of 11 patients, autologous marrow was purged with a combination of monoclonal antibodies in an attempt to remove myeloma cells. Seven patients obtained complete response after treatment with high-dose melphalan and total body irradiation. Three of the seven patients had recurrence of their M protein. Eight patients were alive 9–43 months after transplantation, and four were disease free at 12–29 months.[134]

Thirty-five previously untreated patients with aggressive myeloma received either VAD or vincristine, melphalan, cyclophosphamide, and prednisone. Forty-three percent had a complete response after high-dose melphalan with total body irradiation, followed by infusion of the unpurged autologous bone marrow. The 42-month survival rate was 81%. Best results were achieved in patients who had an initial low β_2-microglobulin level.[135] In another series, 53 newly diagnosed patients with multiple myeloma were treated with high-dose melphalan.[136] Twenty-five patients received a second course of high-dose melphalan and an autologous bone marrow transplant. The median duration of survival of the 53 patients was 37 months.

Fermand et al.[137] treated 43 patients who had multiple myeloma with high-dose chemotherapy, total body irradiation, and autologous peripheral blood stem cell infusion. Twenty-seven patients had refractory disease either in relapse or resistant to conventional therapy. The estimated 4-year survival rate was 73%. The risk of neoplastic cell reinfusion seemed minimal in their experience. Jagannath and Barlogie[138] used "total therapy" consisting of VAD, high-dose cyclophosphamide, etoposide, dexamethasone, cisplatin, cytarabine, and then melphalan (200 mg/m² IV). After recovery, the patients received a second injection of melphalan (200 mg/m² IV). Bone marrow and peripheral blood stem cells were infused after each of the two cycles of high-dose melphalan. The results of this study are not yet available. Previously treated patients may also respond to high-dose cyclophosphamide and melphalan, followed by autologous bone marrow transplantation and administration of peripheral blood stem cells. Satisfactory mobilization of peripheral blood stem cells occurred if the patient had received melphalan for <1 year and was given colony-stimulating factor-granulocyte/macrophage before collection of peripheral blood stem cells. Projected overall survival was about 85% at 1 year.[138]

Management of Complications

The presence of hypercalcemia, which occurs in one-fourth of patients with multiple myeloma, should be suspected if the patient exhibits anorexia, nausea, vomiting, polyuria, polydipsia, increased constipation, weakness, confusion, or stupor. Treatment is urgent because renal insufficiency commonly develops. Hydration, preferably with isotonic saline, is essential. In the elderly patient, caution must be exercised to avoid fluid overload. Furosemide (Lasix) may be useful, but adequate hydration must be maintained. In addition, prednisone in an initial dosage of 25 mg qid should be given, but the dosage must be reduced and the therapy discontinued as soon as possible. If these measures fail, bisphosphonates such as pamidronate disodium (Aredia) or etidronate disodium (Didronel), gallium nitrate, mithramycin, or calcitonin are effective. Because prolonged bed rest often contributes to hypercalcemia, patients with myeloma should be encouraged to be as active as possible.

Renal insufficiency occurs in one-half of patients with multiple myeloma at some time during its course and is associated with shortened survival. It usually develops insidiously but may progress rapidly; it is second only to infection as a leading cause of death. Maintenance of a high urine output (3 L/24 hr) is important in preventing renal failure in patients with Bence Jones proteinuria. Allopurinol is effective for the prevention and treatment of hyperuricemia. Prompt correction of dehydration is of utmost importance. Because metabolic acidosis is usually present, sodium bicarbonate should be administered orally and intravenously in the event of acute renal failure. Loop diuretics such as furosemide are given to maintain a high urine flow rate of 100 ml/hr. Hemodialysis is necessary in the event of renal failure. Plasmapheresis has been reported to be of benefit.[139] In a prospective randomized study by Johnson et al,[140] patients were treated either by forced diuresis and chemotherapy or by forced diuresis, chemotherapy, and plasmapheresis. Patients with severe myeloma cast formation or other irreversible changes were found to be unlikely to benefit from plasmapheresis.[140]

We identify the patient with renal insufficiency as accurately as possible by noninvasive techniques, vigorously treat precipitating factors, promptly initiate chemotherapy with regimens such as VAD, and begin hemodialysis therapy when required. If renal function does not improve and if renal failure is acute or subacute, plasmapheresis is instituted. Dialysis is continued in patients with irreversible renal failure. Renal transplantation for myeloma kidney has been shown to prolong survival.

Prompt and appropriate treatment of bacterial infections is necessary. In patients with recurrent gram-positive infections, penicillin given prophylactically has achieved good results. Intravenously administered γ-globulin is helpful but expensive. Although antibody response is impaired, pneumococcal vaccine and influenza immunization should be provided for all patients.

Skeletal lesions, manifested by pain and fracture, are a major problem. Patients should be encouraged to be as active as possible but to avoid trauma. Fixation of fractures or pending fractures of long bones with an intramedullary rod and methyl methacrylate has given good results. Patients in a prospective study receiving the bisphosphonate clodronate had fewer new lytic lesions and experienced less progression of vertebral fractures, decreased serum calcium and urinary calcium excretion, and less bone pain than did those in the placebo group.[141] Newer oral bisphosphonates are a promising area for the future.

The presence of an extradural plasmacytoma must be suspected in patients with severe back pain, the development of weakness or paresthesias of the lower extremities, or bowel or bladder dysfunction. MRI, CT, or myelography must be performed immediately. Dexamethasone and radiation therapy are usually helpful. If the neurologic deficit worsens, surgical decompression is necessary.

Symptomatic hyperviscosity should be treated by plasmapheresis (see the section Waldenström's Macroglobulinemia). Plasmapheresis relieves the symptoms and should be initiated regardless of the viscosity level if the patient is symptomatic. Anemia during the plateau phase often responds to the administration of erythropoietin.[142]

Prognosis and Staging

The duration of survival of patients with multiple myeloma ranges from a few months to many years; the median is 2.5–3 years. The most important prognostic factors are listed in Table 87–6. The uncorrected β_2-microglobulin level is one of the most powerful prognostic factors. The level of C-reactive protein correlates with the serum IL-6 level, which is a major growth factor for plasma cells. In a survival analysis of 162 patients with multiple myeloma, Bataille et al.[143] reported that

Table 87-6. Adverse Prognostic Factors in Multiple Myeloma

Elevated β_2-microglobulin level

High plasma cell labeling index

Elevated lactate dehydrogenase value

Elevated thymidine kinase level

High C-reactive protein value

Plasmablastic morphology

Hypoalbuminemia

Advanced age

Elevated creatinine concentration

Hypodiploidy, low RNA content of plasma cells

Anemia, hypercalcemia, thrombocytopenia

Primary resistance to therapy and progressive disease

Rapid response to therapy

the median duration of survival was 6 months in patients with high C-reactive protein and β_2-microglobulin levels and 54 months for those who had low levels of both. An elevated lactate dehydrogenase level is also a predictor of poor prognosis. In a study of 391 patients with multiple myeloma,[144] 11% had an elevated lactate dehydrogenase level. This was associated with aggressive disease, a high tumor mass, and a poor response to chemotherapy. The median duration of survival was 9 months. San Miguel et al.[145] reported that CD4 T-cell numbers of $<700 \times 10^6$/L were associated with a higher stage of myeloma and shorter survival.

In a study of 107 consecutive patients with newly diagnosed multiple myeloma at our clinic from 1984 to 1986 (which allows a 5-year follow-up), we found that age, plasma cell labeling index, and levels of thymidine kinase, β_2-microglobulin, serum albumin, and C-reactive protein were all significant univariate prognostic factors. Multivariate analysis revealed that only plasma cell labeling index and β_2-microglobulin level had independent prognostic significance. In patients <65 years, eight of nine (89%) who had a low plasma cell labeling index and a low β_2-microglobulin level were alive almost 6 years after starting chemotherapy.[146] It is important to recognize that identifiable subsets of patients with multiple myeloma will have long survivals. This must be taken into consideration when planning therapy. Patients who respond rapidly to chemotherapy and who have a high plasma cell labeling index have a shorter duration of remission and survival.[147]

The Durie-Salmon[148] clinical staging system is based on a combination of factors that correlate with myeloma cell mass (Table 87-7). The median duration of survival is approximately 5 years for patients with stage IA disease and 14.7 months for

Table 87-7. Clinical Staging System for Multiple Myeloma

Stage	Description
I	Low cell mass ($<0.6 \times 10^{12}$/m^2)
	All of the following:
	Hemoglobin value >10 g/dl; IgG <5 g/dl; IgA <3 g/dl; calcium value normal
	Urinary monoclonal protein value <4 g/24 hr
	No generalized lytic lesions
II	Intermediate (neither stage I nor stage III)
III	High cell mass ($>1.2 \times 10^{12}$/m^2)
	Any one of the following:
	Hemoglobin value <8.5 g/dl; IgG >7 g/dl; IgA >5 g/dl; calcium >12 mg/dl
	Urinary monoclonal protein >12 g/24 hr
	Advanced lytic bone lesions
A	Creatinine level <2 mg/dl
B	Creatinine level ≥2 mg/dl

those with stage IIIB disease. However, this clinical staging system is unreliable and has many shortcomings.

Future Directions

Enhancement of the multidrug-resistant gene is a factor in the resistance to VAD. This phenotype is characterized by the expression of glycoprotein P-170. The expression of P-glycoprotein was noted in 6% of patients with no prior chemotherapy but reached 100% in patients who received high doses of both vincristine and doxorubicin.[149] Response to verapamil, a calcium channel blocker that reverses the resistance to doxorubicin, has been disappointing.[150] A combination of cyclosporine and VAD produced a response in 10 of 21 patients with multiple myeloma refractory to chemotherapy.[151]

The use of a monoclonal antibody to IL-6, a potent growth factor for plasma cells, has produced temporary responses in advanced multiple myeloma and plasma cell leukemia.[152]

The capacity of colony-stimulating factor-granulocyte/macrophage or colony-stimulating factor-granulocyte to shorten the duration of neutropenia after high-dose chemotherapy may be helpful. These growth factors are also useful in the collection of hematopoietic peripheral blood stem cells for autologous stem cell rescue in patients with multiple myeloma after high-dose chemotherapy and total body irradiation.

It is essential to develop more sensitive techniques for the detection of residual myeloma with the advent of aggressive chemotherapy and radiation in an attempt to cure the disease. Even though an M protein is not detected in the serum and urine with immunofixation and the bone marrow contains no identifiable myeloma cells, patients frequently relapse with myeloma of the same isotype that was present initially. Billadeau et al.[153] used oligonucleotide primers to amplify regions of rearranged heavy chain alleles with the polymerase chain reaction from patients with multiple myeloma. These investigators were able to detect 1 myeloma cell in 100,000 cells. By using malignant cells to generate standard curves, the number of residual myeloma cells was determined.

Variant Forms of Multiple Myeloma

Smoldering Multiple Myeloma

The diagnosis of SMM depends on the presence of an M protein level >3 g/dl in the serum and of >10% atypical plasma cells in the bone marrow in the absence of anemia, renal insufficiency, and skeletal lesions.[154] Often a small amount of M protein is found in the urine, and the concentration of uninvolved immunoglobulins in the serum is decreased. The plasma cell labeling index is low. In some patients, symptomatic multiple myeloma has not developed for years. SMM must be recognized because these patients should not be treated unless progression occurs. Biologically, these patients have BMG, but it is difficult to accept this diagnosis initially when the M-protein level is >3 g/dl and the bone marrow contains >10% plasma cells. It has been reported that the presence of a lytic bone lesion, a serum M-protein level >3 g/dl, and Bence Jones protein (>50 mg/day) indicates a shorter median time to progression (10 months), compared with 61 months for patients without any of these factors.[155]

Plasma Cell Leukemia

Patients with plasma cell leukemia have >20% plasma cells in the peripheral blood and an absolute plasma cell count of ≥2,000/mm³. This disorder may be classified as primary when it is diagnosed in the leukemic phase or as secondary when there is leukemic transformation of a previously recognized multiple myeloma. Approximately 60% of patients have the primary form. Compared with patients who have the secondary form, those with primary plasma cell leukemia are younger and have a greater incidence of hepatosplenomegaly and lymphadenopathy, a higher platelet count, fewer lytic bone lesions, a smaller M-protein component, and a longer survival.[156]

Treatment of plasma cell leukemia is unsatisfactory, although melphalan and prednisone may produce remission in the primary form.[157] The response rate is higher with combination chemotherapy than with a single alkylating agent; unfortunately, the survival is still short. Secondary plasma cell leukemia rarely responds to chemotherapy because these patients have already received alkylating agents and are resistant to them.

Nonsecretory Myeloma

Patients with nonsecretory myeloma have no M protein in either the serum or the urine and constitute only 1% of patients with myeloma. For certainty of diagnosis, an M protein must be identified in the plasma cells by immunoperoxidase or immunofluorescence methods. As some patients show no evidence of an M protein within the cells, it is possible that no such protein is synthesized; >12 such patients have been described.[158] Survival similar to that of patients with multiple myeloma[159] or longer[160] has been reported.

Immunoglobulin D Myeloma

IgD myeloma differs sufficiently from IgG and IgA myelomas to warrant mention as a separate entity. The M protein is smaller, and Bence Jones proteinuria of the λ-type is more common. Plasma cell leukemia, amyloidosis, and extramedullary plasmacytomas are more frequent with IgD myeloma. A recent review showed the median survival of patients with IgD myeloma to be less than that of patients with IgG or IgA myeloma, but this may be because IgD myeloma often goes undiagnosed until later in its course.[161]

Osteosclerotic Myeloma

The major clinical feature in osteosclerotic myeloma (POEMS syndrome) is a chronic inflammatory demyelinating polyneuropathy causing predominantly motor disability.[162,163] Presumably, the plasma cells secrete a monoclonal immunoglobulin or other substance that is toxic to peripheral nerves and is also responsible for the endocrine abnormalities in this syndrome. Single or multiple osteosclerotic bone lesions are characteristic.[164] The acronym POEMS (*polyneuropathy, organomegaly, endocrinopathy, M protein, and skin changes*) describes the complete syndrome.[165] In contrast to patients with multiple myeloma, the hemoglobin level of POEMS syndrome patients is usually normal, and in some patients erythrocytosis occurs. Thrombocytosis is common. The bone marrow aspirate usually contains <5% plasma cells, and hypercalcemia and renal insufficiency rarely occur. Most patients have a λ-light chain type of M protein. The protein level of cerebrospinal fluid is elevated, and low velocities in motor nerve conduction are found. Hepatosplenomegaly, hyperpigmentation, gynecomastia, edema, digital clubbing, hypertrichosis, atrophic testes, and impotence may occur. Evidence of Castleman disease may be found.[166] The diagnosis is confirmed by the identification of monoclonal plasma cells at biopsy of an osteosclerotic lesion.

Among patients who have a single lesion or multiple osteolytic lesions in a limited area, more than one-half will obtain substantial improvement of the neuropathy from radiation treatment. If patients have widespread osteosclerotic lesions, chemotherapy with melphalan and prednisone may be helpful.

Solitary Plasmacytoma of Bone

The diagnosis of a solitary plasmacytoma (solitary myeloma) is based on histologic evidence of a tumor consisting of plasma cells and identical to those seen in multiple myeloma. In addition, complete skeletal radiographs must show no other lesions, the bone marrow aspirate must contain no evidence of multiple myeloma, and immunoelectrophoresis or immunofixation of the serum and concentrated urine should show no M protein. Some exceptions to the last-mentioned criterion occur. The most uncertain criterion for the diagnosis is the length of observation necessary before it can be ascertained that the disease will not become generalized. Disease-free survival at 10 years ranges from 15 to 25%,[167,168] and about 50% of patients with solitary plasmacytoma of bone survive 10 years.[168,169] There is no evidence that adjuvant chemotherapy influences the incidence of conversion to multiple myeloma.[170] Myeloma occurs within 3 years in two-thirds of those who have progression.[171] Treatment consists of irradiation within the range of 4,000–5,000 cGy. Electrophoresis, immunoelectrophoresis, and immunofixation of serum and urine are essential in following the course of a patient with an apparently solitary plasmacytoma.

Extramedullary Plasmacytoma

Extramedullary plasmacytoma is a plasma cell tumor that arises outside the bone marrow, most frequently in the upper respiratory tract, including the nasal cavity and sinuses, nasopharynx, and larynx.[172] Extramedullary plasmacytomas also may occur in the gastrointestinal tract, central nervous system, urinary bladder, thyroid, breast, testes, parotid gland, and lymph nodes.[173]

The diagnosis is based on the finding of a plasma cell tumor in an extramedullary site and the absence of multiple myeloma on bone marrow examination, radiography, and appropriate studies of blood and urine. Treatment consists of tumoricidal radiation. The prognosis for extramedullary plasmacytoma is favorable, although experience is limited. In one series, only 5 of 25 patients showed progression of disease, of whom 1 developed a single bony lesion, 2 progressed to multiple myeloma, and 2 developed multiple extramedullary plasmacytomas.[174] In another series, multiple myeloma developed in 4 of 13 patients with extramedullary plasmacytoma, after a mean of 13 months,[175] and in still another series, multiple myeloma developed in 3 of 13 patients.[176] In stage I disease, therapy may be curative.[177]

WALDENSTRÖM'S MACROGLOBULINEMIA (PRIMARY MACROGLOBULINEMIA)

Macroglobulinemia is the result of an uncontrolled proliferation of lymphocytes and plasma cells in which a large monoclonal IgM protein is produced. The condition bears similarities to multiple myeloma, lymphoma, and CLL.

Epidemiology and Etiology

Waldenström's macroglobulinemia is an uncommon disease; at the Mayo Clinic it is one-sixth as common as multiple myeloma. The disease is more frequent in certain families. For example, a father and two children had a monoclonal IgM protein and a lymphoproliferative process, and a third child had Waldenström's macroglobulinemia.[178] Macroglobulinemia also has been found in monozygotic twins.[179] There is only one reported case of Waldenström's macroglobulinemia occurring after radiotherapy; this occurred in a patient treated for ankylosing spondylitis.[180]

Chromosomal abnormalities are frequent, but no specific abnormality has been recognized. In one series, 17 of 19 patients had clonal chromosomal abnormalities, with chromosomes 10, 11, 12, 15, 20, and 21 most commonly involved.[181] In another report, clonal chromosomal changes were detected in 10 of 17 patients, with chromosomes 2, 4, and 5 most frequently involved.[182] Peripheral blood lymphocytes express CD9 (BA-2) and CD24 (BA-1) and stain with a single class of light chain. Reduction in CD4 T cells is common.[183]

Clinical Manifestations

In a series of 71 patients reported by Kyle and Garton,[18] the ages ranged from 30 to 89 years, with a median of 63 years and only 1% of patients <40 years; 62% were men. Weakness, fatigue, and bleeding (especially oozing from the oronasal area) are common presenting symptoms. Blurred or impaired vision, dyspnea, loss of weight, neurologic symptoms, recurrent infections, and congestive heart failure may occur. In contrast to multiple myeloma, bone pain is rare in macroglobulinemia. Physical findings include pallor, hepatosplenomegaly, and lymphadenopathy. Retinal lesions include hemorrhages, exudates, and venous congestion with vascular segmentation ("sausage" formation). Abnormalities in platelet adhesiveness, prothrombin time, and thromboplastin generation play a role in the pathogenesis of the bleeding tendency. Thrombocytopenia from the antiplatelet activity of monoclonal IgM has been reported.[184] Hyperviscosity may contribute to the bleeding diathesis as well. Sudden deafness, progressive spinal muscular atrophy, and multifocal leukoencephalopathy have been reported with macroglobulinemia.

A sensorimotor peripheral neuropathy is common. About one-half of patients with peripheral neuropathy display activity against myelin-associated glycoprotein.[185] Renal insufficiency is uncommon. Deposits of IgM on the endothelial aspect of the basement membrane may become large enough to occlude the capillary lumen. Nephrotic syndrome is rare and, when present, is usually due to amyloidosis. However, nonamyloid nephrotic syndrome has been reported.[186]

Pulmonary involvement is manifested by diffuse pulmonary infiltrates and isolated masses, which may be the major features of the disease, overshadowing the other features of macroglobulinemia.[187] Pleural effusion may occur.[188]

A hyperviscosity syndrome due to an increase of the whole blood viscosity may develop, most commonly manifested by bleeding. Chronic nasal bleeding and oozing from the gums are most frequent, but postsurgical or gastrointestinal bleeding may occur. Flame-shaped retinal hemorrhages are common, and papilledema may be seen. The patient may complain of blurring or a loss of vision. Neurologic symptoms include dizziness, headache, vertigo, nystagmus, hearing loss, ataxia, paresthesias, diplopia, somnolence, and coma. Hyperviscosity can precipitate or aggravate congestive heart failure.[189]

In the Mayo Clinic experience, 15 (29.4%) of 51 patients with Waldenström's macroglobulinemia had a serum viscosity of >4 centipoises (cP) (normal, ≤1.8). Unexpectedly, 5 of the 15 patients had no symptoms related to hyperviscosity. Nine patients had bleeding, and three complained of blurred vision.[18] Crawford et al.[190] reported that six of eight patients with a serum viscosity >5 cP had symptoms. None of their patients had symptoms if the level was <3 cP.

Although most patients have symptoms when the relative viscosity is >4 cP, the relationship between serum viscosity and clinical manifestations is not precise. We have seen a patient with a serum viscosity of 15 cP but no symptoms of the hyperviscosity syndrome.

Laboratory Evaluation

Almost all patients with Waldenström's macroglobulinemia have moderate to severe normocytic normochromic anemia, usually as a result of depression of erythropoiesis and excessive destruction or loss of red cells. A Coombs-positive hemolytic anemia is uncommon. The plasma volume is frequently increased, which reduces the hemoglobin and hematocrit levels independent of change in the red cell mass, resulting in a spurious reduction of hemoglobin and hematocrit. Rouleau formation is striking, and the erythrocyte sedimentation rate is usually greatly increased. Leukocyte and platelet counts are usually normal, but mild decreases may be present. Lymphocytosis or monocytosis is not uncommon, serum cholesterol concentration is often low, and hyperuricemia may be present.

The serum protein electrophoretic pattern of Waldenström's macroglobulinemia is characterized by a tall, narrow peak or dense band, almost always of γ-mobility. This pattern is indistinguishable from that of multiple myeloma. Of the IgM proteins, 75% have a κ-light chain. IgG and IgA levels are frequently reduced. Low-molecular-weight IgM (7S) is present and may account for a large part of the elevated IgM. A monoclonal light chain protein is present in the urine of 80% of cases.

The bone marrow aspirate is often hypocellular, but biopsy specimens are hypercellular and extensively infiltrated with lymphoid cells. The lymphocytes tend to be small, are often basophilic, and resemble plasma cells. The number of plasma cells is always greater than normal, and normal marrow elements are often decreased. The number of mast cells is increased, which can be helpful in differentiating macroglobulinemia from lymphoid myeloma or lymphoma. Lytic bone lesions occur in <5% of cases, but osteoporosis is not uncommon.

Differential Diagnosis

The combination of typical symptoms and physical findings with the presence of a high level (usually >3 g/dl) of monoclonal IgM protein and lymphoid-plasma cell infiltration of the bone marrow provides the diagnosis of Waldenström's macroglobulinemia. Multiple myeloma, CLL, and MGUS of the IgM type must be differentiated.

The presence of a monoclonal IgM protein level of <2 g/dl, the absence of anemia and organomegaly, mild lymphocytosis of the bone marrow, and the absence of symptoms are suggestive of MGUS of the IgM type. These patients should be followed without therapy. Almost 20% of patients with MGUS of the IgM type eventually develop Waldenström's macroglobulinemia, lymphoma, CLL, or amyloidosis.[18]

Patients with IgG or IgA multiple myeloma may have plasmacytoid lymphocytes in the bone marrow and no lytic bone lesions; thus, their disorder may be confused with macroglobulinemia.[191] However, some patients with anemia, oronasal bleeding, blurred vision, and large amounts of IgM protein in the serum may also have lytic bone lesions and plasma cells characteristic of myeloma in the bone marrow; they should be considered to have macroglobulinemia rather than IgM myeloma.[192,193]

Therapy

Patients with Waldenström's macroglobulinemia should not be treated unless they have anemia; constitutional symptoms, such as weakness, fatigue, night sweats, weight loss, or hyperviscosity; or significant hepatosplenomegaly or lymphadenopathy. Patients with MGUS should not be treated but should be followed carefully for the development of symptomatic disease.

Specific therapy should be directed against the abnormal proliferation of lymphocytes and plasma cells. Chlorambucil, in an initial dose of 6–8 mg/day, is a useful agent. The dosage of chlorambucil must be altered depending on the leukocyte and platelet counts. A combination of chlorambucil and prednisone for 1 week every 4–6 weeks is also efficacious.

Combination chemotherapy with BCNU, cyclophosphamide, vincristine, melphalan, and prednisone produced objective response in >80% of patients.[194] IFN-α$_2$ has been reported to be of benefit in macroglobulinemia.[8,195] Fludarabine has produced response in approximately one-half of patients resistant to alkylating agents.[196] 2-Chlorodeoxyadenosine produced a response in all nine previously untreated patients and in 40% of the 20 patients who had failed to respond to previous therapy. Only one of seven patients refractory to chemotherapy responded, as opposed to only one of four resistant to fludarabine.

Since acute leukemia may develop in patients treated with alkylating agents,[197] chemotherapy should be discontinued in patients who have been treated for 2 years in whom the disease has reached a plateau state. Patients should be followed closely and chemotherapy reinstituted when the disease progresses. Corticosteroids have been helpful in patients whose condition is resistant to alkylating agents.[198] The median duration of survival of the 71 patients with Waldenström's macroglobulinemia reported by Kyle and Garton[18] was 5 years.

Transfusions of packed red blood cells should be given for symptomatic anemia. However, one must be aware of the increased plasma volume in many patients with macroglobulinemia and of the spuriously low hemoglobin and hematocrit levels; consequently, transfusions should not be given simply on the basis of a low hemoglobin or hematocrit.

Symptomatic hyperviscosity should be treated with plasmapheresis by daily plasma exchanges of 3,000–4,000 ml, until the patient is asymptomatic. The plasma should be replaced with albumin rather than with plasma.

HEAVY CHAIN DISEASES

The heavy chain diseases (HCDs) are characterized by an M protein that constitutes a portion of the immunoglobulin heavy chain in the serum or urine, or both. These heavy chain proteins are devoid of light chains and represent a lymphoplasma cell proliferative process. Three major types have been identified: γ-, α-, and μ-HCD.[199,200]

γ-Heavy Chain Disease

The abnormal protein consists of a γ-chain with significant deletions of amino acids, including the C$_H$1 domain of the constant region. In one case of γ3-HCD, two deletions and a splice correction were identified.[201] The molecular weight range of the monomeric γ-chain is 27,000–49,000.

The median age of the patient with γ-HCD at onset is approximately 60 years, but it has been recognized in persons <20 years of age. Patients with γ-HCD usually present with a lymphoma-like illness, but the clinical findings are diverse and range from an aggressive lymphoproliferative process to an asymptomatic state.[202] Weakness, fatigue, and fever are common, but other features have been recognized, including parotid gland swelling, severe soreness of the tongue, nodular infiltration of the skin, extranodal non-Hodgkin lymphoma, autoimmune hemolytic anemia, idiopathic thrombocytopenia purpura, rapid enlargement of the thyroid gland, neutropenic from hypersplenism, and an atypical lymphoproliferative process. Hepatosplenomegaly and lymphadenopathy occur in about 60% of patients. Anemia is found in approximately 80% of patients initially and develops in nearly all eventually. Coombs-positive autoimmune hemolytic anemia has been reported in a number of instances. The serum protein electrophoretic pattern may show a broad-based band, more suggestive of a polyclonal than of a monoclonal protein. Some patients have hypogammaglobulinemia and a very small increase in the β-band. The M protein is most often found in the β-area, but its mobility ranges from α_1 to slow γ. The concentration of the M protein varies from trace levels to 9 g/dl. Most of the proteins are IgG_1. The urinary protein concentration ranges from a trace to 20 g/day but is usually <1 g/24 hr. Immunoelectrophoresis or immunofixation is necessary for the detection of the monoclonal γ-heavy chain without an associated light chain.

The bone marrow and lymph nodes contain increased numbers of plasma cells, lymphocytes, or plasmacytoid lymphocytes. The histologic pattern is variable and includes that of generalized or localized lymphoma or myeloma, but some cases show no evidence of a lymphoplasmacytic proliferative process.[203] Osteolytic lesions are rare.[204]

Therapy is indicated only for the symptomatic patient. Many different drugs have been used, including nitrogen mustard, melphalan, cyclophosphamide, prednisone, vincristine, vinblastine, procarbazine, azathioprine, chlorambucil, and doxorubicin. Radiotherapy also has been used. The results have been inconsistent and generally disappointing in that responses are often incomplete or brief. Therapy with cyclophosphamide, vincristine, and prednisone can be tried for patients with symptomatic γ-HCD and evidence of a progressive lymphoid-plasma cell proliferative process. If there is no response to this regimen, doxorubicin should be added.

The clinical course of γ-HCD varies from a rapidly progressive downhill course with death within a few weeks to the asymptomatic presence of a stable monoclonal heavy chain in the serum or urine or both. In one case the monoclonal γ-heavy chain disappeared without therapy, and in another it disappeared after recovery from a serious illness. The clinical course may be prolonged. One patient had had cervical lymphadenopathy for 22 years and hemolytic anemia for 17 years before the diagnosis of γ-HCD was made. The median duration of survival of 49 patients described in the literature was 12 months (range, 1–264 months).[202]

α-Heavy Chain Disease

First described in 1968, α-HCD has become the most frequently reported type of HCD.[205–208] The α-chain displays extensive internal deletions encompassing the V_H region and the entire first constant domain. α-mRNA contains inserted sequences of unknown origin.[209] Most patients are from the Mediterranean region and usually develop the disorder in the second or third decade of life. α-HCD has been found in children[210,211] as well as in the elderly.[212] About 60% of patients are male. Most commonly, gastrointestinal tract involvement occurs, characterized by severe malabsorption, loss of weight, diarrhea, and steatorrhea. Rarely, a patient has respiratory tract involvement when initially seen.

Plasma cell infiltration of the jejunal mucosa, with or without involvement of the mesenteric or para-aortic lymph nodes, is the most frequent pathologic feature.[213] α-HCD may involve the stomach,[214] and α-heavy chains may be found only in the gastric juice and in the cellular infiltrate.[215] The bone marrow is normal.

Immunoproliferative small intestinal disease is characterized by a dense, compact mucosal cellular infiltrate. In addition, a follicular lymphoid pattern may be seen. High-grade lymphoma may be present.[216] The disease is restricted to patients with small intestinal lesions that have the same pathologic pattern associated with α-HCD, but these patients do not synthesize α-heavy chains.[217]

Berger et al[218] found chromosomal abnormalities in three of four patients with α-HCD and a rearrangement of 14q32 in two of the four patients. Rearrangements of both heavy and light chain genes have been reported.[219]

The serum protein electrophoretic pattern is normal in one-half of cases; in the remainder, an unimpressive broad band may appear in the α_2- or β-regions. The diagnosis of α-HCD depends on the recognition of a monoclonal α-heavy chain that is not associated with a light chain.[220] The amount of α-chain in the urine is small, and Bence Jones proteinuria has never been reported. Nonsecretory α-HCD has been described.[221]

Most often α-HCD is progressive and fatal, but remissions and response to antibiotics have been recorded.[222] In patients who do not respond to antibiotics and in those with initially extensive intestinal or mesenteric involvement, combination chemotherapy with cyclophosphamide, doxorubicin (Adriamycin), vincristine, and prednisone should be given.[223]

μ-Heavy Chain Disease

A patient who had μ-HCD associated with CLL and amyloidosis was described in 1970. Seven patients were reported by Franklin[224] in 1975, all but one of whom had CLL. Twenty-eight cases of μ-HCD were recently reviewed.[225] The age range of patients was 15–80 years (median, 57.5 years); two patients were <40 years. One-half were male. Of 27 patients, 22 had an associated lymphoplasma cell proliferative disorder. Hepatosplenomegaly was found in most patients. Increased numbers of lymphocytes and plasma cells were seen in the marrow. More than one-half had vacuolated plasma cells. Lytic bone lesions were found in only 20% of patients. The serum protein electrophoretic pattern was usually normal, except for the presence of hypogammaglobulinemia; an abnormal band was found in only 8 of 19 cases. Bence Jones proteinuria has been recognized in two-thirds of patients, but μ-chain fragments in the urine are rare.

In addition to cases of μ-HCD associated with CLL, patients with μ-HCD have been found who exhibit features resembling lymphoma, multiple myeloma with amyloidosis, nonsecretory myeloma, and benign lymphadenopathy. A patient with systemic lupus erythematosus who had a monoclonal μ-heavy chain and an IgG κ-protein has been reported.[226] We observed an asymptomatic patient with BMG whose clinical course and laboratory findings remained stable for 3 years and who then developed an aggressive lymphoproliferative process ending in death 6 months later.[225] More cases of μ-HCD will be recognized and its clinical spectrum will broaden, as has happened with γ-HCD. The course of μ-HCD is variable, and the duration of survival ranges from a few months to many years. Treatment with corticosteroids and alkylating agents has produced some benefit.

CRYOGLOBULINEMIA

Cryoglobulins are proteins that precipitate when cooled and that dissolve when heated (Fig. 87-9). They are designated as idiopathic or essential when they are not associated with any recognizable disease. Cryoglobulinemia may be classified as type I (monoclonal), type II (mixed), and type III (polyclonal).

In type I, the cryoglobulin is most commonly characterized by IgM or IgG, but IgA and Bence Jones cryoglobulinemias have been reported. Unexpectedly, many patients with large amounts of monoclonal cryoglobulins are completely asymptomatic, whereas others with monoclonal cryoglobulins in the range of 1–2 g/dl experience pain, purpura, Raynaud's phenom-

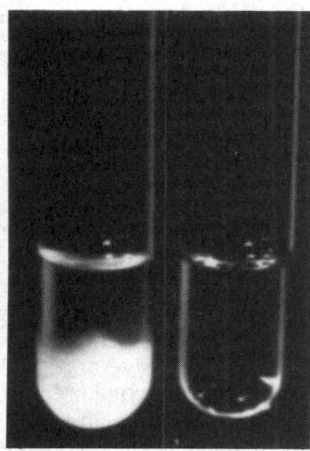

Fig. 87-9. Cryoglobulinemia. **(Left)** Precipitate formed at 1°C. **(Right)** Disappearance of precipitate on heating to 37°C. (From Kyle and Greipp,[243] with permission.)

enon, cyanosis, and even ulceration and sloughing of skin and subcutaneous tissues on exposure to the cold because the cryoglobulins precipitate at high temperatures. The temperature at which the cryoglobulin precipitates is much more important than the amount of protein.[227] Type I cryoglobulins are associated with macroglobulinemia, multiple myeloma, or MGUS. In this type of cryoglobulinemia, the protein itself probably undergoes a temperature-dependent conformational change, which results in polymerization at low temperatures.[228]

Type II (mixed) cryoglobulinemia typically is characterized by monoclonal IgM protein and polyclonal IgG, although monoclonal IgG or monoclonal IgA with polyclonal IgM may be seen as well. Serum electrophoresis usually shows a normal serum electrophoretic pattern or a diffuse hypergammaglobulinemia (polyclonal) pattern. The quantity of mixed cryoglobulin is usually <0.2 g/dl and may not reach maximal amounts for 7 days at 4°C. Patients with mixed cryoglobulinemia frequently have vasculitis, glomerulonephritis, or lymphoproliferative or chronic infectious processes. Purpura and polyarthralgias are common. Involvement of the joints is symmetric and is not migratory; chronic joint deformities rarely develop. Raynaud's phenomenon, necrosis of the skin, and neurologic involvement may be present.[229] Neurologic involvement consists mainly of sensorimotor peripheral neuropathy.[230] Renal involvement is common. In almost 80% of renal biopsy specimens, glomerular damage can be classified as diffuse, proliferative glomerulonephritis with thickening of the glomerular basement membrane.[231,232] The nephrotic syndrome may be seen.[233] However, renal insufficiency and the development of end-stage renal failure are infrequent. Hepatic dysfunction and serologic evidence of previous infection with hepatitis B virus are common in some series.[232,234] Hepatitis C virus is commonly associated with type II mixed cryoglobulinemia.[235,236] Infiltration of liver portal tracts with lymphocytes that stained with the same immunoglobulin type as those in the serum was noted in 9 of 12 cases of essential mixed cryoglobulinemia reported by Monteverde et al.[237] Non-Hodgkin lymphoma developed in 5 of 13 patients with type II essential mixed cryoglobulinemia.[238]

Oral corticosteroids are the most frequent therapeutic agents. If there is no response, cyclophosphamide, chlorambucil, or azathioprine may be useful. Plasmapheresis has been effective in some instances. IFN-α_2 is of considerable benefit. In one series of 21 patients with severe type II essential mixed cryoglobulinemia, it produced a complete remission in 11 patients, partial remission in 5, and minor responses in the remainder.[239] In another series of 22 cases, IFN-α_2 produced encouraging results.[240]

Type III (polyclonal) cryoglobulinemia, which is not associated with a monoclonal component, is found in many patients with infectious or inflammatory diseases.

PYROGLOBULINEMIA

Pyroglobulins are immunoglobulins that precipitate when heated to 56°C and that do not dissolve when cooled.[241] They resemble Bence Jones protein in that they precipitate when heated to 56–60°C, but they can be distinguished easily from the latter by immunoelectrophoresis with appropriate antisera. Pyroglobulins are usually of the IgG class, but IgM and IgA pyroglobulins have been reported.[242] In most cases, pyroglobulinemia is associated with multiple myeloma, but it may also occur in macroglobulinemia, lymphoproliferative syndromes, and other neoplastic diseases. Pyroglobulinemia is not associated with any symptoms and may be regarded as a laboratory curiosity.

REFERENCES

1. Howerton DA, Check IJ, Hunter RL: Densitometric quantitation of high resolution agarose gel protein electrophoresis. Am J Clin Pathol 85:213, 1986
2. Roberts RT: Usefulness of immunofixation electrophoresis in the clinical laboratory. Clin Lab Med 6:601, 1986
3. Keren DF, Warren JS, Lowe JB: Strategy to diagnose monoclonal gammopathies in serum: high-resolution electrophoresis, immunofixation, and κ/λ quantification. Clin Chem 34:2196, 1988
4. Riches PG, Sheldon J, Smith AM, Hobbs JR: Overestimation of monoclonal immunoglobulin by immunochemical methods. Ann Clin Biochem 28:253, 1991
5. Whicher JT, Hawkins L, Higginson J: Clinical applications of immunofixation: a more sensitive technique for the detection of Bence Jones protein. J Clin Pathol 33:779, 1980
6. Axelsson U, Bachmann R, Hällén J: Frequency of pathological proteins (M-components) in 6,995 sera from an adult population. Acta Med Scand 179: 235, 1966
7. Saleun JP, Vicariot M, Deroff P, Morin JF: Monoclonal gammopathies in the adult population of Finistère, France. J Clin Pathol 35:63, 1982
8. Kyle RA, Finkelstein S, Elveback LR, Kurland LT: Incidence of monoclonal proteins in a Minnesota community with a cluster of multiple myeloma. Blood 40:719, 1972
9. Crawford J, Eye MK, Cohen HJ: Evaluation of monoclonal gammopathies in the "well" elderly. Am J Med 82:39, 1987
10. Schechter GP, Shoff N, Chan C et al: Monoclonal gammopathies of undetermined significance in black and Caucasian veterans in a hospital population. p. 83. In Obrams GI, Potter M (eds): Epidemiology and Biology of Multiple Myeloma. Springer-Verlag, Berlin, 1991
11. Singh J, Dudley AW Jr, Kulig KA: Increased incidence of monoclonal gammopathy of undetermined significance in blacks and its age-related differences with whites on the basis of a study of 397 men and one woman in a hospital setting. J Lab Clin Med 116:785, 1990
12. Papadopoulos NM, Elin RJ, Wilson DM: Incidence of γ-globulin banding in a healthy population by high-resolution electrophoresis. Clin Chem 28:707, 1982
13. Sinclair D, Sheehan T, Parrott DMV, Stott DI: The incidence of monoclonal gammopathy in a population over 45 years old determined by isoelectric focusing. Br J Haematol 64:745, 1986
14. De Rossi G, De Sanctis G, Bottari B et al: Surface markers and cytotoxic activities of lymphocytes in monoclonal gammopathy of undetermined significance and untreated multiple myeloma: increased phytohemagglutinin-induced cellular cytotoxicity and inverted helper/suppressor cell ratio are features common to both diseases. Cancer Immunol Immunother 24:133, 1987
15. Van Den Akker TW, Tio-Gillen AP, Solleveld HA et al: The influence of T cells on homogeneous immunoglobulins in sera of athymic nude mice during aging. Scand J Immunol 28:359, 1988
16. Radl J: Benign monoclonal gammopathy is neither a "silent myeloma" nor a premyeloma. p. 127. In Radl J, van Camp B (eds): Proceedings of the Third EURAGE Symposium on Monoclonal Gammopathies: Clinical Significance and Basic Mechanisms. EURAGE Book Service, Leiden, Netherlands, 1991
17. Kyle RA: "Benign" monoclonal gammopathy—after 20 to 35 years of follow-up. Mayo Clin Proc 68:26, 1993

18. Kyle RA, Garton JP: The spectrum of IgM monoclonal gammopathy in 430 cases. Mayo Clin Proc 62:719, 1987
19. Axelsson U: A 20-year follow-up study of 64 subjects with M-components. Acta Med Scand 219:519, 1986
20. Manthorne LA, Dudley RW, Case DC Jr et al: A longitudinal study of monoclonal gammopathy of undetermined significance (MGUS), abstracted. Clin Res 36:414, 1988
21. Giraldo MP, Rubio-Félix D, Perella M et al: Gammapatías monoclonales de significado indeterminado: aspectos clínicos biológicos y evolutivos de 397 casos. Sangre (Barc) 36:377, 1991
22. Blade J, Lopez-Guillermo A, Rozman C et al: Malignant transformation and life expectancy in monoclonal gammopathy of undetermined significance. Br J Haematol 81:391, 1992
23. Peltonen S, Wasastjerna C, Wager O: Clinical features of patients with a serum M component. Acta Med Scand 203:257, 1978
24. Lindström FD, Dahlström U: Multiple myeloma or benign monoclonal gammopathy? A study of differential diagnostic criteria in 44 cases. Clin Immunol Immunopathol 10:168, 1978
25. Greipp PR, Witzig TE, Gonchoroff NJ et al: Immunofluorescence labeling indices in myeloma and related monoclonal gammopathies. Mayo Clin Proc 62:969, 1987
26. Witzig TE, Gonchoroff NJ, Katzmann JA et al: Peripheral blood B cell labeling indices are a measure of disease activity in patients with monoclonal gammopathies. J Clin Oncol 6:1041, 1988
27. Witzig TE, Kyle RA, Greipp PR: Circulating peripheral blood plasma cells in multiple myeloma. Curr Top Microbiol Immunol 182:195, 1992
28. Billadeau D, Quam L, Thomas W et al: Detection and quantitation of malignant cells in the peripheral blood of multiple myeloma patients. Blood 80:1818, 1992
29. Sonneveld P, Durie BGM, Lokhorst HM et al: Analysis of multidrug-resistance (MDR-1) glycoprotein and CD56 expression to separate monoclonal gammopathy from multiple myeloma. Br J Haematol 83:63, 1993
30. Schnur MJ, Appel GB, Bilezikian JP: Primary hyperparathyroidism and benign monoclonal gammopathy. Arch Intern Med 137:1201, 1977
31. Mundis RJ, Kyle RA: Primary hyperparathyroidism and monoclonal gammopathy of undetermined significance. Am J Clin Pathol 77:619, 1982
32. Alexanian R: Monoclonal gammopathy in lymphoma. Arch Intern Med 135:62, 1975
33. Noel P, Kyle RA: Monoclonal proteins in chronic lymphocytic leukemia. Am J Clin Pathol 87:385, 1987
34. Kyle RA, Lust JA: Monoclonal gammopathies of undetermined significance. Semin Hematol 26:176, 1989
35. Zawadzki ZA, Benedek TG: Rheumatoid arthritis, dysproteinemic arthropathy, and paraproteinemia. Arthritis Rheum 12:555, 1969
36. Hurst NP, Smith W, Henderson DR: IgG (kappa) paraproteinaemia and arthritis. Br J Rheumatol 26:142, 1987
37. Kelly JJ Jr, Kyle RA, O'Brien PC, Dyck PJ: Prevalence of monoclonal protein in peripheral neuropathy. Neurology 31:1480, 1981
38. Latov N, Sherman WH, Nemni R et al: Plasma-cell dyscrasia and peripheral neuropathy with a monoclonal antibody to peripheral-nerve myelin. N Engl J Med 303:618, 1980
39. Kelly JJ Jr, Kyle RA, Latov N: Polyneuropathies Associated With Plasma Cell Dyscrasias. Martinus Nijhoff Publishing, Boston, 1987
40. Kyle RA, Dyck PJ: Neuropathy associated with the monoclonal gammopathies. p. 1275. In Dyck PJ, Thomas PK, Griffin JW et al (eds): Peripheral Neuropathy. 3rd Ed. WB Saunders, Philadelphia, 1993
41. Merlini G, Farhangi M, Osserman EF: Monoclonal immunoglobulins with antibody activity in myeloma, macroglobulinemia and related plasma cell dyscrasias. Semin Oncol 13:350, 1986
42. Annesley TM, Burritt MF, Kyle RA: Artifactual hypercalcemia in multiple myeloma. Mayo Clin Proc 57:572, 1982
43. Martin NF, Kincaid MC, Stark WJ et al: Ocular copper deposition associated with pulmonary carcinoma, IgG monoclonal gammopathy and hypercupremia: a clinicopathologic correlation. Ophthalmology 90:110, 1983
44. Kyle RA, Robinson RA, Katzmann JA: The clinical aspects of biclonal gammopathies: review of 57 cases. Am J Med 71:999, 1981
45. Maruta T, Fujita H, Harano H et al: Triclonal gammopathy (IgAκ, IgGκ, and IgMκ) in a patient with plasmacytoid lymphoma derived from a monoclonal origin. Am J Hematol 42:212, 1993
46. Kyle RA, Greipp PR: "Idiopathic" Bence Jones proteinuria: long-term follow-up in seven patients. N Engl J Med 306:564, 1982
47. Kyle RA: History of multiple myeloma. p. 325. In Wiernik PH, Canellos GP, Kyle RA, Schiffer CA (eds): Neoplastic Diseases of the Blood. 2nd Ed. Churchill Livingstone, New York, 1991
48. Turesson I, Zettervall O, Cuzick J et al: Comparison of trends in the incidence of multiple myeloma in Malmö, Sweden, and other countries, 1950–1979. N Engl J Med 310:421, 1984
49. Linos A, Kyle RA, O'Fallon WM, Kurland LT: Incidence and secular trend of multiple myeloma in Olmsted County, Minnesota: 1965–1977. J Natl Cancer Inst 66:17, 1981
50. Kyle RA, Beard CM, O'Fallon WM, Kurland LT: Incidence of multiple myeloma in Olmsted County, Minnesota, 1978 to 1990 with a review of the trends since 1945, abstracted. Blood, suppl. 80:119a, 1992
51. Hansen NE, Karle H, Olsen JH: Trends in the incidence of multiple myeloma in Denmark 1943–1982: a study of 5500 patients. Eur J Haematol 42:72, 1989
52. Bernstein SC, Perez-Atayde AR, Weinstein HJ: Multiple myeloma in a child. Cancer 56:2143, 1985
53. Latreille J, Barlogie B, Johnston D et al: Ploidy and proliferative characteristics in monoclonal gammopathies. Blood 59:43, 1982
54. Tienhaara A, Pelliniemi TT: Flow cytometric DNA analysis and clinical correlations in multiple myeloma. Am J Clin Pathol 97:322, 1992
55. Dewald GW, Kyle RA, Hicks GA, Greipp PR: The clinical significance of cytogenetic studies in 100 patients with multiple myeloma, plasma cell leukemia, or amyloidosis. Blood 66:380, 1985
56. Gould J, Alexanian R, Goodacre A et al: Plasma cell karyotype in multiple myeloma. Blood 71:453, 1988
57. Philip P: Chromosomes of monoclonal gammopathies. Cancer Genet Cytogenet 2:79, 1980
58. Gutensohn K, Weh HJ, Walter TA, Hossfeld DK: Cytogenetics in multiple myeloma and plasma cell leukemia: simultaneous cytogenetic and cytologic studies in 51 patients. Ann Hematol 65:88, 1992
59. Meltzer P, Shadle K, Durie B: Somatic mutation alters a critical region of the c-myc gene in multiple myeloma, abstracted. Blood, suppl. 1. 70:282, 1987
60. Selvanayagam P, Goodacre A, Strong L et al: Alterations of bcl-1 oncogene in human multiple myeloma, abstracted. Proc Am Assoc Cancer Res 28:19, 1987
61. Selvanayagam P, Blick M, Narni F et al: Alteration and abnormal expression of the c-*myc* oncogene in human multiple myeloma. Blood 71:30, 1988
62. Tsuchiya H, Epstein J, Selvanayagam P et al: Correlated flow cytometric analysis of H-ras p21 and nuclear DNA in multiple myeloma. Blood 72:796, 1988
63. Portier M, Molès J-P, Mazars G-R et al: p53 and *RAS* gene mutations in multiple myeloma. Oncogene 7:2539, 1992
64. Durie BGM, Mason DY, Giles F et al: Expression of the BCL-2 oncogene protein in multiple myeloma, abstracted. Blood, suppl 1. 76:347a, 1990
65. Ladanyi M, Wang S, Niesvizky R et al: Proto-oncogene analysis in multiple myeloma. Am J Pathol 141:949, 1992
66. Preudhomme C, Facon T, Zandecki M et al: Rare occurrence of P53 gene mutations in multiple myeloma. Br J Haematol 81:440, 1992
67. Neri A, Baldini L, Trecca D et al: p53 Gene mutations in multiple myeloma are associated with advanced forms of malignancy. Blood 81:128, 1993
68. Barlogie B, Epstein J, Selvanayagam P, Alexanian R: Plasma cell myeloma—new biological insights and advances in therapy. Blood 73:865, 1989
69. Barker HF, Hamilton MS, Ball J et al: Expression of adhesion molecules LFA-3 and N-CAM on normal and malignant human plasma cells. Br J Haematol 81:331, 1992
70. Epstein J: Myeloma phenotype: clues to disease origin and manifestation. Hematol Oncol Clin North Am 6:249, Apr 1992
71. Epstein J, Xiao H, He X-Y: Markers of multiple hematopoietic-cell lineages in multiple myeloma. N Engl J Med 322:664, 1990
72. Caligaris-Cappio F, Gregoretti MG, Ghia P, Bergui L: In vitro growth of human multiple myeloma: implications for biology and therapy. Hematol Oncol Clin North Am 6:257, Apr 1992
73. Bergui L, Schena M, Gaidano G et al: Interleukin 3 and interleukin 6 synergistically promote the proliferation and differentiation of malignant plasma cell precursors in multiple myeloma. J Exp Med 170:613, 1989
74. Kawano M, Yamamoto I, Iwato K et al: Interleukin-1 beta rather than lymphotoxin as the major bone resorbing activity in human multiple myeloma. Blood 73:1646, 1989
75. Hirano T, Yasukawa K, Harada H et al: Complementary DNA for a novel human interleukin (BSF-2) that induces B lymphocytes to produce immunoglobulin. Nature 324:73, 1986
76. Kishimoto T: Factors affecting B-cell growth and differentiation. Annu Rev Immunol 3:133, 1985
77. Rabin EM, Mond JJ, Ohara J, Paul WE: B cell stimulatory factor 1 (BSF-1) prepares resting B cells to enter S phase in response to anti-IgM and lipopolysaccharide. J Exp Med 164:517, 1986
78. Kawano M, Hirano T, Matsuda T et al: Autocrine generation and requirement of BSF-2/IL-6 for human multiple myelomas. Nature 332:83, 1988
79. Bataille R, Jourdan M, Zhang X-G, Klein B: Serum levels of interleukin 6, a

potent myeloma cell growth factor, as a reflection of disease severity in plasma cell dyscrasias. J Clin Invest 84:2008, 1989

80. Zhang XG, Bataille R, Widjenes J, Klein B: Interleukin-6 dependence of advanced malignant plasma cell dyscrasias. Cancer 69:1373, 1992

81. Klein B, Bataille R: The critical role of IL-6 in human multiple myeloma. p. 79. In Radl J, van Camp B (eds): Proceedings of the Third EURAGE Symposium on Monoclonal Gammopathies: Clinical Significance and Basic Mechanisms. EURAGE Book Service, Leiden, Netherlands, 1991

82. Hirano, T, Suematsu S, Matsusaka T et al: The role of interleukin 6 in plasmacytomagenesis. Ciba Found Symp 167:188, 1992

83. Ichimaru M, Ishimaru T, Mikami M, Matsunaga M: Multiple myeloma among atomic bomb survivors in Hiroshima and Nagasaki, 1950–76: relationship to radiation dose absorbed by marrow. J Natl Cancer Inst 69:323, 1982

84. Smith PG, Douglas AJ: Mortality of workers at the Sellafield plant of British Nuclear Fuels. BMJ 293:845, 1986

85. Darby SC, Doll R, Gill SK, Smith PG: Long term mortality after a single treatment course with X-rays in patients treated for ankylosing spondylitis. Br J Cancer 55:179, 1987

86. Aksoy M, Erdem S, Dinçol G et al: Clinical observations showing the role of some factors in the etiology of multiple myeloma: a study in 7 patients. Acta Haematol 71:116, 1984

87. Kagan E, Jacobson RJ: Lymphoid and plasma cell malignancies: asbestos-related disorders of long latency. Am J Clin Pathol 80:14, 1983

88. Riedel DA, Pottern LM: The epidemiology of multiple myeloma. Hematol Oncol Clin North Am 6:225, 1992

89. Cuzick J, De Stavola B: Multiple myeloma—a case-control study. Br J Cancer 57:516, 1988

90. Cohen HJ, Bernstein RJ, Grufferman S: Role of immune stimulation in the etiology of multiple myeloma: a case control study. Am J Hematol 24:119, 1987

91. Maldonado JE, Kyle RA: Familial myeloma: report of eight families and a study of serum proteins in their relatives. Am J Med 57:875, 1974

92. Judson IR, Wiltshaw E, Newland AC: Multiple myeloma in a pair of monozygotic twins: the first reported case. Br J Haematol 60:551, 1985

93. Grosbois B, Gueguen M, Fauchet R et al: Multiple myeloma in two brothers. An immunochemical and immunogenetic familial study. Cancer 58:2417, 1986

94. Bourguet CC, Grufferman S, Delzell E et al: Multiple myeloma and family history of cancer: a case-control study. Cancer 56:2133, 1985

95. Buss DH, Prichard RW, Cooper MR: Plasma cell dyscrasias. Hematol Oncol Clin North Am 2:603, 1988

96. Kyle RA: Monoclonal gammopathies and the kidney. Annu Rev Med 40:53, 1989

97. McCarthy CS, Becker JA: Multiple myeloma and contrast media. Radiology 183:519, 1992

98. Chan KW, Ho FCS, Chan MK: Adult Fanconi syndrome in κ light chain myeloma. Arch Pathol Lab Med 111:139, 1987

99. Alpers CE, Tu W-H, Hopper J Jr, Biava CG: Single light chain subclass (kappa chain) immunoglobulin deposition in glomerulonephritis. Hum Pathol 16:294, 1985

100. Heilman RL, Velosa JA, Holley KE et al: Long-term follow-up and response to chemotherapy in patients with light-chain deposition disease. Am J Kidney Dis 20:34, 1992

101. Brenner B, Nagler A, Viener A et al: Partial response of meningeal myeloma to craniospinal radiotherapy. Scand J Haematol 37:360, 1986

102. Leifer D, Grabowski T, Simonian N, Demirjian ZN: Leptomeningeal myelomatosis presenting with mental status changes and other neurologic findings. Cancer 70:1899, 1992

103. Gutnik SH, Bacon BR: Endoscopic appearance of gastric myeloma. Gastrointest Endosc 31:263, 1985

104. Kyle RA, Schreiman JS, McLeod RA, Beabout JW: Computed tomography in diagnosis and management of multiple myeloma and its variants. Arch Intern Med 145:1451, 1985

105. Daffner RH, Lupetin AR, Dash N et al: MRI in the detection of malignant infiltration of bone marrow. AJR 146:353, 1986

106. Libshitz HI, Malthouse SR, Cunningham D et al: Multiple myeloma: appearance at MR imaging. Radiology 182:833, 1992

107. Shaikh BS, Lombard RM, Appelbaum PC, Bentz MS: Changing patterns of infections in patients with multiple myeloma. Oncology 39:78, 1982

108. Glaspy JA: Disturbances in hemostasis in patients with B-cell malignancies. Semin Thromb Hemost 18:440, 1992

109. Hjorth M, Hellquist L, Holmberg E et al: Initial versus deferred melphalan-prednisone therapy for asymptomatic multiple myeloma stage I—a randomized study. Eur J Haematol 50:95, 1993

110. Holland JF, Hosley H, Scharlau C et al: A controlled trial of urethane treatment in multiple myeloma. Blood 27:328, 1966

111. Lee BJ, Lake-Lewin D, Meyers JE: Intensive treatment of multiple myeloma. p. 61. In Wiernik PH (ed): Controversies in Oncology. John Wiley & Sons, New York, 1982

112. MacLennan ICM, Chapman C, Dunn J, Kelly K: Combined chemotherapy with ABCM versus melphalan for treatment of myelomatosis. Lancet 339:200, 1992

113. Gregory WM, Richards MA, Malpas JS: Combination chemotherapy versus melphalan and prednisolone in the treatment of multiple myeloma: an overview of published trials. J Clin Oncol 10:334, 1992

114. Belch A, Shelley W, Bergsagel D et al: A randomized trial of maintenance versus no maintenance melphalan and prednisone in responding multiple myeloma patients. Br J Cancer 57:94, 1988

115. Kyle RA, Pierre RV, Bayrd ED: Multiple myeloma and acute myelomonocytic leukemia: report of four cases possibly related to melphalan. N Engl J Med 283:1121, 1970

116. Rosner F, Grünwald HW: Simultaneous occurrence of multiple myeloma and acute myeloblastic leukemia: fact or myth? Am J Med 76:891, 1984

117. Rosner F, Grünwald HW: Multiple myeloma and Waldenström's macroglobulinemia terminating in acute leukemia: review with emphasis on karyotypic and ultrastructural abnormalities. NY State J Med 80:558, 1980

118. Cuzick J, Erskine S, Edelman D, Galton DAG: A comparison of the incidence of the myelodysplastic syndrome and acute myeloid leukaemia following melphalan and cyclophosphamide treatment for myelomatosis: a report to the Medical Research Council's working party on leukaemia in adults. Br J Cancer 55:523, 1987

119. Bergsagel DE, Bailey AJ, Langley GR et al: The incidence of acute leukemia in myeloma patients treated with alkylating agents, abstracted. p. 60. In Lecture and Symposium Abstracts. Joint Meeting of the Eighteenth Congress of the International Society of Hematology and Sixteenth Congress of the International Society of Blood Transfusion, Montreal, Quebec, Canada, August 16–22, 1980

120. Kyle RA, Gertz MA: Second malignancies after chemotherapy. p. 689. In Perry MC (ed): The Chemotherapy Source Book. Williams & Wilkins, Baltimore, 1992

121. Avvisati G, Mandelli F: The role of interferon-α in the management of myelomatosis. Hematol Oncol Clin North Am 6:395, 1992

122. Westin J, Rödger S, Turesson I: Interferon alpha-2b as maintenance therapy in multiple myeloma: effect on plateau phase duration and survival, abstracted. p. 71. In the Twenty-fourth Congress of the International Society of Haematology: Book of Abstracts. Blackwell Scientific Publications, London, United Kingdom, 1992

123. Salmon SE, Crowley J: Impact of glucocorticoids (GC) and interferon (IFN) on outcome in multiple myeloma, abstracted. Proc Annu Meet Am Soc Clin Oncol 11:316, 1992

124. Oken MM, Kyle RA, Greipp PR et al: Possible survival benefit with chemotherapy plus interferon (rIFN$_\alpha$2) in the treatment of multiple myeloma, abstracted. Proc Annu Meet Am Soc Clin Oncol 11:358, 1992

125. Österborg A, Björkholm M, Björeman M et al: Natural interferon-α in combination with melphalan/prednisone versus melphalan/prednisone in the treatment of multiple myeloma stages II and III: a randomized study from the Myeloma Group of Central Sweden. Blood 81:1428, 1993

126. Cooper MR, Dear K, McIntyre OR et al: A randomized clinical trial comparing melphalan/prednisone with or without interferon alfa-2b in newly diagnosed patients with multiple myeloma: a Cancer and Leukemia Group B study. J Clin Oncol 11:155, 1993

127. Alexanian R, Dimopoulos MA, Delasalle K, Barlogie B: Primary dexamethasone treatment of multiple myeloma. Blood 80:887, 1992

128. Garton J, Kyle R, Gertz M et al: Treatment of refractory multiple myeloma with high dose intravenous methylprednisolone, abstracted. Proc Annu Meet Am Soc Clin Oncol 11:358, 1992

129. Quesada JR, Gutterman JU: Annotation: alpha interferons in B-cell neoplasms. Br J Haematol 64:639, 1986

130. Buckner CD, Fefer A, Bensinger WI et al: Marrow transplantation for malignant plasma cell disorders: summary of the Seattle experience. Eur J Haematol, suppl. 51. 43:186, 1989

131. Gahrton G, Tura S, Ljungman P et al: Allogeneic bone marrow transplantation in multiple myeloma. N Engl J Med 325:1267, 1991

132. Bensinger WI, Buckner CD, Clift RA et al: Phase I study of busulfan and cyclophosphamide in preparation for allogeneic marrow transplant for patients with multiple myeloma. J Clin Oncol 10:1492, 1992

133. Cunningham D, Milan S, Millar B et al: Strategies for the management of myeloma with conventional chemotherapy and high dose melphalan (HDM) and ABMT-possible roles for verapamil and maintenance interferon. p. 133. In Pileri A, Boccadoro M (eds): Multiple Myeloma from Biology to Therapy: Abstracts Book of the Third International Workshop, Torino, Italy, April 9–12, 1991

134. Anderson KC, Barut BA, Ritz J et al: Monoclonal antibody-purged autologous bone marrow transplantation therapy for multiple myeloma. Blood 77:712, 1991

135. Attal M, Huguet F, Schlaifer D et al: Intensive combined therapy for previously untreated aggressive myeloma. Blood 79:1130, 1992

136. Harousseau JL, Milpied N, Laporte JP et al: Double-intensive therapy in high-risk multiple myeloma. Blood 79:2827, 1992

137. Fermand JP, Chevret S, Levy Y et al: The role of autologous blood stem cells in support of high-dose therapy for multiple myeloma. Hematol Oncol Clin North Am 6:451, 1992

138. Jagannath S, Barlogie B: Autologous bone marrow transplantation for multiple myeloma. Hematol Oncol Clin North Am 6:437, 1992

139. Pasquali S, Cagnoli L, Rovinetti C et al: Plasma exchange therapy in rapidly progressive renal failure due to multiple myeloma. Int J Artif Organs, suppl. 2. 8:27, 1985

140. Johnson WJ, Kyle RA, Pineda AA et al: Treatment of renal failure associated with multiple myeloma: plasmapheresis, hemodialysis, and chemotherapy. Arch Intern Med 150:863, 1990

141. Lahtinen R, Laakso M, Palva I et al: Randomised, placebo-controlled multi-centre trial of clodronate in multiple myeloma. Lancet 340:1049, 1992

142. Garton JP, Kyle RA, Gertz MA et al: A double-blind placebo controlled study of the role of recombinant human erythropoietin (r-HuEPO) for the anemia of multiple myeloma, abstracted. Blood, suppl. 80:84a, 1992

143. Bataille R, Boccadoro M, Klein B et al: C-reactive protein and β_2-microglobulin produce a simple and powerful myeloma staging system. Blood 80:733, 1992

144. Dimopoulos MA, Barlogie B, Smith TL, Alexanian R: High serum lactate dehydrogenase level as a marker for drug resistance and short survival in multiple myeloma. Ann Intern Med 115:931, 1991

145. San Miguel JF, González M, Gascón A et al: Immunophenotypic heterogeneity of multiple myeloma: influence on the biology and clinical course of the disease. Br J Haematol 77:185, 1991

146. Greipp PR, Lust JA, O'Fallon WM et al: Plasma cell labeling index and beta$_2$-microglobulin predict survival independent of thymidine kinase and C-reactive protein in multiple myeloma. Blood 81:3382, 1993

147. Boccadoro M, Marmont F, Tribalto M et al: Early responder myeloma: kinetic studies identify a patient subgroup characterized by very poor prognosis. J Clin Oncol 7:119, 1989

148. Durie BGM, Salmon SE: A clinical staging system for multiple myeloma: correlation of measured myeloma cell mass with presenting clinical features, response to treatment, and survival. Cancer 36:842, 1975

149. Grogan TM, Spier CM, Salmon SE et al: P-glycoprotein expression in human plasma cell myeloma: correlation with prior chemotherapy. Blood 81:490, 1993

150. Salmon SE, Dalton WS, Grogan TM et al: Multidrug-resistant myeloma: laboratory and clinical effects of verapamil as a chemosensitizer. Blood 78:44, 1991

151. Sonneveld P, Durie BGM, Lokhorst HM et al: Modulation of multidrug-resistant multiple myeloma by cyclosporin. Lancet 340:255, 1992

152. Klein B, Wijdenes J, Zhang X-G et al: Murine anti-interleukin-6 monoclonal antibody therapy for a patient with plasma cell leukemia. Blood 78:1198, 1991

153. Billadeau D, Blackstadt M, Greipp P et al: Analysis of B-lymphoid malignancies using allele-specific polymerase chain reaction: a technique for sequential quantitation of residual disease. Blood 78:3021, 1991

154. Kyle RA, Greipp PR; Smoldering multiple myeloma. N Engl J Med 302:1347, 1980

155. Dimopoulos MA, Moulopoulos A, Smith T et al: Risk of disease progression in asymptomatic multiple myeloma. Am J Med 94:57, 1993

156. Noel P, Kyle RA: Plasma cell leukemia: an evaluation of response to therapy. Am J Med 83:1062, 1987

157. Walker JD, Kaczmarski RS: Survival of twenty-two months in a patient with primary plasma cell leukaemia treated with melphalan and prednisolone. Postgrad Med J 64:232, 1988

158. Franchi F, Seminara P, Teodori L et al: The non-producer plasma cell myeloma: report of a case and review of the literature. Blut 52:281, 1986

159. Cavo M, Galieni P, Gobbi M et al: Nonsecretory multiple myeloma: presenting findings, clinical course and prognosis. Acta Haematol 74:27, 1985

160. Dreicer R, Alexanian R: Nonsecretory multiple myeloma. Am J Hematol 13:313, 1982

161. Fibbe WE, Jansen J: Prognostic factors in IgD myeloma: a study of 21 cases. Scand J Haematol 33:471, 1984

162. Kyle RA, Dyck PJ: Osteosclerotic myeloma (POEMS syndrome). p. 1288. In Dyck PJ, Thomas PK, Griffin JW et al (eds): Peripheral Neuropathy. 3rd Ed. WB Saunders, Philadelphia, 1993

163. Waldenström JG: POEMS: a multifactorial syndrome, editorial. Haematologica 77:197, 1992

164. Takatsuki K, Sanada I: Plasma cell dyscrasia with polyneuropathy and endocrine disorder: clinical and laboratory features of 109 reported cases. Jpn J Clin Oncol 13:543, 1983

165. Bardwick PA, Zvaifler NJ, Gill GN et al: Plasma cell dyscrasia with polyneuropathy, organomegaly, endocrinopathy, M protein, and skin changes: the POEMS syndrome. Report on two cases and a review of the literature. Medicine 59:311, 1980

166. Case Records of the Massachusetts General Hospital (Case 10-1987). N Engl J Med 316:606, 1987

167. Bataille R, Sany J: Solitary myeloma: clinical and prognostic features of a review of 114 cases. Cancer 48:845, 1981

168. Frassica DA, Frassica FJ, Schray MF et al: Solitary plasmacytoma of bone: Mayo Clinic experience. Int J Radiat Oncol Biol Phys 16:43, 1989

169. Chak LY, Cox RS, Bostwick DG, Hoppe RT: Solitary plasmacytoma of bone: treatment, progression, and survival. J Clin Oncol 5:1811, 1987

170. Holland J, Trenkner DA, Wasserman TH, Fineberg B: Plasmacytoma: treatment results and conversion to myeloma. Cancer 69:1513, 1992

171. Dimopoulos MA, Goldstein J, Fuller L et al: Curability of solitary bone plasmacytoma. J Clin Oncol 10:587, 1992

172. Wiltshaw E: The natural history of extramedullary plasmacytoma and its relation to solitary myeloma of bone and myelomatosis. Medicine 55:217, 1976

173. Kyle RA, Greipp PR: Plasma cell dyscrasias: current status. CRC Crit Rev Oncol Hematol 8:93, 1988

174. Knowling MA, Harwood AR, Bergsagel DE: Comparison of extramedullary plasmacytomas with solitary and multiple plasma cell tumors of bone. J Clin Oncol 1:255, 1983

175. Kapadia SB, Desai U, Cheng VS: Extramedullary plasmacytoma of the head and neck: a clinicopathologic study of 20 cases. Medicine 61:317, 1982

176. Meis JM, Butler JJ, Osborne BM, Ordóñez NG: Solitary plasmacytomas of bone and extramedullary plasmacytomas: a clinicopathologic and immunohistochemical study. Cancer 59:1475, 1987

177. Soesan M, Paccagnella A, Chiarion-Sileni V et al: Extramedullary plasmacytoma: clinical behaviour and response to treatment. Ann Oncol 3:51, 1992

178. Blattner WA, Garber JE, Mann DL et al: Waldenström's macroglobulinemia and autoimmune disease in a family. Ann Intern Med 93:830, 1980

179. Fine JM, Muller JY, Rochu D et al: Waldenström's macroglobulinemia in monozygotic twins. Acta Med Scand 220:369, 1986

180. Epenetos AA, Rohatiner A, Slevin M, Woothipoom W: Ankylosing spondylitis and Waldenström's macroglobulinaemia: a case report. Clin Oncol 6:83, 1980

181. Palka G, Spadano A, Geraci L et al: Chromosome changes in 19 patients with Waldenström's macroglobulinemia. Cancer Genet Cytogenet 29:261, 1987

182. Carbone P, Caradonna F, Granata G et al: Chromosomal abnormalities in Waldenström's macroglobulinemia. Cancer Genet Cytogenet 61:147, 1992

183. Pilarski LM, Andrews EJ, Serra HM et al: Abnormalities in lymphocyte profile and specificity repertoire of patients with Waldenström's macroglobulinemia, multiple myeloma, and IgM monoclonal gammopathy of undetermined significance. Am J Hematol 30:53, 1989

184. Varticovski L, Pick AI, Schattner A, Shoenfeld Y: Anti-platelet and anti-DNA IgM in Waldenström macroglobulinemia and ITP. Am J Hematol 24:351, 1987

185. Nobile-Orazio E, Marmiroli P, Baldini L et al: Peripheral neuropathy in macroglobulinemia: incidence and antigen-specificity of M proteins. Neurology 37:1506, 1987

186. Hory B, Saunier F, Wolff R et al: Waldenström macroglobulinemia and nephrotic syndrome with minimal change lesion. Nephron 45:68, 1987

187. Winterbauer RH, Riggins RCK, Griesman FA, Bauermeister DE: Pleuropulmonary manifestations of Waldenström's macroglobulinemia. Chest 66:368, 1974

188. Monteagudo M, Lima J, Garcia-Bragado F, Alvarez J: Chylous pleural effusion as the initial manifestation of Waldenström's macroglobulinemia. Eur J Respir Dis 70:326, 1987

189. Bloch KJ, Maki DG: Hyperviscosity syndromes associated with immunoglobulin abnormalities. Semin Hematol 10:113, 1973

190. Crawford J, Cox EB, Cohen HJ: Evaluation of hyperviscosity in monoclonal gammopathies. Am J Med 79:13, 1985

191. Levin AM, Lichtenstein A, Gresik MV et al: Clinical and immunologic spectrum of plasmacytoid lymphocytic lymphoma without serum monoclonal IgM. Br J Haematol 46:225, 1980

192. Zarrabi MH, Stark RS, Kane P et al: IgM myeloma, a distinct entity in the spectrum of B-cell neoplasia. Am J Clin Pathol 75:1, 1981

193. Takahashi K, Yamamura F, Motoyama H: IgM myeloma—its distinction from Waldenström's macroglobulinemia. Acta Pathol Jpn 36:1553, 1986

194. Case DC Jr, Ervin TJ, Boyd MA: Waldenström's macroglobulinemia: long term results with M-2 protocol, abstracted. Blood, suppl 1. 72:239, 1988

195. Rossi JF, Legouffe E, Laporte JPh et al: Treatment of Waldenström's macroglobulinemia (WM) by very low doses of interferon alpha-2A (IFN-2A), abstracted. Blood, suppl. 78:469a, 1991

196. Kantarjian HM, Redman JR, Keating MJ: Fludarabine phosphate therapy in other lymphoid malignancies. Semin Oncol, suppl. 8. 17:66, 1990

197. Horsman DE, Card RT, Skinnider LF: Waldenström macroglobulinemia terminating in acute leukemia: a report of three cases. Am J Hematol 15:97, 1983

198. Jane SM, Salem HH: Treatment of resistant Waldenström's macroglobulinemia with high dose glucocorticosteroids. Aust NZ J Med 18:77, 1988

199. Kyle RA, Greipp PR: Heavy chain diseases. Section III. Myeloma and related disorders. p. 513. In Wiernik PH, Canellos GP, Kyle RA, Schiffer CA (eds): Neoplastic Diseases of the Blood. 2nd Ed. Churchill Livingstone, New York, 1991

200. Fermand J-P, Brouet J-C, Danon F, Seligmann M: Gamma heavy chain "disease": heterogeneity of the clinicopathologic features. Report of 16 cases and review of the literature. Medicine 68:321, 1989

201. Alexander A, Anicito I, Buxbaum J: Gamma heavy chain disease in man: genomic sequence reveals two noncontiguous deletions in a single gene. J Clin Invest 82:1244, 1988

202. Kyle RA, Greipp PR, Banks PM: The diverse picture of gamma heavy-chain disease: report of seven cases and review of literature. Mayo Clin Proc 56:439, 1981

203. Wester SM, Banks PM, Li C-Y: The histopathology of γ heavy-chain disease. Am J Clin Pathol 78:427, 1982

204. Kanoh T, Nakasato H: Osteolytic gamma heavy chain disease. Eur J Haematol 39:60, 1987

205. Seligmann M: Immunochemical, clinical, and pathological features of α-chain disease. Arch Intern Med 135:78, 1975

206. Rambaud JC, Galian A, Matuchansky C et al: Natural history of α-chain disease and the so-called Mediterranean lymphoma. Recent Results Cancer Res 64:271, 1978

207. Asselah F, Slavin G, Sowter G, Asselah H: Immunoproliferative small intestinal disease in Algerians. I. Light microscopic and immunochemical studies. Cancer 52:227, 1983

208. Haghighi P, Wolf PL: Alpha-heavy chain disease. Clin Lab Med 6:477, 1986

209. Fakhfakh F, Dellagi K, Ayadi H et al: α Heavy chain disease α mRNA contain nucleotide sequences of unknown origins. Eur J Immunol 22:3037, 1992

210. Joller PW, Joller-Jemelka HI, Shmerling DH, Skvaril F: Immunological and biochemical studies of an unusual α heavy chain protein in a 9-year-old boy. J Clin Lab Immunol 15:167, 1984

211. Bowie MD, Hill ID: α-Chain disease in children. J Pediatr 112:46, 1988

212. Geraci L, Merlini G, Spadano A et al: Alpha heavy chain disease: report of two cases. Haematologica (Pavia) 70:431, 1985

213. Haghighi P, Kharazmi A, Gerami C et al: Primary upper small-intestinal lymphoma and alpha-chain disease: report of 10 cases emphasizing pathological aspects. Am J Surg Pathol 2:147, 1978

214. Tungekar MF, Omar YT, Behbehani K: Gastric alpha heavy chain disease. Oncology 44:360, 1987

215. Coulbois J, Galian P, Galian A et al: Gastric form of alpha chain disease. Gut 27:719, 1986

216. Price SK: Immunoproliferative small intestinal disease: a study of 13 cases with alpha heavy-chain disease. Histopathology 17:7, 1990

217. Rambaud JC, Halphen M, Galian A, Tsapis A: Immunoproliferative small intestinal disease (IPSID): relationships with α-chain disease and "Mediterranean" lymphomas. Springer Semin Immunopathol 12:239, 1990

218. Berger R, Bernheim A, Tsapis A et al: Cytogenetic studies in four cases of alpha chain disease. Cancer Genet Cytogenet 22:219, 1986

219. Smith WJ, Price SK, Isaacson PG: Immunoglobulin gene rearrangement in immunoproliferative small intestinal disease (IPSID). J Clin Pathol 40:1291, 1987

220. Doe WF, Danon F, Seligmann M: Immunodiagnosis of alpha chain disease. Clin Exp Immunol 36:189, 1979

221. Rambaud J-C, Galian A, Danon FG et al: Alpha-chain disease without qualitative serum IgA abnormality: report of two cases, including a "nonsecretory" form. Cancer 51:686, 1983

222. O'Keefe SJD, Winter TA, Newton KA et al: Severe malnutrition associated with α-heavy chain disease: response to tetracycline and intensive nutritional support. Am J Gastroenterol 83:995, 1988

223. Ben-Ayed F, Halphen M, Najjar T et al: Treatment of alpha chain disease: results of a prospective study in 21 Tunisian patients by the Tunisian-French Intestinal Lymphoma Study Group. Cancer 63:1251, 1989

224. Franklin EC: μ-Chain disease. Arch Intern Med 135:71, 1975

225. Wahner-Roedler DL, Kyle RA: Mu-heavy chain disease: presentation as a benign monoclonal gammopathy. Am J Hematol 40:56, 1992

226. Leach IH, Jenkins JS, Murray-Leslie CF, Powell RJ: μ-Heavy chain and monoclonal IgG κ paraproteinaemia in systemic lupus erythematosus. Br J Rheumatol 26:460, 1987

227. Letendre L, Kyle RA: Monoclonal cryoglobulinemia with high thermal insolubility. Mayo Clin Proc 57:629, 1982

228. Wang A-C: Molecular basis for cryoprecipitation. Springer Semin Immunopathol 10:21, 1988

229. Montagnino G: Reappraisal of the clinical expression of mixed cryoglobulinemia. Springer Semin Immunopathol 10:1, 1988

230. Gemignani F, Pavesi G, Fiocchi A et al: Peripheral neuropathy in essential mixed cryoglobulinaemia. J Neurol Neurosurg Psychiatry 55:116, 1992

231. D'Amico G, Colasanti G, Ferrario F et al: Renal involvement in essential mixed cryoglobulinemia: a peculiar type of immune-mediated renal disease. Adv Nephrol 17:219, 1988

232. D'Amico G, Colasanti G, Ferrario F, Sinico RA: Renal involvement in essential mixed cryoglobulinemia. Kidney Int 35:1004, 1989

233. Tarantino A, De Vecchi A, Montagnino G et al: Renal disease in essential mixed cryoglobulinemia: long-term follow-up of 44 patients. Q J Med 50:1, 1981

234. Gorevic PD, Kassab HJ, Levo Y et al: Mixed cryoglobulinemia: clinical aspects and long-term follow-up of 40 patients. Am J Med 69:287, 1980

235. Misiani R, Bellavita P, Fenili D et al: Hepatitis C virus infection in patients with essential mixed cryoglobulinemia. Ann Intern Med 117:573, 1992

236. Agnello V, Chung RT, Kaplan LM: A role for hepatitis C virus infection in type II cryoglobulinemia. N Engl J Med 327:1490, 1992

237. Monteverde A, Rivano MT, Allegra GC et al: Essential mixed cryoglobulinemia, type II: a manifestation of a low-grade malignant lymphoma? Clinical-morphological study of 12 cases with special reference to immunohistochemical findings in liver frozen sections. Acta Haematol 79:20, 1988

238. Frankel AH, Singer DRJ, Winearls CG et al: Type II essential mixed cryoglobulinemia: presentation, treatment and outcome in 13 patients. Q J Med 82:101, 1992

239. Casato M, Laganà B, Antonelli G et al: Long-term results of therapy with interferon-α for type II essential mixed cryoglobulinemia. Blood 78:3142, 1991

240. Ferri C, Marzo E, Longombardo G et al: Alpha interferon in the treatment of mixed cryoglobulinaemia patients. Eur J Cancer, suppl 4. 27:S81, 1991

241. Dammacco F, Miglietta A, Lobreglio G, Bonomo L: Cryoglobulins and pyroglobulins: an overview. Ric Clin Lab 16:247, 1986

242. Invernizzi F, Cattaneo R, Rosso di San Secondo V et al: Pyroglobulinemia: a report of eight patients with associated paraproteinemia. Acta Haematol (Basel) 50:65, 1973

243. Kyle RA, Greipp PR: The laboratory investigation of monoclonal gammopathies. Mayo Clin Proc 53:719, 1978

244. Kyle RA, Garton JP: Laboratory monitoring of myeloma proteins. Semin Oncol 13:310, 1986

245. Kyle RA: Classification and diagnosis of monoclonal gammopathies. p. 152. In Rose NR, Friedman H, Fahey JL (eds): Manual of Clinical Laboratory Immunology. 3rd Ed. American Society for Microbiology, Washington, DC, 1986

Amyloidosis

88

Robert A. Kyle and Morie A. Gertz

INTRODUCTION

The term *amyloid* was coined in 1838 by Matthias Schleiden, a German botanist, to describe a normal amylaceous constituent of plants. Rudolph Virchow, in 1854, applied the term *amyloid* because it was similar to cellulose.[1]

Amyloid has a homogeneous and amorphous appearance under the light microscope and stains pink with hematoxylin and eosin. Under polarized light, amyloid stained with Congo red produces an apple-green birefringence. The amorphous, hyaline-like appearance of amyloid is misleading because it is a fibrous protein, which on electron microscopy is shown to consist of rigid, linear, nonbranching, aggregated fibrils 7.5–10 nm wide and of indefinite length. All amyloid fibrils display a cross-β-pleated pattern that imparts the optical properties to amyloid. The fibrils are insoluble and generally resist proteolytic digestion. The deposits occur extracellularly and ultimately lead to damage of normal tissue. A classification of amyloidosis is shown in Table 88-1.

BIOLOGIC AND MOLECULAR ASPECTS

The fibrils are composed of various subunits, depending on the type of amyloid, and include monoclonal light chains (κ or λ), protein A, transthyretin (prealbumin), β_2-microglobulin (β_2-M), apolipoprotein A1, gelsolin, cystatin C, (pro)calcitonin, atrial natriuretic peptide, islet amyloid polypeptide, β-protein, or scrapie protein.

Glenner et al.[2] demonstrated that amyloid fibrils from a patient with primary (AL) amyloidosis were virtually identical to the variable portion of a monoclonal light chain (Bence Jones protein). Thus, the variable portion of a monoclonal light chain, or in some instances the intact light chain, constitutes the fibril subunit of AL amyloid. The light chain class is more frequently λ than κ (by a 3:1 ratio) in AL amyloidosis. Solomon et al.[3] found that in 11 of 20 amyloidosis cases (55%), the λ-chains were of the λ_{VI} subclass. In fact, all recognized λ_{VI} monoclonal light chains have been associated with amyloidosis. This finding supports the hypothesis that some light chains possess features that render them "amyloidogenic." Low-molecular-weight immunoglobulin light chain fragments with a lower isoelectric point were more frequently associated with amyloidosis; this finding suggests that these physical properties predict amyloidogenicity of light chains.[4] In 5 of 14 patients with AL amyloidosis, Buxbaum and Hauser[5] demonstrated the synthesis of immunologically identical light chains that were of lower molecular weight than were intact light chains. This suggests that aberrant de novo synthesis of light chains or abnormal proteolytic processing may occur in AL amyloidosis patients. Others have also reported the secretion of free light chains and light chain fragments in such patients.[6]

The mechanism for the deposition of monoclonal light chains as amyloid is unclear. Nomura et al.[7] identified κ light chains and amyloid fibrils in plasma cells. In another report, bone marrow cells cultured from a patient with multiple myeloma and AL amyloidosis revealed Congo red-positive material in macrophages, but not in plasma cells.[8] Recently, an animal model for AL amyloidosis has been reported. Human light chains obtained from the urine of patients with amyloidosis injected into mice produced deposits of typical amyloid in the walls and parenchymal tissue of the kidneys, liver, heart, lungs, and spleen.[9]

Amyloid fibrils consisting of an internally deleted IgG1 heavy chain with total absence of the C_H1, hinge, and C_H2 regions were reported in a patient with systemic amyloidosis who died of hepatic and renal failure. There were no associated light chains; thus, the designation was heavy chain amyloidosis.[10]

In secondary (AA) amyloidosis, the major component of the amyloid fibril is protein A, which has a molecular weight of 8,500, consists of 76 amino acids, and is unrelated to any known immunoglobulin.[11] With the use of an antiserum to amyloid A (AA), an antigenically related larger molecule (molecular weight 12,500), known as serum amyloid A protein (SAA), has been found in the sera of normal patients as well as in those with amyloidosis. SAA has 104 amino acid residues, and the sequence of protein A corresponds to the N terminal of SAA, which provides strong evidence that protein A is derived by proteolytic cleavage of SAA. SAA levels are increased greatly in AA and modestly in AL amyloidosis but are within normal limits in familial (AF) amyloidosis. The SAA level corresponds to the incidence of secondary amyloidosis.[12] Human SAA is polymorphic[13] and exists in three major forms; SAA 1 α is the

Table 88-1. Classification of Amyloidosis

Amyloid Type	Clinical	Protein Precursor	Protein Type or Variant
AL	Primary: no evidence of preceding or coexisting disease, except multiple myeloma	κ, λ (i.e., λ_{VI})	Aκ, Aλ (i.e., $A\lambda_{VI}$)
AA	Secondary: coexistence with other conditions, such as rheumatoid arthritis or chronic infection, familial Mediterranean fever, Muckle-Wells syndrome	SAA	—
AL	Localized: involvement of a single organ without evidence of systemic involvement (e.g., urinary bladder, urethra, ureter, tracheobronchial)	κ, λ	Aκ, Aλ
ATTR (AF)	Familial amyloid polyneuropathy (FAP I) (Portuguese, Swedish, and Japanese)	Transthyretin (prealbumin)	Met 30
	FAP II (Indiana/Swiss, German)	Transthyretin (prealbumin)	Ser 84
	Appalachian	Transthyretin (prealbumin)	Ala 60
AApoA1	FAP III (Iowa, Van Allen)	ApoA1	Arg 26
$A\beta_2$-M	Associated with chronic dialysis	β_2-microglobulin	—

(Modified from Husby et al.,[103] with permission.)

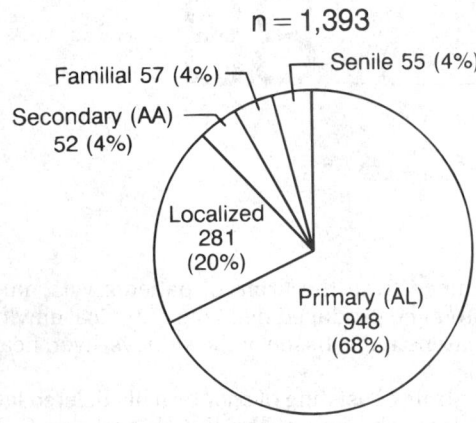

n = 1,393

Familial 57 (4%)
Senile 55 (4%)
Secondary (AA) 52 (4%)
Localized 281 (20%)
Primary (AL) 948 (68%)

Fig. 88-1. Types of amyloid found in 1,393 cases of amyloidosis seen at the Mayo Clinic during 1977–1991.

most common. Interleukin-1 and -6 and tumor necrosis factor play a role in SAA induction.[14] SAA is synthesized by the liver[15] and is found in the rough endoplasmic reticulum and the Golgi apparatus of the hepatocytes. The low prevalence of AA amyloidosis in patients with rheumatoid arthritis and Crohn disease suggests that factors such as amyloid-enhancing factor or the SAA amino acid sequence are important in the development of amyloidosis.

Amyloid P component (AP) is a glycoprotein composed of 10 identical glycosylated polypeptide subunits, each with a molecular weight of 23,500 and arranged as two pentamers. Human serum amyloid P component (SAP), a member of the pentraxin family of plasma proteins, is produced in the liver, is present in normal persons, and shows 50–60% homology with C-reactive protein.[16] SAP is bound to the amyloid fibrils in a calcium-dependent fashion but is not an integral part of the fibrillar structure. It is found in all types of amyloid, including the vessel walls in Alzheimer disease patients.[17] Neither the physiologic function of AP nor its pathologic role in amyloidosis is known.[18] Glycosaminoglycans are present in amyloid deposits,[19] but their role is unknown. Amyloid-enhancing factor accelerates the deposition of AA in the mouse model.[20] It has recently been suggested that amyloid-enhancing factor consists of ubiquitin.[21]

The catabolism or breakdown of amyloid fibrils is an important factor in pathogenesis. Lavie and associates[22] reported that monocytes in patients with amyloidosis failed to degrade AA, suggesting that different patterns of proteolysis may predispose one to the development of amyloidosis. Human neutrophil elastase has been identified on amyloid fibrils of AL, AA, and AF origin, indicating that this enzyme might also play a role in amyloid precursor protein degradation.[23]

Amyloidosis results from the interplay of many factors, including excessive deposition of amyloid and degradation of the amyloid fibrils. The pathogenesis of systemic amyloidosis has been reviewed.[24,25]

PRIMARY AMYLOIDOSIS

Introduction and Epidemiology

During the 15-year period 1977–1991, a total of 1,393 patients with amyloidosis were seen at the Mayo Clinic, of whom more than two-thirds had the primary (AL) form (Fig. 88-1). AL amyloidosis can be divided into two categories (AL and AL with multiple myeloma) on the basis of appearance and number of plasma cells in the bone marrow, amount of monoclonal (M) protein in the serum and urine, and the presence or absence of

skeletal lesions. However, differentiation on the basis of these features is often difficult because of overlap. Furthermore, the amyloid fibrils consist of the N-terminal amino acid residues of the variable portions of a monoclonal immunoglobulin light chain in both AL and AL with myeloma. In both instances, the M protein is the product of the plasma cell, and consequently each condition represents a plasma cell proliferative process. Both categories should be considered together as AL amyloidosis.

AL amyloidosis cannot be differentiated from AA by organ distribution or by electron microscopy. AA rarely produces peripheral neuropathy or symptomatic cardiac involvement, whereas these are common features in AL.

The age- and sex-adjusted annual rate of AL in Olmsted County, MN, is 0.89 per 100,000. Applying this to the U.S. population, one would expect approximately 2,225 new cases annually. The age-adjusted rate in males was more than twice that in females.[26] The median age at diagnosis in 843 cases of AL seen at the Mayo Clinic during 1982–1992 was 62 years. Only 2.5% were <40 years of age.

Clinical Manifestations

Weakness or fatigue and loss of weight are the most frequent symptoms; the median loss of weight in the Mayo Clinic series was 11 kg. Dyspnea, pedal edema, paresthesias, light-headedness, and syncope are frequently seen in patients with congestive heart failure or peripheral neuropathy. Hoarseness or change of voice, as well as jaw claudication, may occur.

Physical Findings

The liver is palpable in about one-fifth of patients, and splenomegaly of modest degree occurs in approximately 5%. Macroglossia is present in only 10% of patients (Figs. 88-2 and 88-3). Purpura commonly involves the neck, face, and eyes (Figs. 88-4 and 88-5). Ankle edema is common, and orthostatic hypotension may be severe. Generalized lymphadenopathy is infrequent but may be the initial manifestation of AL amyloidosis.

Syndromes

Almost one-third of patients have a nephrotic syndrome at the time amyloidosis is diagnosed. Carpal tunnel syndrome, congestive heart failure, peripheral neuropathy, and orthostatic hypotension are other presenting syndromes (Fig. 88-6); congestive heart failure and orthostatic hypotension often develop during the course of the disease. One of these syndromes in conjunction with an M protein in the serum or urine is a strong indication of amyloidosis, but appropriate biopsy specimens must be taken for diagnosis.

Organ System Involvement

Cardiac and Circulatory

Congestive heart failure is present in approximately 20% of patients at diagnosis and develops during the course of the disease in an additional 5%. The electrocardiogram frequently shows either low voltage in the limb leads or characteristics consistent with an anteroseptal infarction (loss of anterior forces), but no evidence of myocardial infarction is present at autopsy.[27] Atrial fibrillation, atrial or junctional tachycardia, ventricular premature complexes, and heart block are common electrocardiographic features.[28]

Echocardiography is a valuable technique for the recognition and evaluation of amyloid heart disease. In approximately 10% of Mayo Clinic patients with systemic amyloidosis, the condition is first recognized by echocardiography (Foley DA, Miller FA Jr, Seward JB et al, unpublished data). The major echocardiographic features are increased thickness of the left and right ventricular walls, abnormal myocardial texture (granular sparkling), atrial enlargement, valvular thickening and regurgitation, pericardial effusion, and abnormal diastolic and finally systolic ventricular function. Initially, abnormal relaxation results in diastolic filling abnormalities. With increased amyloid infiltration, a pattern of restriction occurs. This is associated with marked shortening of the deceleration time and the development of cardiac symptoms.[29] Increased thickness of the left ventricular wall and septum correlates with an increased incidence of congestive heart failure.[30] Preservation of systolic function (normal ejection fraction) persists until late in the disease. Digoxin is not beneficial in these patients because the cardiac failure is predominantly a result of poor diastolic filling. Amyloid infiltration is frequently misinterpreted as left ventricular hypertrophy. Constrictive pericarditis or hypertrophic obstructive cardiomyopathy may be difficult to differentiate from amyloid heart disease. Intermittent claudication of the jaw or upper and lower extremities occurs in almost 10% of patients.[31] Orthostatic hypotension occurs in 15% of patients; it is usually due to involvement of the autonomic nervous system.

Renal

Nephrotic syndrome is present in almost one-third of patients at diagnosis. The degree of proteinuria does not correlate well with the extent of amyloid deposition in the kidneys. Gross hematuria is rare. The kidneys may be enlarged, but they are often of normal size or even small. Nephrogenic diabetes insipidus, adult Fanconi syndrome, priapism, and renal vein thrombosis have been reported in patients with AL. Adrenal insufficiency has been reported in both AL and AA amyloidosis.[32]

Neurologic

Sensorimotor peripheral neuropathy, characterized by dysesthetic numbness involving the lower extremities, occurs in one-sixth of patients.[33] It is very difficult to differentiate AL from AF amyloidosis when peripheral neuropathy dominates

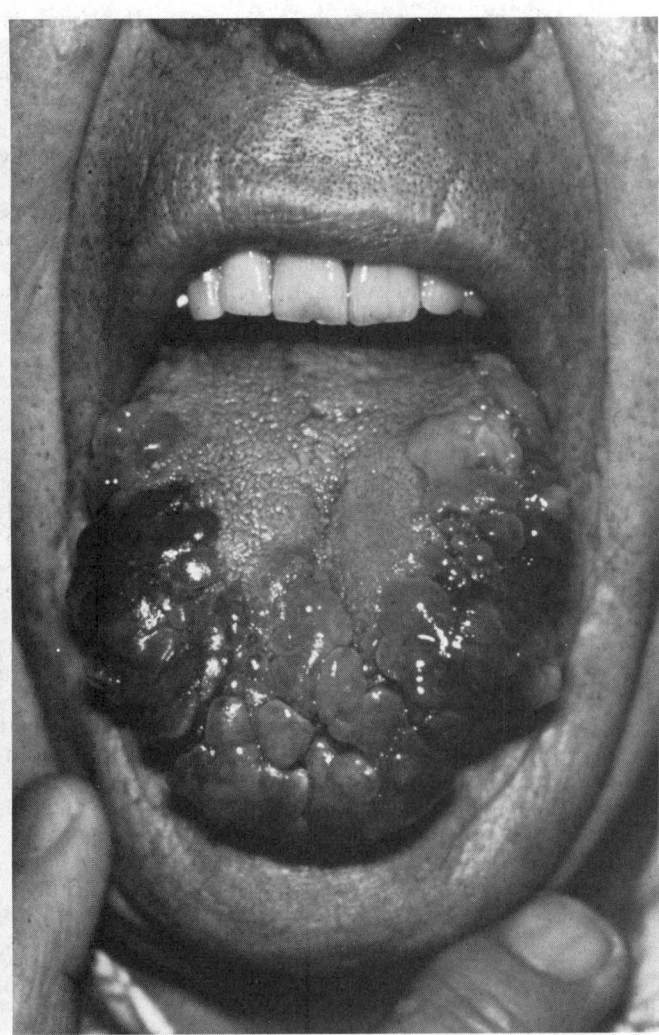

Fig. 88-2. Macroglossia with increased vascularity of the tongue. (From Kyle and Greipp,[99] with permission.)

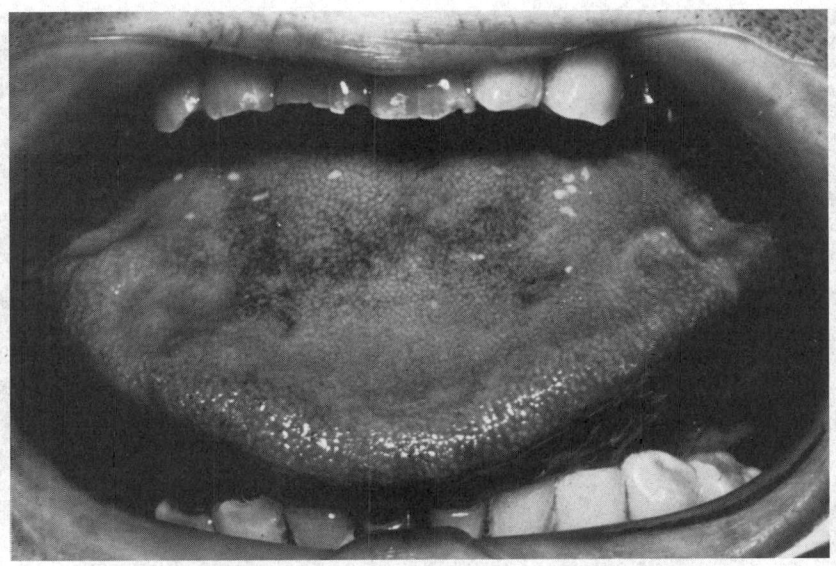

Fig. 88-3. Macroglossia. Note the dental indentations on the dorsum of the tongue.

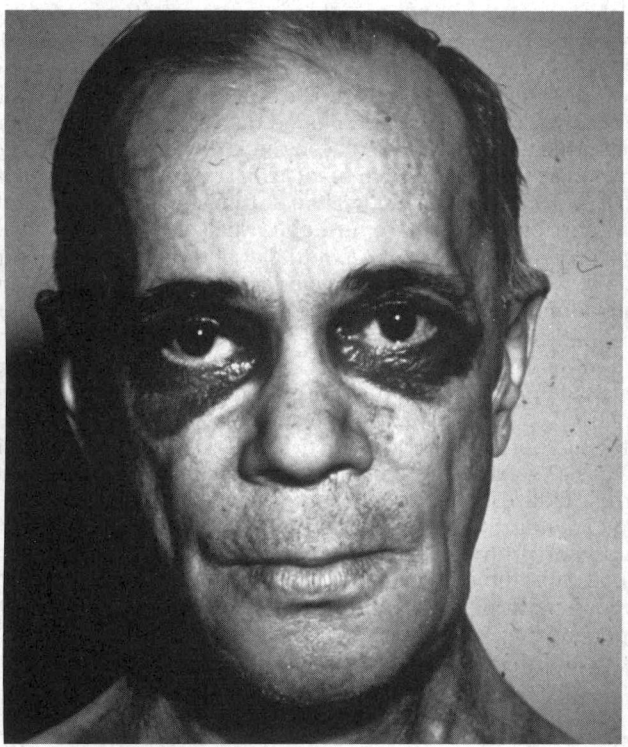

Fig. 88-4. Postproctoscopic periorbital purpura (PPPP). (From Kyle and Bayrd,[100] with permission.)

the clinical picture. Autonomic dysfunction may be a prominent feature and is often manifested by orthostatic hypotension, diarrhea, or impotence. Cranial neuropathy is rare, but it may be the initial manifestation of AL.[34] Carpal tunnel syndrome occurs in almost one-fourth of patients.

Amyloidosis can involve periarticular structures and produce the "shoulder pad" syndrome (Fig. 88-7). Large amyloid deposits (amyloidomas) may produce osteolytic lesions and cause pathologic fractures.[35] Extensive deposits of amyloid produce pseudohypertrophy of skeletal muscles, which may be impressive[36] (Fig. 88-8). Amyloid deposition in the walls of small vessels may cause progressive myopathy from ischemia.[37]

Involvement of the skin in systemic amyloidosis may be manifested by petechiae, ecchymoses, papules, plaques, nodules, tumors, bullous lesions, alopecia, dystrophy of the nails, or skin thickening resembling scleroderma.[38] Rarely, amyloid may be found in the external auditory canal (Fig. 88-9).

Bleeding is rarely a major complication of AL amyloidosis. Decreased vitamin K-dependent clotting factors, increased antithrombin activity, increased fibrinolysis, increased intravascular coagulation, and infiltration by amyloid of small vessels may contribute to bleeding.[39]

Gastrointestinal

Histologic involvement of the gastrointestinal tract occurs in most patients with AL amyloidosis but is usually asymptomatic. Occasionally, malabsorption or pseudo-obstruction of the bowel may be seen and, rarely, amyloidosis of the stomach may present as a gastric mass resembling a carcinoma. Malabsorption occurs in <5% of patients. Ascites may be seen, gastrointestinal bleeding may be present,[40] and hepatic involvement is common, although liver failure is rare.[41]

Pulmonary

Histologic involvement of the pulmonary blood vessels and alveolar septa is common, but dyspnea is rare. Chest radiographs may show interstitial infiltration or a reticular pattern. Tracheobronchial involvement or the presence of amyloid pulmonary nodules remain localized and do not progress to systemic amyloidosis.[42]

Laboratory Findings

Hematologic

Anemia is not a prominent feature in AL amyloidosis. When present, it is usually due to renal insufficiency, multiple myeloma, or gastrointestinal bleeding. Thrombocytosis occurs in about 10% of patients and may be a clue to the diagnosis. Howell-Jolly bodies in the peripheral blood smear are found in one-fourth of patients and are indicative of hyposplenism.[43]

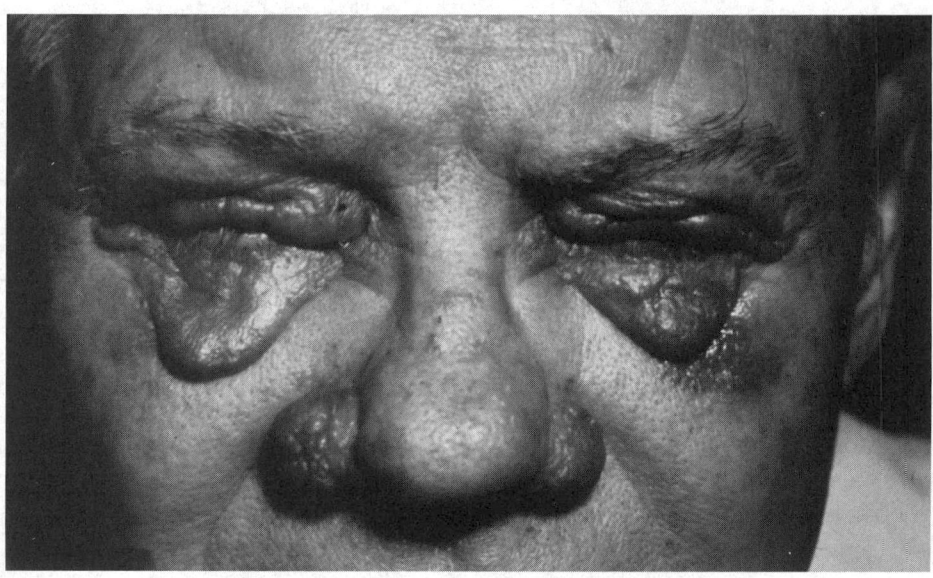

Fig. 88-5. Amyloid involving the upper eyelids, which obstruct the pupils. Note the prominent alae, which were friable.

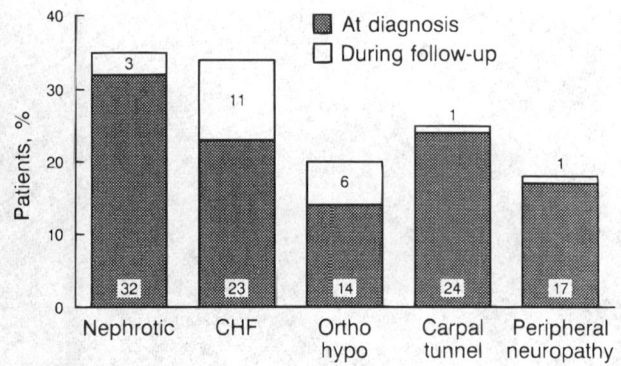

Fig. 88-6. Syndromes seen at diagnosis and during follow-up of patients with primary (AL) amyloidosis. Some patients had more than two syndromes at presentation. (From Kyle and Gertz,[101] with permission.)

Renal

Proteinuria is present in approximately 80% of patients, and renal insufficiency is present initially in almost one-half the patients. In one-fourth of the patients in the Mayo Clinic series, the creatinine level was ≥2 mg/dl at diagnosis. Not infrequently, the first manifestation of AL is a sudden increase in previously normal serum cholesterol or triglyceride values, leading to the recognition of a nephrotic syndrome from AL.

Serum and Urine Protein

The serum protein electrophoretic pattern is one of a localized band or spike (usually of modest size) in slightly less than one-half of cases. Hypogammaglobulinemia is seen in nearly one-fourth of patients. Immunoelectrophoresis or immunofixation reveals a monoclonal protein in two-thirds of patients, and almost 20% have a free monoclonal light chain (Bence Jones proteinemia).

Electrophoresis of a concentrated urine specimen generally shows an albumin peak and a small globulin band. Immunoelectrophoresis or immunofixation of the urine reveals a monoclonal light chain in approximately two-thirds of cases, and an M protein is found in the serum or urine in 90% of patients.

Most of the remaining patients have a demonstrable monoclonal population of plasma cells in the bone marrow. Thus, approximately 98% of patients with AL have an M protein in the serum or urine or a monoclonal plasma cell population in the marrow.

In the patients included in our series, the median percentage of plasma cells in the bone marrow was 7%, and only 14% of patients had >20% plasma cells in the marrow. Radiographs of the bones are normal unless the patient has multiple myeloma.

Other Findings

Levels of serum alkaline phosphatase are increased in about one-fourth of patients. Hyperbilirubinemia is an infrequent finding but when present is an ominous sign. Hypoalbuminemia is associated with the nephrotic syndrome. The prothrombin time is increased in about 15% of patients. Isolated factor X deficiency occurs in <5% of patients, but the thrombin time is prolonged in more than one-half of patients.[44]

Diagnosis and Differential Diagnosis

The possibility of primary systemic (AL) amyloidosis must be considered in every patient who has an M protein in the serum or urine and who has nephrotic syndrome, refractory chronic congestive heart failure, sensorimotor peripheral neuropathy, carpal tunnel syndrome, giant hepatomegaly, or idiopathic malabsorption. The initial diagnostic procedure should be to obtain an abdominal fat aspirate, since this is positive in >80% of patients.[45] Experience in the staining technique and interpretation are important before it can be used routinely. A bone marrow aspirate and biopsy specimen should be obtained to determine the degree of plasmacytosis. Marrow specimens stain for amyloid in slightly more than one-half of patients (Fig. 88-10).

If the abdominal fat and bone marrow biopsy results are negative, a rectal biopsy specimen should be taken, which must include the submucosa; this biopsy is positive in approximately 80% of patients. If these sites are negative, tissue should be obtained from a suspected involved organ. Renal biopsy

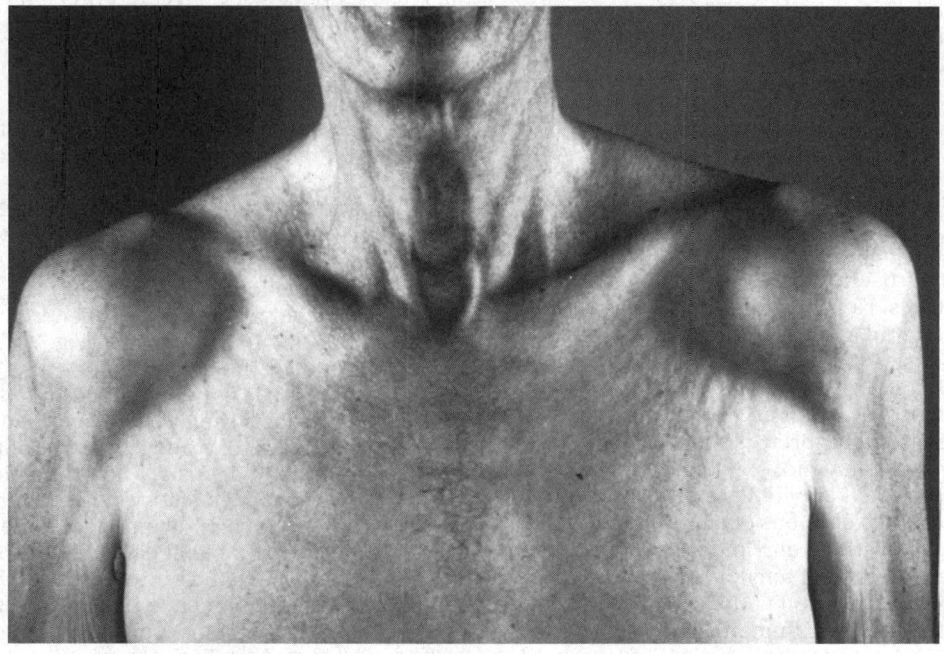

Fig. 88-7. Periarticular infiltration of amyloid, producing the "shoulder pad" syndrome.

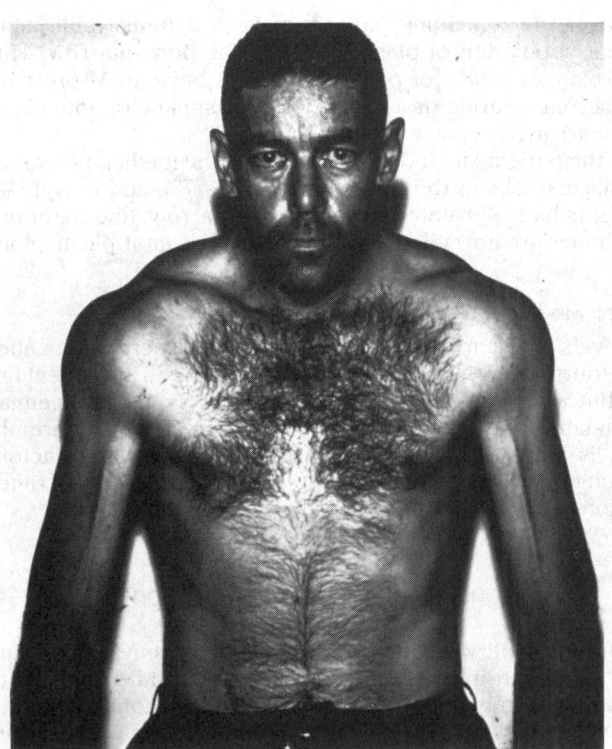

Fig. 88-8. Pseudohypertrophy of skeletal muscles from infiltration by amyloid. (From Kyle and Greipp,[99] with permission.)

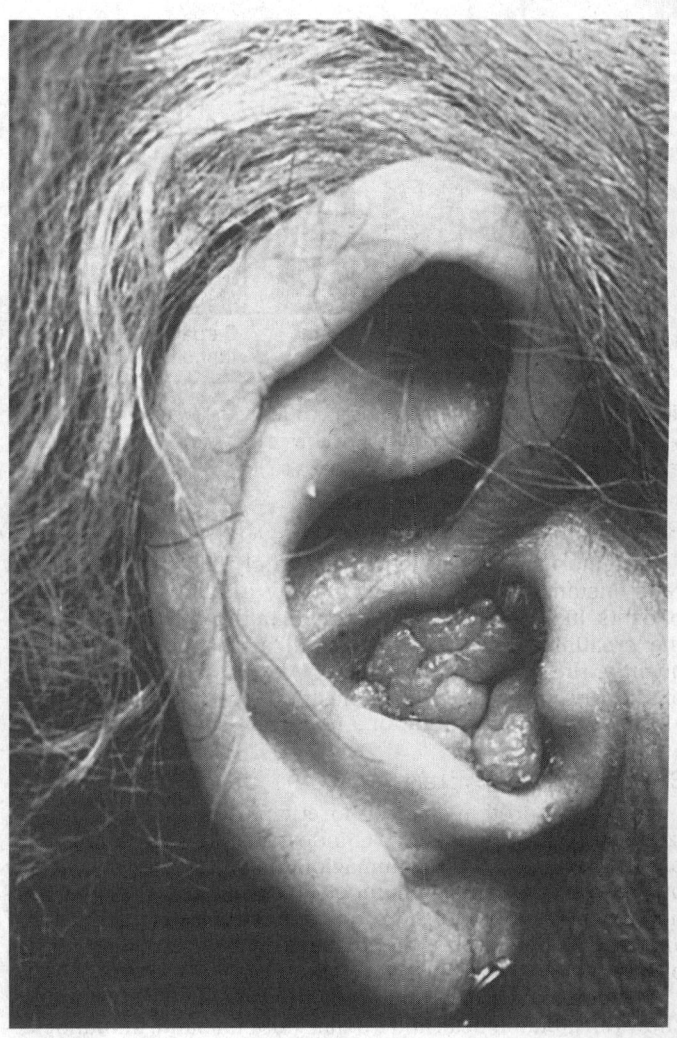

Fig. 88-9. Occlusion of ear canal by nodules of cutaneous amyloid. (From Gertz and Kyle,[102] with permission.)

results in a high incidence of positive findings in patients with nephrotic syndrome or renal insufficiency. Because small deposits of amyloid may be associated with the nephrotic syndrome, renal biopsy specimens that have the appearance of minimal change glomerulopathy must be carefully stained for amyloid. Liver biopsy frequently discloses amyloid. The incidence of bleeding with kidney or liver biopsy is not increased. Tissue obtained at carpal tunnel decompression should always be examined for amyloid because it is positive in a high percentage of patients with AL amyloidosis. The sural nerve is an excellent source of biopsy material in patients with peripheral neuropathy. Endomyocardial biopsy is positive in almost all cases in which it is performed. Biopsy specimens taken from the small intestine, skin, prostate, and gingiva may be positive (Fig. 88-10).

Congo red produces an apple-green birefringence under polarizing light and is the most commonly used stain. Although false-positive and false-negative results may occur, Congo red is a more reliable stain than methyl violet, crystal violet, or thioflavin T. Electron microscopy may be necessary for identification of the typical fibrils. Non-amyloid fibrillar glomerulopathy such as immunotactoid glomerulopathy must be distinguished from amyloidosis.[46] Light chain deposition disease must also be differentiated from amyloidosis.[47]

AA amyloid typically loses its affinity for Congo red and its polarization characteristics after pretreatment with potassium permanganate, whereas AL amyloid, senile systemic amyloid, familial amyloid, and localized amyloid are all resistant to potassium permanganate, but exceptions occur. Antiserum to amyloid P component reacts with all amyloid types and is useful for demonstrating the presence of amyloid. The most reliable approach to histologic classification is the use of specific antisera to AA, κ, λ, transthyretin (prealbumin), and β_2-microglobulin. ^{123}I-labeled serum amyloid P component can be used for locating and monitoring the extent of systemic amyloidosis.[48]

Increased uptake of ^{99m}Tc-pyrophosphate is not a reliable test.[49]

Prognosis

The mean survival after diagnosis in an earlier Mayo Clinic series of 81 patients with primary amyloidosis seen during 1935–1959 was 4.9 months.[50] The median duration of survival of 735 patients with AL seen at the Mayo Clinic during 1982–1991 was 2 years. The longer survival is due to several factors—earlier diagnosis of AL, improved supportive care, and superior chemotherapy. Survival varies greatly, depending on the associated syndrome; it is generally 6 months from the onset of congestive heart failure (Fig. 88-11). Cardiac involvement accounts for the death of more than one-half of patients.

Multivariate analysis was applied to data from 168 patients with AL amyloidosis seen at the Mayo Clinic during 1970–1980 in whom all laboratory and clinical studies were performed within 1 month of diagnosis. The proportional hazard method of Cox showed that congestive heart failure, the presence of a urinary monoclonal light chain, hepatomegaly, and the extent of weight loss had a significant influence on survival during the first year.[51] Elevated serum creatinine level, diagnosis of multiple myeloma, presence of orthostatic hypotension, and the presence of a serum M protein had a significant adverse influence on survival in those who lived >1 year after diagnosis.

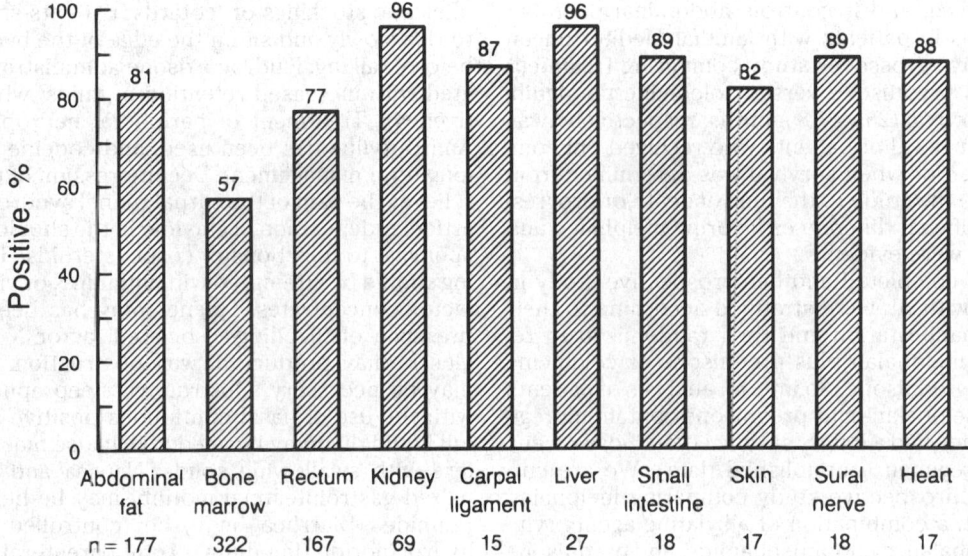

Fig. 88-10. Results of biopsy from sites of involvement in patients with primary (AL) amyloidosis seen at the Mayo Clinic, 1982–1991.

The serum β_2-microglobulin level is a useful prognostic factor. The median duration of survival was 33 months in AL patients with a level of <2.7 μg/ml and 11 months in those with an elevated level. When the analysis was restricted to patients with normal renal function, those with an elevated β_2-microglobulin level also had a significantly shortened survival.[52] Patients who present with a normal serum creatinine level and urinary protein value of <2 g/day are unlikely to require dialysis.[53]

Therapeutic responses in amyloidosis are difficult to evaluate because no method for measuring the amount of amyloid in the body is readily available. Currently, evaluation of response to therapy is limited to measurement of physical findings, evaluation of organ function, and improvement in laboratory test abnormalities. Quantitation of response is easiest to measure in patients with a nephrotic syndrome. The extent of amyloid deposition can be measured with ^{123}I-labeled serum

amyloid P component,[48] but it is not available for widespread use. Survival is the ultimate measure of the efficacy of therapy.

Therapy

Therapy for AL amyloidosis is not satisfactory. Because amyloid fibrils consist of the variable portion of a monoclonal immunoglobulin light chain, treatment should be attempted with alkylating agents that are known to be effective against plasma cell proliferative processes. In a randomized placebo-controlled double-blind study of 55 patients with AL, those who received melphalan and prednisone therapy continued treatment longer and received larger doses than did patients in the placebo group before the code was broken because of progressive disease; the results suggest that the chemotherapy was of some benefit.[54] Survival, however, did not differ significantly between the two groups. Colchicine inhibits casein induction

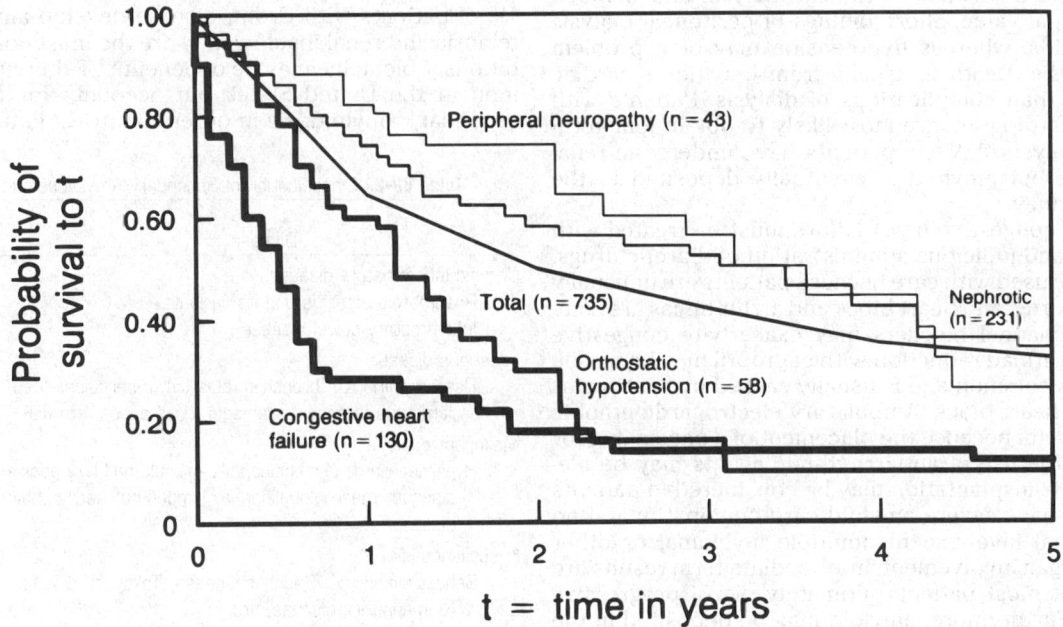

Fig. 88-11. Survival of patients with AL amyloidosis and associated syndromes seen at the Mayo Clinic, 1982–1991.

of amyloidosis in mice, and it controls abdominal pain and prevents amyloidosis in patients with familial Mediterranean fever. In a prospective crossover study comparing treatment with melphalan and prednisone versus colchicine no significant difference in survival (25 vs. 18 months, respectively) was evident. When the survival of patients who received only one regimen was analyzed or when survival was determined from the time of entry into the study to the time of death or progression of disease, significant differences favoring melphalan and prednisone therapy were evident.[55]

We have recently completed another prospective study in which 219 patients with AL were stratified according to their dominant clinical manifestation and then randomized to receive colchicine or melphalan plus prednisone or colchicine plus melphalan and prednisone. An interim analysis of patients receiving the two melphalan- and prednisone-containing regimens showed that they had a longer survival than those receiving the colchicine regimen (unpublished data). We are currently engaged in a prospective study comparing melphalan and prednisone with a combination of alkylating agents (vincristine, BCNU, melphalan, cyclophosphamide, and prednisone [VBMCP]).

The development of a myelodysplastic syndrome or acute myeloid leukemia in patients with AL has been recognized. We found that 10 of 153 patients with biopsy-proven AL who were treated with melphalan developed cytogenetic abnormalities consistent with alkylating agent-induced damage to hematopoietic cells. Of the 10 patients, 8 died as a direct result of their pancytopenia. Four patients had acute myeloid leukemia, five had a myelodysplastic syndrome, and one had a nondiagnostic bone marrow examination. Although 6.5% of the entire group had leukemia or a myelodysplastic syndrome, the actuarial risk in patients surviving 3.5 years was 21%.[56]

Dimethylsulfoxide may degrade amyloid fibrils in vitro and in mice, but the results have been disappointing in humans. α-Tocopherol (vitamin E) has reduced amyloid deposition after the injection of casein in mice, but in a recent study no benefit was seen.[57] Interferon-α$_2$ has not produced objective responses in our hands.[58]

The nephrotic syndrome should be managed with salt restriction and diuretic agents as needed. Albumin infusions have only transient benefit and are not useful for long-term treatment of edema. Chronic renal dialysis is necessary when symptomatic azotemia develops. Peritoneal dialysis and hemodialysis are of equal value. Shortcomings of peritoneal dialysis include peritonitis, whereas hypotension may be a problem with hemodialysis. Death is usually from hepatic or cardiac amyloid rather than complications of dialysis. Patients with a normal echocardiogram are most likely to obtain long-term benefit from dialysis.[53] A few patients have undergone renal transplantation, but amyloid is eventually deposited in the transplanted kidney.

Patients with congestive heart failure must be treated with salt restriction and judicious administration of diuretic drugs. Digitalis must be used with care because patients are unusually sensitive to the drug, and heart block and arrhythmias are common. Calcium channel blockers may exacerbate congestive heart failure. Afterload reduction with captopril may be useful. Sudden death is common and is usually caused by ventricular arrhythmias or heart block. Ambulatory electrocardiographic monitoring is useful because the placement of a pacemaker for heart block or the use of antiarrhythmic agents may be lifesaving. Cardiac transplantation may be considered in patients <60 years who have severe amyloid cardiomyopathy and no evidence of renal involvement, multiple myeloma, or other symptomatic organ involvement. Intermediate-term results are promising,[59] but most patients ultimately die of progressive amyloidosis.[60] Furthermore, amyloid may be deposited in the donor heart within 6 months.[61]

Treatment of orthostatic hypotension may be helped by use of elastic stockings or leotards. Patients should be instructed to rise slowly and sit on the edge of the bed for a few minutes before walking. Fludrocortisone administration is often associated with increased retention of fluids, which limits its effectiveness. Treatment of peripheral neuropathy is ineffective. Amitriptyline has been used, and codeine is often helpful for long-term management. Decompression of the carpal ligament relieves the pain of the carpal tunnel syndrome. Pain from periarticular deposition of amyloid in the shoulders is usually unresponsive to injections of corticosteroids. Treatment of bleeding should be attempted with vitamin K or vitamin K-dependent factor concentrates. Splenectomy has been beneficial in the presence of bleeding-associated factor X deficiency. Macroglossia may produce airway obstruction, and tracheostomy may be necessary. Obstructive sleep apnea may be treated with the use of nasal continuous positive airway pressure. A full liquid diet may be needed because macroglossia can interfere with swallowing solids. Nausea and vomiting from impaired gastrointestinal motility may be helped with metoclopramide. Diarrhea may be controlled with loperamide hydrochloride (Imodium). Total parenteral nutrition has been used when amyloid autonomic neuropathy produces severe pseudo-obstruction. Patients with pseudo-obstruction may mistakenly undergo surgical intervention for suspected mechanical obstruction.

SECONDARY AMYLOIDOSIS

Secondary amyloidosis is associated with an inflammatory process, malignancy, or a wide variety of other conditions (Table 88-2). M protein is not found in the serum or urine. At the Mayo Clinic, only 4% of amyloidosis patients have the AA type, but the incidence depends on the patient population.

Rheumatoid arthritis is the most frequent cause of AA amyloidosis and is found in approximately 4% of patients with long-term rheumatoid arthritis.[62] In 90% of cases, the nephrotic syndrome or renal failure is the major manifestation, but the gastrointestinal tract and thyroid may also be involved. In contrast to AL amyloidosis, the heart is rarely involved.[63] Almost 80% of patients have their rheumatic disorder for >10 years before the development of amyloidosis. Amyloidosis has been associated with ankylosing spondylitis, Still disease, psoriatic arthritis, Reiter syndrome, Sjögren syndrome, and lupus erythematosus. Crohn disease infrequently results in amyloidosis. Almost 1% of patients with Crohn disease develop amyloidosis. Proteinuria and renal insufficiency are the most common manifestations. Colchicine may be of benefit.[64] Tuberculosis is uncommon in the United States but accounts for many cases of secondary amyloidosis in other countries. Patients with para-

Table 88-2. Classification of Secondary Amyloidosis in 64 Patients

Disease	No. of Patients
Chronic inflammatory diseases	
Rheumatoid arthritis and its variants	42
Inflammatory bowel disease	6
Infectious disease	13
Osteomyelitis (5), bronchiectasis (5), tuberculosis, lepromatous leprosy, paraplegia, drug abuse, etc. (3)	
Malignant disease	2
Hypernephroma (1), eosinophilic granuloma (1), Hodgkin disease, macroglobulinemia, lymphoma, heavy chain diseases	
Miscellaneous	0
Behçet syndrome, Gaucher disease, Takayasu disease, Niemann-Pick disease, etc.	
None	1

(Modified from Gertz and Kyle,[63] with permission.)

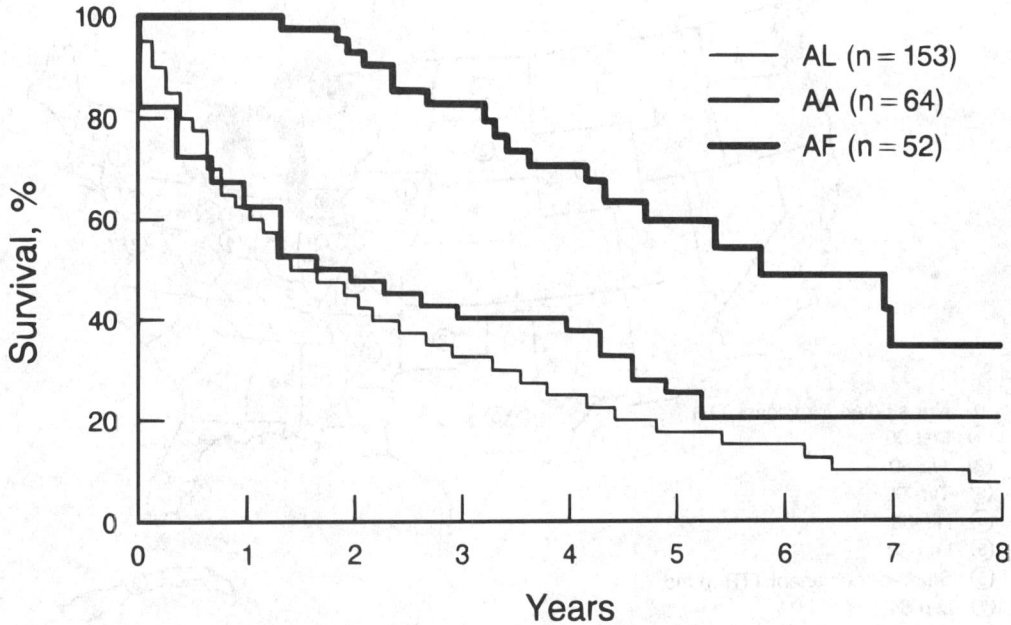

Fig. 88-12. Survival of patients with familial amyloidosis (AF) in comparison with survival for those with primary (AL) and secondary (AA) systemic amyloidosis. (From Gertz et al.,[70] with permission.)

plegia and recurrent infections may develop AA amyloidosis. Bronchiectasis, osteomyelitis, cystic fibrosis, and hypogammaglobulinemia are uncommon causes. Neoplasms, including Hodgkin disease, non-Hodgkin lymphoma, macroglobulinemia, and hypernephroma, have been noted with systemic amyloidosis.

Treatment of AA amyloidosis depends on the underlying disease. Resorption of amyloid after therapy for osteomyelitis, tuberculosis, or empyema has been reported. Nephrectomy for hypernephroma may result in the disappearance of amyloid. Dimethylsulfoxide has apparently helped some patients with rheumatoid arthritis or ankylosing spondylitis. Chlorambucil is beneficial in juvenile chronic arthritis.[65] Renal transplantation may be helpful.[66,67] The duration of survival in AA is similar to that in AL, but both are shorter than the duration of survival in AF amyloidosis (Fig. 88-12).

FAMILIAL AMYLOIDOSIS

Familial or hereditary amyloidosis has been reviewed.[68,69] All forms except familial Mediterranean fever have an autosomal dominant inheritance pattern. In our practice, the geographic distribution of familial amyloidosis is wide and not associated with clustering[70] (Fig. 88-13). More than 30 transthyretin point mutations have been recognized. Clinically, familial amyloidosis can be classified most easily as neuropathic, nephropathic, or cardiopathic.

Neuropathic

Type I familial amyloidosis, described by Andrade,[71] is characterized by a sensorimotor peripheral neuropathy beginning in the lower extremities of persons who are in the third decade of life, as well as by autonomic changes, disturbances of bladder and gastrointestinal function, and vitreous opacities. Death usually results within 10 years. In some patients, symptoms do not begin until the sixth or seventh decade of life. Most cases have been reported from Sweden, Portugal, and Japan. Amyloid fibrils consist of transthyretin (prealbumin) with methionine at position 30 in place of valine.[72]

Type II familial amyloidosis (Indiana) is characterized by development of the carpal tunnel syndrome in persons who are in the fifth or sixth decade of life. Sensorimotor peripheral neuropathy often involves the lower extremities later, but involvement of the autonomic and central nervous system is not a feature. Impotence and vitreous opacities may occur. Involvement of the kidney is not characteristic.

Specific treatment does not exist for familial amyloidosis, and management is limited to symptomatic care. Recently, liver transplantation was reported in four Swedish patients with transthyretin Met 30. The variant transthyretin in serum decreased dramatically after transplantation. Some improvement was apparent in intestinal function.[73]

Nephropathic

Familial Mediterranean fever affects persons of Mediterranean descent and is characterized by recurrent episodes of fever and abdominal pain that begin in childhood.[74] Colchicine is effective in controlling the symptoms and preventing the development of amyloidosis.[75]

Familial amyloidosis involving the kidneys has been reported by Ostertag[76] and more recently by Mornaghi et al.[77] The major features were hypertension and renal insufficiency, which progressed rapidly to end-stage renal failure. Recently, an English family with the Ostertag-type hereditary amyloidosis resulting from an apolipoprotein AI mutation (Arg 60) was recognized.[78]

Cardiopathic

Systemic amyloidosis manifested by progressive congestive heart failure, which begins in persons who are in the fourth or fifth decade of life and leads to death within 2–6 years, has been described in Denmark.[79,80] A large kindred in the Appalachian region of the United States with cardiomyopathy has been reported.[81]

Miscellaneous

Hereditary cerebral hemorrhage with amyloidosis has been recognized in Iceland. It occurs in the third or fourth decade of life and is characterized by cerebral hemorrhage, which may

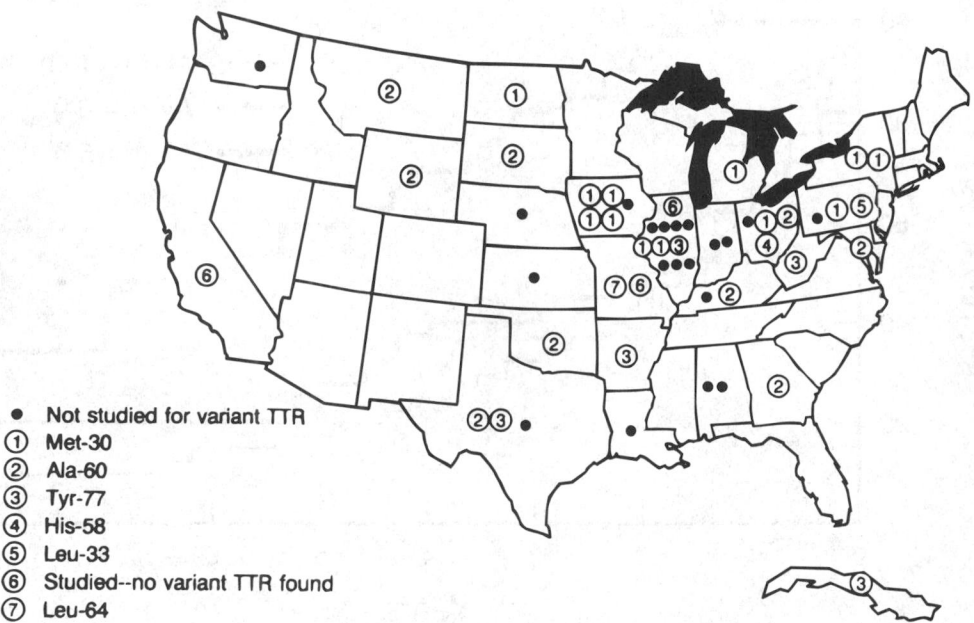

Fig. 88-13. Geographic distribution of 52 North American-born patients with familial amyloidosis. TTR, transthyretin. (From Gertz et al.,[70] with permission.)

cause immediate death or recurrent strokes of varying severity. The amyloid consists of cystatin C (γ trace). This variant of cystatin C has glutamine at position 58 in place of leucine.[82] Hereditary cerebral hemorrhage with amyloidosis—Dutch type—is composed of β-protein.[83]

SENILE AMYLOIDOSIS

Small deposits of amyloid in the brain, heart, aorta, and pancreas of patients >70 years of age are common.[84] Senile cardiac amyloid consists of two types: senile cardiac amyloid (ASC_1), which involves the ventricles, and isolated atrial amyloid (IAA). ASC_1 fibrils consist of transthyretin,[85] whereas IAA fibrils contain atrial natriuretic peptide.[86] In one patient with systemic senile amyloidosis, a single amino acid substitution of isoleucine for valine at position 122 was found.[87] This finding is of interest, although a single amino acid substitution probably is not responsible for a condition as common as senile amyloidosis.

Senile cardiac amyloid has been found in 25% of patients ≥80 years old. Extracardiac involvement is common, but the amounts of amyloid are small.[88] Senile cardiac amyloidosis has been recognized antemortem; it was characterized by congestive heart failure, and the mean survival after diagnosis was 26 months, which is much longer than that seen with cardiac AL amyloidosis.[89] The amyloid fibrils consist of normal transthyretin. No variants have been recognized.

LOCALIZED AMYLOIDOSIS

Localized amyloidosis most commonly involves the lungs, urinary bladder, ureter, urethra, or skin. Although the amyloid fibrils consist of κ or λ light chains, no M protein is in the serum or urine. The amyloidosis never becomes systemic, and treatment is unnecessary unless it causes local symptoms.

Amyloidosis localized to the lung can be classified as tracheobronchial, single or multiple nodular, or diffuse interstitial.[90] In the tracheobronchial form, mucosal amyloid deposits occur and may produce cough, dyspnea, wheezing, and hemop-

PREFERRED APPROACH

When the histologic diagnosis of amyloidosis is made, the clinician must determine the type because all classes of amyloid appear the same when viewed under polarized light after Congo red staining. The first step is a careful history in which the presence of weakness or fatigue, weight loss, purpura (especially periorbital), light-headedness, change in voice or tongue, jaw claudication, paresthesias, dyspnea, and features of steatorrhea is ascertained. It is important to ask about familial involvement. Periorbital purpura, macroglossia, submandibular swelling, hepatomegaly, edema, and orthostatic hypotension are important physical features suggesting systemic amyloidosis. The presence of a nephrotic syndrome, congestive heart failure, carpal tunnel syndrome, sensorimotor peripheral neuropathy, or orthostatic hypotension in conjunction with an M protein in the serum or urine is a strong indication of amyloidosis. Immunofixation is frequently necessary for detection of a small M protein. The diagnosis is confirmed by biopsy. Abdominal fat and bone marrow should be the first tissues to undergo biopsy. If the results are negative, a rectal biopsy specimen, including submucosa, should be obtained. If this is negative, tissue should be obtained from a suspected involved organ.

Treatment of primary (AL) amyloidosis is directed toward reduction in the production of the monoclonal precursor light chain. Currently, we are engaged in a prospective study comparing melphalan and prednisone with a combination of alkylating agents (vincristine, BCNU, melphalan, cyclophosphamide, and prednisone). In the event of secondary amyloidosis, treatment is directed against the underlying disorder. Patients with localized amyloidosis should not be treated unless the amyloid is producing local symptoms. There is no effective treatment for senile amyloidosis. Liver transplantation is beneficial for familial amyloidosis.

tysis. Solitary amyloid nodules may be single or multiple. Amyloid may be confined to the larynx or adjacent structures.[91]

Amyloidosis localized to the urinary bladder frequently produces gross hematuria.[92] Cystoscopy often reveals a tumefactive deposit that is confused with carcinoma. Amyloid may be localized to the ureter and often produces obstruction and hydronephrosis. Amyloid may also be localized to the urethra.

DIALYSIS-ASSOCIATED AMYLOIDOSIS

Patients on long-term hemodialysis often develop a carpal tunnel syndrome with pain involving the shoulders, hands, wrists, hips, and knees.[93] Areas of cystic radiolucency are common in the juxta-articular bones. Pathologic fractures have occurred from large amyloid deposits. The major component of the amyloid is β_2-microglobulin.[94] Usually, the patient has been on hemodialysis with cuprophane membranes for >10 years and has high serum levels of β_2-microglobulin.[95] Systemic amyloid deposits also occur but are of little or no clinical consequence. Amyloidosis is seen with both hemodialysis and peritoneal dialysis. Renal transplantation often leads to dramatic improvement in joint symptoms, and when performed early it is the most effective preventive measure. Clinical trials using a β_2-microglobulin-absorbent column are in progress.[96]

ALZHEIMER DISEASE

A serious form of amyloidosis in the elderly is cerebral amyloidosis associated with Alzheimer disease. Neuropathologic findings include cerebral amyloid angiopathy, senile plaques, and neurofibrillary tangles. The cause of Alzheimer disease is unknown.[97] The major protein component of the cerebrovascular amyloid fibril and the plaque consists of β-protein. The mechanism of amyloid formation is being studied intensely.[98]

ACKNOWLEDGMENT

This work was supported in part by the Quade Amyloidosis Research Fund.

REFERENCES

1. Kyle RA, Gertz MA: Amyloidosis. p. 525. In Wiernik PH, Canellos GP, Kyle RA, Schiffer CA (eds): Neoplastic Diseases of the Blood. 2nd Ed. Churchill Livingstone, New York, 1991
2. Glenner GG, Ein D, Eanes ED et al: Creation of "amyloid" fibrils from Bence Jones proteins in vitro. Science 174:712, 1971
3. Solomon A, Kyle RA, Frangione B: Light chain variable region subgroups of monoclonal immunoglobulins in amyloidosis AL. p. 449. In Glenner GG, Osserman EF, Benditt EP et al (eds): Amyloidosis. Plenum, New York, 1986
4. Bellotti V, Merlini G, Bucciarelli A et al: Relevance of class, molecular weight and isoelectric point in predicting human light chain amyloidogenicity. Br J Haematol 74:65, 1990
5. Buxbaum J, Hauser D: Aberrant immunoglobulin synthesis in light chain amyloidosis: free light chain and light chain fragment production by human bone marrow cells in short-term tissue culture. J Clin Invest 78:798, 1986
6. Preud'homme JL, Ganeval D, Grünfeld JP et al: Immunoglobulin synthesis in primary and myeloma amyloidosis. Clin Exp Immunol 73:389, 1988
7. Nomura S, Kanoh T, Uchino H: Intracellular formation of amyloid fibrils in myeloma: cytochemical, immunochemical and electron microscopic observations. Nippon Ketsueki Gakkai Zasshi 45:615, 1982
8. Durie BGM, Persky B, Soehnlen BJ et al: Amyloid production in human myeloma stem-cell culture, with morphologic evidence of amyloid secretion by associated macrophages. N Engl J Med 307:1689, 1982
9. Solomon A, Weiss DT, Pepys MB: Induction in mice of human light-chain-associated amyloidosis. Am J Pathol 140:629, 1992
10. Eulitz M, Weiss DT, Solomon A: Immunoglobulin heavy-chain-associated amyloidosis. Proc Natl Acad Sci USA 87:6542, 1990
11. Levin M, Franklin EC, Frangione B, Pras M: The amino acid sequence of a major nonimmunoglobulin component of some amyloid fibrils. J Clin Invest 51:2773, 1972
12. De Beer FC, Mallya RK, Fagan EA et al: Serum amyloid-A protein concentra-

tion in inflammatory diseases and its relationship to the incidence of reactive systemic amyloidosis. Lancet 2:231, 1982
13. Kluve-Beckerman B, Dwulet FE, Benson MD: Human serum amyloid A: three hepatic mRNAs and the corresponding proteins in one person. J Clin Invest 82:1670, 1988
14. Skinner M: Protein AA/SAA. J Intern Med 232:513, 1992
15. Kisilevsky R, Benson MD, Axelrad MA, Boudreau L: The effect of a liver protein synthesis inhibitor on plasma SAA levels in a model of accelerated amyloid deposition. Lab Invest 41:206, 1979
16. Prelli F, Pras M, Frangione B: The primary structure of human tissue amyloid P component from a patient with primary idiopathic amyloidosis. J Biol Chem 260:12895, 1985
17. Coria F, Castaño E, Prelli F et al: Isolation and characterization of amyloid P component from Alzheimer's disease and other types of cerebral amyloidosis. Lab Invest 58:454, 1988
18. Pepys MB: Amyloid P component and the diagnosis of amyloidosis. J Intern Med 232:519, 1992
19. Snow AD, Willmer J, Kisilevsky R: Sulfated glycosaminoglycans: a common constituent of all amyloids? Lab Invest 56:120, 1987
20. Kisilevsky R: Proteoglycans, glycosaminoglycans, amyloid-enhancing factor, and amyloid deposition. J Intern Med 232:515, 1992
21. Chronopoulos S, Lembo P, Alizadeh-Khiavi K, Ali-Khan Z: Ubiquitin: its potential significance in murine AA amyloidogenesis. J Pathol 167:249, 1992
22. Lavie G, Zucker-Franklin D, Franklin EC: Degradation of serum amyloid A protein by surface-associated enzymes of human blood monocytes. J Exp Med 148:1020, 1978
23. Skinner M, Stone P, Shirahama T et al: The association of an elastase with amyloid fibrils. Proc Soc Exp Biol Med 181:211, 1986
24. Westermark P, Johnson KH, Pitkänen P: Systemic amyloidosis: a review with emphasis on pathogenesis. Appl Pathol 3:55, 1985
25. Sipe JD: Amyloidosis. Annu Rev Biochem 61:947, 1992
26. Kyle RA, Linos A, Beard CM et al: Incidence and natural history of primary systemic amyloidosis in Olmsted County, Minnesota, 1950 through 1989. Blood 79:1817, 1992
27. Smith TJ, Kyle RA, Lie JT: Clinical significance of histopathologic patterns of cardiac amyloidosis. Mayo Clin Proc 59:547, 1984
28. Roberts WC, Waller BF: Cardiac amyloidosis causing cardiac dysfunction: analysis of 54 necropsy patients. Am J Cardiol 52:137, 1983
29. Klein AL, Hatle LK, Taliercio CP et al: Serial Doppler echocardiographic follow-up of left ventricular diastolic function in cardiac amyloidosis. J Am Coll Cardiol 16:1135, 1990
30. Cueto-Garcia L, Reeder GS, Kyle RA et al: Echocardiographic findings in systemic amyloidosis: spectrum of cardiac involvement and relation to survival. J Am Coll Cardiol 6:737, 1985
31. Gertz MA, Kyle RA, Griffing WL, Hunder GG: Jaw claudication in primary systemic amyloidosis. Medicine 65:173, 1986
32. Danby P, Harris KPG, Williams B et al: Adrenal dysfunction in patients with renal amyloid. Q J Med 76:915, 1990
33. Kyle RA, Dyck PJ: Amyloidosis and neuropathy. p. 1294. In Dyck PJ, Thomas PK, Griffin JW et al (eds): Peripheral Neuropathy. Vol. 2. 3rd Ed. WB Saunders, Philadelphia, 1993
34. Traynor AE, Gertz MA, Kyle RA: Cranial neuropathy associated with primary amyloidosis. Ann Neurol 29:451, 1991
35. Kavanaugh JH: Multiple myeloma, amyloid arthropathy, and pathological fracture of the femur: a case report. J Bone Joint Surg Am 60:135, 1978
36. Whitaker JN, Hashimoto K, Quinones M: Skeletal muscle pseudohypertrophy in primary amyloidosis. Neurology 27:47, 1977
37. Bruni J, Bilbao JM, Pritzker KPH: Myopathy associated with amyloid angiopathy. Can J Neurol Sci 4:77, 1977
38. Piette WW: Myeloma, paraproteinemias, and the skin. Med Clin North Am 70:155, 1986
39. Greipp PR, Kyle RA, Bowie EJW: Factor-X deficiency in amyloidosis: a critical review. Am J Hematol 11:443, 1981
40. Yood RA, Skinner M, Rubinow A et al: Bleeding manifestations in 100 patients with amyloidosis. JAMA 249:1322, 1983
41. Gertz MA, Kyle RA: Hepatic amyloidosis (primary [AL], immunoglobulin light chain): the natural history in 80 patients. Am J Med 85:73, 1988
42. Chen KTK: Amyloidosis presenting in the respiratory tract. Pathol Annu 24 (Pt 1):253, 1989
43. Gertz MA, Kyle RA, Greipp PR: Hyposplenism in primary systemic amyloidosis. Ann Intern Med 98:475, 1983
44. Gastineau DA, Gertz MA, Daniels TM et al: Inhibitor of the thrombin time in systemic amyloidosis: a common coagulation abnormality. Blood 77:2637, 1991
45. Gertz MA, Li C-Y, Shirahama T, Kyle RA: Utility of subcutaneous fat aspira-

tion for the diagnosis of systemic amyloidosis (immunoglobulin light chain). Arch Intern Med 148:929, 1988

46. Korbet SM, Schwartz MM, Lewis EJ: Immunotactoid glomerulopathy. Am J Kidney Dis 17:247, 1991

47. Buxbaum JN, Chuba JV, Hellman GC et al: Monoclonal immunoglobulin deposition disease: light chain and light and heavy chain deposition diseases and their relation to light chain amyloidosis; clinical features, immunopathology. and molecular analysis. Ann Intern Med 112:455, 1990

48. Hawkins PN, Lavender JP, Pepys MB: Evaluation of systemic amyloidosis by scintigraphy with ^{123}I-labeled serum amyloid P component. N Engl J Med 323:508, 1990

49. Gertz MA, Brown ML, Hauser MF, Kyle RA: Utility of technetium Tc 99m pyrophosphate bone scanning in cardiac amyloidosis. Arch Intern Med 147: 1039, 1987

50. Kyle RA, Bayrd ED: "Primary" systemic amyloidosis and myeloma: discussion of relationship and review of 81 cases. Arch Intern Med 107:344, 1961

51. Kyle RA, Greipp PR, O'Fallon WM: Primary systemic amyloidosis: multivariate analysis for prognostic factors in 168 cases. Blood 68:220, 1986

52. Gertz MA, Kyle RA, Greipp PR et al: Beta$_2$-microglobulin predicts survival in primary systemic amyloidosis. Am J Med 89:609, 1990

53. Gertz MA, Kyle RA, O'Fallon WM: Dialysis support of patients with primary systemic amyloidosis: a study of 211 patients. Arch Intern Med 152:2245, 1992

54. Kyle RA, Greipp PR: Primary systemic amyloidosis: comparison of melphalan and prednisone versus placebo. Blood 52:818, 1978

55. Kyle RA, Greipp PR, Garton JP, Gertz MA: Primary systemic amyloidosis: comparison of melphalan/prednisone versus colchicine. Am J Med 79:708, 1985

56. Gertz MA, Kyle RA: Acute leukemia and cytogenetic abnormalities complicating melphalan treatment of primary systemic amyloidosis. Arch Intern Med 150:629, 1990

57. Gertz MA, Kyle RA: Phase II trial of α-tocopherol (vitamin E) in the treatment of primary systemic amyloidosis. Am J Hematol 34:55, 1990

58. Gertz MA, Kyle RA: Phase II trial of recombinant interferon alfa-2 in the treatment of primary systemic amyloidosis. Am J Hematol 44:125, 1993

59. Hosenpud JD, Uretsky BF, Griffith BP et al: Successful intermediate-term outcome for patients with cardiac amyloidosis undergoing heart transplantation: results of a multicenter survey. J Heart Transplant 9:346, 1990

60. Hosenpud JD, DeMarco T, Frazier OH et al: Progression of systemic disease and reduced long-term survival in patients with cardiac amyloidosis undergoing heart transplantation: follow-up results of a multicenter survey. Circulation, Suppl. 3. 84:III-338, 1991

61. Deng M, Park JW, Roy-Chowdury R et al: Heart transplantation for restrictive cardiomyopathy: development of cardiac amyloidosis in preexisting monoclonal gammopathy. J Heart Lung Transplant 11:139, 1992

62. Laakso M, Mutru O, Isomäki H, Koota K: Mortality from amyloidosis and renal diseases in patients with rheumatoid arthritis. Ann Rheum Dis 45:663, 1986

63. Gertz MA, Kyle RA: Secondary systemic amyloidosis: response and survival in 64 patients. Medicine 70:246, 1991

64. Greenstein AJ, Sachar DB, Nannan Panday AK et al: Amyloidosis and inflammatory bowel disease: a 50-year experience with 25 patients. Medicine 71: 261, 1992

65. Deschênes G, Prieur AM, Hayem F et al: Renal amyloidosis in juvenile chronic arthritis: evolution after chlorambucil treatment. Pediatr Nephrol 4:463, 1990

66. Pasternack A, Ahonen J, Kuhlbäck B: Renal transplantation in 45 patients with amyloidosis. Transplantation 42:598, 1986

67. Hartmann A, Holdaas H, Fauchald P et al: Fifteen years' experience with renal transplantation in systemic amyloidosis. Transplant Int 5:15, 1992

68. Varga J, Wohlgethan JR: The clinical and biochemical spectrum of hereditary amyloidosis. Semin Arthritis Rheum 18:14, 1988

69. Jacobson DR, Buxbaum JN: Genetic aspects of amyloidosis. Adv Hum Genet 20:69, 1991

70. Gertz MA, Kyle RA, Thibodeau SN: Familial amyloidosis: a study of 52 North American-born patients examined during a 30-year period. Mayo Clin Proc 67:428, 1992

71. Andrade C: A peculiar form of peripheral neuropathy: familiar atypical generalized amyloidosis with special involvement of the peripheral nerves. Brain 75:408, 1952

72. Costa PP, Figueira AS, Bravo FR: Amyloid fibril protein related to prealbumin in familial amyloidotic polyneuropathy. Proc Natl Acad Sci USA 75:4499, 1978

73. Holmgren G, Steen L, Ekstedt J et al: Liver transplantation in four Swedish FAP met30 patients, abstracted (0.39). In the Second International Symposium on Familial Amyloidotic Polyneuropathy and Other Transthyretin Related Disorders. Skellefteå, Sweden, June 1–3, 1992

74. Sohar E, Gafni J, Pras M, Heller H: Familial Mediterranean fever: a survey of 470 cases and review of the literature. Am J Med 43:227, 1967

75. Zemer D, Pras M, Sohar E et al: Colchicine in the prevention and treatment of the amyloidosis of familial Mediterranean fever. N Engl J Med 314:1001, 1986

76. Ostertag B: Demonstration einer eigenartigen familiären "paraamyloidose," abstracted. Zentralbl Allg Pathol 56:253. 1933

77. Mornaghi R, Rubinstein P, Franklin EC: Familial renal amyloidosis: case reports and genetic studies. Am J Med 73:609, 1982

78. Soutar AK, Hawkins PN, Vigushin DM et al: Apolipoprotein AI mutation Arg-60 causes autosomal dominant amyloidosis. Proc Natl Acad Sci USA 89: 7389, 1992

79. Frederiksen T, Gøtzsche H, Harboe N et al: Familial primary amyloidosis with severe amyloid heart disease. Am J Med 33:328, 1962

80. Ranløv I, Alves IL, Ranløv PJ et al: A Danish kindred with familial amyloid cardiomyopathy revisited: identification of a mutant transthyretin-methionine[111] variant in serum from patients and carriers. Am J Med 93:3, 1992

81. Benson MD, Wallace MR, Tejada E et al: Hereditary amyloidosis: description of a new American kindred with late onset cardiomyopathy: Appalachian amyloid. Arthritis Rheum 30:195, 1987

82. Jensson O, Gudmundsson G, Arnason A et al: Hereditary cystatin C (γ-trace) amyloid angiopathy of the CNS causing cerebral hemorrhage. Acta Neurol Scand 76:102, 1987

83. Castaño EM, Wisniewski T, Frangione B: Inherited amyloids of the nervous system. Curr Opin Neurobiol 1:448, 1991

84. Wright JR, Calkins E, Breen WJ et al: Relationship of amyloid to aging: review of the literature and systematic study of 83 patients derived from a general hospital population. Medicine 48:39, 1969

85. Cornwell GG III, Westermark P, Natvig JB. Murdoch W: Senile cardiac amyloid: evidence that fibrils contain a protein immunologically related to prealbumin. Immunology 44:447, 1981

86. Johansson B, Wernstedt C, Westermark P: Atrial natriuretic peptide deposited as atrial amyloid fibrils. Biochem Biophys Res Commun 148:1087, 1987

87. Gorevic PD, Prelli FC, Wright J et al: Systemic senile amyloidosis: identification of a new prealbumin (transthyretin) variant in cardiac tissue: immunologic and biochemical similarity to one form of familial amyloidotic polyneuropathy. J Clin Invest 83:836, 1989

88. Cornwell GG III, Murdoch WL, Kyle RA et al: Frequency and distribution of senile cardiovascular amyloid: a clinicopathologic correlation. Am J Med 75:618, 1983

89. Olson LJ, Gertz MA, Edwards WD et al: Senile cardiac amyloidosis with myocardial dysfunction: diagnosis by endomyocardial biopsy and immunohistochemistry. N Engl J Med 317:738, 1987

90. Rubinow A, Celli BR, Cohen AS et al: Localized amyloidosis of the lower respiratory tract. Am Rev Respir Dis 118:603, 1978

91. Lewis JE, Olsen KD, Kurtin PJ, Kyle RA: Laryngeal amyloidosis: a clinicopathologic and immunohistochemical review. Otolaryngol Head Neck Surg 106: 372, 1992

92. Khan SM, Birch PJ, Bass PS et al: Localized amyloidosis of the lower genitourinary tract: a clinicopathological and immunohistochemical study of nine cases. Histopathology 21:143, 1992

93. Drüeke TB: Beta-2-microglobulin amyloidosis and renal bone disease. Miner Electrolyte Metab 17:261, 1991

94. Gejyo F, Yamada T, Odani S et al: A new form of amyloid protein associated with chronic hemodialysis was identified as β$_2$-microglobulin. Biochem Biophys Res Commun 129:701, 1985

95. Bardin T, Zingraff J, Shirahama T et al: Hemodialysis-associated amyloidosis and beta-2 microglobulin: clinical and immunohistochemical study. Am J Med 83:419, 1987

96. Gejyo F, Arakawa M: β$_2$-Microglobulin-associated amyloidoses. J Intern Med 232:531, 1992

97. Glenner GG: The pathobiology of Alzheimer's disease. Annu Rev Med 40: 45, 1989

98. Glenner GG: Alzheimer's disease. J Intern Med 232:533, 1992

99. Kyle RA, Greipp PR: Amyloidosis [AL]: clinical and laboratory features in 229 cases. Mayo Clin Proc 58:665, 1983

100. Kyle RA, Bayrd ED: Amyloidosis; review of 236 cases. Medicine 54:271, 1975

101. Kyle RA, Gertz MA: Systemic amyloidosis. CRC Crit Rev Oncol Hematol 10: 49, 1990

102. Gertz MA, Kyle RA: Primary systemic amyloidosis—a diagnostic primer. Mayo Clin Proc 64:1505, 1989

103. Husby G, Araki S, Benditt EP et al: The 1990 guidelines for nomenclature and classification of amyloid and amyloidosis. p. 7. In Natvig JB, Førre Ø, Husby G et al (eds): Amyloid and Amyloidosis 1990. Kluwer Academic, Dordrecht, The Netherlands, 1991

Atypical Immune Proliferations

89

Douglas S. Harrington, Aneal S. Masih, and
David T. Purtilo

INTRODUCTION

The development of modern classification systems for hematologic malignancies resulted from recognition that specific histologic and cytologic patterns correlated with prognosis.[1-3] The Working Formulation for Clinical Usage, which evolved from the earlier Rappaport scheme for non-Hodgkin lymphomas (NHLs), reliably predicts prognosis based on whether malignant infiltrates are composed of small or large cells and whether the pattern is follicular or diffuse.[1] The Rye classification scheme for Hodgkin disease correlates prognosis with histologic features such as the number of Reed-Sternberg cells, the composition of the background lymphoid cells, and the degree and type of sclerosis.[2] The French-American-British (FAB) scheme for leukemias relies on cytologic features for lymphocytic leukemias and a combination of cytologic and cytochemical features for myeloid leukemias.[3]

These systems can be reliably applied to most clinically relevant situations, but some conditions do not neatly fall into these categories. The Working Formulation fails when classifying T-cell lymphomas because the classification is based on histologic evaluation alone and because T-cell lymphomas can present with a wide spectrum of cytologic variation within the same patient over the course of the disease.[4,5] The FAB system for lymphocytic leukemias similarly does not reliably predict prognosis, and immunophenotypic analysis is becoming increasingly more important.[6]

The tremendous diversity of the immune system and its variable responses to challenges has led to recognition of certain hyperplastic responses that are clearly benign and manifest specific histologic patterns if biopsied.[7] Examples of benign hyperplastic immune responses include follicular hyperplasia, in which B-cell areas of the lymph node increase in size and number (Fig. 89-1) and sinus histiocytosis, in which benign histiocytes distend lymph node sinuses[7] (Plate 89-1). Although clearly benign or malignant lesions usually can be easily diagnosed by clinicopathologic correlation, a significant group of patients present with unusual clinical features, and their biopsies result in pathologic diagnoses that prompt use of terms such as "borderline," "atypical," or "uncertain malignant potential," leaving the clinician at a loss as to how to treat the condition. Other disorders present with clinical features that suggest a malignant process but also show characteristic but unusual histologic features that correlate with a benign condi-

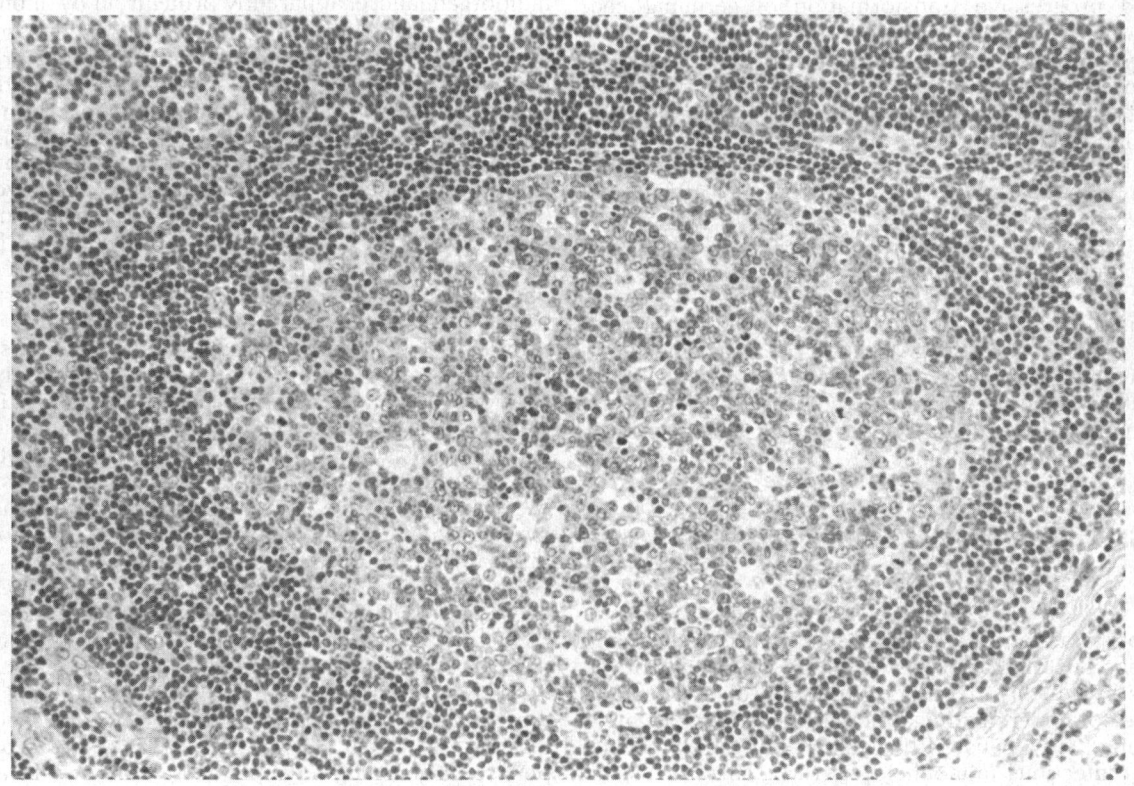

Fig. 89-1. Follicular hyperplasia. Prominent reaction centers with a high mitotic rate and numerous tingible-body macrophages are characteristic of benign follicular hyperplasia. (H&E × 400.)

tion. Most of these processes are related to an abnormal immune response to some inciting stimulus. In some, both the cause of immune dysfunction and the basis for abnormal proliferation are known, whereas in others only circumstantial evidence of an abnormal immune response exists. The more commonly encountered "atypical" responses related to viruses, drugs, and genetic predispositions, as well as certain relevant processes of unknown cause, are discussed.

WHAT CONSTITUTES AN ATYPICAL LYMPHOPROLIFERATION

Most clinical lymphoproliferative disorders are discrete, easily recognizable conditions, which can be diagnosed by paying careful attention to the patient's history, physical examination, and selected laboratory tests. Many of these disorders encompass a spectrum of histologic findings reflecting variable host responses to the underlying etiologic agent. Some of the disorders fall outside of the usually recognized patterns of host response and are therefore considered atypical; some patient biopsies will show characteristic features that are consistent with the suspected disease, whereas others will present histologic patterns that are not clearly benign or malignant or will manifest a malignant pattern that is not easily categorized.

Certain conditions have characteristic clinical features with unusual benign lymph node morphology that suggests a lymphoproliferative process, and that are not associated with progression to frank neoplasia.[7] Conditions of this type include autoimmune disorders such as systemic lupus erythematosus (SLE), drug reactions, fatal infectious mononucleosis (FIM), infection-associated hemophagocytic syndrome, and acquired immunodeficiency syndrome (AIDS) lymphadenopathy.[7-9]

Other benign conditions may present with nonspecific clinical features associated with nodal morphologic atypia.[7-9] Conditions of this type include infectious mononucleosis, Kikuchi disease, and progressive transformation of germinal centers.[7-9]

Another group of lesions is associated with pathologic and clinical features that are "borderline" (i.e., not clearly benign or malignant) and that may resolve spontaneously or progress to frank neoplasia. Conditions in this category include posttransplantation lymphoproliferative disorders, angioimmunoblastic lymphadenopathy with dysproteinemia (AILD), systemic Castleman disease, low-grade (0–1) angiocentric immunoproliferative lesions (AIL), and lymphomatoid papulosis (LP).[7-10] Progression to lymphoma has been documented in AIL and LP.[7-10]

This discussion is confined to those diseases that are considered benign but may sometimes result in the death of the patient either by progression to malignancy or by damage to the immune system. Accurate diagnosis requires careful correlation of immunohistologic, karyotypic, virologic, and genotypic analyses with the clinical findings.

VIRUS-ASSOCIATED ATYPICAL LYMPHOPROLIFERATIONS

Epstein-Barr Virus

The prototypical cause of atypical lymphoproliferations is the ubiquitous Epstein-Barr virus (EBV).[8] A knowledge of the mechanisms by which EBV induces lymphoproliferation provides a model for understanding other virus-associated lymphoproliferations.[8] EBV causes the well-characterized clinical syndrome of infectious mononucleosis (IM). This discussion does not specifically address IM but covers those lesions that fall outside the spectrum that is clinically recognized as IM.

EBV, a large herpesvirus (172,000 base pairs), preferentially infects B cells in humans and causes lifelong infection.[8] The key to understanding atypical responses to EBV involves the relationship established between the virus and the immune system after primary infection.[8] Primary infection by EBV results in two main responses, depending on the age of the individual or the maturity of the immune system.[8] If the primary infection occurs in early childhood, the immune response and clinical symptoms are almost always silent, but about two-thirds of infected older children and adults will develop IM.[8] Once infected by EBV, an individual maintains a lifelong symbiotic relationship with the virus in which a virus-driven B-cell proliferation is kept in check by the host immune surveillance.[8] A low level of virus production occurs in the oropharyngeal region by unknown mechanisms; about 1 in 106 B cells in peripheral blood carries EBV.[8] The intimate association of oropharyngeal epithelium with oropharyngeal lymphoid tissue results in a constant cycle of circulating infected B cells.[8] Disease results when the immune system is depressed, either by iatrogenic means or by concurrent infections with other agents[8] (Fig. 89-2). The resulting immunosuppression allows escape of EBV-infected B cells and resultant lymphoproliferation.[8-12] The self-limited course of IM contrasts with the atypical responses that can occur.[8]

FIM occurs in approximately 1 in 3,000 IM cases, or about 40 cases annually in the United States.[8,11-13] The explosive lymphoproliferation that occurs in FIM mimics that in certain hematologic neoplasms, such as lymphoid leukemia, and can obscure recognition of FIM as a cause of death.[8,11-13] Patients who progress to FIM initially present with the usual signs and symptoms of IM, including fever, sore throat, malaise, anorexia, nausea, vomiting, and a maculopapular rash, but these symptoms are usually more extensive.[11] The median age at presentation is 13 years, with a 1:1 male/female ratio.[11] The median survival time is approximately 4 weeks, and splenic rupture is conspicuously rare as a cause of death in these patients.[8,11] Patients who develop FIM succumb to severe and progressive multiorgan failure, apparently brought on by anomalous killer cell activity, which nonselectively destroys uninfected hepatocytes, bone marrow elements, skin, and other organs during the unrestricted polyclonal immune response initiated by the EBV infection.[8-11] Patients initially manifest an atypical lymphocytosis but subsequently develop severe, persistent pancytopenia, hepatic dysfunction resulting in fulminant hepatitis, meningoencephalitis, and varying degrees of myocarditis[8-11] (Fig. 89-3). FIM is characterized by extensive infiltration of lymphoid and parenchymal organs by polyclonal T and B cells in varying degrees of transformation, resulting in a polymorphous pattern, which contrasts with the monomorphic pattern of malignant infiltrates[8,11-13] (Plate 89-2).

Rarely, elderly patients, malnourished patients, and those with cancer also develop EBV-associated atypical lymphoproliferation.[8,12,13] These patients have a secondary immunodeficiency.[13] Most of them will have had a prior infection with EBV and will have achieved a virus-immune system balance before acquiring an immunodeficiency, which then allows the virus to escape the defective immune surveillance mechanisms.[8,11-13] Lymphoproliferations ranging from IM to FIM to overt lymphoma can then occur.[8,11-13]

Patients with AIDS also experience virus reactivation because the T-cell arm of the immune system is selectively attacked by the AIDS virus, with resulting loss of control over the persistent EBV infection.[8,12-14] Various lesions, including explosive follicular hyperplasia, hairy leukoplakia of the tongue, and lymphoma have all been associated with EBV.[8,12-14] A direct role for EBV in HIV-infected patients with persistent genealogic lymphadenopathy syndrome has been recently challenged.[14] Children with AIDS often develop lymphoid interstitial pneumonitis due to EBV-induced polyclonal B-cell proliferation; adults with AIDS have a 1,000-fold

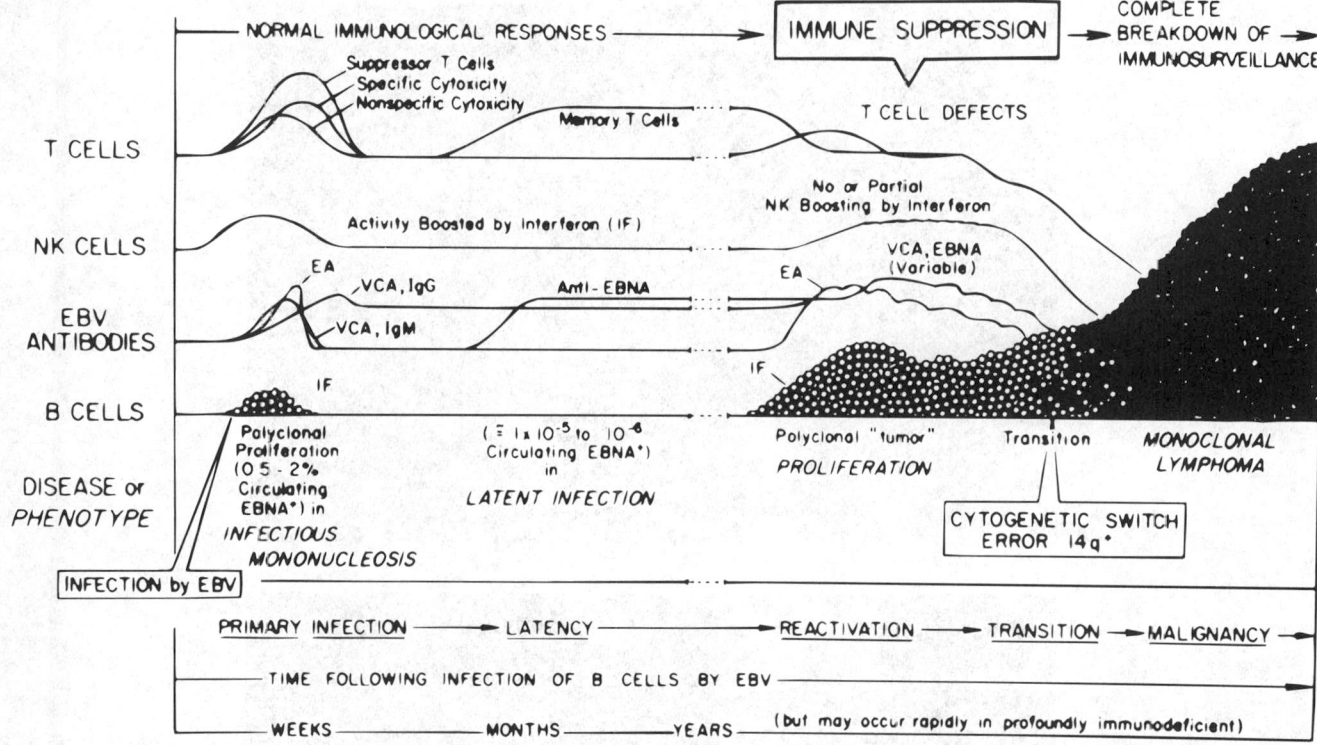

Fig. 89-2. EBV-immune system relationship and the development of lymphoproliferations associated with various immune deficits or diseases.

increased risk of developing malignant lymphomas, most of which probably begin as polyclonal EBV-associated lymphoproliferations and progress to monoclonality owing to lack of adequate control of EBV by the damaged T-cell system and further cytogenetic events.[8,12–14] About 50% of the NHLs in AIDS patients are etiologically linked to EBV.[8,12–14]

The diagnosis of various EBV-associated atypical lymphoproliferations can be difficult because the usual EBV-antibody responses may be lacking or unusually high, and the clinical picture may resemble an acute leukemia, another malignancy, or overwhelming sepsis.[8,11–14] An accurate diagnosis may require performing serologic studies of the EBV-specific antibodies to the viral capsid antigen (VCA), early antigen (EA), and EBV nuclear antigen (EBNA); staining of lymphoid tissue for EBNA; establishment of lymphoblastoid cell lines; and in some cases, molecular analyses, including in situ and Southern blot hybridization or polymerase chain reaction (PCR) studies[8,11–14] (Table 89-1). Because FIM is rare, a search for a heritable immunodeficiency in family members is mandatory.[8,11–13] Association of EBV with other conditions is discussed in the relevant section.

Cytomegalovirus

Cytomegalovirus (CMV), also a herpesvirus, can cause the mononucleosis syndrome but is usually latent until unmasked by immunodeficiency, pregnancy, multiple drug exposures, or immunosuppression.[9,15] CMV causes less of a lymphoproliferative response than EBV, and activation often results in more extensive inflammation and tissue necrosis.[15] Diagnosis is made by appropriate serologic studies, by identification of characteristic T-cell nuclear inclusions in cytologic or tissue biopsy specimens, or by molecular techniques, including in situ hybridization or immunoperoxidase studies[9,15,16] (Plate 89-3).

Human Herpesvirus-6

Human herpesvirus-6 (HHV-6) was isolated from AIDS patients in 1986.[17] The virus is capable of infecting multiple cell types, including T and B lymphocytes, megakaryocytes, and neural cells.[17] The salivary glands are the likely site of persistence and replication. A high degree of DNA sequence homology is found between HHV-6 and CMV.[18] The virus does not appear to be capable of lymphoblastoid cell line immortalization in contrast to EBV.

The HHV-6 infection can be evaluated using immunoassays including enzyme-linked immunosorbent assay, indirect fluorescent antibody tests, neutralization assays, Western blotting, in situ hybridization, PCR, and Southern blot analysis.[17–19] Disease associations are complicated by the fact that approximately 90% of children between 1 and 4 years of age have seroconverted, and an equal number of adults are seropositive.[19] CMV and EBV are able to reactivate the HHV-6 carrier state, yielding titer rises.[17–19]

The HHV-6 virus has been strongly linked only to roseola infantum (exanthem subitum), a short-lived childhood febrile illness, although early reports linked this virus to lymphoma.[17] The HHV-6 virus is capable of causing an IM-like illness that is heterophil-negative in previously healthy individuals.[17] Strong disease associations have also been recently reported for Rosai-Dorfman disease (sinus histocytosis with massive lymphadenopathy) and Kikuchi disease (histiocytic necrotizing lymphadenitis).[17–20] These entities are discussed later. Recently a human β-herpes virus called HHV-7 has been described but little disease correlation is documented.

Infection-Association Hemophagocytic Syndrome

Infection-associated hemophagocytic syndrome (IAHS) is also included in the spectrum of atypical lymphoproliferations and usually occurs in the setting of immunodeficiency.[21] The

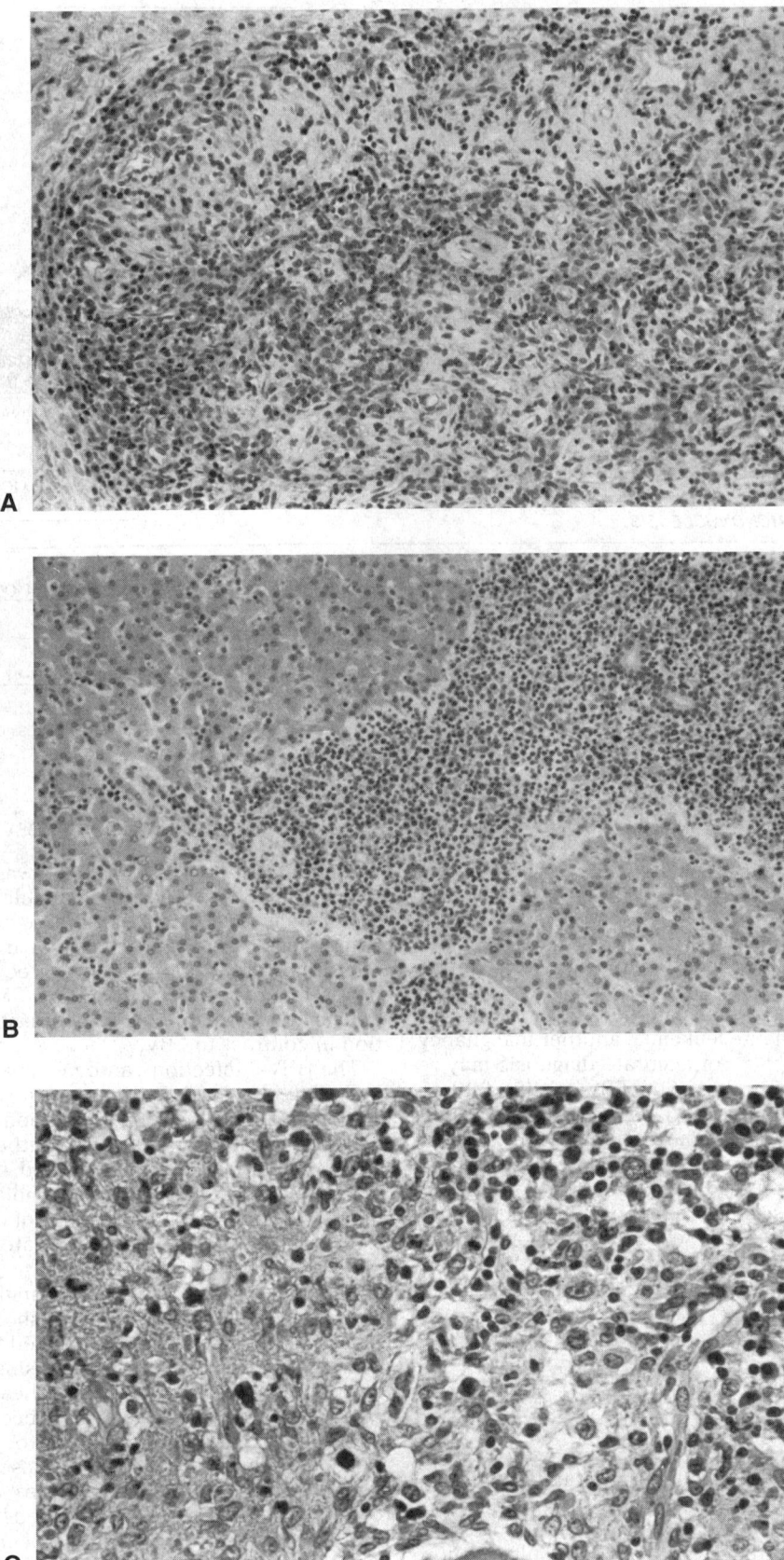

Fig. 89-3. FIM. **(A)** Lymph node biopsy shows depleted lymphoid elements. Note the absence of reaction centers and abundant histiocytes. (H&E × 200.) **(B)** Liver biopsy shows a polymorphous infiltrate of the portal area, which evokes focal necrosis. (H&E × 200.) **(C)** Bone marrow biopsy shows depletion of marrow elements, foci of hemorrhagic necrosis with macrophages, lymphocytes, and immunoblasts. (H&E × 200.)

Table 89-1. EBV Diagnostic Procedures

Parameter Assayed	Method
Infectious (viable) EBV virions	
EBV cytopathic effect	Conventional tissue culture
EBV early antigen detection	Centrifugation culture and direct immunofluorescence
Establishment of EBNA and/or EBV genome-positive lymphoblastoid cell lines	Culture of lymphocytes from peripheral blood or biopsy material; cord-blood lymphocyte transformation by throat washings
Circulating EBV antibodies	
VCA: IgG, IgM, IgA	Indirect immunofluorescence
EA-D: IgG, IgA	Indirect immunofluorescence
EA-R: IgG	Indirect immunofluorescence
EBNA: IgG	Anticomplement immunofluorescence Enzyme-linked immunosorbent assay
Heterophil: IgM	Paul-Bunnell-Davidson test
Monospot	Rapid slide test
EBV protein(s) in tissue	
EBNA	Anticomplement immunofluorescence; immunoblotting (Western blot analysis)
EBV-specific cytotoxic T cell functions	Lymphocytotoxicity assay; regression assay
EBV nucleic acid analysis	
EBV DNA	Dot blot hybridization; Southern blot analysis; in situ hybridization; PCR
EBV RNA	Dot blot hybridization; Northern blot analysis; in situ hybridization
EBV terminal repeat (clonal marker)	Southern blot analysis

syndrome was originally described in patients with viral infections but has subsequently been encountered in patients with fungal, bacterial, and parasitic infections; in immunodeficient patients; and in patients with T-cell lymphomas.[21] Approximately 80% of patients with FIM exhibit clinicopathologic findings consistent with IAHS.[22]

Patients with IAHS present with hepatosplenomegaly, abnormal liver function tests, fever, bilateral pulmonary infiltrates, rashes, lymphadenopathy, and pancytopenia.[9,21,22] Early in the course of IAHS the bone marrow appears normal, but myeloid hyperplasia, lymphocytic infiltration, cellular necrosis, and increased macrophages subsequently appear.[9,21,22] At necropsy activated macrophages, exhibiting phagocytosis, infiltrate areas of hemorrhagic necrosis.[22] A coagulopathy also occurs. Marked sinus histiocytosis with prominent erythrophagocytosis[21,22] (Plate 89-4) is evident throughout the reticuloendothelial system of affected patients, and hyperplasia of the spleen can result in splenic weights in excess of 1 kg.[21,22]

A familial form of hemophagocytic syndrome occurs. Familial erythrophagocytic lymphohistiocytosis is an autosomal recessive condition, which usually presents before 5 years of age with hepatosplenomegaly and fever.[9,23,24] Histologic examination of lymph nodes shows lymphoid proliferation early in the disease, which is followed by lymphoid depletion at later stages. The disease terminates in a hemophagocytic syndrome with pancytopenia, jaundice, and marked erythrophagocytosis. Patients exhibit multiple defects in cellular immunity.[25]

Retroviruses and Lymphoproliferation

During the recent decade, the RNA retroviruses have been implicated in a spectrum of lymphoproliferative disorders.[26] The AIDS retrovirus (human immunodeficiency virus [HIV]) does not transform lymphocytes but selectively destroys helper T cells.[26] During acute HIV infection, a mononucleosis-like syndrome often occurs, and chronic persistent lymphadenopathy may ensue.[26] The T-cell immunodeficiency caused by HIV permits opportunistic viral, bacterial, protozoal, and fungal infections.

The most extensively studied transforming retrovirus is the human T-cell leukemia/lymphoma virus type I (HTLV-I), which is implicated in the endemic form of adult acute T-cell leukemia/lymphoma (ATL) in Japan and the Caribbean basin.[26] This virus has the capacity to selectively immortalize T cells in vitro, but HTLV-I infection alone is insufficient to cause malignancy, as only 1 in 2,500 chronic viral carriers develop T-cell malignancies.[8,26] HTLV-I infection occurs during sexual intercourse or by blood transfusion. The viral infection probably increases the likelihood of further cytogenetic events by stimulating T-cell lymphoproliferation.[26] Seropositive asymptomatic carriers of the virus exhibit subtle signs of immunodeficiency.[8,26] Those who progress to ATL have HTLV-I-positive serology, generalized lymphadenopathy, hepatosplenomegaly, skin lesions, and distinct involvement of peripheral blood by a spectrum of malignant T cells ranging from small lymphocytes to bizarre hyperlobated forms.[26] Not all patients manifest a leukemic phase. ATL only occurs in 2% of infected individuals and can take years to develop.[26] The prognosis is poor, as all patients present with stage IV disease; the median survival is <6 months.[26] Of greater concern in evaluating atypical proliferations is the rare patient who develops a lymphocytosis in association with HTLV-I infection because these must be closely followed.

Of the many HTLV-I-infected patients who do not develop ATL, most are asymptomatic, but a small group develops an early benign transient lymphocytosis; if subacute or chronic lymphocytosis persists, the risk of progression to ATL increases.[26]

DRUG-ASSOCIATED LYMPHOPROLIFERATIVE DISORDERS

Although some drugs permit activation of latent viral infections such as EBV by causing immunosuppression, other drugs cause atypical lymphoid responses by unknown mechanisms. Diphenylhydantoin (Dilantin) is a rare but well-documented cause of such responses.[27–29] The clinical presentation is similar to that of a viral infection and includes fever, rash, lymphadenopathy, and eosinophilia.[27–29] Acquired IgA deficiency may develop. The symptoms usually abate when the drug is stopped.[27–29] Lymph node histology is similar to that in IM; florid follicular hyperplasia or paracortical expansion by a polymorphous immunoblastic infiltrate can efface the nodal architecture[27–29] (Fig. 89-4). Focal necrosis and Reed-Sternberg-like cells may be evident.[27–29] Hodgkin disease and NHL have both been reported in association with diphenylhydantoin therapy.[28]

Other hyperplastic lymphoid responses to drugs have been reported, including pseudoperipheral T-cell lymphoma in association with carbamazepine.[29] The immunosuppressive drugs, including cyclosporine, steroids, antilymphocyte globulin, and cytotoxic agents usually unmask latent viral infections.

A wide range of immunologic abnormalities (Table 89-2) occur in patients taking a spectrum of pharmocologic agents, with the anticonvulsants being the prototypical example[27–29] (Table 89-3).

Familial predisposition to hypersensitivity reactions is well documented.[28] Aromatic anticonvulsants (i.e., phenytoin) produce arene oxide metabolites that these patients are unable to detoxify.[28] Presumably, the metabolites combine with cellular molecules forming neoantigens that provoke an abnormal immune response.[28]

The development of an abnormal immune response in associ-

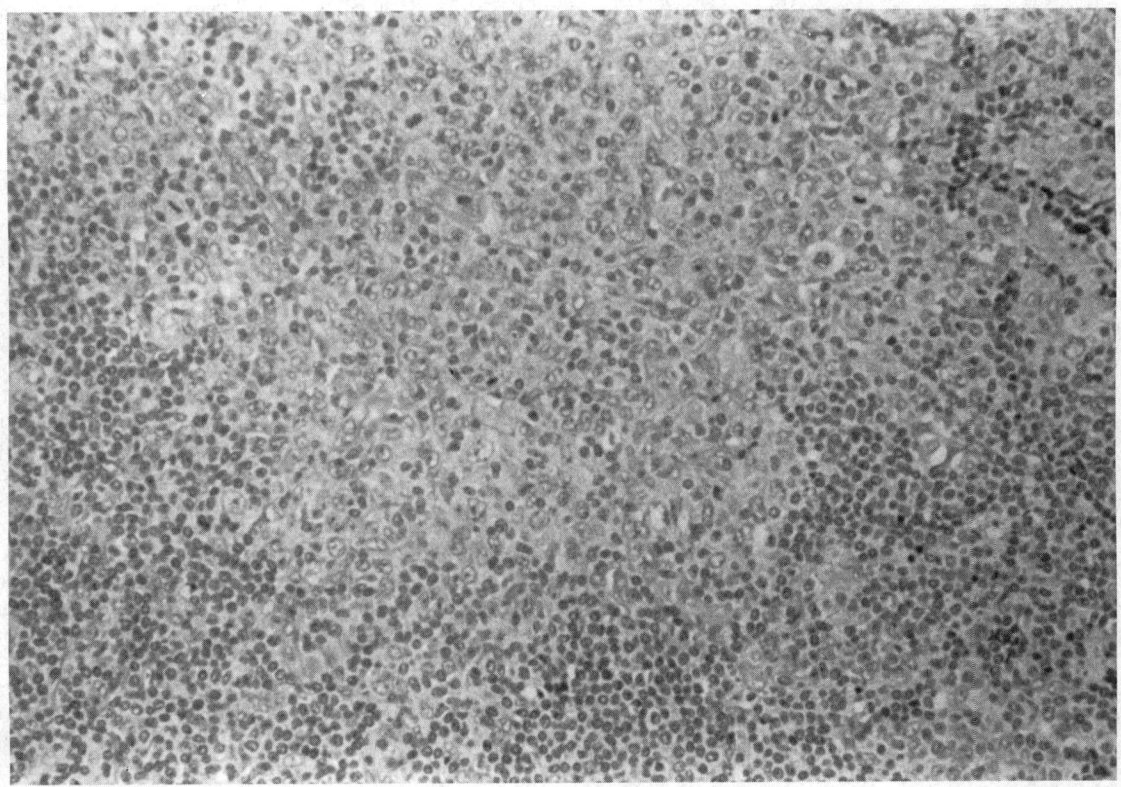

Fig. 89-4. Dilantin-associated florid follicular hyperplasia. Explosive follicular hyperplasia resulted in irregular follicle structures surrounded by mottled paracortex containing immunoblasts. (H&E × 200.)

ation with drug therapy requires withdrawal of the presumed causative agent. If lymphadenopathy or lymphoproliferative disorders are evident, biopsy and evaluation are indicated to rule out malignant processes.[28]

POST-TRANSPLANTATION LYMPHOPROLIFERATIVE SYNDROME

Bone marrow and solid organ transplant recipients are exposed to a variety of immunosuppressive agents, including azothiaprine, prednisone, cyclophosphamide, FK506, antilymphocyte globulin, anti-T-cell monoclonal antibodies, and cyclosporine. These patients are prone to develop a post-transplant lymphoproliferative disorder (PTLD), which includes atypical polyclonal lymphoproliferations and monoclonal NHL.[30–39] The atypical lymphoproliferations can be aggressive with continued immunosuppression but are polyclonal or oligoclonal, as shown by immunoperoxidase and gene rearrangement studies. The clonal ambiguity has led to difficulties in diagnosis and nomenclature.[32] Most PTLDs are associated with EBV.[30–39]

The prevalence and the post-transplantation interval that precedes development of PTLD vary with the type of organ transplanted and the immunosuppressive agents administered.[33] Transplant patients have an overall PTLD prevalence of approximately 2–10%, which is ≤30 times the incidence in the general population.[33] Most (78%) cases are extranodal, the brain and spinal cord being involved in 39% and the allograft itself in 15%. The incidence of PTLD in heart transplant recipients is 13% and in heart-lung recipients 9.5%.[34,35] Among bone marrow transplant recipients, those receiving T-cell-depleted bone marrow allografts appear to be at particularly high risk of EBV-associated lymphoproliferation.[33,36] EBV-genome-positive lymphomas have occurred after intervals of 2–49 months and do not respond to acyclovir or conventional chemotherapy even after immunologic function is restored.[37] Prophylactic acyclovir therapy appears to diminish the prevalence of secondary lymphoid neoplasms in such patients.[37]

PTLD after bone marrow transplantation has been associated with mortality >90%; solid organ transplants (excluding cardiac) ≤50%.[33] Factors associated with prognosis are listed

Table 89-2. Immune Disorders Associated with Drugs

Autoimmune disease
Immune complex disease
Abnormal cellular immune responses
Abnormal humoral immune responses
Hypersensitivity reactions
T-cell quantitative and qualitative abnormalities
Lymphadenopathy
Transient lymphoproliferative disorders
Lymphoma

Table 89-3. Drugs That Can Cause Lymphadenopathy or Atypical Lymphoproliferation

Phenytoin (Dilantin)	Tetracycline
Carbamazepine (Tegretal)	Sulfasalazine
Primidone	Griseofulvin
Phenylbutazone	Para-amino salicylic acid
Aspirin	Calmette-Guérin bacillus
Indomethacin	Antithymocyte globulin
Gold salts	OKT-3
Allopurinol	Halothane
Sulfonamides	Methyldopa; levodopa
Penicillins	Thiouracil compounds
Gentamicin	Iron-dextran
Erythromycin	Insulin

Table 89-4. Prognostic Factors in Post-Transplant Lymphoproliferative Disorders

Favorable	Unfavorable
Clinical	
Infectious mononucleosislike illness	Old age
Lymphadenopathy	Disseminated disease
Multiple organ dysfunction	Systemic symptoms
Single organ involvement	Lymphomatous presentation
Serologic evidence of primary or reactivated EBV infection	Extranodal disease
Pathologic	
Polymorphic	Monomorphic
Monoclonal *weak* banding on Southern analysis	Monoclonal *intense* banding on Southern analysis
Absence of c-*myc* rearrangements	c-*myc* rearrangements
Mixed monoclonal and polyclonal B-cell proliferations	

in Table 89-4. Histopathology and clonality should not be relied on as the sole criteria for clinical behavior because high mortality has been described for all features on some series.[33]

The pathogenesis of PTLD is related to a disruption of the host's EBV immune surveillance by immunosuppression (Fig. 89-2). Impairment of T-cell-mediated responses to EBV leads to a serologic pattern of acute infection, increased oropharyngeal shedding of virus, and increased numbers of EBV-infected B lymphocytes in the peripheral blood. If immunosuppression is continued, EBV-infected B cells proliferate explosively, resulting in multiple independent, EBV-driven B-cell proliferations. Subsequent additional cytogenetic events then allow a dominant clonal population of B lymphocytes to emerge, resulting in the development of lymphoma.

Reduction or removal of immunosuppression is essential in PTLD and usually results in resolution in all patients with nonclonal or mixed polyclonal-monoclonal disease but in only 50% of patients with clonal disease.[33,38,39] Distinguishing between a polyclonal and a monoclonal PTLD often requires molecular analysis, since ≤50% of transplant-associated lymphomas do not express surface immunoglobulin.[31,33]

Treatment of PTLD depends on the extent of disease and the clonality of the lymphoproliferation as well as factors listed in Table 89-4. Localized node-based polyclonal processes usually respond favorably to acyclovir and reduced immunosuppression.[30,32,33] Monoclonal lymphoma and polyclonal proliferations with extensive visceral involvement are usually treated with chemotherapy, but the mortality rate is high (≤80%).[30,32,33] Anti-B-cell monoclonal antibody therapy with CD21 and CD24 can induce partial or complete remissions in poor prognosis groups.[33]

ATYPICAL LYMPHOPROLIFERATIVE DISEASE IN PATIENTS WITH AUTOIMMUNE DISORDERS

Other disorders of immune regulation have an increased prevalence of lymphoid neoplasia. Patients with autoimmune collagen-vascular disease can develop NHLs, which often arise in the setting of reactive lymphadenopathy.[40,41] Rheumatoid arthritis (RA) patients have a specific defect in T-cell inhibition of EBV-induced lymphocyte proliferation and a fivefold increase in the rate of spontaneously transforming B-cell clones in vitro.[42] Individuals with Sjögren syndrome also show a progression of lymphoid hyperplasia to frank neoplasia, with a risk 44 times that observed in the general population.[43] Patients treated for Hodgkin disease have an increased prevalence of secondary lymphoid malignancies.[44] These lymphomas show a predilection for extranodular involvement, particularly of the gastrointestinal tract.[44]

Lymphocytes and lymphoid tissue react similarly in autoimmune diseases and infections. In autoimmune diseases, the inciting stimulus is persistent whereas in infections the stimulus is contained and eliminated.[44] It is the persistence of the stimulus in autoimmunity coupled with underlying immune system abnormalities that results in atypical lymphoproliferations and a predisposition to develop malignant lymphoma.[44]

Rheumatoid Arthritis

Lymphadenopathy occurs in ≤75% of RA patients at some point in their disease.[44] The most striking feature of RA lymphadenopathy is follicular hyperplasia with decreased proliferative activity and increased CD8 cells in germinal centers mimicking follicular lymphoma.[44] However, in most cases the follicles are polyclonal by immunohistochemical studies. Felty syndrome (RA with splenomegaly and neutropenia) can mimic B-cell lymphoproliferations such as hairy cell leukemia. The clinical picture, peripheral blood findings, and sometimes the pathologic examination of the spleen after splenectomy rule out malignancy. The neutropenia in Felty syndrome is most likely due to autoimmune destruction of neutrophils.[44] Overt lymphoid malignancy is rare in RA.[44]

Systemic Lupus Erythematosus and Mixed Connective Tissue Diseases

Mild lymphadenopathy is common in SLE with ≤70% of SLE patients exhibiting clinically apparent lymphadenopathy.[44] Progressive lymph node enlargement, isolated lymphadenopathy, and splenomegaly are uncommon and warrant an evaluation to rule out malignancy, infection, or drug reactions.[40–44]

Sjögren Syndrome

Sjögren syndrome is a chronic autoimmune disorder that causes inflammation of the salivary and lacrimal glands.[43,44] The progressive involvement of the salivary glands leads to pseudolymphomas and myoepithelial sialadenitis (MESA). The lesions of MESA have been shown to contain clonal populations of B cells, indicating that MESA is actually a prelymphoma or lymphoma in situ.[44]

GENETICALLY LINKED IMMUNODEFICIENCY AND LYMPHOPROLIFERATIONS

In 1952 Burton recognized that recurrent and persistent pyogenic infections in a young male patient were due to a lack of antibodies.[12] Subsequently, the triad of autoimmunity, immunodeficiency, and lymphoproliferation has been defined in an increasingly large group of patients with inherited and acquired immunodeficiency disorders.[8,12,14] About six well-defined X-linked immunodeficiency disorders are known,[12,14] and many persons with uncontrolled lymphoproliferations other than these well-defined disorders probably have subclinical or undefined inherited immunodeficiencies. The prevalence of these lymphoproliferative disorders ranges from about 2% in patients with Burton agammaglobulinemia to 25% in males with the X-linked lymphoproliferative (XLP) disease.[12,14] Organ transplant recipients show a similar prevalence.[8,30–39] The lymphoproliferations associated with these immunodeficiency disorders are due predominantly to EBV.[8,30–39]

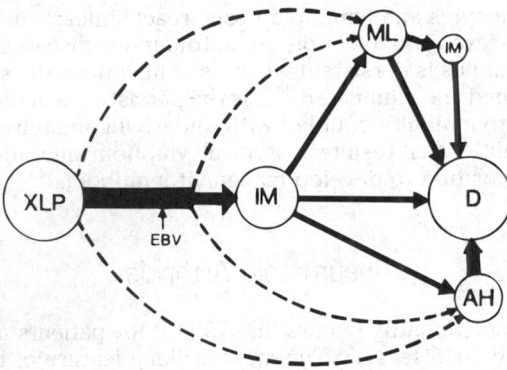

Fig. 89-5. Diagram illustrating the hypothesized temporal events in the natural history of XLP syndrome. The size of the arrows and circles indicates the relative number of patients with each phenotype. About 75% of afflicted males died of FIM by age 10, and all patients died by age 40. ML, malignant lymphoma; D, death. (From Grierson and Purtilo,[76] with permission.)

X-Linked Lymphoproliferative Disease

XLP disease illustrates the spectrum of lymphoproliferations that can occur within the background of hereditary immunodeficiencies. The disorders range from benign or fatal IM to NHL.[8,10–14] After EBV infection, chronic or fatal IM, acquired hypogammaglobulinemia or agammaglobulinemia, pure red cell aplasia, necrotizing lymphoid vasculitis, and/or NHL ensue[8,10–14] (Fig. 89-5).

Patients who develop sporadic FIM are older (median age 13 years) at presentation than males with XLP who develop FIM (median age 2 years).[8,11] The features of FIM occurring in males with XLP are similar to, but more extensive than, those in sporadic FIM.[8,11,12] Both groups of patients fail to control the explosive EBV-driven lymphoproliferation,[8,11,12] which causes extensive tissue destruction at multiple organ sites.[8,11,12] The main differential diagnosis in these patients involves lymphoma versus florid IM. Patients who develop malignant lymphoma present with a localized mass without dissemination at the time of diagnosis.[45] By contrast, patients with severe or fatal IM have a disseminated lymphoproliferation involving multiple organ sites, including skin, liver, spleen, lung, bone marrow, and brain.[8,11–14,45] The localized masses evident in lymphoma are not usually seen in FIM, in which generalized adenopathy is apparent; in malignant lymphoma, an extranodal mass with localized regional adenopathy is evident.[8,11,45]

Males with XLP do not usually have clinical evidence of immunodeficiency before EBV infection, and they are not unduly vulnerable to other infectious agents.[8,11–14,45] Affected males can be identified by pedigree analysis, IgG subclass deficiency, low anti-EBNA titers, and a failure to switch from IgM to IgG antibodies on challenge with bacteriophage φX174.[8,11–14,45] The mutation responsible for the XLP syndrome is genetically linked to a restriction fragment length polymorphism detectable with the DXS42 probe (Xq25).[46] Identification of carrier females and prenatal diagnosis can now be performed. These patients should be treated with prophylactic high EBV-titer immunoglobulin. Mothers of boys with XLP usually have persistently elevated EBV antibody titers.[8,11–14,45] If the XLP patients survive an acute infection with EBV, they often have persistently inverted T-helper/suppressor cell (CD4/CD8) ratios, hypogammaglobulinemia, decreased lymphocyte responses to mitogens, and defective natural killer cell activity.[8,11–14,45] The secondary immune deficits may be due to the extensive necrosis throughout the immune system of XLP patients that occurs during acute infection with EBV.[8,11] The disease should be suspected in families in which maternally related boys develop FIM, acquired hypogammaglobulinemia, agammaglobulinemia, or malignant lymphoma.[8,11–14,45]

Other Heritable Immunodeficiency Diseases with Lymphoproliferations

A complete review of genetically linked diseases manifesting lymphoproliferation is beyond the scope of this discussion, but certain conditions have been sufficiently characterized to allow recognition. Wiskott-Aldrich syndrome has an X-linked inheritance pattern, and is characterized by chronic eczema, chronic suppurative otitis media, anemia, and thrombocytopenic purpura.[8,14] Patients have defective cell-mediated immunity and poor antibody responses to polysaccharide antigens.[8,14] Males with Wiskott-Aldrich syndrome are more immunocompetent than males with XLP, and FIM has not been reported in association with this syndrome.[14] EBV-specific antibody responses are less commonly abnormal in Wiskott-Aldrich patients[14]; however, these patients are more likely to develop widely disseminated malignant lymphoma (50%) than XLP males with the malignant phenotype, who develop localized NHL predominantly in the ileocecal region.[8,14] Because lymphoproliferation in Wiskott-Aldrich syndrome has not been as extensively studied as XLP, the disseminated disease may actually be a manifestation of FIM. The role of EBV and FIM in Wiskott-Aldrich syndrome deserves closer attention.

Ataxia-telangiectasia is an autosomal recessive trait characterized by severe progressive cerebellar ataxia associated with oculocutaneous telangiectasia, sinopulmonary infections, and abnormal eye movements.[8,14] The immune defects involve both T and B cells, and decreased levels of IgA and IgG are frequent.[8,14] EBV reactivation occurs in ataxia-telangiectasia patients but has not been extensively studied. Lymphocytosis associated with chromosome abnormalities may persist for years.[14] Chromosome 14 abnormalities in these patients are associated with a high incidence of chronic T-cell leukemia,[8,14] and preleukemic clonal expansions of cells and full-blown leukemias in these patients often demonstrate the inv(14q)(q11q32) or the t(14;14)(q11;q32) translocation.[47,48] Molecular analysis has shown that the cytogenetic breakpoint at 14q11 occurs in the joining region of the T-cell receptor γ-chain.[47,48] The 14q32 breakpoints appear more heterogeneous and include breaks within the immunoglobulin heavy chain locus and at 14q32.1, the site of TCL1, an oncogene.[47,48] Identical cytogenetic and molecular findings have been detected in T-cell neoplasms not associated with ataxia-telangiectasia.[47,48] The chromosome 14 abnormality involves both the immunoglobulin heavy chain locus and the T-cell receptor α-chain locus.[47,48] The chromosomal location of many of the gene defects in these hereditary illnesses will be mapped in the future and will provide further molecular evidence of the etiology of these diseases.

ATYPICAL LYMPHOPROLIFERATIONS OF UNKNOWN CAUSE

Angiofollicular Lymph Node Hyperplasia

Angiofollicular lymph node hyperplasia (AFH), or Castleman disease, has many other names, including giant lymph node hyperplasia, angiomatous lymphoid hamartoma, lymph nodal hamartoma, and lymph node hyperplasia of Castleman.[49–54] There is no sex or age preference, and most patients present with asymptomatic mediastinal masses, which are discovered on routine chest radiographic examination.[49–54] There are two types of localized AFH: hyaline-vascular (90%) and the plasma cell type.[49–54] The hyaline-vascular type is more common and has a histologic pattern characterized by follicular hyperplasia distributed evenly throughout the lymph node.[49,52] The follicles are unusually small, and their germinal centers are often penetrated by radial capillaries, which are surrounded by collagen or hyaline material[49,52] (Plate 89-5A). The germinal centers are surrounded by multiple concentric layers of lymphocytes. In the plasma cell type, which is less common (10%) and may represent an earlier stage of the lesion, the germinal centers are larger, the peripheral cuffs of mature lymphocytes are not as prominent, and the interfollicular areas are occupied by extensive sheets of plasma cells, occasionally including some atypical forms[49-51] (Plate 89-5B). The plasma cell group tends to affect younger persons and has a higher rate of mesenteric and retroperitoneal tumors.[49-51]

Clinical symptoms associated with the plasma cell type include fever, sweats, weight loss, and fatigue.[49-51] Associated laboratory abnormalities include anemia, an elevated erythrocyte sedimentation rate, hypergammaglobulinemia, hypoalbuminemia, hyperferremia, and hypertransferrinemia.[49]

Multicentric lesions have been identified in a subgroup of patients and may herald a higher risk of subsequent development of overt lymphoma.[49,50]

Most reports in the literature favor the concept that the hyaline-vascular type of AFH is a reactive chronic lymphoid hyperplasia.[51,52] The plasma cell type is considered to have an inflammatory pathogenesis, either through chronic antigenic stimulation (i.e., infection) or via an autoimmune mechanism. Immunohistochemical and gene rearrangement studies have recently identified clonal cell populations in some cases of multicentric AFH.[53,54] A plasma cell dyscrasia associated with polyneuropathy, organomegaly, endocrinopathy, monoclonal gammopathy, and skin changes (POEMS syndrome) is sometimes associated with Castleman disease.[54] There is no apparent clinical value in differentiating the POEMS syndrome from osteosclerotic myeloma with peripheral neuropathy.[54]

A role for interleukin-6 (IL-6) in the pathobiology of Castleman disease has been defined. Culture supernatants of Castleman disease lymph nodes have been shown to produce a B-cell differentiating factor that has been identified as IL-6.[55,56] Immunohistochemical studies with an anti-IL-6 monoclonal antibody have revealed the presence of IL-6 within the lymph nodes of these patients. In addition, a particular interfollicular pattern of IL-6 gene expression has been associated with Castleman disease.[57] Brandt et al.[58] recently reported that mia constitutively producing IL-6 administered after infection of bone marrow with an IL-6 expressing recombinant retrovirus develops a syndrome that closely resembles Castleman disease. IL-6 is a mediator of acute phase reactions and thrombopoiesis.[59] The systemic manifestations of Castleman disease are thought to be a consequence of the dysregulation of IL-6. In fact, Beck et al.[60] have shown that many of the symptoms and laboratory abnormalities associated with Castleman disease were alleviated by infusion of an IL-6 antibody.

Progressively Transformed Germinal Centers

Progressively transformed germinal centers represent a type of follicular hyperplasia that can resemble a variant of Hodgkin disease known as nodular lymphocyte predominance Hodgkin disease[61,62] (Plate 89-6A). Patients usually present with focal lymphadenopathy and are biopsied. Histologically, biopsies show large follicles lacking follicular centers, which are prominent in the central area of the lymph node[61,62] (Plate 89-6B). Progressively transformed germinal centers must be distinguished from nodular lymphocyte-predominant Hodgkin disease (Plate 89-6L–E), and the presence of progressively transformed germinal centers does not imply an increased risk of subsequently developing Hodgkin disease.[61,62]

Angioimmunoblastic Lymphadenopathy with Dysproteinemia

AILD is the preferred term for a condition that occurs more often in elderly patients and is characterized by generalized lymphadenopathy, hepatosplenomegaly, anemia, and hypergammaglobulinemia.[63,64] Other terms for AILD include immunologic aberrations in idiopathic reticuloses, atypical lymph node hyperplasia with fatal outcome (immunodysplastic disease),

diffuse plasmacytic sarcomatosis, chronic pluripotential immunoproliferative syndrome, immunoblastic lymphadenopathy, and lymphogranulomatosis X.[63,64] Biopsies of lymph nodes affected by AILD show complete effacement of the architecture, a prominent vascular proliferation, a florid immunoblastic proliferation, abundant plasma cells in clusters or sheets, burned-out germinal centers, focal necrosis, eosinophilic material, a background of mature lymphocytes, and, occasionally, eosinophils and neutrophils[63,64] (Plate 89-7). The median survival of patients with AILD is 30 months.[63,64] Most patients are treated with prednisone or combination chemotherapy. Randomized prospective treatment trials are needed to determine optimum treatment.

AILD in association with malignant lymphoma is defined by the presence of clusters, islands, or diffuse infiltrates of monomorphic immunoblasts and has a much graver prognosis.[63,64] The most important prognostic factor in AILD is achievement of complete remission.[63,64] Many apparent cases of AILD may actually represent T-cell lymphomas, as clonal populations of T cells have been identified in several cases studied by Southern blot analysis.[65]

A stepwise progression from benign AILD lesions to malignant has been suggested by serial chromosome studies in AILD patients.[65] Approximately 96% of AILD and AILD-like lymphoma specimens have EBV genome detectable by PCR or in situ hybridization.[66] Other angiocentric lymphoproliferations including lethal midline granuloma (polymorphic reticulosis) have had EBV genomes demonstrated by molecular techniques.[67]

Histiocytic Necrotizing Lymphadenopathy

Histiocytic necrotizing lymphadenitis (Kikuchi disease) is a pseudolymphomatous lesion, which presents as cervical lymphadenopathy and occurs predominantly in young women.[9,17,66-68] Patients usually present with a cervical mass, but are otherwise asymptomatic and do not show evidence of IM.[9,68,69] The process usually resolves spontaneously within 1–4 months without further therapy.[68,69] Histologic sections reveal focal aggregates of histiocytes and immunoblasts, which surround necrotic foci lacking granulocytic infiltration (Plate 89-8). These lesions are scattered throughout the cortex and paracortex. The mixture of histiocytes and atypical immunoblasts can lead to a misdiagnosis of malignant lymphoma,[68] but careful attention to histologic detail will usually reveal the correct diagnosis. These patients do not have an increased risk of lymphoma, and surgical excision is curative.

Although the etiology of histiocytic necrotizing lymphadenitis is unknown, its histologic and clinical features are similar to those of SLE,[69] and the disease may, in fact, reflect a self-limited autoimmune condition resembling SLE.[9,17] Other agents associated with this entity include toxoplasma, *Yersinia* species, and HHV-6.[9,17]

Sinus Histiocytosis with Massive Lymphadenopathy

Patients with sinus histiocytosis with massive lymphadenopathy (Rosai-Dorfman disease) usually present with bilateral lymphadenopathy predominantly affecting the cervical region, and they usually exhibit some systemic symptoms, including fever, polyclonal hypergammaglobulinemia, and increased erythrocyte sedimentation rate.[9,70-72] The disease occurs most commonly in black children.[70-72] Biopsies reveal pericapsular fibrosis, dilation of sinuses, numerous intrasinusoidal histiocytes, and abundant plasma cells. The most striking histologic feature is the presence of lymphocytes and other hematopoietic cells within the cytoplasm of the sinus histiocytes (emperipolesis) (Plate 89-9). The disease has a protracted but benign course; spontaneous regression of the lymphadenopathy and total recovery will occur in most cases.[70,71] Clinically most of the patients are thought to have a NHL. Administration of antibiotics, radiation, antituberculous therapy, and/or steroids does not have a major impact on the course of the disease.[70,71] The etiology of the disease remains obscure. A relationship to an underlying immunodeficiency has been postulated.[72]

Reactive Follicular Hyperplasia in the Elderly

Reactive follicular hyperplasia (RFH) is a common finding in the lymph node biopsies from children and young adults. The detection of RFH in patients ≥60 years should be considered an atypical finding requiring close follow-up as the risk of NHL is increased.[73] This is especially true if multiple enlarged nodes are evident.[73]

A GENERAL APPROACH TO THE DIAGNOSIS OF ATYPICAL LYMPHOID HYPERPLASIAS

The accurate diagnosis of atypical lymphoproliferations requires a systemic approach. The history and physical examination often suggest a malignant process, which will require a biopsy for confirmation. The conditions that have a characteristic histologic appearance (e.g., Castleman disease) can be accurately diagnosed with histologic examination alone, but most patients will require application of more sophisticated diagnostic procedures to appropriately prepared specimens (Table 89-1). The use of a protocol in handling hematolymphoid tissue biopsies is mandatory (Table 89-5). If the clinical features and biopsy findings are suggestive of a viral process, serology and virologic assays may be confirmatory, and the patient can be observed without further workup. If the family history and clinical features suggest a heritable immune defect, then pedigree and immunologic analysis of the patient and family members is mandatory. For patients whose condition is still suspect after the routine procedures, specialized procedures such as immunophenotyping (cryostat or flow cytometry), cytogenetics, or Southern blot analysis may be required. These procedures require fresh or specially prepared tissue; the practice of placing the entire biopsy specimen in formalin is to be condemned. Selected specialized procedures useful in the evaluation of atypical lymphoproliferations are discussed in the following section.

Immunoperoxidase Studies

Immunophenotypic analysis has revolutionized the understanding of hematologic lesions and increased diagnostic accuracy. To reliably apply immunophenotypic analysis to diagnostic problems, a thorough understanding of specimen requirements and of the limitations of the procedure is necessary. Immunophenotyping of most hematologic lesions obtained by biopsy requires snap-frozen tissue. Snap freezing is best performed in dry ice-isopentane slurries or in liquid nitrogen. Most antibodies react only to frozen tissue antigens because fixation techniques denature or alter the antigen to the point at which the antibody will no longer react.[74] Cryostat freezing is usually unsatisfactory because it causes extensive artifacts. Recently, antibodies that recognize T and B cells in fixed tissue have been developed, but they lack the specificity of frozen tissue antibodies because cross-phenotypic reactivity ranges between 5% and 15%.[74,75]

A useful criterion for malignancy is the establishment of clonality in lymphoid lesions. The expression of cytoplasmic or surface immunoglobulin by B cells is a clonal marker that can be detected with monoclonal antibodies.[74,75] In a clonal process all the cells will express a single light chain, whereas benign (i.e., nonclonal) lesions will manifest a mixture of κ and λ light chains.[74,75] There are limitations to the usefulness of light chain restriction: many B-cell lymphomas, especially in post-transplant cases, do not express immunoglobulin; the analysis must be performed on snap-frozen tissue unless plasmacytoid differentiation is evident; and a high background may obscure positive staining.[74,75] T cells do not have a clonal marker that can be identified by using monoclonal antibodies.[74,75] The only way to firmly establish clonality in T-cell lymphoproliferations and B-cell processes that do not express immunoglobulins is by Southern blot analysis of immunoglobulin genes and T-cell receptor gene configurations.[75]

Molecular Analysis

The mechanism by which B cells generate antibody diversity remained obscure until gene rearrangement was discovered and applied to the study of antibody formation. B cells rearrange segments of DNA, encoding genes for immunoglobulin proteins, and each individual cell has a unique gene rearrangement, which will be transmitted to all its daughter cells.[75] T cells also rearrange DNA, encoding a receptor found on their cell surface in a manner identical to that of B cells.[75] When T or B cells become malignant, they produce progeny that all carry the same gene rearrangement. Usually, only T cells rearrange T-cell receptor genes, and B cells rearrange immunoglobulin genes.[75] The Southern blot technique is used to analyze the gene configuration of lymphoproliferations and can be applied to peripheral blood, bone marrow, cell suspensions, and tissue biopsies.[75]

Southern blot analysis requires fresh or frozen tissue. DNA is extracted from the tissue; purified; cut with special enzymes, called restriction enzymes, which yield smaller DNA fragments; size-fractionated on agarose gels; transferred to nylon or nitrocellulose membranes; hybridized to radioactively labeled DNA probes specific for the genes of interest; and autoradiographed. Immunoglobulin DNA probes generally only bind to immunoglobulin genes, and T-cell receptor DNA probes only bind to T-cell receptor genes.[75] The autoradiograph yields specific banding patterns based on the restriction enzymes used and whether a clonal population is present. In polyclonal lymphoid populations, the only bands that are visible are germline bands, which originate from stromal cells that do not rearrange lymphoid receptor genes; in material with >1% populations of clonal T or B cells, clonal bands will be observed in positions other than the germline, indicating the presence of a clonal population of lymphoid cells (Fig. 89-6). Lineage and clonality can be determined by whether T- or B-cell probes yield clonal bands. It should be emphasized that identification of a clonal population does not prove that it is malignant. Nevertheless, whenever a clonal proliferation is observed, it is very likely that the clone is a malignant one.

Viral genomes can be demonstrated by in situ hybridization,

Table 89-5. Lymph Node Protocol

Fresh tissue
  Flow cytometric analysis (cell-surface markers, DNA ploidy)
  Microbiologic cultures (sterile)
  Cytogenetic analysis (sterile)
Touch preparations
  Cytomorphologic examination
  Enzyme detection (i.e., terminal deoxynucleotidyl transferase [TdT] (air dry then ethanol fixation)
Flash frozen tissue
  Immunohistochemistry (cell surface markers)
  Molecular biologic analysis (Ig and T cell receptor gene analysis, oncogene expression)
Tissue fixed in formaldehyde and/or mercuric chloride solutions
  Histopathologic examination
  Paraffin immunohistochemistry
Tissue fixed in glutaraldehyde
  Electron microscopic examination

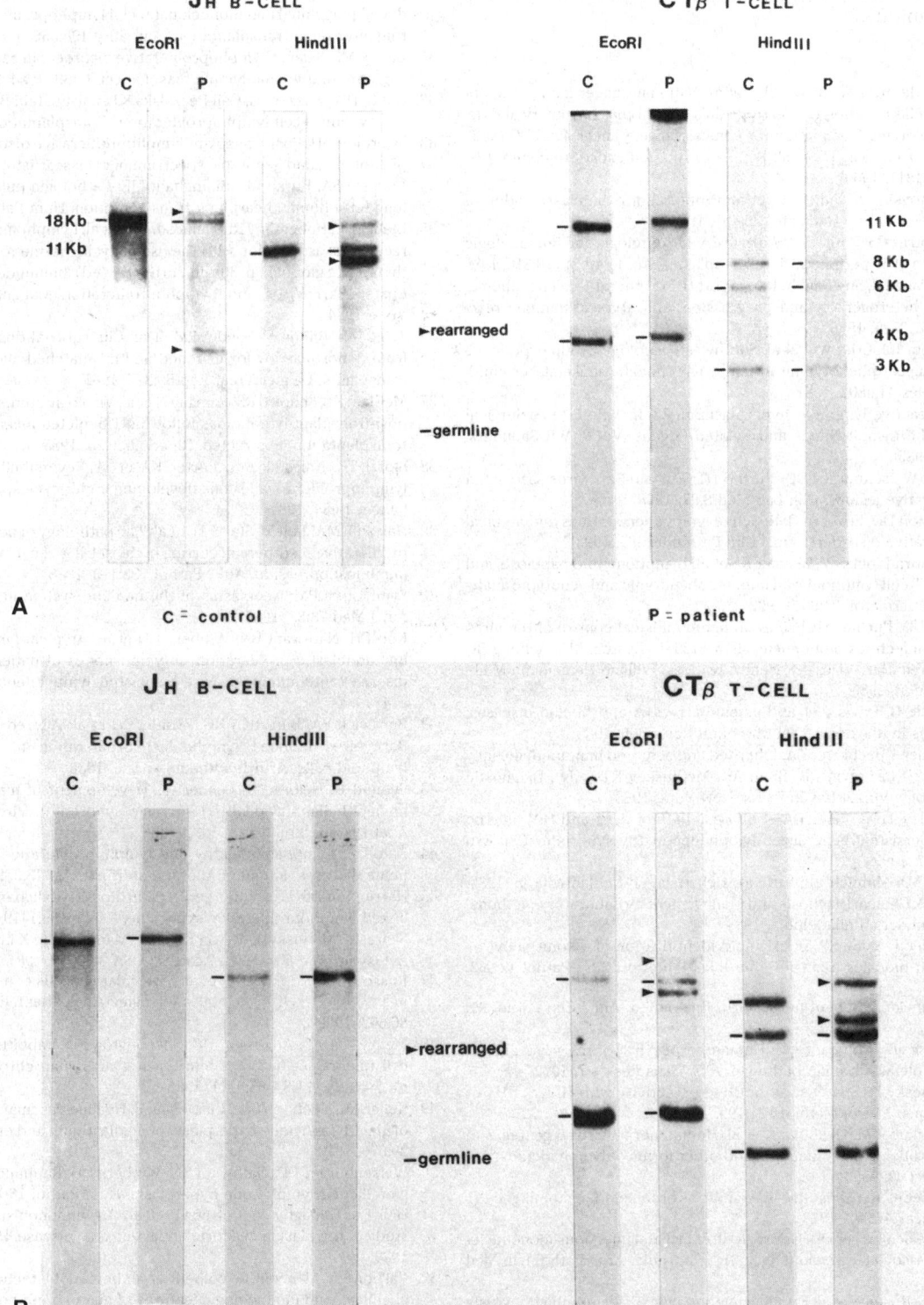

Fig. 89-6. (A) B-cell lymphoma gene rearrangement analysis reveals clonal rearrangements (arrowheads) with the restriction enzymes *Eco*RI and *Hind*III, when an immunoglobulin heavy chain gene probe is used, but only germline bands with a T-cell probe (dashes). **(B)** T-cell lymphoma gene rearrangement analysis reveals clonal bands with the T cell β-chain receptor probe and use of *Eco*RI and *Hind*III restriction enzymes (arrowheads) and germline B-cell genes (dashes). C, control; P, patient.

PCR, or Southern analysis.[67] PCR is particularly sensitive and can amplify viral genomes that are incorporated into nonpathologic cells.[67] When used with in situ hybridization, localization of genomes in neoplastic or hyperplastic cells is stronger evidence of involvement in the process.[67]

CONCLUSION

Atypical lymphoproliferations occur in a variety of clinical settings in response to a variety of stimuli. Accurate diagnosis of these processes is made by careful clinicopathologic correlation and in some cases by genetic, immunologic, virologic, and molecular techniques.

REFERENCES

1. Rosenberg SA, Berard CW, Brown BW et al: National Cancer Institute sponsored study of classification of non-Hodgkin's lymphomas: summary and description of a working formulation for clinical usage. Cancer 49:2112, 1982
2. Lukes RJ, Craver LF, Hall TC et al: Report of the nomenclature committee. Cancer Res 26:1311, 1966
3. Bennet JM, Catovsky D, Daniel MT et al: Proposals for the classification of the acute leukemias. Br J Haematol 33:451, 1976
4. Weiss LM, Crabtree GS, Rouse RV, Warnke RA: Morphologic and immunologic characterization of 50 peripheral T-cell neoplasms. Am J Pathol 118:316, 1985
5. Winberg CD, Krance R, Sheibani K, Rappaport H: Peripheral T-cell lymphoma. Morphological heterogeneity and progression, and atypical immune reactions. Cancer 57:2329, 1986
6. Pullen DJ, Falleta JM, Crist WM et al: Southwest Oncology Group experience with immunological phenotyping in acute lymphocytic leukemia of childhood. Cancer Res 41:4802, 1981
7. Schnitzer B: Reactive lymphoid hyperplasia. p. 22. In Jaffe E (ed): Surgical Pathology of the Lymph Nodes and Related Organs. Vol 2. WB Saunders, Philadelphia, 1985
8. Harrington DS, Weisenburger DD, Purtilo DT: Epstein-Barr virus-associated lymphoproliferative lesions. Clin Lab Med 8:97, 1988
9. Krishnan J, Danon DD, Frizzera G: Reactive lymphadenopathies and atypical lymphoproliferative disorders. Am J Clin Pathol 99:385, 1993
10. Harrington DS, Braddock SW, Blocker KS et al: Lymphomatoid papulosis and progression to T-cell lymphoma: an immunophenotypic and genotypic analysis. J Am Acad Dermatol, 21:951, 1992
11. Weisenburger DD, Purtilo DT: Failure in immunological control of the virus infection: fatal infectious mononucleosis. p. 129. In Epstein MA, Achong BG (eds): The Epstein-Barr Virus—Recent Advances. William Heinemann Medical Books, London, 1986
12. Okano M, Thiele G, Davis J et al: Epstein-Barr virus and human diseases: recent advances in diagnosis. Clin Microbiol Rev 1:300, 1988
13. Purtilo DT, Linder J, Seemayer TA: Inherited and acquired immunodeficiency disorders. p. 121. In Colvin RB, Bhan AK, McCluskey RT (eds): Diagnostic Immunopathology. Vol. 2. Raven Press, New York, 1988
14. Boyle MJ, Sculley TB, Cooper DA et al: Epstein-Barr virus and HIV play no direct role in persistent generalized lymphadenopathy syndrome. Clin Exp Immunol 87:357, 1992
15. Ray CG, Hicks MJ, Minnich LL: Viruses, rickettsia, and chlamydia. p. 1286. In Henry JB (ed): Clinical Diagnosis and Management by Laboratory Methods. Vol. 50. WB Saunders, Philadelphia, 1984
16. Masih AS, Linder J, Shaw BW et al: Rapid identification of cytomegalovirus in liver allograft biopsies by in-situ hybridization. Am J Surg Pathol 12:362, 1988
17. Horowitz C, Beneke J: Human herpesvirus-6 revisited. Am J Clin Pathol 99: 583, 1993
18. Pellett PE, Black JB, Yamamoto M: Human herpesvirus-6: the virus and its search for its role as a human pathogen, Adv Virus Res 41:1, 1992
19. Saxinger C, Polesky H, Eby N et al: Antibody reactivity with HBLV (HHV-6) in US populations. J Virol Methods 21:199, 1988
20. Sumiyoshi Y, Kikuchi M, Ohshima K et al: Human herpesvirus-6 genomes in histiocytic necrotizing lymphadenitis and other forms of lymphadenitis. Am J Clin Pathol 99:609, 1993
21. Risdall RJ, McKenna RW, Nesbitt ME et al: Virus associated hemophagocytic syndrome. Cancer 44:993, 1979
22. Mroczek EC, Weisenburger DD, Grierson HL et al: Fatal infectious mononucleosis and virus-associated hemophagocytic syndrome. Arch Pathol Lab Med 111:530, 1987
23. Soffer D, Okon E, Rosen N et al: Familial hemophagocytic lymphohistiocytosis in Israel. Cancer 54:2423, 1984
24. Perry MC, Harrison EG, Burgert EO et al: Familial erythrophagocytic lymphohistiocytosis. Cancer 38:209, 1976
25. Ladisch S, Poplack D, Holliman B et al: Immunodeficiency in familial erythrophagocytic lymphohistiocytosis. Lancet 1:581, 1978
26. Ehrlich GD, Poiesz BJ: Clinical and molecular parameters of HTLV-I infection. Clin Lab Med 8:65, 1988
27. Abbondanzo SL, Irey NS, Frizzera G: Dilantin-associated lymphadenopathy: spectrum of histopathologic patterns. Proc Int Acad Pathol 74A:431, 1993
28. Segal GH, Clough JD, Tubbs RR: Autoimmune and iatrogenic causes of lymphadenopathy. Semin Oncol 20:611, 1993
29. Severson GS, Harrington DS, Burnett DA, Linder J: Dermatopathic lymphadenopathy associated with carbamazepine: a case mimicking a lymphoid malignancy. Am J Med 83:597, 1987
30. Hanto DW, Gajl-Peczalska KJ, Frizzera G et al: Epstein-Barr virus (EBV) induced polyclonal and monoclonal B-cell lymphoproliferative diseases occurring after renal transplantation. Ann Surg 198:356, 1983
31. Cleary ML, Sklar J: Lymphoproliferative disorders in cardiac transplant recipients are multiclonal lymphomas. Lancet 1:489, 1984
32. Hanto DW, Frizzera G, Gajl-Peczalska KJ et al: Epstein-Barr virus immunodeficiency, and B-cell lymphoproliferation. Transplantation 39:461, 1985
33. Swerdlow SH: Post-transplant lymphoproliferative disorders: a morphologic, phenotypic, and genotypic spectrum of disease. Histopathology 20:373, 1992
34. Yousem SA, Burke CB, Billingham ME: Pathologic pulmonary alterations in long term human heart-lung transplantation. Hum Pathol 16:911, 1985
35. Bieber CP, Hebersling RL, Jamieson SW et al: Lymphoma in cardiac transplant recipients: association with the use of cyclosporine A, prednisone, and antithymocyte globulin. p. 309. In Purtilo DT (ed): Immunodeficiency and Cancer: Epstein-Barr Virus and Lymphoproliferation Malignancies. Plenum, New York, 1984
36. Trigg ME, Billing R, Sondel PM et al: Clinical trial depleting T-lymphocytes from donor marrow for matched and mismatched allogeneic bone marrow transplants. Cancer Treat Rep 69:377, 1985
37. McClain KL, Shapiro RS, Ramsay N et al: Virologic studies in four patients with post-transplant lymphomas following T-depleted mismatched bone marrow transplantation, abstracted. Blood 66:2420, 1985
38. Starzl TE, Nalesnik MA, Porter KA et al: Reversibility of lymphomas and lymphoproliferative lesions developing under cyclosporine-steroid therapy. Lancet 1:584, 1984
39. Nalesnik MA, Jaffe R, Starzl TE et al: The pathology of post-transplant lymphoproliferative disorders occurring in the setting of cyclosporine A-prednisone immunosuppression. Am J Pathol 133:173, 1988
40. Symmons DPM: Neoplasms of the immune system in rheumatoid arthritis. Am J Med 78:22, 1985
41. Koo CH, Nathwani BN, Winberg CD et al: Atypical lymphoplasmacytic and immunoblastic proliferation in lymph nodes of patients with autoimmune disease (autoimmune-disease-associated lymphadenopathy). Medicine 63: 274, 1984
42. Bardwick PA, Bluestein HG, Zvaifler NJ et al: Altered regulation of Epstein-Barr virus induced lymphoblast proliferation in rheumatoid arthritis lymphoid cells. Arthritis Rheum 23:626, 1980
43. Schmid U, Helbran D, Lennert K: Development of malignant lymphoma in myoepithelial sialadenitis (Sjögren's syndrome). Virchows Arch A Pathol Anat Histopathol 395:11, 1982
44. Dale DC: Lymphadenopathy and lymphoproliferative disorders in autoimmune diseases. Immunol Allergy Clin North Am 13:359, 1993
45. Harrington DS, Weisenburger DD, Purtilo DT: Malignant lymphoma in the X-linked lymphoproliferative syndrome. Cancer 59:1419, 1987
46. Skare JC, Milunsky A, Byron KS et al: Mapping the X-linked lymphoproliferative syndrome. Proc Natl Acad Sci USA 84:2015, 1987
47. Russo G, Isobe M, Gatti R et al: Molecular analysis of a t(14;14) translocation in leukemic T-cells of an ataxia telangiectasia patient. Proc Natl Acad Sci USA 86:602, 1989
48. Mengle-Gaw L, Albertson DG, Sherrington PD, Rabbitts TH: Analysis of a T-cell tumor-specific breakpoint cluster at human chromosome 14q32. Proc Natl Acad Sci USA 85:9171, 1988
49. Keller AR, Hochholzer L, Castleman B: Hyaline-vascular and plasma-cell types of giant lymph node hyperplasia of mediastinum and other locations. Cancer 29:670, 1972
50. Weisenburger DD, Nathwani BN, Winberg CD, Rappaport H: Multicentric angiofollicular lymph node hyperplasia. Hum Pathol 16:162, 1985
51. Hall PA, Donaghy M, Cotter FE et al: An immunohistologic and genotypic study of the plasma cell form of Castleman's disease. Histopathology 14:333, 1989
52. Carbone A, Manconi R, Volpe R et al: Immunohistochemical, enzyme histochemical, and immunologic features of giant lymph node hyperplasia of the hyaline-vascular type. Cancer 58:908, 1986
53. Hanson CA, Frizzera G, Patton DF et al: Clonal rearrangement for immunoglobulin and T-cell receptor genes in systemic Castleman's disease. Association with Epstein-Barr virus. Am J Pathol 131:84, 1988
54. Miralles GD, O'Fallon JR, Talley NJ: Plasma cell dyscrasia with polyneuropathy—spectrum of the POEMS syndrome. N Engl J Med 327:1919, 1992
55. Yabahura A, Yanagisawa M, Murata T et al: Giant lymph node hyperplasia (Castleman's disease) with spontaneous production of high levels of B cell differentiation factor activity. Cancer 63:260, 1989
56. Yoshizaki K, Matsuda T, Nishimoto N et al: Pathogenic significance of interleukin 6 (IL-6/BSF-2) in Castleman's Disease. Blood 74:130, 1989
57. Leger-Revet M, Peuchmaur M, Devergne O et al: Interleukin-6 gene expression in Castleman's disease. Blood 78:292, 1991
58. Brandt SJ, Bodine DM, Dunbar CE et al: Dysregulated interleukin-6 expression

produces a syndrome resembling Castleman's disease in mia. J Clin Invest 86:592, 1990

59. Kishimoto T: The biology of interleukin-6. Blood 74:1, 1989
60. Beck JT, Hsu SM, Wijdenes J et al: Alleviation of systemic manifestations of Castleman's disease by monoclonal anti-IL-6 antibody therapy. N Engl J Med (in press)
61. Burns BF, Colby TV, Dorfman RF: Differential diagnostic features of nodular L&H Hodgkin's disease, including progressive transformation of germinal centers. Am J Surg Pathol 8:253, 1984
62. Ferry JA, Zukerberg LR, Harris NL: Florial progressive transformation of germinal centers—a syndrome affecting young men, without early progression to nodular lymphocyte predominance Hodgkin's disease. Am J Surg Pathol 16:252, 1992
63. Ohsaka A, Saito K, Sakai T et al: Clinocopathologic and therapeutic aspects of angioimmunoblastic lymphadenopathy-related lesions. Cancer 69:1259, 1992
64. Brincker J, Birkeland SA: The relationship between disease activity, treatment response, and immunologic reactivity in immunoblastic lymphadenopathy: a longitudinal study of treatment with levamisole and cytostatics. Cancer 47:266, 1981
65. Schlegelberger B, Feller A, Godde E et al: Stepwise development of chromosomal abnormalities in angioimmunoblastic lymphadenopathy. Cancer Genet Cytogenet 50:15, 1990
66. Weiss L, Jaffe ES, Liu X et al: Detection and localization of Epstein-Barr viral genomes in angioimmunoblastic lymphadenopathy and AILD-like lymphoma. Blood 79:1789, 1982
67. Borisch B, Hennig I, Laeng RH et al: Association of the subtype 2 of the Epstein-Barr virus with T-cell non-Hodgkin's lymphoma of the midline granuloma type. Blood 82:858, 1993
68. Pileri S, Kikuchi M, Helbron D, Lennert K: Histiocytic necrotizing lymphadenitis without granulocytic infiltration. Virchows Arch A Pathol Anat Histopathol 340:257, 1982
69. Dorfman RF, Berry GJ: Kukuchi's histiocytic necrotizing adenitis: an analysis of 108 cases with emphasis on differential diagnosis. Semin Diagn Pathol 5:329, 1988
70. Rosai J, Dorfman RF: Sinus histiocytosis with massive lymphadenopathy: a newly recognized benign clinicopathologic entity. Arch Pathol 87:63, 1969
71. Rosai J, Dorfman RF: Sinus histiocytosis with massive lymphadenopathy—a pseudolymphomatous benign disorder: analysis of 34 cases. Cancer 30:1174, 1972
72. Foucar E, Rosai J, Dorfman RF et al: Immunologic abnormalities and their significance in sinus histiocytosis with massive lymphadenopathy. Am J Clin Pathol 5:515, 1984
73. Osborne BM, Butler JJ: Clinical implications of nodal reactive follicular hyperplasia in the elderly patient with enlarged lymph nodes. Mod Pathol 4:24, 1991
74. Linder J, Ye Y, Armitage JO, Weisenburger DD: Monoclonal antibodies marking T- and B-lymphocytes in paraffin-embedded tissue. In McMichael AJ (ed): Leukocyte Typing. Vol. 3. Oxford University Press. Oxford, 1987
75. Cossman J, Uppenkamp M, Sundeen J et al: Molecular genetics and the diagnosis of lymphoma. Arch Pathol Lab Med 112:117, 1988
76. Grierson H, Purtilo DT: Epstein-Barr virus infections in males with the X-linked lymphoproliferative syndrome. Ann Intern Med 106:538, 1987

Systemic Mastocytosis

90

Robert I. Parker and Dean D. Metcalfe

INTRODUCTION

Mastocytosis has been confounding both clinicians and scientists for more than a century. In 1869, Nettleship and Tay[1] described what we now know as urticaria pigmentosa in a 2-year-old girl. In 1877, Paul Ehrlich[2] was the first to describe mast cells in his study of granulated connective tissue cells; he believed that these cells represented overnourished or overfed connective tissue cells and termed them *mastzellen*. That same time, Unna[3] demonstrated mast cells in the skin lesions of urticaria pigmentosa, the term suggested by Sangster[4] the following year. Nearly 50 years later, urticaria pigmentosa was recognized as the characteristic skin lesion of "mastocytosis"[5]; finally, in 1949, the systemic nature of mastocytosis was recognized by Ellis[6] in his report of the autopsy findings of a 1-year-old infant with diffuse organ infiltration by mast cells. This systemic organ infiltration by mast cells often results in protean clinical manifestations that frequently obscure the underlying disease process. While the most commonly involved organ in systemic mastocytosis is the skin, a significant number of cases eventually show mast cell infiltration in multiple organs; it is in this clinical setting that the term disseminated or systemic mastocytosis has generally been used. The classification schema proposed by Travis et al.[7] and modified by Friedman and Metcalf[8] to include lymphadenopathic mastocytosis with eosinophilia, points out the difficulty clinicians and researchers have in classifying this disorder (Table 90-1). Some researchers suggest that mastocytosis can be considered primarily a biochemical disorder that results from the uncontrolled release of mediators contained within the mast cell or induced by mast cell activation[9] (Table 90-2). However, this approach understates the significance of the pathologic effects of the organ infiltration by mast cells and does not adequately

Table 90-1. Mayo Clinic Classification of Mastocytosis

Indolent mastocytosis
    Skin only
        Urticaria pigmentosa
        Diffuse cutaneous mastocytosis
    Systemic
        Marrow
        Gastrointestinal (with or without urticaria pigmentosa)
Mastocytosis with an associated hematologic disorder (with or without urticaria pigmentosa)
    Myelodysplastic disorders
    Myeloproliferative disorders
    Acute myeloid leukemia
    Malignant lymphoma
    Chronic neutropenia
Mast cell leukemia
Lymphadenopathic mastocytosis with eosinophila (with or without urticaria pigmentosa); aggressive mastocytosis

Table 90-2. Mediators in Mastocytosis

Skin specimens
  Histamine
  Leukotriene B_4
  5-hydroxyeicosatetraenoic
  Tryptase
  Chymase
  Heparin
Cutaneous blister fluid
  Histamine
  Prostaglandin D_2
  Platelet-activating factor
Plasma
  Histamine
  Tryptase
Histamine metabolites
  Nτ-methylhistamine
  Nτ-methylimidazole acetic acid
PGD_2 metabolites
  9α-Hydroxy-11,15-dioxo-2,3,4,5-tetra-norprostane-1,20-dioic acid
  9α-Hydroxy-11,15 dioxo-2,3,18,19-tetra-norprost-5-ene-1,20-dioic acid
Cytokines
  TNF-α
  IL-4
  IL-5
  IL-6
  IL-8
Chondroitin sulfate B
Arylsulfatases

address the spectrum of hematologic disorders observed in this disease. A consensus classification schema suggested in 1991[10] (Table 90-3) is proposed as a reasonable approach to the classification, and therefore the diagnosis, of this disease.

BIOLOGY AND PATHOGENESIS OF MAST CELL DISEASE

Mast cells and basophils are recognized as the effector cells of the immediate allergic reaction by virtue of their high-affinity receptors for IgE. The wide distribution of mast cells throughout the human body, especially in proximity to blood vessels in atopic and nonatopic individuals alike, and the recognition of mast cell and basophil activation by nonimmunologic means, suggest that these cells also may be involved in nonatopic conditions. Recent evidence that these cells synthesize and release cytokines in response to IgE and non-IgE-mediated stimuli adds further support to the hypothesis that these cells play a role not only in the pathobiology of several disease processes but also in maintaining homeostasis. Thus, mast cell- and basophil-mediated events have been postulated to play a role in host

Table 90-3. Consensus Revised Classification of Systemic Mastocytosis

Indolent
  Syncope
  Cutaneous disease
  Ulcer disease
  Malabsorption
  Bone marrow mast cell aggregates
  Skeletal disease
  Hepatosplenomegaly
  Lymphadenopathy
Hematologic disorder
  Myeloproliferative
  Myelodysplastic
Aggressive lymphadenopathic mastocytosis with eosinophilia
Mastocytic leukemia

defense against parasitic diseases, in wound healing, in tumor angiogenesis, and in immunoregulation. Furthermore, the early appearance of Fc$_\epsilon$RI during cell differentiation may be important for these cells to respond to IgE-mediated stimuli before granulation, possibly by mediating cytokine production.

Although basophils and mast cells are similar in their ability to bind IgE to their surface and to be stimulated after antigen-mediated cross-linking of surface bound IgE, these cells do not represent blood and tissue forms of the same cell type.[11-13] They differ in significant ways with regard to their morphology, biology, and cell-surface structures[13-17] (Table 90-4). These cells also exhibit significant differences in response to cytokines and the complement system.[13,16-18]

It is now accepted that mast cells are derived from pluripotential hematopoietic cells.[19] This was first demonstrated by Kitamura with in vivo experiments using genetically mast cell-deficient mutant mice and their co-geneic normal littermates. One of the mutants, the WBB6$_{F1}$-W/W^V mouse, is ordinarily devoid of mast cells but can develop mast cells if it receives a bone marrow graft either from its normal littermates (WBB6$_{F1}$- $+/+$ mice) or from semisyngeneic C57BL/6-bg/bg ("beige") mice. These experiments established that mouse mast cells develop from bone marrow precursors. Mast cells originate from a cell more primitive than those precursors committed either to the neutrophil/macrophage or erythroid cell lineages.[20]

In contrast to the WBB6$_{F1}$-W/W^V mouse, the genetically mast cell-deficient WCB6$_{F1}$-Sl/Sl^d mouse fails to develop mature mast cells after either systemic or local injection of WCB6$_{F1}$-$+/+$ cell populations containing mast cell precursors.[21] Sl/Sl^d mouse bone marrow cells can, however, differentiate into tissue mast cells after intravenous injection into W/W^V mice. Taken together, these findings indicate that the mast cell deficiency of the W/W^V mouse reflects an abnormality of the mast cell precursors themselves, whereas the mast cell deficiency of the Sl/Sl^d mouse reflects an abnormality of tissue microenvironmental factors regulating mast cell differentiation. Products of the W or Sl loci that influence mast cell development have been identified. The W locus encodes the c-kit tyrosine kinase receptor,[22] whereas Sl encodes the c-kit ligand often referred to as stem cell factor (SCF).[23-25]

Several molecules are known to promote or augment murine mast cell proliferation: interleukin (IL)-3, IL-4, SCF, IL-9, and IL-10.[26-28] Bone marrow cells cloned in a collagen gel in the presence of IL-3 produced either pure or mixed mast cell colonies.[29] Mouse bone marrow cultured in IL-3 gives rise to cultures that consist of >85% mast cells by 3 weeks. By contrast, colony-stimulating factor-granulocyte/macrophage (CSF-GM) or transforming growth factor-β (TGF-β) inhibit the differentiation of IL-3-dependent mast cells.[30,31] IL-4 has little or no ability to sustain the proliferation of mouse mast cells in the absence of IL-3.[27] In the presence of IL-3, IL-4 promotes mast cell proliferation and maturation in vivo. Anti-IL-4 antibodies administered to mice on days 0 and 7 of infection with *Nippostrongylus brasiliensis* results in a 50% reduction in mucosal mastocytosis.[32] c-kit ligand or SCF can induce the proliferation of mast cells both in vitro[23-25] and in vivo.[33] While SCF alone can increase colony-forming unit-spleen (CFU-S) number in vivo, its capacity to do so in vitro is dependent on its interaction with other growth factors.[34] IL-10, when used in combination with IL-3 or IL-4, also enhances mast cell proliferation. Taken together, these data suggest that IL-3 is both necessary and sufficient for mast cell growth from bone marrow, but SCF and other cytokines are necessary for long-term mast cell survival and maturation. In fact, the removal of IL-3 from cultures of IL-3-dependent murine mast cell cultures leads to apoptosis.[35] These mast cells are "rescued" from apoptosis by the addition of SCF.

The proliferation and differentiation of mast cells may also

Table 90-4. Natural History, Major Mediators, and Surface-Membrane Structures of Human Mast Cells and Basophils

Characteristic	Basophils	Mast Cells
Biology		
Origin of precursor cells	Bone marrow	Bone marrow
Site of maturation	Bone marrow	Connective tissue (a few in bone marrow)
Mature cells in circulation	Yes (usually <1% of blood leukocytes)	No
Mature cells recruited into tissues from circulation	Yes (during immunologic inflammatory responses)	No
Mature cells normal residing in connective tissues	No (not detectable by microscopy)	Yes
Proliferative ability of morphologically mature cells	None reported	Yes (under certain circumstances)
Life span	Days (like other granulocytes)	Weeks to months (according to studies in rodents)
Mediators		
Major mediators stored preformed in cytoplasmic granules	Histamine, chondroitin sulfates, neutral protease with bradykinin-generating activity, β-glucuronidase, elastase, cathepsin G-like enzyme, major basic protein, Charcot-Leyden crystal protein	Histamine, heparin, or chondroitin sulfates; neutral proteases (tryptase with or without chymase); many acid hydrolases; cathepsin G; carboxypeptidase
Major lipid mediators produced on appropriate activation	Leukotriene C_4	Prostaglandin D_2, leukotriene C_4, platelet-activating factor
Cytokines released on appropriate activations	IL-4	TNF-α, IL-4, IL-5, IL-6
Surface structures		
Immunoglobulin receptors	FcεRI, FcγRII (CDw32)	FcεRI, Fcγ RII (CDW32)
Cytokine or growth-factor receptors	Receptors for IL-2 (CD25), -3, -4, -5, and -8 and for SCF (some basophils express low numbers of c-*kit* receptors)	c-*kit* receptor
Cell-adhesion structures	LFA-1 α-chain (CD11a), C43bi receptor (CD11b), gp150,95 (CD11c), LFA-1β chain (CD18), IL-2R (CD25), ICAM-1 (CD54), and CD44	CD11c, CD18, ICAM-1 (CD54), CD44, VLA-4

(Modified from Galli,[13] with permission.)

be influenced by adhesive interactions with components of the marrow matrix. Recently, mast cells have been shown to adhere spontaneously to vitronectin. This interaction increases the proliferative rate of mast cells maximally stimulated by IL-3.[36] Recently, human mast cells have been cultured from blood or bone marrow in sufficient numbers to permit the study of mast cell growth and differentiation. Human bone marrow CD34+ cells maintained in IL-3-containing liquid suspension cultures produced basophils rather than mast cells after 2–3 weeks of incubation.[37] Similarly, single lineage and mixed CFUs containing basophils but not mast cells are observed when mononuclear cells are assayed in semisolid media in the presence of recombinant human IL-3.[38]

As in rodents, c-*kit* and its ligand SCF are involved in the growth and differentiation of mast cells. In the human, SCF is encoded by a gene on chromosome 12. SCF is primarily, but not exclusively, produced by stromal cells. SCF may either be released as a soluble growth factor, or it may be expressed on the cell surface of stromal cells.[23] The membrane-bound form of SCF is determined by tissue-specific alternative splicing and may play a role in stromal-dependent growth and differentiation of hematopoietic cells exposing c-*kit*.

Human SCF acts synergistically with human IL-3 to produce a three- to fivefold increase in total mast cell and basophil numbers over human IL-3 alone.[39] The percentage of cell types in the cultures grown in human IL-3 with or without SCF remain the same, with basophils constituting 18–35%, and mast cells 3% at 3 weeks of culture. In the presence of human IL-3 followed by SCF alone, the percentage of mast cells increases over 6 weeks. Mast cells cultured in the presence of IL-3 plus SCF, but not IL-3 alone, are berberine sulfate positive, suggesting the presence of heparin proteoglycans within granules, which is a

sign of mast cell differentiation. Electron microscopic examination of cultures supplemented with IL-3 and SCF, but not IL-3 alone, also revealed maturational changes in which mast cell granules contain tryptase and exhibited scroll, reticular, and homogeneous patterns as seen in CD34+ cultured over 3T3 fibroblasts.[39] Thus, to produce mast cells from human bone marrow, the optimum conditions require at least a brief exposure of CD34+ cells to IL-3, followed by SCF. By contrast, mast cells may be produced from human fetal liver[40] or from human peripheral blood following the addition of SCF only.[41] Thus, the circulating mast cell precursor no longer requires IL-3 for its differentiation.

While mast cells originate in the bone marrow, they migrate to connective tissue sites and mature. Under normal conditions, mast cells are found throughout connective tissues and are particularly numerous in the epithelial surface of the skin and the respiratory tract, in the gastrointestinal and genitourinary tracts, and in perivascular areas.[11–15,42] At these sites, mast cells exhibit one of two phenotypes, as determined by staining characteristics and granule enzyme content. Mast cells within the skin and other connective tissue sites stain intensely with dyes, probably due to their heparin content. Historically these mast cells have been referred to as "connective tissue" mast cells. Mast cells at mucosal locations, such as the lamina propria of gastrointestinal tract, stain less intensely and are referred to as "mucosal" mast cells. IL-3-dependent murine bone marrow-derived mast cells exposed to IL-4 and IL-10 contain more mouse mast cell protease (MMCP)-2-mRNA, which is more characteristic of the mucosal phenotype.[43] By contrast, murine mast cells exposed to SCF stain more intensely and synthesize heparin,[33] which is more characteristic of the connective tissue mast cell. In humans, the mucosal phenotype contains a specific tryptase, while the connective tissue phenotype contains both this tryptase and a chymotryptase.[44] Both human mast cell phenotypes appear to contain heparin.[45] The human mucosal mast cell is sometimes referred to as the T mast cell for its tryptase content, and the human connective tissue mast cell as a CT mast cell for its content of both tryptase and chymotryptase.

Limited data have been reported on the expression of mast cell adhesion molecules that may be involved in their attachment to connective tissue matrix or to other cell types. Resting murine bone marrow-derived mast cells express intracellular adhesion molecule-1 (ICAM-1) and vascular cell adhesion molecule-1 (VCAM-1). Co-culture of activated murine mast cells and of phorbol myristate acetate stimulated EL4 cells (murine T cell line) results in the formation of heterotypic aggregates. Both the size and the number of aggregates can be reduced by the addition of antibodies directed against ICAM-1, leukocyte function-associated antigen-1 (LFA-1), and VCAM-1.[46] Human lung and uterine mast cells express surface antigens for ICAM-1 and are deficient in CD11a (integrin α_L chain) and CD11b (integrin α_M chain)[47] and therefore do not express LFA-1 ($\alpha_L\beta_2$) or CD11a/CD18 or Mac-1/CR3 ($\alpha_M\beta_2$) or CD11b/CD18, respectively. In contrast to lung mast cells, uterine mast cells express both CD11c (integrin α_x chain) and the β_2 subunit (CD18) and thus express p150,95 ($\alpha_x\beta_2$ or CD11c/CD18). Uterine mast cells also express the VLA-4 ($\alpha_4\beta_1$ or CD49d/CD29), although the presence of this receptor on lung mast cells remains to be determined. These findings suggest that mast cells express functional surface receptors that permit aggregation with other cells.

Mast cell adherence to laminin appears to explain, in part, the distribution of mast cells in tissues. Mast cells accumulate on the undersurface of the endothelial cell basement membrane, which is known to be rich in laminin. Exposure to laminin and its degradation products may promote the migration of mast cells into a wound site with subsequent attachment.[48–50] In addition, mouse bone marrow cells, cultured for 1 week in the presence of IL-3 and sorted on the basis of IgE receptors, adhere to laminin after activation.[52] The ability of such mast cell precursors to adhere to laminin before their expression of mature phenotypic characteristics provides a mechanism by which these cells can be localized. The mast cell precursors may then develop their terminal phenotype dependent on the local tissue environment. Other mast cell adhesion receptors that have recently been defined include an RGD-sensitive fibronectin receptor[52] and vitronectin receptor.

The demonstration of adhesion surface antigens on both human lung and uterine mast cells by immunofluorescence and flow cytometry has provided further insight into possible interactions between mast cells and extracellular matrix that may permit mast cell migration. Uterine mast cells express the γ- and β-subunits of the vitronectin receptor $\alpha_V\beta_3$ (CD51/CD61).[47] The presence of this receptor on lung mast cells remains to be determined. Mast cell migration can be stimulated by IL-3[53] or SCF[54] and further potentiated by the combination of IL-3 and SCF.[55] Finally, mast cells have the ability to exit from tissues to epithelial surfaces. For example, dog mastocytoma cells adhere to tracheal epithelial cells in vitro.[55] Other receptors that direct mast cell precursors to their tissue destination undoubtedly exist, providing a basis for mast cell function in normal tissues.

The pathophysiology of systemic mast cell disease is largely a reflection of normal mast cell responses in abnormal sites or of heightened, unregulated mast cell responses in normal sites. In at least some cases, the focal accumulation of mast cells is the consequence of increased local production of soluble mast cell growth factor (c-kit ligand)[56] and may be a reversible event.[57] While the tissue accumulation of mast cells per se does not induce mast cell activation or degranulation,[57] their presence in large numbers may facilitate dysregulated degranulation.

The granules of human mast cells are known to contain histamine, heparin, neutral proteases, and IL-4; on activation, mast cells release these substances to the surrounding environment. It is believed that many of the manifestations of systemic mastocytosis are the consequence of mast cell degranulation. While early work focused on histamine and other primary mediators released by mast cells, the more recent discovery that mast cells are a potential source of cytokines has suggested new mechanisms by which mast cell activation may result in pathologic responses. It has now been clearly shown that stimulation of mast cells by the Fc$_\epsilon$RI (the high-affinity receptor for the Fc portion of IgE) or by other mechanisms induces mouse mast cells to synthesize increase levels of mRNA or to secrete products for multifunctional proinflammatory or mitogenic cytokines such as IL-1, -3, -4, -5, and -6.[12] In addition, high local levels of CSF-GM, interferon-γ (IFN-γ), tumor necrosis factor-α (TNF-α), and macrophage inflammatory proteins 1α and 1β, T-cell activation antigen 3, and JE are produced in mouse mast cells.[58–64] More recently, human mast cells have been shown to synthesize and release TNF-α, IL-4, IL-5, and IL-6.[65–67] These cytokines play a critical role in the regulation not only of inflammation but also of hemostasis, hematopoiesis, angiogenesis, and tissue remodeling, and potentially have critical roles in tumor development or resistance.[62,63] The recognition that mast cell stimulation results in the initiation of both an acute as well as a sustained inflammatory response has brought us closer to understanding the true nature of the tissue pathology noted in mastocytosis.

PATHOLOGY AND PATHOPHYSIOLOGY

The pathophysiology of mast cell disease can be divided into systemic and local effects. The systemic effects of this disorder arise from the release of significant amounts of mediators into the systemic circulation and can result in either flushing or syncope. The local manifestations of this disease result largely from the effects of focal collections of mast cells. However, other systemic effects of mast cell disease may result largely from the consequences of severe end-organ dysfunction (e.g., cardiomyopathy, bone marrow dysfunction).

The classic pathologic legion of cutaneous mast cell disease is the lesion of urticaria pigmentosa. However, in nearly one-half of cases of systemic mastocytosis, cutaneous lesions are lacking, and other organs need be biopsied to make the diagnosis. The most frequently involved organs in systemic mastocytosis are the bone marrow, skin, lymph nodes, spleen, liver, and gastrointestinal tract; the lungs and kidneys are virtually never involved. It is not the purpose of this chapter to review the histopathology of cutaneous mast cell lesions. However, because of the high frequency of bone marrow involvement and the relatively high value of bone marrow biopsy in the diagnosis of this disorder, we describe the mast cell lesion most frequently found in the bone marrow.

Bone Marrow

Focal mast cell lesions of the bone marrow, identified on bone marrow biopsy specimens, have been reported to be present in ≤90% of adults with systemic mast cell disease[7,68–72] (Table 90-5). The typical bone marrow lesions observed in a bone marrow biopsy are foci of spindle-shaped mast cells in a fibrotic background (Figs. 90-1 and 90-2). Usually there is an abundant admixture of eosinophils and lymphocytes, creating the so-called MEL lesion. These lesions may be located in perivascular, peritrabecular, and intertrabecular sites. They usu-

Table 90-5. Distribution of Mast Cells in Bone Marrow of Patients with Systemic Mastocytosis

Series	Patients (N)	Age Range (yr)	Median Age (yr)	Number (%) with Focal Lesions	Number (%) with Focal Lesions or Increased Mast Cells
Webb et al.[68]	26	32–78	61	21 (84)	25 (100)
Brunning et al.[69]	14	25–88	71	9 (84)	11 (100)
Horny et al.[70]	38	46–72	49	35 (92)	38 (100)
Ridell et al.[72]	18	21–72	49	10 (56)	9 (50)
Travis et al.[7]	58	17–80	60	NA	NA
Lawrence et al.[71]	46	5–76	39	32 (74)	32 (74)

Abbreviation: NA, not available.

ally are characterized by increased reticulin staining; occasionally, Masson trichome staining reveals collagen deposition. Occasional mast cell lesions are infiltrated by normal-appearing small noncleaved lymphocytes or are ringed by a cuff of mature small noncleaved lymphocytes (Fig. 90-3). Frequently, in marrows extensively involved by mast cell lesions, the bony trabeculae are moderately to markedly thickened.

While some studies of adult patients with systemic mast cell disease have reported increased marrow mast cells in the absence of focal mast cell lesions,[68–70] most patient marrows reviewed contain focal mast cell lesions. On hematoxylin and eosin (H&E) staining, the dominant granulated cell in these lesions is often the eosinophil. Eosinophils can be distinguished from mast cells by the presence of round often bilobed, nuclei and abundant deeply granulated cytoplasm. By contrast, the typical mast cell has a spindle-shaped or oval nucleus and fine eosinophilic granules that are generally apparent only at

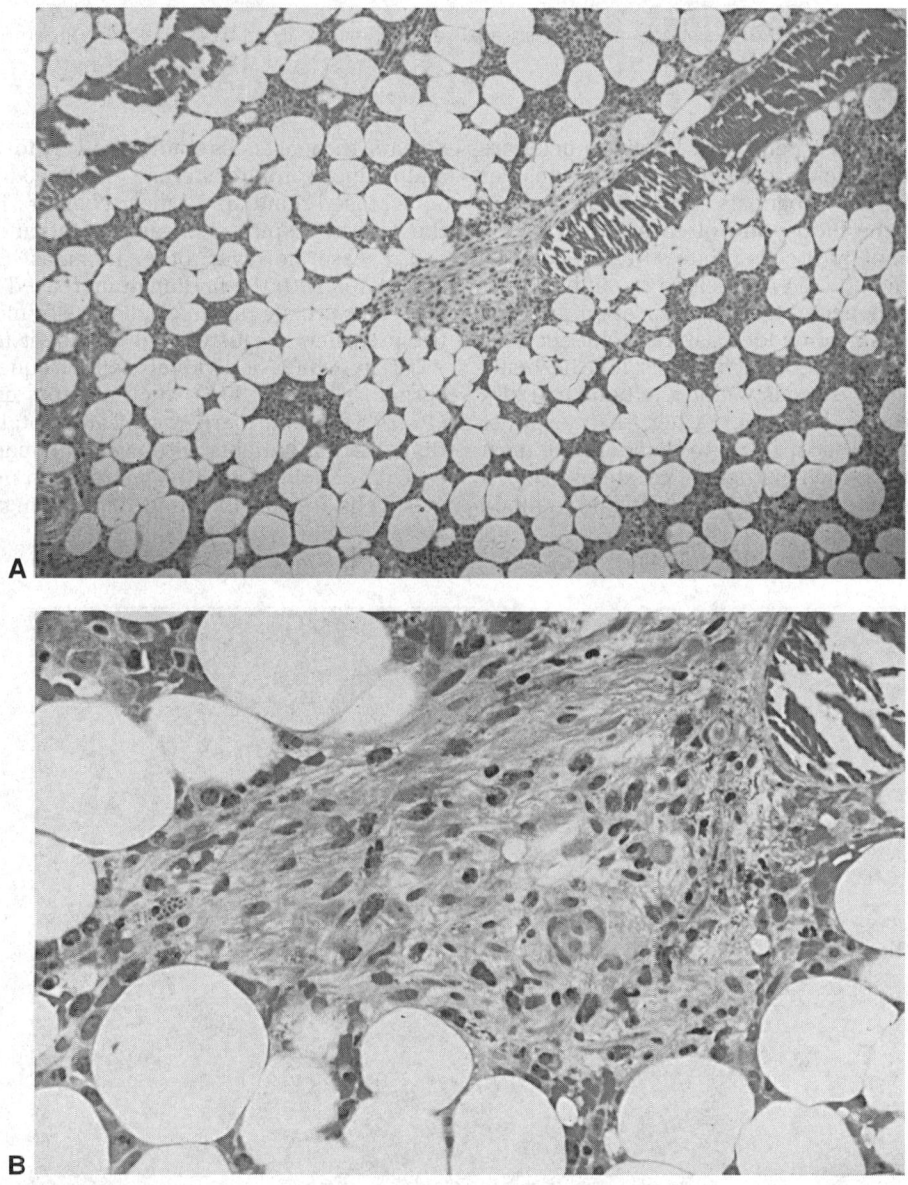

Fig. 90-1. (A) Low power view (× 20) of a small bone marrow mast cell lesion. **(B)** High-power view (× 156) of a marrow mast cell lesion. Note the presence of eosinophils and lymphocytes along with mast cell lesion. (From Parker,[73] with permission.)

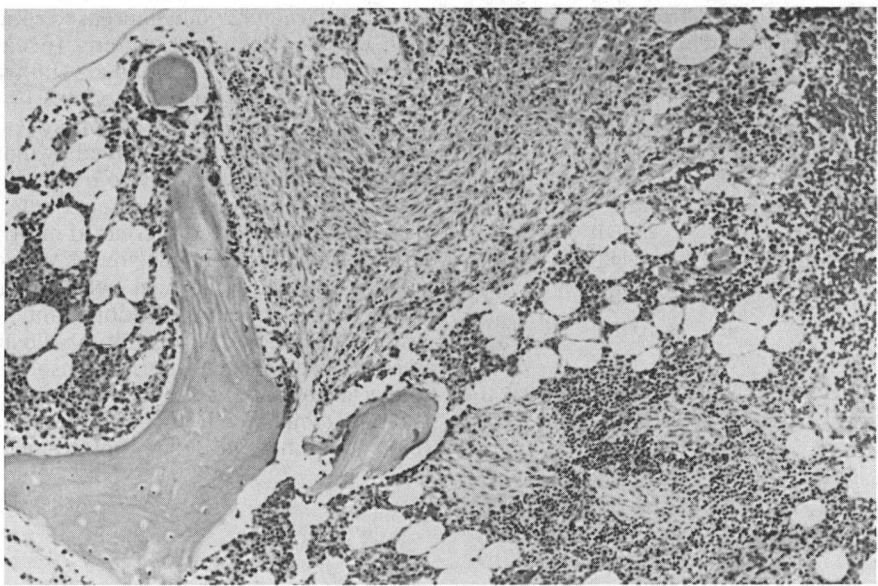

Fig. 90-2. Low-power view (× 20) of a marrow mast call lesion with a fibrotic matrix. (From Travis et al.,[160] with permission.)

high-power magnification. Mast cells with bilobed nuclei are occasionally seen in these lesions; some investigators consider them an indicator of a poor prognosis.[7] Wright-Giemsa and toluidine blue stains of the biopsy are often necessary for a definitive demonstration of mast cells (Plate 90-1). Frequently, these stains are negative on EDTA-decalcified paraffin-embedded material as a consequence of the decalcification process. We therefore prefer paraffin-embedded aspirate clot sections and nondecalcified plastic-embedded biopsies for the histochemical identification of mast cells within the bone marrow. In our experience, marrow biopsies, rather than aspirate smears or clot sections, are most likely to demonstrate mast cell disease in the marrow. When histochemical stains are performed on the plastic-embedded marrow biopsy and in blood smears, the mast cells stain positively for chloracetate esterase and aminocaproate esterase (Table 90-6).

Increased numbers of mast cells are frequently present on the marrow aspirate smears of patients with systemic mast cell disease; however, other non-mast cell disorders may be associated with the finding of increased marrow mast cells as well. In systemic mast cell disease, a more specific finding is the presence of clusters of confluent mast cells (frequently ≥20) in which individual cells frequently cannot be discerned[73,74] (Plate 90-2). Such clusters are seen in a minority (10–30%) of bone marrow aspirates obtained from both pediatric and adult patients with systemic mast cell disease. In diseases producing a reactive increase in marrow mast cells, the mast cells are usually found singly or in small clusters. In com-

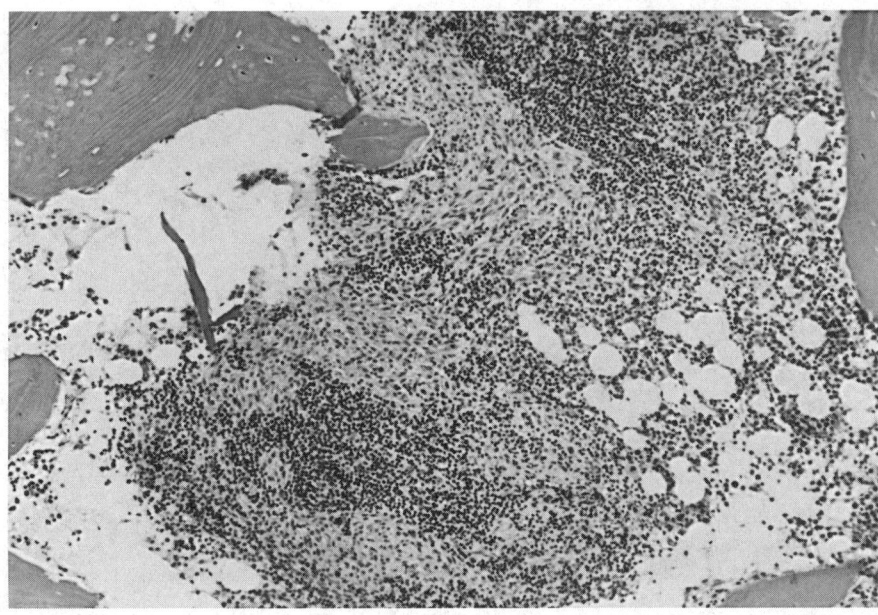

Fig. 90-3. Low-power view (× 20) of marrow mast cell lesion demonstrating infiltration and cuffing by normal small noncleaved lymphocytes.

Table 90-6. Histochemical Stains Useful in Distinguishing Mast Cells and Basophils

Stain	Mast Cells	Basophils	AML-M3[a]
Geimsa	+	+	−
Toluidine blue	+	+	−
Chloroacetate esterase	+	−	−
Aminocaproate esterase	+	−	−
Tartrate-resistant acid phosphate	+	−	−
Peroxidase	−	−	+

[a] Acute myeloid leukemia, FAB acute promyelocytic subclassification.

parison to adults with systemic mast cell disease, marrow involvement in children appears to be much less common.[74] In a study of 19 children with cutaneous or disseminated mast cell disease, only 10 patients demonstrated small focal mast cell lesions in the marrow biopsy and only 5 demonstrated increased mast cells on aspirate smear. In contrast to the focal lesions found in the marrow of adults with systemic mast cell disease, the lesions seen in the children were uniformly small and subtle and were most frequently found in perivascular sites. Aside from the small size, however, these lesions had the other characteristics of the larger lesions seen in adult marrow.[74]

While the typical mast cell lesions in adults with systemic mast cell disease are highly specific for that disorder, they are not necessarily diagnostic; they should only be considered diagnostic of systemic mast cell disease when other clinical and laboratory parameters indicative of a mast cell disorder are present. The finding of clusters of confluent mast cells on aspirate smear appears to be highly specific for systemic mast cell disease, but only a few patients (<30%) manifest this finding. This number may, however, represent a significant underestimation, as the ability to obtain adequate marrow spicules on aspiration in regions of marrow fibrosis is quite variable. The progression of marrow involvement in systemic mast cell disease is unknown. Although many adults appear to have stable, or possibly decreasing, marrow involvement over time,[71] the clinical significance of the extent of marrow involvement by mast cells remains elusive. Studies of children with systemic mast cell disease have not included large enough numbers or extended over a long enough period to justify any statements regarding either the significance of marrow mast cell lesions at initial presentation or the incidence or significance of the progression of mast cell involvement of the marrow.

Lymph Node

While lymph node, liver, and spleen are rarely biopsied in patients with mast cell disease, pathologic studies have documented significant involvement of these organs in patients with systemic involvement.[70,74–77] In reviewing the records of 58 mastocytosis patients followed at the Mayo Clinic, Travis and Li[75] demonstrated peripheral lymphadenopathy in 26% and central lymphadenopathy in 19% of patients at diagnosis. Lymphadenopathy was more pronounced in patients with associated hematologic malignances and aggressive nonleukemic mastocytosis. Within the lymph nodes, mast cell infiltrates were most common in the paracortex, followed by the follicles, the medullary cords, and the sinuses. Early infiltrates were exemplified by clusters of mast cells. Eosinophils accompanied mast cell infiltrates in lymph node tissues in approximately one-half of lymph nodes studied. In an earlier study,[76] dense eosinophilic abscess-like lesions were demonstrated in the lymph nodes of 2 of 19 patients examined. Blood vessel proliferation in the paracortical areas infiltrated by mast cells and

extramedullary hematopoiesis were documented in a few patients. Travis and Li and colleagues noted that mast cell infiltrates in lymph node tissues could resemble T-cell lymphomas in their pericortical distribution, clear cytoplasm of the mast cells in some cases, and an associated vascular proliferation and eosinophilia. When mast cells replaced the lymphoid follicles, the pattern often bore a resemblance to follicular hyperplasia or lymphoma. Lawrence and colleagues[71] found lymphadenopathy in 25% of patients with systemic disease at presentation but in none of the patients in whom the disease was confined to the skin. In a study of 21 patients, Horny et al.[77] demonstrated lymph node involvement in 80%, with the medullary cords and sinuses most often involved.

Spleen

Splenic involvement is also common in mastocytosis, seen in 40–50% of patients with systemic disease at presentation.[71,75] Travis et al.[75] reviewed the pathologic features of 16 spleens; 14 were involved with mast cell disease. All but one spleen showed a paratrabecular distribution of mast cell infiltrates: 10 (64%) perifollicular, 2 (14%) follicular, and 1 (7%) diffuse. Various degrees of trabecular and capsular fibrosis and eosinophilic infiltration were present in biopsies examined; 71% of biopsies revealed extra medullary hematopoiesis. Cross sections of the parenchyma showed multiple 1–2-mm nodular areas attributed to fibrosis or infiltrations. Again, mast cell infiltrations in the spleen produce a lesion that could be confused with T-cell lymphoma, follicular hyperplasia, follicular lymphoma, Kaposi sarcoma, or a granulomatous process. Particularly in the spleen, mast cell infiltrates can resemble a myeloproliferative disorder or hairy cell leukemia. While splenomegaly has been demonstrated in up to three-quarters of patients with systemic mast cell disease, only one-half of patients have been shown to have splenic infiltration by mast cells.[78] Markedly increased splenic weights (>700 g) generally occurred in patients who fit into unfavorable categories of mastocytosis such as aggressive mastocytosis or mastocytosis associated with a hematologic disorder.

Liver

Hepatic fibrosis was the most frequent finding in the liver and was noted in all liver specimens examined in the series reported by Yam et al.[76] Fibrosis was minimal in one patient, mild in six, moderate in four, and severe in two patients. In the latter two patients, the presence of pseudolobes pointed to the diagnosis of cirrhosis. Fibrotic patterns included a periductil pattern and portal-to-portal fibrosis. Five patients had fatty metamorphosis, and sinusoidal dilation was noted in five. A mononuclear cell infiltrate indicative of mild inflammation was commonly present. Cholestasis was noted in only one patient. The usual liver chemistry values (except for alkaline phosphatase) were often normal, despite significant hepatic involvement. In addition, the severity of hepatic involvement did not correlate with the size of the liver or with the liver chemistries.

Organ Fibrosis

The lymph nodes, liver, spleen, and bone marrow are common sites of involvement in mastocytosis. Involvement of these organs is most common in cases in which the disease is aggressive or associated with a hematologic disorder. Fibrosis associated with mast cell proliferation and eosinophilic infiltrations are common accompaniments of the disease process. It is interesting to speculate on the association between mast cells and fibrosis. Fibrosis accompanies mast cell infiltrates, particularly in lymphoid tissue and in the marrow. Mast cells themselves may produce certain connective tissue components, and mast cells synthesize TGF-β and other agents that may promote fibrosis. Indeed, histamine has been shown to promote fibroblast proliferation both in vivo and in vitro in both humans and rats through an H_2-receptor-mediated process.[79,80] Other mast cell constituents have also been implicated in radiation, chemotherapy, inflammation, and injury-induced pulmonary fibrosis.[81–84] Ultimately, in the case of liver disease, fibrosis may lead to ascites requiring aggressive therapy. The association of mast cells and lymphoid tissues may reflect either regional overproduction of growth factors for mast cells or a predisposition for mast cells[56] at certain sites within the body.

CLINICAL MANIFESTATIONS

In discussing the clinical presentation of mast cell disease, one must first become familiar with an appropriate clinical classification schema. We find the consensus revised classification schema[10] clinically useful (Table 90-3). This classification schema divides mast cell disease into four categories of increasing clinical aggressiveness and is adapted from the work of Travis et al.[7] at the Mayo Clinic and the revised classification scheme from the National Institutes of Health. The first category is termed "indolent" mastocytosis. By far, most mastocytosis patients seen will fall into this category. Their disease invariably involves the target organs listed and results in a pathophysiologic process than can be managed successfully for decades and does not appear to shorten life span. Eight manifestations of indolent mastocytosis were proposed and are listed in Table 90-3: (1) hemodynamic instability manifested as repeated episodes of flushing and syncope, (2) cutaneous mast cell disease with clear dermatopathology due to an increase in dermal mast cells, (3) ulcers of the stomach and duodenum associated with increased gastric acid, (4) malabsorption due to mast cell infiltration of the intestine, (5) mast cell infiltration of the bone marrow, (6) skeletal disease due to the activity of mast cells on bony surfaces, (7) hepatosplenomegaly, and (8) lymphadenopathy due to mast cell infiltration. These manifestations do not define subgroups, since a particular patient may have more than one manifestation. The second category consists of mastocytosis associated with a hematologic disorder. Affected patients have increased mast cells in one or more target organs plus a demonstrable bone marrow abnormality such as a myeloproliferative or myelodysplastic disorder; the skin is variably involved. In this category, the prognosis is determined primarily by the associated hematologic disorder. The third category, "aggressive mastocytosis" was previously called lymphadenopathic mastocytosis with eosinophilia. It is typically a rapidly progressive disease involving first the bone marrow and then the gastrointestinal tract, liver, spleen, and lymph nodes. The prognosis is much more guarded than that of the first category. The last category of systemic mastocytosis is mast cell leukemia, a primary leukemic process with increased mast cell burdens in both bone marrow and blood. The prognosis for patients with mast cell leukemia is extremely poor and survivals are typically <1 a year, even with aggressive combination chemotherapy.[85]

The typical clinical presentation for patients with a systemic mast cell disorder is hard to define, given that any patient may have more than one organ involved with mast cells. In addition, many patients exhibit vague or nonspecific constitutional symptoms such as weakness, fatigue, night sweats, and weight loss that cannot be attributed to any particular organ dysfunction. Some patients present primarily with neurologic or neuropsychiatric manifestations such as seizures, alterations in cognitive abilities, or depression that may be related to the underlying disease process or, in the case of neuropsychiatric

abnormalities, to the inability of the medical community to reach a diagnosis. The etiology of these symptoms is unclear, although mediator-induced hypotensive effects on the brain or a mixed organic brain syndrome, or both, have been hypothesized.[86,87] The clinician must consider the possibility of mastocytosis in a patient who presents with vague allergic-type symptoms and a syndrome of neuropsychiatric dysfunction. The following sections describe the more typical organ-specific manifestations of this disorder.

Syncope/Flushing Disorders

Typically, a patient will describe "attacks" characterized by flushing or sensations of warmth, usually accompanied by palpitations, shortness of breath, chest discomfort, nausea and diarrhea, headache, lightheadedness, and occasionally overt syncope. A unique characteristic of this syndrome is that after the episodes, patients may experience fatigue lasting several hours. Syncopal episodes may be precipitated by heat exposure, emotional stress, or physical exertion and may occur premenstrually. Some patients may have a variant of the syncopal disorder manifested solely as hemodynamic abnormalities. During episodes of flushing, many patients experience a significant dramatic decrease of blood pressure accompanied by tachycardia, while other patients may exhibit tachycardia accompanied by an elevation in blood pressure. In this second group of patients, pheochromocytoma must be ruled out. These hemodynamic variants of the mast cell syncope/flushing disorder may be related to mast cell mediator release involving prostaglandin D_2 (PGD$_2$).[9,88] PGD$_2$ is a potent vasodilator metabolized in vivo by 11-ketoreductase to the metabolite 9α,11β,-PGF$_2$, a potent pressor substance.[89] It is attractive to speculate that the hemodynamic instability noted in some patients, and the variation noted among patients, is a consequence of differences in prostaglandin metabolism resulting in marked differences in acute levels of PGD$_2$ relative to its metabolite 9α,11β,-PGF$_2$. Such syncope/flushing in the absence of demonstrable mast cell hyperplasia does not establish the diagnosis of mastocytosis.

Cutaneous Disease

Cutaneous manifestations of systemic mast cell disease may appear early in life. In a series of 112 patients,[90] solitary mastocytomas were present at birth or developed within the first week of life. The multiple lesions of urticaria pigmentosa may also be found at birth or may appear during early childhood. The onset of urticaria pigmentosa follows a biphasic curve with one peak at 2.5 months of age and the second peak at 26.5 years.[91] Lesions are present in 80% of affected children by 6 months of age. The frequency of skin lesions in patients with systemic mastocytosis is 50–100% in various studies.[7,68,69,92–94] However, the true percentage of patients with systemic mastocytosis without dermatologic lesions is unknown. There appears to be no sex predilection, and a familial association is generally not seen. In <50 families, mastocytosis of one form or another has affected more than one family member, including several families with affected twins.[95–98]

Mast cell disease has four cutaneous manifestations: urticaria pigmentosa, mastocytoma, diffuse/erythrodermic disease, and telangiectasia macularis eruptiva perstans. The most common cutaneous mast cell lesion is urticaria pigmentosa, which appears as red-brown macules, papules, and plaques

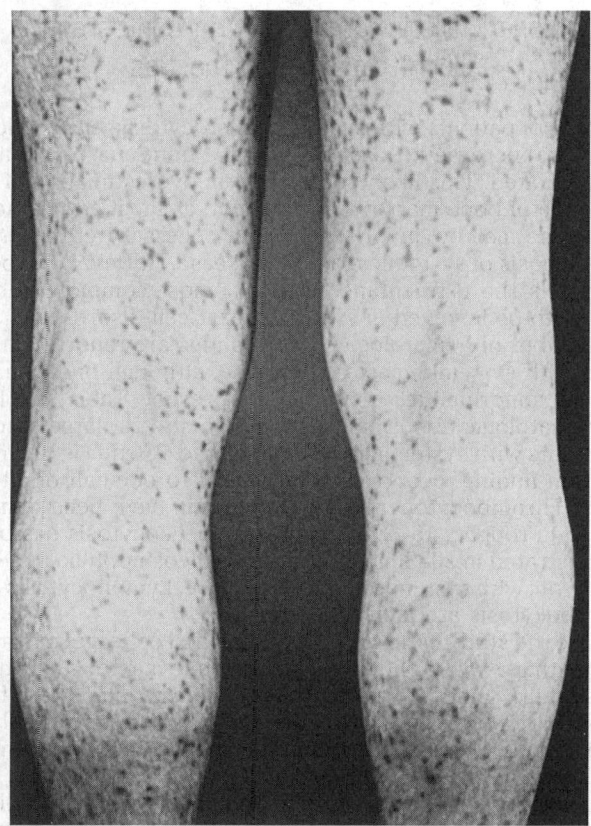

Fig. 90-4. Urticaria pigmentosa. (From Soter,[91] with permission.)

(Fig. 90-4). Lesions occur in a generalized and random distribution and may form clusters with a cobblestone appearance. Erythema, edema, and blister formation with subsequent crusting of the lesions has been reported, particularly in young children. Gross hemorrhage into bullous lesions can occur, presumably secondary to high local levels of heparin released from mast cells. After the age of 10, vesicles generally do not occur, and the lesions tend to be smaller and more numerous. Approximately one-half of patients in whom urticaria appears in infancy or childhood experience resolution by adolescence; in the remainder of patients, only lightly pigmented macules remain.[90,99] Lesions that appear after age 10 tend to persist and remain symptomatic. The lesions of urticaria pigmentosa are usually of the highest density on the trunk, although they may affect all skin areas, including mucous membranes. The palms, soles, face, and scalp are often free of disease or are lightly affected. Telangiectasias, petechiae, or ecchymosis may occur in the lesions or in adjacent clinically normal skin. The most common clinical manifestations include pruritis, dermatographism, and the presence of Darier sign (wheal and erythema occurring after a brisk stroke to a lesion). A positive Darier sign may result in blister formation with hemorrhage, particularly in infants. Flushing has been reported to occur in up to one-third of patients with urticaria pigmentosa. In various retrospective studies, 10–70% of patients with urticaria pigmentosa have been documented as having systemic disease, with the bone marrow the most frequently involved site. However, Travis et al.[7] reported that the absence of urticaria pigmentosa and the absence of skin symptoms are poor prognostic features in patients with systemic disease.

Mastocytomas may be present at birth, although most appear within the first 3 months of life and are rarely described in adults.[69,100,101] Lesions are generally few in number and may be solitary or show focal clustering. The most common presentation is as a macule, plaque, or nodule, but bullous lesions

have been described. Most mastocytomas form on the extremities and rarely involve palms or soles. In most cases, the lesions are thought to involute spontaneously; however, this has not invariably been reported. Rare patients have had systemic manifestations such as flushing.[102]

Diffuse cutaneous mastocytosis is a rare disorder that generally presents before the age of 3 and involves the entire cutaneous integument. The skin may appear normal; more commonly, it has a yellow-red-brown color with a peau d'orange appearance. Yellow to cream-colored papules that resemble xanthomas and pseudoxanthoma elasticum have also been described.[103] A generalized erythroderma form of diffuse cutaneous mastocytosis is manifested by severe edema and a doughy thickening of the skin.[104] Dermatographism with the formation of hemorrhagic blisters is a common finding in this disorder. Extensive bullae with rupture and crusting may be the first presentation in an infant who later develops diffuse cutaneous mastocytosis. Thus, bullous erythrodermic mastocytosis must be included in the differential diagnosis of neonatal blister disorders.[105] Diffuse cutaneous mastocytosis reportedly may resolve spontaneously at age 5–15 months; in other cases the disease persists; however, when present, these children are at risk of complications such as flushing, hypotension, shock, and occasionally death. Diarrhea and other gastrointestinal manifestations are common in this disorder and occasional patients have been demonstrated to have significant gastrointestinal bleeding.[106]

Telangiectasia macularis eruptiva perstans is a rare form of mastocytosis traditionally thought to be limited to the skin. In isolated cases, splenomegaly, increased numbers of mast cells in the bone marrow, and abnormal skeletal radiographs suggest that this form of mastocytosis may have systemic features.[107] Many of the original patients reported with this disorder were obese middle-aged women. However, one pediatric case report involves a 10-year-old girl.[108] The lesions in this disorder are generalized, red, telangiectatic macules on a tan to brown background. Individual lesions are 2–6 mm in diameter and are without sharply defined outlines. Sites become edematous when rubbed. Pruritis, purpura, and blister formation are generally not associated with this disorder. In occasional patients, the lesions may coexist with those of urticaria pigmentosa.[109]

Gastrointestinal Ulcer Disease

Gastrointestinal symptoms have commonly been reported in patients with systemic mastocytosis (Table 90-7). Both retrospective and prospective studies[68,69,110,111] have documented abdominal pain, diarrhea, nausea, vomiting, and peptic ulcer disease in one-fourth to one-half of individuals with systemic mastocytosis. Recent studies with the mast cell-deficient mouse[112] suggest that mast cells may be essential for normal gastric acid secretion. Cherner et al.[113] have demonstrated a broad range of basal acid secretion values in a prospective study of 16 patients with systemic mastocytosis. Six of these patients were shown to have clinically significant acid hypersecretion. The importance of histamine in inducing the acid hypersecretion in these patients was borne out by the finding of low gastrin levels in many of the patients.

Table 90-7. Gastrointestinal Manifestations of Systemic Mastocytosis

Abdominal pain
Diarrhea
Nausea
Peptic ulcer disease
Malabsorption

Gastrointestinal Malabsorption

Up to one-third of patients with systemic mastocytosis have been demonstrated to have some laboratory evidence of fat malabsorption.[113] However, the degree of malabsorption is generally not of clinical importance. While the etiology of this mild malabsorption is unclear, potential explanations include acid hypersecretion and mucosal dysfunction. Shortened intestinal transit time does not appear to contribute to the malabsorption syndrome.[113] Limited studies have indicated that mast cells may be increased in the small intestine of patients with systemic mastocytosis, although a clear correlation between mucosal mast cell numbers and gastrointestinal symptoms has not been noted. Miner[114] evaluated several patients who presented with symptoms of systemic mastocytosis and either urticaria pigmentosa or increased marrow mast cells. Mucosal biopsies from five of these patients demonstrated a variation in mast cell numbers, depending on the site measured. This observation supports the basic premise that the particular symptoms manifested by a patient with systemic mast cell disease is influenced by the site of the local increase in mast cell numbers.

Skeletal Disease

Occasional patients with marked bony infiltration with mast cells have been noted. The most common radiographic abnormality is diffuse osteopenia, which is frequently an incidental finding on radiography.[113,115-118] In some patients, osteoporosis may be the sole initial manifestation of systemic mast cell disease.[119] Both lytic and sclerotic lesions have been described. Bone scans may be normal or may show focal or diffuse abnormalities.[120] In patients with aggressive disease, diffuse bone pain as well as pathologic fractures have been reported.[121]

Visceral/Hepatosplenomegaly

Hepatic involvement with mast cell lesions is a common finding in systemic mastocytosis, although a significant degree of hepatic dysfunction is generally not observed. Alkaline phosphatase is frequently elevated, but this elevation is largely attributable to bone disease. Webb et al.[68] demonstrated hepatomegaly in 45% and splenomegaly in 50% of 26 patients they studied. Rare patients with systemic mastocytosis have been demonstrated to have portal hypertension, and significant splenomegaly may be a contributing factor to the hematologic abnormalities noted in many patients.

Lymphadenopathy

Lymphadenopathy has been demonstrated in ≤60% of patients with systemic mast cell disease.[75] In a review of 58 patients with systemic mastocytosis, Travis et al.[7] demonstrated peripheral lymphadenopathy in 26% of patients and central lymphadenopathy in 19% at of diagnosis. A similar presence of both peripheral and central lymphadenopathy has been demonstrated by Austen and colleagues at the Brigham and Women's Hospital[120] and by the National Institutes of Health group.[71] The presence of lymphadenopathy in and of itself does not signal aggressive disease, and no specific symptoms are referable to lymphadenopathy. However, patients who present with lymphadenopathy and significant hepatosplenomegaly should be followed closely for evolution into a more aggressive systemic disorder.

Bone Marrow Mast Cell Aggregates and Hematologic Abnormalities

In 90% of patients with systemic mastocytosis, either a focal or diffuse increase of mast cells in the bone marrow will be demonstrated. This likely represents an overestimation of the incidence of bone marrow involvement, as most early studies used bone marrow involvement as a necessary criterion for the diagnosis of systemic mast cell disease. However, the bone marrow is the extracutaneous organ most commonly documented to be involved in systemic mast cell disorders.

A number of hematologic abnormalities are reported in patients with systemic mast cell disease, although one or more of these abnormalities is not always present. Table 90-8 lists the hematologic abnormalities noted in several large studies of patients with systemic mast cell disease. Anemia is the most common finding, occurring in one-third to one-half of all patients. Thrombocytopenia and leukopenia have been demonstrated in roughly 15–20% of patients. Leukocytosis has been demonstrated in 20–30% of patients, and eosinophilia in ≤40% of patients with systemic mast cell disease. Lymphocytosis and thrombocytosis are unusual findings.

While the study conducted by Travis and colleagues demonstrated that ≤7% of patients with systemic mastocytosis have a basophilia, and ≤4% have circulating mast cells,[7] these findings have not been universally demonstrated in other similarly large studies. However, monocytosis has been reported in approximately 15% of patients with mastocytosis. Mast cells and basophils are similar but not identical. Although mast cells in the bone marrow are densely granulated cells, when seen in the peripheral blood they frequently have the appearance of atypical monocytes containing scattered large basophilic granules. They also frequently appear somewhat dysplastic, making identification on Wright stain difficult. Frequently, stains specific for mast cells must be performed to identify the cells in the peripheral blood conclusively and to distinguish them from either basophils or hypergranulated monocytes. Table 90-6 lists several histochemical stains used to differentiate mast calls from basophils.

According to the revised consensus classification, the second category of systemic mastocytosis includes those patients who present with systemic disease and a hematologic syndrome resembling a myeloproliferative or myelodysplastic pro-

Table 90–8. Hematologic Abnormalities in Systemic Mast Cell Disease

	Travis et al.[7]	Webb et al.[68]	Brunning et al.[69]	Lawrence et al.[71]
Patients (N)	58	26	14	32
Cytopenias				
Anemia	47%	37%	36%	50%
Thrombocytopenia	16	22	14	19
Leukopenia	16	15	21	9
Lymphopenia	–	–	–	–
Increased white blood elements				
Leukocytosis	19%	29%	21%	31%
Eosinophilia	19	17	43	21
Basophilia	7	0	0	NA
Monocytosis	16	17	0	18
Lymphocytosis	2			
Thrombocytosis	9			
Increased mast cells[a]				
<10%	2	2	0	N/A
>10%	2	2	0	N/A

Abbreviation: NA, not available.
[a] In peripheral blood.

Table 90–9. Systemic Cell Disease:
Malignant/Premalignant Manifestations

Myeloproliferative disorder

Myelodysplastic syndrome

"Lymphadenopathic syndrome"

Non-Hodgkin lymphoma

Mast cell leukemia

Acute leukemia (secondary)

Table 90–10. Consensus Diagnostic Workup

If mastocytosis is suspected on clinical grounds
   Routine
      Examine skin—gross and microscopic
      Bone marrow biopsy and aspiration
      Serum for mast cell tryptase
      24-hr urine for mediators
   Additional studies
      Bone scan/skeletal survey
      Gastrointestinal workup[a]—upper gastrointestinal series, small bowel radiography, computed tomography scan, endoscopy
   Electroencephalography, neuropsychiatric workup

[a] May be adequate criteria for primary diagnosis.

cess. Several premalignant or overtly malignant syndromes have been described with systemic mast cell disease (Table 90-9). A relatively small subgroup of adult patients with systemic mast cell disease has been documented to have either a myeloproliferative or myelodysplastic process.[7,68,71,93,122,123] The peripheral blood picture in these patients may be consistent with that of either chronic myeloid leukemia (CML) or chronic myelomonocytic leukemia. The presence of either of these disorders is associated with a poor prognosis.[71,72] As with primary myeloproliferative and myelodysplastic syndromes, a secondary acute leukemia may develop in patients with systemic mast cell disease. Many of the patients with systemic mast cell disease who are demonstrated to have significant cytopenias on bone marrow examination have had overtly dysplastic myeloid or erythroid maturation. In addition, a small number of patients have developed diffuse fibrosis of the bone marrow with a marked hypocellularity. Those patients with systemic mast cell disease with a CML-like picture are Philadelphia chromosome negative. Surprisingly, the prospective series by Lawrence et al.[71] demonstrated that some patients have decreasing marrow mast cell involvement, in spite of increasing systemic symptomatology.

Lymphadenopathic Mastocytosis with Eosinophilia

A subset of patients with systemic mastocytosis who present with, or subsequently develop, significant lymphadenopathy, hepatosplenomegaly, and peripheral eosinophilia have been described.[7,8,70] Lymph node biopsies in these patients frequently show a hyperplastic picture suggestive of a malignant lymphoproliferative disorder. However, tissue pathology does not support a diagnosis of a non-Hodgkin lymphoma. Clinically, these patients have an aggressive form of the disease with marked visceral and bony involvement and dramatically shortened survival. Many of these patients display a marked eosinophilia on peripheral blood. Frequently, the eosinophils are dysplastic and hypogranular, similar to those seen in the idiopathic hypereosinophilic syndrome.

Mast Cell Leukemia

These cases are characterized by the presence of a large number of atypical-appearing mast cells in the peripheral blood, a leukocytosis and granulocytosis, and a compressed clinical course.[85] Survival with aggressive chemotherapy was 2–9 months, with a mean of <6 months. This syndrome appears to represent the most aggressive form of mast cell disorder and appears to be a de novo malignant proliferation of mast cells.

LABORATORY EVALUATION

A suggested diagnostic evaluation for systemic mast cell disease is presented in Table 90-10. If mastocytosis is suspected on clinical grounds, the routine workup should consist of an examination of the skin, both gross and microscopic; a bone marrow biopsy and aspirate; serum for tryptase levels; and a 24-hour urine for mediators (particularly histamine and/or its metabolites). Additional studies, as suggested by symptomatology or findings during the routine evaluation, would include a bone scan or skeletal survey, or both; a gastrointestinal evaluation involving radiographic studies of the upper gastrointestinal tract and small intestines, computed tomography scan, and endoscopy; and a neuropsychiatric workup with electroencephalography. In all cases, the fundamental requirements for the diagnosis of mastocytosis remains the presence of significant increases in mast cell numbers in one or more target tissues. The classic lesions of mastocytosis, namely, mast cell aggregates, are required for the diagnosis of bone marrow involvement. However, a dramatic increase in mast cells within the lamina propria of the gastrointestinal tract may establish the diagnosis of systemic mast cell disease without evidence of cutaneous, marrow, or other visceral involvement. While it is clear that the symptoms of mast cell disease can reflect local increases of mast cells, slight increases in mast cell numbers in target tissues, such as the skin and bone marrow, are not diagnostic because they may only reflect a normal inflammatory or reactive process. Likewise, while plasma or urinary levels of histamine are frequently increased in systemic mastocytosis,[124] the solitary finding of increased levels of histamine or histamine metabolites may reflect any of a number of other situations, such as anaphylaxis or response to unusual immunologic stimuli. Similarly, serum tryptase may be elevated after anaphylaxis, and may sometimes be normal in spite of a marrow diagnosis. Thus, no single laboratory test can establish the diagnosis of mastocytosis. Rather, the demonstration of mast cell mediators in blood or urine simply prompts the clinician to investigate further for the presence of abnormal collections of mast cells.

DIFFERENTIAL DIAGNOSIS

The differential diagnosis of systemic mast cell disease must be considered on two levels (Table 90-11). The first is that of clinical grounds, where other disease processes that may produce symptoms similar to those seen in systemic mast cell disorders must be excluded. These disorders include allergic or "mediator" diseases such as hyper-IgE syndrome, parasitic infestations of the gastrointestinal tract or viscera, hereditary or acquired angioneurotic edema, idiopathic anaphylaxis, complement disorders, or idiopathic capillary leak syndrome. When episodic hypertension is a major symptom component, pheochromocytoma must be considered; when significant unexplained ulcer disease is present, a Zollinger-Ellison/gastrinoma syndrome must be ruled out.

The second level at which one must consider a differential diagnosis is at the level of histopathology. In this regard, three particular disorders may present with bone marrow lesions

Table 90–11. Differential Diagnosis of Systemic Mastocytosis

Clinical syndrome
  Hyper-IgE syndrome
  Hereditary/acquired angioneurotic edema
  Complement disorders
  Parasitic infestations
  Idiopathic anaphylaxis
  Idiopathic capillary leak syndrome
  Pheochromocytoma
  Zollinger-Ellison syndrome/gastrinoma
Marrow histopathology
  Primary myelofibrosis
  Angioimmunoblastic lymphadenopathy
  Eosinophilic fibrohistiocytoma of bone

Table 90–12. Therapy for Cutaneous Mastocytosis

Mastocytoma
  Not required
  Excision
Urticaria pigmentosa and diffuse and erythrodermic cutaneous mastocytosis
  H₁ antihistamines
  H₁ and H₂ antihistamines
  Ketotifen
  Disodium cromoglycate
  Topical corticosteroids with occlusion
  PUVA
Telangiectasia macularis eruptive perstans
  PUVA

reminiscent of those seen in systemic mastocytosis. These disorders are primary myelofibrosis, angioimmunoblastic lymphadenopathy, and eosinophilic fibrohistiocytoma. The distinction of mastocytosis from these three disorders is generally accomplished by close review of the histopathologic material and correlation with other clinical and laboratory features. When the marrow is diffusely infiltrated with an increased number of mast cells, there is frequently a background of fibrosis to these lesions. In this setting, differentiation from primary myelofibrosis is often difficult.[69,125] In areas of fibrosis, the mast cells are often elongated and relatively agranular on H&E stain. Toluidine blue stain or other stains to bring out the metachromatic granules of the mast cell may be particularly useful in these cases. The differentiation of systemic mastocytosis from angioimmunoblastic lymphadenopathy generally relies on the lack of plasma cells and immunoblasts and the absence of neovascularity in the lesions of mastocytosis. Differentiation of systemic mastocytosis from the bone marrow lesions of fibrohistiocytoma is much more problematic. Large histiocytic cells described in eosinophilic fibrohistiocytic lesions have a striking resemblance to the large mast cells seen in many mastocytosis lesions.[70,126,127] It may be that eosinophilic fibrohistiocytic lesions of the bone represent an indolent form of systemic mast cell disease.[87]

THERAPY

No cure has been found for mastocytosis and little documentation suggests that symptomatic therapy substantially alters the course of disease. A primary concern in therapy for both cutaneous and systemic mast cell disease is the avoidance of triggering factors (which vary from patient to patient) such as temperature extremes, physical exertion, or the ingestion of agents such as ethanol, nonsteroidal anti-inflammatory drugs, or opiate analgesics. Physical trauma to lesions or environmental factors may also trigger acute episodes with reports of anaphylaxis after *Hymenoptera* stings and exposure to iodinated contrast materials in patients with systemic mast cell disease.[128] Epinephrine remains the drug of choice in the treatment of anaphylaxis, either idiopathic or induced by environmental factors. Patients with mast cell disease and a history of anaphylaxis should be advised to carry epinephrine-filled syringes and taught to self-medicate. These patients may also benefit from the concurrent use of H₁ and H₂ antihistimines prophylactically. Tables 90-12 and 90-13 list some of the more common therapeutic modalities used in both cutaneous and systemic mast cell disease.

Classic H₁ antihistamines have been used to decrease the irritability of the skin and mitigate symptoms of pruritis. Amelioration can be achieved through the use of antihitamines, but rarely does total ablation of signs and symptoms occur.

Hydroxyzine and doxepin are two potent H₁ antihistamines found quite useful in our experience. Doxepin is particularly useful for patients who have central nervous system manifestations of mast cell disease. Frequently the dose-limiting side effect of antihistamine therapy is sedation. Patients sensitive to the sedative effects of antihistamines may benefit from the use of newer nonsedative antihistamines, although their use is contraindicated in patients with liver disease. For patients who continue to have significant disease symptoms while on H₁ antihistimes, the combination of H₁ and H₂ antagonists has been shown to be at times effective in relieving pruritis and wheal formation.[129] H₂ antihistamines such as ranitidine and cimetidine have been quite useful in the treatment of gastritis and peptic ulcer disease associated with mastocytosis. Doses of these H₂ antihistamines can be titrated on the basis of symptom control or to a particular level of gastric acid secretion.

Oral administration of disodium cromoglycolate has been reported to reduce pruritis and wheal formation in urticaria pigmentosa in patients with or without systemic disease.[127,130–133] This agent has also been reported to be of benefit in cutaneous mast cell disease in children and infants.[129,130] Oral cromolyn sodium has also proved most useful for the control of gastrointestinal complaints often seen with systemic disease.[114] Sometimes other symptoms such as headache and bone pain have also been reported to improve with the use of cromolyn sodium.

Table 90-13. Therapy for Systemic Mastocytosis

Antihistamine[a]
  H₁ receptor blockade
    Hydroxyzine
    Doxepin
  H₂ receptor blockade
    Ranitidine
    Cimetidine
Epinephrine
Steroids
Cromolyn sodium
Aspirin (if the patient is not sensitive)
Anticholinergics
PUVA
Chemotherapy[b]
Radiotherapy[b]
Splenectomy[b]
Diphosphonate[b]
Interferons, growth factors[b]
Cyclosporin[b]

[a] Representative drugs only.
[b] Use restricted to treatment of aggressive mastocytosis (third major category, Table 90-3) or mastocytosis with an associated hematologic disorder (second major category, Table 90-3).

Ketotifen has been widely used in Europe. It has been reported to prevent mast cell degranulation and to be effective in the relief of pruritis and wheal formation in urticaria pigmentosa and in other forms of diffuse cutaneous mastocytosis.[134–136] One patient has been reported in whom findings of osteoporosis improved after therapy with ketotifen.[137] By contrast, one pediatric study found ketotifen no more effective than hydroxyzine.[138] Similarly, the drug azelastine, an antihistamine with mast cell-stabilizing properties offered little benefit over chlorpheniramine.[139] Diphosphonates have also been reported useful in the treatment of mastocytosis-associated osteopenia.[117]

While systemic corticosteroids have not been shown to be effective in the treatment of cutaneous mastocytosis, topical administration or intralesional injections of corticosteriods have resulted in symptomatic and cosmetic improvement. Caution must be exercised with repeated or extensive application of corticosteroids, as this may result in cutaneous atrophy or adrenocortical suppression.[140] The oral administration of 8-methoxpsoralen plus ultraviolet A (PUVA) photochemotherapy has resulted in a decrease in pruritis and wheal formation in patients with urticaria pigmentosa with or without systemic disease.[141–144] Frequently, prolonged controlled disease results after a single course of PUVA therapy but relapses occurring 3–6 months after cessation of therapy are common. PUVA therapy has been associated with decreased levels of urine and blood mediators.[141,142,145] Occasional patients experience a decrease in cutaneous lesions after exposure to natural sunlight; however, there are no controlled studies using ultraviolet B phototherapy.[91]

Significant malabsorption, hepatic fibrosis, and ascites have been noted in patients with severe mastocytosis.[111,146,147] Systemic corticosteroids have been useful in decreasing the malabsorption and ascites in some of the patients. In adults, oral prednisone (40–60 mg/day) usually results in a decrease in symptoms over a 2–3-week period.[148] After initial improvement, steroids can frequently be tapered to an alternate-day dosing regimen. However, with time, the ascites frequently recurs; it has been suggested that these patients may benefit from a portacaval shunt.[147]

Aspirin and other non-steriodal anti-inflammatory agents have been useful in some patients whose primary manifestation is recurrent episodes of flushing or syncope, or both. The use of these agents may be problematic in patients with significant ulcer disease. Some patients may worsen with aspirin. Calcium channel blockers and platelet-activating factor inhibitors have been effective in anecdotal cases.[149,150]

A small percentage of patients with systemic mast cell disease may have a syndrome mimicking a non-Hodgkin lymphoma, an aggressive myeloproliferative disease, or rarely an overt nonlymphocytic leukemia.[8,71,122,151] Two patients have been reported with systemic mast cell disease associated with primary mediastinal germ cell tumor.[152,153] In this group of patients, traditional chemotherapy directed toward their neoplastic process may be appropriate. Chemotherapy with cyclophosphamide, vincristine, and prednisone has been used in some patients whose clinical picture is that of a non-Hodgkin lymphoma, although the response to chemotherapy is variable.[152] Radiotherapy has been used in limited patients to control local disease.[154]

Splenectomy has been performed on a number of patients with severe aggressive mastocytosis, in an attempt to improve their limiting cytopenias.[155] With splenectomy, survival increased by an average of 12 months. Patients who had undergone splenectomy appeared better able to tolerate chemotherapy. While splenectomy is of no value in the management of indolent mast cell disease, it should be considered in selected patients with more aggressive forms of mastocytosis.

PROGNOSIS

The prognosis of patients with mast cell disorders is clearly related to the extent of the disease. Patients who present with cutaneous disease, flushing disorders, or limited extracutaneous organ involvement frequently have an indolent course requiring chronic medical management. Few if any of these cases have been documented to progress into a more advanced form of the disease.[71,120] In contrast to the clinical course of patients with limited disease, a prospective analysis of 46 patients identified elevated lactate dehydrogenase levels, late age of onset, and the presence of a significant hematologic abnormality (defined as a myeloproliferative, myelodysplastic, or overt leukemic picture) as indicators of a poor prognosis and shortened survival.[71] Of the parameters studied by multivariate analysis, only late age at onset of symptoms and elevated serum lactate dehydrogenase levels were found to be predictive of a poor prognosis. Other groups have also identified the presence of a myeloproliferative or myelodysplastic blood picture as conferring a poorer prognosis.

FUTURE DIRECTIONS

In addition to the therapeutic modalities already mentioned, some innovative therapies on the horizon are worth discussing separately. Mastocytosis involves both mast cell hyperplasia and systemic mediator release. Mast cells release primary mediators that induce the production and secretion of secondary mediators, but these mediators also effect mast cell proliferation and degranulation. An approach using an "antiproliferative" mediator to treat mastocytosis is attractive and may warrant investigation. CSF-GM has been shown to inhibit the growth of IL-3-dependent mast cells in murine bone marrow[156] as does IFN-γ.[157] Recently, a patient with aggressive systemic mastocytosis has shown a significant response to treatment with recombinant human IFN-γ2B.[158] In addition, the use of the T-cell-dependent immunosuppressant cyclosporine also merits investigation. An anti-IgE antibody coupled to an antimitotic agent has been used (without success) to treat a patient with mast cell leukemia.[159] While none of these approaches can be supported with clinical series, and may not be appropriate in patients with indolent mastocytosis, innovative approaches to therapy may be reasonable to consider, given our current inability to affect survival significantly in the more aggressive forms of this disorder.

REFERENCES

1. Nettleship E, Tay W: Rare forms of urticaria. BMJ 2:323, 1869
2. Ehrlich P: Beiträge zur theoretic and Praxis der histologischer Färbung. Doctoral thesis, University of Leipzig, Leipzig, Germany, 1878
3. Unna PG: Beiträge zur Anatomie und Pathogenese der Urticaria Simplex und Pigmentosa. Monatsschr Prakt Dermatol Suppl Dermatol Stud 3:9, 1878
4. Sangster A: An anomalous mottled rash, accompanied by pruritis, factious urticaria and pigmentation, "urticaria pigmentosa (?)." Trans Clin Soc Lond 11:161, 1878
5. Sézary A, Levy-Coblentz G, Chauvillon P: Dermatographisme et mastocytose. Bull Soc Fr Dermatol Syphiligr 43:359, 1936
6. Ellis JM: Urticaria pigmentosa: a report of a case with autopsy. Arch Pathol 48:426, 1949
7. Travis WD, Li C-Y, Bergstralh EF, et al: Systemic mast cell disease. Analysis of 58 cases and literature review. Medicine 67:345, 1988
8. Friedman BS, Metcalfe DD: Mastocytosis. p. 163. In Tauber AI, Wintroub BU, Stolper-Simon A (eds): Biochemistry of the Acute Allergic Reaction. Fifth International Symposium. Alan R Liss, 1989
9. Roberts LJ II, Oates JA: Biochemical diagnosis of systemic mast cell disorders. J Invest Dermatol 96:19S, 1991
10. Metcalfe DD: Clinical advances in mastocytosis—conclusions. J Invest Dermatol 96:64S, 1991
11. Kitamura Y: Heterogeneity of mast cells and phenotypic changes between subpopulations. Annu Rev Immunol 7:59, 1989

12. Galli SJ: New insights into "the riddle of the mast cell": microenvironmental regulation of mast cell development and phenotypic heterogeneity. Lab Invest 62:5, 1990

13. Galli SJ: New concepts about the mast cell. N Engl J Med 328:257, 1993

14. Galli SJ, Dvorak AM, Dvorak HF: Basophils and mast cells: morphologic insights into their biology, secretory patterns, and function. Prog Allergy 34:1, 1984

15. Schwartz LB, Austen KF: Structure and function of the clinical mediators of mast cells. Prog Allergy 34:271, 1984

16. Valent P, Majic O, Maurer D et al: Further characterization of surface membrane structures expressed on human basophils and mast cells. Int Arch Allergy Appl Immunol 91:198, 1990

17. Seder RA, Paul WE, Dvorak AM et al: Mouse splenic and bone marrow cell populations that express high-affinity Fc_ϵ receptions and produce interleukin-4 are highly enriched in basophils. J Immunol 149:599, 1992

18. Columbo M, Horowitz EM, Botana LM et al: The human c-kit receptor ligand, rhSCF, induces mediator release from human cutaneous mast cells and enhances IgE-dependent mediator release from both skin mast cells and peripheral blood basophils. Proc Natl Acad Sci USA 88:2835, 1991

19. Kitamura Y, Go S, Hatanaka S: Decrease of mast cells in W/W^V mice and their increase by bone marrow transplantation. Blood 52:447, 1978

20. Sonoda T, Kitamura Y, Haku Y et al: Mast cell precursors in various hematopoietic colonies of mice produced in vivo and in vitro. Br J Haematol 53:611, 1983

21. Nakano T, Kanakura Y, Nakahata T et al: Genetically mast cell-deficient W/W^V mice as a tool for studies of differentiation and function of mast cells. Fed Proc 46:1920, 1987

22. Geissler EN, Ryan MA, Housman DE: The dominant-white spotting (W) locus of the mouse encodes the c-kit protooncogene. Cell 55:185, 1988

23. Anderson DM, Lyman SD, Baird A et al: Molecular cloning of mast cell growth factor, a hematopoietin that is active in both membrane bound and soluble forms. Cell 63:235, 1990

24. Huang E, Nocka K, Beier DR et al: The hamatopoietic growth factor KL is encoded at the Sl locus and is the ligand of the c-kit receptor, the gene product of the W locus. Cell 63:225, 1990

25. Martin FH, Suggs SV, Langley KE et al: Primary structure and functional expression of rat and human cell factor DNAs. Cell 63.203, 1990

26. Ihle JN, Keller J, Oersolan S et al: Biological properties of homogenous interleukin-3. I. Demonstration of WEHL-3 growth factor activity, mast cell growth-factor activity, P cell-stimulating factor activity and histamine-producing factor activity. J Immunol 131:282, 1993

27. Lee F, Yokota T, Otsuka T et al: Isolation and characterization of a mouse interleukin cDNA clone that expresses B cell stimulatory factor 1 activities and T cell mast cell-stimulating activities. Proc Natl Acad Sci USA 83:2061, 1986

28. Thompson-Sneips L, Dahr V, Bond MW et al: Interleukin 10: a novel stimulatory factor for mast cells and their progenitors. J Exp Med 173:507, 1991

29. Lanotte M, Arock M, Lacaze N et al: Murine basophil-mast differentiation: toward optimal conditions of selective growth and maturation of basophil-mast or allied cells. J Cell Physiol 129:199, 1986

30. Bressler RB, Thompson HL, Keffer JM et al: Inhibition of the growth of IL-3-dependent mast cells from murine bone marrow by recombinant granulocyte macrophage-colony-stimulating factor. J Immunol 143:135, 1989

31. Brodie DH, Wasserman SI, Alvaro-Garcia J et al: Transforming growth factor-beta 1 selectively inhibits IL-3 dependent mast cell proliferation without affecting mast cell function or differentiation. J Immunol 143:1590, 1989

32. Madden KB, Urban JF Jr, Zilgener HJ et al: Antibodies to IL-3 and IL-4 suppress helminth-induced intestinal mastocytosis. FASEB J 5:A1012, 1991

33. Tsai M, Takashi T, Thompson H et al: Induction of mast cell proliferation, maturation, and heparin synthesis by the rat c-kit ligand, stem cell factor. Proc Natl Acad Sci USA 88:6382, 1991

34. Bodine DM, Orlic D, Birket NC et al: Stem cell factor increases colony-forming unit-spleen number in vitro in synergy with interleukin-6, and in vivo in S/S^d mice as a single factor. Blood 79:913, 1992

35. Mekori YA, Oh CK, Metcalfe DD: IL-3 dependent cells undergo apoptosis upon removal of IL-3: prevention of apoptosis by c-kit ligand. J Immunol 151:3775, 1993

36. Bianchine PJ, Burd PR, Metcalfe DD: IL-3 dependent mast cells attach to plate-bound vitronectin: demonstration of augmented proliferation in response to signals transduced via cell surface vitronectin. J Immunol 149:3665, 1992

37. Kirshenbaum AS, Goff JP, Irani A-M et al: Interleukin 3-dependent growth of basophil-like and mast-like cells from human bone marrow. J Immunol 142:2424, 1989

38. Leary AG, Yang Y-C, Clark SC et al: Recombinant gibbon interleukin-3 supports formation of human multilineage colonies in culture: comparison with recombinant human granulocyte-macrophage colony-stimulating factor. Blood 70:1343, 1987

39. Kirshenbaum AS, Goff JP, Kessler SW et al: Effect of IL-3 and stem cell factor on the appearance of human basophils and mast cells from CD34 + pluripotent progenitor cells. J Immunol 148:772, 1992

40. Nilsson G, Irani AA, Ishizaka T, Schwartz LP: Human recombinant stem cell factor (SCF), the ligand for c-kit, induces development of human mast cells whereas IL-3 induces basophil-like cells from fetal liver cells (FLC). FASEB J 6:A1722, 1992

41. Agis H, Wilheim M, Sperr WR et al: Monocytes do not make mast cells when cultured in the presence of SCF. J Immunol 151:4221, 1993

42. Bienenstock J, Blennerhassett M, Kakuta Y et al: Evidence for central and peripheral nervous system interaction with mast cells. p. 275. In Galli SJ, Austen KF (eds): Mast Cell and Basophil Differentiation and Function in Health Disease. Raven Press, New York, 1989

43. Ghidyal N. McNeil HP, Gurish MF et al: Transcriptional regulation of the mucosal mast cell protease, MMCP-2, by IL-3, IL-4, and IL-10. J Allergy Clin Immunol 89:245, 1992

44. Irani AA, Schechter NM, Craig SS et al: Two types of human mast cells that have distinct neutral protease compositions. Proc Natl Acad Sci USA 83:4464, 1986

45. Craig SS, Irani A-M, Metcalfe DD, Schwartz LB: Ultrastructural localization of heparin to human mast cells of the MC_{TC} and MC_T types by labeling with antithrombin III-gold. Lab Invest 69:552, 1993

46. Thompson HL, Chad K, Barbieri S, Metcalfe DD: Mast cells activated through FCεRI exhibit ICAM-1 and VCAM-1 dependent adhesion. J Allergy Clin Immunol 89:377, 1992

47. Guo C, Kagay-Sobotka A, Lichenstein LM, Bochner BS. Unique phenotypic characteristics of human uterine mast cells (UMC). J Allergy Clin Immunol 87:303, 1991

48. Thompson HL, Burbelo PD, Sequi-Real B et al: Laminin promotes mast cell attachment. J Immunol 143:2323, 1989

49. Thompson HL, Burbelo PD, Yamada Y et al: Mast cells chemotax to laminin with enhancement of after IgE-mediated activation. J Immunol 143:4188, 1989

50. Thompson HL, Burbelo PD, Yamada Y et al: Identification of an amino acid sequence in the laminin A chain mediating mast cell attachment and spreading. Immunology 72:144, 1991

51. Thompson HL, Burbelo PD, Metcalfe DD: Regulation of adhesion of mouse bone marrow-derived mast cells to laminin. J Immunol 145:3425, 1990

52. Dastych J, Costa JJ, Thompson HL, Metcalfe DD: Mast cell adhesion to fibronectin. Immunology 73:478, 1991

53. Matsurra N, Zetter BR: Stimulation of mast cell chemotaxis by interleukin 3. J Exp Med 170:1421, 1989

54. Meininger CJ, Yano H, Rottapel R et al: The c-kit receptor ligand functions a a mast cell chemoattractant. Blood 79:958, 1992

55. Varsano S, Lazarus SC, Gold W, Nadel J: Selective adhesion of mast cells to tracheal epithelial cell in vitro. J Immunol 140:2184, 1988

56. Longley BJ Jr, Marganroth GS, Tyrrell L et al: Altered metabolism of mast cell growth factor (c-kit ligand) in cutaneous mastocytosis. N Engl J Med 328:1302, 1993

57. Galli SJ, Iemura A, Garlick DS et al: Reversible expansion of primate mast cell populations in vivo by stem cell factor. J Clin Invest 91:148, 1993

58. Plunt M, Pierce JH, Watson CJ et al: Mast cell lines produce lymphokines in response to cross-linkage of Fcε RI or to calcium ionophores. Nature 339:64, 1989

59. Wodnar-Filipowicz A, Heusser CH, Moroni C: Production of the haemotopoietic growth factors GM-CSF and interleukin-3 by mast cells in response to IgE receptor-mediated activation. Nature 339:150, 1989

60. Burd PR, Rogers HW, Gordon JR et al: Interleukin 3-dependent and independent mast cells stimulated with IgE and antigen express multiple cytokines. J Exp Med 170:245, 1989

61. Gordon JR, Galli SJ: Mast cells as a source of both preformed and immunologically inducible TNF-α/cachectin. Nature 341:274, 1990

62. Gordon JR, Burd PR, Galli SJ: Mast cells as a source of multifunctional cytokines. Immunol Today 11:458, 1990

63. Galli SJ, Gordon JR, Wershil BK: Cytokine production by mast cells and basophils. Curr Opin Immunol 3:865, 1991

64. Gordon JR, Galli SJ: Release of both preformed and newly systhesized tumor necrosis factor (TNF-α)/cachectin by mouse mast cells stimulated by the FcεRI: a mechanism for the sustained action of mast cell-derived TNF-α during IgE-dependent biological responses. J Exp Med 174:103, 1991

65. Walsh LJ, Trinchieri G, Waldorf HA et al: Human dermal mast cells contain and release tumour necrosis factor α, which induces endothelial leukocyte adhesion molecule-1. Proc Natl Acad Sci USA 88:4220, 1990

66. Bradding P, Feather IH, Howarth PH, et al: Interleukin 4 is localized to and released by human mast cells. J Exp Med 176:1381, 1992

67. Bradding P, Feather IH, Wilson S et al: Immunolocalization of cytokines in the nasal mucosa of normal and perennial rhinitic salyicts. J Immunol 151: 3852, 1993

68. Webb TA, Li C-Y, Yam LT: Systemic mast cell disease: a clinical and hematopathologic study of 26 cases. Cancer 49:927, 1982

69. Brunning RD, McKenna RW, Rosai J, Parkin JL, Risdall R: Systemic mastocytosis, extra cutaneous manifestations. Am J Surg Pathol 7:425, 1983

70. Horny H-P, Parwaresch MR, Lennart K: Bone marrow findings in systemic mastocytosis. Hum Pathol 16:808, 1985

71. Lawrence JB, Friedman GB, Travis WD et al: Hematologic manifestations of systemic mast cell disease: a prospective study of laboratory and morphologic features and their relation to prognosis. Am J Med 91:612, 1991

72. Ridell B, Olafsson JH, Roupe G et al: The bone marrow in uriticaria pigmentosa and systemic mastocytosis. Arch Dermatol 122:422, 1988

73. Parker RI: Hematologic aspects of mastocytosis. I. Bone marrow pathology in adult and pediatric systemic mast cell disease. J Invest Dermatol 96:47S, 1991

74. Kettelhut BV, Parker RI, Travis WD, Metcalfe DD: Hematopathology of the bone marrow in pediatric cutaneous mastocytosis: a study of 17 patients. Am J Clin Pathol 91:558, 1989

75. Travis WD, Li C-Y: Pathology of the lymph node and spleen in systemic mast cell disease. Mod Pathol 1:4, 1988

76. Yam LT, Chan CH, Li C-Y: Hepatic involvement in systemic mast cell disease. Am J Med 80:819, 1986

77. Horny H-P, Kaiserling E, Parwaresch MR, Lennert K: Lymph node findings in generalized mastocytosis. Histopathology 21:439, 1992

78. Horny H-P, Ruck MT, Kaiserling E: Spleen findings in generalized mastocytos. Cancer 70:459, 1992

79. Jordana M, Befus AD, Newhouse MT et al: Effect of histamine on proliferation of normal human adult lung fibroblasts. Thorax 43:552, 1988

80. Norrby K: Mast cell histamine: a local mitogen activity via H2-receptors in nearby tissue cells. Virchows Arch A Pathol Anat Histopathol 34:13, 1980

81. Thompson HL, Burbelo PD, Gabriel G et al: Murine mast cells synthesize basement membrane components. A potential role in early fibrosis. J Clin Invest 87:619, 1991

82. Hawkins RA, Claman HR, Clark RAF, Steigerwald J: Increased dermal mast cells proliferation in progressive systematic sclerosis: a link in chronic fibrosis? Ann Intern Med 102:181, 1985

83. Kawanami O, Ferraus VJ, Fulmer JD, Crystal RG: Ultrastructure of pulmonary mast cells in patients with fibrotic lung disorders. Lab Invest 40:717, 1979

84. Aldenborg F, Nilsson K, Jarlshammar B et al: Mast cells and biogennic amines in radiation induced pulmonary fibrosis. Am J Respir Cell Mol Biol 8:112, 1993

85. Travis WD, Li C-Y, Hoagland HC et al: Mast cell leukemia: report of a case and review of the literature. Mayo Clin Proc 61:957, 1986

86. Korenblat PW, Wedner HJ, White MP et al: Systemic mastocytosis. Arch Intern Med 144:2249, 1984

87. Rogers MP, Bloomingdale K. Murawski BJ et al: Mixed organic brain syndrome as a manifestation of systemic mastocytosis. Psychosomat Med 48: 437, 1986

88. Lewis RA, Sote NA, Diamond PT et al: Prostaglandin D_2 generation after activation of rat and human mast cells with anti-IgE. J Immunol 129:1627, 1982

89. Liston TE, Roberts LJ II: Transformation of prostaglandin D_2 to 9α-11β-(15S)-trihydroxy-prosta-(5Z, 13E)-dien-1-oic acid, (9α,11β-prostaglandin F_2): a unique biologically active prostaglandin produced enzymatically in vivo in humans. Proc Natl Acad Sci USA 82:6030, 1985

90. Caplan RM: The natural course of urticaria pigmentosa: analysis and follow-up of 112 cases. Arch Dermatol 87:146, 1963

91. Soter NA: The skin in mastocytosis. J Invest Dermatol 96:32S, 1991

92. Mutter RD, Tannenbaum M, Ultmann JE: Systemic mast cell disease. Ann Intern Med 59:887, 1963

93. Sagher F, Even-Paz Z: Mastocytosis and the Mast Cell. Year Book, Chicago, 1967

94. Demis DJ: The mastocytosis syndrome: clinical and biological studies. Ann Intern Med 59:194, 1963

95. Jelinak JE: Urticaria pigmentosa bei drei leibichen Brüdern. Hautazart 21: 303, 1970

96. Bazex A, Duprét A, Christol B, Andrieu H: Les mastocytosis familiales: présentation de deux observations: revue générale: intérêt nosologique. Ann Dermatol Venereol 98:241, 1971

97. Von Weber K: Urticaria pigmentosa bei eineiigen Zwillingen. Dermatol Monatssschr 159:258, 1973

98. Rockoff AS: Urticaria pigmentosa in identical twins. Arch Dermatol 114:1227, 1978

99. Klaus SN, Winkelmann RK: Course of urticaria pigmentosa in children. Arch Dermatol 86:68, 1962

100. Chagrin L, Sachs P: Urticaria pigmentosa appearing as a solitary nodular lesion. Arch Dermatol 69:345, 1954

101. Johnson WC, Helmig EB: Solitary mastocytosis (urticaria pigmentosa). Arch Dermatol 84:806, 1961

102. Birt AR, Nickerson M: Generalized flushing of the skin with urticaria pigmentosa. Arch Dermatol 80:311, 1959

103. Griffiths WAD, Daneshlob K: Pseudoxanthomatous mastocytosis. Br J Dermatol 93:91, 1975

104. Orkin M, Good RA, Clawson CC et al: Bullous mastocytosis. Arch Dermatol 101:547, 1970

105. Golitz LE, Weston WL, Lane AT: Bullous mastocytosis: diffuse cutaneous mastocytosis with extensive blisters mimicking scalded skin syndrome or erythema multiforme. Pediatr Dermatol 1:288, 1984

106. Smith TF, Welch TR, Allen JB, Sondheimer JM: Cutaneous mastocytosis with bleeding: probable heparin effect. Cutis 39:241, 1987

107. Allen BR: Telangiectasia macularis perstans. Br J Dermatol, suppl. 16. 99: 28, 1978

108. Ball FI: Telangiectasia macularis eruptiva perstans: report of an early stage in a child. Arch Dermatol Syphilol 36:65, 1937

109. Parkes Weber F, Rast H: Telangiectasia macularis eruptiva perstans—a telangiectatic and relatively pigmentless variety of urticaria pigmentosa of adults. Acta Derm Venereol (Stockh) 16:216, 1935

110. Roberts LJ, Fields JP, Oates JA: Mastocytosis without urticaria pigmentosa: a frequently unrecognized cause of recurrent syncope. Trans Assoc Am Physicians 95:36, 1982

111. Debeudkelaere S, Schoors DF, Devis G: Systemic mast cell disease: a review of the literature with special focus on the gastrointestinal manifestations. Acta Clin Belg 46:226, 1991

112. Stechschulte DJ, Morris DC, Jilka RL, Dilecpan KN: Impaired gastric acid secretion in mast cell-deficient mice. Am J Physiol 259:G41, 1990

113. Cherner JA, Jensen RT, Dubois A et al: Gastrointestinal dysfunction in systemic mastocytosis. Gastroenterology 95:657, 1988

114. Miner PB Jr: The role of the mast cell in clinical gastrointestinal disease with special reference to systemic mastocytosis. J Invest Dermatol 91:40S, 1991

115. Fallon MD, Whyte MP, Teitelbaum SL: Systemic mastocytosis associated with generalized osteopenia. Hum Pathol 12:813, 1981

116. Schoenaers P, DeClerk LS, Timmermans U, Stevens WJ: Systemic mastocytosis, an unusual case of osteoporosis. Clin Rheum 6:458, 1987

117. Cundy T, Beneton MNC, Darby AJ et al: Osteopenia in systemic mastocytosis: natural history and responses to treatment with inhibitors of bone resorption. Bone 8:149, 1987

118. Bardin T, Lequesne M: The osteoporosis of heparin therapy and systemic mastocytosis. Clin Rheum, suppl. 2. 8:119, 1989

119. Lidor C, Frisch B, Gazit D et al: Osteoporosis as the sole presentation of bone marrow mastocytosis. J Bone Miner Res 8:871, 1990

120. Horan RF, Austen KF: Systemic mastocytosis: retrospective review of a decade's clinical experience at the Brigham and Women's Hospital. J Invest Dermatol 96:5S, 1991

121. Rafii W, Firooznia H, Golimbu C, Balthazar E: Pathologic fracture in systemic mastocytosis: radiographic spectrum and review of the literature. Clin Orthop 180:260, 1983

122. Travis WD, Li C-Y, Yam LT et al: Significance of systemic mast cell disease with associated hematologic disorders. Cancer 61:965, 1988

123. Horny H-P, Ruck M, Wehrmann M, Kaiserling E: Blood findings in generalized mastocytosis: evidence of frequent simultaneous occurrence of myeloproliferative disorders. Br J Haematol 76:186, 1990

124. Friedman BS, Steinberg S, Meggs WJ et al: Analysis of plasma histamine levels in patients with mast cell disorders. Am J Med 87:649, 1989

125. Udoji WE, Razavi SA: Mast cells and myelofibrosis. Am J Clin Pathol 63:203, 1978

126. Rywlin AM, Hoffman EP, Ortega RS: Eosinophilic fibrohistiocytic lesion of the bone arrow: a distinctive new morphologic finding, probably related to drug hypersensitivity. Blood 40:464, 1972

127. Te Velde J, Vismans FJFE, Leenheers-Binnendijk L et al: The eosinophilic finbohistiocytic lesion of the bone marrow: a mastocellular lesion in bone disease. Vichows Arch A Pathol Anat Histopathol 377:279, 1978

128. Müller UR, Horat W, Wuthrsch B et al: Anaphylaxis after *Hymenoptera* stings in three patients with urticaria pigmentosa. J Allergy Clin Immunol 72:685, 1983

129. Frieri M, Alling DW, Metcalfe DD: Comparison of the therapeutic efficacy of cromolyn sodium with that of combined chlorpheniramine and cimetidine

130. Soter NA, Austen KF, Wasserman ST: Oral disodium cromoglycolate in the treatment of systemic mastocytosis. N Engl J Med 310:465, 1979

131. Czarnetzki BM, Behrendt H: Urticaria pigmentosa clinical picture and response to oral disodium cromoglycolate. Br J Dermatol 105:563, 1981

132. Evans S, Vickers CFH: Bullous urticaria pigmentosa (cutaneous mastocytosis) and sodium cromoglycolate therapy. Acta Derm Venerol (Stockh) 61:572, 1982

133. Welch EA, Alper JC, Bogaars H, Farrell DS: Treatment of bullous mastocytosis with disodium cromoglycolate. J Am Acad Dermatol 9:349, 1983

134. Czarnetzki BM: A double-blind cross-out study of the effect of Ketotifen in urticaria pigmentosa. Dermatologica 166:44, 1983

135. MacPherson JL, Kemp A, Rogers M et al: Occurrence of platelet-activating factor (PAF) and an endogenous inhibitor of platelet aggregation in diffuse cutaneous mastocytosis. Clin Exp Immunol 77:391, 1989

136. Huston DP, Bressler RB, Kaliner M et al: Prevention of mast cell degranulation by Ketotifen in patients with physical urticarias. Ann Intern Med 104:507, 1986

137. Graves L III, Stechschultz DJ, Morris DC, Lukert BP: Inhibition of mediator release in systemic mastocytosis is associated with reversal of bone changes. J Bone Miner Res 5:113, 1990

138. Kettelhut BV, Berkebile C, Bradley D, Metcalfe DD: A double-blind placebo controlled trial of ketotifin versus hydroxyzine in the treatment of pediatric mastocytosis. J Allergy Clin Immunol 83:866, 1989

139. Friedman BS, Santiago ML, Berkebile C, Metcalfe DD: Comparison of azelastine and chlorpheniramine in the treatment of mastocytosis. J Allergy Clin Immunol 92:520, 1993

140. Barton J, Lauker RM, Schecter NM, Lazarus GS: Treatment of urticaria pigmentosa with corticosteroids. Arch Dermatol 121:1516, 1985

141. Czarnetzki PM, Rosenbach T, Kolde G, Frosch PJ: Phototherapy of urticaria pigmentosa: clinical response and changes of cutaneous reactivity, histamine and chemotactic leukotrienes. Arch Dermatol Res 277:105, 1985

142. Granerus G, Roupe G, Swanbeck G: Decreased urinary histamine metabolite after successful PUVA treatment of urticaria pigmentosa. J Invest Dermatol 76:1, 1981

143. Cristophers E, Hönigsmann H, Wolff K: PUVA treatment of urticaria pigmentosa. Br J Dermatol 98:701, 1978

144. Vella Briffa D, Eady RAJ, James MP et al: Photochemotherapy (PUVA) in the treatment of urticaria pigmentosa. Br J Dermatol 109:67, 1983

145. Kolde G, Frosch PJ, Czarnetzki BM: Response of cutaneous mast cells to PUVA in patients with urticaria pigmentosa: histomorphometric, ultrastructural and biochemical investigations. J Invest Dermatol 83:175, 1984

146. Reisberg IR, Oyakawa S: Mastocytosis with malabsorption, myelofibrosis, and massive ascites. Am J Gastroenterol 82:54, 1987

147. Bonnet P, Smadja C, Szekely A-M et al: Intractable ascites in systemic mastocytosis treated with portal diversion. Dig Dis Sci 32:209, 1987

148. Metcalfe DD: The treatment of mastocytosis: an overview. J Invest Dermatol 96:5S, 1991

149. Fairley JA, Pentland AP, Voorhees JJ: Urticaria pigmentosa responsive to nifedipine. J Am Acad Dermatol 11:740, 1984

150. Guinot P, Summerhayes C, Berdah L et al: Treatment of adult systemic mastocytosis with PAF-acether antagonist BN52063, letter. Lancet 2:114, 1988

151. Hutchinson RM: Mastocytosis and co-existent non-Hodgkin's lymphoma and myeloproliferative disorders. Leuk Lymphoma 7:29, 1992

152. Chariot P, Monnet I, LeLong F et al: Systemic mast cell disease associated with primary mediastinal germ cell tumor. Am J Med 90:381, 1991

153. Chariot P, Monnet I, Gaulard P et al: Systemic mastocytosis following mediastinal germ cell tumor: an association confirmed. Hum Pathol 24:111, 1993

154. Janjan NA, Conway P, Lundberg J, DerFus G: Radiation therapy in a case of systemic mastocytosis: evaluation of histamine levels and mucosal effects, Am J Clin Oncol 5:337, 1992

155. Friedman B, Darling G, Norton J et al: Splenectomy in the management of systemic mast cell disease. Surgery 107:94, 1990

156. Bressler RB, Thompson HL, Keffer JM, Metcalfe DD: Inhibition of the growth of IL-3-dependent mast cells from murine bone marrow by recombinant granulocyte macrophage-colony-stimulating factor. J Immunol 143:135, 1989

157. Nafziger J, Arock M, Guillosson J-J, Weitzerbin J: Specific high affinity receptors for interferon-γ on mouse bone marrow-derived mast cells: inhibiting effect of interferon-γ on mast cell precursors. Eur J Immunol 20:113, 1991

158. Kluin-Nelemans HC, Jansen JH, Breukelman H et al: Response to interferon alfa-2b in a patient with systemic mastocytosis. N Engl J Med 329:619, 1992

159. Clancy RL, Gaulde J, Vallieres M et al: An approach to immunotherapy using antibody to IgE in mast cell leukemia. Cancer 37:693, 1976

160. Travis WD, Li C-Y, Yam LT et al: Significance of systemic mast cell disease with associated hematologic disorders. Cancer 62:965, 1988

Clinical Approach to Infections in the Compromised Host

91

Melisse Sloas, Marc Rubin, Thomas J. Walsh, and Philip A. Pizzo

INTRODUCTION

Patients with hematologic disease may be predisposed to the development of infections as a result of a wide array of potential defects in host defenses. Just as the clinical spectrum of hematologic diseases is broad, so is the range of associated abnormalities in host defense. Accordingly, the types of infec- tion encountered in this population as well as their relative severity will vary dramatically.

A wide spectrum of potentially complex issues pertains to infections in compromised patients. While good care demands a broad base of factual knowledge, optimal management mandates evaluation of each patient on an individual basis. Although it is useful, and often appropriate, to draw general guidelines for diagnosis and therapy, decisions should always be placed within the context of each patient's specific, often unique, clinical setting.

TYPES AND SOURCES OF PATHOGENS ENCOUNTERED IN COMPROMISED PATIENTS

The list of predominant pathogens encountered in the compromised host is extensive and includes bacteria, fungi, viruses, and protozoa. The range of potential pathogens in any given patient will depend on the specific perturbations in host defense present in that individual, which in turn will vary according to the underlying disease and its management (Table 91-1). For example, the bacterial pathogens encountered in neutropenic patients with acute myeloid leukemia (AML) will differ dramatically from those commonly encountered in a patient with sickle cell anemia and splenic dysfunction. This chapter

presents detailed analysis of the pathogens associated with specific hematologic disorders.

The epidemiology of most pathogens is well established, but it is often difficult to determine the precise environmental or endogenous origin of organisms isolated from individual infectious episodes. It is clear, however, that most pathogens can generally be found in an endogenous body site at some point before causing infection in compromised patients. Many of these, such as the enteric gram-negative bacteria or *Candida albicans,* may be found in the normal flora of healthy individuals. Others, such as *Pseudomonas aeruginosa* or *Aspergillus* spp., are usually acquired from exogenous sources but cause transient colonization before the development of invasive disease. Still others, such as varicella-zoster virus and *Pneumocystis carinii,* may be present in a latent or subclinical stage for years before the development of significant infection. Ultimately the presence or absence of serious invasive disease will be determined both by the relative virulence of the resident

Table 91-1. Predominant Pathogens in Compromised Patients: Association with Selected Defects in Host Defense

Host-Defense Impairment	Bacteria	Fungi	Viruses	Other

Neutropenia	Gram-negative
	  Enteric organisms (*E. coli, K. pneumoniae, Enterobacter* spp. *Citrobacter* spp.)
	  Pseudomonas aeruginosa
	Gram-positive
	  Staphylococci (coagulase-negative, coagulase-positive)
	  Streptococci (group D, α-hemolytic)
	  Anaerobes (anaerobic streptococci, *Clostridia* spp. *Bacteroids* spp.)
		Candida species (*C. albicans, C. tropicalis,* other species)
		Aspergillus species (*A. fumigatus, A. flavus*)		

Abnormal cell-mediated immunity	*Legionella* *Nocardia asteroides* *Salmonella* spp. Mycobacteria (*M. tuberculosis* and atypical mycobacteria) Disseminated infection from live bacteria vaccine (BCG)	*Cryptococcus neoformans* *Histoplasma capsulatum* *Coccidioides immitis* *Candida*	Varicella-zoster virus Herpes simplex virus Cytomegalovirus Epstein-Barr virus Herpes virus 6 Disseminated infection from live virus vaccines (vaccinia, measles, rubella, mumps, yellow fever, live polio)	*Pneumocystis carinii* *Toxoplasma gondii* *Cryptosporidium* *Strongyloides stercorali*

Immunoglobulin abnormalities	Gram-positive
	  Streptococcus pneumoniae, Staphylococcus aureus
	Gram-negative
	  Haemophilus influenzae
	  Neisseria spp., enteric organisms
			Enteroviruses
			Disseminated infection from live virus vaccines (vaccinia, measles, rubella, mumps, yellow fever, live polio)
				Giardia lamblia

Complement abnormalities				

C3, C5	Gram-positive
	  S. pneumoniae, staphylococci
	Gram-negative
	  Haemophilus influenzae, Neisseria spp., enteric organisms			

C5–C9	*Neisseria* spp. (*N. gonorrhoea, N. meningitides*)			

(Table continues)

Table 91-1. *(Continued)*

Host-Defense Impairment	Bacteria	Fungi	Viruses	Other
Anatomic disruption				
Oral cavity	α-Hemolytic streptococci, oral anaerobes (*Peptococcus, Peptostreptococcus*)	*Candida*	Herpes simplex virus	
Esophagus	Staphylococci, other colonizing organisms	*Candida*	Herpes simplex virus Cytomegalovirus	
Lower gastrointestinal tract	Gram-positive Group D streptococci Gram-negative Enteric organisms Anaerobes (*Bacterioides fragilus, Clostridium perfringens*)	*Candida*		*Strongyloides stercoralis*
Skin (IV catheter)	Gram-positive Staphylococci, streptococci *Coynebacteria, Bacillus* spp. Gram-negative *P. aeruginosa*, enteric organisms Mycobacteria *M. fortuitum, M. chelonei*	*Candida Aspergillus*		
Urinary tract	Gram-positive Group D streptococci Gram-negative Enteric organisms *P. aeruginosa*	*Candida*		
Splenectomy	Gram-positive *S. pneumoniae DF2 bacillus Capnocytophaga canimorsus* Gram-negative *S. pneumoniae H. influenzae Salmonella* (sickle cell disease)			*Babesia*

or colonizing organism and by the severity and type of host impairment (Fig. 91-1). Clinically, it is crucial that potential sources of infection and mechanisms of colonization be identified in order to develop rational strategies for infection prevention in high-risk populations.

Bacteria

Bacteria are responsible for most infections encountered in compromised patients, accounting for the greatest morbidity and mortality. The predominant bacterial pathogens encountered will vary substantially depending on the population at risk. Patients with neutropenia are at high risk of serious infections due to gram-negative pathogens such as *Escherichia coli, Klebsiella pneumoniae,* and *P. aeruginosa. E. coli* and *K. pneumoniae* are Enterobacteriaceae present in the normal gastrointestinal flora, while *P. aeruginosa* is more often acquired from exogenous sources. Other gram-negative bacteria, such as *Haemophilus influenzae, Neisseria* spp., or *Salmonella* spp., are more often encountered in other high-risk patients such as those with dysgammaglobulinemia or those who have just undergone splenectomy. Other important gram-negative bacteria of increasing importance include other Enterobacteriaceae (e.g., *Citrobacter* spp., *Enterobacter* spp., or *Serratia marces-*

cens), *Acinetobacter* spp., non-*aeruginosa* pseudomonads, and *Legionella* spp.

Patients with serious illness may show a dramatic change in the pattern of their colonizing microbial flora after admission to the hospital. Indeed, the most consistent and clinically important change observed is a relative decrease in the organisms comprising the normal flora and a concomitant increase in potentially pathogenic aerobic gram-negative bacteria. These changes have been observed in the noncancer population,[1] as well as in patients with leukemia.[2] In the study by Fainstein et al.[2] the oropharyngeal and fecal flora of 33 leukemic patients was examined serially during the course of hospitalization for intensive chemotherapy. Although most patients had a "normal" pattern of microbial flora on admission, by the completion of the hospital stay 68% of the initial throat isolates and 57% of the fecal isolates had changed. The main shift was due to either the predominance or the acquisition of aerobic gram-negative bacilli (mostly *E. coli, K. pneumoniae, Enterobacter* spp., and *P. aeruginosa*). While these changes were initially seen even before antibiotics were administered, they were clearly accentuated after courses of antibacterial therapy.

In another study addressing this issue, 48 patients with leukemia were followed for 2.5 years with extensive microbiologic surveillance.[3] Again, the culture data and clinical observations indicated that most infections caused by gram-negative bacte-

Exogenous microbial flora ⟶ Colonization ⟶ Endogenous microbial flora

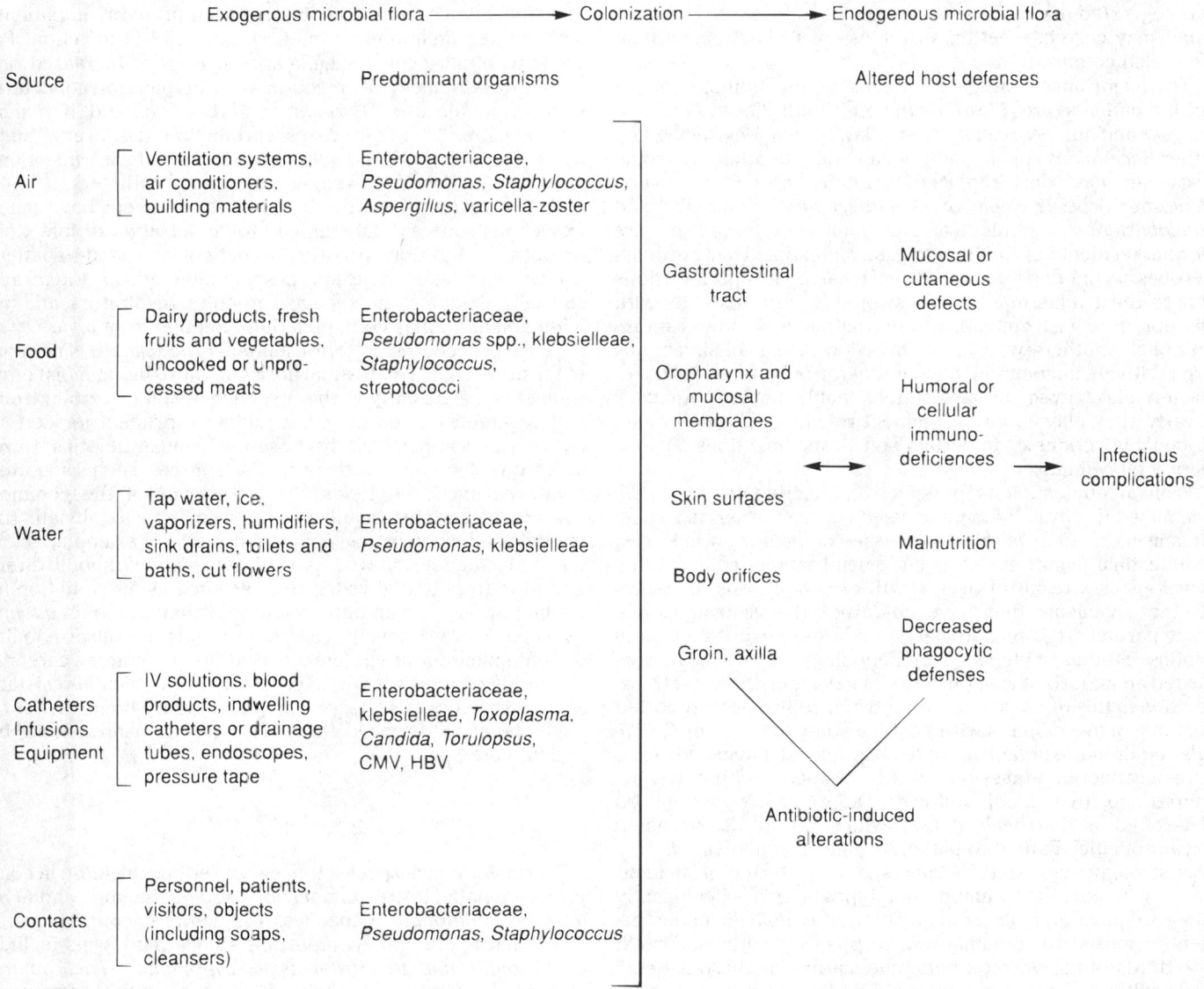

Fig. 91-1. Sources of nosocomial infection in high-risk patients. Interactions between colonization and infection.

ria originated in the endogenous flora. However, 47% of infections were caused by organisms that had colonized the patients only after admission to the hospital. Studies have also suggested that differences may exist among the gram-negative bacteria, not only in their propensity to colonize but also in their ability to produce invasive infection after colonization. For example, certain biotypes of Enterobacteriaceae species have been associated with a particularly high incidence of both colonization and infection in leukemic patients.[4] Nevertheless, most patients who become colonized with enteric gram-negative rods do not develop clinically significant infections. By contrast, other organisms such as *P. aeruginosa* appear to be intrinsically more virulent and are much more likely to cause invasive infection after colonization, especially during periods of severe host impairment, such as profound granulocytopenia.[5]

Over the past 15 years, the incidence of infections due to gram-positive organisms has increased significantly in both compromised and noncompromised patients.[6–13] The most common gram-positive organisms causing infection in almost all groups of immunocompromised patients are the coagulase-positive and coagulase-negative staphylococci (usually *Staphylococcus aureus* and *S. epidermidis,* respectively) and streptococcal species (both enterococci and nonenterococcal

α-hemolytic streptococci). Although relatively uncommon overall, *Streptococcus pneumoniae* is seen with increased frequency in dysgammaglobulinemia or splenectomy patients. Serious infections due to α-hemolytic streptococci may be seen more commonly in patients who have received high doses of cytosine arabinoside (ara-C) and who have mucositis. Streptococcal bacteremia in these patients may be complicated by pulmonary involvement, including adult respiratory distress syndrome.[14] The use of prophylactic fluoroquinolones may be associated with an increased incidence of staphylococcal and streptococcal infection.[15,16] Other potentially important gram-positive bacteria that are encountered less frequently include *Corynebacterium* spp., *Bacillus* spp., and *Listeria monocytogenes*. Some of these organisms, such as *S. pneumoniae,* enterococci, and *S. epidermidis,* are found in almost all healthy individuals as part of the normal gastrointestinal or skin flora. Others, such as methicillin-resistant *S. aureus* or *Corynebacterium jeikeium,* are not commonly found as part of the normal flora but are more often acquired from exogenous sources, particularly in hospitalized patients.[17,18] The increase in bacteremias due to organisms that colonize the skin (e.g., *C. jeikeium* and *S. epidermidis)* is often attributed to the increased use of indwelling intravenous catheters, although not all studies have corroborated this.[12,19] One study by Khabbaz and co-workers[20] has suggested that gastrointestinal colonization with *S. epidermidis* may correlate better with subsequent bacteremia than does skin colonization.

The major anaerobic bacteria causing infection in compromised patients are *Clostridium* spp. (both *Clostridium perfringens* and non-*perfringens* clostridia), *Bacteroides fragilis,* and other *Bacteroides* spp. In addition, a variety of other anaerobic organisms have been reported, including *Fusobacterium* spp., *Peptostreptococcus, Peptococcus, Eubacterium, Veillonella,* and *Bifidobacterium.*[21–24] Most of these anaerobic organisms are normal residents of the human gastrointestinal tract, with anaerobes accounting for about 90% of fecal organisms. Infections due to these anaerobes are most often seen in patients with disruption of gastrointestinal mucosal barriers, often as a result of chemotherapy or tumor invasion. Anaerobic infections are relatively uncommon, accounting for only about 5–10% of bacteremias, even in profoundly neutropenic patients.[25] Clearly, they play a more prominent role in localized intra-abdominal infections or in certain soft tissue infections such as perirectal cellulitis.

From an epidemiologic perspective, infection due to *C. difficile* may differ from infection caused by most other anaerobic organisms. *C. difficile*-related disease (ranging from mild gastrointestinal symptoms to pseudomembranous colitis) often develops as a result of overgrowth of endogenous toxin-producing organisms that have colonized the gastrointestinal tract, particularly after surgical procedures or exposure to antibiotics. Studies addressing epidemiologic issues have suggested an important role for nosocomial acquisition and transmission of this organism. McFarland and colleagues[26] reported that one of five patients with positive stool cultures for *C. difficile* acquired the organism while hospitalized, having been culture-negative on admission. Of these patients with newly acquired positive stool cultures, approximately one-third developed a diarrheal illness, while two-thirds remained asymptomatic. Patient-to-patient transmission of *C. difficile* was strongly suggested by time/space clustering of incident cases with identical immunoblot types and by significantly more frequent and earlier acquisition of *C. difficile* among patients exposed to roommates with positive cultures. Almost two-thirds of the hospital personnel caring for these patients had positive cultures for *C. difficile* from their hands, and significant contamination of the rooms of both symptomatic and asymptomatic patients was found. Clearly, these data may have important implications for the prevention of *C. difficile*-related disease.

Anaerobic bacteria of the gastrointestinal tract may assist in protecting against infections caused by other organisms. The theory of colonization resistance argues, in short, that the large quantity of anaerobic bacteria normally present in the gut produce unfavorable conditions for colonization or overgrowth by other more pathogenic organisms, such as the Enterobacteriaceae or *P. aeruginosa.*[27] Indeed, this concept has been supported by a number of preclinical studies. For example, Van der Waaij and colleagues[28] showed that gastrointestinal colonization could be established in germfree mice by oral administration of small inocula (approximately 10^3 organisms) of gram-negative bacteria. By contrast, $>10^7$ organisms were required to establish colonization in mice with their normal flora intact. Although prophylaxis with fluoroquinolones or trimethoprim-sulfamethoxazole has been shown to decrease the incidence of bacteremia in some studies, the development of resistant organisms has limited its clinical value.

In the past, mycobacterial infections have been relatively uncommon in most immunocompromised populations. Recent data have shown a striking increase in the number of infections due to *Mycobacterium tuberculosis* and, of particular concern, the emergence of multidrug-resistant tuberculosis in the United States.[29,30] Infections due to *M. tuberculosis* as well as

M. avium-intracellulare complex are seen primarily in patients with human immunodeficiency virus-1 (HIV-1) infection. Patients with hairy cell leukemia appear to be at increased risk of the development of infection with atypical mycobacteria such as *M. kansasii, M. fortuitum, M. chelonei,* and *M. avium-intracellulare.*[31–33] In rare cases, certain "rapid growers," such as *M. fortuitum* and *M. chelonei,* cause significant infections around exit sites of indwelling intravenous catheters.

The community and the hospital environment have many exogenous sources that can lead to colonization or infection, or both. In addition to patient-to-patient and staff-to-patient transmission, exogenous sources include food, air, water, and specialized equipment, such as catheters, respirators, and humidifiers, as well as contamination resulting from a variety of invasive procedures.[34,35] For example, *P. aeruginosa* is not part of the normal gastrointestinal flora but flourishes in moist environments, particularly in the presence of soil or certain fruits and vegetables. Accordingly, it might be prudent for certain patients at risk particularly those receiving antibiotics, to restrict direct contact with potential sources such as potted plants or uncooked foods.[36–38] Knowledge of the common sources of certain organisms can also help to obviate the spread of infection or prevent an outbreak. For example, a clustering of infections due to *Legionella pneumophila* should direct attention to potential water sources such as air-conditioning cooling towers[39,40]; an outbreak of infection due to *Pseudomonas cepacia* in an intensive care unit should raise the possibility of contamination of equipment used for respiratory care[41]; a clustering of infection due to *C. difficile* or methicillin-resistant *S. aureus* should raise suspicion of a staff or patient carrier or might point to the need for more rigorous handwashing by patient care staff.

Fungi

The major fungal species that cause serious infection in compromised patients are *Candida* spp., *Aspergillus* spp., and *Cryptococcus neoformans.* Other less frequently encountered, but nevertheless potentially important, fungal pathogens include *Coccidioides immitis, Histoplasma capsulatum, Trichosporon beigelii,* the Zygomycetes (e.g., *Mucor* spp. or *Rhizopus* spp.), *Fusarium* spp., *Drechslera, Malassezia furfur,* and the dematiaceous fungi.[42–47] The predominant fungal pathogens will vary according to the nature of host impairment in any given patient. For example, invasive infections due to *Candida* or *Aspergillus* spp. are most commonly encountered in patients with prolonged episodes of neutropenia. Infections due to *C. neoformans, H. capsulatum,* or *C. immitis* are more often seen in patients having an underlying disease or receiving a therapeutic intervention associated with impaired cell-mediated immunity, such as lymphomas, HIV infection, or corticosteroid treatment.

Overall, *Candida* spp. represent the most common fungal pathogens responsible for serious infection in immunocompromised patients. *C. albicans* may be found as part of the normal human gastrointestinal and cutaneous flora,[48] but certain factors may predispose patients to a change in the patterns of colonization with this fungus. This change is often marked in those receiving broad-spectrum antibiotics, requiring extensive hospitalization, or receiving immunosuppressive agents. Indeed, widespread and even visibly apparent gastrointestinal "overgrowth" can occur in these settings.[49] Gastrointestinal colonization and overgrowth can then provide an ideal setting for the development of invasive disease, which often occurs secondary to intercurrent mucosal disruption as a result of surgery, tumor invasion, or chemotherapy.[45] Certain fungal species appear to be intrinsically more pathogenic than others; colonization with these organisms is more frequently associated with invasive infection. For example, in one series, 16% of cancer patients colonized with *Torulopsis glabrata* developed serious invasive infection[50]; in another study, 14 of 25 patients colonized by *Candida tropicalis* developed an infection with this organism.[51]

Aspergillus spp. constitute the second most common fungal pathogens in immune-compromised hosts. *Aspergillus* spp. are not part of the normal human flora but are usually acquired from exogenous sources in the hospital setting, such as unfiltered air, contaminated ventilation systems, sites of renovation or construction, food, and ornamental plants.[44,52] Air is the principal route of transmission of *Aspergillus* spp. within the hospital environment, and the respiratory tract is the most common entry portal. Upper airway colonization with *Aspergillus* probably precedes most cases of invasive infection; some authorities believe that documentation of nasal carriage of *Aspergillus* may be predictive for the development of aspergillosis in certain high-risk settings.[53] Also, smokers appear to have an increased incidence of colonization with *Aspergillus* spp., but in some studies they do not appear to have an increased incidence of invasive *Aspergillus,* even in the setting of severe immunosuppression.[54,55]

C. neoformans, the third most common pathogenic fungus in the compromised population, is an encapsulated yeast that is ubiquitous in nature. Although pigeon excreta is the classically implicated environmental source, this fungus can be found widely in many types of soil.[56,57] *C. neoformans* does not normally colonize humans. Primary infection is usually not hospital acquired and is often subclinical. Disseminated infection in high-risk patients usually represents reactivation of latent infection.

Viruses

The most significant viral infections seen in immunocompromised patients belong to the herpes group and include herpes simplex virus (HSV), varicella-zoster virus (VZV), and cytomegalovirus (CMV). Serious infections due to these viruses are clearly seen with increased frequency in certain subgroups of immunosuppressed patients, particularly those with impaired cell-mediated immunity. Other viruses can cause serious infection in this population, but their incidence does not appear to be substantially increased compared to a normal population. These include Epstein-Barr virus (EBV); human herpes virus, type 6 (HHV-6); influenza and parainfluenza viruses; respiratory syncytial virus (RSV); measles virus; adenoviruses; and the enteroviruses. In addition to nonhematologic organ toxicity caused by direct viral replication, infection with some viruses, such as parvovirus or HIV-1, may, in certain hosts, result in secondary hematologic abnormalities and further compromise immune function.[58]

Infection due to HSV, VZV, or CMV can result either from primary infection or from reactivation of latent infection. Most serious infections in adults occur as a result of reactivation of infection initially acquired before the onset of impaired immune function.

Both HSV-1 and HSV-2 can lead to significant morbidity in the compromised host. As in immunocompetent individuals, HSV-1 is encountered with greater frequency. Primary infection with HSV-1 usually occurs in childhood between the ages of 2 and 10 and is most often transmitted by contact with oral secretions. HSV-2 infection is usually spread by genital contact, generally acquired after puberty. In adults, the incidence of antibodies to HSV (presumably reflective of prior infection) has been 30–100% in various studies and appears to be higher in groups of lower socioeconomic status.[59–62] In a retrospective review of sera from patients with hematologic diseases presenting for bone marrow transplantation (BMT), 51 of 93 had elevated titers (≥1–8) of anti-HSV antibody.[63] High titers of anti-HSV-1 have been correlated with the development of subsequent infections in immunocompromised patients.[64,65] In addition to reactivation of latent disease, seronegative individuals may acquire primary infection from contact with either asymptomatic execretors or overtly infected persons, although virus titers and transmissibility are greater in the latter group.[59]

In the healthy population, VZV is a highly contagious virus that causes primary infection predominantly in children. Primary varicella infection, or chickenpox, occurs in approximately 50% of children before they enter school, and the vast majority of adults have VZV antibodies as a result of prior clinical or subclinical infection. In immunocompromised patients, both primary disease and reactivation of latent virus are clinically important. In accordance with its prevalence in the healthy population, primary varicella in compromised patients tends to affect children and is responsible for most serious infections in those with hematologic malignancies.[66,67] Adult patients who are seronegative are also at risk.

Person-to-person transmission to other patients at risk of primary varicella can occur after close contacts both in and out of the hospital. Primary varicella is transmitted predominantly by the respiratory route. Secondary varicella infection, or herpes zoster (also known as shingles), can occur in otherwise healthy patients, particularly in the aged, but is more common and usually more severe in immunosuppressed patients.[68–71] In virtually all cases, herpes zoster represents reactivation of latent disease. Little concrete evidence has been found to support its contraction by exposure to other patients with either primary varicella or zoster.[71,72] However, patients at risk of the development of primary varicella may acquire the infection through contact with patients who have zoster or primary disease.

CMV can cause serious infection in a variety of immunocompromised populations, but most notably in the HIV-infected population and in those undergoing allogeneic BMT. Most studies indicate a 60–70% prevalence of antibody to CMV by adulthood in both compromised and noncompromised patients.[73–76] As with HSV, the prevalence of antibodies will vary with the socioeconomic condition, geography, and age of the population studied. A study from Houston found that only about 25% of healthy white subjects aged 18–22 had positive titers, compared with 50% for nonwhite individuals.[77]

In the compromised host, serious CMV infection can occur either by reactivation of latent disease as a result of immunosuppression or through primary infection. Among patients undergoing BMT, it has been clearly demonstrated that the incidence of significant CMV infection (usually pulmonary) is substantially higher for patients who are initially seropositive for anti-CMV antibody than for those who are seronegative. In the study by Meyers et al.,[74] 69% of seropositive patients developed CMV, compared with 36% of seronegative patients. Presumably, most of the seropositive patients underwent reactivation of latent disease, while the seronegative patients acquired primary infection. For this latter group, it was subsequently established that the source of virus was often transfused blood products or bone marrow from seropositive donors. Indeed, the exclusive use of seronegative blood products for seronegative patients has nearly eliminated serious CMV infection in these patients.[78]

Increasing age may be associated with reactivation of CMV. McVoy and Adler[79] used IgM positivity as a marker of reactivation in patients with known positivity for IgG and found an increase in positivity from 15% for those <20 years old to 63% for those >60 years old. Consequently, older patients with hematologic diseases could be at higher risk than younger patients for development of CMV infection.

The development of CMV in high-risk seropositive patients

has been largely assumed to occur as a result of reactivation of endogenous previously acquired virus. Accordingly, blood products for patients who are already seropositive have generally not been screened. However, studies using restriction enzyme digest profiles and strain-specific neutralizing antibody measurements indicate that even seropositive patients can develop symptomatic CMV as a result of reinfection with different donor strains.[80-82] In light of these findings, further studies may be warranted to address the value of exclusive use of seronegative blood products even for seropositive patients.

The respiratory viruses, including RSV, influenza, parainfluenza, and adenovirus, have been increasingly recognized as pathogens in immunocompromised patients over the past decade. RSV is the leading cause of pneumonia and bronchiolitis in young children and is an important cause of nosocomial infection in children's hospitals. A study by Hall et al.[83] found a higher incidence of nosocomial acquisition of RSV, of RSV pneumonia, and of deaths due to RSV in children with cancer than in children with normal immune function.[83] Another study described severe RSV infection in adults with lymphoma and in adults who have had BMT or solid organ transplantation.[84] Prompt identification and isolation of infected patients are mandatory to prevent nosocomial transmission of RSV infection.

Parasites

With the exception of *P. carinii,* parasites are relatively uncommon causes of infection in compromised patients with non-HIV-related diseases. The parasitic infections most commonly encountered include those due to *P. carinii, Toxoplasma gondii, Cryptosporidium,* and *Strongyloides stercoralis* and occur most commonly in patients with altered cell-mediated immunity. When infection develops as a result of these organisms, it usually represents the reactivation of a latent or asymptomatic infection previously acquired outside the hospital setting. Gastroenteritis due to *Cryptosporidium* is an exception, with person-to-person transmission (both in and out of the hospital), as well as large water source outbreaks having been clearly documented.[85-90]

Infections due to *P. carinii* are the most important clinically.[91] Symptomatic infection due to *P. carinii* likely results from reactivation of latent cysts acquired early in life rather than from new acquisition of disease. One study supporting this concept evaluated serum from 600 normal volunteers and used an indirect fluorescent antibody test for detection of anti-*P. carinii* IgG.[92] Of the children tested in this series, significant titers were found in nearly all by the age of 2 years, which implies asymptomatic infection early in life. In addition, the largest published study of a so-called institutional clustering of *P. carinii* infection, which occurred at St. Jude Children's Cancer Research Hospital, failed to corroborate, or even suggest, any patient-to-patient spread.[91]

By contrast, studies of "clusters" of *P. carinii* pneumonia (PCP) have suggested the possibility of person-to-person transmission.[93-95] In the study from Memorial Hospital, 11 cases of PCP were seen in a 3-month period, 10 of them involving patients with leukemia or lymphoma. Epidemiologic analysis indicated that most of the patients had either had extensive contact with each other or were being treated by the same physician before the onset of disease.[94] In a study by Ruebush et al.,[93] 10 cases of PCP were seen in a 10-month period, all in children with acute lymphocytic leukemia (ALL). While their risk of infection appeared to be related to the intensity of chemotherapy, members of the hospital staff who had close contact with these children had significantly higher titers of anti-*P. carinii* antibody than those of other staff members or than parents of the children, suggesting that transmission

could have occurred within the hospital environment. In addition, animal data suggest airborne transmission from infected to uninfected rats.[96] Although these studies are suggestive, person-to-person transmission of *Pneumocystis* has not been clearly documented, even at centers with a large number of cases.

ALTERATIONS IN HOST-DEFENSE-ASSOCIATED PATHOGENS AND MAJOR CLINICAL CORRELATES

The range of abnormalities in host defense that can occur in patients with hematologic diseases and the major associated pathogens are listed in Table 91-2. For any given patient, only rarely is a specific defect in host defense seen in isolation. Nevertheless, certain types or patterns of defects are more often associated with specific underlying diseases or particular therapeutic interventions.

Anatomic Alterations

The skin and mucosal surfaces represent an important primary defense against both endogenous and exogenous sources of infections. Compromised patients frequently have alterations in integumentary and mucosal barriers. Disruption of skin and mucosa may result from invasion by malignant cells, effects of chemotherapy or radiotherapy, use of invasive diagnostic or therapeutic procedures (e.g., intravenous catheters), and effects of locally disruptive infections such as oral HSV. Such mucosal alterations may provide a nidus for microbial colonization, a focus for localized infection, and a portal of entry for systemic invasion.

The types of organisms associated with specific alterations in skin or mucosal surfaces will depend on the site of breakdown as well as the presence or absence of other associated factors. For example, isolated disruption of the skin associated with insertion of an indwelling intravenous catheter primarily increases the risk of infection due to certain gram-positive organisms, usually coagulase-negative staphylococci. However, in patients who have been hospitalized, who are neutropenic, or who have received prior broad-spectrum antibiotics, the "normal flora" of the skin can change, and serious catheter-related infections due to a variety of other organisms can occur. These organisms include other gram-positive bacteria, such as *C. jeikeium* or *Bacillus* spp.[18,97,98]; a variety of gram-negative organisms, including *P. aeruginosa,* non-*aeruginosa* pseudomonads, or enteric gram-negative rods[99-102]; fungi such as *C. albicans* or *Aspergillus* spp.[103-105]; and atypical *Mycobacterium* spp., such as *M. chelonei* or *M. fortuitum.*

Because the gastrointestinal tract is normally colonized by a wide array of aerobic and anaerobic bacteria, as well as by some fungi, disruption of its mucosa can lead to infections by a variety of pathogens, and sometimes to polymicrobial infection. Identification of a specific site of mucosal alteration within the gastrointestinal tract may be helpful in predicting the relative frequency of certain pathogens from knowledge of the normal flora in that area and in guiding empirical therapy, which is started even before isolation of an organism. In addition, isolation of certain organisms from blood cultures often helps direct diagnostic or therapeutic intervention toward specific sites, even in the absence of clinically evident disease. For example, isolation from the blood of organisms normally found in the mouth, such as *Peptococcus* or *Capnocytophaga,* should focus attention on the oral cavity, while cultures growing *B. fragilis* or *Streptococcus bovis* can be clues to pathology originating in the lower gastrointestinal tract.[22,106-108]

One of the most common causes of disruption of the gastrointestinal mucosal integrity is administration of chemotherapeutic agents to patients with malignancy. Those that lead to the most serious problems include ara-C, the anthracyclines (daunorubicin and doxorubicin), methotrexate, mercaptopurine, and fluorouracil. While stomatitis is usually the most clinically recognizable manifestation of gastrointestinal toxicity, the clinician should remember that significant oral mucositis is often only the "tip of the iceberg" and that diffuse gastrointestinal involvement is likely present.

The genitourinary tract may also be affected by tumor, procedures, or cytotoxic therapy, with subsequent colonization and potential for local or invasive infection. The urinary tract pathogens most commonly encountered in these settings are the enteric gram-negative rods, enterococci, and *C. albicans.*

In addition to actual mucosal breakdown, other anatomic alterations can occur in compromised patients, increasing their risk of infection. Mechanical obstruction of body passages by tumor, for example, can greatly increase the risk of serious localized infection. This may be due in part to stasis of local body fluids, with resultant overgrowth of potentially pathogenic colonizing organisms. Common sites of secondary infection due to obstruction include the lung, urinary tract, biliary tract, and auditory tube. An obstructive process should be considered when infection at any of these sites fails to respond to appropriate antibiotics.

Anatomic alteration can also predispose to infection simply by providing a nidus for growth of organisms. It is likely that most healthy individuals experience periodic but uneventful episodes of transient bacteremia (e.g., secondary to toothbrushing). In the setting of altered anatomy or foreign bodies such as prosthetic devices, however, even transient bacteremia can lead to persistent localized infection. Important examples of hematologic diseases associated with such anatomic alterations include sickle cell anemia and hemophilia. In patients with sickle cell disease, macrophage and splenic dysfunction predispose to the development of certain bacteremias, especially by *S. pneumoniae* and *Salmonella* spp.[109–111] Many of these patients have underlying anatomic abnormalities of bones and joints as a result of vaso-occlusive crises causing infarction of bone marrow, bony cortex, or synovium. In turn, these changes may predispose to the development of infection at the sites of anatomic alteration, such as osteomyelitis or arthritis.[112,113] Decreased blood flow to these areas, as well as increased adherence of organisms, may be additional contributing factors. Similarly, hemophiliacs may develop anatomic alterations of joints as a result of repeated episodes of hemarthrosis. Although suppurative arthritis has been less frequently described in hemophiliacs than in patients with sickle cell disease, it can occur and should be considered in the differential diagnosis of any hemophiliac whose articular signs and symptoms fail to improve quickly after administration of appropriate coagulation factors.[114] Patients with chronic hemolytic states may develop gallstones, which can also provide a nidus for infection.

Phagocyte Defects

Quantitative and qualitative defects affecting polymorphonuclear leukocytes (PMNs) and monocytes can occur in compromised patients. While both cell types are important, the contribution of granulocyte abnormalities to the pathogenesis of infectious diseases has been better described and more completely elucidated, primarily because isolated defects in monocytes are relatively rare.

Quantitative Abnormalities

Significance of Neutropenia in Predisposing to Infection

Of the many abnormalities in host defense that potentially affect compromised patients, granulocytopenia is perhaps the most important for two reasons: (1) it predisposes patients

to a wide array of pathogenic organisms, and (2) it may be associated with rapid progression of infection, often in the absence of classic signs and symptoms.

Most clinicians associate granulocytopenia with malignant disease, with which it can occur as a result of either a myelophthisic process or, more commonly, cytotoxic therapy. Indeed, cancer patients account for most cases of neutropenia encountered in the clinical setting. However, it is important to emphasize that many other pathologic processes may be associated with granulocytopenia. Unfortunately, very few data specifically address the relative risks, types, or management of infections in neutropenic patients with nonmalignant diseases. In the absence of these data, the clinician is often forced to extrapolate from the studies in the cancer population.

For cancer patients receiving cytotoxic therapy, the relationship between the development of granulocytopenia and serious infection has been established unequivocally. Bodey et al.[115] followed the course of 34 patients with ALL and 29 patients with acute myeloid leukemia (AML) (age range 1–77 years) and correlated the development of infection with granulocyte counts over the course of treatment (Table 91-3). The salient findings of this study were as follows. First, the incidence of proven infection and the absolute granulocyte level showed a definite relationship. The risk of infection began to increase significantly when granulocyte counts fell to <1,000/ mm^3 and was most marked when the counts were ≤100/mm^3. Second, in addition to the absolute granulocyte count, an important factor in predicting the risk of infection at any level was the duration of granulocytopenia. Thus, counts in the range of 1,000/mm^3 for a short duration (e.g., ≤1 week) were associated with little risk of infection, compared with a significant risk if the counts stayed within that range for ≥4 weeks. By contrast, neutropenia in the range of 100/mm^3, even for a few days, was associated with a significant risk. Third, the incidence of infection was also related to a falling granulocyte count, but the magnitude of the fall was less important than the final granulocyte levels. Fourth, at any granulocyte level, the severe infectious episodes occurred more frequently during relapse than during remission, suggesting that other factors played a role in predisposing to infection.

For practical purposes, granulocytopenia is usually defined as a cell count of <500 PMNs/mm^3 and band forms/mm^3. The absolute granulocyte count, the duration of granulocytopenia, and whether the neutrophil count is falling or rising must all be considered when assessing the risk to any individual patient. Granulocytopenia primarily predisposes patients to bacterial and fungal infection and does not per se appear to increase the incidence or severity of viral and parasitic infections.

Types of Bacterial Infections in Neutropenic Patients

General trends in the frequency of infection caused by certain types of organisms have occurred since the 1950s and 1960s, when aggressive cytotoxic regimens were in early development. In those years, gram-positive bacteria were encountered most commonly.[116–118] However, by the 1970s, gram-negative organisms emerged as the predominant pathogens isolated in neutropenic patients. Interestingly, during the 1980s and 1990s, gram-positive organisms have re-emerged as common bacterial isolates at many centers; at some centers they now represent the most frequently encountered organisms.[8,10,119,120] While an appreciation of these fluctuations can be helpful for the clinician, the potential for institutional variation in the patterns of infection cannot be overemphasized. Indeed, some major centers treating neutropenic patients still see a preponderance of gram-negative organisms.[25] Accordingly, clinicians treating granulocytopenic patients should have a working knowledge of the specific isolates encountered at their own facility.

Disease/Condition	Neutropenia	Phagocyte Dysfunction	Abnormal Cell-Mediated Immunity
			Table 91-2. Selected Hematologic Diseases, Associated Host-Factors Contributing
Acute myeloid leukemia	Major factor	Abnormalities described	May result from therapy (e.g., bone marrow transplantion)
Acute lynmphocytic leukemia	Major factor	Abnormalities described	May result from disease or therapy
Hairy cell leukemia	Major factor (also monocytopenia)	Probably contributes	Probably contributes
Chronic lymphocytic leukemia	Not prominent unless aggressive therapy or end stage	Not prominent	May result from therapy (e.g., steroids)
Chronic myeloid leukemia	Not prominent unless aggressive therapy or end stage	Abnormalities described	Not prominent
Multiple myeloma	Not prominent unless aggressive therapy or end stage	Abnormalities described	Not prominent
Hodgkin disease	May be major factor, depending on therapy	Abnormalities described	Major factor
Myelodysplastic syndromes	Variable	Abnormalities described	No prominent
Aplastic anemia	Major factor	Abnormalties described	May result from therapy (e.g., steroids, antithymocyte globulin, cyclosporine, bone marrow transplantation)
Chronic granulomatous disease	No prominent	Major factor—defective oxidative metabolism	Not prominent
G6PD deficiency	Not prominent	Major factor if severe	No prominent
Myeloperoxidase deficiency	Not prominent	Major factor (usually with little clinical manifestations)	Not prominent
Paraoxysmal nocturnal hemoglobinuria	May contribute	Potentially contributory—deficient Fc receptor	Not prominent
Thalassemia major	Not prominent	Abnormalities described	Abnormalities described
Sickle cell disease	Not prominent unless aplastic crisis	Abnormalities described	Not prominent

Defense Impairment, and Common Pathogens
to Infection

Abnormal Humoral Immunity	Anatomic Disruption	Splenic Dysfunction	Most Common Pathogens
May result from therapy	Often significant, may be caused by therapy, tumor invasion, localized infection	Not prominent	Bacteria 　Gram-positive (staphylococci, streptococci) 　Gram-negative (enteric organisms, *P. aeruginosa*) Fungi 　*Candida* 　*Aspergillus* Viruses 　Herpes simplex 　Varicella-zoster Other 　*P. carinii*
May result from therapy	Often significant (see AML)	Not prominent	See AML, *P. carinii* more common in some centers
Not prominent	Not prominent unless aggressive therapy	Major factor if therapeutic splenectomy	Gram-positive and gram-negative bacteria Atypical Mycobacteria
Major factor	Not prominent unless agressive therapy	Not prominent	Bacteria 　*S. pneumoniae* 　*H. influenzae* 　*Neisseria* spp.
Not prominent	Not prominent unless aggressive therapy	No prominent	Few infections in stable chronic phase Blast crisis (see AML)
Major factor	Not promient	Not prominent	Bacteria 　*S. pneumoniae* 　*H. influenzae* 　*Neisseria* spp. 　Enteric gram-negative
May result from therapy	May be significant depending on therapy	Major factor if diagnostic splenectomy or radiation to splenic bed	See AML—viral and parasitic infections may occur with higher frequency
Not prominent	Not prominent	Major factor if therapeutic splenectomy	Gram-positive and gram-negative bacteria
Not prominent	Not prominent unless agressive therapy	Not prominent	Gram-positive and gram-negative bacteria *Candida Aspergillus* Other depends on therapy
Not prominent	Not prominent	Not prominent	Catalase-positive organisms *S. aureus*, enteric gram-negative bacteria, *P. cepacia*, *Nocardia*, *Aspergillus*
Not prominent	Not prominent	Not prominent	Catalase-positive organisms if severe
Not prominent	Not prominent	Not prominent	Infections rare, possible increase in *Candida* infections
Not prominent	Thromboembolic disease may contribute (intra-abdominal infections)	Not prominent	Bacterial infections
Abnormalities described	Gallstones may serve as nidus	Major if therapeutic splenectomy	Bacteria 　Staphylococci 　Streptococci 　Enteric gram-negative 　*Salmonella*
Probable major factor—complement activation and opsonization	Bone infarctions may serve as nidus	Major factor	Bacteria 　*S. pneumoniae* 　*H. influenzae* 　*Salmonella*

Table 91-3. Association of Granulocyte Level and the Chance of Developing Significant Infection

Granulocyte Level (per mm³)		Percentage of Serious Infections for Different Durations of Granulocytopenia (in wk)							
Initial	Change	1	2	3	4	6	10	12	14
Any level	Any fall	12							
Any level	Fall to 2,000	2							
Any level	Fall to 1,500	5							
Any level	Fall to 1,000	10	30	45	50	65	70	85	100
Any level	Fall to 500	19							
Any level	Fall to <100	28	50	72	85	100			

(Adapted from Bodey et al.,[115] with permission.)

Gram-Negative Bacteria. The relative frequency of infections due to gram-negative organisms has decreased over the past 15 years.[120] *E. coli* and *K. pneumoniae* are the most common gram-negative isolates at most centers. These organisms are frequently isolated from the blood; the most common endogenous source is the gastrointestinal tract. Other common sources include the urinary tract and the respiratory tract, although a precise source of gram-negative bacteremia is identified in only a few cases. In neutropenic patients, gram-negative organisms may be isolated from cultures drawn at the onset of fever or may cause secondary infections in patients already receiving antibiotics. Interestingly, the National Cancer Institute, has had a dramatic decrease in infections due to *P. aeruginosa,* often an extremely virulent pathogen in neutropenic hosts.[120] However, all three organisms can cause rapidly progressive and lethal infection. *Enterobacter* spp., *Citrobacter* spp., and *S. marcescens* are increasingly encountered Enterobacteriaceae that can rapidly become resistant to a broad range of β-lactam antibiotics through the induction of chromosomally mediated β-lactamases.[121] Other less common gram-negative organisms include *Acinetobacter* spp., *Haemophilus* spp., (usually nontypable *H. influenzae*),[122] and non-*aeruginosa* pseudomonads (often catheter related and antibiotic resistant).[101]

Gram-Positive Bacteria. The gram-positive organisms most frequently encountered are the coagulase-negative staphylococci (most commonly *S. epidermidis*), coagulase-positive staphylococci (*S. aureus*), group D streptococci (most commonly *S. faecalis*), and α-hemolytic streptococci (e.g., *S. mutans* or *S. viridans*). They can cause either primary or secondary infection in neutropenic patients. Both coagulase-positive and coagulase-negative staphylococci are most commonly isolated from the blood, and often from patients with indwelling intravenous catheters or skin breakdown from other causes. In addition, both have been well documented to cause infections around catheter sites or foreign bodies, such as prosthetic heart valves or orthopaedic implants. *S. aureus* tends to be significantly more virulent and may cause a picture of rapidly developing septic shock as well as serious deep-seated infections. Most infections due to coagulase-negative staphylococci tend to be relatively indolent compared with *S. aureus*. A picture of septic shock is only rarely, if ever, seen with most coagulase-negative staphylococcal bacteremias, and it has been debated whether these organisms can cause invasive visceral infections (e.g., pneumonia). Both group D and non-group D streptococci are also most commonly isolated from the blood. Group D streptococci are part of the normal gastrointestinal flora, are frequent components of intra-abdominal infections, and are a relatively common cause of urinary tract infections (second to the enteric gram-negative rods). As compared with other streptococci, they are relatively β-lactam-resistant. Of additional concern, isolates of *Enterococcus* that are resistant

to vancomycin have been increasingly observed at some centers. Most α-hemolytic streptococci are part of the normal oral flora and may be seen with increased frequency after chemotherapy that produces significant oral mucosal disruption (e.g., high-dose ara-C).[123,124] Most α-hemolytic streptococci are sensitive to a variety of β-lactam antibiotics. However, recent reports have documented particularly virulent strains of α-hemolytic streptococci that appear to be associated with the use of high-dose ara-C.[123] Other gram-positive bacteria encountered in neutropenic patients include *Bacillus* spp. (often catheter related), *C. jeikeium* (often catheter related and relatively antibiotic resistant), *S. faecium* (a group D *Streptococcus*, which may be resistant to vancomycin), and *Lactobacillus* (which may also be resistant to vancomycin).

Anaerobic Bacteria. Infections due to anaerobic bacteria may also be encountered in neutropenic patients, albeit less commonly than those due to aerobic organisms.[125–127] The anaerobic organisms most frequently encountered are *B. fragilis* and *Clostridium* spp., both of which normally inhabit the human gastrointestinal tract. Infections caused by these organisms are often associated with a concomitant abnormality in gastrointestinal mucosal integrity. While bacteremia may occur, only rarely are anaerobes isolated from cultures drawn at the discovery of initial fever in neutropenic patients. More commonly, they present as secondary infections. Bacteremia due to *C. perfringens* can be a particularly fulminant and rapidly lethal process.[125] By contrast, when bacteremia due to *B. fragilis* occurs, it is often relatively indolent.[127] These anaerobes are most commonly isolated as components of necrotizing gingivitis or of intra-abdominal infections, including peritonitis, intra-abdominal abscesses, and perirectal cellulitis or abscesses.[127] While *B. fragilis* and *C. perfringens* are the most common organisms, other species may be clinically important. These include other species of *Bacteroides*[22] and *Clostridia* (e.g., *C. tertium* or *C. septicum*, which are often clindamycin resistant).[24] *C. difficile* is also a common cause of morbidity in neutropenic patients. It is not associated with bacteremia or invasive disease; rather, it produces a wide range of gastrointestinal pathology due to elaboration of toxins.

Mycobacteria. Infections attributable to *Mycobacterium* spp. are only rarely encountered in neutropenic patients and for the most part are not seen with increased frequency in this population. With the emergence of *M. tuberculosis* in a number of American cities, however, it seems likely that an increase in this infection will be observed in cancer patients. Patients with hairy cell leukemia (HCL) appear to have an increased risk of developing infections with certain atypical mycobacteria. HCL is often associated not only with neutropenia but also with profound monocytopenia, which may be an important risk factor for these infections.[128] Dysfunction of cell-mediated immunity may also be a contributing factor. In addition to the more common bacterial infections seen in other neutropenic hosts, patients with HCL may develop significant infections due to *M. kansasii, M. fortuitum, M. chelonei,* and *M. avium-intracellulare* complex.[31–33] "Fast-growing" mycobacteria (*M. fortuitum* and *M. chelonei*) may also cause persistent exit site or tunnel infections in patients with indwelling intravenous catheters or wound infections after surgery.

Types of Fungal Infection Seen in Neutropenic Patients

The next most common type of organisms encountered in neutropenic patients are the fungi. Although neutropenia per se may predispose the patient to the development of fungal infection, certain subsets of neutropenic patients appear to be at heightened risk, most notably (1) those with prolonged neutropenia (≥ 1 week) and (2) those receiving broad-spectrum antibacterial therapy. In contrast to the bacterial infections often associated with the onset of fever in neutropenic patients, fungal infections only rarely cause primary infection (i.e., initial infection in patients not yet receiving antibiotics). More commonly, fungal infections occur as secondary processes in patients receiving antibacterial drugs. Although a variety of fungal infections can be encountered in the neutropenic host, *Candida* spp. and *Aspergillus* spp. predominate.

Qualitative Abnormalities

A variety of hematologic diseases may be associated with pronounced functional defects in effector cells, which in turn may contribute to the development of infectious complications. The microbicidal activity of granulocytes and monocytes involves complex interactions between the cell and the organism or inflammatory site. Some of the major functions important for microbicidal activity that have been elucidated include migration of the cell to the inflammatory site (chemotaxis), cell activation, phagocytosis, and intra- or extracellular killing by both the oxygen-dependent and oxygen-independent pathways. Clinically important defects in granulocyte function have been more completely delineated than have abnormalities in monocytes, with specific abnormalities described in nearly every measurable function of neutrophils. Problematic are patients with "borderline" granulocyte counts (e.g., absolute granulocyte counts in the range of 500–2,000/mm^3, that are not falling precipitously), most commonly occurring with the myelodysplastic syndromes or newly diagnosed leukemias.

The traditional wisdom has been that cells less mature than the metamyelocyte are deficient in microbicidal activity. This was based largely on early data on white cells obtained from healthy individuals. Subsequently, however, a number of studies have documented significant functional defects in mature PMNs from patients with AML.[129–132] In addition, one study initiated in patients with AML before treatment found a correlation between abnormalities in myeloperoxidase activity of the PMNs and the subsequent development of infectious complications.[133] Although somewhat fewer data are available addressing this issue for patients with ALL, studies have shown evidence of functional deficits in PMNs from these patients.[134,135] Accordingly, it is prudent to approach all patients with acute leukemia and "borderline" granulocyte counts as if they had an absolute neutropenia.

Significant defects in granulocyte function have also been found in PMNs from patients with myelodysplastic syndromes and preleukemic states[136–138]; in some studies, these have correlated with infectious complications.[139] Although it is likely that these functional defects contribute to the increased infections seen in these populations, their effects per se are difficult to establish. The clinician should probably assume that neutrophils from patients with myelodysplastic syndromes or preleukemia are functionally defective. As in the case of AML or ALL, from a clinical perspective, patients with borderline granulocyte counts should be approached as if they had an absolute neutropenia.

Phagocyte dysfunction can also be due to the therapeutic use of pharmacologic agents and radiation for the treatment of the underlying hematologic disease. Again, because most patients receiving these therapies have multiple defects in host defense, the clinical significance of these in vitro findings is often difficult to establish. In addition to pronounced effects on phagocyte function, many of the drugs themselves (e.g., cyclophosphamide) can impair other immune parameters, including the production of quantitative defects, and can cause abnormalities in humoral responses and cell-mediated immunity.

In vitro studies have demonstrated inhibition of a variety of functional granulocyte parameters, including hexose monophosphate shunt activity, superoxide production, phagocytosis, chemotaxis, and microbicidal activity, by antineoplastic agents. The implicated agents have included methotrexate, 6-mercaptopurine, vincristine, vinblastine, anthracyclines, cyclophosphamide, carmustine, and platinum compounds.[140–149]

It is widely accepted that exogenous administration of glucocorticoids leads to increased susceptibility to infection. The major effect of steroids on in vitro measurement of granulocyte function appears to be confined to a decrease in chemotactic activity, which inhibits accumulation of PMNs at the site of infection and decreases the localized inflammatory response.[150] This may in large part account for the clinical observation that the signs and symptoms of even severe infections may be "masked" or greatly reduced in patients receiving steroids. In vitro, steroids may also impair PMN phagocytosis, microbicidal activity, and antibody-dependent cytotoxicity, but often at very high concentrations that some investigators believe to be of little clinical relevance.[151,152] In addition to their effects on granulocytes, steroids may have important effects on the function of circulating monocytes, although the available data are limited. Documented effects have included in vivo monocytopenia, as well as in vitro defects in monocyte chemotaxis, phagocytosis, and killing of bacteria and fungi.[153,154] In addition to their action on granulocytes and monocytes, steroids may enhance susceptibility to infection through other mechanisms, including negative effects on wound healing, skin fragility, lymphocyte function, production of cytokines, and humoral immune responses.

A variety of biologic agents are being employed increasingly in the management of hematologic disorders, among which the colony-stimulating factors (predominantly colony-stimulating factor-granulocyte/macrophage [CSF-GM] and colony-stimulating factor-granulocyte [CSF-G]) and interleukin-2 (IL-2) are most notable. A number of functional parameters may be enhanced by CSF-GM or CSF-G, including oxidative metabolism, phagocytosis, microbicidal activity, and antibody-dependent cytotoxicity. However, recently reported data underscore the potential for inhibition of cell function as well. For example, in autologous BMT patients, impaired in vivo migration of granulocytes during CSF-GM administration has been documented.[155] Impaired granulocyte function has been noted in some patients receiving high doses of IL-2. Patients receiving high-dose IL-2 therapy appeared to have an increased incidence of significant infections due to *S. aureus*.[156,157] Granulocyte function studies from patients receiving IL-2 demonstrated decreased production of superoxide, decreased chemotaxis, and decreased Fc receptor γ-III expression.[157] While the clinical significance of any of these effects on functional parameters has yet to be established, one must keep an open mind to their potential to impair, as well as improve, cell function.

Many other commonly employed drugs have had documented in vitro or in vivo effects on phagocyte function, including nonsteroidal anti-inflammatory drugs,[158–162] opiates and other narcotic analogues,[163–165] ethanol,[166] benzodiazepines,[167] methylxanthines,[168] β-blocking agents,[169] phenytoin,[170,171] inhaled and intravenous anesthetics,[172,173] gold compounds,[174–176] nicotine,[177] allopurinol,[178] cyclosporine,[179,180] heparin,[181] calcium-channel blocking agents, and antibiotics.[182]

Radiotherapy has also been associated with granulocyte dysfunction both in animal studies and in humans. Baehner and colleagues[183] studied granulocyte function in children with ALL. They found significant impairment of bactericidal activity when the cells were obtained during periods of craniospinal irradiation as compared with values before radiotherapy. The effect was transient, and cell function returned to normal 2–4 weeks after completion of radiotherapy.

Defects in Cell-Mediated Immunity

Cellular immune dysfunction may either be primary, as in a number of congenital immunodeficiency states, or secondary to other disorders or therapeutic interventions. Secondary deficiency in cell-mediated immunity (CMI) is most commonly seen in patients with lymphoid malignancies, those with acquired immunodeficiency syndrome (AIDS), recipients of organ transplants, and patients receiving steroids or radiotherapy. The specific pathogens encountered and the spectrum of clinical findings in patients with CMI defects vary with the underlying disease, the degree of immunosuppression, and the presence or absence of other host-defense abnormalities. Defective CMI can lead to infections caused by bacteria, fungi, viruses, and protozoa. For the most part, however, the organisms are distinct from those that cause serious infection in patients with phagocyte abnormalities (Table 91-1). The most frequently encountered pathogens are often characterized as intracellular organisms because they can survive and even replicate inside macrophages in a nonimmune individual or in the absence of T-cell immunity. T-cell function appears to be required for macrophage activation and subsequent microbicidal activity.[184] Among the pathogens are (1) bacteria, including mycobacteria (both *M. tuberculosis* and atypical mycobacteria), *Legionella, Nocardia asteroides,* and *Salmonella* spp.; (2) fungi, including *C. neoformans, H. capsulatum,* and *C. immitis;* (3) viruses, including VZV, HSV, CMV, and EBV; and (4) parasites, including *P. carinii, T. gondii, Cryptosporidium,* and *S. stercoralis.* Patients with CMI deficiency are also at risk of the development of disseminated infection due to live vaccines, even with attenuated organisms. Accordingly, these patients should not receive bacillus Calmette-Guérin (BCG), vaccinia, measles, rubella, mumps, yellow fever, or live polio vaccines. The one exception is that all HIV-infected children, regardless of symptomatology, should receive the measles vaccine. While severe measles infection with high mortality has been reported, little morbidity has been reported from the measles vaccine in this patient population.[185]

Hodgkin disease, followed by the non-Hodgkin lymphomas, is the best characterized and most commonly encountered malignant disorder associated with impaired CMI.[186–188] While the degree of immune impairment may correlate with the extent of disease and is often compounded by the administration of immunosuppressive therapy, both Hodgkin disease and non-Hodgkin lymphoma are associated with intrinsic impairment of CMI, which can persist even after apparent cure. Patients in remission are still at increased risk of the development of certain infections, particularly disseminated VZV infection; the identification of primary chickenpox or even localized zoster in these patients mandates prompt therapy with intravenous acyclovir (see the section Approach to Viral Infections).

Clinically significant intrinsic impairment of CMI has not been well established for other malignancies. CMI defects have been postulated to help explain the incidence of atypical mycobacterial infections in patients with HCL and also occurs in relatively rare T-cell malignancies such as mycosis fungoides or T-cell chronic lymphocytic leukemia (CLL). CMI defects clearly exist in children with ALL, as evidenced by their increased susceptibility to the development of *P. carinii* or disseminated VZV infection, but it is likely that concurrent therapy plays a major role. Similarly, while CMI defects may occur in patients with a variety of other malignancies, they are often explained by the use of therapeutic agents or by concomitant nutritional deficiencies.

Impaired CMI is not a prominent feature of nonmalignant hematologic disorders unless it is associated with therapy or the acquisition of HIV-1 infection. Abnormalities in CMI have been described in patients with hemophilia who have received factor VIII concentrates.[189,190] Clearly, hemophiliacs who have acquired infection with HIV-1 from factor replacement therapy may have severe impairment of CMI. However, some studies have shown that HIV-1-seronegative hemophiliacs who have received factor VIII concentrates, as well as previously untreated hemophiliacs, have immune impairment.[191] Patients with sickle cell anemia have been found to have anergy in association with zinc deficiency and decreased nucleoside phosphorylase activity[192]; CMI defects have been described in patients with thalassemia.[193] Overall, however, the clinical significance of these findings is uncertain.

Pharmacologic agents and radiation are major causes of impaired CMI. Corticosteroids are the pharmacologic agents most often associated with CMI abnormalities, although they may also cause immune suppression through their effects on other host-defense mechanisms.[194] The degree of immunosuppression and the relative risk of infection will depend on the dose and duration of corticosteroids, as well as on the underlying disease. Even when these factors are known, however, infectious complications in patients receiving corticosteroids may be highly variable and difficult to predict on an individual basis.[150] Nevertheless, whether corticosteroid therapy is being used should always be taken into account when one is confronted with potentially infected patients. Those patients about to embark on corticosteroid-containing treatment regimens who have a known history of tuberculosis or positive purified protein derivative should be treated with prophylactic isoniazid to prevent reactivation and potential dissemination of disease.

A number of cytotoxic agents may also be associated with impaired CMI, notably methotrexate, cyclophosphamide, 6-mercaptopurine, and azothioprine.[195,196] Infections due to impaired CMI, such as PCP, have also been associated with certain combination chemotherapeutic regimens more often than with others.[197] In patients with hematologic malignancies, cytotoxic agents are frequently administered in combination with other immunosuppressive therapies, such as corticosteroids or radiotherapy.

Cyclosporine is an immunosuppressant used to suppress transplant rejection and also as a therapeutic modality in aplastic anemia. It is associated with alterations in T-helper cells, effector T cells, and natural killer cells. It has not been established, however, that the use of cyclosporine is associated per se with an increased risk of infection. While there are anecdotal reports of unusual infections in patient receiving cyclosporine, evidence shows that its use can decrease certain infections as compared with other immunosuppressive regimens used for allograft recipients.[198,199]

Radiotherapy can result in impaired CMI, especially when used in combination with other immunosuppressive agents or for the treatment of patients with underlying diseases associated with intrinsic CMI defects (e.g., as a component of the preparatory regimen for BMT or for the treatment of Hodgkin disease). CMI defects may persist for ≤1 year after intensive radiotherapy or after BMT.[200] Accordingly, patients should be considered at risk of the development of certain infections during this period.

A number of infections may themselves result in impaired CMI. Viral infections may affect CMI either directly (e.g., by infecting crucial cellular components such as T lymphocytes or macrophages) or by affecting other immunoregulatory mechanisms.[201] The key viral infection associated with impaired CMI is HIV-1. Patients with AIDS have profound defects in CMI and are susceptible to a wide array of infectious complications. Other viral infections associated with CMI defects include CMV, EBV, RSV, hepatitis B, and influenza. Other nonviral infections that have been variably associated with impaired CMI by in vitro testing have included tuberculosis, leprosy, bacterial pneumonia, *Brucella,* typhoid fever, coccidiomycosis, syphilis, and a variety of parasitic diseases.[202]

Noninfectious disorders linked to abnormal CMI include chronic protein-calorie malnutrition, uremia, diabetes mellitus, sarcoidosis, cystic fibrosis, and other conditions resulting from surgery and the administration of anesthesia.

Abnormalities of Humoral Defense Mechanisms—Immunoglobulins and Complement

Immunoglobulins and complement are among the most important components of the humoral immune system; defects or deficiencies in either may be associated with serious infections. Other proteins classified as part of the humoral defense system include lysozyme and lactoferrin, tuftsin, and fibronectin. Abnormalities in these proteins have been variably associated with infectious complications. Immunoglobulins and complement each have associated opsonic, lytic, and neutralizing activities and function predominantly against bacterial infection. Patients with either primary or secondary defects or deficiencies in these proteins are at highest risk of the development of serious infection due to the encapsulated bacteria and, to a lesser extent, to the enteroviruses and *Giardia lamblia*.

Multiple myeloma is frequently associated with a defect in humoral immunity.[203] The degree of humoral impairment in multiple myeloma is related to the stage of the disease. Malignant plasma cells induce the production of a protein that is synthesized by macrophages and that selectively suppresses B-cell function. CMI remains intact unless patients are treated with corticosteroids or cytotoxic therapy. In addition, myeloma patients with IgG paraprotein have an increased rate of catabolism of both normal and clonal IgG.

Myeloma patients are most susceptible to recurrent pyogenic infections from high-grade polysaccharide-encapsulated bacteria such as *S. pneumoniae, H. influenzae,* or *Neisseria* spp. However, infections due to enteric gram-negative rods and staphylococci are also frequently encountered. In the series by Doughney et al.,[204] the gram-negative bacilli accounted for most isolates. Savage et al.[205] found a biphasic pattern of infection, with infections due to *S. pneumoniae* and *H. influenzae* occurring earlier in the course of disease (i.e., within the first 8 months of diagnosis) or in patients responsive to therapy and those due to gram-negative bacilli occurring more frequently in patients with refractory or advanced disease. The sites of recurrent infection are most often the upper respiratory tract, urinary tract, or skin. Repetitive bouts of infection may herald the diagnosis of multiple myeloma; infection represents the major cause of death.

Because pneumococcal infections are frequent, some studies have explored the potential role of pneumococcal vaccine administration to these patients. Multiple myeloma patients may show a rise in antibody titer after administration of pneumococcal vaccine but, because preimmunization titers are frequently low, postimmunization titers often fail to reach a protective level.[203] In addition, postimmunization antibody levels fall rapidly in this population, in part owing to increased catabolism of immunoglobulins.[200] This is of practical importance, since revaccination with pneumococcal vaccine may be associated with arthus reactions or systemic reactions.[206] Nevertheless, it is currently recommended that patients with multiple myeloma receive pneumococcal vaccine and that revaccination be considered in patients demonstrating a rapid decline in pneumococcal antibody levels.[207] Revaccination should be given no sooner than 6 years after administration of the initial vaccine.[208,209] The efficacy of prophylaxis with passive administration of immunoglobulins has not been established and cannot be recommended.

Patients with B-cell CLL also appear to have an intrinsic defect in the clonal B cells, which leads to unbalanced immunoglobulin chain synthesis and resultant hypogammaglobuli-

nemia. The incidence of infection correlates with the duration and stage of the disease, as well as with the serum levels of immunoglobulins (particularly IgG). Infection is a major cause of morbidity and mortality and may account for $\leq 60\%$ of deaths in certain series.[210] The organisms causing serious infection are often the encapsulated bacteria, although patients are also at risk of infection due to staphylococci and enteric gram-negative bacilli.[211] Upper and lower respiratory tract infections are encountered most commonly, although septicemia and other sites such as urinary tract and skin are frequently involved. Therapeutic administration of corticosteroids or cytotoxic drugs will increase the risk of infection and may dramatically expand the list of potential pathogens.[211,212] It is recommended that patients with CLL receive polyvalent pneumococcal vaccine, although its efficacy in this population has not been demonstrated unequivocally. A multicenter trial demonstrated that prophylaxis with pooled intravenous immunoglobulin decreased the incidence of bacterial infection; however, the decrease was primarily seen in minor or moderately severe infections only.[211] In addition, the cost-effectiveness of immunoglobulin prophylaxis and its effect on the quality of life has recently been questioned.[213]

The precise role of abnormalities in humoral defenses in other malignancies has not been well defined. Observed defects may be due in part to the components of therapy, as opposed to intrinsic defects associated with the underlying disease. Patients with acute leukemia have been found to have lower levels of antibody to the core glycolipid of the Enterobacteriaceae than those of noncancer patients, and their antibody levels are found to fall after cytotoxic therapy.[214] Theoretically, this could contribute to an increased risk of infection with enteric gram-negative bacteria, but this has not been established. Cytotoxic chemotherapy, radiotherapy, and steroids all adversely affect B-cell as well as T-cell functions, which may result in diminished opsonizing activity, inadequate agglutination and lysis of bacteria, and deficient neutralization of bacterial toxins. Cytotoxic therapy can blunt the humoral response to vaccine administration,[215,216] but adequate responses have also been documented for patients in remission on maintenance chemotherapy.[217]

Role of Splenectomy and Splenic Dysfunction

Abnormalities in splenic function may be a prominent part of a number hematologic disorders, as a result of either intrinsic impairment of therapeutic or diagnostic splenectomy. Splenic dysfunction in the absence of splenectomy is crucial in patients with sickle cell disease who lose function presumably as a result of repeated infarctions. Splenectomy can be performed either as a part of staging or as a therapeutic intervention.

The precise reason for enhanced susceptibility to infection in asplenic patients or patients with splenic dysfunction is not entirely clear. The spleen probably plays an adjunctive role in fighting infection in a number of ways. First, it appears to function as a sieve, removing organisms from the blood that have been ineffectively opsonized by complement. In addition, it participates in the primary immunoglobulin response and is involved in the regulation of the alternate complement pathway, with low levels of immunoglobulins and properdin reported in patients after splenectomy.[218,219] A decrease in the opsonic peptide tuftsin has also been reported after splenectomy,[220] and alternate pathway defects may be important in patients with sickle cell disease and splenic dysfunction.[221]

The risk of the development of serious infection, as well as the types of infections, vary somewhat depending on the etiology of the abnormal splenic function and the presence or absence of other immunologic abnormalities. For example, patients who have undergone splenectomy after trauma may be at lower risk of infection than other groups. Increased risk of *Salmonella* infection appears to be unique for the sickle cell population. In general, however, most asplenic patients or splenectomized patients are at increased risk of serious bacterial infection, primarily infection due to *S. pneumoniae* and *H. influenzae* as well as *Neisseria* spp. and *Capnocytophaga canimorsus*. The initial presentation of even overwhelming infection can be deceptively subtle, with fever often the only sign. Accordingly, all asplenic patients with underlying hematologic disease who present with fever should be managed initially as potentially septic. In addition to a detailed physical examination, evaluation should routinely include at least two blood cultures and a urine culture, a culture of any other potentially infected site, and a chest radiograph. For all such patients we first give empirical intravenous antibiotics (even for those who are non-neutropenic) and continue a course of antibiotics for a minimum of 72 hours until the preantibiotic culture results are known. If the cultures are found to be negative and the patient is clinically stable, we often discontinue antibiotics and observe. We do not recommend routine prophylactic antibiotics for asplenic patients. However, most authorities do recommend penicillin prophylaxis for small children.

Because asplenic patients are predisposed to pneumococcal infection, pneumococcal vaccine should be administered ≥ 2 weeks before elective splenectomy.[222] The rationale for this timing of vaccination is twofold. First, evidence shows that splenectomized patients respond less well to pneumococcal polysaccharides than do patients with intact splenic function.[223] However, a 1986 study in patients with Hodgkin disease showed that the antibody response to pneumococcal vaccine was not affected by the timing of immunization relative to splenectomy.[215] Second, and perhaps more importantly, presplenectomy immunization can result in protective titers immediately after splenectomy. Finally, it should be remembered that, although pneumococcal vaccine is effective in these patients, it does not eliminate the risk of serious pneumococcal disease, the possibility of which should be kept in the forefront even in vaccinated patients. Because asplenic patients are at risks of infection with all encapsulated bacteria, they should also be immunized with *H. influenzae* b and the meningococcal vaccines.[224]

PROPHYLAXIS OF INFECTIONS IN HIGH-RISK PATIENTS

Prophylaxis of Bacterial Infections

With bacterial organisms accounting for most infections in compromised patients, trials designed to assess prophylactic strategies have appropriately focused on these pathogens. Strategies assessed fall into several major categories: (1) the use of mechanical techniques to prevent acquisition of new pathogens; (2) the use of various absorbable or nonabsorbable oral antibiotic regimens either to prevent acquisition or to decrease the number of potentially pathogenic colonizing organisms; (3) the use of passive or active immunization; and (4) the use of prophylactic granulocyte transfusions (Tables 91-4 and 91-5). In addition, more recent strategies are evaluating a number of biologic agents (e.g., the CSFs) for the prevention of infection.

However, one strategy in particular that is applicable in almost every setting in which immunocompromised patients are involved is handwashing. While stressing the need of rigorous handwashing may appear somewhat trivial and may be intuitively obvious to many, its importance cannot be overemphasized, particularly in the hospital setting. Organisms of all types can be transmitted on the hands of health care workers or patients. If questioned, most health care workers avidly affirm the importance of handwashing, yet only a few adhere to a

Table 91-4. Methods for Preventing Infection in High-Risk Patients

Prevent Acquisition and/or Suppress or Eliminate Microbial Flora	Improve or Modify Host Defenses
Isolation	Immunization
Simple or reverse isolation	Active
Isolation with HEPA air filtration	*Haemophilus influenzae*
Prophylactic antibiotics	*Pseudomonas*
Nonabsorbable antibiotics	*Pneumococcus*
Trimethoprim sulfamethoxazole,	VZV
erythromycin	Passive
Selective decontamination	J-5 core glycolipid
Quinolones	Pooled immunoglobulins
Prophylactic antivirals	Hyperimmune globulins
Acyclovir	Monoclonal antibodies
Amantadine	Cell component replacement
Prophylactic antifungals	Leukocyte transfusions
Acyclovir	Accelerate granulocyte recovery
Amantadine	Lithium
Prophylactic antifungals	CSF-G
Nystatin	CSF-GM
Imidazoles	
Triazoles	
Amphotericin B	
Prophylactic antiparasitics	
Thiabendazole	
Trimethoprim-sulfamethoxazole	
Combination-comprehensive	
Total protective isolation	

strict policy. In one study of an intensive care unit, health care personnel washed their hands after less than one-half of patient contacts, and physicians specifically did so after less than one-third of contacts.[225] In the high-risk setting, all health care personnel should wash their hands immediately after every patient contact, no matter how brief. In addition, high-risk patients (or their parents or guardians) should be instructed in the importance of handwashing and urged to remind health care workers who inadvertently forget. Physicians, nurses, and other health care workers should not be embarrassed or intimidated by gentle but firm reminders from patients or colleagues that handwashing has been overlooked.

Methods

Mechanical Techniques

A number of so-called mechanical techniques or intervention strategies have been assessed in granulocytopenic patients. Typical "reverse" isolation after the onset of neutropenia has no documented efficacy in preventing infection. First, colonization by potential pathogens is likely to have already occurred by the time granulocytopenia develops. In addition, requiring patients to wear a surgical mask outside of their own rooms will do little to protect against subsequent infection. Likewise, perhaps the only value of having medical personnel "gown, glove, and mask" before entering a patient's room is to heighten their awareness of the importance of other less expensive and more effective measures, such as handwashing.[226] On mostly theoretical grounds, some authorities have recommended that all foods be thoroughly cooked and that fresh fruits or vegetables be avoided to obviate transmission of gram-negative bacteria that can colonize raw or unprocessed food.[36,37] However, the actual value of these measures in preventing infection remains unproven.

The use of a total protective environment (TPE) is a comprehensive anti-infective regimen designed to reduce the patient's endogenous microbial burden, while preventing the acquisi-

Table 91-5. Relative Merits and Deficiencies of Various Strategies to Prevent Infection in Granulocytopenic Patients

	Total Protected Environment	Nonabsorbable Antibiotics	Trimethoprim Sulfamethoxazole	Selective Decontamination	Quinolones
Efficacy					
Reduced infection	Yes	No	±	±	Yes
Decrease in fever	Yes	No	No	No	No
Decrease or shorten need for antibiotics and antifungals	No	No	No	±	Yes
Contribute to survival	No	No	No	No	No
Compliance					
Well tolerated?	No	No	±	±	Yes
Impact on efficacy	Yes	Yes	Yes	±	No
Liabilities					
Emergence of resistant organisms	Yes	Yes	Yes	Yes	Yes
Organ side effects					
Interference with other drugs	Yes	Yes	Yes	No	No
Bone marrow suppression	No	No	Yes	Yes	No
Specific organ toxicity	No	No	Yes	Yes	Yes
Cost					
For the drugs or regimens	Yes	Yes	No	Yes	Yes
For surveillance or monitoring	Yes	Yes	Yes	Yes	Yes
Reducing need for hospitalization or for drugs	No	No	No	±	?

tion of new organisms. A sterile environment is created in a clean-air room with constant positive airflow and is maintained by an aggressive program, including surface decontamination, sterilization of all objects that enter the room, and an intensive regimen to disinfect the patient, including oral nonabsorbable antibiotics, skin antiseptics, antibiotic sprays and ointments, and a low microbial diet. A number of studies have documented that TPE can reduce infections in profoundly granulocytopenic individuals.[227] However, TPE is expensive and, because of improvements in treating established infections and in shortening the duration of neutropenia, it does not offer a survival advantage to most patients. Thus, TPE is not necessary for the routine care of most granulocytopenic patients.

Oral Antibiotic Regimens

The value of oral antibiotic regimens designed to protect the patient against the development of bacterial infections during the course of granulocytopenia has been subject to ongoing debate. The rationale for this approach is based on the observation that most organisms ultimately implicated in infection (particularly the gram-negative bacteria) can be isolated from the patient's own flora.[3] Since the mid-1970s, numerous studies have evaluated a variety of prophylactic oral regimens. These have included nonabsorbable antibiotics (e.g., gentamicin, vancomycin, polymixin, and colistin),[227–234] as well as antibiotics absorbed from the gastrointestinal tract (e.g., trimethoprim-sulfamethoxazole, erythromycin, or quinolones).[229,235–248] The goal of many of the earlier studies employing nonabsorbable agents was total decontamination of the alimentary tract, which met with only marginal success in the absence of strict isolation procedures.[228] The agents were often unpleasant in taste; noncompliance was a major problem, potentially leading to rebound overgrowth of pathogenic organisms.[228]

The use of trimethoprim-sulfamethoxazole, with and without added antibiotics such as erythromycin, was meant primarily to result in selective decontamination of the gastrointestinal tract—in other words, to eliminate the potentially pathogenic aerobic flora (mostly the enteric gram-negative bacteria) while preserving most anaerobic organisms and preserving colonization resistance. Despite the voluminous literature on the subject, a final answer on the efficacy of trimethoprim-sulfamethoxazole in this setting has not been established, and debate as to its value continues.[236,242,249–251] Potential pitfalls associated with the use of trimethoprim-sulfamethoxazole include bone marrow suppression,[236,242,249–251] development of resistant organisms,[228,252] rash,[253] and an increase in fungal colonization.[242]

More recently, the use of fluoroquinolones (chiefly norfloxacin and ciprofloxacin) has received attention in the literature.[243,246–248] Fluoroquinolones offer the advantage of gram-negative coverage, including *Pseudomonas aeruginosa* with preservation of the anaerobic flora. In clinical trials of immunocompromised patients, fluoroquinolones have shown superior efficacy in the prevention of gram-negative bacteremia than either placebo[254] or trimethoprim-sulfamethoxazole[253,255]; they have also been well tolerated. However, studies have demonstrated colonization with resistant gram-negatives during the use of fluoroquinolones as prophylaxis.[256,257] In addition, there has been an increase noted in gram-positive infections in patients on prophylactic fluoroquinolones.[16,255,258,259] Kotilainen et al.[258] documented seven episodes of ciprofloxacin-resistant coagulase-negative staphylococcal infections in neutropenic patients after the introduction of ciprofloxacin onto their ward. In another study, Cruciani et al.[255] compared 21 children given prophylactic norfloxacin to 23 given trimethoprim-sulfamethoxazole; there were four documented streptococcal infections in those treated with norfloxacin compared to only one gram-positive in the trimethoprim-sulfamethoxazole group. The multicenter Italian GIMEMA study is one of the few studies comparing the different fluoroquinolones.[257] In this study, 619 patients were randomized to receive either ciprofloxacin or norfloxacin. Although more benefits were seen with ciprofloxacin, these were only true for those patients who were severely neutropenic for <1 week. Because current information does not definitively support the use of prophylactic antimicrobial agents and because of the disastrous consequences of bacterial resistance, we do not support the use of prophylactic antimicrobial agents.

Growth Factors and Immune Mediators

The development of cytokines in the past decade is allowing clinicians to both influence the most critical factor in susceptibility of infection and neutropenia, and to manipulate the hematopoietic and immune systems. The only commercially available cytokines are CSF-G and CSF-GM, which stimulate the proliferation and maturation of bone marrow progenitor cells.[260] Although CSF-G and CSF-GM do not prevent neutropenia, multiple studies have demonstrated an increase in the neutrophil count and a decrease in the duration of neutropenia after their use.[261–264] There are many reports of CSF-G and CSF-GM use, but these studies have used multiple doses and schedules; patients have had varied underlying malignancies and received different chemotherapeutic regimens, and few studies are randomized or placebo controlled. Crawford et al.[262] randomized 104 patients to receive placebo and 95 patients to receive CSF-G at 230 μg/m²/day after chemotherapy for small cell lung cancer. Patients treated with CSF-G demonstrated a significant decrease in the number of days with a neutrophil count of <500 cells/mm³ (3 days as compared to 6 for placebo patients), and in depth of neutropenia. CSF-G-treated patients also had significantly fewer episodes of fever and neutropenia, and the treatment group had 51% fewer culture-confirmed infections. Other advantages were a 45% reduction in days of hospitalization and a 47% decrease in days of intravenous antibiotic use for the CSF-G cohort. A randomized double-blind placebo-controlled trial of CSF-GM was performed by Nemunaitis et al.[261] in patients with leukemia and lymphoma undergoing autologous BMT. Sixty-five patients were treated with CSF-GM (250 μg/m²/day), while 63 were given placebo. The neutrophil count of CSF-GM-treated patients rose more rapidly to 500 cells/mm³. Although no difference was noted in number of days with fever or percentage of patients with fever between the two groups, patients receiving CSF-GM did have a decrease in number of days of antibiotic therapy and in days of hospitalization. Because of their stimulation of neutrophil and macrophage function, these growth factors may also have a role in the treatment of fungal infection; a study conducted by Roilides et al.[265] found that incubation of neutrophils with CSF-G in vitro produced an increase in the oxidative burst of the neutrophils in response to *C. albicans*. It is unknown whether CSF-G or CSF-GM is helpful in preventing infection or in modifying infectious morbidity in patients who are neutropenic and become febrile. CSF-G has been demonstrated to be of benefit in patients with aplastic anemia,[266] congenital or acquired neutropenia,[267] and HIV infection.[268] However, in addition to their expense, side effects are noted with both agents.[269] Either drug can cause bone pain or an increase in hepatic transaminases. The use of CSF-G can result in Sweet syndrome, while the use of CSF-GM has been complicated by fever, chills, hypoxia, skin rash, fluid retention, and pericarditis.

Other cytokines currently being studied include CSF-M, which stimulates macrophage and monocyte cell lines and augments the immune response to *C. albicans* in vitro. IL-1 affects the immune system at multiple levels, including the stimulation of other cytokines and increasing the number of polymorphonuclear leukocytes.[269] Animal models have shown an increase in survival in mice infected with *Pseudomonas* or *Klebsiella* and then treated with IL-1.[270] IL-3 not only stimulates all cell lines but also enhances the effect of monocytes and eosinophils.[271] Interferon-γ enhances the activity of macrophages against intracellular organisms and protozoa and increases the activity of monocytes and polymorphonuclear leukocytes against some bacteria and fungi.[269,272] It has been shown to decrease the frequency of infection and the need for antibiotics in patients with chronic granulomatous disease.[273] These cytokines are promising agents for future use in bone marrow recovery and in the treatment of bacterial or fungal infection.

Prophylaxis of Fungal Infections

Because of the increasing incidence of invasive mycoses in immunocompromised patients, antifungal prophylaxis has been studied fairly extensively (Table 91-4). The most frequently evaluated antifungal agents have included nystatin, amphotericin B, miconazole, clotrimazole, ketoconazole, and fluconazole. Prophylactic regimens have generally been aimed at reduction of invasive infections due to *Candida,* and by virtue of the antifungal activity of the agents employed they would not be expected to have a significant impact against *Aspergillus* infections or mucormycoses. Strategies designed to prevent infection from *Aspergillus* have largely concentrated on prevention of its acquisition from the environment.

Until recently, several problems with antifungal prophylaxis were noted. First, when an adequate dose of an antifungal agent such as amphotericin B, ketoconazole, or clotrimazole was administered, there was a consistent decrease in fungal colonization but not necessarily a concomitant decrease in invasive fungal infections.[252] Second, several studies employing prophylactic and empiric antifungal regimens reported a shift in the colonization pattern of fungal organisms. In general, these drifts have been toward more resistant fungi. Thus, prophylactic regimens can successfully eradicate the susceptible fungi (particularly *C. albicans*) but can lead to overgrowth and ultimate invasion by more resistant species, especially *Aspergillus.* However, a recent double-blind randomized study of BMT recipients reported by Goodman et al.[274] has shown a decrease in both fungal colonization and infection after antifungal prophylaxis with fluconazole. One hundred seventy-nine patients were treated with 400 mg/day of fluconazole from initiation of chemotherapy until neutrophil counts of 1,000 cells/mm³ were achieved or until drug toxicity or an invasive fungal infection was suspected. As compared to patients given placebo, fluconazole-treated patients had a significant decrease in fungal colonization (67.2% versus 29.6%), superficial fungal infection (33.3% versus 8.4%), and systemic fungal infection (15.8% versus 2.8%). In addition, the number of deaths due to invasive fungal disease in the fluconazole-treated group showed a significant decrease. Although the number of fluconazole-treated patients eliminated from the study because of hepatotoxicity was not significant, the mean increase in alanine aminotransferase was significantly higher in the fluconazole-treated group. Unfortunately fluconazole use did not decrease the need for empirical amphotericin B. Although this study showed no significant increase in *C. krusei* infection in the fluconazole-treated group as compared with the placebo group, a recent study by Wingard et al.[275] revealed a sevenfold increase risk of *C. krusei* infection after fluconazole prophylaxis in BMT and acute leukemia patients. During the time that Wingard et al. used fluconazole as antifungal prophylaxis, *C. krusei* became the most commonly isolated fungal pathogen.

Overall, the potential benefits of prophylactic antifungal therapy must be balanced against the toxicity and relative efficacy of the regimen employed, as well as epidemiologic considerations. Until a clear benefit can be proved, widespread chemoprophylaxis against fungi should not be attempted.

Prophylaxis of Viral Infections

Herpes Simplex Virus

HSV can be a frequent cause of morbidity in compromised patients, particularly those undergoing BMT or renal transplantation or intensive chemotherapy for acute leukemia. In these settings the incidence of reactivation is high (≤80%) in seropositive patients not receiving prophylaxis.[64,65,276,277] Higher antibody titers (≥1:16) appear to be most predictive of subsequent development of clinical infection. Studies employing prophylactic intravenous acyclovir[64,65,278] or oral acyclovir[279,280] in these settings have demonstrated nearly 100% efficacy in the prevention of clinically significant reactivation of HSV. The placebo-controlled study by Saral and co-workers[64] in BMT patients used intravenous acyclovir at a dose of 250 mg/m² tid beginning 3 days before the BMT. None of 10 patients receiving acyclovir developed HSV infection, whereas 7 of 10 patients receiving placebo did. In the study by Wade et al.,[279] oral acyclovir (400 mg five times per day) was begun 1 week before BMT. The results showed that among patients who had a minimum of 40% compliance with the prescribed dose, the prophylaxis was 100% clinically effective. The study by Gluckman and colleagues[280] also showed complete clinical efficacy, but at a lower dose of oral acyclovir (200 mg/m^2 qid). All the studies employing prophylactic acyclovir have demonstrated the absence of significant toxicities in these settings. Recent studies of the prevention of CMV disease with ganciclovir in recipients of allogeneic BMTs have also addressed prophylaxis of HSV infection.[281,282] In one study, high-dose acyclovir was given to patients until marrow engraftment, after which the patients were changed to ganciclovir.[282] None of the ganciclovir recipients excreted HSV, compared to HSV excretion in 14 of 31 controls. In the study by Winston et al.,[281] ganciclovir (2.5 mg/kg tid) was begun pretransplant and continued until day 120 after BMT but held during periods in which the neutrophil count was $<1.0 \times 10^9$/L. In this study, acyclovir was not given. Only 5% of ganciclovir patients excreted HSV compared with 29% of those receiving a placebo; however, there were cases of localized, clinically evident HSV disease. No trials have been conducted to compare acyclovir versus ganciclovir in the prevention of both HSV and CMV in BMT patients. It seems prudent to use either oral or intravenous acyclovir in a prophylactic regimen for several subgroups of high-risk patients: (1) those who are seropositive (with titers of 1:16 or higher) undergoing BMT; on engraftment, these patients may be changed to ganciclovir if CMV positive; (2) those who are seropositive and receiving intensive therapy for acute leukemia; and (3) those with a previous clinical history of HSV infection undergoing these therapies. In addition, it is reasonable to consider prophylactic acyclovir in conjunction with cytoreductive therapy of any type if previous cycles of similar therapy have resulted in clinically significant HSV infection.

Varicella-Zoster Virus

One of the most important and simple methods of preventing VZV infection is isolation of infectious individuals from other high-risk immunosuppressed patients. Infectious patients include any with a diagnosis of either primary VZV (chickenpox) or secondary VZV (zoster). Of these groups those with chickenpox are more highly infectious, the respiratory route being the major mode of transmission. In addition to those with diagnosed VZV infection (i.e., the presence of characteristic lesions), individuals at risk of chickenpox who have had known exposure to the virus (mostly young children) should be considered potentially infectious and kept away from susceptible immunosuppressed patients. The incubation period for chickenpox is 10–21 days, and patients may spread the infection from 2 days before the appearance of lesions until the time of crusting of all lesions. Therefore, any individual who has not had chickenpox but who has been exposed should not be allowed contact with susceptible immunosuppressed patients from 1 week after the initial exposure until at least 3 weeks after the exposure or until complete crusting of any lesions that appear.

Passive immunization with zoster immunoglobulin (ZIG) has been shown to reduce the incidence of pneumonitis and encephalitis and decrease the mortality of chickenpox from 7% to 0.5% in immunocompromised patients. Immunosuppressed children or adults who are seronegative or possess low-titer antivaricella antibody should receive ZIG (1 vial/10 kg) within 72 hours after exposure to a potentially infectious source. One dose should be protective for about 4 weeks.

A live attenuated varicella vaccine will be commercially available soon; so far >9,000 children and 2,000 adults have re-

ceived this vaccine.[283] While 95% of normal children seroconvert after receiving the vaccine, approximately 80% of immunosuppressed children of normal adults will produce antibodies to VZV and 25% will be antibody negative at 1 year.[284] The vaccine has been shown to prevent transmission of chickenpox from normal children to children with leukemia in 85% of cases.[285] Varicella vaccine has also been given to healthy siblings of children with malignancies; of 30 children vaccinated, 6 contracted chickenpox and only 4 transmitted it to their immunocompromised siblings.[286] In spite of the effectiveness of the varicella vaccine, there are still concerns about its use. Most immunocompromised patients have had their chemotherapy interrupted for 1 week before and after vaccine administration. Little data regarding the efficacy and safety of vaccine administration during chemotherapy exists. Arbeter et al.[287] compared 24 children who continued to receive 6-mercaptopurine while the vaccine was administrated with 20 children whose chemotherapy was suspended. Although the number of patients studied was small, there was no difference in antibody response or in vitro lymphocyte proliferation, no difference in side effects, and no difference in breakthrough infection. Approximately 40% of immunocompromised children develop a rash at the vaccine site after immunization. The child is contagious with this rash, will need isolation, and may require therapy with acyclovir. Additionally, rash, viremia, and elevated hepatic transaminases were documented in a vaccinated 4-year-old child with leukemia.[288] Since the clinical picture of varicella is milder in breakthrough infection, there is some concern that vaccine recipients may have an asymptomatic infection and may be infectious without physical signs of varicella. The concern that VZV vaccine would increase the risk of the development of herpes zoster infection in immunocompromised patients has been dismissed by Hardy et al. who demonstrated a lower incidence of zoster in vaccinated children with leukemia (13 children with zoster of 548 vaccinated) than in children who have had natural infection (15 of 96).[289] The varicella vaccine seems better suited to providing herd immunity in the normal population than in protecting those who are immunocompromised.

Cytomegalovirus Infection

Strategies aimed at the prevention of CMV infection in high-risk patients have focused on the use of seronegative blood products in seronegative patients, on passive immunization, and on chemoprophylaxis with acyclovir or ganciclovir. In seronegative patients the exclusive use of seronegative blood products has nearly eliminated serious CMV infection.[78] Additionally, transplanting seronegative recipients with bone marrow and solid organs from seronegative donors also results in a decreased incidence of CMV infection post-transplant.[290,291] The use of high-titer CMV immunoglobulin is controversial in the prevention of CMV disease in BMT recipients but has been shown to be beneficial in CMV-seronegative renal transplant recipients.[78,291,292] Investigations have reported acyclovir to be effective in preventing CMV infection and disease in patients undergoing transplantation of renal allografts from cadavers and in patients following BMT.[75,293] More recently, studies in recipients of allogeneic BMT who are CMV seropositive or who are seronegative with seropositive donors have shown a decreased incidence of CMV infection with prophylactic ganciclovir, whether ganciclovir is given pretransplant or after engraftment.[281,282,294,295] In one study, the primary adverse event associated with ganciclovir was neutropenia requiring interruption of ganciclovir in 58% of patients.[281] However, the increased incidence (relative risk 4.3) of bacterial infection seen during the period of ganciclovir-associated neutropenia in one study is of concern for an already immunocompromised population.[282]

Amantadine, an antiviral with activity against influenza A,

can prevent illness in ≤90% exposed to influenza A. It can also reduce the severity of symptoms if begun within the first 48 hours of illness with influenza A.[296] The use of amantadine should be considered in persons at high risk of severe influenza infection during a community outbreak. However, amantadine causes mild central nervous system disturbances which may be more severe in the elderly or in those with diminished renal function.[296]

Prophylaxis of Parasitic Infections

Strategies aimed at prevention of parasitic diseases in immunosuppressed patients have primarily targeted *P. carinii* (Table 91-4). The agent studied most extensively has been trimethoprim-sulfamethoxazole, which has proved effective in prevention of *P. carinii* in children with leukemia, in patients undergoing BMT, and in AIDS patients. An intermittent (i.e., two or three times weekly) dosage schedule is both effective and less toxic.[297] Although trimethoprim sulfamethoxazole is the drug of choice for PCP prophylaxis in AIDS patients, up to 65% of adults with AIDS have adverse reactions to this drug (primarily dermatologic and hematologic).[298,299] Recent studies have shown aerosolized pentamidine to be less effective but better tolerated.[300] Dapsone may be a useful alternative in the prevention of PCP, but only small numbers of patients have been studied.[301,302] Other agents given for prophylaxis include atovaquone, pyrimethamine with sulfadoxine, and pyrimethamine with dapsone, but data concerning their efficacy are limited.[299] The value of these agents in high-risk groups other than AIDS is only speculative at present.

Active and Passive Immunization for the Prevention of Infections in High-Risk Groups

Active Immunization

In the United States, few eligible adults are actually immunized. Shapiro et al.[303] conducted an investigation showing that only 21% of those with an indication for the pneumococcal vaccine received it, in spite of the evidence of the increasing incidence and severity of pneumococcal infection due to the AIDS epidemic, the growing population >65 years of age, and the increase in penicillin-resistant *Pneumococcus*. The pneumococcal vaccine contains 23 of the serotypes responsible for >88% of pneumococcal bacteremias in the United States; however, it only provides effective protection in 61% of immunocompetent recipients and is less protective in immunocompromised hosts.[304] Despite its varying efficacy, the pneumococcal vaccine is recommended for patients who are asplenic, undergoing transplant, have certain malignancies (Hodgkin disease, lymphoma, and multiple myeloma), or are infected with HIV.[224] Another recently available inactivated vaccine against encapsulated bacteria is the *H. influenzae* b vaccine. Although few data are available in adults, it is recommended for patients with anatomic or functional asplenia and its use should be considered in HIV-infected patients.[224] Yearly vaccination with the influenza vaccine, an inactivated viral vaccine, is recommended for those at increased risk of severe disease with influenza infection; this includes the elderly, persons with chronic cardiac or pulmonary disease, persons immunosuppressed due to malignancy or drug therapy, and those with symptomatic HIV infection, although the protective value in severely immunocompromised patients is suboptimal.[296] It is important for health care workers and family members of immunocompromised persons to receive the influenza vaccine in order to prevent transmission to those at risk of severe disease.

As a general rule, live attenuated viral or bacterial vaccines should not be administered to patients who are immunosuppressed as a result of leukemia, lymphoma, generalized malignancy, symptomatic HIV infection, or therapy with alkylating agents, antimetabolites, radiation, or large amounts of corticosteroids.[209] The only live bacterial vaccine currently available in the United States is BCG. The live viral vaccines that are available include measles, mumps, and rubella vaccines, oral poliovirus vaccine, and yellow fever vaccine. The latest recommendations of the Centers for Disease Control (CDC) state that patients with leukemia in remission whose chemotherapy has been terminated for ≥3 months may be given live virus vaccines. With respect to corticosteroid usage, low- to moderate-dose short-term systemic corticosteroid therapy (<2 weeks), topical steroid therapy, long-term alternate-day treatment with low to moderate doses of short-acting systemic steroids, and intra-articular, bursal, or tendon injection of corticosteroids should not be considered contraindications to live viral vaccine administration.[209] A 1989 study in BMT recipients documented the safety and efficacy of administering measles-mumps-rubella (MMR) vaccine to patients in remission 2 years after transplantation who do not have active graft-versus-host disease.[305] While live vaccines should generally be avoided in patients with symptomatic HIV infection, the CDC recommends that MMR vaccine be administered to all HIV-infected children, even if symptomatic because of the recent resurgence of measles and the potential severity of measles in this population.[185]

Passive Immunization

Passive immunization involves administration of preformed antibodies to high-risk patients, with the goal of either replacing qualitatively or quantitatively defective immunoglobulins and/or attenuating the virulence of pathogenic organisms or their toxic components. Studies have examined the use of a variety of antibody preparations, including pooled immunoglobulins, immunoglobulins collected from individuals with high titers of specific antibodies ("hyperimmune" preparations), and monoclonal antibodies.

Passive immunization with varicella-zoster immunoglobulin is effective in preventing infection and decreasing the incidence of morbidity and mortality associated with primary chickenpox in susceptible hosts. Another "hyperimmune" preparation that has been investigated in high-risk patients consists of the so-called J-5 antisera collected from patients with high titers of antibody directed against the core glycolipid of Enterobacteriaceae. In a clinical trial, J-5 antisera was not shown to reduce the mortality of neutropenic patients with gram-negative infections.[306] A recent randomized double-blind trial of HA-1A, a human monoclonal IgM to the lipid component of endotoxin, demonstrated improved survival in patients with gram-negative bacteremia.[307] However, subsequent follow-up data showed unanticipated toxicity in the HA-1A treated patients, precluding its current use.

Immunoglobulin preparations with high titers against CMV have been used as adjuncts in the prevention and treatment of CMV-associated disease in BMT patients.[78,308,309] CMV-enriched immunoglobulin has been shown to prevent CMV disease but not infection in seronegative recipients of a kidney from a seropositive donor.[291] Pooled immunoglobulin preparations have also been assessed in a number of immunocompromised populations. Both intramuscular and intravenous routes have been studied. In patients with hypo- or dysgammaglobulinemia not associated with malignancy or cytotoxic therapy, administration of pooled immunoglobulins has been effective in preventing infections due to encapsulated bacteria and in the treatment of certain enteroviral infections.[310] In patients with malignancy, the effects of immunoglobulin preparations have been less clear cut. Recently, a randomized placebo-controlled trial of intravenous immunoglobulin in patients with

CLL showed that it was effective in decreasing the incidence of bacterial infections.[212] While some early reports suggest a potential benefit of intravenous immunoglobulin in patients with multiple myeloma, its value in this population remains controversial, and further studies will be needed before firm conclusions can be drawn.[310]

MANAGEMENT OF FEVER AND INFECTION IN NEUTROPENIC PATIENTS

Initial Evaluation of the Febrile Neutropenic Patient

The goal of the initial evaluation of a newly febrile neutropenic patient is to identify potential sources of infection in order to optimize therapy. Ideally we would like to be able to distinguish at the outset those febrile patients with an infection from those who are infection free. In a prospective study from the NCI evaluating >1,000 consecutive episodes of fever and neutropenia, there were no features identified on presentation that reliably distinguished bacteremic patients from those with unexplained fever.[311] Physical examination was helpful only if a specific site of infection (e.g., cellulitis or abscess) was readily detectable. Other measurements that might be predictive in noncompromised patients, including the degree of fever, the presence of chills or rigors, or a "toxic" appearance, were not helpful in this population. Indeed, significant and potentially life-threatening bacteremias were not infrequently present, even in the absence of any symptoms or signs on physical examination. Of the patients with proven bacteremia, 55% had no evidence of infection on physical examination, aside from the presence of fever.

For neutropenic patients with a new fever, the standard initial evaluation should include the following:

1. *Careful physical examination.* Particular attention should be devoted to areas that may "hide" a site of infection unless closely examined, notably the oral cavity and the perianal area. There is some debate as to whether neutropenic patients should have an initial rectal examination because manipulation in this area may lead to bacteremia. It is our policy to first perform a complete external examination of the perirectal area, including deep palpation. Then, only if there are findings suggestive of a localized inflammatory site (e.g., pain or fluctuance) do we perform a careful digital examination. We have found that virtually all perianal or perirectal sites of infection can be detected with this approach.
2. *Blood cultures.* A minimum of two sets of blood cultures should be obtained. If the patient has an indwelling intravenous catheter, at least one set should be drawn through the catheter and another drawn from a peripheral vein. For patients with multilumen intravenous catheters, a culture should be obtained through each lumina, as well as the specific lumen clearly identified on the culture bottle. This is important because catheter infection may be limited to a single lumen.
3. *Urine culture.* Because of the absence of granulocytes, microscopic examination of the urine may be normal even in the presence of a urinary tract infection.
4. *Chest radiograph.*
5. In addition, accessible sites of potential infection should be aspirated or biopsied and appropriate material sent for Gram stain, culture, and histologic examination. Other diagnostic tests directed at certain sites, such as cranial computed tomography (CT) or lumbar puncture, should be reserved for patients who have symptoms or signs referable to those areas.

Even with a comprehensive evaluation, an infectious cause of the initial fever is demonstrated in only 30–50% of patients.

Moreover, definitive diagnosis may take days, presumably because of the relatively low microbial inoculum. This probably reflects the short period that elapses between the onset of fever and the evaluation and initiation of empirical therapy. Even subtle indications of inflammation must be considered as sites of infection in the presence of granulocytopenia. For example, minimal perirectal erythema and tenderness may be the harbinger of a perirectal cellulitis. Minimal erythema or discharge at the exit site of an indwelling intravenous catheter may herald a tunnel or exit-site infection.

Colonization with microorganisms often precedes development of significant infection. Logic has dictated that identification of a specific pathogen during the colonization phase might help guide the clinician toward earlier use of appropriate antimicrobial therapy at the first signs of infection. Accordingly, some investigators have recommended routing serial surveillance culturing in neutropenic patients. To evaluate the clinical value of this concept, an NCI study of 652 febrile granulocytopenic episodes was conducted.[45] Nose, throat, urine, and stool cultures were obtained serially during the neutropenic episode. Of those patients who became septic and from whose blood a specific causative pathogen was isolated, 62% were found to be colonized with the infecting organism. However, the results of the surveillance cultures provided little clinically useful information for the following reasons: (1) no single body site was predictive; (2) other potential pathogens were usually isolated in addition to the organism responsible for infection; and (3) the actual pathogens isolated from the blood cultures were usually known prior to their isolation from the surveillance cultures. Furthermore, the cost of routine surveillance is enormous, and knowledge of the colonizing flora is unlikely to have a significant impact on initial antibiotic management, because most clinicians routinely employ broad-spectrum antibiotics for the empirical treatment of febrile granulocytopenic patients. For these reasons, we do not recommend routine surveillance cultures in neutropenic patients. They can be helpful, however, in certain subgroups of patients, such as those with protracted neutropenia (>3–4 weeks) and those at centers that have a high incidence of particularly virulent or resistant organisms, such as *P. aeruginosa* or *Aspergillus* spp.

Antibiotic Strategies

Empirical Antibiotics

The management of neutropenic cancer patients as compared with nonimmunocompromised patients more frequently involves the use of empirical antibiotics, directed against a wide array of potential pathogens. It has now become well accepted that when a neutropenic patient develops a new fever (fever is usually defined as one oral temperature reading of ≥38.5°C or more than two successive readings of ≥38°C during a 12-hour period), an empirical antibacterial regimen should be started expeditiously. This holds true even in those patients who have no clinically evident source of infection. The rationale for this approach evolved from the observation that bacteremias in neutropenic patients are often rapidly lethal, especially those due to gram-negative organisms.[5,312–315] A delay of even 24–48 hours for the results of initial blood cultures can substantially increase morbidity and mortality. In addition, no reliable way has been found to determine whether an isolated fever in a neutropenic patient is due to an underlying infection. Within that context, even fevers that are temporally associated with the administration of blood products or with fever-producing antineoplastic drugs should be considered potentially infectious in etiology and treated as such. In sum, virtually all new fevers in the neutropenic population warrant careful clinical and microbiologic evaluation, followed by prompt initiation of empirical antibiotic therapy. Conversely, any clinically

Table 91-6. Essential Properties of Empirical Regimens

Broad spectrum of activity that includes *Pseudomonas aeruginosa*
Ability to achieve high serum bactericidal levels
Effective in the absence of netrophils
Low potential for the emergence of resistance
Acceptable toxicity profile

Table 91-7. Aminoglycoside-Based Combination Regimens

Aminoglycoside	+	Antipseudomonal β-Lactam	±	Additional Anti-Gram-Positive
Gentamicin		Extended-spectrum		Isoxozolyl-penicillin
Tobramycin		penicillin		Nafcillin
Amikacin		Carbenicillin		Oxacillin
		Ticarcillin		OR
		Azlocillin		First-generation
		Mezlocillin		cephalosporin
		Piperacillin		Cephalothin
		OR		Cefazolin
		Third-generation		OR
		cephalosporin		Vancomycin
		Ceftazidime		
		Cefoperazone		
		OR		
		Aztreonam		

evident site of potential infection mandates expeditious broad-spectrum therapy, even in the absence of fever.

The goal of empirical antibiotic therapy is to protect against the early morbidity and mortality that results from untreated bacterial infections. Accordingly, regimens have been formulated to maximize activity against organisms that are commonly encountered or particularly virulent, or both. One must remember that empirical regimens cannot realistically be designed to cover every potential bacterial pathogen. Likewise, no regimen is capable of completely eliminating the risk of subsequent development of infections in persistently neutropenic cases. Empirical antibiotic regimens should be individualized at each institution in order to cover those organisms seen at that hospital and to cover organisms associated with certain chemotherapeutic regimens.

Traditionally, gram-negative bacteria have been the most frequently isolated pathogens in the neutropenic population, with *E. coli, K. pneumoniae,* and *P. aeruginosa* the most common. While gram-negative bacteria still predominate at some institutions, the trend in recent years has been toward more gram-positive infections, which now account for most isolates at many centers.[8,10,119,316–321] In general, gram-negative infections tend to be more virulent; early empirical regimens were formulated to provide protection primarily against these organisms while maintaining a broad spectrum of activity against other potential pathogens. Indeed, adequate coverage of these gram-negative organisms is still an essential property of any empirical regimen (Table 91-6).

In order to achieve the desired properties of empirical therapy, it has been necessary to employ combinations of antibiotics. Early experience combining aminoglycosides and an expanded-spectrum penicillin such as carbenicillin resulted in an improved clinical outcome.[322] This combination appeared to obviate both the poor clinical efficacy of aminoglycosides when used alone and the emergence of resistance to the expanded-spectrum penicillins often encountered when used as single agents. In addition, a body of in vitro data emerged showing a synergistic effect of such combinations against the gram-negative bacilli, particularly *P. aeruginosa.*[211,323–332] Such combination regimens are still widely used and represent a standard against which newer regimens are tested.

Many variations of the initial gentamicin-carbenicillin combination have been studied (Table 91-7). These consist of an aminoglycoside at the "core" usually in combination with an extended-spectrum (or antipseudomonal) penicillin and often with an antistaphylococcal β-lactam antibiotic (e.g., nafcillin or a first-generation cephalosporin). Third-generation cephalosporins can also be combined with aminoglycosides, provided that the third-generation cephalosporin has good antipseudomonal activity (e.g., ceftazidime or cefoperazone).[333] In general, no specific combination has been shown to have consistently superior efficacy. If an aminoglycoside-containing combination regimen is to be employed, the choice of specific antibiotics should be based primarily on the institutional antibiotic sensitivity patterns and secondarily on toxicity and cost differences.

In order to avoid the use of aminoglycosides yet retain the theoretical advantages of combination antibiotics, various non-aminoglycoside-containing combination regimens have been devised and studied. For the most part these have consisted of combinations of two β-lactam antibiotics (so-called double β-

lactam regimens), usually consisting of an expanded-spectrum carboxy- or ureidopenicillin and a third-generation cephalosporin (e.g., piperacillin and ceftazidime).[334,335] While double β-lactam combinations may offer some of the potential advantages of other combinations, they also have some of the inherent disadvantages of any combination regimen (see below). In addition, increased β-lactamase induction is a theoretical disadvantage when certain of these agents are combined (thus accelerating the development of resistant organisms).[335]

Monotherapy with an aminoglycoside or an extended-spectrum penicillin is not a viable option. However, since the combination of an aminoglycoside and a β-lactam antibiotic has demonstrable efficacy, one might ask whether there are any valid reasons to consider the use of other single-agent regimens as an alternative. The most important reason for answering this question in the affirmative is that certain antibiotics now offer viable options for such monotherapy.[316,336,337] Of those currently available, the third-generation cephalosporins and the carbapenems are the two classes that include potential candidates for empirical single-agent therapy. Ceftazidime has been the most extensively studied of the third-generation cephalosporins; most other agents in this class exhibit inadequate activity against *P. aeruginosa* for use as monotherapy (*P. aeruginosa* is among the most virulent of the gram-negative organisms). Cefoperazone also has activity against *P. aeruginosa,* but its clinical value in this setting has not been as extensively evaluated. In the carbapenem class, imipenem is the only currently available agent; several trials support its efficacy as monotherapy.[338,339]

Ceftazidime has a broad spectrum of activity, which encompasses the vast majority of bacterial pathogens encountered in neutropenic hosts, including *P. aeruginosa* (Table 91-8). Standard dosing results in serum and tissue levels that are bactericidal for these organisms, and the toxicity profile is similar to that of most β-lactams.

A large randomized study evaluating 550 consecutive episodes of fever and neutropenia conducted at the NCI compared a combination of antibiotics (i.e., cephalothin, gentamicin, and carbenicillin) with ceftazidime as a single agent.[340] The overall results show that monotherapy compared favorably with a standard combination regimen (Table 91-9). Approximately two-thirds of the episodes in both groups were successfully treated for the entire duration of the granulocytopenia without requiring any changes in the initial regimen. Another one-third of the episodes required some change or modification (e.g., addition of an antibacterial, antifungal, or antiviral drug) to ensure a successful outcome (Table 91-10) (see also indications for modifications below), and an equally low number in both

Table 91-8. Activity of Newer Antibiotics Against Pathogens Commonly Encountered in Cancer Patients

Antibiotic	Enteric Gram-Negative	P. Aeruginosa	Coagulase-Positive Staphylococci	Coagulase-Negative Staphylococci	Group D Streptococci	Non-Group D Streptococci	Anaerobes
Ceftazidime	Good	Good	Moderate (poor against methicillin-resistant strains)	Poor against the majority (most are methicillin-resistant)	Poor	Good	Poor
Cefoperazone	Good	Moderate to good	Moderate (poor against methicillin-resistant strains)	Poor against the majority	Poor	Good	Poor
Other third-generation cephalosporins	Good	Poor to moderate	Moderate (poor against methicillin-resistant strains)	Poor against the majority	Poor	Good	Poor to moderate (moxalactam and ceftizoxime have some activity)
Impipenem	Good	Good	Good (poor against methicillin-resistant strains)	Poor against the majority	Good	Good	Good
Quinolones	Good	Good	Good (including most methicillin-resistant strains)	Good (limited clinical experience)	Poor to moderate	Poor to moderate	Poor
Aztreonam	Good	Good	Poor	Poor	Poor	Poor	Poor

groups (about 5%) died of infection. None of the deaths was attributable to a specific deficiency in one regimen that was not present in the other (i.e., an organism sensitive to one regimen but resistant to the other). In addition, the average time to initial defervescence was equivalent for those receiving monotherapy and those treated with combination antibiotics.

Two subgroups of patients identified in this study appeared to require more frequent modifications of the initial regimen in order to achieve a successful outcome: (1) those presenting with a documented source of infection to account for the initial fever, and (2) those having relatively protracted periods of granulocytopenia (>1 week). However, the need for modification in these subgroups was identical for those episodes treated with monotherapy and those treated with combination therapy. In this study, these modifications did not represent a failure of either regimen per se but instead reflected the limita-

Table 91-9. Outcome of 550 Febrile Neutropenic Episodes Randomized to Monotherapy or to Combination Antibiotic Therapy

	Regimen	
	Monotherapy (Ceftazidime)	Combination Therapy (Cephalothin, Gentamicin, Carbenicillin)
No. of episodes	282	268
Success without modification[a]	175 (62%)	180 (67%)
Success with modification[b]	93 (33%)	78 (29%)
Failure[c]	14 (5%)	11 (4%)

[a] Successful treatment not requiring any additions to or changes in the initial antibiotic regimen.
[b] Successful treatment requiring some addition to or change in the initial antibiotic regimen.
[c] Death due to infection.
(Modified from Pizzo et al.,[311] with permission.)

Table 91-10. Modifications of Therapy During the Course of Granulocytopenia

Clinical Event	Possible Modifications of Therapy
Breakthrough bacteremia	If gram-positive isolate (e.g., *S. epidermidis*), add vancomycin
	If gram-negative isolate (i.e., presumably resistant), switch to regimen containing non-cross-resistant antibiotics (e.g., aminoglycoside plus a carbapenem or extended-spectrum penicillin)
Catheter-associated infection	Add vancomycin (as well as gram-negative coverage if not already being given)
Severe oral mucositis or necrotizing gingivitis	Add specific antianaerobic agent (e.g., clindamycin or metronidazole) or change to antibiotic with improved anaerobic coverage (e.g., imipenem)
Esophagitis	Trial of oral clotrimazole, fluconazole, IV amphotericin B, or acyclovir
Pneumonitis, diffuse or interstitial	Trial of trimethoprim sulfamethoxazole and erythromycin (plus broad-spectrum antibiotics, if patient is granulocytopenic)
New infiltrate in a granulocytopenic patient also receiving antibiotics	If granulocyte count is rising, watch and wait
	If granulocyte count is not recovering, biopsy to establish diagnosis, add amphotericin B empirically
Perianal tenderness	If patient is already receiving broad-spectrum antibiotics, add a specific antianaerobic agent
	If patient is not on antibiotics, begin broad-spectrum therapy with anaerobic coverage
Persistent fever and neutropenia	Continue antibiotics after 1 week of persistent fever and neutropenia; add systemic antifungal therapy empirically

tions of any regimen in treating patients at high risk of the development of subsequent infections.

In a recent review of 12 randomized controlled trials comparing ceftazidime as single-agent therapy for febrile, neutropenic patients with combination therapy, Sanders et al.[341] studied 1,077 episodes of fever and neutropenia and 248 episodes of bacteremia. In this meta-analysis, he was unable to demonstrate an advantage of combination therapy over monotherapy with ceftazidime.

Imipenem is a member of the carbapenem class of antibiotics and offers another option for empirical monotherapy. Overall it has the broadest spectrum of activity of any available antibiotic (Table 91-8). Of note is its excellent in vitro activity against group D streptococci and many anaerobes. A large randomized study recently completed at the NCI compared monotherapy with ceftazidime to monotherapy with imipenem (Freifeld A, Pizzo P, unpublished observations). Both drugs showed success without modification in slightly more than 60% of episodes of fever without a known source. In patients with a documented infection, 16% of those receiving imipenem required antibiotic modification, while 27% of those receiving ceftazidime needed a change in antibiotics—usually the addition of anaerobic coverage in patients on ceftazidime. However, more side effects were seen in patients on imipenem, most notably nausea and *Clostridium difficile* colitis. In addition, imipenem could not be used in patients with brain tumors or with a decreased creatinine clearance because of the increased risk of seizures.[342]

Several authorities have raised concerns regarding the use of single-agent therapy for fever and neutropenia. Some of these concerns are purely theoretical; others are based on unique experiences limited to specific centers. However, these issues underscore the appropriateness of maintaining a flexible approach with regard to selection of an empirical regimen, which should be based on individual and institutional experience. Also, regardless of the specific regimen chosen, the clinician must be acutely aware of the potential need for changes in that regimen during the course of granulocytopenia (Table 91-10). This mandates frequent and meticulous clinical evaluation by an experienced supportive care team.

During the late 1980s, gram-positive organisms re-emerged as the most frequently encountered isolates at many centers. While the precise explanation for this shift is unclear, it is evident that many of these gram-positive bacteria (e.g., the enterococci and the coagulase-negative staphylococci) are either resistant to, or poorly covered by, most standard empirical regimens. Some authorities have therefore recommended the addition of vancomycin to empirical regimens. Conversely, it has been argued that because many of these organisms are of relatively low virulence and are often inhibited by the antibiotics (even "suboptimal" antibiotics), vancomycin may be safely withheld until the gram-positive isolate has been identified microbiologically.

In a randomized study of a vancomycin-containing versus a non-vancomycin-containing regimen conducted by Karp et al.,[119] the incidence of secondary gram-positive infections was reduced in the vancomycin-containing group. However, no difference in morbidity was related to gram-positive infections between the two groups, and all the gram-positive infections in the non-vancomycin-treated group were successfully treated by its addition after the organism had been identified and reported by the microbiology laboratory. There also appeared to be less need for amphotericin B in the group that received vancomycin initially. In a more recent study conducted by the European Organization for Research and Treatment of Cancer, 747 patients were randomized to receive ceftazidime and amikacin or ceftazidime, amikacin, and vancomycin.[343] No difference was found in the number of days febrile between the two groups. The group receiving ceftazidime and amikacin did need more antimicrobial modifications, most commonly the addi-

tion of vancomycin, but the group receiving the vancomycin-containing regimen required the addition of antifungal therapy more frequently. Notably, no deaths occurred due to gram-positive infection in the first 3 days of therapy, regardless of the antibiotic regimen.

In addition, a retrospective analysis from the NCI indicated that no excess morbidity resulted when the institution of vancomycin was delayed by waiting for either a microbiologic or clinical indication for its use (i.e., a positive culture for a resistant gram-positive organism or a clinical infection developing in the presence of other antibiotics).[8] All the primary gram-positive isolates (from cultures obtained before empirical therapy) and 82% of the secondary gram-positive isolates (from cultures obtained after institution of antibiotics) were treated successfully with this pathogen-directed approach.

We do not favor routine inclusion of vancomycin in all empirical antibiotic regimens. However, as with all components of these regimens, its use should be guided by institutional experience and sensitivity patterns.

The development of newer broad-spectrum antibiotics has expanded the available options for empirical therapy of fever and neutropenia; both aztreonam and ciprofloxacin present useful additions to the antibiotic armamentarium. Aztreonam, a monobactam active against gram-negative aerobes, including *P. aeruginosa,* should not be used as monotherapy because of its limited spectrum. At the NCI, we use aztreonam in combination with vancomycin in patients with allergies to β-lactam antibiotics. Ciprofloxacin, the most commonly used quinolone, has a distinctive mechanism of action, inhibition of bacterial DNA gyrase. Its spectrum of activity includes many staphylococci and gram-negative organisms, including multiply-resistant *P. aeruginosa, Enterobacter, Serratia,* and *Klebsiella.* However, it has poor streptococcal coverage and is inactive against anaerobes. The use of ciprofloxacin as monotherapy for fever and neutropenia has been complicated by an increase in breakthrough bacteremias with streptococci.[344,345] Although ciprofloxacin can be combined with vancomycin or a penicillin as empirical therapy, we prefer to reserve its use for multiply-resistant gram-negative infections.

In a study by Flaherty et al.,[346] 32 patients were switched to oral ciprofloxacin after a mean of 6 days of intravenous therapy. However, the use of ciprofloxacin alone was associated with a 12% incidence of superinfections and a 9% incidence of breakthrough bacteremia due to *Fusobacterium, S. viridans,* and *S. aureus.* Oral ciprofloxacin was combined with oral clindamycin as empirical therapy in a more recent study by Rubenstein et al.[347] In this prospective study, febrile and neutropenic patients were randomized to treatment with oral clindamycin and ciprofloxacin or with intravenous aztreonam and clindamycin. All patients were treated as outpatients and had to meet strict entry criteria, including the presence of a central venous catheter. Of 83 episodes, 32 were due to a documented infection, and 15 of these were bacteremias. A similar response rate, defined as the resolution of all clinical and laboratory indicators of infection, was seen for both regimens. Response rate did not vary by the initial degree of neutropenia but was decreased when neutrophil recovery was delayed. Of the 40 patients in the oral therapy group, 6 required hospital admission for either treatment failure (3 patients) or drug toxicity (3 patients), while no patient in the intravenous therapy group needed admission. Although this study suggests that a subset of neutropenic patients with fever may be treated with oral therapy, the study was limited by small sample size, the definition of response, and the distribution of underlying malignancy (only 11 patients had leukemia). A large prospective controlled trial comparing oral therapy with amoxicillin/clavulanate with ceftazidime is in progress at the NCI.

Approach to the Patient with Prolonged Granulocytopenia

Length of Antibiotic Therapy

A question of practical importance is the length of time antibiotics should be continued in persistently neutropenic patients. Should they always be continued until the granulocyte count recovers, or can they be safely discontinued before that time? Our overall approach is illustrated in Figure 91-2.

Operationally, it is easiest to approach the question of duration of therapy by placing patients in two categories: (1) those whose initial workup did not reveal the source of infection (i.e., patients with fever of undetermined origin [FUO]), and (2) those whose initial workup revealed a documented infection to account for the fever. Most patients (approximately 60%) at most centers will fall into the FUO category, although this will vary with the institution, therapy, and patient population.

Limited data specifically address the issue of duration of empirical therapy in neutropenic patients presenting with FUO. In a randomized NCI study, patients with FUO and persistent granulocytopenia were assigned either to discontinue antibiotics on day 7 of therapy or to continue them until the resolution of the neutropenia[348] (Table 91-11). A large percentage of afebrile patients who stopped antibiotics developed recurrent fever, and an alarmingly high percentage of persistently febrile patients whose antibiotics were discontinued developed hypotensive episodes. It was concluded that day 7 was too early to discontinue antibiotics in this group.

In a subsequent randomized study conducted at the NCI, persistently neutropenic afebrile patients were assigned either to continue or to discontinue antibiotics on day 14. Preliminary analysis shows no difference between the two groups; approximately one-third of patients became febrile again, regardless of whether they stopped or continued antibiotics. However, those whose fevers recurred after discontinuation of antibiotics responded to a re-institution of their initial regimen, while those remaining on antibiotics required addition of amphotericin B. Currently, for FUO patients who are predicted to have a long duration of neutropenia and who have remained afebrile at day 14 ($\geq$7 days), we discontinue antibiotics and cautiously observe. More recent studies have suggested that antibiotics can also be safely discontinued in afebrile patients who have evidence of bone marrow recovery, even though their neutrophil count is still <500 cells/mm^3.[349,350]

In addition, for persistently neutropenic patients who have had clinical and microbiologic resolution of their infection and who are afebrile at day 14 ($\geq$7 days), we consider discontinuing antibiotics. The final decision as to whether to continue or discontinue antibiotics rests on a number of clinical parameters, such as the degree of or potential for antibiotic toxicity, the predicted duration of neutropenia, the seriousness of the initial infection, and the presence or absence of other factors predisposing to subsequent infection. It should be emphasized that any neutropenic patient whose antibiotics are discontinued requires meticulously careful follow-up evaluation so that any new fevers or infection can be quickly detected.

Modifications of Antibiotic Therapy During the Course of Granulocytopenia

Empirical antibiotics have their greatest impact early in the course of neutropenia. It is during these early days after the initial febrile episode and before results of the initial cultures are known that the antibiotic regimen is truly empirical. One must not assume that the efficacy of an empirical regimen implies that it will suffice as the sole antimicrobial therapy throughout a protracted course of neutropenia. Indeed, it is during a prolonged granulocytopenic episode that the patient is at highest risk of multiple types of secondary infections or

superinfections, as well as for changing clinical parameters, many of which dictate specific types of modifications of the initial regimen to ensure a successful outcome. Only a few secondary infections actually represent a true failure of the initial antibiotics. Rather, they should be viewed as part of the "natural history" of most patients with prolonged neutropenia, and the need for modifications of the initial regimen should be expected and planned for.

Modifications for Resistant Bacterial Isolates

Bacterial isolates resistant to the initial empirical regimen are invariably encountered when managing neutropenic patients. Although their occurrence can be minimized if the initial regimen is selected on the basis of regional sensitivity patterns, the overall incidence of resistant organisms will vary dramatically, depending on the institution, characteristics of the patient population, selection of antibiotics, and unexplained ecologic fluctuations. Clinically, it is important to distinguish between organisms in the environment with intrinsic or de novo antibiotic resistance (primary resistance) and organisms that develop resistance while the patient is receiving antibiotics (secondary resistance). Organisms with primary resistance may cause either initial infection or breakthrough infections, while organisms developing secondary resistance cause infections in patients already being treated with antibiotics.

Primary resistance is predominantly dependent on the institution and/or location and is reflective of a regional "pool" of organisms with similar sensitivity patterns. In addition, individual patients may be colonized with resistant organisms in the absence of an environmental reservoir. For a patient whose site of infection is believed likely to harbor a resistant organism (e.g., coagulase-negative staphylococci from a catheter exit-site infection) or for a patient with a prior history of recurrent infections due to a rare but resistant organism, appropriate modifications of the initial empirical regimen are warranted.

Organisms with intrinsic resistance to most components of standard empirical regimens may also cause secondary or breakthrough infection. Commonly encountered examples include the appearance of breakthrough infections due to methicillin-resistant coagulase-negative staphylococci, enterococci, or anaerobes in patients whose initial regimens do not include antibiotics active against these organisms. Rarer examples would include secondary infections due to non-*aeruginosa* pseudomonads, *C. jeikeium*, or atypical mycobacteria. For patients receiving non-vancomycin-containing empirical regimens, reports from the microbiology laboratory of gram-positive cocci growing from a culture should prompt the addition of vancomycin, with subsequent modifications made on the basis of a final sensitivity determination. If anaerobes are reported, clindamycin or metronidazole should be added.

The appearance of secondary resistance is seen more frequently with certain organisms. For example, *Enterobacter* spp., *Citrobacter* spp., and *Serriatim* spp. harbor inducible β-lactamases; a 1989 report documents the appearance of a clinically significant clustering of resistant *Enterobacter* in a neutropenic population.[351] Accordingly, when these organisms are isolated from a patient, careful observation for the emergence of resistance is warranted, and an aminoglycoside should be added to the regimen of patients receiving monotherapy with a broad-spectrum β-lactam. *P. aeruginosa* may develop resistance to imipenem through a relatively novel mechanism involving change in porins. Hence, for patients receiving single-agent therapy with imipenem who have a documented infection with *P. aeruginosa,* an aminoglycoside should be added to their regimen. Secondary development of resistance among the gram-positive organisms is somewhat rarer, although it has been described. Of note, an increasing number of reports have docu-

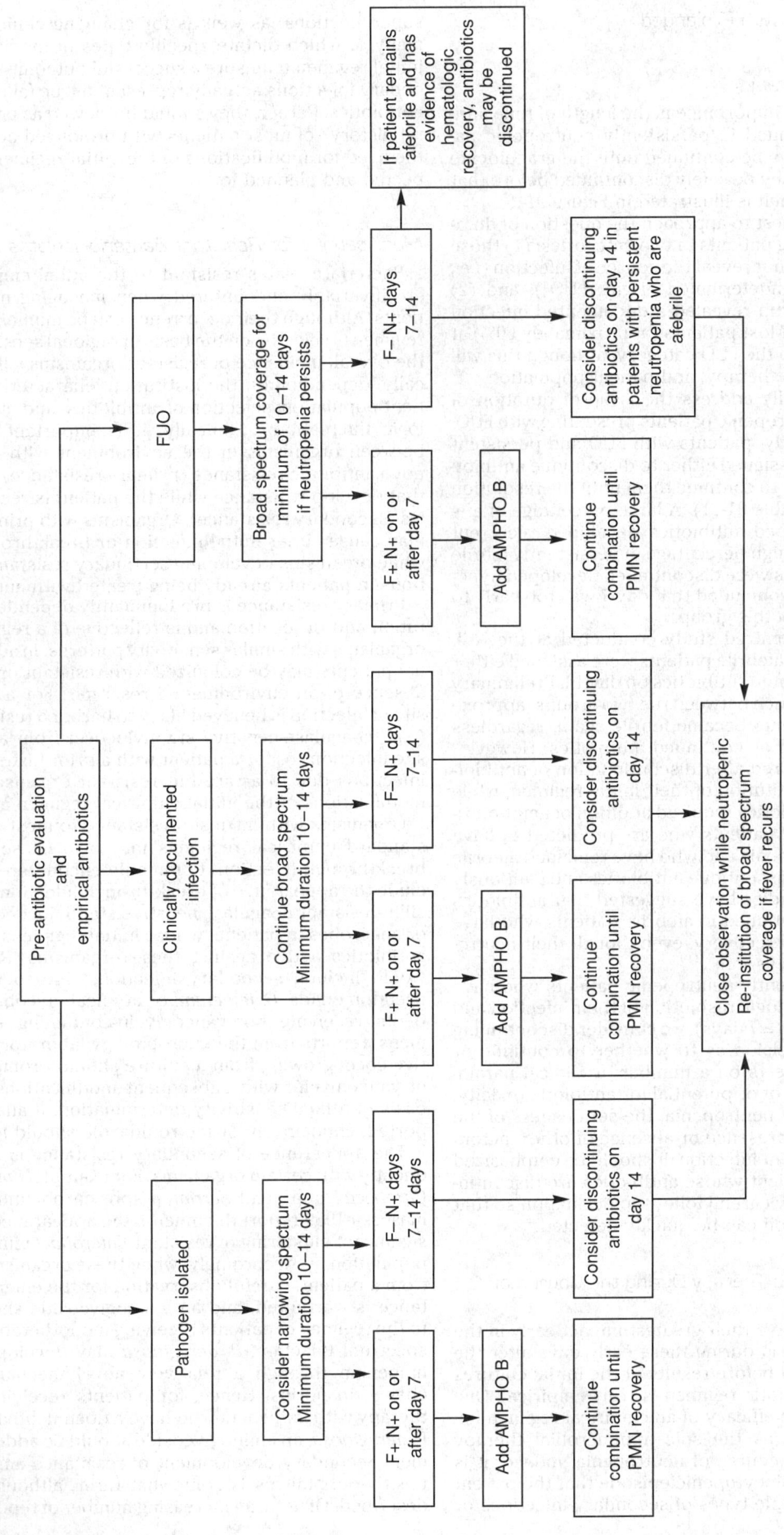

Fig. 91-2. Algorithm for antibiotic management in febrile neutropenic patients. F+ N+, febrile, neutropenic; F− N+, afebrile, neutropenic; FUO, no source of fever on pre-antibiotic evaluation; AMPHO B, amphotericin B.

Table 91-11. Outcome of Patients with Unexplained Fever Who Were Randomized Either to Continue or to Discontinue Empirical Antibiotics When They Remained Persistently Granulocytopenic

	Continue Antibiotics		Discontinue Antibiotics	
	F− G+ (%)	F+ G+ (%)	F− G+ (%)	F+ F+ (%)
Remained afebrile or improved	100	62	59	44
Became febrile or worsened	0	38	41	56
Became hypotensive	0	0	12	38

Abbreviations: F−, reduction of fever; G+, granulocytopenia; F+, continuation of fever.

mented the emergence of vancomycin-resistant coagulase-negative staphylococci and enterococci in patients receiving vancomycin.[352–355]

Modifications Based on Changing Clinical Parameters

For neutropenic patients receiving antibiotics, the appearance of a new clinically documented infection (e.g., cellulitis or pneumonia) or the progression of a previously documented site of infection should raise suspicion of the presence of resistant organisms. Attempts should be made to obtain microbiologic confirmation with appropriate tissue samples. In addition, changes in the empirical regimen should be made to cover the potential for resistant bacteria. The site of infection can be helpful in guiding certain antibiotic choices (Table 91-10).

The development of marginal or necrotizing gingivitis is relatively common in patients who have received intensive cytotoxic therapy (Fig. 91-3). Anaerobic organisms contribute to this process, and an antianaerobic agent such as clindamycin or metronidazole should be added to the empirical regimen if gingivitis is diagnosed.

The most common pathogens contributing to perianal cellulitis (which may be manifest only by localized pain) are the aerobic gram-negative bacilli, enterococci, and bowel anaerobes.[127] Therefore, the appearance of this infection in a patient already receiving broad-spectrum antibiotics will mandate the addition of antianaerobic agents, as well as a change in broad-spectrum coverage. Similarly, any suspected intra-abdominal site of infection should prompt the addition or inclusion of antibiotics active against aerobic gram-negative bacilli, enterococci, and bowel anaerobes.

In febrile and neutropenic patients who demonstrate abdominal pain, the possible development of typhlitis or pseudomembranous colitis should be considered. Typhlitis, a necrotizing inflammation of the cecum, presents as right lower quadrant pain and fullness but may progress to an acute abdomen with decreased bowel sounds, abdominal distension, and rebound.[356] Mortality is high, and the optimal therapy is controversial, but all patients should receive broad-spectrum antibiotics, specifically with coverage of *Enterococcus,* anaerobes, and gram-negative bacteria. Antibiotic-associated colitis has long been associated with the administration of a variety of antibiotics; the risk of its development may also be increased by antineoplastic agents. Consequently, neutropenic patients receiving broad-spectrum antibiotics are at high risk. Most cases are thought to be caused by a toxin produced by *C. difficile.*[357] The spectrum of disease caused by *C. difficile* may range from asymptomatic colonization or mild diarrhea to overt pseudomembranous colitis with peritoneal signs and extensive mucosal erosion.[358] Diagnosis should be made by documentation of toxin production, and therapy should be instituted with either oral vancomycin (125 mg qid) or oral metronidazole (250 mg qid). The treatment of *C. difficile*-associated disease in patients who cannot take oral medications is problematic. Intravenous vancomycin does not achieve sufficient levels within the colon to be effective, but intravenous metronidazole does achieve such concentrations, and successes with the latter approach have been reported.[359,360]

The development of an exit-site infection or cellulitis around an indwelling intravenous catheter is often caused by a gram-positive organism; if such an infection is noted, vancomycin should be added to the regimen, if not already included. Importantly, however, one must remember that neutropenic patients may be infected at any site by "atypical" organisms. Accordingly, for most new or progressive clinically documented infections, empirical changes should usually include modification

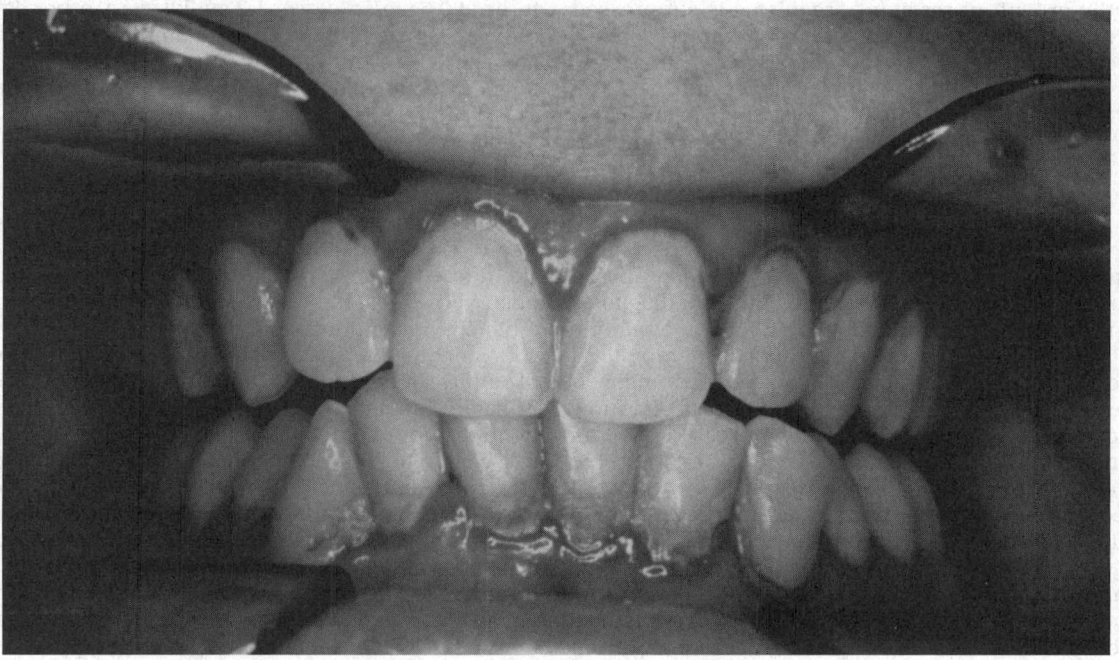

Fig. 91-3. Marginal gingivitis. Note well-demarcated red (dark) border on gingiva.

of the components directed at the gram-positive as well as those directed at the gram-negative bacteria.

The development of a new site of infection may also warrant the addition of other antibiotics directed at fungi, viruses, or parasites. Burning retrosternal pain is frequently an indication of esophagitis, most often caused by cytotoxic therapy, *Candida* infection, or HSV infection. Accordingly, empirical therapy with amphotericin B or acyclovir, or both, may be indicated (see the sections on herpes simplex and *Candida* infections). The development of pulmonary infiltrates might raise suspicion not only of resistant bacteria but also of *P. carinii*, fungi, or a viral pneumonia. In a neutropenic patient receiving broad-spectrum antibiotics who shows a new localized infiltrate, perhaps the first question to ask is whether the granulocyte count is rising. If so, the appearance of the "new" infiltrate may simply represent an inflammatory reaction at a previously unrecognized site of infection, and close observation without any modification may be appropriate.[361] If the granulocyte count is not rising and the patient has been neutropenic for only a short time (≤1 week), a bacterial process is most likely, and changes in the antibacterial coverage should be considered. If the patient has been persistently neutropenic for a more prolonged period, a fungal pneumonia should also be strongly considered and amphotericin B added while a diagnostic workup is initiated. The development of an interstitial infiltrate in a neutropenic patient should raise suspicion of a variety of infectious and noninfectious diagnoses. The most likely infectious causes of interstitial infiltrates are *P. carinii* and CMV, although a variety of other organisms, including bacteria (e.g., *Legionella*), other viruses, and fungi, should be considered. Appropriate modifications of therapy will depend on the presence or absence of other risk factors (e.g., BMT or administration of corticosteroids) and on the availability and feasibility of diagnostic tests such as sputum induction, bronchoalveolar lavage, or open lung biopsy (see Fig. 91-4 for approach to the cancer patient with pulmonary infiltrates).

Patients in whom hypotension develops while receiving broad-spectrum antibiotics should be presumed septic with a resistant organism or breakthrough infection. In these cases, changes in the empirical regimen should be made expeditiously and continued for the duration of treatment if an organism is not recovered. So-called culture-negative sepsis may occur when the growth of resistant organisms is suppressed by marginally effective antibiotics or when the cultures are not drawn during the bacteremic episode. In addition, it is likely that a variety of endogenous mediators (e.g., tumor necrosis factor) play a role in the associated cardiovascular changes, which often persist in the absence of identifiable bacteremia.

Empirical Antifungal Therapy

The rationale for empirical utilization of antifungal compounds is based on several observations. First, the diagnosis of even a disseminated fungal infection is difficult in an immunocompromised patient. Withholding antifungal therapy until a definitive clinical or microbiologic diagnosis is established frequently permits widespread dissemination. Second, it is now possible to identify subgroups of immunosuppressed patients who are at greatest risk of mycotic disease. Thus, neutropenic patients who remain persistently febrile despite a 4–7-day trial of broad-spectrum antibacterial therapy are particularly susceptible to fungal infection.[362,363] Finally, an accumulating body of data suggests that early institution of effective antifungal agents will improve the therapeutic outcome in immunocompromised patients with established mycoses.[364,365] Thus, use of an empirically based antifungal regimen might be expected to have a dual effect: suppression of fungal overgrowth that inevitably accompanies the administration of broad-spectrum

antibacterial agents, and early treatment of subclinical localized mycotic disease before dissemination has a chance to occur. Unfortunately neither the ideal antifungal agent nor the optimal time to initial empirical therapy is known.

Two prospective randomized studies were the first to demonstrate the efficacy of empirical amphotericin B in persistently febrile neutropenic patients.[362,366] In the NCI study,[362] patients who were granulocytopenic and persistently febrile without an identifiable infectious source were randomly assigned after 7 days of broad-spectrum antibacterial therapy to three study arms. In group I, all antibiotic therapy was discontinued; in group II, the broad-spectrum antibacterial agents were continued; and in group III, the antibacterial agents were continued and amphotericin B added (at a dosage of 0.5 mg/kg/day). Clinically or microbiologically proven infections (bacterial and fungal) occurred in 6 of the 16 patients in group I, in 6 of the 16 patients in group II, but in only 2 of the 18 patients in group III. Documented fungal infections occurred in one patient in group I (esophageal candidiasis), in five patients in group II (three with invasive candidiasis, one with disseminated aspergillosis, and one with a disseminated mixed *Candida* and *Aspergillus* infection), and in one patient in group III (a fatal pulmonary infection with *Petriellidium boydii*, an amphotericin B-resistant organism). Further confirmation of the beneficial role of empirical antifungal therapy was provided by consideration of the mean time to defervescence after day 7 randomization. Patients receiving empirical amphotericin B (group III), defervesced within 3–5 days. Patients remaining on antibiotics alone (group II) required 7–8 days to defervescence, while those randomized to discontinue all therapy (group I) required 11–12 days. Thus, this trial strongly suggested a beneficial role for empirical amphotericin B among high-risk patients.

The other randomized trial of empirical amphotericin B was performed by the European International Antimicrobial Therapy Cooperative Group.[366] This randomized multicenter trial examined the use of empirically administered amphotericin B in granulocytopenic patients who remained persistently febrile for 4 days despite administration of antibacterial antibiotics. Patients were divided into two groups: 68 randomly assigned to receive empirical amphotericin B and 64 assigned to continue the protocol antibiotics. Amphotericin B was administered at 0.6 mg/kg/day or 1.2 mg/kg every other day. Abatement of fever occurred in 69% of the amphotericin B-treated group and in 53% of the other group ($P = 0.09$). Six documented fungal infections, four of which were deemed severe, occurred in the 64 patients randomized not to receive empirical amphotericin B in comparison with only 1 patient with fungemia among the 68 treated empirically with amphotericin B ($P = 0.01$). No deaths occurred as a result of fungal infections in those receiving empirical amphotericin B versus four deaths due to fungal infections in those not receiving it ($P = 0.05$). No difference in overall survival between the two groups was observed. Two other retrospective evaluations also reported a benefit for amphotericin B.[363,367]

Despite further support and clinical evidence for the efficacy of empirical therapy with amphotericin B,[368,369] some clinicians remain reluctant to administer a potentially toxic agent to patients in whom a definitive diagnosis of a fungal infection has not been made. Fever, nephrotoxicity, chilling reactions, and electrolyte imbalances (especially hypokalemia) are frequently associated with amphotericin B; anemia, thrombocytopenia, and anaphylaxis have been noted less frequently.

A study at the NCI attempted to avoid the toxicity of amphotericin B yet provide empirical antifungal therapy with ketoconazole.[368] Seventy-two patients who remained neutropenic and febrile after 7 days of antimicrobial therapy were randomized to receive amphotericin B (0.5 mg/kg/day) or ketoconazole (800 mg/kg/day). The results were similar in terms of duration of

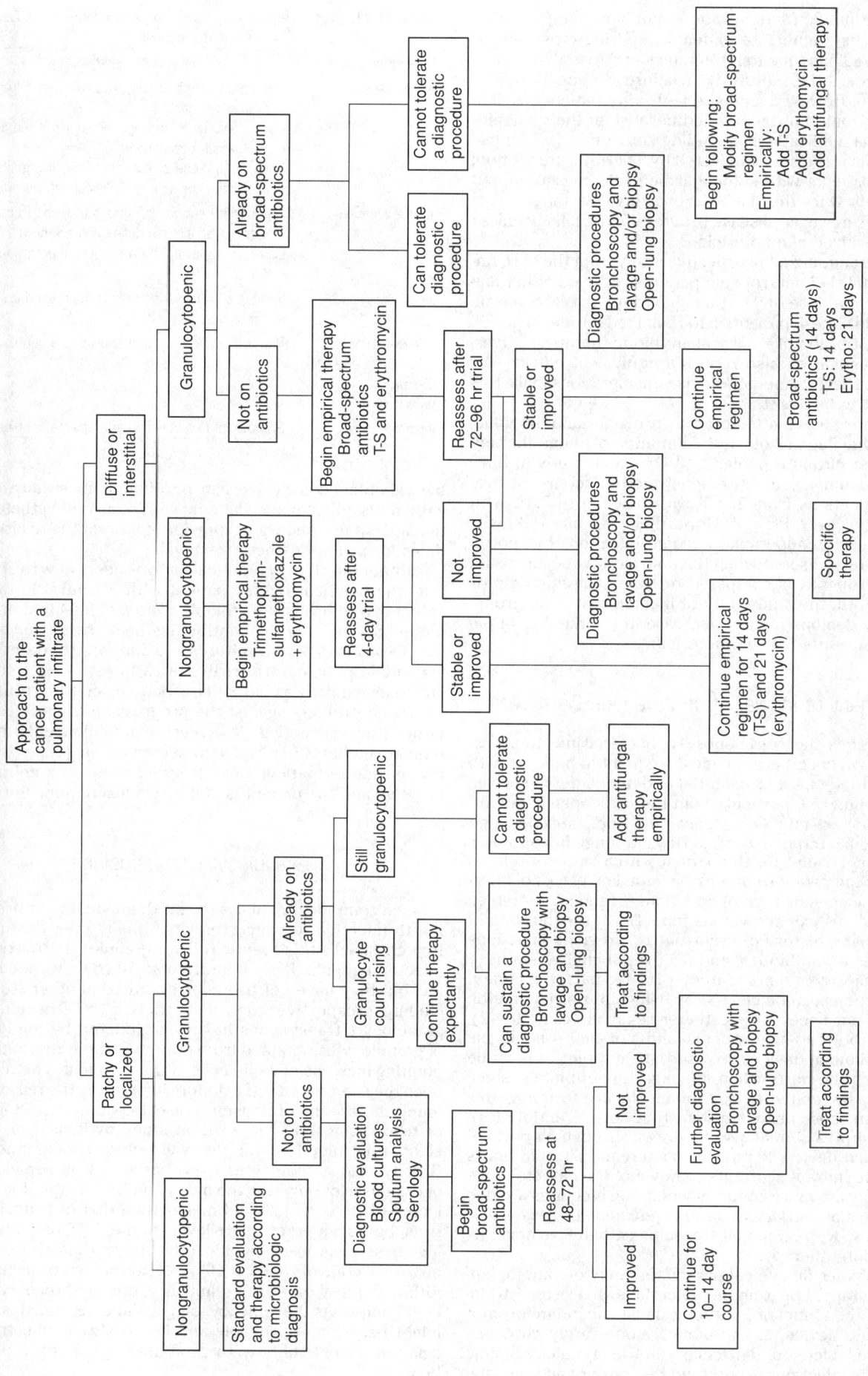

Fig. 91-4. Algorithm for the management of the cancer patient with a pulmonary infiltrate.

fever after antifungal randomization, number of documented fungal infections, number of patients requiring crossover to the alternate regimen due to intolerance, and overall outcome scored as success (i.e., survival) or failure (i.e., death due to fungal disease). However, almost one-third of patients eligible for this study could not be enrolled because of their inability to tolerate oral medications, including ketoconazole. The use of ketoconazole was also complicated by its erratic absorption; only 8 of 12 patients with ketoconazole peaks measured had adequate levels. Once the diagnosis of an invasive fungal infection was made, however, disease progression was likely unless the patient received amphotericin B.

In a similar randomized prospective study from the M.D. Anderson Hospital, 172 neutropenic patients received either amphotericin B (at a dose of 0.6–1.0 mg/kg/day) or ketoconazole (200 mg PO qid); these patients had remained febrile for 72–96 hours after institution of empirical antibiotic therapy.[370] Overall, these investigators also reported equivalent efficacy for both regimens. Several methodologic considerations make this study difficult to interpret.

Several centers have attempted to prevent candidal infections by starting fluconazole at the initiation of chemotherapy or at the onset of neutropenia.[274,371] One such study in BMT patients by Goodman et al.[274] demonstrated a decrease in invasive fungal infections from 15.8% with placebo to 2.8% with fluconazole. However, Philpott-Howard et al.[371] showed a significant decrease in superficial *Candida* infections but not in invasive candidial disease when fluconazole was begun at the onset of neutropenia as compared to either amphotericin or nystatin; or both; the study did not include a placebo group. Neither study demonstrated a decrease in the number of patients requiring empirical amphotericin.

Management of Indwelling Intravenous Catheters

While infections due to gram-positive bacterial infections (especially staphylococci) are the most frequent in patients with indwelling catheters, other bacterial and nonbacterial species are also encountered, particularly in the neutropenic patient. These include resistant *Corynebacterium* spp., *Bacillus* spp., gram-negative bacteria, mycobacteria, and fungi. In approaching management issues for the patient with a catheter-related infection, it is important to process several key pieces of information: (1) the specific type of infection, (2) the location (i.e., bacteremia versus exit site versus tunnel), (3) the duration of infection, (4) any history of recurrent or previous infections and responses to antibiotics, and (5) overall clinical status.

The vast majority of simple catheter-related bacteremias and exit-site infections can be cleared by using appropriate antibiotics and do not necessitate catheter removal (Table 91-12). This applies both to neutropenic and non-neutropenic patients. If multilumen devices are used, the antibiotics must be rotated among the ports when infusing the antibiotics, since infection may be limited to one lumen (failure to follow this procedure can cause persistent infection despite antibiotics). Diagnostic cultures should also be drawn through all ports of any multilumen device. Persistent bacteremia after 48 hours of appropriate therapy warrants removal of the catheter. Failures of therapy are more common when the infections are due to such organisms as *Bacillus* spp., *C. jeikeium*, or *C. albicans*; in these cases, we recommend prompt catheter removal as well as antibiotic therapy.

In addition, specific clinical parameters may dictate the approach to therapy. For example, infections that extend to involvement of the tunnel of a catheter usually mandate prompt removal of the device, as antibiotics alone rarely cure this "closed-space" infection, particularly in the granulocytopenic host. Likewise, infections around the reservoir of an implanta-

Table 91-12. Recommended Approaches to Central Intravenous Catheter-Related Infections

Type of Infection	Management
Most bacteremias	Appropriate antibiotic(s), depending on cultures and granulocyte status
	Rotate antibiotics through all lumina of the catheter if multilumen device used
	Removal of catheter if persistent cultures after 48 hr of therapy, or sooner if clinical deterioration
Exit site infections	Appropriate antibiotics; obtain cultures (remembering that not all exit-site infections are gram-positive)
	Catheter removal if no response or progression after 48 hr
Tunnel infections	Immediate removal of catheter and appropriate antibiotics
Bacillus spp. or *Corynebacterium jeikeium* infections	Removal of catheter and appropirate antibiotics
Fungemia	Removal of catheter and appropirate antibiotics

ble subcutaneous device can be difficult to eradicate if the catheter is still in place. Patients with recurrent catheter infections (despite a history of appropriate therapy) are also candidates for prompt catheter removal.

Another question of practical importance is how to approach a febrile non-neutropenic patient with a central intravenous catheter who has no identifiable source of infection on examination. Should empirical antibiotics be started? Our policy in this setting is to obtain cultures and start appropriate antibiotics; stable patients are treated with intravenous ceftriaxone and followed daily as outpatients pending culture results. This approach protects against the progression of undetected yet virulent infections (e.g., *S. aureus*), can minimize the need for ultimate catheter removal, and decreases hospital costs while maximizing outpatient time. If by 72 hours the cultures are negative and the patient is stable, we discontinue antibiotics.

Granulocyte Transfusions

Since granulocytopenia is the predominant factor predisposing to infection in cancer patients, many investigators have hypothesized a therapeutic role for granulocyte transfusion in infected patients. Early data from small trials were encouraging, but they have not been corroborated in other studies, including prospective controlled trials.[372–375] The efficacy of granulocyte transfusions has been hindered by the low yield of granulocytes obtained from donors and the resultant disappointing increase of white cells in the recipient. The result has been the need for multiple donors, increasing the risk of alloimmunization[376] and of transmission of infections (e.g., CMV[377,378] or toxoplasmosis).[379] In a recent study by Bensinger et al.,[378] eight white blood cell donors were given subcutaneous CSF-G daily, and granulocytes were harvested on a mean of 7.6 occasions. Not only was the mean number of granulocytes collected (41.6×10^9) sixfold higher than that of historical controls, but mean granulocyte levels in the BMT patients receiving these cells were significantly higher than those seen in historical controls (0.95×10^9 at 24 hours post-transfusion).[380] Although these data are preliminary, this method of collection could improve the efficacy of granulocyte transfusion and might permit more reliable and successful administration of cell component therapy to profoundly granulocytopenic patients.[381,382]

APPROACH TO THE NEUTROPENIC PATIENT WITH FEVER AND INFECTION

We define clinically relevant neutropenia as ≤500 polymorphonucleocytes and band forms per microliter or any count that is falling and expected to be <500 within 24 hours. Any fever in this population should be interpreted as potentially indicating serious infection (including those following administration of blood products). Conversely, even in the absence of fever, any subtle indication of infection should be considered potentially serious and treated as such. Fever is defined as one oral temperature reading over 38.5°C or more than two successive readings of ≥38°C in a 12-hour period.

Routine workup should include a complete history and physical examination, with particular attention directed towards sites that may "hide" infection, such as the mouth and perirectal area. At least two sets of blood cultures should be obtained (including one from a peripheral vein), with cultures drawn through each lumen of any multilumen intravenous access device. A urine culture and a chest radiograph should be obtained. Further workup should be delineated by the clinical presentation of the patient.

Empirical antibacterial therapy should be administered to all neutropenic patients with the new onset of fever or with clinical evidence of infection even in the absence of fever. There is no single best regimen; however, there are many inappropriate regimens. At a minimum, regimens should have broad-spectrum activity directed against gram-positive and gram-negative organisms (including *P. aeruginosa*). Aminoglycosides or extended-spectrum penicillins (e.g., ticarcillin, mezlocillin, piperacillin, azlocillin) should never be used as single agents or as the only agents with anti-gram-negative activity.

For most patients, we initiate single-agent empirical therapy (monotherapy). Of the antibiotics that are potentially useful for monotherapy, ceftazidime has been studied most extensively and has the longest track record of efficacy. While development of resistance to these agents has not been reported frequently, it must be monitored if they are used alone. Imipenem appears to be equally efficacious but is often associated with intolerance or toxicity. Nausea and vomiting with higher doses and seizures in susceptible patients have been reported.

The monobactam aztreonam is useful for patients with significant β-lactam allergies who still require the use of an antipseudomonal antibiotic in addition to an aminoglycoside. Accordingly, for patients with significant β-lactam allergies who present with fever and neutropenia we begin a combination of aztreonam plus an aminoglycoside plus vancomycin. Further study is warranted to see if aztreonam can suffice as the only anti-gram-negative component of empirical regimens (thus avoiding the use of an aminoglycoside).

Because the incidence of infection due to gram-positive organisms is increasing, the question of whether vancomycin should be included in the initial empirical regimen has been the subject of considerable debate. We do not routinely include it in initial therapy but reserve its use for specific clinical or microbiologic indications.

Clearly, for certain patients who present with a defined site of infection, the "standard" regimen should be individually modified. For example, for a neutropenic patient presenting with a perirectal abscess, coverage might be extended to include an antianaerobic agent (e.g., metronidazole or clindamycin), as well as an agent active against group D streptococci (e.g., vancomycin); for a neutropenic patient with Hickman catheter exit site infec-

tion, vancomycin might be added to extend gram-positive coverage.

For most neutropenic patients who present with fever, a microbiologically or clinically documented infectious etiology is not identified (i.e., they have FUO). For this group we prefer to continue empirical antibiotics until the resolution of neutropenia. However, this is not always practical, especially for those with prolonged neutropenia. Therefore, for persistently neutropenic patients with FUO who undergo defervescence and remain afebrile from days 7 to 14 (i.e., do not require empirical amphotericin B or other modifications), we discontinue antibiotics on day 14 and carefully observe. Depending on the amount of additional time they remain neutropenic, a substantial number may undergo recrudescence and require prompt resumption of empirical therapy.

For patients who present with a documented infection, we continue therapy for a minimum of 10–14 days, even if the granulocytopenia resolves before this time. If the infection has been identified microbiologically, we switch to narrower-spectrum therapy to complete the course at the resolution of granulocytopenia. However, if no isolate is obtained, we continue broad-spectrum coverage for the duration of treatment.

Common modifications in antibacterials include changes in gram-negative coverage for potentially resistant organisms and addition of intravenous vancomycin for improved gram-positive coverage or of oral vancomycin for *C. difficile,* and addition of clindamycin or metronidazole to improve anaerobic coverage.

For patients with a persistent or new fever after ≥7 days of empirical antibacterial therapy, we begin empirical amphotericin B and continue it along with the antibacterial agents until the resolution of neutropenia. Following an initial test dose of 1 mg over 1 hour, we proceed directly to 0.5 mg/kg/day (without dose escalation). Adequate hydration and diuresis (saliuresis) are important in limiting resultant azotemia. However, patients requiring long courses of amphotericin B will invariably have some rise in BUN and creatinine, which usually stabilizes. Assuming good hydration and no other complicating factors, such modest elevations should not prompt a routine dose reduction in amphotericin B. Most patients will normalize following completion of therapy.

Acyclovir is the most common antiviral agent added in neutropenic patients and may be directed toward HSV or VZV. Trimethoprim sulfamethoxazole is the most common antiparasitic agent added, with activity directed primarily against *P. carinii.*

Although gram-positive organisms will cause most infections associated with central venous catheters, gram-negative organisms are not infrequently encountered. Neutropenic patients who present with even a mild exit site infection should receive broad-spectrum coverage directed at gram-positive and gram-negative organisms, including *P. aeruginosa.*

More than 90% of catheter-related bacteremias can be successfully treated with antibiotics alone without the need for catheter removal. Initial cultures should be drawn through all lumina or any multilumen device, and antibiotic administration should be rotated among the ports. Persistent positive cultures or progression of infection after 24–48 hours of appropriate antibiotics mandates prompt catheter removal. Other indications for initial catheter removal are infection caused by *Bacillus* spp., *Corynebacterium jeikeium,* any tunnel infection (extending to >2 cm from the exit site), and candidemia.

CLINICAL APPROACH TO FUNGAL INFECTIONS IN IMMUNOCOMPROMISED PATIENTS

The most common fungal infections encountered in immuno-compromised patients are those due to *Candida* spp., *Aspergillus* spp., and *C. neoformans*. Serious invasive *Candida* and *Aspergillus* infections are seen most often in granulocytopenic patients, although other populations may also be at risk. Infections due to *C. neoformans* are more common in patients with altered cellular immunity, and HIV-infected patients now constitute the largest group at significant risk of this infection.

Infections Due to *Candida* Species

Oropharyngeal Candidiasis

Of all *Candida* infections seen in the immunosuppressed population, oral candidiasis, or thrush, is most often encountered. Patients with cell-mediated immune deficits are particularly susceptible to the development of oropharyngeal and esophageal candidiasis. The clinical importance of oropharyngeal *Candida* infections in immunocompromised patients is threefold. First, locally invasive disease may be painful, especially when it occurs in association with mucositis or oral HSV infection. Second, oropharyngeal infection may be a harbinger of more serious mucosal disease affecting other sites, including the epiglottis, esophagus, or lower gastrointestinal tract. Finally, it may serve as a nidus for the development of fungemia and disseminated disease, particularly in granulocytopenic patients with concurrent mucosal disruption.

The presumptive diagnosis of oropharyngeal candidiasis is often relatively easy to make by visual examination. In most cases, characteristic creamy white patches appear on the mucosal surfaces, which can be friable and which bleed easily when scraped. Wet-mount examination of scrapings will show typical yeast forms. However, the definitive diagnosis is often elusive because other local processes such as HSV or noninfectious mucositis may be clinically and visually indistinguishable. While oral swabs for microscopic examination or fungal culture are often positive, even patients without thrush are likely to be colonized by *Candida* and to have positive smears or cultures. Similarly, positive oral cultures for HSV do not rule out the potential for concomitant *Candida* infection.

Therapeutic approaches include a number of options. First, for asymptomatic patients at relatively low risk of disseminated *Candida* (e.g., those who are nongranulocytopenic or who have a short expected duration of granulocytopenia), specific therapy may not be warranted. Many of these infections will clear spontaneously after the return of the granulocytes or discontinuation of antibiotic or immunosuppressive therapy, or both. Therapy should be considered for patients who are chronically immunosuppressed (e.g., AIDS patients), who have significant symptoms (usually pain), or who are at relatively high risk of dissemination (e.g., granulocytopenic). Potential therapeutic drugs include oral nonabsorbable antifungal agents (e.g., nystatin or clotrimazole), oral absorbable antifungal agents (e.g., fluconazole, ketoconazole), and amphotericin B. Both nystatin and clotrimazole can be effective in the treatment of thrush, although clotrimazole appears to be better tolerated, and prophylactic studies suggest its superior efficacy.[383–386] Nystatin is usually administered in doses of 100,000 U three to six times per day, and clotrimazole troches are administered five times per day.

If no symptomatic response occurs after a trial of nonabsorbable agents, or if the condition of the patient precludes administration of oral agents, treatment with systemic antifungal agents may be warranted, depending on the severity of the symptoms and the degree of immunosuppression. In addition, failure to respond to nonabsorbable agents with symptomatic

progression should alert the clinician to the potential existence of more serious or more extensive *Candida* infection, as well as to the possibility of nonfungal processes, such as HSV infection or mucositis induced by cytotoxic therapy. Accordingly, appropriate diagnostic studies, including culture of oral lesions for HSV, should be initiated (see the section on approach to viral infections). Certain cases may warrant concomitant empirical antiviral therapy with acyclovir.

Oropharyngeal candidiasis refractory to nonabsorbable agents may be treated with fluconazole or amphotericin B. Fluconazole at a dose of 100 mg qid has been shown to be as effective as ketoconazole but has the advantages of absorption independent of gastric pH and of availability in oral and intravenous formulations.[387] For oropharyngeal candidiasis in granulocytopenic patients that is either severe or unresponsive to other agents, amphotericin B at relatively low doses (e.g., 0.3 mg/kg/day) may be effective. We prefer to administer 0.5–0.6 mg/kg/day in neutropenic patients and to continue therapy until the granulocyte count has resolved.

Esophageal Candidiasis

Esophageal candidiasis is a locally invasive infection of the esophagus caused by *Candida* spp. The infection usually remains localized in nongranulocytopenic patients.[388] Significant granulocytopenia may predispose patients with esophageal candidiasis to submucosal vascular invasion as disseminated disease. The most common site of infection is the distal third of the esophagus, perhaps because *Candida* grows especially well in acidic environments. Many of the principles of diagnosis and management of thrush apply to esophageal candidiasis.

The diagnosis of esophageal candidiasis requires a high index of suspicion in susceptible hosts. Burning pain localized to the retrosternal or epigastric areas is the most commonly reported symptom. Its presence in the appropriate host should alert the clinician to the possibility of this diagnosis. The pain is often aggravated by swallowing and may also be associated with dysphagia localized to the site of maximal involvement. However, even significant esophageal candidiasis may be asymptomatic.[389–391]

The physical examination is usually not helpful in establishing the diagnosis of esophageal candidiasis. While patients often have either visibly apparent or symptomatic oropharyngeal involvement, or both, the absence of thrush does not rule out the diagnosis, since the distal esophagus may be the only focus of disease. Conversely, the presence of even severe thrush in a patient with burning retrosternal pain does not establish the diagnosis of esophageal candidiasis, since other processes could be operative. Signs suggestive of oral HSV infection or of chemotherapy-related mucositis may suggest other etiologies but are not diagnostic and do not rule out the presence of a mixed process. For example, patients may present with severe oral HSV infection and concomitant esophageal candidiasis, or vice versa.

In terms of diagnostic tests, oral smears or cultures for fungus or HSV may be suggestive but are not diagnostic. Mouth cultures for *Candida* are virtually never helpful because of the high rate of colonization, even in the absence of infection. If oral lesions suggestive of HSV infection are apparent, cultures should be obtained. Importantly, positive oral cultures for HSV do not establish the diagnosis of HSV esophagitis, nor do negative cultures rule it out. Barium swallows or upper gastrointestinal series may be helpful in establishing or ruling out certain noninfectious processes, such as gastroesophageal reflux or peptic ulcer disease. They may also reveal mucosal irregularities suggestive of *Candida* esophagitis (e.g., "cobblestoning") but are not helpful in establishing the definitive diagnosis.[392]

Only endoscopic biopsy with culture and histologic tissue examination can establish the diagnosis of esophageal candidiasis with certainty and at the same time diagnose or rule out other processes. Endoscopic examination without biopsy may suggest a diagnosis on the basis of visual appearance and culture results. However, similarities in the visual appearance of different lesions, coupled with the nonspecificity of culture results from specimens obtained noninvasively, detract from the clinical value of this procedure. Unfortunately, not all patients are able to tolerate an endoscopic biopsy. The most clinically relevant complications of esophagoscopy with biopsy are bacteremia and bleeding. Both complications are more common in patients who have received cytotoxic therapy and who are granulocytopenic or thrombocytopenic, or both.

Accordingly, in granulocytopenic patients showing symptoms and signs consistent with esophageal candidiasis, we initiate empirical therapy directed at *Candida* and/or HSV and reserve endoscopic biopsy for patients refractory to therapy or for those in whom empirical therapy with amphotericin B is relatively contraindicated (e.g., patients with renal insufficiency or amphotericin B intolerance). For noncytopenic patients, the decision to employ endoscopic esophageal biopsy should be predicated on the relative risks and benefits of the procedure within the context of the degree of immunosuppression, ease of empirical therapy, and response or lack of response to selected agents. Patients who are granulocytopenic, who are receiving other aggressive immunosuppressive regimens (e.g., corticosteroids, total body irradiation, antithymocyte globulin), or who otherwise have a high propensity for the dissemination of *Candida* and who have documented esophageal candidiasis or have failed an initial empirical trial of oral nonabsorbable agents are candidates for therapy with intravenous amphotericin B. Amphotericin B should be administered intravenously at a dosage of 0.5–0.6 mg/kg/day. For neutropenic patients, it should be continued at least until resolution of neutropenia. In patients in whom resolution of granulocytopenia is unlikely to occur (e.g., patients with aplastic anemia who have not responded to therapy), we administer amphotericin B for ≥2 weeks of therapy (about 500 mg total dose for most adults or 10 mg/kg for children). If symptoms have resolved and the patient is afebrile and clinically stable, we discontinue amphotericin B and watch closely for the return of symptomatology. In high-risk patients, particularly those with fever and granulocytopenia, the clinician should also consider the potential presence of clinically occult diffuse gastrointestinal and/or disseminated candidiasis.

Granulocytopenic patients with clinical symptoms of infective esophagitis who are not candidates for endoscopy are often candidates for presumptive or empirical therapy. At the NCI, if such patients have only mild to moderate symptoms and are clinically stable, a 3-day trial of clotrimazole troches (five times per day) is initiated. In patients with more severe symptoms or those whose symptoms fail to respond to, or worsen with, clotrimazole, amphotericin B is initiated at the doses outlined above. In addition, in patients in whom definitive diagnostic procedures are not feasible, treatment with acyclovir is often initiated as a logical extension of empirical amphotericin B therapy. In patients with active herpetic stomatitis, we usually initiate acyclovir (250 mg/m² tid) simultaneously with empirical antifungal therapy. For those patients without clinical evidence of HSV infection, we begin acyclovir if there is no response to initial antifungal agents.

Symptomatic patients who are not at high risk of disseminated candidiasis but who are unable to swallow oral medications are also candidates for intravenous amphotericin B. Nongranulocytopenic symptomatic patients who are clinically stable and who have no apparent foci of *Candida* beyond the esophageal mucosa may benefit from lower dosages of amphotericin B (0.1–0.3 mg/kg/day).[393] Many can be treated successfully with a total amphotericin dose of only 2–5 mg/kg over 1–2 weeks.

Most ambulatory patients with AIDS, solid tumors, or other non-neoplastic diseases who have esophageal candidiasis respond favorably to fluconazole at oral dosages of 100–200 mg once daily.[394] Nonabsorbable agents such as nystatin and clotrimazole can also be effective in this population.[395] In AIDS patients, esophageal candidiasis is often a chronically recurrent process, as are many of the fungal and protozoal infections. Accordingly, some form of chronic suppressive antifungal therapy is often desirable in this population. Suppressive regimens that can be effective in selected patients include oral fluconazole (50–100 mg/day), nystatin suspension (500,000–1.5 million U, 5–15 ml, PO qid), or clotrimazole troches (10 mg five times a day dissolved slowly in the mouth). Relapse of esophageal candidiasis during maintenance oral therapy may require institution of intravenous amphotericin B and should prompt the physician to consider other causes of infective esophagitis.

Approach to the Patient with Candidemia

Candidemia is associated with high morbidity and mortality and may be a harbinger of disseminated *Candida* infection. Candidemia is seen almost exclusively in patients with significant impairment in host defense. Those at highest risk are neutropenic patients receiving broad-spectrum antibacterial agents. Other populations in whom candidemia and disseminated candidiasis occurs include transplant recipients, postsurgical patients, burn victims, low-birthweight neonates, patients with indwelling intravenous catheters, and those receiving hyperalimentation.[396]

Between 1977 and 1984, the estimated incidence of hospital-acquired bloodstream infections caused by *Candida* spp. tripled in the United States from 0.5 to 1.5 per 10,000 admissions.[397,398] Estimates from large teaching hospitals have been as high as 8.5 per 10,000 admissions, with candidemia accounting for up to 10% of nosocomial bloodstream infections.[399] A study from Memorial Sloan-Kettering Hospital in New York conducted during 1978–1982 showed a 31% increase in fungemia in cancer patients (predominantly due to *Candida* spp.), as compared with the 1974–1977 period.[400] The mortality attributable to candidemia has been 21–52%.[399,401,402] Candidemia increases the average length of hospital stay by 30 days.[399]

Candidemia usually occurs in patients who have been hospitalized for some time. In the study by Horn et al.,[400] the average period of hospitalization before the onset of candidemia was 20 days. In addition, the first positive blood cultures were obtained after a mean of 11.7 days of neutropenia and a mean of 11.8 days of antibiotics. Fever is often the only sign; its presence in a susceptible host, in the absence of other etiologies, should always raise the possibility of fungal infection. Other signs that can occur with early candidemia include embolic skin lesions, which in some series have occurred more commonly with *C. tropicalis,* and diffuse myalgias, which may be indicative of *Candida* myositis.[400,403] A large percentage of immunocompromised patients with candidemia will have disseminated candidiasis; signs referable to involvement of specific organ systems (e.g., eye, central nervous system, heart valves, liver, and spleen) should also be sought.

In an immunosuppressed patient in whom a blood culture is reported positive for *Candida* spp., the following clinical approach seems prudent on the basis of current knowledge. A positive blood culture should rarely, if ever, be considered due to a contaminant. Culture contamination probably occurs far less frequently than does true candidemia in a susceptible host. In addition, even viscerally disseminated candidiasis is associated with a low incidence of positive blood cultures. Accordingly, there is a danger in waiting for a second "confirmatory" culture before taking action, as it can yield negative results in the face of significant disease.

Central venous catheters, arterial catheters for monitoring blood pressure, and hyperalimentation lines have all been associated with increased risk of candidemia and may be considered independent risk factors for disseminated infection.[404-406] If the patient does not have a catheter in place, an endogenous source should be assumed, and the likelihood of disseminated disease can be even higher. These patients should receive antifungal therapy as outlined below. If the patient does have a catheter, it is difficult to determine whether a positive blood culture represents an infection limited to the lumen or to the surface of the catheter itself or whether the organisms were drawn from the circulation. If quantitative culture techniques are available (e.g., the lysis-centrifugation method) and simultaneous cultures have been obtained peripherally and through the catheter, a higher number of colonies obtained through the catheter (or a positive culture exclusively drawn through the catheter) may indicate an infection localized to the catheter. However, because *Candida* adheres avidly to plastic surfaces, an infection that appears to be originating from the catheter could simply represent locally proliferating organisms that adhered to the catheter during a period of candidemia.

The decision as to whether to remove intravascular catheters from patients with candidemia is both difficult and controversial. Although some recommend catheter removal only in cases of thrombophlebitis or disseminated infection, the catheter may represent a nidus for infection and a source for dissemination. In one study, only 11 patients of 155 with fungemia and central intravascular lines were treated without removal of the line; of these, 9 were treatment failures in spite of receiving >500 mg of amphotericin B.[402] In addition, it is difficult to predict which patients can be successfully treated with the catheter in place, and such treatment delays can be costly. Therefore, we favor prompt removal of all indwelling intravenous catheters in this setting.

All patients with impaired host defenses and documented candidemia should undergo evaluation for dissemination of disease. Documentation of disseminated disease will mandate aggressive and often protracted therapy. The most common sites of dissemination are the eye (endophthalmitis), skin, liver, and spleen. Evaluation for disseminated disease should include careful ophthalmologic examination, examination of the skin, and imaging studies of the liver and spleen. It is important to realize that in the neutropenic host, assessment of the eyes, liver, and spleen can show negative results, even in the face of widespread dissemination.[407,408] This presumably reflects that the lesions visualized by direct examination or imaging studies largely represent an inflammatory reaction. Accordingly, meaningful assessment of disseminated disease in neutropenic patients with candidemia is probably best accomplished after recovery of the granulocytes. Patients with candidemia of >7 days' duration should be assumed to have disseminated disease.

The next question to address is whether a patient with candidemia and an indwelling intravenous catheter (but without evidence of dissemination) should receive antifungal therapy after removal of the catheter or whether catheter removal alone will suffice. Most authorities recommend that all episodes of candidemia in this population be treated with a course of antifungal therapy. Data to support this rationale and approach have been reported in retrospective series that have documented an increased incidence of disseminated *Candida* infection at autopsy in patients with prior candidemia who were not treated with amphotericin B, as compared with those who were so treated.[402] In another study, 4 of 33 patients with candidemia that was believed to be catheter related treated only by catheter removal (and not with amphotericin B) developed *Candida* endophthalmitis, diagnosed 8–66 days after the last positive blood culture.

Intravenous amphotericin B is the accepted treatment with the best efficacy in the management of *Candida* bloodstream infections. In patients without evidence of disseminated disease, we administer a test dose of 1 mg and then proceed directly to 0.5 mg/kg/day. Because *C. tropicalis* and *C. parapsolosis* may be more amphotericin B-resistant than other *Candida* spp., if either is isolated we administer amphotericin B at a dose of 1 mg/kg/day and consider the addition of flucytosine. There is no evidence that a stepwise escalation of dose to the targeted daily dose decreases toxicity, and a recent double-blind randomized trial comparing initial full doses with stepwise escalation showed no statistical difference in toxicity between the two regimens.[409] No data are available to delineate the most appropriate duration of therapy. We currently administer a minimal course for a total of 10 mg/kg or about 500 mg (about 2 weeks of therapy in most adults). If the patient is neutropenic at the time the isolate is obtained, we continue amphotericin B at least until recovery of the granulocyte count to $\geq 500/mm^3$, even if the 500 mg total dose is achieved before that time. Neutropenic patients should also be evaluated for disseminated disease ≥ 1 week after recovery of the granulocyte count. Persistent fever, localizing symptoms, or elevation of liver function tests (particularly alkaline phosphatase) after recovery of the granulocyte count should suggest the possibility of disseminated *Candida* infection.

If candidemia continues in spite of amphotericin, we add flucytosine (100–150 mg/kg/day) with careful monitoring of blood levels. There is little evidence that the addition of an azole antifungal agent will be of benefit in this situation, but this may be considered after other treatment options have failed.[410] However, fluconazole may have a role as monotherapy in treatment of patients with candidemia but with a low probability of disseminated *Candida* infection.

Candida Endophthalmitis

Candida endophthalmitis (CE) is a relatively common complication of candidemia. Montgomerie and Edwards[411] found that 5 of 25 patients receiving hyperalimentation developed ocular lesions clinically consistent with CE. The lesions of CE are white, resemble cotton balls in appearance, and involve the chorioretina, from which they rapidly extend into the vitreous. In the appropriate setting, they often indicate not only infection of the eye but also widespread dissemination to other organs, the number of ocular lesions observed funduscopically correlating with the extent of disseminated visceral infection.[412] It must be remembered that eye lesions may not be recognized in granulocytopenic patients.[413] Of the various *Candida* species, *C. albicans* appears to have a predilection for eye involvement.[414] Recognition of these lesions mandates a search for other locations of disseminated disease and expeditious treatment with amphotericin B, since CE can cause irreversible loss of vision or complete blindness in the involved eye. In selected cases, partial vitrectomy may also be helpful both diagnostically and therapeutically.[396] Adult patients with CE should probably receive a minimum total dose of 1.5–2.0 g of amphotericin B, with continuation of therapy at least until resolution of the ophthalmologic findings. Strong consideration should be given to the addition of flucytosine, especially in cases with perimacular involvement. If coexistent disseminated disease is found at other sites, even more prolonged therapy may be required.

Hepatosplenic Candidiasis

Only since about 1980 has hepatosplenic candidiasis or chronic disseminated candidiasis been recognized as an important clinical entity in the immunosuppressed host.[407,415-417] It is most commonly seen in patients who have had prolonged or recurrent episodes of neutropenia. Presumably it results from hematogenous dissemination, and therefore all patients with documented candidemia should be evaluated for hepatosplenic involvement. Importantly, however, only a few patients with documented hepatosplenic candidiasis will have had preceding candidemia. One must be aware of the signs and symptoms suggestive of this diagnosis, even in the absence of positive fungal blood cultures.

Four findings should raise the suspicion of hepatosplenic candidiasis in patients who have, or have recently recovered from, episodes of neutropenia, whether seen alone or in concert[407,416,417]: (1) persistent fever after recovery of the granulocyte count, which is unresponsive to standard antimicrobial therapy; (2) "rebound" leukocytosis; (3) elevated serum alkaline phosphatase; and (4) abdominal pain.

In a 1988 report, Thaler and colleagues[407] reviewed their experience with 8 cases of hepatosplenic candidiasis seen at the NCI, as well as 65 other cases that were diagnosed antemortem and reported in the literature. Of the 73 patients, 68 had been neutropenic. In 87%, the underlying diagnosis was acute leukemia, with only 3 patients having neutropenia due to aplastic anemia. The clinical findings and laboratory abnormalities became apparent only after recovery of the granulocytes to normal levels, and none of the patients was diagnosed while neutropenic. Fever was a presenting symptom in 85% of patients and abdominal pain in 57%. An elevation of the serum alkaline phosphatase was the most consistent biochemical abnormality. Serum transaminases and bilirubin were usually normal. Leukocytosis was present in 31%, and 50% had received prior antifungal therapy. With regard to imaging studies, ultrasound and CT were both helpful in visualizing the lesions, and there was a suggestion that CT might be more sensitive and ultrasound more specific (with the appearance of the characteristic "bullseye" pattern (Fig. 91-5). Magnetic resonance imaging (MRI) may prove more helpful, as even smaller lesions may be detectable.

The definitive diagnosis can be established only by histologic or microbiologic methods. Grossly, the liver and spleen are usually studded with white to yellow nodules of 1–2 cm. The earliest histologic appearance of the invasive *Candida* lesion is an abscess composed of a necrotic center surrounded by an intense acute inflammatory infiltrate. Because the yeast forms and pseudohyphae often are only in the center of the abscess, serial sections and special stains are frequently needed to show their presence. As the lesion ages, the polymorphonuclear inflammatory cells mix with mononuclear cells, and a peripheral fibrous proliferation begins to wall off the lesion. As healing occurs, this proliferation progresses to a well-defined granuloma with occasional giant cells. Because resolved or resolving lesions may coexist with more acute lesions, the absence of organisms on a liver biopsy should not be considered evidence that invasive candidiasis has resolved if there

is clinical evidence to the contrary. It is important to realize that the culture of the liver specimen will often be negative even if yeast and pseudohyphae are visualized. In the review by Thaler et al.,[407] biopsy material was cultured in 45 patients and was negative in 26. Of the 26 patients who received antifungal therapy before the biopsy, cultures were negative in 18. Of the 18 patients who did not receive antecedent antifungal therapy, fungal cultures were negative in 7. Of the 31 *Candida* isolates in this review, 20 were *C. albicans*, 6 were *C. tropicalis*, 1 was *C. pseudotropicalis*, and 1 was *C. stellatoidea*, and in 3 patients the species of *Candida* isolate was not determined. The decision of whether to perform a liver biopsy depends on the ability of the patient to withstand the procedure safely and on the degree of clinical suspicion for the diagnosis of hepatosplenic candidiasis as opposed to other possible diagnoses. In general, we prefer to make a histologic or microbiologic diagnosis, if at all possible.

For the treatment of hepatosplenic candidiasis, amphotericin B, either alone or in combination with 5-flucytosine (5-FC), is the most appropriate therapy. The NCI review found a wide range in the total dose of administered amphotericin B, from 0.7 to >9.0 g.[407] Autopsy data indicated that patients who received <2 g of amphotericin B had residual disease; those receiving more either were living or had no evidence of *Candida* infection on autopsy. Accordingly, we treat all patients with ≥2 g of amphotericin B. In the absence of clearly defined end points, we continue amphotericin B until resolution of all radiographic evidence of disease, performing follow-up studies at monthly intervals, or more frequently if clinically indicated. Fever, leukocytosis, and alkaline phosphatase can also be helpful in assessing response in individual cases. We routinely employ a daily dose of 0.5–1 mg/kg of amphotericin B, with the higher doses used for documented *C. tropicalis*, failure of response to lower doses, or cases in which amphotericin B is used as a single agent (i.e., without concomitant 5-FC). The total amount required will vary dramatically from patient to patient but may be as high as ≥10 g in individual cases. We routinely add 5-FC to the therapy for at least the first month, carefully monitoring serum levels.[418] In patients with normal renal function, we begin with a total daily dose of 100 mg/kg and carefully monitor serum levels to avoid toxicity (aiming for a serum level in the range of 50–100 μg/ml). More recently, studies have suggested that the use of liposomal encapsulated amphotericin B may allow for delivery of larger doses with less toxicity.[419] In one multicenter trial of liposomal amphotericin B, 23 immunocompromised patients who experienced nephrotoxicity with conventional amphotericin or who had baseline renal dysfunction were treated for invasive *Candida* infection with the liposomal form.[420] In 19 (82%) of these patients, the infection was eradicated, and 2 other patients showed improvement.

Although experience is limited, fluconazole has been useful in the treatment of hepatosplenic candidiasis which has been refractory to amphotericin B therapy.[421,422] In one study, six patients with leukemia and hepatosplenic candidiasis who had received ≤4 g of amphotericin without resolution of infection were treated with fluconazole (200–400 mg/day).[421] All patients achieved resolution of fever and of other symptoms within 2–8 weeks and CT scan improvement within 4–8 weeks. A second study of patients who either did not improve with, or who were intolerant of, amphotericin demonstrated response to fluconazole treatment in 14 of 16 cases.[422] Since there is both limited data and reports of treatment failure with the use of fluconazole as the initial treatment of hepatosplenic candidiasis, we initially treat all patients with amphotericin B.[423]

A practical question that often arises with many patients diagnosed as having hepatosplenic candidiasis is whether chemotherapy can be safely continued during the course of antifungal therapy. It is our policy to continue antifungal ther-

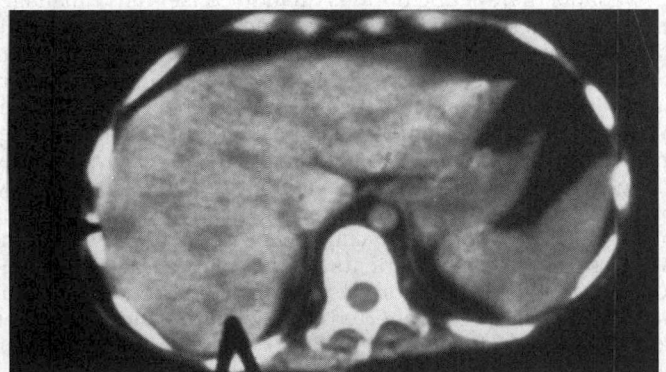

Fig. 91-5. CT scan showing typical lesions of hepatic candidiasis.

apy and chemotherapy cycles simultaneously, watching closely for progression of fungal disease. New fevers during neutropenic episodes are managed in a standard fashion, with the addition of empirical broad-spectrum antibacterial agents. For patients who have completed antifungal therapy (with radiographic resolution of hepatosplenic disease) and who require further chemotherapy, we do not institute amphotericin automatically at the onset of neutropenia. Instead, we begin amphotericin B concomitantly with empirical antibacterial agents at the onset of fever and rigorously observe for signs or symptoms that suggest recrudescence of disseminated disease.

Candida Infections of the Genitourinary Tract

The major risk factors for the development of *Candida* urinary tract infection are the use of an indwelling urinary catheter, administration of broad-spectrum antibiotics, and diabetes mellitus. The kidney was the most frequently involved organ in some autopsy series of disseminated *Candida* infection,[424] and candiduria may be a sign of disseminated disease in the appropriate setting.

Clinically, the most commonly encountered situation is a urinalysis showing yeast or a positive urine culture for *Candida*. In immunocompetent patients without predisposing conditions, this often represents contamination from *Candida* colonizing the external urogenital tract. In addition, *Candida* spp. were isolated from the urine of 8% of normal males and 12% of normal females in one series.[425] In patients with urinary tract symptoms, an indwelling catheter, or immune impairment, the finding of candiduria may be more significant. The most difficult problem is in differentiating between bladder or catheter colonization and true infection. As a general rule, pyuria in non-neutropenic patients and/or symptoms of urinary tract infection in the absence of other etiologies should indicate the potential for true infection due to *Candida*. Quantitative colony counts are of little value in determining the significance of candiduria. No laboratory test definitively distinguishes between upper and lower tract infection, but abdominal CT scans can be helpful and should be done in patients at risk of disseminated disease.

In patients who have indwelling bladder catheters, the simplest and most effective means of eradicating the *Candida* is removal of the catheter. However, certain groups of non-neutropenic patients may benefit from additional therapy aimed at local eradication, including (1) those with symptoms that fail to resolve with catheter removal or for whom catheter removal is not feasible; (2) those with upper urinary tract abnormalities (e.g., history of papillary necrosis or ongoing urinary tract obstruction) in whom there is a more significant risk of the development of ascending infection; (3) those with candiduria who will require urinary tract procedures such as transurethral resection of the prostate or chemotherapy for bladder cancer; and (4) those with persistent candiduria who are about to receive aggressive systemic cytotoxic therapy for ensuing neutropenia. For these patients with disease believed to be confined to the lower urinary tract, amphotericin B bladder washes can prove effective. Doses of 100 mg in 500 ml of D_5W or in sterile water may be instilled and removed once or twice daily. The potential use of a single intravenous dose of amphotericin B in these settings has been suggested, but there are insufficient data to support this approach. The use of 5-FC alone is not recommended because of the potential for the rapid emergence of resistance. Of a fluconazole dose 70% is excreted unchanged into the urine and can provide an alternative to amphotericin in non-neutropenic patients.[426] In addition, the ease of administration and relative lack of toxicity make fluconazole an attractive alternative for chronic suppression of candiduria; however, physicians must be alert for the

potential for *Torulopsis glabrata* superinfection because of its resistance to fluconazole.

Other groups of patients may require systemic amphotericin B. Clearly, patients (usually neutropenic) with renal involvement attributed to hematogenous spread require treatment with intravenous amphotericin B as well as assessment of other sites for disseminated disease. Neutropenic patients with persistent or symptomatic candiduria should also be considered for systemic therapy. In granulocytopenic patients, persistent candiduria may pose a risk of subsequent dissemination or, rarely, may be the first sign of established visceral involvement.

Infections Due to *Aspergillus* Species

In non-HIV-infected immunocompromised patients, *Aspergillus* spp. are the second most commonly encountered fungal pathogens. *A. fumigatus* and *A. flavus* account for the vast majority of human infections, with infections due to *A. niger* or other species reported only rarely. Serious invasive infections due to *Aspergillus* spp. occur most frequently in patients with prolonged granulocytopenia or patients receiving high doses of corticosteroids.[427-430]

Aspergillomas

The term aspergilloma refers to colonization of a pulmonary cavity by *Aspergillus* spp. Aspergillomas can be either primary or secondary. Primary aspergillomas tend to follow granulocyte recovery in patients who have had an episode of invasive pulmonary aspergillosis during a period of granulocytopenia. Pathophysiologically, this results from a walling off of the infection associated with the inflammatory response generated by PMN.

Clinically, the most common symptom encountered is hemoptysis, occurring to some degree in ≤75% of patients.[431] It can range in severity from intermittent blood-tinged sputum to massive pulmonary hemorrhage with exsanguination. In most patients who have not developed the initial infection in the setting of granulocytopenia, the lesions are usually solitary, with radiographs typically demonstrating a round or oval mass overlaid by a crescent of air (Monad's sign)[432] (Fig. 91-6). Sputum cultures may be positive for *Aspergillus* in approximately 50% of cases and may be highly suggestive of the diagnosis in the appropriate setting, but they are neither sensitive nor specific. In patients suspected of having aspergilloma, serum should be sent for determination of *Aspergillus* precipitins, which were positive in 92% of 66 patients tested in one review of 10 reported series.[431] However, serologic tests for the diagnosis of *Aspergillus* remain experimental and are not commercially available.

Available therapeutic options include conservative management (with no surgery and no medication), intracavitary installation of amphotericin B, systemic administration of amphotericin B, and surgical removal of the lesion. Currently, most authorities recommend a conservative approach, when possible.[431,433] Several arguments support conservative management. First, life-threatening bleeding is relatively rare, especially with the first episode of hemoptysis.[434] Second, many patients have underlying diseases associated with significant pulmonary compromise, making them relatively poor operative risks. Third, many patients sustain long relatively asymptomatic periods. In addition, resolutions of aspergillomas without therapy have been reported.[427] Most authorities agree that surgery is indicated for significant recurrent hemoptysis or severe hemoptysis. Clearly, each patient must be approached on an individual basis, and the decision with respect to surgical intervention should be made within the context of the severity

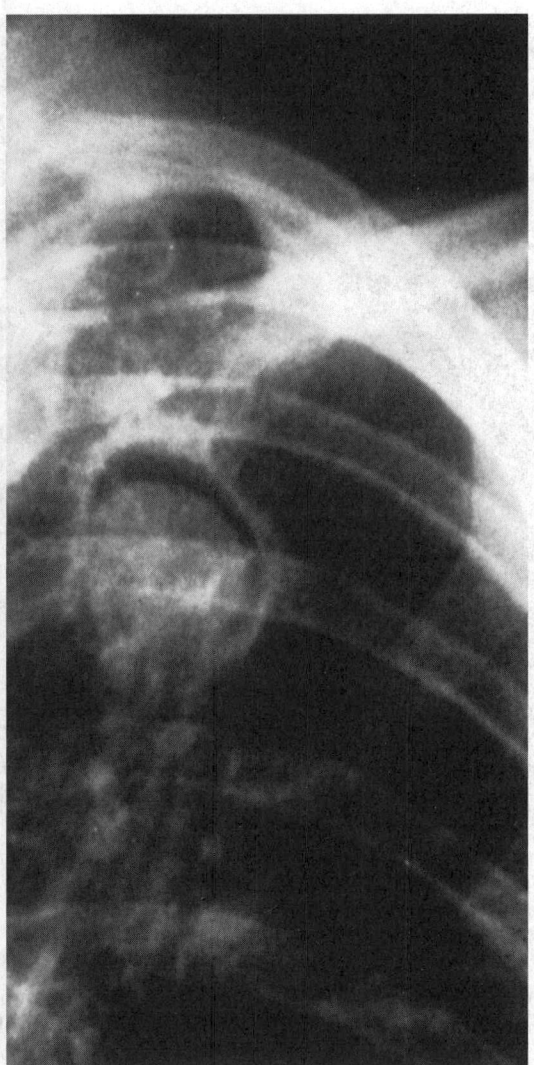

Fig. 91-6. Typical radiographic appearance of aspergilloma.

of the symptoms, the prognosis of the underlying disease, and the relative operative risks.

Because aspergillomas primarily represent colonization within a pre-existing cavity, systemic administration of antifungal therapy is rarely effective.[435] However, in a small percentage of patients who have localized invasive disease surrounding the aspergilloma and also have systemic symptoms (so-called chronic necrotizing pulmonary aspergillosis), intravenous amphotericin B has reportedly been effective.[427,436] Intracavitary amphotericin B has been reported to be effective in stabilizing or improving radiographic findings in small series of patients, but more data will be required to assess its ultimate value.[431,437]

Invasive *Aspergillus* Infections

Of the infections encountered in compromised patients, invasive *Aspergillus* infections are among the most serious because they are often multifocal, are associated with extensive tissue invasion and destruction, and in the absence of appropriate host defenses respond poorly to available antimicrobial therapy. Among cancer patients, those with acute leukemia who are undergoing aggressive cytotoxic therapy appear to be at highest risk.[54] However, in a study by Weinberger et al.,[438] fungal infections were responsible for 72% of deaths from infection, and more than one-half of these fungal infections were

due to *Aspergillus*. Overall, prolonged neutropenia is clearly the most important risk factor predisposing to invasive *Aspergillus* infection.[439]

With rare exception, *Aspergillus* infection is acquired by inhalation of *Aspergillus* conidia. Consequently, invasive infection occurs primarily in the lung, frequently with upper respiratory sites (usually the sinuses) affected as well.[440] The disease is often multifocal, with many patients having concomitant involvement of sinuses as well as multiple lung sites. Within the respiratory tree *Aspergillus* has a predilection for invading blood vessels as well as tissue parenchyma. Tissue infarction and subsequent necrosis often occur, which may lead to rapidly progressive extensive disease (Fig. 91-7). The process often behaves in a "malignant" fashion, extending predominantly by local invasion, with little respect for tissue planes and anatomic boundaries. Extension of primary disease in the sinus or orbit through bone to involve the roof of the mouth or the brain is not uncommon. Disease originating in the lung can extend through the pleura and even involve the chest wall. Hematogenous dissemination to distant organ sites such as the central nervous system, liver, and skin is relatively rare but has been reported.[441]

Since early diagnosis and prompt institution of therapy have been associated with improved outcome,[365] knowledge of the early signs and symptoms of invasive aspergillosis is critical for the clinician caring for patients with prolonged episodes of granulocytopenia. The most common symptom is pleuritic chest pain, which occurs in 100% of patients; in 50% of patients, it develops an average of 6 days before the appearance of pulmonary infiltrates.[437] Pathophysiologically, pleuritic pain probably occurs as a result of tissue infarction, which often extends to involve the pleural surfaces. Cough occurs in 93% of patients and shortness of breath in 27%. With respect to pulmonary signs, rales are most common and are heard in 100% of patients with invasive aspergillosis.

The sinuses are also frequently involved in invasive aspergillosis; they may be the initial or sole site of disease, or sinus involvement may occur concomitantly with pulmonary infection. Signs or symptoms include sinus pain, nasal ulceration or eschar, periorbital edema, epistaxis, and discharge. In a study by Gerson et al.,[439] one-third of patients with invasive pulmonary aspergillosis had microbiologic or pathologic documentation of *Aspergillus* sinus infection. Accordingly, all granulocytopenic patients with suspected or proven invasive aspergillosis should have a clinical and radiographic evaluation of the sinuses. In addition, *Aspergillus* infection in the maxillary sinuses may invade inferiorly into the roof of the hard palate, and initial symptoms may be minimal, even in the presence of bone destruction. A small ulceration of the hard palate may be the first sign of widespread disease (Fig. 91-8A). Sinus infection may also extend directly to involve the central nervous system or the orbit.[440]

A high index of suspicion is critical to the early diagnosis of aspergillosis; this infection should be considered with the appearance of any new abnormality in the chest radiograph of a persistently neutropenic patient with fever. The radiographic appearance of invasive pulmonary aspergillosis can range from discrete or multifocal nodular lesions to patchy densities to diffuse consolidation or even cavitation[439,442] (Fig. 91-8). The appearance can vary dramatically from patient to patient or change dramatically at granulocyte recovery—the ensuing inflammatory response can even give the appearance of worsening disease, when in fact the condition is one of clinical improvement. In our experience at the NCI, the most characteristic finding on chest radiograph is a localized infiltrate extending toward the pleural surface. Standard chest radiographs often underestimate the extent of pulmonary disease, especially if obtained early in the course or while the patient is neutropenic. CT scans of the chest are more accurate

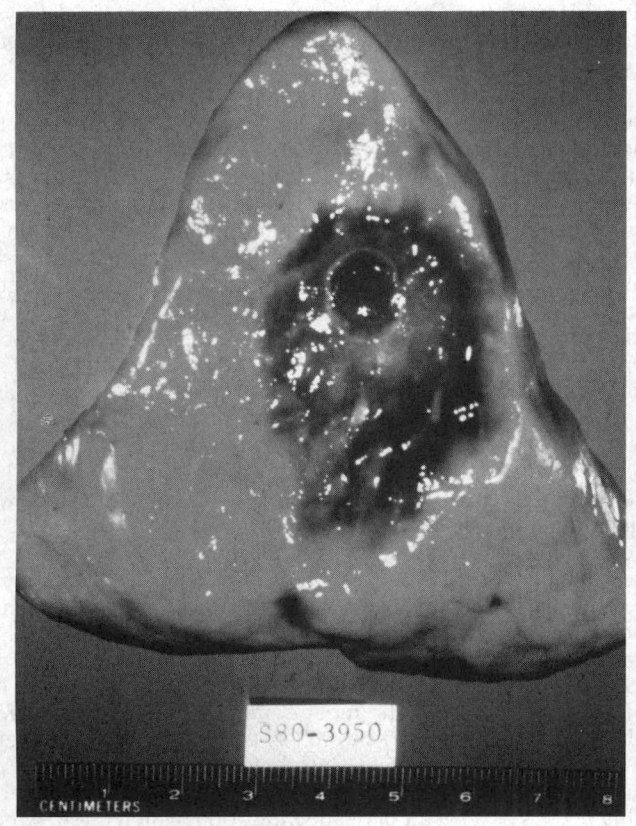 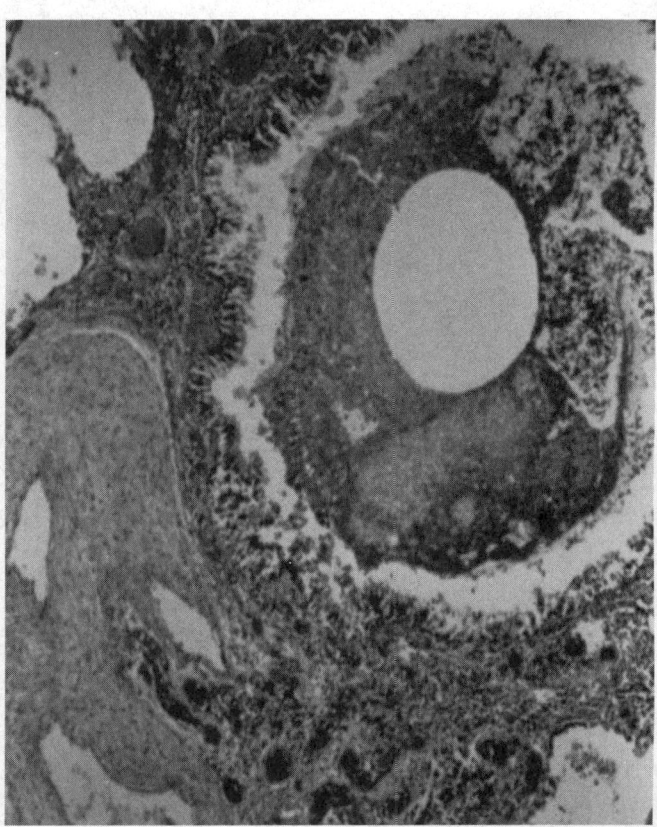

Fig. 91-7. (A) Autopsy specimen of lung from patient with invasive *Aspergillus*. **(B)** Histologic specimen from lung showing invasion of *Aspergillus* around blood vessels.

at defining the extent of disease and often visualize multifocal lesions in the face of single or no lesions on plain chest radiographs[443] (Fig. 91-8C & D). The radiographic appearance of *Aspergillus* sinusitis can range from minimal mucosal thickening to sinus obliteration and extensive bony erosion or destruction.

The only way to achieve a definitive diagnosis of invasive aspergillosis is by biopsy of the involved area, with either histologic or microbiologic confirmation, or both. Unfortunately, invasive procedures such as open lung biopsy or even transbronchial biopsy or sinus aspiration are often impractical or contraindicated in suspected aspergillosis patients, owing to thrombocytopenia, other bleeding abnormalities, or concurrent medical problems. Even a highly directed open biopsy may fail to document the fungal elements and yield only necrotic or infarcted tissue.[444] Therefore, a less invasive means of establishing the diagnosis would be of great practical value. Accordingly, the clinical value of cultures obtained noninvasively (from sputum or nares or from fiberoptic bronchoscopy with brushings or lavage) has been examined in a number of studies.[53,55,445–447] Cumulative data in these studies would suggest that, in a high-risk patient with signs or symptoms consistent with invasive *Aspergillus,* positive cultures from these sites are often predictive of invasive disease. In these patients, directed therapy is often indicated, even in the absence of a definitive diagnosis. However, these data also indicate that negative cultures do not rule out the diagnosis. False-negative culture results may occur in >50% of histopathologically proven cases, even when the specimens are obtained bronchoscopically. Conversely, because *Aspergillus* may colonize the respiratory tract, positive cultures in the absence of signs or symptoms should be interpreted with caution, and directed therapy should rarely be based solely on these results.

Blood cultures are rarely, if ever, positive in invasive asper-

gillosis. The growth of *Aspergillus* spp. in a blood culture is much more likely to represent a contaminant than a clinically significant isolate. Immunodiagnostic assays for the detection of *Aspergillus* antigens in serum and body fluids are promising but are not widely available and require further study.

For granulocytopenic patients with a diagnosis of invasive aspergillosis, therapy with amphotericin B should be initiated promptly, and a workup to determine the extent of disease should be begun simultaneously. This should include a careful physical examination, with special attention to the lungs, hard palate, nares, sinuses, and orbits. A minimal radiographic evaluation should include chest and sinus radiographs. Any suspicious findings or documented abnormalities should be followed by either CT or MRI in order to define the extent of disease more accurately and to provide better guidelines for assessment of subsequent therapeutic response.

Amphotericin B should be administered at a dose range of 0.5–1.5 mg/kg/day. Treatment with empirical amphotericin does not preclude the development of aspergillosis; 22 of 24 patients who were receiving empirical amphotericin developed progressive pulmonary infiltrates ultimately shown to be due to *Aspergillus.*[448] If a persistently neutropenic patient is receiving empirical amphotericin B and has either a clinical picture compatible with aspergillosis or evidence of documented infection, the dosage of amphotericin should be increased to 1.0–1.5 mg/kg.[449] Patients should continue amphotericin B until resolution of clinical and radiographic evidence of disease. At a minimum, a total dose of 2 g should be administered, although many patients will require substantially longer courses. The response to therapy and the ultimate survival of patients with invasive aspergillosis will be critically dependent on recovery from granulocytopenia, decreased dosage of any steroids, and/or removal of other immunologic deficits and may be depen-

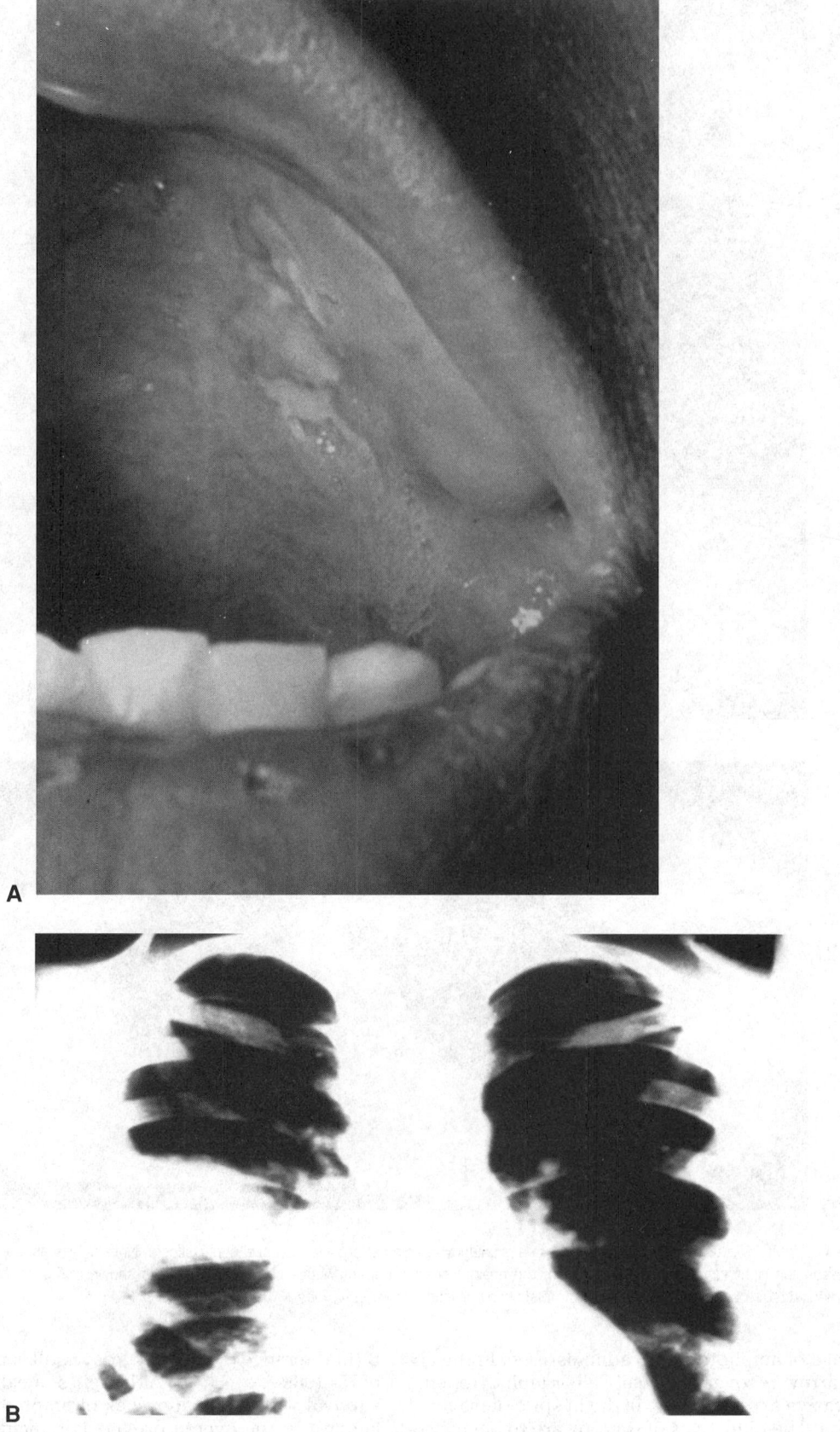

Fig. 91-8. (A) Invasive aspergillosis extending from the maxillary sinuses to involve the hard palate. **(B)** Chest radiograph showing classic appearance of invasive aspergillosis, with wedge-shaped infiltrate extending to the pleura. *(Figure continues.)*

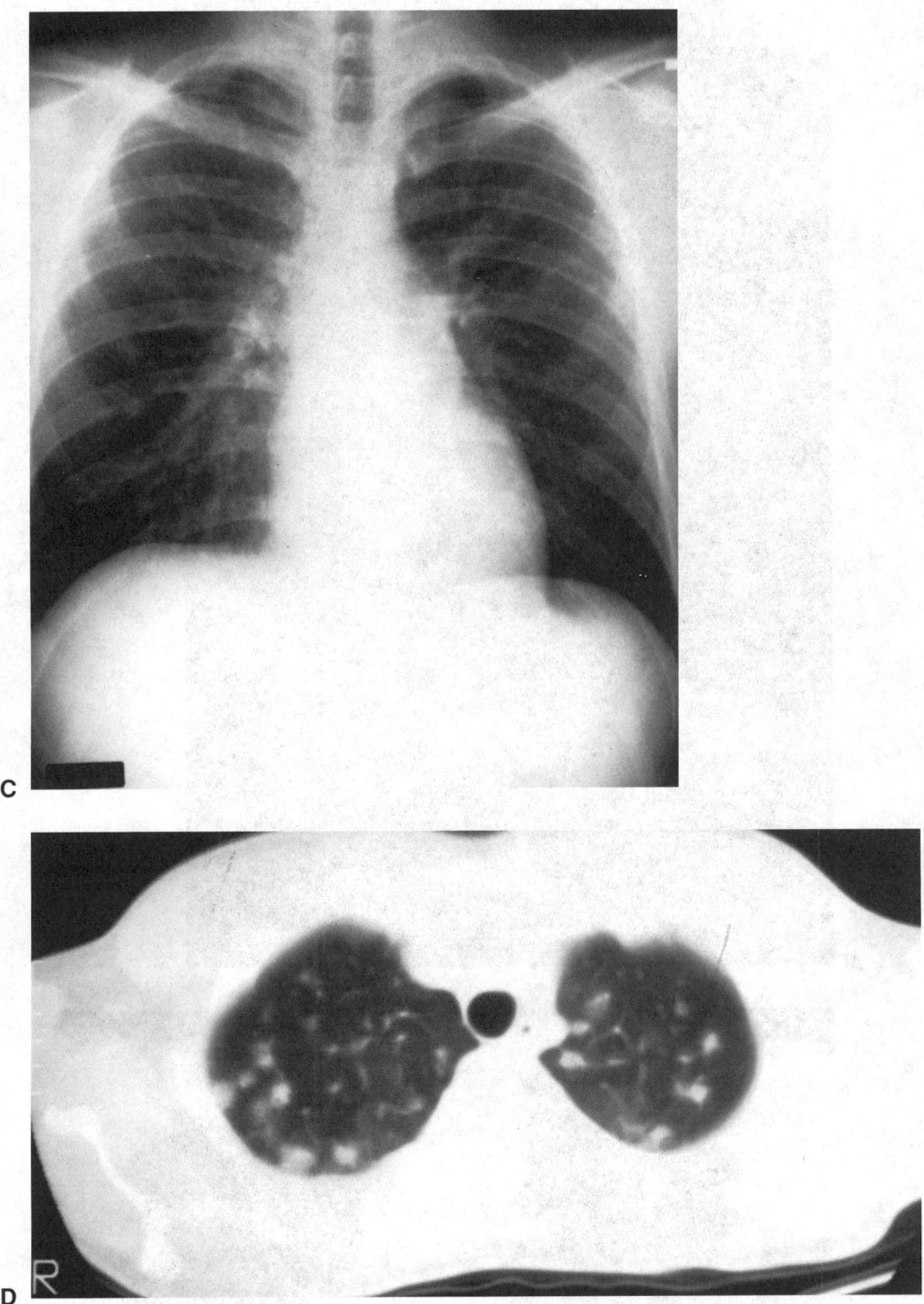

Fig. 91-8 *(Continued)*. **(C)** Chest radiograph from a granulocytopenic patient with invasive aspergillosis. Note subtle appearance of round densities in the right lung field. **(D)** CT scan of the chest from the patient whose chest radiograph is shown in Fig. B. Note extensive involvement despite minimal abnormalities on plain radiograph. *(Figure continues.)*

dent on the dosage of amphotericin B administered. In the absence of bone marrow recovery, virtually all granulocytopenic patients with invasive aspergillosis will die in spite of maximal antifungal therapy. The objectives of therapy are to delay progression and allow time for bone marrow recovery. Adjunctive therapy with granulocyte stimulating factors such as CSF-G and CSF-GM should be considered to hasten bone marrow recovery. Many studies using "standard" dosages of amphotericin

B (in the range of 0.5 mg/kg/day) still reported mortality rates of 75–100%.[364,365,441,450] Although, some data indicate improved survival with higher dosages of amphotericin B (1.0–1.5 mg/kg/day),[451] the overall prognosis remains dismal, as reflected in the recent report by Pannuti et al.,[452] in which *Aspergillus* was the cause of 36% of nosocomial pneumonias after BMT and resulted in the death of 19 of 20 infected patients.

Future therapies for invasive aspergillosis include liposomal

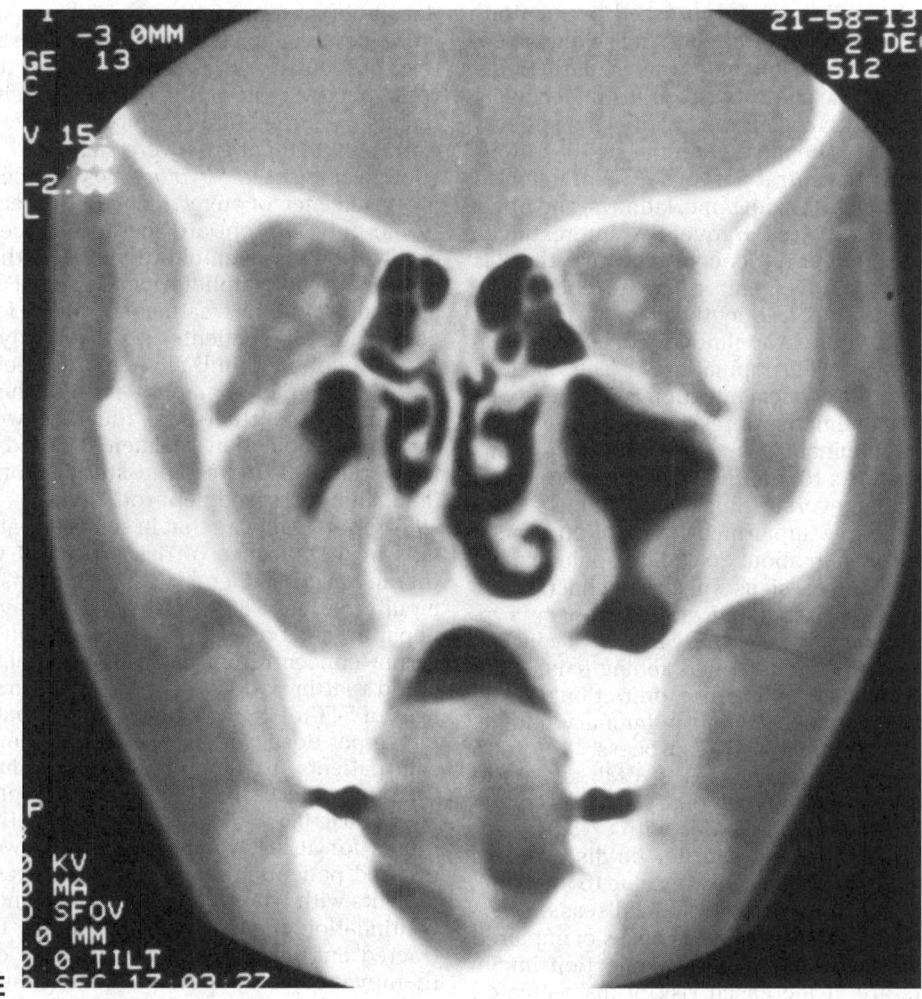

Fig. 91-8 *(Continued)*. **(E)** MRI showing invasive aspergillosis in the maxillary sinus extending through bone to involve the roof of the mouth.

preparations of amphotericin and itraconazole. Liposomal amphotericin has been used to treat immunocompromised patients who have either failed or experienced renal toxicity with conventional amphotericin in several small series.[420,453,454] In these studies, a complete response to liposomal amphotericin was seen in 20 (38%) of 52 patients with proven invasive *Aspergillus* infection; another 8 patients showed improvement with therapy. Of interest, 5 of the 19 patients treated by Lopez-Berestein et al.[454] improved in spite of continued neutropenia. In a report by Denning et al.[455] in 1989, itraconazole therapy of aspergillosis was successful in 7 of 10 immunocompromised patients treated, including 4 of 5 with pulmonary disease. In a larger study from the Mycoses Study Group, 23 (44%) of 52 patients demonstrated clinical or radiographic improvement after 2–3 months of itraconazole treatment; patients with invasive pulmonary aspergillosis responded at a higher rate, with improvement seen in 53% (18 of 34 patients).[456] In general, surgical resection of lesions has little role in treating severely immunocompromised patients with invasive aspergillosis because (1) the disease is often multifocal, and (2) other medical conditions frequently preclude even less invasive procedures. However, resection may be considered in selected patients who are considered good surgical candidates, who are not responding to antifungal therapy, and whose noninvasive evaluation indicates disease confined to a single accessible area. Surgery may also have a role in the treatment for bone and soft tissue extension of infection that develops during antifungal therapy.[449]

A question that often arises is how to approach patients with a previous history of invasive aspergillosis who require subsequent myelosuppressive chemotherapy. That issue was addressed in a study by Karp et al.[457] conducted in 1988, in which 10 patients with AML and a prior history of invasive aspergillosis underwent 14 subsequent courses of chemotherapy. In nine of these patients, prophylaxis with amphotericin B (1 mg/kg/day) plus 5-FC was begun before institution of chemotherapy. All these patients survived the ensuing granulocytopenic episode without evidence of reactivation of invasive aspergillosis. By contrast, the one patient who did not receive prophylactic therapy suffered reactivation of aspergillosis and died. On the basis of these data, prophylaxis with amphotericin B with or without 5-FC seems reasonable in certain high-risk patients. However, more data are needed before firm recommendations can be established.

Infections Due to *Cryptococcus Neoformans*

Cryptococcal infection can cause disease ranging from mild or asymptomatic to life-threatening and affects both immunocompetent and immunosuppressed individuals. Of patients with cryptococcosis in the pre-AIDS era, >50% had no predisposing factors, and white males predominated.[458,459] The recent increase in cases of cryptococcal infection is largely due to the increasing numbers of patients with HIV-1 infection, among whom it represents one of the most common cause of life-threatening infection. Other immunosuppressed populations at risk include patients receiving therapeutic doses of corticosteroids, those with lymphoid malignancies (particularly Hodgkin disease), patients with sarcoidosis (even if not receiving corticosteroids), patients with organ transplants, and patients with diabetes mellitus.[458,459] The most common site of serious *Cryptococcus* infection is the central nervous system followed by the lungs. Other sites, such as skin, bone, kidneys, and other viscera, have been reported less frequently. Interestingly, when central nervous system cryptococcosis occurs, there is no apparent pulmonary involvement in most cases. Conversely, respiratory involvement frequently occurs in isolation, although it often coexists with extrapulmonary disease, particularly in the immunosuppressed population.[460] The onset of central nervous system cryptococcal infection is frequently insidious, although heavily immunosuppressed populations may have an abrupt or even fulminant onset. Typically, symptoms are subtle, evolve over weeks to months, and most frequently include waxing and waning fevers, headaches, dizziness, somnolence, and signs of cognitive impairment. In addition, cranial nerve abnormalities are seen in about 20% and papilledema in ≤30% of cases. Classic meningeal signs, such as nuchal rigidity, are rare. Symptoms and signs associated with pulmonary cryptococcosis are often mild or may be entirely absent. Typically, symptoms, if they occur, may include mild aching pain, scant hemoptysis, and, rarely, pleuritic pain, rales, or friction rubs.[460] Chest radiographs may show an isolated pulmonary nodule, an interstitial infiltrate, or a consolidative process.

In patients with significant deficiencies in CMI, any unexplained central nervous system or pulmonary signs or symptoms should raise the suspicion of infection with *Cryptococcus*. Subtle or intermittent symptoms should not be disregarded. Fever may be absent but may also be the only clue to infection, even with significant central nervous system disease; unexplained fever in patients with AIDS or other causes of impaired CMI should prompt a workup for cryptococcal infection. Immunosuppressed patients are at increased risk of disseminated disease, and this should be investigated even if initial symptoms or signs indicate an isolated site. The appropriate workup includes, at a minimum, cultures of suspected sites, tests for cryptococcal antigen in cerebrospinal fluid and serum, and cerebrospinal fluid examination. If tissue specimens are obtained, diagnosis may also be established histopathologically.

Cerebrospinal fluid examination is helpful in establishing the diagnosis of central nervous system disease. In non-AIDS patients, abnormalities may include elevated opening pressure, low glucose (about 50%), elevated protein, and a mononuclear cell pleocytosis (usually with <500 cells/mm^3).[460,461] Importantly, AIDS patients or patients receiving high doses of corticosteroids may have little or no inflammatory response and consequently have little or no pleocytosis in the face of significant central nervous system disease. This is considered a poor prognostic sign. Overall, mass lesions due to *Cryptococcus* are relatively rare but may occur in 10–25% of patients. If suspected, mass lesions should be ruled out before lumbar puncture.

The latex agglutination test for detection of cryptococcal polysaccharide antigen is >90% sensitive and specific for the diagnosis of cryptococcal disease and should be performed in both serum and cerebrospinal fluid of patients in whom the diagnosis is suspected.[461] False-positive results may occur in the presence of rheumatoid factor (which may be eliminated by digestion with pronase or addition of reducing agents), in some malignancies, or by cross-reactivity with the rarer fungus *Trichosporon beigelii*.[462–464] Approximately 25% of HIV-infected patients will have a false-negative antigen in the cerebrospinal fluid; the yield is often improved with repeated sampling. Specimens for India ink staining and for culture should always be obtained when possible. When the meninges are involved, *Cryptococcus* will usually grow from cerebrospinal fluid specimens.

Results of sputum cultures in pulmonary cryptococcosis are more variable, however. Sputum cultures are frequently negative, particularly if disease is limited to a solitary nodule. A retrospective review from Duke University has shown excellent results from the culture of bronchoalveolar lavage fluid; however, only five patients were sampled.[465] In addition, positive sputum cultures for *Cryptococcus* are occasionally encountered in the absence of any evidence of parenchymal disease.[466]

The only appropriate therapy for central nervous system cryptococcosis is amphotericin B, with or without 5-FC. The combination of amphotericin B and 5-FC for 6 weeks is generally considered the treatment of choice for cryptococcal meningitis in non-AIDS patients. In a 1979 study comparing 0.4 mg/kg/day of amphotericin B alone for 10 weeks with a combination of 0.3 mg/kg/day of amphotericin B plus 5-FC for 6 weeks, no difference in mortality was found between the two regimens, but the combination regimen resulted in higher cure rates, fewer relapses, more rapid sterilization of the cerebrospinal fluid, and decreased nephrotoxicity.[467] More recent data (in a 1987 report) indicate that in selected patients with mild meningitis in the absence of risk factors, 4 weeks of combination therapy might suffice.[468] If 5-FC is used, care must be taken to monitor serum 5-FC levels closely, to avoid toxicity (diarrhea, hepatitis, and bone marrow suppression), maintaining the peak serum concentration at 50–100 µg/ml. We and others have found that in patients with normal renal function, initial dosages of 5-FC of 25 mg/kg qid are adequate (as opposed to 37.5 mg/kg per dose, which is often recommended).

In patients in whom 5-FC is contraindicated or cannot be tolerated, successful therapy with amphotericin alone at dosages of 0.4–0.6 mg/kg/day can be effective and should be continued for at least 6 and perhaps 10 weeks (for immunosuppressed patients, a minimum of 10 weeks is recommended). Patients with lymphoreticular malignancies or those requiring continuation of corticosteroid therapy may require more protracted antifungal regimens; in these cases, the duration of therapy is adjusted according to the results of clinical and laboratory response.

The most appropriate therapy of central nervous system cryptococcosis in AIDS patients has not yet been defined, but it is clear that eradication of the organism is rarely achieved and that long-term suppressive therapy is usually indicated. A retrospective review of treatment of cryptococcosis in AIDS patients, conducted by Chuck and Sande[469] in 1989, indicated that addition of 5-FC to amphotericin B neither enhanced survival nor prevented relapse in this population. In addition, AIDS patients appear to be particularly susceptible to the toxicities of 5-FC, >50% requiring its discontinuation because of secondary cytopenias, according to this study.[469] Because this study was uncontrolled and flucytosine levels were not measured, and because other groups have reported success with the combination of amphotericin B and flucytosine, the role of flucytosine remains controversial.[465] More recent studies prospectively comparing fluconazole and amphotericin B with and without flucytosine have shown varying results; the optimal therapy for cryptococcal infection in HIV-infected patients is unknown.[470,471] The 40–60% rate of relapse after cessation of treatment mandates life-long maintenance therapy for HIV-infected patients. Initially, most patients received weekly amphotericin B, but maintenance with fluconazole has proved more effective with the advantages of fewer side effects and available oral preparations.[472]

Post-therapy, patients should have repeat lumbar punctures performed at least every few months for the first year, as most relapses occur within the first 6 months; a reasonable schedule is at 1, 3, 6, and 12 months after the conclusion of therapy. The cerebrospinal fluid should be followed even if the original disease did not involve the central nervous system, as relapses have been found to occur there. Moreover, central nervous system disease can relapse at extraneural sites.

Other Fungal Infections in Immunosuppressed Patients

Zygomycosis (Mucormycosis)

Infections due to members of the Mucoraceae family are the fourth most commonly encountered fungal infections in compromised patients. The Mucoraceae include *Mucor, Rhizomucor, Rhizopus,* and *Absidia.* Patients at risk of zygomycosis include those with granulocytopenia, diabetic ketoacidosis, or kwashiokor and those receiving deferoxamine. Infections due to these organisms resemble aspergillosis both epidemiologically and clinically. The two most common clinical presentations are rhinocerebral and pulmonary mucormycosis, most commonly seen in patients with uncontrolled ketoacidosis or with granulocytopenia. Early and aggressive surgical debridement, intravenous amphotericin B, and correction of underlying metabolic abnormalities or immunologic deficits are essential for the cure of rhinocerebral mucormycosis. Treatment of pulmonary and disseminated disease requires early initiation of intravenous amphotericin B therapy and reversal of immunologic impairment.[473]

Pseudallescheria boydii

Pseudoallescheria boydii is a soil saprophyte and a common cause of mycetoma. However, various medical centers have increasingly reported *P. boydii* as a cause of lethal disseminated infection in immunocompromised patients.[474] The populations at risk and the clinical and histopathologic manifestations of disseminated pseudallescheriosis are similar to those of disseminated *Aspergillus* infection. However, *P. boydii* is usually resistant to amphotericin B but is susceptible to miconazole. Disseminated infection due to this organism is one of the few remaining indications for intravenous miconazole.[44] Other triazole antifungals, including ketoconazole, itraconazole, and saperconazole, have been used with varying degrees of success.[475–477]

Fusarium Species

Disseminated infections with *Fusarium* spp. may occur in granulocytopenic patients. They are often associated with prominent erythrematous maculopapular to nodular skin lesions. Biopsy will reveal branching septate hyphae invading blood vessels, and the organism can be cultured from the lesions. Amphotericin B is the drug of choice for therapy, although resistance has been reported and mortality is as high as 75%.

Trichosporon beigelii

Disseminated disease due to the yeast *T. beigelii* has been increasingly documented in severely immunosuppressed patients and clinically resembles disseminated candidal disease.[46] Important risk factors for infection include granulocytopenia, corticosteroid use, and the presence of an intravascular catheter.[478] The lungs, kidneys, skin, and eyes are the main sites affected. In untreated patients, serum and cerebrospinal fluid may be falsely positive for cryptococcal antigen.[464] Bone marrow recovery is the most important factor for a favorable outcome. Some *T. beigelii* are resistant to amphotericin B in vivo; the optimal antifungal therapy is unknown, but both anecdotal patient reports and animal data suggest that triazole antifungal agents are effective.[478,479]

CLINICAL APPROACH TO VIRAL INFECTIONS IN IMMUNOCOMPROMISED PATIENTS

Viral infections cause a wide range of disorders in patients with impaired immunity, ranging from subclinical infection to overwhelming disease and death. Of the viruses causing disease in this population, those belonging to the herpes group are encountered most commonly. The human herpes virus group includes HSV, VZV, CMV, EBV, and HHV-6. Almost all these viruses are encountered with greater frequency in patients with immune dysfunction than in normal hosts. Patients with defects in CMI are the major population at risk. CMI impairment that may lead to serious viral infection is seen in patients with hematologic malignancies (particularly Hodgkin disease and the non-Hodgkin lymphomas), those with HIV-1 infection, patients undergoing organ transplantation (e.g., bone marrow, kidney, liver, heart), patients receiving corticosteroids or other aggressive immunosuppressive agents (including many cytotoxic antineoplastic regimens), severely malnourished individuals, and those with primary congenital or acquired CMI defects.

A characteristic shared by each of these viruses is that they can cause disease either at initial exposure (i.e., primary infection) or after reactivation of latent disease. Indeed, latency is the hallmark of herpes virus infections and, by application of current molecular biologic techniques, the mechanism by which these viruses establish and maintain latency as well as undergo reactivation from the latent state are being elucidated.[480]

Infections Due to Herpes Simplex Virus

Infection with HSV may cause significant morbidity but is only rarely fatal in the compromised host. HSV infection usually represents reactivation of latently established disease.

When HSV infection occurs even in the most severely immunocompromised patients, it tends to remain localized and only rarely disseminates to distant sites. Although disseminated HSV infection can lead to death, the morbidity associated with localized HSV infection in compromised patients is a far more clinically relevant issue. The most common sites at which HSV occurs in non-AIDS patients are the mouth and perioral area, the nares, and the esophagus. In addition, a patient with a previous history of genital or perianal HSV may experience reactivation at these sites. Pain is the hallmark of lesions attributable to HSV. As compared with its effects in healthy individuals, the infection in compromised patients causes more symptoms (predominantly pain), is associated with larger and more numerous lesions, and persists for a longer period (Fig. 91-9). Chronic ulcerated lesions (herpes phagedena) in the oral or anogenital region may persist for weeks to months in certain subgroups, such as those with hematologic malignancies or AIDS.[481,482] Esophagitis due to HSV is typically manifested by burning pain on swallowing with or without associated dysphagia and may or may not be associated with visibly apparent oral lesions. HSV esophagitis may be clinically indistinguishable from other causes of similar symptoms in this population, including chemotherapy-induced mucositis, *Candida* esophagitis, and CMV esophagitis.

Mucocutaneous HSV infection may also cause secondary complications such as bleeding or infection. Mucosal disruption may lead to localized secondary bacterial infection and may also provide a portal of entry for bacteria into the bloodstream.

Dissemination beyond the oral, anogenital, nasal, or esophageal mucosa occurs rarely. The incidence of dissemination is not well established but is probably <1%. The the most common sites of dissemination are the skin, lungs, liver, central nervous system, and adrenals. The diagnosis of disseminated HSV should be considered in any patient with CMI defects and unexplained findings referable to these sites.

The diagnosis of localized oral, nasal, or anogenital HSV infection is rarely problematic. Early lesions usually have a characteristic vesicular appearance, and appropriately obtained cultures are usually positive within 48 hours. When obtaining

APPROACH TO FUNGAL INFECTIONS

Candida Infections

In neutropenic patients we first treat symptomatic oral candidiasis with clotrimazole (usually clotrimazole troches, administered five times per day). If there is no improvement, we begin amphotericin B at 0.5 mg/kg/day. We do not routinely use fluconazole for the treatment of candidiasis in neutropenia patients. Symptoms of esophageal candidiasis may be indistinguishable from those caused by chemotherapy, radiotherapy, or HSV infection. For suspected or diagnosed *Candida* esophagitis, we begin amphotericin B. Because of the risks associated with esophagoscopy and biopsy in the neutropenic population, we usually elect to treat empirically and not to perform this procedure.

Isolation of *Candida* from blood cultures has been increasingly achieved owing to changing characteristics of the neutropenic population and improved microbiologic techniques. In a neutropenic patient even a single colony of *Candida* isolated from the blood should be viewed as significant and not discarded as a contaminant. When candidemia occurs, we take the following approach: (1) begin amphotericin B; (2) remove and/or change all intravenous lines; and (3) begin a diagnostic workup to look for disseminated disease, which at a minimum should include follow-up evaluation of blood cultures, measurement of alkaline phosphatase, an ophthalmologic examination, and CT of the liver and spleen. Abnormalities on CT may not become apparent until resolution of granulocytopenia, and imaging studies should be repeated at this time if disseminated disease is suspected.

Hepatosplenic candidiasis is the most common manifestation of disseminated fungal disease in the neutropenic population. Patients with neutropenia of prolonged duration who are receiving broad-spectrum antibacterial agents are at highest risk. Clues to the diagnosis include abdominal pain, "rebound" leukocytosis and persistent fever following recovery of granulocytopenia, and elevated alkaline phosphatase. Ultrasound, CT, and MRI may all be useful in making a presumptive diagnosis. Definitive diagnosis requires histologic and/or microbiologic demonstration of *Candida* from hepatic tissue. However, even when organisms are demonstrated histologically, they rarely grow in culture. We initiate therapy with a combination of amphotericin B (0.5 mg/kg/day) and 5-flucytosine (initially 100 mg/kg/day in four divided doses, assuming normal renal function), carefully monitoring 5-FC levels. Amphtericin B is continued for a minimum total dose of 2 g, although some patients have required ≤9 g. Therapy should be continued until resolution of radiographic abnormalities.

Aspergillus Infection

In most non-neutropenic patients with aspergillomas, we favor a conservative approach, reserving surgical resection for those with recurrent or significant hemoptysis. Surgery should also be considered for patients with isolated aspergillomas about to receive cytotoxic therapy that will place them at increased risk of bleeding.

Invasive aspergillosis occurs most commonly in patients with prolonged periods of granulocytopenia (average time of onset is about 3 weeks in most studies). Fever, cough, and pleuritic chest pain are clues to the diagnosis and may have their onset before the appearance of pulmonary infiltrates. The lungs and sinuses are the sites most commonly affected, and lesions are often multifocal. When invasive aspergillosis is suspected, CT scans of the lungs and sinuses should be performed and may reveal widespread disease in the face of minimal findings on plain radiographs. In the appropriate clinical setting, positive sputum or nasal cultures are highly suggestive of the diagnosis. Surgery has little role in therapy because the disease is usually multifocal and because many patients have concomitant thrombocytopenia. In the absence of granulocyte recovery, invasive aspergillosis is nearly always fatal. The goal of therapy is to stabilize the disease and bide time until resolution of granulocytopenia. We treat patients with high-dose amphotericin B (1.0–1.5 mg/kg/day), and add 5-FC if there is evidence of continued progression. Therapy should continue until resolution of radiographic abnormalities, with a minimum of 2 g of amphotericin B.

cultures for HSV it is important to remember the following steps. False-negative results may be obtained from lesions that appear either very early (i.e., before vesicle formation) or late in the course of evolution (after crusting). Ideally, culture material should consist of serious fluid from vesicles that is obtained after gentle unroofing. Also, specimens should be promptly inoculated into tissue cultures and should not be kept at room temperature for prolonged periods. It is helpful to store frozen culture medium on the hospital floors so that it is readily available to the clinician. Techniques such as direct immunofluorescence, enzyme-linked immunosorbent assays, and monoclonal antibody staining allow for rapid diagnosis.

The definitive diagnosis of HSV esophagitis or disseminated disease may be more elusive. Accordingly, for patients with CMI defects in whom the diagnosis is suspected on clinical grounds, empirical therapy is often instituted. In patients with esophagitis, the simultaneous presence of characteristic oral lesions may point toward the diagnosis but neither confirms nor rules out the presence of other contributing factors. In the absence of oral lesions, positive oral cultures may indicate esophageal infection, but they may also reflect asymptomatic excretion or infection at another site. In these settings, empirical therapy with acyclovir or amphotericin B, or both, may be indicated, and in selected patients esophagoscopy and biopsy may be performed (see also discussion of *Candida* esophagitis).

The diagnosis of HSV pneumonitis presents similar problems. Positive cultures of respiratory secretions may reflect asymptomatic excretion or excretion from another infected site (e.g., oral cavity), or they may indicate lung or tracheobronchial involvement. Lavage fluid showing multinucleated giant cells may be helpful but is not specific. The diagnosis of HSV meningoencephalitis can only be made definitively by brain biopsy. Cerebrospinal fluid findings often show many erythrocytes, and CT, electroencephalographic, or brain scans showing temporal localization may be suggestive, but none are specific for the diagnosis of HSV infection. Even in confirmed cases, the virus is seldom isolated from the cerebrospinal fluid. The development of the polymerase chain reaction (PCR) is a potentially useful test for the diagnosis of HSV.

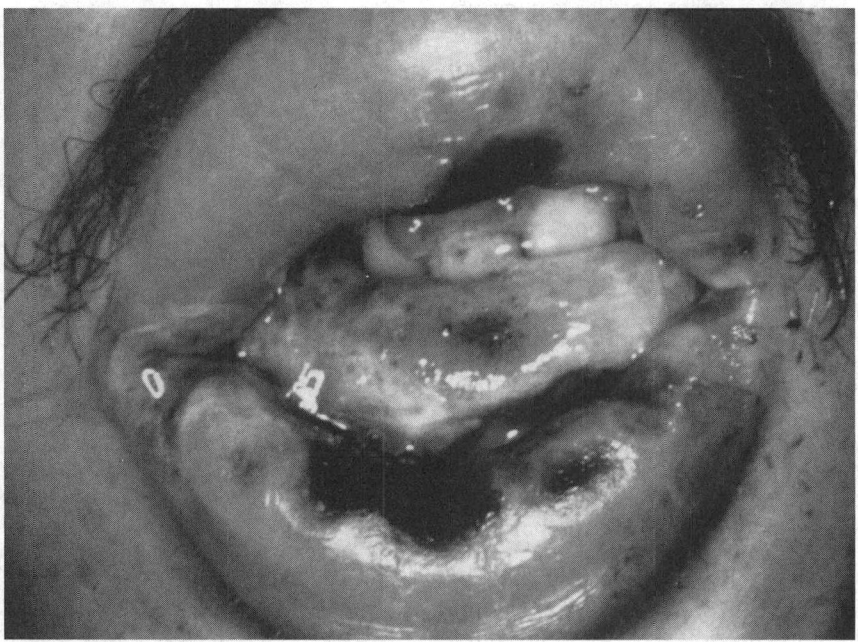

Fig. 91-9. Extensive oral herpes simplex in a granulocytopenic patient with chemotherapy-induced mucositis and oral candidiasis.

Acyclovir is the drug of choice for the treatment of HSV infections in immunosuppressed patients. For mucocutaneous disease, either oral or intravenous acyclovir is effective in shortening the length of symptoms, the time of virus shedding, and the time to healing. Because many patients with oral or esophageal HSV infection have difficulty swallowing, intravenous administration is often more useful. The appropriate intravenous dosage is 250 mg/m^2 (or 5 mg/kg) tid. Therapy should be continued for 1 week or until lesions have crusted. Patients with diagnosed or suspected visceral or central nervous system dissemination should receive intravenous acyclovir at a dosage of 500 mg/m^2 (or 10 mg/kg) tid, and therapy should be continued for ≥10 days. During the past several years, treatment of HSV infections has been increasingly complicated by the emergence of acyclovir-resistant virus. Resistant HSV has primarily been isolated in the most immunosuppressed patients such as those with AIDS or those who have undergone BMT.[483,484] In a review by Englund et al.,[483] 7 patient isolates of 207 were found to be resistant to acyclovir; all 7 of these patients were immunocompromised from BMT (4 cases), solid organ transplantation (2 cases), or AIDS (1 case). Although resistance to acyclovir has been associated with chronic low-dose acyclovir in both animal models and case reports, no specific regimen or dose has been implicated.[485,486] Spontaneous mutations in the viral thymidine kinase lead to a mixed population of HSV, and chronic acyclovir therapy may permit the emergence of the acyclovir-resistant viral population. Resistant HSV is usually susceptible to foscarnet, used for successful treatment of these patients.[484]

Infections Due to Varicella-Zoster Virus

In contrast to HSV infection, VZV infection in compromised patients may be associated with significant morbidity as well as significant mortality. Both primary disease (chickenpox) and reactivation of latent disease (zoster or "shingles") are clinically important in this population.

Primary Varicella Infection (Chickenpox)

In noncompromised patients, chickenpox is a highly contagious, but relatively benign, self-limited disease that requires no therapy. Primary infection usually occurs during childhood (usually by the age of 3 years) and may result in either subclinical or clinically apparent disease. Approximately 90% of individuals have acquired antibodies to VZV (implying primary infection) by the age of 15 years.[487] In healthy children, chickenpox is usually limited to the skin. When it occurs in adults, about 15% also have radiographic evidence of pulmonary involvement, although fewer have pulmonary symptoms, which are usually mild in nature.[487,488] In immunocompetent patients, dissemination is rare, with a self-limited cerebellar ataxia occurring in about 1 in 4,000 children and encephalitis in 0.1–0.2%.[487] By contrast, primary varicella frequently disseminates and can cause serious morbidity and mortality in patients with impaired CMI. Children with immune impairment represent the highest-risk group for primary varicella, which parallels its age distribution in the normal host, with only about 10% of adults at risk of primary disease. However, for patients of any age with a newly diagnosed disease associated with defective CMI (e.g., Hodgkin disease) or for those about to receive therapy that can result in impaired CMI (e.g., intensive chemotherapy or corticosteroids), it is prudent to check for a clinical history of chickenpox or to check serum titers in the absence of clinical information. The absence of VZV antibody titers indicates a significant risk of the acquisition of primary disease, if exposed, and has important implications for management after potential exposure.

Of those seriously immunocompromised children who contract primary varicella and who do not receive either ZIG or early therapy with acyclovir, about one-third will develop visceral dissemination: among these children mortality is in the range of 7–20% (usually due to progressive pulmonary insufficiency).[66] The lung is the major site of dissemination, which occurs 3–7 days after the onset of skin lesions, with chest radiographs classically showing diffuse nodular infiltrates. The central nervous system and liver are two other frequent sites of dissemination. VZV hepatitis in the absence of central nervous system or pulmonary involvement rarely causes death.

Among children, the highest-risk groups for serious disseminated VZV are those with malignancy who are undergoing intensive cytoreductive therapy, those receiving organ transplantation, and those with primary disorders of CMI. Among children being treated for malignancy who develop VZV, those with leukemia and lymphoma represent the largest group, probably because hematologic malignancies are the most common in this age group. Dissemination is more likely in children with ≤ 500 lymphocytes/mm^3 at the onset of disease and in those in whom chemotherapy was continued after the onset of skin lesions.[66] Disseminated VZV occurs more often in patients with advanced disease, although this may be related to the use of more aggressive therapy.[67]

The diagnosis of primary cutaneous chickenpox is usually made relatively easily on clinical grounds from the appearance of the lesions. However, immunosuppressed patients, particularly those with AIDS, occasionally develop atypical lesions such as papules or hyperkeratosis. A high index of suspicion must be maintained in susceptible hosts. Knowledge of antecedent VZV antibody titers or a clinical history of prior infection can be helpful in this setting. A Tzanck smear, performed by scraping the base of the lesion, may show multinucleated giant cells. A positive Tzanck smear is highly suggestive of the diagnosis in the appropriate clinical setting, but it is not diagnostic, as other viral processes such as HSV infection are also associated with multinucleated giant cells. Cultures of skin lesions often yield positive results, but culture for VZV can take up to 10–14 days. Immunofluorescent stains on scrapings from skin lesions are very helpful in early diagnosis and are often more sensitive than culture. Acute and convalescent serum antibody measurements may be helpful in confirming the diagnosis retrospectively.

All immunosuppressed patients with suspected primary VZV infection should undergo a chest radiograph and measurement of liver transaminases in order to establish a baseline and to detect clinically silent disseminated disease. Examination of the sputum in VZV pneumonia, may show multinucleated giant cells, and culture may yield positive results. Central nervous system involvement may be very difficult to diagnose with certainty antemortem; when involved, VZV is usually not cultured from the cerebrospinal fluid.[489]

Patients with confirmed or suspected primary varicella should be placed in immediate isolation to avoid exposure of other susceptible patients. Other immunocompromised patients at risk of acquisition of primary varicella who had contact with the patient during the infectious stage (beginning 48 hours before the appearance of the lesions and lasting until crusting of the lesions) should be contacted and promptly given varicella-zoster immunoglobulin. The incubation period is 10–21 days after exposure; exposed patients should consequently avoid contact with other patients for that period.

Early institution of intravenous acyclovir will dramatically reduce the incidence of visceral dissemination of primary varicella. In a randomized double-blind placebo-controlled trial of acyclovir in immunosuppressed children with primary varicella, pneumonitis developed in 5 of 11 placebo recipients but in 0 of 11 patients who received acyclovir.[490] Vidarabine therapy can also be effective, although it is rarely used, as acyclovir is widely available.[491] Intravenous acyclovir should be instituted at a dose of 500 mg/m^2 (or 10 mg/kg) tid; therapy should be continued for ≥ 7 days, or until all lesions have crusted. Patients receiving this dose of acyclovir should be well hydrated in order to maintain urine flow and avoid renal precipitation and toxicity. Therapy for disseminated disease is identical, although more protracted courses may be required.

Herpes Zoster

Herpes zoster, or shingles, is believed to represent reactivation of latent disease. Although some reports have suggested that zoster can be acquired exogenously, this has not been firmly substantiated, and the vast majority of cases are not temporally associated with antecedent exposure.[69,71,492] Although zoster can occur in healthy individuals, it is clearly

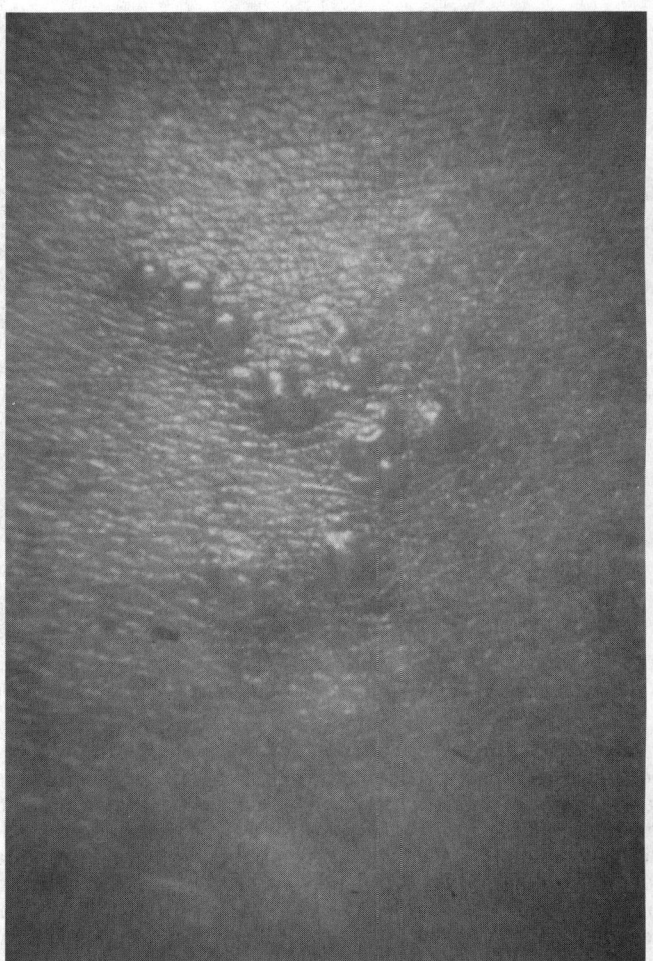

Fig. 91-10. Early lesions of zoster in an immunosuppressed patient.

more common in certain immunosuppressed populations. Patients with malignancy, especially those with Hodgkin disease, are at highest risk (about 15%), followed by patients with non-Hodgkin lymphoma (about 8%), and patients with solid tumors (about 2%).[67,69,489,493–498] Zoster is more common in patients with advanced disease, as opposed to those with limited disease or in remission. However, in certain subgroups (e.g., patients with Hodgkin disease or lymphomas), an increased risk continues even after cure of the malignancy.[499] Zoster is more likely to develop at skin sites that have been previously damaged by tumor or radiotherapy. More intensive immunosuppression is associated with a higher risk of zoster (e.g., patients who receive combinations of chemotherapy and radiotherapy are at greater risk than those who receive either modality alone). Following significant radiotherapy (e.g., for BMT), the increased risk for zoster may last ≤ 1 year.[499] Zoster usually appears unilaterally and follows a dermatomal distribution even in immunosuppressed patients. Early lesions may be very subtle (Fig. 91-10). Rarely, it may present with cutaneous dissemination without a prior history of dermatomal involvement (so-called atypical disseminated zoster or varicelliform zoster, which resembles primary varicella).[69,497,500] Visceral dissemination of zoster occurs somewhat less frequently than does dissemination of primary varicella infection. In immunosuppressed patients, the incidence of dissemination is 24–50%, while visceral dissemination (lungs, central nervous system, liver, and uvea) occurs in 8–19%.[501,502]

Guidelines for the diagnosis of zoster are similar to those for the diagnosis of primary varicella. When an immunosuppressed patient with suspected or diagnosed zoster is encountered, several important questions arise. First, has the patient had significant contact with other patients who may be at risk of the development of primary varicella? Although patients with zoster are less infectious than those with primary varicella, direct contact may spread infection to susceptible individuals, who should receive ZIG. Second, is the disease localized, or is there any evidence of cutaneous or visceral dissemination? All patients at risk of dissemination should have a baseline physical examination, chest radiograph, and measurement of liver transaminases. Third, is the patient a candidate for therapy? Clearly, any patient with disseminated disease is a candidate for therapy with intravenous acyclovir.

In addition, patients with localized disease who are at significant risk of dissemination should be treated. This includes (1) patients with an underlying diagnosis of either Hodgkin disease or non-Hodgkin lymphoma, whether or not undergoing therapy (those receiving therapy will be at higher risk of dissemination); (2) patients with any malignancy who are undergoing aggressive cytotoxic therapy (defined as therapy that produces significant leukopenia); (3) patients who have received total body irradiation or BMT, for ≤1 year after the procedure; (4) patients with AIDS; and (5) other patients with severe congenital or acquired defects in CMI (including those receiving systemic corticosteroids or other immunosuppressive drugs).

Attempts should be made to treat patients as soon after the appearance of the lesions as possible (preferably within 72 hours), even if they are confined to a single dermatome since earlier therapy may result in improved outcome. However, the results of studies summarized below indicate that patients with older lesions that have not healed should also receive therapy.

Although both vidarabine and acyclovir have been shown in controlled trials to be effective for the treatment of zoster in immunocompromised patients, acyclovir has been more effective.[501–504] A 1986 study by Shepp and colleagues[504] compared intravenous acyclovir with vidarabine in compromised patients. Acyclovir was found to be significantly better in preventing disease progression or dissemination, shortening culture positivity, decreasing new lesion formation, and decreasing time to pain resolution and crusting of lesions.

The first randomized, double-blind, placebo-controlled trial of acyclovir for zoster in immunosuppressed patients was reported in 1983 by Balfour and co-workers.[501] A 1-week course of 1,500 mg/m^2/day IV of acyclovir halted significant progression of disease in patients presenting with either localized or cutaneous disseminated disease. For patients who presented with lesions confined to a single dermatome, acyclovir did not prevent local skin progression (i.e., either increase in the rash within the initial dermatome or extension to a new contiguous dermatome). However, it did decrease wider cutaneous spread, as well as visceral dissemination in patients who presented with either localized or disseminated cutaneous disease. Of the four patients randomized to placebo in whom visceral disease developed, three died. Two patients who presented with initial visceral dissemination and received acyclovir both survived. Acyclovir was effective at halting progression of disease even if begun in patients whose rash was >72 hours old at entry.

On the basis of these data, intravenous acyclovir at 1,500 mg/m^2/day tid is the treatment of choice for zoster in immunosuppressed patient. It should be continued for a minimum of 7 days, or until crusting of the lesions is noted. Oral acyclovir, even at high doses, is not appropriate therapy for zoster infections. The bioavailability of oral acyclovir is only about 15%, and systemic concentrations achieved following oral dosing are not sufficient to inhibit VZV replication (VZV is 10–20 times more resistant to acyclovir than is HSV).[505] Clinically significant acyclovir-resistant VZV has become an increasing problem in the AIDS era. Chronic infection, often with atypical lesions and

pain are not uncommon in AIDS patients. As in acyclovir-resistant HSV, resistant VZV is often associated with chronic low-dose acyclovir use.[506,507] In order to decrease the risk of developing resistance, it is best to aggressively treat the original VZV infection with high-dose intravenous acyclovir. Since viral susceptibility patterns are not readily available, treatment decisions must often be based on the clinical response to therapy. Foscarnet is an alternative in most patients with resistant VZV infection.[507] Another antiviral agent with activity against VZV and HSV-1 is BVaraU. BVaraU offers the advantage of being available in an oral form and is currently being studied for treatment and suppression of varicella infection in immunocompromised patients (Freifeld A, personal communication).

Infections Due to Cytomegalovirus

CMV causes a variety of syndromes in both immunocompetent and compromised hosts. The virus is ubiquitous, and most of the population is eventually infected, although clinical disease is relatively rare in healthy individuals. In noncompromised hosts, in addition to subclinical infection it may cause heterophil-negative mononucleosis and has, rarely, been associated with more serious complications, including interstitial pneumonitis, hepatitis, Guillain-Barré syndrome, meningoencephalitis, myocarditis, and hemolytic anemia.

In immunosuppressed patients CMV may cause significant morbidity and mortality. Of patients with hematologic disorders, those who present the highest risk of acquiring serious infection are BMT recipients, particularly those undergoing allogeneic BMT, those who receive total body irradiation as part of the ablative regimen, and those who develop acute graft-versus-host disease after BMT.[508,509] Other patients with hematologic malignancies (e.g., leukemia and lymphoma) are also at risk, although the incidence is lower. Other groups at risk include AIDS patients and recipients of solid organ transplants. In immunocompromised populations, disease may represent either acquisition of primary infection or, more commonly, reactivation of latent infection. Transfusion of seronegative blood products into seronegative recipients can dramatically decrease acquisition of primary disease in selected population.

CMV may infect many organ systems. In compromised patients without AIDS (particularly the BMT population), interstitial pneumonia is the most common and most serious complication. However, clinically important infection of other organ sites has been recognized with increasing frequency, most notably in AIDS patients but in other populations as well. The gastrointestinal tract may be infected at any site from the esophagus to the colon. Submucosal ulcerations are common, and symptoms may range from isolated fever to severe hemorrhage or explosive diarrhea. CMV has also been implicated in development of pancreatitis and cholecystitis.[510,511] CMV retinitis may progress to blindness if untreated and occurs in 10–20% of adult AIDS patients, although it has also been described in other immunosuppressed populations.[512] Central nervous system involvement in non-AIDS patients is probably rare and has been reported only anecdotally. Neurologic complications in HIV infected patients include subacute encephalitis, dementia, and polyradiculopathy.[513] This discussion focuses on CMV pneumonitis, the most commonly encountered serious CMV infection in non-AIDS patients and the most thoroughly studied.

Cytomegalovirus Pneumonitis

Depending on the presence or absence of specific risk factors, up to 50% of allograft BMT recipients develop interstitial pneumonia, and about 70% of these cases will be associated with CMV. Typically, this infection occurs within the first 3

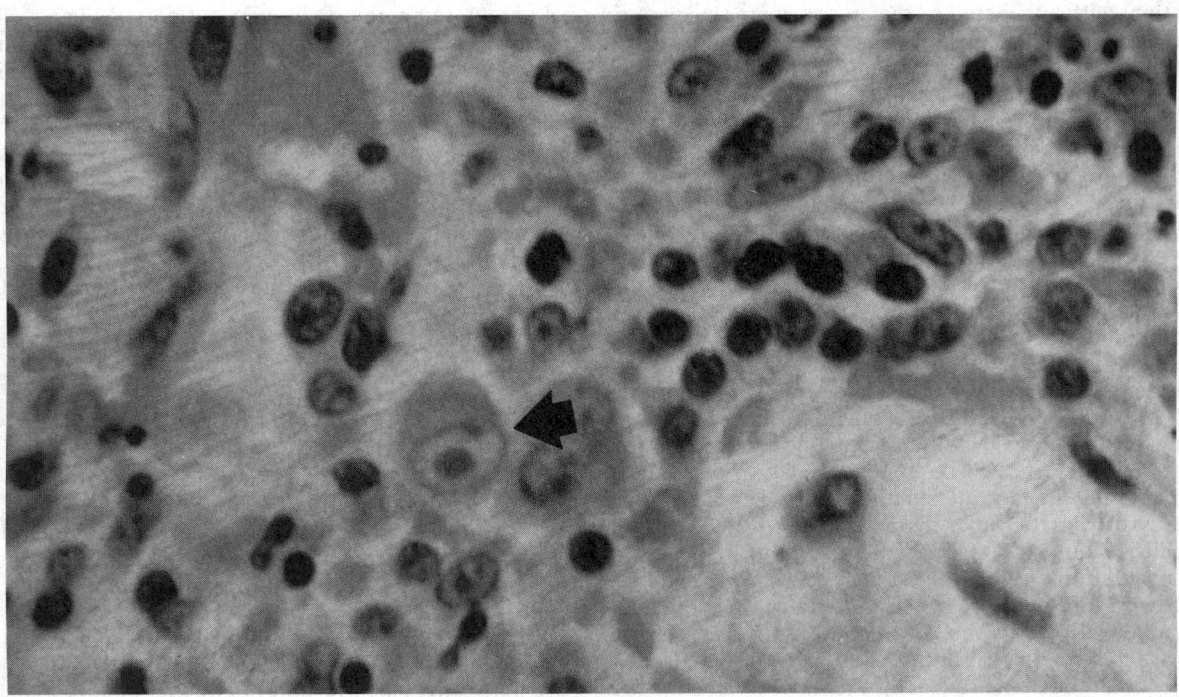

Fig. 91-11. Pulmonary biopsy specimen with cell showing typical intranuclear inclusion of cytomegalovirus (arrow).

months after allogeneic BMT, with a median onset of about 60 days. Cases developing later than 100 days have also been documented, primarily in patients with chronic graft-versus-host disease.[514] Diffuse infiltrates are most common, but localized or nodular infiltrates have been described. Pleural effusions are rare.

CMV pneumonia is clinically indistinguishable from other causes of diffuse infiltrates in the compromised host, especially *P. carinii* infection and specific virologic studies are needed to confirm the diagnosis. While positive cultures from blood, urine, or respiratory secretions may raise suspicion of infection, they do not necessarily correlate with pulmonary infection. Serology for CMV may not be helpful because of false-negative results seen with immunosuppression. To establish the diagnosis, direct examination of pulmonary specimens is required. Although only open-lung biopsy can be considered definitively diagnostic, bronchopulmonary lavage may be of value, particularly in BMT patients. In examining specimens, attempts should be made to employ rapid virologic techniques, since final culture results typically take ≥2–3 weeks to obtain. Techniques that may be helpful include specific immunofluorescence using murine monoclonal antibodies, the use of "shell vial" cultures (involving concentration of specimens and immunofluorescent staining for CMV antigens), in situ nucleic acid hybridization, and the use of the PCR.[515,516] In addition, classic histologic examination may reveal typical intranuclear inclusions of CMV (Fig. 91-11). It should be stressed that even if diagnosis of CMV pneumonia is made or strongly suspected, other potential pathogens should still be sought, as CMV has been identified in association with other organisms.

Therapeutic options for treating serious CMV infection in non-AIDS patients are limited and complicated by serious toxicities. Both foscarnet and ganciclovir appear to be effective in treating CMV infections in patients with AIDS; however, the use of both therapies is limited by toxicity, the need for intravenous dosing, and the emergence of resistant strains of CMV.[517,518] Foscarnet not only has activity against CMV but also shows in vitro inhibition of HIV reverse transcriptase; some studies have suggested improved survival of AIDS patients with CMV retini-

tis treated with foscarnet.[519,520,521] CMV isolates from both AIDS patients and transplant patients have been found to be ganciclovir resistant. The clinical significance is unclear. Resistance has been associated with progressive clinical disease. However, patients may be infected with multiple strains and the virus isolated may not have the same antiviral susceptibilities as the actual infecting strain. It is impossible to make a clinical distinction of progressive CMV disease due to a virulent strain from disease due to a resistant one. While foscarnet has been used to successfully treat patients with ganciclovir-resistant CMV, therapy with both foscarnet and ganciclovir has been beneficial with particularly aggressive disease.[522,523] The neutropenia and thrombocytopenia that often accompany ganciclovir therapy are problematic in patients with bone marrow suppression from chemotherapeutic agents, zidovudine, or their underlying disease.[517] Ganciclovir alone has not been effective in altering the outcome of CMV pneumonia in patients who have received BMT.[524,525] Studies have documented improved outcome in BMT patients with CMV pneumonia who were treated with combinations of ganciclovir (2.5 mg/kg tid or 5 mg/kg bid) and high intravenous doses of immunoglobulin; overall survival improved to 50–70% as compared to <15% survival for historical controls.[526] It should be noted that while AIDS patients frequently appear to respond to ganciclovir or foscarnet therapy, relapse is almost certain when therapy is discontinued. Accordingly, continuous prophylaxis with ganciclovir or foscarnet is required. Immunocompromised patients with CMV disease should also receive maintenance therapy until immune recovery. Potential therapies now being investigated include immunotherapy with CMV-specific CD8-positive lymphocyte subsets and treatment with CMV-specific monoclonal antibody.[527,528]

Infections Due to Respiratory Viruses

The respiratory viruses—RSV, influenza, parainfluenza, and adenovirus—commonly cause upper and lower respiratory tract infections in immunocompetent children and adults. With improved methods of diagnosis and treatment, these viruses are increasingly recognized as important pathogens in immunocompromised patients. RSV is the most frequent cause of lower respiratory tract infection in young children and a common cause of "colds" and tracheobronchitis in older children and adults; in a study from the University of Rochester, RSV pneumonia and prolonged viral shedding were seen more often in children with cancer than in healthy children.[83] In a study of 11 immunocompromised adults with RSV infection conducted by Englund et al.,[84] patients had signs and symptoms similar to those seen in infected children; 6 of 11 adults had RSV pneumonia. Interestingly, 5 patients also had radiographic evidence of sinusitis. Although influenza is the most common cause of viral pneumonia in adults, most information concerning influenza in the immunocompromised host is described in two large pediatric studies.[529,530] In both, children had the same clinical signs and symptoms as the controls. However, clinical illness in children with cancer in the report by Felman et al.[529] was prolonged and resulted in a delay in chemotherapy in 80% of the children studied. Both upper and lower respiratory infections due to parainfluenza have been described in patients after BMT, after solid organ transplantation, with leukemia, and in AIDS patients; rarely, this has resulted in a fatal interstitial pneumonia.[531] Unlike other respiratory viruses, adenovirus may disseminate resulting in pneumonitis, hepatitis, colitis, or hemorrhagic cystitis. In a study by Zahradnik et al.[532] of adenoviral infections in immunocompromised patients, 12 of 15 had pneumonia and 8 hepatitis. Shields et al.[533] reported a 5% incidence of adenoviral infection after BMT. In both studies the adenoviral infection, often a pneumonia, was shown to increase mortality. Advances in culture methodology with the shell vial technique have allowed more rapid microbiologic diagnosis of viral infection. In addition, commercial antigen detection kits permit the diagnosis of RSV within hours; these kits are expected to be available for influenza and parainfluenza in the near future. The antiviral agents ribavarin and amantadine are recommended for certain viral infections in immunocompromised host. Ribavarin is a synthetic nucleoside analogue with in vitro activity against RSV, influenza, parainfluenza, and HIV; but in clinical use it has been found to increase the oxygen saturation and decrease the symptoms in children with RSV only. It is recommended for immunocompromised children with RSV infection. Amantadine is active against only influenza A. No studies have been performed in immunocompromised children or adults, but amantadine has been found to decrease the duration of fever and systemic symptoms in immunocompetent adults with influenza A infection.

CLINICAL APPROACH TO PARASITIC INFECTIONS IN IMMUNOCOMPROMISED PATIENTS

Pneumocystis carinii Pneumonia

PCP is the most common parasitic disease affecting immunocompromised patients. The populations most commonly affected are those with hematologic malignancies (particularly ALL, Hodgkin disease, and non-Hodgkin lymphomas) or AIDS. In addition, however, PCP can occur in patients with solid tumors, transplant patients, and in other immunosuppressed populations, particularly in those receiving therapy associated with impaired CMI (e.g., corticosteroids). Of all the subgroups at risk of PCP, adult AIDS patients have by far the greatest relative risk.

In non-AIDS patients the most common clinical manifestations of PCP include fever, cough, and tachypnea, generally with intercostal retractions and the absence of detectable rales. A chest radiograph typically shows a hazy bilateral alveolar infiltrate, which often begins at the hilus and spreads to the

APPROACH TO VIRAL INFECTIONS

Herpes Simplex Virus

In compromised hosts, HSV is rarely fatal but is a significant cause of morbidity. For treatment of symptomatic infection, either oral acyclovir (200 mg five times per day) or intravenous acyclovir (750 mg/m^2/day in three divided doses) is effective. Patients with persistently compromised immune status (e.g., those with AIDS) may require chronic suppressive treatment. Development of acyclovir resistance can occur.

Varicella-Zoster Virus

Those at risk of primary infection (chickenpox) who are exposed to an infectious source should receive ZIG and be isolated from other susceptible patients. ZIG can decrease both the morbidity and mortality associated with subsequent infection. In seriously compromised cancer patients who develop primary chickenpox (and who do not receive ZIG or early antiviral therapy), visceral dissemination will occur in about one-third, and ≤20% may die. Prompt institution of intravenous acyclovir (1,500 mg/m^3/day in three divided doses) can decrease morbidity and mortality. Acyclovir should be continued for 7 days and until complete crusting of the lesions.

Secondary VZV infection (zoster) can also cause significant morbidity in compromised patients, although dissemination and death are less frequent than for primary disease. Among seriously compromised cancer patients who do not receive antiviral therapy, cutaneous dissemination occurs in 25–50% and visceral dissemination in 8–19%. The lungs and liver are the most common visceral sites of dissemination. Intravenous acyclovir (1,500 mg/m^2/day in three divided doses) can decrease dissemination and hasten healing of lesions and should be administered as soon after the appearance of lesions as possible (preferably within 72 hours). We begin all high-risk patients on intravenous acyclovir—we define as those undergoing neutropenia-producing cytoreductive therapy, those who have received total body irradiation or BMT within the previous year, those with Hodgkin disease or non-Hodgkin lymphoma, those with AIDS, and other patients with significant depression of CMI (e.g., those receiving high doses of corticosteroids). Therapy should continue for 7 days or until the lesions have crusted. We discourage the use of oral acyclovir for prophylaxis or treatment because of the low serum levels attained and the development of resistance. Patients with acyclovir-resistant HSV or VZV infection may be treated with foscarnet.

periphery. Arterial blood gas measurements reveal a low PaO$_2$, normal PaCO$_2$, and alkaline pH. The clinical presentation can be indolent (1–2 months) but is more often rapidly progressive (4–5 days). Chest radiographic findings are occasionally atypical (e.g., lobar consolidation, effusion, or nodular or unilateral pneumocysts); in rare cases, the radiograph may appear normal despite the presence of pneumocysts on biopsy. PCP in cancer patients differs from that in AIDS patients by having a more smoldering and indolent course; the median duration of symptoms is 28 days in AIDS patients but 5 days in non-AIDS

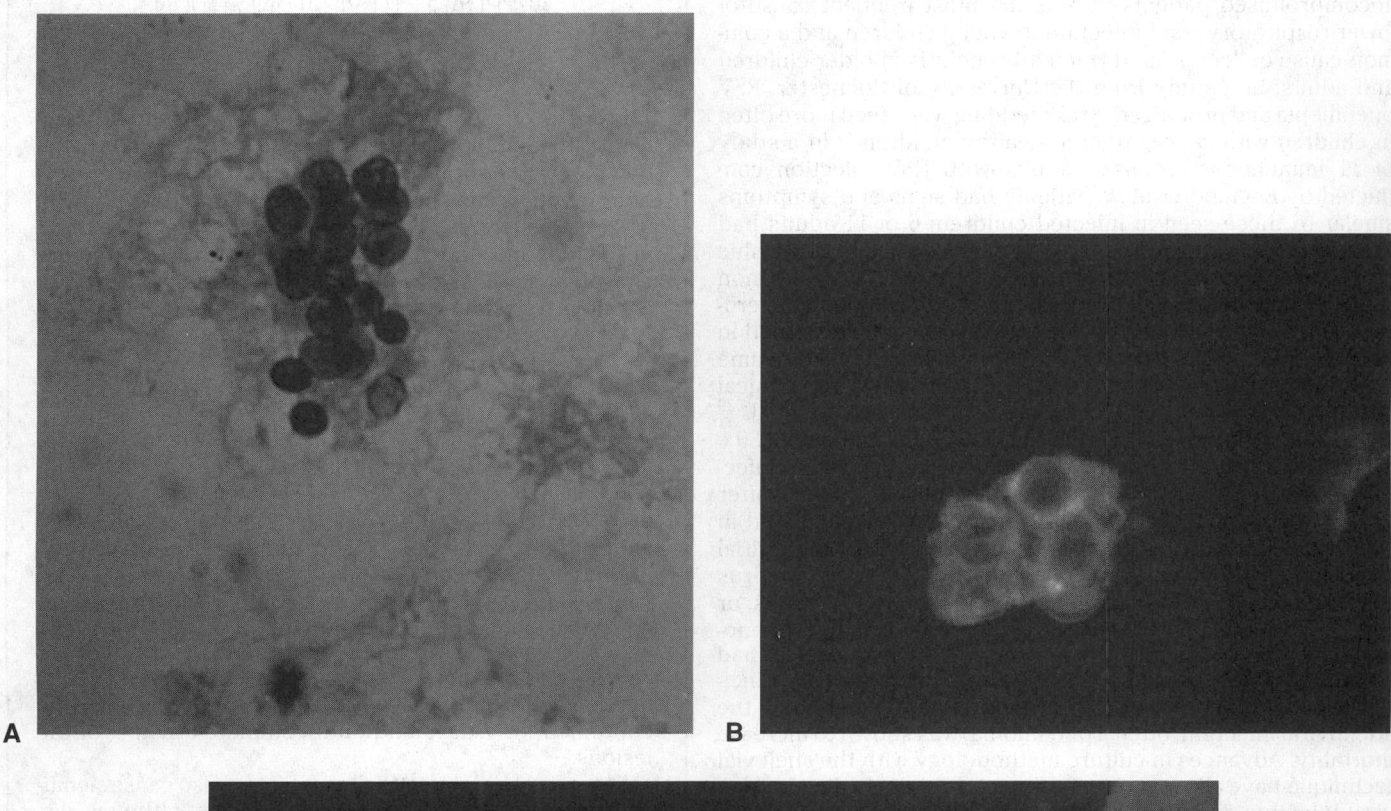

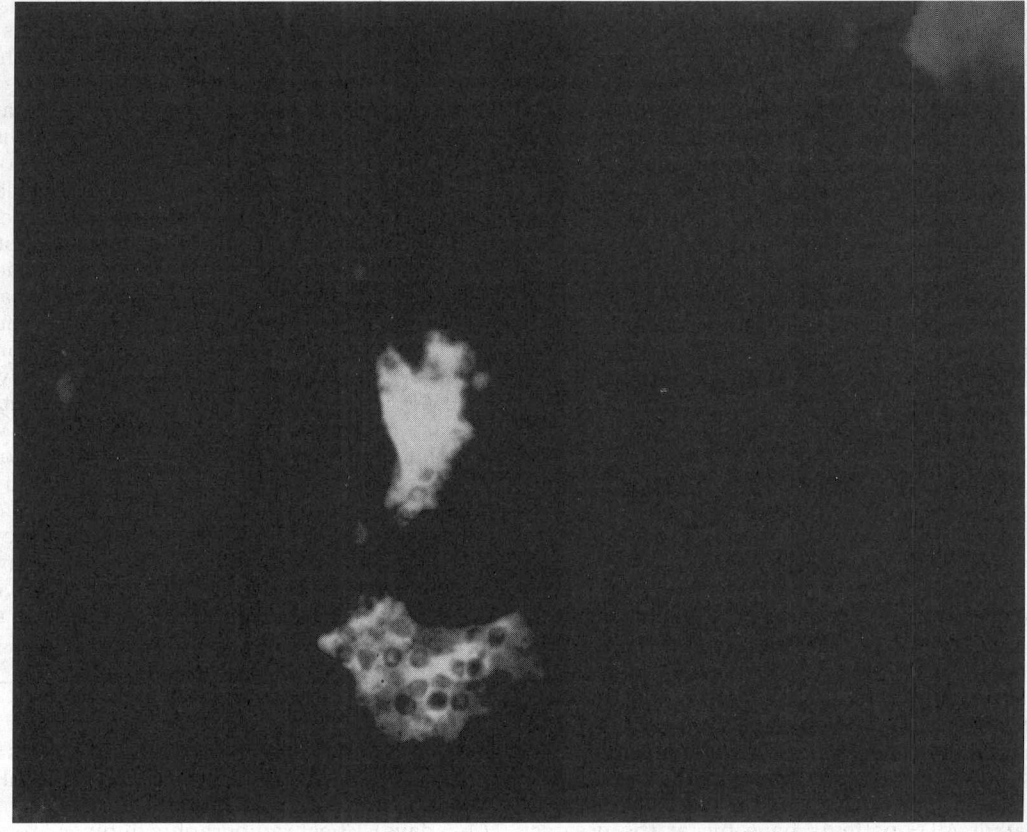

Fig. 91-12. (A) Cluster of *P. carinii* obtained from bronchoalveolar lavage (stained with toluidine blue). **(B & C)** *P. carinii* from induced sputum specimen stained with immunofluorescent monoclonal antibody. (Courtesy of Drs. V. Gill and J. Kovacs, Clinical Center, National Institutes of Health.)

patients.[534] In AIDS patients, disseminated *P. carinii* infections have recently been reported; while the lungs are still the most common site of infection, the lymph nodes, spleen, liver, bone marrow, adrenal glands, kidneys, and gastrointestinal tract are also commonly involved.[535]

The diagnosis of PCP requires demonstration of cysts or trophozoites in pulmonary material from patients with a clinically compatible course; cysts have been found in asymptomatic, previously healthy individuals autopsied after traumatic death. Classically, material obtained from bronchoalveolar lavage or open-lung biopsy and stained with Gomori methenamine-silver nitrate or toluidine blue has been the most reliable for diagnosis. At the NCI, immunofluorescent monoclonal antibody stains on induced sputum specimens have given fast and reliable results[536] (Fig. 91-12). Recent studies using PCR on induced sputum but not on bronchial lavage fluid show an increased sensitivity; in the future PCR may decrease the number of bronchoscopies needed for the diagnosis of PCP.[537]

In clinical situations in which the likelihood of PCP is great, the choice is between proceeding with a diagnostic procedure and administering an empirical course of therapy with trimethoprim-sulfamethoxazole. If techniques for examining induced sputum or bronchoalveolar lavage fluid are readily available, these are initially procedures of choice for establishing the diagnosis. However, if they are not available, or if the patient's clinical or hematologic status does not permit bronchoalveolar lavage, an empirical trial of trimethoprim-sulfamethoxazole (20 mg/kg/day of trimethoprim) plus erythromycin (for *Legionella*) is recommended, rather than proceeding directly to open-lung biopsy. This approach is based on the results of a randomized NCI trial demonstrating that in non-neutropenic patients with diffuse infiltrates, empirical therapy is as safe and effective as is open-lung biopsy.[538] The clinician should realize that a response to therapy may not be apparent for 4–5 days. Indeed, progression over the first few days does not necessarily imply inappropriate or ineffective therapy. It is theorized that this delay in improvement is due to the host's inflammatory response; for this reason, steroids are recommended during the first 72 hours for patients with an arterial oxygen pressure <70 mmHg or an arterial-alveolar gradient of <35 mmHg.[539] If the patient fails to improve (e.g., continued fever, depressed PaO_2, or progressive infiltrates) after 4 days of therapy, modification is then appropriate. In this setting we prefer to add pentamidine (4 mg/kg/day) rather than discontinue the trimethoprim-sulfamethoxazole, since progression may represent slow response rather than true failure.

If a histologic diagnosis is necessary and not achievable by bronchoalveolar lavage, not all procedures, such as transtracheal aspiration, transbronchial biopsy or aspiration, or open-lung biopsy, are of comparable diagnostic accuracy. Burt and colleagues[540] examined each of 17 patients who had undergone open-lung biopsy to evaluate whether the diagnosis of a diffuse interstitial infiltrate could be established with a transthoracic needle aspirate and a transbronchial brush and biopsy. The patients in this unique study served as their own controls. The diagnosis was established from only 30% of the aspirates and from 59% of the transbronchial biopsy samples, suggesting that open-lung biopsy is the procedure of choice. Open-lung biopsy provides the soundest guidance for patient management, especially if the patient is neutropenic and requires multiple antimicrobial agents.

Because patients who are candidates for open-lung biopsy are often thrombocytopenic, appropriate hematologic preparation for surgery is vital. Elevation of the platelet count to a surgically safe level of ≥30,000/mm³ can usually be accomplished by infusion of 4–8 U of platelet concentrates 1 hour before surgery. Maintenance of the platelet count at this level for 24 hours after surgery with additional platelet concentrates minimizes any postoperative bleeding complications.

Because of the importance that *P. carinii* has assumed in patients with AIDS, the search for new therapeutic agents has intensified. Alternative regimens studied have included dapsone alone, trimethoprim with dapsone, clindamycin with primaquine, atovaquone, eflornithine, trimetrexate, and piritrexim.[299] In most cases of PCP in patients who either fail or are unable to tolerate trimethoprim-sulfamethoxazole and pentamidine, we add trimetrexate. The efficacy of trimethoprim-sulfamethoxazole as primary prophylaxis against both PCP and toxoplasmosis in AIDS patients is unknown. A recent French study found that the combination of dapsone and pyrimethamine was as effective as aerosolized pentamidine in preventing PCP and was also effective in the prevention of toxoplasmosis in *Toxoplasma*-antibody-positive patients.[542]

Another clinical dilemma is the treatment of patients who develop PCP while on a preventive regimen. Although it is logical to assume drug failure and change regimens for treatment, there is no data to support this and simply switching to a parenteral route of administration may suffice for treatment.[299]

REFERENCES

1. Johanson WG, Pierce AK, Sanford JP: Changing pharyngeal bacterial flora of hospitalized patients. Emergence of gram-negative bacilli. N Engl J Med 281:1137, 1969
2. Fainstein V, Rodriguez V, Turk M et al: Patterns of oropharyngeal and fecal flora in patients with leukemia. J Infect Dis 144:10, 1981
3. Schimpff SC, Young VM, Greene WH et al: Origin of infection in acute non-lymphocytic leukemia. Ann Intern Med 77:707, 1972
4. Van der Waaij D, Tielemans-Speltie TM, de Roeck-Houben AMJ: Enterobacteriaceae species on leukemic patients. Infection 5:188, 1977
5. Schimpff SC, Greene WH, Young VM, Wiernik PH: Significance of *Pseudomonas aeruginosa* in the patient with leukemia or lymphoma. J Infect Dis, suppl. 130:524, 1974
6. Pizzo PA, Ladisch S, Witebsky FG: Alpha-hemolytic streptococci: clinical significance in the cancer patient. Med Pediatr Oncol 4:267, 1978
7. Pizzo PA, Ladisch S, Simon RM et al: Increasing incidence of gram-positive sepsis in cancer patients. Med Pediatr Oncol 5:241, 1978
8. Rubin M, Hathorn J, Marshall D et al: Gram-positive infections and the use of vancomycin in 550 episodes of fever and neutropenia. Ann Intern Med 108:30, 1988
9. Wade JC, Schimpff SC, Newman KA et al: *Staphylococcus epidermidis:* an increasing cause of infection in patients with granulocytopenia. Ann Intern Med 97:503, 1982
10. Shenep JL, Hughes WT, Roberson PK et al: Vancomycin ticarcillin and amikacin compared with ticarcillin-clavulanate and amikacin in the empirical treatment of febrile neutropenic children with cancer. N Engl J Med 317:1053, 1988
11. Grossi M, Green DM: *Staphylococcus aureus* bacteremia in children and adolescents with acute lymphoblastic leukemia. Oncology 40:321, 1983
12. Winston DJ, Dudnick DV, Chapin M et al: Coagulase-negative staphylococcal bacteremia in patients receiving immunosuppressive therapy. Arch Intern Med 143:32, 1983
13. Friedman LE, Brown AE, Miller DR: *Staphylococcus epidermidis* septicemia in children with leukemia and lymphoma. Am J Dis Child 138:710, 1984
14. Weisman SJ, Scoopo FJ, Johnson GM et al: Septicemia in pediatric oncology patients: the significance of *viridans* streptococcal infections. J Clin Oncol 8:453, 1990
15. Classen DC, Burke JP, Ford CD et al: *Streptococcus mitis* sepsis in bone marrow transplant patients receiving oral antimicrobial prophylaxis. Am J Med 89:441, 1990
16. Trucksis M, Hopper DC, Wolfson JS et al: Emerging resistance to fluoroquinolones in staphylococci: an alert. Ann Intern Med 114:424, 1991
17. Haley RW, Hightower AW, Khabbaz RF et al: Emergence of methicillin-resistant S. aureus infections in United States hospitals. Ann Intern Med 97:297, 1982
18. Gill VJ, Manning C, Lamson M et al: Antibiotic-resistant group JK bacteria in hospitals. J Clin Microbiol 13:472, 1982
19. Rubin M, Todeschini G, Marshall D et al: Does the presence of an indwelling venous catheter affect the type of infections in neutropenic cancer patients (CP)? An analysis of 505 episodes, abstracted (961). p. 264. In Program and Abstracts of Twenty-seventh Interscience Conference on Antimicrobial Agents and Chemotherapy, New York, NY, 1987
20. Khabbaz RF, Cooksey RC, Saba G, Wade JC: The alimentary tract as a source of S. epidermidis (SE) bacteremia in patients with cancer: clues from molecu-

lar epidemiology, abstracted (1036). p. 277. In Program and Abstracts of the Twenty-seventh Interscience Conference on Antimicrobial Agents and Chemotherapy, 1987

21. Kagnoff ME, Armstrong D, Blevins A: Bacteroides bacteremia: experience in a hospital for neoplastic diseases. Cancer 29:245, 1972

22. Fainstein V, Elting LS, Bodey GP: Bacteremia caused by nonsporulating anaerobes in cancer patients. A 12 year experience. Medicine 68:151, 1989

23. Finegold SM, Marsh VH, Bartlett JG: Anaerobic infections in the compromised host. p. 123. In Proceedings of the International Conference on Nosocomial Infections, Centers for Disease Control, Atlanta, 1970

24. Thaler M, Gill V, Pizzo PA: Emergence of Clostridium tertium as a pathogen in neutropenic patients. Am J Med 81:596, 1986

25. Whimbey E, Kiehn TE, Brannon P et al: Bacteremia and fungemia in patients with neoplastic diseases. Am J Med 82:723, 1987

26. McFarland LV, Mulligan ME, Kwok RYY, Stamm WE: Nosocomial acquisition of Clostridium difficile infection. N Engl J Med 320:204, 1989

27. Van der Waaij D: Colonization resistance of the digestive tract: clinical consequences and implications. J Antimicrob Chemother 10:263, 1983

28. Van der Waaij D, Berghuis-de Vries JM, Lekkerkerk-van der Wees JEC: Colonization resistance of the digestive tract in conventional and antibiotic-treated mice. J Hyg (Camb) 69:405, 1971

29. Beck-Sague C, Dooley SW, Hutton MD et al: Hospital outbreak of multidrug-resistant Mycobacterium tuberculosis infections. JAMA 268:1280, 1992

30. Jereb JA, Kelly GD, Dooley SW et al: Tuberculosis morbidity in the United States: final data. MMWR CDC Surveill Summ 40:23, 1991

31. Mackowiak PA, Demian SE, Sutker WS et al: Infections in hairy cell leukemia. Clinical evidence of a pronounced deficit in cell mediated immunity. Am J Med 68:718, 1980

32. Golomb HM, Hadad LJ: Infectious complications in 127 patients with hairy cell leukemia. Am J Hematol 16:393, 1984

33. Weinstein RA, Golomb HM, Grumet G et al: Hairy cell leukemia: association with disseminated atypical mycobacterial infection. Cancer 43:380, 1981

34. Pizzo PA, Myers J: Infections in the cancer patient. p. 2088. In DeVita VT Jr, Hellman S, Rosenberg SA (eds): Cancer, Principles and Practice of Oncology. JB Lippincott, Philadelphia, 1989

35. Maki DG, Alvarado CJ, Hessewer CH et al: Relation of the inanimate hospital environment to endemic nosocomial infection. N Engl J Med 307:1562, 1982

36. Pizzo PA, Purvis D, Waters CW: Microbiological evaluation of food items for patients undergoing gastrointestinal decontamination and protected isolation. J Am Diet Assoc 81:272, 1982

37. Remington JS, Schimpff SC: Please don't eat the salads. N Engl J Med 304:433, 1981

38. Newman KA, Schimpff SC: Hospital hotel services are risk factors for infection among immunosuppressed patients. Rev Infect Dis 9:206, 1987

39. Fraser DW: Legionellosis: evidence of airborne transmission. Ann NY Acad Sci 353:61, 1980

40. Dondero TJ Jr, Rendtorff RC, Mallison GF et al: Outbreak of legionnaire's disease associated with a contaminated air conditioning cooling tower. N Engl J Med 302:365, 1980

41. Henderson DR, Baptiste R, Parillo J, Gill VJ: Indolent epidemic of Pseudomonas cepacia bacteremia and pseudobacteremia in an intensive care unit traced to a contaminated blood-gas analyzer. Am J Med 84:75, 1988

42. Bodey GP: Fungal infections complicating acute leukemia. J Chron Dis 19:667, 1966

43. Hawkins C, Armstrong D: Fungal infections in the immunocompromised host. Baillieres Clin Haematol 13:599, 1984

44. Walsh T, Pizzo PA: Nosocomial fungal infections: a classification for hospital-acquired fungal infections and mycoses arising from endogenous flora or reactivation. Annu Rev Microbiol 42:517, 1988

45. Walsh TJ, Newman KR, Moody M et al: Trichosporinosis in patients with neoplastic disease. Medicine 65:268, 1986

46. Walsh TJ: Trichosporinosis. Infect Dis Clin North Am 3:43, 1989

47. Klotz SA: Malassezia furfur. Infect Dis Clin North Am 3:53, 1989

48. Odds FC: Ecology and epidemiology of Candida species. Zentralbl Mikrobiol 257:207, 1984

49. Kramer BJ, Pizzo PA, Robichaud KJ et al: Role of serial microbiological surveillance and clinical evaluation in the management of cancer patients with fever and granulocytopenia. Am J Med 72:561, 1982

50. Wingard JR, Merz WG, Saral RR: Candida tropicalis: a major pathogen in immunocompromised patients. Ann Intern Med 91:539, 1979

51. Aisner J, Schimpff SC, Sutherland JC et al: Torulopsis glabrata infections in patients with cancer. Increasing incidence and relationship to colonization. Am J Med 61:23, 1976

52. Staib F. Ecological and epidemiological aspects of aspergilli pathogenic for man and animal in Berlin (West). Zentralbl Mikrobiol 257:240, 1984

53. Aisner J, Murillo J, Schimpff S, Steere AC: Invasive aspergillosis in acute

leukemia: correlation with nose culture and antibiotic use. Ann Intern Med 90:4, 1979

54. Gerson SL, Talbot GH, Hurwitz S et al: Prolonged granulocytopenia: the major risk factor for invasive pulmonary aspergillosis in patients with acute leukemia. Ann Intern Med 100:345, 1984

55. Yu VL, Muder RR, Poorsattar A: Significance of isolation of Aspergillus from the respiratory tract in diagnosis of invasive pulmonary aspergillosis. Results from a three-year prospective study. Am J Med 81:249, 1986

56. Emmons CW: Isolation of Cryptococcus neoformans from soil. J Bacteriol 62:685, 1951

57. Ruiz A, Fromtling RA, Bulmer GS: Distribution of Cryptococcus neoformans in a natural site. Infect Immun 31:560, 1981

58. Young N: Hematologic and hematopoietic consequences of B19 parvovirus infection. Semin Hematol 25:159, 1988

59. Hirsch MS: Herpes simplex virus. p. 1334. In Mandell GL, Douglas RG, Bennett JE (eds): Principles and Practice of Infectious Disease. 4th Ed. Churchill Livingstone, New York, 1995

60. Buddingh GJ, Schrum DJ, Lanier JC et al: Studies on the natural history of herpes simplex infection. Pediatrics 11:595, 1953

61. Nahmias AJ, Josey WE, Naib AM et al: Antibodies to herpes virus laminin types 1 and 2 in humans. I. Patients with genital herpes infections. Am J Epidemiol 91:539, 1970

62. Rawls WE, Campione-Piccardo J: Epidemiology of herpes simplex virus type 1 and 2 infections. p. 137. In Nahmias AJ, Dowdle WR, Schinazi RF (eds): The Human Herpes Viruses: An Interdisciplinary Approach. Elsevier, New York, 1981

63. Elfenbein GJ, Saral R: Infectious disease during immune recovery after bone marrow transplantation. p. 157. In Allen JC (ed): Infection and the Compromised Host. Williams & Wilkins, Baltimore, 1981

64. Saral R, Burns WH, Laskin OL et al: Acyclovir prophylaxis of herpes simplex virus infections: a randomized, double-blind controlled trial in bone marrow transplant recipients. N Engl J Med 305:65, 1981

65. Saral R, Ambinder RF, Burns WH et al: Acyclovir prophylaxis against herpes simplex virus infection in patients with leukemia—a randomized, double-blind, placebo-controlled study. Ann Intern Med 99:773, 1983

66. Feldman S, Hughes WJ, Daniel CB: Varicella in children with cancer: seventy-seven cases. Pediatrics 56:388, 1975

67. Reboul F, Donaldson SS, Kaplan HS: Herpes zoster and varicella in children with Hodgkin's disease—an analysis of contributing factors. Cancer 41:95, 1978

68. Ragozzino MW, Melton LJ III, Kurland LT et al: Population-based study of herpes zoster and its sequelae. Medicine 61:310, 1982

69. Schimpff SC, Serpick A, Stoler B et al: Varicella zoster infection in patients with cancer. Ann Intern Med 76:241, 1972

70. Locksley RM, Flournoy N, Sullivan KM et al: Varicella-zoster infection after marrow transplantation. J Infect Dis 132:1172, 1985

71. Miller LH, Brunell PA: Zoster, reinfection or activation of latent virus? Am J Med 49:480, 1970

72. Rado JP, Tako J, Geder L et al: Herpes zoster house epidemic in steroid-treated patients. Arch Intern Med 116:329, 1965

73. Booth JC, Hannington G, Bakir TMF et al: Comparison of enzyme-linked immunosorbent assay, radioimmunoassay, complement fixation, anticomplement immunofluorescence and passive hemagglutination techniques for detecting cytomegalovirus IgG antibody. J Clin Pathol 35:1345, 1982

74. Meyers JD, Flournoy N, Thomas ED: Risk factors for cytomegalovirus infection after human marrow transplantation. J Infect Dis 153:478, 1986

75. Balfour HH, Chase BA, Stapleton JJ et al: A randomized, placebo-controlled trial of acyclovir for the prevention of cytomegalovirus disease in recipients of renal allografts. N Engl J Med 320:381, 1989

76. Drew WL, Mintz L, Miner RC et al: Prevalence of cytomegalovirus infection in homosexual men. J Infect Dis 143:188, 1981

77. White WH, Yow MD, Demmler GJ et al: Prevalence of cytomegalovirus antibody in subjects between the ages of 6 and 22 years. J Infect Dis 159:1013, 1989

78. Bowden RA, Sayers M, Fluornoy N et al: Cytomegalovirus immune globulin and seronegative blood products to prevent primary cytomegalovirus infections after marrow transplantation. N Engl J Med 314:1006, 1986

79. McVoy MA, Adler SP: Immunologic evidence for frequent age-related cytomegalovirus reactivation in seropositive immunocompetent individuals. J Infect Dis 160:1, 1989

80. Chou S: Neutralizing antibody responses to reinfecting strains of cytomegalovirus in transplant recipients. J Infect Dis 160:16, 1989

81. Chou S: Reactivation and recombination of multiple cytomegalovirus strains from individual organ donors. J Infect Dis 160:11, 1989

82. Grundy JE, Lui SF, Super M et al: Symptomatic cytomegalovirus infection

in seropositive kidney recipients: re-infection with donor virus rather than reactivation of recipient virus. Lancet 2:132, 1988

83. Hall CB, Powell KR, MacDonald NE et al: Respiratory synctial viral infection in children with compromised immune function. N Engl J Med 315:77, 1986

84. Englund JA, Sullivan CJ, Jordan MC et al: Respiratory synctial virus infection in immunocompromised adults. Ann Intern Med 109:203, 1988

85. Koch KL, Phillips DJ, Aber RC, Currant WL: Cryptosporidiosis in hospital personnel: evidence for person-to-person transmission. Ann Intern Med 102:593, 1985

86. Navin TR, Juranek DD: Cryptosporidiosis: clinical, epidemiologic, and parasitologic review. Rev Infect Dis 6:313, 1984

87. Soave R, Armstrong D: Cryptosporidium and cryptosporidiosis. Rev Infect Dis 8:1012, 1986

88. Hayes GB, Matte TD, O'Brien TR et al: Large community outbreak of cryptosporidiosis due to contamination of a filtered public water supply. N Engl J Med 320:1372, 1989

89. Kovacs JA, Kovacs AA, Polis M et al: Cryptococcosis in the acquired immunodeficiency syndrome. Ann Intern Med 103:533, 1985

90. Moore AC, Herwaldt BI, Craun GF et al: Surveillance for waterborne disease outbreaks—United States. MMWR CDC Surveill Summ 42:1, 1993

91. Perera DR, Western KA, Johnson HD et al: *Pneumocystis carinii* pneumonia in a hospital for children. JAMA 214:1074, 1970

92. Meuwissen JH, Tauber J, Loewenberg AD et al: Parasitologic and serologic observations of infection with *Pneumocystis* in humans. J Infect Dis 136:43, 1977

93. Ruebush TK, Weinstein RA, Baehner RL et al: An outbreak of *Pneumocystis* pneumonia in children with acute lymphocytic leukemia. Am J Dis Child 132:143, 1978

94. Singer C, Armstrong D, Rosen PP et al: *Pneumocystis carinii* pneumonia: a cluster of eleven cases. Ann Intern Med 82:792, 1975

95. Chave JP, David S, Wauter JP et al: Transmission of *Pneumocystis carinii* from AIDS patients to other immunosuppressed patients: a cluster of *Pneumocystis carinii* pneumonia in renal transplant recipients. AIDS 5:927, 1991

96. Hendley JO, Weller TH: Activation and transmission in rates of infection with *Pneumocystis.* Proc Soc Exp Biol Med 137:1401, 1971

97. Cotton DJ, Gill V, Hiemenz J et al: Bacillus bacteremia in an immunocompromised patient population: clinical features, therapeutic interventions, and relationship to chronic intravenous catheters in sixteen cases. J Clin Microbiol 25:672, 1987

98. Banerjee C, Bustamante CJ, Wharton R et al: *Bacillus* infections in patients with cancer. Arch Intern Med 148:1769, 1988

99. Hiemenz J, Skelton J, Pizzo PA: Perspective on the management of catheter-related infections in cancer patients. Pediatr Infect Dis 5:6, 1986

100. Press OW, Ramsey PG, Larson EB et al: Hickman catheter infections in patients with malignancies. Medicine 63:189, 1984

101. Todeschini G, Rubin M, Gill V et al: Non-*Aeruginosa* bacteremia in cancer patients. Review of 10 year experience at the National Cancer Institute. p. 265. In Proceedings of the Twenty-seventh Interscience Conference on Antimicrobial Agents and Chemotherapy, New York, 1987

102. Viscoli C, Garavente A, Boni L et al: Role of Broviac catheter in infections in children with cancer. Pediatr Infect Dis J 7:536, 1988

103. Allo MD, Miller J, Townsend T, Jan C: Primary cutaneous aspergillosis associated with Hickman intravenous catheter. N Engl J Med 317:1105, 1987

104. Walsh TJ, Bustamante CJ, Vlahov D, Standiford HC: Candidal suppurative peripheral thrombophlebitis: recognition, prevention, and management. Infect Control Hosp Epidemiol 7:16, 1986

105. Rose HD: Venous catheter-associated candidemia. Am J Med Sci 275:265, 1978

106. Forlenza SW, Newman MG, Lipsey AL et al: *Capnocytophaga* sepsis: a newly recognized clinical entity in granulocytopenic patients. Lancet 1:567, 1980

107. Klein RS, Reuco RA, Catalono MT et al: Association of *Streptococcus bovis* with carcinoma of the colon. N Engl J Med 297:800, 1977

108. Steinberg D, Naggar CZ: *Streptococcus bovis* endocarditis with carcinoma of the colon. N Engl J Med 297:1354, 1977

109. Barrett-Connor E: Bacterial infection and sickle cell anemia: an analysis of 250 infections in 166 patients and a review of the literature. Medicine 50:97, 1971

110. Overturf GD, Powars D, Baraff LJ: Bacterial meningitis and septicemia in sickle cell disease. Am J Dis Child 131:784, 1977

111. Hook EW, Kaye D, Gill FA: Factors influencing host resistance to Salmonella infection: the effects of hemolysis and erythrophagocytosis. Trans Am Clin Climatol Assoc 78:230, 1967

112. Syrogiannopoulos GA, McCracken GH, Nelson JD: Osteoarticular infections in children with sickle cell disease. Pediatrics 78:1090, 1986

113. Givner LB, Luddy RE, Schwartz AD: Etiology of osteomyelitis in patients with major sickle hemoglobinopathies. J Pediatr 99:411, 1981

114. Fajardo JE, Mickunas VH, deTriguet JM: Suppurative arthritis and hemophilia. Pediatr Infect Dis 5:593, 1986

115. Bodey GP, Buckley M, Sathe YS et al: Quantitative relationships between circulating leukocytes and infection in patients with acute leukemia. Ann Intern Med 64:328, 1966

116. Levine AS, Schimpff SC, Graw RC et al: Hematologic malignancies and other marrow failure states: progress in the management of complicating infections. Semin Hematol 11:141, 1974

117. McGowan JE: Changing etiology of nosocomial bacteremia and fungemia and other hospital-acquired infections. Rev Infect Dis, suppl. 3. 7:S357, 1985

118. McGowan JE, Barnes MW, Finland M: Bacteremia at Boston City Hospital: occurrence and mortality during 12 selected years (1965–1972) with special reference to hospital acquired cases. J Infect Dis 132:316, 1975

119. Karp JE, Dick JD, Angelopulos C et al: Empiric use of vancomycin during prolonged treatment-induced granulocytopenia: randomized, double-blind, placebo-controlled trial in patients with acute leukemia. Am J Med 81:237, 1986

120. Pizzo PA: Management of fever in patients with cancer and treatment-induced neutropenia. Drug Ther 328:1323, 1993

121. Sanders WE Jr, Sanders CC: Inducible β-lactamases: clinical and epidemiologic implications for use of new cephalosporins. Rev Infect Dis 10:830, 1988

122. Fainstein V, Berkley P, Elting L, Bodey GP: *Haemophilus* species bacteremia in patients with cancer. Arch Intern Med 149:1341, 1989

123. Sotiropoulos SV, Jackson MA, Barker GM et al: Alpha streptococcal sepsis among leukemic children receiving cytosine arabinoside: clinical presentation and prophylaxis, abstracted (601). p. 202. In Program and Abstracts of the Twenty-Ninth Interscience Conference on Antimicrobial Agents and Chemotherapy, Houston, TX, 1989

124. Pizzo PA, Ladisch S, Simon RM et al: Increasing incidence of gram-positive sepsis in cancer patients. Med Pediatr Oncol 5:241, 1978

125. Wynne JW, Armstrong D: Clostridial septicemia. Cancer 29:215, 1972

126. Styrt B, Gorbach SL: Recent developments in the understanding of the pathogenesis and treatment of anaerobic infections. N Engl J Med 321:240, 1989

127. Glenn J, Cotton D, Wesley R et al: Anorectal infections in patients with malignant diseases. Rev Infect Dis 10:42, 1988

128. Seshadri RS, Brown EJ, Zipursky A: Leukemic reticuloendotheliosis: a failure of monocyte production. N Engl J Med 295:181, 1976

129. Cline MJ: A test of individual phagocyte function is a mixed population of leukocytes. Identification of a neutrophil abnormality in acute myelocytic leukemia. J Lab Clin Med 81:311, 1973

130. Bendix-Hansen K: Myeloperoxidase deficient polymorphonuclear leukocytes and leukaemia and allied disorders. Dan Med Bull 35:501, 1988

131. Davey FR, Erba WN, Gatter KC, Mason KY: Abnormal neutrophils in acute myeloid leukemia and myelodysplastic syndrome. Hum Pathol 19:454, 1988

132. Powell BL, Olbrantz P, Bicket D, Bass DA: Altered oxidative product formation is neutrophils of patients recovering from therapy for acute leukemia. Blood 67:1624, 1986

133. Nielsen HK, Bendix-Hansen K: Myeloperoxidase-deficient polymorphonuclear leukocytes (III): relation to incidence of infection in acute myeloid leukemia. Scand J Haematol 33:75, 1984

134. Mazzone A, Ricevuti G, Rossi M, Rizzo SC: Prognostic significance of functional defects of granulocyte in myeloproliferative disease. Oncology 43:176, 1986

135. Pickering LK, Anderson DC, Choi S, Feigin RD: Leukocyte function in children with malignancies. Cancer 35:1363, 1971

136. Martin S, Baldock SC, Ghoneim ATM, Child JA: Defective neutrophil function and microbicidal mechanisms in the myelodysplastic disorders. J Clin Pathol 36:1120, 1983

137. Ruutu P, Ruutu T, Vuopio P et al: Function of neutrophils in preleukemia. Scand J Haematol 18:317, 1977

138. Takahashi I, Inagoki N, Nakada H et al: Superoxide anion production by neutrophils in myelodysplastic syndrome (preleukemia). Acta Med Okayama 42:15, 1988

139. Boogaerts MA, Nelissen V, Roelant C, Goossens W: Blood neutrophil function in primary myelodysplastic syndromes. Br J Haematol 55:217, 1983

140. Pickering LK, Ericsson W, Kohl S: Effect of chemotherapeutic agents on metabolic and bactericidal activity of polymorphonuclear leukocytes. Cancer 42:1741, 1978

141. Van der Nat JM, Beijnen JH, Driebergen RJ et al: *In vitro* immunosuppressive activities of recently developed anthracycline cytostatics. Anticancer Res 8:489, 1989

142. Hyams JS, Donaldson MH, Metcalf JA et al: Inhibition of human granulocyte function by methotrexate. Cancer Res 38:650, 1978

143. MacFadden KD, Saito S, Pruzanski W: The effect of chemotherapeutic agents on chemotaxis and random migration of human leukocytes. J Clin Oncol 3:415, 1985

144. Fumarulo R, Riccardi S, Pantaleo R et al: *In vitro* cisplatin effects on phagocyte functions. Int J Cancer 35:777, 1985

145. Fumarulo R, Riccardi S, Restaino A, Giordano D: Effect of cisplatin on the oxidative metabolism of polymorphonuclear leukocytes in cancer patients. Tumori 70:227, 1984

146. Cream JJ, Pole DS: The effect of methotrexate and hydroxyurea on neutrophil chemotaxis. Br J Dermatol 102:557, 1980

147. Gilbert DN, Starr P, Eubanks N: Inhibition of neutrophil chemotaxis by 4-hydroxy-cyclophosphamide. Cancer Res 37:456, 1972

148. Edelson PJ, Fudenberg HF: Effects of vinblastine on the chemotactic responsiveness of normal human neutrophils. Infect Immun 8:127, 1973

149. Vaudaux P, Kiefer B, Forni M et al: Adriamycin impairs phagocytic function and induces morphologic alterations in human neutrophils. Cancer 54:400, 1984

150. Fauci AS, Dale DC, Balow JE: Glucocorticosteroid therapy. Mechanisms of action and clinical considerations. Ann Intern Med 84:304, 1976

151. Van der Meer JWM: Defense in host-defense mechanisms. p. 41. In Rubin RH, Young LS (eds): Clinical Approach to the Compromised Host. Plenum, New York, 1988

152. Capsoni F, Meroni PL, Zocchi MR et al: Effect of corticosteroids on neutrophil function: inhibition of antibody dependent cell mediated cytotoxicity. J Immunopharmacol 5:217, 1983

153. Rinehart JJ, Sagone AL, Balcerzak SP et al: Effects of corticosteroids on monocyte function. N Engl J Med 292:236, 1975

154. Thompson J, von Furth R: The effect of glucocorticosteroids on the kinetics of mononuclear phagocytes. J Exp Med 131:429, 1976

155. Peters WP, Stuart A, Affronti ML et al: Neutrophil migration is defective during recombinant human-granulocyte-macrophage colony-stimulating factor infusion after autologous bone marrow transplantation. Blood 72:1310, 1988

156. Bock SN, Lee RE, Fisher B et al: A prospective randomized trial evaluating prophylactic antibiotics to prevent catheter-related sepsis in patients treated with immunotherapy. J Clin Oncol 8:161, 1990

157. Jablons D, Bolton E, Mertins S et al: Interleukin 2-based immunotherapy alters circulating neutrophil Fc receptor expression and chemotaxis. J Immunol 144:3630, 1990

158. Colli S, Caruso D, Tremoli E et al: Effect of single oral administration of non-steroidal anti-inflammatory drugs to healthy volunteers on arachidonic acid metabolism in peripheral polymorphonuclear and mononuclear leukocytes. Prostaglandins Leukot Essent Fatty Acids 34:167, 1988

159. Herson VC, Krause PJ, Eisenfeld LI et al: Indomethacin-associated sepsis in very low birth weight infants. Am J Dis Child 142:555, 1988

160. Wildfeuer A: Effects of non-steroidal anti-inflammatory drugs on human leukocytes. Rheumatology 42:16, 1983

161. Kaplan HB, Edelson HS, Korchak et al: Effects of non-steroidal anti-inflammatory agents on human neutrophil functions *in vitro* and *in vivo*. Biochem Pharmacol 33:371, 1984

162. Abramson S, Edelson H, Kaplan H et al: The inactivation of the polymorphonuclear leukocyte by non-steroidal anti-inflammatory drugs. Inflammation, suppl. 8:S103, 1984

163. Ruud B, Benestad HB, Opdahl H: Dual effect of thiopentone on human granulocyte activation. Non-intervention by ketamine and morphine. Acta Anaesthesiol Scand 32:316, 1988

164. Deitch EA, Xu D, Bridges RM: Opioids modulate human neutrophil and lymphocyte function: thermal injury alters beta-endorphin levels. Surgery 104:41, 1988

165. Falke NE, Fischer EG: Cell shape of polymorphonuclear leukocytes is influenced by opioids. Immunology 169:532, 1985

166. MacGregor RR, Safford M, Shalit M: Effect of ethanol on functions required for the delivery of neutrophils to sites of inflammation. J Infect Dis 157:682, 1988

167. Laghi Pasini F, Ceccatelli L, Capecchi PL et al: Benzodiazepines inhibit *in vitro* free-radical formations from human neutrophils induced by FMLP and A23187. Immunopharmacol Immunotoxicol 9:101, 1987

168. Schmeichel CJ, Thomas LC: Methylxanthine bronchodilators potentiate human neutrophil function. J Immunol 138:1896, 1987

169. Straussberg-Djaldetti R, Fishman P, Bessler H et al: The effect of propranalol on protein synthesis and phagocytosis by polymorphonuclear leukocytes from newborn, children, and elderly individuals. Biomed Pharmacother 40:265, 1986

170. Ricevuti G, Marcoli M, Gatti G et al: Assessment of polymorphonucleate leukocyte functions in adult epileptic patients undergoing long-term phenytoin treatment. Hum Toxicol 5:237, 1986

171. Webster RO, Goldstein IM, Flick MR: Selective inhibition by phenytoin of chemotactic factor-stimulated neutrophil functions. J Lab Clin Med 103:22, 1984

172. White IW, Gelb AW, Wexler HR et al: The effects of intravenous anesthetic agents on human neutrophil chemiluminescence. Can J Anaesth 30:506, 1983

173. Welch WD: Effect of enflurane, isoflurane and nitrous oxide on the microbicidal activity of human polymorphonuclear leukocytes. Anesthesiology 61:188, 1984

174. Hafstrøm I: The effect of auranofin on polymorphonuclear granulocytes. Scand J Rheumatol, suppl. 51:36, 1983

175. Kühn SH, Gemperli MB, De Beer FC: Effect of two gold compounds on human polymorphonuclear leukocyte lysosomal function and phagocytosis. Inflammation 9:39, 1985

176. Davis P, Johnston C, Miller CL, Wang K: Effects of gold compounds on the function of phagocytic cells. II. Inhibition of superoxide radical generation by tripeptide-activated polymorphonuclear leukocytes. Arthritis Rheum 26:82, 1983

177. Sasagawa S, Suzuki K, Sakatani T, Fujikura T: Effects of nicotine on the functions of human polymorphonuclear leukocytes *in vitro* and *in vivo*. Scand J Infect Dis, suppl. 41:79, 1983

178. Jones HP, Grisham MB, Bose SK et al: Effect of allopurinol on neutrophil superoxide production, chemotaxis, or degranulation. Biochem Pharmacol 34:3673, 1985

179. Janco RL, English D: Cyclosporine and human neutrophil function. Transplantation 35:510, 1983

180. Weinbaum DL, Kaplan SS, Zdziarski U et al: Human polymorphonuclear leukocyte interaction with cyclosporin A. Infect Immun 43:791, 1984

181. Laghi Pasini F, Pasqui AL, Ceccatelli L et al: Heparin inhibition of polymorphonuclear leukocyte activation *in vitro*. A possible pharmacological approach to granulocyte-mediated vascular damage. Thromb Res 35:527, 1984

182. Kazanjian PH, Pennington JE: Influence of drugs that block calcium channels on the microbicidal function of human neutrophil. J Infect Dis 151:15, 1985

183. Baehner RL, Neiburger RG, Johnson DE, Murrman SM: Transient bactericidal defect of peripheral blood phagocytes from children with acute lymphoblastic leukemia receiving craniospinal irradiation. N Engl J Med 289:1209, 1973

184. Adams DO, Hamilton TA: The cell biology of macrophage activation. Annu Rev Immunol 2:283, 1984

185. Immunization of children infected with human immunodeficiency virus—supplementary ACIP statement. MMWR CDC Surveill Summ 37:181, 1988

186. Twomey JJ, Laughter AH, Farrow S et al: Hodgkin's disease: an immunodepleting and immunosuppressive disorder. J Clin Invest 66:149, 1980

187. Young RC, Corder MP, Haynes HA et al: Delayed hypersensitivity in Hodgkin's disease. A study of 103 untreated patients. Am J Med 52:63, 1972

188. Engleman EJ, Benike CJ, Hoppe RT et al: Autologous mixed lymphocyte reaction in patients with Hodgkin's disease. J Clin Invest 66:149, 1980

189. Lederman MM, Ratnoff OD, Scillian JJ: Impaired cell mediated immunity in patients with classic hemophilia. N Engl J Med 308:79, 1983

190. Menitove JE, Aster RH, Caspar JT et al: T lymphocyte subpopulations in patients with classic hemophilia treated with cryoprecipitate and lyophilized concentrates. N Engl J Med 308:83, 1982

191. Jin ZW, Cleveland RP, Kaufman DB: Immunodeficiency in patients with hemophilia: an underlying deficiency and lack of correlation with factor replacement therapy or exposure to human immunodeficiency virus. J Allergy Clin Immunol 83:165, 1989

192. Ballester OF, Prasad AS: Anergy, zinc deficiency and decreased nucleoside phosphorylase activity in patients with sickle cell anemia. Ann Intern Med 98:180, 1983

193. Fucharoen S, Piankijagum A, Wasi P: Deaths in β-thalassemia/HBG patients secondary to infections. Birth Defects 5A:495, 1988

194. Cupps TR, Fauci AS: Corticosteroid-mediated immunoregulation in man. Immunol Rev 65:134, 1982

195. Balow JE: Cyclophosphamide suppression of established cell mediated immunity. J Clin Invest 56:65, 1975

196. Skinner MD, Schwartz RS: Immunosuppressive therapy. N Engl J Med 217:221, 1972

197. Browne MJ, Hubbard S, Longo D et al: Excess prevalence of *Pneumocystis carinii* pneumonia in patients treated for lymphoma with combination chemotherapy. Ann Intern Med 3:338, 1986

198. Preiksatitis JK, Rosno G, Grumet C et al: Infections due to herpes virus in cardiac transplant recipients. Role of the donor heart and immunosuppressive therapy. J Infect Dis 147:974, 1983

199. Kim JH, Perfect JR: Infection and cyclosporine. Rev Infect Dis 11:677, 1989

200. Witherspoon RP, Lum LG, Storb R: Immunological reconstitution after human marrow grafting. Semin Hematol 21:2, 1984

201. Rouse BT, Horohov DW: Immunosuppression in viral infections. Rev Infect Dis 8:850, 1986

202. Wilson CB: The cellular immune system and its role in host defense. p. 101. In Mandell GL, Douglas RG, Bennett JE (eds): Principles and Practice of Infectious Diseases. 3rd Ed. Churchill Livingstone, New York, 1989

203. Jacobson DR, Zolla-Pazner S: Immunosuppression and infection in multiple myeloma. Semin Oncol 13:282, 1986

204. Doughney KB, Williams DM, Penn RL: Multiple myeloma: infectious complications. South Med J 81:855, 1988

205. Savage DG, Lindenbaum J, Garrett TJ: Biphasic pattern of bacterial infection in multiple myeloma. Ann Intern Med 96:47, 1982

206. Bergens HS, Espersen F, Hertz JB et al: Antibody response to pneumococcal vaccination in patients with myeloma. Scand J Haematol 30:324, 1983

207. Centers for Disease Control: Update: Pneumococcal polysaccharide vaccine usage—United States. Recommendations of the Immunization Practices Advisory Committee. Ann Intern Med 101:348, 1984

208. Immunization Practices Advisory Committee, Center for Disease Control: Recommendations of the Immunization Practices Advisory Committee. Pneumococcal polysaccharide vaccine. MMWR CDC Surveill Summ 5:64, 1988

209. Immunization Practices Advisory Committee, Centers for Disease Control: General recommendations on immunization. Guidelines from the Immunization Practices Committee. Ann Intern Med 111:133, 1989

210. Hanson MM: Chronic lymphocytic leukaemia: clinical studies based on 189 cases followed for a long time. Scand J Haematol, suppl. 18:1, 1973

211. Cooperative Group for the Study of Immunoglobulin in Chronic Lymphocytic Leukemia: Intravenous immunoglobulin for the prevention of infection in chronic lymphocytic leukemia. A randomized, controlled clinical trial. N Engl J Med 319:902, 1988

212. Freeland HS, Scott PP: Recurrent pulmonary infections in patients with chronic lymphocytic leukemia and hypogammaglobulinemia. South Med J 79:1366, 1986

213. Weeks JC, Tierney MR, Weinstein MC: Cost effectiveness of prophylactic intravenous immune globulin in chronic lymphocytic leukemia. N Engl J Med 325:81, 1991

214. Peter G, Pizzo PA, Robichaud KR et al: Possible protective effect of circulating antibodies to the shared glycolipid of Enterobacteriaceae in children with malignancy. Pediatr Res 13:466, 1979

215. Siber GR, Gorham C, Martin P et al: Antibody response to pre treatment immunization and post treatment boosting with bacterial polysaccharide vaccine in patients with Hodgkin's disease. Ann Intern Med 104:467, 1986

216. Gross PA, Gould LA, Brown AE: Effect of cancer chemotherapy on the immune response to influenza virus vaccine: review of published studies. Rev Infect Dis 7:613, 1985

217. Kung FH, Orgel HA, Wallace WW, Hamburger RN: Antibody production following immunization with diphtheria and tetanus toxoids in children receiving chemotherapy during remission of malignant disease. Pediatrics 74:86, 1989

218. Schumacher MJ: Serum immunoglobulin and transferrin levels after childhood splenectomy. Arch Dis Child 45:114, 1970

219. Carlisle HN, Saslaw S: Properdin levels in splenectomized persons. Proc Soc Exp Biol 102:150, 1959

220. Najjar VA, Fridkin M: Antineoplastic, immunogenic and other effects of the tetrapeptide tuftsin: a natural macrophage activator. Ann NY Acad Sci 419: 1, 1983

221. Johnston RB Jr, Newman LS, Struth AG: An abnormality of the alternate pathway of complement activation in sickle cell disease. N Engl J Med 288: 803, 1973

222. Centers for Disease Control: Update on Adult Immunization Recommendations of the Immunization Practices Advisory Committee (ACIP). MMWR CDC Surveill Summ 15(40 RR-12):1, 1991

223. Di Padova F, Dürig M, Harder F et al: Impaired antipneumococcal antibody production in patients without spleens. BMJ 290:14, 1985

224. Recommendations of the Advisory Committee on Immunization Practices (ACIP): Use of vaccines and immune globulins for persons with altered immunocompetence. MMWR CDC Surveill Summ 42(RR-4):1, 1993

225. Albert RK, Condie F: Handwashing patterns in medical intensive care units. N Engl J Med 304:1465, 1981

226. Nauseef WM, Maki DG: A study of the value of simple protective isolation in patients with granulocytopenia. N Engl J Med 304:448, 1981

227. Pizzo PA: Do results justify the expense of protected environments? p. 267. In Wiernik P (ed): Controversies in Oncology. John Wiley & Sons, New York, 1982

228. Verhoef J, Rozenberg-Arska M, Dekker AW: Prevention of bacterial and fungal infections in granulocytopenic patients. Eur J Cancer Clin Oncol 25:1345, 1989

229. Yates JW, Holland JF: A controlled study of isolation and endogenous microbial suppression in acute myelocytic leukemia patients. Cancer 32:1490, 1973

230. Levine AS, Siegel SE, Schreiber AD et al: Protected environment and prophylactic antibiotics: a prospective controlled study of their utility in the therapy of acute leukemia. N Engl J Med 288:477, 1973

231. Levi JA, Vincent PC, Jennis F et al: Prophylactic oral antibiotics in the management of acute leukemia. Med J Aust 1:1025, 1973

232. Schimpff SC, Greene WH, Young VM et al: Infection prevention in acute nonlymphoblastic leukemia: laminar air flow room reverse isolation with nonabsorbable oral antibiotic prophylaxis. Ann Intern Med 82:351, 1975

233. Rodriguez V, Bodey GP, Freireich EJ et al: Randomized trial of protected environment: prophylactic antibiotics in 145 adults with acute leukemia. Medicine 57:253, 1978

234. Storring RA, Jameson B, McElwain TJ et al: Oral non-absorbed antibiotics prevent infection in acute nonlymphoblastic leukemia. Lancet 2:837, 1977

235. Wade JC, Schimpff SC, Hergadon MT et al: A comparison of trimethoprim sulfamethoxazole plus nystatin with gentamicin plus nystatin in the prevention of infections in acute leukemia. N Engl J Med 304:1057, 1981

236. Gurwith MJ, Brunton JL, Lank BA et al: A prospective controlled investigation of prophylactic trimethoprim/sulfamethoxazole in hospitalized granulocytopenic patients. Am J Med 66:248, 1979

237. DeJongh CA, Joshi JH, Newman KA et al: Antibiotic synergism and response in gram negative bacteremia in granulocytopenic cancer patients. Am J Med, suppl. 5C. 80:96, 1986

238. Weiser B, Lange M, Fialk MA et al: Prophylactic trimethoprim-sulfamethoxazole during consolidation chemotherapy for acute leukemia: a controlled trial. Ann Intern Med 95:436, 1981

239. Zinner S, Gaya H, Glauser M et al: Clotrimoxazole and reduction of risk of infection in neutropenic patients: a progress report. p. 795. In Proceedings of the Twenty-first Interscience Conference on Antimicrobial Agents and Chemotherapy, 1981

240. Wilson JM, Guiney DG: Failure of oral trimethoprim-sulfamethoxazole prophylaxis in acute leukemia: isolation of resistance plasmids from strains of Enterobacteriaceae causing bacteremia. N Engl J Med 306:16, 198

241. Wade JC, De Jongh CA, Newman KA et al: Selective antimicrobial modulation as prophylaxis against infection during granulocytopenia: trimethoprim-sulfamethoxazole vs nalidixic acid. J Infect Dis 147:624, 1983

242. Pizzo PA, Robichaud KJ, Edwards BK et al: Oral antibiotic prophylaxis in patients with cancer: a double-blind randomized placebo-controlled trial. J Pediatr 102:125, 1985

243. Rozenberg-Arska M. Dekker AW, Verhoef J: Ciprofloxacin for selective decontamination of the alimentary tract in patients with acute leukemia during remission induction treatment: the effect of fecal flora. J Infect Dis 152:104, 1985

244. Dekker A, Rozenberg-Arska M, Sixma JJ et al: Prevention of infection by trimethoprim sulfamethoxazole plus amphotericin B in patients with acute nonlymphocytic leukemia. Ann Intern Med 95:555, 1981

245. Karp JE, Merz WG, Hendricksen C et al: Infection management during antileukemia treatment-induced granulocytopenia: the role for oral norfloxacin prophylaxis against infections arising from the gastrointestinal tract. Scand J Infect Dis Suppl 48:66, 1986

246. Winston DJ, Ho WG, Nakao SL et al: Norfloxacin versus vancomycin/polymixin for prevention of infections in granulocytopenic patients. Am J Med 80: 884, 1986

247. Bow EJ, Rayner E, Louie TJ: Comparison of norfloxacin with cotrimoxazole for infection prophylaxis in acute leukemia. The trade-off for reduced gram-negative sepsis. Am J Med 84:847, 1988

248. Dekker AW, Rozenberg-Arska M, Verhoef J: Infection prophylaxis in acute leukemia: a comparison of ciprofloxacin with trimethoprim-sulfamethoxazole and colistin. Ann Intern Med 106:7, 1987

249. Tulloch AL: Pancytopenia in an infant associated with sulfamethoxazole-trimethoprim therapy. J Pediatr 88:499, 1976

250. Golde DW, Bersch N, Quan SC: Trimethoprim and sulfamethoxazole inhibition of haematopoiesis in vitro. Br J Haematol 40:343, 1978

251. Deeg HJ, Meyers JD, Storb R et al: Effect of trimethoprim-sulfamethoxazole on hematological recovery after total body irradiation and autologous marrow infusion in dogs. Transplantation 28:243, 1979

252. Meunier F: Prevention of mycoses in immunocompromised patients. Rev Infect Dis 9:408, 1987

253. Liang RS, Yung RW, Chan TK et al: Orfloxacin versus co-trimoxazole for prevention of infection in neutropenic patients following cytotoxic chemotherapy. Antimicrob Agents Chemother 34:215, 1990

254. Karp JE, Merz WG, Hendricksen C et al: Oral norfloxacin for prevention of gram-negative bacterial infections in patients with acute leukemia and granulocytopenia. Ann Intern Med 106:1, 1987

255. Cruciani M, Concia E, Navarra A et al: Prophylactic co-trimoxazole versus norfloxacin in neutropenic children—perspective randomized study. Infection 17:9, 1989

256. Dekker AW, Rozenberg-Arska M, Verhoef J: Infection prophylaxis in acute

leukemia: a comparison of ciprofloxacin with trimethoprim-sulfamethoxazole and colistin. Ann Intern Med 106:7, 1987

257. Del Favero A, Menichetti F, Martino P, Mandelli F: Prevention of bacterial infection in neutropenic patients with hematologic malignancies: a randomized multicenter trial comparing norfloxacin with ciprofloxacin. Ann Intern Med 115:7, 1991

258. Kotilainen P, Nikoskelainen J, Huovinen P: Emergence of ciprofloxacin-resistant coagulase-negative staphylococcal skin flora in immunocompromised patients receiving ciprofloxacin. J Infect Dis 161:41, 1990

259. Oppenheim BA, Hartley JW, Lee W et al: Outbreak of coagulase-negative *Staphylococcus* highly resistant to ciprofloxacin in a leukaemia unit. BMJ 299:294, 1989

260. Liesche GJ, Burgess AW: Granulocyte colony-stimulating factor and granulocyte-macrophage colony-stimulating factor. Drug Ther 327:28, 1992

261. Nemunaitis J, Rabinowe SN, Singer JW, et al: Recombinant granulocyte-macrophage colony-stimulating factor after autologous bone marrow transplantation for lymphoid cancer. N Engl J Med 324:1773, 1991

262. Crawford J, Ozer H, Stoller R et al: Reduction by granulocyte colony-stimulating factor of fever and neutropenia induced by chemotherapy in patients with small-cell lung cancer. N Engl J Med 325:164, 1991

263. Bronchud MH, Scarffe JH, Thatcher N et al: Phase I/II study of recombinant human granulocyte colony-stimulating factor in patients receiving intensive chemotherapy for small cell lung cancer. Br J Cancer 56:809, 1987

264. Vadhan-Raj S, Broxmeyer HE, Hittelman WN et al: Abrogating chemotherapy-induced myelosuppression by recombinant granulocyte-macrophage colony-stimulating factor in patients with sarcoma: protection at the progenitor cell level. J Clin Oncol 10:1266, 1992

265. Roilides E, Uhlig K, Venzon D et al: Neutrophil oxidative burst in response to blastoconidia and pseudohyphae of *Candida albicans*: augmentation by granulocyte colony-stimulating factor and interferon-γ. J Infect Dis 166:668, 1992

266. Kojima S, Fukuda M, Miyajima Y et al: Treatment of aplastic anemia in children with recombinant human granulocyte colony-stimulating factor. Blood 77:937, 1991

267. Bonilla MA, Davis MW, Nakanisi AM et al: A randomized controlled phase III trial of recombinant human granulocyte colony-stimulating factor (filgrastim) for treatment of severe chronic neutropenia. Blood 81:2496, 1993

268. Mueller BU, Jacobsen F, Butler KM et al: Combination treatment with azidothymidine and granulocyte colony-stimulating factor in children with human immunodeficiency virus infection. J Pediatr 121(5 Pt.1):797, 1992

269. Roilides E, Pizzo PA: Biologicals and hematopoietic cytokines in prevention or treatment of infections in immunocompromised hosts. Hematol Oncol Clin North Am 7:841, 1993

270. Ozaki Y, Ohashi T, Minami A et al: Enhanced resistance of mice to bacterial infection induced by recombinant human interleukin-1a. Infect Immun 55:1436, 1987

271. Lopez AF, To LB, Yang YC et al: Stimulation of proliferation, differentiation, and function of human cells by primate interleukin-3. Proc Natl Acad Sci USA 84:2761, 1987

272. Murray HW: Interferon-gamma, the activated macrophage, and host defense against microbial challenge. Ann Intern Med 108:595, 1988

273. The International Chronic Granulomatous Disease Cooperative Study Group: A controlled trial of interferon gamma to prevent infection in chronic granulomatous disease. N Engl J Med 324:509, 1991

274. Goodman JL, Winston DJ, Greenfield RA et al: A controlled trial of fluconazole to prevent fungal infections in patients undergoing bone marrow transplantation. N Engl J Med 326:845, 1992

275. Wingard JR, Merz WG, Rinaldi MG et al: Increase in *Candida krusei* infection among patients with bone marrow transplantation and neutropenia treated prophylactically with fluconazole. N Engl J Med 325:1274, 1991

276. Cheeseman SH, Rubin RH, Stewart JA et al: Controlled clinical trial of prophylactic human leukocyte interferon in renal transplantation: effects on cytomegalovirus and herpes simplex virus infections. N Engl J Med 300:1345, 1979

277. Meyers JD, Flournoy N, Thomas ED: Infection with herpes simplex virus and cell mediated immunity after marrow transplant. J Infect Dis 142:338, 1980

278. Hann IM, Prentice HG, Blackloch HA et al: Acyclovir prophylaxis against herpes-virus infections in severely immunocompromised patients: randomized double blind trial. BMJ 287:384, 1983

279. Wade JC, Newton B, Flournoy N et al: Oral acyclovir for prevention of herpes simplex virus reactivation after marrow transplantation. Ann Intern Med 96:265, 1982

280. Gluckman E, Devergie A, Melo R: Prophylaxis of herpes simplex virus infection after marrow transplant. Ann Intern Med 100:823, 1984

281. Winston DJ, Ho WG, Bartoni K, DuMond C et al: Ganciclovir prophylaxis of cytomegalovirus infection and disease in allogeneic bone marrow transplant recipients. Ann Intern Med 118:179, 1993

282. Goodrich JM, Bowden RA, Fisher L et al: Ganciclovir prophylaxis to prevent cytomegalovirus disease after allogeneic marrow transplant. Ann Intern Med 118:173, 1993

283. Marwick C: Varicella vaccine expected to be ready by 1993. JAMA 268:851, 1992

284. Gershon AA: Human immune responses to live attenuated varicella vaccine. Rev Infect Dis, suppl. 11. 13:S957, 1991

285. Gershon AA: Varicella vaccine: still at the crossroads. Pediatrics 90:144, 1992

286. Diaz PS, Au D, Smith S et al: Lack of transmission of the live attenuated varicella vaccine virus to immunocompromised children after immunization of their siblings. Pediatrics 87:166, 1991

287. Arbeter AM, Granowetter L, Starr SE et al: Immunization of children with acute lymphoblastic leukemia with live attenuated varicella vaccine without complete suspension of chemotherapy. Pediatrics 85:338, 1990

288. Ihara T, Kamya H, Torigoe S et al: Viremic phase in a leukemic child after live varicella vaccination. Pediatrics 89:147, 1992

289. Hardy I, Gershon AA, Steinberg SP et al: The incidence of zoster after immunization with live attenuated varicella vaccine. A study in children with leukemia. N Engl J Med 325:1545, 1991

290. Meyers JD: Prevention of cytomegalovirus infection after marrow transplantation. Rev Infect Dis, suppl. 7. 11:S1691, 1989

291. Syndman DR, Rubin RH, Werner BG: New developments in cytomegalovirus prevention and management. Am J Kidney Dis 21:217, 1993

292. Winston DJ, Ho WG, Lin CH et al: Intravenous immune globulin for prevention of cytomegalovirus infection and interstitial pneumonia after bone marrow transplantation. Ann Intern Med 106:12, 1987

293. Meyers JD, Reed EC, Shepp DH et al: Acyclovir for prevention of cytomegalovirus infection and disease after allogeneic marrow transplantation. N Engl J Med 318:70, 1988

294. Schmidt GM, Horak DA, Niland JC et al: A randomized, controlled trial of prophylactic ganciclovir for cytomegalovirus pulmonary infection in recipients of allogeneic bone marrow transplants. N Engl J Med 324:1005, 1991

295. Goodrich JM, Mori M, Gleaves CA et al: Early treatment with ganciclovir to prevent cytomegalovirus disease after allogeneic bone marrow transplantation. N Engl J Med 325:1601, 1991

296. Centers for Disease Control: Prevention and Control of Influenza Recommendations of the Immunization Practices Advisory Committee (ACIP): MMWR CDC Surveill Summ 41(RR-9):1, 1992

297. Hughes WT, Rivera GK, Schell MJ et al: Successful intermittent chemoprophylaxis for *Pneumocystis carinii* pneumonitis. N Engl J Med 316:1627, 1987

298. Gordon FM, Simon GL, Wofsy CB, Mills J: Adverse reactions to trimethoprim-sulfamethoxazole in patients with the acquired immunodeficiency syndrome. Ann Intern Med 100:495, 1984

299. Masur HM: Prevention and treatment of *Pneumocystis* pneumonia. Drug Ther 327:1853, 1992

300. Schneider ME, Hoepelman IM, Schattenkerk JK et al: A controlled trial of aerosolized pentamidine or trimethoprim-sulfamethoxazole as primary prophylaxis against *Pneumocystis carinii* pneumonia in patients with human immunodeficiency viral infection. N Engl J Med 327:1836, 1992

301. Centers for Disease Control: Guidelines for prophylaxis against *Pneumocystis carinii* pneumonia for children infected with human immunodeficiency virus. MMWR CDC Surveill Summ 40(RR-2):1, 1991

302. Mueller BU, Pizzo PA: Reply to the editor. J Pediatr 122:163, 1993

303. Shapiro ED, Berg AT, Austrian R et al: The protective efficacy of polyvalent pneumococcal polysaccharide vaccine. N Engl J Med 325:1453, 1991

304. Gardner P, Schaffner W: Immunization of adults. N Engl J Med 328:1252, 1993

305. Ljungman P, Fridell E, Lonnqvist B et al: Efficacy and safety of vaccination of marrow transplant recipients with a live attenuated measles, mumps and rubella vaccine. J Infect Dis 159:610, 1989

306. Ziegler EJ, McCutchan JA, Fierer S et al: Successful treatment of gram-negative bacteremia and shock with human antiserum to a UPD-GAL epimerase-deficient mutant *Escherichia coli*. N Engl J Med 307:1225, 1982

307. Ziegler EJ, Fisher CJ Jr, Sprung CL et al: Treatment of gram-negative bacteremia and septic shock with HA-1A human monoclonal antibody against endotoxin. A randomized, double-blind, placebo-controlled trial. N Engl J Med 324:429036, 1991

308. Reed EC, Bowden RA, Dandliker PS et al: Treatment of cytomegalovirus pneumonia with ganciclovir and intravenous cytomegalovirus immunoglobulin in patients with bone marrow transplant. Ann Intern Med 109:783, 1988

309. Emanuel D, Cunningham I, Jules-Elysee K et al: Cytomegalovirus pneumonia after bone marrow transplantation successfully treated with the combina-

tion of ganciclovir and high-dose intravenous immune globulin. Ann Intern Med 109:777, 1988

310. Berkman SA, Lee ML, Gale RP: Clinical uses of intravenous immunoglobulins. Ann Intern Med 112:278, 1990

311. Pizzo PA, Robichaud KJ, Wesley R et al: Fever in the pediatric and young adult patient with cancer. A prospective study of 1001 episodes. Medicine 61:153, 1982

312. Bryant RE, Hood AP, Hood CE et al: Factors affecting mortality of gram negative bacteremia. Arch Intern Med 127:120, 1971

313. Freid MA, Vosti KL: Importance of underlying disease in patients with gram-negative bacteremia. Arch Intern Med 121:418, 1968

314. Umsawasdi T, Middleman EA, Luna M et al: *Klebsiella* bacteremia in cancer patients. Am J Med Sci 265:473, 1973

315. Whitecar JP, Luna M, Bodey GP: *Pseudomonas* bacteremia in patients with malignant disease. Am J Med Sci 260:216, 1970

316. Rubin M, Hathorn JW, Pizzo PA: Controversies in the management of febrile neutropenic patients. Cancer Invest 6:167, 1988

317. Carney N, Fosieck BE Jr, Parker RH et al: Bacteremia due to *Staphylococcus aureus* in patients with cancer: report on 45 cases in adults and review of the literature. Rev Infect Dis 4:1, 1982

318. Kilton LJ, Fosieck BE Jr, Cohen MH et al: Bacteremia due to gram-positive cocci in patients with neoplastic disease. Am J Med 66:596, 1979

319. Ladisch S, Pizzo PA: *Staphylococcus aureus* sepsis in children with cancer. Pediatrics 61:231, 1978

320. Miser JS, Miser AW: *Staphylococcus aureus* sepsis in childhood malignancy. Am J Dis Child 134:831, 1980

321. Sotman SB, Schimpff SC, Young VM: *Staphylococcus aureus* bacteremia in patients with acute leukemia. Am J Med 69:8114, 1980

322. Schimpff SC, Saterlee W, Young VM: Empiric therapy with carbenicillin and gentamicin for febrile patients with cancer and granulocytopenia. N Engl J Med 284:1061, 1971

323. Anderson ET, Young LS, Hewitt WL: Antimicrobial synergism in the therapy of gram negative rod bacteremia. Chemotherapy 24:45, 1978

324. Moellering RC Jr, Eliopoulos GM, Allan JD: Beta-lactam/aminoglycoside combinations: interactions and their mechanisms. Am J Med, suppl. 5C. 80:30, 1986

325. Lyon MD, Smith KR, Saag MS et al: *In vitro* activity of piperacillin, ticarcillin, and mezlocillin alone and in combination with aminoglycosides against *Pseudomonas aeruginosa.* Antimicrob Agents Chemother 30:25, 1986

326. Johnson DE, Thompson B: Efficacy of single agent therapy with azlocillin, ticarcillin, and amikacin and beta-lactam/amikacin combinations for treatment of *Pseudomonas aeruginosa* bacteremia in granulocytopenic rats. Am J Med, suppl. 5C. 80:53, 1986

327. Jawetz E: The use of combinations of antimicrobial drugs. Annu Rev Pharmacol 8:151, 1968

328. Klastersky J, Cappel R, Daneau D: Clinical significance of in vitro synergism between antibiotics in gram-negative infections. Antimicrob Agents Chemother 2:470, 1972

329. Klastersky J, Zinner SH: Synergistic combination of antibiotics in gram-negative bacillary infections. Rev Infect Dis 4:294, 1982

330. Kluge RM, Standiford HC, Tatem BA et al: Comparative activity of tobramycin, amikacin, and gentamicin alone and with carbenicillin against *Pseudomonas aeruginosa.* Antimicrob Agents Chemother 6:442, 1974

331. Reyes MP, El-Khatib MR, Brown WJ et al: Synergy between carbenicillin and an aminoglycoside (gentamicin or tobramycin) against *Pseudomonas aeruginosa* isolated from patients with endocarditis and sensitivity of isolates to normal human serum. J Infect Dis 140:192, 1979

332. Rodriguez V, Whitecar JP, Bodey GP: Therapy of infections with the combination of carbenicillin and gentamicin. Antimicrob Agents Chemother 9:386, 1969

333. Hughes WT, Bodey GP, Meyeres JD et al: Guidelines for the use of antimicrobial agents in neutropenic patients with unexplained fever. J Infect Dis 161:381, 1990

334. Dejace P, Klastersky J: Comparative review of combination therapy: two beta-lactams versus beta-lactam plus aminoglycoside. Am J Med, suppl. 6B. 80:29, 1986

335. Gutman L, Williamson R, Kitzis MD, Acar JF: Synergism and antagonism in double beta-lactam antibiotic combinations. Am J Med, suppl. 5C. 80:21, 1986

336. Hathorn JW, Rubin M, Pizzo PA: Antibiotic therapy in the febrile neutropenic cancer patient: clinical efficacy and impact of monotherapy. Antimicrob Agents Chemother 31:971, 1986

337. Rubin M, Pizzo PA: Monotherapy in neutropenic cancer patients. p. 524. In Peterson PK, Verhoef J (eds): Antimicrobial Agents Annual 3. Elsevier Science Publishers, New York, 1988

338. Rolston KVI, Berkey P, Bodey GP, et al: A comparison of imipenem to ceftazi-

dime with or without amikacin as empiric therapy in febrile neutropenic patients. Arch Intern Med 152:283, 1992

339. Mortimer D, Miller S, Black D et al: Comparison of cefoperazone and mezlocillin with imipenem as empiric therapy in febrile neutropenic cancer patients. Am J Med, suppl. 1A. 85:17, 1988

340. Pizzo PA, Hathorn JW, Heimenz J et al: A randomized trial comparing combination antibiotic therapy to monotherapy in cancer patients with fever and neutropenia. N Engl J Med 315:552, 1986

341. Sanders JW, Powe NR, Moore RD: Ceftazidime monotherapy for empiric treatment of febrile neutropenic patients: A metaanalysis. J Infect Dis 164:907, 1991

342. Calandra G, Lydick E, Carrigan J et al: Factors predisposing to seizures in seriously ill infected patients receiving antibiotics: experience with imipenem/cilastatin. Am J Med 84:911, 1988

343. European Organization for Research and Treatment of Cancer (EORTC) International Antimicrobial Therapy Cooperative Group and the National Cancer Institute of Canada Clinical Trials Group: Vancomycin added to empirical combination antibiotic therapy for fever in granulocytopenic cancer patients. J Infect Dis 163:951, 1991

344. Bayston KF, Want S, Cohen J: A prospective randomized comparison of ceftazidime and ciprofloxacin as initial empiric therapy in neutropenic patients with fever. Am J Med, suppl. 5A. 87:5A-269S, 1989

345. Meunier F, Zinner SH, Gaya H et al: Prospective randomized evaluation of ciprofloxacin versus piperacillin plus amikacin for empiric antibiotic therapy of febrile granulocytopenic cancer patients with lymphomas and solid tumors. Antimicrob Agents Chemother 35:873, 1991

346. Flaherty JP, Watley D, Edlin B et al: Multicenter, randomized trial of ciprofloxacin plus azlocillin versus ceftazidime plus amikacin for empiric treatment of febrile neutropenic patients. Am J Med, suppl. 5A. 87:5A-278S, 1989

347. Rubenstein EB, Rolston K, Benjamin RS et al: Outpatient treatment of febrile episodes in low-risk neutropenic patients with cancer. Cancer 71:3640, 1993

348. Pizzo PA, Robichaud KJ, Gill FA et al: Duration of empiric antibiotic therapy in granulocytopenic cancer patients. Am J Med 67:194, 1979

349. Griffin TC, Buchanan GR: Hematologic predictors of bone marrow recovery in neutropenic patients hospitalized for fever: implications for discontinuation of antibiotics and early discharge from the hospital. J Pediatr 121:28, 1992

350. Mullen CA, Buchanan GR: Early hospital discharge of children with cancer treated for fever and neutropenia: identification and management of the low-risk patient. J Clin Oncol 8:1998, 1990

351. Johnson MP, Ramphal R: Ceftazidime (CAZ) resistant *Enterobacter* bacteremia (B) in febrile neutropenic patients (FNP), abstracted (594). p. 201. In Program and Abstracts of the Twenty-ninth Interscience Conference on Antimicrobial Agents and Chemotherapy, Houston, TX, 1989

352. Schwalbe RS, Stapleton JT, Gilligan PH: Emergence of vancomycin resistance in coagulase-negative staphylococci. N Engl J Med 316:927, 1987

353. Eliopoulos GM: Increasing problems in the therapy of enterococcal infections. Eur J Clin Microbiol Infect Dis 12:409, 1993

354. Handwerger S, Raucher B, Altarac D et al: Nosocomial outbreak due to *Enterococcus faecium* highly resistant to vancomycin, penicillin, and gentamicin. Clin Infect Dis 16:750, 1993

355. Johnson AP, Uttley AH, Woodford N et al: Resistance to vancomycin and teicoplanin: an emerging clinical problem. Clin Microbiol Rev 3:280, 1990

356. Sloas MM, Flynn PM, Kaste SC, Patrick CC: Typhlitis in children with cancer: a 30-year experience. Clin Infect Dis 17:484, 1993

357. Bartlett JG, Change TW, Gurwith M et al: Antibiotic associated pseudomembranous colitis due to toxin producing *Clostridia.* N Engl J Med 298:531, 1978

358. Gerding DN: Disease associated with *Clostridium difficile* infection. Ann Intern Med 110:255, 1989

359. Oliva SL, Guglielmo J, Jacobs R, Pons VG: Failure of intravenous vancomycin and intravenous metronidazole to prevent or treat antibiotic-associated pseudomembranous colitis. J Infect Dis 159:1154, 1989

360. Kleinfeld DI, Sharpe RJ, Donta ST: Parenteral therapy for antibiotic-associated pseudomembranous colitis. J Infect Dis 157:389, 1988

361. Commers JR, Robichaud KJ, Pizzo PA: New pulmonary infiltrates in granulocytopenic patients being treated with antibiotics. Pediatr Infect Dis J 3:423, 1984

362. Pizzo PA, Robichaud KJ, Gill FA et al: Empiric antibiotic and antifungal therapy for cancer patients with prolonged fever and granulocytopenia. Am J Med 72:101, 1982

363. Burke PJ, Braine HG, Rathun HK et al: The clinical significance and management of fever in acute myelocytic leukemia. Johns Hopkins Med J 139:1, 1976

364. Pennington JE: *Aspergillus* pneumonia in hematologic malignancy. Arch Intern Med 137:769, 1977

365. Aisner J, Schimpff SC, Wiernik PH: Treatment of invasive aspergillosis: relation of early diagnosis and treatment to response. Ann Intern Med 86:539, 1977

366. EORTC International Antimicrobial Therapy Cooperative Group: Empiric antifungal therapy in febrile granulocytopenic patients. Am J Med 86:668, 1989

367. Stein RS, Kayser J, Flexner J: Clinical value of empirical amphotericin B in patients with acute myelogenous leukemia. Cancer 50:2247, 1982

368. Walsh TJ, Rubin M, Hathorn J et al: Amphotericin B vs high-dose ketoconazole for empirical antifungal therapy among febrile, granulocytopenic cancer patients. A prospective randomized study. Arch Intern Med 151:765, 1991

369. Walsh TJ, Lee J, Lecciones J et al: Empiric therapy with amphotericin B in febrile granulocytopenic patients. Rev Infect Dis 13:496, 1991

370. Fainstein V, Bodey GP, Elting L et al: Amphotericin B or ketoconazole therapy of fungal infections in neutropenic cancer patients. Antimicrob Agents Chemother 31:11, 1987

371. Philpott-Howard JN, Wade JJ, Mufti GJ et al: Randomized comparison of oral fluconazole versus oral polyenes for the prevention of fungal infection in patients at risk of neutropenia. J Antimicrob Chemother 31:973, 1993

372. Alavi JB, Rost RK, Djerassi I et al: Leukocyte transfusions in acute leukemia. N Engl J Med 296:706, 1977

373. Volger WR, Winton EF: The efficacy of granulocyte transfusions in neutropenic patients. Am J Med 63:548, 1977

374. Herzig R, Herzig G, Graw RG et al: Efficacy of granulocyte transfusion therapy for gram negative sepsis: a prospective randomized controlled study. N Engl J Med 296:701, 1977

375. Winston D, Ho WG, Gale RP: Therapeutic granulocyte transfusions for documented infections. Ann Intern Med 97:509, 1982

376. Schiffer CA, Aisner J, Daly PA et al: Alloimmunization following prophylactic granulocyte transfusions. Blood 54:766, 1979

377. Winston DJ, Winston GH, Howell CL et al: Cytomegalovirus infections associated with leukocyte transfusions. Ann Intern Med 93:671, 1980

378. Hersman J, Meyers JD, Thomas ED et al: The effect of granulocyte transfusions on the incidence of cytomegalovirus infection after allogeneic marrow transplantation. Ann Intern Med 96:149, 1982

379. Roth JA, Siegel SE, Levine AS, Berard CW: Fatal recurrent toxoplasmosis in the patient initially infected via a leukocyte transfusion. Am J Clin Pathol 56:601, 1971

380. Bensinger WI, Price TH, Dale DC et al: The effects of daily recombinant human granulocyte colony-stimulating factor administration on normal granulocyte donors undergoing leukapheresis. Blood 181:1883, 1993

381. Caspar CB, Seger RA, Burger J et al: Effective stimulation of donors for granulocyte transfusions with recombinant methionyl granulocyte colony-stimulating factor. Blood 81:2866, 1993

382. Strauss RG: Therapeutic granulocyte transfusions in 1993. Blood 81:1675, 1993

383. Yeo E, Alvarado T, Fainstein V, Bodey G: Prophylaxis of oropharyngeal candidiasis with clotrimazole. J Clin Oncol 3:1668, 1985

384. DeGregorio MW, Lee WMF, Ries CA: Candida infections in patients with acute leukemia: ineffectiveness of nystatin prophylaxis and relationship between oropharyngeal and systemic candidiasis. Cancer 50:2780, 1982

385. Yap BS, Bodey GP: Oropharyngeal candidiasis treated with a troche form of clotrimazole. Arch Intern Med 139:656, 1979

386. Lawson RD, Bodey GP: Comparison of clotrimazole troche and nystatin vaginal tablet in the treatment of esophageal candidiasis. Curr Ther Res 27:774, 1980

387. Meunier F, Aoun M, Gerard M: Therapy for oropharyngeal candidiasis in the immunocompromised host: a randomized double-blind study of fluconazole vs. ketoconazole. Rev Infect Dis, suppl. 3. 12:S364, 1990

388. Moskowitz L, Hensley GT, Chan JC et al: Immediate causes of death in acquired immunodeficiency syndrome. Arch Pathol Lab Med 109:735, 1985

389. Holmberg K, Meyer RD: Fungal infections in patients with AIDS and AIDS-related complex. Scand J Infect Dis 18:179, 1986

390. Clotet B, Grifol M, Parra O et al: Asymptomatic esophageal candidiasis in the acquired immunodeficiency syndrome-related complex, letter. Ann Intern Med 105:145, 1986

391. Kodsi B, Wickremesinghe P, Koznin PJ et al: Candida esophagitis: a prospective study of 27 cases. Gastroenterology 5:715, 1976

392. Jones JM: Necrotizing Candida esophagitis: failure of symptoms and roentgenographic findings to reflect severity. JAMA 244:2190, 1980

393. Medoff G, Dismukes WE, Meade RH III et al: A new therapeutic approach to candida infections: a preliminary report. Arch Intern Med 130:241, 1972

394. Fazio RA, Wickremesingthe PC, Arsura EL et al: Ketoconazole treatment of Candida esophagitis: a prospective study of 12 cases. Am J Gastroenterol 78:261, 1983

395. Ginsburg CH, Braden GL, Tauber AI et al: Oral clotrimazole in the treatment of esophageal candidiasis. Am J Med 71:891, 1981

396. Crislip MA, Edwards JE: Candidiasis. Infect Dis Clin North Am 3:103, 1989

397. Centers for Disease Control: Nosocomial infection surveillance, 1983. MMWR CDC Surveill Summ 33:9, 1984

398. Morrison AJ, Freer CV, Searcy MA et al: Nosocomial bloodstream infections: secular trends in a statewide surveillance program in Virginia. Infect Control Hosp Epidemiol 7:550, 1986

399. Wey SB, Pfaller MA, Wenzel RP: Attributable mortality and excess length of stay due to nosocomial candidemia. Arch Intern Med 148:2642, 1988

400. Horn R, Wong B, Kiehn TE, Armstrong D: Fungemia in a cancer hospital: changing frequency, earlier onset, and results of therapy. Rev Infect Dis 7:646, 1985

401. Rose R, Hunting KJ, Townsend TR et al: Morbidity/mortality and economics of hospital-acquired bloodstream infections: a controlled study. South Med J 70:1267, 1977

402. Lecciones JA, Lee JW, Navarro EE et al: Vascular catheter-associated fungemia in patients with cancer: analysis of 155 episodes. Clin Infect Dis 14:875, 1992

403. Arena FP, Perlin M, Brahman H et al: Fever, rash, myalgias of disseminated candidiasis during antifungal therapy. Arch Intern Med 141:1233, 1981

404. Curry CR, Quie PG: Fungal septicemia in patients receiving parenteral hyperalimentation. N Engl J Med 285:1221, 1971

405. Lowder NJ, Lazarus HM, Herzig RH: Bacteremia and fungemia in oncologic patients with central venous catheters: changing spectrum of infection. Arch Intern Med 142:1456, 1982

406. Fraser VJ, Jones M, Dunkel J et al: Candidemia in a tertiary care hospital: epidemiology, risk factors, and predictors of mortality. Clin Infect Dis 15:414, 1992

407. Thaler M, Pastakia B, Shawker TH et al: Hepatic candidiasis in cancer patients: the evolving picture of the syndrome. Ann Intern Med 108:88, 1988

408. Henderson DK, Hockey LJ, Vukalcia LJ et al: Effect of immunosuppression on the development of experimental hematogenous Candida endophthalmitis. Infect Immun 27:628, 1980

409. Brock C, Drew R, Pickard W et al: Tolerance of amphotericin B (AmB) infusions when initially administered as full dose versus a stepwise titration, abstracted (76). p. 113. In Program and Abstracts of the Twenty-ninth Interscience Conference on Antimicrobial Agents and Chemotherapy, Houston, TX, 1989

410. Edwards JE, Filler SC: Current strategies for treating invasive candidiasis: emphasis on infections in nonneutropenic patients. Clin Infect Dis, suppl. 1. 14:S106, 1992

411. Montgomerie JZ, Edwards JE Jr: Association of infection due to Candida albicans with intravenous hyperalimentation. J Infect Dis 137:197, 1987

412. Edwards JE Jr, Foos RY, Montgomerie JZ, Guze L: Ocular manifestations of Candida septicemia: review of seventy-six cases of hematogenous Candida endophthalmitis. Medicine 53:47, 1974

413. Edwards JE Jr: Candida endophthalmitis. p. 211. In Bodey GP, Fainstein V (eds): Candidiasis. Raven Press, New York 1985

414. Edwards JE Jr, Montgomerie JZ, Ishida R et al: Experimental hematogenous endophthalmitis due to Candida species. Species variation in ocular pathogenicity. J Infect Dis 35:294, 1977

415. Haron E, Feld R, Tuffnell P et al: Hepatic candidiasis: an increasing problem in immunocompromised patients. Am J Med 83:17, 1987

416. Tashjian LS, Abramson JS, Peacock JE: Focal hepatic candidiasis: a distinct clinical variant of candidiasis in immunocompromised patients. Rev Infect Dis 6:689, 1984

417. Talbot GH, Provencher M, Cassileth PA: Persistent fever after recovery from granulocytopenia in acute leukemia. Arch Intern Med 148:129, 1988

418. Thaler M, Bacher J, O'Leary T, Pizzo PA: Evaluation of single-drug and combination antifungal therapy in an experimental model of candidiasis in rabbits with prolonged neutropenia. J Infect Dis 158:80, 1988

419. Lopez-Berestein G, Bodey GP, Fainstein V et al: Treatment of systemic fungal infections with liposomal amphotericin B. Arch Intern Med 149:2533, 1989

420. Ringden O, Meunier F, Tollemar J et al: Efficacy of amphotericin B encapsulated in liposomes (AmBisome) in the treatment of invasive fungal infections in immunocompromised patients. J Antimicrob Chemother, suppl B. 28:73, 1991

421. Kauffman CA, Bradley SF, Ross SC, Weber DR: Hepatosplenic candidiasis: successful treatment with fluconazole. Am J Med 91:137, 1991

422. Anaissie E, Bodey GP, Kantarjian H et al: Fluconazole therapy for chronic disseminated candidiasis in patients with leukemia and prior amphotericin B therapy. Am J Med 91:142, 1991

423. Evans TG, Mayer J, Cohen S et al: Fluconazole failure in the treatment of invasive mycoses. J Infect Dis 164:1232, 1991

424. Myerwitz RC, Pazin GJ, Allen CM: Disseminated candidiasis: changes in incidence, underlying diseases and pathology. Am J Clin Pathol 48:29, 1977

425. Goldberg PK, Kozinn PJ, Wise GJ et al: Incidence and significance of candiduria. JAMA 241:582, 1979

426. Gubbins PO, Piscitelli SC, Danziger LH: Candidal urinary tract infections: a comprehensive review of their diagnosis and management. Pharmacotherapy 13:110, 1993

427. Levitz SM: Aspergillosis. Systemic fungal infections: diagnosis and treatment. II. Infect Dis Clin North Am 3:11, 1989

428. DeGregorio MW, Lee WMF, Linker CA et al: Fungal infections in patients with acute leukemia. Am J Med 73:543, 1982

429. Gustafson TL, Schaffner W, Lavely GB et al: Invasive aspergillosis in renal transplant recipients. Correlation with corticosteroid therapy. J Infect Dis 148:230, 1983

430. Wajsczuk CP, Dummer JS, Ho M et al: Fungal infections in liver transplant recipients. Transplantation 40:347, 1985

431. Glimp RA, Bayer AS: Pulmonary aspergilloma. Diagnostic and therapeutic considerations. Arch Intern Med 143:303, 1983

432. Goldberg B: Radiologic appearances in pulmonary aspergillosis. Clin Radiol 13:106, 1962

433. Bennett JE: *Aspergillus* species. p. 2304. In Mandell GL, Douglas RG Jr, Bennett JE (eds): Principles and Practice of Infectious Diseases. 4th Ed. Churchill Livingstone, New York, 1995

434. Faulkner SL, Vernon R, Brown PP et al: Hemoptysis and pulmonary aspergilloma: operative versus nonoperative treatment. Ann Thorac Surg 25:389, 1978

435. Hammerman KJ, Sarosi GA, Tosh FE: Amphotericin B in the treatment of saprophytic forms of pulmonary aspergillosis. Am Rev Respir Dis 109:57, 1974

436. Binder RE, Faling LJ, Pugatch RD et al: Chronic necrotizing pulmonary aspergillosis: a discrete clinical entity. Medicine 61:109, 1982

437. Hargis JJ, Bone RC, Stewart J et al: Intracavitary amphotericin B in the treatment of symptomatic pulmonary aspergillomas. Am J Med 68:389, 1980

438. Weinberger M, Elattar I, Marshall D et al: Patterns of infection in patients with aplastic anemia and the emergence of *Aspergillus* as a major cause of death. Medicine 71:24, 1992

439. Gerson SL, Talbot GH, Lusk E et al: Invasive pulmonary aspergillosis in adult acute leukemia: clinical clues to its diagnosis. J Clin Oncol 3:1109, 1985

440. Viollier AF, Peterson DE, de Jongh CA et al: *Aspergillus* sinusitis in cancer patients. Cancer 58:366, 1986

441. Young RC, Bennett JE, Vogel CL et al: Aspergillosis, the spectrum of disease in 98 patients. Medicine 49:147, 1970

442. Orr DP, Myerowitz RL, Dubois PJ: Patho-radiologic correlation of invasive pulmonary aspergillosis in the compromised host. Cancer 44:2028, 1978

443. Walsh TJ: Invasive pulmonary aspergillosis in patients with neoplastic diseases. Semin Respir Infect 5:111, 1990

444. McCabe RE, Brooks RG, Mark JBD et al: Open lung biopsy in patients with acute leukemia. Am J Med 78:609, 1985

445. Treger TR, Visscher DW, Bartlett MS et al: Diagnosis of pulmonary infection caused by *Aspergillus*: usefulness of respiratory cultures. J Infect Dis 152: 572, 1985

446. Kahn FW, Jones JM, England DM: The role of bronchoalveolar lavage in the diagnosis of invasive pulmonary aspergillosis. Am J Clin Pathol 86:518, 1986

447. Nalesnik MA, Myerowitz RL, Jenkins R et al: Significance of *Aspergillus* species isolated from respiratory secretions in the diagnosis of invasive pulmonary aspergillosis. J Clin Microbiol 11:370, 1980

448. Navarro E, Lecciones JA, Lee JW et al: Invasive pulmonary aspergillosis developing during empirical antifungal therapy in febrile cancer patients. (submitted)

449. Walsh TJ: Management of immunocompromised patients with evidence of an invasive mycosis. Infectious complications in the immunocompromised host. II. Hematol Oncol Clin North Am 7:1003, 1993

450. Fisher BD, Armstrong D, Yu B, Gold JWM: Invasive aspergillosis. Progress in early diagnosis and treatment. Am J Med 71:571, 1981

451. Burch PA, Karp JE, Merz WG et al: Favorable outcome of invasive aspergillosis in patients with acute leukemia. J Clin Oncol 12:1985, 1987

452. Pannuti CS, Gingrich RD, Pfaller MA, Wenzel RP: Nosocomial pneumonia in adult patients undergoing bone marrow transplantation: a 9-year study. J Clin Oncol 9:77, 1991

453. Copra R, Blare S, Strang J et al: Liposomal amphotericin B (AmBisome) in the treatment of fungal infections in neutropenia patients. J Antimicrob Chemother, suppl. B. 28:93, 1991

454. Lopez-Berestein G, Bodey GP, Fainstein V et al: Treatment of systemic fungal infections with liposomal Amphotericin B. Arch Intern Med 149:2533, 1989

455. Denning DW, Tucker RM, Hanson LH et al: Treatment of invasive aspergillosis with itraconazole. Am J Med 86:791, 1989

456. Denning DW, Pappas PG, Kauffman JS et al: Oral itraconazole (IZ) therapy of invasive aspergillosis (IA), abstracted. In Thirty-first Interscience Conference on Antimicrobial Agents and Chemotherapy, Chicago, 1991

457. Karp JE, Burch PA, Merz WG: An approach to intensive antileukemia therapy in patients with previous invasive aspergillosis. Am J Med 85:203, 1988

458. Diamond RD, Bennett JE: Prognostic factors in cryptococcal meningitis. A study of 111 cases. Ann Intern Med 80:176, 1976

459. Littman ML, Walter JE: Cryptococcosis: current status. Am J Med 45:922, 1968

460. Diamond RD: *Cryptococcus neoformans*. p. 2329. In Mandell GL, Douglas RG Jr, Bennett JE (eds): Principles and Practice of Infectious Diseases. 4th Ed. Churchill Livingstone, New York, 1995

461. Perfect JR: Cryptococcosis. Infect Dis Clin North Am 3:77, 1989

462. Gordon MA, Lapa EW: Elimination of rheumatoid factor in the latex test of *Cryptococcus*. Am J Clin Pathol 61:488, 1974

463. Stockman L, Roberts GD: Corrected version. Specificity of the latex test for cryptococcal antigen: a rapid, simple method for eliminating interference factors. J Clin Microbiol 17:945, 1983

464. McManus EJ, Jones JM: Detection of a *Trichosporon beigelii* antigen cross reactive with *Cryptococcus neoformans* capsular polysaccharide in serum from a patient with disseminated trichosporon infection. J Clin Microbiol 21:681, 1985

465. Cameron ML, Bartlett JA, Gallis HA, Waskin HA: Manifestations of pulmonary *Cryptococcus* in patients with acquired immunodeficiency syndrome. Rev Infect Dis 13:64, 1991

466. Duperval R, Hermans PE, Brewer NW et al: Cryptococcosis with emphasis on the significance of isolation of *Cryptococcus neoformans* from the respiratory tract. Chest 72:13, 1977

467. Bennett JE, Dismukes WE, Duma RJ et al: A comparison of amphotericin B alone and combined with flucytosine in the treatment of cryptococcal meningitis. N Engl J Med 301:126, 1979

468. Dismukes WE, Cloud G, Gallis HA et al: Treatment of cryptococcal meningitis with combinations amphotericin B and flucytosine for four as compared with six weeks. N Engl J Med 34:334, 1987

469. Chuck SL, Sande MA: Infections with *Cryptococcus neoformans* in the acquired immunodeficiency syndrome. N Engl J Med 321:794, 1989

470. Larsen RA, Leal MAE, Chan LS: Fluconazole compared with amphotericin B plus flucytosine for cryptococcal meningitis in AIDS. A randomized trial. Ann Intern Med 113:183, 1990

471. Saag MS, Powderly WG, Cloud Gretchen AC et al: Comparison of amphotericin B with fluconazole in the treatment of acute AIDS-associated cryptococcal meningitis. N Engl J Med 326:83, 1992

472. Powderly WG, Saag MS, Cloud GA et al: A controlled trial of fluconazole or amphotericin B to prevent relapse of cryptococcal meningitis in patients with the acquired immunodeficiency syndrome. N Engl J Med 326:793, 1992

473. Sugar AM: Mucormycosis. Clin Infect Dis, suppl. 1. 14:S126, 1992

474. Rippon JW: Pseudallescheriasis. p. 651. In Rippon JW (ed): Medical Mycology. WB Saunders, Philadelphia, 1988

475. Hachimi-Idrissi S, Willemsen M, Desprechins B et al: *Pseudallescheria boydii* and brain abscesses. Pediatr Infect Dis J 9:737, 1990

476. Mesnard R, Lamy T, Dauriac C et al: Lung abscess due to *Pseudallescheria boydii* in the course of acute leukemia. Report of a case and review of the literature. Acta Haematol 87:78, 1992

477. Piper J, Golden J, Brown D et al: Successful treatment of *Scedosporium apiospermium* suppurative arthritis with itraconazole. Pediatr Infect Dis J 9: 674, 1990

478. Walsh TJ, Lee JW, Melcher GP et al: Experimental trichosporon infection in persistently granulocytopenic rabbits: implications for pathogenesis, diagnosis, and treatment of an emerging opportunistic mycosis. J Infect Dis 166:121, 1992

479. Anaissie E, Gokaslan A, Hachem R et al: Azole therapy for trichosporonosis: clinical evaluation of eight patients, experimental therapy for murine infection, and review. Clin Infect Dis 15:781, 1992

480. Stevens JG: Human herpes viruses: a consideration of the latent state. Microbiol Rev 53:318, 1989

481. Muller SA, Herrman CC Jr, Winkelmann RK: Herpes simplex infections in hematologic malignancies. Am J Med 52:102, 1972

482. Siegal EP, Lopez C, Hammer GS et al: Severe acquired immunodeficiency in male homosexuals manifested by chronic perianal ulcerative herpes simplex lesions. N Engl J Med 305:1439, 1981

483. Englund JA, Zimmerman ME, Swierkosz EM et al: Herpes simplex virus resistant to acyclovir. Ann Intern Med 112:416, 1990

484. Erlich KS, Mills J, Chatis P et al: Acyclovir-resistant herpes simplex virus infections in patients with the acquired immunodeficiency syndrome. N Engl J Med 320:293, 1989

485. Wade JC, McLaren C, Meyers JD: Frequency and significance of acyclovir-resistant herpes simplex virus isolated from marrow transplant patients receiving multiple courses of treatment with acyclovir. J Infect Dis 148:1077, 1983

486. Field HJ: Development of clinical resistance to acyclovir in herpes simplex virus-infected mice receiving oral therapy. Antimicrob Agents Chemother 21:744, 1982

487. Whitley RJ: Varicella-zoster virus. p. 1343. In Mandell GL, Douglas RG Jr,

Bennett JE (eds): Principles and Practice of Infectious Diseases. 4th Ed. Churchill Livingstone, New York, 1995

488. Triebwasser JS, Harris RE, Bryant RE, Rhoades ER: Varicella pneumonia in adults. Report of seven cases and a review of the literature. Medicine 46: 409, 1967

489. Jemsek J, Greenberg SB, Taber L et al: Herpes zoster-varicella infections in immunocompromised patients. Ann Intern Med 89:375, 1978

490. Prober CG, Kirk LE, Keeney RE: Acyclovir therapy of chicken pox in immuno-suppressed children—a collaborative study. J Pediatr 101:622, 1982

491. Whitley RJ, Hilty M, Haynes R et al: Vidarabine therapy of varicella in immu-nosuppressed patients. J Pediatr 101:125, 1982

492. Berlin BS, Campbell T: Hospital-acquired herpes-zoster following exposure to chicken pox. JAMA 211:1831, 1970

493. Winston DJ, Gale RO, Meyer DW et al: Infectious complications of bone marrow transplantation. Medicine 58:1, 1979

494. Atkinson K, Meyers JD, Storb R et al: Varicella-zoster virus infection after marrow transplantation for aplastic anemia or leukemia. Transplantation 29:47, 1980

495. Manfardini S, Bajetta E, Arnold CA et al: Herpes zoster-varicella in malignant lymphomas. Eur J Cancer Clin Oncol 11:51, 1975

496. Goffinett DR, Glatstein EJ, Merigan TC: Herpes zoster-varicella infections and lymphoma. Ann Intern Med 76:235, 1972

497. Sokal JE, Firat D: Varicella-zoster infection in Hodgkin's disease. Am J Med 39:452, 1965

498. Ruckdeschel JC, Schimpff SC, Smith AC et al: Herpes zoster and impaired cell-associated immunity to the varicella-zoster virus in patients with Hodg-kin's disease. Am J Med 62:77, 1977

499. Hirsch MS: Herpes group virus infections in the compromised host. p. 347. In Rubin RH, Young LS (eds): Clinical Approach to Infections in the Compro-mised Host. Plenum, New York, 1988

500. Dolin R, Reichman RC, Mazur MH et al: Herpes zoster-varicella infections in immunocompromised patients. Ann Intern Med 89:375, 1978

501. Balfour HH Jr, Bean B, Laskin OL et al: Acyclovir halts progression of herpes zoster in immunocompromised patients. N Engl J Med 308:1448, 1983

502. Whitley RJ, Soong SJ, Dolin R et al: Early vidarabine therapy to control the complications of herpes zoster in immunosuppressed patients. N Engl J Med 307:971, 1982

503. Whitley RJ, Chien LT, Dolin R et al: Adenine arabinoside therapy of herpes-zoster in the immunosuppressed. NIAID collaborative antiviral study. N Engl J Med 294:1113, 1976

504. Shepp DH, Dandliker PS, Meyers JD: Treatment of varicella-zoster virus in-fections in severely immunocompromised patients. N Engl J Med 314:208, 1986

505. Balfour HH Jr: Acyclovir. Antimicrob Agents Chemother 3:345, 1988

506. Pahwa S, Biron K, Lim W et al: Continuous varicella-zoster infection associ-ated with acyclovir resistance in a child with AIDS. JAMA 260:2879, 1988

507. Jacobson MA, Berger TG, Fikrig Senih et al: Acyclovir-resistant varicella zoster virus infection after chronic oral acyclovir therapy in patients with the acquired immunodeficiency syndrome (AIDS). Ann Intern Med 112:187, 1990

508. Meyers JD, Fluornoy N, Thomas ED: Nonbacterial pneumonia after alloge-neic marrow transplantation. A review of 10 years' experience. Rev Infect Dis 4:1119, 1982

509. Weiner RS, Bortin MM, Gale RP et al: Interstitial pneumonitis after bone marrow transplantation. Ann Intern Med 104:168, 1986

510. Texidor HS, Hong CL, Norsoph E et al: Cytomegalovirus infection of the alimentary canal: radiologic findings with pathologic correlation. Radiology 163:317, 1987

511. Blumberg RS, Kelsey P, Perrone T et al: Cytomegalovirus- and *Cryptospori-dium*-associated acalculous gangrenous cholecystitis. Am J Med 76:1118, 1984

512. Egbert PR, Pillard RB, Gallagher JB et al: Cytomegalovirus retinitis in immu-nosuppressed hosts. II. Ocular manifestations. Ann Intern Med 93:664, 1980

513. Drew WL: Nonpulmonary manifestations of cytomegalovirus infection in immunocompromised patients. Clin Microbiol Rev 5:204, 1992

514. Wingard JR, Santos GW, Saral R: Late onset interstitial pneumonia following allogeneic bone marrow transplantation. Transplantation 39:21, 1985

515. Crawford SW, Bowden RA, Hackman RC et al: Rapid detection of cytomegalo-virus pulmonary infection by bronchoalveolar lavage and centrifugation culture. Ann Intern Med 108:180, 1988

516. Gleaves CA, Meyers JD: Rapid diagnosis of invasive cytomegalovirus infec-tion by examination of tissue specimens in centrifugation culture. Am J Clin Pathol 88:354, 1987

517. Balfour HH: Management of cytomegalovirus disease with antiviral drugs. Rev Infect Dis, suppl. 7. 12:S849, 1990

518. Drew WL, Miner RC, Busch DF et al: Prevalence of resistance in patients receiving ganciclovir for serious cytomegalovirus infection. J Infect Dis 163: 716, 1991

519. Jabs DA, Davis MD, Meinert CL et al: Mortality in patients with the acquired immunodeficiency syndrome treated with either foscarnet or ganciclovir for cytomegalovirus retinitis. N Engl J Med 326:213, 1992

520. Polis MA, DeSmet MD, Baird BF et al: Increased survival of a cohort of patients with acquired immunodeficiency syndrome and cytomegalovirus retinitis who received sodium phosphonoformate (Foscarnet). Am J Med 94:175, 1993

521. Chrisp P, Clissold SP: Foscarnet: a review of its antiviral activity, pharmaco-kinetic properties and therapeutic use in immunocompromised patients with cytomegalovirus retinitis. Drugs 41:104, 1991

522. Jacobson MA, Drew WL, Feinberg J et al: Foscarnet therapy for ganciclovir-resistant cytomegalovirus retinitis in patients with AIDS. J Infect Dis 163: 1348, 1991

523. Butler KM, DeSmet MD, Husson RN et al: Treatment of aggressive cytomega-lovirus retinitis with ganciclovir in combination with foscarnet in a child infected with human immunodeficiency virus. J Pediatr 120:483, 1992

524. Reed EL, Dandliker PS, Meyers JD: Treatment of cytomegalovirus pneumo-nia with 9-(2-hydroxy-1-(hydroxymethyl)ethoxymethylguanine and high dose corticosteroids. Ann Intern Med 105:214, 1986

525. Shepp DH, Dandliker PS, de Miranda P et al: Activity of 9-(2-hydroxy-1-(hy-droxymethyl)ethoxymethyl)guanine (BW B759U) in the treatment of cyto-megalovirus pneumonia. Ann Intern Med 103:368, 1985

526. Emmanuel D: Treatment of cytomegalovirus disease. Semin Hematol, suppl 1. 27:22, 1990

527. Riddell SR, Reusser P, Greenberg PD: Cytotoxic T cells specific for cytomega-lovirus: a potential therapy for immunocompromised patients. Rev Infect Dis, suppl. 11. 33:S966, 1991

528. Aulitzky WE, Schulz TF, Tilg H et al: Human monoclonal antibodies neutraliz-ing cytomegalovirus (CMV) for prophylaxis of CMV disease: report of a Phase I trial in bone marrow transplant recipients. J Infect Dis 163:1344, 1991

529. Feldman S, Webster RG, Sugg M: Influenza in children and young adults with cancer. 20 cases. Cancer 39:350, 1977

530. Kempe A, Hall CB, MacDonald NE et al: Influenza in children with cancer. J Pediatr 115:33, 1989

531. Whimbey E, Bodey GP: Viral pneumonia in the immunocompromised adults with neoplastic disease: the role of common community respiratory viruses. Semin Respir Infect 7:122, 1992

532. Zahradnik JM, Spencer MJ, Porter DD: Adenovirus infection in the immuno-compromised patient. Am J Med 68:725, 1980

533. Shields AF, Hackman RC, Fife KH et al: Adenovirus infections in patients undergoing bone-marrow transplantation. N Engl J Med 312:529, 1985

534. Kovacs JA, Hiemenz JW, Macher AM et al: *Pneumocystis carinii* pneumonia: a comparison of clinical features in patients with the acquired immune defi-ciency syndrome and patients with other immune diseases. Ann Intern Med 100:663, 1984

535. Cohen OJ, Stoeckle MY: Extrapulmonary *Pneumocystis carinii* infections in the acquired immunodeficiency syndrome. Arch Intern Med 151:1205, 1991

536. Kovacs JA, Gill V, Swan JC et al: Prospective evaluation of a monoclonal antibody in the diagnosis of *Pneumocystis carinii* pneumonia. Lancet 2:1, 1986

537. Lipschik GY, Gill VJ, Lundgren JD et al: Improved diagnosis of pneumocystis carinii infection by polymerase chain reaction on induced sputum and blood. Lancet 340:203, 1992

538. Browne MJ, Potter D, Gress J et al: A randomized trial of open lung biopsy versus empiric antimicrobial therapy in cancer patients with diffuse pulmo-nary infiltrates. J Clin Oncol 8:222, 1990

539. The National Institutes of Health—University of California Expert Panel for Corticosteroids as Adjunctive Therapy for *Pneumocystis* Pneumonia: Special Report: consensus statement on the use of corticosteroids as adjunctive therapy for *Pneumocystis* pneumonia in the acquired immunodeficiency syn-drome. N Engl J Med 323:1500, 1990

540. Burt ME, Flye MW, Webber BI et al: Prospective evaluation of aspiration needle, cutting needle, transbronchial and open lung biopsy in patients with pulmonary infiltrates. Ann Thorac Surg 32:146, 1981

541. Allegra CJ, Chabner BA, Tuazon CU et al: Trimetrexate for the treatment of *Pneumocystis carinii* pneumonia in patients with the acquired immunodefi-ciency syndrome. N Engl J Med 317:978, 1987

542. Girard PM, Landman R, Gaudebout C et al: Dapsone-pyrimethamine com-pared with aerosolized pentamidine as primary prophylaxis against *Pneu-mocystis carinii* pneumonia and toxoplasmosis in HIV infection. N Engl J Med 328:1514, 1993

Nutritional Support of Patients with Hematologic Malignancies

92

Saundra N. Aker and Polly Lenssen

INTRODUCTION

Patients with hematologic malignancies are highly heterogeneous in terms of their nutritional problems and requirement for nutritional intervention. Those patients with aggressive leukemias and lymphomas receive among the most intensive of oncologic therapies and frequently experience significant gastrointestinal and other organ toxicities, decreased dietary intake, and weight loss. Patients with good-risk acute lymphocytic and chronic leukemias less commonly encounter significant nutritional problems.

The advent and widespread use of central venous access devices has helped obviate iatrogenic malnutrition in cancer patients. The use of total parenteral nutrition (TPN), however, has come under increased scrutiny, and among patients with solid tumors has not prolonged survival and may actually increase morbidity.[1,2] This chapter addresses the appropriate use of TPN and other dietary intervention strategies, such as tube feedings and low microbial diets, in patients with hematologic malignancies.

NUTRITIONAL PROBLEMS

Protein-Calorie Malnutrition

Significant weight loss at diagnosis is not a prevalent finding. DeWys et al[3] reported that only 4% of patients with acute myeloid leukemia (AML), 10% with favorable non-Hodgkin lymphoma (NHL), and 15% with unfavorable NHL presented with more than 10% weight loss during the 6 months before initiation of chemotherapy. Among pediatric patients with newly diagnosed acute lymphocytic leukemia (ALL) and AML, only 6% exhibited significant weight loss.[4] The risk of the development of malnutrition subsequent to diagnosis depends on the toxicity of the therapy administered and the progression of the disease. Rickard et al.[5] identified several types of pediatric patients at high risk of nutritional depletion, including patients with NHL involving the gastrointestinal tract, AML, poor-prognosis ALL, and patients who have experienced multiple relapses of their leukemia.[5] By the time patients with acute leukemia become candidates for marrow transplantation, significant weight loss is more prevalent.[6]

Little is known about the effect of protein-calorie malnutrition on outcome in hematologic malignancies. DeWys et al[3] found that weight loss prior to diagnosis had no influence on survival in patients with AML but was associated with a significant decrease in survival in patients with favorable and unfavorable NHL.

Weight loss of 10–15% correlates with a 20% loss of protein mass and clinically significant impairment of physiologic function.[7] The adverse consequences of malnutrition on both cell-mediated and humoral immunities are well described.[8-11] The effects of malnutrition on gastrointestinal function and immunity are particularly relevant in hematologic malignancies. The thinning of mucous membranes, decrease in secretory IgA, and altered gut flora observed in malnutrition have been linked to an increase in gastrointestinal infection.[12,13] Because the gastrointestinal barrier can be breached during intense oncologic therapy, enteric infections are common and are frequently implicated as a source of bacteremias and sepsis.[12,14-16] Short-term protein restriction alone does not result in bacterial transfer across the intestinal mucosa. However, when combined with another insult, such as endotoxin or acute inflammatory responses, invasive bacterial colonization in systemic organs does occur.[17,18] The adequate nourishment of major organs, especially the gastrointestinal tract, seems prudent in immunocompromised patients.

Altered Metabolism

The metabolism of malignant bone marrow is markedly accelerated. Energy expenditure averages 35–50% higher than predicted in both pediatric and adult patients with leukemia.[19-22] Rates of whole-body protein synthesis and breakdown are almost twice normal.[20,22] Similar derangements in energy and protein metabolism have not been found in patients with lymphoma.[22] Energy expenditure decreases in patients with acute leukemia within days of starting chemotherapy[21,23]—further evidence that the leukemia itself induces the high metabolic rate. Analogously, maintenance chemotherapy in children with ALL in remission appears to exert no significant adverse effects on energy metabolism.[24] During induction chemotherapy[21] or marrow transplantation,[25] however, the energy expenditure and protein losses that again increase are attributed to the complications that arise during neutropenia.

Toxicities of Oncologic Treatment

The nutritionally relevant toxicities of oncologic treatment are summarized in Table 92-1. Aggressive multimodal treatment often produces multiple toxicities; when prolonged, it can lead to significant dietary deficits, particularly for children.[26]

Innovative approaches to modifying mucositis include the use of oral forms of antioxidants, such as vitamin E and β-carotene.[27,28] The nutritional consequences of biologic response modifiers have yet to be well described but in general are associated with anorexia and mild to moderate gastrointestinal disturbances.[29,30]

ASSESSMENT OF ALTERED NUTRITION STATUS

Basic Evaluation

Initial and serial nutrition evaluation and screening are indicated in all patients. The degree and time period of any weight loss suggest the severity and chronicity of poor nutrient intake.

Table 92-1. Nutritional Problems Associated with Treatment of Hematologic Malignancies

Treatment	Complications
Chemotherapy	
Alkylating agents[a]	Nausea, vomiting
Antibiotics and antimetabolites[b]	Anorexia, nausea, vomiting, stomatitis
	Esophagitis: doxorubicin, cytarabine
	Gastrointestinal ulceration: doxorubicin, methotrexate
	Hepatotoxic: lomustine, methotrexate
	Nephrotoxic: cisplatin
	Diarrhea: doxorubicin, hydroxyurea, methotrexate
	Constipation: hydroxyurea
Plant alkaloids[c]	Anorexia, nausea, vomiting
	Diarrhea: etoposide
	Stomatitis, constipation, ileus: vinblastine, vincristine
Nitrogen mustard[d]	Anorexia, nausea, vomiting
	Hepatotoxic: chlorambucil, mechlorethamine
	Metallic taste: mechlorethamine
Others[e]	Anorexia, nausea, vomiting
	Stomatitis: mitoxantrone, procarbazine
	Taste disturbances: levamisole
	Xerostomia: procarbazine
	Nephro- and/or hepatotoxic: L-asparaginase
	Diarrhea: levamisole, procarbazine
Steroids	Muscle and bone loss, hypokalemia, fat deposition, fluid retention, glucose intolerance
Radiation	
Head and neck	Stomatitis, xerostomia, odynophagia
Esophageal	Esophagitis, esophageal stricture
Stomach	Anorexia, gastritis
Abdominal	Enteritis, diarrhea, malabsorption, stenosis, obstruction, fistula formation
Total body	Stomatitis, nausea, vomiting, diarrhea, taste alterations, xerostomia, growth failure
Biologicals[f]	Anorexia, nausea, vomiting: interferon, interleukin-2
	Fluid and electrolyte imbalances, diarrhea: interleukin-2
Marrow transplantation	Stomatitis, esophagitis, gastrointestinal ulceration, diarrhea, taste alterations, xerostomia
	Veno-occlusive disease; renal, pulmonary dysfunction; multiple organ failure
	Acute and chronic graft-versus-host disease
	Infectious enteritis

[a] Busulfan, carboplatin, carmustine, cisplatin, cyclophosphamide, dacarbazine, ifosfamide, lomustine, streptozocin, uracil mustard.
[b] Bleomycin, cytarabine, dactinomycin, daunorubicin, doxorubicin, 5-fluorouracil, floxuridine, fludarabine phosphate, hydroxyurea, idarubicin, lomustine, mercaptopurine, methotrexate, mitomycin C, plicamycin, thioguanine.
[c] Etoposide, vinblastine, vincristine.
[d] Chlorambucil, estramustine, mechlorethamine, melphalan, thiotepa.
[e] L-Asparaginase, levamisole, leucovorin, mitoxantrone, pentostatin, procarbazine.
[f] Interferons, interleukins, colony-stimulating factors, including granudocyte and granulocyte/macrophage.
(Data from Cheney and Aker[47]; Charuhas and Aker[30]; and DeLisa et al.[130])

An estimation of ideal body weight provides an index of the adequacy of current tissue stores.

Weight assessment as an index of body composition is of less value in states of fluid imbalance (edema, dehydration, iatrogenic fluid overload) and must be used with caution, especially in critically ill patients, such as those experiencing infectious complications or organ dysfunction with induction therapy or marrow grafting.[31] Actual nutrient intake as can be provided by the dietitian often provides the best guide for judging nutritional adequacy during periods of stress.

Other measures of nutrition assessment, including immune

function tests and serum protein data, have not added to clinical judgment in predicting nutrition-associated complications or survival in surgical patients.[32,33] Similar studies have not been reported in oncology patients. However, measurements of serum albumin, prealbumin, and transferrin seem to reflect metabolic stress, not the adequacy of recent nutrient intake in patients with leukemia undergoing induction chemotherapy[21,34] or marrow transplantation.[35,36]

Pediatric Assessment

Accurate serial weight and height measurements are essential in the assessment of growth and development in children and adolescents. Lack of weight gain in growing children is indicative of nutritional deterioration, while weight loss flags the need for immediate dietary evaluation and intervention. Weight-for-height assessment is the appropriate tool to assess adequacy of body reserves, using standardized charts in prepubertal children[37] and tables in postpubertal adolescents.[38] Van Eys[39] identifies children who are <90% of the standard weight/height ratio (50th percentile) as at risk and those who are <80% as in need of vigorous intervention, whereas Kibirige and coworkers[40] suggest that patients below 95% of standard height/weight ratio may require supplemental nutritional support. Rickard and colleagues[5] define pediatric oncology patients as malnourished if weight-for-height falls below the fifth percentile when height is above the fifth percentile for age, while patients who are below the fifth percentile in both weight and height for age are chronically malnourished.

Serial heights should also be plotted on velocity charts.[41] Decreased height velocity has been observed in children receiving 18 or 24 Gy whole brain irradiation within 6 months of therapy,[42–44] as well as in those undergoing marrow transplantation prepared with total-body irradiation[45] or chemotherapy only.[46] The potential role of chronic nutrient deficits has not been evaluated in poor growth velocity. However, nutrition evaluation is always indicated in children with growth rates below the fifth percentile.

NUTRITIONAL INTERVENTION

Dietary Recommendations and Modifications

Dietary recommendations during periods of treatment toxicities and prolonged anorexia have been extensively reviewed.[30,47,48] Modifications in consistency, texture, and taste of food are required when patients experience mucositis, esophagitis, xerostomia, or dysgeusia.[49,50] Fat and lactose content are often reduced during nausea or diarrhea. A dietitian can recommend appropriate nutritional supplements in patients who exhibit malabsorption or show an inability to gain weight. During hospitalization, a food service that is individualized and that includes frequent follow-up by trained nutrition staff best meets the needs of patients undergoing intense oncologic therapy.[5,51,52]

Low Microbial Diets

The protective benefit of low microbial diets against infection has not been firmly established, owing to lack of controlled trials.[53,54] Nonetheless, the possibility that food will contaminate patients has been shown by reports of pathogenic organisms (*Escherichia coli, Klebsiella* spp., and *Pseudomonas aeruginosa*) in hospital foods.[55–57] Providing a microbial-restricted diet as a means to minimize the acquisition of exogenous organisms is an accepted, noninvasive, and inexpensive preventive

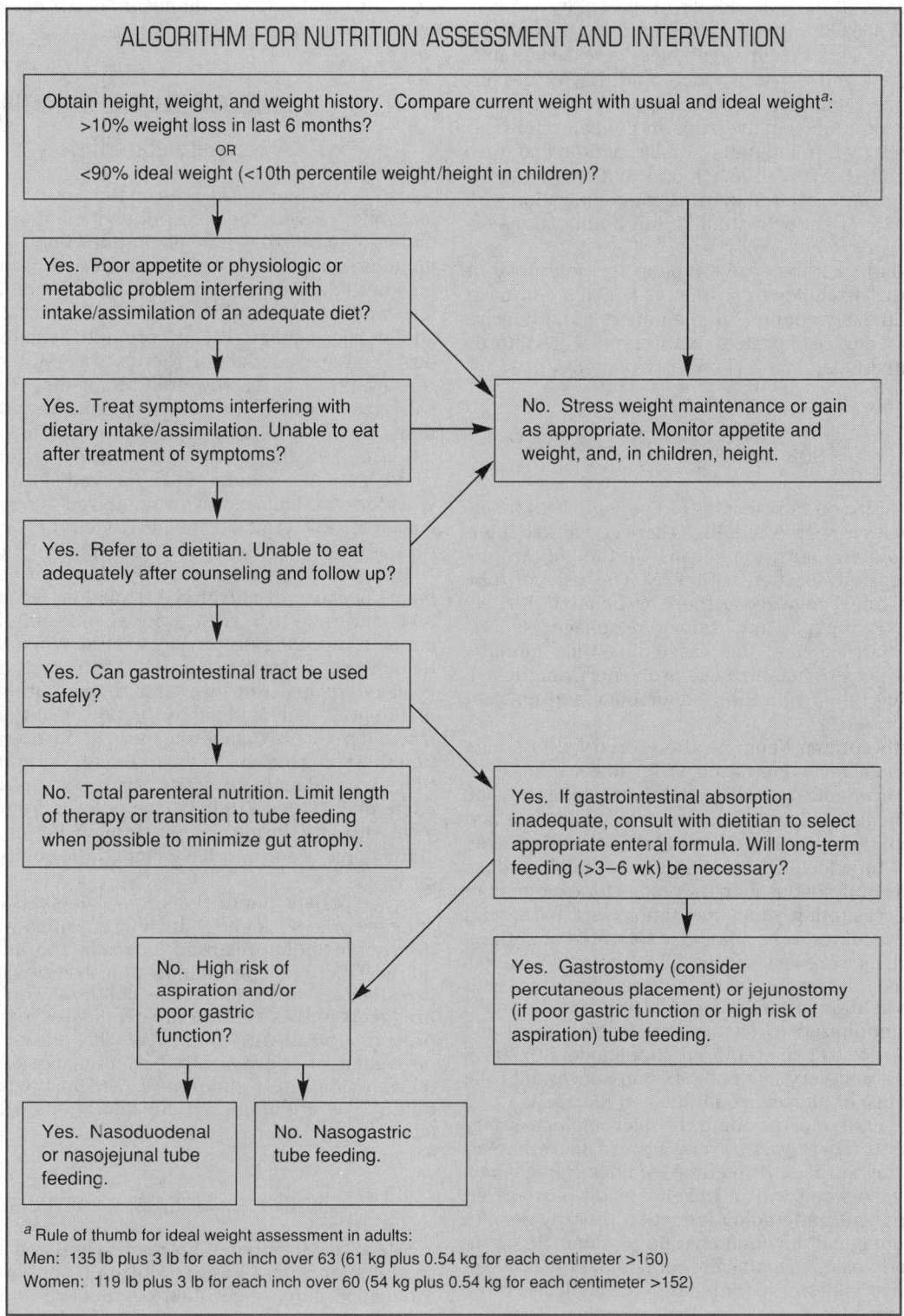

ALGORITHM FOR NUTRITION ASSESSMENT AND INTERVENTION

Obtain height, weight, and weight history. Compare current weight with usual and ideal weight[a]:
>10% weight loss in last 6 months?
    OR
<90% ideal weight (<10th percentile weight/height in children)?

Yes. Poor appetite or physiologic or metabolic problem interfering with intake/assimilation of an adequate diet?

Yes. Treat symptoms interfering with dietary intake/assimilation. Unable to eat after treatment of symptoms?

Yes. Refer to a dietitian. Unable to eat adequately after counseling and follow up?

Yes. Can gastrointestinal tract be used safely?

No. Total parenteral nutrition. Limit length of therapy or transition to tube feeding when possible to minimize gut atrophy.

No. Stress weight maintenance or gain as appropriate. Monitor appetite and weight, and, in children, height.

Yes. If gastrointestinal absorption inadequate, consult with dietitian to select appropriate enteral formula. Will long-term feeding (>3–6 wk) be necessary?

No. High risk of aspiration and/or poor gastric function?

Yes. Gastrostomy (consider percutaneous placement) or jejunostomy (if poor gastric function or high risk of aspiration) tube feeding.

Yes. Nasoduodenal or nasojejunal tube feeding.

No. Nasogastric tube feeding.

[a] Rule of thumb for ideal weight assessment in adults:
Men: 135 lb plus 3 lb for each inch over 63 (61 kg plus 0.54 kg for each centimeter >160)
Women: 119 lb plus 3 lb for each inch over 60 (54 kg plus 0.54 kg for each centimeter >152)

measure. Most hospitals that perform marrow transplantation provide some form of low microbial food service, particularly for patients undergoing gastrointestinal decontamination and treated in ultraisolation laminar airflow or HEPA-filtered environments.[53,54,58,59] Patients with granulocytopenia otherwise not treated with isolation procedures may best be cautioned to avoid most fresh fruits and vegetables, raw or undercooked eggs, meats, and fish, and all but highly processed pasteurized dairy products. The need for a low microbial diet with immunodeficiencies other than granulocytopenia is unknown.

Diets with varying levels of microbial restriction can be char-

acterized as "sterile" diets, "low bacteria" diets, or "cooked food" diets.[53,54,60] A sterile diet, consisting of commercially canned, steam autoclaved, or oven-baked food, requires systematic bacteriologic monitoring, aseptic food preparation, and tray assembly (preferably under a laminar airflow hood in separate kitchen facilities), as well as sterilized utensils, cookware, and tray service items. Sterile diets are used by few institutions because of the high production costs.[58]

Low bacteria diets vary widely in bacterial content and are generally empirically formulated, although some institutions culture foods and assess acceptability when developing such diets.[54,61,62] Moe[54] cultured 198 foods prepared by conventional methods. While 80% of beverages, starches, cooked fresh meats and entrées, and frozen vegetables were acceptable, only 36% of pasteurized dairy products and 42% of dessert and snack items met minimal microbiologic criteria. Up to 17 different species of gram-negative rods in concentrations as high as 10^6/ml colony-forming units in milk, pudding, and ice cream were identified. Ayers et al.[63] found that serving foods containing only *Bacillus* resulted in transient colonization with *Bacillus* spp. in 41% of patients studied, but no infections occurred.

The simplest and least expensive type of low microbial or "cooked food" diet excludes fresh raw vegetables and most raw fruits and will likely contain large numbers of pathogens. It is unknown what degree of protection this type of diet affords for patients treated in laminar airflow environments.

Tube Feedings

Published literature on tube feedings in patients with hematologic malignancies is sparse, although there is renewed interest in the use of enteral nutrition because of the gut atrophy and greater expense associated with TPN. The risks of tube feeding are intuitively recognized as those associated with neutropenia, thrombocytopenia, mucosal and esophageal ulceration, vomiting, diarrhea, and decreased intestinal motility, which may predispose to hemorrhagic problems from the irritation of a feeding tube, aspiration pneumonia, and nutrient malabsorption.

Diarrhea was the primary complication observed in adults with acute leukemia receiving nasogastric tube feedings because of nausea and vomiting during administration of cytosine arabinoside, 6-thioguanine, and daunorubicin.[64] Diarrhea and poor gastric emptying also limited the ability to deliver adequate volumes of tube feeding to patients receiving high-dose chemotherapy and autologous marrow rescue for treatment of solid tumors, necessitating supplementation with parenteral nutrition.[65] Tube feedings were otherwise tolerated in both reports. Tube feedings were less successful in patients with leukemia undergoing allogeneic marrow transplantation with more intensive conditioning, including total body irradiation.[51] Most patients randomized to an "enteral feeding program" were crossed over to TPN or required supplemental intravenous amino acids, and very few patients had successful tube placements because of nausea, vomiting, and diarrhea.

These studies raise concerns about the microbiologic safety of enteral nutrition. There was a trend toward more bacteremias in the autologous patients on tube feedings.[65] *Pseudomonas* sepsis was associated with a hospital-made pasteurized formula in one patient undergoing induction therapy despite selective gastrointestinal decontamination to eliminate gram-negative rods and yeast.[64] Significant contamination can also occur with commercially sterile formulas in the clinical setting, owing to open feeding systems, low osmolar formulas, inadequate hand washing, and prolonged hang times at room temperature.[66–70] Patients receiving antacids, gastric acid inhibitors, H_2-antagonists, antibiotics, steroids, or immunosuppressive therapy may be at increased risk of bacterial colonization during tube feedings.[71]

For the patient who has a functional gastrointestinal tract and who requires nutritional intervention, tube feedings should be considered. Only commercially sterile products should be administered, preferably in a closed feeding system, for a hang time not to exceed 8 hours. In patients with unexplained fever or diarrhea, the enteral feeding should be cultured. Proper tube insertion, formula selection and administration, and monitoring of complications are extensively reviewed by Rombeau and Caldwell.[72]

TOTAL PARENTERAL NUTRITION

Safety and Efficacy

Insufficient literature exists on the use of TPN in hematologic malignancy, with the exception of data regarding patients undergoing marrow transplantation. Popp and co-workers[73] found no difference in long-term survival among patients with advanced diffuse lymphoma undergoing multidrug chemotherapy randomized to adjunctive TPN or to oral nutrition. A few studies suggest that TPN may promote hematopoietic recovery during intensive induction therapy for AML[74] or following marrow grafting.[75] In marrow graft recipients, TPN has been used safely since the 1970s without significant adverse complications, including infection.[75–78] Evidence shows that implementation of TPN during the conditioning regimen in well-nourished patients results in improved long-term survival.[35] Weisdorf and colleagues[35] randomized allogeneic and autologous marrow graft recipients to either TPN or hydration through the first month post-transplant. Of control patients, >60% were crossed over to TPN (median day 21 post-transplant) because of nutritional depletion. Overall survival (Fig. 92-1) and time to relapse were significantly improved in the patients receiving prophylactic TPN. When the autograft patients were analyzed separately, significant differences in survival and relapse rates were not found, but the small numbers of autograft patients limited the power of the study to detect true differences. No differences were observed between nutrition therapies in time to engraftment, duration of hospitalization, or incidences of graft-versus-host disease (GVHD) and bacteremia. Other studies have not confirmed improved survival with TPN during marrow transplantation but, again, small study populations may have limited the ability to detect differences.[51,79]

Other patient populations may benefit from TPN. Rickard and co-workers[80] found that children with advanced malignant disease, including relapsed leukemia and advanced NHL, required TPN to reverse malnutrition. Additionally, these clinical investigators identified those children with AML and poor-prognosis ALL as appropriate candidates for TPN.[81] While improved survival with adjunctive TPN during therapy has not been adequately investigated, maintenance of major organ system function and, in children, growth maintenance and restoration of play are important considerations when oral feedings fail.

Implementation and Formulations

Safe and appropriate TPN may be initiated and monitored in consultation with a hospital nutrition support service or with a nutrition support-certified or oncology dietitian. Adequate delivery of TPN has been enhanced by the use of multilumen central venous access devices.[82] Iatrogenic fluid overload poses a greater risk to patients receiving other multiple intravenous therapies than does inadequate nutrition. Table 92-2 outlines an approach to implementation of TPN.

Research on the pharmacologic applications of nutritional support have intensified as evidence accumulates about the modulation of physiologic, immune, and endocrine functions by nutrients. TPN solutions enriched with branched-chain amino acids have been investigated as a fuel source designed to blunt the muscle catabolism and obligatory nitrogen losses associated with marrow transplantation with mixed success.[36,83] The addition to TPN of glutamine, a nonessential

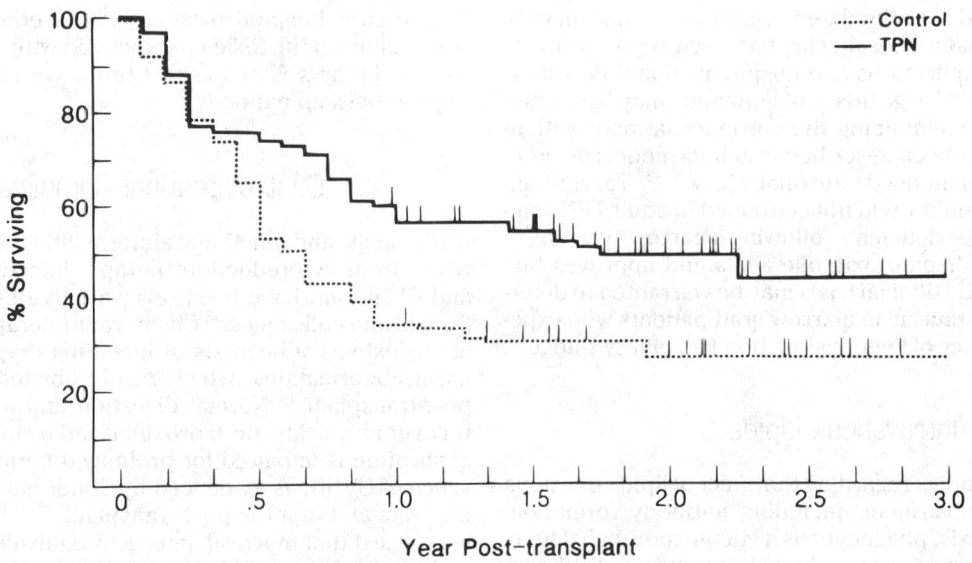

Fig. 92-1. Influence of TPN on overall survival in marrow graft recipients. Life-table curves (Kaplan-Meier plot) show overall survival in TPN prophylaxis versus control groups, $P = 0.011$. Tick marks indicate length of survival at analysis. (From Weisdorf et al.,[35] with permission.)

Table 92-2. Approach to TPN Management

1. Determine macronutrient requirements and distribution of substrates (protein, dextrose, and lipid):

Nutrient	Adult	11–18 yr	7–10 yr	4–6 yr	1–3 yr
Protein (g/kg)					
Maintenance	1.0	1.0	1.2	1.5	1.8
Stress	1.5–2.0	2.0	2.4	3.0	3.0
Energy (kcal/kg)					
Maintenance	30	40–50	50–60	60–70	70–85
Rehabilitation/stress	40–45	45–65	65–75	75–90	90–100
Dextrose (mg/kg/min)[a]	7	10	15	15	15
Lipids	25–30% of total calories; infuse over 12 hours (longer if 3-in-1 delivery system)				
Maintenance fluid[b]	1,500 ml/m²	1,500 ml/m²	100 ml/kg ≤10 kg plus 50 ml/kg for each kg between 11 and 20 kg plus 20 ml/kg for each kg between 21 and 40 kg		

2. Provide electrolytes, vitamins, and trace elements daily, heeding the following special concerns:

	Increased Requirements	Decreased Requirements
Potassium	Amphotericin, thiazide diuretics, steroids, anabolism, GI losses	Spironolactone, renal dysfunction, tumor lysis syndrome
Sodium	GI losses	Pulmonary edema, congestive heart failure, veno-occlusive disease
Calcium		Renal dysfunction, tumor lysis syndrome
Phosphorus	Diuretics, cyclophosphamide, cisplatinum, anabolism	Renal dysfunction
Magnesium	Amphotericin, cyclosporine, GI losses, anabolism	Renal dysfunction, tumor lysis syndrome
Zinc	GI losses, wound healing	
Copper, manganese	GI losses (copper)	Cholestasis

3. Monitor for special management issues (see also the section Nutritional Support in Marrow Transplantation, Organ Complications):

Refractory hyperglycemia	Limit dextrose to <3 mg/kg/min in adults, <10 mg/kg/min in children; increase lipids to 50–60% total kilocalories
Hypertriglyceridemia	>500 mg/dl; limit lipids to 4–8% total kilocalories to provide essential fatty acids
	>2,000 mg/dl; discontinue lipids to decrease risk of pancreatitis
Fluid overload	Provide concentrated dextrose, lipid, amino acid solutions to maximize nutrient support

4. Monitor ability to eat or transition to tube feeding, or both, as soon as feasible.

Abbreviations: TPN, total parenteral nutrition; GI, gastrointestinal.
[a] Recommended maximum dose: to calculate, divide total milligrams dextrose per day by 1,440 min/day/wt in kilograms. Example: 1,700 ml 25% dextrose in a 70-kg patient = 425 g × 1,000 mg/g ÷ 1,440 min/day/70 kg = 4.2 mg/kg/min dextrose.
[b] Account for other sources of fluid to avoid iatrogenic fluid overload.

amino acid oxidized by stimulated lymphocytes and macrophages and intestinal mucosal cells, has been reported to reduce infectious complications and hospitalization time following marrow grafting.[84] Large doses of glutamine may have been more successful in maintaining the gut mucosal barrier than standard TPN, as has been described in animal models of methotrexate or radiation-induced intestinal injury.[85–87] Taurine, another nonessential amino acid not contained in adult TPN solutions, may also be deficient following marrow grafting.[88] Taurine conjugates hepatotoxic bile acids and improves bile acid secretory rates.[89] Clinical trials may be warranted to determine the benefits of taurine in marrow graft patients who experience a high incidence of liver dysfunction and biliary sludge.[90]

Intravenous Lipids

The conflicting studies regarding the effect of lipid emulsions on immunologic impairment, including antibody formation, neutrophil chemotaxis, phagocytosis, reticuloendothelial function, and inflammatory response, have been reviewed.[91,92] Lipids are cleared from the blood by lipoprotein lipase; when this enzyme is saturated, the reticuloendothelial system removes excess lipid. Circulating neutrophils may become lipid laden, exhibiting impaired function. However, a large randomized trial failed to show an association between a dose of lipid routinely used in clinical practice versus a low dose to prevent essential fatty acid deficiency and bacterial and fungal infections during the first hospitalization for marrow grafting in patients with hematologic malignancies.[93] Slow versus bolus infusions are associated with decreased inflammatory response, which may be most relevant to patients with acute pulmonary processes.[91] In general, an infusion of moderate amounts of lipids (25–30% of total calories) over a minimum of 12 hours is considered prudent and safe practice.

NUTRITIONAL SUPPORT IN MARROW TRANSPLANTATION

Standard supportive care during the first month post-transplant has included TPN,[35,82,94,95] and many patients with slow gastrointestinal healing or GVHD have relied on TPN to some

degree after hospital discharge.[96] As other supportive measures diminish the toxicity associated with transplantation, the role of TPN as well as its substitution with enteral feedings will require re-examination.

Gastrointestinal Complications

Histologic and functional abnormalities of the intestinal tract result from cytoreduction therapy, infectious complications, and GVHD and have been reviewed by Beschorner[97] and McDonald and colleagues.[98] Chemoradiotherapy results in moderate to extensive necrosis of intestinal crypts and diffuse mucosal abnormalities, which resolve histologically by day 20 post-transplant.[98] Normal digestion and absorption may not recover as quickly. Both proximal and terminal small intestinal absorption is impaired for prolonged periods, even in the absence of GVHD, as evidenced by abnormal D-xylose and Schilling tests at 4 months post-transplant.[99–101] Permeability studies suggest that mucosal damage is equivalent for conditioning with chemotherapy only and chemoradiotherapy and is greater in patients >30 years old.[102]

Mucosal competence is also impaired. Salivary IgA concentrations are one-half normal levels as late as day 90 post-transplant.[103] Whether IgA secretions at other intestinal sites show similar prolonged immunodeficiency is unknown. The number of immunoglobulin-containing plasma cells in the small intestine decreases after chemoradiotherapy but appears to recover within weeks, provided intestinal GVHD does not develop.[104]

Nausea, vomiting, diarrhea, and oropharyngeal mucositis inhibit oral intake for ≥1 month, as displayed in Figure 92-2. The severity of mucositis is increased in patients treated with total-body irradiation[105] or methotrexate as prophylaxis against GVHD.[106] Limited data are available on the way in which growth factors might influence recovery from mucositis. Nemunaitis and co-workers[107] described no difference in the severity of mucositis in a randomized, double-blinded trial of colony-stimulating factor–rh granulocyte/macrophage in autologous marrow graft recipients, most of whom received total-body irradiation as part of cytoreduction therapy. However, TPN use was decreased and compared with historical controls in patients

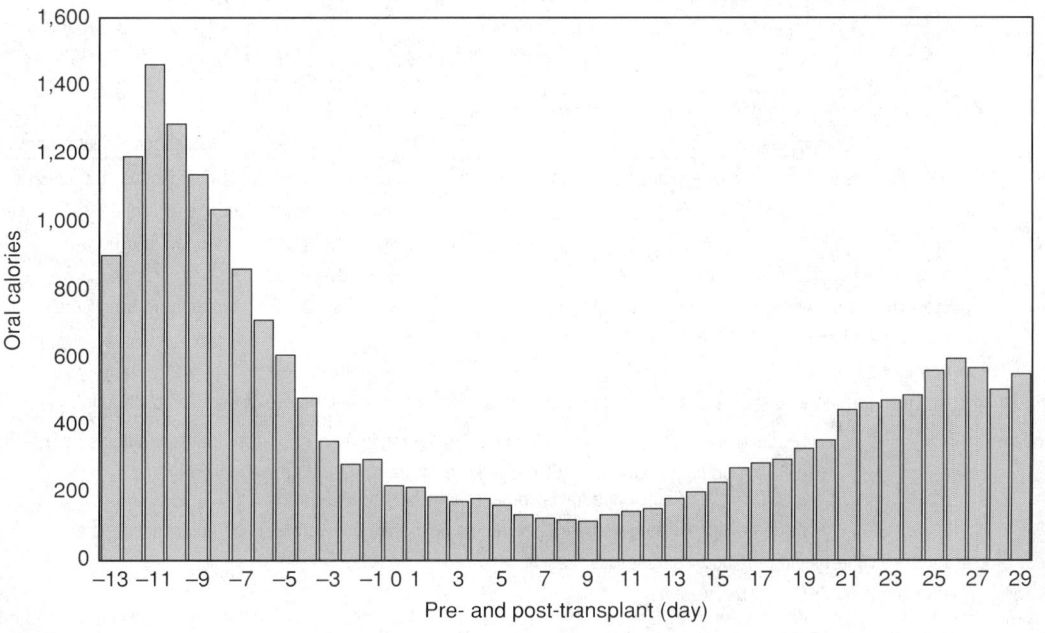

Fig. 92-2. Average daily oral calorie intake in adult marrow transplant recipients (n = 295).

who received colony-stimulating factor-granulocyte after busulfan and cyclophosphamide and autologous marrow grafting.[108]

Organ Complications

Veno-occlusive Disease

Hepatic veno-occlusive disease is characterized by occlusion of small hepatic veins, damaged hepatocytes, fluid retention, ascites, hepatomegaly, and jaundice. The pathophysiology, diagnosis, and treatment at this disease have been reviewed by Shulman and Hinterberger.[109] Insidious weight gain is the first sign of the disorder, and if it progresses, more severe symptoms of liver failure occur, including encephalopathy, coagulopathy, and renal failure.[110-112] Fluid and TPN management are controversial, since limitation of fluids to minimize edema and ascites is frequently complicated by intravascular volume depletion and deterioration of renal function. Conversely, repleting the intravascular space often results in pulmonary edema and massive ascites.

Daily weights and thrice-weekly serum bilirubins in the immediate post-transplant period facilitate early detection of disease in patients at increased risk. In patients with decreased urine output and urinary sodium excretion, restriction of total sodium and use of spironolactone promote negative sodium balance, while reduction of total fluid may decelerate fluid accumulation. Concentrated TPN solutions are indicated if renal perfusion is adequate. The capacity to eliminate intravenous lipids from the bloodstream should be monitored in cases of severe veno-occlusive disease. If encephalopathy develops, the benefits of Hepatamine (an amino acid solution with lower aromatic amino acids, tryptophan, and methionine content) have not been established.[113] Other potential causes of encephalopathy, including poor oxygenation, narcotics, excessive BUN, and sepsis, require correction if an expensive amino acid formulation is considered. In severe disease, the biliary-excreted trace elements, copper and manganese, should be removed from TPN. Measurement of energy needs with indirect calorimetry if available may avert additive hepatotoxicity associated with overfeeding, as well as the risks of debilitation with prolonged underfeeding.

Renal Disease

Hypoperfusion due to capillary leak syndrome to veno-occlusive disease and drug toxicities are implicated most frequently in the etiology of renal failure. Renal damage is suspected when serum creatinine level is twice baseline. An elevated BUN, however, may be partially due to nonrenal factors, including increased protein intake, gastrointestinal bleeding, or hypercatabolism. Prolonged protein restriction to minimize a rise of BUN should be avoided to ensure that adequate calorie and protein support are provided during this catabolic period.

Renal complications are managed by maintaining intravascular volume and correcting electrolyte imbalances. The large fluid load necessitated by TPN is problematic in the oliguric patient and requires daily manipulation, depending on urine output and clinical signs of fluid overload. Hypervolemic hyponatremia is treated with water restriction to prevent congestive heart failure. General indications for hemodialysis are extracellular fluid volume expansion, acidemia, hyperkalemia, and azotemia.

The primary goal of nutritional therapy in acute renal failure is to minimize uremic toxicity and other metabolic derangements and yet prevent malnutrition. Protein levels are typically restricted before dialysis by the TPN volume tolerated. During dialysis, protein intake should meet stress needs as defined in Table 92-2. Serum triglycerides should be monitored weekly since the clearance of intravenous lipids may be reduced.[114] Water-soluble vitamins are lost in the dialysate and should be provided instead of standard intravenous multivitamins, in an effort to prevent excessive serum vitamin A levels.[115]

Pulmonary Disease

The degree of pulmonary edema due to increased capillary permeability induced by cytoreduction therapy may be compounded by iatrogenic fluid overloading. Management includes reducing total sodium from primary sources, including oral intake, TPN, and medications, and using concentrated TPN solutions. During ventilator dependency, adequate TPN should be provided to preserve muscle reserves.

Graft-Versus-Host Disease

Acute Graft-Versus-Host Disease

Minimal to life-threatening skin, liver, and/or intestinal GVHD develops within 10–80 days post-transplant in approximately two-thirds of allogeneic marrow transplant recipients. Patients whose transplants were not fully HLA-compatible are at greater risk.[116] In acute intestinal GVHD, voluminous diarrhea is a prominent manifestation, with the volume corresponding to the extent of mucosal damage.[117] The diarrheal fluid is green and watery, with ropy strands of mucus, protein, and cellular debris, and often contains occult blood. Protein content is high, as evidenced by falling plasma protein levels or by measurements of fecal α_1-antitrypsin in fecal water.[118] Associated symptoms include anorexia, nausea, vomiting, and crampy abdominal pain, which may be related to food ingestion or may occur spontaneously owing to the secretory nature of the diarrhea. Biopsy findings range from necrosis of individual intestinal crypt cells to total mucosal denudation.[119,120] Intestinal function has received limited study, and the characteristics of malabsorption have yet to be determined. There is no evidence that early post-transplant restriction of food protein as potentially antigenic stimulants decreases the risk of acute GVHD.[121]

Weisdorf and colleagues[122] described a syndrome of upper intestinal GVHD presenting clinically as anorexia, dyspepsia, food intolerance, nausea, and vomiting. The clinical picture frequently progressed to symptomatic lower gastrointestinal involvement after failure of immunosuppressive therapy, suggesting that this syndrome may be an early manifestation of a unique intestinal immunopathology. Prolonged nausea and vomiting constitute indication for endoscopic evaluation because of the high incidence of less "classic" intestinal GVHD.[123]

Acute liver GVHD is characterized by abnormal liver function tests, jaundice, and mild hepatomegaly.[98] Hepatic synthesis and enterohepatic circulation of bile salts may be diminished or inhibited, resulting in steatorrhea.

Adequate nutrition is a vital adjunct to immunosuppressive drugs in the treatment of acute GVHD. In severe skin GVHD, energy, protein, and fluid requirements may be high if >50% of total body surface is involved. In intestinal GVHD, the patient is initially dependent on TPN, as complete bowel rest is the only means of decreasing diarrhea.[117] When diarrheal volumes diminish and abdominal pain subsides, isotonic oral liquid supplements are introduced to stimulate intestinal regeneration and assess absorption.[124] Guidelines for the introduction of oral intake have been empirically derived using a five-phase regimen, which emphasizes foods low in lactose, fat, fiber, and total acidity.[124,125] Severe ileal involvement or liver GVHD may necessitate prolonged fat restriction.

Table 92-3. Nutrition-Related Problems 1 Year Post-Bone Marrow Grafting

Sign/Symptom	Chronic Graft-Versus-Host Disease Status[a]		
	None (%)	Limited (%)	Extensive (%)
Weight loss	27	19	33
Weight gain	14	28	34
Oral sensitivity	7	14	41
Xerostomia	10	11	27
Stomatitis	3	3	14
Anorexia	3	6	13
Reflux symptoms	1	6	12
Diarrhea	3	3	12
Steatorrhea	1	0	9
Dysgeusia	0	0	6
Esophageal stricture	0	0	2
Dyspnea	0	0	7
Contractures	0	0	2

[a] Among 192 allogeneic transplant recipients. Percentage of total number of patients is shown.
(Adapted from Lenssen et al.,[131] with permission.)

Chronic Graft-Versus-Host Disease

Chronic GVHD is a multisystem disorder that affects 35–40% of allogeneic marrow graft recipients, presenting 70–400 days post-transplant.[126] Clinical manifestations that may adversely affect nutritional status include anorexia, mucositis, xerostomia, dysphagia, esophageal stricture, cholestatic liver disease, diarrhea or steatorrhea, dyspnea and limited exercise tolerance, restricted joint mobility, and generalized wasting (Table 92-3).

Oral sensitivity is common, with frank stomatitis occurring in a significant portion of patients. Pain, burning, and loss of taste have been described as prodromes of chronic GVHD.[127] In severe cases, only bland liquids and soft foods may be tolerated. Complete nutritional supplements and nutrient-dense carbohydrate polymers are important dietary adjuncts in patients experiencing weight loss.

Esophageal webbing or stricture can result in severe swallowing difficulties.[98] Typical symptoms include pain and difficulty in swallowing food and pills, as well as retrosternal pain caused by esophageal thinning. Webs and strictures are managed with periodic dilation. Diet tolerance varies widely and may be limited to liquids in patient with extensive webbing. Gastrostomy tubes may be indicated when the passage of food is obstructed.

Diffuse intestinal involvement is a rare manifestation of chronic GVHD.[98] Bacterial overgrowth, medications, and chronic liver GVHD may contribute to diarrhea or steatorrhea. A moderate fat restriction, calorie supplementation with medium-chain triglycerides, and mineral and fat-soluble vitamin supplementation may be necessary interim measures.

In patients receiving cyclosporine, magnesium supplementation is necessary in order to correct drug-induced hypomagnesemia and its potential neurologic sequelae.[128,129] Diarrhea can limit the oral magnesium dose, necessitating intravenous replacement. Children with extensive chronic GVHD represent a special risk group. Decreased height velocity has been related to pretransplant cranial irradiation, both chemotherapy-only and total-body irradiation conditioning regimens, and chronic GVHD.[45,46] Although prednisone therapy has been incriminated in growth stunting, catch-up growth has not been observed following cessation of treatment.[45] The contribution of poor nutrient intake as a factor in growth failure after marrow transplantation has not been investigated. Children displaying weight loss, inappropriate weight gain, or growth failure deserve thorough nutritional evaluation to rule out treatable dietary deficiencies.

ACKNOWLEDGMENT

Preparation of this work was supported in part by grant #DK35816 from the Clinical Nutrition Research Units, U.S. Department of Health and Human Services.

REFERENCES

1. Klein S, Simes J, Blackburn GL: Total parenteral nutrition and cancer clinical trials. Cancer 58:1378, 1986
2. McGeer AJ, Detsky AS, O'Rourke K: Parenteral nutrition in cancer patients undergoing chemotherapy: a meta-analysis. Nutrition 6:233, 1990
3. DeWys WD, Begg C, Lavin PT et al: Prognostic effect of weight loss prior to chemotherapy in cancer patients. Am J Med 69:491, 1980
4. Ramirez I, van Eys J, Carr D et al: Malnutrition in children with malignancies. Proc Am Assoc Cancer Res 21:378, 1980
5. Rickard KA, Grosfeld JL, Coates TD et al: Advances in nutrition care of children with neoplastic diseases: a review of treatment, research, and application. J Am Diet Assoc 86:1666, 1986
6. Aker SN, Lenssen P, Darbinian J et al: Nutritional assessment in the marrow transplant patient. Nutr Supp Serv 3:22, 1983
7. Hill G: Body composition research: implications for the practice of clinical nutrition. JPEN J Parenter Enteral Nutr 16:197, 1992
8. Chandra RK: Nutrition, immunity and infection: present knowledge and future directions. Lancet 1:688, 1983
9. Stinnett JD: Nutrition and the Immune Response. CRC Press, Boca Raton, FL, 1983
10. Watson RR: Nutrition, Disease Resistance, and Immune Function. Marcel Dekker, New York, 1984
11. Garre MA, Boles JM, Youinou PY: Current concepts in immune derangements due to undernutrition. JPEN J Parenter Enteral Nutr 11:309, 1987
12. Van Der Meer JWM: Defects in host-defense mechanisms. p. 41. In Rubin RH, Young LS (eds): Clinical Approach to Infection in the Compromised Host. 2nd Ed. Plenum, New York, 1988
13. Chandra RK: Nutritional regulation of immunity and infection in the gastrointestinal tract. J Pediatr Gastroenterol Nutr, suppl 1. 2:S181, 1983
14. Bodey GP, Fainstein V: Infections of the gastrointestinal tract in the immunocompromised patient. Annu Rev Med 37:271, 1986
15. Berg RD: Bacterial translocation from the gastrointestinal tracts of mice receiving immunosuppressive chemotherapeutic agents, abstracted. Curr Microbiol 8:285, 1983
16. Tancrede CH, Andremont AO: Bacterial translocation and gram-negative bacteremia in patients with hematological malignancies. J Infect Dis 152:99, 1985
17. Dietch E, Winterton J, Li M, Berg R: The gut as a portal of entry for bacteremia: role of protein malnutrition. Ann Surg 205:681, 1987
18. Dietch EA, Ma WJ, Ma L et al: Protein malnutrition predisposes to inflammatory-induced gut-origin septic states. Ann Surg 211:560, 1990
19. Young VR: Energy metabolism and requirements in cancer patients. Cancer Res 37:2336, 1977
20. Kien CL, Camitta BM: Close association of accelerated rates of whole body protein turnover (synthesis and breakdown) and energy expenditure in children with newly diagnosed acute lymphocytic leukemia. JPEN J Parenter Enteral Nutr 11:129, 1987
21. Lerebours E, Tilly H, Rimbert A et al: Change in energy and protein status during chemotherapy in patients with acute leukemia. Cancer 61:2412, 1988
22. Humberstone DA, Shaw JHF: Metabolism in hematologic malignancy. Cancer 62:1619, 1988
23. Stallings VA, Vaisman N, Chan HS et al: Energy metabolism in children with newly diagnosed acute lymphoblastic leukemia. Pediatr Res 26:157, 1989
24. Vaisman N, Stallings VA, Chan H et al: Effect of chemotherapy on the energy and protein metabolism of children near the end of treatment for acute lymphoblastic leukemia. Am J Clin Nutr 57:679, 1993
25. Lenssen P, Cheney C, Flournoy N et al: Nitrogen losses associated with marrow transplantation. Clin Nutr, suppl. 4:28, 1984
26. Coates TD, Rickard KA, Grosfeld JL, Weetman RM: Nutritional support of children with neoplastic diseases. Surg Clin North Am 66:1197, 1986
27. Wadleigh RG, Redman RS, Graham MF et al: Vitamin E in the treatment of chemotherapy-induced mucositis. Am J Med 92:481, 1992
28. Mills EED: The modifying effect of beta-carotene on radiation and chemotherapy induced oral mucositis. Br J Cancer 57:416, 1988
29. Krakoff IH: Cancer chemotherapeutic and biologic agents. CA Cancer J Clin 41:264, 1991
30. Charuhas PM, Akar SN: Nutritional implications of antineoplastic chemotherapeutic agents. Clin Appl Nutr 2:20, 1992
31. Cheney CL, Abson KG, Aker SN et al: Body composition changes in marrow

transplant recipients receiving total parenteral nutrition. Cancer 59:1515, 1987

32. Baker JP, Detsky AS, Wesson D et al: Nutritional assessment: a comparison of clinical judgment and objective measurements. N Engl J Med 306:969, 1982

33. Detsky AS, Baker JP, Mendelson RA et al: Evaluating the accuracy of nutritional assessment techniques applied to hospitalized patient: methodology and comparisons. JPEN J Parenter Enteral Nutr 8:153, 1984

34. Merritt RJ, Kalsch M, Roux LD et al: Significance of hypoalbuminemia in pediatric oncology patients—malnutrition or infection? JPEN J Parenter Enteral Nutr 9:303, 1985

35. Weisdorf SA, Lysne J, Wind D et al: Positive effect of prophylactic total parenteral nutrition on long-term outcome of bone marrow transplantation. Transplantation 43:833, 1987

36. Lenssen P, Cheney CL, Aker SN et al: Intravenous branched chain amino acid trial in marrow transplant recipients. JPEN J Parenter Enteral Nutr 11:112, 1987

37. Hamill PVV, Drizd TA, Johnson CL et al: Physical growth: National Center for Health Statistics percentiles. Am J Clin Nutr 32:607, 1979

38. U.S. Vital Health Statistics: Height and Weight of Youths 12–17 Years. Ser 11, No. 124. U.S. Department of Health and Human Services, Washington, DC, 1973

39. Van Eys J: Nutrition in the treatment of cancer in children. J Am Coll Nutr 3:159, 1984

40. Kibirige MS, Morris Jones PH, Stevens RF: Indicators of malnutrition in leukemic children. Arch Dis Child 62:845, 1987

41. Tanner JM, Davies PW: Clinical longitudinal standards for height and height velocity for North American children. Pediatrics 107:317, 1985

42. Starceski PJ, Lee PA, Blatt J et al: Comparable effects of 1800- and 2400-rad (18- and 24-Gy) cranial irradiation on height and weight in children treated for acute lymphocytic leukemia. Am J Dis Child 141:550, 1987

43. Wells RJ, Foster MB, D'Ercole AJ et al: The impact on cranial irradiation on the growth of children with acute lymphocytic leukemia. Am J Dis Child 137:37, 1983

44. Robison LL, Nesbit ME, Sather HN et al: Height of children successfully treated for acute lymphoblastic leukemia: a report from the Late Effects Study Committee of Children's Cancer Study Group. Med Pediatr Oncol 13:14, 1985

45. Sanders JE, Pitchard S, Mahoney P et al: Growth and development following marrow transplantation for leukemia. Blood 68:1129, 1986

46. Wingard JR, Plotnick LP, Freemer CS et al: Growth in children after bone marrow transplantation: busulfan plus cyclophosphamide versus cyclophosphamide plus total body irradiation. Blood 79:1068, 1992

47. Cheney CL, Aker SN: Nutritional care in neoplastic disease. p.625. In Mahan LK, Arlin M (eds): Krause's Food, Nutrition, and Diet Therapy. 8th Ed. WB Saunders, Philadelphia, 1992

48. Bloch AS: Nutrition Management of the Cancer Patient. Aspen, Rockville, MD, 1990

49. Kusler DL, Rambur BA: Treatment for radiation-induced xerostomia. Cancer Nurs 15:191, 1992

50. Boock CA, Reddick JE: Taste alterations in bone marrow transplant patients. J Am Diet Assoc 91:1121, 1991

51. Szeluga DJ, Stuart RK, Brookmeyer R et al: Nutritional support of bone marrow transplant recipients: a prospective, randomized clinical trial comparing total parenteral nutrition to an enteral feeding program. Cancer Res 47:3309, 1987

52. Gauvreau-Stern JM, Cheney CL, Aker SN, Lenssen P: Food intake patterns and foodservice requirements on a marrow transplant unit. J Am Diet Assoc 89:367, 1989

53. Aker SN, Cheney CL: The use of sterile and low microbial diets in ultraisolation environments. JPEN J Parenter Enteral Nutr 7:390, 1983

54. Moe G: Enteral feeding and infection in the immunocompromised patient. Nutr Clin Pract 6:55, 1991

55. Shooter RA, Faiers MC, Cooke EM et al: Isolation of *Escherichia coli Pseudomonas aeruginosa*, and *Klebsiella* from food in hospitals, canteens, and schools. Lancet 2:390, 1971

56. Kominos SD, Copeland CE, Grosiak B, Postic B: Introduction of *Pseudomonas aeruginosa* into a hospital via vegetables. Appl Environ Microbiol 24:567, 1972

57. Subramaniam L, Shriniwas SNV: Food as a likely source of *Pseudomonas aeruginosa*. Indian J Med Res 85:617, 1987

58. Dezenhall A, Curry-Bartley K, Blackburn SA et al: Food and nutrition services in bone marrow transplant centers. J Am Diet Assoc 87:1351, 1987

59. Moe G: Low microbial diets for patients with granulocytopenia. p.125. In Bloch AS (ed): Nutrition Management of the Cancer Patient. Aspen, Rockville, MD, 1990

60. Frankman C, Beck J, Schomberg R: Feeding in protected environments. p. 241. In Rose JC (ed): Handbook for Health Care Food Service Management. Aspen, Rockville, MD, 1984

61. Dong FM, Hashisaka AE, Rasco BA et al: Irradiated or aseptically prepared frozen dairy desserts: acceptability to bone marrow transplant recipients. J Am Diet Assoc 92:719, 1992

62. Pizzo PA, Purvis DS, Waters C: Microbiological evaluation of food items. J Am Diet Assoc 81:272, 1982

63. Ayers LW, Hancock D, Buesching W, Tutschka P: Development and evaluation of diets using non-sterile but controlled microbial content foods for control of nosocomial infections in bone marrow transplant patients. p. 414. L-10. In the Proceedings of the Annual Meeting, American Society of Microbiology, Washington, DC, 1986

64. De Vries EGE, Mulder NH, Houwen B, de Vries-Hospers HG: Enteral nutrition by nasogastric tube in adult patients treated with intensive chemotherapy for acute leukemia. Am J Clin Nutr 35:1490, 1982

65. Mulder POM, Bouman JG, Gietema JA et al: Hyperalimentation in autologous bone marrow transplantation for solid tumors. Comparison of total parenteral versus partial parenteral plus enteral nutrition. Cancer 64:2045, 1989

66. Report of the Ross Workshop on Contamination of Enteral Feeding Products During Clinical Usage. Ross Laboratories, Columbus, OH, 1983

67. Nugent M, Hansell DT, Gray GR: Bacterial contamination of enteral feeds. Clin Nutr 6:21, 1987

68. Bastow MD, Greaves P, Allison SP: Microbial contamination of enteral feeds. Hum Nutr Appl Nutr 36A:213, 1982

69. Fagerman KE, Paauw JD, McCamish MA, Dean RE: Effects of time, temperature, and preservative on bacterial growth in enteral nutrient solutions. Am J Hosp Pharm 41:1122, 1984

70. Schroeder P, Fisher D, Volz M, Paloucek JP: Microbial contamination of enteral feeding solutions in a community hospital. JPEN J Parenter Enteral Nutr 7:364, 1983

71. Anderton A: Microbiological aspects of the preparation and administration of naso-gastric and naso-enteric tube feeds in hospitals—a review. Hum Nutr Appl Nutr 37A:426, 1983

72. Rombeau JL, Caldwell MD: Enteral and Tube Feeding. 2nd Ed. WB Saunders, Philadelphia, 1990

73. Popp MB, Fisher RI, Wesley R et al: A prospective randomized study of adjuvant parenteral nutrition in the treatment of advanced diffuse lymphoma: influence on survival. Surgery 90:195, 1981

74. Hays DM, Merritt RJ, White L et al: Effect of total parenteral nutrition on marrow recovery during induction therapy for acute nonlymphocytic leukemia in childhood. Med Pediatr Oncol 11:134, 1983

75. Weisdorf S, Hofland C, Sharp HL: Total parenteral nutrition in bone marrow transplantation: a clinical evaluation. J Pediatr Gastroenterol Nutr 3:95, 1984

76. Schmidt GM, Blume KG, Bross KJ et al: Parenteral nutrition in bone marrow transplant recipients. Exp Hematol 8:506, 1980

77. Reed MD, Lazarus HM, Herzig RH et al: Cyclic parenteral nutrition during bone marrow transplantation in children. Cancer 51:1563, 1983

78. Sanders JE, Hickman RO, Aker SN et al: Experience with double lumen right atrial catheters. JPEN J Parenter Enteral Nutr 6:95, 1982

79. Lough M, Watkins R, Garden OJ et al: Parenteral nutrition in bone marrow transplant recipients. Clin Nutr, suppl. 5:62, 1986

80. Rickard KA, Grosfeld JL, Kirksey A et al: Reversal of protein-energy malnutrition in children during treatment of advanced neoplastic disease. Ann Surg 190:771, 1979

81. Rickard KA, Coates TD, Grosfeld JL et al: The value of nutrition support in children with cancer. Cancer 58:1904, 1986

82. Aker SN, Cheney C, Sanders JE et al: Nutritional support in marrow graft recipients with single versus double lumen right atrial catheters. Exp Hematol 10:732, 1982

83. Brennan MF, Cerra F, Daly J et al: Report of a research workshop: branched-chain amino acids in stress and injury. JPEN J Parenter Enteral Nutr 10:446, 1986

84. Ziegler TR, Young LS, Benfell K et al: Clinical and metabolic efficacy of glutamine-supplemented parenteral nutrition after bone marrow transplantation. A randomized, double-blind, controlled study. Ann Intern Med 116:821, 1992

85. Fox AD, Kripke SA, DePaula J et al: Effect of a glutamine-supplemented enteral diet on methotrexate-induced enterocolitis. JPEN J Parenter Enteral Nutr 12:325, 1988

86. Klimberg VS, Souba WW, Dolson DJ et al: Prophylactic glutamine protects the intestinal mucosa from radiation injury. Cancer 66:62, 1990

87. Souba WW, Klimberg VS, Hautamaki RD et al: Oral glutamine reduces bacterial translocation following abdominal radiation. J Surg Res 48:1, 1990

88. Desai TK, Maliakkal J, Kinzie JL et al: Taurine deficiency after intensive chemotherapy and/or radiation. Am J Clin Nutr 55:708, 1992

89. Guertin F, Roy CC, Lepage G et al: Effect of taurine on total parenteral nutrition-associated cholestasis. JPEN J Parenter Enteral Nutr 15:247, 1991
90. Frick MP, Snover DC, Feinber SB et al: Sonography of the gallbladder in bone marrow transplant patients. Am J Gastroenterol 79:122, 1984
91. Skeie B, Askanazi J, Rothkopf MM et al: Intravenous fat emulsions and lung function: a review. Crit Care Med 16:183, 1988
92. Wolfe BM, Ney DM: Lipid metabolism in parenteral nutrition. p. 72. In Rombeau JL, Caldwell M (eds): Parenteral Nutrition. WB Saunders, Philadelphia, 1986
93. Lenssen P, Bruemmer B, Aker S et al: Relationship between IV lipid dose and incidence of bacteremia and fungemia in 492 marrow transplant patients, abstracted. JPEN 18:225, 1994
94. Van Lint MT, Zunino P, Mansuino P et al: Total parenteral nutrition following BMT. Bone Marrow Transplant, suppl. 1:222, 1986
95. Yamanaka WK, Tilmont G, Aker SN: Plasma fatty acids of marrow transplant recipients on fat-supplemented parenteral nutrition. Am J Clin Nutr 39:607, 1984
96. Lenssen P, Moe GL, Cheney CL et al: Parenteral nutrition in marrow transplant recipients after discharge from the hospital. Exp Hematol 11:974, 1983
97. Beschorner WE: Destruction of the intestinal mucosa after bone marrow transplantation and graft-versus-host disease. Surv Synth Pathol Res 3:264, 1984
98. McDonald GB, Shulman HM, Sullivan KM, Spencer GD: Intestinal and hepatic complications of human bone marrow transplantation. Parts I and II. Gastroenterology 90:460, 770, 1986
99. Chatti N, Jobin C, Perreault C, Lebrun M: Protein losing enteropathy and malabsorption in patients undergoing allogeneic marrow transplantation. Gastroenterology 86:1045, 1984
100. Guyotat D, Vu Van H, Pigeon R et al: Intestinal absorption tests after bone marrow transplantation. Exp Hematol, suppl 15. 12:118, 1984
101. Milligan DW, Manning A, Quick A, Barnard DL: Vitamin B_{12} absorption following allogeneic bone marrow transplantation. Bone Marrow Transplant, suppl. 1:200, 1986
102. Fegan C, Poynton CH, Whittaker JA: The gut mucosal barrier in bone marrow transplantation. Bone Marrow Transplant 5:373, 1990
103. Izutsu KT, Menard TW, Schubert MM et al: Graft versus host disease-related secretory immunoglobulin A deficiency in bone marrow transplant recipients. Findings in labial saliva. Lab Invest 52:292, 1985
104. Beschorner WE, Yardley JH, Tutschka P, Santos G: Deficiency of intestinal immunity with graft-versus-host disease in humans. J Infect Dis 144:38, 1981
105. Schubert MM, Williams BE, Lloid ME et al: Clinical assessment scale for the rating of oral mucosal changes associated with bone marrow transplantation. Cancer 69:2469, 1992
106. Deeg HJ, Storb R, Thomas ED et al: Cyclosporine as prophylaxis for graft-versus-host disease: a randomized study in patients undergoing marrow transplantation for acute nonlymphoblastic leukemia. Blood 65:1325, 1985
107. Nemunaitis J, Rabinowe SN, Singer JW et al: Recombinant granulocyte-macrophage colony-stimulating factor after autologous bone marrow transplantation for lymphoid cancer. N Engl J Med 324:1773, 1991
108. Sheridan WP, Morstyn G, Wolf M et al: Granulocyte colony-stimulating factor and neutrophil recovery after high-dose chemotherapy and autologous bone marrow transplantation. Lancet 2:891, 1989
109. Shulman HM, Hinterberger W: Hepatic veno-occlusive disease–liver toxicity syndrome after bone marrow transplantation. Bone Marrow Transplant 10:197, 1992
110. Jones RJ, Lee KSK, Beschorner WE et al: Venooclusive disease of the liver following bone marrow transplantation. Transplantation 44:778, 1987
111. McDonald GB, Sharma P, Matthews DE et al: The clinical cource of 53 patients with venocclusive disease of the liver after marrow transplantation. Transplantation 39:603, 1985
112. McDonald GB, Hinds MS, Fisher LD et al: Veno-occlusive disease of the liver and multiorgan failure after bone marrow transplantation: a cohort study of 355 patients. Ann Intern Med 118:255, 1993
113. Lenssen P, Spencer GD, McDonald GB: A randomized trial of Freamine vs. Hepatamine vs. placebo in acute hepatic coma. Gastroenterology 92:1749, 1987
114. Druml W, Fischer M, Sertl S et al: Fat elimination in acute renal failure: long-chain vs. medium-chain triglycerides. Am J Clin Nutr 55:468, 1992
115. Gleghorn EE, Eisenberg LD, Hack S et al: Observations of vitamin A toxicity in three patients with renal failure receiving parenteral alimentation. Am J Clin Nutr 44:107, 1986
116. Witherspoon RP, Storb R: Immunologic aspects of marrow transplantation. Immunol Clin North Am 9:187, 1989
117. Wolford JL, McDonald GB: A problem-oriented approach to intestinal and liver disease after marrow transplantation. J Clin Gastroenterol 10:419, 1988
118. Weisdorf SA, Salati LM, Longsdorf JA et al: Graft-versus-host disease of the intestine: a protein losing enteropathy characterized by fecal alpha 1-antitrypsin. Gastroenterology 85:1076, 1985
119. Sale GE, Shulman HM, McDonald GB, Thomas ED: Gastrointestinal graft-versus-host disease in man. A clinicopathologic study of the rectal biopsy. Am J Surg Pathol 3:291, 1979
120. Snover DC, Weisdorf SA, Vercellotti GM et al: A histopathologic study of gastric and small intestinal graft-versus-host disease following allogeneic bone marrow transplantation. Hum Pathol 16:387, 1985
121. Cheney CL, Weiss NS, Fisher LD et al: Oral protein intake and the risk of acute graft-versus-host disease after allogeneic marrow transplantation. Bone Marrow Transplant 8:203, 1991
122. Weisdorf DJ, Snover DC, Haake R et al: Acute upper gastrointestinal graft-versus-host disease: clinical significance and response to immunosuppressive therapy. Blood 76:624, 1990
123. Spencer GD, Hackman RC, McDonald GB et al: A prospective study of unexplained nausea and vomiting after marrow transplantation. Transplantation 42:602, 1986
124. Gauvreau JM, Lenssen P, Cheney C et al: Nutritional management of patients with acute gastrointestinal graft-versus-host disease. J Am Diet Assoc 79:673, 1981
125. Darbinian J, Schubert M: Special management problems. p. 63. In Lenssen P, Aker SN (eds): Nutritional Assessment and Management During Marrow Transplantation: A Resource Manual. Fred Hutchinson Cancer Research Center, Seattle, WA, 1985
126. Deeg HJ, Storb R: Acute and chronic graft-versus-host disease: clinical manifestations, prophylaxis, and treatment. J Natl Cancer Inst 76:1325, 1986
127. Nims JW, Strom S: Late complications of bone marrow transplant recipients: nursing care issues. Semin Oncol Nurs 4:47, 1988
128. June CH, Thompson CB, Kennedy MS et al: Profound hypomagnesemia and renal magnesium wasting associated with the use of cyclosporine for marrow transplantation. Transplantation 39:620, 1985
129. Thompson C, June CH, Sullivan KM et al: Association between cyclosporine neurotoxicity and hypomagnesemia. Lancet 2:1116, 1984
130. DeLisa AF, Flannelly BP, Gregory RE: Guide for the administration and use of cancer chemotherapeutic agents. Pharm Pract News 19:12, 1992
131. Lenssen P, Sherry ME, Cheney CL et al: Prevalence of nutrition-related problems among long-term survivors of allogeneic marrow transplantation. J Am Diet Assoc 90:835, 1990

Psychosocial Aspects of Hematologic Disorders

93

Jeannie V. Pasacreta and Ruth McCorkle

INTRODUCTION

Major changes in the understanding and treatment of cancer have led to a wider range of treatment options and increasing length of survival from time of diagnosis. While such advances are quite positive, their impact on the emotional lives of patients and families faced with complex treatment decisions as well as the emotional consequences of chronic illness cannot be overlooked.

Hematologic malignancies often carry a large burden of emotional consequences attributable to the chronic nature of the diseases. Involvement with a complicated and fragmented health care delivery system, the need for episodic and aggressive treatment, remissions and exacerbations of acute and uncomfortable symptoms, family separation, financial burden, functional limitations, and role disruptions are but a few of the issues that characterize the life of patient with hematologic malignancies, not to mention the threat to life that these diagnoses impose.

Since hematologic malignancies are known to be fatal when untreated, their diagnosis often leads to fear and intense psychological concerns. Psychosocial issues associated with all cancers may be intensified in patients with hematologic malignancies due to their association with a poor prognosis, a prolonged treatment course often involving numerous hospitalizations, and the systemic nature of the diseases.[1] Death, discomfort from painful medical procedures, body image disturbances secondary to hair loss, central line catheters, sexual dysfunction related to fatigue and fertility, and role and relationship disruptions resulting from lengthy hospitalizations are just a sampling of the issues that confront the patient with hematologic malignancies, highlighting the need for monitoring and attention to the psychosocial needs that accompany all aspects of the illnesses.

The goal of this chapter is to provide information regarding factors that affect psychosocial adjustment among patients with chronic illness, the wide range of psychological responses that are possible throughout the illness trajectory, and the efficacy of various modes of psychosocial intervention in minimizing distress and promoting adaptation. Some practical guidelines regarding patient management and identifying patients that may require formal psychiatric consultation are offered.

CHANGES IN TREATMENT AND SOCIETAL ATTITUDES: ACCOMPANYING TRENDS IN PSYCHOSOCIAL ISSUES

The secrecy that prevailed during the 1960s and prohibited disclosure of a cancer diagnosis by most physicians[2,3] has given way to the practice of imparting the particulars of diagnosis, treatment options, and prognosis on a routine basis. Despite this change, it has been suggested that ongoing fears and concerns among health care providers about cancer have led to a discrepancy between attitude and action resulting in communication of emotionally laden information in a fashion ranging from overprotective and paternalistic to blunt and matter-of-fact.[4,5]

Discrepancies between attitude and practice have also been demonstrated by clinicians who have been found to avoid clear open discussions of topics such as prognosis and death despite consistently expressed beliefs regarding the importance of openness and honesty with all mentally competent patients. Therefore, while the prevailing attitude in health care supports the disclosure of medical information and active involvement of patients in decisions that affect them, the actual behavior of health care providers likely reflects a more limited improvement in patient care.[5]

Clinicians should be mindful of how their personal views and concerns about cancer impact on communication with patients, especially at key decision-making and transition points along the continuum of care. The use of peers and alternate providers to assist patients with issues and concerns that are particularly upsetting for primary clinicians are useful strategies for ensuring maximum support for patients faced with the complex decisions inherent in treatment for hematologic malignancies.

CLINICAL COURSE OF HEMATOLOGIC MALIGNANCIES

In contrast to the treatment of many solid tumor cancers, treatment of hematologic malignancies often involves numerous and lengthy hospitalizations and ongoing outpatient monitoring of the patient's condition. The clinical course of cancer typically follows one of several possible trajectories (Fig. 93-1). A number of patients respond to the curative attempt with long-term remission, remain well, and are, after a period, considered cured. Some patients have a positive response to a curative attempt but then relapse. Other patients begin treatment with a hope for cure but do not respond and progressively decline. In some patients, the disease is too far advanced when diagnosed, and they experience a progression of their disease.[1]

The acute stress response[6] has been described as a usual

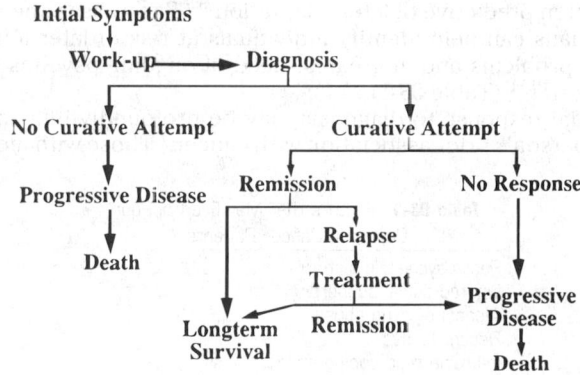

Fig. 93-1. Clinical course of a patient with a hematologic malignancy. (Adapted from Levenson and Lesko,[29] with permission.)

response to the diagnosis of cancer, occurring at each transitional point of illness (beginning treatment, relapse, treatment failure, disease progression). The response is characterized by shock, disbelief, anxiety, depression, sleep and appetite disturbance, and difficulty performing activities of daily living. The acute stress response usually subsides when the medical condition stabilizes and the patient knows what to expect in terms of a treatment plan. Because of the protracted hospitalization associated with the hematologic malignancies and often life-threatening complications such as neutropenia and sepsis, the acute stress response may occur periodically, especially during times of medical crisis or periods associated with excessive physical symptomatology, or both. Emotional support, giving clear information, controlling physical symptoms such as pain and nausea and enhancing patient control over the environment can enhance resolution and inhibit more severe and longstanding emotional sequelae.

Diagnostic Phase

The prediagnostic phase is the time of initial symptom discovery. Systemic symptoms such as weakness and fatigue are often ignored initially; medical advice is usually sought when symptoms persist and worsen. The period of suspicious symptoms associated with a definitive diagnosis is often characterized by fear, shock, and disbelief.

The period from diagnosis through initiation of treatment is characterized by medical evaluation, the development of new relationships with unfamiliar medical personnel, and the need to integrate a barrage of information that is at best frightening and confusing. Within the context of this anxiety-provoking situation, a decision must be made regarding treatment. As one patient aptly stated, "a decision upon which my very life or death might be based." This statement illustrates the tremendous responsibility, concern, and isolation that many people experience during this period.

Because of the particularly poor prognosis often associated with hematologic malignancies by the general public, patients and their families are often particularly anxious when receiving initial information regarding diagnosis and treatment. Consequently, care should be taken to repeat information at several sessions and to inquire about the patient and families' understanding of facts and options.

Weisman and Worden[7] describe the first 100 days after diagnosis as the period of "existential plight in cancer." Patient concerns focus on existential issues of life and death more than on concerns related to health, work, finances, religion, self, or relationships with family and friends. While it is unusual to observe extreme and sustained emotional reactions as the first response to a cancer diagnosis, it remains important to assess the nature of the patients' reaction carefully. Initial reactions are often predictive of later adaptation.[8,9] Early assessment by clinicians can help identify individuals at risk of later adjustment problems and in greatest need of ongoing psychosocial support[10,11] (Table 93-1).

Initial response to diagnosis may be profoundly influenced by a person's prior association with cancer.[1] Those with memories of close relatives with cancer often demonstrate heightened distress, particularly if the relative died or had negative treatment experiences.

During the diagnostic and early treatment period, patients may search for explanations or causes for their cancer and may struggle to give personal meaning to their experience.[12,13] Since many clinicians are guarded about disclosing information until a firm diagnosis is established, patients may develop highly personal explanations that can be inaccurate and provoke intensely negative emotions. Ongoing involvement and accurate information will minimize uncertainty and the development of maladaptive coping strategies based on erroneous beliefs.

While the literature substantiates the devastating emotional impact of a cancer diagnosis, it is also well documented that many individuals cope effectively. Positive coping strategies such as taking action and finding favorable characteristics in the situation have been reported as effective. Maintaining optimism[14] and having an active determination to recover have been associated with positive adjustment. Contrary to the belief of many clinicians, denial has also been found to assist patients in coping effectively with a diagnosis of cancer unless used to an excessive degree.

With the firm establishment of the cancer diagnosis, planning for treatment begins. If patients have been given a clear explanation of their condition while encouraged to maintain hope, the initial reaction of shock, fear, and desperation can give way to a sense of optimism.[6] Health care providers have an important role in monitoring, and possibly mediating, psychosocial adjustment. Keeping patients informed and actively involved in their care and being aware of the unique meaning that individuals may associate with a diagnosis of cancer are vital. Those with pervasive and unyielding negative affect that persists long after that crisis of diagnosis may require ongoing psychosocial intervention throughout treatment and the disease course.

Treatment Decision

Psychosocial factors are critical parameters in considering which treatment is best for a particular patient.[15] The development of a treatment plan should include information about all aspects of the medical/surgical treatments as well as what is known about the psychosocial sequelae.

Often, patients react to a diagnosis of cancer with feelings of fear and helplessness. The patient looks to the primary physician for a curative treatment that will preserve the quality of life. The patient may feel threatened and think nothing can be done but to rely on the doctors. Combating feelings of helplessness during this period can help alleviate painful anxiety. This is best done by a member of the health care team who has established a treatment alliance with the patient. The health care provider should make the person feel like a partner in everything that takes place. This is especially true for the decision about treatment choice.

Decision for Bone Marrow Transplantation

Bone marrow transplantation (BMT) is used increasingly in the treatment of malignant and hematologic disorders. The decision to undergo a BMT is a major life crisis for the patient and family. In addition to the very real threat of death, patients experience social isolation, bodily discomfort, major body image changes, and a sense of loss of control.[14,15] These issues lead to a myriad of emotions, including hope, anger, depression, anxiety, anticipation, guilt, and joy.

Every aspect of the patient's personal and professional life is

Table 93-1. Factors that May Predict Poor Coping in Cancer Patients

Past psychiatric history
Limited social support
Alcohol or drug abuse
Recent losses
Inflexible rigid coping style
Pessimistic outlook on life
Multiple obligations

[Adapted from Rowland,[37] with permission.]

disrupted with BMT.[16-19] The financial burden is tremendous, including medical expenses for the patient and marrow donor in the case of an allogeneic BMT in addition to potential travel expenses and loss of income for other family members. Patients and their immediate families are often far from usual support systems because of the distance to the BMT center.[20] In some cases, family members who have not been close in the past may be forced by the situation to interact with each other, leading to additional stress.

Some preliminary studies have linked negative emotions such as depression with long-term survival among BMT patients.[21] Although such studies have been small and inconclusive and recognize the multiple factors contributing to outcome, further research in this area is needed. Several BMT centers use routine psychosocial screening[22] and follow-up of BMT patients due to the length of the hospitalization, the aggressiveness of the treatment protocols, and the high incidence of complications and physical discomfort. Interventions that maximize patient control have proved useful.[14] Fear of the unknown can be decreased through patient education about procedures and potential complications. Participation in support groups during hospitalization has proved helpful to both patients and family members.[23] In addition to routine psychosocial assessment and follow-up evaluation, routine social work referrals are recommended to assist patients in dealing with the commonplace financial and insurance issues.

Survivorship

The successful treatment of the hematologic malignancies has resulted in cure for many patients and progressively longer lives for others. Longer survival, however, is not without significant emotional sequelae.[24-27] Innovative and new treatments may produce long-term physiologic consequences, such as infertility and organ system failure, that can magnify and exacerbate the psychological aspects initially associated with diagnosis and treatment.[28]

Many patients lack information about what to expect once they are discharged from the hospital. Clinicians need to establish ongoing mechanisms to monitor patients' symptoms, psychosocial status, and the problems they are having in terms of resuming activities and responsibilities. The clinician is then in a position to help the person find the best solution for their situation.

Psychological aspects of survivorship may include concern over termination of treatment, fear of relapse, preoccupation with somatic symptoms, reentry into previous roles, lingering affinity with death, and financial, job, and insurance difficulties.[29] These issues may be manifested in a variety of ways, including denial of past illness, leading to medical compliance issues; ongoing problems with anxiety, panic, and depression; and inability to reenter previous roles. Health care providers should be mindful of psychological sequelae among patients, even within the context of remission and a hopeful prognosis and refer the patient to a specialist, if necessary.

Progressive Disease

The psychosocial issues experienced by the cancer patient depends in part on the clinical course of the disease process. As the disease progresses, the person often reports an upsetting scenario, which includes frequent pain, disability, increased dependence, and diminished functional ability.[6]

The development of a relapse after a disease-free interval can be especially devastating for patients and for those close to them. The medical workup is often difficult and anxiety provoking. Psychosocial problems experienced at diagnosis frequently resurface, often with greater intensity.[6] Shock and depression often accompany relapse and require the person and family to reevaluate the future. In spite of the overwhelming nature of the psychosocial responses, however, most patients do indeed cope effectively with progressive illness, and it is important to recognize that intense emotions are not one and the same with maladaptive coping.

Investigators studying quality of life in cancer patients have demonstrated a clear relationship between an individual's perception of quality of life and the presence of discomfort.[30,31] As uncomfortable symptoms increase, perceived quality of life diminishes. Thus, an important goal in the psychosocial treatment of patients with advanced cancer centers around symptom control.

An issue that surfaces repeatedly among patients, family members, and professional care providers deals with the use of aggressive treatment protocols[32] in the presence of progressive disease. Often patients and families request participation in experimental protocols, even when there is little likelihood of extending survival. Controversy continues about the efficacy of such therapies and the role that health professionals can play in facilitating patient choices about participating.

The need for health care professionals to establish structured dialogue with patients, family members, and health care providers regarding treatment goals and expectations is essential. That certain patients respond to investigational treatment with increased hope, despite progressive illness, should be a consideration in treatment planning. The need to separate and clarify the values, thoughts, and emotional reactions of care providers, patients, and families to these delicate issues is important if individualized care with attention to the people's psychosocial needs is to be provided.

It is beyond the scope of this chapter to present a comprehensive overview of the psychosocial reactions of patients to the process of dying. Once the terminal period has begun, it is not usually the fact of dying, but the quality of dying, that seems to present the overwhelming concern.[33]

FACTORS THAT INFLUENCE PSYCHOSOCIAL ADJUSTMENT

Psychosocial responses to cancer vary widely and are influenced by several factors that clinicians should be mindful of when considering the responses of individual patients. A review of the literature points to key factors that may impact on psychosocial adjustment. These include (1) previous coping strategies and emotional stability and (2) the existence of social support.

Previous Coping Strategies and Emotional Stability

One of the key predictors of psychosocial adjustment to cancer is the coping strategy and emotional stability of the person before diagnosis. Individuals with a history of poor psychosocial adjustment before developing cancer are at highest risk of emotional decompensation and should be monitored closely throughout all phases of treatment.[33] This is particularly true of patients with a history of a major psychiatric syndrome or psychiatric hospitalization, or both.

Since a person's coping style is determined relatively early in life and remains stable over time and across situations, it serves as a useful predictor of adjustment to cancer. Several investigators have found specific personality characteristics, coping strategies, and/or life experiences that either enhance or inhibit positive adjustment to cancer. Those coping strategies found to be most effective have included a "fighting spirit" and having a feeling of control over events, resulting in active participation in treatment. By contrast, poor adjustment has been associated with avoidant coping strategies, prior negative sexual experiences, body image problems, and inhibition in discussing personal and sexual problems.[35]

Existence of Social Support

Social support has consistently been found to influence a person's psychosocial adjustment to cancer. The ability and availability of significant others in dealing with diagnosis and treatment can significantly affect patients' views of themselves. Those diagnosed with all types of life-threatening chronic disorders experience a heightened need for interpersonal support. Those who are able to maintain close connections with family and friends during the course of illness are more likely to cope effectively with the disease than are those who are not able to maintain such relationships.

Living with a chronic illness often requires continuing care and management by a team of specialists. Care is usually provided through follow-up visits to ambulatory or outpatients clinics and consulting rooms, rather than through hospitalization. Historically, patients are often not referred to home nursing care, once they are discharged from the hospital. An initial home nursing visit, however, can be invaluable in assisting the patient and family with the transition, in addition to identifying areas in which ongoing assistance is needed. Homecare referral can assist families who are increasingly relied on within the present health care system to be the major provider of care outside the hospital. The phenomenon of caregiver burden acknowledges that cancer affects not only the patient, but the members of the family as well.[34] The burden that caregiving places on the family highlights the family's needs and the importance of targeting support—information that can help reduce family caregiver burden. Helping to arrange respite care for the patient is also helpful in recognizing caregiver burden.

Differentiating Psychiatric Complications from Expected Psychological Responses

Most patients develop transient psychological symptoms that are responsive to support, reassurance, and information about what to expect regarding the cancer course and its treatment. Some require more aggressive psychotherapeutic intervention, such as pharmacotherapy and ongoing psychotherapy. The following guidelines can assist the clinician in identifying those patients who exhibit behavior suggesting the presence of a psychiatric syndrome.

Most patients do not react to a diagnosis and treatment for cancer by developing a clinically diagnosable psychiatric condition. In some cases, a psychiatric syndrome does occur. If the patient's problems become severe, that is, the provider feels that supportive measures are insufficient and ineffective in controlling emotional distress, referral to a psychiatric clinician is indicated. Factors that can prevent adjustment to cancer illness and treatment include a history of significant depression, manic-depressive illness, schizophrenia, neuroses, organic mental conditions, personality disorders, lack of social support, or inadequate control of physical discomfort.

Since transient symptoms of anxiety and depression are common in patients with cancer, the ability of health care providers to distinguish expected reactions from more severe psychiatric complications is crucial. Anxiety and depression are common symptoms that are particularly evident at transition points during the clinical course of cancer. These symptoms generally subside within 2–4 weeks and are responsive to supportive reassurance and information regarding what to expect during the course of treatment. For a proportion of patients, psychological distress does not subside with the usual interventions. Unfortunately, clinically relevant and severe psychiatric syndromes are often missed by nonpsychiatric care providers. It can be difficult to detect serious psychiatric reactions in pa-

tients because several of the diagnostic criteria used to evaluate the presence of severe depression (e.g., lack of appetite, insomnia, decreased sexual interest, diminished energy) may overlap with the usual disease and treatment effects. Additionally, it is not unusual for health care providers to confuse their own fears about cancer with the emotional reactions of their patients (e.g., "I too would be extremely depressed if I were in a similar situation").

General guidelines designed to assist in distinguishing patients who should be referred for evaluation by a trained psychiatric clinician include the following:

1. Past history of psychiatric hospitalization and/or significant psychiatric/personality disorder
2. Persistent refusal, indecisiveness, or noncompliance with regard to needed treatment
3. Persistent symptoms of anxiety and depression that are unresponsive to usual support from health care providers and/or family members (symptoms may present in the form of constant fear associated with treatment and procedures and/or excessive crying and hopelessness that worsen, rather than improve, with time)
4. An abrupt, unexplained change in mood or behavior
5. Insomnia, anorexia, diminished energy out of proportion to expected treatment effects
6. Persistent suicidal ideation
7. Unusual or eccentric behavior or confusion (may be indicative of an organic mental disorder)
8. Excessive guilt and self-blame for illness

After referral to a psychiatric specialist, one or a combination of several therapeutic modalities may be employed. Cancer and its treatment may precipitate an exacerbation of an underlying mental illness for which the patient was already predisposed and that may require extensive treatment (e.g., hospitalization for a psychosis, ongoing pharmacotherapy or psychotherapy). A discussion of these specialized forms of treatment is not warranted here, but the interested reader can consult appropriate standard texts.[35]

MANAGEMENT OF PSYCHOSOCIAL PROBLEMS

Increased length of survival from time of diagnosis has highlighted the need for psychopharmacologic, psychotherapeutic, and behaviorally oriented interventions to reduce distress, promote adjustment, and improve the quality of life for cancer patients. Numerous studies have documented the efficacy of a variety of modalities in managing psychosocial problems for the cancer patients. Problems that can be managed effectively include emotional distress such as anxiety and depression, sexual dysfunction, body image disturbances, marital and family difficulties, noncompliance, pain, neurologic complications such as delirium and dementia induced by brain metastasis and/or treatment, anticipatory and post-treatment nausea and vomiting, and anorexia and feeding problems.

Pharmacologic Interventions

As an adjunct to one or more of the psychotherapies, pharmacotherapy can be an important aid in bringing psychological symptoms under control. Psychopharmacologic agents for the treatment of psychiatric complications of the hematologic malignancies are briefly reviewed. For a thorough review, as well as expanded treatment guidelines, the reader is referred to a comprehensive discussion by Massie and Lesko.[36]

For patients with excessive anxiety, factors other than a psychological state must first be evaluated. Metabolic abnormalities, pain, hypoxia, and drug withdrawal states can all present as anxiety. Medications such as steroids, antipsychotics often

Table 93-2. Commonly Prescribed Anxiolytics in Cancer Patients

Drug	Starting Dosages (mg PO)	Absorption	Half-life	Comments
Alprazolam (Xanax)	0.25–0.5 t d	Intermediate	Intermediate	Generalized anxiety; panic attacks; mixed anxiety; depression; may be difficult to detoxify
Lorazepam (Ativan)	0.5–1.5 t d	Intermediate	Intermediate	Similar to alprazolam, can produce transient amnesia, which makes it useful with chemotherapy, and before procedures; agent of choice with hepatic impairment
Diazepam (Valium)	2.5–5 tid	Fast	Long	Because of long half-life, not ideal for patients with organic neurologic syndromes
Chlordiazepoxide (Librium)	10–25 tid	Intermediate	Long	Similar to diazepam
Triazolam (Halcion)	0.125–0.5 qhs	Intermediate	Short	Useful for severe initial insomnia; can cause confused state when used in elderly or medically ill

(Adapted freom Levenson and Lesko,[29] with permission.)

used for nausea such as Compazine, and haldol can also cause anxiety characterized by agitation and motor restlessness. After medical or drug-induced causes for anxiety are ruled out, an anxiolytic (e.g., Valium, Ativan, Xanax) is the treatment of choice, with the exception of patients who present with panic episodes, in which case tricyclic antidepressants are most efficacious. Anxiolytic agents are often fast acting and effective. These drugs are most effective when used in adequate dosages and as standing orders. Prescribing anxiolytics on a PRN basis places undue responsibility on patients who are already frightened and anxious. When given orally, these drugs cause minimal respiratory depression. Anxiolytic medication can help patients gain temporary control over agonizing anxiety. The use of these medications may also help the patient make use of psychotherapy, which can provide more permanent control over symptoms. When anxiety develops in the context of the terminal stages of the hematologic malignancies, it is often secondary to hypoxia or to an untreated pain syndrome, or both. Intravenous morphine sulfate is usually effective treatment.[33]

A number of anxiolytics are available for treatment of the cancer patient. These drugs are all similar in their overall clinical effects. Table 93-2 reviews the anxiolytics most often recommended in clinical practice. Because of their shorter half-life, alprazolam and lorazepam have advantages for elderly patients, since toxicity from sedating medications is more common, and withdrawal reactions may occur on abrupt discontinuance, unless the dose is tapered.

It is common for cancer patients to demonstrate depressive symptoms transiently at various points in the illness trajectory. In patients who exhibit prolonged or severe depressive symptomatology, a major depressive illness must be considered. Depression in a cancer population can be related to a recurrence of a past depressive disorder or to the stress associated with cancer treatment or the result of the illness process or treatment agents, or both. Certain medications and cancer treatment agents can produce even severe depressive states (Table 93-3). The diagnosis of major depression in the cancer patient relies heavily on the presence of affective symptoms, such as hopelessness, crying spells, guilt, preoccupation with death and/or suicide, sense of diminished self-worth, and loss of pleasure in most activities, such as being with friends and loved ones. The neurovegetative symptoms that usually characterize depression in physically healthy individuals are not good predictors of depression in the medically ill due to the aspects of the cancer and treatment that also produce these symptoms. A combination of psychotherapy and antidepressant medication will often prove useful in treating major depression in the cancer patient. Commonly used antidepressants and dosages are outlined in Table 93-4. Tricyclic antidepressants are the drugs of choice. The primary medical contraindication to their use is the significant cardiac conduction delays that should be ruled out before the initiation of treatment. These medications are started in low doses (25–50 mg) and are increased slowly, over days to weeks, until symptoms improve. Peak dosages are usually substantially lower than those tolerated by physically healthy individuals. Antidepressant medications may take 2–4 weeks to produce their desired effects. Patients may need ongoing support, reassurance, and monitoring before experiencing the antidepressant effects of medication.

Psychotherapeutic Modalities

Depending on the nature of the problem, the treatment modality may take the form of individual psychotherapy, group therapy, family therapy, marital therapy, behaviorally oriented therapy, or some combination. Table 93-4 outlines the major psychotherapeutic modalities and the advantages goals and indications for each.

CONCLUSIONS

The psychosocial issues faced by persons diagnosed and treated for cancer are influenced by sociocultural, medical, family and individual factors. Although involvement in decision making is clearly a positive aspect of current cancer therapies, great care should be taken to ensure the communication of timely, repeated, and relevant information consistent with patients' needs, tolerance, and comprehension. A multidisciplinary approach is essential to guarantee the communication of comprehensive information to all patients. Patients should be

Table 93-3. Antidepressants Commonly Used in Cancer Patients

Drug	Daily Starting Dosages (mg)	Eventual Therapeutic Range	Sedative Effect	Anticholinergic Effect
Amitryptyline (Elavil)	25	75–150	High	High
Doxepin (Sinequan)	25	75–150	High	Intermediate
Imipramine (Tojranil)	25	75–150	Intermediate	Intermediate
Desipramine (Norpramin)	25	75–150	Low	Low
Nortriptyline (Pamelor)	10–25	50–125	Intermediate	Low
Trazadone (Desyrel)	25	150–250	High	None

(Adapted from Levenson and Lesko,[29] with permission.)

Table 93-4. Psychotherapeutic Modalities in the Oncology Setting

Modality	Indications	Goals and Advantages	Comments
Individual psychotherapy	For patients with prolonged adverse reactions to diagnosis, treatment, and other aspects of chronic illness (i.e., anxiety, depression)	To support patient and enhance their ability to cope with distressing feelings Therapy usually short term, forcused, and goal directed	In some cases, pharmacotherapy and family involvement are useful adjuncts
Support groups	For patients who desire exposure to others who have been through the experience of chronic illness	To support patient and enhance coping ability Usually does not involve a fee Can be beneficial to patient to observe the coping strategies of others	Can benefit patients who have limited support systems by expanding their social network
Family and marital therapy	For patients experiencing sexual problems secondary to illness The illness is leading to increasing family tension and conflict	Can assist couples in clarifying problems and solving them together Can address role changes in family system	Problems and concerns regarding children can be addressed
Progressive muscle relaxation and guided imagery	For patients who desire assistance in enhancing personal control Useful in the management and control of pain and anxiety for some patients Has been useful in controlling anticipatory and post-treatment nausea and vomiting Can control fear assocated with medical procedures	Increases sense of control and participation in treatment Focuses on immediate education of disturbing symptoms Individualized to meet patient's preference and individual circumstances Time limited and goal directed Evaluated in terms of observable changes in symptoms	Realistic goals should be stated explicitly, as some patients expect relaxation and guided imagery to be curative regarding their disease process

given the opportunity to speak with multiple members of the treatment team and with other patients who have experienced similar management and treatment protocols. Care should be taken to provide needed information from a variety of expert perspectives while respecting the unique characteristics, psychosocial profiles, needs, and desires of each individual. In treatment settings with limited resources, every effort should be made to enlist the help and support of providers and services that can assist patients with their complex treatment decisions. Referral to community resources and support services following discharge from the hospital is often helpful, even for patients who cope well with initial treatment.

Most patients undergoing cancer treatment, as well as their families, experience expected periods of emotional turmoil that occur at transition points along the clinical course of cancer. For a small proportion of patients, more severe psychiatric complications may occur, warranting referral to a psychiatric specialist. A variety of psychotherapeutic modalities are useful in helping patients work through the expected emotional responses to cancer, as well as more severe responses. Supportive psychotherapeutic measures should be used routinely as they minimize distress and enhance feelings of control and mastery over self and environment. For these reasons alone, their value in the care of patients with cancer is paramount. Again, for patients who are not responsive to routine support and information, referral to a psychiatric specialist may be indicated.

Throughout the clinical course of cancer, the patient's relationship with health care providers as well as the presence of a supportive social network are important factors in ensuring successful negotiation of the many physical and psychosocial demands imposed by a cancer diagnosis and treatment. Further investigation regarding the utility of systematically tested interventions aimed at promoting psychosocial adjustment to cancer are needed. Investigation aimed at enhancing understanding of the behaviors of individuals experiencing the crisis of cancer and identification of individuals in need of intensive psychosocial support is also needed.

As scientific inquiry continues to produce vast, although sometimes conflicting, information regarding etiology and treatment for cancer, concurrent investigation regarding the psychosocial aspects of the disease are crucial. This line of inquiry will, at the very least, assist in promoting emotional well-being in patients faced with an extreme and unexpected life crisis. At best, expanding the knowledge base relative to the psychosocial aspects of cancer may provide some "missing links" regarding psychosocial adaptation and quality of life and their impact on survival.

REFERENCES

1. Lesko LM: Hematologic malignancies. p. 218. In Holland JC, Rowland JH (eds): Handbook of Psychooncology: Psychological Care of the Patient with Cancer. Oxford University Press, New York, 1989
2. Oken D: What to tell cancer patients: a study of medical attitudes. JAMA 175: 1120, 1961
3. Novack DH, Plumer R, Smith RL, et al: Changes in physicians' attitudes toward telling the cancer patient. JAMA 241:897, 1979
4. Krant MJ: Problems of the physician in presenting the patient with the diagnosis. p. 269. In Cullen JW, Fox BH, Isom RN (eds): Cancer: The Behavioral Dimensions. Raven Press, New York, 1976
5. Dermatis H, Lesko LM: Psychosocial correlates of physician-patient communication at time of informed consent for bone marrow transplantation. Cancer Invest 9:621, 1991
6. Holland J: Clinical course of cancer. p. 75. In Holland JC, Rowland JH (eds): Handbook of Psychooncology: Psychological Care of the Patient With Cancer. Oxford University Press, New York, 1989
7. Weissman A, Worden JW: The existential plight in cancer: significance of the first 100 days. Int J Psychiatry Med 7:1, 1976
8. Graydon JE: Factors that predict patients' functioning following treatment for cancer. Int J Nurs Stud 25:117, 1988
9. Northouse L: The impact of cancer on the family: an overview. Int J Psychiatry Med 14:215, 1984
10. Weisman AD, Worden JW, Sobel HJ: Psychosocial Screening and Intervention with Cancer Patients: Final Report of the Omega Project (CA 19797). National Cancer Institute, Bethesda, 1980
11. Worden JW: Psychosocial screening of cancer patients. J Psychosoc Oncol 1:1, 1983
12. Haberman MR: Psychosocial aspects of bone marrow transplantation. Semin Oncol Nurs 4:55, 1988
13. Steeves RH: Patients who have undergone bone marrow transplantation: their quest for meaning. Oncol Nurs Forum 19:899, 1992
14. Mages NL, Castro JR, Fobair P, et al: Patterns of psychosocial response to cancer: can effective adaptation be predicted? Int J Radiat Oncol Biol Phys 7:385, 1981
15. Richardson JL, Zarnegar Z, Bisno B, Levine A: Psychosocial status at initiation of cancer treatment and survival. J Psychosom Res 34:189, 1990
16. Ferrell B, Grant M, Schmidt GM, et al: The meaning of quality of life for bone marrow transplantation survivors. Part 1. The impact of bone marrow transplant on quality of life. Cancer Nurs 15:153, 1992

17. Baker F, Curbow B, Wingard JR: Role retention and quality of life of bone marrow transplant survivors. Soc Sci Med 32:697, 1991

18. Jenkins PL, Linington A, Whittaker JA: A retrospective study of psychosocial morbidity in bone marrow transplant recipients. Psychosomatics 32:65, 1991

19. Patenaude AF: Psychological impact of bone marrow transplantation: current perspectives. Yale J Biol Med 63:515, 1990

20. Coxon VJ: Subjective perceptions of the demands of hospitalization and anxiety in bone marrow transplant patients. Doctoral dissertation, University of Washington, Seattle, WA, 1989

21. Colon EA, Callies AL, Popkin MK, McGlave PB: Depressed mood and other variable related to bone marrow transplantation survival in acute leukemia. Psychosomatics 32:420, 1991

22. Futterman AD, Wellisch DK, Bond G, Carr CR: The psychosocial levels system. A new rating scale to identify and assess emotional difficulties during bone marrow transplantation. Psychosomatics 32:177, 1991

23. Fobair P, Hoppe RT, Bloom J, et al: Psychosocial problems among survivors of Hodgkin's disease. J Clin Oncol 4:805, 1986

24. Kornblith AB, Anderson J, Cella DF, et al: Comparison of psychosocial adaptation and sexual function of survivors of advanced Hodgkin disease treated by MOPP, ABVD, or MOPP alternating with ABVD. Cancer 70:2508, 1992

25. Lesko LM, Ostroff JS, Mumma GH, et al: Long-term psychological adjustment of acute leukemia survivors: impact of bone marrow transplantation versus conventional chemotherapy. Psychosom Med 54:30, 1992

26. Vose JM, Kennedy BC, Bierman PJ, et al: Long-term sequelae of autologous bone marrow or peripheral stem cell transplantation for lymphoid malignancies. Cancer 69:784, 1992

27. Altmaier EM, Gingrich RD, Fyfe MA: Two-year adjustment of bone marrow transplant survivors. Bone Marrow Transplant 7:311, 1991

28. Wingard JR, Curbow B, Baker F, et al: Sexual satisfaction in survivors of bone marrow transplantation. Bone Marrow Transplant 9:185, 1992

29. Levenson JA, Lesko LM: Psychiatric aspects of adult leukemia. Semin Oncol Nurs 6:76, 1990

30. Ferrell B, Grant M, Schmidt GM, et al: The meaning of quality of life for bone marrow transplant survivors: the impact of bone marrow transplant on quality of life. Part 1. Cancer Nurs 15:153, 1992

31. Ferrell B, Grant M, Schmidt GM, et al: The meaning of quality of life for bone marrow transplant survivors: improving quality of life for bone marrow transplant survivors. Part 2. Cancer Nurs 15:247, 1992

32. Stuber ML, Reed GM: "Never been done before"—consultative issues in innovative therapies. Gen Hosp Psychiatry 13:337, 1991

33. Pasacreta J, McCorkle R, Margolis G: Psychosocial aspects of breast cancer. In Fowble B, Gooddman RL, Glick JH, Rosato EF (eds): Breast Cancer Treatment. Mosby–Year Book, St. Louis, 1991

34. McCorkle R, Yost LS, Jepson C, et al: A cancer experience: relationship of patient psychosocial responses to care-giver burden over time. Psycho-oncology 2:21, 1993

35. Karasu TB (ed): Treatment of Psychiatric Disorders. American Psychiatric Press, Washington, DC, 1989

36. Massie MJ, Lesko LM: Psychopaharmacologic management. p. 470. In Holland JC, Rowland JH (eds): Handbook of Psychooncology: Psychological Care of the Patient With Cancer. Oxford University Press, New York, 1989

37. Rowland JH: Interpersonal resources: coping. p. 53. In Holland JC, Rowland JH (eds): Handbook of Psychooncology: Psychological Care of the Patient With Cancer. Oxford University Press, New York, 1989

Pain Management and Antiemetic Therapy in Hematologic Disorders

94

Janet L. Abrahm

INTRODUCTION

Relieving the pain of patients who have hematologic disorders requires a multifaceted approach.[1,2] An understanding of the transmission of the pain signal and a thorough evaluation of the pain complaint provide a rational basis for treatment decisions. Once the source of the pain has been identified, both nonpharmacologic and pharmacologic therapies can be employed. The neurosurgical methods of pain control are not discussed in this chapter; those interested in these techniques are referred to several excellent reviews.[1–4]

TRANSMISSION OF THE PAIN SIGNAL

For a patient to feel "pain,"[5] a signal arising from a noxious stimulus in the periphery must be transmitted to the centers in the brain that create the experience of pain. Chemicals released at the site of tissue injury initiate or increase the transmission of the signal. Histamine, serotonin, and bradykinin activate local fibers directly, and prostaglandins, which do not themselves activate these fibers, sensitize them to lower levels of mechanical and chemical stimulants.[6]

Following activation of peripheral receptors by chemical, thermal, or mechanical stimuli, the signal passes along myelinated Aδ or unmyelinated C fibers and enters the spinal cord via the dorsal root. Substance P and the excitatory neurotransmitters glutamate, aspartate, and ADP mediate and enhance transmission of this signal.[1] Next, the pain signal usually crosses over and ascends in one of the two contralateral spinothalamic tracts: the paleospinothalamic tract, present in more ancient species, or the neospinothalamic tract. Signals in the paleospinothalamic tract travel via ventromedial thalamic nuclei to the limbic system and hypothalamus, where they transmit the affective (suffering) component of the pain, and of reticular nuclei in the brain stem, where they transmit dull, poorly localized pain. Those in the neospinothalamic tract travel via lateral thalamic nuclear synapses to the somatosensory cortex, where they localize and indicate the intensity of the pain.

Transmission of the pain signal can be inhibited at several sites along this course. The dorsal longitudinal fasciculus is the descending pathway that inhibits transmission of the pain signal as it enters and ascends the spinothalamic tracts. The neurotransmitters involved in this inhibition include dopamine, serotonin, norepinephrine, and the endogenous opioids β-endorphin, enkephalin, and dynorphin.[1] Opiate receptors for both endogenous and exogenous opioids are present in the dorsal horn of the spinal cord, in those ventromedial thalamic nuclei that transmit signals from the paleospinothalamic, but not the neospinothalamic tract, and in the periaqueductal gray matter.[7] Thus, exogenous opiates can provide relief from suffering without affecting the localization of the source of pain. Subpopulations of the receptors (termed μ, δ, κ, σ, and ϵ) are differentially able to induce respiratory depression, physical dependence, and pain relief.[5] New opiate derivatives are therefore being designed to bind receptors that will maximize pain relief and minimize undesirable side effects.[5]

EVALUATION OF THE PAIN COMPLAINT

Initial Evaluation

In evaluating the complaint in patients with hematologic disorders, efforts are initially directed toward determining the cause(s) of the pain: (1) the disease itself, (2) the specific therapy for the disease, and (3) unrelated disorders. Splenomegaly, bone injury (infarction, infection, hemarthroses, infiltration), leptomeningeal infiltration, and spinal cord compression frequently accompany hematologic diseases. Chemotherapy and radiotherapy can cause mucositis, typhlitis, hemorrhagic cystitis, and peripheral neuropathy, and myalgia can follow steroid withdrawal.[8] Immunosuppression, caused by the diseases themselves or by the therapies used to treat them, leads to painful infections such has perirectal abscesses, herpetic or candidal esophagitis, and herpes zoster.

Distress, however, may arise from nonanatomic sources. The pain complaint may represent the patient's only means of expressing nonspecific feelings of distress to the physician. Chapman[9] recognized three categories of this distress: (1) anxiety, arising from fear of disfigurement or of uncontrollable pain, fear of loss of social position or of self-control, or fear of death; (2) anger at the failure of the physicians to provide a cure; and (3) depression from loss of physical ability, a sense of helplessness, and the impact of financial problems. Since these concerns may exacerbate any concomitant painful sensations, alleviating them can significantly reduce distress and decrease the need for pain medications or other interventions.

Furthermore, for the patient whose complaint of pain does not seem to have a straightforward explanation or who has not responded well to the therapeutic maneuvers outlined below, additional questions must be asked to uncover the source of the distress. Patients may deny their disease and use the complaint of pain to justify their incapacity. Their denial is demonstrated by answers to the following types of questions. *How would life be different without the pain?* Such patients will give unrealistic assessments of the extent of their abilities "if only the pain were gone." Hidden fears, resentments, and distrust of the physician may be revealed by answering the question: *What do you think is causing the pain?* Unrealistic expectations of pain treatment may be revealed by answers to the question: *To what extent do you expect your pain to be relieved?* The patient may expect that taking one pill a day will provide total relief, while the physician expects that even a multimodality regimen will relieve only 75% of the pain. A contract fulfilling the expectations of both patient and physician may be formulated once these unspoken assumptions are understood. Finally, other sources of confusion in the way the patient communicates the type of pain experienced can be clarified by the answer to the question: *Do you seem to show your feelings about the pain to the same extent that your family and friends do?* Patients can come from cultural backgrounds different from those of their families, and people with cultural differences often report pain very differently.[10-13] For example, patients of "stoic stock" may not communicate their distress to their spouses,

who may then question the patient's need for narcotic pain medication (i.e., if they themselves were in that much pain, they claim that that would tell their spouses). Clearly, unless the cultural differences are explored, adequate pain control might not be achieved.

Continued Assessment

Effective pain management requires repeated comprehensive assessment of the patient's pain. Pain reports by patients should be believed. The health care provider may not be aware that the clinical presentation of a patient suffering from chronic pain is very different from that of a patient in acute pain. If a patient does not manifest the common autonomic manifestations of acute pain (e.g., tachycardia, sweating, elevated blood pressure) or facial grimacing, the health care provider might doubt that the patient is suffering from severe pain. It must be understood that a patient with severe but chronic pain will not manifest these autonomic findings but will often be withdrawn, quiet, depressed or irritable, and move very little spontaneously but complain of discomfort when moved. When the pain is relieved, these patients often exhibit completely different behaviors, becoming mobile, engaged, and involved with other people. Therefore, the first component in the assessment is to believe the patient's complaint.

Patient reports of pain are valid, reliable, and reproducible.[1] These reports should be used, much as a blood sugar measurement is used in diabetic patients, to monitor the efficacy of the therapy. A variety of assessment tools that can be completed within 5–10 minutes are available.[14-16] They should be used to determine a number of aspects about the pain, including the pain location, intensity, quality, onset, duration; what relieves or exacerbates it; and its functional consequences, including how the pain affects the patient's ability to sleep or eat and how it affects physical activity, relationships with others, emotions, and concentration. The goal is to lower the pain *to a level acceptable to the patient.* If, for example, on a scale of 0 (no pain) to 10 (the worst pain one can imagine), the change in the rating number 1 hour after the patient has been given pain medication will indicate what needs to be done next. Communication between nurse and physician is greatly improved using these tools, as opposed to mere qualitative descriptors, such as "the pain is better," to guide pain management.

THERAPY

A major component of pain therapy is the attempt to reverse the underlying cause of the pain. Surgery, chemotherapy, radiotherapy, and antibiotics may all be employed. However, the pain can still be treated effectively during diagnostic testing to define the cause, during specific therapy, or after all disease-related therapies are exhausted.

The goal of this type of pain management is to relieve pain while preserving the patient's ability to perform normal activities. This requires expertise on the part of health care personnel, who seek to maximize the relief gained while minimizing side effects and alterations in daily routines. A multifaceted approach is required, which includes nonpharmacologic approaches, anesthetic techniques, correct use of a variety of medications that relieve pain with a minimum of side effects, and patient and family education throughout, to foster communication and cooperation with the therapeutic plan.

Nonpharmacologic Methods of Pain Management

Education and Reassurance

Patients with serious hematologic disorders are often required to undergo extensive diagnostic testing, which can include painful procedures. A rehearsal of the planned test or procedure, including the appearance of the room and the length of time to be spent in the test apparatus, can minimize the patient's anxiety. Such explanations offered preoperatively have been shown to lessen the need for postoperative medication and shorten the patient's hospital stay.[17] To divert attention from certain procedures (e.g., bone marrow aspiration or biopsy) that take place in the physician's office or in the patient's room, a pleasant distraction can be very helpful.[18] For example, the physician might encourage the patient to bring in a portable tape player with earphones so that the patient can listen to a favorite piece of music or a book on tape while the procedure is taking place. Alternatively, the physician might turn on the television or radio in the patient's room and encourage the patient to pay attention to that, rather than to the procedure. Patients with good imagination can pretend to be someplace they have previously enjoyed (e.g., a beach or the mountains). They can dissociate themselves[19] by concentrating on those pleasant memories and thereby diminish the painfulness of the procedure.

Hypnosis

Practitioners with formal hypnotic training can make use of more elaborate hypnotic techniques to help their patients deal with painful procedures or conditions.[18,19] Hypnosis takes advantage of the natural ability to enter a trance-like state. An athlete "playing through the pain" is an example of the spontaneous induction of such a state. Patients who are trained to enter a trance at will can modify their perception of pain and diminish sleeplessness, anxiety, and the anticipation of discomfort.[20] Hypnotic training of patients with sickle cell anemia or hemophilia decreases the frequency and pain intensity of painful crises[21] or bleeding episodes,[22,23] respectively.

Even in the absence of a formal hypnotic induction, the words used by the practitioner to describe procedures are very important. For example, the suggestion that hand or arm coolness and numbness will persist after application of an alcohol swab may markedly diminish the discomfort of starting an intravenous line. Using the phrase "You will feel something; I'm not sure what you will feel, as everyone feels this a little differently" in place of "This is going to hurt a lot!" gives the patient permission to alter the sensation and may also diminish the experience of pain.

Transcutaneous Electrical Nerve Stimulation

Transcutaneous electrical nerve stimulation (TENS) devices are indicated for patients with dermatomal pain, such as postherpetic neuralgia (see the section Postherpetic Neuralgia) or radiculopathy from spinal cord compression.[24] For optimal effect, a physiatrist or physical therapist familiar with the device should train the patient in its use.

Anesthetic Techniques

EMLA, a mixture of two topical anesthetic creams (lidocaine 2.5% and prilocaine 2.5%) is used, especially in children, to decrease the pain of superficial cutaneous procedures (e.g., venous cannulation or skin anesthesia prior to lumbar puncture) or bone marrow aspiration or biopsy.[25–27] If anesthesia is to be achieved, the EMLA Cream must be applied in a mound under a semipermeable dressing such as Opsite or Tegaderm ≥85 minutes before the planned procedure.[28,29] When EMLA is used as directed, methemoglobinemia has not been a problem even in children as young as 3 months old[30,31]; skin blanching occurs, sometimes exceeding, but in other studies equaling, the frequency of that found with placebo moisturizing cream placed under the occlusive dressing.[29,32]

Trigger-point injections, nerve blocks, and neurolytic proce-

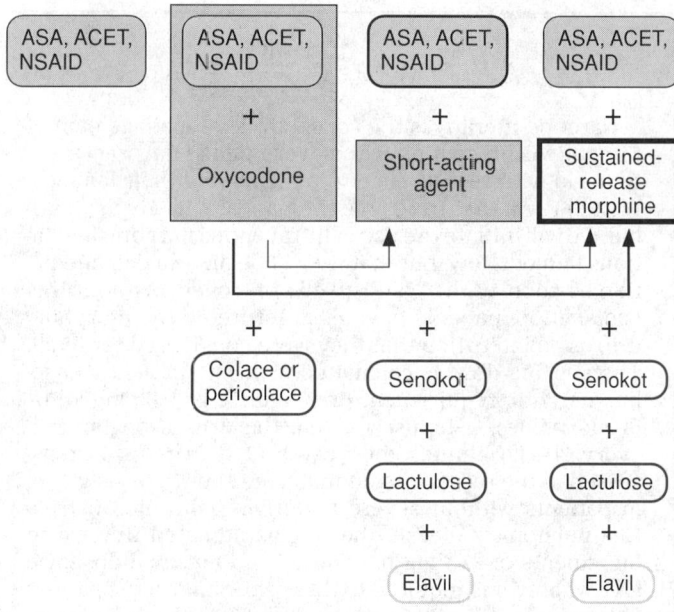

Fig. 94-1. Strategy for pharmacologic management of pain. Multiagent therapy is usually required for optimal pain management. Patients with mild to moderate pain should be started on a non-narcotic analgesic or on a combination of non-narcotic analgesic and a short-acting narcotic. If this combination does not produce adequate relief, or if patients present with severe pain, stronger narcotics, in either short-acting or sustained-release form, should be begun immediately. These patients should also receive non-narcotic analgesics, if indicated. Laxatives are given to all patients receiving narcotics (even for mild pain), and adjuvant tricyclic medications for sleep are offered. Other adjuvant agents should be included as indicated (see text). The drug names given are meant to be illustrative; they are the drugs we commonly use. ⬭, adjuvant drug; ▭, a narcotic; ▭, a short-acting narcotic; ▬, a long-acting narcotic; ⬭, a non-narcotic analgesic (ASA, aspirin; ACET, acetaminophen; NSAID, nonsteroidal anti-inflammatory drug); ⬭, a tricyclic antidepressant; ▯, combination drugs Percodan, Percocet, and Tylox all include both a narcotic and non-narcotic analgesic.

dures are useful for both acute and chronic localized pain. After excisional biopsy of an axillary lymph node, for example, a burning constricting pain in the posterior arm and chest wall may develop; this pain is often promptly relieved by trigger-point injection.[33,34] Lymphoma or myeloma may involve the spine and lead to vertebral collapse or pain from progressive disease that is refractory to antineoplastic therapy. Such pain is often particularly difficult to manage. Insertion of temporary or permanent indwelling epidural or intrathecal catheters to deliver either opiates or local anesthetic agents, or both, can be very effective, especially in relieving lower thoracic or lumbar spine pain, as well as pelvic and lower extremity pain.[35] Those interested in the indications for, and techniques of, the anesthetic and neurolytic procedures are referred to several excellent reviews.[35–38]

Drug Therapy

Drugs useful for pain relief include the non-narcotic analgesics, narcotics, and adjuvant drugs that either potentiate the actions of narcotic analgesics or treat their side effects. Most cases require the use of a combination of medications for optimal pain relief (Fig. 94-1).

Non-narcotic Analgesics

Non-narcotic analgesics should be given to patients with mild to moderate pain. Aspirin, acetaminophen, and nonsteroidal anti-inflammatory drugs (NSAIDs) are especially useful in

MANAGEMENT OF SEVERE PAIN

Narcotic therapy is the cornerstone of management of the patient presenting with severe pain. Our practice is to begin with reassurance to patients and their families. We tell them that to relieve the pain as quickly as possible, we will initiate the use of intravenous narcotic mediations immediately, but that we will begin oral pain mediation as soon as the pain is well controlled. Without this explanation, patients have misinterpreted the morphine drip as an indication that they were considered terminal. The starting dose is calculated from the patient's baseline narcotic requirement or weight (e.g., 0.05 mg/kg/hr of morphine). A bolus is given, the drip is begun, and every 20–30 minutes the degree of pain relief is reassessed. If the relief is inadequate, another bolus is given; in patients without severe underlying chronic obstructive pulmonary diease, the drip is adjusted upward in increments of 2–3 mg/hr. There is no maximal dose; we give whatever is required to relieve the pain. If the patient falls asleep, this is usually an indication that pain relief has been achieved, not that the dose should be lowered. We lower the dose if the respiratory rate falls to <10–12 breaths/min.

Adjuvant agents are begun along with the narcotic (Fig. 94-1). All patients are given Senokot (one or two tablets orally daily or one for every 30 mg morphine up to a maximum 8 pills/day. If more laxative effect is needed, lactulose is added. The starting dose is 15–30 ml PO at bedtime, repeated if necessary in the morning. Lactulose is effective and unlike other agents does not produce either cramping or a feeling of fullness. Amitriptyline (25 or 50 mg PO) is usually ordered as a "patient may refuse" sleep medication. In narcotic-naive patients, Compazine (10 mg PO tid or bid) is given for the first 48 hours to prevent the otherwise common development of nausea. In patients with bone or nerve pain, appropriate adjuvants are added (see text).

When pain relief is adequate, the patient is converted to an equivalent dose of oral narcotic. Three times the parenteral dose is required (Table 94-1). For example, a patient who required 10 mg of morphine per hour (i.e., 240 mg/24 hr IV) will need 720 mg/day of the oral long-acting agent (240 mg × 3). This can be given as 360 mg PO bid or 240 mg PO tid. Two hours after the oral narcotic is begun, the drip is discontinued. Short-acting immediate-release morphine should be available for rescue dosing (see text for dosing recommendations). If the amount of narcotic taken as "rescue dose" is significant, the daily dose of long-acting agent is adjusted upward accordingly.

treating bone pain, as they decrease local prostaglandin release and may thereby reduce the sensitization of pain receptors.[39] It is important to prescribe an adequate dose of the drug at regular intervals, switching to another non-narcotic analgesic only when maximal doses of the first have become ineffective. Since the NSAIDs can cause renal insufficiency in a significant number of patients, renal function should be assessed 1 or 2 weeks after initiation of any of these agents. Keorolac tromethamine (Toradol) is an NSAID of particular value in relieving moderate to severe acute pain. Thirty milligrams of ketorolac intramuscularly equals the pain-relieving potency of 12 mg of morphine intramuscularly.[40] However, ketorolac has all the side effects of the NSAIDs and is not recommended for long-term use. If that degree of pain relief is needed chroni-

cally, a narcotic agent should be substituted. The non-narcotic analgesics should be continued in appropriate cases when narcotic analgesics are added, as they will potentiate the pain-relieving effect of the narcotic[41] (Fig. 94-1).

However, when aspirin is included in a fixed drug combination (e.g., Percodan), salicylate toxicity may develop if the patient takes the pills more often than the prescription indicates. The metabolism of salicylates is limited by the capacity of the hepatic microsomal system. Once that is saturated, salicylate levels are dependent on renal clearance. Thus, small increases in maintenance doses can lead to serious salicylism.[42] Patients with low albumin levels or acid urine are particularly susceptible to the development of salicylate toxicity.[43]

Tricyclic antidepressants (e.g., amitriptyline, nortriptyline), phenytoin, carbamazepine, and steroids are non-narcotic analgesics that demonstrate particular efficacy in relieving pain from nerve injuries. The tricyclic antidepressants are the drugs of choice for painful peripheral neuropathies and for postherpetic neuralgia. Phenytoin and carbamazepine, drugs used to treat trigeminal neuralgia, can also be effective for postherpetic neuralgia.[44,45] Corticosteroids are useful for tumor cell lysis (e.g., in leukemia, lymphoma, and myeloma) and can also provide nonspecific relief for patients with spinal cord compression and plexus infiltrations. Doses of 16–100 mg of dexamethasone are needed to reduce vasogenic edema in spinal cord compression,[46] but lesser doses (6–20 mg/day) can be helpful in patients with plexus injuries.[8]

Narcotic Analgesics

Patient Education

Narcotic analgesics are the mainstay of therapy for moderate to severe pain of malignant or nonmalignant origin. To ensure patient compliance with a narcotic prescription, however, education of other members of the health care team, the patient, and the family is often required to dispel the many misconceptions associated with narcotic therapy. Even physicians who are cancer specialists hesitate to prescribe opiates as needed for patients with severe pain.[47]

Fear of addiction is a common cause of inadequate dispensing of narcotics[48] and a barrier to their acceptance by patients.[47] The physician can increase compliance by providing a full explanation of the differences between addiction and physical dependence, along with reassurance that research has repeatedly indicated that patients with malignancies who take narcotics do not become addicts.[49,50] Patients may also fear that if they take to narcotic medications for moderate pain, these medications will no longer be effective if more severe pain occurs. Since this fear, if unexpressed, can lead to undertreatment, the topic should be addressed even if the patient does not raise the question. A functional goal of therapy, such as returning to a favorite hobby or reinstituting normal activities of everyday life, may enable the patient and the family to accept the narcotic. Finally, misconceptions about religious teachings may prevent health care personnel, patients, and their families from giving or accepting adequate pain medication. Catholics, for example, may not be aware of the Church's position, as stated in the current catechism, that narcotics may be used at the approach of death, even if their use ultimately shortens the patient's life.[51,52] The Church does not consider this use of pain medication to be a means of suicide or euthanasia.[53]

Choice of Medication

Since a wide variety of medications are available, pharmacokinetic considerations and side-effect profiles should be considered when choosing narcotic agent(s). Intermittent moderate to severe pain lasting hours to several days is amenable to

Table 94-1. Relative Potencies of Commonly Used Narcotics

Drug	IM (mg)	PO (mg)
Morphine	10	30
Codeine		188–390
Oxycodone (in Percodan, Tylox)		30
Meperidine (Demerol)	75	300
Levorphanol (Levo-dromoran)	2	4
Hydromorphone (Dilaudid)	1.5	7.5
Methadone	10	20

(Adapted from Foley,[1] with permission.)

oral analgesics with short half-lives (3–4 hours) with appropriate potency. Severe pain of relatively constant intensity should be treated with oral sustained-release morphine (taken bid–tid[54,55]) or transdermal fentanyl (renewed every 48–72 hours).

Drugs with short half-lives should also be used for "rescue doses," given for "breakthrough pain" and for between-doses pain exacerbations. The dose of the rescue medication should be 10% of the total 24-hour dose.[55,56] For example, if a patient is receiving 180 mg of oral sustained-release morphine twice a day, the rescue dose should be 10% of 360 mg, which is 36 mg of short-acting morphine. Agents with short half-lives, such as morphine, hydromorphone, and oxycodone, should also be used in the elderly and in patients with impaired renal or hepatic function.[56] In patients with a previous drug abuse history, agents with longer half-lives, such as methadone or levorphanol, are preferred.

The side-effect profiles of the narcotic agents differ widely. It is often useful, therefore, to switch to another agent if a patient is experiencing dose-limiting side effects with the initial narcotic chosen.[57] For example, if the patient receiving morphine experiences disabling nausea, the substitution of hydromorphone (Dilaudid) at an equianalgesic dose should be considered (Table 94-1). Because of incomplete cross-tolerance, the initial dose for patients on higher doses of narcotics should be only two-thirds to one-half the calculated equianalgesic dose.[56] For example, in the same patient taking morphine (360 mg/day PO), hydromorphone should be begun at 45 or 60 mg/day (one-half or two-thirds the 90-mg dose that would be equianalgesic). For patients receiving even higher doses of narcotic, as little as 20% of the replacement narcotic may be appropriate.[58] The short-acting "rescue" medication (5 or 6 mg hydromorphone) will provide relief if this initial dose does not prove adequate.

Meperidine is the least useful narcotic for patients with long-lasting moderate to severe pain.[59,60] It provides pain relief for only about 1–2 hours[8] and gives rise to an active metabolite, normeperidine, which induces dysphoria, is excitatory to the central nervous system, and can cause seizures.[61] Normeperidine has a half-life of 13–24 hours, which can lengthen with renal failure.[62] Thus, the frequent administration of meperidine required for pain control causes normeperidine levels to rise and increases the likelihood of seizures. The seizure incidence is further increased if the narcotic antagonist naloxone (Narcan) must be given.[63] Other narcotics are therefore better choices for patients with moderate or severe pain who will require days of sustained analgesia. In sickle cell disease, for example, intravenous or oral sustained-release morphine has been shown to be very effective in both inpatient and outpatient pain management.[64] Should hyperirritability or a seizure occur in a patient receiving meperidine, intravenous diazepam (Valium) rather than phenytoin should be used to control the seizure,[1] and morphine should replace the meperidine for pain control.

Routes of Delivery

Narcotics can be delivered noninvasively (orally, rectally, or transdermally) or invasively (subcutaneous/intravenous or by spinal infusion). For patients switched from oral or rectal to parenteral or spinal medication, or vice versa, the dose must be altered accordingly to avoid overdose or undertreatment (Table 94-1). No matter which route is chosen, patients experiencing continuous pain should receive the analgesics regularly and be awakened, if necessary, to administer medications that will prevent recurrence of the pain.[1]

Oral. Most patients will be able to achieve excellent pain relief with either short-acting or sustained-release oral narcotic preparations. In addition, agents have been developed for sublingual or transmucosal use. Buprenorphine tablets are absorbed in 3–5 minutes with 55% bioavailability.[65] Oral transmucosal fentanyl citrate "lollipops" induce rapid analgesia, relieve anxiety, and produce sedation.[66] They are especially useful in the pediatric population and can relieve breakthrough pain in adults.

Rectal. Rectal opiates (morphine, oxymorphone, and hydromorphone) have about the same potency and half-life as orally administered agents[67,68] and must therefore be administered frequently. In single-dose bioavailability studies of sustained-release morphine preparations, despite delayed absorption from the rectal route, total morphine absorption over 24 hours was equivalent, whether the drug was given orally or rectally.[69,70] New sustained-release rectal morphine preparations are also under investigation.[71]

Transdermal. The clinical value of fentanyl in a transdermal delivery system (Duragesic) has now been well established.[72] The transdermal system is a "patch" that adheres to the skin; fentanyl, a very lipophilic opiate, is rapidly absorbed from the contact adhesive into the skin. The drug then diffuses continuously from the patch reservoir into the skin through a rate-controlling membrane and is absorbed from the skin depot into the bloodstream, where it is rapidly metabolized[73] (Figure 94-2). The onset of pain relief is delayed about 12 hours, until an adequate amount of drug is present in the skin reservoir. A relatively constant plasma concentration of fentanyl is not reached until about 14–20 hours after the initial patch is placed.[73] Rescue medication must therefore be provided during the first 48 hours of use of the patch.[74] Converting patients from oral or parenteral medication to the patch is easily accomplished using the table provided in the package insert.[75] Most patients will require dose escalations, as the conversion is a conservative one. A new patch is applied every 72 hours, although a few patients require a new patch every 48 hours.

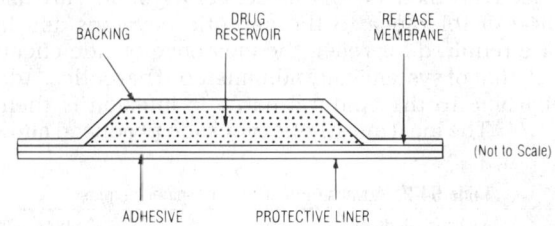

Fig. 94-2. Duragesic is a rectangular transparent unit comprising a protective liner and four functional layers. Proceeding from the outer surface toward the surface adhering to the skin, these layers are (1) a backing layer of polyester film, (2) a drug reservoir of fentanyl and alcohol USP gelled with hydroxyethyl cellulose, (3) an ethylene-vinyl acetate copolymer membrane that controls the rate of fentanyl delivery to the skin surface, and (4) a fentanyl-containing silicone adhesive. Before use, a protective liner covering the adhesive layer is removed and discarded.

The transdermal system is an effective method of delivering pain relief for patients with (1) moderate to severe pain, (2) no oral route available or no desire to take pills, and (3) a stable level of chronic pain. Side effects include those due to the contact adhesive, along with those commonly associated with other opiates.[73,75]

Under certain conditions, the transdermal system should not be used. The delay in achieving effective plasma concentrations and the consequent difficulty of titrating the drug rapidly interfere with the effectiveness of the transdermal delivery system in patients experiencing acute pain or in those with markedly fluctuating narcotic requirements. Another condition militating against the use of the transdermal system is the development of sepsis or of unstable hepatic function because absorption or metabolism of the drug may be affected. When the patient's temperature rises to 40°C, drug absorption from the skin can increase by as much as 35%.[73] If hepatic function is impaired or sepsis or shock develops and blood flow to the liver decreases, plasma concentrations may rise sharply.[73] Because the fentanyl continues to be absorbed from the skin, serum fentanyl levels remain at 50% as long as 14–25 hours after the patch has been removed.[73] Naloxone infusion may be required until drug is eliminated from the skin depot.[76] Lower doses may also be required in elderly patients or in those with respiratory insufficiency.[77]

Subcutaneous and Intravenous. Continuous subcutaneous or intravenous administration of narcotics can provide pain relief in the shortest amount of time, with a minimum of oversedation. The drugs can be delivered by portable infusion pump, initiated or continued in the home.[78–90] Guidelines for their use are available.[81] Patient-controlled analgesia (PCA) systems for subcutaneous or intravenous drug delivery have the advantage of responding to the individual patient's threshold for pain while eliminating delays inherent when nurses must administer supplemental medication.[82] The pumps administer a continuous fixed infusion of the narcotic chosen and allow the patient to self-administer boluses of additional medication at frequencies chosen by the physician. By recording the additional amounts of self-administered medication, the devices also facilitate the adjustment of the continuous dose required for pain relief. The appropriate role of PCA in patients with cancer pain has recently been reviewed.[83]

Spinal. Epidural or intrathecal opioid infusions can be helpful for selected patients with pain below the midthoracic area.[35,84] The infused opioids block pain transmission by binding to receptors in the dorsal horn of the spinal cord.[7,85] Since the drug is being infused in close proximity to the receptors, only a small amount of narcotic is needed and the systemic side effects are reduced. Problems with this delivery system[86] are listed in Table 94-2. If tolerance to the narcotic develops and higher doses are required for relief, the incidence of side effects will approach that of systemically administered narcotics. Addition of bupivicaine to the epidural narcotic infusion is then indicated.[36,87,88] The local anesthetic blockade produced allows for

Table 94-2. Adverse Effects from Spinal Opioids

Narcotic-Induced	Catheter-Related
Pruritis (15%)	Meningitis
Urinary retention (15%)	Epidural hematoma
Nausea and vomiting (15–30% in narcotic-naive patients)	Abscess
Respiratory depression	
Sedation	
Miosis	

(From Reiz and Westberg,[86] with permission.)

fairly rapid lowering of the opiate concentration and re-establishment of opiate sensitivity.

Adjuvant Medications

Adjuvant medications are used both to add to the analgesic effect of the narcotics and to treat the complications they induce.

Adjuvant Analgesics

Adjuvant analgesics enhance the pain-relieving properties of narcotics. Tricyclic antidepressants are among the most effective psychotropic analgesics.[89] It has been suggested that they produce these effects by raising the concentration of the endogenous pain inhibitors serotonin and norepinephrine[90,91] and increase the bioavailability of morphine.[92] These tricyclics act more promptly and at lower levels as opiate adjuvants than they do as antidepressants (e.g., amitriptyline is effective within 2–3 days at 50–100 mg/day).[91]

The addition of dextroamphetamine (2.5–7.5 mg PO or 10 mg IM bid[93]) permits lowering of the narcotic dose by one-third to one-half, while maintaining equivalent analgesia and less sedation.[93] Methylphenidate (10 mg PO with breakfast and 5 mg PO with lunch) can also increase the analgesic effect and reduce sedation in patients receiving narcotics.[94] Pemoline is a chewable psychostimulant that is chemically unrelated to amphetamines but that may be as useful in reversing opiate-induced sedation.[89] Patients are started on one tablet (18.75 mg) in the morning and at noon, and the dose is gradually increased to a total of ≤75 mg/day. These combinations are very useful, for example, in treating neuropenic patients with perirectal abscesses whose severe pain generally occurs as the neutrophil count rises. Tolerance to the amphetamine effect does not develop before 2–3 weeks of therapy, and the abscess pain has usually resolved by then.

Hydroxyzine (25–100 mg PO or IM)[95,96] also has opiate-potentiating abilities, diminishes opiate-induced nausea and vomiting,[96] and is especially useful in patients who might benefit from an anxiolytic agent.

Laxatives

Constipation is the most common narcotic-induced side effect[8] (Fig. 94-1); laxatives should therefore be given routinely, not on a prn basis,[8,59,97] to patients treated with any of the drugs listed in Table 94-1. Detailed bowel preparation recommendations can be found,[8,98,99] but none has been studied in a controlled fashion. If bowel obstruction occurs, pain relief can be maintained with methylphenidate or dextroamphetamine. Alternatively, methotrimeprazine, a phenothiazine, can be substituted for a short time.[100] Single-dose studies of 15 mg IM of methotrimeprazine have shown this drug to be equivalent to 15 mg IM of morphine. The recommended parenteral starting dose is 5–10 mg. Both clonidine[101] and continuous subcutaneous infusion of metoclopramide (60 mg/day)[102] reverse the "narcotic bowel syndrome,"[101] enabling patients to return to oral narcotics.

Sleep Medications

Sleep medications that produce sedation (benzodiazepines, barbiturates, chloral hydrate) are not good choices for patients receiving narcotics, as these drugs will produce excessive daytime sedation. Tricyclic antidepressants (e.g., 25–50 mg of amitriptyline) are preferred as they produce only night-time sedation and act as opiate adjuvants[89,91] (Fig. 94-1).

Naloxone

Naloxone (Narcan) reverses narcotic-induced respiratory depression, although repeated doses are often required.[8] Respiratory depression can occur in patients with mild to moderate pain during the initial use of narcotics, although it is rare in patients with severe pain or in those chronically receiving narcotics. Caution should be exercised before administering naloxone to the patient who is chronically receiving narcotics, to avoid precipitation of severe withdrawal. In such cases, it is inadvisable to administer the usual 0.4-mg/ml dose; rather, 0.4 mg of naloxone should be diluted with 10 ml of saline and only enough given to reverse respiratory depression.[1] In a comatose patient, endotracheal tube placement is recommended to prevent aspiration from the salivation and bronchial spasm that will be induced.[1]

SPECIFIC CLINICAL PROBLEMS

Oral Complications

Oral complications of chemotherapeutic and marrow transplant regimens can be a frequent cause of pain. A thorough dental evaluation and prompt treatment of infections can minimize the discomfort arising from underlying periodontal disease and caries; secondary bacterial, viral, and fungal infections; and mucositis.[103] Sucralfate[104] and colony-stimulating factor-granulocyte[105] diminish the incidence, duration, and intensity of chemotherapy-induced mucositis. Viscous lidocaine (Xylocaine) or a slurry of sucralfate, diclonine, or kaopectate in diphenhydramine provides symptomatic treatment of mucositis pain.[106] For individual lesions, benzocaine in Orabase can be helpful. Milk of magnesia, which dries the mucosa, is not recommended.[103] The more severe cases, occurring in marrow transplant recipients, usually require infusional morphine therapy, delivered by standard drip or PCA.[106]

Coagulation Disorders

Patients with inherited or acquired disorders of coagulation may have excessive risk of bleeding if aspirin-containing pain relievers are used.[107,108] If acetaminophen is not effective, these patients may obtain significant relief from ibuprofen or the non-acetylated salicylates, such as salsalate (Disalcid) or choline magnesium trisalicylate (Trilisate), which do not prolong the bleeding time.[108–110] Since these agents share aspirin's ability to compete with warfarin for albumin binding,[43] careful monitoring of patients' coagulation parameters is recommended when these drugs are started or stopped.

Postherpetic Neuralgia

Postherpetic neuralgia can be a difficult problem for patients with hematologic disorders and has been the subject of several reviews.[111–113] Phenytoin (300 mg/day) or carbamazepine (started at 100 mg/day and slowly titrated to 400–800 mg/day)[44] has some efficacy, but amitriptyline is the agent of choice, having been effective in 60–70% of patients in a randomized double-blind controlled trial.[114,115] Elderly patients, however, do not tolerate the anticholinergic side effects well. Nortriptyline (Pamelor) may be useful in these patients. Topical capsaicin (0.075%), which depletes substance P, has shown efficacy in a multicenter double-blind, randomized placebo-controlled trial.[116] Transdermal lidocaine ointment (2–10%) can also be effective.[1] TENS devices provided relief for 1 year in 50% of postherpetic neuralgia patients, and 30% were pain free at 2 years.[24] Acute herpes zoster pain may respond to sympathetic blockade; postherpetic neuralgia may respond to local anesthetic and steroid block.[117]

Sickle Cell Anemia

Patients with sickle cell anemia suffer from both chronic and episodic pain. Chronic arthritic pain can be treated with physical therapy and full doses of antiarthritic medication, but some patients require low doses of chronic narcotic therapy to maintain independent functioning. Several studies have confirmed the safety and efficacy of long-term opioids in the treatment of pain of nonmalignant origin.[64,118–120] In several cases, joint replacement may be required.

When a patient with sickle cell anemia experiences a severe episode of pain, it is always important to attempt to define the precise cause of the pain before attributing it to a vaso-occlusive crisis. To manage crisis pain, non-narcotic analgesics that treat bone pain, an opiate adjuvant such as amitriptyline, and laxatives should be added to narcotic therapies (Fig. 94-1). Oxygen is not required in the absence of documented hypoxia.[121]

Since intravenous access is often difficult in these patients, narcotics such as morphine can be given orally[122] or by injections on a fixed schedule, with a "patient may refuse" provision. Meperidine should be avoided in this population for the reasons mentioned above. Furthermore, patients with sickle cell anemia absorb intramuscular meperidine poorly.[123] In that minority of patients who require large doses of medication, intravenous morphine delivered by standard drip or PCA is usually effective.[64,124] To dispel any atmosphere of distrust between patient and health care provider,[122,124] a contract agreed to by both provider and patient can be established.[125] The contract describes the dose, duration, and type of analgesics to be used and is updated yearly. When the crisis is resolved, the dose is tapered daily, without lengthening the interval between doses; if necessary, the patient is begun on equivalent doses of oral narcotic medication.

Problems of the Elderly

Pain management in the elderly is complicated by difficulties in pain assessment, as well as by altered pharmacokinetics of narcotics[126] and of psychotropic adjuvant medications.[127] Elderly patients may underreport pain.[128] Physicians may ascribe observed limitations in social contact and physical activity to age-related changes, when in fact they are pain-induced limitations.[129]

Elderly patients are particularly susceptible to the side effects of NSAIDs, and patients taking them should be monitored closely.[130] In elderly patients (age 70–89), the volume of distribution for narcotics is generally smaller, the drugs have a longer plasma half-life, and clearance is decreased, all of which lead to a prolonged duration of effect.[129] Therefore, the effective doses for these patients are one-half to one-quarter of those needed in younger patients.[126,127] Drugs with short half-lives should be used (e.g., oxycodone or hydromorphone), and initial doses should be low.[129] Patients should be monitored carefully for the development of sedation or confusion, especially if they are receiving antihistaminic agents (cimetidine, diphenhydramine) or drugs with anticholinergic activity.

The acute urinary retention due to opiates (especially in patients with prostatic hypertrophy) and the hypotension and tachycardia caused by tricyclic compounds can be more frequent and of more clinical severity in this population. The starting dose should be low (usually 10 mg at bedtime), and the dose should be slowly increased as tolerated. Doxepin, which does not share these side effects, may be a better tolerated opiate adjuvant.[90]

Patients with Opiate Addiction

The physician should be aware that drug requirements may be significantly higher and that dosing intervals are shorter in the addict.[131] In patients on methadone maintenance, therapeutic dosing must be provided over and above their baseline dose.[131] In all cases, the goal should be to deliver adequate medication to relieve the patient's pain. It has been recommended that (1) the physician always work from a written treatment plan, (2) one physician prescribe all psychotropic medication, (3) information about the patient's drug use be obtained from sources in addition to the patient, and (4) when the question of "addiction" first arises, consultation be obtained from an addiction medicine specialist.[132] If narcotics are needed, patients should be given limited quantities of long-acting medications on a scheduled basis.

Both former opiate abusers themselves and the physicians caring for them hesitate to use opiates for pain relief, as they fear inducing a relapse of the addiction.[133] This concern is based on the observation that once a receptor has been habituated to the opioid, it retains its avidity for opioids, even after a long period of abstinence.[131] In addition to those noted above, suggested techniques to minimize these risks include discussion of the individual's concerns and increased involvement by the patients in their recovery programs.[131]

ANTIEMETIC THERAPY

A number of effective antiemetic therapies are used to prevent the nausea and vomiting induced in patients by treatment of their hematologic disorders with chemotherapy or radiotherapy. These antiemetic therapies markedly improve patients' quality of life. Most patients can expect complete control of nausea and vomiting.[134]

Pathophysiology of Vomiting

The means by which chemotherapy agents induce vomiting is still incompletely understood.[135–137] Two areas in the medulla are responsible for emesis: the chemoreceptor trigger zone (CTZ) and the emetic center. Substances in the blood or the cerebrospinal fluid stimulate the CTZ, which then signals the emetic center to induce the various muscular contractions that result in the expulsion of stomach contents.

While the sites of emetic action of the chemotherapeutic agents have not been identified, blocking agents directed against type 3 serotonin receptors (5-HT$_3$ receptors) have been effective in inhibiting chemotherapy-induced nausea and vomiting. Higher centers in the brain, such as the cortex, are also thought to be involved in producing anticipatory nausea and vomiting. Thus, cognitive therapies, as well as antianxiety and amnesic agents, are also effective antiemetics.

Therapy

Anticipatory Nausea and Vomiting

Anticipatory nausea and vomiting (ANV) is thought to be a classic conditioned response.[138] Chemotherapy administration (the unconditioned stimulus) results in nausea and vomiting—the unconditioned response. Clinic sights, smells, and sounds are the conditioned stimulus. After frequent pairings of chemotherapy administration and the clinic sights, smells, and sounds, the response (nausea and vomiting) can be triggered in the absence of any chemotherapy by clinic sights, smells, or sounds or simply by seeing clinic personnel, even at a location distant from the site of treatment.

Patients in whom post-treatment nausea or vomiting never develops do not develop ANV either. Of those who do experience post-treatment nausea and vomiting the risk of developing ANV increases with the increasing frequency, severity, and duration of the symptoms.[138] Other possible predisposing factors include susceptibility to motion sickness,[139] awareness of tastes or odors during infusions, younger age, lengthier infusions, greater autonomic sensitivity, and general anxiety or emotional distress.[138]

The best way to prevent ANV is to give aggressive antiemetic therapy and to treat anxiety with the agents described below. However, in patients for whom this has not been successful and in whom ANV develops, a variety of behavioral techniques have been helpful. These include hypnosis,[140] progressive muscle relaxation with guided imagery,[141] systemic desensitization,[142] and distraction.[143] Results may be optimized if a therapist trained in these techniques works with the patient, but a recent study of progressive muscle relaxation with guided imagery suggests that patients can apply this technique on their own.[138,141]

Two different drug regimens have been shown to reduce ANV. Clonidine can be given for 5 days before chemotherapy.[144] Alternatively, alprazolam can be given the night before, the morning of, and just before chemotherapy, and then qid for 2 days after therapy.[145] Alprazolam significantly reduced ANV compared with placebo, even though it had no effect on anxiety levels.

Antiemetic Agents

Most studies of the newer, more potent antiemetic agents ondansetron and metoclopramide have been conducted in patients receiving therapy with cisplatinum, a drug of high emetic potential. While cisplatinum is not generally used to treat patients with hematologic malignancies, the data are included in the following discussion, as the findings can probably be extrapolated to other drugs of equivalent or less emetogenic potential. When available, data regarding efficacy in patients receiving radiotherapy or emetogenic drugs commonly used to treat hematologic disorders is reviewed.

Choice of Agent

The choice of antiemetic agent(s) depends on (1) the emetogenic potential of the chemotherapy or radiotherapy regimen, (2) the side-effect profile of the antiemetic agent(s), and (3) patient preferences and characteristics.

The emetogenic potential of the drugs is shown in Table 94-3. While most drugs produce emesis 1–2 hours after they are given (in patients who have never before received chemotherapy), the onset of emesis from high-dose intravenous cyclophosphamide is delayed until 9–18 hours after treatment.[146]

The side-effect profiles for the antiemetic agents are discussed below. Past history of alcohol intake and patient age modify certain aspects of the profiles. Patients who have a history of alcohol intake of more than five alcoholic drinks/day (>100 g of alcohol) tend to have less nausea and vomiting. This has been studied carefully in patients receiving high-dose cisplatinum therapy[147,148] but has been anecdotally observed in patients receiving other agents.

Younger patients have a higher incidence of acute dystonic reactions after receiving metoclopramide therapy: trismus or torticollis was seen in only 2% of patients >30 years of age but in 27% of younger patients.[149] Younger patients find cannabinoids more effective than do older patients because they can better tolerate the side effects associated with the therapeutic doses of these agents.[150] No systematic studies of the side effects and efficacy of antiemetics in the geriatric population have been published.

Patient preferences regarding degree of alertness can help

COMBINATION ANTIEMETIC REGIMENS

High to Moderately High Emetogenic Potential

Metoclopramide 2–3 mg/kg IV × 2 doses beginning 30 minutes before chemotherapy, and repeat at 2 hours, plus

Dexamethasone 10–20 mg IV over 15 minutes, plus

Lorazepam 0.5–2 mg IV × 1 (if use low dose, may repeat × 1), plus

Diphenhydramine 50 mg IV (in patients <30 years old or with history of dystonic reaction)

OR

Ondansetron[a] 24 mg IV × 1, plus

Dexamethasone 10–20 mg IV × 1 over 15 minutes

Moderately High to Moderate Emetogenic Potential

Lower the dose of metoclopramide in above regimen to 1–2 mg/kg IV and give 2–3 doses beginning 30 minutes before chemotherapy, repeated q2h

OR

Ondansetron[a] 8–12 mg IV (<60–75-kg patient) or 8 mg PO bid or tid, plus

Dexamethasone 10–20 mg IV

Moderately Low or Low Emetogenic Potential

Dexamethasone 10–20 mg IV over 15 minutes

OR

Prochlorperazine 10 mg PO or 25 mg parenterally q6h prn

OR

(If control is not achieved, or there is past history of inadequate control)

Ondansetron[a] 8–12 mg IV (<60–75-kg patient) or 8 mg PO bid or tid, plus

Dexamethasone 10–20 mg IV

[a] For doses and schedules of other 5-HT$_3$ antagonists, see Gralle.[134]

(Data from Gralle[134] and Beck et al.[194])

Table 94-3. Emetogenic Potential of Drugs Commonly Used to Treat Hematologic Malignancies

Emetogenic Potential	Drug
High (>90%)	DTIC
	High-dose cytarabine (>500 mg/m^2)
	High-dose cyclophosphamide[a]
	Mechlorethamine
Moderately high (60–90%)	Cyclophosphamide (routine dose)
	Hexamethylmelamine
	Methotrexate
	Nitrosoureas
	Procarbazine
Moderate (30–60%)	Asparaginase
	Azacytidine
	Daunorubicin
	Doxorubicin
Moderately low (10–30%)	Bleomycin
	Cytarabine (standard dose)
	Etoposide
	Hydroxyurea
	Melphalan
	Mercaptopurine
	Methotrexate (low dose)
	Thiotepa
	Vinblastine
Low (<10%)	Busulfan
	Chlorambucil
	Corticosteroids
	Thioguanine
	Vincristine

[a] Late-onset emesis.
(Data from Gralla[134] and Merrifield and Chaffee.[135])

regimens that include cyclophosphamide, methotrexate, or doxorubicin showed significant efficacy and superiority of ondansetron over placebo.[151–153] Ondansetron also demonstrates efficacy in patients with emesis (induced by non-cisplatinum chemotherapy) that has been refractory to standard antiemetics, with complete control in 50% of these patients.[154,155]

Ondansetron effectively prevents nausea and vomiting in patients treated with highly emetogenic agents for acute leukemia,[156,157] for multiple myeloma (i.e., high-dose melphalan),[158] or being prepared for bone marrow transplant with cyclophosphamide and total-body irradiation.[159,160] In the transplant patients, 83% of "patient days" were without any vomiting or retching and in a further 10% there were no more than two emetic episodes. Ondansetron is also effective in preventing emesis induced by single- or multiple-fraction radiotherapy.[161,162]

Furthermore, ondansetron is as effective as metoclopramide in preventing nausea induced by cisplatinum[163–165] or by cyclophosphamide alone or with doxorubicin chemotherapy.[166–168] In a recent study, however, ondansetron alone was inferior to metoclopramide plus dexamethasone in patients receiving cyclophosphamide, methotrexate, and 5-fluorouracil therapy for breast cancer.[169]

Ondansetron and the other 5-HT$_3$ receptor antagonists have far fewer side effects than occur with metoclopramide. Reports of extrapyramidal reactions are very rare,[170] and sedation, dystonic reactions, akathisia (severe restlessness, "ants-in-pants" feeling), and tardive dyskinesias do not occur; patients experience only mild headache and develop elevations of transaminases.[134]

Metoclopramide

Metoclopramide is a substituted benzamide capable of blocking the emetic activity of chemotherapy agents by blocking 5-HT$_3$ receptors in the CTZ. Delivery of the drug on a sched-

the health provider chose an antiemetic regimen, as can the level of anxiety the provider observes in the patient. Some patients do very well with regimens that include no antianxiety agents; others may benefit from the inclusion of those agents, despite the somnolence that accompanies their use.

Ondansetron

Ondansetron is the best studied of the 5-HT$_3$ receptor antagonists; this class also includes the drugs dolasetron, granisetron, tropisetron, and RG 12915. Several studies of patients receiving

ule that maintains adequate levels during expected emesis appears to be important.[134]

Metoclopramide is also effective in radiotherapy-induced emesis, possibly because this type of emesis may be induced by serotonin release from the small bowel or by vagal nerve stimulation. Metoclopramide is effective in preventing nausea induced by chemotherapeutic agents, even of high emetogenic potential.[171–175]

However, the side effects, which may be caused by the interaction of metoclopramide with dopamine receptors, can be quite troublesome. They include akathisia, dystonic reactions (age related), sedation, and diarrhea. Benzodiazepines such as lorazepam can prevent or reverse the akathisia, and diphenhydramine or cogentin can prevent or reverse the dystonias.[176] However, these agents induce additional side effects, including dry mouth and sedation. Furthermore, short-term high-dose or long-term use of metoclopramide has been associated with persistent and disabling movement disorders, especially tardive dyskinesias.[177,178]

Steroids

The mechanism of the antiemetic action of corticosteroids remains undefined. Steroids are effective used alone to prevent emesis induced by agents of moderate or low emetogenic potential.[179–181] They are also a useful component of antiemetic therapy regimens that include either ondansetron or metoclopramide and add efficacy to both in randomized controlled trials.[134,182–184] Dexamethasone and methylprednisolone are the best studied agents, but no trials have demonstrated the superiority of one agent over another.

Benzodiazepines

The benzodiazepine lorazepam has only mild antiemetic activity on its own.[176] It markedly decreases the akathisia and anxiety associated with metoclopramide therapy, however, and induces a dose-related memory loss and marked sedation.[176,185,186] Alprazolam is useful in preventing ANV.

Other

Other agents that are more active than placebo include the butyrophenones, haloperidol and droperidol[187]; the phenothiazine, prochlorperazine[188]; and the cannabinoids, dronabinol (THC) and nabilone.[150,189,190] These agents are less effective drugs than the agents mentioned above, and all but prochlorperazine are associated with significant side effects. All cause sedation. In addition, the butyrophenones produce dystonic reactions, akathisia, and occasionally hypotension. The cannabinoids cause ataxia, dry mouth, orthostatic hypotension and dizziness, euphoria or dysphoria, and a feeling of being "high."[191]

Combination Antiemetic Therapy

For drugs of low or moderately low emetogenic potential, no antiemetic drug or dexamethasone alone may be sufficient. For drugs of higher emetogenic potential, however, standard antiemetic treatment usually includes combinations of several antiemetic agents along with agents designed to treat anxiety, provide amnesia, or prevent known side effects. For drugs with high emetogenic potential, it is very important to give antiemetic therapy for an adequate period before administering chemotherapy agents, and to continue to prevent emesis for about 24–48 hours after the drugs have been given. Other agents useful in combination include transdermal scopolamine and metopimazine, a new dopamine D_2 antagonist, which is a phenothiazine derivative. Transdermal scopolamine adds effi-

cacy when added to a standard regimen of metoclopramide and dexamethasone.[192] Metopimazine significantly enhances the efficacy of ondansetron when used twice a day in patients receiving moderately emetogenic drugs.[193]

REFERENCES

1. Foley KM: Management of cancer pain. p. 2417. In DeVita VT, Hellman S, Rosenberg SA (eds): Cancer: Principles and Practice of Oncology. 4th Ed. JB Lippincott, Philadelphia, 1993
2. Spross JA, McGuire DB, Schmitt RM: Oncology Nursing Society position paper on cancer pain. Oncol Nurs Forum 17:595, 751, 943, 1990
3. Wall PD, Melzack R (eds): Textbook of Pain. 3rd Ed. Churchill Livingstone, Edinburgh, 1993
4. Bonica JJ: The Management of Pain. 2nd Ed. Lea & Febiger, Philadelphia, 1990
5. Payne R: Anatomy, physiology, and neuropharmacology of cancer pain. Med Clin North Am 71:153, 1987
6. Yaksh TL, Hammond DL: Peripheral and central subtrates involved in the rostral transmission of nociceptive information. Pain 13:1, 1982
7. Yaksh TL: Spinal opiate analgesia: characteristics and principles of action. Pain 11:3, 1981
8. Levy MH: Pain management in advanced cancer. Semin Oncol 12:394, 1985
9. Chapman CR: Psychologic and behavioral aspects of cancer pain. p. 44. In Bonica JJ, Ventafridda V (eds): Advances in Pain Research and Therapy. Vol. 2. Raven Press, New York, 1979
10. Choiniere M, Melzack R: Acute and chronic pain in hemophilia. Pain 31:317, 1987
11. Wolff BB: Ethnocultural factors influencing pain and illness behavior. Clin J Pain 1:23, 1985
12. Wolff BB, Langley S: Cultural factors and the response to pain: a review. Am Anthropol 70:494, 1968
13. Zborowski M: Cultural components in responses to pain. J Soc Issues 8:16, 1952
14. Donovan MI: Clinical assessment of cancer pain. p. 105. In McGuire DB, Yarbro CH (eds): Cancer Pain Management. WB Saunders, Philadelphia, 1987
15. Syrjala KL: The measurement of pain. p. 133. In McGuire DB, Yarbro CH (eds): Cancer Pain Management. WB Saunders, Philadelphia, 1987
16. McCaffery M, Beebe A: Pain: Clinical Manual for Nursing Practice. CV Mosby, St. Louis, 1989
17. Egbert LD, Battit GE, Welch CE, Bartlett MK: Reduction of postoperative pain by encouragement and instruction of patients. N Engl J Med 270:825, 1964
18. Zeltzer L, LeBaron S: Hypnosis and non-hypnotic techniques for reduction of pain and anxiety during painful procedures in children and adolescents with cancer. J Pediatr 101:1032, 1982
19. Hilgard ER, Hilgard JR: Hypnosis in pain control. p. 63. In: Hypnosis in the Relief of Pain. William Kaufman, Los Altos, CA, 1975
20. Finer B: Hypnotherapy in pain of advanced cancer. Adv Pain Res Ther 2: 223, 1979
21. Zeltzer L, Dash J, Holland JP: Hypnotically induced pain control in sickle cell anemia. Pediatrics 64:533, 1979
22. LaBaw WL: Autohypnosis in haemophilia. Haematologia (Budap) 9:103, 1975
23. Hilgard ER, Hilgard JR: Dentistry. p. 144. In: Hypnosis in the Relief of Pain. William Kaufman, Los Altos, CA, 1975
24. Sjölund BH, Eriksson M, Loeser JD: Transcutaneous and implanted electrical stimulation of peripheral nerves. p. 1852. In Bonica JJ: The Management of Pain. 2nd Ed. Lea & Febiger, Philadelphia, 1990
25. Gunawardene R, Davenport H: Local application of EMLA and glycerol trinitrate ointment before venipuncture. Anaesthesia 45:52, 1990
26. Halperin D, Koren G, Attias D et al: Topical skin anesthesia for venous subcutaneous drug reservoir and lumbar punctures in children. Pediatrics 84:81, 1989
27. Nott M, Peacock J: Relief of injection pain in adults: EMLA cream for five minutes before venipuncture. Anaesthesia 45:772, 1990
28. Lander J, Nazarali S, Friesen E et al: A comparison of topical anesthetics. (under review)
29. Lander J: Reflections about EMLA. APS Bull 1:14, 1993
30. Frayling I, Addison G, Chattergee K, Meakin G: Methaemoglobinaemia in children treated with prilocaine-lignocaine cream. BMJ 301:153, 1990
31. Engberg G, Danielson K, Henneberg S, Nilsson A: Plasma concentrations of prilocaine and lidocaine and methemoglobin formation in infants after epicutaneous application of 5% lidocaine-prilocaine cream (EMLA). Acta Anaesth Scand 31:624, 1987
32. Villada G, Zetlaoui J, Revuz J: Local blanching after epicutaneous application

of EMLA cream: a double-blind randomized study among fifty healthy volunteers. Dermatologica 181:38, 1990

33. Bonica JJ, Sola AF: Chest pain caused by other disorders. p. 1114. In Bonica JJ (ed): The Management of Pain. 2nd Ed. Lea & Febiger, Philadelphia, 1990

34. Bonica JJ, Sola AF: Myofascial pain syndromes. p. 352. In Bonica JJ (ed): The Management of Pain. 2nd Ed. Lea & Febiger, Philadelphia, 1990

35. Ready LB: Regional analgesia with intraspinal opioids. p. 1967. In Bonica JJ (ed): The Management of Pain. 2nd Ed. Lea & Febiger, Philadelphia, 1990

36. Ferrer-Brechner T: Anesthetic management of cancer pain. Semin Oncol 12: 431, 1985

37. Bonica JJ, Buckley FP: Regional analgesia with local anesthetics. p. 1883. In Bonica JJ (ed): The Management of Pain. 2nd Ed. Lea & Febiger, Philadelphia, 1990

38. Bonica JJ, Buckley FP, Moricca G, Murphy TM: Neurolytic blockade and hypophysectomy. p. 1980. In Bonica JJ (ed): The Management of Pain. 2nd Ed. Lea & Febiger, Philadelphia, 1990

39. Galasko CSB: Mechanisms of bone destruction in the development of skeletal metastases. Nature 263:507, 1976

40. Brown CR, Mazzulla JP, Mok MS et al: Comparison of repeat doses of intramuscular ketorolac tromethamine and morphine sulfate for analgesia after major surgery. Pharmacotherapy 10:45S, 1990

41. Beaver WT: Aspirin and acetaminophen as constituents of analgesic combinations. Arch Intern Med 141:293, 1981

42. Levy G, Tsuchiya T: Salicylate accumulation kinetics in man. N Engl J Med 287:430, 1972

43. Stimmel B: Non-narcotic analgesics and nonsteroidal anti-inflammatory drugs. p. 68. In: Pain, Analgesia, and Addiction. The Pharmacologic Treatment of Pain. Raven Press, New York, 1983

44. Gerson GR, Jone RB, Luscombe DR: Studies on concomitant use of carbamazepine and clomipramine for the relief of post-herpetic neuralgia. Postgrad Med J suppl 4. 53:104, 1977

45. Swerdlow M, Cundill JG: Anticonvulsant drugs and chronic pain. Clin Neuropharmacol 7:51, 1984

46. Greenberg HS, Kim J-H, Posner JB: Epidural spinal cord compression from metastatic tumor: results from a new treatment protocol. Ann Neurol 8:361, 1980

47. Von Roenn JH, Cleeland CS, Gonin R et al: Physician attitudes and practice in cancer pain management: a survey from the Eastern Cooperative Oncology Group. Ann Intern Med 119:121, 1993

48. Marks RM, Socahr EJ: Undertreatment of medical inpatients with narcotic analgesics. Ann Intern Med 78:173, 1973

49. Twycross RG: Clinical experience with diamorphine in advanced malignant disease. Int J Clin Pharmacol Ther Toxicol 9:184, 1974

50. Kanner RM, Foley KM: Patterns of narcotic drug use in a cancer pain clinic. Ann NY Acad Sci 362:161, 1981

51. Congregation for doctrine of the faith. Declaration on euthanasia. United States Catholic Conference, Washington, DC, 1980, p. 6

52. John Paul II: Catechism of the Catholic Church, Euthanasia. p. 549, Pauline. St. Paul Books and Media, Libreria Editrice Vaticana, 1994

53. O'Rourke K: Pain relief: the perspective of Catholic tradition. J Pain Sympt Mgmt 7:485, 1992

54. Brescia FJ, Walsh M, Savarese JJ, Kaiko RF: A study of controlled-release oral morphine (MS Contin) in an advanced cancer hospital. J Pain Sympt Mgmt 2:193, 1987

55. Warfield CA: Guidelines for routine use of controlled-release oral morphine sulfate tablets. Semin Oncol 20:36, 1993

56. Portenoy RK: Cancer pain management. Semin Oncol 20:19, 1993

57. Galer BS, Coyle N, Pasternak GW, Portenoy RK: Individual variability in response to different opioids: report of five cases. Pain 49:87, 1992

58. MacDonald N, Der L, Allan S, Champion P: Opioid hyperexcitability: the application of alternate opioid therapy. Pain 53:353, 1993

59. Twycross RG, Lack SA: Symptom Control in Far Advanced Cancer: Pain Relief. Pittman, London, 1983

60. McGivney WT, Crocks GM: The care of patients with severe chronic pain in terminal illness. JAMA 251:1182, 1984

61. Kaiko RF, Foley KM, Grabinski PY et al: Central nervous system excitatory effects of meperidine in cancer patients. Ann Neurol 13:180, 1983

62. Szeto HH, Inturrisi CE, Houde R et al: Accumulation of normeperidine, an active metabolite of meperidine, in patients with renal failure of cancer. Ann Intern Med 86:738, 1977

63. Gilbert PE, Martin WR: The antagonism of the convulsant effects of heroin, d-propoxyphene, meperidine, normeperidine and thebaine by naloxone in mice. J Pharmacol Exp Ther 192:538, 1975

64. Brookoff D, Polomano R: Treating sickle cell pain like cancer pain. Ann Intern Med 116:364, 1992

65. Ventafridda V, De Conno F, Guarise G et al: Chronic analgesic study on buprenorphine action in cancer pain—comparison with pentazocine. Drug Res 33:587, 1983

66. Stanley TH, Ashburn MA: Novel delivery systems: oral transmucosal and intranasal transmucosal. J Pain Sympt Mgmt 7:163, 1992

67. Westerling D, Lindahl S, Anderson KE, Anderson A: Absorption and bioavailability of rectally administered morphine in women. Eur J Clin Pharmacol 23:59, 1982

68. Beaver WT, Feise GA: A comparison of the analgesic effect of oxymorphone by rectal suppository and intramuscular injections in patients with postoperative pain. J Clin Pharmacol 17:276, 1977

69. Kaiko RF, Cronin C, Healey N et al: Bioavailability of rectal and oral MS Contin. Am Soc Clin Oncol Proc 8:336, 1989

70. Kaiko RF, Fitzmartin RD, Thomas GB, Goldenheim PD: The bioavailability of morphine in controlled-release 30 mg tablets per rectum compared with immediate-release 30 mg rectal suppositories and controlled-release 30 mg oral tablets. Pharmacotherapy 12:107, 1992

71. Hanning CD, Vickers AP, Smithe G et al: The morphine hydrogel suppository: a new sustained release rectal preparation. Br J Anaesth 61:221, 1988

72. The role of the fentanyl series for pain management: novel delivery system. J Pain Sympt Mgmt suppl. 7:51, 1992

73. Calis KA, Kohler DR, Corso DM: Transdermally administered fentanyl for pain management Clin Pharm 11:22, 1992

74. Payne R: Transdermal fentanyl: suggested recommendations for clinical use. J Pain Symp Mgmt 7:S40, 1992

75. Bailey PL, Stanley TH: Package inserts and other dosage guidelines are especially useful with new analgesic delivery systems. Anesth Analg 75:873, 1992

76. Goldfrank L, Weisman RS, Errick JK, Lo MW: A nomogram for continuous intravenous naloxone. Ann Emerg Med 15:566, 1986

77. Scott JC, Stanski DR: Decreased fentanyl and alfentanil requirements with age: a simultaneous pharmacokinetic and pharmacodynamic evaluation. J Pharmacol Exp Ther 240:159, 1987

78. Campbell CF, Mason JB, Weiler JM: Continuous subcutaneous infusion of morphine for the pain of terminal malignancy. Ann Intern Med 98:51, 1983

79. Kerr IG, Sone M, DeAngelis C et al: Continuous narcotic infusion with patient-controlled analgesia for chronic cancer pain in outpatients. Ann Intern Med 108:554, 1988

80. Moulin DE, Kreeft JH, Murray-Parsons N, Bouquillon AI: Comparison of continuous subcutaneous and intravenous hydromorphone infusions for management of cancer pain. Lancet 337:465, 1991

81. Portenoy RK, Moulin DE, Rogers A et al: Intravenous infusion of opioids in cancer pain: clinical review and guidelines for use. Cancer Treat Rep 70: 575, 1985

82. White PF: Use of patient-controlled analgesia for management of acute pain. JAMA 259:243, 1988

83. Ferrell BR, Nash CC, Warfield C: The role of patient-controlled analgesia in the managment of cancer pain. J Pain Sympt Mgmt 7:149, 1992

84. Payne R: Role of epidural and intrathecal narcotics and peptides in the management of cancer pain. Med Clin North Am 71:313, 1987

85. Pasternak GW: Multiple opiate receptors. JAMA 2599:1362, 1988

86. Reiz S, Westberg M: Side effects of epidural morphine. Lancet 1:203, 1980

87. Hogan Q, Haddox JD, Abran S et al: Epidural opiates and local anesthetics for the management of cancer pain. Pain 46:271, 1991

88. Cousins MJ, Bridenbaugh PO (eds): Neural blockade in clinical anesthesia and management of pain. 2nd Ed. JB Lippincott, Philadelphia, 1988

89. Breitbart W, Passik SD: Psychiatric approaches to cancer pain management. p. 49. In Breitbart W, Holland JC (eds): Psychiatric Aspects of Symptom Managment in Cancer Patients. American Psychiatric Press, Washington, DC, 1993

90. Stimmel B: Drugs used for affective disorders: the tricyclic antidepressants. p. 202. In Stimmell B (ed): Pain, Analgesia, and Addiction. The Pharmacologic Treatment of Pain. Raven Press, New York, 1983

91. Monks R: Psychotropic drugs. p. 1676. In Bonica JJ (ed): The Management of Pain. 2nd Ed. Lea & Febiger, Philadelphia, 1990

92. Ventafridda V, Ripamonti C, De Conno F et al: Antidepressants increase bioavailability of morphine in cancer patients. Lancet 1:1204, 1987

93. Forrest W, Brown B, Brown C et al: Dextroamphetamine with morphine for the treatment of postoperative pain. N Engl J Med 296:712, 1977

94. Bruera E, Chadwick S, Brennels C et al: Methylphenidate associated with narcotics for the treatment of cancer pain. Cancer Treat Rep 71:67, 1987

95. Beaver WT: Comparison of analgesic effects of morphine sulfate, hydroxyzine and other combinations in patients with postoperative pain. p. 553. In Bonica JJ, Ventafridda V (eds): Advances in Pain Research and Therapy. Raven Press, New York, 1976

96. Benedetti C, Butler SH: Systemic analgesics. p. 1640. In Bonica JJ (ed): The Management of Pain. 2nd Ed. Lea & Febiger, Philadelphia, 1990

97. Ruden RA: Prevention of opiate induced constipation. Curr Concepts Perspect Nutr 2:1, 1983

98. Maguire LC, Yan JL, Mlller E: Prevention of narcotic-induced constipation. N Engl J Med 305:1651, 1981

99. Portenoy RK: Constipation in the cancer patient: causes and management. Med Clin North Am 71:303, 1987

100. Beaver WT, Wallenstein SL, Houde RW, Rogers AG: A comparison of the analgesic effect of methotrimeprazine and morphine in patients with cancer. Clin Pharmacol Ther 7:436, 1983

101. Sandgren JE, McPhee MS, Greenberger NJ: Narcotic bowel syndrome treated with clonidine. Ann Intern Med 101:331, 1984

102. Bruera E, Brenneis C, Michaud M, MacDonald N: Continuous Sc infusion of metoclopramide for treatment of narcotic bowel syndrome. Cancer Treat Rep 71:1121, 1987

103. Peterson DE, Sonis ST (eds): Oral Complications of Cancer Chemotherapy. Marinus Nijhoff, Boston, 1983

104. Pfeiffer P, Hansen SO, Madsen EL, May O: Sucralfate prophylaxis of chemotherapy-induced stomatitis. Am Soc Clin Oncol Proc 8:171, 1989

105. Gabrilove JL, Jakubowski A, Scher H et al: Effect of granulocyte colony-stimulating factor on neutropenia and associated morbidity due to chemotherapy for transitional cell carcinoma of the urothelium. N Engl J Med 318:1414, 1988

106. Hill HF, Mackie AM, Coda BA et al: Patient-controlled analgesia administration: a comparison of steady-state morphine infusions with bolus doses. Cancer 67:873, 1991

107. Kaneshiro MM, Mielke CH, Kasper CK et al: Bleeding time after aspirin in disorders of intrinsic clotting. N Engl J Med 281:1039, 1969

108. Kasper CK, Rapaport SI: Bleeding times and platelet aggregation of analgesics in hemophilia. Arch Intern Med 77:189, 1972

109. Edmiston K, Griffin TW, Rybak ME et al: Hematologic effects of choline magnesium trisalicylate during chemotherapy. Am Soc Clin Oncol Proc 8:339, 1989

110. Thomas P, Hepburn B, Kim HC, Saidi P: Nonsteroidal anti-inflammatory drugs in the treatment of hemophilic arthropathy. Am J Hematol 12:131, 1982

111. Loeser JD: Herpes zoster and postherpetic neuralgia. Pain 25:149, 1986

112. Portenoy RK, Duma C, Foley KM: Acute herpetic and postherpetic neuralgia: clinical review and current management. Ann Neurol 20:651, 1986

113. Watson PB, Evans RJ: Postherpetic neuralgia, a review. Arch Neurol 43:836, 1986

114. Watson CP, Evans RJ, Reed K et al: Amitriptyline versus placebo in postherpetic neuralgia. Neurology 32:670, 1982

115. Max MB, Schafer SC, Culnane M et al: Amitriptyline, but not lorazepam, relieves postherpetic neuralgia. Neurology 38:427, 1988

116. Bernstein JE, Korman NJ, Bickers DR et al: Topical capsaicin treatment of chronic post-herpetic neuralgia. J Am Acad Dermatol 21:265, 1989

117. Mayne GE, Brown M, Arnold P et al: Pain of herpes zoster and postherpetic neuralgia. p. 345. In Raj PP (ed): Practical Management of Pain. Year Book Medical, Chicago, 1986

118. Zenz M, Strumpf M, Tryba M: Long-term oral opioid therapy in patients with chronic nonmalignant pain. J Pain Sympt Mgmt 7:67, 1992

119. Schofferman J: Long-term use of opioid analgesics for the treatment of chronic pain of nonmalignant origin. J Pain Symptom Mgmt 8:279, 1993

120. Portenoy RK, Foley KM: Chronic use of opioid analgesics in non-malignant pain: report of 38 cases. Pain 25:171, 1986

121. Lubin BH, Vichinsky E: Sickle cell anemia. In Brain MC, Carbone PP (eds): Current Therapy in Hematology-Oncology. Vol. 3. BC Decker, Philadelphia, 1988

122. Friedman EW, Webber AB, Osborn HH, Schwartz S: Oral analgesia for treatment of painful crisis in sickle cell anemia. Ann Emerg Med 15:787, 1986

123. Abbuhl S, Jacobson S, Murphy JG, Gibson G: Serum concentration of meperidine in patients with sickle cell crisis. Ann Emerg Med 15:433, 1986

124. Schechter NL, Berrien FB, Katz SM: The use of patient-controlled analgesia in adolescents with sickle cell pain crisis: a preliminary report. J Pain Sympt Mgmt 3:109, 1988

125. Charache S, Lubin B, Reid CD (eds): Management and Therapy of Sickle Cell Disease. U.S. Department of Health and Human Services, Public Health Service, National Institutes of Health, Washington, DC, 1985

126. Kaiko RF, Wallenstein SL, Rogers AG et al: Narcotics in the elderly. Med Clin North Am 66:1079, 1982

127. Thompson TL II, Moran MG, Nies AS: Psychotropic drug use in the elderly. N Engl J Med 308:134; 194, 1983

128. Fields SD: History-taking in the elderly: obtaining useful information. Geriatrics 46:26, 1991

129. Portenoy RK: Pain management in the older patient. Oncology, suppl. 6:86, 1992

130. Schlegel SE, Paulus H: Non-steroidal and analgesic therapy in the elderly. Clin Rheum Dis 12:245, 1986

131. Savage SR: Addiction in the treatment of pain: significance, recognition and management. J Pain Sympt Mgmt 8:265, 1993

132. Wesson DR, Ling W, Smith DE: Prescription of opioids for treatment of pain in patients with addictive disease. J Pain Sympt Mgmt 8:289, 1993

133. Gonzales GR, Coyle N: Treatment of cancer pain in a former opioid abuser: fears of the patient and staff, and their influence on care. J Pain Sympt Mgmt 7:246, 1992

134. Gralla RJ: Antiemetic therapy. p. 2338 In Devita VT, Hellman S, Rosenberg SA (eds): Cancer: Principles and Practice of Oncology. 4th Ed. JB Lippincott, Philadelphia, 1993

135. Merrifield KR, Chaffee BJ: Recent advances in the management of nausea and vomiting caused by antineoplastic agents. Clin Pharm 8:187, 1989

136. Borison HL, McCarthy LE: Neuropharmacology of chemotherapy induced emesis. Drugs 25:8, 1983

137. Borison HL: Role of the area postrema in vomiting and related functions. Rev Pharmacol Clin Exp 3:7, 1986

138. Andrykowski MA, Jacobsen PB: Anticipatory nausea and vomiting with cancer chemotherapy. p. 107. In Breitbart W, Holland JC (eds): Psychiatric Aspects of Symptom Management in Cancer Patients. American Psychiatric Press, Washington, DC, 1993

139. Leventhal H, Easterling DV, Nerenz DR, Love RR: The role of motion sickness in predicting anticipatory nausea. J Behav Med 11:117, 1988

140. Redd WH, Andresen GV, Minagawa RY: Hypnotic control of anticipatory emesis in patients receiving cancer chemotherapy. J Consult Clin Psychol 50:14, 1982

141. Buish TG, Tope DM: Psychological techniques for controlling the adverse side effects of cancer chemotherapy: findings from a decade of research. J Pain Sympt Mgmt 7:287, 1992

142. Morrow GR, Morrell BS: Behavioral treatment for the anticipatory nausea and vomiting induced by cancer chemotherapy. N Engl J Med 307:1476, 1982

143. Redd WH, Jacobsen PB, Die-Trill M et al: Cognitive/attentional distraction in the control of conditioned nausea in pediatric cancer patients receiving chemotherapy. J Consult Clin Psychol 55:391, 1987

144. Fetting JH, Sheidler VR, Stefanek ME et al: Clonidine for anticipatory nausea and vomiting: a pilot study examining dose-toxicity relationships and potential for further study. Cancer Treat Rep 71:409, 1987

145. Greenberg DB, Surman OS, Clarke J et al: Alprazolam for phobic nausea and vomiting related to chemotherapy. Cancer Treat Rep 71:549, 1987

146. Fetting JH, Grochow LB, Folstein MF et al: The course of nausea and vomiting after high-dose cyclophosphamide. Cancer Treat Rep 66:1487, 1982

147. D'Acquisto RW, Tyson LB, Gralla RJ et al: The influence of a chronic high alcohol intake on chemotherapy-induced nausea and vomiting. Proc Am Soc Clin Oncol 5:257, 1986

148. Sullivan JR, Leyten MJ, Bell R: Decreased cisplatin induced nausea and vomiting with alcohol ingestion. N Engl J Med 309:13,796, 1983

149. Kris MG, Tyson LB, Gralla RJ et al: Extrapyramidal reactions with high-dose metoclopramide. N Engl J Med 309:433, 1983

150. Chang AE, Shiling DJ, Stillman RC et al: Delta-9-tetrahydrocannabinol as an antiemetic in cancer patients receiving high-dose methotrexate: a prospective randomized evaluation. Ann Intern Med 91:819, 1979

151. Beck TM, Ciociola AA, Jones SE et al: Efficacy of oral ondansetron in the prevention of emesis in outpatients receiving cyclophosphamide-based chemotherapy. Ann Intern Med 118:407, 1993

152. Campora E, Oliva C, Mammoliti S et al: Oral ondansetron (GR 38032F) for the control of CMF-induced emesis in the outpatient. Br Cancer Res Treat 19:129, 1991

153. Cubeddu LX, Hoffman IS, Fuenmayor NT, Finn AL: Antagonism of serotonin S3 receptors with ondanseron prevents nausea and emesis induced by cyclophosphamide-containing chemotherapy regimens. J Clin Oncol 8:1721, 1990

154. Seynaeve C, de Muider PH, Lane-Allman E et al: The 5-HT3 receptor antagonist ondansetron re-establishes control in refractory emesis induced by non-cis-platin chemotherapy. Clin Oncology 3:199, 1991

155. duBois A, Meerpohl HG, Christmann D et al: Antiemetic therapy with the 5-HT3 antagonist ondansetron in cisplatin-induced vomiting refractory to standard antiemetic regimens. Proc Am Soc Clin Oncol 10:A1235, 1991

156. Carden PA, Mitchell SL, Waters KD et al: Prevention of cyclophosphamide/cytarabine-induced emesis with ondansetron in children with leukemia. J Clin Oncol 8:1531, 1990

157. Braken BJ, Raemaekers JM, Koopmans PP, dePauw BC: Control of nausea and vomiting with ondansetron in patients treated with intensive non-cis-platin chemotherapy for acute myeloid leukemia. Eur J Cancer 29:515, 1993

158. Viner CV, Selby PJ, Zulian GB et al: Ondansetron—a new safe and effective antiemetic in patients receiving high-dose melphalan. Ca Chemother Pharmacol 25:449, 1990

159. Tiley C, Powles R, Catalano J et al: Results of a double blind placebo controlled study of ondansetron as an antiemetic during total body irradiation in patients undergoing bone marrow transplantation. Leuk Lymphoma 7: 317, 1992

160. Hewitt M, Cornish J, Pamphilon D, Oakhill A: Effective emetic control during conditioning of children for bone marrow transplantation using ondansetron, a 5-HT3 antagonist. Bone Marrow Transplant 7:431, 1991

161. Roberts JT, Priestman TJ: A review of ondansetron in the management of radiotherapy-induced emesis. Oncology 50:173, 1993

162. Scarantino CW, Ornitz RD, Hoffman LG, Anderson RF Jr: Radiation-induced emesis: effects of ondanseron. Semin Oncol, 6 suppl. 15. 19:38, 1992

163. Hainsworth J, Harvey W, Pendergrass K et al: A single-blind comparison of intravenous ondanseron, a selective serotonin antagonist, with intravenous metoclopramide in the prevention of nausea and vomiting associated with high-dose cisplatin chemotherapy. J Clin Oncol 9:721, 1991

164. de Mulder PH, Seynaeve C, Vermorken JB et al: Obdansetron compared with high-dose metoclopramide in prophylaxis of acute and delayed cisplatin-induced nausea and vomiting: a multicenter, randomized, double-blind, crossover study. Ann Intern Med 113:834, 1990

165. Marty M, Pouillart P, Scholl S et al: Comparison of the 5-hydroxytryptamine 3 (seotonin) antagonist ondansetron (GR 38032F) with high-dose metoclopramide in the control of cisplatin-induced emesis. N Engl J Med 322:816, 1990

166. Fraschini G, Ciociola A, Esparza L et al: Evaluation of three oral dosages of ondansetron in the prevention of nausea and emesis associated with cyclophosphamide-doxorubicin chemotherapy. J Clin Oncol 9:1268, 1991

167. Kaasa S, Kvaloy S, Dicato MA et al: A comparison of ondansetron with metoclopramide in the prophylaxis of chemotherapy-induced nausea and vomiting: a randomized, double-blind study. International Emesis Study Group. Eur J Cancer 26:311, 1990

168. Bonneterre J, Chevallier B, Metz R et al: A randomized double-blind comparison of ondansetron and metoclopramide in the prophylaxis of emesis induced by cyclophosphamide, fluorouracil, and doxorubicin or epirubicin chemotherapy. J Clin Oncol 8:1063, 1990

169. Levitt M, Warr D, Yelle L et al: Ondansetron compared with dexamethasone and metoclopramide as antiemetics in the chemotherapy of breast cancer with cyclophosphamide, methotrexate, and fluorouracil. N Engl J Med 328:1081, 1993

170. Halperin JHR, Murphy R: Extrapyramidal reaction to ondansetron. Cancer 69:1275, 1992

171. Gralla RJ, Itri LM, Pisko SE et al: Antiemetic efficacy of high-dose metoclopramide: randomized trials with placebo and prochlorperazine in patients with chemotheapy-induced nausea and vomiting. N Engl J Med 305:905, 1981

172. Homesley HD, Gainey JM, Jobson VW et al: Double-blind placebo-controlled study of metoclopramide in cisplatin-induced emesis. N Engl J Med 307:250, 1982

173. Strum SB, McDermed JE, Opfell RW et al: Intravenous metoclopramide: an effective antiemetic in cancer chemotherapy. JAMA 247:2683, 1982

174. Edge SB, Funkhouser WK, Berman A et al: High-dose oral and intravenous metoclopramide in doxorubicin/cyclophosphamide-induced emesis. Am J Clin Oncol 10:257, 1987

175. Taylor W, Bateman DN: Metoclopramide and chemotherapy-induced emesis. Ann Intern Med 101:141, 1984

176. Kris MG, Gralla RJ, Clark RA et al: Antiemetic control and prevention of side-effects of anticancer therapy with lorazepam or diphenhydramine when used in conjunction with metoclopramide plus dexamethasone: a double-blind, randomized trial. Cancer 69:1353, 1987

177. Breitbart W: Tradive dyskinesia associated with high-dose intravenous metoclopramide. N Engl J Med 315:518, 1986

178. Miller LG, Jankovic J: Metoclopramide-induced movement disorders: clinical findings with a review of the literature. Arch Intern Med 149:2486, 1989

179. Markman M, Sheidler V, Ettinger DS et al: Antiemetic efficacy of dexamethasone: randomized, double-blind, crossover study with prochlorperazine in patients receiving cancer chemotherapy. N Engl J Med 311:549, 1984

180. Cassileth PA, Lusk EJ, Torri S et al: Antiemetic efficacy of dexamethasone therapy in patients receiving cancer chemotherapy. Arch Intern Med 143:1347, 1983

181. Lee BJ: Methylprednisolone as an antiemetic. N Engl J Med 304:486, 1981

182. Grunberg SM, Akerley WL, Baker C et al: Comparison of metoclopramide and metoclopramide plus dexamethasone in complete prevention of cisplatinum induced emesis. Proc Am Soc Clin Oncol 4:262, 1985

183. Roila F, Tonato M, Cognetti F et al: Prevention of cisplatin-induced emesis: a double-blind multicenter randomized crossover study comparing ondansetron and ondansetron plus dexamethasone. J Clin Oncol 9:675, 1991

184. Smyth JF, Coleman RE, Nicolson M et al: Does dexamethasone enhance control of acute cisplatin induced emesis by ondansetron? BMJ 303:1423, 1991

185. Laszlo J, Clark RA, Hanson DC et al: Lorazepam in cancer patients treated with cisplatin: a drug having antiemetic, amnesic, and anxiolytic effects. J Clin Oncol 3:864, 1985

186. Gordon CJ, Pazdur R, Ziccarelli A et al: Metoclopramide versus metoclopramide and lorazepam. Superiority of combined therapy in the control of cisplatin-induced emesis. Cancer 63:578, 1989

187. Grossman B, Lessen LS, Cohen P: Droperidol prevents nausea and vomiting from cis-platinum. N Engl J Med 301:47, 1979

188. Wampler G: The pharmacology and clinical effectiveness of phenothiazines and related drugs for managing chemotherapy-induced emesis. Drugs 25:31, 1983

189. Sallan SE, Cronin C, Zelen M, Zinberg NE: Antiemetics in patients receiving chemotherapy for cancer: a randomized comparison of delta-9-tetrahydrocannabinol and prochlorperazine. N Engl J Med 302:135, 1980

190. Orr LE, McKernan JF, Bloone B: Antiemetic effect of tetrahydrocannabinol. Arch Intern Med 140:1431, 1980

191. Colls BM, Ferry DG, Gray AJ et al: The antiemetic activity of tetrahydrocannabinol versus metoclopramide and thiethylperazine in patients undergoing cancer chemotherapy. NZ Med J 91:449, 1980

192. Meyer RB, O'Mara V, Reidenberg MM: A controlled clinical trial of the addition of transdermal scopolamine to a standard metoclopramide and dexamethasone antiemetic regimen. J Clin Oncol 5:1994, 1987

193. Herrstedt J, Sigsgaard T, Boesgaard M et al: Ondansetron plus metopimazine compared with ondansetron alone in patients receiving moderately emetogenic chemotherapy. N Engl J Med 328:1076, 1993

194. Beck TM, Hesketh PJ, Madajewicz S et al: Stratified, randomized, double-blind comparison of intravenous ondansetron administered as a multiple-dose regimen versus two single-dose regimens in the prevention of cisplatin-induced nausea and vomiting. J Clin Oncol 10:1969, 1992

Indwelling Access Devices

95

Janet L. Abrahm and Jane Bradley Alavi

INTRODUCTION

Indwelling devices that permit chronic access to the venous and central nervous systems have permitted novel and more comfortable forms of treatment for both children and adults.

Indwelling central venous access devices are useful for patients who require frequent administration of blood or blood products, peripheral stem cell apheresis, or infusional therapy with medications such as chemotherapeutic agents, deferoxamine, amphotericin, or pain medications. Similarly, through the use of indwelling epidural or intrathecal catheters and Ommaya reservoirs, prolonged access to the cerebrospinal fluid may be obtained for the delivery of chemotherapy, antibiotics, antifungal agents, or pain medications. The choice of the appropriate device and application of careful maintenance procedures can minimize the associated complications and maximize the patient's quality of life.

INDWELLING CENTRAL VENOUS ACCESS DEVICES

Chronic venous access devices can minimize the discomfort of repeated venipuncture; prevent venous thrombosis, phlebitis, and vesicant infiltration; maintain patient mobility; and minimize hospital stays. Certain patients with hematologic diseases are at increased risk of the development of thrombophlebitis from standard (peripheral) intravenous lines and may therefore be best served by an indwelling access device. Factors associated with this increased risk include (1) age of the patient (>60 years); (2) certain characteristics of the solutions being infused (e.g., hypertonicity of the solution, irritating diluents such as alcohol, highly acidic or alkaline pH, particulate matter in the solution); (3) type of drugs infused (vesicant chemotherapy, certain antibiotics, dexamethasone, furosemide, phenytoin); (4) factors associated with the catheter itself and its insertion (size and composition, traumatic insertion, microbial contamination); and (5) duration of infusion (85% of cases of phlebitis occur 24–48 hours after placement of the intravenous line).[1-4] Since patients with these risk factors or with visibly poor peripheral venous access can usually be identified before therapy begins, early placement of an indwelling device is reasonable. To minimize the occurrence of septic episodes, the devices should be placed prior to giving agents that induce neutropenia.[5]

Device Types

Catheters

In all indwelling catheters used for prolonged central venous access, the proximal capped portion of the catheter exits from a subcutaneous tunnel on the chest or abdominal wall while the distal tip is indwelling in a central vein[6] (Fig. 95-1). All catheters are composed of a radiopaque silicone elastomer but differ in type of opening and internal diameter.[7]

Silicone elastomer catheters with a simple opening at the distal tip include a variety of peripherally inserted central catheters (PICCs), placed at the bedside, and the Hickman, Broviac, and apheresis catheters, which are surgically inserted in the operating room or the radiology suite. The PICCs vary in size from 1.9 to 4.8 F (23–16 gauge) and are 40–60 cm in length.[8,9] The 10.8 F Hickman has a larger internal diameter (ID) than that of the Broviac (1.6- versus 1.0-mm bore, respectively). For peripheral stem cell apheresis, a 14.4 F catheter is available in a 90-cm length.[10]

The Groshong catheter, available in a variety of internal diameters, has a three-position valve adjacent to a closed distal tip. The valve remains closed at rest but opens outward for infusion when positive pressure is applied and opens inward for aspiration when negative pressure is applied.[11] Catheters with a Groshong-type opening are available as PICCs or as surgically inserted devices.

All the above-mentioned catheters, except for PICC and apheresis devices, are available with double and triple lumens for patients requiring nutritional support or infusional therapy, along with blood sampling and blood product administration. Double-lumen devices have either 1.3-mm IDs each or 1.0- and 1.6-mm IDs; those with triple lumens have 1.0-, 1.0-, and 1.25-mm IDs (Fig. 95-2).

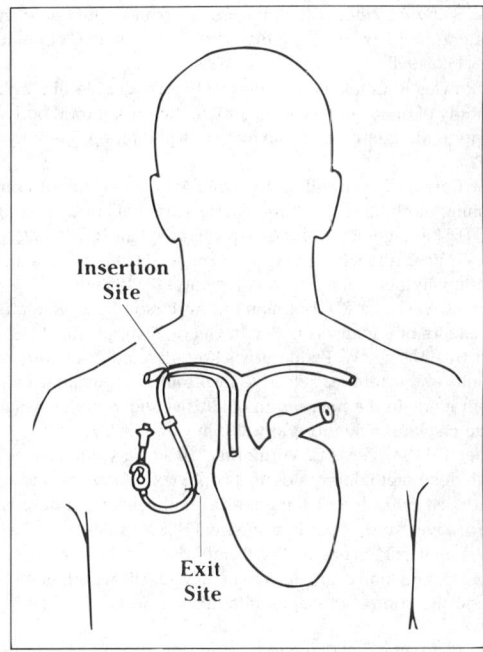

Fig. 95-1. Schematic diagram of an indwelling central venous catheter in place. "Insertion site" refers to the insertion of the proximal end of the catheter into the central vein; the "exit site" is the exit of the distal end of the catheter onto the chest wall. Clamp attached to the catheter is shown next to the Luer-Lok cap at the distal end. (From Hickman Subcutaneous Port, Use and Maintenance, and How to Care for Your Hickman or Broviac Catheter. Davol Inc., Cranston, RI, with permission.)

Implantable Central Venous Devices (Ports)

Totally implantable central venous access devices consist of a port (a self-sealing silicone septum with a body of plastic or metal) connected to a radiopaque silicone elastomer catheter[6] (Fig. 95-3). No portion exits on the chest wall. This port is surgically placed in a subcutaneous pocket, and the catheter is inserted into a central vein. Devices are available with single or double ports connected to catheters with either standard openings or Groshong-type valves. For continuous infusions, these devices require an external infusion pump.

A port that can be placed in the antecubital fossa is also available (the Port-A-Cath P.A.S. Port).[12] Its reservoir is much smaller than the standard port, and the septum has only a 6.6-mm ID. The attached catheter has a 1.0-mm ID, the same size as the Broviac.

Other implantable devices have self-contained pumps. These devices and guidelines for their management are discussed elsewhere.[13-16]

Device Choice

Patient characteristics and preference as well as the duration of use, purposes for which the device is required, and relative complication rates all aid in deciding among the types of catheters and in choosing between catheters and ports[6,17-20] (Table 95-1).

Patient Characteristics and Preference

For female patients, or for any patient being treated in the outpatient setting, peripherally inserted devices (i.e., PICCs or P.A.S. ports) may be the devices of choice, as they have the advantage of eliminating the need for patients to disrobe to access the device. The peripheral devices are also helpful in

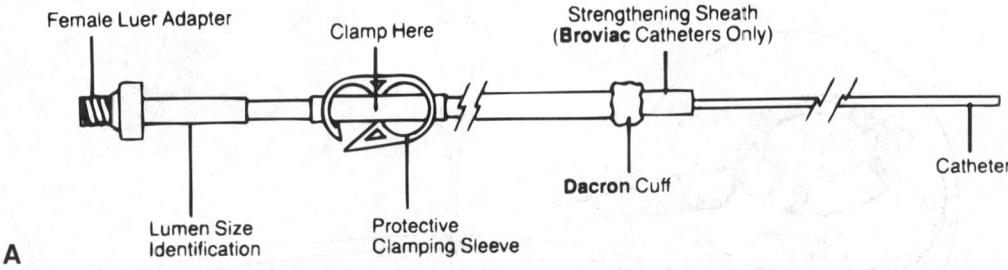

A

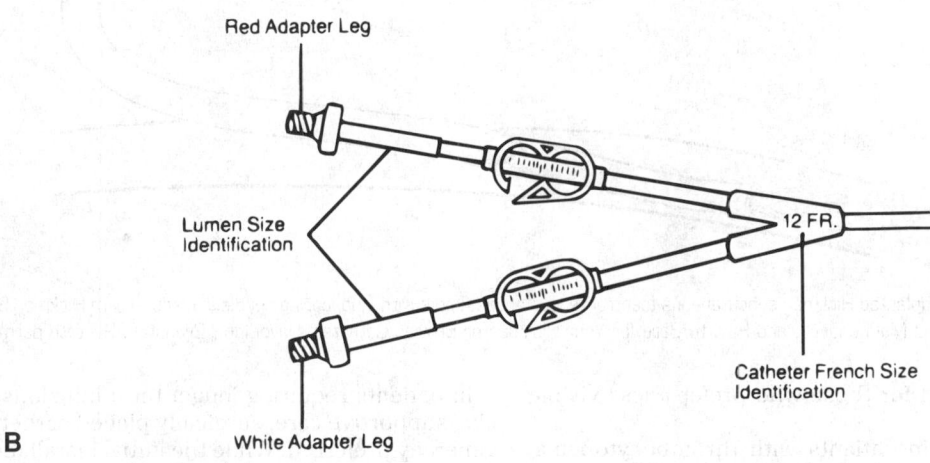

B

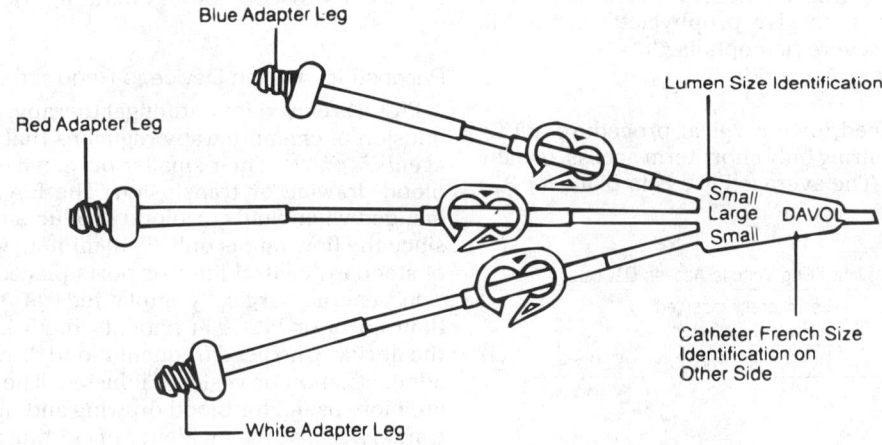

C

Fig. 95-2. Central venous catheters, with built-in clamps. **(A)** Hickman and Broviac single-lumen catheters. **(B)** Hickman and Leonard round dual-lumen catheters. **(C)** Hickman triple-lumen catheters. (From Hickman Subcutaneous Port, Use and Maintenance, and How to Care for Your Hickman or Broviac Catheter. Davol Inc., Cranston, RI, with permission.)

patients with chest wall abnormalities that would preclude the use of centrally placed catheters or ports (e.g., subcutaneous carcinoma of the chest wall, open wounds, tracheostomies, or fibrosis induced by radiotherapy).

A patient who needs a catheter, but who is unable to maintain a Hickman or Broviac catheter at home, could have a catheter with a Groshong-type valve inserted, as those devices require less care.[11,21,22]

Younger patients (children and adolescents) have a lower risk of complications with ports than they do with catheters.[19] While one retrospective study noted no difference in infection rates between Broviac-Hickman catheters and ports,[23] three prospective nonrandomized studies indicated a significantly lower complication rate for the ports than for the catheters, especially in the youngest children.[17,19,23] Ports are also useful for adult patients who are unable to care for a catheter or who

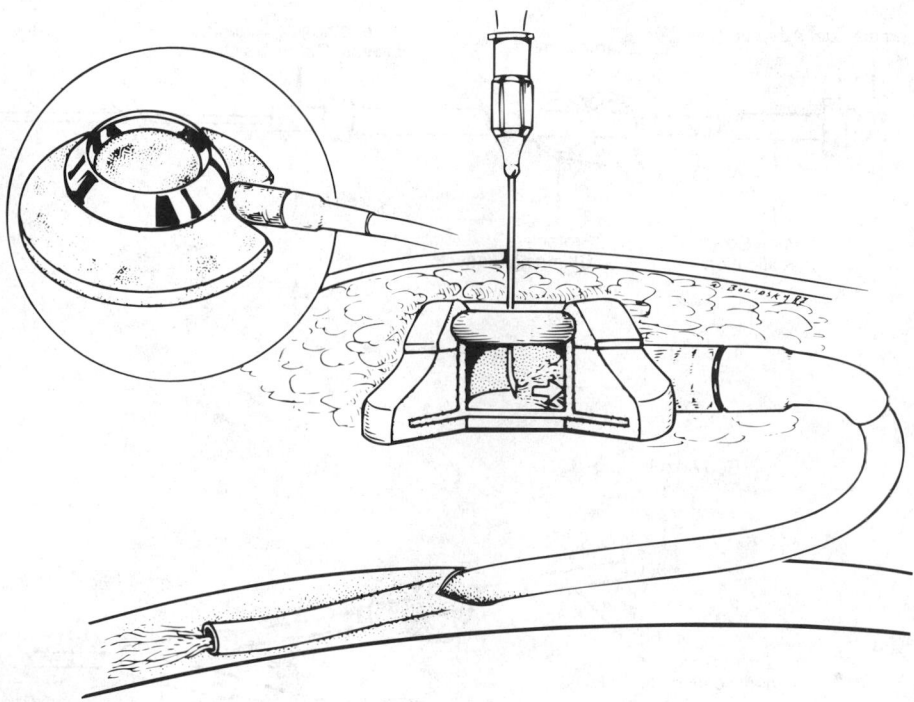

Fig. 95-3. Totally implanted Hickman subcutaneous (central venous access) port with a noncoring needle in place. (From Hickman Subcutaneous Port, Use and Maintenance, and How to Care for Your Hickman or Broviac Catheter. Davol Inc., Cranston, RI, with permission.)

do not wish to do so, and for those who prefer a less visible access device.

In obese patients and in patients with thrombocytopenia, the subcutaneous location of the ports poses a problem. In the obese patient, it may be difficult to find a port placed on the chest wall. For the patient with chronic thrombocytopenia ($<20,000$ platelets/mm^3), neither type of port may be satisfactory because of the risk of hematoma associated with the recurrent needle punctures required for access. Ports have been successfully used, however, to give prophylactic factor VIII therapy to children with severe hemophilia.[24]

Duration of Use

Since they avoid the need for a surgical procedure, PICCs are useful for patients requiring only short-term access, usually several weeks to months. The average PICC is in place for 3–4 weeks.[8,25,26]

Table 95-1. Choice of Indwelling Venous Access Device

	Peripherally Inserted Central Catheter			
	P.A.S	Port	Catheter	Port
Patient characteristics				
Chest wall problem		X		
Outpatient (especially female)		X		
Age				
Child or adolescent				X
Adult			X	X
Obese			X	
Thrombocytopenic			X	
Duration of use				
<3 mo		X		
<6 mo			X	
>6 mo				X
Purpose				
Frequent access			X	
Vesicant infusion			X	

In patients requiring longer-term infusions and more extensive supportive care, surgically placed catheters and ports are generally preferred. While the initial installation cost is greater for the ports than for the catheters, the maintenance costs of the catheter make it more expensive after 6 months of use.[19] Both catheters and ports have remained in place safely for months to years.[27,28] A relatively newer device, the P.A.S. Port is even more cost effective than a standard port as it does not require fluoroscopy or an operating room for placement.[29,30]

Purpose for Which Device is Required

PICCs are used for antifungal therapy, hyperalimentation, or infusion of chemotherapy regimens that may include vesicant agents.[8,9,22,31,32] Their smaller bore makes them less useful for blood drawing or transfusion. The P.A.S. Port is not recommended when fluids or blood products must be given rapidly, since the flow rate is only 6–10 ml/min, which is less than that of standard central lines or ports placed in the chest.[30]

In general, surgically implanted catheters are more useful than ports or PICCs in patients requiring frequent access of the device, who need frequent blood drawing or blood product administration or vesicant infusion. The larger-bore catheters are more useful for blood drawing and blood product administration because the incidence of clotting after such use is lower with them than with smaller-bore devices.[27] Groshong-type catheters, however, may be less useful for patients requiring frequent blood drawing because the valve may make blood aspiration more difficult. If a port or a PICC is chosen, the catheter with the largest bore is recommended. In the larger-gauge PICCs, which collapse easily, blood drawing is usually more successful if a syringe is used instead of a vacuum tube collection system.[31]

Continuous vesicant infusion may be more safely accomplished with catheters, as they avoid the danger of needle dislodgement and disconnection of the catheter from the septum associated with the implanted ports.[33] However, the use of a needle-containing device called a "Gripper," which holds the needle in the port, may decrease the incidence of needle dislodgement.

For support during autologous or allogeneic bone marrow transplantation, double- or triple-lumen catheters are used.[34,35] In those transplant patients undergoing peripheral stem cell apheresis, percutaneously placed translumbar silicone apheresis catheters are preferred, as the internal diameter of the Hickman is often too small.[36]

Relative Complication Rates

Conflicting data have been reported regarding the relative complication rates seen with the two types of devices, although the overall complication rate is probably less for the ports than for the catheters. Of three prospective randomized trials, two showed no significant differences in infection rates.[37,38] The other trial, an investigation of patients with solid tumors, demonstrated a significantly higher rate of infection with the catheters, as well as increased frequency of several other complications when the devices were in place for 6 months.[39] A retrospective matched cohort study of patients with solid tumors also found a significantly higher rate of infection with catheters than with ports.[40] Patients with ports also reported fewer restrictions in activity and hygiene.[39]

In human immunodeficiency virus (HIV)-infected patients, it is not clear whether more complications are caused by ports or by catheters. A large retrospective study of patients with either Hickman or Port-a-Cath devices in place demonstrated no difference in the infection risk for patients with one device versus the other.[41] However, analysis of two other retrospective studies (one of catheter-associated infections[42] and one of port-associated infections[43]) indicates that the rate of device-associated infection in HIV-positive patients with catheters may be higher than in those with ports. In these studies, while the patient characteristics and the purpose for which the device was inserted were comparable, the catheter-associated infection rate was 0.47 per 100 days,[42] and the port-associated infection rate was 0.17 per 100 days.[43]

Device Insertion

Catheters

Catheters can be inserted nonsurgically or surgically. PICCs are placed nonsurgically in the hospital or in the home by appropriately trained physicians or nurses.[22,31] Insertion failure can occur in 8–22% of attempts, although the failure rate decreases with experience.[8,9] After careful skin preparation using sterile technique and, for large-gauge introducers, local anesthesia, the catheter is inserted through the introducer into the basilic vein. The catheter is advanced into the axillary or subclavian vein or superior vena cava and is secured by sutures or sterile tape. If chemotherapy, total parenteral nutrition, or certain hyperosmolar solutions are to be infused, radiologic verification of the catheter tip position in the superior vena cava is recommended.[9]

Hickman, Broviac, and Groshong catheters are inserted surgically in the operating room or the radiology suite[44] under general or local anesthesia. All catheter insertion techniques include (1) creating a subcutaneous tunnel on the anterior chest wall; (2) pulling the catheter up through the tunnel; and (3) positioning the catheter's Dacron cuff(s) in it, leaving its remaining proximal portion, with the Luer-Lok tip, exiting from the tunnel on the chest wall[11,17,45,46] (Fig. 95-1). The distal catheter tip is then usually placed percutaneously into the central circulation through the internal jugular or cephalic vein[15,47] and threaded to the right atrium under fluoroscopic guidance. Its position is confirmed by chest radiography.

No significant difference has been found in time to failure,

infection, or obstruction of catheters inserted percutaneously rather than by direct visualization.[15,48,49] Catheters should be inserted by experienced personnel, however, as complication rates fall as experience in catheter insertion is gained.[27,50,51] If the chest wall or the superior vena cava and subclavian veins are not usable, the best alternate site is the inferior vena cava.[15,36,52,53] Apheresis catheters for peripheral stem cell harvest are preferentially inserted into the inferior vena cava. Techniques for their insertion are reviewed elsewhere.[36]

Ports

Ports are surgically inserted into the antecubital fossa or chest or abdominal wall using local anesthesia.[54] If possible, they should be placed in the nondominant arm or in the side of the chest near it to minimize the probability of needle dislodgement or coring of the port septum during continuous access.[14]

The P.A.S. Port can be inserted at the bedside.[29,30] It consists of an implantable port with an attached radiopaque catheter, the distal tip of which contains an electromagnet. The port is placed percutaneously in a pocket in the antecubital fossa. The venous catheter is introduced using the same techniques as described above for PICCs without attached ports.[29–31] Fluoroscopy is unnecessary, as the progress of the catheter toward the right atrium can be externally tracked with a handheld sensor wand (Cathfinder) that detects the electromagnet in the distal tip. A chest radiograph to verify catheter position is still recommended prior to infusion of certain solutions.[29]

The chest wall ports are placed in the operating room into a subcutaneous pocket in the infraclavicular space, and the attached catheter is placed with the aid of fluoroscopy into the subclavian, jugular, or cephalic vein and is threaded through the superior vena cava to the right atrium (Fig. 95-3). No portion of the device remains visible. For hepatic artery infusion, the catheter is placed during exploratory celiotomy, and the port is placed in the right upper quadrant of the abdominal wall.[33]

Device Management

Catheters

Catheter care is begun by the nurses and later taught to patients and their families. To minimize infectious complications, it is preferable to assign this responsibility (as well as infusions and blood sampling through the catheter) to nurses expert in catheter care and use.[7,17,55–57] Standard procedures are available and should be adopted by each institution, to be followed by all who care for the patient.[22,31,58] The care of PICCs must be especially meticulous, as the risk of infection exceeds that with surgically inserted devices.[6,7] Guidelines for access and maintenance of PICCs are available.[7,22,31,58]

Patient and family education in catheter care is required to maintain patency, to prevent damage to the external portion of the catheter, to prevent air embolization, and to reduce the risk of infection.[11,18,22,31] Instructions should cover permissible activities, techniques of dressing change, heparin instillation, and changing the Luer-Lok plug, as well as emergency care, in the event of damage to the external portion of the catheter. This education program should be begun far enough in advance of patient discharge to ensure patient/family competence and may be reinforced by an educational booklet,[59] by attendance at a "hands-on" class, or by nurses sent into the home, at least initially, to verify compliance with procedures. Patients with catheters or ports in place should be given written documentation about the device,[14] as well as a medical alert card, necklace, or bracelet indicating its location and type of access, as well as the health care personnel to be contacted if problems arise.[22]

Dressing changes for surgically inserted catheters require sterile technique for 2 weeks after insertion, until fibrous growth into the Dacron cuffs is complete.[6,7,18,55] The catheter exit site is cleansed with a povidone-iodine solution. Hydrogen peroxide is also sometimes used, as it prevents scab formation at the site. Sterile dressing changes are made every other day or every third day for 2–3 weeks after insertion, depending on the dressing materials used.[6,7,18] The type of dressing, if any, needed to cover the site is controversial.[7,18,22] One prospective randomized study indicated that when a rigorous cleansing protocol was followed, the incidence of site infection was not different whether standard gauze and povidone-iodine, transparent polyurethane dressings (e.g., Opsite and Tegaderm) that are permeable to water vapor, or no dressing was applied.[60] Another study, however, indicated an increased risk when transparent dressings were used.[61] The advantages and disadvantages of transparent dressings, gauze, or no dressing have recently been reviewed.[22] Moisture-vapor occlusive dressings are strongly recommended for patients with tracheostomies or open wounds near the catheter site. After 2–3 weeks, clean technique is used in some institutions for nonneutropenic patients, and a Band-Aid or small gauze dressing may be used to cover the exit site.[6,62] More complete guidelines for access and maintenance of surgically inserted catheters are available.[58]

The catheter is not usually considered to be securely anchored in place for 10–21 days after catheter placement, although insertion site stitches are usually removed after 10 days.[7] Even then, catheters should not be allowed to hang freely; instead, they should be taped to the chest wall or inserted into a brassiere cup.[22] A clamp should be immediately available in the event of any breaks in the line. Some manufacturers include a clamp placed on the catheter (Fig. 95-2). Patients should be advised to keep the catheter out of the reach of pets or small children, who could dislodge it inadvertently by pulling on it.

Since a thrombus on the catheter tip can be the nidus for a bacterial or fungal infection,[63] every effort should be made to prevent one from forming. In a prospective randomized trial, low-dose coumadin (1 mg/day) beginning 3 days before catheter insertion and continuing for 90 days significantly decreased the number of venogram-proven thromboses from 38% in control patients to 9.5% in those treated with warfarin.[64] In addition, heparin should be instilled in Hickman and Broviac-type catheters after each episode of blood drawing or blood product administration and when the catheters are not being used for intravenous therapy. A minimum of 2.5–4 ml of heparin in saline (100 U/ml) should be instilled in each lumen[7] because such flushes have been shown to reduce bacterial growth on catheter tips.[65] In the outpatient setting, twice-weekly flushes may be adequate.[22] A further decrease in intraluminal infection due to bacteria sensitive to vancomycin may be provided by adding vancomycin (25 μg/ml) to the heparin flush.[66] The line is then plugged with a Luer-Lok injection plug, which is taped in place and changed once per week.[6,7]

It should be remembered, however, that the use of the heparin flush will alter coagulation tests if blood is drawn through the catheter.[67] The first 10-ml sample will have spuriously elevated levels of fibrin degradation products, prothrombin times, and partial thromboplastin times, as well as a spuriously low fibrinogen level. Elevations in prothrombin time and partial thromboplastin time will persist in the second 10-ml sample.

Catheters with Groshong-type valves require less maintenance than do Hickman or Broviac-type catheters. However, they do require a 5-ml saline flush weekly or after use[6,11,21] because the special valve can be kept in the open position by small clots or solid residues from medications, and blood will backflow into the catheter, forming a clot.

For apheresis catheters used for peripheral stem cell harvest, a regimen of 325 mg/day of aspirin, begun the day after catheter placement, led to a greater number of thrombosis-free apheresis procedures than was noted with historical control subjects.[68] More detailed guidelines for nursing education and practice regarding maintenance of catheters are available.[58]

Ports

Ports can be used immediately after insertion. However, because postoperative edema and discomfort often delay any attempts at access for several days, patients should be sent from the operating room with the Huber needle in place and ready for use.[14,22,69]

To access a port that has no needle in place, the skin is prepared with povidone-iodine solution,[70] and a freezing agent (ethylene dichloride) is applied, followed by insertion of a 19–22-gauge Huber needle (depending on the product to be infused)[14] (Fig. 95-3). This steel needle has a deflected point and side opening, designed to prevent coring of the septum.[13] The needle is primed with saline, attached to a saline-containing syringe and connecting tubing, and then inserted perpendicular to the septum.[71] Correct placement in the port can be confirmed by aspiration for blood return. However, blood aspiration is often unsuccessful, usually because the needle is misaligned or a fibrin sheath has formed, creating a ball valve effect. In the absence of swelling after a 10–20-ml saline infusion, the needle can be assumed to be correctly placed and the port safely used.[6] Detailed accessing procedures for drawing blood and for administering drugs and blood products are available.[14,71]

During use, the port is covered with a transparent occlusive sterile dressing, further reinforced by a window frame of paper tape.[13,22,71] The dressing is changed when the needle is changed, as well as when the dressing becomes nonocclusive or wet or evidence of infection or of skin irritation develops. After each use or every 4 weeks, implanted access devices also require heparin instillation (3–5 ml of 100 U/ml heparinized saline solution) or a 20-ml saline flush.[6,13,22] Use and maintenance of the peripheral port are essentially the same as for ports implanted in the chest wall.[12] More detailed guidelines for nursing education and practice regarding the maintenance of implanted ports and reservoirs are available.[69]

Device Removal

Catheters are removed nonsurgically by applying steady tension, so that the catheter is released from the Dacron cuff.[18] For catheters that have been in place for prolonged periods or for cases in which bacterial studies of the internal catheter tip are desired, blunt dissection of the cuff, with transection of the catheter above it and sterile removal of its inner portion, can be performed under local anesthesia.[33,72] Ports are removed surgically under local anesthesia.

Complications

Complications of indwelling vascular access devices include cutaneous reactions to standard-care materials, mechanical problems, phlebitis and infiltration, infection, hemorrhage, catheter occlusion of nonthrombotic or thrombotic etiology, and vesicant drug extravasation.

Cutaneous Reactions

Approximately 5% of patients develop skin reactions to the products used in caring for the devices.[73] These reactions include erythema, urticaria, exanthematous or purpuric eruptions, and skin peeling or abrasion. These skin abnormalities must be distinguished from exit-site infections by appropriate culturing of the site for bacteria. In the uninfected patients, change of the dressing material, tape, and local skin care regimen is effective in reversing the skin abnormalities.[73]

Skin erosion over the implanted ports, either from malnutrition, separated wound edges, local infection, or carcinoma metastatic to the skin, occurs in 3–10% of patients, and removal of the port is always required.[22,74]

Mechanical Problems

Catheters

Damage to the external segment of the catheter includes (1) separation between the Luer-Lok connection and the tubing; (2) cracks caused by repeated cross-clamping, if rubber-tipped forceps are not used; and (3) cuts made by scissors mistaken for clamps.[6] Catheter repair kits should therefore be available on appropriate nursing units. Patients should also be informed to contact their physicians or the oncology nursing staff immediately if the catheter is damaged at home.

Apheresis catheters placed in the inferior vena cava can also develop fractures of the external segment, with visible leakage,[36] and they can be repaired using the kits mentioned above. Fractures of the internal portion of the catheter, however, require catheter removal. Most of these fractures can be detected by injecting radiographic contrast material through them and observing the flow of the dye fluoroscopically.[36]

Ports

The port may "flip" within its pocket because of defective suturing or excessive arm movement, or because of manipulation by the patient.[22,75] This malposition can be surgically corrected.

Phlebitis and Infiltration

Phlebitis and infiltration are uncommon complications associated with properly positioned centrally placed access devices but are noted with PICCs in 13–23% of patients.[31,76] A randomized controlled trial compared the complications associated with steel needles, small-bore short Teflon catheters, and PICCs.[77] PICCs had the highest incidence of phlebitis (27%) and the lowest incidence of infiltration (8.1%); steel needles are associated with the lowest incidence of phlebitis (8%) and the highest incidence of infiltration (45%); and Teflon catheters fell in-between, with a 19–20% incidence of both phlebitis and infiltration. The aseptic phlebitis usually occurs within the first week after PICC insertion. It can be prevented by nonsteroidal anti-inflammatory agents[29] or treated with warm compresses for 48–72 hours.[31] Catheter removal is usually not required.

Infection

Incidence

The incidence of device-associated infection varies depending on the type of device inserted and the medical disorder of the patient. Overall, the incidence of catheter-associated infection is about 1–3 per 1,000 days of patient use.[18] The use of multiple-lumen catheters does not seem to affect this infection rate significantly.[34,35] The infection rate with implanted ports is lower, 0.3 per 1,000 patient days.[18,78] Patients with HIV infection[41,42] or those receiving a bone marrow transplant[34,35,79] have significantly higher rates of both catheter- and port-related infections.

Location

Infections can occur in the skin or in the catheter and vessels themselves. Skin infections include (1) exit-site infections, defined as "erythema, tenderness, induration or purulence within 2 cm of the skin exit site of the catheter or any edge of the port,"[17,28]; (2) tunnel infections, defined as "erythema, tenderness or induration along the subcutaneous tract of the catheter at >2 cm from the skin exit site or port edge, with or without signs of inflammation or purulence at the exit site or surrounding the port"[17,27,80]; and (3) port pocket infections. They are generally prevented by meticulous insertion and maintenance techniques.[55,56] Both retrospective and prospective studies showed exit-site infections to be responsible for 39–45.5% and tunnel infections for 20.3–22% of all catheter-related infections.[27,80] Prophylactic antibiotics have not consistently proved beneficial in preventing these infections.[18,27]

Organisms

The most common infecting organisms are bacterial, with gram-positive organisms more frequent than gram-negative organisms.[18] In patients not infected with HIV, an average of 36% of infections will be due to coagulase-negative staphylococci, 16% to *Staphylococcus aureus,* and 12% to *Streptococcus* spp., with 28% due to gram-negative rods. *Pseudomonas* is found when showering or swimming has been allowed. *Xanthomonas* infections can be particularly troublesome.

A reported 5% of infecting organisms are fungal, mostly *Candida* spp.,[18,27,81,82] although nosocomially acquired cutaneous infections with *Aspergillus flavus* have been noted at the sites of insertion and along the subcutaneous tract of Hickman catheters.[83,84] Septicemia due to catheter infection by either typical or atypical *Mycobacterium* spp. has also been noted.[17,85–88]

In HIV-positive patients, *S. aureus* has been responsible for as many as 87% of Hickman catheter infections,[42] although others have indicated that it accounted for only 35–39%, *S. epidermidis* for 22–26% and *Pseudomonas aeruginosa* for 17–26%.[41,89] In children with HIV who have indwelling catheters, infections due to *Pseudomonas* spp. are becoming an increasing problem.[90–92]

Indications for Removal

Exit-Site and Tunnel Infections

Exit-site infections caused by bacteria rarely require catheter removal for resolution, as most (69–100%) will respond to antibiotics alone.[27,50,51,80] These infections are most often caused by *S. epidermidis.*[15,18] Similarly, with implanted ports, infections of the skin pocket have been found to resolve in about 70% of cases without removal of the device.[17,18,28,54]

Tunnel infections, by contrast, usually do not respond to antibiotics; they have been reported to resolve without catheter removal in only 25–50% of cases.[27,50,51,80] Catheters were removed from all patients with cutaneous *Aspergillus* infection, six of whom recovered after antifungal therapy and local wound care[83] (Table 95-2). Resolution of leukopenia was required for infection resolution. Similarly, *Mycobacterium*[17] and atypical mycobacterial infection of the tunnel or exit site requires catheter removal as well as excision of infected tissue.[88]

Table 95-2. Indications for Catheter Removal

Venous access devices
Exit site infection caused by atypical mycobacteria
Tunnel infections
Bacteremia caused by *Staphylococcus aureus, Xanthomonas, Pseudomonas* spp.
Fungemia
Central nervous system access devices
Deep catheter track or epidural space infection

Septicemia

In a patient with septicemia and a catheter or port in place, it is often difficult to determine whether the catheter itself is truly infected or whether the bacteremia is from another source. Several methods have been proposed to investigate infection of the catheter. Catheters are presumed to be infected, using quantitative blood culture methods, if (1) the colony counts from cultures drawn through the catheter are 5–10-fold greater than the counts from cultures drawn peripherally or (2) the colony count of the blood drawn through the catheter is ≥100 colony-forming units/ml).[22,80,93,94] Another method involves culturing the catheter hub and exit site and comparing the organisms found there with those found in blood cultures. If the organisms are found to be identical, the likelihood is very high that the catheter itself is infected.[95] Moreover, negative cultures from the hub and exit site strongly suggest that the catheter is not infected: all catheters with negative hub and exit-site cultures had negative catheter tip cultures.[95]

In assessing the cause of infection in a patient with a port, care must be taken not to draw blood cultures through a possibly infected port pocket, unless the Huber needle is already in place. Accessing a port through an infected port pocket could introduce organisms into the reservoir and from there into the systemic circulation.[22,96]

When another source is definitely identified, however, the catheters can usually be left in place, since the incidence of hematogenous colonization is low (1%).[27,45] When there is no thrombophlebitis, even when the catheter is believed to be the source of the infection or when no source is clearly identified, resolution of bacterial septicemia occurs in 75% of episodes, without removal of the catheter.[18,93]

The possibility of clearing the infection without catheter removal, however, is much lower in patients with septic thrombophlebitis, occluded catheters, exit-site infections, or bacteremia due to *S. aureus, Xanthomonas,* or *Pseudomonas* species (*aeruginosa* or non-*aeruginosa*), or fungal septicemia.[18,97,98] In one study, children with *Candida* fungemia were treated successfully with the line left in place,[5] but in other studies, children with catheter-related candidemia suffered more treatment failure, secondary complications, and mortality if the catheters were left in place during antifungal treatment.[99,100] In general, catheter removal is recommended in patients with bacteremia due to *S. aureus, Xanthomonas,* or *Pseudomonas* species and in those with fungemia due to either *Aspergillus* or *Candida* spp. (Table 95-2). Replacement of catheters on the contralateral side within 1–3 days after removal is usually not associated with recurrent catheter infection.[45,54]

Hemorrhage

Despite the frequent occurrence of thrombocytopenia in patients requiring indwelling access devices, minimal bleeding complications are associated with their placement or with the placement of the larger apheresis catheters.[10,45,50] Capillary fragility from prolonged steroid therapy, however, may contribute to perioperative hemorrhage.[50] Pressure dressings and platelet transfusions given pre- and postoperatively usually control local oozing.[45] However, in patients with uncontrolled disseminated intravascular coagulation, excessive bleeding has occurred with catheter insertion; many groups consider disseminated intravascular coagulation an absolute contraindication to catheter placement.[18,45,50]

Catheter Occlusion

Nonthrombotic Causes

Inability to aspirate blood from the port or catheter does not necessarily mean that it has clotted. Other causes include a malpositioned Huber needle, catheter abutment against the wall of the vein, catheter kinking, precipitation of drug solutions in the catheter lumen, development of fibrin sheaths, and catheter migration, with resultant malposition of the tip.[22,101] The problem may resolve by changing the patient's position or by performing a Valsalva maneuver, if it is simply due to abutment of the catheter tip against the wall of the vein.[7,14,22] Precipitation of incompatible solutions may be reversed by warm soaks over the tunnel site, but prevention is usually the only effective "remedy."[22]

Occlusion by a fibrin sheath, leading to a ball valve effect,[6,15] occurs in 10–20% of cases.[101,102] The fibrin sleeve itself may embolize as well.[103,104] Techniques using nonlytic and lytic agents to remove the sheaths have been described.[14,22] Lytic therapy is discussed below.

Catheter migration occurs in 5.5–29% of insertions when the subclavian approach is used.[105] Review of the patient's chest radiograph will most commonly show the malpositioned catheter tips to be in the internal jugular vein or in the contralateral brachiocephalic vein. It is important to reposition the catheter, as venous thrombosis can occur as a result of damage to the endothelium, turbulence created by the tip at venous branching points, or insufficient dilution of infusates that cause thrombophlebitis. This can usually be done without catheter removal, using angiographic techniques.[101,105] Migration of the apheresis catheter in the subcutaneous space also manifests as access failure, since the catheter tip is pulled back to the wall of the inferior vena cava or out of the intravascular space.[36] Intravascular malposition can be corrected by tip deflectors or J-wires.[106]

Thrombosis

Thrombosis can occur in the catheter itself or in the superior vena cava or veins of the upper extremity. The thrombus usually results from failure to follow standard flush procedures. Thromboses were seen in 16% of implanted ports.[28] An incidence of 18% is reported with PICCs,[107] but the incidence of thrombosis in patients with properly cared for centrally inserted catheters is only 0–10%.[20,28,108,109] The incidence is equally low in syngeneic and allogeneic marrow transplant patients, despite the use of multiple-lumen catheters.[34–36] In patients undergoing autologous marrow transplant, however, the incidence of thrombosis is 13–20%.[109] This higher incidence may be due to the increased number of patients in this group who have platelet counts of >150,000 mm^3 and to the frequent placement of two catheters at bone marrow harvest.[109]

Noninvasive methods used for diagnosis, including duplex ultrasound,[108,110] magnetic resonance imaging,[111] Doppler,[108,112] and plethysmography,[108] have low sensitivity or have not been reliable, and nuclear scans have been falsely normal because of the development of collateral circulation.[108] Venography is recommended to support the clinical diagnosis.[28,36,108] In patients with prior subclavian catheterization, however, duplex scans may be useful to predict the success of repeat catheter placement.[113]

Therapy

The course of action for those patients undergoing high-intensity antineoplastic therapy in whom asymptomatic subclavian or innominate vein thromboses develop is unclear. Asymptomatic occlusion is seen in 25% of patients undergoing autologous marrow transplantation; partial occlusion develops in an additional 34%.[114] Since the incidence of complications caused by these thrombi is unknown, no therapeutic recommendations can be made.

Patients with symptomatic upper-extremity deep venous thromboses (DVTs), however, probably do require therapy.

They may develop septic thrombophlebitis,[18,27] superior vena cava syndrome, major long-term upper-extremity disability, venous gangrene, and pulmonary emboli. In one retrospective study and review, 12% of patients with catheter-induced upper-extremity DVTs developed pulmonary emboli, 40% of which occurred in patients receiving anticoagulant therapy.[108] A higher incidence of pulmonary emboli was found in a prospective study of patients with upper-extremity DVT, in whom lung scans were performed within 48 hours of venographic diagnosis of the thrombosis. This study found a 20% incidence (4 of 19 patients) of high-probability lung scans in patients with catheter-associated DVT, with a 5% incidence of symptomatic emboli.[115]

There is no consensus about the best therapy for patients with upper-extremity DVTs. Some reports suggest that conservative therapy (heat and elevation) is efficacious, producing resolution of edema and pain and minimal chronic venous insufficiency.[109] Other investigators have recommended anticoagulation with heparin, thrombolysis, or surgical clot removal.[28,36,108,116]

Anticoagulation with heparin, however, has not been consistently successful in preventing pulmonary emboli from subclavian vein thrombi.[105,117] Therefore, bolus or infusional thrombolytic therapy with streptokinase or urokinase is usually considered. Bolus thrombolytic therapy has reopened occluded catheters in 85–90% of episodes, and removal of the catheter is not usually required.[55,116,118–120] One commonly used procedure is to instill 1–3 ml of a solution of streptokinase (750–10,000 IU/ml) or urokinase (5,000 IU/ml) into the catheter or port, leave it in place for 20 minutes to 1 hour, and then to aspirate at 5-minute intervals until the catheter reopens.[58] If the first instillation is ineffective, the procedure can be repeated or the other solution used.[36,118,120,121] Similarly, fibrin sheaths have been dissolved in 87% of patients who had streptokinase (3,000 IU/hr) infused into each catheter lumen for 12–24 hours.[101] No fevers, coagulation abnormalities, or other adverse reactions have been noted with urokinase, but streptokinase can cause mild to moderate systemic reactions (fever and chills) in patients with recent streptococcal infections or in those who have previously received the drug for thrombolysis. Once patency is restored, heparin is usually given for 5–7 days.

For thrombi refractory to streptokinase or urokinase bolus, options to dissolve the thrombus include tissue plasminogen activator[122] or infusions of streptokinase[123] or urokinase through a catheter placed at or within the clot.[116] High-dose streptokinase therapy is effective[123] but expensive and is associated with a high incidence of bleeding. It is not recommended for patients with such bleeding risks are thrombocytopenia or mucositis. Infusion of urokinase for 24–72 hours was found to restore catheter patency in 74% of patients (81% of those with clots present for <7 days and in 56% of those with clots present for >7 days).[116] Infusion into the superficial venous circulation of the involved extremity was not effective. Even though a low infusion concentration was used (5,000 IU/hr streptokinase or 500–2,000 IU/kg/hr urokinase), a systemic lytic state was documented. Therefore, urokinase infusion should not be undertaken in patients with contraindications to systemic fibrinolytic therapy.[124] Another regimen for refractory clots involves an infusion of urokinase (40,000 U/hr) for 6 hours. This regimen achieved a dissolution of thrombi in 90% of patients; a repeat 6-hour infusion raised the dissolution rate to 95%.[125] No bleeding complications were seen. In all patients with incomplete recanalization or residual thrombus, however, the catheter should be removed, to prevent recurrence of thrombosis.[45,116] The same urokinase instillation technique is recommended for patients with occluded ports.[69] Successful clot resolution with urokinase was reported in 50–87% of patients.[17,54]

Vesicant Drug Extravasation

It is very unusual for a spontaneous leak to form in a large-bore catheter, but an attempt to irrigate an occluded catheter with a small syringe can cause a rupture, through which the drug can extravasate.[6,45] Occlusion of the catheter tip by a fibrin sheath may force drug back up the sheath and through the exit site of the catheter.[28]

Leaks may develop if the catheter is disconnected from the reservoir or if the catheter is punctured by mistake by the Huber needle.[22] In addition, outpatients using a port for continuous infusion of chemotherapy can suffer drug extravasation if the Huber needle is dislodged from the septum.[33,126–128] Even usually nonvesicant drugs can produce skin necrosis severe enough to warrant removal of the port.[33] Use of the Port-a-Cath port, which has a thicker septum than the MediPort or Infus-a-Port devices, has been associated with only a 3–4% incidence of extravasation.[54,126–128] The thickness of the septum has been postulated to be responsible for the small incidence of needle displacement noted with the Port-a-Cath,[128] but no randomized trials have compared complications associated with the three devices. Securing the needle to the chest wall with tape has been recommended,[126,127] but the use of a Gripper needle provides much more secure needle placement and may lower the incidence of this complication. If infusion pumps are used, attention must be paid to minimizing tension between the needle and the infusion tubing.

Treatment protocols for vesicant drug extravasation, as recommended by the Oncology Nursing Society,[129–136] are outlined in Table 95-3. In studies of their use (excluding the recom-

Table 95-3. Management of Vesicant Drug Extravasation

| Drug | Therapy | | |
	Antidote Preparation	Method of Administration	Comments
Antibiotics[130,131,136]			
Dactinomycin	None	Apply 1–2 ml of 1 mmol DMSO (50–100%) to an area twice that of the affected area once. Air-dry without a dressing	Apply *cold* packs for 20 minutes, qid, for 72 hours. Elevate extremity for 24–48 hours, then use normally
Mitomycin			
Plicamycin			
Daunorubicin			
Doxorubicin			
Vinca alkaloids[131–133]			
Vinblastine	Add 1 ml preservative-free normal saline to one vial containing 150 U hyaluronidase	Inject five 1-ml doses subcutaneously into site with multiple injections	Apply *warm* compresses for 20 minutes, qid, for 72 hours
Vincristine			
Etoposide			
Alkylators[130,134,135]			
Mechlorethamine	Mix 1.6 ml of 25% sodium thiosulfate with 8.4 ml sterile water for injection	Inject 5 ml IV through existing line	Apply *cold* packs to the site for 20 minutes, qid, for 72 hours

mended therapy with dimethyl sulfoxide [DMSO]), 89% of vesicant extravasations were reported to resolve without additional therapy.[130] However, 30% of anthracycline extravasations progressed to ulceration. A prospective uncontrolled study of anthracycline extravasation showed that the application of DMSO four times a day for 4 days prevented progression to ulceration in all patients.[136]

At many centers, it is recommended that an extravasation kit be kept in units in which vesicant drugs are given. The kit includes the appropriate medications, as well as order sheets preprinted for immediate use. In general, if an antidote is to be administered through the device, as much of the residual drug as possible should be aspirated from the needle, tubing, and tissues, before the antidote is given. If swelling or pain persists for 72–96 hours after drug administration, a plastic surgeon should be consulted.

CENTRAL NERVOUS SYSTEM ACCESS DEVICES

In patients with hematologic disorders, devices that permit chronic access to the central nervous system are useful for a variety of purposes. The available devices include permanent epidural catheters, ports with attached silicone-elastomer catheters, implanted pumps with attached silicone-elastomer catheters, and Ommaya reservoirs.

Catheters

Chronic epidural access has become widely available since the development of a permanent epidural catheter that can be placed percutaneously.[137] The catheters are most commonly used for pain control. The catheter consists of three pieces: two radiopaque silicone-rubber catheters (an epidural segment (1.3-mm outer diameter [OD]) and an exteriorized line (3.1-mm OD, 0.68-mm ID) with an external Luer connector and a subcutaneous Dacron cuff) and a splice segment that joins the two catheter segments.[137]

Insertion

Catheter insertion is done under local anesthesia.[137] A paravertebral incision is made at the level of the L2 dorsal spine, and the epidural portion of the catheter is inserted through a 14-gauge Hustead or Touhy needle to the desired spinal cord level. Epidural placement is verified by fluoroscopy and sensory blackade. The exteriorized line is then tunneled from a subcostal location on the mid-nipple line around to the lower end of the paravertebral incision, and the splice segment is secured to the two catheters and then to the supraspinous tissue to avoid kinking. A Millex-OR 0.22-μm filter is attached to the Luer connector, and a locking Luer injection cap is connected to the filter.

Access and Management

The catheter can be used immediately. Bolus doses can be given from a syringe, or the catheter can be connected to external pumps that deliver continuous infusion opiate with bolus "rescue" doses or combinations of opioids and local anesthetics (see Ch. 94). Only preservative-free solutions can be used. Wound and catheter exit-site cleaning and dressing changes are recommended until the last sutures are removed, usually 3 weeks. After that, the exit site is cleansed daily with hydrogen peroxide and povidone-iodine wash, and the filter

and injection port are changed every 4 days using sterile technique.[137] More detailed nursing protocols for accessing and managing these catheters and for monitoring the patients receiving epidural narcotics are available.[58]

Complications

The catheters can remain safely in place for months.[138] Complications include those attributable to the opioids being infused, pain during injection,[139] myoclonus,[140] obstruction and dislocation,[139,141] and infection.[138,139,142] Exit-site and superficial catheter track infections occurred infrequently (in about 10% of patients).[138,142] The epidural space infection rate was 1 in 1,702 days of catheter use, similar to the infection rate of 1 in 1,045 per days of use associated with the Hickman catheter.[138] S. aureus and S. epidermidis accounted for two-thirds of all the infections.[138] Exit-site and superficial catheter track infections could be cleared without catheter removal,[138,142] but catheter removal was required for patients with deep catheter track or epidural infections[138] (Table 95-2).

Epidural Ports/Implanted Pumps

Epidural ports (e.g., Port-a-Cath) and implanted pumps (e.g., Infusaid) have also been used to deliver bolus or continuous infusions of opiates into the epidural or intrathecal space to relieve pain of malignant or nonmalignant origin.[140,143] Subarachnoid infusions using the implanted pumps are recommended as efficacious and cost effective for patients with relatively long life expectancy (>3 months).[140] The use of implanted pumps has been reviewed elsewhere.[144]

Complications include both those noted above for implanted ports, and also pain on injection of morphine, pump pocket seromas, cerebrospinal fluid leaks, cerebrospinal fluid hygromas, and postspinal headache.[140,145] Removal rates for infection were similar to those of ports used for vascular access (10%).[145] Because the seromas act as growth media for bacterial contamination, they should be monitored carefully. Management of hygromas and postspinal headache is reviewed elsewhere.[140] Detailed access and management procedures for epidural ports and implanted pumps and for monitoring patients receiving opioids through them are available.[16,69]

Ommaya Reservoir

The Ommaya reservoir device was first described in 1963 by Ommaya,[146] and with minimal changes it is still used for access to the spinal fluid within the cerebral ventricle. The reservoir is used to remove cerebrospinal fluid for culture, cytology, or measurement of drug levels; to drain cysts in craniopharyngiomas and astrocytomas; to administer antibiotics or antifungal agents; to administer intraventricular chemotherapy to treat leukemic or carcinomatous meningitis; to administer interferon or lymphokine-activated killer cells directly into a tumor; and to administer opioid pain medications.[147]

The device consists of a dome or mushroom-shaped capsule with a top made of self-sealing silicone elastomer that can be punctured numerous times without leaking. The flat base of the capsule, by contrast, is composed of firm polypropylene and is not easily punctured. An outlet arm connected to a ventricular catheter is attached at the base, either laterally or in the center, extending downward. Capsules range in size from 12 mm in diameter (for babies) to 30 mm. Those commonly used for adults have an internal volume capacity of 1.45–2.4 ml.

Insertion

The Ommaya reservoir is placed subcutaneously by a neurosurgeon.[148] Prior to insertion, a computed tomography scan is generally required to evaluate ventricular size and placement. Presoaking the device in bacitracin to prevent subsequent infection has been advocated.[149] For placement, the ventricular catheter is passed through a burr hole into the frontal horn of the right lateral ventricle or, if necessary, into that of the left lateral ventricle or the ventricle body. The catheter end is connected to the base or side arm of the capsule, which then is fitted into the burr hole or a subgaleal pocket. The Silastic skirt of the reservoir may be sutured to the periosteum. A postoperative computed tomography scan is suggested to verify the catheter tip position.

Accessing the Device

The Ommaya reservoir can be used immediately postoperatively for sampling cerebrospinal fluid or for injection of drugs. Usually, however, it is not accessed until the third postoperative day.[147] The thoroughly cleansed, gently shaved scalp is prepared with three iodine scrubs and, with use of sterile technique, the reservoir is accessed obliquely with a 23-gauge butterfly needle inserted with the bevel downward.[147] The cerebrospinal fluid can be directly aspirated, or antibiotics or chemotherapeutic agents can be administered through a second syringe attached to the butterfly needle. After removal of the needle, the injected medication can be gently pumped into the spinal fluid by emptying the capsule using repeated pressure. Once the incision has healed and the stitches removed, no special local care or flushing is required. The device can remain in place for months or years. More detailed accessing and management guidelines are available.[69]

Complications

Infection

In general, the Ommaya reservoir has proved very safe, with a complication rate of approximately 10–20%,[148–151] although higher rates were reported in the past.[152] The most common complication is infection, seen in about 10–15% of patients,[151] especially those who have undergone radiotherapy or who required a second surgical procedure for revision of the catheter.[148] Most infections have been due to *S. epidermidis,* but infections due to numerous other gram-positive and gram-negative bacteria as well as fungal organisms have been documented.[151,153] In general, the device is not removed, and patients are treated as though they have meningitis. For infections with *S. epidermidis,* vancomycin is given intravenously[154] or, in refractory cases, instilled into the reservoir.[155] Removal of the reservoir is sometimes required.

Miscellaneous

Neurologic complications are rare when the catheter is placed into the nondominant ventricle, but a variety of other complications, which occur infrequently, have been reported. These include (1) intraventricular hemorrhage or subdural hematoma shortly after catheter placement; (2) leakage of cerebrospinal fluid around the catheter, primarily in patients with increased intracranial pressure, which caused backflow of fluid along the catheter and produce a subgaleal collection[152,156]; (3) reservoir leaks after repeated use[150]; (4) occlusion by cellular debris or, when a catheter is placed directly into a tumor, by very proteinaceous tumor fluid[150]; (5) obstruction by lodging of the catheter in brain tissue or abutment against a ventricle wall[150]; (6) seizures immediately following injection of medications[150]; (7) white matter disease (leukoencephalopathy or brain necrosis), most often due to methotrexate injection via the Ommaya device, although found with systemic administration of methotrexate as well[150,157]; and (8) tumor growth around the cannula. In one case, the catheter may have permitted the spread of Burkitt lymphoma cells from the meninges into the cerebral tissue, where the tumor was found.[158]

REFERENCES

1. Faulkner LA, Miller D: An analysis of phlebitis in a 240 bed hospital. NITA 4:274, 1981
2. Larson E, Lunche S, Tran JT: Correlates of IV phlebitis. NITA 7:203, 1984
3. Jemison-Smith P, Thrupp LD: Phlebitis, infections, and filtration. NITA 5:328, 1982
4. Jones ER: Relationship between pH of intravenous medications and phlebitis: an experimental study. NITA 5:273, 1982
5. Hartman GE, Shochat SJ: Management of septic complications associated with Silastic catheters in childhood malignancy. Pediatr Infect Dis J 6:1042, 1987
6. Goodman MS, Wickham R: Venous access devices: an oncology nurse overview. Hosp Pharm 20:495, 1985
7. Simon RC: Small gauge central venous catheters and right atrial catheters. Semin Oncol Nurs 3:87, 1987
8. Markel S, Reynen K: Impact on patient care: 2652 PIC catheter days in the alternative setting. J Intraven Nurs 13:347, 1990
9. Brown JM: Peripherally inserted central catheters—use in home care. J Intraven Nurs 12:144, 1989
10. Lund GB, Lieberman RP, Haire WD et al: Translumbar inferior vena cava catheters for long-term access. Radiology 174:31, 1990
11. Camp LD: Care of the Groshong catheter. Oncol Nurs Forum 15:745, 1988
12. Winters V, Peters B, Coilà S, Jones L: A trial with a new peripheral implanted vascular access device. Oncol Nurs Forum 17:891, 1990
13. Hagle ME: Implantable devices for chemotherapy. Semin Oncol Nurs 3:96, 1987
14. Gallina EJ: Practical guide to chemotherapy administration for physicians and oncology nurses. p. 2570. In DeVita VT, Hellman S, Rosenberg SA (eds): Cancer Principles and Practice of Oncology. 4th Ed. JB Lippincott, Philadelphia, 1993
15. Alexander HR: Vascular access and other specialized techniques of drug delivery. p. 556. In DeVita VT, Hellman S, Rosenberg SA (eds): Cancer Principles and Practice of Oncology. 4th Ed. JB Lippincott, Philadelphia, 1993
16. Oncology Nursing Society: Access Device Guidelines: Module III—Pumps (Infusion Systems). Recommendations for Nursing Education and Practice. 1989
17. Mirro J, Rao BN, Kumar M et al: A comparison of placement techniques and complications of externalized catheters and implantable port use in children with cancer. J Pediatr Surg 25:120, 1990
18. Decker MD, Edwards KM: Central venous catheter infections. Pediatr Clin North Am 35:579, 1988
19. Ross MN, Haase GM, Poole MA et al: Comparison of totally implanted reservoirs with external catheters as venous access devices in pediatric oncologic patients. Surg Gynecol Obstet 167:141, 1988
20. Bottino J, McCredie KB, Groschel DHM, Lawson M: Long-term intravenous therapy with peripherally inserted silicone elastomer central venous catheters in patients with malignant disease. Cancer 43:1937, 1979
21. Shaw C, Newcomer L, Young J: Efficacy of Groshong catheters for oncology patients. Am Soc Clin Oncol Proc 8:335, 1989
22. Lucas AB: A critical review of venous access devices: the nursing perspective. Curr Issues Cancer Nurs Pract 1:1, 1992
23. Wurzel CL, Halom K, Feldman JG, Rubin LG: Infection rates of Broviac-Hickman catheters and implantable venous devices. Am J Dis Child 142:536, 1988
24. Ljung R, Petrini P, Lindgren AK, Berntorp E: Implantable central venous catheter facilitates prophylactic treatment in children with haemophilia. Acta Pediatr 81:918, 1992
25. Goodwin ML: The Seldinger method for PICC insertion. J Intraven Nurs 12:238, 1989
26. Velardi M, France K, Roemeling R et al: Usefulness of Per-Q-Cath as an intermediate access device to facilitate ambulatory chemotherapy. Proc Am Soc Clin Oncol 9:335, 1990
27. Press OW, Ramsey PG, Larson EB et al: Hickman catheter infections in patients with malignancies. Medicine 63:189, 1984
28. Lokich JL, Bothe A, Benotti P, Moore C: Complications and management of implanted venous access catheters. J Clin Oncol 3:710, 1985
29. Finney R, Albrink MH, Hart MB, Rosemurgy AS: A cost-effective peripheral venous port system placed at the bedside. J Surg Res 53:17, 1992

30. Morris P, Buller R, Kendall S, Anderson B: A peripherally implanted permanent central venous access device. Obstet Gynecol 78:1138, 1991

31. Hadaway LC: Evaluation and use of advanced I.V. technology. Part 1: central venous access devices. J Intraven Nurs 12:73, 1989

32. Kyle KS, Myers JS: Peripherally inserted central catheters: development of a hospital-based program. J Intraven Nurs 13:287, 1990

33. Reed WP, Newman KA, Applefeld MM, Sutton FJ: Drug extravasation as a complication of venous access ports. Ann Intern Med 102:788, 1985

34. Moosa HH, Juilian TB, Rosenfeld CS, Shadduck RK: Complications of indwelling central venous catheters in bone marrow transplant recipients. Surg Gynecol Obstet 172:275, 1991

35. Petersen FB, Clift RA, Hickman RO et al: Hickman catheter complications in marrow transplant recipients. JPEN J Parenter Enteral Nutr 10:58, 1986

36. Haire WD: Hickman line management. p. 419. In Armitage JO, Antman KH (eds): High-Dose Cancer Therapy: Pharmacology, Hematopoietins, Stem Cells. Williams & Wilkins, Baltimore, 1992

37. Kappers-Klunne MC, Degener JE, Stijnen T, Abels J: Complications from long-term indwelling central venous catheters in hematologic patients with special reference to infection. Cancer 64:1747, 1989

38. Mueller BU, Skelton J, Callender DPE et al: A prospective randomized trial comparing the infectious and noninfectious complications of an externalized catheter versus a subcutaneously implanted device in cancer patients. J Clin Oncol 10:1943, 1992

39. Carde P, Cosset-Delaigue MF, Laplanche A, Chareau I: Classic external indwelling central venous catheter versus totally implanted venous systems for chemotherapy administration: a randomized trial in 100 patients with solid tumors. Eur J Cancer Clin Oncol 25:939, 1989

40. Pegues D, Axelrod P, McClaren C et al: Comparison of infections in Hickman and implanted port catheters in adult solid tumor patients. J Surg Oncol 49:156, 1992

41. Skoutelis AT, Murphy RL, MacDonnell KB et al: Indwelling central venous catheter infections in patients with acquired immune deficiency syndrome. J Acquir Immune Defic Syndr 3:335, 1990

42. Raviglione MC, Battan R, Pablos-Mendez A et al: Infections associated with Hickman catheters in patients with acquired immunodeficiency syndrome. Am J Med 86:780, 1989

43. van der Pijl H, Frissen PHJ: Experience with a totally implantable venous access device (Port-A-Cath®) in patients with AIDS. AIDS 6:709, 1992

44. Robertson LJ, Mauro MA, Jaques PF: Radiologic placement of Hickman catheters. Radiology 170:1007, 1989

45. Abrahm JL, Mullen JL: A prospective study of prolonged central venous access in leukemia. JAMA 248:2868, 1982

46. Heimbach DM, Ivey TD: Technique for placement of a permanent home hyperalimentation catheter. Surg Gynecol Obstet 143:634, 1976

47. Jansen RF, Wiggers T, van Geel BN, van Putten WLJ: Assessment of insertion techniques and complication rates of dual lumen central venous catheters in patients with hematological malignancies. World J Surg 14:101, 1990

48. Gauderer MWL, Stellato TA: Subclavian Broviac catheters in children—technical considerations in 146 consecutive placements. J Pediatr Surg 20:402, 1985

49. Hawkins J, Nelson EW: Percutaneous placement of Hickman catheters for prolonged venous access. Am J Surg 144:624, 1982

50. Reed WP, Newman KA, deJongh C et al: Prolonged venous access for chemotherapy by means of the Hickman catheter. Cancer 52:185, 1983

51. Newman K, Tenney J, Reed W et al: Infectious and noninfectious complications of Hickman catheters, abstracted (345), p. 156. In Program and Abstracts of the American Society for Microbiology, Twenty-seventh Interscience Conference on Antimicrobial Agents and Chemotherapy, Washington, DC, 1987

52. Torosian MH, Meranze S, Mullen JL, McLean G: Central venous access with occlusive superior central venous thrombosis. Ann Surg 203:30, 1986

53. Williard W, Coit D, Lucas A, Groeger JS: Long-term vascular access via the inferior vena cava. J Surg Oncol 46:162, 1991

54. Bothe A, Piccione W, Ambrosino JJ et al: Implantable central venous access system. Am J Surg 147:565, 1984

55. Hubbard SM, Seipp CA: Administration of cancer treatments: practical guide for physicians and oncology nurses. p. 2189. In Devita VT, Hellman S, Rosenberg SA (eds): Cancer Principles and Practice of Oncology. 2nd Ed. JB Lippincott, Philadelphia, 1985

56. Cairo MS, Spooner S, Sowden L et al: Long term use of indwelling multipurpose silastic catheters in pediatric cancer patients treated with aggressive chemotherapy. J Clin Oncol 4:784, 1986

57. Wagman LD, Kerkemo A, Johnston MR: Venous access: a prospective, randomized study of the Hickman catheter. Surgery 95:303, 1984

58. Oncology Nursing Society: Access Device Guidelines: Module I—Catheters. Recommendations for Nursing Education and Practice. Pittsburgh, PA, 1989

59. Howser DM, Meade CD: Hickman catheter care. Developing organized teaching strategies. Cancer Nurs 10:70, 1987

60. Petrosino B, Becker H, Christian B: Infection rates in central venous catheter dressings. Oncol Nurs Forum 15:709, 1988

61. Conly JM, Grieves K, Peters B: A prospective, randomized study comparing transparent and dry gauze dressings for central venous catheters. J Infect Dis 159:310, 1989

62. Handy C: Vascular access devices: hospital to home care. J Intraven Nurs, suppl. 12:1, 1989

63. Stillman RM, Soliman F, Garcia L, Sawyer FN: Etiology of catheter-associated sepsis: correlation with thrombogenicity. Arch Surg 112:1497, 1977

64. Bern MM, Lokich JJ, Wallach SR et al: Very low doses of warfarin can prevent thrombosis in central venous catheters: a randomized prospective trial. Ann Intern Med 112:423, 1990

65. Bailey MJ: Reduction of catheter-associated sepsis in parenteral nutrition using low-dose intravenous heparin. BMJ 1:1671, 1979

66. Schwartz C, Hendrickson KJ, Roghmann K, Powell K: Prevention of bacteremia attributed to luminal colonization of tunneled central venous catheters with vancomycin-susceptible organisms. J Clin Oncol 8:1591, 1990

67. Barton JC, Poon M-C: Coagulation testing of Hickman catheter blood in patients with acute leukemia. Arch Intern Med 146:2165, 1986

68. Haire WD, Lieberman RP, Lund GB, Kessinger A: Translumbar inferior vena cava catheters. Bone Marrow Transplant 7:389, 1991

69. Oncology Nursing Society: Access Device Guidelines: Module II—Implanted Ports and Reservoirs. Recommendations for Nursing Education and Practice. Pittsburgh, PA, 1989

70. Long MC, Ovaska M: Comparative study of nursing protocols for venous access ports. Cancer Nurs 15:18, 1992

71. Moore CL, Erikson KA, Yanes LB et al: Nursing care and management of venous access ports. Oncol Nursing Forum 13:35, 1986

72. Reed WP, Newman KA, Tenney JH: An improved technique for the removal of longterm implantable central venous access lines. Surg Gynecol Obstet 161:479, 1985

73. Bagnall-Reeb HA, Ruccione K: Management of cutaneous reactions and mechanical complications of central venous access devices in pediatric patients with cancer: algorithms for decision making. Oncol Nurs Forum 17:677, 1990

74. Brothers TE, Von Moll LK, Niederhuber JE et al: Experience with subcutaneous infusion ports in three hundred patients. Surg Gynecol Obstet 166:295, 1988

75. Gerbarski SS, Gerbarski KS: Chemotherapy port "twiddler's syndrome": a need for preinjection radiography. Cancer 54:38, 1984

76. Lawson M, Bottino J, McCredia K: Long-term IV therapy: a new approach. Am J Nurs 79:1100, 1979

77. Williams DN, Gibson J, Vos J, Kind AE: Infusion thrombophlebitis and infiltration associated with intravenous cannula types. NITA 5:379, 1982

78. Groeger JS, Lucas A, Coit D et al: Totally implanted venous access ports in cancer patients: a prospective evaluation of morbidity. Proc Am Soc Clin Oncol 9:320, 1990

79. Ulz L, Petersen FB, Ford R et al: A prospective study of complications in Hickman right-atrial catheters in marrow transplant patients. JPEN J Parenter Enteral Nutr 14:27, 1990

80. Benezra D, Kiehn TE, Gold JWM et al: Prospective study of infections in indwelling central venous catheters using quantitative blood cultures. Am J Med 85:495, 1988

81. Ryan JA, Abel RM, Abbott WM et al: Catheter complications in total parenteral nutrition. N Engl J Med 290:757, 1974

82. Curry CR, Quie PG: Fungal septicemia in patients receiving parenteral hyperalimentation. N Engl J Med 285:1221, 1971

83. Allo MD, Miller J, Towsent T, Tan C: Primary cutaneous aspergillosis associated with Hickman intravenous catheters. N Engl J Med 317:1105, 1987

84. Krol TC, O'Keefe P: Brachial plexus neuritis and fatal hemorrhage following aspergillus infection of a Hickman catheter. Cancer 50:1214, 1982

85. Hoy JH, Rolston KVI, Hopfer RL, Bodey GF: *Mycobacterium fortuitum* bacteremia in patients with cancer and long-term venous catheters. Am J Med 83:213, 1987

86. Svirbely JR, Buesching WJ, Ayers LW et al: *Mycobacterium fortuitum* infection of a Hickman catheter site. Am J Clin Pathol 80:733, 1983

87. Brannan DP, DuBois RE, Ramirez MJ et al: Cefoxitin therapy for *Mycobacterium fortuitum* bacteremia with associated granulomatous. South Med J 77:381, 1984

88. Flynn PM, van Hooser B, Gigliotti F: Atypical mycobacterial infections of Hickman catheter exit sites. Pediatr Infect Dis J 7:510, 1988

89. Nelson MR, Shanson DC, Barter GJ et al: *Pseudomonas* septicaemia associated with HIV. AIDS 5:761, 1991

90. Roilides E, Marshall D, Venzon D et al: Bacterial infections in human immu-

nodeficiency virus type 1-infected children: the impact of central venous catheters and antiretroviral agents. Pediatr Infect Dis J 10:813, 1991

91. Roilides E, Butler KM, Husson RN: *Pseudomonas* infections in children with human immunodeficiency virus infection. Pediatr Infect Dis J 11:547, 1992

92. Johnson PR, Decker MD, Edwards KM et al: Frequency of Broviac catheter infections in pediatric oncology patients. J Infect Dis 154:570, 1986

93. Flynn PM, Shenep JL, Stokes DC, Barrett FF: In situ management of confirmed central venous catheter-related bacteremia. Pediatr Infect Dis J 6:729, 1987

94. Andremont A, Paulet R, Nitenberg G, Hill C: Value of semiquantitative cultures of blood drawn through catheter hubs for estimating the risk of catheter tip colonization in cancer patients. J Clin Microbiol 26:2297, 1988

95. Cercenado E, Ena J, Rodriguez-Creixéms M et al: A conservative procedure for the diagnosis of catheter-related infections. Arch Intern Med 150:1417, 1990

96. Moore CL: Nursing management of infusion catheters. p. 74. In Lokich I (ed): Cancer Chemotherapy by Infusion. Precept Press, Chicago, 1987

97. Dugdale DC, Ramsey PG: *Staphylococcus aureus* bacteremia in patients with Hickman catheters. Am J Med 89:137, 1990

98. Elting LS, Bodey GP: Septicemia due to *Xanthomonas* species and non-*aeruginosa Pseudomonas* species: increasing incidence of catheter-related infections. Medicine 69:296, 1990

99. Eppes SC, Troutman JL, Gutman LT: Outcome of treatment of candidemia in children whose central catheters were removed or retained. Pediatr Infect Dis J 8:99, 1989

100. Dato VM, Dajani AS: Candidemia in children with central venous catheters: role of catheter removal and amphotericin B therapy. Pediatr Infect Dis J 9:309, 1990

101. Cassidy FP, Zajko AB, Bron KM et al: Non-infectious complications of long-term central venous catheters. Radiologic evaluation and management. AJR 149:671, 1987

102. Ellerton J, Myers A, Graze P et al: Development of sheating clots on central venous catheters used for chemotherapy administration and blood drawing. Am Soc Clin Oncol Proc 8:330, 1989

103. Brismar B, Hardstedt C, Jacobson S: Diagnosis of thrombosis by catheter phlebography after prolonged central venous catheterization. Ann Surg 194:779, 1981

104. Ross AH, Griffith CD, Anderson JR, Grieve DC: Thromboembolic complications with silicone elastomer subclavian catheters. JPEN J Parenter Enteral Nutr 6:61, 1982

105. Walker TG, Geller SC, Waltman AC et al: A simple technique for redirection of malpositioned Broviac or Hickman catheters. Surg Gynecol Obstet 167:246, 1988

106. Lois JF, Gomes AS, Pusey E: Nonsurgical repositioning of central venous catheters. Radiology 165:329, 1987

107. Feinberg B, Hill C: The percutaneous peripherally inserted silicone central venous catheter (PPSC): an idea whose time has come. Am Soc Clin Oncol Proc 8:334, 1989

108. Horattas MC, Wright DJ, Fenton AH et al: Changing concepts of deep venous thrombosis of the upper extremity—report of a series and review of the literature. Surgery 104:561, 1988

109. Haire WD, Lieberman RP, Edney J et al: Hickman catheter-induced thoracic vein thrombosis. Cancer 66:900, 1990

110. Haire WD, Lynch TG, Lieberman RP et al: Utility of duplex ultrasound in the diagnosis of asymptomatic catheter-induced subclavian vein thrombosis. J Ultrasound Med 10:493, 1991

111. Haire WD, Lynch TG, Lund GB et al: Limitations of magnetic resonance imaging and ultrasound-directed (duplex) scans in the diagnosis of subclavian vein thrombosis. J Vasc Surg 13:391, 1991

112. Knudson CJ, Weidmeyer DA, Erickson SJ et al: Color Doppler sonographic imaging in the assessment of upper extremity deep venous thrombosis. AJR 154:399, 1990

113. Haire WD, Lynch TG, Lieberman RP, Edney JA: Duplex scans before subclavian vein catheterization predicts unsuccessful catheter placement. Arch Surg 127:229, 1992

114. Haire WD, Lieberman RP, Lund GB et al: Thrombotic complications of silicone rubber catheters during autologous marrow and peripheral stem cell transplantation: a prospective comparison of Hickman and Groshong catheters. Bone Marrow Transplant 7:57, 1991

115. Monreal M, Lafoz E, Ruiz J et al: Upper-extremity deep venous thrombosis and pulmonary embolism. Chest 99:280, 1991

116. Fraschini G, Jadeja J, Lawson M et al: Local infusion of urokinase for the lysis of thrombosis associated with permanent central venous catheters in cancer patients. J Clin Oncol 5:672, 1987

117. Donayre CE, White GH, Mehringer SM, Wilson SE: Pathogenesis determines late morbidity of axillosubclavian vein thrombosis. Am J Surg 152:179, 1986

118. Hurtubise MR, Bottino JC, Lawson M, McCredie KB: Restoring patency of occluded central venous catheters. Arch Surg 115:212, 1980

119. Glynn MFX, Langer B, Jeejeebhoy KN: Therapy for thrombotic occlusion of long term intravenous alimentation catheters. JPEN J Parenter Enteral Nutr 4:387, 1980

120. Lawson M: Partial occlusion of indwelling central venous devices. J Intraven Nurs 14:157, 1991

121. Rubin R: Local instillation of small doses of streptokinase for treatment of thrombotic occlusions of long term access catheters. J Clin Oncol 1:572, 1983

122. Atkinson JB, Bagnall HA, Gomperts E: Investigational use of tissue plasminogen activator (t-PA) for occluded central venous catheters. JPEN J Parenter Enteral Nutr 14:310, 1990

123. Rubenstein M, Creger WP: Successful streptokinase therapy for catheter-induced subclavian vein thrombosis. Arch Intern Med 140:1370, 1980

124. Sharma GVRK, Cella G, Parisi AF, Sasahara AA: Thrombolytic therapy. N Engl J Med 306:1268, 1982

125. Haire WD, Lieberman RP, Lund GB: Obstructed central venous catheters: restoring function with a 12-hour infusion of low-dose urokinase. Cancer 66:2279, 1990

126. Strum SB, McDermed JE: Drug extravasation and the Port-a-Cath system. Ann Intern Med 103:472, 1985

127. Kerr IG, Iscoe N, Sone M, Hanna S: Venous access ports. Ann Inter Med 103:637, 1985

128. Lokich JJ, Moore C: Drug extravasation in cancer chemotherapy. Ann Intern Med 104:124, 1986

129. Dorr RT: Discussion: What is the appropriate management of tissue extravasation by antitumor agents. Plast Reconstr Surg 75:403, 1985

130. Larson DL: What is the appropriate management of tissue extravasation by antitumor agents? Plast Reconstr Surg 75:387, 1985

131. Oncology Nursing Society: Cancer Chemotherapy Guidelines: Module V. Recommendations for the Management of Extravasation and Anaphylaxis. Pittsburgh, PA, 1988

132. Dorr RT, Alberts DS, Woods MW: Vinca alkaloid ulceration: experimental mouse model and effects of local antidotes. Proc Am Assoc Cancer Res 23:109, 1982

133. Dorr RT, Alberts DS: Skin ulceration potential without therapeutic anticancer activity for epipodophyllotoxin commercial diluents. Invest New Drugs 1:151, 1983

134. Owen O, Dellatorre DL, Scott EJ, Cohen MR: Accidental intramuscular injection of mechlorethamine. Cancer 45:2225, 1980

135. Whitehouse MW, Beck FW: Question of cyclophosphamide derived aldehydes and their effect on lymphocyte distribution in vivo: protective effect of thiols and bisulphate ions. Agents Actions 5:541, 1975

136. Olver IN, Aisner J, Hament A et al: A prospective study of topical dimethyl sulfoxide for treating anthracycline extravasation. J Clin Oncol 6:1732, 1988

137. DuPen SL, Peterson DG, Bogosian AC et al: A new permanent exteriorized epidural catheter for narcotic self-administration to control cancer pain. Cancer 59:986, 1987

138. DuPen SL, Peterson DG, Williams A, Bogosian AJ: Infection during chronic epidural catheterization: diagnosis and treatment. Anesthesiology 73:905, 1990

139. Hogan Q, Haddox JD, Abram S: Epidural opiates and local anesthetics for the management of cancer pain. Pain 46:271, 1991

140. Krames ES: Intrathecal infusional therapies for intractable pain: patient management guidelines. J Pain Symptom Mgmt 8:36, 1993

141. Crul BJ, Delhaas EM: Technical complications during the long-term subarachnoid or epidural administration of morphine in terminally ill cancer patients: a review of 140 cases. Reg Anaesth 16:209, 1991

142. Hahn MB, Bettencourt JA, McCrea WB: In vivo sterilization of an infected long-term epidural catheter. Anesth 76:645, 1992

143. Gourlay GK, Plummer JL, Cherry DA et al: Comparison of intermittent bolus with continuous infusion of epidural morphine in the treatment of severe cancer pain. Pain 47:135, 1991

144. Kwan JW: Use of infusion devices for epidural or intrathecal administration of spinal opioids. Am J Hosp Pharm, suppl 1. 47:S18, 1990

145. Plummer JL, Cherry DA, Cousins MJ et al: Long-term spinal administration of morphine in cancer and non-cancer pain: a retrospective study. Pain 44:215, 1991

146. Ommaya AK: Subcutaneous reservoir and pump for sterile access to ventricular cerebrospinal fluid. Lancet 2:983, 1963

147. Sundaresan N, Suite NDA: Optimal use of the Ommaya reservoir in clinical oncology. Oncology 3:15, 1989

148. Machado M, Salcman M, Kaplan RS, Montgomery E: Expanded role of the cerebrospinal fluid reservoir in neurooncology: indications, causes of revision, and complications. Neurosurgery 17:600, 1985

149. Gower DJ, Gower VC: Infected Ommaya reservoirs. Neurosurgery 22:1116, 1988

150. Obbens EAMT, Leavens ME, Beal JW, Lee Y-Y: Ommaya reservoir in 387 cancer patients: a 15 year experience. Neurology 35:1274, 1985

151. Lishner M, Perrin RG, Feld R et al: Complications associated with Ommaya reservoirs in patients with cancer. Arch Intern Med 150:173, 1990

152. Ratcheson RA, Ommaya AK: Experience with the subcutaneous cerebrospinal-fluid reservoir: preliminary report of 60 cases. N Engl J Med 279:1025, 1968

153. Siegal T, Pfeffer MR, Steiner I: Antibiotic therapy for infected Ommaya reservoir systems. Neurosurgery 22:97, 1988

154. Connors JM: Cure of Ommaya reservoir associated *Staphylococcus epidermidis* ventriculitis with a simple regimen of vancomycin and rifampin without reservoir removal. Med Pediatr Oncol 10:549, 1982

155. Sutherland GE, Palitang EG, Marr JJ, Leudke SL: Sterilization of Ommaya reservoir by instillation of vancomycin. Am J Med 71:1068, 1981

156. Wasserstrom WR, Glass JP, Posner JB: Diagnosis and treatment of leptomeningeal metastases from solid tumors: experience with 90 patients. Cancer 49:759, 1982

157. Glass JP, Lee Y-Y, Bruner J, Fields WS: Treatment-related leukoencephalopathy: a study of three cases and literature review. Medicine 65:154, 1986

158. Bleyer WA, Pizzo PA, Spence AM et al: The Ommaya reservoir: newly recognized complications and recommendations for insertion and use. Cancer 41:2431, 1978

HEMOSTASIS
AND
THROMBOSIS

Part VII

Megakaryocyte and Platelet Structure

96

William M. Isenberg and Dorothy Ford Bainton

INTRODUCTION

Circulating platelets—small, anucleate cells derived from megakaryocytes—serve important roles in normal hemostasis. Adequate numbers of these cells (140,000–440,000/mm³) are therefore required in the peripheral blood. At one extreme, when the absolute numbers of platelets in the periphery decrease, petechiae can occur. Alternatively, in other disease states, such as advanced atherosclerosis, inappropriate platelet activation, adhesion, and aggregation can contribute to morbidity and mortality. It is therefore important to understand the numerous basic cell-biologic processes that cells of the megakaryocyte lineage undergo, with the aim of finding ways to encourage hemostasis when needed and to avoid pathologic thrombosis when it poses a threat to the patient. Analysis of the structure of these cell types has provided insight into their functions, which have been further elucidated in studies using basic cell-biologic methods. This chapter discusses megakaryocyte and platelet structure/function relationships, with special emphasis on protein synthesis and packaging (granule formation), adhesive interactions, shape change, and secretion from storage organelles. Figure 96-1 illustrates the major organelles of the circulating unstimulated platelet, the end-stage cell of this lineage.

MEGAKARYOCYTES

Cell Maturation and Ploidy

Bone marrow smears stained with Romanovsky dyes display the following cells of the megakaryocytic series: stage I—deeply basophilic, small (15–50 μm), immature megakaryoblasts, with a rounded or only slightly indented nucleus and numerous nucleoli; stage II—granular, maturing megakaryocytes (20–80 μm), often with lobulated nuclei; and stage III—more azurophilic, mature megakaryocytes (20–150 μm) containing eccentric, distinctly lobulated nuclei. Zucker-Franklin[1] provides a color view of these various stages. With maturation, the nucleus becomes more polyploid, the ploidy increasing from 2N to as high as 64N, with a mean of 16N. Ploidy is classically measured by densitometric analysis of Feulgen-stained cells,[2] although propidium iodide staining followed by fluorescence-activated cell sorting (FACS) analysis has more recently been used.[3–5] There is no distinct correspondence between cytoplasmic maturation and nuclear ploidy, however.[2] Megakaryoblasts tend to be 2–4N and mature megakaryocytes of higher ploidy. However, two cells of identical staining and size may differ in ploidy class. These largest cells of hematopoiesis constitute approximately 0.37% of the bone marrow.[6]

Light microscopic examination shows cells of the megakaryocyte lineage to be negative for peroxidase, Sudan black B, naphthol AS-D chloroacetate esterase, and α-naphthol butyrate esterase. They are positive with periodic acid-Schiff and acid phosphatase stains. They may also be positive for α-naphthyl acetate, the reaction being inhibited by fluoride.[7]

The maturational pathway of the megakaryocyte-platelet lineage is illustrated in Figure 96-2. As shown in the diagram, the burst-forming unit-megakaryocyte (BFU-Mk) cells bear immunologic markers similar to those of other bone marrow progenitor cell types.[8–11] Glycoprotein (GP) IIb/IIIa has been detected in colony-forming unit-megakaryocyte (CFU-Mk) cells and confirms the lineage at that stage.[12] Pluripotent stem cells have been shown to lack the GPIIb subunit.[13] Previously, the megakaryoblast was the earliest identifiable stage, discernable using the cytochemical platelet peroxidase reaction.[14] The megakaryoblast stage of development is important because endomitosis begins during this stage, and the cells begin to accumulate the α-granule proteins von Willebrand factor (vWF), thrombospondin (TSP), platelet factor-4 (PF-4), and β-thromboglobulin (β-TG), as well as the vWF receptor protein GPIb.[10]

Protein Synthesis and Packaging

The ultrastructural features of a maturing megakaryocyte (stage II) are illustrated in Figure 96-3. As is consistent with a high synthetic activity, rough endoplasmic reticulum (RER)

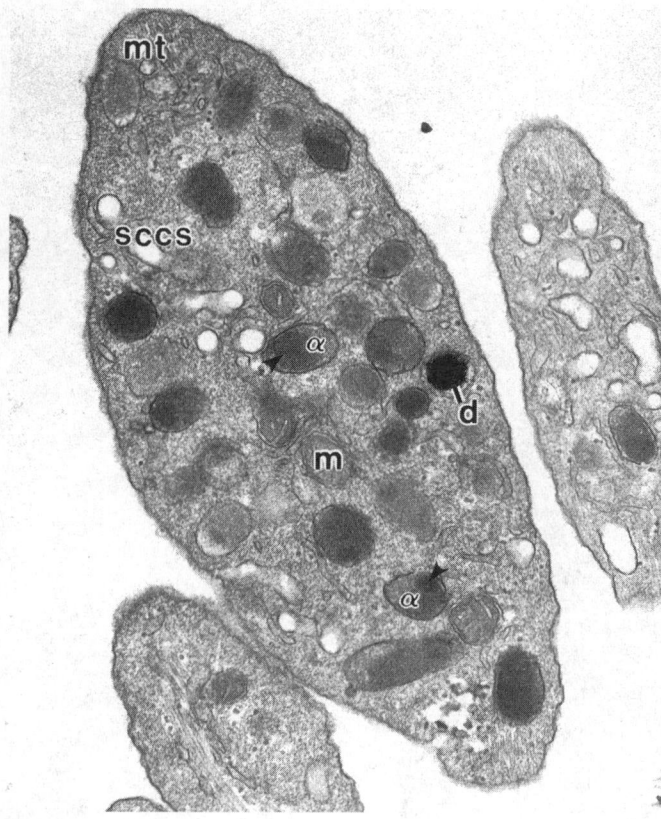

Fig. 96-1. Circulating platelet. Shaped like a disc, platelets contain numerous α-granules (α) with nucleoids (arrowheads), occasional osmiophilic dense bodies (d), and mitochondria (m). Tracer studies demonstrate that the surface-connected canalicular system (sccs) is in continuity with the extracellular milieu. Each platelet contains a circumferential microtubular coil (mt), cut in cross section. (× 37,500.)

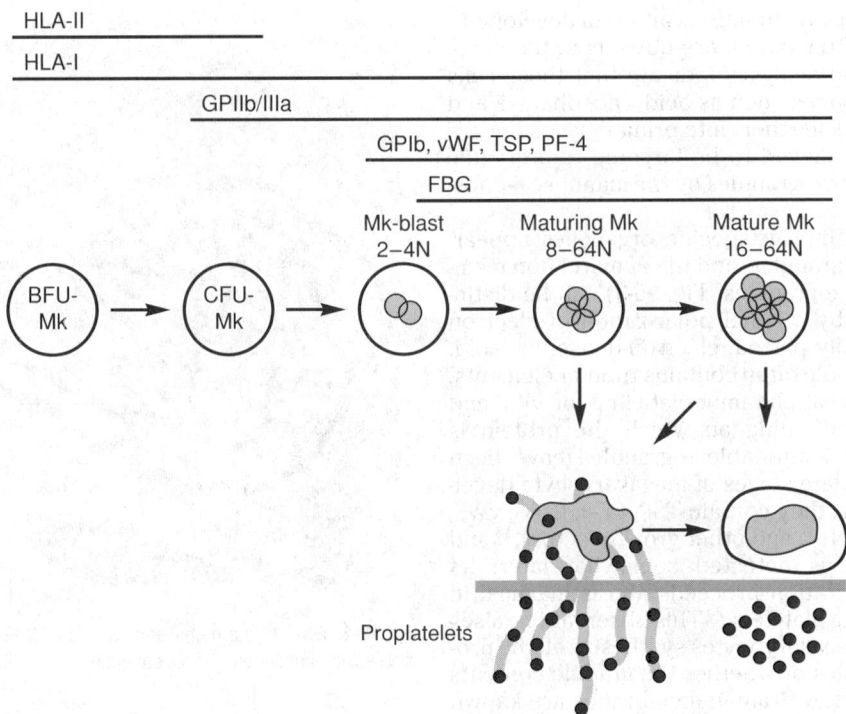

Fig. 96-2. Megakaryocyte maturation. BFU-Mk and CFU-Mk stages are indistinguishable from other bone marrow progenitor cells on morphologic grounds, and cells of both stages bear immunologic markers (HLA-1, -2) of other undifferentiated stem cells. The lineage can be confirmed at the CFU-Mk stage by the appearance of GPIIb/IIIa. GPIb and the α-granule proteins vWF, TSP, PF-4, β-TG, and fibrinogen (FBG) are not detectable until the megakaryoblast stage, and, although detectable earlier, FBG is not conspicuous until the mature megakaryocyte stage. Proplatelets or individual cells may be shed from either maturing or mature megakaryocytes. Once all the platelets have been shed, a bare nucleus remains. (Data from Bessis,[8] Bentfeld-Barker and Bainton,[9] Vainchenker and Kieffer,[10] Hoffman,[11] and Molla et al.[13])

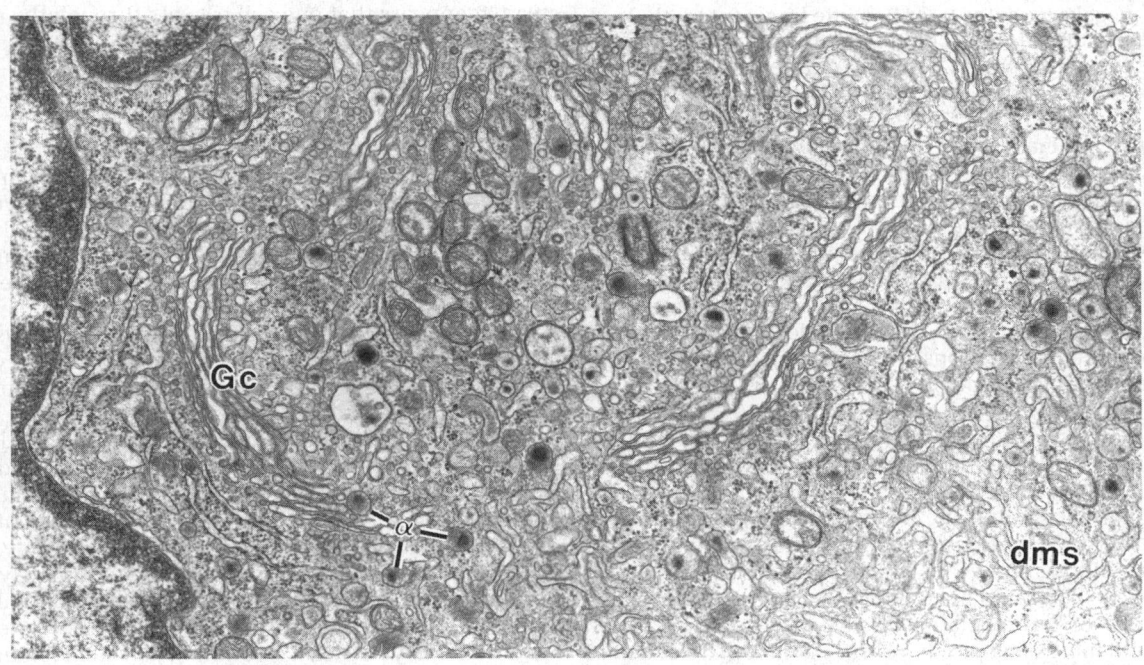

Fig. 96-3. Maturing megakaryocyte. During this stage of maturation, there are numerous Golgi complexes (Gc) with budding vesicles. α-Granules (α) with their dense nucleoids begin to appear. dms, demarcation membrane system. (× 16,000.)

profiles and Golgi cisternae are numerous and well developed.[9] Vesicles, both coated and uncoated, are obvious in the juxta-Golgi region. Cytochemical analyses indicate that these cells synthesize lysosomal enzymes such as acid phosphatase and aryl sulfatase and then package them into primary lysosomes.[15] Lysosomal enzymes are believed to be targeted to a granule population distinct from the α-granules by the mannose 6-phosphate receptor.[16]

With maturation, more lineage-specific organelles appear, namely, α-granules, dense granules, and the demarcation membrane system (DMS). The α-granules (Fig. 96-3) can be distinguished morphologically by a zonal polarization of electron density and an eccentrically placed, electron-dense nucleoid. The more electron-lucent pole often contains tubular elements, found to be sites of preferential immunolabeling for vWF and possibly serving as a scaffolding on which the protein is stored.[17] Morphologically identifiable α-granules have been seen at early, middle, and late stages of megakaryocyte development; at all these stages, they contain TSP, PF-4, β-TG, vWF, platelet-derived growth factor, and other growth factors,[18] and osteonectin.[19] Fibrinogen is detected somewhat later; its amount increases as maturation proceeds and is maximal in the α-granules of circulating platelets.[20] This observation raises the question of whether megakaryocytes synthesize all the proteins contained in α-granules or whether the granule contents are acquired in other ways. α-Granule membranes are known to contain P-selectin.[21,22]

Endocytosis

Although the megakaryocytic synthesis of some platelet α-granule proteins (PF-4, β-TG, vWF, TSP) is well accepted, there is growing controversy regarding fibrinogen.[23–25] Recently, Handagama et al[24] showed that megakaryocytes can endocytose fibrinogen, albumin, and IgG from the plasma and can incorporate these proteins into α-granules. Subsequently, in a series of experiments using kistrin and barbourin (RGD- or KGD-containing peptides purified from snake venoms), Handagama and co-workers[26–28] showed that fibrinogen incorporation into megakaryocyte α-granules is mediated by GPIIb/IIIa. When these megakaryocytes later become fragmented, their α-granules are contained in circulating platelets. Thus, platelet α-granules appear to contain proteins derived from both endogenous synthesis and endocytosis of plasma proteins synthesized by other cell types.[29] The capacity for endocytosis of α-granule proteins makes the megakaryocyte more complex than other cells that produce secretory granules.

Another distinct granule population, the dense granules, also employ an exogenous uptake pathway to incorporate serotonin.[30] These granules also contain adenine nucleotides, pyrophosphate, and calcium and their membranes appear to contain granulophysin and P-selectin.[31–33] Their inherent electron density, with a characteristic peripheral halo, makes them visible in whole-mount preparations. They can be positively identified by the uranaffin reaction.[34,35]

Platelet Formation

An additional lineage-specific ultrastructural specialization of the megakaryocyte is the appearance and proliferation of the DMS. This diffuse organelle, which begins to appear early in maturation, is illustrated in Figure 96–4. The DMS may mark the boundaries of future platelet fields and becomes more prominent with increasing ploidy.[9] Once distinct platelet fields have been sufficiently delineated in the mature megakaryocyte, cytoplasmic fragmentation ensues. It is not clear whether individual platelets break from the megakaryocyte or whether frag-

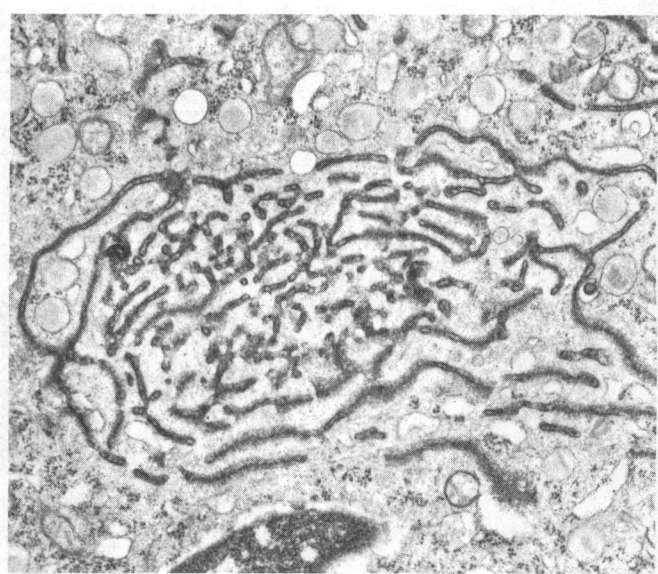

Fig. 96-4. DMS of the megakaryocyte. The DMS, here stained with tannic acid, marks the boundaries of future platelets. (× 12,500.)

mentation proceeds by the morphologically better documented and more widely accepted proplatelet scheme of formation.[36,37] The site of platelet release is also actively contested. Most investigators think that proplatelets are released through the sinus endothelial cells, as depicted in Figure 96–2. However, others postulate that megakaryocytes undergo cytoplasmic fragmentation in the pulmonary capillary beds.[38] Small numbers of megakaryocytes do circulate and, if mature, probably undergo fragmentation in the capillary bed in which they lodge. Whether all megakaryocytes have an obligatory stage of life in the pulmonary vasculature remains to be proved.

Occasionally, other nucleated cells (lymphocytes, neutrophils, erythrocytes) are observed within the megakaryocyte cytoplasm.[8,39] This process, known as emperipolesis, does not represent phagocytosis on the part of the megakaryocyte. Instead, it appears that one cell transits through the megakaryocyte DMS without injuring either cell.

PLATELETS

In normal persons, quiescent discoid platelets spend on average 7–10 days in the circulation before being removed by the reticuloendothelial system. The ultrastructural features of resting platelets are illustrated schematically in Figure 96-5 and pictorially in Figure 96-1. Each cell contains a single peripheral microtubule coil,[40] which, along with a subplasmalemmal actin membrane skeleton,[41] likely serves to control the discoid platelet shape. Peripheral to the microtubule coil, the cytoplasm is poor in organelles, except for the plasma membrane itself and its surface invaginations, the surface-connected canalicular system (SCCS). Both membranes are richly invested by a glycocalyx that can be seen well when tannic acid is added to the fixative. Recall the megakaryocyte in Figure 96-4, in which tannic acid labels the DMS, the membranes of which are destined to become platelet plasma membranes. Presumably, this glycocalyx comprises the several integral membrane glycoproteins such as GPIb/IX, GPIIb/IIIa, and GPIIIb (IV) that participate in platelet adhesion and aggregation. Thus, the platelet plasma membrane plays at least two important hemostatic roles: (1) in cell-cell and cell-matrix interactions, and (2) in aiding fluid-phase coagulation. Although the various components of the enzyme-substrate complexes that constitute the coagulation

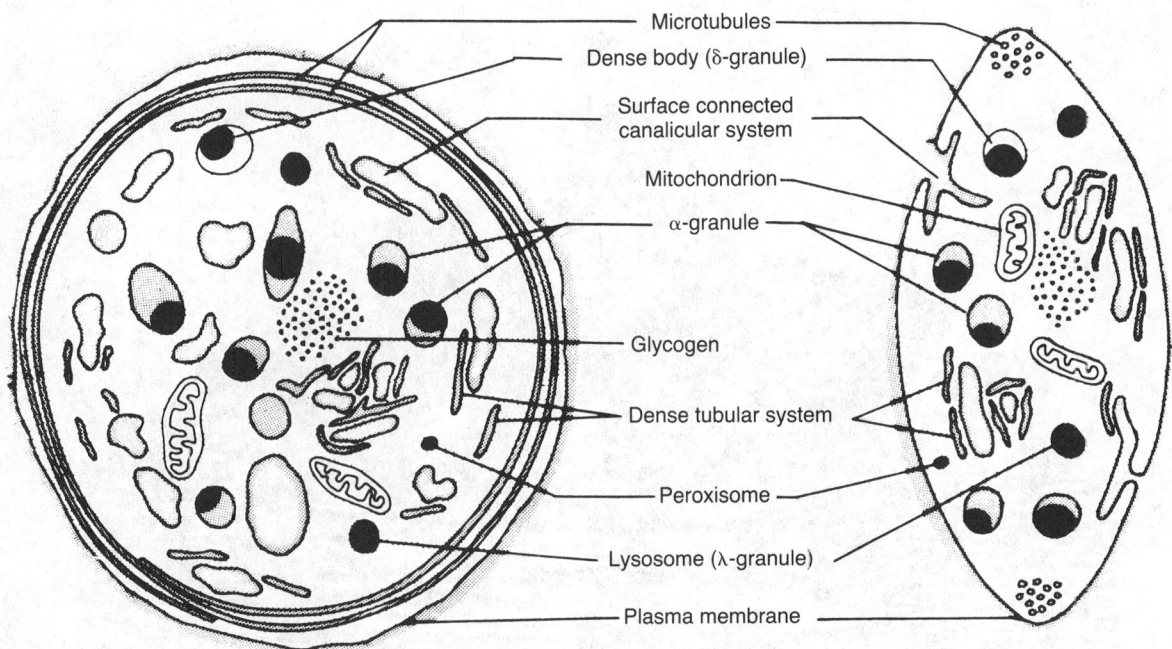

Fig. 96-5. Schematic of platelet organelles. (From Bentfeld-Barker and Bainton,[9] with permission.)

pathway can interact in the fluid phase, the rate of the reaction increases by at least 1,000-fold in the presence of a phospholipid surface.[42] The platelet plasma membrane acts as this surface and serves to enrich the local concentrations of reactants such as factors X, V, and prothrombin (see Ch. 100). In addition, the platelet α-granule contains some factor V, which, when secreted, participates in this process (see the section Secretion).

Within the confines of the microtubular coil, one finds the secretory granules of the platelet, the α- and dense granules; mitochondria, peroxisomes, and lysosomes; glycogen stores; and two membrane systems, the SCCS, and the dense tubular system. The dense tubular system is thought to be a remnant of the megakaryocyte RER, presumably the site of prostaglandin synthesis in platelets[43]; it serves as a storage site for calcium in circulating cells, a function analogous to that of the sarcoplasmic reticulum of skeletal myocytes.[44]

Activation by a platelet agonist, such as ADP, epinephrine, collagen, or thrombin, when bound to its receptor,[45] causes profound biochemical alterations.[46] In addition, activation enhances cell interactions and induces platelet shape change and secretion.

Heterotypic and Homotypic Adhesive Interactions

After a breach of the vasculature, exposing the subendothelium to flowing blood, platelets interact with other cell types or with extracellular matrix material (e.g., immobilized vWF, collagen, laminin, fibronectin) in a series of events referred to as adhesion. The molecular interactions that are believed to account for platelet adhesion are discussed at length in Chapters 97 and 98; important receptors and their respective ligands include GPIb/IX—vWF[47]; GPIa/IIa (VLA-2)—collagen[48]; GPIc/IIa (VLA-5)—fibronectin[49]; and VLA-6—laminin.[50] Distinct from platelet adhesion is aggregation, the process wherein activated platelets participate to form platelet thrombi. The early phase of aggregation is reversible, whereas the later phase is irreversible. The early phase is mediated by the interaction of GPIIb/IIIa with fibrinogen,[49] and the later phase may be mediated by other receptors and ligands.[51] Both platelet adhesion and

aggregation in vivo are illustrated in Figure 96-6. Since platelet aggregation involves changes in platelet shape and secretion of granule contents, these two processes are now described.

Shape Change

The unstimulated platelet, as seen with the scanning electron microscope, is shown in Figure 96-7A. After activation with thrombin, the cells develop numerous long filopodial projections (Fig. 96-7B). This change in shape can be observed in aggregometry tracings as well, as the cells change from a discoid to a more spherical, albeit spiny, morphology. Shape change serves at least two major functions. It not only increases the surface area of the platelet,[55] serving as a membrane reservoir that can be added to the plasma membrane following activation,[56] but also increases the likelihood that portions of adjacent cells will interact and initiate aggregation. The ultrastructural correlates of shape change, as seen in thin sections, are depicted in Figure 96-7C. Initially, filopodial projections of organelle-poor cytoplasm are seen peripheral to the microtubular coil (Fig. 96-7C). The actin cytoskeleton, rather than the microtubular coil, appears to regulate change in shape. Close inspection of Figure 96-7C reveals that filopodia have formed while the coil is still intact. Furthermore, profiles of microtubules cannot be seen in platelet projections by electron microscopy until several minutes after thrombin stimulation.

Secretion

The two major secretory granule populations of the platelet are the α-granules and the dense granules. The ultrastructure of the α-granule is shown in Figure 96-3 and that of the dense granule in Figure 96-1. The contents of these secretory organelles can be identified using immunocytochemical approaches, such as that illustrated in Figure 96-8, showing the α-granular distribution of immunoreactive fibrinogen.[57-59] α-Granule contents and their presumed role(s) are discussed in more detail in Chs. 97 and 98.

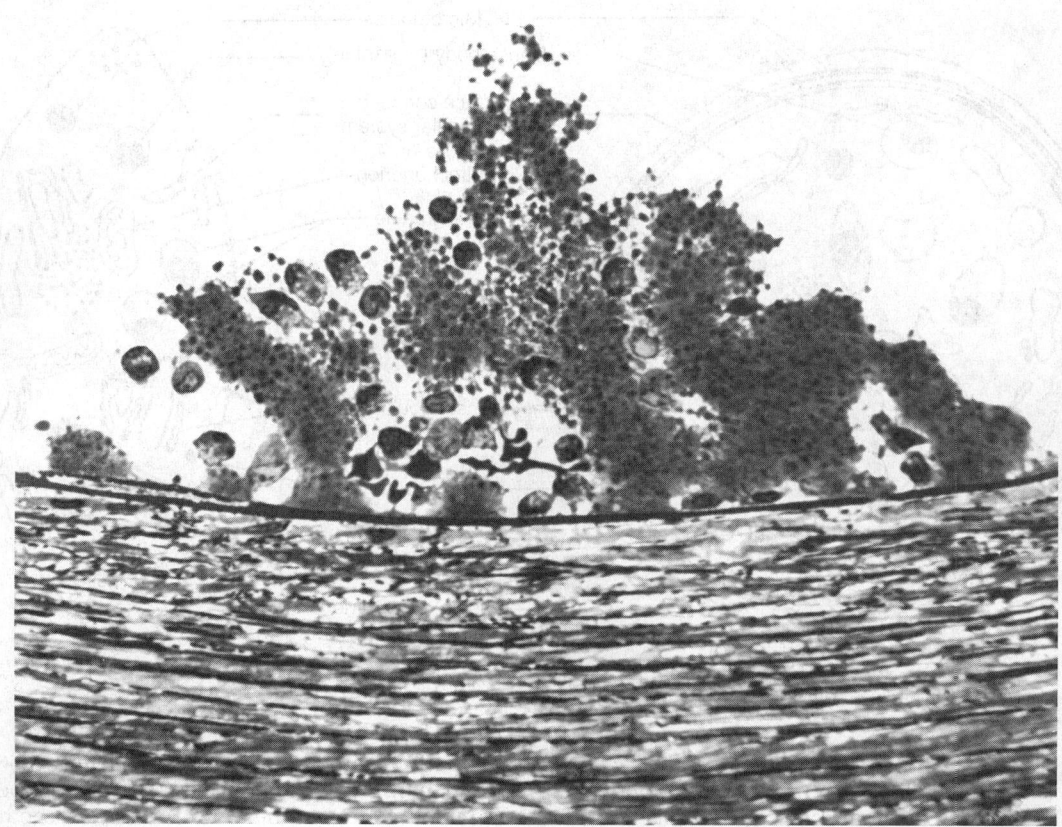

Fig. 96-6. Platelet adhesion and aggregation in vivo. The process of denuding rabbit aorta has initiated both platelet adhesion and platelet aggregation. (× 820.) (From Baumgartner,[52] with permission.)

Several of the interactions between activated platelets and other cells or matrix material appear to be mediated by adhesive proteins bound to receptors on the platelet surface. Many of these ligands are stored in α-granules, which secrete their contents in response to a high dose of a platelet agonist such as thrombin or ADP. The exocytotic pathway in platelets is unusual. As the cell changes in shape, the secretory granules (and other organelles) become increasingly centralized within a constricting microtubular coil (Fig. 96-7C). The α-granules fuse with one another and with the SCCS, which in turn becomes progressively dilated[60] (Fig. 96-7D). α-Granule contents can be detected by immunocytochemical techniques within the dilated SCCS and on the plasma membrane. Secretion from the SCCS to the extracellular fluid is accomplished through a widening of the pores of the SCCS on the plasma membrane.[53] Surface expression of a granule membrane protein of 140 kd (P-selectin) accompanies α-granule secretion.[21,22,61,62] Immunoreactive P-selectin (CD62) is restricted to granule membranes in resting cells (Fig. 96-9). Once secretion has begun, the protein is rapidly and uniformly redistributed to the SCCS and plasma membrane[21,63] (Fig. 96-10).

Analysis of sequence homologies has shown that P-selectin is a member of a new family of lectin-like cell adhesion molecules.[61,64,65] Other family members include the endothelial leukocyte adhesion molecule-1 and the lymphocyte homing receptor, Mel-14 antigen. P-selectin has been shown to bind to human neutrophils and monocytes,[66] as well as to human memory T lymphocytes and natural killer cells.[67] Antibodies directed against P-selectin blocked leukocyte incorporation into a forming thrombus in a baboon model system.[68] In addition, we have recently observed that contact zones of irreversibly aggregated platelets contain immunoreactive P-selectin but lack the integrin GPIIb/IIIa and its ligand fibrinogen. Measurement of P-selectin expression may become a powerful tool in laboratory medicine. Figure 96-11 shows a FACS analysis of platelets, in unstimulated and stimulated states. It is clear that a population of activated platelets (larger volume, surface expression of P-selectin antigen) can be found in the stimulated sample. The full potential of this method of monitoring patients with hypercoagulable states or patients who are predisposed toward pathologic thrombosis has yet to be realized.[69]

Clot Retraction

Once the platelets that have aggregated into a thrombus have successfully closed the defect in the vessel wall, the clot in vivo presumably undergoes the same phenomenon seen in the test tube—clot retraction. When the blood clot retracts, the edges of the wound are drawn together. A restriction of the luminal size of the thrombus also ensures continued patency of the vessel and, thus, perfusion of the tissue served by it. Figure 96-12 shows the complex mosaic that forms after several minutes of thrombin stimulation. This ultrastructural appearance is due to the intricate interactions among several cell projections. Note that the cell cytoplasm is essentially devoid of organelles, the platelets having undergone viscous metamorphosis.[70] This phenomenon, observable only when considerable time has elapsed after stimulation, may be mediated by the interaction of the integrin GPIIb/IIIa with the actin cytoskeleton. Phillips et al[71] showed an association between the fibrinogen receptor and actin in vitro, 30 minutes after stimulation was initiated. Preliminary data from our laboratory indicate that the cytoskeletal protein talin, as well as vinculin, may be involved in this association. Others have shown an analogous interaction among fibronectin, the fibronectin receptor, and talin in the chick fibroblast system.[72]

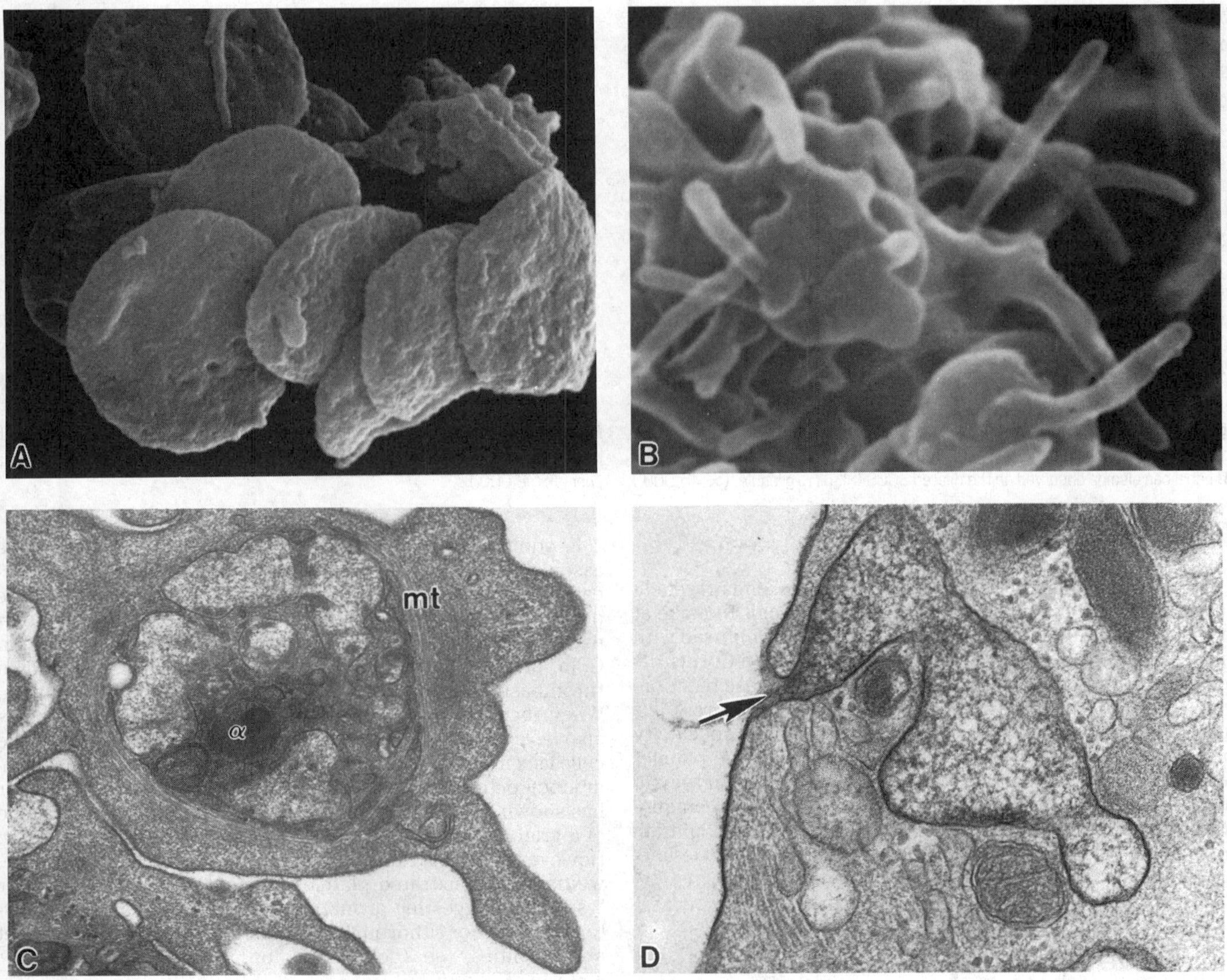

Fig. 96-7. Changes in platelets after activation. **(A)** Resting discoid platelet as seen by scanning electron microscopy (SEM) (× 7,000.) (From Stenberg et al,[53] with permission.) **(B)** Platelet activated with ADP develops long, slender filopodial projections, by SEM. (× 21,000.) **(C)** Similar projections, as well as centralized α-granules (α) and the constricting microtubular coil (mt), seen after thrombin stimulation, by thin-section electron microscopy. (× 32,000.) **(D)** With activation, granules fuse with the dilated SCCS (stained with tannic acid), connected with the cell exterior through narrow pores (arrow). Through such openings, α-granule contents are secreted. (× 65,000.) (From Stenberg et al,[54] with permission.)

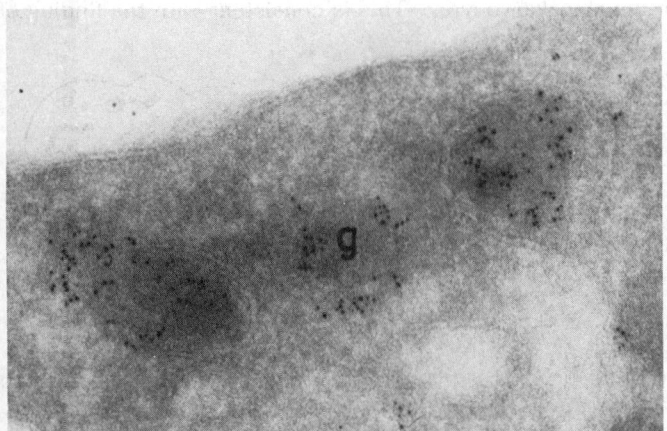

Fig. 96-8. Immunocytochemical localization of fibrinogen in α-granules. Gold-labeled antifibrinogen binds to α, α-granule (g) contents. (× 50,000.)

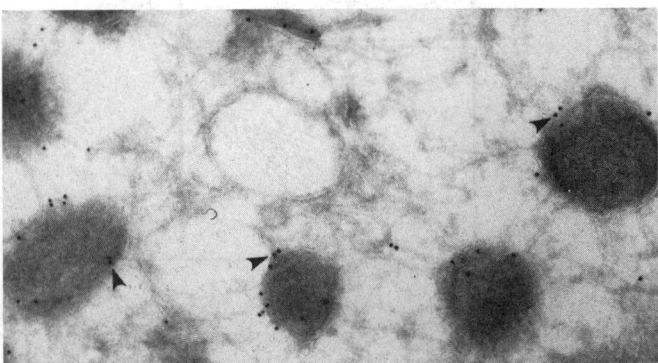

Fig. 96-9. Immunocytochemical localization of P-selectin in platelets. The immunogold label (arrowheads) decorates the α-granule membranes. (× 48,000)

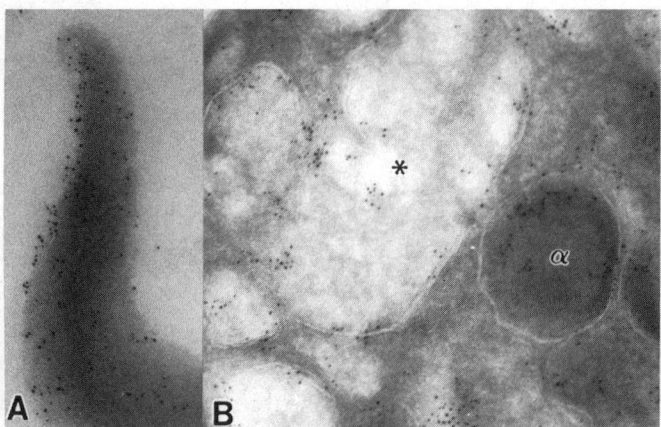

Fig. 96-10. Immunolocalization of P-selectin following platelet activation. **(A)** The immunoprobe is found along the plasma membrane, extending out along filopodia. **(B)** Label can also be observed on the dilated SCCS (*). α, α-granule. (× 45,000.)

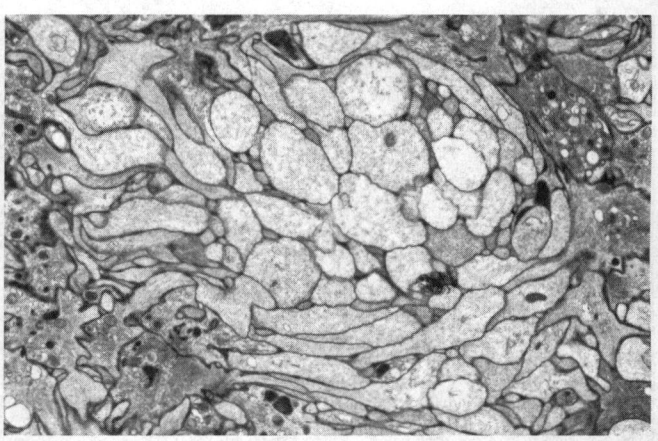

Fig. 96-12. Clot retraction and viscous metamorphosis. Platelets activated with thrombin for 15 minutes form complex interactions, retract, and become organelle poor. (× 2,000.)

Pathology of the Megakaryocytic Lineage

The diagnosis of acute megakaryoblastic leukemia (French-American-British classification M7) can be difficult to make at the light microscopic level, as the cells are often confused with those seen in acute lymphocytic leukemia. Breton-Gorius developed the electron microscopic platelet peroxidase reaction, which positively identifies this lineage in the bone marrow.[14,73] Figure 96-13 contrasts the myeloperoxidase reaction specificity for cells of the myeloid lineage (Fig. 96-13A) with the platelet peroxidase reaction, which is specific for the megakaryocytic lineage (Fig. 96-13B). Currently, this technique has been supplanted by immunocytochemistry for GPIIb/IIIa at the light microscopic level, a specific marker for the megakaryocyte lineage that is also expressed early in maturation.[74,75]

In addition to neoplasia, several congenital conditions are associated with altered platelet morphology. Storage pool disease is a heterogeneous group of disorders in which there are decreased amounts of granule products found in platelets. Bernard-Soulier syndrome, characterized by platelets deficient in GPIb, are also considerably larger than normal. Glanzmann thrombasthenia platelets lack or are deficient in GPIIb/IIIa. When there is a total absence of this integrin, the α-granules also lack fibrinogen. Finally, in the gray platelet syndrome, the cells lack morphologically normal α-granules. Interestingly, immunocytochemical analysis of the cells from this last disorder has shown that they contain P-selectin; therefore, the absence of α-granule formation is not due to the absence of P-selectin. However, in at least one patient with αδ-storage pool disease, we have demonstrated platelet phenotypic heterogeneity for P-selectin, suggesting formation defects during megakaryocytopoiesis.[76] (For a thorough discussion of these several platelet abnormalities, see Zucker-Franklin,[1] Stenberg and Bainton,[57] and Chs. 129 and 130.)

Lastly, thrombocytopenia is among the myriad signs of infection with the human immunodeficiency virus (HIV) (see Ch. 155). The pathogenesis of this decreased platelet count was initially ascribed to an immune-mediated destructive process analogous to that seen in idiopathic thrombocytopenic purpura. However, recent evidence indicates that, although platelet survival in HIV-infected individuals is modestly shortened, there is likely a more basic production abnormality at the level of the megakaryocyte.[77] This is consistent with the finding of

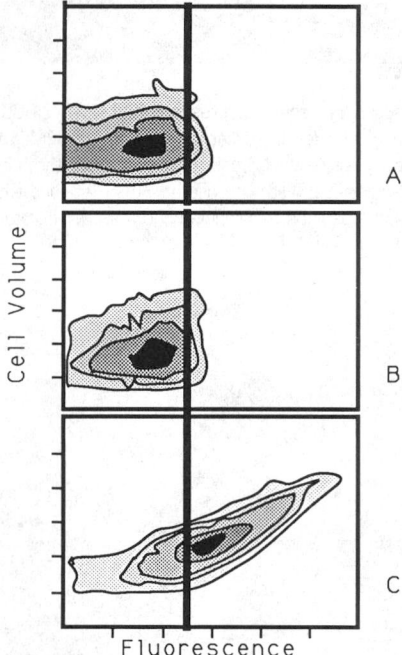

Fig. 96-11. Flow cytometric analysis of activation-dependent change in platelet volume and surface expression of P-selectin. **(A)** Histogram of resting platelets, stained with control antiserum. **(B)** Unstimulated cells stained with anti-P-selectin. **(C)** Stimulated cells stained with anti-P-selectin. (Courtesy of Drs. Laurence Corash and Margaret Rheinschmidt.)

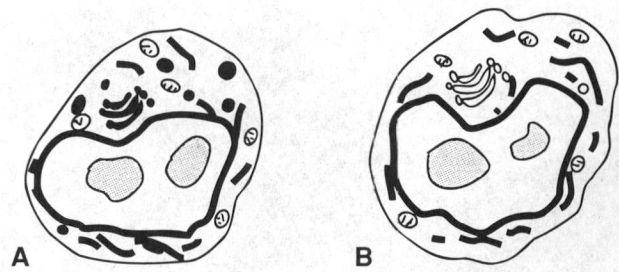

Fig. 96-13. Subcellular distribution of the reaction products for myeloperoxidase and platelet peroxidase. **(A)** Cells of the myeloid lineage have myeloperoxidase activity in the perinuclear cisterna, in the Golgi apparatus, and in azurophilic granules. **(B)** Cells of the megakaryocytic lineage have platelet peroxidase activity in the perinuclear cisternae and endoplasmic reticulum. By contrast, the Golgi complex and any formed granules are peroxidase negative.

HIV RNA in these cells and the demonstration of ultrastructurally abnormal megakaryocytes in bone marrow biopsy specimens of HIV-infected patients.[78] Given that the marrow of such individuals usually contains normal or increased numbers of megakaryocytes, the virus probably interferes with megakaryocyte maturation or platelet fragmentation, or both.

REFERENCES

1. Zucker-Franklin D: Megakaryocytes and platelets. p. 621. In Zucker-Franklin D, Greaves MF, Grossi CE, Marmont AM (eds): Atlas of Blood Cells. Vol 2. 2nd Ed. Lea & Febiger, Philadelphia, 1988
2. Paulus J-M: DNA metabolism and development of organelles in guinea-pig megakaryocytes: a combined ultrastructural, autoradiographic and cytophotometric study. Blood 35:298, 1970
3. Jackson CW, Brown LK, Sommerville BC et al: Two-color flow cytometric measurement of DNA distributions of rat megakaryocytes in unfixed, unfractionated marrow cell suspensions. Blood 63:768, 1984
4. Corash L, Chen HY, Levin J et al: Regulation of thrombopoiesis: effects of the degree of thrombocytopenia on megakaryocyte ploidy and platelet volume. Blood 70:177, 1987
5. Tomer A, Harker LA, Burstein SA: Flow cytometric analysis of normal human megakaryocytes. Blood 71:1244, 1988
6. Levine RF: Isolation and characterization of normal human megakaryocytes. Br J Haematol 45:487, 1980
7. Bennett JM, Catovsky D, Daniel M-T et al: Criteria for the diagnosis of acute leukemia of megakaryocyte lineage (M7). A report of the French-American-British Cooperative Group. Ann Intern Med 103:460, 1985
8. Bessis M: Blood Smears Reinterpreted. Springer International, Berlin, 1977, p. 131
9. Bentfeld-Barker ME, Bainton DF: Ultrastructure of rat megakaryocytes after prolonged thrombocytopenia. J Ultrastruct Res 61:201, 1977
10. Vainchenker W, Kieffer N: Human megakaryocytopoiesis: in vitro regulation and characterization of megakaryocytic precursor cells by differentiation markers. Blood Rev 2:102, 1988
11. Hoffman R: Regulation of megakaryocytopoiesis. Blood 74:1196, 1989
12. Levene RB, Lamaziere JMD, Broxmeyer HE et al: Human megakaryocytes. V. Changes in the phenotypic profile of differentiating megakaryocytes. J Exp Med 161:457, 1985
13. Molla A, Andrieux A, Chapel A et al: Lack of transcription of the αIIb integrin in human early haematopoietic stem cells. Br J Haematol 82:635, 1992
14. Breton-Gorius J, Guichard J: Ultrastructural localization of peroxidase activity in human platelets and megakaryocytes. Am J Pathol 66:277, 1972
15. Bentfeld-Barker ME, Bainton DF: Identification of primary lysosomes in human megakaryocytes and platelets. Blood 59:472, 1982
16. Kornfeld S: Trafficking of lysosomal enzymes. FASEB J 1:462, 1987
17. Cramer EM, Meyer D, LeMenn R et al: Eccentric localization of von Willebrand factor within a tubular structure of platelet α-granules resembling that of Weibel-Palade bodies. Blood 66:710, 1985
18. Aglietti M, Monzeglio C, Apra F et al: In vivo priming of human normal neutrophils by granulocyte-macrophage colony stimulating factor: effect on the production of platelet activating factor. Br J Haematol 75:333, 1990
19. Breton-Gorius J, Clezardin P, Guichard J et al: Localization of platelet osteonectin at the internal face of the α-granule membranes in platelets and megakaryocytes. Blood 79:936, 1992
20. Cramer EM, Debili N, Martin JF et al: Uncoordinated expression of fibrinogen compared with thrombospondin and von Willebrand factor in maturing human megakaryocytes. Blood 73:1123, 1989
21. Stenberg PE, McEver RP, Shuman MA et al: A platelet alpha-granule membrane protein (GMP-140) is expressed on the plasma membrane after activation. J Cell Biol 101:880, 1985
22. Berman CL, Yeo EL, Wencel-Drake JD et al: A platelet alpha granule membrane protein that is associated with the plasma membrane after activation. J Clin Invest 78:130, 1986
23. Leven RM, Schick PK, Budzynski AZ: Fibrinogen biosynthesis in isolated guinea pig megakaryocytes. Blood 65:501, 1985
24. Belloc F, Hourdille P, Fialon P et al: Fibrinogen synthesis by megakaryocyte rich human marrow cell concentrates. Thromb Res 38:341, 1985
25. Uzan G, Courtois G, Stanckovic Z et al: Expression of the fibrinogen genes in rat megakaryocytes. Biochem Biophys Res Commun 140:543, 1986
26. Handagama PJ, Shuman MA, Bainton DF: Incorporation of intravenously injected albumin, immunoglobulin G, and fibrinogen in guinea pig megakaryocyte granules. J Clin Invest 84:73, 1989
27. Handagama P, Bainton DF, Jacques Y et al: Kistrin, an integrin antagonist, blocks endocytosis of fibrinogen into guinea pig megakaryocyte and platelet α-granules. J Clin Invest 91:193, 1993
28. Handagama P, Scarborough RM, Shuman MA et al: Endocytosis of fibrinogen into megakaryocyte and platelet α-granules is mediated by αIIbβ3 (glycoprotein IIb-IIIa) Blood 82:135, 1993
29. Harrison P: Platelet alpha-granular fibrinogen. Platelets 3:1, 1992
30. Atkinson P, White MV, Kaliner MA: Histamine and serotonin. p. 193. In Gallin JI, Goldstein IM, Snyderman R (eds): Inflammation: Basic Principles and Clinical Correlates. 2nd Ed. Raven Press, New York, 1992
31. Holmsen H, Weiss HJ: Secretable storage pools in platelets. Annu Rev Med 30:119, 1979
32. Holmsen H: Platelet secretion. p. 390. In Colman RW, Hirsh J, Marder VJ, Salzman EW (eds): Hemostasis and Thrombosis. JB Lippincott, Philadelphia, 1982
33. Israels SJ, Gerrard JM, Jacques YV et al: Platelet dense granule membranes contain both granulophysin and P-selectin (GMP-140). Blood 80:143, 1992
34. Tranzer JP, DaPrada M, Pletscher A: Storage of 5-hydroxytryptamine in megakaryocytes. J Cell Biol 52:191, 1972
35. Payne CM: A quantitative ultrastructural evaluation of the cell organelle specificity of the uranaffin reaction in normal human platelets. Am J Clin Pathol 81:62, 1984
36. Radley JM, Scurfield G: The mechanisms of platelet release. Blood 56:996, 1980
37. Handagama PJ, Feldman BF, Jain NC et al: Circulating proplatelets: isolation and quantitation in healthy rats and in rats with induced blood loss. Am J Vet Res 48:962, 1987
38. Trowbridge EA, Martin JF, Slater DN: Evidence for a theory of physical fragmentation of megakaryocytes, implying that all platelets are produced in the pulmonary circulation. Thromb Res 28:461, 1982
39. Larsen TE: Emperipolesis of granular leukocytes within megakaryocytes in human bone marrow. Am J Clin Pathol 53:485, 1970
40. Behnke O: Further studies on microtubules: a marginal bundle in human and rat thrombocytes. J Ultrastruct Res 13:469, 1965
41. Fox JEB, Boyles JK, Reynolds CC et al: Actin filament content and organization in unstimulated platelets. J Cell Biol 98:1985, 1984
42. Nesheim ME, Eid S, Mann KG: Assembly of the prothombinase complex in the absence of prothrombin. J Biol Chem 256:9874, 1981
43. Gerrard JM, White JG, Peterson DA: The platelet dense tubular system: its relationship to prostaglandin synthesis and calcium flux. Thromb Haemost 40:224, 1978
44. White JG, Krivit W: The canalicular system of the blood platelet: a possible sarcoplasmic reticulum. J Lab Clin Med 70:999, 1967
45. Coughlin S, Vu TK, Hung DT et al: Characterization of a functional thrombin receptor. Issues and opportunities. J Clin Invest 89:351, 1992
46. Kroll MH, Schafer AI: Biochemical mechanisms of platelet activation. Blood 74:1181, 1989
47. Fujimoto T, Ohara S, Hawiger J: Thrombin induced exposure and prostacyclin inhibition of the receptor for factor VIII/von Willebrand factor on human platelets. J Clin Invest 69:1212, 1982
48. Kunicki TJ, Nugent DJ, Staats SJ et al: The human fibroblast class II extracellular matrix receptor mediates platelet adhesion to collagen and is identical to the platelet glycoprotein Ia-IIa complex. J Biol Chem 263:4516, 1988
49. Wayner EA, Carter WG, Piotrowicz RS et al: The function of multiple extracellular matrix receptors in mediating cell adhesion to extracellular matrix: preparation of monoclonal antibodies to the fibronectin receptor that specifically inhibit cell adhesion to fibronectin and react with platelet glycoproteins Ic-IIa. J Cell Biol 107:1881, 1988
50. Sonnenberg A, Modderman PW, Hogervorst F: Laminin receptor on platelets is the integrin VLA-6. Nature 336:487, 1988
51. Phillips DR, Charo IF, Scarborough RM: GPIIb-IIIa: the responsive integrin. Cell 65:359, 1991
52. Baumgartner HR: The role of blood flow in platelet adhesion, fibrin deposition, and formation of mural thrombi. Microvasc Res 5:167, 1973
53. Stenberg PE, Shuman MA, Levine SP et al: Optimal techniques for the immunocytochemical demonstration of β-thromboglobulin, platelet factor 4, and fibrinogen in the alpha granules of unstimulated platelets. Histochem J 16:983, 1984
54. Stenberg PE, Shuman MA, Levine SP et al: Redistribution of alpha-granules and their contents in thrombin-stimulated platelets. J Cell Biol 98:748, 1984
55. Mosher DF, Pesciotta DM, Loftus JC et al: Secreted alpha granule proteins: the race for receptors. p. 171. In George JN, Nurden AT, Phillips DR (eds): Platelet Membrane Glycoproteins. Plenum, New York, 1985
56. Escolar F, Leistikow E, White JG: The fate of the open canalicular system in surface and suspension-activated platelets. Blood 74:1983, 1989
57. Stenberg PE, Bainton DF: Storage organelles in platelets and megakaryocytes. p. 257. In Phillips DR, Shuman MA (eds): Biochemistry of Platelets. Academic Press, San Diego, 1986

58. Rendu F, Marche P, Maclouf J: Signal transduction in normal and pathological thrombin-stimulated human platelets. Biochimie 68:305, 1987

59. Sixma JJ, Slot JW, Geuze HJ: Immunocytochemical localization of platelet granule proteins. Methods Enzymol 169:301, 1989

60. Morgenstern E, Patscheke H, Mathieu: The origin of the membrane convolute in degranulating platelets. A comparative study of normal and "gray" platelets. Blut 60:15, 1990

61. Bevilacqua M, Butcher E, Furie B et al: Selectins: a family of adhesion receptors. Cell 67:233, 1991

62. Bevilacqua MP, Nelson RM: Selectins. J Clin Invest 91:379, 1993

63. Isenberg WM, McEver RP, Shuman MA et al: Topographic distribution of a granule membrane protein (GMP-140) that is expressed on the platelet surface after activation: an immunogold-surface replica study. Blood Cells 12: 191, 1986

64. Stoolman LM: Adhesion molecules controlling lymphocyte migration. Cell 56:907, 1989

65. Johnston GI, Cook RG, McEver RP: Cloning of GMP-140, a granule membrane protein of platelets and endothelium: sequence similarity to proteins involved in cell adhesion and inflammation. Cell 56:1033, 1989

66. Moore KL, Stults NC, Diaz S et al: Identification of a specific glycoprotein ligand for P-selectin (CD62) on myeloid cells. J Cell Biol 118:445, 1992

67. Moore KL, Thompson LF: P-selectin (CD-62) binds to subpopulations of human memory T lymphocytes and natural killer cells. Biochem Biophys Res Commun 186:173, 1992

68. Palabrica T, Lobb R, Furie BC et al: Leukocyte accumulation promoting fibrin deposition is mediated *in vivo* by P-selectin on adherent platelets. Nature 359:848, 1992

69. Abrams CS, Ellison N, Budzynski AZ et al: Direct detection of activated platelets and platelet-derived microparticles in man. Blood 75:128, 1990

70. White JG, Estensen RD: Degranulation of discoid platelets. Am J Pathol 68: 289, 1972

71. Phillips DR, Jennings LK, Edwards HH: Identification of membrane proteins mediating the interaction of human platelets. J Cell Biol 86:77, 1980

72. Horwitz A, Duggan K, Buck C et al: Interaction of plasma membrane fibronectin receptor with talin—a transmembrane linkage. Nature 320:531, 1986

73. Breton-Gortius J, Reyes F, Duhamel G et al: Megakaryoblastic acute leukemia: identification by the ultrastructural demonstration of platelet peroxidase. Blood 51:45, 1978

74. Stenberg PE, Beckstead JH, McEver RP et al: Immunohistochemical localization of membrane and α-granule proteins in plastic-embedded mouse bone marrow megakaryocytes and murine megakaryocyte colonies. Blood 68:696, 1986

75. Erber WN, Breton-Gorius J, Villeval JL et al: Detection of cells of megakaryocyte lineage in haematological malignancies by immuno-alkaline phosphatase labelling cell smears with a panel of monoclonal antibodies. Br J Haematol 65:87, 1986

76. Lages B, Shattil SJ, Bainton DF et al: Decreased content and surface expression of alpha-granule membrane protein GMP-140 in one of two types of platelet alpha delta storage pool deficiency. J Clin Invest 87:919, 1991

77. Ballem PJ, Belzberg A, Devine DV et al: Kinetic studies of the mechanism of thrombocytopenia in patients with human immunodeficiency virus infection. N Engl J Med 327:1779, 1992

78. Zucker-Franklin DA, Cal YZ: Megakaryocytes of human immunodeficiency virus-infected individuals express viral RNA. Proc Natl Acad Sci USA 86:5595, 1989

Molecular Basis of Platelet Function

97

Edward F. Plow and Mark H. Ginsberg

INTRODUCTION

Platelets ordinarily circulate in blood vessels as individuals entities that do not interact with other platelets or other cell types. A transition from this nonadhesive to an adhesive state can be rapidly initiated if platelets are exposed to an appropriate stimulus. A scenario of the platelet adhesive reactions initiated in response to an injury to a blood vessel wall is illustrated in Figure 97-1. Disruption of the endothelial cell lining of the vessel exposes constituents within the subendothelial matrix, including a variety of adhesive proteins that can support initial platelet attachment. Following attachment, platelets may undergo a spreading reaction in which multiple contacts are formed between the cell surface and the matrix. These additional contacts may be critical in stabilizing the association of the platelets with the matrix in flowing blood. In conjunction with these adhesive reactions, the cells often encounter agonists within the microenvironment that can trigger platelet secretion. The secretory response results in the release of the contents of intracellular storage granules from within the platelet. Granule constituents include substances that can stimulate circulating platelets and cause them to acquire new adhesive properties. These stimulated platelets interact with one another, during platelet aggregation, to form an effective plug to seal the injured vessel wall and prevent excessive blood loss. This series of platelet responses—attachment, spreading, secretion, and aggregation—is essential for the hemostatic function of platelets. These same events, occurring on an injured endothelial cell or on an atherosclerotic plaque, may result in the formation of a platelet-rich thrombus, which can compromise the patency of the blood vessel and lead to thrombosis. At the other extreme, abnormalities in platelet adhesive reactions of either a genetic (e.g., Glanzmann thrombasthenia or Bernard-Soulier syndrome) or an acquired origin can result in lifelong bleeding episodes. Thus, platelet adhesive reactions and secretion are central events in health and disease processes; bleeding, hemostasis, and thrombosis are delicately balanced on these platelet functions.

This chapter addresses the molecular basis of platelet adhesive reactions and secretory responses. Great strides have

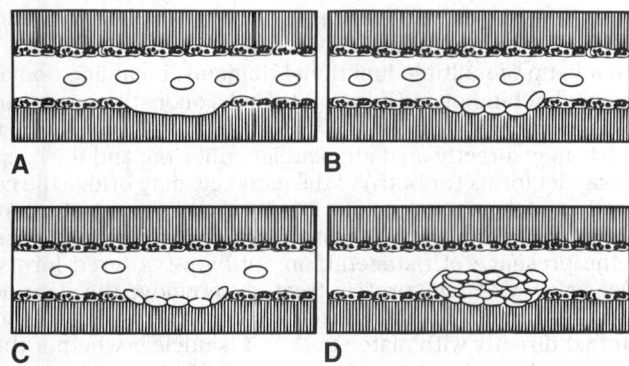

Fig. 97-1. Hemostatic response of platelets to injury. **(A)** Disruption of the endothelial cell lining of the blood vessel exposes constituents of the subendothelial matrix. **(B)** Platelets attach to, and spread on, the matrix constituents. **(C)** Platelet secretion may be initiated. **(D)** Released platelet constituents can activate additional platelets, which aggregate to form a thrombus.

been made in defining the mechanisms that govern these functional responses. At the heart of these platelet responses are ligand-receptor interactions. Indeed, the platelet has often served as a model cell type for studying ligand-receptor interactions and establishing basic mechanisms of cell adhesion and secretion.

MOLECULAR BASIS OF PLATELET ADHESION

Substrates for Platelet Attachment and Spreading

Some of the major subendothelial matrix proteins that support platelet attachment or spreading reactions, or both, are listed in Table 97-1. From the extent of this list, it is clear that the platelet can adhere to a variety of substrates once the endothelium has been disrupted. The endothelium must also create an effective barrier to prevent circulating platelets from reaching the matrix and initiating thrombus formation. In addition to serving as a physical barrier, endothelial cells synthesize and elaborate components, notably prostacyclin (prostaglandin I_2), that prevent platelet activation and impart a nonthrombogenic character to the normal endothelium (see Ch. 99).

Several considerations have an impact on the role of the individual matrix constituents in mediating platelet adhesion.

1. Not all of the adhesive proteins listed in Table 97-1 support the same spectrum of platelet adhesive responses. For example, under some conditions, platelets attach to, but do not spread on, laminin,[1] whereas von Willebrand factor

(vWF) and fibronectin support cell attachment and spreading.[2-4] Collagen not only supports the attachment and spreading of platelets but also can provoke a secretory response.[5] Of the multiple forms of collagen, types I, III, and VI are regarded as being particularly important in supporting platelet adhesion.

2. Evidence is growing that the properties of endothelial cells from different blood vessels vary; it also is likely that the composition of the subendothelial matrix will vary. Thus, certain proteins may play a dominant role in supporting platelet adhesion in certain blood vessels. Moreover, even at the same anatomic location, the nature of the injury will expose different substrata.

3. Shear rate developed by flowing blood varies with vessel caliber and greatly influences platelet adhesion. Shear is particularly important in defining the contribution of vWF to platelet adhesion. Patients with von Willebrand disease (see Ch. 113) have a bleeding diathesis, attesting to the importance of vWF in supporting platelet function. However, in vitro experiments demonstrate that vWF plays a role in platelet adhesion at high but not at low shear rates.[3,6] By contrast, a role for fibronectin in supporting platelet adhesion can be demonstrated at both high and low shear.[7-9]

4. A variety of these adhesive proteins interact. For example, vWF, fibronectin, and thrombospondin all bind to collagen (although they exhibit differential reactivity with different collagen types).[10-12] These interactions may bridge the platelet to a matrix protein or may modulate the adhesive properties of a matrix protein.

5. Several of the adhesive proteins are present in platelet secretory granules or in plasma, or both, as well as being matrix constituents. vWF and fibronectin are present in all three locations, and thrombospondin is a major platelet granule constituent.[13,14] Proteins from all three sources—the matrix, the platelet, and the plasma—contribute to platelet adhesion. The adhesive proteins derived from these different sources may be functionally distinct, since they are not structurally identical. For example, the degree of vWF and fibronectin multimerization differs for molecules derived from plasma and the matrix.

Platelet Adhesion Receptors

The individual adhesive proteins come in contact with the platelet by serving as ligands for specific cell-surface receptors (Table 97-2). Several nomenclature systems have been used to identify the membrane proteins of the platelet, and the same receptor may have multiple designations. The most widely

Table 97-1. Subendothelial Matrix Constituents that Support Platelet Adhesion

Matrix Constituent	Comment
Collagens	Large family of proteins with certain members supporting platelet adhesion, aggregation, and secretion
von Willebrand factor	Large multimeric protein critical for the hemostatic function of platelets
Fibronectin	Dimeric or multimeric protein that supports attachment and spreading of platelets
Thrombospondin	Trimeric protein exhibiting both adhesive and antiadhesive properties
Laminin	A protein supporting platelet attachment
Microfibrils	A fibular bundle of protein constituents found in certain matrices

Table 97-2. Platelet Receptors for Adhesive Proteins

Ligand	Receptor(s)	Other Designations
Collagen	GPIa/IIa	VLA-2, $\alpha_2\beta_1$
	GPIIb/IIIa	$\alpha_{IIb}\beta_3$
	GPIV	GPIIIb, CD36
Fibrinogen	GPIIb/IIIa	$\alpha_{IIb}\beta_3$
Fibronectin	GPIc/IIa	VLA-5, $\alpha_5\beta_1$
	GPIIb/IIIa	$\alpha_{IIb}\beta_3$
Thrombospondin	Vitronectin receptor	$\alpha_v\beta_3$
	GPIV	GPIIIb
Vitronectin	Vitronectin receptor	$\alpha_v\beta_3$
	GPIIb/IIIa	$\alpha_{IIb}\beta_3$
vWF	GPIb/IX	$\alpha_{IIb}\beta_3$
	GPIIb/IIIa	
Laminin	GPIc/IIa region	VLA-6, $\alpha_6\beta_1$

used nomenclature is based on electrophoretic mobility of the membrane proteins on polyacrylamide gel systems in which the higher-molecular-weight proteins move more slowly. This separation gave rise to glycoprotein (GP) I, II, III, and so on, with GPI having the highest molecular weight. As the gel systems employed became more discriminating, several proteins were discerned in the GPI position, hence GPIa, GPIb, and GPIc, and so forth.[15] Further refinement is still required; for example, there are at least three distinct polypeptides in the GPIc position. Several of the membrane proteins exist on the platelet surface as noncovalent complexes; thus, GPIb/IX, GPIc/IIa, and GPIIb/IIIa, can be regarded as single-membrane proteins. Other nomenclature systems have arisen because several platelet membrane proteins are present and have been assigned different names on other cell types. This is the basis for the VLA designations for some of the platelet membrane proteins. Similarly, certain proteins may also have extracellular matrix and leukocyte differentiation antigen (CD) designations, but the later nomenclatures have been used infrequently in the platelet literature. Some receptors have been named on the basis of their function (e.g., the vitronectin and the fibronectin receptors). While functional designations seem highly appropriate from a descriptive standpoint, at least two membrane proteins on platelets can serve as receptors for vitronectin and fibronectin (Table 97-2), and several platelet constituents have been referred to as collagen receptors. Beyond creating a nomenclature complexity, the redundancy of the platelet receptors enables the cell to establish multiple contacts with a single matrix constituent; thus, a single ligand initiates several distinct functional responses by engaging different receptors.

Integrin Family of Adhesion Receptors

Many of the adhesive protein receptors on platelets are members of the integrin family. The integrins are broadly distributed heterodimeric (two subunits) cell-surface molecules that share certain structural, immunochemical, and functional properties.[16-25] The β-subunits, of which eight have currently been identified, are highly homologous, exhibiting ≥35–45% identity at the primary amino acid sequence level. The α-subunits, of which 13 have currently been identified, are also similar to one another but exhibit less extensive sequence identity.[20,26] The α-subunits are synthesized as a single-chain polypeptide; some, such as GPIIb, are proteolytically processed to a two-chain form.[27-30] Each β-subunit combines in a noncovalent complex with an α-subunit to form an adhesive protein receptor. A single β-subunit can combine with several α-subunits. Platelets express two distinct β-subunits, β_1 and β_3 (β_2 is not detected), and five α-subunits (Table 97-3). Of the integrins expressed on blood cells, GPIIb/IIIa is the only one restricted to platelets/megakaryocytes, and its presence may contribute to the association of platelets with tumor cells.[31-33]

Role of GPIb/IX in Platelet Adhesion

GPIb/IX is a notable example of a cell-surface molecule involved in platelet adhesion that is not a member of the integrin family. Platelets from patients with Bernard-Soulier syndrome lack GPIb/IX; these patients have a marked bleeding dia-

thesis[34-36] (see Ch. 129). The role of GPIb/IX in hemostasis can be traced directly to its function as a receptor for vWF. vWF is made up of multiple functional domains, including domains involved in binding to GPIb and to matrix constituents such as collagen and microfibrils[10,37-43] (see Ch. 112). Thus, vWF in the matrix may directly mediate platelet adhesion, and the plasma or platelet forms (or both) of the molecule may bridge the cells to other matrix components. In vitro, vWF does not interact directly with GPIb on platelets. An interaction can be measured in the presence of ristocetin, an antibiotic. Altered forms of vWF, asialo-vWF (the protein treated to remove the sialic acid residues from its carbohydrate moieties) and bovine vWF can interact directly with platelets.[44-46] It is unclear whether there is a physiologic counterpart of ristocetin in humans; the association of vWF with matrix constituents may alter its properties and permit its direct binding to GPIb. In addition, exposure of platelets to increased fluid shear stress also induces the high-affinity interaction of GPIb and vWF.[47] This is of clear potential pathologic significance in narrowed arteries.

GPIb is multifunctional, as it can also serve as a binding site for thrombin.[48,49] It is also a target for certain of the drug-induced platelet antibodies.[50] The full primary structures of both GPIb[51,52] and GPIX[53] have been determined from cDNA cloning approaches. GPIb is composed of a heavy chain and a light chain. The light chain spans the platelet membrane and appears to mediate the association of GPIb with the cytoskeletal architecture within the platelet cytoplasm.[54,55] The heavy chain is highly susceptible to proteolysis, and a large proteolytic fragment, glycocalicin, can be detected in the plasma of some patients with thrombocytopenic disorders.[56] GPIX is a small, single-chain polypeptide with a molecular weight of 20,000. The contribution of GPIX to the function of GPIb/IX is unclear. GPV is also deficient in Bernard-Soulier platelets and may form a loose association with GPIb/IX.[34,35]

PLATELET SECRETION

The foregoing discussion has emphasized the adhesive functions of platelets in mediating the physical closure of breaks in blood vessels. Another important function of platelets is the release of a variety of substances that stimulate or inhibit platelets or other blood and vascular cells. The substances can covalently modify the thrombus to affect its mechanical properties, regulate coagulation, contribute to cell adhesive events, and modulate the growth of cells of the vessel wall. Thus, the platelet is not simply the stop leak of the vasculature, but also has the capacity to signal its presence in a thrombus in a variety of ways.

Most of these substances are actively and selectively secreted from platelets either from preformed storage granules or by being synthesized de novo from membrane phospholipids. There are also factors in the platelet cytoplasm that can affect thrombus structure or vascular cell growth; they are released as a result of minor degrees of platelet lysis during hemostasis. Some of these factors and their intraplatelet sources are illustrated in Figure 97-2. The dense bodies (or granules) (see Ch. 96) and platelet membranes are a source of a group of rapidly secreted, short-acting mediators (i.e., they are either rapidly inactivated or rapidly diffuse away from the site of the thrombus). Their effects are rapid on surrounding cells, and they serve to modulate the behavior of both platelets and vessel wall cells, particularly as regards vascular tone. The platelet dense bodies, the most rapidly secreted of platelet organelles,[57] release ADP, which is a potent agonist for recruiting other platelets, as well as ATP, which is an agonist for other cells of the blood.[58,59] They also release biogenic amines such as serotonin, which can influence vascular tone. The dense bodies are also rich in divalent cations. The physiologic role

Table 97-3. Platelet Integrins

Integrin	Ligand
GPIa/IIa (VLA-2, $\alpha_2\beta_1$)	Collagen
GPIc/IIa (VLA-5, $\alpha_5\beta_1$)	Fibronectin
$\alpha_6\beta_1$ (mobility similar to that of GPIc/IIa)	Laminin
GPIIb/IIIa ($\alpha_{IIb}\beta_3$)	Fibrinogen, fibronectin, vitronectin, vWF
$\alpha_v\beta_3$ (vitronectin receptor)	Fibrinogen, fibronectin, vitronectin, vWF

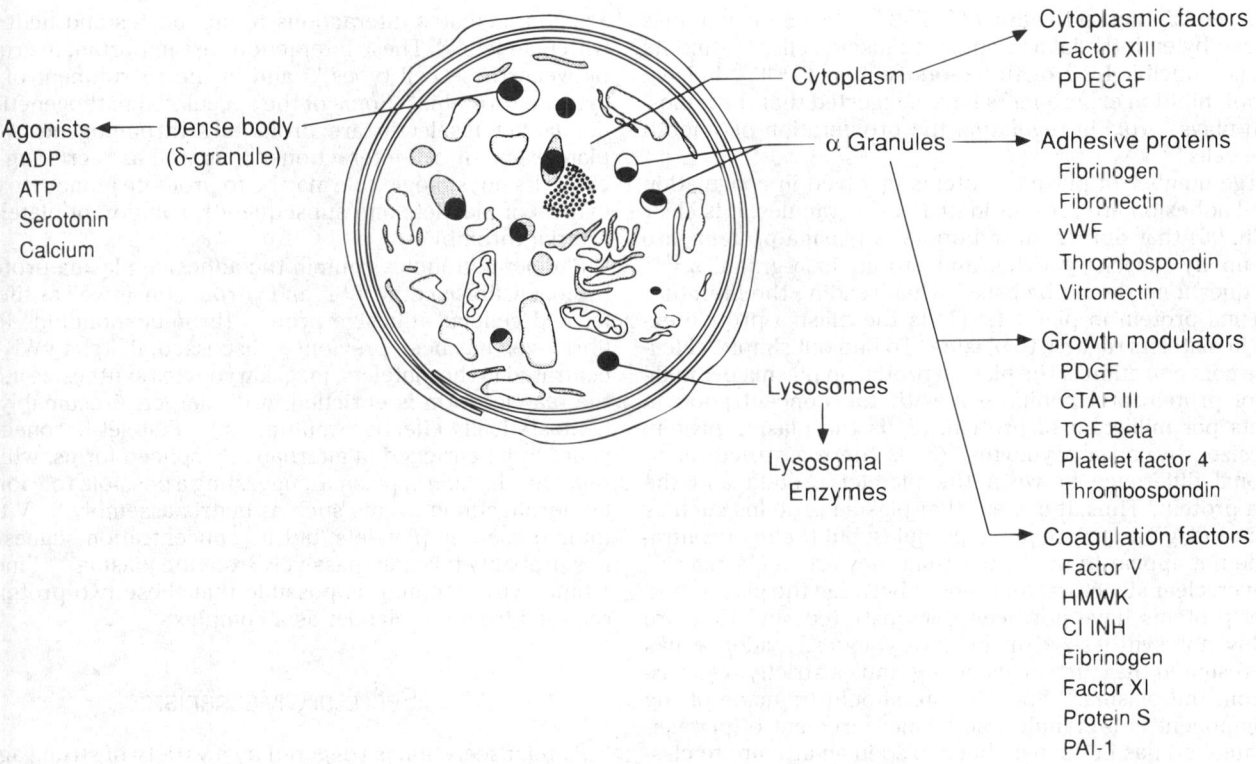

Fig. 97-2. Substances released by platelets and their intraplatelet sources. Illustrated are some of the bioactive substances released from dense bodies, α-granules, lysosomes, the cytoplasm, and the platelet membrane. PDECGF, platelet-derived endothelial cell growth factor; PAF, platelet-activating factor; HETEs, hydroxyeicosatetraenoic acids; HMWK, high-molecular-weight kininogen; C1 INH, C1 inhibitor; PAI-1, plasminogen activator inhibitor-1; VWF, von Willebrand factor; PDGF, platelet-derived growth factor; CTAP, connective tissue-activating peptide; TGF, transforming growth factor.

of released dense body calcium is not clear; however, one could speculate that it serves to ensure adequate calcium for some of the calcium-dependent enzymes involved in coagulation or cross-linking of the thrombus. Finally, dense body membranes contain granulophysin, a membrane protein of unknown function.[60]

Arachidonate-derived mediators such as thromboxane A_2 are generated as a consequence of hydrolysis of membrane phospholipids,[61] their role in recruitment of other platelets and as vasoactive substances is extensively discussed in Chapter 98. Mention should also be made of platelet-activating factor (PAF)[62] (alkyl-2-acetyl-sn-glycero-3-phosphocholine), which was originally described as platelet activator released from stimulated mast cells. It is clear that its biologic effects are greater than simply platelet activation, although its effects on platelets clearly play a role in some of the platelet sequestration that occurs during allergic injury.[63,64] Similarly, it is produced by a variety of cells as well as platelets. It is possible that this important mediator, produced locally, may contribute either to recruitment of other platelets or to some of the vascular phenomena associated with hemostasis.

Platelets contain lysosomes that release enzymes.[65] Compared with neutrophils, platelets are probably a minor source of lysosomal hydrolases in the blood.[65] Nevertheless, mention should be made of platelet-associated heparatinase (probably a lysosomal enzyme), which can cleave a vascular endothelial cell surface glycosaminoglycans to produce an antiproliferative fragment.[66] Factor XIII, a major transglutaminase that catalyzes the formation of isopeptide bonds between the γ-glutaminyl residues and the ε-amino groups of lysines forming stable covalent cross-links between proteins, is contained in the platelet cytosol.[67] Factor XIII functions in the cross-linking of fibrin, as well as in the cross-linking of other components of a throm-

bus such as fibronectin[68] or α_2-antiplasmin[69] to fibrin. Moreover, platelet factor XIII has been suggested to play a role in cross-linking and stabilizing cytoskeletal elements.[70,71] Small quantities of this factor are probably released into thrombi, where it may also affect their stability.

Platelets contain a wide variety of peptides, primarily in α-granules, that can modulate the growth and patterns of gene expression of vessel wall cells. The first peptide to be described was platelet-derived growth factor (PDGF),[72] which has three isoforms and two distinct receptors on smooth muscle cells and fibroblasts.[73] PDGF probably plays an important role in the smooth muscle cell proliferation that may occur consequent to platelet interaction with vessel wall. Its receptors are transmembrane tyrosine kinase-type receptors, and signal transduction from the PDGF receptor is similar to that from other tyrosine kinase receptors such as the insulin and epidermal growth factor receptors.[74] Another α-granule growth factor is connective tissue-activating peptide-III (CTAP-III), which stimulates fibroblast proliferation. CTAP-III is a probable precursor of β-thromboglobulin, and its structure is related to another α-granule protein, platelet factor 4.[75] Both platelet factor 4 and CTAP-III are members of a large protein family involved in growth control and inflammation.[76,77] Interleukin-1 (IL-1) is expressed on the surface of activated platelets, but the mechanism whereby it is found there is unclear.[78] Transforming growth factor-β (TGF-β) was first isolated from platelets, a rich source of this peptide mediator that is a potent stimulus for the biosynthesis of matrix molecules and their receptors.[79] TGF-β has complex effects on cell proliferation, in some cell systems stimulating and in other systems inhibiting cellular proliferation. In addition, thrombospondin, for which platelets are the major source in blood, is a large (around 450 kd) protein that, as noted above, may play a role in platelet aggregation, regulation of angiogenesis, and activation of TGF-β.[80] Thrombospondin is produced by endothelial and smooth muscle cells,[81,82] and its mRNA is inducible by growth factors such as PDGF.[82] Indeed, immunoinhibition experiments have suggested that thrombospondin plays a role in regulating the proliferation of smooth muscle cells.[83]

A large number of plasma proteins involved in coagulation and cell adhesion are present in platelet α-granules. It is clear (see Ch. 96) that during thrombopoiesis plasma proteins are taken up by megakaryocytes and stored in α-granules.[84,85] Three questions should be asked when reading the literature on plasma protein in platelets: (1) Is the plasma protein enriched in platelets relative to plasma? To find out simply, calculate the concentration of the plasma protein in plasma per milligram of protein and compare it with the concentration in platelets per milligram of protein. (2) Is the plasma protein synthesized by megakaryocytes? (3) Is there a structural or functional difference between the platelet protein and the plasma protein? Thus, it is clear that plasma proteins such as albumin and IgG are present in α-granules, but their concentrations do not appear to be greater than they are in plasma.[67,86] Moreover, clear structural differences between the plasma and platelet proteins have not been demonstrated, and they are probably not synthesized in megakaryocytes. Evidence has been presented that they arrive in α-granules strictly by transport from the plasma.[85] Special note should be made of the IgG component in α-granules, since measurement of platelet-associated IgG has in the past been used in an attempt to classify patients with thrombocytopenia. Clearly its presence predominantly in α-granules, rather than on the cell surface, requires a re-evaluation of the significance of this measurement.

With respect to coagulation proteins present in and released by platelets, a wide variety of procoagulant and anticoagulant enzymes and cofactors have been reported in platelets. It is clear that megakaryocytes synthesize factor V,[87,88] and more factor V is present in platelet α-granules[89] than can be accounted for by uptake from plasma. Moreover, platelet factor V plays a clear role in assembling the platelet prothrombinase, which is involved in the final step in blood coagulation (i.e., the generation of thrombin).[90] Megakaryocytes take up fibrinogen, and its biosynthesis by megakaryocytes remains controversial.[85] Platelets also contain protein S[91] and plasminogen activator inhibitor-1 (PAI-1).[92] Protein S is a cofactor for the action of activated protein C, and PAI-1 is an inhibitor of urokinase and tissue plasminogen activators. Thus, the concentration of these proteins in platelets suggests that platelets may be a favored site for the anticoagulant action of protein C, a tempting idea considering the local concentration of factor V, a protein C substrate, on the platelet surface. Similarly, the local release of PAI-1 from platelets may play a role in modulating the fibrinolytic events in the vicinity of thrombi.

Platelets are the major peripheral blood source of β-amyloid precursor protein (APP).[93] APP is a membrane protein, thought to be localized to α-granules, that serves as the precursor of the approximately 40 residue peptides found in amyloid deposits in the brains of Alzheimer disease patients.[94] APP is a protease inhibitor, and it may be released by proteolytic cleavage.[95] Two central questions of current interest are (1) What is the role of APP in platelet function? The recent description of its capacity to inhibit factor Xa suggests the possibility of a natural anticoagulant.[96] The effects of APP on the spectrum of coagulation and fibrinolytic proteases will clearly be of interest. (2) Does platelet-derived APP contribute to deposits of amyloid in the brain?

P-selectin[97-100] (GMP-140, GPIIa, PADGEM, CD62) is an α-granule membrane protein that is absent from the surface of resting platelets. It is structurally similar to the E- and L-selectins,[101] a family of carbohydrate-binding proteins involved in adhesive interactions of circulating leukocytes (see Ch. 5). P-

selectin mediates interactions of monocytes and neutrophils with platelets.[101] These interactions are important in cross-talk between these cell types[102] and in the recruitment of leukocytes to thrombi.[103] Some of the speculated pathogenetic roles of platelet P-selectin are promoting thrombogenesis[103] and platelet-tumor cell interactions,[104] as well as recruiting monocytes. Its physiologic role may be to promote monocyte phagocytosis of platelets and subsequent resolution of platelet-rich arterial thrombi.

Platelet α-granules contain the adhesive plasma proteins fibrinogen, fibronectin, vWF, and vitronectin as well as the platelet and cellular adhesive protein thrombospondin.[14] Platelet fibrinogen has been previously discussed. Platelet vWF is concentrated in the platelets, megakaryocytes synthesize it,[105] and the platelet form is enriched in the larger, presumably more hemostatically effective, multimers.[106] Platelet fibronectin appears to be enriched in alternatively spliced forms, which are relatively lacking in plasma, suggesting a possible role for platelet fibronectin in events such as matrix assembly.[107] Vitronectin is present in platelets, but its concentration suggests that it is probably taken up passively from the plasma.[108] Since PAI-1 binds vitronectin, it is possible that these two proteins are released from the platelet as a complex.[109]

Secretory Mechanisms

Platelet secretion is triggered by a variety of strong agonists such as thrombin. Induction of secretion by weak agonists, such as ADP, occurs when the cells are brought into close contact (i.e., during aggregation).[110] The latter secretory mechanism is clearly dependent on thromboxane A_2, generated as a consequence of arachidonic acid release. A discussion of signaling pathways involved in secretory events is in Chapter 98.

The two morphologically prominent platelet storage granules, α-granules and dense bodies, contain a variety of substances important in platelet function. Since these granules have a limiting membrane, it would seem likely that the final secretory event would involve exocytosis (i.e., fusion of the secretory granule membrane with the plasma membrane).[111] This has been observed in dense body secretion.[112,113]

The incorporation of an α-granule membrane marker into the plasma membrane[114-116] directly established that exocytosis occurs during the secretion of α-granule contents and that simple exocytosis occurs[117] occasionally, as depicted in Figure 97-3A. Nevertheless, in human platelets, most α-granules are seen to move centripetally during secretion and are thus not in a

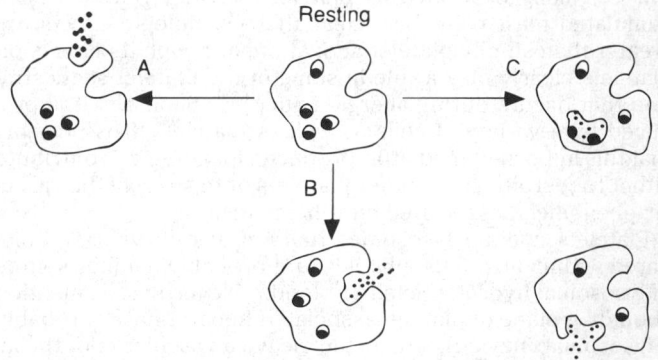

Fig. 97-3. Three possible exocytotic pathways for α-granule contents. **(A)** Simple exocytosis in which the granule membrane fuses with the plasma membrane. **(B)** Fusion of the granule with an invagination of the plasma membrane, the open canalicular system. **(C)** Fusion of granules with each other to form a compound granule that then fuses with the plasma membrane. Note that the final morphologic appearance in Figs. B and C is quite similar.

Table 97-4. Common Platelet-Aggregating Agonists

Agonist	Comment
ADP	Released from platelet α-granule; acts synergistically with many other agonists
Thrombin	Formed by activation of the coagulation system
Collagen	In subendothelial matrix
Epinephrine	May allow for hormonal regulation of hemostasis
Calcium ionophore	Not naturally occurring; mobilizes calcium in platelets
Arachidonate + metabolites	Active metabolites are formed and released from stimulated platelets
Serotonin	Released from platelets, may primarily sensitize platelets to other agonists
Platelet-activating factor	Lipid mediator produced by other cells that can activate a variety of cells, including platelets

locale that would permit fusion with the peripheral plasma membrane.[57,117-120] Two hypotheses, illustrated in Figure 97-3B and C, have been proposed to account for exocytosis when the granules are centralized. The mechanism illustrated in Figure 97-3B suggests that there are invaginations of the plasma membrane deep into the center of the platelet, and that α-granule membranes fuse with these invaginations; the secretory products are then moved to the outside of the cell through a conduit termed the open canalicular system, or surface-connected canalicular system.[121-123] The other mechanism, illustrated in Figure 97-3C, suggests that α-granules fuse with each other or with another cellular compartment to form a compound granule that is morphologically distinct from the α-granule. It is the compound granule that then moves toward and fuses with the plasma membrane.[57,117,124] Whatever the route by which granule components reach the cell surface, it is clear that there is substantial inward membrane traffic in platelets as well.[114,125-127] This inward traffic can serve to clear adhesive and procoagulant proteins from the cell surface and hence limit prothrombotic events.

MOLECULAR BASIS OF PLATELET AGGREGATION

Aggregation Response of Platelets

Platelets in blood, in plasma, or as an isolated cell population do not interact. If an appropriate agonist is added to the cells, however, rapid aggregation can ensue. Thus, a key element of this response is that platelet aggregation is a stimulated event. Some agonists that can initiate this response are listed in Table 97-4. Of particular physiologic relevance are the platelet-derived agonists—ADP, serotonin, platelet-activating factor, and arachidonate metabolites—which provide a means for stimulated platelets to recruit additional cells; collagen, which supports platelet adhesion and secretion as well as aggregation; thrombin, which links platelets and the blood coagulation system in thrombus formation; and epinephrine, which permits hormonal regulation of platelet function. These agonists activate platelets by interacting with specific receptors. Receptor occupancy triggers a complex series of intracellular reactions (see Ch. 98); these reactions ultimately form a set of common steps that permit the cells to aggregate. Platelet aggregation is energy dependent and can be distinguished on this basis from platelet agglutination induced by ristocetin or certain platelet antibodies.

At blood concentrations of $1-3 \times 10^8$/ml, platelet suspensions are opalescent. With addition of an agonist, a stirred suspension of normal platelets will aggregate, and a visible de-

crease in turbidity can be observed. Dedicated instruments (platelet aggregometers) for measuring the changes in light transmission through platelet suspensions are used extensively in clinical laboratories to evaluate platelet function (see Ch. 104). Certain instruments will also provide simultaneous measurements of other platelet functions, such as secretion.[110] While the information gained from aggregometry can be extremely useful, it is important to recognize that aggregation in vitro does not necessarily reflect platelet function in vivo.

A typical aggregometer tracing obtained with a suspension of isolated human platelets is shown in Figure 97-4A. From this pattern, the three essential components required for this functional response can be identified.

1. *Platelet agonist.* The agonist used in Figure 97-4 is ADP. This agonist induces platelet shape change, from discoid to a more spherical form, a transition that can be detected in the aggregometer as a slight decrease in light transmission. This transformation is not a prerequisite for platelet aggregation; epinephrine aggregates platelets but does not cause a shape change that is recordable in most conventional aggregometers.
2. *Divalent cations.* Calcium and magnesium support platelet aggregation. Trace amounts of calcium may be a prerequisite for platelet aggregation under all circumstances, and divalent cations can influence the specificity of GPIIb/IIIa for its ligands.[128]
3. *Fibrinogen.* Fibrinogen is not only a major plasma protein but is also present in, and secreted from, platelets[129,130] (see Chs. 100 and 111). By virtue of its capacity to form fibrin and to support platelet aggregation, fibrinogen plays a dual role in thrombus formation. These activities, as well as the contribution of fibrinogen to blood viscosity, are believed to account for the increased risk of cardiovascular disease associated with elevated levels of fibrinogen.[131] The dependence of platelet aggregation on fibrinogen concentration is evident from the tracings illustrated in Figure 97-4B.

In certain circumstances, vWF may substitute for fibrinogen in supporting platelet aggregation. It is postulated that, at the high shear rates encountered in certain blood vessels, vWF may play a dominant role in aggregation.[132] Certain pathologic circumstances—platelet-type von Willebrand disease and type IIB von Willebrand disease—may also favor a role for this protein in platelet aggregation.[133-137]

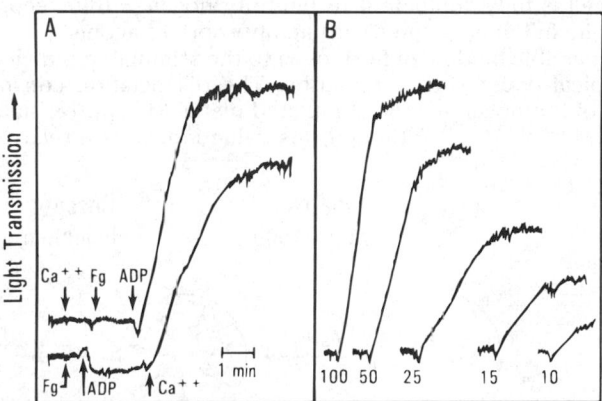

Fig. 97-4. Aggregation response of human platelets. **(A)** In order to aggregate, isolated human platelets require divalent ions (Ca^{2+}), an agonist (ADP), and an adhesive protein (fibrinogen [Fg]). Shape change is observed as a slight decrease in light transmission induced by ADP and is followed by an increase in transmission as the platelets aggregate. **(B)** Both the rate and extent of platelet aggregation are dependent on the concentration of fibrinogen. The concentration of fibrinogen (in microgram per milliliter) is indicated below each tracing.

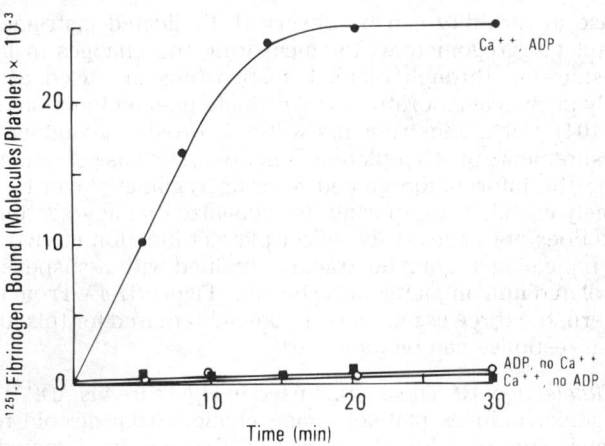

Fig. 97-5. Binding of fibrinogen to human platelets. ^{125}I-fibrinogen binds minimally to platelets in the absence of an agonist but does bind when an agonist such as ADP is added. A divalent ion, calcium, must be present for fibrinogen binding to occur.

Molecular Mechanisms Involved in Platelet Aggregation

The basis for the requisite roles of the agonist, calcium, and fibrinogen in platelet aggregation becomes evident when the direct interaction of fibrinogen with the cell is examined. Little fibrinogen binds to nonstimulated platelets (Fig. 97-5). If an agonist is added, however, time-dependent binding is observed. Stimulated platelets can bind ≥40,000 fibrinogen molecules per cell, a considerable number in view of the small size of platelets.[138-140] If the system is depleted of divalent ions, fibrinogen no longer binds to the stimulated platelets. Thus, the role of the agonist is to induce fibrinogen receptors, and calcium is required to support fibrinogen binding to its receptors.

These series of events define the fibrinogen-dependent pathway of platelet aggregation[141-146] schematically depicted in Figure 97-6. All the platelet agonists listed in Table 97-4 can initiate this pathway of platelet aggregation. The common event triggered by these platelet agonists is receptor induction—the conversion of a latent cell-surface receptor to a state in which it can bind fibrinogen. Receptor induction is very rapid, and the cell is fully competent to bind fibrinogen within seconds after its initial encounter with an appropriate agonist.

Reversible binding of fibrinogen to the stimulated platelet is a typical equilibrium interaction. The dissociation constant (K_d) of fibrinogen for the stimulated platelet is approximately 0.3 μM.[138,139,141-143] Although this value indicates a relatively low-affinity interaction (hormone receptors can often bind their ligands with 10^3–10^6-fold higher affinities), the plasma concentration of fibrinogen (10 μM) exceeds its K_d by approximately 30-fold. These interrelationships indicate that the fibrinogen-binding sites on stimulated platelets can become saturated with the ligand under physiologic circumstances. The reversible binding of fibrinogen to its platelet receptor requires divalent cations. Millimolar concentrations of calcium or magnesium can meet these requirements.[138,139,142,147]

Following reversible fibrinogen binding, the interaction undergoes a time-dependent stabilization.[143,144,147,148] This transition is termed irreversible fibrinogen binding and correlates closely with irreversible platelet aggregation. Conditions that initially dissociate fibrinogen from the cell and disaggregate platelets, such as the removal of divalent ions or the agonist, are no longer effective in removing the bound ligand or dissociating the platelets after a period of time. The molecular basis for irreversible fibrinogen binding is unclear. Either bound fibrinogen remains on the cell surface but its exposure changes considerably,[149] or the ligand/receptor complex is internalized.[125,126] The stability of platelet aggregates imparted by irreversible fibrinogen binding may be important for maintaining a thrombus in a microenvironment in which agents that prevent additional platelet activation and thrombus growth are being generated.

GPIIb/IIIa—Platelet Receptor for Fibrinogen

A single-membrane protein, GPIIb/IIIa, serves as the platelet receptor for fibrinogen[138,150-152]; occupancy of this receptor is essential for platelet aggregation. It is the most abundant cell-surface protein of platelets, accounting for approximately 15% of the protein mass of the platelet membrane. GPIIb/IIIa is also a constituent of platelet α-granule membranes[114]; this internal pool can become surface expressed during platelet activation.[130,131] The resting platelet has 40,000–80,000 copies of GPIIb/IIIa on its surface, and platelet activation can increase this number by 0–100%. Each GPIIb/IIIa is capable of binding one fibrinogen molecule.

GPIIb/IIIa is a member of the integrin family of cell-adhesion receptors. GPIIb, the α-subunit, is largely specific for cells of the platelet/megakaryocyte lineage. GPIIIa, the β-subunit, has been designated β$_3$. This β-subunit is known to complex with a different α-subunit to form the vitronectin receptor, α$_v$β$_3$.[153] α$_v$β$_3$ is expressed by a variety of cell types, including platelets and endothelial cells.[154-156] The complete amino acid sequences of both GPIIb and GPIIIa subunits have been deduced from their cDNAS[28,157]; the carbohydrate side chains and disulfide linkages have also been placed.[158-161] A schematic model illustrating some of the important structural features of the

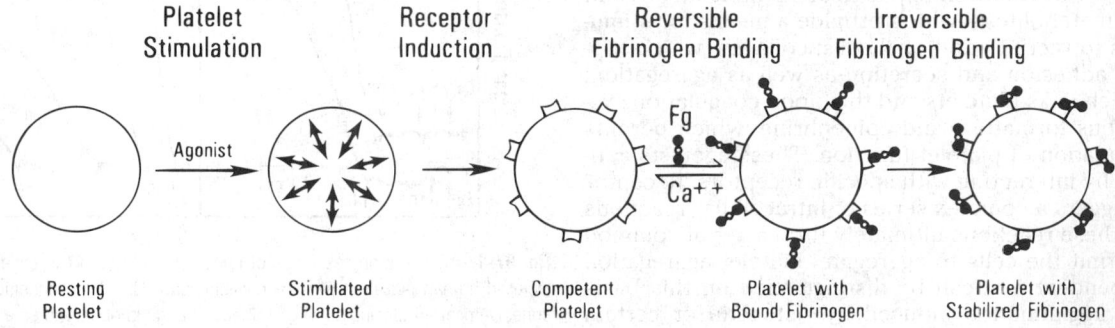

Fig. 97-6. Fibrinogen-dependent pathway of platelet aggregation. Stimulation of platelets with an agonist causes induction of fibrinogen receptors. The reversible binding of fibrinogen to the competent receptor requires divalent ions. Irreversible fibrinogen binding occurs with time as the ligand-receptor interaction becomes nondissociable.

two subunits is illustrated in Fig. 97-7. GPIIb is synthesized in megakaryocytes as a single chain but becomes proteolytically processed to the two-chain form during its transit to the cell surface.[162] The two subunits interact noncovalently in a 1:1 stoichiometry, to form the GPIIb/IIIa complex.[163] Complex formation occurs soon after biosynthesis of the individual subunits and is required for efficient cell-surface expression.[162,164] Micromolar calcium concentrations are required to maintain the subunits in a complex as compared with the millimolar requirements for fibrinogen binding.[165–169] Platelet activation is necessary to transform GPIIb/IIIa to a state in which it is competent to bind ligand. The biochemical basis for this transformation is unknown. At extremes, access of ligand to the receptor could be regulated by a change either directly in GPIIb/IIIa or in its microenvironment. There is support for both possibilities.[170–173]

Several mechanisms can be envisioned to explain how fibrinogen binding to GPIIb/IIIa can result in platelet aggregation. The simplest possibility is that a single fibrinogen molecule, by virtue of its dimeric structure, bridges two GPIIb/IIIa molecules symmetrically on adjacent platelets. Indeed, evidence can be cited to support this possibility.[174–176] As multiple sites within each fibrinogen molecule can be recognized by GPIIb/IIIa, asymmetric variations of direct bridging can be envisioned. Still another possibility is that changes subsequent to fibrinogen binding are required for platelet aggregation. Irreversible fibrinogen binding,[144] conformational changes in bound fibrinogen[177,178] and in occupied GPIIb/IIIa,[179] clustering of fibrinogen/GPIIb/IIIa,[180] and interactions of the receptor with the cytoskeleton of the cells[181–183] occur after the initial binding of fibrinogen to the cells. Whether such postreceptor occupancy events play a direct role in platelet aggregation is unknown. While the exact mechanism of platelet aggregation is not fully resolved, it is clear that occupancy of GPIIb/IIIa by ligand is essential for eliciting the cellular response. Accordingly, antagonists of ligand binding to GPIIb/IIIa provide a means of blocking platelet aggregation and thrombus formation. Antagonists of ligand binding include monoclonal antibodies, small peptide ligands, and nonpeptidic ligand mimetics. Representatives of

Table 97-5. Recognition Peptides of GPIIb/IIIa[a]

Peptide Designation	Structure[b]
Fibrinogen γ-chain	-XXKQAGDV
RGD	RGDX

[a] The naturally occurring sequences in human fibrinogen; S (serine) or F (phenylanine) at the C terminus of the two RGD sequences within the α-chain; and H (histidine)-H-L (leucine)-G-G-A at the N terminus of the γ-chain peptide.

[b] Amino acids: K, lysine; G, glutamine; A, alanine; G, glycine; D, aspartic acid; V, valine; X, one of several amino acids.

these classes of antagonists are currently being evaluated in animal models and in patients as antithrombotic agents.[184–189]

Recognition Specificity of GPIIb/IIIa

Discrete amino acid sequences establish the way in which GPIIb/IIIa recognizes fibrinogen and its other ligands. Two peptides define this recognition specificity of GPIIb/IIIa (Table 97-5). One peptide corresponds to the extreme C terminus of the γ-chain, one of the three constituent chains of fibrinogen.[174,190] The recognized amino acid sequence may be as small as the last six amino acid residues.[191] The second peptide is as small as four amino acids and contains Arg-Gly-Asp (RGD).[192–195] RGD sequences occur in two sites within the Aα chain of fibrinogen.[196] RGD sequences are also found in a variety of other proteins, including several that bind to GPIIb/IIIa. In addition, several other integrin receptors recognize RGD sequences within their ligands.[24,197–202] Thus, the RGD amino acid sequence is a broadly used recognition code in cellular adhesive reactions. By contrast, the γ-chain sequence appears to be unique to fibrinogen. Synthetic peptides containing either the γ-chain peptide sequence or the RGD sequence interact directly with GPIIb/IIIa and bind to the same or mutually exclusive sites within the receptor.[203,204] However, the preponderance of current evidence indicates that it is the C-terminus of the γ-chain that is critical for fibrinogen binding to GPIIb/IIIa.[205–207]

Fibrinogen is not the only ligand that binds to GPIIb/IIIa. Several other adhesive proteins that can serve as ligands are noted in Table 97-2. All these adhesive proteins contain at least one RGD sequence, and RGD peptides interfere with the binding of fibronectin,[192] vWF,[193] and vitronectin[208] to platelets. Since plasma fibrinogen concentrations are 10-fold higher than its K_d for GPIIb/IIIa, under physiologic conditions the receptor is nearly saturated with fibrinogen. Thus, fibrinogen is the dominant ligand for GPIIb/IIIa in this environment. However, all these ligands, except fibrinogen, are present in subendothelial cell matrices, and these other interactions may dominate in this microenvironment. In addition to its role in platelet aggregation, GPIIb/IIIa may also be involved in platelet adhesion, particularly in stabilizing cell-matrix interactions. It may be in this latter function that these other GPIIb/IIIa ligands play a key role. Thrombospondin associates with the surface of resting and stimulated platelets.[209–211] On the surface, it plays an auxiliary role in platelet aggregation by stabilizing platelet aggregates.[212] This activity may arise from its capacity to bind to fibrinogen.[213] Several candidate receptors for thrombospondin have been proposed.[214–218]

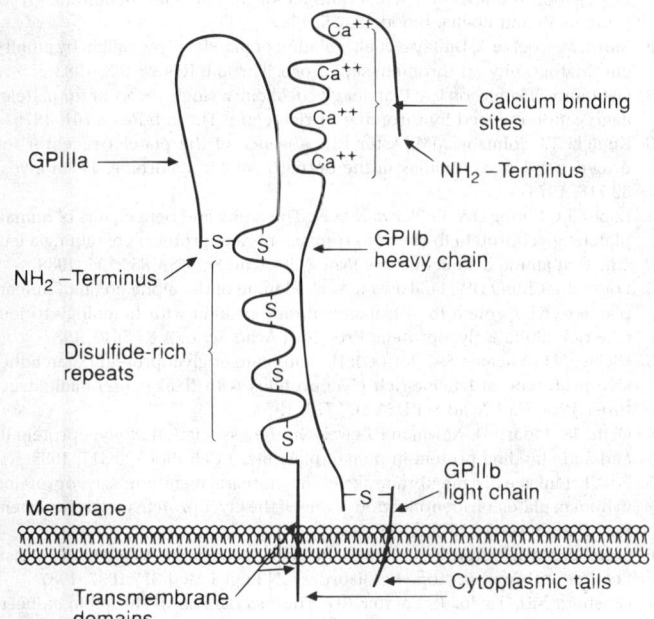

Fig. 97-7. Schematic model illustrating structural features of GPIIb/IIIa, the platelet fibrinogen receptor.

REFERENCES

1. Ill CR, Engvall E, Ruoslahti E: Adhesion of platelets to laminin in the absence of activation. J Cell Biol 99:2140, 1985
2. Leytin VL, Gorbunova NA, Misselwitz F et al: Step-by-step analysis of adhesion of human platelets to a collagen-coated surface defect in initial attach-

ment and spreading of platelets in von Willebrand's disease. Thromb Res 34:51, 1984

3. Sakariassen KS, Bolhuis PA, Sixma JJ: Human blood platelet adhesion to artery subendothelium is mediated by factor VIII-von Willebrand factor bound to the subendothelium. Nature 279:636, 1979

4. Grinnell F, Hays DG: Cell adhesion and spreading factor. Similarity to cold insoluble globulin in human serum. Exp Cell Res 115:221, 1978

5. Brass LF, Bensusan HB: The role of collagen quaternary structure in the platelet: collagen interaction. J Clin Invest 54:1480, 1974

6. Weiss HJ, Turitto VT, Baumgartner HR: Effect of shear rate on platelet interaction with subendothelium in citrated and native blood. 1. Shear rate-dependent decrease of adhesion in von Willebrand's disease and the Bernard-Soulier syndrome. J Lab Clin Med 92:750, 1978

7. Houdijk WPM, Sakariassen KS, Nievelstein PFEM, Sixma JJ: Role of factor VIII-von Willebrand factor and fibronectin in the interaction of platelets in flowing blood with monomeric and fibrillar human collagen types 1 and 111. J Clin Invest 75:531, 1985

8. Houdijk WPM, Sakariassen KS, Sixma JJ: Role of factor VIII-von Willebrand factor and fibronectin in the interaction of platelets in flowing blood with human collagen types I and III. J Clin Invest 1983

9. Houdijk WPM, deGroot PG, Nievelstein PF, Sakariassen KS: Subendothelial proteins and platelet adhesion. von Willebrand factor and fibronectin, not thrombospondin, are involved in platelet adhesion to extracellular matrix of human vascular endothelial cells. Arteriosclerosis 6:24, 1986

10. Santoro SA, Cowan JF: Adsorption of von Willebrand factor by fibrillar collagen—implications concerning the adhesion of platelets to collagen. Coll Relat Res 2:31, 1982

11. Engvall E, Ruoslahti E, Miller EJ: Affinity of fibronectin to collagens of different genetic types and to fibrinogen. J Exp Med: 147:1584, 1978

12. Mumby SM, Raugi GJ, Bornstein P: Interactions of thrombospondin with extracellular matrix proteins: selective binding to type V collagen. J Cell Biol 98:646, 1984

13. Wencel-Drake JD, Plow EF, Zimmerman TS et al: Immunofluorescent localization of adhesive glycoproteins in resting and thrombin-stimulated platelets. Am J Pathol 115:156, 1984

14. Wencel-Drake JD, Painter RG, Zimmerman TS, Ginsberg MH: Ultrastructural localization of human platelet thrombospondin, fibrinogen, fibronectin, and von Willebrand factor in frozen thin section. Blood 65:929, 1985

15. Phillips DR, Agin PP: Platelet plasma membrane glycoproteins. Evidence for the presence of non-equivalent disulfide bonds using non-reduced-reduced two-dimensional gel electrophoresis. J Biol Chem 252:2121, 1977

16. Ginsberg MH, O'Toole TE, Loftus JC, Plow EF: Ligand binding to integrins: dynamic regulation and common mechanisms. Cold Spring Harbor Symp Quant Biol 57:221, 1992

17. Ginsberg MH, Du X, Plow EF: Inside-out integrin signalling. Curr Opin Cell Biol 4:766, 1992

18. Plow EF, D'Souza SE, Ginsberg MH: Consequences of the interaction of platelet membrane glycoprotein GPIIb-IIIa (αIIbβ3), and its ligands. J Lab Clin Med 120:198, 1992

19. Ginsberg MH, Du X, O'Toole TE et al: Platelet integrins. Thromb Haemost 70:87, 1993

20. Hynes RO: Integrins: versatility, modulation, and signalling in cell adhesion. Cell 69:11, 1992

21. Hynes RO: Integrins: a family of cell surface receptors. Cell 48:549, 1987

22. Parise LV: The structure and function of platelet integrins. Curr Opin Cell Biol 1:947, 1989

23. Phillips DR, Charo IF, Parise LV, Fitzgerald LA: The platelet membrane glycoprotein IIb-IIIa complex. Blood 71:831, 1988

24. Ruoslahti E: Integrins. J Clin Invest 87:1, 1991

25. Hemler ME: VLA proteins in the integrin family: structures, functions, and their role on leukocytes. Annu Rev Immunol 8:365, 1990

26. Fitzgerald LA, Poncz M, Steiner B et al: Comparison of cDNA-derived protein sequences of the human fibronectin and vitronectin receptor alpha subunits and platelet glycoprotein IIb. Biochemistry 26:8158, 1987

27. Bray PF, Rosa JP, Lingappa VR et al: Biogenesis of the platelet receptor for fibrinogen: evidence for separate precursors for glycoproteins IIb and IIIa. Proc Natl Acad Sci USA 83:1480, 1986

28. Poncz M, Eisman R, Heidenreich R et al: Structure of the platelet membrane glycoprotein IIb. Homology to the alpha subunits of the vitronectin and fibronectin membrane receptors. J Biol Chem 262:8476, 1987

29. Loftus JC, Plow EF, Frelinger AL III et al: Molecular cloning and chemical synthesis of a region of platelet GPIIb involved in adhesive function. Proc Natl Acad Sci USA 840:7114, 1987

30. Loftus JC, Plow EF, Jennings L, Ginsberg MH: Alternative proteolytic processing of platelet membrane glycoprotein IIb. J Biol Chem 263:11025, 1988

31. Grossi IM, Hatfield JS, Fitzgerald LA et al: Role of tumor cell glycoproteins immunologically related to glycoproteins Ib and IIb/IIIa in tumor cell-platelet and tumor cell-matrix interactions. FASEB J 2:2385, 1988

32. Honn KV, Chen YQ, Timar J et al: Alpha IIb beta 3 integrin expression and function in subpopulations of murine tumors. Exp Cell Res 201:23, 1992

33. Boukerche H, Berthier-Vergnes O, Tabone E et al: Platelet-melanoma cell interaction is mediated by the glycoprotein IIb-IIIa complex. Blood 74:658, 1989

34. Nurden AT, George JN, Phillips DR: Platelet membrane glycoproteins: their structure, function, and modification in disease. p. 160. In Phillips DR, Shuman MA (eds): Biochemistry of Platelets. Harcourt Brace Jovanovich, Orlando, FL, 1986

35. George JN, Nurden AT, Phillips DR: Molecular defects in interactions of platelets with the vessel wall. N Engl J Med 311:1084, 1984

36. Nurden AT, Didry D, Rosa JP: Molecular defects of platelets in Bernard-Soulier syndrome. Blood Cells 9:333, 1983

37. Fauvel F, Grant ME, Legrand YJ et al: Interaction of blood platelets with a microfibrillar extract from adult bovine aorta: requirement for von Willebrand factor. Proc Natl Acad Sci USA 80:551, 1983

38. Mohri H, Fujimura Y, Shima M et al: Structure of the von Willebrand factor domain interacting with glycoprotein Ib. J Biol Chem 263:17901, 1988

39. Fujimura Y, Titani K, Holland LZ et al: von Willebrand factor. A reduced and alkylated 52/48-kDa fragment beginning at amino acid residue 449 contains the domain interacting with platelet glycoprotein Ib. J Biol Chem 261:381, 1986

40. Nokes TJ, Mahmoud NA, Savidge GF et al: von Willebrand factor has more than one binding site for platelets. Thromb Res 34:361, 1984

41. Chopek MW, Girma J-P, Fujikawa K et al: Human von Willebrand factor: a multivalent protein composed of identical subunits. Biochemistry 25:3146, 1986

42. Girma J-P, Chopek MW, Titani K, Davie EW: Limited proteolysis of human von Willebrand factor by *Staphylococcus aureus* V-8 protease: isolation and partial characterization of a platelet-binding domain. Biochemistry 25:3156, 1986

43. Girma J-P, Kalafatis M, Pietu G et al: Mapping of distinct von Willebrand factor domains interacting with platelet GPIb/GPIIIa and with collagen using monoclonal antibodies. Blood 67:1356, 1986

44. Kirby EP: The agglutination of human platelets by bovine factor VIII: J. J Lab Clin Med 100:963, 1982

45. DeMarco L, Girolami A, Russell S, Ruggeri ZM: Interaction of asialo von Willebrand factor with glycoprotein Ib induces fibrinogen binding to the glycoprotein IIb/IIIa complex and mediates platelet aggregation. J Clin Invest 75:1198, 1985

46. Gralnick HR, Williams SB, Coller BS: Asialo von Willebrand factor interactions with platelets. Interdependence of glycoproteins Ib and IIb/IIIa for binding and aggregation. J Clin Invest 75:19, 1985

47. Peterson DM, Stathopoulos NA, Giorgio TD et al: Shear-induced platelet aggregation requires von Willebrand factor and platelet membrane glycoproteins Ib and IIb-IIIa. Blood 69:625, 1987

48. Moroi M, Goetze A, Dubay E et al: Isolation of platelet glycocalicin by affinity chromatography on thrombin-sepharose. Thromb Res 28:103, 1982

49. Okumura T, Jamieson GA: Platelet glycocalicin: a single receptor for platelet aggregation induced by thrombin or ristocetin. Thromb Res 8:701, 1976

50. Kunicki TJ, Johnson MM, Aster RH: Absence of the platelet receptor for drug-dependent antibodies in the Bernard-Soulier syndrome. J Clin Invest 62:716, 1978

51. Lopez JA, Chung DW, Fujikawa K et al: The alpha and beta chains of human platelet glycoprotein Ib are both transmembrane proteins containing a leucine-rich amino acid sequence. Proc Natl Acad Sci USA 85:2135, 1988

52. Lopez JA, Chung DW, Fujikawa K et al: Cloning of the alpha chain of human platelet glycoprotein Ib: a transmembrane protein with homology to leucine-rich alpha 2-glycoprotein. Proc Natl Acad Sci USA 84:5615, 1987

53. Hickey MJ, Williams SA, Roth GJ: Human platelet glycoprotein IX: an adhesive prototype of leucine-rich glycoproteins with flank-center-flank structures. Proc Natl Acad Sci USA 86:6773, 1989

54. Okita JR, Pidard D, Newman PJ et al: On the association of glycoprotein Ib and actin-binding protein in human platelets. J Cell Biol 100:317, 1985

55. Fox JE: Linkage of a membrane skeleton to integral membrane glycoproteins in human platelets: identification of one of the glycoproteins as glycoprotein Ib. J Clin Invest 76:1673, 1985

56. Steinberg MH, Kelton JG, Coller BS: Plasma glycocalicin. An aid in the classification of thrombocytopenic disorders. N Engl J Med 317:1037, 1987

57. Ginsberg MH, Taylor L, Painter RG: The mechanism of thrombin-induced platelet factor 4 secretion. Blood 55:661, 1980

58. Greenberg S, Di Virgilio F, Steinberg TH, Silverstein SC: Extracellular nucleotides mediate Ca^{2+} fluxes in J774 macrophages by two distinct mechanisms. J Biol Chem 263:10337, 1988

59. Sung SS, Young JD, Origlio AM et al: Extracellular ATP perturbs transmembrane ion fluxes, elevates cytosolic [Ca^{2+}], and inhibits phagocytosis in mouse macrophages. J Biol Chem 260:13442, 1985

60. Israels SJ, Gerrard JM, Jacques YV et al: Platelet dense granule membranes contain both granulophysin and P-selectin (GMP-140). Blood 80:143, 1992

61. Kroll MH, Schafer AI: Biochemical mechanisms of platelet activation. Blood 74:1181, 1989

62. Snyder F: Biochemistry of platelet-activating factor: a unique class of biologically active phospholipids. Proc Soc Exp Biol Med 190:125, 1989

63. Page C, Abbott A: PAF: new antagonists, new roles in disease and a major role in reproductive biology. Trends Pharmacol Sci 10:255, 1989

64. Braquet P, Bourgain R, Mencia Huerta JM: Effect of platelet-activating factor on platelets and vascular endothelium. Semin Thromb Hemost 15:184, 1989

65. Bentfeld ME, Bainton DF: Cytochemical localization of lysosomal enzymes in rat megakaryocytes and platelets. J Clin Invest 56:1635, 1975

66. Castellot JJ Jr, Favreau LV, Karnovsky MJ, Rosenberg RD: Inhibition of vascular smooth muscle cell growth by endothelial cell-derived heparin. Possible role of a platelet endoglycosidase. J Biol Chem 257:11256, 1982

67. Sixma JJ, van den Berg A, Schiphorst M et al: Immunocytochemical localization of albumin and factor XIII in thin cryo sections of human blood platelets. Thromb Haemost 51:388, 1984

68. Mosher DF: Action of fibrin-stabilizing factor on cold-insoluble globulin and α2-macroglobulin in clotting plasma. J Biol Chem 251:1639, 1976

69. Tamaki T, Aoki N: Cross-linking of alpha 2-plasmin inhibitor to fibrin catalyzed by activated fibrin-stabilizing factor. J Biol Chem 257:14767, 1982

70. Cohen I, Glaser T, Veis A, Bruner Lorand J: Ca^{2+}-dependent cross-linking processes in human platelets. Biochim Biophys Acta 676:137, 1981

71. Kahn DR, Cohen I: Factor XIIIa-catalyzed coupling of structural proteins. Biochim Biophys Acta 668:490, 1981

72. Ross R: Platelet-derived growth factor. Lancet 1:1179, 1989

73. Heldin CH, Westermark B: Platelet-derived growth factor: three isoforms and two receptor types. Trends Genet 5:108, 1989

74. Williams LT: Signal transduction by the platelet-derived growth factor receptor. Science 243:1564, 1989

75. Wenger RH, Wicki AN, Walz A et al: Cloning of cDNA coding for connective tissue activating peptide III from a human platelet-derived lambda gt11 expression library. Blood 73:1498, 1989

76. Sugano S, Stoeckle MY: Transformation by Rous sarcoma virus induces a novel gene with homology to a mitogenic platelet protein. Cell 49:321, 1987

77. Richmond A, Balentien E, Thomas HG et al: Molecular characterization and chromosomal mapping of melanoma growth stimulatory activity, a growth factor structurally related to beta-thromboglobulin. EMBO J 7:2025, 1988

78. Kaplanski G, Porat R, Aiura K et al: Activated platelets induce endothelial secretion of interleukin-8 in vitro via an interleukin-1-mediated event. Blood 81:2492, 1993

79. Sporn MB, Roberts AB, Wakefield LM, Assoian RK: Transforming growth factor-B: biological function and chemical structure. Science 233:532, 1986

80. Schultz-Cherry S, Murphy-Ullrich JE: Thrombospondin causes activation of latent transforming growth factor-beta secreted by endothelial cells by a novel mechanism. J Cell Biol 122:923, 1993

81. Mosher DF, Doyle MJ, Jaffe EA: Synthesis and secretion of thrombospondin by cultured human endothelial cells. J Cell Biol 93:343, 1982

82. Majack RA, Cook SC, Bornstein P: Platelet-derived growth factor and heparin-like glycosaminoglycans regulate thrombosponding synthesis and deposition in the matrix by smooth muscle cells. J Cell Biol 101:1059, 1985

83. Majack RA, Goodman LV, Dixit VM: Cell surface thrombospondin is functionally essentially for vascular smooth muscle cell proliferation. J Cell Biol 106:415, 1988

84. Handagama PJ, George JN, Shuman MA et al: Incorporation of a circulating protein into megakaryocyte and platelet granules (peroxidase/endocytosis/guinea pig). Proc Natl Acad Sci USA 84:861, 1987

85. Handagama PJ, Shuman MA, Bainton DF: Incorporation of intravenously injected albumin, immunoglobulin G, and fibrinogen in guinea pig megakaryocyte granules. J Clin Invest 84:73, 1989

86. George JN, Saucerman S, Levine SP et al: Immunoglobulin G is a platelet alpha granule-secreted protein. J Clin Invest 76:2020, 1985

87. Nichols WL, Gastineau DA, Solberg LA Jr, Mann KG: Identification of human megakaryocyte coagulation factor V. Blood 65:1396, 1985

88. Chiu HC, Schick PK, Colman RW: Biosynthesis of factor V in isolated guinea pig megakaryocytes. J Clin Invest 75:339, 1985

89. Wencel-Drake JD, Dahlback B, Ginsberg MH: Ultrastructural localization of coagulation factor V in human platelets. Blood 68:244, 1986

90. Mann KG, Nesheim ME, Hibbard LS, Tracy PB: The role of factor V in the assembly of the prothrombinase complex. Ann NY Acad Sci 370:378, 1981

91. Schwarz HP, Heeb MJ, Wencel-Drake JD, Griffin JH: Identification and quantitation of protein S in human platelets. Blood 66:1452, 1985

92. Erickson LA, Ginsberg MH, Loskutoff DJ: Detection and partial characterization of an inhibitor of plasminogen activator in human platelets. J Clin Invest 74:1465, 1984

93. Van Nostrand WE, Schmaier AH, Farrow JS et al: Protease nexin-2/amyloid beta-protein precursor in blood is a platelet-specific protein. Biochem Biophys Res Commun 175:15, 1991

94. Van Nostrand WE, Schmaier AH, Farrow JS, Cunningham DD: Protease nexin-II (amyloid beta-protein precursor): a platelet alpha-granule protein. Science 248:745, 1990

95. Oltersdorf T, Fritz LC, Schenk DB et al: The secreted form of the Alzheimer's amyloid precursor protein with the Kunitz domain is protease nexin-II. Nature 341:144, 1989

96. Komiyama Y, Murakami T, Egawa H et al: Purification of factor XIa inhibitor from human platelets. Thromb Res 66:397, 1992

97. McEver RP: Selectins: novel receptors that mediate leukocyte adhesion during inflammation. Thromb Haemost 65:223, 1991

98. Larsen E, Cell A, Gilbert GE et al: PADGEM protein: a receptor that mediates the interaction of activated platelets with neutrophils and monocytes. Cell 59:305, 1989

99. Stoolman LM: Adhesion molecules controlling lymphocyte migration. Cell 56:907, 1989

100. Buck CA: Immunoglobulin superfamily: structure, function and relationship to other receptor molecules. Semin Cell Biology 3:179, 1992

101. Johnston GI, Cook RG, McEver RP: Cloning of GMP-140, a granule membrane protein of platelets and endothelium: sequence similarity to proteins involved in cell adhesion and inflammation. Cell 56:1033, 1989

102. Nagata K, Tsuji T, Todoroki N et al: Activated platelets induce superoxide anion release by monocytes and neutrophils through P-selectin (CD62). J Immunol 151:3267, 1993

103. Palabrica T, Lobb R, Furie BC et al: Leukocyte accumulation promoting fibrin deposition is mediated in vivo by P-selectin on adherent platelets. Nature 359:848, 1992

104. Stone JP, Wagner DD: P-selectin mediates adhesion of platelets to neuroblastoma and small cell lung cancer. J Clin Invest 92:804, 1993

105. Nachman RL, Levine R, Jaffe EA: Synthesis of factor VIII antigen by cultured guinea pig megakaryocytes. J Clin Invest 60:914, 1977

106. Lopez-Fernandez M, Ginsberg MH, Ruggeri ZM et al: Multimeric structure of platelet factor VIII/von Willebrand factor: the presence of larger multimers and their reassociation with thrombin-stimulated platelets. Blood 60:1132, 1982

107. Paul JI, Schwarzbauer JE, Tamkun JW, Hynes RO: Cell-type-specific fibronectin subunits generated by alternative splicing. J Biol Chem 261:12258, 1986

108. Barnes DW, Silnutzer J, See C, Shaffer M: Characterization of human serum spreading factor with monoclonal antibody. Proc Natl Acad Sci USA 80:1362, 1983

109. Salonen E-M, Vaheri A, Pollanen J et al: Interaction of plasminogen activator inhibitor (PAI-1) with vitronectin. J Biol Chem 264:6339, 1989

110. Charo IF, Feinman RD, Detwiler TC: Interrelations of platelet aggregation and secretion. J Clin Invest 60:866, 1977

111. Palade G: Intracellular aspects of the process of protein synthesis. Science 189:347, 1975

112. Morgenstern E, Edelmann L: Fibrinogen distribution on surfaces and in organelles of ADP stimulated human blood platelets. Eur J Cell Biol 38:292, 1985

113. Allen RD, Zacharski LR, Widirstky ST et al: Transformation and motility of human platelets: details of the shape change and release reaction observed by optical and electron microscopy. J Cell Biol 83:126, 1979

114. Wencel-Drake JD, Plow EF, Kunicki TJ et al: Localization of internal pools of membrane glycoproteins involved in platelet adhesive responses. Am J Pathol 124:324, 1986

115. Berman CL, Yeo EL, Wencel-Drake JD et al: A platelet alpha granule membrane protein that is associated with the plasma membrane after activation. Characterization and subcellular localization of PADGEM glycoprotein. J Clin Invest 78:130, 1986

116. Stenberg PE, McEver RP, Shuman MA et al: A platelet alpha-granule membrane protein (GMP-140) is expressed on the plasma membrane after activation. J Cell Biol 101:880, 1985

117. Morgenstern E, Neumann K, Patscheke H: The exocytosis of human blood platelets. A fast freezing and freeze-substitution analysis. Eur J Cell Biol 43:273, 1987

118. White JG: Current concepts of platelet structure. Am J Clin Pathol 71:363, 1979

119. Stenberg PE, Shuman MA, Levine SP, Bainton DF: Redistribution of alpha-granules and their contents in thrombin-stimulated platelets. J Cell Biol 98:748, 1984

120. Droller MJ: Ultrastructure of the platelet release reaction in response to various aggregating agents and their inhibitors. Lab Invest 29:12015, 1973

121. Leung LL, Kinoshita T, Nachman RL: Isolation, purification, and partial characterization of platelet membrane glycoproteins IIb and IIIa. J Biol Chem 256:1994, 1981

122. White JG: A search for the platelet secretory pathway using electron dense tracers. Am J Pathol 58:31, 1970

123. Behnke O: Electron microscopic observations on the membrane systems of the rat blood platelet. Anat Rec 158:121, 1967

124. Painter RG, Ginsberg MH: Centripetal myosin redistribution in thrombin-stimulated platelets. Relationship to platelet factor 4 secretion. Exp Cell Res 155:198, 1984

125. Wencel-Drake JD, Frelinger AL III, Dieter MG, Lam SC-T: Arg-Gly-Asp-dependent occupancy of GPIIb/IIIa by applaggin: evidence for internalization and cycling of a platelet integrin. Blood 81:62, 1993

126. Wencel-Drake JD: Plasma membrane GPIIb/IIIa: evidence for a cycling receptor pool. Am J Pathol 136:61, 1990

127. Michelson AD, Adelman B, Barnard MR et al: Platelet storage results in a redistribution of glycoprotein Ib molecules. Evidence for a large intraplatelet pool of glycoprotein Ib. J Clin Invest 81:1734, 1988

128. Kirchhofer D, Gailit J, Ruoslahti E et al: Cation-dependent changes in the binding specificity of the platelet receptor GPIIb-IIIa. J Biol Chem 265:18525, 1990

129. Broekman MJ, Handin RI, Cohen P: Distribution of fibrinogen, and platelet factors 4 and XIII in subcellular fractions of human platelets. Br J Haematol 31:51, 1975

130. Gerrard JM, Phillips DR, Rao GH et al: Biochemical studies of two patients with the gray platelet syndrome. Selective deficiency of platelet alpha granules. J Clin Invest 66:102, 1980

131. Ernst E, Resch KL: Fibrinogen as a cardiovascular risk factor: a meta-analysis and review of the literature. Ann Intern Med 118:956, 1993

132. Weiss HJ, Hawiger J, Ruggeri ZM et al: Fibrinogen-independent platelet adhesion and thrombus formation on subendothelium mediated by glycoprotein IIb-IIIa complex at high shear rate. J Clin Invest 83:288, 1989

133. Weiss HJ, Pietu G, Rabinowitz R et al: Heterogeneous abnormalities in the multimeric structure, antigenic properties, and plasma-platelet content of factor VIII/von Willebrand factor in subtypes of classic (type 1) and variant (type 11A) von Willebrand's disease. J Lab Clin Med 101:411, 1983

134. DeMarco L, Mazzucato M, DeRoia D et al: Distinct abnormalities in the interaction of purified types IIA and IIB von Willebrand factor with the two platelet binding sites, glycoprotein complexes Ib-IX and IIb-IIIa. J Clin Invest 86:785, 1990

135. Saba HI, Fujimura Y, Saba SR et al: Spontaneous platelet aggregation in type IIB Tampa von Willebrand disease is inhibited by the 52/48-kDa fragment of normal von Willebrand factor, which contains the GPIb binding domain. Am J Hematol 30:150, 1989

136. Weiss HJ, Meyer D, Rabinowitz R et al: Pseudo-von Willebrand's disease. An intrinsic platelet defect with aggregation by unmodified human factor VIII/von Willebrand factor and enhanced adsorption of its high-molecular-weight multimers. N Engl J Med 306:326, 1982

137. Gralnick HR, Williams SB, McKeown LP et al: Von Willebrand's disease with spontaneous platelet aggregation induced by an abnormal plasma von Willebrand factor. J Clin Invest 76:1522, 1985

138. Bennett JS, Vilaire G: Exposure of platelet fibrinogen receptors by ADP and epinephrine. J Clin Invest 64:1393, 1979

139. Marguerie GA, Plow EF, Edgington TS: Human platelets possess an inducible and saturable receptor specific for fibrinogen. J Biol Chem 254:5357, 1979

140. Mustard JF, Kinlough-Rathbone RL, Packham MA et al: Comparison of fibrinogen association with normal and thrombasthenic platelets on exposure to ADP or chymotrypsin. Blood 54:987, 1979

141. Marguerie GA, Thomas-Maison N, Larrieu M-J, Plow EF: The interaction of fibrinogen with its platelet receptor in the plasma milieu. Blood 59:91, 1982

142. Marguerie GA, Ardaillou N, Cherel G, Plow EF: The binding of fibrinogen to its platelet receptor. J Biol Chem 257:11872, 1982

143. Marguerie GA, Plow EF: Interaction of fibrinogen with its platelet receptor: kinetics and the effect of pH and temperature. Biochemistry 20:1074, 1981

144. Marguerie GA, Edgington TS, Plow EF: Interaction of fibrinogen with its platelet receptor as part of a multistep reaction in ADP-induced platelet aggregation. J Biol Chem 255:154, 1980

145. Plow EF, Marguerie GA: A regulatory role of fibrinogen in platelet aggregation. Circulation 62:131, 1980

146. Plow EF, Marguerie GA: Participation of ADP in the binding of fibrinogen to thrombin-stimulated platelets. Blood 56:553, 1980

147. Peerschke EL, Zucker MB, Grant RA et al: Correlation between fibrinogen binding to human platelets and platelet aggregability. Blood 55:841, 1980

148. Peerschke EI: Irreversible platelet fibrinogen interactions occur independently of fibrinogen alpha chain degradation and are not mediated by intact platelet membrane glycoprotein IIb-IIIa complexes. J Lab Clin Med 111:84, 1988

149. Peerschke EI: Decreased accessibility of platelet-bound fibrinogen to antibody and enzyme probes. Blood 74:682, 1989

150. Bennett JS, Hoxie JA, Leitman SF et al: Inhibition of fibrinogen binding to stimulated human platelets by a monoclonal antibody. Proc Natl Acad Sci USA 80:2417, 1983

151. Bennett JS, Vilaire G, Cines DB: Identification of the fibrinogen receptor on human platelets by photoaffinity labeling. J Biol Chem 257:8049, 1982

152. Parise LV, Phillips DR: Reconstitution of the purified platelet fibrinogen receptor fibrinogen binding properties of the glycoprotein IIb-IIIa complex. J Biol Chem 260:10698, 1985

153. Ginsberg MH, Loftus JC, Ryckwaert J-J et al: Immunochemical and amino-terminal sequence comparison of two cytoadhesins indicates they contain similar or identical beta subunits and distinct alpha subunits. J Biol Chem 262:5437, 1987

154. Lam SC-T, Plow EF, D'Souza SE et al: Isolation and characterization of a platelet membrane protein related to the vitronectin receptor. J Biol Chem 264:3742, 1989

155. Fitzgerald LA, Charo IF, Phillips DR: Human and bovine endothelial cells synthesize membrane proteins similar to human platelet glycoproteins IIb and IIIa. J Biol Chem 260:10893, 1985

156. Charo IF, Fitzgerald LA, Steiner B et al: Platelet glycoproteins IIb and IIIa: evidence for a family of immunologically and structurally related glycoproteins in mammalian cells. Proc Natl Acad Sci USA 83:8351, 1986

157. Fitzgerald LA, Steiner B, Rall SC Jr et al: Protein sequence of endothelial glycoprotein IIIa derived from a cDNA clone. Identity with platelet glycoprotein IIIa and similarity to integrin. J Biol Chem 262:3936, 1987

158. Calvete JJ, Henschen A, Gonzalez-Rodriguez J: Assignment of disulphide bonds in human platelet GPIIIa. A disulphide pattern for the beta-subunits of the integrin family. Biochem J 274:63, 1991

159. Calvete JJ, Henschen A, Gonzalez-Rodriguez J: Complete localization of the intrachain disulphide bonds and the N-glycosylation points in the alpha-subunit of human platelet glycoprotein IIb. Biochem J 261:561, 1989

160. Calvete JJ, Alvarez MV, Rivas G et al: Interchain and intrachain disulphide bonds in human platelet glycoprotein IIb. Localization of the epitopes for several monoclonal antibodies. Biochem J 261:551, 1989

161. Reason AJ, Dell A, Morris HR et al: Characterisation of the N-linked oligosaccharides of the light chain of human glycoprotein IIb by f.a.b.-m.s. Carbohydr Res 221:169, 1991

162. Duperray A, Troesch A, Berthier R et al: Biosynthesis and assembly of platelet GPIIb-IIIa in human megakaryocytes: evidence that assembly between pro-GPIIb and GPIIIa is a prerequisite for expression of the complex on the cell surface. Blood 74:1603, 1989

163. Jennings LK, Phillips DR: Purification of glycoproteins IIb and III from human platelet plasma membranes and characterization of a calcium-dependent glycoprotein IIb-III complex. J Biol Chem 257:10458, 1982

164. O'Toole TE, Loftus JC, Plow EF et al: Efficient surface expression of platelet GPIIb-IIIa requires both subunits. Blood 74:14, 1989

165. Fujimura K, Phillips DR: Calcium cation regulation of glycoprotein IIb-IIIa complex formation in platelet plasma membranes. J Biol Chem 258:10247, 1983

166. Fitzgerald LA, Phillips DR: Calcium regulation of the platelet membrane glycoprotein IIb-IIIa complex. J Biol Chem 260:11366, 1985

167. Steiner B, Parise LV, Leung B, Phillips DR: Ca^{2+}-dependent structural transitions of the platelet glycoprotein IIb-IIIa complex. J Biol Chem 266:14986, 1991

168. Brass LF, Shattil SJ, Kunicki TJ, Bennett JS: Effect of calcium on the stability of the platelet membrane glycoprotein IIb-IIIa complex. J Biol Chem 260:7875, 1985

169. Kunicki TJ, Pidard D, Rosa J-P, Nurden AT: The formation of Ca^{++}-dependent complexes of platelet membrane glycoproteins IIb and IIIa in solution as determined by crossed immunoelectrophoresis. Blood 58:268, 1981

170. Coller BS: Activation affects access to the platelet receptor for adhesive glycoproteins. J Cell Biol 103:451, 1986

171. Sims PJ, Ginsberg MH, Plow EF, Shattil SJ: Effect of platelet activation on the conformation of the plasma membrane glycoprotein IIb-IIIa complex. J Biol Chem 266:7345, 1991

172. O'Toole TE, Loftus JC, Du X et al: Affinity modulation of the $\alpha_{IIb}\beta_3$ integrin (platelet GPIIb-IIIa) is an intrinsic property of the receptor. Cell Regul 1:883, 1990

173. Shattil SJ, Hoxie JA, Cunningham M, Brass LF: Changes in the platelet membrane glycoprotein IIb-IIIa complex during platelet activation. J Biol Chem 260:11107, 1985

174. Kloczewiak M, Timmons S, Lukas TJ, Hawiger J: Platelet receptor recogni-

tion site on human fibrinogen, synthesis and structure-function relationship of peptides corresponding to the carboxy-terminal segment of the gamma chain. Biochemistry 23:1767, 1984

175. Kloczewiak M, Timmons S, Bednarek MA et al: Platelet receptor recognition domain on the gamma chain of human fibrinogen and its synthetic peptide analogues. Biochemistry 28:2915, 1989
176. Gawaz MP, Loftus JC, Bajt ML et al: Ligand bridging mediates integrin $\alpha_{IIb}\beta_3$ (platelet GPIIb-IIIa) dependent homotypic and heterotypic cell-cell interactions. J Clin Invest 88:1128, 1991
177. Zamarron C, Ginsberg MH, Plow EF: A receptor-induced binding site in fibrinogen elicited by its interaction with platelet membrane glycoprotein IIb-IIIa. J Biol Chem 266:16193, 1991
178. Abrams CS, Ellison N, Budzynski AZ, Shattil SJ: Direct detection of activated platelets and platelet-derived microparticles in humans. Blood 75:128, 1990
179. Frelinger AL III, Lam SC-T, Plow EF et al: Occupancy of an adhesive glycoprotein receptor modulates expression of an antigenic site involved in cell adhesion. J Biol Chem 263:12397, 1988
180. Isenberg WM, McEver RP, Phillips DR et al: The platelet fibrinogen receptor: an immunogold-surface replica study of agonist-induced ligand binding and receptor clustering. J Cell Biol 104:1655, 1987
181. Tuszynski GP, Kornecki E, Cierniewski C et al: Association of fibrin with the platelet cytoskeleton. J Biol Chem 259:5247, 1984
182. Painter RG, Ginsberg MH: Concanavalin A induces interactions between surface glycoproteins and the platelet cytoskeleton. J Cell Biol 92:565, 1982
183. Phillips DR, Jennings LK, Edwards HH: Identification of membrane proteins mediating the interaction of human platelets. J Cell Biol 86:77, 1980
184. Yasuda T, Gold HK, Fallon JT et al: Monoclonal antibody against the platelet glycoprotein (GP) IIb/IIIa receptor prevents coronary artery reocclusion after reperfusion with recombinant tissue-type plasminogen activator in dogs. J Clin Invest 81:1284, 1988
185. Shebuski RJ, Berry DE, Bennett DB et al: Demonstration of Ac-Arg-Gly-Asp-Ser-NH$_2$ as an antiaggregatory agent in the dog by intracoronary administration. Thromb Haemost 61:183, 1989
186. Phillips DR, Charo IF, Scarborough RM: GPIIb-IIIa: the responsive integrin. Cell 65:359, 1991
187. Scarborough RM, Rose JW, Naughton MA et al: Characterization of the integrin specificities of disintegrins isolated from American pit viper venoms. J Biol Chem 268:1058, 1993
188. Haskel EJ, Adams SP, Feigen LP et al: Prevention of reoccluding platelet-rich thrombi in canine femoral arteries with a novel peptide antagonist of platelet glycoprotein IIb/IIIa receptors. Circulation 80:1775, 1989
189. Rote WE, Werns SW, Davis JH et al: Platelet GPIIb/IIIa receptor inhibition by SC-49992 prevents thrombosis and rethrombosis in the canine carotid artery. Cardiovasc Res 27:500, 1993
190. Kloczewiak M, Timmons S, Hawiger J: Localization of a site interacting with human platelet receptor on carboxy-terminal segment of human fibrinogen gamma chain. Biochem Biophys Res Commun 107:181, 1982
191. Tranqui L, Andrieux A, Hudry-Clergeon G et al: Differential structural requirements for fibrinogen binding to platelets and to endothelial cells. J Cell Biol 108:2519, 1989
192. Ginsberg MH, Pierschbacher MD, Ruoslahti E et al: Inhibition of fibronectin binding to platelets by proteolytic fragments and synthetic peptides which support fibroblast adhesion. J Biol Chem 260:3931, 1985
193. Plow EF, Pierschbacher MD, Ruoslahti E et al: The effect of Arg-Gly-Asp-containing peptides on fibrinogen and von Willebrand factor binding to platelets. Proc Natl Acad Sci USA 82:8057, 1985
194. Gartner TK, Bennett JS: The tetrapeptide analogue of the cell attachment site of fibronectin inhibits platelet aggregation and fibrinogen binding to activated platelets. J Biol Chem 260:11891, 1985
195. Haverstick DM, Cowan JF, Yamada KM, Santoro SA: Inhibition of platelet

adhesion to fibronectin, fibrinogen, and von Willebrand factor substrates by a synthetic tetrapeptide derived from the cell-binding domain of fibronectin. Blood 66:946, 1985
196. Doolittle RF: Fibrinogen and fibrin. Sci Am 106:126, 1981
197. D'Souza SE, Ginsberg MH, Plow EF: Arginyl-Glycyl-Aspartic Acid (RGD): a cell adhesion motif. TIBS 16:246, 1991
198. Koivunen E, Gay DA, Ruoslahti E: Selection of peptides binding of the $\alpha_5\beta_1$ integrin from phage display library. J Biol Chem 268:20205, 1993
199. Hautanen A, Gailit J, Mann DM, Ruoslahti E: Effects of modifications of the RGD sequence and its context on recognition by the fibronectin receptor. J Biol Chem 264:1437, 1989
200. Ruoslahti E, Pierschbacher MD: New perspectives in cell adhesion: RGD and integrins. Science 238:491, 1987
201. Pytela RP, Pierschbacher MD, Ginsberg MH et al: Platelet membrane glycoprotein IIb/IIIa: member of a family of Arg-Gly-Asp-specific adhesion receptors. Science 231:1559, 1986
202. Ruoslahti E, Pierschbacher MD: Arg-Gly-Asp: a versatile cell recognition signal. Cell 44:517, 1986
203. Lam SC-T, Plow EF, Smith MA et al: Evidence that arginyl-glycyl-aspartate peptides and fibrinogen gamma chain peptides share a common binding site on platelets. J Biol Chem 262:947, 1987
204. Santoro SA, Lawing WJ Jr: Competition for related but nonidentical binding sites on the glycoprotein IIb-IIIa complex by peptides derived from platelet adhesive proteins. Cell 48:867, 1987
205. Farrell DH, Thiagarajan P, Chung DW, Davie EW: Role of fibrinogen alpha and gamma chain sites in platelet aggregation. Proc Natl Acad Sci USA 89:10729, 1992
206. Hettasch JM, Bolyard MG, Lord ST: The residues AGDV of recombinant gamma chains of human fibrinogen must be carboxy-terminal to support human platelet aggregation. Thromb Haemost 68:701, 1992
207. Gartner TK, Amrani DL, Derrick JM et al: Characterization of adhesion of "resting" and stimulated platelets to fibrinogen and its fragments. Thromb Res 71:47, 1993
208. Thiagarajan P, Kelly KL: Exposure of binding sites for vitronectin on platelets following stimulation. J Biol Chem 263:3035, 1988
209. Phillips DR, Jennings LK, Prasanna HR: Ca2+-mediated association of glycoprotein G (thrombin sensitive protein, thrombospondin) with human platelets. J Biol Chem 255:11629, 1980
210. Wolff R, Plow EF, Ginsberg MH: Interaction of thrombospondin with resting and stimulated human platelets. J Biol Chem 261:6840, 1986
211. Aiken ML, Ginsberg MH, Plow EF: Divalent cation dependent and independent surface expression of thrombospondin on thrombin stimulated human platelets. Blood 69:58, 1987
212. Leung LL: Role of thrombospondin in platelet aggregation. J Clin Invest 74:1764, 1984
213. Leung LL, Nachman RL: Complex formation of platelet thrombospondin with fibrinogen. J Clin Invest 70:542, 1982
214. Asch AS, Barnwell J, Silverstein RL, Nachman RL: Isolation of the thrombospondin membrane receptor. J Clin Invest 79:1054, 1987
215. Lawler J, Weinstein R, Hynes RO: Cell attachment to thrombospondin: the role of ARG-GLY-ASP, calcium, and integrin receptors. J Cell Biol 107:2351, 1988
216. Tuszynski GP, Karczewski J, Smith L et al: The GPIIb-IIIa-like complex may function as a human melanoma cell adhesion receptor for thrombospondin. Exp Cell Res 182:473, 1989
217. Karczewski J, Knudsen KA, Smith L et al: The interaction of thrombospondin with platelet glycoprotein GPIIb-IIIa. J Biol Chem 264:21322, 1989
218. Roberts DD, Haverstick DM, Dixit VM et al: The platelet glycoprotein thrombospondin binds specifically to sulfated glycolipids. J Biol Chem 260:9405, 1985

Molecular Basis for Platelet Activation

98

Lawrence F. Brass

INTRODUCTION

Platelets play two related roles in hemostasis. First, by forming multicellular aggregates linked by fibrinogen, platelets help to create a physical barrier that limits the loss of blood from sites of vascular injury. Second, by accelerating the rate at which coagulation proteins are activated, phospholipids on the platelet surface facilitate thrombin generation and fibrin formation. For the purposes of this chapter, platelet activation can be thought of as occurring in three phases: (1) an activating event caused by contact with an agonist such as collagen or thrombin, (2) generation of intracellular second messengers, and (3) a set of responses that include cytoskeletal rearrangements (shape change), storage granule exocytosis (secretion), and platelet-platelet interactions (aggregation). These events mirror those that occur in other hematopoietic cells, but in platelets they are uniquely adapted to the platelet's role in hemostasis.

PLATELET AGONISTS AND THEIR RECEPTORS

A variety of agents have been shown to cause or support platelet activation, including normal constituents of the subendothelial connective tissue matrix (collagen), plasma proteins (von Willebrand factor [vWF]), plasma proteases (thrombin), circulating hormones (epinephrine and vasopressin), and products of platelet metabolism (ADP and thromboxane A_2 [TxA_2]). Under normal conditions, platelet activation begins when vascular damage strips away endothelial cells, exposing the underlying connective tissue layer and tissue factor, and causing platelets to be activated by collagen and thrombin (Fig. 98-1).

Platelet agonists are commonly classified as strong or weak, but the distinctions between them are often blurred. By one definition, strong agonists are those that can trigger granule secretion even when aggregation is prevented. Thrombin and collagen are examples of strong agonists. By contrast, weak agonists, such as ADP and epinephrine, require aggregation for secretion to occur. Presumably the real differences between strong and weak agonists reflect differences in the sets of intracellular effectors that are coupled to their receptors. For example, the strong agonists stimulate phosphoinositide hydrolysis and eicosanoid formation, raise the cytosolic free Ca^{2+} concentration, and cause aggregation and secretion that are relatively unimpaired by inhibitors of TxA_2 formation. This suggests that their receptors are coupled to both phospholipase C and phospholipase A_2. It also suggests that the phosphoinositide hydrolysis pathway is the dominant mediator of platelet responses to strong agonists. The weak agonists, on the other hand, have little or no ability to cause phosphoinositide hydrolysis and are more dependent on TxA_2 formation for their effects. This suggests that their receptors are linked to phospholipase A_2, but not to phospholipase C. In theory, it should be possible to account for all of the effects of different platelet agonists in this manner. However, at the moment this is not possible. There are still too many unexplained differences from agonist to agonist.

For example, although neither ADP nor epinephrine cause phosphoinositide hydrolysis in human platelets, ADP is able to raise the cytosolic free Ca^{2+} concentration while epinephrine does not, probably because of the ability of ADP, but not epinephrine, to allow a rapid influx of Ca^{2+} across the platelet plasma membrane.

The receptors for most, if not all, platelet agonists are formed by plasma membrane proteins with one or more transmembrane domains. Of the receptors that have been fully characterized, five are members of the large superfamily of G-protein-coupled receptors (Fig. 98-2 and Table 98-1). Each of these has a characteristic structure consisting of a single polypeptide with seven transmembrane domains, and each is coupled by G proteins to second messenger generating enzymes such as phospholipase C_β and adenylyl cyclase (Table 98-2).

Thrombin

Thrombin is a serine protease whose natural substrates include fibrinogen, factor V, factor VIII, and protein C. Thrombin is generated in vivo by the sequential activation of the enzymes of the coagulation cascade. Since negatively charged phospholipids on the surface of activated platelets accelerate coagulation factor activation, platelets promote thrombin generation. Since thrombin in turn causes platelet activation, a mutually reinforcing relationship exists that promotes hemostasis. When added to platelets in vitro, thrombin causes phosphoinositide hydrolysis, TXA_2 formation, protein phosphorylation, and an increase in the cytosolic free Ca^{2+} concentration, as well as shape change, granule secretion, and fibrinogen receptor exposure[1-8] (Fig. 98-3). Thrombin also suppresses cAMP synthesis.[9] These responses can be detected at thrombin concentrations as low as 0.1 nM (approximately 0.01 NIH U/ml of highly purified thrombin). Although arachidonate metabolites such as TxA_2 contribute to platelet responses to thrombin, increasing the thrombin concentration overcomes the blockade of platelet activation caused by aspirin, suggesting that TxA_2 formation is helpful, but not necessary, for thrombin-induced platelet activation.

All the platelet responses to thrombin require proteolytically active thrombin, and many, if not all, appear to be mediated by G proteins. Until recently, however, the thrombin receptor had not been identified, and there was no satisfactory explanation for the mechanism of its activation. Binding studies with radioiodinated thrombin suggested that there were approximately 50 high-affinity thrombin-binding sites per platelet with a K_d of 0.3 nM and 1,700 moderate-affinity sites per platelet with a K_d of 11 nM.[10] The high-affinity binding sites are believed to be associated with membrane glycoprotein (GP) Ib,[11] which is itself a substrate for thrombin, along with GPIX and GPV.[12-15]

In 1991 two laboratories using expression cloning in *Xenopus laevis* oocytes independently reported the successful isolation of similar cDNA clones encoding thrombin receptors from the human megakaryoblastic Dami cell line[16] and from hamster fibroblasts.[17] The structure of the Dami cell thrombin receptor is illustrated in Figure 98-4. Structurally, it resembles other re-

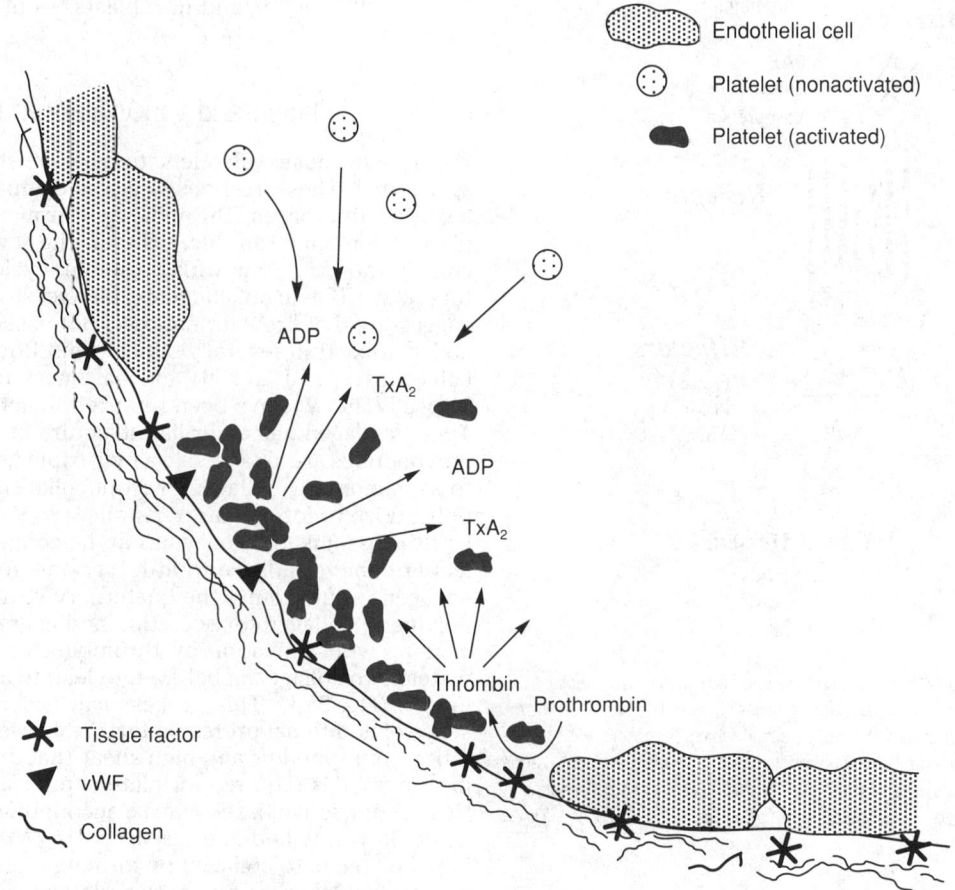

Endothelial cell

Platelet (nonactivated)

Platelet (activated)

ADP

TxA₂

ADP

TxA₂

Thrombin

Prothrombin

✳ Tissue factor

▼ vWF

〜 Collagen

Fig. 98-1. Platelet activation at the vessel wall. Platelet activation begins when vascular damage strips away endothelial cells, exposing collagen and tissue factor. Circulating platelets adhere to the exposed collagen, either directly or via vWF. Others are activated by locally generated thrombin. These events are followed by a change in the platelet's shape, storage granule secretion, and the formation of multicellular aggregates as additional platelets are recruited into the growing platelet plug. The recruitment of nonadherent platelets is facilitated by the release of soluble factors from the platelets, such as ADP and TxA₂. This phase of hemostasis is completed when the platelet plug is stabilized by a meshwork of fibrin.

ceptors that interact with G proteins. In particular, it is comprised of a single polypeptide chain with seven hydrophobic domains, an extracellular N terminus, and sites for post-translational processing including palmitoylation and N-linked glycosylation. Homologies with protein C helped to define a potential site for cleavage by thrombin in the receptor N terminus between residues Arg^{41} and Ser$^{42.}$ Mutations at this site prevented activation of the expressed receptor by thrombin.[16,18]

Based on the existence of a potential thrombin cleavage site within the N terminus of the receptor, it was proposed that the N terminus distal to the point of cleavage forms a tethered ligand capable of activating the receptor.[16] In support of this hypothesis, a 14-residue peptide corresponding to residues Ser^{42}–Phe^{55} (SFLLRNPNDKYEPF) was shown to cause platelet aggregation, and mutations in the tethered ligand domain were found to inhibit activation of the expressed receptor.[16,19] Subsequent studies have shown that receptor-derived peptides can also evoke many, if not all, of the other effects of thrombin on platelets, as well as on other thrombin-responsive cells, including fibroblasts, smooth muscle cells, monocytes, endothelial cells, and some lymphocytes. Thus, a short peptide whose sequence corresponds to a portion of the receptor can reproduce the effects of a 36-kd protease. Extending this concept further, studies from a number of laboratories have now shown that the first five residues of the tethered ligand domain SFLLR are sufficient to activate the receptor[19–21] and that anti-

Table 98-1. Agonist Receptors on Platelets

Agonist	Receptor	Platelets (~N)	Receptor Type	References
Thrombin	Thrombin receptor^a	1,800	G protein coupled	16, 22
TxA₂	TxA₂ receptor	1,000	G protein coupled	74, 78
Epinephrine	α₂-Adrenergic	300	G protein coupled	59, 60, 65
Platelet-activating factor (PAF)	PAF receptor	200–2,000	G protein coupled	246, 247
Vasopressin	V₁ receptor	100	G protein coupled	248–251
ADP	?	?	?	47
Collagen	GPIa/IIa^b	?	Integrin and ?	

^{a} GPIb has also been shown to be a high-affinity binding site for thrombin on platelets (see text), but has not yet been shown to be a functional receptor.
^{b} GPIa/IIa has been shown to bind collagen, but has not yet been shown to be a functional receptor.

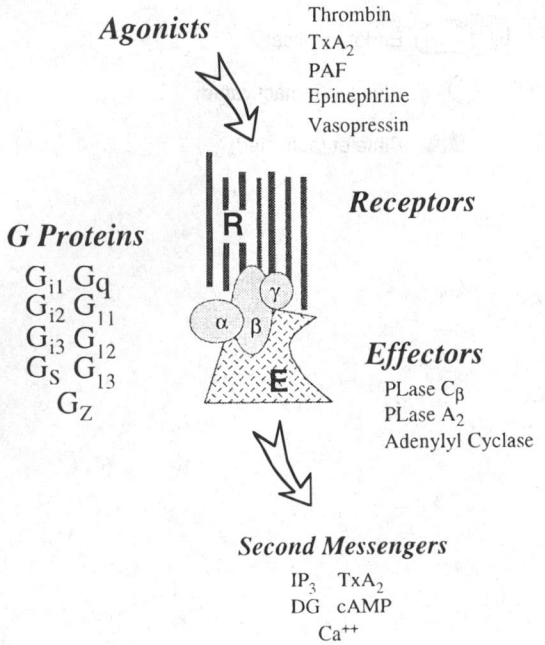

Agonists

Thrombin
TxA_2
PAF
Epinephrine
Vasopressin

Receptors

G Proteins

G_{i1} G_q
G_{i2} G_{11}
G_{i3} G_{12}
G_s G_{13}
G_z

Effectors

PLase C_β
PLase A_2
Adenylyl Cyclase

Second Messengers

IP_3 TxA_2
DG cAMP
Ca^{++}

Fig. 98-2. Platelet activation via a common mechanism involving receptors, G proteins, and second messenger generating enzymes. Five of the agonists known to activate platelets share a common mechanism in which receptors with seven transmembrane domains are coupled to phospholipase C_β, phospholipase A_2, and/or adenylyl cyclase by one or more of the nine G proteins known to be present in platelets. These enzymes determine the concentrations of IP_3, DAG, Ca^{2+}, TxA_2, and cAMP present in the platelets.

bodies directed against this domain can inhibit platelet activation by thrombin.[22,23] Those same antibodies bind to approximately 1,800 sites per platelet,[22] a number in good agreement with the number of moderate-affinity thrombin-binding sites.[10] Present models suggest that, once exposed by thrombin, the tethered ligand domain interacts with as yet unidentified sites in the remainder of the receptor, producing a conformational change that is transmitted across the plasma membrane to the cytosolic domains of the receptor. In turn, this causes an exchange of GDP for GTP on receptor-associated G proteins, leading to an increase in phospholipase C_β activity and suppression of adenylyl cyclase.[24] Each thrombin receptor is thought to produce only a brief burst of activity before the GTP on the G proteins is hydrolyzed back to GDP and the receptors become desensitized.[25–27] As with other G-protein-coupled receptors, desensitization of the thrombin receptor is thought to be due to a combination of receptor phosphorylation and sequestration.[25–28] Internalization of activated thrombin receptors via coated pits in the plasma membrane, followed by intracellular trafficking through endosomes and into lysosomes or back to the cell surface, has been demonstrated in megakaryo-

blastic cell lines[26,27] and fibroblasts,[25] but may not occur on platelets.[29]

Collagen and von Willebrand Factor

Collagen causes platelets to change shape, secrete, and aggregate.[6] These responses are accompanied by phosphoinositide hydrolysis, thromboxane formation, protein phosphorylation, and an increase in the cytosolic free Ca^{2+} concentration.[30–34] As with thrombin, cyclo-oxygenase inhibitors retard, but do not eliminate, platelet responses to collagen, suggesting that TxA_2 formation is not essential.[30–32,34] Human collagen exists in several distinct forms. Both connective tissue collagen (types I and III) and basement membrane collagen (types IV and V) have been reported to activate platelets.[35–37] Type I collagen has a fibrillar structure in which three 100-kd polypeptides are arranged in a long triple-helical array referred to as monomeric collagen or tropocollagen. These monomers polymerize to form a larger parallel array that becomes covalently cross-linked by enzymes in the connective matrix. Platelets are able to adhere to at least some forms of monomeric collagen,[37] but require the quaternary structure presented by polymeric collagen for secretion and aggregation.[38]

Along with activation by thrombin, the initial adhesion of platelets to collagen is believed to lead to aggregate formation in vivo (Fig. 98-1). This process can occur in vitro in the absence of additional protein cofactors. However, under the conditions of rapid flow and high shear that are normally present in vivo, vWF is required for platelet adhesion to the subendothelial connective tissue matrix, accounting for the hemostatic defect in von Willebrand disease.[39–43] vWF supports the binding of platelets to collagen by forming a bridge between collagen and glycoproteins on the platelet surface, particularly GPIb. In addition, there is reason to believe that platelets also express receptors through which they interact with collagen directly. One of these is the GPIa/IIa (integrin $\alpha_2\beta_1$) complex.[44] Two unrelated patients have been described with hemorrhagic disorders and defective platelet responses to collagen. Both proved to have little or no GPIa and reduced amounts of GPIIa.[45,46] Liposomes that contain GPIa and GPIIa have been shown to stick to collagen fibrils in the Mg^{2+}-dependent manner that is characteristic of the platelet-collagen interaction.[47] Therefore, the GPIa/IIa complex appears to be capable of binding to collagen; whether it is also a signal transducing receptor remains to be determined.

ADP

In contrast to thrombin and collagen, ADP can originate from within the platelet, where it is normally stored in the dense secretory granules. Secretion of this ADP, along with TxA_2, helps to recruit additional platelets into a growing platelet plug. When added to platelets in vitro, ADP causes TxA_2 formation,

Table 98-2. G Protein α-Subunits in Platelets[a]

G Protein	kd	Toxin[c]	Phosphorylated?	Enzyme Regulated	Function	References
$G_{i\alpha2}$, $G_{i\alpha3}$, $G_{i\alpha1}$	40–41	Pertussis	No	Adenylyl cyclase, phospholipase C?	↑ cAMP, ↑ IP_3/DAG[b]	85
$G_{z\alpha}$	41	Neither	Yes	?	?	119, 120, 252
$G_{q\alpha}$, $G_{11\alpha}$	42	Neither	No	Phospholipase C	↑ IP_3/DAG	24, 102
$G_{12\alpha2}$, $G_{13\alpha3}$	44	Neither	?	?	?	24
$G_{s\alpha}$	45	Cholera	No	Adenylyl cyclase	↑ cAMP	253

Abbreviation: IP_3/DAG, inositol 1,4,5-triphosphate/diacylglycerol.
[a] The G protein subunits $G_{o\alpha}$ and $G_{16\alpha}$ have been sought in platelets by Western blots, but not detected.[24]
[b] The involvement of the G_i family members as the source of the $G_{\beta\gamma}$ is presumptive, but is based on the absence of any other pertussis toxin-sensitive G proteins in platelets.
[c] "Toxin" refers to whether the α-subunit is a substrate for ADP-ribosylation by pertussis toxin or cholera toxin.

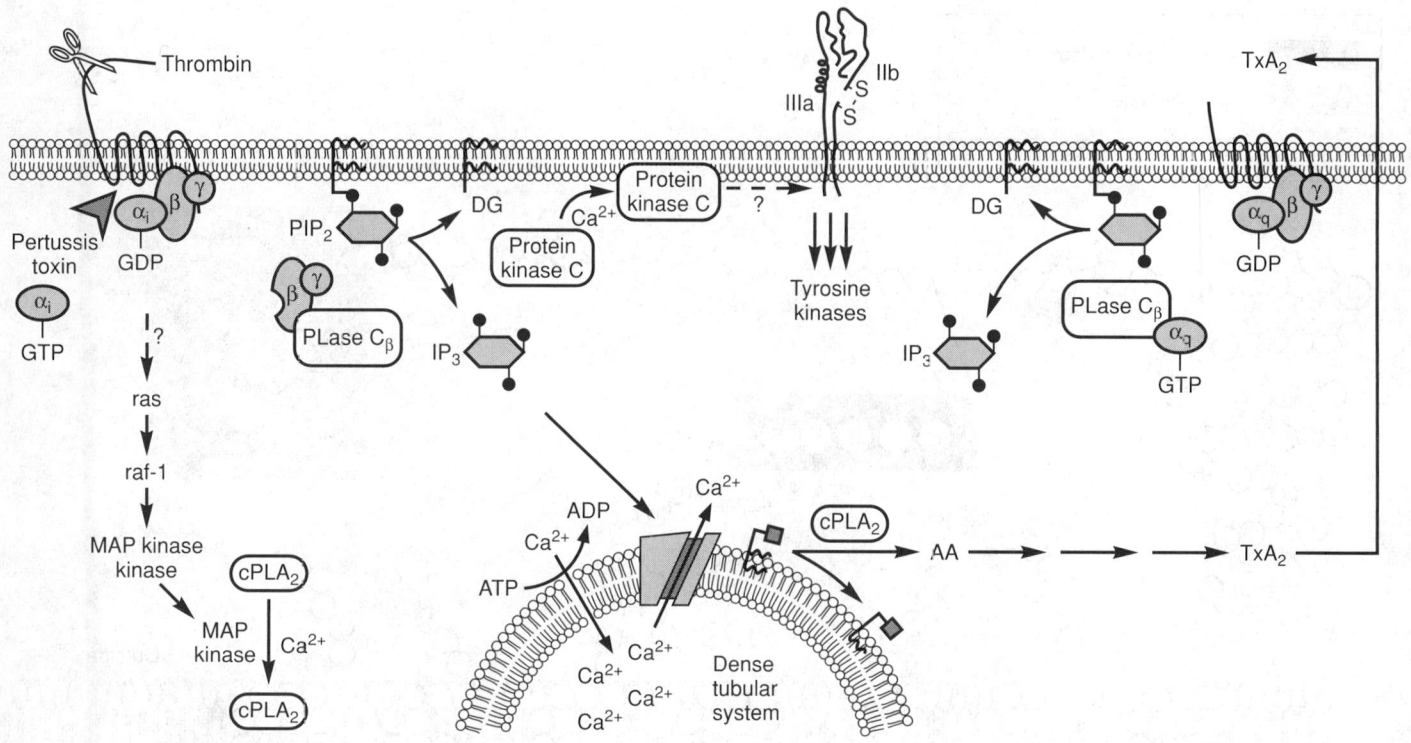

Fig. 98-3. Signal transduction during platelet activation. The binding of agonists to receptors on the platelet surface initiates cascades of intracellular second messengers, including inositol 1,4,5-trisphosphate (IP$_3$) and diacylglycerol (DG) generated through the hydrolysis of phosphatidylinositol 4,5-bisphosphate (PIP$_2$) by phospholipase C$_\beta$ (PLC$_\beta$). In platelets, PLC$_\beta$ is activated in a pertussis toxin-sensitive manner by a G protein possibly G$_{\beta\gamma}$ derived from G$_i$, and in a pertussis toxin-resistant manner by a different G protein, presumably G$_{q\alpha}$ or G$_{11\alpha}$, or both. Once formed, IP$_3$ releases Ca^{2+} from the platelet-dense tubular system, raising the cytosolic free Ca^{2+} concentration. Diacylglycerol activates protein kinase C, triggering granule secretion and fibrinogen receptor exposure on the GPIIb/IIIa complex. Phosphorylation by protein kinase C may also contribute to the activation of mitogen-activated protein (MAP) kinase that occurs in thrombin-treated platelets and is illustrated here as occurring via a member of the ras family of low-molecular-weight GTP-binding proteins, raf-1 kinase, and MAP kinase kinase, as is believed to occur in other cells. At this point, this is still speculative because the link between G-protein-coupled receptors and this pathway remains to be clarified. At the same time, the rising cytosolic free Ca^{2+} concentration facilitates arachidonate (AA) formation by the cytosolic form of phospholipase A$_2$ (cPLA$_2$), possibly by causing its association with cell membranes following phosphorylation by MAP kinase. Although this event is shown as occurring at the dense tubular system, it may also occur at the plasma membrane, and phospholipase A$_2$ may be directly activated by G$_{\beta\gamma}$ derived from one or more G proteins. Arachidonate is metabolized to TxA$_2$, which can interact with receptors on the platelet surface to cause further platelet activation. During this process tyrosine kinases, including members of the *src* family, are activated and phosphorylate multiple platelet proteins, many of which have not been identified. In platelets, tyrosine kinase activation appears to occur predominantly downstream from fibrinogen receptor exposure and platelet aggregation, but can also occur independently of those events.

protein phosphorylation, an increase in the cytosolic free Ca^{2+} concentration, fibrinogen receptor exposure, aggregation, and secretion. ADP also inhibits cAMP formation. These responses are half-maximal at approximately 1 μM ADP and appear to be largely independent of phosphoinositide hydrolysis. ADP is, at most, a weak activator of phospholipase C in human platelets.[48,49] Most of the increase in the cytosolic free Ca^{2+} concentration seen in ADP-stimulated platelets is due to increased Ca^{2+} influx across the plasma membrane rather than to inositol 1,4,5-triphosphate (IP$_3$)-induced of release of Ca^{2+} from the dense tubular system.[50] A number of attempts have been made to characterize platelet ADP receptors. In terms of substrate specificity, these receptors are distinct from those on other cells that recognize adenosine or ATP, neither of which activate platelets.[51] However, binding studies with ^{14}C-labeled ADP have produced variable results and, to date, the ADP receptor has not been conclusively identified.

Epinephrine

In several respects, epinephrine is unique among platelet agonists. Epinephrine causes aggregation and secretion, but not shape change. Epinephrine-induced phospholipase C acti-vation, to the extent that it occurs, appears to be dependent on TxA$_2$ formation and can be suppressed by preincubating the platelet with aspirin.[52] Aspirin also blocks second-wave, or secretion-dependent, platelet aggregation in response to epinephrine. This gives rise to a characteristic aggregometer tracing in which epinephrine-induced primary aggregation is followed by disaggregation of the initially formed platelet clumps. Dependence on TxA$_2$ formation does not adequately account for epinephrine's ability to aggregate platelets, however, since epinephrine can still cause fibrinogen receptor expression in aspirin-treated platelets.[53,54]

These observations suggest that there are other, as yet unknown, mechanisms involved in platelet responses to epinephrine. What might those be? Epinephrine, like thrombin, is a potent inhibitor of cAMP formation. This effect is thought to be mediated by one or more of the forms of the G protein G$_i$ that are present in platelets.[55] However, although elevated cAMP concentrations clearly inhibit platelet activation, it does not appear that a decrease in the basal cAMP concentration can trigger platelet activation. Epinephrine has also been reported to increase the rate of Na$^+$/H$^+$ exchange across the platelet plasma membrane. The increase in the cytosolic pH that this

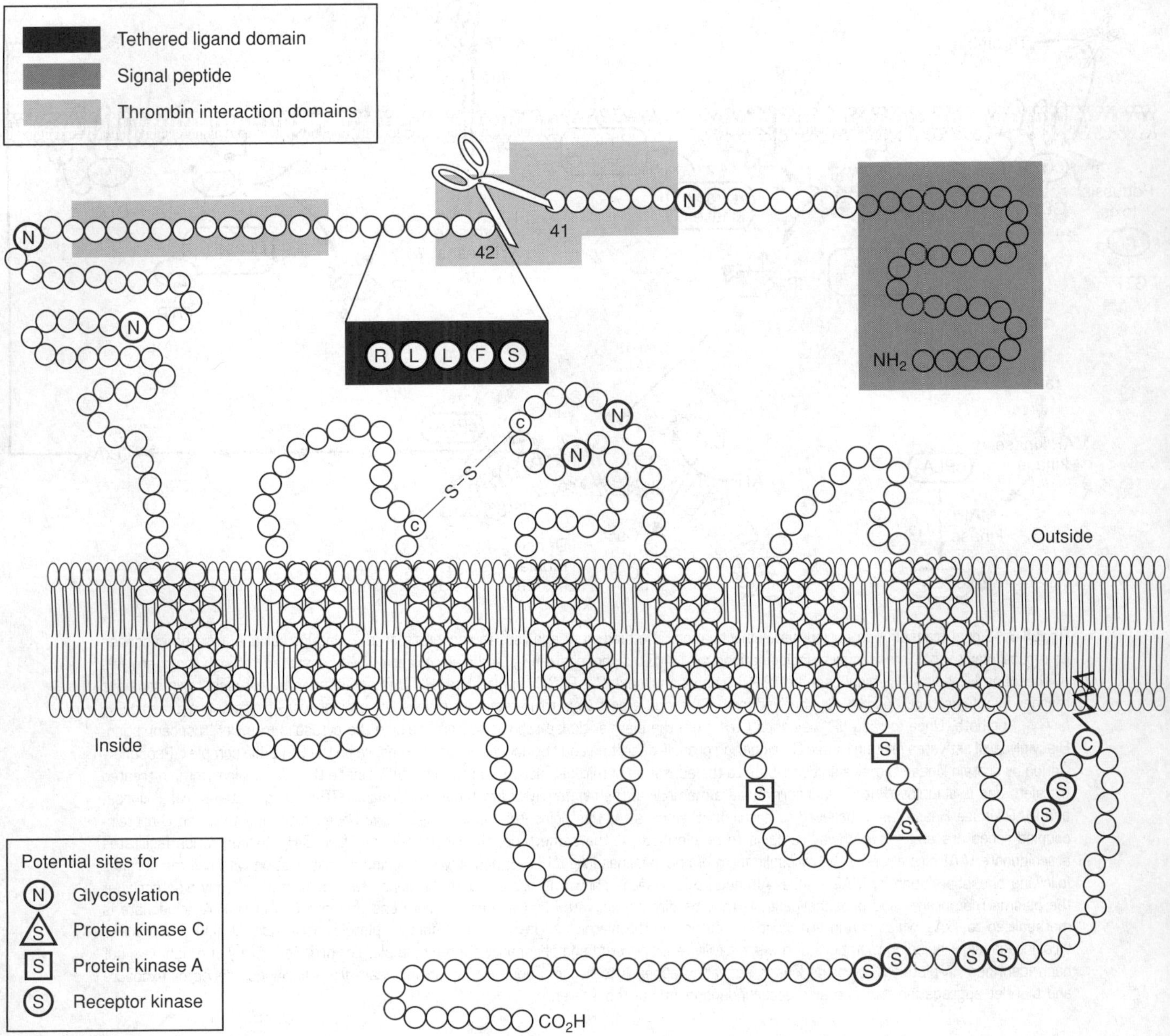

Fig. 98-4. Thrombin receptor structure. Based on a series of studies by Coughlin and co-workers,[254] the platelet thrombin receptor is believed to be a member of the family of G-protein-coupled receptors. Receptor activation is thought to occur when thrombin binds to and cleaves the receptor N terminus between residues Arg 41 and Ser 42, exposing the tethered ligand domain SFLLRN. Some of the putative features of the receptor include a signal peptide presumed to be absent from the mature protein, an internal disulfide bond, palmitoylation of a cysteine residue near the C terminus, and potential sites for phosphorylation by protein kinase C, protein kinase A, and a member of the βARK family of receptor kinases.

would be expected to produce has been linked to the mechanism of phospholipase A_2 activation by epinephrine,[56] although at least one study suggests that this occurs after fibrinogen receptor exposure.[57]

The ability of epinephrine to inhibit adenylyl cyclase, while failing to stimulate phospholipase C, is characteristic of responses that are mediated by α_2-adrenergic receptors. Binding studies with radiolabeled antagonists confirm this classification and show that there are approximately 300 sites per platelet.[58–60] Platelet responses to epinephrine are labile and vary widely from individual to individual. In fact, some otherwise normal platelets fail to respond to epinephrine or do so only after a prolonged delay.[61] The reasons for this variability are not entirely clear, although there are two reports of families

in which a mild bleeding disorder was associated with impaired epinephrine-induced aggregation and a decrease in the number α_2-adrenergic receptors.[62,63] α_2-Adrenergic receptors, including those from platelets, have been isolated, cloned, and sequenced.[64,65] Structurally, they resemble other members of the family of G-protein-coupled receptors, including the thrombin receptor.

Thromboxane A_2

TxA_2 was originally described as a highly potent, but labile, aggregation-stimulating substance. It is now known that TxA_2 is produced by the aspirin-sensitive cyclo-oxygenase pathway from arachidonate via the endoperoxides PGG$_2$ and PGH$_2$. A number of stable endoperoxide/thromboxane analogues have been synthesized. Some of these, such as U46619 and U44069, are platelet agonists. Others, including pinane-thromboxane and 13-azaprostanoic acid, are receptor antagonists and inhibit platelet activation.[66,67] When added to platelets in vitro, endoperoxide/thromboxane agonists cause shape change, aggregation, secretion, phosphoinositide hydrolysis, protein phosphorylation and an increase in the cytosolic free Ca^{2+} concentration, while having little, if any, effect on cAMP formation.[68-72] These responses are detectable at concentrations as low as 10 nM. Similar responses are seen when platelets are incubated with exogenous arachidonic acid.[68] Since the effects of arachidonate can be inhibited with aspirin, they are thought to be largely due to thromboxane formation.[73]

Once formed, TxA$_2$ can diffuse across the plasma membrane and activate other platelets. Like ADP, this amplifies the initial stimulus for platelet activation[74] (Figs. 98-1 and 98-3). This process is effective locally, but is limited by the brief (around 30 seconds) half-life of TxA$_2$ in solution, helping to confine the spread of platelet activation to the original area of injury. The platelet TxA$_2$ receptor was initially characterized by binding studies with radiolabeled agonists and antagonists. Those studies identified approximately 1,000 binding sites for TxA$_2$ per platelet[75] with K$_d$ between 30 and 100 nM.[75-77] In 1991 a TxA$_2$ receptor was cloned and shown to have predicted structure characteristic of the family of G-protein-coupled receptors.[78] Presumably it or a closely related receptor is present in platelets and is coupled to phospholipase C.

G PROTEINS AND COUPLING OF RECEPTORS TO MESSENGER-GENERATING ENZYMES

G proteins are $\alpha\beta\gamma$ heterotrimers that mediate the interaction of cell-surface receptors with cellular effectors, such as phospholipases and ion channels (Fig. 98-2). G protein activity is tightly linked to the binding and hydrolysis of GTP. In the resting state, GDP is bound to the guanine nucleotide binding site on G$_\alpha$. Agonists whose receptors interact with G proteins promote the release of GDP and its replacement with GTP present in the cytosol. At the same time G$_\alpha$ undergoes a conformational change and at least partially dissociates from the heterodimeric $\beta\gamma$ subunit, G$_{\beta\gamma}$. Originally, G$_\alpha$/GTP was thought to be primarily responsible for target regulation, while G$_{\beta\gamma}$ played a subordinate role, helping to anchor the G protein to membranes and limiting G-protein action by capturing free G$_\alpha$. However, it is now clear that G$_{\beta\gamma}$ also serves a primary role, independently activating phospholipases, ion channels, and receptor kinases.[79] At some point after it is bound to G$_\alpha$, GTP is hydrolyzed to GDP by the intrinsic GTPase activity of G$_\alpha$, and G$_\alpha$/GDP recombines with G$_{\beta\gamma}$ until the next cycle of receptor-mediated activation.

Many of the known forms of G$_\alpha$ can be covalently modified by one or more bacterial toxins. G$_{s\alpha}$, for example, is a substrate for ADP ribosylation by cholera toxin, which activates the G protein by inhibiting the hydrolysis of GTP. Other forms of G$_\alpha$, such as G$_{o\alpha}$ and G$_{i\alpha}$, are substrates for a pertussis toxin, which uncouples the G proteins from receptors. G proteins are traditionally thought to regulate events at the plasma membrane, but recent studies have shown that G proteins can be associated with cytoplasmic structures distinct from the plasma membrane as well.[80,81] The role of G proteins at these sites remains to be clarified.

Cloning studies have shown that nearly all of the forms of G$_\alpha$ exist as families of closely related proteins. There are, for example, at least three different forms of G$_{i\alpha}$ that are 85–95% homologous with each other at the amino acid level. To date, $\geq$22 forms of G$_\alpha$, 4 forms of G$_\beta$, and 6 forms of G$_\gamma$ had been described, yielding hundreds of possible combinations, not all

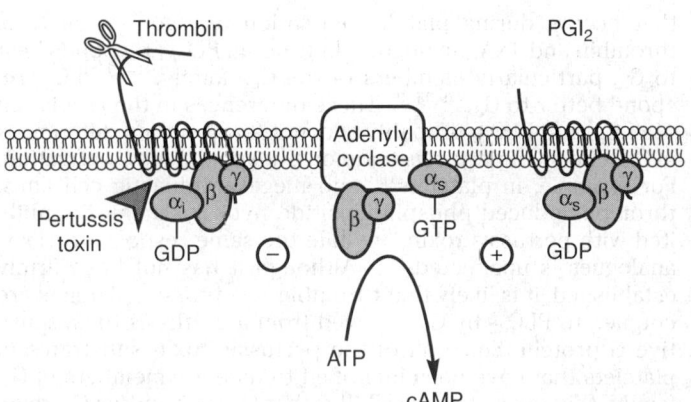

Fig. 98-5. Regulation of adenylyl cyclase in platelets. Elevated cAMP levels inhibit platelet activation. Adenylyl cyclase, the enzyme that catalyzes cAMP formation from ATP in platelets, is subject to dual regulation mediated by different G proteins. PGI$_2$ derived from endothelial cells stimulates adenylyl cyclase via the G protein G$_s$. Agonists such as thrombin inhibit cAMP formation via one or more of the forms of G$_i$ that are present in platelets.

of which exist in nature. G proteins are usually identified according to their α-subunits. The nine forms of G$_\alpha$ that have been reported in platelets are shown in Table 98-2. Known targets for these G proteins include adenylyl cyclase, phospholipase C$_\beta$, and phospholipase A$_2$, but not all of the known G proteins have assigned functions. G-protein structure and function have been recently reviewed.[79,82-84]

G-Protein Regulation of Adenylyl Cyclase

Platelets contain both of the G proteins that are known to regulate cAMP formation by adenylyl cyclase in most mammalian tissues: G$_s$ and G$_i$. G$_{s\alpha}$ is present in at least its 45-kd form. G$_{i\alpha}$ is present in all three of its known forms, with an order of prevalence G$_{i\alpha2}$>>G$_{i\alpha3}$>G$_{i\alpha1}$.[85] Traditionally, agents that increase cAMP levels in platelets, such as prostacyclin (PGI$_2$), are described as having receptors that are coupled to G$_s$, while agonists that suppress cAMP formation, such as thrombin and epinephrine, are described as having receptors coupled to G$_i$ (Fig. 98-5). However, recent studies have shown that adenylyl cyclase exists in at least six forms.[86] Although all are stimulated by G$_{s\alpha}$, they respond differently to the additional presence of G$_{\beta\gamma}$. Some, such as type I (calmodulin-activated) brain adenylyl cyclase, are inhibited by G$_{\beta\gamma}$, while others, such as types II and IV, are stimulated by G$_{\beta\gamma}$.[86] Still others (types III, V, and VI) are unaffected by G$_{\beta\gamma}$, although inhibition by G$_{\beta\gamma}$ can be achieved indirectly by forming complexes with G$_{s\alpha}$. Direct inhibition of type V adenylyl cyclase by G$_{i\alpha}$ has recently been demonstrated.[87] Relatively little information is available about the forms of adenylyl cyclase present in platelets, beyond the absence of type I enzyme.[87] Polymerase chain reaction has been used to detect message encoding adenylyl cyclase in the megakaryoblastic HEL cell line.[88] Types III and VI were detected, as was a novel message encoding a protein with homologies to types II and IV adenylyl cyclase.

G-Protein Regulation of Phospholipase C

Platelets contain at least two of the known families of phospholipase C: PLC$_\beta$ and PLC$_\gamma$. The β-forms are thought to be regulated by G proteins, while the γ-forms are regulated by protein-protein interactions that depend on the state of tyrosine phosphorylation.[89,90] PLC$_\beta$ is thought to be primarily responsible for the rapid burst of phosphoinositide hydrolysis that occurs during platelet activation by agonists such as thrombin and TxA$_2$ analogues. In general, PLC$_{\beta 1}$ responds best to G$_\alpha$, particularly members of the G$_{q\alpha}$ family.[91-95] PLC$_{\beta 2}$ respond better to G$_{\beta\gamma}$.[79,95-99] These differences in the regulation of PLC$_{\beta 1}$ and PLC$_{\beta 2}$ probably account for observed differences in the effects of pertussis toxin on phospholipase C activation. For example, in platelets[100] and megakaryoblastic cell lines, thrombin-induced phosphoinositide hydrolysis can be inhibited with pertussis toxin,[101] while the same response to TxA$_2$ analogues is unaffected.[72,74] Although it has not been firmly established, it is likely that thrombin receptors in platelets are coupled to PLC$_{\beta 2}$ by G$_{\beta\gamma}$ derived from a pertussis toxin-sensitive G protein. Since all of the pertussis toxin substrates in platelets that have been identified to date are members of G$_{i\alpha}$ family, this raises the possibility that G$_{i1}$, G$_{i2}$, and/or G$_{i3}$ regulate phospholipase C as well as adenylyl cyclase. Thromboxane receptors, on the other hand, are apparently coupled to PLC$_{\beta 1}$ by G$_\alpha$ derived from G$_q$ or G$_{11}$, both of which are present in platelets (Table 98-2 and Fig. 98-3). Shenker et al.[102] have shown that an antibody directed against a domain common to G$_{q\alpha}$ and G$_{11\alpha}$ can inhibit TxA$_2$ receptor-stimulated GTPase activity. The reason why these groupings are still tentative is the lack of definitive studies in which complexes containing receptors, G proteins, and phospholipase C are isolated from platelets.

G-Protein Regulation of Phospholipase A$_2$

Phospholipase A$_2$ is the second phospholipid-hydrolyzing enzyme in platelets whose activation may involve G proteins, by several possible mechanisms. One is the indirect activation of phospholipase A$_2$ via an increase in cytosolic Ca^{2+} or mitogen-activated protein (MAP) kinase activity; the other is direct activation by G proteins (Fig. 98-3). Both may occur in platelets. Current evidence suggests that phospholipase A$_2$ is primarily located in the platelet cytosol and that arachidonate release and metabolism occur in the dense tubular system, but these issues need to be readdressed in view of recent information about new forms of phospholipase A$_2$.[103-106] Two families of enzymes with phospholipase A$_2$ activity have now been identified: a low-molecular-weight (14-kd) secreted form that requires mM Ca^{2+} concentrations and a higher molecular weight (85–100-kd) form that is optimally activated by micromolar and submicromolar Ca^{2+} concentrations.[107-111] Of these, the more interesting enzyme for second messenger generation in platelets is the cytosolic form, since it has the potential of being active at the intracellular Ca^{2+} concentrations reached during platelet activation.[110] In cells other than platelets, this enzyme has been shown to be a substrate for phosphorylation by MAP kinase, leading to the suggestion that Ca^{2+} plus phosphorylation lead to the association of phospholipase A$_2$ with cell membranes where its substrates are located.[112] MAP kinase, in turn, is thought to be activated by convergent pathways beginning with either growth factor receptors possessing intrinsic tyrosine kinase activity or G-protein-coupled receptors. How these pathways are regulated by agonists such as thrombin remains to be determined.

In theory, phospholipase A$_2$, like PLC$_\beta$, could be directly regulated by either G$_\alpha$ or G$_{\beta\gamma}$. Most of the limited evidence available points to G$_{\beta\gamma}$.[79,113,114] In platelets GTP and the nonhydrolyzable GTP analogue GTPγS have been shown to cause [^{3}H]-arachidonate release. The extent of release was unaffected by an inhibitor of diacylglycerol (DAG) lipase, suggesting that the arachidonate was derived through the action of phospholipase A$_2$ and not from the DAG produced by phosphoinositide hydrolysis. Thrombin-induced release of [^{3}H]arachidonate from permeabilized platelets appeared to be GTP dependent and was inhibited by pertussis toxin, suggesting that it may also involve G$_{\beta\gamma}$ derived from G$_i$.[115-118] However, at present there

still remains a great deal of uncertainty about the mechanisms by which phospholipase A$_2$ is activated in platelets.

Other G Proteins in Platelets

In addition to G$_s$, G$_i$, G$_q$, and G$_{11}$, platelets also contain G$_z$.[119,120] G$_{z\alpha}$ has a limited tissue distribution and appears to be most abundant in platelets and some neural tissues. G$_{z\alpha}$ is unaffected by pertussis toxin and hydrolyzes GTP to GDP at a rate slower than other G proteins.[121] When protein kinase C (PKC) is activated in platelets, G$_{z\alpha}$, but not G$_{i\alpha}$ or G$_{q\alpha}$ becomes phosphorylated on Ser^{27} with a 1:1 stoichiometry.[119,122,123] The biologic effects of this phosphorylation event are still largely unknown, as is the role of G$_z$ itself. Under certain conditions, G$_{z\alpha}$ has been shown to inhibit cAMP formation.[124] However, it does not appear to perform this role in platelets. In addition to G$_{z\alpha}$, transcripts encoding several other forms of G$_\alpha$ have been described: G$_{12\alpha}$, G$_{13\alpha}$, G$_{14\alpha}$, and G$_{16\alpha}$.[99,125,126] Based on their amino acid sequences, none of these is predicted to be a substrate for pertussis toxin. By RNA analysis, G$_{12\alpha}$, G$_{13\alpha}$, and G$_{14\alpha}$ are widely distributed,[125] while G$_{16\alpha}$ is found predominantly in hematopoietic cells.[126] Peptide-directed antisera show that G$_{12\alpha}$ and G$_{13\alpha}$ are present in platelets, but G$_{16\alpha}$ has not been detected.[24]

SECOND MESSENGERS

In general, agonists cause platelet activation by stimulating the production of one or more cascades of second messenger molecules. Two pathways that are particularly central to this process are the phosphoinositide hydrolysis pathway and the eicosanoid pathway (Fig. 98-3). The phosphoinositide pathway begins when phospholipase C cleaves phosphatidylinositol 4,5-bisphosphate (PIP$_2$) to form IP$_3$ and DAG, both of which serve as second messengers. The eicosanoid pathway begins when arachidonate is released from membrane phospholipids, usually by phospholipase A$_2$. The newly liberated arachidonate is then metabolized to TxA$_2$, which is itself a potent stimulus for platelet activation.

Phosphoinositide Hydrolysis

One of the earliest responses of platelets to agonists is the hydrolysis of membrane PIP$_2$ by phospholipase C to form diacylglycerol and IP$_3$.[7,127,128] DAG, which is hydrophobic, remains associated with the lipid bilayer, where it activates PKC and causes protein phosphorylation, granule secretion, and fibrinogen receptor expression.[129-131] IP$_3$ enters the cytosol, where it triggers Ca^{2+} release from the platelet-dense tubular system and contributes to the increase in the cytosolic free Ca^{2+} concentration that usually accompanies platelet activation.[132-135] The ability of DAG and IP$_3$ to activate PKC and mobilize Ca^{2+} from intracellular sites is a general phenomenon and not one that is unique to platelets.[90,136,137] It is the response to PKC activation and Ca^{2+} mobilization that varies from cell to cell.

Figure 98-6 shows a detailed view of inositol phosphate metabolism. The most abundant of the inositol-containing phospholipids in the platelet membrane is not PIP$_2$, but phosphatidylinositol (PI). A 4-kinase phosphorylates the inositol ring of PI to form phosphatidylinositol 4-phosphate (PIP), which in turn is phosphorylated to form PIP$_2$. The relative abundance of the three phosphoinositides is: PI>PIP>PIP$_2$. Under the appropriate conditions, phospholipase C is able to hydrolyze all three forms of the phosphoinositides, producing DAG in each case.[138] Diacylglycerol can also be formed by hydrolysis of

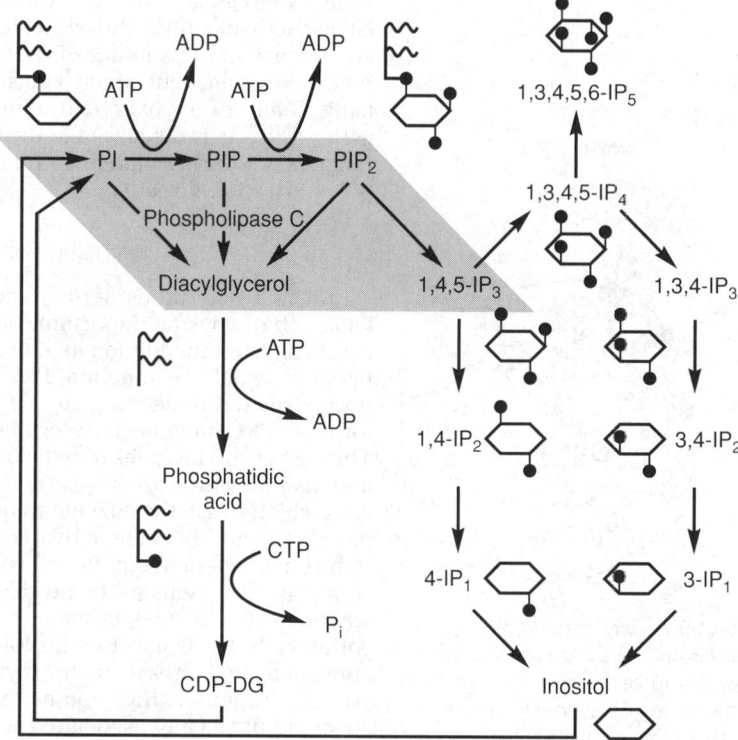

Fig. 98-6. The phosphoinositide pathway. During platelet activation, phospholipase C hydrolyzes the membrane phosphoinositide PIP_2 to form DAG and 1,4,5-IP_3. The further metabolism of 1,4,5-IP_3 to inositol is shown in the right half of the figure. This process involves a series of enzymes that either phosphorylate or dephosphorylate the inositol ring, adding or removing phosphate groups. Of the inositol phosphates shown, only 1,4,5-IP_3 has a clearly established biologic role, serving as the trigger for Ca^{2+} release from the platelet-dense tubular system. The metabolism of DAG is illustrated in the left half of the figure. DAG is formed from PI and PIP, as well as from PIP_2. In addition to stimulating PKC, DAG can serve as a source for arachidonate or can be phosphorylated by DAG kinase to form phosphatidic acid, which in turn is metabolized to CDP-DAG (CDP-DG) and then back to PI. This figure shows only a fraction of the large number of intermediates that exist in this pathway. Additional details can be found in Majerus et al.[138]

other, more abundant, membrane phospholipids, such as phosphatidylcholine. Only the hydrolysis of PIP_2, however, yields 1,4,5-IP_3.

Once formed, 1,4,5-IP_3 can be metabolized in a number of ways, including dephosphorylation to 1,4-IP_2 and phosphorylation to 1,3,4,5-IP_4. Dephosphorylation of 1,3,4,5-IP_4 produces 1,3,4-IP_3 which in turn yields two additional forms of IP_2. Further dephosphorylation produces IP_1 from IP_2, and inositol from IP_1. The inositol is then recycled back into the phosphoinositide pool by reaction with CDP-DAG.[138] The various inositol phosphate isomers present in platelets can be radiolabeled by preincubating the cells with [³H]*myo*-inositol and then separated by high-performance liquid chromatography. 1,4,5-IP_3 can also be quantitated by radioimmunoassay. Studies using these methods have shown that the production of 1,4,5-IP_3 and its subsequent conversion to 1,3,4-IP_3 takes only a few seconds in thrombin-stimulated platelets.[7,139] Since 1,3,4-IP_3 has little if any second messenger activity, this effectively limits the duration of the signal carried by 1,4,5-IP_3.

Cytosolic Calcium

The interlocking mechanisms by which platelets regulate the movements of Ca^{2+} are central to the events of platelet activation. Ca^{2+} serve as intracellular second messengers and, like protein kinases, affects enzyme activity and protein-protein interactions. Based on studies with intracellular probes, the cytosolic free Ca^{2+} concentration in resting platelets is 50–100 nM. In general, this value increases during platelet activation, but the magnitude of the increase depends on the agonist used.

Strong agonists such as thrombin or collagen cause an increase to ≥1 μM, while weaker agonists cause a smaller increase. Epinephrine has no detectable effect on the cytosolic free Ca^{2+} concentration when measured with quin-2 or fura-2, but does cause an increase that can be detected with the photoprotein aequorin.[8,48,140–142]

The ability of resting platelets to maintain a low cytosolic Ca^{2+} concentration is primarily due to the limited permeability of the platelet plasma membrane, which restricts Ca^{2+} influx from plasma (Fig. 98-7A). The permeability of the platelet plasma membrane to Ca^{2+} may be affected by the integrity of the GPIIb/IIIa complex.[143–146] In addition, platelets are able to expel Ca^{2+} from the cytosol—either back across the plasma membrane or into the dense tubular system. The dense tubular system is thought to be a derivative of megakaryocyte endoplasmic reticulum.[147] Like similar structures in other cells, including sarcoplasmic reticulum in muscle, it lies close to the plasma membrane and possesses an inwardly directed Ca^{2+}-Mg^{2+}-ATPase pump that allows it to sequester Ca^{2+}. The capacity of the dense tubular system to store Ca^{2+} is large, but not infinite.[148] To compensate for the steady-state influx of Ca^{2+} across the plasma membrane, platelets also need an outwardly directed Ca^{2+} efflux. In other cells this is accomplished by either a Ca^{2+}/Mg^{2+}-ATPase or by an Na^+/Ca^{2+} exchanger. However, to date there is little evidence that Na^+/Ca^{2+} exchange plays a major role in platelets, and the existence of a plasma membrane Ca^{2+}/Mg^{2+}-ATPase is still debated.

The increase in cytosolic Ca^{2+} that occurs during platelet activation is due partly to the discharge of Ca^{2+} from the dense tubular system and partly to increased Ca^{2+} influx (Fig. 98-7B).

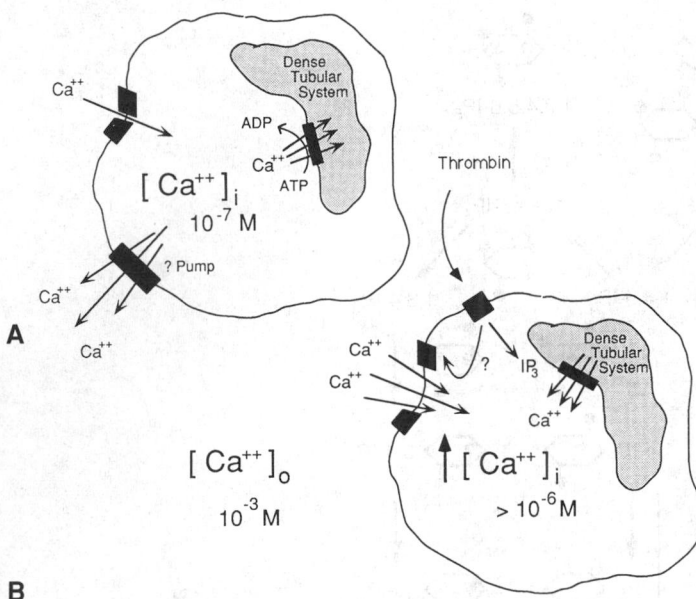

Fig. 98-7. Ca^{2+} homeostasis in platelets. **(A)** Resting platelets maintain their cytosolic free Ca^{2+} concentration at approximately 10^{-7} M by pumping Ca^{2+} out of the cell across the plasma membrane and by sequestering Ca^{2+} within the dense tubular system. Ca^{2+} uptake into the dense tubular system is driven by an ATP-dependent Ca^{2+} pump that resembles that present in muscle. The mechanism that pumps Ca^{2+} out of the cell is unknown. **(B)** When platelets are activated by agonists such as thrombin, collagen, and ADP, but not epinephrine, the cytosolic free Ca^{2+} concentration increases to $>10^{-6}$ M. This is due partly to the IP_3-mediated release of Ca^{2+} from the dense tubular system and partly to increased Ca^{2+} influx across the plasma membrane. The mechanism that triggers Ca^{2+} influx is unknown.

Unlike muscle cells, platelets do not have voltage-gated Ca^{2+} channels.[149–152] Instead, it has been proposed that there are agonist-operated Ca^{2+} channels linked to receptor occupancy, but this remains to be established.[142] The trigger for Ca^{2+} release from the dense tubular system is IP_3,[132–135,153] presumably acting on a combination receptor/channel similar to the ones found in other cells.[154] How does Ca^{2+} cause platelet activation? Part of its effect is exerted through calcium-dependent enzymes that are not optimally active at the free Ca^{2+} concentration present in resting cells, but that become active when the Ca^{2+} concentration rises. These include phospholipases A_2, phospholipase C, calpain, phosphorylase kinase, and myosin light chain kinase plus an unknown number of additional enzymes. The interaction between phospholipase A_2 and Ca^{2+} has already been described. Ca^{2+} affects phospholipase C in at least two ways. First, adding Ca^{2+} to permeabilized platelets or to platelet membranes causes phosphoinositide hydrolysis, suggesting that Ca^{2+} activates the enzyme. Second, Ca^{2+} affects the substrate specificity of phospholipase C. At Ca^{2+} concentrations higher than those present in resting platelets, phospholipase C loses its preference for PIP_2 and hydrolyzes the other phosphoinositides as well.[138]

In addition to these enzymes, platelets also contain two proteases, calpains I and II, which depend on Ca^{2+}, but differ in their absolute Ca^{2+} requirements.[155–157] Neither is active at the Ca^{2+} concentration present in resting platelets. Both are present in the platelet cytosol.[158,159] Known platelet substrates for calpain include actin-binding protein and P235 (talin).[155,160,161] The nature of these substrates and the high concentrations of Ca^{2+} required for calpain activity suggest that calpain participates in the late events of platelet activation, those that follow the agonist-induced increase in the cytosolic free Ca^{2+} concentration.[162,163] Finally, at least two platelet en-

zymes are regulated by Ca^{2+} via calmodulin.[164] Phosphorylase kinase activates phosphorylase, leading to glycogenolysis and an increase in the amount of ATP available for platelet activation.[165] Myosin light chain kinase phosphorylates the 20-kd light chain of myosin and enhances its interaction with actin.[166–168] As is discussed in the section on cytoskeletal rearrangements during platelet activation, Ca^{2+} also affects actin polymerization directly.

Protein Kinase C

PKC is a ubiquitous serine- and threonine-specific protein kinase that plays an important, but still incompletely defined, role in signal transduction in platelets. Like many of the participants in signal transduction, PKC is actually a family of structurally related molecules. At the present time, nine different forms of PKC have been described, falling into two groups.[169] The first group includes α, two splice variants of β (βI and βII), and γ, all of which are regulated by both Ca^{2+} and diacylglycerol, which cause the enzyme to be translocated to the plasma membrane and become activated. The second group appears to be Ca^{2+} independent. Platelets contain at least the α, β, and δ forms.[170] It remains to be determined whether these play distinguishable roles in platelet activation. In platelets, as in other cells, the usual stimulus for PKC activation is DAG formation and an increase in the cytosolic free Ca^{2+} concentration.[130] Together, these activate the enzyme and cause it to become physically associated with the plasma membrane.[171] PKC can also be activated in platelets by phorbol esters and synthetic membrane-permeable DAGs.[130,131,172] Once activated, PKC appears to be involved in a variety of responses in platelets, some of which seem contradictory. These include positive effects, such as aggregation and secretion, as well as negative effects, which emerge when platelets are preincubated with phorbol esters prior to the addition of an agonist. The inhibitory effects are discussed later in this chapter.

Several of the PKC substrates that are phosphorylated during platelet activation have been identified, including pleckstrin (P47), myosin light chain (P20), and the α-subunit of the G protein, G_z. $G_{z\alpha}$ has already been discussed. Phosphorylation of myosin light chain by PKC occurs at a site distinct from myosin light chain kinase and is believed to affect the interaction of myosin with actin.[173] Pleckstrin was cloned for the first time in 1988 using a cDNA library from the myeloid HL60 cell line.[174,175] It has a deduced molecular weight of 40 kd, contains potential sites for Ca^{2+} binding and for phosphorylation by PKC, and appears to be present in many hematopoietic cells, but not in nonhematopoietic cells.[174,176] Its function remains unknown, but several recent reports have pointed out that the first and last 100 residues of pleckstrin are homologous with domains in other molecules, many of which are involved in signal transduction or the regulation of signal transduction events, including low-molecular-weight GTP-binding proteins, β-adrenergic receptor kinase, and PLC_γ.[177,178] It was proposed that the newly recognized pleckstrin homology domains, like src homology domains 2 and 3, mediate protein-protein interactions. If so, then phosphorylation of pleckstrin by PKC may modulate its role in these events. Other PKC substrates that have been identified in platelets include actin-binding protein,[179] myosin light chain kinase and GP180, a transmembrane glycoprotein whose function is unknown.[180] Precisely how the phosphorylation of any of these proteins leads to fibrinogen receptor up-regulation and granule secretion is an important question that remains unanswered.

Thromboxane Formation

The second major pathway for signal transduction in platelets is the eicosanoid pathway. Eicosanoids are formed from arachidonate (5,8,11,14-eicosatetraenoic acid), which is the

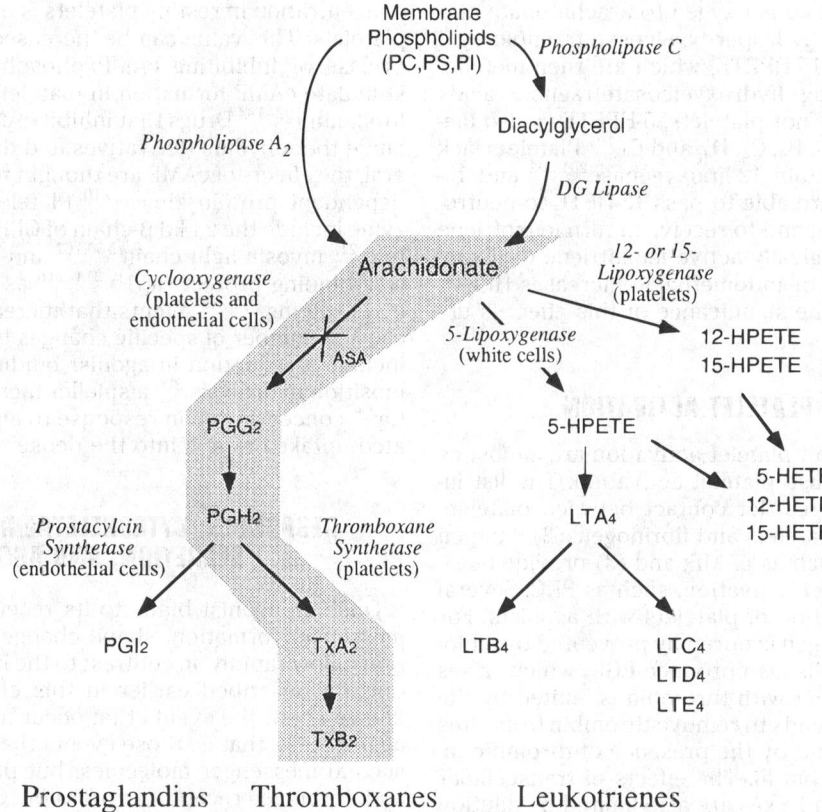

Membrane
Phospholipids
(PC,PS,PI)

Phospholipase C

Phospholipase A₂

Diacylglycerol

DG Lipase

Cyclooxygenase
(platelets and
endothelial cells)

Arachidonate

*12- or 15-
Lipoxygenase*
(platelets)

5-Lipoxygenase
(white cells)

12-HPETE
15-HPETE

ASA

PGG₂

5-HPETE

5-HETE
12-HETE
15-HETE

*Prostacyclin
Synthetase*
(endothelial cells)

PGH₂

*Thromboxane
Synthetase*
(platelets)

LTA₄

PGI₂

TxA₂

LTB₄

LTC₄
LTD₄
LTE₄

TxB₂

Prostaglandins   Thromboxanes   Leukotrienes

Fig. 98-8. Eicosanoid pathways. The formation of arachidonate and its subsequent metabolism to prostaglandins, thromboxanes, and leukotrienes is illustrated. Arachidonate is released from membrane phospholipids such as phosphatidylcholine (PC) and phosphatidylserine (PS) by the direct action of phospholipase A_2 or is formed from phosphatidylinositol (PI) by the sequential action of phospholipase C and diacylglycerol (DG) lipase. Once formed, the arachidonate can be metabolized by any of three sets of molecules, depending on which enzymes are present. In platelets, arachidonate is metabolized by via the aspirin-sensitive cyclo-oxygenase pathway to form TxA_2. In endothelial cells, prostaglandins such as PGI_2 are formed. In white cells, 5-lipoxygenase directs arachidonate metabolism toward leukotriene formation. Platelets also contain 12- and 15-lipoxygenase. The biologic significance of the molecules formed by this pathway is less clear, but platelet 12-HETE can be metabolized to 12,20-DiHETE in neutrophils, where it may competitively inhibit the metabolism of leukotriene B_4. (From Marcus et al.,[255] with permission.)

most abundant unsaturated fatty acid found in platelets (Fig. 98-8). In resting platelets, arachidonate is esterified to the second carbon of the glycerol backbone of phosphatidylcholine, phosphatidylethanolamine, phosphatidylserine, and PI,[181–184] which are predominantly located on the inner leaflet of the plasma membrane.[185] Most platelet agonists cause a rapid release of arachidonate from phospholipids.[186,187] This release is thought to occur either by direct hydrolysis by phospholipase A_2[186,188] or, to a lesser extent, by the sequential hydrolysis of phospholipid by phospholipase C and DAG by a lipase.[189,190] Regulation of the cytosolic forms of phospholipase A_2 is discussed elsewhere in this chapter and is currently thought to involve G proteins, changes in the cytosolic Ca^{2+} concentration and pH, and, perhaps, phosphorylation of the enzyme by MAPK. However, many of the details, particularly as they apply to platelets, remain to be established.

The number of known metabolites of arachidonate is almost as great as the number of inositol phosphates formed via the phosphoinositide hydrolysis pathway. However, a greater percentage appear to have regulatory/second messenger function. Three known families of eicosanoids diverge from each other at the level of the enzyme that oxygenates arachidonate (Fig. 98-8). These are the prostanoids, the leukotrienes, and the epoxides. Which metabolites are formed in a particular cell appears to depend in part on which enzymes are present. The prostanoids are formed by the cyclo-oxygenase pathway and include endoperoxides and thromboxanes, as well as the pros-

taglandins. The leukotrienes are formed via the lipoxygenase pathway and the epoxides by the cytochrome P-450 epoxygenase pathway. All three of these pathways are present in platelets, but the predominant route for arachidonate metabolism is the prostanoid pathway leading to TxA_2 formation.[191]

Prostanoid synthesis begins with the conversion of arachidonate via cyclo-oxygenase to PGH_2. PGH_2 is the parent compound for both the prostaglandins (e.g., PGE_2 and PGI_2) and thromboxane A_2, all of which are biologically active. The prostaglandins suppress platelet activation by stimulating cAMP formation.[192–194] TxA_2 activates platelets.[68–72] Although both arms of this pathway may be present in the same cell, the balance between prostaglandin and thromboxane synthesis varies. For example, platelets synthesize primarily thromboxanes, while endothelial cells synthesize primarily prostaglandins. In platelets, cyclo-oxygenase and thromboxane synthetase have been localized to the platelet dense tubular system, the apparent site of TxA_2 formation.[105] Cyclo-oxygenase is irreversibly inactivated by aspirin,[195,196] which acetylates a serine residue near the C terminus.[197,198] Since platelets lack the ability to synthesize meaningful amounts of protein, inactivation of cyclo-oxygenase by aspirin effectively halts prostanoid synthesis until new platelets are formed. Indomethacin and other nonsteroidal anti-inflammatory agents also inactivate cyclo-oxygenase, but without covalently modifying the enzyme.[199,200]

The formation of leukotrienes from arachidonate begins with lipoxygenase (Fig. 98-8). Three different forms of this enzyme have been described. Each adds oxygen to arachidonate at a different site, producing 5-hydroperoxyeicosatetraenoic acid (5-HPETE), 12-HPETE, and 15-HPETE, which are then metabolized to the corresponding hydroxyeicosatetraenoic acids (HETEs). In leukocytes, but not platelets, 5-HPETE is also metabolized to leukotrienes A4, B4, C4, D4, and E4.[191] Platelets lack 5-lipoxygenase, but do contain 12-lipoxygenase[201,202] and 15-lipoxygenase.[203] Platelets are able to pass 12-HETE to neutrophils for further metabolism and to receive in turn leukotriene A4 for metabolism to biologically active leukotriene C4. Exposure of platelets to aspirin or indomethacin increases HPETE and HETE formation, but the significance of this effect is unknown.

INHIBITION OF PLATELET ACTIVATION

The mechanisms that limit platelet activation are almost as elaborate as those that cause platelet activation. The list includes processes that (1) restrict contact between platelets and agonists or between platelets and fibrinogen; (2) dampen platelet responsiveness, such as cAMP; and (3) provide negative feedback during platelet activation, such as PKC. Several processes limit the interaction of platelets with agonists. For example, contact with collagen is normally prevented by endothelial cells. Endothelial cells also produce PGI_2, which raises platelet cAMP levels. Contact with thrombin is limited by the rapid flow of blood, which tends to remove thrombin from sites of tissue factor exposure and by the presence of thrombin inhibitors such as antithrombin III. The effects of transcellular messengers such as ADP and TxA_2 are also limited by dilution in flowing blood and by their brief half-lives. Other mechanisms exist as well, including tight controls on the free Ca^{2+} concentration in resting platelets and the inability of platelet fibrinogen receptors to bind fibrinogen until they have undergone the transformation that accompanies platelet activation.

Protein Kinase C

Once activated by DAG or phorbol esters, PKC appears able to inhibit, as well as promote, platelet activation. The inhibitory effects emerge when platelets are preincubated with phorbol esters or DAG under conditions in which platelet activation does not occur. If an agonist is added several minutes later, the responses of the platelet to that agonist, especially those dependent on the products of phosphoinositide hydrolysis, are either attenuated or abolished.[204-206] This phenomenon may represent a form of negative feedback. Several different mechanisms have been proposed to underlie this effect. PKC has been shown to phosphorylate platelet IP_3-5'-phosphomonesterase, the enzyme that hydrolyzes IP_3 to $1,4-IP_2$.[207] Phosphorylation accelerates the rate of IP_3 hydrolysis and may limit the duration of the signal for Ca^{2+} release. It has also been shown that phorbol esters can block the ability of platelet agonists to stimulate phosphoinositide hydrolysis and attenuate cAMP formation.[7,208] This finding suggests that PKC may inhibit G proteins or the receptors to which they are normally coupled. However, of the G proteins that are present in platelets, only G_z has been shown unequivocally to be a substrate for PKC, and its role in platelet activation is still unknown. Serine residues in G-protein-coupled receptors can be phosphorylated by PKC. One such potential site in the third cytoplasmic loop of the thrombin receptor is shown in Figure 98-4.

cAMP

The relationship between elevated cAMP levels and suppression of platelet function is better established than that for PKC, but the precise mechanisms are no more certain. The cAMP concentration in resting platelets is normally about 1 pmol/10^8 platelets. This value can be increased by stimulating adenylyl cyclase or inhibiting cAMP phosphodiesterase. Agents that stimulate cAMP formation in platelets include PGI_2, PGE_1, and forskolin.[192-194] Drugs that inhibit cAMP phosphodiesterase include theophylline derivatives and dipyridamole.[192,209] In general, the effects of cAMP are thought to be mediated by a cAMP-dependent protein kinase.[210] Platelet substrates for this enzyme include the 24-kd β-chain of GPIb,[211,212] actin-binding protein,[213] myosin light chain,[166,167] and the-low-molecular weight GTP-binding protein rap1b,[214-216] as well as several unidentified proteins.[217,218] Agents that increase cAMP levels typically cause a number of specific changes in platelet function. These include a reduction in agonist binding,[219] impaired phosphoinositide hydrolysis,[220] a smaller increase in the cytosolic free Ca^{2+} concentration in response to agonists,[221,222] and accelerated uptake of Ca^{2+} into the dense tubular system.[223]

RESPONSES: CYTOSKELETAL REARRANGEMENTS, SECRETION, AND AGGREGATION

Once an agonist binds to its receptor and initiates second messenger formation, shape change, secretion, and aggregation follow rapidly. In contrast to the initial steps of signal transduction described earlier in this chapter, relatively little is known about the events that occur just prior to secretion and aggregation, that is, those events that follow the generation of second messenger molecules, but precede granule extrusion and fibrinogen receptor expression. Clearly, there are changes in the cytosolic Ca^{2+} concentration and in the phosphorylation state of numerous platelet proteins. Previously quiescent enzymes become activated. Precisely how these changes lead to membrane fusion, granule exocytosis, and fibrinogen receptor expression is still unknown.

Cytoskeletal Rearrangements

One of the more dramatic events during platelet activation is the metamorphosis that occurs when nonactivated platelets adhere and spread on exposed collagen fibrils or become activated in the circulation by soluble factors such as thrombin or ADP. In either case, platelets lose their normal discoid shape and acquire an irregular morphology with multiple filopodial projections (see Ch. 96). This transformation is associated with and largely due to cytoskeletal rearrangements within the platelet. The platelet cytoskeleton includes ≥14 different proteins, most of which have counterparts in other cells.[224] The proteins are arranged in three major structures: a cytoplasmic meshwork, the membrane-associated cytoskeleton, and a microtubule coil. Together, these lend support to the platelet plasma membrane and give shape to both resting and activated platelets. Although each of these will be considered separately, it should remembered that in the intact cell they form an integral unit.

The cytoplasmic meshwork is composed of actin filaments and associated proteins. Actin is a globular 42-kd protein that accounts for ≤20% of total platelet protein. In resting platelets, 40-50% of the actin is present as filamentous F-actin. This increases to 70-80% during platelet activation.[225] At the same time, myosin is phosphorylated by myosin light chain kinase[168] and becomes associated with F-actin, forming filaments that are anchored to the platelet plasma membrane by attachment (via actin-binding protein) to the GPIb/IX complex.[226-228] Tension is generated by contraction of the anchored filaments. Anchorage of platelets to extracellular matrix proteins via cell-surface glycoproteins also has parallels with the formation of focal adhesion plaques in fibroblasts. Recent evidence shows that activation of the GPIIb/IIIa complex leads to the phosphorylation on tyrosine of a number of proteins, including the tyrosine kinase pp125[Fak].[229–231] In fibroblasts, pp125[Fak] is localized at sites where transmembrane glycoproteins of the integrin family bind to extracellular matrix proteins, on the one hand, and intracellular cytoskeletal proteins, on the other. These sites are thought to help anchor cells to the surrounding matrix and provide sites at which tension can be applied by contractile elements within the cell, but it is clear that in platelets these events also generate a new round of signaling molecules whose significance is just beginning to be understood.[232]

The membrane-associated cytoskeleton is composed of actin, actin-binding protein, P235 (talin), vinculin, spectrin, α-actinin, and several membrane glycoproteins. Actin-binding protein is an elongated 250-kd protein present in platelets as a dimer.[233,234] Actin-binding protein is able to bind to both actin and the membrane GPIb/IX complex, allowing it to link actin filaments to the platelet plasma membrane.[226–228] In resting platelets, actin-binding protein is part of a semirigid array that helps to maintain the platelet's discoid shape and limits the lateral movement of GPIb. This role is analogous to that performed by spectrin in erythrocytes.[235] When platelets are activated, actin filaments form and attach themselves to actin-binding protein. Later the rising cytosolic Ca^{2+} concentration activates calpain, which cleaves actin-binding protein, severing the link to GPIb.[155,161] Calpain also cleaves P235, a 235-kd protein that is antigenically cross-reactive with talin.[160,161,236]

The third major structural element in platelets is the microtubule coil.[237] This coil is a single tightly wound polymer of tubulin that encircles the platelet perimeter and helps to maintain its discoid shape.[238] During platelet activation, the microtubule coil contracts. At the same time, platelet granules move toward the center of the cell. Initially it was thought the granule centralization was due to coil contraction. However, that view has been challenged.[239] Intriguingly, microtubule coils identical to those in platelets have been observed in megakaryocytes, suggesting that they may be preformed by the megakaryocyte and may participate in platelet formation.[240]

Secretion

Secretion occurs from at least three morphologically distinguishable types of storage granules: dense granules, α-granules, and lysosomal granules (see Chs. 96 and 97). Several of the α- and dense-granule constituents are capable of supporting platelet activation, including ADP, Ca^{2+} vWF, and fibrinogen. Therefore, the release of stored materials, like the formation of TxA_2, helps to recruit additional platelets into expanding platelet aggregates. This phenomenon is readily demonstrated in a platelet aggregometer where an initial "primary" response triggers "secondary" aggregation. This phenomenon is seen particularly well with weak agonists such as epinephrine or with low concentrations of ADP. In general, a maximal platelet response to injury requires granule secretion. Therefore, a defect in either signal transduction leading to secretion or the storage granules themselves adversely effects platelet function.

Aggregation: Fibrinogen Receptor Activation

The hallmark of platelet activation is aggregation. Platelets form aggregates because fibrinogen binds to the platelet surface and acts as a bridge between adjacent platelets. The mechanism by which fibrinogen receptors become activated on the platelet surface remains one of the great unsolved mysteries of platelet biology, although a solution to this problem seems to be drawing closer. As is discussed in Chapter 97, the platelet

fibrinogen receptor is formed from a Ca^{2+}-dependent, heterodimeric complex of membrane GPIIb and -IIIa (the integrin $\alpha_{IIb}\beta_3$). There are 40–50,000 copies of this complex per platelet. Based on the ability of complex-dependent monoclonal antibodies to bind to resting platelets as well as activated platelets, the GPIIb/IIIa heterodimer is thought to be present on resting platelets, but unable to bind fibrinogen. In other words, platelet activation appears to evoke a change in the GPIIb/IIIa complex that renders it competent to bind fibrinogen.[241,242] In support of this model, other monoclonal antibodies have been developed that bind to GPIIb and GPIIIa only after the addition of agonist, suggesting that new antigens have become available as a consequence of activation. This change occurs within seconds of agonist addition. The significance of the fibrinogen receptor to normal platelet function is reflected in the substantial bleeding disorder seen in patients with Glanzmann thrombasthenia whose platelets lack functional GPIIb/IIIa complexes (see Ch. 129).

The complete primary sequences of GPIIb and GPIIIa have been deduced from full-length cDNA clones and the proteins expressed in naive cells. The results suggest that both glycoproteins cross the platelet plasma membrane and have short cytoplasmic extensions. It is reasonable to suppose that intracellular events within the platelet signal fibrinogen receptor expression by interacting with the cytoplasmic domains of one or both molecules. Although Ca^{2+} plays a large role in fibrinogen binding and in the stability of the GPIIb/IIIa complex, fibrinogen receptor expression does not appear to be due to the direct interaction of cytoplasmic Ca^{2+} with either of the two glycoproteins.[129] Instead, the up-regulation of platelet fibrinogen receptors may be due in part to the activation of PKC. Activators of this enzyme, such as phorbol esters, stimulate fibrinogen binding.[129] They also can cause phosphorylation of the cytosolic domain of GPIIIa, but at a stoichiometry of <0.05: 1.[243,244] The results of recent studies in which truncated forms of the glycoproteins were expressed in CHO cells raise the possibility that an unidentified protein may interact with the cytosolic domains of one or both of the two glycoproteins, either preventing fibrinogen receptor exposure in resting platelets or stimulating receptor exposure in activated platelets.[245] However, the nature of the interaction is unknown.

SUMMARY

In summary, platelet activation is currently seen as a tightly regulated series of events beginning with the binding of agonists to receptors on the platelet surface and culminating with secretion and aggregation. These events are linked by at least two major signaling pathways and amplified by the release of several metabolic products and the contents of the platelet storage granules. The structures of the receptors for a number of biologically important platelet agonists have been defined at the molecular level along with the earliest events of platelet activation initiated by receptor occupation. However, the amount that is presently known should not obscure the amount that remains to be determined. It is hoped that by the time this book enters its third edition there will be a better understanding of such key issues as the structure of platelet receptors for agonists such as ADP and collagen, the role of tyrosine kinases in platelet activation before and after fibrinogen binds to GPIIb/IIIa, and the molecular basis for fibrinogen receptor up-regulation and granule exocytosis.

REFERENCES

1. Rittenhouse-Simmons S: Production of diglyceride from phosphatidylinositol in activated human platelets. J Clin Invest 63:580, 1979
2. Bell RL, Majerus PW: Thrombin-induced hydrolysis of phosphatidylinositol in human platelets. J Biol Chem 255:1790, 1980

3. Broekman MJ, Ward JW, Marcus AJ: Phospholipid metabolism in stimulated human platelets. J Clin Invest 66:275, 1980

4. Billah MM, Lapetina EG: Rapid decrease of phosphatidylinositol 4,5-bisphosphate in thrombin-stimulated platelets. J Biol Chem 257:12705, 1982

5. Agranoff BW, Murthy P, Seguin EB: Thrombin-induced cleavage of phosphatidyl bisphosphate in human platelets. J Biol Chem 258:2076, 1983

6. Packham MA, Guccione MA, Greenberg JP et al: Release of ^{14}C-serotonin during initial platelet changes induced by thrombin, collagen or A23187. Blood 50:915, 1977

7. Rittenhouse SE, Sasson JP: Mass changes in myoinositol trisphosphate in human platelets stimulated by thrombin. Inhibitory effects of phorbol ester. J Biol Chem 260:8657, 1985

8. Rink TJ, Smith S, Tsien R: Cytoplasmic free Ca^{2+} in human platelets: Ca^{2+} thresholds and Ca^{2+}-independent activation for shape-change and secretion. FEBS Lett 148:21, 1982

9. Aktories K, Jakobs KH: N_i-mediated inhibition of human platelet adenylate cyclase by thrombin. Eur J Biochem 145:333, 1984

10. Harmon JT, Jamieson GA: Activation of platelets by alpha-thrombin is a receptor-mediated event. J Biol Chem 261:15928, 1986

11. Harmon JT, Jamieson GA: The glycocalicin portion of platelet glycoprotein Ib expresses both high and moderate affinity binding sites for thrombin. J Biol Chem 261:13224, 1986

12. Michelson AD, Barnard MR: Thrombin-induced changes in platelet membrane glycoproteins Ib, IX, and IIb-IIIa complex. Blood 70:1673, 1987

13. McGowan EB, Ding A, Detwiler TC: Correlation of thrombin-induced glycoprotein V hydrolysis and platelet activation. J Biol Chem 258:11243, 1983

14. Bienz D, Schnippering W, Clemetson KJ: Glycoprotein V is not the thrombin activation receptor on human blood platelets. Blood 68:720, 1986

15. Lanza F, Morales M, De la Salle C et al: Cloning and characterization of the gene encoding the human platelet glycoprotein V. J Biol Chem 268:20801, 1993

16. Vu T-KH, Hung DT, Wheaton VI, Coughlin SR: Molecular cloning of a functional thrombin receptor reveals a novel proteolytic mechanism of receptor activation. Cell 64:1057, 1991

17. Rasmussen UB, Vouret-Craviari V, Jallat S et al: cDNA Cloning and expression of a hamster α-thrombin receptor coupled to Ca^{2+} mobilization. FEBS Lett 288:123, 1991

18. Vu T-KH, Wheaton VI, Hung DT et al: Domains specifying thrombin-receptor interaction. Nature 353:674, 1991

19. Scarborough RM, Naughton MA, Teng W et al: Tethered ligand agonist peptides. Structural requirements for thrombin receptor activation reveal mechanism of proteolytic unmasking of agonist function. J Biol Chem 267:13146, 1992

20. Vassallo RR Jr, Kieber-Emmons T, Cichowski K, Brass LF: Structure/function relationships in the activation of platelet thrombin receptors by receptor-derived peptides. J Biol Chem 267:6081, 1992

21. Chao BH, Kalkunte S, Maraganore JM, Stone SR: Essential groups in synthetic agonist peptides for activation of the platelet thrombin receptor. Biochemistry 31:6175, 1992

22. Brass LF, Vassallo RR Jr, Belmonte E et al: Structure and function of the human platelet thrombin receptor: studies using monoclonal antibodies against a defined epitope within the receptor N-terminus. J Biol Chem 267:13795, 1992

23. Hung DT, Vu T-KH, Wheaton VI et al: Cloned platelet thrombin receptor is necessary for thrombin-induced platelet activation. J Clin Invest 89:1350, 1992

24. Brass LF, Hoxie JA, Manning DR: Signaling through G proteins and G protein-coupled receptors during platelet activation. Thromb Haemost 70:217, 1993

25. Ishii K, Hein L, Kobilka B, Coughlin SR: Kinetics of thrombin receptor cleavage on intact cells: relation to signaling. J Biol Chem 268:9780, 1993

26. Hoxie JA, Ahuja M, Belmonte E et al: Internalization and recycling of activated thrombin receptors. J Biol Chem 268:13756, 1993

27. Brass LF, Pizarro S, Ahuja M et al: Changes in the structure and function of the human thrombin receptor during activation, internalization and recycling. J Biol Chem 269:2943, 1994

28. Brass LF: Homologous desensitization of HEL cell thrombin receptors: distinguishable roles for proteolysis and phosphorylation. J Biol Chem 267:6044, 1992

29. Norton KJ, Scarborough RM, Kutok JL et al: Immunologic analysis of the cloned platelet thrombin receptor activation mechanism: evidence supporting receptor cleavage, release of the N-terminal peptide, and insertion of the tethered ligand into a protected environment. Blood 82:2125, 1993

30. Kinlough-Rathbone RL, Cazenave J-P, Packham MA, Mustard JF: Effect of inhibitors of the arachidonate pathway on the release of granule contents from rabbit platelets adherent to collagen. Lab Invest 42:28, 1980

31. Ardlie NG, Garrett JJ, Bell LK: Collagen increases cytoplasmic free calcium in human platelets. Thromb Res 42:115, 1986

32. Watson SP, Reep B, McConnell RT, Lapetina EG: Collagen stimulates [3H]-inositol trisphosphate formation in indomethacin-treated human platelets. Biochem J 226:831, 1985

33. Rittenhouse SE, Allen CL: Synergistic activation by collagen and 15-hydroxy-9 alpha,11 alpha-peroxidoprosta-5, 13-dienoic acid (PGH_2) of phosphatidylinositol metabolism and arachidonic acid release in human platelets. J Clin Invest 70:1216, 1982

34. Lapetina EG, Reep B, Read NG, Moncada S: Adhesion of human platelets to collagen in the presence of prostacyclin, indomethacin and compound BW 755C. Thromb Res 41:325, 1986

35. Barnes MJ, Gordon JL, MacIntyre DE: Platelet aggregating activity of type I and III collagens from human aorta and chicken skin. Biochem J 160:647, 1976

36. Barnes MJ, Gordon JL, MacIntyre DE: Platelet aggregation by basement membrane-associated collagens. Thromb Res 18:375, 1980

37. Santoro SA: Identification of a 160,000 dalton platelet membrane protein that mediates the initial divalent cation-dependent adhesion of platelets to collagen. Cell 46:913, 1986

38. Brass LF, Bensusan HB: The role of collagen quaternary structure in the platelet:collagen interaction. J Clin Invest 54:1480, 1974

39. Tschopp TB, Weiss H, Baumgartner HR: Decreased adhesion of platelets to subendothelium in von Willebrand's disease. J Lab Clin Med 83:296, 1974

40. Sakariassen K, Bolhuis P, Sizma JJ: Human blood platelet adhesion to arterial subendothelium is mediated by factor VIII-von Willebrand factor bound to subendothelium. Nature 279:636, 1979

41. Houdijk WPM, Sakariassen K, Nievelstein P, Sixma JJ: Role of factor VIII-von Willebrand factor and fibronectin in the interaction of platelets in flowing blood with monomeric and fibrillar human collagen types I and III. J Clin Invest 75:531, 1985

42. Santoro SA: Preferential binding of high molecular weight forms of von Willebrand factor to fibrillar collagen. Biochim Biophys Acta 756:123, 1983

43. Gralnick HR, Williams SB, Morisato DK: Effect of multimeric structure of the factor VIII/von Willebrand factor protein on binding to platelets. Blood 58:387, 1981

44. Ginsberg MH, Loftus J, Plow EF: Platelets and the adhesion receptor superfamily. Prog Clin Biol Res 283:171, 1988

45. Nieuwenhuis HK, Akkerman JWN, Houdijk WPM, Sixma JJ: Human blood platelets showing no response to collagen fail to express glycoprotein Ia. Nature 318:470, 1985

46. Kehrel B, Baleisen L, Kokott R et al: Deficiency of intact thrombospondin and membrane glycoprotein Ia in platelets with defective collagen-induced aggregation and spontaneous loss of disorder. Blood 71:1074, 1988

47. Staatz WD, Rajpara SM, Wayner EA et al: The membrane glycoprotein Ia-IIa (VLA-2) complex mediates the Mg^{++}-dependent adhesion of platelets to collagen. J Cell Biol 108:1917, 1989

48. Fisher GJ, Bakshian S, Baldassare JJ: Activation of human platelets by ADP causes a rapid rise in cytosolic free calcium without hydrolysis of phosphatidylinositol-4,5-bisphosphate. Biochem Biophys Res Commun 129:958, 1985

49. Daniel JL, Dangelmaier CA, Selak M, Smith JB: ADP stimulates IP_3 formation in human platelets. FEBS Lett 206:299, 1986

50. Hallam TJ, Sanchez A, Rink TJ: ADP increases cytoplasmic free Ca^{2+} in quin 2-loaded human platelets mainly by influx across the plasma membrane. Thromb Haemost 50:76, 1983

51. Harrison MJ, Brossmer R: Inhibition of ADP-induced platelet aggregation by adenosine tetraphosphate. Thromb Haemost 36:388, 1976

52. Siess W, Weber PC, Lapetina EG: Activation of phospholipase C is dissociated from arachidonate metabolism during platelet shape change induced by thrombin or platelet-activating factor. Epinephrine does not induce phospholipase C activation or platelet shape change. J Biol Chem 259:8286, 1984

53. Bennett JS, Vilaire G, Burch JW: A role for prostaglandins and thromboxanes in the exposure of platelet fibrinogen receptors. J Clin Invest 68:981, 1981

54. Peerschke EI: Induction of human platelet fibrinogen receptors by epinephrine in the absence of released ADP. Blood 60:71, 1982

55. Aktories K, Schultz G, Jakobs KH: Islet-activating protein impairs α_2-adrenoceptor-mediated inhibitory regulation of human platelet adenylate cyclase. Naunyn Schmiedebergs Arch Pharmacol 324:196, 1983

56. Sweatt JD, Connolly TM, Cragoe EJ, Limbird LE: Evidence that Na^+/H^+ exchange regulates receptor-mediated phospholipase A_2 activation in human platelets. J Biol Chem 261:8667, 1986

57. Banga HS, Simons ER, Brass LF, Rittenhouse SE: Activation of phospholipases A and C in human platelets exposed to epinephrine: role of glycoproteins IIb/IIIa and dual role of epinephrine. Proc Natl Acad Sci USA 83:9197, 1986

58. Newman KD, Williams LT, Bishopric NH, Lefkowitz RJ: Identification of α-

adrenergic receptors in human platelets by 3H-dihydroergocryptine binding. J Clin Invest 61:395, 1978

59. Kaywin P, McDonough M, Insel PA, Shattil SJ: Platelet function in essential thrombocythemia: decreased epinephrine responsiveness associated with a deficiency of platelet alpha-adrenergic receptors. N Engl J Med 299:505, 1978

60. Motulsky HJ, Insel PA: [^{3}H]Dihydroergocryptine binding to alpha-adrenergic receptors of human platelets. A reassessment using the selective radioligands [^{3}H]prazosin, [^{3}H]yohimbine, and [^{3}H]rauwolscine. Biochem Pharmacol 31:2591, 1982

61. Scrutton MC, Clare KC, Hutton RA, Bruckdorfer KR: Depressed responsiveness to adrenaline in platelets from apparently normal human donors: a familial trait. Br J Haematol 49:303, 1981

62. Rao AK, Willis J, Kowalska MA, Wachtfogel YT, Colman RW: Differential requirements for platelet aggregation and inhibition of adenylate cyclase by epinephrine. Studies of a familial platelet α_2-adrenergic receptor defect. Blood 71:494, 1988

63. Tamponi G, Pannocchia A, Arduino C et al: Congenital deficiency of α_2-adrenoreceptors on human platelets: description of two cases. Thromb Haemost 58:1012, 1987

64. Regan JW, Nakata H, DeMarinis RM et al: Purification and characterization of the human platelet α_2-adrenergic receptor. J Biol Chem 261:3894, 1986

65. Kobilka BK, Matsui H, Kobilka TS et al: Cloning, sequencing, and expression of the gene coding for the human platelet α_2-adrenergic receptor. Science 238:650, 1987

66. Nicolaou KC, Magolda RL, Smith JB et al: Synthesis and biological properties of pinane-thromboxane A2, a selective inhibitor of coronary artery constriction, platelet aggregation, and thromboxane formation. Proc Natl Acad Sci USA 76:2566, 1979

67. Le Breton GC, Venton DL, Enke SE, Halushka PV: 13-Azaprostanoic acid: a specific antagonist of the human blood platelet thromboxane/endoperoxide receptor. Proc Natl Acad Sci USA 76:4097, 1979

68. Gerrard JM, Carroll RC: Stimulation of protein phosphorylation by arachidonic acid and endoperoxide analog. Prostaglandins 22:81, 1981

69. Pollock WK, Armstrong RA, Brydon LJ et al: Thromboxane-induced phosphatidate formation in human platelets. Biochem J 219:833, 1984

70. Best LC, McGuire MB, Martin TJ et al: Effects of epoxymethano analogues of prostaglandin endoperoxides on aggregation, on release of 5-hydroxytryptamine and on metabolism of 3'5'-cyclic AMP and cyclic GMP in human platelets. Biochim Biophys Acta 583:344, 1979

71. Brace LD, Venton DL, Le Breton GC: Thromboxane A2/prostaglandin H2 mobilizes calcium in human blood platelets. Am J Physiol 249:H1, 1985

72. Brass LF, Woolkalis MJ, Manning DR: Interactions in platelets between G proteins and the agonists that stimulate phospholipase C and inhibit adenylyl cyclase. J Biol Chem 263:5348, 1988

73. Siess W, Siegel FL, Lapetina EG: Arachidonic acid stimulates the formation of 1,2-diacylglycerol and phosphatidic acid in human platelets. Degree of phospholipase C activation correlates with protein phosphorylation, platelet shape change, serotonin release, and aggregation. J Biol Chem 258:11236, 1983

74. Brass LF, Shaller CC, Belmonte EJ: Inositol 1,4,5-triphosphate-induced granule secretion in platelets. Evidence that the activation of phospholipase C mediated by platelet thromboxane receptors involves a guanine nucleotide binding protein-dependent mechanism distinct from that of thrombin. J Clin Invest 79:1269, 1987

75. Hanasaki K, Arita H: Characterization of thromboxane A2/prostaglandin H2 (TXA2/PGH2) receptors of rat platelets and their interaction with TXA2/PGH2 receptor antagonists. Biochem Pharmacol 37:3923, 1988

76. Hung SC, Ghali NI, Venton DL, Le Breton GC: Specific binding of the thromboxane A2 antagonist 13-azaprostanoic acid to human platelet membranes. Biochim Biophys Acta 728:171, 1983

77. Saussy DL Jr, Mais DE, Burch RM, Halushka PV: Identification of a putative thromboxane A2/prostaglandin H2 receptor in human platelet membranes. J Biol Chem 261:3025, 1986

78. Hirata M, Hayashi Y, Ushikubi F et al: Cloning and expression of cDNA for a human thromboxane A2 receptor. Nature 349:617, 1991

79. Clapham DE, Neer EJ: New roles for G-protein $\beta\gamma$-dimers in transmembrane signalling. Nature 365:403, 1993

80. Ercolani L, Stow JL, Boyle JF et al: Membrane localization of the pertussis toxin-sensitive G protein subunits α_{i2} and α_{i3} and expression of a metallothionein-α_{i2} fusion gene in LLC-PK1 cells. Proc Natl Acad Sci USA 87:4635, 1990

81. Lewis JM, Woolkalis MJ, Gerton GL et al: Subcellular distribution of the α subunit(s) of G_i: visualization by immunofluorescent and immunogold labeling. Cell Regul 2:1097, 1991

82. Hepler JR, Gilman AG: G proteins. Trends Biochem Sci 17:383, 1992

83. Conklin BR, Bourne HR: Structural elements of G_α subunits that interact with $G_{\beta\gamma}$, receptors, and effectors. Cell 73:631, 1993

84. Yamane HK, Fung BK-K: Covalent modifications of G-proteins. Annu Rev Pharmacol Toxicol 33:201, 1993

85. Williams A, Woolkalis MJ, Poncz M et al: Identification of the pertussis toxin-sensitive G proteins in platelets, megakaryocytes and HEL cells. Blood 76:721, 1990

86. Iyengar R: Molecular and functional diversity of mammalian G_s-stimulated adenylyl cyclases. FASEB J 7:768, 1993

87. Taussig R, Iniguez-LLuhi JA, Gilman AG: Inhibition of adenylyl cyclase by $G_{i\alpha}$. Science 261:218, 1993

88. Hellevuo K, Yoshimura M, Kao M et al: A novel adenylyl cyclase sequence cloned from the human erythroleukemia cell line. Biochem Biophys Res Commun 192:311, 1993

89. Cockcroft S, Thomas GMH: Inositol-lipid-specific phospholipase C isoenzymes and their differential regulation by receptors. Biochem J 288:1, 1992

90. Berridge MJ: Inositol trisphosphate and calcium signalling. Nature 361:315, 1993

91. Smrcka AV, Hepler JR, Brown KO, Sternweis PC: Regulation of polyphosphoinositide-specific phospholipase C activity by purified G_q. Science 251:804, 1991

92. Taylor SJ, Exton JH: Two α subunits of the G_q class of G proteins stimulate phosphoinositide phospholipase C-β1 activity. FEBS Lett 286:214, 1991

93. Taylor SJ, Chae HZ, Rhee SG, Exton JH: Activation of the β1 isozyme of phospholipase C by α subunits of the G_q class of G proteins. Nature 350:516, 1991

94. Blank JL, Ross AH, Exton JH: Purification and characterization of two G-proteins that activate the β1 isozyme of phosphoinositide-specific phospholipase C. Identification as members of the G_q class. J Biol Chem 266:18206, 1991

95. Smrcka AV, Sternweis PC: Regulation of purified subtypes of phosphatidylinositol-specific phospholipase C_β by G protein α and $\beta\gamma$ subunits. J Biol Chem 268:9667, 1993

96. Blank JL, Brattain KA, Exton JH: Activation of cytosolic phosphoinositide phospholipase C by G-protein $\beta\gamma$ subunits. J Biol Chem 267:23069, 1992

97. Camps M, Carozzi A, Schnabel P et al: Isozyme-selective stimulation of phospholipase C-β2 by G protein $\beta\gamma$-subunits. Nature 360:684, 1992

98. Katz A, Wu D, Simon MI: Subunits $\beta\gamma$ of heterotrimeric G protein activate β2 isoform of phospholipase C. Nature 360:686, 1992

99. Birnbaumer L: Receptor-to-effector signaling through G proteins: roles for $\beta\gamma$ dimers as well as α subunits. Cell 71:1069, 1992

100. Brass LF, Laposata M, Banga HS, Rittenhouse SE: Regulation of the phosphoinositide hydrolysis pathway in thrombin-stimulated platelets by a pertussis toxin-sensitive guanine nucleotide-binding protein. Evaluation of its contribution to platelet activation and comparisons with the adenylate cyclase inhibitory protein, G_i. J Biol Chem 261:16838, 1986

101. Brass LF, Manning DR, Williams A et al: Receptor and G protein-mediated responses to thrombin in HEL cells. J Biol Chem 266:958, 1991

102. Shenker A, Goldsmith P, Unson CG, Spiegel AM: The G protein coupled to the thromboxane A2 receptor in human platelets is a member of the novel G_q family. J Biol Chem 266:9309, 1991

103. Kramer R, Checani G. Deykin A et al: Solubilization and properties of Ca^{2+}-dependent human platelet phospholipase A2. Biochim Biophys Acta 878:394, 1986

104. Yoshimoto T, Yamamoto S, Okuma M, Hayaishi O: Solubilization and resolution of thromboxane synthesizing system from microsomes of bovine blood platelets. J Biol Chem 252:5871, 1977

105. Carey F, Menashi S, Crawford N: Localization of cyclo-oxygenase and thromboxane synthetase in human platelet intracellular membranes. Biochem J 204:847, 1982

106. Laposata M, Krueger CM, Saffitz JE: Selective uptake of [^{3}H]arachidonic acid into the dense tubular system of human platelets. Blood 70:832, 1987

107. Mayer RJ, Marshall LA: New insights on mammalian phospholipase A2(s); comparison of arachidonoyl-selective and nonselective enzymes. FASEB J 7:339, 1993

108. Sharp JD, White DL, Chiou XG et al: Molecular cloning and expression of human Ca($^{2+}$)-sensitive cytosolic phospholipase A2. J Biol Chem 266:14850, 1991

109. Kramer RM, Roberts EF, Manetta J, Putnam JE: The Ca^{2+}-sensitive cytosolic phospholipase A2 is a 100-kDa protein in human monoblast U937 cells. J Biol Chem 266:5268, 1991

110. Takayama K, Kudo I, Kim DK et al: Purification and characterization of human platelet phospholipase A2 which preferentially hydrolyzes an arachidonoyl residue. FEBS Lett 282:326, 1991

111. Glaser KB, Mobilio D, Chang JY, Senko N: Phospholipase A2 enzymes: regulation and inhibition. Trends Pharmacol Sci 14:92, 1993

112. Lin L-L, Wartmann M, Lin AY et al: cPLA$_2$ is phosphorylated and activated by MAP kinase. Cell 72:269, 1993

113. Jelsema CL: Regulation of phospholipase A$_2$ and phospholipase C in rod outer segments of bovine retina involves a common GTP-binding protein but different mechanisms of action. Ann NY Acad Sci 559:158, 1989

114. Kim D, Lewis DL, Graziadei L et al: G-protein βγ-subunits activate the cardiac muscarinic K$^+$-channel via phospholipase A$_2$. Nature 337:557, 1989

115. Nakashima S, Hattori H, Shirato L et al: Differential sensitivity of arachidonic acid release and 1,2-diacylglycerol formation to pertussis toxin, GDPβS and NaF in saponin-permeabilized human platelets: possible evidence for distinct GTP-binding proteins involving phospholipase C and A$_2$ activation. Biochem Biophys Res Commun 148:971, 1987

116. Kajiyama Y, Murayama T, Nomura Y: Pertussis toxin-sensitive GTP-binding proteins may regulate phospholipase A$_2$ in response to thrombin in rabbit platelets. Arch Biochem Biophys 274:200, 1989

117. Silk ST, Clejan S, Witkom K: Evidence of GTP-binding protein regulation of phospholipase A$_2$ activity in isolated human platelet membranes. J Biol Chem 264:21466, 1989

118. Murayama T, Kajiyama Y, Nomura Y: Histamine-stimulated and GTP-binding protein-mediated phospholipase A$_2$ activation in rabbit platelets. J Biol Chem 265:4290, 1990

119. Carlson K, Brass LF, Manning DR: Thrombin and phorbol esters cause the selective phosphorylation of a G protein other than G$_i$ in human platelets. J Biol Chem 264:13298, 1989

120. Gagnon AW, Manning DR, Catani L et al: Identification of G$_{z\alpha}$ as a pertussis toxin-insensitive G protein in human platelets and megakaryocytes. Blood 78:1247, 1991

121. Casey PJ, Fong HKW, Simon MI, Gilman AG: G$_z$, a guanine nucleotide-binding protein with unique biochemical properties. J Biol Chem 265:2383, 1990

122. Lounsbury KM, Casey PJ, Brass LF, Manning DR: Phosphorylation of G$_z$ in human platelets: selectivity and site of modification. J Biol Chem 266:22051, 1991

123. Lounsbury KM, Schlegel B, Poncz M et al: Analysis of G$_{z\alpha}$ by site-directed mutagenesis: sites and specificity of protein kinase C-dependent phosphorylation. J Biol Chem 268:3494, 1993

124. Wong YH, Conklin BR, Bourne HR: G$_z$-mediated hormonal inhibition of cyclic AMP accumulation. Science 255:339, 1992

125. Strathmann MP, Simon MI: G$_{\alpha 12}$ and G$_{\alpha 13}$ subunits define a fourth class of G protein α subunits. Proc Natl Acad Sci USA 88:5582, 1991

126. Amatruda TT III, Steele DA, Slepak VZ, Simon MI: G$_{\alpha 16}$, a G protein α subunit specifically expressed in hematopoietic cells. Proc Natl Acad Sci USA 88:5587, 1991

127. Billah MM, Lapetina EG, Cuatrecasas P: Phospholipase A2 and phospholipase C activity of platelets. J Biol Chem 255:10227, 1981

128. Lapetina EG: Inositol phospholipids and GTP-binding proteins in signal transduction in stimulated human platelets. Adv Prostaglandin Thromboxane Leukot Res 16:217, 1986

129. Shattil SJ, Brass LF: Induction of the fibrinogen receptor on human platelets by intracellular mediators. J Biol Chem 262:992, 1987

130. Kaibuchi K, Takai Y, Sawamura M et al: Synergistic functions of protein phosphorylation and calcium mobilization in platelet activation. J Biol Chem 258:6701, 1983

131. Lapetina EG, Reep B, Ganong BR, Bell RM: Exogenous sn-1,2-diacylglycerols containing saturated fatty acids function as bioregulators of protein kinase C in human platelets. J Biol Chem 260:1358, 1985

132. Brass LF, Joseph SK: A role for inositol triphosphate in intracellular Ca^{2+} mobilization and granule secretion in platelets. J Biol Chem 260:15172, 1985

133. O'Rourke FA, Halenda SP, Zavoico GB, Feinstein MB: Inositol 1,4,5-trisphosphate releases Ca^{2+} from a Ca^{2+}-transporting membrane vesicle fraction derived from human platelets. J Biol Chem 260:956, 1985

134. Adunyah S, Dean W: Inositol triphosphate-induced Ca^{2+} release from human platelet membranes. Biochem Biophys Res Commun 128:1274, 1985

135. Authi KS, Crawford N: Inositol 1,4,5-trisphosphate-induced release of sequestered Ca^{2+} from highly purified human platelet intracellular membranes. Biochem J 230:247, 1985

136. Kikkawa U, Nishizuka Y: The role of protein kinase C in transmembrane signalling. Annu Rev Cell Biol 2:149, 1986

137. Irvine RF: Metabolism and function of inositol phosphates. ISI Atlas of Science. Biochemistry 1:337, 1988

138. Majerus PW, Connolly TM, Bansal VS et al: Inositol phosphates: synthesis and degradation. J Biol Chem 263:3051, 1988

139. Tarver AP, King WG, Rittenhouse SE: Inositol 1,4,5-trisphosphate and inositol 1,2-cyclic 4,5-trisphosphate are minor components of total mass of inositol trisphosphate in thrombin-stimulated platelets. Rapid formation of inositol 1,3,4-trisphosphate. J Biol Chem 262:17268, 1987

140. Johnson PC, Ware JA, Cliveden PB et al: Measurement of ionized calcium in blood platelets with the photoprotein aequorin. Comparison with quin 2. J Biol Chem 260:2069, 1985

141. Ware JA, Johnson PC, Smith M, Salzman EW: Effect of common agonists on cytoplasmic ionized calcium concentration in platelets. Measurement with 2-methyl-6-methoxy 8-nitroquinoline (quin2) and aequorin. J Clin Invest 77:878, 1986

142. Drummond AH, MacIntyre DE: Platelet inositol lipid metabolism and calcium flux. p. 380. In MacIntyre DE, Gordon JL (eds): Platelets in Biology and Pathology. Vol. III. Elsevier Science, New York, 1987

143. Brass LF: Ca^{2+} transport across the platelet plasma membrane. A role for membrane glycoproteins IIb and IIIa. J Biol Chem 260:2231, 1985

144. Powling MJ, Hardisty RM: Glycoprotein IIb-IIIa complex and Ca^{2+} influx into stimulated platelets. Blood 66:731, 1985

145. Rybak ME, Renzulli LA, Bruns MJ, Cahaly DP: Platelet glycoproteins IIb and IIIa as a calcium channel in liposomes. Blood 72:714, 1988

146. Suldan Z, Brass LF: The role of the glycoprotein IIb-IIIa complex in plasma membrane Ca^{++} transport: a comparison of results obtained with platelets and HEL cells. Blood 78:2887, 1991

147. White JG: Interaction of membrane systems in blood platelets. Am J Pathol 66:295, 1972

148. Brass LF: Ca^{2+} homeostasis in unstimulated platelets. J Biol Chem 259:12563, 1984

149. Barnathan ES, Addonizio VP, Shattil SJ: Interaction of verapamil with human platelet α-adrenergic receptors. Am J Physiol 242:H19, 1982

150. Johnson GJ, Leis LA, Francis G: Disparate effects of the calcium-channel blocker, nifedipine and verapamil, on alpha2-adrenergic receptors and thromboxane A2-induced aggregation in human platelets. Circulation 73:847, 1986

151. Doyle VM, Ruegg UT: Lack of evidence for voltage dependent calcium channels on platelets. Biochem Biophys Res Commun 127:161, 1985

152. Motulsky HJ, Snavely MD, Hughes RJ, Insel PA: Interaction of verapamil and other calcium channel blockers with α$_1$ and α$_2$ adrenergic receptors. Circ Res 52:226, 1983

153. Wilson DB, Connolly TM, Bross TE et al: Isolation and characterization of the inositol cyclic phosphate products of polyphosphoinositide cleavage by phospholipase C. Physiological effects in permeabilized platelets and Limulus photoreceptor cells. J Biol Chem 260:13496, 1985

154. Mikoshiba K: Inositol 1,4,5-trisphosphate receptor. Trends Pharmacol Sci 14:86, 1993

155. Tsujinaka T, Sakon M, Kambayashi J, Kosaki G: Cleavage of cytoskeletal proteins by two forms of calcium-activated neutral proteases in human platelets. Thromb Res 28:149, 1982

156. Tsujinaka T, Shiba E, Kambayashi J-I, Kosaki G: Purification and characterization of a low calcium requiring form of calcium-activated neutral protease from human platelets. Biochem Int 6:71, 1983

157. Malik MN, Ramaswamy S, Tuzio H et al: Micromolar calcium requiring protease from human platelets: purification, partial characterization and effect on the cytoskeletal proteins. Life Sci 40:593, 1987

158. Yoshida N, Weksler BB, Nachman RL: Purification of human platelet calcium-activated protease: effect on platelet and endothelial function. J Biol Chem 258:7168, 1983

159. Sakon M, Kambayashi J-I, Ohno H, Kosaki G: Two forms of calcium-activated neutral protease in platelets. Thromb Res 24:207, 1981

160. O'Halloran T, Beckerle MC, Burridge K: Identification of talin as a major cytoplasmic protein implicated in platelet activation. Nature 317:449, 1985

161. Fox JE, Goll DE, Reynolds CC, Phillips DR: Identification of two proteins (actin-binding protein and P235) that are hydrolyzed by endogenous Ca^{2+}-dependent protease during platelet aggregation. J Biol Chem 260:1060, 1985

162. Fox JE, Reynolds CC, Phillips DR: Calcium-dependent proteolysis occurs during platelet aggregation. J Biol Chem 258:9973, 1983

163. Brass LF, Shattil SJ: Inhibition of thrombin-induced platelet activation by leupeptin. Implications for the participation of calpain in the initiation of platelet activation. J Biol Chem 263:5210, 1988

164. Feinstein MB: The role of calmodulin in hemostasis. Prog Hemost Thromb 6:25, 1982

165. Gear ARL, Schneider W: Control of platelet glycogenolysis. Activation of phosphorylase kinase by calcium. Biochim Biophys Acta 392:111, 1975

166. Hathway DR, Adelstein RS: Human platelet myosin light chain kinase requires the calcium-binding protein calmodulin for activity. Proc Natl Acad Sci USA 76:1653, 1979

167. Hallam TJ, Daniel JL, Kendrick Jones J, Rink TJ: Relationship between cytoplasmic free calcium and myosin light chain phosphorylation in intact platelets. Biochem J 232:373, 1985

168. Scholey JM, Taylor KA, Kendrick-Jones J: Regulation of non-muscle myosin assembly by calmodulin-dependent light chain kinase. Nature 287:233, 1980

169. Asaoka Y, Nakamura S, Yoshida K, Nishizuka Y: Protein kinase C, calcium, and phospholipid degradation. Trends Biochem Sci 17:414, 1992

170. Grabarek J, Raychowdhury M, Ravid K et al: Identification and functional characterization of protein kinase C isozymes in platelets and HEL cells. J Biol Chem 267:10011, 1992

171. Salama SE, Haslam RJ: Characterization of the protein kinase activities of human platelet supernatant and particulate fractions. Biochem J 218:285, 1984

172. Siess W, Lapetina EG: Phorbol esters sensitize platelets to activation by physiological agonists. Blood 70:1373, 1987

173. Naka M, Nishikawa M, Adelstein RS, Hidaka H: Phorbol ester-induced activation of human platelets is associated with protein kinase C phosphorylation of myosin light chains. Nature 306:490, 1983

174. Tyers M, Rachubinski RA, Stewart MI et al: Molecular cloning and expression of the major protein kinase C substrate of platelets. Nature 333:470, 1988

175. Tyers M, Haslam RJ, Rachubinski RA, Harley CB: Molecular analysis of pleckstrin: the major protein kinase C substrate of platelets. J Cell Biochem 40:133, 1989

176. Gailani D, Fisher TC, Mills DC, Macfarlane DE: P47 phosphoprotein of blood platelets (pleckstrin) is a major target for phorbol ester-induced protein phosphorylation in intact platelets, granulocytes, lymphocytes, monocytes and cultured leukaemic cells: absence of P47 in non-haematopoietic cells. Br J Haematol 74:192, 1990

177. Haslam RJ, Koide HB, Hemmings BA: Pleckstrin domain homology. Nature 363:309, 1993

178. Musacchio A, Gibson T, Rice P et al: The PH domain: a common piece in the structural patchwork of signalling proteins. TIBS 18:343, 1993

179. Litchfield DW, Ball EH: Phosphorylation of caldesmon77 by protein kinase C in vitro and in intact human platelets. J Biol Chem 262:8056, 1987

180. Bourguignon LYW, Walker G, Bourguignon GJ: Phorbol ester-induced phosphorylation of a transmembrane glycoprotein (GP180) in human blood platelets. J Biol Chem 260:11775, 1985

181. Marcus AJ, Ullman HL, Safier LB: Lipid composition of subcellular particles of human blood platelets. J Lipid Res 10:108, 1969

182. Cohen P, Derksen A: Comparison of phospholipid and fatty acid composition of human erythrocytes and platelets. Br J Haematol 17:359, 1969

183. Bills TK, Smith JB, Silver MJ: Metabolism of ^{14}C-arachidonic acid by human platelets. Biochim Biophys Acta 424:303, 1976

184. Russell FA, Deykin D: The effect of thrombin on the uptake and transformation of arachidonic acid by human platelets. Am J Hematol 1:59, 1976

185. Perret B, Chap HJ, Douste-Blazy L: Asymmetric distribution of arachidonic acid in the plasma membrane of human platelets. Biochim Biophys Acta 556:434, 1979

186. McKean ML, Smith JB, Silver MJ: Formation of lysophosphatidylcholine by human platelets in response to thrombin. J Biol Chem 256:1522, 1981

187. Neufeld EJ, Majerus PW: Arachidonate release and phosphatidic acid turnover in stimulated human platelets. J Biol Chem 258:2461, 1983

188. Bills TK, Smith JB, Silver MJ: Selective release of arachidonic acid from the phospholipids of human platelets in response to thrombin. J Clin Invest 60:1, 1977

189. Bell RL, Kennerly DA, Stanford N, Majerus PW: Diglyceride lipase: a pathway for arachidonate release from human platelets. Proc Natl Acad Sci USA 76:3238, 1979

190. Prescott SM, Majerus PW: Characterization of 1,2-diacylglycerol hydrolysis in human platelets. J Biol Chem 258:764, 1983

191. Smith WL: The eicosanoids and their biochemical mechanisms of action. Biochem J 259:315, 1989

192. Mills DCB, Smith JB: The influence on platelet aggregation of drugs that affect the accumulation of adenosine 3':5' cyclic monophosphate in platelets. Biochem J 121:185, 1971

193. Haslam RJ: Interactions of the pharmacological receptors of blood platelets with adenylate cyclase. Ser Haematol 6:333, 1973

194. Steer ML, Wood A: Regulation of human platelet adenylate cyclase by epinephrine, prostaglandin E1 and guanine nucleotides. J Biol Chem 254:10791, 1979

195. Burch JW, Baenziger NL, Stanford N, Majerus PW: Sensitivity of fatty acid cyclooxygenase from human aorta to acetylation by aspirin. Proc Natl Acad Sci USA 75:5181, 1978

196. Burch JW, Stanford N, Majerus PW: Inhibition of platelet prostaglandin synthetase by oral aspirin. J Clin Invest 61:314, 1978

197. Roth GJ, Machuga ET, Ozols J: Isolation and covalent structure of the aspirin-modified, active-site region of prostaglandin synthetase. Biochemistry 22:4672, 1983

198. DeWitt DL, Smith WL: Primary structure of prostaglandin G/H synthase from sheep vesicular gland determined from the complementary DNA sequence. Proc Natl Acad Sci USA 85:1412, 1988

199. Rome LH, Lands WE: Structural requirements for time-dependent inhibition of prostaglandin biosynthesis by anti-inflammatory drugs. Proc Natl Acad Sci USA 72:4863, 1975

200. Stanford N, Roth GJ, Shen TY, Majerus PW: Lack of covalent modification of prostaglandin synthetase (cyclo-oxygenase) by indomethacin. Prostaglandins 13:669, 1977

201. Hamberg M, Samuelsson B: Prostaglandin endoperoxides. Novel transformations of arachidonic acid in human platelets. Proc Natl Acad Sci USA 71:3400, 1974

202. Fitzgerald LA, Phillips DR: Calcium regulation of the platelet membrane glycoprotein IIb-IIIa complex. J Biol Chem 260:11366, 1985

203. Wong PY, Westlund P, Hamberg M et al: 15-Lipoxygenase in human platelets. J Biol Chem 260:9162, 1985

204. Watson SP, Lapetina EG: 1,2-Diacylglycerol and phorbol ester inhibit agonist-induced formation of inositol phosphates in human platelets: possible implications for negative feedback regulation of inositol phospholipid hydrolysis. Proc Natl Acad Sci USA 82:2623, 1985

205. Zavoico GB, Halenda SP, Shaafi RI, Feinstein MB: Phorbol myristate acetate inhibits thrombin-stimulated Ca^{2+} mobilization and phosphatidylinositol 4,5-bisphosphate hydrolysis in human platelets. Proc Natl Acad Sci USA 82:3859, 1985

206. MacIntyre DE, McNicol A, Drummond AH: Tumour-promoting phorbol esters inhibit agonist-induced phosphatidate formation and Ca^{2+} flux in human platelets. FEBS Lett 180:160, 1985

207. Connolly TM, Lawing WJ Jr, Majerus PW: Protein kinase C phosphorylates human platelet inositol trisphosphate 5'-phosphomonoesterase, increasing the phosphatase activity. Cell 46:951, 1986

208. Jakobs KH, Bauer S, Watanabe Y: Modulation of adenylate cyclase of human platelets by phorbol ester. Impairment of the hormone-sensitive inhibitory pathway. Eur J Biochem 151:425, 1985

209. Alvarez R, Taylor A, Fazzari JJ, Jacobs JR: Regulation of cAMP metabolism in platelets. Sequential activation of adenylate cyclase and cAMP phosphodiesterase by prostaglandins. Mol Pharmacol 20:302, 1981

210. Taylor SS: cAMP-dependent protein kinase. J Biol Chem 264:8443, 1989

211. Fox JEB, Reynolds CC, Johnson MM: Identification of glycoprotein Ibβ as one of the major proteins phosphorylated during exposure of intact platelets to agents that activate cAMP-dependent protein kinase. J Biol Chem 262:12627, 1987

212. Wardell MR, Reynolds CC, Berndt MC et al: Platelet glycoprotein Ibβ is phosphorylated on serine 166 by cyclic AMP-dependent protein kinase. J Biol Chem 264:15656, 1989

213. Wallach D, Davies PJA, Pastan I: Cyclic AMP-dependent phosphorylation of filamin in mammalian smooth muscle. J Biol Chem 253:4739, 1978

214. Matsui Y, Kikuchi A, Kawata M et al: Molecular cloning of smg p21B and identification of smg p21 purified from bovine brain and human platelets as smg p21B. Biochem Biophys Res Commun 166:1010, 1990

215. White TE, Lacal J-C, Reep B et al: Thrombolamban, the 22-kDa platelet substrate of cyclic AMP-dependent protein kinase, is immunologically homologous with the Ras family of GTP-binding proteins. Proc Natl Acad Sci USA 87:758, 1990

216. Fischer TH, Gatling MN, Lacal J-C, White GC, II: Rap1B, a cAMP-dependent protein kinase substrate, associates with the platelet cytoskeleton. J Biol Chem 265:19405, 1990

217. Haslam RJ, Lynham JA, Fox JEB: Effects of collagen, ionophore A23187 and prostaglandin E1 on the phosphorylation of specific proteins in blood platelets. Biochem J 178:397, 1979

218. Kaser-Glanzmann R, Gerber E, Luscher EF: Regulation of the intracellular calcium level in human blood platelets: cAMP dependent phosphorylation of a 22,000 dalton component in isolated Ca2+-accumulating vesicles. Biochim Biophys Acta 558:34, 1979

219. Lerea KM, Glomset JA, Krebs EG: Agents that elevate cAMP levels in platelets decrease thrombin binding. J Biol Chem 262:282, 1987

220. Watson SP, McConnell RT, Lapetina EG: The rapid formation of inositol phosphates in human platelets by thrombin is inhibited by prostacyclin. J Biol Chem 259:13199, 1984

221. Feinstein MB, Egan JJ, Shaafi RI, White J: The cytoplasmic concentration of free calcium in platelets is controlled by stimulators of cyclic AMP production (PGD2, PGE1, forskolin). Biochem Biophys Res Commun 113:598, 1983

222. Sage SO, Rink TJ: Inhibition by forskolin of cytosolic calcium rise, shape change and aggregation in quin2-loaded human platelets. FEBS Lett 188:135, 1985

223. Kaser-Glanzmann R, Jakabova M, George JN, Luscher EF: Stimulation of calcium uptake in platelet membrane vesicles by cAMP and protein kinase. Biochim Biophys Acta 466:429, 1977

224. Fox JEB: The platelet cytoskeleton. p. 175. In Verstraete M, Vermylen J,

Lijnen R, Arnout J (eds): Thrombosis and Hemostasis 1987. Leuven University Press, Leuven, Belgium, 1987

225. Carlsson L, Markey F, Blikstad I et al: Reorganization of actin in platelets stimulated by thrombin as measured by the DNase I inhibition assay. Proc Natl Acad Sci USA 76:6376, 1979

226. Okita JR, Pidard D, Newman PJ et al: On the association of glycoprotein Ib and actin-binding protein in human platelets. J Cell Biol 100:317, 1985

227. Fox JEB: Identification of actin-binding protein as the protein linking the membrane skeleon to glycoproteins on platelet plasma membranes. J Biol Chem 260:11970, 1985

228. Ezzell RM, Kenney DM, Egan S et al: Localization of the domain of actin-binding protein that binds to membrane glycoprotein Ib and actin in human platelets. J Biol Chem 263:13303, 1988

229. Lipfert L, Haimovich B, Schaller MD et al: Integrin-dependent phosphorylation and activation of the protein tyrosine kinase pp125^{FAK} in platelets. J Cell Biol 119:905, 1992

230. Huang M-M, Lipfert L, Cunningham M et al: Adhesive ligand binding to integrin $\alpha_{IIb}\beta_3$ stimulates tyrosine phosphorylation of novel protein substrates before phosphorylation of pp125^{FAK}. J Cell Biol 122:473, 1993

231. Haimovich B, Lipfert L, Brugge JS, Shattil SJ: Tyrosine phosphorylation and cytoskeletal reorganization in platelets are triggered by interaction of integrin receptors with their immobilized ligands. J Biol Chem 268:15868, 1993

232. Shattil SJ: Regulation of platelet anchorage and signaling by integrin $\alpha_{IIb}\beta_3$. Thromb Haemost 70:224, 1993

233. Schollmeyer JV, Rao GHR, White JG: An actin-binding protein in human platelets. Am J Pathol 93:433, 1978

234. Rosenberg S, Stracher A, Lucas RC: Isolation and characterization of actin and actin-binding protein from human platelets. J Cell Biol 91:201, 1981

235. Fox JE, Reynolds CC, Morrow JS, Phillips DR: Spectrin is associated with membrane-bound actin-filaments in platelets and is hydrolyzed by the Ca^{2+}-dependent protease during platelet activation. Blood 69:537, 1987

236. Collier NC, Wang K: Purification and properties of human platelet P235. A high molecular weight protein substrate of endogenous calcium-activated protease(s). J Biol Chem 257:6937, 1982

237. Nachmias VT, Yoshida K: The cytoskeleton of the blood platelet: a dynamic structure. Adv Cell Biol 2:181, 1988

238. Behnke O: Further studies on microtubules. A marginal bundle in human and rat thrombocytes. J Ultrastruct Mol Struct Res 13:469, 1965

239. Behnke O: Effects of some chemicals on blood platelet microtubules, platelet shape and some platelet functions in vitro. Scand J Haematol 7:123, 1970

240. Leven RM, Nachmias VT: Cultured megakaryocytes: changes in the cytoskeleton after adenosine diphosphate-induced spreading. J Cell Biol 92:313, 1982

241. Coller BS: A new murine monoclonal antibody reports an activation-dependent change in the conformation and/or microenvironment of the platelet glycoprotein IIb/IIIa complex. J Clin Invest 76:101, 1985

242. Shattil SJ, Hoxie JA, Cunningham M, Brass LF: Changes in the platelet membrane glycoprotein IIb-IIIa complex during platelet activation. J Biol Chem 260:11107, 1985

243. Parise LV, Criss AB, Nannizzi L, Wardell MR: Glycoprotein IIIa is phosphorylated in intact human platelets. Blood 75:2363, 1990

244. Hillery CA, Smyth SS, Parise LV: Phosphorylation of human platelet glycoprotein IIIa (GPIIIa). Dissociation from fibrinogen receptor activation and phosphorylation of GPIIIa in vitro. J Biol Chem 266:14663, 1991

245. O'Toole TE, Mandelman D, Forsyth J et al: Modulation of the afinity of integrin $\alpha_{IIb}\beta_3$ (platelet GP IIb-IIIa) by the cytoplasmic domain of αIIb. Science 254:845, 1991

246. Chao W, Olson MS: Platelet-activating factor: receptors and signal transduction. Biochem J 292:617, 1993

247. Honda Z, Nakamura M, Miki I et al: Cloning by functional expression of platelet-activating factor receptor from guinea-pig lung. Nature 349:342, 1991

248. Bichet DG, Arthus M-F, Barjon JN et al: Human platelet fraction arginine-vasopressin: potential physiological role. J Clin Invest 79:881, 1987

249. Inaba K, Umeda Y, Yamane Y et al: Characterization of human platelet vasopressin receptor and the relation between vasopressin-induced platelet aggregation and vasopressin binding to platelets. Clin Endocrinol (Oxf) 29:377, 1988

250. Siess W, Stifel M, Binder H, Weber P: Activation of V1-receptors by vasopressin stimulates inositol phospholipid hydrolysis and arachidonate metabolism in human platelets. Biochem J 233:83, 1986

251. Vittet D, Cantau B, Mathieu M-N, Chevillard C: Properties of vasopressin-activated human platelet high affinity GTPase. Biochem Biophys Res Commun 154:213, 1988

252. Lounsbury KM, Brass LF, Manning DR: Phosphorylation of $G_{z\alpha}$ in human platelets: proximity to the amino-terminus of the subunit. J Cell Biol 111:334a, 1990

253. Smith SK, Limbird LE: Evidence that human platelet α-adrenergic receptors coupled to inhibition of adenylate cyclase are not associated with the subunit of adenylate cyclase ADP-ribosylated by cholera toxin. J Biol Chem 257:10471, 1982

254. Coughlin SR, Vu T-KH, Hung DT, Wheaton VI: Characterization of a functional thrombin receptor. Issues and opportunities. J Clin Invest 89:351, 1992

255. Marcus AJ, Safier LB, Ullman HL et al: Platelet-neutrophil interactions (12S)-hydroxyeicosatetraen-1,20-dioic acid: a new eicosanoid synthesized by unstimulated neutrophils from (12S)-20-dihydroxyeicosatetraenoic acid. J Biol Chem 263:2223, 1988

Endothelial Cell Structure and Function

99

Marc A. Shuman

INTRODUCTION

The vascular endothelium, the exclusive interface between the blood and tissues, is a highly complex structure. As such, it serves as a barrier and a transport organ for the multitude of circulating substances. Moreover, it is further specialized to serve different requirements and functions in various organs. An additional level of complexity relates to the location of the vessels lined by endothelium. Endothelium lining vessels in the arterial circulation are exposed to intraluminal pressures far greater than venous endothelium. Similarly, the size and type of vessel (i.e., capillary versus artery) has important consequences on the cellular phenotype. Thus, other types of cells lining the vessel wall as well as the matrix components differ depending on the nature of the vessel. As would be expected, injury or disease affecting the endothelium disrupts the blood interface, allowing undesirable substances to gain entry into the vessel wall and organ parencyhma. On the other hand, injury or disease of the vessel wall can result in expression of a variety of ordinarily latent bioactive substances, or the diminished synthesis and secretion of others, which dramatically alter the interaction of the cellular and plasma components of the blood with the vessel and organ. Examples of such diseases include vasculitis, atherosclerosis, infection, and impaired immune responses. This chapter describes the normal physiology and biochemistry of the vascular endothelium and how it is altered in hematologic and systemic disorders.

ANGIOGENESIS

Formation of blood vessels occurs in two situations: during embryonic development and in a variety of postnatal conditions, including chronic inflammation, cancer, wound healing, and maturation of the corpus luteum. During embryogenesis, endothelial cells originate from angioblasts in the lateral mesoderm.[1,2] Vasculogenesis or blood vessel formation occurs in situ by the aggregation and differentiation of endothelial cells. Initially, the vessels appear as small sacs lined by endothelial cells.[3,4] The type of vessel formed is determined by the local environment, as angioblasts have no regional specificity.[5] The sacs extend to form an interconnecting set of tubes with the heart a highly specialized extension of this process. Following tube formation, smooth muscle cells ensheath the endothelial cells.[6] Additional vessel formation occurs by fusion of existing tubes or by extension of new tubes. The extracellular matrix plays an important role in modulating the endothelial cell phenotype: types IV and V basement membrane collagen induce a tube-like structure, while types I and II collagen induce a flattened proliferative endothelium.[7] Fibronectin modulates endothelial cell shape and proliferation,[8] whereas laminin influences endothelial attachment and differentiation.[9]

While the growth factor(s) responsible for vasculogenesis has not been identified definitively, *flk*-1, a receptor[10,11] for the angiogenic growth factor vascular endothelial growth factor (VEGF),[12] has been identified in the blood islands and endothelial cells of mouse embryos at the earliest stages of blood vessel formation,[11] implying that VEGF may be involved in this process (see below). Whether fibroblast growth factor (FGF) is also required for vascular endothelial growth during embryogenesis is unclear. In vitro basal replication of endothelial monolayers is inhibited by anti-FGF antibodies, as is endothelial cell movement at an artificial wound edge.[13,14]

Postnatal neovascularization occurs in response to cytokines, growth factors, and pathologic stimuli. Capillary formation in the rabbit cornea in response to tumor implants and other stimuli has been used as an experimental model to study neovascularization.[15] The initial changes in limbal vessels occur in the endothelium in venules facing the stimulus, resulting in increased endoplasmic reticulum, free ribosomes, and prominent Golgi.[16,17] Next, the basal lamina of the basement membrane begins to fragment,[18] presumably due to induction of proteases, including plasminogen activators, urokinase and tissue plasminogen activator (u-PA and t-PA), and type IV collagenases.[19,20] Small villous endothelial cytoplasmic processes protrude through these gaps in the lamina.[18] Ultimately, the entire cell migrates through the basement membrane into the perivascular space.[18] This process is repeated by successive endothelial cells with the formation of a capillary sprout. Endothelial cells appear to slide past each other, enclosing a portion of the lumen as other endothelial cells migrate out of the venule, presumably preventing leakage from the parent vessel. Closely following these changes is an increase in DNA synthesis in endothelial cells in the middle of the capillary rather than at the capillary tip.

Table 99-1. Angiogenic Factors

Vascular Growth Factor	In Vitro Effects	In Vivo Effects
VEGF	+	+
PD-ECGF	+	+
FGF	+	+
TNF-α	Inhibitory	+
TGF-α	+	+
TGF-β	Inhibitory	+
Angiogenin	No effect	+
Interleukin-8	+	+

Abbreviations: FGF, fibroblast growth factor; PD-ECGF, platelet-derived endothelial cell growth factor; TGF, transforming growth factor; TNF, tumor necrosis factor; VEGF, vascular endothelial growth factor.

With capillary sprout formation, branching and anastomosis of the tips occurs to form loops.[21] Once loops are formed, blood flows begins. How lumen formation occurs is unclear, but micrographic analysis demonstrates a lumen in capillary sprouts enclosed by a single endothelial cell.[22,23]

Several polypeptide vascular growth factors have been described (Table 99-1). Most stimulate endothelial proliferation in vitro as well as angiogenesis in vivo, while others only have an in vivo effect, suggesting that their effect may be indirect. Some of these growth factors appear to promote growth of endothelial cells only (VEGF, platelet-derived endothelial cell growth factor [PD-ECGF]), whereas others, such as FGF, are mitogenic for several different types of cells.

Vascular Endothelial Growth Factor

Like FGF, VEGF was purified first from bovine pituitary cells.[24] Subsequently it has been identified in guinea pig and murine tumor cell lines.[25,26] VEGF is a specific mitogen for endothelial cells in vitro and a potent angiogenic factor in vivo.[12,27,28] In its active form, VEGF is present as a homodimer, each subunit having a molecular weight of 23,000. In addition to its mitogenic effect, VEGF also increases vascular permeability.[26] VEGF expression has also been noted in human brain tumors, and is believed to be responsible for the marked angiogenesis associated with glioblastoma multiforme tumors.[29,30] *flk*-1 is a high-affinity receptor for VEGF.[11] It is a member of the receptor tyrosine kinase (RTK) subclass III tyrosine kinase family of receptors.[10,31] *flk*-1 is the first angiogenic growth factor receptor to be described in blood vessels during angiogenesis.[11] Receptor mRNA has been identified by in situ hybridization as early as the blood island stage in the yolk sac of 8.5–10.5-day mouse embryos.[11] The mRNA has also been identified in proliferating endothelial cells of vascular sprouts and branching vessels of mouse embryonic and early postnatal brain. These findings suggest that both *flk*-1 and, indirectly, VEGF are likely to be critically involved in angiogenesis. In addition, the *flt*-like tyrosine kinase,[32] *fms* also a subclass III RTK, has been shown to have high-affinity binding for VEGF.[33]

Platelet-Derived Endothelial Cell Growth Factor

As the name implies, PD-ECGF was first described in platelets.[34,35] Subsequently, it has been identified in normal and transformed cell lines.[36] Purification of PD-ECGF and cloning of the cDNA indicate that it is a single polypeptide chain with a molecular weight of 45,000.[35,37,38] It has been reported to be a mitogen specifically for endothelial cells without activity on fibroblasts or other types of cells.[38] Like FGF, PD-ECGF lacks a signal sequence and is not secreted from cells. The nature and specificity of the angiogenic activity of PD-ECGF is unclear, given the observation that it appears to be the product of the same gene as human thymidine phosphorylase.[39] Expression of recombinant PD-ECGF in *Escherichia coli* has confirmed that it has thymidine phosphorylase activity[39] and that this activity is responsible for its endothelial cell mitogenicity.[40]

Fibroblast Growth Factors

FGFs are a family of growth factors that are mitogenic for mesodermally derived tissues. Basic FGFs are found in most tissues that have been studied, while acidic FGFs are primarily found in neural tissues such as the pituitary, brain, hypothalamus, and retina.[41–43] All FGFs share the property of a high affinity for the glycosaminoglycan heparin sulfate.[43–47] The role of endogenous heparans in FGF activity is unclear; however, a heparan sulfate proteoglycan has been found to mediate the binding of basic FGF to the cell surface.[48] Four different receptors for FGFs have been described[49,50]; however, none have been identified in blood vessels in vivo. *flg* and *bek*, FGF receptors 1 and 2, have been sought unsuccessfully in capillary endothelial cells during development.[51,52]

Transforming Growth Factor-α

Transforming growth factor-α (TGF-α) is an in vitro mitogen for endothelial cells as well as a potent in vivo angiogenic stimulus.[53] As TGF-α is a mitogen for a variety of different types of cells, its effect on endothelium is not specific. TGF-α, a 55,000-dalton polypeptide, is produced by transformed fibroblasts as well as a variety of tumor cells lines and macrophages.[54–57] Thus, secretion of TGF-α may be responsible for angiogenic activity observed with certain tumors as well as chronic inflammation. TGF-α utilizes the epidermal growth factor (EGF) receptor for cell signaling.[58,59] While EGF also has partial in vitro mitogenic and in vivo angiogenic activity, it is weak and unlikely to be of significance.[53]

Transforming Growth Factor-β

Like TGF-α, TGF-β actually inhibits endothelial cell growth in vitro.[60,61] However, when injected in vivo, it is a potent angiogenic stimulus.[53,62] The mechanism for this latter activity has not been identified. As TGF-β is a chemoattractant for monocytes and fibroblasts,[63] its effects on neovascularization may be mediated by these cells. TGF-β is found in a variety of tumor cell types as well as normal tissue, including platelets, kidney, placenta, cartilage, and bone.[64,65] TGF-β is synthesized as a 25,000-dalton homodimer[66] and is secreted in an inactive form that must be activated either proteolytically or by acidification.[67,68]

Tumor Necrosis Factor-α

Tumor necrosis factor-α (TNF-α) has potent in vivo angiogenic activity[69]; however, like TGF-β, it inhibits endothelial cell proliferation in vitro.[70,71] TNF-α does, however, stimulate endothelial cell migration and tube formation in vitro.[69] The experimental conditions used in demonstrating the in vivo effects of TNF-α on blood vessels appear to be critical.[72] When injected into a tumor, TNF-α causes necrosis, thrombosis, and hemorrhage. TNF-α is synthesized as a 17,000-dalton polypeptide by a variety of tumor cells and activated macrophages.[73] Thus, its effect on angiogenesis may be limited to inflammatory conditions and neovascularization with certain types of tumors.

Angiogenin

Angiogenin has potent in vivo angiogenic activity.[74] This basic polypeptide (molecular weight 14,400) is produced by a variety of tumors and normal fibroblasts.[75–77] Like TGF-β, it has no effects on endothelial cells in vitro, raising the issue of whether its angiogenic effects are indirect. Moreover, its mode of action on cells is somewhat mysterious. It has partial structural homology with ribonucleases, as well as limited in vitro ribonuclease activity.[78–82] Inhibition of this activity is associated with decreased angiogenic activity.[80] Angiogenin mRNA has been demonstrated in rat liver,[76] which may be the source of the protein found in plasma.[77]

Interleukin-8

Interleukin-8 (IL-8), a macrophage-derived cytokine, stimulates angiogenesis in vivo in a rabbit corneal model.[83] Moreover, it stimulates proliferation of and is chemotactic for human umbilical vein endothelial cells.[83] These data suggest a potential role for IL-8 in inflammatory disorders with a prominent macrophage component such as rheumatoid arthritis. When antibodies against IL-8 were added to the conditioned media of human rheumatoid synovial tissue, angiogenic activity was blocked.[83] Two coagulation proteins, thrombin[84] and fibrin,[85] have been implicated in angiogenesis; however, the mechanism responsible for these effects has not been determined.

ANATOMY

The vascular endothelium has been estimated to represent approximately 6×10^{13} cells or 1 kg of tissue.[86] In surface area, this is equivalent to about 7 m^2. Descriptions of the architecture of vascular endothelium have been based on morphometric studies of cultured cells, tissue explants, and tissue sections. The diversity of endothelial subcellular organelles that have been described relates to the specific requirements of the tissue of origin and the type of vessel from which it is derived. An additional influence is the type of conditions chosen (i.e., media, growth factors, matrix substrate, co-culture with smooth muscle cells, hydrodynamic conditions, and so forth to culture cells. Characteristically, endothelial cells form a single layer in vivo; when they are cultured in vitro, they retain this property, often described as a "cobblestone" appearance. An interesting and unexplained observation is that contact inhibition of cell growth is retained in spite of the addition of endothelial mitogens.

Cell surface receptors involved in endothelial cell-cell, and cell-matrix interactions have been identified. Platelet and endothelial cellular adhesion molecule-1 (PECAM-1), a member of the immunoglobulin gene superfamily[87,88] (see below) of cell adhesion molecules, becomes intensely localized to intercellular junctions when endothelial cells achieve cell-cell contact.[89] By contrast, PECAM-1 is diffusely distributed on the cell surface prior to confluence. In addition, anti-PECAM antibodies prevent the association of endothelial cells in monolayer cultures into the cobblestone appearance.[90] At least 40% of PECAM-1 is composed of complex carbohydrate, and, like other immunoglobulin gene superfamily members, it contains C2 immunoglobulin-like homology units that mediate cell adhesion.

A calcium-dependent intercellular cell adhesion molecule (CAM) has been identified in vascular endothelial cells and termed V-CAD, for vascular cadherin.[91] V-CAD is responsible for the calcium-dependent adherence of endothelial cells to each other. V-CAD has been identified as a 135-kd membrane protein.

The integrins $\alpha_5\beta_1$, and $\alpha_2\beta_1$, and $\alpha_v\beta_3$ have been reported to be organized in focal contacts in both cultures and explants of umbilical vein endothelial cells.[92] Laminin, fibronectin, and type IV collagen, ligands for these integrins, have also been identified in strand-like structures associated with cell-cell borders.[92] Anti-$\alpha_5\beta_1$ antibodies increase the passage of macromolecules across confluent endothelial cell monolayers suggesting that this receptor has an important role in controlling monolayer integrity and permeability.[92]

Junctions between vascular endothelial cells are not as complex as in other types of epithelium.[93] Desmosomes are not present, and tight junctions are limited usually to a few points of membrane contact or fusion, as well as a few strands.[94,95] Striking postsegmental variations occur in postcapillary endothelium,[94] where inflammatory reactions are thought to begin by focal separation of the cells.[96]

Gap junctions are not present in the capillary endothelium or postcapillary endothelial venules, in contrast to endothelium in larger vessels such as veins, arterioles, and arteries.[94] The presence of these junctions appears to reflect a response to the luminal pressures to which the cells are subjected. The association of the junctions with occluding zonules (tight junctions) is likely to reinforce intercellular adhesion and stabilize the integrity of arterial endothelia. In contrast to capillaries, the junctions of endothelium and postcapillary venules are structurally partially open and functionally permeable.[97] Beneath the endothelium is a tight basement membrane divided into leaflets that accommodate pericytes in capillaries and postcapillary venules.

Endothelial cells are further specialized by the presence of numerous 70-nm vesicles termed caveolae or plasmalemmal vesicles associated with the plasmalemma on the luminal and abluminal surfaces. They represent biochemically differentiated distinct microdomains of the endothelial cell surface. In contrast to the remainder of the endothelial cell membrane, plasmalemmal vesicles are devoid of strong anionic sites, and are believed to be involved in the transport of anionic molecules, which represent most plasma proteins. Plasmalemmal vesicles appear to be the major organelle involved in transendothelial exchange (see below). Relatively few plasmalemmal vesicles are present in brain capillaries, whereas they are abundant in cardiac endothelium.

Fenestrae, or 60-nm circular openings, are present in the attenuated periphery of capillary and postcapillary endothelium in mucosal and glandular microvasculature. Transendothelial channels, pores uninterrupted by hydrophobic barriers, are also present in the attenuated regions of endothelial cells; however, their function has not been defined. Endothelial cells also have coated pits and vesicles, the density of which varies with the type of organ from which the cells are derived.

Weibel-Palade bodies, unique rod-shaped, secretory organelles, are associated exclusively with endothelial cells.[98] However, they are not present in endothelial cells in all species. Electron micrographs reveal a single membrane that surrounds a homogeneous matrix and a number of tubular structures. von Willebrand factor (vWF) is contained within Weibel-Palade bodies,[99] and is secreted both constitutively and in response to a variety of agonists[100] (see Ch. 112). It has also been suggested that the multimeric, condensed form of vWF is necessary for Weibel-Palade body formation in endothelial cells.[101] The membrane surrounding Weibel-Palade bodies has been shown to contain P-selectin, which also serves as a transmembrane receptor for leukocytes[102,103] (see the section Adhesion of Neutrophils and Monocytes and Ch. 112). In unstimulated endothelium, P-selectin is limited to Weibel-Palade bodies, but following activation of cells by complement, thrombin, and other stimuli, it becomes expressed on the plasma membrane.

PHYSIOLOGY AND BIOCHEMISTRY

Interaction of Endothelial Cells with Blood Cells

Leukocytes

Normally, leukocytes circulate freely in blood and do not interact with the endothelial surface of the blood vessel. However, following injury, or activation of endothelium, a series of leukocyte reactions are initiated characterized as rolling, adhesion, extravasation, and invasion. These reactions require expression of a number of different cell adhesion receptors on endothelium and their ligands, or counter-receptors on leukocytes (Table 99-2).

Adhesion of Neutrophils and Monocytes

The initial event (rolling) appears as a slowing of leukocyte movement through the vessel lumen, and margination along the endothelial surface.[104,105] This low-affinity reaction requires translocation of P-selectin from Weibel-Palade bodies to the endothelial surface.[102,103,106,107] A variety of agonists, including thrombin, histamine, terminal complement components, hydrogen peroxide, and cytokines,[102,103,108-113] stimulate the rapid (within seconds) but transient appearance of P-selectin on the endothelial cell surface. The surface expression of P-selectin, which is then internalized within minutes, is followed by expression of E-selectin, which is necessary for continued leukocyte adherence.[114,115] E-selectin is not constitutively expressed. Expression requires protein and mRNA synthesis and is induced within 1 hour of exposure to TNF-α, IL-1, and lipopolysaccharide (LPS).[108] Maximal exposure is by 6 hours and declines thereafter over 24 hours.

P- and E-selectin are cell adhesion receptors and members of the selectin gene family,[116,117] which also includes L-selectin (see Ch. 5), a leukocyte adhesion receptor.[118] These three transmembrane proteins contain (sequentially) an N-terminal, a Ca^{2+}-dependent lectin domain, and EGF-like domain, and a complement-binding domain, with the transmembrane and cytoplasmic domain at the carboxyl terminus. Each of these domains correlates closely with the exon-intron structure of each member of this gene family. Moreover, all three genes are tightly clustered on human chromosome 1. It is likely that the three genes arose by exon shuffling and gene duplication.

Sialated Lewis^x (sLe^x), a fucosylated tetrasaccharide [N-acetyl-D-neuraminic acid $\alpha(2,3)$-D-galactose-$\beta(1,4)$-{D-fucose-$\alpha(1-30)$}-N-acetyl-D-glucosamine], binds to P- and E-selectin.[119,120] sLe^x and other fucosylated lactosamines are present in abundance on neutrophils and monocytes.[115,117,119-124] The P-selectin-sLe^x bond acts as a tether, slowing the progress of the neutrophil through the circulation. All three selectins require a sialic acid residue for high-affinity binding.

Table 99-2. Adhesion Receptors on Endothelial Cells and Their Leukocyte Ligands

Endothelial Adhesion Receptor	Leukocyte Ligand
Ig superfamily	
ICAM-1	Integrins $\alpha_L\beta_2$ (CD11a/CD18) and $\alpha_M\beta_2$ (CD11b/CD18)
ICAM-2	$\alpha_L\beta_2$ (CD11a/CD18)
VCAM-1	Integrin $\alpha_4\beta_1$ (VLA-4)
PECAM-1 (CD31)	Unidentified
Selectin	
E-selectin	Sialyl-Lewis antigen
P-selectin	Unidentified
Addressin	
GlyCAM-1	L-selectin

Abbreviations: -CAM, cell adhesion molecule; GlyCAM-1 glycosylation-dependent CAM-1; ICAM, intercellular adhesion molecule; PECAM-1, platelet and endothelial cellular adhesion molecule-1; VCAM-1, vascular CAM-1.

Once leukocyte rolling occurs, β_2 integrins become functionally expressed on the surface of the activated neutrophils. For example, $\alpha_L\beta_2$ (also known as CD11a/CD18 or leukocyte function associated antigen-1 [LFA-1]) binds to the endothelial cell adhesion receptors known as intercellular adherence molecule (ICAM)-1 and -2.[125,126] ICAM-1 is slowly expressed over 24 hours on the surface of vascular endothelium following stimulation by TNF-α, interferon-γ, or IL-1.[127] Expression continues in the presence of the cytokine. Cytokines increase expression of ICAM-1 mRNA.[128,129]

ICAM-1 and -2 are members of the immunoglobulin gene superfamily, containing an extracellular domain with immunoglobulin-like homology units of the C2 subclass that function as CAMs.[128–130] The immunoglobulin domain consists of 90–100 amino acids and has an ellipsoid structure (4 $\times$ 2.5 nm) composed of two antiparallel β-strands, centrally stabilized by a disulfide bond.[131,132] ICAM-1 has the appearance of a bent rod on electron micrographs. Based on structural data, a model of ICAM-1 has been proposed in which the five immunoglobulin domains are unpaired, arranged end to end, and slightly angled to the β-strands.[133] ICAM-2 has two immunoglobulin domains with 35% homology to the corresponding domains on ICAM-1.[133] ICAM-1 and -2 bind leukocyte $\alpha_L\beta_2$ via their first amino terminal immunoglobulin domain.[133] Interestingly, the major group of human rhinoviruses also binds to this immunoglobulin domain.[134] The third immunoglobulin-like domain of ICAM-1 is the binding site for integrin $\alpha_M\beta_2$ (CD11b/CD18 or Mac-1). ICAM-1 and -2 are the products of homologous genes, which are likely to have evolved from a primordial gene.

ICAM-1 is highly inducible in immune and inflammatory reactions on several different types of cells besides endothelium, including lymphocytes, fibroblasts, and epithelial cells,[125,126,135,136] while ICAM-2 is constitutively expressed on endothelium alone. In vivo, ICAM-1 expression has been documented on endothelial cells in hypersensitivity skin reactions, and after IL-1 and interferon-γ administration.[127,137]

Vascular cell adhesion molecule-1 (VCAM-1), an additional member of the immunoglobulin gene superfamily, was first identified on endothelial cells exposed to inflammatory cytokines (IL-1 and TNF) and LPS.[138,139] Several types of leukocytes, including monocytes, T and B lymphocytes, basophils, and eosinophils, bind to VCAM-1. The leukocyte ligand for VCAM-1 is a β_1 integrin, VLA-4.[140] Evidence of the importance of VCAM-1 in the inflammatory response is the demonstration that its expression is increased in postcapillary venular endothelium during cardiac allograft rejection.[141]

Adhesion of activated neutrophils to endothelium is associated with significant cytotoxicity. The pathobiologic basis for vascular injury appears to be a complicated one. That close contact between the leukocyte and endothelium is required was suggested in an experimental model involving neutrophils and rat pulmonary artery endothelial cells in culture. Surface activation of nicotinamide adenine dinucleotide phosphate (NADPH) oxidase and generation of superoxide ion and hydrogen peroxide by the neutrophils was associated with damage to the vascular cells.[142] The pathway for cytotoxicity may involve generation of an oxidant within the endothelium by the ferrous ion, resulting in conversion of hydrogen peroxide to hydrogen radical.[143]

Lymphocyte Adhesion

A large body of evidence supports the concept that lymphocytes recirculate from blood to lymphatic tissues through specialized postcapillary vessels termed high endothelial venules (HEVs).[144,145] "Homing" receptors on lymphocytes target them to HEVs within specific types of lymphoid tissues, including lymph nodes and Peyer's patches.

At least three types of endothelial receptors for T lymphocytes have been described. The lymphocyte-endothelial interaction is an essential first step in the migration of lymphocytes to inflammatory sites. Lymphocyte CD11a/CD18 mediates binding to ICAM-1.[136,146,147] A second pathway of adhesion involves binding of integrin $\alpha_4\beta_1$ (VLA-4) on T lymphocytes to VCAM-1 on endothelial cells.[148] A third endothelial cell receptor for CD4$^+$ memory T cells is E-selectin.[149,150] Thus, it is likely that multiple adhesion pathways are possible for unstimulated lymphocytes.

Receptors involved in binding of activated T-lymphocytes to endothelium appear to be more restricted: lymphocyte CD11a/CD18 binds to ICAM-1 and ICAM-X.[136,146,147] In addition, adhesion of T lymphocytes by the β_1 integrin VLA-4 to VCAM-1 is enhanced by increased expression of the latter on cytokine-activated endothelium.

Two L-selectin-binding sulfated glycoproteins, a major 50-kd species and a minor 90-kd one, were identified in the high endothelial venules of murine peripheral and mesenteric lymph nodes.[151] These vascular addressins[152,153] or tissue-specific adhesion receptors are involved in lymphocyte homing. A cDNA for the 50-kd protein has been isolated and characterized.[154] Approximately 70% of this fucosylated and sulfated glycoprotein is carbohydrate. It is expressed on the luminal surface of peripheral lymph node high endothelial venules. The O-linked carbohydrate is clustered like mucin-like substances, which are richly O-linked glycosylated rod-like proteins. Clustering of the carbohydrate ligand is likely to enhance the avidity of binding to L-selectin. Based on the above consideration, the 50-kd protein has been named GlyCAM-1 (glycosylation-dependent cell adhesion molecule-1).

Platelets

Like neutrophils, platelets do not normally adhere to unstimulated endothelium. However, following injury to endothelium, platelets adhere to the subendothelial extracellular matrix (see Ch. 97). In vessels exposed to high shear stress, $>600^{s-1}$, the primary adhesion protein for platelets within the matrix and basement membrane is vWF.[155] vWF contains binding domains with the potential to interact with collagen[156] and glycosaminoglycans within the subendothelial matrix. vWF synthesized by endothelium[157] is secreted both luminally and abluminally (see Ch. 112). vWF synthesized by megakaryocytes[158] is ultimately secreted by activated platelets. Thus, there are several potential sources of vWF to modulate platelet adhesion. The role of shear stress in binding of vWF to the platelet glycoprotein (GP)Ib/IX complex has not been determined. vWF also binds to integrin $\alpha_{IIb}\beta_3$ on activation of platelets, either after activation of platelets by agonists or after ligation of GPIb/IX by vWF.[159] The significance of this reaction is uncertain. Binding of vWF to $\alpha_{IIb}\beta3$ is not sufficient to compensate for the absence of GPIb/IX, as patients who lack the latter receptor have defective platelet adhesion.

Platelet adhesive interactions in vessels in which shear stress is (e.g., the venous circulation) are not well characterized. A number of vascular endothelial basement membrane and matrix proteins have the potential to serve as adhesive ligands for platelets in vivo. Vascular endothelial cells make several types of collagen (IV,[160] V, and VIII[161,162]), some of which have been documented to be present in blood vessels. Minimal requirements for platelet adhesion include the triple helical structure of native collagen.[163] While the actual vascular form of collagen involved in platelet adhesion has not been well characterized, monomeric collagen supports platelet adhesion.[164] Both Mg^{2+} and Mn^{2+} enhance platelet adhesion to collagen. It is likely that platelets adhere to subendothelial collagen via the $\alpha_2\beta_1$ integrin[165] (see Ch. 97). Initial platelet adhesion to collagen does not appear to require platelet activation, and it results in platelet spreading. Additional, nonintegrin platelet collagen receptors, such as GPIV (CD36) and GPVI have also been described.[166]

Other vascular basement membrane and matrix proteins that are candidate adhesion molecules for platelets are vitronectin and fibronectin (FN). Platelets contain at least two vitronectin receptors, $\alpha_v\beta_3$ and $\alpha_{IIb}\beta_3$, while at least two FN receptors, $\alpha_5\beta_1$ and $\alpha_{IIb}\beta_3$ are present on platelets.[167,168] Both FN receptors require Ca^{2+} for binding. In contrast to $\alpha_{IIb}\beta_3$, $\alpha_5\beta_1$ binds to FN without prior platelet activation.[167,167a] Both receptors appear to recognize the RGD sequence in the cell-binding domain of FN.[168,169] In addition, a third type of FN binding to platelets that does not require Ca^{2+} has been described that is RGD independent and involves the gelatin-binding domain of FN.[170] Platelets also spread on FN; however, spreading is only supported by the cell binding domain. Platelets also adhere to thrombospondin (TSP) through receptors that remain to be fully characterized. TSP is made by vascular endothelium[171] and by megakaryocytes,[172] and is released from the platelet α-granule during platelet secretion.[173]

Platelets also contain an integrin receptor for laminin ($\alpha_6\beta_1$), which co-distributes with type IV collagen.[174]

Interaction of Erythrocytes with Vascular Endothelium

Normally, red blood cells do not interact with the endothelium. However, evidence has been presented that sickled erythrocytes bind to microvascular endothelial cells, and that TSP mediates this adhesion[175] (see Ch. 43).

Activation and Inhibition of the Coagulation System

In an unperturbed state, vascular endothelium does not participate in activation of coagulation.[176] Indeed, endothelium actively inhibits activation of clotting. Vascular endothelium synthesizes and expresses on its surface thrombomodulin,[177] a transmembrane receptor for thrombin that induces a conformational change in the enzyme that results in inhibition of its clotting activity and its ability to activate factor V.[178] Moreover, binding of thrombin to thrombomodulin enhances its ability to activate protein C on the endothelial surface.[179] Activated protein C in turn inactivates factors VIIIa and Va.[180–182] Inactivation of factors Va and VIIIa occurs on the surface of endothelium by a complex of proteins C and S. Specific receptors for protein S have been described on endothelial cells. Activated protein C increases the affinity of protein S binding to endothelium. Protein C binds specifically to endothelial cells in a reaction that requires protein S. Synthesis of protein S by endothelial cells has been reported[183,184] and may be a partial source of the plasma protein in addition to the liver. The activated protein C-protein S complex on endothelial cells provides a potentially important mechanism for inhibiting blood clotting.

Regulation of thrombomodulin activity on endothelium appears to occur in response to mediators of inflammation. Thus, endotoxin, IL-1, and TNF all decrease thrombomodulin activity[185–187] and consequently activation of protein C and inhibition of coagulation. Protein C activation on human umbilical vein endothelial cells is also suppressed by oxidized low-density lipoprotein (LDL).[188]

An additional mechanism for inhibiting clotting relates to the presence on the surface of vascular endothelium of heparan sulfate, a glycosaminoglycan, which binds antithrombin III.[189] Presumably, vascular endothelium is continuously coated with heparin-bound antithrombin III, which is poised to inactivate thrombin, factor Xa, and factor IXa, which are generated at sites of activation of clotting.[190]

Endothelium synthesizes both prostacyclin[191] (prostaglandin I_2 [PGI_2]) and endothelium-derived relaxing factor (EDRF),[192–194] potent anti-platelet antagonists (see below).

Following injury or disease of the vascular wall, a number of changes occur in the endothelium (Fig. 99-1). Perhaps the most important is the expression of tissue factor, a transmembrane glycoprotein that serves as a cofactor for factor VII/VIIa[95–198] on the luminal surface of endothelium. Normally tissue factor is not detectable on endothelial cells, in vitro[199] or in vivo.[200] However, a variety of cytokines such as IL-1, TNF, and endotoxin stimulate expression of tissue factor on endothelium.[201–205] TNF appears to induce tissue factor expression by an indirect mechanism in that it induces release of IL-1, which in turn directly stimulates tissue factor synthesis.[204] In addition, oxidized LDL is a potent inducer of human arterial and venous endothelial cell tissue factor activity.[206]

Virtually instantaneously, factor VII binds to tissue factor, and the resulting complex activates factor X.[207] Factors Xa and Va are then capable of activating prothrombin by either of two pathways, either on the surface of platelets[208] or on endothelium.[209] Endothelial cells contain factor V, which is expressed on their surface.[209] Factor V in turn is activated by either thrombin or an endogenous endothelial enzyme.[210] Factor Xa binds to factor Va on either platelets or endothelium. As this reaction is kinetically more favorable on platelets, prothrombin activation on the endothelium may serve as an auxiliary mechanism for clotting. The factor Xa/Va complex activates prothrombin, thereby leading to thrombin generation and fibrin formation (see Ch. 100).

Receptors for factors IX and IXa have also been described on vascular endothelial cells.[211,212] Addition of factors IXa and VIIIa to endothelial cells results in acceleration of activation of factor X and an increase in the affinity of factor IXa for its receptor on endothelium.[212]

Endothelial cells also synthesize a transglutaminase resembling a previously described guinea pig liver transglutaminase.[213] This enzyme cross-links the α- and γ-chains of fibrin, providing a cellular basis for clot stabilization. In the presence of the plasma transglutaminase (factor XIII), the role of the endothelial enzyme in normal hemostasis is unclear. It may

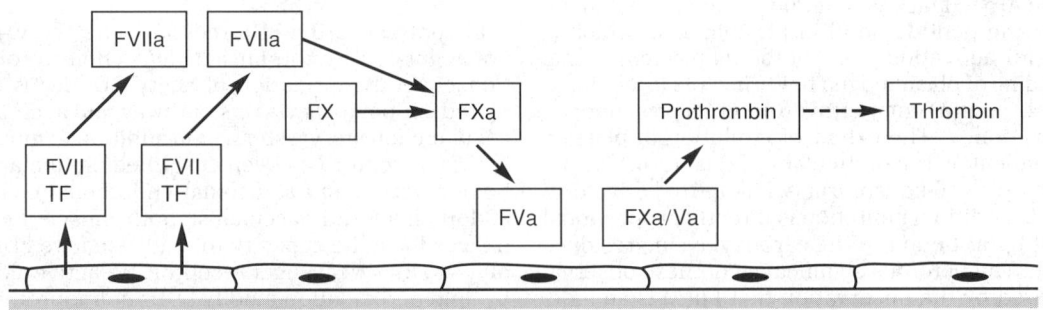

Fig. 99-1. Regulation of activation of coagulation by endothelium. Tf, tissue factor; F, factor.

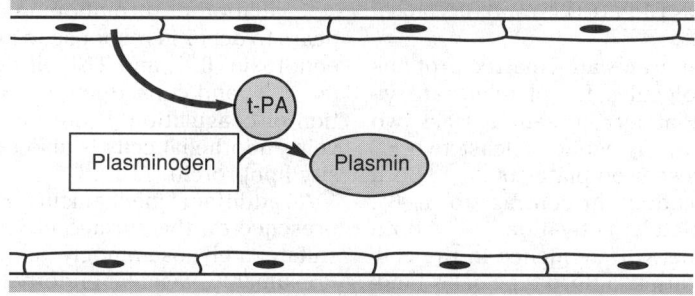

Fig. 99-2. Activation of fibrinolysis of endothelium. Agonist-activated endothelium secretes t-PA, which then activates clot-bound plasminogen, resulting in localized fibrinolysis.

be that the latter cross-links vascular matrix proteins such as vitronectin or fibrin to the endothelial cell surface.

Activation and Inhibition of Fibrinolysis by Vascular Endothelium

Vascular endothelium serves as the principle locale for regulating activation of fibrinolysis (Fig. 99-2). Vascular endothelium synthesizes and secretes both t-PA[214] and plasminogen activator inhibitor-1 (PAI-1).[215] Contact-inhibited, early passaged endothelial cells do not appear to synthesize u-PA; however, when capillary endothelial cells are grown under conditions mimicking angiogenesis, u-PA is synthesized.[216] t-PA is the primary activator of intravascular fibrinolysis (se Ch. 101). A variety of agonists stimulate t-PA expression by vascular endothelium, including thrombin.[217] However, thrombin also stimulates synthesis and secretion of PAI-1.[218] The net effect is inhibition of activation of plasminogen.

In addition to their effect on stimulating expression of endothelial procoagulant proteins, endotoxin and IL-1 promote inhibition of fibrinolysis by stimulating synthesis of PAI-1.[219,220] Treatment of endothelial cells in vitro with endotoxin or injection into animals results in increased PAI-1 on their surface. Thus, in conditions associated with infection and inflammation, the net effect is inhibition of clot dissolution.

Studies of a quantitatively minor lipoprotein called Lp(a) suggest that it may impair fibrinolysis. The amino acid sequence encoded by the cDNA for apolipoprotein a [apo(a)], a constituent of Lp(a), has considerable homology with plasminogen, particularly with the triple-looped, disulfide-bonded kringle 4.[221] Thus apo(a) contains anywhere from 15–40 such structures, which have as much as 75% homology with plasminogen kringle 4.[221] A variety of isoforms of Lp(a) are present in plasma.[222] Moreover, apo(a) contains a single structure homologous to kringle 5 in plasminogen. In addition, apo(a) contains a region that shares 94% homology with the protease domain of plasminogen, including the catalytic triad His-Asp-Ser. However, instead of an Arg 561, apo(a) contains a Ser, in the domain corresponding to the peptide bond in plasminogen, which is the cleavage site for activation, thus inhibiting plasmin formation. Because binding of plasminogen to fibrin clots is mediated by kringles 1 and 4,[223] Lp(a) competitively inhibits plasminogen binding and activation.[224] The extent of inhibition of plasmin formation is dependent on the particular Lp(a) isoform[225]: inhibition is greatest by a 540-kd isoform, while a 610-kd isoform is not inhibitory. In addition, inhibition is directly proportional to the quantity of Lp(a) bound to the carboxyl lysine residues of degraded fibrin. The potential significance of these observations is underscored by the observation that Lp(a) is an independent risk factor of atherosclerosis in coronary artery disease.[226]

METABOLISM AND TRANSPORT OF PLASMA COMPONENTS BY THE ENDOTHELIUM

Physiologic Considerations

In addition to the multiple factors influencing the interactions between plasma proteins and endothelium discussed in the preceding sections, the metabolic requirements and specialized functions of each organ have a significant effect on the ultimate cellular destination of these substances. As described for other types of polarized epithelial cells, transport of plasma molecules across the endothelium occurs by two general processes, endocytosis and transcytosis, by which molecules are transported through the endothelial cell to the target cell.[227] Transcytosis occurs by the same basic mechanisms as endocytosis. at least three mechanisms of transcytotic uptake have been described: (1) receptor-mediated; (2) fluid phase, or bulk uptake of water-soluble molecules not bound to the cell membrane; and (3) non-specific adsorptive, whereby molecules electrostatically bound to the endothelial cell membrane are internalized. In contrast to endocytosis, plasma molecules are transported by transcytosis directly through the cell in vesicles, bypassing the lysosomal compartment. Examples of molecules that are exchanged between the blood and tissues in a receptor-mediated transcytotic pathway are albumin,[228,229] transferrin,[230] insulin,[231,232] LDL,[233] very-low-density lipoprotein (VLDL),[234,235] and ceruloplasmin.[236] In contrast to receptor-mediated endocytosis, low-affinity ligand binding sites are located on uncoated pits and plasmalemmal vesicles. Plasmalemmal vesicles, transendothelial fenestrae, and channels,[237] are the major organelles involved in transcytotic passage of molecules through the endothelium.

In addition to the inherent characteristics of the endothelium of a particular organ, transport of substances from the blood is strongly influenced by hydrostatic and oncotic pressures[238] and the size,[237,239] shape, charge,[240] and concentration of the molecule.

Pathologic Transport by Endothelium

In contrast to the LDL receptor, the acetyl-LDL receptor is not regulated by the intracellular cholesterol concentration. Consequently, formation of acetyl-LDL leads to receptor-mediated endocytosis via this pathway and accumulation of intracellular cholesteryl esters.[241] In addition to monocytes, the acetyl-LDL receptor has been described on human umbilical vein, bovine aortic, and sinusoidal endothelial cells.[188,242,243] Both endothelium and vascular smooth muscle as well as macrophages have the capacity to oxidize native LDL to a form that binds to this "scavenger receptor." Reactive aldehydes derived by lipid peroxidation modify LDL apolipoprotein B, which then can bind to the acetyl-LDL receptor.[244] Indeed, modified forms of LDL have been found in atherosclerotic lesions.[245]

ENDOTHELIUM AND REGULATION OF VASCULAR CONTRACTILITY AND PLATELET ACTIVATION

Endothelial Vasodilators and Platelet Antagonists

Endothelium-Derived Nitric Oxide

Several substances as well as shear stress stimulate the release of a potent vasodilator, EDRF,[246,247] determined to be nitric oxide[248] or a nitrosylated compound, S-nitrocysteine.[249] Nitric oxide synthase is a cytoplasmic endothelial enzyme that forms nitric oxide from L-arginine by oxidation of the guanidine-nitrogen terminal of L-arginine.[250] Nitric oxide synthase requires calmodulin, NADPH, and Ca^{2+}.[250,251] Inhibitors of nitric oxide synthesis such as analogs of L-arginine (L-N^G-mono-methyl-arginine [L-NMMA]) increase blood pressure,[252] indicating that the circulation is basally vasodilated due to continuous nitric oxide release from the endothelium.

EDRF induces vasodilatation by increasing cyclic 3'5'-guanosine monophosphate (cGMP) in vascular smooth muscle.[253] EDRF also stimulates guanylyl cyclase in platelets, resulting in inhibition of platelet activation.[254]

Prostacyclin

Prostacyclin (PGI$_2$), the synthetic product of the endothelial cyclo-oxygenase, is formed from arachidonic acid[255] in response to thrombin,[256] histamine,[257] bradykinin,[258] kallikrein,[259] IL-1,[260] interferon,[261] TNF,[262] high-density lipoprotein,[263] fibrin,[264] activated complement factors,[265] EGF,[266] TGF,[267] shear stress,[268] and a variety of other agents. Compared with EDRF, PGI$_2$ has little effect on endothelium-dependent relaxation.[269]

PGI$_2$ is also a potent platelet antagonist by virtue of its ability to increase platelet cAMP.[270] Platelet endoperoxides are also converted to PGI$_2$ by endothelial cells,[271] suggesting a potential negative feedback regulatory mechanism when activated platelets are in contact with endothelium. PGI$_2$ can be converted to 6-keto-PGI$_1$, also a vasodilator and inhibitor of platelets.[272]

PGI$_2$ synthesis is inhibited by a variety of drugs, most notably aspirin[273] and other nonsteroidal anti-inflammatory agents.[256] The significance of inhibition of PGI$_2$ synthesis or release, or both, by a variety of other pharmacologic agents or substances[274-282] remains to be determined.

In addition to the above vasodilators, endothelium is a source of monoamine oxidase, which deactivates catecholamines and serotonin, potent vasoconstrictors.[283-285]

Endothelial Vasoconstrictors

Endothelin

Endothelin is a potent 21-amino acid polypeptide. Of the three forms identified, endothelial cells appear to synthesize only endothelin-1.[269,286] The effect of endothelin on the vasculature is concentration dependent—at low concentrations it causes vasodilation, and at higher concentrations it is a potent vasoconstrictor.[287] Endothelin-induced contraction of porcine coronary artery smooth muscle indirectly activates voltage-operated Ca^{2+} channels.[288] Synthesis and secretion of endothelin is stimulated by a variety of substances, including thrombin, TGF-β, IL-1, epinephrine, and so forth.[269,289] Synthesis of endothelin is inhibited by both cGMP and cAMP.[289,290] EDRF and atrial naturietic factor inhibit endothelin synthesis by stimulating guanylyl cyclase.[289,291]

Cyclo-oxygenase-Dependent Vasoconstrictors

Thromboxane A$_2$ and endoperoxides (PGH$_2$) are both potent vasoconstrictors that activate vascular smooth muscle and platelets.[292] In addition, superoxide anions, cyclo-oxygenase by-products, induce endothelium-dependent contractions by degradation of nitric oxide and by a direct effect on vascular smooth muscle.[293]

SIGNALING MOLECULES

Leukocyte Activators

Platelet-Activating Factor

Platelet-activating factor (PAF; alkyl-2-acteyl-sn-glycero-3-phosphocholine)[294,295] is not expressed by quiescent endothelial cells; however, after stimulation by thrombin, histamine, TNF, leukotrienes, and other agonists,[296-301] it appears on the cell surface. PAF has diverse biologic activities, including activation of neutrophils via a seven-membrane-spanning G-protein-linked receptor.[302,303] Following activation by PAF, neutrophil expression of the β_2 integrins CD11a/CD18 and CD11b/CD18 is increased, thereby enhancing leukocyte adhesion to endothelium.[303] PAF also activates platelets.[304] Activated endothelial cells metabolize PAF, resulting in its rapid inactivation and reversal of its proadhesive effects.[305] In addition, PGI$_2$ inhibits PAF synthesis.[306]

Interleukin 8

Endothelial cells activated by TNF-α, IL-1, and LPS synthesize and secrete IL-8,[307-310] a leukocyte chemotactic stimulus. In addition, IL-8 stimulates expression of β_2 integrins.[311] However, IL-8 also reduces adhesion of neutrophils to cytokine-activated endothelium, expressing E-selectin by unknown mechanisms.[312]

Colony-Stimulating Factor-Granulocyte/Macrophage

Colony-stimulating factor-granulocyte/macrophage (CSF-GM) stimulates multilineage, hematopoietic progenitor cell growth in addition to burst-forming unit-erythroid (BFU-E) growth and myeloid (polymorphonuclear leukocytes, eosinophils) and macrophage colony growth[313-315] (see Ch. 16). CSF-GM also stimulates the activity of neutrophils, eosinophils, and monocytes/macrophages.[316-318] CSF-GM synthesis has been documented in endothelial cells,[319,320] vascular smooth muscle cells,[321] fibroblasts,[322] monocytes,[323] T cells, mast cells, and thymic epithelial cells. Its synthesis is induced by cytokines, and it in turn can induce the synthesis of IL-1 in neutrophils[324] and TNF-α in monocytes.[325] The extent to which any of these biologic processes is modulated by CSF-GM made by endothelium under normal or pathologic conditions is unclear.

REFERENCES

1. Coffin JD, Poole TJ: Embryonic vascular development: immunohistochemical identification of the origin and subsequent morphogenesis of the major vessel primordia in quail embryos. Development 102:735, 1988
2. Peault B, Coltey M, Le Douarin NM: Ontogenic emergence of quail leukocyte/endothelium cell surface antigen. Cell Differen 23:165, 1988
3. Haar JL, Ackerman GA: A phase and electron micrographic study of vasculogenesis and erythropoiesis in the yolk sac of the mouse. Anat Rec 170:199, 1971
4. Wagner RC. Endothelial cell embryology and growth. Adv Microcirc 9:45, 1980
5. Poole TJ, Coffin JD: Vasculogenesis and angiogenesis: two distinct morphogenetic mechanisms establish embryonic vascular pattern. J Exp Zool 251:224, 1989
6. Girard H: Arterial pressure in the chick embryo. Am J Physiol 224:454, 1973

7. Madri JA, Williams SK: Capillary endothelial cell cultures: phenotypic modulation by matrix components. J Cell Biol 97:153, 1983

8. Ingber DE: Fibronectin controls capillary endothelial cell growth by modulating cell shape. Proc Natl Acad Sci USA 87:3579, 1990

9. Grant DS, Tashiro K-I, Segui-Real B et al: Two different laminin domains mediate the differentiation of human endothelial cells into capillary-like structures in vitro. Cell 58:933, 1989

10. Matthews W, Jordan CT, Gavin M et al: A receptor tyrosine kinase cDNA isolated from a population of enriched primitive hematopoietic cells and exhibiting close genetic linkage to c-kit. Proc Natl Acad Sci USA 88:9026, 1991

11. Millauer B, Wizigmann-Voos S, Schnurch H et al: High affinity VEGF binding and developmental expression suggest Flk-1 as a major regulator of vasculogenesis and angiogenesis. Cell 72:835, 1993

12. Ferrara N, Henze WJ: Pituitary follicular cells secrete a novel heparin-binding growth factor for vascular endothelial cells. Biochem Biophys Res Commun 161:1989

13. Baird A, Ling N: Fibroblast growth factors are present in the extracellular matrix produced by endothelial cells in vitro: implications for a role of heparinase-like enzymes in the neovascular response. Biochem Biophys Res Commun 142:428, 1987

14. Schweigerer L, Neufeld G, Friedman J et al: Capillary endothelial cells express basic fibroblast growth factor, a mitogen that promotes their own growth. Nature 325:257, 1987

15. Gimbrone MA, Cotran RS, Leapman SB, Folkman J: Tumor growth and neovascularization: an experimental model using the rabbit cornea. J Natl Cancer Inst 52:413, 1974

16. Cliff WJ: Observations on healing tissue: a combined light and electron microscopic investigation. Philos Trans R Soc Lond Biol 246:305, 1963

17. Schoefl GI: Studies on inflammation. III. Growing capillaries: their structure and permeability. Virchows Arch A Pathol Anat Histopathol 337:97, 1963

18. Ausprunk DH, Folkman J: Migration and proliferation of endothelial cells in preformed and newly formed blood vessels during tumor angiogenesis. Microvasc Res 14:53, 1977

19. Kalebic T, Garbisa S, Glaser B, Liotta LA: Basement membrane collagen: degradation by migrating endothelial cells. Science 221:281, 1983

20. Pepper MS, Vassalli J-D, Montesano R, Orci L: Urokinase-type plasminogen activator is induced in migrating capillary endothelial cells. J Cell Biol 105:2535, 1987

21. Folkman J, Klagsbrun M: Angiogenic factors. Science 235:442, 1987

22. Paku S, Niedhard P: First steps of tumor-related angiogenesis. Lab Invest 65:334, 1991

23. Folkman J, Haudenschild C: Angiogenesis in vitro. Nature 288:551, 1980

24. Gospodarowicz D, Abraham JA, Schilling J: Isolation and characterization of a vascular endothelial cell mitogen produced by pituitary-derived folliculo stellate cells. Proc Natl Acad Sci USA 86:7311, 1989

25. Levy AP, Tamargo R, Brem H, Nathans D: An endothelial cell growth factor from the mouse neuroblastoma cell line NB41. Growth Factors 2:9, 1989

26. Conelly DT, Heuvelmann DM, Nelson R et al: Tumor vascular permeability factor stimulates endothelial cell growth and angiogenesis. J Clin Invest 84:1470, 1989

27. Plouet J, Schilling J, Gospodarowicz D: Isolation and characterization of a newly identified endothelial cell mitogen produced by AtT-20 cell. EMBO J 8:3801, 1989

28. Conn G: Amino acid and cDNA sequences of a vascular endothelial cell mitogen that is homologous to platelet-derived growth factor. Proc Natl Acad Sci USA 87:2628, 1990

29. Schweiki D, Itin A, Soffer D, Keshet E: Vascular endothelial growth factor induced by hypoxia may mediate hypoxia-initiated angiogenesis. Nature 359:843, 1992

30. Plate KH, Breier G, Weich HA, Risau W: Vascular endothelial growth factor is a potential tumor angiogenesis factor in human gliomas in vivo. Nature 359:845, 1992

31. Ullrich A, Schlessinger J: Signal transduction by receptors with tyrosine kinase activity. Cell 61:203, 1990

32. Shibuya M, Yamaguchi S, Yamane A et al: Nucleotide sequence and expression of a novel human receptor-type tyrosine kinase gene (flt) closely related to the fms family. Oncogene 5:519, 1990

33. Devries C, Escobedo JA, Ueno H et al: The fms-like tyrosine kinase, a receptor for vascular endothelial growth factor. Science 255:989, 1992

34. Clemens DR, Isley WL, Brown MT: Dialysable factor in human serum of platelet origin stimulates endothelial cell replication and growth. Proc Natl Acad Sci USA 80:1641, 1983

35. Miyazono K, Okabe T, Urabe A et al: Purification and properties of an endothelial cell growth factor from human platelets. J Biol Chem 262:4098, 1987

36. Usuki K, Heldin N-E, Miyazono K, et al: Production of platelet-derived endothelial growth factor by normal and human transformed human cell in culture. Proc Natl Acad Sci USA 86:7427, 1989

37. Miyazono K, Heldin C-H: High-yield purification of platelet-derived endothelial cell growth factor: structural characterization and establishment of a specific antiserum. Biochemistry 28:1704, 1989

38. Ishikawa F, Miyazono K, Hellman U et al: Identification of angiogenic activity and the cloning and expression of platelet-derived endothelial cell growth factor. Nature 338:557, 1989

39. Moghaddam A, Bicknell R: Expression of platelet-derived endothelial cell growth factor in Escherichia coli and confirmation of its thymidine phosphorylase activity. Biochemistry 31:12141. 1992

40. Finnis C, Dodsworth N, Pollitt CE et al: Thymidine phosphorylase activity of platelet-derived endothelial cell growth factor is responsible for endothelial cell mitogenicity. Eur J Biochem 212:201, 1993

41. Thomas KA, Rios-Candelore M, Fitzpatrick S: Purification and characterization of acidic fibroblast growth factor from bovine brain. Proc Natl Acad Sci USA 81:357, 1984

42. Esch F, Baird A, Ling N et al: Primary structure of bovine pituitary basic fibroblast growth factor (FGF) and comparison with the amino-terminal sequence of bovine brain acidic FGF. Proc Natl Acad Sci USA 82:6507, 1985

43. Sullivan R, Klagsbrun M: Purification of cartilage-derived growth factor by heparin affinity chromatography. J Biol Chem 260:2399, 1985

44. Baird A, Esch F, Gospodarowicz D, Guillemin R: Inhibition of endothelial cell proliferation by type-β transforming growth factor: interactions with acidic and basic fibroblast growth factors. Biochemistry 67:265, 1986

45. Shing Y, Folkman J, Sullivan R et al: Heparin affinity: purification of a tumor-derived capillary endothelial growth factor. Science 223:1296, 1984

46. Gospodarowicz D, Cheng J, Lui GM et al: Isolation by heparin-sepharose chromatography of brain fibroblast growth factor: identity with pituitary fibroblast growth factor. Proc Natl Acad Sci USA 223:1296, 1984

47. Maciag T, Mehlman T, Freisel R, Schreiber A: Heparin binds endothelial cell growth factor, the principal endothelial cell mitogen in bovine brain. Science 225:932, 1984

48. Kiefer M, Stefhens JC, Crawford K et al: Ligand-affinity cloning and structure of a cell surface heparan sulfate proteoglycan that binds basic fibroblast growth factor. Proc Natl Acad Sci USA 87:6985, 1990

49. Robinson CJ: Multiple receptors for the growing FGF-family. Trends Pharmacol Sci 12:123, 1991

50. Heuer JG, von Bartheld CS, Kinoshita Y et al: Alternating phases of FGF receptor and NGF receptor expression in the developing chicken nervous system. Neuron 5:283, 1990

51. Wanaka A, Milbrandt J, Johnson EM: Expression of FGF receptor gene in rat development. Development 111:455, 1991

52. Peter KG, Werner S, Chen G, Williams LT: Two FGF receptor genes are expressed in epithelial and mesenchymal tissues during limb formation and organogenesis in the mouse. Development 114:233, 1992

53. Schreiber AB, Winkler ME, Derynk R: TGF-α: a more potent angiogenic mediator than epidermal growth factor. Science 232:1250, 1986

54. Todaro GJ, Fryling C, DeLarco JE: Transforming growth factors produced by certain human tumor cells: polypeptides that react with growth factor receptors. Proc Natl Acad Sci USA 77:5258, 1980

55. Anzano MA, Roberts AB, Smith JM et al: Sarcoma growth factor from conditioned media of virally transformed cells is composed of both type α and type β transforming growth factors. Proc Natl Acad Sci USA 80:6264, 1983

56. Madtes DK, Raines EW, Sarakjeassen KS et al: Induction of transforming growth factor-α in activated human alveolar macrophages. Cell 53:285, 1988

57. Rappolee DA, Mark D, Banda MJ, Werb Z: Wound macrophages express TGF-α and other growth factors in vivo: analysis by mRNA phenotyping. Science 241:708, 1988

58. Marquardt H, Hunkapiller MW, Hood LE, Todaro GJ: Rat transforming growth factor type 1: structure and relation to epidermal growth factor. Science 223:1079, 1984

59. DeRynk R, Roberts AB, Winkler ME et al: Human transforming growth factor-α: precursor structure and expression in E. coli. Cell 38:287, 1984

60. Frater-Schroder M, Muller G, Birchmeier W, Bohlen P: Transforming growth factor-β inhibits endothelial cell proliferation. Bichem Biophys Res Commun 137:295, 1986

61. Baird A, Durkin T: Inhibition of endothelial cell proliferation by type β-transforming growth factor: interactions with acidic and basic fibroblasts growth factors. Biochem Biophys Res Commun 138:476, 1986

62. Roberts AB, Sporn M, Assoian RK et al: Transforming growth factor type β: rapid induction of fibrosis and angiogenesis in vivo and stimulation of collagen formation in vitro. Proc Natl Acad Sci USA 83:4167, 1986

63. Wahl SM, Hunt DA, Wakefield LM et al: Transforming factor type β induces monocyte chemotaxis and growth factor production. Proc Natl Acad Sci USA 84:5788, 1987

64. Assoian RK, Komoriya A, Meyers CA et al: Transforming growth factor-β in human platelets. Identification of a major storage site, purification, and characterization. J Biol Chem 258:7155, 1983

65. Roberts AB, Sporn MB: Transforming growth factor β. Adv Cancer Res 51: 107, 1988

66. Sporn MB, Roberts AB, Wakefield LM, DeCrombrugghe B: Some recent advances in the chemistry and biology of transforming growth factor-β. J Cell Biol 105:1039, 1987

67. Lawrence DA, Pircher R, Julien P: Conversion of high molecular weight latent β-TGF from chicken embryo fibroblasts into a low molecular weight active β-TGF under acidic conditions. Biochem Biophys Res Commun 133: 1026, 1985

68. Keski-Oja J, Lyons RM, Moses HL: Inactive secreted forms of transforming growth factor-β (TGFβ): activation of proteolysis. J Cell Biochem, suppl. 11a:60, 1987

69. Leibovich SJ, Polverini PJ, Shepard HM et al: Macrophage-induced angiogenesis is mediated by tumor necrosis factor-α. Nature 329:630, 1987

70. Frater-Schroder MF, Risau W, Hallmann R et al: Tumor necrosis factor type α, a potent inhibitor of endothelial cell growth *in vitro*, is angiogenic *in vivo*. Proc Natl Acad Sci USA 84:5277, 1987

71. Schweigerer L, Malerstein B, Gospodarowicz D: Tumor necrosis factor inhibits the proliferation of cultured capillary endothelial cells. Biochem Biophys Res Commun 143:997, 1987

72. Haranaka KE, Karswell A, Williamson BD et al: Purification, characterization, and antitumor activity of mouse nonrecombinant tumor necrosis factor. Proc Natal Acad Sci USA 83:3949, 1986

73. Sherry B, Cerami A: Cachectin/tumor necrosis factor exerts endocrine, paracrine and autocrine control of inflammatory responses. J Cell Biol 107:1269, 1988

74. Bicknell R, Vallee BL: Angiogenin activates endothelial cell phospholipase C. Proc Natl Acad Sci USA 85:5961, 1988

75. Fett JW, Strydom DJ, Lobb RR et al: Isolation and characterization of angiogenin, an angiogenic protein from human carcinoma cells. Biochemistry 24:5480, 1985

76. Weiner HL, Weiner LH, Swain JL: Tissue distribution and developmental expression of the mRNA encoding angiogenin. Science 237:280, 1987

77. Bond MD, Vallee BL: Isolation of angiogenin using a bovine ribonuclease inhibitor binding assay. Biochemistry 27:6282, 1988

78. Kurachi K, Davie EW, Strydom DJ et al: Sequence of the cDNA and gene for angiogenin, a human angiogenesis factor. Biochemistry 24:5494, 1985

79. Riordan JF, Vallee BL: Human angiogenin, an organogenic protein. Br J Cancer 57:587, 1988

80. Shapiro R, Riordan JF, Vallee BL: Characteristic ribonucleolytic activity of human angiogenin. Biochemistry 25:3527, 1986

81. Rybak M, Vallee BL: Base cleavage specificity of angiogenin: with *Saccharomyces cerevisiae and Escherichia coli* 5S RNAs. Biochemistry 27:2288, 1988

82. Shapiro R, Weremovicz S, Riordan JF, Vallee BL: Ribonucleolytic activity of angiogenin: essential histidine, lysine, and arginine residues. Proc Natl Acad Sci USA 84:8783, 1987

83. Koch AE, Polverini PJ, Kunkel SL et al: Interleukin-8 as a macrophage-derived mediator of angiogenesis. Science 258:1798, 1992

84. Tsopanoglou NE, Pipili-Synetos E, Maragoudakis ME: Thrombin promotes angiogenesis by a mechanism independent of fibrin formation. Am J Physiol 264:C1302, 1993

85. Nagy JA, Brown LF, Senger DR et al: Pathogenesis of tumor stroma generation: a critical role for leaky bloody vessels and fibrin deposition. Biochim Biophys Acta 948:305, 1988

86. Wolinsky H: A proposal linking clearance of circulating lipoproteins to tissue metabolic activity as a basis for understanding atherogenesis. Circ Res 47:301, 1980

87. Newman PJ, Berndt MC, Gorski J et al: PECAM-(CD31) cloning and relation to adhesion molecules of the immunoglobulin gene superfamily. Science 247:1219, 1990

88. Stockinger H, Gadd SJ, Eher R et al: Molecular characterization and functional analysis of the leukocyte surface protein CD31. J Immunol 145:3889, 1990

89. Muller WA, Ratti CM, McDonnell SL, Cohn ZA: A human endothelial cell-restricted externally disposed plasmalemmal protein enriched in intercellular junctions. J Exp Med 170:399, 1989

90. Albelda SM, Oliver PD, Romer LH, Buck CA: Endo-CAM, a novel endothelial cell-cell adhesion molecule. J Cell Biol 110:1227, 1990

91. Heimark RL, Degner M, Schwartz SM: Identification of a Ca^{2+}-dependent cell-cell adhesion molecule. J Cell Biol 110:1745, 1990

92. Lampugnani MG, Resnati M, Dejana E, Marchisio PC: The role of integrins in the maintenance of endothelial monolayer integrity. J Cell Biol 112:479, 1991

93. Palade GE, Simionescu M, Simionescu N. Structural aspects of the permeability of the microvascular endothelium. Acta Physiol Scand 463:11, 1979

94. Simionescu M, Simionescu N, Palade GE: Segmental differentiation of cell junctions in the vascular endothelium: the microvasculature. J Cell Biol 67: 863, 1975

95. Wissig SL: Identification of the small pore in muscle capillaries. Acta Physiol Scand Suppl 463:33, 1979

96. Majno G, Palade GE: Studies on inflammation. I. The effect of histamine and serotonin on vascular permeability: an electron microscopic study. J Biophys Biochem Cytol 11:571, 1961

97. Simionescu N, Simionescu M, Palade GE: Open junctions in the endothelium of the postcapillary venules of the diaphragm. J Cell Biol 79:27, 1978

98. Weibel ER, Palade GE: New cytoplasmic components in arterial endothelia. J Cell Biol 23:101, 1964

99. Wagner DD, Olmsted JB, Marder VJ: Immunolocalization of von Willebrand protein in Weibel-Palade bodies of human endothelial cells. J Cell Biol 95: 355, 1982

100. Sporn LA, Marder VJ, Wagner DD: Differing polarity of the constitutive and regulated secretory pathways of von Willebrand factor in endothelial cells. J Cell Biol 108:1283, 1989

101. Voorberg J, Fontijn R, Calafat J et al: Biogenesis of von Willebrand factor-containing organelles in heterologous transfected CV-1 cells. EMBO J 12: 749, 1993

102. Bonfanti R, Furie BC, Furie B, Wagner DD: PADGEM(GMP 140) is a component of Weibel-Palade bodies of human endothelial cells. Blood 73:1109, 1989

103. McEver RP, Beckstead JH, Moore KL et al: GMP-140, a platelet membrane alpha-granule protein, is also synthesized by vascular endothelial cells and is localized in Weibel-Palade bodies. J Clin Invest 84:92, 1989

104. Ley K, Gaehtgens P, Fennie C et al: Lectin-like cell adhesion molecule 1 mediates leukocyte rolling in mesenteric venules in vivo. Blood 77:2553, 1991

105. von Andrian UH, Chambers JD, McEvoy LM et al: Two-step model of leukocyte-endothelial cell interaction in inflammation: distinct roles for LECAM-1 and the leukocyte β2 integrins in vivo. Proc Natl Acad Sci USA 88:7538, 1991

106. Larsen E, Celi A, Gilbert GE et al: PADGEM protein: a receptor that mediates the interaction of activated platelets with neutrophils and monocytes. Cell 59:305, 1989

107. Geng J-G, Bevilacqua MP, Moore KL et al: Rapid neutrophil adhesion to activated endothelium mediated by GMP-140. Nature 343:77, 1990

108. Weller A, Isenmann S, Vestweber D: Cloning of the mouse endothelial selectins. Expression of both E- and P-selectin is inducible by tumor necrosis factor. J Biol Chem 267:15176, 1992

109. Manning AM, Kukielka GL, Dore M et al: Regulation of GMP-140 mRNA in a canine model of inflammation, abstracted. FASEB J 6:1060A, 1992

110. Sanders WE, Wilson RW, Ballantyne CM, Beaudet AL: Molecular cloning and analysis of in vivo expression of murine P-selectin. Blood 80:975, 1992

111. Hattori R, Hamilton KK, Fugate RD et al: Stimulated secretion of endothelial von Willebrand factor is accompanied by rapid distribution to the cell surface of the intracellular granule membrane protein GMP-140. J Biol Chem 264:7768, 1989

112. Hattori R, Hamilton KK, McEver RP, Sims PJ: Complement proteins C5-9 induce secretion of high molecular weight multimers of endothelial von Willebrand factor and translocation of granule membrane protein GMP-140 to the cell surface. J Biol Chem 264:9053, 1989

113. Patel KD, Zimmerman GA, Prescott SM et al: Oxygen radicals induce human endothelial cells to express GMP-140 and bind neutrophils. J Cell Biol 112: 749, 1991

114. Pober JS, Bevilacqua MP, Mendrick DL et al: Two distinct monokines, interleukin-1, and tumor necrosis factor, each independently induce biosynthesis and transient expression of the same antigen on the surface of cultured human vascular endothelial cells. J Immunol 136:P1680, 1986

115. Bevilacqua MP, Pober JS, Mendrick DL et al: Identification of an inducible endothelial-leukocyte adhesion molecule. Proc Natl Acad Sci USA 84:9238, 1987

116. Bevilacqua MP, Nelson RM: Selectins. J Clin Invest 91:379, 1993

117. Lasky LA: Selectins: interpreters of cell-specific carbohydrate information during inflammation. Science 258:964, 1992

118. Gallatin WM, Weissman IL, Butcher EC: A cell-surface molecule involved in organ-specific homing of lymphocytes. Nature 304:30, 1983

119. Phillips ML, Nudelman E, Gaeta FC et al: ELAM-1 mediates cell adhesion by recognition of a carbohydrate ligand, sial-Le^x. Science 250:1130, 1990

120. Walz G, Aruffo A, Kolanus W et al: Recognition by ELAM-1 of the sialyl-Lex determinant on myeloid and tumor cells. Science 250:1132, 1990

121. Fukuda M, Sooncer E, Oates JE et al: Structure of sialylated fucosyl lactosaminoglycan isolated from human granulocytes. J Biol Chem 259:10925, 1984

122. Symington FW, Hedges DL, Hakamori S: Glycolipid antigens of human polymorphonuclear neutrophils and the inducible HL-60 myeloid leukemia cell line. J Immunol 134:2498, 1985

123. Ohmmori K, Yoneda T, Ishihara G, et al: Sialyl SSEA-1 antigens as a carbohydrate marker of human natural killer cells and immature lymphoid cells. Blood 74:255, 1989

124. Munro JM, Lo SK, Corless C et al: Expression of sialyl-Lewis X, an E-selectin ligand, in inflammation, immune processes, and lymphoid tissue. Am J Pathol 141:1397, 1992

125. Springer TA, Dustin ML, Kishimoto TL, Marlin SD: The lymphocyte function-associated LFA-1, CD2, and LFA-3 molecules: cell adhesion receptors of the immune system. Annu Rev Immunol 5:223, 1987

126. Dustin ML, Staunton DE, Springer TA: Supergene families meet in the immune system. Immunol Today 9:213, 1988

127. Munro JM, Pober JS, Cotran RS: Tumor necrosis and interferon-gamma induce distinct patterns of endothelial activation and associated leukocyte accumulation in skin of *Papio anubis*. Am J Pathol 135:121, 1989

128. Simmons D, Makgoba MW, Seed B: ICAM-1, an adhesion ligand of LFA-1, is homologous to the neural cell adhesion molecule NCAM. Nature 331:624, 1988

129. Staunton DE, Marlin SD, Stratowa C et al: Primary structure of ICAM-1 demonstrates interaction between members of the immunoglobulin and integrin supergene families. Cell 52:925, 1988

130. Staunton DE, Dustin ML, Springer TA: Functional cloning of ICAM-2, a cell adhesion ligand for LFA-1 homologous to ICAM-1. Nature 339:61, 1989

131. Williams AF, Barclay AN: The immunoglobulin superfamily—domains for cell surface recognition. Annu Rev Immunol 6:381, 1988

132. Alzari PM, Lascombe M-B, Poljak RJ: Three-dimensional structure of antibodies. Annu Rev Immunol 6:555, 1988

133. Springer TA: Adhesion receptors of the immune system. Nature 364:425, 1990

134. Staunton DE, Dustin ML, Erickson HP, Springer TA: The arrangement of the immunoglobulin-like domains of ICAM-1 and the binding sites for LFA-1 and rhinovirus. Cell 61:243, 1990

135. Kishimoto TK, Larsonn RS, Corbi AL et al: The leukocyte integrins. Adv Immunol 46:149, 1989

136. Dustin ML, Springer TA: Lymphocyte function-associated antigen-1 (LFA-1) interaction with intercellular adhesion molecule-1 (ICAM-1) is one of at least three mechanisms for lymphocyte adhesion to cultured endothelial cells. J Cell Biol 107:321, 1988

137. Vejlsgaard GL, Ralfkiaer E, Avnstorp C et al: Kinetics and characterization of intercellular adhesion molecule-1 (ICAM-1) expression on keratinocytes in various inflammatory skin lesions and malignant cutaneous lymphomas. J Am Acad Dermatol 20:782, 1989

138. Osborn L, Hession R, Tizard R et al: Direct expression cloning of vascular cell adhesion molecule 1, a cytokine induced endothelial protein that binds to lymphocytes. Cell 59:1203, 1989

139. Rice GE, Munro JM, Bevilacqua MP: Inducible cell adhesion molecules 110 (INCAM-110) is an endothelial receptor for lymphocytes. J Exp Med 171: 1369, 1990

140. Elices MJ, Osborn L, Takada Y et al: VCAM1 on activated endothelium interacts with the leukocyte integrin VLA-4 at a site distinct from VLA-4/fibronectin binding site. Cell 60:577, 1990

141. Briscoe DM, Schoen FJ, Rice GE et al: Induced expression of endothelial-leukocyte adhesion molecules in human cardiac allografts. Transplantation 51:537, 1991

142. Varani J, Fligiel SEJ, Till GO et al: Pulmonary endothelial cell killing by human neutrophils: possible involvement of hydroxyl radical. Lab Invest 53:656, 1985

143. Gannon DE, Varani J, Phan SH et al: Source of iron in neutrophil-mediated killing of endothelial cells. Lab Invest 57:37, 1987

144. Stamper HB Jr, Woodruff JJ: Lymphocyte homing into lymph nodes: in vitro demonstration of the selective affinity of recirculating lymphocytes for high endothelial venules. J Exp Med 144:828, 1976

145. Jalkanen ST, Butcher EC: In vitro analysis of the homing properties of human lymphocytes: developmental regulation of functional receptors for high endothelial venules. Blood 66:577, 1985

146. Hamann A, Jablonski-Westrich D, Duijvestijn A et al: Evidence of an accessory role of LFA-1 in lymphocyte-high endothelium interaction during homing. J Immunol 140:693, 1988

147. Shimizu Y, Newman W, Gopal TV et al: Four molecular pathways of T cell adhesion to endothelial cells: roles of LFA-1, VCAM-1, and ELAM-1 and changes in pathway hierarchy under different activation conditions. J Cell Biol 113:1203, 1991

148. Elices MJ, Osborn L, Takada Y et al: VCAM-1 on activated endothelium interacts with the leukocyte integrin VLA-4 at a site distinct from the VLA-4/fibronectin binding site. Cell 60:577, 1990

149. Shimizu Y, Shaw S, Graber N et al: Activation-independent binding of memory T cells to adhesion molecule ELAM-1. Nature 349:799, 1991

150. Picker LJ, Kishimotom TK, Smith CW et al: ELAM-1 is an adhesion molecule for skin-homing T-cells. Nature 349:796, 1991

151. Imai Y, True DD, Singer MS, Rosen SD: Direct demonstration of the lectin activity gp90^MEL, a lymphocyte homing receptor. J Cell Biol 111:1225, 1990

152. Yednock TA, Rosen SD: Lymphocyte homing. Adv Immunol 44:313, 1989

153. Stoolman LM: Adhesion molecules controlling lymphocyte migration. Cell 56:907, 1989

154. Lasky LA, Singer MS, Dowbenko D et al: An endothelial ligand for L-selectin is a novel mucin-like molecule. Cell 69:927, 1992

155. Turrito VT, Weiss HJ, Zimmerman TS, Sussman II: Factor VIII/von Willebrand factor in subendothelium mediates platelet adhesion. Blood 65:823, 1985

156. Pareti FI, Fujimura Y, Dent JA et al: Isolation and characterization of a collagen binding domain in human von Willebrand factor. J Biol Chem 261:15310, 1986

157. Jaffe EA, Hoyer LW, Nachman RL: Synthesis of von Willebrand factor by cultured human endothelial cells. Proc Natl Acad Sci USA 71:1906, 1974

158. Nachman RL, Levine R, Jaffe EA: Synthesis of factor VIII antigen by cultured guinea pig megakaryocytes. J Clin Invest 60:914, 1977

159. Savage B, Shattil SJ, Ruggeri ZM: Modulation of platelet function through adhesion receptors. A dual role for glycoprotein IIb-IIIa (integrin $\alpha IIb\beta 3$) mediated by fibrinogen and glycoprotein Ib-von Willebrand factor. J Biol Chem 267:11300, 1992

160. Laurie GW, Leblond CP, Martin GR: Localization of type IV collagen, laminin, heparin sulfate proteoglycan, and fibronectin to the basal lamina of basement membrane. J Cell Biol 95:340, 1982

161. Sage H, Trueb B, Bornstein P: Biosynthetic and structural properties of endothelial cell type VIII collagen. J Biol Chem 258:13391, 1983

162. Kittelberger R, Davis PF, Greenhill NS: Immunolocalization of type VIII collagen in vascular tissue. Biochem Biophys Res Commun 159:414, 1989

163. Wilner GD, Nossel HL, LeRoy EC: Aggregation of platelets by collagen. J Clin Invest 47:2616, 1968

164. Santoro SA: Identification of a 160,000 dalton platelet membrane protein that initiates the divalent cation-dependent adhesion of platelets to collagen. Cell 46:913, 1986

165. Staatz WD, Rajpara SM, Wayner EA et al: The membrane glycoprotein Ia-IIa (VLA-2) complex mediates the Mg++-dependent adhesion of platelets to collagen. J Cell Biol 108:1917, 1989

166. Asch AS, Barnwell J, Silverstein RL et al: Isolation of the thrombospondin membrane receptor. J Clin Invest 79:1054, 1987

167. Hynes RO: Fibronectins. Springer-Verlag, New York, 1990

167a.Yamada KM: Adhesive recognition sequences. J Biol Chem 266:12809, 1991

168. Obara M, Kang MS, Yamada KM: Site-directed mutagenesis of the cell-binding domain of human fibronectin: separable, synergistic sites mediate adhesive function. Cell 53:649, 1988

169. Bowditch RD, Halloran CE, Aota S et al: Integrin $\alpha IIb\beta 3$ (platelet GPIIB-IIIa) recognizes multiple sites in fibronectin. J Biol Chem 266:23323, 1991

170. Winters KJ, Walsh JJ, Rubin BG, Santoro SA: Platelet interactions with fibronectin: divalent cation-independent platelet adhesion to the gelatin-binding domain of fibronectin. Blood 81:1778, 1993

171. Mosher DF, Doyle MJ, Jaffe EA: Synthesis and secretion of thrombospondin by cultured endothelial cells. J Cell Biol 93:343, 1982

172. Jaffe EA, Leung LLK, Nachman RL et al: Thrombospondin is the endogenous lectin of human platelets. Nature 295:246, 1982

173. Leung LLK: Role of thrombospondin in platelet aggregation. J Clin Invest 74:1764, 1984

174. Ill CR, Engvall E, Ruoslahti E: Adhesion of platelets to laminin in the absence of activation. J Cell Biol 99:2140, 1985

175. Brittain HA, Eckman JR, Swerlick RA et al: Thrombospondin from activated platelets promotes sickle erythrocyte adherence to microvascular endothelium under physiologic flow: a potential role for platelet activation in sickle cell vaso-occlusion. Blood 81:2137, 1993

176. Rodgers GM, Greenberg CS, Shuman MA: Characterization of the effects of cultured vascular cells on the activation of blood coagulation. Blood 61: 1155, 1983

177. Maruyama I, Bell CE, Majerus PW: Thrombomodulin is found on endothelium of arteries, veins, capillaries, and lymphatics, and on syncytioblast of human placenta. J Cell Biol 101:363, 1985

178. Esmon CT: The role of protein C and thrombomodulin in the regulation of blood coagulation. J Biol Chem 264:4743, 1989

179. Esmon CT, Esmon NL, Harris KW: Complex formation between thrombin and thrombomodulin inhibits both thrombin-catalyzed fibrin formation and factor V activation. J Biol Chem 257:7944, 1982

180. Kisiel W, Canfield WM, Ericssson EH, Davie EW: Anticoagulant properties of bovine plasma protein C following activation by thrombin. Biochemistry 16:5824, 1977

181. Fulcher CA, Gardiner JE, Griffin JH, Zimmerman TS: Proteolytic inactivation of human factor VIII procoagulant protein by activated protein C and its analogy with factor V. Blood 63:486, 1984

182. Walker FJ, Sexton PW, Esmon CT: Inhibition of blood coagulation by activated protein C through selective inactivation of activated factor V. Biochim Biophys Acta 571:333, 1979

183. Fair DS, Marlar RA, Urin EJ: Human endothelial cells synthesize protein S. Blood 67:1168, 1986

184. Stern D, Brett J, Harris K, Nawroth P: Participation of endothelial cells in protein C-protein S anticoagulant pathway: the synthesis and release of protein S. J Cell Biol 102:1971, 1986

185. Moore KL, Andreoli SP, Esmon NL et al: Endotoxin enhances tissue factor and suppresses thrombomodulin expression in vascular endothelium *in vitro*. J Clin Invest 79:124, 1987

186. Nawroth PP, Stern DM: Modulation of endothelial cell hemostatic properties by tumor necrosis factor. J Exp Med 163:740, 1986

187. Nawroth PP, Handley DA, Esmon CT, Stern DM: Interleukin-1 induces endothelial cell procoagulant while suppressing cell surface anticoagulant activity. Proc Natl Acad Sci USA 83:3460, 1986

188. Weis JR, Pitas RE, Wilson BD, Rodgers GM: Oxidized low-density lipoprotein increases cultured human endothelial cell tissue factor activity and reduces protein C activation. FASEB J 5:2459, 1991

189. Marcum JA, Atha DH, Fritze LM et al: Cloned bovine aortic endothelial cells synthesize anticoagulantly active heparan sulfate proteoglycan. J Biol Chem 261:7507, 1986

190. Stern D, Nawroth P, Macrum J et al: Interaction of antithrombin III with bovine aortic segments: role of heparin in binding and enhanced anticoagulant activity. J Clin Invest 75:272, 1985

191. Weksler BB, Marcus AJ, Jaffe EA: Synthesis of prostaglandin I_2 (prostacyclin) by cultured human and bovine endothelial cells. Proc Natal Acad Sci USA 74:3922, 1977

192. Furchgott RF, Zawadski JV: The obligatory role of endothelial cells in the relaxation of arterial smooth muscle by acetylcholine. Nature 288:373, 1980

193. Brenner BM, Troy JL, Ballermann BJ: Endothelium-dependent vascular responses: mediators and mechanisms. J Clin Invest 84:1373, 1989

194. Griffith TM, Edwards DH, Lewis MJ et al: The nature of endothelial-derived vascular relaxant factor. Nature 308:645, 1984

195. Spicer E, Horton R, Bloem L et al: Isolation of cDNA clones for human tissue factor: primary structure of the protein and cDNA. Proc Natl Acad Sci USA 84:5148, 1987

196. Scarpati EM, Wen D, Broze GJ Jr, Sadler JE: Human tissue factor: cDNA sequence and chromosome localization of the gene. Biochemistry 26:5234, 1987

197. Fisher KL, Gorman CM, Vehar GA et al: Cloning and expression of human tissue factor cDNA. Thromb Res 48:89, 1987

198. Morrisey JH, Fakhrai H, Edgington TS: Molecular cloning of the cDNA for tissue factor, the cellular receptor for the initiation of the coagulation protease cascade. Cell 50:129, 1987

199. Rodgers GM, Broze GJ Jr, Shuman MA: The number of receptors for factor VII correlates with the ability of cultured cells to initiate coagulation. Blood 63:434, 1984

200. Wilcox JN, Smith KM, Schwartz SM et al: Localization of tissue factor in the normal vessel wall and in the atherosclerotic plaque. Proc Natl Acad Sci USA 86:2839, 1989

201. Bevilacqua MP, Pober JS, Majeau GR et al: Interleukin-1 (IL-1) induces biosynthesis and cell surface expression of procoagulant activity in human vascular endothelial cells. J Exp Med 160:618, 1984

202. Bevilacqua MP, Pober JS, Majeau GR et al: Recombinant tumor necrosis factor induces procoagulant activity in cultured human vascular endothelium: characterization and comparison with interleukin 1. Proc Natl Acad Sci USA 83:4533, 1986

203. Nawroth PP, Stern DM: Modulation of endothelial cell hemostatic properties by tumor necrosis factor. J Exp Med 163:740, 1986

204. Nawroth PP, Bank I, Handley D et al: Tumor necrosis factor/cachectin interacts with endothelial cell receptors to induce release of interleukin 1. J Exp Med 163:1363, 1986

205. Clozel M, Kuhn H, Baumgartner HR: Procoagulant activity of endotoxin-treated human endothelial cells exposed to native human flowing blood. Blood 73:729, 1989

206. Weis JR, Pitas RE, Wilson BD, Rodgers GM: Oxidized low-density lipoprotein increases cultured human endothelial cell tissue factor activity and reduces protein C activity. FASEB J 5:2459, 1991

207. Nemerson Y: The reaction between bovine brain tissue factor and factors VII and X. Biochemistry 5:601, 1966

208. Miletich JP, Jackson CM, Majerus PW: Interaction of coagulation factor Xa with platelets. Proc Natl Acad Sci USA 74:4033, 1977

209. Rodgers GM, Shuman MA: Prothrombin is activated on vascular endothelial cells by factor Xa and calcium. Proc Natl Acad Sci USA 80:7001, 1983

210. Rodgers GM, Kane WH: Activation of endogenous factor V by a homocysteine-induced vascular endothelial cell activator. J Clin Invest 77:1909, 1986

211. Heimark RL, Schwartz S: Binding of coagulation factors IX and X to the endothelial cell surface. Biochem Biophys Res Commun 11:723, 1983

212. Stern DM, Drillings M, Nossel HL et al: Binding of factors IX and IXa to cultured vascular endothelial cells. Proc Natl Acad Sci USA 80:4119, 1983

213. Greenberg CS, Achyuthan KE, Borowitz MJ, Shuman MA: The transglutaminase in vascular cells and tissues could provide an alternate pathway for fibrin stabilization. Blood 70:707, 1987

214. Levin EG, Loskutoff DJ: Cultured bovine endothelial cells produce both urokinase and tissue-type plasminogen activators. J Cell Biol 94:631, 1982

215. van Mourik JA, Lawrence DA, Loskutoff DJ: Purification of an inhibitor of plasminogen activator (antiactivator) synthesized by endothelial cells. J Biol Chem 259:14914, 1984

216. Gross J, Moscatelli D, Jaffe E, Rifkin D: Plasminogen activator and collagenase production by cultured capillary endothelial cells. J Cell Biol 95:974, 1982

217. Loskutoff DJ: Effect of thrombin on the fibrinolytic activity of cultured bovine endothelial cells. J Clin Invest 64:329, 1979

218. Gelehrter TD, Sznycer-Laszuk R: Thrombin induction of plasminogen activator-inhibitor in cultured human endothelial cells. J Clin Invest 77:165, 1986

219. Crutchley DJ, Conanan LB: Endotoxin induction of an inhibitor of plasminogen activator in bovine pulmonary artery endothelial cells. J Biol Chem 261:154, 1986

220. Bevilacqua MP, Schleef RR, Gimbrone MA, Loskutoff DJ: Regulation of the fibrinolytic system of cultured vascular endothelium by interleukin 1. J Clin Invest 78:587, 1986

221. McClean JW, Tomlinson JE, Kuang WJ et al: cDNA sequence of human apolipoprotein(a) is homologous to plasminogen. Nature 130:132, 1987

222. Utermann G, Menzel H, Kraft H et al: Lp(a) glycoprotein phenotypes: inheritance and relation to Lp(a)-lipoprotein concentrations in plasma. J Clin Invest 80:458, 1987

223. Vali Z, Patthy L: Location of the intermediate and high affinity ω-aminocarboxylic acid-binding sites in human plasminogen. J Biol Chem 257:2104, 1982

224. Harpel PC, Gordon BR, Parker TS: Plasmin catalyses binding of lipoprotein(a) to immobilized fibrinogen and fibrin. Proc Natl Acad Sci USA 86:3847, 1989

225. Rouy D, Grailhe P, Nigon F et al: Lipoprotein(a) impairs generation of plasmin by fibrin bound tissue-type plasminogen activator. Arterioscler Thromb 11:629, 1991

226. Scott JJ: Thrombogenesis linked to atherogenesis at last? Nature 341:22, 1989

227. Simionescu N: The microvascular endothelium: segmental differentiations; transcytosis, selective distribution of anionic sites. p. 61. In Weissmann G, Samuelson B, Paoletti R (eds): Advances in Inflammation Research. Vol. 1. Raven Press, New York, 1979

228. Bignon J, Chahinian P, Feldman G, Sapin C: Ultrastructural immunocytochemical demonstration of autologous albumen in the alveolar capillary membrane and in the alveolar lining material in normal rats. J Cell Biol 64:503, 1975

229. Yokota S: Immunocytochemical evidence for transendothelial transport of albumen and fibrinogen in rat heart and diphragm. Biomed Res 4:577, 1983

230. Tavassoli M, Kishimoto T, Soda R et al: Liver endothelium mediates the uptake of iron-transferrin complex by hepatocytes. Exp Cell Res 165:369, 1986

231. Dernovsek RK, Bar RS, Ginsberg BH, Lioubin MN: Rapid transport of biologically active insulin through cultured endothelial cells. J Clin Endocrinol Metab 58:761, 1984

232. Dernovsek RK, Bar RS: Processing of cell bound insulin by capillary and microvascular endothelial cells in culture. Am J Physiol 248:E244, 1985

233. Vasile E, Simionescu M, Simionescu N: Visualization of the binding, endocytosis, and transcytosis of low-density lipoprotein in arterial endothelium in situ. J Cell Biol 96:1677, 1983

234. Baker DP, Van Lenten BJ, Fogelman AM et al: LDL, scavenger, β-LDL receptors on aortic endothelial cells. Arteriosclerosis 4:248, 1984

235. Vasile E, Popescu G, Simionescu M, Simionescu N: Enhanced transcytosis and accumulation of β-very low density lipoproteins in the aorta of rabbits with experimental hyperlipidemia, abstracted. p. 68. In: XVIth International Congress of the International Academy of Pathology, Vienna, 1986

236. Kataoka M, Tavassoli M: The role of liver endothelium in the binding and uptake of ceruloplasmin. Studies with colloidal gold probe. J Ultrastruct Res 90:194, 1985

237. Renkin EM: Capillary transport of macromolecules: pore and other endothelial pathways. J Appl Physiol 58:315, 1985

238. Chien S, Fan F-C, Lee MAL, Handley DA: Effects of arterial pressure on endothelial transport of macromolecules. Biorheology 21:631, 1984

239. Simionescu N: Cellular aspects of transcapillary exchange. Physiol Rev 63:1536, 1983

240. Curry F-RE: The effect of charge on the transport of intermediate size protein probes across the capillary wall. p. 120. In Lambert PP, Bergmann P, Beauwens R (eds): The Pathogenicity of Cationic Proteins. Raven Press, New York, 1982

241. Goldstein JL, Ho YK, Basu SK, Brown MS: Binding site on macrophages that mediates uptake and degradation of acetylated low density lipoprotein producing massive cholesterol deposition. Proc Natl Acad Sci USA 76:333, 1979

242. Stein O, Stein Y: Bovine aortic endothelial cells display macrophage-like properties towards acetylated ^{125}I-labelled low density lipoprotein. Biochim Biophys Acta 620:631, 1980

243. Nagelkerke JF, Barto KP, van Berkel TJ: In vivo and in vitro uptake and degration of acetylated low density lipoprotein by rat liver endothelial, Kupffer and parenchymal cells. J Biol Chem 258:1221, 1983

244. Steinberg D, Parthasarathy S, Carew TE et al: Beyond cholesterol: modifications of low-density lipoprotein that increase its atherogenicity. N Engl J Med 320:915, 1989

245. Boyd HC, Gown AM, Wolfbauer G, Chait A: Direct evidence for a protein recognized by a monoclonal antibody against oxidatively modified LDL in atherosclerotic lesions from a Watanabe heritable hyperlipidemic rabbit. Am J Pathol 135:815, 1989

246. Rubanyi GM, Romero JC, Vanhoutte PM: Flow-induced release of endothelium-derived releasing factor. Am J Physiol 250:H1145, 1986

247. Furcgott RF, Zawadzki JV: The obligatory role of endothelial cells in the relaxation of arterial smooth muscle by acetylcholine. Nature 299:373, 1980

248. Palmer RMJ, Ferrige AG, Moncada S: Nitric oxide release accounts for the biological activity of endothelium-derived relaxing factor. Nature 327:524, 1987

249. Myers PR, Minor RL Jr, Guerra R Jr et al: Vasorelaxant properties of the endothelium-derived relaxing factor more closely resemble S-nitrosocysteine than nitric oxide. Nature 345:161, 1990

250. Palmer RMJ, Ashton DS, Moncada S: Vascular endothelial cells synthesize nitric oxide from L-arginine. Nature 333:664, 1988

251. Bredt DS, Hwang PM, Glatt CE, Loewenstein C: Cloned and expressed nitric oxide synthase structurally resembles cytochrome P-450 reductase. Nature 351:714, 1991

252. Rees DD, Palmer RMJ, Moncada S: Role of endothelium-derived nitric oxide in the regulation of blood pressure. Proc Natl Acad Sci USA 86:3375, 1989

253. Rapoport RM, Murad F: Agonist-induced endothelium-dependent relaxation in rat thoracic aorta may be mediated through cyclic through cGMP. Circ Res 52:352, 1983

254. Busse R, Luckhoff A, Bassenge E: Endothelium-derived relaxant factor inhibits platelet activation. Naunyn Schmiedbergs Arch Pharmacol 336:566, 1987

255. Marcus AJ, Weksler BB, Jaffe EA: Enzymatic conversion of prostaglandin endoperoxide H2 and arachidonic acid to prostacyclin by cultured human endothelial cells. J Biol Chem 253:7138, 1978

256. Weksler BB, Ley CW, Jaffe EA: Stimulation of endothelial prostacyclin production by thrombin, trypsin, and the ionophore A23187. J Clin Invest 62:923, 1978

257. Baenziger NL, Fogerty FJ, Mertz LF et al: Regulation of histamine-mediated prostacyclin synthesis in cultured human vascular endothelial cells. Cell 24:915, 1981

258. Hong SL: Effect of bradykinin and thrombin on prostacyclin synthesis in endothelial cells from calf and pig aorta and human umbilical vein. Thromb Res 18:787, 1980

259. Moritz I, Kanayasu T, Murota SI: Kallikrein stimulates prostacyclin production in bovine vascular endothelial cells. Biochim Biophys Acta 792:304, 1984

260. Rossi V, Breviario F, Ghezzi P et al: Prostacyclin synthesis induced in vascular cells by interleukin-1. Science 229:174, 1985

261. Eldor A, Fridman R, Vlodavksy I et al: Interferon enhances prostacyclin production by cultured vascular endothelial cells. J Clin Invest 73:251, 1984

262. Endo H, Akahoshi T, Kashiwazaki S: Additive effects of IL-1 and TNF on induction of prostacyclin synthesis in human vascular endothelial cells. Biochem Biophys Res Commun 156:1007, 1988

263. Fleisher LN, Tall AR, Witte LD et al: Stimulation of arterial endothelial cell prostacyclin synthesis by high density lipoproteins. J Biol Chem 257:6653, 1982

264. Kaplan KL, Mather T, DeMarco L et al: Effect of fibrin on endothelial cell production of prostacyclin and tissue plasminogen activator. Arteriosclerosis 9:43, 1989

265. Rampart M, Bult H, Herman AG: Activated complement and anaphylotoxins increase the in vitro production of prostacyclin by rabbit aorta endothelium. Naunyn Schmiedebergs Arch Pharmacol 322:158, 1983

266. Ristimaki A, Ylikorkala O, Perheentupe J et al: Epidermal growth factor stimulates prostacyclin production by cultured human vascular endothelial cells. Thromb Haemost 59:249, 1988

267. Ristimaki A: Transforming growth factor alpha stimulates prostacyclin production by cultured human vascular endothelial cells more potently than epidermal growth factor. Biochem Biophys Res Commun 160:1100, 1989

268. Grabowski EF, Jaffe EA, Weksler BB: Prostacyclin production by cultured endothelial cell monolayers exposed to step increases in shear stress. J Lab Clin Med 105:36, 1985

269. Luscher TF, Vanhoutte PM: The Endothelium Modulator of Cardiovascular Function. CRC Press, Boca Raton, FL, 1990

270. Smith WL: The eicosanoids and their biochemical mechanism of action. Biochem J 259:315, 1989

271. Marcus AJ, Weksler BB, Jaffe EA et al: Synthesis of prostacyclin from platelet-derived endoperoxides by cultured human endothelial cells. J Clin Invest 66:979, 1980

272. Wong PY-K, Lee WH, Chao PH-W et al: Metabolism of prostacyclin by 9-hydroxyprostaglandin dehydrogenase in human platelets. J Biol Chem 255:9021, 1980

273. Jaffe EA, Weksler BB: Recovery of endothelial cell prostacyclin production after inhibition by low doses of aspirin. J Clin Invest 63:532, 1979

274. Brown Z, Neild GH, Lewis GP: Mechanism of inhibition of prostacyclin synthesis by cyclosporine in cultured human umbilical vein endothelial cells. Transplant Proc, suppl 3. 20:654, 1988

275. Hecker M, Ullrich V: Studies on the interaction of minoxidil with prostacyclin synthase in vitro. Biochem Pharmacol 37:3363, 1988

276. Reinders JH, Brinkman HJ, van Mourik JA et al: Cigarette smoke impairs endothelial cell prostacyclin production. Arteriosclerosis 6:15, 1986

277. Busacca M, Balconi G, Pietra A et al: Maternal smoking and prostacyclin production by cultured endothelial cell from umbilical arteries. Am J Obstet Gynecol 148:1127, 1984

278. Bull HA, Pittilo RM, Woolf N et al: The effect of nicotine on human endothelial cell release of prostaglandins and ultrastructure. Br J Exp Pathol 69:413, 1988

279. Sinha AK, Dutta-Roy AK, Chiu HC et al: Coagulant factor Xa inhibits prostacyclin formation in human endothelial cells. Arteriosclerosis 5:244, 1985

280. Hadjiagapiou C, Spector AA: 12-Hydroxyeicosatetraenoic acid reduces prostacyclin production by endothelial cells. Prostaglandins 31:1135, 1986

281. Hullin F, Raynal P, Ragab-Thomas JMF et al: Effect of dexamethasone on prostaglandin synthesis and on lipocortin status in human endothelial cells. Inhibition of prostaglandin I_2 synthesis occurring without alteration of arachidonic acid liberation and of lipocortin synthesis. J Biol Chem 264:3506, 1989

282. Spector AA, Hoak JC, Fry GL et al: Effect of fatty acid modification on prostacyclin production by cultured human endothelial cells. J Clin Invest 65:1003, 1980

283. Shepro D, Dunham B: Endothelial cell metabolism of biogenic amines. Annu Rev Physiol 48:335, 1986

284. Lee SL, Fanburg BL: Serotonin uptake by bovine pulmonary artery endothelial cells in culture. I. Characterization. Am J Physiol 250:C761, 1986

285. Branaczyk Kuzma A, Audus KL, Borchardt RT: Catecholamine-metabolizing enzymes of bovine brain microvessel endothelial cell monolayers. J Neurochem 46:1956, 1986

286. Yanagisawa M, Kurihara H, Kimura S et al: A novel potent vasoconstrictor peptide produced by vascular endothelial cells. Nature 332:411, 1988

287. Kasuya Y, Ishikawa T, Yanagisawa M et al: Mechanism of contraction to endothelin in isolated porcine coronary artery. Am J Physiol 257:H1828, 1989

288. Goto K, Kasuya Y, Matsuki N et al: Endothelin activates the dihydropyridine-sensitive voltage-dependent Ca^{2+} channel in vascular smooth muscle. Proc Natl Acad Sci USA 86:3915, 1989

289. Boulanger C, Luscher TF: Release of endothelin from porcine aorta: inhibition by endothelium-derived nitric oxide. J Clin Invest 85:587, 1990

290. Yokokawa K, Kohno M, Yasunari K et al: Endothelin-3 regulates endothelin-1 production in cultured endothelial cells. Hypertension 18:304, 1991

291. Saijonmaa O, Ristimaki A, Fyhrquist F: Atrial naturietic peptide, nitroglycerine, and nitroprusside reduce basal and stimulated endothelin production from cultured endothelial cells. Biochem Biophys Res Commun 173:514, 1990

292. Yang Z, von Segesser L, Bauer E et al: Different activation of endothelial L-

arginine and cyclooxygenase pathway in human internal mammary artery and saphenous vein. Circ Res 68:52, 1991

293. Katusic ZS, Vanhoutte PM: Superoxide anion is an endothelium-derived contracting factor. Am J Physiol 357:H33, 1988

294. Zimmerman GA, McIntyre TM, Mehra M et al: Endothelial cell-associated platelet-activating factor: a novel mechanism for signaling intercellular adhesion. J Cell Biol 110:529, 1990

295. Hopkins NK, Schaub RG, Gorman RR: Acetyl glyceryl ether phosphorylcholine (PAF-acether) and leukotriene B4-mediated neutrophil chemotaxis through an intact endothelial cell monolayer. Biochim Biophys Acta 805: 30, 1984

296. Prescott SM, Zimmerman GA, McIntyre TM: Human endothelial cells in culture produce platelet-activating factor (1-alkyl-2-acetyl-sn-glycero-3-phosphocholine) when stimulated with thrombin. Proc Natl Acad Sci USA 81: 3534, 1984

297. Camussi G, Aglietta M, Malavasi F et al: The release of platelet-activating factor from human endothelial cells in culture. J Immunol 131:2397, 1983

298. Bussolino F, Camussi G, Baglioni C: Synthesis and release of platelet-activating factor by human vascular endothelial cells treated with tumor necrosis factor or interleukin 1 alpha. J Biol Chem 263:11856, 1988

299. McIntyre TM, Zimmerman GA, Prescott SM: Leukotrienes C4 and D4 stimulate human endothelial cells to synthesize platelet-activating factor and bind neutrophils. Proc Natl Acad Sci USA 83:2204, 1986

300. McIntyre TM, Zimmerman GA, Satoh K et al: Cultured endothelial cells synthesize both platelet-activating factor and prostacyclin in response to histamine, bradykinin, and adenosine triphosphate. J Clin Invest 76:271, 1985

301. Lewis MS, Whatley RE, Cain P et al: Hydrogen peroxide stimulates the synthesis of platelet-activating factor by endothelium and induces endothelial cell-dependent neutrophil adhesion. J Clin Invest 82:2045, 1988

302. Hopkins NK, Schaub RG, Gorman RR: Acetyl glyceryl ether phosphorylcholine (PAF-acether) and leukotriene B4-mediated neutrophil chemotaxis through an intact endothelial cell monolayer. Biochim Ciophys Acta 805: 30, 1984

303. Lorant DE, Patel KP, McIntyre TM et al: Coexpression of GMP-140 and PAF by endothelium stimulated by histamine or thrombin: a juxtacrine system for adhesion and activation of neutrophils. J Cell Biol 115:223, 1991

304. Benveniste J, le Couedic JP, Kamoun P: Aggregation of human platelets by platelet-activating factor. Lancet 1:344, 1975

305. Blank ML, Spector AA, Kaduce TL et al: Metabolism of platelet activating factor (1-alkyl-2-acetyl-sn-glycero-3-phosphocholine) and 1-alkyl-2-acetyl-sn-glycerol by human endothelial cells. Biochim Biophys Acta 876:373, 1986

306. Zimmerman GA, McIntyre TM, Prescott SM: Production of platelet-activating factor by human vascular endothelial cells: evidence for a requirement for specific agonists and modulation by prostacyclin. Circulation 72:718, 1985

307. Strieter RM, Kunkel SL, Showell HJ et al: Endothelial cell gene expression of a neutrophil chemotactic factor by TNF-alpha, LPS, and IL-1 beta. Science 243:1467, 1989

308. Schroder J-M, Christophers EJ: Secretion of novel and homologous neutrophil-activating peptides by LPS-stimulated human endothelial cells. Immunology 142:244, 1989

309. Sica A, Matsushima K, van Damme J et al: IL-1 transcriptionally activates the neutrophil chemotactic factor/IL-8 gene in endothelial cells. Immunology 69: 548, 1990

310. Baggiolini M, Imboden P, Detmers P: Neutrophil activation and the effects of interleukin-8/neutrophil-activating peptide 1(IL-8/NAP-1). Cytokines 4:1, 1992

311. Detmers PA, Lo SK, Olsen-Egbert E et al: Neutrophil-activating protein 1/ interleukin 8 stimulates the binding activity of the leukocyte adhesion receptor CD11b/CD18 on human neutrophils. J Exp Med 171:1155, 1990

312. Gimbrone MA Jr, Obin MS, Brock AF et al: Endothelial interleukin-8: a novel inhibitor of leukocyte-endothelial interactions. Science 246:1601, 1989

313. Clark S, Kamen R: The human hematopoietic colony-stimulating factors. Science 236:1229, 1987

314. Strife A, Lambek C, Wisniewsky D et al: Activities of four purified growth factors on highly enriched human hematopoietic progenitor cells. Blood 69:1508, 1987

315. Metcalf D: The molecular biology and functions of the granulocyte-macrophage colony-stimulating factors. Blood 67:257, 1986

316. Gasson JC, Weisbart RH, Kaufman SE et al: Purified granulocyte-macrophage colony-stimulating factor: direct action on neutrophils. Science 226:1339, 1984

317. Lopez AF, Williamson DJ, Gamble JR et al: Recombinant granulocyte-macrophage colony-stimulating factor stimulates in vitro mature human neutrophil and eosinophil function, surface receptor expression, and survival. J Clin Invest 78:1220, 1986

318. Morrissey PJ, Grabstein KH, Reed SG, Conlon PJ: Granulocyte/macrophage colony-stimulating factor. A potent activation signal for mature macrophages and monocytes. Int Arch Allergy Appl Immunol 88:40, 1989

319. Quesenberry PJ, Gimbrone MA: Vascular endothelium as a regulator of granulopoiesis: production of colony-stimulating factor by cultured human endothelial cells. Blood 56:1060, 1980

320. Broudy VC, Kaushansky K, Harlan JM, Adamson JW: Interleukin-1 stimulates human endothelial cells to produce granulocyte-macrophage colony-stimulating factor. J Immunol 134:464, 1987

321. Schrader JW, Moyer C, Ziltener JH, Reinisch CL: Release of the cytokines colony-stimulating factor-1, granulocyte-macrophage colony-stimulating factor, and IL-6 by cloned murine vascular smooth muscle cells. J Immunol 146:3799, 1991

322. Zucali JR, Dinarello CA, Oblon DJ et al: Interleukin 1 stimulates fibroblasts to produce granulocyte-macrophage colony-stimulating activity and prostaglandin E1. J Clin Invest 77:1857, 1986

323. Sullivan R, Gans PJ, McCarroll LA: The synthesis and secretion of granulocyte-macrophage colony-stimulating by isolated human monocytes: kinetics of the response to bacterial endotoxin. J Immunol 130:800, 1983

324. Lindemann A, Riedel D, Oster W et al: Granulocyte/macrophage colony-stimulating factor induces interleukin-1 production by human polymorphonuclear neutrophils. J Immunol 140:837, 1988

325. Cannistra SA, Rimbaldi A, Spriggs DR et al: Human granulocyte-macrophage colony-stimulating factor induces expression of the tumor necrosis factor gene by the U937 cell line and by normal human monocytes. J Clin Invest 79:1720, 1987

Molecular Basis of Blood Coagulation

100

Bruce Furie and Barbara C. Furie

INTRODUCTION

Blood coagulation is a host-defense system that maintains the integrity of the high-pressure closed circulatory system. After tissue injury, alterations in the capillary bed and laceration of venules and arterioles lead to extravasation of blood into soft tissues or external bleeding. To prevent excessive blood loss, the hemostatic system, which includes platelets, vascular endothelial cells, and plasma coagulation proteins, is called into play. Immediately after tissue injury, a platelet plug is formed through the processes of platelet adhesion and aggregation. Blood coagulation may be considered a mechanism for rapid replacement of an unstable platelet plug with a chemically stable fibrin clot. A series of interdependent enzyme-mediated reactions translate the molecular signals that initiate blood coagulation into a major biologic event, the formation of the fibrin clot.

In vitro the generation of thrombin and the formation of a fibrin clot propagate through two separate pathways, the intrinsic pathway and the extrinsic pathway.[1,2] To generate a clot via the intrinsic pathway, components intrinsic to whole blood are required. To generate a clot via the extrinsic pathway, components intrinsic to whole blood are required along with an activator, tissue factor, which is extrinsic to blood (Table 100-1). Tissue factor, also known as tissue thromboplastin, is a cell-surface protein that comes in contact with the flowing blood on blood vessel injury.

The intrinsic pathway of blood coagulation includes protein cofactors and enzymes (Fig. 100-1). This pathway is initiated by the activation of factor XII by kallikrein on negatively charged surfaces, including glass in vitro. High-molecular-weight kininogen facilitates this activation. The enzyme form of factor XII, factor XIIa, catalyzes the conversion of factor XI, a proenzyme, to its active enzyme form, factor XIa. In the presence of Ca^{2+}, factor XIa activates the proenzyme factor IX to its enzyme form, factor IXa. Factor IXa binds to the cofactor factor VIIIa bound on membrane surfaces in the presence of calcium ions to generate a complex with enzymatic activity known as tenase. This tenase complex converts the proenzyme factor X to its enzyme form, factor Xa. In a parallel series of interactions, factor Xa binds to the cofactor factor Va, bound on membrane surfaces, in the presence of calcium ions to generate a complex with enzymatic activity known as prothrombinase. This complex converts the proenzyme, prothrombin, to its enzyme form, thrombin. Thrombin acts on fibrinogen to generate the fibrin monomer, which rapidly polymerizes to form the fibrin clot. During laboratory analysis of blood clotting, the intrinsic pathway of blood coagulation is evaluated by using the activated partial thromboplastin time (PTT). The clotting of plasma is initiated by the addition of negatively charged particles such as kaolin.

The extrinsic pathway of blood coagulation also includes protein cofactors and enzymes (Fig. 100-1). This pathway is initiated by the formation of a complex between tissue factor on cell surfaces and factor VIIa. Although the mechanism by which a small amount of factor VII is converted to factor VIIa is unknown, in the absence of ongoing blood clotting, plasma contains factor VIIa at levels of 0.5–8.4 ng/ml.[3] When tissue factor is exposed to plasma following injury, this factor VIIa complexes with tissue factor to form an enzyme complex that activates factor X to factor Xa. In turn, factor Xa can feedback to convert more factor VII to factor VIIa,[4] thus accelerating the rate of activation of the extrinsic pathway. Factor VIIa/tissue factor complex, like the tenase complex, converts factor X to its active form, factor Xa, which binds to the cofactor factor V, bound on membrane surfaces in the presence of calcium ions, to generate the prothrombinase complex. This complex converts prothrombin to thrombin, which converts fibrinogen to fibrin to generate the fibrin clot. During laboratory analysis of blood clotting, the extrinsic pathway of blood coagulation is evaluated by using the prothrombin time. The clotting of plasma is initiated by the addition of exogenous tissue factor.

This scheme of blood clotting (Fig. 100-1) remains invaluable for understanding clot formation in vitro, and specifically for laboratory monitoring of anticoagulation therapy for, and diagnosis of, coagulation disorders. Yet, the physiologic pathways relevant to blood coagulation in vivo are clearly different. A scheme of blood coagulation in vivo must consider the following salient features. First, since patients with hereditary factor XII, prekallikrein or high-molecular-weight kininogen deficiency have a markedly prolonged PTT but no bleeding phenotype, these proteins are not likely to be components required to maintain hemostasis in vivo and should not be included in an in vivo model of blood clotting.[5-7] Second, tissue factor, a normal constituent of the surface of nonvascular cells and of stimulated monocytes and endothelial cells, activates blood coagulation. Third, the tissue factor/factor VIIa complex activates not only factor X but factor IX as well, suggesting a central role for factors VIII and IX in coagulation initiated by the tissue factor pathway.[8] Finally, factor XI deficiency is not invariably associated with a bleeding phenotype; as such, the position and prominence of factor IX in the blood coagulation cascade remains uncertain. Figure 100-2 presents one model of blood coagulation that depicts the pathway of sequential reactions that might lead to clot formation in vivo.[9] The key to the initiation of blood coagulation is tissue factor. The exposure of cell surfaces expressing tissue factor to the plasma proteins leads to the binding of factor VIIa to tissue factor. Either this tissue factor/factor VII complex has low but finite coagulant activity[10] or tissue factor complexed to the activated form of factor VII, factor VIIa, activates factors IX and X.[11] The protease responsible for initial activation of factor VII is unknown, but once clotting is activated, several proteases farther down the pathway can activate factor VII. Factors Xa and VIIa both catalyze the activation of factor VII, so a potential mechanism for acceleration of factor VII activation exists.[12] Furthermore, thrombin and factor XIa in the presence of negatively charged surfaces catalyze the activation of factor XI.[13] Once factor XIa is generated, an additional mechanism augments the activation of factor IX. Factor IXa in complex with factor VIIIa on membrane surfaces activates factor X. Factor Xa in complex with factor Va on membrane surfaces activates prothrombin. Thrombin cleaves fibrinogen, yielding monomeric fibrin, which then polymerizes to form the fibrin clot.

Table 100-1. Properties of the Genes, mRNAs, and Gene Products of the Components of the Blood Coagulation Cascade

	Molecular Weight	Gene (kb)	Chromosome[a]	mRNA	Exons	(kb)	Plasma Concentration (μg/ml)	Function
Prothrombin	72,000	21	11p11–q12	2.1	14		100	Protease zymogen
Factor X	56,000	22	13q34	1.5	8		10	Protease zymogen
Factor IX	56,000	34	q26–27.3	2.8	8		5	Protease zymogen
Factor VII	50,000	13	13q34	2.4	8		0.5	Protease zymogen
Factor VIII	330,000	185	q28	9.0	26		0.1	Cofactor
Factor V	330,000	7.0					10	Cofactor
Factor XI	160,000	23			15		5	Protease zymogen
Factor XII	80,000	12	5	2.4	14		30	Protease zymogen
Fibrinogen	340,000						3,000	Structural
Aα chain	66,000		4q26–q28		5	–		
Bβ chain	52,000		4q26–q28		8	–		
γ-chain	46,000		4q26–q28		9	v		
Protein C	62,000	11		1.8	8		4	Protease zymogen
Protein S	80,000			2.4	25			Cofactor
von Willebrand factor	225,000 × n	175	12pter–p12	8.5	52		10	Adhesion
Tissue factor	37,000	12	1pter–p12	2.1	6		0.0	Cofactor/initiator
Factor XIII								Fibrin stabilization

Abbreviation: n, number of subunits, where the subunit M_r is 225,000.
[a] Chromosomal assignments from Royle et al.[107]
(Adapted from Furie and Furie,[263] with permission.)

The blood coagulation cascade proceeds on cell surface membranes. Indeed, only on the membrane surfaces of stimulated cells can the reactions involved in blood clotting proceed efficiently. Tissue factor is an integral membrane protein of known primary structure found on the surface of nonvascular cells.[14–16] This protein binds to factors VII and VIIa, generating the tissue factor/factor VIIa complex on membrane surfaces that activates factor X.[17] In another example of enzyme assembly on membrane surfaces, factors IXa and VIIIa both bind to phospholipid membranes.[18,19] It is envisioned that these two proteins skate about on the membrane, collide, and form the tenase complex, factor IXa/factor VIIIa. This complex has the enzymatic activity to convert factor X, also bound to the cell membrane, to factor Xa. Similarly, factors Xa and Va bind to phospholipid membranes.[20] These two proteins also skate about on the membrane, collide, and form the "prothrombinase" complex, factor Xa/factor Va.[21] This complex has the enzymatic activity to convert prothrombin, also bound to the cell membrane, to thrombin, which is released from the cell surface. In vivo, platelet membranes contribute the critical surface for blood clotting. Activated (but not resting) platelets express a factor VIIIa binding site.[22] During platelet activation in vitro, small microparticles are released from the platelet membrane that are especially rich in receptors for factors VIIIa and Va.[23,24] However, the physiologic relevance of this phenomenon is unknown.

STRUCTURE OF THE BLOOD COAGULATION PROTEINS

Domain Structure

Each of the blood coagulation proteins contains multiple functional units, derived from common ancestral genes (Fig. 100-3). As a rule these functional units, or domains, are encoded by individual exons. Although the domains are not structurally identical, they have sufficient homology in structure to suggest homology of function as well. These domains are responsible for directing protein trafficking and post-translational processing during biosynthesis and for membrane-binding properties, protein complex formation, and enzyme function of the mature protein. In factor IX, for example, these domains are independently folded but give evidence of significant interdomain interaction.[25]

Signal Peptide

The nascent chains of secreted proteins contain a short domain that permits translocation of the growing polypeptide chain into the endoplasmic reticulum. This domain is dominated by hydrophobic amino acids and is usually about 15–30 residues in length. The blood coagulation proteins found in the plasma are initially synthesized with a signal peptide, which is cleaved within the endoplasmic reticulum.

Propeptide/γ-Carboxyglutamic Acid-Rich Domain

The vitamin K-dependent proteins contain a propeptide domain between the signal peptide and the γ-carboxyglutamic acid-rich N-terminal region. This propeptide, known to be 18 residues long in factor IX[26,27] and 24 residues long in protein C,[28] contains a γ-carboxylation recognition site, which directs γ-carboxylation of the vitamin K-dependent proteins after synthesis.[29] Adjacent to the carboxylation recognition site is the γ-carboxyglutamic acid-rich region of these proteins. Glutamic acid residues within this region serve as substrates for the vitamin K-dependent γ-carboxylase. After carboxylation, the propeptide is cleaved from the mature protein in a late post-translational processing step. A single exon in the vitamin K-dependent proteins encodes the propeptide (including the γ-carboxylation recognition site) and the γ-carboxyglutamic acid-rich region of approximately 40 residues. The γ-carboxyglutamic acid domain of the vitamin K-dependent proteins contains 10–12 γ-carboxyglutamic acid residues and is critical to the Ca^{2+}-binding properties of these proteins. This domain is responsible for promoting the calcium-dependent interaction of these proteins with membrane surfaces, a characteristic essential for the function of these proteins.

The three-dimensional structure of the γ-carboxyglutamic acid-rich region in bovine prothrombin fragment 1 is disordered in the absence of Ca^{2+}.[30] In the presence of Ca^{2+} the

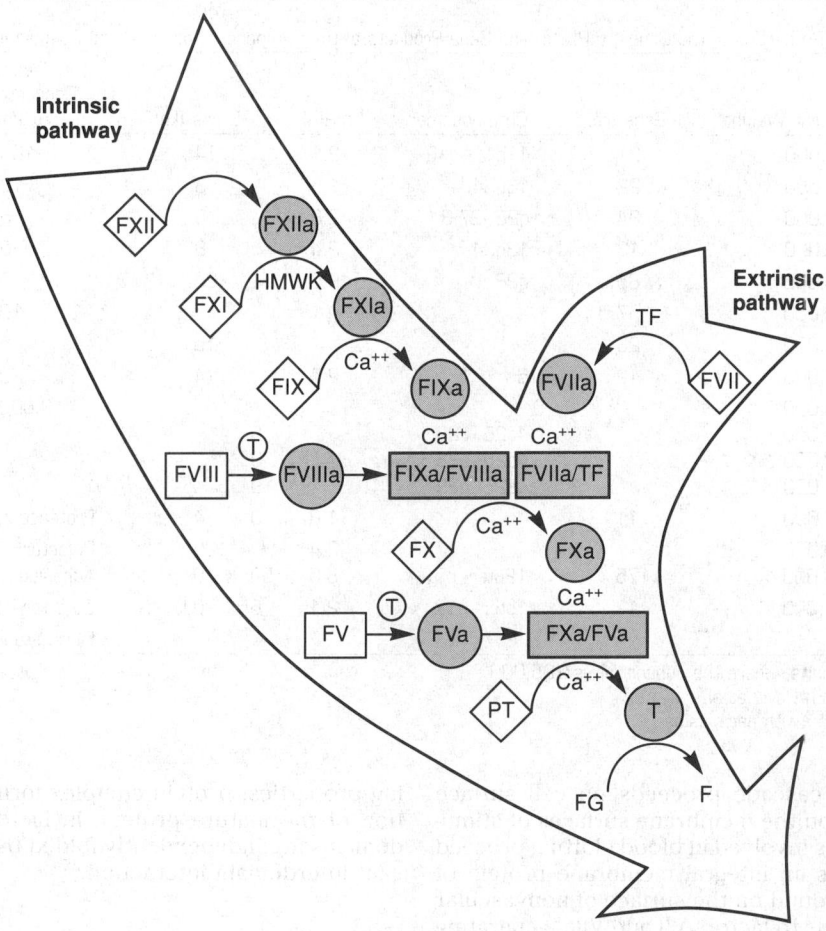

Fig. 100-1. Blood coagulation cascade. Glycoprotein components of the intrinsic pathway include factors XII, XI, IX, VIII, X, and V, prothrombin, and fibrinogen. Glycoprotein components of the extrinsic pathway, initiated by the action of tissue factor located on cell surfaces, include factors VII, X, and V, prothrombin, and fibrinogen. Cascade reactions culminate in the conversion of fibrinogen to fibrin and the formation of a fibrin clot. Certain reactions, including the activation of factor X and prothrombin, take place on membrane surfaces. Proenzymes, diamonds; procofactors, squares; enzymes and cofactors, circles; macromolecular complexes on membrane surfaces, shaded rectangles; FG, fibrinogen; F, fibrin; PT, prothrombin; T, thrombin; TF, tissue factor; HMWK, high-molecular-weight kininogen. (Modified from Furie and Furie,[263] with permission.)

Gla domain assumes a unique structure.[31] Of the 10 γ-carboxy-glutamic acid residues, 4 residues on one side and 2 residues on the other define a carboxylate surface that chelates five Ca^{2+} organized in a linear cluster that extend from one side of the molecule to the other (Fig. 100-4). The NH_2-terminal alanine loops back to form an ion pair with Gla 17, Gla 21 and Gla 27. With the exception of Gla 6, all the γ-carboxyglutamic acid residues are critical for prothrombin function.[32] The mechanism by which this region promotes interaction of the protein with membrane surfaces involves the formation of this unique fold and the expression of a membrane-binding site.

Epidermal Growth Factor Domain

The epidermal growth factor (EGF)-like domain is a common motif found in many proteins, including some of the proteins involved in blood coagulation; in the blood clotting proteins it is highly homologous with the EGF precursor.[33] This domain, about 43–50 amino acid residues in length, contains three disulfide bonds arranged in a characteristic covalent structure. Although the EGF domain in some proteins mediates their interaction with an EGF or EGF-like receptor on cell surfaces, the EGF domains on the blood clotting proteins participate in protein complex formation. A calcium binding site, present in some of the EGF domains of the vitamin K-dependent proteins, is defined by carboxylate groups on aspartic acid.[34] The struc-

tures of the EGF domains of factors IX and X, determined by nuclear magnetic resonance spectroscopy, demonstrate marked homology to the three-dimensional structure of EGF.[35,36] Factors IX, X, and VII contain two adjacent EGF domains (as does protein C, while protein S has four EGF domains). Factor XII contains two nonadjacent EGF domains, while tissue plasminogen activator (t-PA) and prourokinase each have a single EGF domain.

Kringle Domain

Another common motif in proteins is the kringle domain. This region, with a characteristic covalent structure defined by a pattern of three disulfide bonds, is about 100 amino acid residues in length. The three-dimensional structure of the prothrombin kringles reveals an oblate ellipsoid, with folding defined by close contacts between the sulfur atoms of two of the disulfide bridges.[30] Internal structures are well conserved among kringles from various proteins, but molecular surface differences relate to differences in function. The kringle domains play a role in protein complex formation. In prothrombin, kringles play no role in membrane binding,[37] but rather the second kringle domain interacts with factor Va in the prothrombinase complex.[38] Kringles are found in prothrombin,[39] factor XII,[40] plasminogen,[41] prourokinase,[42] and t-PA[43] among the proteins involved in hemostasis.

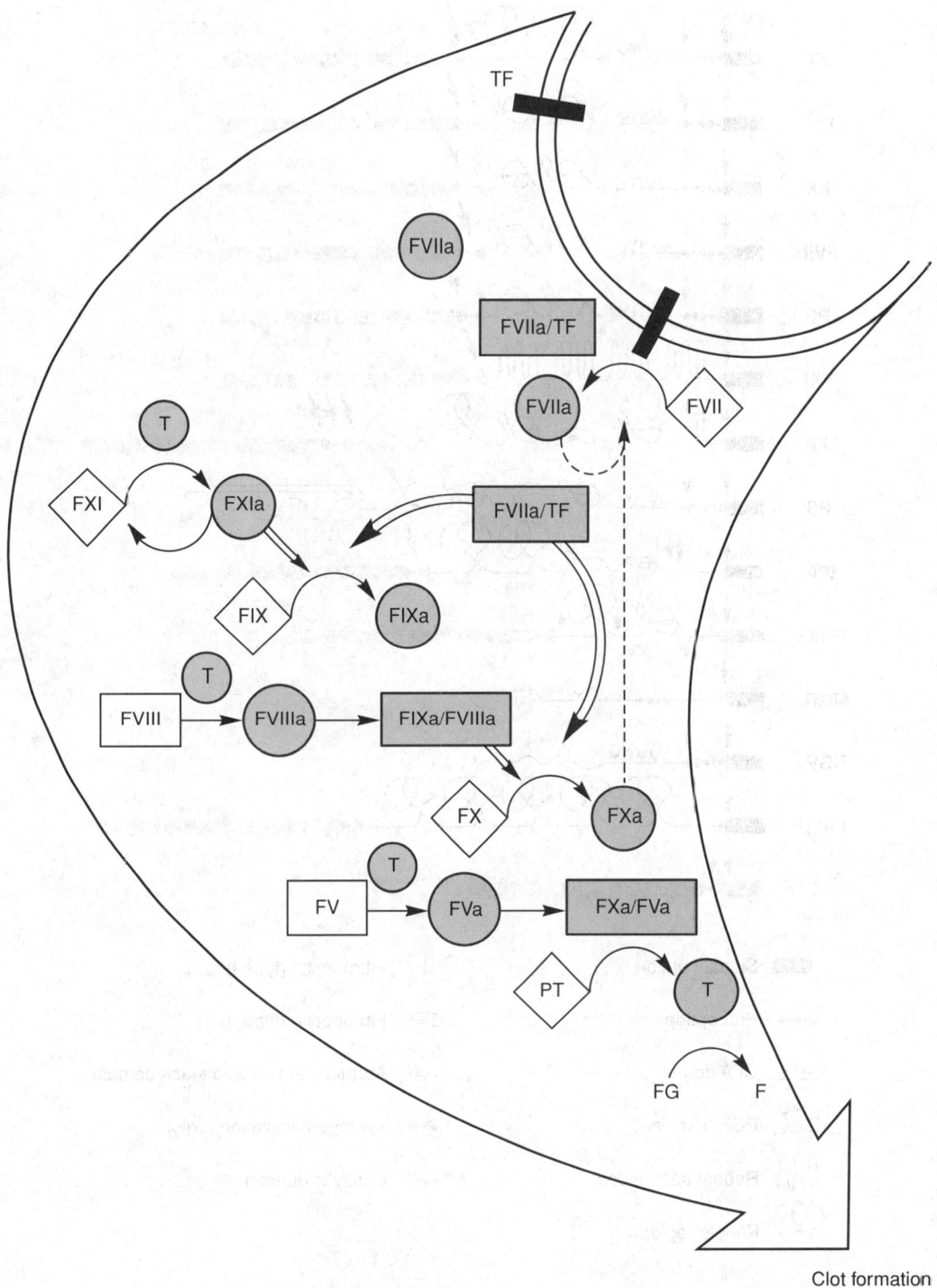

Fig. 100-2. Physiologic pathways of blood coagulation. Blood coagulation is initiated by tissue factor (TF) expressed on cell surfaces. When plasma comes in contact with tissue factor, factor VIIa in plasma binds to this receptor. The factor VIIa/tissue factor complex activates both factor IX and factor X. The proteolytic activation of factor VII to VIIa, factor XI to XIa, factor VIII to VIIIa, and factor V to Va through feedback mechanisms (e.g., thrombin, T or factor XIa) greatly accelerate the rate of blood clotting. The process culminates with the generation of fibrin and its polymerization to form a fibrin clot. (Modified from Furie and Furie,[9] with permission.)

Catalytic Domain

A catalytic domain, highly homologous with the structure of trypsin and chymotrypsin, is common to all the blood-clotting enzymes. This domain includes a site for the conversion of an inactive proenzyme to an active enzyme via cleavage of peptide bonds, a process known as zymogen activation by limited proteolysis. Furthermore, this domain contains the enzymatic ma-

chinery for cleavage of peptide bonds, the specific recognition site for macromolecular substrates, and the site for interaction with specific protein inhibitors that regulate enzymatic activity. The blood-clotting proteases are serine proteases, a class of enzymes with a common mechanism of enzymatic action that requires the catalytic triad of serine, aspartic acid, and histidine within the active site. The catalytic domain of the

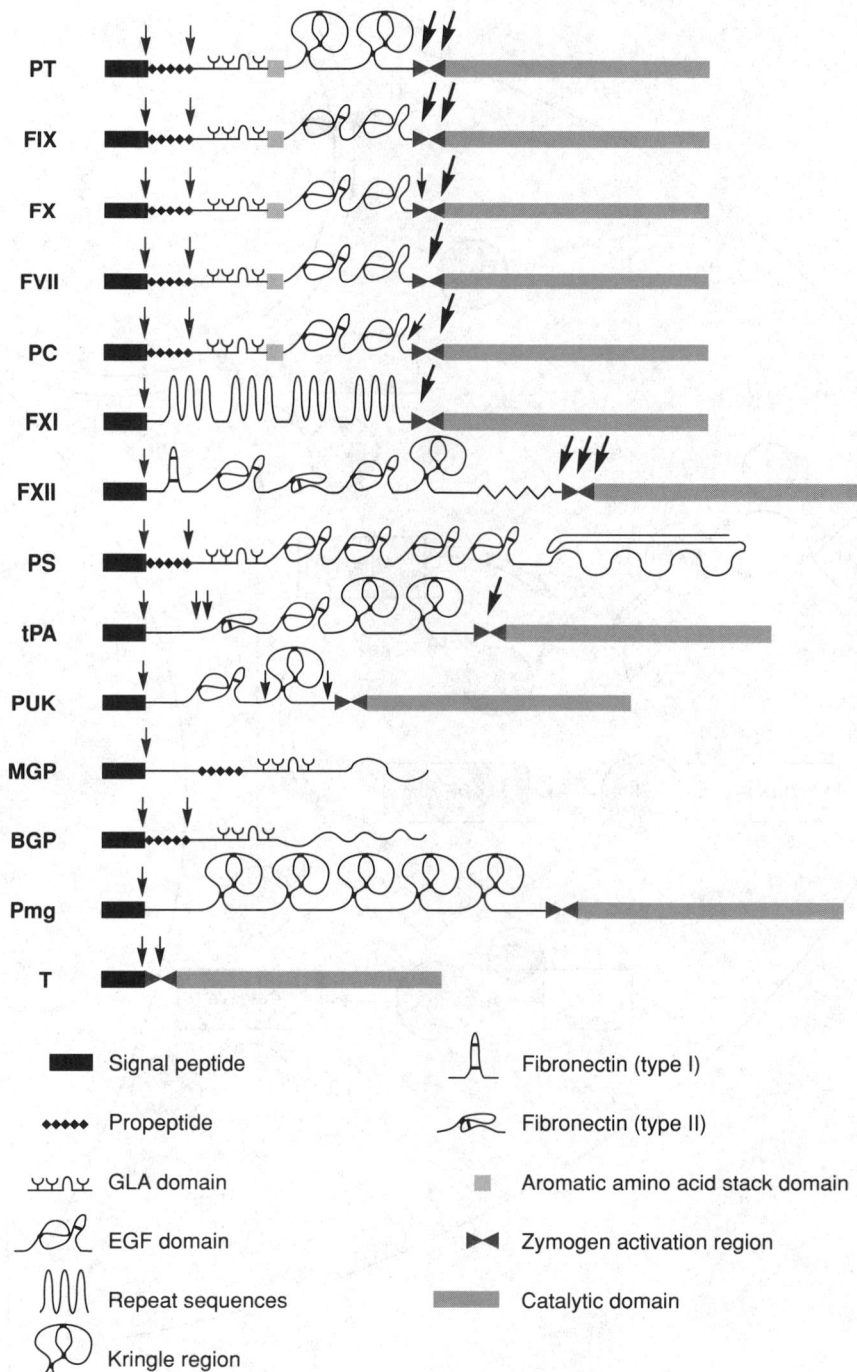

Fig. 100-3. Structural domains of the proteins involved in hemostasis and related proteins. Domains, identified in the key, include signal peptide, propeptide, Gla domain, epidermal growth factor (EGF) domain, repeat sequences, kringle region, fibronectin (type I and II) domains, aromatic amino acid stack, zymogen activation region, and catalytic domain. Sites of proteolytic cleavage associated with synthesis of mature protein are indicated by thin arrows and those associated with zymogen activation by thick arrows. PT, prothrombin[264]; FIX, factor IX[265,266]; FX, factor X[82,94]; FVII, factor VII[99]; PC, protein C[26768]; FXI, factor XI[53]; FXII, factor XII[47,48]; PS, protein S[269]; tPA, tissue plasminogen activator[43]; PUK, prourokinase[42]; MGP, matrix Gla protein[270]; BGP, bone Gla protein[168]; Pmg, plasminogen[41]; T, trypsin. (Modified from Furie and Furie,[263] with permission.)

blood-clotting proteases has an active site and an internal core nearly identical to that of trypsin.[44] The molecular surfaces surrounding the enzyme active site are likely responsible for defining the extended substrate binding site of the enzyme. Indeed, solution of the crystal structure of human α-thrombin has emphasized the structural homology between thrombin and other well-characterized serine proteases, while simultane-

ously providing details of the molecular structure not available from models derived indirectly from other homologous structures.[45] Two patches of positively charged amino acids close to the C-terminal B-chain helix form the presumed heparin binding site and a secondary fibrinogen binding site.[46] The interaction of the A and B chains is stabilized by charged residues. A deep canyon-like active site cleft probably contributes

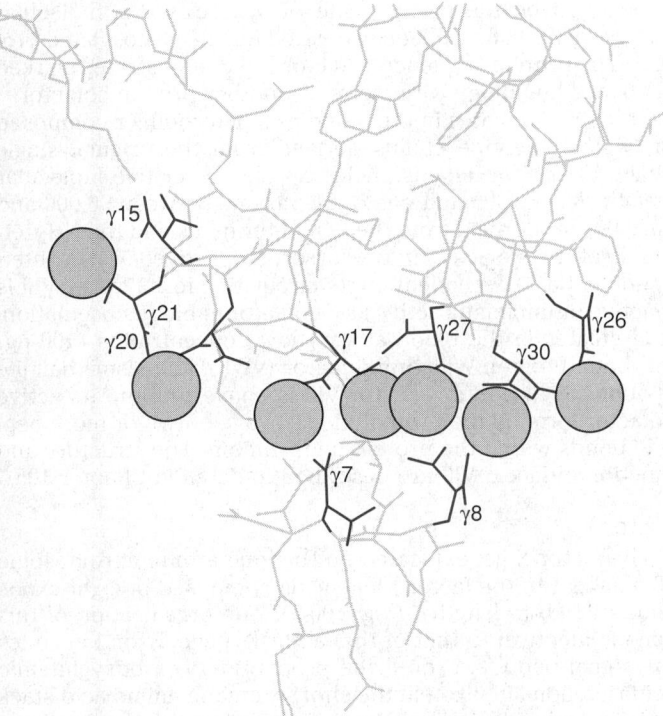

Fig. 100-4. Three-dimensional structure of the γ-carboxyglutamic acid-rich region of prothrombin. This region is responsible for metal binding and membrane-protein interaction. (Modified from Soriano-Garcia et al,[31] with permission.)

significantly to the narrow substrate specificity of thrombin.[45,46]

Other Domains

Other motifs that appear within the proteins involved in hemostasis include the aromatic amino acid stack domain, the repeat regions observed in factor XI and, the fibronectin type I and type II domains. The functions of these domains are unknown.

Components of the Intrinsic and Extrinsic Pathways

Factor XII

The factor XII gene, located on chromosome 5, contains 14 exons and 13 introns[40,47] (Fig. 100-5). Exon I encodes the signal peptide, exon II encodes a segment with no structural homology with other proteins, exons III and IV code for a region homologous with the type II fibronectin structure, exons V and VII each encode EGF domains, exon VI encodes a fibronectin finger domain that intervenes between the EGF domains, and exons VIII and IX each encode a kringle domain. The trypsin-like catalytic domain, including the activation region, is encoded by the remaining exons X–XIV. The gene organization of the catalytic domains parallels that of urokinase, factor XI, and t-PA. The factor XII mRNA is 2.4 kb in length.[47,48] The mature, plasma form of factor XII is composed of 596 amino acids residues in a single polypeptide chain.[40,48]

Factor XII, also known as Hageman factor, is the first component of the intrinsic pathway. As such, it is a component of the contact phase of activation of blood coagulation observed in vitro. This protein does not appear to have a physiologic role in blood coagulation in vivo, as patients lacking this protein do not have a bleeding disorder. The protein circulates in the blood as a single-chain proenzyme of 80,000 molecular weight.[49,50] Factor XII is a glycoprotein, with carbohydrate attached to Asn 230 and Asn 414. Other glycosylation sites include Thr 280, 286, 309, 310, and 318 and Ser 289. The surface binding properties of factor XII, specifically the enhancement of the rate of factor XII activation by negatively charged surfaces, may be mediated by the positively charged amino acid sequence His-Lys-Tyr-Lys, a structure common to factor XII and kininogen.[51] The factor XII concentration in plasma is about 30 μg/ml. Factor XII has a plasma half-life of 2 days.[52]

Factor XI

The gene for factor XI, an intrinsic pathway component, contains 15 exons and 14 intervening sequences[53] (Fig. 100-5). Exon I encodes a 5′ untranslated sequence, while exon 2 encodes a signal peptide. Four repeat sequences are each encoded by two exons: repeat 1 by exons III and IV, repeat 2 by exons V and VI, repeat 3 by exons VII and VIII, and repeat 4 by exons IX

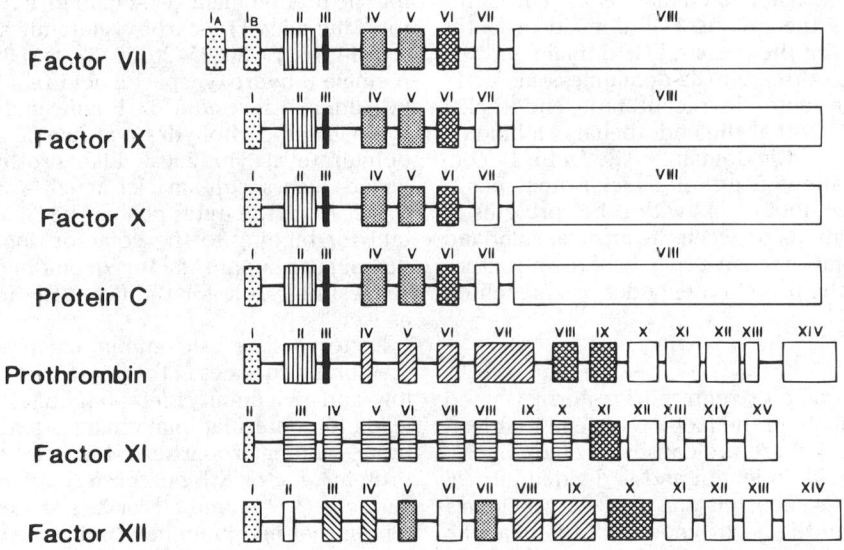

Fig. 100-5. Gene structures among the blood coagulation and regulatory serine proteases. Exons are shown schematically according to scale. Introns (thin lines) are not drawn to scale. Exon codes for most of the individual domains shown in the key for Figure 100-3. (Modified from Furie and Furie,[263] with permission.)

and X. The trypsin-like domain, responsible for the proteolytic function of the enzyme form of the zymogen, is encoded by exons XII–XV. Factor XI has a 160,000 molecular weight[54] and is composed of two identical chains bound together by disulfide bonds.[55] Factor XI circulates in the blood at a concentration of 5 μg/ml. Its biologic half-life is about 3 days.[56,57]

Factor IX

Factor IX plays a critical role in blood coagulation (see Ch. 107). Its gene, adjacent to the factor VIII gene, is located on the X chromosome. Defects in this gene, both major and minor, are the cause of hemophilia B (see Ch. 107). This gene is 34 kb in length, contains eight exons, [58] and has a structure that is highly homologous with the structures of factors VII and X and protein C genes (Fig. 100-5). These genes are sufficiently similar to suggest that they were derived ancestrally from a common related gene. Factor IX is encoded on a 2.8-kb mRNA transcript. The factor IX gene is regulated by a liver-specific cis-activating element that binds to the liver-specific transcription factors CCAAT enhancer-binding protein (NF1-L); the NF1-L binding site is located at -99 to -76 upstream of the transcriptional start site.[59] The EBP binding site is located close to the transcription initiation site. An androgen responsive promoter element in the factor IX gene explains the curious phenotype of factor IX Leyden[60] (see Ch. 107).

The mature protein, with a molecular weight of 56,000, requires vitamin K for its synthesis and contains 12 γ-carboxyglutamic acid residues. The fully carboxylated form of the protein binds to metal ions and to membrane surfaces in the presence of metal ions. Factor IX contains two classes of metal-binding sites, defined by γ-carboxyglutamic acid,[61] and a third class, which is a component of the EGF domain.[62,63] The site within the EGF domain is defined in part by Asp 64, a residue that is partially β-hydroxylated. Factor IX is a glycoprotein contain N- and O-linked sugars. A tetrasaccharide is O-linked to Ser 61 through a fucose.[64] Factors IX and IXa bind to phospholipid membranes composed of phosphatidylserine-phosphatidylcholine.[19,65] This interaction requires both Ca^{2+} and fully carboxylated factor IX.[65] The expression of phospholipid-binding properties involves two metal-dependent conformational transitions.[65] Factors IX and IXa bind to activated platelets but not to resting platelets.[66,67] However, it is not known whether a receptor is present on the platelet surface or the role played by surface phospholipid. Factor IXa, but not factor IX, binds to factor VIIIa on the surface of activated platelets.[68] The factor VIIIa binding site requires the second EGF domain of factor IXa[69] and includes regions of the second EGF domain and the serine protease domain.[70] Although Gla-domainless factor IX was thought to bind to a factor IX receptor on endothelial cells,[71] it appears more likely that the endothelial cell binding site of factor IX resides in the Gla domain.[72] The factor IX concentration in plasma is about 5 μg/ml. This protein has a plasma half-life of about 24 hours.[73] As with other proteins of this molecular size, it partitions between the intravascular and extravascular space. A comprehensive review of the structure of the factor IX gene and the protein it encodes are presented in Chapter 107.

Factor VIII

Factor VIII is a critical cofactor required for normal blood clotting (see Ch. 105). Defects in the factor VIII gene that lead to the deficiency of factor VIII are the cause of hemophilia A. The factor VIII gene is 186 kb in length and is divided into 26 exons[74,75] (see Fig. 105-1). As such, it is one of the largest genes yet discovered. Located on the X chromosome, it is near the locus of the factor IX gene. Factor VIII is synthesized as a single polypeptide chain, including a 19-residue signal peptide; in its mature form, it contains 2,332 amino acid residues.[74,75] Although this factor is synthesized by many cell types, the liver

appears to be the primary site of synthesis.[76] A molecular weight of 330,000 has been estimated for the glycosylated protein. The protein sequence of factor VIII demonstrates marked sequence homology with factor V, another protein cofactor.[77] Factor VIII circulates in the blood as a heterodimer composed of two polypeptide chains derived from the original single chain. These two chains, including one of relative molecular weight (M_r) 80,000 and one of M_r varying between 90,000 and 200,000, are derived from the COOH-terminus and the NH_2-terminus of the single-chain precursor, respectively. Their interaction is Ca^{2+} dependent. In its circulating form, factor VIII is inactive or minimally active as a cofactor in blood coagulation. It circulates in the blood at very low concentration (100 ng/ml) bound to von Willebrand factor (vWF). Its plasma half-life is about 8–12 hours.[78] Factor VIII is converted into its active cofactor form by the proteolytic cleavage of two or more peptide bonds within the protein by thrombin. The structure and function of factor VIII are described in detail in Chapter 105.

Factor X

The factor X gene, located on the long arm of chromosome 13 adjacent to the factor VII gene, is composed of eight exons and is 22 kb in length[79] (Fig. 100-5). The organization of this gene is identical to that of the factor IX gene. Exon I encodes the signal peptide, exon II the propeptide/γ-carboxyglutamic acid-rich domain, exon III the short aromatic amino acid stack domain, exons IV and V the two EGF domains, exon VI the activation region, and exons VII and VIII the catalytic domain. The 5′ end of the factor X gene is linked to the 3′ end of the factor VII gene.[80] A liver-specific promotor element, FXP1 binding site, was located to -63 to -42 bp upstream of the factor X gene, while other promotor elements, FXP2 and FXP3, span -215 to -149 and from -457 to -351, respectively.[80] After transcription, the factor X mRNA of about 1.5 kb includes a short 3′ untranslated region following the stop codon.[81,82] The polyadenylation signal is located within the 3′ end of the coding sequence. Factor X, with a molecular weight of 56,000, is synthesized as a single polypeptide chain.[79,82] However, factor X as isolated from plasma is composed of two polypeptide chains, a heavy chain with a molecular weight of 38,000[83,84,85] and a light chain with an molecular weight of 18,000.[86,87] These chains are linked by a single disulfide bond. The Arg-Lys-Arg sequence at residues 139–141 in the single polypeptide chain appears very susceptible to intracellular or extracellular proteolysis, yielding the predominant two-chain form.[79,82] The light chain of factor X includes 11 γ-carboxyglutamic acid residues at positions 6, 7, 14, 16, 19, 20, 25, 26, 29, 32, and 39 in the human protein.[88] A single β-hydroxyaspartic acid residue is located in the first EGF domain at residue 63. Bovine factor X contains both asparagine-linked carbohydrate at Asn 36 and threonine-linked carbohydrate at Thr 300.[89] Like prothrombin, the asparagine-linked sugars contain NeuAcα2 → 3Galβ1 → 3(NeuAcα2 → 6)GlcNAc in the outer chain. The two EGF domains are important for binding to the cofactor, factor Va. The second EGF domain can support factor Va binding but at reduced affinity,[70] suggesting a role for the first EGF domain in this interaction as well.[90]

Factor X is a calcium-binding protein that interacts with membrane surfaces in the presence of calcium. It contains both low- and high-affinity metal-binding sites,[91] occupancy of which leads to conformational changes and the expression of membrane-binding properties.[92] Like the other vitamin K-dependent proteins, factor X binds preferentially to acidic phospholipid surfaces.[93-95] Bound factor X is an "extrinsic" membrane protein in that no component of it is embedded within the membrane.

The plasma concentration of factor X is maintained at about 10 μg/ml. Its half-life in plasma is about 36 hours.[73] Coagulopoietin X, an activity identified in plasma rendered deficient in factor X, may play a role in the regulation of the plasma concentration of this factor.[96] However, as with the other plasma clotting proteins, the molecular basis of the control of factor X plasma levels is unknown.

Factor VII

The factor VII gene is 13 kb in length[97] and is located on the long arm of chromosome 13, immediately adjacent to the factor X gene.[98] The coding region is found on nine separate exons (Fig. 100-5). Pre-profactor VII is synthesized via two alternate forms. In one form, incorporating exon IB encoding for the signal peptide, factor VII arises from a gene whose gene organization is identical to the factor IX gene. In a second form, exon IA directs the coding of the signal peptide instead of exon IB. In this form, the pre-profactor VII has a polypeptide extension of the NH$_2$-terminus that elongates the signal peptide/propeptide from 38 to 60 residues. Exon II encodes the propeptide and γ-carboxyglutamic acid-carboxyglutamic acid-rich domain, and exon III encodes the short aromatic amino acid stack domain, a segment common to all the vitamin K-dependent proteins. Exons IV and V each encode one of the EGF domains. The catalytic domain is coded by exons VI–VIII, with the activation peptide encoded within exon VI. The mRNA for factor VII is about 2.4 kb in length,[99] with a 3′ untranslated region of 1.0-kb length and a poly(A) tail located after the stop codon.

Factor VII is a component of the extrinsic pathway of blood coagulation and forms a complex with tissue factor to generate an enzyme complex that activates factor X. Human factor VII, with a molecular weight of 50,000, circulates in plasma as a single chain zymogen containing 406 amino acid residues.[99] The NH$_2$-terminal domain includes 11 γ-carboxyglutamic acid residues at positions 6, 7, 14, 16, 19, 20, 25, 26, 29, 34, and 35 in bovine factor VII.[100] Asp 63 is partially β-hydroxylated. Factor VII is a glycoprotein, containing 13% carbohydrate.

In contrast to other proenzymes involved in blood coagulation, factor VII circulates in the blood in two forms: the inactive zymogen factor VII and the enzymatic active factor VIIa.[3] Recent information suggests that factor VII may be a true zymogen, with no enzymatic activity prior to cleavage.[101] The concentration of factor VIIa is low but sufficient to generate significant factor X-activating activity when the factor VIIa forms a complex with newly exposed tissue factor. The factor Xa formed can activate factor VII to factor VIIa, increasing the amount of factor VIIa available during tissue injury. This model would allow significant amplication of thrombin formation via the extrinsic pathway.

Factor V

Factor V is a plasma glycoprotein with a molecular weight of 330,000. This protein is a critical cofactor, which in its activated form facilitates activation of prothrombin by factor Xa. Factor V is a single-chain protein that circulates in the blood in a precursor, inactive cofactor form. The factor V gene, which has not been described, encodes a 7-kb mRNA, which itself encodes a pre-factor V including a 28-amino acid residue signal peptide and a mature protein composed of 2,196 amino acids residues.[102,103] The heavy chain region is composed of two domains with notable structural homology, termed the A domain. The light chain region is composed of another A domain and of two homologous C domains. The heavy chain region and light chain region are joined by a connecting region known as the B domain. The A1-A2-B-A3-Cl-C2 domain structure is also present in factor VIII.[77]

Although the liver appears to be the primary site of synthesis of factor V, megakaryocytes also synthesize this protein. In addition to its presence in plasma, factor V is a component of the α-granules in megakaryocytes and subsequently in plate-

lets[104] and is secreted on platelet stimulation with specific agonists. Factors V and Va bind to two classes of binding sites on the surface of platelets.[105] However, the higher-affinity binding sites interact specifically with factor Va, and not with factor V. The plasma concentration of factor V is 10 μg/ml, and its plasma half-life is about 12 hours.[106]

Prothrombin

The prothrombin gene, located on chromosome 11,[107] is 21 kb in length, and is composed of 14 exons, each encoding all or part of a functional domain of prothrombin[108] (Fig. 100-5): signal peptide (exon I), propeptide/γ-carboxyglutamic acid-rich domain (exon II), aromatic amino acid stack domain (exon III), two kringle domains (exons IV–VII), the activation region (exons VIII and IX), and the catalytic domain (exons X–XIV). The introns vary considerably in size, from 84 bp for the intron between exons VIII and IX to 9,447 bp for that between exons XII and XIII. Although the structure of prothrombin is homologous with those of factors IX, X, and VII and protein C, the prothrombin gene demonstrates only partial homology with the genes of these proteins. Exons I–III are shared by all these proteins, but prothrombin contains exons IV–VII encoding the kringle domains and has a homologous serine protease domain composed of seven exons, in contrast to the two exons found in the factor IX gene family. The prothrombin mRNA is 2.1 kb in length and includes a 5′ untranslated region >150 bp, a 1.8-kb open reading frame, and a 97-bp 3′ untranslated region. The prothrombin gene contains a weak promoter before the transcription initiation site and liver-specific enhancer element spanning about 900 bases upstream from the transcription initiation site. This site interacts with hepatic nuclear factor-1 (HNF-1).[109,110]

Prothrombin is a plasma glycoprotein with a molecular weight of 72,000.[39,111,112] On the basis of direct protein sequence analysis and the predicted sequence based on the nucleotide sequence of the cDNA, the complete amino acid sequence of the human protein is known.[108,111,112] As with all the blood-clotting proteins, prothrombin is synthesized with a hydrophobic signal peptide from residues −43 to −19. After translocation to the rough endoplasmic reticulum, the signal peptide is removed by a signal peptidase. The propeptide, containing the γ-carboxylation recognition site,[29] includes residues −18 to −1. During protein synthesis, but after γ-carboxyglutamic acid carboxylation, this peptide is removed by an intracellular propeptidase. The mature prothrombin that circulates in the plasma is composed of 579 amino acid residues arranged in a single polypeptide chain. The 10 γ-carboxyglutamic acid residues are located in the Gla domain of human prothrombin at residues 6, 7, 14, 16, 19, 20, 25, 26, 29, and 32. Carbohydrate represents about 10% of the mass of prothrombin. *N*-Asparagine-linked carboyhydrate is attached to Asn 78, Asn 100, and Asn 373 in bovine prothrombin,[113] and human prothrombin likely contains carbohydrate at the homologous amino acids. Complex asparagine-linked oligosaccharides include NeuAcα2 → 3Galβ1 → 3(NeuAcα2 → 6)GlcNAc. The short aromatic amino acid stack domain has significant α-helical structure and serves to link the Gla domain to two kringle domains,[30] which are similar to structures found in factor XII, plasminogen, and t-PA and are defined structurally by the pattern of disulfide bonds. The function of these domains is uncertain, but they may be important for protein complex formation with factor Va. The remainder of prothrombin, accounting for approximately one-half the protein structure, represents the catalytic domain. This region includes the activation domain that is critical for the conversion of the zymogen into the active enzyme and the trypsin-like region that possesses the protease activity. Prothrombin has no coagulant activity in its zymogen form and must be converted to thrombin in order to participate in blood coagulation.

The metal-binding properties of prothrombin are conferred by γ-carboxyglutamic acid residues.[114] Abnormal (des-γ—carboxy) prothrombin, lacking γ-carboxyglutamic acid, does not bind to Ca^{2+} and does not interact with membrane surfaces in the presence of calcium.[115,114] Prothrombin binds Ca^{2+} and other metal ions via two classes of metal binding sites[116–119] and, on metal binding, undergoes conformational changes leading to expression of membrane-binding properties.[120–122] Concomitantly, neoantigens are exposed on the metal-stabilized conformers of prothrombin.[123–126] Prothrombin is an extrinsic membrane-binding protein. In the presence of calcium ions, a surface of the prothrombin-metal complex interacts with phospholipid vesicles; a marked preference for acidic phospholipids, specifically phosphatidylserine, has been demonstrated. The N-terminal third of the protein contains the lipid-binding domain.

The plasma concentration of prothrombin is about 100 μg/ml,[127,128] and the plasma half-life of prothrombin is about 3 days.[73,129]

Fibrinogen

Fibrinogen is the most abundant plasma protein involved in blood coagulation. At a plasma concentration of 2–3 mg/ml, it represents about 2% of the total plasma proteins. In addition, platelets contain fibrinogen within their α-granules, but they do not synthesize the protein.[130,131] Although platelet fibrinogen differs structurally and functionally from plasma fibrinogen, both forms are derived from the same genes.[132] Thus, these variant forms likely arise via post-translational modifications or protein degradation. Fibrinogen, unique among the blood-clotting proteins, is encoded by three separate genes, each of which encodes one of the three subunits. These three genes, located on chromosome 4, are clustered on a 50-kb region.[133] The fibrinogen genes are organized with the α-chain gene 10 kb upstream of the γ-chain gene, which in turn is 13 kb upstream of the β-chain gene. The α-, γ-, and β-chain genes contain nine, five, and eight exons, respectively. The regulation of these genes is coordinated at the transcriptional level by the synchronous production of three separate mRNA species.[134]

Fibrinogen is a structural protein that circulates in the plasma in a functionally inert precursor form. Its conversion to fibrin leads to polymerization of fibrin and to formation of a fibrin clot. Human fibrinogen, with a molecular weight of about 340,000, is composed of three pairs of polypeptide chains: two Aα chains, two Bβ chains, and two γ-chains.[135] The α-, β-, and γ-chains demonstrate significant structural homology within their amino acid sequence, suggesting their evolutionary origin from a common ancestral gene.[136–138] The Aα chain has a molecular weight of 63,500 and contains 610 amino acid residues, the Bβ chain has a molecular weight of 56,000 and contains 461 amino acid residues, and the γ-chain has a molecular weight of 47,000 and contains 411 amino acid residues. The Aα, Bβ, and γ-chains are covalently linked through disulfide bonds. The disulfide bonds near the N-terminal regions of these polypeptide chains link the three chains to each other, as well as linking the two Aα chains together and the two γ-chains together. This region is known as the disulfide knot. Electron micrographs of fibrinogen show a trinodular molecule.[139] The plasma half-life of fibrinogen is about 3–5 days.[140,141]

Factor XIII

Factor XIII is a zymogen of a cyteine transglutaminase that circulates in the blood. It is composed of two peptide subunits, the α-chain (M_r 75,000) and the β-chain (M_r 80,000).[142] Factor XIII, with a molecular weight of 320,000, is a tetrameric structure with two α-chains and two β-chains held together noncovalently. After binding to Ca^{2+},[143] factor XIII ($α_2β_2$) is activated to its enzyme form, factor XIIIa ($α_2'β_2$), by thrombin through cleavage of the bond between Arg 37 and Gly 38 in the α-chain, thus releasing an activation peptide with a molecular weight of 4,500. Factor XIIIa contains a free sulfhydryl group at the active site on the α-chain and functions as a transamidase in cross-linking glutamic acids and lysine residues. The concentration of factor XIII in plasma is about 60 μg/ml. Platelet factor XIII is composed of only α-chains in the form of a dimer, $α_2$. Enzymatically, the platelet and plasma form of factor XIIIa are equivalent.

Tissue Factor

Tissue factor is an integral membrane protein with a molecular weight of about 45,000, which is located on the plasma membrane of most vascular cells.[144,145] This protein, a receptor for factor VII, is required for the initiation of blood coagulation through the extrinsic pathway. Factor VII binding to tissue factor is calcium dependent. Tissue factor is a transmembrane protein composed of 263 amino acid residues.[15,16] A short hydrophobic domain of 23 amino acids likely represents the membrane-spanning region (Fig. 100-6). The N-terminal domain of 219 amino acid residues is a dominant component of the protein and is oriented extracellularly. A short 21-residue C-terminal cytoplasmic domain contains palmitate and stearate bound through a thioester bond to a cysteine residue.[146] Although specific glycosylation sites have not been established, tissue factor has multiple potential N- and O-linked sites. Tissue factor is expressed constitutively in most nonvascular cells; in monocytes and endothelial cells, its expression is associated with cell stimulation.[147–149] The tissue factor gene is 12.4 kb in length and is composed of six exons.[150]

von Willebrand Factor

A multimeric glycoprotein, vWF is present in the plasma and within the α-granules of platelets and the Weibel-Palade bodies of endothelial cells (see Ch. 112). The gene for vWF is located on chromosome 12 and is about 176 kb in length.[151] The gene includes 52 exons that encode a signal peptide, a large propolypeptide (M_r 80,000), and the mature vWF monomer (M_r 225,000).[152] A 9-kb mRNA encodes a precursor form of the protein, synthesized as a single polypeptide chain containing 2,813 amino acid residues.[152–155] Pro-vWF undergoes post-translational modification involving initial formation of dimers, which then undergo multimerization via a process that is dependent on the presence of the intact propeptide.[156,157] The high-molecular-weight vWF multimers vary in size up to about 10 million, the largest forms displaying the most potent biologic activity.

Two critical biologic roles are fulfilled by vWF. First, it can mediate platelet aggregation and the adhesion of platelets to the injured vascular wall. Adhesion occurs through simultaneous binding of vWf to its receptor, glycoprotein Ib, on platelet surfaces and to collagen in the subendothelium. In addition to being constitutively secreted from endothelial cells, vWF is stored in the Weibel-Palade bodies of endothelial cells and released on stimulation of granule release.[158] As a plasma carrier protein, vWF binds noncovalently to and stabilize factor VIII and circulates in the blood as a factor VIII/vWF complex. Factor VIII binds stoichiometrically to the vWF subunit.[159] Under physiologic conditions, however, most of the factor VIII binding sites on mature vWf are unoccupied.

SYNTHESIS OF THE BLOOD COAGULATION PROTEINS
Biosynthesis of the Vitamin K-Dependent Blood Clotting Proteins

Six of the plasma proteins involved in blood coagulation or the regulation of blood coagulation (including prothrombin, factors IX, X, and VII, protein C, and protein S) require vitamin

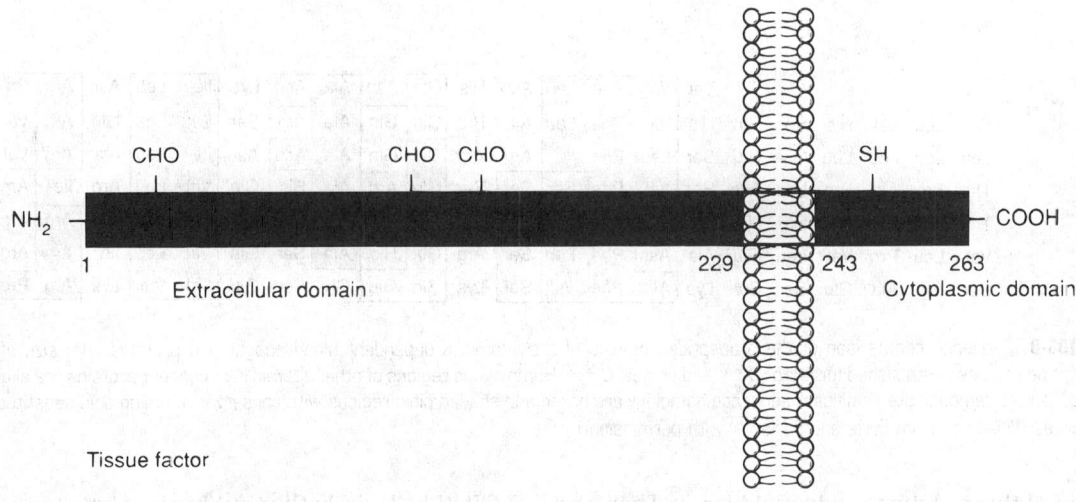

Fig. 100-6. Structure of tissue factor. Extracellular domain extends from residues 1–229. This region contains three potential glycosylation sites (CHO). A short transmembrane domain is rich in hydrophobic amino acids. Cytoplasmic domain, from residues 243–263, contains a free sulfhydryl (SH) group, which undergoes esterification to palmitate or stearate.

K for their synthesis. These proteins contain between 10 and 12 residues of γ-carboxyglutamic acid[160,161] within the first 45 residues of their NH$_2$-termini (Fig. 100-7). They represent a unique class of calcium-binding proteins, which assemble on membrane surfaces in the presence of Ca^{2+}. These proteins are synthesized in a precursor form, which includes a typical signal peptide and a propeptide that intervenes between the signal sequence and the mature NH$_2$-terminus of the protein. Following translocation through the rough endoplasmic reticulum, specific glutamic acid residues in the prozymogen are selectively γ-carboxylated.

Vitamin K-dependent carboxylation is catalyzed by a membrane-bound γ-carboxylase located in the endoplasmic reticulum. In the presence of reduced vitamin K, molecular oxygen, carbon dioxide, and the protein precursor substrate, specific glutamic acids adjacent to the γ-carboxylation recognition site on the propeptide are converted to the corresponding γ-carboxyglutamic acids. A synthetic peptide whose sequence was based on the γ-carboxylation recognition site within the propeptide of prothrombin binds to the carboxylase, offering a strategy for purification of the carboxylase by affinity chromatography.[162] A highly purified carboxylase was obtained by this strategy using the propeptide of factor IX.[163] These enzyme preparations catalyze both the formation of γ-carboxyglutamic acid from glutamic acid and vitamin K epoxide from vitamin

K, which indicates the coupling of these two processes[162,164] (see Ch. 114). The vitamin K-dependent carboxylase is a single-chain protein with a molecular weight of 94,000 composed of a single polypeptide chain of 758 amino acids.[163,165,166] The carboxylase can be expressed in insect cells otherwise lacking carboxylase activity.[167]

The propeptide within the vitamin K-dependent proteins directs γ-carboxylation. This region demonstrates sequence homology among proteins that contain γ-carboxyglutamic acid[168,169] (Fig. 100-8), an observation that has suggested a role for the propeptide in carboxylation. Site-specific mutagenesis has shown that factor IX species lacking the 18-residue propeptide or containing point mutations at conserved residues, -16 or -10, within the propeptide eliminate γ-carboxylation.[29,170] Analogous studies of prothrombin have demonstrated the importance of amino acids at residues -18, -17, -15, and -10 in the propeptide of prothrombin. Deletion mutants of proprotein C lacking residues in the -17 to -12 portion of the propeptide were also associated with impaired γ-carboxylation.[171] These results demonstrate that the propeptide contains a recognition element, termed the γ-carboxylation recognition site, which designates the vitamin K-dependent proteins for γ-carboxylation. This propeptide is required for carboxylation. Furthermore, expression of a cDNA construct in which the propeptide is adjacent to a glutamic acid-rich region of thrombin leads

Residue Number		5		10		15		20		25		30		35		40	
Human prothrombin	A N T - F L γ γ V R K G N L γ R γ C V γ γ T C S Y γ γ A F γ A L γ S S T A T D V F W A
Human factor IX	Y N S G K L γ γ γ F V Q G N L γ R γ C M γ γ K C S F γ γ A R γ V F γ N T γ K T T γ F W K
Human factor X	A N S - F L γ γ M K K G H L γ R γ C M γ γ T C S Y γ γ A R γ V F γ D S D K T N γ F W N
Human factor VII	A N A - F L γ γ L R P G S L γ R γ C K γ γ Q C S F γ γ A R γ I F K D A γ R T K L F W I
Human protein C	A N S - F L γ γ L R H S S L γ R γ C I γ γ I C D F γ γ A K γ I F Q N V D D T L A F W S
Human protein S	A N S - L L γ γ T K Q G N L γ R γ C I γ γ L C N K γ γ A R γ V F γ N D P γ T D Y F Y P

Fig. 100-7. γ-Carboxyglutamic acid-rich domains of the vitamin K-dependent proteins. One-letter amino acid code (see Ch. 3) is employed (γ denotes γ-carboxyglutamic acid). Sequences have been aligned to maximize sequence homology.

	-24						-18								-10									-1	+1
Factor IX							Thr	Val	Phe	Leu	Asp	His	Glu	Asn	Ala	Asn	Lys	Ile	Leu	Asn	Arg	Pro	Lys	Arg	Tyr
Prothrombin	Ser	Leu	Val	His	Ser	Gln	His	Val	Phe	Leu	Ala	Pro	Gln	Gln	Ala	Arg	Ser	Leu	Leu	Gln	Arg	Val	Arg	Arg	Ala
Factor X	Leu	Leu	Leu	Leu	Gly	Glu	Ser	Leu	Phe	Ile	Arg	Arg	Glu	Gln	Ala	Asn	Asn	Ile	Leu	Ala	Arg	Val	Thr	Arg	Ala
Protein C	Thr	Pro	Ala	Pro	Leu	Asp	Ser	Val	Phe	Ser	Ser	Ser	Glu	Arg	Ala	His	Gln	Val	Leu	Arg	Ile	Arg	Lys	Arg	Ala
Factor VII	Trp	Lys	Pro	Gly	Pro	His	Arg	Val	Phe	Val	Thr	Glu	Glu	Glu	Ala	His	Gly	Val	Leu	His	Arg	Arg	Arg	Arg	Ala
Protein S	Val	Leu	Pro	Val	Leu	Glu	Ala	Asn	Phe	Leu	Ser	Arg	Gln	His	Ala	Ser	Gln	Val	Leu	Ile	Arg	Arg	Arg	Arg	Ala
Bone Gla protein	Ser	Gly	Ala	Glu	Ser	Ser	Lys	Ala	Phe	Val	Ser	Lys	Gln	Glu	Gly	Ser	Glu	Val	Val	Lys	Arg	Pro	Arg	Arg	Tyr

Fig. 100-8. Sequence comparison of the propeptide domains of the vitamin K-dependent blood coagulation proteins. The size of the propeptide has been established for factor IX[267] and protein C.[2867] Homologous regions of other vitamin K-dependent proteins are aligned. Residues that demonstrate significant sequence homology are boxed and shaded pink; regions with conservative amino acid substitutions are boxed. (Modified from Furie and Furie,[263] with permission.)

to carboxylation of these glutamic acid residues.[172] Thus, the propeptide is sufficient to support carboxylation, and no other components within the substrate are required, except to improve efficiency of carboxylation.

Peptides containing a complete propeptide sequence and carboxylatable glutamic acid residues are efficiently carboxylated, with a K_m of 3 μM.[172-174] By contrast, peptides without the γ-carboxylation recognition site or with a truncated site are poor substrates for the carboxylase. Glutamic acid, but not aspartic acid, is a substrate for the carboxylase. Based on the predicted structure of the propeptide of factor X, an 18-residue peptide stimulates the carboxylation of the pentapeptide

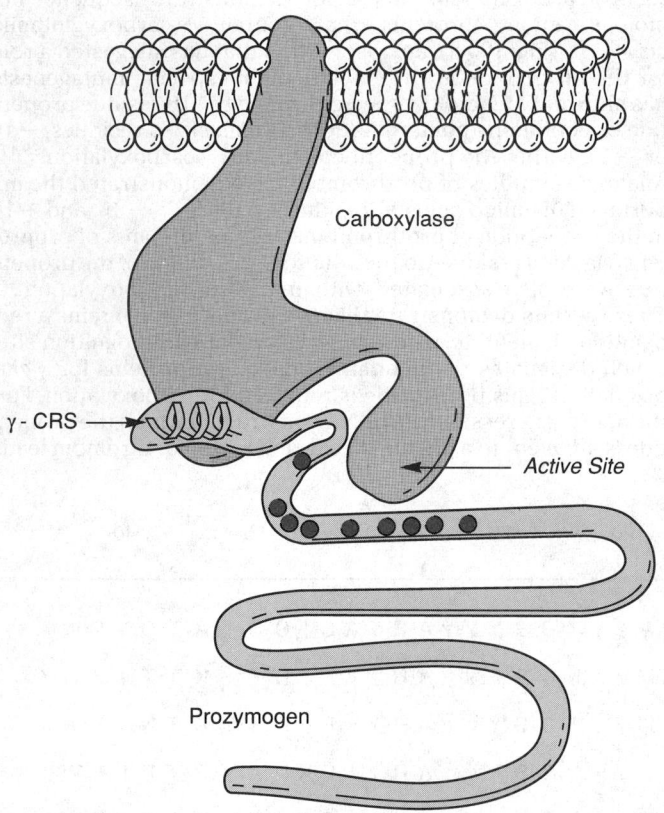

Fig. 100-9. Vitamin K-dependent carboxylase. The precursors of the vitamin K-dependent blood clotting proteins, which contain the γ-carboxylation recognition site (γ-CRS) within the propeptide, bind to the carboxylase through this recognition site. Glutamic acids are converted to γ-carboxyglutamic acids by the carboxylase in the presence of vitamin K, oxygen, and carbon dioxide. (Modified from Furie and Furie,[263] with permission.)

FLEEL (Phe-Leu-Glu-Glu-Leu) by the partially purified carboxylase by about eightfold.[175]

The propeptide of prothrombin contains the carboxylation recognition site on its N-terminus and the propeptide cleavage site at the C-terminus. This peptide incorporates a 10-residue amphipathic α-helix, from residues -3 to -13.[176] This helix serves as a rigid extension to expose the carboxylation recognition site (Fig. 100-9). In contrast to factor IX, profactor IX cannot be activated to its enzymatically active form and does not bind to acidic membranes even though it is fully carboxylated.[177] Thus, the propeptide plays two roles in the synthesis of the vitamin K-dependent proteins: (1) via the γ-carboxylation recognition site, the propeptide signals for carboxylation of adjacent glutamic acid residues; and (2) the propeptide inhibits premature zymogen activation and membrane binding during intracellular processing.

The propeptide contains a sequence adjacent to the sessile bond that is characteristic of many proproteins and prohormones: Arg-X-Arg/Lys-Arg at residues -4 to -1, where propeptide cleavage occurs between -1 and $+1$. The propeptidase enzyme responsible for cleavage is PACE (also known as furin),[178] a constitutively expressed protease located in the trans-Golgi region that cleaves substrates with adjacent basic amino acid residues. A liver endopeptidase with a similar substrate specificity has been purified and cloned, but does not appear to be the propeptide.[179,180] Site-specific mutagenesis of profactor IX has emphasized the importance of Arg -1, the lack of importance of the side chain of residue -3, and the effect of mutation of residue -2 on the efficiency of cleavage.[181]

During synthesis of the vitamin K-dependent proteins, the signal peptide contains a recognition element that directs the partially synthesized protein to the endoplasmic reticulum (Fig. 100-10). With cleavage of the signal peptide, the carboxylation recognition site on the propeptide is expressed. The vitamin K-dependent carboxylase is anchored to this region and modifies all the glutamic acids with a given proximity to the recognition site. After carboxylation, the protein is transported to the Golgi apparatus, where the propeptide undergoes cleavage. Final processing of the protein is completed in the Golgi compartment.

Post-Translational β-Hydroxylation

An unusual amino acid, *erythro*-β-hydroxyaspartic acid, is located in the NH$_2$-terminal EGF domains of protein C[182] and factors IX, X, and VII. In addition, *erythro*-β-hydroxyasparagine has been identified in protein S.[183] These amino acids are formed by post-translational hydroxylation of aspartic acid and asparagine. Their function remains unknown, although it has been suggested that they are involved in defining the metal-binding properties of these proteins.

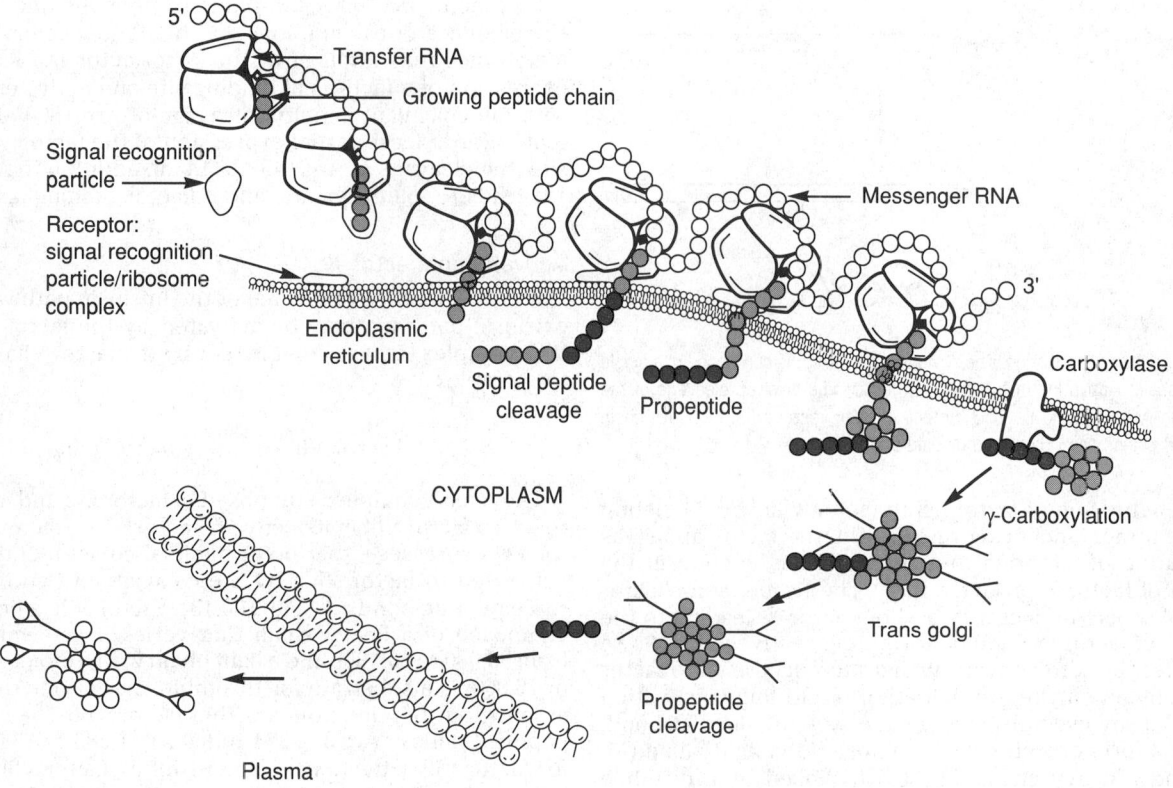

Fig. 100-10. Biosynthesis of the vitamin K-dependent blood coagulation proteins. Signal recognition particle binds to the signal peptide, thus directing this complex to the endoplasmic reticulum. Signal peptide directs translocation to the luminal aspect of the endoplasmic reticulum. After signal peptide cleavage by signal peptidase, propeptide is expressed. This region, containing the γ-carboxylation recognition site, binds to the vitamin K-dependent carboxylase. Specific glutamic acids are converted to γ-carboxyglutamic acids by this enzyme. Propeptide is removed in the trans-Golgi region. (Modified from Furie and Furie,[263] with permission.)

Unlike post-translational γ-carboxylation, β-hydroxylation of factor IX is not directed by the propeptide, nor does this process require vitamin K or concomitant γ-carboxylation. β-Hydroxylation occurs in domains homologous to the EGF precursor in certain vitamin K-dependent proteins,[183] as well as in proteins outside this family, including the complement proteins C1r and C1s, thrombomodulin, uromodulin, and the low-density lipoprotein receptor.[183–185] A consensus sequence encompassing the β-hydroxylated aspartic acid and asparagine residues within a number of EGF domains has been noted by Stenflo et al.[183]

Cys-X-Asp/Asn-X-X-X-X-Phe/Tyr-X-Cys-X-Cys

EGF domains that lack the consensus sequence do not contain this post-translational modification. The hydroxylation is catalyzed by aspartyl β-hydroxylase, an enzyme that requires 2-ketoglutarate and Fe^{2+}.[186] This reaction is blocked by agents that inhibit 2-ketoglutarate-dependent dioxygenases.[187]

von Willebrand Factor Multimerization

vWF is synthesized as a single polypeptide chain containing a signal peptide, a large propolypeptide (M_r 80,000) and the mature vWF (M_r 225,000). During synthesis, the mature vWF forms a dimer, which multimerizes to the high-molecular-weight, biologically active forms critical for cellular adhesion. Synthesis of vWF takes place in endothelial cells and megakaryocytes. In endothelial cells vWF is secreted via a constitutive pathway involving mainly dimeric forms. In addition, the regulated pathway involves storage of vWF in Weibel-Palade bodies,

within which vWF undergoes multimerization and subsequently cleavage of the propolypeptide. Endothelial cells degranulate under specific stimuli, leading to the secretion of vWF. The propolypeptide is required for multimerization[156,157] and is further required for directing vWF to the Weibel-Palade bodies.[188]

ACTIVATION OF BLOOD COAGULATION

Mechanism of Extrinsic Activation

Activation of blood clotting through the extrinsic pathway likely plays a dominant physiologic role in hemostasis. Tissue factor, a cellular receptor for factors VII and VIIa, is present on most cell surfaces. The expression of tissue factor activity is constitutive on most nonvascular cells and is inducible via de novo synthesis in cells within the blood or on the blood vessel wall, including monocytes and endothelial cells. On tissue injury and laceration of blood vessels, nonvascular cells become exposed to blood, leading immediately to the formation of a complex of tissue factor on the cell surface with factor VIIa from the blood. The formation of this complex initiates the tissue factor pathway, culminating in the generation of thrombin and in the formation of a fibrin clot.

$$\text{Factor VII} \xrightarrow{\text{FVIIa/TF}} \text{factor VIIa}$$

Through its extracellular domain, tissue factor forms a catalytic complex with factor VIIa in the presence of Ca^{2+}.[17,145] Low amounts (10–100 pM) of factor VIIa are present in normal plasma.[3] With tissue factor as a cofactor, factor VIIa can autoca-

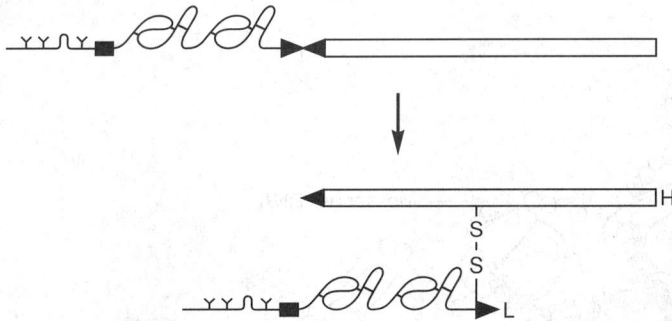

Fig. 100-11. Factor VII activation. The zymogen, factor VII, is composed of a single polypeptide chain. Activation of factor VII to factor VIIa involves cleavage of the bond between Arg 152 and Ile 153 by factor Xa or factor VIIa. Light (L) chain and heavy (H) chains are linked by a disulfide bond.

talyze the activation of factor VII to factor VIIa.[189,190] Deletion of the membrane anchoring region of tissue factor abolishes autoactivation of factor VII but not cofactor function in the activation of factor X or factor IX.[191] The tissue factor/factor VIIa complex acts on factor IX and on factor X, leading to the generation of factor IXa and factor Xa, respectively. Factor Xa is able to feedback to convert further more factor VII to factor VIIa, thereby amplifying the initiation of clotting.[4] Activation of factor VII involves cleavage of the Arg 152–Ile 153 bond, leading to a form of factor VIIa composed of a light chain (M_r 20,000) and a heavy chain (M_r 30,000) linked by a disulfide bond[192–194] (Fig. 100-11). This reaction is greatly enhanced by the presence of tissue factor and phospholipid vesicles.[11,195,196] Activation of factor VII is associated with the expression of the catalytic triad within the heavy chain, His 41, Ser 192, and Asn 90, common to the active site of all serine proteases. Although the potential for factor Xa-mediated and factor VIIa-mediated amplification of this pathway is apparent, the nature of the protease that generates constitutive factor VIIa in plasma is unknown.

Activation of Factor IX

The activation of factor IX proceeds either via the tissue factor pathway or through the intrinsic pathway with factor XIa.

$$\text{Factor IX} \xrightarrow{\text{TF/factor VIIa or factor XIa}} \text{factor IXa}$$

Factor IX can be activated through the extrinsic pathway.[197] The factor VIIa/tissue factor complex activates both factor IX and factor X in reactions that require Ca^{2+}. Although the kinetics of factor IX activation by factor XIa and by factor VIIa/tissue factor differ, both enzymes cleave the same peptide bonds and generate the same structural form of factor IXa.

The activation of factor IX by factor XIa, in contrast to the activation of the other vitamin K-dependent blood clotting proteins or the activation of factor IX by factor VIIa tissue factor (which occur on membrane surfaces), takes place in the solution phase. Membrane surfaces, including those of artificial phospholipid vesicles or platelets, do not accelerate the generation of factor IXa. The reaction has an absolute requirement for Ca^{2+}.[198] Factor IX is activated by the cleavage of two internal peptide bonds, the Arg 145-Ala 146 bond and the Arg 180-Val 181 bond[199,200] (Fig. 100-12). A factor IXa light chain (M_r 18,000), from residues 1–145, and a factor IXa heavy chain (M_r 27,000), from residues 181–416, are generated by the proteolytic activation. These chains remain covalently attached through a single disulfide bond. An activation peptide, from residues 146–180, is cleaved from factor IX during activation.

Like factor IX, factor IXa binds to phospholipid vesicles in the presence of calcium ions and binds to calcium and other metal ions. Activation of factor IX to factor IXa leads to the expression of a factor VIII binding site and active enzyme site with full coagulant activity. Cleavage of Arg 180-Val 181 is required for at least partial expression of the factor VIII binding site; the cleavage of Arg 145-Ala 146 in addition to Arg 180-Val 181 leads to full enzymatic and cofactor binding activity.

Activation of Factor X

Factor X, at the confluence of the intrinsic pathway and the extrinsic pathway, may be activated by the factor IXa/factor VIIIa complex (tenase complex) or by the factor VIIa/tissue factor complex.

$$\text{Factor VIII} \xrightarrow{\text{thrombin}} \text{factor VIIIa}$$

The tenase complex, composed of factor IXa and factor VIIIa, requires factor VIII in its active cofactor form, factor VIIIa. Factor VIII expresses either no or minimal cofactor activity but is converted to factor VIIIa by the cleavage of two or possibly three peptide bonds[201] (Fig. 100-13). Factor VIII, a heterodimer composed of a heavy chain that varies in molecular weight from 90,000 to 200,000 and a light chain with a molecular weight of 76,000, is a substrate for thrombin, an enzyme that cleaves at least four peptide bonds within factor VIII. The cleavage of peptide bonds at Arg 372-373 and at Arg 1,686-1,689 is required for factor VIII activation.[201] The resulting factor VIIIa contains polypeptide chains of 50,000 molecular weight (derived from the heavy chain), of 43,000 molecular weight, and 73,000 molecular weight (derived from the light chain)[202] (see Ch. 105). Factors VIII and VIIIa bind tightly to phospholipid vesicles and to activated platelets.[22,203]

$$\text{Factor X} \xrightarrow{\text{factor IXa/factor VIIIa or factor VIIa/TF}} \text{factor Xa}$$

Factor IXa binds to factor VIIIa that is bound to phospholipid membranes and activated platelets. A possible role for endothelial cell membranes in factor X activation has also been suggested.[204] The formation of this enzyme complex is required for activation of factor X on a physiologically relevant time scale.[205] Alternatively, factor VIIa in complex with tissue factor on cell surfaces can activate factor X on a physiologically relevant time scale. The formation of this complex requires Ca^{2+}.

Factor X, a zymogen with no coagulant activity, is converted to its active enzyme form, factor Xa, by cleavage of a single polypeptide bond between Arg 51 and Ile 52 in the heavy chain (Fig. 100-14). This cleavage is catalyzed either by the complex

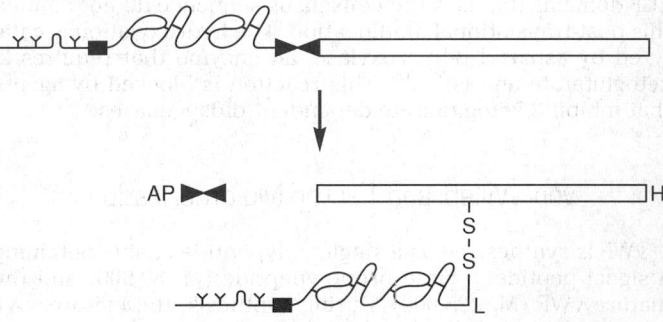

Fig. 100-12. Factor IX activation. The zymogen, factor IX, is composed of a single polypeptide chain. Activation of factor IX to factor IXa involves cleavage of two peptide bonds. Factor IXa contains a light (L) chain and a heavy (H) chain linked by a disulfide bond. An activation peptide (AP) is released during the activation process.

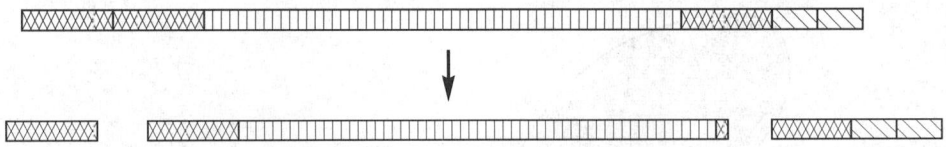

Fig. 100-13. Activation of factor VIII, an inactive cofactor composed of a single polypeptide chain. Factor VIII is converted to its active cofactor form, factor VIIIa, by the cleavage of two, and possibly three, peptide bonds to generate a heavy chain and a light chain noncovalently linked in the presence of Ca^{2+}.

of factor IXa and factor VIIIa on membrane surfaces in the presence of Ca^{2+} or by the complex of factor VIIa and tissue factor on membrane surfaces in the presence of Ca^{2+}.[206,207] An activator without physiologic importance, the coagulant protein of Russell's viper venom, is often used for clinical laboratory measurements in a test known as the Stypven time.[208] The activation peptide remains associated with factor Xa[209] but, with the exception of the C-terminal amino acids, does not contribute to the initial formation of a complex with tenase.[210] Although zymogen activation results in a major functional change in the protein, only subtle structural changes in factor X are associated with the development of enzymatic activity.[211] The expression of enzymatic activity involves the catalytic triad common to all serine proteases—His 93, Asp 138, and Ser 233—in the heavy chain of bovine factor X.

Factor Xa is inhibited by specific plasma protease inhibitors, including antithrombin III and α_2-macroglobulin.[212] These inhibitors are probably scavengers in that they neutralize the potent coagulant activity of any factor Xa that flows passed the site of tissue injury.

The tissue factor pathway is regulated by a protease inhibitor, tissue factor pathway inhibitor (TFPI).[213-216] The gene for this protein is located on chromosome 2 and includes 9 exons.[217,218] This inhibitor, with a molecular weight of 34,000 contains three tandem Kunitz-type protease inhibitor domains.[219] TFPI binds factor Xa directly and inhibits factor VIIa-tissue factor activity in a reaction that appears to involve the formation of a factor Xa/TFPI/factor VIIa/tissue factor complex.[220] The generation of this complex down-regulates the activity of the tissue factor pathway.

Generation of Thrombin: Assembly of the Prothrombinase Complex

The conversion of prothrombin to thrombin is mediated by the enzyme action of factor Xa and the cofactor factor Va in a complex formed on membrane surfaces. The factor Xa/factor Va complex that is formed on membranes in the presence of Ca^{2+} is known as the "prothrombinase" complex, since it serves to act on prothrombin as substrate (Fig. 100-15).

$$\text{Factor V} \xrightarrow{\text{thrombin}} \text{factor Va}$$

The factor Xa/factor Va/membrane complex has many structural and functional parallels with the factor IXa/factor VIIIa/membrane complex. Factors V and Va are extrinsic membrane-binding proteins. The interaction of these factor V forms with membranes is independent of Ca^{2+} or other metal ions. Factor V binds with high affinity to phospholipid vesicles rich in phosphatidylserine,[221-224] to activated platelets,[105,225] and to microparticles derived from activated platelets.[226,227]

Factor V circulates in the blood as an inactive cofactor or as a cofactor with low intrinsic activity. It is converted to its active cofactor form, factor Va, by the hydrolysis of three peptide bonds, Arg 709-Ser 710, Arg 1,018-Thr 1,019, and Arg 1,545-Ser 1,546, by thrombin or factor Xa[228-231] (Fig. 100-16). These cleavages generate a heavy chain (M_r 110,000) and a light chain (M_r 78,000) linked noncovalently in the presence of Ca^{2+}.

$$\text{Prothrombin} \xrightarrow{\text{factor Xa/factor Va}} \text{thrombin}$$

In the presence of Ca^{2+}, a complex of factors Xa and Va forms on phospholipid vesicles. The formation of the prothrombinase complex involves three steps: (1) the binding of factor Va to membrane surfaces; (2) the binding of factor Xa to membrane surfaces; (3) the interaction of membrane-bound factors Va and Xa.[232] Although factor Xa can activate prothrombin directly in the absence of Ca^{2+}, factor Va, and membrane surfaces, the rate of activation is very slow and irrelevant on a physiologic time scale. By contrast, the rate of prothrombin activation by the prothrombinase complex is about 300,000 times as high as the rate of activation by factor Xa.[232]

Although phospholipid vesicles serve as a model system for study of prothrombinase complex formation on platelets, the details of formation of the complex may vary on the two surfaces. Factor Va binds to specific sites on the platelet surface, defining the formation of the prothrombinase complex. Factor Va appears to be the factor Xa receptor on platelets.[233, 234] Factor Xa binds to platelets, leading to the expression of prothrombinase activity.[235] Furthermore, factor Va binds to endothelial cells, monocytes, and lymphocytes, facilitating assembly of the prothrombinase complex.[236-239]

Prothrombin is converted to thrombin by the prothrombinase complex. Although multiple fragments can be generated by the action of prothrombinase on prothrombin, two or possibly three peptide bonds are necessarily cleaved in generating thrombin, a two-chain enzyme with a molecular weight of 38,000[240-243] (Fig. 100-17). Cleavage of the Arg 271-Thr 272 or Arg 286-Thr 287 bond in the presence of plasma proteins yields fragment 1.2 (M_r 43,000) or fragment 1·2·3 (M_r 45,000), respectively, both derived from the NH_2-terminus of human prothrom-

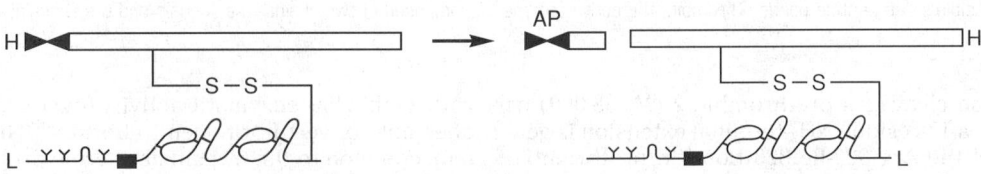

Fig. 100-14. Factor X activation. Factor X is composed of two chains, a heavy (H) chain and a light (L) chain, linked by a disulfide bond. Activation of factor X to factor Xa requires cleavage of a single peptide bond on the heavy chain. AP, activation peptide.

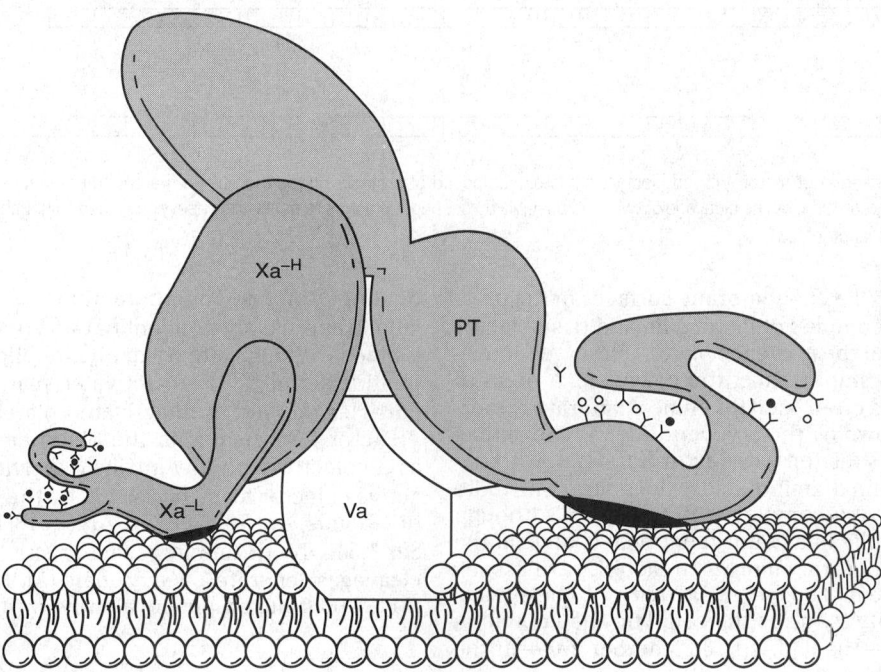

Fig. 100-15. Model for the macromolecular complex associated with zymogen activation. A central feature of the proteins involved in blood coagulation is their assembly on membrane surfaces. Interaction of Ca^{2+} with the γ-carboxyglutamic acids on vitamin K-dependent proteins leads to the exposure of a membrane-binding site on these proteins. Assembly of these proteins on membranes in a geometry defined by the protein cofactor facilitates enzyme-substrate interaction. The protein cofactor likely plays an important regulatory role in this complex. Factor Xa, enzyme (L, light chain; H, heavy chain); prothrombin (PT), substrate; factor Va, cofactor; Ca^{2+}, O; γ-carboxyglutamic acid, Y; lipid-binding site (black). (Modified from Furie and Furie,[263] with permission.)

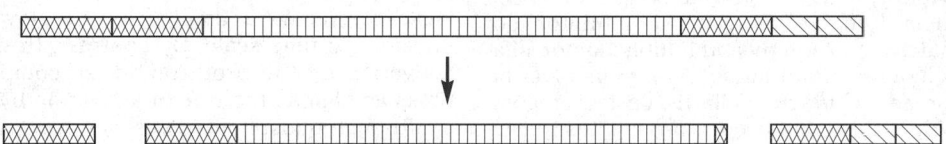

Fig. 100-16. Activation of factor V, an inactive cofactor composed of a single polypeptide chain. Factor V is converted to its active cofactor form, factor Va, by the cleavage of two and possibly three peptide bonds to generate a heavy chain and a light chain noncovalently linked in the presence of calcium ions.

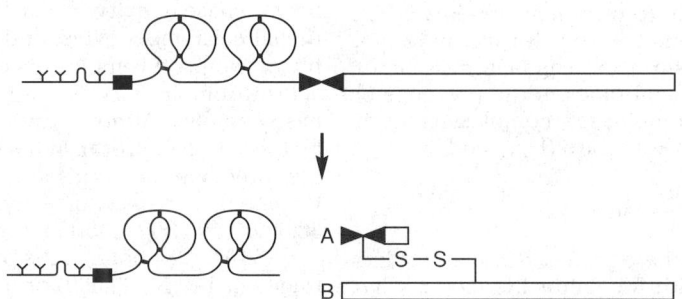

Fig. 100-17. Activation of prothrombin, which is composed of a single polypeptide chain. Its activation to thrombin involves cleavage of two or possible three peptide bonds. Thrombin, the active enzyme, is composed of two chains, the A chain and the B chain, linked by a disulfide bond.

bin.[244,245] With these cleavages prethrombin 2 (M_r 38,000) or prethrombin 2 with a 13-residue NH_2-terminal extension is generated. Cleavage of the Arg 322-Ile 323 bond in prothrombin generates meizothrombin and in prethrombin 2 generates both the A chain (M_r 5,000) and the B chain of thrombin (M_r 32,000) linked by a single disulfide bond. In contrast to thrombin, mei-

zothrombin has enzymatic activity toward small substrates but does not convert fibrinogen to fibrin.[246] The charge relay system, common to the trypsin-like serine proteases, is located at His 365, Asp 419, and Ser 527.

Thrombin is inhibited by antithrombin III. This inhibition is greatly accelerated by heparin (see Ch. 102).

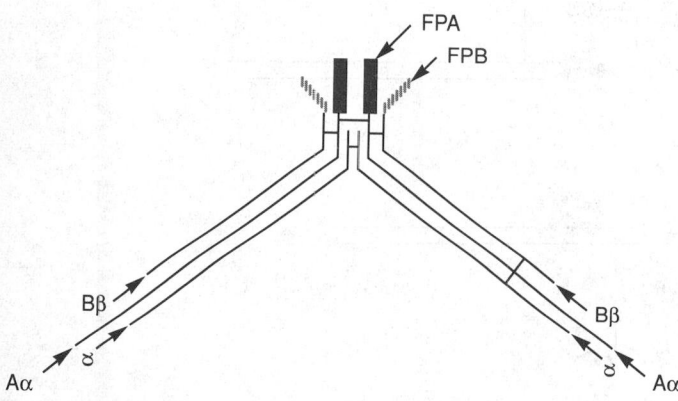

Fig. 100-18. Conversion of fibrinogen to fibrin monomer. Fibrinogen is composed of three chains, the Aα, Bβ, and γ-chains arranged as a heterodimer, $Aα_2Bβ_2γ_2$. The conversion of fibrinogen to fibrin, $α_2β_2γ_2$, requires the cleavage of peptide bonds to release fibrinopeptide A and fibrinopeptide B.

Conversion of Fibrinogen to Fibrin

$$\text{Fibrinogen} \xrightarrow{\text{thrombin}} \text{fibrin} - \text{fibrinopeptide A}$$
$$+ \text{ fibrinopeptide B}$$

Fibrinogen circulates as a plasma protein in a biologically inactive form. It is converted to fibrin as a consequence of the cleavage of peptide bonds in both the Aα and the Bβ chain by the enzyme thrombin (Fig. 100-18). Thrombin is specific for the Arg 16-Gly 17 bond in the Aα chain. Cleavage of this bond releases fibrinopeptide A, a peptide containing 16 amino acid residues from the Aα chain, thereby generating a new amino terminus on the α-chain. Thrombin is also specific for the Arg 14-Gly 15 bond in the Bβ chain, cleavage of which releases fibrinopeptide B, a 14-amino acid peptide, from the Bβ chain, thereby generating a new amino terminus on the β-chain. Thus, the covalent structure of fibrinogen and fibrin are identical except for the removal of two fibrinopeptide A and two fibrinopeptide B fragments from fibrinogen.

The fibrin monomer, on generation, homopolymerizes to form long strands known as protofibrils (Fig. 100-19). Both fi-

brinogen and fibrin are characterized by a trinodal domain structure, with a linear D-E-D domain organization. After removal of the fibrinopeptides, binding sites within the central E domain of the fibrin monomer bind to sites on the D domain of the γ-chain of another fibrin monomer.[247] This yields a half-staggered noncovalent complex between two monomeric units.[248] Addition of a third monomer in a half-staggered orientation facilitates the end-on-end interaction of the D domains of two adjacent monomers. Through these two intermolecular interactions, E domain-D domain and D domain-D domain, two-stranded protofibrils are formed. Only after the protofibrils have become sufficiently long is their lateral association—a necessary event in the formation of thick fibrin fibrils—observed.

The polymerized form of fibrin contains fibrin monomers that are noncovalently bound to each other. As such, the fibrin strands are unstable. Through the action of factor XIIIa, the α- and γ-chains of adjacent fibrin strands are covalently cross-linked to yield a form of fibrin that is not easily disrupted. Factor XIIIa, a transglutaminase, catalyzes the condensation of lysine residues on one chain and glutamic acid residues on a second chain.[249] Factor XIII, an inactive precursor, is a plasma protein that is converted to its active form, factor XIIIa, by the proteolytic action of thrombin.

Although many details of blood coagulation remain unclear, there has been considerable definition of the structure and function of participating components and the special role that cell membranes play in complex formation. The rapid generation of thrombin, with concomitant platelet activation and fibrin clot formation, is localized to the region of tissue injury. The role of cells and soluble proteins in regulating the response to vascular injury is developed in Chapters 97 and 99.

Contact Phase of Blood Coagulation: Activation of Factors XII and XI

Patients with factor XII, prekallikrein, or high-molecular-weight kininogen deficiency have no bleeding phenotype despite prolonged PTTs. These proteins are not required for hemostasis (i.e., the rapid generation of fibrin clot). However, these proteins may play a role in fibrinolysis and in fibrin formation during inflammation and wound healing.

Prekallikrein, with a molecular weight of 100,000, is in part

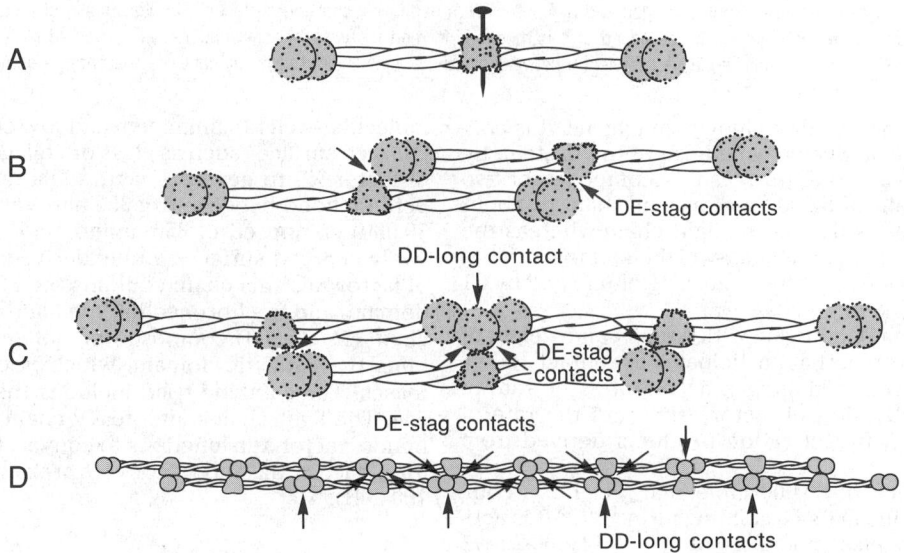

Fig. 100-19. Formation of fibrin strands. **(A)** Fibrin forms **(B)** a staggered dimer. **(C)** The addition of another fibrin monomer end-on-end yields a trimer. **(D)** Continued addition of fibrin monomer generates the fibrin strands.

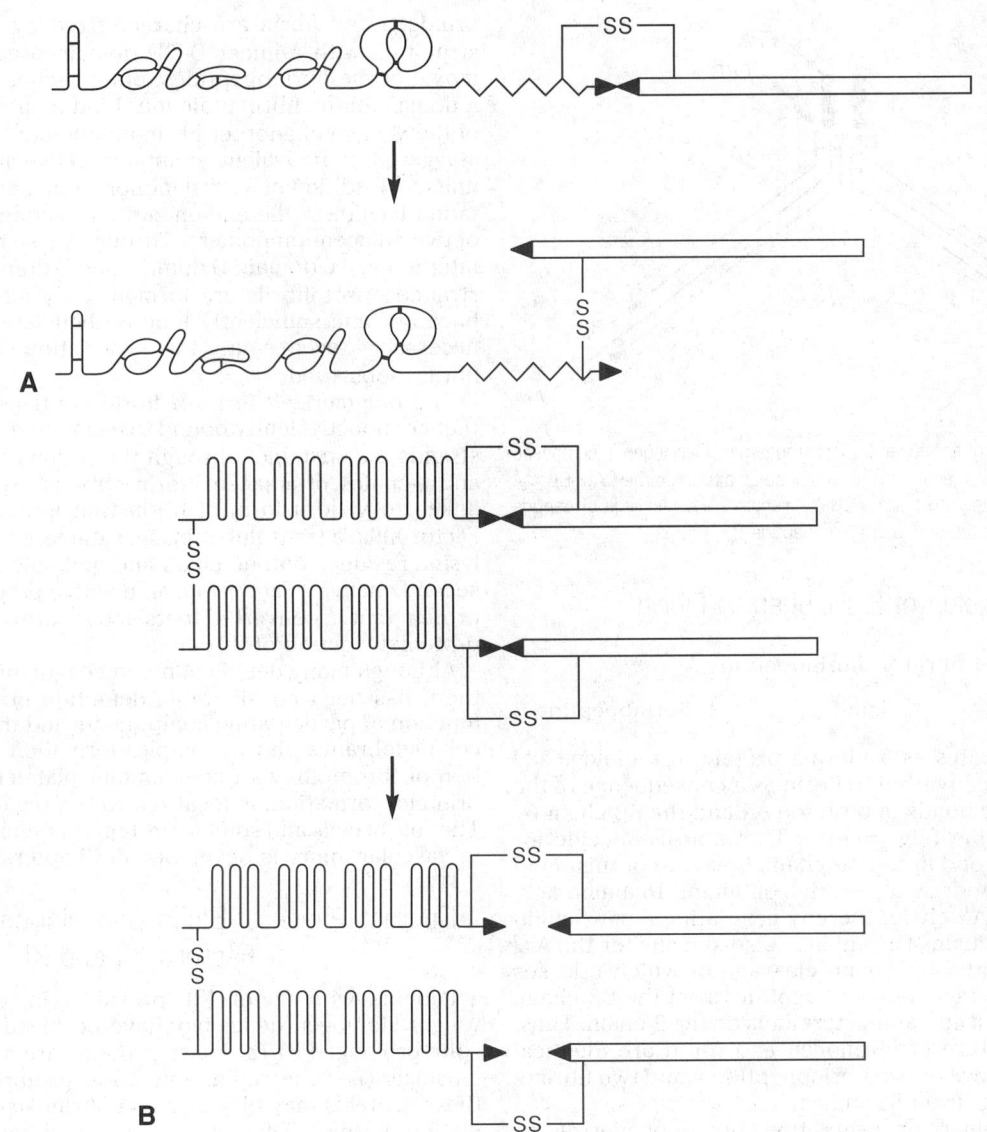

Fig. 100-20. Contact phase of blood coagulation. **(A)** Factor XII, a zymogen composed of a single polypeptide chain, is converted to its active form, factor XIIa, by the cleavage of a single peptide bond. Kallikrein catalyzes this reaction, and the rate of the reaction is greatly accelerated by high-molecular-weight kininogen and by contact with negatively charged surfaces. The light chain of factor XIIa contains the enzyme active site. **(B)** Factor XI, composed of a homodimer formed by two identical subunits, is converted to factor XIa by the enzyme factor XIIa. Each subunit is cleaved to yield a heavy chain and a light chain; the latter contains the enzyme active site.

bound to high-molecular-weight kininogen in plasma. It is converted to kallikrein, the active enzyme form of the protein, by factor XIIa. Kallikrein, a serine protease, is composed of two subunits, a heavy chain of 52,000 and a light chain of about 35,000. The active site resides on the light chain whereas the heavy chain binds to high-molecular-weight kininogen.[250] In plasma, kallikrein is inactivated by α_2-macroglobulin and by C1 inhibitor.[251,252]

High-molecular-weight kininogen, with a molecular weight of 120,000, is a plasma protein that participates in contact activation. High-molecular-weight kininogen accelerates the rate of surface-dependent activation of factor XII[253] and the rate of prekallikrein activation by activation products derived from factor XIIa.[254]

Factor XII, a zymogen of 80,000 molecular weight, is composed of 596 amino acids in its circulating form.[40,47,48] It is activated to factor XIIa by plasma kallikrein[255–257] (Fig. 100-20A).

Factor XII → factor XIIa

This reaction is greatly accelerated by the presence of high-

molecular-weight kininogen and by contact with negatively charged surfaces such as glass or collagen.[258,259] The activation of factor XII to generate factor XIIa involves cleavage of the peptide bond between Arg 353 and Val 354. A heavy chain (M_r 50,000) composed of 353 amino acid residues binds to negatively charged surfaces and is derived from the NH_2-terminus of factor XII. This chain contains the EGF domains, the kringle domain, and the fibronectin type I and type II domains. A light chain (M_r 30,000) composed of 243 amino acid residues contains the catalytic domain, which is common to serine proteases. The catalytic triad includes His 393, Asp 442, and Ser 544. The light chains and heavy chain are linked by disulfide bonds. Factor XIIa functions to convert factor XI to its activated form, factor XIa, and to convert prekallikrein to kallikrein (Fig. 100-20B).

$$\text{Factor XI} \xrightarrow{\text{factor XIIa}} \text{factor XIa}$$

Factor XI is composed of two identical polypeptide chains, each of 80,000 molecular weight, connected by a disulfide bond.

Factor XI is converted to its enzymatic form, factor XIa, by proteolytic cleavage of the Arg 369-Ile 370 bond in each chain (Fig. 100-20B). The heavy chain (M_r 50,000) derived from the amino terminus, and light chain (M_r 30,000) remain attached through a disulfide bond. The catalytic domain of factor XIa resides on the light chain; the catalytic triad common to all serine proteases includes His 44, Asp 93, and Ser 188.

Factors XI and XIa bind to platelets.[260–262] It remains uncertain whether factor XI-platelet interaction has a physiologic role and whether factor XIa on platelets activates factor IX on the solid phase.

REFERENCES

1. Ratnoff OD, Davie EW: Waterfall sequence for intrinsic blood clotting. Science 145:1310, 1964
2. Macfarlane RG: An enzyme cascade in the blood clotting mechanism and its function as a biochemical amplifier. Nature 202:498, 1964
3. Morrissey JH, Macik BG, Neuenschwander PF, Comp PC: Quantitation of activated factor VII levels in plasma using tissue factor mutant selectively deficient in promoting factor VII activation. Blood 81:734, 1993
4. Radcliffe R, Nemerson Y: Activation and control of factor VII by activated factor X and thrombin. Isolation and characterization of a single chain form of factor VII. J Biol Chem 250:388, 1975
5. Ratnoff OD, Colopy JE: A familial hemorrhagic trail associated with a deficiency of a clot-promoting fraction of plasma. J Clin Invest 34:602, 1955
6. Colman RW, Bagdasarian A, Talamo RC et al: Williams trait. Human kininogen deficiency with diminished levels of plasminogen proactivator and prekallikrein associated with abnormalities of the Hageman factor-dependent pathways. J Clin Invest 56:1650, 1975
7. Wuepper KD: Prekallikrein deficiency in man. J Exp Med 138:1345, 1973
8. Osterud B, Rapaport SI: Activation of factor IX by the reaction product of tissue factor and factor VII: additional pathway for initiating blood coagulation. Proc Natl Acad Sci USA 74:5260, 1977
9. Furie B, Furie BC: The molecular and cellular biology of blood coagulation. N Engl J Med 326:800, 1992
10. Zur M, Radcliffe RD, Oberdick J, Nemerson Y: The dual role of factor VII in blood coagulation. Initiation and inhibition of a proteolytic system by a zymogen. J Biol Chem 257:5623, 1982
11. Rao LVM, Rapaport SI: Activation of factor VII bound to tissue factor: a key early step in the tissue factor pathway of blood coagulation. Proc Natl Acad Sci USA 85:6687, 1988
12. Radcliffe R, Nemerson Y: Mechanism of activation of bovine factor VII. Products of cleavage by factor Xa. J Biol Chem 251:4749, 1976
13. Naito K, Fujikawa K: Activation of human blood coagulation factor XI independent of factor XII. Factor XI is activated by thrombin and factor XIa in the presence of negatively charged surfaces. J Biol Chem 266:7353, 1991
14. Bach R, Nemerson Y, Konigsberg W: Purification and characterization of bovine tissue factor. J Biol Chem 256:8324, 1981
15. Spicer EK, Horton R, Bloem L et al: Isolation of cDNA clones coding for human tissue factor: primary structure of the protein and cDNA. Proc Natl Acad Sci USA 84:5148, 1987
16. Morrissey JH, Fakhrai H, Edgington TS: Molecular cloning of the cDNA for tissue factor, the cellular receptor for the initiation of the coagulation protease cascade. Cell 50:129, 1987
17. Guha A, Bach R, Konigsberg W, Nemerson Y: Affinity purification of human tissue factor: interaction of factor VII and tissue factor in detergent micelles. Proc Natl Acad Sci USA 83:299, 1986
18. Gilbert GE, Furie BC, Furie B: Binding of factor VIII to phospholipid vesicles. J Biol Chem 265:815, 1990
19. Jones ME, Griffin MJ, Monroe DM et al: Comparison of lipid binding and kinetic properties of normal, variant, and γ-carboxyglutamic acid-modified human factor IX and factor IXa. Biochemistry 24:8064, 1985
20. Mann KG, Jenny RJ, Krishnaswamy S: Cofactor proteins in the assembly and expression of blood clotting enzyme complexes. Annu Rev Biochem 57:915, 1988
21. Mann KG: Surface-dependent hemostasis. Semin Hematol 29:213, 1992
22. Nesheim ME, Pittman DD, Wang JH et al: The binding of ^{35}S-labeled recombinant factor VIII to activated and unactivated platelets. J Biol Chem 263:16467, 1988
23. Sims PJ, Faioni EM, Wiedmer T, Shattil SJ: J Biol Chem 263:18205, 1988
24. Gilbert GE, Sims PJ, Wiedmer T et al: Platelet-derived microparticles express high affinity receptors for factor VIII. J Biol Chem 266:17261, 1991
25. Vysotchin A, Medved LV, Ingham KC: Domain structure and domain-domain interactions in human coagulation factor IX. J Biol Chem 268:8436, 1993
26. Diuguid DL, Rabiet M-J, Furie BC et al: Molecular basis of hemophilia B: a

27. defective enzyme due to an unprocessed propeptide is caused by a point mutation in the factor IX precursor. Proc Natl Acad Sci USA 83:5803, 1986
27. Bentley AK, Rees DJG, Rizza C, Brownlee GG: Defective propeptide processing of blood clotting factor IX caused by mutation of arginine to glutamine at position -4. Cell 45:343, 1986
28. Foster DC, Yoshitake S, Davie EW: The nucleotide sequence of the gene for human protein C. Proc Natl Acad Sci USA 82, 4673, 1985
29. Jorgensen MJ, Cantor AB, Furie BC et al: Recognition site directing vitamin K-dependent γ-carboxylation resides on the propeptide of factor IX. Cell 48:185, 1987
30. Park CH, Tulinsky A: Three-dimensional structure of the kringle sequence: structure of prothrombin fragment 1. Biochemistry 25:3977, 1986
31. Soriano-Garcia M, Padmanabhan K, de Vos AM, Tulinsky A: The Ca^{2+} ion and membrane binding structure of the Gla domain of Ca-prothrombin fragment 1. Biochemistry 31:2554, 1992
32. Ratcliffe J, Furie B, Furie BC: The importance of specific γ-carboxyglutamic acid residues in prothrombin: evaluation by site-specific mutagenesis. J Biol Chem 268:24339, 1993
33. Gregory H, Preston BM: The primary structure of human urogastrone. Int J Pept Protein Res 9:107, 1977
34. Handford PA, Mayhew M, Baron M, et al: Key residues involved in calcium-binding motifs in EGF-like domains. Nature 351:164, 1991
35. Huang LH, Cheng H, Pardi A et al: Sequence-specific ^{1}H NMR assignments, secondary structure, and location of the calcium binding site in the first epidermal growth factor like domain of blood coagulation factor IX. Biochemistry 30:7402, 1991
36. Ullner M, Selander M, Persson E et al: Three-dimensional structure of the apo form of the N-terminal EGF-like module of blood coagulation factor X as determined by NMR spectroscopy and simulated folding. Biochemistry 31:5974, 1992
37. Kotkow K, Furie B, Furie BC: The interaction of prothrombin with phospholipid membranes is independent of either kringle domains. J Biol Chem 268:15633, 1993
38. Kotkow K, Furie B, Furie BC: Role of prothrombin kringle domains in factor Va binding to prothrombin by the prothrombinase complex. Circulation 86:686, 1992
39. Magnusson S, Petersen TE, Sottrup-Jensen L, Cleays H: Complete primary structure of prothrombin: isolation, structure and reactivity of ten carboxylated glutamic acid residues and regulation of prothrombin activation by thrombin. p. 123. In Reich E, Rifkin DB, Shaw E (eds): Proteases and Biological Control. Cold Spring Harbor Laboratory Press, Cold Spring Harbor, NY, 1973
40. Cool DE, Edgell CJS, Louie GV et al: Characterization of human blood coagulation factor XII gene. J Biol Chem 262:13662, 1987
41. Malinowski DP, Sadler JE, Davie EW: Characterization of a complementary deoxyribonucleic acid coding for human and bovine plasminogen. Biochemistry 23:4243, 1984
42. Holmes WE, Pennica D, Blaber M et al: Cloning and expression of the gene for prourokinase in E. coli. Biotechnology 3:923, 1985
43. Ny T, Elgh F, Lund B: The structure of the human tissue-type plasminogen activator gene: correlation of intron and exon structures to functional and structural domains. Proc Natl Acad Sci USA 81:5355, 1984
44. Furie B, Bing DH, Feldmann RJ et al: Computer-generated models of blood coagulation factor Xa, factor IXa, and thrombin based upon structural homology with other serine proteases. J Biol Chem 257:3875, 1982
45. Bode W, Mayr I, Baumann U et al: The refined 1.9 A crystal structure of human α-thrombin: interaction with D-Phe-Pro-Arg chloromethylketone and significance of the Tyr-Pro-Pro-Trp insertion segment. EMBO J 8:3467, 1989
46. Bode W, Turk D, Karshidov A: The refined 1.9 A x-ray crystal structure of D-Phe-Pro-Arg chloromethylketone-inhibited human α-thrombin: structure analysis, overall structure, electrostatic properties, detailed active-site geometry and structure-function relationships. Protein Sci 1:426, 1992
47. Cool DE, Edgell CJS, Louie GV et al: Characterization of human blood coagulation factor XII cDNA. J Biol Chem 260:13666, 1985
48. Que BG, Davie EW: Characterization of a cDNA coding for human factor XII (Hageman factor). Biochemistry 25:1525, 1986
49. Revak SD, Cochrane CG, Johnston AR, Hugli TE: Structural changes accompanying enzymatic activation of human Hageman factor. J Clin Invest 54:619, 1974
50. Fujikawa K, Walsh KA, Davie EW: Isolation and characterization of bovine factor XII (Hageman factor). Biochemistry 16:2270, 1977
51. Clarke BJ, Cote HCF, Cool DE et al: Mapping of a putative surface-binding site of human coagulation factor XII. J Biol Chem 264:11497, 1989
52. Veltkamp JJ, Loeliger EA, Hemker HC: The biological half-time of Hageman factor. Thromb Haemost 13:1, 1965

53. Asakai R, Davie EW, Chung DW: Organization of the gene for human factor XI. Biochemistry 26:7221, 1987
54. Bouma BN, Griffin JH: Human blood coagulation factor XI: purification, properties and mechanism of activation by activated factor XII. J Biol Chem 252:6432, 1977
55. Fujikawa K, Chung DW, Hendrickson LE, Davie EW: Amino acid sequence of human factor XI, a blood coagulation factor with four tandem repeats that are highly homologous with plasma prekallikrein. Biochemistry 25:2417, 1986
56. Nossel HL, Niemetz J, Sawitsky A: Blood PTA (factor XI) levels following plasma infusion. Proc Soc Exp Biol Med 115:896, 1964
57. Rosenthal RL, Sloan E: PTA (factor XI) levels following plasma infusion. J Lab Clin Med 66:709, 1965
58. Yoshitake S, Schach BG, Foster DC et al: Nucleotide sequence of the gene for human factor IX. Biochemistry 24:3736, 1985
59. Crossley M, Brownlee GG: Disruption of a C/EBP binding site in the Factor IX promotor is associated with hemophilia B. Nature 345:444, 1990
60. Crossley M, Ludwig M, Stowell KM et al: Recovery from hemophilia B Leyden: an Androgen-responsive element in the factor IX promotor. Science 257:377, 1992
61. Amphlett GW, Byrne R, Castellino FJ: The binding of metal ions to bovine factor IX. J Biol Chem 253:6774, 1978
62. Morita T, Isaacs BS, Esmon CT, Johnson AE: Derivatives of blood coagulation factor IX contain a high affinity Ca^{+2} binding site that lacks γ-carboxyglutamic acid. J Biol Chem 259:5698, 1984
63. Rees DJG, Jones IM, Handford PA et al: The role of β-hydroxyaspartate and adjacent carboxylate residues in the first EGF domain of human factor IX. EMBO J 7:2053, 1988
64. Nishimura H, Takao T, Hase S et al: Human factor IX has a tetrasaccharide O-glycosidically linked to serine 61 through the fucose residue. J Biol Chem 267:17520, 1992
65. Liebman HA, Furie BC, Furie B: The factor IX phospholipid-binding site is required for calcium-dependent activation of factor IX by factor IXa. J Biol Chem 262:7605, 1987
66. Rawala R, Ahmad SS, Walsh PN: Factor IXa binding to activated human platelets promotes factor X activation. Blood 70:393a, 1987
67. Ahmad SS, Rawala-Sheikh RR, Walsh PN: Comparative interactions of factor IX and factor IXa with human platelets. J Biol Chem 264:3244, 1989
68. Ben-Tal O, Porter T, Furie B et al: Cleavage of factor IX at arginine 180-valine 181 is required and sufficient for optimal interaction with factor VIIIa in the tenase complex. Thromb Haemost 69:958, 1993
69. Huber P, Ben-Tal O, Gilbert GE et al: The second epidermal growth factor domain of factor IX is required for factor IXa-factor VIIIa complex formation: studies with factor IX-factor X chimeras. Circulation 82:365, 1990
70. Hertzberg M, Furie B, Furie BC: Construction, expression and characterization of a chimera of factor IX and factor X: the role of the second epidermal growth factor domain and the serine protease domain in factor Va binding. J Biol Chem 267:14759, 1992
71. Rimon S, Melamed R, Savion N et al: Identification of a factor IX/factor IXa binding protein on the endothelial cell surface. J Biol Chem 262:6023, 1987
72. Toomey JR, Smith KJ, Roberts HR, Stafford DW: The endothelial cell binding determinant of human factor IX resides in the γ-carboxygluatmic acid domain. Biochemistry 31:1809, 1992
73. Biggs R, Denson KWE: The fate of prothrombin and factors VIII, IX and X transfused to patients deficient in these factors. Br J Haematol 9:532, 1963
74. Gitschier J, Wood WI, Goralka TM et al: Characterization of the human factor VIII gene. Nature 312:326, 1984
75. Toole JJ, Knopf JL, Wozney JM et al: Molecular cloning of a cDNA encoding human antihaemophilic factor. Nature 312:342, 1984
76. Wion KL, Kelly D, Summerfield JA: Distribution of factor VIII mRNA and antigen in human liver and other tissues. Nature 317:726, 1985
77. Church WR, Jernigan RL, Toole J et al: Coagulation factors V and VIII and ceruloplasmin constitute a family of structurally related proteins. Proc Natl Acad Sci USA 81:6934, 1984
78. Bennett B, Ratnoff OD: Studies on the response of patients with classic hemophilia to transfusion with concentrates of antihemophilic factor. J Clin Invest 51:2593, 1972
79. Leytus SP, Foster DC, Kurachi K, Davie EW: Gene for human factor X: a blood coagulation factor whose gene organization is essentially identical with that of factor IX and protein C. Biochemistry 25:5098, 1986
80. Miao CH, Leytus SP, Chung DW, Davie EW: Liver-specific expression of the gene coding for human factor X, a blood coagulation factor. J Biol Chem 267:7395, 1992
81. Leytus SP, Chung DW, Kisiel W et al: Characterization of a cDNA coding for human factor X. Proc Natl Acad Sci USA 81:3699, 1984
82. Fung MR, Hay CW, MacGillivray RTA: Characterization of an almost full-length cDNA coding for human factor X. Proc Natl Acad Sci USA 82:3591, 1985
83. Titani K, Fujikawa K, Enfield DL et al: Bovine factor X_1 (Stuart factor): amino acid sequence of heavy chain. Proc Natl Acad Sci USA 72:3082, 1975
84. Jackson CM: Characterization of two glycoprotein variants of bovine factor X and demonstration that the factor X zymogen contains two polypeptide chains. Biochemistry 11:4873, 1972
85. Fujikawa K, Legaz ME, Davie EW: Bovine factors X_1 and X_2 (Stuart factor): isolation and characterization. Biochemistry 11:4882, 1972
86. Enfield DL, Ericsson LE, Walsh KA et al: Bovine factor X_1 (Stuart factor), primary structure of the light chain. Proc Natl Acad Sci USA 72:16, 1975
87. McMullen B, Fujikawa K, Kisiel W et al: Complete amino acid sequence of the light chain of human blood coagulation factor X: evidence for identification of residue 63 as β-hydroxyaspartic acid. Biochemistry 22:2875, 1983
88. Morris HR, Dell A, Petersen TE et al: Mass spectrometric identification and sequence location of the ten residues of the new amino acid (γ-carboxyglutamic acid) in the N-terminal region of prothrombin. Biochem J 153:663, 1976
89. Mizuochi T, Yamashita K, Fujikawa K et al: The structures of the carbohydrate moieties of bovine blood coagulation factor X. J Biol Chem 255:3526, 1980
90. Rezaie AR, Neuenschwander PF, Morrissey JH, Esmon CT: Analysis of the functions of the first epidermal growth factor-like domain of factor X. J Biol Chem 268:8176, 1993
91. Furie BC, Furie B: Interaction of lanthanide ions with bovine factor X and their use in the affinity chromatography of the venom coagulant protein of *Vipera russelli*. J Biol Chem 250:601, 1975
92. Nelsestuen GL, Broderius M, Martin G: Role of γ-carboxyglutamic acid. Cation specificity of prothrombin and factor X-phospholipid interaction. J Biol Chem 251:6886, 1976
93. Nelsestuen GL, Broderius M: Interaction of prothrombin and blood clotting factor X with membranes. Biochemistry 16:4172, 1977
94. Nelsestuen GL, Lim TK: Equilibria involved in prothrombin and blood clotting factor X-membrane complex. Biochemistry 16:4177, 1977
95. Lim TK, Bloomfield VA, Nelsestuen GL: Structure of the prothrombin- and blood clotting factor X-membrane complex. Biochemistry 16:4177, 1977
96. Trauber D, Hawkins K, Karpatkin M, Karpatkin S: Humoral factor that specifically regulates factor X levels in rabbits (coagulopoietin-X). J Clin Invest 64:1713, 1979
97. O'Hara PJ, Grant FJ, Haldeman BA et al: Nucleotide sequence of the gene coding for human factor VII, a vitamin K-dependent protein participating in blood coagulation. Proc Natl Acad Sci USA 84:5158, 1987
98. Gilgenkrantz S, Briquet ME, Andre E et al: Structural genes of coagulation factors VII and X located on 13q34. Ann Genet 29:32, 1986
99. Hagen FS, Gray CL, O'Hara P et al: Characterization of the cDNA coding for human factor VII. Proc Natl Acad Sci USA 83:2412, 1986
100. Takeya H, Kawabata S-I, Nakagawa K et al: Bovine factor VII. Its purification and complete amino acid sequence. J Biol Chem 263:14868, 1988
101. Williams EB, Krishnaswamy S, Mann KG: Zymogen/enzyme discrimination using peptide chloromethyl ketones. J Biol Chem 264:7536, 1989
102. Kane WH, Ichinose A, Hagen FS, Davie EW: Cloning of cDNAs coding for the heavy chain region and connecting region of human factor V, a blood coagulation factor with four types of internal repeats. Biochemistry 26:6508, 1987
103. Jenny RJ, Pittman DD, Toole JJ et al: Complete cDNA and derived amino acid sequence of human factor V. Proc Natl Acad Sci USA 84:4846, 1987
104. Tracy PB, Eide LL, Bowie EJ, Mann KG: Radioimmunoassay of factor V in human plasma and platelets. Blood 60:59, 1982
105. Tracy PB, Peterson JM, Nesheim ME et al: Interaction of coagulation factor V and factor Va with platelets. J Biol Chem 254:10354, 1979
106. Webster WP, Roberts HR, Penick GD: Hemostasis in factor V deficiency. Am J Med Sci 248:194, 1964
107. Royle NJ, Irwin DM, Koschinsky ML et al: Human genes encoding prothrombin and ceruloplasmin map to 11p11–q12 and 3q21–24 respectively. Somat Cell Mol Genet 13:285, 1987
108. Friezner-Degen SJ, Davie EW: Nucleotide sequence of the gene for human prothrombin. Biochemistry 26:6165, 1987
109. Chow BK, Ting V, Tufaro F, MacGillivray RT: Characterization of a novel liver-specific enhancer in the human prothrombin gene. J Biol Chem 266:18927, 1991
110. Bancroft JD, Schaefer LA, Degen SJF: Characterization of the Alu-rich 5'-flanking region of the human prothrombin-encoding gene. Gene 95:253, 1990
111. Walz DA, Hewett-Emett D, Seegers WH: Amino acid sequence of human prothrombin fragments 1 and 2. Proc Natl Acad Sci USA 74:1969, 1977
112. Butkowski RJ, Elion J, Downing MR, Mann KG: Primary structure of human prethrombin 2 and thrombin. J Biol Chem 252:4942, 1977

113. Mizuochi T, Yamashita K, Fujikawa K et al: The carbohydrate of bovine prothrombin: occurrence of Gal-β-1-3GlcNAc grouping in asparagine-linked sugar chains. J Biol Chem 254:6419, 1979

114. Borowski M, Furie B, Goldsmith GH, Furie BC: Metal and phospholipid binding properties of partially carboxylated variant prothrombins. J Biol Chem 260:9258, 1985

115. Esmon CT, Suttie JW, Jackson CM: The functional significance of vitamin K action. Difference in phospholipid binding between normal and abnormal prothrombin. J Biol Chem 250:4095, 1975

116. Bajaj SP, Butkowski RJ, Mann DG: Prothrombin fragments, Ca^{2+} binding and activation kinetics. J Biol Chem 250:2150, 1975

117. Furie BC, Mann KG, Furie B: Substitution of lanthanide ions for calcium ions in the activation of bovine prothrombin by activated factor X: high affinity metal binding sites of prothrombin and the derivatives of prothrombin activation. J Biol Chem 251:3235, 1976

118. Benarous R, Elion J, Labie D: Ca^{2+} binding properties of human prothrombin. Biochemistry 38:391, 1976

119. Furie BC, Blumenstein M, Furie B: Metal binding sites of a γ-carboxyglutamic acid-rich fragment of bovine prothrombin. J Biol Chem 254:12521, 1979

120. Nelsestuen GL: Role of γ-carboxyglutamic acid. An unusual transition required for calcium-dependent binding of prothrombin to phospholipid. J Biol Chem 251:5648, 1976

121. Prendergast FG, Mann KG: Differentiation of metal ion-induced transitions of prothrombin fragment 1. J Biol Chem 252:840, 1977

122. Bloom JW, Mann KG: Metal ion-induced conformational transitions of prothrombin and prothrombin fragment 1. Biochemistry 17:4430, 1978

123. Furie B and Furie BC: Conformation-specific antibodies as probes of the γ-carboxyglutamic acid-rich region of bovine prothrombin: studies of metal-induced structural changes. J Biol Chem 254:9766, 1979

124. Tai MM, Furie BC, Furie B: Conformation-specific antibodies directed against the bovine prothrombin-calcium complex. J Biol Chem 255:2790, 1980

125. Tai MM, Furie BC, Furie B: Localization of the metal-induced conformational transition of bovine prothrombin. J Biol Chem 259:4162, 1984

126. Borowski M, Furie BC, Bauminger S, Furie B: Prothrombin requires two sequential metal-dependent conformational transitions to bind phospholipid. J Biol Chem 261:14969, 1986

127. Ganrot PO, Nilehn JE: Immunochemical determination of human prothrombin. Scand J Clin Lab Invest 21:238, 1968

128. Blanchard RA, Furie BC, Jorgensen M et al: Acquired vitamin K-dependent carboxylation deficiency in liver disease. N Engl J Med 305:242, 1981

129. Shapiro SS, Martinez J: Human prothrombin metabolism in normal man and in hypocoagulable subjects. J Clin Invest 48:1292, 1969

130. Nachman RL, Mavena AJ, Zucker-Franklin D: Subcellular localization of platelet fibrinogen. Blood 24:853, 1963

131. Ganguly P: Isolation and some properties of fibrinogen from human blood platelets. J Biol Chem 247:1809, 1972

132. Doolittle RF, Takagi T, Cottrell BA: Platelet and plasma fibrinogens are identical gene products. Science 185:368, 1974

133. Kant JA, Fornace AJ Jr, Saxe D et al: Evolution and organization of the fibrinogen locus on chromosome 4: gene duplication accompanied by transposition and inversion. Proc Natl Acad Sci USA 82:2344, 1985

134. Crabtree GR, Kant JA: Coordinate accumulation of the mRNAs for the α-, β-, and γ-chains of rat fibrinogen following defibrination. J Biol Chem 257:7277, 1982

135. McKee PA, Mattock P, Hill RL: Subunit structure of human fibrinogen, soluble fibrin and cross-linked insoluble fibrin. Proc Natl Acad Sci USA 66:738, 1970

136. Crabtree GR, Kant JA: Molecular cloning of cDNA for the α-, β- and γ-chains of rat fibrinogen. A family of coordinately regulated genes. J Biol Chem 256:9718, 1981

137. Chung DW, Chan WY, Davie EW: Characterization of a complementary deoxyribonucleic acid coding for the γ-chain of human fibrinogen. Biochemistry 22:3250, 1983

138. Chung DW, Que BG, Rixon MW et al: Characterization of complementary deoxyribonucleic acid and genomic deoxyribonucleic acid for the beta chain of human fibrinogen. Biochemistry 22:3244, 1983

139. Fowler WE, Erickson HP: Trinodular structure of fibrinogen. Confirmation by both shadowing and negative stain electron microscopy. J Mol Biol 134:241, 1979

140. MacFarlane AS, Todd D, Cromwell S: Fibrinogen catabolism in humans. Clin Sci 26:415, 1964

141. Takeda Y: Studies of the metabolism and distribution of fibrinogen in healthy men with autologous ^{125}I-labeled fibrinogen. J Clin Invest 45:103, 1966

142. Folk JE and Finlayson JS: The ε(γ-glutamyl) lysine crosslink and the catalytic role of transglutaminase. Adv Protein Chem 31:1, 1977

143. Curtis CG, Brown KL, Credo RB et al: Calcium-dependent unmasking of active-center cystein during activation of fibrin stabilizing factor. Biochemistry 13:3774, 1974

144. Bach R, Nemerson Y, Konigsberg W: Purification and characterization of bovine tissue factor. J Biol Chem 256:8324, 1981

145. Broze GJ, Leykam JE, Schwartz BD, Miletich JP: Purification of human brain tissue factor. J Biol Chem 260:10917, 1985

146. Bach R, Konigsberg WH, Nemerson Y: Human tissue factor contains thioester-linked palmitate and stearate on the cytoplasmic half-cystine. Biochemistry 27:4227, 1988

147. Niemetz J: Coagulant activity of leukocytes. Tissue factor activity. J Clin Invest 51:307, 1972

148. Rodgers GM, Greenberg CS, Shuman MA: Characterization of the effects of cultured vascular cells on the activation of blood coagulation. Blood 61:1155, 1983

149. Colucci M, Balconi G, Lounzet R et al: Cultured human endothelial cells generate tissue factor in response to endotoxin. J Clin Invest 71:1893, 1983

150. Mackman N, Morrissey JH, Fowler B, Edgington TS: Complete sequence of the human tissue factor gene, a highly regulated cellular receptor that initiates the coagulation protease cascade. Biochemistry 28:1755, 1989

151. Ginsburg D, Handin RI, Bonthron DT et al: Human von Willebrand factor (vWF): isolation of complementary DNA (cDNA) clones and chromosomal localization. Science 228:1401, 1985

152. Mancuso DJ, Tuley EA, Westfield LA et al: Structure of the gene for human von Willebrand factor. J Biol Chem 264:19514, 1989

153. Bonthron DT, Handin RI, Kaufman RJ et al: Structure of pre-pro-von Willebrand factor and its expression in heterologous cells. Nature 324:270, 1986

154. Verweij CL, Diergaarde PJ, Hart M, Pannekoek H: Full-length von Willebrand factor (vWF) cDNA encodes a highly repetitive protein considerably larger than the mature vWF subunit. EMBO J 5:1839, 1986

155. Shelton-Inloes BB, Titani K, Sadler JE: cDNA sequences for human von Willebrand factor reveal five types of repeated domains and five possible protein sequence polymorphisms. Biochemistry 25:3164, 1986

156. Verweij C, Hart M, Pannekoek H: Expression of variant von Willebrand factor (vWF) cDNA in heterologous cells: requirement of the pro-polypeptide in vWF multimer formation. EMBO J 6:2885, 1987

157. Wise RJ, Pittman DD, Handin RI et al: The propeptide of von Willebrand factor independently mediates the assembly of von Willebrand multimers. Cell 52:229, 1988

158. Wagner DD, Olmsted JB, Marder V: Immunolocalization of von Willebrand protein in Weibel-Palade bodies of human endothelial cells. J Cell Biol 95:355, 1982

159. Lollar P, Parker CG: Stoichiometry of the porcine factor VII-von Willebrand factor association. J Biol Chem 262:17572, 1987

160. Stenflo J, Fernlund P, Egan W, Roepstorff P: Vitamin K-dependent modifications of glutamic acid residues in prothrombin. Proc Natl Acad Sci USA 71:2730, 1974

161. Nelsestuen GL, Zytkovicz TH, Howard JB: The mode of action of vitamin K. Identification of γ-carboxyglutamic acid as a component of prothrombin. J Biol Chem 249:6347, 1974

162. Hubbard BR, Ulrich M, Jacobs M et al: Vitamin K-dependent carboxylase: affinity purification from bovine liver using a synthetic propeptide containing the γ-carboxylation recognition site. Proc Natl Acad Sci USA 86:6893, 1989

163. Wu SM, Cheung WF and Stafford DW: Identification and purification to near homogeneity of the vitamin K-dependent carboxylase. Proc Natl Acad Sci USA 88:2236, 1991

164. Morris DP, Soute BAM, Vermeer C, Stafford DW: Characterization of the purified vitamin K-dependent γ-glutamyl carboxylase. J Biol Chem 268:8735, 1993

165. Wu S-M, Cheung W-F, Frazier DF, Stafford DW: Cloning and expression of the cDNA for human gamma-glutamyl carboxylase. Science 254:1634, 1991

166. Rehemtulla A, Roth DA, Wasley LC et al: In vitro and in vivo functional characterization of bovine vitamin K-dependent γ-carboxylase expressed in Chinese hamster ovary cells. Proc Natl Acad Sci USA 90:4611, 1993

167. Roth DA, Rehemtulla A, Kaufman RJ et al: Expression of vitamin K-dependent carboxylase in baculovirus-infected insect cells. Proc Natl Acad Sci USA 90:8372, 1993

168. Pan LC, Price PA: The propeptide of rat bone γ-carboxygluamic acid protein shares homology with other vitamin K-dependent protein precursors. Proc Natl Acad Sci USA 82:6109, 1985

169. Price PA, Fraser JD, Metz-Virca G: Molecular cloning of matrix Gla protein: implications for substrate recognition by the vitamin K-dependent γ-carboxylase. Proc Natl Acad Sci USA 84:8335, 1987

170. Rabiet MJ, Jorgensen MJ, Furie B, Furie BC: Effect of propeptide mutations on posttranslational processing of factor IX: evidence that β-hydroxylation and γ-carboxylation are independent events. J Biol Chem 262:14895, 1987

171. Foster DC, Rudinski MS, Schach BG et al: Propeptide of human protein C is necessary for γ-carboxylation. Biochemistry 26:7003, 1987

172. Ratcliffe JV, Jorgensen MJ, DiMichelle D et al: Sufficiency of the γ-carboxylation recognition site on the propeptides of the vitamin K-dependent proteins for carboxylation. Blood 78:180A, 1991

173. Ulrich M, Furie B, Jacobs M et al: Vitamin K-dependent carboxylation: a synthetic peptide based upon the γ-carboxylation recognition site sequence of the prothrombin propeptide is an active substrate for the carboxylase in vitro. J Biol Chem 263:9697, 1988

174. Hubbard B, Jacobs M, Ulrich et al: Vitamin K-dependent carboxylation: in vitro modification of synthetic peptides containing the γ-carboxylation recognition site. J Biol Chem 264:14145, 1989

175. Knobloch JE, Suttie JW: Vitamin K-dependent carboxylase: control of enzyme activity by the "propeptide" region of factor X. J Biol Chem 262:15334, 1987

176. Sanford DG, Kanagy C, Sudmeir JL et al: Structure of the propeptide of prothrombin containing the γ-carboxylation recognition site determined by two-dimensional NMR spectroscopy. Biochemistry 30:9835, 1991

177. Bristol JA, Furie BC, Furie B: Profactor IX: carboxylated profactor IX is not a substrate for proteolytic activation and lacks a γ-carboxyglutamic acid-dependent membrane binding site. Blood 82:63A, 1993

178. Wasley LC, Rehemtulla A, Bristol JA, Kaufman RJ: PACE/furin can process the vitamin K-dependent profactor IX precursor within the secretory pathway. J Biol Chem 268:8458, 1993

179. Kawabata S-I, Davie EW: A microsomal endopeptidase from liver with substrate specificity for processing proproteins such as the vitamin K-dependent proteins of plasma. J Biol Chem 267:10331, 1992

180. Kawabata S-I, Nakagawa K, Muta T et al: Rabbit liver microsomal endopeptidase with substrate specificity for processing proproteins is structurally related to rat testes metalloendopeptidase 24.15. J Biol Chem 268:12498, 1993

181. Bristol JA, Furie BC, Furie B: Propeptide processing during factor IX biosynthesis: effect of point mutations adjacent to the propeptide cleavage site. J Biol Chem 268:7577, 1993

182. Drakenberg T, Fernlund P, Roepstorff P, Stenflo J: β-Hydroxyaspartic acid in vitamin K-dependent protein C. Proc Natl Acad Sci USA 80:1802, 1983

183. Stenflo J, Lundwall N, Dahlback B: β-Hydroxyasparagine in domains homologous to the epidermal growth factor precursor in vitamin K-dependent protein S. Proc Natl Acad Sci USA 84:368, 1987

184. Stenflo J, Onlin A-K, Owen WG, Schneider WJ: β-Hydroxyaspartic acid or β-hydroxyasparagine in bovine low density lipoprotein receptor and in bovine thrombomodulin. J Biol Chem 263:21, 1988

185. Przysiecki CT, Staggers JE, Ramjit HG et al: Occurrence of β-hydroxylated asparagine residues in non-vitamin K-dependent proteins containing epidermal growth factor-like domains. Proc Natl Acad Sci USA 84:7856, 1987

186. Gronke RS, VanDusen WJ, Garsky VM et al: Aspartyl β-hydroxylase: in vitro hydroxylation of a synthetic peptide based on the structure of the first growth factor-like domain of human factor IX. Proc Natl Acad Sci USA 86:3609, 1989

187. Derian CK, VanDusen W, Przysiecki CT et al: Inhibitors of 2-ketoglutarate-dependent dioxygenases block aspartyl β-hydroxylation of recombinant human factor IX in several mammalian expression systems. J Biol Chem 264:6615, 1989

188. Wagner DD, Saffaripour S, Bonfanti R et al: Von Willebrand factor propolypeptide directs Weibel-Palade body-like organelle formation in heterologous secretory cells. Blood, suppl. 74:192a, 1989

189. Pederson AH, Lund-Hansen T, Bisgaard-Frantzen H et al: Autoactivation of human recombinant coagulation factor VII. Biochemistry 28:9331, 1989

190. Yamamoto M, Nakagaki T, Kisiel W: Tissue factor-dependent autoactivation of human blood coagulation factor VII. J Biol Chem 267:19089, 1992

191. Neuenschwander PF, Morrissey JH: Deletion of the membrane anchoring region of tissue factor abolishes autoactivation of factor VII but not cofactor function. J Biol Chem 267:14477, 1992

192. Kisiel W, Fujikawa K, Davie EW: Activation of bovine factor VII (proconvertin) by factor XIIa (activated Hageman factor). Biochemistry 16:4189, 1977

193. Radcliffe R, Nemerson Y: Mechanism of action of bovine factor VII: products of cleavage of factor Xa. J Biol Chem 251:4797, 1976

194. Radcliffe R, Bagdassarian A, Colman R, Nemerson Y: Activation of bovine factor VII by Hageman factor fragments. Blood 50:611, 1977

195. Bach R, Gentry R, Nemerson Y: Factor VII binding to tissue factor in reconstituted phospholipid vesicles: induction of cooperativity by phosphatidylserine. Biochemistry 25:4007, 1986

196. Nakagaki T, Foster DC, Berkner KL, Kisiel W: Initiation of the extrinsic pathway of blood coagulation: evidence for the tissue factor dependent autoactivation of human coagulation factor VII. Biochemistry 30:10819, 1991

197. Osterud B, Rapaport SI: Activation of factor IX by the reaction product of tissue factor and factor VII: additional pathway for initiating blood coagulation. Proc Natl Acad Sci USA 74:5260, 1977

198. Byrne R, Amphlett GW, Castellino FJ: Metal ion specificity of the conversion of bovine factors IX, IXα, and IXαα to bovine factor IXaβ. J Biol Chem 255:1430, 1980

199. Fujikawa K, Legaz M, Kato H, Davie EW: The mechanism of activation of bovine factor IX (Christmas factor). Biochemistry 13:4508, 1974

200. DiScipio RG, Kurachi K, Davie EW: Activation of human factor IX (Christmas factor). J Clin Invest 61:1528, 1978

201. Pittman DD, Kaufman RJ: Proteolytic requirements for thrombin activation of antihemophilic factor (factor VIII). Proc Natl Acad Sci USA 85:2429, 1988

202. Lollar P, Parker CG: Subunit structure of thrombin-activated porcine factor VIII. Biochemistry 28:666, 1989

203. Gilbert GE, Furie BC, Furie B: Binding of human factor VIII to phospholipid vesicles. J Biol Chem 265:815, 1990

204. Stern DM, Nawroth PP, Kisiel W et al: A coagulation pathway on bovine endothelial aortic segments leading to generation of factor Xa and thrombin. J Clin Invest 74:1910, 1984

205. Van Dieijen G, Tans G, Rosing J, Hemker HC: The role of phospholipid and factor VIIIa in the activation of bovine factor X. J Biol Chem 256:3433, 1981

206. Radcliffe RD, Barton PD: Comparisons of the molecular forms of activated bovine factor X. J Biol Chem 248:6788, 1973

207. Jesty J, Spencer AK, Nemerson Y: The mechanism of activation of factor X. J Biol Chem 249:5614, 1974

208. Williams WJ, Esnouf MP: The fractionation of Russell's viper (Vipera russelli) venom with special reference to the coagulant protein. Biochem J 84:52, 1962

209. Furie BC, Furie B, Gottlieb AJ, Williams WJ: Activation of bovine factor X by the venom coagulant protein of Vipera russelli: complex formation of the activation fragments. Biochim Biophys Acta 365:121, 1974

210. Duffy EJ, Lollar P: Intrinsic pathway activation of factor X and its activation peptide-deficient derivative, factor X$_{des143-191}$. J Biol Chem 267:7821, 1992

211. Furie B, Furie BC: Spectral changes in bovine factor X associated with activation by the venom coagulant protein of Vipera russelli. J Biol Chem 251:6807, 1976

212. Gitel SN, Medina VM, Wessler S: Inhibition of human activated factor X by antithrombin III and alpha 1-proteinase inhibitor in human plasma. J Biol Chem 259:6890, 1984

213. Sanders NL, Bajaj SP, Zivelin A, Rapaport SI: Inhibition of tissue factor/factor VIIa activity in plasma requires factor X and an additional plasma component. Blood 66:204, 1985

214. Broze GJ Jr, Miletich JP: Characterization of the inhibition of tissue factor in serum. Blood 69:150, 1987

215. Novotny WF, Girard TJ, Miletich JP, Broze GJ: Purification and characterization of the lipoprotein-associated coagulation inhibitor from human plasma. J Biol Chem 264:18832, 1989

216. Rapaport SI: Inhibition of factor VIIa/tissue factor-induced blood coagulation: with particular emphasis upon a factor Xa-dependent inhibitory mechanism. Blood 73:359, 1989

217. Girard TJ, Eddy R, Wesselschmidt RL et al: Structure of the human lipoprotein-associated coagulation inhibitor gene. J Biol Chem 266:5036, 1991

218. Van der Logt CPE, Reitsma PH, Bertina RM: Intron-exon organization of the human gen coding for the lipoprotein-associated coagulation inhibitor: the factor Xa-dependent inhibitor of the extrinsic pathway of blood coagulation. Biochemistry 30:1571, 1991

219. Wun TC, Kretzmer KK, Girard TJ et al: Cloning and characterization of a cDNA coding for the lipoprotein associated coagulation inhibitor shows that it consists of three tandem Kunitz-type inhibitory domains. J Biol Chem 263:6001, 1988

220. Broze GJ Jr, Warren LA, Novotny WF et al: The lipoprotein-associated coagulation inhibitor that inhibits the factor VII-tissue factor complex also inhibits factor Xa: insight into its possible mechanism of action. Blood 71:335, 1988

221. Bloom JW, Nesheim ME, Mann KG: Phospholipid binding properties of bovine factor V and factor Va. Biochemistry 18:4419, 1979

222. Pusey ML, Nelsestuen GL: Membrane binding properties of blood coagulation factor V and derived peptides. Biochemistry 23:6202, 1984

223. Abbott AJ, Nelsestuen GL: Association of a protein with membrane vesicles at the collisonal limit: studies with blood coagulation factor Va light chain also suggest major differences between small and large unilamellar vesicles. Biochemistry 26:7994, 1987

224. Krishnaswamy S, Mann KG: The binding of factor Va to phospholipid vesicles. J Biol Chem 263:5714, 1988

225. Wiedmer T, Esmon CT, Sims PJ: On the mechanism by which complement proteins C5b-9 increase platelet prothrombinase activity. J Biol Chem 261: 14587, 1986

226. Sims PJ, Faioni EM, Wiedmer T, Shattil SJ: Complement proteins C5b-9 cause release of membrane vesicles from platelet surfaces that are enriched in membrane receptors for factor Va and express prothrombinase. J Biol Chem 263:18205, 1988

227. Sims PJ, Wiedmer T, Esmon CT et al: Assembly of the platelet prothrombinase complex is linked to vesiculation of the platelet plasma membrane: studies in Scott syndrome: an isolated defect in platelet procoagulant activity. J Biol Chem 264:17049, 1989

228. Esmon CT: The subunit structure of thrombin-activated factor V. Isolation of activated factor V, separation of subunits, and reconstitution of biological activity. J Biol Chem 254:964, 1979

229. Suzuki K, Dahlback B, Stenflo J: Thrombin-catalyzed activation of human coagulation factor V. J Biol Chem 257:6556, 1982

230. Nesheim ME, Foster WB, Mann KG: Characterization of factor V intermediates. J Biol Chem 259:3187, 1984

231. Odegaard B, Mann KG: Proteolysis of factor Va by factor Xa and activated protein C. J Biol Chem 262:11233, 1987

232. Mann KG, Jenny RJ, Krishnaswamy S: Cofactor proteins in the assembly and expression of blood clotting enzyme complexes. Annu Rev Biochem 57: 915, 1988

233. Kane WH, Lindout MJ, Jackson CM, Majerus PW: Factor Va dependent binding of factor Xa to platelets. J Biol Chem 255:1170, 1980

234. Miletich JP, Jackson CM, Majerus PW: Patients with congenital factor V deficiency have decreased factor Xa binding sites on their platelets. J Clin Invest 62:824, 1978

235. Miletich JP, Jackson CM, Majerus PW: Interaction of coagulation factor Xa with human platelets. Proc Natl Acad Sci USA 74:4033, 1977

236. Rodgers GM, Shuman MA: Prothrombin is activated on vascular endothelium by factor Xa and calcium. Proc Natl Acad Sci USA 80:7001, 1983

237. Maruyama I, Salem H, Majerus PW: Coagulation factor Va binds to human umbilical vein endothelial cells (HUVE) and accelerates protein C activation. J Clin Invest 73:654, 1984

238. Tracy P, Rohrbach MS, Mann KG: Functional prothrombinase complex assembly on isolated monocytes and lymphocytes. J Biol Chem 258:7264, 1983

239. Tracy P, Eide LL, Mann KG: Human prothrombinase complex assembly and function on isolated peripheral blood cell populations. J Biol Chem 260: 2119, 1985

240. Stenn KS, Blout ER: Mechanism of bovine prothrombin activity by an insoluble preparation of bovine factor Xa (thrombokinase). Biochemistry 11:4502, 1972

241. Heldebrant CM, Butkowski RJ, Bajaj SP, Mann KG: The activation of prothrombin. II. Partial reactions, physical and chemical characterization of the intermediates of activation. J Biol Chem 248:7149, 1973

242. Esmon CT, Owen WG, Jackson CM: The conversion of prothrombin to thrombin. I. Characterization of the reaction product formed during activation of bovine prothrombin. J Biol Chem 249:606, 1974

243. Rosenberg JS, Beeler DL, Rosenberg RD: Activation of human prothrombin by highly purified human factors V and Xa in presence of human antithrombin III. J Biol Chem 250:1607, 1975

244. Aronson DL, Stevan L, Ball AP et al: Generation of the combined prothrombin activation peptide (F1·2) during the clotting of blood and plasma. J Clin Invest 60:1410, 1977

245. Rabiet M-J, Blashill A, Furie B, Furie BC: Prothrombin fragment 1·2·3, a major product of prothrombin activation in human plasma. J Biol Chem 261:13210, 1986

246. Rosing J, Zwaal RFA, Tans G: Formation of meizothrombin as intermediate in factor Xa-catalyzed prothrombin activation. J Biol Chem 261:4222, 1986

247. Fowler WE, Hantgan RR, Hermans J, Erickson HP: Structure of the fibrin protofibril. Proc Natl Acad Sci USA 78:4872, 1981

248. Krakow W, Endres GF, Siegel BM, Scheraga HA: An electron microscopic investigation of the polymerization of bovine fibrin monomer. J Mol Biol 71:95, 1972

249. Folk JE, Finlayson JS, Peyton MP: Cross-link fibrin polymerized by factor XIII: ε(γ-glutamyl) lysine. Science 160:892, 1968

250. Van der Graaf FG, Tans G, Bouma BN, Griffin JH: Isolation and functional properties of the heavy and light chains of human plasma kallidrein. J Biol Chem 257:14300, 1982

251. Schapira M, Scott CF, Colman RW: Contribution of plasma protease inhibitors to the inactivation of kallikrein in plasma. J Clin Invest 69:462, 1982

252. Van der Graff F, Koedam JA, Bouma BN: Inactivation of kallikrein in human plasma. J Clin Invest 71:149, 1983

253. Meier HK, Webster ME, Mandle R et al: Enhancement of the surface-dependent Hageman factor activation by high molecular weight kininogen. J Clin Invest 60:18, 1977

254. Griffin JH, Cochrane CG: Mechanisms for the involvement of high molecular weight kininogen in surface-dependent reactions. Proc Natl Acad Sci USA 73:2554, 1976

255. Meier HL, Pierce JV, Colman W, Kaplan AP: Activation and function of human Hageman factor: the role of high molecular weight kininogen and prekallikrein. J Clin Invest 60:18, 1977

256. Griffin JH: Role of surface in surface-dependent activation of Hageman factor (blood coagulation factor XII). Proc Natl Acad Sci USA 75:1998, 1978

257. Fujikawa K, Heimark RL, Kurachi K, Davie EW: Activation of bovine factor XII (Hageman factor) by plasma kallikrein. Biochemistry 19:1322, 1980

258. Ratnoff OD: The biology and pathology of the initial stages of coagulation. Prog Hematol 5:204, 1966

259. Wilner GD, Nossell HL. LeRoy EC: Activation of Hageman factor by collagen. J Clin Invest 12:2608, 1968

260. Lipscomb MS, Walsh PN: Human platelets and factor XI. Localization in platelet membranes of factor XI-like activity and its functional distinction from plasma factor XI. J Clin Invest 63:1006, 1979

261. Greengard JS, Heeb MJ, Ersdal E et al: Binding of coagulation factor XI to washed human platelets. Biochemistry 25:3884, 1986

262. Ahmad SS, Rawala-Sheikh R, Walsh PN: Comparative interactions of factor IX and factor IXa with human platelets. J Biol Chem 264:3244, 1989

263. Furie B, Furie BC: The molecular basis of blood coagulation. Cell 53:505, 1988

264. Degen SJ, MacGillivray RTA, Davie EW: Characterization of the cDNA and gene coding for human prothrombin. Biochemistry 22:2087, 1983

265. Kurachi K, Davie EW: Characterization of a cDNA coding for human factor IX. Proc Natl Acad Sci USA 79:6461, 1982

266. Choo KH, Gould KG, Rees DJG, Brownlee GG: Molecular cloning of the gene for human anti-haemophilic factor IX. Nature 299:178, 1982

267. Foster D, Davie EW: Characterization of a cDNA coding for human protein C. Proc Natl Acad Sci USA 81:4766, 1984

268. Beckmann RJ, Schmidt RJ, Santerre RF: The structure and evolution of a 461 amino acid human protein C precursor and its messenger RNA, based upon the DNA sequence of cloned human liver cDNAs. Nucleic Acids Res 13:5233, 1985

269. Lundwall A, Dackowski W, Cohen E et al: Isolation and sequence of the cDNA for human protein S, a regulator of blood coagulation. Proc Natl Acad Sci USA 83:6716, 1986

270. Price PA, Williamson MK: Primary structure of bovine matrix Gla protein, a new vitamin K-dependent bone protein. J Biol Chem 260:14971, 1985

Molecular and Cellular Basis of Fibrinolysis

101

H. Roger Lijnen and Désiré Collen

INTRODUCTION

The fibrinolytic system in mammalian blood plays an important role in the dissolution of blood clots and in the maintenance of a patent vascular system. The fibrinolytic system (Fig. 101-1) comprises an inactive proenzyme, plasminogen, which can be converted to the active enzyme, plasmin, which degrades fibrin into soluble fibrin degradation products. Two immunologically distinct physiologic plasminogen activators have been identified in blood: tissue plasminogen activator (t-PA) and urokinase plasminogen activator (u-PA). Inhibition of the fibrinolytic system may occur either at the level of the plasminogen activators, by specific plasminogen activator inhibitors (PAI-1 and PAI-2), or at the level of plasmin, by α_2-antiplasmin. Some physicochemical properties of the main components of the fibrinolytic system are summarized in Table 101-1. Plasminogen activation may also be induced by an "intrinsic" pathway involving several proteins, including factor XII, high-molecular-weight kininogen (HMWK), and prekallikrein. Kallikrein, generated from prekallikrein by the action of factor XII and HMWK, may convert single-chain u-PA (scu-PA) to two-chain u-PA (tcu-PA).

Regulation and control of the fibrinolytic system are mediated by specific molecular interactions among its main components and by controlled synthesis and release of plasminogen activators and PAIs, primarily from endothelial cells. Disorders of the fibrinolytic system may result either from impaired activation (thrombotic complications) or from excessive activation (bleeding tendency) of the fibrinolytic system.

PROTEIN STRUCTURE OF THE MAIN COMPONENTS OF THE FIBRINOLYTIC SYSTEM

All the enzymes of the fibrinolytic system are serine proteases (i.e., their active site consists of a catalytic triad composed of the amino acids Ser-Asp-His. This active site is located in the COOH-terminal region of the molecules (serine protease domain), while the NH$_2$-terminal regions contain one or more functional domains, including the finger domain (homologous to the fingers in fibronectin), the epidermal growth factor domain (homologous to growth factors), and kringle domains, which are disulfide-bonded triple-loop structures of about 80 amino acids each. The inhibitors of the fibrinolytic system show significant sequence homology and are grouped into the serpin (serine proteinase inhibitor) superfamily. The COOH-terminal region of these inhibitors contains a specific reactive site peptide bond; when cleaved by their target enzyme, a peptide from the inhibitor is released, forming an inactive enzyme/inhibitor complex. The reactive site of the serpins has a basic amino acid residue (arginine or lysine) in the P_1 position (Arg X or Lys X) (Table 101-1).

Human plasminogen is a 92-kD single-chain glycoprotein, consisting of 791 amino acids; it contains 24 disulfide bridges and 5 homologous kringles[1,2] (Fig. 101-2). Native plasminogen has NH$_2$-terminal glutamic acid (Glu-plasminogen) but is easily converted by limited plasmin digestion to modified forms with NH$_2$-terminal lysine, valine, or methionine, commonly designated Lys-plasminogen. The plasminogen kringles contain lysine binding sites that mediate the specific binding of plasminogen to fibrin and the interaction of plasmin with α_2-antiplasmin; they play a crucial role in the regulation of fibrinolysis.[3]

t-PA is a 70-kD serine protease, originally isolated as a single polypeptide chain of 527 amino acids[4] (Fig. 101-3). Subsequently it was shown that native t-PA contains an NH$_2$-terminal extension of three amino acids (Gly-Ala-Arg-).[5] t-PA is converted by plasmin to a two-chain form (tct-PA) by hydrolysis of the Arg 275-Ile 276 peptide bond. The NH$_2$-terminal region is composed of several domains with homologies to other proteins: a finger domain comprising residues 4–50, a growth factor domain comprising residues 50–87, and two kringles comprising residues 87–176 and 176–262. The region constituted by residues 276–527 represents the serine protease part with the catalytic site, composed of His 322, Asp 371, and Ser 478.[4] These distinct domains in t-PA are involved in several functions of the enzyme, including its binding to fibrin, fibrin-specific plasminogen activation, rapid clearance in vivo, and binding to endothelial cell receptors. Binding of t-PA to fibrin is mediated via the finger and the second kringle domains. Initially, it was proposed that mainly the second kringle of t-PA would be responsible for the stimulatory effect of fibrin on plasminogen activation, although other studies claimed that both kringles are equivalent in their ability to mediate the stimulation of the catalytic efficiency of t-PA by fibrin.[6]

scu-PA is a 54-kD glycoprotein containing 411 amino acids[7] (Fig. 101-4). On proteolytic cleavage of the Lys 158-Ile 159 peptide bond, the molecule is converted to a two-chain derivative (i.e., tcu-PA). The catalytic triad is located in the COOH-terminal polypeptide chain and is composed of Asp 255, His 204, and Ser 356. The NH$_2$-terminal chain contains an epidermal growth factor domain (residues 5–49) and one kringle domain. A low-molecular-weight tcu-PA (33,000) can be generated with plasmin by hydrolysis of the Lys 135-Lys 136 peptide bond following previous cleavage of the Lys 158-Ile 159 bond.

α_2-Antiplasmin is a 70-kD single-chain glycoprotein containing about 13% carbohydrate. The molecule consists of 452 amino acids and contains two disulfide bridges[8] (Fig. 101-5). α_2-Antiplasmin is a serpin with a reactive-site peptide bond Arg 364-Met 365. Its concentration in normal human plasma is about 70 μg/ml (approximately 1 μM). α_2-Antiplasmin is synthesized primarily in a plasminogen-binding form that becomes partly converted in circulating blood to a non-plasminogen-binding form (about 30% of the total), which lacks a 26-residue peptide from the COOH-terminal end.[9] The inhibitor is cross-linked to the fibrin α-chain when blood is clotted in the presence of Ca^{2+} and activated coagulation factor XIII; the glutamine residue in the second position at the NH$_2$-terminal end is involved in cross-linking.[10]

PAI-1 is a 52-kD single-chain glycoprotein consisting of 379 amino acids; it is a serpin with reactive-site peptide bond Arg 346-Met 347.[11] PAI-1 is stabilized by binding to a plasminogen activator binding protein identified as S-protein or vitronectin.[12] PAI-1 is very labile and is found in tissue culture fluid in

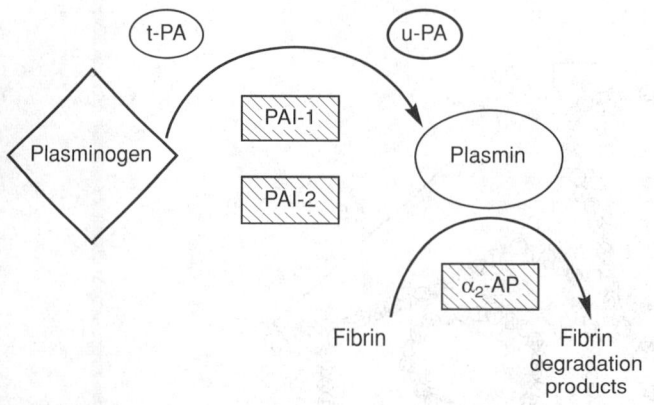

Fig. 101-1. Schematic representation of the fibrinolytic system. t-PA, tissue plasminogen activator; u-PA, urokinase plasminogen activator; PAI-1, PAI-2, plasminogen activator inhibitor -1 and -2; α_2-AP, α_2-antiplasmin.

a "latent" form that can be partly reactivated by treatment with denaturing agents.[13]

PAI-2 exists in two different forms with comparable kinetic properties: a 47-kD intracellular nonglycosylated form with a pI of 5.0, and a 60-kD secreted glycosylated form with a pI of 4.4.[14] PAI-2 is a serpin[15] containing 393 amino acids with reactive-site Arg 358-Thr 359.

GENE STRUCTURE OF THE MAIN COMPONENTS OF THE FIBRINOLYTIC SYSTEM

The human plasminogen gene was mapped to the long arm of chromosome 6 at band q26 or q27[16] (Table 101-2). It spans 52.5 kb of DNA and consists of 19 exons separated by 18 introns.[17] Each of the five kringles is encoded by two separate exons, with a single intron in the middle of each structure. The gene is closely related to that of apolipoprotein (a).[18]

The human t-PA gene has been localized on chromosome 8 (bands 8.p.12 → q.11.2)[19]; >36,000 base pairs (bp) of the human t-PA genomic sequence have been determined.[20] It consists of 14 exons, and the intron/exon organization suggests that the assembly is an example of the "exon shuffling" principle whereby the distinct structural domains are encoded by a single exon or by adjacent exons.[21] The proximal promoter sequences in the human t-PA gene contain typical TATA and CAAT boxes and potential recognition sequences for transcription factors (e.g., AP1, NF1, SP1, AP2) have been identified.[22] A sequence similar to the consensus sequence of the cAMP-responsive element and a sequence homologous with the consensus sequence of the AP2 binding site were recently identified and were suggested to have a cooperative effect on constitutive t-PA gene expression.[23] Allelic dimorphism

has been observed in the human t-PA gene as a result of an Alu insertion/deletion event that occurred early in evolution.[24]

The human u-PA gene is 6.4 kb long and is located on chromosome 10.[19] It contains 11 exons and the intron/exon organization of the gene closely resembles that of the t-PA gene.[25] However, exons III, VIII, and IX of t-PA are totally absent, and exon IV is partially missing in the u-PA gene; this accounts for the absence of a finger domain and a second kringle in u-PA. Exon II of the u-PA gene codes for a signal peptide consisting of 20 amino acids; exons III and IV code for the growth factor domain, and exons V and VI for the kringle region. The 5′-region of exon VII, which codes for the peptide connecting the light chain and the heavy chain, is 39 bp longer than the corresponding exon X of the t-PA gene. The 3′-region of exon VII and exons VIII–XI code for the heavy chain.

The gene for human α_2-antiplasmin is located on chromosome 18, bands p11.1–q11.2.[26] It contains 10 exons and 9 introns, covering approximately 16 kb of DNA.[27] The NH2-terminal region of the protein, comprising the fibrin cross-linking site, is encoded by exon IV, whereas both the reactive site and the plasminogen-binding site in the COOH-terminal region are encoded by exon X.

The PAI-1 gene has been mapped to chromosome 7, bands q21.3–q22.[28] It is approximately 12.2 kb in length and consists of nine exons and eight introns. The PAI-2 gene is located on chromosome 18 q21–q23. It spans 16.5 kb and contains 8 exons; a consensus sequence TATAAAA is found 22 bp 5′ of the proposed transcription initiation site. The structure of the gene is quite different from that of PAI-1 but is similar to that of the chicken ovalbumin gene.[29]

MECHANISM OF ACTIVATION OF PLASMINOGEN TO PLASMIN

Lys-plasminogen is converted to plasmin by cleavage of a single Arg 561-Val 562 peptide bond (the 791-amino acid numbering system is employed). The two-chain plasmin molecule is composed of a heavy chain containing the five kringles (NH2-terminal part of plasminogen) and a light chain, (COOH-terminal part) containing the catalytic triad composed of His 603, Asp 646, and Ser 741.[1,2]

Investigation of the activation pathways of plasminogen with the use of monoclonal antibodies specific for Lys-plasminogen has demonstrated that activation of Glu-plasminogen in human plasma occurs by direct cleavage of the Arg 561-Val 562 peptide bond without generation of Lys-plasminogen intermediates.[30]

MECHANISM OF INHIBITION OF PLASMIN BY α_2-ANTIPLASMIN

α_2-Antiplasmin forms an inactive 1:1 stoichiometric complex with plasmin. The inhibition of plasmin (P) by α_2-antiplasmin (A) can be represented by two consecutive reactions: a fast

Table 101-1. Some Properties of the Main Components of the Fibrinolytic System

	M_r (kd)	Carbohydrate Content (%)	No. of Amino Acids	Catalytic Triad	Reactive Site	Plasma Concentration (mg/L)
Plasminogen	92	2	791 (790)[a]	—	—	200
Plasmin	85	2	±715	His 602, Asp 645, Ser 740	—	—
t-PA	68	7	530 (527)[a]	His 322, Asp 371, Ser 478	—	0.005
scu-PA	54	7	411	His 204, Asp 255, Ser 356	—	0.008
α_2-Antiplasmin	70	13	452	—	Arg 364-Met 365	70
PAI-1	52	ND	379	—	Arg 346-Met 347	0.05
PAI-2	47,60	ND	393	—	Arg 358-Thr 359	<0.005

Abbreviations: t-PA, tissue plasminogen activator; scu-PA, single-chain urokinase plasminogen activator, prourokinase; PAI-1, PAI-2, plasminogen activator inhibitor-1 and -2; ND, not determined.

[a] The numbering of amino acid residues is usually based on these initially determined incorrect values.

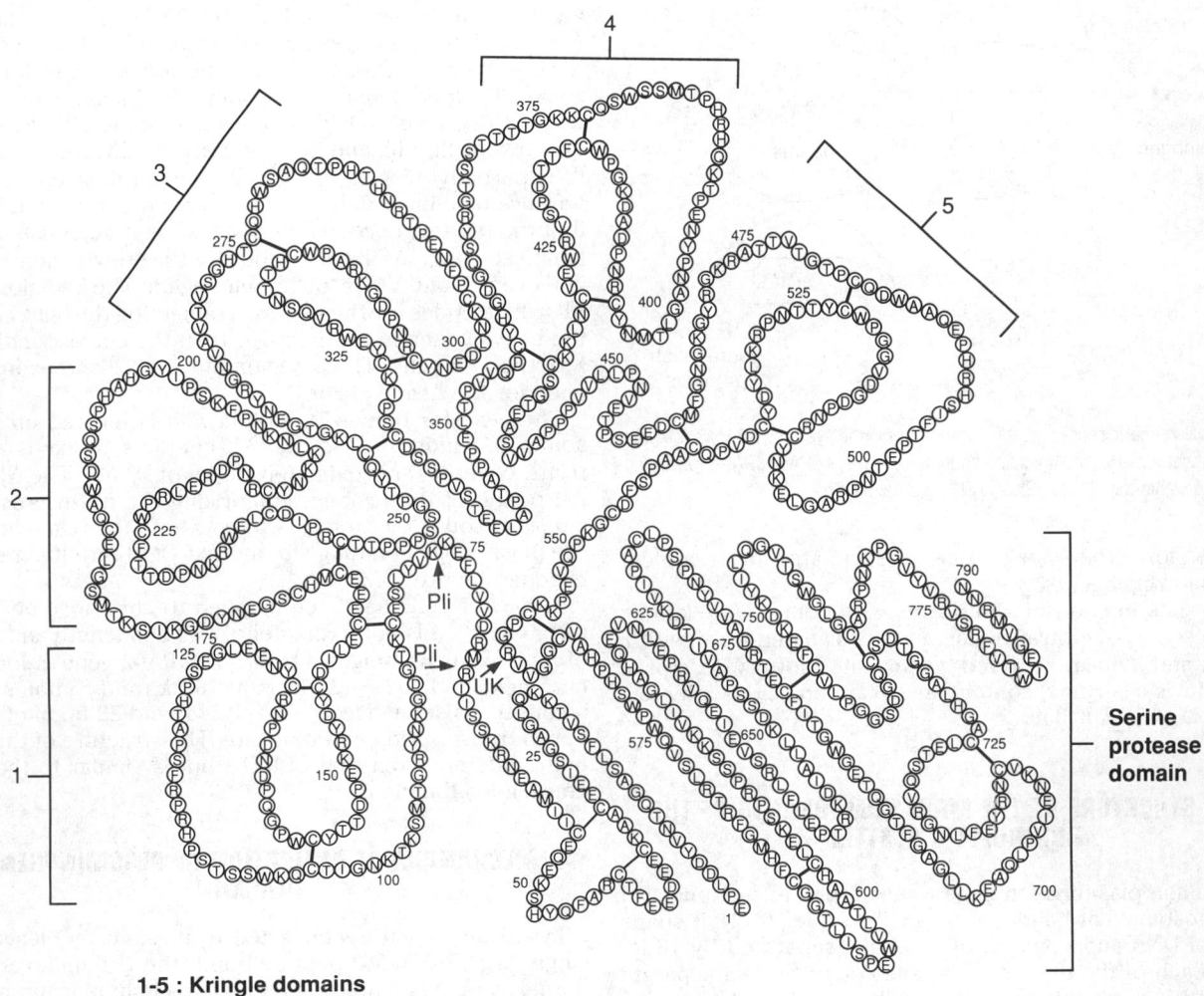

Fig. 101-2. Schematic representation of the primary structure of plasminogen. Pli, plasmic cleavage sites for conversion of Glu-plasminogen to Lys-plasminogen; UK, cleavage site for plasminogen activators, yielding plasmin. (Data from Sottrup-Jensen et al.,[1] with permission.)

second-order reaction producing a reversible inactive complex (PA), followed by a slower first-order transition resulting in an irreversible inactive complex (PA′). This model can be represented by

$$P + A \underset{k_{-1}}{\overset{k_1}{\rightleftharpoons}} PA \overset{k_2}{\rightarrow} PA'$$

The second-order rate constant of the inhibition is very high ($k_1 = 2$–4×10^7 M^{-1}s^{-1}),[31] but this high inhibition rate is dependent both on the presence of free lysine-binding sites and active site in the plasmin molecule and on the availability of a site complementary to the lysine-binding site and of the reactive site peptide bond in the inhibitor (Fig. 101-5). The half-life of plasmin molecules at the fibrin surface, both of whose lysine-binding sites and active site are occupied, is estimated to be two to three orders of magnitude longer than that of free plasmin.[31] Furthermore, the inhibition of plasmin by α_2-antiplasmin is accelerated by lipoprotein (a) [Lp(a)] in the presence of fibrin or fibrinogen fragments, which may result in impairment of fibrinolysis.[32]

MECHANISM OF ACTION OF TISSUE PLASMINOGEN ACTIVATOR

t-PA is a poor enzyme in the absence of fibrin, but the presence of fibrin strikingly enhances the activation rate of plasminogen.[33] In the presence of fibrin, the Michaelis constant for

plasminogen activation by t-PA equals 0.16 μM, as compared with 65 μM in the absence of fibrin. The kinetic data reported by Hoylaerts et al[33] support a mechanism in which fibrin provides a surface to which t-PA and plasminogen adsorb in a sequential and ordered manner, yielding a ternary complex. Fibrin essentially increases the local plasminogen concentration by creating an additional interaction between t-PA and its substrate. The high affinity of t-PA for plasminogen in the presence of fibrin thus allows efficient activation at the fibrin surface (Fig. 101-6). Plasmin formed on the fibrin clot is protected from rapid inhibition by α_2-antiplasmin. Although different kinetic constants for the activation of plasminogen by t-PA have been reported, most studies agree that fibrin stimulates plasminogen activation by t-PA by at least two orders of magnitude. Initial binding of t-PA to fibrin may be governed by the finger domain, and partial degradation of fibrin by plasmin results in enhanced binding of t-PA via kringle 2 to newly exposed COOH-terminal lysine residues.[34] During fibrin clot lysis, sct-PA is converted to tct-PA at the fibrin surface.[35] The physiologic relevance of this conversion remains unclear, although it has been suggested that it may result in enhanced fibrin binding of tct-PA to a large number of low-affinity binding sites.[36] The fibrinolytic process thus seems to be triggered by, and confined to, fibrin.

Direct binding studies, as well as kinetic studies, have shown that Lp(a) competes with plasminogen for binding to fibrin, as a result of binding of Lp(a) to fibrin via its lysine-binding domains.[37–39] Binding of Lp(a) to fibrin is enhanced by partial proteolytic degradation of the fibrin surface.[37] A functional consequence of the competition between Lp(a) and plasminogen for binding to fibrin is the inhibition of fibrin-dependent enhancement of plasminogen activation by t-PA.[38,39] The inhibition constant of Lp(a) for the activation of plasminogen by t-PA (15–22 nM) is of the same order as the physiologic plasma concentration of Lp(a). This suggests that elevated levels of Lp(a), as seen in patients with atherosclerosis, might significantly impair physiologic fibrinolysis.[40]

Over the past several years, a striking analogy between the role of fibrin and of cell surfaces in plasminogen activation has been recognized.[41] Many cell types bind both plasminogen and plasminogen activators, resulting in enhanced plasminogen activation and protection of bound plasmin from inhibition by α_2-antiplasmin.[41]

MECHANISM OF ACTION OF UROKINASE PLASMINOGEN ACTIVATOR

tcu-PA has no fibrin specificity and activates fibrin-bound and circulating plasminogen relatively indiscriminately. Extensive plasminogen activation and depletion of α_2-antiplasmin may occur following treatment of patients with thromboembolic disease with tcu-PA, leading to degradation of several plasma proteins, including fibrinogen and factors V and VIII.

scu-PA, in contrast to tcu-PA, has a significant fibrin specificity. Conversion of scu-PA to tcu-PA during clot lysis appears to constitute a primary positive feedback mechanism for plasminogen activation, whereas binding of plasminogen to fibrin or predigestion of fibrin by plasmin were found to result in some additional acceleration of fibrinolysis.[42] This mechanism of plasminogen activation and fibrin dissolution with scu-PA in a plasma milieu in vitro may, however, not be identical to its physiologic mechanism of action. Indeed, plasmin-resistant mutants of scu-PA (i.e., scu-PA K158E) have only a three- to fivefold lower in vivo thrombolytic potency than wild-type scu-PA,[43] suggesting that for in vivo thrombolysis conversion of scu-PA to tcu-PA may play a less important role. The molecular interactions that regulate the fibrin specificity of scu-PA remain to be further detailed.

MECHANISMS INVOLVED IN THE INHIBITION OF PLASMINOGEN ACTIVATORS

Multiple mechanisms are involved in the rapid inhibition of t-PA in human plasma. PAI-1 is a specific rapid-reacting inhibitor of t-PA, which is present at a low concentration in normal plasma, but at higher concentrations in many clinical conditions (see below).[44] In addition, t-PA is inhibited slowly by α_2-antiplasmin, α_1-antitrypsin, and C_1-inhibitor.[45] The primary mechanism of removal of t-PA from the blood, however, is by clearance via the liver.[46] In healthy volunteers and in patients with acute myocardial infarction, the initial half-life of t-PA was found to be 4–6 minutes.[47,48] Kuiper et al[49] characterized two different recognition systems for removal of t-PA by hepatocytes and by endothelial cells in the liver. Evidence obtained with deletion mutants suggests that the structures involved in the rapid hepatic clearance of t-PA are localized in the NH_2-terminal region, comprising the finger and growth factor domains.[6]

tcu-PA in human plasma is also slowly inhibited by several

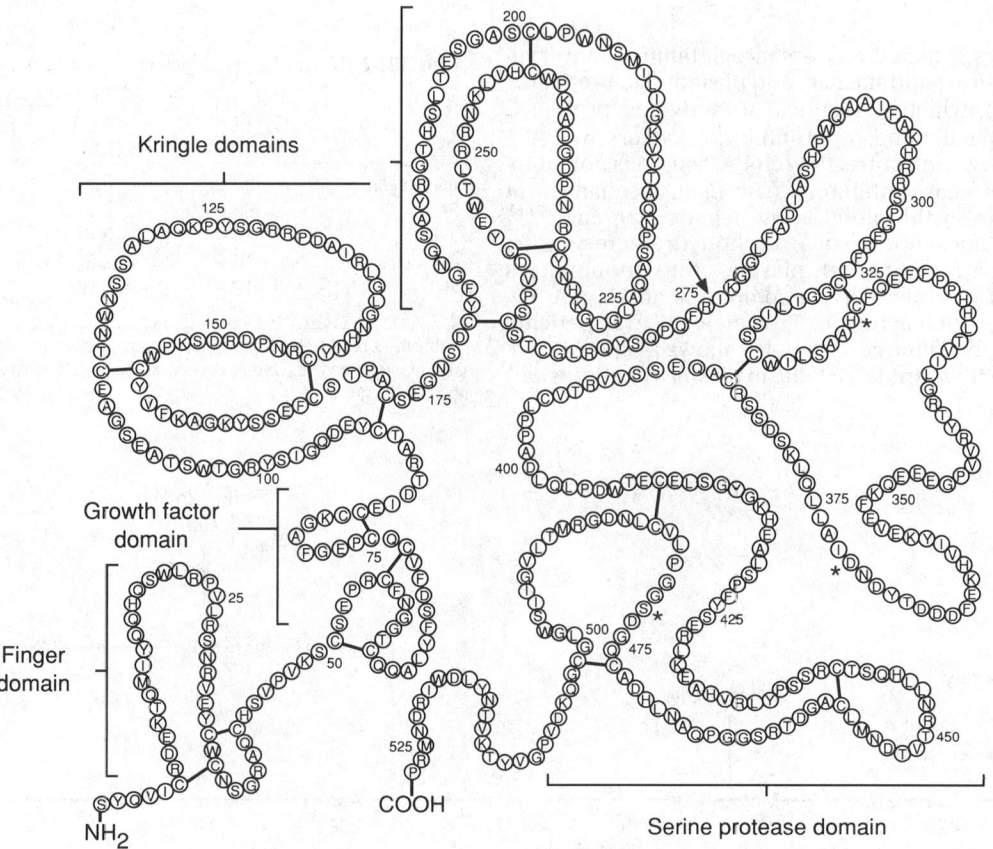

Fig. 101-3. Schematic representation of the primary structure of t-PA. Arrow, cleavage site for plasmin; asterisks, active site residues. (Adapted from Pennica et al.,[4] with permission.)

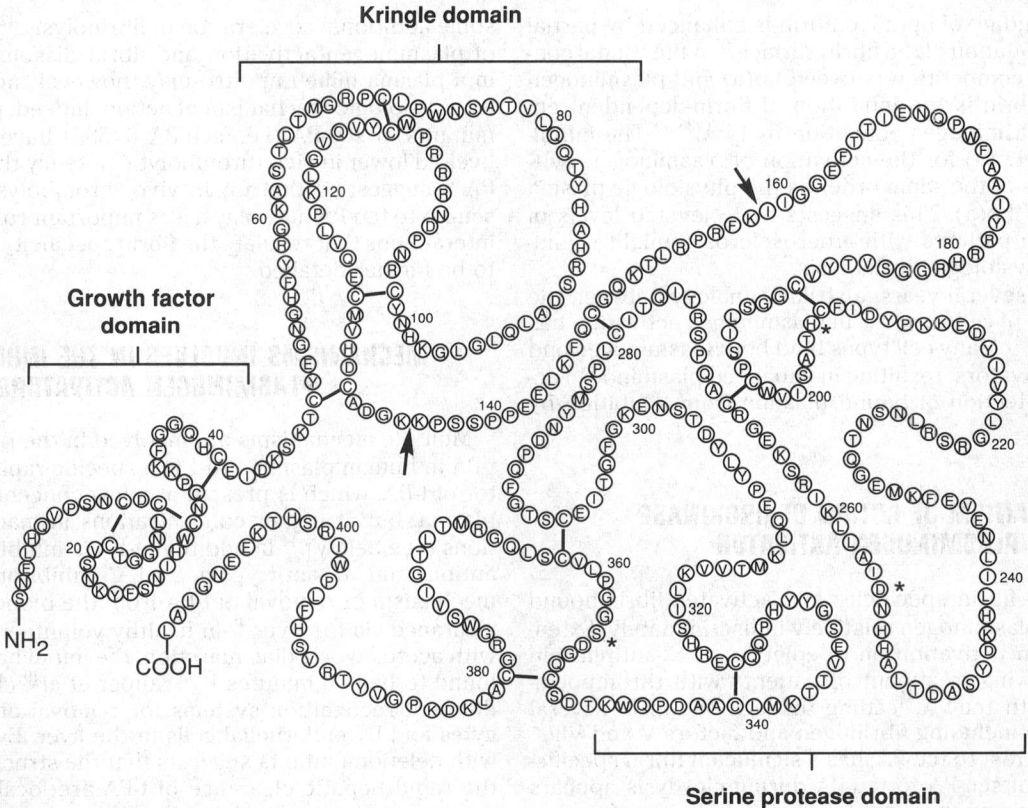

Fig. 101-4. Schematic representation of the primary structure of scu-PA. Arrow, cleavage site for plasmin; asterisks, active site residues. (Adapted from Holmes et al.,[7] with permission.)

protease inhibitors,[50] including α_2-macroglobulin, α_1-antitrypsin, antithrombin III, α_2-antiplasmin, and plasminogen activator inhibitor-3 (PAI-3), which is identical to activated protein C inhibitor. More specific and rapid inhibition occurs by PAI-1 and PAI-2 (see below). In contrast to tcu-PA, scu-PA is not inhibited by plasma protease inhibitors. The main mechanism of removal of u-PA from the blood is by hepatic clearance.[51,52] Rapid clearance does not involve carbohydrate receptors, does not occur via reaction with plasma protease inhibitors followed by rapid clearance of the complexes and is not mediated via the NH_2-terminal region of the molecule.[52] In patients with acute myocardial infarction, scu-PA shows a biphasic disappearance rate with an initial half-life in plasma (postinfusion) of about 4 minutes.[53]

Table 101-2. Some Characteristics of the Genes of the Main Components of the Fibrinolytic System

	Gene Length (kb)	mRNA (kb)	Exons (no.)	Chromosomal Location
Plasminogen	52.5	2.7	19	6
t-PA	36.6	2.7	14	8
scu-PA	6.4	2.4	11	10
α_2-Antiplasmin	16	2.2	10	18
PAI-1	12.2	3.0	9	7
PAI-2	16.5	1.9	8	18

Abbreviations: t-PA, tissue plasminogen activator; scu-PA, single-chain urokinase plasminogen activator, prourokinase; PAI-1, PAI-2, plasminogen activator inhibitor-1 and -2.

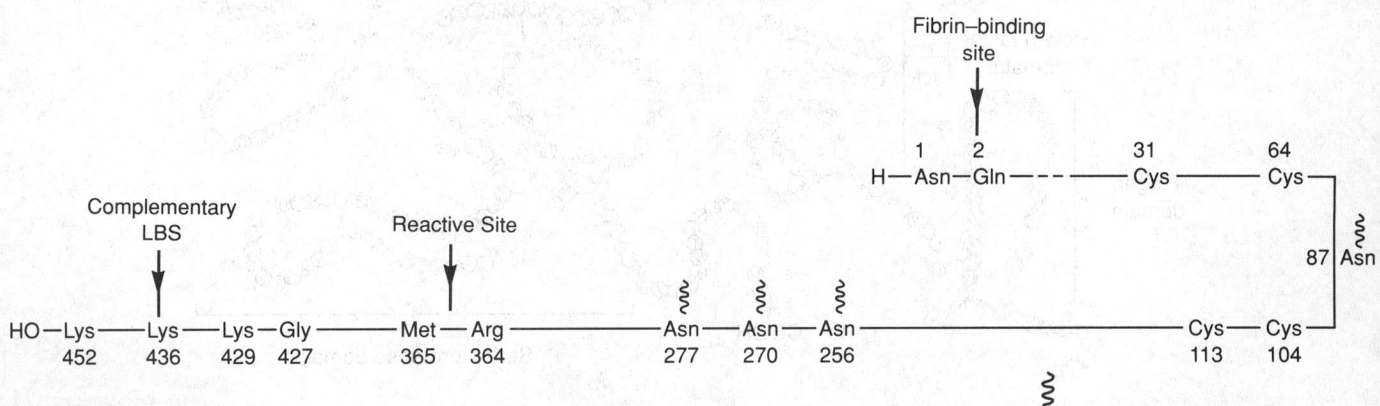

Fig. 101-5. Schematic representation of the primary structure of α_2-antiplasmin. LBS, lysine-binding site; Asn, carbohydrate attached to Asn residues. (Adapted from Holmes et al.,[8] with permission.)

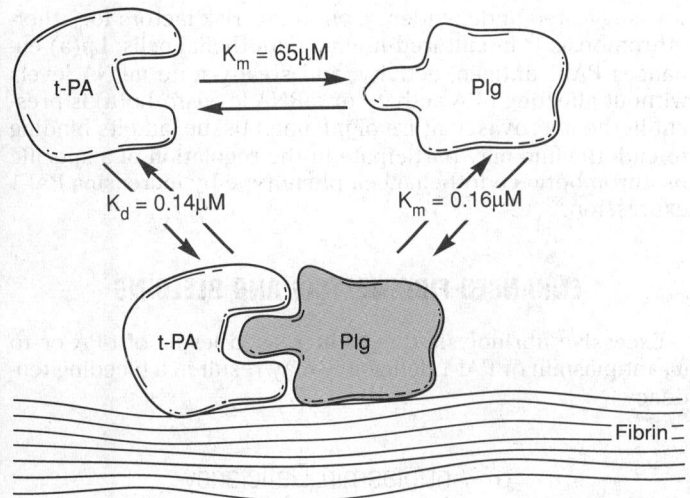

Fig. 101-6. Schematic representation of the molecular interactions that regulate the fibrin-specific activation of the fibrinolytic system by t-PA. t-PA in circulating plasma in the absence of fibrin has a low affinity for its substrate plasminogen ($K_m = 65 \,\mu M$), and no efficient plasminogen activation occurs. t-PA binds specifically to fibrin and the bimolecular t-PA/fibrin complex has a high affinity for plasminogen ($K_m = 0.16 \,\mu M$). Plasminogen binds to the binary t-PA/fibrin complex and is activated to plasmin at the fibrin surface. This in loco-generated plasmin is protected from rapid inactivation by α_2-antiplasmin.

PAI-1 reacts with sct-PA and tct-PA and with tcu-PA, but not with scu-PA or streptokinase.[54] The second-order rate constant for the inhibition of single-chain t-PA by PAI-1 is about 10^7 $M^{-1}s^{-1}$, while inhibition of tct-PA and tcu-PA is even somewhat faster. PAI-1 inhibits its target proteases by formation of a 1:1 stoichiometric reversible complex, followed by covalent binding between the hydroxyl group of the active-site serine residue of the protease and the carboxyl group of the P_1 residue at the reactive center ("bait region") of the serpin. Highly positively charged regions in t-PA (residues 296–304)[55] and in u-PA (residues 179–184)[56] are involved in the rapid interaction. Recently, a molecular form of intact PAI-1 has been isolated that does not form stable complexes with t-PA but is cleaved at the P_1-P_1' peptide bond (substrate PAI-1).[57] Thus, inhibitory PAI-1 may convert not only to latent PAI-1, which can be reactivated, but also to substrate PAI-1, which may be irreversibly degraded by target proteases, including t-PA, u-PA, and thrombin.[57] PAI activity is very rapidly cleared from the circulation via the liver; a half-life of 7 minutes in the rabbit has been reported.[58]

PAI-2 inhibits tcu-PA with a second-order rate constant (k_1) of 9×10^5 $M^{-1}s^{-1}$, which is about 10-fold slower than PAI-1. PAI-2 also efficiently inhibits tct-PA (k_1 of 2×10^5 $M^{-1}s^{-1}$), and inhibits sct-PA (k_1 of 9×10^3 $M^{-1}s^{-1}$) less efficiently; it does not inhibit scu-PA.[54]

PAI-3 (activated protein C inhibitor) inhibits tcu-PA with a second-order rate constant of 8×10^3 $M^{-1}s^{-1}$ in the absence of heparin and of 9×10^4 $M^{-1}s^{-1}$ in the presence of heparin. PAI-3 also inhibits tct-PA, but less efficiently, and it does not inhibit scu-PA.[59]

SYNTHESIS AND SECRETION OF PLASMINOGEN ACTIVATORS AND PLASMINOGEN ACTIVATOR INHIBITORS

The synthesis and secretion of t-PA, u-PA, and PAI-1 by endothelial cells is highly regulated, although some mediators influence the production of plasminogen activators and plasminogen activator inhibitors in parallel. The plasma level of t-PA antigen averages 5 ng/ml. Following stimulation of vascular en-

dothelium by various stimuli, such as venous occlusion, infusion of vasoactive compounds, and physical exercise, a rapid release (within minutes) of t-PA may occur. This response is probably too rapid to represent increased synthesis and may reflect release from cellular storage pools, although these have not been conclusively identified in endothelial cells. A variety of agents increase the synthesis of t-PA by cultured endothelial cells, including thrombin, histamine, butyrate, phorbol myristate acetate (PMA), basic fibroblast growth factor (bFGF), activated protein C, butanol and alcohol derivatives, and retinoids.[60] However, only histamine, butyrate, or a combination of cAMP with protein kinase C agonists were found to stimulate t-PA synthesis without affecting PAI-1 synthesis. The increase of t-PA induced by histamine, thrombin, and PMA in endothelial cells is paralleled by increased levels of t-PA mRNA, as a result of enhanced transcription of the t-PA gene.[60] Overexpression of t-PA in endothelial cells, using a retroviral expression vector, did not alter the morphology, attachment, proliferation, migration, or invasion in in vitro systems.[61] The mechanisms involved in the stimulatory effect of these various agents on t-PA synthesis may be different. Vasoactive substances, such as histamine and thrombin, bind to specific receptors and activate phospholipase C, which acts on phosphatidyl/inositol biphosphate to produce diacylglycerol. Diacyglycerol activates membrane-bound protein kinase C, which plays an important role in the regulation of t-PA synthesis.

While the synthesis of t-PA occurs mainly in endothelial cells, immunocytochemical staining of tissues indicates that many cells of different origin (i.e., fibroblasts and epithelial cells) produce u-PA.[62] The scu-PA concentration in human plasma was reported to range between 2 and 20 ng/ml. Many cells contain a 55-kD receptor that binds u-PA via the amino acid sequence consisting of residues 18–30 in the growth factor domain.[63,64] Membrane-bound u-PA retains its plasminogen activating potential and is protected to some extent from extracellular inhibitors; the presence of u-PA receptors may thus constitute a mechanism involved in breakdown of the extracellular matrix.

Synthesis and secretion of PAI-1 can be modulated by various agonists, such as hormones, growth factors, endotoxin, cytokines, and phorbol esters.[65] PAI-1 mRNA has been demonstrated in a large variety of tissues, suggesting that common cells in these tissues, such as endothelial or smooth muscle cells, may be the site of production. Although post-transcriptional regulation of PAI-1 mRNA levels has been demonstrated, most studies on the regulation of PAI-1 mRNA expression demonstrated effects at the gene transcriptional level. In endothelial cells, PAI-1 gene expression was shown to be stimulated by lipopolysaccharide, interleukin-1, tumor necrosis factor-α, transforming growth factor-β, bFGF, phorbol esters, thrombin, very-low-density-lipoprotein, LP(a), and insulin.[65] PAI-1 mRNA was found to be increased and PAI-1 protein was detected in endothelial cells juxtaposed to thrombi, in smooth muscle cells adjacent to the neointima, and in macrophages. This augmented arterial wall expression of PAI-1 induced by thrombosis may shift the local balance between fibrinolysis and thrombosis toward the latter.[66] Only a few studies have reported downregulation of PAI-1 synthesis in endothelial cells, either by forskolin or by endothelial cell growth factor combined with heparin.[65] Except for platelets, which contain essentially inactive PAI-1, PAI-1 is not stored within cells but is rapidly and constitutively secreted after synthesis.[67]

PAI-2 has been identified in human placenta and in pregnancy plasma; it is also secreted by leukocytes and by fibrosarcoma cells.[54,68] Secretion of PAI-2 is regulated by endotoxin and by phorbol esters that stimulate the gene transcription of PAI-2.[54,68]

IMPAIRED FIBRINOLYSIS AND THROMBOSIS

Impairment of fibrinolysis represents a commonly observed hemostatic abnormality associated with thrombosis. It may be due to defective synthesis or release of t-PA from the vessel wall, or both, or it may be due to increased levels of inhibitors of t-PA or of plasmin.

Deficient Synthesis or Release of Tissue Plasminogen Activator

A deficient fibrinolytic response may be caused by a deficient release of t-PA from the vessel wall or an increased rate of neutralization.[69,70] Juhan-Vague et al[71] investigated 120 patients with spontaneous or recurrent deep vein thrombosis and observed three groups based on their response to venous occlusion. A poor fibrinolytic response (less than twofold increase) to venous occlusion occurred in 35% of these patients, one-fourth of whom had deficient t-PA release and three-fourths of whom had normal t-PA release but increased levels of PAI-1.

Recently, mutant transgenic mice totally lacking functional t-PA were found to lyse experimental pulmonary emboli at a markedly reduced rate. These t-PA knock-out mice, as well as u-PA knock-out mice, however, appeared to be viable, fertile, and healthy under basal conditions.[72] The differential role of t-PA and u-PA in several biologic phenomena, therefore, may need to be re-examined with the use of such in vivo systems.

Enhanced Inhibition of Tissue Plasminogen Activator

The PAI-1 concentration in plasma is very low in healthy subjects (approximately 10–20 ng/ml), but it is increased in several diseases, including venous thromboembolism, obesity, sepsis, and coronary artery disease. Increased PAI-1 levels may promote fibrin deposition in vivo. Mice, transgenic for the human PAI-1 gene, develop venous thrombosis at the tip of the tail within 3 days after birth, but no arterial thrombosis.[73] When endotoxin-treated rabbits, with a markedly increased plasma PAI-1 level, are infused with the defibrinogenating snake venom ancrod, renal fibrin deposits are produced, whereas in normal rabbits ancrod infusion causes hypofibrinogenemia without fibrin deposition.[74] In an experimental rabbit model of jugular vein thrombosis, inhibition of PAI-1 with the use of a monoclonal antibody results in promotion of endogenous thrombolysis and inhibition of thrombus extension.[75] Furthermore, mutant transgenic mice totally lacking functional PAI-1 were shown to lyse experimental pulmonary emboli at a faster rate than occurred in controls.[72]

In patients with ischemic heart disease, including angina pectoris and previous myocardial infarction, a decreased fibrinolytic activity was consistently observed due to increased PAI-1 activity in plasma.[70,76] High PAI-1 activity constitutes an independent risk factor for myocardial reinfarction in young subjects, in whom PAI activity correlates with reinfarction within 3 years, but not with late reinfarction.[70] After successful percutaneous transluminal coronary angioplasty, a decrease in PAI-1 activity was associated with a significantly reduced risk of coronary restenosis.[77] There is a clear correlation between the circadian variation in the time of onset of myocardial infarction, with the highest incidence at about 8 AM, and the circadian rhythm of plasma PAI-1 activity, which is also highest early in the morning.[78] Insulin resistance has been shown to be associated with increased PAI-1 concentration in several populations, and a direct link between insulin and PAI-1 levels

was suggested, independent from other risk factors for atherothrombosis.[79] In cultured human endothelial cells, Lp(a) enhances PAI-1 antigen, activity, and steady-state mRNA levels without affecting t-PA activity or mRNA levels.[80] Lp(a) is present in the microvasculature of inflamed tissue, and its binding to endothelium may participate in the regulation of a specific prothrombotic endothelial cell phenotype by increasing PAI-1 expression.[80]

ENHANCED FIBRINOLYSIS AND BLEEDING

Excessive fibrinolysis due to increased levels of t-PA or to α_2-antiplasmin or PAI-1 deficiency may result in a bleeding tendency.

α_2-Antiplasmin Deficiency

The first patient reported with congenital homozygous α_2-antiplasmin deficiency presented with a severe hemorrhagic diathesis,[81] whereas several cases of heterozygosity have been described with no, or only mild, bleeding symptoms.[69] The α_2-antiplasmin levels in all heterozygotes described thus far are consistently 40–60% of normal. Antigen and activity levels usually correspond well, suggesting that the deficiency is due to decreased synthesis of a normal α_2-antiplasmin molecule. The bleeding tendency in these patients may be due to premature lysis of hemostatic plugs, because in the absence of α_2-antiplasmin, the half-life of plasmin molecules generated on the fibrin surface may be prolonged considerably.

The molecular defect in α_2-antiplasmin Okinawa was identified as a trinucleotide deletion in exon VII leading to deletion of Glu 137 in the protein.[82] In α_2-antiplasmin Nara, the insertion of a cytidine nucleotide at position 1,438 in exon X, leads to deletion of the COOH-terminal 12 amino acids of native α_2-antiplasmin and replacement with 178 unrelated amino acids.[83] It was suggested that these mutations lead to the deficiency by affecting the folding of the protein into the native configuration and thereby blocking its intracellular transport from the endoplasmatic reticulum to the Golgi complex.[82] Acquired α_2-antiplasmin deficiency associated with enhanced fibrinolysis has been reported in liver disease, disseminated intravascular coagulation and/or fibrinolysis and acute promyeolocytic leukemia.[69] α_2-Antiplasmin levels may be significantly reduced in patients undergoing thrombolytic therapy, as a result of systemic activation of the fibrinolytic system.[84] A dysfunctional α_2-antiplasmin molecule (α_2-antiplasmin Enschede), associated with a serious bleeding tendency, has been found in two siblings in a Dutch family. The ability of the protein to bind reversibly to plasmin or to plasminogen was not affected, but it was converted from an inhibitor of plasmin to a substrate.[85] The molecular defect consists of the insertion of an extra alanine residue (GCG insertion) somewhere between amino acid residues 353 and 357 (4 Ala residues), 7–10 positions on the NH$_2$-terminal side of the P$_1$ residue (Arg 364) in the reactive site of α_2-antiplasmin.[86]

Increased Levels of Plasminogen Activator Activity

Excessive fibrinolysis due to increased t-PA activity levels may be associated with a bleeding tendency. A lifelong hemorrhagic disorder associated with enhanced fibrinolysis due to increased levels of circulating plasminogen activator has been described in a few patients.[87,88] Alternatively, excessive fibrinolysis due to decreased PAI-1 levels has been reported in a few cases and was apparently associated with bleeding complications.[89,90] Recently, a complete deficiency of PAI-1 has been reported in a 9-year-old girl who endured several episodes of major hemorrhage, all in response to trauma or surgery.[91] DNA sequence analysis revealed a 2-bp (TA) insertion at the 3' end of exon 4. This mutation results in a shift in the reading frame after the codon for amino acid 210, resulting in a new stop codon. The predicted protein product thus lacks the 169 COOH-terminal amino acids of mature PAI-1, including the Arg 346-Met 347 reactive-site peptide bond.[91]

REFERENCES

1. Sottrup-Jensen L, Petersen TE, Magnusson S: Plasminogen sequence. p. 91. In Dayhoff M (ed): Atlas of Protein Sequence and Structure. Vol 5. Suppl 3. National Biomedical Research Foundation, Washington, DC, 1978
2. Forsgren M, Raden B, Israelsson M et al: Molecular cloning and characterization of a full-length cDNA clone for human plasminogen. FEBS Lett 213:254, 1987
3. Collen D: On the regulation and control of fibrinolysis. Thromb Haemost 43:77, 1980
4. Pennica D, Holmes WE, Kohr WJ et al: Cloning and expression of human tissue-type plasminogen activator cDNA in E. coli. Nature 301:214, 1983
5. Jörnvall H, Pohl G, Bergsdorf N, Wallen P: Differential proteolysis and evidence for a residue exchange in tissue plasminogen activator suggest possible association between two types of protein microheterogeneity. FEBS Lett 156:47, 1983
6. Lijnen HR, Collen D: Strategies for the improvement of thrombolytic agents. Thromb Haemost 66:88, 1991
7. Holmes WE, Pennica D, Blaber M et al: Cloning and expression of the gene for pro-urokinase in Escherichia coli. Biotechnology 3:923, 1985
8. Holmes WE, Nelles L, Lijnen HR, Collen D: Primary structure of human alpha 2-antiplasmin, a serine protease inhibitor (serpin). J Biol Chem 262:1659, 1987
9. Wiman B, Nilsson T, Cedergren B: Studies on a form of alpha 2-antiplasmin in plasma which does not interact with the lysine-binding sites in plasminogen. Thromb Res 28:193, 1982
10. Ichinose A, Tamaki T, Aoki N: Factor XIII-mediated cross-linking of NH2-terminal peptide of alpha 2-plasmin inhibitor to fibrin. FEBS Lett 153:369, 1983
11. Pannekoek H, Veerman H, Lambers H et al: Endothelial plasminogen activator inhibitor (PAI): a new member of the serpin gene family. EMBO J 5:2539, 1986
12. Declerck PJ, De Mol M, Alessi MC et al: Purification and characterization of a plasminogen activator inhibitor-1-binding protein from human plasma. Identification as a multimeric form of S protein (vitronectin). J Biol Chem 263:15454, 1988
13. Hekman CM, Loskutoff DJ: Endothelial cells produce a latent inhibitor of plasminogen activators that can be activated by denaturants. J Biol Chem 260:11581, 1985
14. Genton C, Kruithof EKO, Schleuning WD: Phorbol ester induces the biosynthesis of glycosylated and nonglycosylated plasminogen activator inhibitor 2 in high excess over urokinase-type plasminogen activator in human U-937 lymphoma cells. J Cell Biol 104:705, 1987
15. Ye RD, Wun TC, Sadler JE: cDNA cloning and expression in Escherichia coli of a plasminogen activator inhibitor from human placenta. J Biol Chem 262:3718, 1987
16. Murray JC, Buetow KH, Donovan M et al: Linkage disequilibrium of plasminogen polymorphisms and assignment of the gene to human chromosome 6q26–6q27. Am J Hum Genet 40:338, 1987
17. Petersen TE, Martzen MR, Ichinose A, Davie EW: Characterization of the gene for human plasminogen, a key proenzyme in the fibrinolytic system. J Biol Chem 265:6104, 1990
18. McLean JW, Tomlinson JE, Kuang WJ et al: cDNA sequence of human apolipoprotein(a) is homologous to plasminogen. Nature 330:132, 1987
19. Rajput B, Degen SF, Reich E et al: Chromosomal locations of human tissue plasminogen activator and urokinase genes. Science 230:672, 1985
20. Degen SJF, Rajput B, Reich E: The human tissue plasminogen activator gene. J Biol Chem 261:6972, 1986
21. Patthy L: Evolution of the proteases of blood coagulation and fibrinolysis by assembly from modules. Cell 41:657, 1985
22. Kooistra T, Bosma PJ, Toet K et al: Role of protein kinase C and cyclic adenosine monophosphate in the regulation of tissue-type plasminogen activator, plasminogen activator inhibitor-1, and platelet-derived growth factor mRNA levels in human endothelial cells. Possible involvement of proto-oncogenes c-jun and c-fos. Arterioscler Thromb 11:1042, 1991
23. Medcalf RL, Rueegg M, Schleuning WD: A DNA motif related to the cAMP-responsive element and an exon-located activator protein-2 binding site in the human tissue-type plasminogen activator gene promoter cooperate in

24. basal expression and convey activation by phorbol ester and cAMP. J Biol Chem 265:14618, 1990
24. Ludwig M, Wohn KD, Schleuning WD, Olek K: Allelic dimorphism in the human tissue-type plasminogen activator (tPA) gene as a result of an Alu insertion/deletion event. Hum Genet 88:388, 1992
25. Riccio A, Grimaldi G, Verde P et al: The human urokinase-plasminogen activator gene and its promoter. Nucleic Acids Res 13:2759, 1985
26. Kato A, Nakamura Y, Miura O et al: Assignment of the human alpha 2-plasmin inhibitor gene (PLI) to chromosome region 18p11.1–q11.2 by in situ hybridization. Cytogenet Cell Genet 47:209, 1988
27. Hirosawa S, Nakamura Y, Miura O et al: Organization of the human α_2-plasmin inhibitor gene. Proc Natl Acad Sci USA 85:6836, 1988
28. Klinger KW, Winqvist R, Riccio A et al: Plasminogen activator inhibitor type 1 gene is located at region q21.3–q22 of chromosome 7 and genetically linked with cystic fibrosis. Proc Natl Acad Sci USA 84:8548, 1987
29. Ye RD, Ahern SM, Le Beau MM et al: Structure of the gene for human plasminogen activator inhibitor-2. The nearest mammalian homologue of chicken ovalbumin. J Biol Chem 264:5495, 1989
30. Holvoet P, Lijnen HR, Collen D: A monoclonal antibody specific for Lys-plasminogen. Application to the study of the activation pathways of plasminogen in vivo. J Biol Chem 260:12106, 1985
31. Wiman B, Collen D: On the kinetics of the reaction between human antiplasmin and plasmin. Eur J Biochem 84:573, 1978
32. Edelberg JM, Pizzo SV: Lipoprotein (a) promotes plasmin inhibition by α_2-antiplasmin. Biochem J 286:79, 1992
33. Hoylaerts M, Rijken DC, Lijnen HR, Collen D: Kinetics of the activation of plasminogen by human tissue plasminogen activator. Role of fibrin. J Biol Chem 257:2912, 1982
34. van Zonneveld AJ, Veerman H, Pannekoek H: On the interaction of the finger and the kringle-2 domain of tissue-type plasminogen activator with fibrin. Inhibition of kringle-2 binding to fibrin by ϵ-amino caproic acid. J Biol Chem 261:14214, 1986
35. Rijken DC, Hoylaerts M, Collen D: Fibrinolytic properties of one-chain and two chain human extrinsic (tissue-type) plasminogen activator. J Biol Chem 257:2920, 1982
36. Husain SS, Hasan AAK, Budzynski AZ: Differences between binding of one-chain and two-chain tissue plasminogen activators to non-cross-linked and cross-linked fibrin clots. Blood 74:999, 1989
37. Harpel PC, Gordon BR, Parker TS: Plasmin catalyzes binding of lipoprotein (a) to immobilized fibrinogen and fibrin. Proc Natl Acad Sci USA 86:3847, 1989
38. Loscalzo J, Weinfeld M, Fless GM, Sxanu AM: Lipoprotein (a), fibrin binding and plasminogen activation. Atherosclerosis 10:240, 1990
39. Edelberg JM, Gonzales-Gronow M, Pizzo SV: Lipoprotein (a) inhibition of plasminogen activation by tissue-type plasminogen activator. Thromb Res 57:155, 1990
40. Edelberg JM, Pizzo SV: Lipoprotein (a): the link between impaired fibrinolysis and atherosclerosis. Fibrinolysis 5:135, 1991
41. Plow EF, Felez J, Miles LA: Cellular regulation of fibrinolysis. Thromb Haemost 66:32, 1991
42. Lijnen HR, Van Hoef B, De Cock F, Collen D: The mechanism of plasminogen activation and fibrin dissolution by single chain urokinase-type plasminogen activator in a plasma milieu in vitro. Blood 73:1864, 1989
43. Collen D, Mao JI, Stassen JM et al: Thrombolytic properties of Lys-158 mutants of recombinant single chain urokinase-type plasminogen activator in rabbits with jugular vein thrombosis. J Vasc Med Biol 1:46, 1989
44. Sprengers ED, Kluft C: Plasminogen activator inhibitors. Blood 69:381, 1987
45. Collen D, Lijnen HR: The fibrinolytic system in man. Crit Rev Oncol Hematol 4:249, 1986
46. Korninger C, Stassen JM, Collen D: Turnover of human extrinsic (tissue-type) plasminogen activator in rabbits. Thromb Haemost 46:658, 1981
47. Verstraete M, Su CAPF, Tanswell P et al: Pharmacokinetics and effects of fibrinolytic and coagulation parameters of two doses of recombinant tissue-type plasminogen activator in healthy volunteers. Thromb Haemost 56:1, 1986
48. Garabedian HD, Gold HK, Leinbach RC et al: Comparative properties of two clinical preparations of recombinant human tissue-type plasminogen activator in patients with acute myocardial infarction. J Am Coll Cardiol 9:599, 1987
49. Kuiper J, Otter M, Rijken DC, van Berkel TJC: Characterization of the interaction in vivo of tissue-type plasminogen activator with liver cells. J Biol Chem 263:18220, 1988
50. Lijnen HR, Stump DC, Collen D: Single-chain urokinase-type plasminogen activator: mechanism of action and thrombolytic properties. Semin Thromb Hemost 13:152, 1987
51. Collen D, De Cock F, Lijnen HR: Biological and thrombolytic properties of proenzyme and active forms of human urokinase. II. Turnover of natural and

recombinant urokinase in rabbits and squirrel monkeys. Thromb Haemost 52:24, 1984

52. Stump DC, Kieckens L, De Cock F, Collen D: Pharmacokinetics of single chain forms of urokinase-type plasminogen activator. J Pharmacol Exp Ther 242: 245, 1987

53. Van de Werf F, Nobuhara M, Collen D: Coronary thrombolysis with human single chain urokinase-type plasminogen activator (pro-urokinase) in patients with acute myocardial infarction. Ann Intern Med 104:345, 1986

54. Kruithof EKO: Plasminogen activator inhibitors—a review. Enzyme 40:113, 1988

55. Madison EL, Goldsmith EJ, Gerard RD et al: Serpin-resistant mutants of human tissue-type plasminogen activator. Nature 339:721, 1989

56. Adams DS, Griffin LA, Nachajko WR et al: A synthetic DNA encoding a modified human urokinase resistant to inhibition by serum plasminogen activator inhibitor. J Biol Chem 266:8476, 1991

57. Declerck PJ, De Mol M, Vaughan DE, Collen D: Identification of a conformationally distinct form of plasminogen activator inhibitor-1, acting as a noninhibitory substrate for tissue-type plasminogen activator. J Biol Chem 267: 11693, 1992

58. Colucci M, Paramo JA, Collen D: Generation in plasma of a fast-acting inhibitor of plasminogen activator in response to endotoxin stimulation. J Clin Invest 75:818, 1985

59. Stump DC, Thienpont M, Collen D: Purification and characterization of a novel inhibitor of urokinase from human urine. Quantitation and preliminary characterization in plasma. J Biol Chem 261:12759, 1986

60. Grant PJ, Medcalf RL: Hormonal regulation of haemostasis and the molecular biology of the fibrinolytic system. Clin Sci 78:3, 1990

61. Jaklitsch MT, Biro S, Casscells W, Dichek DA: Transduced endothelial cells expressing high levels of tissue plasminogen activator have an unaltered phenotype in vitro. J Cell Physiol 154:207, 1993

62. Larsson LI, Skriver L, Nielsen LS et al: Distribution of urokinase-type plasminogen activator immunoreactivity in the mouse. J Cell Biol 98:894, 1984

63. Vassalli JD, Baccino D, Belin D: A cellular binding site for the M_r 55,000 form of the human plasminogen activator, urokinase. J Cell Biol 100:86, 1985

64. Nielsen LS, Kellerman GM, Behrendt N et al: A 55,000–60,000 M_r receptor protein for urokinase-type plasminogen activator. Identification in human tumor cell lines and partial purification. J Biol Chem 263:2358, 1988

65. Loskutoff DJ: Regulation of PAI-1 gene expression. Fibrinolysis 5:197, 1991

66. Sawa H, Fujii S, Sobel BE: Augmented arterial wall expression of type-1 plasminogen activator inhibitor induced by thrombosis. Arterioscler Thromb 12: 1507, 1992

67. Loskutoff DJ, van Mourik JA, Erickson LA, Lawrence DA: Detection of an unusually stable fibrinolytic inhibitor produced by bovine endothelial cells. Proc Natal Acad Sci USA 80:2956, 1983

68. Schleef RR, Loskutoff DJ: Fibrinolytic system of vascular endothelial cells. Role of plasminogen activator inhibitors. Haemostasis 18:328, 1988

69. Lijnen HR, Collen D: Congenital and acquired deficiencies of components of the fibrinolytic system and their relation to bleeding or thrombosis. Fibrinolysis 3:67, 1989

70. Wiman B, Hamsten A: The fibrinolytic enzyme system and its role in the etiology of thromboembolic disease. Semin Thromb Hemost 16:207, 1990

71. Juhan-Vague I, Valadier J, Alessi MC et al: Deficient t-PA release and elevated PA inhibitor levels in patients with spontaneous or recurrent deep venous thrombosis. Thromb Haemost 57:67, 1987

72. Carmeliet P, Collen D, Mulligan R: Gene inactivation of the fibrinolytic enzymes tissue-type plasminogen activator, urokinase-type plasminogen activator and plasminogen activator inhibitor-1. Ann Hematol, suppl. I. 66:A-70, 1993

73. Erickson LA, Fici GJ, Lund JE et al: Development of venous occlusions in mice transgenic for the plasminogen activator inhibitor-1 gene. Nature 346: 74, 1990

74. Krishnamurti C, Barr CF, Hassett MA et al: Plasminogen activator inhibitor: a regulator of ancrod-induced fibrin deposition in rabbits. Blood 69:798, 1987

75. Levi M, Biemond BJ, van Zonneveld AJ et al: Inhibition of plasminogen activator inhibitor-1 activity results in promotion of endogenous thrombolysis and inhibition of thrombus extension in models of experimental thrombosis. Circulation 85:305, 1982

76. Prins MH, Hirsh J: A critical review of the relationship between impaired fibrinolysis and myocardial infarction. Am Heart J 122:545, 1991

77. Huber K, Jörg M, Probst P et al: A decrease in plasminogen activator inhibitor-1 activity after successful percutaneous transluminal coronary angioplasty is associated with a significantly reduced risk for coronary restenosis. Thromb Haemost 67:209, 1992

78. Muller JE, Stone PH, Turi ZG et al: Circadian variation in the frequency of onset of acute myocardial infarction. N Engl J Med 313:1315, 1985

79. Juhan-Vague I, Alessi MC, Joly P et al: Plasma plasminogen activator inhibitor-1 in angina pectoris. Influence of plasma insulin and acute-phase response. Arteriosclerosis 9:362, 1989

80. Etingin OR, Hajjar DP, Hajjar KA et al: Lipoprotein (a) regulates plasminogen activator inhibitor-1 expression in endothelial cells. A potential mechanism in thrombogenesis. J Biol Chem 266:2459, 1991

81. Koie K, Ogata K, Kamiya T et al: α_2-Plasmin-inhibitor deficiency (Miyasato disease). Lancet 2:1334, 1978

82. Miura O, Sugahara Y, Aoki N: Hereditary α_2-plasmin inhibitor deficiency caused by a transport-deficient mutation (α_2-PI-Okinawa). Deletion of Glu^{137} by a trinucleotide deletion blocks intracellular transport. J Biol Chem 264: 18213, 1989

83. Miura O, Hirosawa S, Kato A, Aoki N: Molecular basis for congenital deficiency of α_2-plasmin inhibitor. A frameshift mutation leading to elongation of the deduced amino acid sequence. J Clin Invest 83:1598, 1989

84. Collen D, Bounameaux H, De Cock F et al: Analysis of coagulation and fibrinolysis during intravenous infusion of recombinant human tissue-type plasminogen activator in patients with acute myocardial infarction. Circulation 73: 511, 1986

85. Nieuwenhuis HK, Kluft C, Wijngaards G et al: α_2-Antiplasmin Enschede: an autosomal recessive hemorrhagic disorder caused by a dysfunctional α_2-antiplasmin molecule. Thromb Haemost 50:170, 1983

86. Holmes WE, Lijnen HR, Nelles L, et al: α_2-Antiplasmin Enschede: alanine insertion and abolition of plasmin inhibitory activity. Science 238:209, 1987

87. Booth NA, Bennett B, Wijngaards G, Grieve JHK: A new life-long hemorrhagic disorder due to excess plasminogen activator. Blood 61:267, 1983

88. Aznar J, Estellés A, Vila V et al: Inherited fibrinolytic disorder due to an enhanced plasminogen activator level. Thromb Haemost 52:196, 1984

89. Schleef RR, Higgins DL, Pillemer E, Levitt LJ: Bleeding diathesis due to decreased functional activity of type 1 plasminogen activator inhibitor. J Clin Invest 83:1747, 1989

90. Diéval J, Nguyen G, Gross S et al: A lifelong bleeding disorder associated with a deficiency of plasminogen activator inhibitor type 1. Blood 77:528, 1991

91. Fay WP, Shapiro AD, Shih JL et al: Brief report: complete deficiency of plasminogen-activator inhibitor type 1 due to a frameshift mutation. N Engl J Med 327:1729, 1992

Regulatory Mechanisms in Hemostasis: Natural Anticoagulants

102

Charles T. Esmon

INTRODUCTION

A challenge in understanding hemostasis is understanding the mechanisms that serve to localize and limit the clotting response to the immediate area of injury. This chapter has three main goals: to examine the molecular mechanisms by which the natural anticoagulant complexes function to regulate coagulation, to examine how the expression of the anticoagulant complexes may be altered in response to mediators, and to review our current understanding of the physiologic ramifications of the system.

Current information suggests that there are three major natural anticoagulant mechanisms directed at the control of coagulation responses per se: the heparin antithrombin III (AT III) (also called antithrombin) system,[1-3] the protein C anticoagulant pathway,[4-6] and the tissue factor pathway inhibitor[7] formerly referred to as LACI and the extrinsic pathway inhibitor (EPI).[8] These pathways appear to complement each other and to work in concert to exert a potent in vivo anticoagulant response.

INHIBITION OF THE VITAMIN K-DEPENDENT PROTEASES OF THE COAGULATION CASCADE: THE ANTITHROMBIN III/ HEPARIN MECHANISMS

AT III is a glycoprotein inhibitor that functions by neutralizing coagulation proteases by forming a 1:1 complex with the inhibitors:

$$E + AT\ III \rightarrow E \cdot AT\ III$$

This reaction probably accounts for the major mechanism of inhibition of thrombin and factors Xa and XIa,[3] but the reaction is slow in the absence of heparin. Factor VIIa is not inhibited effectively by AT III plus heparin, unless the factor VIIa is complexed to tissue factor.[9,10] Heparin accelerates inhibition of the coagulation proteases about 1,000-fold.[11] As a result, AT III must be present[12] for heparin to function as an effective anticoagulant. With thrombin, optimal rates of inactivation require the simultaneous interaction of heparin with AT III and thrombin.[13,14] Heparin acts to concentrate thrombin and AT III, thereby accelerating their reaction. In addition, the interaction of heparin with AT III alters the conformation of the inhibitor, which presumably makes the protease trap more accessible to thrombin and the other coagulation factors.[3] For factor Xa, the interaction of heparin with factor Xa seems less important.[3,11] With low-molecular-weight heparins, some relative changes in specificities can be obtained with a shift in the relative rates of inactivation for the proteases toward a relatively more rapid inactivation of factor Xa. This is probably due to the observation that factor Xa/heparin interaction plays little role in the inhibition process. The physiologic ramifications of this remain to be fully explored but would be anticipated to increase the half-life of thrombin relative to factor Xa as compared with high-molecular-weight heparins.

Little naturally occurring heparin is found in the blood. The vascular endothelium, and the microvascular endothelium in particular, is rich, however, in anticoagulantly active heparin-like proteoglycans.[15] Based on recent studies in the rat, it is now believed that most of the heparin-like proteoglycans are on the abluminal side of the endothelium.[16] It has been proposed that these proteoglycans accelerate inhibition of some of the coagulation proteases.[17,18] Whether the low concentration of heparin-like proteoglycans on the luminal surface is responsible for the acceleration of thrombin clearance or the larger pool of abluminal proteoglycan can interact with thrombin remains unclear.[16] A model of the mechanisms by which these proteoglycans may function is illustrated in Figure 102-1. Proteoglycans are endothelial cell-associated proteins with heparin/heparan side chains bearing the critical carbohydrate sequences required for AT III recognition. Both thrombin and AT III bind to sulfated carbohydrates and are brought into close proximity to each other. AT III undergoes a conformational change required for rapid inactivation of thrombin. Little evidence exists that thrombin alters its structure on binding, but thrombin interaction with heparin is clearly important.[13,14] Heparin functions catalytically, necessitating the rapid dissociation of the thrombin/AT III complex from the proteoglycan.[14] This critical step is responsible for re-exposure of the heparin sites for binding with other thrombin and AT III molecules.

One important feature of heparin as an anticoagulant is that the molecules are heterogeneous, both structurally and functionally. Less than one-third of the heparin in commercial preparations is catalytically active in accelerating AT III-dependent inhibition of thrombin, and <10% of the naturally occurring heparin-like proteoglycans are anticoagulantly functional.[16] The critical structure responsible for the inhibition of thrombin by AT III is a specific sequence of sulfated sugars corresponding to iduronic acid-N-acetylglucosamine-6-OSO_3-glucuronic acid-N-sulfated glucosamine-6-OSO_3-iduronic acid-2-OSO_3-N-sulfated glucosamine-6-OSO_3-iduronic acid-2-OSO_3-glucuronic acid-6-OSO_3.[3]

The function of other forms of nonanticoagulantly active forms of heparin in commercial heparin preparations is unresolved. Some functions of heparin, such as its potential role in blocking angiogenesis,[19] can be divorced from its role as an anticoagulant.

INHIBITION OF THE EXTRINSIC PATHWAY OF COAGULATION

The AT III/heparin complex accounts for inhibition of all the vitamin K-dependent proteins, except factor VIIa. Although it has long been recognized that the factor VIIa/tissue factor complex is inhibited by serum, factor VIIa alone is remarkably stable both in serum and in vivo.[7] An inhibitor of the extrinsic pathway has been described, recently renamed as tissue factor pathway inhibitor (TFPI). The available evidence suggests a

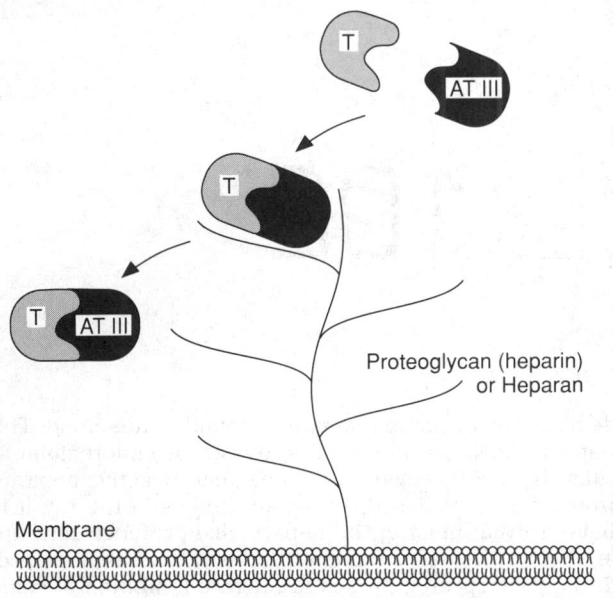

Fig. 102-1. Thrombin inhibition by AT III in the presence of heparan molecules on the endothelial cell surface. The binding of AT III to the heparan results in a conformational change in the AT III that results in rapid inactivation of thrombin. Both thrombin and antithrombin bind to the heparan. After complex formation with AT III, the complex rapidly dissociates from the heparan.

remarkable and novel mechanism of action. The inhibitor forms a complex with factor Xa and inhibits factor Xa activity.[20] How, then, does this serve as the mechanism for inhibition of the tissue factor/factor VIIa complex? Insight into the mechanism comes from structure/function analysis. Binding of the factor Xa to the TFPI is Ca^{2+} independent and does not require the Gla domain of factor Xa.[20] Both Ca^{2+} and the Gla domain are required for factor Xa-dependent inhibition of factor VIIa. Furthermore, once TFPI inhibits the tissue factor/factor VIIa/factor Xa complex, the addition of chelating agents frees factor VIIa from inhibition and dissociates TFPI.[7,21] Thus, the TFPI/factor Xa complex forms first, and this complex combines with the membrane-bound factor VIIa/tissue factor complex (Fig. 102-2). The precise role played by factor Xa in factor VIIa inactivation remains unclear. The model shown in Figure 102-2 hypothesizes a conformational change at the factor VIIa recognition site on the TFPI. Alternatively, the role of factor Xa may

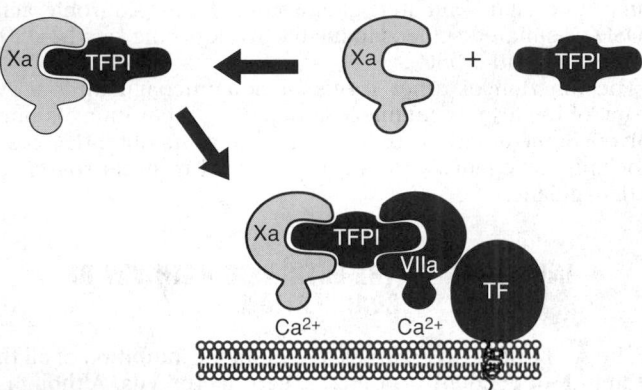

Fig. 102-2. Inhibition of factor VIIa by tissue factor pathway inhibitor (TFPI). In this model, the binding of TFPI to factor Xa results in a conformational change in the TFPI that facilitates the inhibition of factor VIIa, which is complexed to tissue factor (TF).

simply be to concentrate the inhibitor at the membrane surface. Although the model shows the initial event as a solution phase reaction, the possibility exists that the reaction can occur on the membrane surface as well.

Some potential insights into the molecular basis for the capacity of the inhibitor to neutralize two proteases simultaneously can be derived from an analysis of the structure of TFPI. This protein has recently been cloned and a cDNA coding for TFPI characterized.[8] The inhibitor has three tandem repeated domains with strong homology to other basic protease inhibitors of the Kunitz-type (i.e., of the same general class as inter-α-trypsin inhibitor).[7] The repeated inhibitor domains leave open the possibility that factor Xa reacts with one of these sites and factor VIIa binds to a separate site. Binding of factor Xa at one site may alter the conformation of the inhibitor at a second site, thereby "baiting" the trap for factor VIIa. Alternatively, factor Xa may concentrate the inhibitor at the membrane surface, forcing the equilibrium toward factor VIIa neutralization.

One potential advantage of this mechanism is that the inhibition of factor VIIa may be delayed temporally until factor Xa is formed, ensuring that some product can be made when tissue factor is exposed to the blood.[7] This may contribute significantly to the fine-tuning of the regulatory mechanisms.

INHIBITION OF THE REGULATORY PROTEINS (COFACTORS) OF THE BLOOD COAGULATION SYSTEM: THE PROTEIN C ANTICOAGULANT PATHWAY

The third major regulatory mechanism involves the protein C anticoagulant pathway. This pathway differs from the previous two primarily by the nature of the target molecules that it inhibits. Unlike the TFPI and AT III mechanisms directed at the inhibition of the protease components of the coagulation cascade, activated protein C inhibits two of the nonproteolytic regulatory proteins (cofactors) of the blood coagulation cascade: factor Va and factor VIIIa. The components of the pathway are illustrated schematically in Figure 102-3A, which depicts normal physiologic conditions, and in Figure 102-3B, which depicts this pathway after an inflammatory insult.

In this model, thrombin forms at a wound site and excess thrombin moves downstream to bind to thrombomodulin on endothelial cells. This complex activates protein C[22] catalytically, and activated protein C rapidly dissociates from the activation complex. For activated protein C to function effectively, it must interact with protein S bound to cell surfaces.[23–25] This interaction facilitates activated protein C binding to platelet[26] and endothelial cell surfaces,[27] although other cell types may be involved as well.[28,29] The cell-surface-bound complex can then inactivate the target proteins, factors Va and VIIIa.[30] The procofactors factors VIII and V seem relatively resistant to the action of activated protein C.[31,32] Protein S circulates in the blood in at least two forms: (1) as the free protein, and (2) noncovalently associated with a large, multisubunit regulatory protein of the complement system, C4b-binding protein (C4b-BP).[33,34] Only the free form of protein S functions as an active inhibitor in this pathway.[35,36] Recently, protein S has also been proposed to inhibit prothrombin activation directly, probably by binding to factor Va or factor Xa, or both.[37] The relative importance of this direct inhibition versus the cofactor function for activated protein C is unknown, but it seems likely that the cofactor function predominates. In addition to protein S, Dahlbäck et al.[38] have identified patients whose plasma is normal in protein S, but fails to respond to addition of activated protein C, suggesting the possibility of another plasma protein involved in the anticoagulant function of activated protein C.[38] Since its mechanism of action or chemical properties await characterization, the putative cofactor is not included in Figure 102-3A. In the presence of activated protein C, the rate-limiting

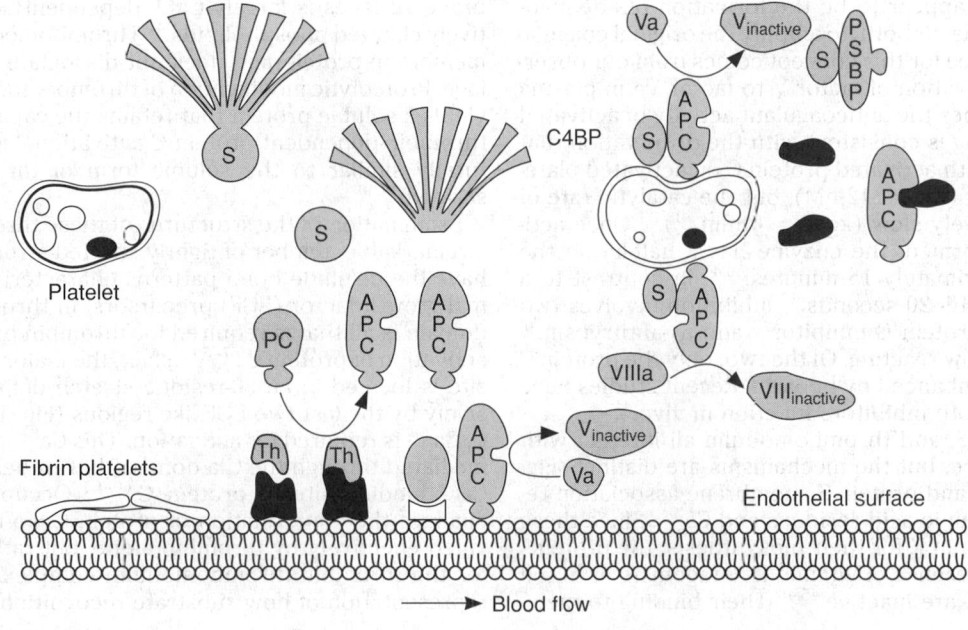

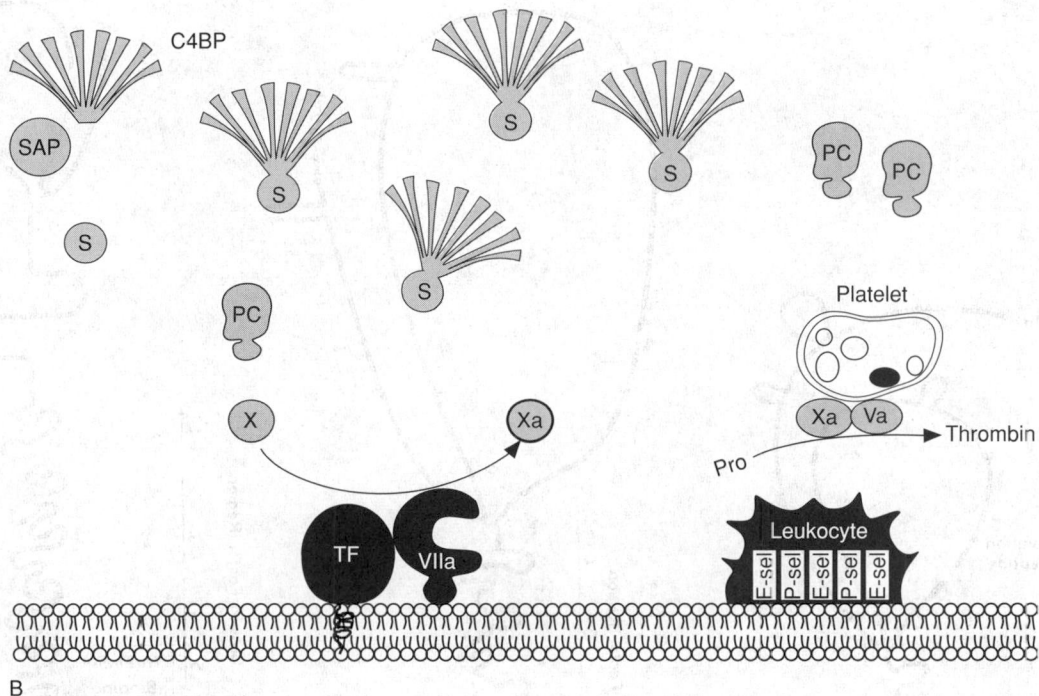

Fig. 102-3. **(A)** Formation and function of activated protein C under basal conditions. A small thrombus containing platelets and fibrin is illustrated on the lining of a small vessel. Thrombin (Th) originating on the surface of the thrombus is carried in a capillary bed by blood flow. On the endothelial cells in the capillaries, thrombin binds to thrombomodulin. The thrombin/thrombomodulin complex rapidly converts protein C (PC) to activated protein C (APC). The APC subsequently functions as an anticoagulant by enzymatically degrading clotting factors Va and VIIIa on membrane surfaces. Protein S (S) is required for these inhibitory steps to occur. Approximately 60% of the protein S is complexed to C4b-binding protein (C4BP) and is not functionally active. C4b-BP also binds serum amyloid P (SAP). APC is inhibited in plasma by protein C inhibitor, which is also known as plasminogen activator inhibitor-3, and by α_1-antitrypsin. (From Esmon,[5] with permission, adapted from Esmon.[124]) **(B)** Inflammation-induced changes in the coagulation system. During inflammation, the thrombomodulin available on the endothelial surface is decreased. This results in decreased activated protein C formation. Tissue factor (TF) is expressed on the cell surface, resulting in increased factor Xa formation, leading to more thrombin formation on the platelet surface. Binding of leukocytes to the endothelial cell surface is increased by the appearance of endothelial leukocyte adhesion molecules (E- or P-selectin) and the bound leukocytes then contribute to local vascular damage. In the plasma, inflammation results in increased levels of C4b-BP. This increase shifts the protein S to the complexed, inactive form; farther down, it regulates the protein C system. These inflammation-induced changes promote thrombus formation.

steps in coagulation appear to be the formation of adequate factor Va or factor VIIIa, or both, to amplify the original coagulation stimulus. Evidence for this concept comes from our observation that prior activation of factor V to factor Va in plasma almost totally abolishes the anticoagulant activity of activated protein C. This finding is consistent with the observation that factor Va interacts with activated protein C on activated platelets with high affinity (Km = 12 nM), but the catalytic rate of inactivation is relatively slow (kcat = 6 min^{-1}).[39] Once activated protein C is formed, the enzyme has a half-life in the circulation of approximately 15 minutes,[40,41] in contrast to a thrombin half-life of 10–20 seconds.[42] Inhibition involves two major inhibitors: a protein C inhibitor[43] and α_1-antitrypsin.[44] Both are relatively slow reacting. Of the two, only the protein C inhibitor activity is enhanced by heparin. Recent studies have demonstrated that both inhibitors function in vivo.[41]

Protein C, protein S, and thrombomodulin all interact with the membrane surface, but the mechanisms are distinct (Fig. 102-4). For protein C and protein S, membrane association requires γ-carboxyglutamic acid residues and Ca^{2+}. Since these proteins require vitamin K for their biosynthesis, the proteins synthesized in the presence of vitamin K antagonists or in the absence of vitamin K are inactive.[45,46] Their binding to membrane surfaces is largely Ca^{2+} dependent and requires negatively charged phospholipids.[47] Thrombomodulin is an integral membrane protein and does not dissociate from the cell surface. Proteolytic modification of thrombomodulin with elastase yields a soluble protein that retains the capacity to accelerate thrombin-dependent protein C activation[48] that may be structurally similar to the soluble form of thrombomodulin described.[49,50]

Examination of the structures of these three proteins shows a remarkable number of tightly knotted structures.[51-56] These have the disulfide bond patterns characteristic of the epidermal growth factor (EGF) precursors. In thrombomodulin, this domain is all that is required for thrombin binding and for the activation of protein C.[57-59] In fact, the major thrombin binding site is located in an 80-residue stretch defined almost exclusively by the last two EGF-like regions (Fig. 102-4C). In protein C, Ca^{2+} is required for activation. This Ca^{2+} dependence is not mediated through the Gla domain, but rather through a single Ca^{2+}-binding site in protein C.[60-62] Occupancy of this site changes the conformation of protein C, so that it is not activated effectively by thrombin alone, but rather is a substrate for the thrombin/thrombomodulin complex.[63,64] A schematic representation of how substrate recognition is defined is pre-

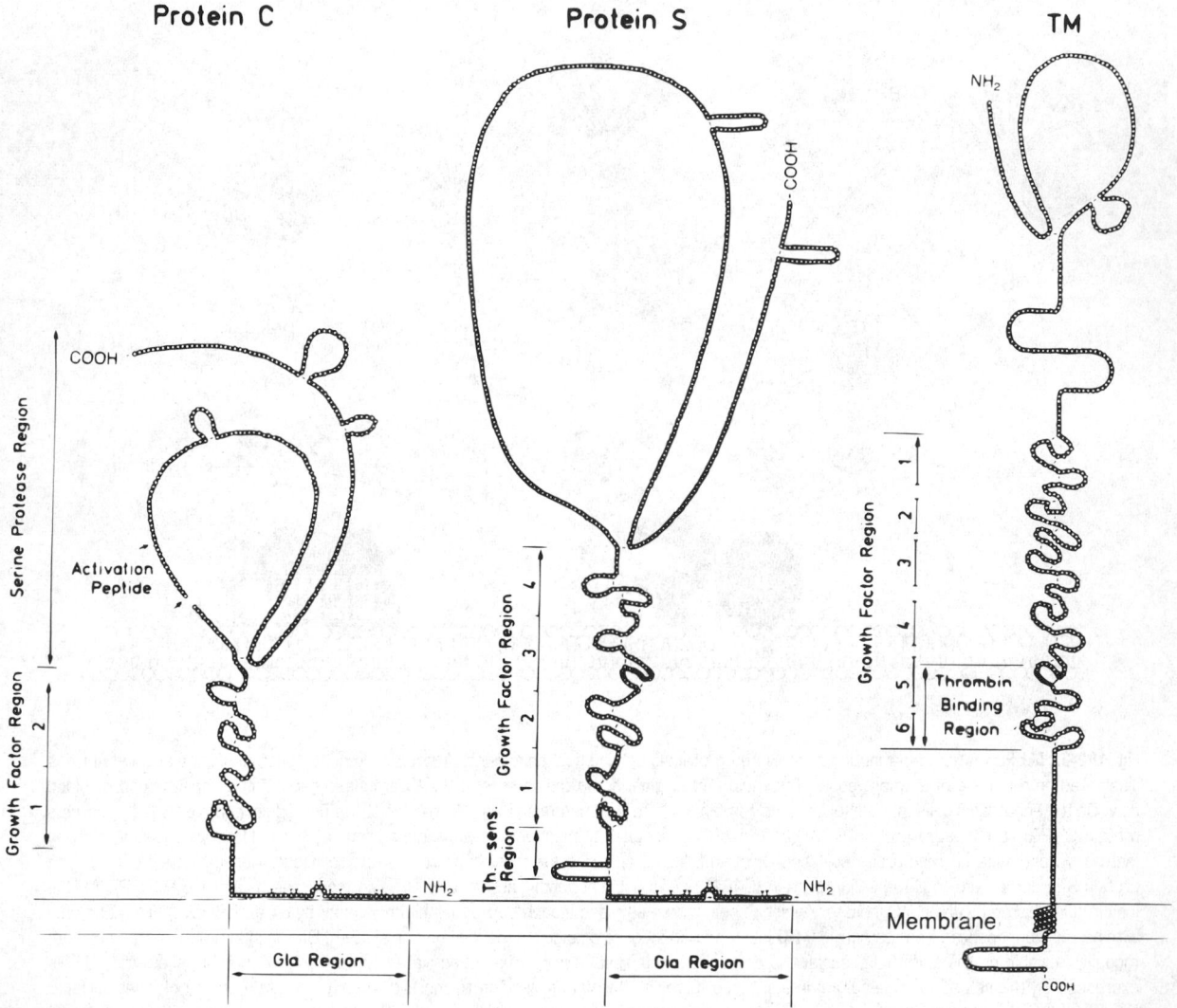

Fig. 102-4. Schematic representation of protein C, protein S, and thrombomodulin. The disulfide bonds in thrombomodulin are predicted by homology. The γ-carboxyglutamic acid residues in protein C and protein S are indicated by small Y-shaped symbols. (From Esmon,[5] with permission.)

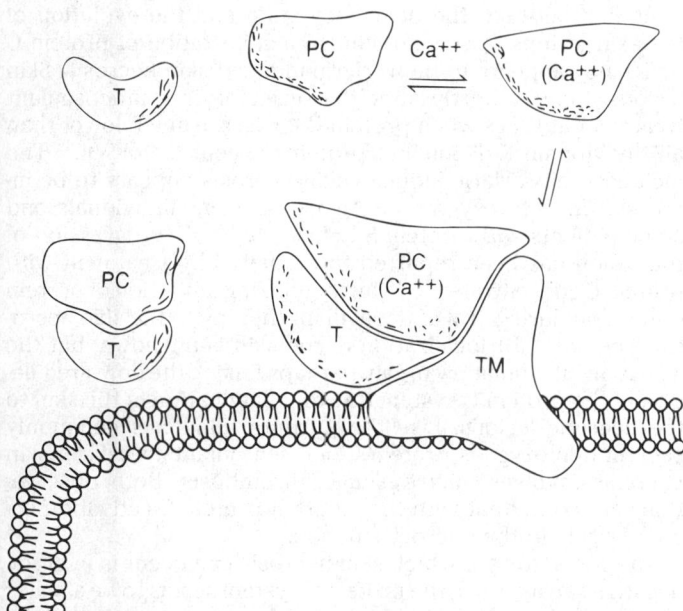

Fig. 102-5. A plausible mechanism for thrombomodulin function. Thrombin (T) can interact with protein C (PC) in the absence of Ca^{2+} (upper left). In the presence of Ca^{2+}, a conformational change in protein C occurs that prevents the interaction with thrombin (upper right). A conformational change occurs in the enzymatic active site of thrombin when thrombin binds to thrombomodulin. This change prevents cleavage of protein C by thrombin in the absence of Ca^{2+} (lower left). However, the change in the binding site of thrombin induced by thrombomodulin results in the binding of the Ca^{2+}-stabilized conformation of protein C (lower right) and the subsequent formation of activated protein C. TM, thrombomodulin. (From Johnson, et al.,[60] with permission.)

sented in Figure 102-5. The β-hydroxy aspartic acid residue in protein C[65] and the three hydroxylated aspartic acid and asparagines in protein S[66] are located within the EGF domains. The role of these hydroxylated residues is unknown, but they appear to be located near the Ca^{2+}-binding site. Substitution of the aspartic acid with glutamic acid interferes with normal Ca^{2+} binding.[55] This observation, coupled with their known role as metal-binding residues in bacterial proteins,[67] suggests that they are involved in Ca^{2+} binding, but recent two-dimensional nuclear magnetic resonance structural studies indicate that these residues are not directly involved in ligating the Ca^{2+}.[68] The hydroxylated residues could be involved with metal-dependent recognition of other proteins. Activated protein C also contains a monovalent ion-binding site that accelerates cleavage of synthetic substrates.[69]

Bovine thrombomodulin has also been shown to contain a β-hydroxy aspartic acid residue.[70] The role in thrombomodulin function remains unknown.

The COOH-terminal regions of the three proteins demonstrate little structural similarity. In protein C, this region contains the serine protease domain that has extensive sequence homology to trypsin.[71] In activated protein C, the protease domain is covalently linked to the EGF and Gla domains by a single disulfide bridge.[71,72] Protein C circulates both as a single-chain and two-chain molecule with a ratio of about 1:3.[73,74] There are also two subforms, referred to as α and β, with the latter appearing somewhat smaller and differing specifically in the heavy chain. The different forms appear to differ in carbohydrate content.

In contrast to protein C, protein S is a single-chain molecule. Consistent with the proposed model as a binding protein (Fig. 102-3), the COOH-terminal domain has no similarity with other proteases. Some sequence similarities have been noted with

steroid-binding proteins.[75] The role of this domain remains uncertain, but evidence suggests that the domain is involved in C4bBP interaction,[76] although this concept would appear to be inconsistent with site specific mutations in this region of protein S that do not influence C4b-BP binding.[77]

In thrombomodulin, the role of the NH_2-terminal domain is also obscure. Limited sequence similarities to some lectins has led to the hypothesis that it may be involved in carbohydrate binding, but no direct evidence for this function exists. This domain is not critical to protein C activation, leaving open the possibility that this receptor may participate in more than one control mechanism.

CONTROL MECHANISMS IN PROTEIN C ACTIVATION

Protein C activation can be controlled by a number of different mechanisms. When thrombin binds to thrombomodulin, several coagulation reactions, including fibrin generation and platelet activation, are inhibited.[78-82] This results in direct inhibition of thrombin function. Bound thrombin reacts with AT III more rapidly than does free thrombin,[80] an acceleration that is dependent on the presence of sulfated galactosaminoglycans (chondroitin sulfate) on the thrombomodulin molecule.[83] The rapid inactivation of thrombomodulin-bound thrombin ensures the termination of protein C activation shortly after thrombin generation has ceased. Thus, the two processes are very tightly coupled. Within this context, thrombomodulin appears to work in concert with vascular heparins to augment thrombin clearance. The relative importance of the role of thrombomodulin and heparin in this process is unknown and may vary within different organs. For instance, thrombomodulin cannot be detected in the microcirculation of the human brain,[84] although low levels are present.[85] Thrombin can be internalized when bound to thrombomodulin,[86] but the extent of internalization is variable, and its importance is controversial.[87] This internalization is much slower than the rate of thrombin inhibition, raising the question of the role of this process in regulation. The thrombin AT III complex dissociates very readily from thrombomodulin, so that neither thrombin nor thrombin/antithrombin clearance via internalization is likely to contribute significantly to overall clearance of either species from the circulation.[83]

INFLAMMATORY MEDIATORS, THROMBOMODULIN, AND THE HEMOSTATIC BALANCE

Under most circumstances, the clotting process is under very tight control, and the in vivo regulatory mechanisms adequately limit the extent of clotting in response to injury. Inflammatory events, such as occur in gram-negative bacterial sepsis, can shift this balance in favor of the clotting response at the expense of the natural anticoagulant mechanisms. A prime target for this modulation appears to be the protein C anticoagulant pathway. A hypothetical depiction of the vasculature following an inflammatory insult is presented in Figure 102-3B. As compared with the normal vasculature, inflammatory mediators depress thrombomodulin, thereby inhibiting protein C activation.[88-91] As a result, more free thrombin is formed. The levels of C4b-BP are elevated[92]; this leads to a shift toward the C4b-BP/protein S complex. Since this complex is not active in supporting activated protein C anticoagulant activity,[35,36] the limited amounts of activated protein C that are formed are not fully functional. Thus, there is a major decrease in the anticoagulant activity of this system.

Not only is the anticoagulant pathway down-regulated, but several procoagulant events ensue essentially simultaneously. Tissue factor synthesis and cell surface expression[93] are initiated, leading to the activation of factors X and XI. This occurs not only on the endothelium (Fig. 102-3B), but on the macrophage/monocytes as well. Leukocytes are also bound to the cell surface.[94] Since these cells release both proteases and active oxygen species, this may contribute to vascular injury. In particular, recent studies have shown that human thrombomodulin is especially sensitive to oxidant damage due to oxidation at Met 388.[95]

Formation of tissue factor and the down-regulation of the protein C pathway is predicted to lead to factor Xa formation and to increased stability of the factor Xa/factor Va complex on the platelet surfaces.

These observations raise the question of why inflammatory stimuli do not lead to even more severe injury. Available evidence suggests that TFPI remains fully active.[7] Little evidence has been presented that vascular heparin-like substances are down-regulated by these stimuli.

WHERE DO ANTICOAGULANT FACTORS FUNCTION? COORDINATED CONTROL OF A COMPLEX PROCESS

As pointed out by Busch et al.,[96] the vasculature presents an unusual feature. As blood moves from the large vessels to the capillaries, the surface area of endothelium in contact with each milliliter of blood rises dramatically. For endothelial cell surface-bound receptors, this translates directly into an increase in the concentration of the regulatory receptor. Thrombomodulin is present at approximately 100,000 copies per endothelial cell. The concentration of thrombomodulin in a vessel about the size of a coronary artery would be approximately 0.1–0.2 nM. Rapid clotting with thrombin occurs at concentrations of approximately 10 nM. Thus, the concentration of regulatory proteins is insufficient to control the process. By contrast, the microcirculation includes a concentration of thrombomodulin of approximately 500 nM. Since the interaction with thrombomodulin is governed by a K_d of ≤ 0.5 nM,[97] virtually no free thrombin would exist in the microcirculation. This assumes that the concentration of the receptor is invariant throughout the vasculature. Certainly, thrombomodulin is present in capillaries, and the available evidence suggests that the concentration per cell is approximately constant.[98,99] If one makes the same assumptions for other regulatory mechanisms of the endothelium, it would appear that the microcirculation may be a major site for the function of vascular heparins, prostacyclin, and plasminogen activator, as well as thrombomodulin.

The heparin and protein C systems do not work in isolation, but rather orchestrate a coordinated control over coagulation events (Fig. 102-1). AT III inhibits many factors in the presence of heparin, but the inactivation of platelet-bound factor Xa/factor Va complex is relatively resistant to the action of heparin and AT III.[100] This complex is also relatively resistant to inactivation by activated protein C.[24,101] Protein S, however, is capable of at least partially overcoming this protection.[39] Thus, activated protein C may be required for factor Xa clearance by the AT III/heparin system. No comparable interplay has yet been elucidated between TFPI and these two anticoagulant systems.

POTENTIAL ROLE OF PROTEIN C IN PREVENTION OF THROMBOSIS AND DISSEMINATED INTRAVASCULAR COAGULATION

Clinical manifestations of impaired functions of the protein C system provide important clues that it is a major inhibitor of coagulation in the microcirculation. Homozygous protein C deficiency is usually manifested by purpura fulminans that results from microvascular thrombosis. This has been effectively treated with protein C concentrate,[102] establishing an unambig-

uous link between the deficiency state and the evolution of the skin lesions. A second clinical manifestation of protein C deficiency appears to be warfarin-induced skin necrosis. Skin lesions appear shortly after the onset of oral anticoagulant treatment at times when protein C levels are much lower than all the vitamin K-dependent proteins except factor VII.[45] The incidence of warfarin-induced skin necrosis appears to be increased in heterozygous protein C-deficient individuals and some patients with protein S deficiency.[103–105] Progression of the lesion has been reported to be halted by treatment with protein C concentrate,[106,107] further linking inhibition of protein C function during oral anticoagulant therapy to the skin necrosis. The basis for localization to the skin is unknown, but the skin is an inflammatory organ, perhaps linking the down-regulation of the protein C system due to inflammation in the skin to the necrotic lesions. Like the purpura fulminans commonly seen in homozygous protein C-deficient infants, warfarin skin necrosis involves microvascular thrombosis. Both observations are consistent with the fact that protein C activation occurs largely in the microcirculation.

Another setting in which skin necrosis can occur is in gram-negative sepsis. Since the protein C system seems to be a major target of inflammatory mediators with respect to the coagulation system, activated protein C might offer protection from gram-negative sepsis. In a baboon model of *Escherichia coli* sepsis, activated protein C blocked both the fibrinogen consumption and the organ damage that ultimately lead to death.[108] Although high levels of activated protein C were required, nevertheless, this approach holds promise as an adjunct therapy for disseminated intravascular coagulation. Despite the bacterial challenge to vascular integrity, no overt bleeding complications were observed with activated protein C treatment of the shock process.

Protein C is also consumed in patients during septic shock.[109] Some of these patients develop severe purpura lesions resembling those of homozygous protein C-deficient infants. It follows that protein C might effectively prevent these lesions from progressing. Based on early, and therefore limited, clinical data, protein C may be effective in treating patients with very low protein C levels and septic shock.[110]

Activated protein C has also been studied for its ability to inhibit fibrinogen accretion on preformed jugular vein thrombi in dogs and rhesus monkeys.[111] Fibrin deposition was decreased approximately 4-fold in dogs and 10-fold in rhesus monkeys relative to a control. Despite the obvious influence on thrombus growth, bleeding at surgical sites was not significantly increased.

Activated protein C has also been tested in a baboon model of platelet-dependent thrombosis,[112] entailing examination of platelet deposition on prosthetic vascular grafts. Under the conditions employed, infusion of activated protein C reduced platelet deposition by $\leq 70\%$. Thus, in this model, activated protein C was an effective antithrombotic and did not alter primary hemostasis. Since activated protein C is generated in response to thrombin/thrombomodulin interaction, it follows that systemic infusion of thrombin, which would lead to protein C activation, might actually retard platelet and fibrin formation on the vascular grafts. Indeed, infusion of thrombin into baboons at 1 or 2 U/kg/min reduced the platelet or fibrin deposition on the graft in a dose-dependent fashion.[113]

Ischemia is another potential setting in which protein C may play a role in preventing injury. Model studies in dogs and pigs demonstrate the rapid activation of protein C in ischemic areas in the heart following ligation of the coronary artery. Blocking this activation impairs recovery of coronary function.[114] Taken together, studies on protein C in the coronary circulation suggest that it might be important in preventing or limiting platelet deposition at sites of arterial injury and, if occlusion should occur, it could play important functions in keeping the coronary microcirculation patent.

GENETICS OF PROTEIN C

Recent advances in genetics have facilitated the analysis of the molecular basis of protein C deficiency. The protein C cDNA and genomic clones have been sequenced.[115–117] Heterozygous protein C-deficient patients usually have no clinical symptoms. In some families, however, the protein C deficiency clearly correlates with an increased risk of thrombosis.[118,119] The genetic basis of these pedigrees has been determined and summarized in a comprehensive review.[118] More than 130 different pedigrees of families with protein C deficiency have now been characterized at the level of mutations within the gene. Of 134 apparently unrelated probands characterized, 99 had low expression levels and 18 had dysfunctional molecules with near-normal antigen levels. Single base-pair substitutions are the most common finding, with 67 different base-pair substitutions now characterized. Three mutations in the promoter have been detected. Deletions within the protein C gene appear to be relatively rare. The available mutations have not provided any striking insights into protein C function, and it is difficult to determine from the limited number of available sequences and patients whether certain mutations carry a greater risk of thrombosis than others.

GENETICS OF PROTEIN S

The protein S gene has been sequenced and characterized,[120–122] revealing a complex gene containing 15 exons. The molecular basis of protein S-deficient patients has been determined in only a relatively few instances. This is in part because of the existence of a pseudo-gene for protein S that complicates the analysis. Furthermore, although protein S is clearly important for the anticoagulant pathway to function in vivo, the ability of protein S to stimulate anticoagulant activity in vitro in purified systems is modest, usually about two- to threefold. Finally, in at least some of the patients with low free protein S, the defect may lie in the C4bBP. For these reasons, too few patients have been characterized to allow any clear picture of the molecular basis of protein S deficiency to emerge. The approaches to protein S gene analysis have been described by Schmeidel et al[123]

SUMMARY

Current information indicates that protein C, protein S, and thrombomodulin are potent inhibitors of the blood coagulation process. The system is down-regulated by inflammatory mediators. Total deficiencies of protein C and S are associated with severe thrombotic complications. Presumably, the down-regulation of the protein C pathway by inflammatory agents decreases the capacity of the system to redirect thrombin from a procoagulant enzyme into the initiator of a potent anticoagulant.

REFERENCES

1. Bauer KA, Rosenberg RD: The pathophysiology of the prethrombotic state in humans: insights gained from studies using markers of hemostatic system. Blood 70:343, 1987
2. Rosenberg RD: Regulation of the hemostatic mechanism. p. 534. In Stamatoyannopoulos G, Nienhuis AW, Leder P, Majerus PW (eds): The Molecular Basis of Blood Diseases. WB Saunders, Philadelphia, 1987
3. Marcum JA, Rosenberg RD: Anticoagulantly active heparin-like molecules. p. 207. In Simionescu N, Simionescu M (eds): Endothelial Cell Biology in Health and Disease. Plenum, New York, 1988
4. Stenflo J: The biochemistry of protein C. p. 21. In Bertina RM (ed): Protein C and Related Proteins. Churchill Livingstone, Edinburgh, 1988
5. Esmon CT: The roles of protein C and thrombomodulin in the regulation of blood coagulation. J Biol Chem 264:4743, 1989
6. Laemmle B, Griffin JH: Formation of the fibrin clot: the balance of procoagulant and inhibitory factors. Clin Haematol 14:281, 1985
7. Rapaport SI: Inhibition of factor VIIa/tissue factor-induced blood coagulation: with particular emphasis upon a factor Xa-dependent inhibitory mechanism. Blood 73:359, 1989
8. Wun T-C, Kretzmer KK. Girard TJ et al: Cloning and characterization of a cDNA coding for the lipoprotein-associated coagulation inhibitor shows that it consists of three tandem Kunitz-type inhibitory domains. J Biol Chem 263:6001, 1988
9. Shigematsu Y, Miyata T, Higashi S et al: Expression of human soluble tissue factor in yeast and enzymatic properties of its complex with factor VIIa. J Biol Chem 267:21329, 1992
10. Lawson JH, Butenas S, Ribarik N, Mann KG: Complex-dependent inhibition of factor VIIa by antithrombin III and heparin. J Biol Chem 268:767, 1993
11. Craig PA, Olson ST, Shore JD: Transient kinetics of heparin-catalyzed protease inactivation by antithrombin III: characterization of assembly, product formation and heparin dissociation in the factor Xa reaction. J Biol Chem 264:5452, 1989
12. Brinkhouse KM, Smith HP, Warner ED, Seegers WH: The inhibition of blood clotting: An unidentified substance which acts in conjunction with heparin to prevent the conversion of prothrombin to thrombin. Am J Physiol 125:683, 1939
13. Hoylaerts M, Owen WG, Collen D: Involvement of heparin chain length in the heparin-catalysed inhibition of thrombin by antithrombin III. J Biol Chem 259:5670, 1984
14. Olson ST: Transient kinetics of heparin-catalyzed protease inactivation by antithrombin III. J Biol Chem 263:1698, 1988
15. Marcum JA, Rosenberg RD: Anticoagulantly active heparin-like molecules from the vascular tissue. Biochemistry 23:1730, 1984
16. de Agostini AI, Watkins SC, Slayter HS et al: Localization of anticoagulantly active heparan sulfate proteoglycans in vascular endothelium: antithrombin binding on cultured endothelial cells and perfused rat aorta. J Cell Biol 111:1293, 1990
17. Hjort PF: Intermediate reaction in the coagulation of blood with tissue thromboplastin. Scand J Clin Lab Invest 9:1, 1957
18. Marcum JA, McKenney JB, Rosenberg RD: The acceleration of thrombin-antithrombin complex formation in hindquarters via naturally occurring heparin-like molecules bound to the endothelium. J Clin Invest 74:341, 1984
19. Folkman J, Weisz PB, Joullie MM et al: Control of angiogenesis with synthetic heparin substitutes. Science 243:1490, 1989
20. Broze GJ, Jr., Warren LA, Novotny WF et al: The lipoprotein-associated coagulation inhibitor that inhibits the factor VII-tissue factor complex also inhibits factor Xa: insight into its possible mechanism of action. Blood 71:335, 1988
21. Rao LVM, Rapaport SI: Studies of a mechanism inhibiting the initiation of the extrinsic pathway of coagulation. Blood 69:335, 1987
22. Esmon CT, Owen WG: Identification of an endothelial cell cofactor for thrombin-catalyzed activation of protein C. Proc Natl Acad Sci USA 78:2249, 1981
23. Walker FJ: Regulation of activated protein C by a new protein: a role for bovine protein S. J Biol Chem 255:5521, 1980
24. Walker FJ: Regulation of activated protein C by protein S: the role of phospholipid in factor Va inactivation. J Biol Chem 256:11128, 1981
25. Hackeng TM, Hessing M, van't Veer C et al: Protein S binding to human endothelial cells is required for expression of cofactor activity for activated protein C. J Biol Chem 268:3993, 1993
26. Harris KW, Esmon CT: Protein S is required for bovine platelets to support activated protein C binding and activity. J Biol Chem 260:2007, 1985
27. Stern DM, Nawroth PP, Harris K, Esmon CT: Cultured bovine aortic endothelial cells promote activated protein C-protein S-mediated inactivation of Factor Va. J Biol Chem 261:713, 1986
28. Furmaniak-Kazmierczak E, Hu CY, Esmon CT: Protein S enhances C4b binding protein interaction with neutrophils. Blood 81:405, 1993
29. Oates AM, Salem HH: The binding and regulation of protein S by neutrophils. Blood Coagul Fibrinolysis 2:601, 1991
30. Fulcher CA, Gardiner JE, Griffin JH, Zimmerman TS: Proteolytic inactivation of human factor VIII procoagulant protein by activated protein C and its analogy with factor V. Blood 63:486, 1984
31. Walker FJ, Sexton PW, Esmon CT: Inhibition of blood coagulation by activated protein C through selective inactivation of activated factor V. Biochim Biophys Acta 571:333, 1979

32. Vehar GA, Davie EW: Preparation and properties of bovine factor VIII (anti-hemophilic factor). Biochemistry 19:401, 1980

33. Dahlbäck B, Stenflo J: High molecular weight complex in human plasma between vitamin K-dependent protein S and complement component C4b-binding protein. Proc Natl Acad Sci USA 78:2512, 1981

34. Dahlbäck B, Smith CA, Muller-Eberhard HJ: Visualization of human C4b-binding protein and its complexes with vitamin K-dependent protein S and complement protein C4b. Proc Natl Acad Sci USA 80:3461, 1983

35. Comp PC, Nixon RR, Cooper MR, Esmon CT: Familial protein S deficiency is associated with recurrent thrombosis. J Clin Invest 74:2082, 1984

36. Dahlbäck B: Inhibition of protein Ca cofactor function of human and bovine protein S by C4b-binding protein. J Biol Chem 261:12022, 1986

37. Heeb MJ, Mesters RM, Tans G et al: Binding of protein S to factor Va associated with inhibition of prothrombinase that is independent of activated protein C. J Biol Chem 268:2872, 1993

38. Dahlbäck B, Carlsson M, Svensson PJ: Familial thrombophilia due to a previously unrecognized mechanism characterized by poor anticoagulant response to activated protein C: prediction of a cofactor to activated protein C. Proc Natl Acad Sci USA 90:1004, 1993

39. Solymoss S, Tucker MM, Tracy PB: Kinetics of inactivation of membrane-bound factor Va by activated protein C. J Biol Chem 263:14884, 1988

40. Comp PC, Jacocks RM, Ferrell GL, Esmon CT: Activation of protein C in vivo. J Clin Invest 70:127, 1982

41. Heeb MJ, Mosher D, Griffin JH: Activation and complexation of protein C and cleavage and decrease of protein S in plasma of patients with intravascular coagulation. Blood 73:455, 1989

42. Lollar P, Owen W: Clearance of thrombin from the circulation in rabbits by high-affinity binding sites on endothelium. J Clin Invest 66:1222, 1980

43. Suzuki K, Deyashiki Y, Nishioka J et al: Characterization of a cDNA for human protein C inhibitor. A new member of the plasma serine protease inhibitor superfamily. J Biol Chem 262:611, 1987

44. Heeb MJ, Griffin JH: Physiologic inhibition of human activated protein C by α_1-antitrypsin. J Biol Chem 263:11613, 1988

45. D'Angelo SV, Comp PC, Esmon CT, D'Angelo A: Relationship between protein C antigen and anticoagulant activity during oral anticoagulation and in selected disease states. J Clin Invest 77:416, 1986

46. D'Angelo A, Vigano-D'Angelo S, Esmon CT, Comp PC: Acquired deficiencies of protein S: Protein S activity during oral anticoagulation, in liver disease and in disseminated intravascular coagulation. J Clin Invest 81:1445, 1988

47. Nelsestuen GL, Kisiel W, DiScipio RG: Interaction of vitamin K-dependent proteins with membranes. Biochemistry 17:2134, 1978

48. Kurosawa S, Galvin JB, Esmon NL, Esmon CT: Proteolytic formation and properties of functional domains of thrombomodulin. J Biol Chem 262:2206, 1987

49. Ishii H, Majerus PW: Thrombomodulin is present in human plasma and urine. J Clin Invest 76:2178, 1985

50. Takano S, Kimura S, Ohdama S, Aoki N: Plasma thrombomodulin in health and diseases. Blood 76:2024, 1990

51. Lundwall A, Dackowski W, Cohen E et al: Isolation and sequence of the cDNA for human protein S, a regulator of blood coagulation. Proc Natl Acad Sci USA 83:6716, 1986

52. Wen D, Dittman WA, Ye RD et al: Human thrombomodulin: complete cDNA sequence and chromosome localization of the gene. Biochemistry 26:4350, 1987

53. Petersen TE: The amino-terminal domain of thrombomodulin and pancreatic stone protein are homologous with lectins. FEBS Lett 231:51, 1988

54. Jackman RW, Beeler DL, Fritze L et al: Human thrombomodulin gene is intron depleted: nucleic acid sequences of the cDNA and gene predict protein structure and suggest sites of regulatory control. Proc Natl Acad Sci USA 84:6425, 1987

55. Öhlin A-K, Linse S, Stenflo J: Calcium binding to the epidermal growth factor homology region of bovine protein C. J Biol Chem 263:7411, 1988

56. Suzuki K, Kusumoto H, Deyashiki Y et al: Structure and expression of human thrombomodulin, a thrombin receptor on endothelium acting as a cofactor for protein C activation. EMBO J 6:1891, 1987

57. Kurosawa S, Stearns DJ, Jackson KW, Esmon CT: A 10-kDa cyanogen bromide fragment from the epidermal growth factor homology domain of rabbit thrombomodulin contains the primary thrombin binding site. J Biol Chem 263:5993, 1988

58. Stearns DJ, Kurosawa S, Esmon CT: Micro-thrombomodulin: residues 310–486 from the epidermal growth factor precursor homology domain of thrombomodulin will accelerate protein C activation. J Biol Chem 264:3352, 1989

59. Suzuki K, Hayashi T, Nishioka J et al: A domain composed of epidermal growth factor-like structures of human thrombomodulin is essential for thrombin binding and for protein C activation. J Biol Chem 264:4872, 1989

60. Johnson AE, Esmon NL, Laue TM, Esmon CT: Structural changes required for activation of protein C are induced by Ca^{2+} binding to a high affinity site that does not contain γ-carboxyglutamic acid. J Biol Chem 258:5554, 1983

61. Öhlin A-K, Landes G, Bourdon P et al: β-Hydroxyaspartic acid in the first epidermal growth factor-like domain of protein C: its role in Ca^{2+} binding and biological activity. J Biol Chem 263:19240, 1988

62. Rezaie AR, Esmon NL, Esmon CT: The high affinity calcium-binding site involved in protein C activation is outside the first epidermal growth factor homology domain. J Biol Chem 267:11701, 1992

63. Esmon NL, DeBault LE, Esmon CT: Proteolytic formation and properties of γ-carboxyglutamic acid-domainless protein C. J Biol Chem 258:5548, 1983

64. Amphlett GW, Kisiel W, Castellino FJ: Interaction of calcium with bovine plasma protein C. Biochemistry 20:2156, 1981

65. Drakenberg T, Fernlund P, Roepstorff P, Stenflo J: β-Hydroxyaspartic acid in vitamin K-dependent protein C. Proc Natl Acad Sci USA 80:1802, 1983

66. Stenflo J, Lundwall A, Dahlbäck B: β-Hydroxyasparagine in domains homologous to the epidermal growth factor precursor in vitamin K-dependent protein S. Proc Natl Acad Sci USA 84:368, 1987.

67. Fowler SA, Paulson D, Owen BA, Owen WG: Binding of iron by factor IX, possible role for beta hydroxyaspartic acid. J Biol Chem 261:4371, 1986

68. Selander-Sunnerhagen M, Ullner M, Persson E et al: How an epidermal growth factor (EGF)-like domain binds calcium: high resolution NMR structure of the calcium form of the NH_2-terminal EGF-like domain in coagulation factor X. J Biol Chem 267:19642, 1992

69. Hill KA, Castellino FJ: The effect of monovalent cations on the pre-steady state reaction kinetics of bovine activated plasma protein C and des-1-41-light chain activated plasma protein C. J Biol Chem 262:140, 1987

70. Stenflo J, Öhlin A-K, Owen WG, Schneider WJ: β-hydroxyaspartic acid or β-hydroxyasparagine in bovine low density lipoprotein receptor and in bovine thrombomodulin. J Biol Chem 263:21, 1988

71. Stenflo J, Fernlund P: Amino acid sequence of the heavy chain of bovine protein C. J Biol Chem 257:12180, 1982

72. Fernlund P, Stenflo J, Roepstorff P, Thomsen J: Vitamin K and the biosynthesis of prothrombin. V. γ-Carboxyglutamic acids, the vitamin K-dependent structures in prothrombin. J Biol Chem 250:6125, 1975

73. Miletich JP, Leykam JF, Broze GJ Jr: Detection of single chain protein C in human plasma. Blood 62:1127, 1983

74. Heeb MJ, Schwarz HP, White T et al: Immunoblotting studies of the molecular forms of protein C in plasma. Thromb Res 52:33, 1988

75. Long GL: Structure and molecular biology of human protein S. p. 153. In Suttie JW (ed): Current Advances in Vitamin K Research. Elsevier, New York, 1988

76. Walker FJ: Characterization of a synthetic peptide that inhibits the interaction between protein S and C4b-binding protein. J Biol Chem 264:17645, 1989

77. Chang GTG, Ploos van Amstel HK, Hessing M et al: Expression and characterization of recombinant human protein S in heterologous cells—studies of the interaction of amino acid residues Leu-608 to Glu-612 with human C4b-binding protein. Thromb Haemost 67:526, 1992

78. Esmon CT, Esmon NL, Harris KW: Complex formation between thrombin and thrombomodulin inhibits both thrombin-catalyzed fibrin formation and factor V activation. J Biol Chem 257:7944, 1982

79. Esmon NL, Carroll RC, Esmon CT: Thrombomodulin blocks the ability of thrombin to activate platelets. J Biol Chem 258:12238, 1983

80. Hofsteenge J, Taguchi H, Stone SR: Effect of thrombomodulin on the kinetics of the interaction of thrombin with substrates and inhibitors. Biochem J 237:243, 1986

81. Jakubowski HV, Kline MD, Owen WG: The effect of bovine thrombomodulin on the specificity of bovine thrombin. J Biol Chm 261:3876, 1986

82. Maruyama I, Salem HH, Ishii H, Majerus PW: Human thrombomodulin is not an efficient inhibitor of procoagulant activity of thrombin. J Clin Invest 75:987, 1985

83. Bourin M-C, Öhlin A-K, Lane DA et al: Relationship between anticoagulant activities and polyanionic properties of rabbit thrombomodulin. J Biol Chem 263:8044, 1988

84. Ishii H, Salem HH, Bell CE et al: Thrombomodulin, an endothelial anticoagulant protein, is absent from the human brain. Blood 67:362, 1986

85. Wong VLY, Hofman FM, Ishii H et al: Regional distribution of thrombomodulin in human brain. Brain Res 556:1, 1991

86. Maruyama I, Majerus PW: Protein C inhibits endocytosis of thrombin-thrombomodulin complexes in A549 lung cancer cells and human umbilical vein endothelial cells. Blood 69:1481, 1987

87. Beretz A, Freyssinet J-M, Gauchy J et al: Stability of the thrombin-thrombomodulin complex on the surface of endothelial cells from human saphenous vein or from the cell line EA.hy 926. Biochem J 259:35, 1989

88. Moore KL, Andreoli SP, Esmon NL et al: Endotoxin enhances tissue factor and suppresses thrombomodulin expression of human vascular endothelium in vitro. J Clin Invest 79:124, 1987
89. Nawroth PP, Handley DA, Esmon CT, Stern DM: Interleukin-1 induces endothelial cell procoagulant while suppressing cell surface anticoagulant activity. Proc Natl Acad Sci USA 83:3460, 1986
90. Nawroth PP, Bank I, Handley D et al: Tumor necrosis factor/cachectin interacts with endothelial cell receptors to induce release of interleukin 1. J Exp Med 163:1363, 1986
91. Moore KL, Esmon CT, Esmon NL: Tumor necrosis factor leads to internalization and degradation of thrombomodulin from the surface of bovine aortic endothelial cells in culture. Blood 73:159, 1989
92. Boerger LM, Morris PC, Thurnau GR et al: Oral contraceptives and gender affect protein S status. Blood 69:692, 1987
93. Bevilacqua MP, Pober JS, Majeau GR et al: Interleukin-1 (IL-1) induces biosynthesis and cell surface expression of procoagulant activity in human vascular endothelial cells. J Exp Med 160:618, 1984
94. Bevilacqua MP, Pober JS, Wheeler ME et al: Interleukin 1 acts on cultured human vascular endothelium to increase the adhesion of polymorphonuclear leukocytes, monocytes, and related leukocyte cell lines. J Clin Invest 76:2003, 1985
95. Glaser CB, Morser J, Clarke JH et al: Oxidation of a specific methionine in thrombomodulin by activated neutrophil products blocks cofactor activity. J Clin Invest 90:2565, 1992
96. Busch C, Cancilla P, DeBault L et al: Use of endothelium cultured on microcarriers as a model for the microcirculation. Lab Invest 47:498, 1982
97. Owen WG, Esmon CT: Functional properties of an endothelial cell cofactor for thrombin-catalyzed activation of protein C. J Biol Chem 256:5532, 1981
98. Maruyama I, Bell CE, Majerus PW: Thrombomodulin is found on endothelium of arteries, veins, capillaries, lymphatics, and on syncytiotrophoblast of human placenta. J Cell Biol 101:363, 1985
99. DeBault LE, Esmon NL, Olson JR, Esmon CT: Distribution of the thrombomodulin antigen in the rabbit vasculature. Lab Invest 54:172, 1986
100. Teitel JM, Rosenberg RD: Protection of factor Xa from neutralization by the heparin-antithrombin complex. J Clin Invest 71:1383, 1983
101. Nesheim ME, Canfield WM, Kisiel W, Mann KG: Studies on the capacity of factor Xa to protect factor Va from inactivation by activated protein C. J Biol Chem 257:1433, 1982
102. Dreyfus M, Magny JF, Bridey F et al: Treatment of homozygous protein C deficiency and neonatal purpura fulminans with a purified protein C concentrate. N Engl J Med 325:1565, 1991
103. Broekmans AW, Bertina RM, Loeliger EA et al: Protein C and the development of skin necrosis during anticoagulant therapy. Thromb Haemost 49:251, 1983
104. McGehee WG, Klotz TA, Epstein DJ, Rapaport SI: Coumarin necrosis associated with hereditary protein C deficiency. Ann Intern Med 100:59, 1984
105. Comp PC, Elrod JP, Karzenski S: Warfarin-induced skin necrosis. Semin Thromb Hemost 16:293, 1990
106. Muntean W, Finding K, Gamillscheg A, Schwarz HP: Multiple thromboses and coumarin-induced skin necrosis in a child with anticardiolipin antibodies: effects of protein C concentrate administration, abstracted. Thromb Haemost 65:2017, 1991

107. Schramm W, Spannagl M, Bauer KA et al: Treatment of coumarin-induced skin necrosis with a monoclonal antibody purified protein C concentrate. Arch Dermatol 129:753, 1993
108. Esman NL, Owen WG, Esmon CT: Isolation of a membrane-bound cofactor for thrombin-catalyzed activation of protein C. J Biol Chem 257:859, 1982
109. Griffin JH, Mosher DF, Zimmerman TS, Kleiss AJ: Protein C, an antithrombotic protein, is reduced in hospitalized patients with intravascular coagulation. Blood 60:261, 1982
110. Gerson WT, Dickerman JD, Bovill EG, Golden E: Severe acquired protein C deficiency in purpura fulminans associated with disseminated intravascular coagulation: treatment with protein C concentrate. Pediatrics 91:418, 1993
111. Emerick SC, Murayama H, Yan SB et al: Preclinical pharmacology of activated protein C. p. 351. In Holcenber JS, Winkelhake JL (eds): The Pharmacology and Toxicology of Proteins. Alan R Liss, New York, 1987
112. Gruber A, Griffin JH, Harker LA, Hanson SR: Inhibition of platelet-dependent thrombus formation by human activated protein C in a primate model. Blood 73:639, 1989
113. Hanson SR, Griffin JH, Harker LA et al: Antithrombotic effects of thrombin-induced activation of endogenous protein C in primates. J Clin Invest 92:2003, 1993
114. Snow TR, Deal MT, Dickey DT, Esmon CT: Protein C activation following coronary artery occlusion in the in situ porcine heart. Circulation 84:293, 1991
115. Foster DC, Yoshitake S, Davie EW: The nucleotide sequence of the gene for human protein C. Proc Natl Acad Sci USA 82:4673, 1985
116. Plutzky J, Hoskins J, Long GL, Crabtree GR: Evolution and organization of the human protein C gene. Proc Natl Acad Sci USA 83:546, 1986
117. Beckmann RJ, Schmidt RJ, Santerre RF et al: The structure and evolution of a 461 amino acid human protein C precursor and its messenger RNA, based upon the DNA sequence of cloned human liver cDNAs. Nucleic Acids Res 13:5233, 1985
118. Reitsma PH, Poort SR, Bernardi F et al: Protein C deficiency: a data base of mutations. For the Protein C & S Subcommittee of the Scientific and Standardization Committee of the International Society on Thrombosis and Haemostasis. Thromb Haemost 69:77, 1993
119. Bovill EG, Tomczak JA, Grant B, et al: Protein C$_{Vermont}$: symptomatic type II protein C deficiency associated with two GLA domain mutations. Blood 79:1456, 1992
120. Schmidel DK, Tatro AV, Phelps LG et al: Organization of the human protein S genes. Biochemistry 29:7845, 1990
121. Edenbrandt C-M, Lundwall A, Wydro R, Stenflo J: Molecular analysis of the gene for vitamin K-dependent protein S and its pseudogene. Cloning and partial gene organization. Biochemistry 29:7861, 1990
122. Ploos van Amstel HK, Reitsma PH, van der Logt CPE, Bertina RM: Intron-exon organization of the active human protein S gene PSα and its pseudogene PSβ: duplication and silencing during primate evolution. Biochemistry 29:7853, 1990
123. Schmidel DK, Nelson RM, Broxson EH Jr et al: A 5.3-kb deletion including exon XIII of the protein Sα gene occurs in two protein S-deficient families. Blood 77:551, 1991
124. Esmon CT: The regulation of natural anticoagulant pathways. Science 235:1348, 1987

Clinical Evaluation of Hemorrhagic Disorders: Bleeding History and Differential Diagnosis of Purpura

103

Barry S. Coller and Paul I. Schneiderman

INTRODUCTION

The initial evaluation of patients with hemorrhagic problems involves obtaining a detailed history of bleeding symptoms and analyzing any current hemorrhagic lesions, which are most often on the skin. This chapter focuses on the bleeding history and the differential diagnosis of purpuric skin lesions that may reflect an underlying hemorrhagic or nonhemorrhagic disorder.

BLEEDING HISTORY

The bleeding history forms the basis of the diagnosis and therapy of hemorrhagic disorders. In order to maximize its value, several basic principles of eliciting and interpreting this information deserve emphasis.

1. Many normal, healthy people consider their bleeding and bruising excessive. For example, using standardized self-administered questionnaires, Miller et al.[1] found that 23% of the normal population had "positive" bleeding histories, and Wahlberg et al.[2] reported that a remarkable 65% of healthy women and 35% of healthy men answered "yes" to the question: "Do you suffer from a bleeding disorder?"[2] (Table 103-1).
2. Patients with profound coagulation disorders invariably have dramatically abnormal bleeding histories, although surprisingly they may not volunteer the information unless specifically questioned.
3. Patients with mild to moderate abnormalities may not be recognized as having excessive bleeding symptoms, even though they are at risk of developing excessive bleeding if exposed to severe hemostatic challenges. In the study by Miller et al.,[1] 35% of patients with heterozygous von Willebrand disease (vWD) had negative bleeding histories, and in the study by Wahlberg et al.,[2] approximately 54% of men and 38% of women with either vWD or a platelet function defect failed to identify themselves as suffering from a bleeding disorder (Table 103-1).

    Identification of the group of patients with milder defects, and distinguishing them from the normal population, requires considerable skill and experience. In fact, given the low frequency of hemorrhagic disorders in the population and the high false-positive rate in the normal population, the task is truly formidable. For example, if one uses the values of 65% for the sensitivity of the bleeding history and 77% for its specificity derived from the study con-

ducted by Miller et al.[1] and assumes a prevalence of 10 patients with vWD in a population of 100,000,[3] the predictive accuracy of a positive history is a dismal 0.03%. Thus, in a population of 100,000 people, seven patients with vWD with positive histories (65% of 10) would have to be differentiated from the 22,998 normal persons with positive histories (23% of 99,990).

4. A search for objective confirmation of subjective symptoms provides important information in assessing the severity of the patient's disorder. This is especially important in obtaining a bleeding history because some patients are extremely cognizant of even minor hemorrhagic problems, whereas others ignore major ones. Specific objective indicators are discussed below with each group of symptoms, but overall indicators would include information concerning (1) visits to other physicians for bleeding problems, along with any laboratory data obtained; (2) previous need for transfusion of whole blood, packed red blood cells, plasma, platelets, or coagulation factor concentrates; and (3) a history of documented anemia or physician-prescribed iron therapy, or both.
5. A medication history is incomplete without specific questions concerning aspirin and other medications available without prescription that may affect platelet function because patients might not recognize these agents as medications. Similarly, it is important to inquire about vitamin tablets that may contain vitamin K in patients taking oral anticoagulants.
6. Although self-administered questionnaires with yes or no answers facilitate data collection and statistical analysis, obtaining the maximal amount of useful information requires a dialogue between patient and physician. This allows the physician a chance to assess whether the patient truly understands what is being asked, to refine the questions in response to the initial answers, and to follow up on potentially important data that become obvious only as the discussion proceeds. In short, good history taking is not a passive process in which boxes are checked off in response to bland and ambiguous questions, but rather an extremely active process of initial data gathering, hypothesis development, construction of questions to test the hypothesis, additional data gathering, and new hypothesis development. Moreover, it is an exhilarating endeavor in which physicians must meld their knowledge of science, medicine, and human behavior into a series of pointed questions that the patient can understand and respond to.
7. The constellation of hemorrhagic symptoms is extremely important in suggesting the etiology of the disorder. Thus,

Table 103-1. Self-Administered Questionnaire for the Diagnosis of Hemorrhagic Disorders

Questions	Males		Females	
	Normals (N = 23)	Patients[a] (N = 24)	(N = 20)	Patients[a] (N = 21)
Do you suffer from a bleeding disorder?	35[b]	46	65	62
Bleeding from the gums?	52	67	50	67
Long bleeding after tooth extraction?	4	21	10	24
Skin bleeding?	0	13	15	10
Long bleeding from small wounds?	13	25	10	10
Tendency to bruises?	22	25	55	62
Spontaneous bruises?	0	4	40	48
Nose bleeding?	57	63	85	57
Blood coughed up or vomited?	9	13	5	10
Metrorrhagia?	—	—	55	42
Muscle bleeding?	4	13	15	0
Blood in the urine?	0	8	10	10
Joint bleeding?	0	0	0	10
Blood in the stool?	13	8	5	10
Treated with vitamin K?	0	4	10	19
Treated with plasma or blood transfusion?	0	4	0	0

[a] The patient group consisted of 16 individuals with von Willebrand disease, 27 individuals with a variety of qualitative platelet abnormalities (including aspirin-like defects (N = 9), isolated abnormal collagen-induced aggregation (N = 12), and isolated abnormal arachidonic acid-induced aggregation (N = 6), and 2 patients with antithrombin III deficiency.

[b] Percentage of normal patients compared with patients with von Willebrand's disease, platelet abnormalities, or antithrombin III deficiency answering "yes" to indicated questions. Subjects were given a choice of "yes," "no," and "don't know." The percentage answering "no" and "don't know" varied considerably from question to question.

(Adapted from Wahlberg et al.,[2] with permission.)

spontaneous hemarthroses and muscle hemorrhages are highly suggestive of severe hemophilia, whereas epistaxis, gingival bleeding, and menorrhagia are more commonly found in patients with thrombocytopenia, platelet disorders, or vWD.

8. Excessive bruising and bleeding may be a manifestation of diseases of the blood vessel rather than diseases of coagulation or platelets. In patients with impressive bleeding histories, but no abnormalities in coagulation or platelets, one needs to have a high index of suspicion for hereditary hemorrhagic telangiectasias, Cushing disease, scurvy, Ehlers-Danlos syndrome, and other systemic disorders. In patients whose hemorrhagic symptoms are confined to the skin, consideration must be given to a wide range of dermatologic disorders.

9. The diagnostic value of any single hemorrhagic symptom varies with the different disorders. Studies of hemophilia carriers by Wahlberg[4] and of patients with vWD or platelet function abnormalities[2] ranked the individual questions on the basis of their ability to discriminate between the patients and normal subjects. The results from the hemophilia carrier study are shown in Table 103-2. Since the patterns of hemorrhage differ with different hemorrhagic disorders, the diagnostic value of any given question will differ as well. For example, in the study on patients with vWD and platelet disorders,[2] prolonged bleeding after tooth extractions (Table 103-1) was a more sensitive discriminator than it was in the study on hemophilia carriers[4] (Table 103-2).

10. A dietary history is extremely important in patients taking oral anticoagulants because the patient's intake of vitamin K will affect the response to the medication. In order to maintain a constant level of anticoagulation, the dietary intake of vitamin K must remain constant. The absolute amount of vitamin K intake is less important, so it is reasonable to permit the patient free choice of diet with the proviso that, once selected, it remain reasonably constant. If the patient wishes to change diets, the level of anticoagulation

must be monitored more carefully. Patients should also be instructed that food additives, such as fish oils, may contain vitamin K. Patients who are not taking food by mouth are at particularly high risk of the development of vitamin K deficiency, especially if they are also taking broad-spectrum antibiotics, since the latter decrease the vitamin K contribution from bacteria in the gastrointestinal tract. This combination of decreased oral intake and antibiotic therapy is quite common in patients with bowel disorders during the preoperative and postoperative periods. It is vital to recognize this scenario because vitamin K is required on a daily basis despite its fat solubility, and significant depression of coagulation factors can occur within just several days.

11. Potentially confounding pharmacologic and medical influ-

Table 103-2. Discriminant Capacity of Questions in Distinguishing Between Normal Persons and Hemophilia Carriers

Questions	Sensitivity[a]	Specificity[b]	Difference Between Carriers and Noncarriers (P)
Tendency to bruises?	50	77	<0.025
Metrorrhagia	44	81	<0.025
Abnormal bleeding at delivery	38	97	<0.005
Abnormal bleeding at operation	35	92	<0.005
Tendency to nosebleeding?	32	87	<0.05
Long bleeding after tooth extraction?	15	98	n.s.
Blood in the urine?	11	98	n.s.
Long bleeding from small wounds	8	96	n.s.
Blood in the stool?	3	100	n.s.

[a] Percentage of positive responses among carriers.
[b] Percentage of negative responses among normals.
(Adapted from Wahlberg[4] with permission.)

ences need to be considered in evaluating the history. Thus, for example, since pregnancy and birth control pills can increase von Willebrand factor (vWF) in some patients with the mild to moderate forms of the disease, this needs to be considered in assessing the bleeding history. The decrease in vWF soon after delivery can lead to prolonged postpartum hemorrhage. Similarly, since the stress of surgery or pregnancy can lead to thrombocytopenia in type IIB vWD, bleeding may be especially severe at these times.[5,6]

12. Assessing excessive bleeding in the newborn is especially difficult. For example, some neonates with Glanzmann thrombasthenia have only minimal symptoms at birth, and the symptoms of vWD may be masked by an increase in vWF as a result of the stress involved in the delivery. Similarly, a significant number of hemophilic neonates do not have hemorrhagic symptoms in the first weeks of life. Large cephalohematomas may be due just to birth trauma, but if they continue to progress after delivery, hemophilia or vitamin K-dependent factor deficiency should be considered. Delayed bleeding from the umbilical stump should raise the possibility of factor XIII deficiency or a fibrinogen abnormality (quantitative or qualitative).

Documenting the History

Table 103-3 shows a bleeding history form. It should be filled out by the physician during discussions with the patient; it is designed specifically not to be self-administered by the patient. The use of the form ensures that the major symptoms are elicited and recorded in a standardized manner. The form itself then can be made a part of the patient's permanent record.

Epistaxis

Bleeding from the nose is one of the most common manifestations of platelet disorders and vWD; it is also the most common symptom of hereditary hemorrhagic telangiectasias. At the same time, a large fraction of the normal population has experienced at least one or more nosebleeds. Thus, when a group of normal subjects are presented with the question, "Nose bleeding?" on a self-administered questionnaire, 57% of the men and 85% of the women answered "yes" (Table 103-1). To obtain more meaningful data, it is important to inquire about the frequency of nosebleeds and whether the nosebleeding occurs spontaneously or only with trauma. The latter may not always be appreciated because some people habitually and unconsciously traumatize their mucous membranes when manually removing crusted secretions from their nose. If the bleeding is confined to a single nostril, it is more likely due to a localized vascular abnormality than to a systemic coagulopathy. In northern locales, nosebleeding from nonhematologic etiologies is more likely to occur in the dry winter months, especially if forced-air heating systems that dry out the mucous membranes are used. It is also important to ascertain the effects of aging on epistaxis, since many people with no discernible abnormalities will have childhood epistaxis that disappears after puberty, whereas patients with hereditary hemorrhagic telangiectasias usually suffer increasingly severe epistaxis with the onset of adulthood, middle age, and old age. It may also be useful to ask women if the nosebleeding is related to their menstrual cycle, since very unusual cases of ectopic uterine tissue in the upper airways or sinuses, or both, have been reported. The length of time for the bleeding to stop will provide valuable insight into the severity of the episodes. Objective information can be obtained by inquiring as to whether the epistaxis was severe enough to require evaluation by a physician, and if so, whether packing, cautery, or transfusions were considered necessary.

Gingival Hemorrhage

Bleeding from the gums is another very common symptom of platelet disorders and vWD. In addition, it is often the first sign of hemostatic compromise in patients in whom thrombocytopenia develops after chemotherapy. Interestingly, patients with long-standing disorders might not recognize that their gingival bleeding is excessive because they assume that everyone bleeds from their gums on a daily basis. In fact, occasional, but not perennial, gum bleeding is very common among the normal population, with 52% of normal males and 50% of normal females answering "yes" to the question, "Bleeding from the gums?" It is therefore important to establish the frequency with which the patient's gum bleeding occurs and whether it is spontaneous, since the vast majority of normal persons will only experience gum bleeding after the trauma of tooth brushing. If spontaneous gum bleeding occurs during the night, patients may notice blood-tinged stains on their pillow cases. Daily gum bleeding with tooth brushing may or may not be abnormal, depending on whether the patient has known gingival disease and on whether a hard bristle or soft bristle tooth brush is used. Since the routine tooth scaling to remove plaque performed by dental workers is a significant hemostatic challenge, it is useful to inquire whether the patient was told that he or she bled excessively after this procedure. This also provides a more objective assessment of the extent of bleeding. Finally, some patients may have oral mucous membrane bleeding in the form of blood blisters as another manifestation of a hemorrhagic diathesis, particularly severe thrombocytopenia, with a predilection for sites at which irregularities in the patient's teeth may traumatize the inner surface of the cheek.

Skin Hemorrhage

Petechial lesions characteristically appear as crops or showers of lesions in dependent portions of the vasculature. However, the integrity of the microvasculature is dependent on a variety of vascular and extravascular factors, so it is not surprising that patients with similar platelet or coagulation disorders show considerable variability in the appearance of petechial lesions. When infants cry, they increase the venous pressure (see below) and this may be sufficient provocation to bring out petechial lesions in patients with platelet disorders such as Glanzmann thrombasthenia.

Bruising is one of the most difficult symptoms to evaluate because patients vary greatly in their recognition and response to the symptom. Patients who always bruise excessively even without trauma may assume that this is normal because they have experienced it all their lives, whereas normal persons who bruise only rarely may grow inordinately concerned about a single large bruise associated with trauma. There is also a clear gender-related difference, with bruising much more common in women than in men. For example, 22% of normal men and 55% of normal women responded affirmatively to the question, "Tendency to bruises?," and no normal men but 40% of normal women indicated that they had "spontaneous bruises." It is necessary, therefore, to try to define the nature of the bruising better so as to render a judgment as to whether it is likely to be part of a hemorrhagic diathesis.

The dermatologic literature recognizes the entity purpura simplex in which women have excessive bruising in relationship to their menstrual cycle, although the time in the cycle when the bruising is excessive may vary from woman to woman. Needless to say, this is a diagnosis that should be entertained only after excluding other etiologies. If no underlying hematologic or nonhematologic causes can be found, it is appropriate to reassure the patient that she is unlikely to be at risk of excessive hemorrhage, even with more severe hemostatic challenges such as surgery. It is inappropriate, however, to tell the patient that nothing is wrong with her, because this

Table 103-3. Bleeding History

1. Epistaxis
   A. Ages when affected
   B. Frequency
   C. Spontaneous
   D. Left, right, or both nostrils
   E. Seasonal correlation
   F. Time to stop
   G. Required
      1. Packing
      2. Cautery
      3. Transfusions
   Comments:
2. Gingival hemorrhage
   A. Frequency
   B. Spontaneous or with tooth brushing
   Comments:
3. Skin hemorrhage
   A. Petechiae
   B. Bruises
      1. Frequency
      2. Relationship to menses
      3. Spontaneous
      4. Exposed sites
         a. Arms
         b. Legs
      5. Unexposed sites
         a. Trunk
         b. Back
      6. Size
      7. Knots in center
      8. Painful
      9. Color
      10. Time to resolution
      11. Number currently
   Comments:
4. Tooth extractions—ages at extractions
   A. Deciduous
   B. Permanent
      Molar
      Other
   C. Duration of bleeding
      1. Packing
      2. Resuturing
      3. Transfusion
   D. Estimated blood loss
   Comments:
5. Bleeding from minor cuts
   A. Blade or electric razor
   B. Approximate time to stop
   C. Requires
      1. Direct pressure
      2. Tissue paper
   Comments:
6. Bleeding from major trauma
   A. Knife wound
   B. Motor vehicle accident
   C. Need for
      1. Sutures
      2. Transfusions
   Comments:

7. Hemoptysis
   A. Spontaneous
   B. Associated with respiratory infection?
   Comments:
8. Hematemesis
   A. Spontaneous
   B. Known increase in portal pressure
   C. Associated with vomiting
      1. Beginning of episode
      2. End of episode
   Comments:
9. Hematuria
   A. Frequency
   B. Gross or microscopic
   C. Related to urinary infection
   D. Duration
   E. Required
      1. Cystoscopy
      2. Transfusion
   Comments:
10. Hematochezia
    A. Frequency
    B. Duration
    C. Known hemorrhoids
    Comments:
11. Melena
    A. Frequency
    B. Duration
    C. Known ulcer disease
    D. Required
       1. Transfusion
       2. Surgery
    E. Documented by tests for occult blood
    Comments:
12. Central nervous system bleeding
    A. Hemorrhagic stroke
    B. Documentation
       1. Computed tomography scan
       2. Magnetic resonance imaging
    Comments:
13. Venipuncture site bleeding
    Comments:
14. Ophthalmic bleeding
    A. Subconjunctival hemorrhage
    B. Retinal hemorrhage
    C. Retrobulbar hemorrhage
    Comments:
15. Menses
    A. Frequency
    B. Duration in days
       1. Heavy flow
       2. Total flow
    C. Comparison to sisters or friends
    D. Required
       1. Transfusion
       2. Iron therapy
       3. Birth control pills
       4. Dilation and curettage
       5. Hysterectomy
    E. Known fibroid tumor
    Comments:

16. Childbirth
    A. Pregnancies
    B. Spontaneous abortions (indicate month of gestation)
    C. Induced abortions
    D. Estimated blood loss
    E. Anemia documented
    F. Required
       1. Transfusion
       2. Dilation and curettage
       3. Hysterectomy
       4. Iron therapy
    Comments:
17. Hemarthroses
    A. Joints
       1. Elbow
       2. Knee
       3. Ankle
       4. Wrist
       5. Shoulder
       6. Other
    B. Frequency
    C. Required
       1. Transfusion
       2. Aspiration
    Comments:
18. Previous surgical procedures
    A. Procedure
    B. Date
    C. Excess bleeding
    D. Required
       1. Whole blood
       2. Plasma
       3. Platelets
       4. Coagulation-factor concentrate
    E. Reoperation
    F. Wound healing
    Comments:
19. Bleeding at circumcision
    Comments:
20. Telangiectasias
    A. Mucous membranes
    B. Skin
    C. Gastrointestinal tract
    Comments:
21. Connective tissue
    A. Double jointedness
    B. Skin hyperextensibility
    C. Fat distribution changes
    Comments:
22. Wound healing
    Comments:
23. Medications
    A. Iron
    B. Birth control pills
    C. Aspirin or other antiplatelet medications
    Comments:
24. Family history of bleeding

(Based on Coller and Hultin, unpublished data.)

can be misinterpreted to suggest that the physician thinks she inappropriately sought medical attention for a trivial matter. These patients clearly do have an abnormality that can be quite frightening, even though the defect has not been identified biochemically.

As with the other symptoms, it is important to try to establish whether the patient's hemorrhagic response is excessive given the inciting trauma. Thus, bruising unassociated with any trauma is most likely to be pathologic, and the patient should be asked specifically whether bruises appeared even without any recognized antecedent trauma. Unfortunately, patients vary significantly in appreciating when they have been traumatized. For example, mothers of children who are old enough to be physically active but still young enough to be held in the mother's arms, often focus on other matters while holding the child and do not realize that they are being repeatedly kicked. Similarly, normal toddlers and youngsters who are physically active commonly have bruises on their legs and arms.

The location of the bruise may offer indirect evidence on the relationship of the bruising to trauma since the vast majority of traumatic events occur to exposed sites on the arms and legs. If the patient suffers repeated bruising on unexposed sites on the trunk or back, this is more likely to be either spontaneous or in response to minimal trauma. The size of the bruise may also give some indication of the extent of bruising. It is best to provide patients with some size standards that they can relate to, such as "dime-sized," "silver-dollar-sized," or "as large as your palm." When assessing size it is important to remember that bruises often spread during the resolution phase. Some idea of the extent of the hemorrhage into the bruise can be obtained by noting whether a darkly discolored and raised "knot" was present in the center of the bruise and whether the bruise was painful.

The color of the bruise may also be quite significant. Bruises associated with hemorrhagic phenomena tend to be the dark purple characteristic "black-and-blue" marks that evolve into shades of yellow-green as they resolve. By contrast, patients with senile purpura or Cushing syndrome commonly have bruises that are much redder in appearance. Since easy bruising may be the presenting symptom of Cushing syndrome, it is important to have a high index of suspicion for this disorder in younger patients whose bruises simulate the appearance of senile purpura. Another color variant worth distinguishing is the jet black central area and violaceous-erythematous surrounding area characteristic of coumadin-induced skin necrosis. This thrombotic disorder, associated in some cases with protein C or protein S deficiency, has a predilection for fatty tissues such as the breasts and is not uncommonly mistaken for a hemorrhagic abnormality because of the bruise-like nature of the lesion and the association with oral anticoagulant use.

Bruises usually take 10–14 days to resolve, depending on the extent of the bruise. When patients indicate that their bruises take months to resolve or that they have required casting of a limb in order for the bruising to stop, consideration should be given to the poorly understood entity of psychogenic purpura.

Tooth Extractions

The patient's bleeding in response to tooth extraction can provide extremely important information. The hemostatic challenge varies, however, with the tooth removed; molar extractions are usually the severest tests of hemostasis. Objective information can be obtained about the duration and extent of bleeding by asking about the need to reconsult the dentist for packing, suturing, or even transfusion of blood products. A deep injection given to achieve anesthesia by nerve block constitutes another hemostatic challenge; hemorrhage that extends down into the neck is especially important to note, since it may compromise the airway.

Bleeding from Minor Cuts

In our society, shaving nicks are the most common minor cuts suffered; patients with platelet disorders or vWD usually bleed excessively from these nicks. If a patient uses an electric razor or a depilatory instead of a razor blade, it is worthwhile asking whether a razor blade was ever used and, if so, why the switch was made. Although it may be difficult to obtain truly objective information about bleeding after razor nicks, it may be helpful to ask whether the patient delays leaving home in the morning because of persistent oozing from these wounds or whether the patient leaves home with small pieces of tissue paper still attached to the bleeding wounds. It is also useful to instruct the patient that direct pressure for 5 minutes is usually much more effective than tissue paper, since rebleeding is very common when the latter is removed. Patients with purpura secondary to amyloidosis (see below) may paradoxically choose to switch from an electric razor to a blade razor because the pressure of the electric razor causes more purpura than occurs with razor nicks.

Hemoptysis

Hemoptysis is virtually never the presenting symptom of a bleeding disorder and is rare even with serious bleeding disorders. Thus, a comprehensive search for an anatomic abnormality or an underlying infectious or neoplastic disease is required, even if the patient has a systemic coagulopathy. Patients with bleeding diatheses may, however, have blood-tinged sputum in association with acute respiratory tract infections. Occasionally, a patient with an upper respiratory tract infection associated with a postnasal drip may also complain of hemoptysis, even though the true source of blood is in the upper airway.

Bleeding from Major Trauma

In the absence of previous surgery, the extent of bleeding in response to major trauma furnishes the most reliable information about the future hemostatic risk. In order to assess the appropriateness of the bleeding, the details of the injury must be determined. The need for sutures and transfusions provides objective information. Excessive bleeding due to thrombocytopenia or platelet dysfunction tends to occur immediately, whereas excessive bleeding due to coagulation abnormalities may be delayed for hours or days. It is especially important to ascertain whether aspirin or other antiplatelet agents were taken at the time of injury to alleviate pain.

Hematemesis

As with hemoptysis, hematemesis is virtually never the presenting symptom of a hemostatic disorder, and thus a search for an anatomic basis is mandatory. Hemostatic defects may, however, contribute significantly to the problem, as in patients with liver disease and esophageal varices, or patients with gastritis secondary to aspirin ingestion.

Hematuria

Urinary tract bleeding is also virtually never the first symptom of a hemostatic disorder, and thus, a full investigation to define an anatomic defect is necessary. Hemostatic defects may, however, exacerbate hematuria caused by other disorders; thus, patients with urinary tract infections, for example, that might ordinarily produce only microscopic hematuria, may suffer from gross hematuria. Normal subjects may also develop gross hematuria with urinary tract infections and, since women are much more likely to contract such infections, it may explain why no normal men but 10% of normal women complained of blood in their urine in the study by Wahlberg et al[2] (Table 103-1). Even among patients with platelet disorders and vWD, however, only 8% of men and 10% of women complained of hematuria[2] (Table 103-1).

Hematochezia

Hemorrhoids are the most common cause of hematochezia, but more serious, less common, causes must be excluded. In the study conducted by Wahlberg et al.,[2] 13% of normal men and 5% of normal women complained of blood in the stool (Table 103-1). Although a systemic coagulopathy may exacerbate hematochezia, the bleeding should not be ascribed to the coagulopathy itself without extensive evaluation. vWD, platelet abnormalities, and both the inherited and acquired forms of angiodysplasia may all be associated with severe recurrent episodes of hematochezia, and the search for discrete bleeding sites is often frustrating and inconclusive. Associations between vWD and both angiodysplasia and hereditary hemorrhagic telangiectasias have been reported, but it is possible that the vWD just makes it more likely that the vascular disorder will be diagnosed, since the hemorrhage is likely to be more severe.

Melena

It is important to make certain that the patient understands precisely what is meant by the term melena, because many patients will answer "yes" to a question about black stools when, on further questioning, it is clear that their stools are really dark brown. The black rubber tubing of a stethoscope is a good visual prompt for making this clear. Objective evidence of gastrointestinal hemorrhage can be obtained by explicitly asking whether the patient's stool ever tested positive for occult blood and whether the patient ever underwent endoscopy. As with the other sources of gastrointestinal bleeding, melena is virtually never the presenting symptom of a congenital hemostatic defect. Recurrent episodes of melena, like hematochezia, do occur in patients with serious hemorrhagic abnormalities or angiodysplasia and on occasion may even be lethal. Objective data on previous hospitalizations, the results of endoscopic studies, and the need for blood replacement should be obtained.

Central Nervous System Bleeding

Severe thrombocytopenia (<5,000 platelets/mm^3) is associated with central nervous system hemorrhage, with both diffuse petechial lesions and gross hemorrhagic strokes. Hemophilia is also associated with spontaneous central nervous system hemorrhage, and it greatly increases the risk of serious hemorrhagic stroke with even minimal head trauma. It is of interest that spontaneous central nervous system hemorrhage is exceedingly rare in Glanzmann thrombasthenia.

Venipuncture Site Bleeding

Patients with diffuse intravascular coagulation, hyperfibrinolysis, thrombocytopenia, or qualitative platelet disorders characteristically bleed for a long time after venipunctures, whereas patients with inherited coagulation disorders do not. Delayed bleeding, however, may occur in the latter group.

Ophthalmic Bleeding

Subconjunctival hemorrhages are associated with both platelet and coagulation abnormalities, especially in young children who cry, leading to increased venous pressure. Severe thrombocytopenia may lead to retinal hemorrhage if not effectively treated for several days to weeks. Orbital hemorrhage is more commonly associated with hemophilia than with platelet disorders.

Menses

Assessing the severity of menstrual flow based on the number of sanitary napkins or tampons used is not reliable because women vary greatly in their hygienic practices. It is usually more helpful to establish the number of days of heavy flow and the total number of days for an average menstrual period; if the former is >3 or the latter is >6 or 7, or both, it is likely that the menstrual bleeding is excessive. It may also help to ascertain whether the bleeding is heavy enough to require especially large sanitary napkins or to require curtailment of ordinary activities. Objective data include whether a physician (1) prescribed birth control pills to control the bleeding, (2) told the patient she was anemic, (3) prescribed iron, (4) performed a dilation and curettage to assess the bleeding, (5) was forced by circumstances to perform an emergency hysterectomy to secure hemostasis, and/or (6) performed an elective hysterectomy or radiation sterilization of the uterus as preventive measures.

Childbirth

A detailed history of bleeding with each pregnancy should be obtained, including objective data regarding the need for transfusions, dilation and curettage, iron therapy, and/or hysterectomy. It is useful to specifically ask if the patient's doctor commented on her bleeding being excessive at delivery, even if none of the objective criteria were met. A history of recurrent spontaneous abortion may be part of the antiphospholipid antibody syndrome, which may include lupus-like anticoagulants, anticardiolipin antibodies, and/or false-positive serologic tests for syphilis. The suspicion of this syndrome should be even greater if the recurrent spontaneous abortions occur after the first trimester. Recurrent spontaneous abortions have also been reported in association with abnormalities of fibrinogen, presumably due to abnormal stability of placental attachment.

Hemarthroses

Joint bleeding is the hallmark of the hemophilias and is extremely rare in all other hemostatic defects except severe vWD. Since joint bleeds are usually not associated with skin discoloration, patients may not appreciate that their symptoms are caused by hemorrhage. It is important, therefore, to inquire specifically about pain, swelling, and limitation of motion, rather than merely asking about bleeding into the joints.

Operations

The details of each surgical procedure should be recorded, including any statements made by the surgeon about the extent of bleeding. In general, excessive bleeding due to coagulation abnormalities may be delayed in time for hours to a day or so, whereas excessive bleeding due to platelet disorders or thrombocytopenia usually occurs immediately. Emphasis should be placed on ascertaining whether any blood products were administered. Specific questioning about tonsillectomy and appendectomy may be required, as patients tend to forget about these operations, especially if they were performed many years before. The hospital records should be secured because they may contain important clinical and laboratory data that the patient never knew or forgot. When hospital records are unavailable, it may help to ask how long the patient was hospitalized, since delayed discharge may have been due to excessive bleeding.

Circumcision

Congenital bleeding disorders, in particular, the hemophilias may cause excessive bleeding at circumcision as their first manifestation. Delayed bleeding from the umbilical stump or after circumcision is said to be particularly suggestive of factor XIII deficiency, but the hemophilias due to factor VIII or to factor IX deficiency are probably equally likely to produce these symptoms.

Telangiectasias

Patients may manifest a wide range of telangiectatic lesions, ranging from pinpoint erythematous dots that blanch when compressed, to classic cherry angiomata that can be up to several centimeters in diameter (see under Differential Diagnosis). The vast majority of the otherwise normal population will demonstrate an increase in skin telangiectasias with aging, associated with the development of papular cherry angiomata. The latter may have a distinctive blue appearance if present in the deeper layers of the skin. Similarly, patients with hereditary hemorrhagic telangiectasias usually have progressively more severe disease as they age. In fact, it is not at all clear what constitutes the minimal criteria for hereditary hemorrhagic telangiectasias; some otherwise normal persons with no clinical manifestations in their early years may develop easy bruising in association with skin telangiectasias in their later years. The classic hallmarks of hereditary hemorrhagic telangiectasias include epistaxis and tongue telangiectasias, but lesions may be present in virtually every organ, manifesting as space-occupying lesions, sources of bleeding, or sources of arteriovenous shunting. On physical examination, the lesions may be much more subtle than the florid examples found in most textbooks; a very careful search of the integument is necessary, focusing on the face, chest, shoulders, legs, and under the nails. Lesions are also commonly found on the vermilion border of the lips and under the tongue, even when the tip of the tongue is not involved. It is important to distinguish the lesions of hereditary hemorrhagic telangiectasias from the spider telangiectasias associated with liver disease. The latter have a more splotchy appearance, are concentrated on the shoulders, chest, and face, and have a more serpiginous quality.

Connective Tissue

If Ehlers-Danlos syndrome is considered in the differential diagnosis, it is useful to inquire specifically as to whether the patient was "double-jointed" as a child or had unusually distensible skin. More obvious abnormalities such as lens dislocations should be apparent. Questions regarding common skin manifestations of Cushing syndrome should also be posed, including rounded faces, purple striae, truncal obesity, or fat deposition in the back of the neck. Old photographs of the patient may be extremely helpful in deciding whether facial changes are new. The full differential diagnosis of disorders affecting the integrity of the blood vessel and supporting tissues is discussed below.

Wound Healing

Although abnormal wound healing is not a common problem in hemostatic disorders, defects have been reported in association with factor XIII deficiency and fibrinogen abnormalities. Patients with Ehlers-Danlos syndrome and Cushing disease are also likely to have had abnormal wound healing.

Medications

The dose of each prescription and nonprescription drug taken by the patient should be recorded. Specific questions should cover aspirin and other antiplatelet agents, birth control pills, vitamins, and food supplements since these may not be appreciated as medications by the patient. Iron therapy in the past should also be noted, since it may provide information on previous episodes of anemia due to blood loss.

Family History

A pedigree going back at least one or two generations should be determined with emphasis on hemorrhagic or thrombotic manifestations, or both, for each member. Details about the cause of death for each deceased person should also be obtained.

Summary

Obtaining the details of the bleeding history requires insight into the mechanisms and manifestations of the different hemorrhagic disorders, as well as an appreciation of the patient's perceptions of symptoms. Whenever possible, objective data should be obtained to provide a more comprehensive and credible picture. Although obtaining a complete bleeding history may seem tedious, it is well worth the effort, since therapeutic decisions should weigh the patient's previous response to the same or similar hemostatic challenges as much or more than the laboratory values. In fact, a recent study showed that routine screening assays of coagulation and platelets failed to detect any clinically significant abnormalities in >100 preoperative patients with normal bleeding histories.[7] Although the clinical value of routine laboratory tests for screening for coagulation abnormalities is still in dispute, this study certainly highlights the central role of the bleeding history in evaluating hemostatic risk.

DIFFERENTIAL DIAGNOSIS OF HEMORRHAGIC DERMATOLOGIC LESIONS

Skin hemorrhage is defined as the indiscriminate extravasation of blood cells out of the vasculature and into the skin or subcutaneous tissue, or both. The amount of blood leaking from the vessel determines the size of the lesion, with minute amounts producing pinpoint red lesions <2 mm in size (petechiae), and larger amounts producing purpuric lesions (2 mm to 1 cm) or frank ecchymoses (>1 cm).[6] Despite these precise definitions, conventional usage often groups purpuric lesions and ecchymoses under the term purpura, and this general group of disorders, including petechiae, is often referred to as the purpuras. All these lesions can be readily differentiated from simple erythema and telangiectasias, in which the blood remains confined within the vasculature, because these latter lesions will blanch if direct pressure is applied to them. This can be easily demonstrated using a glass slide or the tip of a ballpoint pen with the penpoint in the retracted position. True purpura may demonstrate partial blanching with these maneuvers, but a nonblanchable component will remain. The color of the lesion depends on the size and location of the hemorrhage, as well as the time since the extravasation occurred. Initially, superficial lesions are bright red or deep red, and deeper lesions have more of a purple appearance. With time, the lesions evolve into deep purple, brown, orange, or blue-green discolorations.

The general mechanisms by which extravasation of blood from the vasculature can occur is depicted schematically in Figure 103-1. The integrity of the blood vessel depends on (1) the competence of the hemostatic mechanism to combat the basal level of ongoing vascular trauma, (2) the strength of the blood vessel itself and its surrounding tissues, and (3) the transmural pressure gradient tending to drive blood out of the vessel. Even if all these systems are functioning normally, however, serious trauma of diverse etiologies may be sufficient to cause hemorrhagic extravasation.

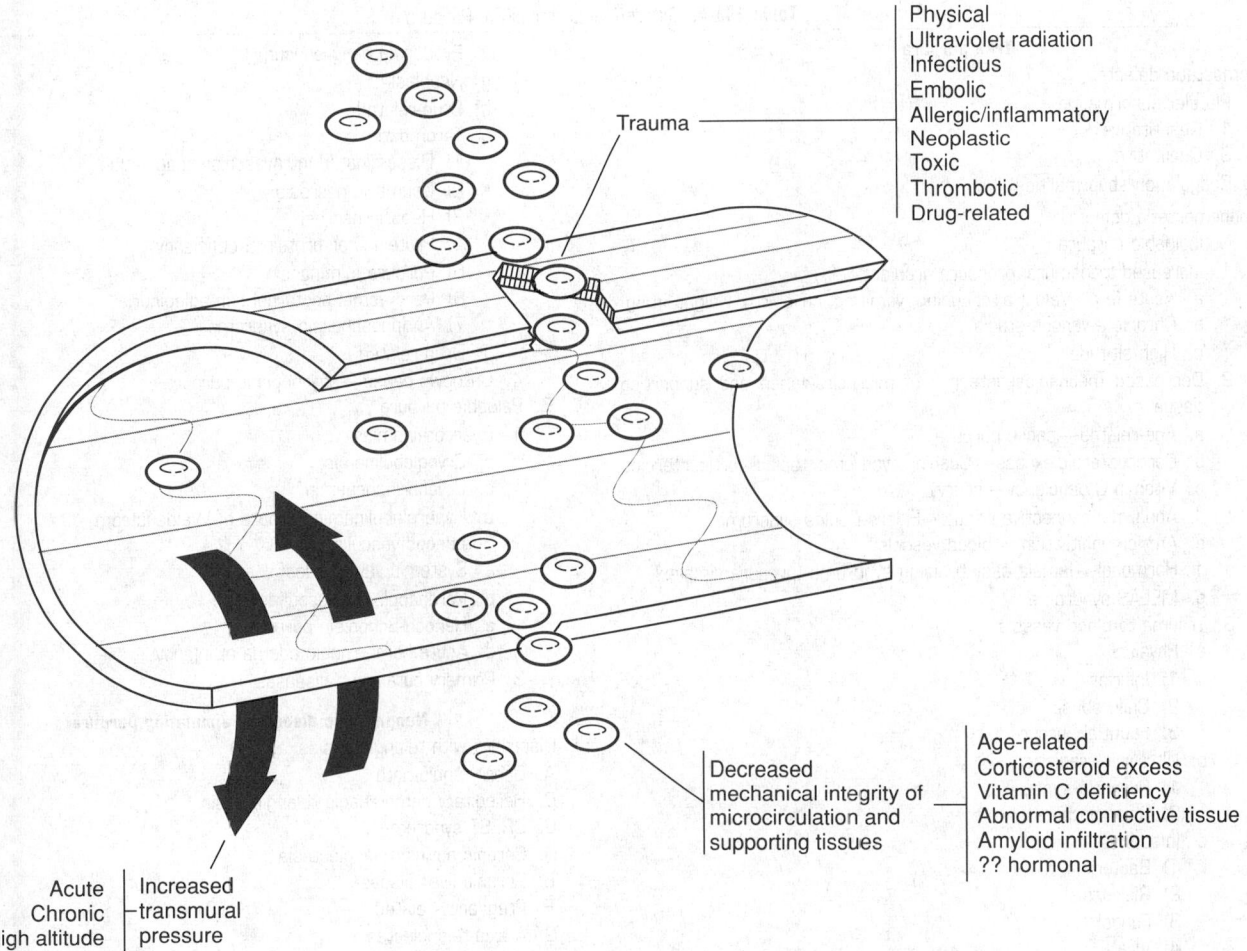

Fig. 103-1. Mechanism of nonpalpable purpura.

A classification of disorders producing skin hemorrhage is given in Table 103-4.[8,9] It is organized primarily according to etiology, but a division is made between lesions that are palpable and those that are not palpable. This is because palpability can be readily determined at the bedside and thus has important practical significance in developing a differential diagnosis. Although the specific mechanism(s) producing palpability is still poorly understood, one hypothesis is that a lesion becomes palpable when a generalized increase in vascular permeability secondary to an inflammatory process results in marked extravasation of plasma proteins with the development of extravascular coagulation leading to fibrin deposition. Support for such a mechanism comes from studies showing that the palpable induration accompanying delayed hypersensitivity reactions can be diminished by administration of oral anticoagulants.[10] Alternatively, palpability may be secondary to extensive cellular infiltration, as in certain inflammatory or malignant disorders.

Purpuric lesions secondary to hemostatic defects were described in the previous section. Among the nonhemostatic defects, those that produce nonpalpable lesions are considered first.

Nonpalpable Purpura

Increased Transmural Pressure

Acute

The clinical picture of minute petechiae of the face (especially the eyelids) (Plate 103-1), neck, and upper chest may be seen after prolonged Valsalva maneuvers, coughing, vomiting, childbirth, or weight lifting.[11,12] A similar syndrome can be found in newborns with umbilical cord strangulation, in children with suction purpura due to suction cups on toys, and in adults with either superior vena cava syndrome or basilar skull fractures.[13] Lesions on the lower extremities, especially in the elderly, may be due to acute venous stasis due to tight clothing or stockings. Occasionally, such dependent purpura may be palpable (Plate 103-2), even in the absence of microscopic evidence of inflammation.

Chronic

Chronic venous stasis of the lower extremity, due to either venous valvular incompetence or to the chronic use of tight-fitting garments, can convert subclinical insults of diverse etiologies into frank purpura. In addition, even the normal hydrostatic pressure head in the legs puts this area at greater risk of the development of extravasation of blood. Thus, it is common, but not universal, for the first petechiae due to hemostatic defects to appear at the ankles. Moreover, other common cutaneous disorders, such as drug rashes, contact dermatitis,[14] and sunburn often progress to become petechial and purpuric over the lower extremities after the first 24 hours. Chronic venous stasis accompanied by recurrent episodes of extravasation of red blood cells leads to the development of purpuric and yellow-brown macules, with the latter due to the persistent presence of hemosiderin.

High-Altitude

An increase in cutaneous petechiae has been noted in mountain climbers ascending >3,800 m above sea level.[15] In this case, the mechanism for purpura may be an increase in

Table 103-4. Differential Diagnosis of Purpura

True purpura

I. Hemostatic defects
   A. Platelet abnormalities
      1. Quantitative
      2. Qualitative
   B. Coagulation abnormalities
II. Nonhemostatic defects
   A. Nonpalpable purpura
      1. Increased transmural pressure gradient
         a. Acute (e.g., Valsalva, coughing, vomiting, childbirth, weight lifting)
         b. Chronic—venous stasis
         c. High altitude
      2. Decreased mechanical integrity of microcirculation and supporting tissue
         a. Age-related—senile purpura
         b. Corticosteroid excess—Cushing syndrome, topical corticsoteroids
         c. Vitamin C deficiency—scurvy
         d. Abnormal connective tissue—Ehlers-Danlos syndrome
         e. Amyloid infiltration of blood vessels[a]
         f. Hormonal—female easy bruising syndrome (purpura simplex)
         g. MELAS syndrome
      3. Trauma to blood vessels
         a. Physical
            1) Injuries
            2) Child abuse
            3) Factitial purpura
         b. Ultraviolet radiation
            1) Purpuric sunburn
            2) Solar purpura
         c. Infectious
            1) Bacterial
            2) Rickettsial
            3) Fungal
            4) Viral
            5) Parasitic
         d. Embolic
            1) Infectious organisms[a]
            2) Atheroemboli (cholesterol crystal emboli)
            3) Fat emboli
            4) Calciphylaxis
         e. Allergic and/or inflammatory
            1) Serum sickness
            2) Contact dermatitis
            3) Pigmented purpuric eruptions

      f. Pyoderma gangrenosum
      g. Neoplastic[a]
      h. Drug-related
      i. Thrombotic
         1) Disseminated intravascular coagulation
         2) Coumarin necrosis
         3) Heparin necrosis
         4) Protein C or protein S deficiency
         5) Purpura fulminans
         6) Paroxysmal nocturnal hemoglobinuria[a]
         7) Antiphospholipid syndrome
      j. Drug-related
      4. Unknown cause—psychogenic purpura
   B. Palpable purpura
      1. Dysproteinemias
         a. Cryoglobulinemia
         b. Cryofibrinogenemia
         c. Hyperglobulinemic purpura of Waldenström
      2. Cutaneous vasculitis
         a. Systemic vasculitides[b]
         b. Paraneoplastic vasculitis
         c. Henoch-Schönlein purpura
         d. Acute hemorrhagic edema of infancy
      3. Primary cutaneous diseases

Nonpurpuric disorders simulating purpura

I. Disorders with telangiectasias
   A. Cherry angiomata
   B. Hereditary hemorrhagic telangiectasia
   C. CREST syndrome
   D. Chronic actinic telangiectasia
   E. Chronic liver disease
   F. Pregnancy-related
   G. Ataxia-telangiectasia
   H. Other
II. Kaposi sarcoma and other vascular sarcomas[c]
III. Fabry disease
IV. Neonatal extramedullary hematopoiesis
V. Angioma serpiginosum

Abbreviation: CREST, calcinosis, Raynaud (phenomenon), esophageal (dysfunction), sclerodactyly, telangiectasia.
[a] May also have a palpable purpuric component.
[b] May also have a nonpalpable purpuric component.
[c] May also have a purpuric component, either nonpalpable or palpable.

transmural pressure due to reduced extravascular pressure, rather than increased intravascular pressure.

Decreased Mechanical Integrity of Microcirculation and Supporting Tissue

Age-Related

Chronic solar damage and decreased collagen, elastin, and ground substance due to aging (senile purpura) may result in characteristic red to purple purpuric patches on the extensor surfaces of the forearms and hands (Plate 103-3). The skin accompanying solar purpura is thin and lacks elasticity, making it particularly susceptible to tears induced by shearing forces.[16] Owing to the decreased healing capacity that accompanies aging, the purpuric changes may take months to resolve. Interestingly, the syndromes of premature aging such as progeria, Werner syndrome, and acrogeria may all give rise to acral purpuric changes identical to those of senile purpura.[17]

Corticosteroid Excess

The patches of purpura in corticosteroid excess (Cushing syndrome, topical corticosteroid use) are classically described as appearing on the extensor surfaces of the forearms, but they may appear on both the flexor and extensor aspects of both the upper and lower extremities. As with senile purpura, the lesions have a very characteristic bright red appearance, and the skin is fragile.[8] Shear stress is often the immediate cause of the purpura, and the patches may last for weeks to months. The use of potent fluorinated topical corticosteroids, either alone or with occlusive dressings, may result in cutaneous atrophy and purpura. Microscopic examination shows a loss of dermal connective tissue with thinning of the epidermis.

Vitamin C Deficiency

Follicular keratosis and perifollicular purpura with entrapped corkscrew hairs are the characteristic findings of vitamin C deficiency (scurvy) (Plate 103-4). Larger ecchymoses on the legs and mucous membranes are seen in more severe cases and may be produced by mild or inapparent trauma. Petechial lesions and hemorrhagic gingivitis or stomatitis may also occur. Scurvy is therefore characterized by the 4H's: hemorrhagic signs, hyperkeratosis of the hair follicles, hypochondriasis (weakness and arthralgias), and hematologic abnormalities.[18]

Abnormal Connective Tissue

Easy bruising is one of the most prominent features of abnormal connective tissue (Ehlers-Danlos syndrome) types IV and V, but bruising may also be seen in the more common types I to III. Milder forms of Ehlers-Danlos syndrome that do not meet the diagnostic criteria for the more classic forms have recently been described, and mild to moderate bruising may be seen in these patients.[19] In evaluating patients for this heterogeneous group of connective tissue disorders, it is important to assess the elasticity of the skin, the extensibility of the joints, and the presence of associated abnormalities, such as high-arched palate and pectus excavatum.

Amyloid Infiltration of Blood Vessels

Cutaneous manifestations may be prominent in primary systemic amyloidosis associated with either mild plasmacytosis or multiple myeloma.[20] Histologic examination demonstrates extensive infiltration of blood vessel walls and/or dermis with amyloid; the vascular deposition is presumably responsible for the increased vascular fragility. As a result, minimal trauma can produce hemorrhagic lesions ("pinch purpura"), and petechiae occur readily when an increase in transmural pressure is present (e.g., after a Valsalva maneuver or after proctoscopy), especially when the amyloidosis involves the eyelids and face. Many different cutaneous lesions can occur, including brown to tan colored translucent papules, plaques, nodules, and bullae; all may become hemorrhagic, either spontaneously or with minimal trauma. An enlarged tongue with peripheral indentations secondary to pressure from the adjacent teeth (scalloped tongue) is also frequently seen in patients demonstrating cutaneous amyloid lesions, whereas alopecia and nail changes are less common manifestations.

Hormonal

The female predominance and the frequent association with phases of the menstrual cycle suggest that the female easy bruising syndrome (purpura simplex) is due to hormonal effects on the blood vessel and/or its surrounding tissues.[8] Concomitant use of nonsteroidal anti-inflammatory drugs may inhibit platelet function and contribute to the severity of the symptoms. Patients complain of frequent purpuric and ecchymotic lesions with minimal trauma. As discussed in the section on history taking, patients with this entity do not appear to be at increased risk of hemorrhage from more severe hemostatic challenges such as surgery.

MELAS Syndrome

Mitochondrial encephalomyopathy encompasses a group of disorders characterized by one or more enzymatic defects of aerobic metabolism leading to morphologic abnormalities of mitochondria in multiple organs. A 6-month-old boy with MELAS syndrome who demonstrated recurrent crops of purpuric macules on the palms and soles has been reported.[21]

Trauma to Blood Vessels
Physical

Any form of injury, if severe enough, can damage blood vessels sufficiently to cause skin hemorrhage. It is thus important to know in detail the extent of the injury before deciding

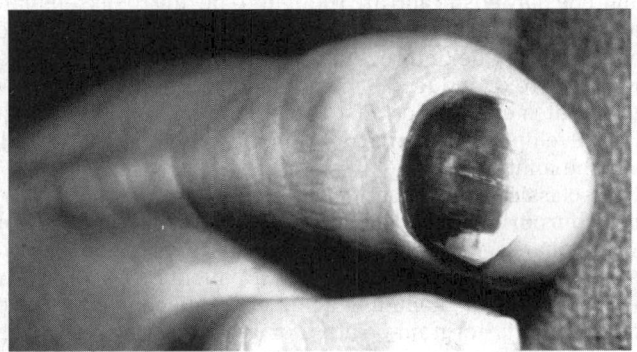

Fig. 103-2. 'Tennis toe' subungual hemorrhage.

whether the skin hemorrhage is consistent with the magnitude of the trauma.[11] Traumatic lesions usually have well-defined margins. Depending on the etiology (e.g., occupational, accidental, recreational), the pattern may be annular or circumferential (e.g., baseball injury), linear or loop shaped (e.g., child beating), or subungal (e.g., running shoe injury) (Fig. 103-2). The lesions associated with child abuse often include both cutaneous purpura and petechiae of the bulbar and palpebral conjunctivae, the latter reflecting strangulation or smothering, or both.[22,23] Patients with factitial, or self-inflicted, purpura usually have medium to large lesions on the lower extremities, but other sites may be involved as well. These patients characteristically express indifference to the bruises.

Ultraviolet Radiation

Acute severe sunburn can have a petechial component if the damage is severe enough. Patients have also been described in whom petechial eruptions developed on the legs and trunk after just brief exposures to natural sunlight. It is hypothesized that their skin is particularly sensitive to long-wave ultraviolet light.[24,25]

Infectious

Bacterial, viral, rickettsial, protozoal, and parasitic infections may all produce purpura as a primary clinical manifestation.[26,27] The pathogenesis of infectious purpura is often complex and may include direct vascular invasion by the organism, diffuse intravascular coagulation, immune complex vasculitis, septic emboli, and/or direct toxic effects on the vasculature. Although characteristic patterns of purpura have been described for the different agents, overlap between the patterns is quite common.

Gram-negative sepsis with *Pseudomonas* sp., *Klebsiella* sp., or *Escherichia coli* produces characteristic lesions of ecthyma gangrenosum, which begin as plaque-like areas of edema and erythema with subsequent nodule formation surmounted by irregular purpura (Plate 103-5). The central area of purpura is often bullous and is surrounded by concentric areas of normal skin and a thin band of erythema. Erosions and ulceration may occur. Lesions may be single or multiple, and the palms and soles are occasionally involved. The differential diagnosis of ecthyma gangrenosum includes fungal sepsis due to Candida species, drug eruptions, cryoglobulinemia, pyoderma gangrenosum, necrotizing vasculitis, polyarteritis nodosa, hyperviscosity syndrome, Sweet syndrome, and leukemic infiltrates.

Meningococcemia initially produces erythematous papules, but these soon evolve into stellate purple to slate-gray purpuric lesions (Plate 103-6). The combination of purulent meningitis and petechiae strongly suggests that *Neisseria meningitides* is the etiologic agent.[28] Acrocyanosis and symmetric peripheral gangrene may ensue and are thought to be due to disseminated intravascular coagulation (DIC). The purpura of meningococcemia may be due to direct vascular invasion by the organism or an endotoxin-induced Schwartzman reaction. In chronic intermittent meningococcemia an immune complex dermatitis may develop, characterized by hemorrhagic papulovesicles over the joints.

The classic rash of scarlet fever characteristically features linear purpuric lines in the skinfolds (Pastia's lines). Streptococcal pharyngitis has been reported to produce perioral, neck, and truncal petechiae in 2% of patients.

Bacterial sepsis, including acute and subacute bacterial endocarditis due to gram-positive or gram-negative organisms, may cause purpuric macules, papules, hemorrhagic bullae, erosions, and/or ulcers (Plate 103-7). The first manifestations of pneumococcal sepsis in asplenic patients may be facial petechiae and purpura, accompanied by acral cyanosis or livedo reticularis.[29,30] The full syndrome of purpura fulminans (see below) has been described following a variety of bacterial and viral infections. Although splinter hemorrhages of the nails occur in subacute bacterial endocarditis, they may also be seen in normal persons following trauma, or in patients with trichinosis, peptic ulceration, hypertension, malignancies, severe rheumatoid arthritis, and a number of dermatologic conditions; thus, the specificity of splinter hemorrhages as a sign of endocarditis is quite limited.[31,32]

Rickettsial infections, including Rocky Mountain spotted fever (Plate 103-8) and epidemic typhus, typically produce an array of cutaneous changes ranging from urticarial macules to petechiae, ecchymoses, and areas of hemorrhagic necrosis. Although the characteristic lesion of Lyme borreliosis is a nonpurpuric annular expanding plaque (erythema migrans), the central aspect of this lesion may contain a purpuric macule, papule, or a hemorrhagic bulla.

Patients with either disseminated fungal infections (e.g., cryptococcosis, zygomycosis, candidemia)[33] or locally invasive fungal diseases (e.g., mucormycosis) may have necrosis, purpura, and/or petechiae early in the course of the illness.[34]

Viral infections may have primary purpuric eruptions as their presenting manifestations. Recently, human parvovirus B19 infection has been described as demonstrating a petechial or confluent purpuric rash on the buttocks, axilla, and/or chest.[35]

Purpura may be the initial manifestation of parasitic infections, especially in the immunocompromised host. Migration of filariform larvae of *Strongyloides stercoralis* typically produces rapidly progressive abdominal thumbprint, linear and reticulated purpura on a background of petechiae; the periumbilical region is usually most severely affected.[36,37] Disseminated *Pneumocystis carinii* infections in patients with acquired immunodeficiency syndrome may demonstrate purpuric papules and nodules that resemble the lesions of Kaposi sarcoma (see below).[38]

Embolic

Atheroemboli with prominent cholesterol crystals, usually originating from atherosclerotic lesions in the aorta, produce a constellation of cutaneous findings, including acral petechiae and purpura, livedo reticularis, nodules, unilateral peripheral ulcers, and bilateral cyanosis and gangrene.[39] Distal pulses are present and occasionally the emboli can actually be seen in the retinal circulation as refractile interruptions in the column of arterial blood. The syndrome is seen most frequently in older men on anticoagulation or after vascular repair procedures. A high predilection for the pancreas makes elevations of serum amylase a common accompanying laboratory finding. The recent recognition that this syndrome is often undiagnosed argues in favor of a high index of suspicion, especially in older men with livedo reticularis.

Fat embolism may occur 2–3 days after severe trauma. The initial findings include upper extremity, thoracic, and/or conjunctival petechiae. The full syndrome consists of hyperthermia, respiratory distress, retinal fat emboli, neurologic symptoms, and pulmonary infiltrates.[40,41] Subcutaneous and vascular calcification in patients with chronic renal failure and secondary hyperparathyroidism (calciphylaxis) may result in cutaneous hemorrhagic necrosis in a vascular (livedoid) pattern.[42]

Allergic and/or Inflammatory

In serum sickness, morbilliform or urticarial eruptions are the most common cutaneous manifestations. Linear or serpiginous bands of erythema along the sides of the hands and feet may be seen at the margins of the palmar or plantar surfaces.[43] If the patients are thrombocytopenic, purpura usually appears within these linear bands. The eruption often heralds the onset of the syndrome. Immunologic evaluation of biopsy material often demonstrates immunoglobulin and complement deposits.

Allergic or irritant contact dermatitis to clothing, rubber, or detergent whiteners may result in purpuric eruptions that may simulate the pigmented purpuric eruptions.[44]

The pigmented purpuric eruptions,[45–48] including Schamberg disease and Majocchi disease, are a poorly understood group of disorders characterized by petechiae and purpura on a background of light to dark brown or orange hyperpigmentation (Plates 103-9 to 103-11); telangiectasias may or may not be present. Occasionally scaling, lichenification, and atrophy are seen. These eruptions characteristically involve the lower extremities, but they may also be seen on either the arms or trunk, or both; on occasion, they may even be found on the palms and soles.[49] They are not associated with any systemic manifestations. There is a great deal of clinical overlap between these disorders, and an individual patient may demonstrate features of more than one pigmented purpuric eruption. Histologically, extravasation of red blood cells, hemosiderin deposits within macrophages, and a perivascular lymphohistiocytic infiltrate with endothelial cell swelling are seen. The pathogenesis of these disorders is not established, but suggested mechanisms include increased capillary fragility with rupture of capillaries in the papillary dermis, aneurysmal dilation of the microvasculature, and abnormal cellular immune responses to an unknown antigen.[50] Cutaneous T-cell lymphoma can produce lesions simulating those found with the pigmented purpuric eruptions,[51] and the differential diagnosis of these disorders should include this possibility.

Pyoderma Gangrenosum

Pyoderma gangrenosum is a destructive, necrotizing ulceration of the skin presenting as a nodule, pustule, or hemorrhagic bulla. The lesions occur on the calves, thighs, buttocks and face. Pyoderma gangrenosum occurs in association with inflammatory bowel disease, rheumatoid arthritis, gammopathies, blood dyscrasias, leukemia, and lymphoma. A superficial hemorrhagic bullous form occurs with acute leukemia or other myeloproliferative disorders.

Neoplastic

Infiltration of the skin in the Langerhans cell histiocytosis group of disorders can result in the development of a papular and crusted dermatitis of the scalp and intertriginious areas (Plates 103-12 and 103-13). These lesions can have both petechial and purpuric features. As indicated above, cutaneous T-cell lymphoma may produce cutaneous lesions similar to those

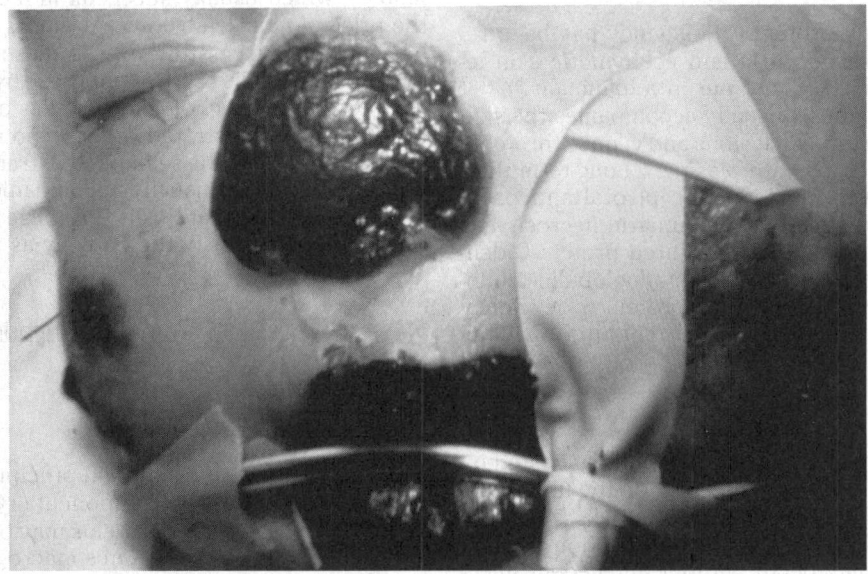

Fig. 103-3. Disseminated intravascular coagulation.

seen in the pigmented purpuric eruptions. Similarly, skin infiltrations in patients with leukemias, lymphomas, and plasma cell disorders can produce red to purple papules that may simulate purpura.[52]

Drug-Related

Petechial and purpuric reactions can be observed after administration of a variety of drugs, including aspirin, alclofenac, allopurinol, atropine, belladonna, bismuth, carbamazepine, carbimazol, carbromal, chloral hydrate, chlordiazepoxide, cimetidine, desipramine, disopyramide doxepin, fenbufen, gold salts, indomethacin, iodides, isoniazide, meclofenamate sodium, mefenamic acid, menthol, mercury, morphine, naproxen, nitrofurantoin, penicillamine, penicillin, phenacetin, phenytoin, piperazine, piroxicam, pyrazolon derivatives, quinine, quinidine, sulfonamides, sulindac, thiouracils, and tolmetin.[53] The mechanism for at least some of these reactions is presumed to be allergic hypersensitivity.

Thrombotic

DIC may result from a variety of different insults, many of which have the common denominator of producing hypotension (see Ch. 116). Since endothelial cells are active metabolically, hypotension can produce widespread ischemia and endothelial cell damage. This damage can expose subendothelial surfaces, which in turn can initiate an uncontrolled thrombotic response that ultimately selectively depletes coagulation factors and platelets. Alternative mechanisms for initiating the process involve the recently described effects of endotoxin and other mediators such as interleukin-1 and tumor necrosis factor on increasing endothelial cell (and monocyte) procoagulant activity. This is achieved, at least in part, by an induction of tissue factor expression, an increase in tissue plasminogen activator inhibitor synthesis, and a decrease in the production of thrombomodulin and tissue plasminogen activator.[54,55] Since there is a potential for both thrombotic and hemorrhagic manifestations, it is not surprising that the skin manifestations are diverse. The most common findings of diffuse intravascular coagulation are acral cyanosis (Plate 103-14) with variably associated petechial, purpuric, and ecchymotic lesions (Fig. 103-3). In the most severe cases, hemorrhagic gangrene of fingers and toes can occur.[26] The presence of peripheral gangrene may

be an important consideration in the often difficult decision as to whether heparin is indicated in controlling the syndrome.

Coumarin Necrosis

Coumarin necrosis affects 0.01–0.1% of all patients receiving coumarin and appears from the second to the fourteenth day (usually days 3–6) of coumarin therapy.[56] Patients who are deficient in protein C or perhaps protein S appear to be at high risk because they are most likely to suffer a temporary imbalance in the reduction of the procoagulant vitamin K factors and the anticoagulant vitamin K factors.[57–60] Coumarin necrosis begins suddenly as painful erythematous patches (Plate 103-15) that become edematous and rapidly progress to irregularly hemorrhagic and necrotic plaques, nodules, and bullae; eventually large tumid indurations and infarcts occur[61] with eschar formation and sloughing[62] (Plate 103-16). This syndrome appears to be more common in women than men and the lesions often develop in the skin overlying fatty areas, such as the buttocks, thighs, and breasts. Men can also be affected, and more acral lesions can occur, as witnessed by the reports of penile involvement.[56] Lesions may be symmetric and widely distributed; on occasion, they may be severe enough to require surgical intervention.[63] Histologically, fibrin and platelet thrombi are observed in the dermal and subcutaneous vasculature. The lesions of coumarin necrosis can be differentiated from hemorrhagic lesions due to excessive coumarin administration by the presence of the nearly black eschar in the center of the necrotic zone and by histologic examination. Ancillary differentiating points in favor of coumarin necrosis including the female sex predilection, the usually normal or near-normal prothrombin time, and the relationship to the onset of therapy.

Heparin Necrosis

Skin necrosis due to subcutaneous or intravenous heparin administration may occur rarely.[64,65] Cutaneous necrosis may occur 6–14 days following initiation of therapy either at the injection site or in a more widespread distribution, and represents a hypersensitivity reaction to heparin. The management of this disorder and its prevention are discussed in Chapter 120.

Protein C Deficiency

Congenital, homozygous protein C deficiency has been reported to produce diffuse purpuric and ecchymotic skin lesions suggestive of chronic DIC and purpura fulminans.[60,66,67] Widespread venous thrombosis usually accompanies the skin lesions. Fortunately, both the skin lesions and venous thrombosis respond rapidly to therapy with plasma.[68] Long-term therapy may require the careful introduction of oral anticoagulants.[69] Cutaneous necrosis similar to coumarin necrosis has also been reported in a patient with acquired protein C deficiency due to the development of an immunoglobulin inhibitor.[70] Several infants with homozygous protein S deficiency have also demonstrated neonatal and recurrent purpura fulminans.[71,72]

Purpura Fulminans

Purpura fulminans defines a syndrome of DIC manifested by massive widespread ecchymoses, especially on the upper and lower extremities, abdomen, thighs, and buttocks[66,67] (Plate 103-17). It may be triggered by any of the infectious agents discussed above[26,73] or may occur without antecedent infections. Homozygous protein C deficiency can produce essentially the same pattern in the neonate.[60,74] Clinically, the syndrome of purpura fulminans is most often characterized by symmetric hemorrhagic necrosis and bulla formation. The lesions enlarge with time and progress to gangrene, often with autoamputation of the digits. Associated symptoms and signs include prostration, fever, and edema of the extremities; death is not uncommon. Histopathology reveals hemorrhagic necrosis of the dermis with thromboses of the capillaries and small blood vessels. Fibrinoid necrosis of vessel walls and perivascular granulocytic infiltrates have been described.

Paroxysmal Nocturnal Hemoglobinuria

Occasional patients with paroxysmal nocturnal hemoglobinuria develop erythematous patches with dusky centers that may enlarge to form painful plaques of erythema with central necrosis.[75] Hemorrhagic bullae, ulcerations, petechiae, ecchymoses, palpable purpura, and eschar formation may also develop. Histologically, intravascular thrombi are seen in the absence of vasculitis.

Phospholipid Antibody Syndrome

Antiphospholipid syndrome is characterized by the variable presence of antibodies to phospholipid/protein complexes, including cardiolipin and those used in coagulation assays (lupus anticoagulant), in association with a tendency to thrombosis and fetal wastage, and/or thrombocytopenia. Antibodies to cardiolipin (or cardiolipin/protein complexes) are often present. Cutaneous manifestations are present in only a few patients, but they may include widespread cutaneous necrosis with thrombi within the microvasculature (similar to that seen in purpura fulminans), livedo reticularis, leg ulcers, and acral red to purple macules.[76]

Unknown Cause

Psychogenic Purpura

Psychogenic purpura (Gardner-Diamond syndrome) is the term given to a poorly understood disorder of severe, recurrent ecchymoses affecting women almost exclusively[77-79] (Plate 103-18). Patients usually experience pain before or at the time the bruise appears, and the bruising is often so extensive that the patient loses the use of the limb during the healing process. In the most severe cases, the patient can become bedridden. In desperation, physicians sometimes cast the affected limb(s), which usually succeeds in facilitating healing, but at the price of muscle atrophy. Attempts to identify the etiology have been unsuccessful. Early studies implicated allergic reactions to blood cells or DNA, but these hypotheses are no longer fully accepted. Psychological profiles of patients with this disorder have demonstrated widespread abnormalities,[78-80] raising the possibility of self-inflicted trauma, a view supported by the healing that usually accompanies casing. It is far from certain, however, that this is the cause in all cases, so it is best to continue to classify the etiology as unknown.

Palpable Purpura

Dysproteinemias

Cryoglobulinemia

Cryoglobulins represent cold-precipitable proteins found in plasma or serum. Single component cryoglobulins may be IgG, IgM, or IgA.[81] These cryoproteins may be idiopathic in origin or may occur with Waldenström's macroglobulinemia, myeloma, lymphoma, or monoclonal gammopathies of unknown significance. Mixed cryoglobulins usually involve rheumatoid factor-like activity and are usually a complex of IgG with IgM molecules having anti-IgG reactivity; less frequently, IgG or IgA antibodies may have anti-IgG activity. Mixed cryoglobulins may be seen as an idiopathic phenomenon or in association with a wide variety of subacute and chronic disorders. Clinical lesions of cryoglobulinemia include the intermittent appearance of acral hemorrhagic necrosis (Fig. 103-4), macular and palpable purpura, livedo reticularis, subungual hemorrhage (Plate 103-19), urticaria, leg ulcerations, Raynaud phenomenon, hemorrhagic pustular folliculitis, and erythema multiforme-like lesions.[82-84] Weakness and arthralgias are prominent noncutaneous symptoms.

Cryofibrinogenemia

Cryofibrinogenemia indicates the presence in the blood of an abnormal cold precipitable protein indistinguishable from fibrinogen or fibrin. Cutaneous manifestations include sensitivity to cold, purpura, livedo reticularis, cyanosis, ulcerations, erythema, hematoma, urticaria, gangrene, acral blisters, and Raynaud phenomenon.[85] Essential (primary) cryofibrinogenemia occurs in association with DIC. Secondary cryofibrinogenemia may occur with neoplastic, thromboembolic, or infectious disorders.

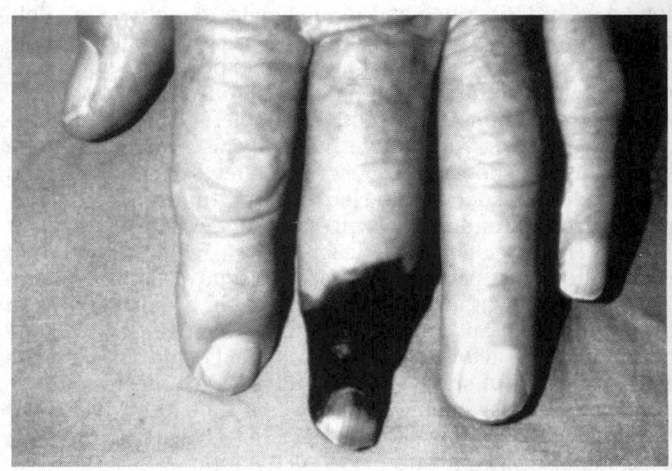

Fig. 103-4. Cryoglobulins.

Hyperglobulinemic Purpura of Waldenström

Macular and papular, discrete or confluent purpuric lesions with hemosiderin staining are the classic cutaneous findings of benign hyperglobulinemic purpura (Plate 103-20), a syndrome that most often occurs on the legs of women aged 20–40 years.[47] Precipitating factors include increased hydrostatic pressure, hyperviscosity, and low temperatures.[86–88] The polyclonal increase in globulins (mostly IgG) can be associated with Sjögren syndrome, systemic lupus erythematosus, polymyositis, rheumatoid arthritis, myeloma, thymoma, sarcoid, or multiple sclerosis. Lesions may be recurrent and the eruption must be differentiated from the pigmented purpuric eruptions. Histologically, acute inflammatory cells, red blood cells, and arteriolar necrosis predominate. Circulating complexes containing IgG anti-IgG or IgA anti-IgG, or both, have been detected.[82]

Cutaneous Vasculitis

Systemic Vasculitides

Patients with collagen vascular diseases, as well as those with systemic large and small vessel vasculitis (including hypocomplementemic vasculitis, polyarteritis nodosa, Wegener's granulomatosis, Churg-Strauss angiitis, rheumatoid vasculitis, or relapsing polychondritis), may have an array of vasculitic purpuric lesions, including petechiae, papules, ecchymoses, hemorrhagic bullae, splinter hemorrhages, and periungual hemorrhages[82,89–92] (Plates 103-21 and 103-22). Nonpurpuric cutaneous lesions may also be present, including ulcers, subcutaneous nodules, livedo reticularis, erythema, erythematous plaques, and telangiectasias.

Paraneoplastic Vasculitis

Paraneoplastic vasculitis is a syndrome of petechiae, palpable purpura, urticaria, maculopapular lesions, leg ulcers, and/or erythema multiforme seen in association with hairy cell leukemia and other lympho- and myeloproliferative disorders.[93–95] Intense pruritus or dysesthesias are prominent symptoms. In some cases, the cutaneous lesions may precede the diagnosis of the malignancy or signal the recurrence of the malignancy. Carcinomas of the breast, lung, colon, cervix, prostate, and kidney have all been reported in association with cutaneous vasculitis.[95,96]

Henoch-Schönlein Purpura

Henoch-Schönlein purpura is a leukocytoclastic vasculitis that usually affects children.[97–99] Palpable purpuric lesions, abdominal pain, and arthritis of the knees and ankles are common findings, but other organs may be involved as well. Acute and chronic renal disease is an important associated finding. There is no sex predilection, but there is a seasonal increase during the winter months. Several precipitating factors have been implicated, including infections, environmental chemicals, toxins, insect bites, physical trauma, complement component C2 deficiency, and malignancies. Clinical presentations include the explosive onset over the legs and buttocks of urticarial papules and plaques, with or without purpura (Plate 103-23), palpable purpura, or hemorrhagic bullae; larger stellate, reticulate and necrotic lesions may also occur (Plate 103-24). Occasionally, ecchymotic lesions resembling child abuse may be present, but unlike the latter, the lesions of Henoch-Schönlein purpura are usually strikingly symmetric. Henoch-Schönlein purpura is thought to be an immune complex disease, with 50% of patients producing IgA rheumatoid factor.[99] IgA containing immune complexes have been detected, especially during the early phases of the syndrome.[100–102]

A recent study reported that 10% of adults with leukocytoclastic vasculitis demonstrate livedoid superficial plaques, with multifocal areas of hemorrhage or necrosis, and reticulate margins connecting adjacent lesions.[103] These lesions contain IgA and C3 deposits in the blood vessel walls. Smooth margined purpuric papules with uniform hemorrhage also showed IgA, but more frequently demonstrated IgG or IgM vascular deposits.

Acute Hemorrhagic Edema of Infancy

Children aged 4 months to 2 years are most likely to acquire this syndrome, which is characterized by fever, tender iris-like or medallion-like large purpuric cutaneous lesions, and edema.[104–106] The lesions occur on the cheeks, eyelids, ears, extremities, and genitalia and must be differentiated from the cutaneous findings of child abuse, Sweet syndrome, Kawasaki disease, and hemorrhagic erythema multiforme.

Primary Cutaneous Diseases

Insect bites (especially blackfly bites), dermatitis herpetiformis, pityriasis rosea, and other primary cutaneous disorders may present with purpuric papules and vesicles mimicking septic and vasculitic lesions. Several patients have been described with symmetrical edema and erythema of the hands, feet, inner thighs, and buttocks, that progressed to petechiae and purpura (papular-purpuric "gloves and socks" syndrome).[107] Recently, parvovirus B19 infection has been documented in a patient with this disorder.

Nonpurpuric Disorders Simulating Purpura

Disorders with Telangiectasias

Cherry Angiomas

Cherry angiomas are the common papular, brightly erythematous lesions seen on the trunk and extremities of middle-aged and older men and women. The lesions are progressive with age and may produce easy bruising, as they tend to bleed excessively with trauma. Pinpoint or smaller cherry angiomas may be present in large numbers and may mimic a petechial eruption. Differentiating this very common disorder from hereditary hemorrhagic telangiectasias may be difficult, and these lesions may, in fact, be part of the continuum of that disorder.

Hereditary Hemorrhagic Telangiectasia

Hereditary hemorrhagic telangiectasia is an autosomal dominant disorder with an estimated frequency of 1 in 50,000, manifested by widespread dermal, mucosal, and visceral telangiectasias. Clinically, venous lakes and papular, punctate, mat-like, and linear telangiectasias appear on all areas of the skin and mucous membranes, with a predominance of lesions under the tongue and on the face, lips (Plate 103-25), perioral region, tongue, nasal mucosa, fingertips, toes, and trunk.[108] Epistaxis is a nearly universal finding in this disorder, with symptoms almost always becoming worse with age. The severity of the disorder can often be gauged by the age at which the nosebleeds begin, with the most severely affected patients developing recurrent epistaxis during childhood. Cutaneous changes usually begin at puberty and progress throughout life. Bleeding can occur in virtually every organ, with gastrointestinal, oral, and urogenital sites most common. Hepatic and splenic arteriovenous fistulas, as well as intracranial, aortic, and splenic aneurysms may occur; pulmonary arteriovenous fistulae have been reported to cause oxygen desaturation. The vessels of hereditary hemorrhagic telangiectasia show a discontinuous endothelium and inadequate smooth muscle. The surrounding stroma lacks elastin. Thus, the bleeding tendencies are attributed to mechanical fragility of the abnormal vessels. The gene responsible for hereditary hemorrhagic telangiectasias has recently been localized to chromosome 9 in several families.[108a,108b]

Chronic Actinic Telangiectasias, Chronic Liver Disease, Pregnancy

Telangiectasias from chronic actinic damage (Plate 103-26), and telangiectatic mats seen in scleroderma (CREST syndrome) (Plate 103-27) may be easily confused with the lesions of hereditary hemorrhagic telangiectasia. Angiokeratoma corporis diffusum, ataxia telangiectasia, and spider telangiectasias from chronic liver disease must also be differentiated. Spider telangiectases have a central, prominent, easily blanchable feeding vessel with several smaller telangiectasias emanating from this central vessel. Spider telangiectasias seen in patients with chronic liver disease are distributed from the head to the nipple line, and correlate with the risk of bleeding from esophageal varices.[109]

Vascular changes in pregnancy, as in chronic liver disease, have been attributed to an increase in circulating estrogens. Two-thirds of white women and one-tenth of black women develop spider angiomas by the third trimester of pregnancy. These are found on the chest and upper arms; they resolve spontaneously after delivery. Unilateral nevoid telangiectasias also may develop during pregnancy, resolving postpartum.

Ataxia-Telangiectasia

Ataxia-telangiectasia (Louis-Bar syndrome) is an autosomal recessive disorder characterized by the appearance of telangiectasias at 3–5 years of age that first develop on the bulbar conjunctivae, then involve the central face, ears, eyelids, and extensor aspects of the forearms. The full syndrome is characterized by progressive cerebellar ataxia beginning during the second year of life, recurrent sinopulmonary infections, and associated abnormalities of humoral and cellular immunity.

Kaposi Sarcoma and Other Vascular Sarcomas

The epidemic form of Kaposi sarcoma found among patients infected with the human immunodeficiency virus is easily confused with purpuric (Plate 103-28) and ecchymotic (Plate 103-29) lesions, as well as some of the pigmented purpuric eruptions[110] (Plate 103-30). Oral lesions of epidemic Kaposi sarcoma may also mimic petechiae and purpura (Plate 103-31). Similarly, angiosarcoma may present as a purple to brown plaque resembling purpura (Plate 103-32).

Fabry Disease

Fabry disease (angiokeratoma corporis diffusum) is an X-linked inherited disorder of glycolipid metabolism with deficiency of the enzyme ceramide trihexosidase.[111] Accumulation of glycolipid throughout the body leads to cutaneous, renal, ophthalmologic, cardiac, and central nervous system manifestations. Angiokeratoma corporis diffusum lesions are pinpoint to 4-mm deep red, blue, or black macules or papules (Plate 103-33). These nonblanchable lesions are distributed over the trunk, extremities, and genitalia. In mild cases, lesions are localized to the thighs, scrotum, or periumbilical region. Grouping of lesions may occur. Superficial corneal dystrophy and varicosities of the bulbar conjunctivum are commonly seen (Plate 103-34).

Neonatal Extramedullary Hematopoiesis

Infants with congenital toxoplasmosis, rubella, or cytomegalovirus infections may have these dark red, blue, or blue-gray macules and/or papules at birth or within the first 48 hours of life.[112] The lesions are most commonly found on the scalp, neck, and trunk but may be widely distributed. These lesions fade into tan or copper-colored macules by 8 weeks of age.

Angioma Serpiginosum

Angioma serpiginosum is a vascular nevoid lesion showing pinpoint vascular ectasias on a background of erythema.[8] The lesion is partially blanchable and is not petechial. Capillary microscopy demonstrates punctate dilated capillaries. This lesion is usually seen on the legs and buttocks of women, but it may occur anywhere and may expand in childhood and regress with age.

REFERENCES

1. Miller CH, Graham JB, Goldin LR, Elston RC: Genetics of classic von Willebrand's disease. II. Optimal assignment of the heterozygous genotype (diagnosis) by discriminant analysis. Blood 54:137, 1979
2. Wahlberg T, Blomback M, Hall P, Axelsson G: Applications of indicators, predictors and diagnostic indices in coagulation disorders. I. Evaluation of a self-administered questionnaire with binary questions. Methods Inf Med 19:194, 1980
3. Rodeghiero F, Castaman G, Dini E: Epidemiologic investigation of the prevalence of vWd. Blood 69:454, 1987
4. Wahlberg T: Carriers and noncarriers of haemophilia A. II. Evaluation of bleeding symptoms registered by a self-administered questionnaire with binary (no/yes) questions. Thromb Res 25:415, 1982
5. Hultin MB, Sussman II: Postoperative thrombocytopenia in type IIB von Willebrand disease. Am J Hematol 33:64, 1990
6. Rick ME, Williams SB, Sacher RA, McKeown LP: Thrombocytopenia associated with pregnancy in a patient with type IIB von Willebrand's disease. blood 69:786, 1987
7. Rohrer MJ, Michelotti MC, Nahrwold DL: A prospective evaluation of the efficacy of preoperative coagulation testing. Ann Surg 208:554, 1988
8. Champion RH: Purpura. p. 1109. In Rook A, Wilkinson DS, Ebling FJG et al (eds): Textbook of Dermatology. Vol. 2. 4th Ed. Blackwell Scientific. Oxford, 1986
9. Crosby WH: Purpura. p. 1. In Demis DJ (ed): Clinical Dermatology. 15th Rev. JB Lippincott, Philadelphia, 1988
10. Edwards RL, Rickles FR: Delayed hypersensitivity in man: effects of systemic anticoagulation. Science 200:541, 1978
11. Rasmussen JE: Puzzling purpuras in children and young adults. J Am Acad Dermatol 6:67, 1982
12. Schachner LA, Hansen RC: Pediatric Dermatology. Churchill Livingstone, New York, 1988, p. 904
13. Metzker A, Merlob P: Suction purpura. Arch Dermatol 128:822, 1992
14. Fisher AA: Purpuric contact dermatitis. Cutis 33:346, 1984
15. Mitchell RE: Chronic solar dermatosis: a light and electron microscopic study of the dermis. J Invest Dermatol 48:203, 1967
16. Beauregard S, Gilchrest BA: Syndromes of premature aging. Dermatol Clin 5:109, 1987
17. Forster PJG: Microvascular fragility at high altitude. Br Med J 296:1004, 1988
18. Wirth PB, Kalb RE: Scurvy. Arch Dermatol 126:385, 1990
19. Holzberg M, Hewan-Lowe KO, Olansky AJ: The Ehlers-Danlos syndrome: recognition, characterization, and importance of a milder variant of the classic form. J Am Acad Dermatol 19:656, 1988
20. Kyle RA: Amyloidosis: review of 236 cases. Medicine 54:271, 1975
21. Horiguchi Y, Fujii T, Imamura S: Purpuric manifestations in mitochondrial encephalomyopathy. J Dermatol 18:295, 1991
22. Ellerse NS: The cutaneous manifestations of child abuse and neglect. Am J Dis Child 133:906, 1979
23. American Medical Association Report of the Council on Scientific Affairs: AMA Diagnostic and Treatment Guidelines Concerning Child Abuse and Neglect. JAMA 254:796, 1985
24. Leung AKC: Purpura associated with exposure to sunlight. J R Soc Med 79: 423, 1986
25. Kalivas L, Kalivas J: Solar purpura. Arch Dermatol 124:24, 1988
26. Kingston ME, Mackey D: Skin clues in the diagnosis of life threatening infections. Rev Infect Dis 8:1, 1986
27. Musher DM: Cutaneous manifestations of bacterial sepsis. Hosp Pract 24: 71, 1989
28. Mancebo J, Domingo P, Blanch L et al: The predictive value of petechiae in adults with bacterial meningitis, letter to editor. JAMA 256:2820, 1986
29. Vanwyck DB: Overwhelming postsplenectomy infection: the clinical syndrome. Lymphology 16:107, 1983
30. Rusonis PA, Robinson HN, Lamberg SI: Livedo reticularis and purpura: presenting features in fulminant pneumococcal septicemia in an asplenic patient. J Am Acad Dermatol 15:1120, 1986

31. Fanning WL, Aronson M: Osler's nodes, Janeway lesions, and splinter hemorrhages. Arch Dermatol 113:648, 1977
32. Braverman IM: Skin Signs of Systemic Disease. 2nd Ed. WB Saunders, Philadelphia, 1981, p. 849
33. Grossman ME, Silvers DN, Walther RR: Cutaneous manifestations of disseminated candidiasis. J Am Acad Dermatol 2:111, 1980
34. Radentz WH: Opportunistic fungal infections in immunocompromised hosts. J Am Acad Dermatol 20:989, 1989
35. Shiraishi H, Umetsu K, Yamamoto H et al: Human parvovirus (HPV/B19) infection with purpura. Microbiol Immunol 33:369, 1989
36. Von Kuster LC, Genta RM: Cutaneous manifestations of strongyloidiasis. Arch Dermatol 124:656, 1988
37. Kalb RE, Grossman ME: Periumbilical purpura in disseminated strongyloidiasis. JAMA 256:1170, 1986
38. Litwin MA, Williams CM: Cutaneous *Pneumocystis carinii* infection mimicking Kaposi sarcoma. Ann Int Med 117:48, 1992
39. Falanga V, Fine MJ, Kapoor WN: The cutaneous manifestations of cholesterol crystal embolization. Arch Dermatol 122:1194, 1986
40. Miller JD: Fat embolism: a clinical diagnosis. Am Family Pract 35:130, 1987
41. Oh WH, Mital MA: Fat embolism: current concepts of pathogenesis, diagnosis, and treatment. Orthop Clin North Am 9:769, 1978
42. Khafif RA, DeLima C, Silverberg A, Frankel R: Calciphylaxis and systemic calcinosis, collective review. Arch Int Med 150:956, 1990
43. Bielory C, Yancey KB, Young NS et al: Cutaneous manifestations of serum sickness in patients receiving antithymocyte globulin. J Am Acad Dermatol 13:411, 1985
44. Calnan CD, Peachey RDG: Allergic contact purpura. Clin Allergy 1:287, 1971
45. Sherertz EF: Pigmented purpuric eruptions. Semin Thromb Hemost 10:190, 1984
46. Randall SJ, Kierland RR, Montgomery H: Pigmented purpuric eruptions. Arch Dermatol 64:177, 1951
47. Newton RC, Raimer SS: Pigmented purpuric eruptions. Dermatol Clin 3:165, 1985
48. Ferriero JE, Pasan G, Queseda R, Gould E: Benign hypergammaglobulinemic purpura of Waldenström associated with Sjögren's syndrome. Case report and review of immunologic aspects. Am J Med 81:734, 1986
49. Geary RC Jr, Marks VJ: Idiopathic pigmented purpuric eruption with palmarplantar involvement. Cutis 40:109, 1987
50. Aiba S, Tagami H: Immunohistologic studies in Schamberg's disease: evidence for cellular immune reaction in lesional skin. Arch Dermatol 124:1058, 1988
51. Barnhill RL, Braverman IM: Progression of pigmented purpura-like eruptions to mycosis fungoides: report of three cases. J Am Acad Dermatol 19:25, 1988
52. Dreizen S, McCredie KB, Keating MJ et al: Leukemia-associated skin infiltrates. Postgrad Med 85:45, 1989
53. Bruinsma W: A Guide to Drug Eruptions. 5th Ed. The Free University, Brussels, The Netherlands, 1990, p 40
54. Bevilacquca MP, Gimbrone MA Jr: Inducible endothelial functions in inflammation and coagulation. Semin Thromb Hemost 13:425, 1987
55. Girardin E, Grau GE, Dayer J-M et al: Tumor necrosis factor and interleukin-1 in the serum of children with severe infectious purpura. N Engl J Med 319:397, 1988
56. Renicu AM: Anticoagulant-induced necrosis of skin and subcutaneous tissues: report of two cases and review of the English literature. South Med J 69:775, 1976
57. Broekmans AW, Bertina RM, Loeliger EA et al: Protein C and the development of skin necrosis during anticoagulant therapy, letter to editor. Thromb Haemost 49:251, 1983
58. Goldberg SL, Orthner CL, Yalisove BL et al: Skin necrosis following prolonged administration of coumarin in a patient with inherited protein S deficiency. Am J Hematol 38:64, 1991
59. Kazmier FJ: Thromboembolism, coumarin necrosis, and protein C. Mayo Clin Proc 60:673, 1985
60. Gladson CL, Groncy P, Griffin JH: Coumarin necrosis, neonatal purpura fulminans, and protein C deficiency. Arch Dermatol 123:1701, 1987
61. Stone MS, Rosen T: Acral purpura: an unusual sign of coumarin necrosis. J Am Acad Dermatol 14:797, 1986
62. Horn JR, Danziger LH, Davis RJ: Warfarin-induced skin necrosis: report of four cases. Am J Hosp Pharm 38:1763, 1981
63. Cole MS, Minifee PK, Wolma FJ: Coumarin necrosis—a review of the literature. Surgery 103:271, 1988
64. White PW, Sadd JR, Neusel RE: Thrombotic complications of heparin therapy including six cases of heparin-induced skin necrosis. Ann Surg 190:595, 1978
65. Rongioletti F, Pisan S, Ciaccio AP et al: Skin necrosis due to intravenous heparin. Dermatologia 178:47, 1989
66. Auletta MJ, Headington JT: Purpura fulminans: a cutaneous manifestation of severe protein C deficiency. Arch Dermatol 124:1387, 1988
67. Spicer TE, Rau JM: Purpura fulminans. Am J Med 61:566, 1976
68. Branson H, Katz J, Marble R, Griffin JH: Inherited protein C deficiency and coumarin-responsive chronic relapsing purpura fulminans syndrome in a neonate. Lancet 2:1165, 1983
69. Sills RH, Marlar RA, Montgomery RR et al: Severe homozygous protein C deficiency. J Pediatr 105:409, 1984
70. Gruber A, Blasko G, Sas G: Functional deficiency of protein C and skin necrosis in multiple myeloma. Thromb Res 42:579, 1986
71. Pegelow CH, Ledford M, Young JN: Severe protein S deficiency in a newborn. Pediatrics 89:674, 1992
72. Mahasandana C, Suvatte V, Chuansumrit A et al: Homozygous protein S deficiency in an infant with purpura fulminans. J Pediatr 117:750, 1990
73. Hautekeete ML, Berneman ZN, Bieger R et al: Purpura fulminans in pneumococcal sepsis. Arch Intern Med 146:497, 1986
74. Griffin JH, Evatt B, Zimmerman TS et al: Deficiency of protein C in congenital thrombotic disease. J Clin Invest 68:1370, 1981
75. Rietschel RL, Lewis CW, Simmons RA, Phyliky RL: Skin lesions in paroxysmal nocturnal hemoglobinuria. Arch Dermatol 114:560, 1978
76. Grob JJ, Bonerand JJ: Thrombotic skin disease as a marker of the anticardiolipin syndrome. J Am Acad Dermatol 20:1063, 1989
77. Gardner FH, Diamond LK: Autoerythrocyte sensitization: a form of purpura producing painful bruising following autosensitization to red blood cells in certain women. Blood 10:675, 1955
78. Ratnoff OD, Agle DP: Psychogenic purpura: a re-evaluation of the syndrome of autoerythrocyte sensitization. Medicine 47:475, 1968
79. Gottlieb AJ: Autoerythrocyte and DNA sensitivity. p. 1369. In Williams JW, Beutler E, Erslev AJ, Lichtman MA (eds): Hematology. McGraw-Hill, New York, 1983
80. McDuffie FC, McGuire FL: Clinical and psychological patterns in autoerythrocyte sensitivity. Ann Intern Med 63:255, 1965.
81. Winfield JB: Cryoglubulinema. Hum Pathol 14:350, 1983
82. Cream JJ: Vasculitis. Curr Probl Dermatol 3:65, 1989
83. Brouet J-C, Clauvel J-P, Danon F et al: Biological and clinical significance of cryoglobulins: a report of 86 cases. Am J Med 57:775, 1974
84. Gorevic PD, Kassab HJ, Levo Y et al: Mixed cryoglublinemia: clinical aspects and long term follow-up of 40 patients. Am J Med 69:287, 1980
85. Bair J-S, Wu Y-C, Lu Y-C: Cryofibrinogenemia: report of a case. J Formoson Med Assoc 90:99, 1991
86. Waldenström J: Clinical methods for determination of hyperproteinemia and their practical value for diagnosis. Nord Med 20:2288, 1943
87. Strauss WG: Purpura hyperglobulinemia of Waldenström. Report of a case and review of the literature. N Engl J Med 260:857, 1959
88. Kyle RA, Gleich GJ, Bayrd ED: Benign hypergammaglobulinemic purpura of Waldenström. Medicine 50:113, 1971
89. Fauci AS, Haynes BF, Katz P: The spectrum of vasculitis. Clinical, pathologic, immunologic, and therapeutic considerations. Ann Intern Med 89:660, 1978
90. Sams WM Jr, Thorne EG, Shore P et al: Leukocytoclastic vasculitis. Arch Dermatol 112:219, 1976
91. Sams WM Jr: Necrotizing vasculitis. J Am Acad Dermatol 3:1, 1980
92. Fauci AS: Vasculitis. J Allergy Clin Immunol 72:211, 1983
93. Cupps TR, Fauci AS: Vasculitis and neoplasm. Major Probl Intern Med 21:116, 1981
94. Longley S, Caldwell JR, Panush RS: Paraneoplastic vasculitis. Unique syndrome of cutaneous angiitis and arthritis associated with myeloproliferative disorders. Am J Med 80:1027, 1986
95. Greer JM, Longley S, Edwards NL et al: Vasculitis associated with malignancy. Experience with 13 patients and literature review. Medicine 67:220, 1988
96. Callen JP: Cutaneous leukocytoclastic vasculitis in a patient with an adenocarcinoma of the colon. J Rheumatol 14:386, 1987
97. Meadow R: Schönlein-Henoch syndrome. Arch Dis Child 54:822, 1979
98. Allen DM, Diamond LK, Howell DA: Anaphylactoid purpura in children (Schönlein-Henoch syndrome). Am J Dis Child 99:833, 1960
99. Macke SE, Jordon RE: Leukocytoclastic vasculitis. A cutaneous expression of immune complex disease. Arch Dermatol 118:296, 1982
100. Saulsbury FT: IgA rheumatoid factor in Henoch-Schönlein purpura. J Pediatr 108:71, 1986
101. Levinsky RJ, Barrett TM: IgA immune complexes in Henoch-Schönlein purpura. Lancet 2:1100, 1979
102. Kawana S, Ohta M, Nishiyama S: Value of the assay for IgA-containing circulating immune compress in Henoch-Schönlein purpura. Dermatologica 172:245, 1986
103. Piette WW, Stone MS: A cutaneous sign of IgA-associated small dermal vessel leukocytoclastic vasculitis in adults (Henoch-Schönlein purpura). Arch Dermatol 125:53, 1989

104. Saraclar Y, Tinaztepe K, Adalioglu G: Acute hemorrhagic edema of infancy (AHEI)—a variant of Henoch-Schönlein purpura or a distinct entity? J All Clin Immunol 86:473, 1990

105. Dubin BA, Bronson JM, Eng AM: Acute hemorrhagic edema of childhood. An unusual variant of leukocytoclastic vasculitis. J Am Acad Dermatol 23: 347, 1990

106. Legrain V, Lejean S, Taieb A et al: Infantile acute hemorrhagic edema of the skin: study of ten cases. J Am Acad Dermatol 24:17, 1991

107. Harma M, Feldmann R, Saurat JH: Papular-purpuric "gloves and socks" syndrome. J Am Acad Dermatol 252:341, 1991

108. Peery WH: Clinical spectrum of hereditary hemorrhagic telangiectasia (Osler-Weber-Rendu disease). Am J Med 82:989, 1987

108a. McDonald MT, Papenberg KA, Ghosh S: A disease locus for hereditary hemorrhagic telangiectasia maps to chromosome 9 of 33–34. Nature Genet 6:197, 1994

108b. Shovlin CL, Hughes JMB, Tuddenham EGD: A gene for hereditary haemorrhagic telangiectasia maps to chromosome 9q3. Nature Genet 6:205, 1994

109. Foutch PG, Sullivan JA, Gaines JA, Sanowski RA: Cutaneous vascular spiders in cirrhotic patients: correlation with hemorrhage from esophageal varices. Am J Gastroenterol 83:723, 1988

110. Fauci AS, Macher AM, Longo DL et al: Acquired immunodeficiency syndrome: epidemiologic, clinical, immunologic, and therapeutic considerations. Ann Intern Med 100:92, 1984

111. Desnick RJ, Sweeley CC: Fabry's disease: alpha-galactosidase A deficiency. p. 906. In Stanbury JB, Wyngaarden JB, Fredrickson DS (eds): The Metabolic Basis of Inherited Disease. 5th Ed. McGraw-Hill, New York, 1983

112. Fine JD, Arndt KA: Torch syndrome. p. 1. In Demis DJ (ed): Clinical Dermatology. 15th Rev. JB Lippincott, Philadelphia, 1988

Laboratory Evaluation of Hemostatic Disorders

104

Samuel A. Santoro and Charles S. Eby

INTRODUCTION

Once the presence of a bleeding disorder has been established or a high level of suspicion is generated by either the history or physical examination, or both (see Ch. 103), laboratory tests are employed to establish the diagnosis. Familiarity with, and rational application of, a few laboratory procedures will enable one to place the defect in one of several broad categories. More specialized tests are subsequently employed to establish a definitive diagnosis.

For diagnostic purposes, the hemostatic system may be somewhat simplistically divided into two parts: the plasma coagulation factors, and platelets. An abnormality in either portion may give rise to a bleeding disorder. Although the history and physical examination may provide clues as to which portion of the hemostatic system is defective, the information is not definitive. Therefore, when faced with a bleeding disorder, the first task is to establish whether the disorder is due to either impairment of the reactions leading to thrombin generation and fibrin clot formation or to inadequate numbers or function of platelets. This is accomplished by performing a prothrombin time (PT), an activated partial thromboplastin time (PTT), a platelet count, and a bleeding time.

SCREENING TESTS OF PLASMA COAGULATION FACTORS

The PT and PTT are employed to assess the function of the plasma coagulation factors, with the notable exception of factor XIII. For diagnostic purposes, it is useful to divide the plasma coagulation reactions into the extrinsic, intrinsic, and common pathways, although recent data from several laboratories have indicated the existence of several interconnections between these pathways. These pathways are diagrammed schematically in Figure 104-1. (See Ch. 100 for a detailed discussion of each of these factors and reactions.) The extrinsic system includes the reactions of tissue factor and factor VII that lead to the conversion of factor X to factor Xa. The intrinsic system is composed of factors VIII, IX, XI, and XII, prekallikrein, and high-molecular-weight kininogen. The common pathway includes factors V and X, prothrombin, fibrinogen, and factor XIII.

Prothrombin Time

A PT is performed by addition of a crude preparation of tissue factor (commonly an extract of brain) to citrate-anticoagulated plasma, recalcification of the plasma, and measurement of the clotting time.[1] It is standard practice to add both thromboplastin (tissue factor preparation) and Ca^{2+} in a single step. It should be apparent from Figure 104-1 that abnormalities of factors VII, V, and X, prothrombin, or fibrinogen may result in prolongation of the PT. The test may be prolonged due to either a deficiency of one or more of the involved factors or to the presence of an inhibitor. The PT is also the most frequently used method to monitor the anticoagulant effect of warfarin, which causes a decrease in the activity of vitamin K-dependent factors VII, IX, and X and prothrombin. Warfarin dosage is typically adjusted to achieve a desired patient/mean normal PT ratio expressed as the International Normalized Ratio (INR) (see Ch. 120).

Commercially available thromboplastins vary in the animal source and method of preparation, resulting in differing sensitivities to factor deficiencies.[2] Although differences in instrumentation, methodology, and control plasmas also contribute to inter- and intralaboratory variability, the lack of a standard thromboplastin is thought to be the most important factor.[3] The World Health Organization has established a reference thromboplastin derived from human brain that has been used

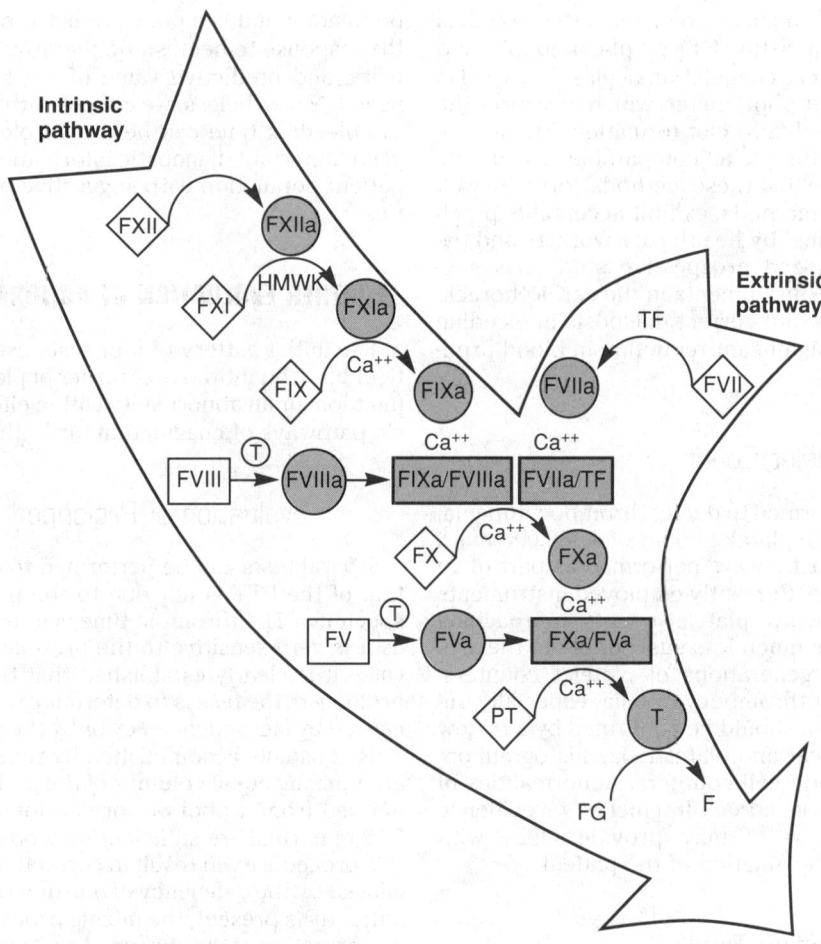

Fig. 104-1. Reactions of coagulation. HMWK, high-molecular-weight kinogen; TF, tissue factor; T, thrombin; PT, prothrombin; FG, fibrinogen; F, fibrin clot (not cross-linked).

to calibrate secondary standards, available to manufacturers and laboratories for the evaluation of thromboplastin reagents.[2] The sensitivity of a thromboplastin is described by the International Sensitivity Index (ISI). Most commercial thromboplastins are less sensitive to factor deficiencies than to the reference standard (ISI = 1.0) and have ISIs of 1.2–2.8.[4]

Some authorities and panels have advocated routine reporting of PTs, especially for anticoagulant monitoring, as an INR.[5,6] The INR converts the PT patient/PT mean normal ratio to the value expected if the test had been performed with the reference thromboplastin and is given by INR = (PT patient/PT mean normal)^{ISI}. Advocates argue that use of the INR would reduce interlaboratory variation in reported PT results and permit the adoption of more uniform and consistent PT target ranges for monitoring oral anticoagulation. The use of recombinant human tissue factor is a potential alternative to the use of the many animal thromboplastins currently in use.[7] When compared to the World Health Organization standard thromboplastin, the ISI of recombinant human tissue factor was 0.96–1.12, with a comparable degree of precision.[8]

The use of sensitive thromboplastins or of the INR, or both, is not without drawbacks, however. Mild deficiencies of extrinsic or common pathway coagulation factors that represent a negligible bleeding risk do not prolong the PT when an insensitive (ISI >2) thromboplastin is used. If, however, the PT ratio is converted to the INR, or if a sensitive thromboplastin is used, more patients, especially those with acquired vitamin K deficiency or liver disease, will be identified with an abnormal coagulation test and will be at risk of receiving unnecessary plasma infusions or for having invasive procedures delayed or canceled. Thus, clinical judgment must be brought to bear in interpreting the INR within a particular clinical context.

Activated Partial Thromboplastin Time

The PTT is performed by the addition of a surface activating agent, such as kaolin, silica, or ellagic acid, and phospholipid to citrate-anticoagulated plasma.[1] After incubation for a period sufficient to provide for the optimal activation of the contact factors, the plasma is recalcified and the clotting time measured. The name of the test emanates from the phospholipid reagents being originally derived from a lipid-enriched extract of complete thromboplastin, hence the term partial thromboplastin. The PTT is dependent on factors of both the intrinsic and common pathways (Fig. 104-1). The PTT may be prolonged due to a deficiency of one or more of these factors or to the presence of inhibitors that affect their function. Although it is commonly stated that decreases in factor levels to approximately 30% of normal are required to prolong the PTT, in practice the variability is considerable in the sensitivity of different commercially available PTT reagents to the various factors. In our experience, the levels vary from 25% to 40%. Since detection of a fibrin clot does not require covalent cross-linking of the fibrin, neither the PT nor the PTT will detect even severe deficiencies of factor XIII.

Recently developed portable instruments offer the potential for rapid determination of the PT and PTT at the bedside or in an outpatient setting.[9–15] Briefly, blood from a finger stick is applied to an opening on a disposable card. The blood flows by capillary action through an enclosed channel that contains either lyophilized thromboplastin (PT) or phospholipid and surface activator (PTT), where coagulation begins. The card is inserted into a portable laser photometer, which measures the time until blood flow stops due to clot formation. The instruments convert the clotting time to a "comparable" PT or PTT result. Early studies indicate that these methods correlate well with traditional laboratory methods, exhibit acceptable precision, and are easily performed by health care workers and patients. One recent randomized prospective study has suggested that the use of these instruments in the cardiothoracic operating room facilitated rapid correct diagnosis in bleeding patients and resulted in a significant reduction in blood product use.[16]

Platelet Count

The platelet count is performed to detect thrombocytopenia, which is usually defined as a platelet count of $<150,000/mm^3$. The procedure is now almost always performed as part of an automated blood cell profile. Currently employed instruments are quite reliable, even down to platelet counts approaching $20,000-30,000/mm^3$, and are much less susceptible to the artifacts that plagued earlier generations of platelet counters. Nevertheless, the finding of thrombocytopenia, especially unexpected thrombocytopenia, should be confirmed by a review of the peripheral blood smear and platelet size histogram obtained from automated blood cell counters. Abnormalities of platelet size, the presence of red cell fragments, or evidence of pseudothrombocytopenia[17-20] may provide clues with which to direct the further evaluation of the patient.

Bleeding Time

The bleeding time is the screening test for platelet function[21-23] (see Ch. 160). The test is not, as its name might imply, a global test of the hemostatic system. The test is not significantly prolonged in most disorders that result in prolongation of the PT or PTT (e.g., deficiencies of factors VIII, IX, or VII). The bleeding time is prolonged not only due to functional defects of platelets per se, but also to deficiencies or functional abnormalities of plasma proteins such as von Willebrand factor (vWF), which are required for normal interactions of platelets with the vessel wall. The bleeding time may also be prolonged in severe hypofibrinogenemia.

The procedure is usually performed with a disposable template device that produces one or two standardized incisions on the volar aspect of the forearm. A sphygmomanometer around the arm is inflated to 40 mmHg to standardize venous pressure. The time required for bleeding to cease is determined by carefully blotting the blood emerging from the wounds with filter paper at 30-second intervals.

The test is influenced by a number of factors, including the depth, location, and direction of the incisions; skin thickness; and skill of the technologist performing the test, in addition to platelet function.[24,25] The bleeding time may be prolonged by some of the many medications known to inhibit platelet function (see Ch. 130). Knowledge of the platelet count is essential for accurate interpretation of the bleeding time. The test is independent of platelet count down to approximately 100,000 platelets/mm^3 and is prolonged in a linear fashion as the platelet count falls from 100,000 to $10,000/mm^3$.[21] Because of this, a bleeding time is generally indicated only when the platelet count is $>100,000/mm^3$. In the presence of thrombocytopenia, a prolonged bleeding time must be interpreted with caution.

Analysis of the performance of the bleeding time indicates that the test functions poorly as a screening test in the general

population and is a poor predictor of surgical bleeding and of the response to hemostatic therapy.[26,27] The sensitivity, specificity, and predictive value of the test have not been established. Nevertheless, we concur with Triplett's conclusion that the bleeding time can be a valuable laboratory test that can yield important diagnostic information when used in a selected patient population with suggestive or positive bleeding histories.[22]

FURTHER EVALUATION OF ABNORMAL SCREENING TESTS

The initial battery of four tests establishes whether the patient has a quantitative disorder of platelets, a defect in platelet function, or an abnormality within either the intrinsic or extrinsic pathways of coagulation, or both.

Evaluation of Prolonged PT and/or PTT

Several tests can be performed to ensure that the prolongation of the PTT is not due to the presence of heparin in the specimen. The thrombin time is a useful test for this purpose, as it is very sensitive to the presence of heparin (see below). Once it is clearly established that the PT or PTT, or both, is prolonged, the task is to determine whether the prolongation is caused by factor deficiency or by the presence of an inhibitor.[28] This is usually accomplished by repeating the determinations after mixing equal volumes of the patient's plasma with plasma derived from a pool of normal donors. Since factor levels of 50% of normal are sufficient to produce a normal PT and PTT, this procedure will result in correction of the abnormality if it is caused by the deficiency of one or more factors. If an inhibitory antibody is present, the mixing procedure will result in little or no correction of the abnormality. Two caveats must be borne in mind. First, relatively low-titer, low-avidity inhibitors producing only modest prolongations of the PT or PTT, or both, may be difficult to detect with the 1:1 mixing procedure. Some authorities have advocated performing inhibitor assays on other than 1:1 mixtures, in an effort to detect weaker inhibitors. In our experience, this procedure has not proved satisfactory and, as often as not, has produced ambiguous results. Second, some classes of inhibitors seen in patients with severe factor VIII deficiency react slowly with factor VIII in the normal plasma on mixing and may not be detected if the mixture is assayed immediately.[29] The latter situation is addressed by assaying the mixture after an incubation of 0.5-2 hours, as well as immediately after mixing.

A series of 100 consecutive patients referred for consultation because of a prolonged PTT demonstrated that in 50% of patients the problem was indicative of a hemostatic defect.[30] Of the hemostatically compromised patients, 81% gave an abnormal hemostatic history. A laboratory approach to evaluating acquired and inherited prolongations of the PT or PTT, or both, is presented in algorithm form. This approach is discussed in greater detail below.

Inhibitors

Factor VIII inhibitors and lupus anticoagulants are the most frequently encountered inhibitors of coagulation. Factor IX inhibitors are encountered much less often; other inhibitors are seen only rarely. A detailed discussion of circulating anticoagulants is presented in Chapter 115. One of the several approaches described below should be employed to establish the presence of the lupus anticoagulant. Assays of specific coagulation factors are employed to document the specificity of inhibitors against individual factors.

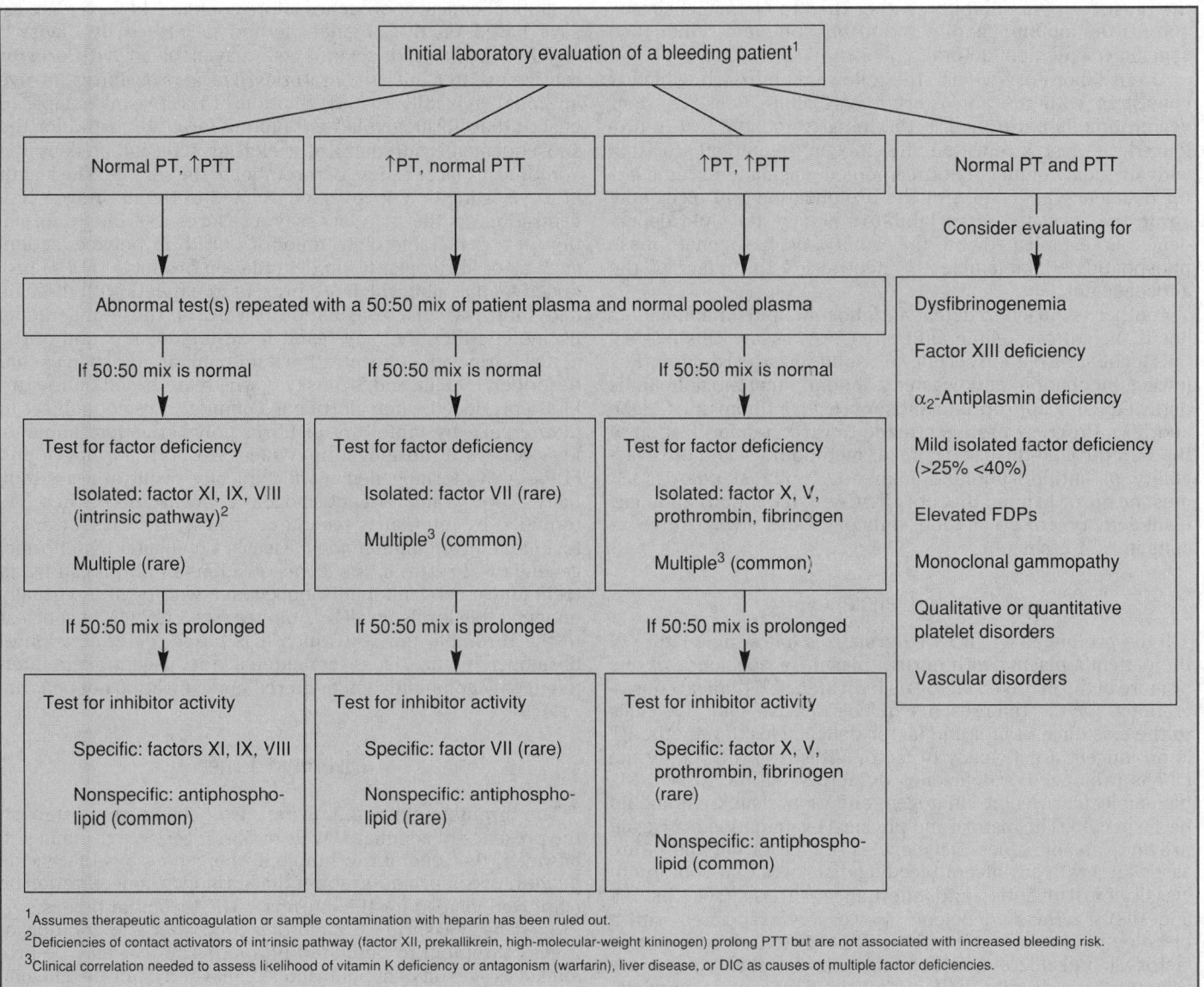

Initial laboratory evaluation of a bleeding patient[1]

| Normal PT, ↑PTT | ↑PT, normal PTT | ↑PT, ↑PTT | Normal PT and PTT |

Consider evaluating for

Abnormal test(s) repeated with a 50:50 mix of patient plasma and normal pooled plasma

If 50:50 mix is normal | If 50:50 mix is normal | If 50:50 mix is normal

Test for factor deficiency

Isolated: factor XI, IX, VIII (intrinsic pathway)[2]

Multiple (rare)

Test for factor deficiency

Isolated: factor VII (rare)

Multiple[3] (common)

Test for factor deficiency

Isolated: factor X, V, prothrombin, fibrinogen

Multiple[3] (common)

Dysfibrinogenemia

Factor XIII deficiency

α_2-Antiplasmin deficiency

Mild isolated factor deficiency (>25% <40%)

Elevated FDPs

Monoclonal gammopathy

Qualitative or quantitative platelet disorders

Vascular disorders

If 50:50 mix is prolonged | If 50:50 mix is prolonged | If 50:50 mix is prolonged

Test for inhibitor activity

Specific: factors XI, IX, VIII

Nonspecific: antiphospholipid (common)

Test for inhibitor activity

Specific: factor VII (rare)

Nonspecific: antiphospholipid (rare)

Test for inhibitor activity

Specific: factor X, V, prothrombin, fibrinogen (rare)

Nonspecific: antiphospholipid (common)

[1]Assumes therapeutic anticoagulation or sample contamination with heparin has been ruled out.

[2]Deficiencies of contact activators of intrinsic pathway (factor XII, prekallikrein, high-molecular-weight kininogen) prolong PTT but are not associated with increased bleeding risk.

[3]Clinical correlation needed to assess likelihood of vitamin K deficiency or antagonism (warfarin), liver disease, or DIC as causes of multiple factor deficiencies.

Quantitation of the level of factor VIII inhibitors may have therapeutic implications.[29] Two common approaches have evolved. In the Bethesda assay, patient plasma or dilutions of patient plasma and normal plasma are incubated for 2 hours at 37°C, after which the residual factor VIII activity is measured.[31,32] One Bethesda unit/ml is the concentration that will neutralize 50% of the added factor VIII during the 2-hour incubation. In the new Oxford assay, the preliminary incubation requires 4 hours. One new Oxford unit/ml is defined as the concentration of inhibitor that will neutralize 50% of the added factor VIII (from a lyophilized concentrate) in 4 hours.[32,33]

Lupus Anticoagulants

The so-called lupus-type anticoagulant is by far the inhibitor most likely to be encountered[34] (see Ch. 115 for a more extensive discussion). Only about one-third of these anticoagulants occur in patients with lupus erythematosus. A review of the literature indicates that this anticoagulant is present in approximately 25% of patients with systemic lupus erythematosus (SLE), if the analysis is restricted to series composed of consecutive or otherwise unselected patients. The lupus anticoagulant is paradoxically associated with an increased occurrence of thrombosis, recurrent fetal loss, and thrombocytopenia.

When these complications are encountered in a lupus anticoagulant-positive patient without SLE, the term primary antiphospholipid syndrome has been applied.[35]

The lupus anticoagulants have been shown to react with anionic phospholipids and may therefore give rise to either a prolonged PTT (common) or prolonged PT (less common), or both. Several different laboratory procedures have been proposed as tests for the lupus anticoagulant. These have included tests based on the PTT, the PT performed with dilute thromboplastin (the tissue thromboplastin inhibition test), the dilute Russell's viper venom time (activation of factor X by venom and subsequent thrombin generation) performed with limiting concentrations of venom and phospholipid, the kaolin clotting time, the plasma clotting time, and platelet or phospholipid neutralization procedures.[36,37] No single test for the detection of lupus anticoagulants has proved entirely satisfactory or gained widespread acceptance. The sensitivity and specificity have not been adequately established for any of these procedures. Problems include patient-to-patient variability due to the heterogeneity of these antibodies, as well as variation in the sensitivity of reagents to inhibitory activity. A set of minimal guidelines have been proposed.[38] These include the demonstration that (1) an abnormality of phospholipid-dependent coagulation reactions is present; (2) the abnormality is due to the presence of an inhibitor, rather than to factor deficiency; and (3) the inhibitor is directed at phospholipid rather than specific coagulation factors.

At our laboratory we use the following approach, which is consistent with the above criteria. A dilute Russell's viper venom time is performed. If the initial screening test is prolonged, the test is repeated after mixing the patient's plasma with an equal volume of normal pooled plasma to exclude factor deficiency as a cause of the prolongation and to demonstrate the presence of an inhibitor. Finally, the lipid dependence is established by the ability of hexagonal phase phosphatidylethanolamine to "neutralize" the effect of the anticoagulant.

Another test used to detect antiphospholipid immunoglobulins is the anticardiolipin antibody (ACA) assay. This test entails incubating patient serum with solid-phase cardiolipin. Following incubation and washing, bound immunoglobulin is detected using appropriate antisera (e.g., antihuman IgG, IgM, and IgA). Progress has been made toward standardization of the ACA through the use of similar methodology and the availability of antiphospholipid immunoglobulin standards.[39] It must be borne in mind that not all ACAs exhibit lupus anticoagulant activity, nor do all lupus anticoagulants give positive results in ACA assays.

Factor Deficiency

If the prolonged PT or PTT normalizes following mixture of the patient's plasma with normal plasma, a deficiency of one or more of the involved factors is indicated.[28,40] Clinical considerations, such as the presence of liver disease, may give clues to the existence of multiple factor deficiencies. If only the PT is prolonged, a deficiency of factor VII is present. If only the PTT is prolonged, a deficiency of factors VIII, IX, XI, and XII, high-molecular-weight kininogen, and/or prekallikrein should be suspected. The history and physical examination may again provide valuable clues. Deficiencies of factors VIII and IX are associated with significant bleeding disorders that conform to classic sex distribution and inheritance patterns (see Chs. 106 and 108). Factor XI deficiency is variably associated with a bleeding diathesis (see Ch. 110). Even severe deficiencies of factor XII, prekallikrein, or high-molecular-weight kininogen are asymptomatic despite the fact that the PTT may be markedly prolonged.

If both the PT and the PTT are prolonged, the patient has either a deficiency of multiple factors affecting both the intrinsic and extrinsic pathways and/or the common pathway or has a selective deficiency of factor V or X, prothrombin, or fibrinogen. In this setting, a concentration of fibrinogen adequate for clot formation should be ensured before other specific factor assays are performed. Fibrinogen levels must fall to the level of 60–80 mg/dl before hypofibrinogenemia can be accepted as the sole explanation for the prolonged PT and PTT. If hypofibrinogenemia is not the cause of the abnormal PT and PTT, specific assays for factors V and X and prothrombin should be performed.

Factors V, VII, and X and prothrombin are usually assayed by determining the ability of dilutions of the patient plasma to correct the PT of a plasma congenitally deficient in the factor to be assayed. The degree of correction is compared to that produced by equivalent dilutions of normal pooled plasma. Factors VIII, IX, XI, and XII are determined in a similar manner, except that the specific factor assays are based on the PTT.

Fibrinogen Determinations

A number of procedures for the determination of fibrinogen have been devised. These include chemical determinations of thrombin-clottable protein, salt precipitation techniques, and immunochemical approaches. More common, however, are assays based on the original method described by Clauss,[41] which is the basis for several assays available in "kit" form for routine use in clinical laboratories. These procedures involve an initial (typically 10-fold) dilution of the plasma sample to ensure that fibrinogen is rate limiting for clotting and for the subsequent measurement of a clotting time initiated by the addition of a large excess of thrombin to the sample. The length of the clotting time is inversely related to the fibrinogen concentration. As this type of assay measures the time to formation of a detectable clot, inhibitors of fibrin polymerization, such as of fibrinogen/fibrin degradation products (FDPs) produced by plasmin, which are present in patients with disseminated intravascular coagulation (DIC) or in those undergoing fibrinolytic therapy, may result in an underestimation of the actual fibrinogen concentration. End-point assays such as that described by Ellis and Stransky,[42] which are based on the turbidity produced when clotting is complete, are not subject to interference by inhibitors of fibrin polymerization. Immunologic assays of fibrinogen may measure both fibrinogen and FDPs. A dysfibrinogenemia will typically result in a substantially lower value for fibrinogen concentration when determined by the Clauss technique than by the Ellis–Stransky technique or by immunologic assays. Congenital hypofibrinogenemia will result in low concentrations of fibrinogen by all techniques; congenital afibrinogenemia will result in virtually undetectable levels by all techniques (see Ch. 111). In contrast to the thrombin time on which it is based, determination of fibrinogen by the Clauss technique is not susceptible to interference by commonly encountered concentrations of heparin.

Thrombin Time

The thrombin clotting time has also been used to establish the presence of adequate levels of fibrinogen. We recommend, however, that one of the simple fibrinogen assays that yields quantitative information about the fibrinogen concentration be employed instead for this purpose. The thrombin time is performed by measuring the clotting time after the addition of excess thrombin to undiluted plasma.[1] The test may be prolonged as a result of hypofibrinogenemia or dysfibrinogenemia; the presence of FDPs, heparin, or an antibody to thrombin; and in amyloidosis.[43,44] Prolongation of the thrombin time due to hyperfibrinogenemia has also been described.[45] The relative sensitivity of the thrombin time to these factors is dependent on the precise configuration of the assay.[40] Correction of a prolonged thrombin time on the addition of protamine sulfate or of a commercially available ion-exchange resin (Heparsorb) is a presumptive test for the presence of heparin or a heparin-like anticoagulant.

Evaluation of Thrombocytopenia

Thrombocytopenia is commonly defined as a platelet count of $<150,000/mm^3$. Thrombocytopenia is a laboratory finding indicative of an underlying disease process, but does not constitute the diagnosis. A number of different conditions may give rise to the finding of thrombocytopenia. Some of the more common causes are listed in Table 104-1. These disorders may be divided into those of decreased platelet production, increased platelet destruction, and splenic pooling due to splenomegaly. Increased platelet destruction is further subdivided into immune-mediated destruction and nonimmune consumption. The causes of thrombocytopenia are considered in detail elsewhere (see Chs. 125–128).

The clinical history and physical examination may provide

Table 104-1. Causes of Thrombocytopenia

Impaired production
  Megakaryocyte hypoplasia
    Chemical and physical agents
    Myelopthisis
    Aplastic anemia and related disorders
  Ineffective thrombopoiesis
    Vitamin B_{12} or folate deficiency
    Myeloproliferative and myelodysplastic disorders
    Paroxysmal nocturnal hemoglobinuria
Enhanced destruction
  Immune-mediated mechanisms
    Autoantibody (idiopathic thrombocytopenic purpura)
    Isoantibody (post-transfusion purpura, neonatal alloimmune thrombocy-
      topenic purpura)
    Drug-induced
    Immune complex disorders
  Nonimmune mechanisms
    Disseminated intravascular coagulation
    Thrombotic thrombocytopenic purpura/hemolytic uremic syndrome
    Dilutional
Splenomegaly and hypersplenism

important clues to the cause of thrombocytopenia. Laboratory evaluation should include a careful examination of the peripheral blood smear, the platelet histogram from the automated blood cell count, and usually the bone marrow. Examination of the marrow is especially important in establishing the presence of decreased platelet production, which is generally associated with diminished numbers of megakaryocytes. The results of these two examinations or of the clinical history, or both, may suggest that other more specialized tests be performed to define the etiology of the thrombocytopenia. These tests include serum B_{12} and folate levels, sucrose or acid hemolysis tests, and tests for the presence of DIC (see below).

The determination of platelet-associated immunoglobulin for the diagnosis of immune-mediated thrombocyotpenias is discussed in Chapter 125. A recent study suggested that measurement of circulating levels of glycocalicin, a proteolytic fragment of platelet glycoprotein Ib (GPIb), may aid in the classification of thrombocytopenia.[46] Plasma glycocalicin concentration may reflect overall platelet turnover, platelet mass, and rate of platelet destruction. Clinical experience with this determination is limited, however, and the test is not widely available.

Artifactual causes of apparent thrombocytopenia must be considered as well. These include pseudothrombocytopenia due to platelet aggregation within the specimen, anticoagulant-induced platelet agglutination, and platelet satellitism.[17–20]

Evaluation of Prolonged Bleeding Time

A bleeding time that is prolonged out of proportion to the platelet count is indicative of a defect in platelet function. Laboratory evaluation of the prolonged bleeding time should not proceed until the history has been thoroughly reviewed to identify drugs or associated clinical conditions that could account for the prolonged bleeding time. (Acquired platelet dysfunction is considered in Chapter 130, inherited disorders in Chapter 129.)

von Willebrand Disease

von Willebrand disease (vWD) is the most likely cause of an inherited prolongation of the bleeding time. It is now believed by some to be the most common of the inherited disorders of hemostasis.[47–49] The prevalence of this disorder was recently

estimated at 0.8% in a population of children in northern Italy.[49] vWD is considered in detail elsewhere (see Chs. 112 and 113). The disorder arises as a consequence of quantitative or qualitative abnormalities of the vWF protein.

Although a prolonged bleeding time is the hallmark of vWD, this laboratory finding is not specific for vWD. Thus, the diagnosis is definitively established by means of additional laboratory tests.[50] These usually include measurements of the amount of vWF protein present in plasma, the functional activity of the vWF, and the procoagulant activity of the associated factor VIII molecule. Analysis of the multimeric structure of vWF is useful in some settings, as described below.

The vWF protein is quantitated by immunochemical procedures. Rocket immunoelectrophoresis (electroimmunoassay) remains the most commonly employed procedure, although other approaches, including immunoradiometric and enzyme-linked immunosorbent assays, have been developed.[1,51] In most patients with vWD, the antigenic level of the von Willebrand protein will be reduced. However, in patients with type II disorders (decreased high-molecular-weight forms), antigenic levels of the protein may be close to, or within, the reference range.

Pregnancy, ingestion of oral contraceptives, or liver disease may elevate the plasma level of vWF and factor VIII coagulant activity, complicating the diagnosis. A recent study demonstrated that levels of vWF are a function of the ABO blood group.[52] Persons with blood group O had significantly lower levels of vWF (75 U/dl) than were found in group A (106 U/dl), group B (117 U/dl), or group AB (123 U/dl) subjects.

The functional activity of vWF is assessed by measurement of the ristocetin cofactor activity of the patient's plasma. This assay determines the ability of vWF in the plasma to agglutinate a standardized suspension of fixed normal platelets in the presence of ristocetin from either the rate or extent of platelet agglutination.[1,53,54] Agglutination is usually measured in a platelet aggregometer, although other approaches have been devised. This activity is usually decreased in plasma from patients with vWD, even in those with types IIb or platelet-type vWD in which enhanced platelet agglutination/aggregation to low concentrations of ristocetin is added to the patient's own platelet-rich plasma. Even in type I disorders, determination of ristocetin cofactor activity by the semiquantitative procedure described above appears to have a greater diagnostic sensitivity than the more qualitative determination of ristocetin-induced platelet aggregation in platelet-rich plasma.[55] This is attributable to the lower concentrations of vWF actually present in the ristocetin cofactor assays.

This functional assay tests only the ristocetin-dependent interaction of vWF with the platelet membrane GPIb/IX complex. Clinically useful tests of the interactions of vWF with the platelet membrane IIb/IIIa complex or with components of the extracellular matrix have not been devised. Defects in these interactions may, at least theoretically, also contribute to bleeding disorders.

Factor VIII procoagulant activity is also typically, but not universally, decreased in vWD. This activity is commonly measured in an assay based on the ability of various dilutions of patient plasma to correct the clotting time of authentic factor VIII-deficient plasma in a PTT-based assay. Although factor VIII levels are commonly reduced in vWD, the level may not be sufficiently low so as to prolong the PTT. Thus, a PTT within the normal range does not permit exclusion of the diagnosis of vWD.

In contrast to the type I forms of vWD, in which a generalized decrease in all multimeric forms of vWF occurs, the type II forms of the disease manifest a selective deficiency of the higher-molecular-weight forms. The deficiency may have a number of causes, including impaired biosynthesis, enhanced proteolysis, or selective adsorption of the high-molecular-weight forms

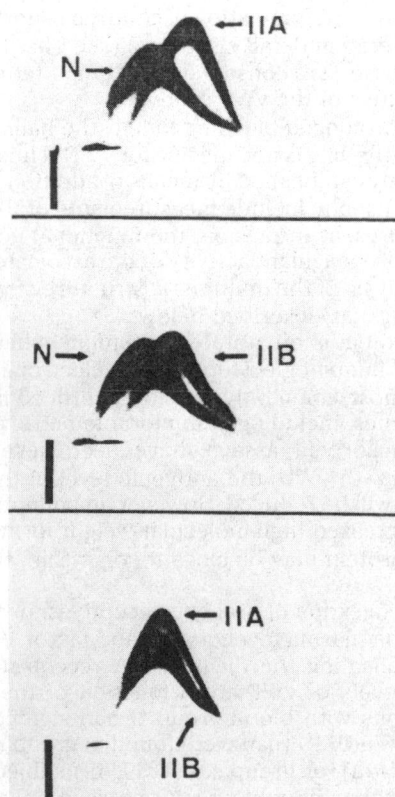

Fig. 104-2. Crossed immunoelectrophoresis of vWF in normal plasma (N) and types IIA and IIB von Willebrand disease. The first dimension sample well is indicated by the vertical line. The direction of electrophoresis (anode) is to the right in the first dimension and to the top in the second. The patterns from different plasmas have been overlaid for comparison. The asymmetric pattern in normal plasma results from the different migration rates of different-size multimers. In types IIA and IIB von Willebrand disease, the largest multimers (slowest migrating) are missing. (From Ruggeri et al.,[58] with permission.)

onto platelets.[48] As the higher-molecular-weight forms account for most of the ristocetin cofactor activity in plasma, a discrepancy between the amount of ristocetin cofactor activity present and the level of vWF antigen should lead to the suspicion of the presence of a type II disorder. Two approaches may be used to confirm this suspicion.

In crossed immunoelectrophoresis, the plasma sample is electrophoresed through agarose in the first dimension to separate the vWF multimers by size and then electrophoresed in the second dimension into agarose containing antibody to vWF. An immunoprecipitate forms, the shape of which is indicative of the distribution of vWF multimers.[56] An example of this technique is shown in Figure 104-2.

Sodium dodecyl sulfate/agarose gel electrophoresis provides a higher-resolution analysis of the multimer distribution but is not yet available in most clinical coagulation laboratories.[57] Following electrophoretic separation in agarose in the presence of sodium dodecyl sulfate, the vWF multimers are detected with either ^{125}I-labeled antibodies or enzyme-linked antibodies to vWF. This technique is illustrated in Figure 104-3.

Establishing the existence of a type II disorder is no longer an academic exercise. Since deamino-D-arginine vasopressin (DDAVP) is now considered front-line therapy for type I vWD but appears to be less effective in the type II disorders and can induce thrombocytopenia in some of the type II variants, this distinction has taken on important therapeutic implications.[47,48]

Although ristocetin-induced platelet aggregation of the patient's own platelet-rich plasma is not recommended as a front-line test for the diagnosis of vWD, it is useful in sorting out type II forms of the disease. Platelets in type IIB disease exhibit enhanced platelet aggregation to low concentrations of ristocetin when platelet-rich plasma is examined, even though the ristocetin cofactor activity of the patient's plasma may be diminished.[58] This is attributed to an exceptionally high affinity of the abnormal vWF for the platelet, resulting in its adsorption from plasma. A similar phenomenon is observed in platelet-type or pseudo-vWD, except that the defect resides in the patient's platelets rather than in the vWF molecule.[59,60]

In trying to establish the diagnosis of vWD, one must be aware that all the laboratory parameters may fluctuate significantly over time.[61] On some occasions, all four major parameters—bleeding time, vWF antigen, vWF activity, and factor VIII activity—may be within the normal range. In the presence of a strong clinical suspicion, repeated testing is warranted to establish the diagnosis. The use of laboratory tests for the diagnosis and classification of vWD is discussed in further detail in Chapter 113.

Platelet Function Testing

A prolonged bleeding time in the presence of a relatively normal platelet count may be due to an inherited defect in platelet function, but less frequently than to vWD. The inherited defects of platelet function include abnormalities or deficiencies of membrane glycoproteins; deficiencies of secretory granules or their contents, or both; and defects in the enzymatic machinery required for secretion. Hereditary disorders of platelet function are considered in Chapter 129. Acquired defects due to associated disease states, such as uremia, multiple myeloma, myeloproliferative disorders, various inhibitory antibodies, or the presence of medications must also be considered. Acquired disorders of platelet function are discussed in Chapter 130.

Review of the peripheral blood smear may provide a clue to the nature of the platelet function defect. In gray platelet syndrome (α-granule deficiency), the characteristic purplish staining of platelets is absent, leaving them with a gray, washed-out appearance. Giant platelets are present in Bernard-Soulier syndrome and in a variety of other inherited disorders associated with thrombocytopenia. If the smear is prepared from fresh blood in the absence of anticoagulant, platelet aggregates are readily apparent in normal individuals. The aggregates are not detectable in Glanzmann's thrombasthenia. None of these observations can be considered definitive. Additional studies are required to establish the diagnosis.

Platelet aggregation studies are the mainstay of platelet function testing in the laboratory.[62-64] Platelet aggregation is monitored by the increase in light transmission through a suspension of platelet-rich plasma as aggregation occurs. Collagen, ADP, epinephrine, arachidonic acid, and ristocetin are commonly used agonists in the clinical laboratory. Studies of platelet aggregation are usually performed in concert with studies of platelet secretion. The secretion of granule contents is usually monitored by following the agonist-induced release of ^{14}C-serotonin from platelet-dense granules or of ATP release by a chemiluminescence procedure. These rather sophisticated evaluations are obviously beyond the scope of most clinical laboratories but are usually available in referral centers.

Platelet aggregation patterns observed in some of the more common, classical inherited abnormalities are shown in Figure 104-4. As more has been learned about platelet function defects and more disorders described, it has become clear that simple examination of the results of the usual set of platelet function studies in many cases does not permit a diagnosis at the molec-

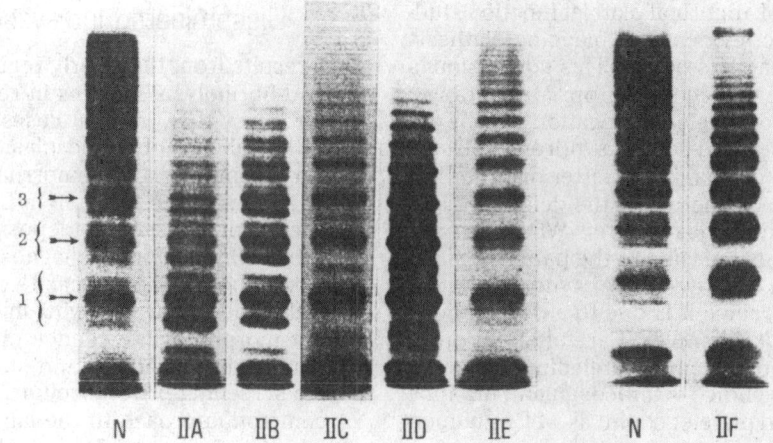

Fig. 104-3. Sodium dodecyl sulfate/agarose multimeric analysis of plasma vWF from a normal subject, compared with vWF of type II vWD variants. The three smallest individual oligomers are indicated by the brackets. Arrows point to the predominant band in each normal oligomer. In types IIA and IIB vWD, the fastest-moving band in each oligomer is increased relative to the predominant band. However, bands with similar mobilities to all normal bands are present. In types IIC, IID, IIE, and IIF, either some normal bands are missing or bands are present that are not seen in normal plasma. (From Berkowitz et al.,[82] with permission.)

ular level. Although some disorders, such as Glanzmann's thrombasthenia (defect in GPIIb/IIIa) or Bernard-Soulier syndrome (defect in GPIb), give rise to unambiguous findings, defects such as storage pool deficiency, cyclo-oxygenase deficiency, or thromboxane synthase deficiency, may give rise to

virtually identical patterns of aggregation with the commonly used agonists. More detailed studies, including analysis of platelet membrane proteins, electron microscopic examination of the platelets, analysis of granule contents, or the analysis of arachidonic acid metabolites, may be required for a definitive

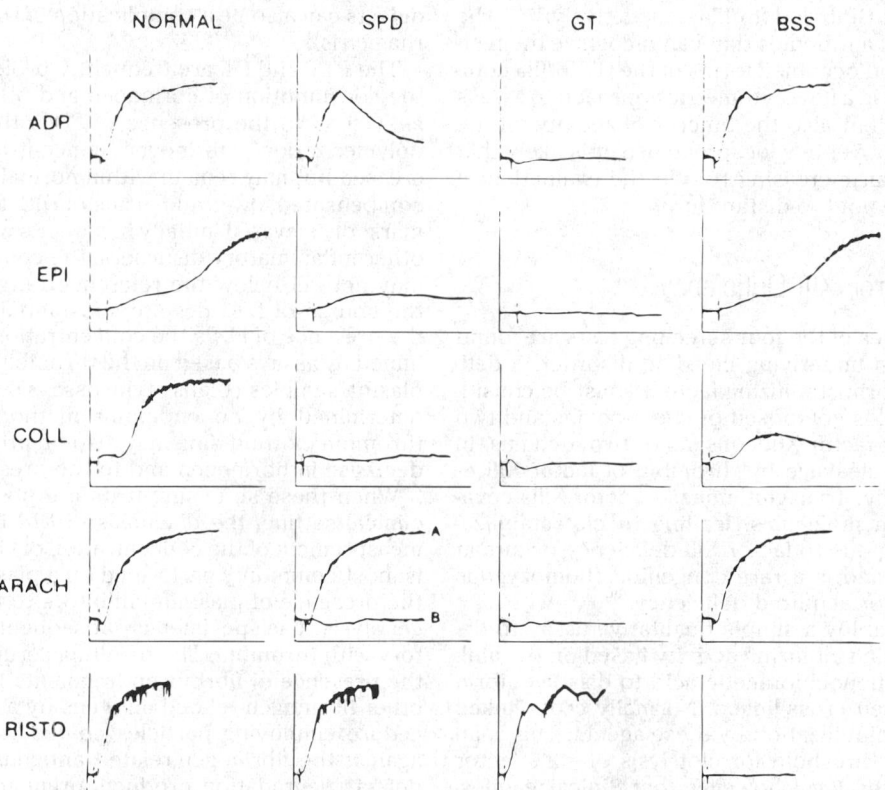

Fig. 104-4. Platelet aggregation patterns in platelet disorders. Representative aggregation patterns in response to ADP, epinephrine (EPI), collagen (COLL), arachidonic acid (ARACH), and ristocetin (RISTO) are shown for a normal subject and for patients with a storage pool defect (SPD), Glanzmann's thrombasthenia (GT), and Bernard-Soulier syndrome (BSS). The characteristic abnormality in patients with release defects is an absent second wave of aggregation with ADP and epinephrine, an absent or greatly diminished aggregation with collagen, and a normal or variably reduced arachidonate aggregation. In Glanzmann's thrombasthenia, the characteristic abnormality is absent aggregation with all agents, except ristocetin. In Bernard-Soulier syndrome, the characteristic abnormality is absent aggregation with ristocetin and a reduced response to collagen, but aggregation with ADP, epinephrine, and arachidonate is normal. (From White et al.,[83] with permission.)

diagnosis. The clinical value of abnormal platelet function studies is that they provide direct evidence of bleeding diathesis as the result of a defect of platelets per se. This conclusion is crucial, as it will guide in the choice of appropriate therapy.

Although ristocetin-induced platelet aggregation may be abnormal both in vWD and in Bernard-Soulier syndrome, plasma ristocetin cofactor activity is normal in the latter disorder but is usually decreased in vWD. Furthermore, the defect in ristocetin-induced platelet aggregation observed in vWD can be corrected by the addition of normal plasma to the patient's platelet-rich plasma. The defect in Bernard-Soulier syndrome is not corrected by normal plasma, since it is due to a deficiency of the platelet membrane GPIb/IX complex. Careful attention to detail is required to obtain reproducible platelet function studies. Results are influenced by choice of anticoagulant, pH, time of storage, rate of stirring, and platelet count, as well as numerous drugs.[63,64]

Several other tests were more commonly used in years past but are less commonly employed today. These include assays of platelet factor 3 activity, clot retraction, and glass bead retention. These procedures lack the diagnostic specificity of the approach to platelet function testing outlined above and are not commonly performed in most diagnostic coagulation laboratories.

The development and characterization of monoclonal antibodies reactive with platelet surface-adhesive receptors have resulted in new approaches to the investigation of platelet function disorders. Assays for the diagnosis of Bernard-Soulier syndrome (GPIb deficiency) and Glanzmann's thrombasthenia (GPIIb/IIIa complex deficiency) have been developed using antibodies directed against GPIb and IIb/IIIa, respectively.[65,66] The availability of a panel of antibodies that can recognize the resting, activated, and ligand-occupied forms of the GPIIb/IIIa complex has been exploited in a flow cytometric approach to assess not only the presence, but also the functional activity, of the complex.[67] Although not yet in widespread use, it is likely that such assays will play an increasing role in the evaluation of platelet function in the not-too-distant future.

Factor XIII Deficiency

When no abnormalities of the four screening tests are found despite suspicion of an underlying bleeding disorder, a deficiency of factor XIII (fibrin stabilizing factor), must be considered. Plasma factor XIII is composed of two α-chains and two β-chains, while platelet factor XIII consists of two α-chains. In the presence of Ca^{2+}, cleavage by thrombin of factor XIII α-chains produces an active transglutaminase. Factor XIIIa covalently cross-links fibrin molecules, leading to clot stabilization.[68] Clinical bleeding due to factor XIII deficiency occurs at levels <2% of normal and is a rare congenital (homozygous recessive inheritance) or acquired deficiency.[68-70]

Most laboratories employ a simple qualitative assay to detect a deficiency of fibrin-stabilizing activity based on the ability of 5 M urea or 1% monochloracetic acid to dissolve fibrin clots that have not been cross-linked. Normally cross-linked clots are resistant to solubilization by these agents. This is an insensitive test with a threshold for clot lysis of <2% factor XIII activity. It is below this level, however, that clinical manifestations of factor XIII deficiency occur.

More quantitative assays of factor XIII transglutaminase activity have been devised.[71,72] These tests are more sensitive and rapid than the clot lysis assay; they can also be automated. However, they are not in widespread use because screening for factor XIII deficiency is rarely clinically indicated. Factor XIII α- and β-subunits can be quantitated by immunologic methods using commercial polyclonal antisera. The determinations may be helpful in characterizing an inherited deficiency.[70]

Disseminated Intravascular Coagulation

DIC results from the poorly regulated activation of coagulation and fibrinolysis systems in response to an underlying illness or injury that, in most cases, is clinically apparent. The generation of thrombin and plasmin predisposes the patient to both thrombotic and hemorrhagic complications. DIC syndrome is considered in detail in Chapter 116.

Detection of diffuse fibrin deposition in the microvasculature would be definitive for the diagnosis of DIC, but obtaining such direct evidence is impractical. Red cell fragmentation on a peripheral blood smear signifying microangiopathic hemolysis is indirect morphologic evidence of DIC. However, this finding lacks sufficient sensitivity and specificity to be considered a reliable screening procedure for DIC.

A common approach to the laboratory investigation of DIC is to employ a battery of relatively simple, rapid procedures to document the activation of both coagulation and fibrinolytic systems.[40,73-75] Interpretation of the test results can be difficult, however, since none of these tests is specific for DIC. In general, screening tests are more sensitive in the setting of acute fulminant DIC than in clinical conditions associated with chronic compensated DIC.

Thrombocytopenia occurs as a result of thrombin generation, platelet activation, and microvascular thrombus formation. Thus, the platelet count is commonly depressed in DIC and is a component of most laboratory DIC profiles. Unfortunately, thrombocytopenia is associated with several of the predisposing conditions for DIC (i.e., liver disease, leukemia, sepsis), even in the absence of DIC. Acquired platelet function defects can also be a complication of DIC, adding to the hemorrhagic risk.

The PTT and PT are frequently prolonged in DIC[74,75] due to the consumption of fibrinogen and other coagulation factors, as well as to the presence of FDPs that interfere with fibrin polymerization. Fibrinogen concentration is frequently decreased but may remain within normal limits in the chronic or compensated low-grade forms of DIC. Since fibrinogen may be markedly elevated initially in patients with sepsis, neoplasia, or other inflammatory disorders, the concentration of fibrinogen may not fall below the reference range, at least early during the course of DIC, despite substantial decreases. Because of the presence of FDPs the concentration of fibrinogen as determined by assays based on the thrombin clotting time of diluted plasma samples (Clauss-type assays) will be lower than those determined by an end-point method (Ellis–Stransky). The thrombin clotting time may also be prolonged due both to the decrease in fibrinogen and to the presence of FDPs.

When these screening tests are positive in an appropriate clinical setting, the diagnosis of DIC is usually confirmed by measurement of the concentration of FDPs. This determination is most commonly performed on a plasma sample collected in the presence of plasmin inhibitors to prevent in vitro fibrinogenolysis. The specimen is subsequently clotted in the laboratory with thrombin. The resulting serum sample is assayed for the presence of fibrinogen fragments D and E and sometimes other fibrinogen-related antigens by a latex agglutination procedure employing particles coated with antibodies directed against the fibrinogen-related antigens. Obviously, the assay detects degradation products originating from either fibrinogen or fibrin, as the antigens are expressed on both. It should also be apparent that samples that clot poorly, for example, due to the presence of a high concentration of heparin or low concentration of fibrinogen, may result in artifactually elevated levels of FDPs.

Several monoclonal antibodies directed against the fibrin-specific degradation product, D-dimer, have been employed in latex agglutination assays similar to those described above. Comparisons of the D-dimer and FDP assays have led to different conclusions. Carr et al[76] believe that the D-dimer assay is more specific but less sensitive than the FDP assay, and they recommend using the D-dimer to confirm a positive FDP result. However, Wilde et al[77] and Boisclair et al[78] concluded that both assays were 100% sensitive in patients fulfilling their clinical criteria for DIC. Finally, Greenberg et al.[79] reported considerable discordance between the results of the two tests in patients suspected of having DIC. Critical evaluation of these studies is hampered by variability in patient selection and by the inconsistent use of immunoblotting as the gold standard for detection of FDP. Neither the D-dimer nor the FDP assay distinguishes between pathologic and physiologic fibrinolysis and may be elevated due to recent trauma, surgery, and thrombotic events. One advantage of the D-dimer assay is the convenience of performing the test on plasma, instead of having to perform the extra step of preparing serum, since fibrinogen and fibrin do not cross-react with the D-dimer monoclonal antibody. In addition to the semiquantitative latex agglutination methods, quantitative and automated assays have been introduced for both the D-dimer and FDP tests.[80,81] No compelling data have been found to support the use of both tests in the laboratory evaluation of a patient with suspected DIC. Cost, convenience, and test volume are appropriate factors to consider when deciding which test and method to implement. Frequently, the results of the first DIC panel are normal or inconclusive. Repetition of the test battery may disclose changes over time (e.g., decreased platelets or fibrinogen) consistent with DIC.

Bleeding due to hyperfibrinogenolysis without thrombin generation is a rare complication of various acute and chronic conditions. Typical laboratory findings are normal platelet count, decreased fibrinogen and plasminogen levels, and shortened euglobulin lysis time. Since fibrinogen degradation is increased, FDP are elevated. However, since fibrin degradation is not increased, D-dimer levels are not increased.

A number of more sophisticated laboratory determinations have been useful in examining and defining the pathophysiology of DIC. These include decreased the plasma concentrations of antithrombin III, α_2-antiplasmin, factors V and VIII, and protein C. However, these determinations are not commonly used clinically to establish the diagnosis of DIC.[40,73] Concentrations of fibrinopeptides A and B increase in DIC, directly reflecting the action of thrombin on fibrinogen. Elevated levels of the fibrinopeptides are not, however, specific for DIC. The role of this determination in the clinical evaluation of suspected DIC has not been established. The unavailability of the results of most of the above tests in a sufficiently short time interval represents a major impediment to their use in the evaluation of DIC.

Paracoagulation tests such as the protamine sulfate precipitation test or the ethanol gelatin test, which detect qualitatively the presence of circulating complexes of fibrinogen, fibrin monomer, and the higher-molecular-weight degradation products, lack sufficient sensitivity and specificity and are not recommended for routine use in the evaluation of suspected DIC.

REFERENCES

1. Miale JB: Laboratory Medicine—Hematology. 6th Ed. CV Mosby, St. Louis, 1982
2. Kirkwood TBL: Calibration of reference thromboplastins and standardisation of the prothrombin time ratio. Thromb Haemost 49:238, 1983
3. Ray MJ, Smith IR: The dependence of the international sensitivity index on the coagulometer used to perform the prothrombin time. Thromb Haemost 63:424, 1990
4. Bussey HI, Force RW, Bianco TM. Leonard AD: Reliance on prothrombin time ratios causes significant errors in anticoagulation therapy. Arch Intern Med 152:278, 1992
5. Hirsh J: Substandard monitoring of warfarin in North America. Time for change. Arch Intern Med 152:257, 1992
6. Poller L, Hirsh J: Special report: a simple system for the derivation of international normalized ratios for the reporting of prothrombin time results with North American thromboplastin reagents. Am J Clin Pathol 92:124, 1989
7. Rehemtulla A, Pepe M, Edgington TS: High level expression of recombinant human tissue factor in Chinese hamster ovary cells as a human thromboplastin. Thromb Haemost 65:521, 1991
8. Tripodi A, Arbini A, Chantarangkul V, Mannucci M: Recombinant tissue factor as substitute for conventional thromboplastin in the prothrombin time test. Thromb Haemost 67:42, 1992
9. Anderson DR, Harrison L, Hirsh J: Evaluation of a portable prothrombin time monitor for home use by patients who require long-term oral anticoagulant therapy. Arch Intern Med 153:1441, 1993
10. Ansell J, Holden A, Knapic N: Patient self-management of oral anticoagulation guided by capillary (fingerstick) whole blood prothrombin times. Arch Intern Med 149:2509, 1989
11. Ansell J, Tiarks C, Hirsh J et al: Measurement of the activated partial thromboplastin time from a capillary (fingerstick) sample of whole blood. A new method for monitoring heparin therapy. Am J Clin Pathol 95:222, 1991
12. Lucas FV, Duncan A, Jay RM et al: A novel whole blood capillary technique for measuring the prothrombin time. Am J Clin Pathol 88:442, 1987
13. White RH, McCurdy SA, van Marensdorff H et al: Home prothrombin time monitoring after the initiation of warfarin therapy: a randomized prospective study. Ann Intern Med 111:730, 1989
14. Oberhardt BJ, Dermott SC, Taylor M et al: Dry reagent technology for rapid convenient measurements of blood coagulation and fibrinolysis. Clin Chem 37:520, 1991
15. Sane DC, Gresalfi NJ, Enney-O'Mara LA et al: Explanation of rapid bedside monitoring of coagulation and fibrinolysis parameters during thrombolytic therapy. Blood Coagul Fibrinolysis 3:47, 1992
16. Despotis GJ, Santoro SA, Spitznagel E et al: Prospective evaluation and clinical utility of on-site monitoring of coagulation in patients undergoing cardiac operation. J Thorac Cardiovasc Surg 107:271, 1994
17. Payne BA, Pierre RV: Pseudothrombocytopenia: a laboratory artifact with potentially serious consequences. Mayo Clin Proc 59:123, 1984
18. Kjeldsberg CR, Swanson J: Platelet satellitism. Blood 43:831, 1974
19. Pegels JG, Bruynes ECE, Engelfriet CP et al: Pseudothrombocytopenia: an immunologic study on platelet antibodies dependent on ethylene diamine tetra-acetate. Blood 59:157, 1982
20. Cunningham VL, Brandt JT: Spurious thrombocytopenia due to EDTA-independent cold-reactive agglutinins. Am J Clin Pathol 97:359, 1992
21. Harker LA, Slichter SJ: The bleeding time as a screening test for evaluation of platelet function. N Engl J Med 287:155, 1972
22. Triplett DA: The bleeding time—neither pariah nor panacea. Arch Pathol Lab Med 113:1207, 1989
23. Burns ER, Lawrence C: Bleeding time—a guide to its diagnostic and clinical utility. Arch Pathol Lab Med 113:1219, 1989
24. Bowie EJW, Owen CA: The bleeding time. Prog Hemost Thromb 2:249, 1974
25. Buchanan GR, Holtkamp CA: A comparative study of variables affecting the bleeding time using two disposable devices. Am J Clin Pathol 91:45, 1989
26. Rogers RPC, Levin J: A critical reappraisal of the bleeding time. Semin Thromb Hemost 16:1, 1990
27. Lind SE: The bleeding time does not predict surgical bleeding. Blood 77:2547, 1991
28. Suchman AL, Griner PF: Diagnostic uses of the activated partial thromboplastin time and prothrombin time. Ann Intern Med 104:810, 1986
29. Kasper CK: Therapy of factor VIII inhibitors. p. 59. In Zimmerman TS, Ruggeri AM (eds): Coagulation and Bleeding Disorders—The Role of Factor VIII and von Willebrand Factor. Marcel Dekker, New York, 1989
30. Kitchens CS: Prolonged activated partial thromboplastin time of unknown etiology: a prospective study of 100 consecutive cases referred for consultation. Am J Hematol 27:38, 1988
31. Kasper CK, Aledort LM, Counts RB et al: A more uniform measurement of factor VIII inhibitors. Thromb Diath Haemorrh 34:869, 1975
32. Kessler CM: An introduction to factor VIII inhibitors: the detection and quantitation. Am J Med, suppl. 5A. 91:15, 1991
33. Rizza CR, Biggs R: The treatment of patients who have factor VIII antibodies. Br J Haematol 24:65, 1973
34. Love PE, Santoro SA: Antiphospholipid antibodies: anticardiolipin and the lupus anticoagulant in systemic lupus erythematosus (SLE) and in non-SLE disorders. Ann Intern Med 112:682, 1990
35. McNeil HP, Chesterman CN, Krilis SA: Anticardiolipin antibodies and lupus anticoagulants comprise separate antibody subgroups with different phospholipid binding characteristics. Br J Haematol 73:506, 1989
36. Gastineau DA, Kazmier FJ, Nichols WL, Bowie EJW: Lupus anticoagulant: an analysis of the clinical and laboratory features of 219 cases. Am J Hematol 19:265, 1985

37. Triplett DA: Coagulation assays for the lupus anticoagulant: review and critique of current methodology. Stroke suppl. 1. 23:11, 1992

38. Exner T, Triplett DA, Taberner D, Machin SJ: Guidelines for testing and revised criteria for lupus anticoagulants. Thromb Haemost 65:320, 1991

39. Harris EN: The Second International Anti-Cardiolipin Standardization Workshop/The Kingston Anti-Phospholipid Antibody Study (KAPS) Group. Am J Clin Pathol 94:476, 1990

40. Ockelford PA, Carter CJ: Disseminated intravascular coagulation: the application and utility of diagnostic tests. Semin Thromb Hemost 8:198, 1982

41. Clauss A: Gerinnungsphysiologische schnell Methods zur Bestimmung des Fibrinogens. Acta Haematol 17:237, 1957

42. Ellis BC, Stransky A: A quick and accurate method for the detection of fibrinogen in plasma. J Lab Clin Med 58:477, 1961

43. Flaherty MJ, Henderson R, Wener MH: Iatrogenic immunization with bovine thrombin: a mechanism of prolonged thrombin times after surgery. Ann Intern Med 1112:631, 1989

44. Gastineau DA, Gertz MA, Daneils TM et al: Inhibitor of the thrombin time in systemic amyloidosis: a common coagulation abnormality. Blood 77:2637, 1991

45. Carr ME, Gabriel DA: Hyperfibrinogenemia as a cause of prolonged thrombin clotting time. South Med J 79:563, 1986

46. Steinberg MH, Kelton JG, Coller BS: Plasma glycocalicin—an aid in the classification of thrombocytopenic disorders. N Engl J Med 317:1037, 1987

47. Bloom AL: von Willebrand factor: clinical features of inherited and acquired disorders. Mayo Clin Proc 66:743, 1991

48. Ruggeri ZM: Structure and function of von Willebrand factor: relationship to von Willebrand's disease. Mayo Clin Proc 66:847, 1991

49. Rodeghiero F, Castaman G, Dini E: Epidemiologic investigation of the prevalence of von Willebrand's disease. Blood 69:454, 1987

50. Triplett DA: Laboratory diagnosis of von Willebrand's disease. Mayo Clin Proc 66:832, 1991

51. Zimmerman TS, Hoyer LW, Dickson L, Edgington TS: Determination of the von Willebrand's disease antigen (factor VIII-related antigen) in plasma by quantitative immunoelectrophoresis. J Lab Clin Med 86:152, 1975

52. Gill JC, Endres-Brooks J, Bauer PJ et al: The effect of ABO blood group on the diagnosis of von Willebrand disease. Blood 69:1691, 1987

53. Weiss HJ, Hoyer LW, Rickles FR et al: Quantitative assay of a plasma factor deficient in von Willebrand's disease that is necessary for platelet aggregation. J Clin Invest 52:2708, 1973

54. Macfarlane DE, Stibbe J, Kirby EP et al: A method for assaying von Willebrand factor (ristocetin cofactor). Thromb Diath Haemorrh 34:306, 1975

55. Weiss HJ: Abnormalities of factor VIII and platelet aggregation—use of ristocetin in diagnosing the von Willebrand syndrome. Blood 45:403, 1975

56. Zimmerman TS, Roberts J, Edgington TS: Factor VIII-related antigen: multiple molecular forms in human plasma. Proc Natl Acad Sci USA 72:5121, 1975

57. Ruggeri ZM, Zimmerman TS: Variant von Willebrand disease: characterization of two subtypes by analysis of multimeric composition of factor VIII/von Willebrand factor in plasma and platelets. J Clin Invest 65:1318, 1980

58. Ruggeri ZM, Pareti FI, Mannucci PM et al: Heightened interaction between platelets and factor VIII/von Willebrand factor in a new subtype of von Willebrand's disease. N Engl J Med 302:1047, 1980

59. Weiss HJ, Meyer D, Rabinowitz R et al: Pseudo-von Willebrand's disease. An intrinsic platelet defect with aggregation by unmodified human factor VIII/von Willebrand factor and enhanced adsorption of its high molecular weight multimers. N Engl J Med 306:326, 1982

60. Miller JL, Castella A: Platelet-type von Willebrand's disease: characterization of a new bleeding disorder. Blood 60:790, 1982

61. Abildgaard CF, Suzuki Z, Harrison J et al: Serial studies in von Willebrand's disease: Variability versus "variants." Blood 56:712, 1980

62. Yardumian DA, Macki IJ, Machin SJ: Laboratory investigation of platelet function: a review of methodology. J Clin Pathol 39:701, 1986

63. Tiffany ML: Technical considerations for platelet aggregation and related problems. CRC Crit Rev Clin Lab Sci 19:27, 1985

64. Williams CE, Entwistle MBP, Short PE: Platelet function tests: a critical review of methods. Med Lab Sci 42:262, 1985

65. Montgomery RR, Kunicki TJ, Taves C et al: Diagnosis of Bernard-Soulier syndrome, and Glanzmann's thrombasthenia with a monoclonal assay on whole blood. J Clin Invest 71:385, 1983

66. Jennings LK, Ashmun RA, Wang WC, Dokter ME: Analysis of human platelet glycoprotein IIb-IIIa and Glanzmann's thrombasthenia in whole blood by flow cytometry. Blood 68:173, 1986

67. Ginsberg MH, Frelinger AL, Lam SC-T et al: Analysis of platelet aggregation disorders based on flow cytometric analysis of membrane GPIIB-IIIa with conformation specific monoclonal antibodies. Blood 76:2017, 1990

68. Lorand L, Losowsky MS, Miloszewski KJM: Human factor XIII: fibrin-stabilizing factor. Prog Hemost Thromb 5:245, 1980

69. Otis PT, Feinstein DI, Rapaport SI, Patch MJ: An acquired inhibitor of fibrin stabilization associated with isoniazid therapy: clinical and biochemical observations. Blood 44:771, 1974

70. Girolami A, Sartori MT, Simioni P: An updated classification of factor XIII defect. Br J Haematol 77:565, 1991

71. Dempfle CE, Harenberg J, Hochreuter K, Heene DL: Microtiter assay for measurement of factor XIII activity in plasma. J Lab Clin Med 119:522, 1992

72. Fickenscher K, Aab A, Stüber W: A photometric assay for blood coagulation factor XIII. Thromb Haemost 65:535, 1991

73. Bick RL: Disseminated intravascular coagulation. Hematol Oncol Clin North Am 6:1259, 1992

74. Kobayashi N, Maekawa T, Takada M et al: Criteria for diagnosis of DIC based on the analysis of clinical and laboratory findings in 345 DIC patients collected by the research committee on DIC in Japan. Bibl Haematol 49:265, 1983

75. Siegal T, Seligsohn U, Aghai E, Modan M: Clinical and laboratory aspects of disseminated intravascular coagulation (DIC): a study of 118 cases. Thromb Haemost 39:122, 1978

76. Carr JM, McKinney M, McDonagh J: Diagnosis of disseminated intravascular coagulation—role of D-dimer. Am J Clin Pathol 91:280, 1989

77. Wilde JT, Kitchen S, Kinsey S et al: Plasma D-dimer levels and their relationship to serum fibrinogen/fibrin degradation products in hypercoagulable states. Br J Haematol 71:65, 1989

78. Boisclair MD, Lane DA, Wilde JT et al: A comparative evaluation of assays for markers of activated coagulation and/or fibrinolysis: thrombin-antithrombin complex, D-dimer and fibrinogen/fibrin fragment E antigen. Br J Haematol 74:471, 1990

79. Greenberg CS, Devine DV, McCrae KM: Measurement of plasma fibrin D-dimer levels with the use of a monoclonal antibody coupled to latex beads. Am J Clin Pathol 87:94, 1987

80. Sigal SH, Cembrowski GS, Shattil SJ et al: Prototypic quantitative assay for fibrinogen/fibrin degradation products. Arch Intern Med 147:1790, 1987

81. Kario K, Matsuo T, Kabayashi H et al: Rapid quantitative evaluation of plasma D-dimer levels in thrombotic states using an automated latex photometric immunoassay. Thromb Res 66:179, 1992

82. Berkowitz SD, Ruggeri ZM, Zimmerman TS: von Willebrand disease. p. 215. In Zimmerman TS, Ruggeri ZM (eds): Coagulation and Bleeding Disorders—The Role of Factor VIII and von Willebrand Factor. Marcel Dekker, New York, 1989

83. White GC, Marder VJ, Colman RW et al: Approach to the bleeding patient. p. 1048. In Colman RW, Hirsh J, Marder VJ, Salzman EW (eds): Hemostasis and Thrombosis—Basic Principles and Clinical Practice. 2nd Ed. JB Lippincott, Philadelphia, 1987

Structure, Biology, and Genetics of Factor VIII

105

Randall J. Kaufman and Stylianos E. Antonarakis

INTRODUCTION

Hemophilia A, a bleeding disorder resulting from a deficiency in factor VIII, was documented >1,700 years ago in the Talmud.[1] The genetics of hemophilia A were described during the early 1800s,[2] and transfusion of whole blood was shown to treat a hemophilia-associated bleeding episode successfully by 1840.[3] The presence of factor VIII in plasma was demonstrated in 1911,[4] and in 1937 Patek and Taylor[5] described its role in hemostasis. However, a detailed structural characterization of the factor VIII gene and protein product was only recently achieved.

Since Hemophilia A and von Willebrand disease are both associated with factor VIII deficiency, their relationship was confused for many years. Early preparations of antihemophilic factor were demonstrated not only to correct the clotting time of hemophilic plasma, but also to restore platelet adhesion and agglutination defects in the plasma from patients with von Willebrand disease. Over the last decade it has been demonstrated that factor VIII and von Willebrand factor (vWF) are two separate proteins that exist as a complex in plasma and that are under separate genetic control. These proteins have distinct biochemical and immunologic properties, as well as unique and essential physiologic functions. Factor VIII is an X-linked gene product that accelerates the activation of factor X by factor IXa in the presence of calcium and phospholipid. vWF is an autosomal gene product that is essential for platelet adhesion to subendothelium and for ristocetin-induced platelet agglutination. Since vWF and factor VIII are found in the plasma as a complex and vWF serves to stabilize factor VIII and regulate its activity, the activities of these two proteins are intimately intertwined. Based on a greater understanding of factor VIII and vWF, in 1985 the Subcommittee on factor VIII and vWF of the International Committee on Thrombosis and Haemostasis formulated nomenclature guidelines[6]: factor VIII protein is designated VIII; factor VIII antigen is designated VIII:Ag; factor VIII procoagulant activity is designated VIII:C; von Willebrand factor is designated vWF; and von Willebrand factor antigen is designated vWF:Ag.

FACTOR VIII FUNCTION

The physiologic response to blood vessel injury is the sequential activation of plasma proteases of the blood coagulation cascade, leading to the localized generation of thrombin and the conversion of fibrinogen to fibrin (see Ch. 100). Thrombin generation requires the interaction of proteases, protein cofactors, and substrate zymogens that assemble on a phospholipid surface or the cell surface. Factor VIII is proteolytically activated by factor Xa or thrombin, or both, to yield factor VIIIa, which serves as a cofactor for factor IXa-mediated activation of factor X.

The mechanism by which factor VIIIa functions in the factor Xa-generating complex is poorly understood. Factor VIII has no enzymatic activity of its own but acts as a cofactor to increase the V_{max} of factor X activation by factor IXa by 10,000-fold in the presence of negatively charged phospholipids and calcium.[7] The mechanism by which factor VIIIa accelerates the proteolysis of factor X by factor IXa likely involves the interaction of factor VIIIa and factor IXa on a phospholipid surface to facilitate a conformational change in the enzyme that favors catalysis.[8]

The reported specific activity of pure factor VIII ranges from 2,300 U/mg[9] to 8,000 U/mg.[10] The definition of factor VIII activity is complicated, since thrombin converts the cofactor into a much more active form. However, for standardization, 1 U of factor VIII is defined as that amount of activity in 1 ml of normal pooled human plasma measured in a factor VIII assay using factor VIII-deficient plasma.[11] For greater convenience and precision, factor VIII activity can be measured by its ability to promote activation of factor X in the presence of factor IXa, phospholipid, and Ca^{2+}. Factor Xa is measured directly by monitoring cleavage of a synthetic chromogenic substrate.[12] Factor VIII antigen can be measured using factor VIII-specific antibodies in specific immunoassays.[13]

Characterization of factor VIII has been hampered by its low concentration in plasma, its heterogeneity in size, and its exquisite sensitivity to degradation. Recent advances in our understanding of factor VIII resulted from the use of immunoaffinity chromatography for the successful purification of factor VIII from porcine[14] and human plasma,[9,15] and from the cloning of the human factor VIII gene and elucidation of the primary structure of factor VIII.[16–18]

FACTOR VIII STRUCTURE

The deduced primary amino acid sequence of human factor VIII determined from the cloned cDNA demonstrated that factor VIII is encoded by a precursor protein of 2,351 amino acid residues from which a 19-amino-acid signal peptide is cleaved. Plasma factor VIII is a heterodimer processed from a larger precursor polypeptide. It consists of a COOH-terminal-derived light chain of 80,000 MW in a metal ion-dependent association with an NH_2-terminal-derived heavy chain fragment of 90,000–200,000 MW.[16,18] In the plasma this complex is stabilized by association through hydrophilic and hydrophobic interactions with a 50-fold excess of vWF. The amino acid sequence revealed an organization of three structural domains that occur in the order A1:A2:B:A3:C1:C2, as shown in Figure 105-1.[16,18] The A1 (amino acid residues 1–329) and A2 (380–711) domains of factor VIII are located in the heavy chain and the A3 (1,649–2,019) domain is located in the light chain. The A domains have 30% homology to each other, to the triplicated A domains of ceruloplasmin and factor V.[16,19,20] The residues implicated for copper binding in ceruloplasmin are conserved in the first and third A domains of factor VIII, suggesting that the A domains of factor VIII may be involved in metal ion binding. However, these residues are not conserved in the A domains of factor V, although copper ions were detected in purified preparations of factor V[21] and factor VIII.[22] The C1 (residues 2,020–2,172) and C2 (residues 2,173–2,332) domains are located in the terminus of the factor VIII light chain and exhibit homology to milk fat globule protein and to A, C, and D chains of discoidin 1, which are all capable of binding glyco-conjugates and negatively charged phospholipids.[23,24] The B

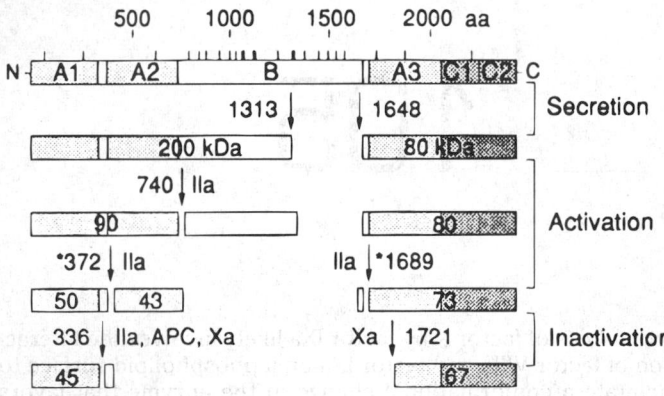

Fig. 105-1. Domain structure and processing of factor VIII. The structural domains of factor VIII are depicted in the top line: (1) a triplicated A domain of 330 amino acids, (2) a unique B domain of 980 amino acids, and (3) a duplicated C domain of 150 amino acids. The hatched areas represent highly acidic regions. The vertical bars represent the position of potential asparagine-linked glycosylation sites. Intracellularly, factor VIII is cleaved within the B domain to generate a 200-kd peptide and the 80-kd light chain polypeptide. The thrombin (IIa), activated protein C (APC), and factor Xa (Xa) cleavage sites are shown. Factor Xa also cleaves at all the thrombin cleavage sites. The two cleavages required for thrombin activation are indicated (*). (From Kaufman,[211] with permission.)

domain is encoded by a single large exon of 3,100 nucleotides, has no known homology to other proteins, and contains 18 of the 25 potential asparagine (N)-linked glycosylation sites within factor VIII. The cloning of the factor V cDNA and gene revealed a high degree of amino acid conservation between the A and C domains with no detectable homology within the B domains,[19] although both B domains are encoded by large single exons. The domain organization and homologies between factors V and VIII suggest that these genes evolved from a primordial ferroxidase gene by triplication of the A domain, insertion of the B domain, and addition of the two C domains. After duplication of the primordial cofactor gene, the factor V and factor VIII genes likely evolved by extensive divergence of amino acid residues within the B domain, while amino acid residues within the A and C domains were conserved.

In addition to the A, B, and C domains, there are three acidic amino acid-rich regions in the factor VIII protein molecule at the junction of the A1/A2 (residues 331–372), A2/B (residues 700–740), and B/A3 (residues 1,649–1,689) domains that are juxtaposed to sites of thrombin cleavage (Fig. 105-1). All these acidic regions also contain the post-translationally modified amino acid tyrosine sulfate at residues 364, 718, 719, 721, 1,664, and 1,680.[25] The murine factor VIII cDNA is highly homologous to the A and C domains of human factor VIII, whereas the acidic regions and B domain show partial homology.[26] However, all thrombin cleavage sites and sulfated tyrosine residues are conserved. The murine factor VIII B domain also contains 19 potential N-linked glycosylation sites, although in different positions than in the human sequence, suggesting that glycosylation in the B domain is important for factor VIII expression or function, or for both.

BIOSYNTHESIS AND METABOLISM OF FACTOR VIII

The natural cell type(s) that produces factor VIII has not been definitively identified. However, evidence obtained from liver transplantation in factor VIII-deficient dogs[27,28] and several hemophiliac patients[29,30] strongly implies that the liver is a major site of factor VIII synthesis. In addition, immunochemical localization by light microscopic[31] or electron microscopic[32] examination detected the factor VIII antigen in hepatocytes.

However, RNA hybridization analysis has detected factor VIII mRNA in hepatocytes and in many other cells and tissues.[33] To date there are no known established cell lines that express factor VIII. Thus, it has not been possible to study the biosynthesis of factor VIII in its natural host cell. However, the expression of factor VIII in mammalian cells transfected with the factor VIII gene allowed analysis of the biosynthesis and processing of this glycoprotein.[34]

Analysis of the expression of factor VIII in Chinese hamster ovary cells provided insights into its probable biosynthetic pathway (Fig. 105-2). On synthesis, factor VIII is translocated into the lumen of the endoplasmic reticulum (ER), where the signal peptide is cleaved. In the ER, addition of high-mannose oligosaccharide to multiple asparagine residues within the factor VIII molecule occurs. A significant portion of the factor VIII in the ER is bound to a resident protein of the ER, the glucose-regulated protein of 78,000 MW (GRP78), also known as immunoglobulin-binding protein, or BiP.[35,36] BiP expression is induced by glucose deprivation, inhibition of N-linked glycosylation, or the presence of malfolded protein within the ER.[37,38] Increased BiP expression inhibits factor VIII secretion.[39] BiP exhibits a peptide-dependent ATPase activity.[40] Dissociation from BiP and secretion of factor VIII require unusually high levels of intracellular ATP.[41] It is speculated that either the BiP-mediated ATP-dependent release assists protein folding or that BiP binding prohibits improperly folded molecules exiting the ER compartment and directs them to degradation. The secretion-competent factor VIII transits to the Golgi apparatus. In the Golgi apparatus, most factor VIII is cleaved at two sites within the B domain after residues 1,313 and 1,648 to generate the heavy chains (90,000–200,000 MW) and the light chain (80,000 MW). Also within the Golgi apparatus, factor VIII is further processed by (1) modification of the asparagine-linked high-mannose-containing oligosaccharides to complex types, (2) addition of carbohydrate to multiple serine and threonine residues within the B domain, and (3) addition of sulfate to six tyrosine residues within the heavy and the light chains.

vWF promotes the association of the light and heavy chains of factor VIII and results in accumulation of stable factor VIII activity in the conditioned medium of factor VIII-producing cells.[34,42] The heavy and light chains of factor VIII synthesized in the absence of vWF in the conditioned medium are secreted as dissociated chains that are subsequently degraded. The effect of vWF in promoting assembly and stable secretion of factor VIII in cell-culture systems may reflect the role of vWF in regulating levels of factor VIII activity in vivo.[43–47] These findings suggest that the reduction in factor VIII levels associated with vWF deficiency may result partly from the inability of factor VIII to be stabilized in the plasma on secretion from the cell.

Factor VIII and vWF are cleared with a half-life of 12 hours on infusion of the factor VIII11/vWF complex into hemophilia patients.[43,46,47] Infusion of pure factor VIII also exhibits clearance kinetics similar to that of factor VIII/vWF complex, presumably due to rapid binding of factor VIII to plasma vWF.[44,45] By contrast, infusion of pure factor VIII into patients with severe von Willebrand disease or into severe vWF-deficient dogs results in rapid clearance (half-life of 2.4 hours).[43,45] These studies establish the stabilizing influence of vWF for factor VIII in the circulation. Autosomally inherited factor VIII deficiency results from genetic defects in vWF that reduce its ability to bind and stabilize factor VIII in plasma.[48,49]

INTERACTIONS OF FACTOR VIII WITH COMPONENTS OF HEMOSTASIS

Binding to von Willebrand Factor

vWF plays a critical role in regulating factor VIII activity by several different mechanisms. vWF stabilizes factor VIII on secretion from the cell[34,42] and is required for its normal survival

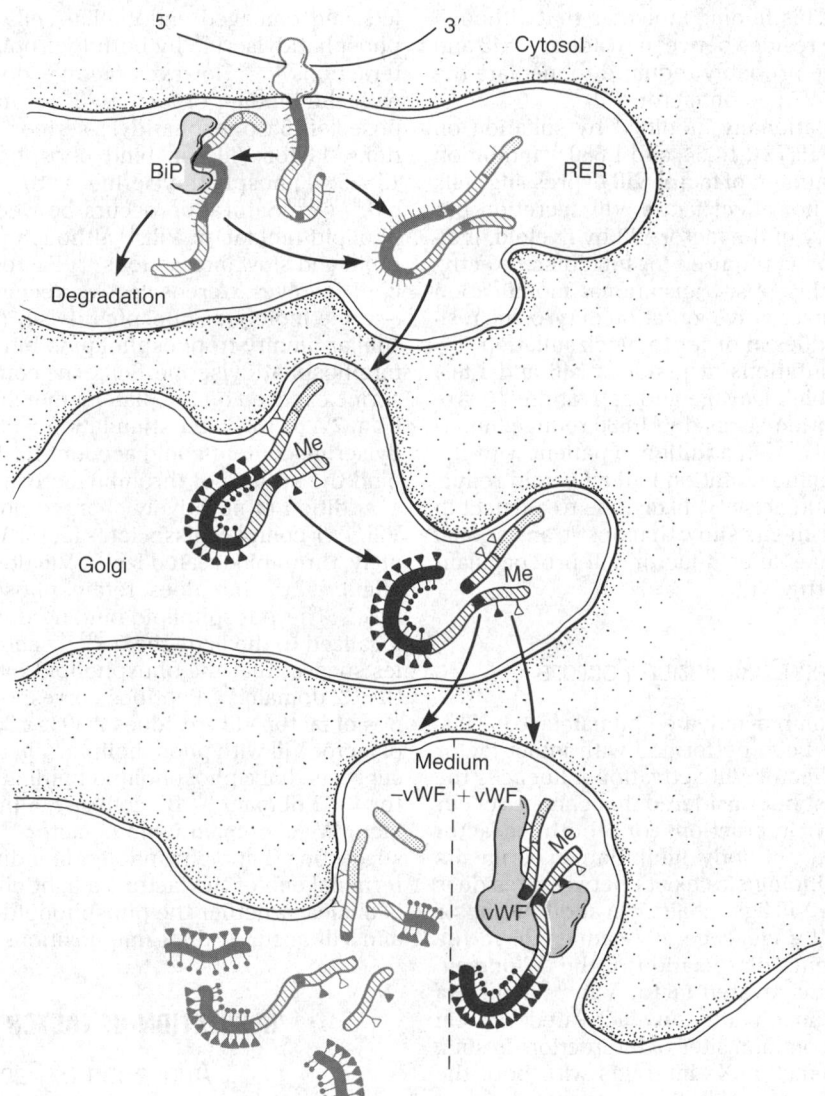

Fig. 105-2. Synthesis, processing, and secretion of factor VIII in mammalian cells. The factor VIII primary translation product is translocated into the lumen of the ER, where asparagine-linked glycosylation occurs. A fraction of factor VIII binds tightly to the glucose-regulated protein of 78 kd (GRP78 or BiP) and is probably destined for degradation. A proportion of the molecules transit to the Golgi apparatus, where complex modification of carbohydrate on asparagine-linked sites (Y), addition of carbohydrate to serine and threonine residues (♥), sulfation of tyrosine residues, and cleavage of the protein to the mature heavy and light chains occur. The presence of vWF in the medium promotes stable secretion of factor VIII. In the absence of vWF, the individual chains are secreted and degraded. The A (crosshatched), B (solid black), and C (dotted) domains are indicated. The acidic regions where tyrosine sulfation occurs adjacent to the A domains are shown (solid black). (From Kaufman et al.,[34] with permission.)

in plasma.[43–47] vWF protects factor VIII from activation by factor Xa[50] and from inactivation by activated protein C[51,52] but does not interfere with activation by thrombin.[53,54] Finally, vWF prevents factor VIII binding to phospholipids[55,56] and activated platelets.[57] Based on these functions, it is proposed that vWF binding to platelet receptor glycoprotein (GP)Ib brings factor VIII to the vicinity of platelets adhering to damaged endothelium.[57]

The interaction of factor VIII with vWF is mediated by a major factor VIII-binding site that resides within the first 272 amino acids of the mature vWF molecule.[58–60] Specific missense mutations within this region of vWF can cause autosomal hemophilia due to a deficiency in factor VIII.[49] Most vWF molecules contain one factor VIII-binding site that can be saturated in vitro.[61] However, the ratio of factor VIII to vWF observed in vivo is 1:50.[44]

The corresponding vWF binding site on factor VIII resides within the NH₂ terminus of the light chain of factor VIII.[62–65] A

vWF-binding site on factor VIII was localized by monoclonal antibody inhibition to residues 1,673 to 1,684.[66,67] This region is composed of a high density of acidic amino acids located at the NH₂ terminus of the factor VIII light chain and is removed by thrombin cleavage at residue 1,689 (Fig. 105-1). Deletion of the acidic region in the NH₂ terminus of the light chain by site-directed mutagenesis yielded a molecule that did not bind vWF with high affinity, although the purified protein had a specific activity similar to wild-type factor VIII.[57] These results demonstrate that the acidic region within residues 1,649–1,689 of the light chain is critical for appropriate interaction with vWF but is not required for cofactor function of factor VIII. It was recently demonstrated that antibodies that bind the factor VIII C2 domain can inhibit binding to vWF and to phosphatidylserine.[68] This observation is consistent with the presence of a phospholipid-binding region between residues 2,303 and 2,332 within the C2 domain[69] and that phospholipid and vWF compete for binding to factor VIII.[55,56] This finding indicates that although a primary vWF-binding site resides between residues 1,648 and 1,689, multiple contacts are probably required to mediate the multitude of effects that vWF has on factor VIII.

Factor VIII is post-translationally modified by sulfation on tyrosine residues 346,718,719,721, 1,664, and 1,680.[25] Inhibition of tyrosine sulfation by treatment of factor VIII-expressing cells with sodium chlorate did not affect factor VIII secretion but reduced the specific activity of the factor VIII by fivefold, indicating that this modification is required for full cofactor activity.[25] The importance of this post-translational modification was also studied by the conservative mutation of tyrosine residues to phenylalanine residues in order to block sulfation. Tyrosine to phenylalanine mutations at residues 346 and 1,664 reduced the rate of thrombin cleavage and activation.[70] Tyrosine to phenylalanine mutation at residue 1,680 reduced interaction with vWF by fivefold.[70,71] In addition, a patient with the 1,680 tyrosine-to-phenylalanine mutation had a fivefold reduction in factor VIII antigen and activity, likely due to a defect in vWF binding.[72] These experiments show that post-translational sulfation of tyrosine residues affects factor VIII procoagulant activity and interaction with vWF.

Binding to Other Coagulation Factors

Due to the lability of thrombin-activated human factor VIIIa, most binding studies have been performed with intact factor VIII. Since it is known that factor VIII activation influences the activity of factor IXa,[8] it must be considered that changes occur in binding affinities or sites of interactions (or in both) on factor VIII activation. Monoclonal antibody inhibition experiments suggest that a factor IXa-binding site exists between residues 1,770 and 1,840 of the factor VIII light chain.[73] In addition, factor IXa inactivates factor VIII by cleavage at residue 336 in the heavy chain[74,75] and prevents dissociation of the A2-domain polypeptide from thrombin-activated factor VIII.[76] Factor IXa protects factor VIII from inactivation by activated protein C,[77-79] indicating possible common sites of interaction. In sum, these results suggest that factor IXa interacts with both the heavy and light chains of factor VIII. Similar characteristics were identified for the binding of enzyme factor Xa to factor Va where both the heavy chain[80,81] and light chain[82,83] contribute to binding. There is suggestive evidence that factor X interacts with factor VIII.[84,85] However, no studies have localized the site of binding. Factor Va mediates binding of the substrate prothrombin via the factor V heavy chain.[80]

In the presence of anionic phospholipids and Ca^{2+}, activated protein C inactivates factors Va and VIIIa.[86] Factor Va is cleaved by activated protein C after residues 506 and 1,765, although cleavage after residue 506 is likely responsible for the loss in cofactor activity.[87] Similarly, activated protein C cleaves factor VIII and factor VIIIa after multiple residues 336, 562, and 740.[88] Inactivation is more closely associated with cleavage after residue 562, the site homologous to residue 506 in factor V. Binding sites for activated protein C were localized to the light chains at residues 1,865–1,874 in factor Va and 2,009–2,010 in factor VIII, which are both localized to a homologous region in the COOH-terminal end of the A3-domain.[89]

Binding to Phospholipids

Phospholipids interact with substrates, enzymes, and cofactors to play a critical role in the assembly and functional activity of the coagulation protease complexes. Negatively charged phospholipids are required for factor VIIIa-mediated enhancement of the activation of factor X.[7,90,91] In vivo, the negatively charged phospholipids are likely provided by activated plate-lets and damaged endothelial cells. Factors VIII and V bind phosphatidylserine by both hydrophobic and electrostatic interactions.[92-98] However, factor V does not efficiently compete with the binding of factor VIII to phospholipid vesicles composed of 15% phosphatidyl-L-serine.[90] Under equilibrium conditions, factor VIII can bind phospholipid vesicles containing 15–25% phosphatidylserine with an apparent K_d of 2–4 nM.[90,99,100] Saturation occurs between 170 and 385 mol phospholipid/mol factor VIII,[90] although the process involves both rapid and slow interactions.[101] Factor VIII binding to phospholipid involves stereoselective recognition of the O-phospho-L-serine moiety of phosphatidylserine.[102] Factor V displays a similar affinity to phospholipids but has a lower requirement for phosphatidylserine. Since the composition of phosphatidylserine exposed on the platelet membrane surface can increase from 2% to 13% after stimulation,[103] the increase in phosphatidylserine content could account for the ability of factor VIII to bind the surface of thrombin-activated platelets specifically.

Addition of negatively charged phospholipids to the factor VIII/vWF complex dissociates factor VIII from vWF.[55,56] Interestingly, thrombin-treated factor VIII does not bind vWF with high affinity[53,62,65] but does retain phospholipid binding properties.[56] The phospholipid-binding domain within factor VIII is localized to the light chain,[104,105] and antibody inhibition studies suggest that the phospholipid binding site likely occurs in the C2 domain.[106] Peptides corresponding to the COOH terminus of factor VIII (residues 2,303–2,332) inhibit the interaction of factor VIII with phospholipid.[69] In addition, deletion analysis suggests that a phospholipid-binding domain resides in the factor V C2 domain.[107] By contrast, a proteolytic fragment of the factor V A3 domain inhibits factor V binding to phospholipid, suggesting that a phospholipid-binding site resides in the NH2-terminal end of the factor Va light chain.[108] Thus, at present it is unclear whether the phospholipid-binding sites of factors V and VIII occur at the same positions within the proteins.

REGULATION OF FACTOR VIII ACTIVITY

Activation of Factor VIII

On treatment of intact factor VIII with thrombin, a rapid 30-fold increase and subsequent first-order decay of procoagulant activity occurs. The activation coincides with proteolysis of both the heavy and light chains of factor VIII (Fig. 105-1). Cleavage within the heavy chain after arginine residue 740 generates a 90,000 MW polypeptide that is subsequently cleaved after arginine residue 372 to generate polypeptides of 50,000 MW and 43,000 MW.[109] Concomitantly, the 80,000 MW light chain is cleaved after arginine residue 1,689 to generate a 73,000 MW polypeptide.[109] Each thrombin cleavage site is bordered by a region rich in acidic amino acids that also contains the post-translationally modified amino acid tyrosine sulfate.[25] The tyrosine sulfate residues enhance thrombin cleavage at adjacent sites,[70] suggesting that these regions interact with the anion binding exosite in thrombin, similar to the thrombin interaction with the COOH-terminal end of hirudin that has acidic amino acids and also contains tyrosine sulfate.[110,111]

Numerous studies correlated the appearance of 90,000, 50,000, 43,000, and 73,000 MW polypeptides with peak factor VIII activity.[109,112,113] Mutagenesis studies showed that cleavages after residues 740 and 1,648 were not required for cofactor activity.[114] By contrast, mutation at either Arg 372 or Arg 1,689 yielded molecules that were not cleaved by thrombin at the mutated site and were not susceptible to thrombin activation.[114,115] Resistance to thrombin cleavage at one site did not alter susceptibility to thrombin cleavage at the other cleavage sites. The importance of cleavage at residues 372 and 1,689 for activation of factor VIII was also elucidated when missense mutations were identified in hemophilia A patients at either residue 372 or residue 1,689.[116,117] In contrast to most hemophilia A patients, these patients have normal levels of circulating factor VIII antigen but no detectable factor VIII activity. These findings indicate that activation requires cleavage at both residues 372 and 1,689, but does not appear to require a specific sequential order for cleavage at these sites. Cleavage at 1,689 releases factor VIII from the inhibitory influence of vWF and accounts for a portion of the increase in factor VIII activity.[118] However, cleavage at 1,689 appears additionally to increase the activity of factor VIII in the absence of vWF.[119]

The B domain, delimited by amino acid residues 740 and 1,648, is cleaved from factor VIII during and activation. Comparison of the deduced amino acid sequence of porcine, murine, and human factor VIII showed a striking divergence within the B domains, whereas the bordering A2 and A3 domains exhibit 80–85% homology.[18,26] Factor VIII molecules constructed to lack most or all of the B domain have specific activities, thrombin cleavage products (except for the B domain), and thrombin activation coefficients similar to the wild-type molecule.[120,121] The B domain deletion molecules exhibit no detectable difference in vWF binding, survival in plasma, and ability to normalize the cuticle bleeding time after infusion into a factor VIII-deficient dog, compared with the wild-type factor VIII.[54] By these analyses, removal of the B domain did not affect in vitro or in vivo procoagulant activity. One notable difference between wild-type and B-domain deleted factor VIII is that the B domain deleted molecule is expressed at 5–10-fold higher levels, exhibits a reduced association with BiP in the endoplasmic reticulum, and is secreted more efficiently.[36,54] This suggests that the B domain may regulate factor VIII biosynthesis. It is also possible that the B domain may have procoagulant, anticoagulant, or vasoactive properties heretofore unknown. For example, a portion of the B domains of factor V and factor VIII can serve as a substrate for transglutaminase activity of factor XIII.[122,123]

Inactivation of Factor VIII

The activity of thrombin-activated factor VIII requires all polypeptides of the heterotrimer composed of the 50,000, 43,000, and 73,000 MW species.[124–126] The 53,000-MW A1 domain is in a metal ion-dependent association with the 73,000-MW light chain. The 43,000-MW A2 domain polypeptide is associated with the A1 domain and 73,000-MW light chain by electrostatic interactions that likely involve residues 336–372 between the A1 and A2 domains.[127,128] A detailed characterization of thrombin-activated factor VIIIa was hampered due to its marked instability. Protein concentration and pH are important factors for isolation of a stable thrombin-activated factor VIIIa.[129] Decay of factor VIII activity after thrombin activation in vitro does not correlate with any specific proteolytic event.[130,131] Loss of procoagulant activity in vitro is due to reversible dissociation of the 43,000-kd A2 domain polypeptide from the heterotrimer that occurs at physiologic pH.[127,132] The specific activity of porcine factor VIII is approximately fivefold greater than human factor VIIIa, which correlates with a lower K_d of the A2 domain polypeptide compared with the thrombin-activated heterotrimer.[132,133] Once activated by thrombin, factor VIIIa is stabilized by the addition of factor X and phospholipid.[134]

Factor VIII is inactivated by proteolytic cleavage. Cleavage after residue 336 is mediated by factor Xa,[109] factor IXa,[74,76] activated protein C,[109,135] and also thrombin in the presence of phospholipid.[25] Additionally, factor Xa and factor IXa cleave the light chain after residue 1719,[74,109] and activated protein C cleaves the heavy chain after residue 562.[88] Because of the multiple cleavages that occur with these enzymes, it is difficult to attribute the significance of any single cleavage to its role in factor VIII inactivation. The activation of protein C by thrombin is subject to regulation by thrombomodulin on the endothelial cell surface and may represent a significant mechanism to prevent factor VIIIa from escaping the localized area of vessel wall damage.[136] Protein C deficiency is associated with severe thrombotic disease, suggesting that this feedback mechanism may be physiologically significant.[137,138] The relative contributions of proteolytic inactivation and chain dissociation in regulating factor VIII activity in vivo are not known. The isolation of thrombin-activated factor VIIIa in a stable form should provide a means of characterizing the inactivation process directly.

Regulation of Factor VIII Activity by Biologic Membranes

Procoagulant activity is profoundly affected by the presence of cellular surfaces. On platelet activation by thrombin, the platelet surface exhibits procoagulant activity. This activity results from the exposure of negatively charged phospholipids and possibly specific receptors for the coagulation factors. Negatively charged phospholipids are usually confined to the inner leaflet of cellular membranes and are exposed on cellular lysis at sites of injury.[139,140] Unactivated platelets exhibit binding sites for factor Va and Xa.[141–143] Platelet activation is associated with exposure of factor VIII and factor IXa binding sites.[144–147] There are approximately 400 factor VIII sites per activated platelet, and factor V cannot compete with factor VIII binding.[144] The specificity in binding of factor VIII suggests that a specific receptor for factor VIII is involved. In addition, the kinetics of thrombin generation mediated by the prothrombinase complex on pure phospholipid surfaces compared with activated platelets suggest that a specific saturable receptor exists for prothrombinase, and probably also for the factor Xa-generating enzyme complex.[148] Platelet binding is mediated by the factor VIII light chain and is inhibited by the presence of vWF. A factor VIII mutant protein that cannot bind vWF with high affinity retains its ability to bind platelets.[57] Thus the vWF-binding site and the platelet-binding site appear to be distinct within the factor VIII molecule. After activation, factor VIIIa is released from vWF and is available to bind to activated platelets. Thus, one result of thrombin-mediated cleavage within the light chain on factor VIII activation is release of factor VIII from vWF to allow binding to platelets.

The anticoagulant properties of the endothelial cell surface is maintained by several independent mechanisms: (1) heparin sulfate on the surface of endothelial cells accelerates the inactivation of thrombin by antithrombin III; (2) thrombomodulin expressed on endothelial cells can alter the proteolytic specificity of thrombin to activate protein C; and (3) endothelial cells secrete prostacyclin, an inhibitor of platelet aggregation, and tissue plasminogen activator, an initiator of fibrinolysis. Endothelium also exhibits dramatic procoagulant activities. Activated endothelial cells induce expression of tissue factor and can mediate the activation of factor X. Endothelial cells contain high-affinity receptors for factor IX or IXa, as well as factor X.[149,150] At present it is not known whether specific binding sites for factor VIII exist on endothelial cells. Thus, the endothelial cell surface may positively or negatively influence factor VIII activity through the generation of activated protein C or by the binding of factor IXa and X to initiate assembly of the factor X-activating complex.

Regulation of Factor VIII Activation

The present understanding of the mechanism by which factor VIII functions is presented in Figure 105-3. The two chains of factor VIII are associated by a divalent metal ion bridge. vWF

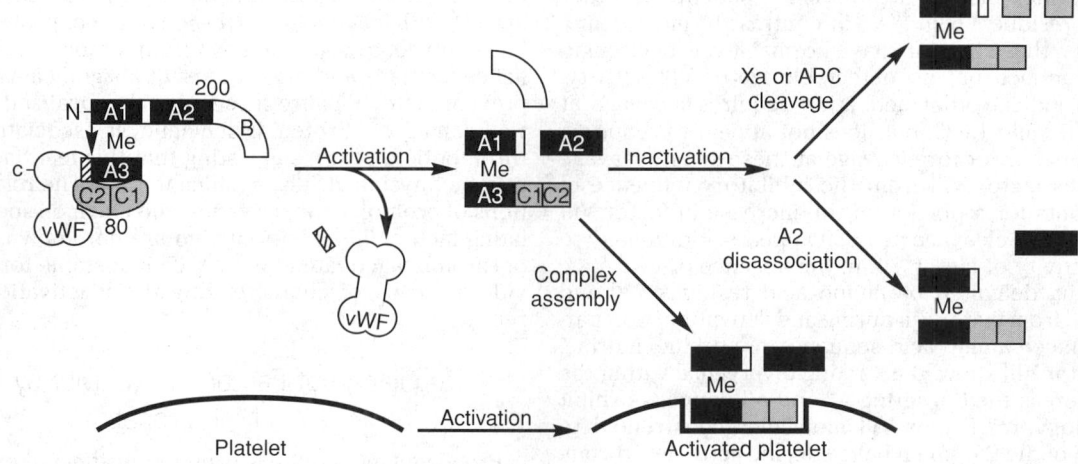

Fig. 105-3. Model for thrombin activation and inactivation of factor VIII. Factor VIII is depicted as two chains in a metal ion (Me) association. vWF ()---() is illustrated to promote association of the light and heavy chains of factor VIII. Thrombin cleavage at residues 336 and 1,689 releases the activated species from the vWF complex. Inactivation may occur through a conformational change (disassociation) or by a specific proteolytic event.

interacts with the NH_2 terminus and the COOH terminus of the light chain. The mechanism by which initial activation of factor VIII occurs is unknown, but recent evidence has accumulated showing that the extrinsic pathway may be the most significant physiologic initiator of factor VIIIa generation.[151] Patients deficient in factor VII have low levels of factor Xa compared with patients who have deficiencies in factor VIII.[152] In addition, infusion of VIIa into a chimpanzee increases the level of circulating factor Xa.[155] These results indicate that the primary mechanism of factor Xa generation in vivo is via the extrinsic pathway. Since patients deficient in factor VIII or factor IX do have a bleeding diathesis, there is a need for an intrinsic pathway for hemostasis in vivo. Two possible mechanisms could explain the need for factors VIII and IX in vivo. First, since factor Xa generation via the tissue factor pathway can bind tissue factor pathway inhibitor (TFPI) and subsequently inhibit the factor VIIa/tissue factor complex, only small amounts of factor Xa can be generated before further extrinsic factor X activation is inhibited.[154,155] Since TFPI does not inhibit the intrinsic formation of factor IXa or its activity, the intrinsic route is required to amplify the response. Alternatively, since the extrinsic pathway can activate factor IX in vitro, this pathway may primarily activate factor IX as opposed to factor X in vivo.[156] Either mechanism could explain the need for factors VIII and IX for effective hemostasis.

Factor VIII activation by thrombin requires cleavage at both residues 372 and 1,689. Cleavage at 1,689 releases activated factor VIII from vWF. Activated factor VIII is a heterotrimer composed of the 50,000 MW, 43,000 MW, and 73,000 MW polypeptides. Activated factor VIII is transferred from vWF to a factor VIII receptor present on activated platelets to participate in assembly of the active factor IXa complex.[57] Activated factor VIII is stabilized by assembly into the factor Xa complex.[134] After activation of factor VIII, there is a first-order decay of activity that, in vitro, likely results from dissociation of the A2 domain. In vivo, inactivation may also occur through proteolytic inactivation by activated protein C, factor Xa, or thrombin at residue 336 or 562, or both.

Activated factor VIII enhances the catalytic efficiency of factor IXa by 10,000-fold. Enhanced efficiency occurs through several mechanisms. Binding of factor VIII induces a conformational change in the factor IXa active site and greatly increases the k_{cat}.[99] The phospholipid membrane also binds factor IXa and factor X so that the enzyme complex and substrate are

concentrated within a two-dimensional surface to reduce the K_m. It is also likely that factor VIIIa interacts with factor X to enhance the extended substrate recognition site of factor IXa, analogous to the interaction of factor Va with meizothrombin.[157] Finally, membrane fluidity may also influence the kinetics of factor X activation, similar to thrombin activation, possibly by influencing the mechanism of catalysis.[158]

HEMOPHILIA A

The gene for factor VIII is on the human X chromosome, and therefore hemophilia A is a classic example of X-linked recessive inheritance. It occurs almost exclusively in males; females with one abnormal copy of the factor VIII gene are carriers because the other X chromosome contains a normal copy of the gene. The frequency of the disorder is 1 in 5,000–10,000 male births, and no particular ethnic group has an unusually lower or higher incidence of the disease. The severity and frequency of bleeding in patients correlate with the factor VIII activity in plasma.[159,160] Of particular interest for the understanding of factor VIII function is a category of patients who have a considerable amount of factor VIII protein in their plasma (≥30% of normal) but whose protein is nonfunctional (i.e., the factor VIII activity is much less than the factor VIII plasma level [usually <2% of normal]). Approximately 5% of patients belong to this category, termed cross-reacting material (CRM) positive.[161] Another category is called CRM reduced: the factor VIII antigen and activity are reduced to approximately the same level.

Before the introduction of modern treatment, severe hemophilia A was a genetically lethal disease in which affected men produced few offspring. Therefore, nearly one-third of the mutant alleles would be lost in each generation. In 1935 Haldane predicted that in order to maintain a constant frequency in the population, about one-third of cases would be the result of novel mutations. The prediction was proved correct, since a large number of different mutations have been found in the factor VIII gene, and many patients have been identified who carry a de novo mutation not present in the X chromosome of their mothers.

FACTOR VIII GENE STRUCTURE AND LOCATION

The factor VIII gene is 186 kb long (approximately 0.1% of the DNA of the X chromosome) and contains 26 exons and 25 introns. The nucleotide sequence of the exons, intron-exon

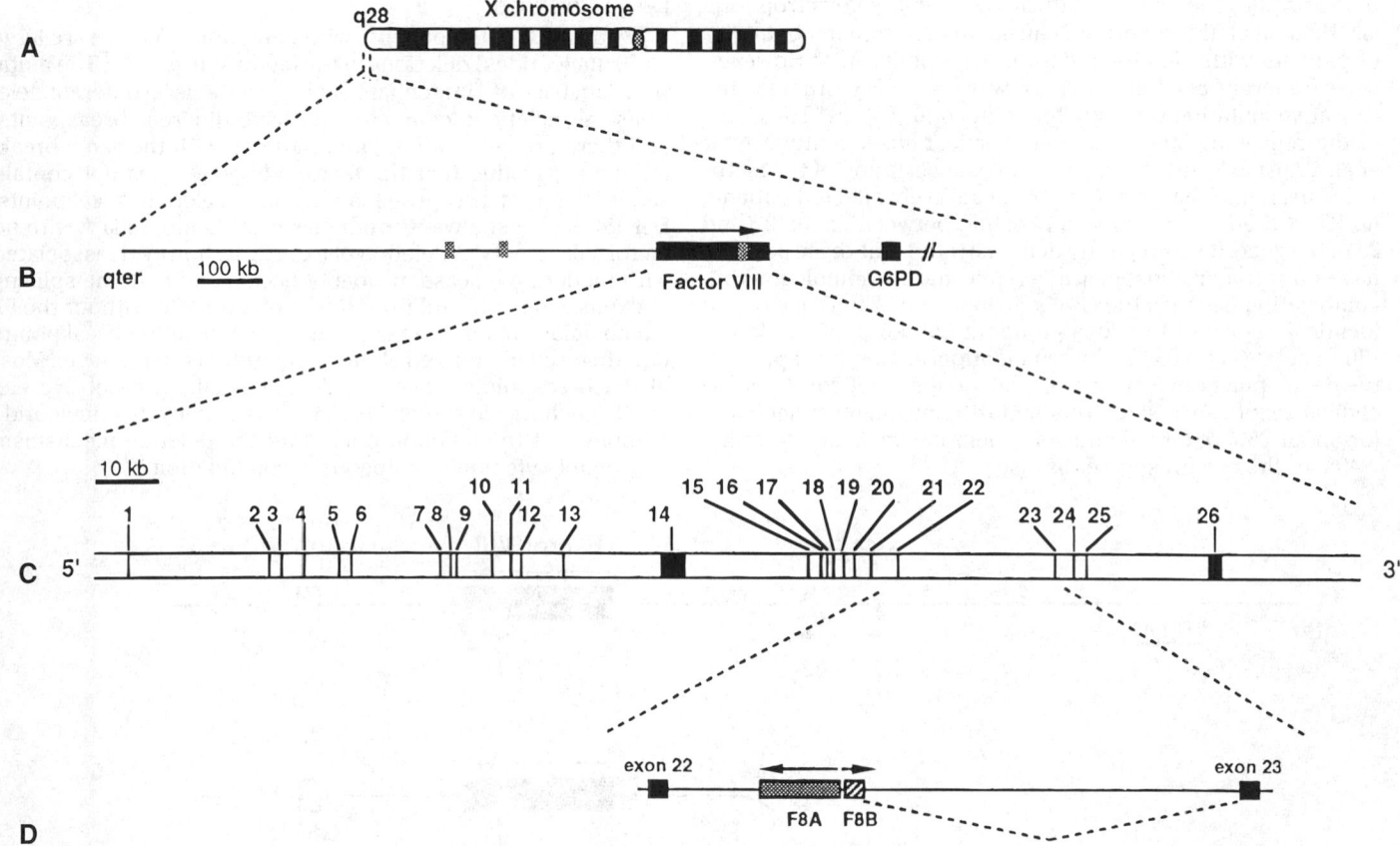

Fig. 105-4. (A–D) Schematic representation of chromosomal localization and structure of the factor VIII gene. The gene is located about 1,000 kb from the Xqter (Fig. B). It is 186 kb long and contains 26 exons (Fig. C). In the large intron 22 there are two nested genes, the intronless F8A and F8B, which utilizes the exon 23 of factor VIII gene as its second exon (Fig. D). There are three copies of the F8A/F8B sequences on Xq28, as shown by the gray boxes of Fig. B. See text for further discussion of the gene structure.

boundaries, and 5′ and 3′ untranslated regions has been determined.[17,18,162] The exon length varies from 69 to 262 nucleotides except for exon 14, which is 3,106 nucleotides, and the last exon 26, which has 1,958 nucleotides (Fig. 105-4). There are some large intervening sequences such as IVS22, which is 32 kb and IVS1, IVS6, IVS13, IVS14, and IVS25, which are 14–23 kb long.

The normal factor VIII mRNA is approximately 9 kb, of which the coding sequence is 7,053 nucleotides. There is a CpG island within IVS22 that is associated with two additional transcripts. One transcript of 1.8 kb is produced abundantly in a wide variety of cells. The orientation of this transcript is opposite to that of factor VIII and contains no intervening sequence.[163] This 1,739-nt-long cDNA has been termed factor VIII-associated gene A (F8A) and is conserved in the mouse.[164] The second transcript of 2.5 kb is transcribed in the same direction as factor VIII; after a short exon that may encode for eight amino acids, it utilizes exons 23–26 of the factor VIII gene.[165] This gene has been termed factor VIII-associated gene B (F8B). The two transcripts (F8A and F8B) originate within 122 bases from each other. The sequences of F8A and F8B along with few kilobases of surrounding DNA are also present in two other areas of the X chromosome approximately 400 kb telomeric to factor VIII gene.[163,166] The function of these transcripts and their potential protein products are unknown.

The factor VIII gene maps on the long arm of the X chromosome, in the most distal band Xq28. Haldane and Smith[167] reported linkage of hemophilia A with color blindness, and Boyer and Graham[168] demonstrated close linkage of hemophilia A with polymorphisms at the glucose-6-phosphate-dehydrogen-

ase (G6PD) locus. Additional studies confirmed the close linkage of factor VIII with G6PD.[169] Patterson et al.[170] showed that G6PD and factor VIII genes lie within 500 kb of each other. Pulsed field gel electrophoresis and physical mapping of Xq28 using yeast artificial chromosomes suggested that the factor VIII gene mapped distal to G6PD.[166,171] The order of these loci and the direction of transcription is Xcen-G6PD-3′F8-5′F8-Xqter.[166,172] The distance from factor VIII gene to the Xq telomere is approximately 1 Mb.

FACTOR VIII GENE DEFECTS

Since the cloning of the factor VIII gene, the DNA of >1,000 hemophilia A patients has been examined for molecular defects. Initially, restriction endonuclease analysis and Southern blot cloning and sequencing were the methods used. The introduction of polymerase chain reaction (PCR) amplification from genomic DNA or from RNA (RT-PCR) revolutionized the mutation detection protocols. Several screening methods for recognition of mutations have been employed, namely, denaturing gradient gel electrophoresis, single-stranded conformational analysis, RNA cleavage analysis, and subsequently direct sequencing of PCR products.

Gross DNA Rearrangements

Common Partial Inversion of Factor VIII

The efforts to characterize all mutations in the factor VIII gene in a defined sample of hemophilia A patients revealed a surprising and unexpected finding. After scanning all the exons of factor VIII gene using denaturing gradient gel electrophoresis, Higuchi et al.[72] found the causative mutation in about 90% of patients with mild-to-moderate hemophilia A.[173] However, when severely affected patients were similarly studied, the causative mutation was only found in about 50%.[174] The cause of the remaining 50% remained elusive. Subsequently Naylor et al.,[175] using RT-PCR of illegitimate transcription of the factor VIII gene, found that in about 40% of severely affected patients no RT-PCR amplification was possible between exons 22 and 23 of the gene. It was recently demonstrated that these patients have an intrachromosomal inversion due to homologous recombination between the F8A gene in intron 22 and one of two identical copies of F8A located about 550 kb 5' of the factor VIII gene[176] (Fig. 105-5). The elucidation of this hot spot and the development of a simple diagnostic test is of considerable clinical significance since this mutation mechanism accounts for about 25% of all patients with hemophilia A and certainly >40% of those with severe disease.

Large Deletions

In about 5% of the patients with hemophilia A there are large (>50 nucleotides) deletions in the factor VIII gene.[177] The mutation data base of Tuddenham et al.[178] contains 59 different deletions. All deletions characterized have different breakpoints, and there are no two unrelated patients with the same breakpoints, suggesting that the factor VIII gene does not contain sequences that are prone to become deletion breakpoints. Deletions almost always produce severe hemophilia A with no factor VIII activity. A deletion of exon 22 is, however, associated with moderate disease, probably because of in-frame splicing of exons 21 and 23 and production of a protein without the 52 amino acids encoded by exon 22.[179] Few deletion breakpoints have been characterized at the nucleotide sequence level. Most of the breakpoints examined do not occur in repetitive elements such as Alu-sequences. There is usually 2–4 nucleotide homology at the junction point, and the deletion mechanism is probably via nonhomologous recombination.[180]

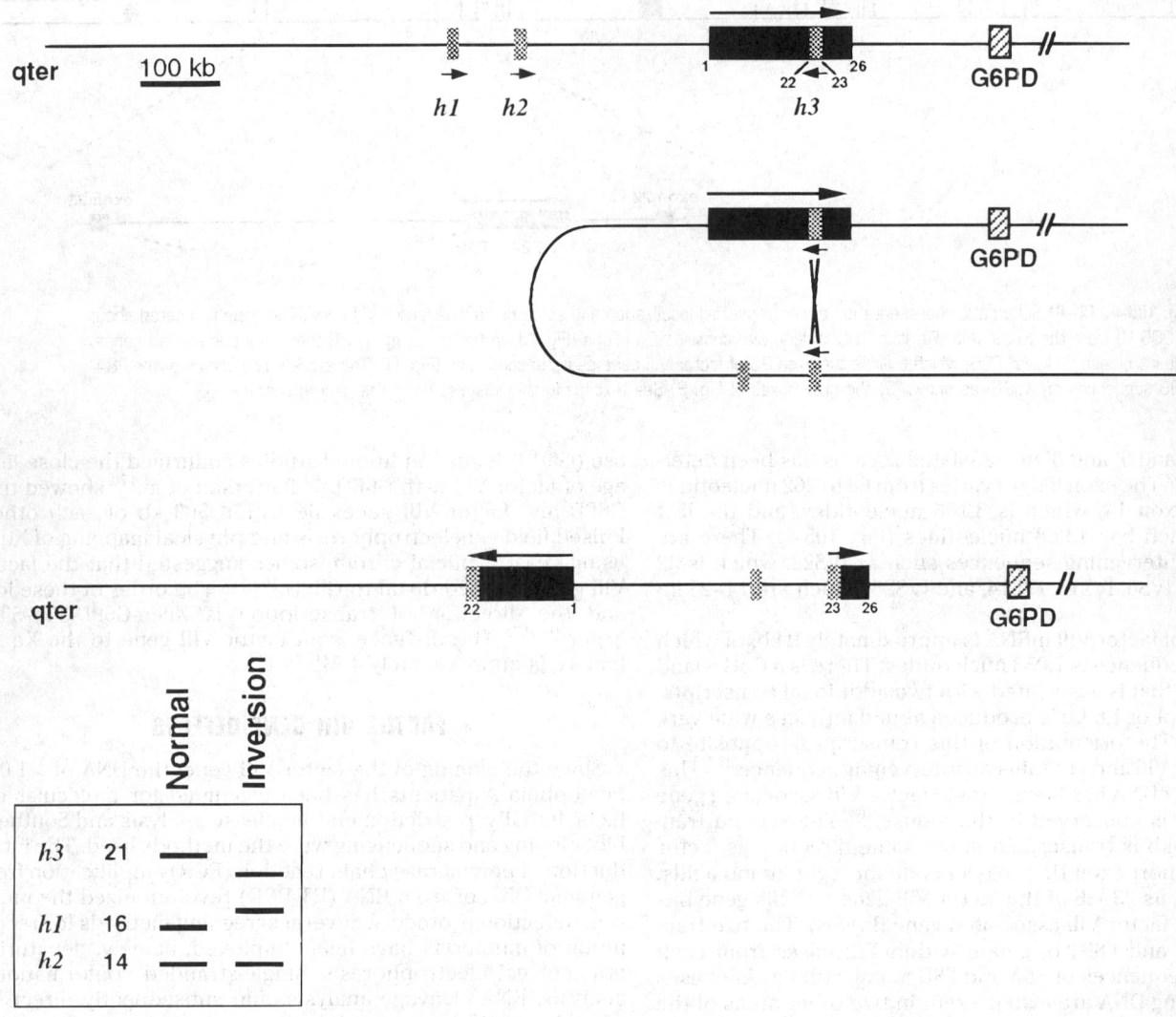

Fig. 105-5. Mechanism of one type of the common inversion of the factor VIII gene. Due to intrachromosomal crossing over between the homologous regions h3 and h4, there is an inversion of factor VIII sequences encompassing exons 1–22. The inversion is easily recognizable after Southern blot analysis using part of the homologous regions as probe.

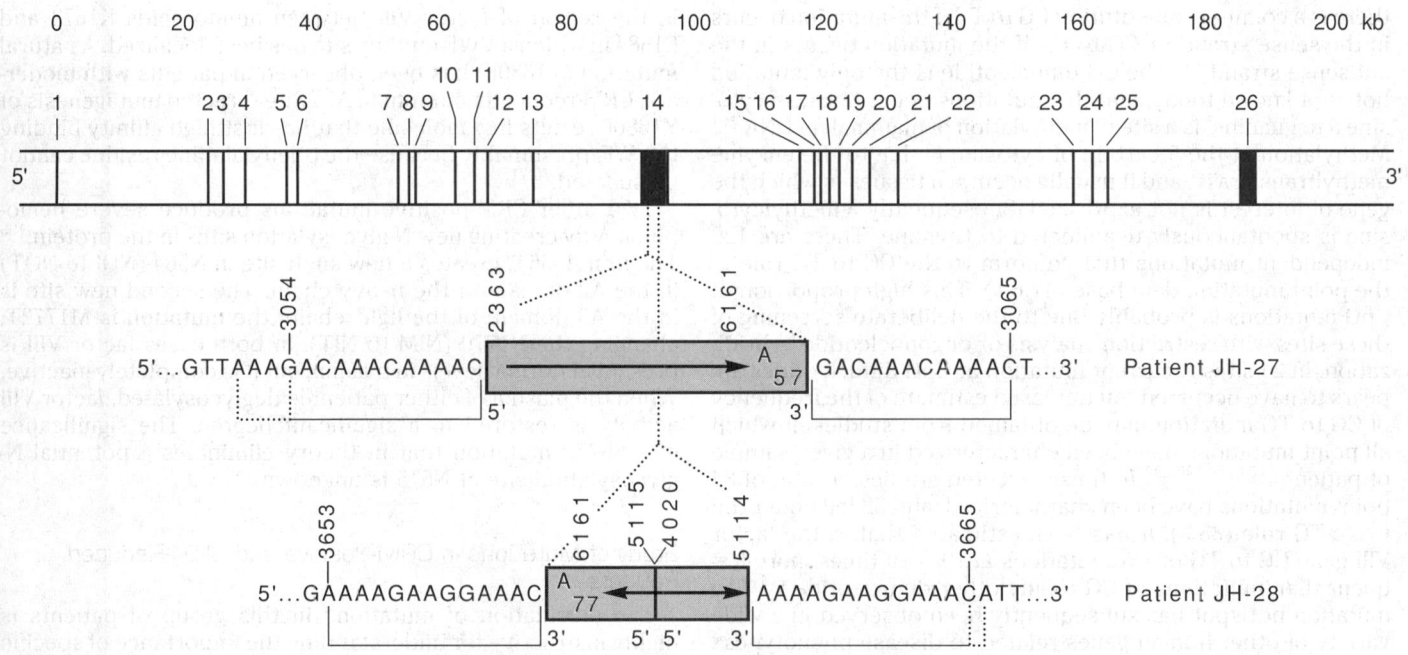

Fig. 105-6. Schematic representation of insertions of LINE retrotrans-posons in exon 14 of factor VIII gene. Filled boxes represent the LINE elements and the arrows within the boxes point toward the 3' end of the sequence. The numbers on the LINE boxes represent the corresponding nucleotides of the consensus LINE sequence. Numbers in italics in the flanking sequences denote the corresponding nucleotides of the factor VIII cDNA. The target site duplication is bracketed. (From Kazazian et al.,[212] with permission.)

Insertion of Retrotransposons

De novo insertion of LINE repetitive elements in the human genome was first reported in the factor VIII gene.[181] In one case of severe hemophilia A, a 3.8-kb portion of a LINE element was inserted in exon 14 of factor VIII. The inserted DNA had a poly-(A)tail, produced a target site duplication, and was inserted in a relatively adenine-rich sequence of exon 14 (Fig. 105-6). The de novo insertion in the second case was a 2.1-kb portion of a LINE element and produced a severe hemophilia A. It occurred in a different site of exon 14 and had all the characteristics of retrotransposition. LINE elements comprise about 5% of the human genome, and there are approximately 10^5 copies.[182] The full length of the element is 6.5 kb, and most of the copies in the human genome are partial and defective. The consensus sequence of LINE element contains two open reading frames, the second of which predicts a protein with amino acid homology with reverse transcriptase. About 3,000 LINE copies are full length and are potential transposable elements. Only a few of these, perhaps those with open reading frames, can produce a new insertion through an RNA intermediate. They are probably transcribed into DNA and then reinserted as double-stranded DNA into a new genomic site.[183] The full-length "active" LINE element responsible for the insertion in the first hemophilia A patient was cloned and characterized. It maps on chromosome 22 and probably encodes for a peptide that has reverse transcriptase activity.[184] A third LINE element insertion in intron 10 has also been observed but, since it did not co-segregate with the hemophilia A phenotype, it represents a recently established private polymorphism.[185] Insertions of LINE or other retrotransposons are not common, since there are only two such examples in >1,000 patients studied.

Duplications

Duplications of parts of human genes are very rare causes of mutations. Two such lesions are described in the factor VIII gene. In one there was a duplication of 23 kb of IVS22 inserted between exons 23–25.[186] This rearrangement, found in two female siblings, was apparently unstable and led to deletion of exons 23–25 in the male offspring of one of the females. In the second case there was an in-frame duplication of exon 13 in a patient with mild hemophilia A.[187]

Point Mutations

Small Deletion/Insertions

Small deletions or insertions in the coding region of factor VIII gene that result in frameshifts have been reported. A compilation of point mutations indicates that there are 21 small deletions (of 1, 2, 4, 11, and 23 nucleotides) among 252 independent mutations recorded (8.3%).[188] The number of small insertions (1 and 10 nucleotides) in the mutation data base is seven (2.8% of the total point mutations). About one-half of the small deletions (10 of 21) or insertions (4 of 7) were found in exon 14. All the mutations that result in translation frameshifts cause severe hemophilia A.

Nonsense Mutations

Sixty-three independent nonsense mutations in 21 different codons are included in the point mutation data base, comprising 25% of the total number of point mutations. This percentage is perhaps biased, since many investigators have used restriction digestion analysis with *TaqI* that recognizes CG to TG mutations, in particular CGA to TGA (Arg to Stop) substitutions.[189] In two samples of 53 severe hemophilia A patients in which all point mutations have been characterized, the number of mutant nonsense codons was 7 (i.e., 13.2% [7 of 53] of the total severe mutations, or 28% [7 of 25] of the point mutations).[173,190] (There are 4 large deletions and 24 inversions in the sample of 53 severe hemophilia A patients).

CpG Dinucleotide Hypermutability

The study of point mutations in factor VIII uncovered two general lessons concerning human mutations. The first was the discovery of a mutation hot spot at CpG dinucleotides in which there is a common substitution CG to TG if the mutation occurs in the sense strand or CG to CA if the mutation occurs in the antisense strand.[189] The CG dinucleotide is the only mutation hot spot known today, and the mutations occur because cytosine 5 to guanine, is a site of methylation of mammalian DNA.[191] Methylation at the 5 carbon of cytosine is due to the enzyme methyltransferase, and it usually occurs in tissues in which the gene of interest is not expressed. Subsequently 5-methylcytosine is spontaneously deaminated to thymine. There are 120 independent mutations that conform to the CG to TG rule in the point mutation data base (47.6%). This high proportion of CpG mutations is probably due to the deliberate screening of these sites with restriction analysis or oligonucleotide hybridization. In 24 sites recurrent mutation at CpG dinucleotides appears to have occurred. An unbiased estimate of the frequency of CG to TG mutation may be obtained from studies in which all point mutations have been characterized in a given sample of patients.[173,174,190,192] In these selected studies, a total of 84 point mutations have been characterized, and 32 fell under the CG-to-TG rule (38%). It has been estimated that in the factor VIII gene CG to TG or CA mutations are 10–20 times more frequent than mutations of CG to any other dinucleotide.[193] The mutation hot spot has subsequently been observed in a wide variety of other human genes related to disease phenotypes.

Exon Skipping due to Nonsense Mutations

An important observation concerning the pathophysiology of nonsense mutations has recently been made in the factor VIII gene and independently in the fibrillin and OAT genes.[190,194] In some cases a nonsense codon mutation can lead to abnormal RNA processing, in which the exon containing the mutation is skipped. This observation was made after the introduction of RT-PCR in the mutation detection methodology. In one case of Glu, 1987 to Stop mutation in exon 19 all detectable RNA lacked the sequences of this exon. In the second case of Arg 2,116 to Stop mutation of exon 22, there was about 50% of RNA without the sequences of exon 22, while the remaining 50% of RNA was of normal size. The junctions of exons 18–20 and 21–23 do not result in translational frameshift. The mechanism, significance, and frequency of the exon skipping due to nonsense mutations are presently unknown.

Missense Mutations

The study of missense mutations (i.e., nucleotide substitutions that result in amino acid substitutions) is important for understanding the function of the protein and the pathophysiology of the disease. A total of 92 mutations leading to amino acid substitutions have been described (Fig. 105-7). These mutations are spread throughout the different domains of the gene except for exon 14; this exon encodes for the B domain which is devoid of amino acid substitutions that cause hemophilia A. In spite of knowledge of amino acid substitutions, the mode of action of most of these mutations in producing reduced factor VIII activity in plasma is unknown. However, several mutations have been identified that alter thrombin cleavage sites or the VWF-binding site, or otherwise introduce or destroy N-linked glycosylation sites.

Natural mutations in patients with CRM-positive hemophilia A affect the thrombin cleavage needed for activation of the molecule. Mutations R372H and R372C have been shown in vitro to abolish the normal cleavage by thrombin in the heavy chain.[195–197] It is not clear whether the S373L mutation has an effect in thrombin cleavage. Mutations R1689C and R1689H abolish thrombin cleavage at the light chain.[173,198] These mutations also lead to CRM-positive hemophilia A in which there is a normal amount of nonfunctional factor VIII in plasma.

Two sulfated tyrosine residues (Y1664 and Y1680) are found in the region of factor VIII between amino acids K1673 and E1684 in which a VWF-binding site has been localized. A natural mutation (Y1680F) has been observed in patients with moderate, CRM-reduced hemophilia A.[72] Site-directed mutagenesis of Y1680F results in a molecule that has lost high-affinity binding to VWF, presumably because the phenylalanine residue cannot be sulfated.[70,71]

Two other CRM-positive mutations produce severe hemophilia A by creating new N-glycosylation sites in the protein.[199] The first, I566T, creates a new such site in N564 (NQI to NQT) in the A2 domain of the heavy chain. The second new site is in the A3 domain of the light chain; the mutation is M1772T, changing the N1770 (NIM to NIT). In both cases factor VIII is present at normal levels in plasma, but it is completely inactive. When the plasma of either patient is deglycosylated, factor VIII activity is restored to a significant degree. The significance of a S577P mutation that in theory eliminates a potential N-glycosylation site at N575 is unknown.

Study of Mutations in CRM-Positive and CRM-Reduced Patients

The elucidation of mutations in this group of patients is highly instructive for understanding the importance of specific amino acid residues. A small number of such mutations have been described.[188] Since about 40% of CRM-positive mutations occur in the A2 domain, which consists of 228 amino acids or about 10% of the coding region of factor VIII, this region must be important in procoagulant activity. Most mutations, however, are CRM negative and probably affect the folding or stability, or both, of the protein. Since these mutations result in absence of secreted factor VIII and the in vitro functional studies depend on the analysis of the protein produced in eukaryotic cells after transfection with factor VIII cDNA, the mechanisms of action of these mutants will be difficult to elucidate.

Other Missense Mutations of Interest

Cases with two different mutations in the same amino acid are also of interest (Fig. 105-6). These are E272G, E272K; Y473C, Y473H; R531C, R531G; V634A, V634M; R1781C, R1781H; N1922D, N1922S; R1941L, R1941Q; R2209L, R2209Q; P2300L, P2300S; and R2307L, R2307Q. Mutations in the last 30 amino acids of factor VIII (C2 domain) may cause reduced phospholipid binding. Candidates are R2304L, R2307L, and R2307Q. The domains of factor VIII for binding to factors IX, X, and others have not been clearly elucidated.

Splicing Errors

A small number of potential splicing errors have been identified.[178] However, no formal proof that the mutations cause abnormal splicing has been obtained. Two mutations in the invariant GA of the acceptor splice site in introns 5 and 6 are associated, as expected, with severe hemophilia A. Four mutations occur in the donor splice site consensus and two in cryptic splice sites. No extensive functional analysis of these mutations has been done. It seems that in spite of the presence of >50 splice junctions in the factor VIII gene, splicing mutants do not account for a sizable fraction of hemophilia patients.

Promoter Mutations

No examples of mutations in the 5' untranslated region of factor VIII gene have been reported to date. If such mutations do occur, they are probably infrequent, since two laboratories failed to find any nucleotide substitutions in 530 nucleotides of the 5' flanking region of factor VIII in 227 patients with hemophilia A[74] (Gitschier J, Kogan S, Levinson B et al., unpublished

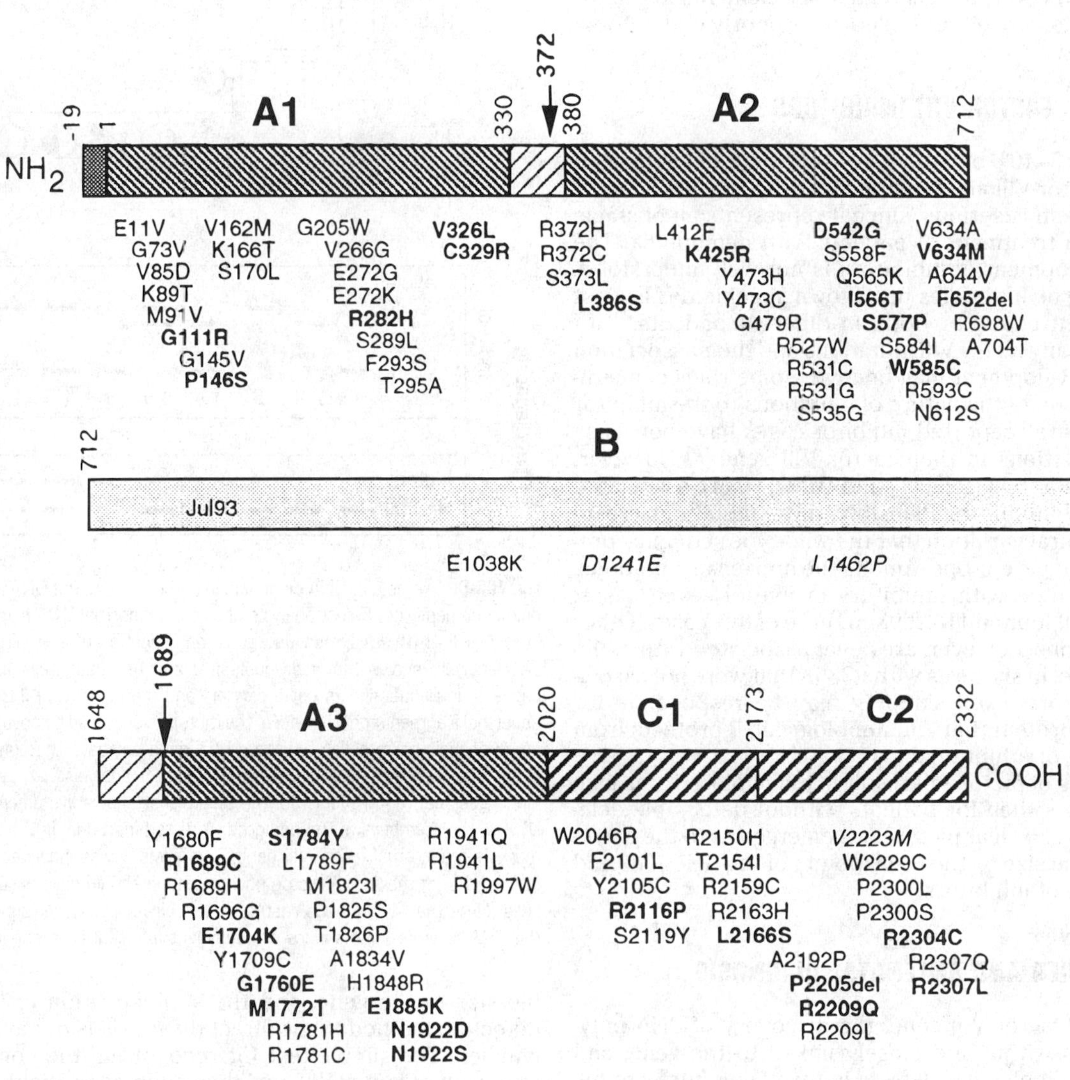

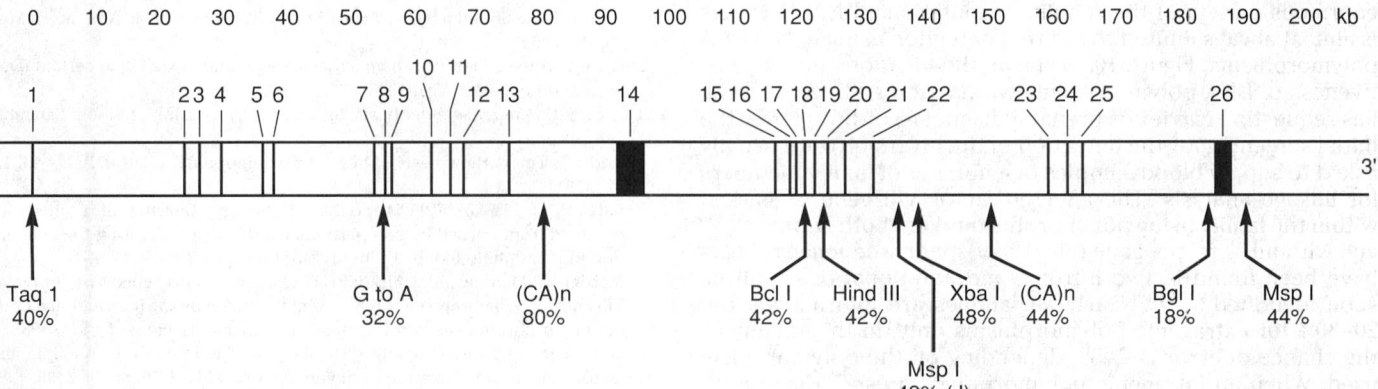

Fig. 105-7. Missense mutations in the factor VIII protein. The structural domains of the protein are shown, and the amino acid substitutions are depicted using the one-letter code for amino acids. For example, E11V indicates a glutamic acid to valine substitution at amino acid residue 11.

Fig. 105-8. DNA polymorphisms within the factor VIII gene. Arrows denote the location of the polymorphisms. Percent numbers represent the observed heterozygosity of each polymorphic system in female individuals. The Msp I site in intron 22 is only polymorphic in Japanese (J). There are two polymorphic (CA)n repeats identified in introns 13 and 22.

data). Notably, however, the cis-regulatory elements for factor VIII gene expression are either unknown or poorly understood.

FACTOR VIII INHIBITORS

Approximately 5–10% of patients with hemophilia A develop antibodies to factor VIII after treatment with exogenous factor VIII.[200] The problem is serious, since it represents an obstacle for the long-term treatment of patients with hemophilia. The etiology of development of inhibitors is not well understood. Epitope mapping of antibodies has shown specificities against the heavy or light chain, or both, in different patients.[201,202] The analysis of many factor VIII mutations and their association with inhibitor development may uncover some rules concerning the contribution of the nature of mutations to the inhibitor formation. Almost all reported inhibitor cases have nonsense mutations or deletions in their factor VIII gene.[174] However, two missense mutations (R2209Q and W2229C) are associated with low levels of inhibitors. Plausibly, these mutations create such local structural variation that the wild-type sequence presents an immunologic epitope. Among the nonsense mutations, R1941X is associated with inhibitors in five of seven cases; R2147X in three of four and R2209X in three of five cases. Other nonsense mutations, however, are never associated with inhibitors. For example, in six cases with R336X that were not associated with inhibitors, exon skipping may be responsible for some factor VIII protein that "immunologically" protects from the development of inhibitors.

Gross deletions of factor VIII result in a fivefold greater incidence of inhibitors than for patients without detectable deletions.[178] However, no clear picture has emerged as to the correlation between the size or the breakpoints of the deletions and the development of inhibitors.

CARRIER AND ANTENATAL DIAGNOSIS

The cloning of factor VIII gene, the discovery of DNA polymorphic markers within and closely linked to the gene, and the elucidation of molecular defects in many patients with hemophilia A dramatically changed the practice of diagnosis of carriers and affected fetuses. The discovery of the common partial inversion of the factor VIII gene provided a means of diagnosis using Southern blot analysis.[176] This defect accounts for approximately 45% of severe hemophilia A. The diagnosis of the exact molecular defect in the remaining families is still not practical even in sophisticated laboratories. Because of the enormous variety of the remaining mutations, DNA diagnosis is almost always limited to indirect detection using linked DNA polymorphisms. Figure 105-8 shows the location and informativeness of DNA polymorphisms within factor VIII gene. Families requesting carrier or prenatal diagnosis, or both (after the initial screening for the detection of the inversion), are usually asked to supply blood samples of a number of family members for linkage analysis. The affected factor VIII gene is marked within the family using polymorphic markers both within[203–206] and without[207,208] the gene (Fig. 105-9). Short sequence repeats have been found in two introns, and additional ones will be soon identified.[209,210] Nearly all families are informative, but 20–30% for extragenic polymorphisms only. In those families the chance of error is 2–5% depending on the polymorphism used. When an intragenic polymorphism is used, the chance or error is negligible (certainly <1%).

The indirect detection of mutant genes is not feasible when only one male offspring is available and the carrier status of the mother is unknown. In these cases direct detection of the molecular defect should be employed. However, because of the large number of different molecular defects, the considera-

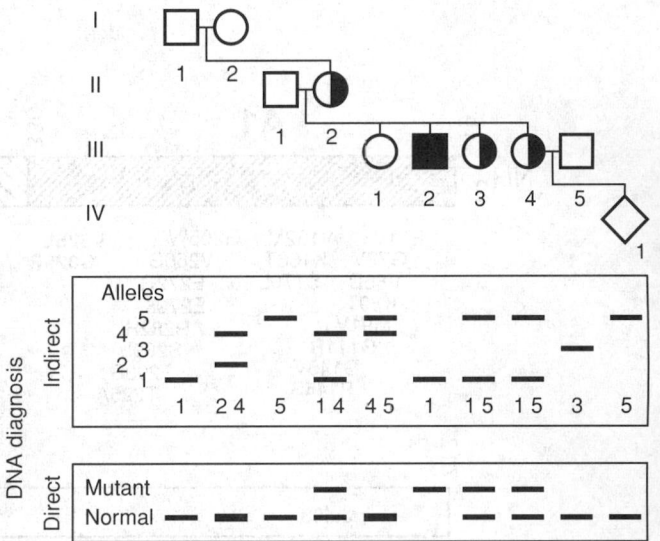

Fig. 105-9. Example of DNA diagnosis in hemophilia A. The DNA analysis is shown below the pedigree. Direct analysis shows an abnormal DNA fragment in affected individual III-2 (this fragment is due to amplification of a small rearrangement). This analysis shows that individuals II-2 and her daughters III-3 and III-4 are carriers, individual III-1 is not a carrier, and the parents of II-2 do not have the abnormal fragment and, therefore, the mutation occurred de novo in one X chromosome of their germ cells. The fetus IV-1 does not have the abnormal factor VIII allele, and therefore he is not affected. Indirect analysis was performed using a highly informative intragenic polymorphism that shows five different alleles in the DNA of the members of the pedigree. Affected individual III-2 has allele 1, which marks his abnormal factor VIII gene. This allele 1 was inherited from his grandfather I-1 and, therefore, the de novo mutation should have occurred in his germ cells. Note that without the results of the direct DNA analysis in this pedigree, the DNA polymorphisms were not sufficient for identifying carriers.

ble size of the gene, and the sophistication of the mutation detection methodology, direct diagnosis is not available for all families. The simple test for recognizing the common partial inversion of factor VIII, which accounts for about 45% of cases of severe hemophilia A, has dramatically changed the situation. Few laboratories will deal with the remaining molecular defects. It seems that the method of choice is the RT-PCR amplification of illegitimate transcripts and their analysis using chemical cleavage or another mutation screening method.

REFERENCES

1. Rosner F: Hemophilia in the Talmud and rabbinic writings. Ann Intern Med 70:833, 1969
2. Otto JE: An account of an hemorrhagic disposition existing in certain families. Med Repository 6:1, 1803
3. Lane S: Haemorrhagic diathesis. Successful transfusion of blood. Lancet 1:185, 1840
4. Addis T: The pathogenesis of hereditary hemophilia. J Pathol Bacteriol 15:427, 1911
5. Patek AJ Jr, Taylor FHL: Hemophilia II. Some properties of a substance obtained from normal human plasma effective in accelerating the coagulation in hemophilic blood. J Clin Invest 16:113, 1937
6. Marder VJ, Mannucci PM, Firkin BG et al: Standard nomenclature for factor VIII and von Willebrand factor: a recommendation by the International Committee on Thrombosis and Haemostasis. Thromb Haemost 54:871, 1985
7. van Dieijen G, Tans G, Rosing J, Hemker HC: The role of phospholipid and factor VIIIa in the activation of bovine factor X. J Biol Chem 256:3433, 1981
8. Mutucumarana VP, Duffy EJ, Lollar P, Johnson AE: The active site of factor IXa is located far above the membrane surface and its conformation is altered upon association with factor VIIIa: a fluorescence study. J Biol Chem 267:17012, 1992
9. Fulcher CA, Zimmerman TS: Characterization of the human factor VIII procoagulant protein with a heterologous precipitating antibody. Proc Natl Acad Sci USA 79:1648, 1982

10. Hamer RJ, Koedam JA, Beeser-Visser NH, Sixma JJ: Human factor VIII: purification from commercial factor VIII characterization, identification and radiolabeling. Biochim Biophys Acta 873:356, 1986

11. Rizza CR, Rhymes IL: Coagulation assay of VIIIc and IXa. p. 18. In Bloom KAL (ed): The Hemophilias. Churchill Livingstone, Edinburgh, 1982

12. Suomela H, Blomback M, Blomback B: The activation of factor X evaluated by using synthetic substrates. Thromb Res 10:267, 1977

13. Nordfang O, Ezban M, Nilsson P, Knudsen JB: Radioimmunoassay for quantitative measurement of factor VIII-heavy chain. Br J Haematol 68:307, 1987

14. Fass DN, Knutson GJ, Katzmann JA: Monoclonal antibodies to porcine factor VIII coagulant and their use in the isolation of active coagulant protein. Blood 59:594, 1982

15. Rotblat F, O'Brien DP, O'Brien FJ et al: Purification of human factor VIII:C and its characterization by Western blotting using monoclonal antibodies. Biochem 24:4294, 1985

16. Vehar GA, Keyt B, Eaton D et al: Structure of human factor VIII. Nature 312:337, 1984

17. Wood WT, Capon DJ, Simonsen CC et al: Expression of active human factor VIII from recombinant DNA clones. Nature 312:330, 1984

18. Toole JJ, Knopf JL, Wozney JM et al: Molecular cloning of a cDNA encoding human antihemophilic factor. Nature 312:342, 1984

19. Jenny RJ, Pittman DD, Toole JJ et al: Complete cDNA and derived amino acid sequence of human factor V. Proc Natl Acad Sci USA 84:4846, 1987

20. Koschinsky ML, Funk WD, von Ooar BA, MacGillivray RTA: Complete cDNA sequence of human preceruloplasmin. Proc Natl Acad Sci USA 83:5086, 1986

21. Mann KG, Lawler CM, Vehar GA, Church WR: Coagulation factor V contains copper ion. J Biol Chem 2259:12949, 1984

22. Bihoreau N, Pin S, Dekersabiec AM et al: Metal identification in human antihemophilic A-factor (factor VIII). C R Acad Sci Serie III Life Sci 316:536, 1993

23. Poole S, Firtel RA, Lamar E, Rowekamp W: Sequence and expression of the discoidin I gene family in dictyostelium discoideum. J Mol Biol 153:273, 1981

24. Stubbs JD, Lekutis C, Singer KL et al: cDNA cloning of a mouse mammary epithelial cell surface protein reveals the existence of epidermal growth factorlike sequences. Proc Natl Acad Sci USA 87:8417, 1990

25. Pittman DD, Wang JH, Kaufman RJ: Identification and functional importance of tyrosine sulfate residues within recombinant factor VIII. Biochemistry 31:3315, 1992

26. Elder B, Lakich D, Gitschier J: Sequence of the murine factor VIII cDNA. Genomics 16:374, 1993

27. Marchioro TL, Hougie C, Ragde H et al: Hemophilia: role of organ homografts. Science 163:188, 1969

28. Webster WP, Zukoski CF, Hutchin P et al: Plasma factor VIII synthesis and control as revealed by canine organ transplantation. Am J Physiol 220:1147, 1971

29. Lewis JH, Bontempo FA, Sperio JA et al: Liver transplantation in a hemophiliac. N Engl J Med 312:1189, 1985

30. Bontempo FA, Lewis JH, Gorenc TJ et al: Liver transplantation in hemophilia A. Blood 69:1721, 1987

31. Kelly DA, Summerfield JA, Tuddenham EGD: Localization of factor VIIIC: antigen in guinea-pig tissues and isolated liver cell fractions. Br J Haematol 56:535, 1984

32. Zelechowska MG, van Mourik JA, Brodniewicz-Proba T: Ultrastructural localization of factor VIII procoagulant antigen in human liver hepatocytes. Nature 317:729, 1985

33. Wion KL, Kelly D, Summerfield JA et al: Distribution of factor VIII mRNA and antigen in human liver and other tissues. Nature 317:726, 1985

34. Kaufman RJ, Wasley LC, Dorner AJ: Synthesis, processing and secretion of recombinant human factor VIII expressed in mammalian cells. J Biol Chem 263:6352, 1988

35. Munro S, Pelham HRB: An Hsp70-like protein in the ER: identity with the 78 Kd glucose-regulated protein and immunoglobulin heavy chain binding protein. Cell 46:291, 1986

36. Dorner AJ, Bole DG, Kaufman RJ: The relationship of N-linked glycosylation and heavy chain-binding protein association with the secretion of glycoproteins. J Cell Biol 105:2665, 1987

37. Lee AS: Coordinated regulation of a set of genes by glucose and calcium ionophores in mammalian cells. Trends Biochem Sci 12:20, 1987

38. Kozutsumi Y, Segal M, Normington K et al: The presence of malfolded proteins in the endoplasmic reticulum signals the induction of glucose-regulated proteins. Nature 332:462, 1988

39. Dorner AJ, Wasley LC, Kaufman RJ: Overexpression of GRP78 blocks stress induction of GRPs and secretion of specific proteins in Chinese hamster ovary cells. EMBO J 4:1563, 1992

40. Flynn GC, Pohl J, Flocco MT, Rothman JE: Peptide-binding specificity of the molecular chaperone BiP. Nature 353:726, 1991

41. Dorner AJ, Wasley LC, Kaufman RJ: Protein dissociation from GRP78 and

42. Wise RJ, Dorner AJ, Krane M et al: The role of von Willebrand factor multimerization and propeptide cleavage in the binding and stabilization of factor VIII. J Biol Chem 266:21948, 1991

43. Tuddenham EGD, Lane RS, Rotblat F et al: Response to infusions of polyelectrolyte fractionated human factor VIII concentrate in human hemophilia A and von Willebrand's disease. Br J Haematol 52:259, 1982

44. Weiss HJ, Sussman JJ, Hoyer LW: Stabilization of factor VIII in plasma by the von Willebrand factor. Studies on posttransfusion and dissociated factor VIII and in patients with von Willebrand's disease. J Clin Invest 60:390, 1977

45. Brinkhous KM, Sandberg H, Garris JB et al: Purified human factor VIII procoagulant protein: comparative hemostasis response after infusions into hemophilic and von Willebrand disease dogs. Proc Natl Acad Sci USA 82:8752, 1985

46. Douglas AS: Antihemophilic globulin assay following plasma infusions in hemophilia. J Lab Clin Med 51:850, 1958

47. Over J, Sixma JJ, Doucet-de-Bruine MHM et al: Survival of [125]iodine-labeled factor VIII in normals and patients with classic hemophilia. J Clin Ivest 62:223, 1978

48. Nishino M, Girma JP, Rothschild C et al: New variant of von Willebrand disease with defective binding to factor VIII. Blood 74:1591, 1989

49. Mazurier C: von Willebrand disease masquerading as haemophilia A. Thromb Haemost 67:391, 1992

50. Koedam JA: Interaction between factor VIII and vWF. PhD thesis, University of Utrecht, The Netherlands, 1989

51. Koedam JA, Meijers JCM, Sixma JJ, Bouma BN: Inactivation of human factor VIII by activated protein C cofactor activity of protein S and protective effect of von Willebrand factor. J Clin Invest 82:1236, 1988

52. Fay PI, Coumans J-V, Walker FJ: von Willebrand factor mediates protection of factor VIII from activated protein C-catalyzed inactivation. J Biol Chem 266:2172, 1991

53. Hamer RJ, Koedam JA, Beeser-Visser NH, Sixma JJ: The effect of thrombin on the complex between factor VIII and von Willebrand factor. Eur J Biochem 167:253, 1987

54. Pittman DD, Alderman EA, Tomkinson KN et al: Biochemical, immunological, and in vivo functional characterization of B-domain deleted factor VIII. Blood 81:2925, 1993

55. Andersson L-O, Brown JE: Interaction of factor VIII-von Willebrand factor with phospholipid vesicles. Biochem J 200:161, 1981

56. Lajmonovich A, Hudry-Clergeon G, Freyssinet J-M, Marguerie G: Human factor VIII procoagulant activity and phospholipid interaction. Biochim Biophys Acta 678:123, 1981

57. Nesheim M, Pittman DD, Fass DN et al: The effect of von Willebrand factor on the binding of factor VIII to thrombin activated platelets. J Biol Chem 266:17815, 1991

58. Foster PA, Fulcher CA, Marti T et al: A major factor VIII binding domain resides within the amino-terminal 272 amino acid residues of von Willebrand factor. J Biol Chem 262:8443, 1987

59. Takahashi Y, Kalafatis M, Girma J-P et al: Localization of factor VIII binding domain on a 34 kilodalton fragment of the N-terminal portion of von Willebrand factor. Blood 70:1679, 1987

60. Bahou WH, Ginsburg D, Sikkink R et al: A monoclonal antibody to von Willebrand factor (vWF) inhibits factor VIII binding. J Clin Invest 84:56, 1989

61. Lollar P, Parker CG: Stoichiometry of the porcine factor VIII-von Willebrand factor association. J Biol Chem 262:17272, 1987

62. Hamer RJ, Koedam JA, Beeser-Visser NH et al: Factor VIII binds to von Willebrand factor via its M_r-80,000 light chain. Eur J Biochem 166:37, 1987

63. Sewerin KI, Larsen K, Sandberg H, Andersson L-O: The binding between factor VIII and von Willebrand factor. Res Clinic Lab 16:235, 1986

64. Ezban M, Nordfang O: Interaction of isolated heavy and light chain of factor VIII:C with the von Willebrand factor. Res Clinic Lab 16:112, 1986

65. Lollar P, Hill-Eubanks DC, Parker CG: Association of the factor VIII light chain with von Willebrand factor. J Biol Chem 263:10451, 1988

66. Foster PA, Fulcher CA, Houghten RA, Zimmerman TS: An immunogenic region within amino acid residues Val[1670]–Glu[1684] of the factor VIII light chain induces antibodies which inhibit binding of factor VIII to von Willebrand factor. J Biol Chem 263:5230, 1988

67. Leyte A, Verbeet MP, Brodneiwicz-Proba T et al: The interaction between human blood-coagulation factor VIII and von Willebrand factor: characterization of a high-affinity binding site on factor VIII. Biochem J 257:679, 1989

68. Shima M, Scandella D, Yoshioka A et al: A factor VIII neutralizing monoclonal antibody and a human inhibitor alloantibody recognizing epitopes in the C2 domain inhibit factor VIII binding to von Willebrand factor and to phosphatidylserine. Thromb Haemost 69:240, 1993

69. Foster PA, Fulcher CA, Houghten RA, Zimmerman TS: Synthetic factor VIII

peptides with amino acid sequences contained within the C2 domain of factor VIII inhibit factor VIII binding to phosphatidylserine. Blood 75:1999, 1990

70. Michnick DA, Pittman DD, Kaufman RJ: Identification of individual tyrosine sulfation sites within factor VIII required for optimal activity and efficient thrombin cleavage. Thromb Haemost 69:1509a, 1993

71. Leyte A, van Schijndel HB, Niehrs C et al: Sulfation of Tyr 1680 of human blood coagulation factor VIII is essential for the interaction of factor VIII with von Willebrand factor. J Biol Chem 266:740, 1991

72. Higuchi M, Wong C, Kochhan L et al: Characterization of mutations in the factor VIII gene by direct sequencing of amplified genomic DNA. Genomics 6:65, 1990

73. Lenting RJ, Donath MJSH, van Mourik JA, Mertens K: Identification of a high affinity binding site for factor IXa on the light chain of human factor VIII. J Biol Chem 269:7150, 1994

74. O'Brien DP, Johnson D, Byfield P Tudendham EGD: Inactivation of factor VIII by factor IXa. Biochem 31:2805, 1992

75. Lamphear BJ, Fay PJ: Proteolytic interactions of factor IXa with human factor VIII and factor VIIIa. Blood 80:3120, 1992

76. Lamphear BJ, Fay PJ: Factor IXa enhances reconstitution of factor VIIIa from isolated A2 subunit and A1/A3-C1-C2 dimer. J Biol Chem 267:3725, 1992

77. Walker FJ, Chavin SI, Fay PJ: Inactivation of factor VIII by activated protein C and protein S. Arch Biochem Biophys 252:322, 1987

78. Bertina RM, Cupers R, van Wijngaarden A: Factor IXa protects activated factor VIII against inactivation by activated protein C. Biochem Biophys Res Commun 125:177, 1984

79. Rick ME, Kriezek DM, Esmon NL: Factor IXa modifies the degradation of factor VIII by activated protein C. Clin Res 36:417a, 1988

80. Guinto ER, Esmon CT: Loss of prothrombin and of factor Xa-factor Va interactions upon inactivation of factor Va by activated protein C. J Biol Chem 259:13986, 1983

81. Annamalai AE, Rao AK, Chiu HC et al: Epitope mapping of functional domains of human factor Va with human and murine monoclonal antibodies. Evidence for the interaction of heavy chain with factor Xa and calcium. Blood 70:139, 1987

82. Tucker MM, Foster WB, Katzmann IA, Mann KG: A monoclonal antibody which inhibits the factor Xa interaction. J Biol Chem 258:1210, 1983

83. Tracy PB, Mann KG: Prothrombinase complex assembly on the platelet surface is mediated through 74,000-dalton component of factor Va. Proc Natl Acad Sci USA 80:2380, 1983

84. Vehar GA, Davie EW: Preparation and properties of bovine factor VIII (anti-hemophilic factor). Biochemistry 19:401, 1980

85. Nordfang O, Ezban M: Generation of active coagulation factor VIII from isolated subunits. J Biol Chem 263:1115, 1988

86. Walker FJ, Fay PJ: Regulation of blood coagulation by the protein C system. FASEB J 6:2561, 1992

87. Odegaard B, Mann KG: Proteolysis of factor Va by factor Xa and activated protein C. J Biol Chem 262:11233, 1987

88. Fay PJ, Smudzin TM, Walker FJ: Activated protein C-catalyzed inactivation of human factor VIII and factor VIIIa. Identification of cleavage sites and correlation of proteolysis with cofactor activity. J Biol Chem 266:20139, 1991

89. Walker FI, Scandella D, Fay PI: Identification of the binding site for activated protein C on the light chain of factors V and VIII. J Biol Chem 265:1484, 1990

90. Gilbert GE, Furie BC, Furie B: Binding of human factor VIII to phospholipid vesicles. Biochemistry 265:815, 1990

91. Kemball-Cook G, Barrowcliffe TW: Interaction of factor VIII with phospholipids: role of composition and negative charge. Thromb Res 67:57, 1992

92. Bloom J, Nesheim ME, Mann KG: Phospholipid-binding properties of bovine factor V and factor Va. Biochem 18:4419, 1979

93. Andersson LO, Thuy LP, Brown JE: Affinity chromatography of coagulation factors II, VIII, IX, and X on matrix-bound phospholipid vesicles. Thromb Res 23:481, 1981

94. van de Waart P, Bruls H, Hemker HC, Lindhout T: Interaction of bovine blood clotting factor V and its subunits with phospholipid vesicles. Biochemistry 22:2427, 1983

95. Pusey ML, Nelsestuen GL: Membrane binding properties of blood coagulation factor V and derived peptides. Biochemistry 23:6202, 1984

96. Krieg UC, Isaacs BS, Yemul SS et al: Interaction of blood coagulation factor Va with phospholipid vesicles examined by using lipophilic photoreagents. Biochemistry 26:103, 1987

97. Lecompte MF, Krishnaswamy S, Mann KG et al: Membrane penetration of bovine facor V and Va detected by labeling with 5-iodonaphthalene-1-azide. J Biol Chem 262:1935, 1987

98. Atkins JS, Ganz PR: The association of human coagulation factors VIII, IXa, and X with phospholipid vesicles involves both electrostatic and hydrophobic interactions. Mol Cell Biochem 112:61, 1992

99. Duffy EJ, Parker ET, Mutucumarana VP et al: Binding of factor VIIIa and factor VIII to factor IXa on phospholipid vesicles. J Biol Chem 267:17006, 1992

100. Gilbert GE, Drirkwater D, Barter S, Clouse SB: Specificity of phosphatidylserine-containing membrane binding sites for factor VIII. Studies with model membranes supported by glass microspheres (liphspheres). J Biol Chem 267:15871, 1992

101. Bardelle C, Furie B, Furie BC, Gilbert GE: Membrane binding kinetics of factor VIII indicate a complex binding process. J Biol Chem 268:8815, 1993

102. Gilbert GE, Drinkwater D: Specific membrane binding of factor VIII is mediated by O-phospho-L-serine, a moiety of phosphatidylserine. Biochemistry 32:9577, 1993

103. Bevers EM, Comfurius P, Zwaal RF: Changes in membrane phospholipid distribution during platelet activation. Biochim Biophys Acta 736:57, 1983

104. Kemball-Cook G, Edwards SJ, Sewerin K et al: The phospholipid-binding site of factor VIII is located on the 80 kD light chain. Thromb Haemost 58:222a, 1987

105. Bloom JW. The interaction of rDNA factor VIII, factor VIIIdes797 1562 and factor VIII$_{des-797-1562}$-derived peptides with phospholipid. Thromb Res 48:439, 1987

106. Arai M, Scandella D, Hoyer LW: Molecular basis of factor VIII inhibition by human antibodies. Antibodies that bind to the factor VIII light chain prevent the interactions of factor VIII with phospholipid. J Clin Invest 83:1978, 1989

107. Ortel TL, Devore-Carter D, Quinn-Allen MA, Kane WH: Deletion analysis of recombinant human factor V. Evidence for a phosphatidylserine binding site in the second C-type domain. J Biol Chem 267:4189, 1992

108. Kalafatis M, Jenny RJ, Mann KG: Identification and characterization of a phospholipid binding site of bovine factor Va. J Biol Chem 265:21580, 1990

109. Eaton D, Rodriguez H, Vehar GA: Proteolytic processing of human factor VIII. Correlation of specific cleavages by thrombin, factor Xa, and activated protein C with activation and inactivation of factor VIII coagulant activity. Biochem 25:505, 1986

110. Rydel TJ, Ravichandran KG, Tulinsky A et al: The structure of a complex of recombinant hirudin and human alpha-thrombin. Science 249:277, 1990

111. Niehrs C, Huttner WB, Carvallo D, Degryse E: Conversion of recombinant hirudin to the natural form by in vitro tyrosine sulfation. Differential substrate specificities of leech and bovine tyrosylprotein sulfotransferases. J Biol Chem 265:9314, 1990

112. Fulcher CA, Roberts JR, Zimmerman TS: Thrombin proteolysis of purified factor VIII. Correlation of activation with generation of a specific polypeptide. Blood 61:807, 1983

113. Fay PJ, Anderson MT, Chavin SI, Marder VJ: The size of human factor VIII heterodimers and the effects produced by thrombin. Biochim Biophys Acta 871:268, 1986

114. Pittman DD, Kaufman RJ: Proteolytic requirements for thrombin activation of anti-hemophilic factor (factor VIII). Proc Natl Acad Sci USA 85:2429, 1988

115. Pittman DD, Kaufman RJ: Structure-function relationships of factor VIII elucidated through recombinant DNA technology. Thromb Haemost 61:161, 1989

116. Gitschier I, Kogan S, Levinson B, Tuddenham EGD: Mutations of factor VIII cleavage sites in hemophilia A. Blood 72:1022, 1988

117. O'Brien DP, Tuddenham EGD: Purification and characterization of factor VIII 1,689-Cys: a nonfunctional cofactor occurring in a patient with severe hemophilia A. Blood 73:2117, 1989

118. Hill-Eubanks DC, Parker CG, Lollar P: Differential proteolytic activation of factor VIII-von Willebrand factor complex by thrombin. Proc Natl Acad Sci USA 86:6508, 1989

119. Aly AM, Hoyer LW: Factor VIII-East Hartford (arginine 1689 to cysteine) has procoagulant activity when separated from von Willebrand factor. J Clin Invest 89:1382, 1992

120. Toole JJ, Pittman DD, Orr EC et al: A large region (~95 kDa) of human factor VIII is dispensable for *in vitro* procoagulant activity. Proc Natl Acad Sci USA 83:5939, 1986

121. Eaton DL, Wood WI, Eaton D et al: Construction and characterization of an active factor VIII variant lacking the central one-third of the molecule. Biochemistry 25:8342, 1987

122. Francis RT, McDonagh I, Mann KG: Factor V is a substrate for the transamidase factor XIIIa. J Biol Chem 261:9787, 1986

123. Brown JE, Bajsarowicz K: Factor VIII can serve as an acceptor for FXIIIa catalyzed incorporation of a pentylamine substrate. Thromb Haemost 69:1089a, 1993

124. Lollar P, Parker CG: Subunit structure of thrombin-activated porcine factor VIII. Biochemistry 28:666, 1987

125. Fay PJ, Haidaris PJ, Smudzin TM: Human factor VIIIa subunit structure. J Biol Chem 266:8957, 1991

126. Pittman DD, Milenssen M, Bauer K, Kaufman RJ: The A2 domain of human

recombinant factor VIII is required for procoagulant activity but not for thrombin cleavage. Blood 79:16467, 1991

127. Fay PJ, Smudzin TM: Characterization of the interaction between the A2 subunit and A1/A3-C1-C2 dimer in human factor VIIIa. J Biol Chem 267:13246, 1992

128. Fay PJ, Haidaris PJ, Huggins CF: Role of the COOH-terminal acidic region of A1 subunit in A2 subunit retention in human factor VIIIa. J Biol Chem 268:17861, 1993

129. Lollar P, Parker CG: pH-dependent denaturation of thrombin-activated porcine factor VIII. J Biol Chem 265:1688, 1990

130. Hultin MB, Jesty J: The activation and inactivation of human factor VIII by thrombin: effect of inhibitors of thrombin. Activation and inactivation of human factor VIII. Blood 57:476, 1981

131. Rick ME, Hoyer LW: Thrombin activation of factor VIII: the effect of inhibitors. Br J Haemotol 36:585, 1977

132. Lollar P, Parker ET: Structural basis for the decreased procoagulant activity of human factor VIII compared to the porcine homolog. J Biol Chem 266:12481, 1991

133. Lollar P, Parker ET, Fay PJ: Coagulant properties of hybrid human/porcine factor VIII molecules. J Biol Chem 267:23652, 1992

134. Lollar P, Knutson GJ, Fass DN: Stabilization of thrombin-activated porcine factor VIII:C by factor IXa and phospholipid. Blood 63:1303, 1984

135. Fulcher CA, Gardiner JE, Griffin JH, Zimmerman TS: Proteolytic inactivation of human factor VIII procoagulant protein by activated protein C and its analogy with factor V. Blood 63:486, 1984

136. Esmon CT: Molecular events that control the protein C anticoagulant pathway. Thromb Haemost 70:29, 1993

137. Griffin JH, Evatt B, Zimmerman TS et al: Deficiency of protein C in congenital thrombolic disease. J Clin Invest 68:1370, 1981

138. Bertina RM, Broekmans AW, van der Linden IK, Mertens K: Protein C deficiency in a Dutch family with thrombolic disease. Thromb Haemost 48:1, 1982

139. Zwaal RF: Membrane and lipid involvement in blood coagulation. Biochim Biophys Acta 515:163, 1978

140. Bevers EM, Comfurius P, Van Rijn JLML et al: Generation of prothrombin-converting activity and the exposure of phosphatidylserine at the outer surface of platelets. Eur J Biochem 122:429, 1982

141. Miletich JP, Jackson CM, Majerus PW: Properties of the factor Xa binding site on human platelets. J Biol Chem 253:6908, 1978

142. Kane WH, Lindhout MJ, Jackson CM, Majerus PW: Factor Va-dependent binding of factor Xa, to human platelets. J Biol Chem 255:1170, 1980

143. Tracy PB, Nesheim ME, Mann KG: Coordinate binding of factor-Va to the unstimulated platelet. J Biol Chem 256:743, 1981

144. Nesheim ME, Pittman DD, Wang JH et al: The binding of ^{35}S-labeled recombinant factor VIII to activated and unactivated human platelets. J Biol Chem 263:16467, 1988

145. Muntean W, Leschnik B, Haas J: Factor VIII coagulant moiety binds to platelets by binding to phospholipids of the platelet membrane. Thromb Res 45:345, 1987

146. Rawala-Sheikh R, Ahmad S, Ashby B, Walsh P: Kinetics of coagulation factor X activation by platelet-bound factor IXa. Biochemistry 29:2606, 1990

147. Gilbert GE, Sims PJ, Wiedmer T et al: Platelet-derived microparticles express high affinity receptors for factor VIII. J Biol Chem 266:17261, 1991

148. Nesheim ME, Furmaniak-Kazmierczak E, Henin C, Cote G: On the existence of platelet receptors for factor V(a) and factor VIII(a). Thromb Haemost 70:80, 1993

149. Stern DM, Drillings M, Kisiel W et al: Activation of factor IX bound to cultured bovine aortic endothelial cells. Proc Natl Acad Sci USA 81:913, 1984

150. Stern DM, Drillings M, Nossel HL et al: Binding of factors IX and IXa to cultured vascular endothelial cells. Proc Natl Acad Sci USA 80:4119, 1983

151. Broze GR Jr: The role of tissue factor pathway inhibitor in a revised coagulation cascade. Semin Hematol 29:159, 1992

152. Bauer KA, Kass BL, ten Cate H et al: Detection of factor X activation in humans. Blood 74:2007, 1989

153. Bauer KA, ten Cate H, Kass BL, Rosenberg RD: Factor IX is directly activated by the factor VII/VIIa-tissue factor mechanism *in vivo*. Blood 76:731, 1989

154. Broze GJ Jr, Warren LA, Novotny WF et al: The lipoprotein-associated coagulation inhibitor that inhibits the factor VIII-tissue factor complex also inhibits factor Xa: insight into its possible mechanism of action. Blood 71:335, 1988

155. Rao LVM, Rapaport SI: Studies of a mechanism inhibiting the initiation of the extrinsic pathway of coagulation. Blood 69:645, 1987

156. Osterud B, Rapaport S: Activation of factor IX by the reaction product of tissue factor and factor VII. Additional pathway for initiating blood coagulation. Proc Natl Acad Sci USA 74:5260, 1977

157. Armstrong S, Husten J, Esmon C, Johnson A: The active site of membrane-bound meizothrombin: a fluorescence determination of its distance from the phospholipid surface and its conformational sensitivity to calcium and factor Va. J Biol Chem 165:6210, 1990

158. Govers-Riemslag JWP, Janssen MP, Zwaal RFA, Rosing J: Effect of membrane fluidity and fatty acid composition on the prothrombin-converting activity of phospholipid vesicles. Biochemistry 31:10000, 1992

159. Rizza CR, Spooner RID: Treatment of haemophilia and related disorders in Britain and Northern Ireland during 1976–80: report on behalf of the Directors of Haemophilia Centres in the United Kingdom. BMJ 1286:929, 1983

160. Hoyer LW: Molecular pathology and immunology of factor VIII (hemophilia A and factor VIII inhibitors). Hum Pathol 18:153, 1987

161. Lazarchick I, Hoyer LW: Immunoradiometric measurement of the factor VIII procoagulant antigen. J Clin Invest 62:1048, 1978

162. Gitschier J, Wood WI, Goralka TM et al: Characterization of the human factor VIII gene. Nature 312:326, 1984

163. Levinson B, Kenwrick S, Lakich D et al: A transcribed gene in an intron of the human factor VIII gene. Genomics 7:1, 1990

164. Levinson B, Bermingham JR, Metzenberg A et al: Sequence of the human factor VIII-associated gene is conserved in mouse. Genomics 13:862, 1992

165. Levinson B, Kenwrick S, Gamel P et al: Evidence for a third transcript from the human factor VIII gene. Genomics 14:585, 1992

166. Freije D, Schlessinger D: A 1.6 nb contig of yeast artificial chromosomes around the human factor VIII gene reveals three regions homologous to probes for the DXS 115 locus and two for the DXYS64 locus. Am J Hum Genet 51:66, 1992

167. Haldane JBS, Smith CAB: A new estimate of the linkage between the genes for colour blindness and haemophilia in man. Ann Eugen 14:10, 1947

168. Boyer SH, Graham JB: Linkage between the X chromosome loci for G6PD electrophoretic variation and hemophilia A. Am J Hum Genet 17:320, 1965

169. Filippi G, Mannucci PM, Coppola R et al: Studies on hemophilia A in Sardinia bearing on the problems of multiple allelism, carrier detection and differential mutation rate in the two sexes. Am J Hum Genet 36:44, 1984

170. Patterson M, Schwartz C, Bell M et al: Physical mapping studies on the human X chromosome in the region Xq27-Xqter. Genomics 1:297, 1987

171. Poustka A, Detrich A, Langenstein G et al: Physical map of Xq27-Xqter: localizing the region of the fragile X mutation. Proc Natl Acad Sci USA 88:8302, 1991

172. Migeon BR, McGinnis MJ, Antonarakis SE et al: Severe hemophilia A in a female by cryptic translocation: order and orientation of factor VIII within Xq28. Genomics 16:20, 1993

173. Higuchi M, Antonarakis SE, Kasch L et al: Towards a complete characterization of mild to moderate hemophilia A: detection of the molecular defect in 25 of 29 patients by denaturing gradient gel electrophoresis. Proc Natl Acad Sci USA 88:8307, 1991

174. Higuchi M, Kazazian HH, Kasch L et al: Molecular characterization of severe hemophilia A suggests that about half the mutations are not within the coding region and splice junctions of the factor VIII gene. Proc Natl Acad Sci USA 88:7405, 1991

175. Naylor JA, Green PM, Rizza CR, Gianelli F: Factor VIII gene explains all cases of haemophilia A. Lancet 340:1066, 1992

176. Lakich D, Kazazian HH, Antonarakis SE, Gitschier J: Inversions disrupting the factor VIII gene as a common cause of severe hemophilia A. Nature Genetics 5:236, 1993

177. Antonarakis SE, Kazazian HH Jr: The molecular basis of hemophilia A in man. Trends Genet 4:233, 1988

178. Tuddenham EGD, Cooper DN, Gitschier J et al: Haemophilia A: database of nucleotide substitutions, deletions, insertions and rearrangements of the factor VIII gene. Nucleic Acid Res 19:4821, 1991

179. Youssoufian H, Antonarakis SE, Aronis S et al: Characterization of five partial deletions of the factor VIII gene. Proc Natl Acad Sci USA 84:3772, 1987

180. Woods-Samuels P, Kazazian HH Jr, Antonarakis SE: Nonhomologous recombination in the human genome: deletions in the human factor VIII gene. Genomics 10:94, 1991

181. Kazazian HH Jr, Wong C, Youssoufian HG et al: A novel mechanism of mutation in man: hemophilia A due to de novo insertion of L1 sequences. Nature 332:164, 1988

182. Fanning TG, Singer MF: LINE-1: a mammalian transposable element. Biochem Biophys Acta 910:203, 1987

183. Kazazian HH Jr, Scott AF: "Copy and paste" transposable elements in the human genome. J Clin Invest 91:1859, 1993

184. Dombroski BA, Mathias SL, Nanthakumar E et al: Isolation of a human transposable element. Science 254:1808, 1991

185. Woods-Samuels P, Wong C, Mathias SL et al: Characterization of a nondeleterious L1 insertion in an intron of the human factor VIII gene and evidence for open reading frames in functional L1 elements. Genomics 4:290, 1989

186. Gitschier J: Maternal duplication associated with gene deletion in sporadic hemophilia. Am J Hum Genet 43:274, 1988

187. Murru S, Casula L, Pecorara M et al: Illegitimate recombination produced a duplication within the factor VIII gene in a patient with mild hemophilia A. Genomics 7:115, 1990

188. McGinniss MJ, Kazazian HH Jr, Hoyer LW et al: Spectrum of mutations in CRM-positive and CRM-reduced hemophilia A. Genomics 15:392, 1993

189. Youssoufian H, Kazazian HH Jr, Phillips DG et al: Recurrent mutations in haemophilia A give evidence for CpG mutations hotspots. Nature 324:380, 1986

190. Naylor JA, Green PM, Rizza CR, Gianelli F: Analysis of factor VIII mRNA reveals defects in every one of 28 haemophilia A patients. Hum Mol Genet 2:11, 1993

191. Cooper DN, Youssoufian H: The CpG dinucleotide and human genetic disease. Hum Genet 74:151, 1988

192. Diamond C, Kogan S, Levinson B, Gitschier J: Amino acid substitutions in conserved domains of factor VIII and related proteins: study of patients with mild to moderately severe hemophilia A. Hum Mut 1:248, 1992

193. Youssoufian H, Antonarakis SE, Bell W et al: Nonsense and missense mutation in hemophilia A: estimate of the relative mutation rate at CpG dinucleotides. Am J Hum Genet 42:718, 1988

194. Dietz HC, Valle D, Francomano CA et al: The skipping of constitutive exons in vivo induced by nonsense mutations. Science 259:680, 1993

195. Gitschier J, Kogan S, Levinson B, Tuddenham EGD: Mutations of factor VIII cleavage sites in hemophilia A. Blood 72:1022, 1988

196. Arai M, Inaba H, Higuchi M et al: Detection of a mutation altering a thrombin cleavage site (arginine-372-histidine). Proc Natl Acad Sci USA 86:4277, 1989

197. O'Brien D, Pattinson JK, Tuddenham EGD: Purification and characterization of factor VIII 372-cys: a hypofunctional cofactor from a patient with moderately severe hemophilia A. Blood 75:1664, 1990

198. Arai M, Higuchi M, Antonarakis SE et al: Characterization of a thrombin cleavage site mutation (Arg 1689 to Cys) in the factor VIII gene of two unrelated patients with cross-reacting material-positive hemophilia. Blood 75:384, 1990

199. Aly AM, Higuchi M, Kasper CK et al: Hemophilia A due to mutations that create new N-glycosylation sites. Proc Natl Acad Sci USA 89:4933, 1992

200. Sultan Y: Prevalence of inhibitors in a population of 3435 hemophilia patients in France. Thromb Hemost 67:600, 1992

201. Fulcher CA, de Graff S, Mahoney S, Zimmerman TS: FVIII inhibitor IgG subclass and FVIII polypeptide specificity determined by immunoblotting. Blood 69:1475, 1987

202. Scandella D, Mattingly M, de Graaf S, Fulcher CA: Localization of epitopes for human factor VIII inhibitor antibodies by immunoblotting and antibody neutralization. Blood 74:1618, 1990

203. Millar DS, Steinbrecher RA, Wieland K et al: The molecular genetic analysis of haemophilia A: characterization of six partial deletions in the factor VIII gene. Hum Genet 86:219, 1990

204. Gitschier J, Drayna D, Tuddenham EGD et al: Genetic mapping and diagnosis of haemophilia A achieved through a BclI polymorphism in the factor VIII gene. Nature 314:738, 1988

205. Antonarakis SE, Waber PG, Kittur SD et al: Hemophilia A: molecular defects and carrier detection by DNA analysis. N Engl J Med 313:843, 1985

206. Wion KL, Tuddenham EGD, Lawn RM: A new polymorphism in the factor VIII gene for prenatal diagnosis of hemophilia A. Nucleic Acids Res 14:4535, 1986

207. Harper K, Winter RM, Pembrey ME et al: A clinically useful DNA probe linked to haemophilia A. Lancet 2:6, 1984

208. Oberle I, Camerino G, Heilig R et al: Genetic screening for hemophilia A (classic hemophilia) with a polymorphic DNA probe. N Engl J Med 312:682, 1985

209. Lalloz MR, McVey IH, Pattison IK, Tuddenham EGD: Haemophilia A diagnosis by analysis of a hypervariable dinucleotide repeat within the factor VIII gene. Lancet 338:207, 1991

210. Peake IR, Lillicrap DP, Boulyjenkov V et al: Report of a joint WHO/WHF meeting on the control of haemophilia: carrier detection and prenatal diagnosis. Blood Coagul Fibrinolysis 4:313, 1993

211. Kaufman RJ: Expression and structure-function properties of recombinant factor VIII. Trans Med Rev 6:235, 1992

212. Kazazian HH Jr, Wong C, Youssoufian H et al: Haemophilia A resulting from de novo insertion of L1 sequences represents a novel mechanism for mutation in man. Nature 332:164, 1988

Clinical Aspects of and Therapy for Hemophilia A

106

Doreen B. Brettler, Elissa M. Kraus, and Peter H. Levine

INTRODUCTION

Hemophilia A, the most common of the true hemophilias, accounts for approximately 85% of cases. It is an X-linked recessive bleeding disorder attributable to decreased plasma levels of properly functioning factor VIII (also known as antihemophilic factor).

Probably originally named haemorrhaphilia, the disease was referred to as hemophilia by Schönlein in the early 1800s.[1] In 1893, Wright[2] noted that blood from patients with hemophilia demonstrated a prolonged clotting time. In 1911, Addis[3] showed that the latter could be corrected in vitro by adding normal plasma. In 1947, both Brinkhouse[4] and Quick[5] independently suggested a role for factor VIII in the generation of plasma thromboplastic activity. That same year, Pavlovsky[6] correctly inferred the presence of multiple types of hemophilia by showing that he could correct the clotting defect in certain hemophilic plasma samples by adding plasma from certain other hemophilic donors.

Lane[7] successfully transfused a patient with hemophilia in 1840, and plasma was first used as therapy in 1923 by Feisly.[8] Due to the minute quantities of factor VIII in plasma, its short half-life, and problems of circulatory volume overload, the vast majority of persons with hemophilia succumbed to hemorrhage early in life during the era of whole blood plasma therapy. In one study from Scandinavia,[9] for example, the mean age of death between the years 1950 and 1959 was 10.2 years for all persons with hemophilia.

In 1964 Pool et al.[10] analyzed the content of the annoying precipitate that formed transiently during the thawing of fresh frozen plasma and found it to contain a disproportionately high amount of factor VIII. Thus, the era of cryoprecipitate therapy began, and this treatment made the first meaningful improvement in life expectancy. For example, in the same Scandinavian study,[9] the average age at death between 1960 and 1969 doubled to 20.1 years.

The late 1960s saw the introduction of partially purified preparations of factor VIII, prepared by glycine precipitation of fresh plasma and later by polyethylene glycol precipitation.[11] More recently, therapeutic products highly purified from human plasma by the use of immunoaffinity chromatography have been available.[12] The first infusion of recombinant factor VIII was reported by White and colleagues in 1988.[13] Subsequently, >100 patients have been studied, all of whom have received recombinant factor VIII without difficulty.[14]

INCIDENCE

Both Hemophilia A and B were studied by the National Heart, Lung, and Blood Institute in 1972.[15] Their estimate of incidence was 25 cases per 100,000 males. Other studies have suggested lower figures, and most experts believe the correct figure to be approximately 20 cases per 100,000 males (1 per 10,000 of the whole population), with factor VIII deficiency accounting for 85% of these. Factor IX deficiency explains 14%, and the remaining cases involve the rare congenital clotting factor factor XI, X, VII, or V deficiencies. There is no reason to believe that the incidence of hemophilia varies in different races or by geographic areas of the world.

Among patients with hemophilia A being treated in the United States, 60% are classified as severe (i.e., have a factor VIII level of <1% of normal). Most of the remainder have moderate disease (factor VIII level >1% of normal). The number of people with mild disease is not known, as many such patients undoubtedly are mild bleeders and escape detection.

CLINICAL SEVERITY

The frequency and severity of bleeding in hemophilia may be predicted from the factor VIII procoagulant level, assayed in comparison to a reference standard that is assumed to have factor VIII levels of 100%, corresponding to a factor VIII activity of 1.0 U/ml. The factor VIII level in normal persons ranges from 50% to 200% (0.50–2.0 U/ml). Those with factor VIII levels ≤1% of normal (≤0.01 U/ml) have hemorrhages requiring therapy two to four times monthly on the average, although the range is large and the episodes are irregularly spaced. Such patients are classified as severe hemophiliacs. Those with factor VIII levels >5% of normal (>0.05 U/ml) are considered mild hemophiliacs and usually hemorrhage only due to trauma or surgery. Some such cases are not diagnosed until adult life. Occasional spontaneous hemarthrosis may occur in such patients, especially in joints damaged by previously undertreated post-traumatic hemorrhage. Patients whose factor VIII levels are between these two ranges are considered moderately severe, and their clinical picture falls between the two extremes. If such patients have had multiple untreated, or suboptimally treated hemarthroses with subsequent joint damage, the anatomic instability of these joints will cause frequent and severe bleeding, and the disease will therefore appear clinically more severe than the factor VIII assay would suggest.

The choice of treatment for factor VIII deficiency depends on its severity. Those with severe or moderate disease are treated with factor concentrate. Patients with mild disease (factor VIII levels >10%) can receive desmopressin (deamino-D-arginine vasopressin [DDAVP]). Cryoprecipitate is also used in some centers to treat mild hemophilia A. However, since it cannot be virally inactivated, most physicians use factor concentrate in patients with mild hemophilia A who do not respond to DDAVP.

Within a given hemophilia kindred, the clinical and laboratory severity of the disorder is relatively consistent. The appearance of a more severe clinical course in a family relative should raise the question of either established anatomic lesions that predispose to frequent or severe hemorrhage, or the development of an inhibitor.

CLINICAL MANIFESTATIONS

The clinical hallmarks of hemophilia A are (1) lack of excessive hemorrhage from minor cuts or abrasions due to the normalcy of platelet function; (2) joint and muscle hemorrhages, which lead to the most difficult and disabling long-term sequelae; (3) easy bruising; (4) prolonged and potentially fatal postoperative hemorrhage; and (5) a panoply of social psychologic, vocational, and economic problems. For many patients treated with blood products prior to 1985, acquisition of human immunodeficiency virus (HIV) exacerbated already severe clinical problems.[16] Finally, slowly progressive hepatocellular disease, mainly attributable to chronic hepatitis C, remains a threat to patients.[17]

Hemarthroses

The joints most frequently involved (in descending order of frequency) are the knees, elbows, ankles, shoulders, hips, and wrists. Bleeding into the hand is rare and usually follows significant trauma, while the spine is rarely, if ever, involved.

The first episodes of acute hemarthrosis occur in childhood, but often not until the child begins to walk. Infants and small children may develop large ecchymoses from being carried or lifted. Hemarthrosis is usually either spontaneous or associated with imperceptible trauma. The onset of hemorrhage is signaled by an "aura," consisting of vague warmth, a tingling sensation, and/or a sense of mild restlessness or anxiety; this aura may last up to 2 hours. Mild discomfort and slight limitation of joint motion occur next, followed (after 1 to several hours) by pain, joint swelling, cutaneous warmth, and eventual severe limitation of motion. Once bleeding has stopped, the blood is reabsorbed, and the joint returns to normal over several days to several weeks.

When pain, swelling, and severe limitation of motion are present, the hemorrhage is far advanced and the process of synovitis begins; this may predispose the joint to further episodes of hemarthrosis and to hemophilic arthropathy[18] (Fig. 106-1). Joint hemorrhage should be treated after the earliest symptoms are noted and before any physician findings to prevent the long-term disabling sequelae. Adults may demonstrate periodic joint pain due to established hemophilic arthropathy rather than bleeding and may have considerable fibrosis of the joint capsule, thus preventing joint swelling. They may develop chronic limitation of motion, removing the value of this finding in diagnosing an acute bleed. Prophylactic correction of the hemostatic defect over several weeks or months can help the patient to differentiate acute hemarthrosis from the background of chronic symptoms and signs.

An episode of bleeding into a joint predisposes to further episodes for at least two possible reasons.[19] First, hemarthrosis stimulates proliferation, chronic inflammation, and hypervascularity of the synovial membrane. Second, hemarthrosis is accompanied by rapid atrophy of the periarticular musculature and a subsequent compromise in joint protection exerted by these muscles (Fig. 106-2).

Chronic Arthritis

Recurrent hemarthrosis may lead to a self-perpetuating condition in which joint abnormalities persist in intervals between bleeding episodes. Clinically, the involved joint is chronically swollen, although painless and slightly warm. There are clinical

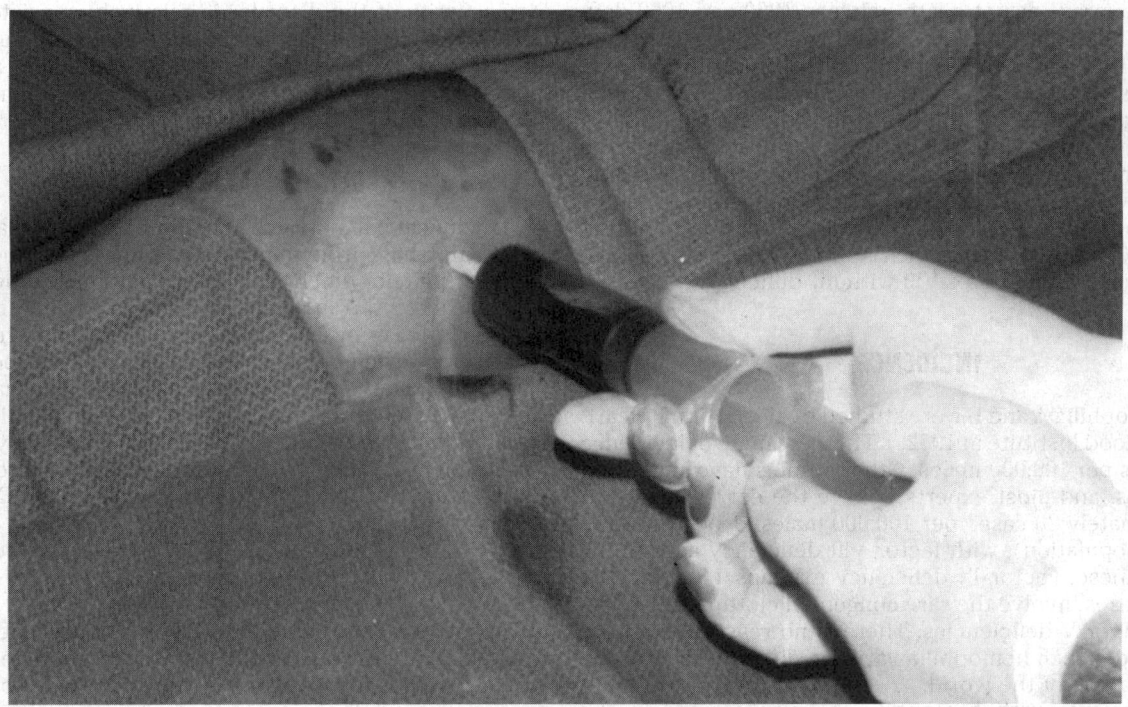

Fig. 106-1. Joint aspiration under sterile conditions of an acute knee hemorrhage.

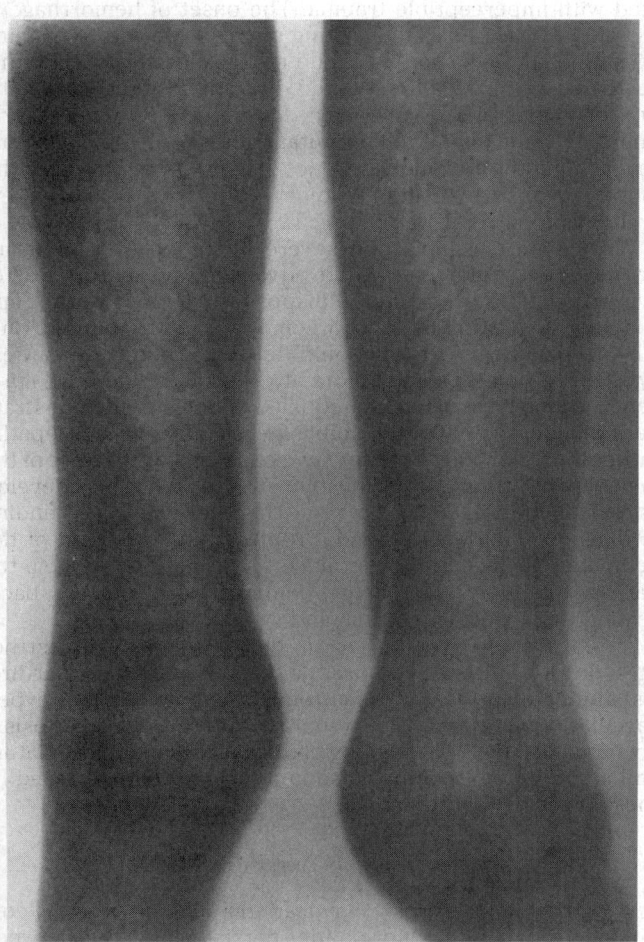

Fig. 106-2. End-stage hemophilic arthropathy of right and left knee with bilateral quadriceps atrophy and valgus external rotation deformity.

findings of chronic synovitis, including prominent synovial bogginess with or without effusion (Fig. 106-3). Mild limitation of motion may be present, often with flexion deformity. Factor replacement does not modify these parameters. The likelihood of developing chronic arthritis is directly related to the overall severity of the underlying coagulation defect. In one study of 139 hemophiliac patients, only 42% were found to have definite and an additional 14% possible hemophilic arthritis, based on clinical and radiographic features.[20] Despite any previous history of hemarthrosis, however, no patient with a factor level >20% had hemophilic arthritis, while up to one-third with levels between 6% and 20% had possible or definite arthritis. In those patients who develop chronic arthritis, it is not clear whether the phenomenon is due to repeated subclinical minor hemorrhage or to irreversible synovial proliferation induced by major hemarthroses. However, it is this clinical state that often progresses to the severe destructive arthritis seen in advanced hemophilic arthropathy. The radiologic changes are seen in Figures 106-4 and 106-5. Nonsteroidal anti-inflammatory agents have been found to offer significant pain relief without routinely causing increased bleeding difficulties.

End-Stage Hemophilic Arthropathy

Long-standing end-stage hemophilic arthropathy has features in common with both degenerative joint disease and advanced rheumatoid arthritis.[18] The radiographic changes are shown in Figures 106-6 and 106-7. Clinically, the joint appears enlarged and "knobby," due to osteophytic bony overgrowth (Fig. 106-2). Synovial thickening and effusion, however, are not prominent. Range of motion is severely restricted, and fibrous, in contrast to bony, ankylosis is frequently seen. Subluxation, joint laxity, and malalignment are common. Hemarthroses, however, decrease in frequency.

Septic Arthritis

Although many diseases such as rheumatoid arthritis and osteoarthritis confer an increased risk of bacterial infection of a previously damaged joint, septic arthritis is a rarely reported complication of hemophilic arthritis. Pyogenic arthritis in he-

abdomen (which mimics appendicitis) or pain referred to the groin (which is mistaken for hemarthrosis of the hip.)[22] Distension of the iliopsoas muscle causes the leg to be held in flexion at the hip, and compression of the femoral nerve causes pain on the anterior surface of the thigh. Increased pressure on the femoral nerve leads to paresthesia, hypesthesia, weakness of the quadriceps muscle, and even permanent paralysis of the thigh flexors.

Other Closed-Space Hemorrhage

Bleeding into the muscles of the forearm may lead to median or ulnar nerve paralysis or Volkmann's ischemic contracture of the hand. Calf lesions may lead to fixed equinovarus deformity at the ankle or to peroneal or other nerve palsies. Less common is wrist bleeding with nerve entrapment syndromes. Spontaneous or traumatic bleeding into the tongue or the mus-

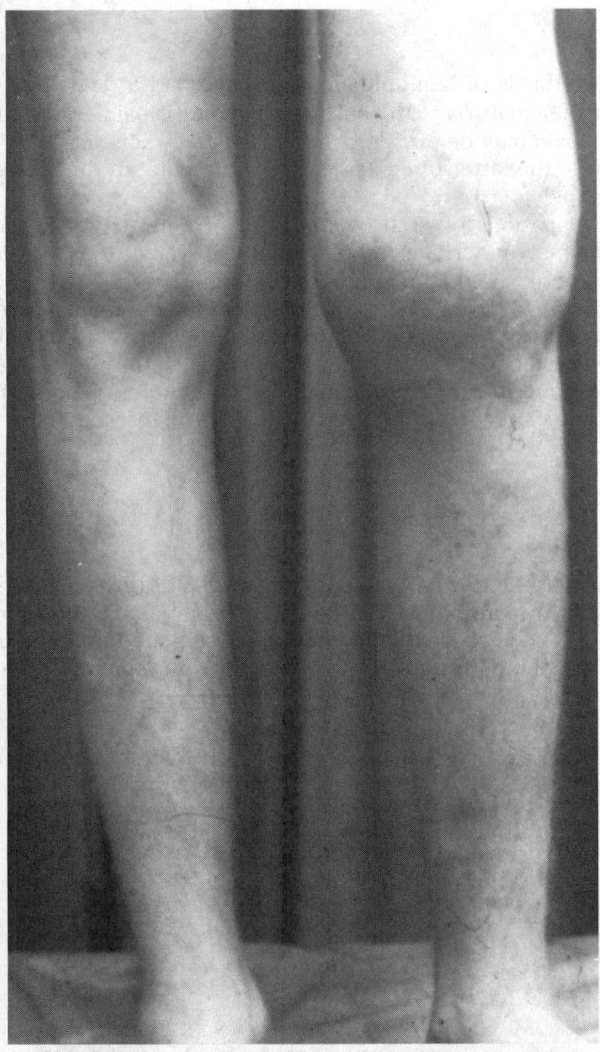

Fig. 106-3. Chronic synovitis of left knee with swelling and warmth on physical examination but absence of pain.

mophiliacs more commonly occurs in adults than in children and is usually monarticular, with a predilection for knee involvement. Compared with spontaneous hemarthrosis, septic arthritis is associated with a fever >38°C within 12 hours of presentation, an increased peripheral leukocyte count, and articular pain that does *not* improve with replacement therapy. A predisposing factor other than hemophilic arthropathy is often identifiable, including previous arthrocentesis, arthroplasty, intravenous drug usage, or immunosuppression secondary to HIV-1 infection. *Staphylococcus aureus* is the most frequently identified organism.[21]

Hematomas

Small intramuscular hematomas are common and may resolve spontaneously, but large hematomas may lead to severe sequelae by way of compression of vital structures. Large hematomas may produce fever, leukocytosis, severe pain, and hyperbilirubinemia due to erythrocyte degradation. Those not adequately treated may result in fibrous organization with contractures. A large hematoma of the back and flank is seen in Figures 106-8 and 106-9.

Psoas Hematoma

Hematoma of the psoas muscle or in the muscles of the retroperitoneum may cause either pain in the lower quadrant of the

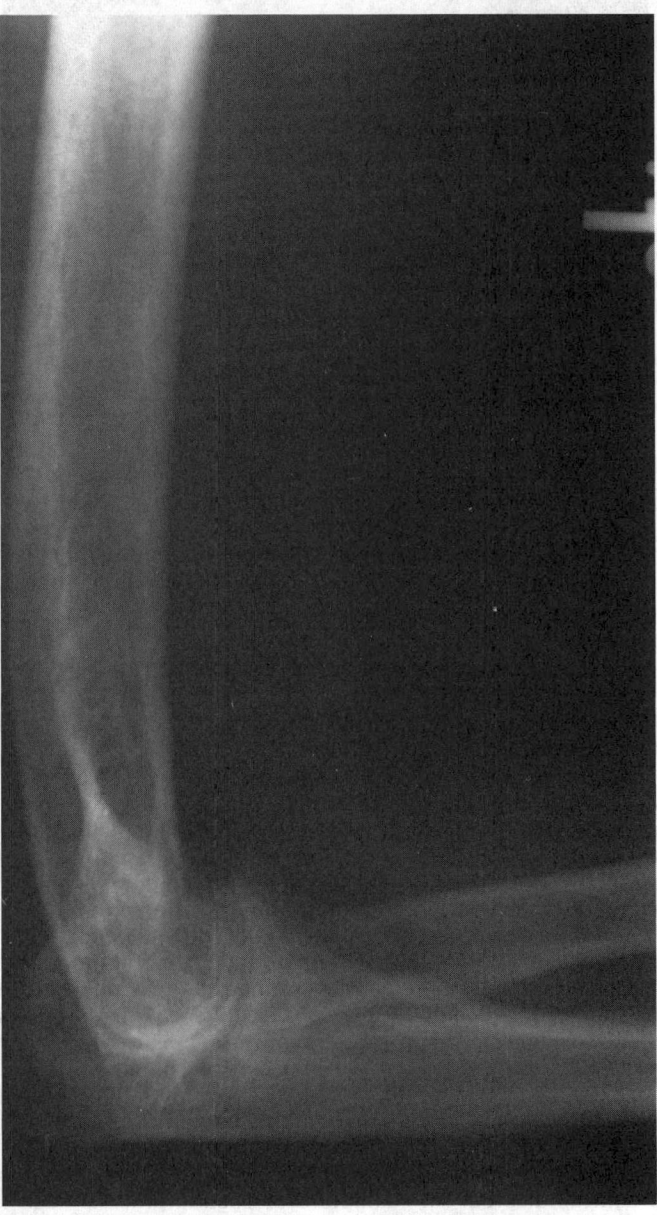

Fig. 106-4. Hemophilic arthropathy of elbow with narrowing of joint space.

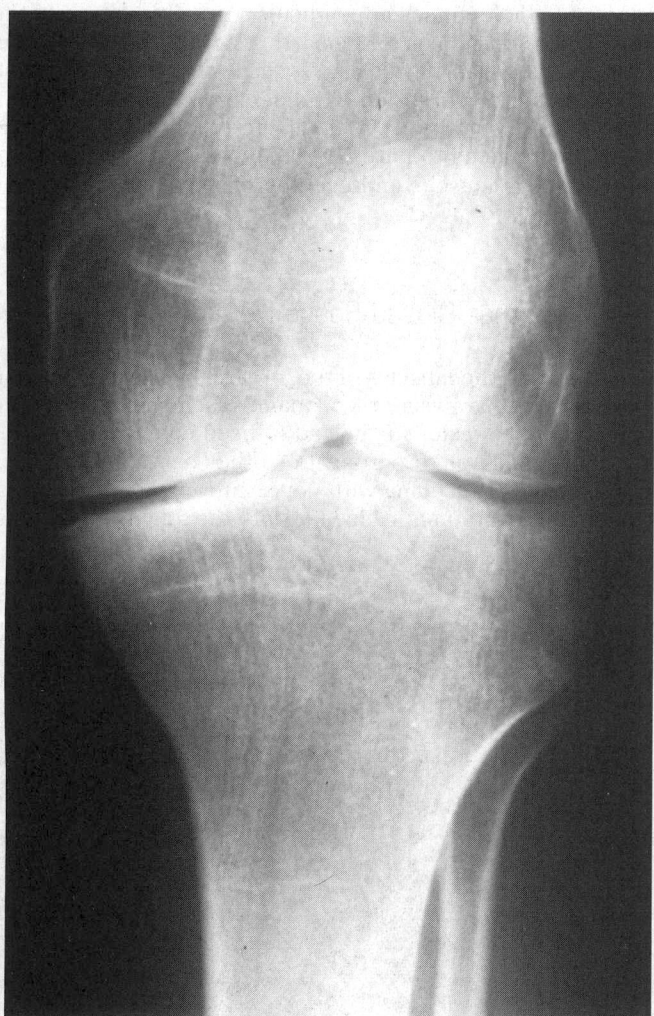

Fig. 106-5. Hemophilic arthropathy of knee with narrowing of joint space, irregularity of articular surfaces, and subchondral sclerosis.

cles or soft tissues of the neck or throat may rapidly obstruct the airway, thereby requiring prompt and vigorous therapy.

Hemophilic Cysts and Pseudotumors

A large intramuscular hemorrhage may uncommonly result in the formation of a simple muscle cyst that clinically appears to be an encapsulated soft tissue area of swelling overlying muscle. Cyst formation in this setting is confined by the muscular fascial plane and results most likely from inadequate resorption of blood and clot. Subperiosteal or intraosseous hemorrhage, by contrast, may lead to a rare skeletal complication of hemophilia, a hemophilic psuedotumor.[22] Hemophilic pseudotumors are of two types: (1) the adult type that occurs proximally, usually in the pelvis or femur, and (2) a childhood type that occurs distal to the elbows or knees and carries a better prognosis than the adult type. Conservative early management of both muscle cysts and psuedotumors is indicated, including immobilization and factor replacement. If these lesions progress, however, surgical removal is indicated to avoid serious complications such as spontaneous rupture, fistula formation, neurologic or vascular entrapment, and fracture of adjacent bone.[23] Aspiration of a pseudotumor or cyst is contraindicated. An example of a pseudotumor is seen in Figure 106-10.

Hematuria

Two-thirds of hemophiliacs will have had at least one episode of hematuria.[24] Most urinary bleeding is painless, but mild flank pain may be present, and occasionally severe renal colic occurs, the latter often associated with a clot in the ureter or renal pelvis.

Explanations of such bleeding vary from a trivial cause to significant underlying renal pathology. Hematuria is treated with increased fluid intake for several days and rest, followed by factor VIII for 2–4 days if the bleeding continues. Use of ϵ-aminocaproic acid should be avoided because of the risk of preventing the lysis of clots that obstruct the ureter. Renal ultrasound or other studies are not done unless hematuria is chronic or recurrent or severe flank pain is present.

Intracranial Bleeding

Intracranial bleeding accounts for 25% of the hemorrhagic deaths in hemophiliacs. Antecedent trauma has occurred in one-half of such deaths. Bleeding may be subdural, epidural, subarachnoid, intracerebral, or (rarely) intraspinal. In one co-

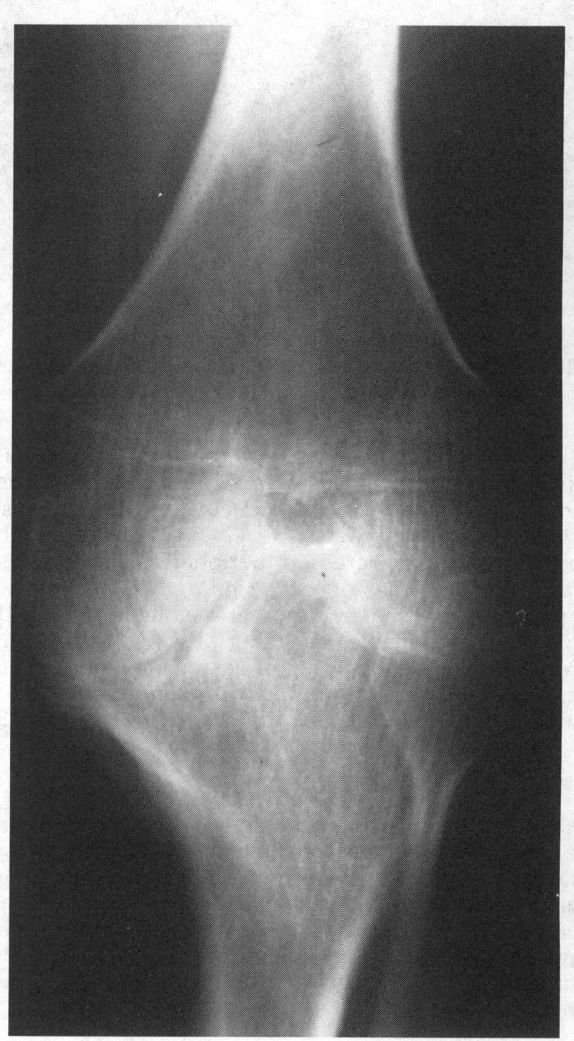

Fig. 106-6. End-stage arthropathy of knee with almost complete obliteration of joint space and bony loss.

CONTROL OF PAIN IN HEMOPHILIA

Pain is an extremely common problem for many persons with hemophilia. The two major causes are pain due to pressure from hemorrhage into joints, muscles, or other tissues and chronic arthritis pain, in which permanent changes have occurred in the anatomy of the joints. The control of pain is a major issue for people with hemophilia, and extensive time and energy should be put into training the patient in this regard. We believe that several general rules are important.

Acute joint pain should always be assumed to be due to bleeding. At the earliest symptom of joint discomfort or limitation of motion, the correct therapy is correction of the clotting factor defect. Early application of infusion therapy prevents pain and long-term joint clotting factor defect. Patients who are taught the general philosophy "when in doubt, infuse" will wind up using less clotting factor concentrate in the long run than those who adopt a "wait and see" attitude. The latter group will have advanced lesions requiring frequent treatment and higher doses and will also develop chronic synovitis requiring many days or weeks of treatment.

Chronic joint pain that fails to respond to infusion of factor VIII or IX may sometimes be arthritic pain. However, this determination should only be made after an attempt has been made to correct the coagulation defect for a period of days. If the pain that persists is accompanied by stiffness and is accentuated early in the day, it is more likely to be arthritic than hemorrhagic. In patients whose pain has hemorrhagic characteristics and who do not respond to correction of the coagulation factor defect, the use of nonsteroidal anti-inflammatory agents may provide considerable benefit. Aspirin must be avoided because of its prolonged antiplatelet effect.

A major problem for most patients with hemophilia prior to the availability of adequate means of correcting the coagulopathy was narcotic addiction. Obviously, the non-narcotic agents should be used whenever possible when analgesics are required. More than 90% of patients treated at our center never use narcotic pain medicines and control their pain only with infusion therapy and the use of acetaminophen. Among older adolescents and adults with established hemarthrosis, the use of nonsteroidal drugs for arthritic pain is helpful, and at any given time between one-third and one-half of our patients in this age group will be using nonsteroidal anti-inflammatory agents.

Patients should be taught that literally hundreds of medications available over the counter contain aspirin. Lists of aspirin-containing compounds are available from a variety of sources including the National Hemophilia Foundation in New York. Our own general rule is that patients with hemophilia take no new medication of any sort until they have checked with the center.

Occasionally the relief of chronic pain in hemophilia will require the use of alternative therapies, such as an exercise program administered by a physical therapist, biofeedback, acupuncture or acupressure, transcutaneous nerve stimulation, or hypnosis. A risk with hypnosis is that the patient may neglect to pay attention to episodes of pain, which indicate new hemorrhage for which the patient should be seeking medical intervention.

In the last analysis the best way to control pain in hemophilia is to prevent it through the early and adequate application of replacement therapy and through the use of home infusion incorporated into a program of patient education and comprehensive hemophilia care.

operative study of 2,500 hemophiliacs studied over 10 years,[25] 71 episodes of central nervous system bleeding were documented; the mortality rate was 34%, and 47% of the survivors were left with mental retardation, seizure disorders, or motor impairment.

Survivors had been treated with sufficient clotting factor concentration to raise the factor VIII level to 30%–50% of normal for ≥10–14 days. Current regimens suggest maintaining levels approaching 100%.

Other Sites of Hemorrhage

Gastrointestinal hemorrhages, manifested by hematemesis, melena, or hematochezia, are unusual in hemophilia. They are usually caused by organic gastrointestinal lesions.

Prolonged gingival oozing is common after shedding of deciduous teeth, eruption of new teeth, or instrumentation. If such oozing is sufficiently prolonged or severe enough to require therapy, several days of ε-aminocaproic acid (Amicar) therapy will usually suffice. Infusion of coagulation factor is only occasionally needed.

Epistaxis is not unusual in the severe hemophiliac, but it is unusual for mild hemophiliacs in the absence of a local nasal lesion. It is largely treated by local measures but may require factor infusion and cauterization.

Post-traumatic hemorrhage requires a special comment. Normal platelet plug formation may initially provide good hemostasis but delayed bleeding usually follows trauma. For this reason, many centers advocate treatment after significant trauma whether or not evidence of hemorrhage is yet apparent.

THERAPY

General Considerations

The many ramifications of this lifelong expensive and crippling illness must be considered or the efficacy of treatment will be impaired and the outcome will be poor. Hemophilia societies are useful sources of paramedical support and information. Many problem areas exist, including the following: (1) interactional difficulties between hemophiliacs and the health care system[26]; (2) psychological sequelae of overprotectiveness, such as the daredevil syndrome[27]; (3) poor adjustment of the hemophilic child to school[28]; (4) the enormous financial cost—in the range of $20,000–100,000/year for each patient depending on weight and severity; (5) important vocational problems in adults with established arthropathy[29]; and finally, (6) a low level of education about hemophilia on the part of health care professionals, owing to the relative rarity of the disease and the pace of recent therapeutic advances.

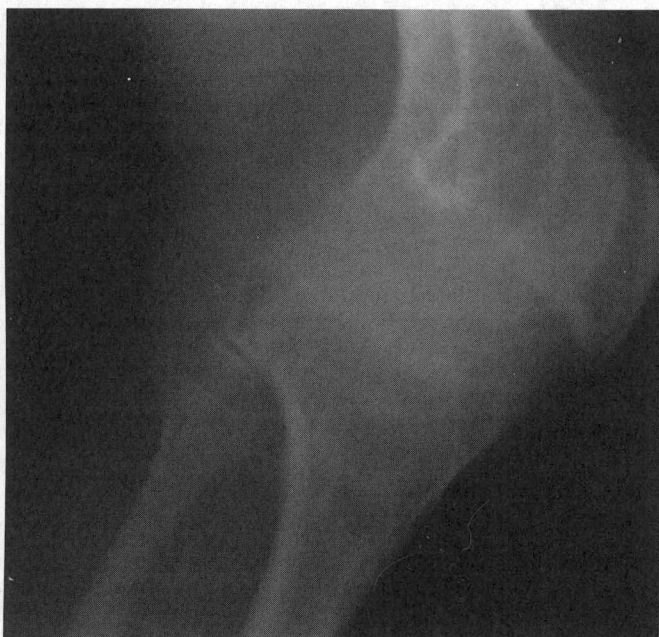

Fig. 106-7. End-stage hemophilic arthropathy with posterior subluxation of the tibia on the femur.

Principles of Replacement Therapy for Factor VIII

The hemostatically effective plasma level for each coagulation factor is different and depends in part on the nature, extent, and duration of the bleeding lesion. The dose of replacement factor is calculated in units: 1 U is the activity of a given coagulation factor found in 1 ml of pooled, citrated fresh frozen human plasma. The factor must be given in sufficient quantity to allow for its clearance, metabolic half-life, and volume of distribution with the body.

The half-life of factor VIII in plasma is between 8 and 12 hours, which includes an initial rapid decline in level owing to diffusion into extravascular pools.[30] The minimum hemostatic level of factor VIII for relatively mild hemorrhages is 30% (0.30 U/ml of plasma), while that for advanced joint or muscle bleeding or for other major hemorrhagic lesions is 50% (0.50 U/ml). One to several days of maintenance therapy is needed for such advanced lesions to resolve. Resolution is achieved by repeating the infusion at 24-hour intervals at approximately 75% of the original dose. For life-threatening lesions or surgery, levels of 80%–100% (0.80–1.00 U/ml) should be achieved and the factor VIII level should be kept above the 30%–50% range by means of appropriate doses of factor VIII infused at intervals of 8–12 hours.[31] This more frequent infusion regimen decreases the incidence of excessively low levels just prior to an infusion and also decreases the total amount of factor needed to maintain given in vivo minimum plasma levels. Constant infusion regimens are another option when levels need to be maintained above a set minimum.[32]

Doses can be calculated by multiplying the recipient plasma volume in milliliters by the desired increment of factor VIII in units per milliliter. A simpler and reproducible dose calculation is that each unit of factor VIII infused per kilogram of body weight yields a 2% rise in plasma factor VIII level (i.e., 0.02 U/ml). An example of therapy for a 50-kg patient with an extensive laceration would include maintenance of a 30% factor VIII level in vivo until healing is complete. This can be accomplished by an initial infusion to the 60% level with 1,500 U (30 × 50 kg) of factor VIII, followed by 750 U every 12 hours thereafter for 7–10 days, with dose adjustments being made every few days as indicated by factor VIII assays.

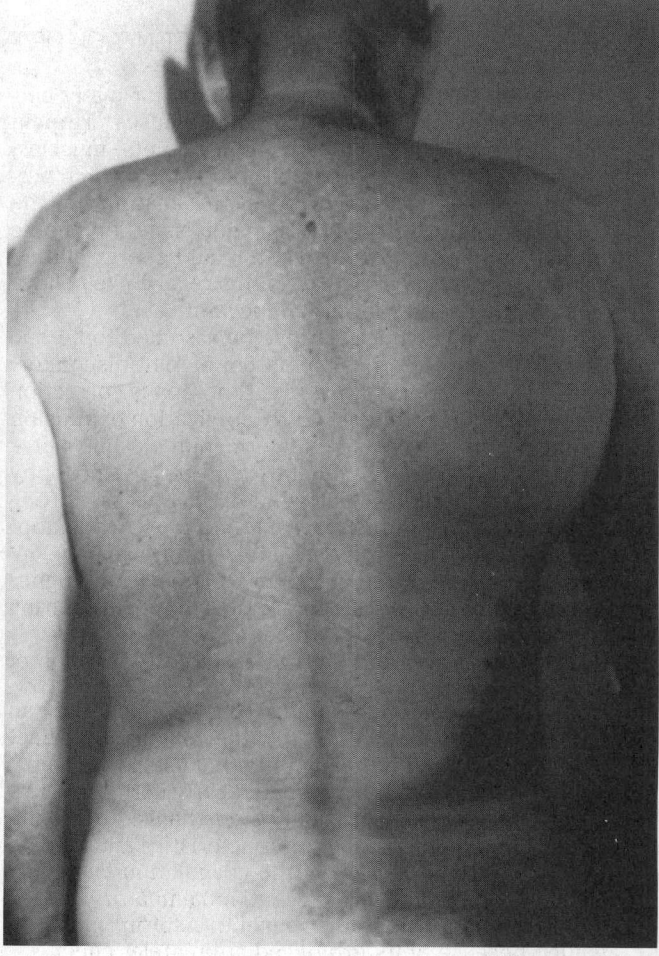

Fig. 106-8. Large hematoma starting in the right scapula region and extending down the right back to the right flank.

For patients with major or life-threatening lesions, the laboratory measurement of in vivo factor VIII activity is advisable because of variations that result from the responses of patients to such infusions.[33] Substitution of the activated partial thromboplastin time or another screening test for a formal factor VIII assay should be avoided because the results may be misleading.

Antihemophilic factor may be given on a variety of schedules to keep the amount of in vivo factor VIII above a fixed level, thus converting a patient with severe deficiency to one with a mild or moderate deficiency. Prophylactic factor used on a regular basis in small children is being explored as a method of preventing later costly joint deterioration. Such a program can dramatically reduce the incidence of hemorrhages, but it can also increase the expense, the drain on plasma resources, and possibly the side effects as well. Indications for such prophylactic use include intensive physical therapy, recurrent hemorrhage in a single joint or chronic synovitis, or learning a new physical activity.

Other Therapeutic Principles

Acute hemarthrosis should be treated with early infusion therapy, which will minimize the risk of chronic synovitis or progressive arthropathy and avoid the need for excessive pain medication or for arthrocentesis. Aspiration of the joint during an acute hemorrhage should be avoided unless the swelling and pain are very severe or a septic joint is suspected. The

INDICATIONS FOR INFUSION

Guidelines for doses of replacement therapy are variable from treater to treater, and there should be room for upward dose modification when the clinician is concerned that lesions are advanced or more threatening than usual. Below is a table of typical initial doses of replacement therapy used at our hemophilia treatment center.

Indications for Therapeutic Infusions	Factor VIII Units[a]
Mild Hemorrhage	15 U/kg: yields 30% level in vivo
Early joint or muscle bleeding severe epistaxis	
Gingival or dental bleeding (unresponsive to ε-aminocaproic acid)	
Hematuria (if persistent)	
Major Hemorrhage[b]	25 U/kg: yields 50% level in vivo
Advanced joint or muscle bleeding	
Neck, tongue, or pharyngeal hematoma	
Severe trauma, no evidence of bleeding	
Severe abdominal pain	
Gastrointestinal hemorrhage	
Life-threatening lesions[c]	40–50 U/kg: yields 80–100% level in vivo
Intracranial hemorrhage	
Surgery	
Major trauma with bleeding	
Retroperitoneal hemorrhage	
Head trauma	

[a] For major hemorrhage, one to several weeks of maintenance of minimum levels will be mandatory.

[b] Subsequent doses will usually be required.

[c] For factor VIII, maintenance is generally given by infusions at least every 12 hours, the half-life being 8–12 hours.

total consumption of factor concentrate and health care costs are the same in patients so treated as in those in whom advanced hemorrhagic lesions develop, and the health of the patient is clearly improved.[34]

Chronic hemophilic arthropathy can improve remarkably from several weeks or months of intensive physical therapy for muscle building and increased joint stability, intervals of avoiding weight bearing to allow for the regression of synovitis, and the correction of flexion contractures by wedging casts, night splints, or traction.[35] Regular prophylactic infusions of factor VIII can also be used to prevent traumatic bleeding.

Chronic synovitis should be treated with intensive factor VIII replacement plus conservative orthopaedic and physical therapy measures, a program that produces a medical synovectomy in about one-half of the treated joints.[36] Surgical synovectomy has been suggested for patients with nonhealing chronic synovitis or with frequently recurring hemarthrosis and the progressive development of severe chronic arthropathy; it has also been successful in preventing long-term sequelae.[37] Surgical synovectomy is associated not only with a marked decrease in the frequency of hemorrhage in the joint, but also with some loss of joint motion, which may not be fully regained despite physical therapy. More recently, radioactive synovectomies, performed by injecting radioactive dysprosium into a joint, have been done successfully. Such a procedure can be considered for patients who are poor surgical risks.

Joint replacement has been performed with excellent results for advanced hip arthropathy.[38] Although total knee replacements have now been performed in many patients, orthopaedists have generally restricted this procedure to patients with such severe knee pain that fusion is the only alternative (Fig. 106-11). Other joint prosthesis procedures, such as total shoulder replacements, are also successfully performed in persons with hemophilia.

Dental care should begin with preventive dentistry early in life to minimize expense and subsequent morbidity. Restorative dentistry can now be performed with adequate local anesthesia, including the use of mandibular block, under coverage of factor VIII replacement.[39] For oral surgery, the use of fibrinolysis inhibitors such as ε-aminocaproic acid or tranexamic acid markedly reduces the amount of coagulation factor replacement needed for hemostasis.[39] When ε-aminocaproic acid is given orally at full therapeutic doses for 7–10 days, a single factor VIII infusion of 40 U/kg just prior to the oral surgery is often sufficient for normal hemostasis. If persistent, severe oozing occurs, another factor VIII infusion may be needed.

Therapy for Mild Hemophilia A

Patients with mild hemophilia A (factor VIII levels >5%) do not bleed spontaneously, but usually only after trauma or surgical procedures. The current treatment of choice for patients with factor VIII levels >10% is DDAVP (Stimate), a synthetic analogue of vasopressin.[40] Although its exact mechanism of action is not understood, it is thought to stimulate release of factor VIII from storage sites.[41] The routine dosage is 0.3 ug/kg in 50 ml of normal saline given intravenously over a period of 30–40 minutes. In a factor VIII-deficient patient, DDAVP will usually increase the factor VIII level threefold.[42] Thus, it may not be helpful in patients with factor VIII levels of <10%.

In order to assess how an individual patient will respond to DDAVP, a staging test should be done. When the patient is not bleeding, a baseline factor VIII level is obtained and then the dose of DDAVP is administered. Thirty to 45 minutes after the infusion stops, a second factor VIII level is checked. The factor VIII level should rise at least threefold. If the levels rise to >80%, the response is adequate for major surgery. In some patients DDAVP can only be used for minor hemorrhages since the factor VIII levels do not rise sufficiently. DDAVP can also be used with factor concentrate in mild hemophiliacs to obtain high levels of factor VIII if needed. When DDAVP is used for major surgery, it should be given 1 hour before surgery and then every 12 hours. Tachyphylaxis may occur after repeated doses secondary to depletion of factor VIII from storage sites.[40] Thus factor VIII levels should be checked frequently after the first 2 days. If tachyphylaxis does occur, factor concentrate must be substituted.

If a patient with mild hemophilia has an inadequate response to DDAVP, cryoprecipitate or factor concentrate must be used when the patient has surgery or encounters trauma. Since plasma-derived concentrates undergo effective virucidal procedures while cryoprecipitate cannot (and recombinant concentrate is now available), the use of factor concentrates is recommended.

Although DDAVP is usually administered in a hospital or emergency room setting, a protocol can be adapted for home use. Equivalent results with subcutaneous DDAVP can be obtained, which would make home therapy much simpler.[43] Unfortunately, no subcutaneous preparation of DDAVP is available in the United States. Intranasal DDAVP in formulations concentrated enough to increase factor VIII levels as efficaciously as intravenous DDAVP is now available, making home management simpler.

The common side effects of DDAVP include facial warmth and flushing during the infusion. Insignificant variations in blood pressure may be noted. Headaches may occur as late as 6–8 hours after the infusion. Abdominal cramping with diar-

SURGERY AND HEMOPHILIA

Both elective and emergency surgery can be done in a patient with hemophilia A unless an inhibitor is present. Before surgery (1) a hematologist and diagnostic coagulation laboratory should be available; (2) the surgeon should feel comfortable handling a patient with a coagulation disorder; (3) there should be a blood bank or pharmacy capable of providing adequate amounts of the appropriate replacement material; (4) an appropriate rehabilitation team should be available for postoperative management, especially with orthopaedic surgery; and (5) no inhibitor should be present. An inhibitor level must be checked immediately prior to surgery. Surgery should be scheduled on Monday or Tuesday to allow for availability of laboratory services for factor level assays and best access to consultants.

Preoperative orders should include "No IM medication" and "No ASA-containing compounds such as Darvon, Empirin or percodan." For major surgery, the factor VIII level should be brought to the 80–100% range (40–50 U/kg) about 1 hour prior to surgery and then kept >30–50% for 10–14 days. The theoretical calculations should be checked every 2–3 days with factor VIII assays and the dose adjusted accordingly.

Postoperatively, pain management should be aggressive, with patient-assisted narcotic delivery systems (PCA) or constant infusional narcotic dosing.

For oral surgery such as impacted wisdom teeth removal, the factor level prior to surgery is raised to 100% with infusions. Postoperatively ε-aminocaproic acid (1 g PO every 4 hours) for 7–10 days is given. If the dental procedure is minor, ε-aminocaproic acid may be used alone.

Patients with mild hemophilia may be able to utilize DDAVP. If there is a poor response to DDAVP, some physicians use cryoprecipitate. However, if DDABP cannot be used, we recommend factor concentrate since it can be treated with viricidal methods and is thus currently safer than cryoprecipitate.

Complications of factor use include hepatitis C, which has largely been eliminated by the new production methods and hemolysis due to anti-A or anti-B in the concentrate preparation. If hemolysis occurs, blood loss should be replaced by type O packed red cells, and concentrates with low isoagglutinin titers should be obtained and utilized.

rhea and generalized myalgias have rarely been noted. In very ill patients, fluid retention resulting in congestive heart failure has been reported.[44] In small children receiving large fluid volumes, seizures induced by severe hyponatremia after DDAVP infusion have recently occurred.[45] In the young pediatric age group serum sodium levels should be monitored and large amounts of intravenous fluid avoided if DDAVP is used, especially if repeated doses are given. Myocardial infarction temporally related to DDAVP infusion has been reported,[46] although whether DDAVP truly causes a hypercoagulable state is unclear. These serious side effects are very uncommon. In summary, DDAVP is the treatment of choice in persons with mild hemophilia A if they respond adequately.

Health Care Delivery

The keystone of therapy in hemophilia is to provide the patient with access to immediate and adequate correction of the hemostatic defect at the earliest symptom suggestive of hemor-

rhage. For most persons with severe and moderately severe hemophilia, the achievement of this goal is through a combination of intensive education of the patient and family, plus the institution of a carefully supervised self-therapy program.

Self-Therapy Program

With the exception of patients with inhibitor antibodies, those who are unreliable or unstable, or children <3 years of age, most patients are candidates for home therapy. The day-to-day supervision of the patient may often be provided by a physician in the patient's immediate geographic vicinity, with subsequent regular visits to a hemophilia center for long-term evaluation and comprehensive care. At most centers, all patients and selected family members receive an individual half-day course on the pathophysiology, diagnosis, and therapy of hemophilia. The first several infusions are administered under medical supervision. If the patient or family demonstrate both proficiency in self-infusion and good grasp of basic principles, maximum independence is allowed.

At some centers, all patients attend biannual comprehensive evaluation sessions as a minimum mandatory requirement for continuation in the program. At each session the patient is evaluated by a hematologist and an orthopaedic surgeon, a nurse, a medical social worker, an oral surgeon, a physical therapist, a vocational counselor, and, when indicated, a genetic counselor and/or a psychologist or psychiatrist. Table 106-1 shows data collected on hemophiliacs treated in traditional outpatient hematology clinics for 1 year and then introduced into the formal comprehensive care program, which includes self-therapy.[47] It should be emphasized that the least important aspect of self-therapy is the teaching of venipuncture. The program achieves its dramatic results through patient education as well as the systematic application of the skills of a variety of appropriate medical personnel who can address the long-term problems of this lifelong disease.

Because of the many problems arising from the introduction of HIV into the blood supply in the 1970s and early 1980s,[15] comprehensive hemophilia care now also involves dealing with the acquired immunodeficiency syndrome (AIDS) and HIV.[48] Patients are examined at more frequent intervals, prophylaxis with antiretroviral agents such as zidovudine is considered, and infectious disease consultation may be obtained. Additionally, intensive counseling sessions with the patient, the family, and a social worker are provided for discussion of issues such as transmission of HIV and the impact of this infection on the life of the patient.

Complications of Therapy

Lyophilized factor concentrates revolutionized the care of persons with hemophilia. Home therapy programs were instituted and thus the long-term effects of hemorrhage were decreased and days lost from work or school lessened.[47] Life span gradually increased until the AIDS era.[9] Lyophilized concentrate is a pooled product made from plasma of between 2,000 and 30,000 donors. Infectious complications from transfusion-transmitted viruses began to be noted in hemophiliacs in the late 1970s and subsequently became a major concern.[49] However, all factor concentrates currently produced are virally inactivated, and thus infectious complications have been greatly decreased. Increased purity of concentrates has also occurred over the ensuing years.

Infectious Complications

Hepatitis

The major hepatitis viruses transmitted through plasma-derived concentrate and cryoprecipitate infusion are hepatitis B (HBV) and C (HCV). Acute HBV infection with elevated liver

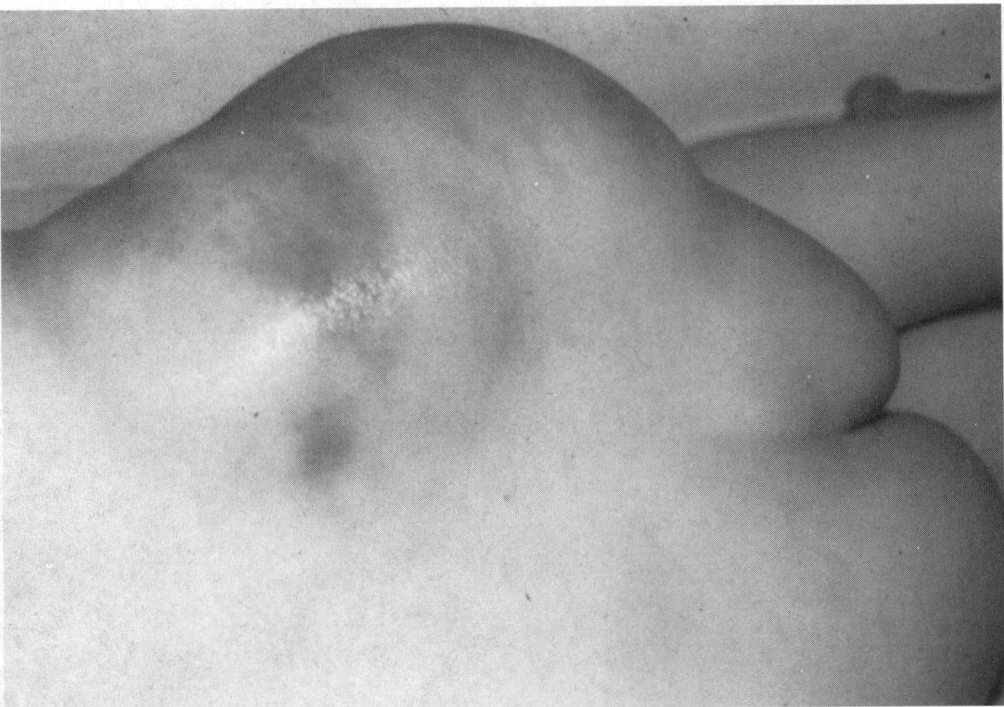

Fig. 106-9. Large hematoma of the right flank.

function tests, jaundice, and fever is uncommon in hemophiliacs, but approximately 90% of patients who were given infused concentrates before the current viral inactivation methods became available have developed antibody to HBV (HBsAb positive), indicating exposure.[50] A small percentage of patients, approximately 5%, have become chronic carriers (HBsAg positive).[51] Chronic carriers may be more prone to the development of symptomatic chronic liver disease or carcinoma of the liver. Delta hepatitis (HDV), a virus that requires the presence of HBV as a carrier, is also a potential risk to hemophilia patients, especially in endemic areas, since coinfection with HDV and HBV may cause fulminant hepatitis.[50] Persons with hemophilia who are chronic HBV carriers may also have antibodies to HDV, indicating exposure to HDV through factor concentrate. Even with virucidal methods used currently to prepare factor concentrate, HBV infections have been reported. Thus,

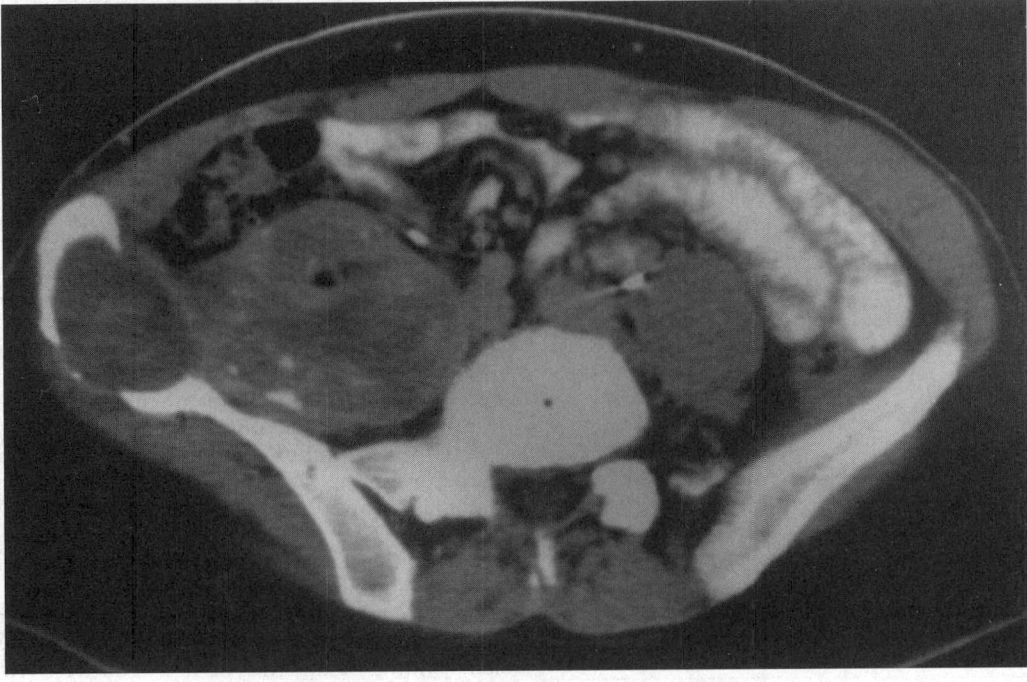

Fig. 106-10. Computed tomography scan showing large pseudotumor involving right psoas muscle with extension into right iliac crest.

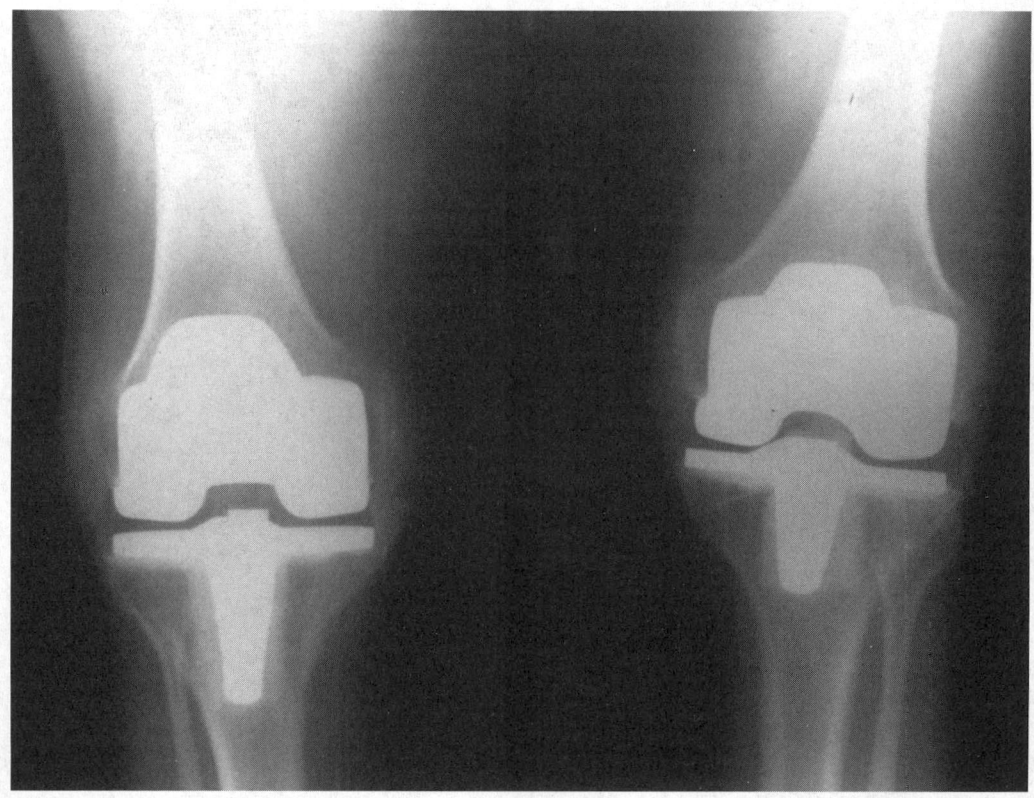

Fig. 106-11. Bilateral total knee replacements in a patient with end-stage hemophilic arthropathy.

all newly diagnosed persons with hemophilia should receive HBV vaccination. In a newly diagnosed infant, the series of three innoculations is started at birth.

HCV has been a common infectious complication of factor infusion. (It was termed non-A, non-B hepatitis in the 1970s.[52]) A serologic marker for HCV is available.[53,54] Data suggest that ≥80% of persons with hemophilia infused before 1985 carry the marker, indicating past exposure to the virus. Approximately 90% of hemophiliacs have either persistently or intermittently elevated liver enzymes, which most likely represents the consequences of HCV exposure.[55] When liver biopsies are done on selected hemophilia patients with abnormal liver enzymes, 20%–30% have shown changes consistent with chronic active hepatitis or cirrhosis.[56] HCV has also been associated with the development of heptacellular carcinoma.[57] Thus, HCV may represent a long-term problem for persons with hemophilia.

Table 106-1. Outcomes of Comprehensive Care of Hemophilia

Outcome Data	Year Before Program	Fifth Year of Program
Patients seen at primary centers (n)	1,783	3,795
Patients seen at affiliate centers (n)	329	1,037
Patients receiving regular comprehensive care (n)	1,333	4,682
Patients on self-infusion ("home care") (n)	514	2,001
Average days/yr lost from work or school	14.5	4.3
Average hospital admission/yr	1.9	0.26
Average days/yr spent as inpatient	9.4	1.8
Patients with third party coverage (%)	74	93
Out-of-pocket expense/patient/yr	$ 850[a]	$ 342
Overall costs of care/patient/yr	$15,800[a]	$5,932
Unemployed adults (%)	36	12.8

[a] These figures represent retrospective estimates from small samples in the case of most centers.

Outbreaks of hepatitis A related to factor concentrate have recently been reported from Europe. As a vaccine for hepatitis A becomes available, newly diagnosed persons with hemophilia should receive it.

Human Immunodeficiency Virus

HIV was introduced into the American blood supply in the 1970s.[58] By the late 1970s, factor concentrate was widely contaminated and by 1982, approximately 50% of persons with hemophilia were infected with HIV.[59] Currently, 70% of American hemophiliacs are HIV antibody positive.[60] Hemophilic patients, especially those infected after the age of 22 years and those who have been HIV seropositive for at least 7 years, have approximately 40% probability of developing symptomatic AIDS.[61] It is not clear why the age of acquisition of infection should influence outcome, but this has now been confirmed in a larger multicenter study.[62] Otherwise, when compared with other high-risk groups, the course of HIV-1 infection in hemophilia is very similar. As in other risk groups, low CD4 lymphocyte levels are strong predictors of which specific person will become symptomatic. *Pneumocystis carinii* pneumonia (Fig. 106-12) was the most common presenting AIDS-defining condition in HIV-seropositive hemophilia patients before the advent of prophylaxis. Other opportunistic infections, such as candida esophagitis and cryptococcal meningitis/septicemia, are reported in this subgroup. Kaposi sarcoma, however, is a very rare presenting condition in persons with hemophilia. Non-Hodgkin lymphoma can occur late in the disease at an incidence of 5.5%.[63]

Currently, as with other HIV-seropositive patients, persons with hemophilia who have CD4 lymphocyte counts <400–500 cells/μl can be considered for prophylactic zidovudine; in those with a count of <200 cells/mm[3], *Pneumocystis* prophylaxis should be added. The use of antiretroviral drugs that are hepatotoxic may be more problematic in persons with hemophilia since many have pre-existing liver disease secondary to

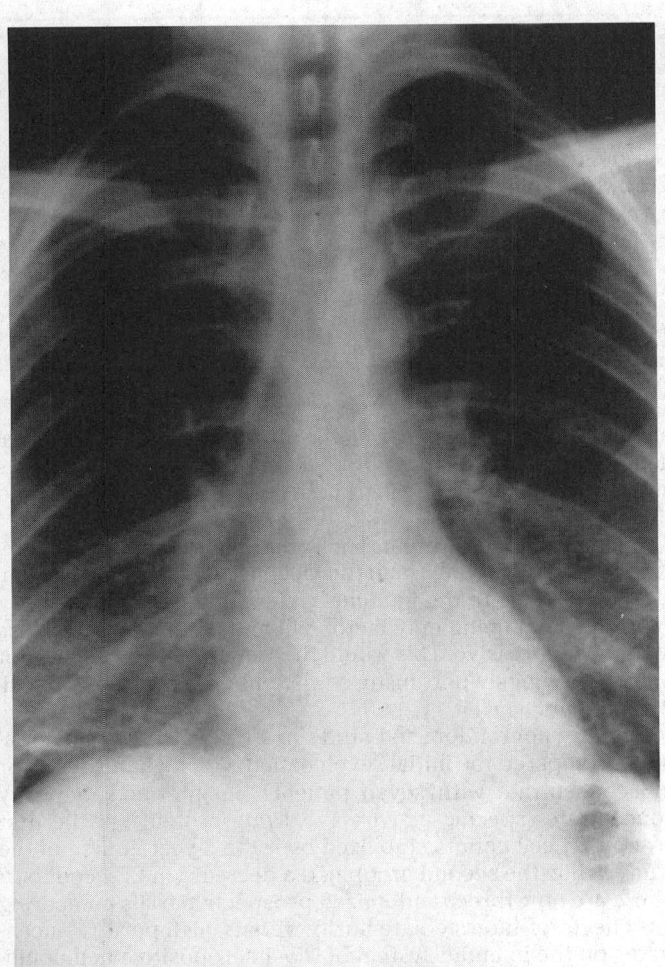

Fig. 106-12. Bilateral interstitial infiltrates in a hemophilic patient with *Pneumocystis carinii* pneumonia.

HCV. Thus, liver chemistries should be monitored carefully, especially in persons on combination antiretroviral therapy.

Virucidal Treatments of Concentrates

There is now a triple barrier to viral transmission through factor concentrates: (1) self-exclusion for donors, (2) donor screening, and (3) viral inactivation procedures. Self-exclusion includes asking the plasma donor detailed questions concerning hepatitis, possible HIV exposure, and general health (to elicit nonspecific symptoms of HIV infection). Donor screening now includes HCV testing, as well as serologic testing for HIV-1 and HBV.

Multiple methodologies for attenuating viruses during processing of factor concentrate have been devised.[64] They include heating the concentrate and the use of solvent/detergent combinations, which disrupt lipid-coated viruses such as HIV and some hepatitis viruses.[65,66]

A third methodology for eliminating virus from concentrate involves affinity chromatography using a murine monoclonal antibody to either von Willebrand factor or factor VIII.[67] Cryoprecipitate is used as the starting material. A much higher purity factor VIII concentrate results (specific activity >3,000 U/mg protein before addition of albumin stabilizer). HIV titers are reduced significantly by this process. The product is either pasteurized in the final stage (Monoclate-P, Rorer) or is initially treated with tri-n-butyl phosphate (TNBP)/Triton X-100 (Hemophil M, Hyland). A summary of these methods and specific concentrates is given in Table 106-2.

Alloantigens in Factor Concentrate

In addition to viral contamination of factor concentrates, it has been shown (beginning in the early 1980s) that intermediate purity concentrate itself may cause immune aberrations in hemophiliacs, perhaps secondary to the presence of multiple foreign proteins.[68] Factor concentrate in vitro may down-regulate Fc receptors on the macrophage[69] or may inhibit the mixed lymphocyte culture reaction[70] or interleukin-2 production by monocytes.[71] Since detailed immunologic studies were not done routinely on the hemophilia population before infection of patients with HIV, information regarding the effect of concentrate on patients is sporadic. In Scotland, in a group of HIV-seronegative hemophiliacs receiving locally produced factor concentrate not contaminated by HIV, approximately 50% demonstrated mildly decreased helper/suppressor T-lymphocyte ratios secondary to depressed CD4 cell levels.[68] These abnormalities appeared to be related to intensity of treatment. Others researchers have also shown that in a group of HIV-seronegative hemophiliacs, CD4 cell levels are mildly reduced when compared with normal controls.[72] Thus, frequent infusions of intermediate purity factor concentrates may lead to mild immune suppression.

Additional Complications

Other complications of treatment with concentrate include urticaria, temperature elevations, and very rarely anaphylaxis. Urticaria and bronchospasm are more commonly seen with infusions of cryoprecipitate. When cryoprecipitate is used, some centers order type-specific products.

Factor concentrates may also contain measurable titers of isoagglutinins (anti-A or anti-B). When concentrate is administered in large amounts, such as postoperatively, to patients with A and B blood types, significant hemolysis may occur.[73] If the patient with this complication requires blood transfusions, type O should be given. Factor concentrate with low isoagglutinin titer can subsequently be obtained from specific manufacturers. Rarer complications of factor concentrate include a syn-

Table 106-2. Factor VIII Concentrates and Viral Inactivation Method Used

Viral Inactivation Method	Name of Concentrate	Manufacturer
Heating		
Super-dry heat: 80°C for 72 hr	8Y	UK National Health Service[a]
Vapor heat	AHF-vapor treated	Immuno[a]
Heating in aqueous solution 60°C for 10 hr (pasteurization)	Humate-P	Behringwerke
Solvent/detergent		
TNBP/cholate	Melate-SD	NY Blood Center
TNBP/polysorbate 80	Profilate OSD	Alpha
TNBP/Tween-80	Koate HP	Miles
Very high purity products		
Purification by affinity chromatography		
Pasteurized	Monoclate P	Rorer
TNBP/Triton X-100 in "wet" state	Hemophil M	Baxter
	ARC–Method M	American Red Cross
Recombinant factor VIII		
Recombinate		Baxter
Kogenate		Miles
Bioclate		Armour

Abbreviations: AHF, antihemophilic factor; TNBP, tri-n-butyl phosphate.
[a] Available in Europe only.

Table 106-3. Infectious Complications of Plasma-Derived Factor Concentrates

	Before 1985	After 1985
Hepatitis B/delta hepatitis	Present	Decreased; all patients should be vaccinated with hepatitis B vaccine
HIV-1	Present	Essentially eliminated
Hepatitis C	Present	Decreased, but cases still occur, even with present methodologies of viral inactivation
Hepatitis A	Not studied	Sporadic cases with specific solvent detergent-treated concentrates
B19 parvovirus	Probably present	Present, but limited
HTLV-1	Limited	Probably eliminated

Abbreviations: HTLV-1, human T-cell leukemia/lymphoma virus 1.

drome of primary pulmonary hypertension described in five patients with severe hemophilia A who used large amounts of concentrate.[74] The mechanism has not been elaborated but may be due to particulate matter or immune complexes being deposited in the lungs. A summary of infectious implications associated with therapy is given in Table 106-3.

Choice of Concentrate

Selection of a factor concentrate depends on efficacy, safety concerning virally transmitted diseases, purity, and cost. Demonstrating that a concentrate is free of harmful viruses is difficult since reliable animal models, especially for HCV, are not available. Human clinical trials are necessary to prove that new factor concentrates are safe. To demonstrate whether a specific concentrate is free of HBV, HCV, or HIV, studies using previously nontransfused patients, primarily newly diagnosed hemophiliac infants, are undertaken. Serologic studies of antiviral antibodies and liver function may be positive if patients are exposed to specific viruses.

Both HCV and HBV are difficult to inactivate. Heating the lyophilized concentrate at 60–68°C for 30–72 hours does not inactivate HCV, although raising the temperature to 80°C for 72 hours does eliminate HCV.[66] Heating the concentrate in solution (60°C for 10 hours of "pasteurization") appears to kill HCV, although there are anecdotal reports that hepatitis B and C have still occurred after pasteurization methods were used.[75,76]

Solvent/detergent-treated concentrates appear to be free of HCV.[77] Of note is that solvent/detergent methods do not inactivate viruses without lipid envelopes. Thus, parvovirus, for example, may not be killed. In Ireland, Italy, Germany, and Belgium a recent outbreak of hepatitis A occurred in 84 hemophilia patients infused exclusively with solvent/detergent-inactivated concentrates purified by ion exchange chromatography.[78]

HIV appears to be easily inactivated by any of the current viral inactivation procedures. In all viral safety trials in which HIV antibody status was studied, which include over 300 subjects, no seroconversions occurred.[64] However, 18 cases of HIV seroconversion have been reported with heat-treated factor VIII concentrate not associated with viral safety trials.[79] Most cases used concentrate that was dry heated at 60°C, a methodology that is no longer used. "Dry heat" at high temperatures for longer periods of time (80° for 72 hours), vapor treatment, or heat treatment in solution ("pasteurization") appear to be efficacious in killing HIV. The solvent/detergent methods, as well as purification by affinity chromatography, also appear safe, vis-à-vis HIV infection.

Highly Purified Concentrate

Concentrates purified using affinity chromatography (Monoclate, Hemophil M) have a final specific factor VIII activity of approximately 3,000 U/mg protein.[67] The purity is significantly

---

PURITY OF FACTOR VIII

It is our opinion that for previously untreated and infrequently treated hemophiliacs and for others who are free of HIV infection, a concentrate that is pasteurized, treated with solvent/detergent, or immunoaffinity purified can be used. It should be virus free, but not necessarily highly purified. For HIV-seropositive patients, highly purified concentrates that are virally inactivated offer theoretical benefits.

---

higher than previously available products, and most extraneous human proteins have been removed. These products are efficacious and appear to be free of hepatitis viruses and HIV.

Since extraneous proteins such as immune complexes, aggregated immunoglobulins, and the killed viruses may be additionally suppressive to the immune system of a hemophiliac, concentrates containing only factor VIII and albumin may be less immunosuppressive. This would theoretically be beneficial not only to previously untransfused patients, but to HIV-seropositive patients as well.

An early nonrandomized study of 14 HIV-1-seropositive patients compared the initial seven patients on high-purity factor VIII concentrate with seven patients on intermediate-purity concentrate (specific activity 1–3 U/mg protein); in the first group CD4 cell counts stabilized over the 3-year course of the study, while the second group had a decrease in CD4 counts.[80] There are now three randomized prospective trials comparing the effects of intermediate-purity versus high-purity concentrates on the immune system of HIV-1 seropositive hemophiliacs.[81] Two studies, using immune affinity-purified factor VIII, have shown independently that HIV-1-seropositive hemophilia patients have a slower decline of CD4 cell counts on the very high-purity concentrate versus the intermediate-purity concentrate.[82,83] In a third study using a less high-purity concentrate, no difference between the two groups could be seen.[84] All studies were performed with small numbers of patients.

Recombinant Factor VIII

Currently, there are three recombinant factor VIII products approved for clinical use, Recombinate (Baxter), Kogenate (Miles), and Bioclate (Armour). The final products are highly purified factor VIII, with a specific activity of approximately 7,000 U/mg protein prior to the addition of human albumin. Recombinant factor VIII has been shown to be safe and as efficacious as plasma-derived factor VIII concentrate, with similar recovery and half-life.[13,14,85] Major surgery has been performed using the concentrate, with excellent hemostasis.

Two ongoing clinical trials are evaluating inhibitor development in persons with hemophilia treated with recombinant factor VIII. The patients in these trials are those most at risk of inhibitor development: persons who have previously been untransfused, mostly infants. To date, 16 of 64 patients developed an inhibitor after a median of 9 exposure days.[86] Although this prevalence is high, in 9 of the 16 patients, inhibitors remained at low titer. In another study, 17 of 69 previously untransfused patients given recombinate by infusion developed inhibitors.[87] It is not clear whether recombinant factor concentrate leads to increased inhibitor development or inhibitor development at an earlier time. Previous studies showing inhibitor prevalences of 10–15% were cross-sectional cohort, not prospective studies in a high-risk group. Also, the patients were not moni-

FACTOR VIII: RECOMBINANT VERSUS PLASMA DERIVED

Who should receive recombinant factor concentrate? There are many different opinions; ours is that this product should be reserved for those persons with hemophilia who are HIV-1 seronegative as well as HCV seronegative (i.e., mostly young children). The product is ≥$0.10/unit more expensive than the most expensive plasma-derived high-purity product. In this era of medical cost containment, price is a large issue. In addition, the possibility of inhibitor development must be discussed with the family or patient who will receive recombinant factor VIII.

tored as closely for inhibitor development. Thus, these studies are difficult to compare.

Cure of Hemophilia A

Liver transplantation currently offers a cure for hemophilia, albeit an impractical one. Persons with hemophilia A have undergone liver transplantation because of end-stage liver disease caused by HBV or HCV. In one of the first series (four patients with hemophilia A), three survived the initial surgery and then normalized their factor VIII levels, requiring no further replacement.[88] Additional patients with hemophilia A have since undergone liver transplantation; of those who survived, factor VIII levels have been normalized. In the future, gene replacement therapy may offer a hope of cure to all persons with hemophilia.

GENETIC COUNSELING AND PRENATAL DIAGNOSIS

The cloning of the factor VIII gene and the determination of its molecular structure allow detection of carriers and accurate prenatal diagnosis. Female relatives of individuals with hemophilia may be carriers of the abnormal gene, and therefore may be at risk of having children with hemophilia. Women who are considered obligate carriers are daughters of individuals with hemophilia and women who have one son and another relative with hemophilia. These women have a 50% risk of each newborn son having hemophilia. Women who have two sons with hemophilia are obligate heterozygotes. However, a small proportion of these women may be either somatic mosaics or germline mosaics.[89] Reproductive risk in these circumstances is difficult to assess and depends on the proportion of ova carrying the abnormal gene.

Other female relatives are considered possible carriers of the gene for hemophilia. This would include women who have one son with hemophilia and no other affected relatives. In these isolated cases, the hemophilia may result from (1) transmission through asymptomatic females, (2) a new mutation in the mother, (3) a new mutation in the individual with hemophilia (a true de novo mutation), or (4) as a result of somatic or germline mosaicism in the mother.[90] The probability for carriership for a mother of an isolated case is estimated to be 0.85.[91]

Carrier Detection

Potential hemophilia A carriers should be offered genetic testing for determination of carrier status. Current methods of carrier detection include standard phenotypic clotting assays, as well as more accurate genotypic analysis. Probability of carriership should first be determined from pedigree data. Information anterior to the proband is used to determine genetic risk. This figure can be modified by Bayesean analysis if the individual has any sons without hemophilia.

Phenotypic assessment of carrier status for hemophilia A is determined by specific assays for factor VIII activity, factor VIII antigen, and von Willebrand factor antigen. In general, women who are carriers of hemophilia A have approximately 50% of the normal level of factor VIII. These values may be affected by various physiologic conditions or medications, or both. Of particular note are the effect of pregnancy (especially after the 22nd week of gestation) and estrogen-containing drugs such as birth control pills, which elevate factor VIII levels.[92,93] The age of the individual being tested and the ABO blood type must also be noted; blood type O is associated with decreased factor VIII levels.[94] Factor VIII concentrations are also influenced by X-chromosome inactivation (the Lyon hypothesis), which may cause false-negative results.[95] Laboratory data are used to determine probability of carriership. The laboratory values can be combined with the pedigree data to give a final probability. For determination of odds ratios favoring carriership in hemophilia A, bivariate linear discriminant analysis using factor VIII, von Willebrand antigen, age, and ABO blood type is recommended.

Determination of carrier status for hemophilia A may also be performed using molecular diagnostic methods. The factor VIII gene is large (see Ch. 105), and the mutations identified to date are heterogeneous. Thus, direct mutational analysis is not available for routine screening. Most genotypic testing employs an indirect marker, restriction fragment length polymorphism (RFLP). Which marker to use for polymorphism analysis is determined by the mutation's location (intragenic versus extragenic), the degree of heterozygosity, and the ethnic origin of the family. Southern blot analysis and polymerase chain reaction are the techniques used for identification of these polymorphisms. For hemophilia A, >95% of females are informative, with the following intragenic markers: the intron 13 CA repeat, the intron 22 CA repeat, BclI, and XbaI. The BglI and the intron 7 polymorphism may be informative in other families. Indirect testing using intragenic markers is >99% accurate. However, there are limitations. For the study to be informative, the marker must be heterozygous. Heterozygosity differs significantly in various ethnic groups, and this must be accounted for when considering which polymorphisms to use in a particular family. Blood samples from several key family members are required for genotypic testing. Blood from an affected male is required. Since many older hemophiliacs are infected with HIV-1 and thus have shortened survival, blood sampling to obtain DNA that can then be frozen for future use in genetic analysis should be encouraged. All family members must agree to genotypic testing, and all family relationships reported must be correct. In some families linked extragenic markers may be informative, but accuracy of the results is decreased due to possible genetic recombination.

When sporadic cases of hemophilia occur in a family, polymorphism testing can only be used to exclude transmission of the mutation because the mutation is not identified by these methods, and therefore its origin is not known. In these families, direct mutation analysis can be considered. Direct screening methods for mutations in these large genes have been developed. Three screening methods are utilized for hemophilia A: denaturing gradient gel electrophoresis, single-stranded conformational polymorphism analysis, and direct sequencing of amplified DNA.[96–100]

Prenatal Diagnosis

Several techniques are available for the prenatal diagnosis of hemophilia. The basic strategy is to determine fetal sex first, and then to determine whether the fetus has the gene for hemophilia. Fetal sex can be determined by ultrasonography and fetal chromosome analysis. Experienced sonographers can determine fetal sex reliably at 16–20 weeks of gestation. Fetal sex, however, is more accurately determined by examination of the fetal chromosomes. Chromosomes can be obtained by amniocentesis or chorionic villus sampling (CVS). Amniocentesis is performed at 15–20 weeks' gestation or at 12–14 weeks' gestation ("early amniocentesis"—risk approximately 1%).[101,102] CVS, by either the transcervical or the transabdominal route, is done at 9–12 weeks' gestation.[103,104] In general, whether amniocentesis or a CVS procedure is chosen depends on patient preferences regarding timing of the procedure, risk to the fetus, and reliability of the results. Reports suggesting an association between CVS and limb reduction defects have raised questions about the risks of this procedure. These risks can be lessened if the CVS procedure is performed after 10 weeks' gestation, and if placental trauma is minimized. The risk of loss of pregnancy may be somewhat higher for CVS compared with amniocentesis.

The diagnosis of hemophilia in a fetus can be accomplished by genotypic analysis of fetal DNA or by phenotypic analysis of fetal blood. Fetal DNA can be extracted from both fetal amniocytes and chorionic villi and analyzed by RFLP of the DNA, as above. If prenatal diagnosis is not possible by DNA analysis, then fetal blood sampling can be done by a cordocentesis. This technique is done from 20–21 weeks' gestation and involves the ultrasound-guided puncture of an umbilical cord vessel.[105] The fetal blood is analyzed by phenotypic clotting assays.

Preimplantation diagnosis after in vitro fertilization has recently been proposed as a method of prenatal testing. Amplification of informative regions of the factor VIII gene by polymerase chain reaction from a single cell has been reported. All women who undergo carrier testing or prenatal diagnosis, or both, for hemophilia should have genetic counseling, preferably before choices regarding carrier testing and prenatal diagnosis must be made. The aims of counseling in these cases are to provide information about genetic risk, determination of carrier status, and prenatal diagnosis as well as to provide psychological and emotional support during the processes.

REFERENCES

1. Brinkhous KM: A short history of hemophilia, with some comments on the word "hemophilia." p. 3. In Brinkhous KM, Hemker KC (eds): Handbook of Hemophilia. American Elsevier, New York, 1975
2. Wright AE: On a method of determining the condition of blood coagulability for clinical and experimental purposes, and on the effect of the administration of calcium salts in haemophilia and actual or threatened haemorrhage. Br Med J 2:223, 1893
3. Addis T: The pathogenesis of hereditary haemophilia. J Pathol Bacteriol 15:427, 1911
4. Brinkhous KM: Clotting defect in hemophilia: deficiency in a plasma factor required for platelet utilization. Proc Soc Exp Biol Med 66:117, 1947
5. Quick AJ: Studies on the enigma of the hemostatic dysfunction of hemophilia. Am J Med Sci 214:292, 1947
6. Pavlovsky A: Contribution to the pathogenesis of hemophilia. Blood 2:185, 1947
7. Haemorrhagic diathesis: successful transfusion of blood. Lancet 1:185, 1840
8. Feisly R: Études sur l'hemophilie. Bull M Soc Med Hop Paris 47:1778, 1923
9. Ramgren O: A clinical and medisocial study of haemophilia in Sweden. J Intern Med 171:759, 1962
10. Pool JG, Hershgold EJ, Pappenhagen AR: High potency antihaemophilic factor concentrate prepared from cryoglobulin precipitate. Nature 203:312, 1964
11. Johnson AJ, Newman J, Howell MB, Puszkin S: Two large scale procedures for purification of human antihemophilic factor (AHF). Blood 28:1011, 1966
12. Levine PH: Factor VIII:C purified from plasma via monoclonal antibodies: human studies. Semin Hematol, Suppl. 25:38, 1988
13. White G, MacMillan C, Kingdon H et al: Recombinant factor VIII. N Engl J Med 320:166, 1989
14. Schwartz RS, Abilgaard CF, Aledort LM et al: Human recombinant DNA derived antihemophilic factor in the treatment of hemophilia A. N Engl J Med 323:1800, 1990
15. Department of Health, Education, and Welfare: National Heart and Lung Institute Blood Resource Studies. Vol. 3. Pilot Study of Hemophilia Treatment in the U.S. US Government Printing Office, Washington, DC, 1972
16. Eyster ME, Mitchell HG, Ballard J et al: Natural history of human immunodeficiency virus infection in hemophiliacs. Ann Intern Med 107:1, 1987
17. Mannucci PM, Capitaneo A, Del Ninno E et al: Asymptomatic liver disease in hemophiliacs. J Clin Pathol 28:620, 1973
18. Upchurch KS, Brettler DB, Levine PH: Hemophilic arthropathy. p. 1509. In Kelley WN, Harris E, Ruddy S, Sledge LB (eds): Textbook of Rheumatology. 4th Ed. WB Saunders, Philadelphia, 1993
19. Hilgartner MW: Hemophilic arthropathy. Adv Pediatr 21:139, 1975
20. Steven MM, Madhok SD, Forbes CO et al: Hemophilic arthritis. Am J Med 58:181, 1986
21. Ellison RT, Reller LB: Differentiating pyogenic arthritis from spontaneous hemarthrosis in patients with hemophilia. West J Med 144:42, 1986
22. Ahlberg A: On the natural history of hemophilic psuedotumor. J Bone Joint Surg 57A:1133, 1975
23. Gilbert MS: Musculoskeletal manifestations of hemophilia. Mt Sinai J Med 44:339, 1977
24. Singher LT: Renal and urological complications of hemophilia. p. 377. In Brinkhouse KM, Hemker HC (eds): Handbook of Hemophilia. American Elsevier, New York, 1975
25. Eyster ME, Gill FM, Blatt PM et al: Central nervous system bleeding in hemophiliacs. Blood 51:1179, 1978
26. Levine PH: Deficiency in current hemophilia therapy: need for factor XIV. JAMA 219:214, 1972
27. Mattsson A, Gross S: Adaptional and defensive behavior in young hemophiliacs and their parents. Am J Psychiatry 122:1349, 1966
28. Connor FP: The hemophilic child in school. Ann NY Acad Sci 240:221, 1975
29. Taylor C: Rehabilitation counseling. p. 127. In Boone DC (ed): Management of Hemophilia. FA Davis, Philadelphia, 1976
30. Shulman NR: Surgical care of patients with hereditary disorders of blood coagulation. p. 61. In Ratnoff OD (ed): Treatment of Hemorrhagic Disorders. Harper & Row, New York, 1968
31. Post M, Telfer MD: Surgery in hemophilic patients. J Bone Joint Surg 57A:1136, 1975
32. Bona RD, Weinstein RA, Weisman ST et al: The use of continuous infusion of factor concentrates in the treatment of hemophilia. Am J Hematol 32:8, 1990
33. Rizza CR: The management of patients with coagulation factor deficiencies. p. 365. In Biggs R (ed): Human Blood Coagulation Haemostatis and Thrombosis. 2nd Ed. Blackwell Scientific Publications, Oxford, 1972
34. Levine PH: Delivery of health care in hemophilia. Ann NY Acad Sci 240:201, 1973
35. Boone DC: Common musculoskeletal problems and their management. p. 52. In Boone DC (ed): Comprehensive Management of Hemophilia. FA Davis, Philadelphia, 1976
36. Levine PH: Unsolved problems with current therapeutic regimens for hemophilia. p. 23. In: Unsolved Therapeutic Problems in Hemophilia. National Heart, Lung, and Blood Institute, US Government Printing Office, Washington, DC, 1976
37. Storti E, Ascari E: Surgical management of advanced hemophilic arthropathy. Clin Orthop 242:60, 1989
38. Luck JV, Kasper CK: Surgical management of advanced hemophilic arthropathy. Clin Orthop 242:60, 1989
39. Evans BE, Aledort LM: Hemophilia and dental treatment. J Am Dent Assoc 96:827, 1978
40. Mannucci PM: Desmopressin: a nontransfusional form of treatment for congenital and acquired bleeding disorders. Blood 72:1449, 1988
41. Mannucci PM, Canciani MT, Rota L et al: Response of factor VIII/von Willebrand factor to desmopressin in healthy subjects and patients with hemophilia A and von Willebrand's disease. Br J Haematol 47:283, 1981
42. Mariani G, Ciavarella N, Mazzuconi MG et al: Evaluation of the effectiveness of DDAVP in surgery and bleeding episodes in hemophilia and von Willebrand's disease. Clin Lab Haematol 6:229, 1984
43. Mannucci PM, Vicente V, Alberca I et al: Intravenous and subcutaneous administration of DDAVP to hemophiliacs: pharmacokinetics and factor VIII responses. Thromb Haemost 58:1037, 1987
44. de la Fuente B, Kasper CK, Rickles FR et al: Response of patients with mild and moderate hemophilia A and von Willebrand's disease to treatment with desmopressin. Ann Intern Med 103:6, 1985
45. Weinstein RE, Bona RD, Altman AJ et al: Severe hyponatremia after repeated intravenous administration of desmopressin. Am J Hematol 32:258, 1989
46. Bond L, Bevan D: Myocardial infarction in a patient with hemophilia treated with DDAVP. N Engl J Med 318:121, 1988
47. Smith PS, Levine PH, Directors of 11 Participating Hemophilia Centers: The

benefits of comprehensive care of hemophilia: a five year study of outcomes. Am J Publ Health 74:616, 1984

48. Levine PH: The implications of acquired immune deficiency syndrome for the management of hemophilia. p. 322. In Seghatchian MJ, Savidge GF (eds): Factor VIII/von Willebrand's factor. CRC press, Boca Raton, FL, 1989

49. Cederbaum AI, Blatt PM, Levine PH: Abnormal serum transaminase levels in patients with hemophilia A. Arch Intern Med 142:481, 1982

50. Jacobson IM, Dienstag JL, Werner BG et al: Epidemiology and clinical impact of hepatitis D (delta) infection. Hepatology 5:188, 1985

51. Allain JP: Transfusion support for haemophiliacs. Clin Haematol 3:99, 1984

52. Levine PH, McVerry BA, Attock B et al: Health of intensively treated hemophiliacs with special reference to abnormal liver chemistries and splenomegaly. Blood 50:1, 1977

53. Choo QL, Kuo G, Wiener AJ et al: Isolation of cDNA clone derived from a blood borne nonA nonB viral hepatitis genome. Science 244:359, 1989

54. Kuo G, Choo QL, Alter HJ et al: An assay for circulating antibodies to a major etiologic virus of human nonA, nonB hepatitis. Science 244:362, 1989

55. Brettler DB, Forsberg AD, Dienstag JL et al: The prevalence of antibody to HCV in a cohort of hemophilic patients. Blood 76:254, 1990

56. Aledort LM, Levine PH, Hilgartner M et al: A study of liver biopsies and liver disease among hemophiliacs. Blood 66:367, 1985

57. Columbo M, Mannucci PM, Brettler DB et al: Hepatocellular carcinoma in hemophilia. Am J Hematol 37:243, 1991

58. Levine PH: The acquired immune deficiency syndrome in persons with hemophilia. Ann Intern Med 103, 723, 1985

59. Eyster EM, Goedert JJ, Sarngadharan MG et al: Development and early natural history of HTLV-III antibodies in persons with hemophilia. JAMA 253: 2219, 1985

60. Centers for Disease Control: HIV/AIDS Surveillance Report. December 1989: 1–16

61. Eyster MG, Mitchell HG, Ballard JO et al: Natural history of human immunodeficiency virus infections in hemophiliacs: effects of T cell subsets, platelet counts, and age. Ann Intern Med 107:1, 1987

62. Goedert JJ, Kessler CK, Aledort LM et al: A prospective study of HIV-1 infection and the development of AIDS in patients with hemophilia. N Engl J Med 321:1141, 1989

63. Ragni MV, Belle SH, Jaffe RA et al: Acquired immunodeficiency syndrome associated non-Hodgkin's lymphomas and other malignancies in patients with hemophilia. Blood 81:1889, 1993

64. Brettler DB, Levine PH: Factor concentrates for treatment of hemophilia. Which one to choose? Blood 73:2067, 1989

65. Prince AM, Horowitz B, Brotman B: Sterilization of hepatitis and HTLV-III viruses by exposure to tri (n-butyl) phosphate and sodium cholate. Lancet 1:706, 1986

66. Mannucci PM: Modern treatment of hemophilia: from the shadows toward the light. Thromb Haemost 70:17, 1993

67. Zimmerman TS: Purification of factor VIII:C by monoclonal antibody affinity chromatography. Semin Hematol 25:25, 1988

68. Carr R, Edmund E, Prescott RJ et al: Abnormalities of circulating lymphocyte subsets in haemophiliacs in the AIDS-free population. Lancet 1:1431, 1984

69. Eibl MM, Ahmad R, Wolf VM et al: A component of factor VIII preparations which can be separated from factor VIII activity down modulates human monocyte functions. Blood 69:1153, 1987

70. Schreiber AB: The preclinical characterization of monoclate factor VIII:C antihemophilic factor (human). Semin Hematol, suppl. 25:25, 1988

71. Thorpe R, Dilger P, Dawson NJ et al: Inhibition of interleukin-2 secretion by factor VIII concentrates: a possible cause of immunosuppression in haemophiliacs. Br J Haematol 71:387, 1989

72. Sullivan JL, Brewster FE, Brettler DB et al: Hemophilic immunodeficiency: influence of exposure to factor VIII concentrate, HTLV-III/LAV, and herpes virus. J Pediatr 104:504, 1986

73. Seeler RA: Hemolysis due to anti-A and anti-B in factor VIII preparations. Arch Intern Med 130:101, 1972

74. Goldsmith GH, Bailey RG, Brettler DB et al: Primary pulmonary hypertension in patients with classical hemophilia. Ann Intern Med 108:797 1988

75. Schimpf K, Mannucci PM, Kreutz W et al: Absence of hepatitis after treatment with a pasteurized factor VIII concentrate in patients with hemophilia and no previous transfusion. N Engl J Med 316:918, 1987

76. Brackmann HH, Egli H: Acute hepatitis B infection after treatment with heat-inactivated factor VIII concentrate. Lancet 2:967, 1988

77. Horowitz MS, Rooks C, Horowitz B et al: Virus safety of solvent/detergent treated antihaemophilic factor concentrate. Lancet 2:186, 1988

78. Mannucci PM: Outbreak of hepatitis A among Italian patients with hemophilia. Lancet 339:819, 1992

79. Centers for Disease Control: Safety of therapeutic products used for hemophilia patients. MMWR 29:441, 1988

80. Brettler DB, Forsberg AD, Levine PH et al: Factor VIII:C purified from plasma via monoclonal antibodies: human studies. Blood 73:1909, 1989

81. Brettler DB: Proposed protocol for the evaluation of the high purity concentrates on the immune system of hemophilia patients. Thromb Hemost 62: 811, 1989

82. DeBiasi R, Rocino A, Miraglea E et al: The impact of a very high purity factor VIII concentrate on the immune system of human immune deficiency virus-infected hemophiliacs: a randomized prospective two year comparison with an intermediate purity concentrate. Blood 78:1919, 1992

83. Seremitis S, Aledort LM, Bona R et al: A three year randomized prospective study of high or intermediate purity factor VIII concentrate in asymptomatic HIV hemophiliacs: effects on immune function. Blood 80:366a, 1992

84. Mannucci PM, Gringeri A, deBiasi R et al: Immune status of asymptomatic HIV-infected hemophiliacs: randomized, prospective two year comparison of treatment with a high purity or an intermediate purity factor VIII concentrate. Thromb Haemost 67:310, 1992

85. Goldsmith JC, the Recombinate Study Group: Clinical trials of Recombinate safety and efficacy of a genetically engineered antihemophilic factor in previously treated patients. Blood 78:64a, 1991

86. Lusher JM, Arkin S, Abilgaard CF et al: Recombinant factor VIII for the treatment of previously untreated patients with hemophilia A. Safety, efficacy and development of inhibitors. N Engl J Med 328: 453, 1993

87. Bray GL, Gomperts EO, Courter S et al: A multicenter study of recombinant factor VIII (Recombinate): safety, efficacy, and inhibitor risk in previously untreated patients with hemophilia A. Blood 83:2428, 1994

88. Bontempo FA, Lewis JH, Gorenc TJ et al: Liver transplantation in hemophilia A. Blood 69:1721, 1987

89. Brocker-Vriends AH, Briet E, Dreesen JC et al: Somatic origin of inherited hemophilia A. Hum Genet 85:288, 1990

90. Gitschier J, Levinson B, Lehesjoki A-E, De La Chapelle A: Mosaicism and sporadic haemophilia: implications for carrier determination. Lancet 1:27, 1989

91. Peake IR, Lillicrap DP, Boulyjenkov V et al: Report of a joint WHO/WFH meeting on the control of haemophilia: carrier detection and prenatal diagnosis. Blood Coagul Fibrinolysis 4:313, 1993

92. Hoyer LW, Carta CA, Mahoney MJ: Detection of hemophilia carriers during pregnancy. Blood 60:1407, 1982

93. Stableforth P, Montgomery DC, Wilson E et al: Effect of oral contraceptives on factor VIII clotting activity and factor VIII related antigen in normal women. J Clin Pathol 28:498, 1975

94. Graham JB, Rizza CR, Chediak J et al: Carrier detection in hemophilia A: a cooperative international study. I. The carrier phenotype. Blood 67:1554, 1986

95. Lyon M: Sex chromatin and gene action in the mammalian X-chromosome. Am J Hum Genet 14:244, 1962

96. Traystman MD, Kiguchi M, Kasper CK et al: Use of denaturing gradient gel electrophoresis to detect point mutations in the factor VIII gene. Genomics 6:293, 1990

97. Orita M, Iwahana H, Kanazawa H et al: Detection of polymorphisms of human DNA by gel electrophoresis as single-strand conformation polymorphisms. Proc Natl Acad Sci 86:2766, 1989

98. Higuchi M, Kochhan L, Schwaab R et al: Molecular defects in hemophilia A: identification and characterization of mutations in the factor VIII gene and family analysis. Blood 74:1045, 1989

99. Higuchi M, Wong C, Kochhan L et al: Characterization of mutations in the factor VIII gene by direct sequencing of amplified genomic DNA. Genomics 6:65, 1990

100. Lakich D, Kazazian HH Jr, Antonarakis SE, Gitschier J: Inversions disrupting the factor VIII gene are a common cause of severe haemophilia A. Nat Genet 5:236, 1993

101. Tabor A, Philip J, Madsen M et al: Randomized controlled trial of genetic amniocentesis in 4606 low-risk women. Lancet 1:1287, 1986

102. Henry GP, Miller WA. Early amniocentesis. J Reprod Med 37:396, 1992

103. Rhoads GG, Jackson LG, Schlesselman EA: The safety and efficacy of chorionic villus sampling for early prenatal diagnosis of cytogenetic abnormalities. N Engl J Med 320:609, 1989

104. Jackson LG, Zachary JM, Fowler SE et al: A randomized comparison of transcervical and transabdominal chorionic villus sampling. N Engl J Med 327: 594, 1992

105. Daffos F, Capella-Pavlovsky M, Forestier F: Fetal blood sampling during pregnancy with use of a needle guided by ultrasound of 606 consecutive cases. Am J Obstet Gynecol 153:655, 1985

Biochemistry of Factor IX and Molecular Biology of Hemophilia B

107

Steven A. Limentani and Bruce Furie

INTRODUCTION

Factor IX is a plasma protein with a molecular weight of 56,000 whose synthesis by the liver requires vitamin K. Factor IX participates in an intermediate phase of the blood coagulation pathway (see Ch. 100). It can be activated by factor XIa or factor VIIa complexed with tissue factor. In complex with factor VIIIa on membrane surfaces, factor IXa then activates factor X. The critical importance of factor IX is emphasized by the phenotype of hemophilia B, an hereditary disease characterized by factor IX deficiency.

In 1952 factor IX was discovered, distinct from factor VIII, in that after mixing two hemophiliac plasmas from unrelated patients, the clotting time of the mixed plasma was corrected.[1,2] Hemophilia B, or Christmas disease, is a sex-linked disorder defined by the congenital decrease in factor IX activity. The molecular defect causing factor IX deficiency in the index patient has recently been shown to be a point mutation causing a change from Cys 206 to serine in the catalytic domain.[3] Hemophilia B accounts for about 12% of the total cases of hemophilia. The disease is variable in phenotype, and the degree of bleeding severity usually correlates with the level of factor IX activity present in the patient's plasma. As anticipated from the variable phenotypes of hemophilia B and the similarity of phenotypes within each particular family, hemophilia B is caused by a variety of genetic defects. It is estimated that one-third of cases of hemophilia B arise from spontaneous mutations.

GENE STRUCTURE AND REGULATION

The factor IX gene is 34 kb in size, but only a limited amount of this DNA encodes the factor IX protein. The gene contains seven introns that range in size from 188 nucleotides to almost 10 kb.[4] The gene is located on the tip of the long arm of the X chromosome at Xq26-27.3, close to the factor VIII gene.[5] The cDNA consists of a 2.8 kb-open reading frame, coding for a 461-amino acid precursor protein.[6,7] The protein is encoded by all eight exons (Fig. 107-1). The first, exon 1, codes for the signal peptide. The second, exon 2, codes for the propeptide and γ-carboxyglutamic acid domain of factor IX. Exon 3 codes for the aromatic amino acid stack domain, a short linking segment common to all of the vitamin K-dependent proteins. Exons 4 and 5, separated by a large intron, each code for the two epidermal growth factor (EGF)-like domains of factor IX. Exon 6 codes for the activation domain of factor IX, while exons 7 and 8 code for the catalytic (serine protease) domain. The factor IX gene was derived ancestrally from a precursor of the prothrombin gene.[8] The genes for factor VII, factor X, and protein C share common splice junctions with the gene for factor IX, demonstrating the close relationship of the vitamin K-dependent proteins.

The regulation of the factor IX gene includes enhancer elements and an androgen-sensitive region. TATA boxes have been proposed at -27,[9] -187,[10] -265,[11] and -411.[11] A CAAT box is located at -238.[10] A transcription initiation site has been defined at $+1$[9] and a transcription start site at -150.[10] Reijnen et al.,[12] using primer extension and SI nuclease mapping, have confirmed possible transcription initiation sites at $+1$, $+4$, and $+30$, but were unable to demonstrate a transcription initiation site at -150. Reverse direction promoter-like activity has been identified in the region between -800 and -750.[10] A silencer has been identified between $-1,600$ and $-1,900$ and may lie at $-1,680$ with the sequence CCTCTCCTA.[10]

Factor IX Leyden is a form of hemophilia B characterized by a severe bleeding disorder during childhood; factor IX activity and antigen levels are <1%.[13] With the onset of puberty or with the administration of androgen therapy,[14] the factor IX levels rise to 30–60% of normal, and the hemophilia phenotype disappears (Fig. 107-2). The mutations in the genes of patients in various pedigrees with the factor IX Leyden phenotype are located at -21, -20, -6, $+6$, $+8$, and $+13$ of the transcriptional start site.[15-19] An additional point mutation causing moderate hemophilia has been described in a 3-year-old patient at -5; the consequence of this mutation during adolescence is as yet unknown.[20] The point mutations that are the basis for hemophilia B Leyden have served to increase understanding of the 5' regulatory region of the factor IX gene. A binding site for the CCAAT/enhancer binding protein (C/EBP) between $+1$ and $+18$ has been identified.[21] C/EBP binding is ablated by the mutation at $+13$, and protein expression is decreased by the mutation at -6. Furthermore, a binding site for nuclear factor-1 liver has been defined between -76 and -99.[21] A mutation at -20, -21, or -26 led to the identification of a binding site for hepatic nuclear factor-4 (HNF-4) between -10 and -34.[15,22,23] In contrast to the factor IX Leyden phenotype, the mutation at -26 does not lead to correction of factor IX levels after puberty[23]; an androgen-responsive element is located between -20 and -36. In normal individuals, factor IX levels increase from 80 U/dl to 99 U/dl after puberty, a change that is statistically significant.[24]

The gene organization of factor IX is nearly identical to that of factor X, factor VII and protein C (see Fig. 100-4). After transcription, a factor IX mRNA is generated that is about 2.8 kb.[6,7] This mRNA includes a 5' untranslated region and a long 3' untranslated region of 1.4 kb. This 3' sequence contains a poly(A) tail nearly 1.4 kb 3' to the stop codon and the typical processing sequence (AATAAA) 16 bp 5' to this polyadenylation site. This leads to a long, noncoding tail in the mRNA.[9,11]

SYNTHESIS OF FACTOR IX

Factor IX is synthesized in the hepatocyte as a precursor protein; it then undergoes a series of intracellular post-translational modifications, leading to the production of mature, fully active factor IX (Fig. 107-3). The coding sequence of the factor

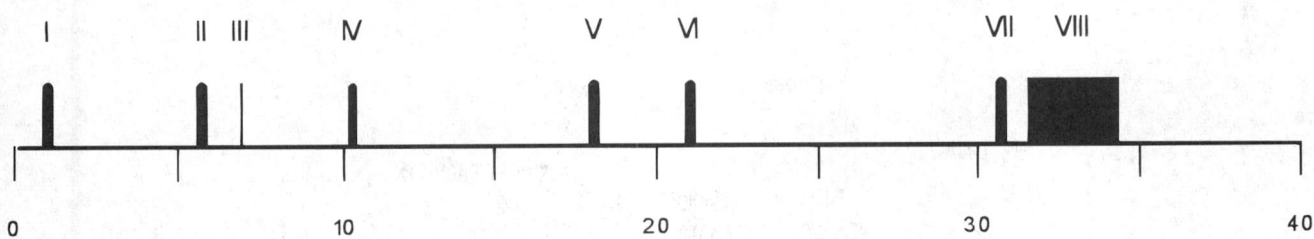

Fig. 107-1. Structure of the factor IX gene. The factor IX gene includes eight exons and seven introns.

IX gene encodes two peptides that are removed prior to secretion of the mature factor IX into the blood: a 28-residue signal peptide that directs the nascent peptide chain to the endoplasmic reticulum and an 18-residue propeptide between the signal peptide and the mature N terminus of factor IX.[7] The signal peptide is cleaved co-translationally by the signal peptidase. The propeptide contains the γ-carboxylation recognition site that directs γ-carboxylation of the adjacent glutamic acid residues in the γ-carboxyglutamic acid domain of mature factor IX. This recognition element is defined by amino acids −18, −17, −16, −14, and −10 toward the N terminus of this region. The vitamin K-dependent carboxylase binds to the γ-carboxylation recognition site within the propeptide.[25,26] The carboxylation reaction, catalyzed by the carboxylase, requires a reduced form of vitamin K (vitamin KH_2), molecular oxygen, carbon dioxide, and the factor IX precursor, uncarboxylated profactor IX, containing glutamic acid residues.[27] The carboxylase is an enzyme with a molecular weight of 94,000 that is sufficient to carboxylate a precursor substrate in the presence of the necessary cofactors.[28–31] The carboxylase is a membrane protein, and its catalytic activity resides on the luminal side of the rough endoplasmic reticulum.[32,33]

In addition, Asp 64 undergoes β-hydroxylation. From the cDNA sequences of factor IX,[6,7] factor X,[34] protein C,[35,36] protein S,[37] and factor VII,[38] it is apparent that specific aspartic acid residues in precursor forms of these proteins undergo β-hydroxylation post-translationally. Stenflo et al.[39] have suggested that a consensus sequence consisting of Cys-X-Asp/Asn-X-X-X-Phe/Tyr-X-Cys-X-Cys signals this event. Factor IX contains about 0.4 mol of β-hydroxyaspartic acid/mol of factor IX.[40,41] This modified amino acid is formed from aspartic acid by a

post-translational process catalyzed by a 2-oxoglutarate-dependent dioxygenase,[42] which has been partially purified from bovine liver.[43] The β-hydroxylase is present within the endoplasmic reticulum.

Bovine and human factor IX are glycoproteins that contain about 17% carbohydrate. Bovine factor IX contains four N-linked glycosylation sites at residues 158, 168, 173, and 261.[44–46] These residues correspond to residues 157, 167, 172, and 261 in human factor IX. However, residue 172 is threonine in human factor IX, and residue 261 lacks the appropriate consensus sequence for N-linked glycosylation. Two O-linked glycosylation sites have been identified in the first EGF domain of factor IX.[47,48] The O-linked sugar at residue 53 is composed of glucose and xylose in equal molar ratios, with the glucose linked to Ser 53. An analogous trisaccharide has been analyzed that is linked to Ser 53 of bovine factor IX and has the structure D-xylose p α 1-3-D-xylose p α 1-3-D-glucose p β I-o-serine-53.[49] The O-linked sugar at residue 61 is composed of equal molar ratios of galactose, fucose, N-acetylglucosamine, and N-acetylneuraminic acid and is linked to Ser 61 through the fucose residue.[48,50]

Profactor IX, including the propeptide and factor IX sequence, undergoes carboxylation in the endoplasmic reticulum. Profactor IX, even in its fully carboxylated form and in contradistinction to factor IX, is not capable of binding to membrane surfaces.[51] Presumably, this feature prevents factor IX from being hung up inside the cell, where high levels of calcium ions within the endoplasmic reticulum could support factor IX-membrane interaction. Profactor IX undergoes additional post-translational processing, including disulfide bond formation and glycosylation, characteristic of other secreted plasma proteins. The propeptide is cleaved as a late processing event.[7,52,53] Furin/PACE cleaves peptide bonds at a site adjacent to the sequence Arg −4:X:Arg −2:Arg −1, where X can be any amino acid.[54] Bristol and colleagues[55] used site-directed mutagenesis to define a hierarchy of the efficiency of cleavage given different paired amino acids at the P1 and P2 positions: Lys-Arg > Arg-Arg > Thr-Arg > Arg-Lys > Lys-Lys ≫ Lys-Thr. γ-Carboxylation precedes propeptide cleavage.[51]

STRUCTURE OF FACTOR IX

Human factor IX is a single-chain glycoprotein composed of 415 amino acids (Fig. 107-4).[6,7,56] It has a molecular weight of 56,000.[57,58]

Propeptide

The propeptide directs γ-carboxylation of profactor IX and then is cleaved to yield factor IX. The propeptide includes an amphipathic α-helix, with a hydrophobic and hydrophilic face.[59] The carboxylation recognition site is located proximal to this helix. Mutations in the propeptide have been documented as the cause of some forms of hemophilia B. Diuguid et al.[52] determined the size of the propeptide of factor IX by analysis of a mutant factor IX, factor IX Cambridge. This mutant

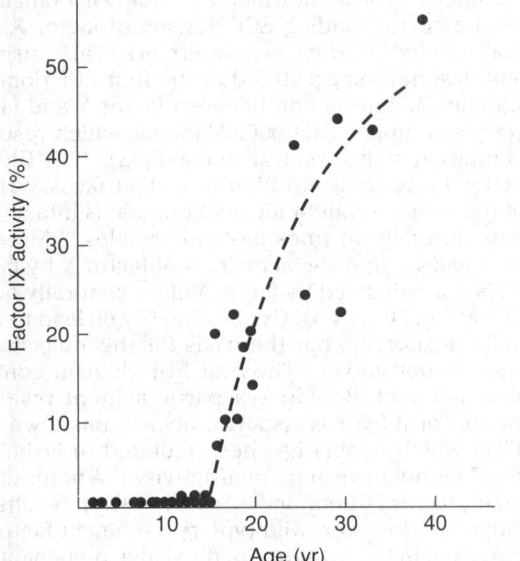

Fig. 107-2. Factor IX Leyden. Changes in the plasma factor IX level as a function of age. (From Briet et al.,[13] with permission.)

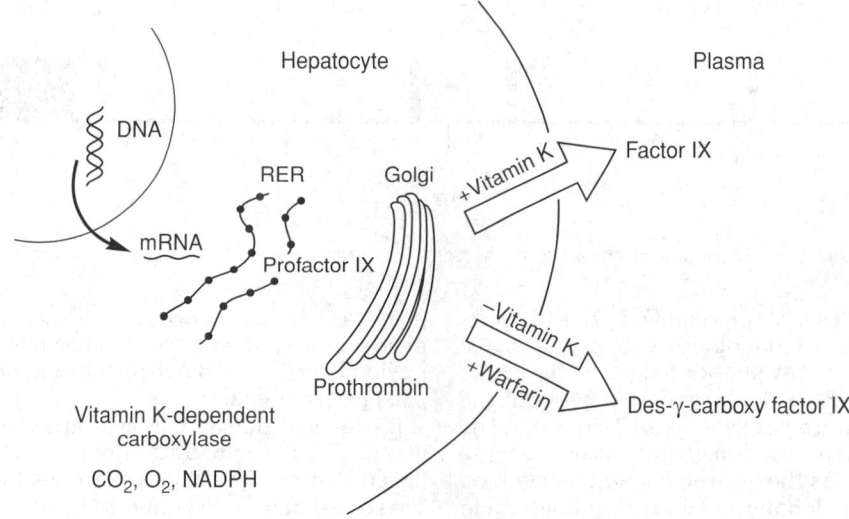

Fig. 107-3. Biosynthesis of factor IX. Factor IX is synthesized in the liver in a precursor form. The signal peptide is responsible for translocation of the nascent peptide chain to the endoplasmic reticulum. Profactor IX undergoes post-translational processing, including γ-carboxylation, glycosylation, β-hydroxylation, disulfide bond formation, and finally propeptide cleavage. γ-Carboxylation requires molecular oxygen, reduced vitamin K, and carbon dioxide in the presence of the vitamin K-dependent γ-carboxylase.

has an 18-residue N-terminal extension due to the mutation of Arg −1 to a serine, precluding propeptide cleavage by a propeptidase with trypsin-like specificity. Concurrently Bentley et al.[53] evaluated factor IX Oxford 3, a mutant factor IX in which Arg −4 is mutated to glutamine; this mutation also prevents propeptide cleavage.[53] Similar mutations have been described: factor IX San Dimas (Arg −4 → Gln),[60] factor IX Troed-Y-Rhiw (Arg −4 → Gln),[61] factor IX London-3 (Arg −4 → Gln), factor IX London-4 (Arg −4 → Gln),[62] factor IX Malmo-6 (Arg −4 → Trp),[62] and factor IX Kawachinagano (Arg −4 → Gln).[63] Each of these mutants is characterized by the complete absence of factor IX activity and the presence of the 18-residue propeptide extension. Of the several proteins studied,[52,60,64] there is a partial defect in γ-carboxylation of factor IX. Because of this defect in γ-carboxylation and because of the failure of propeptide cleavage, these profactor IX mutants cannot bind to phospholipid vesicles, nor can they be activated by factor XIa. These data and the marked sequence homology of this domain in γ-carboxyglutamic acid-containing proteins led to the proposal of a role for the propeptide in designating protein precursors containing this specific propeptide for subsequent γ-carboxylation.[65] Using site-specific mutagenesis and an heterologous mammalian expression system, Jorgensen et al.[26,41] demonstrated that protein-engineered factor IX lacking the 18-residue propeptide was not carboxylated in vivo. Similarly, point mutations at −16 (Phe → Ala) or −10 (Ala → Glu), both positions highly conserved in the propeptides of the vitamin K-dependent proteins, inhibited γ-carboxylation. These results demonstrated that the propeptide contains a recognition element, designated the γ-carboxylation recognition site, which signals for the γ-carboxylation of the vitamin K-dependent proteins during hepatic biosynthesis.

γ-Carboxyglutamic Acid Domain

The NH$_2$ terminal γ-carboxyglutamic acid domain of human factor IX includes 12 γ-carboxyglutamic acid residues located at positions 7, 8, 15, 17, 20, 21, 26, 27, 30, 33, 36, and 40.[66,67] The γ-carboxyglutamic acid domain defines some of the critical calcium-binding sites of the protein and is required for the interaction of factor IX with membrane surfaces in the presence of calcium ions.[68] Naturally occurring point mutations of glu-

tamic acid residues destined to be γ-carboxylated include Glu 7, Glu 8, Glu 17, Glu 21, Glu 27, Glu 30, and Glu 33; patients with these mutations have moderate-to-severe hemophilia, emphasizing the functional importance of these residues.[69] A small loop, formed by cysteine at residues 18 and 23, is common to all of the vitamin K-dependent blood clotting proteins. Point mutations at Cys 18 or Cys 23 result in severe hemophilia.

Epidermal Growth Factor-Like Domains

The γ-carboxyglutamic acid domain is linked to two adjacent EGF domains by a short domain rich in aromatic amino acids. The EGF domains, each characterized by a segment of 53 amino acids and a pattern of disulfide-bonded cysteine residues, have distinct functions. The structure of the first EGF domain has been determined by two-dimensional nuclear magnetic resonance spectroscopy.[70] The first EGF domain may function as a spacer, since factor IX, in which the first EGF domain substitutes for the corresponding EGF domain of factor X, has full functional activity.[71,72] However, Astermark et al.,[73] using inhibitory peptides, have suggested that the first EGF domain may participate in the interaction between factor X and factor IXa in the tenase complex. Factor IX Alabama, which results from a point mutation in the first EGF domain (Asp 47 → Gly),[74] may be defective in its ability to bind to cell surfaces.[75] However, because the γ-carboxyglutamic acid domain is intact, this mutant binds normally to phospholipid vesicles.[76] More recent evidence suggests that the activation of factor X by factor IXa Alabama is not enhanced by factor VIIIa.[77] Naturally occurring mutations at Gln 50, Cys 51, Cys 56, and Gly 60 lead to a severe hemophilia phenotype, but the basis for this defective factor IX function is not known. The first EGF domain contains an unusual amino acid, β-hydroxyaspartic acid, at residue 64.[78] The function of β-hydroxyaspartic acid is unknown. Mutant factor IX in which Asp 64 has been mutated to lysine, valine, or glycine does not have functional activity.[79] A naturally occurring mutant, factor IX London-6 (Asp 64 → Gly), results in mild hemophilia B.[80] However, wild-type recombinant factor IX has been expressed in the presence of dipyridyl, o-phenanthroline, or pyridine 2,4-dicarboxylate, which are inhibitors of 2-ketoglutarate-dependent dioxygenases.[81] The factor IX expressed in this system is fully γ-carboxylated but contains <0.1 mol of

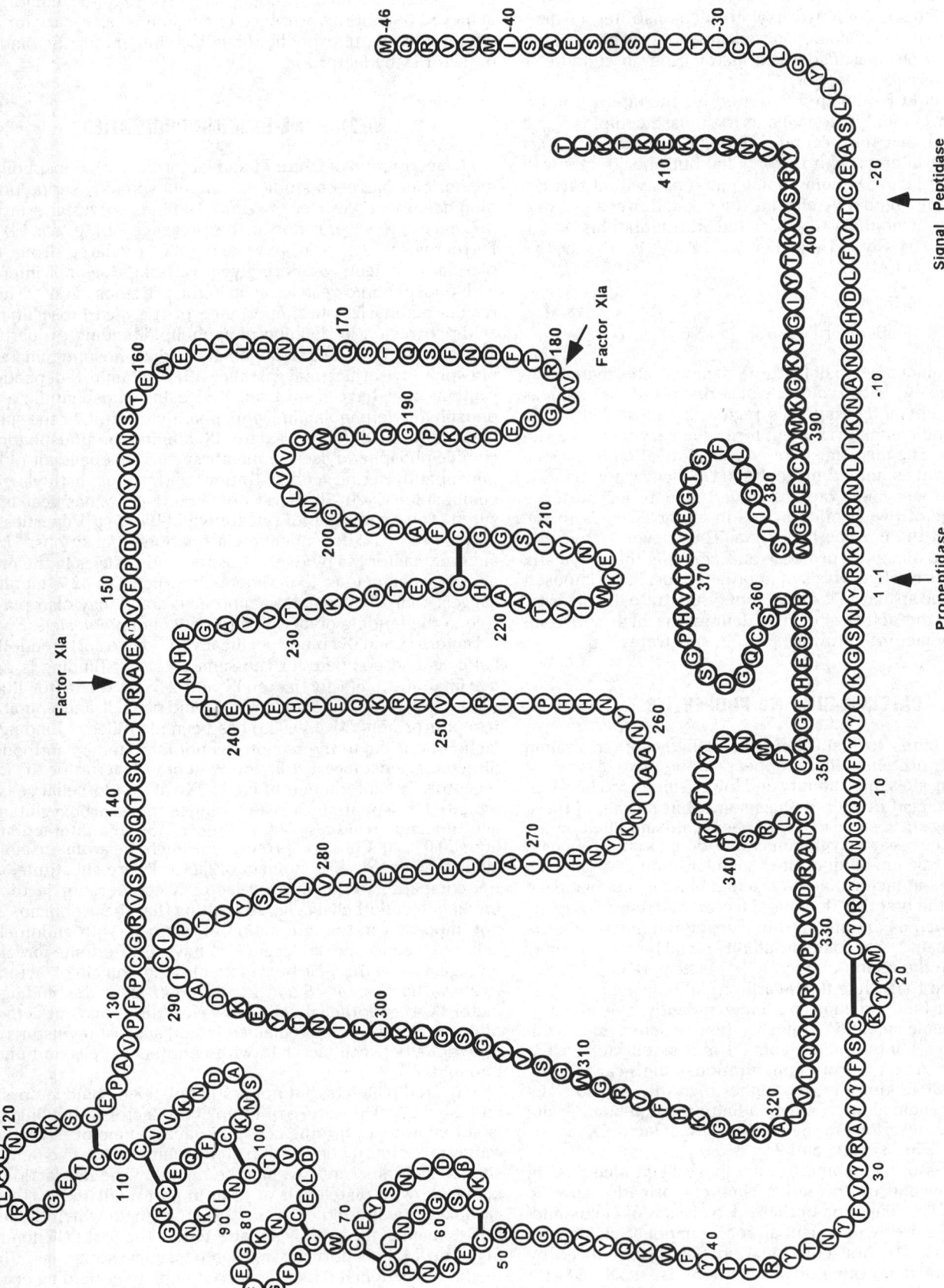

Fig. 107-4. Amino acid sequence of factor IX. The pre-profactor IX sequence includes the signal peptide, propeptide, γ-carboxyglutamic acid domain, aromatic amino acid stack domain, two EGF domains, and the serine protease domain. Amino acids are designated by the one-letter code; γ, γ-carboxyglutamic acid; β, β-hydroxyaspartic acid.

β-hydroxylated aspartic acid/mol of factor IX, compared with 0.5 mol in the factor IX expressed in the absence of inhibitors. The factor IX that is not β-hydroxylated demonstrates full functional activity when evaluated in a coagulant assay and is indistinguishable from plasma-derived factor IX in an endothelial cell-binding assay.

The second EGF domain is required for the interaction between factor IXa and factor VIIIa in the tenase complex.[71,72] It would appear that this second EGF domain contains contact residues that interact with factor VIIIa, but not directly with the substrate factor X. Some point mutations within this domain have only a moderate effect on function. However, moderate-to-severe hemophilia is associated with mutations of Asn 92, Gly 93, Arg 94, Gly 114, Cys 124, Asn 92, Cys 95, Cys 99, Cys 111, Asn 120, and Ala 127.[69]

Serine Protease Domain

The C-terminal portion of factor IX demonstrates marked sequence homology with zymogens of serine proteases, such as trypsin and chymotrypsin. This region is almost 250 amino acids long and contains, in latent form, the enzyme active site of factor IXa. The mechanism of enzyme activation involves a process known as limited proteolysis. On cleavage of peptide bonds, the proenzyme is rapidly converted to its enzyme form. The cleavage of two peptide bonds in factor IX leads to the generation of the enzyme factor IXa. The enzyme active site is common to all serine protease and contains the enzymatic machinery for the hydrolysis of peptide bonds. Superimposed on this generic structure is an extended substrate binding site, surrounding the active site, that defines the high substrate specificity of factor IXa toward protein substrates.

CALCIUM-BINDING PROPERTIES

Factor IX binds to metal ions. As with the other vitamin K-dependent proteins, there appear to be two classes of metal-binding sites: high affinity and lower affinity.[82] The γ-carboxyglutamic acid domain defines some, but not all, of these metal-binding sites, since factor IX chemically modified by the removal of the γ-carboxyglutamic acid domain still retains a high-affinity calcium-binding site.[68] Similar findings have been demonstrated in factor IXa.[83] A calcium-binding site has been localized to the first EGF domain of factor IX.[84] Asp 47, Asp 49, Gln 50, and Asp 64 are involved in calcium binding within the first EGF domain.[85] A second low-affinity metal binding site may be present in the region of Phe 77.[84,85] Astermark et al.[86] have demonstrated that while the γ-carboxyglutamic acid and EGF domains can bind calcium ions independently, the intact γ-carboxyglutamic acid-EGF domains bind calcium ions with higher affinity.[86] Interdomain contact and stabilization were also detected in that thermal denaturation of the γ-carboxyglutamic acid-EGF modules is 10°C higher then the γ-carboxyglutamic acid domain alone.[87] A high-affinity calcium-binding site has also been described in the heavy chain of factor IX involving residues 235, 237, 240, and 245.[88]

Two classes of metal-binding sites have been identified in both factor IX and prothrombin using conformation-specific antibodies.[89,90] Occupation of these two classes of metal-binding sites leads to two sequential conformational changes in these proteins. The first conformational change, induced by magnesium and many other divalent cations, is associated with the quenching of intrinsic fluorescence. The second, metal-selective conformational change is only induced by calcium ions. Fab fragments of the conformation-specific antibodies, directed against factor IX after it has undergone the conformational transition that is calcium ion selective, block the binding of factor IX to phospholipid vesicles and the activation of factor IX by factor XIa. This finding suggests that the conformer achieved only in the presence of calcium is necessary for the expression of a phospholipid-binding site and for the binding of factor IX by factor XIa.

MEMBRANE-BINDING PROPERTIES

The interaction of factor IX and factor IXa with phospholipid membranes has been studied using phosphatidylserine/phosphatidylcholine vesicles.[76] Factor IX binds to vesicles in the presence of Ca^{2+}, but not in the presence of Mg^{2+} or EDTA. Furthermore, des-γ-carboxy factor IX, prepared from the plasma of patients who are given warfarin, does not interact with phospholipid vesicles even in the presence of Ca^{2+}. These results emphasize the importance of the γ-carboxyglutamic acid-rich region in defining phospholipid-binding properties. The specificity of factor IX for an acidic phospholipid (e.g., phosphatidylserine) may parallel other vitamin K-dependent proteins that have been evaluated using phosphatidic acid, phosphatidylethanolamine, phosphatidylinositol, or the specificity may be different. Factor IX affinity for phosphatidylcholine-phosphatidylserine membranes is independent of the phosphatidylserine concentration with phosphatidylserine compositions >20–30%[91]; a K_d of about 1–2 μM has been measured. The expression of phospholipid-binding properties involves two metal-dependent conformational transitions.[89] Like factor IX, factor IXa binds to phospholipid vesicles in the presence of calcium ions. Experiments in which Trp 42 is mutated suggest that the aromatic amino acid stack may also play a role in the binding of factor IX to phospholipid vesicles.[92,93]

Factors IX and IXa bind specifically to bovine aortic endothelial cells and compete for the same site.[94–96] Binding is half-maximal at 2.1 nM for factor IX and 2.5 nM for factor IXa.[94] About 20,000 molecules of factor IX bind per cell, and a putative receptor protein (M_r 140,000) has been identified.[97] Binding of factors IX or IXa to the receptor is not inhibited by antibodies directed against factor VIII, von Willebrand factor, or the EGF receptor. The interaction of factor IX with endothelial cells is inhibited by a peptide corresponding to the γ-carboxyglutamic acid domain (residues 1–42)[98]; the K_i for this interaction is about 0.05 μM. Chimeric proteins in which the aromatic amino acid stack or first EGF domain of factor IX are substituted by the comparable domain from factor X compete for factor IX binding to endothelial cells, suggesting that these domains are not important in the interaction of factor IX with endothelial cells.[99] Cheung and colleagues[100] have utilized site-directed mutagenesis of the γ-carboxyglutamic acid domain of factor IX to show that residues 5 and 10 are required for the binding of factor IX to endothelial cells. However, the coagulant activity of the mutant proteins remained intact, suggesting distinct interactions between factor IX with endothelial cells and phospholipids.[100]

Activated platelets, but not resting platelets, bind factors IX and IXa.[101,102] The nature of the platelet factor IX binding site is not known, nor are the actual surfaces on factor IX that are required for interaction with platelet membranes. The binding site for factors IX and IXa may be distinct. The interaction of factor IXa with platelets is at least in part mediated by the γ-carboxyglutamic acid domain.[103] Factor IXa, in which the first EGF domain of factor IX is substituted by the first EGF domain of factor X, binds normally to platelets, suggesting that either the first EGF domain is not involved in platelet binding or the first EGF domain of factor X is sufficient for this interaction.[104] Factor IXa binds to the factor IX binding site but also binds to additional sites that do not bind factor IX. In the presence of saturating concentrations of factors VIIIa and X, the K_d of factor IXa (K_d = 0.5 nM) binding is five times lower than that of factor

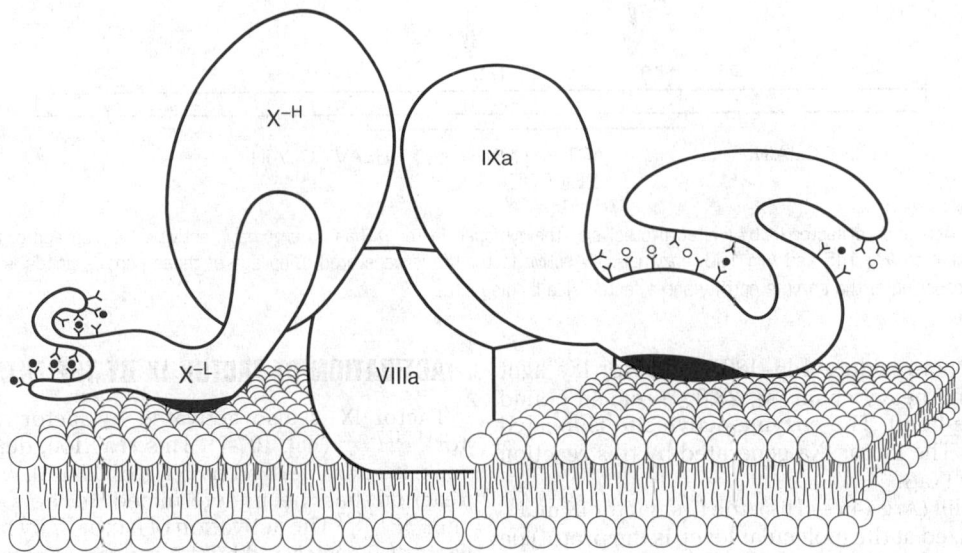

Fig. 107-5. A model of the structure of the tenase complex. The tenase complex (the enzyme complex capable of activating factor X to factor Xa) includes factor IXa as enzyme and factor VIIIa as cofactor bound to the membrane surface. The substrate factor X interacts with factor IXa, factor VIIIa, and the membrane.

IX.[105,106] The importance of factor VIII for factors IX and IXa binding to cell membranes remains uncertain.

Factor IX is activated by factor XIa in a reaction that is independent of membrane surfaces. The rate of factor IX activation is not affected by the binding of factor XIa to platelets.[106]

FORMATION OF THE TENASE COMPLEX

The binding of factor IXa to factor VIII has been studied using both porcine and human factor VIII. Using fluorescence anisotropy to monitor the interaction of porcine factor VIIIa and factor IXa derivatized with a fluorescent label within its active site, Duffy et al.[107] have shown that these proteins interact on phospholipid membrane surfaces with a K_d of 2 nM in 1:1 molar stoichiometry. The factor IXa active site is distinct from the membrane surface, and its structure is perturbed on interaction with factor VIIIa during the formation of the tenase complex.[108] Activation of factor IX to factor IXa leads to the expression of a factor VIII-binding site and active enzyme site with full coagulant activity.[109] Reciprocally, activation of factor VIII by thrombin yields factor VIIIa, which binds more tightly than factor VIII to factor IXa.[107] Cleavage of Arg 180-Val 181 is required for at least partial expression of the factor VIII binding site; the cleavage of Arg 145-Ala 146 in addition to Arg 180-Val 181 leads to full enzymatic and cofactor binding activity.[109]

The binding of factor IXa, factor VIIIa, and phospholipid (the tenase complex) (Fig. 107-5) has been explored with chimeric proteins in which the first and second EGF domains of factor X are substituted for the native domains in factor IX. The chimeras in which the second EGF domain of factor IX has been substituted with the second EGF domain of factor X do not bind significantly in the tenase complex but interact normally with phospholipid.[71] The chimera in which the first EGF domain of factor IX has been substituted with the first EGF domain of factor X has full or nearly full biologic activity, indicating that the first EGF domain is not involved in factor VIIIa binding.[71,72] Furthermore, this form does bind in the tenase complex.[71] This finding suggests that the second EGF domain of factor IX is required for enzymatic activity and that it contains a recognition site for factor VIIIa.[71]

ACTIVATION OF FACTOR IX BY THE INTRINSIC PATHWAY

Factor IX is a proenzyme with no catalytic activity that is activated to factor IXa by factor XIa or by factor VIIa and tissue factor in a reaction that depends on the presence of calcium (Fig. 107-6). The kinetics of factor IX activation by factor VIIa and tissue factor or factor XIa are comparable. Factor IX is converted to its enzyme form, factor IXa, by factor XIa. This reaction requires calcium ions, but takes place in solution. In contrast to the other vitamin K-dependent blood clotting proteins, membrane surfaces, including phospholipid vesicles or cell surfaces, do not enhance factor IX activation. The activation of factor IX by factor XIa is abnormally slow in factor IX New London (Pro 50 → Glu).[110] This implicates the EGF domain in factor IX activation. When factor IX is activated by factor XIa, two peptide bonds are cleaved: one bond is located at Arg 145-Ala 146 and the other bond is at Arg 180-Val 181[111,112] (Fig. 107-7). Factor IX is first cleaved to form factor IXa, in which the Arg-Ala bond at residues 145–146 is cleaved followed by the cleavage of the Arg-Val bond at residues 180–181.[113] With the release of the internal carbohydrate-rich activation frag-

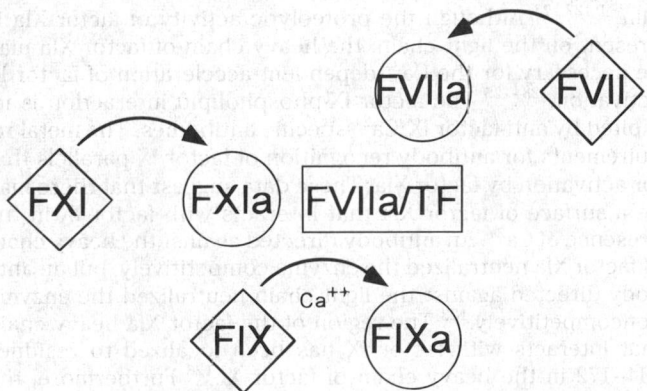

Fig. 107-6. Pathways of factor IX activation. Factor IX is activated independently by either factor XIa or factor VIIa/tissue factor. Factor XIa can activate factor IX in the absence of membrane surfaces, but calcium ions are required. The complex of factor VIIa and tissue factor on membrane surfaces in the presence of calcium ions also converts factor IX to its active enzyme form.

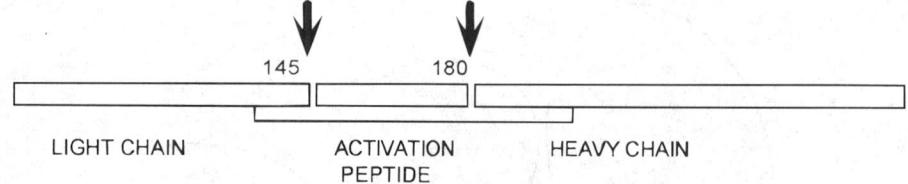

Fig. 107-7. Activation of factor IX by limited proteolysis. The zymogen factor IX has no enzymatic activity. On cleavage of the peptide bonds adjacent to Arg 145 and Arg 180, enzymatically active factor IXa is generated. Cleavage of these peptide bonds is associated with the expression of the enzyme activity and a factor VIIIa binding site.

ment (M_r 11,000), from residues 146–180, the factor IXa light chain (M_r 17,000) and heavy chain (M_r 28,000) remain bound by a single disulfide bond. The enzyme active site is located on the heavy chain. The factor IXa generated by this reaction is designated factor IXaβ.

Factor IX Chapel Hill (Arg 145 → His), the first factor IX mutation to be characterized at the molecular level, is the prototype of a genetic defect in which activation of a zymogen is impaired due to the mutation of an arginine preceding a sessile bond.[114] It has <20% of the coagulant activity when compared with factor IXaβ.[76] Factors IX Chicago-2 (Arg 145 → His)[115] and IX Albuquerque (Arg 145 → Cys)[116] have been found to have mutations at the same site. In each of these mutations, the loss of the arginine at position 145 precludes the cleavage of the sessile bond separating the factor IX light chain from the activation peptide. Failure to cleave this bond results in a molecule that cleaves factor X very slowly. The active site of factor IXa is formed, however, as demonstrated by its ability to cleave synthetic substrate normally.[117] Factor IX mutants at position 180 include factor IX Hilo (Arg 180 → Gln), factor IX Milano (Arg 180 → Gln), factor IX Deventer (Arg 180 → Trp), and factor IX Nagoya (Arg 180 → Trp), all resulting in hemophilia B_M, a type of hemophilia in which the patient's mutant factor IX causes a marked prolongation of the ox brain thromboplastin time due to increased inhibition of the in vitro activation of factor VII.[118,119] Factor IX Novara (Val 181 → Phe) results in the hemophilia B_M phenotype, while factor IX Kashihara (Val 182 → Phe) results in hemophilia B.[119,120]

The activation of factor IX by factor XIa is highly metal selective, with optimal activation only in the presence of Ca^{2+} and suboptimal activation in the presence of Sr^{2+}.[82,121] The K_m for the activation of factor IX by factor XIa without calcium is 18 μM, and the k_{cat} is 2.4 min^{-1}. In the presence of calcium the K_m is decreased to 2 μM, and the k_{cat} is increased to 10.4 min^{-1}.[122,123] Although the proteolytic activity of factor XIa is present on the light chain, the heavy chain of factor XIa may be necessary for the Ca^{2+}-dependent acceleration of factor IX activation.[123–125] The factor IX-phospholipid interaction is inhibited by anti-factor IX/Ca^{2+}-specific antibodies. The metal requirements for antibody recognition of factor IX parallels that for activation by factor XIa. These data suggest that there may be a surface of factor XIa that interacts with factor IX in the presence of Ca^{2+}. An antibody directed against the heavy chain of factor XIa neutralized the enzyme competitively, but an antibody directed against the light chain neutralized the enzyme noncompetitively.[123] The region of the factor XIa heavy chain that interacts with factor IX has been localized to residues 134–172 in the heavy chain of factor XI.[126] Furthermore, the presence or absence of calcium did not change the rate of activation of factor IX by factor XIa light chain.[123] On the basis of these studies and antibody inhibition studies using antibodies to factor IX, the heavy chain of factor XIa has been implicated as specifically interacting with the phospholipid-binding site of factor IX in the presence of Ca^{2+}.

ACTIVATION OF FACTOR IX BY THE EXTRINSIC PATHWAY

Factor IX is also activated by factor VIIa and tissue factor[114,127–129] (Fig. 107-7). This reaction, dependent on calcium ions, is characterized by a K_m of 0.3 μM.[113,127] The k_{cat} for this reaction has been determined to be between 13 and 68 min^{-1}.[113,127] The activation of factor IX by factor VIIa and tissue factor is accelerated by the activation of factor IX to factor IXa by factor Xa.[130]

The relative importance of factor IX activation by factors XIa or VIIa and tissue factor has been evaluated by measuring the factor IX activation peptide in patients with factors VII and XI deficiency.[131] There was a significant reduction in the baseline levels of the factor IX activation peptide in patients with factor VII deficiency but not in patients with factor XI deficiency when compared with normal controls. Furthermore, the administration of recombinant factor VIIa to chimpanzees results in a significant increase in both the factor IX and factor X activation peptides at the same time point.[131] Infusion of recombinant factor VIIa into patients with factor VII deficiency causes an increase in the abnormally low levels of the factors IX and X activation peptides and prothrombin fragment F1·2.[132] These studies suggest that the activation of factor IX by factor VIIa and tissue factor is important in vivo.

Almus et al.[133] have evaluated the activation of factors IX and X by factor VIIa and tissue factor in an umbilical vein model. In this system the activation of factors IX and X occurs at the same rate. These results further substantiate the importance of both of these reactions in the initiation of the extrinsic pathway of blood coagulation.

FACTORS IXa ENZYMATIC ACTIVITY

Once generated, factor IXa forms a complex with factor VIIIa on membrane surfaces in an interaction that is calcium dependent. This complex on the membrane is required for the activation of factor X at rates that are physiologically significant.[134] Factor IXa is inhibited by antithrombin III, which forms a 1:1 stoichiometric complex with factor IXa as well as other activated coagulation factors. This reaction is accelerated approximately 1,000-fold by the addition of heparin.[135–138] Under comparable conditions, antithrombin III neutralizes 57% of factor IXa activity within 30 minutes in the absence of heparin but completely inhibits factor IXa within 15 seconds in the presence of heparin.[135] In contrast to the solution-phase activation of factor IX by factor XIa, factor X is converted to its enzyme form, factor Xa, by factor IXa in complex with factor VIIIa on membrane surfaces. This reaction requires calcium ions. Membrane surfaces, including phospholipid vesicles, activated platelets, or endothelial cells, are required for significant factor X activation. Thus, factor IX is a membrane-binding protein, and the presence of γ-carboxyglutamic acid is intimately related to these membrane-binding properties. These proteins may have two distinct binding domains, one related to zymogen activation and the other to macromolecular assembly of the enzyme in complex with the specific cofactor.

Factor IXa is a serine protease that expresses its activity via the catalytic domain, which resides in the heavy chain. This activity is generated by the classic catalytic triad that in factor IXa is located at His 41, Asp 89, and Ser 185 in the heavy chain.

The activation of factor X by factor IXa has been evaluated under multiple experimental conditions. Calcium by itself accelerates factor IXa activation of factor X, but its more important role is to allow for the formation of the tenase complex on membrane surfaces. The presence of both factor VIIIa and membrane surfaces greatly accelerates the activation of factor X, while the presence of either of these cofactors alone has a minimal effect.[139,140] The K_{cat} for factor X activation by factor IXa in the presence of factor VIIIa but without phospholipid vesicles is 0.058 min^{-1}; the same reaction without factor VIIIa but with phospholipid vesicles (25 μM) has a k_{cat} of 0.095 min^{-1}, whereas in the presence of factor VIIIa and phospholipid vesicles the reaction is greatly accelerated, with a k_{cat} of $1,740 \text{ min}^{-1}$.[101] The activation of factor X by factor IXa is also supported by activated platelets. The k_{cat} for this reaction is $1,240 \text{ min}^{-1}$, which is very close to the k_{cat} for factor X activation in the presence of phospholipid vesicles. These results suggest a physiologic role for platelets in this process.

Factor IXa activates factor X in the presence of both bovine[141] and human umbilical vein[142] endothelial cells. Stern et al.[141] have demonstrated equal binding of factors IX and IXa to bovine aortic endothelial cells. There is an equivalent increase in binding of both factor IX and factor IXa in the presence of activated or unactivated factor VIII. However, when factor X is added to the reaction mixture, a high-affinity binding site with relative specificity for factor IXa is expressed, and the interaction of factor IXa with endothelium is increased 10–40-fold. Factor X does not enhance factor IXa binding without the presence of factor VIII. While similar interactions have been demonstrated for factor IXa, factor VIII, and human umbilical vein endothelial cells, the rate of this reaction did not approach the rate of a control performed with phospholipid vesicles and only reached maximal velocity after a 10–12-minute lag phase.[142]

Factor IX Eagle Rock and factor IX Bergamo are both characterized by the substitution of valine for Gly 363 and are functionally normal except for their inability to bind antithrombin III and their inability to activate factor X.[120,143] This may be due to the location of this mutation next to the active site Ser 365, causing distortion of the specificity pocket of the enzyme.

Defects Affecting Enzymatic Activity

Mutations within the catalytic domain of factor IX may decrease enzymatic activity. A mutation of Ile 397 → Thr has been recognized in multiple hemophilia B families, including factor IX Vancouver,[144] factor IX Long Beach,[145] and factor IX Los Angeles.[143] This lesion is near, but not within, the active site of factor IXa; it may alter the extended substrate binding site for factor X. Factor IX Angers (Gly 396 → Arg) has a mutation within the substrate-binding pocket of factor IXa that disrupts enzymatic activity.[146] Factor IX B$_{m \text{ Lake Elsinore}}$ (Ala 390 → Val)[147] also possesses a mutation within the substrate binding pocket that interferes with enzymatic activity. Factor IX Eagle Rock (Gly 363 → Val)[143] and factor IX Bergamo[119] both have mutations adjacent to Ser 365, the active site serine, that interfere with enzymatic activity. A mutation of Arg 333 also leads to a defect in the ability to catalyze factor X cleavage.

MOLECULAR BASIS OF HEMOPHILIA B

Defects in Gene Structure that Cause Hemophilia B

Gross deletions of the factor IX gene causes severe, antigen-negative hemophilia B[148,149] (Fig. 107-8). These defects have been associated with anti-factor IX antibodies in response to replacement therapy with factor IX.[148] While antibody production may be associated with gross gene deletions, not all such patients have demonstrated such a response.[150,151] In addition, some patients with anti-factor IX antibodies do not possess gross gene deletions,[62,152] and in at least one case antibodies developed in an antigen-positive patient.[152] Thus, the lack of the factor IX gene is not the sole factor controlling the development of an immunologic response to factor IX replacement therapy.

Smaller deletions of the factor IX gene cause hemophilia B. Factor IX Chicago-1 possesses a complex deletion of exons 5, 7, and 8, totaling approximately 25 kb.[153] Factor IX Seattle-1 contains an intragenic deletion of exons 5 and 6 of the factor IX gene,[154] resulting in the production of a truncated factor IX protein of 36,000 MW that is excreted into the urine.[155] Factor IX Yemen[149] and factor IX Tubingen[149] each possess deletions of exons 1–3 of the factor IX gene, with variable amounts of the 5'-flanking sequence also having been deleted. Factor IX Hanover has a deletion of exons 4 and 5 totaling 8 kb.[149] Factor IX Strasbourg contains a 2.8-kb intragenic deletion encompassing exon 4, the exon encoding the first EGF-like domain.[156] Despite possessing 30% of normal factor IX antigen levels, this family displays a severe hemophilic phenotype. Factor IX Ratingen shows a loss of exon 7, with a deletion of 1.5 kb.[149] Factor IX London-10 contains a deletion of the codon for Arg 37,[62] resulting in a severe hemophilic phenotype despite the presence of 12% of normal factor IX antigen levels. Factor IX Seattle-2 contains a deletion of a single adenine nucleotide at position 17,699 (in exon 4) of the factor IX gene, corresponding to residue 85 of the factor IX molecule.[157] This results in a frameshift mutation, creating a stop codon at codon 86. Factor IX London-11 (deletion of bases 31,059–31,060), factor IX London-12 (deletion of nucleotide 6392), and factor IX Malmo-1 (deletion of nucleotides 30,950–30,957) also result in frameshifts leading to premature stop codons.[62] It is unclear whether these mRNAs are processed normally, resulting in a truncated plasma protein secreted in the urine as above, or whether these frameshift mutations result in an unstable mRNA, producing a thalassemia-like syndrome.

In other cases, point mutations can lead to the production of little to no factor IX antigen. Rees et al.[158] and Winship[159] have described point mutations within the obligatory donor splice junction of exons 6 and 3, respectively. These mutations result in the production of an improperly spliced mRNA, causing a defect in transcription that results in no factor IX antigen being produced by these patients. Factor IX Bordeaux (Lys 411 → Stop),[160] factor IX Portland (Arg 252 → Stop),[161] factor IX Malmo-3 (Arg 248 → Stop),[62] Malmo-4 (Arg 29 → Stop),[62] and Malmo-5 (Trp 194 → Stop),[62] factor IX New York (Arg 338 → Stop),[162] factor IX Oxford 11 (Gln 11 → Stop),[163] factor IX Bonn-1 (Arg 338 → Stop),[149] an unnamed mutant (Arg 252 → Stop),[164] and other mutations all possess nonsense mutations resulting in premature stop codons. In each case, the premature stop signal yields an antigen-negative phenotype.

Finally, several missense mutations have been described that result in markedly reduced levels of factor IX antigen (Fig. 107-9). Factor IX London-8 (Cys 336 → Arg) results in the loss of a cysteine that is conserved not only in the coagulation proteases but in the digestive serine proteases as well.[62] This loss disrupts the tertiary structure of the catalytic domain. Factor IX London-9 (Asn 120 → Tyr) also leads to a severe, antigen-negative phenotype.[62] This substitution of a bulky, hydrophobic aromatic ring for the hydrophilic asparagine residue is presumed to yield an unstable protein product. Factor IX Oxford-5 (Gly 114 → Ala),[163] Oxford-8 (Glu 7 → Asp),[163] and Oxford-9 (Ala 291 → Pro)[163] all possess little circulating factor IX antigen.

A gene insertion and a combination of a gene insertion plus gene deletion have been reported to cause hemophilia B. Hemophilia B El Salvador contains a 6.1-kb insertion near exon 4

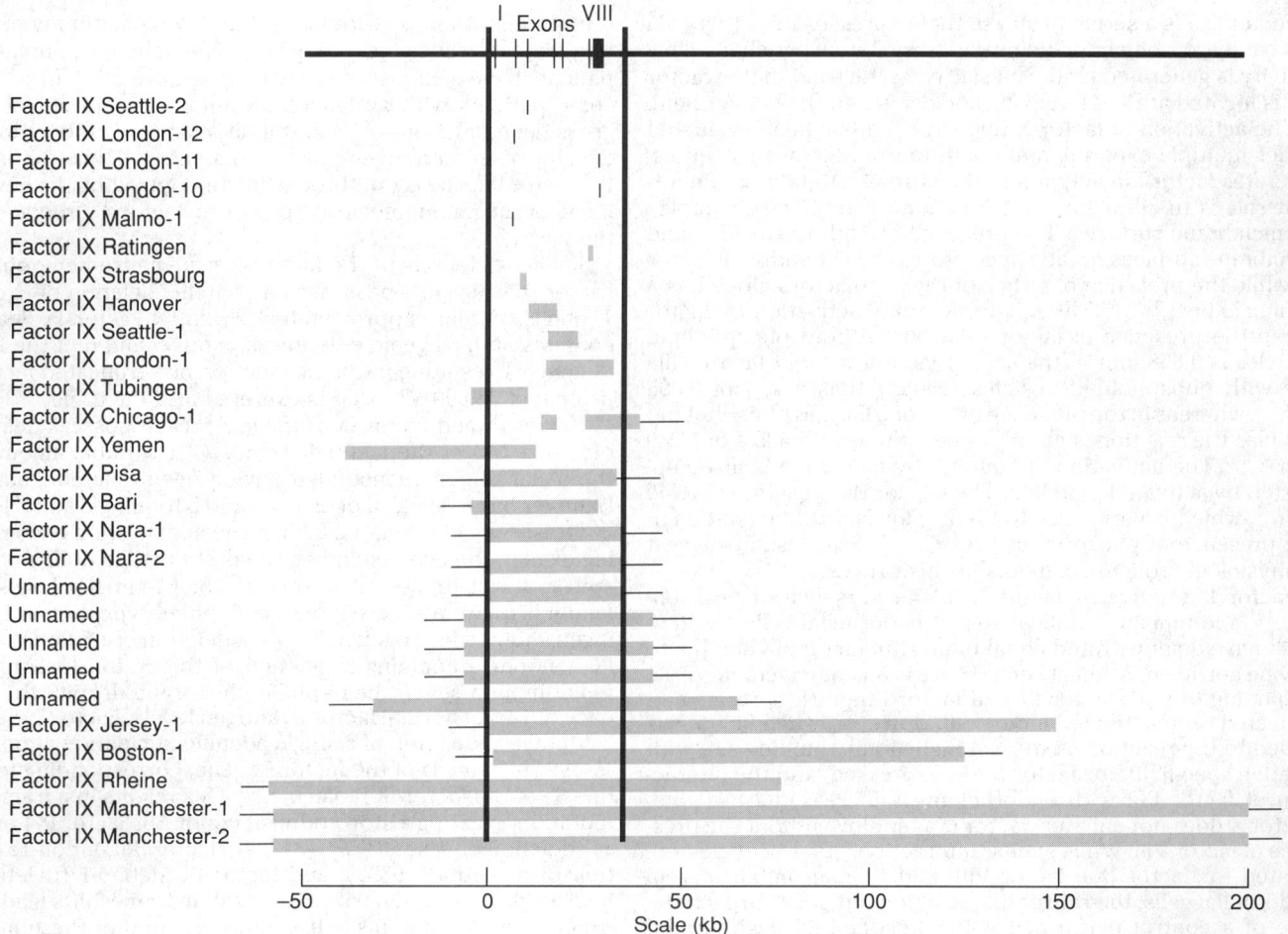

Fig. 107-8. Factor IX gene deletions as a cause of hemophilia B. Deleted portions of factor IX gene, pink rectangles; uncertain extent of deletion, red lines. The factor IX gene (exons 1–8) is shown in black.

of the factor IX gene,[165] resulting in moderate hemophilia, with factor IX activity of 1% and factor IX antigen of 6%. A combination of a 2-kb insertion and a 1-kb deletion mutation in intron 6 results in hemophilia B Sydney, in which there is no circulating factor IX antigen.[166]

Antigen-Positive Hemophilia B

Approximately one-third of the cases of hemophilia B fall within the group termed cross-reactive material positive. Such patients have normal levels of factor IX antigen and variable levels of factor IX activity, due to the presence of a dysfunctional factor IX molecule. Mutations have been described that affect post-translational protein processing, γ-carboxylation, lipid binding, EGF domain function, zymogen activation, and substrate recognition and/or enzymatic activity. In addition, a series of patients has been reported to display the hemophilia B_M phenotype. This has proved to be a heterogeneous set of mutations, as noted below.

A developing theme in understanding the molecular basis of hemophilia B is the discovery of duplicate mutations in apparently unrelated patients. To date, 378 unique point mutations (both missense and nonsense) have been reported.[69] Several groups have postulated that the CpG dinucleotide sequence is a mutational hot spot.[167–169] The CpG sequence is a component of four of the six arginine codons; as a mutational hot spot, it may represent an important cause for the development of spontaneous point mutations. Furthermore, using a mathematical model, the 20 CpG dinucleotides in the factor IX coding

sequence showed an observed mutation rate 150 times the rate that would be expected for the predicted transition rate.[170] Of 51 single base pair substitutions found in one study, 27 were at CpG dinucleotides, which represents a 38-fold excess for mutations at these sites.[171] In another study, point mutations at CpG dinucleotides were estimated to be increased by 77-fold over the expected rate.[172]

In patients with mutant plasma proteins, the mutation of arginine to another amino acid also appears to be a developing theme. Since internal point mutations are likely to destabilize protein structure and lead to markedly diminished circulating protein levels, patients preselected for circulating mutant protein antigen are likely to have amino acid substitutions on the protein surface. Arginines, located on the protein surface, are used by proteases of the trypsin family to hydrolyze adjacent bonds during protein processing and zymogen activation. It would thus appear, given the functional importance of arginines, that their mutation leads to phenotypically obvious defects in protein function.

Molecular Diagnosis

Hemophilia B is diagnosed by the finding of isolated, hereditary factor IX deficiency. Factor IX deficiency may be observed by prolongation of the activated partial thromboplastin time and by failure of plasma from these patients to correct the clotting time of known factor IX-deficient plasma. These findings, combined with a lifelong history of bleeding or a family history of bleeding disorders, secure the diagnosis. The level

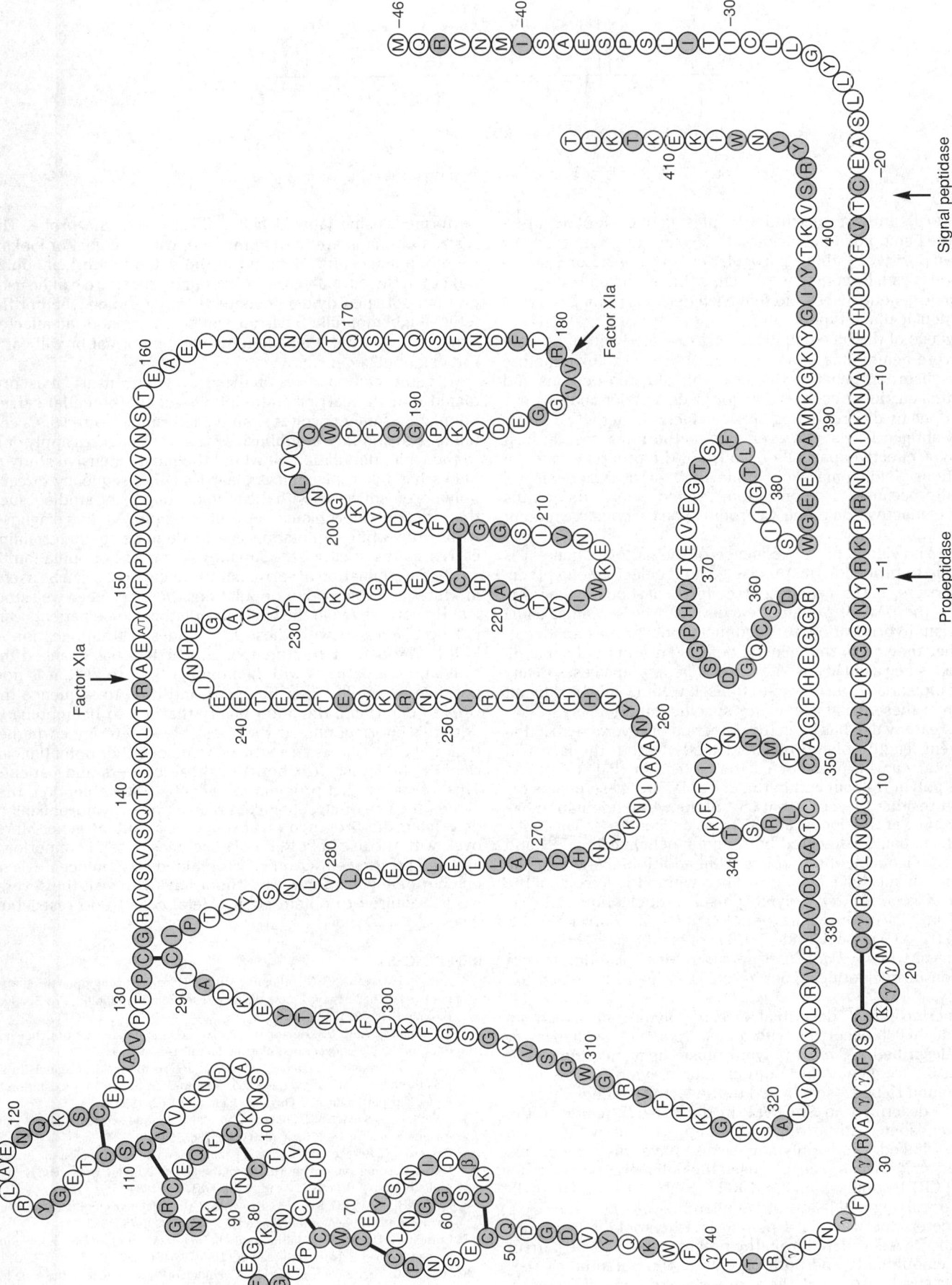

Fig. 107-9. Missense and nonsense mutations in the factor IX amino acid DNA sequence as a cause of hemophilia B. Missense mutations are designated by red shading and nonsense mutations are designated by a red circle. Amino acids are designated by the one-letter code; γ, γ-carboxyglutamic acid;

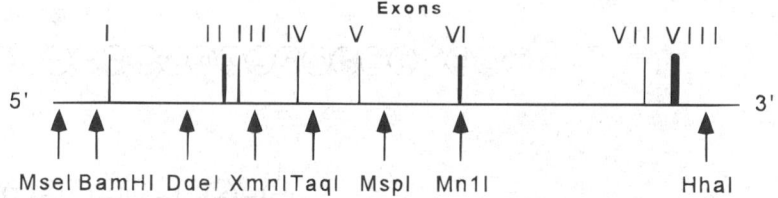

Fig. 107-10. Restriction fragment length polymorphisms in the factor IX gene.

of factor IX antigen present in the plasma of each patient permits the hemophilia to be characterized as antigen negative or antigen positive. Within a particular cohort, the factor IX activity level is usually constant, reflecting that each family displays the same genetic defect and that each defect is associated with a particular phenotype.

Because of the bleeding disorder associated with moderate or severe hemophilia B, and because of the sex-linked nature of the disorder, genetic counseling for affected persons and potential carriers becomes a major issue. Carrier analysis has been done by differentiating between factor IX activity and factor IX antigen levels. However, this method has been at best only 80% effective, partially because of the preponderance of mutations yielding markedly diminished factor IX antigen and partially because of "lyonization," which causes differential levels of inactivation of the X chromosome carrying the mutant gene.[173]

With knowledge of the sequence of the factor IX gene, it is possible to probe for the precise genetic defect among potential carriers. If the genetic defect for a particular cohort is known, the DNA of potential carriers can be screened using stringent hybridization to oligonucleotide probes to detect whether they carry that genetic defect. This method is handicapped, since as many as one-third of hemophilia cases in any generation arise from new mutations. It would likely be difficult to detect these using probes for specific mutations.

Of greater value has been the detection of several restriction fragment length polymorphisms (RFLPs) within the factor IX gene that can be used for carrier detection (Fig. 107-10). A single polymorphism within the factor IX coding sequence occurs at residue 148, such that 65% of the white population has a threonine at that locus, and 35% has an alanine.[174] This polymorphism can be detected both immunochemically[175,176] and through oligonucleotide probes.[174] In addition, five intragenic polymorphisms have been described within the introns of the factor IX gene. A *Taq*I polymorphism at nucleotide 11,111 is found in 35% of the white population.[177] An *Xmn*I polymorphism (G → C) at nucleotide 7,076 is present on 29% of X chromosomes, while a *Dde*I/*Hinf*I polymorphism resulting from a deletion of nucleotides 5,505 to 5,554 is found at a 24% frequency.[178]

Camerino et al.[179] described an *Msp*I polymorphism near nucleotide 16,000 occurring with a 20% frequency, while Hay et al.[180] described a *Bam*HI polymorphism at nucleotide −587, with a 6% frequency. In addition, four polymorphisms have been found to be closely linked to the factor IX gene. Mulligan et al.[181] described an *Sst*I RFLP in the q26-q27 region of the X chromosome with a frequency of approximately 50%. Two closely linked *Taq*I polymorphisms have also been described.[182,183] Winship et al.[184] used the polymerase chain reaction (PCR) to unmask an *Hha*I RFLP 8 kb 3′ to the factor IX gene, occurring in 48% of the population studied.

To determine whether a person is a hemophilia B carrier, genomic DNA is isolated from the potential carrier, the patient with hemophilia B, and both parents of the potential carrier. That DNA is digested with the appropriate restriction enzymes, and the digested DNA is run on an appropriate gel matrix. The DNA is transferred to nitrocellulose, and a Southern blot is performed, using labeled factor IX cDNA as the probe. The restriction maps are then compared, with the goal of looking for any polymorphisms found in the patient with hemophilia but not in the normal parent. The same procedure can be used on DNA obtained by amniocentesis to determine whether the fetus of a hemophilia B carrier will be a normal or an affected male, and whether a female fetus will be normal or will carry the hemophilia gene.

With the combination of these polymorphisms, it is predicted that the carrier status of 89% of the potential carrier population (among whites) can be determined with 99.9% certainty.[163] It should be emphasized that these figures apply only to the white population, in whom the most extensive study of RFLPs has taken place. It is clear that the frequency of each polymorphism varies with the ethnic group being studied, such that the polymorphisms currently employed for diagnosis within the white population are inadequate for determining carrier status in either the Japanese[185] or black population.[186]

The determination of carrier status using RFLPs can be useful in whites and some other populations that have been well studied. However, even in the white population, some patients cannot be diagnosed with these techniques. The application of PCR to the detection of hemophilia carriers has changed the evaluation of patients with hemophilia B. With PCR, it is now possible to amplify specific exons and then to sequence the DNA to determine the abnormality that led to hemophilia B. With this information, it is then possible to determine whether that mutation is present in the genome of either potential carriers or the fetuses (or both) of those carriers and patients. This obviates the problem of genetic recombination that clouds the use of closely linked restriction polymorphisms to determine the presence or absence of a mutant gene. Moreover, with the use of PCR, it now becomes possible to perform antenatal testing either on cells obtained by amniocentesis or on chorionic villus samples without having to wait the several weeks required to obtain enough fetal cells to do restriction digests.

REFERENCES

1. Aggeler PM, White SG, Glendenning MB et al: Plasma thromboplastin component (PTC) deficiency: a new disease resemblig hemophilia. Pro Soc Exp Biol Med 79:692, 1952
2. Schulman I, Smith CH: Hemorrhagic disease in an infant due to deficiency of a previously undescribed clotting factor. Blood 7:794, 1952
3. Taylor SAM, Duffin J, Cameron C et al: Characterization of the original Christmas disease mutation (cysteine 206 → serine): from clinical recognition to molecular pathogenesis. Thromb Haemost 67:63, 1992
4. Yoshitake S, Schach BG, Foster DC et al: Nucleotide sequence of the gene for human factor IX. Biochemistry 24:3736, 1985
5. Camerino G, Grzeschik KH, Jaye M et al: Regional localization on the human X chromosome and polymorphism of the coagulation factor IX gene (hemophilia B locus). Proc Natl Acad Sci USA 81:498, 1984
6. Choo KH, Gould KG, Rees DG, Brownlee GG: Molecular cloning of the gene for human anti-haemophilic factor IX. Nature 299:178, 1982
7. Kurachi K, Davie EW: Isolation and characterization of a cDNA coding for human factor IX. Proc Natl Acad Sci USA 79:6461, 1982
8. Foster DC, Yoshitake S, Davie EW: The nucleotide sequence of the gene for human protein C. Proc Natl Acad Sci USA 82:4673, 1985
9. Anson DS, Choo KH, Rees DJG et al: The gene structure of human anti-haemophilic factor IX. EMBO J 3:1053, 1984

10. Salier J-P, Hirosawa S, Kurachi K: Functional characterization of the 5′-regulatory region of human factor IX gene. J Biol Chem 265:7062, 1990

11. Yoshitake S, Schach BG, Foster DC et al: Nucleotide sequence of the gene for human factor IX. Biochemistry 24:3736, 1985

12. Reijnen MJ, Bertina RM, Reitsma PH: Localization of transcription initiation sites in the human coagulation factor IX gene. FEBS Lett 270:207, 1990

13. Briet E, Bertina RM, Van Tilburg NH, Veltkamp JJ: Haemophilia B Leyden: a sex linked hereditary disorder that improves after puberty. N Engl J Med 306:788, 1982

14. Briet E, Wijnands MC, Veltkamp MD: The prophylactic treatment of hemophilia B Leyden with anabolic steroids. Ann Intern Med 103:225, 1985

15. Reijnen MJ, Peerlinck K, Maasdam D et al: Hemophilia B Leyden: substitution of thymine for guanine at position −21 results in a disruption of a hepatocyte nuclear factor 4 binding site in the factor IX promoter. Blood 82:151, 1993

16. Fahner JB, Salier JP, Landa L et al: Defective promoter structure in a human factor IX Leyden. Blood, suppl. 72:295A, 1988

17. Reitsma PH, Bertina RM, van Amstel P et al: The putative factor IX gene promoter in hemophilia B Leyden. Blood 72:1074, 1988

18. Royle G, Van De Water NS, Berry E et al: Haemophilia B Leyden arising de novo by point mutation in the putative factor IX promoter region. Br J Haematol 77:191, 1991

19. Reitsma PH, Mandalaki T, Kasper CK et al: Two novel point mutations correlate with an altered developmental expression of blood coagulation factor IX (hemophilia B Leyden phenotype). Blood 73:743, 1989

20. Picketts DJ, D'Souza CD, Bridge PJ, Lillicrap D: An A to T transversion at position −5 of the factor IX promoter results in hemophilia B. Genomics 12:161, 1992

21. Crossley M, Brownlee GG: Disruption of a C/EBP binding site in the factor IX promoter is associated with haemophilia B. Nature 345:444, 1990

22. Reijnen MJ, Sladek FM, Bertina RM, Reitsma PH: Disruption of a binding site for hepatocyte nuclear factor 4 results in hemophilia B Leyden. Proc Natl Acad Sci USA 89:6300, 1992

23. Crossley M, Ludwig M, Stowell KM et al: Recovery from hemophilia B leyden: an androgen responsive element in the factor IX promoter. Science 257:377, 1992

24. Sweeney JD, Hoernig LA: Age-dependent effect on the level of factor IX. Am J Clin Pathol 99:687, 1993

25. Hubbard B, Ulrich M, Jacobs M et al: Vitamin K-dependent carboxylase: affinity purification from bovine liver by using a synthetic propeptide containing the γ-carboxylation recognition site. Proc Natl Acad Sci USA 86:6893, 1989

26. Jorgensen MJ, Cantor AB, Furie BC et al: Recognition site directing vitamin K-dependent γ-carboxylation resides on the propeptide of factor IX. Cell 48:185, 1987

27. Suttie JW: Mechanism of action of vitamin K: synthesis of γ-carboxyglutamic acid. CRC Crit Rev Biochem 8:191, 1980

28. Wu SM, Morris DP, Stafford DW: Identification and purification to near homogeneity of the vitamin K-dependent carboxylase. Proc Natl Acad Sci USA 88:2236, 1991

29. Rehemtulla A, Roth DA, Wasley LC et al: In vitro and in-vivo functional characterization of bovine vitamin K-dependent γ-carboxylase expressed in Chinese hamster ovary cells. Proc Natl Acad Sci USA 90:4611, 1993

30. Roth D, Rehemtulla A, Kaufman RJ et al: Expression of vitamin K-dependent carboxylase in baculovirus-infected inset cells. Proc Natl Acad Sci USA 90:8372, 1993

31. Wu S-M, Cheung W-F, Frazier D, Stafford DW: Cloning and expression of the cDNA for human γ-glutamyl carboxylase. Science 254:1634, 1991

32. Wallin R, Prydz H: Studies on a subcellular system for vitamin K-dependent carboxylation. Thromb Haemost 41:529, 1979

33. Carlisle TL, Suttie JW: Vitamin K-dependent carboxylase: subcellular location of the carboxylase and enzymes involved in vitamin K metabolism in rat liver. Biochemistry 19:1161, 1980

34. Leytus SP, Chung DW, Kisiel W et al: Characterization of a cDNA coding for human factor X. Proc Natl Acad Sci USA 81:3699, 1984

35. Beckmann RJ, Schmidt RJ, Santerre RF et al: The structure and evolution of a 461 amino acid human protein C precursor and its messenger RNA, based upon the DNA sequence of cloned human liver cDNAs. Nucleic Acids Res 13:5233, 1985

36. Long GL, Belagaje RM, MacGillivray RTA: Cloning and sequencing of liver cDNA coding for bovine protein C. Proc Natl Acad Sci USA 81:5653, 1984

37. Lundwall A, Dackowski W, Cohen E et al: Isolation and sequence of the cDNA for human protein S, a regulator of blood coagulation. Proc Natl Acad Sci USA 83:6716, 1986

38. Hagen FS, Gray CL, O'Hara P et al: Characterization of the cDNA coding for human factor VII. Proc Natl Acad Sci USA 83:2412, 1986

39. Stenflo J, Lundwall A, Dahlback B: β-Hydroxyasparagine in domains homologous to the epidermal growth factor precursor in the vitamin K-dependent protein S. Proc Natl Acad Sci USA 84:368, 1987

40. Fernlund P, Stenflo J: β-Hydroxyaspartic acid in vitamin K-dependent proteins. J Biol Chem 258:12509, 1983

41. Rabiet M-J, Jorgensen MJ, Furie B, Furie BC: Effect of propeptide mutations on processing of factor IX. J Biol Chem 262:14895, 1987

42. Stenflo J, Holme E, Lindstedt S et al: Hydroxylation of aspartic acid in domains homologous to the epidermal growth factor precursor is catalyzed by a 2-oxoglutarate-dependent dioxygenase. Proc Natl Acad Sci USA 86:4447, 1989

43. Gronke RS, Welsch DJ, VanDusen WJ et al: Partial purification and characterization of bovine liver aspartyl β-hydroxylase. J Biol Chem 265:8558, 1990

44. Fujikawa K, Legaz ME, Kato H, Davie EW: The mechanism of activation of bovine factor IX (Christmas factor) by bovine factor XIa (activated plasma thromboplastin antecedent). Biochemistry 13:4508, 1974

45. Katayama K, Ericsson LH, Enfield DL et al: Comparison of amino acid sequence of bovine coagulation factor IX (Christmas Factor) with that of other vitamin K-dependent plasma proteins. Proc Natl Acad Sci USA 75:4990, 1979

46. Mizuochi T, Taniguchi T, Fujikawa K et al: The structure of the carbohydrate moieties of bovine blood coagulation factor IX (Christmas factor). J Biol Chem 258:6020, 1983

47. Nishimura H, Kawabata S, Kisiel W et al: Identification of a disaccharide (Xyl-Glc) and a trisaccharide (Xyl₂-Glc) O-glycosidically linked to a serine residue in the first epidermal growth factor-like domain of human factor VII and IX and protein Z and bovine protein Z. J Biol Chem 264:20320, 1989

48. Nishimura H, Takao T, Hase S et al: Human factor IX has a tetrasaccharide O-glycosidically linked to serine 61 through the fucose residue. J Biol Chem 267:17520, 1992

49. Hase S, Nishimura H, Kawabata S et al: The structure of (xylose)₂ glucose-O-serine 53 found in the first epidermal growth factor-like domain of bovine blood clotting factor IX. J Biol Chem 265:1858, 1990

50. Harris RJ, van Halbeek H, Glushka J et al: Identification and structural analysis of the tetrasaccharide NeuAcα(2 → 6)Galβ(1 → 4)GlcNAcβ(1 → 3)Fucα1 → O-linked to serine 61 of human factor IX. Biochemistry 32:6539, 1993

51. Bristol JA, Furie BC, Furie B: Profactor IX: carboxylated profactor IX is not a substrate for proteolytic activation and lacks a γ-carboxyglutamic acid-dependent membrane binding site. Blood, suppl. 1. 80:242, 1993

52. Diuguid DL, Rabiet M-J, Furie BC et al: Molecular basis of hemophilia B: a defective enzyme due to an unprocessed propeptide is caused by a point mutation in the factor IX precursor. Proc Natl Acad Sci USA 83:5803, 1986

53. Bentley AK, Rees DJG, Rizza C, Brownlee GG: Defective propeptide processing of blood clotting factor IX caused by mutation of arginine to glutamine at position −4. Cell 45:343, 1986

54. Wasley LC, Rehemtulla A, Bristol JA, Kaufman RJ: PACE/furin can process the vitamin K-dependent pro-factor IX precursor within the secretory pathway. J Biol Chem 268:8458, 1993

55. Bristol JA, Furie BC, Furie B: Propeptide processing during factor IX biosynthesis. J Biol Chem 268:7577, 1993

56. Katayama K, Ericsson L, Enfield D et al: Comparison of amino acid sequence of bovine coagulation factor IX (Christmas factor) with that of other vitamin K-dependent proteins. Proc Natl Acad Sci USA 76:4990, 1979

57. Fujikawa K, Thompson AR, Legaz ME et al: Isolation and characterization of bovine factor IX (Christmas factor). Biochemistry 12:4938, 1973

58. DiScipio RG, Hermodson MA, Yates SG, Davie EW: A comparison of human prothrombin, factor IX (Christmas factor), factor X (Stuart factor) and protein S. Biochemistry 16:698, 1977

59. Sanford DG, Kanagy C, Sudmeir JL et al: Structure of the propeptide of prothrombin containing the γ-carboxylation recognition site determined by two-dimensional NMR spectroscopy. Biochemistry 30:9835, 1991

60. Ware J, Diuguid DL, Liebman HA et al: Factor IX San Dimas: substitution of glutamine for arginine −4 in the propeptide leads to incomplete γ-carboxylation and altered phospholipid binding properties. J Biol Chem 264:11401, 1989

61. Liddell MB, Lillicrap DP, Peake IR, Bloom AL: Defective propeptide processing and abnormal activation underlie the molecular pathology of factor IX Troed-y-Rhiw. Br J Haematol 72:208, 1989

62. Green PM, Bentley DR, Mibashan RS et al: Molecular pathology of haemophilia B. EMBO J 8:1067, 1989

63. Sugimoto M, Miyata T, Kawabata S et al: Factor IX Kawachinagano: impaired function of the Gla domain caused by attached propeptide region due to substitution of arginine by glutamine at position −4. Br J Haematol 72:216, 1989

64. Galeffi P, Brownlee GG: The propeptide region of clotting factor IX is a signal for a vitamin K dependent carboxylase: evidence from protein engineering of amino acid −4. Nucleic Acids Res 15:9505, 1987

65. Pan LC, Price PA: The propeptide of rat bone γ-carboxyglutamic acid protein shares homology with other vitamin K-dependent protein precursors. Proc Natl Acad Sci USA 82:6109, 1985

66. Bucher D, Nebelin E, Thomsen J, Stenflo J: Identification of γ-carboxyglutamic acid residues in bovine factors IX and X, and in a new vitamin K-dependent protein. FEBS Lett 68:293, 1976

67. Fryklund L, Borg H, Andersson L-O: Amino terminal sequence of human factor IX: presence of γ-carboxyglutamic acid residues. FEBS Lett 65:187, 1976

68. Morita T, Isaacs BS, Esmon CT, Johnson AE: Derivatives of blood coagulation factor IX contain a high affinity Ca²⁺ binding site that lacks γ-carboxyglutamic acid. J Biol Chem 259:5698, 1984

69. Gianelli F, Green PM, High KA et al: Haemophilia B: database of point mutations and short additions and deletion—fourth edition, 1993. Nucleic Acids Res 21:3075, 1993

70. Huang LH, Cheng H, Pardi A et al: Sequence-specific ¹H NMR assignments, secondary structure, and location of the calcium binding site in the first epidermal growth factor like domain of blood coagulation factor IX. Biochemistry 30:7402, 1991

71. Huber P, Ben-Tal O, Gilbert G et al: The second factor IX EGF domain is required for complex formation with factor VIIIa. Circulation, suppl. 82:1449, 1990.

72. Lin S-W, Smith KJ, Welsch D, Stafford DW: Expression and characterization of human factor IX and factor IX-factor X chimeras in mouse C127 cells. J Biol Chem 265:144, 1990

73. Astermark J, Hogg PJ, Bjork I, Stenflo J: Effects of γ-carboxyglutamic acid and epidermal growth factor-like modules of factor IX on factor X activation. J Biol Chem 267:3249, 1992

74. Davis LM, McGraw RA, Ware JL et al: Factor IX Alabama: a point mutation in a clotting protein results in hemophilia B. Blood 69:140, 1987

75. Nawroth PP, Wilner GD, Stern DM: The EGF domain of the factor IX molecule is involved in factor IX-endothelial cell interaction, abstracted. Circulation, suppl. 74:II-232, 1986

76. Jones ME, Griffith MJ, Monroe DM et al: Comparison of lipid binding and kinetic properties of normal, variant, and γ-carboxyglutamic acid modified human factor IX and factor IXa. Biochemistry 24:8064, 1985

77. McCord DM, Monroe DM, Smith KJ, Roberts HR: Characterization of the functional defect in factor IX Alabama. Evidence for a conformational change due to high affinity calcium binding in the first epidermal growth factor domain. J Biol Chem 265:10250, 1990

78. McMullen BA, Fujikawa K, Kisiel W: The occurrence of β-hydroxyaspartic acid in the vitamin K-dependent blood coagulation zymogens. Biochem Biophys Res Commun 115:8, 1983

79. Rees DJG, Jones IM, Handford PA et al: The role of β-hydroxyaspartate and adjacent carboxylate residues in the first EGF domain of human factor IX. EMBO J 7:2053, 1988

80. Green PM, Bentley DR, Mibashan RS et al: Molecular pathology of haemophilia B. EMBO J 8:1067, 1989

81. Derian CK, VanDusen W, Przysiecki CT et al: Inhibitors of 2-ketoglutarate-depencent dioxygenases block aspartyl β-hydroxylation of recombinant human factor IX in several mammalian expression systems. J Biol Chem 264:6615, 1989

82. Amphlett GW, Byrne R, Castellino FJ: The binding of metal ions to bovine factor IX. J Biol Chem 253:6774, 1978

83. Morita T, Kisiel W: Calcium binding to a human factor IXa derivative lacking γ-carboxyglutamic acid factor VIII evidence for two high-affinity sites that do not involve β-hydroxyaspartic acid. Biochem Biophys Res Commun 130:841, 1985

84. Handford PA, Baron M, Mayhew M et al: The first EGF-like domain from human factor IX contains a high-affinity calcium binding site. EMBO J 9:475, 1990

85. Handford PA, Mayhew M, Baron M et al: Key residues involved in calcium-binding motifs in EGF-like domains. Nature 351:164, 1991

86. Astermark J, Bjork I, Ohlin AK, Stenflo J: Structural requirements for Ca²⁺ binding to the γ-carboxyglutamic acid and epidermal growth factor-like regions of factor IX. J Biol Chem 266:2430, 1991

87. Vysotchin A, Medved LV, Ingham KC: Domain structure and domain-domain interactions in human factor IX. J Biol Chem 268:8436, 1993

88. Bajaj SP, Sabharwal AK, Gorka J, Birktoft JJ: Antibody-probed conformational transitions in the protease domain of human factor IX upon calcium binding and zymogen activation: putative high-affinity Ca²⁺-binding site in the protease domain. Proc Natl Acad Sci USA 89:152, 1992

89. Liebman HA, Furie BC, Furie B: The factor IX phospholipid-binding site is required for calcium-dependent activation of factor IX by factor XIa. J Biol Chem 262:7605, 1987

90. Borowski M, Furie BC, Bauminger S, Furie B: Prothrombin undergoes two metal-dependent conformational transitions required for phospholipid binding. J Biol Chem 261:14969, 1986

91. Beals JM, Castellino FJ: The interaction of bovine factor IX, its activation intermediate, factor IX alpha, and its activation products, factor IXa alpha and factor IXa beta, with acidic phospholipid vesicles of various compositions. Biochem J 236:861, 1986

92. Liebman HA: The metal-dependent conformational changes in factor IX associated with phospholipid binding. Eur J Biochem 212:339, 1993

93. Liebman HA, Berlin ST, Limentani SA et al: Role of the aromatic amino acid stack domain of factor IX in phospholipid binding. Blood, suppl. 80:1460, 1992

94. Stern DM, Drillings M, Nossel HL et al: Binding of factors IX and IXa to cultured vascular endothelial cells. Proc Natl Acad Sci USA 80:4119, 1983

95. Heimark RL, Schwartz SM: Binding of coagulation factors IX and X to the endothelial cell surface. Biochem Biophys Res Commun 111:723, 1983

96. Stern D, Nawroth P, Handley D, Kisiel W: An endothelial cell-dependent pathway of coagulation. Proc Natl Acad Sci USA 82:2523, 1985

97. Rimon S, Melamed R, Savion N et al: Identification of a factor IX/IXa binding protein on the endothelial cell surface. J Biol Chem 262:6023, 1987

98. Ryan J, Wolitzky B, Heimer E et al: Structural determinants of the factor IX molecule mediating interaction with the endothelial cell binding site are distinct from those involved in phospholipid binding. J Biol Chem 264:20283, 1989

99. Cheung W-F, Straight DL, Smith KJ et al: The role of the epidermal growth factor-1 and hydrophobic stack domains of human factor IX in binding to endothelial cells. J Biol Chem 266:8797, 1991

100. Cheung WF, Hamaguchi N, Smith KJ, Stafford DW: The binding of human factor IX to endothelial cells is mediated by residues 3–11. J Biol Chem 267:20529, 1992

101. Rawala R, Ahmad SS, Ashby B, Walsh PN: Kinetics of coagulation factor X activation by platelet-bound factor IXa. Biochemistry 29:2606, 1990

102. Ahmad SS, Rawala-Sheikh RR, Walsh PN: Comparative interactions of factor IX and factor IXa with human platelets. J Biol Chem 264:3244, 1989

103. Rawala-Sheikh R, Ahmad SS, Monroe DM et al: Role of γ-carboxyglutamic acid residues in the binding of factor IXa to platelets and in factor-X activation. Blood 79:398, 1992

104. Ahmad SS, Rawala-Sheikh R, Cheung W-F et al: The role of the first growth factor domain of human factor IXa in binding to platelets and in factor X activation. J Biol Chem 267:8571, 1992

105. Ahmad SS, Rawala-Sheikh R, Walsh PN: Platelet receptor occupancy with factor IXa promotes factor X activation. J Biol Chem 264:20012, 1989

106. Walsh PN, Sinha D, Koshy A et al: Functional characterization of platelet-bound factor XIa: retention of factor XIa activity of the platelet surface. Blood 68:225, 1986

107. Duffy EJ, Parker ET, Mutucumarana VP et al: Binding of factor VIIIa and factor VIII to factor IXa on phospholipid vesicles. J Biol Chem 267:17006, 1992

108. Mutucumarana VP, Duffy EJ, Lollar P, Johnson AE: The active site of factor IXa is located far above the membrane surface and its conformation is altered upon association with factor VIIIa. A fluorescence study. J Biol Chem 267:17012, 1992

109. Ben-Tal O, Porter TJ, Furie B, Furie BC: Cleavage of factor IX at Arg 180-Val 181 is required and sufficient for optimal interaction with factor VIIIa in the tenase complex. Thromb Haemost 69:1504, 1993

110. Lozier JN, Monroe DM, Stanfield-Oakley S et al: Factor IX New London: substitution of proline for glutamine at position 50 causes severe hemophilia B. Blood 75:1097, 1990

111. DiScipio RG, Kurachi K, Davie EW: Activation of human factor IX (Christmas factor). J Clin Invest 61:1528, 1978

112. Lindquist PA, Fujikawa K, Davie EW: Activation of bovine factor IX (Christmas factor) by factor XIa (activated plasma thromboplastin antecedent) and a protease from Russell's viper venom. J Biol Chem 253:1902, 1978

113. Bajaj SP, Rapaport SI, Russell WA: Redetermination of the rate-limiting step in the activation of factor IX by factor XIa and by factor VIIa/tissue factor. Explanation for different electrophoretic radioactivity profiles obtained on activation of ³H and ¹²⁵I-labeled factor IX. Biochemistry 22:4047, 1983

114. Noyes CM, Griffith MJ, Roberts HR et al: Identification of the molecular defect in factor IX Chapel Hill. Substitution of histidine for arginine at position 145. Proc Natl Acad Sci USA 80:4200, 1983

115. Diuguid DL, Rabiet MJ, Furie BC, Furie B: Molecular defects of factor IX Chicago-2 (Arg 145 → His) and prothrombin Madrid (Arg → Cys): arginine mutations that preclude zymogen activation. Blood 74:193, 1989

116. Toomey JR, Stafford D, Smith K: Factor IX Albuquerque (arginine 145 to cysteine) is cleaved slowly by factor XIa and has reduced coagulant activity, abstracted. Blood, suppl. 72:312a, 1988

117. Braunstein KM, Noyes CM, Griffith MJ et al: Characterization of the defect

in activation of factor IX Chapel Hill by human factor XIa. J Clin Invest 68: 1420, 1981

118. Huang MN, Kasper CK, Roberts HR et al: Molecular defect in factor IX Hilo, a hemophilia B_M variant: Arg → Gln at the carboxy terminal cleavage site of the activation peptide. Blood 73:718, 1989

119. Bertina RM, van der Linden IK, Mannucci PM et al: Mutations in haemophilia B_M occur at the Arg^{180}-Val activation site or in the catalytic domain of factor IX. J Biol Chem 265:10876, 1990

120. Sakai T, Yoshioka A, Yamamoto K et al: Blood clotting factor IX Kashihara: amino acid substitution of valine-182 by phenylalanine. J Biochem 105:756, 1989

121. Byrne R, Amphlett GW, Castellino FJ: Metal on specificity of the conversion of bovine factors IX, IXa, and IXa to bovine factor IXa. J Biol Chem 255:1430, 1980

122. Bajaj SP: Cooperative Ca^{2+} binding to human factor IX: Effects of Ca^{2+} on the kinetic parameters of the activation of factor IX by factor XIa. J Biol Chem 257:4127, 1982

123. Sinha D, Seaman FS, Walsh PN: Role of calcium ions and the heavy chain of factor IXa in the activation of human coagulation factor IX. Biochemistry 26:3768, 1987

124. van der Graaf F, Greengard JS, Bouma BN et al: Isolation and functional characterization of the active light chain of activated human blood coagulation factor XI. J Biol Chem 258:9669, 1983

125. Sinha D, Koshy A, Seaman FS, Walsh PN: Functional characterization of human blood coagulation factor XIa using hybridoma antibodies. J Biol Chem 260:10714, 1985

126. Baglia FA, Jameson BA, Walsh PN: Identification and chemical synthesis of a substrate-binding site for factor IX on coagulation factor XIa. J Biol Chem 266:24190, 1991

127. Morrison SA, Jesty J: Tissue factor-dependent activation of tritium-labeled factor IX and factor X in human plasma. Blood 63:1338, 1984

128. Osterud B, Rapaport SI: Activation of factor IX by the reaction product of tissue factor and factor VII: Additional pathway for initiating blood coagulation. Proc Natl Acad Sci USA 74:5260, 1977

129. Zur M, Nemerson Y: Kinetics of factor IX activation via the extrinsic pathway: dependence of K_m on tissue factor. J Biol Chem 255:5703, 1980

130. Lawson JH, Mann KG: Cooperative activation of human factor IX by the human extrinsic pathway of blood coagulation. J Biol Chem 266:11317, 1991

131. Bauer KA, Kass BL, ten Cate H et al: Factor IX is activated in vivo by the tissue factor mechanism. Blood 76:731, 1990

132. Bauer KA, Mannucci PM, Gringeri A et al: Factor IXa-factor VIIa-cell surface complex does not contribute to the basal activation of the coagulation mechanism in vivo. Blood 79:2039, 1992

133. Almus FE, Rao LVM, Fleck RA, Rapaport SI: Properties of factor VIIa/tissue factor complexes in an umbilical vein model. Blood 76:354, 1990

134. van Dieigen G, Tans G, Rosing J, Hemker HC: The role of phospholipid and factor VIIIa in the activation of bovine factor X. J Biol Chem 256:3433, 1981

135. Rosenberg JS, McKenna P, Rosenberg RD: Inhibition of human factor IXa by human antithrombin-heparin cofactor. J Biol Chem 250:8883, 1975

136. Kurachi F, Fujikawa K, Schmier G, Davie EW: Inhibition of bovine factor IXa and factor Xa by antithrombin III. Biochemistry 15:373, 1976

137. Jordan RE, Oosta GM, Gardner WT, Rosenberg RD: The binding of low-molecular-weight heparin to hemostatic enzymes. J Biol Chem 255:10073, 1980

138. Jordan RE, Oosta GM, Gardner WT, Rosenberg RD: The kinetics of hemostatic enzyme-antithrombin interactions in the presence of low-molecular-weight heparin. J Biol Chem 255:10081, 1980

139. Beals JM, Chibber AK, Castellino FJ: The kinetic assembly of the intrinsic bovine factor X activation system. Arch Biochem Biophys 268:485, 1989

140. Mertens K, vanWijngaarden A, Bertina RM: The role of factor VIII in the activation of human blood coagulation factor X by activated factor IX. Thromb Haemost 54:654, 1985

141. Stern DM, Nawroth PP, Kisiel W et al: The binding of factor IXa to cultured bovine aortic endothelial cells: induction of a specific site in the presence of factors VIII and X. J Biol Chem 260:6717, 1985

142. Varadi K, Elodi S: Formation and functioning of the factor IXa-factor VIII complex on the surface of endothelial cells. Blood 69:442, 1987

143. Spitzer SG, Warn-Cramer BJ, Kasper CK, Bajaj SP: Replacement of isoleucine-397 by threonine in the clotting proteinase factor IXa (Los Angeles and Long Beach variants) affects macromolecular catalysis but not L-tosylarginine methyl ester hydrolysis. Biochem J 265:219, 1990

144. Geddes VA, LeBonniec BF, Louie GV et al: A moderate form of hemophilia B is caused by a novel mutation in the protease domain of factor $IX_{Vancouver}$. J Biol Chem 264:4689, 1989

145. Ware J, Davis L, Frazier D et al: Genetic defect responsible for the dysfunctional protein factor $IX_{Long Beach}$. Blood 72:820, 1988

146. Vidaud M, Attree O, Schaad O et al: Self-inhibition of factor IX by a Gly to

147. Spitzer SG, Pendurthi UR, Kasper CK, Bajaj SP: Molecular defect in factor $IX_{Bm Lake Elsinore}$. J Biol Chem 263:10545, 1988

148. Gianelli F, Choo KH, Rees DJG et al: Gene deletions in patients with haemophilia B and anti-factor IX antibodies. Nature 303:181, 1983

149. Ludwig M, Schwab R, Eigel A et al: Identification of a single nucleotide C-to-T transition and five different deletions in patients with severe hemophilia B. Am J Hum Genet 45:115, 1989

150. Taylor SAM, Lillicrap DP, Blanchette V et al: A complete deletion of the factor IX gene and new *TaqI* variant in a hemophilia B kindred. Hum Genet 79:273, 1988

151. Wadelius C, Blomback M, Pettersson U: Molecular studies of haemophilia B in Sweden. Hum Genet 81:13, 1988

152. Ludwig M, Schwaab R, Olek K et al: Haemophilia B+ with inhibitor. Thromb Haemost 59:340, 1988

153. Matthews RJ, Anson DS, Peake IR, Bloom AL: Heterogeneity of the factor IX locus in nine hemophilia B inhibitor patients. J Clin Invest 79:746, 1987

154. Chen SH, Yoshitake S, Chance PF et al: An intragenic deletion of the factor IX gene in a family with hemophilia B. J Clin Invest 76:2161, 1985

155. Bray GL, Thompson AR: Partial factor IX protein in a pedigree with hemophilia B due to a partial gene deletion. J Clin Invest 77:1194, 1986

156. Vidaud M, Chabret C, Gazengel C et al: A *de novo* intragenic deletion of the potential EGF domain of the factor IX gene in a family with severe hemophilia B. Blood 68:961, 1986

157. Schach BG, Yoshitake S, Davie EW: Hemophilia B (factor $IX_{Seattle-2}$) due to a single nucleotide deletion in the gene for factor IX. J Clin Invest 80:1023, 1987

158. Rees DJG, Rizza CR, Brownlee GG: Haemophilia B cause by a point mutation in a donor splice junction of the human factor IX gene. Nature 316:643, 1985

159. Winship PR: Carrier detection and patient studies in hemophilia B. D. Phil thesis. Oxford University, Oxford, 1986

160. Attree O, Vidaud D, Vidaud M et al: Mutations in the catalytic domain of human coagulation factor IX: rapid characterization by direct genomic sequencing of DNA fragments displaying an altered melting temperature. Genomics 4:266, 1989

161. Chen SH, Scott CR, Schoof J et al: Factor IX Portland: a nonsense mutation (CGA to TGA) resulting in hemophilia B. Am J Hum Genet 44:567, 1989

162. Driscoll MC, Bouhassira E, Aledort LM: A codon 338 nonsense mutation in the factor IX gene in unrelated hemophilia B patients: factor $IX_{338, New York}$. Blood 74:737, 1989

163. Winship PR: Characterization of the molecular defect in haemophilia B patients using the polymerase chain reaction procedure, abstracted. Thromb Haemost, suppl. 62:465, 1989

164. Siguret V, Amselem S, Vidaud M et al: Identification of a CpG mutation in the coagulation factor IX gene by analysis of amplified DNA sequences. Br J Haematol 70:411, 1988

165. Chen SH, Scott CR, Edson JR, Kurachi K: An insertion within the factor IX gene: hemophilia B El Salvador. Am J Hum Genet 42:581, 1988

166. Trent RJ, Wallace RC, Rickard KA: Deletion/insertion of DNA in an intron of the factor IX gene produces severe hemophilia B−, abstracted. Blood, suppl. 72:312a, 1988

167. Gitschier J, Wood WI, Shuman MA, Lawn RM: Identification of a missense mutation in the factor VIII gene of a mild hemophiliac. Science 232:1415, 1986

168. Youssoufian H, Kazazian HH Jr, Phillips DG et al: Recurrent mutations in haemophilia A give evidence for CpG mutation hotspots. Nature 324:380, 1986

169. Coulondre C, Miller JH, Farabaugh PJ, Gilbert W: Molecular basis of base substitution hotspots in *Escherichia coli*. Nature 274:775, 1978

170. Sved J, Bird A: The expected equilibrium of the CpG dinucleotide in vertebrate genomes under a mutation model. Proc Natl Acad Sci USA 87:4692, 1990

171. Green PM, Montandon AJ, Bentley DR et al: The incidence and distribution of CpG → TpG transitions in the coagulation factor IX gene. A fresh look at CpG mutational hotspots. Nucleic Acids Res 18:3227, 1990

172. Koeberl DD, Bottema CDK, Buerstedde J-M et al: Functionally important regions of the factor IX gene have a low rate of polymorphism and a high rate of mutation in the dinucleotide CpG. Am J Hum Genet 45:448, 1989

173. Kasper CK, Osterud B, Minami JY et al: Hemophilia B: characterization of genetic variants and detection of carriers. Blood 50:351, 1977

174. McGraw RA, Davis LM, Noyes CM et al: Evidence for a prevalent dimorphism in the activation peptide of human coagulation factor IX. Proc Natl Acad Sci USA 82:2847, 1985

175. Wallmark A, Ljung R, Nilsson IM et al: Polymorphism of normal factor IX detected by mouse monoclonal antibodies. Proc Natl Acad Sci USA 82:3839, 1985

176. Smith KJ: Monoclonal antibodies to coagulation factor IX define a high frequency polymorphism by immunoassays. Am J Hum Genet 37:668, 1985

177. Camerino G, Grzeschik KH, Jaye M et al: Regional localization on the human X chromosome and polymorphism of the coagulation factor IX gene (hemophilia B locus). Proc Natl Acad Sci USA 81:498, 1984

178. Winship PR, Anson DS, Rizza CR, Brownlee GG: Carrier detection in haemophilia B using two further intragenic restriction fragment length polymorphisms. Nucleic Acids Res 12:8861, 1984

179. Camerino G, Oberle I, Drayna D, Mandel JL: A new MspI restriction fragment length polymorphism in the hemophilia B locus. Hum Genet 71:79, 1985

180. Hay CW, Robertson KA, Yong SN et al: Use of BamHI polymorphism in the factor IX gene for the determination of hemophilia B carrier status. Blood 67:1508, 1986

181. Mulligan L, Holden JJA, White BN: A DNA marker closely linked to the factor IX (haemophilia B) gene. Hum Genet 75:381, 1987

182. Drayna D, Davies K, Hartley D et al: Genetic mapping of the human X chromosome using restriction fragment length polymorphisms. Proc Natl Acad Sci USA 81:2836, 1984

183. Arveiler B, Oberle I, Vincent A et al: Genetic mapping of the Xq27-q28 region: new RFLP markers useful for diagnostic applications in fragile-X and hemophilia-B families. Am J Hum Genet 42:380, 1988

184. Winship PR, Rees DJG, Alkan M: Detection of polymorphisms at cytosine phosphoguanadine dinucleotides and diagnosis of haemophilia B carriers. Lancet 1:631, 1989

185. Kojima T, Tanimoto M, Kamiya T et al: Possible absence of common polymorphisms in coagulation factor IX gene in Japanese subjects. Blood 69:349, 1987

186. Zhang M, Chen SH, Scott CR, Thompson AR: The factor IX BamHI polymorphism: T-to-G transversion at the nucleotide sequence −561. Hum Genet 82:283, 1989

Clinical Aspects of and Therapy for Hemophilia B

108

Harold R. Roberts and T. Flint Gray III

INTRODUCTION

Hemophilia B is a hereditary hemorrhagic disorder characterized by genetic mutations leading to deficiency of factor IX coagulant activity. Clinically, the disease is manifested by excessive or even spontaneous bleeding, most often affecting the weight-bearing joints, soft tissues, or mucous membranes.

The basis for distinguishing hemophilia B from hemophilia A was provided by the observations of the Argentinian hematologist Pavlovsky[1] in 1947. He observed that mixing blood of certain pairs of hemophilic patients in vitro normalized the clotting time, and that transfusion of blood between such a pair of subjects decreased the clotting time of the recipient for >24 hours.[1] These findings were not initially understood, but their significance was clarified in 1952 when several investigators showed that although hemophilia A and B are clinically identical, the defect in hemophilia B was due to the deficiency of a factor distinct from factor VIII.[2,3] In contrast to factor VIII, the new factor was found to be present in normal serum and adsorbable by barium sulfate. Aggeler et al.[2] referred to the missing factor as plasma thromboplastin component (PTC) and to the disease state as PTC deficiency. Shortly thereafter, Biggs et al.[4] described a family with the surname Christmas possessing a deficiency similar to that described by Aggeler, hence the trivial name Christmas disease. PTC was termed factor IX in 1959 by the International Committee on Nomenclature of Coagulation Factors.

GENETICS

Hemophilia B occurs in approximately 1 in 30,000 live male births, significantly less frequently than hemophilia A.[5] Since the disease displays X-linked recessive inheritance, females are very rarely affected. When females are affected, it is usually the result of (1) extreme lyonization, or (2) abnormalities of the X chromosome such as Turner syndrome (45,XO karyotype), XO mosaicism, or other rare abnormalities of the sex chromosome.[6,7] It is possible that disease in females could result from mating between a hemophilia B father and a hemophilia B carrier mother. Hemophilia in females is rare but has been described in human as well as animal models.[8]

The following generalizations are applicable to the inheritance of hemophilia B: (1) all female offspring of a hemophilic father are obligatory carriers for the hemophilic trait (46,XX[h]); (2) all male offspring of a hemophilic father will be normal (46,XY); (3) female offspring of hemophilia B carriers will have a 50% chance of being carriers themselves; and (4) male offspring of carriers will have a 50% chance of being afflicted with hemophilia B (Fig. 108-1). Carriers usually have about 50% levels of factor IX but occasionally are symptomatic and have circulating factor IX levels of <20% of normal. If one carrier in a kindred has low levels of factor IX as the result of extreme lyonization, other carriers in the same kindred may be similarly affected. Symptomatic hemophilia B carriers may be more common than symptomatic hemophilia A carriers.

About one-third of all cases of hemophilia B are the result of de novo mutations, as might have been predicted on the basis of observations by Haldane[9] with regard to hemophilia A. The incidence of mutations involving CpG dinucleotides in the DNA sequence is higher in general and for hemophilia A and B in particular.[10–12]

Although carriers may be detected by pedigree analysis or phenotypic evaluation (e.g., measurement of factor IX activity), the sensitivity of such testing is mediocre due to the variability of X-chromosome inactivation.[13] Linkage studies using restric-

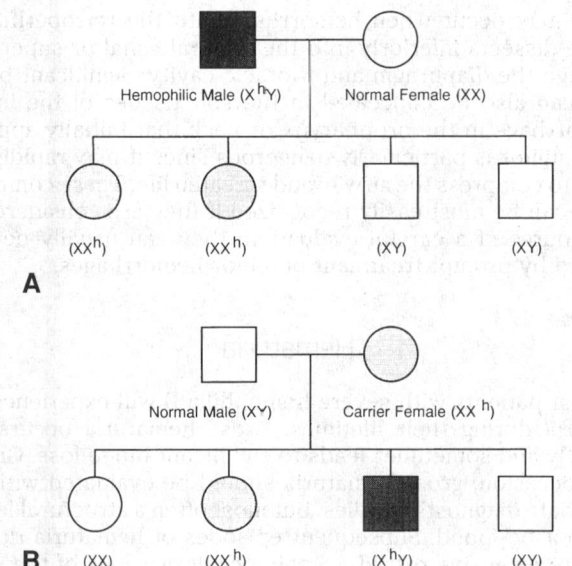

Fig. 108-1. Inheritance patterns for hemophilia B. (**A**) Results of mating between a hemophilic male and a normal female. (**B**) Results of mating between a female carrier for hemophilia B and a normal male. X, normal X chromosome; Y, normal Y chromosome; X^h, X-chromosome-bearing hemophilia B mutation; XY, normal male phenotype; XX, normal female phenotype; XX^h, female carrier for hemophilia; X^hY, hemophilic male.

tion fragment length polymorphism analysis have demonstrated the potential to assign carriership with increased sensitivity.[13,14] More recently, the polymerase chain reaction combined with high-performance liquid chromatography has been used to detect heterozygosity.[15] The analysis by immunoassay of the phenotypic expression of an exonic polymorphism affecting the factor IX protein has also been used to detect the carrier status.[16] The standardization of these techniques should allow more accurate carrier detection and improved genetic counseling.

ETIOLOGY AND PATHOGENESIS

Hemophilia B is heterogeneous in both its clinical severity and molecular pathogenesis (see Ch. 107). Clinical severity (mild, moderate, or severe bleeding) roughly correlates with the level of factor IX activity, as shown in Table 108-1. The decreased factor IX activity results from decreased production of factor IX or production of a defective molecule deficient in enzymatic activity, or both. For example, the genetic defect in factor IX Chapel Hill causes defective activation, a lesion that results in mild hemophilia B.[17] In factor IX Alabama the genetic

Table 108-1. Clinical Classification of Hemophilia B

Classification	Factor IX Activity	Clinical Manifestations
Severe	<1% of normal (0.1 U/ml)	Spontaneous hemorrhage from early infancy
		Frequent spontaneous hemarthroses and other hemorrhages, requiring clotting factor replacement
Moderate	1–5% of normal (0.01–0.05 U/ml)	Hemorrhage secondary to trauma or surgery
		Occasional spontaneous hemarthroses
Mild	5–25% of norma (0.05–0.25 U/ml)	Hemorrhage secondary to trauma or surgery
		Rare spontaneous hemarthroses

defect causes defective interaction with activated factor VIII, such that moderate hemophilia B ensues.[18] The genetic defect in factor IX Lake Elsinore alters the catalytic region of the factor IX molecule and leads to severe hemophilia B.[19] These variants of hemophilia B each exhibit a different structural alteration in the factor IX molecule, leading to a variable decrease in function and clinical severity. In some hemophilia B patients, factor IX molecules are undetectable; these patients are invariably severely affected. A particularly interesting variant is hemophilia B Leiden.[20] At birth these patients have severe disease with <1% factor IX activity, but beginning in adolescence, the factor IX levels gradually rise to ≥50% of normal. The mutations responsible for hemophilia B Leiden occurs in the promoter region of the factor IX gene 5' to the initiation site. The promoter region contains an androgen response element that is thought to stimulate transcription and subsequent synthesis of factor IX. When treated in preadolescence with exogenous androgen, these patients exhibit gradual increases in factor IX levels mimicking that seen in adolescence.

CLINICAL MANIFESTATIONS

General Considerations

Clinical manifestations of hemophilia B, which are indistinguishable from those of hemophilia A, are sometimes noted at the time of circumcision, but excessive bleeding following this event is less frequent than commonly believed. More often, easy bruising and frequent hematomas are noted by mothers of affected infants. Hematomas and hemarthroses are characteristic of factor IX and other procoagulant deficiencies and distinguish them from bleeding resulting from qualitative and quantitative platelet disorders.

Bleeding in hemophilia B is sometimes delayed and may not become noticeable until several days after minor trauma. Hematomas in patients with hemophilia tend to dissect through tissues along fascial planes. For example, a small hematoma originating in the buttock after an intramuscular injection may dissect to involve muscles of the back and leg and may even become life-threatening.

Hemarthroses

The hallmark of severe hemophilia is repeated hemarthroses, resulting in chronic, crippling hemophilic arthropathy.[21] In decreasing order of frequency, the most commonly involved joints are the knee, elbow, ankle, shoulder, wrist, and hip. The first indication of a joint hemorrhage is a sensation of intra-articular burning, followed by a sensation of fullness, tightness, swelling, and increasing pain leading to limitation of motion. Although the intra-articular space is enclosed by a synovial lining that limits the extent of bleeding, joint swelling may be severe enough to compromise neurovascular function. Involuntary muscle splinting due to pain leads to joint immobilization and initiates a vicious cycle of atrophy and contracture. Repeated bleeding into a joint results in deposition of hemosiderin, which contributes to synovial inflammation and increased vascularity, predisposing to further bleeding. Joints with a chronically inflamed and hypertrophic synovium are referred to as "target joints" and are susceptible to recurrent hemarthroses unless treated for several weeks with factor IX replacement therapy. With repeated bleeding, destruction of intra-articular cartilage and adjacent bone occurs and leads to progressive deterioration of joint function with further muscle atrophy and contracture. The joint deformity that occurs in severe hemophilia is so characteristic that it is virtually diagnostic of hemophilia A or B. A detailed radiologic classification of hemophilic arthropathy based on eight criteria and level of severity has been used for initial orthopaedic evaluation and to evaluate the effect of prophylactic therapy.[22]

Pseudotumors

Pseudotumors are cystic lesions that arise in patients with clotting factor deficiencies, most commonly hemophilia A or B. The cysts arise from hematomas and may begin in the subperiosteal area of bone or in soft tissue. Once formed, the lesions tend to expand, probably due to repeated bleeding and osmosis. When the cystic lesions become sufficiently large, they are referred to as pseudotumors, which may be lobulated and consist of a thick, brownish necrotic core of debris surrounded by a thick fibrous wall. Expansion may lead to obstruction or compression of adjacent organs, or rupture through the skin or into nearby viscera. Such complications may be accompanied by infection. Surgical resection is the therapy of choice, but may be unsuccessful when a pseudotumor becomes unduly large. For this reason, surgical excision is suggested early in the course of development of pseudotumors. Other types of treatment, such as radiation, drainage, or factor IX replacement therapy, are not effective.

Neurologic Symptoms

Intracranial hemorrhage is one of the major causes of death in hemophilia B and may occur even in the absence of recognizable trauma. However, few hemophilic infants have intracranial hemorrhage as a complication of vaginal delivery. Because intracranial hemorrhage is often catastrophic, such bleeding must be prevented if possible. Any sign or symptom suggestive of intracranial hemorrhage should be treated as a potential medical emergency. For example, any unusual or peculiar headache in a hemophilic patient should be considered due to an intracranial hemorrhage until proven otherwise. Thus, prompt treatment with factor IX concentrate is indicated prior to any diagnostic procedures such as computed tomography scans, skull radiographs, or other procedures. Appropriate diagnostic tests should be obtained only after the patient's clotting defect is corrected. Intracranial bleeding exemplifies the shortcomings of current replacement therapy of hemophilia B and points out the need for a continuous level of factor IX (such as that provided by prophylactic therapy), since hemorrhage into the central nervous system may result in serious or fatal complications before "on demand" treatment can be instituted. Other bleeding complications affecting nervous tissue include neuropathies that result from compression of nerves by hematomas or intraneural bleeding, or both. Peripheral nerve compression by a hematoma is a particularly common problem, as exemplified by femoral nerve palsy secondary to retroperitoneal hematoma that dissects into and compresses the femoral canal. The prognosis for recovery after prolonged nerve compression is poor, again necessitating an aggressive treatment approach based on clinical suspicion.

Soft Tissue Hemorrhage

Soft tissue hemorrhage in hemophilia B may be mild and uncomplicated, as in a small localized hematoma, but must be treated with care due to the risk of progression via dissection and resultant serious complications. Large dissecting hematomas can occur rapidly in a matter of hours or slowly over a period of days. Soft tissue hemorrhages may be particularly dangerous when occult dissection into enclosed areas occurs. For example, major blood loss and compromise of vital structures may occur when hemorrhage into the retroperitoneal space dissects inferiorly into the femoral canal or superiorly through the diaphragm and thoracic cavity. Significant blood loss can also be concealed in the soft tissues of the limbs. Hemorrhage in the oropharynx or neck that initially appears to be minor is particularly dangerous since it may rapidly enlarge to compress the airway and threaten life. These complications can be most easily recognized if they are considered in the course of a careful evaluation; they can usually be prevented by prompt treatment of minor hemorrhages.

Hematuria

Most patients with severe hemophilia B will experience hematuria during their lifetimes. Gross hematuria occurs frequently and sometimes leads to significant blood loss. On the first occasion, gross hematuria should be evaluated with appropriate diagnostic studies, but most often a structural lesion will not be found. Subsequent episodes of hematuria do not require extensive restudy. Small, occult erosions of the renal pelvis may sometimes cause such hematuria. The most common complication of hematuria is renal colic caused by ureteral obstruction with clots. Hematuria is sometimes self-limited to a few days, but it may persist for weeks or months if untreated.

LABORATORY EVALUATION AND DIFFERENTIAL DIAGNOSIS

The clinical diagnosis of hemophilia B should be considered in any male with a lifelong history of crippling hemarthroses and in any infant with evidence of abnormal bleeding. Mild or moderate hemophilia B should be considered in any person with abnormal surgical bleeding or hematoma formation out of proportion to injury. Hemarthrosis in a patient with a prolonged partial thromboplastin time (PTT) suggests the diagnosis of either hemophilia A or hemophilia B. Definitive diagnosis of hemophilia B requires a specific assay for factor IX. The prothrombin time (PT), thrombin time, and bleeding time are usually normal. However, there is a variant of hemophilia B, termed hemophilia B_M (subscript referring to the index family surname, Martin), characterized by an abnormal ox-brain PT as well as a prolonged PTT.[23] The usual PT, performed with rabbit or human brain thromboplastin, is normal or only slightly prolonged. The molecular biology of this variant has been well studied, suggesting that the prolonged ox-brain PT may result from competitive inhibition of factor VII by factor IX for the substrate, factor X.[24-26]

Screening tests of coagulation may be normal in mild or even moderate hemophilia B since as little as 20–30% of normal levels of factor IX activity may be sufficient to yield a normal PTT. Thus, the patient's clinical and family history of hemorrhage, with particular attention to a history of bleeding after surgical procedures and dental extractions, is a more reliable indicator of a bleeding disorder than screening tests of clotting function (such as the PTT and PT). Hemophilia B is distinguished from acquired coagulopathies on the basis of its lifelong symptoms and its sex-linked transmission within an involved kindred. A lack of family history does not rule out the diagnosis, however, since approximately one-third of mutations occur de novo.

The level of factor IX activity usually correlates well with the observed clinical severity. In severe hemophilia B patients, the factor IX levels are usually <1% of normal and are associated with frequent "spontaneous" bleeding episodes, so called because the patient can recall no specific trauma. Factor IX levels of 1–5% are usually associated with moderate disease, while levels of >5% are usually predictive of mild hemophilia B. Overlap between these categories is common. Table 108-1 describes the features of mild, moderate, and severe hemophilia B. Spontaneous bleeding is uncommon with factor IX levels of >25–30% of normal, although excessive bleeding may occur with trauma or surgery. A normal PTT does not alone guarantee levels of factor IX activity sufficient to prevent abnormal surgical bleeding.

THERAPY

General Considerations

Replacement therapy is dictated by the location of bleeding and whether it is mild, moderate, or severe.[27] 1-Deamino-8-arginine vasopressin (DDAVP) is of no value in hemophilia B. Antifibrinolytic agents such as ϵ-aminocaproic acid and tranexamic acid are useful following dental extractions but are of no value in treating hemarthroses. These agents should never be used to treat hematuria because of the chance of developing ureteral clots with subsequent obstruction and, on occasion, renal failure.[28] Aspirin should be avoided in hemophilia B. The pain of hemophilic arthropathy can be treated with acetaminophen or nonsteroidal anti-inflammatory drugs. The latter may enhance the bleeding tendency; therefore, different ones should be tried in an attempt to find the one best tolerated by the patient. Because of the danger of addiction in patients with frequent painful bleeding episodes, it is wise to avoid using narcotics (codeine, morphine, meperidine) for chronic pain, although the fear of addiction should not deter the physician from using narcotics when appropriate for acute presentations. Narcotic use in hemophilic patients should be closely monitored and the dangers of addiction openly and frankly discussed with the patient (see Ch. 107).

Dosage in Replacement Therapy

One unit of factor IX is defined as the amount of factor IX activity present in 1 ml of pooled normal human plasma and is equivalent to 100% activity. The dose of factor IX needed to achieve a desired level of activity can be calculated based on estimation of the patient's plasma volume and knowledge of factor IX kinetics.

Plasma volume may be estimated as 5% of body weight or 50 ml/kg body weight. Thus the plasma volume of a 70-kg patient is approximately 3,500 ml. By definition, for such a patient to have 100% factor IX activity, 1 U/ml or a total of 3,500 U of factor IX must be present in this plasma volume. If severe hemophilia B is present, it may be assumed the initial factor IX activity is zero. Thus, to obtain 100% activity ≥3,500 U of factor IX must be administered. Because of rapid redistribution into the extravascular space and adsorption onto endothelial cells of vessel walls, however, only about 50% of the infused factor IX remains in circulation after a short period. In this hypothetical patient, therefore, the initial dose to obtain 100% activity must be 7,000 U. To generalize to any size patient with any initial factor IX level and any desired target level, infusion of 1 U/kg body weight of factor IX will raise the factor IX level approximately 1%. For example, a dose of 1,750 U would raise a 50-kg patient from a starting factor IX level of 15% to a target of 50% activity.

After its initial rapid redistribution, factor IX has a second phase half-life of approximately 18–24 hours.[29] Because the variability in this measurement is significant, it is best determined in each individual patient to allow proper dosing. Based on these data, the factor IX level of a patient raised to 100% activity would be expected to decay to 50% by approximately 24 hours after infusion of the initial dose. A second bolus one-half the amount of the first should then raise the level from

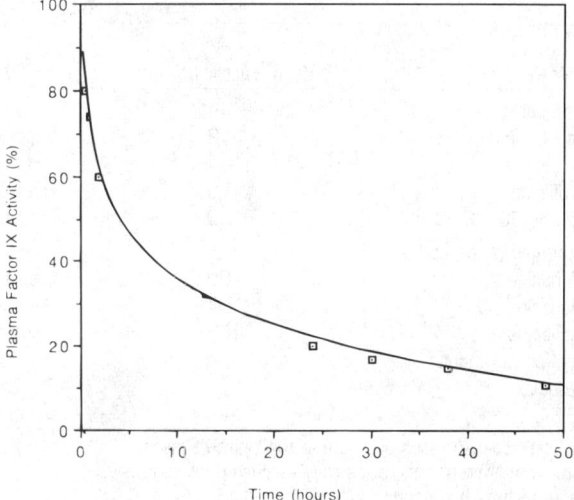

Fig. 108-2. Kinetics of factor IX activity decay following factor IX infusion in hemophilia B. Note the initial rapid decrease due to extravascular redistribution and endothelial adsorption, and the slower second phase decay. (Adapted from Goldsmith et al.,[36] with permission.)

50% to 100% factor IX activity. Factor IX is commonly administered in boluses every 12–24 hours. Figure 108-2 illustrates the kinetics of factor IX decay. It is generally recommended that factor IX levels be monitored after the initial bolus and then daily (initially with peak and trough measurements) to allow individual adjustment in dosing in the treatment of significant bleeding, or in surgical patients. The use of a constant infusion of factor IX to maintain a steady-state level, as has been done with factor VIII concentrates, has not been reported with the recently available highly purified factor IX preparations. Constant infusion of crude factor IX concentrates is not recommended.

Plasma

Fresh frozen plasma or the supernatant from cryoprecipitated plasma can be used as a source of factor IX replacement. However, plasma therapy is limited by the volumes that must be administered, since each milliliter contains only 1 U factor IX activity. It is difficult to achieve increments in factor IX activity >10–15% of normal with plasma alone. Thus, plasma therapy is not generally recommended since highly purified preparations free of transmissible viruses are now available. In the absence of factor IX concentrates, however, adult patients can tolerate a loading dose of plasma of about 20 ml/kg body weight, followed by 3–6 ml plasma/kg body weight every 8–12 hours. The use of purified factor IX preparations in all hemophilia B patients without inhibitors is now the treatment of choice.

Factor IX Concentrates

When factor IX levels higher than can be achieved with plasma are needed, factor IX concentrates are used.[30-33] Until recently, pure preparations of factor IX were not available, and crude preparations referred to as prothrombin complex concentrates (PCCs) were used. PCCs are obtained from DEAE Sephadex adsorption of the supernatant from cryoprecipitated plasma and contain variable quantities of factors VII, IX, and X, prothrombin, protein C, and protein S. The purity of these products is in the range of 1–5 U factor IX activity/mg protein.[33] The presence of these other factors allows the use of these preparations as replacement therapy for other factor deficiencies (see Ch. 110). Table 108-2 describes selected PCCs containing factor IX. These products are now considered safe in regard

Table 108-2. Factor IX Concentrates[a]

Product	Purity (U of Factor IX/mg)	Viral Inactivation	Other Factors IX Ratio[b] II	VII	X	Manufacturer
Crude preparations						
Bebulin VH	2	Vapor heat	1.00	0.01	0.14	Immuno
Proplex	4	Dry heat 60°C	1.70	2.10	1.50	Baxter/Hyland
Profilnine	5	Heat 60°C/heptane	1.10	0.40	0.51	Alpha
Konyne 80	1–3	Dry heat 80°C	0.70	0.07	0.85	Bayer/Miles
Highly purified preparations						
Alphanine	69	Heat 60°C/heptane	0.01	0.01	0.05	Alpha
Alphanine SD	>150	Solvent/detergent	—	—	—	Alpha
Mononine	188	Thiocyanate, ultrafiltration	Undetectable			Armour
Activated preparations						
Autoplex	—	Dry heat 60°C	—	—	—	Baxter
FEIBA	—	Vapor heat	1.23	0.76	0.43	Immuno

[a] Factor IX concentrates available in the United States.
[b] Data from limited lots; ratios may vary from lot to lot.
(Adapted from Thompson,[33] with permission.)

to human immunodeficiency virus (HIV) and hepatitis virus transmission.

Despite their utility, PCCs have been less than ideal therapy for hemophilia B due to the presence of clotting factors other than factor IX, which are unnecessary for the treatment of hemophilia B and may contribute to the risk of thromboembolic phenomena (e.g., deep venous thrombosis, disseminated intravascular coagulation [DIC]), which have been associated with use of these products. For this reason, dosing with crude preparations to raise factor IX activity to >50% of normal has been recommended only with great caution. Recently, highly purified factor IX concentrates have become available, allowing safer and more liberal therapy. Purified factor IX is prepared by improved chromatographic procedures that allow better separation of factor IX from the other clotting factors. The purity of the factor IX obtained is 2 orders of magnitude higher than with the crude preparations and contains 50–200 U factor IX/mg protein. Multiple studies have documented the clinical efficacy, lack of thrombogenicity, and viral safety of the purified preparations.[33–37] The decreased risk of thrombosis permits dosing to 100% activity. The currently available purified factor IX preparations are listed in Table 108-2, and they are now the treatment of choice for hemophilia B patients.

CURRENT APPROACH TO THERAPY FOR HEMOPHILIA B

The use of prophylactic therapy should now be strongly considered for new severely affected patients with hemophilia B. Twice weekly dosing with 25–40 U/kg highly purified factor IX should prevent spontaneous bleeding and the development of chronic joint disease. If prophylactic therapy is not possible, prompt "on demand" therapy should be available. When life-threatening hemorrhage is suspected, such as in the central nervous system or near the airway, factor IX should be administered immediately before any diagnostic procedures are performed. Antifibrinolytic agents are helpful in preventing bleeding following dental procedures, but are not recommended for treatment of other hemorrhagic events in patients without inhibitors. These agents are contraindicated in the treatment of hematuria due to the risk of ureteral obstruction.

Presentations

Hemarthroses/Superficial Hematomas

Most hemarthroses can be treated with one or two doses of factor IX with a goal of reaching plasma factor IX levels of about 25–30% of normal. Typically this involves the administration of about 30 U factor IX/kg body weight. The same dose may be repeated, if needed, at 24-hour intervals. Similar doses are given for superficial and small hematomas. Should hematomas appear to be dissecting at the time of diagnosis, factor IX should be administered until the dissection ceases and resolution of the hematoma begins.

Major Bleeding

Major bleeding episodes (i.e., those involving the gastrointestinal tract or central nervous system, or life-threatening bleeding in or around the airway or retroperitoneal space) should be treated with factor IX in doses sufficient to achieve levels of ≥50% of normal; usually higher levels are indicated. Levels of 100% can be achieved using the pure factor IX preparations with minimal risk of thrombosis. Treatment should be continued for ≤7–10 days, or until the bleeding episode is controlled and resolution of the hematoma begins. Therapeutic recommendations are summarized in Table 108-3.

Monitoring Therapy

Factor IX therapy lasting <1 or 2 days or given for a hemarthrosis need not be monitored by factor IX assays as long as the patient does not have an inhibitor and is known to respond to conventional doses of factor IX. When factor IX is administered for serious bleeding, assays for factor IX immediately after the initial dose and on a daily basis thereafter are indicated to maintain peak levels of 50–100% and minimum levels of 25–50%. Replacement therapy with crude factor IX concentrates for >5–7 days should be monitored carefully in light of the potential for thrombotic complications.

Complications

Viral Hepatitis and HIV Infection

The success of treatment of hemophilia with clotting factor concentrates has been tempered first by the transmission of viral hepatitis and, more recently, by HIV transmission.

Most patients who received factor IX concentrates before

Table 108-3. Guidelines for Replacement Therapy in Hemophilia B

Type of Hemorrhage	Desired Factor IX Activity[a] (%)	Duration of Therapy (days)
Minor		
Uncomplicated hemarthrosis	20–30	1–2
Superficial hematoma	20–30	1–2
Moderate		
Hematoma with dissection	25–50	3–7
Oral mucosa, epistaxis	25–50	2–5
Hematuria	25–50	3–7
Major		
Pharyngeal/retropharyngeal	50–100	7–10
Retroperitoneal	50–100	7–10
Gastrointestinal bleeding	50–100	5–10
Central nervous system	50–100	7–10
Dental extraction	25–50	2–5
Surgery	50–100	7–10

[a] These are guidelines; therapy should be individually tailored, in both dose and duration. Doses are administered every 12–24 hours; see text for methods of calculating dose. The use of purified factor IX preparations is encouraged, especially when achieving levels >50% due to the risk of thrombotic complications with crude factor IX preparations.

1984 show evidence of hepatitis B infection.[38] Many of these patients have chronic hepatitis, and a proportion have developed cirrhosis, which can be of particular concern in the hemophilic population due to the risk of bleeding from varices. Hepatitis C, which accounts for most non-A, non-B hepatitis, is now thought to be the major cause of chronic liver disease in these patients. Efforts to decrease the risk of hepatitis in donated blood began with screening for hepatitis B surface antigen in 1972. Before the recent introduction of a test for hepatitis C antibody, elevated alanine aminotransferase and hepatitis B core antibody were used as surrogate markers of hepatitis C infection. The use of the hepatitis C virus antibody test should further decrease the risk of contamination of plasma-derived products with hepatitis C virus.

In addition to screening of the blood supply, the availability of the hepatitis B vaccine since the 1980s has allowed further means to decrease the risk of hepatitis B infection. All hemophilic patients not previously infected with hepatitis B should be vaccinated. Hepatitis C vaccines are not presently available.

The problem of hepatitis infection led to the addition of viral inactivation steps to the manufacture of clotting factor concentrates beginning in 1983. The methods used include dry heating, heating in solution or in solvent-suspension, treatment with solvent/detergents, and immunoaffinity chromatography and ultrafiltration.[39]

In retrospective studies, HIV seropositivity was detected in blood samples from multitransfused hemophilic patients from as early as 1978. AIDS was first reported in hemophilic patients in 1982, but most seroconversions probably occurred between 1981 and 1983.[40] AIDS has now exceeded hemorrhagic complications as the most common cause of death in the hemophilic population. HIV infection rates have been significantly lower for patients treated with factor IX concentrates (30–50%) compared with those treated with factor VIII concentrates (70–90%), probably due to the additional steps in manufacture of factor IX concentrates.[38,42] Fortunately, all current clotting factor concentrates appear to be safe in terms of transmission of viral disease. However, because clotting factor concentrates are prepared from pooled human plasma from as many as 20,000–30,000 donors, the possibility exists for contamination with new pathogenic viruses resistant to current inactivation practices. There is also a remote possibility of breakdown in the manufacturing process that could result in viral contamination of clotting factor preparations. The development of recom-binant methods for production of factor IX may decrease the risk of these potential problems.[42]

Disseminated Intravascular Coagulation and Thromboembolism

Thromboembolic complications, including DIC, deep venous thrombosis, and pulmonary embolism have been associated with the use of crude factor IX concentrates.[43–45] In an early series of 13 hemophilia B patients undergoing surgery, 6 patients had significant postoperative thrombosis, including 3 with deep vein thromboses and 3 with pulmonary emboli (one fatal).[46] Similar complications have occurred in nonsurgical settings, although perhaps not as frequently. In addition to thromboembolic phenomena, there are several reports of myocardial infarction occurring in young patients following the use of crude concentrates.[46–48] Diffuse thrombosis and a peculiar myocardial necrosis have been documented on autopsy in a few patients treated with crude factor IX products.[49] Most patients had no sign of atherosclerosis or other cardiac disease.

Different mechanisms have been proposed for the complications of DIC or thrombosis, or both, that occur when PCCs are used. Since many of these complications are seen in patients with liver disease, it is possible that failure of the liver to clear activated clotting factors from the circulation predisposes to thrombosis. Factors VIIa, IXa, and Xa are known to be present in some but not all the products.[50–52] Factor VIIa, with a half-life of 2–4 hours, is a potential thrombogenic agent, although factor Xa-phospholipid complexes are also suspect.[53] These findings contrast with the absence of activated factors in the highly purified factor IX concentrates[33–37] (Fig. 108-3). Clinical trials of purified factor IX, including use in surgical settings, have been notable for a lack of thrombosis, validating the advantage of the pure preparations.[34–38]

Inhibitors

Inhibitors to factor IX are observed in about 2–4% of severely affected hemophilia B patients, a lower prevalence than factor VIII inhibitors in hemophilia A.[54,55] They are highly restricted polyclonal alloantibodies (usually IgG4-κ) and occur frequently in patients who have undetectable factor IX antigen.[56] Hemophilia B patients with inhibitors frequently exhibit partial or complete deletions in the factor IX gene, although patients with measurable but abnormal factor IX antigen also develop inhibitors.[57–59]

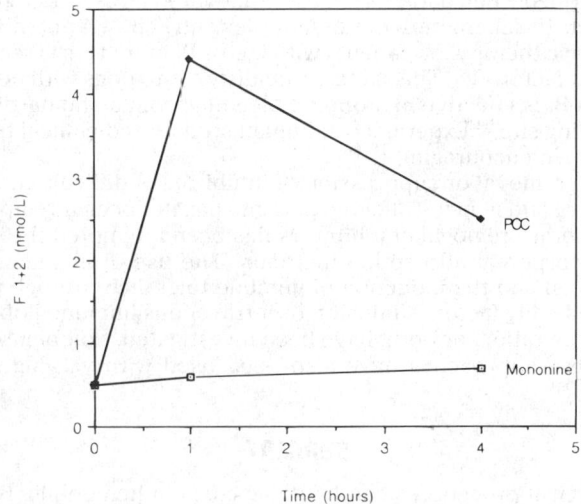

Fig. 108-3. Purified factor IX versus PCC. Prothrombin activation fragment (F_{1+2}) measured before and after infusions of Mononine and PCC. (Adapted from Kim et al.,[34] with permission.)

Inhibitors are quantified by measurement of factor IX activity in mixes of serial dilutions of inhibitor-containing plasma with pooled normal human plasma (containing factor IX). The strength of inhibition of factor IX activity is expressed in Bethesda inhibitor units (BIU).[60,61] One BIU is defined as a 50% reduction in the activity of factor IX in the mixture under standard conditions of time and temperature. Inhibitors complicate the treatment of hemophilia B and preclude the use of conventional therapy. It is possible to overcome low titers of inhibitor (<10 BIU) with increased doses of factor IX, while in the case of high-titer inhibitor (>10 BIU) this is not possible. Therefore, the treatment of patients with inhibitors can be divided into three approaches: (1) overcoming low-titer inhibitors with increased factor IX doses, (2) providing factor IX "bypassing" activity in patients with high-titer inhibitors, and (3) removing or suppressing the inhibitor.

In the case of patients with low-titer inhibitors, higher than normal doses of purified factor IX can be administered in an effort to achieve a measurable circulating level of factor IX. If satisfactory levels of factor IX are not achieved, a trial of PCC administration (in the range of 75–100 U/kg body weight every 8–12 hours) may be of value since these crude preparations contain putative inhibitor "bypassing" activity. The risk of thrombosis related to the use of PCCs is presumably decreased by the anti-factor IX antibody, although this has not been proved. If satisfactory amounts of factor IX overcome the inhibitor, an anamnestic response may be induced so that the antibody titer increases to levels much >10 BIU. Anamnesis may occur within 5 days after initiation of treatment. An anamnestic response of >10 BIU defines a high responder patient. Those who do not respond to factor IX with an anamnestic increase in antibody are termed low responders.

Hemophilia B patients with high-titer inhibitors may be treated with activated prothrombin complex concentrates such as Autoplex or FEIBA. Although these preparations contain factor IX, its presence in this setting is irrelevant due to the excess of inhibitor; the utility of these products derives from their ability to provide activated clotting factors that "bypass" factor IX. Therefore, monitoring of factor IX activity is not warranted, and the preparations are dosed empirically. Thromboembolic events, including DIC, have been reported with FEIBA and Autoplex.[62] The administration of activated concentrates in the setting of a high-titer inhibitor does not guarantee adequate hemostasis, which is achieved in only 60–80% of cases. For this reason, close monitoring is required in treatment of hemorrhage. Elective surgery should not be performed when patients are using activated PCCs. Table 108-3 depicts the characteristics of Autoplex and FEIBA. A potentially effective therapy for patients with factor IX inhibitors is recombinant factor VIIa. This factor, administered to dogs with hemophilia B, is effective in stopping bleeding from a standardized bleeding site.[64] Experience in human studies and clinical trials has been encouraging.[64–66]

The removal or suppression of inhibitors is difficult and expensive and in many affected patients has not been attempted. Temporary removal of inhibitors has been attempted through extracorporeal adsorption methods. The use of immunosuppression and the induction of immune tolerance through prolonged daily factor IX infusion or intravenous immunoglobulin administration, or both, have been investigated. Combinations of these approaches have also been used with varying success.[66–68]

SURGERY

Surgical procedures can be done safely in hemophilia B patients who are undergoing factor IX replacement therapy, except when high-titer inhibitors are present.[36,69] Factor IX levels should be raised to 100% of normal with a purified factor IX concentrate before surgery and maintained by infusions of factor IX every 12–24 hours for 7–10 days, depending on the type of surgery.

PROGNOSIS AND FUTURE DIRECTIONS

Before the era of effective therapy for hemophilia B, the life expectancy of a patient was 11 years.[70] When factor IX concentrates became available, life expectancy was dramatically improved despite the ensuing epidemic of hepatitis. The introduction of HIV infection into more than one-half of the patients between 1978 and 1983 has resulted in increased mortality from the acquired immunodeficiency syndrome. However, the availability of concentrates free of HIV and hepatitis viruses holds the promise of a virtually normal life span for new patients and those who have avoided HIV infection. The recent introduction of purified factor IX products has freed hemophilia B patients from the risks of iatrogenic thrombosis and suboptimal treatment present with crude factor IX preparations. Previously untreated patients, or those treated since 1985 may expect a normal life span in the absence of central nervous system bleeding, provided that factor IX concentrates are readily available.

In addition to "on demand," therapy, prophylactic therapy of hemophilia B is now possible. Continued regularly scheduled factor IX infusions once or twice weekly may prevent the development of hemarthroses in very young patients and allow a more active life style with decreased complications in patients of all ages. Although prophylactic therapy is expensive, consideration should be given to the potential savings gained from a decreased complication rate and increased productivity of patients so treated.

The most exciting prospect for treatment of hemophilia B is the possibility of cure through gene therapy. Since the determination of the factor IX gene structure, rapid progress has been made in developing methods to transfer and maintain the gene, first in in vitro cell cultures and more recently directly into animals.[14,71,72] Refinement of gene transfer techniques may lead to the ability to provide low-cost, safe, prophylactic therapy to hemophilic patients in the future, allowing them to lead a normal life.

REFERENCES

1. Pavlovsky A: Contribution to the pathogenesis of hemophilia. Blood 2:185, 1947
2. Aggeler PM, White SG, Glendenning MB et al: Plasma thromboplastin component (PTC) deficiency: a new disease resembling hemophilia. Proc Soc Exp Biol Med 79:692, 1952
3. Schulman I, Smith CH: Hemorrhagic disease in an infant due to deficiency of a previously undescribed clotting factor. Blood 7:795, 1952
4. Biggs R, Douglas AS, Macfarlane RG et al: Christmas disease. Br Med J 2: 1378, 1952
5. McGraw RA, Davis LM, Lundblad RL et al: Structure and function of factor IX: defects in hemophilia B. Clin Haematol 14:359, 1985
6. Gartler SM, Riggs AD: Mammalian X chromosome inactivation. Annu Rev Genet 17:155, 1983
7. Taylor SAM, Deugau KV, Lillicrap DP: Somatic mosaicism and female-to-female transmission in a kindred with hemophilia B (factor IX deficiency). Proc Natl Acad Sci USA 88:39, 1991
8. Brinkhous KM, Davis PD, Graham JB, Dodd WJ: Expression and linkage of genes for X-linked hemophilia A and B in the dog. Blood 41:577, 1973
9. Haldane JBS: The rate of spontaneous mutation of a human gene. J Genet 31:317, 1935
10. Youssoufian H, Kazazian HH Jr, Phillips DG et al: Recurrent mutations in haemophilia A give evidence for CpG mutation hotspots. Nature 324:380, 1986
11. Barker D, Schafer M, White R: Restriction sites containing CpG show a higher frequency of polymorphism in human DNA. Cell 36:131, 1984
12. Bird AP: CpG-rich islands and the function of DNA methylation. Nature 321: 209, 1986
13. Mariani G, Chistolini A, Hassan HJ et al: Carrier detection for hemophilia B: evaluation of multiple polymorphic sites. Am J Hematol 33:1, 1990

14. Brocker-Vriends AHJT, Bakker E, Kanhai HHH et al: The contribution of DNA analysis to carrier detection and prenatal diagnosis of hemophilia A and B. Ann Hematol 64:2, 1992

15. Asakawa JI, Satoh C, Yamasaki Y, Chen SH: Accurate and rapid detection of heterozygous carriers of a deletion by combined polymerase chain reaction and high-performance liquid chromatography. Proc Natl Acad Sci USA 89:9126, 1992

16. Thompson AR, Chen SH, Smith KJ: Diagnostic role of an immunoassay-detected polymorphism of factor IX for potential carriers of hemophilia B. Blood 72:1633, 1988

17. Chung KS, Madar DA, Goldsmith JC et al: Purification and characterization of an abnormal factor IX (Christmas factor) molecule: factor IX Chapel Hill. J Clin Invest 62:1078, 1978

18. Davis LM, McGraw RA, Ware JW et al: Factor IX Alabama. A point mutation in a clotting protein results in hemophilia B. Blood 69:140, 1987

19. Usharani P, Warn-Cramer BJ, Kasper CK, Bajaj SP: Characterization of three abnormal factor IX variants (B$_M$, Lake Elsinore, Long Beach, and Los Angeles) of hemophilia B. Evidence for defects affecting the latent catalytic site. J Clin Invest 75:76, 1985

20. Briet E, Bertina RM, van Tilberg RH, Veltkamp JJ: Hemophilia B Leyden. A sex linked hereditary disorder that improves after puberty. N Engl J Med 306:788, 1982

21. Arnold WD, Hilgartner MW: Hemophilic arthropathy. Current concepts of pathogenesis and management. J Bone Joint Surg 59A:287, 1977

22. Pettersson H, Ahlberg A, Nilsson IM: A radiologic classification of hemophilic arthropathy. Clin Orthop 149:153, 1980

23. Hougie C, Twomey JJ: Hemophilia B$_M$: a new type of factor IX deficiency. Lancet 1:698, 1967

24. Huang MN, Kasper CK, Roberts HR et al: Molecular defect in factor IX$_{Hilo}$, a hemophilia B$_M$ variant: Arg→Gln at the carboxy terminal cleavage site of the activation peptide. Blood 73:718, 1989

25. Bertina RM, van der Linden IK: factor IX Deventer: evidence for heterogeneity of hemophilia B$_M$. Thromb Haemost 47:136, 1982

26. Vidaud M, Attrel O, Schaad O et al: Self-inhibition of factor IX by a Gly to Arg mutation at the substrate binding pocket is linked to severe hemophilia B, abstracted. Blood 72, suppl. 1:313a, 1988

27. Kasper CK, Dietrich SL: Comprehensive management of hemophilia. Clin Haemost 14:489, 1985

28. Pitts TO, Spero JA, Bontempo FA, Greenberg A: Acute renal failure due to high-grade obstruction following therapy with epsilon-aminocaproic acid. Am J Kidney Dis 8:441, 1986

29. Smith KJ, Watt GW, Thompson AR: Labeled factor IX kinetics in patients with hemophilia B. Blood 58:625, 1981

30. Tullis JL, Melin M, Jurigian P: Clinical use of human prothrombin complexes. N Engl J Med 273:667, 1965

31. Hoag S, Johnson FF, Robinson JA, Aggeler PM: Treatment of hemophilia B with a new clotting-factor concentrate. N Engl J Med 280:581, 1969

32. Menache D: Factor IX concentrates. Thromb Diathes Hemorr 33:600, 1975

33. Thompson AR: Factor IX concentrates for clinical use. Semin Thromb Hemost 19:25, 1993

34. Kim HC, McMillan CW, White GC et al: Purified factor IX using monoclonal immunoaffinity technique: clinical trials in hemophilia B and comparison to prothrombin complex concentrates. Blood 76:568, 1992

35. Kim HC, McMillan CW, White GC et al: Clinical experience of a new monoclonal antibody purified factor IX: half-life, recovery and safety in patients with hemophilia B. Semin Hematol, suppl. 2. 27:30, 1990

36. Goldsmith JC, Kasper CK, Blatt PM et al: Coagulation factor IX: successful surgical experience with a purified factor IX concentrate. Am J Hematol 40:210, 1992

37. Mannucci PM, Bauer KA, Gringeri A et al: Thrombin generation is not increased in the blood of hemophilia B patients after the infusion of a purified factor IX concentrate. Blood 76:2540, 1990

38. Roberts HR, Macik BG: Factor VIII and IX concentrates: clinical efficacy related to purity. p. 583. In Verstraete M, Vermylen J, Lijnen R, Arnout J (eds): Thrombosis and Haemostasis. Leuven University Press, Leuven, Belgium, 1987

39. Fricke WA, Lamb MA: Viral safety of clotting factor concentrates. Semin Thromb Hemost 19:54, 1993

40. Ragni MV, Tegtmeier GE, Levy JA et al: AIDS retrovirus antibodies in hemophiliacs treated with factor VIII or factor IX concentrates, cryoprecipitate, or fresh frozen plasma: prevalence, seroconversion rate, and clinical correlations. Blood 67:592, 1986

41. Goedert JJ, Kessler CM, Aledort LM et al: A prospective study of human immunodeficiency virus type I infection and the development of AIDS in subjects with hemophilia. N Engl J Med 321:1141, 1989

42. Limentani SA, Roth DA, Furie BC, Furie B: Recombinant blood clotting proteins for hemophilia therapy. Semin Thromb Hemost 19:62, 1993

43. Cederbaum AI, Blatt PM, Roberts HR: Intravascular coagulation with use of human prothrombin complex concentrates. Ann Intern Med 84:683, 1976

44. Conlan MG, Hoots WK: Disseminated intravascular coagulation and hemorrhage in hemophilia B following elective surgery. Am J Hematol 35:203, 1990

45. Kasper CK: Postoperative thromboses in hemophilia B. N Engl J Med 289:160, 1973

46. Fuerth JH, Mahrer P: Myocardial infarction after factor IX therapy. JAMA 245:1455, 1981

47. Agrawal BL, Zelkowitz L, Hletko P: Acute myocardial infarction in a young hemophiliac patient during therapy with factor IX concentrate and epsilon aminocaproic acid. J Pediatr 98:931, 1981

48. Sullivan DW, Purdy LJ, Billingham M, Glader BE: Fatal myocardial infarction following therapy with prothrombin complex concentrates in a young man with hemophilia A. Pediatrics 74:279, 1984

49. Gruppo RA, Bove KE, Donaldson VH: Fatal myocardial necrosis associated with prothrombin-complex-concentrate therapy in hemophilia A. N Engl J Med 309:242, 1983

50. Blatt PM, Lundblad RL, Kingdon HS et al: Thrombogenic materials in prothrombin complex concentrates. Ann Intern Med 81:766, 1974

51. Hultin MB: Activated clotting factors in factor IX concentrates. Blood 54:1028, 1979

52. Seligsohn U, Kasper CK, Osterud B, Rapaport SI: Activated factor VII: presence in factor IX concentrates and persistence in the circulation after infusion. Blood 53:828, 1979

53. Giles AR, Nesheim ME, Hoogendoorn H et al: The coagulant-active phospholipid content is a major determinant of in vivo thrombogenicity of prothrombin complex (factor IX) concentrates in rabbits. Blood 59:401, 1982

54. Roberts HR: Overview of inhibitors to factor VIII and IX. p. 1. In Hoyer LW (ed): Factor VIII Inhibitors. Alan R Liss, New York, 1984

55. Sultan Y, the French Hemophilia Study Group: Prevalence of inhibitors in a population of 3435 hemophilia patients in France. Thromb Haemost 67:600, 1992

56. Orstavik KH, Miller CH: IgG subclass identification of inhibitors to factor IX in haemophilia B patients. Br J Haematol 68:451, 1988

57. Ludwig M, Schwaab R, Olek K et al: Haemophilia B$^+$ with inhibitor, letter. Thromb Haemost 59:340, 1988

58. Matsushita T, Tanimoto M, Yamamoto K et al: DNA sequence analysis of three inhibitor-positive hemophilia B patients without gross gene deletion: identification of four novel mutations in factor IX gene. J Lab Clin Med 116:492, 1990

59. Matthews RJ, Anson DS, Peake IR, Bloom AL: Heterogeneity of the factor IX locus in nine hemophilia B inhibitor patients. J Clin Invest 79:746, 1987

60. Kasper CK, Aledort LM, Counts RB et al: A more uniform measurement of factor VIII inhibitors, letter, Thromb Diasthes Haemorrh 34:869, 1975

61. Gadarowski JJ, Czapek EE, Ontiveros JD, Pedraza JL: Modification of the Bethesda assay for factor VIII or IX inhibitors to improve efficiency. Acta Haematol 80:134, 1988

62. Mizon P, Goudemand J, Jude B, Marey A: Myocardial infarction after FEIBA therapy in a hemophilia-B patient with a factor IX inhibitor. Ann Hematol 64:309, 1992

63. Brinkhous KM, Hedner U, Garris JB et al: Effect of recombinant factor VIIa on the hemostatic defect in dogs with hemophilia A, hemophilia B, and von Willebrand's disease. Proc Natl Acad Sci USA 86:1382, 1989

64. Hedner U, Glazer S, Falch J: Recombinant activated factor VII in the treatment of bleeding episodes in patients with inherited and acquired bleeding disorders. Transfus Med Rev 7:78, 1993

65. Schmidt ML, Smith HE, Gamerman S et al: Prolonged recombinant activated factor VII (rfVIIa) treatment for severe bleeding in a factor-IX-deficient patient with an inhibitor. Br J Haematol 78:460, 1991

66. Hedner U, Glazer S: Management of hemophilia patients with inhibitors. Hematol Oncol Clin North Am 6:1035, 1992

67. Nilsson IM, Berntorp E, Freiburghaus C: Treatment of patients with factor VIII and IX inhibitors. Thromb Haemost 70:56, 1993

68. Bloom AL: Management of factor VIII inhibitors: evolution and current status. Haemostasis 22:268. 1992

69. Kitchens CS: Surgery in hemophilia and related disorders. A prospective study of 100 consecutive procedures. Medicine 65:34, 1986

70. National Heart, Lung and Blood Institute: Summary report: NHLBI's blood resource studies. DHEW publ no. (NIH) 73-416. Bethesda, National Heart, Lung and Blood Institute, MD, 1972

71. Palmer TD, Thompson AR, Miller AD: Production of human factor IX in animals by genetically modified skin fibroblasts. Blood 73:438, 1989

72. Kay MA, Rothenberg S, Landen CN et al: In vivo gene therapy of hemophilia B: sustained partial correction in factor IX-deficient dogs. Science 262:117, 1993

Donald I. Feinstein

INHIBITORS IN HEMOPHILIA A

Factor VIII inhibitors are antibodies that develop in patients with hemophilia A in response to factor VIII contained in various blood products. Most of these antibodies neutralize factor VIII coagulant activity. Although they do not increase the frequency of bleeding episodes, they make treatment of bleeding much more difficult. The incidence of factor VIII inhibitors complicating hemophilia A is approximately 5–10% of all patients with hemophilia A and 10–15% of those with severe hemophilia A.[1,2] However, in more recent studies of inhibitor formation in previously untreated patients receiving highly purified plasma derived factor VIII, the incidence of inhibitors was 18–35%,[3–5] and with intermediate purity factor VIII concentrates the incidence was 25–52%.[6–8] In prospective studies using recombinant factor VIII, the incidence was approximately 20%.[7,8] In most of these prospective studies, the inhibitors were detected early, with a median number of exposure days before inhibitor formation of 9–11,[7,8] and about 50% were low titer and transient. Thus, most patients with severe hemophilia who are destined to develop an inhibitor do so early after exposure to factor VIII.[7–9] The reason for the variable incidence with newer and more purified concentrates is not explained.

Although the great majority of inhibitors develop in severe or moderate forms of hemophilia A, well-documented cases include patients with mild hemophilia A.[2,10–14] In general, these patients develop only low-titer inhibitors following exposure to factor VIII. After abstinence from products containing factor VIII, the inhibitors disappear after 4–12 weeks, and the inhibitors do not necessarily reappear on re-exposure.

Patients with low-titer inhibitors (3–5 Bethesda units) that do not rise after further exposure to factor VIII are known as low responders (approximately 25% of hemophiliacs with inhibitors), whereas those that rise markedly with further exposure to factor VIII (anamnestic response) are known as high responders (approximately 75% of hemophiliacs with inhibitors).[15] Inhibitor titers usually begin to rise 2–3 days after exposure to factor VIII, reach a maximum within 7–21 days, and then decrease very slowly (Fig. 109-1). Once formed, high-titer inhibitors tend to persist for long, although variable periods, and detectable levels of inhibitor may be present 1–2 years later without re-exposure to factor VIII. By contrast, low-titer inhibitors in low responders occasionally disappear and may not reappear with exposure to factor VIII.

Pathophysiology

The reasons for the development of inhibitors in a minority of patients with hemophilia A remain unknown. Brother pairs have a higher-than-expected incidence or absence of inhibitors.[9,16] Another factor suggesting genetic susceptibility is the finding of a lesser incidence of HLA-A1 and a higher incidence of certain complement components located close to HLA-DR in hemophiliacs with inhibitors.[17] By contrast, no correlation exists between factor VIII gene deletions and the development of factor VIII inhibitors.[18,19] Shapiro and Hultin[10] suggested that immune tolerance might be involved to explain the develop-

ment of inhibitors in patients with hemophilia A. Since factor VIII does not cross the placenta, tolerant hemophiliacs could be exposed to factor VIII in utero only as a result of maternal-fetal hemorrhage. Thus, according to this hypothesis, only non-tolerant hemophiliacs would develop inhibitors following exposure to factor VIII. Induction of tolerance in hemophiliacs with inhibitors results in the disappearance of the inhibitor in a significant number of patients, which supports this theory.[20–22]

Characterization and Properties of Inhibitors

Factor VIII inhibitors in hemophilia A are IgG. Although light chain and heavy chain subtyping has demonstrated restricted heterogeneity,[23–30] heavy chain subtyping of these antibodies has shown a significant predominance of the IgG4 subtype.[25,28,31] IgG4 does not fix complement, which might explain why hemophiliacs do not develop immune complex disease. Factor VIII inhibitors show species specificity, both in vitro and in vivo, in that human factor VIII is usually neutralized to a greater extent than is bovine or porcine factor VIII, and infusion of porcine factor VIII into a patient with an inhibitor often raises the factor VIII level.

The reaction between factor VIII and inhibitors is time and temperature dependent. Two different patterns of antigen/antibody reaction have been described. In the type I pattern, characteristic of most alloantibodies, as seen in hemophiliacs, factor VIII is completely inactivated in the presence of excess inhibitor,[32–34] whereas in the type II pattern characteristic of many autoantibodies, the inhibitor frequently does not completely inactivate factor VIII in vitro in the presence of excess inhibitor.[23,35–37] In the latter cases, despite the demonstration of a significant amount of residual factor VIII activity in vitro, the patient bleeds as if there were no coagulant function in vivo.[38,39]

The antigenic regions on the factor VIII molecule to which neutralizing factor VIII inhibitors bind have been identified.[40–43] Interestingly, the epitopes to which allo- or autoantibodies are directed are limited to certain areas of the factor VIII light or heavy chains, or both[40–43] (Fig. 109-2). Immunoblotting and binding studies with fragments of factor VIII have shown that plasma from approximately 50% of inhibitor patients contain at least two different neutralizing antibodies directed at both the light and heavy chain, whereas the other 50% bind to only the light chain.[43] In addition, it has been noted that the inhibitor produced by a given patient may change over the course of time and a few non-neutralizing antibodies may occur as well.[40–44]

Laboratory Evaluation and Quantification of Inhibitor Titer

The presence of an inhibitor to factor VIII should be suspected in a hemophiliac if transfused factor VIII appears either to have a short half-life or is not efficacious in achieving hemostasis, or both. This can be suspected in the laboratory whenever the partial thromboplastin time of a mixture of patient's

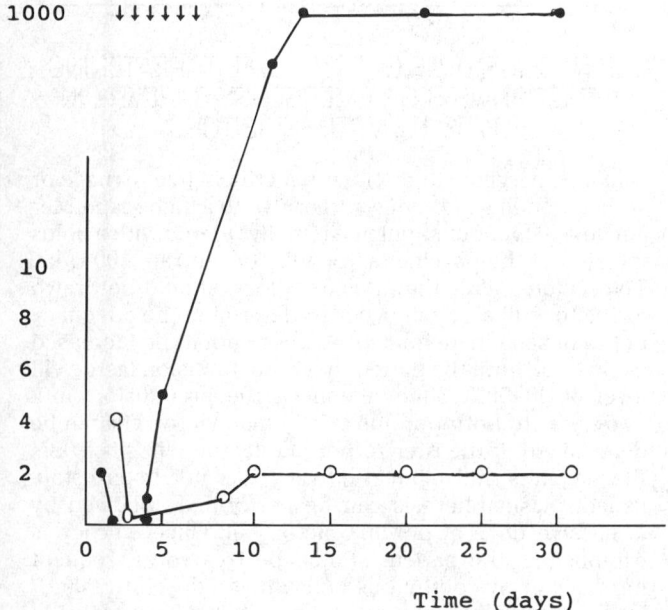

Fig. 109-1. Inducible and noninducible factor VIII inhibitors. Solid circles, high responder; open circles, low responder; arrows, factor VIII concentrate.

plasma and normal plasma, after incubation for 2 hours at 37°C, is longer than that of a mixture of patient plasma and hemophilic plasma known not to contain an inhibitor. The sensitivity of this assay can be markedly increased by using a 4:1 patient/normal plasma mixture and incubating with kaolin/cephalin suspension for 2 hours at 37°C.[45,46] As these tests lack specificity, in order to confirm that an inhibitor acts specifically with factor VIII, a dilution of the patient's plasma must be incubated with an equal volume of normal plasma and factor VIII levels measured in subsamples removed immediately and after 60 and 120 minutes. If the inhibitor is specific for factor VIII, factor VIII will decrease over time in the incubation mixture. Other methods, using nephelometry,[47] inhibition of coagulation in agarose gel,[48,49] and immunoradiometry,[50-52] have been described but have not been adopted for widespread use.

Most centers in the United States use the Bethesda assay for quantification of factor VIII inhibitors.[53] Factor VIII assays are done on 2-hour incubation mixtures of various dilutions of patient's plasma with normal plasma. A test sample producing a residual factor VIII activity of 50% of normal is considered to contain 1 Bethesda unit of inhibitor per milliliter, and the inhibitor titer equals the reciprocal of the dilution of inhibitor plasma that neutralizes 50% of normal factor VIII. In England, the New Oxford Method is used to quantitate factor VIII inhibitors.[54]

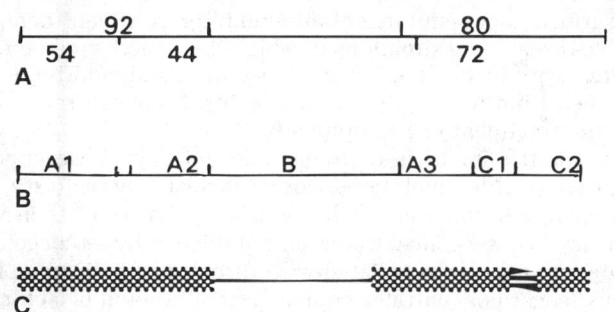

Fig. 109-2. Localization of factor VIII inhibitor epitopes. **(A)** Thrombin cleavage fragments, **(B)** factor VIII domains, **(C)** inhibitor epitopes. Hatched bar, inhibitor.

One Bethesda unit equals 1.21 times 1 Oxford unit.[54] An inhibitor unit does not imply that any specific number of factor VIII units infused into the patient will neutralize any specific number of inhibitor units.

Therapy

General Considerations

The presence of an inhibitor in a hemophiliac, the titer of that inhibitor, and whether the patient is a low responder or high responder are important determinants of immediate and future therapy. Minor hemorrhage may respond to conservative measures, such as immobilization and compression. For a hemorrhage requiring blood product therapy, two possible choices are available: (1) raise the factor VIII level by infusion of human or porcine factor VIII and, if the inhibitor titer is moderately high, precede this therapy by maneuvers to lower the titer; or (2) infuse an agent that bypasses the need for factor VIII, such as factor IX complex concentrates or factor VIIa.

High-Purity Human Factor VIII Concentrate

High-purity human factor VIII may be used successfully in the treatment of critical hemorrhages in either low or high responders with low inhibitor levels (<5 Bethesda units) and in patients with moderate inhibitor levels (10–30 Bethesda units) after reduction of the inhibitor level by plasmapheresis or immunoadsorption. In order to neutralize the inhibitor and achieve a hemostatic level of 30–50 U/ml, an adult patient is given an initial bolus of factor VIII of 5,000–10,000 U, followed by a continuous infusion of 300–1,000 U/hr. Alternatively, a large amount of factor VIII can be given every 1–4 hours (20 U of factor VIII for each Bethesda unit plus an additional 40 U/kg).[59] Since the dose of factor VIII concentrate needed to neutralize inhibitors and provide a hemostatic level of factor VIII cannot be predicted by the inhibitor level, factor VIII levels need to be assayed frequently in order to monitor the plasma factor VIII level achieved in vivo. However, although blood drawn for assay even a few minutes later may not have a measurable factor VIII level by the time the blood is processed and the assay completed, the infused factor VIII may achieve in vivo hemostasis before it is inactivated.

In patients who are high responders and who sustain a critical hemorrhage, hemostasis should be achieved early, before the anamnestic response occurs. As the factor VIII inhibitor level rises after several days of factor VIII therapy, factor VIII should be continued at a frequent interval or continuously—hemostasis can be maintained because of the slow neutralization rate of factor VIII.[32]

Porcine Factor VIII Concentrate

The suitability of a patient for porcine factor VIII depends partially on the degree of cross-reactivity of the patient's inhibitor with porcine factor VIII. The level of inhibitor to porcine factor VIII can be determined in the Bethesda test or the Oxford test by substituting porcine factor VIII for human factor VIII. Although the degree of cross-reactivity can vary widely from 0% to 75%,[60-63] on average it is usually about 25% (i.e., about 1 U of antiporcine factor VIII equals 4 U of antihuman factor VIII[60] (Kasper CK, personal communication). After treatment with porcine factor VIII, the degree of cross-reactivity increases. Thus, measurements of cross-reactivity are useful in predicting efficacy before the use of the porcine concentrate.

Although dosage is relatively arbitrary, in patients with inhibitor titers of <5 Bethesda units, 50 U of porcine factor VIII/kg should be given initially, and in patients with >5 Bethesda units, 50–150 U/kg[60,63] (Kasper CK, personal communication).

FACTORS TO BE CONSIDERED IN SELECTING A BLOOD PRODUCT FOR A BLEEDING EPISODE

1. Patients known to be high responders should not receive blood products containing factor VIII to treat minor hemorrhages, so as to avoid an anamnestic response (unless they are undergoing induction of immune tolerance). Conservative measures combined with the administration of factor IX complex concentrate is frequently adequate, since only a few inhibitor titers rise on exposure to the small amount of factor VIII coagulant antigen that may contaminate such concentrates.
2. If a hemorrhage is critical, an attempt should be made to raise the plasma factor VIII level into the hemostatic range of 30 to 50 U/ml.
3. In those patients with a serious hemorrhage who are either low responders or high responders with a low inhibitor level (<5 Bethesda units), high-purity human factor VIII can be given initially in an initial large bolus of 5,000–10,000 U, followed by a continuous infusion of 1,000 U/hr. Alternatively porcine factor VIII can be used. By contrast, the same type of patient (low inhibitor level of <5 Bethesda units) with a minor hemorrhage can be most easily managed with factor IX complex concentrate in doses of 75–100 U/kg repeated once or twice at 8–12-hour intervals as necessary. Factor IX complex concentrate has only trace amounts of factor VIII antigen and only rarely causes an anamnestic response.[55]
4. If the level of inhibitor against human factor VIII is >10 Bethesda units but the level of inhibitor against porcine factor VIII is much <10 Bethesda units, a large dose of porcine factor VIII should be tried.
5. If a patient has a moderately high inhibitor level of 10–30 Bethesda units to both porcine and human factor VIII, the inhibitor level may be lowered by about 50–66% by a 1.5-vol plasmapheresis[56] or extracorporeal immunoadsorption,[57,58] after which a large infusion of factor VIII concentrate may achieve hemostatic levels. Alternatively, patients with moderately high inhibitor levels can be treated with factor IX complex or with the porcine factor VIII concentrate (particularly if the level of inhibitor against porcine factor VIII is <10 Bethesda units).
6. If a patient has a very high inhibitor level (>30 Bethesda units), the only alternatives are factor IX complex concentrates or the porcine concentrate.

MANAGEMENT OF CRITICAL, LIFE-THREATENING HEMORRHAGES OR EMERGENCY SURGERY IN PATIENTS WITH INHIBITORS

In an emergent situation with a critical hemorrhage or with impending lifesaving surgery, both a high responder and low responder should be initially treated with a bolus infusion of the porcine factor VIII concentrate 100 U/kg. Ten minutes after the infusion, blood should be drawn for factor VIII assay in order to determine the adequacy of the dose; if inadequate, the dose should be increased by 50 U/kg, until the patient has a postinfusion factor VIII level of 30–50%. Simultaneously, the preinfusion antibody titer to both porcine and human factor VIII can be determined. If the titer to porcine factor VIII is >10 Bethesda units and clinical efficacy has not been established, plasmapheresis can be performed, followed by a massive dose of porcine factor VIII. Once efficacy is established, the patient should be treated at frequent intervals or by continuous infusion at a dose of 1,000 U/hr. Factor VIII levels should be monitored frequently. As long as hemostatic levels are achieved, the porcine concentrate should be continued for several days. If the inhibitor titer begins to rise and hemostatic levels can no longer be achieved, anti-inhibitor coagulant complex concentrate or factor IX complex concentrate should be used for several days.

If the patient does not respond initially to porcine factor VIII, anti-inhibitor complex concentrate may be administered, starting at a dose of 100 U/kg. Factor VIIa is currently available on a compassionate basis on research protocol by the manufacturer.

Factor IX Complex Concentrate

If human factor VIII cannot be used because the inhibitor level is too high (>30 Bethesda units), an attempt may be made to bypass the need for factor VIII, by giving a factor IX complex concentrate.[65–72] These concentrates contain phospholipids, prothrombin, and factors VII, IX, and X, but the substance(s) responsible for factor VIII bypassing activity remain(s) unknown.[73,74] These concentrates are of two types: unactivated intermediate-purity factor IX complex concentrates; and activated concentrates, so-called anti-inhibitor coagulant complex. The activated concentrates (Autoplex [Baxter]; FEIBA [Immuno]), contain a greater amount of the factor VIII bypassing material and are specifically designed for patients with factor VIII inhibitors. Both types of concentrates have proved efficacious in controlled clinical trials,[70,71] and no significant differences have been demonstrated. However, some patients have described successful use of anti-inhibitor coagulant complex in life-threatening situations in which the unactivated concentrates were ineffective. These concentrates should be distinguished from the highly purified factor IX concentrates used for the treatment of hemophilia B.

In addition to their unpredictable efficacy, these concentrates have other limitations. Dosage is relatively arbitrary, and no reliable in vitro method is available that reflects in vivo efficacy. These concentrates also induce a hypercoagulable state and may be associated with thromboembolic complications. These concentrates contain a small amount of factor VIII antigen and can induce an anamnestic response after their use. If selected for use in critical situations, these concentrates should be used early in the course of the bleeding episode.[55]

It is very important to monitor the level of factor VIII achieved in vivo following the infusion to determine the adequacy of the dose administered; if the initial dose is inadequate, rapid upward titration of the dose is important.

Several patients have had multiple courses of therapy with the porcine concentrate without loss of efficacy. In only the occasional patient have heterologous antibodies to porcine factor VIII developed. Classic anamnestic responses to porcine factor VIII occasionally occur, particularly in high responders who are infrequently treated.[61] In addition, a few cases of thrombocytopenia in response to the porcine concentrate have been reported,[63,64] as has the occasional anaphylactic reaction. Mild febrile reactions are common and are easily modulated with prophylactic antihistamine and acetaminophen.

Human Factor VIIa Concentrate

Purified components of the prothrombin complex have recently been used to treat hemorrhages in patients with inhibitors. A highly purified concentrate containing factor VIIa achieved good hemostasis[75] and more recently, a recombinant preparation of human factor VIIa has shown significant efficacy in patients with inhibitors.[63,76] Recombinant factor VIIa is currently an experimental drug.

Suppression of Inhibitors

Long-term goals in the management of these patients should be aimed at the prevention of anamnesis and suppression of further antibody production. Immunosuppressive therapy has been attempted in many patients, with variable and unpredictable results.[10,26,77-82] In general, with few exceptions, corticosteroid therapy alone is not efficacious in patients with hemophilia A and inhibitors.[82] By contrast, Dormandy and Sultan[83] collected the experience of many investigators using cyclophosphamide and factor VIII. Some degree of success was achieved on 40 occasions in 18 of 45 patients. The data reported by Hultin et al.[82] are in agreement with these observations. Although total elimination of antibody occurs very rarely, immunosuppressive therapy may be helpful in patients requiring factor VIII infusion, particularly low responders with low inhibitor titers.[82] Rarely, treatment of inhibitors soon after their appearance and before re-exposure to factor VIII may be an important determinant of successful outcome.[82] Despite these encouraging reports, the use of immunosuppressive drugs has not gained wide acceptance.

The induction of immune tolerance by the frequent regular infusions of factor VIII has become increasingly accepted, but the financial implications of this therapy are great.[20,61] A patient who is a high responder with a high-titer inhibitor is given daily or alternate-day infusions of various amounts of human factor VIII.[20,61] Following chronic administration of factor VIII, the inhibitor titer first increases and then progressively decreases, with most patients achieving either a very low titer (<2.5 U), or the inhibitor is undetectable. Moreover, the patient no longer has anamnesis with continued exposure to factor VIII. Similar results have been achieved at some centers, either with less amounts of factor VIII[21,61,84-86] or by giving factor VIII repeatedly but at irregular intervals.[87] Immune tolerance usually must be maintained by giving low doses of factor VIII every few days.

Successful outcomes of the induction of tolerance occur in about 75% of patients and appear to be more common in patients <20 years of age, in patients who are low responders, and in those receiving higher doses of factor VIII (≥50 U/kg/day). Human immunodeficiency virus status does not appear to affect outcome (Kasper CK, personal communication, 1993).

Successful regimens using factor VIII infusions combined with immunosuppressive drugs appear to shorten the induction of immune tolerance significantly, attaining remission at a much lower cost.[88]

In recent studies,[89,90] high-dose intravenous immunoglobulin given together with high-dose factor VIII and cyclophosphamide appeared to have a synergistic effect in achieving a state of immune tolerance. Intravenous IgG may have both a short- and long-term immunosuppressive effect.[91-93] Anti-idiotypic antibodies are present in the IgG preparations[94-96]; the emergence of anti-idiotypic antibodies may be the explanation for the occasional occurrence of spontaneous remission and some instances of remission induced by immunosuppressive agents.[95,97,98]

Inhibitors in Hemophilia B

Inhibitors to factor IX occur in hemophilia B secondary to alloimmunization following transfusion similar to hemophilia A. Although the overall incidence of inhibitors complicating hemophilia B is only 2.4-2.8%,[10,99] the incidence in patients with severe hemophilia B is approximately 12%.[10] Patients with major gene deletions who do not have demonstrable factor IX protein in their plasma may be especially susceptible to the development of factor IX antibodies,[100] but more recent observations have not supported this conclusion.

Like factor VIII inhibitors, factor IX inhibitors are IgG.[10,101-103] Some have restricted light chain and heavy chain heterogeneity,[102,104] whereas others are polyclonal.[103,105] The kinetic behavior of factor IX inhibitors differs from that of factor VIII inhibitors in that factor IX inhibitors produce an immediate loss of factor IX activity, with no progressive loss on further incubation.[10,101]

Laboratory Evaluation and Quantification

Factor IX inhibitors should be suspected in a hemophiliac if transfused factor IX either appears to have a short half-life or is not efficacious in achieving hemostasis, or both. This can be suspected in the laboratory whenever a partial thromboplastin time of a mixture of the patient's plasma and normal plasma is longer than that of a mixture of patient plasma and factor IX-deficient plasma known not to contain an inhibitor. Specificity can be determined by doing factor IX assays of an incubation mixture of patient plasma and normal plasma over time. A modification of the Bethesda assay is used to quantitate the inhibitor level.[53]

Therapy

In patients with hemophilia B who have inhibitors, the clinical course is not different from that seen in those with hemophilia A with inhibitors. Most of these cases can be managed with factor IX complex concentrates or the anti-inhibitor/coagulant complex. Whether the efficacy of these concentrates is due to neutralization of the inhibitor or to bypassing activity similar to that observed in hemophilia A, or both, is unknown. In addition, the induction of immunotolerance has been achieved in hemophilia B patients with the infusion of high doses of intravenous IgG in combination with cyclophosphamide and factor IX concentrates.[106]

REFERENCES

1. Kasper CK: Incidence and course of inhibitors among patients with classic hemophilia. Thromb Diath Haemorrh 30:264, 1973
2. Biggs R: Complications of treatment. p. 181. In Biggs R, Macfarlane RG (eds): Treatment of Hemophilia A and B and von Willebrand's Disease. Blackwell, London, 1978
3. Lusher JM, Salzman PM, Monoclate Study Group: Viral safety and inhibitor development associated with factor VIIIC ultra-purified from plasma in hemophiliacs previously unexposed to factor VIIIC concentrates. Semin Hematol 27:1, 1990
4. Lusher JM: Viral safety and inhibitor development associated with monoclonal antibody-purified F VIII C. Ann Hematol 63:138, 1991
5. Addiego JE Jr, Gomperts E, Liu S-L et al: Treatment of hemophilia A with a highly purified factor VIII concentrate prepared by anti-FVIIIc immunoaffinity chromatography. Thromb Haemost 67:19, 1992
6. Ehrenforth S, Kreuz W, Scharrer I et al: Incidence of development of factor VIII and factor IX inhibitors in hemophiliacs. Lancet 339:594, 1992
7. Lusher JM, Arkin S, Abildgaard CF et al: Recombinant factor VIII for the treatment of previously untreated patients with hemophilia A. N Engl J Med 328:453, 1993
8. Lusher J, Warrier I: Incidence of inhibitor development in infants and children with hemophilia A. Clin Res 41:275A, 1993
9. McMillan OW, Shapiro SS, Whitehurst D et al: The natural history of factor VIII:C inhibitors in patients with hemophilia A. A national cooperative study. II. Observations on the initial development of factor VIII:C inhibitors. Blood 71:344, 1988

10. Shapiro SS, Hultin M: Acquired inhibitors to the blood coagulation factors. Semin Thromb Hemost 1:336, 1975
11. Beck P, Giddings JC, Blood AL: Inhibitor of factor VIII in mild haemophilia. Br J Haematol 17:283, 1969
12. Crowell EB: A factor VIII inhibitor in a mild hemophiliac. Am J Med Sci 260:261, 1970
13. Lechner K, Ludwig E, Niessner H, Thaler E: Factor VIII inhibitor in a patient with mild haemophilia A. Hemostasis 1:261, 1972/73
14. Robboy SJ, Lewis EJ, Schur PH, Colman RW: Circulating anticoagulants to factor VIII. Am J Med 49:742, 1970
15. Allain JP, Frommel D: Antibodies to factor VIII. Patterns of immune response to factor VIII in hemophilia A. Blood 47:973, 1976
16. Frommel D, Allain JP: Genetic predisposition to develop factor VIII antibody in classic hemophilia. Clin Immunol Immunopathol 8:34, 1977
17. Alper CA, Raum DD, Awdeh ZL et al: Major histocompatibility complex (MHC)-linked complement alleles as markers for the development of anti factor VIII in hemophiliacs. Prog Clin Biol Res 150:141, 1984
18. Antonarakis WE, Waber PG, Kittur SD et al: Hemophilia A: Detection of molecular defects and of carriers by DNA analysis. N Engl J Med 313:842, 1985
19. Gitschier J, Wood WI, Tuddenham EGD et al: Detection and sequence of mutations in the factor VIII gene of hemophiliacs. Nature 315:427, 1983
20. Brackmann HH: Induced immunotolerance in factor VIII inhibitor patients. Prog Clin Biol Res 150:181, 1984
21. Ewing N, Sanders NL, Dietrich S, Kasper CK: Induction of immune tolerance to factor VIII in hemophiliacs with inhibitors. JAMA 259:65, 1988
22. Sultan Y, White GC, Aronstam A et al: Hemophilic patients with an inhibitor to factor VIII treated with high dose factor VIII concentrate: results of a collaborative study for the evaluation of factor VIII inhibitor titer, recovery and half life of infused factor VIII. Nouv Rev Fr Hematol 28:85, 1986
23. Feinstein DI, Rapaport SI: Acquired inhibitors of blood coagulation. Prog Hemost Thromb 1:75, 1972
24. Shapiro SS, Hulten M: Acquired factor VIII antibodies: further immunologic and electrophoretic studies. Science 160:786, 1968
25. Anderson BR, Terry WD: Gamma G_4-globulin antibody causing inhibition of clotting factor VIII. Nature 217:174, 1968
26. Feinstein DI, Rapaport SI, Chong MMY: Immunologic characterization of 12 factor VIII inhibitors. Blood 34:85, 1969
27. Poon MC, Wine AC, Ratnoff OD, Berier GM: Heterogeneity of human circulating anticoagulants against antihemophilic factor (factor VIII). Blood 46:409, 1975
28. Hultin MB, London FS, Shapiro SS, Yount Y: Heterogeneity of factor VIII antibodies: further immunochemical and biologic studies. Blood 49:807, 1977
29. Kavanaugh ML, Wood CN, Davidson JF: The immunological characterization of human antibodies to factor VIII isolated by immunoaffinity chromatography. Thromb Haemost 45:60, 1981
30. Allain JP, Gallandre A, Lee H: Immunochemical characterization of human antibodies to factor VIII in hemophilic and nonhemophilic patients. J Lab Clin Med 97:791, 1981
31. Lavergne JM, Meyer D, Reisner H: Characterization of human anti-factor VIII antibodies purified by immune complex formation. Blood 48:931, 1976
32. Shapiro SS: The immunologic character of acquired inhibitors of antihemophilic globulin (factor VIII) and the kinetics of their interaction. J Clin Invest 46:147, 1967
33. Biggs R, Austen DEG, Denson DWE et al: The mode of action of antibodies which destroy factor VIII. I. Antibodies which have second-order concentration graphs. Br J Haematol 23:125, 1972
34. Leitner A, Bidwell E, Dike GWR: An antihemophilic globulin (factor VIII inhibitor): purification, characterization and reaction kinetics. Br J Haematol 9:245, 1963
35. Green D: Spontaneous inhibitors of factor VIII. Br J Haematol 15:57, 1968
36. Biggs R, Austen DEG, Denson DWE et al: The mode of action of antibodies which destroy factor VIII. II. Antibodies which give complex concentration graphs. Br J Haematol 23:137, 1972
37. Feinstein DI: Acquired inhibitors against factor VIII and other clotting proteins. p. 825. In Coleman RW, Hush J, Marder VJ, Salzman EW (eds): Hemostasis and Thrombosis. JB Lippincott, Philadelphia, 1987
38. Gawryl MS, Hoyer LW: Inactivation of factor VIII procoagulant activity by two different types of human antibodies. Blood 60:1103, 1982
39. Herbst KD, Rapaport SI, Kenoyer DG et al: Syndrome of an acquired inhibitor of factor VIII responsive to cyclophosphamide and prednisone. Ann Intern Med 95:575, 1981
40. Fulcher CA, de Graaf MS, Roberts JR et al: Localization of human factor FVIII inhibitor epitopes to two polypeptide fragments. Proc Acad Sci USA 82:7728, 1985
41. Fulcher CA, Lechner K, de Graaf MS: Immunoblot analysis shows changes in factor VIII inhibitor chain specificity in factor VIII inhibitor patients over time. Blood 72:1348, 1988
42. Fulcher CA, de Graaf MS, Zimmerman TS: FVIII inhibitor IgG subclass and FVIII polypeptide specificity determined by immunoblotting. Blood 69:1475, 1987
43. Scandella D, Timmons L, Mattingly M et al: A soluble recombinant factor VIII fragment containing the A2 domain binds to some human anti-factor VIII antibodies that are not detected by immunoblotting. Thromb Haemost 67:665, 1992
44. Nilsson IM, Berntorp E, Zettervail O, Dahlbäck B: Noncoagulation inhibitory factor VIII antibodies after induction of tolerance to factor VIII in hemophilia A patients. Blood 75:378, 1990
45. Lossing T, Kasper CK, Feinstein DI: Detection of factor VIII inhibitors with the activated partial thromboplastin time. Blood 49:493, 1977
46. Ewing WP, Kasper CK: In vitro detection of mild inhibitors to factor VIII in hemophilia. Am J Clin Pathol 77:749, 1982
47. Malagon F, Elorza FL, Martin E, Jiminez A: Quantification of antibodies against factor VIII by an immunonephelometric method in a continuous flow system. Ann Clin Biochem 17:256, 1980
48. Bird P: Coagulation in an agarose gel and its application to the detection and measurement of factor VIII antibodies. Br J Haematol 29:329, 1975
49. Coots Mc, Glueck HI, Miller MA: Agarose gel method: its usefulness in assaying factor VIII inhibitors, evaluating treatment, and suggesting a mechanism of action for factor IX concentrates. Br J Haematol 60:735, 1985
50. Furlong RA, Peake IR, Bloom AL: Factor VIII-clotting antigen (VIII:CAg) in hemophilia measured by two immunoradiometric assays (IRMA) using different antibodies, and measurement of inhibitors to procoagulant factor VIII (VIII:C) by IRMA. Br J Haematol 48:643, 1981
51. Hellings JA, van Leeuwen FR, Over J, Mourik JA: Immunoradiometric assay of vIII:CAg, a potential tool to detect human anti-VIII:C antibodies. Thromb Res 26:297, 1982
52. Ljung R, Holmberg L: Immunoradiometric assay of inhibitors of antihaemophilic factor A. Acta Paediatr Scand 71:1019, 1982
53. Kasper CK, Aledort LM, Counts RB et al: A more uniform measurement of factor VIII inhibitors. Thromb Diath Haemorrh 34:869, 1975
54. Austen DE, Lechner K, Rizza CR, Rhymes IL: A comparison of the Bethesda and New Oxford methods of a factor VIII antibody assay. Thromb Haemost 47:72, 1982
55. Kasper CK and the Hemophilia Study Group: Effect of prothrombin complex concentrates on factor VIII inhibitor levels. Blood 54:1358, 1979
56. Francesconi M, Korniger C, Tholer E et al: Plasmapheresis: its value in the management of patients with antibodies to factor VIII. Hemostasis 11:79, 1982
57. Nilsson IM, Jonsson S, Sundqvist SB et al: A procedure for removing high titer antibodies by extracorporeal protein A-Sepharose absorption in hemophilia. Blood 58:38, 1981
58. Uehlinger J, Button GR, McCarthy J et al: Immunoadsorption for coagulation factor inhibitors: Transfusion 31:265, 1991
59. Kasper CK: Complications of hemophilia A treatment: factor VIII inhibitors. Ann NY Acad Sci 97, 1991
60. Kernoff PBA, Thomas ND, Lilley PA et al: Clinical experience with polyelectrolyte-fractionated porcine factor VIII concentrate in the treatment of hemophiliacs with antibodies to factor VIII. Blood 63:31, 1984
61. Kasper CK: The therapy of factor VIII inhibitors. Prog Hemost Thromb 9:57, 1989
62. Gatti L, Manucci PM: Use of porcine factor VIII in the management of seventeen patients with factor VIII antibodies. Thromb Haemost 51:379, 1984
63. Brettler DB, Forsberg AD, Levine PH et al: The use of porcine factor VIII concentrate (Hyate:C) in the treatment of patients with inhibitor antibodies to factor VIII. Arch Intern Med 149:1381, 1989
64. Green D, Tuite GF: Declining platelet counts and platelet aggregation during porcine factor VIII:C infusions. Am J Med 86:222, 1989
65. Bloom AL: Clotting factor concentrates for resistant haemophilia. Br J Haematol 40:21, 1978
66. Roberts HR: Hemophiliacs with inhibitors, therapeutic options. N Engl J Med 305:757, 1981
67. Editorial: Factor VIII inhibitors in hemophilia. Lancet 1:742, 1983
68. Kasper CK: Prothrombin complex concentrates and inhibitors: a reappraisal. JAMA 251:68, 1984
69. Lusher JM, Shapiro SS, Palascak JE et al: Efficacy of prothrombin-complex concentrates in hemophiliacs with antibodies to factor VIII: a multicenter therapeutic trial. N Engl J Med 303:421, 1980
70. Sjamsoedin LJM, Heijnen L, Mauser-Bunschoten EP et al: The effect of activated prothrombin-complex concentrate (FEIBA) on joint and muscle bleeding in patients with hemophilia A and antibodies to factor VIII: a double blind clinical trial. N Engl J Med 305:717, 1981

71. Lusher JM, Blatt PM, Penner JA et al: Autoplex versus proplex: a controlled, double-blind study of effectiveness in acute hemarthrosis in hemophiliacs with inhibitors to factor VIII. Blood 62:1135, 1983

72. Hilgartner MW, Knatterud GL and the FEIBA study group: The use of factor VIII inhibitor by-passing activity (FEIBA IMMUNO) product for treatment of bleeding episodes in hemophiliacs with inhibitors. Blood 61:35, 1983

73. Seligsohn U, Kasper C, Osterud B, Rapaport SI: Activated factor VII: presence in factor IX concentrates and persistence in the circulation after infusion. Blood 53:828, 1979

74. Hultin MB: Studies of factor IX concentrate therapy in hemophilia. Blood 62:677, 1983

75. Hedner U, Kisiel W: Use of human factor VIIa in the treatment of two hemophilia A patients with high titer inhibitors. J Clin Invest 71:1836, 1983

76. Macik BG, Hohneker J, Griffin A, Roberts HL: Use of recombinant FVIIa for treatment of a hemophilic patient with a high titer inhibitor, abstracted. Blood, suppl. 72:302a, 1988

77. Hruby MA, Schulman I: Failure of combined factor VIII and cyclophosphamide to suppress antibody to factor VIII in hemophilia. Blood 42:919, 1973

78. Stein RS, Colman RW: Hemophilia with factor VIII inhibitor: elimination of anamnestic response. Ann Intern Med 79:84, 1973

79. Nilsson IM, Hedner U, Holmberg L: Suppression of factor VIII antibody by combined factor VIII and cyclophosphamide. Acta Med Scand 195:65, 1974

80. Stein RS: Hemophilia: cyclophosphamide and factor VIII concentrate. Ann Intern Med 81:706, 1974

81. Green D: Factor VIII antibodies: immunosuppressive therapy. Ann NY Acad Sci 240:389, 1975

82. Hultin MB, Shapiro SS, Bowman HS et al: Immunosuppressive therapy of factor VIII inhibitors. Blood 48:95, 1976

83. Dormandy KM, Sultan Y: The suppression of factor VIII antibodies in hemophilia. Pathol Biol (Paris), suppl. 23:17, 1975

84. Wensley RT, Burn AM, Reading OM: Induction of tolerance to factor VIII in hemophilia A with inhibitors using low doses of human factor VIII, abstracted. Thromb Hemost 54:227, 1985

85. Aznar JA, Jarquera JI, Peiro A: Suppression of inhibitors in hemophilia with corticoids and factor VIII. Thromb Haemost 49:241, 1983

86. Van Leeuwen EP, Mauser-Bunschoten EP, Van Dijken AJ et al: Disappearance of factor VIII:C antibodies in patients with hemophilia A upon frequent administration of factor VIII in intermediate or low-dose. Br J Haematol 64:291, 1986

87. Rizza CR, Matthews JM: Effect of frequent factor VIII replacement on the level of factor VIII antibodies in hemophilics. Br J Haematol 52:13, 1982

88. Hedner U, Tengborn L: Management of hemophilia A with antibodies: the effect of combined treatment with factor VIII, hydrocortisone, and cyclophosphamide. Thromb Haemost 54:776, 1985

89. Nilsson IM, Berntorp E, Zettervall O: Induction of immune tolerance in patients with hemophilia A and antibodies to factor VIII by combined treatment with intravenous IgG, cyclophosphamide, and factor VIII. N Engl J Med 318:947, 1988

90. Nilsson IM, Berntorp E: Induction of immune tolerance in hemophiliacs with inhibitors by combined treatment with i.v. IgG, cyclophosphamide and factor VIII or IX. Prog Clin Biol Res 324:69, 1990

91. Gianelli-Borradori A, Hirt A, Luthy HP et al: Haemophilia due to factor VIII inhibitors in a patient suffering from a autoimmune disease: treatment with intravenous immunoglobulin. Blut 48:303, 1984

92. Zimmerman R, Kommerell B, Harenber J et al: Intravenous IgG for patients with spontaneous inhibitor to factor VIII. Lancet 1:273, 1985

93. Carreras LO, Perez GN, Xavier DL et al: Autoimmune factor VIII inhibitor responsive to gamma globulin without in vitro neutralization. Thromb Haemost 60:343, 1988

94. Sultan Y, Maisonneuve P, Kazatchkine MD, Nydegger UE: Anti-idiotypic suppression of autoantibodies to factor VIII (anti-haemophilic factor) by high-dose intravenous gammaglobulin. Lancet 2:765, 1984

95. Tiarks C, Pechet L, Humphreys RE: Development of anti-idiotypic antibodies in a patient with a factor VIII autoantibody. Am J Hematol 32:217, 1989

96. Rossi F, Dietrich G, Kazatchkine MD: Antiidiotypic suppression of autoantibodies with normal polyspecific immunoglobulins. Res Monogr Immunol 140:19, 1989

97. Frommel D: Anti-idiotypic suppression of antibodies to factor VIIIc. Lancet 2:1210, 1984

98. Moffat EH, Furlong RA, Dannatt AHG et al: Anti-idiotypes to factor VIII antibodies and their possible role in the pathogenesis and treatment of factor VIII inhibitors. Br J Haematol 71:85, 1989

99. Biggs R: Jaundice and antibodies directed against factors VIII and IX in patients treated for haemophilia or Christmas disease in the United Kingdom. Br J Haematol 26:313, 1974

100. Gianelli F, Choo KH, Rees DJG et al: Gene deletions in patients with hemophilia B and anti-factor IX antibodies. Nature 303:181, 1983

101. Lechner K: Factor IX inhibitors: Report of two cases and a study of the biological, chemical, and immunological properties of the inhibitors. Thromb Diath Haemorrh 25:447, 1971

102. Pike IM, Yount WJ, Puritz EM, Roberts HR: Immunochemical characterization of a monoclonal gamma G4-lambda human antibody to factor IX. Blood 50:11, 1977

103. Reisner MM, Roberts HR, Krumholz S, Young WJ: Immunochemical characterization of a polyclonal human antibody to factor IX. Blood 50:11, 1977

104. Giddings JC, Bloom AL, Kelly MA, Spratt HC: Human factor IX inhibitors: Immunochemical characteristics and treatment with activated concentrate. Clin Lab Haematol 5:165, 1983

105. Orstavik KH: Alloantibodies to factor IX in hemophilia B characterized by crossed immunoelectrophoresis and enzyme-conjugated antisera to human immunoglobulins. Br J Haematol 48:15, 1981

106. Nilsson IM, Berntorp E, Zitterval O: Induction of split tolerance and clinical cure in high responding hemophiliacs with factor IX antibodies. Proc Natl Acad Sci USA 83:9169, 1986

Factor XI and Other Clotting Factor Deficiencies

110

Harold R. Roberts and T. Flint Gray III

INTRODUCTION

This chapter describes the biology and clinical manifestations of deficiencies in prothrombin, factors V, VII, X, XI, XII, and XIII, as well as familial multiple clotting factor deficiencies. Table 110-1 lists the deficiencies and some of their characteristics.

PROTHROMBIN DEFICIENCY (HYPOPROTHROMBINEMIA AND DYSPROTHROMBINEMIA)

History and Epidemiology

At the turn of the century (1905), Morawitz formulated a basic theory of coagulation in which fibrinogen was converted

Table 110-1. Clotting Factor Deficiencies: General Information

Factor Deficient	Human Gene Location	Normal Circulating Half-Life (hr)	Incidence	Bleeding Severity[a]
Prothrombin	11p11-q12	72	Very rare	Moderate[b]
V	1q21-q25	36	1:1 million	Moderate
VII	13q34	3–6	1:500,000	Severe
VIII	Xq28	12	1:10,000 (male)	Severe
IX	Xq27	24	1:30,000 (male)	Severe
X	13q34	40	1:500,000	Severe
XI	4q32-q35	80	Rare[c]	Mild-moderate
XII	5q33-qter	50–70	?	No bleeding
XIII	A subunit:6p24–p25	9 days	<1:1 million	Moderate-severe
	B subunit: 1q31–q32			

[a] Bleeding severity in the most severely affected patients.
[b] The most severely affected patients studied retain some thrombin activity; total deficiency may be incompatible with life.
[c] Rare except in those of Ashkenazi Jewish descent.

to fibrin by a substance he called *fibrin ferment*, or thrombin.[1] In his hypothesis, a precursor molecule (prothrombin) was activated by a hypothetical enzyme (thrombokinase) to yield thrombin. Morawitz's cascade theory was simpler than the one accepted today, but it was essentially correct. True congenital hypoprothrombinemia or dysprothrombinemia is exceedingly rare, and < 30 kindred have been well studied.[1] Hypoprothrombinemia or dysprothrombinemia has no known predilection for any racial or ethnic group.

Genetics and Molecular Biology

The prothrombin gene consists of 14 exons and occupies approximately 24 kb of DNA near the centromere of chromosome 11.[2] The gene codes for signal peptide, a propeptide region, a γ-carboxyglutamic acid domain (that depends on vitamin K for post-translational γ-carboxylation of 10 glutamic acid residues), two kringle regions, a light chain, and a catalytic domain[3] (See Ch. 100). Prothrombin is a single-chain glycoprotein synthesized in the liver and normally present in the plasma at a concentration of 100 μg/ml. Prothrombin undergoes cleavage at several sites to yield thrombin, which consists of an A chain linked to a B chain by a disulfide bridge. The proteolytic conversion of prothrombin to thrombin requires factor Xa, calcium, and phospholipids and is accelerated 300-fold by the presence of activated factor V.[4] Thrombin performs a multitude of functions. Its procoagulant actions include proteolysis of fibrinopeptides A and B from fibrinogen; activation of factors V, VIII, and XIII; and induction of platelet aggregation. These functions are balanced by thrombin-mediated activation of protein C, which inhibits coagulation by degrading factors Va and VIIIa. Thrombin functions as an anticoagulant when complexed with thrombomodulin on the endothelial cell surface. The complex activates protein C, which in turn inhibits coagulation by degrading factors Va and VIIIa. Thrombin also promotes proliferation of fibroblasts and endothelial cells and function as a signal in chemotaxis.

Pathogenesis

A variety of mutations in the prothrombin gene have been discovered. These mutations cause either decreased production or stability of prothrombin, or production of dysfunctional molecules with reduced activity. The subsequent decrease in thrombin activity results in absent or defective clot formation, defective platelet aggregation, and defects in other pathways normally activated by thrombin. The clinical severity of bleeding depends on the particular defect. Table 110-2 depicts some of the known variants of prothrombin, which are inherited in an autosomal fashion.[5–25]

Clinical Manifestations

Bleeding associated with prothrombin deficiency typically consists of easy bruising, epistaxis, soft tissue hemorrhage, postoperative bleeding, and, in women, menorrhagia or metrorrhagia, or both. Hemarthroses have also been described, but are not common.[26] The correlation between prothrombin levels and severity of bleeding is poor. For example, there are asymptomatic patients with prothrombin activities of 15% of normal (e.g., prothrombin Salatka), while patients with prothrombin San Juan are symptomatic with prothrombin activities in the 25% range.[27] Since all known cases of congenital hypo- or dysprothrombinemia have detectable prothrombin levels, it is possible that complete absence of prothrombin activity is incompatible with life.

Laboratory Evaluation

Congenital prothrombin deficiency is marked by prolongation of the prothrombin time (PT) and the partial thromboplastin time (PTT). The bleeding time is normal. The prolonged PT and PTT are corrected if the patient's plasma is mixed with equal amounts of normal plasma. In true hypoprothrombinemia, both the functional and antigenic assays for prothrombin reveal decreased levels. Dysprothrombinemia results in decreased prothrombin activity, but the prothrombin antigen level may be normal or only slightly decreased. Specific diagnosis of prothrombin defects rests on functional and antigenic assays.

Differential Diagnosis

Patients with a bleeding tendency and prolongation of the PT and PTT may be suspected of having a deficiency of prothrombin, but deficiencies of factors V and X and multiple factor deficiencies should also be considered. A definitive diagnosis of hereditary prothrombin deficiency requires a specific assay for prothrombin and demonstration that levels of other clotting factors are normal.

Acquired prothrombin deficiency of liver disease, vitamin K deficiency, or warfarin effect can be distinguished by demonstrating low levels of all the vitamin K-dependent factors.

The lupus anticoagulant is an anti-phospholipid antibody

Table 110-2. Selected Prothrombin Variants[a]

Variant	Mutation	Activity (%)	Antigen (%)	Dysfunction
Homozygous				
Barcelona	CGT to TGT; R 271 to C	5	100	Activation by Xa
Madrid	CGT to TGT; R 271 to C	3	103	Activation by Xa
Segovia		7–20	100	
Salatka	GAG to GCG; Q 466 to A	15–17	100	Substrate binding
Poissy		2	50	
Perija		2	70	
Denver		<1	13	
Heterozygous				
Brussels		20–35	71	
Cardeza		40	100	Activation by Xa
Padua		52	100	
Clamart		50	100	Activation by Xa
Magdeburg		45	100	
Compound heterozygous				
Quick I	GGC to TGC; R 382 to C	<2	34	Fibrinogen binding and platelet aggregation
Quick II	GGC to GTC; G 558 to V	<1	—	Substrate binding
San Juan		7–25	25	
Mexico City		10	<10	Normal function?
Himi I	ATG to ACG; M 337 to T	—	—	
Himi II	CGC to CAC; R 388 to H	—	—	Fibrinogen binding
Habana		1–10	50	
Metz		10	50	Thrombin domain
Molise		10	45	Thrombin domain
Tokushima	CGG to TGG; R 418 to W, and frameshift	—	—	Fibrinogen binding and platelet aggregation
Uncharacterized genetics				
Gainesville		25	72	
Houston		5	52	
Corpus Christi		<1	25	

[a] In this and subsequent tables, amino acids are designated by a single letter: A, alanine; C, cysteine; D, aspartic acid; E, glutamic acid; F, phenylalanine; G, glycine; H, histidine; I, isoleucine; K, lysine; L, leucine; M, methionine; N, asparagine; P, proline; Q, glutamine; R, arginine; S, serine; T, threonine; V, valine; W, tryptophan; Y, Tyrosine.
(Data from references 3 and 5–25.)

that results in a prolonged PTT in vitro. These antibodies are rarely associated with clinical bleeding; however, a small subset of these antibodies recognize an epitope at the C terminus of the prothrombin molecule, resulting in acquired deficiency of prothrombin.[28,29] In these cases the PT is also prolonged. Although these antibodies do not inhibit prothrombin activity in vitro, it is thought that the antibody/prothrombin complex is cleared by the reticuloendothelial system, resulting in a true prothrombin deficiency. The hypoprothrombinemia acquired in this syndrome may be associated with bleeding, particularly soft tissue hemorrhage.

Therapy

Because prothrombin has a long half-life (about 3 days), most patients can be treated with plasma in doses of 15–20 ml/kg body weight as a loading dose, followed by 3 ml/kg body weight every 12–24 hours. Plasma levels of ≥30% of normal are usually sufficient to treat bleeding episodes. Plasma exchange may be employed to achieve higher levels before surgery. Because of potential thromboembolic complications, crude factor IX concentrates, which contain prothrombin, should be reserved for treatment of major hemorrhage or in anticipation of major surgery. Highly purified factor IX concentrates do not contain significant amounts of prothrombin and should not be used to treat prothrombin deficiency. Table 110-3 lists some of the crude factor IX concentrates and the amount of prothrombin contained in each. Highly purified prothrombin concentrates are not presently available.

Table 110-3. Composition of Selected Factor IX Concentrates

Product (Manufacturer)	Relative Amount of Factor[a]			
	II (Prothrombin)	VII	IX	X
Prothrombin complex concentrates				
Bebulin VH (Immuno)	120	13	100	139
Proplex T (Baxter/Hyland)	50	400	100	50
Profilnine HT (Alpha)	148	11	100	64
Konyne 80 (Bayer/Miles)	100	20	100	140
Highly purified factor IX concentrates				
Alphanine (Alpha)	<5	<5	100	<20
Mononine (Armour)	0	0	100	0
Activated prothrombin complex concentrates				
Autoplex T (Baxter/Hyland)	Variable amounts of Factors II, VII, IX, and			
FEIBA (Immuno)	X, and activated factors VIIa, IXa, and Xa			

[a] Data expressed in units of activity normalized to the amount of factor IX present.

FACTOR V DEFICIENCY

History and Epidemiology

As early as 1939, it was known that clotting factors other than prothrombin influenced the PT. In 1943, Quick[30] found that the PT of aged plasma was prolonged; he postulated that a "labile" factor was present in plasma that was different from prothrombin but that was required for a normal PT. At about the same time, Dr. Paul Owren,[31] a Norwegian hematologist, studied a woman with a lifelong history of bleeding and concluded that she was deficient in a factor present in plasma, which, in contrast to prothrombin, was not adsorbed to aluminum hydroxide. Owren's studies[31] were carried out during the Nazi occupation of Norway, and he was unable to report his studies until 1947. Eventually it was found that Owren's patient was deficient in "labile factor," now known as factor V.

Deficiency of factor V is a rare condition with an incidence of approximately 1 in 1 million persons.[32] There is no known predilection for members of any racial or ethnic group. Consanguinity has frequently been observed in the families of affected patients.

Genetics and Molecular Biology

Factor V deficiency is inherited as an autosomal recessive trait, with a gene frequency of $5-10 \times 10^{-4}$.[33] The factor V gene is located at 1q21-25, near genes coding for the selectin leukocyte adhesion molecules.[34] The sequence of the cDNA for human factor V reveals a domain structure similar to that of factor VIII, including three A domains, one B domain, and two C domains.[34] The molecular defects responsible for factor V deficiency are not yet well characterized.[4]

The factor V glycoprotein (335,000 MW, 13% carbohydrate) is primarily synthesized in both the liver (plasma factor V) and the megakaryocytes (platelet factor V), although other tissues are thought to be capable of synthesizing small amounts (e.g., vascular endothelium, monocytes). Plasma factor V circulates at a concentration of about 7μg/ml.[35] Platelet factor V is identical to plasma factor V and accounts for 20% of total body factor V. For full activity, the protein must be activated by thrombin or factor Xa. The active molecule, containing a light and heavy chain linked by Ca^{2+}, serves as an essential cofactor for factor Xa conversion of prothrombin to thrombin. The phospholipid and cell-surface binding sites of factor Va are located on the light chain, while the heavy chain is thought to bind prothrombin. Factor Va is ultimately inactivated by activated protein C, a reaction that requires protein S as a cofactor.

Pathogenesis

The hemorrhagic tendency in factor V deficiency is a direct consequence of the lack of its activity in both plasma and platelets. Some deficient patients have normal levels of antigen but low levels of functional activity. Patients severely deficient in plasma factor V are generally deficient in platelet factor V as well. There is one variant of factor V deficiency, factor V Quebec, in which a brother and sister with abnormal bleeding had moderately reduced plasma levels (40% of normal), but severely reduced platelet factor V (2–4% of normal).[36] The defect in this family points to the importance of platelet factor V for hemostasis.

Clinical Manifestations

Severe factor V deficiency presents with abnormal bruising, epistaxis, soft tissue hemorrhages, and occasional hemarthroses. Crippling hemophilic arthropathy is not usually seen, but hemorrhage involving the central nervous system has been noted. Bleeding from the umbilical stump is frequent. Women commonly experience abnormal menstrual bleeding and postpartum hemorrhage. About one-half of patients are diagnosed in adulthood. Even though severe hemorrhage may occur in

Table 110-4. Typical Laboratory Values for Factor V-Deficient Patients

Assay	Moderate	Severe	Normal
Prothrombin time (sec)	15	65	12
PTT (sec)	40	60	26
Thrombin time (sec)	11	11	11
Bleeding time (min)	7	7 to >15	3–9
Factor V (% normal)	27	<1	100

patients with <1% factor V, bleeding is not as frequent as that seen in severely affected hemophilia A patients. Mild and moderate forms of factor V deficiency have also been reported and most likely reflect genetic heterogeneity of the disorder.

Laboratory Evaluation

Laboratory features of severe deficiency are shown in Table 110-4. Both the PT and the PTT are prolonged, while the thrombin time is normal. The bleeding time may be prolonged in severe factor V deficiency since platelet factor V is virtually undetectable in severely affected patients. Conclusive diagnosis of the deficiency requires a specific factor V activity assay.

Differential Diagnosis

Hereditary factor V deficiency must be distinguished from a combined deficiency of factors V and VIII, which is also inherited. In the latter condition, both factor V and factor VIII levels are about 15–20% of normal. Acquired factor V deficiency occurs in patients with liver disease. It is also reduced in patients with disseminated intravascular coagulation. Inhibitors to factor V occur in some patients with congenital factor V deficiency and rarely in otherwise normal patients, who develop these inhibitors spontaneously. The latter event has been documented in association with the use of topical bovine thrombin preparations (which contain bovine factor V) in cardiac surgery, and in patients treated with antibiotics such as streptomycin (see Ch. 115).[37,38] Inhibitors to factor V can be detected by showing that the patient's plasma inhibits factor V activity in normal plasma.

Therapy

Fresh frozen plasma is the mainstay of treatment for bleeding episodes in deficient patients. No factor V concentrates are commercially available, and cryoprecipitate is not rich in this protein. While platelets contain factor V and can correct the bleeding defect in deficient patients, platelet transfusions are not the treatment of choice because of the possible induction of antiplatelet isoantibodies. However, transfusions of normal platelets may be useful in patients with circulating inhibitors to factor V, since platelet factor V may be available in a milieu protected from inhibitors.[39]

There is not a great deal of experience in the treatment of factor V deficiency; therefore, proposed hemostatic levels are conjectural. Levels of 25% of normal are usually sufficient for many mild or moderate bleeding episodes.[40] This level can be achieved by the use of plasma at an initial dose of 15–20 ml/kg body weight, followed by 3–6 ml/kg body weight daily for 7 days postsurgery. Care must be taken to monitor for evidence of volume overload when large amounts of plasma are infused. Daily plasma infusions for surgery seem reasonable, since the half-life of factor V is about 36 hours.[40]

FACTOR VII DEFICIENCY

History and Epidemiology

The first reported case of factor VII deficiency was described by Alexander et al.[41] in 1951. In the index case, plasma from a child with congenital bleeding displayed a prolonged PT that could be corrected by aged serum, but not by barium sulfate-adsorbed plasma. Factor VII deficiency is inherited as an autosomal recessive trait and affects males and females equally, with an incidence of 1 in 500,000.

Genetics and Molecular Biology

The gene for factor VII is found on chromosome 13, adjacent to the gene for factor X.[42] There is evidence for a regulatory element on chromosome 8 that controls factor VII expression in the liver.[43] As a vitamin K-dependent factor, factor VII contains γ-carboxyglutamyl residues that are necessary for calcium-dependent lipid binding, as well as two epidermal growth factor (EGF)-like regions (EGF domains) and a catalytic domain with typical serine protease features (see Ch. 100).[44]

Factor VII circulates in the plasma at a concentration of 0.5 μg/ml. Tissue factor, a membrane-associated glycoprotein, and calcium are required for activation of factor VII in vivo, an event that may initiate the coagulation cascade.[45,46] Activated factor VII then activates factor X (the extrinsic coagulation pathway) and also activates factor IX. Feedback activation of factor VII by factor Xa amplifies coagulation.

Pathogenesis

Factor VIIa is a critical component of the extrinsic coagulation pathway, in which it activates factor X in the presence of tissue factor and calcium. The factor VIIa/tissue factor complex also activates factor IX, contributing to the activation of the intrinsic pathway. Thus, a deficiency of factor VII is associated with significant clinical manifestations. The relative importance and the interconnections between the extrinsic and intrinsic pathways of coagulation are discussed in Chapter 100.

Factor VII deficiency is heterogeneous, as reflected by variable ratios of factor VII coagulant and antigenic activity and by variable factor VII activity in the presence of tissue factor from different species (Table 110-5). In most cases the pathogenesis of factor VII deficiency is related to normal or reduced production of an abnormal factor VII molecule, presumably due to point mutations or partial gene deletions. Diminished availability or defective function of tissue factor has never been documented as a cause of decreased factor VII activity.

Clinical Manifestations

Factor VII deficiency commonly presents as easy bruising, soft tissue hemorrhage, epistaxis, and, in women, menorrhagia and metrorrhagia. Hemarthroses and crippling hemophilic arthropathy occur in severely affected patients (<1% activity) and may be as severe as that seen in hemophilia A and B.[47] Bleeding in factor VII deficiency is usually easier to control than that seen in hemophilia A and B. Intracranial hemorrhage has been reported, especially in neonates after vaginal delivery. One series cites a 16% incidence of intracranial bleeding in 75 patients with factor VII deficiency, a complication frequently associated with a fatal outcome.[48] Postpartum hemorrhage is seen in patients with factor VII levels <10–20% of normal. Postoperative bleeding is more likely in severely affected patients.

Laboratory Evaluation

Factor VII deficiency is the only hereditary clotting factor deficiency that causes an isolated prolonged PT in the presence of a normal PTT. Occasionally patients deficient in factor VII do have a prolonged PTT, but this is very rare. The bleeding time is usually normal. A specific factor VII activity assay is required to confirm the diagnosis. Typical laboratory features of factor VII deficiency are presented in Table 110-5. The activity can vary dramatically, depending on the source of tissue factor used in the assay. Variants of factor VII deficiency, which are distinguished on the basis of their reactivity toward tissue factors of different animal species are listed in Table 110-5 (High K, personal communication).[49-56]

Antigenic measurements, in conjunction with factor VII functional activity, reveal three patterns of deficiency: those without activity or antigen (antigen negative); those with partial activity and partial antigen (antigen reduced); and those with

Table 110-5. Factor VII Deficiency: Typical Laboratory Values and Activity of Different Variants with Different Tissue Factors

Typical Laboratory Values for Severe Factor VII Deficiency

Assay	Severe	Normal
PT (sec)	36	100
PTT (sec)	28	26
Thrombin time (sec)	11	11
Factor VII (%)	<1	100

Factor VII Activity and Mutations of Selected Variants[a]

Variant	Factor VII Antigen (%)	Activity (%) measured using			Mutation
		Rabbit Tissue Factor	Ox Tissue Factor	Human Tissue Factor	
Padua 1	100	11	105	30–38	
Padua 2	50	40	20	20	
Verona	50	25	45	20	
Hamilton	—	—	—	—	D 57 to N
Kansas	—	0	—	—	Q 100 to R; R 304 to Q
Little Rock	67	6.7	—	16	R 304 to Q
Watanabe	76	20	—	—	R 79 to Q
Unnamed	19	<1	—	—	K 137 to E
Unnamed	52	10	—	—	R 79 to W

[a] Data from references 49–56.

decreased coagulant activity and normal antigen levels (antigen positive). The first of these groups is the most frequent.[52]

Differential Diagnosis

Hereditary factor VII deficiency may be suspected in any male or female patient with a lifelong history of excessive bleeding, whether spontaneous or traumatic, especially in those with isolated prolongation of the PT. Factor X deficiency, and some variants of factor IX deficiency (hemophilia B$_M$), may also exhibit prolonged PTs, but, in contrast to factor VII deficiency, the PTT is also prolonged in the latter two conditions.

Liver disease, warfarin ingestion, or vitamin K deficiency may mimic factor VII deficiency. These disorders may be distinguished from hereditary deficiency by measuring other vitamin K-dependent factors. There is an inherited combined deficiency of prothrombin and factors VII, IX, and X (familial multiple factor deficiency, type III). In some reported cases of this syndrome, factor VII levels are lower than those of other vitamin K-dependent factors.

Therapy

Factor VII deficiency is treated with fresh frozen plasma or crude factor IX concentrates that contain factor VII (Table 110-3). Because the half-life of factor VII is about 3–6 hours, it is difficult to maintain normal levels with plasma replacement therapy alone. Fortunately, it is not usually necessary to raise factor VII levels to 100% to achieve adequate hemaostasis. Although the minimum hemostatic level is not known, an increase to 15–25% of normal generally results in normal hemostasis, even as prophylaxis for surgery. Replacement therapy given every 6–12 hours is satisfactory for most hemorrhagic episodes despite the short in vivo half-life of factor VII.

For spontaneous hemorrhage or mild trauma, factor VII levels of 5–10% are sufficient to stop bleeding. This can be achieved by administering plasma at a dose of 5–10 ml/kg body weight and repeating the dose every 8–12 hours for 1–2 days. For major hemorrhage or surgery, plasma may be given as a loading dose of 20 ml/kg body weight and followed by 3–6 ml/kg body weight every 8–12 hours until healing of surgical wounds occurs. This may require 5–7 days of treatment.

The use of plasma carries with it the risk of transmission of viral diseases, particularly hepatitis C. Other disadvantages of plasma are the potential for volume overload and the inability to achieve high levels of factor VII. For these reasons, intermediate purity factor IX concentrates containing factor VII may be useful. The successful use of factor IX concentrate at a dose of 50 U/kg body weight every 8 hours for 24 hours followed by plasma infusions thereafter has been reported for major orthopaedic surgery.[57]

Specific factor VII concentrates have been described and used in patients with bleeding or as prophylaxis for surgery or childbirth, but these products are not widely available.[58,59] Pure recombinant activated factor VII has been studied in clinical trials as a treatment for hemophilia A and B complicated by inhibitors, but recombinant factor VIIa has been used successfully in limited numbers of factor VII-deficient patients. There is considerable diversity of opinion with regard to the amount of factor VII replacement required for surgery; some investigators have even suggested that replacement is not routinely necessary for surgery.[60] However, most evidence supports the position that patients with a severe or moderate deficiency of factor VII do require replacement therapy before surgery.

FACTOR X DEFICIENCY

History and Epidemiology

During the 1950s, two groups of researchers independently discovered factor X. The index patient, Mr. Rufus Stuart, was originally thought to have factor VII deficiency, but his plasma was later shown to correct the defect in the plasma from the original factor VII-deficient patient.[61] A British group simultaneously studied a factor X-deficient subject named Prower, leading to the original designation of factor X as Stuart-Prower factor. Factor X deficiency has no predilection for any particular racial or ethnic group and is found worldwide. The incidence is estimated at 1 in 500,000. Consanguinity has been shown in a number of families with factor X deficiency, including that of Mr. Stuart, whose mother and father were aunt and nephew.

Genetics and Molecular Biology

Factor X deficiency is transmitted as an autosomal recessive trait. The gene encoding factor X has been localized to chromosome 13 at position 13q34, <3 kb from the gene for factor VII. It consists of eight exons arranged in a fashion similar to the genes of factor IX and factor VII.[62,63] Expression of the factor X gene is restricted to the liver.[64] The mature factor X protein consists of a light chain and a heavy chain, with a γ-carboxyglutamic acid domain containing 11 γ-carboxyglutamyl residues, two EGF-like domains, an activation peptide region, and a catalytic domain typical of serine proteases (see Ch. 100). Factor Xa, in the presence of its cofactors (factor Va, calcium, and phospholipids), converts prothrombin to thrombin.

Pathogenesis

The molecular defect has been identified in some patients with factor X deficiency. Four point mutations involving CpG dinucleotides in the DNA sequence have been described. These include the defect in the original Stuart factor (Val 104 to Met); the defective factor X Vorarlberg (Glu 14 to Lys); factor X San Antonio (Arg 336 to Cys); and factor X Santa Domingo, in which a glycine in the leader peptide is substituted with arginine.[65–67] One small deletion in the factor X gene has been described in a patient with the factor X Friuli defect.[68,69] Other factor X variants have also been described (Table 110-6).

Clinical Manifestations

Hemarthroses, retroperitoneal hematomas and other soft tissue hemorrhages, hematuria, pseudotumors, and menorrhagia are observed in patients with severe factor X deficiency. Severe bleeding episodes comparable to those seen in classic hemophilia A may occur. Crippling hemophilic arthropathy is seen, but is not as severe as in hemophilia A or B. Excessive bleeding is uncommon in mild disease. Patients with levels of factor X ≥15% usually have few hemorrhagic episodes, although bleeding may occur with major surgery or trauma.

Laboratory Evaluation

Typical laboratory findings in factor X deficiency are depicted in Table 110-7. In screening tests of coagulation, the PT and the PTT are prolonged, while the thrombin time is normal. The Russell's viper venom time, which activates factor X directly, is also prolonged. A specific factor X activity assay is

Table 110-6. Activity of Factor X Variants, Measured by Various Assay Systems

Variant	Factor X Antigen	PT	PTT	Russell Viper Venom Time
Stuart	<1	<1	<1	<1
Prower	85	8	—	7
Friuli	100	4	6	80
Padua	100	25–30	90	88
Melbourne	120	100	9	105
Roma	80	30–50	3	100
Vorarlberg	20	<1	32	15
Santo Domingo	5	1	1.5	1
San Antonio	36	14	—	—
Malmo	—	35	43	—
Vienna	5	1	1	—
Vicenza I	80	13	18	25
Vicenza II	72	20	34	54

(Data from references 65–73 and Davie EW, personal communication.)

required for the diagnosis. Typically, the bleeding time is normal even in severely affected patients.

The in vitro assays for factor X activity reflect the heterogeneity of factor X deficiency. The original Stuart plasma demonstrated no detectable activity of factor X by the PT, PTT, or Russell's viper venom-based assays. In other variants of factor X deficiency, the level of measurable factor X activity depends on whether the assay is based on the PT, the PTT, or the Russell's viper venom time[65-73] (Table 110-6).

Differential Diagnosis

Acquired factor X deficiency occurs in liver disease, and as a result of warfarin ingestion or vitamin K deficiency. In these instances other vitamin K-dependent factors are also reduced. Acquired factor X deficiency may accompany amyloidosis.[74] In this setting, essentially no recovery of transfused factor X occurs, as if a circulating inhibitor to factor X were present; however, in vitro mixing assays show no inhibitor in the plasma. Factor X deficiency in amyloidosis is a consequence of adsorption of factor X by extracellular amyloid. Replacement therapy is futile, and improvement is most often seen during therapy of the underlying cause for amyloidosis.[75,76] Splenectomy has been reported to be of value in correcting the factor X deficiency of amyloidosis, presumably via the resultant debulking of splenic amyloid.[77] Hereditary factor X deficiency must be distinguished from various hereditary combined deficiencies of clotting factors. Inhibitors of factor X are very rare.[78]

Therapy

Transfusion with fresh frozen plasma may be used to treat patients with congenital factor X deficiency. Plasma can be given as an initial dose of 15–20 ml/kg body weight, followed

Table 110-7. Typical Laboratory Values for Severe Factor X Deficiency

Assay	Factor X Deficiency	Normal
PT (sec)	>30	12
PTT (sec)	60	29
Thrombin time (sec)	11	11
Bleeding time (min)	6	<10
Factor X (%)	<1	100

by 3–6 ml/kg body weight every 24 hours. The biologic half-life of factor X is about 40 hours; thus, administration of plasma every 12 hours results in a progressive increase in factor X concentration. About 80% of administered factor X remains intravascularly shortly after infusion. Intermediate purity factor IX concentrates, rich in factor X, have been used to prepare patients for surgery or to treat serious bleeding from trauma or surgery. Table 110-3 displays the proportion of factor X present in selected factor IX concentrates.

Factor X levels of about 10–15% provide adequate hemostasis for hemarthroses and uncomplicated soft tissue hemorrhage. Because of the risk of thromboembolism and DIC with high doses or prolonged administration of prothrombin complex concentrates containing factor X, it is not recommended that factor X levels of >50% of normal be exceeded unless absolutely necessary.

FACTOR XI DEFICIENCY

History and Epidemiology

Factor XI deficiency was first recognized as an inherited blood-clotting factor deficiency by Rosenthal and colleagues[79] in 1953. These workers described three related patients, one male and two females, who had a history of bleeding after dental extraction. The observation that plasma from the affected patients corrected the clotting defects of plasma from patients known to be deficient in other clotting factors implied the absence of a previously undescribed coagulation factor, later designated factor XI.

Factor XI deficiency occurs most often in Ashkenazi Jews and only rarely in non-Jewish populations.[80] The calculated gene frequency for factor XI deficiency among Ashkenazi Jews is 4.3%, so appreciable numbers of homozygous patients may be expected.[81]

Genetics and Molecular Biology

Factor XI deficiency is inherited as an autosomal recessive trait. The gene contains 15 exons and is located on chromosome 4q32-q35.[82] After secretion as a homodimer from the liver, factor XI circulates in plasma at a concentration of approximately 5 μg/ml. It is composed of two identical disulfide-linked monomers of 80,000 molecular weight that exhibit significant homology with prekallikrein.[83] In the intrinsic pathway, factor XI is activated by factor XIIa, which cleaves the Arg 369-Ile 370 bond in each monomeric unit, yielding two N-terminal heavy chains, each of molecular weight 50,000, and two C-terminal light chains, each of molecular weight 30,000. Each heavy chain is composed of four tandem repeats designated apple domains. Apple domain-1 binds high-molecular-weight kininogen; apple domain-2 is the factor IX binding site, while apple domain-4 functions to bind the factor XI monomers together for homodimerization (Fujikawa K, Chung DW, personal communication).[84,85] The light chains are homologous with other serine proteases, and each contains a catalytic site for activation of factor IX. Factor XII circulates in a complex with high-molecular-weight kininogen (HMWK), which enhances the activation of factor XI by factor XIIa. Since it is known that patients with undetectable factor XII have no bleeding, it is probable that alternative mechanisms of activating factor XI are important in vivo. Activated factor VII, kallikrein, and thrombin have each been demonstrated to activate factor XI, but the relative importance of the different activation pathways is uncertain.

Table 110-8. Factor XI Levels in Homozygous or Heterozygous Factor XI Deficiency[a]

Mutation Type			
Allele 1	Allele 2	Factor XI Level (%)	PTT (sec)
II	II	1.2	108
III	III	9.7	85
II	III	3.3	67
II	—	52	39
III	—	67	36
—	—	>100	32

[a] Dashes refer to normal allele; standard deviation data not shown.
(Adapted from Seligsohn,[81] with permission.)

Pathogenesis

Presently, three different point mutations account for most analyzed cases of factor XI deficiency.[86,87] Type I mutations occur at the splice junction boundary of the last intron, resulting in either disruption of mRNA splicing or premature translation termination. A mutation in exon 5 resulting in a premature stop codon has been designated the type II mutation. The type III mutation in the exon 9 causes substitution of leucine for phenylalanine at position 238. In small population studies it appears that type II and III mutations are the most common, and compound heterozygosity (type II/III) is found frequently in affected patients. Although genotype appears to correlate with the factor XI levels observed (Table 110-8), a clear correlation of genotype with bleeding tendency has not been established.

Very low factor XI levels are not always associated with a bleeding tendency, an observation that has not been adequately explained. Evidence shows that factor XI-like activity exists on platelet membranes, and it has been suggested that such activity may compensate for deficiency of plasma factor XI.[88] Platelet factor XI has a lower molecular weight and a different electrophoretic migration than that of plasma factor XI, although the two activities cannot be distinguished immunologically.

Clinical Manifestations

Affected patients can be divided into those with major deficiency (≤20% of normal) and those with minor deficiency.[89] Patients with major deficiency may experience excessive bleeding and are usually homozygous or compound heterozygous. Patients with minor deficiencies have little or no bleeding and are usually heterozygous for the disorder. Although hemorrhagic symptoms do not always strictly correlate with the factor XI level, patients with a family history of bleeding in affected relatives will probably have similar experiences. Similarly, patients without a history of bleeding usually do not experience hemorrhage even after trauma.

Those patients who do bleed usually do so only after trauma. Even patients with very low factor XI levels do not have hemorrhagic episodes as frequently or prominently as those seen in hemophilia A and B. Epistaxis, soft tissue hemorrhage, and bleeding after dental extractions may occur. Hemarthroses are very uncommon, and chronic disabling joint disease is not seen. Affected women may experience menorrhagia. Postoperative bleeding may be seen in severely affected patients.

Laboratory Evaluation

The PTT is prolonged in factor XI deficiency, while the PT and thrombin time are normal. A specific assay of factor XI activity is necessary to confirm the diagnosis. Assays of other clotting factors may be necessary to exclude a combined hereditary deficiency of factor XI and other factors as described below. Plasma for factor XI assays should be drawn into nonwettable tubes and assayed as soon as possible. It is reported that the clotting defect in factor XI deficiency cannot always be detected when plasma is exposed to glass or if it is assayed after the plasma is frozen and thawed.

Differential Diagnosis

Factor XI deficiency should be suspected in any patient with a prolonged PTT, especially if the family history suggests a mild-to-moderate lifelong bleeding disorder that affects both males and females. Factor XI deficiency has been described in a familial multiple factor deficiency syndrome (type V) in which factors VIII, IX, and XI are decreased. This syndrome has been described for five patients worldwide, which is more than predicted on the basis of coincidence alone. A combined factor XI/factor IX deficiency has also been described as part of type VI familial multiple factor deficiency.[90]

Acquired factor XI deficiency occurs in patients who develop inhibitors to factor XI. Anti-factor XI antibodies occur in patients with systemic lupus erythematosus and other immunologic diseases (see Ch. 115). Acquired deficiency can be distinguished from the hereditary form on the basis of a history of recent onset and the presence of inhibitory activity in the patient's plasma. Factor XI deficiency has been described as a common finding in patients with Noonan syndrome, which is characterized by congenital cardiac abnormalities, short stature, and mental retardation.[91,92]

Therapy

Soft tissue bleeding may not require treatment. When therapy is required, fresh frozen plasma or the supernatant from cryoprecipitate-poor plasma is used. Commercially available factor XI concentrates are of limited availability.[93] Plasma exchange may be required if the hemorrhage cannot be controlled with plasma alone. The plasma half-life of factor XI is approximately 80 hours. Plasma can be administered as a loading dose of 15–20 ml/kg body weight, followed by 3–6 ml/kg/body weight every 12 hours until hemostasis is achieved. Factor XI levels of 30–40% have been reported with plasma replacement therapy. The risk of hepatitis, especially hepatitis C, is proportional to the number of units of plasma infused.

Surgical procedures performed on factor XI patients vary from cataract surgery to open heart surgery.[94,95] These have been safely carried out with plasma replacement therapy. Bleeding following prostatectomy has been difficult to control even with aggressive plasma therapy. The administration of antifibrinolytic agents such as ε-aminocaproic acid or tranexa-

---

USE OF ANTIFIBRINOLYTIC THERAPY IN CLOTTING FACTOR DEFICIENCY

Patients who undergo dental procedures may be successfully treated with antifibrinolytic agents such as ε-aminocaproic acid or tranexamic acid. This treatment decreases the need for extensive replacement therapy and in some cases, such as factor VII and factor XI deficiencies, may obviate the need for any blood product replacement.

mic acid usually is sufficient to prevent hemorrhage after dental extractions.

Despite observations that some factor XI-deficient patients may not bleed during surgery, the physician may have no way to ascertain which patients will not bleed. A history of past significant surgery without therapy, uncomplicated by bleeding, strongly suggests but does not guarantee satisfactory hemostasis with subsequent surgery. When in doubt, factor XI-deficient patients with levels <10% of normal may be treated with plasma prior to surgery, or plasma may be infused during surgery, if needed.

Alloantibodies to factor XI have been described and are most likely to occur in severely affected patients. These antibodies inhibit factor XI activity and represent a major complication of therapy. One patient with a factor XI inhibitor and severe bleeding failed to respond to maximal plasma therapy but responded dramatically to infusions of an activated factor IX concentrate.[96]

DEFICIENCY OF THE "CONTACT" FACTORS

Factor XII, prekallikrein (PK), and HMWK, in addition to factor XI, are the major factors involved in the "contact" phase of coagulation. Subjects with a deficiency of factor XII, PK, or HMWK have no bleeding, but do exhibit a prolonged PTT. These factors are thought to be important as mediators of various host-defense mechanisms including inflammation, fibrinolysis, and control of blood pressure.[97] Their role in coagulation is related to activation of factor XI. Even though deficiencies of factor XII, PK, and HMWK are not associated with abnormal bleeding, it is important to distinguish deficiency of these contact factors from deficiencies of factors VIII, IX, and XI, which are accompanied by defective hemostasis.

Factor XII Deficiency

Factor XII (Hageman factor) deficiency was first described by Ratnoff and Colopy[98] in 1955. The original patient, Mr. John Hageman, had no history of excessive bleeding; his in vitro clotting abnormality was discovered during a preoperative evaluation. Factor XII levels are lower in patients of Oriental descent than in other ethnic groups. There has been no convincing report of excessive bleeding, even with major surgical procedures. Although activated factor XII had been thought to be the physiologic activator of factor XI, there is no evidence of a decreased factor XI coagulant function in factor XII-deficient patients. Controversy exists regarding the possibility that decreased plasminogen activator activity described in factor XII-deficient patients may be associated with defective fibrinolysis and an increased risk of thromboembolism.[99] Activated factor XII is inhibited by antithrombin III, α_2-antiplasmin, and C1-inhibitor.[100]

The hallmark of severe factor XII deficiency is a markedly prolonged PTT (usually >100 seconds) in a patient with no history of bleeding. The prothrombin and thrombin clotting times are normal. In most patients the bleeding time is normal, although exceptions have been noted. A specific factor XII activity assay is required to confirm the diagnosis.

Prekallikrein Deficiency

PK deficiency (Fletcher factor deficiency) was first described in 1965 by Hathaway et al.,[101] who observed patients with a markedly prolonged PTT who had no history of abnormal bleeding. The disorder is inherited in an autosomal recessive pattern. Plasma from affected patients corrected the clotting defect of plasma deficient in all other known clotting factors including factors XI and XII. In addition, the prolonged PTT of PK-deficient plasma was corrected by exposure to glass. The hallmark of PK deficiency is a markedly prolonged PTT, corrected by exposure to glass, in patients with no bleeding tendencies.[101] A specific assay is required for diagnosis.

High-Molecular-Weight Kininogen Deficiency

Patients with HMWK deficiency (Williams, Fleaujeac, or Fitzgerald factor deficiency) also exhibit a prolonged PTT, but have no bleeding abnormality. The disorder is inherited as an autosomal recessive characteristic. Some patients are also deficient in low-molecular-weight kininogen. Both factor XI and PK circulate in a complex with HMWK, a necessary cofactor for activation of factor XII as well as PK and factor XI.

FACTOR XIII DEFICIENCY

History and Epidemiology

The existence of factor XIII (fibrin-stabilizing factor) was first postulated by Robbins[102] in 1944 when he showed that fibrin formed from purified components was soluble in weak acids, while fibrin formed in the presence of serum or plasma resulted in formation of an insoluble clot. In 1960 Duckert et al.[103] described the first recognized case of a clinical bleeding diathesis due to congenital deficiency of this protein. Fibrin-stabilizing factor was given the designation factor XIII in 1963. Since its first description, >100 cases of factor XIII deficiency have been reported. No racial or ethnic group is disproportionately affected, and the incidence is estimated at one in several million.

Genetics and Molecular Biology

Factor XIII deficiency is inherited as an autosomal recessive trait. Heterozygotes are not affected with bleeding, although it is thought that heterozygous women may have a higher than normal incidence of spontaneous abortions than do normal women. The gene for the A subunit is reported to be at 6p24-25, near the HLA locus; the gene for the B subunit is located at 1q31-32.1.[104–107]

Factor XIII circulates in the plasma at a concentration of 10–20 μg/ml.[98] The protein exists in plasma as a tetramer consisting of two A subunits and two B subunits; each subunit has a molecular weight of about 85,000, and the complete protein has a molecular weight of approximately 330,000. Factor XIII catalyzes the cross-linkage between the γ-glutamyl and ε-lysyl groups of different fibrin strands, rendering the fibrin mesh rigid and insoluble. The catalytic activity of factor XIII resides in the A subunits. Although plasma factor XIII is synthesized in the liver, a dimer of the two A subunits (lacking the *B* unit but retaining activity) is produced in megakaryocytes and placental tissue. The A subunits of factor XIII from all cell lines are thought to be identical in structure and activity. The amino acid sequence of the A subunit and the nucleotide sequence of its complementary DNA have been determined.[108,109] Biochemical studies of the A subunit reveal that a reactive thiol group is unmasked by thrombin cleavage at the N terminus, and further thrombin cleavage at the C terminus inactivates the enzyme by disrupting a calmodulin-like calcium-binding site. The protein sequence and complementary DNA sequence of the B subunit, which has no enzymatic activity, reveals 10 repeating homologous domains that resemble those of β_2-glycoprotein I.[110] The B subunits are thought to act as carriers for the A subunits in plasma factor XIII.

Pathogenesis

Factor XIII deficiency correlates directly with the absence of A subunit activity. Two forms of factor XIII deficiency are known. In type I deficiency, both the A and B subunits are lacking, while in type II deficiency, the A subunit is lacking but the B subunit is present in nearly normal amounts.[111] The genetic mechanisms of these two patterns are unknown. Isolated deficiency of the B subunit has not been reported. Factor XIII deficiency has been reported as the result of acquired inhibitory antibodies; these have been reported most frequently in association with isoniazid use.[112]

Clinical Manifestations

The hallmarks of severe factor XIII deficiency are umbilical stump bleeding in the neonatal period; intracranial hemorrhage with little or no trauma; recurrent soft tissue hemorrhage with a tendency to form hemorrhagic cysts (pseudotumors); and, in women, recurrent spontaneous abortion. Men may also show oligospermia and infertility. The bleeding associated with factor XIII deficiency is usually associated with trauma, except in the case of intracranial hemorrhage, which may occur in the absence of known trauma. Intracranial hemorrhage is reported in ≤25% of patients in some series.[113] Surprisingly, bleeding at the time of surgery is not excessive, although delayed bleeding can occur. Poor wound healing is a common, characteristic feature of this disease. Unlike hemophilia A or B, hemarthroses do not occur.

Laboratory Evaluation

Factor XIII deficiency is marked by normal coagulation screening tests (PT, PTT, thrombin time, and bleeding time) despite a convincing history of bleeding. The most useful assays for factor XIII activity exploit the solubility of non-cross-linked fibrin clots in 5 M urea or weak organic acids. Clots formed in factor XIII-deficient plasma are soluble within minutes in such solutions, whereas normal clots remain insoluble for ≥24 hours. The test of solubility in 2% acetic acid is said to be more sensitive than solubility in 5 M urea, although the latter is more specific for factor XIII deficiency.[114] Other tests for factor XIII activity use measurements of incorporation of fluorescent amino acids into casein, or ammonia production by the amidase activity of factor XIII.[114]

Differential Diagnosis

The clinical presentation of factor XIII deficiency may be confused with abnormalities of fibrinogen that may also present with umbilical stump bleeding, soft tissue hemorrhage, and recurrent abortions. These two conditions may be readily distinguished on the basis of simple screening tests of coagulation, which are all abnormal with fibrinogen defects but normal with factor XIII deficiency. Specific factor XIII assays confirm the diagnosis.

Acquired partial factor XIII deficiency has been reported as a common feature associated with exacerbations of Henoch-Schönlein purpura. The deficiency of factor XIII seems to correlate with abdominal pain and bloody diarrhea. Infusions of factor XIII not only restore normal factor XIII levels, but also decrease the severity and duration of these symptoms during exacerbations.[115]

Therapy

Treatment of factor XIII deficiency is simplified because factor XIII has a long half-life (9 days) and minimal factor XIII activity (perhaps as little as 5%) is required to prevent bleeding complications.[116] Prophylactic therapy is practical for these reasons and is advisable due to the significant risk of intracranial hemorrhage in these patients. Prophylaxis can be accomplished by the use of fresh frozen plasma, given as 1 or 2 U (250–500 ml) every 4–6 weeks, or by administration of a factor XIII concentrate.[93] In one report, soft tissue hemorrhage occurred when the interval between prophylactic transfusions was >6 weeks.[116] There is a report of a factor XIII-deficient patient who suffered repeated spontaneous abortions until started on prophylactic plasma transfusions every 14 days or infusions of a commercial factor XIII concentrate every 21 days. The two pregnancies that followed were uncomplicated.[117] Long-term therapy with purified concentrates of factor XIII has been successful in the prevention of hemorrhagic complications.[93]

FAMILIAL MULTIPLE FACTOR DEFICIENCIES

A number of familial multiple factor deficiencies have been described (Table 110-9). Two of these syndromes (combined factor V/factor VIII deficiency and combined deficiency of factors II, VII, IX, and X) have been well characterized.[90,118]

Combined Factor V/Factor VIII Deficiency

In this syndrome factor V and VIII levels range between 5% and 15% of normal. Careful analysis of affected members of a number of different kindred suggests that the combined defect is due to a single genetic defect. It was initially proposed that the combined deficiency is due to a reduced level of protein C inhibitor, which permitted uncontrolled proteolysis of factor V and VIII by activated protein C. Subsequently, it has been shown that levels of the protein C inhibitor are normal in this disorder.[119] The specific genetic defect resulting in this syndrome is unknown.

Deficiency of Factors II, VII, IX, and X

There are several reports of patients with a combined congenital deficiency of factors II, VII, IX, and X. One of the first patients reported had a severe bleeding tendency requiring treatment with high doses of vitamin K.[120] In the one patient tested, protein C was also reduced. Malabsorption and other causes of vitamin K deficiency or surreptitious warfarin ingestion were convincingly excluded. Parents of affected children

Table 110-9. Familial Multiple Coagulation Factor Deficiencies

Type	Deficient Factors
I	V, VIII
II	VIII, IX
III	II, VII, IX, X
IV	VII, VIII
V	VIII, IX, XI
VI	IX, XI

have not been clinically affected, but parents of one affected child had markedly decreased urinary excretion of γ-carboxyglutamic acid, suggesting a defect in vitamin K-dependent carboxylation of glutamic acid residues in the vitamin K-dependent factors. The clotting defect in some patients has been partially corrected by vitamin K administration, although in other patients vitamin K has had no effect. The precise molecular defect responsible is unknown, but the available evidence suggests a genetic abnormality affecting hepatocyte vitamin K reductase or carboxylase, or defects in vitamin K transport or utilization.

REFERENCES

1. Shapiro SS, McCord S: Prothrombin. p. 177. In Spaet TH (ed): Progress in Hemostasis and Thrombosis. Grune & Stratton, Orlando, FL, 1978
2. Royle NJ, Irwin DM, Koschinsky ML et al: Human genes encoding prothrombin and ceruloplasmin map to 11p11-q12 and 3q21-q24, respectively. Somat Cell Mol Genet 13:285, 1987
3. Degen SJF: The prothrombin gene and its liver-specific expression. Semin Thromb Hemost 18:230, 1992
4. Kane WH, Davie EW: Blood coagulation factors V and VIII: structure and functional similarities and their relationship to hemorrhagic and thrombotic disorders. Blood 71:539, 1988
5. Rabiet MJ, Furie BC, Furie B: Molecular defect of prothrombin Barcelona. J Biol Chem 261:15045, 1986
6. Diuguid D, Rabiet MJ, Furie BC, Furie B: Molecular defects of factor IX Chicago-2 (Arg145 to His) and prothrombin Madrid (Arg271 to Cys): arginine mutations that preclude zymogen activation. Blood 74:193, 1989
7. Rocha E, Paramo JA, Bascones C et al: Prothrombin Segovia: a new congenital abnormality of prothrombin. Scand J Haematol 36:444, 1986
8. Miyata T, Aruga R, Umegama H et al: Prothrombin Salakta: substitution of glutamic acid-466 by alanine reduces the fibrinogen clotting activity and the esterase activity. Biochemistry 31:7457, 1992
9. Ruiz-Saez A, Luengo J, Rodriguez A et al: Prothrombin Perija: a new congenital dysprothrombinemia in an Indian family. Thromb Res 44:587, 1986
10. Kahn MJP, Govaerts A: Prothrombin Brussels, a new congenital defective protein. Thromb Res 5:141, 1974
11. Shapiro SS, Martinez J, Holburn RR: Congenital dysprothrombinemia: an inherited structural disorder of human prothrombin. J Clin Invest 48:2251, 1969
12. Girolami A, Bareggi G, Brunetti A, Sticchi A: Prothrombin Padua: a "new" congenital dysprothrombinemia. J Lab Clin Med 84:654, 1974
13. Huisse MG, Dreyfus M, Guillin MC: Prothrombin Clamart: prothrombin variant with defective Arg 322-Ile cleavage by factor Xa. Thromb Res 44:11, 1986
14. Lutzke G, Fricke U, Topfer G, Urban H: Hereditaine dysprothrombinamie mit geringen Blutunsneigung Prothrombin Magdeburg. Dtsch Med Wochenschr 114:288, 1989
15. Henriksen RA, Mann KG: Identification of the primary structural defect in the dysthrombin Quick I: substitution of cysteine for arginine-382. Biochemistry 279:9160, 1988
16. Henriksen RA, Mann KG: Substitution of valine for glycine 558 in the congenital dysthrombin Quick II alters primary substrate specificity. Biochemistry 28:2078, 1989
17. Valls-de-Ruiz M, Ruiz-Arguelles A, Ruiz-Arguelles GJ, Ambriz R: Prothrombin "Mexico City," an asymptomatic autosomal dominant prothrombin variant. Am J Hematol 24:229, 1987
18. Morishita E, Saito M, Kumabashiri I et al: Prothrombin Himi: a compound heterozygote for two dysfunctional prothrombin molecules (Met337 to Thr and Arg388 to His). Blood 80:2275, 1992
19. Rubio R, Almagro D, Cruz A, Corral JF: Prothrombin Habana: a new dysfunctional molecule of human prothrombin associated with a true prothrombin deficiency. Br J Haematol 54:553, 1983
20. Rabiet MJ, Jandrot-Periss M, Boissel JP et al: Thrombin Metz: characterization of the dysfunctional thrombin derived from a variant of human prothrombin. Blood 63:927, 1984
21. Rabiet MJ: Prothrombin Molise: a mutant prothrombin characterized by a defect in the thrombin domain. Thromb Haemost 54:46, 1985
22. Miyata T, Morita T, Inomoto T et al: Prothrombin Tokushima, a replacement of arginine-418 by tryptophan that impairs the fibrinogen clotting activity of derived thrombin Tokushima. Biochemistry 26:1117, 1987
23. Iwahana H, Yoshimoto K, Shigekiyo T et al: Molecular and genetic analysis of a compound heterozygote for dysprothrombinemia of a prothrombin Tokushima and hypothrombinemia. Am J Hum Genet 51:1386, 1992
24. Smith LG, Coone LAH, Kitchens CS: Prothrombin Gainesville. A dysprothrombinemia in a pair of identical twins. Am J Hematol 11:223, 1981
25. Weinger RS, Rudy C, Moake JL et al: Prothrombin Houston: a dysprothrombin identifiable by crossed immunoelectrofocusing and abnormal *Echis carinatus* venom activation. Blood 55:811, 1980
26. Baudo F, de Cataldo F, Josso F, Silvello L: Hereditary hypoprothrombinaemia. True deficiency of factor II. Acta Haematol 47:243, 1972
27. Guillin MC, Bezeaud A, Rabiet M-J, Elion J: Congenitally abnormal prothrombin and thrombin. Ann NY Acad Sci 485:56, 1986
28. Fleck RA, Rapaport SI, Rao LVM: Anti-prothrombin antibodies and the lupus anticoagulant. Blood 72:512, 1988
29. Bajaj SP, Rapaport SI, Barclay S, Herbst KD: Acquired hypoprothrombinemia due to nonneutralizing antibodies to prothrombin: mechanism and management. Blood 65:1538, 1985
30. Quick AJ: On the constitution of prothrombin. Am J Physiol 140:212, 1943
31. Owren PA: Parahaemophilia. Hemorrhagic diathesis due to absence of a previously unknown clotting factor. Lancet 1:446, 1947
32. Seeler RA: Parahemophilia. Factor V deficiency. Med Clin North Am 56:119, 1972
33. WHO Scientific Group: Inherited blood clotting disorders. Tech Rep Ser WHO 504:1, 1972
34. Cripe LD, Moore KD, Kane WH: Structure of the gene for human coagulation factor V. Biochemistry 31:3777, 1992
35. Tracy PB, Eide LL, Bowie EJW, Mann KG: Radioimmunoassay of factor V in human plasma and platelets. Blood 60:59, 1982
36. Tracy PB, Giles AR, Mann KG et al: Factor V (Quebec): a bleeding diathesis associated with a qualitative platelet factor V deficiency. J Clin Invest 74:1221, 1984
37. Rapaport SI, Zivelin A, Minow RA et al: Clinical significance of antibodies to bovine and human thrombin and factor V after surgical use of bovine thrombin. Am J Clin Pathol 97:84, 1991
38. Cmolik BL, Spero JA, Magovern GJ, Clark RE: Redo cardiac surgery: late bleeding complications from topical thrombin-induced factor V deficiency. J Thorac Cardiovasc Surg 105:222, 1993
39. Chediak J, Ashenhurst JB, Garlick I, Desser RK: Successful management of bleeding in a patient with factor V inhibitor by platelet transfusions. Blood 56:835, 1980
40. Webster WP, Roberts HR, Penick GD: Hemostasis in factor V deficiency. Am J Med Sci 248:194, 1964
41. Alexander B, Goldstein R, Landwehr G, Cook CD: Congenital SPCA deficiency: a hitherto unrecognized coagulation defect with hemorrhage rectified by serum and serum fractions. J Clin Invest 30:596, 1951
42. de Grouchy J, Dautzenberg M-D, Turleau C et al: Regional mapping of clotting factors VII and X to 13q34. Expression of factor VII through chromosome 8. Hum Genet 66:230, 1984
43. Fagan K, Wilkinson J, Allen M, Brownlee S: The coagulation factor VII regulator is located on 8p23.1. Hum Genet 79:365, 1988
44. O'Hara PJ, Grant FJ, Haldeman BA et al: Nucleotide sequence of the gene coding for human factor VII, a vitamin K-dependent protein participating in blood coagulation. Proc Natl Acad Sci USA 84:5158, 1987
45. Nemerson Y: Tissue factor and hemostasis. Blood 71:1, 1988
46. Rao LV, Rapaport SI: Activation of factor VII bound to tissue factor: a key early step in the tissue factor pathway of blood coagulation. Proc Natl Acad Sci USA 85:6687, 1988
47. Briet E, Onvlee G: Hip surgery in a patient with severe factor VII deficiency. Haemostasis 17:273, 1987
48. Ragni MV, Lewis JH, Spero JA, Hasiba U: Factor VII deficiency. Am J Hematol 10:79, 1981
49. Girolami A, Dal Bo Zanon R, Zanella F et al: Factor VII Padua defect: the heterozygote population. Acta Haematol 68:34, 1982
50. Girolami A, Cattarozzi G, Dal Bo Zanon R et al: Factor VII Padua$_2$: another factor VII abnormality with defective ox brain thromboplastin activation and a complex hereditary pattern. Blood 54:46, 1979
51. Girolami A, Falezza G, Patrassi G et al: Factor VII Verona coagulation disorder: double heterozygosis with an abnormal factor VII and heterozygous factor VII deficiency. Blood 50:603, 1977
52. Triplett DA, Brandt JT, Batard MA et al: Hereditary factor VII deficiency: heterogeneity defined by combined functional and immunochemical analysis. Blood 66:1284, 1985
53. Chen Q, Clarke BJ, Blajchman MA, Ofosu FA: Factor VII Hamilton: a novel type 2 mutation located at residue 57 in the first EGF domain of human factor VII, abstracted (2679). Thromb Haemost 69:1291, 1993
54. Kuppuswamy MN, Sabharwal AK, Birktoft JJ, Bajaj SP: Molecular characterization of human factor VII$_{Kansas}$ (GK 704): substitution of Gln^{100} by Arg in one allele and of Arg^{304} by Gln possibly in the other allele, abstracted (2680). Thromb Haemost 69:1292, 1993

55. James HL, Fink LM, Fair DS: Factor VII_{Little Rock} is dysfunctional due to an Arg^{304} to Gln substitution, abstracted (2683). Thromb Haemost 69:1292, 1993

56. Takamiya O, McVey JH, Kemball-Cook G, Tuddenham EGD: Dysfunctional human factor VII variants: detection of missense mutations by PCR and single-strand conformational polymorphisms (SSCP), abstracted (2687). Thromb Haemost 69:1291, 1993

57. Greene WB, McMillan CW: Surgery for scoliosis in congenital factor VII deficiency. Am J Dis Child 136:411, 1982

58. Ferster A, Capouet V, Deville A et al: Cardiac surgery with extracorporeal circulation in severe factor VII deficiency. Haemostasis 23:65, 1993

59. Robertson LE, Wasserstrum N, Banez E et al: Hereditary factor VII deficiency in pregnancy: peripartum treatment with factor VII concentrate. Am J Hematol 40:38, 1992

60. Yorke AJ, Mant MJ: Factor VII deficiency and surgery. Is preoperative replacement therapy necessary? JAMA 238:424, 1977

61. Hougie C, Barrow EM, Graham JB: Stuart clotting defect. I. Segregation of an hereditary hemorrhagic state from the heterogeneous group heretofore called "stable factor" (SPCA, proconvertin, factor VII) deficiency. J Clin Invest 36:485, 1956

62. Leytus SP, Foster DC, Kurachi K, Davie EW: Gene for human factor X: a blood coagulation factor whose gene organization is essentially identical with that of factor IX and protein C. Biochemistry 25:5098, 1986

63. Scambler PJ, Williamson R: The structural gene for human coagulation factor X is located on chromosome 13q34. Cytogenet Cell Genet 39:231, 1985

64. Miao CH, Leytus SP, Chung DW et al: Liver-specific expression of the gene coding for human factor X, a blood coagulation factor. J Biol Chem 267:7395, 1992

65. Watzke HH, Lechner K, Roberts HR et al: Molecular defect (Gla^{+14} to Lys) and its functional consequences in a hereditary factor X deficiency (Factor X "Vorarlberg"). J Biol Chem 265:11982, 1990

66. Reddy SV, Zhou Z-Q, Rao KJ et al: Molecular characterization of mutations causing human factor X_{SanAntonio}. Blood 74:1486, 1989

67. Watzke HH, Hilgartner M, Reddy SV et al: Factor X_{Santo Domingo}: a mutation in the signal peptide resulting in a severe bleeding diathesis. Blood 74:134a, 1989

68. Bernardi F, Marchetti G, Patracchini P et al: Partial gene deletion in a family with factor X deficiency. Blood 73:2123, 1989

69. Telfer TP, Denson KW, Wright DR: A "new" coagulation defect. Br J Haematol 2:308, 1956

70. Fair DS, Revak DJ, Hubbard JG, Girolami A: Isolation and characterization of the factor X Friuli variant. Blood 73:2108, 1989

71. Parkin JD, Madaras F, Sweet B, Castaldi PA: A further inherited variant of coagulation factor X. Aust NZ J Med 4:561, 1974

72. Girolami A, Vicarioto M, Ruzza G et al: Factor X Padua: a "new" congenital factor X abnormality with a defect only in the extrinsic system. Acta Haematol 73:31, 1985

73. De Stafano V, Leone G, Ferrelli R et al: Factor X Roma: a congenital factor X variant defective at different degrees in the intrinsic and extrinsic activation. Br J Haematol 69:387, 1988

74. Furie B, Greene E, Furie BC: Syndrome of acquired factor X deficiency in systemic amyloidosis. N Engl J Med 297:81, 1977

75. Camoriano JK, Greipp PR, Bayer GK, Bowie EJ: Resolution of acquired factor X deficiency and amyloidosis with melphalan and prednisone therapy. N Engl J Med 316:1133, 1987

76. Schwarzinger I, Stain-Kos M, Bettelheim P et al: Recurrent, isolated factor X deficiency in myeloma with repeated normalization of factor X levels after cytostatic chemotherapy followed by late treatment failure associated with development of systemic amyloidosis. Thromb Haemost 68:648, 1992

77. Greipp PR, Kyle RA, Bowie EJ: Factor X deficiency in primary amyloidosis: resolution after splenectomy. N Engl J Med 301:1050, 1979

78. Lankiewicz MW, Bell WR: A unique circulating inhibitor with specificity for coagulation factor X. Am J Med 93:343, 1992

79. Rosenthal RL, Dreskin OH, Rosenthal N: New hemophilia-like disease caused by deficiency of a third plasma thromboplastin factor. Proc Soc Exp Biol Med 82:171, 1953

80. Asakai R, Chung DW, Davie EW et al: Factor XI deficiency in Ashkenazi Jews. N Engl J Med 325:155, 1991

81. Seligsohn U: High gene frequency of factor XI (PTA) deficiency in Ashkenazi Jews. Blood 51:1223, 1978

82. Kato A, Asakai R, Davie EW et al: Factor XI gene (F11) is located on the distal end of the long arm of chromosome 4. Cytogenet Cell Genet 52:77, 1989

83. Fujikawa K, Chung DW, Hendrickson LE, Davie EW: Amino acid sequence of human factor XI, a blood coagulation factor with four tandem repeats that are highly homologous with plasma prekallikrein. Biochemistry 25:2417, 1986

84. Baglia FA, Jameson BA, Walsh PN: Fine mapping of the high molecular weight kininogen site on blood coagulation factor XI through the use of rationally designed synthetic analogs. J Biol Chem 267:4247, 1992

85. Baglia FA, Jameson BA, Walsh PN: Identification and chemical synthesis of a substrate-binding site for factor IX on coagulation factor XIa. J Biol Chem 266:24190, 1991

86. Asakai R, Chung DW, Ratnoff OD, Davie EW: Factor XI (plasma thromboplastin antecedent) deficiency in Ashkenazi Jews is a bleeding disorder that can result from three types of point mutations. Proc Natl Acad Sci USA 86:7667, 1989

87. Hancock JF, Wieland K, Pugh RE et al: A molecular genetic study of factor XI deficiency. Blood 77:1942, 1991

88. Lipscomb MS, Walsh PN: Human platelets and factor XI. Localization in platelet membranes of factor XI-like activity and its functional distinction from plasma factor XI. J Clin Invest 63:1006, 1979

89. Bolton-Maggs PHB, Wan-Yin BY, McCraw AH et al: Inheritance and bleeding in factor XI deficiency. Br J Haematol 69:521, 1988

90. Soff GA, Levin J, Bell WR: Combined factor IX and factor XI deficiency; familial multiple factor deficiency VI (FMFD VI). Semin Thromb Hemost 7:162, 1981

91. Kitchens CS, Alexander JA: Partial deficiency of coagulation factor XI as a newly recognized feature of Noonan syndrome. J Pediatr 102:224, 1983

92. Sharland M, Palton MA, Talbot S et al: Coagulation factor deficiencies and abnormal bleeding in Noonan's syndrome. Lancet 339:19, 1992

93. Stirling D, Ludlam CA: Therapeutic concentrates for the treatment of congenital deficiencies of factors VII, XI, XIII. Semin Thromb Hemost 19:48, 1993

94. Blatt PM, McFarland DH, Eifrig DE: Ophthalmic surgery and plasma thromboplastin antecedent (factor XI) deficiency. Arch Ophthalmol 98:863, 1980

95. Vander-Woude JC, Milam JD, Walker WE et al: Cardiovascular surgery in patients with congenital plasma coagulopathies. Ann Thorac Surg 46:283, 1988

96. Stern DM, Nossel HL, Owen J: Acquired antibody to factor XI in a patient with congenital factor XI deficiency. J Clin Invest 69:1270, 1982

97. Kaplan AP, Silverberg M: The coagulation-kinin pathway of human plasma. Blood 70:1, 1987

98. Ratnoff OD, Colopy JE: A familial hemorrhagic trait associated with a deficiency of a clot-promoting fraction of plasma. J Clin Invest 34:602, 1955

99. Lammle B, Wailleman WA, Huber I et al: Thromboembolism and bleeding tendency in congenital FXII deficiency—a study on 74 subjects from 14 Swiss families. Thromb Haemost 65:117, 1991

100. Donaldson VH, Mitchell BH, Everson B, Ratnoff O: Interactions of C1-inhibitors from normal persons and patients with type II hereditary angioneurotic edema with purified activated Hageman factor (factor XIIa). Blood 75:911, 1990

101. Hathaway WE, Belhasen LP, Hathaway HS: Evidence for a new plasma thromboplastin factor I. Case report, coagulation studies and physicochemical properties. Blood 26:521, 1965

102. Robbins KC: A study on the conversion of fibrinogen to fibrin. Am J Physiol 142:581, 1944

103. Duckert F, Jung E, Schmerling DH: A hitherto undescribed congenital haemorrhagic diathesis probably due to fibrin-stabilizing factor deficiency. Thromb Diath Haemorrh 5:179, 1960

104. Board PG, Webb GC, McKee J, Ichinose A: Localization of the coagulation factor XIII A subunit gene (F13A) to chromosome bands 6p24-p25. Cytogenet Cell Genet 28:25, 1988

105. Webb GC, Coggan M, Ichinose A, Board PG: Localization of the coagulation factor XIII B subunit gene (F13B) to chromosome bands 1q31-q32.1 and restriction fragment length polymorphism at the locus. Hum Genet 81:157, 1989

106. Ichinose A, Davie EW: Characterization of the gene for the a subunit of human factor XIII (plasma transglutaminase), a blood coagulation factor. Proc Natl Acad Sci USA 85:5829, 1988

107. Bottenus RE, Ichinose A, Davie EW: Nucleotide sequence of the gene for the B subunit of human factor XIII. Biochemistry 29:11195, 1990

108. Grundmann U, Amann E, Zettlmeissl G, Kupper HA: Characterization of cDNA coding for human factor XIIIa. Biochemistry 83:8024, 1986

109. Takahashi N, Takahashi Y, Putnam FW: Primary structure of blood coagulation factor XIIIa (fibrinoligase, transglutaminase) from human placenta. Proc Natl Acad Sci USA 83:8019, 1986

110. Lozier JN, Takahashi N, Putnam FW: Complete amino acid sequence of human beta$_2$ glycoprotein I. Proc Natl Acad Sci USA 81:3640, 1984

111. Girolami A, Cappellato MG, Lazzaro AR, Boscaro M: Type I and type II disease in congenital factor XIII deficiency. A further demonstration of the correctness of the classification. Blut 53:411, 1986

112. Graham JE, Yount WJ, Roberts HR: Immunochemical characteristics of a human antibody to factor XIII. Blood 41:661, 1973

113. Duckert F: Documentation of the plasma factor XIII deficiency in man. Ann NY Acad Sci 202:190, 1972

114. Francis JL: The detection and measurement of factor XIII activity: a review. Med Lab Sci 37:137, 1980

115. Hamitsuji H, Tani K, Yasui M et al: Activity of blood coagulation factor XIII as a prognostic indicator in patients with Henoch-Schönlein purpura. Eur J Pediatr 146:519, 1987

116. Fear JD, Miloszewski KJA, Losowsky MS: The half life of factor XIII in the management of inherited deficiency. Thromb Haemost 49:102, 1983

117. Rodeghiero F, Castaman GC, Di Bona E et al: Successful pregnancy in a woman with congenital factor XIII deficiency treated with substitutive therapy. Blut 55:45, 1987

118. Soff GA, Levin J: Familial multiple coagulation factor deficiencies. I. Review of the literature: differentiation of single hereditary disorders associated with multiple factor deficiencies from coincidental concurrence of single factor deficiency states. Semin Thromb Hemost 7:112. 1981

119. Canfield WN, Kisiel W: Evidence of normal levels of activated protein C inhibitor in combined factor V/VIII deficiency disease. J Clin Invest 70:1260, 1982

120. McMillan CW, Roberts HR: Congenital combined deficiency of coagulation factors II, VII, IX, and X. Report of a case. N Engl J Med 274:1313, 1966

Quantitative and Qualitative Disorders of Fibrinogen

111

José Martinez

INTRODUCTION

Human fibrinogen is a 340-kd glycoprotein that circulates in plasma at a concentration of approximately 300 mg/dl. The fibrinogen molecule is a dimer consisting of two identical halves, each composed of three nonidentical polypeptides termed the Aα, Bβ and γ-chains (Fig. 111-1). The halves of the molecule are connected at the amino-terminal central domain (N-terminal) by three interchain disulfide bonds, one linking the Aα chains and two linking the γ-chains. The two γ-chains are linked in an antiparallel manner.[1,2] The three polypeptides of each half of the fibrinogen molecule are also connected by a series of disulfide bridges.[1,2] Elucidation of the amino acid sequence of each chain[1-3] has shown the Aα chain to consist of 610, the Bβ chain of 461, and the γ-chain of 411 amino acids. Attached to the Bβ and γ-chains are four carbohydrate side chains, linked through N-acetylglucosamine to asparagine 52 of each γ-chain and Asn 364 of each Bβ chain; the Aα chain does not contain carbohydrate.[4] The molecular masses of the Aα, Bβ, and γ-chains (including amino acid and carbohydrate components) are 66.5, 54.3, and 48.5 kd, respectively.[2] Electron microscopic examination has revealed a trinodular structure with a central nodule linked through two thin rods to two peripheral nodules[5,6] (Fig. 111-1). This structure is consistent with results obtained by proteolytic cleavage of fibrinogen with cyanogen bromide or plasmin,[7,8] a process that yields a central dimeric fragment (fragment E) corresponding to the central nodule, and two peripheral monomeric fragments (fragments D) corresponding to the peripheral nodules visualized by electron microscopy (Fig. 111-1).

Plasma fibrinogen is synthesized exclusively by the hepatocyte,[9,10] and the synthesis of the three chains is under the coordinated control of three separate genes localized on chromosome 4.[11-14] Subsequent to assembly of the constituent polypeptide chains and the addition of carbohydrate side chains, the mature molecule is secreted into the circulation, where it manifests a half-life of 4 days and a fractional catabolic rate of 25%/day.[15,16]

Fibrinogen plays a central role in three major functional processes: (1) the soluble fibrinogen molecule is converted into insoluble fibrin during the process of blood coagulation; (2) the polymerized fibrin serves as a template for the localized assembly and activation of the fibrinolytic system, which modulates fibrin deposition and clot dissolution; and (3) fibrinogen binds to vascular cells such as platelets, where it supports platelet aggregation, and to endothelial cells, where it participates in tissue repair. The conversion of fibrinogen into insoluble fibrin can be divided into three distinct phases: (1) enzymatic cleavage of fibrinopeptides by thrombin, (2) fibrin polymerization, and (3) fibrin stabilization via covalent cross-linking by factor XIIIa. In the first phase, thrombin cleaves the Arg 16-Gly 17 bond of the Aα chain and the Arg 14-Gly 15 bond of the Bβ chain, resulting in the release of two molecules of fibrinopeptide A (FPA) and two of fibrinopeptide B (FPB) per molecule of fibrinogen.[17-19] Fibrinopeptide release from the constituent Aα and Bβ chains of fibrinogen results in the formation of fibrin monomer, the constituent chains of which are now referred to as the α-, β-, and γ-chains. Although the proteolytic cleavage of FPA and FPB by thrombin appears to be simultaneous, the cleavage of FPA actually occurs prior to, and more rapidly than, that of FPB.[17-19] Moreover, the cleavage of FPA is sufficient to induce clot formation, whereas the exclusive cleavage of FPB does not lead to fibrin formation under physiologic conditions.[20] This has been demonstrated by the use of specific snake venom enzymes, such as Arvin and reptilase, which cleave only FPA, and a copperhead venom enzyme that releases only FPB.[17-20] These enzymes are commonly used to study the functional properties of both normal and abnormal fibrinogens. The association of thrombin with fibrinogen is, in part, mediated through its catalytic site, as shown by nuclear magnetic resonance (NMR) and x-ray crystallographic studies of thrombin bound to a discrete segment of the N-terminal of the Aα chain. However, thrombin also binds to fibrin(ogen)

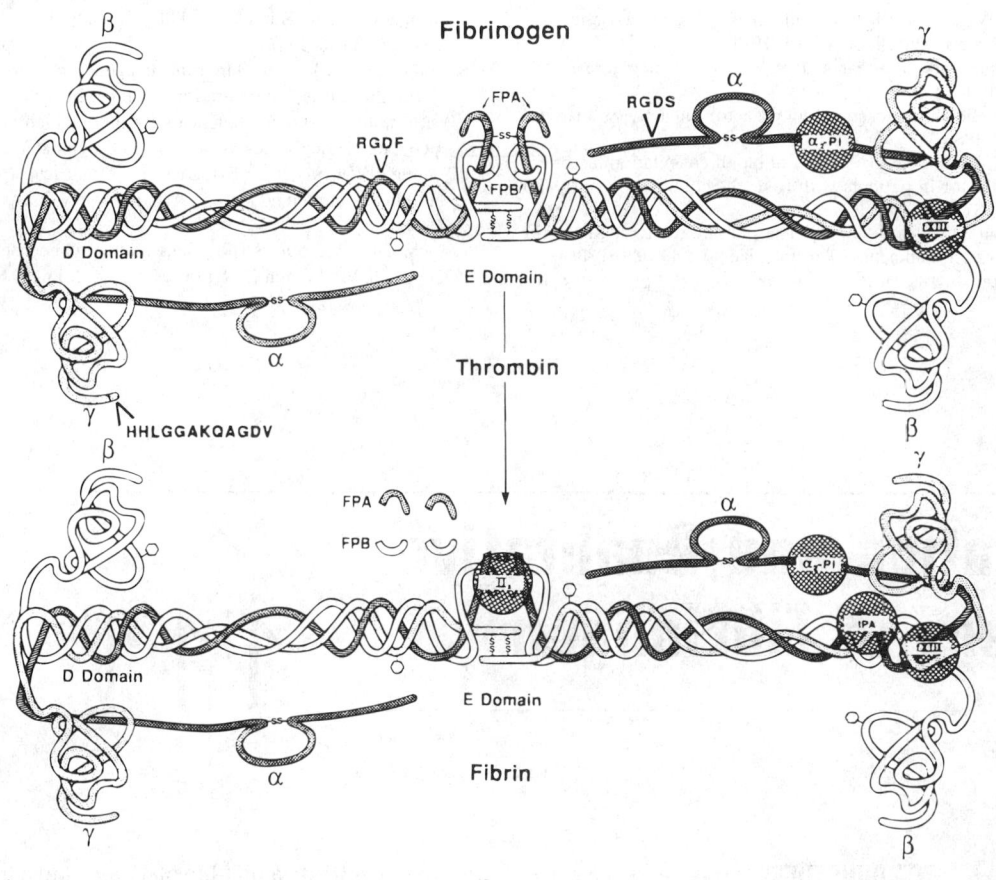

Fig. 111-1. Model of human fibrinogen and fibrin. Each half of the molecule is composed of three chains: Aα, Bβ, and γ. The NH2-terminal regions of the six chains are linked in the central domain (E domain) by disulfide bonds that form the dimer. In this region, fibrinopeptides A and B are cleaved from the Aα and Bβ chains, respectively, by thrombin, which converts fibrinogen into fibrin monomer. The two nodular regions at the C-terminal (D domain) contain the complementary binding sites for the central determinants exposed on release of the fibrinopeptides. Depicted are also segments of the fibrinogen molecule that bind t-PA, α2-antiplasmin, factor XIII, and of thrombin (IIa) to fibrin. The C-terminal γ-peptide and/or the RGD peptide of the C-terminal of the Aα chain intervene in the binding of fibrinogen with platelets and other cells. (Adapted from Mosesson,[23] with permission).

through a noncatalytic site called the fibrinogen recognition site, which binds to a locus formed by the N-terminus of the α-chain (α 27–50) and the N-terminus of the β-chain (β 15–42 and Ala 68).[20] This association is also abnormal in several fibrinogen mutants.[20]

In intact fibrinogen, the negatively charged fibrinopeptides play a role in maintaining the dispersion of individual fibrinogen molecules, because subsequent to their cleavage by thrombin the resulting fibrin monomers polymerize spontaneously. The polymerization process involves the reciprocal noncovalent interaction of molecular determinants in the fragment E region of the molecule, which are exposed by the removal of FPA, with complementary binding sites located in the fragment D region of an adjacent fibrin monomer. The resulting dimer, which is arranged in a half-staggered overlap (Fig. 111-2), continues to grow in length by the staggered addition of fibrin monomers, resulting in the formation of a two-stranded, half-staggered polymer referred to as a protofibril, the basic structural unit of the fibrin clot.[21–23] The half-staggered polymerization process brings two D domains of longitudinally aligned fibrin molecules of each row of the protofibril into close contact with one another, resulting in further stabilization of the noncovalently associated fibrin protofibril (Fig. 111-2). Polymerization continues with the formation of long, double-stranded protofibrils that ultimately associate laterally to form thick fibrin bundles.[22,23] The cleavage of FPB occurs mainly during the ini-

tial phase of fibrin polymerization and exposes determinants that are complementary with binding sites located in the C-terminal region of the α-chain.[23] This interaction seems to increase the rate of formation of thin fibrils, as well as the lateral aggregation to form thick fibrin fibers.[22–24] The three-dimensional fibrin matrix is completed by branching of the fibers at specific contact points located in the fiber bundles.[23] Several of the polymerization sites within fibrin have been identified. The N-terminus of the fibrin α-chain (α 17–20; GPRV) participates in the interaction of the A determinant with the complementary binding site located in fragment D, where a segment of the γ-chain 337–379 is known to participate in fibrin polymerization.[1,23,25] In addition, the N-terminus of the fibrin β-chain participates in the assembly of fibrin by binding to a complementary site located in the C-terminus of the Aα chain.[1,23]

The final stage of fibrin formation is characterized by the factor XIIIa-mediated formation of covalent amide bonds between the ε-amino groups of specific lysine residues and γ-CONH2 groups of certain glutamine residues[26] (see Ch. 100). These covalent bonds are first formed at the DD contact between the γ-chains of two molecules. The dimerization of the γ-chain formed by bridges between Lys 406 of one γ-chain and Gln 398 or 399 of another is then followed by progressive covalent cross-linking of multiple α-chains.[23,26,27] Cross-linking at branch points also produces D-trimers or D-tetramers.[23] As a result of this covalent stabilization, the clot is rendered more

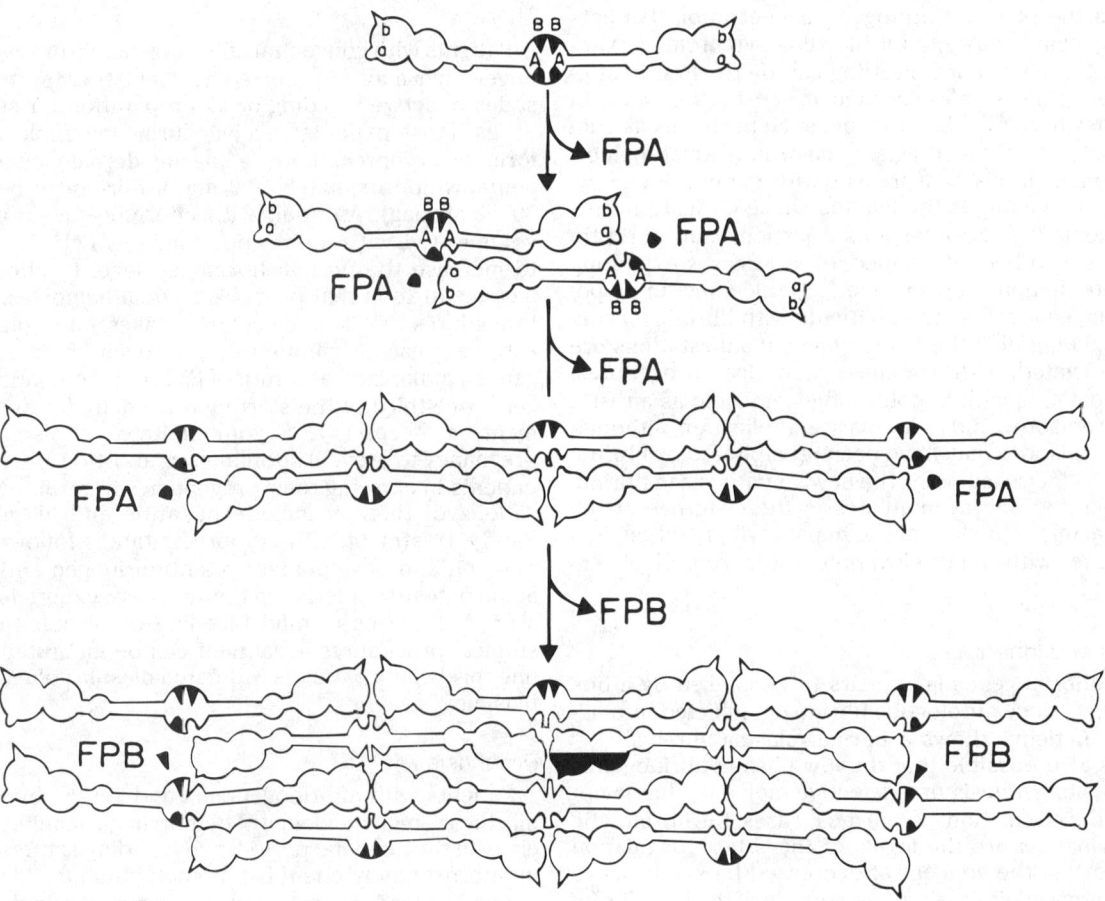

Fig. 111-2. Model of fibrin assembly showing two sets of complementary binding sites. The FPAs are represented by semicircles and the FPBs by triangles. After cleavage of the fibrinopeptides, the binding sites are exposed, the A site is represented by a circular hole and the B site by a triangular. Complementary to these sites in the E domain are those located in the D domain, represented by knobs; α-sites are circular knobs, while β-sites are triangular. After cleavage of fibrinopeptide A (FPA), the A site of the E domain of one molecule interacts with the a site of the D domain of another molecule forming a half-staggered overlap dimer. Additional fibrin monomer units associate through the CD contacts. The protofibril is formed by two rows linked by DD contacts, where the monomers of one row are arranged in a half-staggered overlap with respect to the monomers of the other row. Removal of FPB exposes the Bβ-sites, and this interaction promotes the lateral association of protofibrils into fibrin fibers. (Adapted from Weisel,[246] with permission.)

compact and resistant to both mechanical disruption and dissolution by plasmin.[28]

In addition to plasma fibrinogen, the circulating blood contains a very small pool of fibrinogen, which is present within the platelet α-granules. Some studies have shown that fibrinogen is synthesized by the megakaryocyte,[29] but more recent investigations have demonstrated that both megakaryocytes and platelets are capable of internalizing fibrinogen from plasma via a process mediated by glycoprotein IIb/IIIa.[30,31] Plasma fibrinogen exhibits γ-chain heterogeneity due to differential splicing of the hepatic mRNA.[3] This heterogeneity is manifested by the presence of a minor component, termed γ′, in which the last four amino acids of the γ-chain are replaced by an extended COOH-terminal sequence.[3] The γ′-chain is not present in platelet fibrinogen[32] and does not support platelet aggregation, probably due to the lack of interaction of γ′ with glycoprotein IIb/IIIa of the platelet.[23,33–35] Studies of families with various genetic dysfibrinogenemias have provided conflicting results concerning the presence of the mutant fibrinogen within the platelet. While fibrinogen Paris I was not found in platelets,[36] fibrinogen Oslo I was.[37] However, the discrepancy between the molecular and functional properties of plasma and platelet fibrinogen in these variants could depend on the ability of the platelet and megakaryocyte to internalize the abnormal fibrinogen. Platelet fibrinogen is secreted after stimulation and plays a role in supporting hemostasis.[38]

CLASSIFICATION OF FIBRINOGEN ABNORMALITIES

Fibrinogen abnormalities can be classified as being either congenital or acquired, with both groups manifesting quantitative defects (i.e., afibrinogenemia, hypofibrinogenemia, or hyperfibrinogenemia) or qualitative alterations of the fibrinogen molecule (dysfibrinogenemia). In a few instances, both quantitative and qualitative abnormalities can be present in the same patient (e.g., hypodysfibrinogenemia). The congenital disorders of fibrinogen are reviewed first, after which the acquired disorders are considered.

CONGENITAL DISORDERS

Afibrinogenemia and Hypofibrinogenemia

Congenital afibrinogenemia has been described in approximately 150 families,[39] but low levels of fibrinogen may have been undetected owing to the insensitivity of the methods used to quantitate the fibrinogen concentration. Less frequently, families with subnormal amounts of fibrinogen have been reported, and it is possible that the low fibrinogen concentration in some of these cases may have been associated with the presence of an abnormal molecule (i.e., hypodysfibrinogenemia).

Clinical manifestations in patients with fibrinogen disorders are related to the plasma fibrinogen concentration. Patients with afibrinogenemia may exhibit bleeding symptoms of variable severity. Umbilical cord bleeding can be the first hemorrhagic manifestation of this disorder; it can be the cause of death in the newborn.[39-41] Later in life, such problems as gum bleeding, epistaxis, menorrhagia,[42] gastrointestinal hemorrhage, and hemarthrosis can present with varying intensity, but intracranial bleeding is the leading cause of death in this group of patients.[40-43] Spontaneous abortions and abruptio placentae have also been described, even in cases exhibiting only moderate hypofibrinogenemia.[44-47] Bleeding in hypofibrinogenemia usually occurs in patients with fibrinogen concentrations <50 mg/dl[39]; the hemorrhagic manifestations are generally associated with trauma or surgical procedures. Oddly, some patients with hypofibrinogenemia die as a result of thrombotic episodes and pulmonary embolization, although some of these episodes may have been precipitated by fibrinogen infusions.[48-50] Occasionally, the newly synthesized fibrinogen is not secreted and accumulates in the cisternae of the rough endoplasmic reticulum of the hepatocyte, resulting in a storage disease with mild elevations of serum liver enzymes.[51-53]

Pathogenesis and Inheritance

Congenital afibrinogenemia appears to be caused by a biosynthetic defect, since autologous fibrinogen injected into afibrinogenemic patients shows a normal plasma survival.[54-56] However, it is also possible that the low plasma fibrinogen is caused by the biosynthesis of a defective molecule that is not secreted into the circulation.[51-53] In most cases, the fibrinolytic system is normal, as are the levels of the other coagulation factors, supporting the concept of decreased biosynthesis as opposed to increased utilization as the cause of the hypofibrinogenemia.

Afibrinogenemia is inherited as an autosomal recessive disorder; consanguinity is common in these families.[39,40] The inheritance pattern of hypofibrinogenemia is more complicated. In some families, the abnormality is present in only one parent, and inheritance seems to be dominant. In other families, low levels of fibrinogen in both parents suggest a recessive mode of transmission.[39,40] Analysis of the Aα-, Bβ-, and γ-chain genes in two families with afibrinogenemia failed to indicate any gross abnormalities such as deletions or gross rearrangements of these genes.[57]

Laboratory Findings

All tests based on the appearance of a fibrin clot are abnormal in those patients with afibrinogenemia and severe hypofibrinogenemia. These include the whole blood clotting time, the plasma recalcification time, the partial thromboplastin time (PTT), the prothrombin time (PT), and especially the thrombin time (TT) and reptilase time. These abnormalities can be corrected by addition of either normal plasma or purified normal fibrinogen. The definitive diagnosis is made by immunologic measurements of the fibrinogen concentration, which are sufficiently sensitive to detect nanogram quantities of fibrinogen per milliliter of plasma.[58,59] Measurements of fibrinogen as clottable protein are unreliable, since some abnormal fibrinogens do not convert into fibrin. In most cases of congenital afibrinogenemia, the platelet α-granules are also devoid of fibrinogen.[58] Other coagulation abnormalities in these patients include a prolonged bleeding time and abnormal platelet aggregation, especially with epinephrine and suboptimal concentrations of ADP.[59-61] Prolongation of the bleeding time and the defect in platelet aggregation can be corrected by the infusion of plasma or fibrinogen.[59-61] Mild thrombocytopenia has also been observed in a few families with congenital afibrinogenemia.[62]

Therapy

Patients with congenital afibrinogenemia or severe hypofibrinogenemia may require replacement therapy to control episodes of active bleeding or as preparation for surgical procedures. Most patients receive fibrinogen replacement in the form of cryoprecipitate, a plasma-derived concentrate that contains approximately 300 mg of fibrinogen per unit (i.e., a 30–50-ml bag). An adult with afibrinogenemia and a plasma volume of 3 L will require approximately 12 U of cryoprecipitate to increase the plasma fibrinogen level to about 100 mg/dl, a concentration that provides normal hemostasis for surgical procedures.[63,64] This calculation takes into consideration an extravascular distribution of fibrinogen of 30%. Since fibrinogen is catabolized at a rate of 25%/day, the patient should receive one-third of the starting dose daily for as long as treatment is necessary. Cryoprecipitate is also used during pregnancy to prevent spontaneous abortion and to assist these patients in carrying their pregnancies to term.[65] Major complications of therapy include hepatitis and allergic reactions. Rarely, treatment with cryoprecipitate is followed by allergic reaction and development of antifibrinogen antibodies.[40,42,66] Some patients undergoing therapy have experienced thrombosis.[48-50] In cases of mild bleeding or bleeding during minor surgical procedures, treatment can be instituted by replacing one-third of the patient's estimated plasma volume with normal plasma.

Prognosis

Patients with afibrinogenemia and severe hypofibrinogenemia have a high incidence of hemorrhagic manifestations, especially in the neonatal period; and bleeding is the cause of death in approximately one-third of such patients.[40] Full-term pregnancy is rare[40] except in those cases in which replacement therapy was instituted.[65] The availability of plasma and fibrinogen concentrates in the form of cryoprecipitate and the prompt treatment of bleeding complications should improve the survival of these patients; unfortunately some of these patients can develop antibodies to fibrinogen, rendering the treatment ineffective.

Congenital Dysfibrinogenemia

Congenital dysfibrinogenemia is characterized by the biosynthesis of a structurally abnormal fibrinogen molecule that exhibits altered functional properties and commonly exhibits an abnormal thrombin-mediated conversion to fibrin. The various mutants described carry the name of the city of origin of the patient initially affected with a particular dysfibrinogenemia.[67] Since the description of the first family with dysfibrinogenemia, fibrinogen Paris,[68] in 1964, >300 families with abnormal fibrinogens have been reported.[69,70] Roughly 60% of all cases exhibit no clinical manifestations, while hemorrhage occurs in 28%, thrombosis in about 20%, and hemorrhage and thrombosis in approximately 2% of cases. The abnormal fibrinogen has been rarely associated with impaired wound healing or spontaneous abortion.[69,73]

In >80 of these fibrinogen mutants, the molecular structural defect has been identified.[69,70] Approximately 55 mutations involve FPA and FPB and areas surrounding their cleavage sites, and approximately 20 variants involve the polymerization region of the γ-chain. In another 5 mutations, other regions of the fibrinogen molecule are involved.[69,70] One of the aims of the study of dysfibrinogenemias is to correlate structural abnormalities of the fibrinogen molecule with functional alterations that may or may not exhibit clinical symptoms. However, this type of correlation is often hampered by inadequate knowledge concerning the molecular aberration of fibrinogen. Furthermore, clinical manifestations such as mild post-traumatic bleeding or single episodes of thrombosis may be unrelated to the presence of the abnormal fibrinogen.

Functional abnormalities are usually reflected as abnormalities in one or more phases of the fibrinogen-to-fibrin conversion. These include (1) impaired release of fibrinopeptides, (2) defects in fibrin polymerization, or (3) failure of the polymerized fibrin to undergo normal covalent stabilization by factor XIIIa. In addition, abnormal fibrinogens that do not support proper assembly of the fibrinolytic system or that interact abnormally with platelets, endothelial cells, or calcium have also been described (see below).

The following discussion classifies congenital fibrinogen disorders on the basis of the most prominent functional abnormalities of the mutant molecules. Only those abnormal fibrinogens with known structural defects and/or very distinct functional or clinical properties are discussed. For a more complete listing of the many dysfibrinogenemias described, the reader is referred to several recent reviews.[69]

Biochemical Abnormalities and Clinical Manifestations

Abnormal Fibrinopeptide Release

The proteolytic phase of fibrinogen conversion to fibrin can be studied by a detailed analysis of the rate of release of FPA and FPB by thrombin or by snake venom enzymes which specifically cleave either FPA or FPB. The rates of cleavage can be followed by radioimmunoassays specific for each fibrinopeptide or by high-performance liquid chromatography. The isolation of proteolytic peptides by this technique, followed by peptide sequencing has allowed the characterization of structural

abnormalities of the fibrinopeptides and of other areas of the fibrinogen molecule. DNA sequencing also plays an important role in the identification of mutations of the three genes of fibrinogen. In some of the abnormal fibrinogens, FPA is not released by thrombin or is released at a slow rate; in others, the cleaved fibrinopeptide is structurally abnormal.[70] In addition to abnormal fibrinopeptide release, some congenital dysfibrinogenemias exhibit secondary delays in fibrin polymerization.

Fibrinogen Bethesda was the first mutant fibrinogen described as showing impaired release of fibrinopeptides associated with a mild bleeding disorder.[71] Fibrinogen Detroit was the first abnormal fibrinogen in which a specific amino acid substitution was identified.[72] The most common mutation site in the fibrinogen molecule is Arg 16 of the Aα chain (Table 111-1). Since thrombin cleaves the Arg 16-Gly 17 bond, the release of fibrinopeptide A from these mutant molecules is impaired. Two different substitutions have thus far been reported to occur at this position. Most commonly, Arg 16 is replaced by histidine forming a bond that is not cleaved by reptilase. Almost as frequent, Arg 16 is substituted by cysteine, and this bond is resistant to thrombin cleavage (Table 111-1). The replacement of arginine by cysteine changes the structure of the N-terminus of the mutant by forming an additional intramolecular Aα Cys 16-Aα Cys 16 disulfide bond.[103]

Most patients with Arg 16 substitutions are heterozygous. However, homozygous cases involving the two different substitutions at the arginine thrombin cleavage site manifest hemorrhagic disorders,[73,74] as exemplified by fibrinogens Metz,[92-94]

Table 111-1. Dysfibrinogenemias with Fibrinopeptide Release Abnormalities and a Known Structural Defect

												Aα-Chain Defects								
1 Ala	2 Asp	3 Ser	4 Gly	5 Glu	6 Gly	7 **Asp**	8 Phe	9 Leu	10 Ala	11 **Glu**	12 **Gly**	13 Gly	14 Gly	15 Val	16 **Arg**	17 **Gly**	18 Pro	19 **Arg**	20 Val

	Structural Defect	Clinical Data	Ref.			Structural Defect	Clinical Data	Ref.
Lille	Aα 7 Asp-Asn	Negative	82		Metz[a]	Aα 16 Arg-Cys	Bleeding	92–94
Mitaka II	Aα 11 Glu-Gly	Negative	84		Frankfurt II, III	Aα 16 Arg-Cys	Bleeding	80
Rouen	Aα 12 Gly-Val	Negative	83		Homburg III	Aα 16 Arg-Cys	Bleeding	69, 97
Bicêtre[a]	Aα 16 Arg-His	Bleeding	78		Ledyard	Aα 16 Arg-Cys	Bleeding[a]	98
Giessen I[a]	Aα 16 Arg-His	Bleeding	75, 76		Hershey II	Aα 16 Arg-Cys	Thrombosis?	99
Louisville	Aα 16 Arg-His	Bleeding	77		Amsterdam I	Aα 16 Arg-Cys	Negative	69, 80
Birmingham	Aα 16 Arg-His	Bleeding	79		Zürich I	Aα 16 Arg-Cys	Negative	69, 78
Chapel Hill II	Aα 16 Arg-His	Bleeding and thrombosis	80, 81		Stony Brook I	Aα 16 Arg-Cys	Negative	100
					Bergamo I	Aα 16 Arg-Cys	Negative	101
Barcelona II	Aα 16 Arg-His	Bleeding	85		Kawaguchi	Aα 16 Arg-Cys	Negative	102, 103
Stony Brook II	Aα 16 Arg-His	Bleeding	69, 86		Osaka I	Aα 16 Arg-Cys	Negative	102, 103
Petoskey	Aα 16 Arg-His	Negative	87		Bremen	Aα 17 Gly-Val	Bleeding	247
White Marsh	Aα 16 Arg-His	Negative	88		Detroit[a]	Aα 19 Arg-Ser	Bleeding	17, 72
Manchester	Aα 16 Arg-His	Negative	89		Munich I	Aα 19 Arg-Asn	Bleeding	78, 104
New Albany	Aα 16 Arg-His	Negative	69, 78		Mannheim I	Aα 19 Arg-Gly	Bleeding	105
Sydney I, II	Aα 16 Arg-His	Negative	69, 90		Aarhus[a]	Aα 19 Arg-Gly	Negative	106, 107
Bergamo III	Aα 16 Arg-His	Negative	91					
Amiens I	Aα 16 Arg-His	Negative	92					
Bern II	Aα 16 Arg-His	Negative	95					
Seattle II	Aα 16 Arg-His	Negative	96					

				Bβ-Chain Defects				
New York I	Deletion Bβ 9-27	Thrombosis	109, 110		Ise I	Bβ 15 Gly-Cys	Negative	114
Ijmuiden I	Bβ 14 Arg-Cys	Thrombosis	69, 111		Naples[a]	Bβ 68 Ala-Thr	Thrombosis	115–117
Christchurch II	Bβ 14 Arg-Cys	Negative	112					
Seattle I	Bβ 14 Arg-Cys	Negative	113					

[a] Homozygous.

Giessen I,[75,76] and Bicêtre.[78] Some heterozygous individuals also have had bleeding symptoms due, for example, to fibrinogens Birmingham and Chapel II, but the first mutant was associated with abnormal von Willebrand factor,[79] and in the second case other defects such as impaired cross-linking could have contributed to the hemorrhagic tendency.[80,81] Heterozygous individuals with approximately 50% normal fibrinogen should not have bleeding manifestations, but most of these mutants inhibit the conversion of the normal fibrinogen to fibrin, and this inhibition may play a role in the bleeding tendency.

Fibrinogens Detroit[17,72] and Munich[78,104] involve substitutions at Aα Arg 19 by serine and asparagine, respectively, while in two other mutants—fibrinogens Mannheim[105] and Aarhus[106,107]—Aα Arg 19 is substituted by glycine. With the exception of patients with fibrinogen Aarhus, substitutions at Aα Arg 19 are associated with hemorrhagic tendency (Table 111-1).

Since this area of the α-chain is involved in fibrin polymerization subsequent to FPA release, these mutants show a marked delay in the rate of fibrin polymerization. The delayed release of FPB reported for fibrinogen Detroit probably occurs secondary to defective polymerization related to the Arg 19 substitution.[17] Similarly, fibrinogens Aarhus and Mannheim, which involve a glycine substitution at Arg 19, display a defective release of fibrinopeptides and impaired polymerization.[105-107] Three mutants with substitutions within FPA (Table 111-1)—fibrinogens Lille, Rouen, and Mytaka II—manifest defective cleavage of FPA,[82-84] which is probably due to impaired binding of thrombin to this region of the Aα chain.[108]

Abnormal cleavage of fibrinopeptides has also been observed in fibrinogen mutations involving the N-terminal region of the Bβ chain. A unique abnormality is present in fibrinogen New York, characterized by the slow release of fibrinopeptide A and by a 50% decrease in total release of FPB, associated with delayed polymerization. The biochemical defect is a deletion of amino acids 9–72 of the Bβ chain, a segment that includes part of FPB (amino acids 1–14) and of a plasmin-derived peptide (amino acids 1–42). Transcriptionally, the deleted segment of the polypeptide corresponds to exon 2 of the Bβ-chain gene.[110] The clinical expression of this abnormal fibrinogen is a tendency to thrombosis[109] (see below). Fibrinogens Christchurch II,[112] Seattle I, [113] and Ijmuiden[111] have a substitution at the thrombin cleavage site Arg 14-Gly 15 of the Bβ chain. In these cases, Arg 14 is replaced by cysteine, resulting in a 50% decrease in total FPB release, indicating a heterozygous condition. In fibrinogen Ijmuiden, the additional cysteines present in the mutant either form disulfide bridges between fibrinogen and albumin or remain as free sulfhydryl groups.[111] These mutants show delayed fibrin polymerization, which confirms a role for the exposure of a polymerization site in the Bβ chain subsequent to the cleavage of FPB.[17] The examples described above illustrate the relationship between cleavage of fibrinopeptides and fibrin polymerization. In addition, fibrinogen Ijmuiden seems to exhibit an impaired activation of plasminogen by tissue plasminogen activator (t-PA).[69,111] In fibrinogen Ise (Bβ Gly 15-Cys), the release of fibrinopeptide B is markedly impaired, and this mutant, which is clinically silent, also shows defective polymerization.[114] Several members of fibrinogen Naples (same family as Milano II) were affected by venous and arterial thromboses. Characterization of the abnormal fibrinogen by DNA analysis shows a GCT-to-ACT mutation, which results in the substitution of Bβ Ala 68 by threonine. The possible correlation between defective thrombin binding and thrombosis is discussed below.[115-117]

Other mutants functionally characterized by impaired fibrinopeptide release (but with unknown structural defects) may also express clinical bleeding or thrombosis, or both.[69,74] For example, fibrinogens Bethesda I,[71] Cleveland II,[118] and New Orleans[119] show an increased tendency to bleed. Fibrinogen St. Louis was associated, in the propositus, with hemophilia A; however, the abnormal fibrinogen did not induce a bleeding disorder in other family members.[120] By contrast, other mutants, such as fibrinogen Charlottesville,[121] show a tendency to thrombosis exclusively.

Polymerization Defects

In patients with polymerization defects, the abnormal fibrinogens exhibit a primary delay in fibrin polymerization without an obvious abnormality in fibrinopeptide release. Although the patients show an increased tendency to hemorrhage, some present with thrombosis, spontaneous abortion, or rarely, wound dehiscence. The structural aberrations usually occur in the N- or C-terminal regions of the Aα and Bβ chains or toward the C-terminal regions of the γ-chains (Table 111-2). The first group is exemplified by fibrinogens Kyoto II and Kanazawa, in which the Aα Pro 18 is replaced by leucine.[122,123] Mutations toward the C-terminus affect fibrin polymerization as shown in fibrinogen Lima, a homozygous Aα Arg 141-Ser mutant that is associated with a mild bleeding disorder.[124] Fibrinogen Lima represents one of several dysfibrinogenemias where an amino acid substitution results in the formation of a new consensus sequence for the attachment of an additional N-linked oligosaccharide (Table 111-2). In the case of fibrinogen Lima, the polymerization defect appears to be due to an increased content of sialic acid, since the removal of this monosaccharide markedly improved the rate of fibrin polymerization. Increased content of sialic acid, although without additional N-linked oligosaccharides, has been previously demonstrated to be responsible for the functional abnormality of the dysfibrinogenemia of liver disease (see the section Acquired Abnormalities of Dysfibrinogenemias). In fibrinogen Dusart (Paris V), the Aα Arg 554 is replaced by cysteine, resulting in the formation of disulfide bonds, which link fibrinogen to albumin.[126] The linkage of albumin to fibrinogen may be responsible for inhibition of fibrin polymerization, decrease in plasminogen binding, and results in defective t-PA-induced activation of bound plasminogen.[127,128] It is likely that the defect in the assembly and activation of the fibrinolytic system on the mutant fibrinogen is responsible for the severe thrombotic tendency of affected individuals.[126-128]

Fibrinogens Nijmegen and Pontoise involve mutations of the Bβ chain. In fibrinogen Nijmegen, Bβ Arg 64 is replaced by cysteine, resulting in complexation with albumin and other proteins. A portion of mutant molecules contain free sulfhydryl groups.[111] The formation of fibrinogen/protein complexes along with the free sulfhydryl groups could account for the observed alterations in fibrin polymerization and t-PA-induced activation of plasminogen bound to the mutant.[129] In fibrinogen Pontoise, Bβ Ala 335 is replaced by threonine,[78,130] resulting in the expression of a new N-linked glycosylation site since asparagine is present at position 333.[130]

Mutations in the γ-chain are more common than mutations of the Bβ chain. These include an Arg 275 substitution for histidine, which occurs in six abnormal fibrinogens (Table 111-2). Of these mutants, fibrinogen Haifa exhibits bleeding and thrombosis,[131,132] while fibrinogen Bergamo II has been associated with thrombosis.[133] In the four other dysfibrinogenemias, fibrinogen Tochigi,[135] Osaka III,[132] Baltimore IV,[137] and Tokyo II,[138,139] Arg 275 of the γ-chain is replaced by cysteine, but the affected members were asymptomatic. In fibrinogen Kyoto I, γ Asn 308 is substituted by lysine, resulting in the formation of a new plasmin cleavage and shortening of the γ-chain.[140,141] Although fibrinogens Milano I,[142] Baltimore III,[143] Kyoto III,[144] and Nagoya[145] manifest different amino acid substitutions at the C-terminus of the γ-chain (Table 111-2), causing a defect in fibrin polymerization, each of these mutants is clinically silent. Mutation at γ Met 310 with threonine in fibrinogen Asahi I introduces a new consensus for an additional N-linked glycosylation site at Asn 308.[146,157] The bleeding disorder may be due to the additional oligosaccharide that could be responsible for inhibiting fibrin polymerization and cross-linking.[146,157] Fibrinogen

Table 111-2. Dysfibrinogenemias with Polymerization Abnormalities and Known Structural Defect

	Structural Defect	Clinical Data	Ref.		Structural Defect	Clinical Data	Ref.
				Aα Chain Defects[b]			
Kyoto II	Aα 18 Pro-Leu	Bleeding?	122	Caracas II	Aα 434 Ser-Asn	Negative	125
Kanazawa	Aα 18 Pro-Leu	Negative	123		Additional N-linkage of oligosaccharide		
Lima[a]	Aα 141 Arg-Ser Additional N-linkage of oligosaccharide	Bleeding	124	Dusart (Paris V)	Aα 554 Arg-Cys	Thrombosis	126–128
				Bβ Chain Defects			
Nijmegen	Bβ 64 Arg-Cys	Thrombosis	111, 129	Pontoise	Bβ 335 Ala-Thr Additional N-linkage of oligosaccharide	Negative	78, 130
				γ-Chain Defects			
Haifa	γ 275 Arg-His	Bleeding, thrombosis	69, 131	Baltimore I	γ 292 Gly-Val	Bleeding, thrombosis	67, 147, 148
Bergamo II	γ 275 Arg-His	Thrombosis	133	Baltimore III	γ 308 Asn-Ile	Negative	69, 143
Essen	γ 275 Arg-His	Negative	133	Kyoto I	γ 308 Asn-Lys with new plasmin cleavage and shortening of chain	Negative	140, 141
Perugia	γ 275 Arg-His	Negative	133	Nagoya	γ 329 Gln-Arg	Negative	145
Saga	γ 275 Arg-His	Negative	134	Milano I	γ 330 Asp-Val	Negative	142
Osaka III	γ 275 Arg-Cys	Negative	132	Kyoto III	γ 330 Asp-Tyr	Negative	144
Baltimore IV	γ 275 Arg-Cys	Negative	137	Asahi I	γ 310 Met-Thr Additional N-linkage of oligosaccharide	Bleeding	146, 157
Osaka II	γ 275 Arg-Cys	Unknown	136				
Tochigi	γ 275 Arg-Cys	Negative	135	Bern I	γ 337 Asn-Lys	Negative	248
Tokyo II	γ 275 Arg-Cys	Negative	138, 139	Vlissingen I	γ-Deletion 319–320	Thrombosis	151
				Paris I	γ-Chain elongation	Wound dehiscence	69, 149, 150

[a] Homozygous.
[b] Includes abnormal fibrinogen Aα 526 Val-Glu, which demonstrates normal clotting and is clinically manifested by hereditary renal amyloidosis.[249]

Baltimore I, one of the first dysfibrinogenemias described,[67] is functionally characterized by a decrease in fibrin polymerization due to γ Gly 292-to-Val substitution.[147,148] Certain dysfibrinogenemias are structurally characterized by deletions or elongation of the γ-chain. The prototype of this group is fibrinogen Paris I, a mutant in which the elongated γ-chain is responsible both for delayed polymerization and for abnormal factor XIIIa-mediated cross-linking.[68,149,150] Fibrinogen Vlissingen is structurally characterized by a six-base deletion encoding amino acids γ Asn 319 and Asp 320.[151] This mutant exhibits defects in fibrin polymerization and calcium binding. Clinically, it appears to be associated with thrombotic tendency.[151]

Some abnormal fibrinogens that exhibit defective fibrin monomer polymerization but for which the structural defects are unknown may be associated with bleeding, thrombosis, delayed wound healing, repeated spontaneous abortions, or combinations of these manifestations. For example, fibrinogens Houston[152] and Montreal II[153] are associated with bleeding tendency. Fibrinogen Houston, in addition to exhibiting abnormal fibrin monomer polymerization, also manifests deficient factor XIIIa-mediated cross-linking of α-chains and a circulating inhibitor, which may play a role in the hemorrhagic disorder observed in the patient.[152] Bleeding and delayed wound healing occur in patients with fibrinogen Caracas I.[154]

It is interesting to note that several mutants which are functionally characterized by impaired fibrin polymerization display an increased tendency to thrombosis. Among these are fibrinogen Chapel Hill III[155] and Pamploma II,[156] which also exhibit impaired release of FPB. The possible mechanisms responsible for thrombosis are discussed below.

Defective Cross-linking

Although no abnormal fibrinogens are characterized exclusively by defective factor XIIIa-mediated cross-linking, several mutants exhibit defective cross-linking in addition to abnormal-

ities of fibrinopeptide release or fibrin polymerization. A noted example is fibrinogen Paris I, which exhibits defective γ-chain cross-linking along with delayed polymerization. Both of these functional abnormalities are the result of the extended γ-chain.[149,150] Fibrinogen Asahi I contains additional N-linked carbohydrate in the C-terminus of the γ-chain and also shows a delay in the formation of γ-chain cross-linking.[146,157] Fibrinogen Oklahoma was initially reported to be a mutant with a defect in cross-linking[158]; however, recent studies have shown fibrinogen Oklahoma to have a normal fibrin cross-linking pattern along with an increased sensitivity of clots to plasmin degradation.[159]

Hypodysfibrinogenemias

Congenital hypodysfibrinogenemia includes those cases in which structurally abnormal fibrinogens with altered functional activity are present with total plasma fibrinogen concentrations arbitrarily defined as <150 mg/dl, as measured immunologically or by other physicochemical methods. Measurements of clottable protein are not reliable, since the abnormal molecules do not always incorporate into the clot. About 15 hypodysfibrinogenemias have been fairly well characterized (Table 111-3). In the first clear case of hypodysfibrinogenemia, involving fibrinogen Parma,[160] the patient had a severe bleeding disorder that was corrected by the infusion of normal fibrinogen, which seemed to exhibit a normal plasma survival (Table 111-3). By contrast, fibrinogens Philadelphia[16] and Bethesda III[161] have almost identical properties, including normal fibrinopeptide release, defective fibrin polymerization, and increased catabolic rate of the autologous protein, but normal survival of the homologous protein. These findings indicate that an intrinsic molecular defect of the mutant fibrinogen is responsible for the observed hypercatabolism leading to the hypofibrinogenemia.[17,161]

By contrast, patients with fibrinogen Giessen II show de-

Table 111-3. Congenital Hypodysfibrinogenemias

	Plasma Fibrinogen Concentration (mg/dl)	Fibrinogen Half-life (hr)		Functional Defect(s)	Clinical Data	Reference
		Homologous	Autologous			
Parma	60–75	Probably normal	—	Unknown	Bleeding	160
Philadelphia I	45–78	72	38	Polymerization	Bleeding	16
Bethesda III	100–120	80	34	Polymerization	Bleeding, abortions	161
Giessen II	50	56	—	FPA release, polymerization	Bleeding	162
Chapel Hill I	115–131	65	72	Polymerization	Bleeding	163
Baltimore II	62–96	90	81	FPB release	Negative	164
Malmöe	70	67	—	FPA, FPB release, polymerization	Thrombosis	165
Grand Rapids	120	—	—	FPA, FPB release, polymerization	Negative	167
Adelaide	120–114	—	—	Polymerization?	Bleeding	168
San Juan	50–74	—	—	Unknown	Mild bleeding, von Willebrand disease	169
Valencia	87–90	—	—	Unknown	Bleeding	170
Marburg[a,b]	60	—	—	Polymerization	Thrombosis	166
London II	130	—	—	Polymerization	Thrombosis	172
Alba/Geneva	15–60	—	—	Polymerization	Negative	69, 173
Bern I	140	—	—	Polymerization	Negative	174
Argenteuil	120–150	—	—	FBA release	Thrombosis, protein C deficiency	171
Normal	190–400	72–90	72–90			

[a] Homozygous.
[b] Deletion Aα 461–610.

creased survival of the homologous (normal) protein, indicating an extrinsic (plasmin-like) factor is responsible for mediating the hypercatabolism of fibrinogen.[162] Fibrinogens Chapel Hill I[163] and Baltimore II[164] also show normal survival of both the homologous and autologous proteins, indicating that either a low biosynthetic rate or impaired secretion, or both, are responsible for the hypofibrinogenemia. Fibrinogen Marburg is structurally characterized by deletion of amino acids 461–610 of the Aα chain as the result of a single-base substitution A to T, forming TAA stop codon.[166] The mutant fibrinogen exhibits delayed fibrin polymerization and appears to be disulfide linked to albumin. The abnormal protein did not support the attachment of endothelial cells, suggesting that the RGD peptide of the C-terminus of the normal Aα chain is important in this process.[166]

The functional defect in hypodysfibrinogenemias is heterogeneous; delayed fibrin polymerization is the predominant defect, but abnormal release of fibrinopeptides is also seen (Table 111-3). The major clinical expression in hypodysfibrinogenemia is bleeding, but repeated spontaneous abortions and thrombosis have also been reported (Table 111-3).

Pathogenesis of Thrombosis and Delayed Wound Healing

Approximately 45 dysfibrinogenemias that predispose to arterial or venous thrombosis, or both, have been described. Although some of the affected individuals experienced isolated thrombotic episodes, these may have been unrelated to the abnormal fibrinogen.[73,74] In other cases, frequent episodes of arterial and/or venous thrombosis in a particular patient or in several of the affected family members suggest a causal relationship. Although the mechanisms by which the abnormal fibrinogens promote thrombus formation are largely unknown, analysis of the biochemical properties of the mutant molecules may offer some clues. Fibrinogen Oslo I, in contradistinction to other mutants causing dysfibrinogenemia, exhibits a shortened TT and also renders platelets hyperaggregatable in response to ADP stimulation.[175,176] Several mutant fibrinogens have an impaired ability to bind thrombin, and the excess free thrombin

is available to interact with normal fibrinogen molecules and/ or to induce platelet activation, leading to the formation of platelet aggregates. Fibrinogens New York,[109,110] Malmöe,[165] Naples,[115–117] and Pamplona II,[156] which also exhibits impaired release of FPB, belong to this group. In other cases, increased thrombosis may be the result of defective fibrinolysis as a result of impaired plasminogen activation or increased resistance of the mutant molecule to cleavage by plasmin. Indeed, fibrinogens Dusart,[126–128] Nijmegen,[111,129] Ijmuiden,[111] and Pamplona II[156] exhibit decreased plasminogen binding and defective t-PA activation of the bound plasminogen. Although these mutants also show abnormal conversion of fibrinogen to fibrin, their thrombotic tendency may be related to the defective assembly or activation of the fibrinolytic system. Mutant fibrinogens that exhibit increased resistance to plasmin proteolysis include fibrinogens Chapel Hill II and Chapel Hill III.[80,81,155] Two fibrinogens with substitutions at γ Arg 275 by histidine, fibrinogens Haifa[69,131] and Bergamo II,[133] also manifest thrombotic complications. Furthermore, the plasmic derivative fragment D derived from fibrinogen Haifa is abnormal, which raises the possibility of abnormal fibrinolysis.[69,131]

Other clinical manifestations of dysfibrinogenemias include delayed wound healing and wound dehiscence, as reported for fibrinogens Paris I,[69,149,150] Cleveland I,[177] Caracas I,[154] and Buenos Aires I.[178] The abnormal factor XIIIa-mediated cross-linking of these mutants and the resulting decreased strength of the clots may be responsible for the healing abnormalities. Patients with factor XIII deficiency also manifest defects of the healing process. Recurrent spontaneous abortions (mainly in the first trimester) associated with bleeding or thrombosis have also been reported in several dysfibrinogenemias (Tables 111-1 to 111-3).

Inheritance

Although the vast majority of dysfibrinogenemias are heterozygous, the homozygous condition with no normal fibrinogen has been documented in approximately 11 families. In the case of fibrinogen Metz, the parents were consanguineous and the condition in the propositus was homozygous.[92–94] Similar findings have been reported for fibrinogen Detroit[17,72] among others (Tables 111-1 to 111-3). Some mutants release only 50% of either FPA or FPB[69,70]; in other instances, the amino acid substitution is also present in one-half the molecules.[69,70] Using immunologic, electrophoretic, and chromatographic methods, two distinct populations of fibrinogen have been identified in several mutants.[69]

Laboratory Evaluation

Abnormalities in routine coagulation assays, particularly the PT or PTT, usually provide the first evidence for the presence of an abnormal fibrinogen. The PT is more sensitive than the PTT, but an even more sensitive and specific test is the TT, which in some patients is so prolonged that a visible clot never forms. The reptilase and ancrod times are also useful diagnostic tests when dysfibrinogenemia is suspected, frequently being more abnormal than the TT.[69,73,74] This prolongation occurs uniformly among the dysfibrinogenemias, with the outstanding exception of fibrinogen Oslo I, which shows a shortened TT.[175] Measurement of the plasma fibrinogen concentration in patients with dysfibrinogenemia can give variable results, depending on the type of analytic method used. Frequently, the fibrinogen concentration appears low when measured as clottable protein, especially when methods based on the rate of fibrin formation are used.[73,74] This may be because several of the abnormal fibrinogens have an inhibitory effect on the clotting of normal plasma. Furthermore, because the abnormal fibrinogen may not be incorporated into the clot, the soluble molecules that remain in serum can be mistaken for fibrin degradation products, which thereby leads to the misdiagnosis of an active fibrinolytic system, as in disseminated intravascular coagulation (DIC). In most cases of dysfibrinogenemia, the plasma fibrinogen concentration is actually normal when measured immunologically, and the discrepancy between clottable protein and immunologically measured fibrinogen is a characteristic feature of dysfibrinogenemia. In some instances, however, the abnormal fibrinogen is in fact present in low amounts, as in the hypodysfibrinogenemias. Although the levels of other coagulation factors are usually normal, some dysfibrinogenemias are associated with defects in other specific coagulation factors. For example, fibrinogen St. Louis is associated with factor VIII deficiency,[120] fibrinogens San Juan and Birmingham with deficiency of von Willebrand factor,[79,169] fibrinogen Chapel Hill III with a modest reduction in factor XIII,[155] and fibrinogen Argenteuil with decreased levels of protein C.[17] These associated deficiencies can be clinically important, since hemorrhagic and/or thrombotic manifestations may actually be independent of the abnormal fibrinogen. Accordingly, therapeutic measures should be directed toward correction of the concomitant coagulation abnormalities.

Therapy and Prognosis

Most patients with congenital dysfibrinogenemia are asymptomatic and do not require treatment. Active bleeding can be corrected with replacement therapy; and in those patients with a history of bleeding, replacement therapy can be instituted before surgery or procedures that involve a high risk of hemorrhage. Replacement therapy using plasma or cryoprecipitate can be prescribed according to the guidelines outlined in the afibrinogenemia section. It appears that thrombotic complications were responsible for the death of several patients. In those patients who present with thrombosis, anticoagulant therapy should be recommended on the basis of criteria similar to those of other hypercoagulable states. Recurrent spontaneous abortions have been reported in several families, but continuous replacement of fibrinogen in the form of cryoprecipitate may permit full-term pregnancy.

ACQUIRED ABNORMALITIES OF FIBRINOGEN

Acquired abnormalities of fibrinogen may be classified into three groups: (1) hyperfibrinogenemia, (2) hypofibrinogenemia and (3) dysfibrinogenemia.

Hyperfibrinogenemia

Plasma fibrinogen levels increase significantly with age, with life-style habits such as cigarette smoking, and in certain pathologic conditions, such as hypertension, obesity, and diabetes mellitus.[179-184] However, even among normal individuals, the plasma fibrinogen concentration varies and, although the exact regulatory mechanism is unknown, recent studies indicate that fibrinogen levels may be genetically controlled. For example, high plasma fibrinogen concentrations have been observed in normal individuals exhibiting a specific nucleotide sequence polymorphism at the 5' untranslated region of the Bβ gene.[185,186] Because synthesis of the Bβ chain seems to be a rate-limiting step in fibrinogen biosynthesis,[187] increased transcription of this gene is likely to result in higher levels of fibrinogen. However, this polymorphic site is present in only a minority of the population.[185,186] By contrast, in most individuals fibrinogen behaves as an acute-phase reactant protein; therefore, its concentration is sensitive to inflammatory responses.[188] In this process, the release of interleukin-6 by macrophages leads to an increase in transcription of the Bβ gene, resulting in elevated levels of fibrinogen.[189,190] It is also possible that a genetic polymorphism distinct from that in the 5'-untranslated region described above and located within the interleukin-6-responsive element may play an important role in setting the level of fibrinogen in different individuals.[191]

The concentration of plasma fibrinogen has important clinical implications, as indicated by several studies demonstrating that hyperfibrinogenemia is an independent risk factor in stroke and in ischemic heart disease.[192-195] For example, plasma fibrinogen concentrations in the upper third of the population increased the risk of ischemic heart disease threefold as compared with those in the lower third of the population.[192] Even small increments in the level of fibrinogen such as 1 SD (0.6 mg/ml) above the mean markedly increase the risk of ischemic heart disease.[192] When other risk factors for ischemic heart disease and stroke such as hypertension, serum cholesterol, age, diabetes, and smoking were considered, high levels of fibrinogen were still evident as an important risk factor.[192-195] The pathophysiologic mechanisms by which elevated fibrinogen causes vascular damage is unknown,[196,197] and it is possible that the high concentration of plasma fibrinogen may be due to cytokines released from areas of vascular damage. In this case, hyperfibrinogenemia can be considered a marker of the disease and may not play a role as a causative agent in the development of vascular damage.[196,197] The development of drugs that specifically decrease the level of plasma fibrinogen could clarify whether high levels of fibrinogen play a role in the pathogenesis of atherosclerotic cardiovascular disease.[196,197]

Hypofibrinogenemia

Low levels of plasma fibrinogen can be caused by a relative decrease in biosynthesis of this protein by the hepatocyte or by an increased rate of its catabolism. In some clinical disorders, both mechanisms may be involved in the development of hypofibrinogenemia. Normal or increased levels of plasma fibrinogen are common in liver disease, but moderate hypofibrinogenemia (i.e., a fibrinogen level of <100 mg/dl) may be present in fulminant hepatic failure or in decompensated liver cirrhosis.[198,199] The low levels of fibrinogen correlate with mucosal hemorrhage, which is unrelated to esophageal varices typically present in these patients.[200] In addition, severe hypofibrinogenemia usually carries a poor prognosis.[198,199] The origin of hypofibrinogenemia in this group of patients is multifactorial. In addition to impaired hepatic fibrinogen synthesis,[201] increased catabolism has been observed.[202-205] These studies demonstrated decreased fibrinogen half-life and an increased catabolic rate in patients with a variety of hepatocellular disorders, suggesting that fibrinogen is consumed as part of an intravascular coagulation process in these patients. Indeed, prolongation of fibrinogen survival and an increase in the plasma fibrinogen concentration after administration of heparin are consistent with the occurrence of intravascular coagulation.[202-205] Although these studies, according to some investigators, offer ambiguous results,[210] more recent fibrinogen and prothrombin turnover studies[206,207] confirmed the increased consumption reported by previous investigators. It is interesting that some patients exhibit a low level of antithrombin III in plasma, and the infusion of this coagulation inhibitor increased fibrinogen survival and slowed the catabolic rate, which lends support to the concept that intravascular coagulation may be the cause of hypofibrinogenemia.[207] An active fibrinolytic system does not seem to play a crucial role in the development of hypofibrinogenemia, since the treatment of these patients with fibrinolytic inhibitors does not significantly change the rate of fibrinogen catabolism.[202] These findings, along with an increase of FPA level and fibrinogen/fibrin degradation products and the presence of fibrin deposition in some organs at autopsy,[208-211] indicate that DIC is a contributing factor in the hypofibrinogenemia of some patients with liver disease. Hypofibrinogenemia is also present in patients with acute or chronic DIC of different etiologies, and a low fibrinogen level should alert the physician about this possibility (see Ch. 116).

Other causes of low plasma fibrinogen concentration include the administration of certain drugs; for example, L-asparaginase can induce a severe hypofibrinogenemia, which in infrequent cases causes bleeding manifestations.[212-215] Although the treatment with L-asparginase leads to a decrease in the concentration of several plasma proteins, such as albumin,[214] insulin,[213] plasminogen, and antithrombin III,[216] the levels of fibrinogen are markedly decreased, frequently to <20 mg/dl.[212,215] By contrast, the concentration of other coagulation factors is normal or slightly decreased.[214,215] Some clinical studies and experimental work in rabbits indicate that impaired synthesis, rather than increased catabolism, is the cause of the hypofibrinogenemia in this group of patients.[217,218] Mild decrease of plasma fibrinogen concentration has also been reported in patients treated with valproic acid.[219]

Dysfibrinogenemia

Diverse diseases affecting the liver parenchyma not only produce quantitative alterations of plasma fibrinogen but may also induce dysfibrinogenemia (see Ch. 147). The alteration of functional properties of fibrinogen is the most common cause of dysfibrinogenemia. In severe liver diseases of varied etiology, including liver cirrhosis and viral and toxic hepatitis, approximately 50% of patients exhibit the characteristic dysfibrinogenemia of liver disease.[220-223] Patients with hepatoma exhibit the same abnormality.[224-226] The abnormal fibrinogen is characterized functionally by impaired polymerization of fibrin, which explains the prolongation of the TT. Both the cleavage of fibrinopeptides and the cross-linking of fibrin are normal.[220-226] The structural defect of this abnormal fibrinogen is an increased content of carbohydrate, particularly of sialic acid.[227] An increase in galactose and N-acetylglucosamine with normal mannose is consistent with increased branching of the oligosaccha-

rides rather than the presence of new carbohydrate linkages.[228] Normalization of the TT and of fibrin monomer polymerization is observed after enzymatic removal of the sialic acid from the abnormal fibrinogen.[227,228]

An increase in the content of carbohydrate has also been described with other plasma proteins in patients with liver disease, including hepatocellular carcinoma.[226,229] It is interesting that normal fetal fibrinogen exhibits biochemical and functional properties similar to those described in the abnormal fibrinogen of liver disease,[230] suggesting the possibility that activation of dormant carbohydrate enzymes in the diseased liver is a factor involved in the increase in carbohydrate content.[229] Other alterations of the fibrinogen molecule, such as the partial cleavage of the Aα chain possibly by plasmin, may also play a role in the prolongation of the TT of plasma from some patients with liver disease.[231] An abnormal fibrinogen with biochemical and functional properties similar to those found in patients with liver disease has been described in hypernephroma as part of the paraneoplastic syndrome; this abnormality abated after removal of the tumor but appeared again with the presence of metastasis.[232]

Functional abnormalities of fibrinogen can be secondary to fibrinogen autoantibodies. An inhibition of the release of fibrinopeptides by thrombin or FPA by reptilase was described in a young female with a mild bleeding disorder. The isolated inhibitor was identified as an antibody of the IgG class with κ- and λ-light chains that specifically interfered with the interaction of thrombin with fibrinogen but did not interfere with other functional activities of this enzyme.[233] Antibodies of the IgG class that are able to impair the polymerization of fibrin monomers have been described in association with systemic lupus erythematosus and also in a patient with ulcerative colitis and postnecrotic liver cirrhosis or without underlying disorder.[234-236] While some of these patients exhibit bleeding manifestations,[233,235,236] in others the presence of the antibody was found to be associated with thrombosis[234]; however, in these cases the thrombosis could be related to some other coagulation abnormality, such as lupus anticoagulant, rather than to the fibrinogen antibody.[234] Similarly, thrombotic episodes have been observed in several patients with systemic lupus erythematosus and prolonged TT.[73] A third type of an IgG antibody with specificity against the cross-linking sites of fibrinogen and normal factor XIII activity was described in a patient with sarcoidosis treated with isoniazid. This antibody appeared to be responsible for the patient's mild bleeding disorder.[237]

The monoclonal immunoglobulin of multiple myeloma can prolong the TT by inhibiting fibrin monomer polymerization.[238-241] Although this effect is mediated by the F(ab)₂ fragment of the monoclonal protein, a specific antibody/antigen reaction between the monoclonal and fibrinogen has not been demonstrated. Thus, in addition to acting as specific antibodies to fibrinogen,[237] immunoglobulins might also act by some other undefined mechanism.[238-241] Some of these interactions may lead to clinical manifestations, but most frequently they are clinically silent.

In patients with active bleeding due to paraproteinemias, extensive plasma exchange appears to improve the hemorrhagic tendency.[241] Abnormal fibrinogens showing defective fibrinopeptide release should be differentiated from clinical conditions in which plasma factor interferes with the fibrinogen-to-fibrin conversion. Abnormal thrombin- or reptilase-induced clottability of fibrinogen has been noted in about 40% of patients with systemic light chain amyloidosis.[242] The isolated fibrinogen molecule demonstrated normal clotting ability, and an unidentified factor unrelated to the paraproteinemia was found to be responsible for inhibiting the conversion of fibrinogen to fibrin.[242] Defective formation of fibrin by thrombin is also present in patients found to have circulating heparin or heparin-like substance. However, in these cases, the addition of protamine to the patient's plasma shortens the TT; in addition, the reptilase time is close to normal.[243-245] The identification of plasma factors that interfere with the thrombin clotting ability of fibrinogen leading to dysfibrinogenemia can be clearly made by examining the functional properties of purified patient fibrinogen.

REFERENCES

1. Doolittle RF: Fibrinogen and fibrin. Annu Rev Biochem 53:195, 1984
2. Henschen A, Lottspeich F, Kehl M. Southan C: Covalent structure of fibrinogen. Ann NY Acad Sci 408:28, 1983
3. Mosesson MW: Fibrinogen heterogeneity. Ann NY Acad Sci 408:97, 1983
4. Townsend RR, Hilliker E, Li YT et al: Carbohydrate structure of human fibrinogen. J Biol Chem 257:9704, 1982
5. Slayter HS: Electron microscopic studies of fibrinogen structure: historical perspectives and recent experiments. Ann NY Acad Sci 408:131, 1983
6. Erickson HP, Fowler WE: Electron microscopy of fibrinogen, its plasmic fragments and small polymers. Ann NY Acad Sci 408:146, 1983
7. Blombäck B, Blombäck M, Henschen A et al: N-Terminal disulfide knot of human fibrinogen. Nature 218:130, 1968
8. Lucas MA, Fretto LJ, McKee PA: The relationship of fibrinogen structure to plasminogen activation and plasmin activity during fibrinolysis. Ann NY Acad Sci 408:71, 1983
9. Barnhart MI, Cress DC, Noonan SM, Walsh RT: Influence of fibrinolytic products on hepatic release and synthesis of fibrinogen. Thromb Haemost, suppl. 39:143, 1970
10. Fuller GM, Nickerson JM, Adams MA: Translation and cotranslational events in fibrinogen synthesis. Ann NY Acad Sci 408:440, 1983
11. Chung DW, Rixon MW, Que BG, Davie EW: Cloning of fibrinogen genes and their cDNA. Ann NY Acad Sci 408:449, 1983
12. Crabtree GR, Kant JF, Forance AJ Jr et al: Regulation and characterization of the mRNAs for the Aα, Bβ, and γ chains of fibrinogen. Ann NY Acad Sci 408:457, 1983
13. Olaisen B, Teissberg P, Gedde-Dahl T Jr: Fibrinogen γ chain locus is on chromosome 4 in man. Hum Genet 61:24, 1982
14. Kant J, Forance AJ, Saxe D et al: Organization and evolution of the human fibrinogen locus on chromosome four. Proc Natl Acad Sci USA 82:2344, 1985
15. Collen D, Tytgat GN, Claeys H, Piessens R: Metabolism and distribution of fibrinogen. I. Fibrinogen turnover in physiological conditions in humans. Br J Haematol 22:681, 1972
16. Martinez J, Holburn RR, Shapiro SS, Erslev AJ: Fibrinogen Philadelphia. A hereditary hypodysfibrinogenemia characterized by fibrinogen hypercatabolism. J Clin Invest 53:600, 1974
17. Blombäck B, Hessel B, Hogg D et al: A two-step fibrinogen-fibrin transition in blood coagulation. Nature 275:501, 1978
18. Nossel HL, Hurlet-Jensen A, Liu CY et al: Fibrinopeptide release from fibrinogen. Ann NY Acad Sci 408:269, 1983
19. Shainoff JR, Dardik BN: Fibrinopeptide release from fibrinogen. Ann NY Acad Sci 408:254, 1983
20. Binnie CG, Lord ST: The fibrinogen sequences that interact with thrombin. Blood 81:3186, 1993
21. Ferry JD: The mechanism of polymerization of fibrin. Proc Natl Acad Sci USA 38:566, 1952
22. Hermans J, McDonagh J: Fibrin: structure and interactions. Semin Thromb Hemost 8:11, 1982
23. Mosesson MW: The roles of fibrinogen and fibrin in hemostasis and thrombosis. Semin Hematol 29:177, 1992
24. Siebenlist KR, DiOrio JP, Budzynski AZ, Mosesson MW: The polymerization and thrombin-binding properties of Des-(Bβ1–42)-fibrin. J Biol Chem 265:18650, 1990
25. Shimizu A, Nagel GM, Doolittle RF: Photoaffinity labeling of the primary fibrin polymerization site: isolation and characterization of a labeled cyanogen bromide fragment corresponding to γ-chain residues 337-379. Proc Natl Acad Sci USA 89:2888, 1992
26. Pisano JJ, Finlayson JS, Peyton MP: Cross-link fibrin polymerized by factor XIII: (γ-glutamyl)lysine. Science 160:892, 1968
27. McKee PA, Mattock P, Hill RL: Subunit structure of human fibrinogen, soluble fibrin, and cross-linked insoluble fibrin. Proc Natl Acad Sci USA 66:738, 1970
28. McDonagh RP Jr, McDonagh J, Duckert F: The influence of fibrin cross-linking on the kinetics of urokinase-induced clot lysis. Br J Haematol 21:323, 1971
29. Leven RM, Schick PK, Budzynski AZ: Fibrinogen biosynthesis in isolated guinea pig megakaryocytes. Blood 65:501, 1985
30. Harrison P, Wilbourn B, Debili N et al: Uptake of plasma fibrinogen into the alpha granules of human megakaryocytes and platelets. J Clin Invest 84:1320, 1989
31. Handagama P, Scarborough RM, Shuman MA, Bainton DF: Endocytosis of fibrinogen into megakaryocyte and platelet α-granules is mediated by α$_{IIb}$β$_3$ (glycoprotein IIb-IIIa). Blood 82:135, 1993
32. Mosesson MW, Homandberg GA, Amrani DL: Human platelet fibrinogen gamma chain structure. Blood 63:990, 1984
33. Haidaris PJ, Francis CW, Sporn LA et al: Megakaryocyte and hepatocyte origins of human fibrinogen biosynthesis exhibit hepatocyte-specific expression of gamma chain-variant polypeptides. Blood 74:743, 1989
34. Amrani DL, Newman PJ, Meh D et al: The role of fibrinogen A chains in ADP-induced platelet aggregation in the presence of fibrinogen molecules containing γ' chains. Blood 72:919, 1988
35. Peerschke EIB, Francis CW, Marder VJ: Fibrinogen binding to human blood platelets: effect of γ chain carboxyterminal structure and length. Blood 67:385, 1986
36. Jandrot-Perrus M, Mosesson MW, Denninger MH et al: Studies on platelet fibrinogen from a subject with a congenital plasma fibrinogen abnormality (fibrinogen Paris I). Blood 54:1109, 1979
37. Teige B, Gogstad G, Brosstad F et al: Common structural genes for platelet and plasma fibrinogen. Blood 65:120, 1985
38. Kunicki TJ, Newman PJ, Amrani DL, Mosesson MW: Human platelet fibrinogen: purification and hemostatic properties. Blood 66:808, 1985
39. Mammen EF: Fibrinogen abnormalities. Semin Thromb Hemost 9:1, 1983
40. Ménaché D: Congenital fibrinogen abnormalities. Ann NY Acad Sci 408:121, 1983
41. Girolami A, Zacchello G, D'Elia R: Congenital afibrinogenemia. A case report with some considerations on the hereditary transmission of this disorder. Thromb Haemost 25:460, 1971
42. Egbring R, Andrassy K, Egli H, Meyer-Lindenberg J: Diagnostische und therapeutische Probleme bei kongenitaler Afibrinogenämie. Blut 22:175, 1971
43. Montgomery R, Natelson SE: Afibrinogenemia with cerebral hematoma. Am J Dis Child 131:555, 1977
44. Fried K, Kaufman S: Congenital afibrinogenemia in 10 offspring of uncle-niece marriages. Clin Genet 17:223, 1980
45. McRoyan DK, McRoyan CJ, Kitay DZ, Liu PI: Constitutional hypofibrinogenemia associated with third trimester hemorrhage. Ann Clin Lab Sci 16:52, 1986
46. Prichard JA: Chronic hypofibrinogenemia and frequent placental abruption. Obstet Gynecol 18:146, 1961
47. Ness PM, Budzynski AZ, Olexa SA, Rodvien R: Congenital hypofibrinogenemia and recurrent placental abruption. Obstet Gynecol 61:519, 1983
48. Caen J, Faur J, Ineeman S et al: Nécrose ischémique bilatérale dans un cas de grande hypofibrinogénémie congénitale. Nouv Rev Fr Hematol 4:321, 1964
49. Ingram GIC, McBrien DJ, Spencer H: Fatal pulmonary embolus in congenital fibrinopenia. Report of two cases. Acta Haematol 35:56, 1966
50. MacKinnon HH, Fekete JF: Congenital afibrinogenemia: vascular changes and multiple thromboses induced by fibrinogen infusions and contraceptive medication. Can Med Assoc J 140:597, 1971
51. Pfeifer U, Ormanns W, Klinge O: Hepatocellular fibrinogen storage in familial hypofibrinogenemia. Virchows Arch B Cell Pathol 36:247, 1981
52. Wehinger L, Klinge O, Alexandrakis E et al: Hereditary hypofibrinogenemia with fibrinogen storage in the liver. Eur J Pediatr 141:109, 1983
53. Callea F, Tortora O, Kojima T et al: Hypofibrinogenemia and fibrinogen storage disease. p. 247. In Mosesson MW, Amrani DL, Siebenlist KR, Diorio JP (eds): Fibrinogen. 3. Biochemistry, Biological Functions, Gene Regulation and Expression. Elsevier Science BV, New York, 1988
54. Hardisty RM, Pinniger JL: Congenital afibrinogenaemia: further observations on the blood coagulation mechanism. Br J Haematol 2:139, 1956
55. Gitlin D, Borges WH: Studies on the metabolism of fibrinogen in two patients with congenital afibrinogenemia. Blood 8:679, 1953
56. Tytgat GN, Collen D, Vermylen J: Metabolism and distribution of fibrinogen. II. Fibrinogen turnover in polycythaemia, thrombocytosis, haemophilia A, congenital afibrinogenaemia and during streptokinase therapy. Br J Haematol 22:701, 1972
57. Uzan G, Courtois G, Besmond C et al: Analysis of fibrinogen genes in patients with congenital afibrinogenemia. Biochem Biophys Res Commun 120:376, 1984
58. Base W, Barsigian C, Schaeffer A et al: Influence of branched-chain amino acids and branched-chain keto acids on protein synthesis in isolated hepatocytes. Hepatology 7:324, 1987
59. Cattaneo M, Bettega D, Lombardi R et al: Sustained correction of the bleeding time in an afibrinogenaemic patient after infusion of fresh frozen plasma. Br J Haematol 82:388, 1992
60. Weiss HJ, Rogers J: Fibrinogen and platelets in the primary arrest of bleeding: studies in two patients with congenital afibrinogenemia. N Engl J Med 285:369, 1971
61. Girolami A, De Marco L, Virgolini L et al: Platelet adhesiveness and aggregation in congenital afibrinogenemia. An investigation of three patients with

post-transfusion cross-correction studies between two of them. Blut 30:87, 1975

62. Bommer W, Kunzer W, Schroer H: Kongenitale Afibrinogenämie. Teil II. Ann Paediatr 200:180, 1963

63. Salzman EW: Hemostatic problems in surgical patients. p. 920. In Colman RW, Hirsch J, Marder VJ, Salzman ED (eds): Hemostasis and Thrombosis: Basic Principles and Clinical Practice. 2nd Ed. JB Lippincott, Philadelphia, 1987

64. Mason DY, Ingram GIC: Management of the hereditary coagulation disorders. Semin Hematol 8:158, 1971

65. Inamoto Y, Terao T: First report of case of congenital afibrinogenemia with successful delivery. Am J Obstet Gynecol 153:803, 1985

66. De Vries A, Rosenberg T, Kochwa S, Boss JH: Precipitating antifibrinogen antibody appearing after fibrinogen infusions in a patient with congenital afibrinogenemia. Am J Med 30:486, 1961

67. Beck EA, Charache P, Jackson DP: A new inherited coagulation disorder caused by an abnormal fibrinogen (fibrinogen Baltimore). Nature 208:143, 1965

68. Ménaché D: Constitutional and familial abnormal fibrinogen. Thromb Haemost, suppl. 13:173, 1964

69. Ebert RF: Index of Variant Human Fibrinogens. CRC Press, Boca Raton, FL, 1991

70. Henschen AH: Human fibrinogen—structural variants and functional sites. Thromb Haemost 70:42, 1993

71. Gralnick HR, Givelber HM, Shainoff JR, Finlayson JS: Fibrinogen Bethesda: a congenital dysfibrinogenemia with delayed fibrinopeptide release. J Clin Invest 50:1819, 1971

72. Blombäck M, Blombäck B, Mannen EF, Prasad AS: Fibrinogen Detroit—a molecular defect in the N-terminal disulphide knot of human fibrinogen? Nature 218:134, 1968

73. Galanakis DK: Fibrinogen anomalies and disease. A clinical update. Hematol Oncol Clin North Am 6:1171, 1992

74. Galanakis DK: Dysfibrinogenemia: a current perspective. Clin Lab Med 4: 395, 1984

75. Alving BM, Henschen AH: Fibrinogen Giessen I: a congenital homozygously expressed dysfibrinogenemia with Aα 16 Arg → His substitution. Am J Hematol 25:479, 1987

76. Krause WH, Heene DL, Lasch HG: Congenital dysfibrinogenemia (fibrinogen Giessen). Thromb Haemost 29:547, 1973

77. Galankis DK, Henschen A, Keeling M et al: Fibrinogen Louisville: an Aα16 Arg → His defect that forms no hybrid molecules in heterozygous individuals and inhibits aggregation of normal fibrin monomers. Ann NY Acad Sci 408:644, 1983

78. Henschen A, Kehl M, Southan C et al: Genetically abnormal fibrinogens—some current characterisation strategies. p. 125. In Haverkate F, Henschen A, Nieuwenhuizen W, Straub PW (eds): Fibrinogen—Structure, Functional Aspects, Metabolism. Walter de Gruyter, Berlin, 1983

79. Siebenlist KR, Prchal JT, Mosesson MW: Fibrinogen Birmingham: a heterozygous dysfibrinogenemia (Aα Arg → His) containing heterodimeric molecules. Blood 71:613, 1988

80. Henschen A, McDonagh J: Fibrinogen, fibrin and factor XIII. p. 209. In Zwaal RFA, Hemker HC (eds): Blood Coagulation. Elsevier Science BV, Amsterdam, 1986

81. Carrell M, McDonagh J: Fibrinogen Chapel Hill II: defective in reactions with thrombin, factor XIIIa and plasmin. Br J Haematol 52:35, 1982

82. Morris S, Denninger MH, Finlayson JS, Ménaché D: Fibrinogen Lille-Aα-Asp → 7Asn, abstracted. Thromb Haemost 46:104, 1981

83. Kehl M, Lottspeich F, Henschen A: Genetically abnormal fibrinogens releasing abnormal fibrinopeptides as characterized by high-performance liquid chromatography. p. 183. In Haverkate F, Henschen A, Nieuwenhuizen W, Straub PW (eds): Fibrinogen—Structure, Functional Aspects, Metabolism. Walter de Gruyter, Berlin, 1983

84. Niwa K, Wada Y, Asakura S et al: Fibrinogen Mitaka II: a new type of hereditary abnormal fibrinogen with an Aα Glu-11 to Gly substitution characterized by impaired binding with thrombin, abstracted. Thromb Haemost 69: 962, 1993

85. Borrell M, Vila L, Solá J et al: Fibrinogen Barcelona II: a new case of Aα 16 Arg → His substitution. Haemostasis 20:1, 1990

86. Galankis DK, Hultin M: Fibrinogen Stony Brook II: partial characterization of a heterozygously transmitted peptide A anomaly. Blood Coagul Fibrinolysis 1:567, 1990

87. Higgins DL, Shafer JA: Fibrinogen Petoskey: a dysfibrinogenemia characterized by replacement of Arg A alpha 16 by a histidyl residue: evidence for thrombin-catalyzed hydrolysis at a histidyl residue. J Biol Chem 256:12013, 1981

88. Carr Jr ME, Dastgir Qureshi G: The impact of delayed fibrinopeptide—a release on fibrin structure. J Biol Chem 262:15568 1987

89. Lane DA, Southan C, Ireland H et al: Delayed release of an abnormal fibrino-

peptide A from fibrinogen Manchester: effect of the A alpha 16 Arg leads to His substitution upon fibrin monomer polymerization and the immunological crossreactivity of the peptide. Br J Haematol 53:587, 1983

90. Southan C, Lane DA, Bode W, Henschen A: Thrombin-induced fibrinopeptide release from a fibrinogen variant (fibrinogen Sydney I) with an Aα Arg-16 → His substitution. Eur J Biochem 147:593, 1985

91. Reber P, Furlan M, Beck EA et al: Fibrinogen Bergamo III and fibrinogen Torino: two further variants with hereditary molecular defects in fibrinopeptide A. Thromb Res 46:163, 1987

92. Soria J, Soria C, Samama M, Caen J: Study of 10 cases of congenital dysfibrinogenemia: clinical, molecular, biological aspects. p. 165. In Henschen A, Hessel B, McDonagh J, Saldeen T (eds): Fibrinogen: Structural Variants and Interactions. Walter de Gruyter, Berlin, 1985

93. Soria J, Soria C, Samama M et al: Detection of fibrinogen abnromality in dysfibrinogenemia: special report on fibrinogen Metz characterized by an amino acid substitution located at the peptide bond cleaved by thrombin. p. 129. In Henschen A, Graeff H, Lottspeich F (eds): Fibrinogen—Recent Biochemical and Medical Aspects. Walter de Gruyter, Berlin, 1982

94. Mosesson, MW, DiOrio JP, Muller MF et al: Studies on the ultrastructure of fibrin lacking fibrinopeptide B (β-fibrin). Blood 69:1073, 1987

95. Rupp C, Sievi R, Furlan M, Beck EA: Fibrinogen Bern II: Fibrinogen Erbvariante mit dem Aminosaurenaustausch Arginin Histidin in Position 16 der Aa Kette. Schweiz Med Wochenschr 113:1460, 1983

96. Ebert RF, Schreiber WE, Bell WR: Fibrinogen Seattle II: congenital dysfibrinogenemia with an Arg (Aα₁₆) → His substitution. Thromb Res 43:7, 1986

97. Miyashita C, Schwamborn J, von Blohn G et al: Preliminary report concerning two new cases of congenital dysfibrinogenemia (Homburg II and Homburg III). p. 237. In Henschen A, Hessel B, McDonagh J, Saldeen T (eds): Fibrinogen—Structural Variants and Interactions. Walter de Gruyter, Berlin, 1985

98. Lee MH, Kaczmarek E, Chin DT et al: Fibrinogen Ledyard (AαArg₁₆ → Cys): biochemical and physiologic characterization. Blood 78, 1991

99. Galanakis DK, Henschen A, Schubach W et al: Determination of abnormal structure and heterozygosity by amplification of genomic DNA using the polymerase chain reaction and by amino acid sequence analyses. p. 173. In Matsuda M, Iwanaga S, Takada A, Henschen A (eds): Fibrinogen 4. Current Basic and Clinical Aspects. Elsevier Science BV, Amsterdam, 1990

100. Galanakis DK, Henschen A, Peerschke EIB, Kehl M: Fibrinogen Stony Brook, a heterozygous Aα16Arg T Cys dysfibrinogenemia. J Clin Invest 84:295, 1989

101. Reber P, Furlan M, Beck EA et al: Fibrinogen Bergamo I (Aα16Arg → Cys): susceptibility towards thrombin following aminoethylation, methylation or carboxyamidomethylation of cysteine residues. Thromb Haemost 53:390, 1985

102. Matsuda M, Saeki E, Kasamatsu A et al: Fibrinogen Kawaguchi: an abnormal fibrinogen characterized by defective release of fibrinopeptide A. Thromb Res 37:379, 1985

103. Miyata T, Terukina S, Matsuda M et al: Fibrinogens Kawaguchi and Osaka: an amino acid substitution of Aα arginine-16 to cysteine which forms an extra interchain disulfide bridge between the two Aα chains. J Biochem 102: 93, 1987

104. Marx R, Schramm W: On dysfibrinogenemia. p. 153. In Henschen A, Graeff H, Lottspeich F (eds): Fibrinogen—Recent Biochemical and Medical Aspects. Walter de Gruyter, Berlin, 1982

105. Dempfle CEH, Henschen A: Fibrinogen Mannheim I—identification of an Aα19 Arg → Gly substitution in dysfibrinogenaemia associated with bleeding tendency. p. 159. In Matsuda M, Iwanaga S, Takada A, Henschen A (eds): Fibrinogen 4. Current Basic and Clinical Aspects. Elsevier Science BV, Amsterdam, 1990

106. Hessel B, Adamson L, Procyk R, Therkildsen et al: Fibrinogen Aarhus and factor XIII induced polymerization and gel formation. Br J Haematol 66:355, 1987

107. Blombäck B, Hessel B, Fields R, Procyk R: Fibrinogen Aarhus: an abnormal fibrinogen with Aα 19 Arg → Gly substitution. p. 263. In Mosesson MW, Amrani DL, Siebenlist KR, DiOrio JP (eds): Fibrinogen 3: Biochemistry, Biological Functions, Gene Regulation and Expression. Elsevier Science BV, Amsterdam, 1988

108. Ni F, Konishi Y, Bullock LD et al: High-resolution NMR studies of fibrinogen-like peptides in solution: structural basis for the bleeding disorder caused by a single mutation of Gly(12) to Val(12) in the Aα chain of human fibrinogen Rouen. Biochemistry 28:3106, 1989

109. Al-Mondhiry HAB, Bilezikiant SB, Nossel H: Fibrinogen "New York"—an abnormal fibrinogen associated with thromboembolism: functional evaluation. Blood 45:607, 1975

110. Liu CY, Koehn JA, Morgan FJ: Characterization of fibrinogen New York I. J Biol Chem 260:4390, 1985

111. Koopman J, Haverkate F, Grimbergen J et al: Abnormal fibrinogens Ijmuiden (BβArg₁₄ → Cys) and Nijmegen (Bβ Arg₄₄ → Cys) form disulfide-linked fibrinogen-albumin complexes. Proc Natl Acad Sci USA 89:3478, 1992

112. Kaudewitz H, Henschen A, Soria C et al: Molecular defect of the genetically abnormal fibrinogen Christchurch II. p. 31. In Muller-Berghaus G, Scheefers-Borchel G, Selmayr E, Henschen A (eds): Fibrinogen and Its Derivatives: Biochemistry, Physiology and Pathophysiology. Excerpta Medica, Amsterdam, 1986

113. Pirkle H, Kaudewitz H, Henschen A et al: Substitution of Bβ14 arginine by cyst(e)ine in fibrinogen Seattle I. p. 49. In Lowe GDO, Douglas JT, Forbes CD, Henschen A (eds): Fibrinogen 2: Biochemistry, Physiology and Clinical Relevance. Excerpta Medica, Amsterdam, 1987

114. Yoshida N, Wada H, Morita K et al: A new congenital abnormal fibrinogen Ise characterized by the replacement of Bβ glycine-15 cysteine. Blood 77: 1958, 1991

115. Haverkate F, Koopman J, Kluft C et al: Fibrinogen Milano II: a congenital dysfibrinogenaemia associated with juvenile arterial and venous thrombosis. Thromb Haemost 55:131, 1986

116. Di Minno G, Martinez J, Cirillo F et al: A role for platelets and thrombin in the juvenile stroke of two siblings with defective thrombin-adsorbing capacity of fibrin(ogen). Arterioscler Thromb 11:785, 1991

117. Koopman J, Grimbergen J, Lord ST et al: The functional and structural defect of fibrinogen Naples and its relation with thrombosis, abstracted. In the Tenth Fibrinogen Workshop, Rouen, 1990

118. Crum ED, Shainoff JR, Graham RC, Ratnoff OD: Fibrinogen Cleveland II: an abnormal fibrinogen with defective release of fibrinopeptide A. J Clin Invest 53:1308, 1974

119. Abe Andes W, Chavin SI, Beltram G, Stuckey WJ: Fibrinogen New Orleans: hereditary dysfibrinogenemia with an Aα chain abnormality. Thromb Res 25:41, 1982

120. Sherman LA, Gaston LW, Kaplan ME, Spivack AR: Fibrinogen St. Louis: a new inherited fibrinogen, coincidentally associated with Hemophilia A. J Clin Invest 51:590, 1972

121. Laugen RH, Bithell TC: Hereditary dysfibrinogenemia characterized by slow fibrinopeptide release and competitive inhibition of thrombin. Acta Haematol 71:150, 1984

122. Yoshida N, Okuma M, Hirata H et al: Fibrinogen Kyoto II, a new congenitally abnormal molecule, characterized by the replacement of Aα proline-18 by leucine. Blood 78:149, 1991.

123. Uotani C, Miyata T, Kumabashiri I et al: Fibrinogen Kanazawa: a congenital dysfibrinogenaemia with delayed polymerization having a replacement of proline-18 by leucine in the Aα-chain. Blood Coagul Fibrinolysis 2:413, 1991

124. Maekawa H, Yamazumi K, Muramatsu S et al: Fibrinogen Lima: a homozygous dysfibrinogen with an Aα-arginine-141 to serine substitution associated with extra N-glycosylation at Aα-asparagine-139. J Clin Invest 90:67, 1992

125. Maekawa H, Yamazumi K, Muramatsu S et al: An Aα Ser-434 to N-glycosylated Asn substitution in a dysfibrinogen, fibrinogen Caracas II, characterized by impaired fibrin gel formation. J Biol Chem 266:11575, 1991

126. Soria J, Soria C, Caen JP: A new type of congenital dysfibrinogenaemia with defective fibrin lysis—Dusard syndrome: possible relation to thrombosis. Br J Haematol 53:575, 1983

127. Siebenlist KR, Mosesson MW, DiOria JP et al: The polymerization of fibrinogen Dusart (Aα 554 Arg → Cys) after removal of carboxy terminal regions of the Aα-chains. Blood Coagul Fibrinolysis 4:61, 1993

128. Koopman J, Haverkate F, Grimbergen J et al: Molecular basis for fibrinogen Dusart (Aα 554 Arg → Cys) and its association with abnormal fibrin polymerization and thrombophilia. J Clin Invest 91:1637, 1993

129. Engesser L, Koopman J, de Munk G et al: Fibrinogen Nijmegen: congenital dysfibrinogenemia associated with impaired t-PA mediated plasminogen activation and decreased binding of t-PA. Thromb Haemost 60:113, 1988

130. Kaudewitz H, Henschen A, Soria J, Soria C: Fibrinogen Pontoise—a genetically abnormal fibrinogen with defective fibrin polymerization but normal fibrinopeptide release. p. 91. In Lane DA, Henschen A, Jasani MK (eds): Fibrinogen-Fibrin Formation and Fibrinolysis. Vol. 4. Walter de Gruyter, Berlin, 1986

131. Soria J, Soria C, Samama M et al: Fibrinogen Haifa: fibrinogen variant with absence of protective effect of calcium in plasmin degradation of γ chain. Thromb Haemost 57:310, 1987

132. Yoshida N, Imaoka S, Hirata H et al: Heterozygous abnormal fibrinogen Osaka III with the replacement of γ arginine-275 by histidine has an apparently higher molecular weight γ-chain variant. Thromb Haemost 68:534, 1992

133. Reber P, Furlan M, Henschen A et al: Three abnormal fibrinogen variants with the same amino acid substitution (γ 275 Arg → His): fibrinogens Bergamo II, Essen and Perugia. Thromb Haemost 56:401, 1986

134. Yamazumi K, Terukina S, Onohara S, Matsuda M: Normal plasmic cleavage of the γ-chain variant of "fibrinogen Saga" with an Arg-275 to His substitution. Thromb Haemost 60:476, 1988

135. Yoshida N, Ota K, Moroi M, Matsuda M: An apparently higher molecular weight γ-chain variant in a new congenital abnormal fibrinogen Tochigi

136. Terukina S, Matsuda M, Hirata H et al: Substitution of γArg-275 by Cys in an abnormal fibrinogen "fibrinogen Osaka II." J Biol Chem 263:13579, 1988

137. Schmelzer CH, Ebert RF, Bell WR: Fibrinogen Baltimore IV: congenital dysfibrinogenemia with a γ275 (Arg → Cys) substitution. Thromb Res 56:307, 1989

138. Matsuda M, Baba M, Morimoto K, Nakamikawa C: "Fibrinogen Tokyo II." An abnormal fibrinogen with an impaired polymerization site on the aligned DD domain of fibrin molecules. J Clin Invest 72:1034, 1983

139. Matsuda M, Nakamikawa C, Baba M, Morimoto K: Fibrinogen Tokyo II: an abnormal fibrinogen with an impaired polymerization site on the aligned DD domain of fibrin molecules. p. 213. In Henschen A, Hessel B, McDonagh J, Saldeen T (eds): Fibrinogen—Structural Variants and Interactions. Walter de Gruyter, Berlin, 1985

140. Yoshida N, Okuma M, Moroi M, Matsuda M: A lower molecular weight γ-chain variant in a congenital abnormal fibrinogen (Kyoto). Blood 68:703, 1986

141. Yoshida N, Terukina S, Okuma M et al: Characterization of an apparently lower molecular weight γ-chain variant in fibrinogen Kyoto I. J Biol Chem 263:13848, 1988

142. Reber P, Furlan M, Rupp C et al: Characterization of fibrinogen Milano I: amino acid exchange γ330Asp → Val impairs fibrin polymerization. Blood 67:1751, 1986

143. Bantia S, Bell WR, Dang CV: Polymerization defect of fibrinogen Baltimore III due to a γAsn308 → Ile mutation. Blood 75:1659, 1990

144. Terukina S, Yamazumi K, Okamoto K et al: Fibrinogen Kyoto III: a congenital dysfibrinogen with a γ aspartic acid-330 to tyrosine substitution manifesting impaired fibrin monomer polymerization. Blood 74:2681, 1989

145. Miyata T, Furukawa K, Iwanaga S et al: Fibrinogen Nagoya, a replacement of glutamine-329 by arginine in the γ-chain that impairs the polymerization of fibrin monomer. J Biochem (Tokyo) 105:10, 1989

146. Yamazumi K, Shimura K, Terukina S et al: A γ methionine-310 to threonine substitution and consequent N-glycosylation at γ asparagine-308 identified in a congenital dysfibrinogenemia associated with posttraumatic bleeding, fibrinogen Asahi. J Clin Invest 83:1590, 1989

147. Bantia S, Mane SM, Bell WR, Dang CV: Fibrinogen Baltimore I: polymerization defect associated with a γ292Gly → Val (GGC → GTC) mutation. Blood 76: 2279, 1990

148. Beck EA, Shainoff JR, Vogel A, Jackson DP: Functional evaluation of an inherited abnormal fibrinogen: fibrinogen "Baltimore." J Clin Invest 50:1874, 1971

149. Budzynski AZ, Marder VJ, Ménaché D, Guillin M-C: Defect in the gamma polypeptide chain of a congenital abnormal fibrinogen (Paris I). Nature 252: 66, 1974

150. Mosesson MW, Amrani DL, Ménaché D: Studies on the structural abnormality of fibrinogen Paris I. J Clin Invest 57:782, 1976

151. Koopman J, Haverkate F, Briët E, Lord ST: A congenitally abnormal fibrinogen (Vlissingen) with a 6-base deletion in the γ-chain gene, causing defective calcium binding and impaired fibrin polymerization. J Biol Chem 266:13456, 1991

152. Weinger RS, Rudy C, Moake JL et al: Fibrinogen Houston: a dysfibrinogen exhibiting defective fibrin monomer aggregation and α-chain cross linkages. Am J Hematol 9:237, 1980

153. D'Angelo G, Lacombe M, Lemay et al: A new congenital dysfibrinogenemia with hemorrhagic diathesis (Montreal II). Thromb Haemost 29:35, 1975

154. De Bosch NB, Arocha-Pinango CL, Soria J et al: An abnormal fibrinogen in a Venezuelan family. Thromb Res 1:253, 1977

155. Carrel NM, Gabriel N, Blatt PM et al: Hereditary dysfibrogenemia in a patient with thrombotic disease. Blood 62:439, 1983

156. Fernandez J, Paramo JA, Cuesta B et al: Fibrinogen Pamplona: a new congenital dysfibrinogenemia with abnormal fibrin-enhanced plasminogen activation and defective binding of thrombin to fibrin. p. 25. In Muller-Berghaus G (ed): Fibrinogen and Its Derivatives. Elsevier, New York, 1986

157. Yamazumi K, Shimura K, Mackawa H et al: Delayed intermolecular γ-chain cross-linking by factor XIIIa in fibrinogen Asahi characterized by a γ-Met-310 to Thr substitution with an N-glycosylated γ-Asn-308. Blood Coagul Fibrinolysis 1:557, 1990

158. Hampton JW, Morton RO: Fibrinogen Oklahoma—recharacterization of a familial bleeding diathesis, abstracted. p. 313 In the Thirteenth International Congress of Hematology, 1970

159. Finlayson JS: "Fibrinogen Oklahoma": a study of interactions. Ann NY Acad Sci 408:577, 1983

160. Imperato C, Dettori AG: Ipofibrinogenemia congenita con fibrinoastenia. Helv Paediatr Acta 4:380, 1958

161. Gralnick HR, Coller BS, Fratantoni JC, Martinez J: Fibrinogen Bethesda III: a hypodysfibrinogenemia. Blood 53:28, 1979

162. Krause WH, Heene DL, Lasch HG, Huth K: Kongenitale Dysfibrinogenamie: Fibrinogen Gieben II. Verh Dtsch Ges Inn Med 82:1646, 1976

163. McDonagh RP, Carrell NA, Roberts HR et al: Fibrinogen Chapel Hill: hypodys-

fibrinogenemia with a tertiary polymerization defect. Am J Hematol 9:23, 1980

164. Ebert RF, Bell WR: Fibrinogen Baltimore II: congenital hypodysfibrinogenemia with delayed release of fibrinopeptide B and decreased rate of fibrinogen synthesis. Proc Natl Acad Sci USA 80:7318, 1983

165. Soria J, Soria C, Hedner U et al: Episodes of increased fibronectin level observed in a patient suffering from recurrent thrombosis related to congenital hypodysfibrinogenaemia (fibrinogen Malmöe). Br J Haematol 61:727, 1985

166. Koopman J, Haverkate F, Grimbergen J et al: Fibrinogen Marburg: a homozygous case of dysfibrinogenemia, lacking amino acids Aα 461-610 (Lys 461 AAA → stop TAA). Blood 80:1972, 1992

167. Higgins DL, Lewis SD, Penner JA, Shafer JA: A kinetic method for characterization of heterogeneous fibrinogen and its application to fibrinogen Grand Rapids, a congenital dysfibrinogenemia. Thromb Haemost 48:182, 1982

168. Exner T, Barber S, Sage RE, Kronenberg H: Fibrinogen Adelaide: a familial hypofibrinogenaemia associated with abnormal alpha chains. Br J Haematol 56:95, 1984

169. Owen Jr CA, Bowie EJW, Fass DN et al: Hypofibrinogenemia-dysfibrinogenemia and von Willebrand's disease in the same family. Mayo Clin Proc 54: 375, 1979

170. Aznar J, Fernandez-Pavon A, Reganon E et al: Fibrinogen Valencia: a new case of congenital dysfibrinogenemia. Thromb Haemost 32:564, 1974

171. Gandrille S, Priollet P, Capron L et al: Association of inherited dysfibrinogenaemia and protein C deficiency in two unrelated families. Br J Haematol 68: 329, 1988

172. Lane DA, Ireland H, Thompson E et al: Fibrinogens London I–IV, Manchester, Sydney I and II. Cleavage of fibrinopeptides by thrombin and expression of their polymerization abnormalities. p. 197. In Henschen A, Hessel B, McDonagh J, Saldeen T (eds): Fibrinogen—Structural Variants and Interactions. Walter de Gruyter, Berlin, 1985

173. Aguercif M, Anner R, Ritschard J et al: [Syndromes of congenital and familial disfibrinogenemia. Apropos of 2 additional families.] Pediatrie 27:317, 1972

174. Rupp C, Kuyas C, Häberli A et al: [Fibrinogen Bern I and fibrinogen Bern II: 2 hereditary fibrinogen variants with diverse biochemical properties.] Schweiz Med Wochenschr 111:1543, 1981

175. Egeberg O: Inherited fibrinogen abnormality causing thrombophilia. Thromb Haemost 17:176, 1967

176. Thorsen LI, Stormorken H, Brosstad F et al: A dysfibrinogen, Oslo I, acting as more efficient cofactor in ADP-stimulated platelet aggregation than normal fibrinogen, abstracted. Thromb Haemost 50:202, 1983

177. Forman WB, Ratnoff OD, Boyer MH: An inherited qualitative abnormality in plasma fibrinogen: fibrinogen Cleveland. J Lab Clin Med 72:455, 1968

178. Buraschi JA, Sack ES, Quiroga E, Hendler H: A new fibrinogen anomaly: fibrinogen Buenos Aires, abstracted. Thromb Haemost 34:570, 1975

179. Grannis GF: Plasma fibrinogen: determination, normal values, physiopathologic shifts, and fluctuations. Clin Chem 16:486, 1970

180. Meade TW, Imeson J, Stirling Y: Effects of changes in smoking and other characteristics on clotting factors and risk of ischaemic heart disease. Lancet 2:986, 1987

181. Balleisen L, Bailey J, Epping PH et al: Epidemiology study on factor VII, factor VIII and fibrinogen in an industrial population: I. Baseline data on the relation to age, gender, body weight, smoking, alcohol, pill using and menopause. Thromb Haemost 54:475, 1985

182. Kanell WB, Wolf PA, Castelli WP, D'Agostino RB: Fibrinogen and risk of cardiovascular disease: the Framingham Study. JAMA 258:1183, 1987

183. Abbot RD, Yin Yin MA, Reed DM, Yano K: Risk of stroke in male cigarette smokers. N Engl J Med 315:717, 1986

184. Di Minno G, Mancini M: Measuring plasma fibrinogen to predict stroke and myocardial infarction. Atherosclerosis 10:1, 1990

185. Humphries SE, Cook M, Dubovitz M et al: Role of genetic variation at the fibrinogen locus in determination of plasma fibrinogen concentrations. Lancet 1:1452, 1987

186. Thomas AE, Green FR, Kelleher CH et al: Variation in the promoter region of the β fibrinogen gene is associated with plasma fibrinogen levels in smokers and non-smokers. Thromb Haemost 65:487, 1991

187. Roy SM, Mukhopadtyay G, Redman CM: Regulation of fibrinogen assembly. Transfection of HepG2 cells with Bβ cDNA specifically enhances synthesis of the three component chains of fibrinogen. J Biol Chem 256:6389, 1990

188. Baumann H, Gauldie J: Regulation of hepatic acute phase plasma protein genes by hepatocyte stimulating factors and other mediators of inflammation. Mol Biol Med 7:147, 1990

189. Evans E, Courtois GM, Kilian P et al: Induction of fibrinogen and a subset of acute phase response genes involves a novel monokine which is mimicked by phorbol esters. J Biol Chem 262:10850, 1987

190. Huber P, Laurent M, Dalmon J: Human β fibrinogen gene expression. Upstream sequences involved in its tissue specific expression and its dexametazone and interleukin-6 stimulation. J Biol Chem 265:5695, 1990

191. Baumann RE, Henschen AH: Genetic variation in human Bβ fibrinogen gene promoter influences formation of a specific DNA-protein complex with the interleukin 6 response element, abstracted. Thromb Haemost 69:961, 1993

192. Meade TW, Mellows W, Brozovic M et al: Haemostatic function and ischemic heart disease: principal results of the Northwick Park Heart Study. Lancet 2:533, 1986

193. Wilhelmsen L, Svärdsudd K, Korsan-Bengtsen K et al: Fibrinogen as a risk factor for stroke and myocardial infarction. N Engl J Med 311:501, 1984

194. Kannel WB, D'Agostino RB, Belander AJ: Fibrinogen, cigarette smoking, and risk of cardiovascular disease: insights from the Framingham Study. Am Heart J 113:1006, 1987

195. Balleisen L, Schulte H, Assman G et al: Coagulation factors and the progress of coronary heart disease. Lancet 1:461, 1987

196. Cook NS, Ubben D: Fibrinogen as a major risk factor in cardiovascular disease. Trends Pharmacol Sci 11:444, 1990

197. Eber B, Schumacher M: Fibrinogen: its role in the hemostatic regulation in atherosclerosis. Semin Thromb Hemost 19:104, 1993

198. Lechner K, Niessner H, Thaler E: Coagulation abnormalities in liver disease. Semin Thromb Hemost 4:40, 1977

199. Flute PT: Clotting abnormalities in liver disease. Prog Liver Dis 6:301, 1979

200. Boks AL, Brommer EJ, Schalm SW, Van Vliet HHDM: Hemostasis and fibrinolysis in severe liver failure and their relation to hemorrhage. Hepatology 6: 79, 1986

201. Straub PW: Diffuse intravascular coagulation in liver disease? Semin Thromb Hemost 4:29, 1977

202. Tytgat GN, Collen D, Verstraete M: Metabolism of fibrinogen in cirrhosis of the liver. J Clin Invest 50:1690, 1971

203. Rake MO, Pannell G, Flute PT, William R: Intravascular coagulation in acute hepatic necrosis. Lancet 1:533, 1970

204. Clark RD, Gazzard BG, Lewis ML et al: Fibrinogen metabolism in acute hepatitis and active chronic hepatitis. Br J Haematol 30:95, 1975

205. Coleman M, Finlayson N, Bettigole RE et al: Fibrinogen survival in cirrhosis: improvement by "low dose" heparin. Ann Intern Med 83:79, 1975

206. Collen D, Rouvier J, Chamone DAF et al: Turnover of radiolabelled plasminogen and prothrombin in cirrhosis of the liver. Eur J Clin Invest 8:185, 1978

207. Schipper G, Cate JWT: Antithrombin III transfusion in patients with hepatic cirrhosis. Br J Haematol 52:25, 1982

208. Coccheri S, Mannucci PM, Palareti G et al: Significance of plasma fibrinopeptide A and high molecular weight fibrinogen in patients with liver cirrhosis. Br J Haematol 52:503, 1982

209. Cordova C, Musca A, Violi F et al: Improvement of some blood coagulation factors in cirrhotic patients treated with low doses of heparin. Scand J Haematol 29:235, 1982

210. Paramo JA, Rifon J, Fernandez J et al: Thrombin activation and increased fibrinolysis in patients with chronic liver disease. Blood Coagul Fibrinolysis 2:227, 1991

211. Oka K, Tanaka K: Intravascular coagulation in autopsy cases with liver diseases. Thromb Haemost 42:564, 1979

212. Ramsay NKC, Coccia PF, Krivit W et al: The effect of L-asparaginase on plasma coagulation factors in acute lymphoblastic leukemia. Cancer 40: 1398, 1977

213. Capizzi RL, Bertino JR, Skeel RT et al: L-Asparaginase: clinical biochemical, pharmacological, and immunological studies. Ann Intern Med 74:893, 1971

214. Whitecar JP Jr, Bodey GP, Harris JE, Freireich EJ: L-Asparaginase. N Engl J Med 282:732, 1970

215. Gralnick HR, Henderson E: Hypofibrinogenemia and coagulation factor deficiencies with L-asparaginase treatment. Cancer 27:1313, 1971

216. Priest JR, Ramsay NK, Bennett AJ et al: The effect of L-asparaginase on antithrombin, plasminogen and plasma coagulation during therapy for acute lymphoblastic leukemia. J Pediatr 100:990, 1982

217. Bettigole RE, Himelstein ES, Oettgen HF, Clifford GO: Hypofibrinogenemia due to L-asparaginase: studies of fibrinogen survival using autologous ^{131}I-fibrinogen. Blood 35:195, 1970

218. Alving BM, Barr CF, Tang DB: L-Asparaginase: acute effects on protein synthesis in rabbits with normal and increased fibrinogen production. Blood 63:823, 1984

219. Dale BM, Purdie GH, Rischbieth RH: Fibrinogen depletion with sodium valproate, letter. Lancet 1:1316, 1978

220. Soria J, Soria C, Ryckewaert JJ et al: Study of acquired dysfibrinogenemia in liver disease. Thromb Res 19:29, 1980

221. Green G, Thomson JM, Dymock IW, Poller L: Abnormal fibrin polymerization in liver disease. Br J Haematol 34:427, 1976

222. Lane DA, Scully MF, Thomas DP et al: Acquired dysfibrinogenaemia in acute and chronic liver disease. Br J Haematol 35:301, 1977

223. Palascak JE, Martinez J: Dysfibrinogenemia associated with liver disease. J Clin Invest 60:89, 1977

224. Von Felten A, Straub PW, Grick PG: Dysfibrinogenemia in a patient with primary hepatoma. N Engl J Med 280:405, 1969

225. Verhaeghe R, van Damme B, Molla A, Vermylen J: Dysfibrinogenaemia associated with primary hepatoma. Scand J Haematol 9:451, 1972

226. Gralnick HR, Givelber H, Abrams E: Dysfibrinogenemia associated with hepatoma. N Engl J Med 299:221, 1978

227. Martinez J, Palascak JE, Kwasniak D: Abnormal sialic acid content of the dysfibrinogenemia associated with liver disease. J Clin Invest 61:535, 1978

228. Martinez J, Keane PM, Gilman PB: Carbohydrate composition of normal fibrinogen compared to the abnormal fibrinogen of liver disease. Ann NY Acad Sci 408:655, 1983

229. Martinez J, Barsigian C: Carbohydrate abnormalities of N-linked plasma glycoproteins in liver disease. Lab Invest 57:250, 1987

230. Galanakis DK, Martinez J, McDevitt C, Miller F: Human fetal fibrinogen: its characteristics of delayed fibrin formation, high sialic acid and AP peptide content are more marked in pre-term than in term samples. Ann NY Acad Sci 408:640, 1983

231. Weinstein MJ, Deykin D: Quantitative abnormality of an A chain molecular weight form in the fibrinogen of cirrhotic patients. Br J Haematol 40:617, 1978

232. Dawson NA, Barr CF, Alving BM: Acquired dysfibrinogenemia. Am J Med 78:682, 1985

233. Marciniak E, Greenwood MF: Acquired coagulation inhibitor delaying fibrinopeptide release. Blood 53:81, 1979

234. Galanakis DK, Ginzler EM, Fikrig SM: Monoclonal IgG anticoagulants delaying fibrin aggregation in two patients with systemic lupus erythematosus (SLE). Blood 52:1037, 1978

235. Hoots WK, Carrell NA, Wagner RH et al: A naturally occurring antibody that inhibits fibrin polymerization. N Engl J Med 304:857, 1981

236. Ghosh S, McEvoy P, McVerry BA: Idiopathic autoantibody that inhibits fibrin monomer polymerization. Br J Haematol 53:65, 1983

237. Rosenberg RD, Colman RW, Lorand L: A new haemorrhagic disorder with defective fibrin stabilization and cryofibrinogenaemia. Br J Haematol 26: 269, 1974

238. Soria J, Soria C, Samama M et al: Analysis of a fibrin formation abnromality in a case of multiple myeloma. Br J Haematol 15:207, 1975

239. Coleman M, Vigliano EM, Weksler ME, Nachman RL: Inhibition of fibrin monomer polymerization by lambda myeloma globulins. Blood 39:210, 1972

240. Vigliano EM, Horowitz HL: Bleeding syndrome caused by interaction of IgA myeloma: interaction of protein and connective tissue, abstracted. Blood 26:880, 1965

241. Frick PG: Inhibition of conversion of fibrinogen to fibrin by abnormal proteins in multiple myeloma. Am J Clin Pathol 25:1263, 1955

242. Gastineau DA, Gertz MA, Daniels TM et al: Inhibitor of thrombin time in systemic amyloidosis: a common coagulation abnormality. Blood 77:2637, 1991

243. Khoory MS, Nesheim ME, Bowie EJW, Mann KG: Circulating heparan sulfate proteoglycan anticoagulant from a patient with a plasma cell disorder. J Clin Invest 65:666, 1980

244. Palmer RN, Rick ME, Rick PD et al: Circulating heparan sulfate anticoagulant in a patient with a fatal bleeding disorder. N Engl J Med 310:1696, 1984

245. Tefferi A, Owen BA, Nichols WL et al: Isolation of a heparin-like anticoagulant from the plasma of a patient with metastatic bladder carcinoma. Blood 74: 252, 1989

246. Weisel JW: Fibrin assembly. Lateral aggregation and the role of the two pairs of fibrinopeptides. Biophys J 50:1079, 1986

247. Wada Y, Niwa K, Maekawa H et al: A new type of congenital dysfibrinogen, fibrinogen Bremen, with an Aα Gly-17 to Val substitution associated with hemorrhagic diathesis and delayed wound healing. Thromb Haemost 70: 397, 1993

248. Steinmann C, Reber P, Jungo M et al: Fibrinogen Bern I: substitution γ 337 Asn → Lys is responsible for defective fibrin monomer polymerization. Blood 82:2104, 1993

249. Uemichi T, Liepnieks JJ, Benson MD: Hereditary renal amyloidosis with a novel variant fibrinogen. J Clin Invest 93:731, 1994

Structure, Biology, and Genetics of von Willebrand Factor

112

Denisa D. Wagner and David Ginsburg

INTRODUCTION

The adhesive glycoprotein von Willebrand factor (vWF) was named after Dr. Erich von Willebrand, who described in 1926 a new bleeding disorder distinct from hemophilia.[1] This disorder was later recognized to be caused by decreased synthesis or defects in vWF.[2] vWF circulates in plasma at concentrations ranging between 5 and 10 μg/ml. Some of the molecules are complexed with factor VIII, apparently protecting factor VIII against degradation.[3] vWF is synthesized by only two cell types: endothelial cells and megakaryocytes.[4-6] Besides plasma, vWF is found in platelets, in endothelial cells, and in the basement membrane of blood vessels.[7] All these pools of vWF contribute to the protein's main function: to promote attachment of platelets to areas of vessel injury. To optimize the availability of vWF at the site of injury, a highly active form of the protein is stored in secretory granules of platelets and of endothelial cells.[8] When these cells sense tissue injury (e.g., by contact with thrombin) they instantly mobilize the stored protein. The released vWF binds to glycoprotein Ib (GPIb) on the platelet surface[9-12] and to components of the basement membrane,[13] forming a bridge that can withstand high sheer stress of blood flow. vWF is necessary for this initial attachment step of platelets to the injured area. Together with other adhesive proteins, such as fibrinogen, fibronectin, and thrombospondin, vWF interacts with the GPIIb/IIIa on activated platelets

vWF gene (51 introns, 178 kb) [chromosome 12]

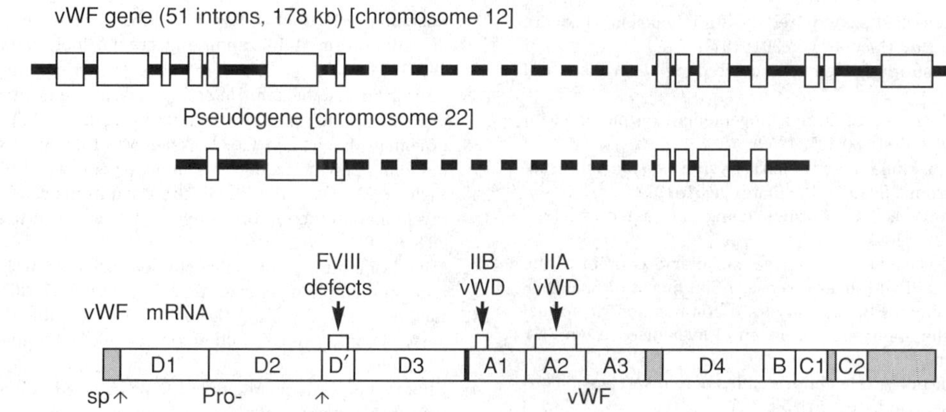

Pseudogene [chromosome 22]

vWF mRNA

FVIII defects   IIB vWD   IIA vWD

| sp↑ | | D1 | D2 | D′ | D3 | A1 | A2 | A3 | D4 | B | C1 | C2 |

Pro- ↑   vWF

Fig. 112-1. Structure of the vWF gene and mRNA. The structures of the vWF gene and pseudogene are indicated schematically at the top of the figure. The corresponding mRNA is also depicted, including the homologous repeat domain structure. The localization within vWF of point mutations associated with von Willebrand disease (vWD) variants are also indicated. [Adapted from Ginsburg and Bowie,[98] with permission.]

and contributes to platelet spreading and aggregation.[14,15] vWF is a large protein composed of many subunits held together covalently by disulfide bonds.[16] In this way, the protein acquires multiple binding sites for platelets and the basement membrane, which may strengthen its interactions during hemostasis.

The vWF Gene

vWF cDNA was independently cloned by four groups in 1985.[17–20] The full-length cDNA sequence predicts a protein of 309,000 molecule weight (2,813 amino acids). In addition, the location of N- and O-linked glycosylation sites within the mature vWF subunit have been determined by direct protein analysis.[21] Comparison of the cDNA and primary amino acid sequences identified a large propeptide (741 amino acids) preceding the mature vWF subunit sequence. This propeptide is identical to a previously observed immunologic activity in plasma termed vW antigen II. This propeptide plays an important role in vWF multimer assembly processing but has no known function after secretion. The vWF gene is located on the short arm of human chromosome 12,[17,19] and a partial, nonfunctional duplication of the gene, termed a pseudogene, is on human chromosome 22.[22] The structures of the unusually large vWF gene and pseudogene are shown schematically in Figure

112-1.[23,24] The gene is composed of 52 exons spanning a total of approximately 180 kb of the human genome. It is similar in size to the factor VIII gene (see Ch. 105) and >100 times larger than the gene for β-globin (see Ch. 35). The vWF gene accounts for approximately 0.1% of human chromosome 12. The vWF pseudogene duplicates the middle portion of the gene from exon 23 to 34, including the intervening sequences. The pseudogene is approximately 97% homologous to the authentic gene, indicating that it has arisen fairly recently in evolution.[24]

Analysis of the vWF amino acid sequence identifies a pattern of homologous repeated segments, designated by the letters A to D in Figures 112-1 and 112-2. This pattern suggests that the vWF gene arose by a complex series of partial gene duplications. The expression of the vWF gene is tightly regulated and restricted exclusively to endothelial cells and megakaryocytes. For this reason, vWF is frequently used as a primary histochemical marker to identify cells of endothelial cell origin. Although potential regulatory DNA sequences upstream of the vWF gene have been analyzed, the molecular basis for the exquisite tissue specificity of vWF gene expression remains to be elucidated. As in the case of β-globin, another highly tissue-specific regulated gene (see Ch. 35), critical transcription regulatory sequences could exist a great distance from the 5′ end of the vWF gene.

Comparison of the vWF DNA sequence to that of other known genes identifies only limited potential relationships. A super-

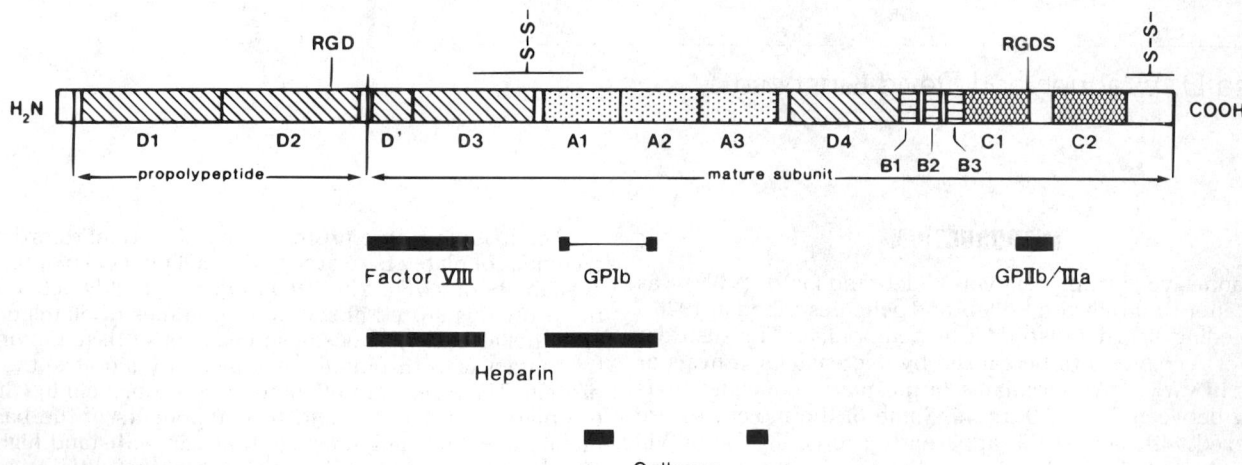

Fig. 112-2. Domain structure of pro-vWF. Binding site locations for other molecules are indicated by black rectangles and those of interchain disulfide bones by -s-s-. [Adapted from Baruch et al.,[124] with permission.]

family of proteins sharing sequence similarity with vWF A domains has been identified[25]; this family contains a number of proteins associated with the extracellular matrix, hemostasis, and cell adhesion. Adhesive functions have also been localized to the vWF A domains. A possible relationship between the C repeats of vWF and segments of thrombospondin and procollagen has also been noted.[26] vWF exons range in size from 40 base pairs to 1.4 kb for exon 28, one of the larger known single exons. This latter exon encompasses most of the A1 and A2 homologous repeats, a region containing several important vWF functional domains, as well as a large number of human mutations associated with types IIA and IIB von Willebrand disease (vWD).

DOMAIN STRUCTURE

vWF exists as a series of multimers varying in molecular weight between 0.5 (dimer) and 20 million (multimer). Electron microscopic observations of the vWF molecules revealed that they are filamentous and contain subunits arranged in a head-to-head and tail-to-tail configuration.[27,28] The building block of multimers is a dimer, held together by disulfide bond(s) located near the C-terminal end of each subunit. The dimers are joined to each other by disulfide bonds located near the N-terminal end of the mature subunit.[29] The mature subunit has a mass of about 270 kd and contains 18.7% carbohydrate.[21] N- and O-linked carbohydrate are found clustered at both ends of the subunit; Cys 169 residues (8.2%) are all involved in interchain and intrachain disulfide bonds.[30,31] Two Arg-Gly-Asp (RGD) sequences were found in pro-vWF (Fig. 112-2). The one on vWF is a part of the binding site for the platelet integrin receptor GPIIb/IIIa.[15] The significance of the other Arg-Gly-Asp sequence located on the propeptide is not known (Fig. 112-2).

Several functional domains in vWF have been identified on the vWF subunit[32] (Fig. 112-2). Two collagen-binding sites are located on the mature vWF subunit[33,34] (Fig. 112-2). The corresponding homologous vWF fragments bind fibrillar collagen only in their native state, not when reduced and alkylated. There may be a third binding site for collagen located on the propeptide.[35] vWF also has at least two binding sites for heparin and may interact with heparin-like molecules in the basement membrane.[36,37] The factor VIII-binding domain is located in the N-terminal portion of the vWF subunit,[38] and the interaction is with the N-terminal portion of the factor VIII light chain[39,40] (see Ch. 105). vWF also has affinity for two platelet receptors. Its binding to GPIb plays a pivotal role in the early events of hemostasis, leading to the attachment of platelets to the area of injury.[10] Several potential, short binding sequences for GPIb on vWF have been identified, all localized to a large disulfide loop contained within the vWF A1 repeat[41,42] (Fig. 112-2). This site appears to interact with the N-terminal portion of the α-chain of GPIb.[43] The binding region of vWF to GPIIb/IIIa on activated platelets is located in the C-terminal portion of the mature subunit. This recognition site can be specifically inhibited by the Arg-Gly-Asp sequence contained within peptides[44] and is therefore likely to include the Arg-Gly-Asp-Ser sequence.[15,45] vWF (with other adhesive proteins such as fibrinogen and fibronectin) may compete for binding to this glycoprotein.

BIOSYNTHESIS

The processing steps leading to the formation of mature vWF multimers have been studied chiefly in endothelial cells,[46] but evaluation of megakaryocyte biosynthesis indicates an identi-

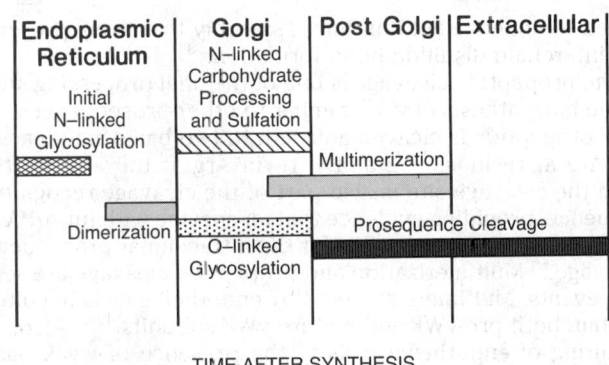

Fig. 112-3. Map of processing steps in the biosynthesis of vWF. Interchain disulfide bonds are formed in two steps (dimerization and multimerization, pink). The propeptide is cleaved late in vWF processing (prosequence cleavage, red). (Adapted from Handin and Wagner,[7] with permission.)

cal pattern of synthesis[6] (Fig. 112-3). vWF is first synthesized as pro-vWF monomer.[47–49] Co-translationally, high-mannose carbohydrate is added to the polypeptide chain. There are 13 potential N-linked glycosylation sites on the mature vWF and 4 on the propeptide. While residing within the endoplasmic reticulum, the C-termini of the pro-vWF subunits are linked together by an unknown number of disulfide bonds.[50] If initial glycosylation is inhibited by the drug tunicamycin, the protein remains monomeric. The monomeric protein synthesized in the presence of tunicamycin is internally degraded and is not secreted from the cells.[51] Only dimeric molecules are transported to the Gogli apparatus, where their processing continues. In the Golgi apparatus, common modifications, including the addition of O-linked carbohydrate, high-mannose carbohydrate processing, and sulfation, take place (Fig. 112-3). In addition, a unique processing event includes the multimerization of dimers by disulfide bond formation.[7] vWF is the only protein known that has disulfide bonds formed late in protein synthesis, as disulfide bonds are usually formed in the endoplasmic reticulum. The latter process is catalyzed by the enzyme disulfide isomerase.[52] The contents of the last compartment of the Golgi apparatus (trans-Golgi) and the post-Golgi secretory vesicles are slightly acidic.[53] It is likely that multimerization takes place in these acidic compartments, since this process can be completely inhibited by culturing cells in the presence of a weak base[51] that increases the pH of acidic cellular compartments. The vWF propeptide plays an active role in the interdimer disulfide bond formation. This conclusion is supported by several experimental observations. When prepro-vWF cDNA is expressed in COS (a monkey kidney cell line) or other cells that normally do not synthesize vWF, these cells are capable of supporting vWF multimerization. By contrast, if pre-vWF cDNA (with the cDNA coding for the propeptide deleted) is expressed in these cells, only dimeric molecules are synthesized and secreted.[54,55] In in vitro multimerization experiments, pro-vWF dimers spontaneously form large multimers, while vWF mature dimers remain dimeric. The in vitro multimerization is promoted by a slightly acidic environment (optimal pH is about 5.8) and will not occur at a neutral or basic pH.[56] Under these acidic pH conditions the propeptide may catalyze the disulfide bond formation among the mature vWF subunits. The propeptide contains sequences similar to those found at the active site of protein disulfide isomerase. These are cysteines separated by two amino acids that readily interchange with disulfide bonds in the substrate. When an additional amino acid was inserted between the cysteines of the propeptide by site specific mutagenesis, vWF expressed did not form multimers.[57] During the biosynthesis of vWF multimers, the propeptide does self-associate, but it is not known whether this association is linked to noncovalent multimer assembly that likely precedes the interchain disulfide bond formation.[58]

The propeptide cleavage is one of the final processing steps in the biosynthesis of vWF. Similar to other prosequences, the vWF propeptide is cleaved adjacent to two basic amino acids, Lys-Arg at residues -2 and -1. An Arg at the -4 position from the cleavage site is also part of the cleavage recognition sequence, providing evidence that an enzyme with furin/PACE-like specificity is responsible for the intracellular prosequence cleavage.[59] Multimerization and propeptide cleavage are separate events. Multimers secreted by endothelial cells in culture contain both pro-vWF and mature vWF subunits.[49,60] Also, the culturing of endothelial cells in the presence of weak bases inhibits multimerization completely, while propeptide cleavage is only slightly affected.[51] Finally, site-specific mutagenesis of the cleavage site inhibits propeptide cleavage, but the expressed protein has a normal multimeric composition.[61]

Although vWF processing is chiefly intracellular, some modifications to the protein likely occur after secretion. Cleavage of the propeptide, which begins in the trans-Golgi compartment, may continue extracellularly. This hypothesis is based on the observation that vWF in normal plasma is composed of only mature subunits, while vWF secreted constitutively from endothelial cells in culture contains both pro-vWF and mature subunits.[49,60] The largest vWF multimers found in plasma are smaller than those found in endothelial cells.[62] A likely possibility is that these unusually large multimers undergo limited proteolysis in the circulation, reducing them to smaller species. Cleavage products of vWF are present in normal plasma, and their amount is further increased in some patients lacking the large multimers (type IIA vWD).[63] Endothelial cells from one patient with type IIA disease were found to produce fewer large multimers, with a concomitant increase in amounts of the proteolytic fragments. In this patient, the primary defect was in the vWF molecule, resulting in a higher sensitivity to proteolysis.[64]

VON WILLEBRAND FACTOR STORAGE AND SECRETION

vWF is the only known adhesive protein that is stored and undergoes regulated secretion from cells other than platelets.[46] Both the platelet pool and the endothelial pool of vWF are important physiologically, as suggested by the observation that a transplant of a normal bone marrow into a pig with severe vWD only partially corrected the hemostatic defects.[65] In platelets, vWF is present in the α-granules along with many other stored proteins. In the Weibel-Palade bodies of endothelial cells, only vWF and its propeptide are found.[66–68] In both organelles, the stored vWF molecules appear to form tubular structures, 150 Å in diameter.[69,70] These tubules are absent in the α-granules of pigs with vWD.[71] A transmembrane glycoprotein of the α-granule, P-selectin (also known as PADGEM,[72] GMP-140,[73] CD62), is a component of the Weibel-Palade body membrane.[74] Like vWF, the biosynthesis of this protein is restricted to endothelial cells and to megakaryocytes. When expressed on the plasma membrane, P-selectin promotes the adhesion of monocytes, neutrophils, and some other subsets of leukocytes.[75,76] The only other recognized component of Weibel-Palade bodies is CD63, a highly glycosylated protein found in lysosomes, which is also expressed on activated platelets.[77,78] Weibel-Palade bodies originate from the Golgi apparatus. They are up to 4-μm long and 0.1-μm thick (Fig. 112-4) and are found in endothelial cells of virtually all blood vessel types. There is, however, variation in the number of Weibel-Palade bodies in each cell in endothelia of different origins.[8]

Fully processed vWF is secreted from cultured endothelial cells by one of two pathways.[79] The constitutive pathway is directed coupled to vWF synthesis and occurs without stimulation. The regulated pathway, involving vWF stored in Weibel-Palade bodies, is initiated by the action of secretagogues. The two pathways differ in that the regulated pathway depends on

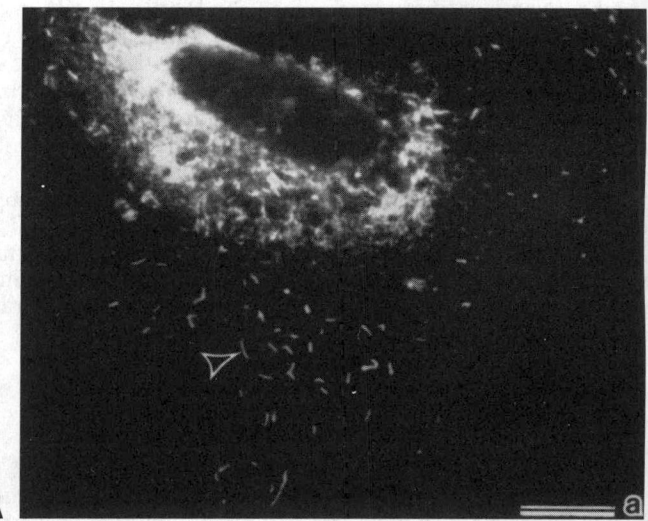

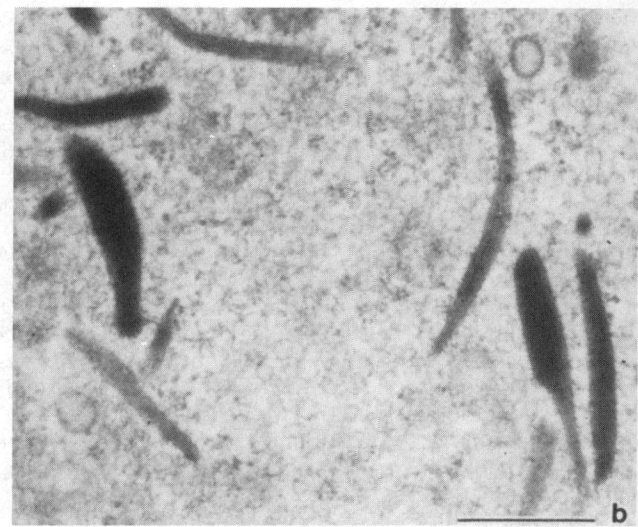

Fig. 112-4. Weibel-Palade bodies of endothelial cells. **(A)** Immunofluorescence staining of a human umbilical vein endothelial cell with anti-vWF antiserum. vWF is present in the perinuclear region, where it is synthesized, and in the Weibel-Palade bodies (arrowhead) throughout the cytoplasm. Bar = 10 μm. **(B)** Electron micrograph of Weibel-Palade bodies of the same origin. Bar = 0.5 μm.

the microtubular cytoskeleton, while the constitutive secretion continues even from cells with depolymerized microtubules.[80] The constitutive secretion occurs evenly into the apical and basolateral direction. By contrast, the release from Weibel-Palade bodies is highly polarized in the basolateral direction. Formation of thrombin and fibrin during vascular injury disrupts the endothelial monolayer, which may lead to the release of stored vWF into the lumen.[81] Another important difference between the two pathways is the biologic activity of the vWF secreted. While mostly small multimers are secreted constitutively, only the largest, biologically most potent, multimers are stored in Weibel-Palade bodies[68,82] (Fig. 112-5). It is not known whether the large multimers are selected for storage or whether the conditions found in the Weibel-Palade body promote multimer assembly. The vWF stored in platelet α-granules is also enriched in large multimers.[83] All the N-terminal D domains (D1–D3) appear to be necessary for vWF storage. Deletions of these individual domains lead to constitutive secretion of the expressed protein.[84,85] Although the propolypeptide remains in the Weibel-Palade bodies noncovalently associated

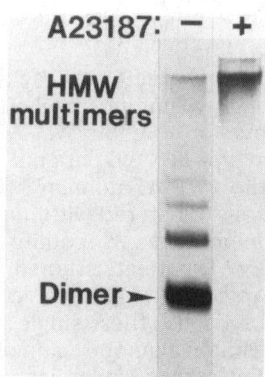

A23187: − +

HMW
multimers

Dimer ▶

Fig. 112-5. Multimeric composition of vWF secreted by endothelial cells in culture. Human umbilical vein endothelial cells were metabolically labeled with ³⁵S-methionine and the constitutively secreted protein (−) and that released during a 10-minute treatment with the secretagogue A23187(+) were purified and analyzed nonreduced on an agarose gel. The autoradiograph of the gel is shown. The protein secreted constitutively is composed predominantly of small multimers, while the vWF secreted from Weibel-Palade bodies is only of high molecular weight (HMW multimers). (Adapted from Sporn et al.,[82] with permission.)

with the mature subunit (Vischer and Wagner, unpublished observations), cleavage of the prosequence has to occur for efficient formation of the storage granules.[86] The biologic function of the two secretory pathways may be different. The small multimers secreted constitutively may be used as carrier proteins for factor VIII; the largest multimers released from Weibel-Palade bodies at the time of vascular injury may act to attach platelets and the injured endothelium to the vessel wall. Some of the released large vWF molecules remain associated with the endothelial membrane,[82] likely interacting with integrin-type receptors.[87] The functional significance of this transient membrane pool of vWF is unknown.

Several secretagogues for vWF that may be of physiologic importance include thrombin,[88] fibrin,[89] histamine,[90] and the terminal complement proteins C5b-9.[91] The release of Weibel-Palade bodies appears to be coupled to Ca²⁺ influx. Thrombin activity as a secretagogue is related to its proteolytic activity and the cleavage of a specific receptor.[79,88,92] Interaction with a cellular receptor is a likely mechanism for fibrin release of vWF. A specific N-terminal fragment of the fibrin β-chain appears to interact with the endothelium.[93] Histamine-induced release can be blocked by histamine H_1-receptor antagonists.[90] Surprisingly, none of the vasoactive agents that cause the rapid rise in levels of vWF in plasma, including 1-deamino-8-D-arginine-vasopressin (DDAVP), causes vWF release from endothelial cells in vitro.[94] It is likely that these agents act through an as yet unknown intermediate. This hypothesis is supported by the observation that plasma from DDAVP-treated normal subjects stimulates release of vWF from cultured endothelial cells.[95] vWF is an unusual molecule in that it interacts specifically with two types of transmembrane receptors: the GPIb receptor of platelets and the integrin-type receptors, such as the GPIIb/IIIa complex on platelets and the vitronectin receptor on endothelial cells. Binding to these receptors is enhanced by the presence of large numbers of binding sites on the vWF multimers. The adhesive activity of the very large multimers is so great that they are kept sequestered in storage organelles and are rapidly released locally at the site of vascular injury.

VON WILLEBRAND DISEASE

Molecular Genetics

With the availability of vWF cDNA and genomic sequences, a molecular genetic approach to the characterization of vWD became possible. Initial Southern blot analysis identified large

gene deletions as the molecular basis of the disease in a small subset of severe, or type III patients.[22,96,97] With the advent of the polymerase chain reaction, extensive direct DNA sequence analysis has been conducted on material from patients with a variety of vWD variants, using platelets as a source for vWF mRNA, or by direct analysis of genomic DNA. Rapid progress has been made over the past few years, and a large number of human mutations have been catalogued.[98,99] As in the case of thalassemia (see Ch. 42), molecular genetic analysis has shed important light on the molecular pathogenesis of vWD and promises to improve diagnosis. For some vWD variants, mutations have been identified in the majority of patients studied, and precise diagnosis and classification by DNA screening may soon become practical.

vWD can be divided into two general categories: those variants due to a pure quantitative deficiency and those due to a qualitative structural or functional abnormality within the vWF protein. This is similar to the distinction in the hemoglobinopathies between quantitative abnormalities of globin synthesis (thalassemia) and qualitative structural or functional abnormalities within the protein subunit, such as in the other hemoglobinopathies. Total disruption of gene function by deletion of a segment of the gene or a nonsense mutation (abrupt termination of the protein by insertion of a stop codon into the coding sequence) generally results in quantitative vWF abnormalities. Conversely, the vast majority of qualitative variants are due to mutations, which result in single amino acid substitutions that interfere with protein structure or function.

Types I and III

Quantitative vWF abnormalities can be either mild or pronounced. Type III (severe vWD) patients suffer from a profound bleeding disorder (see Ch. 113) with very little or no detectable plasma or platelet vWF. Type III vWD is a relatively rare disease, with an incidence of approximately 1 per 1 million.[100] By contrast, type I is the most common form of vWD, accounting for 70–80% of cases; it is associated with a mild-to-moderate quantitative decrease in vWF (levels in the range of 20% to 50% of normal). Type III vWD appears to result from the inheritance of a dysfunctional vWF gene from both parents. Gene deletions varying from 2.3 kb to >180 kb have been identified in several patients and may be associated with an increased risk of developing vWF inhibitor antibodies.[22,96,97] Several other defects resulting in complete loss of vWF function have been identified in type III vWD patients, including nondeletion defects resulting in loss of mRNA expression[101] and recently, specific nonsense mutations or frameshift mutations resulting in gross disruption of the vWF protein coding sequence.[99] Although a limited number of mutations may account for a high percentage of type III vWD patients in Scandinavia, the genetic background of this disorder in other populations appears to be more diverse.[102] This latter observation may make routine DNA diagnosis for this disorder difficult.

In the most straightforward model, type I vWD would simply represent the heterozygous form of type III vWD. However, there is some controversy on this point. Type III vWD has classically been defined as "recessive" in inheritance and parents, who are obligate carriers for the defect, are often completely asymptomatic, with normal laboratory numbers.[22,96,97] However, in other cases, parents are affected with classic type I vWD. The reported prevalence of type I vWD (≤1% of the population[103]) would predict a much higher frequency of type III vWD (1:40,000) than is observed (1:1 million). Thus, the possibility of locus heterogeneity (i.e., defects in other genes giving rise to a disorder clinically indistinguishable from vWD) has been proposed.[98] Consistent with this idea, an animal model for human type I vWD was recently described in the RIIS/J mouse,[104] and preliminary genetic analysis suggests that the defect in this mouse model is in another gene, outside of vWF.[105] However, all genetic analysis of human vWD to date has been consistent with linkage to the vWF gene,[98,99] and the relevance of this mouse model for human vWD remains to be determined.

Type IIA

Type IIA is the most common qualitative abnormality of vWF and is associated with selective loss of large and intermediate-sized vWF multimers (see Ch. 113). Direct sequence analysis from platelet mRNA and genomic DNA has identified a panel of mutations within vWF exon 28 accounting for most type IIA vWD patients.[98,99] Nearly all of these mutations are clustered within the vWF A2 repeat (Fig. 112-1). One particular mutation (Arg 834→Trp) may account for approximately one-third of type IIA vWD cases around the world. In vitro analysis of recombinant vWF containing type IIA vWD mutations suggests that two distinct mechanisms contribute to the pathogenesis of this disorder[106] (Fig. 112-6). In the first group, the single amino acid substitution results in a defect in vWF intracellular processing, with retention of the abnormal vWF in the endoplasma reticulum. In the second subgroup, vWF synthesis and processing in vitro appears to be normal, and the loss of multimers is presumed to occur via increased sensitivity to proteolysis in plasma.[107] Indeed, a 176-kd vWF fragment, due to a single proteolytic cleavage between Tyr 842 and Met 853, is present in the plasma of normal individuals and is markedly increased in the plasma of some type IIA vWD patients.[108] This proteolytic site is located in the middle of the type IIA vWD mutation cluster. A single case of an unusual type II vWD variant has recently been reported in which internal deletion of a segment of vWF protein results from removal of exons 26–33 by a genomic DNA deletion.[109] Whether this unique, internally deleted protein produces loss of vWF multimers via disruption of intracellular vWF multimer assembly or via increased sensitivity to proteolysis has not yet been determined.

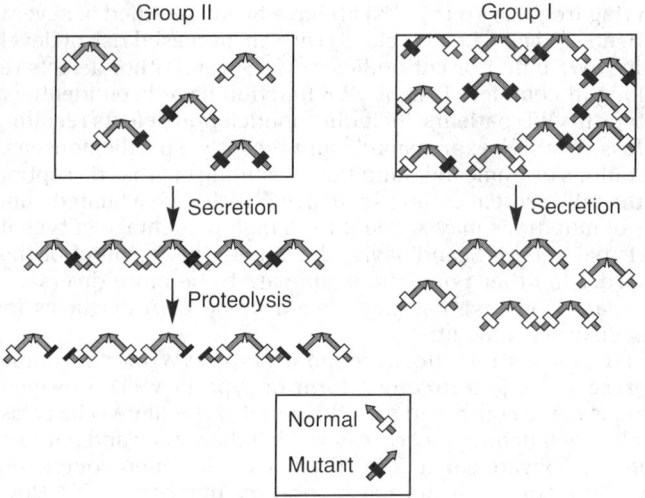

Fig. 112-6. Two mechanisms for the molecular pathogenesis of type IIA vWD. Each vWF monomer is indicated as a gray arrow with the normal sequence indicated by white boxes and mutant sequence by black boxes. Within the cell, mixed dimers are formed, as well as homodimers of mutant and wild-type monomers. In group II, full-size multimers are assembled and proteolyzed after secretion. In group I, mutant subunits are held up in the endoplasmic reticulum; only homomultimers of normal subunits are secreted, predominantly of small size.

Type IIB

Type IIB vWD is also characterized by a loss of large vWF multimers but through a unique mechanism, distinct from those described above for type IIA vWD. A panel of mutations has been identified in type IIB vWD patients, all clustered within a short stretch of the vWF A1 domain[98,99,110,111] (Fig. 112-1). Four of these mutations, clustered within a 35-amino-acid segment of the 2,813-amino acid vWF coding sequence, account for >90% of type IIB vWD patients studied.[99] This observation identifies a critical region of vWF involved in binding to the platelet GPIb receptor. Each of these single amino acid substitutions is thought to result in a unique "gain of function," leading to spontaneous binding of vWF to platelets.[112,113] Under normal conditions, plasma vWF is inert in its interaction toward platelets until it encounters an exposed subendothelial surface. Binding of vWF to collagen or other ligands within the vessel wall at sites of vascular injury presumably results in a secondary conformational change, which then facilitates binding to the GPIb platelet receptor. In type IIB vWD, the mutant vWF is capable of spontaneously binding to GPIb in the absence of a subendothelial contact. The large multimers appear to have the highest affinity for GPIb (presumably because of multivalency) and are rapidly cleared from plasma, along with the platelets, resulting in the characteristic loss of large multimers as well as thrombocytopenia. Screening for this panel of mutations should detect >90% of type IIB vWD patients and should provide precise and rapid DNA diagnosis for this disorder.

Defects in vWF/Factor VIII Binding

Recently, a unique variant of vWD has been defined that has important implications for the differential diagnosis of hemophilia and provides an instructive example of genetic locus heterogeneity. Rare cases of "autosomal" hemophilia have been reported in the past, in which deficiencies in factor VIII activity were inherited in an apparently autosomal manner.[114,115] More recently, biochemical analysis in several families identified a defect residing within the patient's plasma vWF, interfering with its ability to bind and stabilize factor VIII.[116,117] DNA sequence analysis in a number of these patients has identified several mutations, all clustered in a region at the N terminus of vWF, previously shown to be important for factor VIII binding[99] (Fig. 112-1). One of these mutations, Arg 91→Gln, appears to be particularly common.[118] These mutations are generally clinically silent in the heterozygote. However, when coinherited with another abnormal vWF allele, such defects can be associated with moderate deficiency in factor VIII. This variant, often termed vWD Normandy after the province of origin of one of the first patients, should be considered in the differential diagnosis of mild-to-moderate hemophilia, particularly in a female patient or in the context of other features suggesting an autosomal pattern of inheritance.[119]

Prenatal Diagnosis

With the advent of molecular analysis of vWD, prenatal diagnosis has become possible and has been applied in a select number of cases.[120–122] Given the generally mild clinical manifestations of most vWD variants, prenatal diagnosis is generally not indicated. However, in the case of type III or severe vWD, the indications for prenatal diagnosis are similar to those of severe hemophilia. For those vWD variants for which the mutation is known, direct analysis of chorionic villus samples or amniotic fluid can be performed rapidly by polymerase chain reaction and can be expected to provide a highly accurate, specific, and rapid diagnosis.[99] For vWD families in which the specific mutation is unknown, genetic linkage analysis can be performed using a large panel of highly informative restriction fragment length polymorphisms.[123] One particularly useful polymorphism is a highly variable TCTA repeat in intron 40, which has been reported to have over 100 distinct alleles.[123] While all cases of vWD analyzed to date appear to be linked to defects within the vWF gene, the possibility of locus heterogeneity (i.e., involvement of other genes outside of vWF) should be considered when performing this kind of analysis.

Thus, in summary, a large number of mutations have recently been identified in vWD patients, and the list can be expected to grow considerably over the coming years.[99] In addition to providing powerful new tools for the diagnosis and classification of vWD, these mutations have provided important insights into structure and function relationships within this complex protein. The vWF Normandy mutations have helped to map the region of vWF critical for binding to factor VIII, and type IIB and IIA mutations have contributed to the localization of other important vWF functional domains. Recent rapid advances in vWF molecular genetics will eventually lead to a simplified classification of vWD based on molecular pathogenesis to replace the current classification scheme.

REFERENCES

1. von Willebrand EA: Hereditär Pseudohemofili. Finska Läkarsällskapetes Handl 67:7, 1926
2. Berkowitz SD, Ruggeri ZM, Zimmerman TS: von Willebrand Disease. p. 215. In Zimmerman TS, Ruggeri ZM (eds): Coagulation and Bleeding Disorders. The Role of Factor VIII and von Willebrand Factor. Marcel Dekker, New York, 1989
3. Weiss HJ, Sussman II, Hoyer LW: Stabilization of factor VIII in plasma by the von Willebrand factor. Studies on posttransfusion and dissociated factor VIII and in patients with von Willebrand disease. J Clin Invest 60:390, 1977
4. Jaffe EA, Hoyer LW, Nachman RL: Synthesis of antihemophilic factor antigen by cultured human endothelial cells. J Clin Invest 52:2757, 1973
5. Nachman R, Levine R, Jaffe EA: Synthesis of factor VIII antigen by cultured guinea pig megakaryocytes. J Clin Invest 60:914, 1977
6. Sporn LA, Chavin SI, Marder VJ, Wagner DD: Biosynthesis of von Willebrand protein by human megakaryocytes. J Clin Invest 76:1102, 1985
7. Handin RI, Wagner DD: Molecular and cellular biology of von Willebrand factor. Prog Hematol 9:233, 1989
8. Wagner DD: Storage and secretion of von Willebrand factor. p. 161. In Ruggeri ZM, Zimmerman TS (eds): Coagulation and Bleeding Disorders: The Role of Factor VIII and von Willebrand factor. Marcel Dekker, New York, 1989
9. Weiss JH, Turitto VT, Baumgartner HR: Effect of shear rate on platelet interaction with subendothelium in citrated and native blood. I. Shear rate-dependent decrease of adhesion in von Willebrand's disease and the Bernard-Soulier syndrome. J Lab Clin Med 92:750, 1978
10. Clemetson KJ, McGregor JL, James E et al: Characterization of the platelet membrane glycoprotein abnormalities in Bernard-Soulier syndrome and comparison with normal by surface-labeling techniques and high-resolution two-dimensional gel electrophoresis. J Clin Invest 70:304, 1982
11. Coller BS, Peerschke EI, Scudder LE, Sullivan CA: Studies with a murine monoclonal antibody that abolishes ristocetin-induced binding of von Willebrand factor to platelets: additional evidence in support of GPIb as a platelet receptor for von Willebrand factor. Blood 61:99, 1983
12. Wicki AN, Clemetson KJ: The glycoprotein Ib complex of human blood platelets. Eur J Biochem 163:4, 1987
13. Rand JH, Sussman II, Gordon RE et al: Localization of factor-VIII-related antigen in human vascular subendothelium. Blood 55:752, 1980
14. Ruggeri ZM, De Marco L, Gatti L, et al: Platelets have more than one binding site for von Willebrand factor. J Clin Invest 72:1, 1983
15. Plow EF, McEver RP, Coller BS et al: Related binding mechanisms for fibrinogen, fibronectin, von Willebrand factor, and thrombospondin on thrombin-stimulated human platelets. Blood 66:724, 1985
16. Ruggeri ZM, Zimmerman TS: Variant von Willebrand disease: characterization of two subtypes by analysis of multimeric composition of factor VIII/von Willebrand factor in plasma and platelets. J Clin Invest 65:1318, 1980
17. Ginsburg D, Handin RI, Bonthron DT et al: Human von Willebrand factor (vWF): isolation of complementary DNA (cDNA) clones and chromosomal localization. Science 228:1401, 1985
18. Lynch DC, Zimmerman TS, Colins CJ et al: Molecular cloning of cDNA for human von Willebrand factor: authentication by a new method. Cell 41:49, 1985
19. Verweij CL, de Vries CJM, Distel B et al: Construction of cDNA coding for human von Willebrand factor using antibody probes for colony-screening and mapping of the chromosomal gene. Nucleic Acids Res 13:4699, 1985
20. Sadler JE, Shelton-Inloes BB, Sorace JM et al: Cloning and characterization of two cDNAs coding for human von Willebrand factor. Proc Natl Acad Sci USA 82:6394, 1985
21. Titani K, Kumar S, Takio K et al: Amino acid sequence of human von Willebrand Factor. Biochemistry 25:3171, 1986
22. Shelton-Inloes BB, Chehab FF, Mannucci PM et al: Gene deletions correlate with the development of alloantibodies in von Willebrand Disease. J Clin Invest 79:1459, 1987
23. Mancuso DJ, Tuley EA, Westfield LA et al: Structure of the gene for human von Willebrand factor. J Biol Chem 264:19514, 1989
24. Mancuso DJ, Tuley EA, Westfield LA et al: Human von Willebrand factor gene and pseudogene: structure analysis and differentiation by polymerase chain reaction. Biochemistry 30:253, 1991
25. Colombatti A, Bonaldo P: The superfamily of proteins with von Willebrand factor type A-like domains: one theme common to components of extracellular matrix, hemostasis, cellular adhesion, and defense mechanisms. Blood 77:2305, 1991
26. Hunt LT, Barker WC: von Willebrand factor shares a distinctive cysteine-rich domain with thrombospondin and procollagen. Biochem Biophys Res Commun 144:876, 1987
27. Fowler WE, Fretto LJ, Hamilton KK et al: Substructure of human von Willebrand factor. J Clin Invest 76:1491, 1985
28. Slayter H, Loscalzo J, Bockenstedt P, Handin RI: Native conformation of human von Willebrand protein. Analysis by electron microscopy and quasielastic light scattering. J Biol Chem 260:8559, 1985
29. Marti T, Rosselet SJ, Titani K, Walsh KA: Identification of disulfide-bridged substructures within human von Willebrand factor. Biochemistry 26:8099, 1987
30. Legaz ME, Schmer G, Counts RB, Davie EW: Isolation and characterization of human factor VIII (antihemophilic factor). J Biol Chem 248:3946, 1973
31. Kirby EP, Mills DCB: The interaction of bovine factor VIII with human platelets. J Clin Invest 56:491, 1975
32. Ruggeri ZM, Ware J: The structure and function of von Willebrand factor. Thromb Haemost 67:594, 1992
33. Kalafatis M, Takahashi Y, Girma J-P, Meyer D: Localization of a collagen-interactive domain of human von Willebrand factor between amino acid residues Gly 911 and Glu 1, 365. Blood 70:1577, 1987
34. Pareti FI, Niiya K, McPherson JM, Ruggeri ZM: Isolation and characterization of two domains of human von Willebrand factor that interact with fibrillar collagen types I and III. J Biol Chem 262:13835, 1987
35. Takagi J, Sekiya F, Kasahara K et al: Inhibition of platelet-collagen interaction by propolypeptide of von Willebrand factor. J Biol Chem 264:6017, 1989
36. Fretto LJ, Fowler WE, McCaslin DR et al: Substructure of human von Willebrand factor: proteolysis by V8 and characterization of two functional domains. J Biol Chem 261:15679, 1986
37. Fujimura Y, Titani K, Holland LZ et al: A heparin-binding domain of human von Willebrand factor. Characterization and localization to a tryptic fragment extending from amino acid residue Val^{449} to Lys^{728}. J Biol Chem 262:1734, 1987
38. Foster PA, Fulcher CA, Marti T et al: A major factor VIII binding domain resides within the amino-terminal 272 amino acid residues of von Willebrand factor. J Biol Chem 262:8443, 1987
39. Foster PA, Fulcher CA, Houghten RA, Zimmerman TS: An immunogenic region within residues Val^{1670}-Glu^{1684} of the factor VIII light chain induces antibodies which inhibit binding of factor VIII to von Willebrand factor. J Biol Chem 263:5230, 1986
40. Lollar P, Hill-Eubanks DC, Parker CG: Association of the factor VIII light chain with von Willebrand factor. J Biol Chem 263 10451, 1988
41. Berndt MC, Ward CM, Booth WJ et al: Identification of aspartic acid 514 through glutamic acid 542 as a glycoprotein Ib-IX complex receptor recognition sequence in von Willebrand factor. Mechanism of modulation of von Willebrand factor by ristocetin and botrocetin. Biochemistry 31:11144, 1992
42. Mohri H, Fujimura Y, Shima M et al: Structure of the von Willebrand factor domain interacting with glycoprotein Ib. J Biol Chem 263:17901, 1988
43. Vicente V, Kostel PJ, Ruggeri ZM: Isolation and functional characterization of the von Willebrand factor-binding domain located between residues His^{1}-Arg^{293} of the α-chain of glycoprotein Ib. J Biol Chem 263:18473, 1988
44. Ruoslahti E, Pierschbacher MD: Arg-Gly-Asp: a versatile cell recognition signal. Cell 44:517, 1986
45. Haverstick DM, Cowan JF, Yamada KM, Santoro SA: Inhibition of platelet adhesion to fibronectin, fibrinogen, and von Willebrand factor substrates by

a synthetic tetrapeptide derived from the cell-binding domain of fibronectin. Blood 66:946, 1985

46. Wagner DD: Cell biology of von Willebrand factor. Annu Rev Cell Biol 6:217, 1990

47. Wagner DD, Marder VJ: Biosynthesis of von Willebrand protein by human endothelial cells. J Biol Chem 258:2065, 1983

48. Lynch DC, Williams R, Zimmerman TS et al: Biosynthesis of the subunits of factor VIIIR by bovine aortic endothelial cells. Proc Natl Acad Sci USA 80: 2738, 1983

49. Wagner DD, Marder VJ: Biosynthesis of von Willebrand protein by human endothelial cells: processing steps and their intracellular localization. J Cell Biol 99:2123, 1984

50. Wagner DD, Lawrence SO, Ohlsson-Wilhelm BM et al: Topology and order of formation of interchain disulfide bonds in von Willebrand factor. Blood 69:27, 1987

51. Wagner DD, Mayadas T, Marder VJ: Initial glycosylation and acidic pH in the Golgi apparatus are required for multimerization of von Willebrand factor. J Cell Biol 102:1320, 1986

52. Freedman RB: Native disulphide bond formation in protein biosynthesis: evidence for the role of protein disulphide isomerase. Trends Biochem Sci 9:438, 1984

53. Anderson RG, Pathak RK: Vesicles and cisternae in the trans Golgi apparatus of human fibroblasts are acidic compartments. Cell 40:635, 1985

54. Verweij CL, Hart M, Pannekoek H: Expression of variant von Willebrand factor (vWF) cDNA in heterologous cells: requirement of the pro-polypeptide in vWF multimer formation. EMBO J 6:2885, 1987

55. Wise RJ, Pittman DD, Handin RI et al: The propeptide of von Willebrand factor independently mediates the assembly of von Willebrand multimers. Cell 52:299, 1988

56. Mayadas TN, Wagner DD: In vitro multimerization of von Willebrand factor is triggered by low pH: importance of the propolypeptide and free sulfhydryls. J Biol Chem 264:13497, 1989

57. Mayadas TN, Wagner DD: Vicinal cysteines in the prosequence play a role in von Willebrand factor multimer assembly. Proc Natl Acad Sci USA 89: 3531, 1992

58. Wagner DD, Fay PJ, Sporn LA et al: Divergent fates of von Willebrand factor and its propolypeptide (von Willebrand antigen II) after secretion from endothelial cells. Proc Natl Acad Sci USA 84:1955, 1987

59. Rehemtulla A, Kaufman RJ: Preferred sequence requirements for cleavage of pro-von Willebrand propeptide-processing enzymes. Blood 79:2349, 1992

60. Lynch DC, Zimmerman TS, Ling EH, Browning PJ: An explanation for minor multimer species in endothelial cell-synthesized von Willebrand factor. J Clin Invest 77:2048, 1986

61. Verweij CL, Hart M, Pannekoek H: Proteolytic cleavage of the precursor of von Willebrand factor is not essential for multimer formation. J Biol Chem 263:7921, 1988

62. Moake JL, Rudy CK, Troll JH et al: Unusually large plasma factor VIII: von Willebrand factor multimers in chronic relapsing thrombotic thrombocytopenic purpura. N Engl J Med 307:1432, 1982

63. Zimmerman TS, Dent JA, Ruggeri ZM, Hannini LH: Subunit composition of plasma von Willebrand factor. J Clin Invest 77:947, 1986

64. Levene RB, Booyse FM, Chediak JR et al: Expression of abnormal von Willebrand factor by endothelial cells from a patient with type IIA von Willebrand disease. Proc Natl Acad Sci USA 84:6550, 1987

65. Bowie EJW, Solberg LA Jr, Fass DN et al: Transplantation of normal bone marrow into a pig with severe von Willebrand disesae. J Clin Invest 78:26, 1986

66. Wagner DD, Olmsted JB, Marder VJ: Immunolocalization of von Willebrand protein in Weibel-Palade bodies of human endothelial cells. J Cell Biol 95: 355, 1982

67. McCarroll DR, Levin EG, Montgomery RR: Endothelial cell synthesis of von Willebrand antigen II, von Willebrand factor, and von Willebrand factor/von Willebrand antigen II complex. J Clin Invest 75:1089, 1985

68. Ewenstein BM, Warhol MJ, Handin RI, Pober JS: Composition of the von Willebrand factor storage organelle (Weibel-Palade body) isolated from cultured human umbilical vein endothelial cells. J Cell Biol 104:1423, 1987

69. Weibel ER, Palade GE: New cytoplasmic components in arterial endothelia. J Biol Chem 23:101, 1964

70. Cramer EM, Meyer D, le Menn R, Breton-Gorius J: Eccentric localization of von Willebrand factor in an internal structure of platelet alpha-granule resembling that of Weibel-Palade bodies. Blood 66:710, 1985

71. Cramer EM, Caen JP, Drouet L, Breton-Gorius J: Absence of tubular structures and immunolabeling for von Willebrand factor in the platelet alphagranules from porcine von Willebrand disease (published erratum appears in Blood 69:707, 1987). Blood 68:774, 1986

72. Hsu-Lin S, Berman CL, Furie BC et al: A platelet membrane protein expressed

during platelet activation and secretion. Studies using a monoclonal antibody specific for thrombin-activated platelets. J Biol Chem 259:9121, 1984

73. McEver RP, Martin MN: A monoclonal antibody to a membrane glycoprotein binds only to activated platelets. J Biol Chem 259:9799, 1984

74. Bonfanti R, Furie BC, Furie B, Wagner DD: PADGEM (GMP140) is a component of Weibel-Palade bodies of human endothelial cells. Blood 73:1109, 1989

75. Larsen E, Celi A, Gilbert GE et al: PADGEM protein: a receptor that mediates the interaction of activated platelets with neutrophils and monocytes. Cell 59:305, 1989

76. Geng J-G, Bevilacqua MP, Moore KL et al: Rapid neutrophil adhesion to activated endothelium mediated by GMP-140. Nature 343:757, 1990

77. Metzelaar MJ, Wijngaard PLJ, Peters PJ et al: CD63 antigen: a novel lysosomal membrane glycoprotein, cloned by a screening procedure for intracellular antigens in eukaryotic cells. J Biol Chem 266:3239, 1991

78. Vischer UM, Wagner DD: CD63 is a component of Weibel-Palade bodies of human endothelial cells. Blood 82:1184, 1993

79. Loesberg C, Gonsalves MD, Zandbergen J et al: The effect of calcium on the secretion of factor VIII-related antigen by cultured human endothelial cells. Biochim Biophys Acta 763:160, 1983

80. Sinha S, Wagner DD: Intact microtubules are necessary for complete processing, storage and regulated secretion of von Willebrand factor by endothelial cells. Eur J Cell Biol 43:377, 1987

81. Sporn LA, Marder VJ, Wagner DD: Differing polarity of the constitutive and regulated secretory pathways for von Willebrand factor in endothelial cells. J Cell Biol 108:1283, 1989

82. Sporn LA, Marder VJ, Wagner DD: Inducible secretion of large, biologically potent von Willebrand factor multimers. Cell 46:185, 1986

83. Fernandez MF, Ginsberg MH, Ruggeri ZM et al: Multimeric structure of platelet factor VIII/von Willebrand factor: the presence of larger multimers and their reassociation with thrombin-stimulated platelets. Blood 60:1132, 1982

84. Wagner DD, Saffaripour S, Bonfanti R et al: Induction of specific storage organelles by von Willebrand factor propolypeptide. Cell 64:403, 1991

85. Voorberg J, Fontijn R, Calafat J et al: Biogenesis of von Willebrand factor-containing organelles in heterologous transfected CV-1 cells. EMBO J 12: 749, 1993

86. Journet AM, Saffaripour S, Cramer EM et al: von Willebrand factor storage requires intact prosequence cleavage site. Eur J Cell Biol 60:31, 1993

87. Cheresh DA: Human endothelial cells synthesize and express an Arg-Gly-Asp-directed adhesion receptor involved in attachment to fibrinogen and von Willebrand factor. Proc Natl Acad Sci USA 84:6471, 1987

88. Levine JD, Harlan JM, Harker LA et al: Thrombin-mediated release of factor VIII antigen from human umbilical vein endothelial cells in culture. Blood 60:531, 1982

89. Ribes JA, Francis CW, Wagner DD: Fibrin induces release of von Willebrand factor from endothelial cells. J Clin Invest 79:117, 1987

90. Hamilton KK, Sims PJ: Changes in cytosolic Ca^{2+} associated with von Willebrand factor release in human endothelial cells exposed to histamine. Study of microcarrier cell monolayers using the fluorescent probe indo-1. J Clin Invest 79:600, 1987

91. Hattori R, Hamilton KK, McEver RP, Sims PJ: Complement proteins C5b-9 induce secretion of high molecular weight multimers of endothelial von Willebrand factor and translocation of granule membrane protein GMP-140 to the cell surface. J Biol Chem 264:9053, 1989

92. Vu TH, Hung DT, Wheaton VI, Coughlin SR: Molecular cloning of a functional thrombin receptor reveals a novel proteolytic mechanism of receptor activation. Cell 64:1057, 1991

93. Erban JK, Wagner DD: A 130-kDa protein on endothelial cells binds to amino acids 15–42 of the Bβ chain of fibrinogen. J Biol Chem 267:2451, 1992

94. Mannucci PM, Aberg M, Nilsson IM, Robertson B: Mechanism of plasminogen activator and factor VIII increase after vasoactive drugs. Br J Haematol 30:81, 1975

95. Hashemi S, Tackaberry ES, Palmer DS et al: DDAVP-induced release of von Willebrand factor from endothelial cells in vitro: the effect of plasma and blood cells. Biochim Biophys Acta 1052:63, 1990

96. Ngo KY, Glotz VT, Koziol JA et al: Homozygous and heterozygous deletions of the von Willebrand factor gene in patients and carriers of severe von Willebrand disease. Proc Natl Acad Sci USA 85:2753, 1988

97. Peakae IR, Liddell MB, Moodie P et al: Severe type III von Willebrand's disease caused by deletion of exon 42 of the von Willebrand factor gene: family studies that identify carriers of the condition and a compound heterozygous individual. Blood 75:654, 1990

98. Ginsburg D, Bowie EJW: Molecular genetics of von Willebrand disease. Blood 79:2507, 1992

99. Ginsburg D, Sadler JE: von Willebrand disease: a database of point mutations, insertions, and deletions. Thromb Haemost 69:177, 1993

100. Weiss HJ, Ball AP, Mannucci PM: Incidence of severe von Willebrand disease. N Engl J Med 307:127, 1982
101. Nichols WC, Lyons SE, Harrison JS et al: Severe von Willebrand disease due to a defect at the level of von Willebrand factor mRNA expression: detection by exonic PCR-restriction fragment length polymorphism analysis. Proc Natl Acad Sci USA 88:3857, 1991
102. Zhang ZP, Falk G, Blombäck M et al: A single cytosine deletion in exon 18 of the von Willebrand factor gene is the most common mutation in Swedish vWD type III patients. Hum Mol Genet 1:767, 1992
103. Rodeghiero F, Castaman G, Dini E: Epidemiological investigation of the prevalence of von Willebrand's disease. Blood 69:454, 1987
104. Sweeney JD, Novak EK, Reddington M et al: The RIIIS/J inbred mouse strain as a model for von Willebrand disease. Blood 76:2258, 1990
105. Nichols WC, Cooney KA, Yang A et al: von Willebrand disease (vWD) in the RIIIS/J mouse is due to a defect outside of the von Willebrand factor (vWF) gene, abstracted. Blood, suppl. 1. 80:74a, 1992
106. Lyons SE, Bruck ME, Bowie EJW, Ginsburg D: Impaired intracellular transport produced by a subset of type IIA von Willebrand disease mutations. J Biol Chem 267:4424, 1992
107. Dent JA, Galbusera M, Ruggeri ZM: Heterogeneity of plasma von Willebrand factor multimers resulting from proteolysis of the constituent subunit. J Clin Invest 88:774, 1991
108. Dent JA, Berkowitz SD, Ware J et al: Identification of a cleavage site directing the immunochemical detection of molecular abnormalities in type IIA von Willebrand factor. Proc Natl Acad Sci USA 87:6306, 1990
109. Bernardi F, Patracchini P, Gemmati D et al: In-frame deletion of von Willebrand factor A domains in a dominant type of von Willebrand disease. Hum Mol Genet 2:545, 1993
110. Cooney KA, Nichols WC, Bruck ME et al: The molecular defect in type IIB von Willebrand disease. Identification of four potential missense mutations within the putative GpIb binding domain. J Clin Invest 87:1227, 1991
111. Randi AM, Rabinowitz I, Mancuso DJ et al: Molecular basis of von Willebrand disease type IIB. Candidate mutations cluster in one disulfide loop between proposed platelet glycoprotein Ib binding sequences. J Clin Invest 87:1220, 1991

112. Ware J, Dent JA, Azuma H et al: Identification of a point mutation in type IIB von Willebrand disease illustrating the regulation of von Willebrand factor affinity for the platelet membrane glycoprotein Ib-IX receptor. Proc Natl Acad Sci USA 88:2946, 1991
113. Cooney KA, Lyons SE, Ginsburg D: Functional analysis of a type IIB von Willebrand disease missense mutation: increased binding of large von Willebrand factor multimers to platelets. Proc Natl Acad Sci USA 89:2869, 1992
114. Veltkamp JJ, van Tilburg NH: Autosomal haemophilia: a variant of von Willebrand's disease. Br J Haematol 26:141, 1974
115. Graham JB, Barrow ES, Roberts HR et al: Dominant inheritance of hemophilia A in three generations of women. Blood 46:175, 1975
116. Nishino M, Girma J-P, Rothschild C et al: New variant of von Willebrand disease with defective binding to factor VIII. Blood 74:1591, 1989
117. Mazurier C, Diéval J, Jorieux S et al: A new von Willebrand factor (vWF) defect in a patient with factor VIII (FVIII) deficiency but with normal levels and multimeric patterns of both plasma and platelet vWF. Characterization of abnormal vWF/FVIII interaction. Blood 75:20, 1990
118. Eikenboom JCJ, Reitsma PH, Peerlinck KMJ, Briët E: Recessive inheritance of von Willebrand's disease type I. Lancet 341:982, 1993
119. Mazurier C: von Willebrand disease masquerading as haemophilia A. Thromb Haemost 67:391, 1992
120. Peake IR, Bowen D, Bignell P et al: Family studies and prenatal diagnosis in severe von Willebrand disease by polymerase chain reaction amplification of a variable number tandem repeat region of the von Willebrand factor gene. Blood 76:555, 1990
121. Mannhalter C, Kyrle PA, Brenner B, Lechner K: Rapid neonatal diagnosis of type IIB von Willebrand disease using the polymerase chain reaction. Blood 77:2538, 1991
122. Bignell P, Standen GR, Bowen DJ et al: Rapid neonatal diagnosis of von Willebrand's disease by use of the polymerase chain reaction. Lancet 336:638, 1990
123. Sadler JE, Ginsburg D: A database of polymorphisms in the von Willebrand factor gene and pseudogene. Thromb Haemost 69:185, 1993
124. Baruch D, Bahnak B, Girma JP, Meyer D: von Willebrand factor and platelet function in platelet disorders. In Caen JP (ed): Clinical Hematology. Ballieres Clin Haematol 2:627, 1989

Clinical Aspects of and Therapy for von Willebrand Disease

113

Gilbert C. White II and Robert R. Montgomery

INTRODUCTION

von Willebrand disease (vWD) is a genetically and clinically heterogeneous inherited hemorrhagic disorder caused by a deficiency or abnormality of von Willebrand factor (vWF), a large adhesive glycoprotein in plasma, platelets, and endothelial cells. As a result, the interaction of blood platelets with the vessel wall is defective and primary hemostasis is impaired. Along with hemophilia A and hemophilia B, it is one of the most common inherited coagulation disorders.

vWD was first reported in 1926 by Erik von Willebrand,[1] who described a 5-year old Finnish girl from the Åland Islands with a bleeding disorder that could be distinguished from classic hemophilia by an autosomal pattern of inheritance, mucocutaneous hemorrhage rather than joint and soft tissue hemorrhage, a prolonged bleeding time, and normal clot retraction. Of 66 family members, 23 had a similar hemorrhagic diathesis. Two years later, George Minot[2] reported a similar bleeding disorder in five patients and described the intermittent nature of the bleeding disorder. von Willebrand originally attributed the bleeding defect in his patients to either a platelet defect or abnormal capillaries.[3-5] In 1953, three independent groups reported deficiency of factor VIII in vWD,[6-8] and in 1957, Nilsson and co-workers[9] showed that the infusion of fraction I-0 from normal human plasma led to a greater than expected increase in factor VIII levels in patients with vWD, suggesting that the defect might be found in the plasma. More importantly, the infusion of fraction I-0 from hemophilic plasma also led to a greater than expected rise in factor VIII, indicating that the plasma component was something other than factor VIII.[10]

The abnormal interaction between platelets and the vessel wall in vWD was first demonstrated in 1960 by Borchgrevink[11] and was confirmed by numerous workers.[12–15] The next major discovery was the observation by Zimmerman et al.[16] that an antigen associated with factor VIII was decreased in patients with vWD. This antigen is now known as vWF and is a protein distinct from factor VIII. The in vitro measurement of vWF activity was further facilitated by the observation by Howard and Firkin[17] that ristocetin, an antibiotic isolated from the actinomycete species *Nocardia lurida,* induced agglutination of platelets in the presence of vWF. The primary structure of vWF was determined in 1985 when the gene for vWF was independently cloned and sequenced by four groups.[18–21]

PREVALENCE

Population studies indicate that the prevalence of vWD in the general population is 0.82–1.6%.[22] However, this is probably an underestimate of the true prevalence because of difficulties in the laboratory diagnosis of the disease. Severe, type III vWD is much rarer, with a prevalence of approximately 1 in 1 million.

GENETICS

vWD is inherited in an autosomal manner. Males and females are affected approximately equally, and each child of an individual heterozygous for a vWF abnormality has a 50% chance of inheriting the abnormal gene (Fig. 113-1). In classic autosomal recessive disorders, heterozygous offspring are phenotypically normal, whereas in dominant disorders, heterozygous offspring are phenotypically affected. Most patients with vWD show an autosomal dominant pattern of inheritance, although the variability of the laboratory findings and the variability of the clinical expression of the disease implies that penetrance is often incomplete. While most cases of vWD occur as autosomal dominants, recent studies, including most type I and II cases, recent studies suggest that autosomal recessive vWD may be more common than previously recognized. The two reported families with type IIC vWD appear to fit this pattern,[23,24] and reports of recessive inheritance in type IIA[25] and type I[26] disease have appeared. This recessive inheritance may account for some of

the laboratory variability in vWD described above. Some patients with severe type III disease also show recessive genetics, as evidenced by asymptomatic consanguineous parents. However, other patients with type III disease appear to be homozygotes or compound heterozygotes for type I genetic defects, inheriting a different abnormal symptomatic gene from each parent. The severity of the disease in the latter is related to the inheritance of a double gene defect and not to a recessive defect.

CLASSIFICATION

Attempts to classify vWD have been complicated by variability in symptoms and laboratory tests among and within affected individuals. In early reports, patients with severe disease and <1% vWF could be distinguished clinically from patients with milder disease. With the recognition that the factor VIII-related antigen was the abnormal protein in vWD, it became possible to use specific antibodies to examine the molecular defects involved. Initial studies using crossed immunoelectrophoresis showed that some patients had an electrophoretically abnormal protein, so it became possible to classify patients based on the presence or absence of such an abnormal molecule.[27–30] By this technique, approximately 10–15% of patients were shown to have an electrophoretically abnormal vWF protein.

The classification of vWD was greatly advanced by the development of techniques for separating vWF into its multimeric components (see Ch. 112) using sodium dodecyl sulfate (SDS)-agarose electrophoresis[31]; this technique now forms the basis for the clinical classification.[32] In normal human plasma, vWF is present as a series of repeating subunits, which represent multimers of the approximately 300-kd vWF protein. These multimers range in size from a dimer of 600 kd to over 20,000 kd in increments of 600 kd (Fig. 113-2). The highest molecular weight multimers are the ones that mediate platelet adhesion and are best characterized using 0.65% agarose.[33] On gels containing 2–3% agarose, the multimeric subunits appear in three or more discrete bands.[34] On SDS-agarose gels with higher amounts of agarose, fewer multimers are visible, while on gels of lower agarose content all the multimers may be visualized but the resolution is reduced, so that only one band is present for each multimer.

Platelet aggregation or agglutination with ristocetin or botrocetin, a protein isolated from the venom of *Bothrops jararaca,*[35] is also useful for classification. Both compounds aggregate

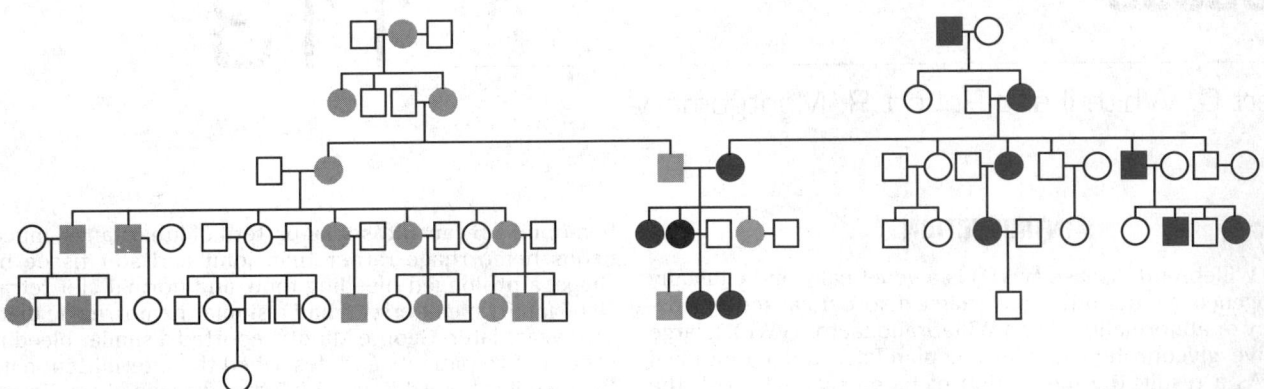

Fig. 113-1. Autosomal pattern of inheritance typical of vWD. In this hypothetical pedigree two families with different defects in the vWF gene are illustrated. The pattern of inheritance is a typical autosomal dominant pattern in which individuals inheriting an abnormal gene from either parent express the defect. A double heterozygote, who would have severe, type III vWD is illustrated. White symbols indicate normal individuals; pink symbols indicate heterozygote for defect I; red symbols indicate heterozygote for defect II; and black symbols indicate a double heterozygote.

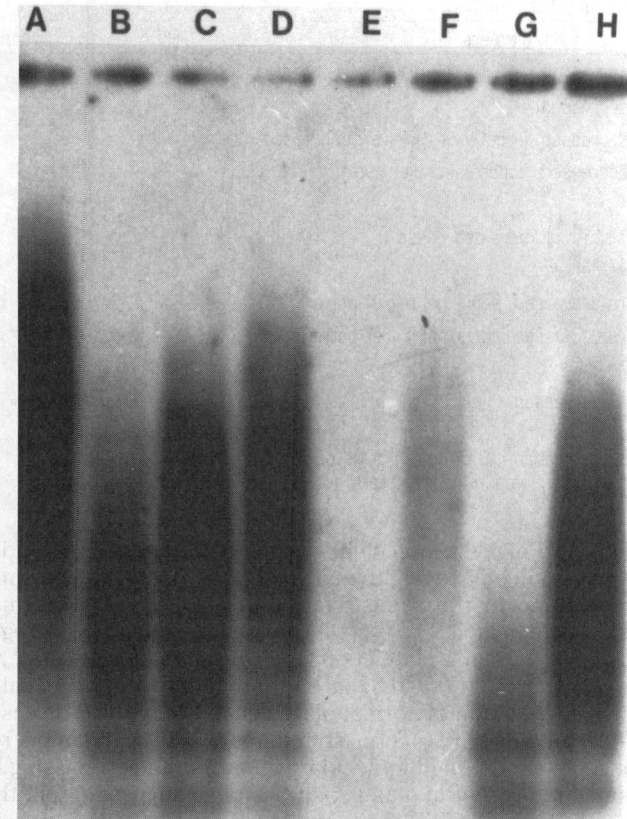

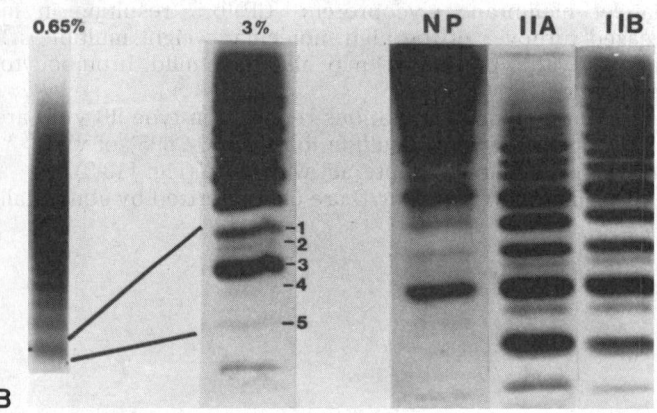

Fig. 113-2. vWF multimers. vWF multimers can be studied in low (0.65%) and high (2–3%) concentrations of agarose. The lower concentration is preferable to evaluate high molecular weight multimers, while the separation of complex multimers requires the high concentrations of agarose. **(A)** Illustration of 0.65% agarose separation of vWF multimers. Samples include plasma from patients with thrombotic thrombocytopenic purpura (lane A), diffuse intravascular coagulation (lane B), ventricular septal defects (lane C), normal plasma (lane D), severe, type III vWD (lane E), type I vWD (lane F), type IIA vWD (lane G), and type IIB vWD (lane H). **(B)** Complex multimer separation. Each multimer seen in 0.65% agarose can be resolved into three to five bands using the higher concentrations of agarose. Plasma from patients with types IIA and IIB vWD has an increase in the more rapidly moving satellite band (satellite band 5). (Courtesy of R. R. Montgomery.)

platelets in a vWF-dependent manner, although they interact with different sequences of the vWF molecule.[36] At 0.3–0.5 mg/ml, ristocetin will cause aggregation of platelet-rich plasma from patients with type IIB and platelet type pseudo-vWD but will not cause aggregation of platelet-rich plasma from normal patients or from patients with type I vWD.

Multimer analysis and platelet aggregation with ristocetin have been used to characterize three general types of vWD (Table 113-1).

Type I

In type I vWD a quantitative abnormality is present, with reduced levels of functional vWF. This is the most commonly diagnosed type, accounting for approximately 70–80% of cases. Multimer analysis shows that all multimers are present in plasma and are in the same relative proportion as in normal plasma. For most patients with type I disease, the concentration of each multimer is reduced compared with normal plasma, but the reduction is variable among patients, is variable on different occasions in any given patient, and may be normal. Plasma levels of factor VIII, vWF, and vWF:Ag may be reduced, usually concordantly, but also may be normal, and the bleeding time may be either prolonged or normal. The partial thromboplastin time may also be normal. Thus, a normal bleeding time and partial thromboplastin time do not rule out the diagnosis of vWD.

Patients with type I vWD have been further subclassified on the basis of the pattern of multimeric subunits, platelet aggregation response to ristocetin, or platelet multimeric pattern.* Based on multimeric pattern, three subtypes of type I vWD have been identified.[37,38] Patients with type IA have all the multimers present in normal relative proportion and represent the largest percentage of type I patients. In patients with type IB disease, all the multimeric subunits of vWF are present, but the amounts of the larger ones are relatively decreased. In type IC all the multimers are present, but the individual multimers are abnormal. Patients with larger than normal multimers have also been reported.[39] Subtypes based on platelet vWF have also been described as platelet-normal, platelet-low, and platelet-discordant.[40,41] Recent studies suggest that platelet vWF may correlate more strongly with bleeding tendency, and this may provide an important clinical distinction. Finally, subtypes based on ristocetin response have been described, including type I$_{New York}$, in which the multimer pattern is normal but the response to ristocetin is heightened.[42,43] In some cases, these subtypes are represented by single case reports.

Given the size of the vWF gene and the structural complexity of the protein, it is likely that multiple gene defects producing the type I phenotype will be found. In some patients with type I disease, silent alleles that produce undetectable or greatly reduced amounts of mRNA for vWF have been demonstrated.[44–46] Point mutations producing premature truncation of the vWF protein and missense mutations within functional domains of vWF have also been demonstrated.[26,47]

Type II

In type II vWD, a qualitative abnormality of vWF is present, which results in defective platelet-vWF-vessel wall interaction. These variants account for 15–30% of cases. The multimeric

---

* The Scientific and Standardization Committee on von Willebrand Factor of the International Society of Thrombosis and Hemostasis has recently proposed an alteration (Sadler JE, personal communication) in the classification system so that type 1 vWD (previously type I) will include only those with normal distribution of vWF multimers and a parallel reduction in vWF activity and vWF:Ag. Patients with type IIA and IIB vWD will be reclassified as type 2A and 2B. Others, previously classified as type I variants and type II variants other than type IIA and IIB, will be classified as miscellaneous type 2 variants (type 2M). The Normandy variant will be referred to as type 2N.

Table 113-1. Classification of vWD

Type	vWF	vWF:Ag	Factor VIII	Multimers	RIPA[a]	Cryoppt[b]
I						
IA	↓	↓	↓	All multimers decreased	−	−
IB	↓	↓	↓	All multimers decreased, large ones relatively decreased	−	−
IC	↓	↓	↓	All multimers decreased, abnormal triplet pattern	−	−
II						
IIA	↓	↓	↓	Large and midsized multimers decreased	−	−
IIB	↓	↓	↓	Large multimers decreased	+	−
IIC	↓	↓	↓	Large multimers decreased, abnormal triplet pattern	−	−
IID	↓	↓	↓	Large multimers decreased, abnormal triplet pattern	−	−
III	↓↓	↓↓	↓↓	All multimers absent	−	−
Platelet-type	↓	↓	↓	Large multimers decreased	+	+

Abbreviation: RIPA, ristocetin-induced platelet aggregation.
[a] Ristocetin-induced aggregation of the patient's platelets in patient plasma with low concentrations (0.5 mg/ml) of ristocetin.
[b] Cryoppt refers to platelet aggregation in patient platelet-rich plasma after addition of normal human cyroprecipitate.

pattern is distinctly abnormal, with absence of the high molecular weight multimers. Plasma levels of factor VIII and vWF activity are usually reduced and the vWF activity is typically lower than the vWF antigen (vWF:Ag), which may be quantitatively normal.

In type IIA vWD, the high and middle molecular weight multimers are absent in plasma and in platelets. Platelet aggregation in response to ristocetin is reduced in proportion to the deficiency of vWF. In some type IIA patients, platelet vWF multimers may be normal, suggesting that two distinct mechanisms could account for the IIA phenotype: (1) abnormal cellular assembly of vWF multimers, and (2) increased susceptibility of vWF to proteolysis in vivo.[48,49] In the latter group of type IIA patients, platelet vWF multimers may be normal.

Evaluation of platelet mRNA from individuals with type IIA vWD[50–54] has demonstrated missense mutations in the A2 domain (Fig. 113-3). Expression of the cDNA for these defects in COS cells resulted in the suspected abnormal vWF multimers in some individuals but normal multimers in others.[50]

Type IIB vWD is characterized by the absence from plasma

of only the highest molecular weight multimers. The middle and low molecular weight multimers are present in normal amounts and in the same relative proportion as in normal plasma. The hallmark of type IIB vWD is an enhanced aggregation of the patient's platelets in the presence of ristocetin. At a concentration of 0.3–0.5 mg/ml, ristocetin does not usually induce aggregation of normal platelets, but in type IIB disease, 0.3–0.5 mg/ml of ristocetin stimulates a full aggregation response. Since the high molecular weight multimers missing in plasma are present in platelets, it has been suggested that the defect in type IIB vWD is an increased affinity of the highest molecular weight multimers for cellular binding sites, such as platelet membrane glycoprotein (GP)lb,[55] resulting in increased turnover of the high molecular weight multimers.[56] Patients with type IIB vWD may also have mild thrombocytopenia.

Most of the known mutations reported in type IIB vWD are within or very near a disulfide loop (C509-C695) of vWF[57–61] that has been shown to interact with GPlb (Fig. 113-3).

Other forms of type II vWD are characterized by abnormali-

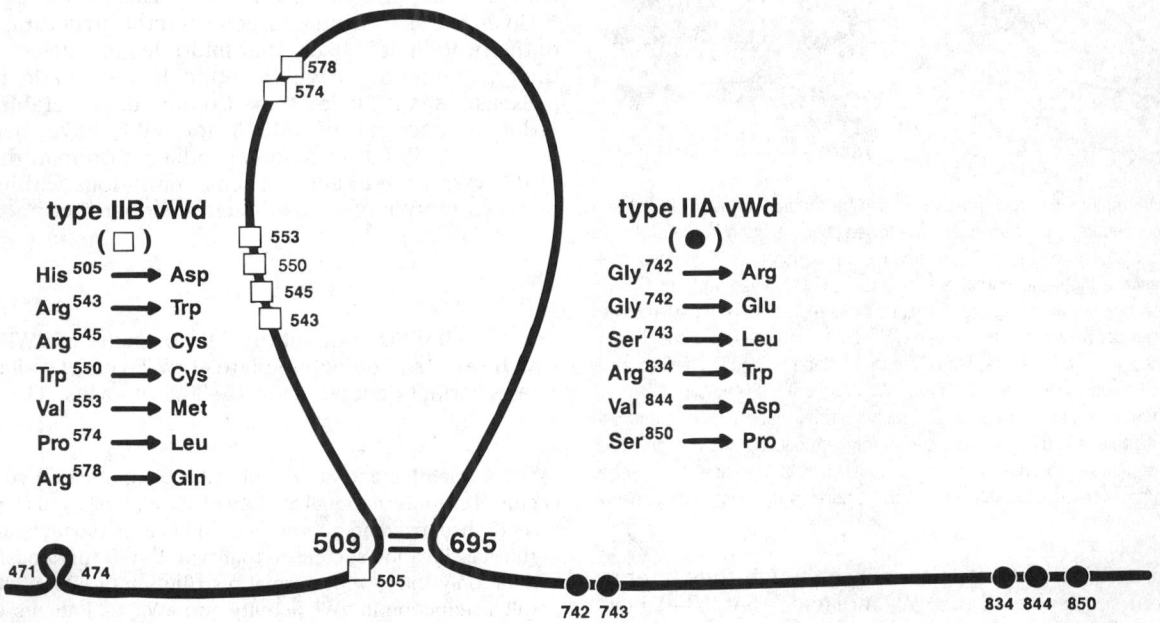

Fig. 113-3. Molecular defects in types IIA and IIB vWD. Schematic drawing of the A1 and A2 domains of vWF that lie within exon 28 and form the GPlb-binding domain of vWF. Type IIA mutations are indicated by closed circles. Type IIB mutations are indicated by open squares. The mutations shown are those that have been established by in vitro expression. (Courtesy of R. R. Montgomery.)

ties in the triplet pattern of multimers. In general, these have been named alphabetically (i.e., IIC, IID, IIE, IIF, IIG, and IIH).[62–66] Plasma levels of factor VIII, vWF, and vWF:Ag are variably decreased. Ristocetin-induced platelet aggregation is reduced.

Type III (Severe Type)

Type III is a severe form of vWD, with markedly decreased plasma and platelet levels of vWF. Usually vWF activity and vWF:Ag are undetectable, and factor VIII levels are typically markedly reduced (to <10%). The bleeding time is prolonged, usually to >15 minutes. Multimeric analysis of plasma from patients with type III disease shows essentially no multimers because of the marked reduction in vWF. This severe form of vWD may be the result of a homozygous defect or of compound heterozygosity.[67]

Four families with severe type III vWD have been found to have deletions of the vWF gene.[68,69] Three families in Italy, one the product of a consanguineous marriage, were shown to have a homozygous deletion of the entire vWF gene, while a family in Wales was found to be homozygous for a 2.3-kb frameshift deletion that includes exon 42. In all four families severe vWD was associated with the development of alloantibody inhibitors to vWF. Another family was identified in whom there was a complete heterozygous deletion of the vWF gene in the proband and one asymptomatic parent, suggesting that a different genetic abnormality was inherited from the second parent and that the proband was a compound heterozygote for vWF defects. An additional 20 patients with severe type III vWD were studied and had no evidence of a deletion.

Platelet-Type Pseudo-von Willebrand Disease

Platelet-type pseudo-vWD, first described by Miller and Castella[70] and by Weiss and co-workers,[71] is a primary platelet disorder involving the platelet receptor for vWF. Phenotypically, patients with platelet-type pseudo-vWD are similar to patients with type IIB disease: multimeric analysis reveals absence of the highest molecular weight multimers; factor VIII, vWF activity, and vWF:Ag are variably reduced; and bleeding time is prolonged. Aggregation is enhanced in response to low concentrations of ristocetin (0.5 mg/ml), and mild thrombocytopenia is commonly present. However, in contrast to type IIB vWD, in which the abnormality is in the vWF itself, the defect in platelet-type pseudo-vWD is in the platelet receptor for vWF, which has an increased affinity for normal vWF. The deficiency of the high molecular weight multimers is thought to occur as a result of increased utilization secondary to the increased affinity of platelets for vWF. Platelet-type pseudo-vWD can be distinguished from type IIB disease by addition of normal human cryoprecipitate to the patient's platelet-rich plasma.[72] In platelet-type disease the cryoprecipitate will induce platelet aggregation, while in type IIB disease it will not. Platelet-type pseudo-vWD can also be distinguished from type IIB disease by the differential binding of the patient's plasma vWF to formalin-fixed platelets. Unlike the response to cryoprecipitate, this method can be performed with previously frozen plasma.[73]

The molecular causes of this disorder have yet to be clearly defined. A putative mutation at position 233 of the GPIb α-chain, resulting in a substitution of a valine for a glycine, has been reported.[74]

von Willebrand Disease Normandy

The Normandy variant of vWD masquerades as an autosomal form of hemophilia A.[75,76] Also termed type IIN vWD, patients with this variant have reduced levels of factor VIII, typically 5–15%, with normal levels of vWF and vWF:Ag. The bleeding time is normal. The molecular defect in vWD Normandy is in the region of vWF involved in binding factor VIII and results in impaired formation of the vWF/factor VIII complex.[77–80] As a result, the half-life of factor VIII in the circulation is markedly shortened and factor VIII levels are reduced. The phenotypic expression of the Normandy variant only occurs if the individual is homozygous for the defect or if the other allele is a second vWD allele with reduced or absent levels of normal vWF such that only the abnormal factor VIII binding allele is predominantly expressed.

CLINICAL MANIFESTATIONS

The hemorrhagic tendency in vWD is highly variable and depends on the type and severity of disease. Patients with types I and II disease may have mild bleeding symptoms characterized by hemorrhage from delicate mucocutaneous tissues. Epistaxis, easy bruising, and gastrointestinal bleeding are common. Delayed hematoma formation and hemarthroses, characteristic of hemophilia A, are not a feature in these patients. In women the most frequent symptom is menorrhagia, which may be severe and out of proportion to other hemorrhagic symptoms. Untreated, menorrhagia may lead to iron deficiency and anemia. Menorrhagia probably accounts for the disproportionate number of women who seek medical attention. Post-traumatic, postsurgical, and dental bleeding may be severe and can be the presenting manifestation. Interestingly, pregnancy in women with vWD is usually tolerated well because plasma vWF and factor VIII levels increase during pregnancy, reaching a peak in the third trimester and falling rapidly postpartum. In patients with type I vWD, this rise is associated with a reduction in hemorrhagic symptoms. However, in patients with variants such as type IIB or platelet-type pseudo-vWD, the elevated levels of abnormal vWF may increase the spontaneous binding to platelets and result in marked thrombocytopenia. Similarly, levels of vWF and factor VIII are elevated in the newborn infant, particularly with vaginal delivery. This increase probably reduces the likelihood of bleeding but makes the diagnosis of vWD difficult in the newborn.

While characteristic bleeding symptoms occur in patients with vWD, the absence of bleeding symptoms does not rule out this diagnosis. In the studies of Goldin and co-workers,[81] Miller and co-workers,[82] and Abildgaard and co-workers,[83] approximately one-half of patients with documented type I or II vWD had no history of bleeding despite reduced factor VIII or vWF levels on at least some occasions.

Patients with severe, or type III, vWD have a severe hemorrhagic tendency. Spontaneous hemorrhage from mucous membranes and the gastrointestinal tract can be frequent and may be life-threatening. Usually, hemorrhage after dental and other surgical procedures can be controlled only by replacement therapy. Perhaps because of the low factor VIII levels, deep hematoma and joint hemorrhages similar to those in hemophilia may occur. In women, menorrhagia is severe and, before hormonal therapy was available, often required extreme treatment such as ovarian ablation by radiation, a practice not currently recommended.

Angiodysplasia refers to small telangiectasias in the wall of the small intestine and colon that occur in some patients with vWD,[84–86] more commonly in those >50 years of age and typically in those with type III disease. Although it is not clear that these are linked disorders, the presence of angiodysplasia in vWD can be a serious and disabling complication. Bleeding from angiodysplasia may present as melena or occult gastrointestinal bleeding, but typically presents with recurrent episodes of acute blood loss. Cycles of hematochezia resulting in hypotension and cessation of bleeding, followed days to weeks later by hematochezia, hypotension, and cessation of bleeding, may occur. Colonoscopy may reveal a bleeding site but more often shows multiple telangiectasias without a defined source of bleeding. Rarely, bleeding can be brisk enough to be visible by angiography. Operative intervention is not recommended unless a source of recurrent bleeding has been definitively identified. Estrogen therapy may be effective.[87]

Mitral valve prolapse has been reported to occur with increased frequency in vWD, perhaps as a linked mesenchymal disorder.[88,89] However, a recent report describes a normal frequency of mitral valve prolapse in patients with vWD.[90]

Inhibitors to vWF in patients with vWD are alloantibodies, usually IgG, which inhibit the hemostatic function of vWF. They are uncommon and occur only in patients with severe type III disease,[91] among whom the prevalence of inhibitors has been estimated to be 7–8%. There is almost always a prior history of exposure to exogenous vWF, as either plasma, cryoprecipitate, or factor VIII concentrates. Patients with deletion of the vWF gene as the cause of their disease may be at higher risk of the development of inhibitors.[68,69] A familial tendency to inhibitor formation has also been noted.[92] The presence of an inhibitor to vWF in a patient with vWD is suggested by the failure to respond clinically to replacement therapy, by decreased recovery of infused vWF, and by lack of correction of the bleeding time. Confirmation of the presence of an antibody requires the demonstration of an inhibitor of ristocetin-induced platelet aggregation in the patient's plasma. In most cases, antibodies to vWF also appear to inhibit factor VIII activity.[93] Alternatively, some antibodies may not inhibit function but promote accelerated clearance of transfused vWF. Those antibodies must be demonstrated by mixing the patient's antibody with normal vWF and demonstrating antigen-antibody binding.[91]

LABORATORY DIAGNOSIS

The standard laboratory workup for vWD consists of five tests: vWF activity, vWF antigen, factor VIII activity, vWF multimeric analysis, and bleeding time (Table 113-2). Analysis of the multimeric composition of vWF is required for accurate classification of vWD subtypes (see Ch. 104).

Ristocetin Cofactor Activity (vWF Activity)

Ristocetin cofactor activity is a functional assay for vWF that measures the vWF-supported agglutination of human platelets by ristocetin. Several methods of quantifying vWF activity have been described.[94–96] In most, ristocetin is added to a suspension of washed formalin- or paraformaldehyde-fixed platelets in the presence of patient plasma as a source of vWF, and agglu-

Table 113-2. Laboratory Tests in vWD

Function	Test[a]
vWF activity	Ristocetin-induced platelet agglutination (vWF:RCoF)
	Ristocetin-induced platelet aggregation
	Botrocetin-induced platelet agglutination
	Glass bead retention
vWF antigen	Laurell immunoassay
	Enzyme-linked immunosorbent assay
Factor VIII	Coagulation assay
Bleeding time	

[a] Ristocetin is a glycopeptide derived from the actinomycete *Nocardia lurida*. Botrocetin is derived from the venom of *Bothrops jararaca* and other *Bothrops* spp.

tination is assessed macroscopically or in an aggregometer. The initial rate of agglutination is proportional to the concentration of plasma vWF. The vWF activity is compared with the activity of normal plasma (assigned an arbitrary activity of 1 U/ml) and expressed in units per deciliter or as a percentage of the activity in normal plasma. Normal plasma levels of vWF are 50–200 U/dl. The vWF activity may be decreased artifactually in individuals with ristocetin-binding proteins in plasma (e.g., vancomycin).[97]

In some laboratories, vWF activity is measured by using platelet-rich plasma from the patient and performing ristocetin-induced platelet aggregation. Since this assay utilizes the patient's own platelets, it will give abnormal results in conditions in which interaction of vWF with platelet membrane GPIb (its receptor on the platelet surface) is impaired. Thus, in patients with Bernard-Soulier syndrome, a disorder in which there is a congenital absence of GPIb, ristocetin-induced platelet aggregation is absent.[98] However, ristocetin cofactor assay with fixed normal platelets is normal in the plasma of patients with Bernard-Soulier syndrome.

von Willebrand Factor Antigen

The substance formerly called factor VIII-related antigen (VIII:RAg) is now referred to as vWF:Ag. The assay is usually performed with use of a rabbit antibody to vWF by either quantitative immunoassay (Laurell technique) or enzyme-linked immunosorbent assay.[99,100] Since vWF is a very large glycoprotein, Laurell quantitative immunoelectrophoresis must be performed slowly (12–18 hours) or the assay will be too sensitive to the smallest multimers of vWF, which migrate faster. The Laurell technique may overestimate the smaller molecular weight multimers, resulting in a false elevation of vWF:Ag in type IIA vWD. The levels of vWF:Ag are compared with a normal human plasma pool and expressed as units per deciliter. Normal values are 50–200 U/dl. Blood type significantly affects the normal level of vWF protein, type AB plasma having up to twice the vWF:Ag level as type O plasma. Some laboratories have developed different normal ranges for each blood type.[101] Since vWF is an acute-phase reactant, levels are increased during stress, pregnancy, and in the newborn after vaginal delivery. Reduced plasma vWF may be found in patients who are hypothyroid, but their levels return to normal when they become euthyroid.[102]

Factor VIII Activity

Factor VIII coagulant activity is usually measured by a single-stage assay using human factor VIII-deficient plasma as substrate.[103] Substrates that have been immunodepleted of factor VIII have also been used but may give different results because vWF is also removed during the immunodepletion. Normal factor VIII levels are 60–150%. Factor VIII levels may also be reduced in patients with hemophilia A, factor VIII inhibitors, diffuse intravascular coagulation, and severe forms of liver disease.

Bleeding Time

The bleeding time is a general test of platelet-vessel wall interactions[104] (see Ch. 160).

Quick[105] observed that the bleeding time in vWD was sensitive to aspirin and that 650 mg of aspirin would prolong the bleeding more in a patient with vWD than in normal individuals.[105] He proposed the aspirin tolerance test as a diagnostic

DIAGNOSTIC DIFFICULTIES IN VON WILLEBRAND DISEASE

Test	1	2	3	4	5	6
Factor VIII	89%	94%	67%	71%	35%	81%
vWF	101%	88%	81%	62%	55%	78%
vWF:Ag	95%	92%	75%	65%	52%	75%
Bleeding time	6½	8	8	9	11½	8

This table illustrates the difficulties that may be encountered in the diagnosis of vWD. The patient, a 34-year-old woman with a mild bleeding disorder characterized by excessive bleeding following wisdom tooth extraction but no bleeding following an automobile accident complicated by a fractured femur, was tested on six occasions over a 2-year period. Her blood type was A, and she was not on oral contraceptives at any time during the testing period. The initial testing was normal, and multimeric analysis showed a normal pattern. Subsequent testing 6 months later was again within normal limits. Testing on a third occasion 3 months later showed a borderline factor VIII level and bleeding time but was otherwise normal. Repeat tests 1 month later were normal, although the vWF and vWF:Ag were borderline. Testing performed 8 months later before dental work was abnormal and consistent with a diagnosis of vWD. Her last tests, 1 year after dental work, were again normal.

test for vWD, although it is no longer used since it is also prolonged in a variety of platelet function defects.

Other Tests

Platelet adherence to columns containing glass beads is reduced in vWD.[106] Although this test is not specific and is rarely used today, it was at one time the most reliable diagnostic

test. Another useful diagnostic test is the response to plasma infusion of normal or hemophilic plasma. In a patient with vWD this results in a sustained rise in factor VIII activity, which contrasts with the shorter biologic half-life that is observed when normal plasma is transfused in patients with hemophilia.[10] This phenomenon, called de novo synthesis, may also have therapeutic benefits but is no longer used as a diagnostic test for ethical reasons.

Differential Diagnosis

Diagnosis is confirmed by finding reduced plasma levels of vWF activity, vWF:Ag, factor VIII, and/or a prolonged bleeding time. In the classic case, all four laboratory tests are abnormal and the diagnosis is not difficult. However, in many cases all four tests are normal, while in others, only one of the four is abnormal. When only the factor VIII is abnormal, vWD can be confused with hemophilia A, and when only the bleeding time is abnormal, it can be confused with a primary platelet disorder. The difficulty in diagnosing vWD has been emphasized by Goldin et al,[81] Miller and co-workers,[82] and Abildgaard and co-workers.[83]

Repeated testing may be necessary to establish the diagnosis of vWD. In the studies by Goldin and co-workers and Miller and co-workers of two large kindreds with vWD, vWF activity, vWF:Ag, factor VIII, and bleeding time were determined and correlated with bleeding symptoms. The results indicated two important facts. First, within each kindred, whose affected members all possessed the same genetic defect, there was remarkable diversity in the phenotype, with 8 different combinations of abnormal test results out of a possible 16 in one family and 10 in the other. Second, of 26 individuals who were genetically affected as determined by pedigree analysis, 11 had a normal panel of tests. Thus, normal values do not exclude a diagnosis of vWD. This conclusion is supported by the studies of Abildgaard and co-workers, who found a normal panel of tests in 29 of 202 tests performed on 50 patients with confirmed vWD. In addition, they confirmed the phenotypic diversity observed by Goldin et al. and Miller et al. with all 16 possible combinations of abnormal findings in their population of patients. Finally, they showed that when patients with vWD

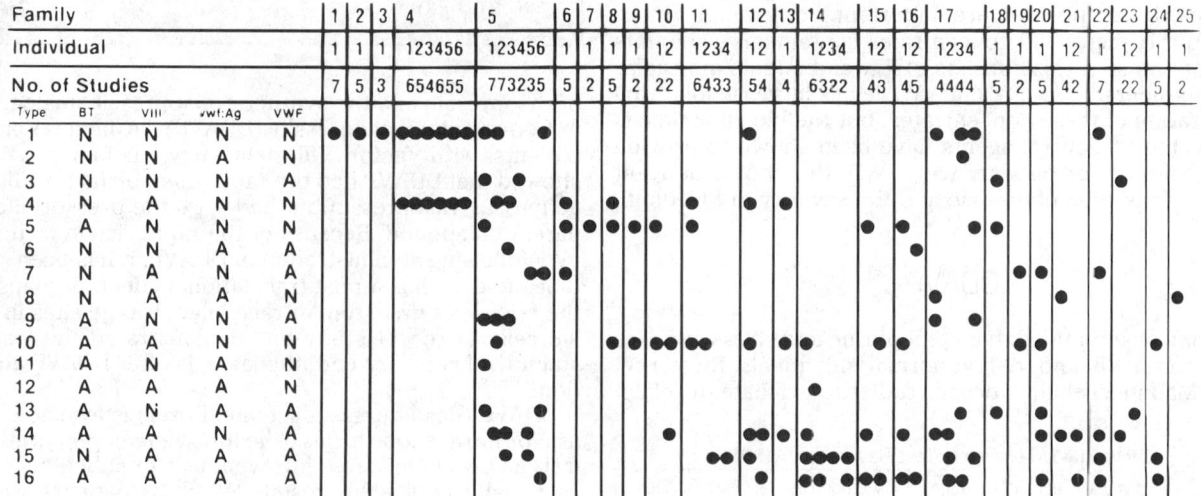

Fig. 113-4. Pattern of abnormalities in vWD. From 25 families with vWD, 50 affected individuals were tested on a total of 202 occasions. The pattern of results in each individual is shown by the dots in the column below that person. For example, in family 7, individual 1 was studied twice and showed an abnormal bleeding time and normal VIII, vWf, and vWf:Ag on both occasions. In family 5, individual 1 was studied on seven occasions and showed six different patterns of results, including all normal, isolated vWf abnormality, isolated bleeding time abnormality, bleeding time and vWF abnormality, bleeding time and vWF:Ag abnormality, and bleeding time, vWF, and vWF:Ag abnormality. BT, bleeding time; VIII, factor VIII activity; vWF, vWF activity. (From Abildgaard et al.,[83] with permission.)

were followed with serial tests, the pattern of abnormality could change, sometimes within a matter of weeks, and that an individual with vWD may demonstrate five or six different patterns[83] (Fig. 113-4).

A recent study by Eikenboom and co-workers[26] may provide an explanation for some of the variability in vWD. They found that within a given kindred the variability in laboratory findings could be roughly correlated with the gene defect, and that differences between individuals with the same gene defect within the kindred roughly correlated with blood group type. In addition, allelic interplay may account for some of the variability in vWD phenotype. For example, in one of Eikenbloom's kindred, the phenotypic expression of the Normandy defect was affected by a second abnormal vWF allele. This suggests that the underlying gene defect in vWD along with other factors such as allelic interplay, blood type, pregnancy, and stress play an important role in the phenotypic expression in the disease.

Since the factor VIII level is variably reduced in vWD, the activated partial thromboplastin time, which is typically prolonged only when that factor VIII level is <30%, is often normal in vWD. The prothrombin time and thrombin clotting time are normal, and the platelet count is normal in most patients but may be reduced in patients with type IIB or platelet-type vWD.

vWD can usually be distinguished from classic hemophilia (Table 113-3). The vWF activity, vWF:Ag, and bleeding time are normal in hemophilia. However, since some patients with vWD may present with an isolated factor VIII deficiency, it is important to take a careful family history to exclude an X-linked pattern of inheritance. Repeated testing may also be required to distinguish vWD from hemophilia. Qualitative platelet defects (i.e., defects due to aspirin ingestion) should also be considered in the differential diagnosis of vWD. A careful drug history may help to distinguish patients with drug-related platelet defects.

THERAPY

The aim of therapy in vWD is correction of both the bleeding time and coagulation abnormalities. This is generally accomplished by raising plasma levels of vWF and factor VIII to normal. Since the bleeding time is sensitive to only the highest molecular weight multimeric forms, the source of the vWF and its multimeric composition are important. For example, intermediate-purity factor VIII concentrates contain large amounts of vWF, but most of this consists of low and middle molecular weight multimers.[107] As a result, vWF levels increase following administration of these concentrates, but the bleeding time is not corrected.[108] Several agents have been shown to provide effective therapy for patients with vWD; the choice of agent depends on the type of disease and the severity of bleeding.

DDAVP

Following observations that epinephrine and stress increase levels of factor VIII and vWF in normal individuals, Ruggeri et al.[92] and Mannucci et al.[109] began studies to evaluate the effect

Table 113-3. Laboratory Test Results in vWD

	von Willebrand Disease	Hemophilia	Platelet Defect
Factor VIII	↓ or nl	↓	nl
vWF	↓ or nl	nl	nl
vWF:Ag	↓ or nl	nl	nl
Bleeding time	↑	nl	↑

Abbreviations: nl, normal test results; ↓, decreased test result; ↑, increased test result.

SURGERY IN VON WILLEBRAND DISEASE

Surgical and dental procedures, including major surgical procedures, may be safely undertaken in patients with most types of vWD. In patients with type I disease, treatment with DDAVP starting 1 hour before surgery and once a day thereafter for 2–3 days will usually suffice for minor procedures such as dental extraction. For more extensive surgery DDAVP may also be used, but cryoprecipitate or Humate-P should be available should DDAVP fail to control hemostasis. Baseline factor VIII and bleeding time should be determined within 1 week of surgery. Approximately 1–2 hours before surgery, DDAVP is given at a dose of 0.3 µg/kg body weight. If the baseline factor VIII or bleeding time is abnormal, these should be repeated 30–60 minutes after DDAVP and shown to be normal before proceeding with surgery. Postoperatively, DDAVP may be given once a day until wound healing is complete. Factor VIII and vWF activity should be determined 30–60 minutes after each dose of DDAVP.

In patients with type II vWD, the approach to surgery is similar to that in type I disease except that replacement therapy with blood products will usually be required. Because it is subjected to virucidal treatment, Humate-P is preferred by some physicians, although cryoprecipitate at a dose of 10–12 bags every 12 hours will also provide adquate hemostasis. Baseline factor VIII and bleeding time are determined within 1 week of surgery. Replacement therapy is started 1–2 hours before surgery at a dose calculated to correct the factor VIII level, and the factor VIII and bleeding time determinations are repeated to ensure correction prior to surgery. Postoperatively, treatment is given every 12 hours until wound healing is complete. Factor VIII and vWF activity are determined daily.

In patients with type III (severe) vWD, replacement therapy with Humate-P or cryoprecipitate with or without DDAVP aimed at correction of the bleeding time and the factor VIII level is required for minor and major procedures. For minor procedures treatment should be continued for 2–3 days; for major surgery it should be continued for 5–10 days.

---

of vasopressin and the synthetic vasopressin analog, 1-desamino-8-D-arginine vasopressin (DDAVP) on factor VIII levels in patients with factor VIII deficiency, including vWD. They showed that DDAVP had the same effect on factor VIII and vWF activity as vasopressin but had <1% the pressor effect of the parent compound. Because of the rapid rise in factor VIII and vWF following administration of DDAVP, it has been suggested that the drug has a post-translational effect, perhaps through the release of vWF from intracellular storage sites in endothelial cells. A recent study has demonstrated the loss of vWF staining of capillary endothelial cells after DDAVP administration.[110]

DDAVP (desmopressin acetate, Rorer) is available in intranasal or intravenous forms. The intravenous preparation (4 µg/ml) can be administered intravenously or subcutaneously with essentially equivalent results.[111–113] In patients with type I vWD, a reproducible two- or threefold increase in vWF activity (and factor VIII) and shortening of the bleeding time occur within 15–30 minutes of DDAVP administration. The dose of DDAVP is 0.2–0.3 µg/kg body weight IV in a volume of 50–100 ml over 30 minutes. For subcutaneous administration, the intravenous DDAVP preparation is used at the same dose with injection of ≤1.5 ml/site (a single treatment may require three or four subcutaneous injections). Two intranasal preparations are available, one of which, a dilute solution (100 μg/ml) used for patients with diabetes insipidus, does not consistently raise plasma levels of vWF or factor VIII and should not be used in vWD. A more concentrated (1.5 mg/ml) intranasal preparation of DDAVP has completed clinical trials and at a dose of 150 μg (75 μg/nostril) produces results equivalent to 0.2 μg/kg IV of DDAVP.[114,115]

Because it stimulates a reproducible increase in vWF activity and is a synthetic product with none of the viral risks of plasma-derived products, DDAVP has become the treatment of choice in most patients with vWD. It is effective for most patients with type I disease, who have reduced amounts of a functionally normal vWF molecule. The effective response to DDAVP should preferably be demonstrated by carrying out a therapeutic trial infusion prior to the time when emergency or surgical use is required. Since it increases plasma levels of vWF by releasing endogenous stores, it is not generally effective in patients with types II or III disease, who either synthesize an abnormal protein or who do not produce functional vWF. However, in type III disease, DDAVP may enhance the response to cryoprecipitate and may be useful when full correction of the bleeding time is required.[116] In type IIB and platelet-type pseudo-vWD, the administration of DDAVP is contraindicated and may result in increased thrombocytopenia.[117]

Plasma Products

Humate-P, a pasteurized intermediate-purity factor VIII concentrate, has been reported to contain some of the large molecular weight vWF multimers and has been used to treat patients with vWD successfully, with correction of factor VIII, vWF, and bleeding time.[118] Other intermediate-purity factor VIII concentrates contain appreciable amounts of vWF, but only the middle and low molecular weight multimers are present (Fig. 113-5). Treatment with these concentrates can raise factor VIII and vWF:Ag levels, but the bleeding time may remain uncorrected. High-purity plasma factor VIII concentrates and recombinant factor VIII concentrates contain little or no vWF.

Cryoprecipitate is a plasma fraction that contains factor VIII, vWF, fibrinogen, and fibronectin, which is obtained by harvesting the precipitate that forms when frozen plasma is warmed to 4°C. The yield of factor VIII and vWF in cryoprecipitate can be increased two- to fivefold by administration of DDAVP to the blood donor prior to plasmapheresis. The full range of plasma vWF multimers is present in cryoprecipitate. Cryoprecipitate is now prepared from donors screened for antibody to human immunodeficiency virus type I (HIV-1), so that the risk of HIV transmission with cryoprecipitate is low. Nevertheless, cryoprecipitate has been reported to transmit both hepa-

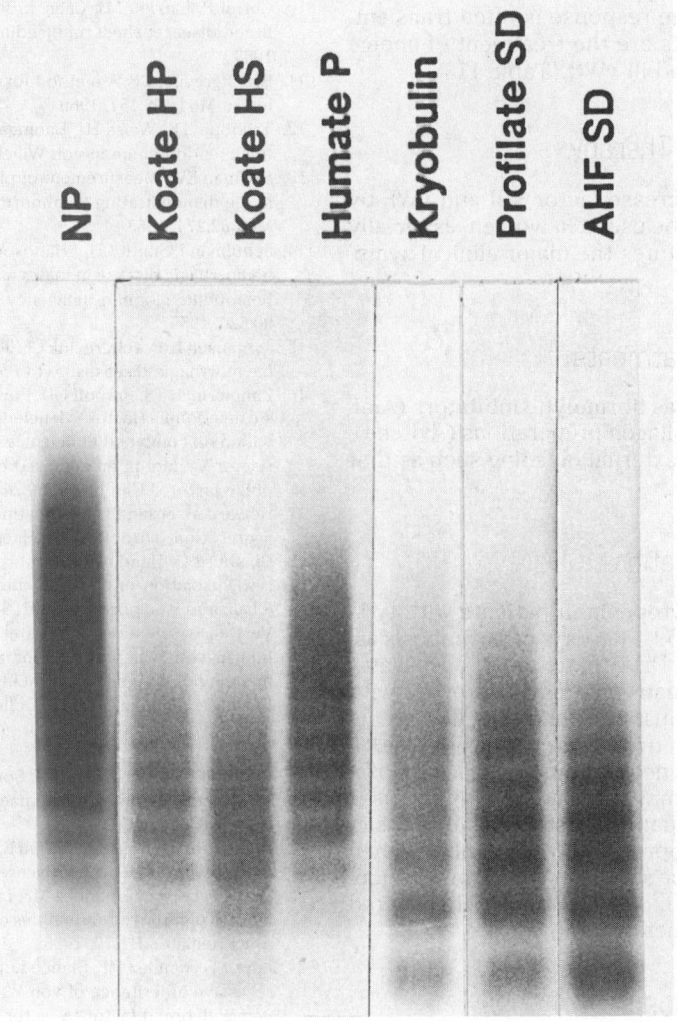

Fig. 113-5. vWF multimers in commercial factor VIII concentrates. Multimer gel is run with 0.65% agarose. The lanes contain normal plasma (NP) and various commercial factor VIII concentrates: Koate-HP, Koate-HS, Humate-P, Kryobulin, Profilate-SD, and AHF-SD. The high molecular weight multimers are variably deficient in all of the concentrates. (Courtesy of R. R. Montgomery.)

Table 113-4. Therapy for vWD

Type	Treatment
I	
IA	DDAVP
IB	DDAVP?
IC	DDAVP?
II	
IIA	Humate-P or cryoprecipitate
IIB	Humate-P or cryoprecipitate
Other type II	Humate-P or cryoprecipitate
III	Humate-P or cryoprecipitate plus DDAVP
Platelet-type	Platelet concentrates

titis B and hepatitis C, and since there is no virus inactivation step, there is a small but finite risk of HIV-1 transmission. The risk of viral transmission can be further reduced by using cryoprecipitate from parents or family members.[119] Each bag of cryoprecipitate contains approximately 100 U of factor VIII and 100 U of vWF activity. Since vWF levels are reduced in individuals with type O blood, plasma from donors with type A, B, and AB blood is preferred as the source of vWF.[120] Like DDAVP, cryoprecipitate may induce thrombocytopenia in patients with platelet-type pseudo-vWD.

Although some patients with type IIA vWD have been reported to respond to DDAVP, the response is often transient. For this reason, plasma products are the treatment of choice in most patients with types II and III vWD (Table 113-4).

Hormonal Therapy

Oral progestational agents increase factor VIII and vWF by unclear mechanisms. They may be useful in women, especially when menstrual bleeding constitutes the major clinical symptoms.

Other Treatments

Local hemostatic agents such as fibrinolytic inhibitors (Amicar, tranexamic acid), fibrillar collagen preparations (Avitene), and fibrin glue may be useful in external bleeding such as that due to dental procedures.

Complications

DDAVP may cause thrombocytopenia in patients with type IIB and platelet-type pseudo-vWD.[117] Reports of thrombosis associated with administration of DDAVP are rare.[121,122] Water intoxication with extreme hyponatremia may also occur with DDAVP, and intravenous fluids must be administered with caution in individuals receiving this drug.[123] Because of these effects on water balance, DDAVP is not recommended in children <1 year of age. Cryoprecipitate may transmit hepatitis viruses and, rarely, HIV-1. The risk of hepatitis must always be considered, and patients should be appropriately immunized when indicated. Humate-P appears to be safe from viral transmission. Inhibitors to vWF develop only in the most severely affected individuals undergoing replacement therapy.

PROGNOSIS

The prognosis in mild forms of vWD is excellent. Bleeding is typically mild, and life-threatening episodes of bleeding are rare. The risk of severe hemorrhage is greatly decreased by accurate diagnosis of the disease and education of both the patient and physician with respect to treatment. Patients with mild forms of vWD can expect a normal life span, but the prognosis in severe, type III vWD is more guarded; in the latter situation, life-threatening hemorrhage may occur despite the safe and effective forms of treatment currently available. The appearance of inhibitors in patients with severe vWD causes additional complications, often preventing adequate treatment.

REFERENCES

1. von Willebrand EA: Hereditär pseudohemofi. Finska Lak Handl 68:87, 1926
2. Minot GR: A familial hemorrhagic condition associated with prolongation of the bleeding time. Am J Med Sci 175:301, 1928
3. von Willebrand EA: Über hereditäre pseudohämophilie. J Intern Med 76:521, 1931
4. von Willebrand EA, Jürgens R: Über eine neue Bluterkrankheit, die konstitutionelle Thrombopathie. Klin Wochenschr 12:414, 1933
5. von Willebrand EA, Jürgens R: Über eine neues vererbbares Blutungsübel: die konstitutionelle Thrombopathie. Dtsch Arch Klin Med 175:453, 1933
6. Alexander B, Goldstein R: Dual hemostatic defect in pseudohemophilia. J Clin Invest 32:551, 1953
7. Larrieu MJ, Soulier JP: Déficit en facteur antihémophilique A chez une fille, associé à un trouble du saignement. Rev Hematol 8:361, 1953
8. Quick AJ, Hussey CV: Hemophilic condition in the female. J Lab Clin Med 42:929, 1953
9. Nilsson IM, Blombäck M, Jorpes E et al: V Willebrand disease and its correction with human plasma fraction I-O. J Intern Med 159:179, 1957
10. Cornu P, Larrieu MJ, Caen J, Bernard J: Transfusion studies in von Willebrand disease: effect on bleeding time and factor VIII. Br J Haematol 9:189, 1963
11. Brochgrevink CF: A method for measuring platelet adhesiveness in vivo. J Intern Med 168:157, 1960
12. Tschopp TB, Weiss HJ, Baumgartner HR: Decreased adhesion of platelets to subendothelium in von Willebrand disease. J Lab Clin Med 83:276, 1974
13. Salzman EW: Measurement of platelet adhesiveness: a simple in vitro technique demonstrating an abnormality in von Willebrand disease. J Lab Clin Med 62:274, 1963
14. Schulman I, Smith CH, Erlandson M, Fort E: Vascular hemophilia: a familial hemorrhagic disease in males and females characterized by combined antihemophilic globulin deficiency and vascular abnormality. Am J Dis Child 90:526, 1955
15. Jorgensen L, Borchgrevink CF: The haemostatic mechanism in patients with haemorrhagic diseases. Acta Pathol Microbiol Scand 60:55, 1964
16. Zimmerman TS, Ratnoff OD, Powell AE: Immunologic differentiation of classic hemophilia (factor 8 deficiency) and von Willebrand disease, with observation on combined deficiencies of antihemophilic factor and proaccelerin (factor V) and on an acquired circulating anticoagulant against antihemophilic factor. J Clin Invest 50:244, 1976
17. Howard M, Firkin BG: Ristocetin—a new tool in the investigation of platelet aggregation. Thromb Diath Haemorrh 26:362, 1971
18. Ginsburg D, Handin RI, Bonthron DT et al: Human von Willebrand factor (vwf): isolation of complementary DNA (cDNA) clones and chromosomal localization. Science 228:1401, 1985
19. Verweij CL, de Vries CJ, Distel B et al: Construction of cDNA coding for human von Willebrand factor antibody probes for colony-screening and mapping of the gene. Nucl Acids Res 13:4699, 1985
20. Lynch DC, Zimmerman TS, Collins CJ et al: Molecular cloning of cDNA for human von Willebrand factor: authentication by a new method. Cell 41:49, 1985
21. Sadler JE, Shelton-Inloes BB, Sorace JM et al: Cloning and characterization of two cDNAs coding for human von Willebrand factor. Proc Natl Acad Sci USA 82:6394, 1985
22. Rodeghiro F, Castaman G, Dini E: Epidemiological investigation of the prevalence of von Willebrand disease. Blood 69:454, 1987
23. Battle J, Lopez Fernandez MF, Lasierra J et al: von Willebrand disease type IIC with different abnormalities of von Willebrand factor in the same sibship. Am J Hematol 21:177, 1986
24. Lopez Fernandez MF, Blanco Lopez MJ, Castineira MP: Further evidence for recessive inheritance of von Willebrand disease with abnormal binding of von Willebrand factor to factor VIII. Am J Hematol 40:20, 1992
25. Asakura A, Harrison J, Gomperts E, Abildgaard C: Type IIA von Willebrand disease with apparent recessive inheritance. Blood 69:1419, 1987
26. Eikenboom JCJ, Reitsma PH, Peerlinck KMJ, Briët E: Recessive inheritance of von Willebrand's disease type I. Lancet 341:982, 1993

27. Zimmerman TS, Roberts J, Edgington TS: Factor VIII related antigen: multiple molecular forms in human plasma. Proc Natl Acad Sci USA 72:5121, 1975

28. Gralnick HR, Sultan Y, Coller BS: von Willebrand disease: combined qualitative and quantitative abnormalities. N Engl J Med 296:1024, 1977

29. Sixma JJ, Over J, Bouma BN et al: Predominance of normal low molecular weight forms of factor VIII in "variant" von Willebrand disease. Thromb Res 12:929, 1978

30. Sultan Y, Simeon J, Caen JP: Electrophoretic heterogeneity of normal factor VIII/von Willebrand protein, and abnormal electrophoretic mobility in patients with von Willebrand disease. J Lab Clin Med 87:185, 1976

31. Ruggeri ZM, Zimmerman TS: Variant von Willebrand disease. Characterization of two subtypes by analysis of multimeric composition of factor VIII/von Willebrand factor in plasma and platelets. J Clin Invest 65:1318, 1980

32. Ruggeri ZM, Zimmerman TS: Classification of variant von Willebrand disease subtypes by analysis of functional characteristics and multimeric composition of factor VIII/von Willebrand factor. Ann NY Acad Sci 370:205, 1981

33. Gill JC, Wilson AD, Endres-Brooks J, Montgomery RR: Loss of the largest von Willebrand factor multimers from the plasma of patients with cardiac defects. Blood 67:758, 1986

34. Ruggeri ZM, Zimmerman TS: The complex multimeric composition of factor VIII/von Willebrand factor. Blood 57:1140, 1981

35. Read MS, Shermer RW, Brinkhous KM: Venom coagglutinin: an activator of platelet aggregation dependent on von Willebrand factor. Proc Natl Acad Sci USA 75:4514, 1978

36. Sugimoto M, Mohri H, McClintock RA, Ruggeri ZM: Identification of discontinuous von Willebrand factor sequences involved in complex formation with botrocetin. A model for the regulation of von Willebrand factor binding to platelet glycoprotein Ib. J Biol Chem 266:18172, 1991

37. Ciavarelli G, Ciavarelli N, Antoncecchi S et al: High-resolution analysis of von Willebrand factor multimer composition defines a new variant of type I von Willebrand disease with aberrant structure by presence of all size multimers (type IC). Blood 66:1423, 1985

38. Takahashi H, Hayashi N, Shibata A: Type IB von Willebrand disease and pregnancy: comparison of analytical methods of von Willebrand factor for classification. Thromb Res 50:409, 1988

39. Mannucci PM, Lombardi R, Castaman G et al: von Willebrand disease "Vicenza" with larger-than-normal (supranormal) von Willebrand factor multimers. Blood 71:65, 1988

40. Gralnick HR, Rick ME, McKeown LP et al: Platelet von Willebrand factor: an important determinant of the bleeding time in type I von Willebrand disease. Blood 68:58, 1986

41. Rodeghiro F, Castaman G, Di Bona E et al: Hyperresponsiveness to DDAVP for patients with type I von Willebrand disease and normal intraplatelet von Willebrand. Eur J Haematol 40:163, 1988

42. Weiss HJ, Sussman II: A new von Willebrand variant (type I, New York): increased ristocetin-induced platelet aggregation and plasma von Willebrand factor containing the full range of multimers. Blood 68:149, 1986

43. Holmberg L, Berntorp E, Donner M, Nilsson IM: von Willebrand disease characterized by increased ristocetin sensitivity and the presence of all von Willebrand factor in plasma. Blood 68:668, 1986

44. Eikenboom JCJ, Ploos van Amstel HK, Reitsma PH, Briët E: Mutations in severe, type III von Willebrand's disease in the Dutch population: candidate missense and nonsense mutations associated with reduced levels of von Willebrand factor messenger RNA. Thromb Haemost 68:448, 1992

45. Peerlinck K, Eikenboom JCJ, Ploos van Amstel HK et al: A patient with von Willebrand's disease characterized by a compound heterozygosity for a substitution of Arg854 by Gln in the putative factor VIII-binding domain of von Willebrand factor (vWF) on one allele and very low levels of mRNA from the second vWF allele. Br J Haematol 80:358, 1992

46. Nichols WC, Lyons SE, Harrison SJ et al: Severe von Willebrand disease due to a defect at the level of von Willebrand factor mRNA expression: detection by exonic PCR-restriction fragment length polymorphism analysis. Proc Natl Acad Sci USA 88:3857, 1991

47. Holmberg L, Dent JA, Schneppenheim R et al: von Willebrand factor mutation enhancing interaction with platelets in patients with normal multimeric structure. J Clin Invest 91:2169, 1993

48. Gralnick HR, Williams SB, McKeown LP et al: In vitro correction of the abnormal multimeric structure of von Willebrand factor in type IIA von Willebrand disease. Proc Natl Acad Sci USA 82:5968, 1985

49. Berkowitz SD, Dent J, Roberts J et al: Epitope mapping of the von Willebrand factor subunit distinguishes fragments present in normal and type IIA von Willebrand disease from those generated by plasmin. J Clin Invest 79:524, 1987

50. Ginsberg D, Konkle BA, Gill JC et al: Molecular basis of human von Willebrand disease: analysis of platelet von Willebrand factor mRNA. Proc Natl Acad Sci USA 86:3723, 1989

51. Inbal A, Seligsohn U, Kornbrot N et al: Characterization of three mutations causing von Willebrand disease type IIa in five unrelated families. Thromb Haemost 67:618, 1992

52. Sugiura I, Matsushita T, Tanimoto M et al: Three distinct candidate point mutations of the von Willebrand factor gene in four patients with type IIa von Willebrand disease. Thromb Haemost 67:612, 1992

53. Ribba AS, Voorberg J, Meyer D et al: Characterization of recombinant von Willebrand factor corresponding to mutations in type IIa and type IIB von Willebrand disease. J Biol Chem 267:23209, 1992

54. Pietu G, Ribba AS, de Paillette L et al: Molecular study of von Willebrand disease: identification of potential mutations in patients with type IIA and type IIB. Blood Coagul Fibrinolysis 3:415, 1992

55. Ruggeri ZM, Pareti FI, Mannucci PM et al: Heightened interaction between platelets and factor VIII/von Willebrand factor in a new subtype of von Willebrand disease. N Engl J Med 302:1047, 1980

56. Ruggeri ZM, Mannucci PM, Lombardi R et al: Multimeric composition of factor VIII/von Willebrand factor following administration of DDAVP: implications for pathophysiology and therapy of von Willebrand disease subtypes. Blood 59:1272, 1985

57. Kroner PA, Kluessendorf ML, Scott JP, Montgomery RR: Expressed full-length von Willebrand factor containing missense mutations linked to type IIB von Willebrand disease show enhanced binding to platelets. Blood 79:2048, 1992

58. Cooney KA, Lyons SE, Ginsburg D: Functional analysis of a type IIB von Willebrand disease missense mutation: increased binding of large von Willebrand factor multimers to platelets. Proc Natl Acad Sci USA 89:2869, 1992

59. Ware J, Dent JA, Azuma H et al: Identification of a point mutation in type IIB von Willebrand disease illustrating the regulation of von Willebrand factor affinity for the platelet membrane glycoprotein Ib-IX receptor. Proc Natl Acad Sci USA 88:2946, 1991

60. Cooney KA, Nichols WC, Bruck ME et al: The molecular defect in type IIB von Willebrand disease. Identification of four potential missense mutations within the putative GPIb binding domain. J Clin Invest 87:1227, 1991

61. Randi AM, Rabinowitz I, Mancuso DJ, Mannucci PM: Molecular basis of von Willebrand disease type IIB. Candidate mutations cluster in one disulfide loop between proposed glycoprotein Ib binding sequences. J Clin Invest 87:1220, 1991

62. Mannucci PM, Abildgaard CF, Gralnick HR et al: Multicenter comparison of von Willebrand factor multimer sizing techniques. Report of the factor VIII and von Willebrand Factor Subcommittee. Thromb Haemost 54:873, 1982

63. Ruggeri ZM, Nilsson IM, Lombardi R, Holmberg L: Aberrant multimeric structure of von Willebrand factor in a new variant of von Willebrand disease (type IIC). J Clin Invest 70:1124, 1982

64. Kinoshita S, Harrison J, Lazerson J, Abildgaard CF: A new variant of dominant type II von Willebrand disease with aberrant multimeric pattern of factor VIII-related antigen (type IID). Blood 63:1369, 1984

65. Mannucci PM, Lombardi R, Federici AB et al: A new variant of type II von Willebrand disease with aberrant multimeric structure of plasma but not platelet von Willebrand factor (type IIF). Blood 68:269, 1986

66. Federici AB, Mannucci PM, Lombardi R et al: Type IIH von Willebrand disease: new structural abnormality of plasma and platelet von Willebrand factor in a patient with prolonged bleeding time and borderline levels of ristocetin cofactor activity. Am J Hematol 32:287, 1989

67. Bloom AL, Peake IR: Apparent 'dominant' and 'recessive' inheritance of von Willebrand disease within the same kindreds. Possible biochemical mechanisms. Thromb Res 15:505, 1979

68. Shelton-Inloes BB, Chehab FF, Mannucci PM et al: Gene deletions correlate with the development of alloantibodies. J Clin Invest 79:1459, 1987

69. Ngo KY, Glotz VT, Koziol JA et al: Homozygous and heterozygous deletions of the von Willebrand gene in patients and carriers of severe von Willebrand disease. Proc Natl Acad Sci USA 85:2753, 1988

70. Miller JL, Castella A: Platelet-type von Willebrand disease: characterization of a new bleeding disorder. Blood 60:790, 1982

71. Weiss HJ, Meyer D, Rabinowitz R et al: Pseudo-von Willebrand disease. An intrinsic platelet defect with aggregation by unmodified human factor VIII/von Willebrand factor and enhanced adsorption of its high-molecular-weight multimers. N Engl J Med 306:326, 1982

72. Miller JL, Kupinski JM, Castella A, Ruggeri ZM: Von Willebrand factor binds to platelet and induces aggregation. J Clin Invest 72:1532, 1983

73. Scott JP, Montgomery RR, Zumwalt KL: A rapid von Willebrand factor (vWf) binding technique that distinguishes type IIB from platelet-type von Willebrand disease (vWd). Clin Res 36:418a, 1988

74. Pincus MR, Dykes DC, Carty RP, Miller JL: Conformational energy analysis of the substitution of Val for Gly 233 in a functional region of platelet GPIb alpha in platelet-type von Willebrand disease. Biochim Biophys Acta 1097:133, 1991

75. Mazurier C, Jorieux S, Diéval J: Evidence for an abnormal FVIII/von Willebrand factor interaction in a patient presenting as a lifelong bleeding diathesis associated with FVIII deficiency. Thromb Haemost 62:472, 1989

76. Nishino M, Girma JP, Rothschild C et al: A new variant of von Willebrand disease with defective binding to factor VIII. Blood 74:1591, 1989

77. Kroner PA, Friedman KD, Fahs SA, Scott JP: Abnormal binding of factor VIII is linked with the substitution of glutamine for arginine 91 in von Willebrand factor in a variant form of von Willebrand disease. J Biol Chem 266:19146, 1991

78. Gaucher C, Mercier B, Jorieux S et al: Identification of two point mutations in the von Willebrand factor gene of three families with the 'Normandy' variant of von Willebrand disease. Br J Haematol 78:506, 1991

79. Tuley EA, Gaucher C, Jorieux S et al: Expression of von Willebrand factor 'Normandy': an autosomal mutation that mimics hemophilia A. Proc Natl Acad Sci USA 88:6377, 1991

80. Cacheris PM, Nichols WC, Ginsburg D: Molecular characterization of a unique von Willebrand disease variant. A novel mutation affecting von Willebrand factor/factor VIII interaction. J Biol Chem 266:13499, 1991

81. Goldin LR, Elston RC, Graham JB, Miller CH: Genetic analysis of von Willebrand disease in two large pedigrees: a multivariate approach. Am J Med Genet 6:279, 1980

82. Miller CH, Graham JB, Goldin LR, Elston RC: Genetics of classic von Willebrand disease: I. Phenotypic variation within families. Blood 54:117, 1979

83. Abildgaard CF, Suzuki Z, Harrison J, et al: Serial studies in von Willebrand disease: variability versus "variants." Blood 56:712, 1980

84. Quick AJ: Telangiectasia: its relationship to the Minot-von Willebrand syndrome. Am J Med Sci 254:585, 1967

85. Ahr DJ, Rickles FR, Hoyer LW et al: von Willebrand disease and hemorrhagic telangiectasia: association of two complex disorders resulting in life threatening hemorrhage. Am J Med 62:452, 1977

86. Ramsey RM, MacLeod DAD, Buist TAS, Heading RC: Persistent gastrointestinal bleeding due to angiodysplasia of the gut in von Willebrand's disease. Lancet 2:275, 1975

87. Chey WD, Hasler WL, Bockenstedt PL: Angiodysplasia and von Willebrand's disease type IIB treated with estrogen/progesterone therapy. Am J Hematol 41:276, 1992

88. Pickering NJ, Brody JI, Barrett MJ: von Willebrand syndromes and mitral-valve prolapse: linked mesenchymal dysplasias. N Engl J Med 305:131, 1981

89. Froom P, Margulis T, Grenadier E et al: von Willebrand factor and mitral valve prolapse. Thromb Haemost 60:230, 1981

90. Kuhsel LC, Polster J, Rudiger HW: An investigation into the frequency of mitral valve prolapse in von Willebrand disease. Clin Genet 24:128, 1983

91. Lopez-Fernandez MF, Martin R, Lopez Berges C et al: Further specificity characterization of von Willebrand factor inhibitors developed in two patients with severe von Willebrand disease. Blood 72:116, 1988

92. Ruggeri ZM, Ciavarelli N, Mannucci PM et al: Familial incidence of precipitating antibodies in von Willebrand disease: a study of four cases. J Lab Clin Med 94:60, 1979

93. Fricke WA, Brinkhous KM, Garris JB, Roberts HR: Comparison of inhibitory and binding characteristics of an antibody causing acquired von Willebrand syndrome: an assay for von Willebrand factor binding by antibody. Blood 66:562, 1985

94. Weiss HJ, Hoyer LW, Rickles FR et al: Quantitative assay of a plasma factor deficient in von Willebrand disease that is necessary for platelet aggregation. Relationship to factor VIII procoagulant activity and antigen content. J Clin Invest 52:2708, 1973

95. Meyer D, Jenkins CSP, Dreyfus MD et al: Willebrand factor and ristocetin. II. Relationship between Willebrand factor, Willebrand antigen and factor VIII activity. Br J Haematol 28:579, 1974

96. Sarji KE, Stratton RD, Wagner RH, Brinkhous KM: Nature of von Willebrand factor: a new assay and a specific inhibitor. Proc Natl Acad Sci USA 71:2937, 1974

97. Coller BS: Polybrene-induced platelet agglutination and reduction in electrophoretic mobility: enhancement by von Willebrand factor and inhibition by vancomycin. Blood 55:276, 1980

98. Caen JP, Nurden AT, Jeanneau C et al: Bernard-Soulier syndrome: a new platelet glycoprotein abnormality. Its relationship with platelet adhesion to subendothelium and with the factor VIII/v on Willebrand factor. J Lab Clin Med 87:586, 1976

99. Zimmerman TS, Hoyer LW, Dickson L, Edgington TS: Determination of the von Willebrand disease antigen (factor VIII-related antigen) in plasma by quantitative immunoelectrophoresis. J Lab Clin Med 86:152, 1975

100. Short PE, Williams CE, Enayat MS et al: Lack of correlation between factor VIII related antigen analysis pattern and parallel or non-parallel dose response in an ELISA factor VIII related antigen assay. J Clin Pathol 37:194, 1984

101. Gill JC, Endres-Brooks J, Bauer PJ et al: The effect of ABO blood group on the diagnosis of von Willebrand disease. Blood 69:1691, 1987

102. Dalton RG, Dewar MS, Savidge GF et al: Hypothyroidism as a cause of acquired von Willebrand disease. Lancet 1:1007, 1987

103. Simone JV, Vanderheiden J, Abildgaard CF: A semiautomatic one-stage factor 8 assay with a commercially prepared standard. J Lab Clin Med 69:706, 1967

104. Harker LA, Slichter SJ: The bleeding time as a screening test for evaluation of platelet function. N Engl J Med 287:155, 1972

105. Quick AJ: Salicylates and bleeding: the aspirin tolerance test. Am J Med Sci 252:265, 1966

106. Zucker MB, Brownlea S, McPherson J: Insights into the mechanism of platelet retention in glass bead columns. Ann NY Acad Sci 516:398, 1987

107. Lopez-Fernandez MF, Lopez Berges C, Corral M et al: Assessment of multimeric structure and ristocetin-induced platelets of von Willebrand factor present in cryoprecipitate and different factor VIII concentrates. Vox Sang 52:15, 1987

108. Blatt PM, Brinkhous KM, Culp HR et al: Antihemophilic factor concentrate therapy in von Willebrand disease. Dissociation of bleeding-time factor and ristocetin-cofactor activities. JAMA 236:2770, 1976

109. Mannucci PM, Canciani MT, Rota L, Donovan BS: Response of factor VIII/von Willebrand factor to DDAVP in healthy subjects and patients with hemophilia A and von Willebrand disease. Br J Haematol 47:283, 1981

110. Takeuchi M, Nagura H, Kaneda T: DDAVP and epinephrine-induced changes in the localization of von Willebrand factor antigen in endothelial cells of human oral mucosa. Blood 72:850, 1988

111. Kohler M, Hellstern P, Tarrach H et al: Subcutaneous injection of desmopressin (DDAVP): evaluation of a new, more concentrated preparation. Haemostasis 19:38, 1989

112. Ghirardini A, Chistolini A, Tirindelli MC et al: Clinical evaluation of subcutaneously administered DDAVP. Thromb Res 49:363, 1988

113. Kohler M, Hellstern P, Miyashita C et al: Comparative study of intranasal, subcutaneous and intravenous administration of desamino-D-arginine vasopressin (DDAVP). Thromb Haemost 55:108, 1986

114. Harris AS, Ohlin M, Svensson E et al: Effect of viscosity on the pharmacokinetics and biological response to intranasal desmopressin. J Pharm Sci 78:470, 1989

115. Lethagen S, Harris AS, Sjorin E, Nilsson IM: Intranasal and intravenous administration of desmopressin: effect on factor VIII/vWF, pharmacokinetics and reproducibility. Thromb Haemost 58:1033, 1987

116. Cattaneo M, Moia M, Delle-Valle P et al: DDAVP shortens the prolonged bleeding times of patients with severe von Willebrand disease treated with cryoprecipitate. Evidence for a mechanism of action independent of released von Willebrand factor. Blood 74:1972, 1989

117. Holmberg L, Nilsson IM, Borge L et al: Platelet aggregation induced by 1-desamino-8-D-arginine vasopressin (DDAVP) in type IIB von Willebrand disease. N Engl J Med 309:816, 1983

118. Berntorp E, Nilsson IM: Use of a high-purity factor VIII concentrate (Hemate-P) in von Willebrand disease. Vox Sang 56:212, 1989

119. McLeod BC, Sassetti R, Cole ER, Scott JP: A high potency, single-donor cryoprecipitate of known factor VIII content dispensed in vials. Ann Intern Med 106:35, 1987

120. Tomasulo PA, Richards W, Bailey M et al: Preselection of donors to improve the quality of cryoprecipitate. Am J Hematol 8:191, 1980

121. Bond L, Bevan D: Myocardial infarction in a patient with hemophilia treated with DDAVP. N Engl J Med 318:121, 1988

122. Mannucci PM, Lusher JM: Desmopressin and thrombosis. Lancet 2:675, 1989

123. Smith TJ, Gill JC, Ambruso DR, Hathaway WE: Hyponatremia and seizures in young children given DDAVP. Am J Hematol 31:199, 1989

Vitamin K: Metabolism and Disorders

114

Barbara C. Furie and Bruce Furie

INTRODUCTION

Vitamin K plays a critical role in the post-translational modification of the blood coagulation proteins, factors VII, IX, and X, and prothrombin, and of the plasma regulatory proteins, proteins C and S. Vitamin K serves as a cofactor for an enzymatic reaction that converts glutamic acid residues in the NH_2-termini of these proteins into γ-carboxyglutamic acid residues[1,2] (Fig. 114-1). The γ-carboxyglutamic acid residues confer essential metal binding properties on the vitamin K-dependent proteins.[3,4] If γ-carboxylation is impaired either as a result of vitamin K deficiency or through pharmacologic intervention, the vitamin K-dependent proteins will be secreted into the blood in their des-γ-carboxy or "abnormal" forms. The des-γ-carboxylated proteins cannot bind Ca^{2+}, and the physiologically important metal ion-mediated binding to phospholipid vesicles or cell membranes does not occur.[5] Since many critical enzymatic reactions of blood coagulation proceed on such surfaces, coagulation and its regulation are impaired. Therefore, vitamin K metabolism is essential to normal hemostatic and antithrombotic mechanisms and it is a key point of intervention in anticoagulant therapy.

MECHANISM OF ACTION OF VITAMIN K

In its role as a cofactor for the vitamin K-dependent carboxylase, vitamin K participates in a series of linked enzyme reactions that result in the generation of γ-carboxyglutamic acid and the regeneration of active cofactor. This series of reactions is known as the vitamin K cycle (Fig. 114-2). In addition to the enzyme, the reduced form of vitamin K and a glutamic acid-containing polypeptide substrate, the reactions require carbon dioxide and molecular oxygen. In the first reaction in the cycle (Fig. 114-2), a H^+ is abstracted from the γ-carbon of the glutamyl residue and a carboxyl group is added. Concomitantly, the cofactor, vitamin K, is converted from the reduced to the epoxide form.[6,7] The enzyme that catalyzes these reactions is the vitamin K-dependent carboxylase, which catalyzes both carboxylation and epoxide formation. These two activities were predicted to be dependent on the same enzyme.[8] The vitamin K-dependent carboxylase has recently been significantly purified, and that prediction is supported by experiments with purer forms of this enzyme.[9,10] The vitamin K-dependent carboxylase is a single-chain protein with a molecular weight of 94,000 composed of a single polypeptide chain of 758 amino acids.[10,11] This enzyme is an integral membrane protein that binds directly to the γ-carboxylation recognition site on the precursor forms of the vitamin K-dependent proteins. The recombinant protein can be expressed in mammalian cells, with the carboxylase activity superimposed on the endogenous activity of the cell.[10,11] However, direct proof that the carboxylase cDNA encodes this carboxylase activity is based on the expression of this enzyme in insect cells that lack endogenous carboxylase.[12]

As epoxidation occurs concomitant with carboxylation and because vitamin K either from dietary sources or gut flora is in the quinone form,[13] tissues in which γ-carboxylation takes place must have a mechanism for generating the reduced form of vitamin K. Several enzymes have been identified that perform this function. Vitamin K epoxide reductase, a dithiol requiring enzyme, reduces vitamin K epoxide to vitamin K quinone[14,15] (Fig. 114-2). Two enzymatic activities have been identified that convert vitamin K quinone to the biologically active hydroquinone (Fig. 114-2). These activities are supported by different cofactors. One enzyme requires a dithiol cofactor and may be the same that reduces the epoxide to the quinone.[16-18] The second enzyme, requiring nicotinamide adenine dinucleotide phosphate (NADPH) as a cofactor, may be a homologue of a liver cytosolic oxidoreductase, DT-diaphorase.[19,20] It is the two dithiol-requiring reductase activities that are inhibited by the coumarins, a family of frequently used oral anticoagulants.[21-23] Coumarins act by preventing the recycling of vitamin K to the reduced form (see Ch. 120). The NADPH-dependent reduction of the quinone form of the vitamin to the hydroquinone appears to be little affected by coumarin anticoagulants.[24]

The mechanism by which vitamin K functions as a cofactor with the γ-carboxylase remains to be elucidated. In one proposal, the activation of molecular oxygen occurs by the formation of a 3-hydroperoxy adduct of dihydrovitamin K, which then acts as a base to abstract the γ-methylene proton from glutamate, thus forming a glutamate carbanion intermediate.[25,26] Alternatively the carboxylase may operate as a dioxygenase during carboxylation and epoxide formation.[27,28]

NATURE OF THE SUBSTRATE

Although many tissues contain the enzymes to carry out γ-carboxylation and the reactions of the vitamin K cycle,[29] the primary site of synthesis of the vitamin K-dependent proteins of the blood is the liver. These proteins are synthesized with both a signal sequence and a propeptide. The canonical leader sequences provide the signal that indicates that the protein is to be secreted and thus allows the growing polypeptide chain to be transferred across the membrane of the rough endoplasmic reticulum.[30] All sequences of the propeptides of the vitamin K-dependent proteins are highly homologous and unique to this class of proteins.[31] These propeptides serve as recognition signals that designate these proteins as substrates for the vitamin K-dependent carboxylase.[32] The γ-carboxylation recognition site resides on the N-terminus of the propeptide. It is extended by a 10-residue amphipathic α-helix.[33]

VITAMIN K

Forms and Distribution

The vitamin K family of chemical compounds has many members. Vitamin K_1 (2-methyl-3-phytyl-1,4-naphthoquinone) is the major form of the vitamin found in plants. Animal tissue and bacteria produce menaquinones, a series of vitamin K forms

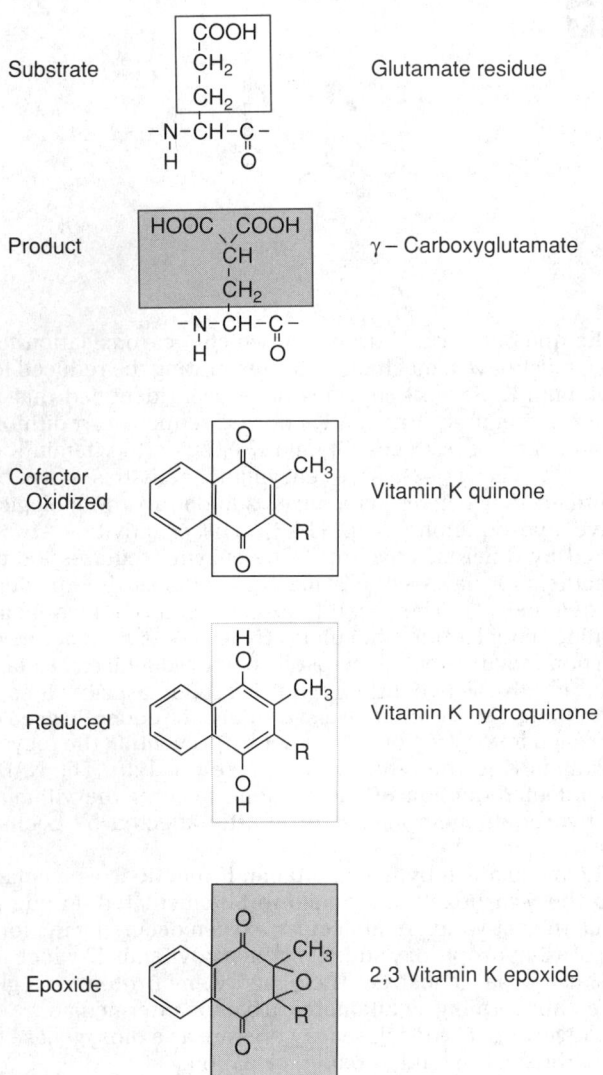

Fig. 114-1. Reactants in the vitamin K-dependent carboxylation pathway.

similar in structure to vitamin K_1 but with varying lengths of unsaturated polyprenyl groups at the 3 position.

Nutritional Sources

Vitamin K is an essential fat-soluble vitamin. The diet is the primary source of vitamin K in humans. Leafy green vegetables, in particular, are a good source of vitamin K_1,[34] although vitamin K_1 is widely distributed in the normal human diet. A contribution to adequate vitamin K intake in humans may be provided by the vitamin K_2 synthesized by intestinal bacteria.[35] The daily dietary requirement for the vitamin has been estimated to be 100–200 μg/day.[36]

Physiology

Vitamin K is absorbed in the ileum. The presence of bile salts and normal fat absorption are required for effective uptake. The storage pool of vitamin K is modest. In the absence of a dietary source of the vitamin, this storage pool can be exhausted within 1 week in an otherwise normal person. Such a deficiency does not generally lead to clinical manifestations, as the vitamin K synthesized by gut flora is available to provide

suboptimal but adequate synthesis of vitamin K-dependent proteins.

VITAMIN K DISORDERS

Hemorrhagic Disease of the Newborn

Hemorrhagic disease of the newborn, due to vitamin K deficiency, develops during the first week of life, usually between days 2 and 7[37–39] (see Ch. 118). Clinical manifestations include bleeding in the skin or from mucosal surfaces, circumcision, and venopuncture sites.[39] Rarely, internal bleeding, including retroperitoneal or intracranial hemorrhage, are the primary manifestations of hemorrhagic disease of the newborn. These ominous complications are the rationale for the use of vitamin K prophylaxis in neonates.

Almost all neonates are vitamin K deficient, presumably as a result of deficient vitamin K nutriture in the pregnant mother during the third trimester and because of the lack of colonization of the colon by bacteria that produce vitamin K in the neonate.[40,41] However, this deficiency is further aggravated in some patients due to inadequate dietary intake of vitamin K. This disorder is more prevalent in breast-fed babies, since human milk, in contrast to cow's milk, contains only 15 μg/L of vitamin K.[42–44]

Neonates with hemorrhagic disease of the newborn have prolonged prothrombin time (PT) and partial thromboplastin time (PTT). However, it remains critical to distinguish whether the prolongation of these coagulation studies is a manifestation of the deficiency of the vitamin K-dependent proteins due to vitamin K deficiency or to decreased synthetic capacity of the liver in newborns. Elevation of the abnormal (des-γ-carboxy) prothrombin (PIVKA-II) antigen level is indicative of vitamin K deficiency, since this form of prothrombin appears only when post-translational γ-carboxylation is impaired, but not when protein synthesis is impaired.[37,38] Administration of vitamin K (100 μg) corrects the deficiency state and usually does not need to be repeated in the otherwise healthy infant.[36]

Prophylactic vitamin K has been in use for inhospital births for the past 30 years. Vitamin K (100 μg to 1 mg) is administered intramuscularly to the newborn immediately after birth. At these doses, vitamin K carries little morbidity and can prevent hemorrhagic disease of the newborn.

Acquired Vitamin K Deficiency

Dietary Deficiency States and Antibiotics

The requirement for vitamin K is sufficiently low relative to the vitamin K content of a normal diet that clinically significant vitamin K deficiency does not occur as a result of inadequate dietary intake. Although sensitive markers of vitamin K deficiency, such as abnormal (des-γ-carboxy) prothrombin antigen,[45] indicate that diet truly depleted of vitamin K can lead to mild vitamin K deficiency, no evidence shows that an inadequate diet alone can have clinical manifestations. Bacteria in the large intestine produce functional forms of vitamin K. In the absence of dietary vitamin K, small amounts of vitamin K in the large intestine are absorbed passively and prevent severe vitamin K deficiency. In patients medicated with antibiotics that destroy the intestinal flora, this vitamin K source is eliminated. Thus, a common setting of vitamin K deficiency is the case of inadequate or minimal dietary intake treated simultaneously with antibiotics (Fig. 114-3). This form of vitamin K deficiency occurs within 1–3 weeks, after depletion of body stores of vitamin K.[46]

Malabsorption syndromes are commonly associated with vitamin K deficiency. Defects in the enterohepatic circulation

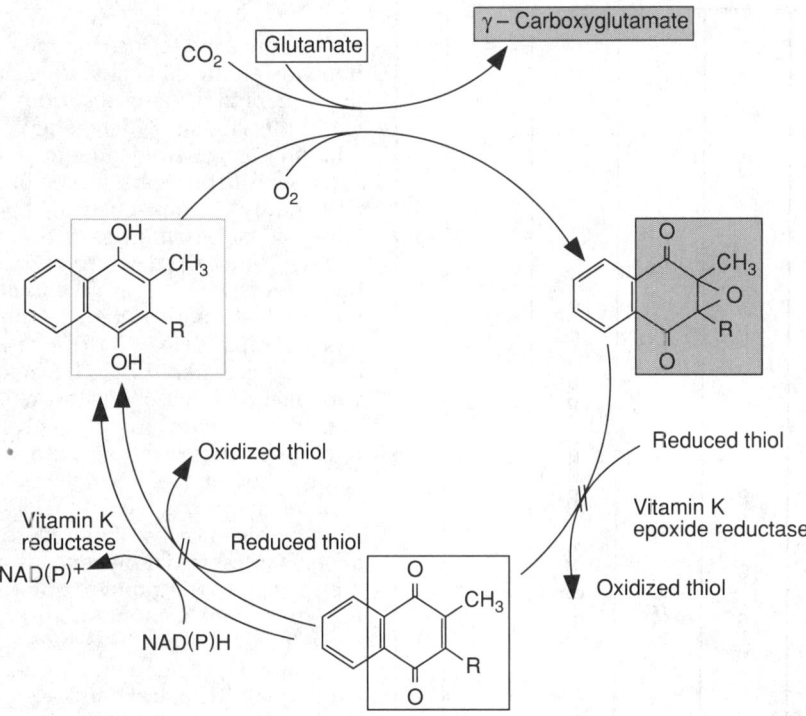

Fig. 114-2. The vitamin K cycle. Reduced vitamin K, the hydroquinone form, is a cofactor for the conversion of glutamate to γ-carboxygluta-mate by the vitamin K-dependent carboxylase, also known as the vitamin K epoxidase. Concomitant with conversion of glutamate to γ-carboxyglutamate, the hydroquinone is converted to 2,3-vitamin K epoxide. The epoxide can be converted to vitamin K quinone by the vitamin K epoxide reductase. Vitamin K quinone can be reduced by two pathways to the vitamin K hydroquinone, completing the cycle.

due to biliary disease interfere with absorption of fat-soluble vitamins in the ileum. Primary biliary cirrhosis,[47] cholestatic hepatitis, and other causes of cholestasis may lead to impaired absorption of vitamin K. Furthermore, intestinal malabsorption, as in sprue or regional enteritis, impairs vitamin K utilization. Older adults also have evidence of mild vitamin K deficiency, presumably because of intestinal malabsorption.[48]

Vitamin K Antagonists

Drugs that inhibit the reutilization of vitamin K lead to a buildup of vitamin K epoxide at the expense of vitamin K hydroquinone. Warfarin and related vitamin K antagonists, whether ingested accidentally, factitiously, or as an overdose of oral anticoagulant therapy, lead to a deficiency of the vitamin K-dependent proteins, prolongation of the PT and PTT, and clinical bleeding manifestations.[49-51] Although such patients are not vitamin K deficient, the clinical and laboratory manifestations due to vitamin K antagonists are identical to those of vitamin K deficiency. Factitious warfarin ingestion may be seen as a component of a major psychiatric disturbance. Despite repeated denials of use of such medications by suspect patients, this diagnosis must be considered in all patients with *acquired* deficiency of all the vitamin K-dependent proteins. Measurement of serum warfarin level can confirm such suspicions. With the introduction of second-generation rodenticides that inhibit vitamin K action, including brodifacoum, cases of factitious ingestion and accidental poisonings have been increasingly reported.[52-58] These long-acting poisons, now widely available (e.g., D-Con), can lead to prolongation of the PT 1 year after a single dose; fatalities have been reported.[59] Chemically distinct from warfarin, these compounds are not detected in serum warfarin assays. Specific assays have been developed[60,61] but are not generally available.

Other drugs cause a vitamin K deficiency-like state as well and respond to vitamin K therapy. Excessive doses of aspirin cause hypoprothrombinemia,[62] presumably due to oxidation of vitamin K. Although the mechanism is not completely understood, certain antibiotics, such as moxalactam and cefamandole, cause hypoprothrombinemia.[63-66] Malnourished patients, even those with initially normal PT, often develop vitamin K deficiency after intravenous antibiotic therapy.[67]

Hereditary Defects of Vitamin K Utilization

Hereditary combined deficiencies of the vitamin K-dependent proteins, including prothrombin, factor IX, factor X, and factor VII, have been documented in six pedigrees.[68-72] Although the molecular basis for this phenotype is unknown, defects in the absorption and transport of vitamin K might be anticipated to manifest this clinical presentation. In addition, abnormalities of the vitamin K-dependent carboxylase or other enzymes within the vitamin K cycle would lead to a deficiency of these proteins. Some patients have been responsive to high daily doses of vitamin K.[56] Other patients have been resistant to vitamin K therapy, emphasizing the heterogeneity of this disorder.

Therapy for Vitamin K Deficiency

Vitamin K deficiency is treated by the administration of vitamin K_1. The preferred route of administration depends on the urgency for correcting the bleeding tendency and on the risk of inducing local hematoma formation. If the bleeding is severe or life-threatening, fresh frozen plasma should be administered. Because of the risk of transmission of viral infection, the

VITAMIN K DEFICIENCY

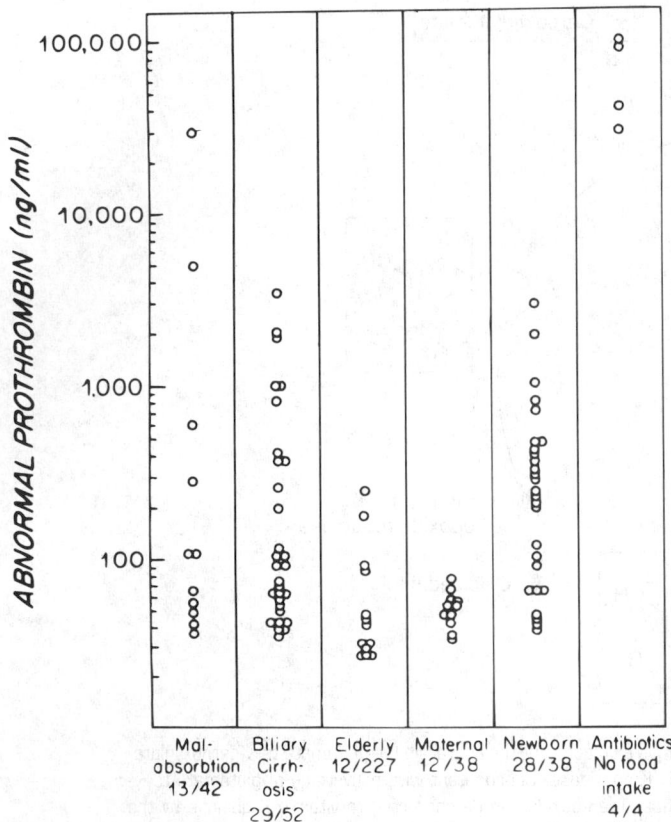

Fig. 114-3. Abnormal (des-carboxy) prothrombin antigen as a marker for vitamin K deficiency. Normal subjects have no detectable abnormal prothrombin. Vitamin K deficiency arises as a result of disorders of absorption, including mild abnormalities in otherwise normal elderly subjects, or because of impaired intake.

THERAPY FOR VITAMIN K DEFICIENCY

The approach to the treatment of vitamin K deficiency depends on the clinical setting and the severity of bleeding. Except in the face of serious internal bleeding, reversal of the vitamin K deficiency by the administration of vitamin K is generally adequate. If the PT is significantly prolonged to indicate a bleeding complication may be induced by intramuscular injection, that route of administration of vitamin K_1 (Aquamephyton) should be avoided. Since the delivery of vitamin K by the subcutaneous route is variable, intravenous vitamin K_1 (Aquamephyton) (10–15 mg) is the recommended approach, as it ensures rapid delivery. However, intravenous vitamin K_1 does require monitoring, because of early reports of severe allergic reactions with the intravenous route of administration; care must be given to initiate rapid reversal of an untoward reaction. With vitamin K, the PT should return toward the normal range within 12 hours and should have corrected within 24–48 hours. Serious bleeding complications attributed to vitamin K deficiency, such as intracranial bleeding, must be reversed immediately. Despite the rapid action of vitamin K, administration of vitamin K should be preceded by the infusion of fresh frozen plasma. This blood component contains all the vitamin K-dependent blood-clotting proteins. In sufficient quantities, fresh frozen plasma can correct, or nearly correct, the PT, as well as the bleeding tendency.

Patients with vitamin K deficiency without bleeding manifestations can be treated with oral vitamin K or, as in patients with chronic vitamin K deficiency secondary to malabsorption syndromes, with subcutaneous vitamin K.

use of blood products must be weighted carefully. There is no role for currently available concentrates of the vitamin K-dependent proteins because of the risk of transmission of viral disease.

REVERSAL OF LONG-ACTING VITAMIN K ANTAGONISTS ("SUPERWARFARINS")

The long-acting vitamin K antagonists employed as rodenticides lead to pronounced bleeding syndromes following factitious or accidental ingestion of these compounds. After diagnosis and confirmation of the diagnosis, treatment can remain challenging because the inhibition of the complete synthesis of the vitamin K-dependent proteins may continue for months after initial exposure, even in the absence of re-exposure. Fresh frozen plasma is used routinely to treat major bleeding complications, but this therapy is associated with a risk of blood-borne infection. Although it is desirable to correct or partially correct the PT, the use of prophylactic fresh frozen plasma chronically carries significant risks and expense. Because of the potency of the second-generation rodenticides and their fat solubility, vitamin K_1 at normal doses of administration is ineffective. However, daily doses of 100–150 mg of vitamin K_1 administered orally have been effective in normalizing the PT. Over time, the dose of vitamin K_1 needed to correct the PT can be adjusted downward, so that only the required amounts of vitamin K are employed.

REFERENCES

1. Stenflo J, Fernlund P, Egan W, Roepstorff P: Vitamin K dependent modification of glutamic acid residues in prothrombin. Proc Natl Acad Sci USA 71: 2730, 1974
2. Nelsestuen GL, Zytkovicz TH, Howard JB: The mode of action of vitamin K. Identification of γ-carboxyglutamic acid as a component of prothrombin. J Biol Chem 249:6347, 1974
3. Sperling R, Furie BC, Blumenstein M et al: Metal binding properties of γ-carboxyglutamic acid. Implications for the vitamin K-dependent blood coagulation proteins. J Biol Chem 253:3898, 1978
4. Furie BC, Blumenstein M, Furie B: Metal binding sites of a γ-carboxyglutamic acid-rich fragment of bovine prothrombin. J Biol Chem 254:12521, 1979
5. Esmon CT, Suttie JW, Jackson CM: The funtional significance of vitamin K action. Difference in phospholipid binding between normal and abnormal prothrombin. J Biol Chem 250:4095, 1975
6. Suttie JW, Hageman JM, Lehrman SR, Rich DH: Vitamin K-dependent carboxylase. Development of a peptide substrate. J Biol Chem 251:5827, 1976
7. Friedman PA, Shia MA, Gallop PM, Griep AE: Vitamin K-dependent gamma-carbon hydrogen bond cleavage and nonmandatory concurrent carboxylation of peptide-bound glutamic acid residues. Proc Natl Acad Sci USA 76: 3126, 1979
8. Larson AE, Friedman PA, Suttie JW: Vitamin K-dependent carboxylase. Stoichiometry of carboxylation and vitamin K 2,3-epoxide formation. J Biol Chem 256:11032, 1981
9. Hubbard BR, Ulrich MMW, Jacobs M et al: Vitamin K-dependent carboxylase: affinity purification from bovine liver using a synthetic propeptide containing the γ-carboxylation recognition site. Proc Natl Acad Sci USA 86:6893, 1989
10. Wu S-M, Cheung W-F, Frazier DF, Stafford DW: Cloning and expression of the cDNA for human γ-glutamyl carboxylase. Science 254:1634, 1991

11. Rehemtulla A, Roth DA, Wasley LC et al: In vitro and in vivo functional characterization of bovine vitamin K-dependent γ-carboxylase expressed in Chinese hamster ovary cells. Proc Natl Acad Sci USA 90:4611, 1993

12. Roth DA, Rehemtulla A, Kaufman RJ et al: Expression of vitamin K-dependent carboxylase in baculovirus-infected insect cells. Proc Natl Acad Sci USA 1993 (in press)

13. Suttie JW: Vitamin K. p. 147. In Machlin L (ed): Handbook of Vitamins. Marcel Dekker, New York, 1984

14. Matschiner JT, Zimmerman A, Bell RG: The influence of warfarin on vitamin K epoxide reductase. Thromb Haemost, suppl. 57:45, 1974

15. Zimmerman A, Matschiner JT: Biochemical basis of hereditary resistance to warfarin in the rat. Biochem Pharmacol 23:1033, 1974

16. Whitlon DS, Sadowski JA, Suttie JW: Mechanism of coumarin action: significance of vitamin K epoxide reductase inhibition. Biochemistry 17:1371, 1978

17. Fasco MJ, Principe LM: Vitamin K_1 hydroquinone formation catalyzed by a microsomal reductase system. Biochem Biophys Res Commun 97:1487, 1980

18. Sherman PA, Sander EG: Vitamin K epoxide reductase: evidence that vitamin K dihydroquinone is a product of vitamin K epoxide reduction. Biochem Biophys Res Commun 103:997, 1981

19. Wallin R, Gebhardt O, Prydz H: NAD(P)H dehydrogenase and its role in the vitamin K (2-methyl-3-phytyl-1,4-naphthaquinone)-dependent carboxylation reaction. Biochem J 169:95, 1978

20. Wallin R: No strict coupling of vitamin K_1 (2-methyl-3-phytyl-1,4-naphthoquinone)-dependent carboxylation and vitamin K_1 epoxidation in detergent-solubilized microsomal fractions from rat liver. Biochem J 178:513, 1979

21. Bell RG: Metabolism of vitamin K and prothrombin synthesis: anticoagulants and the vitamin K-epoxide cycle. Fed Proc 37:2599, 1978

22. Fasco MJ, Principe LM: R- and S-warfarin inhibition of vitamin K and vitamin K_2, 3-epoxide reductase activities in the rat. J Biol Chem 257:4894, 1982

23. Fasco MJ, Hildebrandt EF, Suttie JW: Evidence that warfarin anticoagulant action involves two distinct reductase activities. J Biol Chem 257:11210, 1982

24. Wallin R: Vitamin K antagonism and coumarin anticoagulant drugs. A study of an enzymatic pathway in rat liver that is responsible for the antagonistic effect, abstracted. Thromb Haemost 54:150, 1985

25. Suttie SW, Larson AE, Canfield LM, Carlisle TL: Relationship between vitamin K-dependent carboxylation and vitamin K epoxidation. FASEB J 37:2605, 1978

26. Dubois J, Gaudry M, Bory S et al: Vitamin K-dependent carboxylation. Study of the hydrogen abstraction stereochemistry with gamma-fluoroglutamic acid-containing peptides. J Biol Chem 258:7897, 1983

27. Dowd P, Ham SW, Hershime R: Role of oxygen in the vitamin K-dependent carboxylation reaction: incorporation of a second atom 18O from 18O2. J Am Chem Soc 114:7613, 1992

28. Kuliopulos A, Hubbard BR, Lam Z et al: Dioxygen transfer during vitamin K dependent carboxylase catalysis. Biochemistry 31:7722, 1992

29. Vermeer C, DeBoer-VanDen Berg MAG: Vitamin K-dependent carboxylases. Haematologia (Budap) 18:71, 1985

30. Helgeland L: The submicrosomal site for the conversion of prothrombin precursor to biologically active prothrombin in rat liver. Biochim Biophys Acta 499:181, 1977

31. Furie B, Furie BC: Molecular basis of blood coagulation. Cell 53:505, 1988

32. Jorgensen M, Cantor A, Furie BC et al: Recognition site directing vitamin K-dependent γ-carboxylation resides on the propeptide of factor IX. Cell 48:185, 1987

33. Sanford DG, Kanagy C, Sudmeir JL et al: Structure of the propeptide of prothrombin containing the γ-carboxylation recognition site determined by two-dimensional NMR spectroscopy. Biochemistry 30:9835, 1991

34. Almquist HJ, Stokstad ELR: Hemorrhagic chick disease of dietary origin. J Biol Chem 111:105, 1935

35. McKee RW, Binkley SB, Thayer SA et al: The isolation of vitamin K_2. J Biol Chem 131:327, 1939

36. Frick PG, Riedler G, Brogli H: Dose response and minimal daily requirement for vitamin K in man. J Appl Physiol 23:387, 1967

37. Brinkhous KM, Smith HP: Plasma prothrombin level in normal infancy and in hemorrhagic disease of the newborn. Am J Med Sci 193:475, 1937

38. Dam H, Dyggve H: Relation of vitamin K deficiency to hemorrhagic disease of the newborn. Adv Pediatr 5:129, 1952

39. Sutherland JM, Glueck HI, Glesser G: Hemorrhagic disease of the newborn. Am J Dis Child 113:524, 1967

40. Shearer MJ, Rahim S, Stimmler L et al: Plasma vitamin K_1 in mothers and their newborn babies. Lancet 2:460, 1982

41. Blanchard RA, Furie BC, Barnett J et al: Vitamin K deficiency in newborns and their mothers. Thromb Haemost 54:226, 1985

42. Keenan WJ, Jewett T, Glueck HI: Role of feeding and vitamin K in hypoprothrombinemia of the newborn. Am J Dis Child 121:271, 1971

43. Schneider DL, Fluckiger HB, Manes JD: Vitamin K content of infants formula products. Pediatrics 53:273, 1974

44. Committee on Nutrition, American Academy of Pediatrics: Vitamin K supplementation for infants receiving milk substitute infant formulas and for those with fat malabsorption. Pediatrics 48:483, 1972

45. Blanchard RA, Furie BC, Jorgensen MJ et al: Acquired vitamin K-dependent carboxylation deficiency in liver disease. N Engl J Med 305:242, 1981

46. Ansell JE, Kumar R, Deykin D: The spectrum of vitamin K deficiency. JAMA 237:40, 1977

47. Kaplan MM, Elta GH, Furie B et al: Fat soluble vitamin K nutriture in primary biliary cirrhosis. Gastroenterology 95:787, 1988

48. Krasinsky SD, Russell RM, Furie BC et al: The prevalence of vitamin K deficiency in chronic gastrointestinal disorders. Am J Clin Nutr 41:639, 1985

49. O'Reilly RA, Aggeler PM: Covert anticoagulant ingestion: Study of 25 patients and review of world literature. Medicine 55:389, 1976

50. O'Reilly RA, Aggeler PM, Gibbs JO: Hemorrhagic state due to surreptitious ingestion of bishydroxycoumarin. N Engl J Med 267:19, 1962

51. Bowie EJW, Todd M, Thompson JH Jr et al: Anticoagulant malingeers ("the dicoumarol-eaters"). Am J Med 39:855, 1965

52. Lipton RA, Klass EM: Human ingestion of a "superwarfarin" rodenticide resulting in a prolonged anticoagulant effect. JAMA 252:3004, 1984

53. Chong LL, Chau WK, Ho CH: A case of "superwarfarin" poisoning. Scand J Haematol 36:314, 1986

54. Weitzel JN, Sadowski JA, Furie BC et al: Hemorrhagic disorder caused by surreptitious ingestion of a long-acting vitamin K antagonist/rodenticide, brodifacoum. Blood 76:2555, 1990

55. Barnett VT, Bergmann F, Humphrey H, Chediak J: Diffuse alveolar hemorrhage secondary to superwarfarin ingestion. Chest 102:1301, 1992

56. Routh CR, Triplett DA, Murphy MJ et al: Superwarfarin ingestion and detection. Am J Hematol 36:50, 1991

57. Watts RG, Castleberry RP, Sadowski JA: Accidental poisoning with a super warfarin compound (brodifacoum) in a child. Pediatrics 86:883, 1990

58. Babcock J, Hartman K, Pedersen A et al: Rodenticide-induced coagulopathy in a young child. A case of Munchausen syndrome by proxy. Am J Pediatr Hematol Oncol 15:126, 1993

59. Druse JA, Carlson RW: Fatal rodenticide poisoning with brodifacoum. Ann Emerg Med 21:331, 1992

60. Mount ME, Kurth MJ, Jackson DY: Production of antibodies and development of an immunoassay for the anticoagulant diphacinone. J Immunoassay 9:69, 1988

61. Chalermchaikit T, Felice LJ, Murphy MJ: Simultaneous determination of eight anticoagulant rodenticides in blood serum and liver. J Anal Toxicol 17:56, 1993

62. Goldsweig HG, Kapusta M, Schwartz J: Bleeding, salicylates and prolonged prothrombin time: three case reports and a review of the literature. J Rheumatol 3:37, 1976

63. Uotila L, Suttie JW: Inhibition of vitamin K-dependent carboxylase in vitro by cefamandole and its structural analogs. J Infect Dis 148:571, 1983

64. Bang NU, Tessler SS, Heidenreich RO et al: Effects of moxalactam on blood coagulation and paltelet function. Rev Infect Dis 4:S546, 1982

65. Barza M, Furie B, Brown AE, Furie BC: Defects in vitamin K-dependent carboxylation associated with moxalactam treatment. J Infect Dis 153:1166, 1986

66. Lipsky JJ: Mechanism of the inhibition of the γ-carboxylation of glutamic acid by N-methylthiotetrazole-containing antibiotics. Proc Natl Acad Sci USA 81:2893, 1984

67. Cohen H, Scott SD, Mackie IJ et al: The development of hypoprothrombinaemia following antibiotic therapy in malnourished patients with low serum vitamin K_1 levels. Br J Haematol 68:63, 1988

68. McMillan CW, Roberts HR: Congenital combined deficiency of coagulation factors II, VII, IX, X. N Engl J Med 274:1313, 1979

69. Chung KS, Bezeaud A, Goldsmith JC et al: Congenital deficiency of blood clotting factors II, VII, IX and X. Blood 53:776, 1979

70. Johnson CA, Chung HS, McGrath KM et al: Characterization of a variant prothrombin in a patient congenitally deficient in factor II, VII, IX and X. Br J Haematol 44:461, 1980

71. Goldsmith GH Jr, Pence RE, Ratnoff OD et al: Studies on a family with combined functional deficiencies of vitamin K-dependent coagulation factors. J Clin Invest 69:1253, 1982

72. Vicente V, Maia R, Alberca I et al: Congenital deficiency of vitamin K-dependent coagulation factors and protein C. Thromb Haemost 51:343, 1984

Inhibitors of Blood Coagulation

115

Donald I. Feinstein

INTRODUCTION

Acquired inhibitors of blood coagulation, also known as circulating anticoagulants, are pathologic macromolecules in blood that directly inhibit clotting factors or their reactions. The vast majority have been characterized as antibodies. These inhibitors arise secondary to transfusion of plasma proteins in patients with hereditary bleeding disorders (see Ch. 101) or may arise de novo in patients with previously normal hemostatic mechanisms.

ACQUIRED INHIBITORS OF FACTOR VIII

Clinical Setting

Virtually all inhibitors of factor VIII are recognized because of their interference or neutralization of factor VIII activity. They occur in four clinical situations: alloantibody inhibitors in hemophilia A, postpartum, in association with certain immunologic diseases, and without any associated disorder.

In 1981, Green and Lechner[1] surveyed 215 patients found to have factor VIII inhibitors, in an effort to gather demographic information regarding spontaneously arising inhibitors to factor VIII. The gender incidence was about equal, and most patients were in the seventh decade of life. No associated disease was found in 50% of patients, but rheumatoid arthritis, systemic lupus erythematosus (SLE), drug reactions, and different types of malignancies were seen in 5–8% of the total group. In 7% of cases, disorders occurred during the postpartum period. Overall mortality was 22%. About 38% showed eventual spontaneous disappearance of the inhibitor. The spontaneous remission rate was confirmed by Lottenberg et al.,[2] who reported that among 16 patients receiving no immunosuppressive therapy, 5 had spontaneous remissions.

Factor VIII Inhibitors Occurring in Patients with Immunologic Disorders and in Patients without Underlying Disease

Disorders associated with factor VIII inhibitors include rheumatoid arthritis,[3,4] SLE,[3–5] penicillin allergy,[6] asthma,[3,4] inflammatory bowel disease,[4] erythema multiforme,[4] and dermatitis herpetiformis.[4] Occasionally, factor VIII inhibitors are associated with monoclonal gammopathies. Most patients have no underlying disease.

Factor VIII Inhibitors Occurring Postpartum

Factor VIII inhibitors can occur during the postpartum period in the absence of an underlying disorder.[3–5,7,8] Most often, the inhibitor occurs after the birth of the first child. Although a bleeding tendency may become evident immediately or after a prolonged interval, there is usually a 2–5-month delay before the diagnosis is made. The course in these patients is variable, but the inhibitor disappears spontaneously in most patients after 12–18 months.[7]

In patients who became pregnant again following the occurrence of a postpartum factor VIII inhibitor,[8] none of the patients in remission had a recurrence. The inhibitor actually disappeared during a subsequent pregnancy in patients not in remission.[8]

The cause of these postpartum inhibitors is unknown. The hypothesis that the mother becomes sensitized to allotypic determinants inherited by the fetus and that the antibodies so formed cross-react with the patient's factor VIII has not been substantiated.[8]

Properties of Spontaneously Acquired Factor VIII Inhibitors

With rare exceptions, factor VIII inhibitors are IgG antibodies. These inhibitors have restricted heterogeneity, as many possess either κ or λ light chains by immune neutralization techniques.[3–5,9–15] These inhibitors frequently contain mixtures of heavy-chain subclasses. Hultin et al.[13] found that both hemophilic and nonhemophilic inhibitors contain mixtures of IgG1 and IgG4 subclasses. The high incidence of factor VIII inhibitors containing a subpopulation of IgG4 is significant, as this subclass constitutes <4% of plasma IgG. The inhibitors are specific for factor VIII activity and in general do not interfere with the activities of von Willebrand factor (vWF) within the factor VIII/vWF complex. vWF antigen and function are normal in patients with such inhibitors. Factor VIII inhibitors do not participate in complement fixation[4,5]; they show species specificity both in vitro and in vivo in that human factor VIII is generally neutralized to a greater extent than is bovine or porcine factor VIII. However, infusion of bovine or porcine factor VIII into a patient with an inhibitor often raises the factor VIII level.[16]

The kinetics of the reaction between factor VIII and most hemophilic inhibitors is first order with respect to both factor VIII and inhibitor.[17,18] The inhibitor can be completely neutralized by excess factor VIII.[17,19] A time dependence of the neutralization of factor VIII sometimes requires 1–2 hours to reach equilibrium at low inhibitor concentrations.[17,18] Neutralization occasionally takes place in an initial rapid phase, followed by a slow second phase.[20–23] By contrast, inhibitors arising in nonhemophilic patients frequently differ in their reaction kinetics from inhibitors arising in hemophilic patients.[21,24,25] A linear relationship between the inhibitor concentration and the amount of factor VIII inactivated is observed with hemophilia inhibitors, but not with spontaneous inhibitors. Although most factor VIII inhibitor patients have no factor VIII in the plasma, the occasional patient exhibits some plasma factor VIII activity.[5,22,25,26] Gawryl and Hoyer[25] suggest that this antibody may react with factor VIII in such a way that the vWF protein partially shields factor VIII epitopes.

The epitopes to which allo- or autoantibodies to factor VIII are directed are limited to certain areas of the factor VIII light or heavy chains, or both.[27–30] Immunoblotting and binding studies with fragments of factor VIII demonstrate that plasma from approximately 50% of inhibitor patients contain at least two different neutralizing antibodies directed at both the light and heavy chain, whereas the other 50% bind to only the light chain.[30] In addition, the inhibitor produced by a given patient may change over time; a few non-neutralizing antibodies have also been found.[28,31]

Recognition, Identification, and Quantification of Factor VIII Inhibitors

The presence of a factor VIII inhibitor should be suspected whenever a patient with no prior bleeding history presents with spontaneous massive bruising or a hematoma. The partial thromboplastin time (PTT) is prolonged, whereas the prothrombin time (PT) and thrombin time (TT) are normal. The PTT of a mixture of the patient's plasma and normal plasma is also prolonged, although inactivation of factor VIII may require preincubation for 1–2 hours.[20,21,32,33] Confirmation that an inhibitor acts specifically with factor VIII requires incubating the patient's plasma diluted with an equal volume of normal plasma and performing assays of factors VIII, IX, XI, and XII at 0, 60, and 120 minutes. If the inhibitor is specific for factor VIII, only factor VIII decreases over time. A technique that uses the PTT rather than a factor VIII assay detects weak inhibitors of <0.4 Bethesda units.[32,33]

Quantitative inhibitor measurements are important in the emergency management of hemorrhage and for evaluation of long-term therapy. A standard unit of measurement, termed the Bethesda unit,[34] is best suited for the measurement of inhibitors arising in hemophiliacs, but the complexity of reaction kinetics and variations in antibody affinities for factor VIII, particularly in nonhemophiliac inhibitors with high residual factor VIII, limit standardization. In England, the New Oxford method is used to quantitate factor VIII inhibitors,[35] with 1 Bethesda unit equaling approximately 1.21 times 1 New Oxford unit.

Therapy for Patients with Factor VIII Inhibitors

When a patient with an inhibitor hemorrhages, conservative measures, including immobilization, compression, and possibly ε-aminocaproic acid, should be considered, along with additional therapies. The use of intramuscular injections or aspirin-containing compounds is contraindicated.

The indication for the use of factor VIII concentrate or factor IX complex concentrate is serious active bleeding. If the patient is not actively bleeding, transfusion is unnecessary. Unlike inhibitors associated with hemophilia A, most spontaneously acquired inhibitors are not inducible when the patient is re-exposed to factor VIII. However, these patients, unlike hemophiliacs, have not been previously exposed to virus-contaminated blood products. Thus, porcine factor VIII (Hyate-C, Porton-Speywood, Ltd.)[36] or highly purified factor VIII free of viral contaminants or recombinant factor VIII is indicated. In addition, the human autoantibodies usually have less affinity for porcine factor VIII than for human factor VIII.[36] Consequently, less concentrate is necessary to achieve effective hemostasis.[16,36,37]

An important parameter in determining the amount of factor VIII to be infused is the titer of the inhibitor and its reactivity to porcine factor VIII. If the titer is low (<5 Bethesda units), a large dose of factor VIII sufficient to neutralize all the circulating inhibitor and provide enough excess factor VIII to achieve a plasma factor VIII of ≥0.3 U/ml can be given. This can usually be achieved with the rapid infusion of porcine factor VIII (50–100 U/kg) or human factor VIII (150 U/kg), followed by a continuous infusion at 1,000 U/hr. If a patient has a moderately high inhibitor level of 5–30 Bethesda units, the inhibitor level may be lowered by about 50–65% by plasmapheresis or, alternatively, using one of several methods of extracorporeal immu-

noadsorption.[38,39] Following apheresis or immunoadsorption, the patient is given a bolus of either porcine factor VIII or human factor VIII, followed by a continuous infusion. If the patient has a high-titer inhibitor of >30 Bethesda units, it is impossible to achieve hemostasis, except with porcine factor VIII or factor IX complex concentrate (75 U/kg). Inhibitor plasma should be tested against porcine factor VIII in vitro before its use; continuous use or repeated infusions over an extended time may result in the development of antibodies to the porcine or human factor VIII.[36] In the occasional patient, allergic reactions or thrombocytopenia complicates therapy with porcine factor VIII.[36,40]

Factor VIII levels must be assayed frequently in order to monitor the plasma factor VIII level achieved in vivo, particularly after infusion of a factor VIII concentrate. The infused factor VIII may be efficacious in vivo before it is inactivated, but blood drawn for assay even a few minutes later will not have a measurable factor VIII level.

Factor IX complex concentrates are used to control bleeding in patients with factor VIII inhibitors.[41–45] These concentrates exhibit a procoagulant activity that bypasses the factor VIII-dependent clotting reactions, but the nature of this bypassing activity is unknown.[46] Two types of factor IX complex concentrate have been used in the treatment of patients with factor VIII inhibitors: (1) unactivated factor IX complex concentrates (e.g., Konyne, Proplex), which are used for the treatment of hemophilia B; and (2) activated concentrates (e.g., Autoplex and FEIBA), which contain a higher concentration of activated clotting factor, developed for use in patients with inhibitors. The efficacy of both types of concentrate in hemophiliacs with inhibitors has been demonstrated.[41–44] These concentrates are also effective in achieving hemostasis in patients with high-titer spontaneously acquired inhibitors.

A highly purified concentrate containing factor VIIa was found to achieve good hemostasis in patients with inhibitors[47]; more recently, a recombinant preparation of human factor VIIa has shown significant efficacy.[48]

Long-term goals in the management of these patients should be aimed at immunosuppression of autoantibody production. Assessment of immunosuppressive therapy is difficult because inhibitors occasionally disappear spontaneously.[1] Many patients respond to corticosteroids alone; in one report of 16 patients receiving only steroids,[49] 7 were complete responders, 4 partial responders, and 5 nonresponders. The time to response averaged about 16 days. In their 1981 survey, Green and Lechner[1] found that inhibitors disappeared in 22 of 41 steroid-treated patients. Certain subsets of patients responded better to steroids—particularly childhood and postpartum inhibitors—whereas inhibitors that developed in patients with rheumatoid arthritis were often resistant to steroid therapy. In patients resistant to steroids, the use of cytotoxic agents—particularly cyclophosphamide either alone or in combination with corticosteroids—can be efficacious. Patients with inhibitors who have relatively high residual factor VIII levels in vitro (0.04–0.34 U/ml) respond well.[26] Whether cyclophosphamide should be given daily (1–2 mg/kg) or by intermittent intravenous infusion (500–750 mg/m²) every 3 weeks with or without concomitant factor VIII concentrate is unknown.

The use of factor VIII concentrate infusion before immunosuppressive therapy was first proposed by Green.[50] The hypothesis proposed that the factor VIII concentrate infusion stimulates the abnormal clone of immune cells responsible for autoantibody synthesis and results in a greater cytotoxic effect by the immunosuppressive therapy. A combination of cyclophosphamide, vincristine, and prednisone every 3 weeks, preceded by an infusion of factor VIII concentrate (50–100 U/kg) resulted in complete disappearance of the inhibitor in 11 of 12 patients.[51] The responses occurred rapidly, usually within only two or three courses, and remissions in all patients were dura-

MANAGEMENT OF SPONTANEOUSLY ACQUIRED FACTOR VIII INHIBITORS

Conservative Measures

When a patient with an inhibitor suffers a hemorrhage, conservative hemostatic measures should be used to complement whatever other therapy is used. These measures include immobilization, compression, local application of hemostatic agents, and, on occasion, administration of ε-aminocaproic acid. The patient should not receive intramuscular injections, unnecessary venipunctures, or aspirin-containing compounds.

Selection of a Blood Product

The indication for the use of factor VIII concentrate or factor IX concentrate is active bleeding. If the patient is not actively bleeding, transfusion with factor VIII or IX is unnecessary. Unlike inhibitors associated with hemophilia A, most spontaneously acquired inhibitors do not increase in titer following exposure to factor VIII. Thus, this consideration should not impede tranfusion therapy. However, unlike hemophiliacs, these patients have not been previously exposed to virus-contaminated blood products. Thus, if a factor VIII concentrate is to be used, it is preferable to use porcine factor VIII (Hyate-C, Porton-Speywood, Ltd.) or highly purified human factor VIII. Human autoantibodies usually have less affinity for porcine factor VIII than for human factor VIII, and less porcine factor VIII concentrate is necessary to achieve effective hemostasis. Clearly, porcine factor VIII has certain advantages over human factor VIII in the treatment of this disorder.

The titer of the inhibitor and its reactivity to porcine factor VIII determine the amount of factor VIII to be used. If the titer is low (<5 Bethesda units), a large dose of factor VIII sufficient to neutralize all of the circulating inhibitor and provide enough excess factor VIII to achieve a plasma factor VIII of ≥0.3 U/ml (30%) can be given. This can usually be achieved by giving a rapid infusion of porcine factor VIII of about 75 U/kg, or alternatively by giving 150 U/kg of human factor VIII concentrate followed by a continuous infusion of 1,000 U/hr. If a patient has a moderately high inhibitor level of 5–30 Bethesda units, the inhibitor level may be lowered by about 50–65% by a 1.5-volume plasmapheresis, or alternatively by using one of several methods of extracorporeal immu-

noadsorption. Following apheresis or immunoadsorption, the patient is initially given either porcine factor VIII or human factor VIII, followed by a continuous infusion in the same doses noted above. If the patient has a very high titer inhibitor (>30 Bethesda units), it is impossible to achieve hemostatic levels of factor VIII except by using porcine factor VIII or by bypassing the site of inhibitor action with factor IX complex concentrate with a dose of 75 U/kg. The inhibitor plasma should be tested against porcine factor VIII in vitro prior to its use, and continuous use of repeated infusions over an extended period may result in the development of antibodies to the porcine factor VIII, resulting in a lack of efficacy. In an occasional patient, thrombocytopenia complicates therapy with the porcine concentrate.

Immunosuppression of the Inhibitor

The long-term goal in the management of these patients should be aimed at immunosuppression of the autoantibody production. Although many immunosuppressive regimens have proved efficacious, we initiate therapy with intravenous IgG (1 g/kg) for 2 days. If the inhibitor titer does not significantly decrease after 1 week, immunosuppressive therapy with prednisone (80 mg/day PO) and cyclophosphamide (2 mg/kg/day PO) may be initiated. CBCs are done weekly, and inhibitor titers are determined every 2 weeks. This regimen is continued for 8–10 weeks. If no significant decrease in titer occurs, the regimen is discontinued. A similar immunosuppressive regimen is repeated preceded by an infusion of factor VIII. Human factor VIII (50–100 U/kg) is followed by prednisone (100 mg/day for 5 days), cyclophosphamide (500 mg/m² IV on day 1), and vincristine (2 mg IV on day 1). This regimen is repeated at 3–4 weeks. If the neutrophil nadir is >2500, then the cyclophosphamide dose is increased to 750 mg/m². The patient is encouraged to force oral fluids during and just after cyclophosphamide therapy so as to minimize the risk of hemorrhagic cystitis. If the inhibitor titer is not decreased after three cycles, the regimen is discontinued.

If the above regimen is unsuccessful, the patient is placed on azathioprine (2 mg/kg) and serial CBCs and inhibitor titers are performed. If no significant response occurs within 8 weeks, the regimen is discontinued.

---

ble over 2–5 years. The initial inhibitor titer may be an important prognostic factor in the treatment of these patients.[52] Patients with inhibitor titers of <5–10 Bethesda units respond rapidly, whereas those with higher titers fail to respond.

Azathioprine in doses of 100–200 mg/day has also proved effective; Green and Lechner[1] found 19 of 28 patients to respond completely.

Any response to immunosuppressive therapy will generally occur within 12 weeks. If the titer has not decreased significantly within that period, such therapy should be discontinued.

Spontaneously acquired factor VIII inhibitors may respond to high-dose IgG.[53] The mechanism by which patients with inhibitors respond to intravenous IgG is unknown. However, IgG may have both a short- and long-term immunosuppressive effect.[54–56] Anti-idiotypic antibodies are present in the IgG prepa-

rations[57–59]; evidence shows that the emergence of anti-idiotypic antibodies may be the explanation for the occasional spontaneous remission and some instances of remission induced by immunosuppressive agents.[58,60,61]

The administration of deamino-D-arginine vasopressin (DDAVP) can briefly raise the factor VIII level in patients who have very low inhibitor titers and whose antibodies have type II reaction kinetics.[62]

ACQUIRED INHIBITORS OF VON WILLEBRAND FACTOR

Patients with von Willebrand disease (vWD) may develop inhibitors following plasma transfusion. Moreover, an acquired syndrome similar to hereditary vWD with onset later in life has been well described.[63-74] This acquired syndrome may occur in previously healthy persons, or it may be associated with SLE, lymphoproliferative disorders, or myeloproliferative disorders. The presence of the inhibitor is frequently associated with a monoclonal immunoglobulin, but whether the serum M component had inhibitory activity has not been determined unequivocally.[69,70,72,73] The clinical course in these patients has been variable, from mild to severe and life-threatening bleeding.

Laboratory studies usually show a reduction of ristocetin cofactor activity, vWF antigen, factor VIII activity, and a prolonged bleeding time. In some cases, the patient's plasma impairs ristocetin cofactor activity of normal plasma[65,70-72] or results in a decreased level of vWF in normal plasma. With few exceptions,[66] none of the inhibitors has had inhibitory activity in vitro against factor VIII activity.

Usually, no inhibitory activity is found in the patients' plasma.[70-73] In one patient,[67] correction of the abnormality followed radiation therapy for lymphoma; in another patient, who had Waldenström's macroglobulinemia,[69] vWF was detected on the monoclonal lymphocyte surface. These findings would suggest that in some patients with this syndrome, vWF can bind to cellular surfaces.

Multimer analysis of plasma from patients with acquired vWD has yielded variable results. Seven patients,[70] showed no alteration of multimeric structure (similar to type I vWD), whereas 10 other patients[72-74] lacked high-molecular-weight multimers (similar to type II vWD). These findings would suggest that these antibodies are heterogeneous and are directed against different epitopes of the vWF molecule.

Thus, acquired vWD may result from several different pathophysiologic mechanisms. In one type, the inhibitor inactivates the biologic activity of vWF. In a second type, the inhibitor binds to a site on the vWF molecule lacking biologic activity, causing rapid clearance of vWF from the circulation because of the formation of immune complexes. In a third type, vWF binds to cellular surfaces. In the second and third types, no inhibitor activity against vWF can be demonstrated in vitro.

Infusion of plasma or cryoprecipitate in patients with acquired vWD does not result in the expected increase in vWF activity. The secondary rise in factor VIII activity, characteristically seen in transfused patients with hereditary vWD, does not occur. Despite these findings, transfusion of cryoprecipitate or factor VIII concentrate containing vWF activity (Humate-P) in a bleeding patient may result in effective hemostasis. In two patients,[74] DDAVP resulted in a transient improvement. Two cases of acquired vWD were reported[74] that responded rapidly and completely to high-dose intravenous IgG (1 g/kg × 2 days). Although the inhibitor recurred in one patient within 2–3 weeks, repeated response to intravenous IgG could be attained.

ACQUIRED INHIBITORS OF FACTOR V

Spontaneous factor V inhibitors occur in older previously normal patients in the absence of a common underlying disease.[75-86] The degree of clinical bleeding in these patients varies considerably, in contrast to the uniformly severe bleeding in patients with factor VIII inhibitors. This extreme variability—from no clinical sequelae to fatal hemorrhage—can possibly be explained by the accessibility of platelet factor V to the antibody.[85,86] Studies conducted by Nesheim et al.[85] on a patient with a factor V inhibitor suggest that platelet factor V is relatively protected from an antifactor V antibody in whole blood, even though plasma factor V is completely neutralized. Thus, platelet factor V may play a key role in maintaining hemostatic competency in the presence of a factor V inhibitor. This hypothesis is supported by the efficacy of platelet concentrates in a factor V inhibitor patient.[80] Fresh frozen plasma

failed to effect hemostasis, but on four separate occasions, effective hemostasis was achieved with platelet transfusions. Two other patients responded to platelet transfusions, but others were not responsive. The course of the factor V inhibitor is short-lived in most patients, disappearing within 10 weeks. Whether steroids or other immunosuppressive agents influence the natural history of the inhibitors is unclear. The inhibitor may disappear with immunosuppressive therapy,[80,83,84] or it may disappear spontaneously without specific therapy.[75,79]

The laboratory identification of a factor V inhibitor is based on coagulation assays. Both the PTT and PT are prolonged, and normal plasma fails to correct these assays. These findings in the presence of a normal TT should strongly suggest the presence of a factor V inhibitor.[75] The demonstration that a mixture of the patient's plasma and normal plasma specifically lacks factor V clotting activity is required for a definitive diagnosis. Most of the factor V inhibitors are polyclonal IgG, but one was identified as both IgM and IgG, and another as both IgA and IgG.[79]

The mechanism for the development of these frequently transient factor V antibodies remains obscure. In the single patient with hereditary factor V deficiency, the appearance of the inhibitor was related to transfusion. In patients with spontaneously acquired inhibitors, no common underlying disease was found, except for tuberculosis and fractured femurs.[75,85] However, a variety of temporal associations with these inhibitors have been noted, including drugs, operative procedures, transfusions, and infections.[75,85] Except for occasional patients who have received streptomycin, gentamicin or penicillin, the most common temporal association was a recent operative procedure.[75,85] Patients who had a previous history of surgery displayed a significant reactivity to bovine factor V, whereas patients who had factor V antibodies without a history of previous surgery did not.[87] This finding suggested the possible exposure of the postsurgical patients to bovine factor V. This exposure would account for the immunization to bovine factor V. The resultant factor V antibody cross-reacted with human factor V and led to bleeding.

Indeed, bovine thrombin is used as a topical hemostatic agent in surgical procedures; it contains detectable amounts of factor V.[88] Thus, the development of antibodies to factor V in postsurgical patients is a response to antigen challenge by factor V contamination of the bovine thrombin preparations.

ACQUIRED INHIBITORS OF FACTORS VII, IX, AND X AND PROTHROMBIN

Except for the prothrombin antibody associated with the lupus anticoagulant, spontaneously acquired inhibitors to factors VII, IX, and X or prothrombin are rare. Bajaj et al.[89] described a patient in whom hypoprothrombinemia developed due to an antibody that bound to a prothrombin epitope without inhibition of coagulant activity. Unlike the hypoprothrombinemia associated with the lupus anticoagulant, this patient's plasma did not contain antibody activity against anionic phospholipids, and the antibody bound to the NH_2-terminal end of the prothrombin molecule.

Hawiger et al.[90] described a patient with SLE and severe thrombocytopenia in whom spontaneous bleeding from multiple sites developed, whose plasma contained an antibody that reacted with bovine thrombin. Scully et al.[91] reported a patient who bled excessively after dental extraction and from the gastrointestinal tract. This patient had a prolonged PTT, PT, and TT and a normal reptilase time, and the immunoglobulin fraction of her plasma bound to both thrombin and prothrombin. Barthels and Heimburger[92] described a patient with cirrhosis and bleeding who had a prolonged PTT, PT, and TT. The patient's IgG prolonged the TT but did not affect fibrin polymerization. Stricker et al.[93] described three postsurgical patients with prosthetic cardiac valves in whom antibodies to human and bovine thrombin developed. All three patients had prolonged PTT and TT. The TT did not correct on mixing with normal plasma or protamine, but the reptilase time was normal.

Two patients in whom IgG autoantibodies to factor VII developed had a prolonged PT but a normal PTT.[94,95] Weisdorf et al.[96] described a patient with severe aplastic anemia who had acquired factor VII deficiency. A factor VII-binding immunoglobulin in the patient's plasma bound to factor VII, resulting in rapid clearance of the immune complex.

Spontaneously acquired factor IX inhibitors are extremely rare.[97-101] The clinical setting in which these inhibitors occur is similar to that associated with the development of factor VIII inhibitors. Three were associated with SLE and two with the postpartum state. Most seem to disappear within 1–7 months with onset, but whether immunosuppressive therapy alters the natural history is unknown.

Only one documented case of a factor X inhibitor has been reported.[102] This occurred in an elderly patient with no underlying disease. It was characterized as an IgG autoantibody and disappeared spontaneously without specific therapy.

ACQUIRED INHIBITORS OF FACTOR XI AND XII

Inhibitors directed against factors XI or XII have been reported.[103-109] These were detected in patients with hereditary factor XI deficiency following transfusions, whereas most occurred in patients with SLE. Many of these patients also had low factor XII levels. Zucker et al.[106] studied several patients on long-term chlorpromazine therapy in whom asymptomatic IgM inhibitors of the intrinsic phase of blood coagulation developed. The inhibitor resulted in decreased measurements of all the plasma clotting factors in the intrinsic pathway and was shown to interfere with the coagulant activity of contact product. These inhibitors may be similar to those described by Canoso et al.[110] in patients on long-term high-dose phenothiazine therapy. Except for those with hereditary factor XI deficiency, none of the patients who developed inhibitors to the contact system has had excessive bleeding.

ACQUIRED INHIBITORS THAT AFFECT FIBRIN STABILIZATION, FIBRINOGEN, OR FIBRIN POLYMERIZATION

The terminal phase of blood coagulation is characterized by the cleavage of fibrinopeptides A and B from fibrinogen, polymerization of fibrin monomers, and the covalent cross-linking of the α- and γ-chains of fibrin by factor XIIIa (see Ch. 100). Spontaneously acquired inhibitors of each of these reactions have been described.

Inhibitors of fibrinogen have occurred in patients with hereditary afibrinogenemia following transfusion.[111] In addition, Marciniak and Greenwood[112] reported a patient in whom a polyclonal IgG antibody developed that caused a delay in the release of fibrinopeptide A from normal fibrinogen reacting with thrombin, which retarded the onset of clot formation. This patient had a prolonged PTT, PT, TT, and reptilase time. The isolated inhibitor prolonged the TT of normal plasma.

A high incidence of prolonged TT has been observed in patients with SLE. Galanakis et al.[113] found that two such patients had monoclonal antibodies that reacted with different parts of fibrin and fibrinogen, delaying fibrin polymerization. In addition, patients have developed autoantibodies that inhibit fibrin monomer polymerization.[114,115]

Although a variety of abnormalities of hemostasis are associated with monoclonal gammopathies,[116] isolated M proteins can interfere with the conversion of fibrinogen to fibrin monomer or with the aggregation of fibrin monomers into polymers.[116-118] Coleman et al.[118] provided indirect evidence that at least some M proteins act as antibodies, since Fab fragments of IgG monoclonal proteins were more inhibiting than intact protein, the isolated chains, or the Fc fragments. Spontaneous inhibitors of fibrin stabilization can lead to severe hemorrhagic complications, some fatal.[4,6,119-128] Of the 14 reported patients, 6 showed the development of an inhibitor while taking isoniazid.

Since non-cross-linked fibrin clots could result from neutralization of factor XIII by (1) inhibition of activation to factor XIIIa, (2) inhibition of factor XIIIa, or (3) interference with the cross-linking sites on fibrinogen, the inhibitors may have more than one site of action. A patient who had been taking isoniazid for 8 years, described by Rosenberg et al.,[126] was shown to have an antibody directed against the cross-linking sites on fibrinogen; factor XIII levels were normal. By contrast, an inhibitor prevented the activation of factor XIII by thrombin but did not bind factor XIIIa.[122,125] In other cases, the inhibitor interfered directly with factor XIIIa activity.

A classification scheme for the three types of factor XIII inhibitor is based on the step of the reaction sequence that is inhibited. Type I inhibitors are directed against the activation of the factor XIII zymogen but do not interfere with transamidase activity. Type II inhibitors impair the transamidase activity of factor XIIIa. Type III inhibitors block the reactivity of the fibrin substrate toward factor XIIIa. A fourth type of inhibitor was recently reported,[129] whereby the antibody inhibited factor XIII activity by binding to the fibrin binding site on factor XIII. Characterized as an IgG antibody, this inhibitor disappeared with immunosuppressive therapy.

HEPARIN-LIKE ANTICOAGULANTS

The development of spontaneously acquired heparin-like anticoagulants has been reported in patients with neoplasms or in those undergoing suramin therapy for the treatment of adrenocortical carcinoma.[130-136] Reports of anticoagulants associated with neoplastic disorders[130-132,134-136] include cases of a plasma cell malignancy and a severe hemorrhagic disorder.[129,130,133] Coagulation studies were characterized by a prolonged TT that fails to correct with the addition of normal plasma. However, the prolonged TT can be corrected by the addition of protamine sulfate, toluidine blue, or heparinase to the patient's plasma. Each of these inhibitors possesses biochemical and physicochemical properties of glycosaminoglycans. One patient treated intravenously with protamine sulfate showed an improvement in his laboratory studies, as well as decreased bleeding.[134]

A complex coagulopathy was reported in three women receiving suramin for adrenocortical carcinoma.[133] The severe hepatocellular dysfunction that developed accounted for some of the coagulopathy. In addition, each patient acquired a potent inhibitor of the TT, which increased markedly during exacerbations of hepatic injury. Anticoagulant activity was eliminated in vitro by a combination of heparitinase and chondroitinase ABC, suggesting that the activity was mediated by heparan sulfate and dermatan sulfate. Since suramin inhibits enzymes that normally degrade glycosaminoglycans, hepatic injury was hypothesized to cause the release of glycosaminoglycans, which then accumulate because of failure of degradation.

LUPUS ANTICOAGULANT

General Considerations

The lupus anticoagulant is an IgG or IgM antibody that prolongs phospholipid-dependent coagulation in vitro by binding to epitopes within the phospholipid component of the complex

DIAGNOSTIC APPROACH TO INHIBITORS

The approach to patients with abnormal coagulation tests should initially include a complete history regarding excessive bleeding, particularly as it relates to hemostatic challenges and thrombotic problems, either venous or arterial. Initial laboratory studies should include a repeat of the abnormal coagulation test on a mixture of the patient's plasma and normal plasma. Correction of the abnormal test indicates a "deficiency" state, whereas poor correction indicates the presence of an inhibitor.

Approach to Inhibitors Associated with Bleeding

Patients who present with an acquired bleeding disorder and in whom an inhibitor is demonstrated most often will have antibodies to a specific clotting factor. Subsequent laboratory evaluation should attempt to demonstrate the specific coagulation factor to whch the antibody is directed and to determine the specificity of the antibody. The former is done by doing a specific assay for the coagulation factor suspected of being affected, and the latter is done by doing a specific assay for the coagulation factor of a mixture of various dilutions of patient's plasma (antibody) and normal plasma (antigen) over time. If the inhibitor is specific for a single clotting factor, procagulant activity of that coagulation factor will be neutralized over time, whereas other clotting factor assays will be unaffected. For example, if an acquired inhibitor of factor VIII is suspected and the factor VIII assay is low, a factor VIII assay of a mixture of the patient's plasma and normal plasma should demonstrate a progressive decrease in factor VIII activity from immediately after the mixture was made to 1–2 hours later. By contrast, if factor IX and XI assays were done on the same mixture, factors IX and XI would be unaffected.

Rarely, a spontaneously acquired autoantibody will react with a noncoagulant epitope of a specific hemostatic factor (e.g., prothrombin in the lupus anticoagulant-hypoprothrombinemia syndrome) or a specific clotting factor will be adsorbed to cellular surfaces (e.g., vWF) or to amyloid (e.g., factor X). In these patients, the addition of normal plasma to the patient's plasma will result in correction of the abnormality. In these patients, the in vivo half-life of the affected hemostatic factor will be shortened significantly because of rapid clearance of the antigen/antibody complex or by adsorption of the clotting factor to a pathologic surface.

Spontaneously acquired heparin-like anticoagulants differ from the inhibitors described above in that they are not immunoglobulins, and they do not specifically affect one specific clotting factor. These anticoagulants are easily recognized because their major effect is on the thrombin time, but the reptilase time is normal.

Approach to Inhibitors Not Associated with Excessive Bleeding

If the patient has a history of thrombotic disease or repeated episodes of fetal loss, the patient should be evaluated for the lupus anticoagulant. Most commonly, these patients will have a prolonged PTT and a normal or slightly prolonged PT. However, on occasion, the PT may be more prolonged than usual even in the absence of an associated prothrombin deficiency. If the patient is suspected of having a lupus anticoagulant, several relatively simple tests can be used to confirm the diagnosis. For sensitivity, we favor the kaolin clotting time as modified by Exner and, for specificity, we favor correction of the PTT with phospholipid as described by Rosove or Triplett. In the presence of a lupus anticoagulant with a prolonged PTT, specific intrinsic clotting factor assays are frequently low but will increase with increasing dilution of test plasma. For example, assays for factor IX would be 5%, factor XI 8%, factor XI 9%, and factor XII 10%, and all would progressively increase with increasing dilution of the test plasma. Thus, the lupus anticoagulant will affect all the specific assays, in contrast to an antibody to a specific clotting factor, for which a single assay shows irreversible inactivation of that clotting factor. In the latter case, dilution would not result in an increase in the level of that clotting factor.

of factors Xa and Va, phospholipid, and calcium.[6,137] It was given this name in 1972 because clear proof of its site of action was lacking and because the anticoagulant had been recognized in patients with SLE.[6] It is clearly a misnomer, since the lupus anticoagulant is more frequently encountered in patients without lupus[6,137] and is associated with thrombosis rather than with bleeding.[6,137] Immunoglobulins reacting with other hemostatic factors, such as vWF,[138] factors VIII,[139] IX, and XI, and inhibitors of fibrin polymerization, have also been described in patients with SLE, but they are rare compared with the lupus anticoagulant.

Patients with the lupus anticoagulant who do not have established SLE fall into several different categories: (1) patients with "lupus-like" chronic autoimmune disorders but without findings that fit the criteria for the diagnosis of SLE[140–142]; (2) patients with other chronic systemic autoimmune disorders; (3) patients presenting with a venous or arterial thrombotic event for which no underlying cause may be apparent[143–148]; (4) patients receiving certain drugs, including procainamide[149] and phenothiazines[110,150] (a high prevalence of the lupus anticoagulant and a positive antinuclear antibody test are ob-

served in psychotic patients receiving long-term chlorpromazine therapy[150]; other drugs that can induce the lupus anticoagulant include hydralazine and quinidine); (5) patients with a recent acute viral infection,[151,152] in whom the antibody is usually transient; (6) patients with human immunodeficiency virus infection[153–156]; (7) women with recurrent fetal wastage[141,157–164]; and (8) patients seeking medical attention for a variety of disorders in whom the lupus anticoagulant is discovered as an incidental finding (frequently, such cases are discovered because of a prolonged PTT performed as a routine preoperative evaluation of hemostasis).

The prevalence of the lupus anticoagulant in patients with SLE in which the PTT test was used for its detection is approximately 10%.[6,165] However, a higher prevalence of approximately 50% is found when a modified PTT with a reduced concentration of phospholipid is used to detect the anticoagulant.[141] Moreover, when using the kaolin clotting time—a test with increased sensitivity for detecting low-titer lupus anticoagulants because it contains no added exogenous phospholipid—evidence of inhibitor activity can be demonstrated in the plasma of 30–50% of randomly selected patients with SLE.[166] This percentage approximates the 42–44% incidence of the frequency of anticardiolipin antibodies (ACAs) in patients with SLE.[167]

Properties, Epitope Specificity, Mechanism of Action, and Relationship to Anticardiolipin Antibodies

The lupus anticoagulant is an immunoglobulin. In some patients, for example, those in whom it arises secondary to long-term chlorpromazine therapy, it is IgM[150]; in other patients, it is IgG,[137] and in still others, it may be both IgG and IgM.[137] Although IgA ACAs have been well described, IgA anticoagulant activity has never been investigated. Transplacental transfer of the inhibitor has been reported,[168] which would be compatible with an IgG inhibitor.

The immunoglobulins responsible for the lupus anticoagulant effect react in in vitro assay systems against anionic phospholipids. Reducing the phospholipid component of clotting mixtures amplifies the effect of the inhibitor. Thus, the most sensitive tests for detecting the inhibitor contain only limited amounts of procoagulant phospholipid: the recalcification time of platelet-free plasma,[169] the kaolin clotting time of platelet-poor plasma,[166,170,171] and the PT performed with very dilute tissue factor (the tissue thromboplastin inhibition [TTI] test).[140,171] The addition of an exogenous source of phospholipid corrected the prolonged prothrombin consumption test of blood containing the lupus inhibitor.[172] The addition of liposomes containing phosphatidylserine,[173] rabbit brain phospholipid,[174] or freeze-thawed platelets[175,176] markedly shortens the prolonged PTT of plasma containing the lupus anticoagulant.

Thiagajaran et al.[177] provided direct evidence that a lupus anticoagulant can react with phospholipid in studies of a patient with macroglobulinemia and a monoclonal IgM that behaved as a lupus anticoagulant. The purified immunoglobulin gave precipitin lines in a double immunodiffusion system with phosphatidylserine, phosphatidylinositol, and phosphatidic acid and inhibited calcium-dependent binding of prothrombin and factor X to phospholipid vesicles. Shapiro and Thiagajaran[177] also refer to further studies in which plasma from 17 patients with the lupus anticoagulant had precipitin activity against anionic phospholipids on analysis by double diffusion, whereas the plasma from none of 22 control patients with SLE but without the lupus anticoagulant exhibited such activity.

Phospholipid participates in coagulation in vitro at several known steps: as a component of the prothrombinase complex, as a cofactor with factor VIIIa for factor IXa in the tenase complex, as a cofactor with protein S for activated protein C's proteolytic inactivation of factor Va and factor VIIIa, and as a cofactor for activation of factor X by factor VIIa. The lupus anticoagulant may impede each of these reactions of blood coagulation. The anticoagulant is able to inhibit the binding of both factor X and prothrombin to the negatively charged phospholipid surface.[167,177,178] Whether the lupus anticoagulant can interfere with the procoagulant activity of activated platelets continues to be debated.[179] However, recent studies suggest that the anticoagulant is capable of affecting platelet-dependent prothrombinase activity, particularly when platelets are present in reduced numbers.[179]

Patients with the lupus anticoagulant also have evidence of plasma immunoglobulin reacting with the phospholipid, cardiolipin. This was first recognized as a high prevalence of an associated chronic biologic false-positive test for syphilis,[137,169,180] a test in which cardiolipin is the antigen. With the use of a sensitive quantitative radioimmunoassay for ACAs, most patients with the lupus anticoagulant have elevated levels of ACAs in their plasma.[181]

Although most patients with elevated levels of ACAs also test positive for lupus anticoagulant activity, considerable data support lupus anticoagulant activity and ACAs as distinct subgroups of antibodies that can be separated by affinity or physicochemical methods.[182,183] Purified ACAs fail to bind to immobilized anionic phospholipid and require the presence of β_2-glycoprotein I (GPI), also known as apolipoprotein H.[184,185] Thus, the interaction of ACA with anionic phospholipid requires the presence of a plasma protein cofactor β_2-GPI. Since ACAs do not react with either isolated phospholipid or purified β_2-GPI, ACAs react with either epitopes of the complex or a cryptic epitope on β_2-GPI after it binds to phospholipid.

Whether β_2-GPI is the same cofactor that in normal plasma potentiates lupus anticoagulant in clotting assays has not been clearly established. In fact, when the lupus anticoagulant activity was separated from ACA, prolongation of clotting times in the presence of isolated lupus anticoagulant required the presence of both anionic phospholipid and human prothrombin.[186] Bevers et al.[186] hypothesized that the lupus anticoagulant is an antibody directed to a human prothrombin/phospholipid complex analogous to ACAs directed toward a β_2-GPI/phospholipid complex. These data would corroborate previous studies suggesting that the antibodies responsible for lupus anticoagulant activity exhibit reactivity for both prothrombin and phospholipid.[187,188] These studies strongly suggest that the activity in normal plasma that causes further prolongation of the clotting time when added to plasma containing the lupus anticoagulant reacts only with the complex of phospholipid and prothrombin.

Mechanism of Hypoprothrombinemia in the Hypoprothrombinemia-Lupus Anticoagulant Syndrome

A subset of patients with the lupus anticoagulant will also have a specific deficiency of prothrombin. The plasma of such patients does not contain an antibody that neutralizes prothrombin activity,[189] and the prothrombin antigen is decreased to the same extent as prothrombin activity.[190,191] Bajaj et al.[192] demonstrated that the plasma from patients with the hypoprothrombinemia-lupus anticoagulant syndrome contains antibodies that bind prothrombin without neutralizing its in vitro coagulant activity. The decreased concentration of plasma prothrombin in patients with this syndrome results from the rapid removal of prothrombin/prothrombin antibody complexes. In addition, altered mobility of prothrombin antigen on crossed immunoelectrophoresis indicative of the presence of plasma prothrombin antigen/antibody complexes has been demonstrated in 66–75% of patients with the lupus anticoagulant in whom plasma prothrombin activity was not substantially decreased.[193]

Laboratory Evaluation

The results of coagulation tests usually found in patients with the lupus anticoagulant include a prolonged PTT, which is prolonged when the patient's plasma is mixed with equal parts of normal plasma. The PT is minimally to moderately prolonged (0.5–3 seconds), but occasionally it is normal. However, the PT is prolonged more than normal plasma when diluted tissue factor is used as in the TTI test.[140] The TT is normal. The sensitivity of the PTT for lupus anticoagulant detection varies with different commercial reagents used for the test,[194–196] probably reflecting, at least in part, the variation in the phospholipid composition of these reagents.[196]

The prevention of platelet activation in plasma samples is crucial, since phospholipid, either in the patient plasma or in the normal plasma used for mixing studies, may neutralize weak lupus coagulant activity.[197,198] It is therefore recommended that test plasmas and normal plasma be initially centrifuged at 5,000–15,000g for 10–15 minutes and/or filtered through 0.22-μm screens to remove platelets prior to freezing.[198]

Confirmation of the Diagnosis

The pattern of abnormality of the lupus anticoagulant is often indistinguishable from that of an anticoagulant directed against any one of the several clotting factors that influence the result of the PTT, but not the PT. Therefore, further tests are needed to confirm that the prolonged PTT of a mixture of patient's plasma and normal plasma results from the lupus anticoagulant. It is particularly important to rule out a factor VIII anticoagulant, which, in contrast to the lupus anticoagulant, frequently causes serious bleeding.

Tests based on the observation that excess phospholipid substantially shortens the prolonged PTT of lupus anticoagulant plasma have been advocated as a means of differentiating the lupus anticoagulant from other inhibitors. The excess phospholipid has been added as either freeze-thawed platelets,[176] liposomes containing phosphatidylserine,[173] platelet-derived microvesicles[199] or rabbit brain phospholipid.[174] Correction of prolonged clotting times by excess phospholipid significantly increases specificity, and false-positive results are only encountered for heparinized patients. However, no positive results are obtained from patients with clotting factor inhibitors, congenital factor deficiencies, or hepatic insufficiency or in patients receiving warfarin therapy.

Another diagnostic approach designed to confirm the diagnosis is to perform several of the specific one-stage clotting factor assays based on the PTT technique. The following pattern of results is frequently found: (1) low values for several clotting factors (artifactually decreased values reflecting the ability of the lupus anticoagulant in the test sample to impair the reactivity of the phospholipid reagent common to each assay system); and (2) increasing values for each clotting factor with increasing dilution of the test plasma in the assay system (reflecting a decreased carryover of the lupus anticoagulant into the assay system with a higher dilution of the patient's plasma).

PT tests using dilute tissue thromboplastin have also been used to confirm the presence of the lupus anticoagulant.[140,200] The dilute Russell's viper venom time test, in particular, is a simple, sensitive, relatively specific assay for the detection of the lupus anticoagulant.[201] By contrast, the TTI test is less sensitive and specific.[170,171,174,200]

Detection of Low-Titer Lupus Anticoagulants

The PTT may be normal in patients with a low-titer lupus anticoagulant. Since the recognition of a lupus anticoagulant is important in the management of patients who experience thrombotic events without an underlying disorder, a normal PTT does not preclude a low-titer inhibitor in such patients. Laboratory evaluation should include examination of clotting time in a more sensitive system containing limited amounts of phospholipid and ACAs. Although testing for the latter is standardized, tests for lupus anticoagulant activity have not been standardized, hence the absence of an established reliable method for their quantitation. The most sensitive assay for detecting the presence of the lupus anticoagulant is the kaolin clotting time mixture test as described by Exner et al.[166] and

---

---

the dilute phospholipid PTT described by Alving et al.[202,203] Both assays are also useful in identifying patients with the lupus anticoagulant who are anticoagulated with warfarin.[202,203] In direct comparisons with the TTI test, the dilute Russell's viper venom test, and PTT with and without high concentrations of phospholipid, the assay described by Exner is most sensitive in detecting very low titers of the lupus anticoagulant.[200]

Lupus anticoagulant activity can vary over time.[157,158,204] Therefore, testing 2–4 months apart is important in establishing a persistent abnormality.

Laboratory Recognition of the Hypothrombinemia-Lupus Anticoagulant Syndrome

Although minimal to moderate prolongation of the PT, up to about 3 seconds beyond a control value, can be accounted for by the lupus anticoagulant, the finding of a substantially prolonged PT (e.g., 18–20 seconds) represents presumptive evidence of an associated specific prothrombin deficiency. One may demonstrate three additional findings: (1) a mixture of equal parts of patient's plasma and normal plasma gives the expected value calculated from the mean of the levels in individual plasmas, (2) prothrombin activity and prothrombin antigen are concordantly decreased, or (3) prothrombin has abnormal mobility on crossed immunoelectrophoresis.[187,188]

Clinical Relationships of Lupus Anticoagulant and Anticardiolipin Antibodies

ACAs are detected by solid-phase immunoassay, whereas the lupus anticoagulant is measured as an activity that prolongs lipid-dependent clotting reactions. Both antibodies are antiphospholipid antibodies frequently associated with thrombosis, fetal wastage, or thrombocytopenia with or without autoimmune disorders. Some investigators[206,207] have renamed this clinical entity the antiphospholipid syndrome. In contrast to the antiphospholipid syndrome, the primary antiphospholipid syndrome is defined as either venous or arterial thrombotic disease, or both, or as recurrent fetal wastage associated with elevated levels of antiphospholipid antibodies in the absence of any definite autoimmune disease.[207] The latter patients do not demonstrate any other clinical or serologic evidence of autoimmune disease, except for occasional low-titer (<1:160) antinuclear antibodies. An occasional patient with high-titer ACAs can present with fulminant disease with multiorgan system involvement (e.g., lung, kidney, brain), hypertension, and microvascular and macrovascular thrombosis. As these patients have a high mortality, they require aggressive treatment.

ACAs and lupus anticoagulants are related groups of antibodies.[177,208,209] Most patients who test positive for the lupus anticoagulant have elevated levels of ACA. However, although the correlation between the two is significant, many patients showing positivity for lupus anticoagulant activity do not have elevated levels of ACA or other antiphospholipid antibodies, and vice versa.[210–213] Moreover, ACAs and lupus anticoagulants comprise separate antibody subgroups that can be isolated from one another in vitro; they also possess different phospholipid binding characteristics.[182,183]

Since ACA levels can fluctuate significantly,[214] a negative test for both the lupus anticoagulant and ACA does not completely rule out the presence of phospholipid antibodies. This is particularly true during an acute thrombotic episode, when antiphospholipid antibody titers may transiently decline to normal.[215]

Recent studies[158,204] suggest that when tests for the lupus anticoagulant and ACAs are performed at two separate time intervals (8–16 weeks), a statistically significant association can be shown between persistently positive tests and prior thromboembolic events and fetal loss. The strength of this association is much reduced when transiently positive patients are included. Furthermore, the presence of persistent test positivity for ACA was more strongly associated with previous thromboembolic events and fetal loss than the presence of persistent positivity for the lupus anticoagulant. These studies also showed that a combination of tests for detecting lupus anticoagulant activity is superior to a single test. However, the number of patients who tested positive for lupus anticoagulant activity was small, and tests were considered negative when they were <2 SD above normal.[157]

A false-positive Venereal Disease Research Laboratory test in low titer (1:4–1:8) can be demonstrated in ≤30% of patients with the lupus anticoagulant or ACAs. These cross-reacting antibodies differ from reagin, the antibody responsible for the Wasserman reaction in patients with syphilis.

Relationship of Lupus Anticoagulant and Anticardiolipin Antibodies to Other Antibodies

Subjects with the lupus anticoagulant and ACAs have been shown to have antibodies against other anionic phospholipids (phosphatidylserine, phosphatidylinositol, and phosphatidic acid) but not against neutral or positively charged phospholipids (phosphatidylcholine and phosphatidylethanolamine).[177,216] This finding suggests that lupus anticoagulant and ACAs recognize epitope(s) associated with the negatively charged phosphodiester group in anionic phospholipids that is either blocked or not expressed when the phosphodiester group is linked to a neutral or positively charged compound (choline or ethanolamine).

The phosphoserine groups on serine-phosphorylated proteins are structurally very similar to the phosphodiester/serine moiety on phosphatidylserine, suggesting that antiphospholipid antibodies have the potential to cross-react with serine-phosphorylated proteins. This is supported by the finding that some hybridoma lupus autoantibodies react not only with phospholipids and DNA, but also with cytoskeletal proteins, which are known to be serine phosphorylated.[217] Other studies have demonstrated significant cross-reactivity of anti-DNA anti-

bodies with cell-surface proteins on platelets and other cells.[218–220] These data, along with data indicating that lupus anticoagulant activity and ACAs do not bind to phospholipid without binding to another protein, suggest that these antibodies are members of a larger class of antibodies directed to cryptic epitopes in proteins after binding to phospholipid or to epitopes on the protein/phospholipid complex, or to both.

Correlation Between Clinical Findings and Antiphospholipid Antibodies

Bleeding

Most patients with the lupus anticoagulant do not bleed abnormally. Patients with the lupus anticoagulant have undergone needle biopsy of the kidney and the severe hemostatic challenges of major surgery,[137,143,221] including prostatectomy[137] and open heart surgery,[137] without excessive postoperative bleeding.

Nevertheless, patients with the lupus inhibitor may have clinically significant bleeding. In all but a few, the bleeding can be attributed to some abnormality other than the lupus inhibitor,[6,169] such as depressed prothrombin activity.[168,191,222] The combination of the lupus anticoagulant and a prothrombin coagulant activity below about 20% has resulted in severe and even fatal bleeding. In other patients, thrombocytopenia, alone or in combination with moderate prothrombin deficiency, accounted for the bleeding tendency. The hemorrhagic manifestations may be related to severe uremia.[172]

Evaluation of the risk of abnormal bleeding in patients with the lupus anticoagulant includes establishing the presence of prothrombin deficiency, thrombocytopenia, or uremia. In the absence of these coexisting risk factors, abnormal bleeding is minimal even after trauma or surgery.[143,221,223,224] In summary, most patients with the isolated finding of lupus anticoagulant will not experience abnormal bleeding. Nevertheless, excessive postoperative bleeding has been attributed to the lupus anticoagulant on rare occasions.[225,226]

Thrombosis

Since the initial observation by Bowie et al.[172] in 1963, it has become clear that thrombosis is a major concern in patients with the lupus anticoagulant. The incidence has varied from 17% to 71%, averaging about 30–40%.[141,143,167,224,227] Because of the strong correlation between the occurrence of the lupus anticoagulant and an elevated level of ACA, a high incidence (approximately 40%) of thrombotic disease is reported in patients with elevated ACA levels.[167,206,228] Thrombosis (and fetal loss and thrombocytopenia) are more frequent as the level of ACA increases and very high titers (>7 SD above the normal mean) are associated with thrombotic events. In addition, although some investigators believe that elevated levels of IgG or IgA isotypes are more common than IgM in patients with complications,[229,230] this has not been clearly established. Moreover, the lupus anticoagulant or increased levels of ACA must be persistently present on more than one occasion, since the incidence of thrombotic complications is almost the same in patients with transiently positive test as in patients with negative tests at two different time intervals.[157,158,204] Moreover, the persistent presence of elevated levels of ACA has been shown to be associated with indices of in vivo coagulation activation. In a recent study of patients with SLE[231] who were either persistently ACA⁺ versus patients who were transiently positive or persistently negative, ACA⁺ patients had a higher mean level of F_{1+2} and fibrinopeptide A than that of patients who were either transiently positive or persistently negative or on warfarin therapy. The differences remained significant even if patients with prior thromboembolism were excluded from the analysis. These results suggest that the presence of persistently elevated levels of ACA in SLE patients is associated with an ongoing prothrombotic state.

Thrombosis may be either venous or arterial,[206] with events occurring nearly equally in the arterial and venous circulation. Venous thrombosis is usually manifested as deep venous thrombosis of the lower extremities with or without pulmonary emboli. In addition, unusual sites of venous thrombosis, such as hepatic veins, inferior vena cava, mesenteric veins, renal veins, cerebral venous sinuses, and axillary veins, have occasionally been reported.[206] Arterial thrombosis is manifested as stroke[206,232] or transient ischemic attacks,[233] but myocardial infarction has also been reported.[234] Also, unusual presentations, such as gangrene of the extremities and digits, multi-infarct dementia, and bowel infarction, have also been observed.[235] Thromboembolic pulmonary hypertension with or without SLE can occur in association with the lupus anticoagulant or with elevated levels of ACA, or both.[206,236,237]

Nonbacterial mitral and aortic endocardial valve lesions, with or without SLE, accompanied by thromboembolic transient ischemic attacks and strokes associated with lupus anticoagulant activity and/or elevated levels of ACA have also been reported.[238] Livedo reticularis and cerebrovascular disease (Sneddon syndrome)[207] and giant cell arteritis[239] have also been associated with the presence of these antibodies.

Although thrombosis is supposedly not associated with the lupus anticoagulant or ACA induced by infection or drugs, there have been several reports of human immunodeficiency virus or drug-associated thrombosis.[143,240]

Patients who are persistently positive for the lupus anticardiolipin or who have persistently elevated levels of ACA and suffer a thromboembolic event have a recurrence rate of approximately 50%.[241] In addition, recurrences tend to occur (approximately 90%) on the same side of the circulation as the initial event—venous recurrences after an initial venous event and arterial recurrences after an initial arterial event.[241]

Thrombocytopenia and Other Associations

Thrombocytopenia is a frequent finding in patients with the lupus anticoagulant or ACA. Patients with SLE or related autoimmune disorders show an increased incidence of thrombocytopenia associated with these antiphospholipid antibodies.[242] Moreover, the incidence of these antibodies is increased (approximately 30%) in patients with idiopathic thrombocytopenic purpura. Other occasional associations with antiphospholipid antibodies include migraine, chorea, transverse myelopathy, and Guillain-Barré syndrome.[206]

Fetal Loss

Another major clinical manifestation associated with the lupus anticoagulant or ACA is fetal loss.[141,157,158,160–164,206,224,230,243] Fetal wastage may occur at any time during pregnancy.[162,163,206] Any patient with a history of recurrent first-trimester abortion, second- or third-trimester intrauterine death, or intrauterine growth retardation should be tested for the lupus anticoagulant and ACA. This syndrome occurs in patients with or without SLE; thrombosis of placental vessels and placental infarction are thought to be the mechanisms by which fetal loss occurs.[161,164,206] The high incidence of thrombotic disease in these patients lends further support to this hypothesis.

Pathophysiologic Mechanism(s) of Thrombosis

The nature of the association between thrombosis and antiphospholipid antibodies such as the lupus anticoagulant and ACA is uncertain. Since many subjects with antiphospholipid antibodies never experience thrombosis, it is not clear whether antiphospholipid antibodies are direct causative factors for thrombosis or represent secondary consequences of thrombosis with no direct pathophysiologic role. A third possibility is that antiphospholipid antibodies are markers for the presence of underlying hypercoagulable states that give rise to both thrombosis and antiphospholipid antibodies. Each of these possibilities is discussed below.

Antiphospholipid Antibodies as Direct Causative Factors for Thrombosis

Antiphospholipid antibodies could directly contribute to thrombosis by altering platelet activity, procoagulant or anticoagulant pathways, and/or vascular endothelial function. Several considerations support a possible role for platelet activation in the pathogenesis of antiphospholipid antibody-associated thrombosis. First, many subjects with antiphospholipid antibody-associated thrombosis have some degree of thrombocytopenia,[143,145,223,224] presumably immune in origin. Second, there is an association between antiphospholipid antibodies and antiplatelet antibodies.[242,243] Indeed, antiphospholipid antibodies may directly cross-react with platelets.[244,245] The third consideration is the occurrence of arterial as well as venous thrombotic episodes. Platelet activation is thought to play a role in the pathogenesis of arterial thrombotic disease, whereas other causes of increased thrombotic risk, such as deficiencies of antithrombin III, protein C, or protein S, predispose primarily to increased venous thrombotic risk. A recent study demonstrated increased levels of a urinary metabolite of thromboxane A_2 in patients with phospholipid antibodies.[246] By contrast, another study showed that although phospholipid antibodies could bind to circulating platelets, no evidence of measurable platelet activation was found.[244] Fourth, serum of purified IgG from subjects with antiphospholipid antibodies inhibits the release of the platelet inhibitor, prostacyclin, from vascular segments or cultured vascular endothelial cells.[247–250] This finding suggests that in some subjects with antiphospholipid antibodies, impaired prostacyclin release might lead to excessive platelet activity, resulting in thrombosis. Platelets from subjects with antiphospholipid antibody-associated thrombosis are more resistant to in vitro inhibition by the inhibitory prostaglandin, PGE_1, than are normal platelets. However, except for one study,[251] the correlation between in vitro inhibition of prostacyclin release and thrombosis in subjects with antiphospholipid antibodies has been poor.[248,250]

Several abnormalities of natural anticoagulant pathways have also been reported in subjects with antiphospholipid antibody-associated thrombosis. Serum and purified IgG impair activation of protein C by thrombin complexed to the endothelial cofactor, thrombomodulin,[252,253] and impair the phospholipid-dependent anticoagulant action of activated protein C and its cofactor, protein S.[254–256] Reduced plasma levels of free protein S are observed in subjects with antiphospholipid antibody-associated thrombosis.[240,247,257] However, a close correlation between abnormalities of natural anticoagulant mechanisms and thrombosis in subjects with antiphospholipid antibodies has not been demonstrated.

The recent finding that ACAs are directed against a complex phospholipid and β_2-GPI[182,183] suggests that possibly the antihemostatic effect is due to inhibition of β_2-GPI function. Although patients with severe β_2-GPI deficiency have not been shown to have thromboembolic problems,[258] the presence of anti-β_2-GPI antibodies are associated with lupus anticoagulant activity, ACAs, and thromboembolic complications in patients with SLE.[259]

Impaired fibrinolysis may contribute to thrombosis in subjects with antiphospholipid antibodies.[260,261] However, active SLE[261,262] is independently associated with impaired fibrinolysis.[263] More recent studies of subjects with antiphospholipid antibody-associated thrombosis without SLE have failed to document either impaired fibrinolysis in vivo[264] or any effect of plasma containing antiphospholipid antibodies on in vitro endothelial secretion of either tissue plasminogen activator or plasminogen activator inhibitor-1.[265]

Antibodies against endothelial cells have been reported in some subjects with antiphospholipid antibody-associated thrombosis.[266] These antibodies could conceivably cause thrombosis by directly damaging endothelial cells; by impairing endothelial, antiplatelet, and/or anticoagulant activities; or by bringing about procoagulant changes in endothelial function such as expression of tissue factor.[267,268] Antiphospholipid antibody-containing sera from patients with SLE and thrombosis induced a small but significant increase of endothelial tissue factor activity. When added in combination with a low dose of tumor necrosis factor, a synergistic enhancement of tissue factor activity was found.[268] In addition, these antiphospholipid antibody-containing sera lead to enhanced thrombosis formation in an in vitro thrombosis model. By contrast, non-antiphospholipid antibody-containing sera from patients with SLE did not generate tissue factor activity, nor did the sera produce enhanced thrombus formation.

Antiphospholipid Antibodies as a Secondary Consequence of Thrombosis

Antiphospholipid antibodies are directed against procoagulant anionic phospholipids, which are normally not exposed in the outer membrane leaflet of unactivated platelets and other blood cells, but rather are sequestered in the inner or cytoplasmic leaflet.[269] Conceivably, antiphospholipid antibodies in some subjects with thrombosis arise as an immune response to increased exposure of normally hidden procoagulant anionic phospholipids. Some support for this hypothesis is provided by the finding of antiphospholipid antibodies in subjects with sickle cell anemia, who have abnormal exposure of anionic phospholipids in the external leaflet of the red blood cell membrane as a result of sickling.[270] It is also conceivable that antiphospholipid antibodies that originally arise as a secondary

---

THERAPY FOR PATIENTS WITH THE LUPUS ANTICOAGULANT AND/OR AN INCREASED LEVEL OF ANTICARDIOLIPIN ANTIBODIES

The lupus anticoagulant persists in most untreated adults. Often it disappears spontaneously when it occurs in children in whom an anticoagulant develops after a viral infection, and it may be transient in adult patients without SLE, thromboembolic disorders, or fetal loss.

When the lupus anticoagulant or increased level of ACAs are found in patients with underlying autoimmune disease, treatment of the underlying disease with immunosuppressive therapy frequently results in reduction or disappearance of the antibody. When the lupus anticoagulant is found in association with severe prothrombin deficiency or severe thrombocytopenia ($<20,000/mm^3$), treatment with adrenal corticosteroids is indicated, beginning with a dose of 60–80 mg of prednisone. However, when the lupus anticoagulant or increased level of ACAs is discovered as an isolated finding and not associated with thrombosis or fetal loss, treatment is not indicated.

Therapy for thrombosis associated with the lupus anticoagulant or ACAs should be guided by the knowledge that recurrence is common. Interestingly, the site of the first event (arterial or venous) tends to predict the site of subsequent events. It is recommended that patients with venous thrombosis receive long-term anticoagulation with warfarin at a sufficient dose to maintain an INR of 2.0–3.0. Because of the efficacy of warfarin therapy in preventing recurrence of venous thrombosis, the use of corticosteroids and other immunosuppressive agents to suppress antibody production in the absence of autoimmune disease is not recommended.

In contrast to venous thrombosis, treatment for arterial thrombosis is unknown. Although there are few reports of the efficacy of antithrombotic treatment in these patients, current evidence strongly suggests that intermediate- to high-intensity warfarin therapy (INR = 3.0–3.5) is useful in patients with arterial thrombosis.

A pregnant patient with or without SLE with the lupus anticoagulant and/or ACAs associated with a history of recurrent fetal wastage should be treated either with an adjusted dose of heparin or with prednisone and aspirin.

The average dose of subcutaneous heparin is 12,000 U SC bid. In the presence of a prolonged PTT due to a lupus anticardiolipin, there is no standard method of measuring the heparin effect on the PTT 6 hours after injection. However, several options are available:

1. The preferred method is to use a specific heparin assay.
2. Add the same concentration of phospholipid that corrected the patient's PTT so that the PTT is prolonged 1.5–2.0 times the patient's control values with high concentration of phospholipid.
3. Use a partial thromboplastin that is little affected by the lupus anticoagulant and prolong the PTT to 1.5–2.0 times the patient's control value.

If the prednisone and aspirin regimen is to be used, the starting dose of prednisone should be 40 mg/day for 4 weeks, tapering the dose by 10 mg/day every 4 weeks, to a final maintenance dose of 5 mg/day. Throughout pregnancy, 80 mg of aspirin (1 baby aspirin) should be given daily.

For the patient who becomes pregnant and who has not had a prior thromboembolic event, no treatment is indicated. If the patient has suffered only one fetal loss, particularly in the second and third trimester, with no evidence of placental infarction, the patient should be treated with heparin or prednisone and aspirin as noted above. If the patient shows the persistent presence of ACA or the lupus anticardiolipin, or both, but has not suffered any clinical problems, and requires a major surgical procedure, prophylactic heparin and intermittent pneumatic compression should be used.

For the patient who presents with the catastrophic antiphospholipid syndrome, the favored regimen consists of aggressive therapy with daily plasmapheresis, heparin anticoagulation, pulse high-dose medrol 2 g/day IV × 3 days, and cyclophosphamide 750 mg/m² on day 1.

consequence of thrombosis may then induce abnormalities of hemostasis.

Therapy for Patients with the Lupus Anticoagulant

The lupus anticoagulant usually persists in the untreated adult patient. However, it frequently disappears spontaneously when it occurs in children in whom the anticoagulant develops after a viral infection and may be transient in adult patients without SLE, thromboembolic disorders, or fetal loss.

When either the lupus anticoagulant or ACA, or both, is found in patients with underlying autoimmune disease, treatment of the underlying disease with immunosuppressive therapy frequently results in reduction or disappearance of the antibody.[180,189,222,271] When the anticoagulant is found in association with severe prothrombin deficiency or severe thrombocytopenia ($<20,000/mm^3$), treatment with adrenal corticosteroids is indicated. However, when the lupus anticoagulant and/or ACA is discovered as an isolated finding not associated with thrombosis or fetal loss, treatment is not indicated.

Therapy for thrombosis associated with the lupus anticoagulant or ACA should be guided by the knowledge that recurrence is common.[241] Venous recurrence usually occurs in patients who have an initial venous event, whereas arterial recurrences occur in patients who sustain an initial arterial event.[241] Therefore, it is recommended that patients with venous thrombosis receive long-term anticoagulation with oral anticoagulants. Because of the efficacy of warfarin therapy in preventing recurrence of venous thrombosis, the use of corticosteroids and other immunosuppressive agents to suppress antibody production in the absence of autoimmune disease is not recommended.

In contrast to venous thrombosis, the optimal treatment for arterial thrombosis is unknown. Despite few reports of the efficacy of antithrombotic treatment in these patients, a recent report by Rosove et al.[241] strongly suggests that intermediate- to high-intensity warfarin therapy (International Normalized Ratio [INR] = 3.0–3.5) is useful in patients with arterial thrombosis. Whether venous events require the same degree of anticoagulation is unresolved, but low to intermediate warfarin prophylaxis in these patients is favored (INR = 2–3). There is little evidence that either low-intensity warfarin (INR = 1–1.9) or aspirin alone is efficacious in preventing thrombotic events.[241]

A pregnant patient with or without SLE with the lupus anticoagulant or ACA associated with a history of recurrent fetal wastage should be treated. However, the precise regimen to be followed has not been established. Lubbe et al.[272] described a successful pregnancy outcome in a patient with the lupus anticoagulant and fetal wastage who was treated with prednisone and low-dose aspirin. Subsequently, the same regimen led to successful pregnancy outcomes in 10 of 16 pregnancies in 12 patients, some of whom had lupus.[273] Other investigators, using a similar regimen in patients without lupus, also reported a decrease in fetal wastage in a significant number of patients.[245,271] However, long-term high-dose corticosteroids during pregnancy may be associated with significant side effects. However, in a recent study,[271] prednisone and low-dose aspirin given to 11 patients with recurrent fetal wastage (32 previous fetal losses and 5 live-born babies) resulted in 100% live-born babies (12 pregnancies and 12 live-born babies), and no significant adverse effects to either mother or babies. The prednisone regimen consisted of a starting dose of 40 mg/day for 4 weeks, with the dose tapered by 10 mg/day every 4 weeks to a final maintenance dose of 5 mg/day. The levels of ACA decreased in the great majority of patients.

Wallenberg and Rotmans[274] used low-dose aspirin and dipyridamole in 37 patients with obstetric histories similar to those

with antiphospholipid antibodies, with a 93% success rate. Unfortunately, these patients were not systematically examined for the presence of antiphospholipid antibodies. Similarly, Elder et al.[275] reported similar success using low-dose aspirin alone in 42 patients of whom 16 had SLE (13 with antiphospholipid antibodies). However, Lockshin et al.[276] have cast significant doubt regarding the efficacy of aspirin with or without corticosteroids in high-risk patients with high-titer ACAs. In 11 pregnancies receiving corticosteroids and low-dose aspirin, there were 9 fetal losses, whereas in 10 pregnancies receiving aspirin alone or no therapy there were 5 fetal losses. Rosove et al.[277] reported 14 of 15 successful pregnancy outcomes in 14 patients (5 with lupus), using adjusted full-dose heparin therapy throughout pregnancy. None of the patients was treated with aspirin, and only 1 patient received a short course of corticosteroids for a lupus flare.

Thus, different therapeutic regimens in uncontrolled trials have resulted in a decrease in fetal wastage. The most efficacious regimen appears to be either adjusted-dose heparin or prednisone and low-dose aspirin with a prednisone-tapering regimen as described by Silveira et al.[271] However, a randomized prospective trial in such patients is necessary to determine the optimum therapeutic regimen.[278]

REFERENCES

1. Green D, Lechner K: A survey of 215 non-hemophilic patients with inhibitors to factor VIII. Thromb Hemost 45:200, 1981
2. Lottenberg R, Kentro TB. Kitchens CB: Acquired hemophilia. A natural history study of 16 patients with factor VIII inhibitors receiving little or no therapy. Arch Intern Med 147:1077, 1987
3. Margolius A, Jackson DP, Ratnoff OD: Circulating anticoagulants: a study of 40 cases and a review of the literature. Medicine 40:145, 1961
4. Shapiro SS, Hultin M: Acquired inhibitors to the blood coagulation factors. Semin Thromb Hemost 1:336, 1975
5. Robboy SJ, Lewis EJ, Schur PH, Colman RW: Circulating anticoagulants to factor VIII. Am J Med 49:742, 1970
6. Feinstein DI, Rapaport S: Acquired inhibitors of blood coagulation. Prog Hemost Thromb 1:75, 1972
7. Voke J, Letsky E: Pregnancy and antibody to factor VIII. J Clin Pathol 30:928, 1977
8. Coller BS, Hultin MB, Hoyer LW et al: Normal pregnancy in a patient with a prior postpartum factor VIII inhibitor: with observations on pathogenesis and prognosis. Blood 58:619, 1981
9. Shapiro SS, Carroll KS: Acquired factor VIII antibodies: further immunologic and electrophoretic studies. Science 160:786, 1968
10. Anderson BR, Terry WD: Gamma G4-globulin antibody causing inhibition of clotting factor VIII. Nature 217:174, 1968
11. Feinstein DI, Rapaport SI, Chong MMY: Immunologic characterization of 12 factor VIII inhibitors. Blood 34:85, 1969
12. Poon MC, Wine AC, Ratnoff OD, Bernier GM: Heterogeneity of human circulating anticoagulants against antihemophilic factor (factor VIII). Blood 46:409, 1975
13. Hultin MB, London FS, Shapiro SS, Yount W: Heterogeneity of factor VIII antibodies: further immunochemical and biologic studies. Blood 49:807, 1977
14. Kavanaugh ML, Wood CN, Davidson JF: The immunological characterization of human antibodies to factor VIII isolated by immunoaffinity chromatography. Thromb Haemost 45:60, 1981
15. Allain JP, Gaillandre A, Lee H: Immunochemical characterization of antibodies to factor VIII in hemophilic and non-hemophilic patients. J Lab Clin Med 97:791, 1981
16. Kernoff PB, Thomas ND, Lilley PA et al: Clinical experiences with polyelectrolyte-fractionated porcine factor VIII concentrate in the treatment of hemophiliacs with antibodies to factor VIII. Blood 63:31, 1984
17. Shapiro SS: The immunologic character of acquired inhibitors of antihemophilic globulin (factor VIII) and the kinetics of their interaction with factor VIII. J Clin Invest 46:147, 1967
18. Biggs R, Bidwell E: A method for the study of antihemophilic globulin inhibitors with reference to six cases. Br J Haematol 5:379, 1959
19. Leitner A, Bidwell E, Dike GWR: An antihemophilic globulin (factor VIII) inhibitor: purification, characterization and reaction kinetics. Br J Haematol 9:245, 1963
20. Biggs R, Austen DEB, Denson DWG et al: The mode of action of antibodies

which destroy factor VIII. I. Antibodies which have second-order concentration graphs. Br J Haematol 23:125, 1972

21. Biggs R, Austen DEG, Denson DWE et al: The mode of action of antibodies which destroy factor VIII. II. Antibodies which give complex concentration graphs. Br J Haematol 23:137, 1972

22. Allain JP, Frommell D: Antibodies to factor VIII: variations in stability of antigen-antibody complexes in hemophilia A. Blood 42:437, 1973

23. Allain JP, Frommell D: Antibodies to factor VIII: specificity and kinetics of iso- and hetero-antibodies in hemophilia A. Blood 44:313, 1974

24. Rizza CR, Biggs R: The treatment of patients who have factor VIII antibodies. Br J Haematol 24:65, 1973

25. Gawryl MS, Hoyer LW: Inactivation of factor VIII procoagulant activity by two different types of human antibodies. Blood 60:1103, 1982

26. Herbst KD, Rapaport SI, Kenoyer DG et al: Syndrome of an acquired inhibitor of factor VIII responsive to cyclophosphamide and prednisone. Ann Intern Med 95:575, 1981

27. Fulcher CA, deGraaf Mahoney S, Roberts JR et al: Localization of human factor FVIII inhibitor epitopes to two polypeptide fragments. Proc Natl Acad Sci USA 82:7728, 1985

28. Fulcher CA, Lechner K, deGraaf Mahoney S: Immunoblot analysis shows changes in factor VIII inhibitor chain specificity in factor VIII inhibitor patients over time. Blood 72:1348, 1988

29. Fulcher CA, deGraaf Mahoney S, Zimmerman TS: FVIII inhibitor IgG subclass and FVIII polypeptide specificity determined by immunoblotting. Blood 69:1475, 1987

30. Scandella D, Timmons L, Mattingly M et al: A soluble recombinant factor VIII fragment containing the A2 domain binds to some human anti-factor VIII antibodies that are not detected by immunoblotting. Thromb Haemost 67:665, 1992

31. Nilsson IM, Berntorp E, Zettervall O, Dahlback B: Noncoagulation Inhibitory factor VIII antibodies after induction of tolerance to factor VIII in hemophilia A patients. Blood 75:378, 1990

32. Lossing T, Kasper CK, Feinstein DI: Detection of factor VIII inhibitors with the activated partial thromboplastin time. Blood 49:493, 1977

33. Ewing NP, Kasper CK: In vitro detection of mild inhibitors to factor VIII in hemophilia. Am J Clin Pathol 77:749, 1982

34. Kasper CK, Aledort LM, Counts RB et al: A more uniform mesurement of factor VIII inhibitors. Thromb Haemost 34:869, 1975

35. Austen DE, Lechner K, Rizza CR, Rhymes IL: A comparison of the Bethesda and New Oxford methods of a factor VIII antibody assay. Thromb Haemost 47:72, 1982

36. Morrison AE, Ludlam CA, Kessler C: Use of porcine factor VIII in the treatment of patients with acquired hemophilia. Blood 81:1513, 1993

37. Kasper CK: The therapy of factor VIII inhibitors. Prog Hemost Thromb 9:57, 1989

38. Nilsson IM, Jonsson S, Sundqvist SB et al: A procedure for removing high titer antibodies by extracorporeal protein A-sepharose adsorption in hemophilia. Blood 58:38, 1981

39. Uehlinger J, Button GR, McCarthy J et al: Immunoadsorption for coagulation factor inhibitors. Transfusion 31:265, 1991

40. Green D, Tuite GF: Declining platelet counts and platelet aggregation during porcine factor VIII:C infusions. Am J Med 86:222, 1989

41. Roberts HR: Hemophiliacs with inhibitors, therapeutic options. N Engl J Med 305:757, 1981

42. Lusher JM, Shapiro SS, Palascak et al: Efficacy of prothrombin-complex concentrates in hemophiliacs with antibodies to factor VIII: a multicenter therapeutic trial. N Engl J Med 303:421, 1980

43. Sjamsoedin LJM, Heijnen L, Mauser-Bunschoten EP et al: The effect of activated prothrombin-complex concentrate (FEIBA) on joint and muscle bleeding in patients with hemophilia A and antibodies to factor VIII: a double blind clinical trial. N Engl J Med 305:717, 1981

44. Lusher JM, Blatt PM, Penner JA et al: Autoplex versus Proplex: a controlled, double-blind study of effectiveness in acute hemarthrosis in hemophiliacs with inhibitors to factor VIII. Blood 62:1135, 1983

45. Hilgartner MW, Knatterud GL, the FEIBA study group: The use of factor VIII inhibitor by-passing activity (FEIBA IMMUNO) product for treatment of bleeding episodes in hemophiliacs with inhibitors. Blood 61:35, 1983

46. Hultin MB: Studies of factor IX concentrate therapy in hemophilia. Blood 62:677, 1983

47. Hedner U, Kisiel W: Use of human factor VIIa in the treatment of two hemophilia A patients with high titer inhibitors. J Clin Invest 71:1836, 1983

48. Macik BG, Hohneker J, Griffin A, Roberts HR: Use of recombinant FVIIa for treatment of a hemophilic patient with a high titer inhibitor, abstracted. Blood, suppl. 72:302a, 1988

49. Spero JA, Lewis JH, Hasiba JH: Corticosteroid therapy for acquired factor VIII:C inhibitors. Br J Haematol 48:635, 1981

50. Green D: Suppression of an antibody to factor VIII by a combination of factor VIII and cyclophosphamide. Blood 37:381, 1971

51. Lian EC-Y, Larcada AF, Chiu Ay-Z: Combination immunosuppressive therapy after factor VIII infusion for acquired factor VIII inhibitor. Ann Intern Med 110:774, 1989

52. Green D, Schuette PT, Wallace WH: Factor VIII antibodies in rheumatoid arthritis: effect of cyclophosphamide. Arch Intern Med 140:1232, 1980

53. Green D, Kwaan HC: An acquired factor VIII inhibitor responsive to high-dose gamma globulin. Thromb Haemost 58:1005, 1987

54. Gianelli-Borradori A, Hirt A, Luthy A et al: Haemophilia due to factor VIII inhibitors in a patient suffering from an autoimmune disease: treatment with intravenous immunoglobulin. Blut 48:303, 1984

55. Zimmerman R, Kommerell B, Harenber J et al: Intravenous IgG for patients with spontaneous inhibitor to factor VIII. Lancet 1:273, 1985

56. Carreras LO, Perez GN, Xavier DL et al: Autoimmune factor VIII inhibitor responsive to gamma globulin without in vitro neutralization. Thromb Haemost 60:343, 1988

57. Sultan Y, Maisonneuve P, Kazatchkine MD, Nydegger UE: Anti-idiotypic suppression of autoantibodies of factor VIII (anti-haemophilic factor) by high-dose intravenous gamma globulin. Lancet 2:765, 1984

58. Tiarks C, Pechet L, Humphreys RE: Development of anti-idiotypic antibodies in a patient with a factor VIII autoantibody. Am J Hematol 32:217, 1989

59. Rossi F, Dietrich FG, Kazatchkine MD: Anti-idiotypic suppression of autoantibodies with normal polyspecific immunoglobulins. Res Monogr Immunol 140:19, 1989

60. Frommel D: Anti-idiotypic suppression of antibodies to factor VIIIc. Lancet 2:1210, 1984

61. Moffat EH, Furlong RA, Dannatt AHG et al: Anti-idiotypes to factor VIII antibodies and their possible role in the pathogenesis and treatment of factor VIII inhibitors. Br J Haematol 71:85, 1989

62. de la Fuente B, Panek S, Hoyer LW: The effect of I-deamino 8D-arginine vasopressin (DDAVP) in a nonhaemophilic patient with an acquired type II factor VIII inhibitor. Br J Haematol 59:127, 1985

63. Ingram GIC, Kingston PJ, Leslie J, Bowie EJW: Four cases of acquired von Willebrand's syndrome. Br J Haematol 21:189, 1971

64. Ingram GIC, Prentice CRM, Forbes CD, Leslie J: Low factor VIII-like antigen in acquired von Willebrand's syndrome and response to treatment. Br J Haematol 25:137, 1973

65. Handin RI, Martin V, Moloney WC: Antibody-induced von Willebrand's disease; a newly defined inhibitor syndrome. Blood 48:393, 1976

66. Stableforth P, Tamagnin GL, Dormandy KM: Acquired von Willebrand syndrome with inhibitors both to factor VIII clotting activity and ristocetin-induced platelet aggregation. Br J Haematol 33:565, 1976

67. Joist JH, Kowan JF, Zimmerman TS: Acquired von Willebrand's disease: evidence for quantitative and qualitative factor VIII disorder. N Engl J Med 298:988, 1978

68. McGrath KM, Johnson CA, Stuart JI: Acquired von Willebrand's disease associated with an inhibitor to factor VIII antigen and gastrointestinal telangectasia. Am J Med 67:693, 1979

69. Brody JL, Harder ME, Rossman RE: A hemorrhagic syndrome in Waldenström's macroglobulinemia secondary to immunoadsorption of factor VIII. N Engl J Med 300:408, 1979

70. Manucci PM, Lombardi R, Bader R et al: Studies of the pathophysiology of acquired von Willebrand's disease in seven patients with lymphoproliferative disorders or benign monoclonal gammapathies. Blood 64:614, 1984

71. Fricke WA, Brinkous KM, Garris JB, Roberts HR: Comparison of inhibitory and binding characteristics of an antibody causing acquired von Willebrand syndrome: an assay for von Willebrand factor binding by antibody. Blood 66:562, 1985

72. Macik BG, Gabriel DA, White II GC et al: The use of high-dose intravenous gamma-globulin in acquired von Willebrand syndrome. Arch Pathol Lab Med 112:143, 1988

73. Goudemand J, Samor B, Caron C et al: Acquired type II von Willebrand's disease: demonstration of a complexed inhibitor of the von Willebrand factor-platelet interaction and response to treatment. Br J Haematol 68:227, 1988

74. Ball J, Malia RG, Greaves M, Preston FE: Demonstration of abnormal factor VIII multimers in acquired von Willebrand's disease associated with a circulating inhibitor. Br J Haematol 65:95, 1987

75. Feinstein DI: Acquired inhibitors of factor V. Thromb Haemost 39:663, 1978

76. Grace CS, Wolf P: A high-titer circulating inhibitor of human factor V: clinical, biochemical and immunological features and its treatment by plasmapheresis. Thromb Haemost 34:322, 1975

77. Bryning K, Leslie J: Factor V inhibitor and bullous pemphigoid. BMJ 6088:677, 1977

78. Coots MC, Muhleman F, Glueck HI: Hemorrhagic death associated with a high titer factor V inhibitor. Am J Hematol 4:193, 1978
79. Lane TA, Shapiro SS, Burka ER: Factor V antibody and disseminated intravascular coagulation. Ann Intern Med 89:182, 1978
80. Chediak J, Ashenhurst JB, Garlick I, Desser RK: Successful management of bleeding in a patient with factor V inhibitor by platelet transfusion. Blood 56:835, 1980
81. Feinstein DI, Rapaport SI, McGehee WG, Patch MJ: Factor V anticoagulants: clinical, biochemical and immunological observations. J Clin Invest 49:1578, 1970
82. Onoura CA, Lindenbaum J, Nossel HJ: Massive hemorrhage associated with circulating antibodies to factor V. Am J Med Sci 265:407, 1973
83. Chiu HC, Rao AK, Beckett C, Coleman RW: Immune complexes containing factor V in patient with an acquired neutralizing antibody. Blood 65:810, 1985
84. Vickars LM, Coupland RW, Naiman SC: The response of an acquired factor V inhibitor to activated factor IX concentrate. Transfusion 25:51, 1985
85. Nesheim ME, Nichols WL, Cole TK et al: Isolation and study of an acquired inhibitor of human coagulation factor V. J Clin Invest 77:405, 1986
86. Miletich JP, Majerus DW, Majerus PW: Patients with congenital factor V deficiency have decreased factor Xa binding sites on their platelets. J Clin Invest 62:824, 1978
87. Lawson JH, Pennell BJ, Olson JD, Mann KG: Isolation and characterization of an acquired antithrombin antibody. Blood 76:2249, 1990
88. Jehnder JL, Leung LLK: Development of antibodies to thrombin and factor V with recurrent bleeding in a patient exposed to topical bovine thrombin. Blood 76:2011, 1990
89. Bajaj SP, Rapaport SI, Barclay S, Herbst KD: Acquired hypoprothrombinemia due to non-neutralizing antibodies to prothrombin: mechanism and management. Blood 65:1538, 1985
90. Hawiger J, Hariclei Z, Struzik T: On the immunologic nature of antithrombin in the course of lupus erythematosus disseminatus. Acta Med Pol 5:53, 1964
91. Scully MF, Ellis V, Kakkar VV et al: An acquired coagulation inhibitor to factor II. Br J Haematol 50:655, 1982
92. Barthels M, Heimburger N: Acquired thrombin inhibitor in a patient with liver cirrhosis. Hemostasis 15:395, 1985
93. Stricker RB, Lane PK, Leffert JD et al: Development of antithrombin antibodies following surgery in patients with prosthetic cardiac valves. Blood 4:1375, 1988
94. Campbell E, Sanal S, Mattson J et al: Factor VII inhibitor. Am J Med 68:962, 1980
95. Delmer A, Horellou MH, Andreu G et al: Life threatening intracranial bleeding associated with the presence of an antifactor VII autoantibody. Blood 74:229, 1989
96. Weisdorf D, Hasegawa D, Fair DS: Acquired factor VII deficiency associated with aplastic anaemia: correction with bone marrow transplantation. Br J Haematol 71:409, 1989
97. Largo R, Sigg P, von Felten A, Straub PW: Acquired factor-IX inhibitor in a nonhaemophilic patient with autoimmune disease. Br J Haematol 26:129, 1974
98. Miller K, Neeley JE, Drivit W et al: Spontaneously acquired factor IX inhibitor in a nonhemophiliac child. J Pediatr 93:232, 1978
99. Lechner K: Factor IX inhibitors: report of two cases and a study of the biological, chemical and immunological properties of the inhibitors. Thromb Haemost 25:447, 1971
100. Pike IM, Yount WJ, Puritz EM, Roberts HR: Immunochemical characterization of a monoclonal gamma G_4 lambda human antibody to factor IX. Blood 50:11, 1977
101. Reisner MM, Roberts HR, Krumholz S, Young WJ: Immunochemical characterization of a polyclonal human antibody to factor IX. Blood 50:11, 1977
102. Lankiewicz MW, Bell WR: A unique circulating inhibitor with specificity for coagulation factor X. Am J Med 93:343, 1992
103. Josephson AM, Lisker R: Demonstration of a circulating anticoagulant in plasma thromboplastin antecedent deficiency. J Clin Invest 37:148, 1958
104. Castro O, Farber LW, Clyne LP: Circulating anticoagulants against factors IX and XI in systemic lupus erythematosus. Ann Intern Med 77:543, 1972
105. Krieger H, Breckenridge RT: Circulating anticoagulant interfering with the action of factor XIa in lupus. Blood 42:1002, 1973
106. Zucker S, Zarrabi MH, Roman GS, Miller F: IgM inhibitors of the contact activation phase of coagulation in chlorpromazine-treated patients. Br J Haematol 40:447, 1978
107. Reece EA, Clyne LP, Romero R, Hobbins JC: Spontaneous factor XI inhibitors: seven additional cases and a review of the literature. Arch Intern Med 144:525, 1984
108. Poon MC, Saito H, Koopman WJ: A unique precipitating autoantibody against plasma thromboplastin antecedent associated with multiple apparent plasma clotting factor deficiences in a patient with systemic lupus erythematosus. Blood 63:1309, 1984
109. Goldsmith GH Jr, Silverman P: Inhibitors of plasma thromboplastin antecedent (factor XI): studies on mechanism of inhibition. J Lab Clin Med 106:279, 1985
110. Canoso RT, Hutton D, Deykin D: A chlorpromazine-induced inhibitor of blood coagulation. Am J Hematol 2:183, 1977
111. De Vries A, Rosenberg T, Kochwa S, Boss J: Precipitating antifibrinogen antibody appearing after fibrinogen infusions in a patient with congenital afibrinogenemia. Am J Med 30:486, 1961
112. Marciniak E, Greenwood MF: Acquired coagulation inhibitor delaying fibrinopeptide release. Blood 53:81, 1979
113. Galanakis DK, Ginzler EM, Fikrig SM: Monoclonal IgG anticoagulants delaying fibrin aggregation in two patients with systemic lupus erythematosus (SLE). Blood 52:1037, 1978
114. Hoots WK, Carrell NA, Wagner RH et al: A naturally occurring antibody that inhibits fibrin polymerization. N Engl J Med 304:857, 1981
115. Ghosh S, McEvoy P, McVerry BA: Idiopathic autoantibody that inhibits fibrin monomer polymerization. Br J Haematol 53:65, 1983
116. Lackner H: Hemostatic abnormalities associated with dysproteinemias. Semin Hematol 10:125, 1973
117. Cohen I, Amier J, Ben-Shaul Y et al: Plasma cell myeloma associated with an unusual myeloma protein causing impairment of fibrin aggregation and platelet function in a patient with multiple malignancies. Am J Med 48:766, 1970
118. Coleman M, Viglian EM, Weksler ME, Nachman RL: Inhibition of fibrin polymerization by lambda myeloma globulins. Blood 39:210, 1972
119. Lorand L, Jacobson A, Bruner-Lorand J: A pathological inhibitor of fibrin cross-linking. J Clin Invest 47:268, 1968
120. Lorand L, Urayama T, De Kiewiet JWC, Nossel HL: Diagnostic and genetic studies on fibrin-stabilizing factor with a new assay based on amine incorporation. J Clin Invest 48:1054, 1969
121. McDevitt NB, McDonagh J, Taylor HL, Roberts HR: An acquired inhibitor to factor XIII. Arch Intern Med 130:772, 1972
122. Lorand L, Maldonado N, Fradera J et al: Haemorrhagic syndrome of autoimmune origin with a specific inhibitor against fibrin stabilizing factor (factor XIII). Br J Haematol 23:17, 1972
123. Graham JE, Yount WJ, Roberts HR: Immunochemical characterization of a human antibody to factor XIII. Blood 41:661, 1973
124. Otis PT, Feinstein DI, Rapaport SI, Patch MJ: An acquired inhibitor of fibrin stabilization. Blood 44:771, 1974
125. Lopaciuk S, Bykowska K, McDonagh JM et al: Difference between type 1 autoimmune inhibitors of fibrin stabilization in two patients with severe hemorrhagic disorder. J Clin Invest 61:1196, 1978
126. Rosenberg RD, Colman RW, Lorand L: A new haemorrhagic disorder with defective fibrin stabilization and cryofibrinogenaemia. Br J Haematol 26:269, 1974
127. Lorand L, Velasco PT, Rinne JR et al: Autoimmune antibody (IgG Kansas) against the fibrin stabilizing factor (factor XIII) system. Proc Natl Acad Sci USA 1:232, 1985
128. Nakamura S, Kato A, Sakata Y et al: Bleeding caused by IgG inhibitor to factor XIII treated successfully with cyclophosphamide. Br J Haematol 68:313, 1988
129. Fukue H, Anderson K, McPhedran P et al: A unique factor XIII inhibitor to a fibrin-binding site on factor XIIIa. Blood 79:65, 1992
130. Khoory MS, Nesheim ME, Bowie EJW, Mann KJ: Circulating heparan sulfate proteoglycan anticoagulant from a patient with a plasma cell disorder. J Clin Invest 65:666, 1980
131. Palmer RN, Rick ME, Rick PD et al: Circulating heparan sulfate anticoagulant in a patient with a fatal bleeding disorder. N Engl J Med 310:1696, 1984
132. Chapman GS, George CB, Danley DL: Heparin-like anticoagulant associated with plasma cell myeloma. Am J Clin Pathol 83:764, 1985
133. Horne MK, Stein CA, Renato V et al: Circulating glycosaminoglycan anticoagulants associated with suramin treatment. Blood 71:273, 1988
134. Kaufman PA, Gockerman JP, Greenberg CS: Production of a novel anticoagulant by neoplastic plasma cells: report of a case and review of the literature. Am J Med 86:612, 1989
135. Tefferi A, Owen BA, Nichols WL et al: Isolation of a heparin-like anticoagulant from the plasma of a patient with metastatic bladder carcinoma. Blood 74:252, 1989
136. Tefferi A, Nichols WL, Bowie EJW: Circulating heparin-like anticoagulants: report of five consecutive cases and a review. Am J Med 88:184, 1990
137. Shapiro SS, Thiagarajan P: Lupus anticoagulants. Prog Hemost Thromb 6:263, 1982
138. Simone JV, Cornet JA, Abildgaard CF: Acquired von Willebrand's syndrome in systemic lupus erythematosus. Blood 31:803, 1968

139. Robbey SJ, Lewis EJ, Schur PH, Colman RW: Circulating anticoagulants to factor VIII. Am J Med 49:575, 1957

140. Schleider MA, Nachman RL, Jaffe EA, Coleman M: A clinical study of the lupus anticoagulant. Blood 48:499, 1976

141. Boey ML, Colaco CB, Gharavi AE et al: Thrombosis in systemic lupus erythematosus: striking association with the presence of circulating lupus anticoagulant. Br Med J 287:1021, 1983

142. Calaco CB, Elkin KB: The lupus anticoagulant. Arthritis Rheum 28:67, 1985

143. Mueh JR, Herbst KD, Rapaport SI: Thrombosis in patients with lupus anticoagulant. Ann Intern Med 92:156, 1980

144. Hart RG, Miller VT, Coull BM, Bril V: Cerebral infarction associated with lupus anticoagulants—preliminary report. Stroke 15:114, 1984

145. Gardlund B: The lupus inhibitor in thromboembolism disease and intrauterine death in the absence of systemic lupus. J Intern Med 215:293, 1984

146. Bernstein ML, Salusins M, Bellefle M, Esseltin DW: Thrombotic and hemorrhagic complications in children with the lupus anticoagulant. Am J Dis Child 138:1132, 1984

147. Pomeroy C, Knodell RG, Swaim WR et al: Budd-Chiari syndrome in a patient with the lupus anticoagulant. Gastroenterology 86:158, 1984

148. Glueck HI, Kant KS, Weiss MA et al: Thrombosis in systemic lupus erythematosus. Relation to the presence of circulating anticoagulants. Arch Intern Med 145:1389, 1985

149. Bell WR, Boss GR, Wolfson JS: Circulating anticoagulant in the procainamide-induced lupus syndrome. Arch Intern Med 137:1471, 1977

150. Zarrabi MH, Zucker S, Miller F et al: Immunologic and coagulation disorders in chlorpromazine-treated patients. Ann Intern Med 91:194, 1979

151. Beck DW, Strauss RG, Kisker T, Henriksen RA: An intrinsic coagulation pathway inhibitor in a 3-year-old child. Am J Clin Pathol 71:470, 1979

152. Brodeur GM, O'Neill PJ, Williams JA: Acquired inhibitors of coagulation in nonhemophiliac children. J Pediatr 96:439, 1980

153. Cohen AJ, Philips TM, Kessler CM: Circulatory coagulating inhibitors in the acquired immunodeficiency syndrome. Ann Intern Med 104:175, 1985

154. Bloom EJ, Abrams DI, Rodgers G: Lupus anticoagulant in acquired immunodeficiency syndrome. JAMA 256:491, 1986

155. Cohen AJ, Philips TM, Kessler CM: Circulating coagulation inhibitors in the acquired immunodeficiency syndrome. Ann Intern Med 104:175, 1986

156. Canoso RT, Zon LI, Groopman JE: Anticardiolipin antibodies associated with HTLV-III infection. Br J Haematol 65:495, 1987

157. Feinstein D: Lupus anticoagulant, anticardiolipin antibodies, fetal loss, and systemic lupus erythematosus. Blood 80:859, 1992

158. Ginsberg JS, Brill-Edwards P, Johnston M et al: Relationship of antiphospholipid antibodies to pregnancy loss in patients with systemic lupus erythematosus: a cross-sectional study. Blood 80:859, 1992

159. Infante-Rivard C, David M, Gauthier R, Rivard GE: Lupus anticoagulants, anticardiolipin antibodies, and fetal loss. N Engl J Med 325:1063, 1991

160. Nilsson IM, Astedt B, Hedner U, Berezin D: Intrauterine death and circulating anticoagulant, "antithromboplastin." J Intern Med 197:153, 1975

161. De Wolf F, Carreras LO, Moerman P et al: Decidual vasculopathy and extensive placental infarction in a patient with repeated thromboembolic accidents, recurrent fetal loss, and a lupus anticoagulant. Am J Obstet Gynecol 142:829, 1982

162. Derue GJ, Englert HJ, Harris EN, Hughes GRV: Fetal loss in systemic lupus erythematosus: association with anticardiolipin antibodies. J Obstet Gynaecol 91:356, 1985

163. Branch WD, Scott JR, Kochenour NK et al: Obstetric complications associated with the lupus anticoagulant. N Engl J Med 313:1322, 1985

164. Lockshin MD, Druzin ML, Goei S et al: Antibody to cardiolipin as a predictor of fetal distress or death in pregnant patients with systemic lupus erythematosus. N Engl J Med 313:152, 1985

165. Regan MG, Lackner H, Karpatkin S: Platelet function and coagulation profile in lupus erythematosus. Studies in 50 patients. Ann Intern Med 81:462, 1974

166. Exner T, Rickard KA, Kronenberg BH: A sensitive test demonstrating lupus anticoagulant and its behavioral patterns. Br J Haematol 40:143, 1978

167. Love PE, Santoro SA: Antiphospholipid antibodies: anticardiolipin and the lupus anticoagulant in systemic lupus erythematosus (SLE) and in non-SLE disorders. Ann Intern Med 112:682, 1990

168. Frick PG: Acquired circulating anticoagulants in systemic "collagen disease": autoimmune thromboplastin deficiency. Blood 10:691, 1955

169. Margolius A Jr, Jackson DP, Ratnoff OD: Circulating anticoagulants: a study of 40 cases and review of the literature. Medicine 40:145, 1961

170. Exner T: Similar mechanisms of lupus anticoagulants. Thromb Haemost 53:15, 1985

171. Exner T: Comparison of two simple tests for the lupus anticoagulant. Am J Clin Pathol 83:215, 1985

172. Bowie EJ, Thompson JH Jr, Pascuzzi CA, Owen CA Jr: Thrombosis in systemic lupus despite circulating anticoagulants. J Lab Clin Med 62:416, 1963

173. Kelsey PR, Stevenson KJ, Poller L: The diagnosis of lupus anticoagulant by the activated partial thromboplastin time—the central role of phosphatidyl serine. Thromb Haemost 52:172, 1984

174. Rosove MH, Ismail M, Koziol BJ et al: Lupus anticoagulants: improved diagnosis with a kaolin clotting time using rabbit brain phospholipid in standard and high concentrations. Blood 68:472, 1986

175. Howard MA, Firkin BG: Investigations of the lupus-like inhibitor by-passing activity of platelets. Thromb Haemost 50:775, 1983

176. Triplett DA, Brandt JT, Kaczor D, Schaeffer J: Laboratory diagnosis of lupus inhibitors: a comparison of the tissue thromboplastin inhibition procedure with a new platelet neutralization procedure. Am J Clin Pathol 79:68, 1983

177. Thiagajaran P, Shapiro SS, De Marco L: Monoclonal immunoglobulin M lambda coagulation inhibitor with phopspholipid specificity. Mechanism of lupus anticoagulant. J Clin Invest 66:397, 1980

178. Pengo V, Thiagarajan P, Shapiro SS, Heine MJ: Immunological specificity and mechanism of action of IgG lupus anticoagulants. Blood 70:69, 1987

179. Galli R, Beguin S, Lindhout T et al: Inhibition of phospholipid and platelet-dependent prothrombinase activity in the plasma of patients with lupus anticoagulants. Br J Haematol 72:549, 1989

180. Laurell AB, Malmquist J: Hypergammaglobulinemia, circulating anticoagulant, and biologic false positive Wassermann reaction: a study in two cases. J Lab Clin Med 49:694, 1957

181. Harris EN, Boey ML, Mackworth-Young CG et al: Anticardiolipin antibodies: detection by radioimmunoassay and association with thrombosis in systemic lupus erythematosus. Lancet 2:211, 1983

182. McNeil HP, Chesterman CN, Krilis SA: Anticardiolipin antibodies and lupus anticoagulants comprise separate antibody subroups with different phospholipid binding characteristics. Br J Haematol 73:506, 1989

183. Exner T, Sahman N, Trudinger B: Separation of anticardiolipin antibodies from lupus anticoagulant on a phospholipid-coated polystyrene column. Biochem Biophys Res Commun 155:1001, 1988

184. McNeil HP, Simpson RJ, Chesterman CN, Krilis SA: Antiphospholipid antibodies are directed against a complex antigen that includes a lipid-binding inhibitor of coagulation: β_2-glycoprotein I (apolipoprotein H). Proc Natl Acad Sci USA 87:4120, 1990

185. Galli M, Comfurius P, Maasen C et al: Anticardiolipin antibodies (ACA) directed not to cardiolipin but to a plasma protein cofactor. Lancet 335:1544, 1990

186. Bevers EM, Galli M, Barbui T et al: Lupus anticoagulant IgG's (LA) are not directed to phospholipid only, but to a complex of lipid-bound human prothrombin. Thromb Haemost 66:629, 1991

187. Edson JR, Vogt JM, Hasegawa DK: Abnormal prothrombin crossed-immunoelectrophoresis in patients with lupus inhibitors. Blood 64:807, 1984

188. Fleck RA, Rapaport SI, Rao LVM: Anti-prothrombin antibodies and the lupus anticoagulant. Blood 72:512, 1988

189. Rapaport SI, Ames SB, Duvall BJ: A plasma coagulation defect in systemic lupus erythematosus arising from hypothrombinemia combined with antiprothrombinase activity. Blood 15:212, 1960

190. Natelson EA, Cyprus GS, Hettig RA: Absent factor II in systemic lupus erythematosus: immunologic studies and response to corticosteroid therapy. Arthritis Rheum 19:79, 1976

191. Lillquist KB, Dyerberg J, Krogh-Jensen M: The absence of factor II in a child with systemic lupus erythematosus. Acta Pediatr Scand 67:533, 1978

192. Bajaj SP, Rapaport SI, Fierer DS et al: A mechanism for the hypoprothrombinemia of the acquired hypoprothrombinemia-lupus anticoagulant syndrome. Blood 61:684, 1983

193. Edson JR, Vogt JM, Hasegawa DK: Abnormal prothrombin crossed-immunoelectrophoreis in patients with lupus inhibitors. Blood 64:807, 1984

194. Mannucci PM, Canciani MT, Mari D, Meucci P: The varied sensitivity of partial thromboplastin and prothrombin time reagents in the demonstration of the lupus-like anticoagulant. Scand J Haematol 22:423, 1979

195. Mohammad SF, Martin BA, Hershgold EJ: The importance of reagents in the laboratory detection of lupus anticoagulants. Thromb Haemost 54:82, 1985

196. Stern W, MacDonald VE: Factors affecting the sensitivity of APTT reagents to lupus inhibitors (LI). Thromb Haemost 54:146, 1985

197. Exner T, Triplett DA, Taberner DA: Comparison of test methods for the lupus anticoagulant: international survey on lupus anticoagulants-I (ISLA-1). Thromb Haematol 64:478, 1990

198. Exner T, Triplett DA, Taberner DA, et al: Guidelines for testing and revised criteria for lupus anticoagulants. Thromb Haemost 65:320, 1991

199. Arnout J, Huybrechts E, Vanrusselt M, Vermylen J: A new lupus anticoagulant neutralization test based on platelet-derived vesicles. Br J Haematol 80:341, 1992

200. Lesperance B, David M, Rauch J et al: Relative sensitivity of different tests in the detection of low titer lupus anticoagulants. Thromb Haemost 60:217, 1988

201. Thiagarajan P, Pengo V, Shapiro SS: The use of the dilute Russell viper venom time for the diagnosis of lupus anticoagulants. Blood 68:869, 1986

202. Alving BM, Baldwin PE, Richards RL, Jackson BJ: The dilute phospholipid APTT: a sensitive assay for verification of lupus anticoagulants. Thromb Haemost 54:709, 1985

203. Alving BM, Barr CF, Johansen LE, Tang DB: Comparison between a one-point dilute phospholipid APTT and the dilute Russell viper venom time for verification of lupus anticoagulants. Thromb Haemost 67:672, 1992

204. Long AA, Ginsberg JA, Brill-Edwards P et al: The relationship of antiphospholipid antibodies to thromboembolic disease in systemic lupus erythematosus: a cross-sectional study. Thromb Haemost 66:520, 1991

205. Exner T, Triplett DA, Taberner DA et al: Guidelines for testing and revised criteria for lupus anticoagulants. Thromb Haemost 65:320, 1991

206. Harris EN, Asherson RA, Hughes GRV: Antiphopholipid antibodies—autoantibodies with a difference. Annu Rev Med 39:261, 1988

207. Asherson RA, Khamashta MA, Gil A et al: Cerebrovascular disease and antiphospholipid antibodies in systemic lupus erythematosus, lupus-like disease, and the primary antiphospholipid syndrome. Am J Med 86:391, 1989

208. Harris EN, Gharavi Ae, Tincani A et al: Affinity purified anti-cardiolipin antibodies. J Clin Lab Immunol 17:155, 1985

209. Harris EN, Gharavi AE, Laizou S et al: Cross-reactivity of antiphospholipid antibodies. J Clin Lab Immunol 16:1, 1985

210. Lockshin MD: Anti-cardiolipin antibody. Arthritis Rheum 30:471, 1987

211. Derksen RHWM, Beisma D, Bouma BN et al: Discordant effects of prednisone on anti-cardiolipin antibodies and the lupus anticoagulant. Arthritis Rheum 29:1295, 1986

212. Rosove MH, Brewer PMC, Runge A, Kirji K: Simultaneous lupus anticoagulant and anticardiolipin assays and clinical detection of antiphospholipids. Am J Hematol 32:148, 1989

213. Triplett DA, Brandt JT, Musgrave KA, Orr CA: The relationship between lupus anticoagulants and antibodies to phospholipid. JAMA 259:550, 1988

214. Kalunian KC, Peter JB, Middlefauf HR et al: Clinical significance of a single test for anticardiolipin antibodies in patients with systemic lupus erythematosus. Am J Med 85:602, 1988

215. Drenkard C, Sanchez-Guerrero J, Alarcon-Segovia D: Fall in antiphospholipid antibody at time of thromboocclusive episodes in systemic lupus erythematosus. J Rheumatol 16:614, 1989

216. Triplett DA, Brandt JT, Musgrave KA: The relationship between lupus anticoagulants and antibodies to phospholipid. JAMA 259:550, 1988

217. Vandre DD, Davis FM, Rao PN et al: Distribution of cytoskeletal proteins sharing a conserved phosphorylated epitope. Eur J Cell Biol 41:72, 1986

218. Jacob L, Lety MA, Bach JF et al: Human systemic lupus erythematosus sera contain antibodies against cell-surface protein(s) that share(s) epitope(s) with DNA. Proc Natl Acad Sci USA 83:6970, 1986

219. Asano T, Furie BC, Furie B: Platelet binding properties of monoclonal lupus autoantibodies produced by human hybridomas. Blood 66:1254, 1985

220. Jacob L, Lety MA, Louvard D et al: Binding of a monoclonal anti-DNA autoantibody to identical protein(s) present at the surface of several human cell types involved in lupus pathogenesis. J Clin Invest 75:315, 1985

221. Boxer M, Ellman L, Carvalho A: The lupus anticoagulant. Arthritis Rheum 19:1244, 1976

222. Corrigan JJ Jr, Patterson JH, May NE: Incoagulability of the blood in systemic lupus erythematosus. A case due to hypoprothrombinemia and a circulating anticoagulant. Am J Dis Child 119:365, 1970

223. Waddell CC, Brown JA: The lupus anticoagulant in 14 male patients. JAMA 248:2493, 1982

224. Elias M, Eldor A: Thromboembolism in patients with the lupus type circulating anticoagulant. Arch Intern Med 144:510, 1984

225. Manoharan A, Gottlieb P: Bleeding in patients with lupus anticoagulant. Lancet 2:171, 1984

226. Ordi J, Vilardel M, Oristrell J et al: Bleeding in patients with lupus anticoagulant. Lancet 2:868, 1984

227. Lechner K, Pabinger-Fasching I: Lupus anticoagulant and thrombosis. A study of 25 cases and review of the literature. Hemostasis 15:254, 1985

228. Harris EN, Boey ML, Mackworth-Young CG et al: Anticardiolipin antibodies: detection by radioimmunoassay and association with thrombosis in systemic lupus erythematosus. Lancet 2:1211, 1983

229. Kalunian KC, Peter JB, Middlekauf HR et al: Clinical significance of a single test for anticardiolipin antibodies in patients with systemic lupus erythematosus. Am J Med 85:602, 1988

230. Firkin BG, Howard MA, Radford N: Possible relationship between lupus inhibitor and recurrent abortion in young women. Lancet 2:366, 1980

231. Ginsberg JS, Demeers C, Brill-Edwards P et al: Increased thrombin generation and activity in patients with systemic lupus erythematosus and anticardiolipin antibodies: evidence for a prothrombotic state. Blood 81:2958, 1993

232. Harris EN, Gharavi AE, Asherson RA et al: Cerebral infarction in systemic lupus: association with anticardiolipin antibodies. Clin Exp Rheumatol 2:47, 1984

233. Landi G, Calloni MV, Sabbadini MG: Recurrent ischemic attacks in young adults with the lupus anticoagulant. Stroke 14:377, 1983

234. Hamsten A, Norbert R, Bjorkholm M et al: Antibodies to cardiolipin in young survivors of myocardial infarction: an association with recurrent cardiovascular events. Lancet 1:113, 1986

235. Jindal BK, Martin MF, Gouyer A: Gangrene developing after minor surgery in a patient with undiagnosed systemic lupus erythematosus and lupus anticoagulant. Ann Rheum Dis 42:847, 1983

236. Asherson RA, Mackworth CG, Boey ML et al: Pulmonary-hypertension in systemic lupus erythematosus. Br Med J 287:1024, 1983

237. Anderson NE, Ali MR: The lupus anticoagulant, pulmonary thromboembolism, and fatal pulmonary hypertension. Ann Rheum Dis 43:760, 1984

238. Anderson D, Bell D, Lodge R, Grant E: Recurrent cerebral ischemia and mitral valve vegetation in a patient with phospholipid antibodies. J Rheumatol 14:839, 1987

239. Espinoza LR, Jara LJ, Silveira LH: Anticardiolipin antibodies in polymyalgia rheumatica-giant cell arteritis: association with severe vascular complications. Am J Med 90:474, 1991

240. Stahl CP, Wideman CS, Spira TJ et al: Protein S deficiency in men with long-term human immunodeficiency virus infection. Blood 81:1801, 1993

241. Rosove MH, Brewer PM: Antiphospholipid thrombosis: clinical course after the first thrombotic event in 70 patients. Ann Intern Med 117:303, 1992

242. Harris EN, Asherson RA, Gharavi AE et al: Thrombocytopenia in SLE and related autoimmune disorders: association with anticardiolipin antibody. Br J Haematol 59:227, 1985

243. Harris EN, Gharavi AE, Hegde U et al: Anticardiolipin antibodies in autoimmune thrombocytopenic purpura. Br J Haematol 59:231, 1985

244. Out HJ, deGroot PG, Vliet MV et al: Antibodies to platelets in patients with antiphospholipid antibodies. Blood 77:2655, 1991

245. Hasselaar P, Derkeen RHWM, Blokziji L et al: Cross-reactivity of antibodies directed against cardiolipin, DNA, endothelial cells and blood platelets. Thromb Haemost 63:169, 1990

246. Lellouche F, Martinuzzo M, Said P et al: Imbalance of thromboxane/prostacyclin biosynthesis in patients with lupus anticoagulant. Blood 78:2894, 1991

247. Walker TS, Triplett DA, Javed N et al: Evaluation of lupus anticoagulants: antiphospholipid antibodies, endothelium associated immunoglobulin, endothelial prostacyclin secretion, and antigenic protein S levels. Thromb Res 51:267, 1988

248. Carreras LO, Defrey NG, Machin SJ et al: Arterial thrombosis, intrauterine death and "lupus" anticoagulant: detection of immunoglobulin interfering with prostacyclin formation. Lancet 1:244, 1981

249. Carreras LO, Vermylen JG: Lupus anticoagulant and thrombosis: possible role of inhibition of prostacyclin formation. Thromb Haemost 48:38, 1982

250. Schorer AE, Wickman NWR, Watson KV: Lupus anticoagulant induces a selective defect in thrombin-mediated endothelial prostacylin release and platelet aggregation. Br J Haematol 71:399, 1989

251. Watson KV, Schorer AE: Lupus anticoagulant inhibition of in vitro prostacyclin release is associated with a thrombosis-prone subset of patients. Am J Med 90:47, 1991

252. Comp PC, DeBault LE, Esmon NL et al: Human thrombomodulin is inhibited by IgG from two patients with nonspecific anticoagulants, abstracted. Blood, suppl 1. 62:299a, 1983

253. Cariou R, Tobelem G, Belluci S et al: Effect of lupus anticoagulant on antithrombogenic properties of endothelial cells: inhibition of thrombomodulin-dependent protein C activation. Thromb Haemost 60:54, 1988

254. Marciniak E, Romond EH: Impaired catalytic function of activated protein C: a new in vitro manifestation of lupus anticoagulant. Blood 74:2426, 1989

255. Malia RG, Kitchen S, Greaves M et al: Inhibition of activated protein C and its cofactor protein S by antiphospholipid antibodies. Br J Haematol 76:101, 1990

256. Borrell M, Sala N, deCastellarnau C et al: Immunoglobulin fractions isolated from patients with antiphospholipid antibodies prevent the inactivation of factor Va by activated protein C on human endothelial cells. Thromb Haemost 68:268, 1992

257. Parke AL, Weinstein RE, Bona RD et al: The thrombotic diathesis associated with the presence of phospholipid antibodies may be due to low levels of free protein S. Am J Med 93:49, 1992

258. Bancsi LFJMM, van der Linden IK, Bertina RM: β_2-Glycoprotein I deficiency and the risk of thrombosis. Thromb Haemost 67:649, 1992

259. Viard JP, Amoura Z, Bach JF: Association of anti-β_2-glycoprotein I antibodies with lupus-type circulating anticoagulant and thrombosis in systemic lupus erythematosus. Am J Med 93:181, 1992

260. Tsakeris DA, Marbet GA, Makris PE et al: Impaired fibrinolysis as essential

contribution to thrombosis in patients with lupus anticoagulant. Thromb Haemost 61:175, 1989

261. Angeles-Cano E, Sultan Y, Clauvel JP: Predisposing factors to thrombosis in systemic lupus erythematosus. Possible relation to endothelial cell damage. J Lab Clin Med 94:312, 1979

262. Jurado M, Paramo JA, Gutierrez-Pimentel M, Rocha E: Fibrinolysis potential and antiphospholipid antibodies in systemic lupus erythematosus and other connective tissue disorders. Thromb Haemost 68:516, 1992

263. Glas-Greenwalt P, Kant S, Allen C et al: Fibrinolysis in health and disease: severe abnormalities in systemic lupus erythematosus. J Lab Clin Med 104:962, 1984

264. Francis RB Jr, McGehee WG, Feinstein DI: Entothelial-dependent fibrinolysis in subjects with the lupus anticoagulant and thrombosis. Thromb Haemost 59:412, 1988

265. Francis RB Jr, Neely S: Effect of the lupus anticoagulant on endothelial fibrinolysis activity in vitro. Thromb Haemost 61:314, 1989

266. Cines DB, Lyss AP, Reeber M et al: Presence of complement-fixing anti-endothelial cell antibodies in systemic lupus erythematosus. J Clin Invest 73:611, 1984

267. Tannenbaum SH, Finko R, Cines DB: Antibody and immune complexes induce tissue factor production by human endothelial cells. J Immunol 137:1532, 1986

268. Oosting JD, Deerksen RHWM, Blokziji L et al: Antiphospholipid antibody positive sera enhance endothelial cell procoagulant activity—studies in a thrombosis model. Thromb Haemost 68:278, 1992

269. Op den Kamp JAF: Lipid asymmetry in membranes. Annu Rev Biochem 48:47, 1979

270. Chiu D, Lubin B, Roelofsen B et al: Sickled erythrocytes accelerate clotting in vitro: an effect of abnormal membrane lipid asymmetry. Blood 58:398, 1981

271. Silveira LH, Hubble CL, Jara LJ et al: Prevention of anticardiolipin antibody-related pregnancy losses with prednisone and aspirin. Am J Med 93:403, 1992

272. Lubbe WF, Palmer SJ, Butler WS, Liggins GC: Fetal survival after prednisone suppression of maternal lupus anticoagulant. Lancet 1:1361, 1983

273. Lubbe WF, Pattison N, Liggins G: Antiphospholipid antibodies and pregnancy. N Engl J Med 313:1351, 1985

274. Wallenberg HCS, Rotmans N: Prophylactic low-dose aspirin and dipyridamole in pregnancy. Lancet 1:939, 1988

275. Elder MG, de Swiet M, Robertson A et al: Low-dose aspirin in pregnancy. Lancet 1:410, 1988

276. Lockshin MD, Druzin ML, Quamar T: Prednisone does not prevent recurrent fetal death in women with antiphospholipid antibody. Am J Obstet Gynecol 160:439, 1989

277. Rosove MH, Tabsh K, Wasserstrum N et al: Heparin therapy for pregnant women with lupus anticoagulants or anticardiolipin antibodies. Obstet Gynecol 75:630, 1990

278. Feinstein DI: Lupus anticoagulant, thrombosis, and fetal loss. N Engl J Med 313:1348, 1985

Disseminated Intravascular Coagulation

116

Eliot C. Williams and Deane F. Mosher

INTRODUCTION

Disseminated intravascular coagulation (DIC) is a syndrome characterized by excessive protease activity in the blood, resulting in formation of soluble fibrin and accelerated fibrinolysis. The causes of DIC are many (Table 116-1), and its consequences are varied and often unpredictable. DIC is an epiphenomenon, almost always caused by a serious illness. On occasion DIC itself may become life-threatening.

PATHOPHYSIOLOGY

Physiologic blood coagulation and fibrinolysis are the result of a balanced interplay among sets of proteolytic enzymes, enzyme cofactors, and inhibitors. DIC occurs when the hemostatic regulatory systems break down.[1] The central feature common to almost all forms of DIC is the generation of thrombin and plasmin (the proteases responsible for fibrin formation and fibrinolysis, respectively) in large amounts and in a nonlocalized pattern. This may occur as a result of massive activation of coagulation or fibrinolysis, or both, that overwhelms normal control mechanisms. Less intense, sustained protease formation may gradually deplete protease inhibitors, leading to uncontrolled proteolysis. Imbalances among protease and inhibitor activities in the blood may lead to pathologic enzyme-substrate or enzyme-inhibitor interactions. Physiologic sequences of enzyme reactions may thus not only be enhanced but also grossly distorted. For example, enzymes in the coagulation cascade may activate proteases or neutralize inhibitors normally associated with the fibrinolytic, complement, or kinin systems. Degradation of membrane proteins may interfere with the normal functioning of platelets, leukocytes, or endothelial cells.[2,3]

Initiation

DIC is usually initiated by exposure of blood to tissue factor (Fig. 116-1). Tissue factor on cell surfaces surrounds blood vessels; tissues such as brain and placenta are especially rich in tissue factor.[4] The blood may be exposed to enough tissue factor to cause DIC as a result of trauma, obstetric accident, diffuse vascular injury, or increased endothelial permeability.[5] DIC may also result from expression of tissue factor by circulating cancer cells or cytokine-stimulated monocytes.

The role of procoagulants other than tissue factor in initiation of DIC is less clear. Activation of the contact system of coagulation may produce shock and other cardiovascular manifestations that often accompany DIC, but the contact system has not been shown to make an important contribution to the coagulopathy itself.[6] Proteolytic enzymes such as neutrophil

Table 116-1. Some Causes of DIC

Infection
  Gram-negative bacteria
    Meningococcus
    Enterobacteriaciae
    Salmonella
    Hemophilus
    Pseudomonas
  Gram-positive bacteria
    Pneumococcus
    Staphylococci
    Hemolytic streptococci
  Anaerobes
    Clostridia spp.
  Mycobacterium tuberculosis
  Bacterial meningitis
  Septic shock
  Postsplenectomy sepsis
  Toxic shock syndrome
  Fungi
    Aspergillus
    Histoplasma
    Candida
  Rocky Mountain spotted fever
  Viruses: many
  Protozoa: malaria
Neoplasia
  Solid tumors
    Adenocarcinoma
    Lymphoma
  Leukemia
    Promyelocytic
    Acute myeloid
    Chronic myeloid
    Acute lymphocytic
Vascular disease
  Aortic aneurysm
  Giant hemangioma (Kasabach-
    Merritt syndrome)
  Vascular tumor
  Multiple telangiectasias
  Acute myocardial infarction
  Intracardiac tumor and
    thrombus
  Aortic balloon pump
  Vasculitis
Liver disease
  Fulminant hepatic failure
  Cirrhosis
  Reye syndrome
  Biliary obstruction
Obstetric complications
  Amniotic fluid embolism
  Abruptio placentae
  Midtrimester abortion
  Septic abortion
  Uterine rupture
  Retained dead fetus
  Toxemia of pregnancy
  Hydatidiform mole

Transfusion reactions
  Acute hemolytic transfusion
    reaction
  Massive transfusion
Surgery
  Vascular surgery
  Cardiac bypass surgery
  Liver transplantation
  Peritoneovenous shunt
Envenomation
  Rattlesnakes, other vipers
  Other snakes
  Insects
Trauma and tissue injury
  Brain injury/stroke
  Crush injury
  Burns
  Hyperthermia
  Hypothermia
  Asphyxia/hypoxia
  Ischemia/infarction
  Rhabdomyolysis
  Fat embolism
Shock
Respiratory distress syndromes
Inherited disorders
  Familial antithrombin III deficiency
  Homozygous protein C deficiency
  Hyperlipoproteinemia types II, IV
Drugs/therapeutic agents
  Fibrinolytic agents
  Heparin-associated
    thrombocytopenia
  Ancrod
  Warfarin (in Trousseau syndrome,
    protein C deficiency)
  Intravenous lipid emulsion
  Clotting factor concentrates—factor
    IX, activated factor IX
  Immune drug reaction
Miscellaneous
  Amyloidosis
  Inflammatory bowel disease
  Acute intravascular hemolysis
  Histiocytic disorders
  Sarcoidosis
  Anaphylaxis
  Kawasaki disease
  Pancreatitis

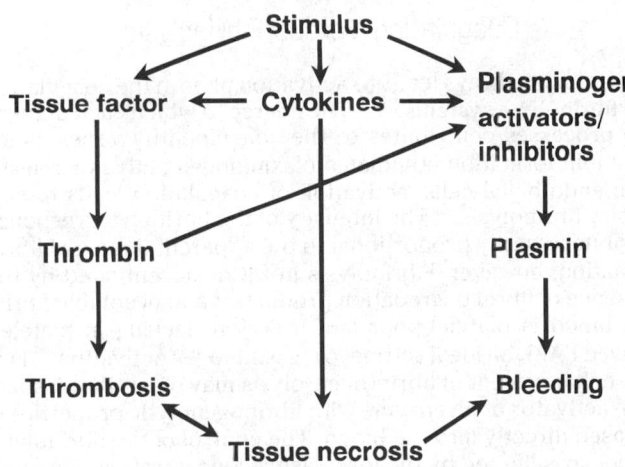

Fig. 116-1. Pathophysiology of DIC. The amounts of tissue factor, cytokines, and plasminogen activators to which the blood and endothelium are exposed depend on the nature and intensity of the stimulus.

ous vipers contain a variety of proteases and other substances that may cause a DIC-like state.

Role of Endothelium

The functional status of the vascular endothelium plays an important role in determining the severity and clinical course of DIC. Normal endothelium regulates clot formation and lysis in a variety of ways (Fig. 116-1), such as by secretion or cell surface expression of heparan sulfate proteoglycan, thrombomodulin, prostacyclin, von Willebrand factor, tissue factor, tissue plasminogen activator, and plasminogen activator inhibitor-1 (PAI-1). Physical damage, infection with viruses or other intracellular pathogens, or exposure to toxins or inflammatory mediators, such as bacterial endotoxin, activated complement, interleukin-1 (IL-1), tumor necrosis factor (TNF), or neutrophil proteases, may lead to loss or perturbation of these regulatory functions.[1,10,11] Such changes may themselves cause DIC or may lower the threshold for DIC in response to a subsequent triggering stimulus.

Role of Leukocytes and Their Secreted Products

Activated monocytes and granulocytes make important contributions to the pathogenesis of DIC, illustrated by experimental animals being protected from endotoxin-induced DIC when they are rendered leukopenic.[12] Monocytes promote coagulation by providing a surface for assembly of the prothrombinase complex.[13] In addition, monocytes secrete mediators of inflammation including TNF, IL-1, and platelet activating factor in response to stimuli such as activated complement and bacterial endotoxin. TNF and IL-1 increase expression of plasminogen activators, tissue factor, and PAI-1 by various cell types (Fig. 116-1) and reduce protein C activation by inhibiting endothelial cell thrombomodulin expression.[14-16] Platelet activating factor activates platelets and increases vascular permeability.[17] The net effect of these molecules is to promote coagulation and down-regulate fibrinolysis.[18-20] Activated granulocytes produce elastase and other proteases that can damage endothelium and promote coagulation and fibrinolysis by neutralizing or degrading proteins that inhibit these processes.[7,8] Leukocytes provide an important link between inflammation and coagulation.

elastase and pancreatic trypsin may in some circumstances contribute to DIC by activating clotting factors, degrading fibrinogen, or neutralizing inhibitors of coagulation and fibrinolysis.[7,8] Some malignant cells produce a cysteine protease that activates factor X ("cancer procoagulant") and that may contribute to DIC.[9] The venoms of rattlesnakes and other poison-

Coagulation Versus Fibrinolysis

DIC almost always leads to activation of both the coagulation and fibrinolytic systems.[21,22] The degree to which each of these two processes contributes to the coagulopathy varies. Since thrombin formation stimulates plasminogen activator release from endothelial cells, activation of coagulation leads to secondary fibrinolysis.[23] The intensity of the fibrinolytic response is not necessarily proportional to the apparent degree of fibrin formation, however. Fibrinolysis in DIC is accentuated by the presence of fibrin degradation products[24] and of soluble fibrin. The blood is platelet-poor and therefore lacking in platelet-derived PAI-1, an ideal setting for plasminogen activation.[25] Further enhancement of fibrin(ogen)olysis may occur if a plasminogen activator or an enzyme with fibrinogenolytic properties is released directly into the blood. The control of the fibrinolytic response is limited by the low plasma concentration of α_2-antiplasmin; when this inhibitor is depleted the systemic effects of plasmin are magnified.[26] The term *primary fibrinolysis* has been applied to states in which the laboratory and clinical findings are dominated by the effects of fibrinolysis and fibrinogenolysis.[21,22] This pattern is probably best considered as representing one end of the spectrum of DIC rather than a different syndrome.

Rarity of Thrombosis

Most patients with acute DIC have little clinical or pathologic evidence for the formation of stable fibrin clots, despite the high level of thrombin activity in their blood.[27,28] Fibrin formation and platelet activation in DIC are poorly localized and usually accompanied by a vigorous fibrinolytic response. Thrombosis tends to be associated with endothelial damage or an intravascular catheter site where adherent platelets can provide a nucleus for stable clot formation.[29] DIC associated with sepsis is characterized by minimal plasmin activity in comparison with the amount of thrombin generated,[30] and thus a higher risk of thrombosis. This is probably a consequence of the procoagulant, antifibrinolytic activities of inflammatory cytokines. Thrombosis may occur after treatment of DIC with inhibitors of fibrinolysis such as ε-aminocaproic acid.[29] Thrombosis is relatively common in association with chronic DIC caused by some types of cancer (Trousseau syndrome).[31]

Tissue Necrosis

Hemorrhagic necrosis of the skin, extremities (purpura fulminans),[32] kidneys, or adrenal glands (Waterhouse-Friderichsen syndrome)[33] may accompany severe DIC. DIC-induced thrombosis of small blood vessels may contribute to these phenomena. However, tissue necrosis can also occur independently of DIC in severe infection and other inflammatory states, possibly via the toxic effects of activated leukocytes and cytokines such as IL-1 and TNF on the endothelium.[34,35] Tissue necrosis may be exacerbated by kinin formation and consequent hypotension, and by iatrogenic peripheral vasoconstriction caused by administration of vasopressors.[36] Animal experiments have shown that specific coagulation inhibitors can prevent endotoxin-induced DIC without affecting tissue necrosis.[37]

Protein C may play an important role in preventing purpura fulminans in infections and other inflammatory states. Administration of activated protein C prevents both tissue necrosis and DIC in experimental animals injected with *Escherichia coli*.[38] Purpura fulminans occurs spontaneously in infants with severe congenital protein C deficiency,[39] and acquired deficiencies of proteins C and S have been found in patients with purpura fulminans associated with bacterial sepsis.[40-42]

Purpura fulminans and other manifestations of tissue necrosis are most often seen in association with overwhelming bacterial sepsis.[43] In children, purpura fulminans also occurs following streptococcal or upper respiratory infections.[44,45] The pathogenesis of postinfectious purpura fulminans is unknown.

Hyperfibrinolysis and Bleeding

Coagulation defects that promote bleeding in DIC include hyperfibrinolysis, depletion of clotting factors and platelets, and inhibition of fibrin polymerization by fibrin degradation products (FDP).[46] Evidence of rapid fibrinolysis is the most important predictor of bleeding risk. Little spontaneous bleeding occurs in conditions in which clotting factor depletion occurs without excessive fibrinolysis (e.g., liver disease or the administration of fibrinogenolytic venoms),[47] which contrasts with the high bleeding incidence following administration of recombinant tissue plasminogen activator. Clinical studies of patients with DIC suggest that the degree of fibrinolytic activation is a major determinant of bleeding risk.[26,48]

Role of Liver and Bone Marrow

The severity of DIC is greater when the ability to compensate for accelerated coagulation and fibrinolysis is diminished. The most important compensatory factors are the synthetic capacities of the liver,[49-51] which must replace clotting factors and inhibitors as they are consumed, and the bone marrow, which must generate platelets. In addition, sufficient quantities of vitamin K and folic acid must be available to support production of clotting factors and platelets.

Acute Versus Chronic DIC

The spectrum of DIC includes acute and chronic syndromes. In acute DIC, activation of coagulation or fibrinolysis, or both, is so rapid and extensive as to cause depletion of coagulation factors and inhibitors. This usually results in bleeding or, less commonly, thrombosis; occasionally both occur simultaneously. In chronic DIC, intravascular coagulation and fibrinolysis do not proceed fast enough to outstrip the rate of synthesis of clotting factors or inhibitors. This may simply reflect a low-grade stimulus, in which case DIC is often mild and asymptomatic. However, DIC may remain compensated despite extensive thrombin formation if production of clotting factors is increased and fibrinolysis is down-regulated. Under these circumstances thrombosis is more likely than bleeding.[31]

The course of DIC thus depends on the intensity of the stimulus and the status of the endothelium, liver, and bone marrow. The balance between coagulation and fibrinolysis, which largely determines whether thrombosis or bleeding will result, is a function of the nature of the stimulus and the integrity of the physiologic anticoagulant and antifibrinolytic systems. The underlying disease may cause bleeding or thrombosis via effects on other organ systems. For example, in septic shock, cytokines act on endothelial cells to promote hemorrhagic tissue necrosis, azotemia secondary to acute tubular necrosis causes platelet dysfunction, and bleeding may be caused by anatomic lesions such as stress ulcers in the upper gastrointestinal tract.

DIAGNOSIS

No single laboratory finding or combination of findings is sensitive or specific enough to allow the construction of a reliable formula for diagnosing DIC. However, as described in Table

Table 116-2. Differential Diagnosis

Condition	Elevated FDP	Prolonged PT	Decreased Platelets	Decreased Fibrinogen	Decreased Antithrombin and/or Antiplasmin	Elevated F1·2 or TAT	Soluble Fibrin
DIC	Yes	Common	Common	Variable	Variable	Yes	Common
Vitamin K deficiency	No	Yes	No	No	No	No	No
Thrombocytopenia of sepsis	No	No	Yes	No	No	No	No
Liver disease	Variable	Common	Variable	Common	Common	Variable	No
Localized coagulation	Yes	Rare	Rare	Rare	Rare	Common	No
Microangiopathy	Minimal	No	Yes	No	No	Variable	No
Lupus anticoagulant	Variable	Yes	Variable	No	No	Variable	No
Hemodilution	No	Yes	Yes	Yes	Yes	No	No

Abbreviations: FDP, fibrin degradation products; PT, prothrombin time; TAT, thrombin/antithrombin III complex.

116-2, the diagnosis can usually be made without ambiguity by careful consideration of both the clinical situation and the laboratory data.[52] DIC is probably present if accelerated fibrinolysis is evident, accompanied by platelet or clotting factor consumption (or both), in a patient with a disorder known to cause DIC.

Screening Tests

The most sensitive standard screening test for DIC is the level of FDP. Since DIC is almost always accompanied by accelerated fibrinolysis, it is probably not present if the FDP level is not elevated. The prothrombin time and the fibrinogen concentration are good screens for clinically significant clotting factor deficiency. The partial thromboplastin time is less useful,[53,54] since it is normal (or shorter than normal) in many patients. The presence of thrombocytopenia or a falling platelet count is neither sensitive nor specific for DIC, although a stable platelet count suggests that thrombin formation has not

been extensive. The presence of schistocytes in the blood smear is a frequent but nonspecific finding, and its absence does not exclude DIC.[55,56] Tests for circulating fibrin are among the most specific for DIC, but they are insensitive and not well standardized.[54,55,57,58]

Indicators of Accelerated Coagulation

A low level of antithrombin III (AT III) suggests DIC, particularly if the liver has normal synthetic capacity and the value declines over time.[55] Levels of most clotting factors drop in acute DIC; activities of the components of the extrinsic coagulation pathway (factors VII, X, V and prothrombin) are particularly likely to be low.[21,35] By contrast, the measured factor VIII activity is often high.[55,59]

Information about the dynamics of DIC can be obtained by measuring the products of coagulation factor activation (Fig. 116-1). The plasma level of fibrinopeptide A, which reflects the rate of fibrin formation, is quite sensitive for DIC but not very specific. Levels of prothrombin activation peptide (F1·2), and thrombin-antithrombin complexes are indicators of the rate of thrombin formation and are also very sensitive tests for DIC.[60]

Indicators of Accelerated Fibrinolysis

The level of circulating FDP is a sensitive measure of fibrinolytic activity. The FDP level is also influenced by the rate at which FDP are cleared by the liver and kidneys. The D-dimer assay measures the subpopulation of FDP derived from crosslinked fibrin (Fig. 116-2). This assay offers an advantage over standard FDP assays in that it may be performed on plasma and is not susceptible to artifacts caused by incomplete clotting of plasma samples.[61] It is somewhat less sensitive than the serum FDP assay, however. The presence of low or falling levels of plasminogen and α_2-antiplasmin activity suggests hyperfibrinolysis. Extreme hyperfibrinolysis does not generally occur until circulating α_2-antiplasmin has been depleted, creating a milieu in which plasmin can act without much opposition.[26,62] More specific but less widely available tests include assays for peptides formed by the action of plasmin on fibrin (Bβ15–42 peptide) or fibrinogen (Bβ1–42 peptide) (Fig. 116-2) and for circulating complexes of plasmin with α_2-antiplasmin or α_2-macroglobulin.[63,64]

Differential Diagnosis

Diseases or syndromes in which either the laboratory or clinical manifestations, or both, resemble those in DIC are shown in Table 116-2.

Vitamin K deficiency[55,66] or immune-mediated thrombocyto-

DIAGNOSIS

The diagnosis of clinically significant DIC is not usually difficult. If a patient has a significantly elevated FDP titer plus evidence of depletion of clotting factors and platelets (a prolonged prothrombin time and low or falling levels of fibrinogen and platelets), the diagnosis can be made with reasonable certainty, particularly if the patient has a disorder known to cause DIC. The best screening tests for DIC are measurements of the FDP, prothrombin time, fibrinogen level, and platelet count. If the FDP titer is normal, DIC is unlikely. If screening tests suggest the presence of DIC, useful additional information can often be obtained by measuring plasma antithrombin III (AT III), plasminogen, and α_2-antiplasmin (α_2-PI) activity. These provide an index of severity (generally, high-grade DIC is associated with AT III and plasminogen activities <60% of normal) and of the balance between coagulation and fibrinolysis, as reflected in the degree of AT III and α_2-PI depletion, respectively.

The presence of liver failure causes the most difficulty in diagnosing DIC, because it also results in deficiency of clotting factors and inhibitors, moderate thrombocytopenia, and delayed clearance of FDP, causing mild to moderate elevation of the FDP titer. When liver failure is present, serial testing may be required; if significant DIC is present, the coagulation abnormalities will become progressively more severe.

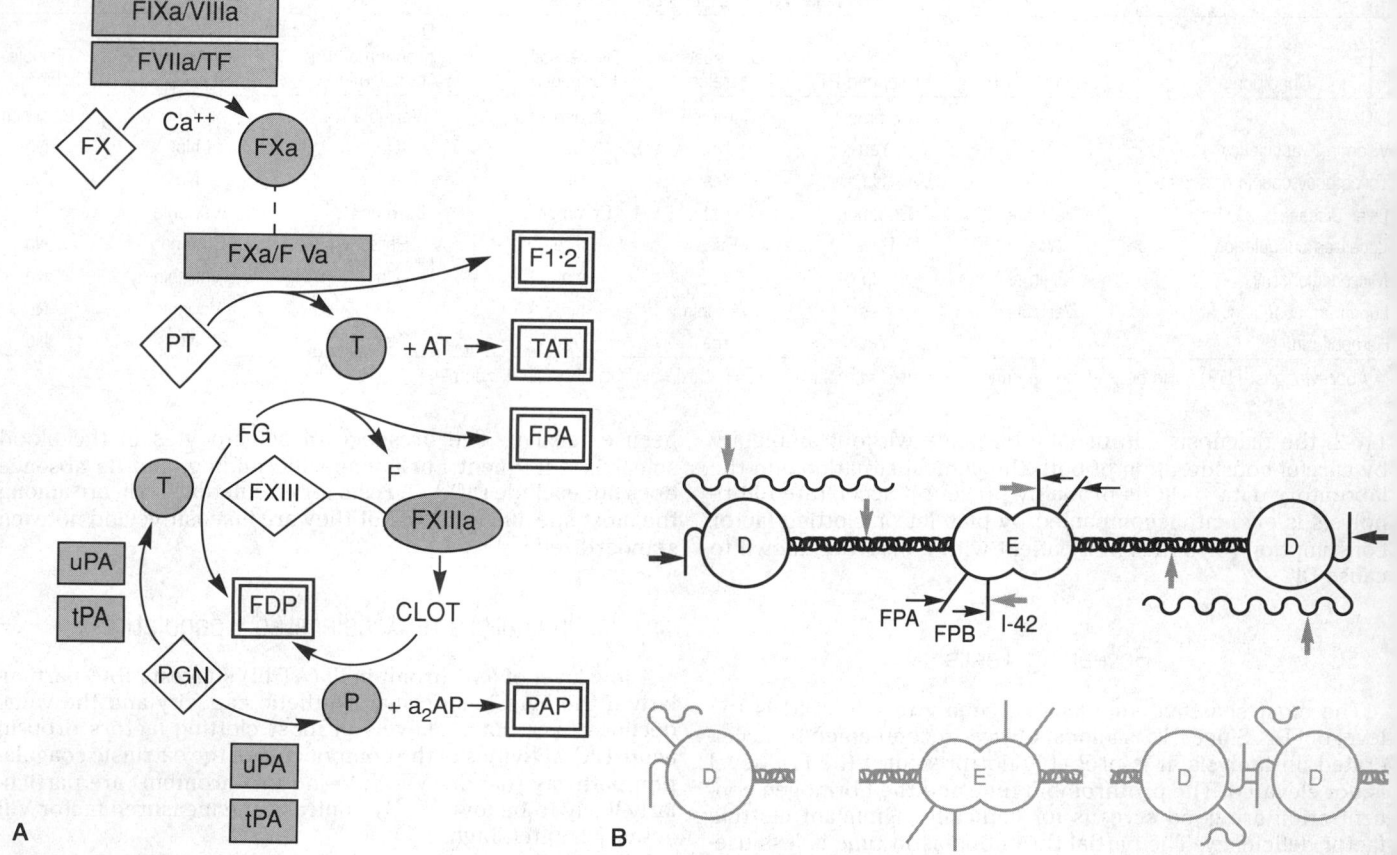

Fig. 116-2. Analytes indicative of DIC. **(A)** Products generated during blood coagulation and fibrinolysis. Products include fragment 1·2 (FI·2), a peptide cleaved from prothrombin (PT) during its conversion to thrombin (T) by factor Xa (FXa), the complex of thrombin and antithrombin III (TAT), fibrinopeptide A (FPA) released from fibrinogen (FG) as it is converted to fibrin (F), fibrinogen or fibrin degradation products (FDP) generated by the action of plasmin (P) on fibrinogen or fibrin, and the complex of plasmin and α₂-antiplasmin (PAP). TF, tissue factor; PGN, plasminogen; u-PA and t-PA, urokinase and tissue plasminogen activator. **(B)** Fibrinogen and its derivatives. Fibrinogen consists of a central globular E domain attached by helical connectors to two globular D domains. Thrombin converts fibrinogen to fibrin by catalyzing release of fibrinopeptides A and B (FPA and FPB) from the surface of the E globule. Plasmin attacks fibrinogen or fibrin at several points: the β-chain in the E globule to release either the 1–42 peptide (also called Bβ1–42 peptide) from fibrinogen or the analogous peptide lacking the FPB portion (Bβ15–42; not shown) from fibrin, the helical connectors to generate D and E fragments, and the L chain on the D globule. Factor XIIIa catalyzes the cross-linking of γ-chains on the surfaces of the D globules. Thus, plasminolysis of cross-linked fibrin generates D dimers rather than single D globules. Black arrows, thrombin; gray arrows, plasmin; red arrows, FXIIIa.

penia[67,68] associated with infection are easily distinguished from DIC by laboratory evaluation (Table 116-2). When these conditions coexist with DIC, they may result in overestimation of its severity. Localized thrombosis produces laboratory findings similar to those of mild DIC, but it can usually be distinguished from DIC on clinical grounds. Microangiopathic disorders such as thrombotic thrombocytopenic purpura may be confused with DIC, since they produce acute illness with multiorgan dysfunction and rapid platelet consumption. However, they do not cause consumption of clotting factors or hyperfibrinolysis.[22,69] Prolonged clotting times, hypofibrinogenemia, and thrombocytopenia due to simple hemodilution may follow hemorrhagic shock, massive transfusion, or cardiopulmonary bypass surgery.[70,71]

The coagulopathy associated with hepatic failure may be difficult to distinguish from DIC.[72] Its features include thrombocytopenia due to platelet sequestration in the spleen or portal circulation, low levels of most coagulation factors and inhibitors, and elevated levels of FDP and protease-inhibitor complexes due to delayed hepatic clearance. In some cases, it may be possible to diagnose DIC in the presence of liver disease only by performing serial measurements, which in the event of acute DIC usually reveal a rapidly changing coagulopathy.[61]

Elevated levels of FDP are often present in patients with renal failure, but this is due primarily to delayed clearance rather than to increased production.[73] Latex bead immunoassays for FDP may give false-positive reactions in the presence of rheumatoid factor,[74] or because of incomplete removal of fibrinogen from the test sample caused by heparin[75] or dysfibrinogenemia.[72,76]

CLINICAL SYNDROMES

Infectious Diseases

Infection is probably the most common cause of DIC.[55,77] DIC may complicate a variety of bacterial, fungal, and viral infections (Table 116-1). The risk of DIC is greatest in meningococcemia and other gram-negative infections that are accompanied by high-grade endotoxemia, or when clearance of the responsible organism from the circulation is impaired, as in asplenic[78,79] or cirrhotic patients. Patients with these conditions are more likely than other patients with DIC to suffer thrombosis or tissue necrosis (purpura fulminans). Conversely, hyperfibrinolysis and severe bleeding are not often found in sepsis.[26,55,80] DIC is a common early manifestation of Rocky Mountain spotted fever, a consequence of rickettsial infection of endothelial cells.[81] Infection of endothelial cells may also underlie DIC caused by certain viral infections.

Cancer

Fibrinogen turnover and levels of circulating fibrinopeptides and FDP are often high in patients with cancer.[21,82–84] This is presumably due to procoagulant and profibrinolytic activity associated with malignant cells and reflects a combination of extravascular activation of coagulation and fibrinolysis and, if malignant cells enter the circulation, DIC.[85–87]

DIC caused by carcinoma is often compensated or "chronic." Carcinomas may cause bleeding, particularly prostate carcinoma,[88] or recurrent deep and superficial venous thrombosis (Trousseau syndrome).[31] Fibrin deposits may develop on cardiac valves (marantic endocarditis) and lead to arterial embolism. There may be an associated microangiopathic hemolytic anemia.[89] Chronic DIC in malignancy often improves with low-dose heparin therapy[31,90] (Fig. 116-3) but responds unpredictably to warfarin. For unknown reasons, dramatic deterioration may occur in patients treated with warfarin alone.[91]

Acute Leukemia

Acute leukemia is accompanied by laboratory evidence of DIC in many patients.[92,93] Leukemic blasts can promote intravascular thrombin formation by expressing procoagulant enzymes[94,95] or cytokines.[96] They also frequently have strong profibrinolytic properties, mediated by urokinase or tissue plasminogen activator[97,98] and other proteolytic enzymes (e.g., elastase) that degrade fibrinogen and inhibitors of fibrinolysis and activate plasminogen.[99] The highest incidence of DIC is found in acute promyelocytic leukemia (APML) [M3, acute myeloid leukemia with t(15;17)].[100,101] A combination of DIC with predominant fibrinolysis and severe thrombocytopenia due to impaired bone marrow function creates a high risk of bleeding in promyelocytic leukemia.[102] Treatment of leukemia may lead to worsening of DIC as leukemic cells lyse and release procoagulant and profibrinolytic substances.[103] DIC in APML has been treated successfully with heparin,[100,104] although there are a number of reports of bleeding associated with hyperfibrinolysis in patients treated with heparin.[101] Such patients may benefit from antifibrinolytic agents given with[101] or without[105] heparin or may be treated with aggressive clotting factor replacement alone.[106]

Vascular Disorders

Disease that involves a large area of endothelium may result in chronic or acute DIC. Usually coagulation and fibrinolysis are not really disseminated but instead are localized in abnormal vessels. In extreme cases, progression to uncompensated acute or subacute DIC occurs. This phenomenon has been reported with large aortic aneurysms,[107] giant hemangiomas,[108,109] multiple telangiectasias,[110] and intracardiac tumors or thrombi.[111]

"Primary" Fibrinolysis

Administration of thrombolytic drugs in sufficient doses results in proteolytic destruction of circulating fibrinogen and in consumption of plasminogen and α_2-antiplasmin.[22,62] Platelet survival is not affected,[22] and thrombin formation and AT III

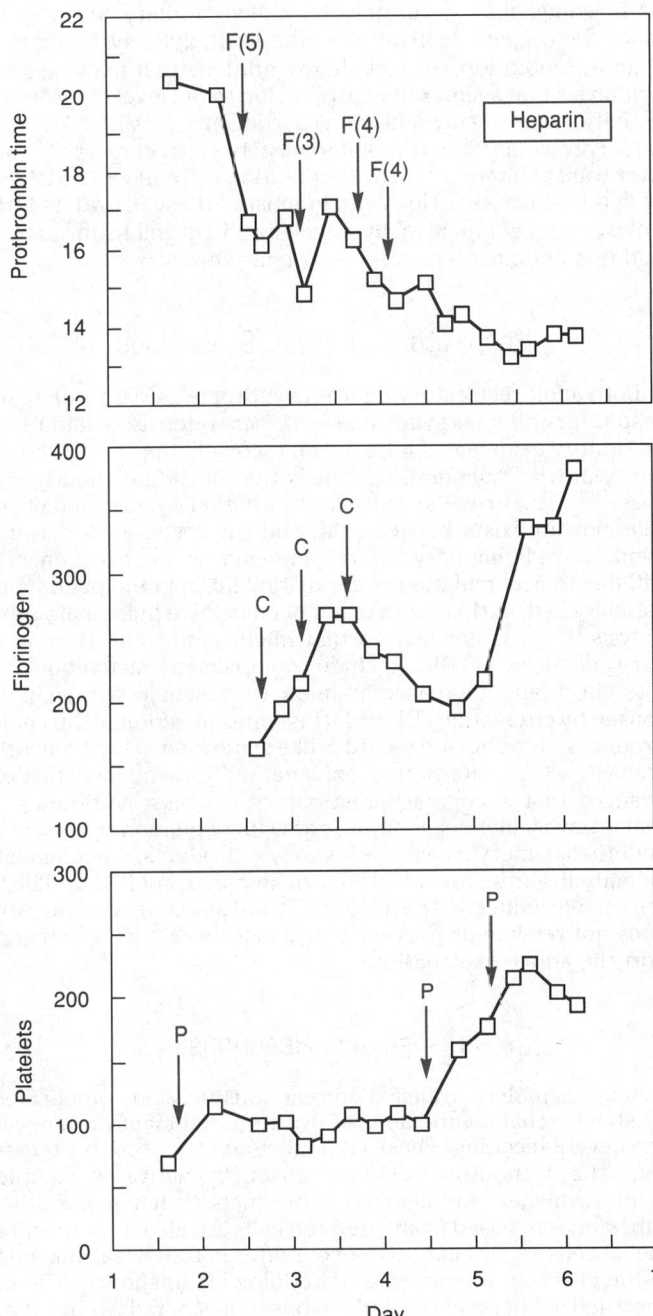

Fig. 116-3. Course of DIC and its response to treatment in a 61-year-old man with widely metastatic prostate carcinoma. The patient presented with spontaneous intracranial hemorrhage. The prothrombin time was prolonged, with borderline thrombocytopenia and fibrinogenopenia. Fibrin degradation product titer was markedly elevated (1 : 160). Plasma α_2-plasmin inhibitor activity was undetectable, whereas antithrombin III was normal (116%), and plasminogen activity was moderately decreased (63%), suggesting predominant activation of fibrinolysis. Fresh frozen plasma (F, with the number of units), cryoprecipitate (C, 10 U), and platelets (P, 10 U) were given, with improvement in the laboratory values as shown. Low-dose heparin therapy (500 U/hr IV) was begun on day 5 and was associated with improvement in laboratory parameters without further transfusion. However, the α_2-plasmin inhibitor activity remained <25% of normal, and the patient died at the end of day 6 of a second intracranial hemorrhage. Prothrombin times are given in seconds, fibrinogen levels in milligrams per deciliter, and platelets in thousands per cubic millimeter.

consumption are minimal. This state, which carries a high risk of bleeding, may accurately be called primary fibrinolysis, since the trigger is activation of the fibrinolytic system rather than thrombin formation. Other conditions that may cause fibrinolysis that seems out of proportion to the level of thrombin activity include acute leukemia (particularly APML),[98,101] prostate carcinoma,[88] cardiopulmonary bypass surgery,[112] and liver transplantation.[113] These conditions also have a relatively high bleeding risk.[26] However, in most of these disorders fibrinolysis is accompanied by accelerated thrombin formation, and it is not clear which is the primary process.[60]

Respiratory Distress Syndromes

Both adult respiratory distress syndrome (ARDS) and infant respiratory distress syndrome (IRDS) are often associated with laboratory evidence of intravascular coagulation,[114–117] the severity of which generally parallels that of the pulmonary disease.[114,118] Controversy exists as to whether a cause-and-effect relationship exists between DIC and the respiratory distress syndromes. Pulmonary failure can occur as a consequence of DIC due to accumulation of circulating fibrin in the pulmonary capillary bed, perhaps as a result of ineffective pulmonary fibrinolysis.[119–121] Other factors that might contribute to pulmonary damage in DIC include complement activation by plasmin[122] and increased pulmonary vascular permeability caused by circulating FDP.[123] Intravenous injection of thrombin produces both DIC and an ARDS-like syndrome in experimental animals.[124] An alternative explanation for the coagulation changes that accompany respiratory distress syndromes is that intravascular coagulation is a result of pulmonary vascular endothelial injury caused by leukocyte products, complement, fat emboli, and so forth.[125,126] Fibrin deposits in ARDS and IRDS are usually limited to the lungs[116,127] and anticoagulant therapy does not reverse or prevent either disorder,[117,128] which support the above explanation.

Transfusion Reactions

Acute hemolytic transfusion reactions may be complicated by shock, renal failure, and DIC with predominant fibrinolysis and severe bleeding. These complications are probably due to generalized endothelial injury caused by activated complement, cytokines, and neutrophil products[129]; heme and other substances released from lysed red cells are also toxic to endothelial cells.[130] DIC may also occur after massive transfusions, in the absence of hemolysis; its etiology is unknown.[131] In an anesthetized patient, the sudden onset of generalized bleeding may be the first sign of an acute transfusion reaction.

Envenomation

The venoms of snakes and other poisonous animals are complex mixtures that have many effects on the coagulation system.[132,133] The bites of rattlesnakes and other vipers are particularly likely to produce coagulopathy.[134] The venoms of these snakes contain toxins that cause vasodilation, increased vascular permeability, generalized endothelial cell damage, and myonecrosis; phospholipases that may release arachidonic acid from cell membranes; and proteases with direct procoagulant and fibrinogenolytic activity. Tissue necrosis localized to the area of the bite is the primary cause of DIC in many cases.[135] Prolongation of clotting times occurs in about one-third of patients following rattlesnake bites, and thrombocytopenia in about one-half.[136] The most dangerous snakes in the United States are the eastern and western diamondback rattlesnakes;

bites from these species frequently cause prolonged fibrinogenolysis and afribrinogenemia.[137–139] Fortunately, clinical bleeding following envenomation is often less severe than would be predicted from the laboratory findings. Antivenin may lessen the severity of envenomation coagulopathy,[134,135,138] but heparin therapy does not seem to be beneficial.[140]

Obstetric Complications

In normal pregnancy, levels of most clotting factors and inhibitors of fibrinolysis increase, and levels of plasminogen activators decrease. The net effect of these changes is to perturb the equilibrium of the coagulation system to promote clot formation and retard clot lysis.[141–143] This change in hemostatic equilibrium presumably reduces the risk of parturient bleeding. However, it also sets the stage for DIC, if uterine contents rich in tissue factor and other procoagulants gain access to the circulation.[144] Severe DIC frequently accompanies abruptio placentae[145] and amniotic fluid embolism, and may also complicate midtrimester abortions.[146] In such obstetric catastrophes, DIC is usually acute and, if the patient survives the initial crisis, self-limited. Delivery of the fetus is the most effective therapy. Replacement therapy with plasma or cryoprecipitate is indicated, but no evidence supports the routine use of heparin or antifibrinolytic drugs. Intrauterine fetal death may produce chronic DIC, particularly if the fetus is retained for several weeks. In such instances coagulation parameters can be normalized prior to uterine evacuation by giving heparin.[147,148] Septic abortion and other high-grade infections during pregnancy may also cause DIC.[149]

Toxemia of pregnancy is associated with microvesicular fatty degeneration of the liver[150,151] and with local to generalized endothelial damage. Clinical syndromes accompanying these phenomena include acute fatty liver of pregnancy and a form of microangiopathy that has been called the HELLP syndrome (hemolysis, elevated liver enzymes, low platelets).[152] Secondary DIC may occur,[153–155] but it is generally not severe unless hepatic failure is present.[153,156] In severe DIC, plasma and cryoprecipitate therapy should be given. No data support the use of heparin in toxemic coagulopathy.

Microangiopathic Disorders

In several diseases presumed to result from endothelial cell damage or dysfunction, intravascular coagulation plays an important pathogenic role. These include thrombotic thrombocytopenic purpura,[157] hemolytic uremic syndrome,[158] vasculopathies associated with systemic lupus erythematosus and progressive systemic sclerosis, toxemia of pregnancy, renal allograft rejection, and heparin-induced thrombotic thrombocytopenia. Although intravascular deposits containing platelets and fibrin occur in each of these conditions, biochemical evidence of plasma protease activation is usually minimal, and laboratory manifestations of DIC such as fibrinogenopenia, soluble fibrin, and high levels of FDP are often absent.[22,69] It seems likely that coagulation is driven by events at the endothelial cell surface that promote platelet aggregation and shift the cell toward a procoagulant and away from a profibrinolytic state, rather than by generation of large amounts of circulating thrombin or other proteases.[159,160] DIC, if it occurs at all, is a secondary phenomenon. Anticoagulants are of little or no benefit in microangiopathic diseases.[69,161]

Postsurgical DIC

Many patients have evidence of subclinical DIC after major surgery, and acute DIC can be a result of operative complications such as shock, sepsis, or hemolytic transfusion reaction.[162] Several surgical procedures may directly cause acute DIC. In liver transplantation fibrinolytic activity in blood is usually high during the anhepatic phase, and frank DIC may occur with hepatic reperfusion.[113] This coagulopathy is probably responsible for the high risk of intracranial hemorrhage after liver transplantation.[163] DIC is common after peritoneovenous shunt placement, presumably due to the presence of procoagulant and profibrinolytic substances in ascitic fluid.[164] Increased blood fibrinolytic activity is often present during cardiopulmonary bypass,[165] and an occasional patient develops frank DIC.[166] However, most of the coagulation changes after cardiopulmonary bypass seem to be due to hemodilution,[70,167] and bleeding is usually due to a surgically correctable lesion rather than coagulopathy.[168]

DIC of Unknown Etiology

The causes of DIC are usually made apparent by its clinical setting. If bleeding or thrombosis due to DIC is the presenting feature of an illness, the underlying cause (e.g., sepsis) usually makes itself known quickly. Some disorders can cause DIC or hyperfibrinolysis, yet elude quick diagnosis. These include occult malignancy (especially prostate carcinoma[169]), hepatic cirrhosis, large abdominal aortic aneurysms,[107] toxic shock syndrome,[170] Kawasaki disease,[171] postinfectious purpura fulminans,[44] and amyloidosis.[172] DIC for which no cause can be found after thorough investigation is rare but has been described.

THERAPY

The mortality rate in severe DIC exceeds 80% in some series.[28,173] Since death is usually caused by progression of the underlying disease rather than DIC per se,[28] elimination or amelioration of the cause, as well as measures to maintain circulation and oxygenation, must be the first priority in any patient with DIC. Occasionally, however, treating the causative disease alone is not enough to prevent serious bleeding or thrombosis. In such instances treatment of the coagulopathy can be lifesaving. The indications for such therapy depend on the nature and treatability of the underlying disease and on the severity of DIC and its complications. Two treatment options are available: replacement of clotting factors and platelets, and use of pharmacologic inhibitors of coagulation and/or fibrinolysis.[174]

Replacement Therapy

Clotting factors and inhibitors can be replaced by giving fresh frozen plasma.[175] The prothrombin time provides a rough indication of the degree to which the components of the extrinsic pathway have been depleted and is the best single parameter to use as a guide for plasma replacement. Patients with hyperfibrinolysis and disproportionate consumption of fibrinogen can be detected and followed by the quantitative fibrinogen assay. They may be given cryoprecipitate, which has a 5- to 10-fold higher fibrinogen concentration than whole plasma. Replacement of plasma factors and fibrinogen is particularly important in patients with liver disease, because in such patients the combination of increased consumption and decreased synthesis may cause rapid depletion of coagulation factors. Theoretical concern that replacement of clotting factors might lead to organ damage by fueling the coagulopathy has not been borne out in clinical practice.[106] Indeed, plasma infusion probably does as much to retard coagulation and fibrinolysis, through replacement of inhibitors, as to promote them. Thrombocytopenia in DIC is not usually severe,[55,173] and most patients

do not require platelet transfusions unless platelet production is impaired (e.g., in leukemia). The potential for volume overload and transmission of blood-borne viral infection must be kept in mind whenever blood products are given.

Pharmacologic Inhibitors

The uses of heparin and antifibrinolytic agents in DIC are controversial. Such treatments have not been shown conclusively to improve survival in DIC and may exacerbate bleeding (heparin) or thrombosis (antifibrinolytic agents).[39,176,177] The evidence that heparin is beneficial in acute DIC is primarily anecdotal.[90,101] Some authorities have advocated giving heparin to treat or prevent tissue necrosis (e.g., purpura fulminans) in acute DIC.[178] However, the rationale for this therapy is questionable, since tissue necrosis may occur despite inhibition of

---

APPROACH TO THERAPY FOR DIC IN SEPTICEMIA

In any patient with DIC, primary consideration must be given to treating the underlying diease. A septic patient must be given appropriate antibiotics, and immediate measures should be taken to eradicate the source of the infection (e.g., drainage of an abscess or removal of an infected intravascular catheter). Care should be given in an intensive care unit equipped to monitor oxygenation and hemodynamic parameters. High-grade DIC that persists once such treatment has been given is an ominous sign.

Therapy for DIC may minimize or prevent either of two complications that result from uncontrolled coagulation and fibrinolysis: thrombosis and bleeding. Although thrombosis is unusual in severe DIC, it occurs more often in the septic form than in other varieties. Thrombosis may occur in veins, particularly around indwelling catheters, or in small and medium-size arteries, causing gangrene of digits or extremities (purpura fulminans). No specific laboratory findings predict these occurrences, although depressed protein C is associated with purpura fulminans in patients with meningococcemia. Since peripheral vasoconstriction may precipitate or exacerbate tissue necrosis in sepsis, blood pressure should be maintained by aggressive fluid administration rather than α-adrenergic agents when possible. When clinical evidence of thrombosis is present, therapy with heparin may be beneficial. The optimal dose has not been established, but it is reasonable to begin with a relatively low dose (5–10 U/kg/hr) to reduce the risk of bleeding. The possibility of associated hemorrhagic necrosis of the adrenal glands, which may lead to life-threatening adrenal insufficiency, should be kept in mind in any patient with sepsis and high-grade DIC.

If significant depletion of clotting factors and inhibitors has occurred, as evidenced by a prothrombin time >1.3–1.5 times control, plasma replacement therapy may reduce the bleeding risk. Patients with extreme hyperfibrinolysis, in whom the bleeding risk is greatest, may also benefit from cryoprecipitate therapy to replace fibrinogen. When the fibrinogen is <100 mg/dl, 10 U of cryoprecipitate for each 2–3 U of plasma will generally be adequate. Prophylactic platelet transfusions may benefit patients who are severely thrombocytopenic (platelet count <20,000/mm³), and platelets should be given to bleeding patients if the platelet count is <50,000/mm³.

REPLACEMENT THERAPY IN DIC

General guidelines for replacement therapy are to give fresh frozen plasma and cryoprecipitate (usually in a ratio of about 10 U of cryoprecipitate for every 2 or 3 U of plasma) to achieve a prothrombin time within 2–3 seconds of the control value, and a fibrinogen level >100 mg/dl. Platelet transfusions (usually 1–3 U/10 kg/day) are appropriate if the platelet count is <10,000–20,000/mm^3 or if bleeding is major and the platelet count is <50,000/mm^3. AT III concentrate ameliorates experimental DIC, and reports suggest that it may be of some clinical benefit in humans. Patients with DIC are at risk of vitamin K and folate deficiency, and empirical administration of these vitamins is advisable in most cases.

USE OF HEPARIN IN THE THERAPY FOR DIC

Heparin may be beneficial in DIC associated with APML or carcinoma and in any case of DIC associated with thrombosis. In the absence of large vessel thrombosis, a low dose of heparin (5–10 U/kg/hr) may be effective. DIC associated with APML often becomes worse during anti-leukemic therapy, an occurrence generally associated with evidence of marked hyperfibrinolysis. If this occurs in a heparinized patient, heparin may be combined with an antifibrinolytic agent such as ε-aminocaproic acid. In patients with carcinoma and DIC (Trousseau syndrome), low-dose heparin may produce improvement in the laboratory and clinical picture, even if the patient is bleeding and the laboratory findings suggest a predominantly fibrinolytic state. Higher doses of heparin in patients with DIC are associated with a higher risk of bleeding and in most cases are of questionable therapeutic value. An exception is the patient with chronic DIC associated with large vessel thrombosis (e.g., Trousseau syndrome), in whom heparin should be given in doses sufficient to prolong the activated partial thromboplastin time to at least 1.5 times control, as is generally done in the treatment of deep venous thrombosis.

thrombin formation,[37] and evidence for efficacy of heparin in established purpura fulminans is unimpressive. The most convincing reports of improvement with heparin treatment have involved patients with chronic DIC. Heparin is often beneficial in patients with DIC associated with carcinoma, even when the laboratory findings suggest a predominantly fibrinolytic state[31,179] (Fig. 116-3). Chronic DIC in other disorders (e.g., retained dead fetus, vascular disorders) may also improve with heparin therapy.[174] Improvement often occurs with a heparin dose of 5–10 U/kg/hr, which is significantly lower than that normally used for anticoagulation.[90,174,176] Heparin should be given by continuous intravenous infusion whenever possible.

ε-Aminocaproic acid and tranexamic acid are lysine analogues that block binding of plasmin to specific lysine residues on fibrin and fibrinogen, thereby inhibiting fibrinolysis. These drugs can reduce bleeding from a variety of causes.[180] However, they may occasionally unmask underlying coagulation and convert a bleeding disorder into a thrombotic condition.[177] They should therefore be used with caution when increased thrombin and fibrin formation is present, as in DIC. When used to treat DIC, antifibrinolytic drugs are usually given in conjunction with heparin to minimize the potential for thrombosis. Patients who may benefit from the use of antifibrinolytic drugs include those in whom there is laboratory evidence of hyperfibrinolysis with depletion of physiologic plasmin inhibitors (i.e., α_2-antiplasmin) and who bleed despite vigorous replacement therapy.[26] ε-Aminocaproic acid in combination with low-dose heparin[101] and tranexamic acid without heparin[105] have been shown to be useful adjuncts in the treatment of the coagulopathy caused by APML. Antifibrinolytic agents without heparin have been beneficial in patients with chronic DIC due to giant hemangiomas (Kasabach-Merritt syndrome)[108,109] and in those with hyperfibrinolysis caused by prostate cancer[88] or peritoneovenous shunt placement for cirrhotic ascites.[164]

New or Experimental Therapy

Broad-spectrum protease inhibitors such as gabexate, nafamostat, and trasylol have been used to treat experimental and clinical DIC.[107,181–183] Preliminary data suggest that they may reduce bleeding and reverse laboratory signs of DIC in some patients. Aprotinin, another protease inhibitor with broad specificity, is of some benefit in experimental DIC[184] and in clinical situations in which there is hyperfibrinolysis and bleeding.[180] AT III concentrates are effective in experimental DIC[185,186] and may be of clinical benefit in patients.[41,187,188] A genetically engineered protease inhibitor, α_1-antitrypsin Pittsburgh, which inhibits thrombin, factor XIIa, factor XIa, and kalli-

krein, improves survival in experimental DIC.[189] Protein C concentrate has been used to treat purpura fulminans associated with meningococcemia and acquired protein C deficiency.[42] Administration of a monoclonal antibody to bacterial endotoxin was associated with faster resolution of DIC in patients with gram-negative sepsis in a large controlled study.[190] Recombinant thrombomodulin[191] and tissue factor pathway inhibitor[192] improve outcome in experimental DIC. The further development of specific inhibitors mediating the regulatory pathways that are altered in DIC offers promise.

REFERENCES

1. Müller-Berghaus G: Pathophysiologic and biochemical events in disseminated intravascular coagulation: dysregulation of procoagulant and anticoagulant pathways. Semin Thromb Hemost 15:58, 1989
2. Schafer A, Adelman B: Plasmin inhibition of platelet function and of arachidonic acid metabolism. J Clin Invest 75:456, 1985
3. Brower M, Levin R, Garry K: Human neutrophil elastase modulates platelet function by limited proteolysis of membrane glycoproteins. J Clin Invest 75:657, 1985
4. Drake T, Morrissey J, Edgington T: Selective cellular expression of tissue factor in human tissues. Implications for disorders of hemostasis and thrombosis. Am J Pathol 134:1087, 1989
5. Iijima K, Fukuda C, Nakamura K: Measurements of tissue factor-like activity in plasma of patients with DIC. Thromb Res 61:29, 1991
6. Pixley RA, De La Cadena R, Page JD et al: The contact system contributes to hypotension but not disseminated intravascular coagulation in lethal bacteremia. J Clin Invest 91:61, 1993
7. Plow EF: Leukocyte elastase release during blood coagulation. A potential mechanism for activation of the alternative fibrinolytic pathway. J Clin Invest 69:564, 1982
8. Higuchi DA, Wun T-C, Likert KM, Broze GJ: The effect of leukocyte elastase on tissue factor pathway inhibitor. Blood 79:1712, 1992
9. Gordon SG, Cross BA: A factor X-activating cysteine protease from malignant tissue. J Clin Invest 67:1665, 1981
10. Moore K, Andreoli S, Esmon N et al: Endotoxin enhances tissue factor and suppresses thrombomodulin expression of human vascular endothelium in vitro. J Clin Invest 79:124, 1987
11. Archipoff G, Beretz A, Freyssinet J-M et al: Heterogeneous regulation of constitutive thrombomodulin or inducible tissue-factor activities on the surface of human saphenous-vein endothelial cells in culture following stimulation by interleukin-1, tumor necrosis factor, thrombin or phorbol ester. Biochem J 273:679, 1991

12. Horn RG, Collins RD: Studies on the pathogenesis of the generalized Shwartzman reaction. Lab Invest 18:101, 1968
13. Robinson RA, Worfolk L, Tracey PB: Endotoxin enhances the expression of monocyte prothrombinase activity. Blood 79:406, 1992
14. Bevilacqua MP, Pober JS, Majeau GR et al: Recombinant tumor necrosis factor induces procoagulant activity in cultured human vascular endothelium: characterization and comparison with the actions of interleukin 1. Proc Natl Acad Sci USA 83:4533, 1986
15. Nawroth PP, Stern DM: Modulation of endothelial cell hemostatic properties by tumor necrosis factor. J Exp Med 163;740, 1986
16. Scarpati EM, Sadler JE: Regulation of endothelial cell coagulant properties. Modulation of tissue factor, plasminogen activator inhibitors, and thrombomodulin by phorbol 12-myristate acetate and tumor necrosis factor. J Biol Chem 264:20705, 1989
17. Morrison D, Ryan J: Endotoxins and disease mechanisms. Annu Rev Med 38:417, 1987
18. Suffredini AF, Harpel PC, Parrillo JE: Promotion and subsequent inhibition of plasminogen activation after administration of intravenous endotoxin to normal subjects. N Engl J Med 320:1165, 1989
19. van der Poll T, Buller HR, ten Cate H et al: Activation of coagulation after administration of tumor necrosis factor to normal subjects. N Engl J Med 322:1622, 1990
20. Bauer KA, ten Cate H, Barzegar S et al: Tumor necrosis factor infusions have a procoagulant effect on the hemostatic mechanism of humans. Blood 74: 165, 1989
21. Merskey C, Johnson AJ, Kleiner G, Wohl H: The defibrination syndrome: clinical features and laboratory diagnosis. Br J Haematol 13:528, 1967
22. Harker L, Slichter S: Platelet and fibrinogen consumption in man. N Engl J Med 287:999, 1972
23. Levin EG, Marzec U, Anderson J, Harker LA: Thrombin stimulates tissue plasminogen activator release from cultured human endothelial cells. J Clin Invest 74:1988, 1984
24. Weitz JI, Leslie B, Ginsberg J: Soluble fibrin degradation products potentiate tissue plasminogen activator-induced fibrinogen proteolysis. J Clin Invest 87:1082, 1991
25. Keijer J, Linders M, van Zonneveld A-J et al: The interaction of plasminogen activator inhibitor 1 with plasminogen activators (tissue-type and urokinase-type) and fibrin: localization of interaction sites and physiologic relevance. Blood 78:401, 1991
26. Williams E: Plasma α-2 antiplasmin activity: role in the evaluation and management of fibrinolytic states and other bleeding disorders. Arch Intern Med 149:1769, 1989
27. McKay D, Müller-Berghaus G: Therapeutic implications of disseminated intravascular coagulation. Am J Cardiol 20:392, 1967
28. Mant M, King E: Severe, acute disseminated intravascular coagulation. A reappraisal of its pathophysiology, clinical significance and therapy based on 47 patients. Am J Med 67:557, 1979
29. Robboy SJ, Colman RW, Minna JD: Pathology of disseminated intravascular coagulation. Analysis of 26 cases. Hum Pathol 3:327, 1972
30. Kario K, Matsuo T, Kodama K et al: Imbalance between thrombin and plasmin activity in disseminated intravascular coagulation. Haemostasis 22: 179, 1992
31. Sack G, Levin J, Bell W: Trousseau's syndrome and other manifestations of chronic disseminated coagulopathy in patients with neoplasms: clinical, pathophysiologic, and therapeutic features. Medicine 56:1, 1977
32. Francis RB: Acquired purpura fulminans. Semin Thromb Hemost 16:310, 1990
33. Margaretten W, Nakai H, Landing B: Septicemic adrenal hemorrhage. Am J Dis Child 105:64, 1963
34. Argenbright LW, Barton RW: Interactions of leukocyte integrins with intercellular adhesion molecule 1 in the production of inflammatory vascular injury in vivo. The Shwartzman reaction revisited. J Clin Invest 89:259, 1992
35. Johnson CS, Chang M-J, Braunschweiger PG, Furmanski P: Acute hemorrhagic necrosis of tumors induced by interleukin-1α: effects independent of tumor necrosis factor. J Natl Cancer Inst 83:842, 1991
36. Hayes MA, Yau EHS, Hinds CJ, Watson JD: Symmetrical peripheral gangrene: association with noradrenaline administration. Intensive Care Med 18:433, 1992
37. Taylor FB, Chang ACK, Peer GT et al: DEGR-factor Xa blocks disseminated intravascular coagulation initiated by *Escherichia coli* without preventing shock or organ damage. Blood 78:364, 1991
38. Taylor FB, Chang A, Esmon CT et al: Protein C prevents the coagulopathic and lethal effects of *Escherichia coli* infusion in the baboon. J Clin Invest 79:918, 1987
39. Marciniak E, Wilson H, Marlar R: Neonatal purpura fulminans: a genetic disorder related to the absence of protein C in the blood. Blood 65:15, 1985
40. Powars D, Rodgers Z, Patch M et al: Purpura fulminans in meningococcemia: association with acquired deficiencies of proteins C and S. N Engl J Med 317:571, 1987
41. Fourrier F, Lestavel P, Chopin C et al: Meningococcemia and purpura fulminans in adults: acute deficiencies of proteins C and S and early treatment with antithrombin III concentrates. Intensive Care Med 16:121, 1990
42. Gerson WT, Dickerman JD, Bovill EG, Golden E: Severe acquired protein C deficiency in purpura fulminans associated with disseminated intravascular coagulation: treatment with protein C concentrate. Pediatrics 91:418, 1993
43. Hautekeete M, Berneman Z, Bieger R et al: Purpura fulminans in pneumococcal sepsis. Arch Intern Med 146:497, 1986
44. Antley R, McMillan C: Sequential coagulation studies in purpura fulminans. N Engl J Med 276:1287, 1967
45. Spicer T, Rau J: Purpura fulminans. Am J Med 61:566, 1976
46. Alkjaersig N, Fletcher A, Sherry S: Pathogenesis of the coagulation defect developing during pathological plasma proteolysis ("fibrinolytic") states. II. The significance, mechanism and consequences of defective fibrin polymerization. J Clin Invest 41:917, 1962
47. Latallo Z: Retrospective study on complications and adverse effects of treatment with thrombin-like enzymes—a multicenter trial. Thromb Haemost 50:604, 1983
48. Stump DC, Taylor FB, Nesheim ME et al: Pathologic fibrinolysis as a cause of clinical bleeding. Semin Thromb Hemost 16:260, 1990
49. Fletcher A, Biederman O, Moore D et al: Abnormal plasminogen-plasmin system activity (fibrinolysis) in patients with hepatic cirrhosis: its cause and consequences. J Clin Invest 43:681, 1964
50. Stein S, Harker L: Kinteic studies of platelets, fibrinogen, and plasminogen in patients with hepatic cirrhosis. J Lab Clin Med 99:217, 1982
51. Hersch S, Kunelis T, Francis R: The pathogenesis of accelerated fibrinolysis in liver cirrhosis: a critical role for tissue plasminogen activator inhibitor. Blood 69:1315, 1987
52. Cembrowski G, Griffin J, Mosher D: Diagnostic efficacy of six plasma proteins in evaluating consumptive coagulopathies. Arch Intern Med 146:1997, 1986
53. Colman R, Robboy S, Minna J: Disseminated intravascular coagulation: an approach. Am J Med 52:679, 1972
54. Colman R, Robboy S, Minna J: Disseminated intravascular coagulation: a reappraisal. Annu Rev Med 30:359, 1979
55. Spero J, Lewis J, Hasiba U: Disseminated intravascular coagulation. Findings in 346 patients. Thromb Haemost 43:28, 1980
56. Visudhiphan S, Piankijagum A, Sathayapraseart P, Mitrchai N: Erythrocyte fragmentation in disseminated intravascular coagulation and other diseases. N Engl J Med 309:113, 1983
57. Halvorsen S, Skjønsberg OH, Ruyter R, Godal HC: Comparison of methods for detecting soluble fibrin in plasma. An in vitro study. Thromb Res 57: 489, 1990
58. Halvorsen S, Skjønsberg OH, Godal HC: The stimulatory effect of soluble fibrin on plasminogen activation by tissue plasminogen activator as studied by the Coa-set fibrin monomer test. Thromb Res 61:453, 1991
59. Lombardi R, Mannucci P, Seghatchian M et al: Alterations of factor VIII von Willebrand factor in clinical conditions associated with an increase in its plasma concentration. Br J Haematol 49:61, 1981
60. Bauer K, Rosenberg R: Thrombin generation in acute promyelocytic leukemia. Blood 64:791, 1984
61. Carr JM, McKinney M, McDonagh J: Diagnosis of disseminated intravascular coagulation. Role of D dimer. Am J Clin Pathol 91:280, 1989
62. Collen D, Verstraete M: α₂-Antiplasmin consumption and fibrinogen breakdown during thrombolytic therapy. Thromb Res 14:631, 1979
63. Harpel P: α-2-Plasmin inhibitor and α-2-macroglobulin-plasmin complexes in plasma. J Clin Invest 68:46, 1981
64. Weitz J, Koehn J, Canfield R et al: Development of a radioimmunoassay for the fibrinogen-derived peptide Bβ1-42. Blood 67:1014, 1986
65. Corrigan V: Vitamin K-dependent coagulation factors in gram-negative septicemia. Am J Dis Child 138:240, 1984
66. Alperin J: Coagulopathy caused by vitamin K deficiency in critically ill, hospitalized patients. JAMA 258:1916, 1987
67. Neame P, Kelton J, Walker I et al: Thrombocytopenia in septicemia: the role of disseminated intravascular coagulation. Blood 56:88, 1980
68. Poskitt T, Poskitt P: Thrombocytopenia of sepsis. The role of circulating IgG-containing immune complexes. Arch Intern Med 145:891, 1985
69. Jaffe E, Nachman R, Merskey C: Thrombotic thrombocytopenic purpura—coagulation parameters in twelve patients. Blood 42:499, 1973
70. Mammen E, Koets M, Washington B et al: Hemostasis changes during cardiopulmonary bypass surgery. Semin Thromb Hemost 11:281, 1985
71. Hewson JR, Neame PB, Kumar N et al: Coagulopathy related to dilution and hypotension during massive transfusion. Crit Care Med 13:387, 1985

72. Vandewater L, Carr J, Aronson D, McDonagh J: Analysis of elevated fibrin(o-gen) degradation product levels in patients with liver disease. Blood 67: 1468, 1986

73. Lane D, Ireland H, Knight I et al: The significance of fibrinogen derivatives in plasma in human renal failure. Br J Haematol 56:251, 1984

74. Rutstein J, Holahan J, Lyons R, Pope R: Rheumatoid factor interference with the latex agglutination test for fibrin degradation products. J Lab Clin Med 92:529, 1978

75. Connaghan D, Francis C, Ryan D, Marder V: Prevalence and clinical implications of heparin-associated false positive tests for serum fibrin(ogen) degradation products. Am J Clin Pathol 86:304, 1986

76. Wilde J, Thomas W, Lane D et al: Acquired dysfibrinogenemia masquerading as disseminated intravascular coagulation in acute pancreatitis. J Clin Pathol 41:615, 1988

77. Bone RC: Modulators of coagulation. A critical appraisal of their role in sepsis. Arch Intern Med 152:1381, 1992

78. Bisno A, Freeman J: The syndrome of asplenia, pneumococcal sepsis, and disseminated intravascular coagulation. Ann Intern Med 72:389, 1970

79. Zarrabi M, Rosner F: Serious infections in adults following splenectomy for trauma. Arch Intern Med 144:1421, 1984

80. Kreger B, Craven D, McCabe W: Gram-negative bacteremia. IV. Re-evaluation of clinical features and treatment in 612 patients. Am J Med 68:344, 1980

81. Rao A, Schapira M, Clements M et al: A prospective study of platelets and plasma proteolytic systems during the early stages of Rocky Mountain spotted fever. N Engl J Med 318:1021, 1988

82. Peck S, Reiquam C: Disseminated intravascular coagulation in cancer patients: supportive evidence. Cancer 31:1114, 1973

83. Peuscher F, Cleton F, Armstrong L et al: Significance of plasma fibrinopeptide A (fpA) in patients with malignancy. J Lab Clin Med 96:5, 1980

84. Rickles F, Edwards R, Barb C, Cronlund M: Abnormalities of blood coagulation in patients with cancer: fibrinopeptide A generation and tumor growth. Cancer 51:301, 1983

85. Mombelli G, Roux A, Haeberli A, Straub P: Comparison of ^{125}I-fibrinogen kinetics and fibrinopeptide A in patients with disseminated neoplasias. Blood 60:381, 1982

86. Pineo G, Regoeczi E, Hatton M, Brain M: The activation of coagulation by extracts of mucus: a possible pathway of intravascular coagulation accompanying adenocarcinomas. J Lab Clin Med 82:255, 1973

87. Rickles F, Edwards R: Activation of blood coagulation in cancer: Trousseau's syndrome revisited. Blood 62:14, 1983

88. Cooper DL, Sandler AB, Wilson LD, Duffy TP: Disseminated intravascular coagulation and excessive fibrinolysis in a patient with metastatic prostate cancer. Response to epsilon-aminocaproic acid. Cancer 70:656, 1992

89. Murgo A: Thrombotic microangiopathy in the cancer patient including those induced by chemotherapeutic agents. Semin Hematol 24:161, 1987

90. Gurewich V, Lipinski B: Low-dose heparin in the treatment of disseminated intravascular coagulation. Am J Med Sci 274:83, 1977

91. Bell W, Starksen N, Tong S, Porterfield J: Trousseau's syndrome: devastating coagulopathy in the absence of heparin. Am J Med 79:423, 1985

92. Myers T, Rickles F, Barb C, Cronlund M: Fibrinopeptide A in acute leukemia: relationship of activation of blood coagulation to disease activity. Blood 57: 518, 1981

93. Sarris AH, Kempin S, Berman E et al: High incidence of disseminated intravascular coagulation during remission induction of adult patients with acute lymphoblastic leukemia. Blood 79:1305, 1992

94. Andoh K, Kubota T, Takada M et al: Tissue factor activity in leukemic cells. Special reference to disseminated intravascular coagulation. Cancer 59:748, 1987

95. Falanga A, Alessio M, Donati M, Barbui T: A new procoagulant in acute leukemia. Blood 71:870, 1988

96. Cozzolino F, Torcia M, Miliani A et al: Potential role of interleukin-1 as the trigger for diffuse intravascular coagulation in acute nonlymphoblastic leukemia. Am J Med 84:240, 1988

97. Wilson EL, Jacobs P, Dowdle E: The secretion of plasminogen activators by human myeloid leukemic cells in vitro. Blood 61:568, 1983

98. Bennett B, Booth N, Croll A, Dawson A: The bleeding disorder in acute promyelocytic leukaemia: fibrinolysis due to u-PA rather than defibrination. Br J Haematol 71:511, 1988

99. Eckhardt T, Koch M: Fibrinogen-proteolysis in acute myelogenous leukemia. Blut 53:39, 1986

100. Collins A, Bloomfield C, Peterson B et al: Acute promyelocytic leukemia. Management of the coagulopathy during daunorubicin-prednisone remission induction. Arch Intern Med 138:1677, 1978

101. Schwartz B, Williams E, Conlan M, Mosher D: Epsilon-aminocaproic acid in the treatment of patients with acute promyelocytic leukemia and acquired alpha-2-plasmin inihbitor deficiency. Ann Intern Med 105:8732, 1986

102. Tallman MS, Kwaan HC: Reassessing the hemostatic disorder associated with acute promyelocytic leukemia. Blood 79:543, 1992

103. Velasco F, Torres A, Andres P et al: Changes in plasma levels of protease and fibrinolytic inhibitors induced by treatment in acute myeloid leukemia. Thromb Haemost 52:81, 1984

104. Hoyle C, Swirsky D, Freedman L, Hayhoe F: Beneficial effect of heparin in the management of patients with APL. Br J Haematol 68:283, 1988

105. Avvisati G, ten Cate J, Büller H, Madelli F: Tranexamic acid for control of haemorrhage in acute promyelocytic leukaemia. Lancet 2:122, 1989

106. Goldberg M, Ginsburg D, Mayer R et al: Is heparin necessary during induction chemotherapy for patients with acute promyelocytic leukemia? Blood 69:187, 1987

107. Mukaiyama H, Shionoya S, Ikezawa T et al: Abdominal aortic aneurysm complicated with chronic disseminated intravascular coagulopathy: a case of surgical treatment. J Vasc Sug 6:600, 1987

108. Neidhart J, Roach R: Successful treatment of skeletal hemangioma and Kasabach-Merritt syndrome with aminocaproic acid. Am J Med 73:434, 1982

109. Warrell R, Kempin S: Treatment of severe coagulopathy in the Kasabach-Merritt syndrome with aminocaproic acid and cryoprecipitate. N Engl J Med 313:309, 1985

110. Bick R: Hereditary hemorrhagic telangiectasia and disseminated intravascular coagulation: a new clinical syndrome. Ann NY Acad Sci 370:851, 1981

111. McIlraith DM, Mant M, Brien W: Chronic consumptive coagulopathy due to intracardiac thrombus. Am J Med 82:135, 1987

112. Bick R: Disseminated Intravascular Coagulation and Related Syndromes. CRC Press, Boca Raton, FL, 1983

113. Porte RJ, Knot EAR, Bontempo FA: Hemostasis in liver transplantation. Gastroenterology 97:488, 1989

114. Bone R, Francis F, Pierce A: Intravascular coagulation associated with the adult respiratory distress syndrome. Am J Med 61:585, 1976

115. Fowler A, Hamman R, Good J et al: Adult respiratory distress syndrome: risk with common predispositions. Ann Intern Med 98:593, 1983

116. Hathaway W, Mull M, Pechet G: Disseminated intravascular coagulation in the newborn. Pediatrics 43:233, 1969

117. Gross S, Filston H, Anderson J: Controlled study of treatment for disseminated intravascular coagulation in the neonate. J Pediatr 100:445, 1982

118. Bell R, Coalson J, Smith J, Johanson W: Multiple organ system failure and infection in adult respiratory distress syndrome. Ann Intern Med 99:293, 1983

119. Hardaway RM: Disseminated intravascular coagulation as a possible cause of acute respiratory failure. Surg Gynecol Obstet 137:419, 1973

120. Saldeen T: The microembolism syndrome. Microvasc Res 11:227, 1976

121. Seeger W, Neuhof H, Hall J, Roka L: Pulmonary vasoconstrictor response to soluble fibrin in isolated lungs: possible role of thromboxane generation. Circ Res 62:651, 1988

122. Malik A, Horgan M: Mechanisms of thrombin-induced lung vascular injury and edema. Am Rev Respir Dis 138:467, 1987

123. Luterman A, Manwaring D, Curreri PW: The role of fibrinogen degradation products in the pathogenesis of the respiratory distress syndrome. Surgery 82:703, 1977

124. Johnson A, Tahamont M, Malik A: Thrombin-induced lung vascular injury. Roles of fibrinogen and fibrinolysis. Am Rev Respir Dis 128:38, 1983

125. Idell S, Gonzalez K, Bradford H et al: Procoagulant activity in bronchoalveolar lavage in the adult respiratory distress syndrome. Contribution of tissue factor associated with factor VII. Am Rev Respir Dis 136:1466, 1987

126. Quinn D, Carvalho A, Geller E te al: 99 mTc-fibrinogen scanning in adult respiratory distress syndrome. Am Rev Respir Dis 135:100, 1987

127. Greene R, Zapol W, Snider M et al: Early bedside detection of pulmonary vascular occlusion during acute respiratory failure. Am Rev Respir Dis 124: 593, 1981

128. Rinaldo JE, Rogers RM: Adult respiratory-distress syndrome. Changing concepts of lung injury and repair. N Engl J Med 306:900, 1982

129. Butler J, Parker D, Pillai R et al: Systemic release of neutrophil elastase and tumor necrosis factor alpha following ABO incompatible blood transfusion. Br J Haematol 78:525, 1991

130. Goldfinger D: Acute hemolytic transfusion reactions—a fresh look at pathogenesis and considerations regarding therapy. Transfusion 17:85, 1977

131. Clavarella D, Reed R, Counts R et al: Clotting factor levels and the risk of diffuse microvascular bleeding in the massively transfused patient. Br J Haematol 67:165, 1987

132. Markland FS: Inventory of alpha- and beta-fibrinogenases from snake venoms. Thromb Haemost 65:438, 1991

133. Pirkle H, Stocker K: Thrombin-like enzymes from snake venoms: an inventory. Thromb Haemost 444, 1991

134. Lwin M, Phillips R, Pe T et al: Bites by Russell's viper (*Viperia russelli siam-*

ensis) in Burma: haemostatic, vascular, and renal disturbances and response to treatment. Lancet 2:1259, 1985

135. Simon T, Grace T: Envenomation coagulopathy in wounds from pit vipers. N Engl J Med 305:443, 1981

136. Russell FE: The clinical problem of crotalid snake venom poisoning. p. 978. In Lee C-Y (ed): Snake Venoms. Springer-Verlag, New York, 1979

137. Weiss H, Allan S, Davidson E, Kochwa S. Afibrinogenemia in man following the bite of a rattlesnake (*Crotalus adamanteus*). Am J Med 47:625, 1969

138. Kitchens C, Van Mierop L: Mechanism of defibrination in humans after envenomation by the eastern diamondback rattlesnake. Am J Hematol 14:345, 1983

139. Budzynski A, Pandya B, Rubin R et al: Fibrinogenolytic afibrinogenemia after envenomation by western diamondback rattlesnake (*Crotalus atrox*). Blood 63:1, 1984

140. Swe TN, Lwin M, Han KE et al: Heparin therapy in Russell's viper bite victims with disseminated intravascular coagulation: a controlled trial. Southeast Asian J Trop Med Public Health 23:282, 1992

141. Stirling Y, Woolf L, North WRS et al: Haemostasis in normal pregnancy. Thromb Haemost 52:176, 1984

142. de Boer K, ten Cate J, Sturk A et al: Enhanced thrombin generation in normal and hypertensive pregnancy. Am J Obstet Gynecol 160:95, 1989

143. Bremme K, Östlund E, Almqvist I et al: Enhanced thrombin generation and fibrinolytic activity in normal pregnancy and the puerperium. Obstet Gynecol 80:132, 1992

144. Boulton FE, Letsky E: Obstetric haemorrhage: causes and management. Clin Haematol 14:683, 1985

145. Pritchard J, Brekken A: Clinical and laboratory studies on severe abruptio placentae. Am J Obstet Gynecol 97:681, 1967

146. White PF, Coe V, Dworsky WA, Margolis A: Disseminated intravascular coagulation following midtrimester abortions. Anesthesiology 58:99, 1983

147. Romero R, Duffy TP, Berkowitz RL et al: Prolongation of a preterm pregnancy complicated by death of a single twin in utero and disseminated intravascular coagulation. N Engl J Med 310:772, 1984

148. Hatch RL, Barke JI, Barke MW: Coagulopathy associated with dilatation and evacuation for intrauterine fetal death. Obstet Gyncol 66:463, 1985

149. Swingler GR, Bigg MA, Hewitt BG, McNulty CAM: Disseminated intravascular coagulation associated with group A streptococcal infection in pregnancy. Lancet 1:1456, 1988

150. Kaplan M: Acute fatty liver of pregnancy. N Engl J Med 313:367, 1983

151. Minakami H, Oka N, Sato T et al: Preeclampsia: a microvesicular fat disease of the liver? Am J Obstet Gynecol 159:1043, 1988

152. Weinstein L: Syndrome of hemolysis, elevated liver enzymes, and low platelet count: a severe consequence of hypertension in pregnancy. Am J Obstet Gynecol 142:159, 1982

153. Lopez-Llera M, Espinosa M, De Leon M, Linares G: Abnormal coagulation and fibrinolysis in eclampsia. A clinical and laboratory study. Am J Obstet Gynecol 124:681, 1976

154. Saleh A, Bottoms S, Norman G et al: Hemostasis in hypertensive disorders of pregnancy. Obstet Gynecol 71:719, 1988

155. Van Dam P, Renier M, Baekelandt M: Disseminated intravascular coagulation and the syndrome of hemolysis, elevated liver enzymes, and low platelets in severe preeclampsia. Obstet Gynecol 73:97, 1989

156. Liebman H, McGehee W, Patch M, Feinstein D: Severe depression of antithrombin III associated with disseminated intravascular coagulation in women with fatty liver of pregnancy. Ann Intern Med 98:330, 1983

157. Ridolfi R, Bell W: Thrombotic thrombocytopenic purpura. Report of 25 cases and review of the literature. Medicine 60:413, 1981

158. Kaplan B, Proesmans W: The hemolytic uremic syndrome of childhood and its variants. Semin Hematol 24:148, 1987

159. Brain M, Dacie J, Hourihane D: Microangiopathic haemolytic anaemia: the possible role of vascular lesions in pathogenesis. Br J Haematol 8:358, 1962

160. Kelton J, Moore J, Santos A, Sheridan D: Detection of a platelet-agglutinating factor in thrombotic thrombocytopenic purpura. Ann Intern Med 101:589, 1984

161. Brain M, Baker L, McBride J et al: Treatment of patients with microangiopathic haemolytic anaemia with heparin. Br J Haematol 15:603, 1968

162. Dyke C, Sobel M: The management of coagulation problems in the surgical patient. Adv Surg 24:229, 1991

163. Estol CJ, Pessin MS, Martinez AJ: Cerebrovascular complications after orthotopic liver transplantation: a clinicopathologic study. Neurology 41:815, 1991

164. Leveen H, Ahmed N, Hutto R et al: Coagulopathy post Leveen shunt. Ann Surg 205:305, 1987

165. Kucuk O, Kwaan HC, Frederickson J et al: Increased fibrinolytic activity in patients undergoing cardiopulmonary bypass operation. Am J Hematol 23:223, 1986

166. Al-Mondihry H, Pierce WS, Richenbacher W, Bull A: Hemostatic abnormalities associated with prolonged ventricular assist pumping: analysis of 24 patients. Am J Cardiol 53:1344, 1984

167. Woodman RC, Harker LA: Bleeding complications associated with cardiopulmonary bypass. Blood 7:1680, 1990

168. Bachmann F, McKenna R, Cole ER, Najafi H: The hemostatic mechanism after open-heart surgery. I. Studies on plasma coagulation factors and fibrinolysis after extracorporeal circulation. J Thorac Cardiovasc Surg 70:76, 1975

169. Lowe F, Somers W: The use of ketoconazole in the emergency management of disseminated intravascular coagulation due to metastatic prostatic cancer. J Urol 137:1000, 1987

170. Risher RF, Goodpasture HC, Peterie JD, Voth DW: Toxic shock syndrome in menstruating women. Ann Intern Med 94:156, 1981

171. Burns JC, Glode MP, Clarke SH et al: Coagulopathy and platelet activation in Kawasaki syndrome: identification of patients at high risk for development of coronary artery aneurysms. Pediatrics 105:206, 1984

172. Meyer K, Williams EC: Fibrinolysis and acquired alpha-2 plasmin inhibitor deficiency in amyloidosis. Am J Med 79:394, 1985

173. Rosner F, Ritz N: The defibrination syndrome. Arch Intern Med 117:17, 1966

174. Feinstein D: Treatment of disseminated intravascular coagulation. Semin Thromb Hemost 14:351, 1988

175. Fresh-frozen plasma. Indications and risks. NIH consensus conference. JAMA 253:551, 1985

176. Feinstein D: Diagnosis and management of disseminated intravascular coagulation: the role of heparin therapy. Blood 60:284, 1982

177. Charytan C, Purtilio D: Glomerular capillary thrombosis and acute renal failure after epsilon-amino caproic acid therapy. N Engl J Med 280:1102, 1969

178. Rubin RN, Colman RW: Disseminated intravascular coagulation. Approach to treatment. Drugs 44:963, 1992

179. Straub P, Riedler G, Frick P: Hypofibrinogenemia in metastatic carcinoma of the prostate: suppression of systemic fibrinolysis by heparin. J Clin Pathol 20:152, 1967

180. Verstraete M: Clinical applications of inhibitors of fibrinolysis. Drugs 29:237, 1985

181. Imaoka S, Ueda T, Shibata H et al: Fibrinolysis in patients with acute promyelocytic leukemia and disseminated intravascular coagulation during heparin therapy. Cancer 58:1736, 1986

182. Umeki S, Adachi M, Watanabe M et al: Gabexate as a therapy for disseminated intravascular coagulation. Arch Intern Med 148:1409, 1988

183. Imaoka S, Ueda T, Shibata H et al: Fibrinolysis with acute promyelocytic leukemia and disseminated intravascular coagulation during heparin therapy. Cancer 58:1736, 1986

184. Svartholm E, Haglund U, Ljungberg J, Hedner U: Influence of aprotinin, a protease inhibitor, on porcine *E. coli* shock. Studies on coagulation, fibrinolytic and hemodynamic response. Acta Chir Scand 155:7, 1989

185. Mammen E, Miyakawa T, Phillips T et al: Human antithrombin concentrates and experimental disseminated intravascular coagulation. Semin Thromb Hemost 11:373, 1985

186. Redens TB, Emerson TE: Antithrombin-III treatment limits disseminated intravascular coagulation in endotoxemia. Circ Shock 28:49, 1989

187. Schipper H, Jenkins C, Kahle L, Ten Cate J: Antithrombin-III transfusion in disseminated intravascular coagulation. Lancet 1:854, 1978

188. Delshammar M, Lasson A, Nilsson I-M et al: Abnormal proteolysis (DIC)—successful treatment with antithrombin III concentrate and a concentrate containing fXIII and native von Willebrand factor. J Intern Med 225:21, 1989

189. Colman R, Flores D, De La Cadena R et al: Recombinant α-1-antitrypsin Pittsburg attenuates experimental gram-negative septicemia. Am J Pathol 130:418, 1989

190. Greenman RL, Schein RMH, Martin MA et al: A controlled clinical trial of E5 murine monoclonal IgM antibody to endotoxin in the treatment of gram-negative sepsis. JAMA 266:1097, 1991

191. Maruyama I: Therapeutic evaluation of recombinant thrombomodulin. Jpn J Clin Med 50:2561, 1992

192. Day KC, Hoffman LC, Palmier MO et al: Recombinant lipoprotein-associated coagulation inhibitor inhibits tissue thromboplastin-induced intravascular coagulation in the rabbit. Blood 76:1538, 1990

Hemostatic Defects Associated with Dysproteinemias

117

Howard A. Liebman

INTRODUCTION

Acquired coagulation abnormalities are frequently observed in patients with dysproteinemias.[1,2] Most of these patients do not manifest bleeding, and the hemostatic abnormalities are usually detected only on laboratory evaluation. However, 10% of patients have clinical evidence of bleeding.[3,4] In most cases, bleeding is mild, consisting of purpura, epistaxis, or hematuria. However, occasional severe bleeding and fatal hemorrhages are observed. The reported hemostatic abnormalities are varied and involve both coagulation and platelet dysfunction.

The pathophysiologic mechanism responsible for these coagulation defects is an abnormal interaction between a hemostatic component and a plasma paraprotein (Fig. 117-1). Paraproteins are monoclonal immunoglobulins associated with plasma cell dyscrasias and lymphoid neoplasms, such as multiple myeloma, plasma cell leukemia, Waldenström's macroglobulinemia, lymphoma, and primary (AL) amyloidosis. The circulating paraprotein may consist of the complete immunoglobulin, the immunoglobulin light chain, or other immunoglobulin fragments. The abnormal immunoglobulin does not have to be present in high concentrations in the circulation but can be expressed on the surface of the malignant lymphocyte or deposited in the extracellular matrix. The serendipitous synthesis of an immunoglobulin by the malignant lymphocyte that possesses a structure that binds with a component of the platelet surface or coagulation proteins can lead to inhibition of function or to accelerated clearance of the platelet or coagulation protein.

The hemostatic defects associated with dysproteinemias include (1) coagulation abnormalities that result from plasma paraproteins that bind hemostatic components and inhibit their function; (2) abnormalities secondary to the increased clearance of coagulation proteins by forming complexes with circulating paraproteins, binding to cell-surface immunoglobulins or binding to immunoglobulin fragments deposited in the extracellular matrix; and (3) hemostatic abnormalities observed in association with dysproteinemias for which no clear pathophysiologic mechanism linking the paraprotein and the hemostatic defect can be found.

HEMOSTASIS INHIBITORS

A prolonged bleeding time with a normal or a moderately decreased platelet count is a common hemostatic defect in dysproteinemias.[5-9] In a prospective study of coagulation abnormalities associated with dysproteinemias, 45% of patients had an abnormal bleeding time.[2] In patients who hemorrhaged, a prolonged bleeding time was observed in 67%. An abnormal bleeding time was also observed in one-third of patients who did not exhibit bleeding.

The prolonged bleeding time in these patients is associated with abnormalities of in vitro platelet function. Abnormalities include decreased platelet adhesiveness,[2,10,11] impaired platelet aggregation,[7,9,10] and reduced platelet factor 3 availability.[9-11] Abnormal platelet function studies are more frequent with higher concentrations of the paraprotein and with increased plasma viscosity. A paraprotein concentration of >5 g/dl is frequently associated with defective platelet function.

Several investigators have studied the effect of purified paraproteins on platelet function.[9,11] Depressed platelet function was observed after the addition of the paraprotein to normal platelet-rich plasma. The resulting defects have been attributed to the nonspecific adsorption of the paraprotein to the platelet surface, resulting in defective platelet surface function.

A severe hemorrhagic disorder due to the development of a thrombasthenic-like platelet defect has also been reported.[12] This patient exhibited high-affinity binding of the monoclonal paraprotein to glycoprotein IIIa on the platelet surface. The immunoglobulin completely inhibited platelet aggregation by preventing fibrinogen binding to the platelet surface.

Since markedly elevated plasma concentrations of paraproteins are more commonly associated with defective platelet function, plasmapheresis has been used in the treatment of hemorrhage.[2,7,9,10,13] No clinical signs or laboratory assays are predictive of the response to plasmapheresis. However, resolution of bleeding has been reported in some cases.

Most patients have other coagulation assay abnormalities in addition to an abnormal bleeding time.[2] Approximately 50% of patients with multiple myeloma and macroglobulinemia have a prolonged thrombin time (TT),[2] associated with the appearance of an abnormal fibrin clot.[5,10,14-20] Transparent gelatin-like fibrin clots formed in the presence of the paraprotein display poor retraction. Electron microscopic studies of fibrin clots from these patients show a structure that is poorly branched with narrowed fibrin strands.[10,20]

The effect of paraproteins on fibrinogen cleavage and fibrin clot formation has been studied extensively. Early investigators suggested that the prolonged TT resulted from paraprotein inhibition of thrombin cleavage of fibrinogen.[14-17] Early reports referred to these paraproteins as antithrombin V.[15,16] However, subsequent studies have failed to demonstrate antithrombin activity.[10,18,20]

Inhibition of fibrin polymerization by the paraprotein accounts for the prolonged TT and abnormal clot formation.[18-23] Studies using purified monoclonal immunoglobulins have shown that these proteins inhibit polymerization of fibrin monomer. Paraproteins of all immunoglobulin subtypes can inhibit polymerization.[21] Using proteolytic immunoglobulin fragments, the inhibitory activity is found to reside on the $F(ab')_2$ or Fab portions of the molecule.[19,21,23] This finding would suggest that the antigen-binding domain of the monoclonal immunoglobulin may be responsible for fibrin/fibrinogen binding. However, direct binding of the inhibitory immunoglobulins to fibrin or fibrinogen has not been demonstrated under the conditions employed.[10,22,23] Therefore, the inhibitory

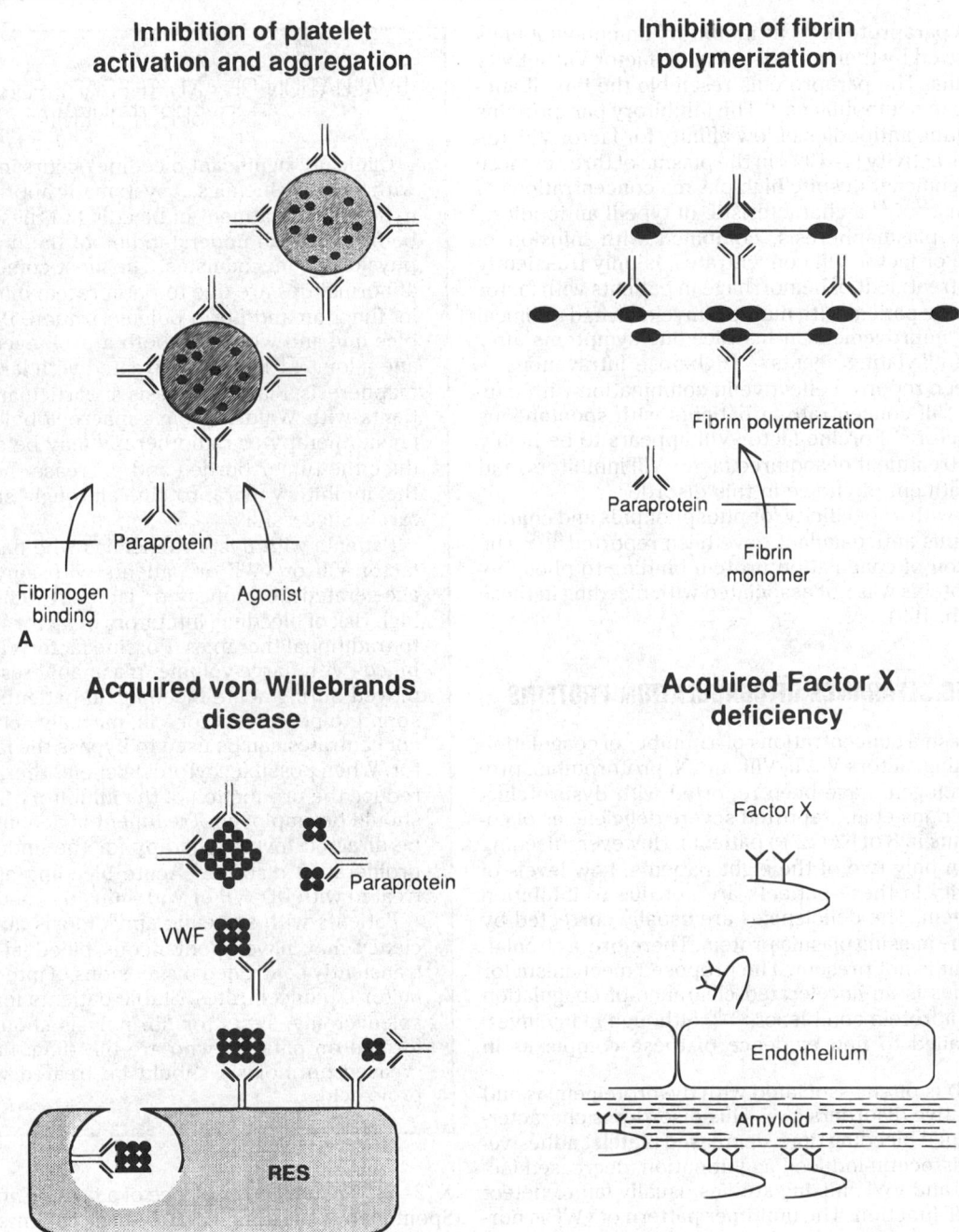

Fig. 117-1. Schematic representation of the pathophysiologic mechanisms responsible for hemostatic abnormalities in patients with dysproteinemias. **(A)** Paraproteins bind to platelets or to fibrinogen/fibrin and inhibit their function. **(B)** Circulating paraproteins bind to von Willebrand protein (vWF), resulting in increased clearance by the reticulendothelial system (RES). Factor X is rapidly cleared from plasma by binding to paraproteins deposited in the subendothelium as amyloid.

immunoglobulins and fibrin may exhibit low-affinity interactions, and not typical antigen-antibody interactions.

Despite the abnormal TT, bleeding is rarely observed in patients with inhibitors of fibrin polymerization. In patients who hemorrhage, other associated hemostatic defects are usually observed. Abnormalities of platelet function are frequently present. Large-volume plasmapheresis has been effective in controlling hemorrhage in selected patients.[6,9,10,13] Fibrinogen, given as fresh frozen plasma or cryoprecipitate, is not helpful. In fact, most patients have elevated plasma fibrinogen concentrations.[24]

Circulating paraproteins that inhibit the function of von Willebrand factor (vWF)[25,26] and factor VIII[28-31] have been de-scribed. Unlike the inhibitors that interfere with fibrin polymerization, these inhibitors are associated with clinical bleeding syndromes. Two patients with IgG multiple myeloma had circulating paraproteins that inhibited ristocetin-induced platelet agglutination and decreased platelet adhesiveness.[25,26] These paraproteins bound vWF when studied by crossed immunoelectrophoresis. Unlike patients with acquired von Willebrand disease (vWD), both patients had increased plasma von Willebrand antigen and normal factor VIII activity.

Four patients with paraproteins that inhibit factor VIII coagulant activity have been reported. The patients had IgA multiple myeloma,[27] Waldenström's macroglobulinemia,[28] chronic lymphocytic leukemia with an IgM paraprotein,[29] and amyloidosis with an IgA paraprotein.[30] The inhibitory immunoglobulins were characterized by their ability to inhibit factor VIII activity in normal plasma. The paraproteins resemble the type II antibody inhibitors in hemophiliacs.[31] The inhibitory paraproteins were slow-reacting antibodies of low affinity for factor VIII. Residual factor VIII activity (7–10%) in the plasma of three of these patients was significant despite high plasma concentrations of the paraproteins,[27,28,30] a characteristic of type II antibodies.

Large-volume plasmapheresis, combined with infusion of cryoprecipitate or factor VIII concentrates, is only transiently effective in the treatment of hemorrhage in patients with factor VIII inhibitors. One patient with multiple myeloma had a clinical remission with improvement in his bleeding symptoms after treatment with alkylating agents.[27] High-dose intravenous γ-globulin has been reported effective in combination with infusions of factor VIII concentrate in patients with spontaneous inhibitors to factor.[32] Porcine factor VIII appears to be highly effective in the treatment of acquired factor VIII inhibitors, and may be the treatment of choice in this disorder.[33]

Paraproteins with a specificity for phospholipids and characteristics of a lupus anticoagulant have been reported.[34,35] The in vitro inhibition of coagulation protein binding to phospholipid by paraproteins was not associated with bleeding in these patients (see Ch. 109).

ACCELERATED CLEARANCE OF COAGULATION PROTEINS

Decreased plasma concentrations of a number of coagulation proteins, including factors V, VII, VIII, and X, prothrombin, protein C, and fibrinogen, have been reported with dysproteinemias.[2,24,36–38] Perkins et al.[2] reported severe deficiencies of coagulation proteins in 8 of 62 (12%) patients. However, bleeding was observed in only two of the eight patients. Low levels of coagulant activity in these patients are not due to inhibition by the paraprotein. The deficiencies are usually corrected by transfusion of the missing plasma protein. Therefore, a circulating anticoagulant is not present. The proposed mechanism for these deficiencies is an accelerated clearance of coagulation protein and paraprotein complexes,[36–38] although many investigators have failed to find evidence of these complexes in plasma.[2,11]

Acquired vWD is often associated with dysproteinemias and lymphoproliferative disorders.[39–45] This disorder is characterized by a prolonged bleeding time, decreased platelet adhesiveness, reduced ristocetin-induced agglutination, decreased factor VIII activity, and vWF. Mixing studies usually fail to detect inhibition of vWF function. The multimer pattern of vWF is normal, although the concentration of all multimers is decreased.[45]

Patients treated with infusions of cryoprecipitate have an appropriate rise in plasma von Willebrand antigen and factor VIII activity.[40,41,43] No secondary postinfusion rise of factor VIII activity occurs, as seen in congenital vWD.[40,43] A rapid clearance of the von Willebrand protein, necessary for stabilization of plasma factor VIII, accounts for this loss of the secondary rise in factor VIII coagulant activity. Patients treated with deamino-D-arginin vasopressin (DDAVP) have an appropriate rise in vWF antigen and activity, followed by an accelerated disappearance of the protein from plasma.[44,45]

Brody et al.[42] reported on a patient with Waldenström's macroglobulinemia and acquired vWD who achieved a remission of his bleeding disorder after splenectomy. Immunofluorescence of the patient's malignant lymphocytes demonstrated surface-bound vWF. Brody and co-workers proposed that vWF preferentially bound the monomeric IgM on the surface of the malignant cell.

More than 40 patients with systemic amyloidosis have been reported with an acquired deficiency in factor X.[46–52] This disorder is characterized by variable deficiencies in plasma factor

---

EVALUATION OF AND THERAPY FOR BLEEDING IN DYSPROTEINEMIAS

Clinically significant bleeding occurs in 10% of patients with dysproteinemias. A systematic approach to the evaluation and treatment of bleeding in these patients must be based on an understanding of the underlying pathophysiologic mechanisms. The most common hemostatic abnormalities are due to paraprotein inhibitors of platelet function and fibrin polymerization. Patients who are bleeding and who have both a prolonged bleeding time and a long TT should be treated with large-volume plasmapheresis. Plasmapheresis is particularly helpful in patients with Waldenström's macroglobulemia. Cytotoxic chemotherapy or radiotherapy may be employed to reduce the tumor burden and decrease the production of the inhibitory paraprotein, although such therapy is rarely successful.

Patients with dysproteinemias who have inhibitors of factor VIII or vWF or patients with amyloid who have accelerated fibrinolysis or factor X deficiency are at a high risk of bleeding. Inhibitors of factor VIII are resistant to traditional therapies. Porcine factor VIII alone or combined with large-volume plasmapheresis can be employed during acute bleeding. In patients who fail to respond to porcine factor VIII, partially activated factor IX concentrates can be used to bypass the factor VIII inhibitor. When possible, cytotoxic chemotherapy designed to reduce the production of the inhibitory immunoglobulin should be employed. Treatment of acquired vWD should be directed toward therapy for the underlying lymphoproliferative disorder. Acute bleeding episodes can be treated with DDAVP or with infusions of cryoprecipitate.

Patients with systemic amyloidosis and factor X deficiency may have spontaneous bleeding, which is only transiently controlled by infusions of intermediate-purity factor IX concentrates. Stable patients may benefit from splenectomy. Tests for fibrinolysis should also be performed on patients who are bleeding. Patients with increased fibrinolysis should be treated with ε-aminocaproic acid.

X (2–50%) and by no evidence of a factor X inhibitor in plasma. Spontaneous bleeding can occur in patients with severe deficiencies (<10 percent) and occasionally precedes the diagnosis of amyloidosis. The clinical course and survival of these patients are variable. Although death usually results from progressive amyloidosis, fatal hemorrhages do occur.

Infusion of large volumes of plasma or factor IX concentrates results in only transient elevations of factor X. Howell[47] proposed that the factor X deficiency results from factor X binding to amyloid deposits. Furie et al.[52] demonstrated rapid clearance of infused ^{131}I-labeled factor X from the circulation of a patient with this disorder. The disappearance half-time was <30 seconds compared with a half-time of 1.5–3 hours in normal subjects. Total-body scans of the patient showed diffuse uptake of radioactivity, but the highest concentrations were seen over the involved liver and spleen. In fact, remissions in factor X deficiency were observed in two patients following splenectomy.[53,54] Extensive amyloid involvement of the spleen is observed in only 9% of patients with primary amyloidosis but is reported in 40% of patients with acquired factor X deficiency.[51] Therefore, an enlarged spleen infiltrated with amyloid may be a major site for factor X clearance.[53–55] While chemotherapy is usually ineffective in the treatment of systemic amyloidosis, a remission of acquired factor X deficiency was reported in one patient treated with melphalan and prednisone.[56]

Using a method of quantitative affinity chromatography, factor X has been shown to bind to amyloid fibrils.[57] No difference in factor X binding to fibrils taken from patients with or without factor X deficiency was found in this study. Factor IX and prothrombin bound the fibrils to a lesser extent. Combined deficiencies of other vitamin K-dependent proteins along with factor X have been reported with amyloidosis.[53,54,58] Also, patients may have decreased functional activity of their residual plasma factor X,[55,59] the etiology of which is unclear.

HEMOSTATIC DEFECTS UNRELATED TO PARAPROTEINEMIA

Patients with multiple myeloma and plasma cell dyscrasias may have a bleeding disorder secondary to a heparin-like anticoagulant.[60-63] Affected patients have a markedly prolonged TT that can be corrected by the addition of protamine sulfate or platelet factor 4. The anticoagulant is an effective cofactor for the inhibition of thrombin in assays using the purified antithrombin III and is destroyed by treatment with heparinase. Continuous infusion of protamine sulfate successfully controlled bleeding in one patient.[63]

A prolonged TT is the most frequent hemostatic assay abnormality observed in patients with AL-type amyloidosis.[64] The presence of a plasma inhibitor of both the thrombin time and reptilase assays has been described in a number of patients with AL amyloid.[65] However, the presence of this inhibitor does not appear to be associated with an increased risk of bleeding.[64,65]

A syndrome of pathologic and excessive fibrinolysis has been reported in 12 patients with systemic amyloidosis.[66-72] All patients had a bleeding diathesis characterized by increased fibrinolytic activity documented by a shortened euglobulin clot lysis test, whole blood lysis time, or positive fibrin plate assay. Fibrinogen levels were moderately reduced and fibrin/fibrinogen degradation products were elevated; no evidence of intravascular coagulation was found. The pathophysiology of this disorder remains unclear. Patients have decreased plasma concentration of α_2-antiplasmin inhibitor,[69] but this is secondary to complex formation with plasmin.[70] Abnormalities have been reported with increased tissue plasminogen activator activity[70] and decreased plasminogen activator inhibitor activity. Elevated plasma urokinase-type activity has been reported in two patients with this disorder.[71,72] Increased fibrinolytic activity in one patient was associated with elevated plasma levels of single-chain urokinase plasminogen activator.[72] Treatment with ε-aminocaproic acid effectively controlled bleeding in 10 patients.

REFERENCES

1. Lackner H: Hemostatic abnormalities associated with dysproteinemias. Semin Hematol 10:125, 1973
2. Perkins HA, MacKenzie MR, Fudenberg HH: Hemostatic defects in dysproteinemias. Blood 35:695, 1970
3. Bayrd ED, Heck FJ: Multiple myeloma. A review of 83 proved cases. JAMA 133:147, 1947
4. Cohen RJ, Bohannon RA, Wallerstein RO: Waldenström's macroglobulinemia. A study of ten cases. Am J Med 41:274, 1966
5. Frick PG: Inhibition of conversion of fibrinogen to fibrin by abnormal proteins in multiple myeloma. Am J Clin Pathol 25:1263, 1955
6. Borchgrevink CF: Platelet adhesion in vivo in patients with bleeding disorders. Acta Med Scand 170:231, 1961
7. Vigliano EM, Horowitz HL: Bleeding syndrome in a patient with IgA myeloma: interaction of protein and connective tissue. Blood 29:823, 1967
8. Nilehn J-E, Nilsson IM: Coagulation studies in different types of myeloma. Acta Med Scand, suppl. 445. 179:194, 1966
9. Penny R, Castaldi PA, Whitsed HM: Inflammation and haemostasis in paraproteinaemias. Br J Haematol 20:35, 1971

10. Cohen I, Amir J, Ben-Shaul Y et al: Plasma cell myeloma associated with an unusual myeloma protein causing impairment of fibrin aggregation and platelet function in a patient with multiple malignancy. Am J Med 48:766, 1970
11. Pachter MR, Basinski DH: The effect of macroglobulins and their dissociation units on release of platelet factor 3. Thromb Haemost 3:501, 1959
12. DiMinno G, Coraggio F, Cerbone A et al: A myeloma paraprotein with specificity for platelet glycoprotein IIIa in a patient with a fatal bleeding disorder. J Clin Invest 77:157, 1986
13. Godal HC, Borchgrevink CF: The effect of plasma pheresis on the hemostatic function in patients with macroglobulinemia Waldenström and multiple myeloma. Scand J Clin Lab Invest, suppl. 84. 17:133, 1965
14. Craddock CG, Adams WS, Figueroa WG: Interference with fibrin formation in multiple myeloma by an unusual protein found in blood and urine. J Lab Clin Med 42:847, 1953
15. Loeliger A, Hers JF: Chronic antithrombinaemia (antithrombin V) with hemorrhagic diathesis in a case of rheumatoid arthritis with hypergammaglobulinemia. Thromb Haemmost 1:499, 1957
16. Verstraete PM, Vermylen C: Recherches sur l'antithrombine V dans la maladie de kahler. Acta Haematol 2:240, 1959
17. Gabriel DA, Carr ME, Cook L, Roberts HR: Spontaneous antithrombin in a patient with benign paraprotein. Am J Hematol 25:85, 1987
18. Glueck HI, Makenzie MR, Glueck CJ: Crystalline IgG protein in multiple myeloma. Identification effects on coagulation and on lipoprotein metabolism. J Lab Clin Med 79:731, 1972
19. Coleman M, Vigliano EM, Weksler ME, Wachman RL: Inhibition of fibrin monomer polymerization by Lambda myeloma globulins. Blood 39:210, 1972
20. Lackner H, Hunt V, Zucker MB, Pearson J: Abnormal fibrin ultrastructure, polymerization and clot retraction in multiple myeloma. Br J Haematol 18:625, 1970
21. Wisloff F, Michaelsen TE, Godal HC: Inhibition or acceleration of fibrin polymerization by monoclonal immunoglobulins and immunoglobulin fragments. Thromb Res 35:81, 1984
22. Gabriel DA, Smith LA, Folds JD et al: The influence of immunoglobulin (IgG) on the assembly of fibrin gels. J Lab Clin Med 101:545. 1983
23. Wisloff F, Michaelsen TE, Kierulf P, Godal HC: The molecular localization of the ability of certain monoclonal immunoglobulins to interfere with fibrin polymerization. Thromb Res 40:473, 1985
24. Sanchez-Avolos J, Soong BCF, Miller SP: Coagulation disorders in multiple myeloma. Cancer 23:1388, 1969
25. Bovill EG, Ershler WB. Golden EA et al: A human myeloma-produced monoclonal protein directed against the active subpopulation of von Willebrand factor. Am J Clin Pathol 85:115, 1985
26. Mohri H, Noguchi T, Hodama F et al: Acquired von Willebrand disease due to inhibitor of human myeloma protein specific for von Willebrand factor. Am J Clin Pathol 87:663, 1987
27. Glueck HI, Hong R: A circulating anticoagulant in IgA-multiple myeloma: its modification by penicillin. J Clin Invest 44:1866, 1965
28. Castaldi PA, Penny R: A macroglobulin with inhibitory activity against coagulation factor VIII. Blood 35:370, 1970
29. Kelsey PR, Leyland MJ: Acquired inhibitor to human factor VIII associated with paraproteinemia and subsequent development of chronic lymphotic leukemia. Br Med J 285:174, 1982
30. Glueck HI, Coots MC, Benson M et al: A monoclonal immunoglobulin A (K) factor VIII: C inhibitor associated with primary amyloidosis: identification and characterization. J Lab Clin Med 113:267, 1989
31. Gawryl MS, Hoyer LW: Inactivation of factor VIII coagulant activity by two different types of human antibodies. Blood 60:1103, 1982
32. Sultan Y, Maisonneuve P, Kazatchkine MD, Nydegger UE: Anti-idiotypic suppression of autoantibodies to factor VIII (antihaemophilic factor) by high-dose intravenous gammaglobulin. Lancet 2:765, 1984
33. Morrison AE, Ludlam CA, Kessler C: Use of porcine factor VIII in the treatment of patients with acquired hemophilia. Blood 81:1513, 1993
34. Thiagarajan P, Shapiro SS, De Marco L: Monoclonal immunoglobulin MX coagulation inhibitor with phospholipid specificity. J Clin Invest 66:397, 1980
35. Goldsmith GH, Saito H, Muir WA: Labile anticoagulant in a patient with lymphoma. Am J Hematol 10:305, 1981
36. Henstell HH, Kligerman M: A new theory of interference with the clotting mechanism: the complexing of euglobulin with factor V, factor VII and prothrombin. Ann Intern Med 49:371, 1958
37. Hurley R, Shaw S: Observation on the haemorrhagic diathesis in multiple myeloma. Postgrad Med J 39:480, 1963
38. Gruber A, Blasko G, Sas G: Functional deficiency of protein C and skin necrosis in multiple myeloma. Thromb Res 42:579, 1986
39. Simone JV, Cornet JA, Abildgaard CF: Acquired von Willebrand's syndrome in systemic lupus erythematosus. Blood 31:806, 1968

40. Mant MJ, Hirsh J, Gauldie J et al: Von Willebrand's syndrome presenting as an acquired bleeding disorder in association with a monoclonal gammopathy. Blood 42:429, 1973
41. Joist JH, Cowan JF, Zimmerman TS: Acquired von Willebrand's disease. Evidence for a quantitative and qualitative factor VIII disorder. N Engl J Med 298:988, 1978
42. Brody KI, Haidar ME, Rossman RE: A hemorrhagic syndrome in Waldenström's macroglobulinemia secondary to immunoadsorption of factor VIII. N Engl J Med 300:408, 1979
43. Handin RI, Martin V, Moloney WC: Antibody-induced von Willebrand's disease: a newly defined inhibitor syndrome. Blood 48:393, 1976
44. Mannucci PM, Lombardi R, Bader R et al: Studies of the pathophysiology of acquired von Willebrand's disease in seven patients with lymphoproliferative disorders or benign monoclonal gammopathies. Blood 64:614, 1984
45. Takahashi H, Nagayama R, Tanabe Y et al: DDAVP in acquired von Willebrand syndrome associated with multiple myeloma. Am J Hematol 22:421, 1986
46. Korsan-Bengtsen K, Hjort PF, Ygge J: Acquired factor X deficiency in a patient with amyloidosis. Thromb Haemost 7:558, 1962
47. Howell M: Acquired factor X deficiency associated with systematized amyloidosis. A report of a case. Blood 21:739, 1963
48. Pechet L, Kastrul J: Amyloidosis associated with factor X (Stuart) deficiency. Case report. Ann Intern Med 61:315, 1964
49. Berhart B, Calletta M, Brook J, Lejnieks I: Amyloidosis with factor X deficiency. Am J Med Sci 264:411, 1972
50. Galbraith PA, Sharma N, Parker WL, Kilgour JM: Acquired factor X deficiency. Altered plasma antithrombin activity and associations with amyloidosis. JAMA 230:1658, 1974
51. Greipp PR, Kyle RA, Bowie EJ: Factor X deficiency in amyloidosis: a critical review. Am J Hematol 11:443, 1981
52. Furie B, Greene E, Furie BC: Syndrome of acquired factor X deficiency and systemic amyloidosis. In vivo studies of the metabolic fate of factor X. N Engl J Med 297:81, 1977
53. Greipp PR, Kyle RA, Bowie EJ: Factor X deficiency in primary amyloidosis. Resolution after splenectomy. N Engl J Med 301:1050, 1979
54. Rosenstein ED, Itzkowitz SH, Penziner AS et al: Resolution of factor X deficiency in primary amyloidosis following splenectomy. Arch Intern Med 143:597, 1983
55. Lucas FV, Fishleder AJ, Becker RC et al: Acquired factor X deficiency in systemic amyloidosis. Cleve Clin J Med 54:399, 1987
56. Camoraino JK, Greipp PR, Bayer GK, Boure EJ: Resolution of acquired factor X deficiency and amyloidosis with melphalan and prednisone therapy. N Engl J Med 316:1133, 1987
57. Furie B, Voo L, McAdam KPW, Furie BC: Mechanism of factor X deficiency in systemic amyloidosis. N Engl J Med 304:817, 1981
58. McPerson RA, Onstad JW, Ugoretz RJ, Wolf PL: Coagulopathy in amyloidosis: combined deficiency of factors IX and X. Am J Hematol 3:225, 1977
59. Fair DS, Edgington TS: Heterogeneity of hereditary and acquired factor X deficiencies by combined immunochemical and functional analysis. Br J Haematol 59:235, 1985
60. Khoory MS, Nesheim ME, Bowie EJW, Mann KG: Circulating heparan sulfate proteoglycan anticoagulant from a patient with a plasma cell disorder. J Clin Invest 65:666, 1981
61. Palmer RN, Rich ME, Rick PD et al: Circulating heparan sulfate anticoagulant in a patient with a fatal bleeding disorder. N Engl J Med 310:1696, 1984
62. Chapman GS, George CB, Donley DL: Heparin-like anticoagulant associated with plasma cell myeloma. Am J Clin Pathol 83:764, 1984
63. Kaufman PA, Gockerman JP, Greenberg CS: Production of a novel anticoagulant by neoplastic plasma cells: report of a case and review of the literature. Am J Med 86:612, 1989
64. Yood RA, Skinner M, Rubinow A et al: Bleeding manifestations in 100 patients with amyloidosis. JAMA 11:443, 1983
65. Gastineau DA, Gerrtz MA, Daniels TM et al: Inhibitor of the thrombin time in systemic amyloidosis: a common coagulation abnormality. Blood 77:2637, 1991
66. Redleaf PD, David RB, Kucinski C et al: Amyloidosis with an unusual bleeding diathesis: observations on the use of epsilon aminocaproic acid. Ann Intern Med 58:347, 1963
67. Millard LG, Rowell NR: Primary amyloidosis and myelomatosis associated with excessive fibrinolytic activity. Br J Dermatol 94:569, 1976
68. Liebman H, Chinowsky M, Valdin J et al: Increased fibrinolysis and amyloidosis. Arch Intern Med 143:678, 1983
69. Myer K, Williams EC: Fibrinolysis and acquired alpha-2-plasmin inhibitor deficiency in amyloidosis. Am J Med 79:394, 1985
70. Takahashi H, Koike T, Yoshida N et al: Excessive fibinolysis in suspected amyloidosis: demonstrations of plasmin-α-2-plasmin inhibitor complex and von Willebrand factor fragment in plasma. Am J Hematol 23:153, 1982
71. Sane DC, Pizzo SV, Greenberg CS: Elevated urokinase-type plasminogen activator level and bleeding in amyloidosis: case report and literature review. Am J Hematol 31:53, 1989
72. Liebman HA, Carfagno MK, Weitz I et al: Excessive fibrinolysis in amyloidosis resulting from elevated plasma single chain urokinase. Am J Clin Pathol 98:534, 1992

Neonatal Hemostatic Disorders

118

Marilyn J. Manco-Johnson and Rachelle Nuss

INTRODUCTION

The unique physiology and developmental changes that occur in the human fetus and newborn infant are reflected in the hemostatic system. An understanding of these findings is a prerequisite to a discussion of the hemorrhagic and thrombotic disorders that occur in the term and preterm infant. Table 118-1 displays the means and lower limits for coagulation factors in normal infants at various gestational ages.[1-3] Many of the proteins, including the vitamin K-dependent proteins, contact factors, antithrombin III (AT III), plasminogen, and factor XIII show a distinct gestational age dependency and often do not approximate normal adult levels until several months after birth. Other plasma proteins are normal (fibrinogen, factor V, α_2-antiplasmin) or increased (factor VIII, von Willebrand factor) relative to adult normal levels. Most of the developmental change is an increase in protein quantity; however, evidence is good that select coagulation proteins change from a distinct fetal form to the adult form. Fetal fibrinogen contains increased sialic acid[4] and phosphorus,[5] resulting in altered migration on two-dimensional isoelectric focusing, and reflected in formation of a more friable clot and prolongation of the thrombin time.

Fetal plasminogen has also been reported to differ in glycosylation.[6] Isolated fetal plasminogen activated by either urokinase or streptokinase has a specific activity of 18% and 12%, respectively, relative to that of the adult molecule.[7,8] Clinically the newborn infant is resistant to fibrinolytic therapy and has required ≤10 times the adult dose.[9] Protein C has been studied in an ovine model, where it shows an increased molecular weight in association with increased carbohydrate content.[10,11] The processing and regulation of the transition from fetal to adult levels and forms is currently unknown. It is possible that delayed transition in infants born prematurely may account for the susceptibility of the preterm infant to hemorrhage and thrombosis.

Fetal von Willebrand factor is comprised of an excess of large molecular weight multimers similar to the pattern reported in thrombotic thrombocytopenic purpura.[12] The larger multimers are associated with increased platelet adhesion and may account for the shorter bleeding time reported in the normal term neonate.[13,14]

Coagulation screening test results in the healthy infant are different from those of adults. Related primarily to low levels of contact system proteins, the partial thromboplastin time (PTT) is prolonged by 2–3 seconds in the term infant and may be more than twice the adult value in the extremely premature infant. On day 1 of life, the prothrombin time (PT) is prolonged by 1 second in the normal term infant and ≤3 seconds in the healthy preterm baby. The PT of well infants prolongs postnatally, with the longest values seen at approximately 3 days of age and normalization by day 5 of life[15]; this physiologic prolongation is not affected by vitamin K administration but is associated with an increase in descarboxy proteins and has been related to a decrease in the activity in hepatic reductase.[16] A prolonged thrombin time (if performed without calcium) reflects fetal fibrinogen; normal values are achieved by 3 weeks of age. The prolonged values are found in healthy infants and vary slightly according to technique and reagents, but are not associated with any bleeding tendency.[17,18]

Platelet number is within the normal adult range from 20 weeks of gestation onward. Platelet aggregation to epinephrine, low-dose ADP, and collagen is slightly decreased, while platelet adhesion, thrombin-induced platelet aggregation, and ristocetin-induced agglutination are normal to increased.[19] The bleeding time is shortened in healthy term and preterm infants.[20,21]

HEREDITARY COAGULATION DISORDERS

Bleeding secondary to severe deficiencies of factors VIII, IX, V, VII, X, and XIII, as well as of prothrombin, fibrinogen, and α_2-antiplasmin may occur in the neonatal period. Affected infants present with ecchymoses, cephalohematomas, umbilical cord stump oozing, and gastrointestinal, abdominal, or intracranial bleeding. Infants may show persistent oozing after routine heel puncture or circumcision. Persistent umbilical cord bleeding is a characteristic of homozygous factor XIII deficiency and should be excluded by laboratory testing. Intracranial bleeding in a term infant should always raise the suspicion of a congenital bleeding disorder, even if family history is unrevealing or if other bleeding manifestations are not seen.[22,23]

When hemophilia is suspected before delivery, efforts should be made to ascertain the diagnosis as soon as possible to guide decisions around labor and delivery. Diagnosis can be made with restriction fragment length polymorphism for most families with factor VIII deficiency (see Ch. 113) and with specific gene probes for factor IX mutations using samples ob-

tained from chorionic villus sampling or amniocentesis.[24] The fetal factor VIII level can be obtained through periumbilical aspiration at 18 weeks. Care must be taken not to contaminate the fetal blood sample with procoagulant amniotic fluid. The physiologic low levels of factor IX in the fetus make interpretation of this test difficult in mild-to-moderate factor IX deficiency. Plans should be made to obtain an umbilical cord blood sample for specific factor assay at delivery and to have a safe transfusion product available for treatment of hemorrhage if necessary.[1] The mode of delivery should be as atraumatic to the infant as possible.

Laboratory tests to establish the diagnosis should always include specific factor assays. Reliance on screening tests, such as the PTT or PT, does not permit a precise diagnosis. Less severe disorders, such as von Willebrand disease or mild deficiencies of factor IX or XI, may be difficult to diagnose during the neonatal period because of overlap with normal infant values; repeat studies at a later date (3–6 months) will usually confirm the diagnosis.

Detailed treatment guidelines for the hemophilias are discussed elsewhere (see Chs. 106 and 108). It is important to use the safest transfusion product available. Only products that have been shown to be free of human immunodeficiency virus, (HIV), hepatitis B, and hepatitis C should be used. In the near future, it is hoped that factor concentrates will also be free of hepatitis A and parvovirus. Coagulation proteins produced by recombinant technology should be used if available. Single donor products (fresh frozen plasma, cryoprecipitate) that have been screened for HIV, hepatitis B, hepatitis C, and cytomegalovirus may be used if safer products are not available.

HEMORRHAGIC DISEASE OF THE NEWBORN

Hemorrhagic disease of the newborn, the bleeding syndromes due to vitamin K deficiency, remains of concern to pediatricians throughout the world.[25] Three syndromes in the newborn and young infant have been described. Early hemorrhagic disease of the newborn presents at or shortly after birth with a bleeding tendency manifested by ecchymoses, bleeding from skin punctures, or intracranial hemorrhage. Frequently a history of maternal use of antibiotics or anticonvulsants can be elicited, although many cases are idiopathic.[26,27] Classic hemorrhagic disease of the newborn usually presents at 2–7 days of age in infants with poor oral intake or exclusive breast feeding.[28] Late hemorrhagic disease of the newborn is a distinct bleeding syndrome occurring in infants 1–3 months of age who are usually exclusively breast fed; associated causes include malabsorption, cholestasis, or liver disease.[29] The usual manifestation of classic hemorrhagic disease of the newborn is severe intracranial hemorrhage.

Infants with hemorrhagic disease of the newborn have low blood levels of vitamin K_1, increased amounts of circulating des-γ-carboxy forms of vitamin K-dependent clotting factors VII, IX, X, prothrombin, protein C, and protein S, as well as prolonged PTs. The diagnosis can be presumptively made if bleeding ceases and the PT shortens within 4–6 hours of intravenous administration of 1 mg of vitamin K. The diagnosis is confirmed by assaying plasma vitamin K as well as des-γ-carboxy forms of vitamin K-dependent clotting factors.[30,31] Because prothrombin circulates with a half-life of 60 hours, evidence of uncarboxylated prothrombin can be sought, even after administration of vitamin K.[32] Most cases of hemorrhagic disease of the newborn occur in infants who have not received vitamin K replacement at birth. The cord blood concentration of vitamin K is approximately 10% that found in maternal plasma, while concentrations of vitamin K in breast milk (1.5 mg/L) are 15% that found in cow's milk. Administration of 10 mg of vitamin K_1/day PO to the mother for 10–14 days prior

Table 118-1. Coagulation Factor Concentrations

Subject	Fibrinogen (mg/dl)	Prothrombin	Favor V	Factor VII	Factor VIII	vWF (Antigen)	Factor IX	Factor X	Factor XI
Fetus (≈20 wk)	96 (40)	0.16 (0.10)	0.70 (0.40)	0.21 (0.12)	0.50 (0.23)	0.65 (0.40)	0.10 (0.05)	0.19 (0.15)	—
Preterm newborn (25–32 wk)	250 (100)	0.32 (0.18)	0.80 (0.43)	0.37 (0.24)	0.75 (0.40)	1.50 (0.90)	0.22 (0.17)	0.38 (0.20)	0.20 (0.12)
Preterm newborn (33–36 wk)	300 (120)	0.45 (0.26)	0.82 (0.48)	0.59 (0.34)	0.93 (0.54)	1.66 (1.35)	0.41 (0.20)	0.44 (0.21)	—
Term newborn (37–41 wk)	240 (150)	0.52 (0.25)	1.00 (0.54)	0.57 (0.35)	1.50 (0.55)	1.60 (0.84)	0.35 (0.15)	0.45 (0.30)	0.42 (0.20)
Older infant (age and level when adult value is approximated)	340 (21 days)	0.97 (45–60 days)	1.00 (1 day)	0.90 (21 days)	0.93 (1–2 days)	1.13 (1 wk)	0.70 (6 mo)	0.55 (6 wk)	0.52 (6 wk)

Abbreviations: Prek, prekallikrein; HMWK, high-molecular-weight kininogen; vWF, von Willebrand factor.

[a] Values (functional activity unless otherwise indicated) are expressed in U/ml compared with normal adult subject reference plasma (100% = 1 U/ml); the mean and a lower limit of range (−2 SD) are shown.

(Adapted from Hathaway and Bonnar,[1] with permission.)

to delivery increases cord blood as well as breast milk concentrations of vitamin K and probably serves as adequate prophylaxis to the infant.[33,34] The need for continued postnatal vitamin K supplementation of breast-feeding mothers is currently unknown. Alternatively, the administration of 1 mg IM of vitamin K to the newborn prevents early, classic, and late hemorrhagic disease of the newborn in most infants.[35] Oral vitamin K administration to the newborn is probably effective if repeated weekly or at least every 2 weeks for the first 6 weeks of life. In a preliminary report, intramuscular administration of neonatal vitamin K prophylaxis was associated with a twofold risk of childhood cancer.[36] The high concentrations of vitamin K achieved with parenteral administration may be mutagenic in the neonate. However, two studies failed to confirm any danger of parenteral vitamin K.[37,38] Because 1 mg IM of vitamin K appears to be effective, this remains the current standard recommended by the American Academy of Pediatrics.[39]

LIVER DISEASE

The coagulopathy of severe liver disease is complex and includes consumption of clotting factors and platelets (due to tissue necrosis, endothelial cell damage, disseminated intravascular coagulation (DIC), increased fibrinolysis, and hypersplenism) as well as failure to synthesize procoagulant and anticoagulant proteins. Severe hepatic disease is seen in neonates with viral hepatitis, fetal hydrops due to erythroblastosis fetalis (Rh incompatibility), shock liver (after severe asphyxia), metabolic disorders (including hereditary fructose intolerance, tyrosinemia, and galactosemia), cirrhosis due to α_1-antitrypsin deficiency or cystic fibrosis, and cholestatic jaundice. Bleeding, especially related to surgery, may be severe. Laboratory tests assessing the severity and mechanism of coagulopathy include platelet count, bleeding time, fibrinogen, PT, thrombin time, fibrin degradation products, and D dimer. Specific assays that may guide therapy include factor V, factor VII and AT III.

Treatment for clinical bleeding or preparation for liver biopsy consists of replacement infusions of fresh frozen plasma, cryoprecipitate, and platelet concentrates. In severe cases, all of these agents may be needed to achieve hemostasis. Alternatively, exchange transfusions followed by platelet concentrates can be used to obtain hemostasis. After aggressive replacement, low-dose heparin may be given to retard consumption of coagulation factors, especially while preparing for definitive therapy such as liver transplantation. AT III concentrate is available for infusion into severely deficient infants to prevent thrombosis of central lines or vascular grafts.

THROMBOCYTOPENIA

Thrombocytopenia is commonly seen during the neonatal period, especially in infants admitted to a neonatal intensive care unit.[40] Although many etiologies have been determined for neonatal thrombocytopenia (Table 118-2), the vast majority of infants have thrombocytopenia due to conditions associated with increased destruction of circulating platelets. These conditions include bacterial and viral infection, pulmonary syndromes (infant respiratory distress syndrome, meconium and amniotic fluid aspiration, pneumonia, and pulmonary hypertension), DIC, localized intravascular consumptive coagulopathies (such as necrotizing enterocolitis, hemangiomas, placental chorangiomas, large vessel thrombosis, and hemangiomas), complicated heart lesions, hyperviscosity, and intrauterine growth retardation. Treatment of the thrombocytopenia is related to management of the underlying disease. Sick, thrombocytopenic infants, especially preterm infants, are vulnerable to intracranial hemorrhage and should be supported with platelet transfusions to maintain a platelet count >30,000/mm³. Efforts should be made to maintain a platelet count of >50,000/mm³ for sick infants undergoing surgery or invasive procedures.

Not infrequently, preterm infants in the recovery stage of respiratory distress syndrome manifest persistent or recurrent thrombocytopenia. Recent evidence shows that the lung is an

---

PREVENTION OF HEMORRHAGIC DISEASE OF THE NEWBORN

1. High-risk mother (mothers receiving antibiotics, anticonvulsants, or warfarin): Vitamin K_1 (10 mg/day PO) for 2 weeks prior to delivery. The baby should receive vitamin K_1 1 mg parenterally as soon as possible after birth or 2 mg PO at birth, 1 week, and 2–4 weeks later. (The American Academy of Pediatrics' current recommendation is for parenteral administration of vitamin K.)
2. Normal pregnancy and delivery: The baby should receive vitamin K_1 1 mg IM as soon as possible after birth or 2 mg PO at birth, 1 week, and 2–4 weeks later.

for the Fetus and Newborn Infants[a]

Factor XII	Prek	HMWK	Factor XIII	Plasminogen	α_2-Antiplasmin	AT III	Protein C (Antigen)	Protein S (Antigen)	Heparin Cofactor II
—	—	—	≈0.30	—	—	0.23	0.10	0.38	0.3
						(0.12)	(0.06)	(0.17)	(0.18)
0.22	0.26	0.28	0.11–0.40	0.35	0.74	0.35	0.29	0.48	—
(0.09)	(0.14)	(0.20)		(0.20)	(≈.50)	(0.20)	(0.21)	(0.27)	
0.25	0.33	0.40	—	0.38	0.73	0.40	0.38	0.26	0.29
(0.09)	(0.23)	(0.10)		(0.26)	(≈.50)	(0.25)	(0.23)	(0.14)	(0.07)
0.44	0.35	0.64	0.61	0.49	0.83	0.56	0.50	0.37	0.49
(0.16)	(0.16)	(0.50)	(0.36)	(0.25)	(≈65)	(0.32)	(0.30)	(0.10)	(0.36)
1.00	0.86	0.82	1.0	1.00	1.0	0.82	0.82	0.80	96
(14 d)	(6 mo)	(6 mo)	(1 mo)	(6 mo)	(1 wk)	(3–6 mo)	(24 mo)	(6 mo)	(6 mo)

Table 118-2. Causes of Neonatal Thrombocytopenia

Infection
  Bacterial: sepsis, congenital syphilis
  Viral: cytomegalovirus, herpes simplex virus, rubella syndrome, enterovirus, HIV
  Other: toxoplasmosis

Immune disorders
  Alloimmunization (NAIT)
  Maternal antibody induced: SLE, ITP

Pulmonary syndromes
  Respiratory distress syndrome
  Meconium and amniotic fluid aspiration
  Pneumonia
  Pulmonary hypertension

Intravascular coagulation syndromes
  DIC
  Major vessel thrombosis: renal vein, aorta
  Necrotizing enterocolitis
  Placental chorangioma
  Chorionic vessel thrombosis

Excessive peripheral utilization
  Giant hemangioma
  Hyperviscosity syndrome
  Erythroblastosis fetalis
  Congenital heart disease

Bone marrow abnormality
  Congential megakaryocytic hypoplasia
  Absent radii (TAR) syndrome
  Phocomelia syndrome
  Fanconi's pancytopenia
  Aplastic anemia
  Trisomy syndromes
  Osteopetrosis
  Congenital leukemia

Sex-linked: Wiskott-Aldrich syndrome and variants

Autosomal recessive: associated with renal diseases and deafness

Autosomal dominant: May-Hegglin anomaly

Other causes
  Postexchange transfusion
  Maternal hyperthyroidism
  Metabolic disorders: hyperglycinemia, cirrhosis, mucolipidosis
  Thrombotic thrombocytopenia purpura
  Postmature and SGA infants (often with maternal hypertension)
  Neonatal neuroblastoma
  Neonatal cold injury

Abbreviations: SLE, systemic lupus erythematosus; ITP, idiopathic thrombocytopenic purpura; TAR, thrombocytopenia with absent radii, SGA, small-for-gestational age.

(Adapted from Hathaway and Bonnar,[1] with permission.)

---

important site of megakaryocytopoiesis.[41] Impaired platelet production secondary to megakaryocyte damage in addition to nutritional deficiencies often aggravates increased platelet destruction in these infants. Often, recurrent thrombocytopenia is the presenting sign of large-vessel thrombosis (particularly catheter-related), bowel ischemia, or incipient sepsis in a preterm infant. The evaluation of thrombocytopenia in a preterm infant should include ultrasound evaluation of the central vessels for thrombosis as well as appropriate bacterial and viral cultures.

Thrombocytopenia in otherwise well term infants is frequently immune mediated. Since the classic paper of Pearson et al.,[42] neonatal alloimmune thrombocytopenia (NAIT) has been recognized with increasing frequency and clinical concern. NAIT is caused by fetomaternal incompatibility for platelet-specific antigens, usually PL^A1 (Zwa).[43,44] Eighty-five percent of whites are PL^A1 positive, and 2% are homozygous for PL^A2. Other platelet antigens may also be involved in NAIT. PLA^5b (BAKa) accounts for 19% of NAIT and is most prevalent among persons of Asian extraction.[45] Other platelet antigens (Pen and Yuk) account for a smaller number of affected neonates. Recent studies suggest the incidence of NAIT is 1 in 1,000–2,000 newborn babies[43]; the first pregnancy is affected in about 50% of cases. NAIT is a serious bleeding disorder with a 25% incidence of intracranial hemorrhage or death. About one-half of the intracranial hemorrhages occur in utero.[46]

The diagnosis of NAIT is made following exclusion of other causes of fetal or neonatal thrombocytopenia. Serologic confirmation should include platelet typing of both parents as well as evidence of maternal antibody directed against paternal platelets; a reference laboratory experienced in evaluation of NAIT should be used for diagnostic studies. Fetal platelet count can be determined using periumbilical vascular sampling by 18 weeks' gestation. Weekly maternal infusions of intravenous γ-globulin in doses of 1 g/kg have been effective in raising the fetal platelet count.[47,48] Also, infusions of washed, pheresed maternal platelets have been given to affected fetuses with good clinical results. Corticosteroids have been used prenatally, but fetal toxicity manifested as oligohydramnios is a concern.[48] When the diagnosis of NAIT is known or highly suspected, the infant should be delivered by cesarean section. After delivery, affected infants may be treated with infusions of PL^A2 platelets (maternal or donor) and/or intravenous γ-globulin 1 g/kg/day given for 1–3 days until the platelet count is >50,000/mm³. The risk of thrombocytopenia in subsequent fetuses is 75–97%.[49]

Autoimmune thrombocytopenia due to passively transferred antibodies from mothers with immune thrombocytopenic purpura or systemic lupus erythematosus may produce varying degrees of thrombocytopenia in the infant.[50] The platelet count

Table 118-3. Coagulation Regulation in the Neonate

Component	Neonatal Functions	Effect on Coagulation
Reticuloendothelial system	Functionally hyposplenic	Delayed clearance of activated coagulation products leading to further activation
Native coagulation inhibitors	↓ AT III ↓ Protein C ↓ Protein S	Diminished capacity to inhibit activated coagulation proteins May promote thrombus formation
Fibrinolysis	↓ Plasminogen ↓ t-PA, normal PAI, slower plasmin generation rates	Decreased response to pharmacologic fibrinolysis Diminished native fibrinolysis in sick infants
Endothelial cells	Largely unknown	Unknown
Production of platelets and synthesis of coagulation proteins	↓ Capacity for compensatory increase in production rate during consumption	Early depletion of platelets and coagulation proteins leading to bleeding complications

Abbreviations: T-PA, tissue plasminogen activator; PAI, plasminogen activator inhibitor.

Table 118-4. Conditions Associated with Neonatal DIC

Obstetric complications
  Abruptio placentae
  Placenta accreta
  Chorioamnionitis
  Fetal demise of one twin
  Pre-eclampsia
  Acute fatty liver of pregnancy
Neonatal infections
  Rubella
  Herpes
  Cytomegalovirus
  Enterovirus
  Systemic candidiasis
  Bacteria, especially gram-negative
Respiratory distress syndrome
Cardiovascular disorders
  Congestive heart failure
  Shock
  Lactic acidosis
  Massive thrombosis
  Placental chorangiomas
  Kasabach-Merritt syndrome (giant hemangioma)
  Rh isoimmunization
  Nonimmune hydrops
Severe liver disease
Severe cold stress

often falls after birth to a nadir on days 1–3. Normal platelet counts are often achieved within 1 or 2 weeks, but ≤4 months may be required for full recovery. In mild cases, no specific treatment is necessary. Infants with symptomatic bleeding or very low platelet counts (<50,000/mm³) may be treated with γ-globulin (1 g/kg/day IV for 1–3 days) or a short course of prednisone (2 mg/kg/day PO) for 1–2 weeks.[47] γ-globulin will produce the most rapid response and should be used for severe bleeding. Platelet transfusions are rarely helpful unless antibody is removed by prior exchange transfusion.

Metabolic, chromosomal, and bone marrow abnormalities causing neonatal thrombocytopenia are rare, but should be evaluated based on appropriate clinical indication (Table 118-2). Many sick neonates are exposed to heparin. A recent report suggested that heparin-induced thrombocytopenia may occur in the neonatal period.[51] This finding has not yet been confirmed.

NEONATAL DISSEMINATED INTRAVASCULAR COAGULATION

DIC is the second most frequent coagulopathy in the neonate after thrombocytopenia (see Ch. 116). Uncontrolled intravascular thrombin generation results when coagulation activation triggered by acidosis, poor perfusion, or endotoxin overwhelms the native regulatory mechanisms. Several components of the neonate's developmentally immature hemostatic system may contribute to the neonate's susceptibility to DIC and are summarized in Table 118-3. Neonatal DIC is associated with a wide variety of conditions (Table 118-4).

Clinically, an infant with DIC manifests poor perfusion, oozing from puncture sites, intracranial, pulmonary, and gastrointestinal hemorrhage, and occasionally large-vessel thrombosis. Characteristic laboratory findings include decreased platelet count, diminished concentrations of fibrinogen, factor V, and factor VIII; increased fibrin degradation products; decreased levels of vitamin K-dependent factors; and a microangiopathic hemolytic anemia. A simple but helpful screening panel includes the platelet count, fibrinogen concentration, D-dimer assay of cross-linked fibrin, and PT. These tests can all be performed on capillary blood specimens and give an estimate of both ongoing activation and bleeding potential. AT III and protein C are often decreased to critical levels (<20% of normal adult levels) and convey a poor prognosis.[52] Other specific factor assays provide confirmatory information but neither increase diagnostic sensitivity nor aid in clinical management.

Therapy for neonatal DIC is primarily directed at reversing the etiologic trigger. Appropriate management with ventilation, intravascular volume support, and antibiotics generally results in normalization of coagulation screening tests within 24–48 hours. Infants with DIC who are actively bleeding should be supported with transfusions to maintain a platelet count of ≥50,000/mm³ and a fibrinogen level ≥100 mg/dl (Table 118-5). Transfusion therapy in babies without bleeding signs may be reserved for a platelet count <20,000/mm³ and a fibrinogen level <50 mg/dl. In infants suffering life-threatening hemorrhage, hemostasis may be achieved more quickly with a two-volume exchange transfusion. Occasionally an infant with DIC manifests large-vessel thrombosis or circulatory impairment caused by diffuse microthrombi, for which low-dose heparin therapy is appropriate. The recent availability of safe (from virus) concentrates of AT III and the anticipated availability of protein C concentrate afford newer, potentially more specific therapy for neonatal DIC. Replacement of AT III has shown promise in one small clinical trial in neonates.[53]

Table 118-5. Therapy for Acquired Hemostatic Defects in the Newborn

Indication	Product	Dosage Guideline
Thrombocytopenia	Platelet concentrate	10 ml/kg will raise platelet count by 75–100 × 10³/mm³
Coagulopathy (DIC, liver disease)	Fresh frozen plasma	10–15 ml/kg will raise factor level by 0.2 U/ml
Severe fibrinogen depletion	Cryoprecipitate	1 U/3 kg will raise fibrinogen level to >100 mg/dl

NEONATAL PURPURA FULMINANS

A unique clinical syndrome of neonatal DIC and purpura fulminans has been recognized and is related to the complete
absence of protein C or protein S in the plasma.[54–56] Babies
born with homozygous deficiency of either protein C or protein
S present within a few hours to days of birth with rapidly progressive skin lesions and diffuse oozing from skin puncture
sites. The skin lesions often begin at heel or venous puncture
sites. These lesions, which are initially red and flat, quickly
become indurated and necrotic, form an eschar, and result in
gangrene. Coagulation screening tests, which may be normal
initially, will subsequently reveal typical evidence of DIC. Family studies document heterozygous deficiency of protein C or
protein S in both parents (typically asymptomatic), while the
infant has undetectable protein by immunologic or functional
assay. DIC and purpura fulminans associated with homozygous
deficiency of protein C or protein S respond quickly and dramatically to fresh frozen plasma.[55] If administered before the
development of tissue necrosis, the lesions will begin to regress
within a few hours. Most episodes of purpura fulminans require
infusion of protein C concentrate (50–100 U/kg) or fresh frozen
plasma (10–15 ml/kg) every 8–12 hours until tissue healing
has occurred, typically 7–10 days.[56] While heparin alone is not
effective, the adjuvant value of heparin is unknown. Before
withdrawing the protein C replacement, oral anticoagulation
with warfarin should be therapeutic so as to avoid skin necrosis. Most children can be maintained on intense oral anticoagulation (International Normalized Ratio 3.0–3.5) for life and do
well. One infant with homozygous protein S deficiency has been
maintained on infusions of cryoprecipitate.[57]

NEONATAL THROMBOSIS

Thrombosis occurs with an increased incidence during the
perinatal period. Risk factors for the development of neonatal
thromboses include indwelling vascular catheters, asphyxia,
poor perfusion, maternal diabetes, polycythemia, congenital
deficiencies of AT III, protein C, and protein S, and intrauterine
growth retardation. A predilection for major vessels and involvement of the arterial circulation is frequent. Most neonatal
thromboses occur on indwelling arterial and venous catheters,
where the pathophysiology includes endothelial damage, mechanical obstruction to blood flow, activation of coagulation,
and an immature coagulation regulatory system. Spontaneous
thromboses do occur and most frequently involve the inferior
vena cava and renal vein; the aorta, renal, and femoral arteries;
and the cerebral arteries and veins.[58]

The diagnosis of neonatal thrombosis can be made by demonstration with an imaging technique or by direct visualization
at surgery. In the past, contrast angiography has been the reference standard for in vivo diagnosis. In this technique, a clot
is visualized by rapid injection of nonionic contrast media or
renographin during radiography. Angiography with ionic contrast media is contraindicated in infants with renal failure or
gut ischemia. Recent improvements in high-resolution real-
time ultrasound have established this technique as standard
for visualization of thrombi in the aorta, inferior vena cava,
and iliac arteries. Doppler ultrasound, with or without color,
has extended noninvasive imaging to the intrarenal arteries
and veins as well as the portal vein, hepatic arteries and veins,
and cerebral arteries of the neonate.[59] Magnetic resonance imaging has demonstrated particular value in visualization of cerebral vascular thrombosis.[60]

When vascular perfusion is significantly impaired by an indwelling catheter, diagnostic studies should be performed expeditiously, and consideration should be given to immediate
use of the catheter for delivery of local fibrinolytic therapy.
After delivery of fibrinolytics, the catheter should be removed
promptly. Nonspecific measures, such as warming of the in-

HEPARIN INFUSION DOSAGE

Age	Bolus (U/kg)	Maintenance (U/kg/hr)
Preterm (28 weeks)	25	15
Preterm (28–36 weeks)	50	20
Full term	100	25–40

volved or contralateral limb, are sometimes helpful. Surgical
thrombectomy must be guided by accessibility and local expertise. When there is recent or progressive thrombosis and organ
dysfunction, either anticoagulant or fibrinolytic therapy must
be carefully considered. Heparin clearance is accelerated in
the neonate, partly due to neonatal differences in plasma volume and liver metabolism and partly due to the lower neonatal
level of AT III.[61] Monitoring heparin therapy using a factor Xa
inhibition assay is preferable because of the baseline physiologic prolongation of the PTT in the preterm infant. The dose
of heparin should be targeted to achieve a plasma level of
0.3–0.6 U/ml. Continuous heparin infusions are far more satisfactory than intermittent bolus infusion in babies.[62] Heparin
therapy should be initiated in the neonate using a bolus of 50
U/kg for preterm and 100 U/kg for term infants. A continuous
infusion should be started at 20–25 U/kg/hr. An extremely preterm infant may require only 15 U/kg/hr, while it is not uncommon for an asphyxiated term infant to require 40–50 U/kg/hr.
Bleeding complications are rare in infants with a heparin level
of <0.8 U/ml.

Fibrinolytic therapy has recently been applied to the treatment of neonatal thrombosis. In vitro and in vivo clinical experience suggests that the neonatal fibrinolytic system is less susceptible to activation by tissue plasminogen activator,
urokinase, or streptokinase, resulting in requirements of ≤10
times the adult dose of 0.1 mg/kg/hr of tissue plasminogen activator or 4,400 U/kg/hr of urokinase.[63] Preliminary reports have
shown a superiority of fibrinolytic therapy over anticoagulation in the treatment of renal vein thrombosis as well as in
maintaining the patency of central venous catheters.[64,65] Cranial sonography should be performed on all neonates prior
to initiation of heparin anticoagulation or fibrinolytic therapy.
Intracranial hemorrhage or ischemic infarction can be exacerbated by these therapies.

During heparin or fibrinolytic therapy, platelet or plasma
transfusion should be given as needed to achieve and maintain
a platelet count of ≥50,000/mm^3, a fibrinogen level of ≥100 mg/
dl, and a PT of <15 seconds. Heparin should be given until the
clot is cleared by imaging examination, usually 3–14 days.
Long-term anticoagulation with warfarin is rarely indicated in
the infant. Fibrinolytic therapy can be given concomitantly with
low-dose heparin (10 U/kg/hr) for 48 hours. Thereafter, fibrinolytic therapy is stopped and heparin is continued at full therapeutic dosage for 2–5 additional days to prevent clot recurrence or progression.[66]

Genetic deficiencies of coagulation regulatory or fibrinolytic
proteins should be suspected in well infants with spontaneous
thromboses. Determination of plasma concentrations of AT III,
protein C, protein S, and plasminogen may be useful to guide
acute therapy. The exclusion of genetic disease, however, is
best accomplished at 6 months of age after maturation of fetal
coagulation proteins. The diagnosis of heterozygous protein C
deficiency may be difficult to determine without family studies,
owing to the late physiologic maturation of this protein in adolescence.

REFERENCES

1. Hathaway WE, Bonnar J: Hemostatic Disorders of the Pregnant Woman and Newborn Infant. pp. 58–59. Elsevier Science Publishing, New York, 1987
2. Toulon P, Rainaut M, Aiach M et al: Antithrombin III (ATIII) and heparin cofactor II (HCII) in normal human fetuses (21st–27th week). Thromb Haemost 56:237, 1986
3. Melissari E, Nicolaides KH, Scully MF et al: Protein S and C4b-binding protein in fetal and neonatal blood. Br J Haematol 70:199, 1988
4. Francis JL, Armstrong DJ: Sialic acid and enzymatic desialation of cord blood fibrinogen. Haemostasis 11:223, 1982
5. Hamulyák K, Nieuwenhuizen W, Devilée PP et al: Reevaluation of some properties of fibrinogen, purified from cord blood of normal newborns. Thromb Res 32:301, 1983
6. Edelberg JM, Enghild JJ, Pizzo SV et al: Neonatal plasminogen displays altered cell surface binding and activation kinetics. J Clin Invest 86:107, 1990
7. Estelles A, Aznar J, Gilabert J et al: Dysfunctional plasminogen in full-term newborn. Pediatr Res 14:1180, 1980
8. Benavent A, Estellés A, Aznar J et al: Dynfunctional plasminogen in full term newborn-study of active site plasmin. Thromb Haemost 51:67, 1984
9. Delaplane S: Urokinase therapy for a CR right atrial thrombosis. J Pediatr 100:149, 1982
10. Manco-Johnson M, Spidelle S, Peters M: Maturation of protein C in the ovine fetus: developmentally linked transition to the adult form. Pediatr Res (in press)
11. Manco-Johnson M, Krugman S, Jacobson L: Identification of a unique form of protein C in the ovine fetus. Pediatr Res (in press)
12. Katz JA, Moake JL, McPherson PD et al: Relationship between human development and disappearance of unusually large von Willebrand factor multimers from plasma. Blood 73:1851, 1989
13. Andrew M, Castle V, Mitchell L et al: Modified bleeding time in the infant. Am J Hematol 30:190, 1989
14. Andrew M, Paes B, Johnston M: Development of the hemostastic system in the neonate and young infant. Am J Pediatr Hematol Oncol 12:95, 1990
15. Aballi, AJ, De Lamerens S: Coagulation changes in the neonatal period and in early infancy. Pediatr Clin North Am 9:785, 1962
16. Bovill EG, Soll, RF, Bhushan F et al: Vitamin K1 metabolism and the production of des-carboxy prothrombin and protein C in the term and premature neonate. Blood 81:77, 1983
17. Andrew M, Paes B, Millner R et al: Development of the human coagulation system in the full-term infant. Blood 70:165, 1987
18. Andrew M, Paes B, Millner R et al: Development of the human coagulation system in the healthy premature infant. Blood 72:1651, 1988
19. Mull MM, Hathaway WE: Altered platelet function in newborns. Pediatr Res 4:229, 1970
20. Feusner JH: Normal and abnormal bleeding times in neonates and young children utilizing a fully standardized template technic. Am J Clin Pathol 74:73, 1980
21. Andrew M, Paes B, Bowker J et al: Evaluation of an automated bleeding time device in the newborn. Am J Hematol 35:275, 1990
22. Yoffe G, Buchanan GR: Intracranial hemorrhage in newborn and young infants with hemophilia. J Pediatr 113:333, 1988
23. Kletzel M, Miller CH, Becton DL et al: Post delivery head bleeding in hemophilic neonates: causes and management. Am J Dis Child 143:1107, 1989
24. Manco-Johnson M: Coagulation disorders. Curr Opin Pediatr 4:102, 1992
25. Hathaway WE: New insights on vitamin K. Hematol Oncol Clin North Am 1:367, 1987
26. Monslet U, Hansen ES: A review of vitamin K: epilepsy and pregnancy. Acta Neurol Scand 85:39, 1992
27. Cornelissen M, Steegers-Theunissen R, Kollée L et al: Supplementation of vitamin K in pregnant women receiving anticonvulsant therapy prevents neonatal vitamin K deficiency. Am J Obstet Gynecol 168:884, 1993
28. Olson JA: Recommended dietary intakes (RDI) of vitamin K in humans. Am J Clin Nutr 45:687, 1987
29. Hogenbirk K, Peters M, Bouman P et al: The effect of formula versus breast feeding and exogenous vitamin K1 supplementation on circulating levels of vitamin K1 and vitamin K-dependent clotting factors in newborns. Eur J Pediatr 152:72, 1993
30. von Kries R, Greer FR, Suttie JW: Assessment of vitamin K status of the newborn infant. J Pediatr Gastroenterol Nutr 16:231, 1993
31. Bovill EG, Soll RF, Lynch M et al: Vitamin K1 metabolism and the production of des-carboxy prothrombin and protein C in the term and premature neonate. Blood 81:77, 1993
32. Shapiro AD, Jacobson LJ, Armon ME et al: Vitamin K deficiency in the newborn infant: prevalence and perinatal risk factors. J Pediatr 109:675, 1986
33. Motohara K, Takagi S, Endo F et al: Oral supplementation of vitamin K for pregnant women and effects on levels of plasma vitamin K and PIVKA-II in the neonate. J Pediatr Gastroenterol Nutr 11:32, 1990
34. Anai, T, Hirota Y, Yoshimatsu J et al: Can prenatal vitamin K1 (Phylloquinone) supplementation replace prophylaxis at birth? Obstet Gynecol 81:251, 1993
35. Cornelissen EA, Kollée LA, De Abreu RA: Effects of oral and intramuscular vitamin K prophylaxis on vitamin K1, PIVKA-II, and clotting factors in breast fed infants. Arch Dis Child 67:1250, 1992
36. Golding J, Greenwood R, Birmingham K et al: Childhood cancer, intramuscular vitamin K, and pethidine given during labour. Br Med J 305:341, 1992
37. Read JS, Mills JL, Shiono PH: The risk of childhood cancer after neonatal exposure to vitamin K. N Engl J Med 329:905, 1993
38. Ekelund H, Finnstrom O, Gunnarskog J et al: Administration of vitamin K to newborn infants and childhood cancer. Br Med J 307:89, 1993
39. American Academy of Pediatrics Vitamin K Ad Hoc Task Force: Controversies concerning vitamin K and the newborn. Pediatrics 91:1001, 1993
40. Castle V, Andrew M, Kelton J et al: Frequency and mechanism of neonatal thrombocytopenia. J Pediatr 108:749, 1986
41. Yamamoto R, Lin LS, Lowe R: The human lung fibroblast cell line, MRC-5, produces multiple factors involved with megakaryocytopoiesis. J Immunol 144:1808, 1990
42. Pearson HA, Shulman NR, Marder VJ et al: Isoimmune neonatal thrombocytopenic purpura clinical and therapeutic considerations. Blood 23:154, 1964
43. Meuller-Eckhardt C, Grubert A, Weisheit M et al: 348 Cases of suspected neonatal alloimmune thrombocytopenia. Lancet 1:363, 1989
44. Taaning E, Antonsen H, Petersen S et al: HLA antigens and maternal antibodies in alloimmune neonatal thrombocytopenia. Tissue Antigens 21:351, 1983
45. Kaplan C, Morel-Kopp, MC, Kroll H et al: HPA-5b (BAK(a)) neonatal alloimmune thrombocytopenia: clinical and immunological analysis of 39 cases. Br J Haematol 78:425, 1991
46. Bussel JP, Berkowitz RL, McFarland JG et al: Antenatal treatment of neonatal alloimmune thrombocytopenia. N Engl J Med 319:1374, 1988
47. Bussel J, Kaplan C, McFarland J et al: Recommendations for the evaluation and treatment of neonatal autoimmune and alloimmune thrombocytopenia. Thromb Haemost 65:631, 1991
48. Lynch L, Bussel JB, McFarland JG et al: Antenatal treatment of alloimmune thrombocytopenia. Obstet Gynecol 80:67, 1992
49. Seidman DS, Chayen B, Kuint J et al: Neonatal alloimmune thrombocytopenia in consecutive pregnancies. J Perinat Med 19:465, 1991
50. Samuels P, Bussel J, Braitman L et al: Estimation of the risk of thrombocytopenia in the offspring of pregnant women with presumed ITP. N Engl J Med 323:229, 1990
51. Spadone D, Clark F, James E et al: Heparin-induced thrombocytopenia in the newborn. J Vasc Surg 15:306, 1992
52. Manco-Johnson MJ, Abshire TC, Jacobson LJ et al: Severe neonatal protein C deficiency: prevalence and thrombotic risk. J Pediatr 119:793, 1991
53. von Kries R, Stannigel H, Göbel U: Anticoagulant therapy by continuous heparin-antithrombin III infusion in newborns with disseminated intravascular coagulation. Eur J Pediatr 144:191, 1985
54. Branson HE, Marble R, Katz J et al: Inherited protein C deficiency and coumarin-responsive chronic relapsing purpura fulminans in a newborn infant. Lancet 11:1165, 1983
55. Marlar RA, Montgomery RR, Broekmans AW et al: Diagnosis and treatment of homozygous protein C-deficient children. J Pediatr 114:528, 1989
56. Dreyfuss M, Magny J, Bridey F et al: Treatment of homozygous protein C deficiency and neonatal purpura fulminans with a purified protein C concentrate. N Engl J Med 325:1565, 1991
57. Mahasandana C, Suvatte V, Varlar RA et al: Neonatal purpura fulminans associated with homozygous protein S deficiency. Lancet 335:61, 1990
58. Manco-Johnson MJ: Diagnosis and management of thrombosis in the perinatal period. Semin Perinatol 14:393, 1990
59. Visser M, Leighton J, van de Bor M et al: Renal blood flow in the neonates: quantification with color flow and pulsed doppler US. Radiology 183:441, 1992
60. Medlock MD, Olivero WC, Hanigan WC et al: Children with cerebral venous thrombosis diagnosed with magnetic resonance imaging and magnetic resonance angiography. Neurosurgery 31:870, 1992
61. McDonald MM, Jacobson LJ, Hay WW et al: Heparin clearance in the newborn. Pediatr Res 15:1015, 1981
62. McDonald MM, Hathaway WE: Anticoagulant therapy by continuous heparinization in newborn and older infants. J Pediatr 101:451, 1982
63. Corrigan JJ: Neonatal thrombosis and the thrombolytic system: pathophysiology and therapy. Am J Pediatr Hematol Oncol 10:83, 1988
64. Nowak-Göttl U, Schwabe D, Schneider W et al: Thrombolysis with recominant tissue-type plasminogen activator in renal venous thrombosis in infancy. Lancet 340:1105, 1992
65. Nuss, R, Hays T, Manco-Johnson MJ: Heparin anticoagulation does not prevent long-term renal dysfunction following renal vein thrombosis. Thromb Haemost 69:1311, 1993
66. Schmidt B, Andrew M: Report of scientific and standardization subcommittee on neonatal hemostasis diagnosis and treatment of neonatal thrombosis. Thromb Haemost 67:381, 1992

INTRODUCTION

Patients clinically suspected of having a hypercoagulable state can be divided into two categories.[1] The first group consists of the inherited thrombotic disorders or primary hypercoagulable states (Table 119-1). In these instances, a specific defect in one of the major natural anticoagulant mechanisms, namely the heparin-antithrombin III (AT III) and protein C anticoagulant pathways, have been identified (Fig. 119-1). The second category consists of a heterogenous group of disorders in which there is an apparent increased risk of developing thrombotic complications as compared with the general population (Table 119-2), and can be referred to as the acquired or secondary hypercoagulable states. The pathophysiologic basis for the hypercoagulable state in most of these situations is not known with certainty. Due to their complex pathophysiology, it is unlikely that defects in merely a single component of the hemostatic mechanism will account for the thrombotic tendency in most of these conditions.

INHERITED THROMBOTIC DISORDERS

In patients <45 years of age referred for evaluation with venous thrombosis, investigators[2-4] have found a combined prevalence of approximately 15 percent for hereditary deficiencies of AT III, protein C, and protein S. These three disorders occur with roughly equal frequency and are less frequent in older patients with venous thrombosis. Abnormalities of plasminogen were found in 2%, and dysfibrinogenias were present in 1%.

In a prospective study of Dutch outpatients of all ages with venographically proved deep vein thrombosis, the prevalence of deficiencies of AT III, protein C, protein S, or plasminogen was 8.3% as compared with 2.2% in controls.[5] Furthermore, the positive predictive values for the presence of one of these deficiency states in patients with either a history of recurrent, familial, or juvenile (<41 years old) thrombosis were only 9%, 16%, and 12%, respectively.

Thus, with tests for AT III, protein C, and protein S, one can anticipate being able to make a diagnosis of a hereditary disorder in only 5–15% of young patients with venous thromboembolism. The following clinical features, however, should suggest the presence of one of these diagnoses and should prompt a screening laboratory evaluation (Table 119-3): thrombosis occurring at an early age, a family history of thrombotic disease, thrombosis occurring at unusual sites (e.g., mesenteric venous thrombosis, cerebral venous thrombosis), recurrent thrombosis with or without apparent precipitating factors, recurrent thrombosis during anticoagulant therapy, and/or warfarin-induced skin necrosis.

It has recently been discovered that many patients with unexplained venous thrombosis demonstrate a poor anticoagulant response to activated protein C in an activated partial thromboplastin time (PTT) assay (see below). This syndrome of resistance to activated protein C has been identified in 20–50% of patients with unexplained venous thrombosis, and appears to be 5–10 times more common than a deficiency of AT III, protein C, or protein S. Resistance to activated protein C has an autosomal dominant mode of inheritance.

Individuals with thrombosis in association with congenital deficiencies of AT III, protein C, protein S, or resistance to activated protein C are usually afflicted with venous thromboembolic disease. Arterial thrombotic events in such patients have been reported, but the pathogenetic role of the deficiency state in such cases is not yet firmly established. The reasons for the relatively low incidence of arterial thrombosis in these disorders are unknown.

There have been reports of thrombosis in patients with hereditary deficiencies of heparin cofactor II, plasminogen, and factor XII. However the causal association between these genetic abnormalities and an increased risk of thrombosis has not been clearly defined. Thus, screening for these deficiencies is not recommended as part of the initial laboratory evaluation of patients suspected of having an inherited thrombotic disorder.

Antithrombin III Deficiency

In 1965, Egeberg[6] reported a Norwegian family, the members of which had plasma AT III concentrations that were 40–50% of normal in association with a history of recurrent thrombotic events. Subsequently, other investigators described additional families with a similar constellation of clinical and laboratory abnormalities.[7-11]

AT III deficiency is inherited in an autosomal dominant fashion, and thus, affects both sexes equally. Initial estimates of the prevalence of AT III deficiency in the general population were cited to be 1 in 2,000–5,000.[12,13] However, studies using functional assays that measure AT III-heparin cofactor activity have found that the prevalence of the deficiency state in the general population is 0.2–0.4%.[14]

Approximately 55% of patients with familial AT III deficiency experience venous thrombotic episodes.[15,16] The initial clinical manifestations occur spontaneously in about 42% of subjects, but are related to pregnancy, delivery, oral contraceptive ingestion, surgery, or trauma in the remaining 58%.[15] The most common sites of disease are the deep veins of the leg and mesenteric veins. Approximately 60% of individuals develop recurrent thrombotic episodes, and clinical signs of pulmonary embolism are evident in 40%.[15] Although cases have been reported in which AT III-deficient infants sustain cerebral venous thrombosis,[11,17] affected children rarely develop thrombotic episodes at any sites before puberty. At this time thrombotic events start to occur with some frequency, and the risk of thrombosis increases substantially with advancing age.[15]

Two major types of inherited AT III deficiency (Table 119-4) have been delineated.[18,19] The classic deficiency state (type I) is a result of the reduced synthesis of biologically normal protease inhibitor molecules.[20] In these cases, the antigenic and functional activity of AT III in the blood is reduced in parallel. The molecular basis of this disorder is either a deletion of a segment of the gene or, more commonly, the occurrence of small deletions, insertions, or single base substitutions leading to a nonsense mutation. The second type of AT III deficiency is produced by a discrete molecular defect within the protease inhibitor (type II). The plasma levels of AT III are greatly reduced, as judged by functional activity measurements, whereas the immunologic determinations of this inhibitor are essentially normal. Among 9 AT-deficient patients derived from a cohort of 210 patients presenting with a history of venous thromboembolism before the age of 40 years or recurrent venous thrombosis, 4 were found to have a type II deficiency.[28]

The first family with a functional deficiency of AT III was

Table 119-1. Inherited Alterations of Coagulation Proteins that Have Been Clearly Associated with a Prethrombotic State

Antithrombin III deficiency
Protein C deficiency
Protein S deficiency
Resistance to activated protein C
Dysfibrinogenemias

reported by Sas and co-workers[29] in many families in 1974. This type of deficiency state has now been reported and further subcategorized on the basis of two different functional assays of AT III activity. The first is the AT III-heparin cofactor assay, which measures the ability of heparin to bind to lysyl residues on the inhibitor and catalyze the neutralization of coagulation enzymes such as thrombin and factor Xa. Another protein in human plasma that exhibits heparin cofactor activity is termed heparin cofactor II.[30] In contrast to AT III, this inhibitor requires concentrations of heparin of ≥ 1 U/ml in the reaction mixture to function as an efficient inhibitor of thrombin and therefore probably plays a minimal role when heparin is used clinically as an anticoagulant.[31] As many functional AT III assays employ heparin concentrations of >1 U/ml, an assay based on factor

Xa inhibition is likely to be more reliable than one based on thrombin inhibition to identify patients with a congenital deficiency of AT III.[32] Heparin cofactor II does not interact with other serine proteases generated by the coagulation cascade. Another mucopolysaccharide, dermatan sulfate, can dramatically accelerate the neutralization of thrombin by this inhibitor. Several patients have been described with inherited deficiencies of heparin cofactor II and thrombotic phenomena, but the causal relationship remains uncertain.[33,34] The second test is the progressive AT III activity assay, which quantifies the capacity of this inhibitor to neutralize the enzymatic activity of thrombin in the absence of heparin.

These two functional assays have identified AT III-deficient patients with reductions in heparin cofactor activity with or without concordant decrements in progressive AT III activity. Several abnormal AT III molecules have been identified with reductions in only heparin cofactor activity that have defects at a heparin-binding site (Table 119-5). These variants generally have mutations at the N-terminal end of the molecule.[35-40] In one of these variants, the substitution of asparagine for Ile 7 produces a new glycosylation site, and the resultant protein has a reduced affinity for heparin. Variants with decreased activity in both AT III activity assays generally have mutations near the thrombin-binding site at the C-terminal end of the

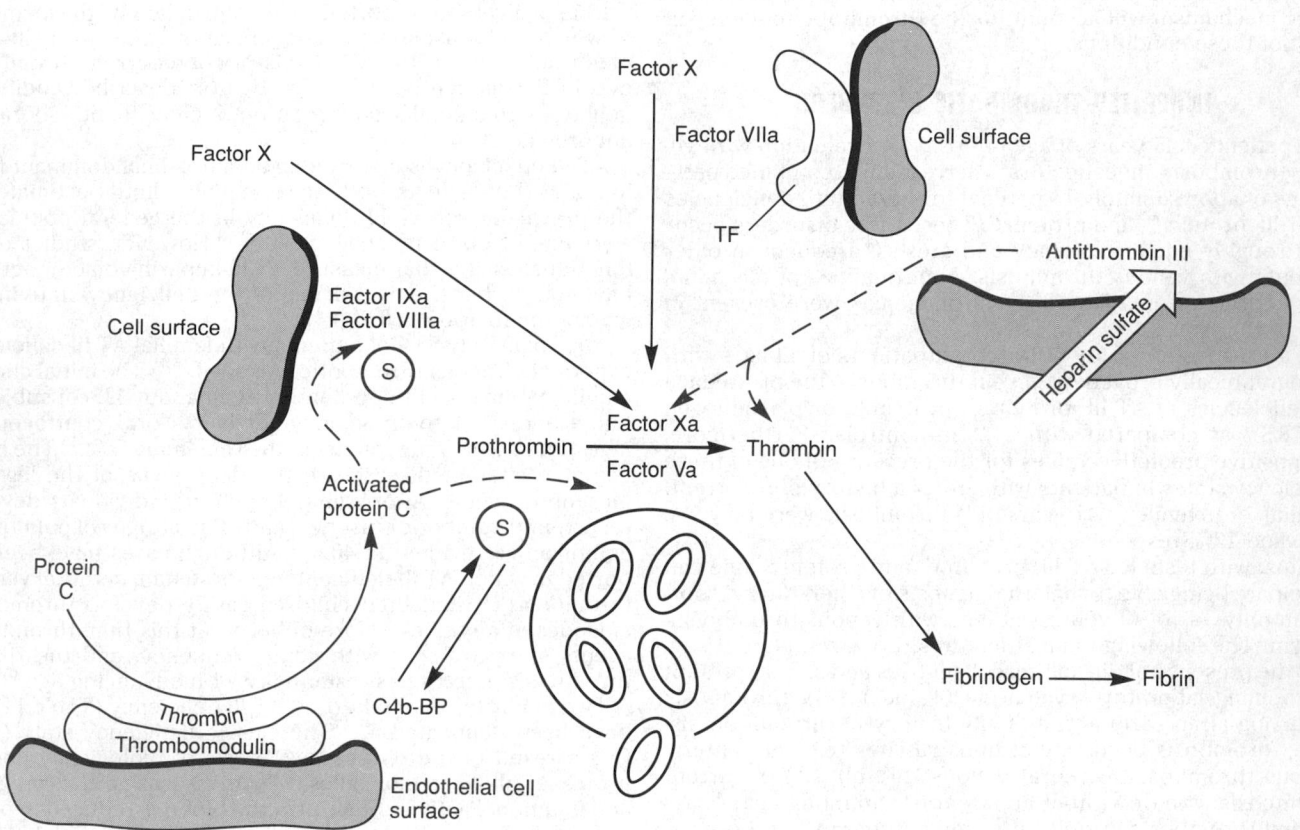

Fig. 119-1. Schematic of the pathways that generate factor Xa and thrombin, and the natural anticoagulant mechanisms that regulate the activity of these enzymes. Factor X can be activated by the extrinsic (factor VIIa/tissue factor [TF]) or the intrinsic (factor IXa/factor VIIIa-activated cell surface complex) pathways. Factor Xa binds to factor Va on activated platelets and mediates the conversion of prothrombin to thrombin under physiologic conditions. During this process, the inactive F_{1+2} fragment is released from the N terminus of prothrombin. Thrombin is then able to act on fibrinogen to form a fibrin clot; the initial step in this conversion results in the liberation of fibrinopeptide A. Thrombin and factor Xa are inactivated by AT III bound to heparan sulfate molecules associated with the vascular endothelium, resulting in the formation of factor Xa/AT III and thrombin/AT III complexes. Protein C is activated by thrombin bound to the endothelial cell receptor thrombomodulin, releasing a small peptide of approximately 1,400 molecular weight. Once activated, protein C functions as a potent anticoagulant by inactivating factors VIIIa and Va. Protein S enhances the binding of activated protein C to phospholipid-containing membranes and is able to accelerate the inactivation of factors VIIIa and Va by this enzyme. The complement component, C4b-binding protein (C4b-BP), forms complexes with protein S, which results in a reduction of its functional activity.

Table 119-2. Acquired or Secondary Hypercoagulable States

Diseases or Syndromes
  Lupus anticoagulant
  Malignancy
    Disease-related: includes migratory superficial thrombophlebitis (Trousseaus syndrome), nonbacterial thrombotic endocarditis, thrombosis associated with chronic disseminated intravascular coagulation
    Treatment-related: associated with the administration of various chemotherapeutic agents (L-asparaginase, mitomycin, adjuvant programs for breast cancer)
  Estrogen administration: associated with oral contraceptives, treatment of prostate cancer with diethylstilbestrol
  Infusion of prothrombin complex concentrates
  Nephrotic syndrome
  Heparin-induced thrombocytopenia
  Thrombotic thrombocytopenic purpura
  Myeloproliferative disorders
  Paroxysmal nocturnal hemoglobinuria
  Hyperlipidemia
  Diabetes mellitus
  Homocystinuria
  Hyperviscosity
  Congestive heart failure
Physiologic factors
  Pregnancy (especially during the postpartum period)
  Postoperative state
  Immobilization
  Advancing age
  Obesity

Table 119-4. Assay Measurements in Heterozygous AT III Deficiency

Type	Antigen	Activity Heparin Cofactor	Activity Progressive AT III
I (Classic)	Low	Low	Low
II			
Active site defect	Normal	Low	Low
Heparin-binding site defect	Normal	Low	Normal

Table 119-5. Point Mutations in AT III Deficiency (Type II)

City or Region of Propositus	Substitution	Effect of Mutation
Rouen 3	Ile 7 → Asn	Defective heparin binding, new carbohydrate attachment site
Rouen 4	Arg 24 → Cys	Defective heparin binding
Basel,[40] Clichy,[36] Dublin II, Franconville	Pro 41 → Leu	Defective heparin binding
Toyama,[35] Tours, Alger, Paris 1,[36] Paris 2,[36] Barcelona 2, Kumamoto, Padua 2, Amiens	Arg 47 → Cys	Defective heparin binding
Rouen 1,[37] Padua 1, Bligny	Arg 47 → His	Defective heparin binding
Rouen 2[38]	Arg 47 → Ser	Defective heparin binding
Budapest 3	Leu 99 → Phe	Defective heparin binding
Geneva[39]	Arg 129 → Gln	Defective heparin binding
Hamilton, Glasgow-II	Ala 382 → Thr	Defective serine protease inhibition
Charleville,[36] Cambridge 1, Vicenza, Sudbury	Ala 384 → Pro	Defective serine protease inhibition
Cambridge 2	Ala 384 → Ser	Defective serine protease inhibition
Stockholm	Gly 392 → Asp	Defective serine protease inhibition
Glasgow, Sheffield, Chicago, Waikato, Avranches[36]	Arg 393 → His	Defective serine protease inhibition
Northwick Park, Milano 1, Frankfurt 1	Arg 393 → Cys	Defective serine protease inhibiton
Pescara	Arg 393 → Pro	Defective serine protease inhibition
Denver, Milano 2	Arg 394 → Ser	Defective serine protease inhibition
Rosny	Phe 402 → Cys	
Torino	Phe 402 → Ser	These mutations result in the presence of trace amounts of the abnormal AT III in patient's plasma
Oslo	Ala 404 → Thr	
Kyoto	Arg 406 → Met	
Utah	Pro 407 → Leu	
Budapest[48]	Pro 429 → Leu	Mutation produces altered conformation of AT III, resulting in abnormal heparin binding and reduced thrombin inhibitory activity

molecule[36,41,42] (Table 119-5). However, all AT III variants cannot be neatly characterized by this schema, as single amino acid substitutions can affect both functional domains of the molecule. This is perhaps best illustrated by a mutation in which Arg 393 is replaced by histidine.[36,42] This reactive site mutation markedly decreases the ability of the protein to inhibit thrombin, but also leads to a conformational alteration such that the abnormal molecule has increased heparin affinity.

Another type of mutation has been described at the C-terminal end of the AT III molecule. In the plasma of AT III-deficient patients derived from a large Utah family, trace amounts of an electrophoretically and functionally abnormal inhibitor molecule have been identified.[43] It was determined that leucine is substituted for Pro 407 in the affected members of this kindred.[44,45] Small amounts of an electrophoretically abnormal inhibitor species have been observed in the plasma of AT III-deficient members of the Oslo kindred[46] first reported by Egeberg.[6] Threonine replaces Ala 404 in the abnormal protein. Mutations at positions 402 and 406 apparently also lead to a similar type of defect.[47] The AT III-deficient subjects in the Utah and Oslo pedigrees appear, however, to have a type I deficiency

Table 119-3. Screening Laboratory Evaluation for Patients Suspected of Having an Inherited Thrombotic Disorder

Functional assay of AT III (heparin-cofactor assay)
Immunologic and functional assays of protein C
Immunologic assays of total and free protein S, functional assay of protein S
Anticoagulant response to activated protein C in an activated partial thromboplastin time assay (test for resistance to activated protein C)
Screen for dysfibrinogenemias (Immunologic and functional assays of fibrinogen, thrombin time)

state as determined by routine laboratory testing. The similarity in characteristics of these mutations suggests that the region of residues 402–407 is important for the maintenance of normal plasma levels of AT III antigen.[45] The mutant inhibitor molecules synthesized by the liver of these deficient individuals may be susceptible to increased intracellular degradation, decreased extracellular export, or increased clearance on entry into the circulation. Finally, the mutation in the AT III variant Budapest has recently been identified.[29] The replacement of a Pro 429 by leucine leads to a molecular defect that can affect both the heparin- and thrombin-binding sites.[48]

The prevalence of thrombosis is different in patients with the two types of functional AT III deficiency. Heterozygous individuals with plasma AT III-heparin cofactor activity of approximately 50% and normal progressive AT III activity have infrequent thrombotic episodes.[37,38] Several of these cases were brought to clinical attention when young children of these heterozygous subjects developed severe venous or arterial thrombosis, or both, accompanied by plasma AT III-heparin cofactor levels of <10%. In each instance, there was a history of parental consanguinity and these children were homozygous for an AT III molecular defect. By contrast, heterozygous type II patients with both diminished progressive AT III activity and AT III-heparin cofactor activity sustain venous thromboembolism as often as type I patients.

The mean concentration of AT III in normal pooled plasma is approximately 140 μg/ml. In plasma from normal individuals, the range of AT III concentrations as determined by immunologic or functional tests is narrow. Most laboratories report a normal range between 80% and 120% for AT III-heparin cofactor determinations[49] and a somewhat wider range for immunoassay results.[50] The AT III-heparin cofactor assay will detect all the different subtypes of the familial deficiency state and is therefore the best single laboratory screening test for the disorder.

Healthy newborns have about one-half the normal adult concentration[51,52] and gradually reach the adult level by 6 months of age.[53] The levels may be considerably lower in infants born after 30–36 weeks of gestation.[53] In the absence of heparin, AT III contributes about 80% of the thrombin-neutralizing capacity of normal adult plasma.[54,55] The levels of a second thrombin inhibitor, α_2-macroglobulin, are higher during the first 2 decades of life than in adults, and this may lessen the risk of thromboembolic complications in AT III-deficient patients during childhood.[56]

A variety of pathophysiologic conditions can reduce the concentration of AT III in the blood. While acute thrombosis will infrequently lower AT III levels substantially,[57] disseminated intravascular coagulation (DIC) usually reduces the level of this inhibitor.[58] Lowered AT III concentrations occur in patients with liver disease (mainly cirrhosis) due to decreased protein synthesis, in patients with the nephrotic syndrome as a consequence of urinary excretion,[59] in users of oral contraceptives, and in individuals receiving estrogen for other purposes.[15,60] The levels of AT III do not change substantially during normal pregnancies but may decrease significantly in women with pregnancy-induced hypertension, pre-eclampsia, or eclampsia. L-Asparaginase can substantially lower the plasma concentration of this inhibitor.[61] Heparin decreases plasma AT III levels, presumably on the basis of accelerated in vivo clearance of the inhibitor.[62] Evaluation of plasma samples from patients suspected of having congenital AT III deficiency during a period of heparinization can therefore potentially lead to an erroneous diagnosis of the disorder.

Due to the number of clinical disorders that can be associated with reductions in the plasma concentration of AT III, definitive diagnosis of the hereditary deficiency state is often difficult. While an AT III level in the normal range drawn on clinical presentation is usually sufficient to exclude the presence of the disorder, low levels should be confirmed by obtaining another sample at a subsequent time. This determination is ideally performed when the patient is no longer receiving oral anticoagulants, as these medications may raise plasma AT III concentrations into the normal range in individuals with the hereditary deficiency state.[7] Clinical assessment of the individual's risk of recurrent thrombosis will determine whether this approach is feasible. In most AT III-deficient subjects, however, this effect of oral anticoagulants is not of sufficient magnitude to obscure the diagnosis.[63] The hereditary nature of the disorder requires the investigation of other family members. Diagnosis of other biochemically affected family members also allows for appropriate counseling regarding the need for prophylaxis against venous thrombosis.

The indications for thrombolytic therapy in patients with heterozygous AT III deficiency are similar to those in other populations with acute venous thromboembolic episodes. These individuals can usually be treated successfully with intravenous heparin, although unusually high doses of the drug may rarely be required to achieve adequate anticoagulation. Indeed, the diagnosis of AT III deficiency is usually considered in the differential diagnosis of "heparin resistance."

In AT III-deficient patients receiving heparin for the treatment of acute thrombosis, the adjunctive role of AT III concentrate purified from human plasma is not clearly defined, as controlled trials have not been performed. However, based on the available data, administration of this product should be administered when difficulty is encountered in achieving adequate heparinization or recurrent thrombosis is observed despite adequate anticoagulation. It is also reasonable to treat AT III-deficient subjects with concentrate before major surgery or in obstetric situations in which the risks of bleeding from anticoagulation are unacceptable. The manufacturing processes used to prepare AT III concentrate result in a product that is >95% pure and inactivates the hepatitis B virus and human immunodeficiency virus-1.[64] Hence, it is preferable to administer AT III concentrate rather than fresh frozen plasma.

The biologic half-life of AT III is approximately 48 hours.[20] The infusion of 50 U/kg body weight of AT III concentrate (1 U is defined as the amount of AT III in 1 ml normal human plasma) will usually raise the plasma AT III level to approximately 120% in a congenitally deficient individual with a baseline level of 50%.[64,65] Plasma levels should be monitored to ensure that plasma levels remain >80% and the administration of 60% of the initial dose at 24-hour intervals is recommended to maintain inhibitor levels within the normal range.[65]

Oral anticoagulants are highly effective in the management of patients with AT III deficiency. Warfarin should be continued indefinitely in patients with recurrent venous thrombosis. Asymptomatic AT III individuals from thrombophilic kindreds are not generally anticoagulated prophylactically unless they are exposed to situations that predispose them to developing thrombosis (e.g., prolonged immobilization, surgery, pregnancy, etc.).[16]

The management of pregnancies in women with congenital AT III deficiency poses special problems. During pregnancy, adjusted-dose heparin administered by the subcutaneous route is the antithrombotic regimen of choice.[66] AT III-deficient patients with a history of previous thrombotic episodes should receive treatment throughout pregnancy, while biochemically affected women who have not yet experienced such events should probably receive treatment. In women who are on chronic oral anticoagulants, several approaches can be taken to minimize the risk of thrombotic complications as well as warfarin embryopathy. One approach is to stop warfarin and commence subcutaneous heparin therapy; this potentially exposes the patient to many months of heparin therapy while she is trying to conceive. Another approach is to use replacement therapy with AT III concentrates until conception. This product, however, needs to be administered intravenously at frequent intervals and is costly. Finally, warfarin therapy could be continued with the performance of pregnancy tests on a frequent basis. As soon as pregnancy is diagnosed, and prior to the sixth week of gestation, oral anticoagulants must be discontinued and heparin therapy initiated. Although the risk of warfarin embryopathy appears to be quite small during the first 6 weeks of pregnancy, even the small risk of this complication makes this the least preferable of the three approaches.[67]

Anabolic steroids such as stanazolol and danazol raise plasma AT III levels in individuals with normal as well as with reduced levels of this inhibitor.[68] In spite of this effect, these drugs have not been shown to prevent thrombosis in patients with hereditary AT III deficiency.[68]

Protein C Deficiency

In 1981, Griffin et al.[69] described the first kindred in which several individuals had plasma levels of protein C antigen of approximately 50% of normal and a history of recurrent thrombotic events. Subsequently, other investigators[70–73] have reported numerous other families with this disorder. This biochemical deficiency state is inherited in an autosomal dominant fashion and has clinical features that are similar to those of hereditary AT III deficiency. In severely affected families, about 75% of protein C-deficient individuals experienced one or more thrombotic events. The initial episode occurs spontaneously in approximately 70%, with the remaining 30% having associated risk factors at the time they develop acute thrombotic events (e.g. pregnancy and delivery, contraceptive pill ingestion, surgery, or trauma). However, most patients are asymptomatic until their early twenties, with increasing numbers of individuals experiencing thrombotic events as they reach the age of 50. The most common sites of disease are the deep veins of the legs, the iliofemoral veins, and the mesenteric veins. Approximately 63% of the affected patients develop recurrent venous thrombosis, with about 40% exhibiting signs of pulmonary embolism. Investigators have noted a high frequency of superficial thrombophlebitis of the leg veins[71] as well as several cases of cerebral venous thrombosis in protein C-deficient patients.[74] There have also been reports of nonhemorrhagic arterial stroke in young adults with hereditary protein C deficiency.[75]

Other kindreds have been reported in which individuals who are heterozygous for protein C deficiency have minimal or no symptoms. Two lines of evidence support this observation.

First, in the homozygous or doubly heterozygous state, newborns develop a syndrome of purpura fulminans and laboratory evidence of DIC in association with protein C antigen levels of <1% of normal.[76–80] However, the heterozygous parents of these infants have only infrequently had thromboses, in contrast to the patients with thrombotic histories and a hereditary partial deficiency of protein C. Second, Miletich et al.[81] observed that the frequency of heterozygous protein C deficiency is as high as 1 in 200 in a healthy adult population and that many biochemically affected individuals had not yet developed thromboses. These data suggest that other, as yet undefined factors, are likely to modulate the phenotypic expression of heterozygous protein C deficiency.

Coumarin-induced skin necrosis has been associated with the presence of heterozygous protein C deficiency.[82] This syndrome typically occurs during the first several days of warfarin therapy, often in association with the administration of large loading doses of the medication. The skin lesions occur on the extremities, breasts, and trunk, as well as the penis, and marginate over a period of hours from an initial central erythematous macule. If vitamin K or a product containing protein C is not rapidly administered, the affected cutaneous areas become edematous, develop central purpuric zones, and ultimately become necrotic. Biopsies demonstrate fibrin thrombi within cutaneous vessels with interstitial hemorrhage. The dermal manifestations of coumarin-induced skin necrosis are clinically and pathologically similar to those seen in infants with purpura fulminans due to severe protein C deficiency.

The pathogenesis of coumarin-induced skin necrosis is attributable to the emergence of a transient hypercoagulable state. The initiation of the drug at standard doses leads to a decrease in protein C anticoagulant activity levels to approximately 50% of normal within 1 day.[83] While the factor VII half-life parallels that of protein C, the levels of the other vitamin K-dependent-factors decline at slower rates consistent with their longer half-lives (Fig. 119-2). Increased thrombin generation has been documented in patients during this early phase of warfarin therapy utilizing an assay for fragment F_{1+2}, an index of the in vivo activation of prothrombin mediated by factor Xa.[84] During this period, the drug's suppressive effect on protein C has a greater influence on the hemostatic mechanism then its action on factor VII. These effects are likely to be exaggerated when high doses of warfarin are initially used or the

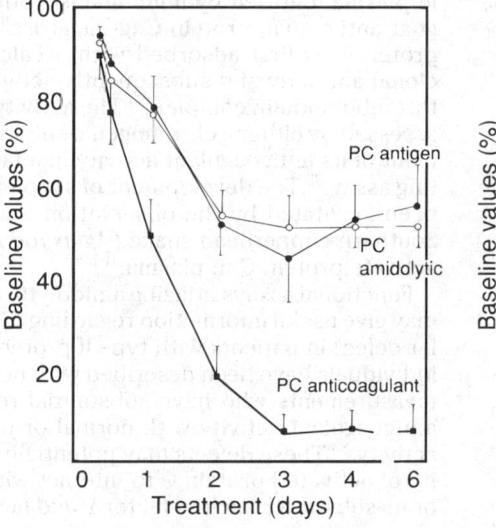
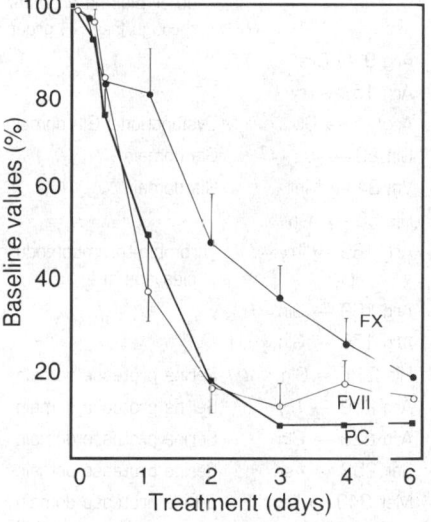

Fig. 119-2. Mean levels of protein C (PC) anticoagulant activity, factor VII (FVII) activity, factor X (FX) activity, protein C amidolytic activity, and protein C antigen following the initiation of warfarin therapy in patients with deep venous thrombosis. Patients were maintained on heparin infusions, and 10 mg of warfarin was administered for the first 3 days. Dosages were subsequently adjusted based on the prothrombin time. Measurements are expressed as percentages of prewarfarin levels. (From D'Angelo et al.,[83] with permission.)

Table 119-6. Assay Measurements in Heterozygous Protein C Deficiency

Type	Antigen	Activity	
		Amidolytic	Coagulant
I (Classic)	Low	Low	Low
II			
	Normal	Low	Low
	Normal	Normal	Low

patient has an underlying hereditary deficiency of protein C, or both. Only approximately one-third of patients with warfarin-induced skin necrosis have an underlying inherited deficiency of protein C, and this complication is infrequent among individuals with the heterozygous deficiency state. A case report has also described this syndrome in association with an acquired functional deficiency of protein C.[85]

Two major subtypes of heterozygous protein C deficiency have been delineated using immunologic and functional assays (Table 119-6). The classic or type I deficiency state is the most common form and is characterized by a reduction in both the immunologic and biologic activity of plasma protein C to approximately 50% of normal. The genetic defects in symptomatic type I-deficient families include a large number of different mutations in the protein C gene, but the missense or nonsense types are most common.[86-88] Other types of mutations resulting in type I protein C deficiency include promoter mutations, splice site abnormalities, in-frame deletions, frameshift deletions, in-frame insertions, and frameshift insertions.[88] In families with a type II deficiency state, affected individuals have normal protein C levels on immunologic examination, yet possess lowered functional levels.[83,89-91] The point mutations that have been identified in patients with type II protein C deficiency are shown in Table 119-7.[88,92-94]

Newborns develop purpura fulminans in association with protein C antigen levels that are <1% of normal.[76-80] In some

Table 119-7. Point Mutations in Protein C Deficiency (Type II)

City or Country of Propositus	Substitution	Effect of Mutation
Paris[94]	Arg −5 → Try	
Malakoff[94]	Arg −1 → His	Propeptide cleavage site
Paris[94]	Arg −1 → Cys	Complex formation with other plasma proteins through free SH group
Spain	Arg 9 → Cys	
Netherlands,[88] Paris	Arg 15 → Try	
Yonago	Arg 15 → Gly	Dysfunctional Gla domain
Vermont I[93]	Gln 20 → Ala	Gla domain
Vermont I[93]	Val 34 → Met	Gla domain
La Jolla I	His 66 → Asn	
Japan,[97] London I	Arg 169 → Try	Thrombin-thrombomodulin cleavage site
Austria[88]	Arg 169 → Gln	
Spain	Arg 178 → Gln	
Austria[88]	His 211 → Gln	Serine protease domain
Spain	Arg 229 → Try	Serine protease domain
Marseille[94]	Arg 229 → Gln	Serine protease domain
Paris[94]	Ser 252 → Asn	Serine protease domain
Austra[88]	Met 343 → Ileu	Serine protease domain
Netherlands[88]	Arg 353 → Try	Serine protease domain
Netherlands,[88] La Jolla II	Asp 359 → Asn	Serine protease domain
Italy[88]	Gly 381 → Ser	Serine protease domain
Purmerend[88]	Gly 391 → Ser	Serine protease domain

instances, a history of consanguinity in the family makes it likely that the affected infants were homozygous for the deficiency state.[77,79,80] These newborns can also be double heterozygotes, as in a patient who had a 5-nucleotide deletion in one protein C allele and a missense mutation in the other.[95] However, a number of case reports have documented homozygous or doubly heterozygous protein C deficiency in which neonatal purpura fulminans is not present. These individuals generally have protein C levels of <20% of normal in the absence of oral anticoagulant therapy, and their clinical presentation is similar to that of severely affected subjects from thrombophilic kindreds with the heterozygous deficiency state.[96,97] Genotyping of such homozygous individuals has led to the identification of missense mutations in the protein C gene; the variant protein C molecules produced by these individuals are either synthesized at a decreased rate or rapidly cleared from the circulation. The parents of these subjects have a type I deficiency state, as do those of infants with purpura fulminans. In addition, patients have been identified who are doubly heterozygous for both type I and type II alleles that were inherited separately from each of the parents.[92] In one of these cases, the type II defect resulted from the replacement of Arg 12 by tryptophan in the heavy chain. This residue is the site at which protein C is activated by the thrombin/thrombomodulin complex.[92] This mutation has been detected in another patient with protein C deficiency.

In patients with heterozygous type I protein C deficiency, the genetic differences between symptomatic and asymptomatic individuals have been evaluated. A common mutation among symptomatic Dutch patients has been found in an asymptomatic Swedish person[87] who is a parent of a doubly heterozygous child. While unique mutations have been reported in three asymptomatic kindreds with heterozygous protein C deficiency initially identified by Miletich et al.,[81] it seems unlikely that genotype will explain the phenotypic variability in patients with type I protein C deficiency.

A variety of immunologic and functional techniques have been developed to measure protein C levels in plasma samples. The most common procedures for antigen determinations are electroimmunoassay,[69,70] enzyme-linked immunosorbent assay,[98] or radioimmunoassay.[99,100] Functional assays have utilized either thrombin[89] or the thrombin/thrombomodulin complex[90] to activate protein C. Other methods have used the thrombin/thrombomodulin complex first to activate protein C in plasma followed by immunoadsorption of the enzyme with goat anti-human protein C IgG-agarose[90] or, alternatively, the protein C is first adsorbed with a calcium-dependent monoclonal antibody and subsequently activated by the thrombin/thrombomodulin complex.[83] The activity of the enzyme is then assessed by either a chromogenic substrate[89,90] or by measurement of its anticoagulant activity in a factor Xa one-stage clotting assay.[83] The development of simpler functional assays has been facilitated by the observation that the venom from the Southern copperhead snake (*Agkistrodon contortrix*) is able to activate protein C in plasma.[101]

Functional assays utilizing amidolytic and clotting end points may give useful information regarding the nature of the molecular defect in patients with type II protein C deficiency. Several individuals have been described with normal protein C antigen measurements who have substantial reductions in protein C anticoagulant activity with normal or near normal amidolytic activity.[83] These defects may potentially reflect a reduced ability of activated protein C to interact with platelet membranes or its substrates such as factor V and factor VIII. The molecular abnormality in one of these families has been determined and is characterized by two γ-carboxyglutamic acid domain mutations (Glu 20 to Ala and Val 34 to Met).[93] By contrast, abnormal protein C molecules that are normally activated by the thrombin-thrombomodulin complex but fail to exhibit proteolytic activity as measured by amidolytic or anticoagulant assays, suggest that the mutations reside near the active site of the proteins.[91]

Protein C circulates in human plasma at 4 μg/ml. The levels of protein C antigen in healthy adults are log normally distributed, with 95% of the values ranging from 70% to 140%.[81] Gender dependence is not significant, but mean protein C concentrations increase by approximately 4% per decade. The relatively wide normal range of protein C measurements in the general population occasionally makes it difficult to identify definitively a given individual as having heterozygous protein C deficiency. If medical and pharmacologic causes of low levels are excluded (see below), patients with a protein C value of <55% are very likely to have the genetic abnormality, while levels of 55–65% are consistent with either a deficiency state or the lower end of the normal distribution.[81] To document the presence of protein C deficiency with confidence, it is therefore useful to obtain repeat laboratory determinations as well as to perform family studies to identify an autosomal dominant inheritance pattern.

Protein C levels in newborns are 20–40% of normal adult levels,[102] and preterm infants have even lower levels.[103] Acquired protein C deficiency occurs in liver disease,[83,102,104] severe infection and septic shock, DIC,[83,102,104,105] adult respiratory distress syndrome,[102] the postoperative state,[102] breast cancer patients receiving cyclophosphamide, methotrexate, and 5-fluorouracil,[106] and in association with L-asparaginase therapy.[107] A particularly severe form of acquired protein C deficiency has been reported in association with purpura fulminans and DIC in patients with acute viral or bacterial infections.[108,109] In contrast to AT III, the antigenic concentrations of vitamin K-dependent plasma proteins, including protein C, may be elevated in patients with the nephrotic syndrome.[110,111] Most uremic patients have low levels of protein C anticoagulant activity, but normal levels of protein C amidolytic activity and antigen.[112] This is due to a dialyzable moiety in uremic plasma.[112]

Warfarin therapy reduces functional[83,89] and, to a lesser extent, immunologic measurements of protein C,[69,70] making it difficult to diagnose individuals with heterozygous protein C deficiency. A reduced ratio of protein C antigen to prothrombin or factor X antigen can identify patients with a type I deficiency state.[69,70] This approach, however, can only be used in subjects in a stable phase of oral anticoagulation, and the diagnostic criteria for the disorder vary with the intensity of warfarin therapy.[70] Other groups have successfully used protein C activity assays in conjunction with functional measurements of factor VII, a vitamin K-dependent zymogen with a similar plasma half-life. In practice, it is preferable to investigate patients suspected of having the deficiency state after oral anticoagulation has been discontinued for ≥1 week and to perform family studies. If it is not possible to discontinue warfarin due to the severity of the thrombotic tendency, such individuals can be studied while receiving heparin therapy, which does not alter plasma protein C levels.

An acquired inhibitor of protein C has been documented in an Australian patient.[113] This individual had a bleeding diathesis for several years and developed purpura fulminans prior to his death. An autopsy showed arterial and venous thrombi in many organs. Laboratory evaluation demonstrated the presence of chronic DIC. The IgG fraction of the patient's plasma completely inhibited the functional anticoagulant activity of activated protein C.

The acute management of thromboembolic events in heterozygous protein C-deficient patients is similar to that of subjects without this disorder. It is advisable to keep the patient fully anticoagulated with heparin during the initiation of oral anticoagulation, and large loading doses of the warfarin should clearly be avoided, as has been recommended in other patient populations. Oral anticoagulants are effective in managing individuals with protein C deficiency, and the recommendations

for its use in such patients who have either sustained recurrent venous thrombosis or are asymptomatic are similar to those in patients with congenital AT III deficiency. Many of the general guidelines for the management of pregnancies in women with this latter disorder are also relevant to this situation in protein C-deficient women.

Stanazolol and danazol raise protein C levels substantially in heterozygous patients with type I protein C deficiency.[114,115] Danazol treatment resulted in a rise in protein C antigen concentration from 66% to 98%, but no change in anticoagulant activity in a subject who is doubly heterozygous for both the type I and II deficiency states. However, these drugs do not prevent thrombosis in patients with this disorder,[115] and an increase in fragment F_{1+2} levels, a measure of the in vivo activity of factor Xa on prothrombin, has been observed in conjunction with the rise in protein C levels in two protein C-deficient patients who received stanazolol for 4 weeks.[114]

As coumarin-induced skin necrosis is a rare complication, therapy has been guided primarily by knowledge regarding its pathogenesis. The diagnosis should be suspected in patients with painful, red skin lesions developing within a few days after the initiation of the drug and immediate intervention is required to prevent progression and reduce complications. Therapy should consist of immediate discontinuation of warfarin, administration of vitamin K, and infusion of heparin at therapeutic doses. Lesions, however, have been reported to progress despite adequate anticoagulation with heparin. In patients with hereditary protein C deficiency, the administration of protein C should be considered, as in other patients with warfarin-induced skin necrosis who will invariably have low plasma levels of functional protein C at the onset of the skin lesions. Fresh frozen plasma has been used, but improved results can be expected with the administration of a highly purified protein C concentrate, which facilitates the rapid and complete normalization of plasma protein C levels.[116]

The infrequent occurrence of warfarin-induced skin necrosis, the relatively high frequency of asymptomatic hereditary protein C deficiency, and the diagnostic difficulty in making a rapid and definitive laboratory diagnosis of the deficiency state are arguments against the routine measurement of plasma protein C levels in all individuals with thrombosis before the initiation of oral anticoagulants. If, however, one is starting oral anticoagulants in a patient who is already known or likely to be protein C deficient, it is prudent to start the drug under the cover of heparin and also to increase the dose of warfarin gradually, starting from a relatively low level (e.g., 2 mg for the first 3 days and then increasing in increments of 2–3 mg until therapeutic anticoagulation is achieved). A case report has reported the successful oral anticoagulation of a subject with heterozygous protein C deficiency and a prior history of warfarin-induced skin necrosis. Therapeutic doses of heparin as well as protein C replacement in the form of fresh frozen plasma were used to prevent the development of this complication.

The management of neonatal purpura fulminans in association with severe protein C deficiency is more complicated. Heparin therapy as well as antiplatelet agents have not been shown to be effective.[76,78,79] The administration of a source of protein C appears to be critical in the initial treatment of these patients. Fresh frozen plasma has been used successfully in these infants. However, the half-life of protein C in the circulation is only about 6–16 hours, and the administration of plasma on a frequent basis is limited by the development of hyperproteinemia, hypertension, loss of venous access, and the potential for exposure to infectious viral agents.[83] Protein C concentrate has recently been successfully used in this disorder, and highly purified concentrates of this protein are currently undergoing clinical trials for this indication.[117] Warfarin has been administered to these infants without the redevelopment of skin necrosis during the phased withdrawal of fresh frozen plasma infusions, and this medication has been used chronically to control the thrombotic diathesis.[76,80] Finally, there has been a report of a 20-month-old child with liver failure and homozygous protein C deficiency undergoing successful liver transplantation.[118] This procedure normalized protein C levels and resolved the thrombotic diathesis.

Protein S Deficiency

In 1984, members from several kindreds who exhibited reduced levels of protein S were described who had a striking history of recurrent venous thrombotic disease.[119,120] Subsequently, many additional families with this disorder have been reported.[121] The clinical presentation of patients with heterozygous protein S deficiency is similar to that of AT III or protein C deficiency. Among 71 protein S-deficient members from 12 pedigrees, 74%, 72%, and 38% of the individuals have sustained deep venous thrombosis, superficial thrombophlebitis, and/or pulmonary emboli, respectively.[122] The mean age of the first thrombotic event was 28 years with a range of 15–68; 56% of the episodes were spontaneous, and the remainder were precipitated by an identifiable factor. Thrombosis has also been reported in the axillary, mesenteric, and cerebral veins.

Young patients with arterial thrombosis and hereditary protein S deficiency have been described. In a cohort of 37 consecutive young adults (<45 years of age) presenting with arterial occlusive disease, 3 persons were discovered with hereditary protein S deficiency.[123] However, the occurrence of arterial thromboembolic events was not increased in protein S-deficient relatives of these people as compared with their unaffected family members.

Under normal conditions, approximately 60% of the total protein S antigen in plasma is complexed to a complement component, C4b-binding protein. Only the free 40% is functionally active as a cofactor in mediating the anticoagulant effects of activated protein C.[121] This observation has led to the development of methods for measuring total and free protein S antigen.[120,124,125] The most reliable measurements of total protein S antigen are usually by radioimmunoassay or enzyme-linked immunosorbent assay techniques.[124–126] After removing protein S/C4b-binding protein complexes from plasma, free protein S may be quantified by immunoassay. Functional assays are based on the ability of protein S to serve as a cofactor for the anticoagulant effect of activated protein C.[119,127,128]

The classic deficiency state is associated with approximately 50% of the normal total S antigen level,[120] and more marked reductions in free protein S antigen and protein S functional activity (Table 119-8). The molecular genetic analysis of mutations in patients with protein S deficiency is complicated by the presence of a protein S pseudogene.[129–132] Molecular analysis of the classic type of deficiency state has identified partial protein S gene deletions.[133] The point mutations that have been identified in these patients include missense or nonsense mutations, single base pair insertions, propeptide mutations, and splice site abnormalities. Another pattern of the hereditary deficiency state is seen when total protein S antigen measurements are in the normal range, but levels of free protein S and protein S functional activity are disproportionately reduced to <40% of normal (Table 119-8). The pathogenetic basis for this type of defect is unknown, but possible explanations include a molecular abnormality in either protein S or C4b-binding protein that leads to a shift of the free protein S pool into the bound form.[119]

Recurrent venous thromboembolic disease can occur in association with doubly heterozygous or homozygous protein S deficiency.[121] The parents of these individuals were asymptomatic and had laboratory studies consistent with the classic protein S-deficient state. In addition, a case report has recently described neonatal purpura fulminans in association with homozygous protein S deficiency.[134]

The average concentration of total protein S antigen in normal adults is 23 μg/ml.[124] The levels increase with advancing age and are significantly lower and more variable in females than males.[135] These factors have confounded the reliable estimation of the prevalence of heterozygous protein S deficiency in the normal population. The resampling of patients as well as family studies are usually required to establish the diagnosis firmly.

Acquired protein S deficiency occurs during pregnancy[126] and in association with the use of oral contraceptives.[135] Reduced protein S levels have been noted in patients with DIC[127,136] and acute thromboembolic disease.[127] C4b-binding protein is an acute-phase protein, and the declines in protein S activity in the latter two conditions as well as in other inflammatory disorders is attributable to a shift of the protein to the complexed, inactive form.[127] The levels of total and free protein S are reduced in men with human immunodeficiency virus infection.[137] Total protein S antigen measurements are generally increased in patients with the nephrotic syndrome, although functional assays give reduced values.[110,111,138] This is, in part, due to the loss of free protein S in the urine and elevations in C4b-binding protein levels. Total and free protein S antigen concentration are moderately decreased in liver disease[125,127] and in association with L-asparaginase chemotherapy.[107] Total protein S antigen values in healthy newborns at term are 15–30% of normal, while C4b-binding protein is markedly reduced to <20%. Thus, the free form of the protein predominates in this setting, and functional levels are only slightly reduced as compared with those in normal adults.[128,139] Interpretation of protein S measurements in individuals on oral anticoagulants is complicated inasmuch as the antigenic and functional levels of the protein are decreased. A few groups have used a strategy similar to that described for protein C-deficient subjects.[120]

In a patient with thromboembolic disease recovering from chickenpox, a transient isolated deficiency of protein S has been reported due to the presence of an autoantibody.[140] Cutaneous necrosis in association with an acquired severe deficiency of protein S has also been described.[141]

The recommendations for the treatment of protein S-deficient patients with anticoagulants and thrombolytic agents are similar to those in individuals without this disorder. Heparin therapy is generally effective for the acute treatment of thrombotic episodes, and standard warfarin schedules appear to be effective in preventing recurrent venous thromboembolism. Anabolic steroids such as danazol or stanazolol have not been shown to have a role in the treatment of protein S-deficient patients.

Inherited Resistance to the Anticoagulant Activity of Activated Protein C

In 1993, Dahlback and colleagues[142] reported the identification of individuals with unexplained personal and familial histories of venous thromboembolism whose plasma exhibited a poor response to activated protein C in an PTT assay. Other clinically affected relatives of the proband demonstrated resistance to the action of activated protein C, and poor anticoagulant responses were also demonstrable in factor IXa- and factor Xa-based assays. Based on these observations, it was initially hypothesized that an additional plasma cofactor, besides protein S, is normally required to support the anticoagulant activity of activated protein C.

Table 119-8. Assay Measurements in Heterozygous Protein S Deficiency

Antigen		Protein S Activity
Total Protein S	Free Protein S	
Classic low	Low	Low
Normal	Low	Low
Normal	Normal	Low

Among 104 consecutive Swedish patients with venous thrombosis referred for evaluation, Svensson and Dahlback[145] found that plasmas from 33% of the subjects showed resistance to the action of activated protein C in a PTT-based assay (i.e., an anticoagulant response below the fifth percentile of controls). Precipitating factors for thrombosis, such as pregnancy and the use of oral contraceptives, were identified in 60% of these patients. Family studies revealed that relatives with resistance to activated protein C had a significantly higher frequency of thrombosis than relatives without the defect. In 25 American patients <50 years of age with unexplained venous thromboembolic disease, this defect was found in approximately 50%.[143] Other groups have reported on similar cohorts of patients with resistance to activated protein C.

A group of Dutch investigators detected resistance to activated protein C in 21% of 301 unselected consecutive patients <70 years old sustaining a first episode of deep venous thrombosis.[144] Patients with this defect were calculated to have a sevenfold increased risk of venous thrombosis as compared with controls. The lower frequency of resistance to activated protein C in this study is primarily attributable to the different selection criteria that was employed to select the thrombosis cohorts.

A defect in factor V involving the mutation of Arg 506 to Gln 506 (Arg 506 Gln) is most often the cause of activated protein C-resistance.[144a,145a] This is the site at which activated protein C cleaves factor Va, and this sequence alteration makes the mutant factor Va molecule biochemically resistant to inactivation by activated protein C. The Arg 506 Gln substitution has been found to be the cause of activated protein C-resistance in 80% of Dutch patients with a poor response to activated protein C in the PTT assay. The defect has an autosomal dominant inheritance pattern.[144,145] Interestingly, its prevalence in healthy controls in approximately 2–5%, and homozygous patients have been identified.[144,145,145a]

Laboratory tests for resistance to activated protein C must be carefully standarized. The level of activated protein C, the activated PTT reagent, and the instrumentation can affect the performance characteristics of the assay. Patients must be investigated when they are not receiving anticoagulants as these drugs will produce marked prolongations in clotting time in the presence of activated protein C. Some functional assays for protein S in plasma are sensitive to activated protein C resistance, thereby leading to low results and an erroneous diagnosis of functional protein S deficiency.

DYSFIBRINOGEMIAS

Qualitative abnormalities of fibrinogen are usually inherited in an autosomal dominant manner. The dysfibrinogenemias are a heterogenous group of clinical disorders that may present with either no clinical symptoms, a bleeding diathesis, or a history of recurrent venous or arterial thromboembolism (see also Ch. 137). Fewer than 20 cases of variant fibrinogens have been reported to be associated with thrombotic complications. These defects can be discovered by screening patients with thrombin and reptilase times, which are often prolonged in these patients, and also by performing fibrinogen assays. In one instance, the thrombin time has been substantially shortened.[147] Functional fibrinogen measurements are usually substantially lower than antigenic measurements in the plasma of these individuals. An occasional individual with a dysfibrinogemia may have a prolonged prothrombin time or PTT, and the inability of some abnormal fibrinogens to clot completely in vitro can result in false-positive results in fibrin(ogen) degradation product tests.

The functional and biochemical defects of a number of abnormal fibrinogens associated with thromboembolic disease have been characterized. The conversion of fibrinogen to fibrin by thrombin results in the proteolytic cleavage of fibrinopeptides A and B from the molecule. Defects in the release of these two

peptides[148,149] or abnormalities in fibrin polymerization[150] have been reported. Such functional defects do not, however, offer a ready explanation for the thrombotic diathesis seen in these subjects. Abnormalities in thrombin binding to fibrin have also been found in some dysfibrinogenemias.[146,151] In one of these kindreds, three homozygous siblings with a β chain substitution of alanine by threonine at position 68 have a severe clinical phenotype sustaining both arterial and venous thrombosis at a young age.[146] The decreased binding of thrombin by this mutant fibrinogen may lead to the presence of excessive thrombin in the circulation and the occurrence of thrombosis. Other fibrinogen mutants have been shown to cause abnormal fibrin polymerization.[150] The fibrin formed from fibrinogen Chapel Hill III has been demonstrated to be abnormally resistant to lysis by plasmin.[150] By contrast, it has been shown that plasminogen activation is decreased in the presence of the fibrin formed from fibrinogen Dusard, in spite of normal tissue plasminogen activator binding to the substrate.[152,153] These abnormalities have the potential for decreasing fibrinolytic activity in vivo, which could result in a familial thrombotic diathesis in biochemically affected persons.

INHERITED ABNORMALITIES OF FIBRINOLYSIS

Dysfunction of fibrinolytic system certainly plays an important role in thrombus formation. Dysplasminogenemia or hypoplasminogenemia has been reported in approximately 20 individuals with thromboembolic disease.[154–157] In the first case of an abnormal plasminogen, the propositus had a history of recurrent thrombosis, and family studies demonstrated that the biochemical abnormality followed an autosomal dominant inheritance pattern.[154] Despite the hereditary nature of the defect, none of the other biochemically affected members of the kindred had sustained thrombotic events. Other Japanese pedigrees have been described with the same biochemical defect,[156] and the gene frequency of this abnormality in Japan is 0.018.[158] Population studies in the United States have not uncovered any cases of this dysplasminogenemia. A study of two unrelated Japanese families with reduced functional and antigenic levels of plasminogen was unable to demonstrate a significant correlation between the deficiency state and thrombosis.[159] The non-Japanese cases of dysplasminogenemias and hypoplasminogenemias have also been remarkable for the lack of thrombotic episodes in biochemically affected family members other than the propositi.

A few reports have documented the existence of thrombophilic families with inherited abnormalities of fibrinolysis.[160] Individuals from these kindreds were initially observed to have reduced fibrinolytic potential after venous occlusion and have subsequently been documented to have high levels of plasminogen activator inhibitor. Re-evaluation of two of these families[160] has recently demonstrated the presence of hereditary protein S deficiency and no association between plasminogen activator inhibitor-1 activity and a history of thrombosis.[161] These data provide further evidence that the association between defective fibrinolysis and familial thrombosis has not been established.[4,162]

Immunochemical methods for the measurement of tissue plasminogen activator and functional assays for its inhibitors have been applied to the study of patients with documented venous thromboembolism. Defective synthesis, or release of tissue plasminogen activator as well as an increased concentration of the inhibitor of this serine protease may be important pathogenetic factors in as many as one-third of these individuals.[163–166] Reduced fibrinolytic activity due to increased plasma levels of a rapid inhibitor of tissue plasminogen activator has been found in young survivors of myocardial infarction.[167,168] The measurements of this inhibitor correlated strongly with serum concentrations of triglycerides.

MANAGEMENT DECISIONS IN PATIENTS WITH AN INHERITED THROMBOTIC DISORDER

When a patient with one of the inherited thrombotic disorders is discovered, family studies should be conducted, since approximately one-half of the members of a given kindred may be affected. Affected individuals should receive counseling on the implications of the diagnosis and advice on the symptoms that require immediate medical attention. In women of child-bearing age, oral contraceptives are contraindicated, in view of the increased thrombotic risk associated with the use of these mediations. All biochemically affected individuals should be carefully evaluated before surgical, medical, or obstetric procedures that carry an increased thrombolic risk. These patients should then receive appropriate prophylactic anticoagulation regimens. If specific concentrates are available for a patient with a particular deficiency state, these can also be administered to raise the plasma levels of the protein to the normal range during the perioperative period. All women with previous thrombotic episodes should receive prophylactic anticoagulants throughout pregnancy, and asymptomatic women should also generally receive such treatment.

In patients with an inherited thrombotic disorder, the occurrence of two or more spontaneously occurring thromboembolic episodes should lead to the continuation of oral anticoagulants for life. Chronic warfarin therapy is generally not recommended until an individual has had at least one documented thrombotic episode.

While it is clear that inherited deficiencies of AT III, protein C, and protein S can be associated with thrombophilia, it should be kept in mind that the reported rates of thrombosis likely represent overestimates. This is due to a diagnostic bias on the part of the physicians and a reporting bias in the literature for those individuals from families with the most severe thrombotic diatheses. In addition, some of the reported episodes of venous thrombosis were not confirmed by objective tests, and it is known that the clinical diagnosis of such events is highly nonspecific. Thus, given that future events in an asymto-matic patient or in an individual with only one prior thrombotic episode cannot currently be accurately predicted and also that there is a finite risk of bleeding associated with warfarin therapy, recommendations relating to long-term anticoagulation are individualized. The clinical features that should be considered in making this decision include the following:

1. The number, sites, and severity of thrombosis (e.g., a patient who previously sustained a massive pulmonary embolus is more likely to receive long-term warfarin than a subject who developed deep venous thrombosis in a calf vein unless symptoms or signs of a significant post-phlebitic syndrome are present)
2. Whether the thrombotic episodes were spontaneous or whether precipitating factors were present (e.g., if a precipitant such as a major abdominal operation was present, it would be reasonable to manage the patient without long-term oral anticoagulation after the acute episode was adequately treated)
3. The sex and life style of the individual (e.g., situations in which these factors may influence the decision-making process as to long-term anticoagulation include women of child-bearing age planning to conceive, occupations that entail prolonged periods of immobilization and thereby might be associated with an increased risk of thromboembolism, and jobs with higher than average chance of trauma that might lead to thrombotic or bleeding complications, or both)
4. A history of thromboembolism in other biochemically affected members of the family (e.g., while marked intra- and interfamilial heterogeneity has been observed in the phenotypic expression of the inherited thrombotic disorders, it is not unreasonable to place asymptomatic, biochemically affected patients from severely affected kindreds on oral anticoagulants starting at puberty)

Factor XII Deficiency

Factor XII is a zymogen of a serine protease that is involved in contact activation and intrinsic blood coagulation in vitro but probably plays no physiologic role in hemostasis (see Ch. 100).

The first patient with factor XII, or Hageman factor, deficiency was reported by Ratnoff and Colopy[169] in 1955. Subjects with severe factor XII deficiency (factor XII activity <1% of normal) have markedly prolonged PTTs, but do not exhibit a bleeding diathesis. However, there have been a number of cases of venous thromboembolism or myocardial infarction in factor XII-deficient patients,[170] including the initial patient described with the abnormality.[171] This thrombophilic tendency has been attributed to reduced plasma fibrinolytic activity. Patients with factor XII deficiency have been reported to have an 8% incidence of thromboembolism, and myocardial infarctions have occurred in relatively young individuals.[170] In families with factor XII deficiency, 2 of 18 homozygous or doubly heterozygous patients had sustained deep venous thrombosis, although each occurred at a time that other predisposing thrombotic risk factors were present.[172] Among heterozygotes with factor XII deficiency, only 1 of 45 heterozygotes had a possible history of venous thrombosis. These investigators concluded that heterozygous factor XII deficiency does not constitute a major thrombotic risk factor, while a severe deficiency may predispose some affected persons to venous thrombosis. Other groups have found a 10–20% incidence of thrombotic episodes in heterozygotes. In summary, it remains uncertain whether an increased thrombotic risk is associated with factor XII deficiency.

LUPUS ANTICOAGULANTS AND THE ANTICARDIOLIPIN SYNDROME

Lupus anticoagulants are antibodies (usually IgG, IgM, or both) that prolong phospholipid-dependent clotting assays in vitro. Paradoxically, the presence of lupus anticoagulants increases the apparent risk of both arterial and venous thromboembolism.[173,174] About one-third of patients with such inhibitors will have thrombotic events (see Ch. 115).

The relationship between the presence of lupus anticoagulants, antiphospholipid antibodies, and a thrombotic predisposition are complex. A study by Triplett et al.[175] demonstrated that antiphospholipid antibodies are not present in all patients with lupus anticoagulants, and the presence of such immuno-globulins does not necessarily confer an increased thrombotic risk on these individuals. However, in patients with systemic lupus erythematosus (SLE), persistently elevated levels of IgG anticardiolipin antibodies appear to correlate more strongly with thrombosis and fetal loss than do abnormalities in clotting assays for lupus anticoagulants.[176,177] Additional evidence that the presence of IgG anticardiolipin antibodies constitutes a thrombotic risk factor comes from a case-control study of healthy adult men participating in the Physicians Health Study.[178] An antibody titer above the 95th percentile was a significant risk factor for venous thromboembolism, but not for ischemic stroke.

Numerous different mechanisms have been implicated in the pathogenesis of thrombosis in these subjects. Some studies have demonstrated alterations in the function of the natural anticoagulant mechanisms of the endothelium, as phospholipids are essential components of vascular cell membranes. IgG from the plasma of a patient with arterial thrombosis and a lupus anticoagulant inhibited prostacyclin production by endothelial cells.[179] Others have reported that immunoglobulins from such patients either increase prostacyclin production or have no effect.[180] However, a recent study of patients with the lupus anticoagulant provided evidence that excessive platelet activation can occur without a compensatory increment in the vascular biosynthesis of prostacyclin.[181] Immunoglobulins from some patients with lupus anticoagulants inhibit protein C activation mediated by the thrombin/thrombomodulin complex on endothelial cell surfaces.[180,182] Abnormalities of the heparin sulfate-AT III or fibrinolytic mechanisms have also been suggested as explanations for the thrombotic tendency associated with lupus anticoagulants.[183]

The management of acute venous thromboembolism in patients with lupus anticoagulants is similar to that of other individuals without this laboratory abnormality. However, the initial treatment of such subjects is complicated because the PTT cannot reliably be used to monitor heparin dosage unless proper in vitro calibration studies are done by spiking known amounts of heparin into plasma samples and measuring the response of the PTT. Thus, it is preferable to monitor anticoagulant therapy in these individuals by performing plasma heparin measurements using either factor Xa or thrombin along with a suitable chromogenic substrate.

The clinical heterogeneity of the patient populations that develop lupus anticoagulants makes it difficult to generalize regarding the long-term antithrombotic management of such individuals. While the relationship between thrombosis and the lupus anticoagulant appears to be strong in patients with SLE,[176] the significance of the association in patients without this disorder is more ambiguous.[184] Indeed, patients who develop transient lupus anticoagulants in association with infections do not usually sustain thromboembolic episodes, and it is unclear whether drug-associated lupus anticoagulants are associated with thrombosis. Thus, the presence of persistent lupus anticoagulant or a high-titer antiphospholipid antibody, or both, in an asymptomatic subject with no prior thrombotic history is not currently an indication for anticoagulant or anti-platelet medications. However, inasmuch as it is not possible to determine the risk of thrombosis reliably in an asymptomatic patient with these laboratory abnormalities, all such individuals should receive appropriate prophylaxis in conjunction with major surgical procedures, or a prolonged period of immobilization, unless there is a strong contraindication to such treatment. Corticosteroids can normalize clotting assay times or reduce antiphospholipid antibody titers in patients with lupus anticoagulants. However, these and other immunosuppressive medications do not prevent recurrent thrombosis.

MARKERS OF COAGULATION ACTIVATION IN PATIENTS WITH INHERITED THROMBOTIC DISORDERS AND LUPUS ANTICOAGULANTS

Advances in our understanding of the biochemistry of the hemostatic mechanisms has also led to the development of sensitive immunochemical methods for measuring peptides or enzyme inhibitor complexes that are liberated with the activation of the coagulation and fibrinolytic systems in vivo.[185–191] Assays for the protein C activation peptide[100] and the F_{1+2} fragment[187,192] measure the scission of protein C by the thrombin/thrombomodulin complex and the cleavage of the prothrombin molecule by factor Xa, respectively. Immunoenzymatic procedures have also recently been established that directly quantify activated protein C in blood.[193] The fibrinopeptide A assay quantifies the cleavage of fibrinogen by thrombin.[189] Studies employing these markers indicate that a biochemical imbalance between procoagulant and anticoagulant mechanisms can be detected in the blood of humans prior to the appearance of thrombotic phenomena.[96]

In asymptomatic people with heterozygous deficiencies of protein C or protein S, the mean F_{1+2} level is significantly increased as compared with age-matched controls.[96,194] Approximately one-third of patients have levels greater than the upper normal limit of normal controls (defined as the mean +2 SD).[96,194] The elevated F_{1+2} concentrations are not due to diminished clearance of the fragment.[96] Fibrinopeptide A levels were elevated in approximately 20% of subjects.[96,194]

Protein C activation as measured by the protein C activation peptide or activated protein C assay is reduced to about 50% of normal in asymptomatic persons with heterozygous protein C deficiency.[96,193] In two adult patients with homozygous protein C deficiency, diminished protein C activation and increased thrombin generation can be normalized by administration of a monoclonal antibody-purified protein C concentrate.[195] Thus, it has been shown that augmented activity of the protein C anticoagulant pathway can inhibit thrombin generation in vivo, and that the activation of protein C by the thrombin/thrombomodulin complex is a tonically active mechanism in the regulation of coagulation system activation.

In asymptomatic patients with hereditary AT III deficiency, it was initially reported that F_{1+2} levels are frequently increased compared with age-matched unaffected siblings.[196] Fibrinopeptide A measurements were similar in both groups. The plasma AT III concentrations were reduced to about 50% of normal in the 22 affected people. Subsequently it was shown that the high concentrations of the fragment resulted from an in vitro anticoagulant effect resulting from the action of low amounts of heparin (final concentration of 4 U/ml) in the presence of reduced blood levels of AT III.[197]

A recent study of 26 AT III-deficient subjects from Italy did not demonstrate significant elevations in plasma F_{1+2} or fibrinopeptide A levels.[194] Another cross-sectional study of asymptomatic persons from a single large family with functional AT III deficiency (AT III Hamilton, a type II mutation with diminished serine protease reactivity) found significantly higher results in affected family members.[198] However, the mean F_{1+2} value was within the normal range and most had normal levels. The mean levels of fibrinopeptide A were not significantly different between the AT III-deficient people and their unaffected family members.[198]

Ginsberg and colleagues[199] have determined that the presence of anticardiolipin antibodies in patients with SLE is associated with a prothrombotic state as measured by the F_{1+2} and fibrinopeptide A assays. In patients who were not receiving warfarin, the mean levels of the markers were significantly higher in SLE patients with anticardiolipin antibodies than in those without, and this relationship was maintained after excluding from analysis those individuals with prior thrombotic histories.

The continuing application of biochemical, molecular biologic, and clinical approaches to the investigation of the hemostatic system will lead to a greater appreciation of the molecular defects that cause venous and arterial vascular disorders in humans. This new information should allow us to identify more precisely individuals who are entering a clinically relevant hypercoagulable state, and to intervene with appropriate therapy before the onset of overt thrombotic disease.

REFERENCES

1. Nachman RL, Silverstein RL: Hypercoagulable states. Ann Intern Med 119: 819, 1993
2. Gladson CL, Scharrer I, Hach V et al: The frequency of type I heterozygous protein S and protein C deficiency in 141 unrelated patients with venous thrombosis. Thromb Haemost 59:18, 1988
3. Ben-Tal O, Zivelin A, Seligsohn U: The relative frequency of hereditary thrombotic disorders among 107 patients with thrombophilia in Israel. Thromb Haemost 61:50, 1989
4. Malm J, Laurell M, Nilsson IM, Dahlback B: Thromboembolic disease—critical evaluation of laboratory investigation. Thromb Haemost 68:7, 1992
5. Heijboer H, Brandjes DPM, Buller HR et al: Deficiencies of coagulation-inhibiting and fibrinolytic proteins in outpatients with deep venous thrombosis. N Engl J Med 323:1512, 1990
6. Egeberg O: Inherited antithrombin deficiency causing thrombophilia. Thromb Diath Haemorrh 13:516, 1965
7. Marciniak E, Farley CH, DeSimone PA: Familial thrombosis due to antithrombin III deficiency. Blood 43:219, 1974
8. Carvalho A, Ellman L: Hereditary antithrombin III deficiency: effect of antithrombin III deficiency on platelet function. Am J Med 61:179, 1976
9. Mackie M, Bennett B, Ogston D, Douglas AS: Familial thrombosis: inherited deficiency of antithrombin III. Br Med J 1:136, 1978
10. Gyde OHB, Middleton MD, Vaughan GR, Fletcher DJ: Antithrombin III deficiency, hypertriglyceridaemia and venous thrombosis. Br Med J 1:621, 1978
11. Ambruso DR, Jacobson LJ, Hathaway WE: Inherited antithrombin III deficiency and cerebral thrombosis in a child. Pediatrics 65:125, 1980
12. Rosenberg RD: Actions and interaction of antithrombin and heparin. N Engl J Med 292:146, 1975
13. Odegard OR, Abildgaard U: Antithrombin III: critical review of assay methods. Significance of variations in health and disease. Haemostasis 7:127, 1978
14. Meade TW, Dyer S, Howarth DJ et al: Antithrombin III and procoagulant activity; sex differences and effects of the menopause. Br J Haematol 74: 77, 1990
15. Thaler E, Lechner K: Antithrombin III deficiency and thromboembolism. Clin Haematol 10:369, 1981
16. Demers C, Ginsberg JS, Hirsh J et al: Thrombosis in antithrombin-III-deficient persons. Report of a large kindred and literature review. Ann Intern Med 116:754, 1992
17. Brenner B, Fishman A, Goldsher D et al: Cerebral thrombosis in a newborn with a congenital deficiency of antithrombin III. Am J Hematol 27:209, 1988
18. Lane DA, Ireland H, Olds RJ et al: Antithrombin III: a database of mutations. Thromb Haemost 66:657, 1991
19. Lane DA, Olds RJ, Boislair M et al: Antithrombin III mutation database: first update. Thromb Haemost 70:361, 1993
20. Ambruso DR, Leonard BD, Bies RD et al: Antithrombin III deficiency: decreased synthesis of a biochemically normal molecule. Blood 60:78, 1982
21. Prochownik EV, Antonarkis S, Bauer KA et al: Molecular heterogeneity of inherited antithrombin III deficiency. N Engl J Med 308:149, 1983
22. Bock SC, Prochownik EV: Molecular genetic survey of 16 kindreds with hereditary antithrombin III deficiency. Blood 70:1273, 1987
23. Olds RJ, Lane DA, Finazzi G et al: A frameshift mutation leading to type I antithrombin deficiency and thrombosis. Blood 76:2182, 1990
24. Olds RJ, Lane DA, Ireland H et al: Novel point mutations leading to type I antithrombin deficiency and thrombosis. Br J Haematol 78:408, 1991
25. Gandrille S, Vidaud D, Emmerich J et al: Molecular basis for hereditary antithrombin III quantitative deficiencies: a stop codon in exon IIIa and a frameshift in exon VI. Br J Haematol 78:414, 1991
26. Grundy CB, Thomas F, Millar DS et al: Recurrent deletion in the human antithrombin III gene. Blood 78:1027, 1991
27. Vidaud D, Emmerich J, Sirieix ME et al: Molecular basis for antithrombin III type I deficiency: three novel mutations located in exon IV. Blood 78:2305, 1991
28. Harper PL, Luddington RJ, Daly M et al: The incidence of dysfunctional antithrombin variants: four cases in 210 patients with thromboembolic disease. Br J Haematol 77:360, 1991
29. Sas G, Blasko G, Banhegyi D et al: Abnormal antithrombin III (antithrombin III "Budapest") as a cause of familial thrombophilia. Thromb Diath Haemorrh 32:105, 1974
30. Tollefsen DM, Blank MK: Detection of a new heparin-dependent inhibitor of thrombin in human plasma. J Clin Invest 68:589, 1981
31. Tollefsen DM, Majerus DW, Blank MK: Heparin cofactor II. Purification and properties of a heparin-dependent inhibitor of thrombin in human plasma. J Biol Chem 257:2162, 1982
32. Demers C, Henderson P, Blajchman MA et al: An antithrombin III assay based on factor Xa inhibition provides a more reliable test to identify congenital antithrombin III deficiency than an assay based on thrombin inhibition. Thromb Haemost 69:231, 1993
33. Sie P, Dupout D, Pichon J, Boneu B: Constitutional heparin cofactor II deficiency associated with recurrent thrombosis. Lancet 2:414, 1985
34. Tran TH, Marbet GA, Duckert F: Association of hereditary heparin cofactor II deficiency with thrombosis. Lancet 2:413, 1985
35. Koide T, Odani S, Takahashi K et al: Antithrombin III Toyama: replacement of arginine-47 by cysteine in hereditary abnormal antithrombin III that lacks heparin-binding ability. Proc Natl Acad Sci USA 81:289, 1984
36. Molho-Sabatier P, Alach M, Gaillard I et al: Molecular characterization of antithrombin III (ATIII) variants using polymerase chain reaction. Identification of the ATIII Charleville as an Ala 384 Pro mutation. J Clin Invest 84: 1236, 1989
37. Owen M, Borg J, Soria J et al: Heparin binding defect in a new antithrombin III variant: Rouen, 47 Arg to His. Blood 69:1275, 1987
38. Borg JY, Owen MC, Soria C et al: Proposed heparin binding site in antithrombin based on arginine 47. A new variant Rouen-II, 47 Arg to Ser. J Clin Invest 81:1292, 1988
39. Gandrille S, Aiach M, Lane DA et al: Important role of Arg 129 in heparin binding site of antithrombin III: identification of a novel mutation Arg 129 to Gln. J Biol Chem 265;18997, 1990
40. Chang JY, Tran TH: Antithrombin III Basel. Identification of a Pro-Leu substitution in a hereditary abnormal antithrombin with impaired heparin cofactor activity. J Biol Chem 261:1174, 1986
41. Sambrano JE, Jacobson LJ, Reeve EB et al: Abnormal antithrombin III with defective serine protease binding (antithrombin III "Denver"). J Clin Invest 77:877, 1986
42. Bauer KA, Ashenhurst JB, Chediak J, Rosenberg RD: Antithrombin "Chicago": a functionally abnormal molecule with increased heparin affinity causing familial thrombophilia. Blood 62:1242, 1983
43. Cosgriff TM, Bishop DT, Hershgold EJ et al: Familial antithrombin III deficiency: its natural history, genetics, diagnosis and treatment. Medicine 62: 209, 1983
44. Bock SC, Harris JF, Schwartz CE et al: Hereditary thrombosis in a Utah kindred is caused by a dysfunctional antithrombin III gene. Am J Hum Genet 37:32, 1985
45. Bock SC, Marrinan JA, Radziejewska E: Antithrombin III Utah: proline-407 to leucine mutation in a highly conserved region near the inhibitor reactive site. Biochemistry 27:6171, 1988
46. Hultin MB, McKay J, Abildgaard U: Antithrombin Oslo: type Ib classification of the first reported antithrombin-deficient family, with a review of hereditary antithrombin variants. Thromb Haemost 59:468, 1988
47. Nakagawa M, Tanaka S, Tsuji H et al: Congenital antithrombin deficiency (ATIII Kyoto): identification of a point mutation altering arginine-406 to methionine behind the reactive site. Thromb Res 64:101, 1991
48. Olds RJ, Lane DA, Caso R et al: Antithrombin III Budapest: a single amino acid substitution (429Pro to Leu) in a region highly conserved in the serpin family. Blood 79:1206, 1992
49. Odegard OR, Lie M, Abildgaard U: Heparin cofactor activity measured with an amidolytic method. Thromb Res 6:287, 1975
50. Fagerhol M, Abildgaard U: Immunological studies on human antithrombin III. Influence of age, sex and use of oral contraceptives on serum concentration. Scand J Haematol 1:10, 1970
51. McDonald M, Hathaway W, Reeve E, Leonard B: Biochemical and functional study of antithrombin III in newborn infants. Thromb Haemost 47:56, 1982
52. Andrew MB, Milner R, Johnston M et al: Development of the human coagulation system in the full-term infant. Blood 70:165, 1987
53. Andrew M, Paes B, Milner R et al: Development of the human coagulation system in the healthy premature infant. Blood 72:1651, 1988
54. Rosenberg RD, Damus PS: The purification and mechanism of action of human antithrombin-heparin cofactor. J Biol Chem 248:6490, 1973
55. Downing MR, Bloom JW, Mann KG: Comparison of the inhibition of thrombin by three plasma protease inhibitors. Biochemistry 17:2649, 1978
56. Mitchell L, Piovella F, Ofosu F, Andrew M: α-2-Macroglobulin may provide protection from thromboembolic events in antithrombin III-deficient children. Blood 78:2299, 1991
57. de Boer A, van Riel L, den Ottolander G: Measurement of antithrombin III, α_2-macroglobulin and α_1-antitrypsin in patients with deep venous thrombosis and pulmonary embolism. Thromb Res 15:17, 1979
58. Damus PS, Wallace GA: Immunologic measurement of antithrombin III-heparin cofactor and α_2-macroglobulin in disseminated intravascular coagulation and hepatic failure coagulopathy. Thromb Res 6:27, 1989
59. Kauffman RH, Veltkamp JJ, Van Tilburg NH, Van Es LA: Acquired antithrom-

bin III deficiency and thrombosis in the nephrotic syndrome. Am J Med 65: 607, 1978

60. Caine YG, Bauer KA, Barzegar S et al: Coagulation activation following estrogen administration to postmenopausal women. Thromb Haemost 68:392, 1992

61. Buchanan GR, Holtkamp CA: Reduced antithrombin III levels during L-asparaginase therapy. Med Pediatr Oncol 8:7, 1980

62. Marciniak E, Gockemen JP: Heparin-induced decrease in circulating antithrombin III. Lancet 2:581, 1978

63. Kitchens CS: Amelioration of antithrombin III deficiency by coumarin administration. Am J Med Sci 293:403, 1987

64. Menache D, O'Malley JP, Schorr JB et al: Evaluation of the safety, recovery, half-life, and clinical efficacy of antithrombin III (human) in patients with hereditary antithrombin III deficiency. Blood 75:33, 1990

65. Schwartz RS, Bauer KA, Rosenberg RD et al: Clinical experience with antithrombin III concentrate in treatment to congenital and acquired deficiency of antithrombin. Am J Med 87:53S, 1989

66. Ginsberg JS, Hirsh J: Anticoagulants during pregnancy. Annu Rev Med 40: 79, 1989

67. Iturbe-Alessio I, Fonseca MC, Mutchinik O et al: Risks of anticoagulant therapy in pregnant women with artificial heart valves. N Engl J Med 315:1390, 1986

68. Winter J, Fenech A, Bennett B, Douglas A: Prophylactic antithrombotic therapy with stanazolol in patients with familial antithrombin III deficiency. Br J Haematol 57:527, 1984

69. Griffin JH, Evatt B, Zimmerman TS et al: Deficiency of protein C in congenital thrombotic disease. J Clin Invest 68:1370, 1981

70. Bertina RM, Broekmans AW, van der Linden IK, Mertens K: Protein C deficiency in a Dutch family with thrombotic disease. Thromb Haemost 45:237, 1982

71. Broekmans AW, Veltkamp JJ, Bertina RM: Congenital protein C deficiency and venous thromboembolism: a study of three Dutch families. N Engl J Med 309:340, 1983

72. Horellou MH, Conard J, Bertina RM, Samama M: Congenital protein C deficiency and thrombotic disease in nine French families. Br Med J 289:1285, 1984

73. Bovill EG, Bauer KA, Dickerman JD et al: The clinical spectrum of heterozygous protein C deficiency in a large New England kindred. Blood 73:712, 1989

74. Wintzen A, Broekmans A, Bertina R et al: Cerebral hemorrhagic infarction in young patients with hereditary protein C deficiency: evidence for "spontaneous" cerebral venous thrombosis. Br Med J 290:350, 1985

75. Camerlingo M, Finazzi G, Casto L et al: Inherited protein C deficiency and nonhemorrhagic arterial stroke in young adults. Neurology 41:1371, 1991

76. Branson HE, Katz J, Marble R, Griffin JH: Inherited protein C deficiency and coumarin-responsive chonic relapsing purpura fulminans in a newborn infant. Lancet 2:1165, 1983

77. Seligsohn U, Berger A, Abend M et al: Homozygous protein C deficiency manifested by massive venous thrombosis in the newborn. N Engl J Med 310:559, 1984

78. Sills RH, Marlar RA, Montgomery RR et al: Severe homozygous protein C deficiency. J Pediatr 105:409, 1984

79. Marciniak E, Wilson HD, Marlar RA: Neonatal purpura fulminans: a genetic disorder related to the absence of protein C in blood. Blood 65:15, 1985

80. Peters C, Casella J, Marlar R et al: Homozygous protein C deficiency: observations on the nature of the molecular abnormality and the effectiveness of warfarin therapy. Pediatrics 81:272, 1988

81. Miletich JP, Sherman L, Broze GJJ: Absence of thrombosis in subjects with heterozygous protein C deficiency. N Engl J Med 317:991, 1987

82. McGehee WG, Klotz TA, Epstein DJ, Rapaport SI: Coumarin necrosis associated with hereditary protein C deficiency. Ann Intern Med 100:59, 1984

83. D'Angelo SV, Comp PC, Esmon CT, D'Angelo A: Relationship between protein C antigen and anticoagulant activity during oral anticoagulation and in selected disease states. J Clin Invest 77:416, 1986

84. Conway EM, Bauer KA, Barzegar S, Rosenberg RD: Suppression of hemostatic system activation by oral anticoagulants in the blood of patients with thrombotic diatheses. J Clin Invest 80:1535, 1987

85. Teepe R, Broekmans A, Vermeer B et al: Recurrent coumarin-induced skin necrosis in a patient with an acquired functional protein C deficiency. Arch Dermatol 122:1408, 1986

86. Romeo G, Hassan H, Staempfli S et al: Hereditary thrombophilia: identification of nonsense and missense mutations in the protein C gene. Proc Natl Acad Sci USA 84:2829, 1987

87. Reitsma PH, Poort SR, Allaart CF et al: The spectrum of genetic defects in a panel of 40 Dutch families with symptomatic protein C deficiency type I: heterogeneity and founder effects. Blood 78:890, 1991

88. Reitsma PH, Poort SR, Bernardi F et al: Protein C deficiency: a database of mutations. Thromb Haemost 69:77, 1993

89. Bertina RM, Broekmans AW, Krommenhoek-van Es C, van Winhgaarden A: The use of a functional and immunologic assay for plasma protein C in

90. Comp PC, Nixon RR, Esmon CT: Determination of functional levels of protein C, an antithrombotic protein, using thrombin-thrombomodulin complex. Blood 63:15, 1984

91. Faioni E, Esmon C, Esmon N, Mannucci P: Isolation of an abnormal protein C molecule from the plasma of a patient with thrombotic diathesis. Blood 71:940, 1988

92. Matsuda M, Sugo T, Sakata Y et al: A thrombotic state due to an abnormal protein C. N Engl J Med 319:1265, 1988

93. Bovill EG, Tomczak JA, Grant B et al: Protein $C_{Vermont}$: symptomatic type II protein C deficiency associated with two GLA domain mutations. Blood 79: 1456, 1992

94. Gandrille S, Alhenc-Gelas M, Gaussem P et al: Five novel mutations located in exons III and IX of the protein C gene in patients presenting with defective protein C anticoagulant activity. Blood 82:159, 1993

95. Sugahara Y, Miura O, Yuen P, Aoki N: Protein C deficiency Hong Kong 1 and 2: hereditary protein C deficiency caused by two mutant alleles. a 5-nucleotide deletion and a missense mutation. Blood 80:126, 1992

96. Bauer KA, Broekmans AW, Bertina RM et al: Hemostatic enzyme generation in the blood of patients with hereditary protein C deficiency. Blood 71:1418, 1988

97. Melissari E, Kakkar VV: Congenital severe protein C deficiency in adults. Br J Haematol 72:222, 1989

98. Boyer C, Rothschild C, Wolf M et al: A new method for the estimation of protein C by ELISA. Thromb Res 36:579, 1984

99. Epstein D, Begum P, Bajaj S, Rapaport S: Radioimmunoassays for protein C and factor X. Plasma antigen levels in abnormal hemostatic states. Am J Clin Pathol 82:573, 1984

100. Bauer KA, Kass BL, Beeler DL, Rosenberg RD: Detection of protein C activation in humans. J Clin Invest 74:2033, 1984

101. Francis R Jr, Seyfert U: Rapid amidolytic assay of protein C in whole plasma using an activator from the venom of agkistrodon contortrix. Am J Clin Pathol 87:619, 1987

102. Mannucci PM, Vigano S: Deficiencies of protein C, an inhibitor of blood coagulation. Lancet 2:463, 1982

103. Karpatkin M, Mannucci PM, Bhogal M et al: Low protein C in the neonatal period. Br J Haematol 62:137, 1986

104. Griffin JH, Mosher DF, Zimmerman TS, Kleiss AJ: Protein C, an antithrombotic protein, is reduced in hospitalized patients with intravascular coagulation. Blood 60:261,1982

105. Marlar RA, Endres-Brooks J, Miller C: Serial studies of protein C and its plasma inhibitor in patients with disseminated intravascular coagulation. Blood 66:59, 1985

106. Rogers JI, Murgo A, Fontana J, Raich P: Chemotherapy for breast cancer decreases plasma protein C and protein S. J Clin Oncol 6:276, 1988

107. Pui CH, Chesney CM, Bergum PW et al: Lack of pathogenic role of protein C and S in thrombosis associated with asparaginase-prednisone-vincristine therapy for leukemia. Br J Haematol 64:283, 1986

108. Auletta MJ, Headington JT: Purpura fulminans. A cutaneous manifestation of severe protein C deficiency. Arch Dermatol 124:1387, 1988

109. Gerson WT, Dickerman JD, Bovill EG, Golden E: Severe acquired protein C deficiency in purpura fulminans associated with disseminated intravascular coagulation: treatment with protein C concentrate. Pediatrics 91:418, 1993

110. Vigano-D'Angelo S, D'Abgelo A, Kaufman C Jr et al: Protein S deficiency occurs in the nephrotic syndrome. Ann Intern Med 107:42, 1987

111. Cosio FG, Harker C, Batard MA et al: Plasma concentrations of the natural anticoagulants protein C and protein S in patients with proteinuria. J Lab Clin Med 106:218, 1985

112. Faioni E, Franchi F, Krachmalnicoff A et al: Low levels of the anticoagulant activity of protein C in patients with chronic renal insufficiency: an inhibitor of protein C is present in uremic plasma. Thromb Haemost 66:420, 1991

113. Mitchell CA, Rowell JA, Hau L et al: A fatal thrombotic disorder associated with an acquired inhibitor of protein C. N Engl J Med 317:1638, 1987

114. Broekmans AW, Conard J, van Weyenberg RG et al: Treatment of hereditary protein C deficiency with stanazolol. Thromb Haemost 57:20, 1987

115. De Stefano V, Leone G, Teofili L et al: Transient ischemic attack in a patient with congenital protein-C during treatment with stanazolol. Am J Haematol 29:120, 1988

116. Schramm W, Spannagl M, Bauer KA et al: Treatment of coumarin-induced skin necrosis with a monoclonal antibody purified protein C concentrate. Arch Dermatol 129:753, 1993

117. Dreyfus M, Magny JF, Bridey F et al: Treatment of homozygous protein C deficiency and neonatal purpura fulminans with a purified protein C concentrate. N Engl J Med 325:1565, 1991

118. Casella J, Lewis J, Bontemp F et al: Successful treatment of homozygous protein C deficiency by hepatic transplantation. Lancet 1:435, 1988

119. Comp PC, Esmon CT: Recurrent venous thromboembolism in patients with a partial deficiency of protein S. N Engl J Med 311:1525, 1984

the study of the heterogenecity of congenital protein C deficiency. Thromb Haemost 51:1, 1984

120. Schwarz HP, Fischer M, Hopmeier P et al: Plasma protein S deficiency in familial thrombotic disease. Blood 64:1297, 1984
121. Comp PC, Nixon RR, Cooper MR, Esmon CT: Familial protein S deficiency is associated with recurrent thrombosis. J Clin Invest 74:2082, 1984
122. Engesser L, Broekmans A, Briet E et al: Hereditary protein S deficiency: clinical manifestations. Ann Intern Med 106:677, 1987
123. Allaart CF, Aronson DC, Ruys T et al: Hereditary protein S deficiency in young adults with arterial occlusive disease. Thromb Haemost 64:206, 1990
124. Fair D, Revak DJ: Quantitation of human protein S in the plasma of normal and warfarin-treated individuals by radioimmunoassay. Thromb Res 36:527, 1984
125. Bertina RM, van Wijngaarden A, Reinalda-Poot J et al: Determination of plasma protein S-the protein factor of activated protein C. Thromb Haemostas 53:268, 1985
126. Comp PC, Thurnau GR, Welsh J, Esmon CT: Functional and immunologic protein S levels are decreased during pregnancy. Blood 68:881, 1986
127. D'Angelo A, Vigano-D'Angelo S, Esmon CT, Comp PC: Acquired deficiencies of protein S. Protein S activity during oral anticoagulation, in liver disease, and in disseminated intravascular coagulation. J Clin Invest 81:1445, 1988
128. Schwarz HP, Muntean W, Watzke H et al: Low total protein antigen but high protein S activity due to decreased C4B-binding protein in neonates. Blood 71:562, 1988
129. Ploos van Amstel HK, van der Zanden AL, Bakker E et al: Two genes homologous with protein S cDNA are located on chromosome 3. Thromb Haemost 58:982, 1987
130. Schmidel DK, Tataro AV, Phelps LG et al: Organization of the human protein S genes. Biochemistry 29:7845, 1990
131. Ploos van Amstel HK, Reitsma PH, van der Logt CPE, Bertina RM: Intronexon organization of the active protein S gene PS alpha and its pseudogene PSb: duplication and silencing during primate evolution. Biochemistry 29:7853, 1990
132. Edenbrandt C, Lundwall A, Wydro R, Stenflo J: Molecular analysis of the gene for vitamin K-dependent protein S and its pseudogene. Cloning and partial gene organization. Biochemistry 29:7861, 1990
133. Schmidel DK, Nelson RM, Broxson EHJ et al: A 5.3-kb deletion including exon XIII of the protein S a gene occurs in two protein S-deficient families. Blood 77:551, 1991
134. Mahasandana C, Suvatte V, Chuansumrit A et al: Homozygous protein S deficiency in an infant with purpura fulminans. J Pediatr 117:750, 1990
135. Boerger LM, Morris PC, Thurnau GR et al: Oral contraceptives and gender affect protein S status. Blood 69:692, 1987
136. Heeb MJ, Mosher D, Griffin JH: Activation and complexation of protein C and cleavage and decrease of protein S in plasma of patients with disseminated intravascular coagulation. Blood 73:455, 1989
137. Stahl CP, Wideman CS, Spira TJ et al: Protein S deficiency in men with long-term human immunodeficiency virus infection. Blood 81:1801, 1993
138. Gouault-Heilmann M, Gadelha-Parente T, Levent M et al: Total and free protein S in nephrotic syndrome. Thromb Res 49:37, 1988
139. Malm J, Bennhagen R, Holmberg L, Dahlback B: Plasma concentrations of C4b-binding protein and vitamin K-dependent protein S in term and preterm infants: low levels of protein S-C4b-binding protein complexes. Br J Haematol 68:445, 1988
140. D'Angelo A, Valle PD, Crippa L et al: Brief report: autoimmune protein S deficiency in a boy with severe thromboembolic disease. N Engl J Med 328:1753, 1993
141. Alessi MC, Aillaud MF, Boyer-Neumann C et al: Cutaneous necrosis associated with severe protein S deficiency. Thromb Haemost 69:524, 1993
142. Dahlback B, Carlsson M, Svensson PJ: Familial thrombophilia due to a previously unrecognized mechanism characterized by poor anticoagulant response to activated protein C: prediction of a cofactor to activated protein C. Proc Natl Acad Sci USA 90:1004, 1993
143. Griffin JH, Evatt B, Wideman C, Fernandez JA: Anticoagulant protein C pathway defective in majority of thrombophilic patients. Blood 82:1989, 1993
144. Koster T, Rosendaal FR, de Rorde H et al: Venous thrombosis due to poor anticoagulant response to activated protein C: Leiden thrombophilia study. Lancet 342:1503, 1993
144a. Dahlback B, Hildebrand B. Inherited resistance to activated protein C is corrected by anticoagulant cofactor activity found to be a property of factor V. Proc Natl Acad Sci USA 91:1396, 1994
145. Svensson PJ, Dahlback B: Resistance to activated protein C as a basis for venous thrombosis. N Engl J Med 330:517, 1994
145a. Bertina RM, Koeleman BPC, Koster T et al: Mutation in blood coagulation factor V associated with resistance to activated protein C. Nature 369:64, 1994
146. Haverkate F, Koopman J, Kluft C et al: Fibrinogen Milano II: a congenital dysfibrinogenemia associated with juvenile arterial and venous thrombosis. Thromb Haemost 55:131, 1986
147. Egeberg O: Inherited fibrinogen abnormality causing thrombophilia. Thromb Diath Haemorrh 17:175, 1967
148. Beck E, Charache P, Jackson D: A new inherited coagulation disorder caused by an abnormal fibrinogen (fibrinogen "Baltimore"). Nature 208:143, 1965
149. Beck E, Shainoff J, Vogel A, Jackson D: Functional evaluation of an inherited abnormal fibrinogen: fibrinogen Baltimore. J Clin Invest 50:1874, 1971
150. Carrell N, Gabriel DA, Blatt PM et al: Hereditary dysfibrinogenemia in a patient with thrombotic disease. Blood 62:439, 1983
151. Al-Mondhiry HAB, Bilezikian SB, Nossel HL: Fibrinogen "New York"—an abnormal fibrinogen associated with thromboembolism: functional evaluation. Blood 45:607, 1975
152. Soria J, Soria C, Caen JP: A new type of congenital dysfibrinogenemia with defective fibrin lysis-Dusard syndrome: possible relation to thrombosis. Br J Haematol 53:575, 1983
153. Koopman J, Haverkate F, Grimbergen J et al: Molecular basis for fibrinogen Dusart (Aα 554 Arg-Cys) and its association with abnormal fibrin polymerization and thrombophilia. J Clin Invest 91:1637, 1993
154. Aoki N, Moroi M, Sakata Y et al: Abnormal plasminogen. A hereditary abnormality found in a patient with recurrent thrombosis. J Clin Invest 61:1186, 1978
155. Sakata Y, Aoki N: Molecular abnormality of plasminogen. J Biol Chem 255:5442, 1980
156. Miyata T, Iwanaga S, Sakata Y, Aoki N: Plasminogen Tochigi: inactive plasmin resulting from replacement of alanine-600 by threonine in the active site. Proc Natl Acad Sci USA 79:6132, 1979
157. Azuma H, Uno Y, Shigekiyo T, Saito S: Congenital plasminogen deficiency caused by a Ser^{572} to Pro mutation. Blood 475, 1993
158. Aoki N, Tateno K, Sakata Y: Differences of frequency distributions of plasminogen phenotypes between Japanese and American populations: new methods for the detection of plasminogen variants. Biochem Genet 22:871, 1984
159. Shigekiyo T, Uno Y, Tomonari A et al: Type I congenital plasminogen deficiency is not a risk factor for thrombosis. Thromb Haemost 67:189, 1992
160. Jorgensen M, Mortensen JZ, Madsen AG et al: A family with reduced plasminogen activator activity in blood associated with recurrent venous thrombosis. Scand J Haematol 29:217, 1982
161. Bolan CD, Krishnamurti C, Tang DB et al: Association of protein S deficiency with thrombosis in a kindred with elevated levels of plasminogen activator-1. Ann Intern Med 119:779, 1993
162. Prins MH, Hirsh J: A critical review of the evidence supporting a relationship between impaired fibrinolytic activity and venous thromboembolism. Arch Intern Med 151:1721, 1991
163. Nilsson I, Ljungner H, Tengborn L: Two different mechanisms in patients with venous thrombosis and defective fibrinolysis: low concentration of plasminogen activator or increased concentration of plasminogen activator inhibitor. Br Med J 290:1453, 1985
164. Juhan-Vague I, Valadier J, Alessi MC et al: Deficient t-PA release and elevated PA inhibitor levels in patients with spontaneous or recurrent deep venous thrombosis. Thromb Haemost 57:67, 1987
165. Nguyen G, Horellou M, Kruithof E et al: Residual plasminogen activator activity after venous stasis as a criterion for hypofibrinolysis: a study in 83 patients with confirmed deep venous thrombosis. Blood 72:601, 1988
166. Engesser L, Brommer E, Kluft C, Briet E: Elevated plasminogen activator inhibitor (PAI), a cause of thrombophilia? A study in 203 patients with familial or sporadic venous thrombophilia. Thromb Haemost 62:673, 1989
167. Hamsten A, Wiman B, de Faire U, Blomback M: Increased plasma levels of a rapid inhibitor of tissue plasminogen activator in young survivors of myocardial infarction. N Engl J Med 313:1557, 1985
168. Hamsten A, Walldius G, Szamosi A et al: Plasminogen activator inhibitor in plasma: risk factor for recurrent myocardial infarction. Lancet 2:3, 1987
169. Ratnoff OD, Colopy JE: Familial hemorrhagic trait associated with deficiency of clot-promoting fraction of plasma. J Clin Invest 34:602, 1955
170. Goodnough LT, Saito H, Ratnoff OD: Thrombosis or myocardial infarction in congenital clotting factor abnormalities and chronic thrombocytopenias: a report of 21 patients and a review of 50 previously reported cases. Medicine 62:248, 1983
171. Ratnoff OD, Busse RJ, Sheon RP: The demise of John Hageman. N Engl J Med 279:760, 1968
172. Lammie B, Wuillemin W, Huber I et al: Thromboembolism and bleeding tendency in congenital factor XII deficiency—a study on 74 subjects from 14 Swiss families. Thromb Haemost 65:117, 1991
173. Mueh J, Herbst K, Rapaport S: Thrombosis in patients with the lupus anticoagulant. Ann Intern Med 92:156, 1980
174. Gastineau DA, Kazmier FJ, Nichols WL, Bowie EJW: Lupus anticoagulants: an analysis of the clinical and laboratory feature of 219 cases. Am J Hematol 19:265, 1985
175. Triplett DA, Brandt JT, Musgrave KA, Orr CA: The relationship between lupus anticoagulants and antibodies to phospholipid. JAMA 259:550, 1988
176. Long AA, Ginsberg JS, Brill-Edwards P et al: The relationship of antiphospholipid antibodies to thromboembolic disease in systemic lupus erythematosus: a cross-sectional study. Thromb Haemost 66:520, 1991
177. Ginsberg JS, Brill-Edwards P, Johnston M et al: Relationship of antiphospholipid antibodies to pregnancy loss in patients with systemic lupus erythematosus: a cross-sectional study. Blood 80:975, 1992
178. Ginsburg KS, Liang MH, Newcomer L et al: Anticardiolipin antibodies and

the risk for ischemic stroke and venous thrombosis. Ann Intern Med 117: 997, 1992

179. Carreras LO, Defreyn G, Machin SJ et al: Arterial thrombosis, intrauterine death and "lupus" anticoagulant: detection of immunoglobulin interfering with prostacyclin production. Lancet 1:244, 1981

180. Cariou R, Tobelem G, Bellucci S et al: Effect of lupus anticoagulant on antithrombogenic properties of endothelial cells—inhibition of thrombomodulin-dependent protein C activation. Thromb Haemost 60:54, 1988

181. Lellouche F, Martinuzzo M, Said P et al: Imbalance of thromboxane/prostacyclin biosynthesis in patients with lupus anticoagulant. Blood 78:2894, 1991

182. Freyssinet J, Wiesel M, Gauchy J et al: An IgM lupus anticoagulant that neutralizes the enhancing effect of phospholipid on purified endothelial thrombomodulin activity—a mechanism for thrombosis. Thromb Haemost 55:309, 1986

183. Faaber P, Rijke T, Van de Putte L et al: Cross reactivity of human and murine anti-DNA antibodies with heparan sulfate. J Clin Invest 77:1824, 1986

184. Love PE, Santoro SA: Antiphospholipid antibodies: anticardiolipin and the lupus anticoagulant in systemic lupus erythematosus (SLE) and in non-SLE disorders. Ann Intern Med 682, 1990

185. Bauer KA, Kass BL, ten Cate H et al: Detection of factor X activation in humans. Blood 74:2007, 1989

186. Bauer KA, Kass BL, ten Cate H et al: Factor IX is activated in vivo by the tissue factor mechanism. Blood 76:731, 1990

187. Teitel JM, Bauer KA, Lau HK, Rosenberg RD: Studies of the prothrombin activation pathway utilizing radioimmunoassays for the F_2/F_{1+2} fragment and thrombin-antithrombin complex. Blood 59:1086, 1982

188. Pelzer H, Schwarz A, Heimburger N: Determination of human thrombin-antithrombin III complex in plasma with an enzyme-linked immunosorbent assay. Thromb Haemost 59:101, 1988

189. Nossel H, Yudelman I, Canfield R et al: Measurement of fibrinopeptide A in human blood. J Clin Invest 54:43, 1974

190. Nossel H, Wasser J, Kaplan K et al: Sequence of fibrinogen protolysis and platelet release after intrauterine infusion of hypertonic saline. J Clin Invest 64:1371, 1979

191. Weitz JI, Koehn JA, Canfield RW et al: Development of a radioimmunoassay for the fibrinogen-derived peptide Bb1-42. Blood 67:1014, 1986

192. Pelzer H, Schwart A, Stuber W: Determination of human prothrombin activation fragment 1 + 2 in plasma in plasma with an antibody against a synthetic peptide. Thromb Haemost 65:153, 1991

193. Gruber A, Griffin JH: Direct detection of activated protein C in blood from human subjects. Blood 79:2340, 1992

194. Mannucci PM, Tripodi A, Bottasso B et al: Markers of procoagulant imbalance in patients with inherited thrombophilic syndromes. Thromb Haemost 67:200, 1992

195. Conard J, Bauer KA, Gruber A et al: Normalization of markers of coagulation activation with a purified protein C concentrate in adults with homozygous protein C deficiency. Blood 82:1159, 1993

196. Bauer KA, Goodman TL, Kass BL, Rosenberg RD: Elevated factor Xa activity in the blood of asymptomatic patients with congenital antithrombin deficiency. J Clin Invest 76:826, 1985

197. Bauer K, Barzegar S, Rosenberg R: Influence of anticoagulants used for blood collection on plasma prothrombin fragment F_{1+2} measurements. Thromb Res 63:617, 1991

198. Demers C, Ginsberg JS, Henderson P et al: Measurements of markers of activated coagulation in antithrombin III deficient subjects. Thromb Haemost 67:542, 1992

199. Ginsberg JS, Demers C, Brill-Edwards P et al: Increased thrombin generation and activity in patients with systemic lupus erythematosus and anticardiolipin antibodies: evidence for a prothrombotic state. Blood 81:2958, 1993

Oral Anticoagulant Therapy 120

Bruce Furie

STRUCTURE OF ORAL ANTICOAGULANTS

The vitamin K antagonists were discovered as the result of an intensive investigation into the etiology of a hemorrhagic disease of cattle that plagued farmers in the Great Plains during the 1920s. This disorder, characterized by hypoprothrombinemia, was associated with the ingestion of spoiled sweet clover hay contaminated with specific toxins.[1,2] Campbell and Link[3] purified 3,3'-methylene-bis-4-hydroxycoumarin from bacterial contaminants in the spoiled hay and discovered that this compound caused a syndrome similar to vitamin K deficiency. Bishydroxycoumarin, a vitamin K antagonist, was introduced into clinical practice as an anticoagulant during the 1940s[4] and is prescribed as dicumarol. Other structurally related vitamin K antagonists with varying pharmacologic properties were developed (Fig. 120-1). The most important vitamin K antagonist used clinically in the United States is warfarin sodium.

MECHANISM OF ACTION OF WARFARIN

As a vitamin K antagonist, warfarin inhibits the synthesis of the vitamin K-dependent blood-clotting proteins, including prothrombin and factors VII, IX, and X, required for normal blood coagulation.[5] In addition, the vitamin K-dependent regulatory proteins, proteins C and S, are also affected due to a decrease in vitamin K-dependent post-translational modifications. The anticoagulant effect of warfarin depends on the reduction in the synthesis of biologically active vitamin K-dependent blood-clotting proteins and the normal clearance from the circulation of fully active vitamin K-dependent blood-clotting proteins synthesized before the introduction of the vitamin K antagonist. Importantly, the administration of warfarin does not lead to instantaneous anticoagulation. Rather, warfarin must be administered for 4–5 days before the anticoagulant effect can be considered therapeutic.

During the synthesis of the vitamin K-dependent proteins, the post-translational modification of glutamic acid to γ-carboxyglutamic acid is catalyzed by the vitamin K-dependent carboxylase.[6] γ-Carboxyglutamic acid is required in these proteins to permit calcium-dependent protein-membrane interaction and for the expression of full biologic activity.[7–9] The carboxylase is an integral membrane protein[10] requiring carbon dioxide, molecular oxygen, and the hydroquinone form of vitamin K to convert glutamic acid to γ-carboxyglutamic acid.[6] During this reaction, a γ-hydrogen on glutamic acid residues on the precursor protein is extracted, and carbon dioxide reacted to form the new carboxyl group. The vitamin K hydroquinone is converted to vitamin K epoxide in a reaction that is closely linked to the carboxylase activity. Although some vitamin K antago-

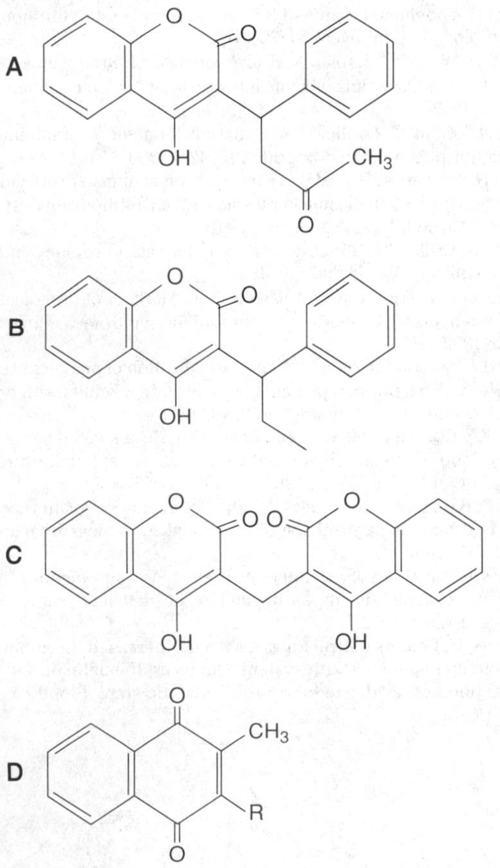

Fig. 120-1. Structure of the oral anticoagulants and their relationship to vitamin K. Chemical structures include **(A)** warfarin, **(B)** phenprocoumon, **(C)** dicoumarol, and **(D)** vitamin K. Vitamin K and the coumarin anticoagulants share a common ring structure, shown in red.

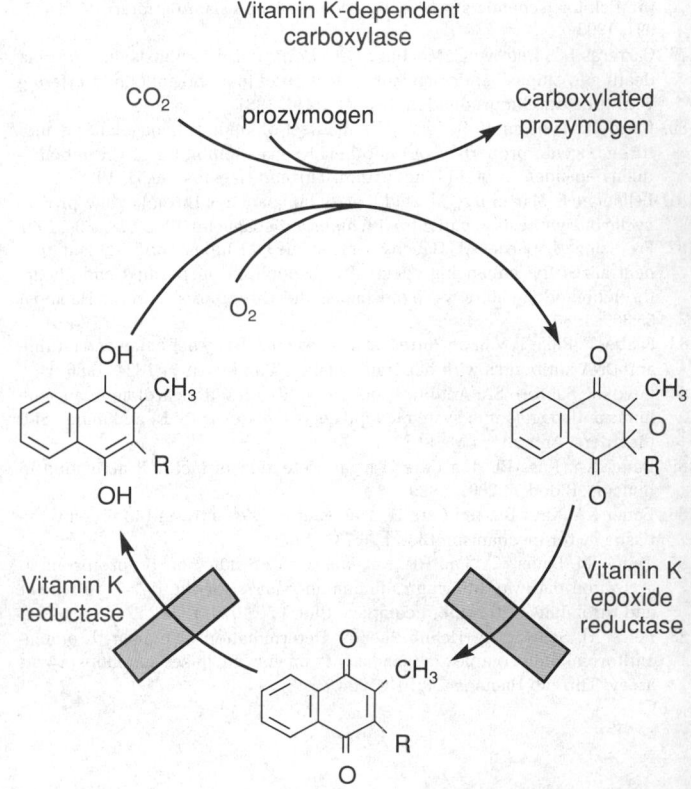

Fig. 120-2. Vitamin K cycle and its inhibition by warfarin. Vitamin K is reduced to the vitamin K hydroquinone by a vitamin K reductase inhibited by warfarin. The vitamin K hydroquinone is a cofactor for the vitamin K-dependent carboxylase. In this reaction, the hydroquinone is oxidized to the vitamin K epoxide and glutamic acid is converted to γ-carboxyglutamic acid. The carboxylase is not inhibited by warfarin. The vitamin K epoxide is salvaged by a vitamin K epoxide reductase, an enzyme sensitive to warfarin inhibition, and is recycled back to vitamin K.

nists inhibit the carboxylase directly, warfarin does not inhibit the vitamin K-dependent carboxylase, except at very high concentration,[11] and is thus not a direct competitor of the action of vitamin K.

Inhibition of γ-carboxylation of the vitamin K-dependent proteins by warfarin yields proteins in the plasma that are partially carboxylated.[12,13] With but a single exception, the elimination of even a single γ-carboxyglutamic acid significantly disables the function of these proteins; some γ-carboxyglutamic acid residues are so critical that their absence abolishes biologic activity of the protein.[14] Therefore, the induction of acarboxy- and des-γ-carboxyprothrombin, for example, in the plasma of patients treated with warfarin, yields primarily functionally inert vitamin K-dependent blood-clotting proteins. The coagulant activity correlates closely with the quantity of fully carboxylated proteins that remain in the plasma of patients treated with warfarin.[15]

The vitamin K cycle represents a metabolic pathway for the utilization and recovery of vitamin K after its participation in vitamin K-dependent carboxylation reactions (Fig. 120-2) (see Ch. 114). Warfarin inhibits some of the enzymes involved in this cycle, blocking the availability of the proper form of vitamin K for participation as a cofactor in the reaction catalyzed by the carboxylase.[16-18] Vitamin K is reduced to the vitamin K hydroquinone by a vitamin K reductase. This enzyme is inhibited by warfarin. The vitamin K hydroquinone is the cofactor for the carboxylase. During carboxylation of glutamic acid residues by the carboxylase, the vitamin K hydroquinone is oxidized to the vitamin K epoxide. Warfarin has no effect on this reaction, except at very high concentration. The vitamin K epoxide is

recycled to vitamin K via a pathway that requires the vitamin K epoxide reductase. This reaction is inhibited by warfarin,[16] leading to increased plasma levels of vitamin K_1 epoxide.

PHARMACOLOGY

Warfarin sodium is administered by the oral route, hence its role in a class of compounds known as oral anticoagulants. Warfarin is nearly completely absorbed, although considerable variation remains in the individual absorption patterns. Peak warfarin levels are observed at 0.5–4 hours after oral administration.[19] Warfarin circulates in the blood bound to albumin. With 97% of warfarin bound to albumin, only small amounts of warfarin circulate free in plasma.[20] However, it is this free warfarin that is biologically active. The mean half-life of warfarin in the blood is 44 hours, but this varies widely in different subjects from 15 to 48 hours.[21] This plasma half-life depends on the rate of warfarin absorption and on the rate of warfarin degradation. The individual variation in the half-life of this drug is dominated by the variability of the degradation rate. Renal clearance of warfarin is low, as most of the warfarin is bound to albumin. Warfarin is metabolized in the liver to yield a series of inactive metabolites that are recovered in the urine.[22] Oxidation of warfarin is associated with the hepatic cytochrome P-450 complex.

The biologic effect of warfarin, the decrease in the plasma activity of the vitamin K-dependent proteins, lags behind the peak plasma warfarin concentration. The coagulant activity of each of these proteins in plasma represents a balance between

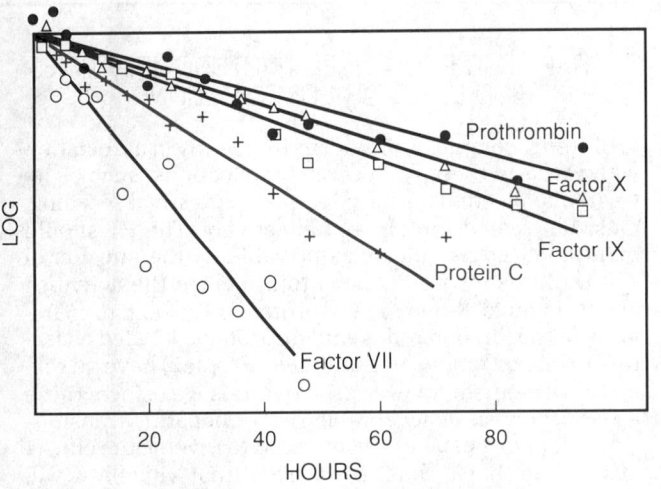

Fig. 120-3. The reduction of the activities of the vitamin K-dependent blood clotting proteins by warfarin. Warfarin (10 mg) was administered to a normal subject on 4 consecutive days. The activities of factors VII, X, and IX and prothrombin are presented as a function of time after the initiation of the medication. Factor VII activity disappears most rapidly, while prothrombin activity decreases more slowly. Factor IX and X activity decreases at an intermediate rate. Because the prothrombin time is so sensitive to the factor VII concentration, with the initiation of warfarin therapy the prothrombin time can be disproportionately prolonged before the levels of factors IX and X and prothrombin are reduced sufficiently to promote an antithrombotic effect.

the synthesis of the protein in a completely active form and its utilization and metabolism. The administration of warfarin impairs the complete synthesis of the vitamin K-dependent proteins by inhibiting γ-carboxylation but does not affect the plasma half-life of these proteins. Thus, the disappearance of factors VII, X, and IX and prothrombin coagulant activities from the plasma is related to the half-life of each of these proteins. Factor VII activity disappears most rapidly with a half-life of about 6 hours (Fig. 120-3). Factors X and IX have half-lives of about 24 hours; these activities decrease less rapidly from the plasma than that of factor VII. Prothrombin has a half-life of about 72 hours, disappearing at the slowest rate of the vitamin K-dependent blood-clotting proteins.

INDICATIONS FOR THERAPY

Warfarin and related oral anticoagulants are employed for the prevention of thromboembolic disorders in patients at risk.[23,24] Because of the 5–6% incidence of systemic embolization associated with atrial fibrillation and valvular heart disease, chronic warfarin therapy is routinely employed in this clinical setting. More recently, oral anticoagulants have been advocated in all patients with atrial fibrillation.[25,26] Patients with prosthetic heart valves, particularly of the mechanical type, require chronic warfarin administration to prevent embolism of formed thrombi. Other patients, such as the family members of patients with serious thromboembolic disorders secondary to defects in the proteins that regulate blood coagulation, may be placed on oral anticoagulant therapy if they also demonstrate a deficiency in these activities and are considered at risk of thromboembolic disease. Warfarin is effective in decreasing the incidence of venous thrombosis after hip surgery[27,28] and has also been employed at low fixed doses in patients with indwelling catheters.[29]

Warfarin is also used to prevent the recurrence of thromboembolic disease. After the acute treatment of thromboembolic diseases, such as pulmonary embolism and deep venous thrombosis, with heparin or fibrinolytic agents, patients are routinely maintained on warfarin for 3–6 months. The decision

to extend treatment for longer periods depends on an analysis of benefit versus risk. Risk factors for recurrent thromboembolic disease include specific abnormalities of coagulation or regulatory proteins, a history of recurrent thromboembolism, and a family history positive for thromboembolism (see Ch. 119). Other uses of warfarin therapy are more controversial. Despite the widespread use of warfarin for more than four decades for the prevention of second myocardial infarction as well as pooled data showing a statistically significant, albeit modest, effect, definitive clinical evidence that warfarin alters the incidence of reinfarction is lacking.[30,31] A recent trial, however, has reopened this question in that high-intensity warfarin therapy was shown to cause a reduction of recurrent infarction, stroke, and mortality.[32] Despite these results, warfarin has not found a major application in patients with myocardial infarction. Nevertheless, anticoagulant therapy, including heparin and warfarin, does play a role in preventing the arterial and venous thromboembolic complications that may occur during the immediate postinfarction period. It is currently recommended that patients with an anterior myocardial infarction, a subset at high risk of thromboembolism, be treated with prophylactic anticoagulants.[33,34] The role of warfarin in the treatment of stroke is unclear.

CONTRAINDICATIONS

Warfarin is contraindicated in patients who fail to comply with the routine administration of the drug and in patients who are unable to obtain regular measurements of the prothrombin time (PT). Furthermore, oral anticoagulants should not be used in patients with either hereditary or acquired bleeding disorders or in patients with anatomic lesions that predispose them to serious bleeding (e.g., active duodenal ulcer). Warfarin crosses the placenta in pregnant women. Because it is teratogenic and has been associated with a fetal warfarin syndrome,[35] warfarin use is contraindicated during pregnancy. Other anticoagulants, such as subcutaneous heparin, are used preferentially instead of warfarin to prevent thromboembolism in pregnant women at risk of thromboembolism.

REGULATION OF THERAPY

The PT is routinely used for monitoring therapy with the oral anticoagulants, including warfarin. The PT is a biologic test in which recalcified, citrated patient plasma is clotted by the addition of a crude preparation of tissue factor and lipid, also known as thromboplastin. Thromboplastin is an extract of either brain or lung tissue, or a mixture of both. Tissue factor initiates the extrinsic pathway of blood coagulation, including factors VII, X, and V, prothrombin, and fibrinogen. Decreases in the activities of three vitamin K-dependent proteins, factors VII and X, and prothrombin, prolong the PT. The patient's PT is usually reported as the clotting time, in seconds, and is compared with the PT of a normal plasma sample. Warfarin is administered to prolong the PT from the normal level (about 12 seconds) into the therapeutic range. More recently, the use of the International Normalized Ratio (INR) is also reported in order to correct for the variation in potency of different thromboplastins (see below). The warfarin dose is adjusted to obtain the recommended therapeutic INR for a given indication. Because factor VII is at the beginning of the extrinsic pathway and factor VII has the shortest half-life of the vitamin K-dependent blood coagulation proteins, the PT is very sensitive to the factor VII level; furthermore, the factor VII level is suppressed more quickly than the other vitamin K-dependent proteins. The optimal therapeutic range varies with the indication for warfarin anticoagulation[36] (see Chs. 123 and 124). Standard intensity

INITIATION OF WARFARIN THERAPY

When warfarin therapy is planned for the chronic anti-coagulation of patients following pulmonary embolism or deep venous thrombosis, patients are routinely treated with heparin during the acute phase of anticoagulation. Heparin is usually administered by continuous intravenous infusion for a period of 7–14 days. Because warfarin will not prolong the PT for 1 or 2 days after the initiation of therapy and because the anticoagulant action of warfarin is adequate only after 4 or 5 days of therapy, warfarin and heparin are given simultaneously for 4 or 5 days. A large loading dose of warfarin is unnecessary. Warfarin therapy (5 mg/day) can be instituted at the initiation of heparin therapy. Subsequently, the warfarin dose can be adjusted to optimize the prolongation of the PT. When adequate control has been established, heparin therapy may be discontinued.

Warfarin is also employed for the initiation of anticoagulant therapy without prior overlapping heparin therapy. A typical example is a patient with valvular heart disease with atrial fibrillation who requires prophylaxis with antithrombotic agents. Although warfarin-induced necrosis is a rare disorder, the prevalence of heterozygous protein C deficiency has been estimated to be 1 in 300 in the United States. To lower the risk of warfarin-induced necrosis, consideration may be given to either the measurement of the functional protein C level in the plasma of a patient to be treated for the first time with warfarin or to the co-administration of subcutaneous heparin therapy for the first 4 or 5 days of warfarin therapy.

warfarin therapy includes a therapeutic PT prolongation of 1.5–2.0 times the control PT value using the thromboplastin preparations currently used in the United States. When the anticoagulant effect is aimed at this level, bleeding complications of about 10–20% occur, with about one-half when the PT is within the therapeutic range. Low-intensity therapy, with a PT of 1.3–1.8 times control, has been shown to be associated with a significantly lower incidence of bleeding.[37,38] For these reasons, lower-intensity therapy, with a PT of 1.3–1.5 times the control PT, appears reasonable in the clinical setting of deep venous thrombosis. However, whether low-intensity therapy provides adequate prophylaxis of thromboembolic disease comparable to standard-dose warfarin therapy in other clinical situations has not been definitely demonstrated. Clinicians should use the INR value in making therapeutic decisions regarding the appropriate dose of warfarin.

International Normalized Ratio

Thromboplastins employed for PT measurements are derived from a variety of tissues, including brain and lung, and various species, including rabbit, bovine, and human. To standardize the potency of these different thromboplastin reagents, these reagents were calibrated using the standardized human brain thromboplastin reagent, the Manchester comparative reagent, as an international reference preparation. A calibration system, based on the linear relationship of the logarithm of the PT of the patient compared to the logarithm of the PT of control plasma, yields the INR:

$$\text{INR} = \left(\frac{\text{patient PT}}{\text{control PT}}\right)^c$$

where the ratio of the patient PT to the control PT is the ob-

THERAPY FOR PROLONGED PROTHROMBIN TIMES AND BLEEDING COMPLICATIONS

Bleeding complications occur frequently in association with warfarin therapy. Severe complications, such as intracranial bleeding or massive gastrointestinal bleeding, must be treated rapidly and effectively. The PT should be normalized as quickly as possible by the infusion of 2–3 U of fresh frozen plasma to replenish the activities of the vitamin K-dependent proteins. Current preparations of the vitamin K-dependent proteins labeled as factor IX concentrations (e.g., Konyne, Proplex) have no role in the treatment of warfarin overdosage, since these agents carry an unacceptable risk of hepatitis transmission. Vitamin K can be administered to reverse the effects of warfarin, but it must be realized that vitamin K will not be effective until 12–36 hours later. Patients given vitamin K may be refractory to the action of warfarin for a period of time after anticoagulant therapy is reinstituted.

Moderate complications, such as hematomas, hemarthrosis, or mild gastrointestinal bleeding, may be treated by the discontinuation of warfarin therapy and the administration of vitamin K. Vitamin K_1 (Aquamephyton) can be administered intravenously (with appropriate caution and monitoring of severe allergic reactions) at a dose of 10 mg. The PT will return toward the normal range within 24 hours.

Mild complications, such as purpura, ecchymoses, or epistaxis, can be treated by withholding or reducing warfarin therapy until the PT returns into the therapeutic range. In this situation, fresh frozen plasma carries an unnecessary risk of viral infection and vitamin K administration greatly complicates reinstitution of anticoagulant therapy with warfarin.

served ratio, and c represents the international sensitivity index. Since each thromboplastin yields a unique c value, PTs obtained using different thromboplastins can be compared, hence the INR. Currently, all commercially available thromboplastins are calibrated with regard to the International Sensitivity Index (ISI), and individual laboratories can report both the PT and the INR for a given sample. The ISI varies, at 1.0–1.2

MANAGEMENT OF CHRONIC WARFARIN THERAPY IN PATIENTS REQUIRING MINOR SURGERY

In patients requiring chronic anticoagulation for such conditions as heart valve prostheses or protein C deficiency, warfarin therapy may need to be discontinued briefly to permit the safe performance of surgical procedures. Warfarin therapy may be stopped 1 week prior to surgery and anticoagulation begun using subcutaneous heparin. With a normal diet, the PT will return to the normal range within the week. Heparin can be discontinued just before surgery. Either heparin and warfarin, or warfarin alone, can be reinstituted after the successful completion of surgery. The period between surgery and the reinitiation of anticoagulants depends on the balance between the risk of bleeding and the risk of thromboembolic disease.

Intensity of Anticoagulant Therapy: Recommended INR Values	
Prevention of	
Deep vein thrombosis	2.0–3.0
Subclavian vein thrombosis	2.0–3.0
Pulmonary embolism	2.0–3.0
Prophylaxis against systemic thromboembolic disease	
Atrial fibrillation	2.0–3.0
Cardiac valve replacement	
Mechanical valves	2.5–3.5
Tissue valves	2.0–3.0

in thromboplastins used in Europe to 1.8–2.8 for the North American thromboplastins.[39,40]

An independent method of monitoring warfarin anticoagulation has been undergoing clinical evaluation.[15,41] This method does not rely on the PT or the use of thromboplastins. By monitoring the level of fully γ-carboxylated prothrombin, or native prothrombin, by immunoassay, it has been possible to identify a therapeutic range of 12 to 24 μg/ml in which bleeding complications are minimized and at which the warfarin dosage is adequate to prevent thromboembolic disease.[42,43] This method has been further evaluated in patients undergoing hip replacement.[44]

Low-dose or minidose warfarin therapy in fixed-dose regimens has been advocated for general prophylaxis of thromboembolic disease following surgery as well as to prevent thrombosis in central venous catheters.[45,46] Because of the highly individual rates of absorption, utilization, and degradation of warfarin, fixed warfarin doses have variable potencies in different patients. However, the PT is insensitive to low-intensity warfarin therapy. The native prothrombin assay may offer an alternative method to monitor low-intensity therapy, as it is sensitive to small amounts of warfarin, permitting adjusted low-dose therapy.

COMPLIANCE

Because of the low toxic/therapeutic ratio, the risk of bleeding associated with warfarin therapy is highest in patients who are not carefully monitored. Therefore, only patients who are willing to subject themselves to the regular inconvenience of the PT measurement should be treated with warfarin. During the initiation of therapy, PTs may be required two or three times a week, then once weekly, until an adequate dosage is determined. Patients treated chronically with warfarin who have had stable PT measurements require a PT every 3 or 4 weeks. Furthermore, only reliable patients who will take their medication regularly should be considered for warfarin therapy.

DIET AND DRUG INTERACTION

Both diet and the co-administration of certain drugs can have a marked effect on the magnitude of warfarin action[47,48] (Table 120-1). Certain drugs diminish the pharmacologic response to warfarin. Barbiturates induce hepatic microsomal enzymes, enhancing the degradation of warfarin. Vitamin K antagonizes the inhibitory effect of warfarin on the synthesis of vitamin K-dependent proteins. Whether vitamin K is administered parenterally or orally, or in excess because of dietary intake, the effect is a blunting of the anticoagulant effect of warfarin. A common mechanism for the enhancement of warfarin action is the displacement of warfarin bound to albumin by other drugs that

Table 120-1. Effect of Drugs on Warfarin Response

Medications that Potentiate the Effect of Warfarin

Acetaminophen	Isoniazid
Acetohexamide	Mefenamic acid
Allopurinol	Methimazole
Androgenic and anabolic steroids	Methotrexate
α-Methyldopa	Methylphenidate
Antibiotics that disrupt intestinal	Nalidixic acid
flora (tetracyclines, streptomycin,	Nortriptyline
erythromycin, kanamycin, nalidixic	Oxyphenbutazone
acid, neomycine)	p-Aminosalicyclic acid
Cephaloridine	Paromomycin
Chloramphenicol	Phenylbutazone
Chlorpromazine	Phenytoin
Chlorpropamide	Phenyramidol
Chloral hydrate	Propylthiouracil
Cimetidine	Quinidine
Clofibrate	Salicylate
Diazoxide	Sulfinpyrazone
Disulfiram	Sulfonamides
Ethacrynic acid	Thyroid hormone
Glucagon	Tolbutamide
Guanethidine indomethacin	

Medications that Depress the Effect of Warfarin

Antipyrine	Glutethimide
Barbiturates	Griseofulvin
Carbamazepine	Haloperidol
Chlorthalidone	Oral contraceptives
Cholestyramine	Phenobarbital
Digitalis	Prednisone
Ethanol	All vitamin preparations containing
Ethchlorvynol	vitamin K

compete for this albumin-binding site. Albumin-binding drugs displace warfarin, thereby increasing the amount of free warfarin in the plasma. It is the free form of warfarin that is pharmacologically active, enhancing warfarin inhibition of vitamin K action. Because the clearance of warfarin from the blood is also a function of the free warfarin level, enhancement of the biologic action of warfarin is followed several days later by a reduction in warfarin action. Numerous drugs displace warfarin from albumin, but model examples include phenylbutazone and chloral hydrate. Chloramphenicol inhibits liver microsomal enzyme synthesis, reducing the normal rate of degradation of warfarin and leading to the enhancement of the effect of a particular warfarin dose.

It is good practice to stabilize the PT on a given dose of warfarin while avoiding changes in medications or diet, including alcohol consumption. In addition to the drugs listed in Table 120-1, a large number of drugs are known to perturb the PT of patients treated with warfarin. Some drug interactions have not been clearly defined. For these reasons, the introduction of a new medication in a patient on stable warfarin therapy requires careful monitoring of the PT during the transition period so as to permit adjustments of the warfarin dosage to accommodate the effects of the new medication. Other anticoagulants or antiplatelet drugs should be avoided during warfarin administration. For example, aspirin has been shown to increase bleeding complications during warfarin therapy.

WARFARIN RESISTANCE

Warfarin resistance is an occasional problem in some patients who have previously taken warfarin but are now refractory to normal doses and in other patients who are refractory to warfarin from the onset of therapy. The consideration of warfarin resistance is usually reserved for patients who require in excess of 15–20 mg/day of warfarin to maintain the PT within the therapeutic range.

The molecular basis of warfarin resistance is unknown in most patients. Patients unknowingly supplemented with vitamin K, such as those undergoing parenteral nutrition or feedings with enteral nutrition products, are resistant to the action of vitamin K antagonists administered at customary doses.[49] Patients with unusual dietary intake, including large amounts of cruciferous vegetables, such as spinach, cabbage, or broccoli, may also be resistant to warfarin because of the large quantities of vitamin K in these foods.[50,51] Once excess vitamin K intake has been ruled out, the mechanism of warfarin resistance remains speculative. There are no proven examples of antibodies arising to warfarin. A rare condition, hereditary warfarin resistance is characterized by the absence of warfarin effect on the synthesis of the vitamin K-dependent blood-clotting proteins despite the achievement of very high plasma warfarin levels.[52,53] Based on the study of the warfarin-resistant rat, it appears that the vitamin K epoxide reductase from these rats is less sensitive to warfarin than is the normal enzyme.[54,55]

Patients resistant to the effects of warfarin can still be treated with warfarin, but higher doses are necessary. With appropriate care, the warfarin dose can be gradually increased until the PT prolongs into the therapeutic range. In these patients, the warfarin dosage threshold at which the PT becomes unacceptably long is higher than in normal persons, but these patients are just as brittle. Small increases in the warfarin dose can prolong the PT significantly beyond the therapeutic range. Treatment with large doses of warfarin (e.g., >50 mg/day) may have toxicities not observed at conventional doses, so the treating physician may elect to use alternative therapies, such as subcutaneous heparin.

COMPLICATIONS

Bleeding complications are observed in 10–20% of patients treated with warfarin therapy.[37,38,42,56–60] About one-half of these complications occur when the therapeutic range of the PT has been exceeded, but one-half occur despite a PT within the therapeutic range. These may be mild, such as epistaxis, purpura, or hematuria, or they may be more serious, such as retroperitoneal bleeding, the formation of large hematomas, or significant gastrointestinal bleeding. Life-threatening bleeding, such as intracranial bleeding, does occur, and patients should be warned of the symptoms of such an event so that they can seek medical attention immediately.

Warfarin-induced skin necrosis is a rare complication. During the onset of warfarin therapy, usually between days 2 and 7, the patient develops a bluish purple lesion on the thigh, breast, buttock, or toes. This lesion is characterized by a clear line of demarcation between the affected area and surrounding tissue. Over several days, this lesion becomes increasely necrotic, while the surrounding area becomes erythematous and inflamed. The histology of the lesion reveals thrombi in the microvasculature. This syndrome is often due to the exaggeration of protein C deficiency by warfarin in a patient who has hereditary heterozygous protein C deficiency.[61] Protein C, a regulatory plasma protein that serves as a natural anticoagulant, requires vitamin K for its complete synthesis (see Ch. 102). Because protein C has a relatively short plasma half-life (Fig. 120-3) warfarin induces a relative protein C deficiency before it reduces the activity of the vitamin K-dependent blood-clotting proteins to an anticoagulant level. Since patients with heterozygous protein C deficiency are especially susceptible to this complication, they should only be treated with warfarin when heparin is employed simultaneously during the first 4 or 5 days of therapy. Warfarin-induced skin necrosis has also been reported in rare cases of hereditary protein S deficiency.

REVERSAL OF WARFARIN EFFECT

Overdosage of warfarin is a common problem that occasionally leads to serious bleeding manifestations. Although generally observed in patients being treated for thromboembolism, warfarin overdosage may also be seen after accidental or surreptitious ingestion. Proper therapy is dependent on the level of bleeding complications. In patients with prolongation of the PT without signs of bleeding, warfarin can be withheld until the PT approaches the therapeutic range. Patients with life-threatening bleeding disorders, including intra-abdominal or intracranial hemorrhage, require urgent, immediate correction of the PT. These patients must be treated with fresh frozen plasma (2–3 U) as a source of the vitamin K-dependent blood coagulation proteins. Because fresh frozen plasma carries the risk of infection, the severity of the bleeding episode must be balanced against the hepatitis risk. Factor IX concentrates include the vitamin K-dependent blood-clotting proteins in a partially purified form. However, because current products essentially ensure the transmission of hepatitis to patients who lack immunity to hepatitis, they are contraindicated. Improvements in the large-scale preparation of purified vitamin K-dependent proteins may offer new agents that will prove useful.[62–64] Vitamin K can be administered to reverse the effects of warfarin. However, the response to vitamin K is delayed for 12–24 hours due to the requirement for de novo synthesis of the vitamin K-dependent blood-clotting proteins. Furthermore, vitamin K administration usually results in normalization of the PT and will interfere with re-anticoagulation with vitamin K antagonists. Furthermore, patients treated with vitamin K may be resistant to warfarin action once warfarin therapy is reinitiated. For these reasons, vitamin K therapy is best reserved for patients with serious bleeding complications initially treated with fresh frozen plasma and whose anticoagulant management can be approached with alternative methods (e.g., heparin). Because the absorption of oral vitamin K, vitamin K_1 (Aquamephyton), is variable, the treatment of warfarin overdosage best involves administration of intravenous vitamin K_1.

REFERENCES

1. Schofield FW: A brief account of a disease in cattle simulating hemorrhagic septicemia due to feeding sweet clover. Can Vet Rec 3:74, 1922
2. Roderick LM: A problem in the coagulation of the blood "sweet clover" disease of cattle. Am J Physiol 96:413, 1931
3. Campbell HA, Link KP: Studies on the hemorrhagic sweet clover disease. IV. The isolation and crystallization of the hemorrhagic agent. J Biol Chem 138: 21, 1941
4. Bingham JB, Meyer OO, Pohle FJ: A preparation from spoiled sweet clover (3,3'-methylene-bis(4-hydroxycoumarin). I. Its effect on the prothrombin and coagulation time of the blood of dogs and humans. Am J Med Sci 202:563, 1941
5. Furie B, Furie BC: Molecular basis of blood coagulation. Cell 53:505, 1988
6. Furie B, Furie BC: The molecular basis of vitamin K-dependent γ-carboxylation. Blood 75:1753, 1990
7. Nelsestuen GL, Zytkovicz TH, Howard JB: The mode of action of vitamin K. Identification of γ-carboxyglutamic acid as a component of prothrombin. J Biol Chem 249:6347, 1974
8. Stenflo J, Fernlund P, Egan W, Roepstorff P: Vitamin K dependent modifications of glutamic acid residues in prothrombin. Proc Natl Acad Sci USA 71: 2730, 1974
9. Esmon CT, Suttie JW, Jackson CM: The functional significance of vitamin K action. Difference in phospholipid binding between normal and abnormal prothrombin. J Biol Chem 250:4095, 1975
10. Wu S-M, Cheung W-F, Frazier D, Stafford DW: Cloning and expression of the cDNA for human γ-glutamyl carboxylase. Science 254:1634, 1991
11. Morris DP, Soute BAM, Vermeer C, Stafford DW: Characterization of the purified vitamin K-dependent γ-glutamyl carboxylase. J Biol Chem 268:8735, 1993
12. Friedman PA, Rosenberg RD, Hauschka PV et al: A spectrum of partially carboxylated prothrombins in the plasmas of coumarin treated patients. Biochim Biophys Acta 494:271, 1977
13. Blanchard RA, Furie BC, Furie B: Antibodies specific for bovine abnormal (des-γ-carboxy) prothrombin. J Biol Chem 254:12513, 1979

14. Ratcliffe J, Furie B, Furie BC: The importance of specific γ-carboxyglutamic acid residues in prothrombin: evaluation by site-specific mutagenesis. J Biol Chem 268:24339, 1993
15. Blanchard RA, Furie BC, Kruger SF et al: Immunoassays of human prothrombin species which correlate with functional coagulant activities. J Lab Clin Med 101:242, 1983
16. Whitlon DS, Sadowski JA, Suttie JW: Mechanism of coumarin action: significance of vitamin K epoxide reductase inhibition. Biochemistry 17:1371, 1978
17. Matschiner JT, Bell RG, Amelotti JM, Knauer TE: Isolation and characterization of a new metabolite phylloquinone in the rat. Biochim Biophys Acta 201:309, 1970
18. Fasco MJ, Hildebrandt EF, Suttie JW: Evidence that warfarin anticoagulant action involves two distinct reduction activities. J Biol Chem 257:11210, 1982
19. Breckenridge AM, Orme MLE: Kinetics of warfarin absorption in man. Clin Pharmacol Ther 14:955, 1973
20. Kelly JG, O'Malley KO: Clinical pharmacokinetics of oral anticoagulants. Clin Pharmacokinet 4:1, 1979
21. O'Reilly RA, Aggeler PM, Leong LS: Studies on coumarin anticoagulant drugs: pharmacodynamics of warfarin in man. J Clin Invest 42:1542, 1963
22. Park BK: Warfarin: metabolism and mode of action. Biochem Pharmacol 37:19, 1988
23. Wessler S, Gitel SN: Warfarin. N Engl J Med 311:645, 1984
24. Hirsh J: Mechanism of action and monitoring of anticoagulants. Semin Thromb Hemost 1:1, 1986
25. Peteersen P, Boysan G, Godtfredsen J et al: Placebo-controlled randomized trial of warfarin and aspirin for prevention of thromboembolic complications in chronic atrial fibrillation: the Copenhagen AFASAK study. Lancet 1:175, 1989
26. Boston Area Anticoagulation Trial for Atrial Fibrillation Investigators: The effect of low dose warfarin on the risk of stroke in patients with nonrheumatic atrial fibrillation. N Engl J Med 323:1505, 1990
27. Francis CW, Marder VJ, Evarts CM et al: Two-step warfarin therapy: prevention of postoperative venous thrombosis without excessive bleeding. JAMA 249:374, 1983
28. Powers PJ, Gent M, Jay RM et al: A randomized trial of less intense postoperative warfarin or aspirin therapy in the prevention of venous thromboembolism after surgery for fractured hip. Arch Intern Med 149:771, 1989
29. Bern MM, Lokich JJ, Wallach SR et al: Very low dose of warfarin can prevent thrombosis in central venous catheters. Ann Intern Med 112:423, 1990
30. Gifford RH, Feinstein AR: A critique of methodology in studies of anticoagulant therapy for acute myocardial infarction. N Engl J Med 280:351, 1969
31. Goldman L, Feinstein AR: Anticoagulants in acute myocardial infarction: the problems of pooling, drowning and floating. Ann Intern Med 90:92, 1979
32. Smith P, Arnesen H, Holme I: The effect of warfarin on mortality and reinfarction after myocardial infarction. N Engl J Med 323:147, 1990
33. Weinreich DJ, Burke JF, Pauletto FJ: Left ventricular mural thrombi complicating acute myocardial infarction. Ann Intern Med 100:789, 1984
34. Stratton JR, Richie JL: The effects of antithrombotic drugs in patients with left ventricular thrombi. Circulation 69:561, 1984
35. Oakley C: Pregnancy in patients with prosthetic heart valves. Br Med J 286:1680, 1983
36. Hirsh J, Dalen JE, Deykin D, Poller L: Oral anticoagulants. Mechanism of action, clinical effectiveness and optimal therapeutic range. Chest, suppl. 102:312, 1992
37. Hull R, Hirsh J, Jay R et al: Different intensities of oral anticoagulant therapy in the treatment of proximal vein thrombosis. N Engl J Med 307:1676, 1982
38. Turpie AGG, Gunstensen J, Hirsh J et al: Randomised comparison of two intensities of oral anticoagulant therapy after tissue heart valve replacement. Lancet 1:1242, 1988
39. Bussey HI, Force RW, Bianco TM, Leonard AD: Reliance on prothrombin time ratios causes significant errors in anticoagulation therapy. Arch Intern med 152:278, 1992
40. Taberner DA, Poller L, Thomson JM et al: The effect of the international sensitivity index (ISI) of thromboplastin on the precision of international normalised ratios (INR). J Clin Pathol 42:92, 1989
41. Blanchard RA, Furie BC, Jorgensen M et al: Acquired vitamin K-dependent carboxylation deficiency in liver disease. N Engl J Med 305:242, 1981
42. Furie B, Liebman HA, Blanchard RA et al: Comparison of the native prothrombin antigen and the prothrombin time for monitoring oral anticoagulant therapy. Blood 64:445, 1984
43. Furie B, Diuguid C, Jacobs M et al: Randomized prospective trial comparing the native prothrombin antigen and the prothrombin time for monitoring oral anticoagulant therapy. Blood 75:344, 1990
44. Kornberg A, Francis CW, Pellegrini VD Jr, et al: Comparison of native prothrombin antigen with the prothrombin time for monitoring oral anticoagulant prophylaxis. Circulation 88:454, 1993
45. Bern MM, Lokich JJ, Wallach SR et al: Very low doses of warfarin can prevent thrombosis in central venous catheters. Ann Intern Med 112:423, 1990
46. Poller L, McKernan A, Thomson JM et al: Fixed minidose warfarin: a new approach to prophylaxis against venous thrombosis after major surgery. Br Med J 295:1309, 1987
47. Koch-Weser J, Sellers EM: Drug interaction with coumarin anticoagulants. N Engl J Med 285:487, 1971
48. Koch-Weser J, Sellers EM: Drug interaction with coumarin anticoagulants. N Engl J Med 285:547, 1971
49. Howard PA, Hannaman KN: Warfarin resistance linked to enteral nutrition products. J Am Diet Assoc 85:713, 1985
50. Kempin SJ: Warfarin resistance caused by broccoli. N Engl J Med 308:1229, 1983
51. Ovesen L, Lyduch S, Idorn ML: The effect of a diet rich in brussels sprouts on warfarin pharmacokinetics. Eur J Clin Pharmacol 34:521, 1988
52. O'Reilly RA, Aggeler PM, Hoag MS et al: Hereditary transmission of exceptional resistance to coumarin anticoagulant drugs: the first reported kindred. N Engl J Med 271:809, 1964
53. Alving BM, Strickler MP, Knight RD et al: Hereditary warfarin resistance. Investigation of a rare phenomenon. Arch Intern Med 145:499, 1985
54. Zimmerman A, Matschiner JT: Biochemical basis of hereditary resistance to warfarin in the rat. Biochem Pharmacol 23:1033, 1974
55. Hildebrandt EF, Suttie JW: Mechanism of coumarin action: sensitivity of vitamin K metabolizing enzymes of normal and warfarin-resistant rat liver. Biochemistry 21:2406, 1982
56. Hull R, Delmore T, Carter C et al: Adjusted subcutaneous heparin versus warfarin sodium in the long-term treatment of venous thrombosis. N Engl J Med 306:189, 1982
57. Forfar JC: Prediction of hemorrhage during long-term oral coumarin anticoagulation by excessive prothrombin ratio. Am Heart J 103:445, 1982
58. Coon WW, Willis PW: Hemorrhagic complications of anticoagulant therapy. Arch Intern Med 133:386, 1974
59. Levine MN, Raskob G, Hirsh J: Hemorrhagic complications of long-term anticoagulant therapy. Chest, suppl. 2. 89:16, 1986
60. Hull R, Delmore T, Genton E et al: Warfarin sodium versus low dose heparin in the long term treatment of venous thrombosis. N Engl J Med 301:855, 1979
61. McGehee WG, Klotz TA, Epstein DJ, Rapaport SI: Coumarin necrosis associated with hereditary protein C deficiency. Ann Intern Med 101:59, 1984
62. Liebman HA, Limentani SA, Furie BC, Furie B: Immunoaffinity purification of factor IX (Christman factor) using conformation-specific antibodies directed against the factor IX-metal complex. Proc Natl Acad Sci USA 82:3879, 1985
63. Limentani SA, Furie BC, Poiesz BJ et al: Separation of human plasma factor IX from HTLV-I or HIV by immunoaffinity chromatography using conformation-specific antibodies. Blood 70:1312, 1987
64. Smith KJ: Immunoaffinity purification of factor IX from commercial concentrates and infusion studies in animals. Blood 72:1269, 1988

Heparin

121

Douglas M. Tollefsen and Morey A. Blinder

INTRODUCTION

Heparin is a sulfated glycosaminoglycan isolated from mammalian tissues that are rich in mast cells. When administered intravenously, heparin binds to a plasma protein, antithrombin (also called antithrombin III), leading to rapid inhibition of proteases of the coagulation pathways. This interaction produces a potent anticoagulant effect. Endogenous heparin-like molecules appear to be involved in the inhibition of coagulation within normal blood vessels and may have a variety of other biologic functions. Although heparin is an effective agent for the treatment and prevention of venous thromboembolic disease, it occasionally produces life-threatening bleeding or triggers thrombocytopenia associated with arterial thrombosis.

In 1923, Howell[1] used the term heparin to describe an aqueous extract of canine liver that inhibited coagulation of blood in vitro. During the next decade, similar extracts were shown to consist of mixtures of sulfated polysaccharides containing uronic acid and glucosamine.[2] The suggestion that heparin might be used to treat thromboembolism was initially greeted with skepticism because of the fear that patients given heparin would bleed to death. According to Jaques,[3] this fear was allayed by a dramatic demonstration conducted by Best at the University of Toronto in 1937:

> Best asked me [Jaques] to anesthetize a dog, prepare it for laparotomy, and inject heparin intravenously. When the most illustrious surgeons in the world arrived, Best explained what I had done (a blood sample which I had taken was incoagulable). Best then picked up a scalpel and handed it to Dr. Balfour with the request that he make a midline incision. The surgeons, properly dressed in their morning suits, jumped back, whereupon Best made the incision and I applied haemostats to two tiny bleeding points and showed a clean dry incision. Within months of this demonstration, surgeons all over the world took up heparin enthusiastically.

In 1939, investigators in Canada and Sweden reported the successful use of heparin as a treatment for recurrent thrombosis and pulmonary embolism.[2,4] The indications for heparin were soon expanded to include vascular surgical procedures, extracorporeal circulation, and prophylaxis of thromboembolism. Despite the widespread clinical use of heparin, its mechanism of action remained obscure until recently.

STRUCTURE AND BIOSYNTHESIS

Heparin

Heparin is found in the secretory granules of mast cells. It is synthesized from uridine diphosphate-sugar precursors as a polymer of alternating D-glucuronic acid (linked $\beta1\rightarrow4$) and N-acetyl-D-glucosamine (linked $\alpha\rightarrow4$)[5] (Fig. 121-1). The glycosaminoglycan chains are built on a core structure consisting of one xylose and two galactose residues covalently attached to serine in a polypeptide backbone. About 10–15 glycosaminoglycan chains, each containing 200–300 monosaccharide units, are attached to a single core protein to yield a proteoglycan with a molecular weight of 750,000–1,000,000.

Once the glycosaminoglycan chains have formed, they rapidly undergo a series of modification reactions that include the following: (1) N-deacetylation of glucosamine residues, followed by sulfation of virtually all the free amino groups to yield N-sulfo-D-glucosamine; (2) epimerization at the C-5 position of D-glucuronic acid to yield L-iduronic acid; (3) O-sulfation of iduronic acid residues at the C-2 position; and (4) O-sulfation of glucosamine residues at the C-6 position (C_2, C_5, and so on, refer to specific carbon atoms in the monosaccharide units as indicated in Fig. 121-2). In addition to these major modifications, several minor but biologically important reactions also occur, including O-sulfation of glucuronic acid at C-2 and C-3 and of glucosamine at C-3.

The reactions that modify the glycosaminoglycan chain appear to be catalyzed by membrane-bound enzymes in the endoplasmic reticulum or Golgi apparatus of the mast cell and are completed within minutes of protein synthesis. After the heparin proteoglycan has been transported to the mast cell granule, an endo-β-D-glucuronidase catalyzes partial degradation of the glycosaminoglycan chains to 5,000–30,000-MW fragments over a period of hours.

Many of the biosynthetic reactions are regulated by modifications that have occurred elsewhere in the heparin chain.[5] For example, N-sulfation stimulates N-deacetylation of nearby residues; epimerization of a glucuronic acid residue requires that the adjacent glucosamine attached at C-4 be N-sulfated and that the glucosamine attached at C1 not be 6-O-sulfated; also, 2-O-sulfation of iduronic acid is inhibited by the presence of a 6-O-sulfate group on the adjacent glucosamine residue. Thus, the final structure obtained is limited by the substrate specificities of the enzymes involved in heparin biosynthesis. Furthermore, all the reactions, with the exception of N-sulfation, are incomplete (e.g., note the potential O-sulfation sites in Figure 121-1 that have remained unmodified), yielding heterogeneous oligosaccharide structures within the glycosaminoglycan chain. In general, iduronic acid residues and O-sulfate groups accumulate in regions of the polymer that have become N-sulfated.

Related Glycosaminoglycans

Two other glycosaminoglycans, heparan sulfate and dermatan sulfate, also have anticoagulant activity.[6] Heparan sulfate is closely related to heparin and is found on the surface of most eukaryotic cells and in the extracellular matrix. Heparan sulfate proteoglycans vary considerably in structure. In general, they are smaller than the heparin proteoglycan and contain fewer glycosaminoglycan chains linked to a larger and more complex core protein. In some cases, the core protein has a hydrophobic domain that anchors the proteoglycan to the cell membrane. Heparan sulfate is synthesized from the same repeating disaccharide unit (D-glucuronic acid linked to N-acetyl-D-glucosamine) as heparin.[7] However, heparan sulfate undergoes less polymer modification than heparin and therefore contains higher proportions of glucuronic acid and N-acetylglucosamine and fewer sulfate groups.

Dermatan sulfate is a repeating polymer of L-iduronic acid and N-acetyl-D-galactosamine.[7] O-sulfation of iduronic acid residues at the C-2 position and of galactosamine residues at the C-4 and C-6 positions occurs to a variable extent. Like heparan

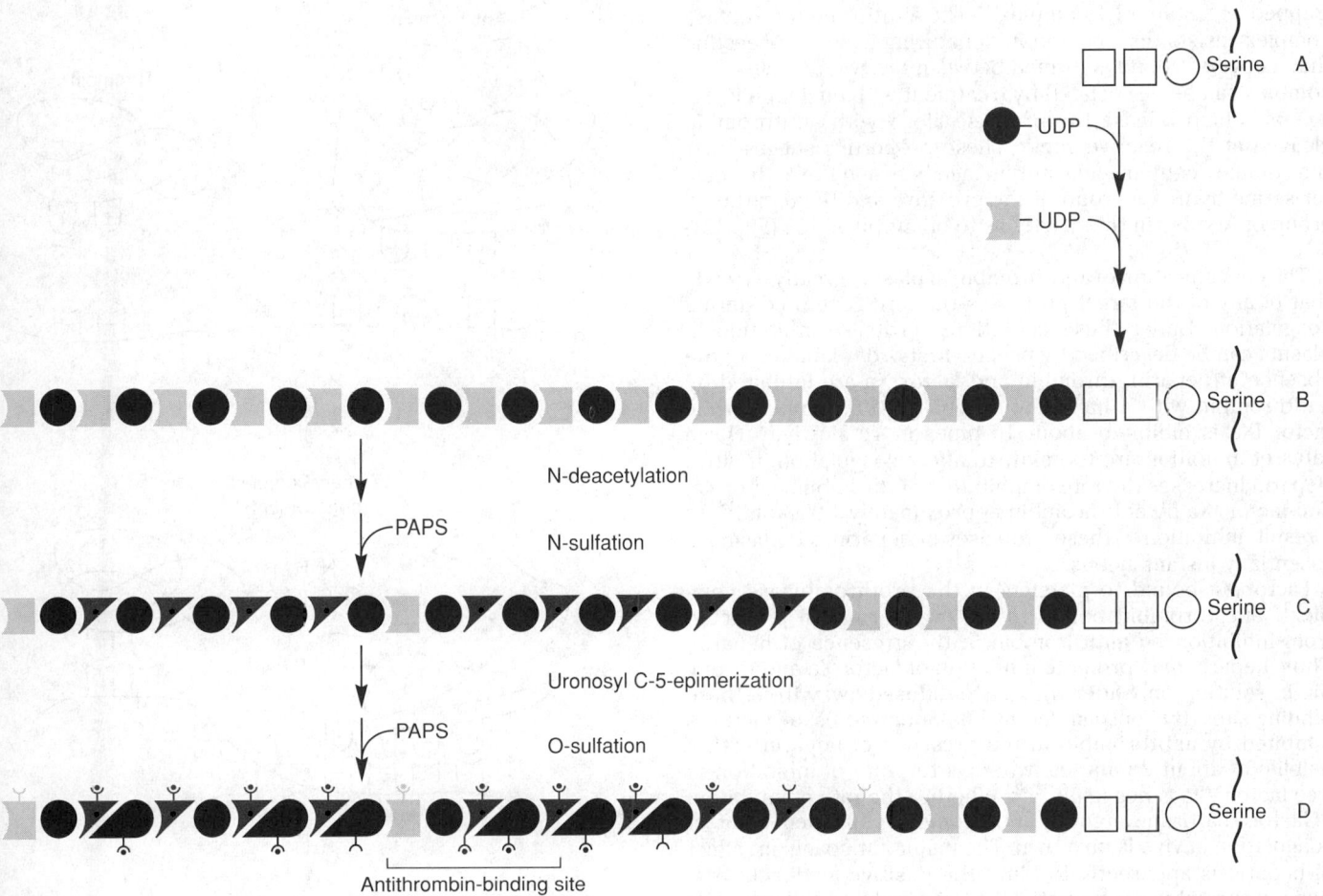

Fig. 121-1. Biosynthesis of the heparin proteoglycan. **(A)** N-acetyl-D-glucosamine and D-glucuronic acid are transferred from uridine diphosphate-sugar precursors to a trisaccharide structure linked to a serine residue in the core protein, **(B)**, forming the unmodified glycosaminoglycan chain. **(C)** N-deacetylation of some of the *N*-acetyl-D-glucosamine residues then occurs, followed by N-sulfation of the free amino groups. **(D)** Epimerization of D-glucuronic to L-iduronic acid and O-sulfation occur to a limited extent to yield the final product, which is then transported to the mast cell secretory granule. Symbols: □, galactose; ⬠, *N*-acetyl-D-glucosamine; ▼, *N*-sulfo-D-glucosamine; •, O-sulfate group; ○, xylose; ●, D-glucuronic acid; ◢, L-iduronic acid; Y, potential O-sulfation site; PAPS, 3′ phosphoadenyolsine-5′-phosphosulfate (sulfate donor). (Modified from Lindahl et al.,[5] with permisison.)

sulfate, dermatan sulfate is a component of proteoglycans on the cell surface and in the extracellular matrix.

ANTICOAGULANT ACTIVITY

Antithrombin

Studies by Brinkhous et al.[8] in 1939 indicated that the anticoagulant effect of heparin is mediated by an endogenous plasma component, termed heparin cofactor. Thirty years later, antithrombin was purified from plasma and shown to have heparin cofactor activity, that is, the ability to inhibit thrombin rapidly only in the presence of heparin.[9,10] Antithrombin is an M_r 58,000 single-chain glycoprotein that is homologous to members of the α_1-antitrypsin family of serine protease inhibitors (serpins).[11-13] It is synthesized in the liver and circulates in plasma at a concentration of $2.6 \pm 0.4 \ \mu M$ (mean ± 2 SD).[14] Antithrombin inhibits activated coagulation factors of the intrinsic and common pathways, including thrombin, factor Xa, and factor IXa, but has relatively little activity against factor VIIa.[15]

Antithrombin acts as a suicide substrate for its target proteases. Inhibition occurs when a protease attacks the reactive site Arg 393-Ser 394 peptide bond in antithrombin and becomes

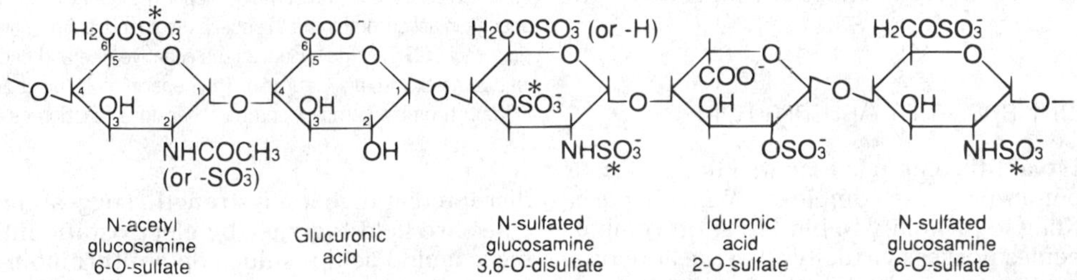

Fig. 121-2. Structure of the antithrombin-binding pentasaccharide of heparin. The sulfate groups marked with asterisks are essential for high-affinity binding.

trapped as a stable 1:1 complex.[16] The antithrombin/protease complex resists dissociation in denaturing agents, suggesting that a covalent bond is formed between the two proteins. The complex can be dissociated by treatment with nucleophilic reagents, which release the protease along with antithrombin cleaved at the reactive site.[17] These properties suggest that the complex contains an ester linkage between the active center serine hydroxyl group of the protease and the α-carbonyl group of Arg 393 in the reactive site of antithrombin (Fig. 121-3C).

The concentration of antithrombin in plasma greatly exceeds that of any of the target proteases that are generated during coagulation. Under these conditions, protease inhibition in plasma can be described by pseudo-first-order kinetics. In the absence of heparin, thrombin and factor Xa are inhibited by antithrombin with a half-life of about 0.5–1.5 minutes, while factor IXa is inhibited about 10 times more slowly.[18] These rates of inhibition are too slow to affect coagulation in vitro. Heparin increases the rate of inhibition of thrombin, factor Xa, and factor IXa by antithrombin approximately 1,000-fold.[18] As a result, inhibition of these proteases in heparinized plasma is essentially instantaneous.

Factor Xa bound to platelets in the prothrombinase complex[19] and thrombin bound to fibrin[20,21] are both protected from inhibition by antithrombin in the presence of heparin. Thus, heparin may promote inhibition of factor Xa and thrombin in solution only after they have diffused away from these binding sites. By contrast, factor VIIa bound to tissue factor is inhibited by antithrombin in the presence of heparin with a half-life of about 2 minutes, whereas the rate of inhibition of free factor VIIa is negligible.[22,23] Whether the rate of inhibition of factor VIIa/tissue factor by antithrombin is sufficient to affect coagulation in vivo is unknown. The major anticoagulant effect of heparin is apparently to blunt the positive feedback reactions of thrombin on activation of factors V and VIII and thus to decrease the rate of thrombin generation.[24–26]

When heparin is added to plasma at a therapeutic concentration (0.1–1.0 U/ml), factors IXa and Xa and thrombin are inhibited almost exclusively by antithrombin. In the presence of higher concentrations of heparin or dermatan sulfate, thrombin is inhibited primarily by heparin cofactor II.[27,28] Heparin also stimulates inhibition of thrombin by plasminogen activator inhibitor 1 (PAI-1),[29] protein C inhibitor,[30] and protease nexin-1 (glia-derived nexin)[31] and inhibition of factor Xa by tissue factor pathway inhibitor (TFPI).[32,33] The latter four inhibitors are present in plasma at less than one-hundredth the concentration of antithrombin. Intravenous infusion of heparin increases the level of circulating TFPI several-fold, presumably by causing release of TFPI from binding sites on the endothelium.[34]

Heparin accelerates plasminogen activation by tissue plasminogen activator (t-PA) or urokinase (u-PA) but decreases the stimulatory effect of fibrin on t-PA activity.[35] Inhibition of t-PA or u-PA by PAI-1 is unaffected by heparin.[36] The net effect of an intravenous infusion of heparin may be to enhance fibrinolysis mediated by endogenous t-PA.[37] However, heparin does not appear to enhance the thrombolytic effect of exogenously administered t-PA.[38]

Binding of Heparin to Antithrombin

Binding of heparin to antithrombin is essential to accelerate formation of antithrombin/protease complexes. When heparin is fractionated according to its ability to bind to antithrombin, the high-affinity molecules possess virtually all of the anticoagulant activity of the starting material, while the low-affinity molecules are inactive.[39–41] Heparin binds to antithrombin with a dissociation constant (K_d) of 2×10^{-8} M.[42] The binding is

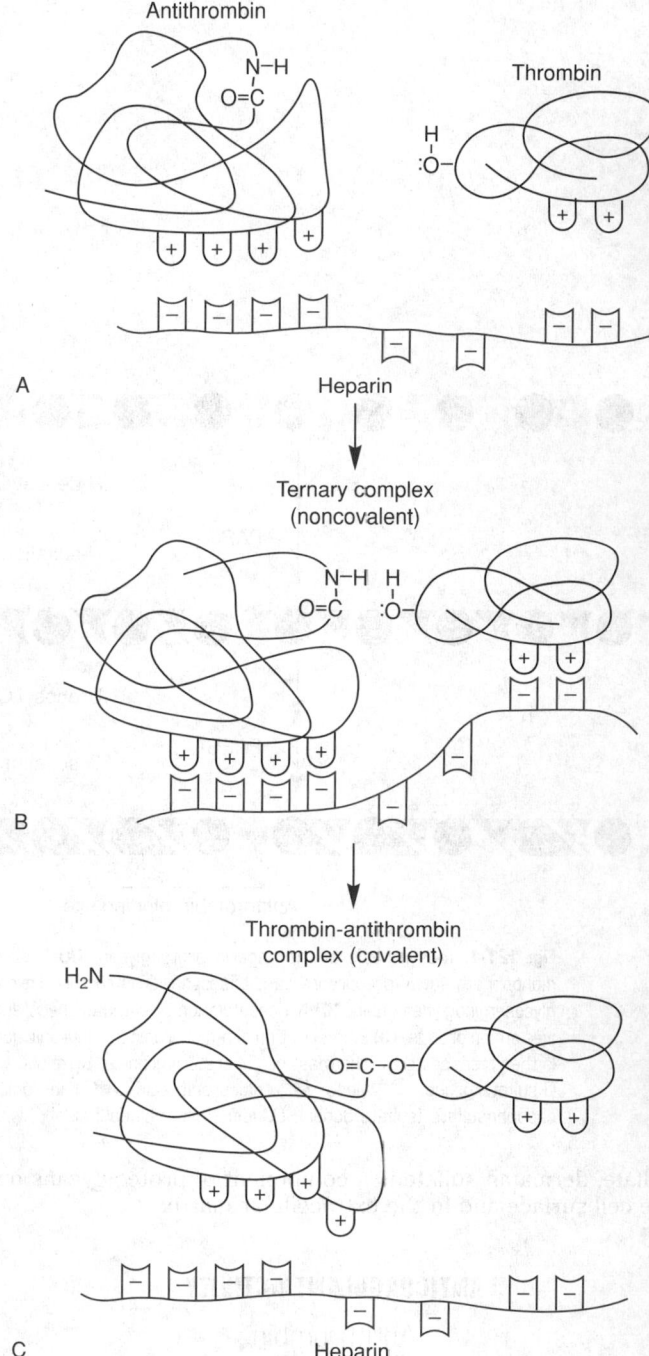

Fig. 121-3. Model for catalysis of the thrombin-antithrombin reaction. **(A)** Thrombin and antithrombin bind simultaneously to a single heparin molecule to form a noncovalent ternary complex. **(B)** The serine hydroxyl group (-OH) in the active site of thrombin is brought into close approximation with the reactive site peptide bond (-CONH-) of antithrombin. Heparin binding also induces a conformational change in antithrombin that renders the reactive site more accessible to proteolytic attack. **(C)** Thrombin cleaves the reactive site and becomes trapped in a covalent complex with antithrombin. The heparin molecule is released from the thrombin/antithrombin complex and can therefore function as a catalyst.

disrupted at high ionic strength, suggesting that the two molecules are held together by electrostatic interactions between basic amino acid residues on antithrombin and sulfate or carboxylate groups on heparin (Fig. 121-3B).

The high-affinity binding site for antithrombin within a heparin chain is the pentasaccharide structure shown in Figure 121-

2.[43-45] This structure contains a 3-O-sulfate group that appears to be unique to the high-affinity binding site for antithrombin. Several of the sulfate groups within the pentasaccharide (marked by asterisks) are essential for binding to antithrombin, while others do not appear to be required. In commercial heparin preparations, approximately 30% of the molecules contain this structure and bind to antithrombin with high affinity.[39-41] An identical structure is thought to arise during the biosynthesis of heparan sulfate chains, although at a much lower frequency. Heparan sulfate chains that contain this structure bind to antithrombin and stimulate protease inhibition. Other glycosaminoglycans that lack the specific pentasaccharide structure (e.g., dermatan sulfate, chondroitin-4-sulfate, or chondroitin-6-sulfate) do not interact with antithrombin.[28]

Heparin binding induces a conformational change in antithrombin that appears to lock the glycosaminoglycan into place on the surface of the inhibitor.[42] The heparin/antithrombin complex then reacts rapidly with a target protease. Interaction with a protease reduces the affinity of antithrombin for heparin, allowing the antithrombin/protease complex to dissociate from the glycosaminoglycan chain.[46] Thus, a single heparin molecule can catalyze the formation of many antithrombin/protease complexes (Fig. 121-3C).

Catalytic Mechanism

Two models have been proposed to explain the catalysis of antithrombin-protease reactions by heparin. In the first model, heparin binding induces a conformational change in the reactive site of antithrombin that allows a target protease to interact more efficiently with this site.[10,18] In the second model, the heparin chain functions as a template that binds antithrombin and the target protease simultaneously to form a ternary complex, and catalysis occurs mainly by an approximation effect.[47] Current evidence suggests that both mechanisms are valid but differ in their relative importance depending on the target protease.

The balance between the two mechanisms may explain differences in the rate enhancement for inhibition of thrombin and factor Xa produced by heparin chains of varying length (Table 121-1). For example, the synthetic pentasaccharide that contains only the antithrombin binding site of heparin increases the rate of inhibition of factor Xa about 270-fold but has relatively little effect on the rate of inhibition of thrombin.[48] Because an oligosaccharide of this size is unlikely to function as a template, induction of a conformational change in antithrombin may be sufficient to catalyze inhibition of factor Xa. Longer heparin chains produce an additional twofold increase in the rate of factor Xa inhibition, which may represent the contribution of the template mechanism. Stimulation of the thrombin-antithrombin reaction requires heparin molecules that contain ≥18 sugar residues (MW approximately 5,400), which is the smallest chain able to form a ternary complex with antithrombin and thrombin.[49] The factor IXa-antithrombin reaction has a similar requirement for longer heparin chains. Therefore, inhibition of thrombin and factor IXa may depend primarily on the template mechanism.

Thrombin binds to heparin with a K_d of $6-10 \times 10^{-6}$ M under physiologic conditions.[50] An increase in the NaCl concentration from 0.15 to 0.30 M causes parallel 20- to 30-fold reductions in the affinity of thrombin for heparin and in the rate of inhibition of thrombin by antithrombin in the presence of full-length heparin.[47,48] By contrast, the thrombin-antithrombin reaction in the absence of heparin is much less dependent on ionic strength. Chemical modifications of thrombin that decrease its affinity for heparin greatly reduce the ability of heparin to stimulate the thrombin-antithrombin reaction.[51] Factor Xa also binds to heparin, but with a much lower affinity in comparison with thrombin. Inhibition of factor Xa by antithrombin in the presence or absence of heparin is unaffected by changes in ionic strength or by chemical modification of factor Xa to reduce its affinity for heparin.[48,52] These observations suggest that catalysis of the reaction between antithrombin and thrombin, but not factor Xa, requires binding of heparin both to antithrombin and to the protease.

At low heparin concentrations, the rate of inhibition of thrombin or factor Xa is proportional to the concentration of heparin/antithrombin complexes present in the incubation.[18,53] The rate of inhibition plateaus at a concentration of heparin in the micromolar range, which is sufficient to saturate the antithrombin. Higher concentrations of heparin decrease the rate of inhibition of thrombin, presumably by favoring the binding of thrombin and antithrombin to separate heparin chains, but do not decrease the rate of inhibition of factor Xa.[18,53] These observations are consistent with the template mechanism for catalysis of the thrombin-antithrombin reaction.[47]

Heparin Cofactor II

Heparin cofactor II (M_r 66,000) is a single-chain glycoprotein that is about 30% identical in amino acid sequence to antithrombin.[54-56] It is present in plasma at a concentration of 1.2 ± 0.4 µM (mean ± 2 SD). Heparin cofactor II inhibits thrombin but is inactive with other proteases generated during coagulation or fibrinolysis.[57] The reactive site of heparin cofactor II contains the sequence Leu 444-Ser 445.[58] Since coagulation proteases generally attack Arg-X peptide bonds in their substrates, the presence of leucine at the P1 position of the reactive site may explain the inability of most of these proteases to react with heparin cofactor II. In contrast to antithrombin, heparin cofactor II also inhibits chymotrypsin-like proteases, albeit slowly.[57,59]

The affinity of heparin cofactor II for heparin is lower than that of antithrombin. Therefore, an approximately 10-fold higher concentration of heparin is necessary to accelerate thrombin inhibition by heparin cofactor II in plasma.[28] Heparin cofactor II requires heparin molecules ≥26 residues in length (MW approximately 7,800) to catalyze thrombin inhibition but does not require the specific antithrombin-binding pentasaccharide.[60-62] By contrast, the activity of heparin cofactor II is stimulated approximately 1,000-fold by dermatan sulfate, which has no effect on the activity of antithrombin.[28] Heparin cofactor II preferentially binds to a high-affinity site in dermatan sulfate that consists of a tandem repeat of three iduronic acid 2-sulfate→N-acetylgalactosamine 4-sulfate disaccharides.[63] The stimulatory effect of heparin and dermatan sulfate depends on the presence of an acidic polypeptide region near the N terminus of heparin cofactor II.[64,65] This region apparently occupies the glycosaminoglycan binding site in the native inhibitor. Heparin and dermatan sulfate appear to displace the acidic region, enabling it to bind to the fibrinogen recognition site (anion binding exosite I) of thrombin and thereby facilitate the interaction of thrombin with the reactive site of heparin cofactor II.[65-67]

Table 121-1. Second-Order Rate Constants for Inhibition of Proteases by Antithrombin/Heparin Complexes

	Thrombin ($\times 10^6$ $M^{-1}sec^{-1}$ [fold-increased])	Factor Xa
Antithrombin	0.0087	0.0023
Antithrombin + pentasaccharide	0.0146 (1.7)	0.61 (270)
Antithrombin + full-length heparin[a]	37 (4300)	1.3 (570)

[a] 24–28 monosaccharide units in length.
(Data from Olson et al.[48])

Addition of dermatan sulfate to plasma causes prolongation of the thrombin time and activated partial thromboplastin time (PTT),[6] and intravenous infusion of dermatan sulfate produces an antithrombotic effect in experimental animals[68–72] and humans.[73–75] These effects appear to be mediated primarily by heparin cofactor II.[28,76,77] Several other natural or synthetic polyanions, including pentosan polysulfate,[78] fucoidan,[79] and chondroitin sulfate E,[80] have been reported to stimulate inhibition of thrombin by heparin cofactor II; these compounds also appear to have some activity with antithrombin.

PHYSIOLOGIC FUNCTIONS

Vascular Heparan Sulfate

Because of the dramatic effect of heparin on the activity of antithrombin in vitro, it has been assumed that an endogenous heparin-like substance must stimulate antithrombin in vivo. Current evidence suggests that heparan sulfate proteoglycans anchored in the vessel wall interact with circulating antithrombin to produce an antithrombotic effect.

Glycosaminoglycans extracted from cloned endothelial cells have anticoagulant activity, and de novo biosynthesis of heparan sulfate proteoglycans has been demonstrated by culturing endothelial cells in the presence of [^{35}S]sulfate.[81,82] Approximately 1–10% of the labeled heparan sulfate from endothelial cells binds to immobilized antithrombin with high affinity. This fraction possesses essentially all the anticoagulant activity of the cell extract and contains the 3-O-sulfated glucosamine residue that is characteristic of the antithrombin-binding pentasaccharide of heparin.

Antithrombin binds to cultured bovine aortic endothelial cells (about 60,000 sites per cell) with a K_d of 12×10^{-9} M, and binding is diminished by pretreatment of the cells with heparinase.[82] Electron microscopic autoradiography of ^{125}I-labeled antithrombin bound to endothelial cells in culture or after perfusion of segments of rat aorta ex vivo indicates that >90% of the antithrombin is associated with the extracellular matrix located in the subendothelium.[83] Binding of antithrombin to the subendothelial matrix of the aorta is greatly increased after crush injury, which causes detachment of most of the endothelial cells. Interaction of coagulation proteases with antithrombin bound to subendothelial heparan sulfate proteoglycans may inhibit thrombosis.[83] Interleukin-1 and tumor necrosis factor decrease heparan sulfate biosynthesis by cultured endothelial cells and reduce the amount of antithrombin that can be bound per cell by about 50%.[84] This mechanism may contribute to the increased thrombogenicity of the endothelium induced by cytokines.

When a trace amount of thrombin is injected into the circulation, the thrombin appears to become bound initially to thrombomodulin on the endothelial cell surface.[85] In comparison with free thrombin, thrombin bound to thrombomodulin reacts less rapidly with fibrinogen and heparin cofactor II, more rapidly with protein C, and at about the same rate with antithrombin.[86] The net effect of these changes in substrate specificity may be a small increase (about threefold) in the rate of the thrombin-antithrombin reaction because of diminished competition from other substrates. After the thrombomodulin has become saturated with thrombin, the excess thrombin may be inhibited rapidly by antithrombin bound to heparan sulfate proteoglycans.[87] Platelet factor 4, released from the α-granules during platelet aggregation, competitively inhibits binding of antithrombin to heparan sulfate and may promote local clot formation at the site of hemostasis.[88]

Evidence for the physiologic importance of the antithrombin-heparan sulfate hemteraction is derived from analysis of certain natural variants of antithrombin, including antithrombin$_{Toyama}$

(Arg 47→Cys)[89] and antithrombin$_{Fontainebleau}$ (mutation unknown).[90] These variants react normally with thrombin and factor Xa in the absence of heparin but have greatly diminished heparin-binding affinities and are not stimulated by heparin in vitro. Because these variants were discovered in homozygous patients with severe venous thromboembolic disease, the normal antithrombotic mechanism appears to depend on the presence of an intact heparin binding site in antithrombin.

Mast Cell Heparin

Heparin binds cationic molecules such as histamine and neutral proteases to form crystalline arrays within the secretory granules of mast cells,[91] but its physiologic function is otherwise unknown. Under normal circumstances, heparin is not released from mast cells into the circulation and cannot be detected in plasma. However, a small amount of heparin may appear in the circulation of patients with systemic mastocytosis and produce mild prolongation of the PTT.[92]

Tumor-Derived Heparan Sulfate

Circulating heparan sulfate, apparently released from tumor cells, has been reported to cause marked prolongation of the thrombin time and PTT and to cause bleeding in a few severely ill patients with malignancies.[93–96] Protamine neutralizes the heparan sulfate anticoagulant in vitro and may be an effective treatment for patients with this type of anticoagulant.[96,97] A coagulopathy associated with circulating heparan sulfate and dermatan sulfate has also been observed in a few patients who were treated with high-dose suramin for metastatic adrenocortical carcinoma.[98]

Inhibition of Cell Proliferation

Heparin inhibits growth of a variety of cultured cells, including endothelial cells, vascular smooth muscle cells, and renal mesangial cells. In addition, heparin prevents the extraordinary proliferation of vascular smooth muscle cells that follows damage to the endothelium in vivo, as demonstrated in the rat carotid artery.[99] These effects are independent of the anticoagulant activity of heparin.[100] Heparan sulfate proteoglycans synthesized by postconfluent vascular smooth muscle cells and endothelial cells also have antiproliferative activity and can be removed from the cells by a platelet heparitinase.[101] This phenomenon suggests that smooth muscle cell proliferation in a damaged blood vessel might be triggered by heparitinase in combination with growth factors released from the platelets. The mechanism by which heparin and heparan sulfate suppress cell growth appears to involve inhibition of a protein kinase C-dependent signaling pathway early in the cell cycle.[102]

Angiogenesis

Acidic and basic fibroblast growth factors (aFGF and bFGF) bind to heparin with very high affinity.[103] These growth factors are mitogens for endothelial cells, smooth muscle cells, and other mesenchymal cells, and they induce angiogenesis. Although heparin inhibits growth of capillary endothelial cells in vitro, it potentiates the growth-promoting effect of aFGF on these cells.[104] This effect depends on the size and degree of sulfation of the heparin molecule but not on its anticoagulant activity. Heparan sulfate proteoglycans in the extracellular matrix bind and stabilize bFGF and may serve as a reservoir from which the growth factor can be released by an excess of heparin or digestion with heparitinase.[105] Heparan sulfate provides a low-affinity binding site for bFGF on the surface of target mesenchymal cells. Furthermore, cell surface heparan sulfate or exogenous heparin promotes the binding of bFGF to its high-affinity receptor (a transmembrane protein with tyrosine kinase activity) and is required for the biologic activity of bFGF.[106,107] Highly sulfated oligosaccharides that bind bFGF have been isolated from heparin or heparan sulfate.[108,109]

CLINICAL APPLICATIONS

Pharmacologic Effects

Heparin produces an immediate anticoagulant effect when administered intravenously. At a plasma concentration of 0.1–1.0 U/ml, heparin causes thrombin and factor Xa to be inhibited very rapidly (half-lives <0.1 second) by antithrombin. Higher concentrations of heparin (>5 U/ml), which may be present transiently after a bolus intravenous infusion, may also stimulate thrombin inhibition by heparin cofactor II.[27] These effects result in prolongation of the PTT and the thrombin time. Although the prothrombin time may also be prolonged, it is affected to a lesser degree by heparin. Low-molecular-weight heparin and dermatan sulfate have substantial antithrombotic activity at doses that do not significantly affect the PTT.[68,110] These findings have provoked considerable debate about the mechanism of the antithrombotic effect and which in vitro test, if any, is correlated with this effect.

Heparin clears lipemic plasma in vivo by causing the release of lipoprotein lipase from the endothelium into the circulation. Lipoprotein lipase hydrolyzes triglycerides present in chylomicrons and very-low-density lipoproteins to glycerol and free fatty acids.[111] The clearing of lipemic plasma may occur at a dose of heparin below that which produces an anticoagulant effect, and rebound hyperlipemia may occur after heparin is discontinued. The effects of heparin on lipid metabolism are striking but have no obvious clinical importance.

Preparations

Heparin for therapeutic use is commonly extracted from porcine intestinal mucosa or bovine lung. During the isolation of heparin from these sources, the core protein is removed and the glycosaminoglycan chains become degraded slightly to yield a heterogeneous mixture of fragments with a mean molecular weight of 12,000 (range 5,000–30,000). These preparations may also contain small amounts of other glycosaminoglycans.[112] Despite the heterogeneity in source and composition among different commercial heparin preparations, their biologic activities are similar (approximately 150 USP U/mg).

The USP unit is defined as the quantity of heparin that will prevent 1.0 ml of citrate-anticoagulated sheep plasma from clotting for 1 hour after the addition of 0.2 ml of 1% calcium chloride. Standard heparin extracted from porcine intestinal mucosa or bovine lung is available as the sodium salt in aqueous solutions of 10–40,000 USP U/ml. The calcium salt of heparin from porcine intestinal mucosa has been associated with a lower frequency of local hematoma when injected subcutaneously and is used commonly in Europe in a low-dose regimen for prevention of thromboembolism.[113]

Low-molecular-weight heparins (mean MW 4,000–6,500) are isolated from standard heparin by gel filtration chromatography or by precipitation with ethanol.[114] Alternatively, they can be produced by partial depolymerization with nitrous acid or by other chemical techniques. Low-molecular-weight heparin preparations accelerate factor Xa inhibition at a dosage similar to that of standard heparin but have greatly reduced thrombin inhibitory activities. The ratio of antithrombin to anti-factor

Xa activity of a given preparation depends largely on the percentage of molecules that are of sufficient length to accelerate the thrombin-antithrombin reaction.[115] Low-molecular-weight heparin preparations differ in chemical composition and molecular weight and cannot be standardized easily. In general, they produce a minimal effect on in vitro clotting tests. In clinical trials, low-molecular-weight heparin is often prescribed in units of anti-factor Xa activity. It cannot be assumed, however, that the same anti-factor Xa dose of two low-molecular-weight heparin preparations will produce equivalent antithrombotic effects.

The "heparinoid" Org 10172 (Orgaran) is a mixture of several types of nonheparin glycosaminoglycans (80% heparan sulfate, 10% dermatan sulfate, 10% others) extracted from porcine intestinal mucosa. This preparation has been used successfully as a replacement for heparin in patients with heparin-induced thrombocytopenia.[116,117]

Absorption and Pharmacokinetics

Heparin is not absorbed through the gastrointestinal mucosa and, therefore, must be given parenterally. It is administered by continuous intravenous infusion, intermittent intravenous injection, or deep subcutaneous injection. Heparin has an immediate onset of action when given intravenously. The onset of action of subcutaneous heparin generally occurs within 20–60 minutes. Although patient-to-patient variation in the bioavailability of standard heparin given by the subcutaneous route is considerable, low-molecular-weight heparins are absorbed more uniformly.[114]

Following a bolus intravenous injection, elimination of heparin activity from the blood can be described by first-order kinetics. However, the half-life of standard heparin varies with the dose administered.[118] As shown in Figure 121-4, the half-life of the anticoagulant activity in humans is approximately 1, 1.5, and 2.5 hours at doses of 100, 200, and 400 U/kg, respectively. Heparin appears to be cleared and degraded primarily by the reticuloendothelial system. A small amount of undegraded heparin is excreted in the urine. The half-life of heparin may be shortened in patients with pulmonary embolism and prolonged in patients with hepatic cirrhosis or end-stage renal disease.[119] Low-molecular-weight heparins have longer biologic half-lives than standard heparin preparations.[120]

Administration and Dosage

Continuous intravenous infusion is the usual method of administration of full-dose heparin, because the incidence of bleeding complications is lower in comparison with intermit-

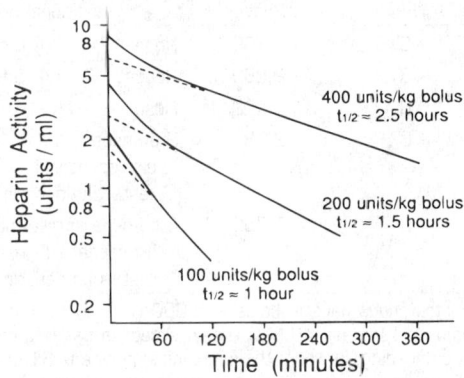

Fig. 121-4. Kinetics of elimination of heparin from the circulation. Bolus injections of heparin were administered intravenously to normal volunteers, whose blood was sampled at various time points thereafter. The heparin activity in the plasma was determined by a thrombin inhibition assay. (From McAvoy,[118] with permission.)

tent infusions.[121] Heparin therapy can be initiated with a bolus injection of 5,000 U followed by 1,000–2,000 U/hr delivered by an infusion pump. Adjusted-dose subcutaneous administration can be used for the long-term management of patients in whom warfarin is contraindicated (e.g., during pregnancy).[122] A daily dose of 15,000–30,000 U given as divided doses every 8–12 hours is usually sufficient to achieve a therapeutic effect similar to that of intravenous heparin. Low-dose heparin prevents thromboembolism in certain high-risk patients.[121] A current regimen for low-dose heparin is 5,000 U given subcutaneously every 8–12 hours. Low-molecular-weight heparin has the potential advantage that it may be given subcutaneously only once a day because of its long half-life.[114]

Laboratory Monitoring

Therapy with standard heparin is usually monitored with a global test of coagulation such as the whole blood clotting time, whole blood recalcification time, or PTT. Because of its convenience and rapid turnaround time, the PTT is the most widely used test. Prolongation of the PTT to >1.5 times the mean control value is effective in preventing recurrent venous thromboembolism; the risk of recurrence is greater in patients who do not achieve this level of anticoagulation.[123] Prevention of recurrence is unrelated to the means of delivery (subcutaneous versus intravenous) or to the total heparin dose administered.[123,124] A PTT of 2.0–2.5 times the mean control value is generally considered to be the upper limit of the therapeutic range. However, major bleeding complications can occur even though the PTT is within the therapeutic range.[124–126]

Because of the fear of bleeding from overdosage, intuitive adjustments in the heparin infusion rate often result in subtherapeutic PTTs during the first 24–48 hours of treatment.[126] Recent prescription guidelines for continuous intravenous heparin (Table 121-2) have reduced the incidence of a subtherapeutic PTT to <2% of patients during the first 24 hours. Supratherapeutic PTT occurred in about two-thirds of patients who received warfarin simultaneously, but the risk of bleeding was not increased in these patients.[126]

Laboratory monitoring of low-dose subcutaneous heparin is unnecessary, since the PTT is not prolonged by this regimen. Similarly, low-molecular-weight heparin has little effect on the PTT at doses that provide therapeutic anticoagulation. The level of low-molecular-weight heparin in plasma can be determined as anti-factor Xa activity. However, preliminary studies in which low-molecular-weight heparin was used to treat deep vein thrombosis suggest that laboratory monitoring is unnecessary.[114]

Heparin Resistance

The dose of heparin required to produce a therapeutic PTT varies from patient to patient. The variability may be due to differences in the plasma concentrations of heparin-binding proteins such as histidine-rich glycoprotein, vitronectin, and platelet factor 4, which competitively inhibit binding of heparin to antithrombin.[88,127,128] In patients with venous thromboembolism, the therapeutic dose is usually <35,000 U/day. Occasionally, the PTT will fail to become prolonged unless a very high dose (>50,000 U/day) of heparin is administered. The level of heparin in these patients may be "therapeutic" at the usual dose when measured by other tests (e.g., anti-factor Xa activity or protamine sulfate titration). These patients may have very short pretreatment PTTs due to the presence of increased levels of factor VIII and may not be truly heparin resistant.[119] Other patients require large doses of heparin because of accelerated clearance of the drug, as may occur with massive pulmonary embolism.[119] Patients with inherited antithrombin deficiency ordinarily have 40–60% of the normal plasma concentration of this inhibitor, and the PTT responds normally to heparin in most of these patients.[129,130] However, acquired antithrombin levels <25% of normal may occur in patients with hepatic cirrhosis,[131] nephrotic syndrome,[132] or disseminated intravascular coagulation (DIC)[133]; in these instances, large doses of heparin may not prolong the PTT. Heparin itself can cause a modest (approximately 15%) decrease in the circulating antithrombin concentration, but this effect is unlikely to have clinical significance.[134]

Indications for Therapy

Venous Thromboembolism

Heparin is used in the initial treatment of venous thromboembolic disease because of its rapid onset of action. In patients with deep vein thrombosis, initial treatment with a vitamin K antagonist alone is inferior to the combination of heparin plus a vitamin K antagonist in preventing further thromboembolic complications.[135] The incidence of recurrent venous thromboembolism within the first 3 months of follow-up is similar (about 7%) in patients who initially receive heparin for 5 or 10 days.[136] The shorter duration of therapy is preferred because it may reduce the length of hospitalization and the incidence of heparin-induced thrombocytopenia. Recent studies have shown that low-molecular-weight heparin is as effective as standard heparin in the treatment of uncomplicated proximal deep vein thrombosis.[137–139] Since low-molecular-weight heparin is administered in a fixed dose regimen without monitoring, it is possible that certain patients with deep vein thrombosis could be treated in the outpatient setting. However, the safety and efficacy of outpatient treatment of deep vein thrombosis remains to be established. Low-dose subcutaneous heparin (5,000 U given every 8–12 hours) and low-molecular-weight heparin are equally effective in prevention of thromboembolism in high-risk patients.[114]

Disseminated Intravascular Coagulation

Patients with acute promyelocytic leukemia frequently have bleeding associated with laboratory evidence of DIC (see Ch. 116). In the past, low-dose heparin by continuous infusion has

Table 121-2. Intravenous Heparin Dose-Titration Nomogram[a]

| PTT[c] (sec) | Intravenous Infusion[b] | | Additional Action |
	Rate Change (ml/hr)	Dose Change (U/day)	
≤45	+6	+5,760	Repeat PTT in 4–6 hr
46–54	+3	+2,880	Repeat PTT in 4–6 hr
55–85	0	0	None
86–110	−3	−2,880	Stop heparin treatment for 1 hr; repeat PTT 4–6 hr after restarting heparin treatment
>110	−6	−5,760	Stop heparin treatment for 1 hr; repeat PTT 4–6 hr after restarting heparin treatment

[a] The initial intravenous heparin bolus is 5,000 U. A continuous intravenous infusion is begun at 42 ml/hr (40,320 U/day) except in patients considered to be at high risk of bleeding, in whom the initial infusion rate is 31 ml/hr (29,760 U/day). The PTT is obtained 4–6 hr after beginning the infusion. Thereafter, the PTT is obtained once a day unless dosage adjustments are required according to the nomogram.

[b] Heparin concentration = 20,000 U in 500 ml (40 U/ml).

[c] PTT determined with Actin-FS thromboplastin reagent (Dade, Mississauga, Ontario, Canada).

(From Hull et al.,[126] with permission.)

been recommended for these patients. Recently, this recommendation has come into question, as several studies have shown no significant difference in remission rate or incidence of bleeding in patients treated with or without heparin.[140-142] High doses of heparin (>15,000 U/day) are associated with an increased incidence of hemorrhagic deaths and are not recommended in this setting.

Trousseau syndrome is an uncommon complication of malignancy characterized by venous thromboembolism, arterial embolic disease, and nonbacterial endocarditis. Laboratory findings are usually consistent with chronic DIC (see Ch. 116). Since warfarin is usually insufficient to prevent recurrence of the thromboembolic manifestations of this syndrome, full-dose heparin administered either intravenously or subcutaneously is recommended.[143,144] The role of heparin in DIC of other etiologies has yet to be established.

Coronary Artery Thrombosis

Heparin treatment of coronary artery disease and myocardial infarction remains controversial. An overview of the data has suggested that subcutaneous or intravenous heparin reduces mortality, reinfarction rate, pulmonary embolism, and stroke in patients with acute myocardial infarction who are not receiving thrombolytic therapy.[145] High-dose subcutaneous heparin seems to be effective in prevention of left ventricular mural thrombosis in patients with acute anterior myocardial infarction and may thereby decrease the incidence of cerebral embolism.[146]

In patients receiving thrombolytic therapy for acute myocardial infarction, heparin (12,500 U twice a day) does not increase the risk of stroke.[147] Whether heparin helps to maintain coronary artery patency after thrombolytic therapy of an acute myocardial infarction is controversial. Heparin may be used in the treatment of unstable angina, but its discontinuation has been associated with reactivation of the angina and myocardial infarction.[148]

Cerebrovascular Thromboembolism

Anticoagulant therapy of ischemic stroke is, for the most part, empirical. Nonambulatory patients may benefit from low doses of heparin to prevent venous thromboembolism. Heparin and low-molecular-weight heparin do not appear to improve the outcome of patients with partial stable or complete stroke.[149] The use of heparin to treat patients with acute embolic stroke of cardiac origin, usually in the presence of nonrheumatic atrial fibrillation, remains controversial because the risk of central nervous system bleeding appears to be high in this situation.[150] Heparin therapy in the management of transient ischemic attacks has not been shown to offer improved survival or a reduced incidence of subsequent strokes.[149]

Other Indications

Heparin (100 U/kg/day) has been used in the prevention of hepatic veno-occlusive disease after bone marrow transplantation. A prospective, randomized study found this regimen to be highly effective in the prevention of veno-occlusive disease, but other studies have been less successful.[151,152]

Heparin has been proposed for the treatment of exercise-induced asthma. The beneficial effect of heparin is not dependent on its anticoagulant properties. Inhaled, heparin at high doses (1,000 U/kg) had no effect on systemic coagulation as measured by the PTT.[153]

Toxicities

Bleeding

Bleeding is the principal toxicity of heparin. Major bleeding has been reported to occur in 1–33% of patients receiving various forms of heparin therapy, and fatal bleeding occurred in 3 of 647 patients treated with heparin in one series.[154] Often an underlying cause for bleeding is present, such as recent surgery, trauma, peptic ulcer disease, or platelet dysfunction. Heparin can interfere with platelet function and prolong the bleeding time, but it is unclear to what extent the the antiplatelet effect contributes to the hemorrhagic complications of heparin therapy.[155]

Four randomized studies have compared the incidence of bleeding during intermittent and continuous intravenous infusion of heparin. Two of the studies demonstrated a significantly lower incidence of bleeding in the patients receiving continuous intravenous infusions (0–1% versus 9–33%),[125,156] and a third study reported a similar trend.[157] However, the total dose of heparin administered by intermittent infusion was higher than that administered by continuous infusion. When the same doses were used in one study, the incidence of bleeding was identical, implying that bleeding was related to the dosage and not to the method of administration.[158] In a study in which patients considered to be at high risk of bleeding were initially treated with a lower dose of heparin (30,000 U/day) than those at low risk for bleeding (40,000 U/day), the incidence of major bleeding was 11% in the high-risk group compared with 1% in the low-risk group.[159] Taken together, these studies suggest that the incidence of bleeding depends both on the total daily dose of heparin and on the presence of underlying risk factors.

Several randomized studies have compared a continuous intravenous infusion of standard heparin with a fixed dose of subcutaneous low-molecular-weight heparin in treatment of venous thrombosis.[137-139] The incidence of major bleeding appears to be lower during therapy with low-molecular-weight heparin.

Thrombocytopenia

Two forms of acute, heparin-induced thrombocytopenia have been reported.[160] Mild thrombocytopenia occurs in about 25% of patients 2–15 days after initiation of full-dose heparin therapy. The platelet count usually remains >100,000/mm^3, and heparin therapy can be continued without undue risk of bleeding. This common form of thrombocytopenia appears to result directly from the induction of platelet aggregation by heparin.[149] A platelet count of <100,000/mm^3 occurs in about 5% of patients treated with bovine heparin and about 1% of patients treated with porcine heparin.[161,162] Much less frequently, thrombocytopenia apparently mediated by an immune mechanism occurs 7–14 days after initiation of full-dose or low-dose heparin therapy. If the patient has been exposed to heparin previously, the thrombocytopenia may occur within the first day of re-exposure. The thrombocytopenia usually resolves within several days after the discontinuation of heparin. Paradoxically, the severe form of heparin-induced thrombocytopenia has been associated in some patients with acute arterial thrombosis manifested by myocardial infarction, cerebrovascular occlusion, skin necrosis, or limb ischemia. Laboratory studies indicate that plasma from such patients often contain IgG molecules that bind heparin, forming immune complexes that activate platelets by binding to Fc receptors on the platelet surface.[163,164] It is not clear whether the presence or absence of these antibodies can be used to predict the recurrence of thrombocytopenia during subsequent heparin administration. Thrombocytopenia may also occur after administration of low-molecular-weight heparin.[114]

Osteoporosis

Radiographic evidence of osteopenia has been reported in 17% of women treated with heparin throughout pregnancy.[165] In most cases, the osteopenia resolves within 1 year after delivery. Spontaneous osteoporotic vertebral fractures occur in

HEPARIN-INDUCED THROMBOCYTOPENIA

Initiation of heparin therapy should be preceded by a platelet count to determine the baseline level. Heparin-induced thrombocytopenia is suggested when the platelet count declines to $<100,000/mm^3$ from a normal pretreatment level in the absence of another cause of thrombocytopenia (for example, sepsis, other drugs, or DIC). Laboratory tests to confirm the diagnosis are occasionally helpful, but action is usually required before the results are available. The diagnosis is more likely when a patient receiving heparin develops symptoms of arterial insufficiency such as limb ischemia, stroke, or skin necrosis that are otherwise unexplained.

In the setting of an unexplained acute arterial thrombosis in a patient on heparin, all heparin should be discontinued immediately. Occasionally, thrombosis may precede the development of thrombocytopenia. The optimal therapy for this condition is uncertain. Fibrinolytic therapy or surgical embolectomy should be considered for arterial thrombosis affecting a limb. The use of an alternative anticoagulant will be dictated by its availability. Initial clinical experience with the heparinoid Org 10172 has been favorable in quickly reversing the thrombocytopenia while establishing effective anticoagulation. A low-molecular-weight heparin preparation may be effective in reversing the thrombocytopenia while maintaining therapeutic anticoagulation, but in some patients the outcome is unfavorable. Treatment with the snake venom protease ancrod, which lowers the fibrinogen concentration, has also been used with some success. Platelet transfusions are not helpful in the treatment of heparin-induced thrombocytopenia.

When thrombocytopenia (platelet count $100,000/mm^3$) is observed in the absence of arterial thrombosis and heparin is considered as the cause, further heparin exposure should be limited to the shortest possible time and the platelet count should be monitored several times per day. If bovine heparin is being used, a switch to porcine heparin may correct the problem. If the platelet count continues to fall, all heparin should be discontinued; in patients with indwelling vascular access, all heparin flushes should be replaced by saline flushes. In patients who are already therapeutically anticoagulated or approaching adequate anticoagulation with a vitamin K antagonist when thrombocytopenia develops, discontinuing the heparin may be sufficient. If further anticoagulation is deemed necessary, one of the alternative anticoagulant agents mentioned above may be used.

2–3% of pregnant women receiving heparin.[165,166] High-dose heparin and prolonged duration of treatment appear to enhance the risk of osteoporosis. Several pregnant patients with thrombembolism have been treated successfully with low-molecular-weight heparin, but the relative risk of osteoporosis in comparison with standard heparin is unknown.[114] The risk of osteoporosis in nonpregnant patients receiving long-term heparin has not been established.

Other Toxicities

Abnormalities in liver function tests occur frequently in patients receiving intravenous or subcutaneous heparin. Mild elevations of the SGOT (AST) and SGPT (ALT) occur without a concomitant increase in serum bilirubin or alkaline phosphatase.[167] Cutaneous allergic reactions to subcutaneous heparin occur rarely.

Use in Pregnancy

In contrast to warfarin, heparin does not cross the placenta and has not been associated with fetal malformations. Therefore, despite the risk of osteoporosis, heparin is the drug of choice for the prophylaxis and treatment of venous thromboembolism during pregnancy.[168] Heparin may also prevent thromboembolic complications associated with mechanical heart valves.[168] Heparin can be administered either by intermittent adjusted-dose subcutaneous injections or by continuous intravenous infusion. Ambulatory management may be facilitated by the use of implantable intravenous ports and indwelling subcutaneous catheters. It has been recommended that pregnant patients with venous thromboembolism be anticoagulated throughout the course of pregnancy and for approximately 1 month following delivery.[168]

An elevated PTT may be associated with increased bleeding at the time of delivery. In the nonpregnant patient, a single dose of subcutaneous heparin is usually cleared within 12 hours, but during the third trimester of pregnancy the PTT may remain prolonged as long as 28 hours after a subcutaneous dose of heparin.[169] It has been recommended that heparin be discontinued ≥24 hours before induction of delivery or immediately at the onset of labor.

Antagonist

The anticoagulant effect of heparin disappears within hours after discontinuation of the drug, and mild bleeding due to heparin can usually be controlled without administration of an antagonist. If life-threatening hemorrhage occurs, the effect of heparin can be reversed quickly by intravenous infusion of the sulfate salt of protamine, a mixture of basic polypeptides isolated from salmon sperm. Protamine binds tightly to heparin in vitro and thereby neutralizes its anticoagulant effect. Protamine may also be used to reverse the action of low-molecular-weight heparin. The typical dose of protamine sulfate is 1 mg/100 U of heparin. Neither the route (intravenous or arterial) nor the rate of administration of protamine has been found to be of clinical importance.[170]

Protamine is used routinely to reverse the anticoagulant effect of heparin following cardiac surgery and other vascular procedures. An antibody-mediated anaphylactic reaction may occur within minutes after receiving the antagonist. This complication occurs in approximately 1% of patients with diabetes mellitus who have received protamine-containing insulin (neutral protein Hagedorn insulin or protamine zinc insulin) but is not limited to this group.[171] This reaction can be fatal.[172] A less common nonimmunologic reaction consisting of pulmonary vasoconstriction, right ventricular dysfunction, and systemic hypotension associated with transient neutropenia may also occur after administration of protamine.[173,174]

REFERENCES

1. Howell WH: Heparin as an anticoagulant. Am J Physiol 63:434, 1923
2. Jorpes E: Heparin: Its Chemistry, Physiology, and Application in Medicine. Oxford University Press, London, 1939
3. Jaques LB: The Howell theory of blood coagulation: a record of the pernicious effects of a false theory. Can Bull Med Hist 5:143, 1988
4. Murray DWG: Heparin in thrombosis and embolism. Br J Surg 27:567, 1939
5. Lindahl U, Kusche M, Lidholt K, Oscarsson L-G: Biosynthesis of heparin and heparan sulfate. Ann NY Acad Sci 556:36, 1989
6. Teien AN, Abildgaard U, Höök M: The anticoagulant effect of heparan sulfate and dermatan sulfate. Thromb Res 8:859, 1976

7. Conrad HE: Structure of heparan sulfate and dermatan sulfate. Ann NY Acad Sci 556:18, 1989

8. Brinkhous KM, Smith HP, Warner ED, Seegers WH: The inhibition of blood clotting: an unidentified substance which acts in conjunction with heparin to prevent the conversion of prothrombin to thrombin. Am J Physiol 125: 683, 1939

9. Abildgaard U: Highly purified antithrombin III with heparin cofactor activity prepared by disc electrophoresis. Scand J Clin Lab Invest 21:89, 1968

10. Rosenberg RD, Damus PS: The purification and mechanism of action of human antithrombin-heparin cofactor. J Biol Chem 248:6490, 1973

11. Peterson TE, Dudeck-Wojciechowska G, Sottrup-Jensen L, Magnusson S: Primary structure of antithrombin III (heparin cofactor): partial homology between alpha 1-antitrypsin and antithrombin III. p. 43. In Collen D, Wiman B, Verstraete M (eds): The Physiological Inhibitors of Blood Coagulation and Fibrinolysys. Elsevier/North Holland Biomedical Press, Amsterdam, 1979

12. Bock SC, Wion KL, Vehar GA, Lawn RM: Cloning and expression of the cDNA for human antithrombin III. Nucleic Acids Res 10:8113, 1982

13. Carrell RW, Travis J: α1-Antitrypsin and the serpins: variation and counter-variation. Trends Biochem Sci 10:20, 1985

14. Conrad J, Brosstad F, Lie-Larson M et al: Molar antithrombin concentration in normal human plasma. Haemostasis 13:363, 1983

15. Rosenberg RD: Biologic actions of heparin. Semin Hematol 14:427, 1977

16. Björk I, Jackson CM, Jörnvall H et al: The active site of antithrombin. Release of the same proteolytically cleaved form of the inhibitor from complexes with factor IXa, factor Xa, and thrombin. J Biol Chem 257:2406, 1982

17. Fish WW, Björk I: Release of a two-chain form of antithrombin from the antithrombin-thrombin complex. Eur J Biochem 101:31, 1979

18. Jordan RE, Oosta GM, Gardner WT, Rosenberg RD: The kinetics of hemostatic enzyme-antithrombin interactions in the presence of low molecular weight heparin. J Biol Chem 255:10081, 1980

19. Teitel JM, Rosenberg RD: Protection of factor Xa from neutralization by the heparin-antithrombin complex. J Clin Invest 71:1383, 1983

20. Hogg PJ, Jackson CM: Fibrin monomer protects thrombin from inactivation by heparin-antithrombin III: implications for heparin efficacy. Proc Natl Acad Sci USA 86:3619, 1989

21. Weitz JI, Hudoba M, Massel D et al: Clot-bound thrombin is protected from inhibition by heparin-antithrombin III but is susceptible to inactivation by antithrombin III-independent inhibitors. J Clin Invest 86:385, 1990

22. Lawson JH, Butenas S, Ribarik N, Mann KG: Complex-dependent inhibition of factor VIIa by antithrombin III and heparin. J Biol Chem 268:767, 1993

23. Rao LVM, Rapaport SI, Hoang AD: Binding of factor VIIa to tissue factor permits rapid antithrombin III/heparin inhibition of factor VIIa. Blood 81: 2600, 1993

24. Ofosu FA, Sié P, Modi GJ et al: The inhibition of thrombin-dependent positive-feedback reactions is critical to the expression of the anticoagulant effect of heparin. Biochem J 243:579, 1987

25. Béguin S, Lindhout T, Hemker HC: The mode of action of heparin in plasma. Thromb Haemost 60:457, 1988

26. Ofosu FA, Hirsh J, Esmon CT et al: Unfractionated heparin inhibits thrombin-catalysed amplification reactions of coagulation more efficiently than those catalysed by factor Xa. Biochem J 257:143, 1989

27. Tollefsen DM, Blank MK: Detection of a new heparin-dependent inhibitor of thrombin in human plasma. J Clin Invest 68:589, 1981

28. Tollefsen DM, Pestka CA, Monafo WJ: Activation of heparin cofactor II by dermatan sulfate. J Biol Chem 258:6713, 1983

29. Gebbink RK, Reynolds CH, Tollefsen DM et al: Specific glycosaminoglycans support the inhibition of thrombin by plasminogen activator inhibitor 1. Biochemistry 32:1675, 1993

30. Pratt CW, Church FC: Heparin binding to protein C inhibitor. J Biol Chem 267:8789, 1992

31. Wallace A, Rovelli G, Hofsteenge J, Stone SR: Effect of heparin on the glia-derived-nexin—thrombin interaction. Biochem J 257:191, 1989

32. Broze GJ Jr, Warren LA, Novotny WF et al: The lipoprotein-associated coagulation inhibitor that inhibits the factor VII-tissue factor complex also inhibits factor Xa: insight into its possible mechanism of action. Blood 71:335, 1988

33. Wesselschmidt R, Likert K, Girard T et al: Tissue factor pathway inhibitor: the carboxy-terminus is required for optimal inhibition of factor Xa. Blood 79:2004, 1992

34. Novotny WF, Brown SG, Miletich JP et al: Plasma antigen levels of the lipoprotein-associated coagulation inhibitor in patient samples. Blood 78:387, 1991

35. Andrade-Gordon P, Strickland S: Interaction of heparin with plasminogen activators and plasminogen: effects on the activation of plasminogen. Biochemistry 25:4033, 1986

36. Keijer J, Linders M, Wegman JJ et al: On the target specificity of plasminogen activator inhibitor 1: the role of heparin, vitronectin, and the reactive site. Blood 78:1254, 1991

37. Agnelli G, Borm J, Cosmi B et al: Effects of standard heparin and a low molecular weight heparin (Kabi 2165) on fibrinolysis. Thromb Haemost 60: 311, 1988

38. Agnelli G, Pascucci C, Cosmi B, Nenci GG: Effects of therapeutic doses of heparin on thrombolysis with tissue-type plasminogen activator in rabbits. Blood 76:2030, 1990

39. Lam LH, Silbert JE, Rosenberg RD: The separation of active and inactive forms of heparin. Biochem Biophys Res Commun 69:570, 1976

40. Höök M, Björk I, Hopwood J, Lindahl U: Anticoagulant activity of heparin: separation of high-activity and low-activity species by affinity chromatography on immobilized antithrombin. FEBS Lett 66:90, 1976

41. Andersson L-O, Barrowcliffe TW, Holmer E et al: Anticoagulant properties of heparin fractionated by affinity chromatography on matrix-bound antithrombin III and by gel filtration. Thromb Res 9:575, 1976

42. Olson ST, Srinivasan KR, Björk I, Shore JD: Binding of high affinity heparin to antithrombin III. Stopped flow kinetic studies of the binding interaction. J Biol Chem 256:11073, 1981

43. Atha DH, Lormeau JC, Petitou M et al: Contribution of monosaccharide residues in heparin binding to antithrombin III. Biochemistry 24:6723, 1985

44. Choay J, Petitou M, Lormeau JC et al: Structure-activity relationship in heparin: a synthetic pentasaccharide with high affinity for antithrombin III and eliciting high anti-factor Xa activity. Biochem Biophys Res Commun 116: 492, 1983

45. Lindahl U, Thunberg L, Bäckström G et al: Extension and structural variability of the antithrombin-binding sequence in heparin. J Biol Chem 259:12368, 1984

46. Olson ST, Shore JD: Transient kinetics of heparin-catalyzed protease inactivation by antithrombin III. The reaction step limiting heparin turnover in thrombin neutralization. J Biol Chem 261:13151, 1986

47. Olson ST, Björk I: Predominant contribution of surface approximation to the mechanism of heparin acceleration of the antithrombin-thrombin reaction. Elucidation from salt concentration effects. J Biol Chem 266:6353, 1991

48. Olson ST, Björk I, Sheffer R et al: Role of the antithrombin-binding pentasaccharide in heparin acceleration of antithrombin-proteinase reactions. Resolution of the antithrombin conformational change contribution to heparin rate enhancement. J Biol Chem 267:12528, 1992

49. Danielsson Å, Raub E, Lindahl U, Björk I: Role of ternary complexes, in which heparin binds both antithrombin and proteinase, in the acceleration of the reactions between antithrombin and thrombin or factor Xa. J Biol Chem 261:15467, 1986

50. Olson ST, Halvorson HR, Björk I: Quantitative characterization of the thrombin-heparin interaction. Discrimination between specific and nonspecific binding models. J Biol Chem 266:6342, 1991

51. Pomerantz MW, Owen WG: A catalytic role for heparin. Evidence for a ternary complex of heparin cofactor, thrombin and heparin. Biochim Biophys Acta 535:66, 1978

52. Owen BA, Owen WG: Interaction of factor Xa with heparin does not contribute to the inhibition of factor Xa by antithrombin III-heparin. Biochemistry 29:9412, 1990

53. Jordan R, Beeler D, Rosenberg R: Fractionation of low molecular weight heparin species and their interaction with antithrombin. J Biol Chem 254: 2902, 1979

54. Tollefsen DM, Majerus DW, Blank MK: Heparin cofactor II. Purification and properties of a heparin-dependent inhibitor of thrombin in human plasma. J Biol Chem 257:2162, 1982

55. Ragg H: A new member of the plasma protease inhibitor gene family. Nucleic Acids Res 14:1073, 1986

56. Blinder MA, Marasa JC, Reynolds CH et al: Heparin cofactor II: cDNA sequence, chromosome localization, restriction fragment length polymorphism, and expression in *Escherichia coli*. Biochemistry 27:752, 1988

57. Parker KA, Tollefsen DM: The protease specificity of heparin cofactor II. Inhibition of thrombin generated during coagulation. J Biol Chem 260:3501, 1985

58. Griffith MJ, Noyes CM, Tyndall JA, Church FC: Structural evidence for leucine at the reactive site of heparin cofactor II. Biochemistry 24:6777, 1985

59. Church FC, Noyes CM, Griffith MJ: Inhibition of chymotrypsin by heparin cofactor II. Proc Natl Acad Sci USA 82:6431, 1985

60. Hurst RE, Poon MC, Griffith MJ: Structure-activity relationships of heparin. Independence of heparin charge density and antithrombin-binding domains in thrombin inhibition by antithrombin and heparin cofactor II. J Clin Invest 72:1042, 1983

61. Maimone MM, Tollefsen DM: Activation of heparin cofactor II by heparin oligosaccharides. Biochem Biophys Res Commun 152:1056, 1988

62. Bray B, Lane DA, Freyssinet J-M et al: Anti-thrombin activities of heparin.

Effect of saccharide chain length on thrombin inhibition by heparin cofactor II and by antithrombin. Biochem J 262:225, 1989

63. Maimone MM, Tollefsen DM: Structure of a dermatan sulfate hexasaccharide that binds to heparin cofactor II with high affinity. J Biol Chem 265:18263, 1990

64. Ragg H, Ulshöfer T, Gerewitz J: Glycosaminoglycan-mediated leuserpin-2/thrombin interaction. Structure-function relationships. J Biol Chem 265:22386, 1990

65. Van Deerlin VMD, Tollefsen DM: The N-terminal acidic domain of heparin cofactor II mediates the inhibition of α-thrombin in the presence of glycosaminoglycans. J Biol Chem 266:20223, 1991

66. Rogers SJ, Pratt CW, Whinna HC, Church FC: Role of thrombin exosites in inhibition by heparin cofactor II. J Biol Chem 267:3613, 1992

67. Sheehan JP, Wu Q, Tollefsen DM, Sadler JE: Mutagenesis of thrombin selectively modulates inhibition by serpins heparin cofactor II and antithrombin III. Interaction with the anion-binding exosite determines heparin cofactor II specificity. J Biol Chem 268:3639, 1993

68. Fernandez F, van Ryn J, Ofosu FA et al: The haemorrhagic and antithrombotic effects of dermatan sulfate. Br J Haematol 64:309, 1986

69. Maggi A, Abbadini M, Pagella PG et al: Antithrombotic properties of dermatan sulphate in a rat venous thrombosis model. Haemostasis 17:329, 1987

70. Merton RE, Thomas DP: Experimental studies on the relative efficacy of dermatan sulphate and heparin as antithrombotic agents. Thromb Haemost 58:839, 1987

71. Van Ryn-McKenna J, Gray E, Weber E et al: Effects of sulfated polysaccharides on inhibition of thrombus formation initiated by different stimuli. Thromb Haemost 61:7, 1989

72. Cadroy Y, Hanson SR, Harker LA: Dermatan sulfate inhibition of fibrin-rich thrombus formation in nonhuman primates. Arterioscler Thromb 13:1213, 1993

73. Agnelli G, Cosmi B, Di Filippo P et al: A randomised, double-blind, placebo-controlled trial of dermatan sulphate for prevention of deep vein thrombosis in hip fracture. Thromb Haemost 67:203, 1992

74. Lane DA, Ryan K, Ireland H et al: Dermatan sulphate in haemodialysis. Lancet 339:334, 1992

75. Cofrancesco E, Boschetti C, Leonardi P, Cortellaro M: Dermatan sulphate in acute leukaemia. Lancet 339:1177, 1992

76. Ofosu FA, Modi GJ, Smith LM et al: Heparan sulfate and dermatan sulfate inhibit the generation of thrombin activity in plasma by complementary pathways. Blood 64:742, 1984

77. Sié P, Ofosu F, Fernandez F et al: Respective role of antithrombin III and heparin cofactor II in the in vitro anticoagulant effect of heparin and of various sulphated polysaccharides. Br J Haematol 64:707, 1986

78. Scully MF, Ellis V, Kakkar VV: Pentosan polysulphate: activation of heparin cofactor II or antithrombin III according to molecular weight fractionation. Thromb Res 41:489, 1986

79. Church FC, Meade JB, Treanor RE, Whinna HC: Antithrombin activity of fucoidan. The interaction of fucoidan with heparin cofactor II, antithrombin III, and thrombin. J Biol Chem 264:3618, 1989

80. Scully MF, Ellis V, Seno N, Kakkar VV: The anticoagulant properties of mast cell product, chondroitin sulphate E. Biochem Biophys Res Commun 137:15, 1986

81. Marcum JA, Rosenberg RD: Heparin-like molecules with anticoagulant activity are synthesized by cultured endothelial cells. Biochem Biophys Res Commun 126:365, 1985

82. Marcum JA, Atha DH, Fritze LMS et al: Cloned bovine aortic endothelial cells synthesize anticoagulantly active heparan sulfate proteoglycan. J Biol Chem 261:7507, 1986

83. de Agostini AI, Watkins SC, Slayter HS et al: Localization of anticoagulantly active heparan sulfate proteoglycans in vascular endothelium: antithrombin binding on cultured endothelial cells and perfused rat aorta. J Cell Biol 111:1293, 1990

84. Kobayashi M, Shimada K, Ozawa T: Human recombinant interleukin-1β- and tumor necrosis factor α-mediated suppression of heparin-like compounds on cultured porcine aortic endothelial cells. J Cell Physiol 144:383, 1990

85. Lollar P, Owen WG: Clearance of thrombin from the circulation in rabbits by high-affinity binding sites on the endothelium. Possible role in the inactivation of thrombin by antithrombin III. J Clin Invest 66:1222, 1980

86. Jakubowski HV, Kline MD, Owen WG: The effect of bovine thrombomodulin on the specificity of bovine thrombin. J Biol Chem 261:3876, 1986

87. Marcum JA, McKenney JB, Rosenberg RD: Acceleration of thrombin-antithrombin complex formation in rat hindquarters via heparinlike molecules bound to the endothelium. J Clin Invest 74:341, 1984

88. Lane DA, Pejler G, Flynn AM et al: Neutralization of heparin-related saccharides by histidine-rich glycoprotein and platelet factor 4. J Biol Chem 261:3980, 1986

89. Koide T, Odani S, Takahashi K et al: Antithrombin III Toyama: replacement of arginine-47 by cysteine in hereditary abnormal antithrombin III that lacks heparin-binding ability. Proc Natl Acad Sci USA 81:289, 1984

90. Boyer C, Wolf M, Vedrenne J et al: Homozygous variant of antithrombin III: AT III Fontainebleau. Thromb Haemost 56:18, 1986

91. Caulfield JP, Lewis RA, Hein A, Austen KF: Secretion in dissociated human pulmonary mast cells. Evidence for solubilization of granule contents before discharge. J Cell Biol 85:299, 1980

92. Nenci GG, Berrettini M, Parise P, Agnelli G: Persistent spontaneous heparinaemia in systemic mastocytosis. Folia Haematol (Leipz) 109:453, 1982

93. Khoory MS, Nesheim ME, Bowie EJW, Mann KG: Circulating heparan sulfate proteoglycan anticoagulant from a patient with a plasma cell disorder. J Clin Invest 65:666, 1980

94. Palmer RN, Rick ME, Rick PD et al: Circulating heparan sulfate anticoagulant in a patient with a fatal bleeding disorder. N Engl J Med 310:1696, 1984

95. Bussel JB, Steinherz PG, Miller DR, Hilgartner MW: A heparin-like anticoagulant in an 8-month-old boy with acute monoblastic leukemia. Am J Hematol 16:83, 1984

96. Tefferi A, Nichols WL, Bowie EJW: Circulating heparin-like anticoagulants: report of five consecutive cases and a review. Am J Med 88:184, 1990

97. Kaufman PA, Gockerman JP, Greenberg CS: Production of a novel anticoagulant by neoplastic plasma cells: report of a case and review of the literature. Am J Med 86:612, 1989

98. Horne MK III, Stein CA, LaRocca RV, Myers CE: Circulating glycosaminoglycan anticoagulants associated with suramin treatment. Blood 71:273, 1988

99. Clowes AW, Karnovsky MJ: Suppression by heparin of smooth muscle cell proliferation in injured arteries. Nature 265:625, 1977

100. Wright TC Jr, Castellot JJ Jr, Petitou M et al: Structural determinants of heparin's growth inhibitory activity. Interdependence of oligosaccharide size and charge. J Biol Chem 264:1534, 1989

101. Fritze L, Reilly C, Rosenberg R: An antiproliferative heparan sulfate species produced by postconfluent smooth muscle cells. J Cell Biol 100:1041, 1985

102. Pukac LA, Ottlinger ME, Karnovsky MJ: Heparin suppresses specific second messenger pathways for protooncogene expression in rat vascular smooth muscle cells. J Biol Chem 267:3707, 1992

103. Vlodavsky I, Folkman J, Sullivan R et al: Endothelial cell-derived basic fibroblast growth factor: synthesis and deposition in subendothelial extracellular matrix. Proc Natl Acad Sci USA 84:2292, 1987

104. Sudhalter J, Folkman J, Svahn CM et al: Importance of size, sulfation, and anticoagulant activity in the potentiation of acidic fibroblast growth factor by heparin. J Biol Chem 264:6892, 1989

105. Bashkin P, Doctrow S, Klagsbrun M et al: Basic fibroblast growth factor binds to subendothelial extracellular matrix and is released by heparitinase and heparin-like molecules. Biochemistry 28:1737, 1989

106. Yayon A, Klagsbrun M, Esko JD et al: Cell surface, heparin-like molecules are required for binding of basic fibroblast growth factor to its high affinity receptor. Cell 64:841, 1991

107. Rapraeger AC, Krufka A, Olwin BB: Requirement of heparan sulfate for bFGF-mediated fibroblast growth and myoblast differentiation. Science 252:1705, 1991

108. Turnbull JE, Fernig DG, Ke Y et al: Identification of the basic fibroblast growth factor binding sequence in fibroblast heparan sulfate. J Biol Chem 267:10337, 1992

109. Tyrrell DJ, Ishihara M, Rao N et al: Structure and biological activities of a heparin-derived hexasaccharide with high affinity for basic fibroblast growth factor. J Biol Chem 268:4684, 1993

110. Carter CJ, Kelton JG, Hirsh J et al: The relationship between the hemorrhagic and antithrombotic properties of low molecular weight heparin in rabbits. Blood 59:1239, 1982

111. Eckel RH: Lipoprotein lipase. A multifunctional enzyme relevant to common metabolic diseases. N Engl J Med 320:1060, 1989

112. Neville GA, Mori F, Holme KR, Perlin AS: Monitoring the purity of pharmaceutical heparin preparations by high-field 1H-nuclear magnetic resonance spectroscopy. J Pharm Sci 78:101, 1989

113. Hirsh J, O'Sullivan EF, Gallus AS, Martin M: Evaluation of subcutaneous calcium heparin therapy in the treatment of thrombo-embolic disease. Med J Aust 1:15, 1970

114. Hirsh J, Levine MN: Low molecular weight heparin. Blood 79:1, 1992

115. Barrowcliffe TW, Thomas DP: Anticoagulant activities of heparin and fragments. Ann NY Acad Sci 556:132, 1989

116. Ortel TL, Gockerman JP, Califf RM et al: Parenteral anticoagulation with the heparinoid Lomoparan (Org 10172) in patients with heparin induced thrombocytopenia and thrombosis. Thromb Haemost 67:292, 1992

117. Chong BH, Ismail F, Cade J et al: Heparin-induced thrombocytopenia: studies with a new low molecular weight heparinoid, Org 10172. Blood 73:1592, 1989

118. McAvoy TJ: Pharmacokinetic modeling of heparin and its clinical implications. J Pharm Biopharm 7:331, 1979

119. Hirsh J, van Aken WG, Gallus AS et al: Heparin kinetics in venous thrombosis and pulmonary embolism. Circulation 53:691, 1976

120. Bara L, Samama M: Pharmacokinetics of low molecular weight heparins. Acta Chir Scand Suppl 543:65, 1988

121. Hyers TM, Hull RD, Weg JG: Antithrombotic therapy for venous thromboembolic disease. Chest, suppl. 89:26, 1986

122. Doyle DJ, Turpie AG, Hirsh J et al: Adjusted subcutaneous heparin or continuous intravenous heparin in patients with acute deep vein thrombosis. A randomized trial. Ann Intern Med 107:441, 1987

123. Hull RD, Raskob GE, Hirsh J et al: Continuous intravenous heparin compared with intermittent subcutaneous heparin in the initial treatment of proximal-vein thrombosis. N Engl J Med 315:1109, 1986

124. Basu D, Gallus A, Hirsh J, Cade J: A prospective study of the value of monitoring heparin treatment with the activated partial thromboplastin time. N Engl J Med 287:324, 1972

125. Salzman EW, Deykin D, Shapiro RM, Rosenberg R: Management of heparin therapy: controlled prospective trial. N Engl J Med 292:1046, 1975

126. Hull RD, Raskob GE, Rosenbloom D et al: Optimal therapeutic level of heparin therapy in patients with venous thrombosis. Arch Intern Med 152:1589, 1992

127. Preissner KT, Muller-Berghaus G: S protein modulates the heparin-catalyzed inhibition of thrombin by antithrombin III. Evidence for a direct interaction of S protein with heparin. Eur J Biochem 156:645, 1986

128. Young E, Prins M, Levine MN, Hirsh J: Heparin binding to plasma proteins, an important mechanism for heparin resistance. Thromb Haemost 67:639, 1992

129. Leclerc JR, Geerts W, Panju A et al: Management of anti-thrombin III deficiency during pregnancy without administration of anti-thrombin III. Thromb Res 41:567, 1986

130. Nielsen LE, Bell WR, Borkon AM, Neill CA: Extensive thrombus formation with heparin resistance during extracorporeal circulation. A new presentation of familial antithrombin III deficiency. Arch Intern Med 147:149, 1987

131. Knot E, ten-Cate JW, Drijfhout HR et al: Antithrombin III metabolism in patients with liver disease. J Clin Pathol 37:523, 1984

132. Kauffmann RH, Veltkamp JJ, van Tilburg NH, van Es LA: Acquired antithrombin III deficiency and thrombosis in the nephrotic syndrome. Am J Med 65:607, 1978

133. Spero JA, Lewis JH, Hasiba U: Disseminated intravascular coagulation. Findings in 346 patients. Thromb Haemost 43:28, 1980

134. Holm HA, Kalvenes S, Abildgaard U: Changes in plasma antithrombin (heparin cofactor activity) during intravenous heparin therapy: observations in 198 patients with deep venous thrombosis. Scand J Haematol 35:564, 1985

135. Brandjes DPM, Heijboer H, Büller HR et al: Acenocoumarol and heparin compared with acenocoumarol alone in the initial treatment of proximal-vein thrombosis. N Engl J Med 327:1485, 1992

136. Hull RD, Raskob GE, Rosenbloom D et al: Heparin for 5 days as compared with 10 days in the initial treatment of proximal venous thrombosis. N Engl J Med 322:1260, 1990

137. Hull RD, Raskob GE, Pineo GF et al: Subcutaneous low-molecular-weight heparin compared with continuous intravenous heparin in the treatment of proximal-vein thrombosis. N Engl J Med 326:975, 1992

138. Prandoni P, Lensing AW, Büller HR et al: Comparison of subcutaneous low-molecular-weight heparin with intravenous standard heparin in proximal deep-vein thrombosis. Lancet 339:441, 1992

139. Simonneau G, Charbonnier B, Decousus H et al: Subcutaneous low-molecular-weight heparin compared with continuous intravenous unfractionated heparin in the treatment of proximal deep vein thrombosis. Arch Intern Med 153:1541, 1993

140. Stone RM, Mayer RJ: The unique aspects of acute promyelocytic leukemia. J Clin Oncol 8:1913, 1990

141. Goldberg MA, Ginsburg D, Mayer RJ et al: Is heparin administration necessary during induction chemotherapy for patients with acute promyelocytic leukemia? Blood 69:187, 1987

142. Rodeghiero F, Avvisati G, Castaman G et al: Early deaths and anti-hemorrhagic treatments in acute promyelocytic leukemia. A GIMEMA retrospective study in 268 consecutive patients. Blood 75:2112, 1990

143. Bell WR, Starksen NF, Tong S, Porterfield JK: Trousseau's syndrome: devastating coagulopathy in the absence of heparin. Am J Med 79:423, 1985

144. Callander N, Rapaport SI: Trousseau's syndrome. West J Med 158:364, 1993

145. Vaitkus PT, Berlin JA, Schwartz S, Barnathan ES: Stroke complicating acute myocardial infarction. A meta-analysis of risk modification by anticoagulation and thrombolytic therapy. Arch Intern Med 152:2020, 1992

146. Turpie AGG, Robinson JG, Doyle DJ et al: Comparison of high-dose with low-dose subcutaneous heparin to prevent left ventricular mural thrombosis in patients with acute transmural anterior myocardial infarction. N Engl J Med 320:352, 1989

147. Maggioni AP, Franzosi MG, Santoro E et al: The risk of stroke in patients with acute myocardial infarction after thrombolytic and antithrombotic treatment. N Engl J Med 327:1, 1992

148. Théroux P, Waters D, Lam J et al: Reactivation of unstable angina after the discontinuation of heparin. N Engl J Med 327:141, 1992

149. Rothrock JF, Hart RG: Antithrombotic therapy in cerebrovascular disease. Ann Intern Med 115:885, 1991

150. Cerebral Embolism Study Group: Cardioembolic stroke, early anticoagulation, and brain hemorrhage. Arch Intern Med 147:636, 1987

151. Attal M, Huguet F, Rubie H et al: Prevention of hepatic veno-occlusive disease after bone marrow transplantation by continuous infusion of low-dose heparin: a prospective, randomized trial. Blood 79:2834, 1992

152. Marsa-Vila L, Gorin NC, Laporte JP et al: Prophylactic heparin does not prevent liver veno-occlusive disease following autologous bone marrow transplantation. Eur J Haematol 47:346, 1991

153. Ahmed T, Garrigo J, Danta I: Preventing bronchoconstriction in exercise-induced asthma with inhaled heparin. N Engl J Med 329:90, 1993

154. Levine MN, Hirsh J: Hemorrhagic complications of anticoagulant therapy. Semin Thromb Hemost 12:39, 1986

155. Schulman S, Johnsson H: Heparin, DDAVP and the bleeding time. Thromb Haemost 65:242, 1991

156. Glazier RL, Crowell EB: Randomized prospective trial of continuous or intermittent heparin therapy. JAMA 236:1365, 1976

157. Wilson JR, Lampman J: Heparin therapy: a randomized prospective trial. Am Heart J 97:155, 1979

158. Mant MJ, O'Brien BD, Thong KL et al: Haemorrhagic complications of heparin therapy. Lancet 1:1133, 1977

159. Gallus A, Jackaman J, Tillett J et al: Safety and efficacy of warfarin started early after submassive venous thrombosis or pulmonary embolism. Lancet 2:1293, 1986

160. Bell WR: Heparin-associated thrombocytopenia and thrombosis. J Lab Clin Med 111:600, 1988

161. Warkentin TE, Kelton JG: Heparin-induced thrombocytopenia. Annu Rev Med 40:31, 1989

162. Rao AK, White GC, Sherman L et al: Low incidence of thrombocytopenia with porcine mucosal heparin: a prospective multicenter study. Arch Intern Med 149:1285, 1989

163. Kelton JG, Sheridan D, Santos A et al: Heparin-induced thrombocytopenia: laboratory studies. Blood 72:925, 1988

164. Adelman B, Sobel M, Fujimura Y et al: Heparin-associated thrombocytopenia: observations on the mechanism of platelet aggregation. J Lab Clin Med 113:204, 1989

165. Dahlman T, Lindvall N, Hellgren M: Osteopenia in pregnancy during long-term heparin treatment: a radiological study post partum. Br J Obstet Gynaecol 97:221, 1990

166. Dahlman TC: Osteoporotic fractures and the recurrence of thromboembolism during pregnancy and the puerperium in 184 women undergoing thromboprophylaxis with heparin. Am J Obstet Gynecol 168:1265, 1993

167. Dukes GEJ, Sanders SW, Russo JJ et al: Transaminase elevations in patients receiving bovine or porcine heparin. Ann Intern Med 100:646, 1984

168. Ginsberg JS, Hirsh J: Anticoagulants during pregnancy. Annu Rev Med 40:79, 1989

169. Anderson DR, Ginsberg JS, Burrows R, Brill-Edwards P: Subcutaneous heparin therapy during pregnancy: a need for concern at the time of delivery. Thromb Haemost 65:248, 1991

170. Arén C: Heparin and protamine therapy. Semin Thorac Cardiovasc Surg 2:364, 1990

171. Weiss ME, Nyhan D, Peng ZK et al: Association of protamine IgE and IgG antibodies with life-threatening reactions to intravenous protamine. N Engl J Med 320:886, 1989

172. Gupta SK, Veith FJ, Ascer E et al: Anaphylactoid reactions to protamine: an often lethal complication in insulin-dependent diabetic patients undergoing vascular surgery. J Vasc Surg 9:342, 1989

173. Lowenstein E, Johnston WE, Lappas DG et al: Catastrophic pulmonary vasoconstriction associated with protamine reversal of heparin. Anesthesiology 59:470, 1983

174. Hobbhahn J, Conzen PF, Habazettl H et al: Heparin reversal by protamine in humans—complement, prostaglandins, blood cells, and hemodynamics. J Appl Physiol 71:1415, 1991

Fibrinolytic Therapy: Indications and Management

122

William R. Bell

INTRODUCTION

Therapeutic utilization of fibrinolysis was first made possible by the discovery that β-hemolytic streptococci secrete a substance, streptokinase (SK), that activates this system.[1] This agent was initially employed for the resolution of pulmonary consolidation associated with a variety of disease processes. When its properties were better understood, SK was then employed for the dissolution of thrombi and emboli.[2,3] Human urine contains an endogenous tissue plasminogen activator, urokinase (UK), that also activates the fibrinolytic system.[4–6] Tissue plasminogen activator (t-PA), an endogenous fibrinolytic agent, was found to be a secretory product of Bowes melanoma cells. This enzyme was isolated and purified and its cDNA cloned, permitting expression of the recombinant protein designated tissue plasminogen activator (rt-PA) in heterologous cells, including *Escherichia coli*, human fibroblasts, and Chinese hamster ovary cells.[7]

Thrombolytic agents, in contrast to anticoagulants, digest and dissolve arterial and venous thrombi and emboli. As thrombi and emboli are dissolved by these agents, blood flow is reinstituted distal to the site of obstruction. This facilitates prompt return of nutrients and oxygen to tissues deprived of blood flow by the obstructing thrombus. Anticoagulants prevent thrombus formation and the extension and propagation of the preformed thrombus, but they do not induce its dissolution. Fibrinolytic agents offer an important approach to the management of thrombotic diseases.

THROMBOLYTIC AGENTS

Currently, four different thrombolytic agents have been approved for clinical use: SK, UK, rt-PA, and acylated lys-plasminogen-streptokinase activator complex (APSAC). SK is purified from secretory products of β-hemolytic streptococci.[2,3] As a pharmacologic agent, this material leads to the expression of plasmin activity. Plasmin dissolves the fibrin clot and also acts to degrade fibrinogen. However, as a foreign antigen, SK and APSAC stimulate an immune response. Antibodies peak in titer in the circulating blood 2–3 weeks after treatment and gradually disappear 3–4 months after completion of treatment. Human UK, plasminogen activator initially purified from human urine, is currently prepared from transformed fetal renal parenchymal cells in tissue culture and by heterologous mammalian cells transfected with the UK cDNA.[8] Recombinant UK is currently in clinical trial. Human t-PA (rt-PA) is also isolated from the tissue culture supernatant of heterologous mammalian cells transfected with rt-PA cDNA.[7,9] Neither UK nor rt-PA is antigenic when employed therapeutically. The properties of these thrombolytic agents are compared in Table 122-1. Although modest differences characterize these agents, all interact with plasminogen to generate the proteolytic enzyme plasmin. None of the currently available agents activates or interacts with plasminogen only at the site of thrombus formation. All of these thrombolytic agents, employed at doses that induce resolution of thrombi and emboli, induce systemic fibrinolysis. The degree of systemic fibrinolysis induced by these agents varies and is directly dependent on the agent, dose, rate of infusion, and duration of therapy. The structure and biochemical interaction of these agents with the plasminogen-plasmin proteolytic enzymes are considered in Chapter 101. Additional agents for activating the fibrinolytic system that are undergoing clinical evaluation include single-chain urokinase plasminogen activator or pro-urokinase, and three antibody-directed (containing antifibrin antibodies) agents, Fab-urokinase, Fab-streptokinase, and Fab-rt-PA.[10–12] Polyethylene glycol attached to any of these agents may possibly prolong their circulation time and reduce the antigenicity observed with SK or SK-containing compounds. However, these agents have not been studied sufficiently in animal models or humans to predict their future clinical value. The development of new agents is directed toward activation of the fibrinolytic system only at the site of thrombus formation, thereby eliminating systemic fibrinolysis. Although a large number of mutational analogs of the expressed rt-PA compound have been prepared, none have more activity than the original wild-type form.

METHODS OF ADMINISTRATION

Thrombolytic agents are administered by intravenous systemic infusion and by local intravenous or intra-arterial perfusion. Both methods are therapeutically efficacious (Table 122-2). Thrombolytic therapy should be initiated as close to diagnosis as possible. If there are no contraindications, prompt administration of thrombolytic therapy is associated with great success in all forms of thrombotic disease. However, excellent results have been observed repeatedly in appreciable numbers of patients when the thrombus and thrombi have been angiographically documented to be present for several weeks to months.[13] Since the thrombus or components of the thrombus are in a dynamic state (e.g., growing and dissolving), the chronicity of the thrombus should not automatically preclude thrombolytic therapy, particularly if no other alternative therapies exist. Before institution of thrombolytic therapy, the diagnosis of thromboembolic disease should be firmly established. A major issue centers about whether angiography should be performed before treatment with thrombolytic agents. If the clinical features of the history, the physical examination, and the arterial blood-gas studies strongly indicate the diagnosis of pulmonary embolism, if the lung perfusion/ventilation scan is "high probability," and if the patient is a nonsmoker aged ≤35 years, treatment with thrombolytic therapy can reasonably be initiated without performing pulmonary angiography.

Thrombolytic therapy is more than, or is as efficacious as, heparin; if there are no contraindications, the frequency of bleeding with thrombolytic therapy is no greater than with heparin.[14–16] Whenever the clinical situation is complex, the diagnosis uncertain, or relative contraindications exist, angiography should be obtained. Noninvasive magnetic resonance

Table 122-1. Properties of Thrombolytic Agents

	SK	UK	rt-P/A	APSAC
Source	Streptococcal culture	Heterologous mammalian tissue culture	Heterologous mammalian tissue culture	Streptococcal culture
Molecular weight	47,000	32,000–54,000	70,000	131,000
Type of agent	Bacterial proactivator	t-PA	t-PA	Bacterial proactivator
Plasma clearance (min)	12–18	15–20	2–6	40–60
Fibrinolytic activation	Systemic	Systemic	Systemic	Systemic
Fibrin specificity	Minimal	Moderate	Moderate	Minimal
Antigenic	Yes	No	No	Yes
Allergic reactions	Yes	No	No	Yes

imaging or computed tomography are not as accurate diagnostic approaches to pulmonary thromboembolism.

If the thromboembolic disease is arterial, angiography should be performed before initiating therapy. If the thrombus is in the peripheral venous circulation, venography or a noninvasive technique (e.g., Doppler) established at the local institution to have the same accuracy as venography should be performed before initiation of therapy. Recently the development of Spiral computed tomography has been helpful in the diagnosis of central venous thrombotic disease that cannot be diagnosed by standard venography (mesenteric veins, portal vein, splenic veins, and so forth) (Fig. 122-1). If the defect is located in the central nervous system, angiography should also be performed before initiating thrombolytic therapy.

Currently available thrombolytic agents can be given either intravenously or intra-arterially. Forearm venous infusion is the site of choice for most thrombotic states employing standard systemic doses of the thrombolytic agent. When local perfusion of the thrombus is desired, a catheter is placed adjacent to, or directly into, the substance of the thrombus. With this local perfusion technique, the greatest frequency of success has been achieved on the arterial side of the circulation.[17] In some regimens employing the local perfusion technique, significantly lower doses of thrombolytic agents are used, while in other regimens the total dose employed is not significantly different from systemic dose therapy.[17] When employing low dosage schedules (5,000–7,500 U/hr SK; 15,000–20,000 U/hr UK), significant systemic effects may not be observed until after 6–8 hours of infusion. Thereafter systemic activation of fibrinolysis comparable to standard systemic thrombolytic therapy is routinely noted. The high success rate experienced with the local perfusion technique is in part due to the mechanical alterations of the thrombus directly by the catheter. Although not rigorously established, delivery of the highest possible concentration of the thrombolytic agent directly to the thrombus will maximize activation of plasminogen bound to the fibrin thrombus and will optimize diffusion into the thrombus. In some anatomic locations, this is best achieved with the local perfusion technique, while in others this is best achieved with a forearm vein systemic infusion. In the treatment of pul-

Table 122-2. Indications: Dosage of Thrombolytic Agents

	SK		UK		rt-PA[a]	
Indication	IV Systemic	Local	IV Systemic	Local	IV Systemic	APSAC
Pulmonary emboli						
Loading dose	250,000 U (30 min)	[b]	4,000 U/kg (30 min)	[b]		
Maintenace dose	100,000 U/hr		4,000 U/kg/hr			
Duration	12–48 hr		12–48 hr			
Deep vein thrombosis						
Loading dose	250,000 U (30 min)	[c]	4,000 U/kg (30 min)	[c]		
Maintenance dose	100,000 U/hr		4,000 U/kg/hr			
Duration	24–72 hr		24–72 hr			
Peripheral arterial occlusion						
Loading dose	250,000 U (30 min)		4,000 U/kg (30 min)			
Maintenance dose	100,000 U/hr	10,000 U/hr	4,000 U/kg/hr	4,000–1,000 U/min		
Duration	24–72 hr	12–72 hr	24–72 hr	8–24 hr		
Indwelling catheter, external arteriovenous shunt						
Loading dose		25,000 U		5,000 U		
Repeat dose 1–5 times		Yes		Yes		
Duration		1–2 hr		1–2 hr		
Acute myocardial infarction						
Loading dose					6 mg 1–3 min	
					54 mg/57 min	
Maintenance dose	1,500,000 U	3,000 U/min	1–3,000,000 U	10,000 U/min	20 mg/60 min	30 U
					20 mg/60 min	
Duration	60 min	15–120 min	60 min	30–120	3 hr	5 min

[a] With this agent, it is important to avoid a total dose of >100 mg.
[b] Both SK and UK can be infused directly into the pulmonary artery, but they become systemic in distribution immediately.
[c] Local infusion therapy for deep vein thrombosis is frequently not possible, particularly in the lower extremities, because of the presence of venous valves. However, it may be helpful to infuse the thrombolytic agent into the involved extremity distal to the site of thrombus formation.

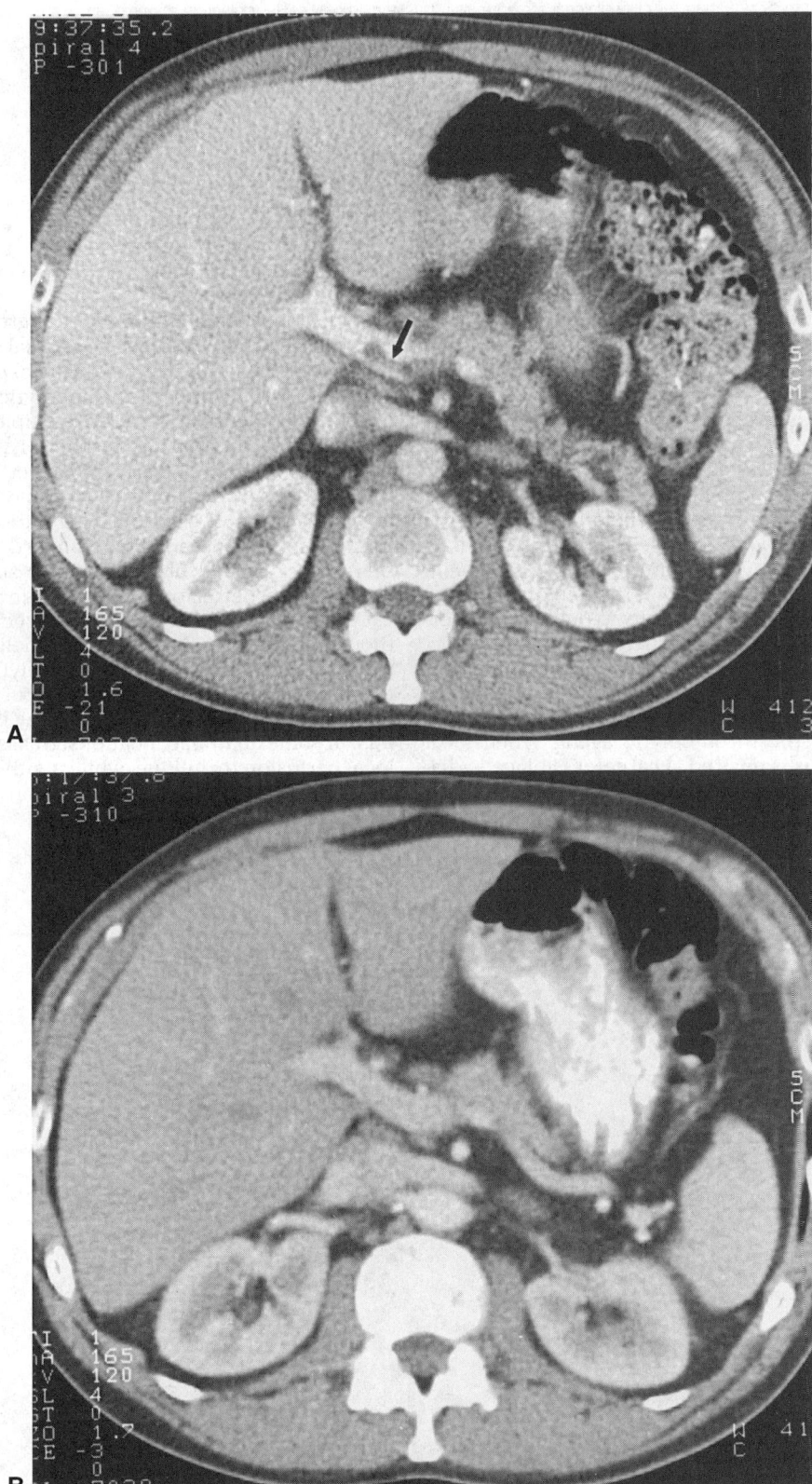

Fig. 122-1. **(A)** Spiral computed tomographic scan of the abdomen reveals the presence of thrombus formation in the portal vein (arrow) before treatment. **(B)** Following thrombolytic therapy with urokinase, the thrombus in the portal vein has disappeared because of lysis.

monary emboli, an angiocatheter can deliver the thrombolytic agent directly into the pulmonary artery. However, this vessel receives nearly 30% of the cardiac output. Thus, any agent delivered locally in this vessel will extend immediately into the systemic circulation. When treating venous thrombosis in the lower or upper extremities, the agent is best administered directly into the involved extremity as close as possible to the site of thrombus formation via a small percutaneous catheter in an accessible superficial vein. With thrombosis associated with indwelling catheters, if the thrombus formation is within the lumen of the catheter or if it is adjacent to and distal to the catheter tip, the infusion should be made directly into the indwelling catheter.[18] If the thrombus is limited to the confines of the catheter lumen, the agent should be placed in the obstructed catheter and allowed to incubate for 2–3 hours. After this time interval, the contents of the catheter can be aspirated and patency restored. This process may have to be repeated one to five times before the catheter can be completely cleared of obstructing thrombus. If the catheter-associated thrombus extends both proximal and distal to the catheter tip, forearm vein infusion on the side nearest the location of the catheter is the optimal technique for treatment.

The bolus infusion technique, in which a large quantity of the thrombolytic agent is infused during a short (15–30 minutes) interval, is most applicable for treatment of acute myocardial infarction. The total dose is infused into a forearm vein to facilitate treatment, as expediently as possible.

The initial dose of SK is larger than the sustaining dose and is given over a shorter time interval. The rationale is to give sufficient SK to overcome inhibition of antibody in the blood. By convention, a loading dose is also used with UK, without

rationale. There is no need for a loading dose when rt-PA is employed.

INDICATIONS FOR THROMBOLYTIC THERAPY

The presence of thrombi that interfere significantly with normal blood flow on either the venous or arterial side of the circulation is an indication for the use of thrombolytic therapy. An exception to this general statement may be thrombus formation in blood vessels that directly connect with the central nervous system. In the brain, prompt restoration of blood flow may possibly be associated with additional damage to the central nervous system tissue as blood under pressure returns to fragile ischemic or infarcted neural tissue.[19]

Pulmonary Thromboembolic Disease

Pulmonary thromboembolism was the first major thrombotic disease in which thrombolytic therapy was demonstrated to be efficacious. Since the original reports demonstrating efficacy with UK and SK,[20–26] several additional reports have appeared.[20–42] Substantial data clearly demonstrate the efficacy in the treatment of pulmonary emboli in the following categories: (1) massive emboli, defined as two lobar arteries completely obstructed with thrombus or several smaller thrombosed vessels the sum of which equal two lobar arteries or greater; (2) massive emboli, with shock; and (3) submassive emboli superimposed on previously existing chronic cardiopulmonary disease, a situation in which even small emboli result in hemodynamic decompensation. In these situations, the initial treatment of choice is thrombolytic therapy (Fig. 122-2).

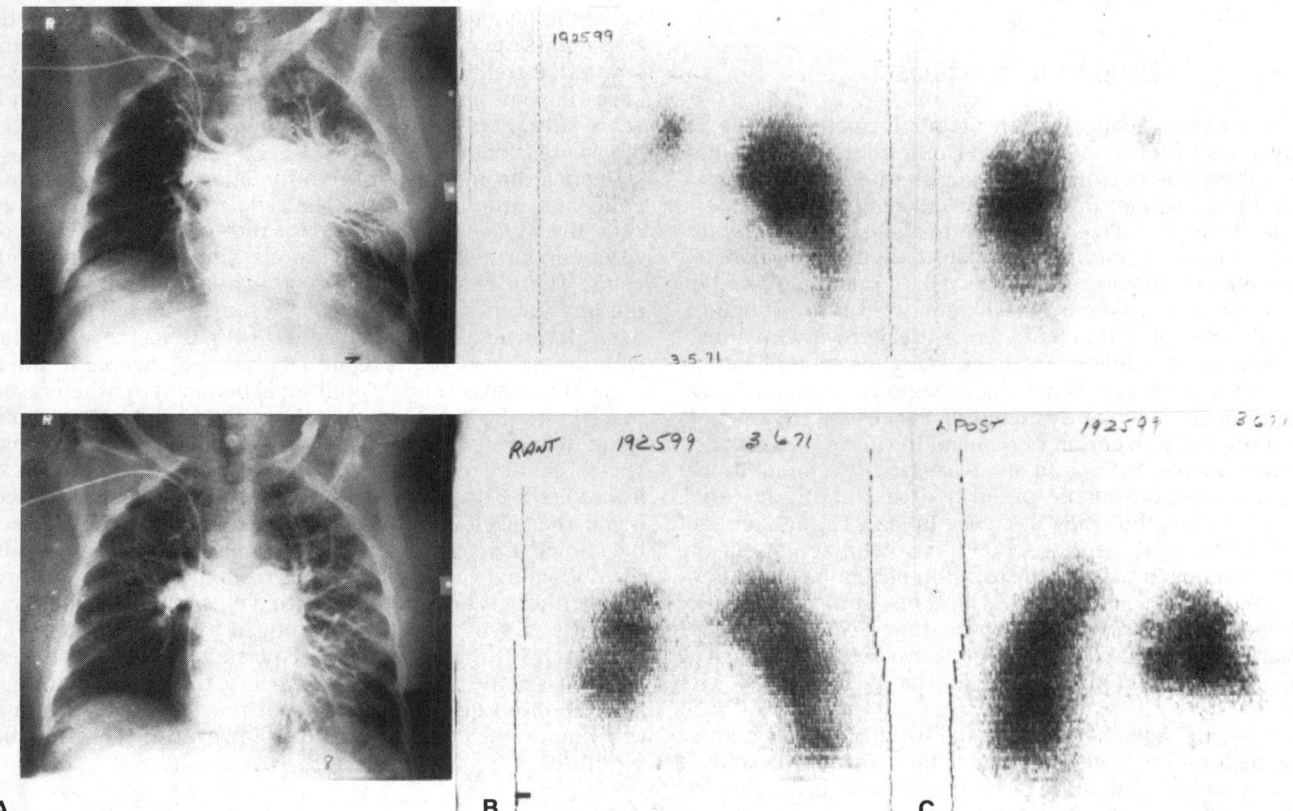

Fig. 122-2. (Upper panel) Matched pulmonary **(A)** angiogram and **(B)** anterior and **(C)** posterior views of a lung perfusion scan revealing massive emboli in the right main and associated pulmonary arteries. (Lower panel) Studies 1 hour following a 24-hour infusion of thrombolytic therapy showing resolution of thromboemboli and return of pulmonary blood flow to normal.

The overall success rates of resolution of pulmonary thromboemboli with SK or UK in the three categories above varies from 80% to 90%.[20–41] The optimal treatment requires immediate infusion on diagnosis. Typical treatment includes a forearm vein infusion of SK at a 250,000-U loading dose over 30–45 minutes, followed by a 100,000-U/hr sustaining dose for a duration of 24–48 hours. Alternatively, UK is infused at 4,000 U/kg over 30–45 minutes, followed by 4,000 U/kg/hr for 24–48 hours. The duration of treatment depends on the total amount and age of the emboli material in the pulmonary arterial circuit. Newly formed thrombi recently embolized to the pulmonary circulation may undergo dissolution by thrombolytic therapy in 2–6 hours.

Recently new therapeutic schedules have employed large doses of thrombolytic agents, "front-loading" in patients with massive pulmonary emboli who acutely experience severe adverse hemodynamic compromise.[43] When these unusually large doses are employed over 60–120 minutes, there frequently is prompt establishment of some blood flow to decrease hemodynamic compromise. These large doses given for 60–120 minutes do not eliminate the need to treat with thrombolytic therapy for the 24–36 hours that is required to dissolve all thromboembolic material and return of hemodynamics to normal.

If thrombolytic therapy is chosen at the time of pulmonary angiography, the catheter in the pulmonary artery may be used to infuse the thrombolytic agent. The angiographic catheter is repositioned from the pulmonary artery into the right atrium. This catheter serves as an excellent path for circulatory access, should it be needed during the treatment procedure. One hour after completion of the infusion of the thrombolytic agent, the catheter is removed before heparin anticoagulation is instituted. In one small study, rt-PA was successfully employed in the treatment of pulmonary emboli.[42]

Deep Vein Thrombosis

The major complications of thrombus formation in the venous systems of the upper or lower extremities or the intra-abdominal venous network, including the inferior vena cava, are subsequent venous insufficiency and acute pulmonary emboli. The objectives of treatment are to alleviate promptly discomfort, pain, and edema of the involved area. In addition, the initial treatment should reduce the risk of pulmonary emboli and the postphlebitic syndrome, including chronic discomfort, edema, skin discoloration, cutaneous breakdown with subsequent ulceration, cellulitis, and necrosis. These complications arise from venous insufficiency due to venous valvular damage with consequent valvular dysfunction. Successful treatment is directed toward prevention of damage to the venous valves.

The anticoagulants heparin and warfarin prevent additional thrombus formation on the preformed thrombotic material. The existing thrombus may decrease in size, retract, and act as a substrate for the endogenous fibrinolytic activity in the area of thrombus formation. Restoration of venous blood flow, a decrease or disappearance of symptoms, and prevention of emboli may result. However, after treatment with heparin venous valve function and venous pressure seldom normalize. These abnormalities predispose to the postphlebitic syndrome.

Thrombolytic agents dissolve the preformed thrombus. Prompt restoration of venous flow, elimination of the risk of pulmonary emboli, reduction of venous hypertension, restoration of normal lymphatic drainage, and preservation of venous valve function follow their successful use. These results have been verified in prospective randomized, blinded, and controlled studies comparing anticoagulation with thrombolytic therapy.[44–74] In these studies, the success rate with thrombolytic therapy is 55–85%, contrasted with 10% with heparin anticoagulation.

As soon as the diagnosis of venous thrombosis is established, thrombolytic therapy should be initiated at a site as close as possible to the thrombus. If the upper extremity is involved (forearm, arm, axillary or subclavian veins), infusion into the ipsilateral forearm is recommended (Fig. 122-3). If the lower extremity is involved, infusion into the ankle or dorsum of the foot of the involved leg should be employed. With SK, the dose is 250,000 U over 30–45 minutes and 100,000 U/hr for 48–72 hours. For UK, the dose is 4,000 U/kg over 30–45 minutes, followed by 4,000 U/kg/hr for 48–72 hours. If the thrombus is large, the area of involvement extensive, and the infusion well tolerated, continuation of the infusion for ≤5–7 days may be useful in order to resolve the thrombotic process.

Since the volume and rate of blood flow in the veins of the lower and upper extremities is much less than other areas, resolution of deep vein thrombosis with thrombolytic therapy is often inadequate. Current practice is to position an infusion catheter through the involved vein, placing the catheter into the substance of the thrombus for direct infusion of the thrombolytic agent. This approach provides mechanical disruption of the thrombus and its surface by the catheter, allows delivery of high concentrations of the thrombolytic agents into the immediate environment, and facilitates rapid resolution of the obstructing thrombus and presentation of normal venous valve function.

The optimal duration of thrombolytic therapy for venous thrombosis has not been established. The time required to resolve venous thrombi must be individualized for optimal results. If success has not been achieved by 5–7 days of continuous intravenous infusion of either SK or UK, treatment should be discontinued and heparin therapy instituted. Studies with long-term follow-up evaluation have demonstrated significant benefit in patients receiving thrombolytic therapy, in contrast to patients receiving heparin alone.[59] These studies demonstrate that treatment with thrombolytic therapy increases the percentage of patent veins with normal valvular function 6–7 years later. Patients treated with heparin may incur irreversible valvular damage.

Venous thrombi also form in the inferior vena cava, the hepatic veins, the portal vein, the renal vein, the superior vena cava, the subclavian veins, and the intracranial veins, including cerebral cortical veins, cavernous sinus veins, and retinal veins. There is some experience in the use of thrombolytic therapy for these conditions,[75–91] but no large studies have been performed. The greatest success is usually associated with the delivery of the agent as close as possible to the site of the thrombus. There is additional benefit if a catheter can be placed into the substance of a thrombus and the thrombolytic agent delivered directly. For treatment of intracranial thrombi, special caution must be exercised. If no other alternatives exist, if irreversible damage has not occurred, and if no evidence of hemorrhage is found, thrombolytic therapy may be a reasonable choice in selected patients. Chronic venous thrombosis of the abdominal venous network is usually refractory to thrombolytic therapy. When the hepatic veins or portal vein are involved, the synthesis of plasminogen by the liver is compromised, and the plasma level of plasminogen is often low. If infusion is made into the hepatic artery, the thrombolytic agent is catabolized in the liver before it reaches plasminogen and the venous thrombus formation. However success has been reported.[92–99]

Arterial Thromboembolic Occlusion

Arterial occlusive disorders, whether they take place gradually over time or whether they are embolic, present with the acute clinical manifestations of pain, decline in temperature

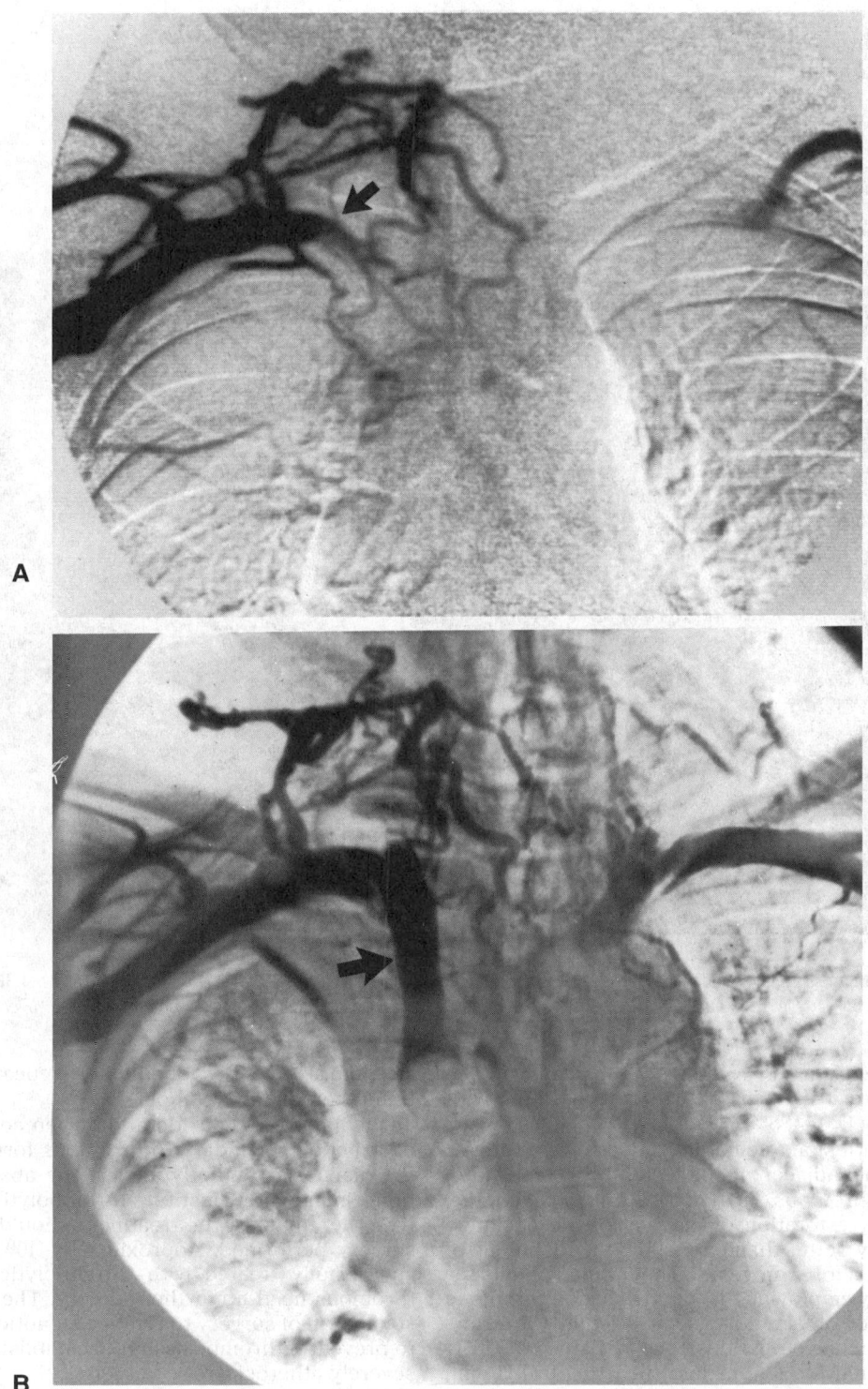

Fig. 122-3. **(A)** Angiogram of the right subclavian vein with cessation of blood flow by obstructing thrombus formation (arrow). **(B)** Repeat angiogram after a 24-hour infusion of thrombolytic therapy into a right forearm vein, demonstrating reconstitution of normal blood in the right subclavian vein and superior vena cava (arrow) into the right atrium.

distal to the occlusion, and discoloration of the involved area. Immediate attention must be given to prevent severe damage or irreversible loss of all tissue distal to the site of occlusion. Until the advent of thrombolytic therapy, these problems were approached surgically. Surgical treatment of arterial vascular occlusion is still indicated in patients with large extensive thrombi or emboli in large proximal arteries and when ischemia is far advanced and sufficient time does not permit thrombo-

lytic therapy. However, thrombolytic therapy by itself or in conjunction with surgery provides improved management for these problems. Unless contraindications exist, thrombolytic therapy may be the initial treatment of choice.

When clinical diagnosis of an arterial thrombotic or embolic vascular occlusion is substantiated by contrast studies, thrombolytic therapy should be promptly initiated. There are two recognized and accepted techniques for infusion of thrombo-

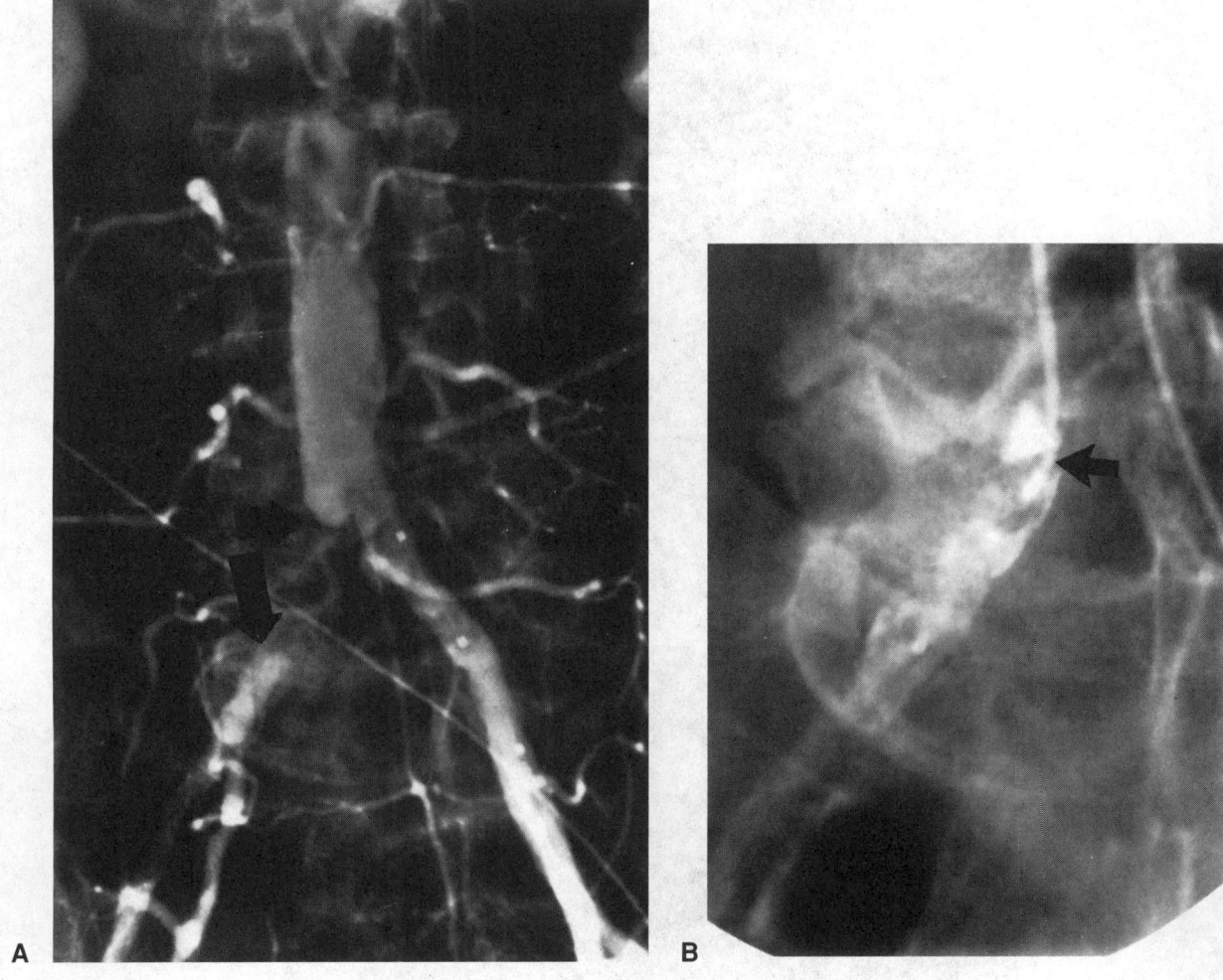

Fig. 122-4. **(A)** Angiography of abdominal aorta demonstrating complete occlusion of the right iliac artery at origin (arrows). **(B)** Angiocatheter tip placed directly into the substance of the thrombus in the right iliac artery for infusion of thrombolytic agent. *(Figure continues.)*

lytic agents: local perfusion and systemic venous infusion. The overall success rate of treatment of arterial occlusions with thrombolytic therapy is 45–85%.[100–123]

With the local perfusion technique, an arterial catheter should be placed either adjacent to, or preferably directly into, the substance of the thrombus (Fig. 122-4). With this technique, the success rate for restoration of patency of the occluded artery is considerably better than employing the technique of systemic infusion via a forearm vein.[17] The optimal results for restoration of patency employing the local perfusion technique have been reported for UK at a dose of 4,000 U/min, until antegrade blood flow is achieved. At this time, the dose of UK is reduced to 2,000 U/min for 1 hour and then to 1,000 U/min, until the intraluminal area has returned to normal. The total duration of therapy is usually 12–18 hours. The resolution time of arterial thrombus formation may be shortened with the use of the pulse spray technique.[124] This technique employs a multi-side-hole catheter that is inserted into the thrombus and perfused with high-dose thrombolytic therapy in bursts. This simultaneously attacks multiple areas in the thrombus with high concentrations of the thrombolytic agent.

Should local perfusion neither be possible nor desirable, intravenous forearm vein infusion should be considered, using the standard doses for systemic therapy (see Table 122-2). The duration of therapy is usually 24 hours. However, in patients in whom there is extensive obstruction involving many vessels, it may be necessary, particularly if there is evidence of progres-

sive improvement as identified by repeat angiography, to continue therapy for ≥48 hours.

The important consideration when confronted with arterial obstruction secondary to thrombus formation is to establish the diagnosis promptly and, in the absence of contraindications, immediately institute thrombolytic therapy. If thrombolytic therapy fails, the treatment should be discontinued and surgery performed. Approximately 40% of patients who are successfully treated with thrombolytic therapy for arterial thrombus need no further surgery. The remainder may need some form of surgery to remove stenotic lesions in an attempt to prevent rethrombosis and to establish long-term patency of severely atherosclerotic vessels.

Although the peripheral arterial system is the most accessible location on the arterial side, certain central sites are amenable to thrombolytic therapy. These include external arteriovenous shunts,[18,125–130] prosthetic heart valves,[131–138] cardiac chamber thrombi,[139–142] retinal artery,[141,142] and cerebral arterial network.[19,143–154]

The resolution of thrombi with thrombolytic therapy has been successful for external arteriovenous shunts, for thrombi associated with prosthetic cardiac valves, and for ventricular thrombi following myocardial infarction. Although no large multicenter study has been conducted, several groups have reported success without experiencing fragmentation of thrombi from valves or mural locations that would then embolize distally, inducing obstruction of smaller arteries with re-

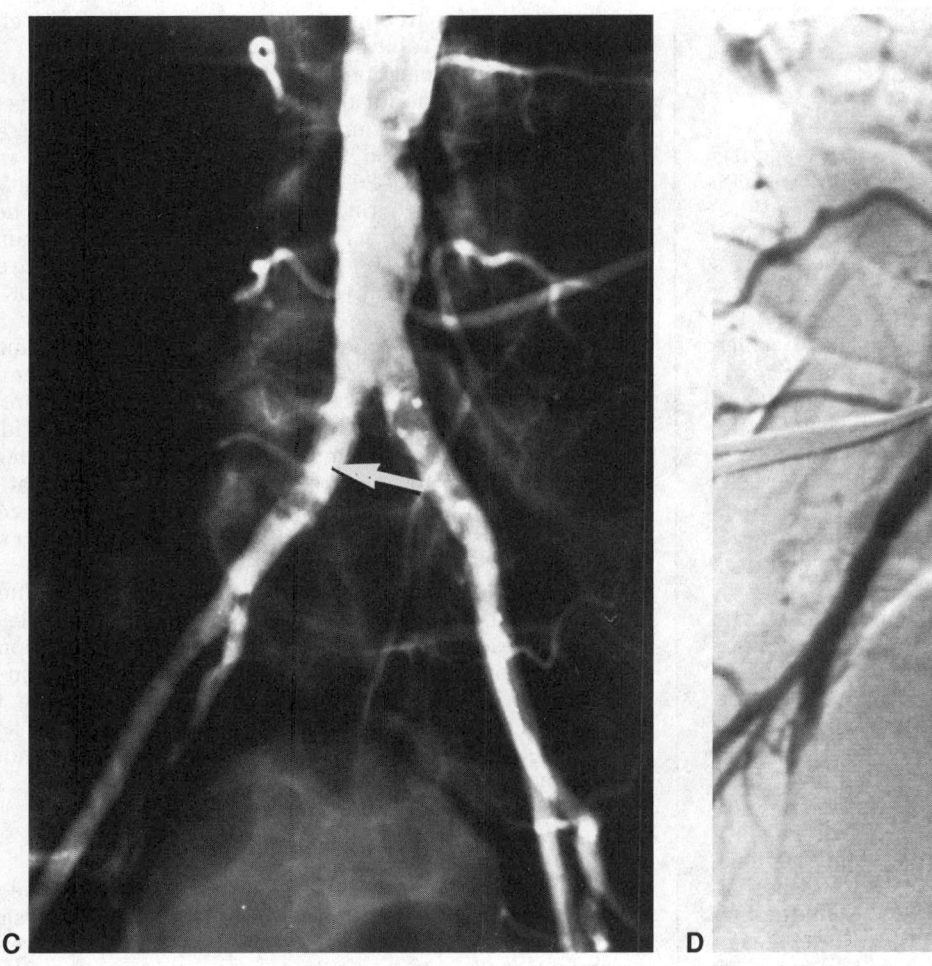

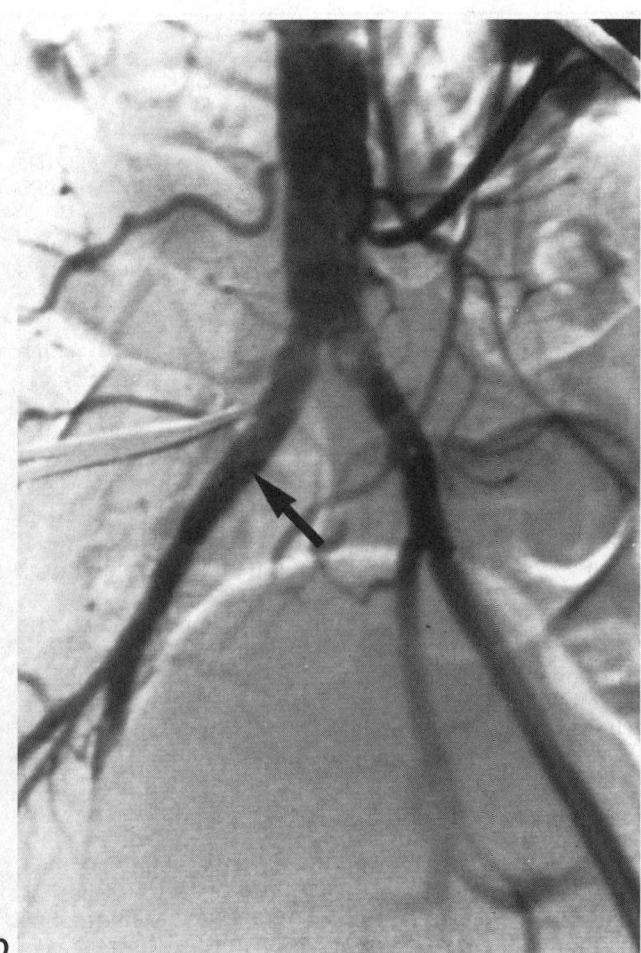

Fig. 122-4 *(Continued).* **(C)** Repeat angiography demonstrating reconstitution of blood flow in the right iliac artery (arrow). Note extensive atheromatous plaque formation now visible in the right iliac artery distal to the arrow. **(D)** After performance of intravascular arthrectomy and removal of the plaque formation (arrow), returning the iliac artery lumen approaches the normal cross section.

sultant extensive damage. This is a serious problem if it occurs within the central nervous system. In resolving thrombi that nearly completely occlude cardiac valve prostheses, there is considerable benefit for the patient who otherwise could not survive because of an inadequate cardiac output. Alternative surgical intervention is not possible because the severely reduced cardiac output precludes cardiac bypass. Because of the possibility of systemic arterial embolization, including the central nervous system, witnessed informed verbal and written consent from patient and family should be obtained before instituting thrombolytic therapy.

Benefit following central retinal artery or retinal vein thrombolysis has not been reliably demonstrated. In this compartment it is apparent that blood flow must be reinstituted within 1–2 hours from the time of vessel obstruction to preserve function of the optic nerve and retinal tissue.

Studies evaluating the efficacy of thrombolytic therapy in the treatment of arterial obstruction of major vessels directly connecting to the brain are in progress.[19,155–164] Until further data are available, extreme caution must be exercised in the use of thrombolytic therapy for this indication.

Acute Myocardial Infarction

Coronary artery occlusion was one of the first thrombotic disorders to be treated with thrombolytic therapy,[165] mostly because nearly 90% of patients with transmural myocardial in-

farction have thrombus occluding one or more of the coronary arteries.[166] Although a small percentage of patients may experience some endogenous spontaneous thrombolysis or spasmolysis, nearly all patients require treatment to establish reperfusion of the myocardium.

After results showing that patency could be established by the infusion of thrombolytic agents directly into the infarct-associated coronary artery, several studies demonstrated the high frequency of reperfusion to the myocardium.[167,168] To salvage the jeopardized ischemic myocardium and reduce mortality from myocardial infarction, rapid dissolution of coronary thrombi was necessary. If reperfusion to the myocardium was re-established within 6 hours from the onset of symptomatic myocardial ischemia, myocardial tissue could be salvaged, left ventricular function normalized, and mortality reduced. For these reasons, rapid systemic thrombolytic therapy has replaced local infusion of fibrinolytic agents through a catheter placed in the coronary artery.

Several randomized, controlled, prospective studies have been completed using a forearm vein infusion of SK, UK, APSAC, rt-PA, and placebo as soon as the patient reached medical attention[169–190] (Fig. 122-5). A significant reduction in mortality in the treated patients compared with placebo-treated patients was demonstrated. The reperfusion rate with any of these three thrombolytic agents varied between 55% and 85%. Reocclusion rates within the first 5 days were between 5% and 15%. Mortality reduction varied among the different studies but in general

SURGERY AS AN ADJUNCT TO THROMBOLYTIC THERAPY

On presentation of arterial obstruction, the diagnosis should be promptly established. Angiography permits immediate diagnosis, provides information on the precise anatomic location of the lesion and on the status of adjacent vessels, and identifies whether the lesion is secondary to thrombus formation or is exacerbated by atherosclerotic disease.

During the initial angiographic study, it may become evident that surgery is not a viable alternative. Such is the case when there is only small vessel involvement and there is no evidence of adequate blood flow distal to the locus of obstruction. If there are massive amounts of thrombus involving predominantly large arterial vessels, if ischemic has advanced so that inadequate time exists for successful thrombolysis, or if there is severe arterial stenosis secondary to athermatous disease, surgery is the preferred treatment.

On the venous side of the circulation, thrombolytic therapy is nearly always the treatment of choice for thrombus formation. Only if the patient is allergic to thrombolic therapy, if there is concommitment hemorrhage, or if there is intravascular obstruction, such as neoplasm, is surgery indicated.

In the absence of contraindications, thrombolytic therapy should be instituted immediately. The local perfusion technique, in which a catheter is placed directly into the substance of the thrombus, permits prompt administration of UK or SK. Relatively high doses of UK are initially employed (4,000 U/min). When successful therapy is apparent on repeat angiography, the dose is decreased to 2,000 U/min, and then to 1,000 U/min. As the thrombus undergoes dissolution, the catheter is advanced into the remaining thrombus until complete resolution occurs. If thrombolytic therapy fails, it is discontinued and surgery performed. Because of the practical problems of assembling the surgical team in an available operating room, thrombolytic therapy can usually be evaluated during the presurgical period. Thus, the adminstration of thrombolytic therapy does not add additional time that might jeopardize tissue recovery. If the thrombolytic therapy is successful, the need for surgery is obviated Following successful thrombolytic therapy, anticoagulation therapy should be given for 4–6 weeks or possibly longer.

If thrombolytic therapy fails, the agent should be discontinued and the surgical option pursued. Before surgery the patient should receive a single intravenous dose of ϵ-aminocaproic acid (5 g) over 45 minutes. The prothrombin time, partial thromboplastin time, and fibrinogen level should then be measured. If the fibrinogen level is <75 mg/dl, the patient should be given either fresh frozen plasma or cryoprecipitate, to increase the plasma fibrinogen to >100 mg/dl. If the prothrombin time and the partial thromboplastin time are significantly prolonged, they should be rechecked after the fibrinogen level is >100 mg/dl.

was 30–55%. Such survival benefits have been statistically established at 6 months and 1 year. These studies have established that thrombolytic therapy is the initial treatment of choice in acute myocardial infarction. Current recommendations of doses, schedule, technique, and duration of infusion of these agents for treatment of acute myocardial infarction are summarized in Table 122-2.

A current timely question is whether one of the three thrombolytic agents is superior to the others in treatment of acute myocardial infarction. From available data, SK, UK, APSAC, and rt-PA induce reperfusion at approximately the same rate, within the range of 50–80%.[176–189] Reduction in mortality is greatest with SK and UK. Undesirable side effects, such as hemorrhage, particularly intracranial hemorrhage, and rethrombosis following successful reperfusion, may be highest during and following rt-PA treatment. rt-PA is more costly than UK or SK.[189,190]

Following successful reperfusion of the myocardium, immediate antithrombotic therapy is needed to prevent rethrombosis. The optimal agent or combination of agents to maintain patency of the reperfused coronary vessels have not been identified. One study with a 3-year follow-up has demonstrated warfarin to be superior to aspirin or aspirin plus other antiplatelet agents. When severe residual stenosis exists following successful thrombolysis, then angioplasty, vessel bypass, or direct surgical repair are indicated.

Only preliminary data are available on the clinical value of thrombolytic therapy in the treatment of angina, unstable angina, and crescendo angina.[191,192] If pain in this condition is secondary to ischemia resulting from blood flow reduction because of thrombus formation progressively occluding the lumen, then thrombolytic therapy may be indicated. The same doses and schedule used to treat myocardial infarction should be employed.

MONITORING THROMBOLYTIC THERAPY

Thrombolytic therapy requires close monitoring of the patient during the administration of fibrinolytic agents. Vital signs should be monitored regularly at 4-hour intervals. However, movement of the patient to the intensive care unit need not be synonymous with institution of thrombolytic therapy. If a stable patient is treated with thrombolytic therapy for venous thrombosis, routine care should be adequate. For the patient who is unstable or requires continuous instrument monitoring, regardless of the condition being treated, the intensive care unit is the optimal location.

Thrombolytic agents activate the fibrinolytic system to generate plasmin. The action of plasmin on plasma substrates may be used to quantitate fibrinolytic activity.[193–195] Single or repeated measurements of fibrinogen or plasminogen, are difficult to interpret (in the absence of synthetic production turnover studies) and may not be informative for dose management. The measurement of levels of specific plasma proteins altered by activation of the fibrinolytic system does not directly correlate with the success or failure of thrombus dissolution and is not predictive of untoward side effects. However, assay of plasmin in the circulating blood may prove indicative of inadequate or excessive fibrinolysis. Measurement of fibrinogen/fibrin degradation products does not provide significant predictive assistance in patient management.

The thrombin time (TT) provides a reasonable approximation of the activity of the fibrinolytic system. Although no study has established the TT as the optimal measure of thrombolytic therapy monitoring, it can serve as a guideline. If, 3–4 hours after institution of thrombolytic therapy, the TT reveals no prolongation compared with initial baseline measurements, dissolution of the thrombus is unlikely. Thrombolytic therapy has failed to activate the fibrinolytic system and an alternative treatment plan should be considered. If it is greater than seven times the normal baseline value, the risk of bleeding is greatly enhanced. If activation has been adequate (i.e., a TT of 1.5–5 times baseline values), the TT is repeated every 12 hours for the duration of treatment.

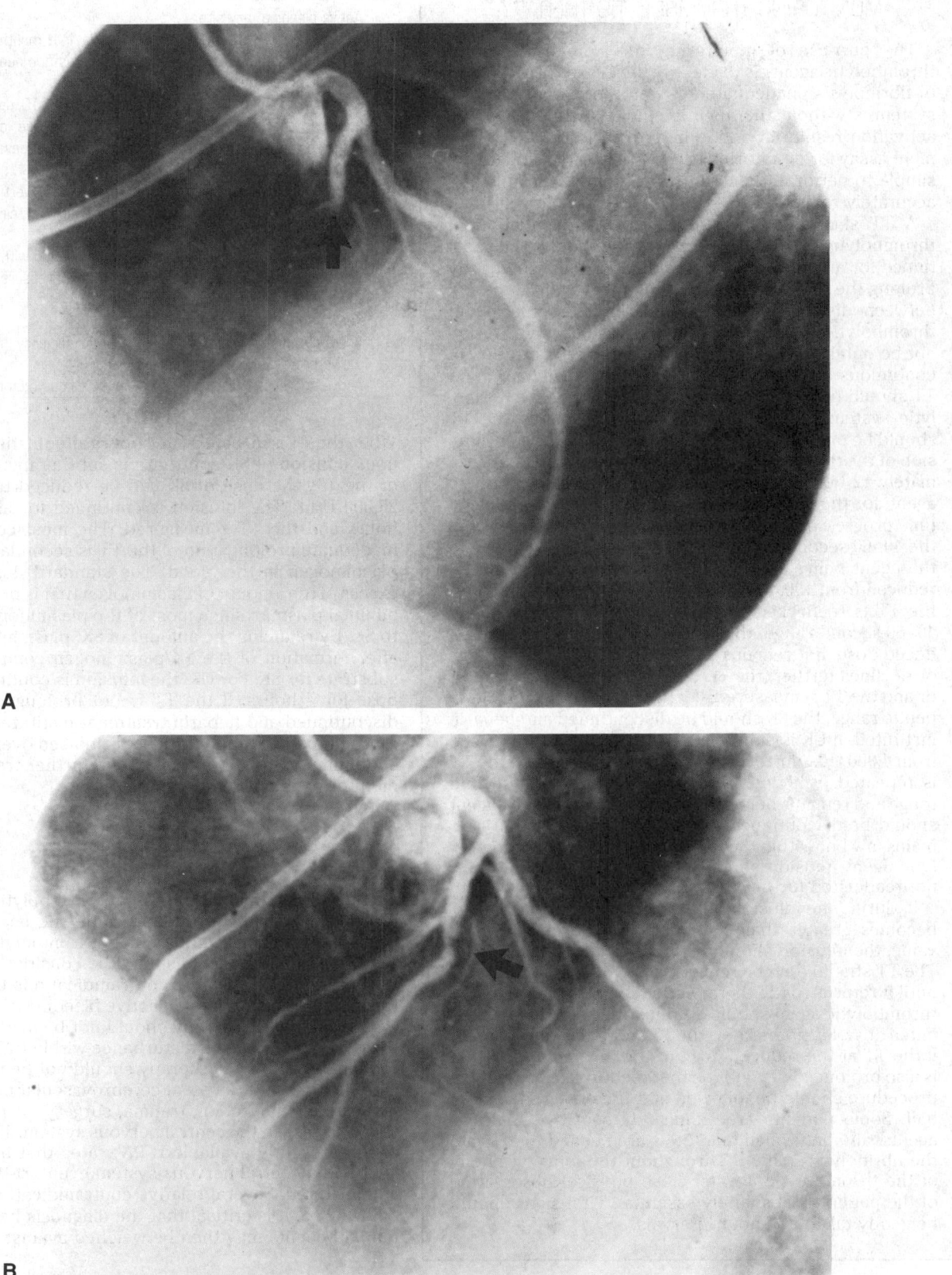

Fig. 122-5. **(A)** Angiography of the coronary arteries reveals occlusion of the left anterior descending vessel with cessation of blood flow (arrow). **(B)** Repeat study after 60 minutes of thrombolytic therapy given intravenously demonstrates reconstitution of blood flow in the left anterior descending vessel with evident residual severe stenotic lesion (arrow).

MONITORING THROMBOLYTIC THERAPY

The purpose of monitoring the administration of thrombolytic agents is to identify the degree of activation of fibrinolysis. Inadequate activation of the fibrinolytic system is without therapeutic efficacy, while excessive activation results in undue hemorrhagic risk. A convenient assay for monitoring is the TT. The TT is relatively simple to perform; the results are rapidly available and accurately reflect the activity of the fibrinolytic system.

A TT should be measured before the initiation of thrombolytic therapy. Heparin therapy should be discontinued for an appropriate interval, as it will significantly prolong the TT. If the situation is urgent and the period between discontinuation of heparin and initiation of thrombolytic therapy must be short, a baseline TT cannot be obtained. Three to four hours after institution of continuous infusion of the thrombolytic agent, a second TT should be obtained to ascertain whether the fibrinolytic system has been activated. At this time, the TT should be prolonged 1.5–5 times the baseline value, infusion of the thrombolytic agent should continue. Approximately 12 hours after the initiation of the thrombolytic agent, for the duration of the infusion. If, as the infusion time progresses, the TT declines significantly (e.g., from the 40–60-second range to the 20–30-second range) and the agent being used is SK, the dose of SK should be reduced from 100,000 U/hr to 50,000 U/hr; 6 hours later, the TT is rechecked. If it has moved back toward the 40–60-second range, the infusion is continued at the reduced dose. If it remains within the 20–30-second range or declines further, the SK dose is reduced to 25,000 U/hr and the TT remeasured. If it has fallen below the therapeutic range, the SK should be discontinued and heparin instituted. If UK is employed, the dose can be increased from 4,000 U/kg/hr to 5,000 U/kg/hr; 6 hours later, the TT is repeated. If it does not return to the 40–60-second range and remains below the therapeutic range, the agent should be discontinued and heparin instituted. If it remains low but within the therapeutic range, the thrombolytic agent infusion should be continued and the dose not readjusted further.

If, during the infusion of a thrombolytic agent, the TT becomes greater than five times the normal baseline value, the infusion should be immediately discontinued. The TT should then be remeasured at 2–4-hour intervals until it returns to the therapeutic range. At that time, the thrombolytic agent should be reinstituted at one-half the initial dose. Six hours later, the TT should be remeasured. If the TT at the reduced dose of the thrombolytic agent is also prolonged beyond the therapeutic range, the same procedure should be followed and the dose reduced by half. Some patients are exquisitely sensitive to these agents, and only small quantities are needed to activate the fibrinolytic system. Throughout the infusion of any of the thrombolytic agents, close physical observation of the patient is absolutely essential. Vital signs should be gently taken at 4-hour intervals.

If, during therapy with either SK or UK, the TT is prolonged to more than five times the normal baseline value, the thrombolytic agent should be discontinued and a repeat thrombin time obtained at 2–3-hour intervals. When the TT returns to 1.5–5 times the normal baseline value and bleeding is absent, thrombolytic therapy can be reinstituted at one-half the initial dose.

Table 122-3. Contraindications to Thrombolytic Therapy

Absolute contraindications
    Active bleeding: any site
    Central nervous system pathology (within 1–2 months): infarction, hemorrhage, trauma, surgery, primary or metastatic neoplastic disease
Relative contraindications
    Surgical procedures or internal trauma within 10 days, including invasive biopsy, thoracentesis, external cardiac massage, paracentesis
    Internal arterial diagnostic procedures within 10 days, excluding uncomplicated arterial blood gas studies
    Gastrointestinal tract ulcers, ulcerative colitis, diverticulitis
    Defective hemostasis: coagulation factor deficiency, circulating anticoagulant (nonlupus type), severe thrombocytopenia
    Subacute bacterial endocarditis, atrial fibrillation with intracardiac thrombi
    Severe arterial hypertension, diastolic blood pressure >125 mmHg
    Pregnancy or first 10 days postpartum
    Known severe allergy to agent
    Acute chronic progressive hepatorenal insufficiency
    Active progressive cavitating lung disease
    Active aggressive ulcerating cutaneous/mucous membrane lesions

When the TT is measured 3–4 hours after institution of a continuous infusion of SK and there is subtherapeutic prolongation of the TT, the dose of SK can be reduced to 50,000 U/hr or 25,000 U/hr. The infusion is continued for an additional 3–4 hours and the TT remeasured. The most common cause of inadequate prolongation of the TT is secondary to inadequate plasminogen in the blood. The standard doses of SK are in excess of the amount of plasminogen that is present, producing minimal plasmin, since most of the plasminogen is complexed to SK. By reducing the amount of SK, plasminogen is available after formation of the SK/plasminogen complex, to serve as substrate for SK. For UK, the infusion is continued at the same dose for 4 hours. If the TT is not prolonged, UK should be discontinued and heparin treatment instituted.

When the thrombolytic agent is infused over a short interval of 30 minutes to 2–3 hours and no further treatment is given, monitoring is not required.

CONTRAINDICATIONS

Contraindications to the use of thrombolytic agents overlap in general with those that preclude the use of heparin and warfarin. Before institution of any thrombolytic agent, the potential risks and benefits should be considered.

There are two absolute contraindications to the use of any thrombolytic agent. First, if active bleeding of any type is present, thrombolytic therapy should not be instituted. Second, if there is any damage or disturbance within the central nervous system, thrombolytic therapy should not be instituted. These conditions include a recent cerebrovascular accident, cerebral hemorrhagic infarction, trauma, surgery, or primary or metastatic disease in the central nervous system. The manufacturer of the presently available rt-PA states that if the patient has ever had a central nervous system event, rt-PA should not be administered. Several relative contraindications are shown in Table 122-3. It is critical that the diagnosis be secure. The potential benefits may then be weighed against the risks.

COMPLICATIONS OF THROMBOLYTIC THERAPY AND MANAGEMENT

The most frequent and serious side effect of thrombolytic agents is bleeding. The frequency of bleeding in reported series varies from <5% to 40%. The frequency of major bleeding

(>10% decline in hematocrit value, requiring red cell transfusion) is 5–12%.

The available data indicate that the frequency of bleeding associated with thrombolytic therapy is not significantly different from that seen with heparin anticoagulation.[11,12,196,197] However, if thrombolytic therapy is incorrectly employed, such as immediately following extensive surgery or in the presence of active gastrointestinal hemorrhage, the associated hemorrhage will be more severe than seen with heparin.

The most common location of bleeding during the infusion of any thrombolytic agent is at the placement of diagnostic angiographic catheters, intracatheters, sheaths, vessel cutdown sites, arterial puncture sites for blood-gas determinations, a recent surgical incision, or intramuscular or subcutaneous injection sites. The most detrimental bleeding occurs within the central nervous system. In those patients who experience bleeding in association with thrombolytic therapy, 60–85% of such instances occur at an invaded site. The frequency of central nervous system bleeding is 0–2%. Available data concerning central nervous system hemorrhage indicate that it is lowest with UK, next lowest with SK, and highest during and immediately following rt-PA and APSAC therapy.

When superficial bleeding at an invaded site occurs, the bleeding can often be controlled with pressure dressings and the thrombolytic therapy continued. If the bleeding occurs at a noninvaded site or in a less accessible location, thrombolytic therapy should immediately be stopped and the thrombin time checked. If the TT is beyond the therapeutic range, the thrombolytic therapy must be withheld and the thrombin time rechecked until it has returned to the lower end of the therapeutic range. If the bleeding has been minimal or has ceased and the indications for treatment are significant, it is reasonable to restart the thrombolytic therapy at one-half the initial dose, without a loading dose. The previous sites of bleeding must be closely monitored and the TT rechecked at 12-hour intervals. If the TT is in the therapeutic range at the time of bleeding from a noninvaded site, the thrombolytic therapy must be discontinued and not restarted.

If surgical intervention is deemed necessary during thrombolytic therapy, the therapy should be promptly discontinued. After an interval of 1–2 hours, the prothrombin time, activated partial thromboplastin time, and fibrinogen concentration can be measured. If these studies are prolonged and the fibrinogen <75 mg/dl, the patient should be given 3–6 U of fresh frozen plasma or 10–15 U of cryoprecipitate before surgery. If any evidence remains for continued activation of the fibrinolytic system, a single 5-g dose of ε-aminocaproic acid (Amicar) may be given intravenously over approximately 45 minutes. This agent inhibits plasmin and prevents further activation of the fibrinolytic system.

Additional complications include fever, embolization of thrombi, and allergic reactions. Febrile reactions are more common with SK, followed by rt-PA, and lowest in frequency with UK. Fever is the direct result of the disease process. Thus, it is difficult to be certain that the febrile reaction is secondary to the therapeutic agent. In most instances, the fever seen with thrombolytic therapy is mild. If it is desirable to reduce the fever, acetaminophen, propoxyphene, or a nonsteroidal anti-inflammatory drug can be given. True allergic reactions that result in immune complexes in the circulating blood are rare. Febrile reactions are seen with equal frequency with all three agents. The use of corticosteroids is not indicated, as they are not helpful in preventing or alleviating the reaction.[198] The offending agent must be discontinued.

Embolization from a dissolving thrombus is infrequent. If it occurs, in either the arterial or venous circulation, the thrombolytic agent infusion should be continued. With therapy, these embolic fragments will usually undergo complete dissolution.

The frequency of embolization of intrachamber cardiac thrombi during thrombolytic therapy appears to be low.[140]

Thrombocytopenia is associated with treatment with rt-PA in approximately 10% of patients.[183] This has not been observed with SK or UK. If the platelet count falls to <75,000/mm³, the agent should be discontinued. A few rare complications, including femoral neuropathy, arthralgia, cutaneous bulbi, impairment of wound healing, serum sickness, renal failure, and mild hepatic dysfunction, have been reported.

Rethrombosis may confound successful thrombolytic therapy. Although the pathogenesis of the development of rethrombosis is complex, the predominant responsible feature is the re-exposure of a damaged endothelial surface that originally initiated thrombus formation. This re-exposed surface may consist of denuded endothelium with collagen at the blood interface, endothelium covered with atheromatous plaque formation, or a damaged endothelial surface covered with partially resolved thrombus. The presence of unresolved thrombus as such is thrombogenic. If circulating platelets are damaged or activated by a thrombolytic agent, the thrombogenicity of the effected area could be considerably enhanced. Plasmin alters some plasma proteins and specifically activates factor V.[199] The generation of procoagulant activity can amplify fibrin formation and initiate renewed thrombosis. Vessel spasm may also contribute to rethrombosis. The coronary vascular endothelium is already damaged at the site of thrombotic obstruction, and additional damage by interventional techniques or by the thrombolytic agent itself would predispose to rethrombosis. The rt-PA binds to endothelial cells and may lead to the release of von Willebrand factor.[200] This adhesive protein facilitates the binding of platelets to exposed subendothelial collagen.

SK and UK administered in the standard doses for the treatment of acute myocardial infarction significantly reduce whole blood and plasma viscosity.[201] When rt-PA is given in the approved dose and schedule for acute myocardial infarction, no significant reduction in blood or plasma viscosity occurs. These observations may explain the greater rate of reocclusion of the coronary arterial system following treatment with rt-PA in contrast to other thrombolytic agents. Reduction in blood viscosity may be an important factor in perfusion of the microcirculation of the myocardium.

Treatment with thrombolytic therapy initially promotes the dissolution of preformed thrombi but, on completion, may induce conditions that favor thrombus formation. Prevention or inhibition of this thrombogenic potential is of considerable concern since available anticoagulants and antiplatelet agents are suboptimal.

REFERENCES

1. Tillet WS, Garner RL: The fibrinolytic activity of hemolytic streptococci. J Exp Med 58:485, 1933
2. Jackson KW, Tang J: Complete amino acid sequence of streptokinase and its homology with serine proteases. Biochemistry 21:6620, 1982
3. Chibber BAK, Castellino FJ: Regulation of the streptokinase mediated activation of human plasminogen by fibrinogen and chloride ions. J Biol Chem 261:5289, 1986
4. Johansson F: Uber die tryptische Verdawing durch den Harn. Hoppe Seylers Z Biol Chem 85:72, 1913
5. Biggs R, MacFarland RG, Pilling J: Observations on fibrinolysis. Experimental activity produced by exercise or adrenaline. Lancet 1:402, 1947
6. Williams JRB: The fibrinolytic activity of the urine. Br J Exp Pathol 32:500, 1951
7. Pennica D, Holmes WE, Kohr WJ et al: Cloning and expression of human tissue-type plasminogen activator cDNA in E. coli. Nature 301:214, 1983
8. Ratzkin B, Lee SG, Schrenk WJ et al: Expression in Escherichia coli of biologically active enzyme by a DNA sequence coding for the human plasminogen activator urokinase. Proc Natl Acad Sci USA 78:3313, 1981
9. Rijken DC, Collen D: Purification and characterization of the plasminogen activator secreted by human melanoma cells in cultures. J Biol Chem 256:7035, 1981

10. Harris JJR: Second-generation plasminogen activators. Protein Eng 1:449, 1987

11. Marder VJ, Sherry S: Thrombolytic therapy: current status. N Engl J Med 318:1512, 1988

12. Loscalzo J, Braunwald E: Tissue plasminogen activator. N Engl J Med 319:925, 1988

13. van Breda A, Katzen B: Thrombolytic therapy of peripheral vascular disease. Semin Int Radiol 2:354, 1985

14. Sherry S, Bell WR, Duckert FH et al: Thrombolytic therapy in thrombosis: a National Institutes of Health Consensus Development Conference. Ann Intern Med 93:141, 1980

15. Keith DS, Phillips SJ, Whisnant SJ et al: Heparin therapy for recent transient focal cerebral ischemia. Mayo Clin Proc 62:1101, 1987

16. Wheeler AP, Jaquiss RDB, Newman JH: Physician practices in the treatment of pulmonary embolism and deep vein thrombosis. Arch Intern Med 148:1321, 1988

17. McNamara TO, Fischer JR: Thrombolysis of peripheral arterial and graft occlusions: improved results using high dose urokinase. AJR 144:769, 1985

18. Bartholomew JR, Bell WR: Thrombolytic therapy in the management of venous catheters. Nutr Int 2:115, 1986

19. del Zeppo GJ, Ferbert A, Otis S et al: Local intra-arterial fibrinolytic therapy in acute carotid artery stroke. Stroke 19:307, 1988

20. Hirsh J, Hale GS, McDonald IGM et al: Resolution of acute massive pulmonary embolism after pulmonary arterial infusion of streptokinase. Lancet 2:593, 1967

21. Hirsh J, Hale GS, McDonald IG et al: Streptokinase therapy in acute major pulmonary embolism: effectiveness and problems. Br Med J 4:729, 1968

22. Urokinase-pulmonary embolism trial: phase I results. JAMA 214:2163, 1970

23. Miller GAH, Sutton GC, Kerr IH et al: Comparison of streptokinase and heparin in treatment of isolated acute massive pulmonary embolism. Br Med J 2:681, 1971

24. Tibbutt DA, Davies JA, Anderson JA et al: Comparison by controlled clinical trial of streptokinase and heparin in treatment of life-threatening pulmonary embolism. Br Med J 1:343, 1974

25. Ruel GJ, Beall AC Jr: Emergency pulmonary embolectomy for massive pulmonary embolism. Circulation, suppl. II. 49/50:236, 1974

26. Urokinase-streptokinase pulmonary embolism trial (phase II) results: a cooperative study. JAMA 229:1606, 1974

27. Sasahara AA, Bell WR, Simon TL et al: The phase II urokinase-streptokinase pulmonary embolism trial. Thromb Diath Haemorrh 33:464, 1975

28. Alpert JS, Smith RE, Ockene IS et al: Treatment of massive pulmonary embolism: the role of pulmonary embolectomy. Am Heart J 89:413, 1975

29. Bell WR: Urokinase in the treatment of pulmonary thromboemboli. p. 153. In Paoletti R, Sherry S (eds): Thrombosis and Urokinase. Academic Press, San Diego, 1977

30. Simon TL: Thrombolytic therapy in pulmonary embolism. Vasc Surg 11:349, 1977

31. McTaggart DR, Ingram TG: Massive pulmonary embolism during pregnancy treated with streptokinase. Med J Aust 1:18, 1977

32. Miller GAH, Hall RJC, Paneth M: Pulmonary embolectomy, heparin, and streptokinase: their place in the treatment of acute massive pulmonary embolism. Am Heart J 93:568, 1977

33. Ly B, Arnesen H, Eie H, Hol R: A controlled clinical trial of streptokinase and heparin in the treatment of major pulmonary embolism. J Intern Med 203:465, 1978

34. Genton E: Thrombolytic therapy of pulmonary thromboembolism. Prog Cardiovasc Dis 21:333, 1979

35. Bitzauw J, Vejlsted H, Albrechtsen O: Pulmonary embolectomy using extra-corporeal circulation. Thorac Cardiovasc Surg 29:320, 1981

36. Etude multicentrique sur deux protocoles d'urokinase dans l'embolie pulmonaire grave: Groupe de Recherche Urokinase; Embolie Pulmonaire. Arch Mal Coeur 77:773, 1984

37. Petipretz P, Simmoneau G, Cerrina J et al: Effects of a single bolus of urokinase in patients with life-threatening pulmonary emboli: a descriptive trial. Circulation 70:861, 1984

38. Woods BO, Beamis JF Jr, Bettencourt PE, Persson AV: Subacute massive thromboembolic occlusion of a main pulmonary artery: report of a case successfully treated by thrombolytic therapy and review of the literature. Angiology 36:58, 1985

39. Lohri A, Lammle B, Marbet GA et al: Fibrinolysetherapie bei massiver Lungenembolie: erfahrungen bei 10 Patienten 1982–1984. Schweiz Med Wochenschr 115:1074, 1985

40. Bell WR, Bartholomew JR: Pulmonary Thromboembolic Disease. Current Problems in Cardiology. Vol. 10. Year Book Medical Publishers, Chicago, 1985

41. Mohr DN, Ryn JH, Litin SC et al: Recent advances in the management of venous thromboembolism. Mayo Clin Proc 63:281, 1988

42. Anderson DR, Levine MN: Thrombolytic therapy for the treatment of acute pulmonary embolism. Can Med Assoc J 146:1317, 1992

43. Goldhaber SZ, Kessler CM, Heit J et al: Randomized controlled trial of recombinant tissue plasminogen activator versus urokinase in the treatment of acute pulmonary embolism. Lancet 2:293, 1988

44. Goldhaber SZ, Kessler CM, Heit JA et al: Recombinant tissue-type plasminogen activator versus a normal dosing regimen of urokinase in acute pulmonary embolism: a randomized controlled multicenter trial. J Am Coll Cardiol 20:24, 1992

45. Hess H: Symposium uber Thrombolyse-Therapie, Munchen. Springer-Verlag, Stuttgart, 1967

46. Robertson BR, Nilsson IM, Nylander G, Olow B: Effect of streptokinase and heparin on patients with deep vein thrombosis. Acta Chir Scand 133:205, 1967

47. Browse NL, Thomas ML, Pim HP: Streptokinase and deep vein thrombosis. Br Med J 3:717, 1968

48. Robertson BR, Nilsson IM, Nylander G: Value of streptokinase and heparin in treatment of acute deep venous thrombosis. Acta Chir Scand 134:203, 1968

49. Kakkar VV, Howe CT, Laws JW, Flanc C: Late results of treatment of deep vein thrombosis. Br Med J 1:810, 1969

50. Kakkar VV, Flanc C, Howe CT et al: Treatment of deep vein thrombosis: a trial of heparin, streptokinase, and Arvin. Br Med J 1:806, 1969

51. Kakkar VV, Flanc C, O'Shea MJ et al: Treatment of deep vein thrombosis with streptokinase. Br J Surg 56:178, 1969

52. Robertson BR, Nilsson IM, Nylander G: Thrombolytic effect of streptokinase as evaluated by phlebography of deep venous thrombi of the leg. Acta Chir Scand 136:173, 1970

53. Kakkar VV: Treatment of deep vein thrombosis: a comparative study of heparin, streptokinase and Arvin. Bull Swiss Acad Med Sci 29:253, 1973

54. Tsapogas MJ, Peabody RA, Wu KT et al: Controlled study of thrombolytic therapy in deep vein thrombosis. Surgery 74:973, 1973

55. Tibbutt DA, Williams EW, Walker MW et al: Controlled trial of ancrod and streptokinase in the treatment of deep vein thrombosis of lower limb. Br J Haematol 27:407, 1974

56. Duckert F, Muller G, Nyman D et al: Treatment of deep vein thrombosis with streptokinase. Br Med J 1:479, 1975

57. Seaman AJ, Common HH, Rosch J et al: Deep vein thrombosis treated with streptokinase or heparin. Angiology 27:549, 1976

58. Common HH, Seaman AJ, Rosch J et al: Deep vein thrombosis treated with streptokinase or heparin: follow-up of a randomized study. Angiology 27:645, 1976

59. Rogers LQ, Lutcher CL: Streptokinase therapy for deep vein thrombosis: a comprehensive review of the English literature. Am J Med 88:389, 1990

60. Bieger R, Boekhout-Mussert RJ, Hohmann F, Loeliger EA: Is streptokinase useful in the treatment of deep vein thrombosis? J Intern Med 199:81, 1976

61. Sharma GVRK, O'Connell DJ, Belko JS, Sasahara AA: Thrombolytic therapy in deep vein thrombosis. p. 181. In Paoletti R, Sherry S (eds): Thrombosis and Urokinase. Academic Press, San Diego, 1977

62. Marder VJ, Soulen RL, Atichartakarn V et al: Quantitative venographic assessment of deep vein thrombosis in the evaluation of streptokinase and heparin therapy. J Lab Clin Med 89:1018, 1977

63. Arnesen H, Heilo A, Jakobsen E et al: A prospective study of streptokinase and heparin in the treatment of deep vein thrombosis. J Intern Med 203:457, 1978

64. Elliot MS, Immelman EJ, Jeffrey P et al: A comparative randomized trial of heparin versus streptokinase in the treatment of acute proximal venous thrombosis: an interim report of a prospective trial. Br J Surg 66:838, 1979

65. Marder VJ: Guidelines for thrombolytic therapy of deep-vein thrombosis. Prog Cardiovasc Dis 21:327, 1979

66. Elliot MS, Immelman EJ, Jeffrey P et al: The role of thrombolytic therapy in the management of phlegmasia caerulea dolens. Br J Surg 66:422, 1979

67. Watz R, Savidge GF: Rapid thrombolysis and preservation of valvular venous function in high deep vein thrombosis. J Intern Med 205:293, 1979

68. Weimer W, Stibbe J, van Seyen AJ et al: Specific lysis of an iliofemoral thrombus by administration of extrinsic (tissue-type) plasminogen activator. Lancet 2:1018, 1981

69. van de Loo JC, Kreissmann A, Trubestein G et al: Controlled multicenter pilot study of urokinase, heparin and streptokinase in deep vein thrombosis. Thromb Haemost 50:660, 1983

70. Bonnet J, Colle JP, Lonent-Roudaut MF et al: Efficacité et intérêt des fibrinolytiques dans les thrombes veineuses anciennes proximales des membres inférieurs. Arch Mal Coeur 77:1033, 1984

71. Kakkar VV, Lawrence D: Hemodynamic and clinical assessment after ther-

apy for acute deep vein thrombosis: a prospective study. Am J Surg 150: 54, 1985

72. Sherry S: Thrombolytic therapy for deep venous thrombosis. Semin Int Radiol 2:331, 1985

73. Ott P, Eldrup E, Oxholm P et al: Streptokinase therapy in the routine management of deep venous thrombosis in the lower extremities. J Intern Med 219: 295, 1986

74. Lewis JD: The management of the limb in acute venous thrombosis. Blood Rev 1:230, 1987

75. Rowe JM, Rasmussen RL, Mader SL et al: Successful thrombolytic therapy in two patients with renal vein thrombosis. Am J Med 77:1111, 1984

76. Crowley JP, Matarese RA, Quevedo SF, Garella S: Fibrinolytic therapy for bilateral renal vein thrombosis. Arch Intern Med 144:159, 1984

77. Burrow CR, Walker WG, Bell WR, Gatewood OB: Streptokinase salvage of renal function after renal vein thrombosis. Ann Intern Med 100:237, 1984

78. Wagoner RD, Stanson AW, Holley KE, Winter CS: Renal vein thrombosis in idiopathic membranous glomerulopathy and nephrotic syndrome: incidence and significance. Kidney Int 23:368, 1983

79. Llach F, Papper S, Massry SG: The clinical spectrum of renal vein thrombosis: acute and chronic. Am J Med 69:819, 1980

80. Farrer JF, Goodwin WE: Treatment of priapism: comparison of methods in 15 cases. J Urol 86:768, 1961

81. King LM, McCune DP, Harris JJ, Buck RL: Fibrinolysin therapy for thrombosis of priapism. J Urol 92:692, 1964

82. Marx FJ: Zur Therapie des Priapismus. Urologe A 20:353, 1981

83. Drance SM: An ophthalmologist's approach to fibrinolysis. Angiology 12: 149, 1961

84. Den Ottolander GJH, Craandijk A: Treatment of thrombosis of the central retinal vein with streptokinase. Thromb Diath Haemorrh 20:415, 1968

85. Rakusin W: Urokinase in the management of traumatic hyphema. Br J Ophthalmol 55:826, 1971

86. Forrester JV, Williamson J: Lytic therapy in vitreous hemorrhage. Trans Ophthalmol Soc UK 94:583, 1974

87. Holmes-Selora PJ, Kanskii JJ, Watson DM: Intravitreal urokinase in the management of vitreous hemorrhage. Trans Ophthalmol Soc UK 94:591, 1974

88. Kohner EM, Pettit JE, Hamilton AM et al: Streptokinase in central retinal vein occlusion: a controlled clinical trial. Br Med J 1:550, 1976

89. Kwaan HC, Dobbie JG, Fetkenhour CL: The use of anticoagulants and thrombolytic agents in occlusive retinal vascular disease. p. 191. In Paoletti R, Sherry S (eds): Thrombosis and Urokinase. Academic Press, San Diego, 1977

90. Chapman-Smith JS, Crock GW: Urokinase in the management of vitreous hemorrhage. Br J Ophthalmol 61:500, 1977

91. Nagpal RD: Dural sinus and cerebral venous thrombosis. Neurosurg Rev 6: 155, 1983

92. Ostering H, Brunner G, Heimburg P et al: Thrombolysis in the Budd-Chiari syndrome induced by partial thromboses of the inferior vena cava and the hepatic veins. Dtsch Med Wochenschr 96:1532, 1971

93. Warren RL, Schlant RC, Wenger NK: Treatment of Budd-Chiari syndrome with streptokinase. Gastroenterology 64:200, 1973

94. Cameron JL, Herlong HF, Sanfey H et al: The Budd-Chiari syndrome: treatment by mesenteric-systemic venous shunts. Ann Surg 198:335, 1983

95. Greenwood LH, Yrizzarry JM, Hallett GW Jr et al: Urokinase treatment of Budd-Chiari syndrome. AJR 141:1057, 1983

96. McDermott WV, Stone MD, Bothe A Jr, Trey C: Budd-Chiari syndrome: historical and clinical review with an analysis of surgical corrective procedures. Am J Surg 147:463, 1984

97. Segadal L, Arnesj JB, Halvorsen JF et al: Budd-Chiari syndrome with obstruction of the inferior caval vein: successful treatment by cavosplenoatrial shunt. Surgery 98:63, 1985

98. Sholar PW, Bell WR: Thrombolytic therapy of inferior vena cava thrombosis in paroxysmal nocturnal hemoglobinuria. Ann Intern Med 103:539, 1985

99. McKee CM, Crothers JG, Mayne EE, Callender ME: Budd-Chiari syndrome treated with acylated streptokinase-plasminogen complex. J R Soc Med 78: 768, 1985

100. Hess H, Seitz W (eds): Collective statistics in thrombolytic therapy. p. 101. In: Symposium der Deutsche Gesellschaft für Angiologie, München, 1966. Springer-Verlag, Stuttgart, 1967

101. Poliwoda H, Alexander K, Buhl V et al: Treatment of chronic arterial occlusions with streptokinase. N Engl J Med 280:689, 1969

102. Samama M, Cormier JM, Abastado M et al: La thrombolyse par la streptokinase. II. A propos de soixante six observations. Coagulation 2:221, 1969

103. Hume M, Gurewich V, Thomas DP, Dealy JB Jr: Streptokinase for chronic arterial occlusive disease. Arch Surg 101:653, 1970

104. Chesterman CN, Briggs JC: Thrombolytic therapy with streptokinase. Med J Aust 57:839, 1970

105. Amery A, Deloof W, Vermylen J, Verstraete M: Outcome of recent thrombo-

106. Salmon J: Treatment fibrinolytique: Résultats obtenus au cours d'une expérience interessant 200 patients. p. 113. In Guillaume J (ed): Colloque International sur la Streptokinase. SPEI, Lyon, 1970

107. Martin M, Schoop W, Zietler E: Streptokinase in chronic arterial occlusive disease. JAMA 211:1169, 1970

108. Verstraete M, Vermylen J, Donati MB: The effect of streptokinase infusion on chronic arterial occlusions and stenosis. Ann Intern Med 74:377, 1971

109. Deutsch E, Ehringer H: Thrombolytic therapy in chronic arterial occlusion. J Clin Pathol 25:644, 1972

110. LeVeen HH, Diaz CA: Venous and arterial occlusive disease treated by enzymatic clot lysis. Arch Surg 105:927, 1972

111. Poliwoda H: Treatment of chronic arterial occlusion with streptokinase. J Clin Pathol 25:642, 1972

112. Heinrich F: Ziel und Aufbau der Studie. p. 1. In Heinrich F (ed): Streptokinase-Therapie bei chronischer arterieller Verschlusskrankheit. Medizinische Verlazsges, Marburg, 1975

113. Fiessinger JN, Aiach M, Lagneau M et al: The indications for streptokinase in arterial occlusions of the limbs. Coeur Med Intern 15:453, 1976

114. Martin M: Thrombolytic therapy in arterial thromboembolism. Prog Cardiovasc Dis 21:351, 1979

115. Conard J, Samama M, Milochevitch R et al: Complications hemorrhagiques au cours de 98 traitements par la streptokinase: place de la surveillance biologique. Nouv Presse Med 8:1319, 1979

116. Kakkasseril JS, Cranley JJ, Arbaugh JJ et al: Efficacy of low-dose streptokinase in acute arterial occlusion and graft thrombosis. Arch Surg 120:427, 1985

117. Hallett JW Jr, Greenwood LH, Yrizarry JM et al: Statistical determinants of success and complications of thrombolytic therapy for arterial occlusion of lower extremity. Surg Gynecol Obstet 161:431, 1985

118. Pernes JM, Brenot P, Raynaud A et al: Results of in situ arterial thrombolysis by the combination of urokinase and lysyl plasminogen in acute arterial occlusive diseases of the lower limb. J Radiol 66:385, 1985

119. Goldberg L, Ricci MT, Sauvage LR et al: Thrombolytic therapy for delayed occlusion of knitted Dacron bypass grafts in the axillofemoral, femoropopliteal and femorotibial positions. Surg Gynecol Obstet 160:491, 1985

120. Graor RA, Risius B, Danny KM et al: Local thrombolysis in the treatment of thrombosed arteries, bypass grafts, and arteriovenous fistulas. J Vasc Surg 2:406, 1985

121. Hallett JW Jr, Greenwood LH, Yrizarry JM et al: Statistical determinants of success and complications of thrombolytic therapy for arterial occlusion of lower extremity. Surg Gynecol Obstet 161:431, 1985

122. Belkin M, Belkin B, Bickman CA et al: Intra-arterial fibrinolytic therapy. Arch Surg 121:769, 1986

123. Lammer J, Pilger E, Neumayer K: Intra arterial fibrinolysis: long-term results. Radiology 161:159, 1986

124. Valji K, Roberts AC, Davis GB, Bookstein JJ: Pulsed spray thrombolysis of arterial and bypass graft occlusions. AJR 156:617, 1991

125. Austen M, Kadir S, Mitchell SE et al: Iliac artery occlusion: management with intrathrombus streptokinase infusion and angioplasty. Radiology 153: 385, 1984

126. Anderson DC, Martin AM, Clunie GJA et al: Eight months' experience in the use of streptokinase for de-clotting arteriovenous cannulae. Proc Eur Dial Transplant Assoc 4:55, 1967

127. Cocke TB, Burgos-Calderon RA, Gonzalez F: The use of streptokinase infusions for arterovenous shunt declotting. Trans Am Soc Artif Intern Organs 16:292, 1970

128. Watt DAL, Dunn BP, Livingstone WR, Macdougall AL: Declotting of Quinton-Scribner shunts. Am Heart J 81:292, 1971

129. Arisz L, Tegzess AM, Donker AJM: The use of streptokinase in obstructed arterio-venous shunts. Postgrad Med J, Aug suppl. J 49:99, 1973

130. Goldberg JP, Contiguglia SR, Mishell JL, Klein MH: Intravenous streptokinase for thrombolysis of occluded arteriovenous access: its use in patients undergoing hemodialysis. Arch Intern Med 145:1405, 1985

131. Luluaga IT, Carrera D, Oliveria J et al: Successful thrombolytic therapy after acute tricuspid-valve obstruction. Lancet 1:1067, 1971

132. Inberg MV, Havia T, Arstila M: Thrombolytic treatment for thrombotic complications of valve prosthesis after tricuspid valve replacement. Scand J Thorac Cardiovasc Surg 11:195, 1977

133. Baglin JY, Diebold B, Henin D et al: Thrombose de prothèse valvulaire: embolie cérébrale mortelle lors du traitement thrombolytique. Arch Mal Coeur 76:1077, 1983

134. Gagnon RM, Beaudet R, Lemire J et al: Streptokinase thrombolysis of chronically thrombosed mitral prosthetic valve. Cathet Cardiovasc Diagn 10:5, 1984

135. Tasrini J, Scheffer J, Vaislic C et al: Place du traitement thrombolytique dans les thromboses des protheses valvulaires: à propos de 2 cas et revue de la littérature mondiale. Arch Mal Coeur 77:1108, 1984

136. Marx JD, Kleynhans PH, Otto AC: Lysis of a coronary embolus by intracoronary streptokinase: a case report. S Afr Med J 68:346, 1985

137. Roudaut M, Ledain L, Roudaut R et al: Thrombolytic treatment of acute thrombotic obstruction with disk valve prosthesis: specimens with 26 cases. Semin Thromb Hemost 13:201, 1987

138. Kurzrok S, Singh AK, Most AS: Thrombolytic therapy for prosthetic cardiac valve thrombosis. J Am Coll Cardiol 9:592, 1987

139. Hecker SP, Zweng HC: Central retinal artery occlusion successfully treated with plasmin. JAMA 176:1067, 1961

140. Kremer P, Fiebig R, Tilsner V et al: Lysis of left ventricular thrombi with urokinase. Circulation 72:112, 1985

141. Hecker SP, Zweng HC: Central retinal artery occlusion successfully treated with plasmin. JAMA 176:1067, 1961

142. Annonier P, Sobel J, Wenger JJ et al: Treatment fibrinolytique local dans les occlusions de l'artère centrale de la rétine. J Fr Ophtalmol 7:771, 1984

143. Schmidt D, Schumacher M, Wakhloo AK: Microcatheter urokinase infusion in central retinal artery occlusion. Am J Ophthalmol 113:429, 1992

144. Clarke RL, Clifton EE: The treatment of cerebrovascular thrombosis and embolism with fibrinolytic agents. Am J Cardiol 6:546, 1960

145. Meyer JS, Gilroy J, Barnhart MI, Johnson JF: Therapeutic thrombolysis in cerebral thromboembolism: double-blind evaluation of intravenous plasmin therapy in carotid and middle cerebral arterial occlusion. Neurology 13:927, 1963

146. Atkin N, Nitzberg S, Dorsey J: Lysis of intracerebral thromboembolism with fibrinolysin. Angiology 15:436, 1964

147. del Zoppo GJ, Copeland BR, Anderchek K et al: Hemorrhagic transformation following tissue plasminogen activator in experimental cerebral infarction. Stroke 21:596, 1990

148. Hanaway J, Torack R, Fletcher AP, Landau WM: Intracranial bleeding associated with urokinase therapy for acute ischemic hemispheral stroke. Stroke 7:143, 1976

149. Fletcher AP, Alkjaersig N, Lewis M, et al: A pilot study of urokinase therapy in cerebral infarction. Stroke 7:135, 1976

150. Fletcher AP, Allkjaersig N: Use of urokinase therapy in cerebrovascular disease. p. 203. In Paoletti R, Sherry S (eds): Thrombolysis and Urokinase. Academic Press, San Diego, 1977

151. Larcan A, Laprevote-Heully MC, Lambert H et al: Indications des thrombolytiques au cours des accidents vasculaires cérébraux thrombosants traités par ailleurs par O. H. B (2 ATA). Therapie 32:259, 1977

152. Labauge R, Blard J-M, Salvaing P et al: Traitement fibrinolytique et anticoagulant des 37 cas d'occlusions artérielles: cérévicocérébrales d'origin thrombe-embolique. p. 362. In Proceedings of the Fifth International Congress on Thromboembolism, Bologna, 1978. Quaderni della Coagulazione, Pisa, 1980

153. Nenci GG, Gresele P, Taramelli M et al: Thrombolytic therapy for thromboembolism of vertebrobasilar artery. Angiology 34:561, 1983

154. del Zeppo GJ: Thrombolytic therapy in cerebrovascular disease. Curr Concept Cerebrovasc Stroke 23:7, 1988

155. Mori E, Tabuchi M, Yoshida T, Yamadori A: Intracarotid urokinase with thromboembolic occlusion of the middle cerebral artery. Stroke 19:802, 1988

156. Theron J, Courtheoux P, Casasco A et al: Local intraarterial fibrinolysis in the carotid territory. Am J Neuroradiol 10:753, 1989

157. Pessin MS, Del Zoppo GJ, Estol CJ: Thrombolytic agents in the treatment of stroke. Clin Neuropharmacol 13:271, 1990

158. Sipos EP, Kirsch JR, Bell WR et al: Intra-arterial urokinase for treatment of retrograde thrombosis following resection of an arteriovenous malformation. J Neurosurg 76:1004, 1992

159. Brott TG, Haley EC, Levy DE et al: Urgent therapy for stroke. Part I & Part II. Stroke 23:632 and 641, 1992

160. Haley EC Jr, Levy DE, Brott TG et al: Urgent therapy for stroke. Part II. Pilot study of tissue plasminogen activator administered 91–180 minutes from onset. Stroke 23:641, 1992

161. von Kummer R, Hacke W: Safety and efficacy of intravenous tissue plasminogen activator and heparin in acute middle cerebral artery stroke. Stroke 23:646, 1992

162. Tsai FY, Higashida RT, Matovich V, Alfieri K: Acute thrombosis of the intracraniel dural sinus: direct thrombolytic treatment. Am J Neuroradiol 13:1137, 1992

163. Mori E, Yoneda Y, Tabuchi M et al: Intravenous recombinant tissue plasminogen activator in acute carotid artery territory stroke. Neurology 42:976, 1992

164. del Zoppp GJ, Poeck K, Pessin MS et al: Recombinant tissue plasminogen activator in acute thrombotic and embolic stroke. Ann Neurol 32:78, 1992

165. Sherry S: The maintenance of a sustained thrombolytic state in man. II. Clinical observations on patients with myocardial infarction and other thromboembolic disorders. J Clin Invest 38:1111, 1959

166. DeWood MA, Spores J, Notske R et al: Prevalence of total coronary occlusion during the early hours of transmural myocardial infarction. N Engl J Med 303:897, 1980

167. Rentrop KP, Blanke H, Karsch KR et al: Acute myocardial infarction: intracoronary application of nitroglycerin and streptokinase. Clin Cardiol 2:354, 1979

168. Rentrop P, Blanke H, Karsch KR et al: Selective intracoronary thrombolysis in acute myocardial infarction and unstable angina pectoris. Circulation 63:307, 1981

169. Van de Werf F, Ludbrook PA, Bergmann SR et al: Coronary thrombolysis with tissue-type plasminogen activator in patients with evolving myocardial infarction. N Engl J Med 310:609, 1984

170. Collen D, Topol EJ, Tiefenbrunn AJ et al: Coronary thrombolysis with recombinant human tissue-type plasminogen activator: a prospective, randomized, placebo-controlled trial. Circulation 70:1012, 1984

171. The TIMI Study Group: Thrombolysis in myocardial infarction trial (TIMI) trial: phase I findings. N Engl J Med 312:932, 1985

172. Verstraete M, Bernard R, Borg M et al: Randomized trial of intravenous recombinant tissue-type plasminogen activator versus intravenous streptokinase in acute myocardial infarction: report from the European Cooperative Study Group for Recombinant Tissue-type Plasminogen Activator. Lancet 1:842, 1985

173. Verstraete M, Bleifeld W, Brower RW et al: Double-blind randomised trial of intravenous tissue-type plasminogen activator versus placebo in acute myocardial infarction. Lancet 2:965, 1985

174. Chesbro JH, Knatterud G, Roberts R et al: Thrombolysis in myocardial infarction (TIMI) trial, phase I: a comparison between intravenous tissue plasminogen activator and intravenous streptokinase: clinical findings through hospital discharge. Circulation 76:142, 1987

175. Mueller HS, Rao AK, Forman SA: TIMI investigators. Thrombolysis in myocardial infarction (TIMI): comparative studies of coronary reperfusion and systemic fibrinogenolysis with two forms of recombinant tissue-type plasminogen activator. J Am Coll Cardiol 10:479, 1987

176. White HD, Norris RM, Brown MA et al: Effect of intravenous streptokinase on left ventricular function and early survival after acute myocardial infarction. N Engl J Med 317:850, 1987

177. Gruppo Italiano per lo Studio della Streptochinasi nell'Infarto Miocardico (GISSI): Effectiveness of intravenous thrombolytic treatment in acute myocardial infarction. Lancet 1:397, 1986

178. Jang I-K, Vanhaecke J, De Geest H et al: Coronary thrombolysis with recombinant tissue-type plasminogen activator: patency rate and regional wall motion after 3 months. J Am Coll Cardiol 8:1455, 1986

179. Topol EJ, Bates ER, Walton JA et al: Community hospital administration of intravenous tissue plasminogen activator in acute myocardial infarction: improved timing, thrombolytic efficacy and ventricular function. J Am Coll Cardiol 10:1173, 1987

180. Topol EJ, Morris DC, Smalling RW et al: A multicenter, randomized, placebo-controlled trial of a new form of intravenous recombinant tissue-type plasminogen activator (activase) in acute myocardial infarction. J Am Coll Cardiol 9:1205, 1987

181. Guerci A, Gerstenblith G, Brinker JA et al: A randomized trial of intravenous tissue plasminogen activator for acute myocardial infarction with subsequent randomization to elective coronary angioplasty. N Engl J Med 317:1613, 1987

182. ISIS-2 Collaborative Group: Randomized trial of intravenous streptokinase, oral aspirin, both, or neither among 17187 cases of suspected acute myocardial infarction: ISIS-2. Lancet 2:349, 1988

183. Rao AK, Pratt C, Berke A et al: Thrombolysis in Myocardial Infarction (TIMI) Trial—Phase I: hemorrhagic manifestations and changes in plasma fibrinogen and the fibrinolytic system in patients treated with recombinant tissue plasminogen activator and streptokinase. J Am Coll Cardiol 11:1, 1988

184. Wilcox RG, von der Lippe G, Olsson CG et al: Trial of tissue plasminogen activator for mortality reduction in acute myocardial infarction. Lancet 2:525, 1988

185. National Heart Foundation of Australia Coronary Thrombolysis Group: Coronary thrombolysis and myocardial salvage by tissue plasminogen activator given up to 4 hours after onset of myocardial infarction. Lancet 1:203, 1988

186. O'Rourke M, Baron D, Keogh A et al: Limitation of myocardial infarction by early infusion of recombinant tissue-type plasminogen activator. Circulation 77:1311, 1988

187. Von de Werf F, Arnold AER: Intravenous tissue plasminogen activator and

size of infarct, left ventricular function, and survival in acute myocardial infarction. Br Med J 297:1374, 1988

188. Magnani B: Plasminogen Activator Italian Multicenter Study (PAIMS): comparison of intravenous recombinant single-chain human tissue-type plasminogen activator (rt-PA) with intravenous streptokinase in acute myocardial infarction. J Am Coll Cardiol 13:19, 1989

189. White HD, Rivers JT, Maslouski AV et al: Effect of intravenous streptokinase as compared with that of tissue plasminogen activators on left ventricular function after first myocardial infarction. N Engl J Med 320:817, 1989

190. Rapaport E: Thrombolytic agents in acute myocardial infarction. N Engl J Med 320:861, 1989

191. A symposium: Thrombosis and thrombolysis in unstable agina. Am J Cardiol 68:1B, 1991

192. van den Brand M, van Zijl A, Geuskens R et al: Tissue plasminogen activator in refractory unstable angina. Eur Heart J 12:1208, 1991

193. Shafer KE, Santoro SS, Sobel BE et al: Monitoring activity of fibrinolytic agents. Am J Med 76:879, 1984

194. Vernon SK: A rapid simple method for monitoring fibrinolysis in vitro. Thromb Res 52:349, 1988

195. Hoffmann JJML, Verhoppen MAL: Automated nephelometry of fibrinogen: analytical performance and observations during thrombolytic therapy. Clin Chem 34:2135, 1988

196. Keith DS, Phillips SJ, Whisnant SJ et al: Heparin therapy for recent transient focal cerebral ischemia. Mayo Clin Proc 62:1101, 1987

197. Wheeler AP, Jaquiss RDB, Newman JH: Physician practices in the treatment of pulmonary emboli and deep vein thrombosis. Arch Intern Med 148:1321, 1988

198. Dykewicz MS, McGrath KG, Davison R et al: Identification of patients at risk for anaphylaxis due to streptokinase. Arch Intern Med 146:305, 1986

199. Lee CD, Mann KS: The activation of human coagulation factor V by plasmin. Blood, suppl. 1. 70:389a, 1987

200. Topol EJ, Bell WR, Weisfeldt ML: Coronary thrombolysis with recombinant tissue-type plasminogen activator. A hematologic and pharmacologic study. Ann Intern Med 103:837, 1985

201. Jan K, Reinhart W, Chien S et al: Altered rheological properties of blood following administration of tissue, plasminogen activator and streptokinase in patients with acute myocardial infarction. Circulation 72:111, 1985

Venous Thromboembolism

123

Jack Hirsh and Jeffrey I. Weitz

INTRODUCTION

Although venous thrombosis can occur in any vein in the body, it occurs most commonly in the lower limbs. Thrombosis of the superficial veins of the legs frequently occurs in varicosities and is usually benign and self-limiting. In contrast to superficial thrombosis, involvement of the deep veins of the leg is a more serious condition. Thrombi localized to the deep veins of the calf are less serious than those involving the proximal (popliteal, femoral, or iliacs) veins because they are often smaller, hence, less commonly associated with long-term disability or clinically important pulmonary embolism. By contrast, proximal vein thrombosis is a serious disorder, as it is frequently complicated by pulmonary embolism. In addition, extensive damage to the valves in the vein often leads to chronic disability from the postphlebitic syndrome.

Venous thrombosis and its major complication, pulmonary embolism, are important causes of morbidity and mortality in hospitalized patients. However, venous thromboembolism also occurs in ambulant patients. The diagnosis of venous thromboembolism is more frequently made in the outpatient setting because of the increased availability of reliable noninvasive diagnostic tests. The result has been increased awareness that patients with leg symptoms can have serious deep vein thrombosis (DVT) and has consequently led to an increase in the rate of referral of ambulant patients for diagnostic testing. The trend for early hospital discharge of postsurgical patients who may not have received in-hospital prophylaxis or for whom it was terminated at discharge despite a continued risk of venous thrombosis has increased the prevalence of venous thrombosis in outpatients.

Although pulmonary embolism is the most feared complication of venous thrombosis, the postphlebitic syndrome is responsible for much greater morbidity because it is a long-term complication that occurs in approximately 60% of patients with proximal vein thrombosis.

PATHOGENESIS OF VENOUS THROMBOEMBOLISM AND CLINICAL RISK FACTORS

Venous thrombi are composed predominantly of fibrin and red cells.[1] They usually arise in the large venous sinuses in the calf, in the valve cusp pockets in the deep veins of the calf, or at sites of vessel damage. Venous thrombosis occurs when activation of blood coagulation exceeds the ability of the natural anticoagulant mechanisms and the fibrinolytic system to prevent fibrin formation.[1] Activation of blood coagulation is usually initiated by tissue or vascular trauma or by inflammation and is augmented by venous stasis. Vascular wall damage is an important predisposing factor to venous thrombosis after major hip or knee surgery.[1]

Under normal circumstances, activated coagulation factors are diluted in the flowing blood and are neutralized by inhibitors on the surface of endothelial cells or by circulating antiproteinases.[2] However, activated clotting factors that escape regulation can trigger the coagulation system leading to fibrin formation. In turn, the fibrinolytic system is activated, with the release of tissue plasminogen activator (t-PA) from endothelial cells[3] and of urokinase (u-PA) from monocytes and leukocytes, which are attracted to the thrombus by released fibrinopeptides and platelet products.

Thrombogenic Factors

Activation of Blood Coagulation

A low level of activation of blood coagulation occurs continuously in normal subjects[4] (Table 123-1). In vivo activation is reduced in patients with hemophilia and is increased to above-

Table 123-1. Thrombogenesis

Stimulation	Inhibition
Activation of coagulation	Circulating inhibitors (antithrombin III, protein C, protein S)
Vessel damage	Endothelial cell components (Heparan sulfate, thrombomodulin)
Stasis	Fibrinolytic system (t-PA, plasminogen)

normal levels in some patients with hereditary deficiencies of antithrombin III (AT III), protein C, and protein S.[4] Activation of blood coagulation also increases with age in patients 45 years of age.

The intrinsic pathway may be activated by contact of factor XII with collagen on exposed subendothelium of damaged vessels or by contact with prosthetic surfaces. Coagulation is further augmented by activated platelets. The extrinsic pathway may be activated by the exposure of blood to tissue factor made available locally as a result of vascular wall damage,[5] by activation of endothelial cells by cytokines, and by activated leukocytes that migrate to areas of vascular injury.[6] Factor X can be activated directly by extracts of malignant cells that contain a cysteine protease.[7] This may be one of the mechanisms by which thrombosis is induced in patients with malignant disease. A factor elaborated by hypoxic endothelial cells can also directly activate factor X[8] and could lead to thrombosis in patients with severe venous stasis, in which stagnant hypoxia occurs in the valve cusps.

Clinical risk factors that predispose to venous thromboembolism by activating blood coagulation include extensive surgery, trauma, burns, infusion of concentrates of prothrombin that contain activated clotting factors, disseminated malignant disease, myocardial infarction, and possibly local hypoxia produced by venous stasis.[8]

Venous Stasis

Venous return from the legs is enhanced by contraction of the calf muscles, propelling blood upward from the extremities. Venous stasis contributes to thrombogenesis by allowing activated coagulation factors to locally accumulate. In addition, stagnation of the blood could lead to local hypoxia, stimulating endothelial cell release of an activator of factor X.[8] Venous stasis is produced by immobility, venous obstruction, increased venous pressure, venous dilation, and increased blood viscosity. Each of these is briefly discussed.

Immobility

Venous thrombosis occurs in immobilized patients because blood pools in the intramuscular sinuses of the calf, which are dilated during recumbency. Many clinical examples highlight the role of stasis in the pathogenesis of venous thrombosis. Thus, the prevalence of venous thrombosis found at autopsy is markedly increased in patients who are confined to bed for >1 week before death. Furthermore, preoperative immobility is associated with a higher frequency of perioperative venous thrombosis, after surgery, patients remain at risk of venous thromboembolism for as long as they are immobile. Finally, immobility contributes to the high incidence of postoperative venous thrombosis in patients undergoing hysterectomy, transabdominal prostatectomy, hip surgery, knee surgery, or surgery for fractures of the lower limb. The effect of immobility on thrombosis is well illustrated by comparing the location of thrombosis in paraplegics with that in stroke patients. Whereas thrombosis occurs with equal frequency in both legs in paraplegics, it occurs more frequently in the paralyzed limb in stroke patients.

Venous Obstruction

Another important cause of venous stasis is venous obstruction. This process contributes to the risk of venous thrombosis in patients with pelvic tumor and to recurrent venous thrombosis in patients with persistent obstruction due to proximal vein thrombosis. Raised central venous pressure produces venous stasis in the extremities, which may explain the high prevalence of venous thrombosis in patients with heart failure.

Increased Blood Viscosity and Venous Dilation

Venous stasis can also result from increased blood viscosity or venous dilation. The blood viscosity can be increased by an elevated hematocrit (polycythemia vera and erythrocytosis), by hypergammaglobulinemia (dysproteinemias), or by an increased fibrinogen concentration (chronic inflammatory or malignant diseases). Stasis due to venous dilation could contribute to the increased risk of thrombosis in patients with varicose veins and in elderly patients, particularly in those who are bedridden. Since estrogens can cause venous dilation, this may explain the increased prevalence of thrombosis during pregnancy,[9] and in woman taking estrogen-containing oral contraceptive pills.[9]

Vessel Wall Damage

Although the normal endothelium is nonthrombogenic, damage or perturbation can trigger the activation of platelets and coagulation. Thus, vascular injury leads to the expression of tissue factor, either directly by endothelial cells or by activated leukocytes attracted to the site of damage. In addition, the exposure of blood to subendothelium leads to platelet adhesion and aggregation.

The vascular endothelium can be damaged by direct trauma, or it can be perturbed by exposure to endotoxin, to inflammatory cytokines such as interleukin-1 and tumor necrosis factor, thrombin, or low oxygen tension. Perturbed endothelial cells synthesize tissue factor and plasminogen activator inhibitor-1 and internalize thrombomodulin—changes that promote thrombogenesis.[10]

Direct venous damage may lead to venous thrombosis in patients undergoing hip surgery, knee surgery, or varicose vein stripping and in patients with severe burns or lower limb trauma. Perturbation of vascular endothelium by exposure to thrombin or inflammatory mediators probably contributes to the thrombosis that occurs after tissue damage, such as surgery or trauma, and in patients with acute or chronic inflammatory states.

Protective Mechanisms

Endothelial-Bound Protective Mechanisms

Normal vascular endothelium is nonthrombogenic to flowing blood. This occurs because endothelial cell-surface glycosaminoglycans and thrombomodulin are potent inhibitors of coagulation, whereas vessel wall generation of prostacyclin and nitric oxide and synthesis of plasminogen activators limit platelet aggregation and fibrin deposition, respectively.

Generation of plasminogen activators[11] by vascular wall cells limits fibrin deposition, while platelet aggregation is inhibited by the release of prostacyclin and endothelium-derived relaxing factor.[12] Endothelial cell affinity for t-PA, plasminogen, and activated protein C and protein S may also contribute to the thromboresistance of the vessel wall.[2] Plasminogen binds to the cell surface, where it can be activated to plasmin by t-PA, thereby promoting local fibrinolytic activity, whereas bound activated protein C and protein S have a potent anticoagulant function.

Inhibitors of Blood Coagulation

Activated coagulation factors are serine proteases and their activity is modulated by several naturally occurring plasma inhibitors. The key inhibitors of the blood coagulation system are AT III, protein C, and protein S.[2] An inherited deficiency of one of these three proteins is found in about 15% of patients who present with venous thrombosis <45 years of age.[13] Some congenital dysfibrinogenemias can also predispose to thrombosis, as can congenital deficiency of plasminogen. Deficiency of heparin cofactor II, a secondary inhibitor of thrombin, has been associated with thrombosis, but a clear causal relationship has yet to be established.

Fibrinolytic System

The basic reaction of the plasma fibrinolytic system is the conversion of plasminogen to the active enzyme, plasmin, by a limited cleavage produced by a variety of plasminogen activators. Two endogenous plasminogen activators, t-PA and u-PA, are synthesized by and released from endothelial cells. u-PA is also synthesized by monocytes. Plasmin hydrolyzes fibrin. Like the coagulation system, the activity of the fibrinolytic system is modulated by inhibitors that regulate both the plasminogen activators and the proteolytic effect of plasmin.[14]

Decreased fibrinolytic activity occurs during the early postoperative period,[15] in women taking oral contraceptives,[16] during the last trimester of pregnancy,[16] and in obese subjects.[17] Fibrinolytic activity in the leg veins is less than that in arm veins, partly explaining the greater tendency for venous thrombosis to occur in the lower extremities. The relative reduction of fibrinolytic activity in the leg veins is more marked in the elderly, which may partly explain why the risk of thrombosis increases with age.

Evidence shows that impaired fibrinolysis predisposes to postoperative venous thrombosis and possibly to coronary artery thrombosis in patients with coronary artery disease.[15] Most of the data suggest that the impaired fibrinolytic activity reported in patients with venous thrombosis is acquired, and is caused by increased levels of plasminogen activator inhibitor.[15] However, occasional cases of familial abnormalities of the fibrinolytic system in association with venous thrombosis are reported.[18,19]

NATURAL HISTORY

Most thrombi are asymptomatic and are confined to the intramuscular veins of the calf. These calf vein thrombi often undergo spontaneous lysis and rarely, if ever, produce long-term sequelae.[20] By contrast, complete lysis of proximal vein thrombosis is uncommon even when heparin treatment is given.[21]

The symptoms and signs of venous thromboembolism are caused by obstruction to venous outflow, inflammation of the vessel wall or perivascular tissues, or by embolization of thrombus into the pulmonary circulation. Asymptomatic pulmonary embolism is detected by perfusion lung scanning in about 50% of patients with documented proximal vein thrombosis.[22] Most clinically significant and fatal emboli probably arise from thrombi in the proximal veins of the legs. Although pulmonary emboli may also complicate calf vein thrombosis, these emboli tend to be smaller in size and occur less commonly than in patients with proximal vein thrombosis.[22] Asymptomatic venous thrombosis is found in 70% of patients who present with confirmed pulmonary embolism.[23] These thrombi are usually large and involve the proximal veins.

Extensive venous thrombosis causes venous valvular damage, which leads to the postphlebitic syndrome.[24] In addition, a previous history of venous thrombosis is associated with an increased risk of further episodes, particularly when patients are exposed to high-risk situations.[25]

Prognosis of Venous Thrombosis

Untreated or inadequately treated venous thrombosis is associated with a high complication rate, which can be decreased markedly by adequate anticoagulant therapy. About 20% of untreated silent calf vein thrombi, and 20–30% of untreated symptomatic calf vein thrombi extend into the popliteal vein. When extension occurs, it is associated with a 40–50% risk of clinically detectable pulmonary embolism.[20] Patients with proximal vein thrombosis who are inadequately treated[26] have a 47% frequency of recurrent venous thromboembolism over 3 months, and patients with symptomatic calf vein thrombosis treated with a 5-day course of intermittent intravenous heparin without continuing oral anticoagulants have a recurrence rate >20% over the next 3 months.[27]

By contrast, clinically detectable recurrence occurs in <2% of patients with proximal vein thrombosis during the initial period of heparin therapy[22] if an adequate anticoagulant response is achieved, and a 2–4% recurrence rate during the subsequent 3 months of treatment with oral anticoagulants or moderate doses of subcutaneous heparin.[26,28,29] After 3 months of anticoagulant therapy, the recurrence rate is 5–10% in the subsequent year.[26,28,29] Patients whose first episode of venous thrombosis was idiopathic, and those who have ongoing risk factors, such as prolonged immobilization or cancer, are at higher risk of recurrence.

Postphlebitic Syndrome

The postphlebitic syndrome is caused by venous hypertension, which is usually the result of valve destruction, but occasionally can be produced by large proximal vein thrombi that block overflow.[30] Valve destruction results in malfunction of the muscular pump mechanism that leads to an increased ambulatory pressure in the deep calf veins. The high pressure ultimately renders the perforating veins of the calf incompetent, so that blood flow is directed from the deep veins into the superficial venous system during muscular contraction. This leads to edema and to impaired viability of subcutaneous tissues, and in its most severe form, to venous ulceration. Outflow obstruction may initially be bypassed by the development of collateral veins, but with time the veins distal to the obstruction become dilated, and their valves become incompetent.

In patients whose thrombosis extends into the iliofemoral veins, the swelling may never disappear. By contrast, the swelling may subside after initial treatment, but recur months or years later in patients with less extensive proximal vein thrombosis. Other symptoms and signs of the postphlebitic syndrome may be delayed for 5–10 years after the initial thrombotic event. These symptoms include pain in the calf, which is relieved by rest and leg elevation; pigmentation and induration around the ankle and lower third of the calf; and ulceration, which usually occurs in the region of the medial malleolus.

Patients with extensive thrombosis involving the iliofemoral vein frequently have greater disability and may even have venous claudication, characterized by incapacitating bursting pain with exercise.[31] This complication rarely occurs in patients with thrombosis involving the more distal veins.

DIAGNOSIS OF VENOUS THROMBOSIS

The approach to the diagnosis of venous thrombosis has changed radically over the past 20 years. It is now accepted that clinical diagnosis of venous thrombosis is nonspecific[32] and that objective tests are required to confirm the diagnosis. This concept has led to three new developments: (1) the widespread use of venography to confirm a clinical suspicion of venous thrombosis, (2) an improvement in the technique and safety of venography, and (3) the development and careful evaluation of two noninvasive tests to replace venography, namely, impedance plethysmography (IPG) and venous ultrasonography.

Although IPG and venous ultrasonography are sensitive and specific for proximal vein thrombosis (thrombosis of the popliteal or more proximal veins) in symptomatic patients, these techniques are insensitive to calf vein thrombosis. Since venous ultrasonography has greater sensitivity and specificity, it has replaced IPG at most centers. Venous ultrasonography is limited in its ability to detect calf vein thrombosis. This problem can be circumvented by repeating the test 7 days later if the initial result is normal, in order to detect the 10–30% of calf vein thrombi that extend proximally. If the test remains negative after 7 days, the risk of clinically important proximal extension is negligible, and it is safe to withhold treatment.[33-36]

Clinical Diagnosis

Although clinical diagnosis is nonspecific, careful documentation of clinical symptoms and signs is helpful in ruling out venous thrombosis when an alternative cause is identified (e.g., sciatica, cellulitis, ruptured Baker cyst, ruptured muscle or tendon, cutaneous vasculitis, or arthritis). In addition, patients can be classified into high-, intermediate-, and low-probability groups based on their clinical manifestations and the presence or absence of risk factors such as recent immobilization, hospitalization within the past 6 months, or malignancy.[37] Patients with classic symptoms and signs of DVT (e.g., localized pain, tenderness, swelling, and discoloration) who have at least one risk factor had a 78% probability of venous thrombosis, while those with atypical symptoms and no risk factors had only a 5% probability of venous thrombosis. These low and high pretest probabilities can be combined with the results of objective noninvasive tests to make clinical decisions. Thus, a low pretest clinical probability and a negative noninvasive test can be used to exclude a diagnosis of venous thrombosis, obviating the need for further testing. By contrast, a high pretest clinical probability and a negative noninvasive test should prompt further investigation with venography.

In about 70% of patients referred for clinically suspected venous thrombosis the diagnosis will not be confirmed by objective tests.[33,34] Of the 30% of patients who have venous thrombosis, about 85% have proximal vein thrombosis. The remainder have thrombosis confined to the calf.[33,34] The conditions that most frequently simulate venous thrombosis are a ruptured Baker cyst, cellulitis, muscle tear, muscle cramp, muscle hematoma, external venous compression, superficial thrombophlebitis, and the postphlebitic syndrome.

Objective Diagnostic Tests

Both invasive and noninvasive tests are useful for the diagnosis of venous thrombosis. Venography is the only invasive test of proven value, whereas the noninvasive studies that are considered useful are IPG and venous ultrasonography. Since venous ultrasonography is the most sensitive and specific noninvasive test, it is considered the test of choice. Unlike venography, neither of the noninvasive tests is sensitive to calf vein thrombosis, but both detect thrombosis of the proximal venous system (Fig. 123-1).

Venography

Venography remains the reference standard for the diagnosis of venous thrombosis.[38] It is technically difficult, and the proper execution and interpretation require considerable experience. With good technique, ascending venography outlines the entire deep venous system of the lower extremities, including the external and common iliac veins. Venography may produce superficial phlebitis, and can even cause DVT in 1–4% of patients.[38]

Impedance Plethysmography

IPG is a noninvasive test that uses electrical resistance (impedance) to detect blood volume changes in the calf produced by inflation and deflation of a pneumatic thigh cuff. The changes in blood volume are reduced if the popliteal or more proximal veins are obstructed.

The impedance test does not distinguish between thrombotic and nonthrombotic obstruction to venous outflow. Thus, false-positive results may be obtained if a patient is positioned incorrectly or inadequately relaxed, if the vein is compressed by an extravascular mass, or if venous outflow is impaired by raised central venous pressure. Reduced arterial inflow to the limb due to severe obstructive arterial disease can also lead to reduced outflow, producing a false-positive result.

The reported sensitivities and specificities for the diagnosis of symptomatic proximal venous thrombosis range from as low as 65% to as high as 95%.[33,37,39-42] The test may not detect nonocclusive proximal vein thrombi and fails to detect most thrombi within the calf veins.

In patients with proximal vein thrombosis, the IPG returns to normal in about 30% of patients by 3 weeks, in 60% of patients at 6 weeks and at 3 months, in 80% of patients at 6 months, and in 90% of patients at 1 year.[41] Information on the status of the IPG findings is clinically useful if the patient returns with recurrent symptoms. In patients whose IPG returned to normal after an episode of venous thrombosis, a positive IPG together with appropriate clinical symptoms is highly suggestive of recurrent venous thrombosis.

Venous Ultrasonography

Venous ultrasonography is performed using a high-resolution real-time scanner equipped with a 5-MHz electronically focused linear-array transducer. The common femoral vein and femoral artery are first located in the groin with the patient in a supine position. The superficial femoral vein is then examined along its course. The patient is then placed in the prone position and the popliteal vein is located and examined down to the level of the trifurcation. At each of these locations, the vein being examined is compressed gently but firmly with the transducer probe, and the results are observed on the monitor. Freeze-frame images of both stages of the procedure are obtained.

Venous ultrasonography is accurate for the detection of proximal vein thrombosis in symptomatic patients but is relatively insensitive to calf vein thrombosis. By extending the field of examination to the distal popliteal vein and the proximal deep calf veins, venous ultrasonography detects about 50% of calf vein thrombi in symptomatic patients.[43,44] Potential limitations of venous ultrasonography are its inability to visualize the iliac veins and the segment of the superficial femoral vein within the femoral canal. These are not serious limitations because isolated thrombi within the femoral canal or the iliac vein rarely occur.[45] Furthermore, the obstruction produced by iliac vein thrombi often limits the compressibility of the common femoral vein segment and hence will be detected with this technique.

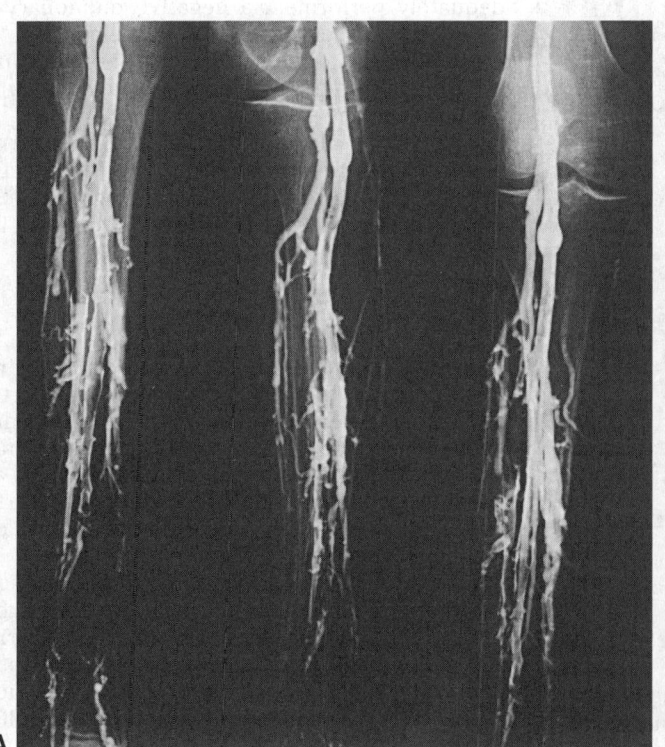
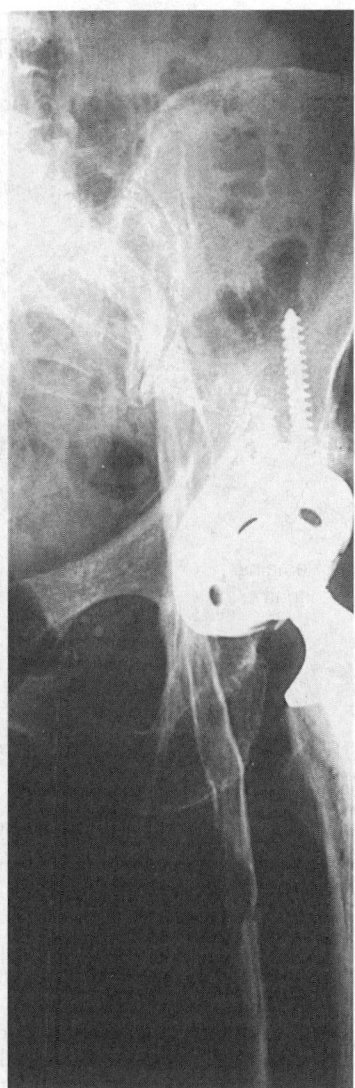

Fig. 123-1. (A) Intraluminal filling defect in both peroneal veins. **(B)** Intraluminal filling defect in proximal superficial femoral and common femoral veins.

Diagnostic Approach

Venous ultrasonography is the noninvasive method of choice because it is the most sensitive and specific. Although it is relatively insensitive to calf vein thrombosis, this shortcoming can be overcome by repeating the test after 5–7 days.

A diagnostic algorithm for the noninvasive diagnosis of clinically suspected venous thrombosis is shown. If venous ultrasonography is not available, an IPG should be done, or the diagnosis should be confirmed with ascending venography. If IPG is used, a negative test result should be confirmed with venography in patients with a high clinical suspicion because about 50% of these patients have venous thrombosis.

DIAGNOSIS OF PULMONARY EMBOLISM

The clinical diagnosis of pulmonary embolism is as nonspecific as the diagnosis of venous thrombosis, necessitating objective tests. However, pulmonary embolism is more difficult to diagnose than venous thrombosis. The diagnosis is confirmed in less than one-half of patients with clinically suspected pulmonary embolism.[23,46]

The chest radiograph is not specific for pulmonary embolism and may show no abnormality. However, it is useful to exclude other causes for the presenting symptoms (e.g., pneumothorax) and is essential for interpreting the lung scan findings. Like the chest radiograph, the electrocardiogram (ECG) is frequently normal or shows nonspecific abnormalities. However in the appropriate clinical setting, ECG evidence of right ventricular strain is strongly suggestive of pulmonary embolism.

Perfusion lung scanning is useful because a normal scan excludes the diagnosis of pulmonary embolism, whereas a large perfusion defect that is not matched on the ventilation scan is highly suggestive of pulmonary embolism. Other lung scan findings, which are seen in about 70% of patients with abnormal perfusion scans, cannot be used either to rule out or to rule in pulmonary embolism. It is these patients who require pulmonary angiography or objective tests for venous thrombosis. Tests for venous thrombosis are useful because 70% of pulmonary emboli are associated with venographically detected DVT of the legs.

Clinical Manifestations

Most pulmonary emboli are clinically silent. Dyspnea is the most frequently reported symptom.[46,47] Chest pain is common and is usually pleuritic in nature, but it may be substernal and

CLINICALLY SUSPECTED VENOUS THROMBOSIS

A practical noninvasive approach for the diagnosis of clinically suspected deep vein thrombosis (DVT) using serial venous ultrasonography.[a]

Venous ultrasound (VUS)

Negative → Positive

Negative → Repeat VUS

Positive → Treatment

Repeat VUS → Becomes positive / Remains negative

Becomes positive → Treatment

Remains negative → Clinically significant DVT excluded

[a]If noninvasive testing is unavailable, venography should be performed.

compressing. Hemoptysis is a less frequent feature of pulmonary embolism.[23,46,47]

The physical signs of pulmonary embolism are nonspecific. Syncope is usually associated with massive pulmonary embolism and is caused by a reduction in cardiac output. This in turn results in hypotension and transient impairment of cerebral blood flow.

Although 70% of patients with pulmonary embolism have venographic evidence of thrombosis at presentation,[23] <20% of these patients have leg symptoms.[23] Massive pulmonary embolism causes tachypnea, tachycardia, cyanosis, and hypotension. Cardiac examination may indicate a right ventricular heave, a loud pulmonary second sound, and a gallop rhythm. Physical examination of the chest may be normal, or nonspecific abnormalities may be detected. Patients with pulmonary infarction or atelectasis may have reduced movement of the affected portion of the chest. Signs of pulmonary consolidation or atelectasis, a pleural friction rub, crackles or a pleural effusion may be evident, and low-grade fever may be present.

Differential Diagnosis

The differential diagnosis of shortness of breath includes atelectasis, pneumothorax, pneumonia, acute bronchitis, acute bronchiolitis, acute bronchial obstruction due to mucous plugging or bronchoconstriction, and acute pulmonary edema. The differential diagnosis of pleuritic chest pain includes pneumonia, viral pleurisy, chest wall pain from trauma or viral infection, pericarditis, and pleural inflammation caused by an immune disorder.

Diagnostic Tests

The diagnostic tests for pulmonary embolism include pulmonary angiography and ventilation/perfusion lung scanning.

Pulmonary Angiography

Pulmonary angiography is the reference standard for establishing the presence or absence of pulmonary embolism.[48] Selective angiography and magnification views improve resolution and reduce the risk associated with the procedure.[48] When adequately performed, a negative pulmonary angiogram excludes the diagnosis of pulmonary embolism.[48] However, unless the tertiary pulmonary arteries are visualized in a patient with a small perfusion defect, the diagnosis of pulmonary embolism cannot be excluded.

Arrhythmias, cardiac perforation, cardiac arrest, and hypersensitivity reactions to contrast medium occur in ≤3–4% of patients undergoing pulmonary angiography.[49] Patients with a history of allergy to radiopaque dye should not undergo pulmonary angiography.

Lung Scan

The lung scan consists of both a perfusion and a ventilation component. For the perfusion component, particles of isotopically labeled microaggregates of human albumin are injected intravenously and become trapped in the pulmonary capillary bed. Their distribution reflects lung blood flow and is recorded with an external photoscanner. A normal perfusion scan excludes pulmonary embolism, while an abnormal perfusion scan is nonspecific.[23,47,50]

Ventilation lung scanning is performed using either radioactive gases or aerosols that are inhaled and exhaled by the patient, while a gamma camera records the distribution of radioactivity within the alveolar gas exchange units. The purpose of ventilation imaging is to improve the specificity of perfusion scanning for the diagnosis of pulmonary embolism. When ventilation scanning was initially introduced, it was assumed that ventilation would be preserved in areas of reduced perfusion caused by pulmonary embolism (so-called ventilation/perfusion mismatch), whereas ventilation would be abnormal when perfusion defects occur as a consequence of primary abnormalities of ventilation (ventilation/perfusion match). This assumption has proved to be only partially correct.[23,47,50]

Diagnostic Approaches

Patients with large perfusion defects (one or more segments or more extensive defects) and a ventilation mismatch have a 90% probability of pulmonary embolism (Fig. 123-2). However, the frequency of pulmonary embolism is not sufficiently low to rule out pulmonary embolism in patients with a large ventilation/perfusion match, and in those with small perfusion defects.[23,47,50] As a result, patients with these lung scan findings require further investigation with either pulmonary angiography or an objective test for venous thrombosis. Although a positive venogram or compression ultrasound can be used to make the diagnosis of venous thromboembolism in a patient with an abnormal perfusion scan, a negative result cannot be used to exclude venous thrombosis because the thrombus may have completely embolized to the lungs.[23,47]

A diagnostic algorithm for the management of clinically suspected pulmonary embolism is shown. Following a history and physical examination, ECG, and chest radiograph, all patients should undergo ventilation/perfusion lung scanning. A negative

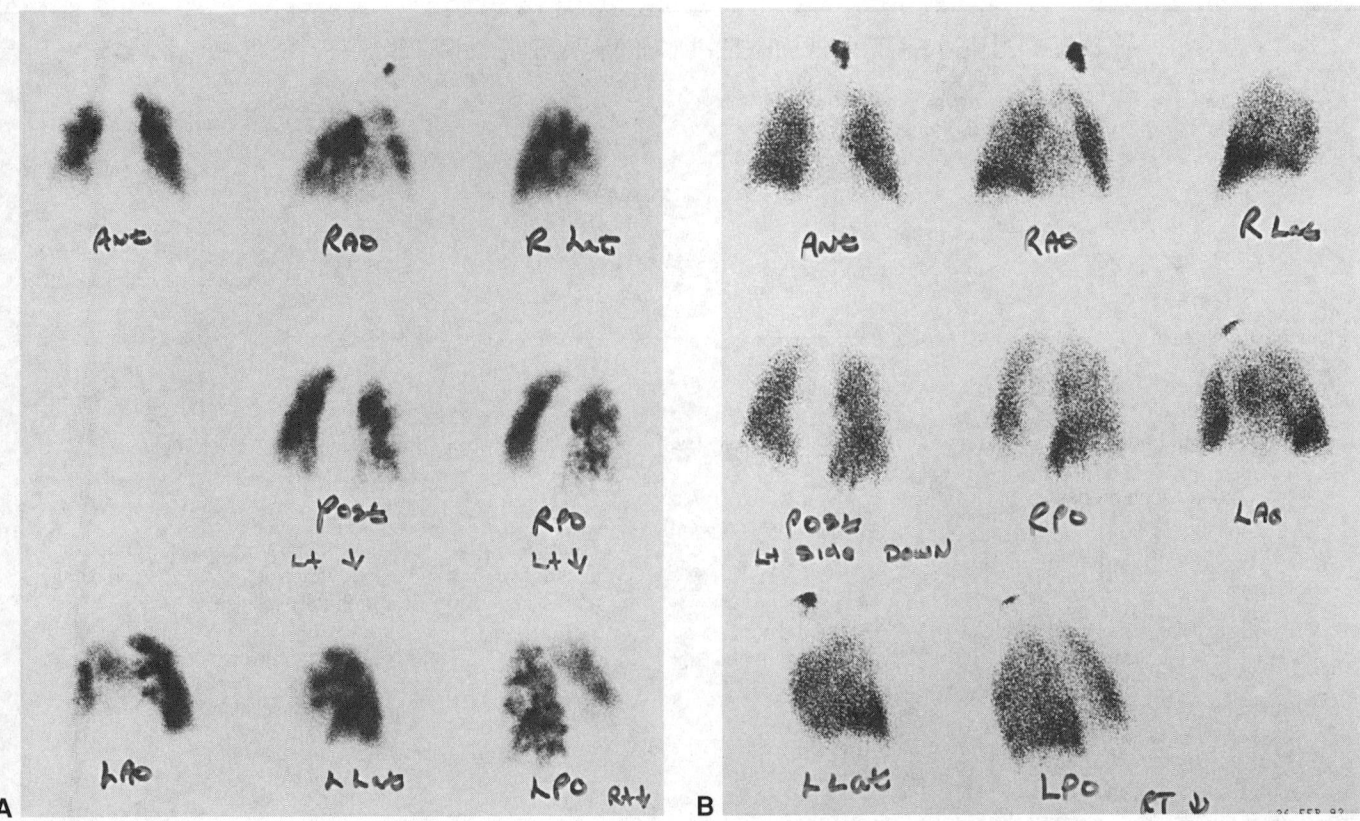

Fig. 123-2. (A & B) Multiple segmental and subsegmental defects. Perfusion scans that are unmatched by the ventilation scan suggest high probability of pulmonary embolism. *(Figure continues.)*

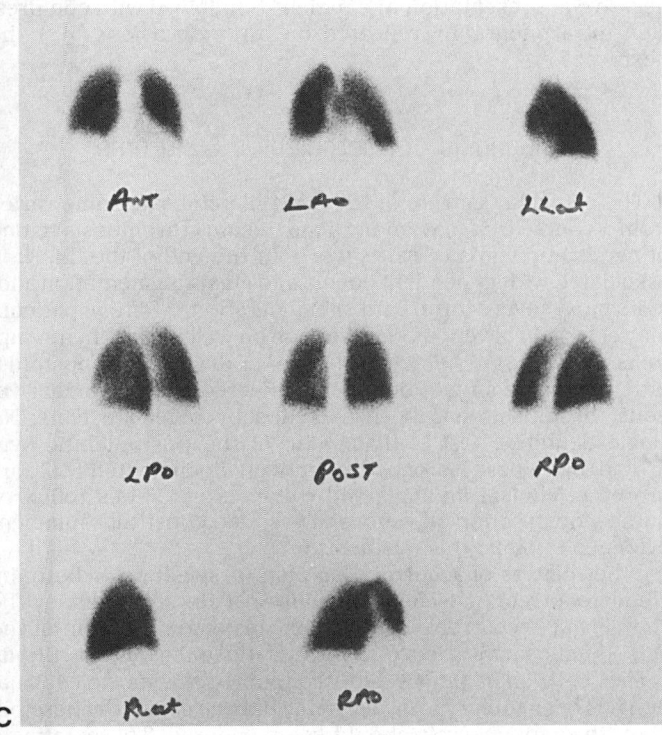

Fig. 123-2 *(Continued).* **(C)** Normal perfusion scan.

perfusion lung scan rules out clinically significant pulmonary embolism, and anticoagulant therapy is withheld. If the perfusion scan demonstrates one or more segmental (or larger) defects, and ventilation to these regions is normal, the diagnosis of pulmonary embolism is made. Although a ventilation/perfusion mismatch supports a diagnosis of pulmonary embolism, a ventilation/perfusion match does not exclude pulmonary embolism, and further objective testing is required in these patients. Similarly, the diagnosis of pulmonary embolism cannot be excluded in patients with small perfusion defects (one or more subsegmental defects) or in those with indeterminate lung scan findings (where the perfusion defects correspond to abnormalities on chest radiograph). In these cases, bilateral venography, venous ultrasonography, or IPG could be performed. If DVT is documented, anticoagulant therapy can be started, obviating the need for pulmonary angiography. However, if these tests are negative, pulmonary angiography is required in patients with a high clinical suspicion of pulmonary embolism. For those with a lower pretest likelihood of pulmonary embolism, an alternative strategy is to withhold anticoagulants and to perform serial noninvasive tests to detect ongoing venous thrombosis.

DIAGNOSIS OF RECURRENT VENOUS THROMBOSIS AND THE POSTPHLEBITIC SYNDROME

Most patients with a past history of venous thrombosis in whom new-onset leg pain develops do not have recurrent DVT when investigated with the appropriate diagnostic tests. Some of these patients have the postphlebitic syndrome, while in others the pain is unrelated to venous thrombosis.[51]

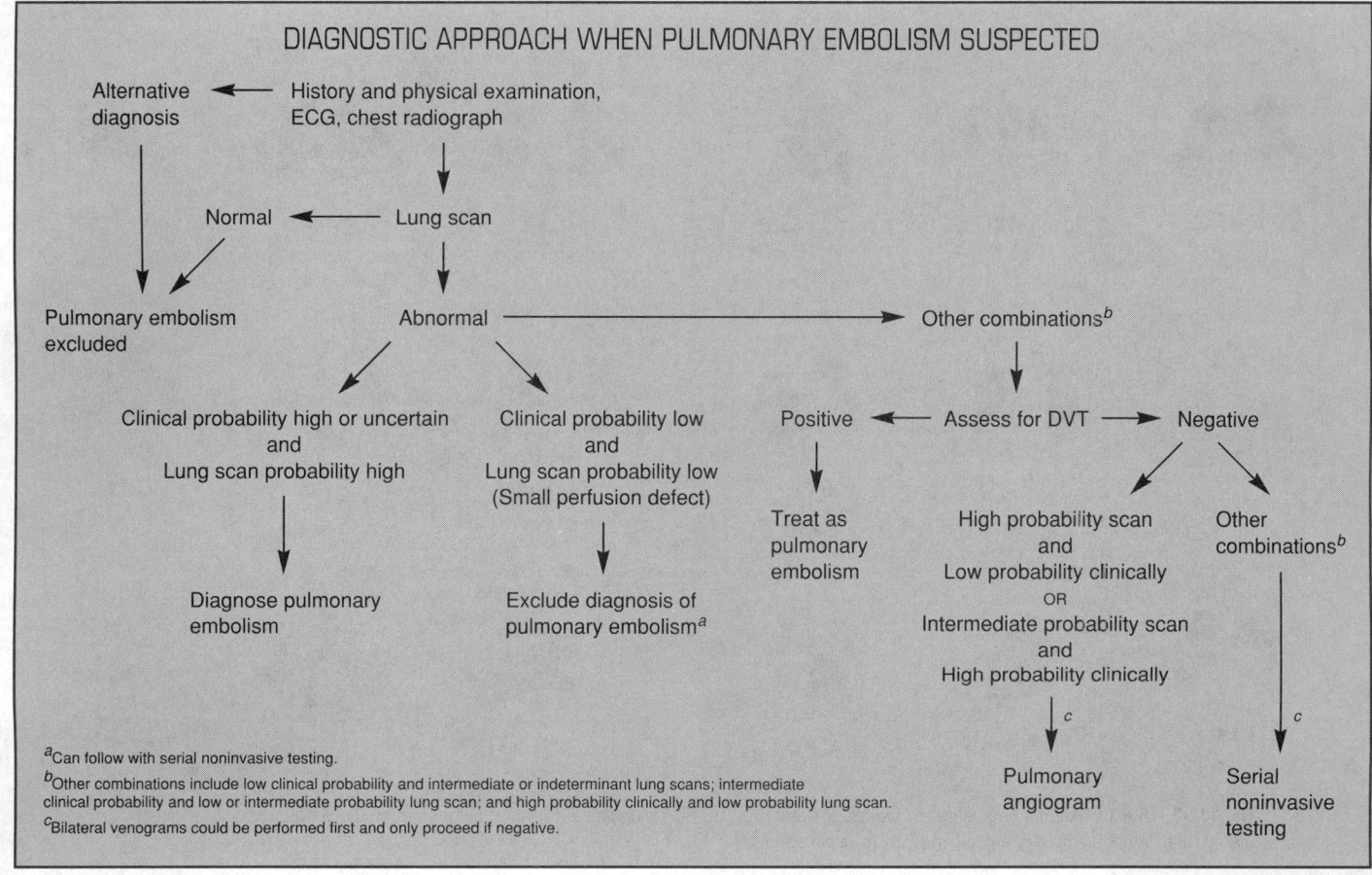

DIAGNOSTIC APPROACH WHEN PULMONARY EMBOLISM SUSPECTED

[a]Can follow with serial noninvasive testing.
[b]Other combinations include low clinical probability and intermediate or indeterminant lung scans; intermediate clinical probability and low or intermediate probability lung scan; and high probability clinically and low probability lung scan.
[c]Bilateral venograms could be performed first and only proceed if negative.

Diagnosis of Acute Recurrent Venous Thrombosis

The diagnosis of acute recurrent venous thrombosis is difficult because the clinical manifestations of recurrence are nonspecific. In addition, all of the validated diagnostic tests for acute venous thrombosis have limitations in this setting because the venous occlusion produced by the initial episode of venous thrombosis makes it difficult to identify new abnormalities.

Our approach to the diagnosis of clinically suspected recurrent venous thrombosis is to use a combination of IPG, compression ultrasonography, and venography. Once anticoagulants are discontinued, the patient undergoes serial IPG and compression ultrasonography at 3–6-month intervals until the tests normalize. Although the IPG normalizes more frequently than venous ultrasonography, both tests are useful because they provide results that can be used for comparison, should the patient present with recurrent symptoms.

The diagnostic algorithm for patients with suspected recurrent venous thrombosis is shown. Both IPG and compression ultrasonography are performed. If either test is positive, and the previous result was negative, the diagnosis of recurrence is made. Similarly, if venous ultrasonography shows more extensive thrombosis than that seen on previous examinations, the diagnosis of recurrent disease can also be established. However, if both IPG and venous ultrasonography are positive, and the previous tests were positive as well, a venogram is performed. If this shows a new intraluminal filling defect or evidence of thrombus extension when compared with the previous venogram, a diagnosis of recurrence is made. However, if no new defect is found, the diagnosis is based on clinical features. Finally, if both the IPG and venous ultrasound are negative at presentation, the patient is followed with compression ultrasonography repeated on three occasions over the next week.

Diagnosis of Postphlebitic Syndrome

The clinical spectrum of the postphlebitic syndrome varies from a course that may mimic acute venous thrombosis to one of persistent leg pain that is worse at the end of the day. It is associated with dependent edema and stasis pigmentation and, in its most severe form, with skin ulceration.[52] Rarely, patients may complain of venous claudication on walking.[53] When symptoms are acute or subacute in onset, a diagnosis of postphlebitic syndrome should only be considered after recurrent venous thrombosis has been excluded by objective tests. No single definitive test is diagnostic of the postphlebitic syndrome, but a past history of objectively documented DVT, appropriate clinical findings, and evidence of venous reflux or outflow obstruction on venous ultrasound constitute sufficient evidence to make this diagnosis.

Other causes of recurrent leg pain or swelling, or both, include recurrent muscle strain, internal derangement of the knee or hip, recurrent cellulitis, extrinsic compression of the vein, lumbosacral disc disease, sciatic pain, and factitious causes of leg pain and swelling. For some patients, no explanation has been found for the leg pain; in these cases, the possibility of thromboneurosis should be considered. These patients may complain of leg pain and tenderness that is disproportionate to the physical findings, or they may present with highly atypical symptoms. In its most severe form, thromboneurosis may be incapacitating because of fear of recurrent venous

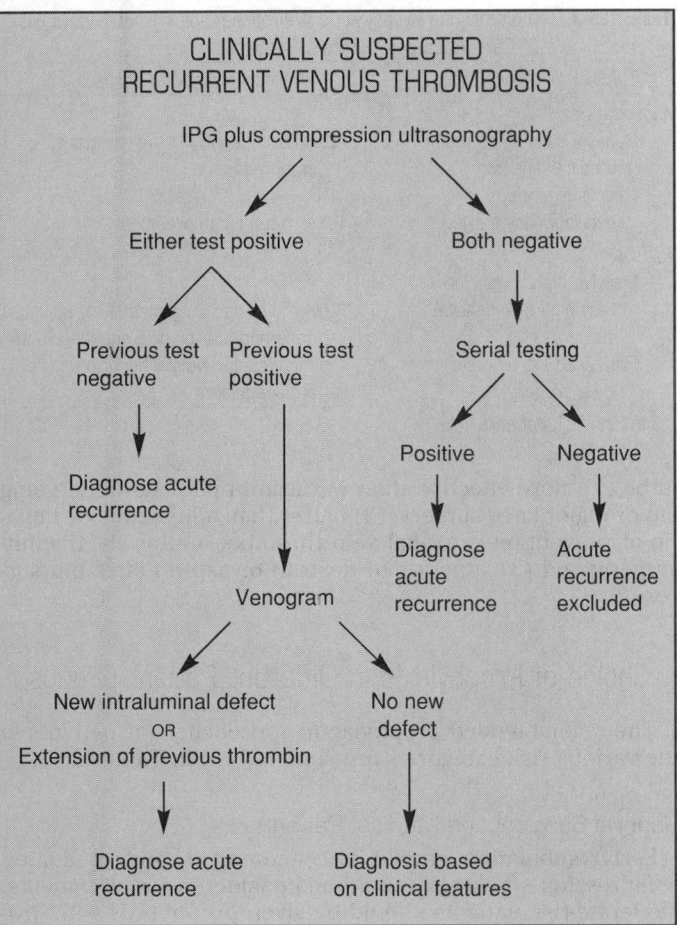

CLINICALLY SUSPECTED
RECURRENT VENOUS THROMBOSIS

IPG plus compression ultrasonography

Either test positive · Both negative

Previous test negative · Previous test positive · Serial testing

Diagnose acute recurrence

Venogram

Positive · Negative

Diagnose acute recurrence · Acute recurrence excluded

New intraluminal defect OR Extension of previous thrombin · No new defect

Diagnose acute recurrence · Diagnosis based on clinical features

Table 123-2. Risk Categories for Venous Thromboembolism

Risk Category	Risk of Venous Thromboemblism (%)		
	Calf Vein Thrombosis	Proximal Vein Thrombosis	Fatal Pulmonary Embolism
High risk	40–80	10–20	1–5
General surgery in patients >40 years with recent history of DVT or pulmonary embolism			
Extensive pelvic or abdominal surgery for malignant disease			
Major orthopaedic surgery of lower limbs			
Moderate risk[a]	10–40	2–10	0.1–0.7
General surgery in patients >40 years lasting ≥30 min			
Immobilization with major medical illness, including stroke cardiac disease, chronic respiratory disease, bowel disease and malignancy			

[a] Risk is increased by advancing age, malignancy, prolonged immobility, varicose veins, and cardiac failure.

compression stockings,[57,60] oral anticoagulants,[54,57,58] intravenous dextran,[54] adjusted-dose subcutaneous heparin,[59] or low-molecular-weight heparins.[58,61] Antiplatelet agents, such as aspirin, are relatively ineffective for preventing venous thromboembolism.[54,57,58]

Prophylactic Therapy

Low-Dose Subcutaneous Heparin

Heparin prevents thrombosis by catalyzing the inhibition of thrombin and factor Xa by AT III (see Ch. 121). Heparin is given subcutaneously at a dose of 5,000 U 2 hours prior to surgery and is then continued postoperatively at a dose of 5,000 U bid–tid. Low-dose heparin prophylaxis does not require laboratory monitoring and is simple and convenient to administer. It is the method of choice for moderate-risk general surgical and medical patients and it reduces the risk of venous thromboembolism by 50–70%.[54,56–58] When used in these doses, heparin is safe and free of serious bleeding complications but, because of the potential for minor bleeding, it should not be used in patients undergoing cerebral, eye, or spinal surgery. Although low-dose heparin is effective in patients undergoing elective hip surgery and reduces the incidence of venous thrombosis by about 40%, it is less effective than warfarin, adjusted-dose heparin,[59] and low-molecular-weight heparin.[58,61] Low-dose heparin has not been shown to be effective in patients with hip fracture or in those undergoing major knee surgery.

Intermittent Pneumatic Compression

Intermittent pneumatic compression of the legs enhances blood flow in the deep veins and increases blood fibrinolytic activity.[54] It is the method of choice for preventing venous thrombosis in patients undergoing neurosurgery[60] and prostatic surgery,[62] is effective in patients undergoing major knee surgery,[63] and is as effective as low-dose heparin in patients undergoing abdominal surgery.[57] Intermittent pneumatic leg

thrombosis or death. Frequently, these patients have a history of multiple hospital admissions for treatment of recurrent venous thrombosis; many are on long-term anticoagulant therapy, and some have had caval interruption procedures. Thromboneurosis may have an iatrogenic component, as the fear of recurrent thrombosis is reinforced each time the attending physician admits the patient to hospital and orders treatment on the basis of clinical suspicion alone. To prevent this problem, it is important to confirm clinical suspicion of acute venous thrombosis (either the first episode or recurrent episodes) by appropriate objective tests. For some patients, the fear of thrombosis is only relieved after suspected recurrent episodes of venous thrombosis have been excluded by appropriate tests on multiple occasions.

VENOUS THROMBOEMBOLISM PROPHYLAXIS

Pulmonary embolism is the most common preventable cause of death in hospital.[54] Hospitalized patients can be classified as either at low, moderate, or high risk of the development of venous thromboembolism[54] (Table 123-2). In the absence of prophylaxis, the frequency of postoperative fatal pulmonary embolism ranges from 0.1–0.8% in patients undergoing elective general surgery, to 0.3–1.7% in patients undergoing elective hip surgery, and to 4–7% in patients undergoing emergency hip surgery.[54] Effective prophylaxis is available for most high-risk groups, and is very cost effective.[55]

Prophylaxis is directed at either suppressing activation of blood coagulation or preventing venous stasis. These objectives can be achieved by using one of several proven prophylactic approaches: low-dose subcutaneous heparin,[54,56,57] intermittent pneumatic compression of the legs,[54,57] graduated

compression is virtually free of clinically important side effects and is particularly useful in patients at high risk of bleeding.

Graduated Compression Stockings

Graduated compression stockings also reduce venous stasis in the legs and are effective for preventing postoperative venous thrombosis in general surgical patients,[57] and in medical or surgical patients with neurologic disorders, including paralysis of the lower limbs.[60] In surgical patients, the combination of graduated compression stockings and low-dose heparin is significantly more effective than low-dose heparin alone.[64,65] Graduated compression stockings are inexpensive and should be considered in all high-risk surgical patients, even if other forms of prophylaxis are used.

Oral Anticoagulants

When administered in doses that prolong the prothrombin time to an International Normalized Ratio (INR) of 2.0, oral anticoagulants effectively prevent postoperative venous thromboembolism in all risk categories.[54,58] Oral anticoagulants can be given preoperatively, at operation, or in the early postoperative period. When begun at surgery or during the early postoperative period, the anticoagulant effect is not achieved until the third or fourth postoperative day. Nevertheless, when used in this fashion, oral anticoagulants are effective in very high-risk patient groups, including patients with hip fractures.[66] However, prophylaxis with oral anticoagulants is relatively inconvenient because careful laboratory monitoring is necessary.

Intravenous Dextran

Dextran 40 is usually given intravenously at a daily dose of 500 ml over 4–6 hours. Treatment is started at surgery and is continued for 2–5 days postoperatively.[54,58] Although an effective form of prophylaxis, dextran is inconvenient, can cause fluid overload in patients with cardiovascular impairment, and increases the risk of postoperative bleeding. In addition, dextran is less effective than warfarin[67] and low-molecular-weight heparin.[68] Given these limitations, dextran is rarely used for prophylaxis.

Adjusted-Dose Subcutaneous Heparin

In this regimen, heparin is given subcutaneously at a dose of 3,500 U tid and is started 2 days prior to surgery. The heparin dose is then adjusted to maintain the activated partial thromboplastin time (PTT) at the upper limit of the normal range. Leyvarz and associates[59] and Green and associates[69] have reported that adjusted-dose heparin regimens are more effective than fixed low-dose heparin in patients undergoing elective hip surgery and in those with spinal cord injury. When the heparin dose was adjusted to prolong the postoperative PTT into the upper normal range, no increase in bleeding was apparent.[59] However, a heparin dose that prolonged the PTT to 1.5 times normal did cause excessive bleeding.[69]

Low-Molecular-Weight Heparins

Although the low-molecular-weight heparins are widely used in Europe, they have only recently been approved in the United States and Canada. Low-molecular-weight heparin is an effective and safe form of prophylaxis in certain high-risk groups[61]: elective hip surgery,[61] hip fracture, major general surgery, major knee surgery, spinal injury, and stroke. Low-molecular-weight heparin is more effective than standard low-dose heparin in general surgical patients, in patients undergoing elective hip surgery, and in patients with stroke or spinal injury.[61] In addition, low-molecular-weight heparin has also been shown

Table 123-3. Recommended Prophylactic Approaches for the Alternative Risk Categories and Different Surgical Groups

Risk Category	Recommended Approaches[a]
Moderate risk	
General surgery or major medical illness	Low-dose heparin or intermittent compression
Neurosurgery or genitourinary surgery	Intermittent compression
High risk[a]	
Elective hip surgery or very high risk general surgery	Low-molecular-weight heparin, adjusted dose heparin, or oral anticoagulants
Fractured hip or major knee surgery	Low-molecular-weight heparin or oral anticoagulants

[a] In high-risk patients.

to be (1) more effective than warfarin in patients undergoing hip or major knee surgery, (2) better than adjusted-dose heparin at preventing proximal vein thrombosis after elective hip surgery, and (3) superior to dextran or aspirin after hip surgery.[61]

Choice of Prophylaxis in Different Patient Groups

The recommended prophylactic approaches for patients in the various risk categories are summarized in Table 123-3.

General Surgical and Medical Patients

Early ambulation should be encouraged, and graduated compression stockings should be considered for all patients. Moderate-risk patients should be given prophylaxis with low-dose heparin. If anticoagulants are contraindicated because of an unusually high risk of bleeding, intermittent pneumatic compression should be used. Patients at very high risk (e.g., those with recent venous thrombosis) should receive low-molecular-weight heparin, oral anticoagulants, or adjusted-dose heparin.

Hip Surgery

Low-molecular-weight heparin, oral anticoagulants, or adjusted-dose heparin is effective in patients undergoing hip surgery. In direct comparisons, low-molecular-weight heparin is more effective than warfarin in preventing thrombosis, and is better than adjusted-dose heparin at preventing proximal vein thrombosis.

Major Knee Surgery

Although low-molecular-weight heparin and intermittent pneumatic compression are effective in preventing venous thrombosis in patients undergoing major knee surgery, low-molecular-weight heparin is more convenient and will probably become the treatment of choice.

Genitourinary Surgery, Neurosurgery, and Ocular Surgery

Intermittent pneumatic compression, with or without static graduated compression stockings, is effective and does not increase the risk of bleeding.

Stroke and Spinal Injury

Low-molecular-weight heparin is more effective than low-dose standard heparin in these patient groups. It is the prophylactic method of choice.

THERAPY FOR VENOUS THROMBOEMBOLISM

The objectives of treating patients with venous thromboembolism are to prevent death from pulmonary embolism, to reduce morbidity from the acute event, to minimize postphlebitic symptoms, and to prevent thromboembolic pulmonary hypertension. All of these goals can be accomplished by adequate anticoagulant therapy.

Preventing Complications of Venous Thromboembolism

Death Due to Pulmonary Embolism

Anticoagulants are effective in reducing mortality from pulmonary embolism.[70] Vena caval interruption, usually with an inferior vena caval filter, should be considered when anticoagulant therapy is contraindicated because of the risk of previous or life-threatening hemorrhage.[70] Far less commonly, caval interruption is used when anticoagulant therapy has failed.

Thrombolytic therapy with streptokinase, u-PA, or t-PA is more effective than heparin alone in improving the angiographic defects produced by pulmonary emboli[70] and may be better than heparin at preventing death in patients with massive pulmonary embolism associated with shock.[71,72] On the basis of these findings, thrombolytic therapy is the treatment of choice for patients with massive pulmonary embolism or in those with underlying cardiac or pulmonary disease in whom even a small or moderate embolus may be life-threatening.

Thromboendarterectomy is effective in selected cases of chronic thromboembolic pulmonary hypertension with proximal pulmonary arterial obstruction.[73] Urgent pulmonary embolectomy is usually reserved for patients with a saddle embolism lodged in the main pulmonary artery or for those with massive embolism whose blood pressure cannot be maintained despite thrombolytic therapy and vasopressor agents.[70]

Anticoagulant Therapy

Anticoagulants are the mainstay of treatment for most patients with venous thromboembolism. A recent study in patients with proximal vein thrombosis highlights the importance of early heparin therapy.[74]

Prospective randomized trials have compared the safety and effectiveness of heparin given by either continuous intravenous infusion, intermittent intravenous injection, or subcutaneous injection. Although continuous intravenous heparin infusion[70] produces less bleeding than occurs with intermittent intravenous injections, heparin delivery by intermittent subcutaneous injections appears to be as safe and efficacious as continuous intravenous heparin infusion for the treatment of patients with venous thrombosis.[70,75] Regardless of whether heparin is given by continuous intravenous infusion or by subcutaneous injection, the doses must be sufficient to produce an adequate anticoagulant response.

Heparin has a half-life that varies considerably among different individuals.[76] After a single intravenous injection, an initial rapid disappearance occurs due to a saturable clearance mechanism, followed by a more gradual linear clearance[77] with a mean heparin half-life of approximately 60 minutes. Whereas intravenous heparin produces an immediate anticoagulant effect, peak heparin levels are not achieved until 3 hours after subcutaneous injection, but the levels will remain therapeutic for ≥12 hours, depending on the dose.

Heparin therapy can be monitored using global tests of blood coagulation, such as the activated clotting time and the PTT, or by heparin assays that measure the ability of heparin to accelerate the inactivation of factor Xa or thrombin. It is important to achieve an adequate anticoagulant response because

the risk of recurrent venous thromboembolism is increased if insufficient heparin is given. Accordingly, the PTT should be maintained above a ratio equivalent to a heparin level of 0.3 U/ml as determined by measuring the anti-factor Xa activity. For most currently used PTT reagents, this is equivalent to an PTT ratio of 1.8 times the control value. Thus, the recommended therapeutic range is a PTT ratio of 1.8 to 2.5.[78] Although higher heparin doses can be used, the upper limit of the therapeutic range should not be exceeded because there is a direct relationship between the daily heparin dose and the risk of bleeding.[79]

Heparin was previously administered for a period of 7–10 days. Oral anticoagulants were started after 3–5 days and overlapped with heparin for 4–5 days. The period of overlap is necessary because the antithrombotic effects of oral anticoagulants are delayed.[80,81] Two recent studies have demonstrated that 9–10 days of heparin therapy is no better than a 4–5-day course of heparin with overlapping warfarin.[79] Since neither study included many patients with major pulmonary embolism or extensive ileofemoral vein thrombosis, it would be prudent to use heparin for ≥7 days in these patients.

After an initial course of heparin therapy, patients with venous thromboembolism require continuing anticoagulant therapy for weeks or months to prevent recurrence.[26,27] Both therapeutic doses of subcutaneous heparin and oral anticoagulants are effective for this indication. Although adjusted-dose heparin produces less bleeding than full-dose warfarin (target INR of 3.5–5.0) in this setting,[28] less intense warfarin therapy (target INR of 2.0–3.0) is just as effective as the higher-intensity regimen but produces significantly less bleeding.

Preventing Morbidity from the Postphlebitic Syndrome

The postphlebitic syndrome is a major cause of morbidity. Thus, at long-term follow-up, ≤50% of patients with a history of proximal vein thrombosis develop postphlebitic syndrome. Surgical thrombectomy does not prevent the disorder because most thrombi recur after surgical removal.[70,82] The ability of thrombolytic therapy to prevent the postphlebitic syndrome has been evaluated to a limited extent. Streptokinase treatment produces complete lysis of acute venous thrombi in 30–40% of cases, and causes partial lysis in an additional 30%.[70] By contrast, complete lysis of venous thrombi occurs in <10% of patients treated with heparin.[70] It is estimated that thrombolysis occurs 3.7 times more often in patients treated with streptokinase than in those given heparin, but major bleeding occurs 2.9 times more frequently with streptokinase.[70] Although five randomized studies have reported that the frequency of the postphlebitic syndrome is significantly higher in patients treated with heparin than in those given streptokinase,[70] one trial[83] reported that streptokinase- and heparin-treated patients had similar manifestations of the postphlebitic state after 5 years of follow-up management.

Two recent studies have reported that the incidence of the postphlebitic syndrome is reduced by the early use of graduated compression stockings.[70] Accordingly, patients with proximal vein thrombosis should be encouraged to wear these stockings at the first sign of leg swelling.

Prevention of Late Effects of Pulmonary Embolism

Clinically significant pulmonary hypertension is an uncommon complication of pulmonary embolism. In randomized trials comparing heparin with either streptokinase or u-PA for the treatment of patients with acute pulmonary embolism, thrombolytic therapy produced greater improvement in lung

THERAPY FOR VENOUS THROMBOSIS

Most patients with proximal vein thrombosis, calf vein thrombosis, and pulmonary embolism should be treated with high-dose heparin followed by less intense oral anticoagulant therapy (INR of 2.0–3.0) for a total of 3 months. High-dose heparin can be given either by continuous intravenous infusion or by twice-daily subcutaneous injection. For intravenous heparin therapy, a bolus of 5,000 U should be followed by a continuous intravenous infusion at a dose of 1,300 U/hr. The initial dose of subcutaneous heparin should be 35,000 U/day given in two divided doses. Because of its delayed onset of action after subcutaneous injection, a 5,000 U IV bolus of heparin should be given together with the first subcutaneous injection in high-risk patients. Heparin should be administered for at total of 4–7 days, and 10 mg of coumadin should be given 24–48 hours after starting heparin treatment.

The dose of heparin should be adjusted to maintain the PTT at 1.8–2.5 times control. To monitor heparin given by continuous intravenous infusion, the PTT should be measured 6 hours after the bolus dose, so that it reflects the anticoagulant effects of the infusion. If twice daily subcutaneous heparin is given, a mid-interval PTT should be measured (i.e., 6 hours after the injection).

The INR is used to monitor oral anticoagulant therapy, and the dose of warfarin should be adjusted to achieve an INR of 2.0–3.0. Heparin can be discontinued when the INR has been therapeutic for 2 successive days.

Indefinite anticoagulant therapy should be considered for patients with continuing risk factors or for those with recurrent venous thromboembolism. Thrombolytic therapy is indicated in patients with major pulmonary embolism (i.e., those with hemodynamic compromise) and in patients with recent proximal vein thrombosis in whom there are no contraindications. If thrombolytic therapy is limited to these indications, about 10% of patients who present with acute venous thromboembolism will be eligible.

scan-detected perfusion defects than heparin during the first week. However, no differences were apparent in the lung scan findings at 2 weeks, 3 months, and 1 year.[84] Subsequent long-term follow-up evaluation in small subgroups of these patients reported that pulmonary capillary blood volume and both pulmonary vascular resistance and functional status were significantly better in patients treated with fibrinolytic therapy than in those given heparin.[70]

Moser and colleagues[73] have reported their experience with surgical pulmonary endarterectomy in carefully selected patients with chronic thromboembolic pulmonary hypertension. Most patients with obstruction of their proximal pulmonary arteries show impressive improvement following endarterectomy.

Side Effects, Cost, and Clinical Value of Thrombolytic Therapy

Bleeding occurs more frequently with thrombolytic therapy than with heparin.[70,85] The risk of hemorrhage increases with the duration of thrombolytic infusion and usually occurs at a site of previous surgery or trauma. Intracranial hemorrhage occurs in about 1% of patients at risk—about twice as frequently as with heparin treatment.

VENOUS THROMBOSIS IN UNUSUAL SITES

Subclavian or Axillary Vein Thrombosis

Although thrombosis of the subclavian or axillary veins most frequently occurs as a complication of a chronic indwelling catheter, it may also occur as a consequence of local malignancy, and is a well-documented complication of mastectomy and radiotherapy.[86] In many cases the cause is uncertain, and idiopathic subclavian or axillary vein thrombosis often occurs in young muscular subjects and may be preceded by repetitive, strenuous activity that involves the affected arm. Some of these patients have a fixed stenosis of the subclavian vein at the level of the inferior border of the clavicle that can be caused by external compression of the subclavian vein by the clavicle and the subclavius muscle or the costocoracoid ligament. Occasionally, subclavian or axillary vein thrombosis occurs in patients with congenital deficiency of AT III, protein C, or protein S or in patients with antiphospholipid antibodies. Finally, thrombosis of the axillary or subclavian vein, or the superior vena cava is a rare complication of perivenous endocardial pacing using an implantable system[87,88] and may lead to fatal pulmonary embolism.[88]

Patients with subclavian or axillary thrombosis develop pain in the axilla as well as edema and cyanosis of the arm. If thrombosis extends into the superior vena cava, the result can be edema and cyanosis of the face, neck, and upper extremities. Dilated superficial veins on the chest and arms appear after a number of days. Occasionally, asymptomatic thrombosis of the internal jugular vein accompanies subclavian vein thrombosis. The definitive diagnosis is made by venography, although venous ultrasonography may also be useful.

Subclavian or axillary vein thrombosis is usually treated with anticoagulants. Thrombolytic therapy also is effective and should be considered because it is estimated that more than two-thirds of patients with subclavian vein thrombosis will have persistent symptoms in the affected arm. However, subclavian vein stenosis that persists after lytic therapy may predispose to recurrence, limiting the benefits of this treatment modality.[89]

Mesenteric Vein Thrombosis

Mesenteric vein thrombosis is uncommon. In an extensive literature review,[90] only 367 patients with mesenteric vein thrombosis were identified. The disorder occurs most commonly in the sixth and seventh decades of life and affects segments of the small bowel (rarely the colon), leading to hemorrhagic infarction rather than gangrene. Bowel infarction often produces bloody ascites and adhesions frequently develop between the involved bowel and the omentum.

Many affected patients have associated disorders, such as thrombosis at other sites, inflammatory bowel disease, recent abdominal surgery, malignant disease, and portal hypertension. Mesenteric vein thrombosis may also complicate hypercoagulable states (such as AT III, protein C, or protein S deficiency), polycythemia vera, and the use of the oral conceptive pill[91] and it has also been reported in late pregnancy. In about 20% of cases, no underlying cause is found.

The clinical manifestations of mesenteric vein thrombosis include intermittent abdominal pain, abdominal distension in the later stages of the disorder, vomiting, diarrhea and melena. Although the diagnosis is often difficult, blood-stained ascitic fluid on abdominal paracentesis, and hemorrhagic bowel infarcts at peritoneoscopy are characteristic findings.

Management includes supportive care, and surgical resection followed by anticoagulant therapy. The mortality rate is about 20%, and recurrence occurs in ≤20% of cases.

Renal Vein Thrombosis

Renal vein thrombosis can occur as a complication of the nephrotic syndrome, possibly because AT III is lost in the urine, and is commonly seen in association with membranous glomerulonephritis.[92] Patients may be asymptomatic, present with mild symptoms of abdominal or back pain, or can develop severe flank pain and tenderness. Pulmonary embolism has been described as a relatively common complication of renal vein thrombosis. Anticoagulant therapy leads to gradual improvement in renal function tests, although patients may suffer from long-standing proteinuria. Thrombolytic therapy has been used successfully in a small number of patients with renal vein thrombosis.[93]

REFERENCES

1. Freiman DG: The structure of thrombi. p. 1123. In Colman RW, Hirsh J, Marder V, Salzman EW (eds): Hemostasis and Thrombosis: Basic Principles and Clinical Practice. 2nd Ed. JB Lippincott, Philadelphia, 1987
2. Esmon CT: Protein C: The regulation of natural anticoagulant pathways. Science 235:1348, 1987
3. Wiman B, Ljungberg B, Chmielewska J et al: The role of the fibrinolytic system in deep vein thrombosis. J Lab Clin Med 105:265, 1985
4. Bauer KA, Goodman TL, Kass BL et al: Elevated factor Xa activity in the blood of asymptomatic patients with congenital antithrombin deficiency. J Clin Invest 76:826, 1985
5. Bauer KA, Kass BL, ten Cate H et al: Factor IX is activated in vivo by the tissue factor mechanism. Blood 76:731, 1990
6. Stewart GJ, Ritchie WG, Lynch PR: Venous endothelial leukocytes. Am J Pathol 74:507, 1974
7. Gordon SG, Franks C, Lewis B: Cancer procoagulation A: a factor X activating procoagulant from malignant tissue. Thromb Res 6:127, 1975
8. Ogawa S, Gerlach H, Eposito C et al: Hypoxia mediates the barrier and coagulant function of cultured bovine endothelium. Increased monolayer permeability and induction of procoagulant properties. J Clin Invest 85:1090, 1990
9. Goodrich SM, Wood JE: Peripheral venous distensivity and velocity of venous blood flow during pregnancy or during oral contraceptive therapy. Am J Obstet Gynecol 90:740, 1964
10. Dittman WA, Majerus PW: Structure and function of thrombomdulin: a natural anticoagulant. Blood 75:329, 1990
11. Loskutoff DJ, Edgington TS: Synthesis of a fibrinolytic activator and inhibitor by endothelial cells. Proc Natl Acad Sci USA 74:3903, 1977
12. Moncada S, Palmer RMJ, Higgs EA: Prostacyclin and endothelium-derived relaxing factor: biological interactions and significance. p. 597. In Verstraete M, Vermylen J, Lijnen R, Arnout J (eds): Thrombosis and Haemostasis. International Society on Thrombosis and Haemostasis. Leuven University Press, Leuven, 1987
13. Heijboer H, Brandjes DPM, Buller HR et al: Deficiencies of coagulation-inhibiting and fibrinolytic proteins in outpatients with deep vein thrombosis. N Engl J Med 323:1512, 1990
14. Collen D: On the regulation and control of fibrinolysis. Thromb Haemost 43: 77, 1980
15. Prins MH, Hirsh J: A critical review of the evidence supporting a relationship between impaired fibrinolysis and venous thromboembolism. Arch Intern Med 151:1721, 1991
16. Menon IS, Peberdy M, Rannie RH et al: A comparative study of blood fibrinolytic activity in normal women, pregnant women and women on oral contraceptives. J Obstet Gynaecol Br Commonw 77:752, 1970
17. Ogston D, McAndrew GM: Fibrinolysis in obesity. Lancet 2:1205, 1964
18. Wille-Jorgensen M, Mortensen JZ, Madsen AG, Thorsen S: A family with reduced plasminogen activator activity in blood associated with recurrent venous thrombosis. Scand J Haematol 29:217, 1982
19. Johansson L, Hedner U, Nilsson IM: A family with thromboembolic disease associated with deficient fibrinolytic activity in vessel wall. J Intern Med 203: 477, 1978
20. Kakkar VV, Flanc C, Howe CT et al: Natural history of postoperative deep vein thrombosis. Lancet 2:230, 1969
21. Hirsh J, Lensing AWA: I. Natural history of minimal calf deep vein thrombosis. II. Rationale and results of thrombolytic therapy. J Vasc Surg (in press)
22. Doyle DJ, Turpie AGG, Hirsh J et al: Adjusted subcutaneous heparin or continuous intravenous heparin in patients with acute deep vein thrombosis: a randomized trial. Ann Intern Med 107:441, 1987
23. Hull RD, Hirsh J, Carter C et al: Pulmonary angiography, ventilation lung scanning and venography for clinically suspected pulmonary embolism with abnormal perfusion lung scan. Ann Intern Med 98:891, 1983
24. Shull KC, Nicolaides AN, Fernandes F et al: Significance of popliteal reflux in relation to ambulatory venous pressure and ulceration. Arch Surg 114:1304, 1979
25. Kakkar VV, Howe CT, Nicolaides AN et al: Deep vein thrombosis of the leg. Is there a "high risk group"? Am J Surg 120:527, 1970
26. Hull RD, Delmore T, Genton E et al: Warfarin sodium versus low-dose heparin in the long-term treatment of venous thrombosis. N Engl J Med 301:855, 1979
27. Lagerstadt CI, Fagher BO, Olsson CG et al: Need for long-term anticoagulant treatment in symptomatic calf-vein thrombosis. Lancet 2:515, 1985
28. Hull RD, Delmore T, Carter C et al: Adjusted subcutaneous heparin vs. warfarin sodium in the long-term treatment of venous thrombosis. N Engl J Med 306:189, 1982
29. Hull RD, Hirsh J, Jay RM et al: Different intensities of anticoagulation in the long-term treatment of proximal vein thrombosis. N Engl J Med 307:1676, 1982
30. Negus D: The post thrombotic syndrome. Ann R Coll Surg Engl 47:92, 1970
31. Cockett FB, Lea Thomas M, Negus D: Iliac vein compression—its relation to iliofemoral thrombosis and the post-thrombotic syndrome. Br Med J 2:14, 1967
32. Forbes CD, Lowe GDO: Clinical diagnosis. p. 9. In Hirsh J (ed): Venous Thrombosis and Pulmonary Embolism: Diagnostic Methods. Vol. 18. Churchill Livingstone, New York, 1987
33. Huisman MV, Buller HR, ten Cate CJ et al: Serial impedance plethysmography for suspected deep venous thrombosis in outpatients: the Amsterdam general practitioner study. N Engl J Med 314:823, 1986
34. Hull RD, Hirsh J, Carter C et al: Diagnostic efficacy of impedance plethysmography for clinically suspected deep-vein thrombosis: a randomized trial. Ann Intern Med 102:21, 1985
35. Heijboer H, Brandjes D, Lensing AWA et al: Efficacy of real-time B-mode ultrasonography versus impedance plethysmography in the diagnosis of deep vein thrombosis in symptomatic outpatients. Thromb Haemost 65:436, 1991
36. Heijboer H, Jongbloets LMM, Büller HR et al: The clinical utility of real-time compression ultrasound in the diagnostic management of patients with recurrent venous thrombosis. Acta Radiol Scand 33:297, 1992
37. Wells PS, Anderson DR, Lensing AWA et al: Evaluation of the accuracy of impedance plethysmography (IPG) and compression ultrasound (CUS) in outpatients with suspected deep vein thrombosis (DVT): a prospective paired design, abstracted. In the Fourteenth Congress of International Society on Thrombosis and Hemostasis, New York, July 4–9, 1993
38. Bettmann MA: Contrast phlebography. p. 20. In Hirsh J (ed): Venous Thrombosis and Pulmonary Embolism: Diagnostic Methods. Vol. 18. Churchill Livingstone, New York, 1987
39. Hull RD, van Aken WG, Hirsh J et al: Impedance plethysmography using the occlusive cuff technique in the diagnosis of venous thrombosis. Circulation 53:696, 1976
40. Wheeler HB, Pearson D, O'Connell D, Mullick SC: Impedance phlebography: technique, interpretation and results. Arch Surg 104:164, 1972
41. Hirsh J: Clinical utility of impedance plethysmography in the diagnosis of recurrent deep-vein thrombosis. Arch Intern Med 148:519, 1988
42. Anderson DR, Lensing AWA, Wells PS et al: Limitations of impedance plethysmography in the diagnosis of clinically suspected deep-vein thrombosis. Ann Intern Med 118:25, 1993
43. Lensing AWA, Prandoni P, Brandjes D et al: Detection of deep-vein thrombosis by real-time B-mode ultrasonography. N Engl J Med 320:342, 1989
44. Comerota AJ, Katz ML, Greenwald LL et al: Venous duplex imaging: should it replace hemodynamic tests for deep venous thrombosis? J Vasc Surg 11: 53, 1990
45. Cogo A, Lensing AWA, Prandoni P, Hirsh J: The distribution of thrombosis in patients with symptomatic deep-vein thrombosis: implications for simplifying the diagnostic process with compression ultrasonography. Arch Intern Med 153:2777, 1993
46. Bell WR, Simon TL, Demets DL: The clinical features of submissive and massive pulmonary emboli. Am J Med 62:355, 1977
47. Hull RD, Hirsh J, Carter C et al: Diagnostic value of ventilation-perfusion in patients with suspected pulmonary embolism and abnormal perfusion lung scans. Chest 88:819, 1985
48. Hirsh J, Bettman M. Coates G, Hull RD: Diagnosis of pulmonary embolism. p. 1322. In Colman RW, Hirsh J, Marder VJ, Salzman EW (eds): Hemostasis and Thrombosis: Basic Principles and Clinical Practice. 3rd Ed. JB Lippincott, Philadelphia, 1994
49. Mills SR, Jackson DC, Older RA, Heaston DK, Moore AV: The incidence, etiologies, and avoidance of complications of pulmonary angiography in a large series. Radiology 136:295, 1980
50. PIOPED Investigators: Value of the ventilation/perfusion scan in acute pulmo-

nary embolism: results of the prospective investigation of pulmonary embolism diagnosis (PIOPED). JAMA 263:2753, 1990

51. Hull RD, Carter C, Jay RM et al: The diagnosis of acute recurrent deep-vein thrombosis: a diagnostic challenge. Circulation 67:901, 1983

52. Owens JC: The post-phlebitic syndrome: management by conservative means. p. 369. In Bergman JJ, Yao JST (eds): Venous Problems. Year Book, Chicago, 1978

53. Tripolitis AJ, Milligan EG, Bodily KC et al: The physiology of venous claudication. Am J Surg 139:447, 1980

54. Gallus AS, Salzman EW, Hirsh J, Marder VJ: Prevention of venous thromboembolism. p. 1331. In Colman RW, Hirsh J, Marder VJ, Salzman EW (eds): Hemostasis and Thrombosis: Basic Principles and Clinical Practice. 3rd Ed. JB Lippincott, Philadelphia, 1994

55. Salzman EW, Davies GC: Prophylaxis of venous thromboembolism: analysis of cost effectiveness. Ann Surg 191:207, 1980

56. Collins R, Scrimgeour A, Yusuf S et al: Reduction in fatal pulmonary embolism and venous thrombosis by perioperative administration of subcutaneous heparin: overview of the results of randomized trials in general, orthopedic, and urologic surgery. N Engl J Med 318:1162, 1988

57. Colditz GA, Tuden RL, Oster G: Rates of venous thrombosis after general surgery: combined results of randomized clinical trials. Lancet 2:744, 1986

58. Hirsh J, Levine MN: Prevention of venous thrombosis in patients undergoing major orthopedic surgical procedures. Br J Clin Pract, suppl. 65. 43:2, 1989

59. Leyvarz PF, Richard J, Bachmann F et al: Adjusted versus fixed dose subcutaneous heparin in the prevention of deep vein thrombosis after total hip replacement. N Engl J Med 309:954, 1983

60. Turpie AGG, Hirsh J, Gent M et al: Prevention of deep vein thrombosis in potential neurosurgical patients: a randomized trial comparing graduated compression stockings alone or graduated compression stockings plus intermittent pneumata compression with control. Arch Intern Med 149:679, 1989

61. Hirsh J, Levine MN: Low molecular weight heparin. Blood 79:1, 1992

62. Coe NP, Collins REC, Klein LA et al: Prevention of deep vein thrombosis in urological patients: a controlled, randomized trial of low dose heparin and external pneumatic compression boots. Surgery 83:230, 1978

63. Hull RD, Delmore TJ, Hirsh J et al: Effectiveness of intermittent pulsatile elastic stockings for the prevention of calf and thigh vein thrombosis in patients undergoing elective knee surgery. Thromb Res 16:37, 1979

64. Wille-Jorgensen P, Thorup J, Fischer A et al: Heparin with and without graded compression stockings in the prevention of thromboembolic complications of major abdominal surgery: a randomized trial. Br J Surg 72:579, 1985

65. Wille-Jorgensen P, Winter CS, Bjerg-Nielsen A et al: Prevention of thromboembolism following elective hip surgery. The value of regional anesthesia and graded compression stockings. Clin Orthop 247:163, 1989

66. Powers PJ, Gent M, Jay RM et al: A randomized trial of post-operative less-intense warfarin or acetylsalicylic acid in the prevention of venous thromboembolism. Arch Intern Med 149:771, 1989

67. Francis CW, Marder VJ, McCollister-Evarts C, Yaukoolbodi S: Two step warfarin therapy: prevention of postoperative venous thrombosis without excessive bleeding. JAMA 249:374, 1983

68. Eriksson BI, Zachrisson BE, Teger-Nilsson A-C et al: Thrombosis prophylaxis with low molecular weight heparin in total hip replacement. Br J Surg 75: 1053, 1988

69. Green D, Lee MY, Ito VY et al: Fixed- vs adjusted-dose heparin in the prophylaxis of thromboembolism in spinal cord injury. JAMA 260:1255, 1988

70. Hirsh J, Salzman EW, Marder VJ: Treatment of venous thromboembolism. p. 1347. In Colman RW, Hirsh J, Marder VJ, Salzman EW (eds): Hemostasis and Thrombosis: Basic Principles and Clinical Practice. 3rd Ed. JB Lippincott, Philadelphia, 1994

71. Tibbutt DA, Davies JA, Anderson JA et al: Comparison by controlled clinical trial of streptokinase and heparin in treatment of life-threatening pulmonary embolism. Br Med J 1:343, 1974

72. Miller GAH, Sutton GC, Kerr IH et al: Comparison of streptokinase and heparin in the treatment of isolated acute massive pulmonary embolism. Br Med J 2:681, 1971

73. Moser KM, Spragg RG, Utley J et al: Chronic thrombotic obstruction in major pulmonary arteries. Results of thromboendarterectomy in 15 patients. Ann Intern Med 99:299, 1983

74. Brandjes DPM, Heijboer H, Buller HR et al: Acenocoumarol and heparin compared with acenocoumarol alone in the initial treatment of proximal vein thrombosis. N Engl J Med 327:1485, 1992

75. Pini M, Pattacini C, Quintavalla R et al: Subcutaneous vs intravenous heparin in the treatment of deep venous thrombosis—a randomized clinical trial. Thromb Haemost 64:222, 1990

76. Hirsh J, van Aken WG, Gallus AS et al: Heparin kinetics in venous thrombosis and pulmonary embolism. Circulation 53:691, 1976

77. Boneu B, Caranobe C, Gabaig AM et al: Evidence for a saturable mechanism of disappearance of standard heparin in rabbits. Thromb Res 46:835, 1987

78. Hirsh J: Heparin. N Engl J Med 324:1565, 1991

79. Hirsh J, Dalen JE, Deykin D, Poller L: Heparin: mechanism of action, pharmacokinetics, dosing considerations, monitoring, efficacy and safety. Chest 102: 337S, 1992

80. Hirsh J, Dalen JE, Deykin D, Poller L: Oral anticoagulants; mechanisms of action, clinical effectiveness, and optimal therapeutic range. Chest 102:312S, 1992

81. Hirsh J: Oral anticoagulant drugs. N Engl J Med 324:1865, 1991

82. Lensing AWA, Hirsh J, Buller HR: Diagnosis of venous thrombosis. p. 1297. In Colman RW, Hirsh J, Marder VJ, Salzman EW (eds): Hemostasis and Thrombosis: Basic Principles and Clinical Practice. 3rd Ed. JB Lippincott, Philadelphia, 1994

83. Kakkar VV, Lawrence D, Fok J, Djazaeri B: Objective assessment of late results of treatment of deep vein thrombosis, abstracted. Br J Surg 68:807, 1981

84. Urokinase Streptokinase Embolism Trial: Phase II Results: a Cooperative Study. JAMA 229:1606, 1974

85. Goldhaber SZ, Buring JE, Lipnick RJ et al: Pooled analysis of randomized trials of streptokinase and heparin in phlebographyically documented acute deep vein thrombosis. Am J Med 76:393, 1984

86. Mavor GE, Kasenally AT, Harper DR, Woodruff PWH: Thrombosis of the subclavian-axillary artery following radiotherapy for cancer of the breast. Br J Surg 60:983, 1973

87. Fritz T, Richeson JF, Fitzpatrick P et al: Venous obstruction: potential complication of transvenous pacemaker electrons. Chest 83:534, 1983

88. Sidd JJ, Stellar LE, Gryska PF, O'Dea AE: Thrombus formation on a transvenous pacemaker electro. N Engl J Med 280:877, 1969

89. Wyles PG, Birtwell AJ, Davis JA, Chennells P: Subclavian vein notch: a phlebographic abnormality associated with subclavian-axillary vein thrombosis. Br J Hosp Med 37:349, 1987

90. Abdu RA, Zakhour B, Dallis JH: Review of mesenteric vein thrombosis—1911 to 1984. Surgery 101:383, 1987

91. Nesbit RR, DeWsse JA: Mesenteric vein thrombosis and oral contraceptives. South Med J 70:360, 1977

92. Llach F, Pappei S, Massry SG: The clinical spectrum of renal vein thrombosis: acute and chronic. Am J Med 69:819, 1980

93. Burrow CR, Walker JEG, Bell JR et al: Streptokinase of renal function after renal vein thrombosis. Ann Intern Med 100:237, 1984

Arterial Thromboembolism

124

Jack Hirsh and Jeffrey I. Weitz

INTRODUCTION

Arterial thrombosis usually occurs as a complication of atherosclerosis. Atherosclerosis is the most common underlying cause of coronary heart disease, cerebrovascular disease, and peripheral arterial disease and, as such, is the single most common cause of mortality and morbidity in the Western population. Arterial narrowing due to atherosclerosis limits blood flow and causes ischemic symptoms when the oxygen requirements are increased by exercise. For example, angina pectoris occurs when the coronary arteries cannot supply sufficient blood flow to meet the demands of the myocardium when its workload is increased by exercise. Similarly, intermittent claudication reflects ischemia of the leg muscles as a result of an imbalance between arterial blood supply and the demands of the exercising muscles, whereas intestinal angina occurs after a large meal, when the blood supply to the gut is insufficient to meet the requirements.

Whereas arterial insufficiency leads to ischemia, tissue infarction occurs when the arterial supply is completely occluded for a critical period of time. Arterial occlusion usually is the result of the rupture or fissuring of an atherosclerotic plaque that exposes thrombogenic material and triggers the formation of a platelet-fibrin thrombus.

PATHOGENESIS OF ATHEROSCLEROSIS

The term atherosclerosis was introduced by Marchand, who recognized the association of fatty degeneration and vessel stiffening.[1] Atherosclerosis affects medium and large arteries and is characterized by patchy intramural thickening of the subintima that encroaches on the arterial lumen and eventually leads to vascular obstruction. The earliest lesion of atherosclerosis is the fatty streak, which is due to an accumulation of lipid-laden foam cells in the intimal layer of the artery. With time, the fatty streak evolves into the fibrous plaque that is the hallmark of established atherosclerosis.

Atherosclerotic lesions are composed of three major components. The first is a cellular component with increased numbers of intimal smooth muscle cells and an accumulation of macrophages. The second component is connective tissue matrix, large amounts of which are produced by the proliferating smooth muscle cells, and extracellular lipid. The third component is lipid, which accumulates within the smooth muscle cells and the macrophages thereby converting them into foam cells. Thus, the development of atherosclerotic lesions involves proliferation of smooth muscle cells, synthesis of connective tissue matrix, and accumulation of macrophages and lipid.

Over the years, two main hypotheses have been proposed to explain the pathogenesis of the atherosclerotic process: the lipid hypothesis[2,3] and the chronic endothelial injury hypothesis.[4] Experimentally, atherosclerosis can be produced by cholesterol feeding[2] or by chronic endothelial injury.[4]

Lipid Hypothesis

The lipid hypothesis postulates that with increased levels of low-density lipoproteins (LDL), lipid accumulates in smooth muscle cells and macrophages as the LDL penetrates the arterial wall. LDL is oxidized in the presence of endothelial cells and in its oxidized form becomes more atherogenic. Thus, oxidized LDL causes endothelial damage[5] and is chemotactic for monocyte/macrophages. The monocytes first adhere to the altered endothelium by interacting with surface adhesion molecules and then migrate through the endothelium and basement membrane by elaborating hydrolases that degrade connective tissue matrix. As these cells accumulate, they take up lipid and are converted to foam cells. Macrophages bind intraintimal LDL via a family of novel receptors known as scavenger receptors, which recognize LDL only after it has been oxidized. Oxidation affects both lipid and apoprotein moieties of the LDL molecule; the lecithin component of LDL phospholipid undergoes conversion to lysolecithin, which is chemotactic for monocytes.[5] In addition, the uptake of oxidized LDL renders the macrophages less mobile, thereby promoting the accumulation of these lipid-laden cells in the intima.

An experimental model of atherosclerosis has been carefully studied in monkeys fed a diet rich in cholesterol.[2] Within 2 weeks of inducing hypercholesterolemia, monocytes become attached to the surface of the arterial endothelium, migrate into the subendothelium, and accumulate lipid, which gives them the appearance of foam cells. Proliferating smooth muscle cells then emerge, also accumulating lipid. As the fibrous plaque enlarges, the endothelial cells retract, exposing the subendothelium to the blood and triggering the formation of platelet-fibrin thrombi. The release of platelet-derived growth factor (PDGF) leads to further smooth muscle proliferation, as described in the response-to-injury hypothesis. Support for the important role of oxidized LDL in atherogenesis comes from several sources. Thus, administration of antioxidants to hyperlipidemic rabbits inhibits the formation of fatty streaks. Oxidized LDL can be extracted from human lesions, and many humans have circulating antibodies specific for epitopes of oxidized LDL.[6]

Chronic Endothelial Injury Hypothesis

The response to injury hypothesis has been reviewed by Ross.[4] It postulates that endothelial injury results in loss of endothelium, adhesion of platelets to subendothelium, aggregation of platelets, release of PDGFs, and elaboration of chemotactic factors that attract leukocytes, which in turn release other growth factors. The growth factors induce replication and migration of smooth muscle cells into the intima and result in the formation of a fibrous plaque. The smooth muscle cells synthesize and secrete connective tissue matrix containing collagen, proteoglycans, and elastic fibers, contributing to the mass of the lesion. Plaque fissure or rupture may trigger the formation of a platelet-fibrin plug, which is then incorporated into the lesion. Repeated injury causes further intimal proliferation and progressive narrowing of the lumen.

The lipid hypothesis and the endothelial injury hypothesis are closely linked. Oxidized LDL is cytotoxic to cultured endothelial cells; it may cause endothelial injury, attract monocytes, and stimulate smooth muscle growth. Modified LDL is also a potent inhibitor of macrophage mobility. Stimulated macrophages release growth factors that promote the proliferation and migration of smooth muscle cells. The smooth muscle cells in turn elaborate a monocyte chemotactic factor and synthesize connective tissue matrix.

The development of atherosclerosis is accompanied by impaired regulation of vascular tone. This is due, at least in part, to decreased production of endothelial-derived relaxing factor (EDRF). In experimental animal models of atherosclerosis, impaired EDRF synthesis can be reversed by lowering the cholesterol level.

Atherosclerotic lesions can develop in the absence of endothelial denudation and without the involvement of PDGFs.[2] Thus, smooth muscle hyperplasia occurs in hypertension without associated endothelial cell loss[7-10] and persists long after platelet interaction with the vessel wall has ceased.[11-13] Cells other than platelets produce growth factors,[14] including macrophages,[15] endothelial cells,[16] and arterial smooth muscle cells[17]; these may contribute to the growth of the atherosclerotic plaque.[4] Within this context, local synthesis of PDGF has been demonstrated in human atherosclerotic plaques removed at surgery.[18]

Growth of Atherosclerotic Plaque

The atherosclerotic plaque grows slowly over a period of years. It can produce severe stenosis or even total vascular occlusion. The mature plaque consists of a fibrous cap composed of collagen, a lipid core containing intracellular and extracellular lipid, and areas of calcification. Lipid-rich plaques are susceptible to spontaneous fissuring or rupture when exposed to high shear stress at sites of stenosis and arterial branching. Two forms of plaque injury are recognized: superficial and deep. Superficial injury produces areas of focal endothelial denudation that can enlarge and lead to the formation of mural or even occlusive thrombi. Plaques that are capped with superficial collagen fibers separated by large number of lipid-filled macrophages tend to predispose to superficial injury.[19,20]

Deep intimal injury is characterized by a split or tear that extends from the luminal surface of a plaque deep down into the plaque substance. This type of injury, which tends to occur in plaques that contain a large lipid-rich pool, exposes blood to the highly thrombogenic contents of the plaque and leads to intraluminal and extraluminal thrombosis. Intraluminal thrombi become incorporated into, and increase the size of, the atherosclerotic plaque, while extraluminal thrombi can be partly or completely occlusive.[21]

PATHOGENESIS OF ARTERIAL THROMBOSIS: THROMBOGENIC FACTORS

Arterial thrombi form under conditions of high flow and are composed mainly of platelet aggregates held together by fibrin strands. Thrombosis is initiated by rupture of the atherosclerotic plaque, exposing thrombogenic material in the subendothelium to the blood.[21,22] If the thrombus is nonocclusive and blood flow remains rapid, the thrombi may organize and become incorporated into the atherosclerotic plaque.[22] With more marked arterial narrowing, shear rates increase and promote more extensive platelet and fibrin deposition, which can result in the formation of an occlusive thrombosis.

Thrombosis occurs when the balance between thrombogenic factors and protective mechanisms is perturbed. The protective mechanisms include the nonthrombogenic properties of intact endothelial cells, fluid-phase antiproteases, and the dissolution of fibrin by the fibrinolytic system, whereas the thrombogenic stimuli include perturbation or loss of endothelial cells and activation of platelets and coagulation.

Nonthrombogenic Properties of Endothelial Cells

The fluidity of blood in vivo is enhanced by the thromboresistant properties of intact vascular endothelium and threatened by damage to the vessel wall.[23] Endothelial cell-surface glycosaminoglycans and thrombomodulin are potent inhibitors of coagulation, while vessel wall generation of prostacyclin and nitric oxide, as well as plasminogen activators, limit platelet aggregation and fibrin deposition, respectively.[24]

Damage to the Vessel Wall

Thrombogenesis is promoted by loss of endothelium, which may be caused by direct physical damage such as occurs with angioplasty, hemodynamic stress, tobacco products, high blood cholesterol, or enzymes released from platelets and leukocytes.[14] The shedding of endothelial cells exposes the subendothelium to platelets and blood coagulation factors. Platelets that adhere to the subendothelium undergo a shape change, aggregate, and secrete their granular contents, thereby recruiting more platelets. At physiologic shear rates, platelet adhesion to subendothelial collagen is mediated by von Willebrand factor and possibly by other adhesive proteins, which bind to a glycoprotein receptor (GPIb) on the platelet surface,[25] as well as to subendothelial proteins.

Although endothelial cell loss represents the most severe form of vascular damage, more subtle injury may also promote thrombogenesis. Thus, endothelial cells exposed to endotoxin, cytokines such as interleukin-1 and tumor necrosis factor, thrombin, hypoxia, or increased shear stress synthesize tissue factor and internalize thrombomodulin, promoting coagulation. In addition, these perturbed cells produce plasminogen activator inhibitor-1, which impairs fibrinolysis, and acquire receptors to which leukocytes and platelets adhere.[24] Finally, the altered endothelial cells synthesize factors that regulate local blood flow. These include vasoconstrictors known as endothelins, as well as vasodilators such as prostacyclin and EDRF.[24]

Platelet Activation

Platelets adhering to collagen undergo a shape change, secrete their granular contents, and aggregate. A variety of other agonists, including thrombin, epinephrine, and thromboxane A_2 (TXA_2), promote platelet aggregation as well.[26] Whereas all these agents stimulate the synthesis of TXA_2, collagen, thrombin, and TXA_2 also induce the release of ADP from platelet granules, which amplifies the aggregation process. In addition to these pathways, thrombin-induced platelet aggregation occurs by means of a third mechanism that may involve the activation of platelet calpain.[27]

Virtually all agonists that induce platelet aggregation act through a common pathway that involves the accumulation of ionized calcium within the platelet cytoplasm either by mobilization of calcium from the dense tubular system[27] or by increased transport across the membrane. This in turn results in the surface exposure of the platelet glycoprotein GPIIb/IIIa, which serves as a receptor for fibrinogen and other Arg-Gly-Asp-containing adhesive proteins such as fibronectin, von Willebrand factor, and thrombospondin.[27] Binding of fibrinogen to GPIIb/IIIa is essential for platelet aggregation because the dimeric fibrinogen bridges the platelets together.

An increase in platelet cAMP levels reduces the calcium-mobilizing effect of all agonists. Prostacyclin produced by endothelial cells inhibits platelet aggregation by activating platelet adenylate cyclase thereby elevating cAMP levels.[28]

Activation of Coagulation

Damage to the vessel wall activates the blood coagulation pathway by exposing blood to tissue factor and by activating platelets. Stimulated platelets promote further activation of coagulation by providing a phospholipid surface on which efficient assembly of coagulation factor complexes can occur. Thrombin formed as a result of these processes then serves to convert fibrinogen to fibrin, stabilizing the platelet aggregates.

PREVENTION AND EPIDEMIOLOGY OF ATHEROSCLEROSIS

The most effective means of preventing arterial thrombosis is to prevent atherosclerosis. The proven risk factors for atherosclerosis are hypercholesterolemia, hypertension, cigarette smoking, obesity, physical inactivity, family history, diabetes, and male gender. The first five of these risk factors are potentially reversible, and there is evidence that their reversal reduces the complications of atherosclerosis.

Cholesterol and Lipids

The plasma level of cholesterol is determined by genetic factors, by the type and amount of fat in the diet, and by other factors, such as obesity, physical activity, and disease states. The results of animal studies, epidemiologic data, and interventional studies have provided good evidence of an association between hypercholesterolemia and atherosclerosis.

Of the three major classes of lipoproteins, very low-density lipoproteins, LDLs, and high density lipoproteins (HDLs), LDLs contain 60–70% of the total serum cholesterol and are the most atherogenic. By contrast, the levels of HDL are inversely correlated with the risk of coronary heart disease.

The association between serum cholesterol and the risk of coronary heart disease is continuous.[29,30] Familial hypercholesterolemia, a disorder caused by an absent or defective LDL receptor, causes premature coronary heart disease.[31,32] In the heterozygous form of this disorder, which occurs in 1 in 500 people, the total cholesterol is usually >300 mg/dl. Approximately 5% of all patients who present with acute myocardial infarction before the age of 60 have heterozygous familial hypercholesterolemia. The homozygous form of familial hypercholesterolemia occurs in 1 in 10^6 subjects. These patients have cholesterol levels ranging from 600 to 1,000 mg/dl; severe coronary heart disease usually develops <20 years of age.

Reduced levels of HDL cholesterol appear to be associated with an increased risk of coronary heart disease. The main causes of reduced HDL cholesterol include cigarette smoking, obesity, physical inactivity, androgenic and related steroids (including anabolic steroids), β-blocking agents, hypertriglyceridemia, and genetic factors. By contrast, weight reduction and exercise elevate HDL cholesterol levels.

Both the cholesterol level and the prevalence of coronary heart disease are influenced by environmental factors that include diet. Thus, people who immigrate from countries in which the prevalence of coronary heart disease and the serum cholesterol levels are low to a country with a high prevalence of coronary heart disease will often sustain increases both in serum cholesterol levels and in rates of coronary heart disease.

Evidence that decreasing serum cholesterol levels with cholesterol-lowering drugs or dietary modification slows or reverses the progression of coronary atherosclerosis[33,34] and reduces coronary events[35] comes from >20 randomized trials that included almost 40,000 subjects.[33,35–37] Lowering the serum cholesterol with diet or drug therapy also slows the progression of angiographically documented coronary atherosclerosis in patients with arterial bypass grafts.[33] Modifying several risk factors such as lowering the serum cholesterol, the blood pressure, and the levels of LDL cholesterol, and cessation of smoking[35] reduce the risk of ischemic heart disease.[38,39] Patients with several risk factors benefit most from these measures.[40]

Smoking

Cigarette smoking increases the risk of coronary heart disease, peripheral arterial disease, cerebrovascular disease, and graft occlusion following reconstructive arterial surgery. It is particularly hazardous in those with a poor cardiovascular risk profile and in women taking estrogens; there is a dose relationship between the risk of coronary heart disease and the number of cigarettes smoked daily.[41] Those who stop smoking have only one-half the risk of those who continue to smoke, regardless of how long they had smoked. Cessation of smoking also reduces mortality after coronary bypass surgery, reduces morbidity and mortality in patients with peripheral vascular disease, and decreases mortality after myocardial infarction.

Although the mechanism by which smoking increases the risk of atherosclerosis is uncertain, there are several possibilities. Thus, cigarette smoking decreases the levels of HDL, increases LDL cholesterol, and, by raising the levels of carbon dioxide, leads to hypoxia, perturbing the anticoagulant properties of the endothelium. In addition, smoking increases platelet reactivity and by elevating the plasma fibrinogen and the hematocrit increases blood viscosity.

Hypertension

Hypertension is a risk factor for stroke, myocardial infarction, and cardiac and renal failure.[42] There is good evidence that treatment of hypertension reduces the incidence of stroke and lowers overall mortality, but evidence that it affects coronary events is less convincing.[43] Pooled analysis of all studies examining the effects of lowering the blood pressure shows a 10% risk reduction for mortality and a 40% risk reduction for stroke. However, the risk reduction for fatal and nonfatal myocardial infarction is only 8%, a difference that is not statistically significant.

Physical Inactivity

Those who exercise regularly have been reported to have a lower incidence of myocardial infarction and death,[44] but it is uncertain whether the association is causal or whether it merely reflects that healthier people are more likely to exercise. In patients who have recovered from an acute myocardial infarct,[45] exercise produces a 19% reduction in the risk of recurrent infarction or death. Regular exercise may exert these protective effects by increasing the levels of HDL cholesterol and lowering the blood pressure.[46,47]

Obesity

Although some observational studies[48] have suggested that obesity is an independent risk factor for coronary heart disease, this has not been a universal finding.

NONSURGICAL THERAPY FOR ARTERIAL THROMBOEMBOLISM

Treatment of atherosclerosis and its thromboembolic complications includes surgical procedures such as endarterectomy, embolectomy, arterial bypass surgery, and angioplasty, as well as medical management. This section discusses the medical treatment of the thrombotic complications of atherosclerosis and the prevention and treatment of systemic embolism from a presumed cardiac source. The measures that can be taken to prevent or delay the progression of atherosclerosis are outlined in the previous section.

The three forms of medical therapy of proven effectiveness in the treatment of arterial thrombosis are antiplatelet agents, thrombolytic agents, and anticoagulants.

Antiplatelet Agents

Two antiplatelet agents, aspirin and ticlopidine, have been shown to be effective for the prevention and treatment of arterial thrombosis.[49] In addition, agents that inhibit the interaction between fibrinogen and its receptors on platelets show great promise.

Aspirin

The antithrombotic effects of aspirin reflect its ability to inhibit the synthesis of TXA_2, a potent inducer of platelet aggregation and vasoconstriction, by inactivating platelet cyclo-oxygenase. Aspirin is rapidly absorbed from the gastrointestinal tract, with peak levels reached 15–20 minutes after ingestion. Despite its rapid clearance from the circulation, the inhibitory effects of aspirin persist for the life span of the platelets because the drug irreversibly acetylates cyclo-oxygenase. To achieve rapid and complete inhibition of TXA_2 production (e.g., in a patient with an evolving myocardial infarct), the recommended dose is a 325-mg tablet of non-enteric-coated aspirin. However, lower aspirin doses can be used for maintenance treatment,[50] with as little as 80 mg/day sufficient to maintain the inhibition of TXA_2 synthesis.

Aspirin reduces the incidence of myocardial infarction and death in several groups of patients: men and asymptomatic women >50 years old and patients with asymptomatic myocardial ischemia, stable angina, unstable angina with or without non-Q-wave infarction, acute myocardial infarction, or cerebrovascular disease. Aspirin also reduces the risk of stroke in patients with cerebral ischemia and decreases the risk of acute thrombosis after either aortocoronary bypass surgery or coronary angioplasty. Finally, aspirin has been shown to lower the incidence of nonfatal myocardial infarction, in a study of healthy U.S. physicians.[49]

The side effects of aspirin therapy are primarily gastrointestinal; gastrointestinal hemorrhage can occur in some cases. These complications are dose related and are reduced if enteric-coated aspirin is used. Aspirin is contraindicated in patients with active peptic ulcer disease or with aspirin-induced asthma; it should be discontinued if gastrointestinal side effects are severe.

In most randomized studies, patients with a history of active peptic ulcer disease were excluded, and the beneficial effects of aspirin occurred without hemorrhagic complications.[51] However, in the U.S. Physicians Study the use of aspirin was associated with an increased incidence of cerebral hemorrhage,[52] a finding not observed in the thousands of symptomatic patients treated with aspirin to prevent the complications of atherosclerosis.[51,53] The preoperative use of aspirin in patients undergoing bypass surgery was associated with an increased incidence of operative bleeding, which probably reflects the combined antiplatelet effect of aspirin and the anticoagulant activity of high-dose heparin used during cardiac surgery.[54]

In studies in which aspirin alone was compared with the combination of aspirin and dipyridamole, no additional benefit was observed from the addition of dipyridamole.[51] However, there is evidence that, like aspirin, dipyridamole augments the

Table 124-1. Thrombotic Disorders for Which Aspirin or Ticlopidine Has Been Shown to be Effective

	Effective	
Indication	Aspirin (Minimum Effective Dose)	Ticlopidine (250 mg bid)
Asymptomatic males and females >50 years old	Yes (325 mg every second day)	—
Silent myocardial ischemia	Yes (75 mg)	—
Stable angina	Yes (325 mg every second day)	—
Unstable angina	Yes (75 mg)	Yes
Acute myocardial infarction	Yes (160 mg)	—
Aortocoronary bypass surgery	Yes (100–325 mg)	Yes
Acute occlusion following coronary angioplasty	Yes (650 mg)	Yes
Peripheral vascular disease	Yes (325 mg)	Yes
Transient cerebral ischemia and incomplete stroke	Yes (30 mg)	Yes
Complete stroke	No evidence	Yes
Placental insufficiency	Yes (60–150 mg)	—
Atrial fibrillation	Yes (325 mg)[a]	—
Prosthetic heart valves	Yes (100 mg)[b]	—

[a] In combination with warfarin.
[b] Not as effective as warfarin.

(From Hirsch J: Thrombolytic agents. Ch. 3. Decker Periodicals, Hamilton, Ontario, Canada, 1993, with permission.)

antithrombotic effect of oral anticoagulants in patients with mechanical prosthetic valves.[55]

Ticlopidine

Ticlopidine is an antiplatelet drug that works through an unknown mechanism[56] and inhibits platelet aggregation induced by a variety of agonists. Unlike aspirin, the inhibitory effects of ticlopidine on platelet function are delayed for 24–48 hours after administration, suggesting that active metabolites are responsible for its activity. The delayed onset of ticlopidine limits its potential value when a rapid antithrombotic effect is required.

Ticlopidine has been shown to be significantly more effective than aspirin in reducing stroke in patients who have sustained transient cerebral ischemia or a minor stroke.[49] Ticlopidine is also effective[49] in (1) reducing the risk of the combined outcome of stroke, myocardial infarction, or vascular death in patients with thromboembolic stroke; (2) decreasing vascular death and myocardial infarction in patients with unstable angina; (3) reducing acute occlusion of coronary bypass grafts; and (4) improving walking distance and decreasing vascular complications in patients with peripheral vascular disease.[49]

The most common side effects of ticlopidine are diarrhea and skin rash, whereas the most serious complication is neutropenia, which is sometimes irreversible. Nevertheless, ticlopidine should be considered in place of aspirin in patients who are allergic or intolerant to aspirin or who have had a vascular event despite the use of aspirin.

The thromboembolic disorders for which aspirin or ticlopidine are effective are listed in Table 124-1. Ticlopidine is more effective than aspirin in patients with who have experienced transient cerebral ischemia and incomplete stroke, but aspirin is much safer and less expensive.

Thrombolytic Therapy

Thrombolytic therapy is useful in the treatment of arterial thrombosis because rapid clot lysis and restoration of blood flow prevents permanent tissue damage. More than 80% of patients with acute myocardial infarction have thrombotic occlusion of the infarct-related coronary artery,[57] and thrombolytic agents produce rapid lysis of these thrombi in 50–75% of cases.[57] Tissue plasminogen activator (t-PA) is more effective than streptokinase in achieving early coronary lysis,[58] but both agents improve left ventricular function and reduce mortality. Streptokinase and t-PA decrease mortality by approximately 25%[57,59] when used without adjunctive aspirin or intravenous heparin, reducing mortality by 40–50% when either agent is combined with aspirin.[57] In the GUSTO study, an accelerated t-PA regimen combined with high-dose intravenous heparin produced a 14% greater reduction in mortality than was achieved with streptokinase. This difference was most evident in patients treated within 4 hours of the onset of symptoms.

Following successful thrombolysis, the reocclusion rate is 10–20% and the reinfarction rate 3–4%.[57] Aspirin reduces the incidence of reinfarction.[53] Full-dose heparin appears to be an important adjunct to t-PA but does not improve the results with streptokinase. Presumably, heparin works by limiting reocclusion after successful thrombolysis. Reocclusion is less common with streptokinase than with t-PA because streptokinase causes extensive plasma proteolysis, and the resultant fibrinogen degradation products produce a systemic anticoagulant state. Preliminary evidence indicates that direct thrombin inhibitors, such as hirulog and hirudin, are more effective than heparin in preventing reocclusion after coronary thrombolysis.

Anticoagulants

The role of anticoagulant therapy in the treatment of arterial thrombosis is controversial.[60,61] As discussed above, aspirin is widely used in patients with atherosclerotic disease. When used alone, heparin is effective in the short-term treatment of unstable angina,[60] but a rebound effect is seen when the drug is stopped. Aspirin appears to prevent the cluster of ischemic events that occur when heparin is discontinued. The addition of heparin to aspirin has been suggested to improve short-term outcome in patients with unstable angina, but it is uncertain whether this effect is sustained.

In patients with acute myocardial infarction, heparin has been reported to reduce reinfarction and death.[60] Moderate doses of heparin (12,500 U SC bid) also reduce the incidence of mural thrombosis detected by two-dimensional echocardiography, a particular problem in patients with anterior infarction.

Heparin prevents early reocclusion of the infarct-related artery after successful thrombolysis with t-PA and probably reduces mortality when used in combination with t-PA. However, the effectiveness of heparin in preventing reinfarction or death after thrombolysis with streptokinase is less certain.

Oral anticoagulants are effective for the treatment of arterial thrombosis.[60] Two recent studies have shown that oral anticoagulants are effective in the long-term treatment of patients with myocardial infarction.[62,63] Both studies used higher-intensity coumadin regimens (International Normalized Ratio [INR] 2.7–4.5 and 2.8–4.8, respectively), and the risk of bleeding was increased with anticoagulants.

Atrial Fibrillation

Patients with nonvalvular atrial fibrillation are at increased risk of stroke, which occurs at a frequency of 5%/yr.[64–68] The risk of stroke increases with age[69,70] and is increased by a number of associated cardiac disorders, including a history of myocardial infarction, angina, heart failure, or thromboembolic event, and the presence of left atrial dilation, left ventricular dysfunction, mitral calcification, or hypertension.

In patients with nonvalvular atrial fibrillation, a moderate dose of warfarin (INR 2.0–3.0) is associated with a 60–80% reduction in the risk of stroke, with only a modest increase in bleeding complications.[64–68] Therefore, warfarin is indicated for an associated cardiac abnormality when anticoagulants are not contraindicated.

Aspirin also is reported to be effective in patients with atrial fibrillation; although it may be less effective than warfarin, aspirin should be used in patients at high risk of stroke, when warfarin is contraindicated. Patients >75 years of age appear to be at increased risk of cerebral hemorrhage with moderate doses of warfarin. These patients should either be treated with a less intense warfarin regimen (INR 1.5–2.0) or with aspirin. The risk of stroke is only about 1%/yr in patients without clinical or echocardiographic risk factors. On the basis of these findings, it would be reasonable to use aspirin rather than warfarin in this patient group.

Mechanical and Bioprosthetic Valves

Patients with prosthetic heart valves are at risk of systemic embolism, which most often manifests as a stroke. The embolic risk is greater with mechanical than with bioprosthetic valves, with prosthetic mitral rather than aortic valves, and is higher with associated atrial fibrillation.[71] For patients with tissue prosthetic valves who are in sinus rhythm, the risk of embolism

Table 124-2. Indications for Anticoagulant Therapy and Aspirin in Arterial Thromboembolism

Indication	Anticoagulants Effective	Aspirin Effective	Drug of Choice
Acute myocardial infarction			
Prevent systemic embolism	Yes[a]	No	Anticoagulants
Prevent reinfarction	Yes[a]	Yes[a]	Either
Prevent death	Yes[a]	Yes[a]	Aspirin
Angina			
Unstable angina	Yes[a]	Yes[a]	Both
Stable angina	No	Yes[a]	Aspirin
Coronary artery bypass graft	?	Yes	Aspirin
Atrial fibrillation			
Prevent systemic embolism	Yes[a]	Yes	Anticoagulants
Treat systemic embolism (including stroke)	Yes[a]	No	Anticoagulants
Valvular heart disease			
Prosthetic	Yes[a]	(Augment effect of anticoagulants)	Anticoagulants
Rheumatic	Yes	No	Anticoagulants
Systemic embolism			
Prevention	Yes	No	Anticoagulants
Treatment	Yes	No	Anticoagulants
Peripheral arterial disease	No	?	Aspirin
Cerebrovascular disease	No	Yes[a]	Aspirin

[a] Evidence from randomized clinical trials.

is largely confined to the first 3 months after valve insertion,[71] whereas patients with mechanical prosthetic valves (particularly in the mitral position) are at lifelong risk of systemic embolism.[71]

Randomized trials in patients with mechanical prosthetic valves have shown that warfarin is effective in reducing the risk of systemic embolism, even when given at a lower intensity than that used in the past.[72,73] For this reason, an INR of 2.5–3.5 is recommended for these patients.[71]

The risk of thromboembolism is lower with uncomplicated bioprosthetic valves than with mechanical valves. In the absence of complications, warfarin should be given for 3 months[71,74] in patients with mitral bioprosthetic valves (INR 2.0–3.0).

The relative effectiveness of anticoagulants and aspirin in the treatment of arterial thromboembolism is summarized in Table 124-2.

REFERENCES

1. Aschoff L: Introduction. p. 1. In Cowdry EV (ed): Arteriosclerosis: A Survey of the Problem. MacMillan, New York, 1933
2. Walker LN, Reidy MA, Bowyer DE: Morphology and cell kinetics of fatty streak lesion formation in the hypercholesterolemia rabbit. Am J Pathol 125:450, 1986
3. Malinow MR, Brown BG, Wissler RW et al: Atherosclerosis regression, arterial wall cell interactions and atherogenic lipoproteins. Arteriosclerosis 3:627, 1983
4. Ross R: The pathogenesis of atherosclerosis—an update. N Engl J Med 314:488, 1986
5. Steinberg D, Parthasarathy S, Carew T et al: Beyond cholesterol. Modifications of low-density lipoprotein that increases its atherogenicity. N Engl J Med 320:915, 1989
6. Wltztum JL: Role of oxidized low density lipoprotein in atherogenesis. Br Heart J, Suppl. 69:S12, 1993
7. Owens GK, Rabinovitch PS, Schwartz SM: Smooth muscle hypertrophy versus hyperplasia in hypertension. Proc Natl Acad Sci USA 78:7759, 1981
8. Owens GK, Schwartz SM: Alterations in vascular smooth muscle mass in the spontaneously hypertensive rat. Role of cellular hypertrophy and hyperplasia. Circ Res 51:280, 1982
9. Limas C, Westrum B, Limas CJ: The evolution of vascular changes in the spontaneously hypertensive rat. Am J Pathol 98:357, 1980
10. Haudenschild CC, Prescott MF, Chobanian AV: Effects of hypertension and its reversal on aortic intimal lesions of the rat. Hypertension 2:33, 1980
11. Clowes AW, Reidy MA, Clowes MM: Kinetics of cellular proliferation after arterial injury. I. Lab Invest 49:327, 1983
12. Clowes AW, Reidy MA, Clowes MM: Kinetics of cellular proliferation after arterial injury. III. Endothelial and smooth muscle growth in chronically denuded vessels. Lab Invest 54:295, 1986
13. Groves HM, Kinlough-Rathbone RL, Richardson M et al: Platelet interaction with damaged rabbit aorta. Lab Invest 40:194, 1979
14. Ross R: The pathogenesis of atherosclerosis—a perspective for the 1990s. Nature 362:801, 1993
15. Shimokado KE, Raines EW, Madtes DK et al: A significant part of macrophage-derived growth factor consists of at least two forms of PDGF. Cell 43:277, 1985
16. DiCorletto PE: Cultured endothelial cells produce multiple growth factors for connective tissue cells. Exp Cell Res 153:167, 1984
17. Walker LN, Bowen-Pope DF, Ross R et al: Production of platelet-derived growth factor-like molecules by cultured arterial smooth muscle cells accompanies proliferation after arterial injury. Proc Natl Acad Sci USA 83:7311, 1986
18. Barrett TB, Benditt EP: Sis (PDGF-B) gene transcript levels are elevated in human atherosclerotic lesions compared to normal artery. Proc Natl Acad Sci USA 84:1099, 1987
19. Davies MJ, Woolif N, Rowles P et al: Morphology of the endothelium over atherosclerotic plaques in human coronary arteries. Br Heart J 60:459, 1988
20. Davies MJ: A macroscopic and microscopic view of coronary thrombi. Circulation 82:1138, 1990
21. Davies MJ, Thomas AC: Plaque fissuring: the cause of acute myocardial infarction, sudden ischaemic death, and crescendo angina. Br Heart J 53:363, 1985
22. Fuster V, Badimon L, Cohen M et al: Insights into the pathogenesis of acute ischemic syndromes. Circulation 77:1213, 1988
23. Vasiliev JM, Gelfand IM: Mechanism of non-adhesiveness of endothelial and epithelial surfaces. Nature 274:710, 1978
24. Harker LA, Gent M: Antiplatelet agents in the management of thrombotic disorders. p. 1506. In Colman RW, Hirsh J, Marder VJ, Salzman EW (eds): Hemostasis and Thrombosis: Basic Principles and Clinical Practice. 3rd Ed. JB Lippincott, Philadelphia, 1994
25. Sakariassen KS, Bolhuis PA, Sixma JJ: Human blood platelet adhesion to artery subendothelium is mediated by factor VIII-VWF bound to the subendothelium. Nature 279:636, 1979
26. Holmsen H: Platelet secretion. p. 524. In Colman RW, Hirsh J, Marder VJ, Salzman EW (eds): Hemostasis and Thrombosis: Basic Principles and Clinical Practice. 3rd Ed. JB Lippincott, Philadelphia, 1994
27. Hawiger J, Brass LF, Salzman EW: Signal transduction and intracellular regulatory processes in platelets. p. 603. In Colman RW, Hirsh J, Marder VJ, Salzman EW (eds): Hemostasis and Thrombosis: Basic Principles and Clinical Practice. 3rd Ed. JB Lippincott, Philadelphia, 1994
28. Salzman EW: Cyclic AMP and platelet function. N Engl J Med 286:358, 1972
29. Martin MJ, Hulley SB, Browner WS et al: Serum cholesterol, blood pressure, and mortality: implications from a cohort of 361,662 men. Lancet 2:933, 1986
30. Stamler J, Wentworth D, Neaton J: Is the relationship between serum cholesterol and risk of death from CHD continuous and graded? JAMA 256:2823, 1986
31. Schaefer EJ, Levy RI: Pathogenesis and management of lipoprotein disorders. N Engl J Med 312:1300, 1985
32. Brown MS, Goldstein JL: Receptor-mediated pathway for cholesterol homeostasis. Science 232:34, 1986
33. Blankenhorn DH, Nessim SA, Johnson RL et al: Beneficial effects of combined colestipol-niacin therapy on coronary atherosclerosis and coronary venous bypass grafts. JAMA 257:3233, 1987
34. Brensike JF, Levy RI, Kelsey SF et al: Effects of therapy with cholestyramine on progression of coronary arteriosclerosis: results of NHLBI Type II Coronary Intervention Study. Circulation 69:313, 1984
35. Yusuf S, Wittes J, Friedman L: Overview of results of randomized clinical trials in heart disease. II. Unstable angina, heart failure, primary prevention with aspirin, and risk factor modification. JAMA 260:2259, 1988
36. Frick MH, Elo O, Haapa K et al: Helsinki Heart Study: primary prevention trial with gemfibrozil in middle aged men with dyslipidemia. N Engl J Med 317:1237, 1987
37. Committee of Principal Investigators: WHO cooperative trial on primary prevention of ischemic heart disease using clofibrate to lower cholesterol: mortality follow-up. Lancet 2:379, 1980
38. Lipids Research Clinics Program: The Lipid Research Clinics Coronary Primary Prevention Trial Results. I. Reduction in the incidence of coronary heart disease. JAMA 251:351, 1984
39. Canner PL, Berge KG, Wenger NK et al: Fifteen-year mortality in Coronary Drug Project patients: long-term benefit with niacin. J Am Coll Cardiol 8:1245, 1984
40. Lipid Research Clinics Program: The Lipid Research Clinics Coronary Primary Prevention Trial results. II. The relationship of reduction in incidence of coronary heart disease to cholesterol lowering. JAMA 251:365, 1984
41. Rogot E, Murray JL: Smoking and causes of death among U.S. veterans: 16 years of observation. Public Health Rep 95:213, 1980
42. MacMahon SW, Cutler JA, Neaton JD et al: Relationship of blood pressure to coronary and stroke morbidity and mortality in clinical trials and epidemiological studies. J Hypertens, suppl. 6. 4:S14, 1986
43. MacMahon SM, Cutler JA, Furberg CD et al: The effects of drug treatment for hypertension on morbidity and mortality from cardiovascular disease. Prog Cardiovasc Dis, suppl. 1. 29:99, 1986
44. Paffenbarger RS, Hyde RT: Exercise as protection against heart attacks. N Engl J Med 302:1026, 1980
45. Collins R, Yusuf S, Peto R: Exercise after myocardial infarction reduces mortality: evidence from randomized controlled trials, abstracted. J Am Coll Cardiol 3:622A, 1984
46. Bonanno JA, Lies JE: Effects of physical training on coronary risk factors. Am J Cardiol 33:760, 1974
47. Goldberg L, Elliott DL, Schutz RW et al: Changes in lipid and lipoprotein levels after weight training. JAMA 252:504, 1984
48. Hubert HB, Feinleib M, McNamara PM et al: Obesity as an independent risk factor for cardiovascular disease: a 26-year follow-up of participants in the Framingham Heart Study. Circulation 67:968, 1983
49. Hirsh J, Salzman EW, Harker L et al: Aspirin and other platelet active drugs: relationship among dose, effectiveness, and side effects. Chest 102:327S, 1992
50. Kearon C, Hirsh J: Optimal dose for starting and maintaining low-dose aspirin. Arch Intern Med 153:700, 1993
51. Antiplatelet Trialists' Collaboration: Secondary prevention of vascular disease by prolonged antiplatelet treatment. Br Med J 296:320, 1988
52. The Steering Committee of the Physicians Health Study Research Group: Special report: preliminary report: findings from the aspirin component of the ongoing physicians' health study. N Engl J Med 318:262, 1988
53. ISIS-2 Collaborative Group: Randomised trial of intravenous streptokinase,

oral aspirin, both or neither among 17,187 cases of suspected acute myocardial infarction; ISIS-2. Lancet 2:349, 1988

54. Goldman S, Copeland J, Moritz T et al: Effect of antiplatelet therapy on early graft patency after coronary artery bypass grafting: VA Cooperative Study #207, abstracted. J Am Coll Cardiol 9:125A, 1987

55. Stein PD, Kantrowitz A: Antithrombotic therapy in mechanical and biological prosthetic heart valves and saphenous vein bypass grafts. Chest 95:107S, 1989

56. Saltiel E, Ward A: Ticlopidine. A review of its pharmacodynamic and pharmacokinetic properties and therapeutic efficacy in platelet dependent disease states. Drugs 34:222, 1987

57. Cairns JA, Collins R, Fuster V et al: Coronary thrombolysis. Chest 102:482S, 1992

58. TIMI Study Group: The thrombolysis in myocardial infarction (TIMI) trial. N Engl J Med 312:932, 1985

59. Yusuf S, Wittes J, Friedman L: Overview of results of randomized clinical trials in heart disease. I. Treatments following myocardial infarction. JAMA 260:2088, 1988

60. Cairns JA, Hirsh J, Lewis D et al: Antithrombotic agents in coronary artery disease. Chest 102:456S, 1992

61. Chalmers TC, Matta RJ, Smith H Jr et al: Evidence favoring the use of anticoagulants in the hospital phase of acute myocardial infarction. N Engl J Med 297:1091, 1977

62. Sixty-Plus Reinfarction Study Group: A double-blind trial to assess long-term oral anticoagulants therapy in elderly patients after myocardial infarction. Lancet 2:989, 1980

63. Smith P, Arnesen H, Holme I: The effect of warfarin on mortality and reinfarction after myocardial infarction. N Engl J Med 323:147, 1990

64. Petersen P, Boysen G, Godtfredsen J et al: Placebo-controlled, randomised trial of warfarin and aspirin for prevention of thromboembolic complications

in chronic atrial fibrillation: the Copenhagen AFASAK study. Lancet 1:175, 1989

65. The Stroke Prevention in Atrial Fibrillation Investigators: The stroke prevention in atrial fibrillation trial.: final results. Circulation 84:527, 1991

66. The Boston Area Anticoagulation Trial for Atrial Fibrillation Investigators: The effect of low-dose warfarin on the risk of stroke in patients with nonrheumatic atrial fibrillation. N Engl J Med 323:1505, 1990

67. Connolly SJ, Laupacis A, Gent M et al: Canadian Atrial Fibrillation Anticoagulation (CAFA) Study. J Am Coll Cardiol 18:349, 1991

68. Ezekowitz MD, Bridgers SL, James KE et al and Veterans Affairs Stroke Prevention in Nonrheumatic Atrial Fibrillation Investigators (SPINAF): Warfarin in the prevention of stroke associated with nonrheumatic atrial fibrillation. N Engl J Med 327:1406, 1992

69. The Stroke Prevention in Atrial Fibrillation Investigators: Predictors of thromboembolism in atrial fibrillation. I. Clinical features of patients at risk. Ann Intern Med 116:1, 1992

70. The Stroke Prevention in Atrial Fibrillation Investigators: Predictors of thromboembolism in atrial fibrillation. II. Echocardiographic features of patients at risk. Ann Intern Med 116:6, 1992

71. Stein PD, Alpert JS, Copeland J et al: Antithrombotic therapy in patients with mechanical and biological prosthetic heart valves. Chest 102:445S, 1992

72. Saour JN, Sieck JO, Rahim Mamo LA et al: Trial of different intensities of anticoagulation in patients with prosthetic heart valves. N Engl J Med 322:428, 1990

73. Altman R, Rouvier J, Gurfinkel E et al: Comparison of two levels of anticoagulant therapy in patients with substitute heart valves. J Thorac Cardiovasc Surg 101:427, 1991

74. Turpie AGG, Gunstensen J, Hirsh J et al: Randomised comparison of two intensities of oral anticoagulant therapy after tissue heart valve replacement. Lancet 1:1242, 1988

Immune Thrombocytopenic Purpura, Neonatal Alloimmune Thrombocytopenia, and Post-Transfusion Purpura

125

James Bussel and Douglas Cines

IMMUNE THROMBOCYTOPENIC PURPURA

Immune thrombocytopenic purpura (ITP) is one of the most common causes of thrombocytopenia encountered in medical practice. The actual incidence of ITP has not been determined precisely, but the disorder has been estimated to affect approximately 1 in 10,000 in the general population and to account for 0.18% of the hospital admissions in one study.[1] However, ITP is much more prevalent in the outpatient practices of most hematologists. The disorder is caused by autoreactive antibodies that bind to platelets and shorten their life span. The clinical presentation of the disease varies widely, from the acute onset of petechiae and severe thrombocytopenia to the incidental discovery of asymptomatic mild thrombocytopenia. ITP may accompany other systemic diseases having more than one cause of thrombocytopenia, in which case recognition and treatment of the autoimmune component may have an important impact on morbidity. Recognition and management of ITP during pregnancy presents the additional challenge of reducing the risk of neonatal bleeding. In this chapter we separate our discussion of ITP in adults and children so as to emphasize the diagnostic and treatment issues pertinent to each age group (see Chs. 126–129 for a discussion of other causes of thrombocytopenia).

ITP in Adults

Clinical Manifestations

Among adults, ITP occurs most commonly in women during the third and fourth decades of life, but the disorder may occur in either sex and at any age.[2,3] Most patients come to medical attention because they develop petechiae or purpura over the course of several days. On occasion, evidence of cutaneous bleeding may be widespread and accompanied by bleeding from mucosal sites such as epistaxis, gingival bleeding, hematuria, menorrhagia, or, less commonly, melena. Rarely, patients present with signs of intracranial hemorrhage or bleeding from other internal sites. However, it is not uncommon for patients to have a history of easy bruisibility for several months or longer prior to an acute exacerbation. In contrast to children, few adults give a history of a systemic viral illness in the weeks preceding the onset of bleeding. A few others have evidence of a pre-existing systemic disorder such as systemic lupus erythematosus (SLE), chronic lymphocytic leukemia (CLL), or human immunodeficiency virus (HIV) infection. However, the typical patient is entirely well with the exception of bleeding.

Differential Diagnosis

ITP is the most common cause of *isolated* thrombocytopenia in an otherwise healthy young adult. Other disorders that need to be considered include familial thrombocytopenia, hypersplenism, mild SLE, drug-induced thrombocytopenias, and HIV infection. During pregnancy, the differential diagnosis also includes gestational thrombocytopenia and pre-eclampsia. Other causes of thrombocytopenia are less common and are generally evident from the initial presentation. Among older adults, the major additional consideration is myelodysplasia, in which thrombocytopenia may precede other manifestations of the disease by months to years.[4]

Initial Evaluation

The physical examination, if abnormal at all, reveals only signs of bleeding. Splenomegaly suggests another diagnosis or an underlying illness with secondary immune thrombocytopenia. The blood counts are normal, with the exception of the platelet count, unless there has been significant bleeding. Thrombocytopenia determined by automated analyzer must be confirmed by a thorough examination of the peripheral smear. This will exclude the diagnosis of pseudothrombocytopenia and other common hematologic conditions, which generally affect multiple cell lines. The mean platelet size is increased in most, but not all patients, but platelets approaching the size of erythrocytes are more typical of some hereditary thrombocytopenias.[5] Coagulation tests to exclude a diagnosis of disseminated intravascular coagulation are rarely needed other than in patients who present during pregnancy. Patients with anemia should be evaluated for evidence of bleeding and immune hemolysis. Bone marrow aspiration and biopsy are generally performed to exclude other causes of thrombocytopenia, but are rarely revealing when the presentation is typical. Erythroid and myeloid development should be normal. Megakaryocytes are generally normal or increased in number.[5] Dysplastic features, including megakaryocyte clumping, suggest a myelodysplastic condition. ITP thus remains a clinical diagnosis of exclusion, and no additional diagnostic studies are required in the typical case.

Pseudothrombocytopenia

As noted above, the blood smear of every patient must be analyzed before making a diagnosis of ITP, both to exclude another cause of thrombocytopenia and to exclude pseudothrombocytopenia. Failure to diagnose pseudothrombocytopenia may lead to serious errors in management.[6] Pseudothrombocytopenia is an in vitro artifact of automated cell counting that occurs with a frequency of between 1 in 1,000 and 1 in 10,000 blood specimens collected in EDTA.[7-9] The phenomenon occurs when platelets are agglutinated by IgG, and less commonly IgM or IgA, autoantibodies or monoclonal proteins[10-12], that bind to a divalent cation-dependent conformer of the platelet glycoprotein (GP)IIb/IIIa complex[13,14] or another cryptic antigen[12] induced by a low concentration of ionized calcium attained only in vitro. In some cases, a direct effect of EDTA on antibody binding has been suggested.[15] The diagnosis should be suspected by finding platelet clumping on a blood smear made from EDTA-anticoagulated blood.[7,16] In some patients, the clumping is extensive enough to cause a spurious leukocytosis.[8,9,17] The diagnosis is confirmed by demonstrating that the platelet count is substantially higher when measured in citrated or heparinized blood, or blood obtained without an anticoagulant. The in vitro clumping occurs at body temperature, which distinguishes this phenomenon from in vitro platelet clumping caused by cold agglutinins,[7,18] although the two phenomena may coexist.[10,13,19] Less commonly, the peripheral blood smear may also show platelets adherent to[8,20] or, rarely, within[21,22] granulocytes or monocytes, a phenomenon known as platelet satellitism. Occasionally, pseudothrombocytopenia may be observed when giant platelets are excluded from automated analysis.[23] Because pseudothrombocytopenia and ITP, or other causes of thrombocytopenia, can coexist, the blood smear of patients with ITP must be analyzed to confirm the automated platelet count before changes in therapy are made.[24]

Pathogenesis

Prior to 1950 the pathogenesis of ITP remained a matter of debate. An immunologic cause was suspected by many investigators based on the prevalence of neonatal thrombocytopenia during prior or subsequent pregnancies in affected women, the frequency of coexisting immune hemolysis, and the clinical response to steroids and splenectomy. However, it was not until the studies of Harrington et al.,[25] showing that infusion of plasma from most ITP patients induced transient thrombocytopenia in normal recipients, that the importance of platelet autoantibodies was generally accepted. This observation was followed by efforts to isolate the autoantibodies and to identify the platelet antigens recognized.[26] The cumulative efforts of many investigators have provided definitive evidence that ITP is caused by platelet-reactive autoantibodies, but the nature of the derangement that leads to autoantibody production remains unknown.

Platelet life span is reduced in essentially all patients with ITP[27,28] due to the clearance of antibody-coated platelets by tissue macrophages.[29,30] The extent of clearance may vary among individuals[31] and may be modulated by cytokines that activate macrophages.[32] The contribution of intravascular destruction, if any, has not been established, but the possibility has been suggested because platelet-derived microparticles[33,34] and antibodies to cytoplasmic components of platelet glycoproteins are found in the plasma of some patients.[35] Nevertheless, the results of treatment, especially the rapid response to such measures as intravenous immunoglobulin (IVIg), anti-D, and splenectomy, suggest that extravascular clearance is the major cause of thrombocytopenia in most patients.

The extent of compensatory platelet production in ITP is a matter of contention. Initial studies were consistent with the notion that platelet production increased by as much as fivefold in most patients in response to the shortened platelet survival.[27,28] This conclusion was in keeping with the increased number of megakaryocytes in the bone marrow and the larger, presumably younger, platelets seen on peripheral smear. In addition, bleeding time studies suggested enhanced hemostatic effectiveness of the residual platelets, consistent with their presumed younger age. However, the results of several recent studies, in which the survival of autologous rather than homologous platelets was studied, indicate that platelet production may be more heterogeneous than previously appreciated.[36-38] Impaired platelet production has been reported in as many as one-half the cases, presumably secondary to destruction of antibody-coated platelets by intramedullary macrophages[39] or a direct effect of autoantibodies on megakaryocyte demarcation.[40] The effect of ITP antibodies on platelet function is discussed in Chapter 130.

Laboratory Evaluation

IgG and/or IgM antibodies against platelet glycoprotein complexes, including GPIIb/IIIa, GPIb/IX, GPV,[41] GPIa/IIa, GPIV,[42] and other specific platelet glycoproteins,[43,44] have been identified on the platelets or in the plasma of most ITP patients using recently developed techniques. These tests are based on the principle of antigen capture, in which a monoclonal antibody to a cell-specific glycoprotein is immobilized on a solid support to which a lysate of the patient's platelets or normal platelets sensitized with the patient's plasma is added. This step enables the antigen, and any associated human antibody, to be captured onto the solid support, where it can then be detected with an appropriately tagged anti-human immunoglobulin by radioimmunoassay or enzyme-linked immunosorbent assay. These assays have largely replaced antiglobulin tests, which had a high incidence of false-positive results. However, antiplatelet antibodies are not detected in approximately 10–30% of typical cases of ITP, even with the use of these newly developed techniques. False-negative test results may be caused by competition between the monoclonal and human antibodies for the same epitope on the platelet. For this reason it is advisable that at least two monoclonal antibodies that recognize distinct epitopes on the same glycoprotein complex be used. Antibodies may also dissociate from the antigen during test performance due to either low affinity or loss of the epitope during solubilization of the platelet. It should also be pointed out that there is little published information on the incidence of "false positives" (i.e., specific antiplatelet glycoprotein antibodies) in disorders that are hard to distinguish from ITP clinically, including myelodysplasia, pre-eclampsia, chronic liver disease, sepsis, and so forth, in which negative test results would be expected to provide the most benefit. Therefore, ITP remains a clinical diagnosis of exclusion, and it is still premature to confirm or to exclude the diagnosis using available platelet antibody tests.

Emergency Therapy

Emergency treatment is indicated for internal or widespread mucocutaneous bleeding. Most patients presenting with platelet counts of <10,000/mm^3 and certainly <5,000/mm^3 should be hospitalized until a beneficial effect of treatment can be documented, although it is possible to administer treatment on an outpatient basis in select cases. General measures to reduce the risk of bleeding should be instituted, including avoidance of drugs that interfere with platelet function, control of blood pressure and other medical conditions that inhibit coagulation, and measures to minimize the risk of trauma. Platelet transfusions are indicated only if there is evidence of major or life-threatening hemorrhage and may be surprisingly effective in this setting,[60,61] especially when given in conjunction with other therapies.[62] Treatment should be initiated with either IVIg (1 g/kg/day for 2 days) or intravenous methylpred-

nisolone (1–2 g/day for 1–3 days),[63] or both.[64] Emergency splenectomy should be reserved for the rare patient who fails to respond and requires additional treatment (e.g., prior to emergency craniotomy for intracranial hemorrhage).

Splenectomy

Although there is no evidence that the duration of treatment with glucocorticoids alters the clinical course of responding patients, it is the practice of most hematologists to taper prednisone over a period of 3–6 months. Despite this approach, most adults relapse whenever the decision to taper or discontinue prednisone is made, at which time splenectomy is considered. In general, splenectomy is the treatment of choice in any ITP patient who requires additional medical treatment to maintain a platelet count of >30,000/mm^3 and who is capable of undergoing the procedure.

Some investigators have reported a correlation between response to splenectomy and prior response to steroids,[65,66] but others have not, and splenectomy should not be excluded from consideration based on any combination of clinical or laboratory parameters.[48,49,51,67] Approximately two-thirds of adults will have a complete response to splenectomy, and another 15% will have a stable partial response.[2,47–49,51,52,65,67] Approximately 10–15% of responding patients will relapse either soon after splenectomy or many years later.[2,48,49,51,52,65] Splenic irradiation and embolization have been used successfully in a few patients in whom splenectomy was judged to be medically hazardous.[68] Severe bleeding is rarely encountered even when the patient is severely thrombocytopenic, and the practice of prophylactic platelet transfusions prior to splenectomy is to be discouraged. The major risk of the procedure after the operative period is overwhelming bacterial sepsis, which has been estimated to occur in 1% of adults who have undergone splenectomy for a variety of reasons. The incidence is lower in adults with uncomplicated ITP managed appropriately.[69] Patients should be immunized with polyvalent pneumococcal vaccine prior to splenectomy, if possible, and periodically thereafter. It is also our practice to have our patients seek urgent medical attention and begin antibiotics immediately at the onset of a systemic febrile illness.

Therapy for Splenectomy Failures

Approximately 10–20% of adults require additional treatment to maintain their platelet counts above 20,000–30,000/mm^3 after splenectomy, although the response rate may be lower in patients with Evans syndrome or SLE.[2,49] Although spontaneous remissions may still occur,[70] it is far more typical for thrombocytopenia to persist, and a mortality rate approaching 5% has been reported in this setting.[1,2,46–49,51,71]

The initial approach to patients with recurrent bleeding or severe thrombocytopenia after splenectomy is the same as that for patients who present with severe acute ITP: the diagnosis must be confirmed, measures to limit bleeding instituted, and treatment with corticosteroids resumed, even if they were ineffective prior to splenectomy. Once the platelet count has been increased to a safe level, the process of tapering steroids is resumed. An occasional patient will prove to be manageable with alternate-day corticosteroids or sufficiently low daily doses of prednisone (5–10 mg) to permit long-term use, but almost all patients will then require one or more of the treatments described below. When long-term treatment with even low doses of corticosteroids is being contemplated, it is important to monitor patients for development of cataracts and to consider measures to prevent osteoporosis.

Multiple treatment options are available. However, it is important to be clear that the goals of therapy for splenectomy failures differ from those on initial presentation, because the chance of inducing a durable, complete, and unmaintained remission is much lower. Treatment must therefore be individualized, with the aim of achieving a platelet count sufficient to prevent spontaneous bleeding as well as protection from injury or other emergencies, if possible. This risk depends not only on the platelet count itself, but on the patient's age, bleeding history, and co-morbid conditions.[72,73] Assessment of bleeding risk must be balanced against a similar estimate of potential complications resulting from each form of treatment. Therefore, no single treatment paradigm is applicable to all patients.

Search for an Accessory Spleen

The presence of an accessory spleen should be sought in any patient who has relapsed and is likely to require additional treatment, since antibody-coated platelets may be removed even if all Howell-Jolly bodies are not.[49,74–77] Most accessory spleens can be detected using ^{99m}Tc sulfur colloid, although more sensitive radionucleotide imaging techniques involving the use of antibody-coated or heat-damaged red cells, or computed tomography or magnetic resonance imaging scanning

may be required in select cases.[75–77] Neither the size of the accessory spleen nor any other characteristic has been useful in predicting a response to surgery. The reported response rates to removal of an accessory spleen vary widely, but are probably about 30%.[49,74,76–78]

Agents that Impair Platelet Clearance

Most patients do not have accessory spleens, and they require doses of corticosteroids to maintain adequate platelet counts that are poorly tolerated. The options for treatment in this setting are described below. Although each is discussed as a sole modality of therapy, we would emphasize that it is often possible to use these agents in combination at lower doses or at less frequent intervals with synergistic benefits and reduced toxicity.

Intravenous Immunoglobulin. A major treatment advance was made in 1981, when Imbach and co-workers[79] observed an increase in the platelet count of a child with immunodeficiency who had been treated with IVIg for infection. Within a few years, IVIg was being used extensively in otherwise healthy children and in adults with acute or chronic ITP. In a recent review of 28 published reports involving treatment of 282 patients with IVIg, >83% achieved a platelet count >50,000/mm^3, and 64% reached >100,000/mm^3 after the initial course of therapy.[80] IVIg is given by intermittent intravenous infusion over 1–5 days in total doses ranging from 500 mg/kg to 2 g/kg/course, with comparable response rates.[81] The infusions are generally repeated as needed every 10–21 days, consistent with the half-life of IgG in the circulation, although unexpectedly high rates of durable complete responses have been reported after IVIg was given on a fixed schedule.[82]

IVIg impairs the clearance of IgG-coated platelets, presumably by competing for binding to tissue macrophage Fc$_\gamma$ receptors.[83] The biologically "active" fraction of IVIg is unknown (i.e., it is uncertain whether monomeric IgG competes directly with antibody-coated platelets for binding to macrophages, or whether IgG aggregates in the preparations or cell-associated or soluble immune complexes formed in the recipient are responsible for the drug's effectiveness). Anti-idiotypic antibodies that interfere with binding or formation of antiplatelet autoantibodies may contribute in the occasional patients who develop long-term remissions,[84] but the observation that Fc$_\gamma$ fragments are as effective, as well as the comparable efficacy of anti-D, suggests that Fc$_\gamma$-receptor blockade is of prime importance in the initial response to IVIG in most patients.[85] There is no evidence that currently available commercial preparations differ in their efficacy or toxicity other than in the rare patient with IgA deficiency and anti-IgA antibodies.

Toxicity is generally mild and self-limited. As many as one-half the patients complain of headache (most often during the initial infusion), which is responsive to oral analgesics and to slowing the rate of administration. Occasional patients experience a more severe, but self-limited, migraine syndrome beginning 1–2 days after infusion; it may be associated with a pleocytosis in the cerebrospinal fluid.[86,87] Positive direct antiglobulin tests occur commonly,[88] and overt hemolytic anemia has occasionally developed from infusion of high-titer isoagglutinins in some preparations,[89,90] as has the formation of red cell isoagglutinins due to transfer of blood group A substance.[91] Other rare side effects include thrombosis,[92] pulmonary or renal failure,[93,94] and anaphylaxis in IgA-deficient patients with anti-IgA antibodies, in whom IgA-depleted preparations should be used.[95,96] Antiviral antibodies are passively acquired after administration of IVIg, but seroconversion to HIV-1 has not been seen, and there are no documented cases of HIV, hepatitis, or other infections having been acquired as a result of treatment,[97] although this has recently been called into question.[97a]

The major limitations of IVIg treatment have been the need for repeated intravenous infusion and its high cost, which averages almost $3,000/course in adults. Complete remissions and the development of a refractory state have each been reported in approximately one-third of patients receiving multiple courses of IVIg.[98] Whether maintenance treatment alters the natural history of chronic ITP remains open to question. In the absence of a controlled study the major indications for IVIg are (1) treatment of medical emergencies, (2) preparation for splenectomy in patients intolerant or resistant to corticosteroids, (3) as a means to defer splenectomy in young children or debilitated adults, (4) during pregnancy when potentially teratogenic drugs must be avoided, (5) chronic management of the rare patient who is refractory to other measures, or (6) while awaiting a response to a slower acting agent such as azathioprine or danazol.

Anti-D. Salama and Mueller-Eckhardt and co-workers[99] proposed that induction of a mild hemolytic anemia by infusing anti-D into Rh(D)+ individuals might inhibit macrophage Fc_γ-receptor function and clearance of antibody-coated platelets to the same extent as infusion of large amounts of nonspecific IgG. Indeed, nearly comparable response rates are seen after administration of 1/1,000 as much IgG given as anti-D compared with the amount given in a typical course of IVIg.[100] Treatment requires approximately 5 minutes and is far less expensive; the systemic side effects of IVIg are also avoided. The limitations of anti-D treatment include its inapplicability to Rh(D)− individuals, slower onset of response, lower increments in the platelet count, limited efficacy in splenectomized individuals, and dose-limiting hemolytic anemia.[100] The indications for its use are the same as those for IVIg.

Danazol. The impeded androgen danazol, given at a dose of 10–15 mg/kg/day, is effective in most adults according to some reports,[101–103] as well as in some children and patients with secondary immune thrombocytopenia.[104,105] Danazol may impair macrophage-mediated clearance of antibody-coated platelets initially,[106] but inhibition of antibody production[102,107] may contribute to its effectiveness after several months of use. Despite these favorable reports, the efficacy of danazol in refractory patients remains a matter of controversy.[103,108–112] The variation in the observed response rates may in part be due to differences in the duration of treatment.[109] In one series, the mean duration of treatment was 2.7 months, but some individuals required as much as 6 months until a response was seen.[102] In our experience, the major indications for danazol are to defer splenectomy and as a corticosteroid-sparing drug. Although an occasional patient will experience an extended, unmaintained remission after a prolonged course, more commonly responses can be maintained at much lower daily doses[113]; relapses typically occur weeks to months after therapy is stopped entirely. Danazol shares with other androgens the potential for causing hepatic injury, including cholestatic hepatitis,[114] peliosis,[115] and neoplasia[116] as its most serious side effect. Thrombocytopenia was reported as a complication of danazol in a few patients treated for disorders other than ITP.[117]

Vinca Alkaloids. Vincristine and vinblastine bind avidly to platelet microtubules.[118,119] This property may permit the drugs to be delivered by antibody-coated platelets to tissue macrophages, thereby inhibiting their phagocytic capabilities.[106,120] Vincristine (0.025 mg/kg; not to exceed 2 mg) and vinblastine (4–6 mg/m²; not to exceed 10 mg) can be administered by injection or slow infusion; the latter method is reported to be somewhat more efficacious.[121] Reported response rates in patients with chronic ITP vary widely. In contrast to

initially favorable reports,[122–125] the results of more recent and larger series indicate that the response rate to either drug is closer to 10–20% among patients with chronic refractory ITP, consistent with our experience, and sustained complete remissions are rare.[26,52,71,122,123] Treatment generally has to be given every 2–4 weeks for an indefinite period, and many patients become refractory or treatment has to be stopped because of neurologic or hematologic toxicity, especially in the elderly or those with mild, pre-existing neurologic impairment.

Immunosuppressants

The immunosuppressive drugs azathioprine or cyclophosphamide are generally reserved for patients who are refractory or intolerant of the above-mentioned treatments. However, the proper place of these drugs in the treatment of refractory patients has recently been reassessed. Of the patients treated with azathioprine, 25–40% attain a complete remission, and an additional 10–20% have a partial response in the experience of some investigators,[52,70,126,127] although lower response rates have been noted by others.[52,128] The variable outcomes reported may again reflect differences in the intensity or duration of treatment. For example, the median time to response among patients in one study was 4 months, and maximal benefit was not achieved in some cases until 7–8 months of treatment.[127] Responses were generally durable and, at least in some patients, persisted after treatment was discontinued. Side effects were rare and predominantly limited to reversible elevations of serum transaminases. Comparable or only slightly lower response rates have been reported with the use of cyclophosphamide as a single agent.[52,128,129] However, since cyclophosphamide may cause infertility[130] or leukemia,[131] its use should be restricted, especially among younger patients. The combination of cyclophosphamide and prednisone with one of a number of additional agents has been effective in a small number of refractory patients with acceptable toxicity.[132,133] A few patients have been treated successfully with cyclosporine,[58,134,135] with a monoclonal antilymphocyte antibody,[136] or with pulsed, high-dose dexamethazone therapy.[57a]

Treatment Whose Mechanism of Action Is Unknown

A few patients with chronic refractory ITP have been treated by incubating their plasma with staphylococcal protein A, with an overall response rate approaching 30%.[137] The mechanism of action is likely to be more complex than simply removal of immune complexes, since the volume of plasma that is generally treated is far less than the amount of antibody removed by plasma exchange, which is rarely effective in chronic ITP.[138] Remarkably, >80% of the reported responses were maintained without additional therapy, with a mean follow-up of 8 months. Approximately one-third of the patients developed an acute hypersensitivity-type reaction, necessitating discontinuation of treatment in 5%.[137,139] Cases of hypotension and fatal anaphylaxis have been reported in patients treated for other disorders.[139] More experience with protein A pheresis will be required before its proper place in the treatment of ITP is clarified. Dapsone[140–142] and colchicine[143,144] have been reported to be effective in a limited number of patients. Their mechanism of action is unknown, and the response rates in refractory patients have not been studied prospectively. Recently, some adults and children with ITP have been treated successfully with recombinant interferon-α_{2b}[145–148] although the efficacy has not been confirmed in other studies, and worsening of thrombocytopenia has been noted on occasion.[149–152] Additional information will be needed before its use can be recommended.

Secondary Thrombocytopenias

Secondary immune thrombocytopenias now comprise ≤40% of the cases of ITP in some series.[153,154] The reason for the increased recognition of secondary ITP is not apparent, other than the recent epidemic of HIV-1 infection (see Ch. 155). However, this incidence needs to be considered when deciding which patients with ITP should be investigated for an underlying disorder and when to treat a patient with a systemic illness for presumed secondary ITP when other causes of thrombocytopenia may be more frequent or may coexist. Since ITP remains a diagnosis of exclusion, the accuracy of these decisions requires familiarity with the prevalence, implications, and proper management of secondary immune thrombocytopenia in each associated condition.

Systemic Lupus Erythematosus
Presentation

Approximately 15–25% of patients with SLE develop thrombocytopenia during the course of their illness, although in only 5–10% of cases is the problem severe enough to require treatment.[2,155–158] Thrombocytopenia may precede the diagnosis of SLE by months to years,[158,159] but such progression occurs in <2% of all patients with classic ITP.[2,160,161] Although SLE may occur more commonly among patients with high titers of certain antinuclear antibodies, the great majority of ITP patients with positive antinuclear antibodies do not develop the disease, and serologic evaluation should be restricted to patients who show additional evidence of the disorder.[159,161,162]

The prognostic significance of thrombocytopenia in patients with SLE depends on the clinical context. Four clinical presentations have been described. The clinical course of patients who develop immune thrombocytopenia without a worsening of other disease manifestations is essentially identical to patients with ITP.[2,155,158,163,164] By contrast, severe thrombocytopenia that develops during a systemic exacerbation of vasculitis may have a different pathogenesis (see below) and carries a poorer prognosis.[155,157,164,165] Thrombocytopenia also occurs in patients with antiphospholipid antibodies, who may be at a somewhat higher risk of thrombosis and recurrent spontaneous abortions.[166–168] Finally, amegakaryocytic thrombocytopenia has been detected in several patients with SLE and should be considered a separate entity.[169,170]

Pathogenesis

The pathogenesis of thrombocytopenia in SLE patients may be multifactorial. Circulating platelet-reactive antibodies with diverse specificities have been identified, including some that bind to different proteins,[171–173] phospholipids,[174–176] and complexes of proteins and phospholipids,[177,178] among others. Which of these antibodies cause thrombocytopenia is unknown. Both DNA and DNA-anti-DNA complexes have been detected on patient platelets, as well.[179] However, since such complexes are found in many patients with SLE, including those in whom thrombocytopenia is absent or mild,[180,181] their importance in accelerating platelet clearance or altering platelet function[182,183] remains to be demonstrated. Platelet clearance may be influenced not only by the composition of these immune complexes, which are undoubtedly heterogeneous, but also by impaired macrophage IgG Fcγ-receptor-mediated clearance due to the underlying disease and its treatment.[184] Finally, when severe thrombocytopenia occurs as part of a systemic relapse, platelet activation and deposition may also occur within vessels involved by vasculitis, such as the kidney.[185] Thrombocytopenia caused by vascular injury may not respond to measures that suffice to manage ITP.

Management

Treatment of thrombocytopenic episodes in patients with SLE is more complicated than the management of classic ITP for several reasons. First, thrombocytopenia caused by platelet-specific antibodies must be distinguished from that caused by systemic vasculitis. In extreme cases, the distinction may be relatively straightforward. At one end of the spectrum, patients with severe thrombocytopenia in whom there is no other evidence of active SLE should be treated as if they had ITP. At the other extreme, it is generally necessary to control the systemic vasculitis before thrombocytopenia will improve. However, in many patients the contribution of vasculitis is not apparent and may vary. Second, since patients with SLE may experience multiple episodes of thrombocytopenia, treatment should only be used when a risk of bleeding exists, to avoid excessive use of corticosteroids in these heavily treated patients. Third, attempts to induce long-term remission with splenectomy should be tempered by the knowledge that many patients continue to require corticosteroids to control the underlying disease. Therefore, management decisions should be based on the extent to which thrombocytopenia per se is the predominant reason for treatment and the likelihood that systemic vasculitis or arthritis will require treatment in the future.

When thrombocytopenia occurs in the absence of a systemic flare, the short-term response to corticosteroids, danazol, IVIg, and immunosuppression in patients with SLE and classic ITP are comparable.[186–191] The role of splenectomy remains controversial. Variation in long-term response rates is undoubtedly influenced by differences in the severity of the underlying disease.[158,192–196] In our opinion, splenectomy is indicated only when thrombocytopenia is severe and persistent, is the predominant reason for treatment, and when systemic manifestations of the SLE are otherwise well controlled, in which situation the procedure is as effective as in ITP. Profound thrombocytopenia that occurs during the course of a systemic exacerbation of SLE may require pulses of high-dose corticosteroids[197,198] or cyclophosphamide,[199] or both.

Lymphoproliferative Disorders
Chronic Lymphocytic Leukemia

Thrombocytopenia caused by marrow and splenic infiltration is a common feature of advanced CLL[200] and is associated with a mean survival of about 19 months.[201] By contrast, immune thrombocytopenia, which occurs in approximately 2% of CLL patients,[202–204] does not confer a poor prognosis[205–207] and requires separate treatment. ITP may precede the diagnosis of CLL or develop at any stage.[206,208,209] The pathophysiology of autoantibody production in CLL and its relationship to the clonal B-cell proliferation has been the subject of recent reviews.[210,211]

The diagnosis of antibody-mediated thrombocytopenia must be made on clinical grounds alone, since platelet antiglobulin tests may be positive in CLL patients in the absence of thrombocytopenia.[212] ITP should be suspected in patients with early-stage CLL whose bone marrow contains "adequate" numbers of megakaryocytes or in patients with a more advanced stage in whom the severity of thrombocytopenia is disproportionate to the extent of marrow infiltration or splenomegaly. The concurrent development of autoimmune hemolytic anemia may suggest the diagnosis as well.[206,209] The cause of thrombocytopenia may be difficult to establish in patients who have a significant tumor burden, and a short course of therapy for ITP, such as IVIg, may be indicated. Although most patients with CLL and immune thrombocytopenia respond to corticosteroids or splenectomy,[205–207,209] cytotoxic or immunosuppressive therapy that may inhibit B-cell proliferation as well as antibody production has been required in some cases.[205–208]

Hodgkin Disease and Non-Hodgkin Lymphomas

ITP occurs in approximately 1% of patients with Hodgkin disease.[2,154,202,213–215] In three-fourths of the reported cases, ITP was diagnosed an average of 52 months (1 month to 22 years) after Hodgkin disease was detected.[216] Hodgkin disease was discovered at the time of splenectomy for ITP in a few patients.[2,217,218] In most of the remaining cases ITP preceded the diagnosis of Hodgkin disease, although in some instances the interval was so long as to place in doubt the significance of the association.[215,216,219-221] A persistent dilemma is whether the development of ITP signals a recurrence of the lymphoma. Although such cases have been reported,[154,216-219,222] approximately two-thirds of the patients did not have evidence of active Hodgkin disease.[214-216,220,223,224] Virtually all patients in whom there was no evidence of recurrent Hodgkin disease responded to some combination of corticosteroids,[216,219,221,224] splenectomy[213,215,217,218] and azathioprine.[215,224] Treatment of active Hodgkin disease has been required in some patients before the thrombocytopenia resolved.[206,218,220]

The association between immune thrombocytopenia and non-Hodgkin lymphomas appears coincidental, and few generalizations can be made from available case reports.[154,215,225-228] The histologic type of lymphoma and extent of the underlying disease has varied widely. In most cases, thrombocytopenia was difficult to manage unless the underlying malignancy responded to chemotherapy.

Leukemia of Large Granular Lymphocytes

The term leukemia of large granular lymphocytes (LGL) is applied to two disorders that can be distinguished by the phenotype of the clonally expanded cell population.[229] Thrombocytopenia occurs in both forms of the disease, although the pathogenesis and treatment differ. In >90% of patients there is a clonal expansion of $CD3^+$, $CD16^+$ T cells (T-LGL), and the natural history is generally one of stability or slow expansion of this cell population. In the remaining patients, the LGL cells express a natural killer (NK) cell phenotype ($CD3^-$, $CD16^+$, $CD57^+$). NK-LGL is typically aggressive, and severe thrombocytopenia, caused by marrow replacement and splenic infiltration, may develop over several months.[229]

Most patients with T-LGL come to medical attention because of recurrent infections due to neutropenia.[230] Thrombocytopenia, which occurs in 5–20% of the patients, is generally mild and may be secondary to splenic enlargement, but occasional patients present with severe thrombocytopenia and a clinical picture compatible with ITP.[230-233] The diagnosis of LGL should be suspected in a patient with thrombocytopenia accompanied by neutropenia, splenomegaly, arthralgias, or a positive test for rheumatoid factor. On occasion, the number of LGL cells is increased only modestly,[229] making it hard to distinguish this disorder from severe ITP, in which an increase in the $CD56^+$, $CD3^-$ NK cell population has also been observed.[234] There are insufficient data to indicate whether the response to treatment of immune thrombocytopenia in patients with T-LGL differs from typical ITP.

Miscellaneous Disorders

Mild thrombocytopenia attributed to hypersplenism occurs commonly in patients with autoimmune hyperthyroidism, resolving slowly with return of the euthyroid state.[235,236] Immune thrombocytopenia probably occurs more commonly in these patients than in the general population as well.[235-239] While most patients respond to measures effective in ITP, others require control of the hyperthyroid state before the thrombocytopenia abates.[236,237,240] In patients with sarcoidosis, immune platelet destruction may be superimposed on thrombocytopenia caused by splenic and marrow infiltration with granulomas.[241-243] ITP has also been reported in patients with myasthenia gravis[244] and in patients with a variety of benign and malignant neoplasms, most of whom responded to conventional treatment for ITP.[228,245-247] Thrombocytopenia occurs commonly after allogeneic bone marrow transplantation in the setting of graft-versus-host disease, in which platelet autoantibodies, vascular injury, and hypersplenism may contribute to accelerated platelet destruction.[248-251] Both transient and persistent immune thrombocytopenias have also been reported after organ and bone marrow allografts donated by patients with presumed compensated ITP.[252-255] Thrombocytopenia associated with HIV infection is discussed in Chapter 155.

ITP in Childhood

The approach to the child with ITP differs substantially from that for adults with respect to the differential diagnosis that must be considered at presentation, the high frequency of spontaneous remission, and, therefore, the greater delay before splenectomy is considered.

Clinical Manifestations

As in adults, children with acute ITP typically present with the sudden onset of petechiae and platelet counts <20–30,000/mm[3.] The relationship between the risk of bleeding and the platelet count appears to be the same as in adults. However, intracranial hemorrhage has been reported in approximately 0.5–1% of the children, an incidence that is higher than in adults.[256] Both sexes are affected with equal frequency. The peak incidence occurs between the ages of 3 and 5.[257] Although many patients have a history of nonspecific viral infection in the weeks prior to development of symptoms, such symptoms are common in children, and a relationship of preceding infection to the development of ITP is hard to document. Occasional patients present with ITP during or ≤4 weeks after an otherwise typical systemic viral infection caused by Epstein-Barr virus,[258,259] varicella,[260,261] cytomegalovirus,[262,263] rubella,[264,265] hepatitis A, B, or C,[266,267] or occasionally other infections,[268,269] or after vaccination with attenuated live virus.[270,271] The parents and pediatrician are usually more concerned than the child, who continues to feel and act completely well. As in adults, the physical examination is notable only for signs of bleeding and the absence of hepatomegaly or lymphadenopathy. Mild splenomegaly is detectable in <10% of children.[160] The CBC should be within normal limits for age, with the exception of the platelet count. This includes the white blood cell differential, which normally has more lymphocytes than neutrophils in children <4–5 years of age.[272,273]

Evaluation

To experienced pediatric hematologists, this constellation of findings (i.e., an otherwise healthy child with isolated thrombocytopenia on CBC and a physical examination notable only for bruising or petechiae) is sufficient to make a diagnosis of ITP, which is by far the most common cause (>95%) of isolated thrombocytopenia in childhood. In general, no additional testing is required if the presentation is typical, although an unresolved issue is the utility of a bone marrow examination in this setting. Specifically, a recent survey showed that many pediatric hematologists no longer believe that examination of the bone marrow is necessary to make a diagnosis of ITP when the presentation is typical, but that such an examination is required (1) when abnormalities of the physical examination or in nonplatelet components of the CBC are seen; (2) in patients who do not respond to treatment; or (3) in those whose initial treatment will be corticosteroids.[272] A response to IVIg in this setting is essentially diagnostic of ITP as well.[273] The outcome of cooperative childhood cancer study group trials, which included thousands of children, demonstrated that it is extremely unlikely (<0.1%) for childhood acute leukemia to present with isolated thrombocytopenia, an otherwise normal blood count and smear, and the absence of hepatosplenomegaly or lymphadenopathy.[256,274] HIV testing should be performed if there is any suspicion that the child or mother is in a defined at-risk group, including ex-premature infants who have received transfusion, or when significant adenopathy is detected.[275,276]

Differential Diagnosis

Once thrombocytopenia is documented in a healthy child and no abnormalities other than bleeding manifestations are detected on physical examination or CBC, the first consideration is to exclude familial, nonimmune thrombocytopenias. These disorders are seen in 2–10% of the children presenting with isolated thrombocytopenia,[277] and they appear to occur far more commonly than does familial ITP.[278,279] Precise diagnostic tests are lacking. A bone marrow examination will not help to differentiate ITP from these inherited syndromes. The utility of testing for platelet antibodies in this setting is uncertain. The diagnosis may not be suspected despite careful questioning, since other affected family members may be asymptomatic. On occasion, an inherited cause of thrombocytopenia may only be suspected after the child has failed to respond to treatment for ITP, at which time the diagnosis may be established by demonstrating thrombocytopenia in parents or siblings. Fortunately, most children with inherited thrombocytopenias have mild-to-moderate thrombocytopenia (40–100,000/mm³) and do not have symptoms or require treatment other than when platelet production is further impaired, such as during infection. The specific inherited thrombocytopenic syndromes are considered in detail in Chapter 129. Hypomegakaryocytic thrombocytopenia may be indistinguishable from ITP on presentation, and the diagnosis may be considered only when the child fails to respond to treatment. Too few cases have been reported to determine the long-term outcome and frequency of response in children to danazol, immunosuppressive therapy, or bone marrow transplantation.

The second consideration is to exclude an underlying disorder associated with ITP. Only HIV (see Ch. 155), SLE, and humoral immunodeficiency states occur with sufficient frequency in childhood to merit consideration. HIV as a cause of ITP in childhood is being seen with increased frequency. Usually the diagnosis is readily apparent by maternal history or from the initial examination of the child. Maternal-child transmission in utero is the most common means of transmission, although occasional cases due to transfusion have been reported. Affected children generally have axillary adenopathy, hepatosplenomegaly, and/or an abnormal hemoglobin, total white blood cell count, or differential. Although the CD4/CD8 ratio is of less use in this age group, HIV testing is reliable in children >6–12 months of age. SLE may develop in as many as 5% of female adolescents who present with ITP. This concern has led some pediatricians to an inappropriate search for antinuclear antibodies in every child with ITP. A positive antinuclear antibody test neither predicts for the development of SLE nor correlates with disease severity, responsiveness, or the incidence of spontaneous remission in otherwise healthy children.[280] Therefore, testing for antinuclear antibodies should only be performed if additional symptoms or laboratory findings suggest the diagnosis. Humoral immunodeficiency is found in 1–2% of children with ITP, most commonly due to IgA deficiency.[281] However, ITP occurs in ≥5% of children with common variable hypogammaglobulinemia.[282] This incidence may be sufficiently high to warrant measuring immunoglobulin levels and documenting response to polyvalent pneumococcal vaccine prior to splenectomy.[283] Immunoglobulin measurements are also indicated in children receiving IVIg, since the use of IgA-depleted preparations may prevent formation of anti-IgA antibodies and is effective when such antibodies already exist.[284]

Third, additional diagnoses must be considered if other cytopenias are present. For example, the finding of severe anemia even if there has been significant epistaxis, should lead to an investigation of alternative diagnoses such as aplastic anemia, myelodysplasia, and disorders associated with accelerated erythrocyte and platelet destruction such as thrombotic thrombocytopenic purpura and Evans syndrome.[285] The diagnosis of the latter may be complicated if the patient has recently been treated either with IVIg, which may contain anti-A or -B isohemagglutinins, or with anti-D, since both therapies may cause a positive direct antiglobulin test.[286]

Management of Chronic ITP After 6 Months

Most pediatric hematologists delay recommending splenectomy for ≥1 year for two reasons. First, children who have platelet counts >20–30,000/mm³ and who are asymptomatic can be followed safely without treatment. Our experience and that of others is that the platelet count generally improves over time.[304] However, the platelet count may fall at the time of puberty in previously stable patients, and mennorhagia can be a complicating feature during this period. Second, the risk of postsplenectomy sepsis may be as high as 2% in children and higher in those <1–2 years of age.[69] Indeed, the risk of sepsis in children may approximate the risk of severe bleeding, and there have been as many reported deaths from infection as from bleeding in this age group.[305,306] It remains to be determined whether this risk is reduced substantially by the use of pneumococcal and H. Flu B vaccines in conjunction with prophylactic antibiotics, which is the standard of care. The interval between repeat vaccinations and the value of prophylactic antibiotics remain unsettled. We currently recommend that Pneumovax be given every 5–10 years but do not administer hepatitis vaccine unless a special risk is identified. We recommend that prophylactic antibiotics be used for the first year after splenectomy and thereafter that they be given immediately for any infection; antibiotics should be given intravenously with a fever >102°C. No other long-term health risks have been identified in children who have been splenectomized for ITP.

Therefore, most pediatric hematologists prefer waiting until a child has reached 5 years of age before recommending splenectomy because of the frequency of infection and high fevers in this population, although there are insufficient data on the risk of sepsis after the age of 2 to make firm recommendations. In the youngest children it may be wise to document protective titers of antibody to the most common pneumococcal serotypes before proceeding to splenectomy. Durable clinical remission occurs in 70–90% of children with typical ITP after splenectomy.[304] Among the few children refractory to splenectomy, alternate diagnoses should be reinvestigated. Few children have significant bleeding problems even if they remain thrombocytopenic, which must be borne in mind when recommending potentially toxic forms of treatment. The rare, symptomatic, refractory pediatric patient should be approached in the same manner as the comparable adult, although the potential side effects of each drug may differ depending on the age of the child.

Immune Thrombocytopenia During Pregnancy

Since ITP occurs commonly in young women, hematologists are often asked to manage this disorder during pregnancy. The incidence is approximately 1–2 in 1,000 deliveries in referral institutions but is likely to be lower in the general community.[307] The proper management of ITP in pregnancy requires awareness of the incidence and consequences of neonatal thrombocytopenia due to transplacental passage of maternal

MANAGEMENT OF CHILDHOOD ITP

The issue of which children with acute ITP should be treated remains unresolved. The major reason to initiate treatment in severely thrombocytopenic children is to prevent intracranial hemorrhage (ICH) or life-threatening hemorrhage,[287] since ≥80% of affected individuals will recover spontaneously, many within the first 2 months.[288,289] Because the incidence of ICH is too low to perform a comprehensive analysis of treatment outcome,[290] experienced pediatric hematologists continue to disagree as to whether the incidence of ICH is sufficient to justify treating all children with severe thrombocytopenia[291] and whether such treatment decreases the risk of severe hemorrhage.[292]

Our recommendations concerning treatment, detailed below, are based on four considerations. First, ICH is rarely, if ever, seen in children with platelet counts >20,000/mm³. Second, 9 of the 18 well-documented cases of ICH reported prior to 1983 occurred >6 weeks after diagnosis, and hemorrhage may occur after initiation of treatment that ultimately succeeds in raising the platelet count.[287] Third, ICH may occur in the absence of other signs of bleeding.[287] Fourth, there is currently no means to identify the subset of children who will develop chronic ITP and no evidence that the incidence is altered by treatment.

IVIg has become the treatment of choice for producing a rapid response,[293,294] although infusion of intravenous methylprednisolone (30 mg/kg/day for 1–3 days) may be as effective and less expensive.[295] The combination of IVIg and corticosteroids may be synergistic.[296] Platelet transfusions should be reserved for ongoing or imminent major hemorrhage.[61] We recommend that all severely thrombocytopenic children with acute ITP (platelet counts <20,000/mm³) be treated with a combination of IVIg (1 g/kg/day for 1–3 days) and intravenous methylprednisolone (30 mg/kg/day) until a platelet count >20,000/mm³ is achieved, and there is no evidence of bleeding. Lessening the risk of hemorrhage and the need to restrict the child's physical activity is associated with considerable relief of parental anxiety as well. The diagnosis of ITP should be reconsidered in the rare situation in which a child fails to demonstrate even a partial response to IVIg or methyprednisolone, or both. Occasionally the addition of plasma exchange, a vinca alkaloid, or intravenous anti-D to the treatment regimen may be required.

Management of Acute ITP After the First Week

The goal of treatment is to maintain a platelet count at >20–30,000/mm³ with a minimum of toxicity. Drugs containing aspirin and glycerol guaiacolate should be avoided. Guidelines must be set for physical activity. It is our policy to preclude competitive contact sports, es-pecially contact football or basketball, lacrosse, soccer, and hockey, for children with platelet counts of <30,000/mm³ but not to restrict other physical activities, including track, swimming, bicycling, baseball, and tennis, although such decisions need to be individualized. In general, activity should be encouraged.

Primary reliance is often placed on prednisone because it is relatively inexpensive, can be given orally, and the toxicity is tolerable when the duration of treatment is limited. One approach is to taper the dose of prednisone over 1–3 months, although there is no evidence that any specific duration of treatment increases the probability of sustained complete remission. An attempt should be made to administer prednisone on an alternate-day regimen to avoid toxicity, including osteoporosis, which may be the most medically significant long-term side effect of corticosteroids in children.

We recommend the use of IVIg[293,294,297,298] or intravenous anti-D (Winthro-SD)[100,299] for children who require >0.33–0.5 mg/kg of prednisone every other day as their initial treatment or when >2–3 months of treatment is required. Both IVIg and anti-D are generally administered on an as-needed basis rather than at fixed intervals. The combination of prednisone with IVIg (and probably anti-D) may be synergistic. Treatment should be continued for ≥3–6 months if a response is seen since spontaneous remissions occur even many months after presentation. With this combination of drugs, few children require splenectomy for acute ITP. Treatment with vinca alkaloids,[125,300] azathioprine, or danazol[301] may be required in a few children in order to defer splenectomy. Since the disease will remit between the first and twelfth month in >80% of children with typical ITP, splenectomy should be deferred, if at all possible, for ≥12 months from the time of diagnosis.

The advantage of IVIg in managing children includes its lack of toxicity, its high rate of efficacy, and the possibility of curative effects.[273,292] The disadvantages are that it must be given intravenously for hours, that optimal use in maintenance depends upon the platelet count (making scheduling difficult), that postinfusion headaches are common, and that its cost is high.[302] In contrast to adults, few pediatric patients become refractory to prolonged treatment with IVIg. There is no evidence that any of the commercially available products differ in clinical effectiveness. Intravenous anti-D is still experimental but should be licensed before the end of 1994. Over 500 patients have been treated in Europe and the United States. Anti-D, which appears to be as safe and effective as IVIg for Rh+ patients who have not undergone splenectomy, may become the treatment of choice in this setting. The cost is considerably less, and infusion is complete within minutes.[100] Whether early treatment with IVIg or anti-D will alter the incidence of chronic ITP remains to be determined.[297,298,303]

autoantibodies, as well as the risks and benefits to the fetus of maternal therapy, invasive monitoring, and surgical delivery. The reader is referred to a recent comprehensive review of thrombocytopenia in pregnancy.[308]

It may be difficult to diagnose ITP when a women presents near term with no prior platelet counts. The most common condition that must be distinguished from ITP is gestational thrombocytopenia, which occurs in approximately 4% of preg-nant women at term (see Ch. 128). The diagnosis of gestational thrombocytopenia is simple when an otherwise entirely healthy woman known to have a normal platelet count in the recent past develops mild thrombocytopenia (>100,000/mm³) during the third trimester of an uncomplicated pregnancy. The importance of making the distinction from ITP is that severe neonatal thrombocytopenia is rare in presumed gestational thrombocytopenia and there is no indication for additional diagnostic or therapeutic intervention.[307] However, gestational thrombocytopenia and ITP are both diagnoses of exclusion. Although the incidence of gestational thrombocytopenia in the typical setting vastly exceeds all other causes of thrombocytopenia combined, on occasion a previously healthy woman will present at term for the first time with mild-to-moderate ITP, early pre-eclampsia, type IIb von Willebrand disease, or a congenital thrombocytopenic condition. The frequency of these other disorders is likely to be higher among women with platelet counts $<75,000/mm^3$ and when thrombocytopenia is detected before the third trimester. The situation is made more complicated because platelet antiglobulin tests do not distinguish ITP from gestational thrombocytopenia,[309–312] and severe neonatal thrombocytopenia has been reported in the offspring of women with presumed gestational thrombocytopenia.[313] Moreover, we and others[310,311] have observed an increase in platelet count after IVIg or corticosteroids

in women whose platelet counts fell to $<50,000/mm^3$ who had a presumptive diagnosis of gestational thrombocytopenia based on clinical criteria; whether these women actually had ITP is unknown. Therefore, all causes of thrombocytopenia in pregnancy should be considered before a diagnosis of gestational thrombocytopenia is assumed.

NEONATAL ALLOIMMUNE THROMBOCYTOPENIA

Presentation

Neonatal alloimmune thrombocytopenia (NAIT) is the platelet analogue of hemolytic disease of the newborn, although there are important differences in natural history and management. NAIT occurs in about 1 in 2,000 term pregnancies (about 800–2,000 cases per year in the United States),[349,350] accounting

---

THERAPY FOR ITP DURING PREGNANCY

Most women with ITP can be managed without difficulty during pregnancy. The only contraindication to pregnancy is treatment with cytotoxic drugs during the first trimester.[314] Only occasional patients experience severe exacerbations during successive pregnancies. Pregnancy does not alter the indications for maternal treatment, since platelet counts of $50–100,000/mm^3$ suffice for cesarean section.[315] Corticosteroids are the mainstay of treatment and appear to have a relatively low incidence of adverse effects in the fetus,[316] although adverse effects have been noted in some experimental and clinical studies.[317–320] Refractory patients and those intolerant of prednisone during pregnancy can generally be managed with IVIg.[321] Splenectomy has been performed successfully during pregnancy, but should be avoided, if possible.[322,323] There is limited experience with azathioprine during pregnancy,[324] although teratogenoic complications have been reported.[325,326] Other drugs, including danazol, should also be avoided if possible, because far less is known about potential effects on the fetus.

The major concern comes at the time of delivery. The goal is to prevent intracranial hemorrhage from occurring in a severely thrombocytopenic neonate during a difficult vaginal delivery.[327,328] However, there is no generally accepted noninvasive means to identify neonates at risk, the benefits of cesarean section are unproved and the relative risks of newer interventional diagnostic and therapeutic measures have not been established.[329,330] Therefore, the best approach to managing delivery in women with ITP remains controversial and continues to evolve.

Initial studies suggested that women with ITP were at high risk of severe neonatal theombocytopenia.[327] However, women with severe ITP and those first diagnosed after delivering a clinically affected child may have been overrepresented in these series.[327,331] Studies performed since the advent of automated platelet counts suggest that the risk is much lower. However, these series may have underestimated the risk by including women with gestational thrombocytopenia. More recently, three prospective studies involving 178 women with ITP diagnosed prior to pregnancy indicate that the incidence of severe neonatal thrombocytopenia (i.e., platelet counts at birth of $<50,000/mm^3$) is approximately 10–15%.[307,311,315]

There were no documented cases of antenatal ICH, arguing against a role for therapeutic intervention, as proposed for alloimmune thrombocytopenia. In addition, ICH occurred in only 2 of 128 neonates. Similarly, in a recent retrospective review, 25% of 474 infants were born with platelet counts $<100,000/mm^3$, among whom the incidence of ICH was 3%.[330]

Unfortunately, no noninvasive means by which the fetal platelet count can be predicted presently exist, and no significant correlation can be seen between fetal and maternal platelet counts either before or after treatment.[313,315,332–336] Severely thrombocytopenic neonates have been born to mothers with normal platelet counts (i.e., previously undiagnosed, presumed compensated ITP),[337] as well as to women with complete clinical responses to splenectomy,[323,338,339] corticosteroids, or IVIg.[313,333,340,341] A report that the risk of neonatal thrombocytopenia is low in women without circulating platelet antibodies requires confirmation.[311] It is now possible to measure the neonatal platelet count directly before delivery by means of fetal scalp sampling[342,343] or percutaneous umbilical blood sampling.[313] However, in inexperienced hands, determination of neonatal platelet counts by fetal scalp sampling is often complicated by falsely low values due to platelet clumping, leading to unnecessary emergency cesarean sections.[335,344] The risk to the fetus of percutaneous umbilical blood sampling depends on the skill of the operator and may be comparable to that of ICH.[311,313,315,345–347] The role of fetal percutaneous blood sampling and cesarean section remains unsettled.[313,329,330,335,348]

The neonatal platelet count commonly falls in the first few days postpartum, possibly because of the maturation of the fetal reticuloendothelial cell system.[331,332] The fall is transient and infrequently requires treatment. Affected neonates will generally respond to IVIg or corticosteroids. To diagnose or exlude ICH, it is mandatory to obtain a radiologic investigation such as an ultrasound as soon after birth as possible in all severely thrombocytopenic neonates. Management with repeated platelet transfusions combined with corticosteroids and IVIg should be instituted emergently if there is any suspicion of bleeding, even in the absence of signs of neurologic impairment.

for about 10–20% of the total number of cases of neonatal thrombocytopenia.[351,352] The actual incidence is likely to be higher as additional cases are identified (by recently developed serologic techniques) in neonates born with moderate thrombocytopenia. In contrast to hemolytic disease of the newborn, almost one-half of the cases of NAIT occur during the first term pregnancy,[349,353] although the incidence of prior miscarriage in these women is unknown.[349,354] Typically, the diagnosis is suspected when bleeding and severe thrombocytopenia occur in a neonate born after an otherwise uneventful pregnancy. Internal bleeding (10–30%) and intracranial hemorrhage (10–20%) are common. The mortality rate may be as high as 4% among index cases.[349,351,353–355] The affected child may show signs and symptoms of hydrocephalus or porencephaly due to hemorrhage in utero.[349,353,356,357] Thus, in contrast to neonatal thrombocytopenia caused by maternal ITP, NAIT is often severe and potentially life-threatening.[358] The platelet count may continue to fall, and bleeding may occur during the first several days after delivery, necessitating prompt diagnosis and management.[349,359] Thrombocytopenia typically persists for several days to 3 weeks if left untreated.[351]

Pathogenesis

NAIT is caused by transplacental passage of maternal alloantibodies against platelet antigens shared by the father and fetus (see Ch. 132). Shed fetal platelet antigens may pass into the maternal circulation by the fourteenth week of gestation,[360,361] at which time the placenta has the capacity to transport maternal antibodies to the fetus. Severe fetal thrombocytopenia has been detected by the twentieth week of gestation.[362–364] Antenatal intracranial hemorrhage has been detected in as many as 10% of all cases, on occasion before the thirtieth week.[349,353,356,357,365,366]

Several biallelic antigen systems have been implicated in the development of these alloantibodies. Most identified cases in whites occur in homozygous HPA-1b (PI^{A2}/PI^{A2}) mothers.[349] NAIT caused by maternal anti-HPA-1a antibodies is frequently complicated by intracranial hemorrhage or other evidence of neonatal bleeding. The few cases attributable to alloantibodies against other determinants on platelet GPIIIa (i.e., anti-HPA-1b[367] and anti-HPA-4 [Yuk^a/Pen][368–370]) and GPIIb (i.e., anti-HPA-3a [Bak^a/Lek][371]) were severe as well. The clinical picture is somewhat more variable in NAIT caused by anti-HPA-5a (Br^a), the second most commonly identified antigen mismatch, which accounts for 15–20% of the cases of NAIT in Europe.[349,359] Platelets express far fewer copies of the GPIa/IIa complex on which the HPA-5 alleles are located than they do GPIIb/IIIa. This difference may contribute to the observation that more index cases of NAIT caused by anti-HPA-5b (Br^a) occur in second or subsequent pregnancies and that as many as 60% of the neonates are asymptomatic at birth,[359] although fatal cases have been reported.[349,354] The HPA-1B allele in extremely rare in Orientals, in whom Yuk-B (HPA-4) is the most commonly identified abnormality. Too few cases of NAIT due to antibodies to PI^{E2},[372] HPA-5a (Br^b),[373] HPA-2 (Ko),[374,375] Sr^a,[376] Gov^a,[377] Nak^a,[378] and other antigens have been described to define the risk of intracranial hemorrhage. Anti-ABO and HLA antibodies have never been proved to be the cause of NAIT,[349,364,379–381] although an association between anti-HLA antibodies and neonatal amegakaryocytic thrombocytopenia has been reported.[351,382] It is likely that additional novel alloantibodies specificities will be identified in the future, some of which may be associated with milder forms of the disease. These advances place additional demands on referral laboratories to acquire and maintain the appropriate reference sera and DNA-based techniques.

Additional genetic factors modify the risk of NAIT in homozygous HPA-1b mothers. For instance, neonatal thrombocytopenia occurs in only 1–6% of women who are homozygous for the HPA-1b allele and who carry an HPA-1a fetus.[349,350] Production of anti-HPA-1a antibodies occurs predominantly in women with the HLA supertypic determinant DRw52a,[383–388] in whom the incidence of NAIT exceeds 25%,[350] a relative risk 10–100-fold above HPA-1b/1b women with other HLA haplotypes. Genetic restriction in the development of anti-HPA-5a antibodies may exist as well.[389] These genetic linkages may have important implications in the management of relatives of affected women, as discussed below.

MANAGEMENT OF THE AFFECTED CHILD WITH NAIT

The index case can be devastating and typically occurs without warning. Since ICH develops in ≥10% of neonates during the peripartum period and may extend in those with antenatal hemorrhage, immediate diagnosis and treatment are mandatory. The maternal platelet count should be documented as normal, although NAIT can occur coincidentally with gestational thrombocytopenia, ITP, or other causes of neonatal thrombocytopenia.[390,391] Any neonate with severe thrombocytopenia who has an otherwise normal physical examination and no evidence of bacterial sepsis, disseminated intravascular coagulation, or congenital viral (herpes, cytomegalovirus, varicella, rubella) or toxoplasma infection should be presumed to have NAIT and therapy should begin immediately.

The treatment of choice is administration of compatible, usually maternal, platelets.[392] Although theoretically platelets should be washed to remove alloantibody and resuspended in AB-positive plasma, in actual practice maternal platelets can be administered safely after centrifugation. The platelets should be irradiated to lessen the risk of graft-versus-host disease.[393] A rise in the platelet count should be verified. Random donor platelets have been transiently effective, especially in cases shown subsequently to be due to anti-HPA-5b (Br^a), since approximately 80% of the population lack this antigen. IVIg is often effective as well, but responses generally take 1–3 days, which may be too late to treat ongoing hemorrhage.[349,394–396] Corticosteroids provide marginal, if any, benefit and should not be used as the sole modality of treatment.[349,354]

Serologic studies should be performed on the *parents* to confirm the diagnosis because of the implications for subsequent pregnancies and genetic counseling of family members. Maternal antibodies that react with paternal platelets are generally demonstrable, although on occasion they may be undetectable, presumably because of adsorption by fetal platelets. Indeed, alloantibodies may not be detected in as many as 15% of typical cases.[349] To confirm the diagnosis, the specificity of maternal antibody should be determined using reference platelets known to carry or lack commonly implicated antigens and the maternal platelet phenotype determined using reference antisera. These studies should only be performed in a laboratory with extensive experience in platelet phenotyping. Newly developed techniques to phenotype platelets using the polymerase chain reaction may eventually make routine testing for the HPA-1 phenotype of all women feasible and cost-effective.[397]

Management of Subsequent Pregnancies

The introduction of fetal blood sampling (FBS) has permitted children at risk of severe thrombocytopenia and hemorrhage to be identified, thereby dramatically changing the management of subsequent pregnancies. An invasive approach is warranted for several reasons: (1) severe thrombocytopenia occurs in >99% of subsequent pregnancies with antigen-positive fetuses[398]; (2) neither the presence nor the absence of alloantibody in the mother, nor a change in antibody titer, clearly predicts the neonatal platelet count[350,353,354,384]; (3) approximately one-half the cases of intracranial hemorrhage occur antenatally and would not be prevented by cesarean section at term; (4) platelet counts commonly fall during gestation so that a single determination early in pregnancy does not suffice to define risk[362]; and (5) effective antenatal treatment is available.

NAIT caused by anti-HPA-1a antibodies will be used as an example because it is the best studied and most common cause of severe disease. The neonatal platelet count and phenotype can and should be determined by FBS as early as 20 weeks' gestation in women with a history of NAIT, in their HPA-1a-negative sisters,[360] and in any HPA-1a-negative, HLA-Dw52A-positive woman when the child's father is HPA-1a positive, even during a first pregnancy. Fetal genotypes can now be determined at 10–18 weeks' gestation using the polymerase chain reaction with DNA from cells obtained by chorionic villous sampling or amniocentesis.[399–401]

Two approaches to antenatal management of thrombocytopenic fetuses have been studied. The more aggressive approach, pursued primarily in several European centers, involves weekly transfusion of washed, irradiated, maternal platelets in utero[354,362,363,402] starting as early as 26–30 weeks' gestation.[364,403,404] This approach requires matched donors in addition to the mother because of the transfusion frequency, although frozen maternal platelets have been used successfully.[405] Each procedure also carries a risk of fetal exsanguination and side effects from transfusion[406] and is labor intensive and costly. In the United States, it has become the practice to administer IVIg (1 g/kg/wk) to the mother once an HPA-1a-positive fetus has been identified or thrombocytopenia has been documented, or both. FBS is repeated 4–6 weeks later and immediately prior to delivery to evaluate response,[354,407] which occurs in about 75% of cases (mean increase about 70,000/mm³).[408,409] In utero transfusion of maternal platelets is restricted to nonresponders.[362,402,403,408] IVIg has also been administered directly to the fetus in utero with variable success.[410,411] In our experience, intracranial hemorrhages were not detected in any of the 72 fetuses managed in this way, compared with a 25% incidence during the index pregnancies.

POST-TRANSFUSION PURPURA

Post-transfusion purpura (PTP) is an uncommon, acquired thrombocytopenia that develops approximately 1 week after blood transfusion. Plasma from affected individuals contains alloantibodies to antigens expressed on intact platelets or on platelet membranes in the transfused blood. Through a mechanism yet to be defined, isoantibody production is accompanied by destruction of the recipient's platelets. The temporal association of thrombocytopenia with blood transfusion was first described by Zucker et al.[412] and by van Loghen et al.[413] A relationship between the development of platelet-specific isoantibodies and the consumption of host platelets was first suggested by Shulman et al.[414] The clinical course of untreated PTP is typically severe and protracted and may end fatally from hemorrhage. However, therapy is rapidly effective in almost all cases, making an early, accurate diagnosis of this disorder imperative.

Clinical Manifestations

The prototypic clinical presentation of PTP is now well defined. The typical patient is a multiparous middle-aged female who presents with an acute onset of bleeding due to severe thrombocytopenia 1 week after the administration of a blood product containing platelet material. This may include fresh or stored whole blood, packed or washed red blood cells, or fresh or frozen plasma. In a recent retrospective analysis 99 of 104 affected individuals were women with a mean age of 58.4 years.[415] Thrombocytopenia was first noted a mean of 6–8 days (range, 1–14 days) after transfusion, and platelet counts were found to be <10,000/mm³ in >80% of cases at presentation.[415] Only one-third of the patients reported having had chills or fever after the transfusion. In the absence of prior pregnancies, almost all of the remaining patients had a history of prior blood transfusions,[398,416–419] suggesting that PTP almost always occurs as an anamnestic immune response. PTP is therefore exceptionally rare in males or in nulliparous females who have no history of prior transfusion.[415,417,418,420,421] In this unusual setting, the onset may be delayed (24 days), consistent with a primary immune response.[420] Subclinical cases have been reported, but the actual incidence of asymptomatic, milder forms of PTP is unknown.[422,423] On rare occasions, thrombocytopenia has developed within hours after transfusion of plasma, whole blood, or packed red blood cells.[424–427] In these cases, isoantibodies reactive with recipient platelets have been identified in the transfused blood product. In each case, the donor was a multiparous female, homozygous for an allele not found on the recipients platelets.

Pathogenesis

The pathogenesis of PTP remains unclear. The enigma is why the recipient's platelets are destroyed by alloantibodies directed at a determinant they seemingly do not express. Any proposed explanation must also account for the low incidence in susceptible individuals exposed to blood products known to contain the provoking antigen, the absence of PTP in women whose pregnancies are complicated by NAIT due to alloantibodies with the same apparent specificity, the prolonged duration of the thrombocytopenia, the reported lack of response to transfusion with antigen-negative platelets,[428] and that the syndrome may or may not recur after inadvertent or deliberate re-exposure to antigen-mismatched blood products.[398,422,429]

Serum from >90% of patients with PTP contains antibodies to the platelet antigen PlA1 (HPA-1a), which is expressed on the platelets of 97–98% of the white population. The remaining cases have been associated with antibodies to the PlA2 (HPA-1b) allele[415,420,430] and other epitopes on platelet GPIIb-IIIa,[415,430–435] or, less commonly, on other surface proteins.[436] Although only antibodies directed to HLA determinants were detected in a few patients,[415,437,438] it is uncertain whether these were the actual cause of the syndrome.[439] Despite the ease with which these isoantibodies are demonstrated in essentially every patient with PTP, their role in the destruction of autologous platelets is unproved. Indeed, in at least one instance, reinfusion of plasma obtained during the period of severe thrombocytopenia did not reproduce the syndrome.[414] Moreover, while alloantibodies with the same apparent specificity circulate in many women with NAIT, PTP has never developed concomitantly.

Another unanswered question is why PTP is rare. Anti-HPA-1a antibodies would be expected to develop after 1–3% of random donor transfusions based on the frequency of HPA-1b homozygous individuals. One factor is the genetic restriction on the production of anti-HPA-1a antibodies. Development of PTP and NAIT is closely linked to the HLA-B8 and -DRw52 loci,[350,383,384,387,440] yet only a single instance each of sisters with PTP[441] and PTP occurring in a woman with a history of NAIT has been reported.[442] Therefore, additional factors, including the specifics of the anamnestic response, may be involved.

No single theory satisfactorily addresses all of these questions. Platelet eluates containing immunoglobulin with anti-HPA-1a reactivity have been detected as long as 100 days after the acute episode.[443–446] In some cases, binding of eluted immunoglobulin to autologous and other HPA-1-negative platelets has been noted.[443,447–449] However, the antigenic specificity of these antibodies has not been determined. Shulman and co-workers[414] initially proposed that donor platelets were lysed by alloantibody (e.g., anti-HPA-1a) in a complement-dependent reaction. The release of antigen-antibody complexes from the lysed platelets might perpetuate the destructive process by binding to Fc_γ receptors on HPA-1a-negative host platelets, reactivating the complement system. However, there has been no direct evidence that HPA-1a/anti-HPA-1a complexes volley between rapidly destroyed platelets and their replacements for several weeks without themselves being cleared from the circulation. More recently, it has been proposed that soluble or particulate HPA-1a antigen is released from lysed donor platelets and binds specifically to antigen-negative platelets, permitting immune complexes to form in situ.[450–453] Only during an anamnestic response would sufficient alloantibody and donor platelet antigens be present coincidentally to initiate the syndrome. It has been deduced that binding of <5% of the amount of soluble HPA-1a antigen estimated to be present in a 1 U of blood would permit sufficient alloantibody to bind and destroy all circulating platelets in vivo. After the first round of destruction, sufficient antigen/antibody complexes might be released to sensitize the markedly reduced number of residual platelets.[454,455] A third possibility is that a subset of anti-HPA-1a antibodies cross-reacts with a determinant on HPA-1b/1b platelets[456] or that autoantibodies develop coincidentally in a small proportion of sensitized individuals.[447–449,457] This is consistent with the generation of autoreactive antierythrocyte antibodies in some individuals after transfusion[458–461] or experimental sensitization[462,463] that may persist beyond the anticipated life span of the transfused red cells.[461,464] In the best-studied example, a substantial proportion of marmosets sensitized to platelets from another species develop acute, persistent (30 to >100 days) immune thrombocytopenia several weeks after immunization. Platelet eluates from the affected animals contain both autoreactive as well as antidonor-specific antibodies.[465]

Diagnosis

The key to diagnosis is suspecting PTP in any patient who develops severe thrombocytopenia approximately 1 week after transfusion. Suspicion is heightened if the patient's plasma is capable of lysing platelets from random normal donors, because there are few other conditions, other than quinidine purpura, associated with lytic antibodies. Treatment must be initiated immediately based on clinical criteria, because it generally

THERAPY FOR PTP

The clinical course of untreated or nonresponsive patients is typically prolonged. In the series cited earlier, bleeding lasted a mean of 10.2 days.[415] It took a mean of 14.6 days until the platelet count was >50,000/mm³ (range 3–90) and 19.5 days until it was >100,000/mm³ (3–130 days). Thrombocytopenia has been reported to last as long as 60–120 days on occasion.[422,440,466] Fatality rates as high as 10% were reported before effective therapy was identified.[398,428,467–470] Therefore, immediate diagnosis and intervention must be made once the disorder is suspected clinically.

The treatment of choice is IVIg 1 g/kg/day for 2 days, although a second course may be required in some patients.[471] Over 90% of the reported patients have responded, generally beginning within the first 2–3 days of treatment.[415,466,471–474] Therefore, IVIg has replaced plasmapheresis[475,476] and exchange transfusion[414,477] as the initial treatment of choice, both because of its somewhat higher response rate and its ease of administration. Although occasional patients respond to corticosteroids given as a single agent,[418,437,478,479] most do not,[415,469] and steroids should be considered to have an adjunctive role, if any, in treatment. A single response to splenectomy in a refractory patient has been reported.[480] Recurrent thrombocytopenia may occur within days of stopping treatment; however, these relapses are generally milder and more easily managed than the initial episode.[455,466,471,472]

The role of prophylactic platelet transfusions in patients with profound thrombocytopenia but non-life-threatening bleeding is unclear. Sera from affected patients commonly contain antibodies to multiple HLA determinants, making provision of antigen-matched platelets problematic. Administration of random donor platelets, which is commonly associated with moderate-to-severe transfusion reactions, including bronchospasm and hypotension, rarely succeeds in raising the platelet count and theoretically may perpetuate the disease.[412–415,474,481,482] Even when antigen-matched platelets can be procured in time, they may[398,428,483] or may not[484,485] suffer the same fate as the patient's own, antigen-negative cells.

Anti-HPA-1a antibodies may persist for >1 year after the initial episode.[486] It has been theorized by some that persistence of high antibody titers may protect against recurrence by immediately destroying potentially sensitizing platelets, thereby precluding coincidence of circulating antigen at the time of an anamnestic response.[398] Exposure[446] or re-exposure[414,455] to blood products containing the relevant antigen does not invariably provoke PTP, but recurrences have been reported.[422,429,455,487] Therefore, most experts recommend limiting the exposure of affected individuals by transfusing only antigen-matched (including autologous) blood products on subsequent occasions.[415] Whether current techniques of washing and filtering erythrocytes or the use of frozen, thawed, and washed red cells remove sufficient platelet antigen to prevent recurrence is unknown.[487,488] It is not known whether the risk of PTP developing in unaffected multiparous or previously transfused siblings that share HLA haplotypes is sufficient to recommend similar restrictions on the source of transfused blood products. The risk of PTP developing in women whose pregnancies were complicated by NAIT appears sufficiently low that only awareness and close monitoring of platelet counts after transfusion appears warranted.

takes several days until the results of confirmatory tests become available.

Alloantibodies to platelet proteins can be demonstrated by Western blotting or an antigen-capture assay. The diagnosis is generally confirmed by demonstrating that serum from the affected patient contains antibodies to a specific alloantigen (i.e., binding of antibody to platelets containing but not those lacking a specific antigen). This is generally accomplished by either an antiglobulin test such as immunofluorescence assay or enzyme-linked immunosorbent assay, or by demonstrating lysis of stored, frozen platelets obtained from known antigen-positive donors. On recovery, the patient's platelets can be phenotyped using reference sera that contain antibodies of known specificity. Typically, platelets obtained from the patient on recovery will not aggregate or lyse when incubated with plasma obtained during the acute phase. This inability to reproduce the syndrome in vitro, the sina qua non of PTP, is the basis of the uncertainty as to its pathogenesis. It is likely that in the future, PCR-based assays will be used to identify rapidly HPA-Ib/Ib-positive individuals and others at risk of developing PTP.

REFERENCES

1. Berchtold P, McMillan R: Therapy of chronic idiopathic thrombocytopenic purpura in adults. Blood 74:2309, 1989
2. Doan CA, Bouroncle BA, Wiseman BK; Idiopathic and secondary thrombocytopenic purpura: clinical study and evaluation of 381 cases over a period of 28 years. Ann Intern Med 53:861, 1960
3. Mueller-Eckhardt C: Idiopathic thrombocytopenic purpura. Clinical and immunologic considerations. Semin Thromb Hemost 3:125, 1977
4. Najean Y, Lecompte T: Chronic pure thrombocytopenia in elderly patients. An aspect of the myelodysplastic syndrome. Cancer 64:2506, 1989
5. Garg SK, Amarosi EL, Karpatkin S: Use of the megakaryocyte as an index of megakaryocyte number. N Engl J Med 284:11, 1971
6. Berkman N, Michaeli Y, Or R, Eldor A: EDTA-dependent pseudothrombocytopenia: a clinical study of 18 patients and a review of the literature. Am J Hematol 36:195, 1991
7. Mant MJ, Doery JCG, Gauldie J, Sims H: Pseudothrombocytopenia due to platelet aggregation and degranulation in blood collected in EDTA. Scand J Haematol 15:161, 1975
8. Savage RA: Pseudoleukocytosis due to EDTA-induced platelet clumping. Am J Clin Pathol 81:317, 1984
9. Payne BA, Pierre RV: Pseudothrombocytopenia: a laboratory artifact with potentially serious consequences. Mayo Clin Proc 59:123, 1984
10. Hoyt RH, Durie BGM: Pseudothrombocytopenia induced by a monoclonal IgM kappa platelet agglutinin. Am J Hematol 31:50, 1989
11. Imai H, Nakamoto Y, Miki K et al: Pseudothrombocytopenia and IgA-related platelet agglutinin in a patient with IgA nephritis. Nephron 34:154, 1983
12. de Caterina M, Fratellanza G, Grimaldi E et al: Evidence of a cold immunoglobulin M autoantibody against 78-kD platelet glycoprotein in a case of EDTA-dependent pseudothrombocytopenia. Am J Clin Pathol 99:163, 1993
13. Pegels JG, Bruynes ECE, Engelfriet CP, von dem Borne AEGKr: Pseudothrombocytopenia: an immunological study on platelet antibodies dependent on ethylene diamine tetra-acetate. Blood 59:159, 1982
14. van Vliet HHD, Kappers-Klunne MC, Abels J: Pseudothrombocytopenia: a cold autoantibody against platelet glycoprotein GP IIb. Br J Haematol 52:501, 1986
15. Onder O, Weinstein A, Hoyer LW: Pseudothrombocytopenia caused by platelet agglutinins that are reactive in blood anticoagulated with chelating agents. Blood 56:177, 1980
16. Shreiner DP, Bell WR: Pseudothrombocytopenia: manifestation of a new type of platelet agglutinin. Blood 42:541, 1973
17. Solanki DL, Blackburn BC: Spurious leukocytosis and thrombocytopenia. A dual phenomenon caused by clumping of platelets in vitro. JAMA 250:2514, 1983
18. Watkins SP Jr, Shulman NR: Platelet cold agglutinins. Blood 36:153, 1970
19. Veenhoven WA, van der Schans GS, Huiges W, et al: Pseudothrombocytopenia due to platelet agglutinins. Am J Clin Pathol 72:1005, 1979
20. Ziegler Z: In vitro granulocyte-platelet rosette formation mediated by an IgG immunoglobulin. Haemostasis 3:282, 1974
21. Griepp PR, Gralnick HR: Platelet to leukocyte adherence phenomena associated with thrombocytopenia. Blood 47:513, 1976
22. Bizzaro N: Platelet satellitosis to polymorphonuclears: cytochemical, immunological, and ultrastructural characterization of eight cases. Am J Hematol 36:235, 1991
23. Kjedsberg CR, Hershgold EJ: Spurious thrombocytopenia. JAMA 227:628 1974
24. Forscher CA, Sussman II, Friedman EW et al: Psudothrombocytopenia masking true thrombocytopenia. Am J Hematol 18:313, 1985
25. Harrington WJ, Minnich V, Hollingsworth JW, Moore CV: Demonstration o a thrombocytopenic factor in the blood of patients with thrombocytopenic purpura. J Lab Clin Med 38:1, 1951
26. Karpatkin S: Autoimmune thrombocytopenic purpura. Blood 56:329, 1980
27. Harker LA: Thrombokinetics in idiopathic thrombocytopenic purpura. Br . Haematol 19:95, 1970
28. Branehog I, Kutti J, Weinfeld A: Platelet survival and platelet production ir idiopathic thrombocytopenic purpura. Br J Haematol 27:127, 1974
29. Chang C-S, Li C-Y, Cha SS: Chronic idiopathic thrombocytopenic purpura Splenic pathologic features and their clinical correlation. Arch Pathol Lat Med 117:981, 1993
30. Neiman JC, Mant MJ, Shnitka TK: Phagocytosis of platelets by Kupffer cells in immune thrombocytopenia. Arch Pathol Lab Med 111:563, 1987
31. Kelton JG, Carter CJ, Rodger C et al: The relationship among platelet-associated IgG, platelet lifespan, and reticuloendothelial cell function. Blood 63: 1434, 1984
32. Ziegler ZR, Rosenfeld CS, Nemunaitis JJ et al: Increased macrophage colony-stimulating factor levels in immune thrombocytopenic purpura. Blood 81: 1251, 1993
33. Zucker-Franklin D, Karpatkin S: Red cell and platelet fragmentation in idiopathic thrombocytopenic purpura. N Engl J Med 297:517, 1977
34. Jy W, Horstmann LL, Arce M, Ahn YS: Clinical significance of platelet microparticles in autoimmune thrombocytopenia. J Lab Clin Med 119:324, 1992
35. Fujisawa K, O'Toole TE, Tani P et al: Autoantibodies to the presumptive cytoplasmic domain of platelet glycoprotein IIIa in patients with chronic immune thrombocytopenic purpura. Blood 77:2207, 1991
36. Bellem PJ, Segal GM, Stratton JR et al: Mechanisms of thrombocytopenia in chronic autoimmune thrombocytopenic purpura: evidence of both impaired platelet production and increased platelet clearance. J Clin Invest 80:33, 1987
37. Heyns A duP, Bradenhorst PN, Lotter MG et al: Platelet turnover and kinetics in immune thrombocytopenic purpura: results with autolgous ^{111}In-labeled platelets and homologous ^{51}Cr-labeled platelets differ. Blood 67:86, 1986
38. Seigel RS, Rae JR, Barth S et al: Platelet survival and turnover: important factors in predicting response to splenectomy in immune thrombocytopenic purpura. Am J Hematol 30:206, 1989
39. Gernsheimer T, Stratton J, Ballem PJ, Slichter SJ: Mechanisms of response to treatment in autoimmune thrombocytopenic purpura. N Engl J Med 320: 974, 1989
40. McMillan R, Luiken GA, Levy R et al: Antibody against megakaryocytes in idiopathic thrombocytopenic purpura. JAMA 239:2460, 1978
41. Kunicki TJ, Newman PJ: The molecular immunology of human platelet proteins. Blood 80:1386, 1992
42. Beer JH, Rabaglio M, Berchtold P et al: Autoantibodies against the platelet glycoproteins (GP) IIb/IIIa, Ia/IIa, and IV and partial deficiency in GPIV in a patient with a bleeding disorder and a defective platelet collagen interaction. Blood 82:820, 1993
43. Deckmyn H, Van Houtte E, Vermylen J: Disturbed platelet aggregation to collagen associated with an antibody against an 85- to 90-Kd platelet glycoprotein in a patient with prolonged bleeding time. Blood 79:1466, 1992
44. Sugiyama T, Okuma M, Ushikibi F et al: A novel platelet aggregating factor found in a patient with defective collagen-induced platelet aggregation and autoimmune thrombocytopenia. Blood 69:1712, 1987
45. Bellucci S, Charpak Y, Chastang C et al: Low dose v conventional doses of corticoids in immune thrombocytopenic purpura (ITP): results of a randomized clinical trial in 160 children, 223 adults. Blood 71:1165, 1988
46. Thompson RL, Moore RA, Hess CE et al: Idiopathic thrombocytopenic purpura. Long-term results of treatment and prognostic significance of response to corticosteroids. Arch Intern Med 130:730, 1972
47. JiJi RM, Firozvi T, Spurling CL: Chronic idiopathic thrombocytopenic purpura: treatment with steroids and splenectomy. Arch Int Med 132:380, 1973
48. Jacobs P, Wood L, Dent SM: Results of treatment in immune thrombocytopenia. Q J Med 58:153, 1986
49. DiFino SM, Lachant NA, Kirshner JJ, Gottlieb AJ: Adult idiopathic thrombocytopenic purpura: clinical findings and response to therapy. Am J Med 69: 430, 1980
50. Myers MC: Results of treatment in 71 patients with idiopathic thrombocytopenic purpura. Am J Med Sci 242:295, 1961
51. den Ottolander GJ, Gratama JW, de Koning J, Brand A: Long-term follow-up study of 168 patients with immune thrombocytopenia: implications for therapy. Scand J Haematol 32:101, 1984
52. Pizzuto J, Ambriz R: Therapeutic experience on 934 adults with idiopathic

thrombocytopenic purpura: multicentric trial of the cooperative Latin American Group on Hemostasis and Thrombosis. Blood 64:1179, 1984

53. Shulman NR, Weinrach RS, Libre EP, Andrews HL: The role of the reticuloendothelial system in the pathogenesis of idiopathic thrombocytopenic purpura. Trans Assoc Am Physicians 78:374, 1965

54. Handin RI, Stossel TP: Effect of corticosteroid therapy on the phagocytosis of antibody-coated platelets by human leukocytes. Blood 51:77, 1978

55. McMillan R, Longmire RL, Tavassoli M et al: In vitro platelet phagocytosis by splenic leukocytes in idiopathic thrombocytopenic purpura. N Engl J Med 290:249, 1974

56. Berchtold P, Wenger M: Autoantibodies against platelet glycoproteins in autoimmune thrombocytopenic purpura: their clinical significance and response to treatment. Blood 81:1246, 1993

57. Fujisawa K, Tani P, Piro L, McMillan R: The effect of therapy on platelet-associated autoantibody in chronic immune thrombocytopenic purpura. Blood 81:2872, 1993

57a. Andersen JC: Response of resistant idiopathic thrombocytopenic purpura to pulsed high-dose dexamethasone therapy. N Engl J Med 330:1560, 1994

58. Kelsey PR, Schofield KP, Geary CG: Refractory idiopathic thrombocytopenic purpura (ITP) treated with cyclosporine. Br J Haematol 60:197, 1985

59. Kitchens CS, Pendergast JF: Human thrombocytopenia is associated with structural abnormalities of the endothelium that are ameliorated by glucocorticosteroid administration. Blood 67:203, 1986

60. McMillan R: Chronic idiopathic thrombocytopenic purpura. N Engl J Med 304:1135, 1981

61. Carr AM, Kruskal M, Kaye J, Robinson S: Efficacy of platelet transfusions in immune thrombocytopenia. Am J Med 80:1051, 1986

62. Baumann MA, Menitove JE, Aster RH, Anderson T: Urgent treatment of idiopathic thrombocytopenic purpura with single-dose gammaglobulin infusion followed by platelet transfusion. Ann Int Med 104:808, 1986

63. Akoglu T, Paydas S, Bayik M et al: Megadose methylprednisolone pulse therapy in adult idiopathic thrombocytopenic purpura. Lancet 337:56, 1991

64. von dem Borne AEGKr, E. Vos JJ, Pegels JG et al: High dose intravenous methylprednisolone or high dose intravenous gammaglobulin for autoimmune thrombocytopenia. BMJ 296:249, 1988

65. Thompson RL, Moore RA, Hess CE et al: Idiopathic thrombocytopenic purpura. Long term results of treatment and the prognostic significance of response to corticosteroids. Arch Int Med 130:730, 1972

66. Brennan MF, Rappaport JM, Maloney WC, Wilson RE: Correlation between response to corticosteroids and splenectomy for adult idiopathic thrombocytopenic purpura. Am J Surg 129:490, 1975

67. Julia A, Araguas C, Rossello J et al: Lack of useful clinical predictors of response to splenectomy in patients with chronic idiopathic thrombocytopenic purpura. Br J Haematol 76:250, 1990

68. Calverley DC, Jones GW, Kelton JG: Splenic radiation for corticosteroid-resistant immune thrombocytopenia. Ann Intern Med 116:977, 1992

69. Lortan JE: Management of asplenic patients. Br J Haematol 84:566, 1993

70. Picozzi VJ, Roeske WR, Creger WP: Fate of therapy failures in adult idiopathic thrombocytopenic purpura. Am J Med 69:690, 1980

71. den Ottolander GJ, Gratama JW, de Koning J, Brand A: Long-term follow-up study of 168 patients with immune thrombocytopenic purpura. Scand J Haematol 32:101, 1984

72. Cortelazzo S, Finazzi G, Buelli M et al: High risk of severe bleeding in aged patients with chronic idiopathic thrombocytopenic purpura. Blood 77:31, 1991

73. Gutherie TH, Brannan DP, Prisant LM: Idiopathic thrombocytopenic purpura in the older patient. Am J Med Sci 296:17, 1988

74. Verheyden CN Jr, Beart RW, Clifton MD, Phyliky RL: Accessory splenectomy in management of recurrent idiopathic thrombocytopenic purpura. Mayo Clin Proc 53:442, 1978

75. Davis HH II, Varki A, Heaton A, Siegel BA: Detection of accessory spleens with Indium 111-labeled autolgous platelets. Am J Hematol 8:81, 1980

76. Wallace D, Fromm D, Thomas D: Accessory splenectomy for idiopathic thrombocytopenic purpura. Surgery 91:134, 1982

77. Facon T, Caulier MT, Fenaux P et al: Accessory spleen in recurrent chronic immune thrombocytopenic purpura. Am J Hematol 41:184, 1992

78. Pawelski S, Konopka L, Zdziechowska H: Recurrence of thrombocytopenia in patients splenectomized for idiopathic thrombocytopenic purpura. Blut 43:355, 1981

79. Imbach P, Barandun S, D'Apuzzo V et al: High-dose intravenous gammaglobulin for idiopathic thrombocytopenic purpura in childhood. Lancet 1:1228, 1981

80. Bussel JB, Pham LC: Intravenous treatment with gammaglobulin in adults with immune thrombocytopenic purpura: review of the literature. Vox Sang 51:264, 1987

81. Bussel JB, Fitzgerald-Pedersen J, Feldman C: Alternation of two doses of intravenous gammaglobulin in the maintenance treatment of patients with immune thrombocytopenic purpura. Am J Hematol 33:184, 1990

82. Godeau B, Lesage S, Divine M et al: Treatment of adult chronic autoimmune thrombocytopenic purpura with repeated high-dose intravenous immunoglobulin. Blood 82:1415, 1993

83. Fehr J, Hoffman V, Kappeler U: Transient reversal of thrombocytopenia in idiopathic thrombocytopenic purpura by high dose intravenous immunoglobulin. N Engl J Med 306:1242, 1982

84. Berchtold P, Dale GL, Tani P, McMillan R: Inhibition of autoantibody binding to platelet glycoprotein IIb/IIIa by anti-idiotypic antibodies in intravenous gammaglobulin. Blood 74:2414, 1989

85. Debre M, Bonnet MC, Fridman WH et al: Infusion of Fcγ-fragments for treatment of children with acute immune thrombocytopenia. Lancet 342:945, 1993

86. Vera-Ramirez M, Charlet M, Parry GJ: Recurrent aseptic meningitis complicating intravenous immunoglobulin therapy for chronic inflammatory demyelinating polyradiculoneuropathy. Neurology 42:1636, 1992

87. Mitterer M, Pescota N, Vogetseder W et al: Two episodes of aseptic meningitis during intravenous immunoglobulin therapy of idiopathic thrombocytopenic purpura. Ann Hematol 67:151, 1993

88. Whitsett CF, Pierce JA, Daffin LE: Positive direct antiglobulin tests associated with intravenous gammaglobulin use in bone marrow transplant recipients. Transplantation 41:663, 1986

89. Copelan EA, Strohm PL. Kennedy MS, Tutschka PJ: Hemolysis following intravenous immune globulin therapy. Transfusion 26:410, 1986

90. Brox AG, Cournoyer D, Sternbach M, Sprull G: Hemolytic anemia following intravenous gamma globulin administration. Am J Med 82:633, 1987

91. Potter M, Stockley R, Storry J, Slade R: ABO alloimunization after intravenous immunoglobulin infusion. Lancet 1:932, 1988

92. Woodruff RK, Grigg AP, Firkin FC, Smith IL: Fatal thrombotic events during treatment of autoimmune thrombocytopenia with intravenous immunoglobulin in elderly patients. Lancet 2:217, 1986

93. Rault R, Piraino B, Johnston JR, Oral A: Pulmonary and renal toxicity of intravenous immunoglobulin. Clin Nephrol 36:83, 1991

94. Phillips AO: Renal failure and intravenous immunoglobulin. Clin Nephrol 37:217, 1992

95. Burks AW, Sampson HA, Buckley RH: Anaphylactic reactions after gamma globulin administration in patients with hypogammaglobulinemia. Detection of IgE antibodies to IgA. N Engl J Med 314:560, 1986

96. Cunningham-Rundles C, Zhou C, McKarious S, Courter S: Long term use of IgA-depleted intravenous immunoglobulin in immunodeficiency subjects with anti-IgA antibodies. J Clin Immunol 13:271, 1992

97. Garcia L, Huh YO, Fisher HE, Lichtiger B: Positive immunohematologic and serologic test results due to high-dose intravenous immune globulin administration. Transfusion 27:503, 1987

97a. Pawlotsky J-M, Bovier M, Deforges L et al: Chronic hepatitis C after high-dose intravenous immunoglobulin. Transfusion 34:86, 1994

98. Bussel JB, Pham LC, Aledort L, Nachman R: Maintenance treatment of adults with chronic refractory immune thrombocytopenic purpura using repeated intravenous infusions of gammaglobulin. Blood 72:121, 1988

99. Becker T, Kuenzlen E, Salama A et al: Treatment of childhood idiopathic thrombocytopenic purpura with rhesus antibodies (anti-D). Eur J Pediatr 145:166, 1986

100. Bussel JB, Graziano JN, Kimberly RP et al: IV anti-D treatment of immune thrombocytopenic purpura: analysis of efficacy, toxicity, and mechanism of effect. Blood 77:1884, 1991

101. Ahn YS, Harrington WJ, Simon SR et al: Danazol for the treatment of idiopathic thrombocytopenic purpura. N Engl J Med 308:1396, 1983

102. Ahn YS, Rocha R, Mylvaganam R et al: Long-term danazol therapy in autoimmune thrombocytopenia: unmaintained remission and age-dependent response in women. Ann Intern Med 111:723, 1989

103. Buelli M, Cortelazzo S, Viero P et al: Danazol for the treatment of idiopathic thrombocytopenic purpura. Acta Haematol 74:97, 1985

104. Weinblatt ME, Kochen J, Ortega J: Danazol for children with immune thrombocytopenic purpura. Am J Dis Child 142:1317, 1988

105. Marino C, Cook P: Danazol for lupus thrombocytopenia. Arch Intern Med 2251:2252, 1985

106. Schreiber AD, Chien P, Tomaski A, Cines DB: Effect of danazol and vinblastine in idiopathic thrombocytopenic purpura. N Engl J Med 316:503, 1987

107. Mylvaganam R, Ahn YS, Harrington WJ, Kim CI: Immune modulation by danazol in autoimmune thrombocytopenia. Clin Immunol Immunopathol 42:281, 1987

108. McVerry BA, Auger M, Bellingham AJ: The use of danazol in the management of chronic immune thrombocytopenic purpura. Br J Haematol 61:145, 1985

109. Ahn YS: Efficacy of danazol in hematologic disorders. Acta Haematol 84:122, 1990

110. Fenaux P, Quiquandon I, Huart JJ et al: The role of danazol in the treatment of refractory idiopathic thrombocytopenic purpura. A report of 22 cases. Nouv Rev Fr Hematol 32:143, 1990

111. Mazzucconi MG, Francesconi M, Falcione E et al: Danazol therapy in refractory chronic immune thrombocytopenic purpura. Acta Haematol 77:45, 1987
112. Nalli G, Sajeva R, Maffe GC, Ascari E: Danazol therapy for idiopathic thrombocytopenic purpura (ITP). Haematol 73:55, 1988
113. Ahn YS, Mylvaganam R, Garcia RO et al: Low-dose danazol therapy in idiopathic thrombocytopenic purpura. Ann Intern Med 107:177, 1987
114. Boue F, Coffin B, Delfraissy JF: Danazol and cholestatic hepatitis. Ann Intern Med 105:139, 1986
115. Nesher G, Dollberg L, Zimran A, Hershko C: Hepatosplenic peliosis after danazol and glucocorticoids for ITP. N Engl J Med 312:242, 1985
116. Kahn H, Manzarbeitia C, Theise N et al: Danazol-induced hepatocellular adenomas. A case report and review of the literature. Arch Pathol Lab Med 115:1054, 1991
117. Arrowsmith JB, Dreis M: Thrombocytopenia after treatment with danazol. N Engl J Med 315:585, 1986
118. Gout PW, Wijcik LL, Beer CT: Differences between vinblastine and vincristine in distribution in the blood of rats and binding by platelets and malignant cells. Eur J Cancer 14:1167, 1978
119. Kelton JG, McDonald JWD, Barr RM et al: The reversible binding of vinblastine to platelets: implications for therapy. Blood 57:431, 1981
120. Ahn YS, Byrnes JJ, Harrington WJ et al: The treatment of idiopathic thrombocytopenia with vinblastine-loaded platelets. N Engl J Med 298:1101, 1978
121. Ahn YS, Harrington WJ, Mylvaganam R et al: Slow infusion of vinca alkaloids in the treatment of idiopathic thrombocytopenic purpura. Ann Intern Med 100:192, 1984
122. Cervantes F, Montserrat E, Rozman C: Treatment of idiopathic thrombocytopenic purpura. N Engl J Med 305:830, 1981
123. Fenaux P, Quiquandon I, Caulier MT et al: Slow infusions of vinblastine in the treatment of adult idiopathic thrombocytopenic purpura: a report of 43 cases. Blut 60:238, 1990
124. Manoharan A: Targeted-immunosuppression with vincristine infusion in the treatment of immune thrombocytopenia. Aust NZ J Med 21:405, 1991
125. Massimo L, Genova R, Marchi A et al: More on vincristine treatment of ITP in children. N Engl J Med 297:397, 1977
126. Bouroncle BA, Doan CA: Treatment of refractory idiopathic thrombocytopenic purpura. JAMA 207:2049, 1969
127. Quiquandon I, Fenaux P, Caulier MT et al: Re-evaluation of the role of azathioprine in the treatment of adult chronic idiopathic thrombocytopenic purpura: a report on 53 cases. Br J Haematol 74:223, 1990
128. Finch SC, Castro O, Cooper M et al: Immunosuppressive therapy of chronic idiopathic thrombocytopenic purpura. Am J Med 56:4, 1974
129. Verlin M, Laros RK Jr, Penner JA: Treatment of refractory thrombocytopenic purpura with cyclophosphamide. Am J Hematol 1:97, 1976
130. Boumpas DT, Austin HA III, Vaughan EM et al: Risk for sustained amenorrhea in patients with systemic lupus erythematosus receiving intermittant pulse cyclophosphamide therapy. Ann Intern Med 119:366, 1993
131. Krause JR: Chronic idiopathic thrombocytopenic purpura (ITP): development of acute non-lymphocytic leukemia subsequent to treatment with cyclophosphamide. Med Pediatr Oncol 10:61, 1982
132. Lacey JV, Penner JA: Management of idiopathic thrombocytopenic purpura in the adult. Semin Thromb Hemost 3:160, 1977
133. Figueroa M, Gehlsen J, Hammond D et al: Combination chemotherapy in refractory immune thrombocytopenic purpura. N Engl J Med 328:1226, 1993
134. Velu TJ, Debusscher L, Stryckmans PA: Cyclosporine for the treatment of refractory idiopathic thrombocytopenic purpura. Eur J Haematol 38:95, 1987
135. Matsumura O, Kawashima Y, Kato S et al: Therapeutic effect of cyclosporine in thrombocytopenia associated with autoimmune disease. Transplant Proc 20:317, 1988
136. Lim SH, Hale G, Marcus RE et al: CAMPATH-1 monoclonal antibody therapy in severe refractory autoimmune thrombocytopenic purpura. Br J Haematol 84:542, 1993
137. Snyder HW Jr, Cochran SK, Balint JP Jr et al: Experience with protein A-immunoadsorption in treatment-resistant adult immune thrombocytopenic purpura. Blood 79:2237, 1992
138. Williams C, Buskard N, Bussel J: Plasma exchange in idiopathic thrombocytopenic purpura. p. 131. In Nydegger, UE (ed): Current Studies in Hematology and Blood Transfusion. S Karger, Basel, 1990
139. Ilstrup S, Perry L, Howe R, Christie D: A 5 year experience with protein A-immunoadsorbtion treatment. Blood 79:222(A), 1992
140. Moss C, Hamilton PJ: Thrombocytopenia in systemic lupus erythematosus responsive to dapsone. BMJ 297:266, 1988
141. Durand JM, Levevre P, Hovette P et al: Dapsone for idiopathic autoimmune thrombocytopenic purpura in elderly patients. Br J Haematol 78:459, 1991
142. Godeau B, Oksenhendler E, Bierling P: Dapsone for autoimmune thrombocytopenic purpura. Am J Hematol 44:70, 1993
143. Strother SV, Zuckerman KS, Lo Buglio AF: Colchicine therapy for refractory idiopathic thrombocytopenic purpura. Arch Intern Med 144:2198, 1984
144. Baker RI, Manoharan A: Colchicine therapy for idiopathic thrombocytopenic purpura—an inexpensive alternative. Aust NZ J Med 19:412, 1989
145. Ellis ME, Neal KR, Leen CLS, Newland AC: Alpha-2a recombinant interferon in HIV associated thrombcytopenia. BMJ 295:1519, 1987
146. Lever AML, Brook MG, Yap I, Thomas HC: Treatment of thrombocytopenia with alfa interferon. BMJ 295:1519, 1987
147. Proctor SJ, Jackson G, Carey P et al: Improvement of platelet counts in steroid-unresponsive idiopathic immune thrombocytopenic purpura after short-course therapy with recombinant α 2b interferon. Blood 74:1894, 1989
148. Cohn RJ, Schwyzer R, Hesseling PB et al: α-Interferon therapy for severe chronic idiopathic thrombocytopenic purpura in children. Am J Hematol 43:246, 1993
149. Belluci S, Bordessoulle D, Coiffer B, Tabah I: Interferon alpha-2b therapy on adult chronic thrombocytopenic purpura. Br J Haematol 73:578, 1989
150. Hurtado R, Pita L, Karpovitch XL et al: Recombinant interferon alfa-2B in refractory idiopathic immune thrombocytopenia. Blood 75:1744, 1990
151. Christolini A, Mazzucconi MG, Dragoni F, et al: Recombinant alpha 2b interferon in the treatment of refractory autoimmune thrombocytopenic purpura. Br J Haematol 80:416, 1992
152. Hudson JG, Yates P, Scott GL: Further concern over use of alpha-interferon in immune thrombocytopenic purpura. Br J Haematol 82:630, 1992
153. Helmerhorst FM, van Leeuwen EF, Pegels JG et al: Primary and secondary autoimmune thrombocytopenia: a serological and clinical analysis. Scand J Haematol 28:319, 1982
154. Hedge UM, Zuiable A, Ball S, Roter BLT: The relative incidence of idiopathic and secondary autoimmune thrombocytopenia: a clinical and serologic evaluation in 508 patients. Clin Lab Haematol 7:7, 1985
155. Nossent JC, Swaak AJG: Prevalence and significance of haematological abnormalities in patients with systemic lupus erythematosus. Q J Med 80:605, 1991
156. Gladman DD, Urowitz MB, Tozman EC, Glynn MFX: Haemostatic abnormalities in systemic lupus erythematosus. Q J Med 52:424, 1983
157. Pistiner M, Wallace DJ, Nessim S et al: Lupus erythematosus in the 1980's: a survey of 570 patients. Semin Arthritis Rheum 21:55, 1991
158. Rabinowitz Y, Dameshek W: Systemic lupus erythematosus after acute "idiopathic" thrombocytopenic purpura: a review. Ann Intern Med 52:1, 1960
159. Perez HD, Katler E, Embury S: Idiopathic thrombocytopenic purpura with high-titer speckled pattern antinuclear antibodies: possible markers for systemic lupus erythematosus. Arthr Rheumat 28:596, 1985
160. McClure PD: Idiopathic thrombocytopenic purpura in children. Diagnosis and management. Pediatrics 55:68, 1975
161. Panzer S, Penner E, Graninger W et al: Antinuclear antibodies in patients with chronic idiopathic autoimmune thrombocytopenia followed 2–30 years. Am J Hematol 32:100, 1989
162. Anderson MJ, Peebles CL, McMillan R, Curd JG: Fluorescent antinuclear antibodies and anti-SSA/Ro in patients with immune thrombocytopenia subsequently developing systemic lupus erythematosus. Ann Intern Med 103:548, 1985
163. Alger M, Alarcon-Segovia D, Rivero SJ: Hemolytic anemia and thrombocytopenic purpura: two related subsets of systemic lupus erythematosus. J Rheumatol 4:351, 1977
164. Miller MH, Urowitz MB, Gladman DD: The significance of thrombocytopenia in systemic lupus erythematosus. Arthritis Rheum 26:1181, 1983
165. Reveille JD, Bartolucci A, Alarcon GS: Prognosis in systemic lupus erythematosus. Negative impact of increasing age at onset, black race, and thrombocytopenia, as well as causes of death. Arthritis Rheum 33:37, 1990
166. Alarcon-Segovia D, Deleze M, Oria CV et al: Antiphospholipid antibodies and the antiphospholipid syndrome in systemic lupus erythematosus. A prospective analysis of 500 consecutive patients. Medicine 68:353, 1989
167. Harris EN, Chan JKH, Asherson EA et al: Thrombosis, recurrent fetal loss, thrombocytopenia: predictive value of IgG anti-cardiolipin antibodies. Arch Intern Med 146:2153, 1986
168. Love PE, Santoro SA: Antiphospholipid antibodies: anticardiolipin and lupus anticoagulant in systemic lupus erythematosus (SLE) and not-SLE disorders. Ann Intern Med 112:682, 1990
169. Griner PF, Hoyer LW: Amegakaryocytic thrombocytopenia in systemic lupus erythematosus. Arch Intern Med 125:328, 1970
170. Nagasawa T, Sakurai T, Kashiwagi H, Abe T: Cell-mediated amegakaryocytic thrombocytopenia associated with systemic lupus erythematosus. Blood 67:479, 1986
171. Kaplan C, Champeix P, Muller JY, Cartron JP: Platelet antibodies in systemic lupus erythematosus. Br J Haematol 67:89, 1987
172. Howe SE, Lynch DM: Platelet antibody binding in systemic lupus erythematosus. J Rheumatol 14:482, 1987

173. Rupin A, Gruel Y, Poumier-Gaschard P et al: Thrombocytopenia in systemic lupus erythematosus: association with antiplatelet and anticardiolipin antibodies. Clin Immunol Immunopathol 55:418, 1990

174. Rauch J, Tannenbaum M, Tannenbaum H et al: Human hybridoma lupus anticoagulants distinguish between lamellar and hexagonal phase lipid systems. J Biol Chem 261:9672, 1986

175. Out HJ, De Groot PG, Van Vliet M et al: Antibodies to platelets in patients with anti-phospholipid antibodies. Blood 77:2655, 1991

176. Murakami H, Lam Z, Furie BC et al: Sulfated glycolipids are the platelet autoantigens for human platelet-binding monoclonal anti-DNA autoantibodies. J Biol Chem 266:15414, 1991

177. Shi E, Chong BH, Chesterman CN: β_2-glycoprotein I is a requirement for anticardiolipin antibodies binding to activated platelets: differences with lupus anticoagulants. Blood 81:1255, 1993

178. Galli M, Bevers EM, Comfurius P et al: Effect of antiphospholipid antibodies on procoagulant activity of activated platelets and platelet-derived microvesicles. Br J Haematol 83:466, 1993

179. Clark WF, Tevaarwerk GJM, Reid BD: Human platelet-immune complex interaction in plasma. J Lab Clin Med 100:917, 1982

180. Mulshine J, Lucas FV, Clough JD: Platelet-bound IgG in systemic lupus erythematosus with and without thrombocytopenia. J Immunol Methods 45:275, 1981

181. Bonacossa IA, Chalmers IM, Rayner HL, Hunter T: Platelet bound IgG levels in patients with systemic lupus erythematosus. J Rheumatol 12:78, 1985

182. Dorsch CA, Meyehoff J: Mechanisms of abnormal platelet aggregation in systemic lupus erythematosus. Arthritis Rheum 25:966, 1982

183. Karpatkin S, Lackner HL: Association of antiplatelet antibody with functional platelet disorders. Autoimmune thrombocytopenic purpura, systemic lupus erythematosus and thrombopathia. Am J Med 59:599, 1975

184. Frank MM, Hamburger MI, Larley TJ et al: Defective reticuloendothelial system Fc-receptor function in systemic lupus erythematosus. N Engl J Med 300:518, 1979

185. Clark WF, Lewis ML, Cameron JS, Parsons V: Intrarenal platelet consumption in the diffuse proliferative nephritis of systemic lupus erythematosus. Clin Sci Mol Med 49:247, 1975

186. Roach BA, Hutchinson GJ: Treatment of refractory systemic lupus erythematosus-associated thrombocytopenia with intermittent low-dose intravenous cyclophosphamide. Arthritis Rheum 36:682, 1993

187. West SG, Johnson SC: Danazol for the treatment of refractory autoimmune thrombocytopenia in systemic lupus erythematosus. Ann Intern Med 108:703, 1988

188. Maier WP, Gordon DS, Howard RF, et al: Intravenous immunoglobulin therapy in systemic lupus erythematosus-associated thrombocytopenia. Arthritis Rheum 33:1233, 1990

189. ter Borg EJ, Kallenberg CGM: Treatment of severe thrombocytopenia in lupus erythematosus with intravenous immunoglobulin. Ann Rheum Dis 51:1149, 1992

190. Goebel KM, Gassel WD, Goebel FD: Evaluation of azathioprine in autoimmune thrombocytopenia and systemic lupus erythematosus. Scand J Haematol 10:28, 1973

191. Ahn YS, Harrington WJ, Seelman RC, Eytel CS: Vincristine therapy of idiopathic and secondary thrombocytopenias. N Engl J Med 291:376, 1974

192. Breckenridge RT, Moore RD, Ratnoff OD: A study of thrombocytopenia. New histologic criteria for the differentiation of idiopathic thrombocytopenia associated with disseminated lupus erythematosus. Blood 30:39, 1967

193. Homan WP, Dineen P: The role of splenectomy in the treatment of thrombocytopenic pupura due to systemic lupus erythematosus. Ann Surg 187:52, 1978

194. Rivero SJ, Alger M, Alcarcon-Segovia D: Splenectomy for hemocytopenia in systemic lupus erythematosus. A controlled appraisal. Arch Intern Med 139:773, 1979

195. Hall S, McCormick JL Jr, Griepp PR et al: Splenectomy does not cure the thrombocytopenia of systemic lupus erythematosus. Ann Intern Med 102:325, 1985

196. Jacobs P, Wood L, Dent DM: Splenectomy and the thrombocytopenia of systemic lupus erythematosus. Ann Intern Med 105:971, 1985

197. Lurie DP, Kahaleh MB: Pulse corticosteroid therapy for refractory thrombocytopenia in systemic lupus erythematosus. J Rheumatol 9:311, 1982

198. Mackworth-Young CG, Walport MJ, Hughes GR: Thrombocytopenia in a case of systemic lupus erythematosus: repeated administration of "pulse" methyl prednisolone. Br J Rheum 23:298, 1984

199. Boumpas DT, Barez S, Klippel JH, Balow JE: Intermittent cyclophosphamide for the treatment of autoimmune thrombocytopenia in systemic lupus erythematosus. Ann Intern Med 112:674, 1990

200. Hansen MM: Chronic lymphocytic leukaemia. Clinical studies based on 189 cases followed for a long time. Scand J Haematol, suppl. 18:1, 1973

201. Rai KR, Sawitsky A, Cronkite EP et al: Clinical staging of chronic lymphocytic leukemia. Blood 46:219, 1975

202. Duhrsen U, Augener W, Zwinger T, Brittinger G: Spectrum and frequency of autoimmune derangements in lymphoproliferative disorders: analysis of 637 cases and comparison with myeloproliferative diseases. Br J Haematol 67:235, 1987

203. Hamblin TJ, Oscier DG, Young BJ: Autoimmunity in chronic lymphocytic leukemia. J Clin Pathol 39:713, 1986

204. Lischner M, Prokocimer M, Zolberg A, Shaklai M: Autoimmunity in chronic lymphocytic leukemia. Postgrad Med J 64:590, 1988

205. Carey RW, McGinnis A, Jacobson BM, Carvalho A: Idiopathic thrombocytopenic purpura complicating chronic lymphocytic leukemia. Management with sequential splenectomy and chemotherapy. Arch Intern Med 136:62, 1976

206. Kaden BR, Rosse WF, Hauch TW: Immune thrombocytopenia in lymphoproliferative diseases. Blood 53:545, 1979

207. Rubinstein DB, Longo DL: Peripheral destruction of platelets in chronic lymphocytic leukemia: recognition, prognosis and therapeutic implications. Am J Med 71:729, 1981

208. Wang G, Ahn YS, Whitcomb CC, Harrington WJ: Development of polycythemia vera and chronic lymphocytic leukemia during the course of refractory idiopathic thrombocytopenic purpura. Cancer 53:1770, 1984

209. Ebbe S, Wittels B, Dameshek W: Autoimmune thrombocytopenic purpura ("ITP" type) with chronic lymphocyte leukemia. Blood 19:23, 1962

210. Kipps TJ, Carson DA: Autoantibodies in chronic lymphocytiuc leukemia and related systemic autoimmune diseases. Blood 81:2475, 1993

211. Sthroeger ZM, Shtoeger D, Shtalrid M et al: Mechanism of autoimmune hemolytic anemia in chronic lymphocytic leukemia. Am J Hematol 43:259, 1993

212. de Rossi G, Granati L, Girelli G et al: Incidence and prognostic significance of autoantibodies against erythrocytes and platelets in chronic lymphocytic leukemia (CLL). Nouv Rev Fr Hematol 30:403, 1988

213. Razis DV, Diamond HD, Craver LF: Hodgkin's disease associated with other malignant tumors and certain neoplastic diseases. Am J Med Sci 238:327, 1959

214. Xiros N, Binder T, Anger B et al: Idiopathic thrombocytopenic purpura and autoimmune hemolytic anemia in Hodgkin's disease. Eur J Haematol 40:437, 1988

215. Jones SE: Autoimmune disorders and malignant lymphoma. Cancer 31:1092, 1973

216. Kirshneer JJ, Zamkoff KW, Gottlieb AJ: Idiopathic thrombocytopenic purpura and Hodgkin's disease: report of two cases and a review of the literature. Am J Med Sci 280:21, 1980

217. Rudders RA, Aisenberg AC, Schiller AL: Hodgkin's disease presenting as "idiopathic" thrombocytopenic purpura. Cancer 30:220, 1972

218. Hamilton PJ, Dawson AA: Thrombocytopenic purpura as the sole manifestation of a recurrence of Hodgkin's disease. J Clin Pathol 26:70, 1973

219. Eisner E, Ley A, Mayer K: Coombs' positive hemolytic anemia in Hodgkin's disease. Ann Intern Med 66:258, 1967

220. Fink K, Al-Mondhiry H: Idiopathic thrombocytopenic purpura in lymphoma. Cancer 37:1999, 1976

221. Pedro-Botet J, Estruch R, Montserrat E et al: Thrombocytopenic purpura as the first manifestation of an inapparent Hodgkin's disease. Scand J Haematol 36:408, 1986

222. Hussein KK, Shaw MT, Oleinick SR: Autoimmune thrombocytopenia and peripheral neuropathy heralding Hodgkin's disease. South Med J 68:1414, 1975

223. Kedar A, Khan AB, Mattern JQA II et al: Autoimmune disorders complicating adolescent Hodgkin's disease. Cancer 44:112, 1979

224. Cohen JR: Idiopathic thrombocytopenic purpura in Hodgkin's disease. A rare occurrence of no prognostic significance. Cancer 41:743, 1978

225. Aghai E, Quitt M, Lurie M et al: Primary hepatic lymphoma presenting as symptomatic immune thrombocytopenic purpura. Cancer 60:2308, 1987

226. Lin M-T, Shen M-C, Su I-J et al: Peripheral Tg/d lymphoma presenting with idiopathic thrombocytopenic purpura-like picture. Br J Haematol 78:280, 1991

227. Lehman HA, Lehman LO, Rustagi PK: Complement-mediated autoimmune thrombocytopenia. Monoclonal IgM antiplatelet antibody associated with lymphoreticular malignant disease. N Engl J Med 316:194, 1987

228. Kim HD, Boggs DR: A syndrome resembling idiopathic thrombocytopenic purpura in 10 patients with diverse forms of cancer. Am J Med 67:371, 1979

229. Snowdon N, Bhavnani M, Swinson DR et al: Large granular T lymphocytes, neutropenia and polyarthropathy: an underdiagnosed syndrome? Q J Med 78:65, 1991

230. Loughran TP Jr, Kadin ME, Starkebaum G et al: Leukemia of large granular lymphocytes: association with clonal chromosomal abnormalities and auto-

immune neutropenia, thrombocytopenia, and hemolytic anemia. Ann Intern Med 102:169, 1985

231. Reynolds CW, Foon KA: T$_\gamma$-lymphoproliferative disease and related disorders in humans and experimental animals: a review of the clinical, cellular and functional characteristics. Blood 64:1146, 1984

232. Loughran TP Jr: Clonal diseases of large granular lymphocytes. Blood 82:1, 1993

233. Saway PA, Prasthofer EF, Barton JC: Prevalence of granular lymphocytic proliferation in patients with rheumatoid arthritis and neutropenia. Am J Med 86:303, 1989

234. Garcia-Suarez J, Prieto A, Reyes E et al: Severe chronic autoimmune thrombocytopenic purpura is associated with an expansion of CD56$^+$CD3$^-$ natural killer cells subset. Blood 82:1538, 1993

235. Kurata Y, Nishioeda Y, Tsubakio T, Kitani T: Thrombocytopenia in Graves' disease: effect of T$_3$ on platelet kinetics. Acta Haematol 63:185, 1980

236. Adrouny A, Sandler RM, Carmel R: Variable presentation of thrombocytopenia in Graves' disease. Arch Intern Med 142:1460, 1982

237. Resnitzky P, Scholfeld S, Daasa H: Effect of Graves' disease on idiopathic thrombocytopenic purpura. Arch Intern Med 139:483, 1979

238. Marshall JS, Weisberger AS, Levy RP, Breckenridge RT: Coexistent idiopathic thrombocytopenic purpura and hyperthyroidism. Ann Intern Med 67:411, 1967

239. Hymes K, Blum M, Lackner H, Karpatkin S: Easy bruising, thrombocytopenia, and elevated platelet immunoglobulin G in Graves' disease and Hashimoto's thyroiditis. Ann Intern Med 94:27, 1981

240. Herman J, Resnitzky P, Fink A: Association between thyrotoxicosis and thrombocytopenia. J Med Sci 14:469, 1978

241. Mayock RL, Bertran P, Morrison CE, Scott JH: Manifestations of sarcoidosis: analysis of 145 patients, with a review of nine series selected from the literature. Am J Med 35:67, 1963

242. Dickerman JD, Holbrook PR, Zinkham WH: Etiology and therapy of thrombocytopenia associated with sarcoidosis. J Pediatr 81:758, 1972

243. Lawrence HJ, Greenberg BR: Autoimmune thrombocytopenia in sarcoidosis. Am J Med 79:761, 1985

244. Anderson MJ Jr, Woods VL, Tani P et al: Autoantibodies to platelet glycoprotein IIb/IIIa and to the acetylcholine receptor in a patient with chronic idiopathic thrombocytopenic purpura and myasthenia gravis. Ann Intern Med 100:829, 1984

245. Schwartz KA, Schlicter SJ, Harker LA: Immune-mediated platelet destruction and thrombocytopenia in patients with solid tumors. Br J Haematol 51:17, 1982

246. Bellone JD, Kunicki TJ, Aster RH: Immune thrombocytopenia associated with carcinoma. Ann Intern Med 99:470, 1983

247. Garnick MB, Griffin JD: Idiopathic thrombocytopenia in association with extragonadal germ cell cancer. Ann Intern Med 98:926, 1983

248. Anasetti C, Rybka W, Sullivan KM et al: Graft-v-host disease is associated with autoimmune-like thrombocytopenia. Blood 73:1054, 1989

249. First LR, Smith BR, Lipton J et al: Isolated thrombocytopenia after allogeneic bone marrow transplantation: existence of transient and chronic thrombocytopenic syndromes. Blood 65:368, 1985

250. Anasetti C, Rybka W, Sullivan KM et al: Graft-v-host disease is associated with autoimmune-like thrombocytopenia. Blood 73:1054, 1989

251. Spruce W, Forman S, McMillarm R et al: Idiopathic thrombocytopenic purpura following bone marrow transplantation. Acta Haematol 69:47, 1983

252. Minchinton RM, Kendram J, Waters AH, Barrett AJ: Autoimmune thrombocytopenia acquired from an allogeneic bone-marrow graft. Lancet 2:627, 1982

253. Waters AH, Metcalfe P, Minchinton RM et al: Autoimmune thrombocytopenia acquired from allogeneic bone-marrow graft: compensated thrombocytopenia in bone marrow donor and recipient. Lancet 2:430, 1983

254. Minchinton RM, Waters AH: Autoimmune thrombocytpenia and neutropenia after bone marrow transplantation. Blood 66:752, 1985

255. Friend PJ, McCarthy LJ, Filo RS et al: Transmission of idiopathic (autoimmune) thrombocytopenic purpura by liver transplantation. N Engl J Med 323:807, 1990

256. Schulman I: Idiopathic (immune) thrombocytopenic purpura in children: pathogenesis and treatment. Pediat Rev 5:173, 1983

257. Lusher JM, Rathi I: Idiopathic thrombocytopenic purpura in children. Semin Thromb Hemost 3:175, 1977

258. Krishamurthy M, Lee CK, Dosik H: Infectious mononucleosis and severe thrombocytopenia. Am J Med Sci 272:221, 1976

259. Kappers-Klunne MC, van Vliet HHDM: IgM and IgG platelet antibodies in a case of infectious mononucleosis and severe thrombocytopenia. Scand J Haematol 32:145, 1984

260. Feusner JH, Schlichter SJ, Harker LA: Mechanisms of thrombocytopenia in varicella. Am J Hematol 7:255, 1979

261. Hara T, Mizuno Y, Igarashi H, Ueda K: Intravenous gamma globulin therapy for thrombocytopenic purpura associated with active varicella infection. Eur J Pediatr 146:531, 1987

262. Fiala M, Kattlove H: Cytomegalovirus mononucleosis with severe thrombocytopenia. Ann Intern Med 79:450, 1973

263. Harris AI, Meyer RJ, Brody EA: Cytomegalovirus mononucleosis with severe thrombocytopenia. Ann Intern Med 83:670, 1975

264. Morse EE, Zinkham WH, Jackson DP: Thrombocytopenic purpura following rubella infection in children and adults. Arch Intern Med 117:573, 1966

265. Ozsoylu S, Kanra G, Savas G: Thrombocytopenic purpura related to rubella infection. Pediatrics 62:567, 1978

266. Ibarra H, Zapata C, Inostroza J et al: Immune thrombocytopenic purpura associated with hepatitis A. Blut 52:371, 1986

267. Durand JM, Lefevre P, Telle H et al: Thrombocytopenic purpura and hepatitis C infection. Haematology (Pavia) 78:135, 1993

268. Lefrere JJ, Couruce AM, Kaplan C: Parvovirus-associated thrombocytopenia. Lancet 1:730, 1989

269. Whitaker JA III, Hardison JE: Severe thrombocytopenia after generalized herpes simplex virus-2 (HSV-2) infection. South Med J 71:864, 1978

270. Bachand AJ, Rubenstein J, Morrison AN: Thrombocytopenic purpura following lives measles vaccination. Am J Dis Child 113:283, 1967

271. Nieminen U, Peltola H, Syrjala MT et al: Acute thrombocytopenic purpura following measles, mumps and rubella vaccination. A report on 23 patients. Acta Paediatr 82:267, 1993

272. Dubanski AS, Oski FA: Controversies in the management of acute idiopathic thrombocytopenic purpura: survey of specialists. Pediatrics 77:49, 1986

273. Bussel JB, Goldman A, Imbach P et al: Treatment of acute ITP in childhood with intravenous infusions of gammaglobulin. J Pediatr 106:886, 1985

274. McIntosh N: Is bone marrow investigation required in isolated childhood thrombocytopenia? Lancet 1:956, 1982

275. Elaurie M, Burns ER, Bernstein LJ et al: Thrombocytopenia and human immunodeficiency virus in children. Pediatrics 82:905, 1988 908.

276. Rigaud M, Leibovitz E, Quee CS et al: Thrombocytopenia in children infected with human immunodeficiency virus long-term follow-up and therapeutic considerations. J Acquir Immune Defic Syndr 5:450, 1992

277. Greinacher A, Mueller-Eckhard C: Hereditary types of thrombocytopenia; an important differential diagnosis in chronic thrombocytopenia. In Sutor AH, Thomas KB (eds): Thrombocytopenia in Childhood. Schattauer, Stuttgart, 1994

278. Najean Y: The congenital thrombocytopenias due to production defect. In Sutor AH, Thomas KB (eds): Thrombocytopenia in Childhood. Schattauer, Stuttgart, 1994

279. Shimizu K, Katsuta I, Uchikawa T: Familial lupoid thrombocytopenia. Am J Hematol 44:9, 1993

280. Bussel JB, Benedetto P, Lee S, Elkon K: Is ITP more severe with a positive ANA? Blood 72:957, 1988

281. Piller F, Le Deist F, Weinberg KI et al: Altered O-glycan synthesis in lymphocytes from patients with Wiskott-Aldrich syndrome. J Exp Med 173:1501, 1991

282. Cunningham-Rundles C: Clinical and immunologic analysis of 103 patients with common variable immunodeficiency. J Clin Immunol 9:1, 1989

283. Bussel JB, Morell A, Skvaril F: IgG2 deficiency in autoimmune cytopenia. Monogr Allergy 20:11, 1986

284. Cuningham-Rundles C, Zhou C, McKarious S, Courter S: Long term use of IgA depleted intravenous immunoglobulin in immunodeficiency subjects with anti-IgA antibodies. J Clin Immunol 13:271, 1993

285. Wang WC: Evans syndrome in childhood: pathophysiology, clinical course in treatment. Am J Pediatr Hematol Oncol 10:330, 1988

286. Gordon J, Cohen O, Finlayson JS: Levels of anti-A and anti-B in commercial immune globulins. Transfusion 20:90, 1980

287. Woerner SJ, Abildgaard CF, French BN: Intracranial hemorrhage in children with idiopathic thrombocytopenic purpura. Pediatrics 67:453, 1981

288. Walker RW, Walker W: Idiopathic thrombocytopenia: initial illness and long term follow-up. Arch Dis Child 59:316, 1984

289. Lusher JM, Zueltzer WW: Idiopathic thrombocytopenic purpura in childhood. J Pediatr 68:971, 1966

290. Krivit W, Tate D, White JG et al: Idiopathic thrombocytopenic purpura and intracranial hemorrhage. Pediatrics 67:570, 1981

291. Buchanan GR: The nontreatment of childhood idiopathic thrombocytopenic purpura. Eur J Pediatr 146:107, 1987

292. Bussel JB: Treatment of acute idiopathic thrombocytopenic purpura, editorial correspondence. J Pediatr 108:326, 1986

293. Imbach P, Barandun S, D'Appuzzo V et al: High-dose intravenous gammaglobulin for idiopathic thrombocytopenic purpura in childhood. Lancet 1:1228, 1981

294. Imbach P, Wagner JP, Berchtold W et al: Intravenous immunoglobulin ver-

sus oral corticosteroids in acute immune thrombocytopenic purpura in childhood. Lancet 2:464, 1985

295. Van Hoff J, Ritchey K: Pulse methylprednisolone therapy for acute childhood idiopathic thrombocytopenic purpura. J Pediatr 113:563, 1988

96. Hara T, Soshida Miyazaki N, Goya N: High dose of gammaglobulin and methyprednisolone therapy for idiopathic thrombocytopenic purpura in children. Eur J Pediatr 144:240, 1985

297. Bussel JB, Schulman I, Hilgartner MW, Barandun S: Intravenous use of gammaglobulin in the treatment of chronic immune thrombocytopenic purpura as a means to defer splenectomy. J Pediatr 103:651, 1983

298. Imholz B, Imbach P, Baumagartner C et al: Intravenous immunoglobulin (i.v. IgG) for previously treated acute or chronic idiopathic thrombocytopenic purpura (ITP) in childhood a prospective multicenter study. Blut 52:63, 1988

299. Andrew M, Blanchette VS, Adams M et al: A multicenter study of the treatment of childhood chronic idiopathic thrombocytopenic purpura with anti-D. J Pediatr 120:522, 1992

300. Higsonmex G, Ozoylu S: Vincristine for treatment of chronic thrombocytopenia in children. N Engl J Med 296:454, 1977

301. Hilgartner MW, Lanzkowski P, Smith CH: The use of azathioprin in refractory idiopathic thrombocytopenic purpura in children. Acta Pediatr Scand 59: 409, 1970

302. Hollenberg JP, Subak LL, Ferry JJ, Bussel JB: Cost effectiveness of splenectomy versus intravenous gammaglobulin in the treatment of chronic immune thrombocytopenic purpura in childhood. J Pediatr 112:530, 1988

303. Salama A, Mueller-Eckhart C, Kiefel V: Effect of intravenous immunoglobulin in immune thrombocytopenia. Lancet 2:193, 1983

304. Ramos MEG, Newman AJ, Fross S: Chronic thrombocytopenia in childhood. J Pediatr 92:584, 1978

305. Erickson WD, Burgert EO, Lynn HB: The hazard of infection following splenectomy in children. Am J Dis Child 116:1, 1968

306. Singer DB: Post-splenectomy sepsis. p. 253. In Rosenberg HS, Bolande RP (eds): Perspectives in Pediatric Pathology. Year Book Medical Publishers, Chicago, 1973

307. Burrows RF, Kelton JG: Fetal thrombocytopenia and its relation to maternal thrombocytopenia. N Engl J Med 329:1463, 1993

308. McCrae KR, Samuels P, Schreiber AD: Pregnancy-associated thrombocytopenia: pathogenesis and management. Blood 80:2697, 1992

309. Hart D, Dunetz C, Nardi M et al: An epidemic of maternal thrombocytopenia associated with elevated antiplatelet antibody. Platelet count and antiplatelet antibody in 116 consecutive pregnancies: relationship to neonatal platelet count. Am J Obstet Gynecol 154:878, 1986

310. Matthews JH, Benjamin S, Gill DS, Smith NA: Pregnancy-associated thrombocytopenia: definition, incidence and natural history. Acta Haematol 84:24, 1990

311. Samuels P, Bussel JB, Braitman LE et al: Estimation of the risk of thrombocytopenia in the offspring of pregnant women with presumed immune thrombocytopenic purpura. N Engl J Med 323:229, 1990

312. Coppelstone JA: Fetal platelet counts in thrombocytopenic pregnancy. Lancet 336:1375, 1990

313. Kaplan C, Daffos F, Forestier F et al: Fetal platelet counts in thrombocytopenic pregnancy. Lancet 336:979, 1990

314. Ostensen M: Treatment with immunosuppressive and disease modifying drugs during pregnancy and lactation. Am J Reprod Immunol 28:148, 1992

315. Moutet A, Fromont P, Farcet J-P et al: Pregnancy in women with immune thrombocytopenic purpura. Arch Intern Med 150:2141, 1990

316. Rayburn WF: Glucocorticoid therapy for rheumatic diseases: maternal, fetal, and breast-feeding considerations. Am J Reprod Immunol 28:138, 1992

317. Warrell DW, Taylor R: Outcome for the foetus of mothers receiving prednisolone during pregnancy. Lancet 1:117, 1968

318. Schatz M, Patterson R, Zeitz S et al: Corticosteroid therapy for the pregnant asthmatic patient. JAMA 233:804, 1975

319. Schmand B, Neuvel J, Smolders-de Haas H et al: Psychological development of children who were treated antenatally with corticosteroids to prevent respiratory distress syndrome. Pediatrics 86:58, 1990

320. Reinisch JM, Simon NG, Karow WG, Gandelman R: Prenatal exposure to prednisone in humans and animals retards intrauterine growth. Science 202:436, 1976

321. Sacher RA, King JC: Intravenous gamma-globulin in pregnancy: a review. Obstet Gynecol Surv 44:25, 1988

322. Jones WR, Storey B, Norton G, Neische FW Jr: Pregnancy complicated by acute idiopathic thrombocytopenic purpura. A report of two patients treated by simultaneous caesarean section and splenectomy. J Obstet Gynecol 81:330, 1974

323. FitzGerald G, McCarthy D, O'Connell LG, McCann SR: Hyperimmune thrombocytopenia in pregnancy treated by splenectomy. Acta Haematol 59:315, 1978

324. Ramsey-Goldman R, Mientus JM, Kutzer JE et al: Pregnancy outcome in women with systemic lupus erythematosus treated with immunosuppressive drugs. J Rheumatol 20:1152, 1993

325. Williamson RA, Karp LE: Azathioprine teratogenicity: review of the literature and case report. Obstet Gynecol 58:237, 1981

326. DeWitte DB, Buick MK, Cyran SE, Maisels MJ: Neonatal pancytopenia and severe combined immunodeficiency associated with antenatal administration of azathioprine and prednisone. J Pediatr 105:625, 1984

327. Territo M, Finklestein J, Oh W et al: Management of autoimmune thrombocytopenia in pregnancy and in the neonate. Obstet Gynecol 145:932, 1983

328. Cines DB, Dusak B, Tomaski A et al: Immune thrombocytopenic purpura and pregnancy. N Engl J Med 99:796, 1983

329. Browning JJ, James DK: Immune thrombocytopenia in pregnancy. Fetal Med Rev 2:47, 1990

330. Cook RL, Miller RC, Katz VL, Cefalo RC: Immune thrombocytopenic purpura in pregnancy: a reappraisal of management. Obstet Gynecol 78:578, 1991

331. Karpatkin M, Porges RF, Karpatkin S: Platelet counts in infants of women with autoimmune thrombocytopenia. Effect of steroid administration to the mother. N Engl J Med 305:936, 1981

332. Kelton JG: The management of the pregnant patient with autoimmune thrombocytopnic purpura. Ann Intern Med 99:796,

333. Bohm R, Hofstaetter C, Brield RC: High-dose intravenous IgG in pregnant women with autoimmune thrombocytopenia: a cautionary note. Blut 48: 469, 1984

334. Scott JR, Rote NS, Cruikshank DP: Antiplatelet antibodies and platelet counts in pregnancies complicated by autoimmune thrombocytopenia. Am J Obstet Gynecol 145:932, 1983

335. Burrows RF, Kelton JG: Low fetal risks in pregnancies associated with idiopathic thrombocytopenic purpura. Am J Obstet Gynecol 163:1147, 1990

336. Christians GCML, Nieuwenhuis HK, von dem Borne AEGK et al: Idiopathic thrombocytopenic purpura in pregnancy: a randomized trial on the effect of antenatal low dose corticosteroids on neonatal platelet count. Br J Obstet Gynecol 97:893, 1990

337. Tchernia G, Morel-Kopp MC, Yvart J, Kaplan C: Neonatal thrombocytopenia and hidden maternal autoimmunity. Br J Haematol 84:457, 1993

338. Heys RF: Child bearing and idiopathic thrombocytopenic purpura. J Obstet Gynaecol Br Comm 73:205, 1966

339. O'Reilly RA, Taber B-Z: Idiopathic thrombocytopenic purpura and pregnancy. Six new cases. Obstet Gynecol 51:590, 1978

340. Pappas C: Placental transfer of immunoglobulin in immune thrombocytopenic purpura. Lancet 1:389, 1986

341. Davies SV, Murray JA, Gee H, Giles H McC: Transplacental effect of high-dose immunoglobulin in idiopathic thrombocytopenia (ITP). Lancet 1:1098, 1986

342. Ayrmlooi J: A new approach to management of immunologic thrombocytopenia in pregnancy. Am J Obstet Gynecol 130:235, 1978

343. Scott JR, Cruiksnak DP, Kochenour NK et al: Fetal platelet counts in the obstetric management of immunologic thrombocytopenic purpura. Am J Obstet Gynecol 136:495, 1980

344. Christiaens GCML, Helmerhorst FM: Validity of intrapartum diagnosis of fetal thrombocytopenia. Am J Obstet Gynecol 157:864, 1987

345. Ghidini A, Sepulveda W, Lockwood CJ, Romers R: Complications of fetal blood sampling. Am J Obstet Gynecol 168:1339, 1992

346. Segal M, Manning FA, Harman CR, Menticoglous S: Bleeding after intravascular transfusion: experimental and clinical observations. Am J Obstet Gynecol 165:1414, 1991

347. Weiner CP, Wenstrom KD, Sipes SL, Williamson RA: Risk factors for cordocentesis and fetal intravascular transfusion. Am J Obstet Gynecol 165:1010, 1991

348. Tschernia G, Kaplan C, Daffos F et al: Autoimmune thrombocytopenic purpura and pregnancy: from threat to routine, a new danger? p. 315. In Kaplan-Gouet C, Schlegel N, Salmon C, McGregor J (eds): Platelet Immunology: Fundamental and Clinical Aspects. Colloque INSERM/John Libbey Eurotext, London, 1991

349. Mueller-Eckhardt C, Grubert A, Weisheit M et al: 348 cases of suspected neonatal allo-immune thrombocytopenia. Lancet 1:363, 1989

350. Blanchette VS, Chen L, de Friedberg ZS et al: Alloimmunization to the PI^{A1} platelet antigen: results of a prospective study. Br J Haematol 74:209, 1990

351. Pearson HA, Shulman NR, Marder VJ, Cone TE Jr: Isoimmune neonatal thrombocytopenic purpura. Clinical and therapeutic considerations. Blood 23:154, 1964

352. Blanchette VS, Peters MA, Pegg-Feige K: Alloimmune thrombocytopenia. Review from a neonatal intensive care unit. p. 87. In Hassig A (ed): Current Studies in Hematology and Blood Transfusion. S. Karger, Basel, 1986

353. Reznikoff-Etievant MF: Management of alloimmune neonatal and antenatal thrombocytopenia. Vox Sang 55:193, 1988

354. Kaplan C, Daffos F, Forestier F et al: Current trends in neonatal alloimmune thrombocytopenia: diagnosis and therapy. p. 267. In Kaplan-Gouet C, Schlegel N, Salmon C, McGregor J (eds): Platelet Immunology: Fundamental and Clinical Aspects. Colloque INSERM/John Libbey Eurotext, London, 1991

355. Bussel JB, Neonatal Immune Thrombocytopenia Study Group: Neonatal alloimmune thrombocytopenia: a prospective case accumulation study, abstracted. Pediatr Res 23:337A, 1988

356. De Vries LS, Connell J, Bydder GM et al: Recurrent intracranial haemorrhages in utero in an infant with alloimmune thrombocytopenia: case report. Br J Obstet Gynaecol 95:299, 1988

357. Naidu S, Messmore H, Caserta V, Fines M: CNS lesions in neonatal isoimmune thrombocytopenia. Arch Neurol 40:552, 1983

358. Jocelyn LJ, Casiro OG: Neurodevelopmental outcome of term infants with intraventricular hemorrhage. Am J Dis Child 146:194, 1992

359. Kaplan C, Morel-Kopp M-C, Kroll H et al: HPA-5b (Brᵃ) neonatal alloimmune thrombocytopenia: clinical and immunological analysis of 39 cases. Br J Haematol 78:425, 1991

360. Kaplan C, Patereau C, Reznikoff-Etievant MF et al: Antenatal Pl^{A1} typing and detection of gp IIb-IIIa complex. Br J Haematol 60:584, 1985

361. Gruel Y, Boizard B, Daffos F et al: Determination of platelet antigens and glycoproteins in the human fetus. Blood 68:488, 1986

362. Kaplan C, Daffos F, Forestier F et al: Management of alloimmune thrombocytopenia: antenatal diagnosis and in utero transfusion of maternal platelets. Blood 72:340, 1988

363. Nicolini U, Rodeck CH, Kichenour NK et al: In utero platelet transfusion for alloimmune thrombocytopenia. Lancet 2:506, 1988

364. Waters A, Murphy M, Hambley H, Nioclaides K: Management of alloimmune thrombocytopenia in the fetus and neonate. p. 155. In Nance ST (ed): Clinical and Basic Science Aspects of Immunohematology. American Association of Blood Banks, Arlington, VA, 1991

365. Herman JH, Jumbelic MI, Ancona RJ, Kickler TS: In utero cerebral hemorrhage in alloimmune thrombocytopenia. Am J Pediatr Hematol Oncol 8:312, 1986

366. Giovangrandi Y, Daffos F, Kaplan C et al: Very early intracranial haemorrhage in alloimmune fetal thrombocytopenia. Lancet 2:310, 1990

367. Mueller-Eckhardt C, Becker T, Weisheit M et al: Neonatal alloimmune thrombocytopenia due to fetomaternal Zwᵇ incompatibility. Vox Sang 50:94, 1986

368. Shibata Y, Matsuda I, Miyaji T, Ichikawa Y: Yukᵃ, a new platelet antigen involved in two cases of neonatal alloimmune thrombocytopenia. Vox Sang 50:177, 1986

369. Morel-Kopp M-C, Blanchard B, Kiefel V et al: Anti-HPA-4b (anti-Yukᵃ) neonatal alloimmune thrombocytopenia: first report in a Caucasian family. Transfus Med 2:273, 1992

370. Friedman JM, Aster RH: Neonatal alloimmune thrombocytopenic purpura and cogenital porencephaly in two siblings associated with a "new" maternal antiplatelet antibody. Blood 65:1412, 1985

371. von dem Borne AEGK, von Reisz E, Vergeugt FWA et al: Bakᵃ, a new platelet-specific antigen involved in neonatal alloimmune thrombocytopenia. Vox Sang 39:113, 1980

372. Hiller MC, Shulman NR: Characteristics of leukocyte and platelet antigens shared by non-human primates and man. Ann NY Acad Sci 162:429, 1969

373. Kiefel V, Schechter Y, Atias D et al: Neonatal alloimmune thrombocytopenia due to anti-Brᵇ(HPA-5a). Report of three cases in two families. Vox Sang 60:244, 1991

374. Bizzaro N, Dianese G: Neonatal alloimmune amegakaryocytosis. Case report. Vox Sang 54:112, 1988

375. Grenet P, Dausset J, Dugas M et al: Purpura thrombopenique neonatal avec isoimmunisation foeto-maternelle anti-Koᵃ. Arch Fr Pediatr 22:1165, 1965

376. Kroll H, Kiefel V, Santosos S, Mueller-Eckhardt C: Srᵃ, a private platelet antigen on glycoprotein IIIa associated with neonatal alloimmune thrombocytopenia. Blood 76:2296, 1990

377. Kelton JG, Smith JW, Horsewood P: Govᵃ/ᵇ alloantigen system on human platelets. Blood 75:2172, 1990

378. Ikeda H, Mitani T, Ohnuma M et al: A new platelet-specific antigen, Nakᵃ, involved in the refractoriness of HLA-matched platelet transfusion. Vox Sang 57:213, 1989

379. Skacel PO, Stacey TE, Tidmarsch EF, Contreras M: Maternal alloimmunization to HLA, platelet and granulocyte-specific antigens during pregnancy: its influence on cord blood granulocyte and platelet counts. Br J Haematol 71:118, 1989

380. Huang ST, Lin J, McKenzie LL, McGowan EI: Severe alloimmune neonatal thrombocytopenia due to HLA A2 antibody, abstracted. Transfusion 27:513, 1987

381. Chow MP, Sun KJ, Yung CH et al: Neonatal alloimmune thrombocytopenia due to HLA-A2 antibody. Acta Haematol 87:153, 1992

382. Evans DI: Immune amegakaryocytic thrombocytopenia of the newborn: association with anti-HLA-A2. J Clin Pathol 40:258, 1987

383. Reznikoff-Etievant MF, Dangu C, Lobet R: HLA-B8 antigen and anti-Pl^{A1} alloimmunization. Tissue Antigens 18:66, 1981

384. Mueller-Eckhardt C, Mueller-Eckhardt G, Willen-Ohff H et al: Immunogenicity of an immune response to the human platelet antigen Zwᵃ is strongly associated with HLA-B8 and DR3. Tissue Antigens 26:71, 1985

385. Decary F: Is HLA-DR3 a risk factor in Pl^{A1}-negative pregnant women? p. 78. In Hassig A (ed): Current Studies in Hematology and Blood Transfusion. S Karger, AG, Basel, 1986

386. Valentin N, Vergracht A, Bignon JD et al: HLA-DRw52a is involved in alloimmunization against PL-A1 antigen. Hum Immunol 27:73, 1990

387. de Waal LP, van Dalen CM, Engelfriet CP, von dem Borne AEGK: Alloimmunization against the platelet-specific Zwᵃ antigen, resulting in neonatal alloimmune thrombocytopenia or posttransfusion purpura, is associated with the supertypic DRw52 antigen, including DR3 and DRw6. Hum Immunol 17:45, 1986

388. Mueller-Eckhardt C, Mueller-Eckhardt G: Alloimmunization against the platelet specific Zwᵃ antigen associated with HLA-Drw52 and/or DRw6. Hum Immunol 18:181, 1987

389. Mueller-Eckhardt C, Kiefel V, Kroll H, Mueller-Eckhardt G: HLA-DRw6, a new immune response marker for immunization against the platelet alloantigen Brᵃ. Vox Sang 57:90, 1989

390. Burrows RF, Kelton JG: Alloimmune neonatal thrombocytopenia associated with incidental maternal thrombocytopenia. Am J Hematol 35:43, 1990

391. van Leeuwen EF, von dem Borne AE, Oudesluijs-Murphy AM et al: Neonatal alloimmune thrombocytopenia complicated by maternal autoimmune thrombocytopenia. Br Med J 281:27, 1980

392. Adner MM, Fisch GR, Starobin SG, Aster RH: Use of "compatible" platelet transfusions in treatment of congenital isoimmune thrombocytopenic purpura. N Engl J Med 280:244, 1969

393. Martin B, Robin H, Williams R, Ornelias W: Neonatal graft vs. host disease following transfusion of maternal platelets, abstracted. Transfusion, suppl. 23:417, 1983

394. Sidiropolis D, Straume B: The treatment of neonatal isoimmune thrombocytopenia with intravenous immunoglobulin (IgG i.v.). Blut 48:383, 1984

395. Buseel JB, Berkowitz RL, McFarland JG et al: Antenatal treatment of neonatal alloimmune thrombocytopenia. N Engl J Med 319:1374, 1988

396. Mueller-Eckhardt CM, Kiefel V, Grubert A: High-dose IgG treatment for neonatal alloimmune thrombocytopenia. Blut 59:146, 1989

397. Gafni A, Blanchette VS: Screening for neonatal thrombocytopenia: an economic perspective. p. 140. In: Current Studies in Hematology and Blood Transfusion. S Karger AG, Basel, 1988

398. Shulman NR, Jordan JV: Platelet Immunology. JB Lippincott, Philadelphia, 1982

399. McFarland JG, Aster RH, Bussel JB et al: Prenatal diagnosis of neonatal alloimmune thrombocytopenia using allele-specific oligonucleotide probes. Blood 78:2276, 1991

400. Kuijpers RWAM, Faber NM, Kanhair HHH, von dem Borne AEGK: Typing of fetal platelet alloantigens when platelets are not available. Lancet 336:1319, 1990

401. Madsen H, Taaning E, Georgsen J et al: PCR for fetal platelet HPA-1 alloantigen typing. Lancet 227:493, 1991

402. Waters AH, Mibashan RS, Nicolaides KH et al: Management of fetal alloimmune thrombocytopenia: the place of intrauterine platelet transfusions. p. 279. In Kaplasi-Gouet C, Schlegel N, Salmon C, McGregor J (eds): Platelet Immunology: Fundamental and Clinical Aspects. Colloque INSERM/John Libbey Eurotext, London, 1991

403. Nicolini U, Tannirandorn Y, Gonzalez P et al: Continuing controversy in alloimmune thrombocytopenia: fetal hyperimmunoglobulinemia fails to prevent thrombocytopenia. Am J Obstet Gynecol 163:1144, 1990

404. Mueller-Eckhardt C, Kiefel V, Jovanovic V et al: Perinatal treatment of fetal alloimmune thrombocytopenia. Lancet ii:910, 1988

405. McGill M, Mayhaus C, Hoff R, Carey P: Frozen maternal platelets for neonatal thrombocytopenia. Transfusion 27:347, 1986

406. Kay HH, Hage ML, Kurtzberg J, Dunsmore KP: Alloimmune thrombocytopenia may be associated with systemic disease. Am J Obstet Gynecol 166:110, 1991

407. Levine AB, Berkowitz RL: Neonatal alloimmune thrombocytopenia. Semin Perinatol, suppl. 2. 15:35, 1991

408. Wenstrom KD, Weiner CP, Williamson RA: Antenatal treatment of fetal alloimmune thrombocytopenia. Obstet Gynecol 80:433, 1990

409. Lynch L, Bussel JB, McFarland JG et al: Antenatal treatment of alloimmune thrombocytopenia. Obstet Gynecol 80:67, 1992

410. Zimmerman R, Huch A: In-utero fetal therapy with immunoglobulin for alloimmune thrombocytopenia. Lancet 340:606, 1992

411. Bowman J, Harman C, Mentigolous S, Pollock J: Intravenous fetal transfusion of immunoglobulin for alloimmune thrombocytopenia. Lancet 340:1034, 1992

412. Zucker MB, Ley AB, Borrelli J et al: Thrombocytopenia with a circulating platelet agglutinin, platelet lysin and clot retraction inhibitor. Blood 14:148, 1959

413. van Loghen JJ Jr, Dorfmeiher H, van der Hart M: Serologic and genetic studies on a platelet antigen (Zw). Vox Sang 4:161, 1959

414. Shulman NR, Aster RH, Leitner A, Hiller MC: Immunoreactions involving platelets. V. Post-transfusion purpura due to a complement-fixing antibody against a genetically controlled platelet antigen. A proposed mechanism for thrombocytopenia and its relevance in "autoimmunity." J Clin Invest 40:1597, 1961

415. Mueller-Eckhardt C, Kroll H, Kiefel V et al: Posttransfusion purpura. p. 249. In Kaplan-Gouet C, Schlegel N, Salmon C, McGregor J (eds): Platelet Immunology: Fundamental and Clinical Aspects. Colloque INSERM/John Libbey Eurotext, London, 1991

416. Taaning E, Killmann S-A, Morling N et al: Post-transfusion purpura (PTP) due to anti-Zw^b (-PI^{A2}): the significance of IgG$_3$ antibodies in PTP. Br J Haematol 64:217, 1986

417. Zeigler Z, Murphy S, Gardner FH: Post-transfusion purpura: a heterogeneous syndrome. Blood 45:529, 1975

418. Seidenfeld AM, Owen J, Glynn MFX: Post-transfusion purpura cured by steroid therapy in a man. Can Med Assoc J 118:1285, 1978

419. Bracey AW, Shulman NR: Effect of plasma exchange on an unusual case of post-transfusion purpura, abstracted. Transfusion suppl. 23:428, 1983

420. Taaning E, Morling N, Ovesen H, Svejgaard A: Post transfusion purpura and anti-Zw^b (-PI^{A2}). Tissue Antigens 26:143, 1985

421. Mueller-Eckhard CM: Post-transfusion purpura. Br J Haematol 64:419, 1986

422. Soulier J, Patereau C, Gobert N et al: Post-transfusional immunologic thrombocytopenia. A case report. Vox Sang. 37:21, 1979

423. Kirmani S, Geier LJ, Gandara DR: Post-transfusion purpura and isoimmune neonatal thrombocytopenia in the same family. A case report, abstracted. Blood 62:245a, 1983

424. Ballem PJ, Buskard NA, Decary F, Doubroff P: Post-transfusion purpura secondary to passive transfer of anti-PI^{A1} by blood transfusion. Br J Haematol 66:113, 1987

425. Nijjar TS, Bonacosa IA, Israels LG: Severe acute thrombocytopenia following infusion of plasma containing anti-PI^{A1}. Am J Hematol 25:219, 1987

426. Scott EP, Moilan-Bergeland J, Dalmasso AP: Posttransfusion thrombocytopenia associated with passive transfusion of a platelet-specific antibody. Transfusion 28:73, 1988

427. Warkentin TE, Smith JW, Hayward CPM et al: Thrombocytopenia caused by passive transfusion of anti-glycoprotein Ia/IIa alloantibody (anti-HPA-5b). Blood 79:2480, 1992

428. Gerstner JB, Smith MJ, Davis KD et al: Post-transfusion purpura: therapeutic failure of PI^{A1}-negative platelet transfusion. Am J Hematol 6:71, 1979

429. Budd JL, Wiegers SE, O'Hara JM: Relapsing post-transfusion purpura. A preventable disease. Am J Med 78:-32768, 1985

430. Chapman JF, Murphy MF, Berney SI et al: Post-transfusion purpura associated with anti-Bak^a and anti-PI^{A2} platelet antibodies and delayed haemolytic transfusion reaction. Vox Sang 52:313, 1987

431. Wautier JL, Boizard B, Lecharny B et al: Purpura post-transfusionnel: identification d'un nouvel antigene plaquettaire Lek^a. Presse Med 13:657, 1984

432. Keimowitz RM, Collins J, Davis K, Aster RH: Post-transfusion purpura associated with alloimmunization against the platelet-specific antigen, Bak^a. Am J Hematol 21:79, 1986

433. Kickler TS, Herman JH, Furihata K et al: Identification of Bak^b, a new platelet-specific antigen associated with posttransfusion purpura. Blood 71:894, 1988

434. Simon TL, Collins J, Kunicki TJ et al: Posttransfusion purpura associated with alloantibody specific for the platelet antigen, Pen^a. Am J Hematol 29:38, 1988

435. Kiefel V, Santoso S, Glockner WM et al: Posttransfusion purpura associaed with an anti-Bak^b. Vox Sang 56:93, 1989

436. Christie DJ, Pulkrabek S, Putnam JL et al: Posttransfusion purpura due to an alloantibody reactive with glycoprotein Ia/IIa (anti-HPA-5b). Blood 77:2785, 1991

437. Vaughan-Neil EF, Ardeman S, Bevan G et al: Post-transfusion purpura associated with unusual platelet antibody (anti-PI-B^1). BMJ 1:436, 1975

438. Hoak JC, Aster RH, Fry GL et al: Post-transfusion purpura (PTP)—a multifaceted enigma, abstracted. Clin Res 27:510A, 1979

439. Dunstan RA, Rosse WF: Post-transfusion purpura: report of a case with anti-PI^{A1} masked by HLA antibodies. Transfusion 25:219, 1985

440. Mueller-Eckhardt C, Kiefel V, Mueller-Eckhardt G et al: Posttransfusion purpura. A survey of 13 cases. Klin Wochenschr 64:1198, 1986

441. Chaplin H, Aster RH, Morgan LK et al: First example of familial posttransfusion purpura in two PI^{A1}-negative sisters. Transfusion 28:326, 1988

442. Cobos E, Gandara DR, Geier LJ, Kirmani S: Post-transfusion purpura and isoimmune neonatal thrombocytopenia in the same family. Am J Hematol 32:235, 1989

443. Pegels JG, Bruynes ECE, Engelfriet CP, von dem Borne AEGK: Post-transfusion purpura: a serological and immunochemical study. Br J Haematol 49:521, 1981

444. Taaning E, Skov F: Elution of anti-Zw^a (PI^{A1}) from autolgous platelets after normalization of platelet count in post-transfusion purpura. Vox Sang 60:40, 1991

445. von dem Borne AEGK, van der Plas-van Dalen CM: Further observations of post-transfusion purpura (PTP). Br J Haematol 61:374, 1985

446. von dem Borne AEGK, van der Plas-van Dalen CM: Further observations on post-transfusion purpura (PTP). Br J Haematol 61:374, 1985

447. Kickler TS: Elevated platelet-associated IgG in PI^{A1}-negative mothers following sensitization to the PI^{A1} antigen during pregnancy. Vox Sang 63:210, 1992

448. Stricker RB, Lewis BH, Corsh L, Shuman MA: Post-transfusion purpura associated with an autoantibody directed against a previously undefined platelet antigen. Blood 69:1458, 1987

449. Minchinton RM, Cunningham I, Cole-Sinclair M et al: Autoreactive platelet antibody in post-transfusion purpura. Aust NZ J Med 20:111, 1990

450. Kickler TS, Ness PM, Herman JH, Bells WR: Studies on the pathophysiology of posttransfusion purpura. Blood 68:347, 1986

451. Dieleman LA, Brand A, Class FHJ et al: Acquired Zw^a antigen on Zw^a negative platelets demonstrated by Western blotting. Br J Haematol 72:539, 1989

452. Ehmann WC, Dancis A, Ferziger R, Karpatkin S: Posttransfusion purpura: conversion of PI^{A1} negative platelets to the PI^{A1}-positive phenotype by stored plasma is not due to the presence of soluble PI^{A1} antigen. Proc Soc Exp Med Biol 195:192, 1990

453. Warejcka D, Janson M, Aster RH: The PI^{A1} antigen, but not HLA-antigens, can be acquired by platelets from plasma, abstracted. Blood 66:109a, 1985

454. Shulman NR, Reid DM, Jones CE et al: Evidence that adsorption of alloantigen-antibody complexes is the basis for posttransfusion purpura, abstracted. Blood, suppl. 1. 75:390a, 1990

455. Shulman NR: Posttransfusion purpura: clinical features and the mechanism of platelet destruction. p. 137. In Nance SJ (ed): Clinical and Basic Aspects of Immunohematology. American Association of Blood Banks, Arlington, VA, 1991

456. Morris FS, Mollison PL: Post-transfusion purpura. N Engl J Med 275:243, 1966

457. Berney SI, Metcalfe P, Wathen NC, Waters AH: Post-transfusion purpura responding to high dose intravenous IgG: further observations on pathogenesis. Br J Haematol 61:627, 1985

458. Fudenberg HH, Rosenfeld RE, Wasserman LR: Unusual specificity of autoantibody in auto-immune hemolytic disease. J Mt Sinai Hosp 25:324, 1958

459. Polesky HF, Bove JR: A fatal hemolytic transfusion reaction with acute autohemolysis. Transfusion 4:285, 1964

460. Salama A, Mueller-Eckhardt C: Delayed hemolytic transfusion reactions. Evidence for complement activation involving allogeneic and autolgous red cells. Transfusion 24:188, 1984

461. Salama A, Berghofer H, Mueller-Eckhardt C: Red blood cell transfusion in warm-type autoimmune haemolytic anemia. Lancet 340:1515, 1992

462. Zmijewski CM: The production of erythrocyte autoantibodies in chimpanzees. J Exp Med 121:657, 1965

463. Cook IA: Primary rhesus immunization of male volunteers. Br J Haematol 21:369, 1971

464. Ness PM, Shirey RS, Thoman SK, Buck SA: The differentiation of delayed serologic and delayed hemolytic transfusion reactions: incidence, long-term serologic findings and clinical significance. Transfusion 30:688, 1990

465. Gengozian N, Ostby DA: Antibodies selectively reactive to autologous and host-type platelets are obtained following interspecies immunizations in marmosets. Clin Exp Immunol 43:128, 1981

466. Chong BH, Cade J, Smith JA, Tatoulis J: An unusual case of post-transfusion purpura: good transient response to high-dose immunoglobulin. Vox Sang 51:182, 1986

467. Boizard N, Wautier J-L: Lek^a, a new platelet antigen absent in Glanzmann's thrombasthenia. Vox Sang 46:47, 1984

468. Gockerman JP, Shulman NR: Isoantibody specificity in post-transfusion purpura. Blood 41:817, 1973

469. Vogelsang G, Kickler TS, Bell WR: Post-transfusion purpura: a report of five patients and a review of the pathogenesis and management. Am J Hematol 21:259, 1986

470. Eisenberg PD, Abramson N: Post-transfusion purpura revisited. N Engl J Med 296:515, 1977

471. Mueller-Eckhardt C, Kiefel V: High-dose IgG for post-transfusion purpura-revisited. Blut 570:163, 1988

472. Mueller-Eckhardt C, Kuenzlen E, Thilo-Korner D, Pralle H: High-dose intravenous immunoglobulin for post-transfusion purpura. N Engl J Med 308:287, 1983

473. Berney SI, Metcalfe P, Wathen NC, Waters AH: Post-transfusion purpura responding to high dose intravenous IgG: further observations on pathogenesis. Br J Haematol 61:627, 1985

474. Walker WS, Yap PL, Kilpatrick DC et al: Post-transfusion purpura following open heart surgery: management by high dose intravenous immunoglobulin infusion. Blut 57:323, 1988

475. Abramson N, Isenberg PD, Aster RH: Post-transfusion purpura: Immunologic aspects and therapy. N Engl J Med 291:1163, 1974

476. Laurensen B, Morling N, Rosenkvist J et al: Post-transfusion purpura treated with plasma exchange by Haemonetics cell separator. J Intern Med 203:539, 1978

477. Cimo PL, Aster RH: Post-transufsion purpura: successful treatment by exchange transfusion. N Engl J Med 287:290, 1972

478. Slichter SJ: Post-transfusion purpura: response to steroids and association with red blood cell and lymphocytotoxic antibodies. Br J Haematol 50:599, 1982

479. Weisberg LJ, Linker CA: Prednisone therapy of post-transfusion purpura. Ann Intern Med 100:76, 1984

480. Cunningham CC, Lind SE: Apparent reponse of refractory post-transfusion purpura to splenectomy. Am J Hematol 30:112, 1989

481. Morse EE: Post-tranfusion thrombocytopenic purpura. Johns Hopkins Med J 121:365, 1968

482. Howard JE, Glassberg AB, Perkins HA: Post-transfusion thrombocytopenic purpura: a case report. Am J Hematol 1:339, 1976

483. Glud TK, Rosthoj S, Jensen MK et al: High-dose intravenous immunoglobulin for post-transfusion purpura. Scand J Haematol 31:495, 1983

484. Lippman SM, Lizak GE, Foung SKH, Grumet FC: The efficacy of PI^{A1}-negative platelet transfusion therapy in posttransfusion purpura. West J Med 148:86, 1988

485. Brecher ME, Moore SB, Letendre L: Posttransfusion purpura: the therapeutic value of PI^{A1}-negative platelets. Transfusion 30:433, 1990

486. Lau P, Sholtis CM, Aster RH: Post-transfusion purpura. An enigma of alloimmunization. Am J Hematol 9:331, 1980

487. Godeau B, Fromont P, Bettaieb A et al: Relapse of posttransfusion purpura after transfusion with frozen-thawed red cells. Transfusion 31:189,

488. Kalish RI, Jacobs B: Post-transfusion purpura: initiation by leukocyte-poor red cells in a polytransfused woman. Vox Sang 53:169, 1987

Thrombocytopenia Due to Decreased Platelet Production

126

Samuel A. Burstein

INTRODUCTION

An estimated 15×10^6 megakaryocytes/kg body weight averaging 12×10^3 fl in volume produce about 1,000–1,500 platelets each.[1] When measured as platelet turnover (calculated by dividing the platelet count by the platelet survival time and correcting for splenic pooling), most of the megakaryocyte cytoplasm is delivered to the circulation as platelets (effective platelet production)[2]. Physiologically, decreased platelet production is due to a decrease in the megakaryocyte mass (virtually always a decrease in the number of megakaryocytes) or to a failure of delivery of an appropriate number of viable platelets by an adequate megakaryocyte cytoplasmic mass, a process termed ineffective platelet production[2] (Fig. 126-1). Table 126-1 shows typical kinetic characteristics for some of these disorders.

A decrease in numbers of megakaryocytes may be due to direct toxicity or damage to their immediate progenitors, the colony-forming unit-megakaryocyte (CFU-Mk) or their precursors, the burst-forming unit-megakaryocyte (BFU-Mk) (see Ch. 19). Abnormalities of growth factors that promote commitment, proliferation, or differentiation of BFU-Mk, CFU-Mk, or their progeny may also be involved in the pathogenesis of platelet production abnormalities; however, there is little evidence that such abnormalities occur frequently.[3] Damage to more primitive stem cells (or to the regulatory mechanisms promoting their growth) would give rise to multilineage cytopenias (see Chs. 21 and 22).

ACQUIRED PRODUCTION DISORDERS

Platelet production abnormalities may be divided arbitrarily into acquired and hereditary disorders.

Marrow Infiltration

Production disorders are commonly observed when the marrow is involved with metastatic cancer, lymphoma, or leukemia. Table 126-2 categorizes the infiltrative processes associated with thrombocytopenia. Although physical replacement of marrow is the etiology of the thrombocytopenia in many cases, it is also possible that inhibitory factors produced by the infiltrating cells are toxic to the cells of the megakaryocytic lineage or interfere with normal regulatory mechanisms. The diagnosis of infiltrative disease is made by marrow examination, although clues to the diagnosis are usually provided by history, physical examination, and a leukoerythroblastic blood smear. The marrow shows decreased megakaryocytes, which may be large due to a compensatory physiologic response to

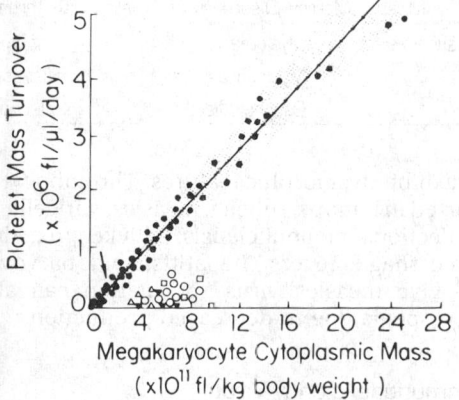

Fig. 126-1. Ineffective platelet production. In thrombocytopenia, the relationship between marrow megakaryocyte cytoplasmic mass and the turnover of platelet mass in the peripheral blood is usually direct. Platelet mass turnover represents the product of the mean megakaryocyte cytoplasmic volume multiplied by the total number of marrow megakaryocytes. The results in normal subjects are indicated by the arrow, and the stippled area represents 95% confidence limits in thrombocytopenic patients with effective production. Ineffective thrombocytopoiesis is identified as a disparity between available marrow substrate (megakaryocyte cytoplasmic mass) and delivery of platelet mass to the peripheral blood (platelet mass turnover). Results in patients with autosomal dominant thrombocytopenia (open circles), Wiskott-Aldrich syndrome (open triangles), megaloblastic anemia (open squares), and preleukemia (closed triangles) are characterized by ineffective platelet production. (From Thompson and Harker,[150] with permission.)

the thrombocytopenia. The treatment approach is specific to the infiltrative process.

Chemotherapy and Irradiation

Direct destruction of megakaryocytes or their progenitors, or both, can be observed following administration of chemotherapeutic agents or irradiation. Thrombocytopenia is one of the most frequent adverse effects of total body irradiation.[4] Following either allogeneic or autologous marrow transplantation, thrombocytopenia may persist despite resolution of leukopenia and anemia. The etiology of prolonged thrombocytopenia after transplantation is unclear; it may be multifactorial (graft-versus-host disease, infections), but decreased production is likely important in some cases.[5]

Agents that are more likely to induce leukopenia generally induce thrombocytopenia as well. Alkylating agents in general produce more prolonged thrombocytopenia than do antimetabolites. Although it has been claimed that some alkylating agents are sparing of the megakaryocytes (e.g., cyclophosphamide), this is a relative phenomenon; conceivably, agents such

as busulfan, the nitrosoureas, or platinum cause cumulative damage in the more primitive progenitors. Other chemotherapeutic agents, such as the vinca alkaloids, may not decrease the platelet count significantly. Reducing the intensity of the chemotherapy dose is currently the most appropriate approach to management, although in the near future it is likely that hematopoietic growth factors that enhance thrombocytopoiesis will prove to be of value in these patients. Agents such as interleukin-1 (IL-1),[6] IL-6,[7] and IL-3/colony-stimulating factor-granulocyte/macrophage (GM-CSF) fusion protein (PIXY-321)[8] have been shown to enhance the platelet count in patients receiving chemotherapy.

Ethanol-Related Disorders

In one analysis, alcohol was a contributing factor in 26% of patients admitted to hospitals with a platelet count of <100,000/mm³, and thrombocytopenia is the most common hematologic abnormality in severe alcoholism[9] (Ch. 147). Alcohol abuse may result in thrombocytopenia due to several mechanisms, including ineffective production related to folate deficiency and increased splenic pooling due to portal hypertension. Ingestion of alcohol inhibits the expected response to thrombocytopenia induced by plateletpheresis.[10] A mild shortening of platelet survival has been reported.[11] However, ethanol itself can be directly toxic to the marrow.[12–15] In vitro studies have shown that alcohol concentrations achievable in vivo inhibit megakaryocyte maturation but do not inhibit megakaryocyte colony formation.[13,15] Megakaryocyte numbers usually are normal, but markedly decreased megakaryocytes have been observed. In one such case, labeling with platelet-specific antibodies demonstrated that numerous small unidentifiable cells were immature megakaryocytes.[13] Rarely, marrow panhypoplasia has been observed in association with alcohol ingestion.[16] Anemia and macrocytosis accompanied by megaloblastic changes and ringed sideroblasts in the erythroid marrow are commonly noted with in association ethanol abuse. However, the severity of the anemia shows no correlation with the thrombocytopenia.[9] Treatment consists of withdrawal of ethanol and administration of a normal diet. Recovery of the platelet count, often with a rebound thrombocytosis, usually occurs within 2 weeks.

Viruses

Mild thrombocytopenia is frequently associated with viral infection. Although the pathophysiologic mechanisms have not been systematically sought, a production deficit is probably important in the etiology of many of the cases. Megakaryocytes are capable of harboring a variety of viruses, and these infected

Table 126-1. Typical Kinetic Profiles in Patients with Thrombocytopenia Due to Production Abnormalities

Category	Megakaryocytes			Platelets			
	Cell No. ($\times 10^6$/kg)	Cytoplasmic Volume (fl)	Cytoplasmic Mass ($\times 10^{11}$ fl/kg)	Concentration (platelets/mm³)	Volume (fl)	Survival (days)	Mass Turnover ($\times 10^5$ fl/mm³/day)
Normal	15 ± 4	12,000 ± 1700	1.8 ± 0.4	250,000 ± 40,000	8.7 ± 0.8	9.6 ± 0.6	3.2 ± 0.5
Decreased megakaryocytopoiesis— damaged marrow	2	14,000	0.3	22,000	9.1	5.2	0.7
Ineffective production							
Autosomal dominant	49	9,400	4.6	64,000	8.9	8.4	1.1
Wiscott-Aldrich syndrome	20	9,000	1.8	40,000	4.0	5.0	0.4
Vitamin B₁₂ deficiency	51	8,900	4.5	62,000	8.5	8.4	0.8
Preleukemia	18	13,300	2.4	16,000	9.0	6.7	0.4

(Adapted from Thompson and Harker,[150] with permission.)

Table 126-2. Infiltrative Marrow Disorders Associated with Thrombocytopenia

Metastatic cancer	Myeloma	Osteopetrosis
Leukemia	Myelofibrosis	Histiocytosis
Lymphoma	Gaucher disease	Infectious processes

INVESTIGATION OF DECREASED PLATELET PRODUCTION

Suspicion of thrombocytopenia due to decreased production should be provoked by a history of irradiation or chemotherapy, thrombocytopenia present at birth or in early infancy in the presence of a normal maternal platelet count, a family history of thrombocytopenia, concurrent anemia or leukopenia, or both, and alcohol abuse. A careful physical examination may suggest a production disorder if signs of alcohol-related liver disease or a hematologic malignancy are present. Although the thrombocytopenia due to splenomegaly is not related to a production abnormality, splenomegaly is often observed as a feature of portal hypertension, lymphoma, or other processes associated with marrow damage, and it may be a concurrent pathophysiologic mechanism of the thrombocytopenia.

The peripheral blood smear is critical to rule out pseudothrombocytopenia (see Ch. 125). Moreover, the blood smear provides additional clues to both the pathophysiologic mechanism of the thrombocytopenia and the diagnosis. For example, giant platelets suggest a hereditary or myelodysplastic syndrome; oval macrocytosis and hypersegmented neutrophils suggest folate or vitamin B_{12} deficiency; and a leukoerythroblastic smear points to an infiltrative process.

A marrow examination is required to evaluate the megakaryocytes. A biopsy is more reliable than an aspirate to determine whether megakaryocytes are decreased. However, an aspirate showing abundant megakaryocytes in the presence of thrombocytopenia is sufficient to suggest platelet destruction or ineffective production. Unfortunately, no clear guidelines are available to determine precisely what defines a decreased or increased number of megakaryocytes. Megakaryocyte morphology is occasionally valuable. The normal compensatory response to thrombocytopenia is enlargement of the cells with increased ploidy. Small, micro-, or hypolobulated megakaryocytes may be seen in myelodysplastic syndromes. Dysmorphic megakaryocytes may be also observed in viral infections, including human immunodeficiency virus. In the future, flow cytometry may provide a more precise analysis of megakaryocytes.

Establishment of the pathologic process of ineffective production is one of exclusion. The marrow examination reveals quantitatively normal megakaryocytes, and the apparent absence of peripheral platelet destruction together with the appropriate clinical circumstances (e.g., folate or vitamin B_{12} deficiency) often points to this mechanism. The bleeding time, although not a useful measurement to predict the propensity for bleeding, may be helpful in distinguishing ineffective production from platelet destruction. In destructive processes such as immune thrombocytopenia, the bleeding time may be shorter than predicted on the basis of the platelet count alone, while in ineffective platelet production, the bleeding time is more often related to the platelet count. In complex cases, platelet survival studies may be necessary to show that consumption or splenic pooling are not significant contributors to the thrombocytopenia; however, survival studies are rarely required for clinical purposes.

cells may exhibit dysmorphic features. Thrombocytopenia has been reported in mumps, rubella, measles, varicella, cytomegalovirus, infectious mononucleosis, chickenpox, dengue and other hemorrhagic fevers, hepatitis, and parvovirus infections.[17-27] Live measles virus vaccination can also induce thrombocytopenia due to decreased production.[28]

Human Immunodeficiency Virus

The thrombocytopenia associated with human immunodeficiency virus (HIV) may be due both to immune mechanisms and to a decrease in platelet production (see Ch. 155). Platelet kinetic studies have shown that patients infected with HIV have a moderate reduction in platelet survival, but all have decreased platelet production irrespective of the degree of thrombocytopenia.[29] HIV has been shown to infect megakaryocytes directly, perhaps via megakaryocyte surface CD4,[30] and HIV mRNA has been detected in megakaryocyte cytoplasm.[31,32] Morphologic abnormalities of megakaryocytes[33] together with growth anomalies of progenitor cells in culture have also been observed in patients with HIV,[34,35] supporting a direct effect of the virus on megakaryocytopoiesis. Isolated amegakaryocytic thrombocytopenia has been observed in a child with HIV.[36] Treatment with zidovudine has been shown to increase platelet production in patients with HIV.[37-39]

Drug-Related Disorders

A variety of drugs and toxins have been implicated in the etiology of aplastic anemia (see Chs. 21 and 22); several have been implicated in isolated thrombocytopenia believed to be due to a production deficit. Estrogen was reported to decrease platelet counts, but detailed thrombokinetic studies have not been carried out, and little work has subsequently been done in this area.[40] Thrombocytopenia due to thiazide diuretics has been reported frequently.[41] Although the etiology in most cases is probably destructive, decreased megakaryocytes have been noted.[42] Chemotherapy may result in prolonged thrombocytopenia that may be isolated.[43] Interferons and IL-2 may induce thrombocytopenia, perhaps the result of inhibited megakaryocytic colony formation.[44,45] IL-2 may induce thrombocytopenia in leukemic patients by enhancing the development of tumor necrosis factor-producing lymphokine-activated killer cells.[45] Anti-tumor necrosis factor antibodies reverse the lymphokine-activated killer cell-dependent inhibition of growth of megakaryocytic progenitors in culture; by contrast, IL-2 itself does not inhibit colony formation. Anagrelide, an agent used to lower the platelet count in patients with malignant thrombocytosis, appears to operate by reducing megakaryocyte size and ploidy, and by disrupting maturation.[46]

Folate and Vitamin B_{12} Deficiency

Varying degrees of thrombocytopenia may be observed with either folate or vitamin B_{12} deficiency; in some cases it may be severe.[47,48] The pathophysiologic mechanism is ineffective production,[1] since megakaryocyte numbers are normal or increased in the marrow, and platelet survival is normal or slightly shortened.[49] Amegakaryocytic thrombocytopenia has been reported in vitamin B_{12} deficiency.[50] Folate deficiency is frequently associated with ethanol abuse; the etiology of the thrombocytopenia may be more complex in these patients.

The blood may show macrocytosis and hypersegmented neutrophils in addition to the thrombocytopenia. Platelets are morphologically normal, but the count is variably decreased. Extremely severe thrombocytopenia may be observed. Often (but not necessarily), the marrow shows megaloblastic changes in the erythroid and myeloid lineages, as well as normal numbers of megakaryocytes, some of which may appear large. Although multiple disconnected nuclear lobulations have been described,[51] distinctive morphologic abnormalities of the megakaryocytes are not often apparent. Rapid recovery of the platelet count can be achieved with administration of the appropriate vitamin or by abstention from ethanol intake.

Iron Deficiency

Although most patients with iron deficiency develop thrombocytosis for unclear reasons, rare cases will show the development of thrombocytopenia,[52] which in even fewer instances is accompanied by decreased megakaryocytes.[53] Recovery of the platelet count has been observed with iron replacement,[53-55] while induction of thrombocytopenia during iron therapy has been reported.[56] Hypotheses have been presented concerning the role of iron in platelet production,[57] but little investigation has been performed in this area.

Acquired Aplastic Anemia

Aplastic anemia involves multiple hematopoietic lineages, although isolated thrombocytopenia can be the presenting feature.[25] Many of the same pathogenetic mechanisms seem to be operative in aplastic anemia and isolated amegakaryocytic thrombocytopenia (see below). (Aplastic anemia is discussed in Ch. 22.)

Paroxysmal Nocturnal Hemoglobinuria

Approximately 25% of patients with paroxysmal nocturnal hemoglobinuria (PNH) have significant marrow aplasia.[58] Megakaryocyte progenitors show increased sensitivity to complement and fail to produce colonies following complement exposure.[59] Since platelet survival is usually normal in PNH,[60] the mechanism of the thrombocytopenia is decreased or ineffective production. (PNH is discussed in Ch. 25.)

Acquired Pure Amegakaryocytic Thrombocytopenic Purpura

Acquired pure amegakaryocytic thrombocytopenic purpura is a rare disorder that may be analogous to other isolated unicellular marrow aplasias. The pathognomonic finding is a normal bone marrow biopsy with markedly decreased or absent megakaryocytes. Platelet survival is normal in these patients, and the platelet counts reflect the degree of megakaryocytic hypoplasia. Amegakaryocytic thrombocytopenia may be a harbinger of aplastic anemia. The pathogenetic mechanisms underlying this disorder are diverse and may be related to drugs or toxins, viruses, cytokine anomalies, and humoral or cell-mediated megakaryocyte suppression.[61-63]

Patients present with bleeding manifestations due to severe thrombocytopenia. Macrocytosis is seen in almost all patients, presumably due to reticolocytosis, but other abnormalities of the peripheral blood are not typically seen. The marrow shows normal cellularity, except for the absence of megakaryocytes.

A decrease in megakaryocytic colony growth may be noted; it is corrected by removal of an inhibitory cell population or antibody.[64]

Since the causes of this disorder are multiple, the natural history and therapeutic approach depend on the specific etiology. Determination of the pathophysiologic mechanisms with megakaryocyte progenitor cell assays may be useful in guiding treatment, as humoral or cell-mediated abnormalities may be discerned with these methods.[3,64] In the absence of these uncommonly available laboratory studies, management is approached on an empirical basis.

If the etiology is viral, intravenous IgG, or anti-HIV therapies are indicated.[61] In the rare patient with isolated amegakaryocytic thrombocytopenia due to ethanol or drugs, avoidance of the offending agent is indicated. Cytotoxic antibodies directed toward the CFU-Mk may be approached with corticosteroids, plasmapheresis, intravenous IgG, danazol, cyclosporine, or cyclophosphamide.[61] In a patient in whom an IgG antibody was found to be blocking CSF-GM action, a complete response to cyclophosphamide was observed.[3] Patients with T-cell-mediated inhibition of megakaryocytopoiesis may respond to antithymocyte globulin, cyclosporine, or hematopoietic growth factors.[61]

Refractory Thrombocytopenia Due to Myelodysplasia

A small proportion of patients (as low as 0.6%) with the myelodysplastic syndrome present with isolated thrombocytopenia—designated refractory thrombocytopenia.[65] Clonal chromosomal abnormalities are required to confirm the diagnosis, with chromosomes 3, 5, 8, or 20 most commonly involved. The usual laboratory findings include macrocytosis of platelets and red cells. Abnormal megakaryocyte morphology, typically mononuclear megakaryocytes, are often observed.[65] Dysmorphic erythroblasts or myeloid cells may also be noted. The clinical course of these patients is the progressive development of additional cytopenias and the myelodysplastic syndrome, with a significant number evolving into acute myeloid leukemia.[65] Therapy has not been shown to be beneficial. Since some of these cases have been misdiagnosed and treated for idiopathic thrombocytopenic purpura (ITP), recognition of this uncommon syndrome is important.

Cyclic Thrombocytopenia

Cyclic oscillations in the platelet count have been observed occasionally. Predominantly occuring in women, these fluctuations can result in thrombocytopenia sufficiently severe to result in bleeding.[66] Most frequently, the cycling occurs in association with the menstrual cycle. It is likely that a production abnormality is not the pathophysiologic mechanism for the thrombocytopenia in this disorder.[67] However, in two males, decreased megakaryocytes were observed, suggesting that decreased production does occur, albeit rarely.[68,69]

CONGENITAL OR HEREDITARY PRODUCTION DISORDERS

Thrombocytopenia due to decreased platelet production in the newborn is uncommon, accounting for <5% of neonatal thrombocytopenia.[70] Most of the thrombocytopenic disorders that are referred to as congenital have a genetic basis, although some may be acquired in the perinatal period (e.g., congenital rubella.[71]

Congenital Aplastic Anemia Syndromes

Congenital aplastic anemia, Fanconi's anemia, and other syndromes associated with failure of several hematopoietic lineages are discussed in Chapters 21–26. These syndromes occasionally present with thrombocytopenia,[72] but it soon becomes apparent that other lineages are involved.

Congenital Amegakaryocytic Thrombocytopenia

Congenital amegakaryocytic thrombocytopenia is a rare disorder of infancy and early childhood of unknown etiology. The inheritance pattern is mixed, with some of the cases being X-linked; others are autosomal recessive.[72] About 40% of affected patients have somatic anomalies fitting no other congenital syndrome.[72] Patients present with isolated severe thrombocytopenia with normal marrow cellularity, but scant or no megakaryocytes. Platelet survival is normal. Anemia and macrocytosis are commonly observed; occasionally hemoglobin F is elevated.[73] In four of five cases so analyzed, CFU-Mk-derived colonies were very low in number, but increased in the presence of IL-3 or CSF-GM, or both although not to normal levels.[74] The natural history of the disorder is not well defined but most patients with isolated thrombocytopenia either die of bleeding complications, progress to aplastic anemia, or develop leukemia.[72] Projected survival is poor—6 years for those who do not have associated physical anomalies and 2 years for those who do.[72]

Treatment with corticosteroids with or without androgens have been useful in some cases, but most patients relapse.[72] Splenectomy is ineffective. Marrow transplantation is appropriate if a donor is available. IL-3, but not CSF-GM, was shown to augment the platelet count and to decrease bleeding complications in five patients to whom the cytokine was administered.[74]

Thrombocytopenia with Absent Radius Syndrome

Thrombocytopenia with absent radius syndrome (TAR) is an autosomal recessive disorder manifest by hypomegakaryocytic thrombocytopenia and absent radii. The general lack of consanguinity for this uncommon syndrome suggests that the gene may be more prevalent than previously suspected or that other modes of inheritance occur.[75–77] Chromosomal abnormalities are absent. Bone marrow culture studies of a patient with TAR showed absence of megakaryocyte colony formation accompanied by high levels of megakaryocyte colony-stimulating activity.[78] This activity declined as the patient's platelet count increased, accompanied by an increase in megakaryocytic colonies. No significant abnormalities of colony formation or colony-stimulating activity were observed in the patient's parents.[78]

Absence of the radii with thumbs present is pathognomonic (Fig. 126-2), and the diagnosis should not be considered unless present.[76] The muscles that normally attach to the radius are inserted into the carpal bones. Short stature accompanied by other skeletal malformations, including absence or malformation of the ulnar bones, and abnormalities of the humerus, shoulder joint, and lower extremities, are frequent.[72] Tetralogy of Fallot and atrial septal defects occur in one-third of patients.[79] Symptomatic milk allergy has been observed frequently and may cause severe bloody diarrhea.[76,80]

Thrombocytopenia is noted at birth, at which time it is most severe, ranging from 15 to 30,000/mm^3. Infection, surgery, gastrointestinal disturbances, and other types of stress are related to even lower counts, and these are often accompanied by a myeloid leukemoid reaction, noted in two-thirds of patients. Eosinophilia, seen in one-half of the patients, is common in those with milk allergy.[76] Many patients have anemia related to bleeding and hemolysis, the latter observed in the first year of life. The bone marrow shows decreased or absent megakaryocytes, sometimes accompanied by erythroid hyperplasia. Megakaryocytes are often small, basophilic, and vacuolated.[76]

The diagnosis is suspected by the typical somatic abnormalities. TAR is distinguished from Fanconi syndrome by the presence of the thumbs and by the lack of chromosomal abnormalities. The platelet count and clinical course of these patients tend to improve with age. If patients survive the initial 1–2 years of life, survival appears to be normal.[76] Thrombocytopenia is best managed by platelet transfusions; orthopaedic surgery should be postponed during the first few years of life. Steroids, splenectomy, and intravenous IgG treatments are usually ineffective.[79,81] Rarely, thrombocytopenia will develop when the patient is an adult; in such cases, splenectomy may be effective.[82,83] Marrow transplantation is an option for the

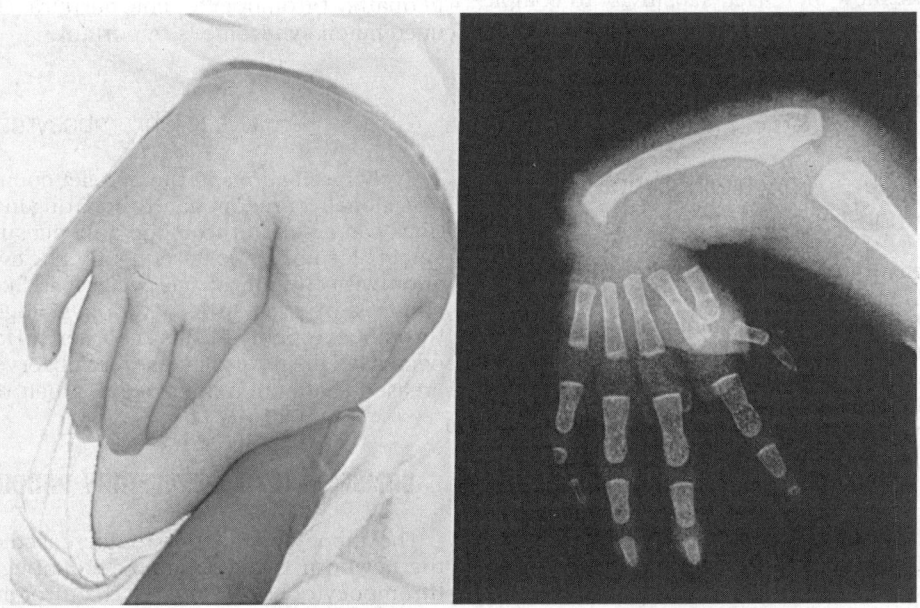

Fig. 126-2. Thrombocytopenia with absent radius syndrome. **(Left)** A typical upper extremity deformity. **(Right)** Radiograph showing complete absence of the radius. (Adapted from Hoffbrand and Pettit,[151] with permission.)

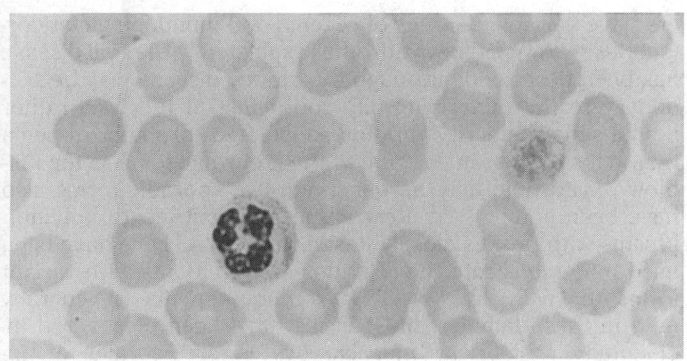

Fig. 126-3. Peripheral blood in the May-Hegglin anomaly. Note the giant platelet and the typical basophilic inclusion in the neutrophil. (Adapted from Hoffbrand and Pettit,[151] with permission.)

rare patients who continue to remain severely thrombocytopenic with bleeding symptoms throughout childhood.[84]

Other Autosomal Recessive Thrombocytopenias

Bernard-Soulier syndrome and gray platelet syndrome are associated with moderate thrombocytopenia. It is not clear whether a production deficit is involved in the etiology of the thrombocytopenia, since platelet survival studies may be shortened or normal in patients with Bernard-Soulier syndrome,[85,86] while megakaryocyte numbers have been reported to be increased or decreased.[85,87] Platelet functional defects are likely more important in the pathogenesis of bleeding in these disorders (see Ch. 129).

Autosomal Dominant Thrombocytopenias

May-Hegglin Anomaly

May-Hegglin anomaly is an autosomal dominant disorder characterized by giant platelets, moderate thrombocytopenia $(40,000–80,000/mm^3)$, and leukocyte inclusion bodies[88] (Fig. 126-3). Patients may have easy bruising or menorrhagia, but 40% are asymptomatic. No deaths due to bleeding have been reported.[89] A variety of overlap syndromes manifest characteristics of Alport syndrome[90,91] (see below).

The pathognomonic feature is the Döhle-body-like inclusion bodies found in neutrophils and eosinophils and occasionally in monocytes. These bright blue spindle-shaped inclusions are composed of parallel 7–10-nm filaments.[89] The platelets are large but exhibit no intrinsic structural abnormalities and have normal surface membrane proteins.[92] Platelet volume may exceed that of red cells, with one-third 30–80 fl.[92] The mechanism by which the giant platelets are formed in the May-Hegglin anomaly and in other macrothrombocytopenias is unknown. Bleeding times are variable.[89,93] Since marrow megakaryocytes appear normal and platelet survival has been shown to be normal or modestly decreased in most cases,[86,93,94] ineffective production is the likely etiology of the thrombocytopenia.

Owing to the modest thrombocytopenia, treatment is not generally required. Platelet transfusions have frequently been given for thrombocytopenia, but their requirement is not clear.[89,94–96] Two patients with symptomatic thrombocytopenia underwent splenectomy without significant response.[97] The leukocyte inclusions do not increase the risk of infection in these patients.[89]

Alport Syndrome Variants

The syndrome of hereditary interstitial nephritis, cataracts, and high-frequency sensorineural deafness, designated Alport syndrome,[98] has been associated with thrombocytopenia and

giant platelets in a number of families, referred to as Epstein syndrome.[99] This syndrome has been seen in association with leukocyte inclusions resembling those in the May-Hegglin anomaly in a pedigree, designated Fechtner syndrome.[100] The Sebastian platelet syndrome is a variant of Fechtner syndrome without the other defects seen in the Alport syndrome.[101] The genetic defects in Alport syndrome are deletions or rearrangements in the α5(IV) collagen gene located on Xq22[102,103] and may be involved in the abnormalities in some Alport variants. However, whether the platelet abnormality is related to this gene defect is unknown.

In these autosomal dominant disorders, platelet counts are variable, although thrombocytopenia to levels of $20,000/mm^3$ may be seen. The mean platelet volume ranges between 20 and 27 fl.[99,100,104] Platelet ultrastructure is normal, as is the bleeding time.[99,104–106] Platelet aggregation has been claimed to be normal in some reports and abnormal in another.[99,100,105] Marrow megakaryocytes are normal, but one report suggests that this may not always be the case.[99,104–107]

Cases are most often diagnosed in adult patients. Many were frequently misdiagnosed as having ITP, and failed to respond to treatment with corticosteroids or splenectomy.[99,104–107] Bleeding tends to be mild or moderate and is manifested as bleeding after dental extraction, easy bruising, postoperative bleeding and hematoma formation, and postpartum hemorrhage.[108] Fatalities have been observed in patients with Sebastian syndrome.[101] Nevertheless, renal failure, rather than thrombocytopenia, is the usual etiology of the morbidity and mortality in Alport syndrome variants.

Other Autosomal Dominant Thrombocytopenias

Thrombocytopenia without other congenital abnormalities has been reported in a number of kindreds with an autosomal dominant inheritance pattern.[109,110] Most of these patients have modest thrombocytopenia with few clinical symptoms, normal platelet morphology, and normal megakaryocytes, but there are exceptions.[1,109,111–114] Some families exhibit macrothrombocytopenia.[114,115] Platelet function is variable.[109,110,112,113,115] Platelet survival has been reported to be normal in most families, suggesting ineffective production.[1,109] However, in one kindred, platelet survival was short; this was demonstrated to be an intrinsic platelet abnormality.[112] In one pedigree with macrothrombocytopenia, an abnormality of glycoprotein IV (CD36) was identified.[116] Mediterranean macrothrombocytopenia has been defined as a syndrome of asymptomatic thrombocytopenia and large platelets in people of Mediterranean descent.[117,118] Their inheritance pattern is not well defined, and little published information is available.[117,118]

Patients with autosomal dominant thrombocytopenia may be relatively more common than previously believed. Most cases are not diagnosed until adulthood; these patients are generally asymptomatic, although exceptions have been reported.[110] Many may be misdiagnosed as having ITP and treated for that disorder.[111,113] Family studies of 54 patients referred with the diagnosis of refractory ITP showed that these patients had autosomal dominant thrombocytopenia with large platelets, normal megakaryocytes, and normal platelet survival.[119] Treatment is usually not indicated. Corticosteroids are ineffective, although splenectomy occasionally results in a modest response.[112] Conceivably, the poor responses to standard therapy in some patients with presumed ITP may reflect the possibility that some of those patients have misdiagnosed hereditary thrombocytopenia.

Wiskott-Aldrich Syndrome

The syndrome of immunodeficiency, microthrombocytopenia, and eczema defines the Wiskott-Aldrich syndrome (WAS), a rare X-linked disorder.[120] One-third of cases have no family history. Although heterozygotes have no abnormalities, a girl was reported with isolated thrombocytopenia believed to be due to random X-chromosomal inactivation of the megakaryocytic lineage.[121] Family studies of a girl with the phenotype of the WAS suggested an autosomal recessive mode of inheritance.[122] The gene involved in the pathogenesis of the syndrome has been identified to be on the short arm of the X chromosome (X p11.2), but the precise gene involved is unknown.[120] However, the X-chromosomal inactivation pattern can be used for prenatal diagnosis and for detection of the carrier state.[123]

A defect in O-glycosylation has been demonstrated to result in abnormalities of the membrane glycoprotein CD43. This may in part be responsible for the T-cell abnormality in these patients,[124] although patients have a defect in both cellular and humoral immunity. The primary defective molecule in WAS has been proposed to be a cytoplasmic molecule with a role in cytoskeletal interactions or Ca^{2+} regulation and calpain activation.[125]

Platelet survival time in these patients is about half-normal[126,127]; however, this moderately reduced survival time does not explain the degree of thrombocytopenia. Platelet turnover is about one-fourth normal and is associated with a normal megakaryocyte mass[1,128]; thus, ineffective production appears to be the major pathophysiologic defect. Since splenectomy results in improvement of the platelet count in many patients so treated, other mechanisms (e.g., a superimposed autoimmune process) may contribute to the thrombocytopenia.

Platelets are abnormally small, about one-half normal size,[126,129] but thrombocytopenia is usually moderate. Platelet function is variable[127,130,131]; an abnormality of glycoprotein Ib may be observed in some patients, but not in others.[132,133] Megakaryocytes are normal or increased in number.[1,128] Immunologic abnormalities include low or absent anti-A and anti-B titers, reflecting the low serum IgM concentrations, and increased IgA and IgE and normal IgG.[120] Peripheral B cells are nonresponsive to polysaccharide antigens and show reduced numbers of cells expressing the membrane glycoprotein CD23.[134]

Patients usually present with bleeding within the first few months of life. Bloody diarrhea and epistaxis are the common manifestations, but intracranial hemorrhage may also occur. Within 6 months, eczema and infections ensue. Beyond the complications of infections and bleeding, there is a 2%/yr risk of the development of a malignancy.[135] Acute myeloblastic leukemia and non-Hodgkin lymphomas of the large cell type, often occurring in the brain and gastrointestinal tract, are the malignancies usually observed. Enlarged lymph nodes and hepatosplenomegaly resulting from lymphoid hyperplasia occur commonly and must be distinguished from the development of a lymphoid malignancy. One-half of deaths associated with this syndrome are infectious, one-fourth related to hemorrhage, and 5% to malignancy.[135] Life expectancy is generally <10 years.

Corticosteroids are of no benefit and may be deleterious because of the propensity for recurrent infections. Patients that exhibit significant bleeding have benefitted from splenectomy, which has been shown to augment platelet number, size, and function in some cases[129,136]; nevertheless, thrombocytopenia recurs in a number of patients. Intravenous γ-globulin is useful in preventing infections but generally does not improve the thrombocytopenia. Should a donor be available, allogeneic marrow transplantation is the most appropriate therapy.[137]

Wiskott-Aldrich Syndrome Variants and Other X-Linked Recessive Thrombocytopenias

A number of kindreds with X-linked thrombocytopenia have been described.[123,138–145] Some of these have X-linked microthrombocytopenia and no associated abnormalities, while oth-

ers have variable degrees of eczema and immunologic abnormalities.[145] A WAS-like syndrome associated with renal disease has been described, although the kidney disease may be secondary to the underlying immune defect of the WAS rather than a separate entity.[140] X-linked isolated thrombocytopenia that maps to the same region of the X chromosome as the full-blown syndrome may be observed, but sporadic forms also have been noted.[146–149] Restriction fragment length polymorphisms with probes closely linked to the WAS gene have been used to demonstrate the relationship of patients with variant forms to WAS.[123,146,147] The thrombocytopenia is generally mild in these families; most cases have been discovered incidentally.[146] Marrow megakaryocytes are normal or increased.[138,142,143] In those few patients reported in whom thrombocytopenia was severe and associated with bleeding, responses to splenectomy have been noted.[138,142]

REFERENCES

1. Slichter SL, Harker LA: Thrombocytopenia: mechanisms and management of defects in platelet production. Clin Haematol 7:523, 1978
2. Harker LA, Finch CA: Thrombokinetics in man. J Clin Invest 48:963, 1969
3. Hoffman R, Briddell RA, van Besien K et al: Acquired cyclic amegakaryocytic thrombocytopenia associated with an immunoglobulin blocking the action of granulocyte-macrophage colony-stimulating factor. N Engl J Med 321:97, 1989
4. Mendehall NP, Noyes WD, Million RR: Total body irradiation for stage II–IV non-Hodgkin's lymphoma: ten-year follow-up. J Clin Oncol 7:67, 1989
5. Adams JA, Gordon AA, Jiang YZ et al: Thrombocytopenia after bone marrow transplantation for leukemia: changes in megakaryocyte growth and growth-promoting activity. Br J Haematol 75:195, 1990
6. Smith JW, Longo DL, Alvord WG et al: The effects of treatment with interleukin-1 alpha on platelet recovery after high-dose carboplatin. N Engl J Med 328:756, 1993
7. Chang A, Mittelman A, Boros L et al: Phase I study of interleukin-6 (IL-6) in cancer patients treated with ifosfamide, carboplatin and etoposide (ICE). (abstracted). Blood 80:89a, 1992
8. Jakubowski A, Raptis G, Gilewski T et al: A phase I/II trial of PIXY 321 (PIXY) in patients (pts) with metastatic breast cancer receiving doxorubicin and thiotepa. Blood, suppl. 1. 80:88a, 1992
9. Cowan DH: Effect of alcoholism on hemostasis. Semin Hematol 17:137, 1980
10. Sullivan LW, Adams WH, Liu YK: Induction of thrombocytopenia by thrombopheresis in man: patterns of recovery in normal subjects during ethanol ingestion and abstinence. Blood 49:197, 1977
11. Cowan DH: Thrombokinetic studies in alcohol-related thrombocytopenia. J Lab Clin Med 81:64, 1973
12. Lindenbaum J: Thrombocytopenia in alcoholics. Ann Intern Med 68:526, 1968
13. Gewirtz AM, Hoffman R: Transitory hypomegakaryocytic thrombocytopenia: etiological association with ethanol abuse and complications regarding regulation of human megakaryocytopoiesis. Br J Haematol 62:333, 1986
14. Cowan DH, Graham RC: Studies on the platelet defect in alcoholism. Throm Haemost 33:310, 1975
15. Levine RF, Spivak JL, Meagher RC et al: Effect of ethanol on thrombopoiesis. Br J Haematol 62:345, 1986
16. Nakao S, Harada M, Kondo K et al: Reversible bone marrow hypoplasia induced by alcohol. Am J Hematol 37:120, 1991
17. Ninomiya N, Maeda T, Matsuda I: Thrombocytopenic purpura occurring during the early phase of a mumps infection. Helv Paediatr Acta 32:87, 1977
18. Bayer WL, Sherman FE, Michaels RH et al: Purpura in congenital and acquired rubella. N Engl J Med 273:1362, 1965
19. Hudson JB, Weinstein L, Chang TW: Thrombocytopenic purpura in measles. J Pediatr 48:48, 1956
20. Espinoza C, Kuhn C: Viral infection of megakaryocytes in varicella with purpura. Am J Clin Pathol 61:203, 1974
21. Verdonck LF, van Heugten H, de Gast GC: Delay in platelet recovery after bone marrow transplantation: impact of cytomegalovirus infection. Blood 66:921, 1985
22. Angle RM, Alt HL: Thrombocytopenic purpura complicating infectious mononucleosis. Blood 5:499, 1950
23. Wyler DC, Butterton JR: Case records of the Massachusetts General Hospital: a 40 year old man with headache, fever, rash, and thrombocytopenia after a Caribbean trip. N Engl J Med 321:957, 1989
24. Young N, Mortimer P: Viruses and bone marrow failure. Blood 63:729, 1984
25. Slater LM, Kat ZJ, Walter B et al: Aplastic anemia occurring as amegakaryo-

cyte thrombocytopenia with and without an inhibitor of granulopoiesis. Am J Hematol 18:251, 1985

26. Ueda K, Akeda H, Tokugawa K et al: Human parvovirus infection. N Engl J Med 314:645, 1986

27. Srivastava A, Bruno E, Briddell R et al: Parvovirus B19-induced perturbation of human megakaryocytopoiesis in vitro. Blood 76:1997, 1990

28. Oski FA, Naiman JL: Effects of live measles vaccine on the platelet count. N Engl J Med 275:352, 1966

29. Ballem PJ, Belzberg A, Devine DV et al: Kinetic studies of the mechanism of thrombocytopenia in patients with human immunodeficiency virus infection. N Engl J Med 327:1779, 1992

30. Basch RS, Kouri YH, Karpatkin S: Expression of CD4 by human megakaryocytes. Proc Natl Acad Sci USA 87:8085, 1990

31. Zucker-Franklin D, Cao YZ: Megakaryocytes of human immunodeficiency virus-infected individuals express viral RNA. Proc Natl Acad Sci USA 86:5595, 1989

32. Louache F, Bettaieb A, Henri A et al: Infection of megakaryocytes by human immunodeficiency virus in seropositive patients with immune thrombocytopenic purpura. Blood 78:1697, 1991

33. Zucker-Franklin D, Termin CS, Cooper MC: Structural changes in the megakaryocytes of patients infected with the human immune deficiency virus (HIV-1). Am J Pathol 134:1295, 1989

34. Stella CC, Bergamaschi G, Nalli G et al: "In vitro" megakaryocytopoiesis in patients with HIV-related thrombocytopenic purpura. Haematologica 73:25, 1988

35. Zauli G, Re MC, Davis B et al: Impaired in vitro growth of purified (CD34+) hematopoietic progenitors in human immunodeficiency virus-1 seropositive thrombocytopenic individuals. Blood 79:2680, 1992

36. Weinblatt ME, Scimeca PG, James-Herry AG et al: Thrombocytopenia in an infant with AIDS. Am J Dis Child 141:15, 1987

37. Hymes KB, Greene JB, Karpatkin S: The effect of azidothymidine on HIV related thrombocytopenia. N Engl J Med 318:516, 1988

38. The Swiss Group for Clinical Studies on the Acquired Immunodeficiency Syndrome (AIDS): Zidovudine for the treatment of thrombocytopenia associated with human immunodeficiency virus (HIV): a prospective study. Ann Intern Med 109:718, 1988

39. Pottage JC, Benson CA, Spear JB et al: Treatment of human immunodeficiency virus-related thrombocytopenia with zidovudine. JAMA 260:3045, 1988

40. Cooper BA, Bigelow FS: Thrombocytopenia associated with the administration of diethylstibesterol in man. Ann Intern Med 52:907, 1960

41. Böttiger LE, Westerholm B: Thrombocytopenia II. Drug-induced thrombocytopenia. J Intern Med 191:541, 1972

42. Rodriguez SU, Leikin S, Hiller MC: Neonatal thrombocytopenia associated with antepartum administration of thiazide drugs. N Engl J Med 270:881, 1964

43. Hadjiyanni M, Valianatou K, Tsilianos M et al: Prolonged thrombocytopenia after procarbazine "overdose." Eur J Cancer 28A:1299, 1992

44. Gugliotta L, Bagnara GP, Catani L et al: In vivo and in vitro inhibitory effect of α-interferon on megakaryocyte colony growth in essential thrombocythaemia. Br J Haematol 71:177, 1989

45. Guarini A, Sanavio F, Novarino A et al: Thrombocytopenia in acute leukaemia patients treated with IL2: cytolytic effect of LAK cells on megakaryocytic progenitors. Br J Haematol 79:451, 1991

46. Mazur EM, Rosmarin AG, Sohl PA et al: Analysis of the mechanism of anagrelide-induced thrombocytopenia in humans. Blood 79:1931, 1992

47. Stabler SP, Allen RH, Savage DG et al: Clinical spectrum and diagnosis of cobalamin deficiency. Blood 76:871, 1990

48. Beck WS, Ferry JA: Megaloblastic anemia: case records of the Massachusetts General Hospital. N Engl J Med 325:1791, 1991

49. Kotilainen M: Platelet kinetics in normal subjects in haematological disorders. Scand J Haematol, suppl. 5:1, 1969

50. Ghosh K, Sarode R, Varma N: Amegakaryocytic thrombocytopenia of nutritional vitamin B12 deficiency. Trop Geogr Med 40:158, 1988

51. Kass L: Bone Marrow Interpretation. 2nd Ed. JB Lippincott, Philadelphia, 1985, p. 312

52. Lopas H, Rabiner SF: Thrombocytopenia associated with iron deficiency anemia. 1. The response to oral and pareneral iron. Clin Pediatr 5:609, 1966

53. Berger M, Brass LF: Severe thrombocytopenia in iron deficiency anemia. Am J Hematol 24:425, 1987

54. Scher H, Silber R: Iron responsive thrombocytopenia. Ann Intern Med 84:571, 1976

55. Sonneborn D: Thrombocytopenia and iron deficiency. Ann Intern Med 80:111, 1974

56. Soff GA, Levin J: Thrombocytopenia associated with repletion of iron in iron-deficiency anemia. Am J Med Sci 295:35, 1988

57. Karpatkin S, Garg SK, Freedman ML: Role of iron as a regulator of thrombopoiesis. Am J Med 57:521, 1974

58. Forman K, Sokol RJ, Hewitt S et al: Paroxysmal nocturnal hemoglobinuria. A clinicopathological study of 26 cases. Acta Haematol 71:217, 1984

59. Dessypris EN, Gleaton JH, Clark DA: Increased sensitivity to complement of megakaryocyte progenitors in paroxysmal nocturnal hemoglobinuria. Br J Haematol 69:305, 1988

60. Aster RH, Enright S: A platelet and granulocyte membrane defect in paroxysmal nocturnal hemoglobinuria: usefulness for the detection of platelet antibodies. J Clin Invest 48:1199, 1969

61. Hoffman R: Acquired pure amegakaryocytic thrombocytopenic purpura. Semin Hematol 28:303, 1991

62. Stoll DB, Blum S, Pasquale D et al: Thrombocytopenia with decreased megakaryocytes. Ann Intern Med 94:170, 1981

63. Hoffman R, Bruno E, Elwell J: Acquired amegakaryocytic thrombocytopenic purpura: a syndrome of diverse etiologies. Blood 60:1173, 1982

64. Gewirtz AM, Sacchetti MK, Bien R et al: Cell-mediated suppression of megakaryocytopoiesis in acquired amegakaryocytic thrombocytopenic purpura. Blood 68:619, 1986

65. Menke DM, Colon-Otero G, Cockerill KJ et al: Refractory thrombocytopenia: a myelodysplastic syndrome that may mimic immune thrombocytopenic purpura. Am J Clin Pathol 98:502, 1992

66. Cohen T, Cooney DP: Cyclic thrombocytopenia. Case report and review of literature. Scand J Haematol 12:9, 1974

67. Tomer A, Schreiber AD, McMillan R et al: Menstrual cyclic thrombocytopenia. Br J Haematol 71:519, 1989

68. Bernard J, Caen J: Purpura thrombopénique et megacaryocytopénie cyclique mensuelle. Nouv Rev Fr Hematol 2:378, 1962

69. Engstrom K, Linquist A, Soderstrom N: Period thrombocytopenia or platelet dysgenesis occurring in a man. Scand J Haematol 3:290, 1966.

70. Andrew M: The hemostatic system in the infant. p. 115. In Nathan DG, Oski FA (eds): Hematology of Infancy and Childhood. 4th Ed. WB Saunders, Philadelphia, 1993

71. Berge T, Brunnhage F, Nisson LR: Congenital thrombocytopenia in rubella embryopathy. Acta Paediatr Scand 52:349, 1963

72. Alter BP, Young NS: The bone marrow failure syndromes. p. 216. In Nathan DG, Oski FA (eds): Hematology of Infancy and Childhood. 4th Ed. WB Saunders, Philadelphia, 1993

73. Van Oostrom CG, Wilms RHH: Congenital thrombocytopenia, associated with raised concentrations of haemoglobin F. Helv Paediatr Acta 33:59, 1978

74. Guinan EC, Lee YS, Lopez KD et al: Effects of interleukin-3 and granulocyte-macrophage colony-stimulating factor on thrombopoiesis in congenital amegakaryocytic thrombocytopenia. Blood 81:1691, 1993

75. Edelberg SB, Cohn J, Brandt NJ: Congenital hypomegakaryocytic thrombocytopenia associated with bilateral absence of the radius—the TAR syndrome: intra-family variation of the clinical picture. Hum Hered 27:147, 1977

76. Hall JG: Thrombocytopenia and absent radius (TAR) syndrome. J Med Genet 24:79, 1987

77. Hedberg VA, Lipton JM: Thrombocytopenia with absent radii. A review of 100 cases. Am J Pediatr Hematol Oncol 10:51, 1988

78. Homans AC, Cohen JL, Mazur EM: Defective megakaryocytopoiesis in the syndrome of thrombocytopenia with absent radii. Br J Haematol 70:205, 1988

79. Hall JG, Levin J, Kuhn JP et al: Thrombocytopenia with absent radius (TAR). Medicine 48:411, 1969

80. Whitfield MF, Barr DG: Cow's milk allergy in the syndrome of thrombocytopenia with absent radii. Arch Dis Child 51:337, 1976

81. Sopo SM, Pesaresi MA, Celestini E et al: Intravenous immunoglobulins in thrombocytopenia with absent radii. Acta Haematol 85:105, 1991

82. Armitage JO, Hoak JC, Elliott TE et al: Syndrome of thrombocytopenia and absent radii: qualitatively normal platelets with remission following splenectomy. Scand J Haematol 20:25, 1978

83. Fayen WT, Harris JW: Case report: thrombocytopenia with absent radii (the TAR syndrome). Scand J Haematol 280:95, 1980

84. Brochstein JA, Shank BR, Kernan NA et al: Marrow transplantation for thrombocytopenia-absent radii syndrome. J Pediatr 121:587, 1992

85. Cullum C, Cooney DP, Schrier SL: Familial thrombocytopenic thrombocytopathy. Br J Haematol 13:147, 1967

86. Heyns AP, Badenhorst PN, Wessels P et al: Kinetics, in vivo redistribution and sites of sequestration of indium-111-labelled platelets in giant platelet syndromes. Br J Haematol 60:323, 1985

87. Myllylä G, Pelkonen R, Ikkala E et al: Hereditary thrombocytopenia: report of three families. Scand J Haematol 4:441, 1967

88. Greinacher A, Bux J, Kiefel V et al: May-Hegglin anomaly: a rare cause of thrombocytopenia. Eur J Pediatr 151:668, 1992

89. Lusher JM, Schneider J, Mizukami I et al: The May-Hegglin anomaly: platelet function, ultrastructure, and chromosome studies. Blood 32:950, 1968

90. Brivet F, Girot R, Barbanel C: Hereditary nephritis associated with May-Hegglin anomaly. Nephron 29:59, 1981

91. Nel N, Van Rensburg BWJ, Du Plessis L et al: Coincidental finding of May-Hegglin anomaly in a patient with end-stage renal failure. Am J Hematol 40:216, 1992

92. Coller BS, Zarrabi MH: Platelet membrane studies in the May-Hegglin anomaly. Blood 58:279, 1981

93. Goodwin HA, Ginsburg AD: May-Hegglin anomaly: a defect in megakaryocyte fragmentation? Br J Haematol 26:117, 1974

94. Hamilton RW, Shaikh BS, Ottie JN: Platelet function, ultrastructure, and survival in the May-Hegglin anomaly. Am J Clin Pathol 74:663, 1980

95. Gausis N, Fortune DW, Whiteside MG: The May-Hegglin anomaly: a case report and chromosome studies. Br J Haematol 16:619, 1969

96. Chatwani A, Bruder N, Shapiro T et al: May-Hegglin anomaly: a rare case of maternal thrombocytopenia in pregnancy. Am J Obstet Gynecol 166:143, 1992

97. Oski FA, Naiman JL, Allen DM et al: Leukocyte inclusions—Döhle bodies associated with platelet abnormality (the May-Hegglin anomaly). Report of a family and review of the literature. Blood 20:657, 1962

98. Alport CA: Hereditary familial congenital haemorrhagic nephritis. Br Med J 1:504, 1927

99. Epstein CJ, Sahud MA, Piel CF et al: Hereditary macrothrombocytopathia, nephritis, and deafness. Am J Med 52:299, 1972

100. Peterson LC, Rao KV, Crosson JT, White JG: Fechtner syndrome—a variant of Alport's syndrome with leukocyte inclusions and macrothrombocytopenia. Blood 65:397, 1985

101. Greinacher A, Nieuwenhuis HK, White JG: Sebastian platelet syndrome: a new variant of hereditary macrothrombocytopenia with leukocyte inclusions. Blut 61:282, 1990

102. Boye E, Vetrie D, Flinter F et al: Major rearrangements in the α5(IV) collagen gene in three patients with Alport syndrome. Genomics 11:1125, 1991

103. Tryggvason K: Cloning of the Alport syndrome gene. Ann Med 23:237, 1991

104. Clare NM, Montiel MM, Lifschitz MD et al: Alport's syndrome associated with macrothrombopathic thrombocytopenia. Am J Clin Pathol 71:111, 1979

105. Eckstein JD, Filip DF, Watts JC: Hereditary thrombocytopenia, deafness and renal disease. Ann Intern Med 82:639, 1975

106. Bernheim J, Dechavanne M, Bryon PA: Thrombocytopenia, macrothrombocytopathia, nephritis, and deafness. Am J Med 61:145, 1976

107. Parsa KP, Lee DBN, Zamboni L et al: Hereditary nephritis, deafness and abnormal thrombopoiesis: study of a new kindred. Am J Med 60:665, 1976

108. Greinacher A, Mueller-Eckhardt C: Hereditary types of thrombocytopenia with giant platelets and inclusion bodies in the leukocytes. Blut 60:53, 1990

109. Dowton SB, Beardsley D, Jamison D et al: Studies of a familial platelet disorder. Blood 65:557, 1985

110. Quick AJ, Hussey CV: Hereditary thrombopathic thrombocytopenia. Am J Med Sci 245:643, 1963

111. Bithell TC, Didisheim P, Cartwright GE et al: Thrombocytopenia inherited as a autosomal dominant trait. Blood 25:231, 1965

112. Murphy S, Oski FA, Gardner FH: Hereditary thrombocytopenia with an intrinsic platelet defect. N Engl J Med 281:857, 1969

113. Majado MJ, Gonzalez C, Tamayo M et al: Effective splenectomy in familial isolated thrombocytopenia. Am J Hematol 39:70, 1992

114. Greaves M, Pickering C, Martin J et al: A new familial "giant platelet syndrome" with structural, metabolic and functional abnormalities of platelets due to a primary megakaryocyte defect. Br J Haematol 65:429, 1987

115. Ardlie NG, Coupland WW, Schoefl GL: Hereditary thrombocytopenia: a familial bleeding disorder due to impaired platelet coagulant activity. Aust NZ J Med 6:37, 1976

116. Yufu Y, Ideguchi H, Narishige T: Familial macrothrombocytopenia associated with decreased glycosylation of platelet membrane glycoprotein IV. Am J Hematol 33:271, 1990

117. von Behrens WE: Splenomegaly, macrothrombocytopenia and stomatocytosis in healthy Mediterranean subjects. Scand J Haematol 14:258, 1975

118. Paulus JM, Casals FJ: Platelet formation in Mediterranean macrothrombocytosis. Nouv Rev Fr Hematol 20:151, 1978

119. Najean Y, Lecompte T: Genetic thrombocytopenia with autosomal dominant transmission: a review of 54 cases. Br J Haematol 74:203, 1990

120. Peacocke M, Siminovitch KA: Wiskott-Aldrich syndrome: new molecular and biochemical insights. J Am Acad Dermatol 27:507, 1992

121. Notarangelo LD, Parolini O, Porta F: Analysis of X-chromosome inactivation and presumptive expression of the Wiskott-Aldrich syndrome (WAS) gene in hematopoietic cell lineages of a thrombocytopenic carrier female of WAS. Hum Genet 88:237, 1991

122. Conley ME, Wang WC, Parolini O, et al: Atypical Wiskott-Aldrich syndrome in a girl. Blood 80:1264, 1992

123. De Saint-Basile G, Schlegel N, Caniglia M et al: X-linked thrombocytopenia and Wiskott-Aldrich syndrome: similar regional assignment but distinct X-inactivation pattern in carriers. Ann Hematol 63:107, 1991

124. Remold-O'Donnell E, Kenney DM, Parkman R et al: Characterization of a human lymphocyte surface sialoglycoprotein that is defective in Wiskott-Aldrich syndrome. J Exp Med 159:1705, 1984

125. Remold-O'Donnell E, Van Brocklyn J, Kenney DM: Effect of platelet calpain on normal T-lymphocyte CD43: hypothesis of events in the Wiskott-Aldrich syndrome. Blood 79:1754, 1992

126. Murphy S, Oski FA, Naiman L et al: Platelet size and kinetics in hereditary and acquired thrombocytopenia. N Engl J Med 286:499, 1972

127. Grottum KA, Hovig T, Holmsen H: Wiscott-Aldrich syndrome: qualitative platelet defects and short platelet survival. Br J Haematol 17:373, 1969

128. Ochs HD, Slichter SJ, Harker LA: The Wiskott-Aldrich syndrome: studies of lymphocytes, granulocytes, and platelets. Blood 55:243, 1980

129. Corash L, Shafer B, Blaese RM: Platelet-associated immunoglobulin, platelet size, and the effect of splenectomy in the Wiscott-Aldrich syndrome. Blood 65:1439, 1985

130. Marone G, Albini F, Di Martino L et al: The Wiskott-Aldrich syndrome: studies of platelets, basophils and polymorphonuclear leucocytes. Br J Haematol 62:737, 1986

131. Verhoeven AJM, van Oostrum IEA, van Haarlem H et al: Impaired energy metabolism in platelets from patients with Wiskott-Aldrich syndrome. Thromb Haemost 61:10, 1989

132. Parkman R, Remold-O'Donnell E, Kenney DM: Surface protein abnormalities in the lymphocytes and platelets from patients with the Wiskott-Aldrich syndrome. Lancet 1:1387, 1981

133. Pidard D, Didry D, Le Deist F: Analysis of the membrane glycoproteins of platelets in the Wiskott-Aldrich syndrome. Br J Haematol 69:529, 1988

134. Simon HU, Higgins EA, Demetriou M et al: Defective expression of CD23 and autocrine growth stimulation in Epstein-Barr virus (EBV)-transformed B cells from patients with Wiskott-Aldrich syndrome (WAS). Clin Exp Immunol 91:43, 1991

135. Perry GS, Spector BD, Schuman LM: The Wiskott-Aldrich syndrome in the United States and Canada (1892–1979). J Pediatr 97:72, 1980

136. Lum LG, Tubergen DG, Corash L et al: Splenectomy in the management of the thrombocytopenia of the Wiskott-Aldrich syndrome. N Engl J Med 302:892, 1980

137. Parkman R, Rappeport S, Geha R: Complete correction of the Wiskott-Aldrich syndrome by allogeneic bone-marrow transplantation. N Engl J Med 298:921, 1978

138. Ata M, Fisher OD, Holman CA: Inherited thrombocytopenia. Lancet 1:119, 1965

139. Canales ML, Mauer AM: Sex-linked hereditary thrombocytopenia as a variant of the Wiscott-Aldrich syndrome. N Engl J Med 277:899, 1967

140. Gutenberger J, Trygstad CW, Stiehn ER: Familial thrombocytopenia, elevated serum IgA levels, and renal disease. Am J Med 49:729, 1970

141. Moore GR: X-linked thrombocytopenia. Clin Genet 5:344, 1974

142. Cohn J, Hauge M, Andersen V et al: Sex-linked hereditary thrombocytopenia with immunological defects. Hum Hered 25:309, 1975

143. Thompson AR, Wood WG, Stamatoyannopoulos G: X-linked syndrome of platelet dysfunction, thrombocytopenia, and imbalanced globin-chain synthesis with hemolysis. Blood 50:303, 1977

144. Chiaro JJ, Dharmkrong-at A, Bloom GE: X-linked thrombocytopenic purpura. Am J Dis Child 123:565, 1972

145. Stomorken H, Hellum B, Egeland T et al: X-linked thrombocytopenia and thrombocytopathia: attenuated Wiskott-Aldrich syndrome. Functional and morphological studies of platelets and lymphocytes. Thromb Haemost 65:300, 1991

146. Donner M, Schwartz M, Carlsson KU et al: Hereditary X-linked thrombocytopenia maps to the same chromosomal region as the Wiskott-Aldrich syndrome. Blood 72:1849, 1988

147. O'Marcaigh AS, Smithson WA, Sachs MI et al: Linkage analysis using M27B, p8 and L1.28 probes in hereditary X-linked thrombocytopenia, abstracted. Blood 80:501a, 1992

148. Notarangelo LD, Parolini O, Faustini R et al: Presentation of Wiskott Aldrich Syndrome as isolated thrombocytopenia. Blood 77:1125, 1991

149. Puck JM, Sminovitch KA, Ponca M et al: Atypical presentation of Wiskott-Aldrich syndrome: diagnosis in two unrelated males based on studies of maternal T cell X chromosome inactivation. Blood 75:2369, 1990

150. Thompson AR, Harker LA: Quantitative platelet disorders. p. 65. In: Manual of Hemostasis and Thrombosis. 3rd Ed. FA Davis, Philadelphia, 1983

151. Hoffbrand AV, Pettit JE: Sandoz Atlas of Clinical Hematology. Gower Medical, London, 1988

Thrombotic Thrombocytopenic Purpura and the Hemolytic Uremic Syndrome

127

Joel L. Moake

INTRODUCTION

The dramatic intravascular platelet clumping disorders thrombotic thrombocytopenic purpura (TTP) and hemolytic uremic syndrome (HUS) were initially reported by Moschcowitz[1] in 1924 and by Gasser et al[2] in 1955. The clinical, pathophysiologic, and therapeutic relationship between these two thrombotic microangiopathies has now been debated for almost 40 years.

In both TTP and HUS, platelets aggregate and occlude arterioles and capillaries of the microcirculation. In TTP, aggregates of platelets reversibly obstruct the arterioles and capillaries of various organs and produce fluctuating ischemia (and sometimes infarction). The microcirculation of the brain is involved in 50–71% of TTP episodes.[3,4] In the closely related HUS, platelet-fibrin thrombi obstruct predominantly (but not exclusively) the vasculature of the kidneys, with associated acute renal failure.[5–9] In both syndromes, the degree of thrombocytopenia reflects the extent of intravascular platelet clumping. Platelet counts are often <10,000/mm^3 during acute episodes of TTP. Erythrocyte fragmentation occurs in both disorders, and schistocytes on peripheral blood films are characteristic (Fig. 127-1). The hemolysis is predominantly intravascular and, along with tissue damage, results in increased serum levels of lactate dehydrogenase. Thrombocytopenia, microangiopathic hemolytic anemia, and LDH elevations are present but are usually less profound in HUS than during episodes of TTP.

The variability of organ dysfunction in TTP (including renal abnormalities in 50–75% of episodes[3,4]) and the occasional extrarenal manifestations in HUS can make the two syndromes difficult to distinguish.[4–9] Rigid compartmentalization is further confounded by observations that (1) either TTP or HUS can occur in different members of the same family[6]; (2) TTP, as well as HUS, can follow hemorrhagic colitis produced by cytotoxin-producing *Escherichia coli* of serotype 0157:H7[10,11]; and (3) both TTP and HUS are associated, on rare occasions, with other conditions (e.g., pregnancy, cancer chemotherapy, or human immunodeficiency virus infection). Many hematologists consider the two disorders to represent various etiologic routes to a common (or at least related) mechanism of intravascular platelet aggregation differing mainly in extent.

EPIDEMIOLOGY

TTP occurs in about 1 in 500,000 population per year. The incidence (or awareness) is, apparently, increasing. Women are affected about twice as often as men. Peak incidence is in the fourth decade, and 90% of patients are <60 years of age. TTP occurs uncommonly in the elderly and in infants. No racial or seasonal predisposition is known. With the exception of occasional reports, as of a husband and wife, case clustering is rare (in contrast to HUS).[12] TTP sometimes presents during the third trimester of pregnancy, and either TTP or HUS can develop in the puerperal period.

Although first described and most often encountered in children, HUS also occurs in adults.[2,5–7,13] There are several strong associations that represent etiologic or pathogenetic clues. The predominant type of childhood HUS is usually preceded by gastroenteritis caused by cytotoxin (Shiga toxin or verotoxin)-producing strains of *Shigella* or *E. coli* (e.g., 0157:H7).[8,9,14] HUS or, less frequently, TTP also develops following therapy with mitomycin C,[15] cyclosporine,[16] or multiple chemotherapeutic agents,[17] which may injure or alter renal (or other) endothelial cells.

PATHOBIOLOGY

Thrombotic Thrombocytopenic Purpura

TTP was first recognized by Moschcowitz in 1924[1] in a 16-year-old girl who had abrupt onset of fever, anemia, renal dysfunction, central nervous system impairment, and cardiac failure, and who died in 2 weeks. At necropsy, hyaline thrombi were found in terminal arterioles and capillaries. It was subsequently determined that thrombocytopenia with adequate numbers of megakaryocytes in the bone marrow was characteristic of the disorder, and that the microvascular thrombi that Moschcowitz described as "hyaline" were composed of aggregated platelets with some fibrin polymers.[18] The characteristic systemic microvascular thrombotic occlusions are seen in virtually all organs, including the lungs and eyes. The brain, heart, spleen, kidneys, pancreas, and adrenals are most frequently involved.

Early vascular lesions in the brain consist almost exclusively of intraluminal platelet thrombi, without perivascular inflammation.[19] The pathologic and clinical findings in TTP suggest that the process results form direct, potentially reversible, platelet aggregation in the microcirculation of multiple organs concurrently. Immunochemical studies of TTP thrombi have revealed an abundance of von Willebrand factor (vWF), with little fibrinogen/fibrin.[20] (The opposite findings are characteristic of thrombotic lesions in disseminated intravascular coagulation.[20]) As discussed later in this chapter, the vWF multimers within these thrombi may function as multimeric bridges promoting platelet-platelet cohesion (aggregation).

Severe thrombocytopenia, intravascular hemolysis with many fragmented erythrocytes (schistocytes) on blood films ("microangiopathic" hemolytic anemia), and neurologic symp-

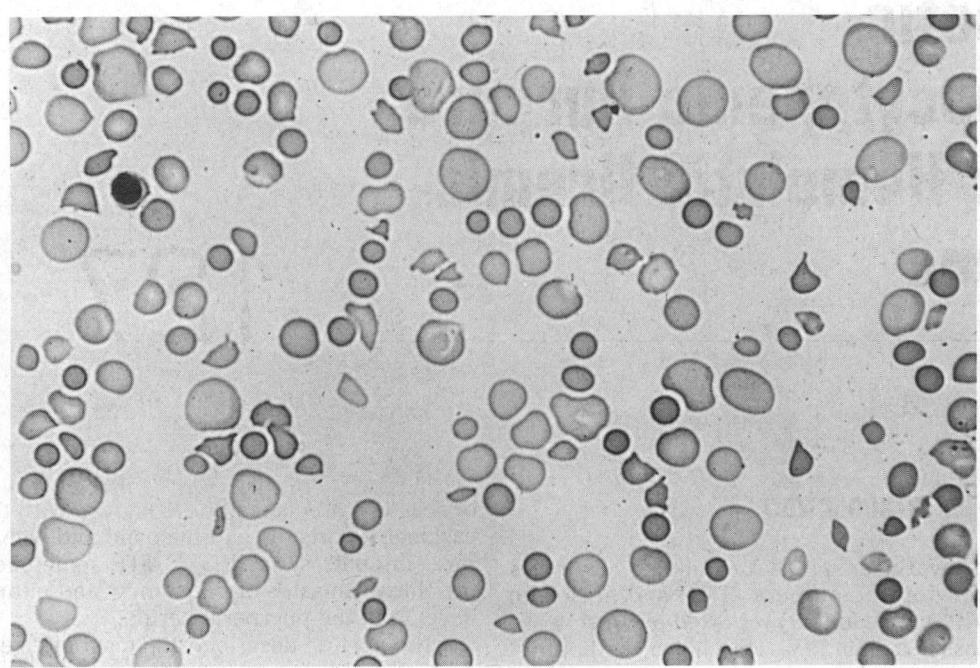

Fig. 127-1. Peripheral blood smear from a patient with TTP.

toms and signs constitute the characteristic TTP clinical triad. The latter may range from transitory bizarre mentation and behavior with sensorimotor deficits or aphasia to seizures and coma. The peripheral blood smear typically also shows reticulocytosis (polychromatophilic erythrocytes) and nucleated red blood cells, both a reflection of the intense hemolytic process. Some patients have fever and renal dysfunction, including proteinurea, hematuria, and azotemia. Symptoms and signs of ischemia in the retinae (visual defects), coronary microvasculature (conduction abnormalities), and mesenteric circulation (abdominal pain) may be present.

Both TTP and HUS are clinical diagnoses. Tissue obtained from the biopsy of bone marrow, gingiva, or kidney may show platelet thrombi; however, it may be obtained at a moment when no arterial thrombi are in the microvessels of the area sampled. Biopsies are not considered necessary (or even, in some cases, safe).

Since the general application of plasma manipulation therapy during the late 1970s, many patients have survived episodes of TTP. Before that time, almost all patients with TTP died of their illness within days to weeks. It has now become apparent that several types of the disorder exist.[13] Single-episode TTP never recurs if the patient recovers. In 10–30% of patients who survive the initial TTP episode, subsequent relapses occur at either occasional or infrequent intervals (intermittent TTP). In the rarest type, chronic relapsing TTP, frequent episodes occur at regular (approximately monthly) intervals. Chronic relapsing TTP usually begins in infancy or childhood.

Hemolytic Uremic Syndrome

HUS was described by Gasser et al.[2] in 1955 as a triad of thrombocytopenia, acute renal failure, and intravascular hemolysis with schistocytosis. Severe renal dysfunction is a prominent feature of HUS. By contrast, abnormal kidney function is generally not as extreme in TTP. Proteinuria and hematuria are present in all patients, and the acute renal failure often requires dialysis. Chronic renal failure is a consequence of HUS in some patients, whereas this is uncommon in individuals who recover from episodes of TTP. The mortality in HUS is much less than in TTP. HUS is, however, a relatively common cause of chronic renal failure in childhood.

The lesions in HUS indicate that renal endothelial cell injury is likely to be the primary etiologic event. Endothelial cells are swollen, and subendothelial spaces are widened. Swelling of the mesangial matrix (i.e., the area between the glomerular capillaries) and hypertrophy of mesangial cells also occurs.[21] These alterations cause narrowing of glomerular capillary lumina. Intraluminal platelet thrombi, accompanied by some fibrin polymers, occlude the narrowed glomerular capillaries and afferent arterioles in diarrhea-associated HUS.[21] (In HUS that is not associated with diarrhea, thrombosis is more impressive in renal arterioles and small arteries.[21])

The histopathologic abnormalities, along with the inevitable thrombocytopenia, suggest the possibility that renal endothelial cell perturbation in HUS is associated predominantly with direct platelet aggregation in the renal microvasculature. That is, aggregation may occur even in the absence of overt endothelial cell desquamation, subendothelial exposure, and platelet-subendothelial adhesion. The thrombocytopenia, along with the absence of consistent clotting abnormalities, suggests that intravascular platelet aggregation is a critical pathophysiologic event, and that activation of coagulation and fibrin generation is secondary and limited in extent.

As endothelial cell swelling and intravascular platelet aggregation leads to the complete obstruction of renal microvessels, the danger increases that irreversible glomerular and tubular necrosis will occur in the involved nephrons. The extent of this glomerular involvement in biopsy specimens (obtained when the disorder has stabilized and platelets have increased to levels >100,000/mm^3) correlates directly with the likelihood of subsequent hypertension or end-stage renal failure. In some cases of HUS, other organs in addition to the kidney (especially the brain, heart, colon, or pancreas) may be affected by microvascular thrombosis and local infarction.[21]

HUS almost always occurs as a single, nonrecurrent episode, although relapses of the disease have been reported in occasional patients.[6]

ETIOLOGY AND PATHOGENESIS

Thrombotic Thrombocytopenic Purpura

TTP is believed to be a consequence of the intrusion into the circulation of one or more platelet-aggregating agents. The aggregating substance has variously been reported to be (1) proteins of 37,000[22] or 59,000 daltons[23]; (2) a calcium-activated protease (calpain) that has cysteine as part of its active enzyme site and the capacity to cleave vWF multimers into fragments with increased platelet-binding capacity[24]; or (3) unusually large vWF multimeric forms[25,26] that may be released into the circulation from endothelial cells damaged or stimulated by autoantibodies, immune complexes, or toxins.

vWF monomers are linked by disulfide bonds into multimers of varying sizes that range into the millions of daltons.[27] vWF multimers are produced within megakaryocytes and endothelial cells and are stored within the α-granules of platelets and the Weibel-Palade bodies of endothelial cells (see Ch. 112). The predominant sources of plasma vWF multimers are apparently endothelial cells. The entire constellation of vWF multimers found in the normal circulation is produced within both megakaryocytes and endothelial cells.[27] Both cell types construct, in addition, vWF multimeric forms that are even greater in size that those found in normal plasma.[28,29] These unusually large (UL)vWF multimers are more effective than the largest plasma vWF forms at binding in flowing systems to fluid shear stress-altered platelet glycoprotein (GP)Ib/IX and subsequently to GPIIb/IIIa complexes, after which they induce aggregation.[28,29] A substance in normal plasma is responsible for reducing the size of ULvWF multimeric forms secreted into the vascular lumen to the somewhat smaller vWF multimers ordinarily in circulation.[30] This substance, which may be a limited disulfide bond reductase, does not have access to the ULvWF forms secreted in the retrograde direction from endothelial cells into the vascular subendothelium. If endothelial cells are damaged and desquamated, platelet GPIb/IX receptors may adhere most effectively (under arterial flow conditions) to ULvWF forms in the subendothelium.

In many patients with a single episode of TTP, ULvWF multimers have been found in plasma during the episode[26] (Fig. 127-2), presumably because of systemic endothelial cell injury or intense stimulation and ULvWF release that "overwhelms" plasma ULvWF-processing capacity. (Platelet aggregation and α-granule release do not account for the appearance of ULvWF multimeric forms in the plasma, probably because any released ULvWF multimers attach tenaciously to GPIb/IX and GPIIb/IIIa vWF receptors on the external surface of platelet membranes.[29]) Serial study of plasma samples from patients during single episodes of TTP has shown that the ULvWF multimers, and often the largest plasma vWF forms, disappear from some patient plasma samples as the TTP episode continues and thrombocytopenia worsens (or remains extreme).[26] Immunohistochemical evidence (mentioned previously) suggests that this is because large and ULvWF forms become attached to platelets during the intravascular aggregation that characterizes the syndrome.[20]

If a TTP patient survives, and suffers no subsequent relapse, vWF multimeric forms in recovery samples are almost always normal. If, however, ULvWF multimers are found in plasma samples after recovery, then the likelihood is considerable that endothelial cell perturbation is persisting and that the patient will have recurrent episodes of TTP. The recurrences may be at irregular, infrequent intervals (intermittent TTP) or, espe-

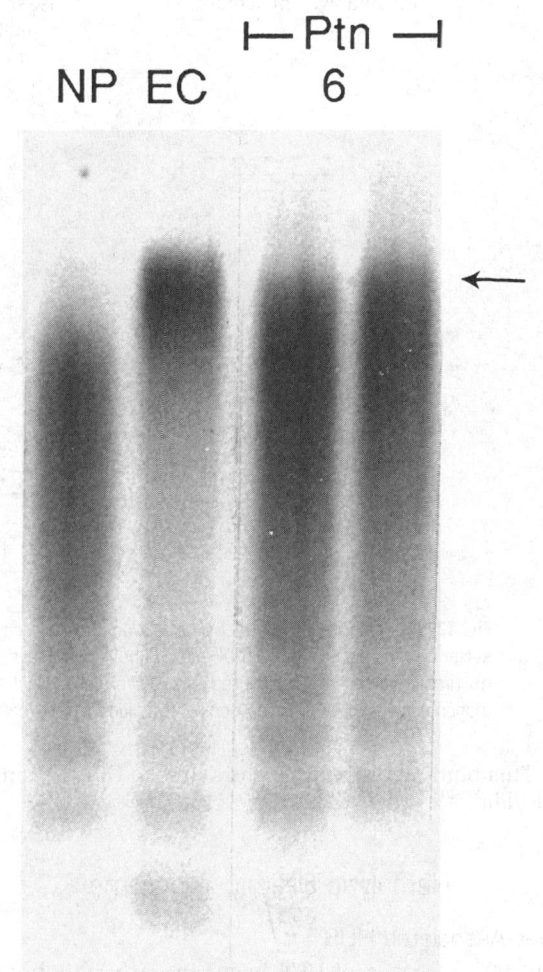

Fig. 127-2. vWF abnormalities in a patient with thrombotic microangiopathy associated with chemotherapy, bone marrow transplantation for refractory lymphoma, and Cyclosporin A. ULvWF forms (arrow) in EDTA-plasma samples obtained 90 minutes apart on the day of death are displayed on this autoradiogram of an unreduced sodium dodecyl sulfate (SDS)-1% agarose gel. The vWF antigen levels in the plasma samples were 225% and 210%, respectively, before they were diluted to 15% and mixed with SDS-urea-EDTA-Tris for electrophoresis. NP, normal pooled platelet-poor plasma; EC, supernatant of cultured human umbilical vein endothelial cells containing ULvWF forms.

cially if they begin in infancy or early childhood, at frequent and regular intervals (chronic relapsing TTP).[25,26] During recurrences of intermittent or chronic relapsing TTP, the ULvWF multimers disappear from patient plasma. This often occurs in association with the disappearance of the largest plasma vWF multimeric forms, as can also be observed in the plasma of other patients during the course of a single episode of TTP.[25,26]

These observations suggest that TTP may be a disorder associated with excessive release of ULvWF multimeric forms from systemic endothelial cells that are perturbed either transiently (single-episode TTP) or occasionally (intermittent TTP). In chronic relapsing TTP of infancy and childhood, a congenital defect in the control of ULvWF release may cause the accumulation of vWF forms in the circulation that periodically exceeds a threshold level required for intravascular aggregation. Elevated levels of fluid shear stress (i.e., the relative parallel motion between fluid planes during flow) in the microcirculation may be necessary during episodes of TTP of all types in order to induce the attachment of ULvWF multimers, as well as the largest plasma vWF forms, to shear-altered platelet vWF recep-

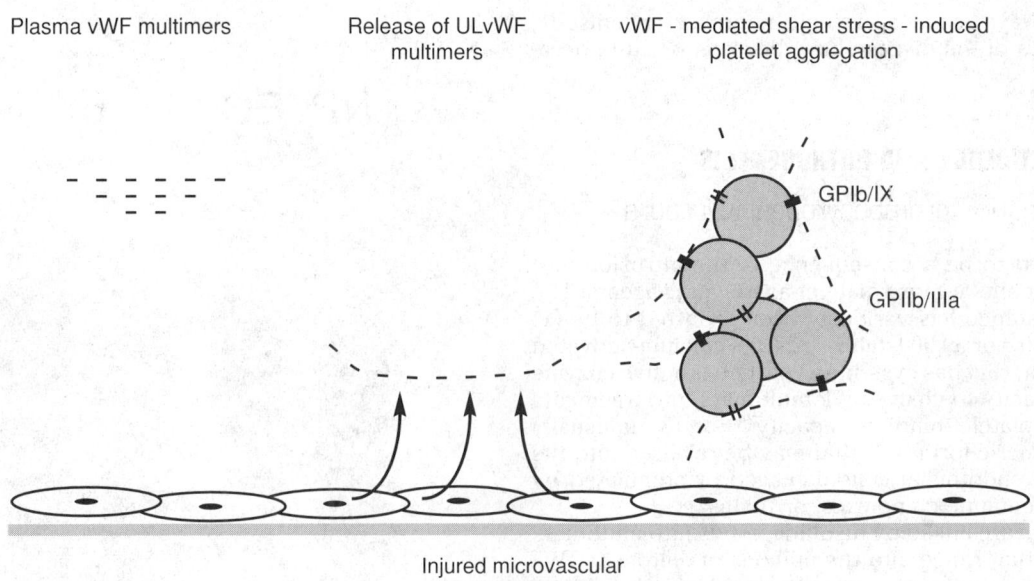

Plasma vWF multimers   Release of ULvWF   vWF - mediated shear stress - induced
                              multimers   platelet aggregation

Fig. 127-3. Hypothetical platelet aggregation in the lumen of a microvessel. Increased fluid shear stresses alter the exposure of platelet surface vWF receptors (GPIb/IX and GPIIb/IIIa), and lead to aggregation mediated by the binding to these altered receptors of ULvWF multimers released from injured endothelial cells. Dashed lines, vWF multimers and ULvWF multimers composed of individual vWF monomers linked by disulfide bonds. (Modified from Moake,[49] with permission.)

tors.[31] This binding probably occurs first to GPIb/IX, and then to GPIIb/IIIa[28,29,32] (Fig. 127-3).

Hemolytic Uremic Syndrome

Diarrhea-Associated HUS

About 90% of cases of HUS occur in early childhood (i.e., after the age of 6 months) and are preceded by bloody diarrhea caused by *Shigella dysenteriae* serotype I or, more commonly in Great Britain and North America, various *E. coli* serotypes.[8] These organisms can sometimes, but not always, be cultured from stool samples.[5-9] The offending enterohemorrhagic *E. coli* are endemic to Buenos Aires and Calgary, among other locales, where HUS is a relatively common cause of acute renal failure in children.[8] Characteristic of these particular bacteria is the capacity to produce one or more structurally similar forms of a powerful exotoxin that can be detected in fecal material.[7-9,33] The protype of this 70,000-dalton protein from *S. dysenteriae* is *Shiga toxin,* which is encoded in *S. dysenteriae* DNA.[33,34] Shiga-like toxin-1 (SLT-1) and -2 (SLT-2) are closely related exotoxins encoded in the DNA of bacteriophages; this DNA becomes incorporated into the genome of a restricted number of *E. coli* OH serotypes.[33,34] Of these, the most frequently associated with HUS is *E. coli* 0157:H7 (about 50% of cases).[8,9]

SLT-1 differs from Shiga toxin by only one amino acid in the A subunit, and the two are antigenically cross-reactive.[33,34] SLT-2 is less homologous in structure and is antigenically distinct from Shiga toxin and SLT-1.[33,34] (SLT-2 may actually be several exotoxin forms that differ slightly from each other.) The *E. coli* serotypes associated with HUS may be capable of producing SLT-1 alone, SLT-2 alone, or both exotoxins. The response of normal humans to the Shiga toxins is to generate increasing titers of toxin-neutralizing antibodies.[7-9]

The prototype, Shiga toxin, is composed of one A subunit (31,500 daltons) and five B subunits (7,700 daltons each) (Fig. 127-4).[8,9,33,34] The structural genes for one A and one B subunit are adjacent in the DNA of *S. dysenteriae,* or in the incorporated bacteriophage DNA of enterohemorrhagic *E. coli.* More efficient translation of B subunit mRNA compared with A subunit mRNA

may account for the relatively greater number of B subunits produced.[33]

Each of the B subunits is capable of binding with high affinity to an unusual disaccharide linkage (galactose α1-4 galactose) in the terminal trisaccharide sequence of the predominant membrane glycophospholipid receptor for the Shiga toxins, globotriosyl ceramide (Gb_3)[33,35] (Fig. 127-4). Although Gb_3 is a component of the membranes of renal glomerular capillary endothelial cells, as well as the membranes of other types of endothelial cells,[33] the precise reason for the predominant kidney damage in diarrhea-associated HUS is not known.

The A subunit of Shiga toxin is internalized by endocytosis and, following the fusion of endosomes and lysosomes, undergoes partial proteolysis and disulfide bond reduction to generate an active intracellular enzyme (27,000 daltons) capable of cleaving the *N*-glycoside bond in one adenosine position of the 28S ribosomal RNA that comprises 60S ribosomal subunits.[33,34] This attack on a single adenine nucleotide is sufficient to inhibit the elongation factor-dependent binding to ribosomes of aminoacyl-bound transfer RNA molecules.[33,34] Peptide chain elongation is truncated, and overall protein synthesis is suppressed.

Ingestion of Shiga toxin-producing *S. dysenteriae,* or of an *E. coli* serotype that produces SLT-1 or SLT-2, or both, can occur by eating contaminated food (e.g., undercooked beef or poultry).[7,8] The enterohemorrhagic microbes then (1) colonize the large intestine; (2) adhere to mucosal epithelial cells; (3) invade, replicate, and destroy colonic cells; and (4) damage the underlying tissue and vasculature, possibly by both exotoxin- and endotoxin-related mechanisms.[7-9,33,34] The patient develops bloody diarrhea. Laboratory evidence indicates that Shiga toxin (from *S. dysenteriae*), or SLT-1 or SLT-2, or both (from enterohemorrhagic *E. coli*), then enter the circulation and attach to Gb_3 molecules on renal glomerular capillary endothelial cells (and, in some patients, probably also to endothelial cell Gb_3 receptors in other organs).[8,33,35,36] The involved endothelial cells become swollen and release ULvWF and other components.

In addition to Gb_3, the Shiga toxins also bind to galabiosylceramide (galactose α1-4 galactose ceramide [Ga_2]) and to the

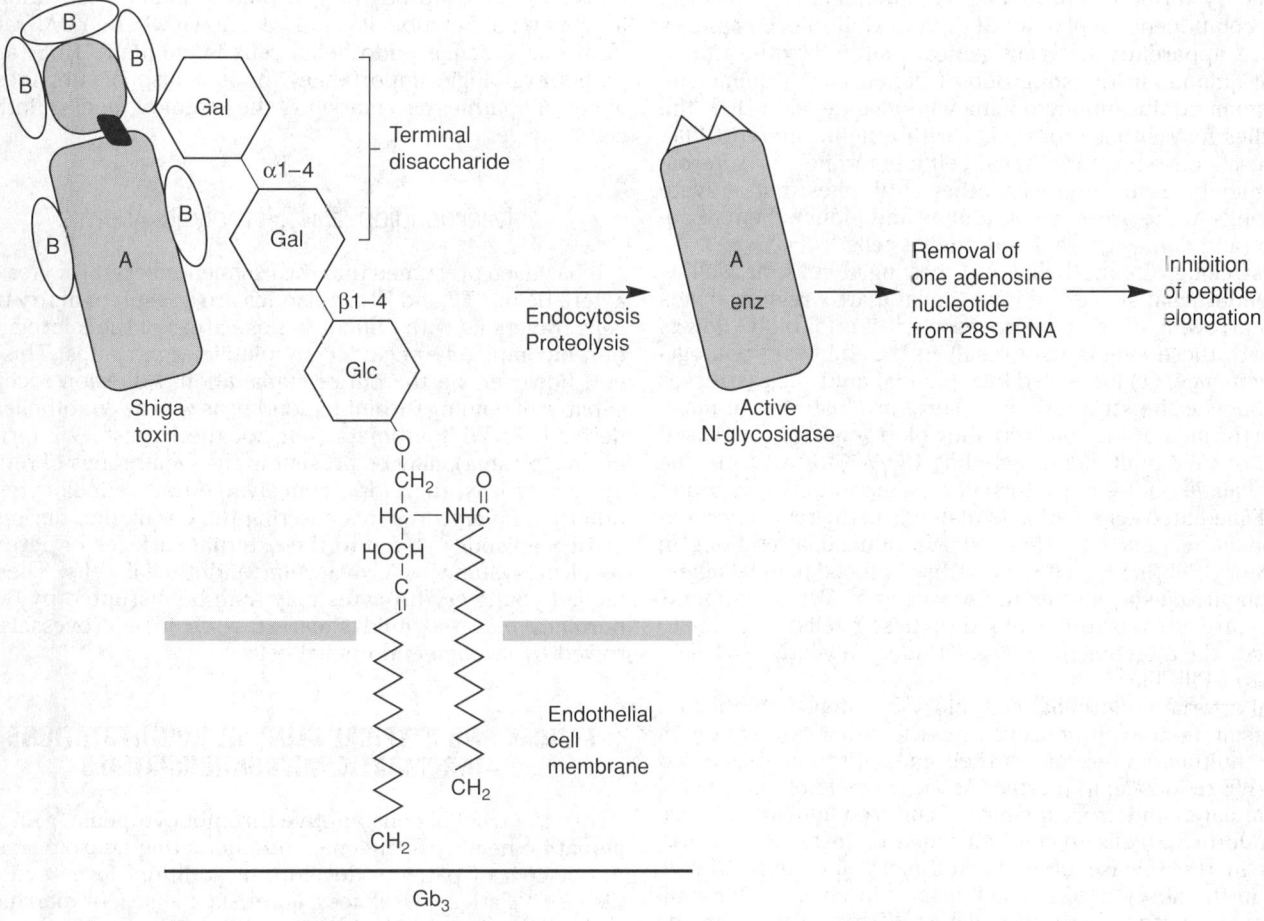

Fig. 127-4. Binding of the B subunits of Shiga toxins to renal microvascular endothelial cell via the disaccharide portion of Gb$_3$ receptors. The A subunit then enters the cell, is activated, and inhibits protein synthesis. (Modified from Moake,[49] with permission.)

erythrocyte P$_1$ antigen.[37] P$_1$ is a pentosyl ceramide molecule that terminates, as does Gb$_3$, in the galactose α1-4 galactose disaccharide recognized by B subunits of the Shiga toxins. Whether or not P$_1$ is also expressed on renal (or other) microvascular endothelial cells, and contributes to the pathogenesis of HUS, has not been resolved. It is also not yet known if weak P$_1$ expression on the red cells of certain individuals decreases competition for the binding of Shiga toxins to Gb$_3$ on renal glomerular and arteriolar endothelial cells, with a consequent increase in the risk of diarrhea-associated HUS in these persons.[37]

In vitro, Shiga toxin, SLT-1, and SLT-2 are directly cytotoxic to proliferating human umbilical vein endothelial cells.[33] The extent of toxin binding may be affected by other substances that up-regulate endothelial cell Gb$_3$ levels. Furthermore, other agents may potentiate the injurious effects of the Shiga toxins on renal (or other) endothelial cells.[38] Candidate substances to produce these potentiating effects include endotoxin lipopolysaccharide (a component of both *S. dysenteriae* and enterohemorrhagic *E. coli*)[33,38]; the cytokines interleukin-1α and -1β and tumor necrosis factor-α and -β (released from monocytes, macrophages and, possibly, renal mesangial cells exposed to endotoxin)[33,38]; or complement-fixing antibodies formed against antigens with altered structure or exposure (and suppressible by interferon-γ) on injured renal endothelial cell surfaces.[39] Compounds released from interleukin-8-activated neutrophils (oxygen-derived free radicals and hydrogen peroxide; elastase and other proteases)[40–42] may also contribute to endothelial cell damage and may account for the relationship between the level of neutrophilia in diarrhea-associated HUS and the extent of irreversible renal damage.[43]

Drug- and Pregnancy-Associated HUS

In addition to HUS associated with diarrhea, the administration of *mitomycin* C,[15] *cyclosporine*,[16] and cancer *chemotherapeutic agents* in combination (sometimes with *total body irradiation*)[17] has been associated with the subsequent development of thrombotic microangiopathy (especially in adults). The syndrome often more closely resembles HUS than TTP and usually develops weeks to months after exposure.[17] If the underlying problem is neoplasia, it may be under relatively good control when the thrombotic microangiopathy occurs. Because chemotherapeutic drugs often cause marrow suppression and thrombocytopenia, as well as renal toxicity, detection of HUS (or TTP) may be delayed. It is not known whether drug metabolites, perhaps including free radicals, may be involved in the putative initial direct damage to the endothelial cells of renal arteries and arterioles that is characteristic of this type of HUS. It is also not known whether the delayed development of thrombotic microangiopathy relates to altered antigenic expression on renal (or other) endothelial cells, with subsequent antiendothelial cell antibody production in these clinical situations.

The formation of endothelial cell autoantibodies associated with immune dysregulation during *pregnancy* or oral contraceptive use might explain the occasional association between these conditions and thrombotic microangiopathy. (The role, if any, of enteropathigenic *E. coli*[8] or antiphospholipid antibodies[44] in these cases is not yet known.)

Further support for the possibility of antiendothelial cell antibody involvement in HUS comes from observations that *quinine*-induced immune thrombocytopenia can also be associated with HUS.[45] Quinine-induced immune thrombocytopenia is caused by antibodies produced by patients taking this drug against components of platelet GPIb/IX or GPIIb/IIIa complexes that have, apparently, been antigenically altered by the attachment of quinine. In the subgroup of patients with quinine-induced immune thrombocytopenia who also develop HUS, the antibodies may either cross-react with quinine-altered GPIIIa molecules[46] on renal endothelial cell membranes, or, alternatively, may be associated with other antibodies that activate neutrophils in the presence of quinine and induce them to adhere to (and damage) renal endothelial cells.[47]

The swelling of endothelial and mesangial cells, as well as of subendothelial spaces and mesangial matrix regions, leads to the narrowing of renal microvessels.[21] If total blood flow is unaltered, these events may result in the following pathogenetic sequence: (1) increased intraluminal fluid shear stresses that influence the structure, exposure, or clustering of molecules in the membranes of circulating blood cells; (2) increased release of vWF multimers, including ULvWF forms, from the Weibel-Palade bodies of perturbed renal endothelial cells; and (3) vWF-mediated aggregation of platelets in the renal microcirculation in response to shear stress-induced alterations in GPIb/IX or GPIIb/IIIa.[28,29,48] Shear stress-induced platelet aggregation in vitro also requires the presence of ADP (from platelets, erythrocytes, or other blood or tissue cells) in order to potentiate the attachment of large or unusually large vWF multimers to GPIIb/IIIa.[29]

Renal arterial endothelial cell injury or intense stimulation may result in the outpouring into the renal circulation of ULvWF multimers in excess of their capacity to be processed by ULvWF reductase in plasma. As an example of endothelial cell stimulation in vitro, exposure of cultured human umbilical vein endothelial cells to purified Shiga toxin for 30 minutes results in the release of vWF multimers, including ULvWF forms, in the absence of any cell lysis.[49] In vivo, ULvWF multimers, along with the largest plasma vWF forms, may then be induced to attach to platelet GPIb/IX and GPIIb/IIIa receptors by the elevated fluid shear stresses in those glomerular capillaries and arterioles that are narrowed by swollen endothelial cells. The result, in this hypothetical series of events, would be aggregated platelets in the renal microcirculation[28,29,31,48] (Fig. 127-3).

If this scenario is, in fact, related to in vivo events, then either ULvWF forms or a relative absence of the largest plasma vWF multimers might be expected in different plasma samples of at least some HUS patients during their acute episodes. Indeed, children with diarrhea-associated HUS and adults with drug-associated HUS have had ULvWF forms in their plasma during the episodes[17,39,50] (Fig. 127-2). In addition, other children and adults have had a relative decrease in their largest plasma vWF multimeric forms when platelet counts were lowest.[17,51,52] (It is possible, however, that ex vivo proteolysis may have contributed to the latter finding in some HUS patients.[50])

Whether or not renal endothelial cell damage compromises the local breakdown of ADP by endothelial cell surface ADPase is not known.[53] The pathophysiologic importance of the following is also not clear: a relative reduction in renal endothelial cell production of prostaglandin I_2 (prostacyclin),[54] which normally suppresses platelet aggregation induced by either chemical agonists or shear stress[55]; a possible increase in tissue factor exposure on renal endothelial cell surfaces, followed by local coagulation activation and fibrin polymer formation[56]; or the release of renal endothelial cell plasminogen activator inhibitor type 1 in excess of tissue plasminogen activator and urokinase, thereby possibly impairing local renal microvascular fibrinolysis.[57]

Platelet-activating factor ([PAF] 1-O-alkyl,2-O-acetyl, glycerol-3-phosphorylcholine), which is released from injured renal endothelial cells, has recently been found to be excreted in increased amounts in the urine of children during the acute phase of HUS.[58] Although PAF promotes platelet activation and impairs renal function, it is not yet known whether PAF release from real vascular endothelial cells is unique to HUS (and of pathophysiologic importance), or if it also occurs in other glomerulopathies as a marker of the extent of renal endothelial cell damage.

Microangiopathic Hemolytic Anemia

It has been presumed that the fragmented erythrocytes characteristic of TTP and HUS episodes are a result of injury to red cells traversing with difficulty those areas of the microcirculation incompletely occluded by platelet aggregates. This may not, however, be the entire explanation. Adhesion receptors capable of binding thrombospondin, as well as endothelial cell-derived ULvWF multimers (but not the largest vWF forms in normal plasma), may be present in the membranes of reticulocytes.[59-61] It is, therefore, conceivable that reticulocytes and other young erythrocytes entering the circulation during TTP or HUS episodes attach to the external surfaces of perturbed renal or systemic microvascular endothelial cells. These attached young erythrocytes may than be disrupted by the abnormally elevated fluid shear stresses in microvessels narrowed by swollen endothelial cells.

TYPICAL AND ATYPICAL CLINICAL MANIFESTATIONS OF THROMBOTIC MICROANGIOPATHIES

TTP is a triad of consumptive thrombocytopenia,[62] microangiopathic hemolytic anemia, and fluctuating neurologic signs. About 40% of patients develop, in addition, fever and renal disease.[63] Fatigue, weakness, anorexia, nausea, or diarrhea are present in some combination in most patients.

Intravascular platelet aggregation results in organ ischemia and severe thrombocytopenia. Platelet counts are <20,000/mm^3 in >50% of patients, and bone marrow megakaryocytes are increased. Bleeding into the skin is common.

Hemolysis is usually severe, with 90% of patients having initial hemoglobin values <10 g/dl. Reticulocytosis, increased erythroid precusors in the bone marrow, and circulating nucleated red blood cells in patients with more extensive hemolysis reflect the compensatory marrow response to the shortened red blood cell survival. Blood films always show extensive poikilocytosis and erythroid fragmentation. (Rarely, schistocytes may appear a few days after the onset of thrombocytopenia and clinical symptoms or signs.) Serum lactate acid dehydrogenase is always increased, often to levels 5–10 times normal. Unconjugated bilirubin may be increased, depending on the extent of hemolysis and the capacity of the liver to accelerate

---

LABORATORY EVALUATION OF THROMBOTIC MICROANGIOPATHY

Hematocrit/hemoglobin
Platelet and leukocyte counts
Peripheral blood smear
Lactate dehydrogenase
Creatinine/blood urea nitrogen
Coagulation studies (prothrombin time, partial thromboplastin time, fibrinogen/fibrin degradation products or D-dimer, fibrinogen)
± Bilirubin/SGOT/SGPT/alkaline phosphatase
± Haptoglobin

the uptake of this substance from the bloodstream. Haptoglobin is usually absent (and always, at least, decreased).

Neurologic abnormalities, which may be transient, occur in 50–71% of patients during acute TTP episodes.[3,4] These may include headache, paresthesias, pareses, aphasia or dysphasia, seizures, visual disturbances, or coma. These symptoms and signs are the result of thrombotic occlusion or bleeding into the brain or retinae, or both. Retinal detachment may occur acutely as a result of thrombi in choroid capillaries or vitreous hemorrhage, or subsequently because of neovascularization.[64,65] Lumbar punctures should be done with extreme caution in severely thrombocytopenic patients and are usually not indicated in TTP. Computed tomography or magnetic resonance imaging can more reliably and safely detect intracerebral hemorrhage or infarction.

Renal dysfunction is present in 50–75% of TTP patients during acute episodes.[3,4] Hematuria and proteinuria are common. A few patients have severe renal failure, with creatinine values >5 mg/dl.[66]

Symptoms of myocardial ischemia are unusual in the absence of underlying cardiac or coronary artery pathology, unless the acute hemolytic anemia is profound. Angina, congestive heart failure with pulmonary edema, or conduction disturbances may occur in severely ill patients, however.[67] Pulmonary vascular thrombi or hemorrhage may uncommonly produce hypoxemia, tachypnea, and infiltrates on chest radiographs that mimic the adult respiratory distress syndrome.[68]

Gastrointestinal bleeding of variable severity occurs frequently in association with the severe thrombocytopenia.[69] Abdominal pain is occasionally the initial symptom of TTP, presumably because of occlusion in mesenteric microvessels. Acute pancreatitis occurs infrequently.[70]

Although thrombi can be observed in the adrenal microvasculature, adrenal insufficiency is not often detected clinically (glucocorticoid administration is a recommended therapy, as discussed below). Thrombosis is common in the microvessels of the spleen and gums, but is less frequently found in the bone marrow.

Most patients who develop TTP have no known underlying disorder or condition. Perhaps one-half of TTP patients have a nonspecific history suggestive of a prodromal viral-like illness.[66] TTP has been reported, rarely, following influenza or polio vaccinations, or influenza, herpes simplex, or coxsackie B virus infections.[62,71–74] Whether or not viruses (or other microbes) are etiologic agents in some cases of TTP is unknown.

TTP has occurred, uncommonly, in patients with immune dysregulation or autoimmunity (acquired immunodeficiency syndrome, systemic lupus erythematosus, idiopathic thrombocytopenic purpura).[74–84] TTP (or HUS) during the third trimester or puerperal period of pregnancy accounts for a small percentage of patients with thrombotic microangiopathy. Fetal death is common, probably as a result of thromboses in the placenta. Thrombotic lesions are absent in the fetus.[85] Of the few healthy infants delivered, none has developed TTP as a neonate. Both improvement and deterioration have occurred in mothers with TTP following delivery.

Distinguishing TTP from HUS may be difficult. Epidemiology and clinical features usually permit distinction, however. Thrombocytopenia and intravascular hemolysis are usually considerably worse in TTP than in HUS. HUS is more common in children and, in contrast to TTP, is inevitably associated with acute, severe renal dysfunction. Symptoms and signs of microthrombi in the brain and other organs are less common and usually less threatening in HUS, compared with TTP, although these may need to be distinguished from neurologic manifestations due to uremia. The frequent clustering of cases, often preceded by bloody diarrhea caused by SLT-producing

---

DIFFERENTIAL DIAGNOSIS OF THROMBOCYTOPENIA AND MICROANGIOPATHIC HEMOLYSIS

The constellation of thrombocytopenia and microangiopathic hemolysis also occurs in disseminated intravascular coagulation (DIC); pre-eclampsia/eclampsia; the HELLP syndrome (pre-eclampsia-associated *h*emolysis, *e*levated *l*iver enzymes, and *l*ow *p*latelets); malignant hypertension; gastric carcinoma, or other types of metastatic neoplasms associated with vascular invasion; and severe vasculitides (e.g., systemic lupus erythematosus or scleroderma). After information is obtained by history and physical examination, the most frequently troublesome diagnostic dilemma is between TTP or HUS and DIC.

Thrombocytopenia, microangiopathic hemolytic anemia, and schistocytosis are more extreme in TTP and HUS than in DIC. In contrast to DIC, coagulation screening studies (prothrombin time, partial thromboplastin time, fibrinogen) are usually normal in TTP and HUS. In contrast to DIC, fibrinogen/fibrin degradation products and D-dimer levels are usually normal in TTP and HUS; however, these may become modestly elevated if the necrosis of cerebral or other tissue results in the activation of coagulation and secondary fibrinolysis.

The distinction between TTP or HUS and DIC caused by a variety of obstetrical crises (premature separation of the placenta, amniotic fluid embolism, retained dead fetus, pre-eclampsia/eclampsia, fatty liver of pregnancy), can also be difficult during the last trimester of pregnancy or the puerperal period. It is the extent of the thrombocytopenia, hemolysis, and schistocytosis, along with the magnitude of the neurologic or renal abnormalities, that will usually point toward a diagnosis of TTP or HUS. Furthermore, in contrast to TTP and HUS, delivery is more predictably effective in reversing the hematologic abnormalities associated with these obstetric emergencies (see Ch. 149).

Patients with the uncommon Evans syndrome (i.e., coincident autoimmune hemolytic anemia and autoimmune thrombocytopenia) may have both spherocytes and a few schistocytes on the peripheral blood smear. This condition can be quickly differentiated from a thrombotic microangiopathy: Evans syndrome displays a positive direct antiglobulin (Coombs) test.

---

enterohemorrhagic *E. coli* species,[7,8,14] is especially prominent in HUS.

THERAPY AND PROGNOSIS

Thrombotic Thrombocytopenic Purpura

In many patients with TTP episodes (71–91% in two recent large series),[3,4] the process can be reversed by intensive plasma manipulation.[3,4,13,84,86–88] This is most effectively done using plasma exchange (i.e., the combination of plasmapheresis and plasma infusion with normal fresh frozen platelet-poor plasma [3–4 L/day]). It is presumed that platelet-aggregating substances (possibly ULvWF multimers and/or other cofactors, aggregating proteins, or enzymes) are being removed by plasmapheresis and that normal plasma is providing some antiaggregating agent that is present in patient plasma in inadequate amounts (ULvWF "reductase" or some other type of aggregation inhibitor?). If plasma exchange is not immediately available, the administration of glucocorticoids (see below) and the infusion of normal fresh frozen plasma at the rate of about 30 ml/kg/day can be used initially. (This is less total daily normal plasma than is provided during plasma exchange.[3]) Plasma exchange should then be arranged as quickly as possible in all newly diagnosed seriously ill patients.[3,4,13,86–88] TTP patients with neurologic abnormalities, cardiac failure, or renal dysfunction should be treated by plasma exchange commencing immediately after diagnosis, if possible.

Relapses in some chronically relapsing TTP patients (especially children) respond to, or can be prevented by periodic transfusion of normal fresh frozen plasma alone (in quantities varying from one to several units) without the need for concurrent plasmapheresis.[13,88–90]

Some patients have recovered from TTP episodes without receiving glucocorticoids, and others with relatively milder presentations have been reported to recover in association with glucocorticoid therapy alone.[4,13,86,91] This latter observation is the basis for recommending that all patients with an acute TTP episode receive pharmacologic doses of a glucocorticoid compound.[4] The apparent usefulness of this treatment may relate to an underlying autoimmune pathogenesis in some TTP patients. In a recent long-term study,[4] prednisolone was started immediately following diagnosis in a dosage of 200 mg/day intravenously. Glucocorticoid therapy should continue, along with plasma exchange (the primary therapeutic maneuver), until the patient recovers.[4]

Depending on the hemoglobin level and intensity of hemolysis, red blood cell transfusions may be required. If the platelet count is very low and bleeding is a primary problem, or if intracranial bleeding is demonstrated by computed tomography or magnetic resonance imaging, platelet transfusions will be necessary. In a few reported patients, however, the transfusion of platelets has been temporally associated with exacerbation of the thrombotic process in the cerebral microcirculation.[13,92]

Although it is not known for certain, plasma exchange should be continued daily for a minimum of about 5 days in patients who respond completely (i.e., attain a normal neurologic status, platelet count $>150,000/mm^3$, rising hemoglobin, and normal serum LDH levels). It is not known whether there is any therapeutic benefit to tapering plasma exchange, or instituting a tapering period of plasma infusion after recovery, in an effort to lessen the possibility of incomplete remission. If the patient is, indeed, in incomplete remission and quickly relapses, the same treatment protocol should be repeated. In patients who achieve only a partial response, but with either some improvement or (at least) stabilization of their clinical condition, plasma exchange should be continued for a period of a few to many additional days in an effort to achieve a complete remission.

If a patient does not respond within the first 5 days of therapy, or deteriorates within the first 2 or 3 days, other forms of therapy should be tried. Options include addition of vincristine ($1.4 mg/m^2$, but not >2 mg total dosage, given by intravenous push on day 1, followed by 1 mg on days 4, 7, and 10)[93]; substitution in the plasma exchange procedures of cryosupernatant (plasma from which the cryoprecipitate portion enriched in fibrinogen, fibronectin, and the largest plasma vWF multimeric forms has been removed) for fresh frozen plasma[94,95]; splenectomy (perhaps in association with glucocorticoids and dextran)[84]; the use of staphylococcal protein A columns (removal through attachment to the Fc portion of IgG antibodies that are bound in immune complexes to platelet or endothelial cell antigens)[96,97]; or addition of azathioprine (Imuran) or other immunosuppressive agents.[13,98]

The use of aspirin and dipyridamole is controversial.[92,99,100] Aspirin may exacerbate hemorrhagic complications, especially in severely thrombocytopenic patients.[99] Neither drug has been unequivocally demonstrated to be useful. The same comments pertain to intravenous prostacyclin, heparin, and fibrinolytic agents.[13] Transfusions or exchange transfusions with fluids other than plasma or its cryosupernatant fraction are almost always ineffective (e.g., albumin, γ-globulin).[13,88,101]

When a patient achieves remission and the plasma exchanges have been discontinued for about 1 week, the platelet count should be monitored regularly. Patients with a protracted and incompletely remitted initial episode usually relapse within days to weeks of the discontinuation of therapy. In about 11–28% of patients who attain a complete remission, the disorder may recur intermittently at intervals of months to years.[3,4,26] Rarely, especially in children, TTP may recur about every 3–4 weeks as a true chronic relapsing disorder with predictable periodicity.

Detection of ULvWF multimers in patient plasma samples obtained after complete and sustained recovery from an initial episode of TTP has accurately predicted subsequent recurrence[13,26] in >90% of the >100 patients tested as of mid-1993. In about 10 patients, subsequent disappearance of ULvWF multimers (either spontaneously or during Imuran therapy) from serially acquired plasma samples has been associated with the absence of additional TTP recurrences. The role of this test in the routine management of TTP remains to be determined.

Hemolytic Uremic Syndrome

There has been considerable controversy concerning the management of patients with HUS. The variability of the disorder explains the difficulty in determining the effectiveness of any specific form of therapy. The severity of renal involvement, reflected by the duration of oliguria, generally correlates with the rate of recovery in both adults and children. In mildly affected children in whom anuria is present for <24 hours, careful attention to fluid and electrolytes is sufficient. In more severely affected children, dialysis is frequently required, and its early institution has resulted in improved survival. HUS in children is, however, associated with some mortality and often with residual renal dysfunction that may progress to hypertension or severe renal failure. Additional forms of therapy have, therefore, been investigated. There is no consensus on any value of anticoagulants, fibrinolytic therapy, or antiplatelet agents in the treatment of HUS.[13]

Management of HUS in adults has generally been similar to that in children. Renal impairment is, however, often more severe in adults than in children, and hemodialysis is generally required.

Based on the value of plasma therapy in TTP, this form of treatment has been tried in HUS with conflicting results.[102,103] Patients have been treated by the initial infusion of 30–40 ml/kg, followed by 15–20 ml/kg/day, in association with hemodialysis. Controlled trials of plasma infusion with hemodialysis, or of plasma infusion with plasmapheresis (plasma exchange) have not been conducted in any of the various forms of HUS. These will be necessary in order to establish with certainty whether either of these management strategies is effective. It will also be important to determine conclusively whether any of the following has a place in the treatment or prophylaxis of the various types of HUS: antibiotics, or vaccination, against *S. dysenteriae* type I or various species of enterhemorrhagic *E. coli* (including 0157:H7, the most common pathogen)[104,105]; interferon-γ, which is capable of suppressing in vitro the interaction between putative autoantibodies and renal endothelial cells[39]; and plasmapheresis over columns of staphylococcal protein A (to which the Fc portions of IgG in immune complexes attach). This latter approach has been used with some apparent success in some patients whose HUS is associated with mitomycin C, cyclosporine, or multiple chemotherapeutic agents.[97,106]

FUTURE DIRECTIONS

In addition to continuing efforts to define precisely the pathophysiologic basis for HUS and the different types of TTP, including the development of animal models, new approaches to treatment can be anticipated. These approaches are likely to include clinical trials of the infusion of ULvWF "reductase"[30,107] purified from normal human plasma, in place of whole fresh frozen plasma or cryosupernatant, as therapy or prophylaxis for TTP (or HUS) episodes.

Derivatives of a chemical, aurin tricarboxylic acid (ATA),[108,109] may ultimately be tried in the treatment or prophylaxis of TTP and HUS. ATA reversibly binds to vWF multimers. It prevents ULvWF multimers and the largest plasma vWF forms from attaching to platelet GPIb molecules. The binding of large vWF forms to both types of platelet surface vWF receptors (GPIb/IX and GPIIb/IIIa complexes) is required for platelet aggregation in fluid shear fields (as in partially obstructed microvessels with high blood flow rates).[28,29,31,48] Other agents that may be subjected to clinical trials in the future as potential treatment of refractory or relapsing TTP (or HUS) include a recombinant fragment of the human vWF monomer that attaches tenaciously to platelet GPIb and blocks GPIb binding of ULvWF and large plasma vWF multimers[110,111]; a monoclonal antibody against the Arg-Gly-Asp (RGD) sequence of the vWF monomer that is involved in binding of vWF multimeric forms to platelet GPIIb/IIIa; either a monoclonal antibody[111] or a small Arg (or Lys)-Gly-Asp-containing peptide[112] capable of blocking the binding of ligands to GPIIb/IIIa; staphylococcal protein A columns that remove circulating IgG-containing immune complexes)[96,97,106]; and solvent/detergent-treated plasma depleted of large vWF multimers and devoid of hepatitis B and C viruses, human immunodeficiency virus and other viruses with lipid envelopes.[31]

REFERENCES

1. Moschcowitz E: Hyaline thrombosis of the terminal arterioles and capillaries: a hitherto undescribed disease. Proc NY Pathol Soc 24:21, 1924
2. Gasser C, Gautier E, Steck A et al: Hamolytisch-uramische Syndrome: Bilaterale Nierenrindennekrosen bei akuten erworbenen hamolytischen Anamien. Schweiz Med Wochensch 85:905, 1955
3. Rock GA, Sumak KH, Buskard NA et al: Comparison of plasma exchange with plasma infusion in the treatment of thrombotic thrombocytopenic purpura. N Engl J Med 325:393, 1991
4. Bell WR, Braine HG, Ness PM, Kickler TS: Improved survival in thrombotic thrombocytopenic purpura-hemolytic-uremic syndrome—clinical experience in 108 patients. N Engl J Med 325:398, 1991
5. Neild G: The haemolytic-uraemic syndrome. Q J Med 63:367, 1987
6. Kaplan BS, Proesmans W: The hemolytic uremic syndrome of childhood and its variants. Semin Hematol 24:1480, 1987
7. Cleary TG: Cytotoxin producing E. coli and the hemolytic uremic syndrome. Pediatr Clin North Am 35:485, 1988
8. Karmali MA: The association of verotoxins and the classical hemolytic uremic syndrome. p. 199. In Kaplan BS, Trompeter RS, Moake JL (eds): Hemolytic-Uremic Syndrome and Thrombotic Thrombocytopenic Purpura. Marcel Dekker, New York, 1992
9. Ashkenazi S: Role of bacterial cytotoxins in hemolytic uremic syndrome and thrombotic thrombocytopenic purpura. Annu Rev Med 44:11, 1993
10. Morrison DM, Tyrell DLJ, Jewell LD: Colonic biopsy in verotoxin-hemorrhagic colitis and thrombotic thrombocytopenic purpura (TTP). Am J Clin Pathol 86:108, 1985
11. Kovacs MJ, Roddy J, Gregoire S et al: Thrombotic thrombocytopenic purpura following hemorrhagic colitis due to E. coli 0157:H7. Am J Med 88:177, 1980
12. Watson CG, Cooper WM: Thrombotic thrombocytopenic purpura-concomitant occurrence in husband and wife. JAMA 215:1821, 1971
13. Byrnes JJ, Moake JL: Thrombotic thrombocytopenic purpura and the hemo-lytic-uremic syndrome: evolving concepts of pathogenesis and therapy. Clin Haematol 15:413, 1986
14. Karmali MA, Petric M, Linn C et al: The association between idiopathic hemolytic uremic syndrome and infection by verotoxin-producing Escherichia coli. J Infect Dis 151:775, 1985
15. Cantrell JE, Phillips TM, Schein PS: Carcinoma-associated hemolytic-uremic syndrome: a complication of mitomycin C chemotherapy. J Clin Oncol 3: 723, 1985
16. Atkinson K, Biggs JC, Hayes J et al: Cyclosporin A associated nephrotoxicity in the first 100 days after allogeneic bone marrow transplantation: three distinct syndromes. Br J Haematol 54:59, 1983
17. Charba D, Moake JL, Harris MA, Hester JP: Abnormalities of von Willebrand factor multimers in drug-associated thrombotic microangiopathies. Am J Hematol 42:268, 1993
18. Baehr G, Klemperer P, Schifrin A: An acute febrile anemia with thrombocytopenic purpura with diffuse platelet thrombosis of capillaries and arterioles. Trans Assoc Am Physicians 65:43, 1936
19. Harkness DR, Byrnes JJ, Lian EC-Y et al: Hazard of platelet transfusion in thrombotic thrombocytopenic purpura. JAMA 246:1931, 1981
20. Asada Y, Sumiyoshi A, Hayashi T et al: Immunohistochemistry of the vascular lesion in thrombotic thrombocytopenic purpura, with special reference to factor VIII related antigen. Thromb Res 38:469, 1985
21. Habib R: Pathology of the hemolytic uremic syndrome. p. 315. In Kaplan BS, Trompeter RS, Moake JL (eds): Hemolytic-Uremic Syndrome and Thrombotic Thrombocytopenic Purpura. Marcel Dekker, New York, 1992
22. Siddiqui FA, Lian EC-Y: Novel platelet-agglutinating protein from a thrombotic thrombocytopenic purpura plasma. J Clin Invest 76:1330, 1985
23. Cheng SH, Lian EC-Y: Purification and some properties of a 59 kda platelet-aggregating protein from the plasma of a patient with thrombotic thrombocytopenic purpura. Thromb Hemost 62:568, 1989
24. Moore JC, Murphy WG, Kelton JG: Calpain proteolysis of von Willebrand factor enhances its binding to platelet membrane glycoprotein IIb/IIIa: an explanation for platelet aggregation in thrombotic thrombocytopenic purpura. Br J Haematol 74:457, 1990
25. Moake JL, Rudy CK, Troll JH et al: Unusually large plasma factor VIII:von Willebrand factor multimers in chronic relapsing thrombotic thrombocytopenic purpura. N Engl J Med 307:1432, 1982
26. Moake JL, McPherson PD: Abnormalities of von Willebrand factor multimers in thrombotic thrombocytopenic purpura and the hemolytic-uremic syndrome. Am J Med 87:3-9N, 1989
27. Ruggeri ZM, Zimerman TS: von Willebrand factor and von Willebrand disease. Blood 70:895, 1987
28. Moake JL, Turner NA, Stathopoulos NA et al: Involvement of large plasma von Willebrand factor (vWF) multimers and unusually large vWF forms derived from endothelial cells in shear stress-induced platelet aggregation. J Clin Invest 78:1456, 1986
29. Moake JL, Turner NA, Stathopoulos NA et al: Shear-induced platelet aggregation can be mediated by vWF released from platelets, as well as by exogenous large or unusually large vWF multimers, requires adenosine diphosphate, and is resistant to aspirin. Blood 71:1366, 1988
30. Frangos JA, Moake JL, Nolasco L et al: Cryosupernatant regulates accumulation of unusually large vWF multimers from endothelial cells. Am J Physiol 256:H1635, 1989
31. Chintagumpala M, Moake JL, Turner N et al: Transfusion with fresh-frozen plasma or solvent/detergent-treated plasma reverses both thrombocytopenia and excessive von Willebrand factor-mediated shear-induced platelet aggregation in chronic relapsing thrombotic thrombocytopenic purpura (TTP). Blood 1994 (in press)
32. Chow TW, Hellums JD, Moake JL, Kroll MH: Shear stress-induced von Willebrand factor binding to platelet glycoprotein Ib initiates calcium influx associated with aggregation. Blood 80:113, 1992
33. Obrig TG: Pathogenesis of Shiga toxin (verotoxin)-induced endothelial cell injury. p. 405. In Kaplan BS, Trompeter RS, Moake JL (eds): Hemolytic-Uremic Syndrome and Thrombotic Thrombocytopenic Purpura. Marcel Dekker, New York, 1992
34. O'Brien AD, Holmes RK: Shiga and Shiga-like toxins. Microbiol Rev 51:206, 1987
35. Lindberg AA, Brown JE, Stromberg N et al: Identification of the carbohydrate receptor for Shiga toxin produced by Shigella dysenteriae type I. J Biol Chem 262:1779, 1987
36. Boyd B, Lingwood CA: Verotoxin receptor glycolipid in human renal tissue. Nephron 51:207, 1989
37. Taylor CM, Milford DV, Rose PE et al: The expression of blood group P₁ in post-enteropathic hemolytic uremic syndrome. Paediatr Nephrol 4:59, 1990
38. van de Kar NCAJ, Monnens LAH, Karmali MA, van Hinsbergh VWM: Tumor necrosis factor and interleukin-1 induce expression of the verocytotoxin

receptor globotriaosylceramide on human endothelial cells: implication for the pathogenesis of the hemolytic uremic syndrome. Blood 80:2755, 1992

39. Leung DYM, Moake JL, Havens PL et al: Lytic anti-endothelial cell antibodies in hemolytic-uremic syndrome. Lancet 2:183, 1988

40. Weiss SJ: Tissue destruction by neutrophils. N Engl J Med 320:365, 1989

41. Milford DV, Taylor CM, Rafaat F et al: Neutrophil elastase and haemolytic uraemic syndrome. Lancet 2:1153, 1989

42. Fitzpatrick MM, Shah V, Trompeter RS et al: Interleukin-8 and polymorphonuclear leukocyte activation in hemolytic-uremic syndrome of childhood. Kidney Int 42:951, 1992

43. Walters MDS, Matthei IU, Kay R et al: The polymorphonuclear leucocyte count in childhood haemolytic uraemic syndrome. Paediatr Nephrol 3:130, 1989

44. Kniaz D, Eisenberg GM, Elrad H et al: Postpartum hemolytic uremic syndrome associated with antiphospholipid antibodies. Am J Nephrol 12:126, 1992

45. Gottschall JL, Elliot W, Lianos E et al: Quinine-induced immune thrombocytopenia associated with hemolytic-uremic syndrome: a new clinical entity. Blood 77:306, 1991

46. Pfueller SL, Bilston RA, Jane S, Gibson J: Expression of the drug-dependent antigen for quinine-dependent antiplatelet antibodies on GPIIIa, but not on GPIb, IIb or IX on human endothelial cells. Thromb Haemost 63:279, 1990

47. Stroncek DF, Vercellotti GM, Hammerschmidt DE et al: Characterization of multiple quinine-dependent antibodies in a patient with episodic hemolytic-uremic syndrome and immune agranulocytosis. Blood 80:241, 1992

48. Peterson DM, Stathopoulos NA, Giorgio TD et al: Shear-induced platelet aggregation requires von Willebrand factor and platelet membrane glycoproteins Ib and IIb/IIIa. Blood 69:625, 1987

49. Moake JL: Haemolytic uraemic syndrome: basic science. Lancet 343:393, 1994

50. Mannucci PM, Lombardi R, Lattuada A et al: Enhanced proteolysis of plasma von Willebrand factor (vWF) in thrombotic thrombocytopenic purpura (TTP) and the hemolytic uremic syndrome. Blood 74:978, 1989

51. Moake JL, Byrnes JJ, Troll JH et al: Abnormal VIII: von Willebrand factor patterns in the plasma of patients with the hemolytic-uremic syndrome. Blood 64:592, 1984

52. Rose PE, Enayat MS, Sunderland R et al: Abnormalities of factor VIII related protein multimers in the haemolytic uraemic syndrome. Arch Dis Child 59:1135, 1984

53. Marcus AJ, Safier LB, Hajjar KA et al: Inhibition of platelet function by an aspirin-insensitive endothelial cell ADPase. Thromboregulation by endothelial cells. J Clin Invest 88:1690, 1991

54. Noris M, Benigni A, Siegler R et al: Renal prostacyclin biosynthesis is reduced in children with hemolytic-uremic syndrome in context of systemic platelet activation. Am J Kidney Dis 20:144, 1992

55. Hardwick RA, Hellums JD, Peterson DM et al: The effect of PGI$_2$ and theophylline on the response of platelets subjected to shear stress. Blood 58:678, 1981

56. Schorer AE, Rick PD, Swam WR, Moldow CF: Structural features of endotoxin required for stimulation of endothelial cell tissue factor production; exposure of preformed tissue factor after oxidant-mediated endothelial cell injury. J Lab Clin Med 106:38, 1985

57. Bergstein JM, Kuederli U, Bang NU: Plasma inhibitor of glomerular fibrinolysis in the hemolytic-uremic syndrome. Am J Med 73:322, 1982

58. Benigni A, Boccardo P, Noris M et al: Urinary excretion of platelet-activating factor in haemolytic uraemic syndrome. Lancet 1:835, 1992

59. Wick TM, Moake JL, Udden MM et al: Unusually large von Willebrand factor multimers increase adhesion of sickle erythrocytes to human endothelial cells under controlled flow conditions. J Clin Invest 80:905, 1987

60. Wick TM, Moake JL, Udden MM, McIntire LV: Unusually large von Willebrand factor multimers preferentially promote young sickle and non-sickle young erythrocyte adhesion to endothelial cells. Am J Hematol 42:284, 1993

61. Sugihara K, Sugihara T, Mohandas N, Hebbel RP: Thrombospondin mediates adherence of CD36$^+$ sickle reticulocytes to endothelial cells. Blood 80:2634, 1992

62. Berberich PR, Cuene SA, Chard RL et al: Thrombotic thrombocytopenic purpura: three cases with platelet and fibrinogen survival studies. J Pediatr 84:503, 1974

63. Ridolfi RL, Bell WR: Thrombotic thrombocytopenic purpura: report of 25 cases and review of the literature. Medicine 60:413, 1981

64. Lewellan DR, Singerman LJ: Thrombotic thrombocytopenic purpura with optic disk neovascularization, vitreous hemorrhage, retinal detachment and optic atrophy. Am J Ophthalmol 89:840, 1980

65. Percival SPB: Ocular findings in thrombotic thrombocytopenic purpura (Moschcowitz's disease). Br J Ophthal 54:73, 1970

66. Amorosi EL, Ultmann JE: Thrombotic thrombocytopenic purpura: report of 16 cases and review of the literature. Medicine 45:139, 1966

67. Ridolfi RL, Hutchins GM, Bell WR: The heart and conductive system in thrombotic thrombocytopenic purpura. Ann Intern Med 91:357, 1979

68. Bone RC, Henry JE, Patterson J et al: Respiratory dysfunction in thrombotic thrombocytopenic purpura. Am J Med 65:262, 1978

69. Hellstrom HR, Nash EC, Fischer ER: TTP as a cause of massive gastrointestinal hemorrhage: report of a case. Gastroenterology 36:132, 1959

70. Hamson HN: Thrombotic thrombocytopenic purpura occurring in the puerperium associated with pancreatic islet cell necrosis. Arch Intern Med 102:124, 1958

71. Brown RC, Blecher TE, French EA et al: Thrombotic thrombocytopenic purpura after influenza vaccination. Br Med J 2:303, 1973

72. Blecher TE, Raper AB: Early diagnosis of thrombotic microangiopathy by paraffin sections of aspirated bone marrow. Arch Dis Child 42:158, 1967

73. Neame PD: Immunologic and other factors in thrombotic thrombocytopenic purpura (TTP). Semin Thromb Hemost 6:416, 1980

74. Myers TJ, Wakem CJ, Ball ED, Tremont ST: Thrombotic thrombocytopenic purpura: combined treatment with palsmapheresis and antiplatelet agents. Ann Intern Med 92:149, 1980

75. Dekker A, O'Brien ME, Cammarata RJ: The association of thrombotic thrombocytopenic purpura with systemic lupus erythematosus. Am J Med Sci 267:243, 1974

76. Case records of the Massachusetts General Hospital. N Engl J Med 269:1195, 1963

77. Morey DA, White JB, Daily WM: Thrombotic thrombocytopenic purpura diagnosed by random lymph node biopsy. Arch Intern Med 98:821, 1956

78. Steinberg AD, Green WT, Talal N: Thrombotic thrombocytopenic purpura complicating Sjögren's syndrome. JAMA 215:757, 1971

79. Benitez L, Mathews M, Mallory GK: Platelet thrombosis with polyarteritis nodosa: report of a case. Arch Pathol 77:116, 1964

80. McLeod BC, Wu KK, Knospe WH: Plasmapheresis in thrombotic thrombocytopenic purpura. Arch Intern Med 140:1059, 1980

81. Zacharski LR, Lustad D, Glick JL: Thrombotic thrombocytopenic purpura in a previously splenectomized patient. Am J Med 60:1061, 1976

82. Leaf AN, Laubenstein LJ, Raphael B et al: Thrombotic thrombocytopenic purpura associated with immunodeficiency virus type I (HIV-1) infection. Ann Intern Med 109:194, 1988

83. Nair JM, Bellevue R, Bertoni M, Dosik H: Thrombotic thrombocytopenic purpura in patients with the acquired immunodeficiency syndrome (AIDS)-related complex: a report of two cases. Ann Intern Med 109:209, 1988

84. Thompson CE, Damon LE, Ries CA, Linker CA: Thrombotic microangiopathies in the 1980s: clinical features, response to treatment, and the impact on the human immunodeficiency virus epidemic. Blood 80:1890, 1992

85. Wurzel JM: TTP lesions in placenta but not fetus. N Engl J Med 301:503, 1979

86. Bukowski RM, Hewlett JS, Reimer RR et al: Therapy of thrombotic thrombocytopenic purpura: an overview. Semin Thromb Hemost 7:1, 1981

87. Shepard KV, Bukowski RM: The treatment of thrombotic thrombocytopenic purpura with exchange transfusions, plasma infusions, and plasma exchange. Semin Hematol 24:178, 1987

88. Byrnes JJ: Plasma infusion in the treatment of thrombotic thrombocytopenic purpura. Semin Thromb Hemost 7:9, 1981

89. Miura M, Koizumi S, Nakamura K et al: Efficacy of several plasma components in a young boy with chronic thrombocytopenia and hemolytic anemia who responds repeatedly to normal plasma infusions. Am J Hematol 17:307, 1984

90. Chintagumpala M, Hurwitz R, Moake J et al: Thrombotic thrombocytopenic purpura in two children: fresh frozen plasma prevents recurrence. J Pediatr 120:49, 1991

91. Petitt RM: Thrombotic thrombocytopenic purpura: a thirty-year review. Semin Thromb Hemost 6:350, 1980

92. Gordon LI, Kwaan HC, Rossi EC: Deleterious effects of platelet transfusions and recovery thrombocytosis in patients with thrombotic microangiopathy. Semin Hematol 24:194, 1987

93. Gutterman LA, Stevenson TD: Treatment of thrombotic thrombocytopenic purpura with vincristine. JAMA 247:1433, 1982

94. Moake JL, Byrnes JJ, Troll JH et al: Effects of fresh-frozen plasma and its cryosupernatant fraction on von Willebrand factor multimeric forms in chronic relapsing thrombotic thrombocytopenic purpura. Blood 65:1232, 1985

95. Byrnes JJ, Moake JL, Panpit K, Periman P: Effectiveness of the cryosupernatant fraction of plasma in the treatment of refractory thrombotic thrombocytopenic purpura. Am J Hematol 34:169, 1990

96. Snyder HW Jr, Seawell BW, Cochran SK et al: Specificity of antibody re-

sponses affected by extracorporeal immunoadsorption on plasma over columns of protein A silica. J Clin Apheresis 7:110, 1992

97. Snyder HW Jr, Mittleman A, Oral A et al: Treatment of cancer chemotherapy-associated thrombotic thrombocytopenic purpura/hemolytic uremic syndrome by protein A immunoadsorption of plasma. Cancer 71:1882, 1993

98. Moake JL, Rudy CK, Troll JH et al: Therapy of chronic relapsing thrombotic thrombocytopenic purpura with prednisone and azathioprine. Am J Hematol 20:73, 1985

99. Rosove MH, Ho WG, Goldfinger D: Ineffectiveness of aspirin and dipyridamole in the treatment of thrombotic thrombocytopenic purpura. Ann Intern Med 96:27, 1982

100. del Zoppo GJ: Antiplatelet therapy in thrombotic thrombocytopenic purpura. Semin Hematol 24:130, 1987

101. Finazzi G, Bellavita P, Falanga A: Inefficacy of intravenous immunoglobulin in patients with low-risk thrombotic thrombocytopenic pupura/hemolytic-uremic syndrome. Am J Hematol 41:165, 1992

102. Misiani R. Apiani AC, Eedefonti A et al: Haemolytic ureamic syndrome: therapeutic effect of plasma infusion. Br Med J 285:1304, 1982

103. Sheth KJ, Gill JC, Hanna J, Leichter HE: Failure of fresh frozen plasma infusions to alter the course of hemolytic-uremic syndrome. Child Nephrol Urol 9:38, 1988

104. Waltersoiel JN, Ashkenazi S, Marrow AL, Cleary TG: Effect of subinhibitory concentrations of antibiotics on extracellular Shiga-like toxin I. Infection 20:25, 1992

105. Bitzan M, Muller-Wiefel DE, Schwarzkopf A, Karch H: The role of antibiotics in the management of verotoxin-associated hemolytic anemia syndrome. Immun Infekt 20:168, 1992

106. Korec S, Schein PS, Smith FP et al: Treatment of cancer-associated hemolytic-uremic syndrome with staphylococcal protein A immunoperfusion. J Clin Oncol 4:210, 1986

107. Phillips MD, Moake JL, Nolasco L, Garcia R: Plasma von Willebrand factor processing activity functions like a disulfide bond reductase: reversible decrease of multimer size, abstracted. Presented at the Fourteenth Congress of the International Society on Thrombosis and Haemostasis, July, 1993

108. Phillips MD, Moake JL, Nolasco LH et al: Aurin tricarboxylic acid: a novel inhibitor of platelet-von Willebrand factor association. Blood 72:1898, 1988

109. Weinstein M, Vosburgh E, Phillips M: Isolation from commercial aurin tricarboxylic acid (ATA) of the most effective polymeric inhibitors of von Willebrand factor interaction with platelet glycoprotein Ib. Comparison with other polyanonic polymers. Blood 78:2291, 1991

110. Sugimoto M, Ricca G, Hrinda ME et al: Functional modulation of the isolated glycoprotein Ib-binding domain on von Willebrand factor expressed in *Escherichia coli.* Biochemistry 30:5202, 1991

111. Alevriadou BR, Moake JL, Ruggeri ZM et al: Real-time analysis of shear dependent thrombus formation and its blockade by inhibitors of von Willebrand factor binding to platelets. Blood 81:1263, 1993

112. Scarborough RM, Naughton MA, Teng W et al: Design of potent and specific integrin antagonists. Peptide antagonists with high specificity for glycoprotein IIb-IIIa. J Biol Chem 268:1066, 1993

Thrombocytopenia Due to Platelet Destruction and Hypersplenism

128

Theodore E. Warkentin, Malcolm S. Trimble, and John G. Kelton

INTRODUCTION

Thrombocytopenia is defined as a platelet count below the lower limit of the normal range (150×10^9/L). Sometimes an expanded definition of thrombocytopenia may be appropriate. For example, an abrupt drop in the platelet count can signify the onset of a platelet-destructive process such as heparin-induced thrombocytopenia or bacteremia even if the platelet count remains $>150 \times 10^9$/L.

When a clinician is faced with a thrombocytopenic patient, three questions must be answered immediately. First, could the patient have pseudothrombocytopenia? Second, what is the clinical severity of the thrombocytopenia? Third, what is the cause of the thrombocytopenia?

Thrombocytopenia can be caused by four general mechanisms: (1) platelet underproduction, (2) increased platelet destruction, (3) platelet sequestration, and (4) hemodilution. Thrombocytopenia caused by increased platelet destruction develops when the rate of platelet destruction surpasses the ability of the bone marrow to produce platelets. Platelets can be destroyed by either immune or nonimmune mechanisms (Table 128-1). Immune-mediated platelet destruction is caused by antibody binding (usually IgG) that results in the clearance of the platelets by the reticuloendothelial system. Nonimmune platelet destruction encompasses all those conditions (for example, disseminated intravascular cogulation [DIC]) that cause platelet destruction independent of immune-mediated platelet clearance. Thrombocytopenia caused by platelet sequestration involves platelet redistribution, usually due to an increase in the splenic platelet pool. Platelet underproduction often occurs with underproduction of other blood cell lines. Hemodilution is characterized by a generally predictable decrease in the red cells, white cells, and platelets caused by the administration of colloids, crystalloids, or blood products.

This classification is useful for all thrombocytopenic patients, including thrombocytopenia in pregnancy and in the newborn. However, in pregnancy and in the newborn, the differential diagnosis must be expanded to include causes unique to these patients (Table 128-2) (see Ch. 125).

Table 128-1. General Mechanisms of Platelet Destruction

Type of Thrombocytopenia	Special Examples
Immunologic	
Definite immune-mediated thrombocytopenia	Autoantibodies
	ITP
	Alloantibodies
	Neonatal alloimmune thrombocytopenia[a]
	Post-transfusion purpura[a]
	Alloimmunization to platelet transfusions[a]
	Antibody-mediated but probably not caused by antiplatelet auto- or alloantibodies
	Drug-induced thrombocytopenia
	Malignancy-associated thrombocytopenia
Probable immune-mediated thrombocytopenia	Bacterial: septicemia
	Parasitic: malaria
	Viral: infectious mononucleous,[a] human immunodeficiency virus
Nonimmunologic	
Thrombin	Disseminated intravascular coagulation[a]
"Platelet activation" or damage	Thrombotic thrombocytopenic purpura[a]
	Hemolytic uremic syndrome[a]
	Renal transplant rejection
	Bone marrow transplantation-associated thrombocytopenia
	Cardiopulmonary bypass surgery
	Cardiopulmonary disorders

[a] See other chapters in this book for a discussion of thrombocytopenia in these disorders.

APPROACH TO THE THROMBOCYTOPENIC PATIENT

Clinical Presentation

Most patients whose platelet count is $>50 \times 10^9$/L have no symptoms, but once the platelet count falls to <10–20×10^9/L, spontaneous bleeding can occur. The signs of platelet bleeding include petechiae and purpura (see Ch. 103). Petechiae first appear on the dependent regions of the body or on traumatized areas. Spontaneous mucous membrane bleeding (wet purpura), epistaxis, and gastrointestinal bleeding indicate more serious hemostatic defects.

History

Many thrombocytopenic patients have a negative history, but certain questions should be asked, including (1) the location and severity of bleeding (if any); (2) the temporal profile of the illness (acute, chronic, or relapsing); (3) symptoms of a secondary illness, such as a neoplasm, infection, and systemic lupus erythematosus (SLE); and (4) a history of recent medication use, alcohol ingestion, or a transfusion (see Ch. 125).

Physical Examination

Signs of bleeding should be sought, as well as the presence of hepatosplenomegaly or lymphadenopathy.

Laboratory Evaluation

The laboratory tests used for the investigation of a patient with thrombocytopenia are summarized in Table 128-3. The blood film is examined to exclude pseudothrombocytopenia, which is characterized by in vitro platelet clumping. This phe-

Table 128-2. Differential Diagnosis of Neonatal Thrombocytopenia and Thrombocytopenia with Pregnancy

Causes of neonatal thrombocytopenia
    Alloimmune neonatal thrombocytopenia
    Maternal autoimmune thrombocytopenia
    Birth asphyxia
    Prematurity
    Neonatal enterocolitis
    Hereditary thrombocytopenia
    Maternal drug ingestion
    Catheter-associated thrombosis (renal vein, inferior vena cava)
    Erythroblastosis fetalis
    Exchange transfusions
Causes of thrombocytopenia associated with pregnancy
    Incidental thrombocytopenia of pregnancy
    Pre-eclampsia/eclampsia[a]
    Thrombotic thrombocytopenic purpura[a]
    Disseminated intravascular coagulation (DIC) due to endometritis, amniotic fluid embolism, retained fetus, abruptio placentae, and pre-eclampsia/eclampsia

[a] Most cases are not associated with overt DIC.

nomenon is usually caused by antibodies that agglutinate platelets in the presence of the anticoagulant EDTA.[1] The platelet aggregates are not counted by the electronic particle counter so the automated platelet count appears falsely low. The correct platelet count can usually be determined by collecting the blood into sodium citrate or heparin anticoagulants or performing a count of non-anticoagulated finger prick samples. Another less common pseudothrombocytopenic disorder is platelet satellitosis, in which rosette-like clusters of platelets are seen around neutophils and monocytes.[2] Pseudothrombocytopenia has resulted in inappropriate therapy[1]; therefore, all thrombocytopenic patients should have their blood film reviewed (see Ch. 125).

Assuming the patient has true thrombocytopenia, the mean platelet volume (MPV) can be helpful in classifying the mechanism of the thrombocytopenia. The presence of large (young) platelets (MPV >12 fL) suggests destructive thrombocytopenia or some form of hereditary thrombocytopenia. Normal or small platelets suggest underproduction or sequestration.

The bone marrow examination is helpful in assessing platelet production, particularly if megakaryocytes are reduced or abnormal in appearance. Examination of the bone marrow can be diagnostic in many disorders (e.g., leukemia, metastatic tumor, megaloblastic anemia, and so forth).

Most patients with immune thrombocytopenia have elevated platelet-associated IgG (PAIgG). Unfortunately, many patients with nonimmune thrombocytopenic disorders also have elevated PAIgG.[3–5] Furthermore, none of the standard PAIgG assays can reliably distinguish nonimmune from immune thrombocytopenic disorders.[5] The recently introduced platelet antibody assays that detect IgG on individual platelet glycoproteins[6–9] may prove more useful diagnostic tests for immune thrombocytopenic disorders.

In patients in whom the mechanism of chronic thrombocytopenia is unclear, we perform an ^{111}In-labeled autologous platelet survival study. Three patterns can be seen: (1) a normal platelet survival and recovery (underproduction); (2) a marked reduction in the platelet life span (increased destruction); and (3) a reduced recovery, but a normal or near normal life span (sequestration). ^{111}In-labeled platelets can also be used to image accessory splenic tissue in patients with idiopathic thrombocytopenic purpura (ITP) who fail splenectomy or a develop postsplenectomy relapse.

Therapy

The bleeding risk for thrombocytopenic patients can be reduced by avoiding drugs that can impair hemostatis (e.g., alcohol, antiplatelet agents, anticoagulants) and invasive proce-

Table 128-3. Laboratory Tests that Can Be Used to Investigate a Thrombocytopenic Patient

Test	Rationale
Routine tests	
CBC	Isolated thrombocytopenia is usually caused by increased platelet destruction, whereas involvement of all cell lines suggests underproduction or sequestration
Examination of the blood film	To exclude pseudothrombocytopenia
	Toxic changes and "left shift" suggest septicema
	Atypical lymphocytes suggest viral infection
	Microangiopathic hemolysis
	Parasites
Blood cultures	To exclude bacteremia, fungemia
Antinuclear antibody (anti-Ro if ANA negative)	To exclude SLE
Thyroid tests (TSH)	Thyroid dysfunction can accompany ITP
Direct antiglobulin test	To exclude coexisting immune hemolytic anemia and immune thrombocytopenia (Evans syndrome)
Monospot, viral serology	Infectious mononucleosis
	Other viral illness
Coagulation	
Activated partial thromboplastin time, prothrombin time, thrombin time, fibrinogen, protamine sulfate	DIC
Antiphospholipid antibodies	Antiphospholipid syndrome
Quantitative immunoglobulins	Gammopathy
HIV serologic testing, T4/T8 ratio	HIV-associated thrombocytopenia
Bone marrow aspiration and biopsy	To assess megakaryocyte number and morphology; to exclude a primary marrow disorder
Platelet antibody testing (many methods)	Sensitive for immune-mediated platelet destruction, but not specific for ITP
Specialized tests	
Drug-dependent antibody testing	Idiosyncratic drug-induced thrombocytopenia
Serotonin platelet release assay	Heparin-induced thrombocytopenia
HLA typing	DR3-B8 in gold-induced thrombocytopenia
Measurement of platelet life span with ^{111}In-labeled platelets	To define the mechanism of thrombocytopenia
	To identify accessory splenic tissue postsplenectomy
vWF multimers, calpain	Thrombotic thromboctyopenic purpura or hemolytic uremic syndrome

Abbreviations: HIV, human immunodeficiency virus; vWF, von Willebrand factor.

dures (intramuscular injections). As many medications as possible should be stopped, because many drugs cause thrombocytopenia or platelet dysfunction. Life-threatening bleeding episodes should be treated with platelet transfusions regardless of the mechanism of the thrombocytopenia.

The role of prophylactic platelet transfusions is controversial.[10–13] As a general rule, patients with chronic thrombocytopenic disorders characterized by increased platelet destruction (e.g., chronic ITP) or chronic underproduction (e.g., aplastic anemia, myelodysplasia) can often tolerate long periods of severe thrombocytopenia without major bleeding episodes. In addition, a prophylactic transfusion can trigger platelet alloimmunization and thereby jeopardize future therapeutic platelet transfusions. Therefore, prophylactic platelet transfusions are seldom indicated for these patients. For patients with a major hemostatic risk such as a significant head injury or trauma or following major surgery, it is reasonable to maintain the platelet count at $>50 \times 10^9$/L. Invasive procedures such as thoracentesis, paracentesis, and liver biopsy are not associated with excess bleeding if the platelet count is $>50 \times 10^9$/L.[14,15] Although a platelet count trigger of 20×10^9/L has traditionally been used at many centers to guide prophylactic platelet transfusions in leukemic and other patients, recent data suggest that a considerably lower platelet count threshold may be acceptable[16] (see Ch. 135).

Prophylactic platelet transfusions should not be given to patients with heparin-induced thrombocytopenia, thrombotic thrombocytopenic purpura, or hemolytic uremic syndrome, since serious bleeding complications are relatively uncommon, and platelet transfusions could exacerbate platelet-mediated thrombotic complications.

ANATOMY AND PHYSIOLOGY

The Spleen: Anatomy and Function

The spleen is a small, well-perfused organ receiving about 5% of the cardiac output.[17] Its anatomy is uniquely suited for its function; the progressive branching of the splenic artery into the trabecular and then central arteries helps separate the plasma from the cellular elements[17] (see Ch. 15). The central arteries arise perpendicularly from the trabecular arteries and skim off the plasma layer from the cells. Soluble antigens in the plasma are delivered to the white pulp, where phagocytic cells process the antigens and initiate antibody production.

The cellular-rich hemoconcentrated fraction of the blood is delivered to the red pulp. A small percentage of this blood flows directly to the splenic veins (the closed system), but most moves into the splenic cords (the open system). Here the cellular elements percolate through a meshwork of reticulum fibers, reticuloendothelial cells, and supporting cells, to reach the splenic sinuses. The cells enter the sinuses by passing through the fenestrations in the basement membrane of the endothelial cells lining the sinuses. The blood exits through the splenic vein into the portal system. Since the veins in the portal system lack valves, any increase in portal pressure is transmitted to the splenic microcirculation.

The spleen has a number of important roles.[17] It is the largest lymphoid organ in the body and plays a pivotal role in host defense by clearing microorganisms and antibody-coated cells. The spleen is also important for antibody synthesis, especially against soluble antigens. The filtering function of the spleen includes (1) culling (removal of damaged or senescent cells and bacteria), (2) pitting (removal of the red cell inclusions and parasites), and (3) remodeling (reticulocyte sequestration and maturation). The spleen also acts as a reservoir for platelets and contains a large exchangeable platelet pool.[18] In humans, the spleen contains <2% of the total red blood cell mass. In some animals (dogs and cats), the spleen is a much more important reservoir for red cells.

Physiologic Platelet Sequestration

Radiolabeled platelets have provided physicians with important information concerning mechanisms of platelet destruction.[19] Until recently, ^{51}Cr was the radiolabel most frequently used, but now ^{111}In is primarily used. [111]In has a much higher binding efficiency for platelets, has a shorter half-life, and can be used for imaging. This permits more accurate studies of platelet localization.

Approximately 30% of the total platelet mass exists as a freely exchangeable pool in the spleen.[18] Since the normal platelet life span is 9–10 days, a platelet spends about one-third of its life, or 3 days, within the spleen. In patients with hypersplenism, as many as 90% of platelets can be found in the spleen. The lowest percentage of platelet recovery occurs in patients with the largest spleens.

After the labeled platelets are injected, accumulation is apparent in both the liver and spleen.[20-22] An initial, irreversible phase of hepatic uptake occurs. This equilibrates during the first 5 minutes and may reflect hepatic clearance of platelets damaged in the labeling procedure. Simultaneously, there is a slow rise in activity over the spleen that peaks in about 20 minutes. Splenic platelet uptake is thus dependent on input (spleen blood flow) and output (clearance).

The splenic platelet pool size can be decreased and the platelet count increased with intravenous infusions of epinephrine in normal individuals and patients with splenomegaly.[18] By contrast, isoprenaline (a β_1- and β_2-agonist) increases the pool size.[23,24] Splenic blood flow increases with increasing spleen size, although perfusion (flow per unit tissue volume) probably falls.[25-27] Blood flow can be increased in some inflammatory disorders (e.g., SLE) without an increase in spleen size. A marked increase or decrease in splenic perfusion alters the proportion of platelets within the spleen.

The most important determinant of the splenic platelet pool is the spleen size.[25,26] The measurement of spleen size can thus be helpful in predicting the degree of thrombocytopenia expected from excess platelet pooling in the spleen. For example, if the splenic platelet pool is 90% (i.e., 10% outside the spleen), the platelet count will be reduced by a factor of 7 (since normally 70% of platelets lie outside the spleen). Consequently, and as a general rule, the spleen must be massively enlarged to produce severe thrombocytopenia.[19] On the other hand, moderate splenomegaly can cause moderate thrombocytopenia.

PATHOLOGIC PLATELET SEQUESTRATION: HYPERSPLENISM

Definition

Hypersplenism is a syndrome characterized by splenomegaly and any or all of the following cytopenias: anemia, leukopenia, or thrombocytopenia. Implicit in the definition is that the cytopenias will correct following splenectomy. Although splenomegaly is almost always present in hypersplenism, most patients with splenomegaly do not have hypersplenism. Almost always, the hypersplenism is the result of an identifiable pathologic process, but in some cases the cause of the splenomegaly remains elusive and is termed *primary*.

Table 128-4. Differential Diagnosis of Splenomegaly and Hypersplenism

Infections
  Acute
    Viral (hepatitis, infectious mononucleosis, cytomegalovirus)
    Bacterial (salmonellosis, septicemia[a])
    Parasite (toxoplasmosis)
  Subacute and chronic
    Subacute bacterial endocarditis
    Tuberculosis
    Malaria[a]
    Fungal disease
Inflammation
  Felty syndrome
  SLE[a]
  Serum sickness
  Sarcoidosis
Congestive splenomegaly
  Intrahepatic
    Cirrhosis[a]
  Extrahepatic
    Portal vein obstruction
    Splenic vein obstruction
    Hepatic vein occlusion (Budd-Chiari syndrome)
  Chronic passive congestion
    Heart failure
Hematologic disorders
  Red cell disorders[a] (hemolytic anemias)
Tumors
  Malignant
    Myeloproliferative disorders
      Myeloid metaplasia[a]
      Polycythemia rubra vera
      Thrombocythemia
    Chronic leukemia
      Chronic myeloid leukemia[a]
      Chronic lymphocytic leukemia
      Hairy cell leukemia[a]
    Lymphoma
    Acute leukemia
    Metastatic solid tumors
  Benign
    Hamartoma
Storage disease
  Gaucher disease[a]
Miscellaneous
  Amyloidosis
  Cysts

[a] Disorders in which hypersplenism commonly occurs.

Pathogenesis

A list of the common disorders producing splenomegaly and hypersplenism is presented in Table 128-4. An increase in the size of the spleen can be caused by several mechanisms. An increase in the workload of the spleen can be due to immunologic stress (infection, inflammation, or an autoimmune disorder) or to increased red cell removal (red cell membrane disorders, hemoglobinopathies). Decreased venous drainage due to portal hypertension will also increase the size of the spleen and is termed congestive splenomegaly. Benign and malignant infiltrative disorders can also increase splenic size (infiltrative splenomegaly) and cause hypersplenism. Some of these disorders produce thrombocytopenia by more than just hypersplenism. These include marrow replacement by tumor, immune-mediated platelet clearance, and drug-induced marrow aplasia. Thus, the demonstration of an enlarged spleen by itself does not necessarily indicate hypersplenism.

Thrombocytopenia

The thrombocytopenia of hypersplenism is caused primarily by increased splenic platelet pooling.[18,25] A massively enlarged spleen can hold 90% of the total platelet mass. In the absence of pathologic platelet overproduction, the total body platelet mass is usually normal and the platelet life span is near-normal.[18] Usually, the splenic transit time remains normal (approximately 10 minutes), but the absolute number of platelets retained within the enlarged spleen is increased. All these platelets remain part of the exchangeable pool. In hypersplenism, the platelet count is usually $50-150 \times 10^9$/L, and only rarely $<20 \times 10^9$/L. Most patients are asymptomatic. Plasma volume expansion occurs in hypersplenism, but hemodilution plays a relatively minor role in the thrombocytopenia. Similarly, some patients have evidence of marrow suppression, but, again, its contribution to the thrombocytopenia tends to be modest.

Anemia

Sequestration and hemodilution combine to produce the anemia of hypersplenism.[28,29] An expansion of the plasma volume accompanies hypersplenism; the degree of expansion is proportional to the size of the spleen.[29-31] In the absence of persistent portal hypertension, this expansion can be improved or corrected by splenectomy.[31]

Neutropenia

The neutropenia of hypersplenism is caused by an increase in the marginated granulocyte pool, a portion of which is located in the spleen.[32-34] The neutropenia of hypersplenism is usually moderate in severity and, therefore, asymptomatic.

Diagnosis

The diagnosis of thrombocytopenia of hypersplenism is made by documenting a group of physical and laboratory findings. Splenomegaly is usually present, but may not be detectable by physical examination. An imaging technique should be used to confirm the splenomegaly. The thrombocytopenia is rarely severe and can be associated with a slight decrease in the MPV.[35] However, often the MPV is normal, and it can even be increased. An ^{111}In-labeled platelet survival study can be diagnostic of hypersplenism, demonstrating reduced platelet recovery and a normal platelet life span. Determining the cause of the splenomegaly is the most important issue.

Therapy

The choice of therapy is determined by three factors: (1) whether the hematologic abnormalities are solely due to the large spleen; (2) the symptomatic state of the patient; and (3) the underlying illness. Thrombocytopenia due to hypersplenism rarely causes bleeding and by itself seldom requires treatment. Indications for treatment other than bleeding include symptomatic anemia with transfusion dependence; recurrent infection due to neutropenia; or mechanical symptoms such as pain or early satiety that are related to the enlarged spleen.

Successful medical treatment of the primary disorder can lead to regression of the hypersplenism without the need for surgery. Examples include chemotherapy for a hematologic malignancy, antibiotics for an infection, and immunosuppression for autoimmune or inflammatory disorders. In congestive splenomegaly, the symptoms of hypersplenism are usually not the primary problem. Correction of the portal hypertension may not be possible without decompressive shunt surgery. In fact, shunt surgery without splenectomy can correct the cytopenias of congestive hypersplenism.[36]

Table 128-5. Considerations for Splenectomy in Hypersplenism

Hypersplenism is the principal cause of the thrombocytopenia.
The thrombocytopenia warrants treatment, and medical treatment will not correct the hypersplenism.
The splenomegaly is causing intractable local symptoms.
The cause of the splenomegaly is unknown.
The surgical risks are acceptable.

Splenectomy

Splenectomy is rarely done for hypersplenism per se, but some patients may benefit from splenectomy; the preoperative considerations are summarized in Table 128-5. A good result from splenectomy would consist of the relief of clinical symptoms due to the hypersplenism in conjunction with minimal morbidity as a result of the procedure. Symptomatic relief includes improved hemostasis and decreased infections, transfusions, and pain. Short-term complications from splenectomy include infections, bleeding, and thromboembolism. The major long-term risk of splenectomy is overwhelming septicemia, which can be reduced by vaccination.

Conditions in which the hypersplenism should be managed by splenectomy include Gaucher disease,[37] chronic hemolytic disorders (hereditary spherocytosis and certain hemoglobinopathies),[38,39] and rarely hairy cell leukemia (selected patients).[40-42] Many patients with hairy cell leukemia will ultimately require systemic therapy despite splenectomy, and chemotherapy is very effective (see Ch. 84). Hence, the role of splenectomy in hairy cell leukemia is diminishing.[43] Splenectomy can also be used to obtain a diagnosis, particularly if an isolated splenic lymphoma is suspected.[44]

Splenectomy has been used to improve the efficacy of other treatments. For example, splenectomy has been used in chronic myeloid leukemia for patients undergoing bone marrow transplantation. Earlier recovery of both platelet and granulocyte counts and a reduction in the number of transfusions were seen in the patients who had splenectomy.[45] No difference in survival between the two groups could be demonstrated.

Splenomegaly can be massive in certain myeloproliferative disorders, particularly myeloid metaplasia. Almost all patients with advanced disease have portal hypertension and painful splenomegaly. Although surgery has a beneficial effect on the symptoms of pain, less than one-half of the patients will have a significant improvement in the thrombocytopenia and anemia.[46] Furthermore, splenectomy is associated with a high morbidity (50%) and mortality (15%) in this disorder.[46,47] Consequently, splenectomy in myeloid metaplasia should be regarded as a palliative procedure with significant risks.

Splenectomy for congestive hypersplenism in the setting of portal hypertension has a high morbidity and mortality.[36,38] Consequently, the procedure is generally considered contraindicated in these patients.

Splenectomy in Gaucher disease usually corrects the cytopenias, relieves abdominal discomfort, and in children improves growth.[48] The issue of whether splenectomy can result in the increased deposition of glucocerebroside in bones instead of the spleen remains unresolved. Hence, some physicians have attempted to preserve residual splenic tissue by partial splenectomy or splenic embolization.[49-55] Experience with these approaches is limited, so they should be considered experimental. The impact of enzyme replacement therapy for Gaucher disease may alter its natural history and reduce the morbidity from hypersplenism (see Ch. 57).

DRUG-INDUCED THROMBOCYTOPENIC SYNDROMES

Many drugs and their metabolites can cause thrombocytopenia. Some drugs cause predictable thrombocytopenia via myelosuppressive (e.g., anticancer chemotherapy) or other

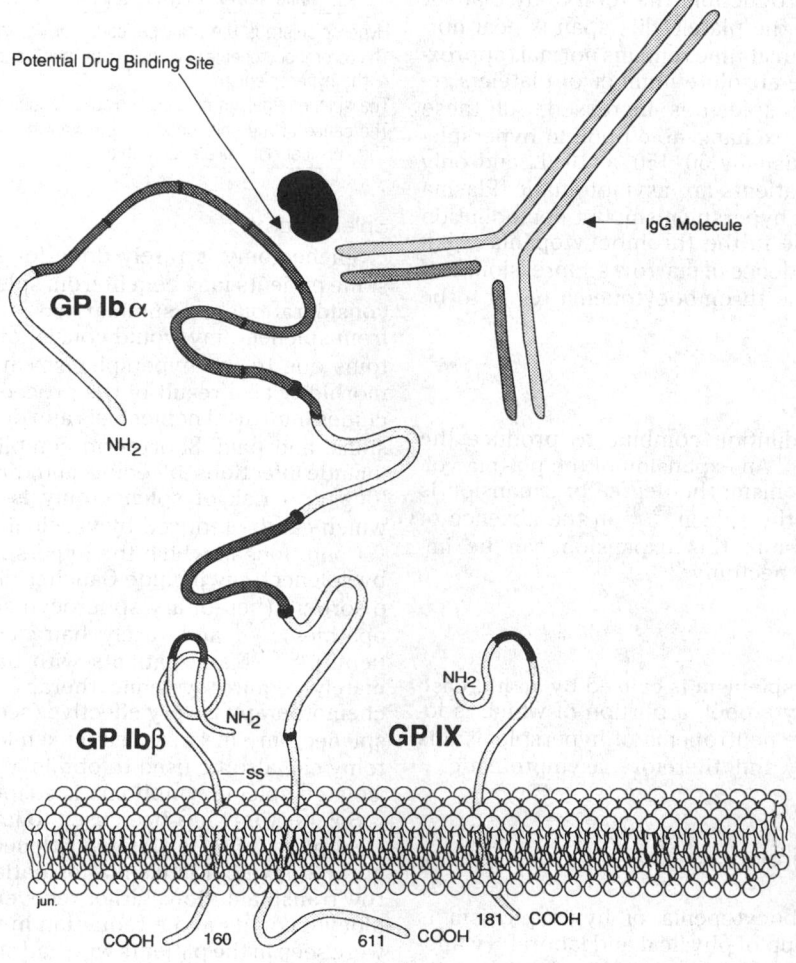

Fig. 128-1. Proposed binding of quinine/quinidine-induced thrombocytopenia.

mechanisms (e.g., ristocetin-induced platelet agglutination). However, an important disorder encountered by hematologists is unexpected thrombocytopenia caused by immunologic (idiosyncratic) mechanisms. The frequency of these reactions varies dramatically among drugs, and can be extremely rare for commonly used medicines such as acetaminophen, more frequent for agents such as quinine and quinidine, and surprisingly common for other drugs such as heparin and valproic acid.

Immunologic drug-induced thrombocytopenia can be divided into two general categories. The one group, which to date represents the largest number of drugs studied, but which may be clinically less important, is exemplified by quinine- and quinidine-induced thrombocytopenia. These disorders are mediated by the binding of the Fab terminus of IgG to a complex comprised of drug (or drug metabolite) and a platelet membrane component (typically platelet GPIb/IX or GPIIb/IIIa) (Fig. 128-1). The Fc portions of the immunoglobulin molecules are not involved in the binding to platelets and presumably are available for the Fc receptors on the phagocytic cells. Typically, moderate-to-severe thrombocytopenia with a platelet count often $<10 \times 10^9/L$ is observed in these patients, and they usually present with the abrupt onset of bleeding.

The other general type of drug-induced thrombocytopenia is exemplified by heparin-induced thrombocytopenia. The Fab portion of the IgG binds to a complex on the platelet surface comprised of heparin and platelet factor 4 (Fig. 128-2). The Fc portion of the IgG binds to the platelet Fc receptor, triggering platelet activation. Because the Fc portions of the IgG mole-

cules are bound to the platelet Fc receptors, they may not be available to the Fc receptors of the reticuloendothelial system, which may explain the less severe thrombocytopenia that characterizes heparin-induced thrombocytopenia.

Heparin-Induced Thrombocytopenia

Heparin is the most important cause of idiosyncratic drug-induced thrombocytopenia for several reasons. First, heparin is a widely used anticoagulant with an immediate onset of action, which makes it effective for the treatment and prophylaxis of thromboembolic disease; consequently, many patients receive this drug (see Chs. 121, 123, and 124). Second, heparin-induced thrombocytopenia (HIT) is relatively common, occurring in about 5% of patients who receive therapeutic doses of heparin for 5–14 days.[56] Finally, HIT can be complicated by arterial and venous thrombosis, which itself often is limb- or life-threatening.[56]

Pathogenesis

Heparin binds reversibly and saturably to platelets and can weakly activate platelets in vitro.[57] However, these nonidiosyncratic effects have not been linked to any clinical sequelae, although some believe they may be responsible for the early and mild platelet count falls that sometimes occur in patients receiving heparin. In general, the platelet-activating effects are proportional to the size and degree of sulfation of the heparin.

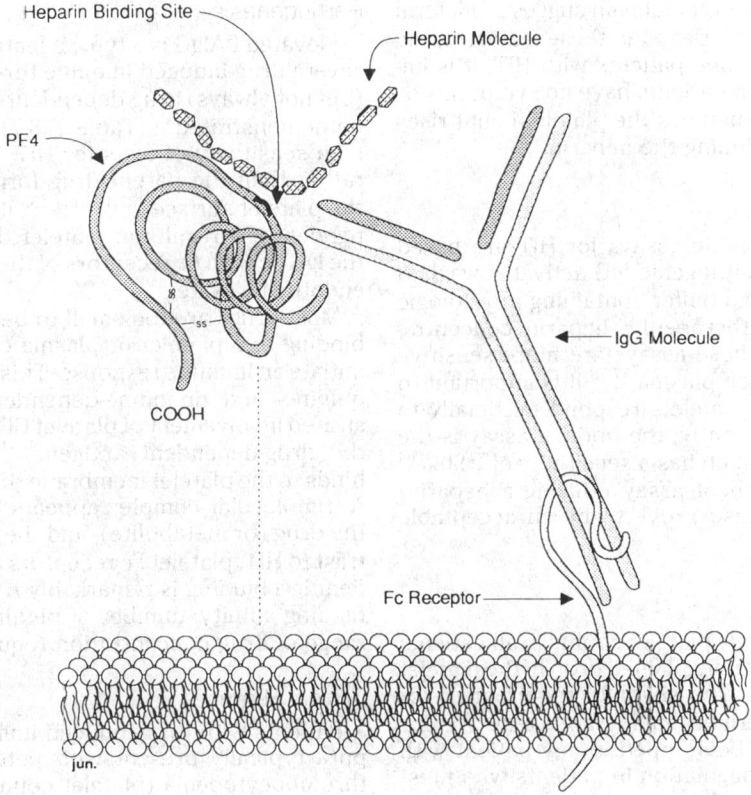

Fig. 128-2. Proposed binding of HIT.

HIT is caused by heparin-dependent IgG that activates platelets via their Fc receptors.[58,59] Work several years ago suggested that the antigen was a complex between heparin and a platelet component.[60] More recent studies indicate that the antigenic target may be a complex of heparin and platelet factor 4.[61-63] A unique laboratory characteristic of HIT is that large heparin concentrations (10–100 U/ml) inhibit platelet activation by the pathogenic IgG,[64] possibly by displacing the pathogenic IgG from surface-bound heparin/platelet factor 4 complex. This laboratory feature is exploited in diagnostic testing for HIT (see the section Diagnosis).

Potential explanations for the thrombotic complications seen in this syndrome include in vivo platelet activation and aggregation (including the generation of procoagulant microparticles[65]), activation of endothelial cells via cross-reactivity with endothelial heparan sulfate,[66] and neutralization of the anticoagulant effects of heparin. Recent studies suggest that the marked differences in clinical sequelae could be caused by platelet variability to Fc receptor stimuli[67,68] and comorbid clinical factors.[69]

A similar syndrome of thrombocytopenia and paradoxical thrombosis can also be caused by low-molecular-weight heparin,[70] as well as other high-sulfated polysaccharides such as pentosan polysulfate[71] and polysulfated chondroitin sulfate (Arteparon).[72]

Clinical Features

Most patients with HIT develop mild-to-moderate thrombocytopenia. The mean platelet count nadir in many series is approximately $50 \times 10^9/L$.[73] Rarely, the platelet count is as low as $10–20 \times 10^9/L$. DIC and mild red cell fragmentation can occur in these patients with severe thrombocytopenia. A high heparin requirement to maintain a therapeutic partial thromboplastin time (heparin resistance) is an occasional, but nonspecific, finding in patients with HIT.

The thrombocytopenia usually begins 5–10 days after the initiation of heparin therapy.[74] As many as 10–30% of the thrombocytopenic patients develop thrombotic complications,[73] usually during the initial phases of the thrombocytopenia. Both venous (deep vein thrombosis, pulmonary embolism, venous limb gangrene) and arterial (especially aortic and iliofemoral arterial thrombosis, cerebrovascular accidents, myocardial infarctions) thrombi have been described (Table 128-6). Other complications include dermal erythema or necrosis at the sites of subcutaneous heparin injection, and acute inflammatory[75] or transient memory disturbances[76] following heparin bolus injections to sensitized individuals (Table 128-6).

Table 128-6. Clinical Sequelae Associated with Heparin-Induced Thrombocytopenia

Venous thrombosis
   Deep vein thrombosis
   Phlegmasia cerulea dolens
   Venous gangrene of a limb[a]
   Pulmonary embolism
   Cerebral sinus thrombosis[b]
Arterial thrombosis
   Iliofemoral artery thrombosis
   Aortic thrombosis (may present with spinal cord infarction)
   Cerebral artery thrombosis (stroke syndrome)
   Myocardial infarction
   Miscellaneous thrombotic events (e.g., occlusion of mesenteric, renal, or spinal arteries)
Dermal manifestations
   Localized skin reactions at heparin injection sites
   Skin necrosis[a]
Sequelae of heparin intravenous bolus administration
   Acute systemic inflammatory reactions
   Transient global amnesia

[a] May be related to concomitant warfarin-induced necrosis.
[b] Associated with pregnancy.

Unexplained hypotension or abdominal pain suggests bilateral adrenal infarction/hemorrhage. Despite, these catastrophic thrombotic complications in some patients with HIT, it is important to emphasize that most patients have no symptoms or residual problems. Indeed, sometimes the platelet count rises to normal levels despite continuing the heparin.

Diagnosis

The most sensitive and specific assays for HIT are based on the observation that the pathogenic IgG activates washed normal platelets suspended in a buffer containing physiologic calcium concentrations and therapeutic heparin concentrations (0.05–0.3 U/ml).[64,67,77] These assays are more sensitive than use of citrated platelet-rich plasma.[77,78] It is important to select platelet donors whose platelets respond maximally to Fc receptor stimulation.[67] Currently, the optimal assay is the ^{14}C-serotonin release assay, which has a sensitivity of ≥90%.[64] An enzyme-linked immunosorbent assay utilizing a heparin/platelet factor 4 target may also prove to be an acceptable diagnostic test.[61]

Management

We recommend obtaining daily platelet counts in all patients receiving heparin therapy. Any unexplained drop in the platelet count should be investigated. The absolute requirement for anticoagulation should be verified angiographically. We believe that the heparin should be stopped in any patient with HIT. However, alternate anticoagulation in patients who must be anticoagulated is uncertain. Many physicians use warfarin, but disadvantages include slow onset of anticoagulant effect and possible initiation of warfarin-induced thrombotic complications in some patients with heparin-induced thrombocytopenia. We have used ancrod (Arvin, Knoll Pharmaceuticals), a defibrinogenating snake venom, for patients with HIT.[79] When ancrod is used, the warfarin should not be used until the clinical syndrome of HIT (thrombocytopenia) is resolving. The heparinoid Org 10172 (Orgaran, Organon-Teknika) has been used successfully in >200 patients with HIT.[80] In vitro cross-reactivity of the heparin-dependent IgG for the heparinoid is a potential disadvantage observed in approximately 10% of patients, although in vivo cross-reactivity (persisting thrombocytopenia, new or progressive thrombosis) may be less common. Low-molecular-weight heparin, which is usually cross-reactive in vitro for heparin-dependent IgG, has been associated with progressive thrombocytopenia and thrombosis in some patients with HIT, and its use cannot be recommended for the treatment of heparin-induced thrombocytopenia.[81]

The patient with a past history of HIT who requires future anticoagulation presents a problem, since the precise risk of recurrence is uncertain. If the heparin-dependent IgG is no longer detectable using sensitive testing, it may be acceptable to use heparin for a brief indication (e.g., open heart surgery using cardiopulmonary bypass).[82] Patients requiring immediate heart surgery have undergone surgery using alternate anticoagulants (ancrod,[83] Org 10172,[84] heparin/iloprost[85]), but each approach has certain drawbacks.

Drug-Induced Immune Thrombocytopenic Purpura

A large number of drugs can produce a syndrome that mimicks acute ITP[86–92] (Table 128-7[93–222]). Typically, these patients develop severe thrombocytopenia (platelet count usually <20 × 10^9/L) together with petechiae and purpura usually within weeks, but occasionally within years of starting drug therapy. These syndromes are much less common than HIT. For example, it is estimated that 1 in 1,000 patients exposed to quinine or quinidine will develop quinine-induced thrombocytopenia.[93]

Pathogenesis

Elevated PAIgG is a typical feature of almost all patients with severe drug-induced immune thrombocytopenia.[87] Sometimes (but not always) drug-dependent binding of IgG to platelets can be demonstrated[87] (Table 128-7). Contrast this with the very high sensitivity of tests for HIT. Sometimes drug metabolites rather than the parent drug form the antigenic structure on the platelet surface.[137,146,151,155] It is believed that the drug-dependent IgG results in platelet destruction via interaction of the IgG Fc with Fc receptors of the macrophages of the reticuloendothelial system.

Most drugs are too small to be immunogenic, and therefore binding to a platelet or plasma component may be critical to initiate an immune response. This is suggested by studies using quinine- and quinidine-dependent IgG, which have demonstrated involvement of platelet GPIIb/IIIa and GPIb/IX in forming the drug-dependent antigen.[97–100] The drug-dependent IgG binds to the platelet membrane through the Fab terminus.[101,102] A trimolecular complex appears to be formed among IgG-Fab, the drug (or metabolite), and the platelet glycoprotein. In contrast to HIT, platelet Fc receptors are not involved. Drug-dependent IgG binding is remarkably heterogeneous with respect to binding affinity, number of binding sites per platelet, and the range of drug concentration required.[103,104]

Clinical Features

Patients with drug-induced immune thrombocytopenic purpura typically present with petechiae, purpura, and severe thrombocytopenia (platelet count often <20 × 10^9/L). Sometimes systemic symptoms such as fever and chills occur in patients with abrupt-onset thrombocytopenia. Some drugs typically produce thrombocytopenia after the first week (sulfa drugs) or several weeks (carbamazepine) of therapy, but drug-induced thrombocytopenia can occur even after several years on a drug. Usually the platelet count begins to rise within a few days of discontinuing the implicated drug, but occasionally several weeks are required for recovery, possibly because of generation of drug-independent IgG (platelet autoantibodies).[87,111]

Diagnosis

A high index of clinical suspicion is often required to make the diagnosis. Quinine is an almost ubiquitous substance found in tonic water, aperitifs, soft drinks, and various over-the-counter medications. Clinicians must consider that patients can inadvertently or surreptitiously be exposed to prescription[107] or illicit drugs.[96,211,212]

Demonstration of drug-dependent binding of IgG to platelets in vitro is the preferred method of diagnosis. Use of labeled immunoglobulin-specific probes (phase II assays) or glycoprotein capture techniques (phase III assays) are preferable to the older, immunoglobulin-nonspecific assays such as platelet factor 3 generation (phase I assays). There are certain caveats in diagnostic testing. First, various metabolites rather than parent drug must sometimes be used to detect the IgG. Second, wash buffer in these assays must include the target drug (or metabolite). Third, even despite these maneuvers, the sensitivity of in vitro assays is relatively low, and the diagnosis of drug-induced thrombocytopenia should be based on clinical grounds, with laboratory confirmation, when possible. Sometimes, inadvertent or deliberate re-exposure to the suspected drug is diagnostic. However, deliberate drug rechallenge should not be performed because of the potential hazard.

Management

As many drugs as possible should be discontinued in patients with suspected drug-induced thrombocytopenia. If further drug treatment is necessary, an alternate, immunologi-

Table 128-7. Drug-Induced Immune Thrombocytopenic Purpura[a]

	Platelet Count <20 × 10⁹/L	Drug Rechallenge	Drug-Dependent in Vitro Testing	References
Quinine/quinidine group				
Quinine	Y	Y	Y(I, II, III)	93–104
Quinidine	Y	Y	Y(I, II, III)	93, 97–111
Gold salts				
Gold sodium thiomalate	Y	Y	Y(III)	87, 112–117
Auranofin (oral gold)	Y	Y	Y(II)	114, 118
Aurothioglucose	Y			119, 120
Antimicrobials				
Antimony-containing antimicrobials				
Stibophen	Y	Y	Y(I)	121
Sodium stibogluconate		Y		122
Cephalosporins				
Cefotetan	Y		Y(II)	123
Cephalothin sodium	Y	Y	Y(I)	124, 125
Cephamandole	Y		Y(III)	126
Gentamicin	Y	Y	Y(I)	127
Nalidixic acid	Y	Y		128
Penicillins				
Ampicillin	Y		Y(II)	87
Apalcillin	Y			129
Methicillin	Y	Y	Y(I)	130
Penicillin	Y		Y(II)	87, 131, 132
Piperacillin	Y	Y		133
Rifampin	Y	Y	Y(I, II)	134, 135
Sulfa antibiotics[b]				
Sulphamethoxazole	Y		Y(I, II)	136, 137
Sulphamethoxypyridazine	Y			138, 139
Sulphisoxazole	Y		Y(I)	92, 140
Suramin	Y			141
Trimethoprim	Y		Y(II)	142
Vancomycin	Y	Y	Y(III)	143, 144
Anti-inflammatory drugs				
Acetaminophen	Y	Y	Y(I)	145, 146
Salicylates				
Acetylsalicylic acid	Y		Y(I)	147, 148
Diflunisal	Y		Y(I)	149
Sodium para-aminosalicyclic acid	Y	Y	Y(I)	150, 151
Sulfasalazine	Y	Y		152
Other nonsteroidal anti-inflammatory drugs				
Diclofenac	Y			153
Fenoprofen	Y			154
Ibuprofen			Y(II)	155
Indomethacin	Y			156
Meclofenamate	Y	Y		157
Oxyphenbutazone	Y			158–160
Phenylbutazone				161, 162
Piroxicam	Y		Y(III)	163
Sulindac				164
Tolmetin	Y	Y	Y(I)	165
Cardiac and antihypertensive drugs				
Positive inotropic drugs				
Amrinone		Y		166, 167
Digitoxin		Y	Y(I)	168
Digoxin		Y	Y(I)	169
Antiarrhythmic drugs				
Amiodarone	Y	Y		170
Procainamide	Y	Y		171, 172
Quinidine (see above)				
β-Blockers				
Alprenolol	Y	Y		173, 174
Oxprenolol	Y	Y		175, 176

(Table continues)

Table 128-7. *(Continued)*

	Platelet Count <20 × 10⁹/ L	Drug Rechallenge	Drug-Dependent in Vitro Testing	References
Miscellaneous antihypertensive agents				
Captopril	Y			177
Diazoxide[c]		Y		178, 179
α-Methyldopa	Y	Y	Y(I)	180
Diuretics				
Acetazolamide[d]	Y		Y(I)	181
Chlorothiazide	Y	Y	Y(I)	91, 182
Chlorthalidone			Y(I)	90
Furosemide	Y	Y	Y(I)	183
Hydrochlorothiazide	Y	Y	Y(I)	184
Spironolactone	Y		Y(I)	91
Benzodiazepines				
Diazepam	Y	Y	Y(I, II)	92, 185
Antiepileptic drugs				
Carbamazepine	Y		Y(I)	186, 187
Diphenylhydantoin	Y		Y(I)	92
Valproic acid	Y	Y		188–190
H₂-antagonists				
Cimetidine	Y	Y	Y(II)	87, 191, 192
Ranitidine			Y(II)	193, 194
Sulfonylurea hypoglycemic drugs				
Chlorpropamide	Y			195, 196
Glibenclamide (glyburide)	Y			197
Iodinated contrast agents				
Diatrizoate sodium/meglumine	Y	Y		198, 199
Iocetamic acid	Y			200
Iopanoic acid	Y	Y	Y(I)	201–230
Sodium ipodate	?	?	?	204
Retinoids				
Isotretinoin	Y	Y		205, 206
Etretinate				207
Antihistamines				
Antazoline	Y	Y	Y(I)	208, 209
Chlorpheniramine	Y	Y	Y(I)	210
Illicit drugs				
Cocaine	Y			211
Heroin	Y	Y		212
Quinine contaminant ("filler")	Y		Y(I, II)	96
Antidepressants				
Tricyclic antidepressants				
Amitriptyline	Y			213
Desipramine			Y(I)	214
Doxepin	Y			213
Imipramine			Y(I)	90
Tetracyclic antidepressants				
Mianserin	Y	Y	Y(I)	215
Antineoplastic drugs				
Actinomycin D	Y	Y		216
Aminoglutethimide	Y	Y		217
Miscellaneous drugs				
Danazol	Y	Y		218
Desferrioxamine		Y		219
Lidocaine	Y	Y	Y(I)	220
Morphine	Y		Y(I)	221
Ticlopidine			Y(II)	222

[a] Some of the evidence implicating the drugs is shown, including severity of the thrombocytopenia, drug rechallenge, and in vitro testing. In vitro testing is classified as phase I (IgG-nonspecific end points such as platelet aggregation, platelet factor 3 generation, clot retraction inhibition, and so forth), phase II (drug-dependent platelet-associated IgG), and phase III (drug-dependent binding to specific platelet glycoproteins). Note that this table excludes drugs of historical importance that are no longer clinically used (e.g., Sedormid[88,89]).

[b] Several other sulfa antibiotics have also been reported to cause immune thrombocytopenia.

[c] Although classified here as an antihypertensive, note that diazoxide is a thiazide derivative.

[d] Although classified here as a diuretic, note that acetazolamide is a sulfonamide derivative.

ally non-cross-reactive substitute should be prescribed. Platelet transfusions should be given to patients with life-threatening bleeding. The transfused platelets will be rapidly destroyed but may be clinically effective before their destruction. In addition, the transfused platelets may facilitate the clearance of the circulating drug-dependent antibody. High-dose intravenous γ-globulin (1 mg/kg given over 6–8 hours) or two consecutive days, is a generally effective treatment for drug-induced immune thrombocytopenia.[108,109]

Gold-Induced Thrombocytopenia

Gold-induced immune thrombocytopenic purpura is a relatively common complication of gold therapy (approximately 1–3% of treated patients).[112] The incidence may be lower with the oral gold preparation.[118] A genetic predisposition to gold-induced thrombocytopenia is suggested by the association with HLA-DR3, which is found in approximately 85% of these patients.[112,113]

The thrombocytopenia typically occurs during the first 20 weeks of therapy, before 1,000 mg of gold has been given.[112] However, in some patients gold-induced thrombocytopenia begins several years into treatment, or even several months after discontinuation of the gold.[117] Although the onset of thrombocytopenia is typically abrupt,[113] regular platelet count monitoring is important since an early diagnosis can be made in some patients.

An important treatment consideration is that the thrombocytopenia often persists for several months despite discontinuation of the gold. It is debated whether this is caused by gold-induced autoimmune thrombocytopenia[119] or whether prolonged release of gold from tissue stores permits a long-term drug-dependent thrombocytopenia[87,114] to occur. Most patients respond to corticosteroids. Immediate, usually transient correction of severe thrombocytopenia can often be achieved with high-dose intravenous γ-globulin.[115] Some patients with persisting thrombocytopenia benefit by splenectomy or gold-chelating agents (dimercaprol, N-acetylcysteine).

Drug-Induced Thrombotic Microangiopathy

Several drugs can trigger a syndrome of thrombocytopenia, fragmentation hemolysis, and renal failure (drug-induced hemolytic uremic syndrome) (see Ch. 127). This syndrome has been best established for quinine[223–226]; some investigators have detected quinine-dependent antigranulocyte[224,225] and antiendothelial IgG[226] in addition to platelet-reactive IgG. Although a similar syndrome appears to be caused by mitomycin C,[227,228] cyclosporine,[229] and penicillamine,[230] it should be noted that many patients who receive these drugs have underlying illness (gastric adenocarcinoma, bone marrow transplantation, collagen vascular disease, respectively) that are themselves associated with hemolytic uremic syndrome. It is possible that thrombotic thrombocytopenic purpura can be caused by the antiplatelet drug ticlopidine.[231] Plasma exchange may be needed for some patients with severe drug-induced hemolytic uremic syndrome (see Ch. 127).[223]

MISCELLANEOUS DRUG-INDUCED THROMBOCYTOPENIC SYNDROMES

Drug-Induced Immune Bicytopenia and Pancytopenia

Rarely, drug-dependent IgG can cause peripheral destruction of red or white cells in addition to platelets. In some cases, investigators have demonstrated distinct drug-dependent IgG

(e.g., both platelet- and leukocyte-reactive quinidine-dependent IgG for quinidine-induced bicytopenia[110]). In other cases, immune mechanisms are capable of injuring a pluripotent hematopoietic stem cell, resulting in pancytopenia accompanied by marrow aplasia or hypoplasia (e.g., gold-induced pancytopenia, carbamazepine-induced pancytopenia, quinidine-induced pancytopenia[232]). A bone marrow aspirate should be performed in patients with suspected drug-induced bicytopenia or pancytopenia, as a hypoplastic marrow can indicate the serious complication of drug-induced aplastic anemia.

Nonidiosyncratic Drug-Induced Pancytopenia

Most antineoplastic drugs produce a dose-dependent pancytopenia caused by nonidiosyncratic injury to hematopoietic cells, including megakaryocytes and their progenitor cells. Typically, the platelet count nadir occurs at a predictable period following treatment and then quickly recovers. Unexpectedly severe or prolonged thrombocytopenia in patients receiving chemotherapy should suggest alternate explanations for the thrombocytopenia.[143,216]

Immediate Drug-Induced Thrombocytopenia

Some drugs result in immediate but generally mild and transient drops in the platelet count. These agents include heparin,[233] protamine,[234] bleomycin,[235] hematin,[236,237] ristocetin[238] (no longer clinically used), desmopressin (particularly in patients with type IIb von Willebrand disease[239]), and porcine factor VIII.[240] For some of these drugs, mild platelet activation/agglutination has been described. However, no clinically adverse sequelae to these effects have been established. In our experience, some immediate thrombocytopenic reactions to heparin were proved to be IgG-mediated HIT in patients who were recently sensitized to heparin via occult heparin exposure (e.g., uncharted intraoperative catheter flushes with heparin).

Drug Hypersensitivity Reactions

Mild-to-moderate thrombocytopenia is sometimes observed in patients with systemic drug hypersensitivity reactions. Comorbid clinical features can include generalized rashes, fever, cholestasis, and leukopenia. Allopurinol,[241] isoniazid,[242] sulphasalazine,[243] and phenothiazine drugs,[244,245] among others, have been implicated in these reactions.

Immune Thrombocytopenia Secondary to Biologic Response Modifiers

Use of purified or recombinant biologic response modifiers such as interferon,[246,247] interleukin-2,[248–250] and certain colony-stimulating factors[251,252] has resulted in some patients developing severe, reversible, destructive thrombocytopenia. An immune mechanism for interferon-induced thrombocytopenia is suggested by elevated platelet-associated IgG levels. Antilymphocyte globulins can also produce severe thrombocytopenia in some patients.[253,254]

OTHER CAUSES OF DESTRUCTIVE THROMBOCYTOPENIA

Incidental Thrombocytopenia of Pregnancy

Maternal thrombocytopenia occurs in 5–7% of pregnancies.[255,256] Most of these women are healthy, have no prior history of thrombocytopenia, and are incidentally detected by routine blood testing. The cause of the mild reduction in platelet count (usually $100–150 \times 10^9$/L) is unknown. This condition is entirely benign, without an increased risk of maternal bleeding or neonatal thrombocytopenia.[255–258] Accordingly, no special obstetric maneuvers are indicated in these women (see Ch. 125).

Pre-eclampsia/Eclampsia

Pre-eclampsia is a disorder unique to pregnancy, characterized by the onset of hypertension and proteinuria, especially in a primigravida near term.[259] It complicates approximately 5% of pregnancies.[259] Pre-eclampsia is often associated with subclinical or clinical evidence of hemostatic and hepatic abnormalities. Thrombocytopenia occurs in 15–20% of pre-eclamptic patients and in about 40–50% of eclamptic patients.[260–261] In addition, some pre-eclamptic patients have evidence of a platelet function defect, exhibiting a prolonged bleeding time despite a normal platelet count.[262]

A subset of patients with pre-eclampsia have microangiopathic hemolysis, elevated liver enzymes, and low platelets.[263,264] This condition usually indicates severe pre-eclampsia and may be associated with a higher risk of maternal and fetal complications.[265,266] Repeated clinical and laboratory assessment of these patients is important, as this syndrome can mimic other life-threatening complications of pregnancy, such as overt DIC, thrombotic thrombocytopenic purpura, septicemia, or acute fatty liver of pregnancy.[267,268]

Although several studies[269–271] have suggested that increased platelet destruction is the mechanism for the thrombocytopenia, the pathogenesis remains controversial. Using sensitive measures of thrombin generation, our group did not find evidence of DIC in a prospective study of 61 pre-eclamptic patients.[272] However, some investigators have demonstrated elevated levels of D dimer[261,273,274] and thrombin/antithrombin complexes,[273,275] together with reduced antithrombin III levels,[273,275,276] in pre-eclamptic patients. Moreover, the highest D-dimer levels tended to occur in the patients with the most severe pre-eclampsia and thrombocytopenia and were associated with increased maternal and neonatal morbidity.[274] Together, these studies suggest that in a few patients, thrombin generation may contribute to the thrombocytopenia, but it is unlikely to be the major mechanism in most patients.

Elevated PAIgG is found commonly in pre-eclampsia-associated thrombocytopenia,[272,277] suggesting that immune mechanisms could contribute to the platelet destruction. However, it is also possible that elevated PAIgG is a nonspecific marker for increased platelet turnover.[278] Decreased endothelial prostacyclin synthesis[279] is a potential explanation for increased platelet activation and turnover[280] in pre-eclampsia. Also consistent with in vivo platelet activation are studies indicating that low-dose aspirin can prevent pre-eclampsia in high-risk patients.[281,282]

Delivery is the treatment of choice for pre-eclampsia and will usually result in resolution of the thrombocytopenia within a few days. Because of the associated hemostatic defects, some physicians recommend demonstrating a normal bleeding time in moderately thrombocytopenic patients before performing epidural anesthesia in this group of patients.[261] In those patients in whom delivery is not an option (i.e., premature fetus), treatment with bed rest and aggressive antihypertensive therapy has been reported to lead to an improvement in the platelet count. However, the clinical course is markedly variable, and some patients develop life-threatening organ failure or bleeding complications or fetal/neonatal morbidity and mortality.[265,283]

Infection

Infection is a common cause of thrombocytopenia, occurring in approximately 50–75% of patients with bacteremia or fungemia, and almost 100% of patients with septic shock or DIC.[284–288] Thrombocytopenia also complicates many viral and parasitic infections. Most often, the thrombocytopenia is mild-to-moderately severe, and is not accompanied by coagulation abnormalities or bleeding complications. However, the likelihood of laboratory or clinical evidence for DIC increases as the platelet count falls to $<50 \times 10^9$/L.

The thrombocytopenia is caused by increased platelet destruction, evidenced by reduced platelet survival,[284] increased numbers of marrow megakarocytes,[286] and large platelets observed in the peripheral blood film. PAIgG levels are usually elevated[3,284,289,290] and are inversely proportional to the platelet count.[284] Some investigators have reported increased levels of circulating immune complexes[291] and platelet-reactive autoantibodies in patients with septicemia.[292] Evidence for the adsorption of microbial antigens to the platelet membrane with subsequent antibody binding by the Fab terminus has been shown in the thrombocytopenia of malaria.[293]

In a subset of patients with severe infection-induced thrombocytopenia, thrombin (DIC) contributes to the platelet destruction. However, thrombin-dependent platelet destruction is not the primary mechanism in most patients.[285] Other potential explanations for thrombocytopenia include endothelial injury resulting in increased platelet consumption, platelet activation by endogenous mediators of inflammation (e.g., platelet-activating factor[294]), microbe-induced platelet activation,[295,296] dimished marrow platelet production, and hypersplenism.

Unexplained thrombocytopenia in any hospitalized patient should prompt a search to exclude a focus of infection, including blood cultures. Prompt recognition and treatment of the infection is the most important therapy. Recovery of the platelet count tends to parallel the resolution of the infection. Prophylactic platelet transfusions are generally not required unless the platelet count falls to $<10–20 \times 10^9$/L, or unless comorbid clinical features increase the likelihood of serious bleeding (e.g., concomitant coagulopathy, invasive procedure, uremic or antibiotic-induced platelet dysfunction). The use of heparin for patients with septic shock or DIC is controversial (see Ch. 116). However, heparin may benefit a subset of patients with clinical evidence of DIC and microvascular thrombosis[287] (e.g., meningococcemia with acral tissue necrosis), and we would use it in these patients.

Systemic Lupus Erythematosus

Thrombocytopenia is a common feature of SLE, occurring in as many as 25% of patients.[297–299] Some patients who are initially considered to have ITP subsequently are shown to have SLE.[300] They can be identified by a high titer of antinuclear antibody and possibly by reactivity to nuclear antigens such as SS-A.[301]

The thrombocytopenia of SLE is immune mediated. However, many different types of platelet-IgG interactions are described (antiglycoprotein,[302,303] antiglycolipid,[304] antiphospholipid,[305] platelet-reactive immune complexes[306]), and the predominant explanation for thrombocytopenia is unknown. Elevated PAIgG, usually with a normal platelet life span, is also observed in some SLE patients with normal platelet counts.[90,307,308] This can be explained by the impaired reticuloendothelial function in SLE, which reduces clearance of IgG-sensitized platelets.[309–311]

Several thrombocytopenic syndromes are seen in SLE patients. For many patients, the thrombocytopenia is chronic, resembling ITP, and is the predominant clinical manifestation of the lupus.[298] Bleeding symptoms may be more frequent in a subgroup of patients with prolonged bleeding times and platelet function abnormalities despite relatively mild thrombocytopenia.[312] Some thrombocytopenic SLE patients have antiphospholipid antibodies and are at increased risk of thrombotic rather than bleeding complications.[313,314] Acute, severe thrombocytopenia can be a prominent feature of patients with a severe multisystem exacerbation of lupus.[298] Rarely, patients with SLE develop an illness that resembles thrombotic thrombocytopenic purpura.[315–317]

Treatment of the thrombocytopenia of SLE is similar to that of ITP (see Ch. 125). Corticosteroids are the first line of therapy, but many patients do not respond or require high doses. This can produce serious adverse effects such as avascular necrosis of the femoral head. Before proceeding to splenectomy, we usually try danazol (an attenuated androgen), in doses of 200–1,200 mg/day.[318–320] This agent reduces phagocytic cell Fc receptor expression.[321] Sometimes several weeks are required to see a benefit. The efficacy of splenectomy in SLE is controversial. Although many patients respond, the overall success rate appears to be lower than for ITP, with a higher operative morbidity.[322–324] Patients with refractory thrombocytopenia can benefit from more aggressive therapies, including high-dose intravenous γ-globulin,[325,326] azathioprine,[327] plasmapheresis,[328] cyclophosphamide plus plasmapheresis,[329] and cyclosporine.[330]

Antiphospholipid Antibody Syndrome

The antiphospholipid antibody syndrome is a clinicopathologic disorder characterized by a wide spectrum of clinical events (particularly thrombosis and recurrent miscarriages) associated with antibodies that recognize a complex of negatively charged phospholipid and a protein cofactor known as β_2-glycoprotein I[331–335] (see Ch. 119). Many patients with this syndrome have thrombocytopenia, which is typically mild and intermittent. The antiphospholipid antibody syndrome should be considered in patients who develop unexplained, multiple, or unusual large vessel thrombosis (e.g., involving cardiac valves,[336] mesenteric vessels,[337] or large limb arteries[338]) or microvascular thrombosis (e.g., nonblanching red or blue macules on hands and feet, symmetric digital gangrene, cutaneous ulcers, livedo reticularis).[339–341]

Antiphospholipid antibodies are usually identified using solid-phase enzyme-linked immunoassays with purified phospholipids (usually cardiolipin) as target antigens, or via the inhibition of certain phospholipid-dependent coagulation assays (lupus anticoagulant). The protein cofactor for the lupus anticoagulant has been identified as prothrombin.[342] Although antiphospholipid antibodies are frequently detected in patients with SLE, they can also be found in patients with other autoimmune disorders, malignancy, or infections, or as a complication of certain drugs. Often no associated condition is identified (primary antiphospholipid antibody syndrome).[343]

The mechanism of the prothrombotic tendency remains elusive, but interference with endothelial prostacyclin formation,[344] impaired fibrinolysis,[345] impaired protein C activation[346] or activity,[347] and antibody binding to platelets[348,349] have all been described. It is not known whether the antiphospholipid antibodies or other factors mediate the increased platelet destruction.[350]

Specific treatment for the thrombocytopenia is usually not required. For many patients, long-term anticoagulant or antiplatelet therapy, or both, are needed to prevent recurrent thromboses (see Ch. 119). Some clinical observations suggest that corticosteroid treatment may exacerbate certain thrombotic complications.[351] Others have noted a benefit from corticosteroid therapy. At present, anticoagulant therapy for asymptomatic patients without a prior history of thrombosis is not indicated.

Malignancy

Thrombocytopenia complicating malignant disorders most frequently results from antineoplastic treatment or marrow replacement by tumor. However, certain thrombocytopenic syndromes have been associated with malignancy, including autoimmune thrombocytopenia, DIC, and thrombotic microangiopathy.

Immune thrombocytopenia has been described in patients with Hodgkin disease,[352] non-Hodgkin lymphoma,[353] and chronic lymphocytic leukemia.[354] Platelet glycoprotein-reactive autoantibodies have been identified in some patients.[355] Sometimes the thrombocytopenia responds to treatment of the neoplasm, although in some patients (particularly those with Hodgkin disease) the thrombocytopenia is indistinguishable from ITP and is not related to the activity of the lymphoma (see Ch. 125).

Chronic DIC occurs in certain malignancies, particularly adenocarcinomas of the pancreas, stomach, lung, colon, breast, and prostate.[356–358] Some patients present with venous or arterial thrombosis, and in these patients the presence of thrombocytopenia is an important clue that should prompt specific investigations for DIC. In our experience, the platelet count typically rises to normal or even elevated levels during heparin therapy; however, recurrent thrombosis and relapse of the thrombocytopenia can occur within hours or days of discontinuing the heparin therapy, even with a therapeutic warfarin effect. DIC with hemorrhagic is more characteristically seen in acute leukemia (especially French-American-British classification subtypes M3, M4, and M5[359]) and in prostate adenocarcinoma.

A destructive thrombocytopenic disorder that resembles hemolytic uremic syndrome or thrombotic thrombocytopenic purpura has been described in patients with adenocarcinoma of the breast and colon.[227,228] It can occur either during remission or with active disease. This syndrome has a high female prevalence with a frequent history of therapy with mitomycin C. DIC is not usually present. Some patients respond to plasmapheresis or protein A immunoadsorption.[360]

Hemophagocytic Syndrome

The hemophagocytic syndrome is characterized by pancytopenia and morphologic evidence of phagocytosis of red cells, granulocytes, and platelets by reactive macrophages. Some patients have an illness characterized by high fever, weight loss, prominent hepatosplenomegaly, severe pancytopenia, elevated liver enzymes, and a terminal infection.[361,362] T-cell lymphomas are the usual explanation for this dramatic illness.[361–364] However, similar patients with fulminant illness have been described following otherwise unremarkable bacterial[365] or viral infections (particularly the Epstein-Barr virus[366–368]). In some cases, the viral infection could have initiated a lymphoma[367]; in others, the infection may represent the initial manifestation of a lymphoma accompanied by a severe immunocompromised state. Re-evaluation of archival tissue suggests that many patients initially diagnosed as having histiocytic medullary reticulosis[369] may have had hemophagocytosis associated with T-cell lymphoma.[362]

Severe, but reversible, hemophagocytosis can be seen in patients with certain unusual infections (e.g., babesiosis,[370,371] ehrlichiosis[372]). Hemophagocytosis has also been observed in patients with SLE,[373] Still disease,[374] and infection with the human immunodeficiency virus.[375] Treatment should be directed at the underlying illness, with blood product support as needed.

Renal Transplantation

Thrombocytopenia can occur during episodes of renal allograft rejection.[376] It is possible that platelet activation and deposition in the renal vasculature contribute to the rejection process.[377] Destructive thrombocytopenia can also complicate the administration of antithymocyte globulin used in the treatment of renal transplant rejection.[254] Immunosuppressive agents such as azathioprine can cause thrombocytopenia by marrow suppression.

Bone Marrow Transplantation

Early, severe thrombocytopenia caused by marrow-ablative therapy invariably accompanies allogeneic and autologous bone marrow transplantation (BMT). In addition, several thrombocytopenic syndromes can occur later in the post-transplant course. The first is a transient decline in the platelet count that occurs within the first 2 months following an initially normal pattern of platelet count recovery.[378,379] Adverse effects of drugs (e.g., trimethoprim-sulfamethoxazole),[378] transient infections, and autoimmune platelet destruction accompanying the initial donor immune system engraftment[379] have been implicated.

A second type of BMT-related thrombocytopenia, which occurs in approximately 25% of bone marrow recipients, is characterized by chronic thrombocytopenia, which persists despite recovery of the other cell lines.[378,380] Often there is associated graft-versus-host or veno-occlusive disease, and the prognosis is poor.[378,380,381] Immune platelet destruction has also been implicated in this disorder.[378,380] The thrombocytopenia sometimes responds to increased immunosuppressive drugs, but many patients succumb to graft-versus-host disease.[380]

Less common is a syndrome of chronic, isolated thrombocytopenia, which begins several months after normal peripheral blood counts have been established. Immune platelet destruction has been demonstrated in several patients and can respond to corticosteroids, intravenous γ-globulin, and splenectomy.[382] Rarely, alloimmune platelet destruction can be caused by residual recipient lymphoid cells that recognize the Pl[A1] alloantigen on donor marrow-derived platelets.[383]

A syndrome of thrombocytopenia, red cell fragmentation, and renal impairment can occur in as many as 10% of BMT patients, usually beginning 3–12 months following transplantation (BMT-associated hemolytic uremic syndrome).[384] The hematologic abnormalities can be mild and remit spontaneously, although patients often have residual azotemia and hypertension. More severely affected patients can benefit from plasma exchange. Unfortunately, the syndrome has a poor overall prognosis and many patients will die irrespective of any intervention.

Cardiopulmonary Bypass Surgery

Excess bleeding is an important problem in patients who undergo heart surgery utilizing cardiopulmonary bypass.[385] Most of these patients receive blood transfusions, and approximately 5% require urgent reoperation for postoperative bleeding.[385]

Thrombocytopenia and transient platelet dysfunction is characteristically seen. Typically, the platelet count falls by 33–50%, primarily due to hemodilution,[386] but also secondary to bleeding and contact with the extracorporeal perfusion device.[387] The bleeding time rises markedly during heart surgery (>30 minutes), but usually improves to <15 minutes shortly after surgery, and to normal several hours later.[386] By contrast, the thrombocytopenia persists for 3–4 days, followed by recovery of the platelet count to values exceeding the preoperative baseline.

The pathogenesis and clinical significance of platelet dysfunction in these patients remains controversial. Several studies have implicated a transient, *intrinsic* defect in platelet function[386,388] (see Ch. 130). For example, decreased in vitro platelet aggregation,[386,388,389] decreased platelet surface membrane proteins,[390–392] selective depletion of platelet α-granules,[386] and evidence for in vivo platelet activation[386,390,393] and platelet vesiculation[390,394] have been described. However, a recent study suggested that the prolonged bleeding times in heart surgery patients could be attributed to an *extrinsic* platelet defect resulting from thrombin inhibition by the high doses of heparin.[395] The issue is further complicated by the potential role of other factors in explaining bleeding in some patients, including hyperfibrinolysis,[388] dilutional coagulopathy,[386] residual heparin effect (including heparin rebound), and preoperative use of aspirin.[396] Treatment of platelet dysfunction after cardiopulmonary bypass surgery is discussed in Chapter 130.

Thrombocytopenia Associated with Cardiovascular Disease

Congenital Cyanotic Heart Disease

Thrombocytopenia caused by a decrease in platelet life span occurs in some patients with severe cyanotic congenital heart disease.[397–399] Bleeding occurs in a few patients and can be related to platelet function defects,[397,400] coagulopathy,[401,402] or hyperfibrinolysis.[403] Reducing the hematocrit by phlebotomy and plasma infusion has been reported to improve the hemostatic defects.[402,404]

Valvular Heart Disease

Although increased platelet turnover is common in valvular heart disease,[405] mild thrombocytopenia occurs infrequently.[406] The pathogenesis of the platelet consumption is not well understood but could be related to increased platelet-von Willebrand factor interactions at high shear.[407] Indeed, high-molecular-weight multimers of von Willebrand factor are reduced in some of these patients,[408] suggesting a possible explanation for the characteristic bleeding from gastrointestinal angiodysplasia observed in some patients with aortic stenosis or hypertrophic cardiomyopathy.[409]

Pulmonary Vascular Disorders

Disorders characterized by pulmonary hypertension can be accompanied by thrombocytopenia, the pathogenesis of which is poorly defined.[410,411] Thrombocytopenia has also been reported to occur in association with occult pulmonary embolism,[412,413] possibly as a result of mild DIC, and in adult respiratory distress syndrome.[414]

REFERENCES

1. Berkman N, Michaeli Y, Or R, Eldor A: EDTA-dependent pseudothrombocytopenia: a clinical study of 18 patients and a review of the literature. Am J Hematol 36:195, 1991
2. Bizzaro N: Platelet satellitosis to polymorphonuclears: cytochemical, immunological, and ultrastructural characterization of eight cases. Am J Hematol 36:235, 1991
3. Mueller-Eckhardt C, Kayser W, Mersch-Baumert K et al: The clinical significance of platelet associated IgG: a study on 298 patients with various disorders. Br J Haematol 46:123, 1980
4. Kelton JG, Powers PJ, Carter CJ: A prospective study of the usefulness of the measurement of platelet-associated IgG for the diagnosis of idiopathic thrombocytopenic purpura. Blood 60:1050, 1982
5. Kelton JG, Murphy WG, Lucarelli A et al: A prospective comparison of four techniques for measuring platelet-associated IgG. Br J Haematol 71:97, 1989
6. Kiefel V, Santoso S, Weisheit M, Mueller-Eckhardt C: Monoclonal antibody-specific immobilization of platelet antigens (MAIPA): a new tool for the identification of platelet-reactive antibodies. Blood 70:1722, 1987

7. Kiefel V: The MAIPA assay and its applications in immunohaematology. Transf Med 2:181, 1992

8. Woods VL Jr, Oh EH, Mason D, McMillan R: Autoantibodies against the platelet glycoprotein IIb/IIIa complex in patients with chronic ITP. Blood 63:368, 1984

9. Woods VL Jr, Kurata Y, Montgomery RR et al: Autoantibodies against platelet glycoprotein Ib in patients with chronic immune thrombocytopenic purpura. Blood 64:156, 1984

10. Beutler E: Platelet transfusions: the 20,000/μL trigger. Blood 81:1411, 1993

11. Schiffer CA: Prophylatic platelet transfusion. Transfusion 32:295, 1992

12. Baer MR, Bloomfield CD: Controversies in transfusion medicine. Prophylatic platelet transfusion therapy: pro. Transfusion 32:377, 1992

13. Patten E: Controversies in transfusion medicine. Prophylatic platelet transfusion revisited after 25 years: con. Transfusion 32:381, 1992

14. McVay PA, Toy PTCY: Lack of increased bleeding after liver biopsy in patients with mild hemostatic abnormalities. Am J Clin Pathol 94:747, 1990

15. McVay PA, Toy PTCY: Lack of increased bleeding after paracentesis and thoracentesis in patients with mild coagulation abnormalities. Transfusion 31:164, 1991

16. Gmür J, Burger J, Schanz U, Fehr J, Schaffner A: Safety of stringent prophylactic platelet transfusion policy for patients with acute leukaemia. Lancet 338:1223, 1991

17. Sills RH: Splenic function: physiology and splenic hypofunction. CRC Crit Rev Oncol Hematol 7:1, 1987

18. Aster RH: Pooling of platelets in the spleen: role in the pathogenesis of "hypersplenic" thrombocytopenia. J Clin Invest 45:645, 1966

19. Peters AM: Splenic blood flow and blood cell kinetics. Clin Haematol 12: 421, 1983

20. Wadenvik H, Jacobsson S, Kutti J, Syrjälä M: In vitro and in vivo behavior of ^{111}In-labelled platelets: an experimental study of healthy male volunteers. Eur J Haematol 38:415, 1987

21. Peters AM, Klonizakis I, Lavender JP, Lewis SM: Use of [111]Indium-labelled platelets to measure spleen function. Br J Haematol 46:587, 1980

22. Peters AM, Walport MJ, Bell RN, Lavender JP: Methods of measuring splenic blood flow and platelet transit time with In-111-labeled platelets. J Nucl Med 25:86, 1984

23. Wadenvik H, Kutti J: The effect of an isoprenaline infusion on the splenic blood flow and intrasplenic platelet kinetics. Eur J Haematol 39:7, 1987

24. Fredén K, Olsson L-B, Suurküla M, Kutti J: The exchangeable splenic platelet pool in response to intravenous infusion of isoprenaline. Scand J Haematol 20:335, 1978

25. Wadenvik H, Denfors I, Kutti J: Splenic blood flow and intrasplenic platelet kinetics in relation to spleen volume. Br J Haematol 67:181, 1987

26. Peters AM, Saverymuttu SH, Wonke B et al: The interpretation of platelet kinetic studies for the identification of sites of abnormal platelet destruction. Br J Haematol 57:637, 1984

27. Peters AM, Lavender JP: Factors controlling the intrasplenic transit of platelets. Eur J Clin Invest 12:191, 1982

28. Sills RH: Hypersplenism. p. 167. In Pochedly C, Sills RH, Schwartz AD (eds): Disorders of the Spleen. Pathophysiology and Management. Marcel Dekker, New York, 1989

29. Bowdler AJ: Splenomegaly and hypersplenism. Clin Haematol 12:467, 1983

30. McFadzean AJS, Todd D, Tsang KC: Observations on the anemia of cryptogenetic splenomegaly. II. Expansion of the plasma volume. Blood 13:524, 1958

31. Blendis LM, Banks DC, Ramboer C, Williams R: Spleen blood flow and splanchnic haemodynamics in blood dyscrasia and other splenomegalies. Clin Sci 38:73, 1970

32. Schaffner A, Augustiny N, Otto RC, Fehr J: The hypersplenic spleen. A contractile reservoir of granulocytes and platelets. Arch Intern Med 145:651, 1985

33. Brubaker LH, Johnson CA: Correlation of splenomegaly and abnormal neutrophil pooling (margination). J Clin Lab Med 92:508, 1978

34. Joyce RA, Boggs DR, Hasiba U, Srodes CH: Marginal neutrophil pool size in normal subjects and neutropenic patients as measured by epinephrine infusion. J Clin Lab Med 88:614, 1976

35. Karpatkin S, Freedman ML: Hypersplenic thrombocytopenia differentiated from increased peripheral destruction by platelet volume. Ann Intern Med 89:200, 1978

36. El-Khishen MA, Henderson JM, Millikan WJ Jr et al: Splenectomy is contraindicated for thrombocytopenia secondary to portal hypertension. Surg Gynecol Obstet 160:233, 1985

37. Shiloni E, Bitran D, Rachmilewitz E, Durst AL: The role of splenectomy in Gaucher's disease. Arch Surg 118:929, 1983

38. Ziemski JM, Rudowski WJ, Jaskowiak W et al: Evaluation of early postsplenectomy complications. Surg Gynecol Obstet 165:507, 1987

39. Emond AM, Morais P, Venugopal S et al: Role of splenectomy in homozygous sickle cell disease in childhood. Lancet 1:88, 1984

40. Coon WW: Splenectomy for thrombocytopenia due to secondary hypersplenism. Arch Surg 123:369, 1988

41. Coon WW: The limited role of splenectomy in patients with leukemia. Surg Gynecol Obstet 160:291, 1985

42. Garrison RN, McCoy M, Winkler C et al: Splenectomy in hematologic malignancy. Am Surg 50:428, 1984

43. Saven A, Piro LD: Treatment of hairy cell leukemia. Blood 79:1111, 1992

44. Morel P, Dupriez B, Gosselin B et al: Role of early splenectomy in malignant lymphomas with prominent splenic involvement (primary lymphomas of the spleen). Cancer 71:207, 1993

45. Banaji M, Bearman SI, Buckner CD et al: The effects of splenectomy on engraftment and platelet transfusion requirements in patients with chronic myelogenous leukemia undergoing marrow transplantation. Am J Hematol 22:275, 1986

46. Benbassat J, Gilon D, Penchas S: The choice between splenectomy and medical treatment with advanced agnogenic myeloid metaplasia. Am J Hematol 33:128, 1990

47. Benbassat J, Penchas S, Ligumski M: Splenectomy in patients with agnogenic myeloid metaplasia: an analysis of 321 published cases. Br J Haematol 42: 207, 1979

48. Zimran A, Kay A, Gelbart T et al: Gaucher disease. Clinical, laboratory, radiologic, and genetic features of 53 patients. Medicine 71:337, 1992

49. Rubin M, Yampolski I, Lambrozo R et al: Partial splenectomy in Gaucher's disease. J Pediatr Surg 21:125, 1986

50. Bar-Maor JA, Govrin-Yehudain J: Partial splenectomy in children with Gaucher's disease. Pediatrics 76:398, 1985

51. Morgenstern L, Phillips EH, Fermelia D, Weinstein IM: Near-total splenectomy for massive splenomegaly due to Gaucher disease: a new surgical approach. Mt Sinai J Med 53:501, 1986

52. Kumpe DA, Rumack CM, Pretorius DH et al: Partial splenic embolization in children with hypersplenism. Radiology 155:357, 1985

53. Yoshioka H, Kuroda C, Hori S et al: Splenic embolization for hypersplenism using steel coils. AJR 144:1269, 1985

54. Mozes MF, Spigos DG, Pollak R et al: Partial splenic embolization, an alternative to splenectomy—results of a prospective, randomized study. Surgery 96:694, 1984

55. Tchernia G, Gauthier F, Mielot F et al: Initial assessment of the beneficial effect of partial splenectomy in hereditary spherocytosis. Blood 81:2014, 1993

56. Warkentin TE, Kelton JG: Heparin-induced thrombocytopenia. Prog Hemost Thromb 10:1, 1991

57. Warkentin TE, Kelton JG: Heparin and platelets. Hematol Oncol Clin North Am 4:243, 1990

58. Kelton JG, Sheridan D, Santos A et al: Heparin-induced thrombocytopenia: laboratory studies. Blood 72:925, 1988

59. Chong BH, Fawaz I, Chesterman CN, Berndt MC: Heparin-induced thrombocytopenia: mechanism of interaction of the heparin-dependent antibody with platelets. Br J Haematol, 73:235, 1989

60. Green D, Harris K, Reynolds N et al: Heparin immune thrombocytopenia: evidence for a heparin-platelet complex as the antigenic determinant. J Lab Clin Med 91:167, 1978

61. Amiral J, Bridey F, Dreyfus M et al: Platelet factor 4 complexed to heparin is the target for antibodies generated in heparin-induced thrombocytopenia, letter. Thromb Haemost 68:95, 1992

62. Kelton JG, Smith JW, Warkentin TE et al: Immunoglobulin G from patients with heparin-induced thrombocytopenia binds to a complex of heparin and platelet factor 4. Blood 83:3232, 1994

63. Greinacher A, Michels I, Liebenhoff U et al: Heparin-associated thrombocytopenia: immune complexes are attached to the platelet membrane by the negative charge of highly sulphated oligosaccharides. Br J Haematol 84:711, 1993

64. Sheridan D, Carter C, Kelton JG: A diagnostic test for heparin-induced thrombocytopenia. Blood 67:27, 1986

65. Warkentin TE, Santos AV, Hayward CPM et al: Platelet-derived microparticles are produced by heparin-induced thrombocytopenia sera and other platelet Fc receptor stimuli, abstracted. Blood, suppl. 1. 78:343a, 1991

66. Cines DB, Tomaski A, Tannenbaum S: Immune endothelial-cell injury in heparin-associated thrombocytopenia. N Engl J Med 316:581, 1987

67. Warkentin TE, Hayward CPM, Smith CA et al: Determinants of donor platelet variability when testing for heparin-induced thrombocytopenia. J Lab Clin Med 120:371, 1992

68. Chong BH, Pilgrim RL, Cooley MA, Chesterman CN: Increased expression of platelet IgG Fc receptors in immune heparin-induced thrombocytopenia. Blood 81:988, 1993

69. Boshkov LK, Warkentin TE, Hayward CPM et al: Heparin-induced thrombocytopenia and thrombosis: clinical and laboratory studies. Br J Haematol 84:322, 1993

70. Eichinger S, Kyrle PA, Brenner B et al: Thrombocytopenia associated with low-molecular-weight heparin, letter. Lancet 337:1425, 1991

71. Follea G, Hamandjian I, Trzeciak MC et al: Pentosane polysulfate associated thrombocytopenia. Thromb Res 42:413, 1986

72. Greinacher A, Michels I, Schäfer M et al: Heparin-associated thrombocytopenia in a patient treated with polysulphated chondroitin sulphate: evidence for immunological crossreactivity between heparin and polysulphated glycosaminoglycan. Br J Haematol 81:252, 1992

73. Warkentin TE, Kelton JG: Interaction of heparin with platelets, including heparin-induced thrombocytopenia. p. 75. In Bounameaux H (ed): Low-Molecular-Weight Heparins in Prophylaxis and Therapy of Thromboembolic Diseases. Marcel Dekker, New York, 1994

74. King DJ, Kelton JG: Heparin-associated thrombocytopenia. Ann Intern Med 100:535, 1984

75. Warkentin TE, Soutar RL, Panju A, Ginsberg JS: Acute systemic reactions to intravenous bolus heparin therapy: characterization and relationship to heparin-induced thrombocytopenia, abstracted. Blood, suppl. 1. 80:160a, 1992

76. Warkentin TE, Hirte HW, Anderson DR et al: Transient global amnesia associated with acute heparin-induced thrombocytopenia. Am J Med (in press)

77. Greinacher A, Michels I, Kiefel V, Mueller-Eckhardt C: A rapid and sensitive test for diagnosing heparin-associated thrombocytopenia. Thromb Haemost 66:734, 1991

78. Kelton JG, Sheridan D, Brain H et al: Clinical usefulness of testing for a heparin-dependent platelet-aggregating factor in patients with suspected heparin-associated thrombocytopenia. J Lab Clin Med 103:606, 1984

79. Demers C, Ginsberg JS, Brill-Edwards P et al: Rapid anticoagulation using ancrod for heparin-induced thrombocytopenia. Blood 78:2194, 1991

80. Magnani HN: Heparin-induced thrombocytopenia (HIT): an overview of 230 patients treated with Orgaran (Org 10172). Thromb Haemost 70:554, 1993

81. Warkentin TE, Kelton JG: Heparin-induced thrombocytopenia. Annu Rev Med 40:31, 1989

82. Olinger GN, Hussey CV, Olive JA, Malik MI: Cardiopulmonary bypass for patients with previously documented heparin-induced platelet aggregation. J Thorac Cardiovasc Surg 87:673, 1984

83. Zulys VJ, Teasdale SJ, Michel ER et al: Ancrod (Arvin^R) as an alternative to heparin anticoagulation for cardiopulmonary bypass. Anesthesiology 71:870, 1989

84. Doherty DC, Ortel TL, De Bruijn N et al: "Heparin-free" cardiopulmonary bypass: first reported use of heparinoid (Org 10172) to provide anticoagulation for cardiopulmonary bypass. Anesthesiology 73:562, 1990

85. Kappa JR, Fisher CA, Todd B et al: Intraoperative management of patients with heparin-induced thrombocytopenia. Ann Thorac Surg 49:714, 1990

86. Hackett T, Kelton JG, Powers P: Drug-induced platelet destruction. Semin Thromb Hemost 8:116, 1982

87. Kelton JG, Meltzer D, Moore J et al: Drug-induced thrombocytopenia is associated with increased binding of IgG to platelets both in vivo and in vitro. Blood 58:524, 1981

88. Ackroyd JF: Allergic purpura, including purpura due to foods, drugs and infections. Am J Med 14:605, 1953

89. Ackroyd JF: The pathogenesis of thrombocytopenic purpura due to hypersensitivity to Sedormid (allyl-isopropyl-acetyl-carbamide). Clin Sci 7:249, 1949

90. Karpatkin M, Siskind GW, Karpatkin S: The platelet factor 3 immunoinjury technique re-evaluated. Development of a rapid test for antiplatelet antibody. Detection in various clinical disorders, including immunologic drug-induced and neonatal thrombocytopenias. J Lab Clin Med 89:400, 1977

91. Karpatkin S: Drug-induced thrombocytopenia. Am J Med Sci 262:68, 1971

92. Cimo PL, Pisciotta AV, Desai RG et al: Detection of drug-dependent antibodies by the ⁵¹Cr platelet lysis test: documentation of immune thrombocytopenia induced by diphenylhydantoin, diazepam, and sulfisoxazole. Am J Hematol 2:65, 1977

93. Danielson DA, Douglas SW III, Herzog P et al: Drug-induced blood disorders. JAMA 252:3257, 1984

94. Belkin GA: Cocktail purpura. An unusal case of quinine sensitivity. Ann Intern Med 66:583, 1967

95. Siroty RR: Purpura on the rocks—with a twist. JAMA 235:2521, 1976

96. Christie DJ, Walker RH, Kolins MD et al: Quinine-induced thrombocytopenia following intravenous use of heroin. Arch Intern Med 143:1174, 1983

97. Berndt MC, Chong BH, Bull HA et al: Molecular characterization of quinine/quinidine drug-dependent antibody platelet interaction using monoclonal antibodies. Blood 66:1292, 1985

98. Chong BH, Du X, Berndt MC et al: Characterization of the binding domains on platelet glycoproteins Ib-IX and IIb/IIIa complexes for the quinine/quinidine-dependent antibodies. Blood 77:2190, 1991

99. Christie DJ, Mullen PC, Aster RH: Quinine- and quinidine platelet antibodies can react with GPIIb/IIIa. Br J Haematol 67:213, 1987

100. Visentin GP, Newman PJ, Aster RH: Characteristics of quinine-and quinidine-induced antibodies specific for platelet glycoproteins IIb and IIIa. Blood 77:2668, 1991

101. Christie DJ, Mullen PC, Aster RH: Fab-mediated binding of drug-dependent antibodies to platelets in quinidine- and quinine-induced thrombocytopenia. J Clin Invest 75:310, 1985

102. Smith ME, Reid DM, Jones CE et al: Binding of quinine- and quinidine-dependent drug antibodies to platelets is mediated by the Fab domain of the immunoglobulin G and is not Fc dependent. J Clin Invest 79:912, 1987

103. Christie DJ, Weber RW, Mullen PC et al: Structural features of the quinidine and quinine molecules necessary for binding of drug-induced antibodies to human platelets. J Lab Clin Med 104:730, 1984

104. Christie DJ, Diaz-Arauzo H, Cook JM: Antibody-mediated platelet destruction by quinine, quinidine, and their metabolites. J Lab Clin Med 112:92, 1988

105. Bolton FG, Dameshek W: Thrombocytopenic purpura due to quinidine. Clinical studies. Blood 11:527, 1956

106. Garty M, Ilfeld D, Kelton JG: Correlation of a quinidine-induced platelet-specific antibody with development of thrombocytopenia. Am J Med 79:253, 1985

107. Reid DM, Shulman NR: Drug purpura due to surreptitious quinidine intake. Ann Intern Med 108:206, 1988

108. Redell MA, Moore BR, Fass L: Use of i.v. immune globulin for presumed quinidine-induced thrombocytopenia, letter. Clin Pharm 8:89, 1989

109. Ray JB, Brereton WF, Nullet FR: Intravenous immune globulin for the treatment of presumed quinidine-induced thrombocytopenia. DICP 24:693, 1990

110. Chong BH, Berndt MC, Koutts J, Castaldi PA: Quinidine-induced thrombocytopenia and leukopenia: demonstration and characterization of distinct antiplatelet and antileukocyte antibodies. Blood 62:1218, 1983

111. Nieminen U, Kekomäki R: Quinidine-induced thrombocytopenic purpura: clinical presentation in relation to drug-dependent and drug-dependent platelet antibodies. Br J Haematol 80:77, 1992

112. Adachi JD, Bensen WG, Kassam Y et al: Gold-induced thrombocytopenia. 12 cases and a review of the literature. Semin Arthritis Rheum 16:287, 1987

113. Coblyn JS, Weinblatt M, Holdsworth D, Glass D: Gold-induced thrombocytopenia. A clinical and immunogenetic study of twenty-three patients. Ann Intern Med 95:178, 1981

114. Kosty MP, Hench PK, Tani P, McMillan R: Thrombocytopenia associated with auranofin therapy: evidence for a gold-dependent immunologic mechanism. Am J Hematol 30:236, 1989

115. Goldstein R, Blanchette VS, Huebsch LB, McKendry RJR: Treatment of gold-induced thrombocytopenia by high-dose intravenous gamma globulin. Arthritis Rheum 29:426, 1986

116. Price AE, Leichtentritt B: Gold therapy in rheumatoid arthritis. Ann Intern Med 19:70, 1943

117. Saphir JR, Ney RG: Delayed thrombocytopenic purpura after diminutive gold therapy. JAMA 195:162, 1966

118. Heuer MA, Pietrusko RG, Morris RW, Scheffler BJ: An analysis of worldwide safety experience with Auranofin. J Rheumatol 12:695, 1985

119. Von dem Borne AEG Jr, Pegels JG, Van der Stadt RJ et al: Thrombocytopenia associated with gold therapy: a drug-induced autoimmune disease? Br J Haematol 63:509, 1986

120. Deren B, Masi R, Weksler M, Nachman RL: Gold-associated thrombocytopenia. Arch Intern Med 134:1012, 1974

121. Kahn HR, Brod RC: Thrombocytopenia due to stibophen. Arch Intern Med 108:218, 1961

122. Braconier JH, Miörner H: Recurrent episodes of thrombocytopenia during treatment with sodium stibogluconate. J Antimicrob Chemother 31:187, 1993

123. Christie DJ, Lennon SS, Drew RL, Swinehart CD: Cefotetan-induced immunologic thrombocytopenia. Br J Haematol 70:423, 1988

124. Sheiman L, Spielvogel AR, Horowitz HI: Thrombocytopenia caused by cephalothin sodium. JAMA 203:601–603, 1968

125. Gralnick HR, McGinniss M, Halterman R: Thrombocytopenia with sodium cephalothin therapy. Ann Intern Med 77:401, 1972

126. Lown J, Barr A: Immune thrombocytopenia induced by cephalosporins specific for thiomethyltetrazole side chain, letter. J Clin Pathol 40:700, 1987

127. Chen J-H, Wiener L, Distenfeld A: Immunologic thrombocytopenia. Induced by gentamicin. NY State J Med 80:1134, 1980

128. Meyboom RHB: Thrombocytopenia induced by nalidixic acid. Br Med J 289:962, 1984

129. Lee M, Sharifi R: Severe thrombocytopenia due to apalcillin. Urol Int 42:313, 1987

130. Schiffer CA, Weinstein HJ, Wiernik PH: Methicillin-associated thrombocytopenia, letter. Ann Intern Med 85:338, 1976

131. Murphy MF, Riordan T, Minchinton RM et al: Demonstration of an immune-mediated mechanism of penicillin-induced neutropenia and thrombocytopenia. Br J Haematol 55:155, 1983

132. Salamon DJ, Nusbacher J, Stroupe T et al: Red cell and platelet-bound IgG penicillin antibodies in a patient with thrombocytopenia. Transfusion 24:395, 1984

133. Olivera E, Lakhani P, Watanakunakorn C: Isolated severe thrombocytopenia and bleeding caused by piperacillin. Scand J Infect Dis 24:815, 1992

134. Blajchman MA, Lowry RC, Pettit JE, Stradling P: Rifampicin-induced immune thrombocytopenia. Br Med J 3:24, 1970

135. Kakaiya RM, Dehertogh D, Walker FJ et al: Rifampin-induced immune thrombocytopenia. A case report. Vox Sang 57:185, 1989

136. Schwartz RH, Rodriguez WJ, Luban NLC: Thrombocytopenia associated with PF_3 antiplatelet activity against the sulfa component of trimethoprim-sulfamethoxazole. South Med J 74:640, 1981

137. Kiefel V, Santoso S, Schmidt S et al: Metabolite-specific (IgG) and drug-specific antibodies (IgG, IgM) in two cases of trimethoprim-sulfamethoxazole-induced immune thrombocytopenia. Transfusion 27:262, 1987

138. Janovsky RC: Fatal thrombocytopenic purpura after administration of sulfamethoxpyridazine. JAMA 172:155, 1960

139. Thomas TF: Thrombocytopenic purpura secondary to sulfamethoxypyridazine. NY State J Med 63:2554, 1963

140. Hamilton HE, Sheets RF: Sulfisoxazole-induced thrombocytopenic purpura. Immunologic mechanism as cause. JAMA 239:2586, 1978

141. Seidman AD, Schwartz M, Reich L, Scher HI: Immune-mediated thrombocytopenia secondary to suramin. Cancer 71:851, 1993

142. Claas FHJ, Van der Meer JWM, Langerak J: Immunological effect of co-trimoxazole on platelets. Br Med J 2:898, 1979

143. Christie DJ, van Buren N, Lennon SS, Putnam JL: Vancomycin-dependent antibodies associated with thrombocytopenia and refractoriness to platelet transfusion in patients with leukemia. Blood 75:518, 1990

144. Zenon GJ, Cadle RM, Hamill RJ: Vancomycin-induced thrombocytopenia. Arch Intern Med 151:995, 1991

145. Heading RC: Purpura and paracetamol, letter. Br Med J 3:743, 1968

146. Eisner EV, Shahidi NT: Immune thrombocytopenia due to a drug metabolite. N Engl J Med 287:376, 1972

147. D'Eshougues JR, Griguer P, Smadja A, Bensaïd J: Purpura thrombocytopénique aigu par sensibilisation ai l'aspirine. Nouv Rev Franc Hématol 1:609, 1961

148. Garg SK, Sarker CR: Aspirin-induced thrombocytopenia on an immune basis. Am J Med Sci 267:129, 1974

149. Bobrove AM: Diflunisal-associated thrombocytopenia in a patient with rheumatoid arthritis, letter. Arthritis Rheum 31:149, 1988

150. Gregg JA, Mayock RL: Thrombocytopenia induced by administration of sodium para-aminosalicylate. JAMA 172:1909, 1960

151. Eisner EV, Kasper K: Immune thrombocytopenia due to a metabolite of para-aminosalicylic acid. Am J Med 53:790, 1972

152. Peña JM, Gonzalez-Garcia JJ, Garcia-Alegria J et al: Thrombocytopenia and sulfasalazine, letter. Ann Intern Med 102:277, 1985

153. Kramer MR, Levene C, Hershko C: Severe reversible autoimmune haemolytic anaemia and thrombocytopenia associated with diclofenac therapy. Scand J Haematol 36:118, 1986

154. Simpson RE III, Goldstein DJ, Hjelte GS, Evans ER: Acute thrombocytopenia associated with fenoprofen, letter. N Engl J Med 298:629, 1978

155. Meyer T, Herrmann C, Wiegand V et al: Immune thrombocytopenia associated with hemorrhagic diathesis due to ibuprofen administration. Clin Invest 71:413, 1993

156. Camba L, Joyner MV: Acute thrombocytopenia following ingestion of indomethacin. Acta Haematol 71:350, 1984

157. Schimizzi GF, Graehl PM, Michalski JP: Severe, reversible thrombocytopenia associated with meclofenamate. Arthritis Rheum 25:359, 1982

158. Armstrong FB, Scherbel AL: Review of toxicity of oxyphenbutazone. Report of a case of thrombocytopenic purpura. JAMA 175:614, 1961

159. Handley AJ: Thrombocytopenia and L.E. cells after oxyphenbutazone, letter. Lancet 1:245, 1971

160. Fireman Z, Yust I, Abramov AL: Lethal occult pulmonary hemorrhage in drug-induced thrombocytopenia. Chest 79:358, 1981

161. Stephens CAL Jr, Yeoman EE, Holbrook WP et al: Benefits and toxicity of phenylbutazone (Butazolidin^R) in rheumatoid arthritis. JAMA 150:1084, 1952

162. Davidson C, Manohitharajah SM: Drug-induced antiplatelet antibodies, letter. Br Med J 3:545, 1973

163. Giordano N, Sancasciani S, Cantore M et al: Thrombocytopenic purpura associated with piroxicam, letter. Clin Exp Rheumatol 5:298, 1987

164. Stambaugh JE Jr, Gordon RL, Geller R: Leukopenia and thrombocytopenia secondary to clinoril therapy, letter. Lancet 2:594, 1980

165. Stefanini M, Nassif RI: Acute thrombocytopenic purpura traced to tolmetin-related antibody. Va Med 109:171, 1982

166. Kinney EL, Ballard JO, Carlin B, Zelis R: Amrinone-mediated thrombocytopenia. Scand J Haematol 31:376, 1983

167. Ansell J, Tiarks C, McCue J et al: Amrinone-induced thrombocytopenia. Arch Intern Med 144:949, 1984

168. Young RC, Nachman RL, Horowitz HI: Thrombocytopenia due to digitoxin. Demonstration of antibody and mechanisms of action. Am J Med 41:605, 1966

169. Pirovino M, Ohnhaus EE, von Felten A: Digoxin-associated thrombocytopenia. Eur J Clin Pharmacol 19:205, 1981

170. Weinberger I, Rotenberg Z, Fuchs J et al: Amiodarone-induced thrombocytopenia. Arch Intern Med 147:735, 1987

171. Rosenstein R, Kosfeld RE, Leight L, Liu YK: Procainamide-induced thrombocytopenia. Am J Hematol 16:181, 1984

172. Meissner DJ, Carlson RJ, Gottlieb AJ: Thrombocytopenia following sustained-release procainamide. Arch Intern Med 145:700, 1985

173. Caviet NL, Klaassen CHL: Thrombocytopenie veroorzaakt door Alprenolol. Ned Tijdschr Geneesk 123:18, 1979

174. Magnusson B, Rödjer S: Alprenolol-induced thrombocytopenia. J Intern Med 207:231, 1980

175. Dodds WN, Davidson RJL: Thrombocytopenia due to slow-release oxprenolol, letter. Lancet 2:683, 1978

176. Patrassi GM, Casonato A, Fabris F, Girolami A: Thrombocytopenia secondary to oxprenolol, a β-blocking agent. Acta Haematol 68:75, 1982

177. Pujol M, Duran-Suarez JR, Martín Vega C et al: Autoimmune thrombocytopenia in three patients treated with captopril, letter. Vox Sang 57:218, 1989

178. Combs JT, Grunt JA, Brandt IK: Hematologic reactions to diazoxide. Pediatrics 40:90, 1967

179. Wales JK, Wolff F: Haematological side-effects of diazoxide, letter. Lancet 1:53, 1967

180. Marcus GJ, Stevenson M, Brown T: Alpha-methyldopa-induced immune thrombocytopenia. Report of a case. Am J Clin Pathol 64:113, 1975

181. Reisner EH Jr, Morgan MC: Thrombocytopenia following acetazolamide (Diamox) therapy. JAMA 160:206, 1956

182. Nordqvist P, Cramér G, Björntorp P: Thrombocytopenia during chlorothiazide treatment. Lancet 1:271, 1959

183. Duncan A, Moore SB, Barker P: Thrombocytopenia caused by frusemide-induced platelet antibody, letter. Lancet 1:1210, 1981

184. Eisner EV, Crowell EB: Hydrochlorothiazide-dependent thrombocytopenia due to IgM antibody. JAMA 215:480, 1971

185. Conti L, Gandolfo GM: Benzodiazepine-induced thrombocytopenia. Demonstration of drug-dependent platelet antibodies in two cases. Acta Haematol 70:386, 1983

186. Kornberg A, Kobrin I: IgG antiplatelet antibodies due to carbamazepine. Acta Haematol 68:68, 1982

187. Tohen M, Castillo J, Cole JO et al: Thrombocytopenia associated with carbamazepine: a case series. J Clin Psychiatry 52:496, 1991

188. Morris N, Barr RD, Pai KRM, Kelton JG: Valproic acid and thrombocytopenia. Can Med Assoc J 125:63, 1981

189. Barr RD, Copeland SA, Stockwell ML et al: Valproic acid and immune thrombocytopenia. Arch Dis Child 57:681, 1982

190. Mattson RH, Cramer JA, Collins JF: A comparison of valproate with carbamazepine for the treatment of complex partial seizures and secondarily generalized tonic-clonic seizures in adults. N Engl J Med 327:765, 1992

191. Mann HJ, Schneider JR, Miller JB, Delaney JP: Cimetidine-associated thrombocytopenia. Drug Intell Clin Pharm 17:126, 1983

192. Glotzbach RE: Cimetidine-induced thrombocytopenia. South Med J 75:232, 1982

193. Gibson PR, Pidcock ME: Immune-mediated thrombocytopenia associated with ranitidine therapy. Med J Aust 145:661, 1986

194. Gafter U, Zevin D, Komlos L et al: Thrombocytopenia associated with hypersensitivity to ranitidine: possible cross-reactivity with cimetidine. Am J Gastroenterol 84:560, 1989

195. Grace WJ: Thrombocytopenia in a patient taking chlorpropamide. N Engl J Med 260:711, 1959

196. FitzPatrick WJ: Thrombocytopenia occurring during chlorpropamide therapy. Diabetes 12:457, 1963

197. Israeli A, Matzner Y, Or R, Raz I: Glibenclamide causing thrombocytopenia and bleeding tendency: case reports and a review of the literature. Klin Wochenschr 66:223, 1988

198. Shojania AM: Immune-mediated thrombocytopenia due to an iodinated contrast medium (diatrizoate). Can Med Assoc J 133:123, 1985

199. Lacy J, Bober-Sorcinelli KE, Farber LR, Glickman MG: Acute thrombocytopenia induced by parenteral radiographic contrast medium. AJR 146:1298, 1986

200. Insausti CLG, Lechin F, Van der Dijis B: Severe thrombocytopenia following oral cholecystography with iocetamic acid. Am J Hematol 14:285, 1983

201. Bishopric GA: Athrombocytosis following oral cholecystography. JAMA 189: 169, 1964

202. Hysell JK, Hysell JW, Gray JM: Thrombocytopenic purpura following iopanoic acid ingestion. JAMA 237:361, 1977

203. Curradi F, Abbritti G, Agnelli G: Acute thrombocytopenia following oral cholecystography with iopanoic acid. Clin Toxicol 18:221, 1981

204. Stacher A: Schwerste Thrombopenie durch ein perorales trijodiertes Gallenkontrastmittel. Wien Klin Wochenschr 78:286, 1966

205. Johnson TM, Rapini RP: Isotretinoin-induced thrombocytopenia, letter. J Am Acad Dermatol 17:838, 1987

206. Hesdorffer CS, Weltman MD, Raftopoulos H et al: Thrombocytopenia caused by isotretinoin, letter. S Afr Med J 70:705, 1986

207. Liang R: Thrombocytopenia associated with etretinate therapy. Acta Haematol 79:112, 1988

208. Ackroyd JF: Thrombocytopenic purpura due to hypersensitivity to the antihistaminic drug antazoline. Sang 26:115, 1955

209. Nielsen JL, Dahl R, Kissmeyer-Nielsen F: Immune thrombocytopenia due to antazoline (Antistina^R). Allergy 36:517, 1981

210. Eisner EV, LaBocki NL, Pinckney L: Chlorpheniramine-dependent thrombocytopenia. JAMA 231:735, 1975

211. Koury MJ: Thrombocytopenic purpura in HIV-seronegative users of intravenous cocaine. Am J Hematol 35:134, 1990

212. Moss RA, Okun DB: Heroin-induced thrombocytopenia. Arch Intern Med 139:752, 1979

213. Nixon D: Thrombocytopenia following doxepin treatment, letter. JAMA 220: 418, 1972

214. Rachmilewitz EA, Dawson RB Jr, Rachmilewitz B: Serum antibodies against desipramine as a possible cause for thrombocytopenia. Blood 32:524, 1968

215. Stricker BHC, Barendregt JNM, Claas FHJ: Thrombocytopenia and leucopenia with mianserin-dependent antibodies. Br J Clin Pharm 19:102, 1985

216. Hodder FS, Kempert P, McCormack S et al: Immune thrombocytopenia following actinomycin-D therapy. J Pediatr 107:611, 1985

217. Ardman B, Rudders R: Aminoglutethimide-induced thrombocytopenia, letter. Cancer Treat Rep 66:1785, 1982

218. Rabinowe SN, Miller KB: Danazol-induced thrombocytopenia, letter. Br J Haematol 65:383, 1987

219. Walker JA, Sherman RA, Eisinger RP: Thrombocytopenia associated with intravenous desferrioxamine. Am J Kidney Dis 6:254, 1985

220. Stefanini M, Hoffman MN: Studies on platelets: XXVIII: Acute thrombocytopenic purpura due to lidocaine (Xylocaine^R)-mediated antibody. Report of a case. Am J Med Sci 275:365, 1978

221. Cimo PL, Hammond JJ, Moake JL: Morphine-induced immune thrombocytopenia. Arch Intern Med 142:832, 1982

222. Claas FHJ, de Fraiture WH, Meyboom RHB: Thrombopénie causée par des anticorps induits par la Ticlopidine. Nouv Rev Fr Hematol 26:323, 1984

223. Gottschall JL, Elliot W, Lianos E et al: Quinine-induced immune thrombocytopenia associated with hemolytic uremic syndrome: a new clinical entity. Blood 77:306, 1991

224. Stroneck DF, Vercellotti GM, Hammerschimdt DE et al: Characterization of multiple quinine-dependent antibodies in a patient with episodic hemolytic uremic syndrome and immune agranulocytosis. Blood 80:241, 1992

225. Maguire RB, Stroneck DF, Campbell AC: Recurrent pancytopenia, coagulopathy, and renal failure associated with multiple quinine-dependent antibodies. Ann Intern Med 119:215, 1993

226. Neahring BJ, Scott JP, Visentin GP et al: Quinine-dependent anti-endothelial cell antibodies in plasma of patients with hemolytic-uremic syndrome (HUS), abstracted. Thromb Haemost 69:641, 1993

227. Murgo AJ: Thrombotic microangiopathy in the cancer patient including those induced by chemotherapeutic agents. Semin Hematol 24:161, 1987

228. Lesesne JB, Rothschild N, Erickson B et al: Cancer-associated hemolyticuremic syndrome: analysis of 85 cases from a National Registry. J Clin Oncol 7:781, 1989

229. Shulman H, Striker G, Deeg HJ et al: Nephrotoxicity of cyclosporin A after allogeneic marrow transplantation: glomerular thromboses and tubular injury. N Engl J Med 305:1392, 1981

230. Speth PAJ, Boerbooms AMT, Holdrinet RSG et al: Thrombotic thrombocytopenic purpura associated with D-penicillamine treatment in rheumatoid arthritis, letter. J Rheumatol 9:5, 1982

231. Page Y, Tardy B, Zeni F et al: Thrombotic thrombocytopenic purpura related to ticlopidine. Lancet 337:774, 1991

232. Kelton JG, Huang AT, Mold N et al: The use of in vitro technics to study drug-induced pancytopenia. N Engl J Med 301:621, 1979

233. Gollub S, Ulin AW: Heparin-induced thrombocytopenia in man. J Lab Clin Med 59:430, 1962

234. Wakefield TW, Bouffard JA, Spaulding SA et al: Sequestration of platelets in the pulmonary circulation as a consequence of protamine reversal of the anticoagulant effects of heparin. J Vasc Surg 5:187, 1987

235. Hilgard P, Hossfeld DK: Transient bleomycin-induced thrombocytopenia. A clinical study. Eur J Cancer 14:1261, 1978

236. Glueck R, Green D, Cohen I, Ts'ao CH: Hematin: unique effects on hemostasis. Blood 61:243, 1983

237. Neely SM, Gardner DV, Reynolds N et al: Mechanism and characteristics of platelet activation by haematin. Br J Haematol 58:305, 1984

238. Escolar G, Monteagudo J, Villamor N et al: Ristocetin induced platelet aggregation: a morphological demonstration. Br J Haematol 69:379, 1988

239. Holmberg L, Nilsson IM, Borge L et al: Platelet aggregation induced by 1-desamino-8-D-arginine vasopressin (DDAVP) in type IIB von Willebrand's disease. N Engl J Med 309:816, 1983

240. Green D, Tuite GF Jr: Declining platelet counts and platelet aggregation during porcine VIII:C infusions. Am J Med 86:222, 1989

241. Rosenbloom D, Gilbert R: Reversible flu-like syndrome, leukopenia, and thrombocytopenia induced by allopurinol. Drug Intell Clin Pharm 15:286, 1981

242. Hansen JE: Hypersensitivity to isoniazid with neutropenia and thrombocytopenia. Am Rev Respir Dis 83:744, 1961

243. Farr M, Tunn E, Bacon PA, Smith DH: Hypogammaglobulinemia and thrombocytopenia associated with sulphasalazine therapy in rheumatoid arthritis, letter. Ann Rheum Dis 44:723, 1985

244. Holt RJ: Fluphenazine decanoate-induced cholestatic jaundice and thrombocytopenia. Pharmacotherapy 4:227, 1984

245. McFarland RB: Fatal drug reaction associated with prochlorperazine (compazine). Report of a case characterized by jaundice, thrombocytopenia, and agranulocytosis. Am J Clin Pathol 40:284, 1963

246. McLaughlin P, Talpaz M, Quesada JR et al: Immune thrombocytopenia following α-interferon therapy in patients with cancer. JAMA 254:1353, 1985

247. Abdi EA, Brien W, Venner PM: Auto-immune thrombocytopenia related to interferon therapy. Scand J Haematol 36:515, 1986

248. Paciucci PA, Mandeli J, Oleksowicz L et al: Thrombocytopenia during immunotherapy with interleukin-2 by constant infusion. Am J Med 89:308, 1990

249. Guarini A, Sanavio F, Novarino A et al: Thrombocytopenia in acute leukemia patients treated with IL2: cytolytic effect of LAK cells on megakaryocytic progenitors. Br J Haematol 79:451, 1991

250. Fleischmann JD, Shingleton WB, Gallagher C et al: Fibrinolysis, thrombocytopenia, and coagulation abnormalities complicating high-dose interleukin-2 immunotherapy. J Lab Clin Med 117:76, 1991

251. Yoshida Y, Hirashima K, Asano S, Takaku F: A phase II trial of recombinant human granulocyte colony-stimulating factor in the myelodysplastic syndromes. Br J Haematol 78:378, 1991

252. Praloran V: Structure, biosynthesis and biological roles of monocyte-macrophage colony stimulating factor (CSF-1 or M-CSF). Nouv Rev Fr Hematol 33: 323, 1991

253. Gratama JW, Brand A, Jansen J et al: Factors influencing platelet survival during antilymphocyte globulin treatment. Br J Haematol 57:5, 1984

254. Madaio MP, Spiegel JE, Levey AS: Life-threatening thrombocytopenia complicating antithymocyte globulin therapy for acute kidney transplant rejection. Transplantation 45:647, 1988

255. Burrows RF, Kelton JG: Incidentally detected thrombocytopenia in healthy mothers and their infants. N Engl J Med 319:142, 1988

256. Burrows RF, Kelton JK: Thrombocytopenia at delivery: a prospective survey of 6715 deliveries. Am J Obstet Gynecol 162:731, 1990

257. Aster RH: Gestational thrombocytopenia. A plea for conservative management. N Engl J Med 323:264, 1990

258. Matthews JH, Benjamin S, Gill DS, Smith NA: Pregnancy-associated thrombocytopenia: definition, incidence and natural history. Acta Haematol 84:24, 1990

259. Barron WM: The syndrome of preeclampsia. Gastroenterol Clin N Am 21: 851, 1992

260. Gibson B, Hunter D, Neame PB, Kelton JG: Thrombocytopenia in preeclampsia and eclampsia. Semin Thromb Hemost 8:234, 1982

261. Schindler M, Gatt S, Isert P et al: Thrombocytopenia and platelet function defects in pre-eclampsia: implications for regional anesthesia. Anaesth Intens Care 18:169, 1990

262. Kelton JG, Hunter DJS, Neame PB: A platelet function defect in preeclampsia. Obstet Gynecol 65:107, 1985

263. Weinstein L: Syndrome of hemolysis, elevated liver enzymes, and low platelet count: a severe consequence of hypertension in pregnancy. Am J Obstet Gynecol 142:159, 1982

264. Barton JR, Sibai BM: Care of the pregnancy complicated by HELLP syndrome. Obstet Gynecol Clin North Am 18:165, 1991

265. Sibai BM, Taslimi MM, El-Nazer A et al: Maternal-perinatal outcome associated with the syndrome of hemolysis, elevated liver enzymes, and low platelets in severe pre-eclampsia. Am J Obstet Gynecol 155:501, 1986

266. Romero R, Mazor M, Lockwood CJ et al: Clinical significance, prevalence, and natural history of thrombocytopenia in pregnancy-induced hypertension. Am J Perinatol 6:32, 1989

267. Goodlin RC: Preeclampsia as the great imposter. Am J Obstet Gynecol 164:1577, 1991

268. Martin JN Jr, Stedman CM: Imitators of preeclampsia and HELLP syndrome. Obstet Gynecol Clin North Am 18:181, 1991

269. Giles C, Inglis TCM: Thrombocytopenia and macrothrombocytosis in gestational hypertension. Br J Obstet Gynaecol 88:1115, 1981

270. Rákóczi I, Tallián F, Bagdány S, Gáti I: Platelet life-span in normal pregnancy and pre-eclampsia as determined by a non-radioisotope technique. Thromb Res 15:553, 1979

271. Stubbs TM, Lazarchick J, Van Dorsten JP et al: Evidence of accelerated platelet production and consumption in nonthrombocytopenic preeclampsia. Am J Obstet Gynecol 155:263, 1986

272. Burrows RF, Hunter DJS, Andrew M, Kelton JG: A prospective study investigating the mechanism of thrombocytopenia in preeclampsia. Obstet Gynecol 70:334, 1987

273. Kobayashi T, Terao T: Preeclampsia as chronic disseminated intravascular coagulation. Study of two parameters: thrombin-antithrombin II complex and D-dimers. Gynecol Obstet Invest 24:170, 1987

274. Trofatter KF Jr, Howell ML, Greenberg CS, Hage ML: Use of the fibrin D-dimer in screening for coagulation abnormalities in preeclampsia. Obstet Gynecol 73:435, 1989

275. Weiner CP: The mechanism of reduced antithrombin III activity in women with preeclampsia. Obstet Gynecol 72:847, 1988

276. Ho C-H, Yang Z-L: The predictive value of the hemostasis parameters in the development of preeclampsia. Thromb Hemost 67:214, 1992

277. Samuels P, Main EK, Tomaski A et al: Abnormalities in platelet antiglobulin tests in preeclamptic mothers and their neonates. Am J Obstet Gynecol 157:109, 1987

278. George JN: Platelet immunoglobulin G: its significance for the evaluation of thrombocytopenia and for understanding the origin of α-granule protein. Blood 76:859, 1990

279. Goodman RP, Killam AP, Brash AR, Branch RA: Prostacyclin production during pregnancy: comparison of production during normal pregnancy and pregnancy complicated by hypertension. Am J Obstet Gynecol 142:817, 1982

280. Socol ML, Weiner CP, Louis G et al: Platelet activation in preeclampsia. Am J Obstet Gynecol 151:494, 1985

281. Benigini A, Gregorini G, Frusca T et al: Effect of low-dose aspirin on fetal and maternal generation of thromboxane by platelets in women at risk for pregnancy-induced hypertension. N Engl J Med 321:357, 1989

282. Schiff E, Peleg E, Goldenberg M et al: The use of aspirin to prevent pregnancy-induced hypertension and lower the ratio of thromboxane A_2 to prostacyclin in relatively high risk pregnancies. N Engl J Med 321:351, 1989

283. Sibai BM, Spinnato JA, Watson DL et al: Pregnancy outcome in 303 cases with severe preeclampsia. Obstet Gynecol 64:319, 1984

284. Kelton JG, Neame PB, Gauldie J, Hirsh J: Elevated platelet-associated IgG in the thrombocytopenia of septicemia. N Engl J Med 300:760, 1979

285. Neame PB, Kelton JG, Walker IR et al: Thrombocytopenia in septicemia: the role of disseminated intravascular coagulation. Blood 56:88, 1980

286. Iberti TJ, Benjamin E, Berger SR et al: Thrombocytopenia following peritonitis in surgical patients. Ann Surg 204:341, 1986

287. Corrigan JJ Jr, Jordan CM: Heparin therapy in septicemia with disseminated intravascular coagulation: effect on mortality and on correction of hemostatic defects. N Engl J Med 283:778, 1970

288. Kreger BE, Craven DE, McCabe WR: Gram-negative bacteremia. IV. Re-evaluation of clinical features and treatment in 612 patients. Am J Med 68:344, 1980

289. Tate DY, Carlton GT, Johnson D et al: Immune thrombocytopenia in severe neonatal infections. J Pediatr 98:449, 1981

290. Kekomäki R, Kekomäki M, Elfving J: Platelet-associated IgG in septicemia, letter. N Engl J Med 301:271, 1979

291. Poskitt TR, Poskitt PKF: Thrombocytopenia of sepsis. Spurious thrombocytopenia produced by the interaction of rheumatoid factor with antiplatelet antibody. Am J Hematol 18:207, 1985

292. Van der Lelie J, Van der Plas-Van Dalen CM, Von dem Borne AEG Jr: Platelet autoantibodies in septicaemia. Br J Haematol 58:755, 1984

293. Kelton JG, Keystone J, Moore J et al: Immune-mediated thrombocytopenia of malaria. J Clin Invest 71:832, 1983

294. Diez FL, Nieto ML, Fernandez-Gallardo S et al: Occupancy of platelet receptors for platelet activating factor in patients with septicemia. J Clin Invest 83:1733, 1989

295. Csako G, Suba EA, Elin RJ: Endotoxin-induced platelet activation in human whole blood in vitro. Thromb Haemost 59:378, 1988

296. Arvand M, Bhakdi S, Dahlbäck B, Preissner KT: *Staphylococcus aureus* α-toxin attack on human platelets promotes assembly of the prothrombinase complex. J Biol Chem 265:14377, 1990

297. Tan EM, Cohen AS, Fries JF et al: The 1982 revised criteria for the classification of systemic lupus erythematosus. Arthritis Rheum 25:1271, 1982

298. Miller MH, Urowitz MB, Gladman DD: The significance of thrombocytopenia in systemic lupus erythematosus. Arthritis Rheum 26:1181, 1983

299. Budman DR, Steinberg AD: Hematologic aspects of systemic lupus erythematosus. Current concepts. Ann Intern Med 86:220, 1977

300. Doan CA, Bouroncle BA, Wiseman BK: Idiopathic and secondary thrombocytopenic purpura: clinical study and evaluation of 381 cases over a period of 28 years. 53:861, 1960

301. Anderson MJ, Peebles CL, McMillan R, Curd JG: Fluorescent antinuclear antibodies and anti-SS-A/Ro in patients with immune thrombocytopenia subsequently developing systemic lupus erythematosus. Ann Intern Med 103:548, 1985

302. Kaplan C, Champeix P, Blanchard D et al: Platelet antibodies in systemic lupus erythematosus. Br J Haematol 67:89, 1987

303. Jouhikainen T, Kekomäki R, Leirisalo-Repo M et al: Platelet autoantibodies detected by immunoblotting in systemic lupus erythematosus: association with the lupus anticoagulant, and with history of thrombosis and thrombocytopenia. Eur J Haematol 44:234, 1990

304. Murakami H, Lam Z, Furie BC et al: Sulfated glycolipids are the platelet autoantigens for human platelet-binding monoclonal anti-DNA autoantibodies. J Biol Chem 266:15414, 1991

305. Khamashta MA, Harris EN, Gharavi AE et al: Immune mediated mechanism for thrombosis: antiphospholipid antibody binding to platelet membranes. Ann Rheum Dis 47:849, 1988

306. Pfueller SL, Firkin BG, McGrath KM, Logan: Analysis of immunoglobulins that bind to platelets from serum of patients with immune thrombocytopenia: molecular weight distribution. Thromb Res 47:305, 1987

307. Kelton JG, Carter CJ, Rodger C et al: The relationship among platelet associated IgG, platelet life span and reticuloendothelial cell function. Blood 63:1434, 1984

308. Bergström A-L, Olsson L-B, Kutti J: Platelet survival and platelet production in systemic lupus erythematosus (SLE). Scand J Rheumatol 9:209, 1980

309. Frank MM, Hamburger MI, Lawley TJ et al: Defective reticuloendothelial system Fc-receptor function in systemic lupus erythematosus. N Engl J Med 300:518, 1979

310. Kelton JG, Singer J, Rodger C et al: The concentration of IgG in the serum is a major determinant of Fc-dependent reticuloendothelial cell function. Blood 66:490, 1985

311. Kabbash L, Esdaile J, Shenker S et al: Reticuloendothelial system Fc receptor function in systemic lupus erythematosus: effect of decreased sensitization on clearance of autologous erythrocytes. J Rheumatol 14:487, 1987

312. Weiss HJ, Rosove MH, Lages BA, Kaplan KL: Acquired storage pool deficiency with increased platelet-associated IgG. Report of five cases. Am J Med 69:711, 1980

313. Derksen RHWM, Bouma BN, Kater L: The prevalence and clinical associations of the lupus anticoagulant in systemic lupus erythematosus. Scand J Rheumatol 16:185, 1987

314. Love PE, Santoro SA: Antiphospholipid antibodies: anticardiolipin and the lupus anticoagulant in systemic lupus erythematosus (SLE) and in non-SLE disorders. Ann Intern Med 112:682, 1990

315. Fox DA, Faix JD, Coblyn J et al: Thrombotic thrombocytopenic purpura and systemic lupus erythematosus. Ann Rheum Dis 45:319, 1986

316. Devinsky O, Petito CK, Alonso DR: Clinical and neuropathological findings in systemic lupus erythematosus: the role of vasculitis, heart emboli and thrombotic thrombocytopenic purpura. Ann Neurol 23:380, 1988

317. Hess DC, Sethi K, Awad E: Thrombotic thrombocytopenic purpura in systemic lupus erythematosus and antiphospholipid antibodies: effective treatment with plasma exchange and immunosuppression. J Rheumatol 19:1474, 1992

318. Morely KD, Parke A, Hughes GRV: Systemic lupus erythematosus: two patients treated with danazol. Br Med J 284:1431, 1982

319. Marino C, Cook P: Danazol for lupus thrombocytopenia. Arch Intern Med 145:2251, 1985

320. West SG, Johnson SC: Danazol for the treatment of refractory autoimmune

thrombocytopenia in systemic lupus erythematosus. Ann Intern Med 108: 703, 1988

321. Schreiber AD, Chien P, Tomaski A, Cines DB: Effect of danazol in immune thrombocytopenic purpura. N Engl J Med 316:503, 1987

322. Coon WW: Splenectomy for cytopenias associated with systemic lupus erythematosus. Am J Surg 155:391, 1988

323. Homan WP, Dineen P: The role of splenectomy in the treatment of thrombocytopenic purpura due to systemic lupus erythematosus. Ann Surg 187:52, 1978

324. Hall S, McCormick JL, Greipp PR et al: Splenectomy does not cure the thrombocytopenia of systemic lupus erythematosus. Ann Intern Med 102:325, 1985

325. Newland AC, Treleaven HG, Minchinton RM, Waters AH: High-dose intravenous IgG in adults with autoimmune thrombocytopenia. Lancet 1:84, 1983

326. Maier WP, Gordon DS, Howard RF et al: Intravenous immunoglobulin therapy in systemic lupus erythematosus-associated thrombocytopenia. Arthritis Rheum 33:1233, 1990

327. Goebel KM, Gassel WD, Goebel FD: Evaluation of azathioprine in autoimmune thrombocytopenia and lupus erythematosus. Scand J Haematol 10: 28, 1973

328. Wall BA, Weinblatt ME, Agudelo CA: Plasmapheresis in the treatment of resistant thrombocytopenia in systemic lupus erythematosus. South Med J 75:1277, 1982

329. Schroeder JO, Euler HH, Löffler H: Synchronization of plasmapheresis and pulse cyclophosphamide in severe systemic lupus erythematosus. Ann Intern Med 107:344, 1987

330. Matsumura O, Kawashima Y, Kato S et al: Therapeutic effect of cyclosporine in thrombocytopenia associated with autoimmune disease. Transplant Proc 20:317, 1988

331. McNeil HP, Simpson RJ, Chesterman CN, Krilis SA: Antiphospholipid antibodies are directed against a complex antigen that includes a lipid-binding inhibitor of coagulation: β$_2$-glycoprotein I (apolipoprotein H). Proc Natl Acad Sci USA 87:4120, 1990

332. Galli M, Comfurius P, Maassen C et al: Anticardiolipin antibodies (ACA) are directed not to cardiolipin but to a plasma protein cofactor. Lancet 335: 1544, 1990

333. Bowles CA: Vasculopathy associated with the antiphospholipid antibody syndrome. Rheum Dis Clin North Am 16:471, 1990

334. Harris EN: Annotation: antiphospholipid antibodies. Br J Hematol 74:1, 1990

335. Triplett DA: Antiphospholipid antibodies and thrombosis. A consequence, coincidence, or cause? Arch Pathol Lab Med 117:78, 1993

336. Young SM, Fisher M, Sigsbee A, Errichetti A: Cardiogenic brain embolism and lupus anticoagulant. Ann Neurol 26:390, 1989

337. Sánchez-Guerrero J, Reyes E, Alarcón-Segovia D: Primary antiphospholipid syndrome as a cause of intestinal infarction. J Rheumatol 19:623, 1992

338. Shapiro LS: Large vessel arterial thrombosis in systemic sclerosis associated with antiphospholipid antibodies. J Rheumatol 17:685, 1990

339. Grob JJ, Bonerandi JJ: Cutaneous manifestations associated with the presence of the lupus anticoagulant. A report of two cases and a review of the literature. J Am Acad Dermatol 15:211, 1986

340. Grob JJ, Bonerandi JJ: Thrombotic skin disease as a marker of the anticardiolipin syndrome. Livedo vasculitis and distal gangrene associated with abnormal serum antiphospholipid activity. J Am Acad Dermatol 20:1063, 1989

341. Grob JJ, San Marco M, Aillaud MF et al: Unfading acral microlivedo. A discrete marker of thrombotic skin disease associated with antiphospholipid antibody syndrome. J Am Acad Dermatol 24:53, 1991

342. Bevers EM, Galli M, Barbui T et al: Lupus anticoagulant IgGs (LA) are not directed to phospholipids only, but to a complex of lipid-bound human prothrombin. Thromb Haemost 66:629, 1991

343. Asherson RA, Khamashta MA, Ordi-Ros J et al: The "primary" antiphospholipid syndrome: major clinical and serological features. Medicine 68:366, 1989

344. Carreras LO, Defreyn G, Machin SJ et al: Arterial thrombosis, intrauterine death and "lupus" anticoagulant: detection of immunoglobulin interfering with prostacyclin formation. Lancet 1:244, 1981

345. Keeling DM, Campbell SJ, Mackie IJ et al: The fibrinolytic response to venous occlusion and the natural anticoagulants in patients with antiphospholipid antibodies both with and without systemic lupus erythematosus. Br J Haematol 77:354, 1991

346. Cariou R, Tobelem G, Bellucci S et al: Effect of lupus anticoagulant on antithrombogenic properties of endothelial cells—inhibition of thrombomodulin-dependent protein C activation. Thromb Haemost 60:54, 1988

347. Malia RG, Kitchen S, Greaves M, Preston FE: Inhibition of activated protein C and its cofactor protein S by antiphospholipid antibodies. Br J Haematol 76:101, 1990

348. Out HJ, de Groot PG, van Vliet M et al: Antibodies to platelets in patients with anti-phospholipid antibodies. Blood 77:2655, 1991

349. Shi W, Chong BH, Chesterman CN: β$_2$-Glycoprotein I is a requirement for anticardiolipin antibodies binding to activated platelets: differences with lupus anticoagulants. Blood 81:1255, 1993

350. Galli M, Cortelazzo S, Viero P et al: Interaction between platelets and lupus anticoagulant. Eur J Haematol 41:88, 1988

351. Davies GE, Triplett DA: Corticosteroid-associated blue toe syndrome: role of antiphospholipid antibodies. Ann Intern Med 113:893, 1990

352. Sonnenblick M, Kramer MR, Hershko C: Corticosteroid responsive immune thrombocytopenia in Hodgkin's disease. Oncology 43:349, 1986

353. Fink K, Al-Mondhiry H: Idiopathic thrombocytopenic purpura in lymphoma. Cancer 37:1999, 1976

354. Carey RW, McGinnis A, Jacobson BM. Carvalho A: Idiopathic thrombocytopenic purpura complicating chronic lymphocytic leukemia. Management with sequential splenectomy and chemotherapy. Arch Intern Med 136:62, 1976

355. Berchtold P, Harris JP, Tani P et al: Autoantibodies to platelet glycoproteins in patients with disease-related immune thrombocytopenia. Br J Haematol 73:365, 1989

356. Sack GH Jr, Levin J, Bell WR: Trousseau's syndrome and other manifestations of chronic disseminated coagulopathy in patients with neoplasms: clinical, pathophysiologic, and therapeutic features. Medicine 56:1, 1977

357. Colman RW, Rubin RN: Disseminated intravascular coagulation due to malignancy. Semin Oncol 17:172, 1990

358. Bick RL: Coagulation abnormalities in malignancy: a review. Semin Thromb Hemost 18:353, 1992

359. Tallman MS, Kwaan HC: Reassessing the hemostatic disorder associated with acute promyelocytic leukemia. Blood 79:543, 1992

360. Synder HW Jr, Mittleman A, Oral A et al: Treatment of cancer chemotherapy associated thrombotic thrombocytopenic purpura/hemolytic uremic syndrome by protein a immunoadsorption of plasma. Cancer 71:1882, 1993

361. Jaffe ES, Costa J, Fauci AS et al: Malignant lymphoma and erythrophagocytosis simulating malignant histiocytosis. Am J Med 75:741, 1983

362. Falini B, Pileri S, De Solas I et al: Peripheral T-cell lymphoma associated with hemophagocytic syndrome. Blood 75:434, 1990

363. Gonzales CL, Medeiros LJ, Braziel RM, Jaffe ES: T-cell lymphoma involving subcutaneous tissue. A clinicopathologic entity commonly associated with hemophagocytic syndrome. Am J Surg Pathol 15:17, 1991

364. Chubachi A, Imai H, Nishimura S et al: Nasal T-cell lymphoma associated with hemophagocytic syndrome. Immunochemical and genotypic studies. Arch Pathol Lab Med 116:1209, 1992

365. De la Serna FJ, Lopez JI, Garcia-Marcilla A et al: Hemophagocytic syndrome causing complete bone marrow failure. Report of an extreme case of a reactive histiocytic disorder. Acta Haematol 82:197, 1989

366. Chen RL, Su IJ, Lin KH et al: Fulminant childhood hemophagocytic syndrome mimicking histiocytic medullary reticulosis. An atypical form of Epstein-Barr virus infection. Am J Clin Pathol 96:171, 1991

367. Craig FE, Clare CN, Sklar JL, Banks PM: T-cell lymphoma and the virus-associated hemophagocytic syndrome. Am J Clin Pathol 97:189, 1992

368. Henter JI, Ehrnst A, Andersson J, Göran E: Familial hemophagocytic lymphohistiocytosis and viral infections. Acta Paediatr 82:369, 1993

369. Scott RB, Robb-Smith AHT: Histiocytic medullary reticulosis. Lancet 2:194, 1939

370. Zuazu JP, Duran JW, Julia AF: Hemophagocytosis in acute brucellosis, letter. N Engl J Med 301:1185, 1979

371. Auerbach M, Haubenstock A, Soloman G: Systemic babesiosis. Another cause of the hemophagocytic syndrome. Am J Med 80:301, 1986

372. Abbott KC, Vukelja SJ, Smith CE et al: Hemophagocytic syndrome: a cause of pancytopenia in human ehrlichiosis. Am J Hematol 38:230, 1991

373. Wong K-F, Hui P-K, Chan JC et al: The acute lupus hemophagocytic syndrome. Ann Intern Med 114:387, 1991

374. Morris JA, Adamson AR, Holt PJL, Davson J: Still's disease and the virus-associated hemophagocytic syndrome. Ann Rheum Dis 44:349, 1985

375. Rule S, Reed C, Costello C: Fatal haemophagocytic syndromes in HIV-antibody positive patient. Br J Haematol 79:127, 1991

376. Pillay VKG, Kurtzman NA, Manaligod JR, Jonasson O: Selective thrombocytopenia due to localised microangiopathy of renal allografts. Lancet 2:988, 1973

377. Leithner C, Sinzinger H, Schwarz M: Treatment of chronic kidney transplant rejection with prostacyclin—reduction of platelet deposition in the transplant; prolongation of platelet survival and improvement of transplant function. Prostaglandins 22:783, 1981

378. First LR, Smith BR, Lipton J et al: Isolated thrombocytopenia after allogeneic bone marrow transplantation: existence of transient and chronic thrombocytopenic syndromes. Blood 65:368, 1985

379. Minchinton RM, Waters AH, Malpas JS et al: Platelet- and granulocyte-specific antibodies after allogeneic and autologous bone marrow grafts. Vox Sang 46:125, 1984

380. Anasetti C, Rybka W, Sullivan KM et al: Graft-v-host disease is associated with autoimmune-like thrombocytopenia. Blood 73:1054, 1989

381. Rio B, Andreu G, Nicod A et al: Thrombocytopenia in veno-occlusive disease after bone marrow transplantation or chemotherapy. Blood 67:1773, 1986

382. Spruce W, Forman S, McMillan R et al: Idiopathic thrombocytopenic purpura following bone marrow transplantation. Acta Haematol 69:47, 1983

383. Panzer S, Kiefel V, Bartram CR et al: Immune thrombocytopenia more than a year after allogeneic marrow transplantation due to antibodies against donor platelets with anti-P1^{A1} specificity: evidence for a host-derived immune reaction. Br J Haematol 71:259, 1989

384. Rabinowe SN, Soiffer RJ, Tarbell NJ et al: Hemolytic-uremic syndrome following bone marrow transplantation in adults for hematologic malignancies. Blood 77:1837, 1991

385. Woodman RC, Harker L: Bleeding complications associated with cardiopulmonary bypass. Blood 76:1680, 1990

386. Harker LA, Malpass TW, Branson HE et al: Mechanisms of abnormal bleeding in patients undergoing cardiopulmonary bypass: acquired transient platelet dysfunction associated with selective α-granule release. Blood 56:824, 1980

387. Hope AF, Heyns A du P, Lotter MG et al: Kinetics and sites of sequestration of indium 111-labeled human platelets during cardiopulmonary bypass. J Thorac Cardiovasc Surg 81:880, 1981

388. Holloway DS, Summaria L, Sandesara J et al: Decreased platelet number and function and increased fibrinolysis contribute to postoperative bleeding in cardiopulmonary bypass patients. Thromb Haemost 59:62, 1988

389. Mammen EF, Koets MH, Washington BC et al: Hemostasis changes during cardiopulmonary bypass surgery. Semin Thromb Hemost 11:281, 1985

390. George JN, Pickett EB, Saucerman S et al: Platelet surface glycoproteins. Studies on resting and activated platelets and platelet membrane microparticles in normal subjects, and observations in patients during adult respiratory distress syndrome and cardiac surgery. J Clin Invest 78:340, 1986

391. Dechavanne M, French M, Pages J et al: Significant reduction in the binding of a monoclonal antibody (LYP 18) directed against the IIb/IIIa glycoprotein complex to platelets of patients having undergone extracorporeal circulation. Thromb Haemost 57:106, 1987

392. Rinder CS, Mathew JP, Rinder HM et al: Modulation of platelet surface adhesion receptors during cardiopulmonary bypass. Anesthesiology 75:563, 1991

393. Addonizio VP Jr, Smith JB, Strauss JF III et al: Thromboxane synthesis and platelet secretion during cardiopulmonary bypass with bubble oxygenator. J Thorac Cardiovasc Surg 79:91, 1980

394. Abrams CS, Ellison N, Budzynski AZ, Shattil SJ: Direct detection of activated platelets and platelet-derived microparticles in humans. Blood 75:128, 1990

395. Kestin AS, Valeri CR, Khuri SF et al: The platelet function defect of cardiopulmonary bypass. Blood 82:107, 1993

396. Goldman S, Copeland J, Moritz T et al: Improvement in early saphenous vein graft patency after coronary artery bypass surgery with antiplatelet therapy: results of a Veterans Administration Cooperative Study. Circulation 77:1324, 1988

397. Wedemeyer AL, Edson JR, Krivit W: Coagulation in cyanotic congenital heart disease. Am J Dis Child 124:656, 1972 158

398. Goldschmidt B: Platelet functions in children with congenital heart disease. Acta Paediatr Scand 63:271, 1974

399. Waldman JD, Czapek EE, Paul MH et al: Shortened platelet survival in cyanotic heart disease. J Pediatr 87:77, 1975

400. Maurer HM, McCue CM, Caul J, Still WJS: Impairment in platelet aggregation in congenital heart disease. Blood 40:207, 1972

401. Henriksson P, Varendh G, Lundstrom NR: Haemostatic defects in cyanotic congenital heart disease. Br Heart J 41:23, 1979

402. Wedemeyer AL, Lewis JH: Improvement in hemostasis following phlebotomy in cyanotic patients with heart disease. J Pediatr 83:46, 1973

403. Gralnick HR: ε-Aminocaproic acid in preoperative correction of haemostatic defects in cyanotic congenital heart disease. Lancet 1:1204, 1970

404. Maurer HM, McCue CM, Robertson LW, Haggins JC: Correction of platelet dysfunction and bleeding in cyanotic congenital heart disease by simple red cell volume reduction. Am J Cardiol 35:831, 1975

405. Jacobson RJ, Rath CE, Perloff JK: Intravascular hemolysis and thrombocytopenia in left ventricular outflow obstruction. Br Heart J 35:849, 1973

406. Steele PP, Weily HS, Davies H, Genton E: Platelet survival in patients with rheumatic heart disease. N Engl J Med 290:537, 1974

407. O'Brien JR: Shear-induced platelet aggregation. Lancet 335:711, 1990

408. Gill JC, Wilson AD, Endres-Brooks J, Montgomery RR: Loss of the largest von Willebrand factor multimers from the plasma of patients with congenital cardiac defects. Blood 67:758, 1986

409. Warkentin TE, Moore JC, Morgan DG: Aortic stenosis and bleeding gastrointestinal angiodysplasia: is acquired von Willebrand's disease the link? Lancet 340:35, 1992

410. Edwards BS, Weir EK, Edwards WD et al: Coexistent pulmonary and portal hypertension: morphologic and clinical features. J Am Coll Cardiol 10:1233, 1987

411. Terai M, Nakazawa M, Takao A, Imai Y: Thrombocytopenia in patients with aortopulmonary transposition and an intact ventricular septum. Br Heart J 57:371, 1987

412. Stahl RL, Javid JP, Lackner H: Unrecognized pulmonary embolism presenting as disseminated intravascular coagulation. Am J Med 76:772, 1984

413. Mustafa MH, Mispireta LA, Pierce LE: Occult pulmonary embolism presenting with thrombocytopenia and elevated fibrin split products. Am J Med 86:490, 1989

414. Schneider RC, Zapol WM, Carvalho AC: Platelet consumption and sequestration in severe acute respiratory failure. Am Rev Respir Dis 122:445, 1980

Hereditary Disorders of Platelet Function

129

Joel S. Bennett

INTRODUCTION

The presence of a prolonged bleeding time in a patient with a normal platelet count suggests a disorder of platelet function, either hereditary or acquired. The acquired disorders are discussed in Chapter 130. The hereditary platelet disorders can be subclassified into disorders of platelet adhesion, aggregation, secretion, or procoagulant activity, according to the predominant phase of platelet function affected. Studies of these conditions have given explanations for the clinical disorders of hemostasis and also provided a framework on which much of our current understanding of normal platelet function is based.

DISORDERS OF PLATELET ADHESION

Bernard-Soulier Syndrome

The Bernard-Soulier syndrome (glycoprotein [GP]Ib/IX deficiency), described in 1948, is a rare congenital platelet function disorder manifested by a prolonged bleeding time, very large platelets, and thrombocytopenia.[1] The functional defect of Bernard-Soulier platelets is their inability to participate in von Willebrand factor (vWF)-dependent adhesion to the subendothelial matrix[2] (Fig. 129-1); their biochemical defect is deficiency or dysfunction of the GPIb/IX complex that mediates this process.[3,4]

Biologic and Molecular Aspects

Following vascular trauma, circulating platelets make contact with and adhere to exposed subendothelial connective tissue. However, the requirements for platelet adherence differ according to the shear rate of the flowing blood.[5] Under low shear conditions, platelets adhere to subendothelial collagen, fibronectin, or laminin. Under high shear conditions, like those found in arterioles and in the microcirculation, platelet adhesion requires the presence of subendothelial vWF.[6,7] vWF is an elongated multimeric glycoprotein, each monomer of which contains two domains that interact with platelets.[8,9] One domain interacts with the GPIIb/IIIa complex after agonist-induced platelet activation.[10] The other interacts with the platelet GPIb/IX complex and is the domain responsible for activation-independent platelet adhesion at high shear.[11] Normally, soluble vWF does not bind to platelets. In vitro, exposure of platelets to the antibiotic ristocetin induces vWF binding to GPIb/IX.[12] However, the factors that induce vWF binding to GPIb/IX in vivo are unknown. One possibility is that changes occur in the conformation of vWF in the subendothelium that allows it to interact with GPIb/IX.[7,13,14] A second, but not mutually exclusive, possibility is that shear stress generated in circulating blood induces vWF binding to GPIb/IX by changing the conformation of either GPIb/IX or vWF.[15-17] Nonetheless, absence of GPIb/IX complexes on the surface of Bernard-Soulier platelets precludes the ability of these platelets to bind to subendothelial vWF under high shear conditions.

The GPIb/IX complex is a 1:1 noncovalent complex of the heavily glycosylated 165,000-MW GPIb with the 20,000-MW GPIX.[15] Both GPIb and GPIX are embedded in the platelet membrane,[18] and the cytoplasmic portion of GPIb is associated with the platelet cytoskeleton[19] through an interaction with actin-binding protein.[20] There are approximately 25,000 copies of GPIb/IX on the platelet surface.[15]

GPIb is composed of a 143,000-MW α-subunit GPIbα disulfide-linked to a 22,000-MW β-subunit GPIbβ.[15] GPIbα is susceptible to cleavage by a calcium-dependent platelet protease and by trypsin, giving rise to a heavily glycosylated 135,000-MW N-terminal fragment termed glycocalicin[15] and a 25,000-MW remnant that remains disulfide-linked to GPIbβ and associated with GPIX.[18] The N-terminal portion of glycocalicin contains binding sites for vWF and thrombin,[15] while the C-terminal portion contains most of the carbohydrate found on GPIb, consisting of

sialic acid-rich hexasaccharides O-linked to serine and threonine residues.[21] GPIbβ contains a serine residue (Ser 166) that can be phosphorylated by the cAMP-dependent protein kinase[22] and may contribute to inhibition of collagen-induced platelet actin polymerization.[23] Both GPIbβ and GPIX are acylated with palmitic acid through thioester linkages, probably at a free cysteine residue in the cytoplasmic portion of each protein.[24] The fatty acid acylation may stabilize their interaction with the membrane lipid bilayer or with other membrane proteins.

Analyses of the amino acid sequences of GPIbα, GPIbβ, and GPIX reveal that each contains leucine-rich amino acid stretches with the consensus sequence L-L—N-L—LPPGLL-G—L-.[21,25,26] Similar sequences were noted first in the plasma protein leucine-rich α_2 glycoprotein and have been observed in 13 other proteins.[15] There are seven tandem leucine-rich (LRG) repeats in GPIbα, while GPIbβ and GPIX each contain a single sequence. The amino acids flanking the repeats have also been conserved.[15] The function of the LRG repeats is not known. The presence of multiple leucine residues suggests that the repeats could act like the leucine zippers that are involved in the dimerization of the oncogenes *fos* and *jun*.[15] However, the leucine zipper motif consists of an amphipathic α-helix, while the LRG may exist as an amphipathic β-sheet.[27] Moreover, the LRG repeats in GPIbα, GPIbβ, and GPIX are not located in regions of each molecule involved in known intermolecular associations.[15] However, they could be involved in intramolecular associations that contribute to the tertiary structure of each molecule. Studies of the biosynthesis and intracellular assembly of recombinant GPIb/IX complexes indicate that each component of the complex (GPIbα, GPIbβ, and GPIX) must be present for the efficient expression of the complex on the cell surface.[28] Accordingly, these studies predict that the lack of GPIb/IX expression in the Bernard-Soulier syndrome could be the result of mutations in any one of the components of the complex.

Etiology and Pathogenesis

The structural defect in Bernard-Soulier platelets is deficiency or dysfunction of the GPIb/IX complex. In most instances, the deficiency is absolute, but in a few instances, 7–47% residual GPIb or GPIb/IX has been detected.[3,29,30] Bernard-Soulier platelets also lack a fourth protein, the 82,000-MW GPV.[3,29] GPV is a substrate for thrombin, which cleaves a soluble 69,000-MW. GPV fragment from the surface of normal but not Bernard-Soulier, platelets.[31,32] GPV cleavage is not involved in platelet activation, however, because prevention of the cleavage with anti-GPV antibodies does not prevent thrombin-induced platelet activation.[32] The amino acid sequence of GPV contains 15 tandem LRG repeats homologous to those of GPIbα, GPIbβ, and GPIX,[33] GPV forms a noncovalent complex with GPIb/IX[34], and, like GPIbα, GPIbβ, and GPIX, the LGR repeats do not appear to be involved in the formation of a GPIb/IX/V complex.[34] There are twice as many GPIb/IX complexes on the platelet surface as there are GPV molecules, suggesting that not all GPIb/IX complexes also contain GPV. Consistent with this observation, studies of GPIb/IX biosyn-

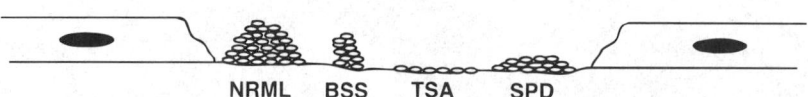

Fig. 129-1. Formation of platelet thrombi on a subendothelial surface. Following the exposure of circulating blood to an exposed subendothelial surface, normal platelets (NRML) cover the exposed surface and aggregate to form platelet thrombi. Bernard-Soulier platelets (BSS), because they cannot bind to subendothelial vWF, fail to cover the endothelial surface, but retain the ability to aggregate and form thrombi. By contrast, thrombasthenia platelets (TSA) retain the ability to cover the exposed subendothelium, but cannot aggregate. δ-Storage pool-deficient platelets (SPD) cover the subendothelial surface and aggregate to form thrombi. However, the size of the thrombi they form is decreased in proportion to the extent of their storage pool deficiency.

thesis suggest that GPV is not required for GPIb/IX expression on the platelet surface.[28] Nonetheless, the basis for the GPV in the Bernard-Soulier syndrome is not known.

The GPIb/IX deficiency in Bernard-Soulier platelets has consequences other than an inability to adhere to vWF. Most Bernard-Soulier platelets are large when observed on peripheral blood smears. However, there is conflicting evidence regarding the size of the platelets in the circulation. It has been reported that circulating Bernard-Soulier platelets are of normal size[35] but have increased membrane, perhaps located in the surface-connected open-canalicular system and extruded when platelets spread during the preparation of a blood smear.[36] Others have found that circulating Bernard-Soulier platelets have an increased volume,[37] a more spherical shape,[37] and a more deformable membrane than normal platelets.[38] The serum prothrombin time has been reported to be shortened in the Bernard-Soulier syndrome[39] and collagen-induced platelet procoagulant activity and factor XI binding to be absent.[40] However, prothrombin consumption measured by a two-stage assay is normal,[41] and the expression of platelet factor 3[41] and prothrombinase activity by Bernard-Soulier platelets is increased,[42] related perhaps to increased membrane surface area or to abnormalities in the distribution of membrane phospholipids.[43] A unexplained decrease in the activity of phospholipase C stimulated by thrombin, trypsin, or the thromboxane analogue U46619 has also been reported in the platelets of the three Bernard-Soulier patients.[44] GPIb/IX has been found to be a target for the drug-dependent antiplatelet antibodies induced by quinidine and quinine,[45–47] and it has been observed that these antibodies fail to bind to Bernard-Soulier platelets.[48]

Genetic Aspects

The Bernard-Soulier syndrome is an autosomal recessive disorder.[49] When it has been possible to study heterozygotes for the syndrome, most have had platelets that were larger than normal, with a GPIb content intermediate between normal and affected individuals.[29,50] Consistent with the rarity of the syndrome, consanguinity has often been noted in patient families.

The GPIbα gene is located on chromosome 17p12-ter,[51] the GPIbβ gene on chromosome 22 (Roth G, Deaven L: personal communication), and the GPIX gene on chromosome 3.[52] The GPIbα gene consists of two exons, with the entire coding unit of the gene contained within the second exon.[51,53] The 5′ flanking region of the gene does not contain the commonly observed TATA or CAAT promoter elements, but does contain the GATA element that is present in genes specifically expressed in megakaryocytes.[54] The GPIbβ gene has not been cloned, but a partial sequence for the GPIX gene has been determined.[55] This gene consists of three exons and two introns that span 1.6 kb, with the reading frame encoding GPIX in the third exon.[55] Like the GPIbα gene, the GPIX gene lacks TATA or CAAT elements and contains a GATA sequence.[55] The latter is located in proximity to the sequence ACTTCCT, which interacts with the *ets* family of transcription factors and is also present in the genes for GPIIb, platelet factor-4 (PF-4), and β-thromboglobulin (β-TG).[55]

Mutations responsible for the Bernard-Soulier syndrome have been determined in a few instances. Their consequences are consistent with the scheme for GPIb/IX biosynthesis described above.[28] One patient whose platelets failed to express GPIbα on their surface was found to be a compound heterozygote for a nonsense mutation in the codon for residue 343 (Trp→stop) that resulted in the synthesis of a 40,000-MW GPIbα fragment.[56] The identity of the other GPIbα mutation was not determined. In a kindred that included three affected siblings whose platelets expressed little GPIb, no abnormalities in the GPIbα or GPIbβ genes were detected.[57] However, the patients were compound heterozygotes for two missense mutations in the coding region for GPIX (Asp 21→Gly, Asn 45→Ser),

confirming that the inability to synthesize GPIX precludes the normal expression of GPIb/IX. Similarly, restriction fragment length polymorphism analysis of the DNA of two affected members of another family indicated that their disease was not linked to the GPIbα loci and that the responsible mutations involved either GPIbβ or GPIX.[58]

Variants of the Bernard-Soulier syndrome have been described that result from qualitative, rather than quantitative, abnormalities in GPIb/IX. A patient with the Bolzano variant whose platelets contain close to 50% of the normal amount of GPIb was found to have an Ala 156→Val substitution in the sixth LRG of GPIbα.[59,60] The inability of a recombinant GPIbα fragment containing this mutation to bind vWF confirmed that it is responsible for the patient's platelet function disorder.[60] A Leu 57→Phe substitution of one GPIbα allele was detected in the affected members of another family who presented with a moderate bleeding diathesis.[61] Although the affected family members were thrombocytopenic and had large platelets, their platelets contained normal amounts of GPIb/IX and agglutinated to a variable extent in the presence of ristocetin. In contrast to the classical Bernard-Soulier syndrome, however, the bleeding disorder in this family was inherited as an autosomal dominant. Why these heterozygous individuals have a bleeding diathesis, whereas the usual Bernard-Soulier heterozygotes are asymptomatic, is also unexplained.

Clinical Manifestations

The Bernard-Soulier syndrome presents in infancy or childhood with bleeding characteristic of defective platelet function: ecchymoses, epistaxis, and gingival bleeding.[49] Later manifestations include menorrhagia and postpartum, gastrointestinal, and post-traumatic hemorrhage.[62,63] Hemarthroses and expanding hematomas are unusual. Although the severity of hemorrhages among affected individuals is variable, it is often sufficient to require frequent transfusions and suppression of menses. In one report of 59 cases, there were 10 deaths.[64] However, in some patients the severity of hemorrhage inexplicably declines over the course of the disease.[64] A patient has been reported with well-documented Bernard-Soulier syndrome who developed severe coronary atherosclerosis and unstable angina, requiring coronary artery bypass surgery.[65] This suggests that the defective platelet function in the Bernard-Soulier syndrome is not sufficient to protect against the development of atherosclerotic vascular disease.

Laboratory Evaluation

The bleeding time in patients with the Bernard-Soulier syndrome is markedly prolonged to >20 minutes.[41] Platelet counts are variable within kindreds and may vary in a given patient. Most patients are thrombocytopenic to some degree, and patients with platelet counts of <20,000/mm^3 have been reported.[66] Platelets seen on stained peripheral blood smears are large, with 30–80% having a mean diameter >3.5 μm.[50] Occasional platelets as large as 20–30 μm in diameter are also present. The red blood cells and white blood cells are normal, and distinctive abnormalities have not been observed in marrow megakaryocytes by light microscopy,[67] although abnormalities in the demarcation membrane system have been observed by electron microscopy.[68] The laboratory tests that distinguish Bernard-Soulier from normal platelets show failure of Bernard-Soulier platelets to agglutinate in the presence of ristocetin and decreased[69] or absent agglutination[70] after exposure to the pit viper venom protein botrocetin. In contrast to von Willebrand disease, these abnormalities cannot be corrected by the addition of normal plasma containing vWF.[66] Absence of ristocetin-induced agglutination and normal platelet aggregation can be reproduced in the whole blood aggregom-

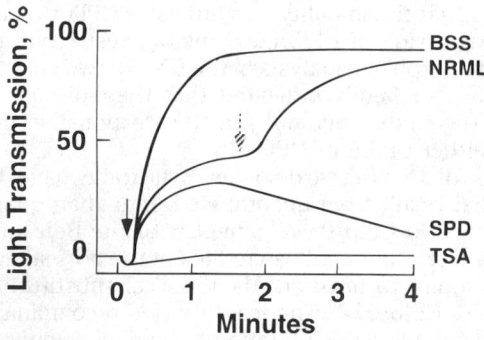

Fig. 129-2. Platelet aggregation in response to ADP. Following the addition of ADP to stirred aliquots of platelet-rich plasma in an aggregometer, there is a brief decrease in light transmission, indicated by the solid arrow, due to platelet shape change. When normal (NRML) or Bernard-Soulier platelets (BSS) are examined, shape change is followed by either a single continuous wave of aggregation at high ADP concentrations or two waves of aggregation at lower ADP concentrations. The hatched arrow at the inflection point between the first and second waves of aggregation is the point at which platelet secretion occurs. δ-Storage pool-deficient platelets (SPD) generally undergo only a first wave of aggregation, and the aggregates may dissociate. Thrombasthenic platelets (TSA) undergo shape change, but do not aggregate.

eter, obviating the difficulty of preparing platelet-rich plasma containing a sufficient number of platelets for conventional aggregometry from Bernard-Soulier blood.[71] Aggregation of Bernard-Soulier platelets induced by agonists such as ADP, collagen, thrombin, and epinephrine is normal (Fig. 129-2).[49] Although a defect in prothrombin consumption, manifested by a short serum prothrombin time, has been reported, expression of PF-3 activity by Bernard-Soulier platelets is normal or increased.[41]

Differential Diagnosis

Other conditions associated with thrombocytopenia and large platelets can be differentiated from the Bernard-Soulier syndrome by the failure of Bernard-Soulier platelets to agglutinate in the presence of ristocetin. Giant platelets, thrombocytopenia, and Döhle bodies in leukocytes are seen in the May-Hegglin anomaly.[72] The function and membrane proteins of May-Hegglin platelets are normal.[73] When hemorrhage does occur in these patients, it correlates with the extent of the thrombocytopenia.[72] Autosomal dominant hereditary nephritis and sensorineural deafness has been associated with large platelets and thrombocytopenia (Epstein syndrome).[74] Although platelet function in some affected individuals is normal,[75,76] in others platelet aggregation and secretion induced by ADP, collagen, and epinephrine is defective.[74,77] Gray platelet syndrome is due to a deficiency of platelet α-granules and is associated with large platelets and thrombocytopenia.[78] In contrast to Bernard-Soulier platelets, these platelets are pale gray on Wright-stained blood smears due to the lack of α-gran-

ules, and they agglutinate normally in the presence of ristocetin.[79] In the autosomal dominant Montreal platelet syndrome giant platelets, thrombocytopenia, and a prolonged bleeding time are associated with spontaneous aggregation at pH 7.4 and normal agonist-induced platelet aggregation.[80] So-called Mediterranean macrothrombocytopenia is not a unique entity, but refers to a putative difference in platelet count and platelet size among Europeans of Northern and Mediterranean origin.[81] There are also anecdotal reports of thrombocytopenia and giant platelets, often associated with a mild bleeding diathesis, but lacking the features of either Bernard-Soulier syndrome or the May-Hegglin anomaly.[82–84]

Acquired Bernard-Soulier-like disorders can be differentiated from the congenital Bernard-Soulier syndrome by history. Antibodies to GPIb occur in some patients with idiopathic thrombocytopenic purpura,[85–87] but it has been difficult to determine whether the antibodies are responsible for bleeding because of the concomitant thrombocytopenia. Two patients with myelodysplasia and an acquired Bernard-Soulier-like syndrome have been reported. One 5-year-old patient had a population of large platelets that agglutinated poorly in response to ristocetin and lacked a GPIb/IX complex.[88] The second patient was a 75-year-old woman who developed an autoantibody against GPIX that inhibited the interaction of her platelets with vWF.[89] A patient has also been reported with a lymphoproliferative disorder and clinical bleeding who had a prolonged bleeding time, a normal platelet count and platelet morphology, and a circulating IgG antibody that inhibited ristocetin-induced platelet agglutination but was directed against an unidentified 210,000-MW platelet protein.[90]

Therapy

Treatment of hemorrhage in patients with the Bernard-Soulier syndrome usually requires platelet transfusion (Table 129-1). Hormonal control of menses has been effective in managing menorrhagia.[91] In several instances splenectomy has been tried in an attempt to increase the platelet count.[92] This has resulted in only transient increases in the platelet count and has not ameliorated the platelet function defect. The use of corticosteroids is not beneficial in this disorder. Desmopressin acetate (DDAVP) has been reported to shorten the bleeding time in several affected individuals.[93–95] The efficacy of DDAVP in Bernard-Soulier patients with hemorrhage has not been reported.

Deficiency of Platelet Collagen Receptors

At low shear, platelets adhere to collagen, fibronectin, and laminin and contain receptors for each of these proteins.[96] However, the interaction of platelets with collagen is unique because collagen not only supports platelet adhesion, but is also a platelet agonist. Several platelet proteins that interact with collagen have been identified, including GPIIb,[97] GPIV,[98] GPVI,[99] the GPIa/IIa complex,[100] a 65,000-MW protein that binds

Table 129-1. Therapy for Inherited Disorders of Platelet Function

Disorder	Defect in Platelet Function	Structural Defect	Treatment Options		
			Platelet Transfusion	DDAVP	Corticosteroids
Bernard-Soulier syndrome	Adhesion	GPIb/IX deficiency	Y	?	N
Thrombasthenia	Aggregation	GPIIb/IIIa deficiency	Y	N	N
Gray platelet syndrome	Secretion	α-Granule deficiency	Y	Y	?
Storage pool disease	Secretion	δ-Granule deficiency	Y	Y	?
Primary secretion defects	Secretion	Defective signal transduction	Y	Y	?
Scott syndrome	Procoagulant activity	Decreased exposure of anionic phospholipids	Y	N	N

Abbreviations: Y, yes; N, No; ?, may be effective in some cases; DDAVP, desmopressin.

to a component of chick skin collagen,[101] and a protein similar but not identical to GPIV.[102] Which of these proteins are collagen receptors is not clear, but clinical data suggest that GPIa/IIa, GPVI, and the GPIV-like protein function in this manner.

GPIa/IIa

The GPIa/IIa heterodimer is indistinguishable from the lymphocyte VLA-2 complex (integrin $\alpha_2\beta_1$)[96,103] and functions as a Mg^{2+}-dependent collagen receptor for a number of cell types,[104] including platelets.[100,105,106] For unexplained reasons, the number of copies of GPIa/IIa per platelet varies from individual to individual, ranging from close to 900 to close to 3,000.[107]

Two patients with histories of bleeding have been reported whose platelets either failed to aggregate in response to collagen[108] or failed to respond to low collagen concentrations, but responded to higher concentrations.[109] The platelets of the first patient contained about 15–25% of the normal amount of GPIa and failed to adhere to collagen under static conditions[108] and to spread and aggregate on collagen under flow conditions.[110] The platelets of the second patient completely lacked GPIa, plus the α-granule protein thrombospondin, and adhered normally to, but failed to spread on, collagen-coated surfaces. Aggregation in response to collagen was restored by the addition of purified thrombospondin. Mysteriously, the patient's bleeding diathesis and the GPIa and thrombospondin deficiencies disappeared at the time of menopause.

GPVI

A deficiency of GPVI, a 61,000-MW platelet membrane protein, has been reported in two patients with histories of purpura and epistaxis.[99,111] The platelets of these patients failed to adhere to and aggregate in response to collagen, despite the presence of normal amounts of GPIa/IIa. Additional support for a role for GPVI in collagen-induced platelet function came from the detection of an antibody against GPVI in a patient with ITP that inhibited collagen-induced platelet function.[99,112]

GPIV

GPIV, also known as CD36, is a single-chain 88,000-MW protein that has been identified on the surface of a variety of cells.[113] GPIV has been found to be an endothelial receptor for red cells parasitized by *Plasmodium falciparum*,[114] a binding site for thrombospondin,[115,116] a receptor for oxidized low-density lipoprotein,[117] and a signal transduction molecule.[118] GPIV has also been purported to be a platelet collagen receptor because Fab fragments of GPIV antibodies inhibit collagen-mediated platelet adhesion and activation and because purified GPIV binds to collagen and inhibits collagen-induced platelet aggregation.[98] GPIV carries the platelet antigen Nak[a],[119] and platelets of Nak[a]-negative individuals lack GPIV.[120] However, Nak[a]-negative individuals are asymptomatic, and their platelets interact with collagen,[121] albeit slightly less well than Nak[a]-positive platelets.[122,123] Thus, a role of GPIV in collagen-mediated platelet function remains to be clarified.

DISORDERS OF PLATELET AGGREGATION

Glanzmann Thrombasthenia

Glanzmann thrombasthenia (GPIIb/IIIa deficiency) is a rare hemorrhagic disorder characterized by a prolonged bleeding time, a normal platelet count, and absent macroscopic platelet aggregation.[49] Thrombasthenia was originally described by Glanzmann in 1918[124] as a bleeding disorder associated with a normal platelet count and abnormal clot retraction. The defect in platelet function responsible for Glanzmann thrombasthenia is the inability of thrombasthenic platelets to aggregate (Fig. 129-1); their structural defect is deficiency or dysfunction of the platelet membrane GPIIb/IIIa complex.[125]

Biologic and Molecular Aspects

Following platelet adhesion to sites of vascular damage, circulating platelets aggregate on the layer of adherent platelets to form hemostatic plugs.[126] Platelet aggregation requires the agonist-induced exposure of binding sites for soluble fibrinogen or vWF, or both, on the platelet membrane GPIIb/IIIa complex.[127–131] Fibrinogen or vWF (or both) bound to GPIIb/IIIa then cross-link adjacent platelets into occlusive platelet plugs. Although GPIIb/IIIa is normally present on the surface of resting platelets, its ligand binding sites are not exposed until platelets are activated by agonists such as thrombin or ADP.[127,132] In addition to interacting with soluble proteins, GPIIb/IIIa can bind to subendothelial vWF and fibronectin, allowing adherent platelets to spread on the subendothelial matrix.[133,134] Following ligand binding, the cytoplasmic domains of GPIIb/IIIa associate with submembranous actin filaments via intermediary cytoskeletal proteins.[135–138] This interaction likely provides a mechanism for transmitting the force of cytoskeletal contraction to the fibrin in a clot, resulting in clot retraction.[139,140] There are approximately 50,000 GPIIb/IIIa complexes on the surface of normal unactivated platelets,[141] and additional complexes, present in the membrane of the platelet α-granules, can be translocated to the platelet surface by platelet activation.[142,143] Glanzmann thrombasthenia results when platelets lack sufficient numbers of functional GPIIb/IIIa complexes on their surface to support platelet aggregation.[125] Because the platelets of obligate heterozygotes for thrombasthenia aggregate normally, but contain one-half the normal number of GPIIb/IIIa complexes, at most 25,000 normal GPIIb/IIIa complexes per platelet are sufficient to support normal platelet aggregation.[144]

The GPIIb/IIIa complex is calcium-dependent heterodimer and dissociates into GPIIb and GPIIIa monomers in the presence of calcium chelators.[145] When examined by electron microscopy, GPIIb/IIIa appears as a 12×8-nm globular head with two 18-nm tails extending from one side.[146,147] When incorporated into phospholipid vesicles, the globular head extends about 20 nm above the vesicle surface, and the tips of the tails are inserted into the phospholipid.[148] This finding suggests that the globular head contains the domains that interact with protein ligands and that the tails contain its membrane anchors.

GPIIb is a two-chain protein with a molecular weight of 136,000 and is composed of disulfide-linked heavy (GPIIbα) and light (GPIIbβ) chains with molecular weights of 125,000 and 23,000, respectively.[145] The light chain contains a transmembrane anchor,[149] while the heavy chain contains domains that interact with GPIIIa.[150,151] GPIIb is synthesized as single-chain 1,008 amino acid precursor, pro-GPIIb.[149,152] In the endoplasmic reticulum (ER), pro-GPIIb pairs with GPIIIa, and the complex is transported to the Golgi apparatus, where pro-GPIIb is cleaved into heavy and light chains.[153] The most notable feature of the GPIIb sequence is the presence of four heavy chain domains that are similar to calcium-binding domains in troponin C and calmodulin[149] and are capable of binding calcium.[154] Moreover, a region proximal to the second calcium-binding domain, extending from residues 294–314, has been chemically cross-linked to a peptide corresponding to the N terminus of the γ-chain of fibrinogen, suggesting that this portion of GPIIb/IIIa is a ligand-binding site.[155–157]

GPIIIa is a cysteine-rich single-chain protein with an apparent molecular weight of 90,000 on unreduced sodium dodecyl sulfate gels that increases to 110,000 following disulfide bond reduction.[145] It contains 736 amino acids and is anchored in the platelet membrane by a domain located near its C terminus.[158-160] The most striking feature of the GPIIIa sequence is the presence of 56 cysteine residues and 28 disulfide bonds.[158,159,161] The disulfide bonds are distributed in three regions in the extracellular portion of the molecule: a cysteine-rich, protease-resistant N terminus (residues 1–62), a protease-sensitive central region (residues 101–422), and a disulfide-rich, protease-resistant core (residues 423–622).[161] In addition, there is a long-range disulfide bond between Cys residues 5 and 435 that produces a large protease-sensitive loop in the molecule.[161-163]

GPIIb and GPIIIa are assembled into heterodimers in the calcium-rich environment of the ER.[164-168] In the absence of heterodimer formation, neither GPIIb nor GPIIIa leave the ER, and each is eventually degraded in this organelle.[168] The factors responsible for the retention of GPIIb and GPIIIa, but not GPIIb/IIIa heterodimers, in the ER are not known. However, it is also apparent that the formation of GPIIb/IIIa heterodimers alone is not sufficient to guarantee egress of GPIIb/IIIa from the ER since mutations that distort the conformation of the complex result in its retention in the ER.[168,169]

Complexes similar to GPIIb/IIIa are present on the surface of most cells. These complexes, named integrins, are members of a superfamily of receptors that mediate a variety of cell-cell and cell-extracellular matrix interactions.[170] Like GPIIb/IIIa, integrins are $\alpha\beta$ heterodimers with α-subunits similar to GPIIb and β-subunits similar to GPIIIa. Currently, 16 integrin α-subunits and 8 β-subunits have been identified, as have several alternatively spliced α- and β-subunit variants.[171] Because each integrin β-subunit interacts with a restricted number of α-subunits, the integrins can be subclassified into subfamilies based on the usage of a particular β-subunit.[170] GPIIb/IIIa belongs to a small subfamily consisting of GPIIb/IIIa, also known as $\alpha_{IIb}\beta_3$, and a receptor for vitronectin, $\alpha_v\beta_3$. While $\alpha_v\beta_3$ is found on a variety of cells, including endothelium and platelets, GPIIb/IIIa expression is normally restricted to cells of the megakaryocytic lineage because the gene for GPIIb is only active in these cells.[159]

Etiology and Pathogenesis

The inability of thrombasthenic platelets to aggregate is due to a deficiency of functional GPIIb/IIIa complexes. This deficiency is also responsible for a number of other platelet abnormalities. First, thrombasthenic platelets fail to spread normally on the subendothelial matrix following initial contact,[133,172] a finding consistent with a role of GPIIb/IIIa in this aspect of platelet adhesion. Second, the fibrinogen content of the α-granules in thrombasthenic platelets is either decreased or absent.[173] Because megakaryocytes do not synthesize fibrinogen,[174-176] its presence in the α-granule results from the endocytosis of plasma fibrinogen, perhaps by a receptor-mediated process.[177,178] Kistrin and barbourin, snake venom proteins that inhibit fibrinogen binding to GPIIb/IIIa, block the endocytosis of fibrinogen by guinea pig megakaryocytes.[179,180] Thus, it is likely that GPIIb/IIIa is involved in the endocytosis of fibrinogen, and the absence of functional GPIIb/IIIa in thrombasthenia accounts for the deficit in α-granule fibrinogen. Third, clot retraction in blood containing thrombasthenic platelets is either absent or reduced.[181] This finding is consistent with a role for GPIIb/IIIa in linking the fibrin clot to the contractile elements of the platelet cytoskeleton.[139,140] Fourth, a number of platelet alloantigens are located on the GPIIb/IIIa complex and have been reported to be absent from thrombasthenic platelets. These include the Bak^a (Lek^a) alloantigen present on GPIIb[182,183] and the PI^{A1}/PI^{A2} and Pen^a/Pen^b alloantigens present on GPIIIa.[184,185]

Those aspects of platelet function that do not depend on GPIIb/IIIa are normal in thrombasthenic platelets. Thrombas-

thenic platelets interact with collagen fibrils[181] and undergo secretion when stimulated by "strong agonists" such as thrombin.[173] vWF binds to GPIb/IX when thrombasthenic platelets are incubated with ristocetin,[12] and thrombasthenic platelets adhere to vWF in the subendothelium.[133,172] Thrombasthenic platelets also express a normal amount of procoagulant activity following lysis,[42] but procoagulant activity is decreased when measured under conditions that require platelet aggregation.[173]

Before the GPIIb/IIIa deficiency in thrombasthenia was recognized, the disease was classified into types I and II according to the presence or absence of clot retraction and α-granule fibrinogen.[173] In type I thrombasthenia, clot retraction and platelet α-granule fibrinogen are absent, while in type II disease, clot retraction is present, but decreased, and α-granule fibrinogen is present. Subsequently, it was found that type I platelets contain <5% of the normal amount of GPIIb/IIIa, while type II platelets contain 10–20%.[186] The residual GPIIb/IIIa in some type II patients may be capable of binding fibrinogen[187] and of supporting limited platelet aggregation that can be detected in whole blood as the loss of single platelets or visualized by light microscopy.[188] "Variant" thrombasthenia has also been described in which the platelet content of GPIIb/IIIa is $\geq$50% of normal and the abnormality in GPIIb/IIIa is qualitative, rather than quantitative.[186]

Genetic Aspects

Glanzmann thrombasthenia is inherited as an autosomal recessive disorder with prominent clusters of the disease in populations with consanguinity.[189-191] The genes for GPIIb and GPIIIa have been cloned and characterized, making it possible to determine the genetic basis for the disease in a number of cases. Because the expression of GPIIb/IIIa on the megakaryocyte surface requires the presence of both GPIIb and GPIIIa,[166] a mutation in the gene for either protein can produce the disease. It has often been possible to determine which gene is affected by measuring the number of vitronectin receptors ($\alpha_v\beta_3$) per platelet, since they may be increased when the GPIIb gene is affected and decreased when the GPIIIa (β_3) gene is affected.[192]

The genes for GPIIb and GPIIIa are both located on the long arm of chromosome 17 at q21$\rightarrow$23[160,193,194] and may reside within 260 kb of each other.[195] The gene for GPIIb spans about 18 kb and is located in a region of chromosome 17 that contains least seven complete and three incomplete Alu-repeats.[152] The gene consists of 30 exons ranging in size from 46–220 bp.[152] Although the organization of exons in many genes reflects the distribution of functional domains in the proteins they encode,[196] this does not appear to be true for the GPIIb gene. The 5′ flanking region of the GPIIb gene lacks TATA or CAAT boxes, much like known housekeeping genes.[197] While it is not yet clear why GPIIb expression is restricted to megakaryocytes, the 5′ flanking region of the gene has been found to contain sequences that are recognized by the GATA-binding transcription factors present in erythroid, megakaryocytic, and mast cell precursors[54,198] and by the *ets* transcription factor that is present in megakaryocytes.[199] The gene for GPIIIa spans >40 kb and contains $\geq$14 exons.[200,201] However, the exons encoding the 5′ untranslated region and the signal peptide have yet to be identified. Like the gene for GPIIb, there is little relationship between the organization of the GPIIIa exons and known functional domains in the protein.

Seven GPIIb mutations have been identified in kindreds with thrombasthenia. One mutation, a 4.5-kb deletion that includes exons 2–9, produced an mRNA that terminated GPIIb translation shortly after the signal peptide.[202] Although the breakpoint at the 5′ end of the deletion was located within an Alu-repeat, the 3′ breakpoint was not, indicating that nonhomologous crossing over involving Alu-repeats could not explain the deletion. Two mutations have been identified that have either altered[203] or deleted[204] a splice acceptor site in the GPIIb gene, resulting in alternative mRNA splicing and aberrant GPIIb proteins. A C→T transition in the codon for Arg 584 has also been reported independently from Japan[203] and China.[202] This transition results in a premature termination codon in the GPIIb mRNA and the synthesis of a truncated GPIIb protein. Three missense mutations (Gly 273→Asp, Gly 418→Asp, Arg 327→His) are of particular interest because they do not prevent the assembly of GPIIb/IIIa complexes but alter the conformation of these complexes sufficiently to impair their transport from the ER to the Golgi apparatus.[169,205,206]

Nine mutations in the GPIIIa gene have been reported. One complex mutation, a 15-kb inversion and a 1-kb deletion, resulted from homologous recombination among three Alu sequences[207] and either led to the synthesis of an unstable GPIIIa mRNA or severely impaired transcription of the GPIIIa gene.[208] Two mutations have been detected that introduce a premature termination codon into the GPIIIa mRNA by shifting the GPIIIa reading frame: one mutation, identified in Iraqi Jews in Israel, was the result of an 11-base deletion in exon xii of the GPIIIa gene[204]; the second mutation, a G→T transition at the intron i-exon i boundary, eliminated the GT splice donor site and resulted in the deletion of exon i by abnormal splicing.[209] In a fourth mutant, exon ix was deleted from the GPIIIa mRNA by alternative splicing,[210] and in a fifth, identified in a patient from China, a G→A transition in the codon for Cys 374 converted it to a codon for tyrosine.[211] The four remaining mutations are missense mutations that have produced variant thrombasthenia, a type of thrombasthenia in which platelets contain nearly normal amounts of nonfunctional GPIIb/IIIa. In one kindred, a C→T transition converted Ser 752 in the cytoplasmic domain of GPIIIa to proline and prevented GPIIb/IIIa activation by cellular agonists.[212] In each of the remaining kindreds, a charged amino acid in the extracellular domain of GPIIIa was converted to an uncharged residue. These mutations (Asp 119→Tyr[213]; Arg 214→Trp[214]; Arg 214→Gln[215]) are located in regions of GPIIIa that have been implicated in ligand binding,[216,217] perhaps explaining the impaired function of the affected complexes.

Additional patients with thrombasthenia have been reported in whom abnormalities in GPIIb/IIIa structure and distribution have been detected, but the responsible mutations have not yet been identified. Three patients with variant thrombasthenia were found to have GPIIb/IIIa complexes that dissociated abnormally in the presence of low concentrations of EDTA.[218–220] The GPIIb/IIIa complex of another patient was not only more sensitive to EDTA, but also failed to react with a anti-GPIIb/IIIa monoclonal antibody, suggesting that the conformation of the complex was abnormal.[221] Two patients from Japan have also been reported with unexplained abnormalities in GPIIb/IIIa structure: one patient had variant thrombasthenia attributed to abnormal GPIIb/IIIa glycosylation,[222] and the platelets of the second patient contained an abnormal form of GPIIb.[223] Finally, the platelets of a patient with a mild thrombasthenia-like illness were found to aggregate poorly in response to ADP and other agonists and to have a deficit in the surface pool, but not the internal pool, of GPIIb/IIIa.[224]

Clinical Manifestations

A review of the clinical manifestations of thrombasthenia in 177 patients, including a cohort of 64 patients followed in Paris over a period of 33 years, has been published.[186] Thrombasthenia typically presents with mucocutaneous bleeding in the neonatal period or infancy, occasionally with bleeding following circumcision. Spontaneous petechiae are uncommon, and bleeding generally results from a condition that would cause

bleeding in an otherwise normal individual. Next to purpura, epistaxis is the most frequent type of bleeding, especially in childhood. Gingival bleeding, often related to poor dental hygiene, and menorrhagia are frequent. Bleeding at menarche may be particularly severe and may require transfusion. Similarly, parturition represents a severe hemorrhagic risk. Other hemorrhagic manifestations include gastrointestinal bleeding and hematuria, while the hemarthroses and deep hematomas characteristic of coagulation disorders are unusual. Serious bleeding may follow trauma or surgery in patients not prepared with normal platelets. The severity of the hemorrhagic diathesis is not predictable, even within single kindreds, and does not correlate with the extent of the GPIIb/IIIa deficiency. Thus, one sibling may experience life-threatening bleeding requiring frequent transfusion, while another will suffer only mild bruising and epistaxis. The apparent decline in the clinical severity of thrombasthenia with age is likely due to a decrease in the incidence of conditions such as epistaxis with aging.

Laboratory Evaluation

Platelet counts and platelet morphology on peripheral blood smears are normal. However, the bleeding times of affected individuals are markedly prolonged.[181,189,190] A diagnosis of thrombasthenia is usually suspected after platelet aggregometry. Normally, the addition of agonists (except for epinephrine) to a stirred suspension of platelets results in an immediate decrease in light transmission corresponding to platelet shape change, followed by a rapid increase in light transmission due to the formation of platelet aggregates. By contrast, stimulation of thrombasthenic platelets results in only platelet shape change, and platelet aggregation is absent[49] (Fig. 129-2). Platelet secretion following platelet stimulation with strong agonists such as thrombin is normal, but secretion in response to weak agonists such ADP and epinephrine is absent. Coagulation tests, such as the prothrombin time and the partial thromboplastin time, are normal in thrombasthenia. Clot retraction in the presence of thrombasthenic platelets is either absent or reduced.

Differential Diagnosis

A history of lifelong bleeding, a prolonged bleeding time, and the absence of platelet aggregation are diagnostic of thrombasthenia and differentiate it from other disorders of platelet adhesion and secretion. Instances of acquired thrombasthenia have been reported and can be differentiated from congenital thrombasthenia by history. Although autoantibodies against GPIIb/IIIa have been detected frequently in patients with idiopathic thrombocytopenic purpura,[225,226] autoantibodies that induce a thrombasthenic-like state are unusual.[227–229] A patient with multiple myeloma has also been reported whose IgG1-κ paraprotein was directed against GPIIIa and inhibited GPIIb/IIIa function.[230] Administration of the drug ticlopidine induces a functional thrombasthenic-like state in normal platelets.[231] Congenital afibrinogenemia may be also associated with a prolonged bleeding time and decreased in vitro platelet aggregation.[232] These findings are due to the absence of sufficient fibrinogen to support platelet aggregation adequately and can be corrected by infusions of fibrinogen.

Therapy

Bleeding in thrombasthenia requires the transfusion of normal platelets[186] (Table 129-1). Because bleeding is a lifelong problem, the use of HLA-matched platelets should be considered to lessen the chance of refractoriness to transfusion due to platelet alloimmunization. In rare instances, thrombasthenic patients have developed antibodies against normal GPIIb and GPIIIa following transfusion.[233,234] Such antibodies could potentially limit the effectiveness of transfused platelets. Oral contraceptives have been useful in controlling menorrhagia. Regular dental care is essential in minimizing gingival bleeding, and fibrinolytic inhibitors such as ε-aminocaproic acid, in addition to platelet transfusions, may be useful in controlling bleeding after dental extractions. Corticosteroids have not proved efficacious in managing bleeding in thrombasthenic patients.[181] Although DDAVP was reported to shorten the bleeding time in a patient with thrombasthenia and to have a beneficial effect during minor dental surgery,[93] this is the only report of an effect of DDAVP in thrombasthenia.[235] In one severely affected child, bone marrow transplantation was performed using marrow from an HLA-identical sibling who was a thrombasthenic heterozygote and completely corrected the platelet function abnormality.[236]

DISORDERS OF PLATELET SECRETION

The platelet cytoplasm contains four types of granules: dense granules containing ADP, ATP, calcium, serotonin, and pyrophosphate; α-granules containing a variety of proteins, some derived from the plasma, others synthesized by the megakaryocyte; lysosomes containing acid hydrolases; and microperoxisomes containing a peroxidase activity.[237] Following platelet activation, the contents of these granules are extruded from the platelet interior by a process known as platelet secretion. Inherited disorders of platelet secretion result from a deficiency of one or more of the types of platelet granules or from abnormalities in the platelet secretory mechanism. Secretion disorders are a frequent cause of mild-to-moderate bleeding manifested by easy bruising, menorrhagia, and excessive postoperative and postpartum blood loss.[238] In one group of 145 patients presenting with these symptoms, 18% were found to have a deficiency of platelet granules, 19% to have an abnormality in the platelet secretory mechanism, and 36% to have von Willebrand disease.[239] No explanation for the bleeding diathesis could be found in 27% of the patients. Patients with disorders of platelet secretion usually have a prolonged bleeding time, absence of the second wave of platelet aggregation when platelets are stimulated by ADP and epinephrine, and decreased aggregation when platelets are stimulated by collagen.[238] These disorders must be differentiated from the acquired abnormalities of platelet secretion induced by drugs such as aspirin or systemic diseases such as uremia and multiple myeloma (see Ch. 130) and from the various types of von Willebrand disease (see Ch. 113).

Disorders of Secretion Due to Deficiency of Platelet Granules

α-Granule Deficiency (Gray Platelet Syndrome, α-Storage Pool Disease)

The gray platelet syndrome, described by Raccuglia in 1971,[78] is a rare disorder that results from the specific absence of morphologically recognizable α-granules in the platelets of affected individuals.

Biologic and Molecular Aspects

Normal platelets contain about 50 spherical or elongated structures termed α-granules that contain a variety of proteins, some of which are specific or relatively specific for platelets and others that are also found in plasma.[240] The former include PF-4, β-TG, platelet-derived growth factor (PDGF), and thrombospondin (TSP); the latter include fibrinogen, vWF, albumin, coagulation factor V, IgG, fibronectin, and a number of protease inhibitors.[237,240,241] The platelet-specific proteins and several

of the plasma proteins (vWF,[242] factor V[243]) are synthesized by megakaryocytes. The others reach the α-granules via endocytosis of circulating protein.[174,177,178] Three proteins have been identified in the α-granule membrane (GPIIb/IIIa,[244] P-selectin [CD62, GMP-140, PADGEM],[245,246] and osteonectin[247]); each can be translocated to the platelet surface following platelet activation.[142,143,245] The GPIIb/IIIa functions as a receptor for fibrinogen,[142] P-selectin mediates the interaction of platelets with various leukocytes,[248] and osteonectin can interact with secreted thrombospondin.[247] GPIIb/IIIa on the platelet surface and in the α-granule membrane may also be involved in the endocytosis and the concentration of plasma fibrinogen in the α-granule.[179,180]

Etiology and Pathogenesis

Electron micrographs of megakaryocytes and platelets from patients with the gray platelet syndrome reveal the absence of normal α-granules and the presence of vacuoles and small α-granule precursors containing material that stains for vWF and fibrinogen.[249,250] The other types of platelet granules are present in normal numbers.[249] The outer membranes of the vacuoles and the small α-granule precursors contain P-selectin and GPIIb/IIIa,[244,251] which can be translocated to the platelet surface after thrombin stimulation.[251] These observations indicate that α-granules are in fact present in gray platelets and suggest that the abnormality responsible for the gray platelet syndrome is the inability to target proteins to these structures. Accordingly, the inability to package and retain PF-4, β-TG, and PDGF in α-granules would account for the elevated plasma concentrations of PF-4 and β-TG and the bone marrow fibrosis observed in patients with the syndrome.[252] Furthermore, the abnormality responsible for the gray platelet syndrome appears to be restricted to megakaryocytes since electron micrographs of endothelial cells from affected patients reveal typical Weibel-Palade bodies, suggesting that these cells are capable of packing vWF normally.[253]

Clinical Manifestations and Laboratory Evaluation

Patients with the gray platelet syndrome present with a lifelong history of mild mucocutaneous bleeding,[78,79,253] although one patient developed subgaleal and epidural hematomas following head trauma.[254] Patients also exhibit variably prolonged bleeding times, moderate thrombocytopenia, reticulin fibrosis of the bone marrow, and large platelets whose gray appearance on a Wright-stained blood smear gives the name to the disorder.[78,79,253] Platelet counts vary from 25,000/mm³ to 150,000/mm³, but generally range between 60,000/mm³ and 100,000/mm³. Studies of platelet aggregation have produced variable results. Aggregation induced by ADP, epinephrine, arachidonic acid, and the calcium ionophore A23187 has generally been normal or nearly normal,[78,252] but collagen-induced aggregation has been decreased to absent in some cases[79,252] and normal in others.[78,254] Responses to thrombin have also been variable, with reports of decreased sensitivity to low thrombin concentrations,[79,252] impaired increments in intracellular calcium,[255] and decreased generation of inositol 1,4,5-triphosphate (IP₃).[256] Gray platelets agglutinate normally when exposed to ristocetin. The contents of their dense granules are normal.[79,257] As expected, the PF-4, β-TG, fibrinogen, vWF, factor V, fibronectin, and TSP content of their α-granules is markedly decreased. Surprisingly, gray platelets contain substantial quantities of albumin and IgG, proteins normally present in α-granules.[251,258] The PF-4 and β-TG concentrations in the plasma of affected individuals are normal or elevated.[79,252]

Genetic Aspects

The mode of inheritance of the gray platelet syndrome is uncertain, but the presence of the disorder in a brother and sister suggests it is an autosomal disease.[257] A disorder resembling the gray platelet syndrome is present in the Wistar Furth strain of rat and is inherited in an autosomal recessive fashion.[259]

Therapy

Treatment of bleeding episodes, if severe, may require the transfusion of normal platelets[254] (Table 129-1). DDAVP was found to shorten the bleeding time in one patient and was used as successful prophylaxis for a dental extraction.[260]

Dense Granule Deficiency (δ-Storage Pool Disease)

Biologic and Molecular Aspects

Normal platelets contain three to six 200–300-nm dense or δ-granules that serve as intracellular storage sites for ADP, ATP, calcium, pyrophosphate, and serotonin.[261] Because of their high calcium content, δ-granules can be visualized in electron micrographs of unfixed, unstained platelet whole mounts.[261] They can also be visualized by electron microscopy of thin sections of fixed platelets after staining with uranyl ions (uranaffin reaction) and by fluorescence microscopy after staining the platelets with mepacrine (quinacrine).[261] The δ-granule membrane contains a 40,000-MW protein called granulophysin that may be related to the synaptosomal membrane protein synaptophysin.[262] Granulophysin is translocated to the platelet surface following platelet activation.[263] The membrane may also contain P-selectin.[263] δ-Granules undergo exocytosis during platelet secretion, coincident with the second wave of platelet aggregation.[264] Although secreted ADP is thought to be involved in the propagation of the primary platelet response, the function of the other δ-granule contents is not known.[265,266] The biogenesis of δ-granules in megakaryocytes is poorly understood. δ-Storage-pool deficiency occurs in two syndromes of tyrosinase-positive albinism in humans,[267,268] in several pigment dilution syndromes in mice[269] and rats,[270] and as part of a Chediak-Higashi-like syndrome in cattle,[271] cats,[272] mink,[273] and foxes.[274] This suggests that the biogenesis of dense granules, melanosomes, and lysosomes is somehow related. The mechanism by which dense granules accumulate ATP and ADP is also not known. It is clear, however, that two pools of adenine nucleotides exist in normal platelets that exchange very slowly, if at all.[275] One pool is a metabolic nongranule pool in which the ATP/ADP ratio is 8–10:1. The second pool is present in the δ-granules and contains 65% of the platelet adenine nucleotides, with an ATP/ADP ratio of 2:3. Thus, in normal platelets, the whole platelet ATP/ADP ratio is <2.5. On the other hand, serotonin is not synthesized by megakaryocytes, but is taken up from the plasma and stored in the δ-granules, where it is protected from platelet monoamine oxidase.[276]

Etiology and Pathogenesis

δ-Storage pool disease represents a heterogeneous group of disorders with δ-granule abnormalities as the common feature.[261] The disorder can be subdivided into deficiency states associated with albinism and those in otherwise normal individuals. δ-Storage pool disease has also been observed in some patients with the Wiskott-Aldrich syndrome,[277] the syndrome of thrombocytopenia with absent radii,[278] the Ehlers-Danlos syndrome,[279] and osteogenesis imperfecta.[280] δ-Storage pool disease is sometimes associated with albinism, as in the Hermansky-Pudlack syndrome (oculocutaneous tyrosinase-positive albinism, platelet dense-granule deficiency, and ceroid-like inclusions in cells of the reticuloendothelial system),[267] and the Chédiak-Higashi syndrome (partial oculocutaneous albinism, frequent pyogenic infections, and giant lysosomal granules in cells of hematologic and nonhematologic origin)[281]; in such cases a quantitative δ-granule deficiency exists.[261,282] In the platelets of nonalbinos, however, the number of uranaffin-positive and mepacrine-positive granules is normal to only slightly decreased, suggesting an inability to package the δ-granule contents in these patients.[261] The platelet content of granulophysin also parallels the apparent number of δ-granules in storage pool-deficient patients, being low in patients with the Hermansky-Pudlack and Chédiak-Higashi syndromes, but normal in nonalbinos.[282] In some nonalbino patients, the δ-granule abnormality is associated with a variable deficiency of α-granules (αδ storage pool disease).[283,284] The nature of the α-granule deficiency in these patients is also heterogeneous. For example, in one patient with severe αδ storage pool disease, a decrease in the platelet content of P-selectin suggested that a defect in α-granule formation accompanied the deficit in δ-granules. In a family with less severe disease, however, the platelet content of P-selectin was normal, suggesting that the α-granule abnormality might be similar to that seen in the gray platelet syndrome.[284] The content of lysosomal acid hydrolases in platelets from patients with δ-storage pool disease is normal,[266] but thrombin-induced acid hydrolase secretion may be impaired in severely affected individuals, an abnormality that can be corrected in vitro by the addition of ADP.[266] The ability of δ-storage pool-deficient platelets to form thrombi on subendothelium has been studied ex vivo under various conditions of shear.[172] It was found that thrombus dimensions were reduced in proportion to the magnitude of the dense-granule deficit and were reduced even further when αδ storage pool disease platelets were examined (Fig. 129-1). These studies suggest that the contents of the δ- and α-granules either potentiate the growth of thrombi on the subendothelium or help to stabilize the thrombi in the presence of high shear stress.

Clinical Manifestations and Laboratory Evaluation

Patients with δ-storage pool disease present with a mild-to-moderate bleeding diathesis characteristic of patients with platelet secretion defects.[238] Platelet counts and morphology are usually normal, but bleeding times are usually, but not always, prolonged.[239] Moreover, the volume of blood that emerges from the bleeding time wounds in these patients is increased over normal, particularly at early time points, suggesting that δ-granule contents are involved in the contraction that follows vascular transection.[285] The quantity of thromboxane B_2 (TxB_2), a metabolite of thromboxane A_2 (TxA_2), in the collected blood is also decreased, especially in patients with αδ storage pool disease, a finding consistent with the impaired agonist-induced prostaglandin and thromboxane synthesis often detected in these platelets.[286] In the aggregometer, δ-storage pool-deficient platelets usually lack a second wave of aggregation when stimulated by agonists such as ADP and epinephrine[287] (Fig. 129-2). Responses to low concentrations of collagen are also diminished to absent, but responses to high collagen concentrations may be normal or nearly normal.[287,288] While this pattern of aggregation is typical for δ-storage pool disease, patients have been reported with normal aggregation studies.[239] Although the steady-state serotonin content of δ-storage pool-deficient platelets is decreased, the rate of uptake of serotonin is normal.[275] Without storage sites, however, the serotonin either leaks out of the platelet or is metabolized by platelet monoamine oxidase.[288,289] In δ-storage pool deficiency, the dense-granule pool of ADP no longer contributes to the whole platelet content of ADP, and the ATP/ADP ratio of δ-storage pool deficient platelets is ≥3.[238] This alteration in ATP/ADP ratio is extremely helpful in the diagnosis of δ-storage pool deficiency, especially when typical aggregation abnormalities are absent.[239]

Genetic Aspects

The Hermansky-Pudlak and Chédiak-Higashi syndromes are inherited as autosomal recessive disorders.[267,281] Although studies of the inheritance of δ-storage pool disease in patients without albinism are limited, examination of three generations of one family with this disorder suggests that it is transmitted in autosomal dominant fashion.[290] The nature of the mutations responsible for δ-storage pool disease are not known. Twelve independent murine mutations result in the disorder, indicating that multiple genetic loci are involved.[269,291–294] The murine *pallid* mutation has been mapped to the gene for protein 4.2.[295] How mutation of this protein, also present in the cytoskeleton of erythrocytes, results in δ-storage pool deficiency is not clear.

Therapy

Bleeding can be controlled by the transfusion of normal platelets (Table 129-1). This is seldom, if ever, necessary, however, because the potential risks of platelet transfusion far outweigh the benefits when bleeding is not life-threatening. Moreover, other methods to improve hemostasis readily without the risks of transfusion are available. Bleeding has been controlled by the administration of cryoprecipitate[296] or DDAVP.[297,298] Because the latter avoids the transfusion of blood products, it should be regarded as the initial therapy of choice. DDAVP is a vasopressin analogue whose pressor effects (V_1 vasopressin receptors) are substantially less than its antidiuretic effects (V_2 vasopressin receptors). Infusion of the drug releases large multimers of vWF and tissue plasminogen activator from tissue stores, and the released vWF accounts for the beneficial effect of the drug on the bleeding time in some forms of von Willebrand disease.[299] However, the precise mechanism of its ability to shorten the bleeding time in patients with disorders of platelet function remains to be determined. In several series of patients with platelet disorders, shortening the bleeding time in response to DDAVP occurred in 43–100% of patients.[297,298] This variability in response rate indicates that if DDAVP is to be used for surgical prophylaxis, a bleeding time must be obtained after the DDAVP infusion to ensure that the bleeding time has responded.

DDAVP is usually administered intravenously in a dose of 0.3 mg/kg over 15–30 minutes (maximum dose, 20 μg), but it is also effective at this dose when given subcutaneously.[15,231,300] The drug can be given intranasally, but absorption by this route may be erratic.[164,166] Beneficial effects are noted within 30–60 minutes and may persist for 4 hours. In some patients, the drug has been given repeatedly at 12–24-hour intervals, although tachyphylaxis can occur.[158] Administration of DDAVP at the recommended dose is generally without serious side effects. Side effects when they occur are mild and uncommon and include a 10–15% decrease in mean arterial pressure, a 20–30% increase in pulse rate, facial flushing, water retention, and hyponatremia leading to seizures, the latter more commonly after repeated administration and when fluids are given freely.[301] A small number of more serious side effects have been reported. DDAVP should be used with caution in children <2 years of age, since hyponatremia with seizures has been reported in such patients.[302] In addition, there are two reports of arterial thrombosis and one of venous thrombosis in patients who had received DDAVP.[303–305] Because the patients who experienced arterial thrombosis were elderly, these reports suggest that DDAVP should be administered cautiously to such patients.

Corticosteroids have also been used to improve hemostasis in patients with inherited platelet disorders. They have been given prophylactically to patients, with shortening of bleeding times and improvement in surgical hemostasis. In a single study, prednisone at doses of 20–50 mg for 3–4 days was given to 14 patients with prolonged bleeding times thought to be due to defective platelet secretion.[306] In each case, the bleeding time corrected, and surgery was performed without excessive bleeding. Shortening of the bleeding time was seen within 3 days and persisted for ≤3–7 days after the prednisone was stopped. Thus, for a patient with a primary platelet function disorder and no contraindications to the use of corticosteroids a 3-day trial of prednisone at a dose of 20–40 mg may be considered. However, prednisone treatment has been ineffective in shortening the bleeding time in patients with thrombasthenia[181] or in normal individuals given aspirin.[307] Failure to respond adequately to corticosteroids does not preclude a trial of DDAVP.

Disorders of Secretion Due to an Abnormal Secretory Mechanism

Platelet function in this group of disorders resembles that of individuals who have been given platelet-inhibitory drugs such as aspirin.[308] Thus, marked impairment of aggregation and secretion responses can be seen with weak platelet agonists such as ADP, epinephrine, and low concentrations of collagen, while responses to stronger agonists such as higher concentrations of collagen may normal or near normal. The bleeding time of patients with this type of secretion defect is usually prolonged. However, when it is normal or only slightly prolonged, it may become markedly prolonged 2 hours after the ingestion of 3 aspirin tablets.[309]

Biologic and Molecular Aspects

Platelets secrete the contents of their cytoplasmic granules following stimulation by a process that involves granule convergence at the center of the platelet, fusion of the granule membranes with the membranes of the surface-connected open canalicular system, and extrusion of the contents of the granules into the platelet's external environment.[310,311] This process requires the activation of signal transduction pathways that generate second messengers to couple agonist receptors on the platelet surface and the effector systems responsible for platelet aggregation and secretion. These pathways are discussed in detail in Chapter 98. Briefly, platelet stimulation results in the activation of the phospholipases C and A_2 and the serine/threonine kinases protein kinase C, calcium-calmodulin-dependent protein kinase, and myosin light chain kinase.[312] Platelets also contain high levels of the protein tyrosine kinase pp60[c-src],[313] the src-related kinases Fyn, Lyn, Hck, and Yes,[314] and the protein kinases p72[syk] and CPTK71.[315] Phospholipase C activation in platelets is a G-protein-mediated process[312] and generates diacylglycerol and IP_3 from phosphotidylinositol 4,5-bisphosphate.[316] Diacylglycerol is a protein kinase C activator, and IP_3 is responsible for the rise in intracellular calcium that accompanies platelet activation induced by most platelet agonists.[317] Platelet activation also results in the phosphorylation of a number of intracellular proteins on serine, threonine, and tyrosine residues.[318–320] Whether any of these phosphorylated proteins are directly involved in platelet secretion remains to be determined.

Etiology and Pathogenesis

These disorders constitute a heterogeneous collection of abnormalities of stimulus-response coupling in platelets. In many of the reported cases, however, the evidence linking the observed biochemical abnormalities to defective platelet secretion is not definitive. Patients have been reported whose platelets display abnormalities in arachidonic acid metabolism, including deficient liberation of arachidonic acid from phospholipids,[321] impaired coupling of the TxA_2 receptor and phospholipase C,[322] and deficiencies of cyclo-oxygenase,[323–328] and thromboxane synthetase.[329,330] Diminished platelet responsiveness to endogenous and exogenous TxA_2 has also been reported and is attributed to abnormalities of platelet endoperoxide/TxA_2 receptors.[331,332] Abnormalities in platelet calcium metabolism have been observed, such as impaired responsiveness to the ionophores A23187[332,333] and ionomycin[334] and diminished agonist-induced calcium mobilization,[335] perhaps due to decreased formation of platelet IP_3.[336,337] Patients have been reported whose platelets respond poorly or not at all to one or more agonists, such as ADP,[338] epinephrine,[339–341] and platelet-aggregating factor.[341,342] In one group of 11 patients with impaired platelet responses to low concentrations of collagen, 8 were noted to have abnormal responses to other weak agonists, such as ADP, epinephrine, TxA_2, and the prostaglandin endoperoxide analogue U44069, but normal responses to strong agonists such as thrombin and high concentrations of collagen.[343] This suggests a defect in coupling stimulation by weak agonists to secretion, rather than a defect in the secretory mechanism itself. In remaining patients, responses to strong agonists were abnormal, and the platelets appeared unable to synthesize TxA_2. Finally, in patients with the neuropsychiatric attention deficit disorder and easy bruising, abnormal dense-granule and lysosome secretion was inexplicably observed when gel-filtered platelets, but not platelets in platelet-rich plasma, were stimulated with thrombin or the ionophore A23187.[344]

Genetic Aspects

Most reports have been of individual patients, so determination of the mode of inheritance has not been possible. When families have been studied, the mode of inheritance appeared to be autosomal dominant.[325,327,330,331,339]

Therapy

The approach to therapy in patients with these disorders is identical to that described above for patients with storage pool disease (Table 129-1).

DISORDERS OF PLATELET PROCOAGULANT ACTIVITY

The plasma membrane of activated platelets provides a surface for the assembly of the tenase and prothrombinase complexes that activate coagulation factor X and prothrombin, respectively (see Ch. 100). This property of platelets was previously termed platelet factor-3. The membrane structures that contribute to platelet procoagulant activity have not been completely defined. Although prothrombinase and tenase assemble on phospholipid vesicles that contain anionic phospholipids, little, if any, anionic phospholipid is present in the outer leaflet of the plasma membrane of unstimulated platelets.[345] Thus, it has been postulated that platelet activation by agonists such as thrombin or collagen either reorients the membrane phospholipids and exposes anionic phospholipids on the platelet surface or induces membrane vesiculation and the concomitant expression of procoagulant activity.[346]

Isolated deficiency of platelet procoagulant activity is exceedingly rare. In one well-studied patient who presented with bleeding after surgery and dental procedures and a spontaneous retroperitoneal hematoma, normal prothrombin and partial thromboplastin times, bleeding times, and platelet function studies were found (Scott syndrome).[347] However, serum prothrombin times were short, and the patient's platelets were unable to express normal procoagulant activity. Moreover, although the patient's platelets secreted normal quantities of factor Va activity, they expressed only 20–25% of the normal number of factor Xa binding sites.[348] In addition, factor X activation by factors IXa and VIIIa was impaired, suggesting a concomitant deficiency of factors IXa or VIIIa binding sites (or both).[349] Finally, when stimulated with the combination of thrombin and collagen, there was decreased exposure of anionic phospholipids on the surface of the platelets,[350] and there was decreased membrane vesiculation.[351] Because a decrease in vesiculation and procoagulant activity was also observed when the patient's erythrocytes were treated with the ionophore A23187, it is likely that the abnormality responsible for the Scott syndrome is intrinsic to either the patient's blood cell membranes or their cytoskeletons.[352]

REFERENCES

1. Bernard J, Soulier JP: Sur une nouvelle variété de dystrophie thrombocytaire hemarroagipare congénitale. Semin Hop Paris 24:3217, 1948
2. Weiss HJ, Tschopp TB, Baumgartner HR et al: Decreased adhesion of giant (Bernard-Soulier) platelets to subendothelium. Further implications on the role of von Willebrand factor in hemostasis. Am J Med 57:920, 1974
3. Clemetson KJ, McGregor JL, James E et al: Characterization of the platelet membrane glycoprotein abnormalities in Bernard-Soulier syndrome and comparison with normal by surface-labeling techniques and high-resolution two-dimensional gel electrophoresis. J Clin Invest 70:304, 1982
4. Hagen I, Nurden A, Bjerrum OJ et al: Immunochemical evidence for protein abnormalities in platelets from patients with Glanzmann's thrombasthenia and Bernard-Soulier syndrome. J Clin Invest 65:722, 1980
5. Baumgartner HR: The role of blood flow in platelet adhesion, fibrin deposition, and formation of mural thrombi. Microvasc Res 5:167, 1973
6. Weiss JH, Turrito VT, Baumgartner HR: Effect of shear rate in platelet interaction with subendothelium in citrated native blood. Shear-dependent increase in adherence in von Willebrand's disease and the Bernard-Soulier syndrome. J Lab Clin Med 92:750, 1978
7. Turrito VT, Weiss HJ, Zimmerman TS, Sussman II: Factor VIII/von Willebrand factor in subendothelium mediates platelet adhesion. Blood 65:823, 1985
8. Girma J-P, Meyer D, Verweij CL et al: Structure-function relationship of human von Willebrand factor. Blood 70:605, 1987
9. Ruggeri ZM, Zimmerman TS: von Willebrand factor and von Willebrand disease. Blood 70:895, 1987
10. Ruggeri ZM, DeMarco L, Gatti L et al: Platelets have more than one binding site for von Willebrand factor. J Clin Invest 72:1, 1983
11. Coller BS, Peerschke EI, Scudder LE, Sullivan CA: Studies with a murine monoclonal antibody that abolishes ristocetin-induced binding of von Willebrand factor to platelets: additional evidence in support of GPIb as a platelet receptor for von Willebrand factor. Blood 61:99, 1983
12. Howard MA, Firkin BG: Ristocetin—a new tool in the investigation of platelet aggregation. Thromb Diath Haemorrh 26:362, 1971
13. Stel HV, Sakariassen KS, de Groot PG et al: von Willebrand factor in the vessel wall mediates platelet adherence. Blood 65:95, 1985
14. Savage B, Shattil SJ, Ruggeri ZM: Modulation of platelet function through adhesion receptors. A dual role for glycoprotein IIb-IIIa (integrin $\alpha_{IIb}\beta_3$) mediated by fibrinogen and glycoprotein Ib-von Willebrand factor. J Biol Chem 267:11300, 1992
15. Roth GJ: Developing relationships: arterial platelet adhesion, glycoprotein Ib, and leucine-rich glycoproteins. Blood 77:5, 1991
16. Ikeda Y, Handa M, Kawano K et al: The role of von Willebrand factor and fibrinogen in platelet aggregation under varying shear stress. J Clin Invest 87:1234, 1991
17. Alevriadou BR, Moake JL, Turner NA et al: Real-time analysis of shear-dependent thrombus formation and its blockade by inhibitors of von Willebrand factor binding to platelets. Blood 81:1263, 1993
18. Fox JEB, Aggerbeck LP, Berndt MC: Structure of the glycoprotein Ib-IX complex from platelet membranes. J Biol Chem 263:4882, 1988
19. Fox JEB: Linkage of a membrane skeleton to integral membrane glycoproteins in human platelets. J Clin Invest 76:1673, 1985
20. Andrews RK, Fox JEB: Identification of a region in the cytoplasmic domain of the platelet membrane glycoprotein Ib-IX complex that binds to purified actin-binding protein. J Biol Chem 267:18605, 1992
21. Lopez JA, Chung DW, Fujikawa K et al: Cloning of the α chain of human platelet glycoprotein Ib: a transmembrane protein with homology to leucine-rich α_2 glycoprotein. Proc Natl Acad Sci USA 84:5615, 1987
22. Wardell MR, Reynolds CC, Berndt MC et al: Platelet glycoprotein Ibα is phosphorylated on serine 166 by cyclic AMP-dependent protein kinase. J Biol Chem 264:15656, 1989
23. Fox JE, Berndt MC: Cyclic AMP-dependent phosphorylation of glycoprotein Ib inhibits collagen-induced polymerization of actin in platelets. J Biol Chem 264:9520, 1989
24. Muszbek L, Laposata M: Glycoprotein Ib and glycoprotein IX in human plate-

lets are acylated with palmitic acid through thioester linkages. J Biol Chem 264:9716, 1989

25. Lopez JA, Chung DW, Fujikawa K et al: The α and β chains of human platelet glycoprotein Ib are both transmembrane proteins containing a leucine-rich amino acid sequence. Proc Natl Acad Sci USA 85:2135, 1988

26. Hickey MJ, Williams SA, Roth GJ: Human platelet glycoprotein IX: an adhesive prototype of leucine-rich glycoproteins with flank-center-flank structures. Proc Natl Acad Sci USA 86:6773, 1989

27. Krantz DD, Zidovetzki R, Kagan BL, Zipursky SL: Amphipathic β structure of a leucine-rich repeat peptide. J Biol Chem 266:16801, 1991

28. Lopez JA, Leung B, Reynolds CC et al: Efficient plasma membrane expression of a functional platelet glycoprotein Ib-IX complex requires the presence of its three subunits. J Biol Chem 267:12851, 1992

29. Berndt MC, Gregory C, Chong BH et al: Additional glycoprotein defects in Bernard-Soulier's syndrome: confirmation of genetic basis by parental analysis. Blood 62:800, 1983

30. Drouin J, McGregor JL, Parmentier S et al: Residual amounts of glycoprotein Ib concomitant with near-absence of glycoprotein IX in platelets of Bernard-Soulier patients. Blood 72:1086, 1988

31. Berndt MC, Phillips DR: Purification and preliminary physicochemical characterization of human platelet membrane glycoprotein V. J Biol Chem 256:59, 1981

32. Bienz D, Schnippering W, Clemetson KJ: Glycoprotein V is not the thrombin activation receptor on human blood platelets. Blood 68:720, 1986

33. Hickey MJ, Hagen FS, Yagi M, Roth GJ: Human platelet glycoprotein V: characterization of the polypeptide and the related Ib-V-IX receptor system of adhesive, leucine-rich glycoproteins. Proc Natl Acad Sci USA 90:8327, 1993

34. Modderman PW, Admiraal LG, Sonnenberg A, von dem Borne AE: Glycoproteins V and Ib-IX form a noncovalent complex in the platelet membrane. J Biol Chem 267:364, 1992

35. Frojmovic MM, Milton JG, Caen JP, Tobelem G: Platelets from "giant platelet syndrome (BSS)" are discocytes and normal sized. J Lab Clin Med 91:109, 1978

36. Milton JG, Frojmovic MM: Invaginated plasma membrane of human platelets: evagination and measurement in normal and "giant" platelets. J Lab Clin Med 93:162, 1979

37. McGill M, Jamieson GA, Drouin J et al: Morphometric analysis of platelets in Bernard-Soulier syndrome: size and configuration in patients and carriers. Thromb Haemost 52:37, 1984

38. White JG, Burris SM, Hasegawa D, Johnson M: Micropipette aspiration of human blood platelets: a defect in Bernard-Soulier's syndrome. Blood 63:1249, 1984

39. Caen J, Bellucci S: The defective prothrombin consumption in Bernard-Soulier syndrome. Blood Cells 9:389, 1983

40. Walsh PN, Mills DCB, Pareti FI et al: Hereditary giant platelet syndrome. Absence of collagen-induced coagulant activity and deficiency of factor-XI binding to platelets. Br J Haematol 29:639, 1975

41. Bithell TC, Parekh SJ, Strong RR: Platelet-function studies in the Bernard-Soulier syndrome. Ann NY Acad Sci 201:145, 1972

42. Bevers EM, Comfurius P, Nieuwenhuis HK et al: Platelet prothrombin converting activity in hereditary disorders of platelet function. Br J Haematol 63:335, 1986

43. Perret B, Levy-Toledano S, Plantavid M et al: Abnormal phospholipid organization in Bernard-Soulier platelets. Thromb Res 31:529, 1983

44. McNicol A, Drouin J, Clemetson KJ, Gerrard JM: Phospholipase C activity in platelets from Bernard-Soulier syndrome patients. Arterioscler Thromb 13:1567, 1993

45. Stricker RB, Shuman MA: Quinidine purpura: evidence that glycoprotein V is a target platelet antigen. Blood 67:1377, 1986

46. Visentin GP, Newman PJ, Aster RH: Characteristics of quinine- and quinidine-induced antibodies specific for platelet glycoproteins IIb and IIIa. Blood 77:2668, 1991

47. Chong BH, Du X, Berndt MC et al: Characterization of the binding domains on platelet glycoproteins Ib-IX and IIb/IIIa for the quinine/quinidine-dependent antibodies. Blood 77:2190, 1991

48. Kunicki TJ, Johnson MM, Aster RH: Absence of the platelet receptor for drug-dependent antibodies in the Bernard-Soulier syndrome. J Clin Invest 62:716, 1978

49. George JN, Nurden AT, Phillips DR: Molecular defects in interactions of platelets with the vessel wall. N Engl J Med 311:1084, 1984

50. George JN, Reimann TA, Moake JL et al: Bernard-Soulier disease: a study of four patients and their parents. Br J Haematol 48:459, 1981

51. Wenger RH, Wicki AN, Kieffer N et al: The 5′ flanking region and chromosomal localization of the gene encoding human platelet membrane glycoprotein Ibα. Gene 85:517, 1989

52. Hickey MJ, Deaven LL, Roth GJ: Human platelet glycoprotein IX. Characterization of cDNA and localization of the gene to chromosome 3. FEBS Lett 274:189, 1990

53. Wenger RH, Kieffer N, Wicki AN, Clemetson KJ: Structure of the human platelet membrane glycoprotein Ibα gene. Biochem Biophys Res Commun 156:389, 1988

54. Orkin SH: GATA-binding transcription factors in hematopoietic cells. Blood 80:575, 1992

55. Hickey MJ, Roth GJ: Characterization of the gene encoding human platelet glycoprotein IX. J Biol Chem 268:3438, 1993

56. Ware J, Russell SR, Vicente V et al: Nonsense mutation in the glycoprotein Ib alpha coding sequence associated with Bernard-Soulier syndrome. Proc Natl Acad Sci USA 87:2026, 1990

57. Wright SD, Michaelides K, Johnson DJ et al: Double heterozygosity for mutations in the platelet glycoprotein IX gene in three siblings with Bernard-Soulier syndrome. Blood 81:2339, 1993

58. Finch CN, Miller JL, Lyle VA, Handin RI: Evidence that an abnormality in the glycoprotein Ib alpha gene is not the cause of abnormal platelet function in a family with classic Bernard-Soulier disease. Blood 75:2357, 1990

59. De Marco L, Mazzucato M, Fabris F et al: Variant Bernard-Soulier syndrome type bolzano. A congenital bleeding disorder due to a structural and functional abnormality of the platelet glycoprotein Ib-IX complex. J Clin Invest 86:25, 1990

60. Ware J, Russell SR, Marchese P et al: Point mutation in a leucine-rich repeat of platelet glycoprotein Ib alpha resulting in the Bernard-Soulier syndrome. J Clin Invest 92:1213, 1993

61. Miller JL, Lyle VA, Cunningham D: Mutation of leucine-57 to phenylalanine in a platelet glycoprotein Ib alpha leucine tandem repeat occurring in patients with an autosomal dominant variant of Bernard-Soulier disease. Blood 79:439, 1992

62. Peaceman AM, Katz AR, Laville M: Bernard-Soulier syndrome complicating pregnancy: a case report. Obstet Gynecol 73:457, 1989

63. Peng TC, Kickler TS, Bell WR, Haller E: Obstetric complications in a patient with Bernard-Soulier syndrome. Am J Obstet Gynecol 165:425, 1991

64. Bellucci S, Tobelem G, Caen JP: Inherited platelet disorders. Prog Hematol 13:223, 1983

65. Humphries JE, Yirinec BA, Hess CE: Atherosclerosis and unstable angina in Bernard-Soulier syndrome. Am J Clin Pathol 97:652, 1992

66. Howard MA, Hutton RA, Hardisty RM: Hereditary giant platelet syndrome: a disorder of a new aspect of platelet function. BMJ 4:586, 1973

67. Maldonado JE, Gilchrist GS, Brigden LP, Bowie EJW: Ultrastructure of platelets in Bernard-Soulier syndrome. Mayo Clin Proc 50:402, 1975

68. Hourdille P, Pico M, Jandrot Perrus M et al: Studies on the megakaryocytes of a patient with the Bernard-Soulier syndrome. Br J Haematol 76:521, 1990

69. Howard MA, Perkin J, Salem HH, Firkin BG: The agglutination of human platelets by botrocetin: evidence that botrocetin and ristocetin act at different sites on the factor VIII molecule and platelet membrane. Br J Haematol 57:25, 1984

70. Nishio K, Fujimura Y, Niinomi K et al: Enhanced botrocetin-induced type IIB von Willebrand factor binding to platelet glycoprotein Ib initiates hyper-agglutination of normal platelets. Am J Hematol 33:261, 1990

71. Nichols WL, Kaese SE, Gastineau DA et al: Bernard-Soulier syndrome: whole blood diagnostic assays of platelets. Mayo Clin Proc 64:522, 1989

72. Godwin HA, Ginsburg AD: May-Hegglin anomaly: a defect in megakaryocyte fragmentation? Br J Haematol 26:117, 1974

73. Coller BS, Zarrabi MH: Platelet membrane studies in the May-Hegglin anomaly. Blood 58:279, 1981

74. Epstein CJ, Sahud MA, Piel CF et al: Hereditary macrothrombocytopenia, nephritis, and deafness. Am J Med 52:299, 1972

75. Peterson LC, Pao FV, Crosson JT, White JG: Fechtner syndrome—a variant of Alport's syndrome with leukocyte inclusions and macrothrombocytopenia. Blood 65:397, 1985

76. Eckstein JD, Filip DJ, Watts JC: Hereditary thrombocytopenia, deafness, and renal disease. Ann Intern Med 82:639, 1975

77. Bernheim J, Dechavanne M, Bryon PA et al: Thrombocytopenia, macrothrombocytopathia, nephritis and deafness. Am J Med 61:145, 1976

78. Raccuglia G: Gray platelet syndrome. A variety of qualitative platelet disorder. Am J Med 51:818, 1971

79. Gerrard JM, Phillips DR, Rao GHR et al: Biochemical studies of two patients with the gray platelet syndrome. Selective deficiency of platelet alpha granules. J Clin Invest 66:102, 1980

80. Milton JG, Hutton RA, Tuddenham EGD, Frojmovic MM: Platelet size and shape in hereditary giant platelet syndromes on blood smear and in suspension: evidence for two types of abnormalities. J Lab Clin Med 106:326, 1985

81. von Behrens WE: Mediterranean macrothrombocytopenia. Blood 46:199, 1975

82. Beck EA: Idiopathic thrombocytopenia with giant platelets. Johns Hopkins Med J 146:281, 1980

83. Yuyu Y, Ideguchi H, Narishige T et al: Familial macrothrombocytopenia associated with decreased glycosylation of platelet membrane glycoprotein IV. Am J Hematol 33:271, 1990

84. AAkhus AM, Stavem P, Hovig T et al: Studies on a patient with thrombocytopenia, giant platelets and a platelet membrane glycoprotein Ib with reduced amount of sialic acid. Br J Haematol 74:320, 1990

85. Devine DV, Currie MS, Rosse Wendell F, Greenberg CS: Pseudo-Bernard-Soulier syndrome: thrombocytopenia caused by autoantibody to platelet glycoprotein Ib. Blood 70:428, 1987

86. Szatkowsi NS, Kunicki TJ, Aster RH: Identification of glycoprotein Ib as a target for autoantibody in idiopathic (autoimmune) thrombocytopenic purpura. Blood 67:310, 1986

87. Kunicki TJ, Newman PJ: The molecular immunology of human platelet proteins. Blood 80:1386, 1992

88. Berndt MC, Kabral A, Grimsley P et al: An acquired Bernard-Soulier-like platelet defect associated with juvenile myelodysplastic syndrome. Br J Haematol 68:97, 1988

89. Varon D, Gitel SN, Varon N et al: Immune Bernard Soulier-like syndrome associated with anti-glycoprotein-IX antibody. Am J Hematol 41:67, 1992

90. Stricker RB, Wong D, Saks SR et al: Acquired Bernard-Soulier syndrome: evidence for the role of a 210,000-molecular weight protein in the interaction of platelets with von Willebrand factor. J Clin Invest 76:1274, 1985

91. Sharma JB, Buckshee K, Sharma S: Puberty menorrhagia due to Bernard Soulier syndrome and its successful treatment by 'Ovral' hormonal tablets. Aust NZ J Obstet Gynaecol 31:369, 1991

92. Gottum KA, Solum NO: Congenital thrombocytopenia with giant platelets: a defect in the platelet membrane. Br J Haematol 16:277, 1969

93. DiMichele D, Hathaway WE: Use of DDAVP in inherited and acquired platelet dysfunction. Am J Hematol 33:39, 1990

94. Waldenstrom E, Holmberg L, Axelsson U et al: Bernard-Soulier syndrome in two Swedish families: effect of DDAVP on bleeding time. Eur J Haematol 46:182, 1991

95. Cuthbert RJ, Watson HH, Handa SI et al: DDAVP shortens the bleeding time in Bernard-Soulier syndrome. Thromb Res 49:649, 1988

96. Hemler ME, Crouse C, Takada Y, Sonnenberg A: Multiple very late antigen (VLA) heterodimers on platelets. Evidence for distinct VLA-2, VLA-5 (fibronectin receptor), and VLA-6 structures. J Biol Chem 263:7660, 1988

97. Shadle PJ, Ginsberg MH, Plow EF, Barondes SH: Platelet-collagen adhesion: inhibition by a monoclonal antibody that binds glycoprotein IIb. J Cell Biol 99:2056, 1984

98. Tandon NN, Kralisz U, Jamieson GA: Identification of glycoprotein IV (CD36) as a primary receptor for platelet-collagen adhesion. J Biol Chem 264:7576, 1989

99. Moroi M, Jung SM, Okuma M, Shinmyozu K: A patient with platelets deficient in glycoprotein VI that lack both collagen-induced aggregation and adhesion. J Clin Invest 84:1440, 1989

100. Kunicki TJ, Nugent DJ, Staats SJ et al: The human fibroblast class II extracellular matrix receptor mediates platelet adhesion to collagen and is identical to the platelet glycoprotein Ia-IIa complex. J Biol Chem 263:4516, 1988

101. Chiang TM, Kang AH: Isolation and purification of collagen α1(I) receptor from human platelet membrane. J Biol Chem 257:7581, 1982

102. Deckmyn H, Van Houtte E, Vermylen J: Disturbed platelet aggregation to collagen associated with an antibody against an 85- to 90-Kd platelet glycoprotein in a patient with prolonged bleeding time. Blood 79:1466, 1992

103. Pischel KD, Bluestein HG, Woods VL Jr: Platelet glycoproteins Ia, Ic, and IIa are physicochemically indistinguishable from the very late activation antigens adhesion-related proteins of lymphocytes and other cell types. J Clin Invest 81:505, 1988

104. Elices MJ, Hemler ME: The human integrin VLA-2 is a collagen receptor on some cells and a collagen/laminin receptor on others. Proc Natl Acad Sci USA 86:9906, 1989

105. Staatz WD, Rajpara SM, Wayner EA et al: The membrane glycoprotein Ia-IIa (VLA-2) complex mediates the Mg^{++}-dependent adhesion of platelets to collagen. J Cell Biol 108:1917, 1989

106. Polanowska Grabowska R, Gear AR: High-speed platelet adhesion under conditions of rapid flow. Proc Natl Acad Sci USA 89:5754, 1992

107. Kunicki TJ, Orchekowski R, Annis D, Honda Y: Variability of integrin $\alpha_2\beta_1$ activity on human platelets. Blood 82:2693, 1993

108. Nieuwenhuis HK, Akkerman JWN, Houdijk WPM, Sixma JJ: Human blood platelets showing no response to collagen fail to express surface glycoprotein Ia. Nature 318:470, 1985

109. Kehrel B, Balleisen L, Kokott R et al: Deficiency of intact thrombospondin and membrane glycoprotein Ia in platelets with defective collagen-induced aggregation and spontaneous loss of disorder. Blood 71:1074, 1988

110. Nieuwenhuis HK, Sakariassen KS, Houdijk WPM et al: Deficiency of platelet membrane glycoprotein Ia associated with a decreased platelet adhesion to subendothelium: a defect in platelet spreading. Blood 68:692, 1986

111. Ryo R, Yoshida A, Sugano W et al: Deficiency of P62, a putative collagen receptor, in platelets from a patient with defective collagen-induced platelet aggregation. Am J Hematol 39:25, 1992

112. Sugiyama T, Okuma M, Ushikubi F et al: A novel platelet aggregating factor found in a patient with defective collagen-induced platelet aggregation and autoimmune thrombocytopenia. Blood 69:1712, 1987

113. Greenwalt DE, Lipsky RH, Ockenhouse CF et al: Membrane glycoprotein CD36: a review of its roles in adherence, signal transduction, and transfusion medicine. Blood 80:1105, 1992

114. Oquendo P, Hundt E, Lawler J, Seed B: CD36 directly mediates cytoadherence of *Plasmodium falciparum* parasitized erythrocytes. Cell 58:95, 1989

115. Asch AS, Barnwell J, Silverstein RL, Nachman RL: Isolation of the thrombospondin membrane receptor. J Clin Invest 79:1054, 1987

116. Li WX, Howard RJ, Leung LL: Identification of SVTCG in thrombospondin as the conformation-dependent, high affinity binding site for its receptor, CD36. J Biol Chem 268:16179, 1993

117. Endemann G, Stanton LW, Madden KS et al: CD36 is a receptor for oxidized low density lipoprotein. J Biol Chem 268:11811, 1993

118. Huang MM, Bolen JB, Barnwell JW et al: Membrane glycoprotein IV (CD36) is physically associated with the Fyn, Lyn, and Yes protein-tyrosine kinases in human platelets. Proc Natl Acad Sci USA 88:7844, 1991

119. Tomiyama Y, Take H, Ikeda H et al: Identification of the platelet-specific alloantigen, Nak^a, on platelet membrane glycoprotein IV. Blood 75:684, 1990

120. Yamamoto N, Ikeda H, Tandon NN et al: A platelet membrane glycoprotein (GP) deficiency in healthy blood donors: Naka– platelets lack detectable GPIV (CD36). Blood 76:1698, 1990

121. Yamamoto N, Akamatsu N, Yamazaki H, Tanoue K: Normal aggregations of glycoprotein IV (CD36)-deficient platelets from seven healthy Japanese donors. Br J Haematol 81:86, 1992

122. Tandon NN, Ockenhouse CF, Greco NJ, Jamieson GA: Adhesive functions of platelets lacking glycoprotein IV (CD36). Blood 78:2809, 1991

123. Diaz Ricart M, Tandon NN, Carretero M et al: Platelets lacking functional CD36 (glycoprotein IV) show reduced adhesion to collagen in flowing whole blood. Blood 82:491, 1993

124. Glanzmann E: Hereditäre hämorrhagische Thrombasthenie. Ein Beitrag zur Pathologie dur Blutplättchen. J Kinderkr 88:1, 1918

125. Phillips DR, Agin PP: Platelet membrane defects in Glanzmann's thrombasthenia. J Clin Invest 60:535, 1977

126. Sixma JJ, Wester J: The hemostatic plug. Semin Hematol 14:265, 1977

127. Bennett JS, Vilaire G: Exposure of platelet fibrinogen receptors by ADP and epinephrine. J Clin Invest 64:1393, 1979

128. Marguerie GA, Plow EF, Edgington TS: Human platelets possess an inducible and saturable receptor specific for fibrinogen. J Biol Chem 254:5357, 1979

129. Ruggeri ZM, Bader R, DeMarco L: Glanzmann thrombasthenia; deficient binding of von Willebrand factor to thrombin-stimulated platelets. Proc Natl Acad Sci USA 79:6038, 1982

130. Fujimoto T, Hawiger J: Adenosine diphosphate induces binding of von Willebrand factor to human platelets. Nature 297:154, 1982

131. Bennett JS, Vilaire G, Cines DB: Identification of the fibrinogen receptor on human platelets by photoaffinity labeling. J Biol Chem 257:8049, 1982

132. Hawiger J, Parkinson S, Timmons S: Prostacyclin inhibits mobilisation of fibrinogen-binding sites on human ADP-and thrombin-treated platelets. Nature 283:1980

133. Sakariassen KS, Nievelstein PFEM, Coller BS, Sixma JJ: The role of platelet membrane glycoproteins Ib and IIb-IIIa in platelet adhesion to human artery subendothelium. Br J Haematol 63:681, 1986

134. Weiss HJ, Hawiger J, Ruggeri ZM et al: Fibrinogen-independent platelet adhesion and thrombus formation on subendothelium mediated by glycoprotein IIb-IIIa complex at high shear rate. J Clin Invest 83:288, 1989

135. Horwitz A, Duggan K, Buck C et al: Interaction of plasma membrane fibronectin receptor with talin-a transmembrane linkage. Nature 320:531, 1986

136. O'Halloran T, Beckerle MC, Burridge K: Identification of talin as a major cytoplasmic protein implicated in platelet activation. Nature 317:449, 1985

137. Phillips DR, Jennings LK, Edwards HH: Identification of membrane proteins mediating the interaction of human platelets. J Cell Biol 86:77, 1980

138. Wheeler ME, Cox AC, Carrol RC: Retention of the glycoprotein IIb-IIIa complex in the isolated platelet cytoskeleton. Effects of separable assembly of platelet psuedopodal and contractile cytoskeletons. J Clin Invest 74:1080, 1984

139. Cohen I, Burk DL, White JG: The effect of peptides and monoclonal antibodies that bind to platelet glycoprotein IIb-IIIa complex on the development of clot tension. Blood 73:1880, 1989

140. Gartner KT, Ogilvie ML: Peptides and monoclonal antibodies which bind to

platelet glycoproteins IIb and/or IIIa inhibit clot retraction. Thromb Res 49: 43, 1988

141. Bennett JS, Hoxie JA, Leitman F et al: Inhibition of fibrinogen binding to stimulated human platelets by a monoclonal antibody. Proc Natl Acad Sci USA 80:2417, 1983

142. Niiya K, Hodson E, Bader R et al: Increased surface expression of the membrane glycoprotein IIb/IIIa complex induced by platelet activation. Relationship to the binding of fibrinogen and platelet aggregation. Blood 70:475, 1987

143. Woods VL Jr, Wolff LE, Keller DM: Resting platelets contain a substantial centrally located pool of glycoprotein IIb-IIIa complex which may be accessible to some but not other extracellular protein. J Biol Chem 261:15242, 1986

144. McEver RP, Baenziger NL, Majerus PW: Isolation and quantitation of the platelet membrane glycoprotein deficient in thrombasthenia using a monoclonal hybridoma antibody. J Clin Invest 66:1311, 1980

145. Jennings LK, Phillips DR: Purification of glycoproteins IIb and III from human platelet plasma membranes and characterization of a calcium-dependent glycoprotein IIb-III complex. J Biol Chem 257:10458, 1982

146. Weisel JW, Nagaswami C, Vilaire G, Bennett JS: Examination of the platelet membrane glycoprotein IIb/IIIa complex and its interaction with fibrinogen and other ligands by electron microscopy. J Biol Chem 267:16637, 1992

147. Carrell NA, Fitzgerald LA, Steiner B et al: Structure of human platelet membrane glycoproteins IIb and IIIa as determined by electron microscopy. J Biol Chem 260:1743, 1985

148. Parise LV, Phillips DR: Reconstitution of the purified platelet fibrinogen receptor. J Biol Chem 260:10698, 1985

149. Poncz M, Eisman R, Heidenreich R et al: Structure of the platelet membrane glycoprotein IIb. J Biol Chem 262:8476, 1987

150. Lam Stephen C-T: Isolation and characterization of a chymotryptic fragment of platelet glycoprotein IIb-IIIa retaining Arg-Gly-Asp binding activity. J Biol Chem 267:5649, 1992

151. Lam SC-T, Plow EF, Ginsberg MH: Platelet membrane glycoprotein IIb heavy chain forms a complex with glycoprotein IIIa that binds Arg-Gly-Asp peptides. Blood 73:1513, 1989

152. Heidenreich R, Eisman R, Surrey S et al: Organization of the gene for platelet glycoprotein IIb. Biochemistry 29:1232, 1990

153. Kolodziej MA, Vilaire G, Gonder D et al: Study of the endoproteolytic cleavage of platelet glycoprotein IIb using oligonucleotide-mediated mutagenesis. J Biol Chem 266:23499, 1991

154. Gulino D, Boudignon C, Zhang L et al: Ca^{2+}-binding properties of the platelet glycoprotein IIb ligand-interacting domain. J Biol Chem 267:1001, 1992

155. Kloczewiak M, Timmons S, Lukas TJ, Hawiger J: Platelet receptor recognition site on human fibrinogen. Synthesis and structure-function relationships of peptides corresponding to the carboxy-terminal segment of the γ chain. Biochemistry 23:1767, 1984

156. D'Souza SE, Ginsberg MH, Burke TA, Plow EF: The ligand binding site of the platelet integrin receptor GPIIb-IIIa is proximal to the second calcium binding domain of its α subunit. J Biol Chem 265:3440, 1990

157. D'Souza SE, Ginsberg MH, Matsueda GR, Plow EF: A discrete sequence in a platelet integrin is involved in ligand recognition. Nature 350:66, 1991

158. Fitzgerald LA, Steiner B, Rall SC Jr et al: Protein sequence of endothelial glycoprotein IIIa derived from a cDNA clone. J Biol Chem 262:3936, 1987

159. Zimrin AB, Eisman R, Vilaire G et al: Structure of platelet glycoprotein IIIa. J Clin Invest 81:1470, 1988

160. Rosa J-P, Bray PF, Gayet O et al: Cloning of glycoprotein IIIa cDNA from human erythroleukemia cells and localization of the gene to chromosome 17. Blood 72:593, 1988

161. Calvette JJ, Henschen A, Gonzalez-Rodriguez J: Assignment of disulphide bonds in human platelet GPIIIa. Biochem J 274:63, 1991

162. Beer J, Coller BS: Evidence that platelet glycoprotein IIIa has a large disulfide-bonded loop that is susceptible to proteolytic cleavage. J Biol Chem 264:17564, 1989

163. Niewiarowski S, Norton KJ, Eckardt A et al: Structural and functional characterization of major platelet membrane components derived by limited proteolysis of glycoprotein IIIa. Biochim Biophys Acta 983:91, 1989

164. Rosa J-P, McEver RP: Processing and assembly of the integrin, glycoprotein IIb-IIIa, in HEL cells. J Biol Chem 264:12596, 1989

165. Duperray A, Berthier R, Chagnon E et al: Biosynthesis and processing of platelet GPIIb-IIIa in human megakaryocytes. J Cell Biol 104:1665, 1987

166. O'Toole TE, Loftus JC, Plow EF et al: Efficient surface expression of platelet GPIIb-IIIa requires both subunits. Blood 74:14, 1989

167. Bodary SC, Napier MA, McLean JW: Expression of recombinant platelet glycoprotein IIbIIIa results in a functional fibrinogen-binding complex. J Biol Chem 264:18859, 1989

168. Kolodziej MA, Vilaire G, Rifat S et al: Effect of deletion of glycoprotein IIb

169. Poncz M, Salahandrin R, Coller BS et al: Glanzmann thrombasthenia secondary to a GLY273-ASP mutation adjacent to the first calcium-binding domain of platelet glycoprotein IIb. J Clin Invest 93:172, 1994

170. Hynes RO: Integrins: A family of cell surface receptors. Cell 48:549, 1987

171. Hynes RO: Integrins: versatility, modulation, and signaling in cell adhesion. Cell 69:11, 1991

172. Weiss HJ, Turitto VT, Baumgartner HR: Platelet adhesion and thrombus formation on subendothelium in platelets deficient in glycoproteins IIb-IIIa, Ib, and storage granules. Blood 67:322, 1986

173. Caen J: Glanzmann thrombasthenia. Clin Haematol 1:383, 1972

174. Handagama P, Rappolee DA, Werb Z et al: Platelet a-granule fibrinogen, albumin, and immunoglobulin G are not synthesized by rat and mouse megakaryocytes. J Clin Invest 86:1364, 1990

175. Louache F, Debili N, Cramer E et al: Fibrinogen is not synthesized by human megakaryocytes. Blood 77:311, 1991

176. Lange W, Luig A, Dolken G et al: Fibrinogen γ-chain mRNA is not detected in human megakaryocytes. Blood 78:20, 1991

177. Handagama PJ, Shuman MA, Bainton DF: Incorporation of intravenously injected albumin, immunoglobulin G, and fibrinogen in guinea pig megakaryocyte granules. J Clin Invest 84:73, 1989

178. Harrison P, Willbourn B, Debili N et al: Uptake of plasma fibrinogen into the alpha granules of human megakaryoctes and platelets. J Clin Invest 84: 1320, 1989

179. Handagama P, Bainton DF, Jacques Y et al: Kistrin, an integrin antagonist, blocks endocytosis of fibrinogen into guinea pig megakaryocyte and platelet α-granules. J Clin Invest 91:193, 1993

180. Handagama P, Scarborough RM, Shuman MA, Bainton DF: Endocytosis of fibrinogen into megakaryocyte and platelet alpha-granules is mediated by alpha IIb beta 3 (glycoprotein IIb-IIIa). Blood 82:135, 1993

181. Caen JP, Castaldi PA, Leclerc JC et al: Congenital bleeding disorders with long bleeding time and normal platelet count. 1. Glanzmann's thrombasthenia (report of fifteen cases). Am J Med 41:4, 1966

182. Boizard B, Wautier J-L: Lek^a, a new platelet antigen absent in Glanzmann's thrombasthenia. Vox Sang 46:47, 1984

183. van Leeuwen EF, von dem Borne AEGK, von Riesz LE et al: Absence of platelet-specific alloantigens in Glanzmann's thrombasthenia. Blood 57:49, 1981

184. Kunicki TJ, Pidard D, Cazenave J-P et al: Inheritance of the human platelet alloantigen, PI^{A1}, in type I Glazmann's thrombasthenia. J Clin Invest 67:717, 1981

185. Furihata K, Nugent DJ, Bissonette A et al: On the association of the platelet-specific alloantigen, Pen^a, with glycoprotein IIIa. J Clin Invest 80:1624, 1987

186. George JN, Caen JP, Nurden AT: Glanzmann's thrombasthenia: the spectrum of clinical disease. Blood 75:1383, 1990

187. Lee H, Nurden AT, Thomaidis A, Caen JP: Relationship between fibrinogen binding and the platelet glycoprotein deficiencies in Glanzmann's thrombasthenia type I and type II. Br J Haematol 48:47, 1981

188. Burgess-Wilson ME, Cockbill SR, Johnston GI, Heptinstall S: Platelet aggregation in whole blood from patients with Glanzmann's thrombasthenia. Blood 69:38, 1987

189. Khanduri U, Pulimood R, Sudarsanam A et al: Glanzmann's thrombasthenia. A review and report of 42 cases from South India. Thromb Haemost 46:717, 1981

190. Reichert N, Seligsohn U, Ramot B: Clinical and genetic aspects of Glanzmann's thrombasthenia in Israel. Report of 22 cases. Thromb Diath Haemorrh 34:806, 1975

191. Awidi AS: Increased incidence of Glanzmann's thrombasthenia in Jordan as compared with Scandinavia. Scand J Haematol 30:218, 1983

192. Coller BS, Cheresh DA, Asch E, Seligsohn U: Platelet vitronectin receptor expression differentiates Iraqi-Jewish from Arab patients with Glanzmann thrombasthenia in Israel. Blood 77:75, 1991

193. Sosnoski DM, Emanuel BS, Hawkins AL et al: Chromosomal localization of the genes for the vitronectin and fibronectin receptors α subunits and for platelet glycoproteins IIb and IIIa. J Clin Invest 81:1993, 1988

194. Bray PF, Rosa J-P, Johnston GI et al: Platelet glycoprotein IIb: chromosomal localization and tissue expression. J Clin Invest 80:1812, 1987

195. Bray PR, Barsh G, Rosa J-P et al: Physical linkage of the genes for platelet membrane glycoproteins IIb and IIIa. Proc Natl Acad Sci USA 85:8683, 1988

196. Nojima H, Sokabe H: Structure of a gene for rat calmodulin. J Mol Biol 193: 439, 1987

197. Luo X, Kim K-H: An enhancer element in the house-keeping promoter for acetyl-CoA carboxylase gene. Nucleic Acids Res 18:3249, 1990

198. Martin F, Prandini M-H, Thevenon D et al: The transcription factor GATA-

exon 28 on the expression of the platelet glycoprotein IIb/IIIa complex. Blood 78:2344, 1991

1 regulates the promoter activity of the platelet glycoprotein IIb gene. J Biol Chem 268:21606, 1993

199. Lemarchandel V, Ghysdael J, Mignotte V et al: GATA and Ets cis-acting sequences mediate megakayocyte-specific expression. Mol Cell Biol 13:668, 1993

200. Zimrin AB, Gidwitz S, Lord S et al: The genomic organization of platelet glycoprotein IIIa. J Biol Chem 265:8590, 1990

201. Lanza F, Kieffer N, Phillips DR, Fitzgerald LA: Characterization of the human platelet glycoprotein IIIa gene. Comparison with the fibronectin receptor β-subunit gene. J Biol Chem 265:18098, 1990

202. Gu J-M, Xu W-F, Wang X-D et al: Identification of a nonsense mutation at amino acid 584-arginine of platelet glycoprotein IIb in patients with type I Glanzmann thrombasthenia. Br J Haematol 83:442, 1993

203. Kato A, Yamamoto K, Miyazaki S et al: Molecular basis for Glanzmann's thrombasthenia (GT) in a compound heterozygote with glycoprotein IIb gene: a proposal for the classification of GT based on the biosynthetic pathway of glycoprotein IIb-IIIa complex. Blood 79:3212, 1992

204. Newman PJ, Seligsohn U, Lyman S, Coller BS: The molecular genetic basis of Glanzmann thrombasthenia in the Iraqi-Jewish and Arab populations in Israel. Proc Natl Acad Sci USA 88:3160, 1991

205. Wilcox DA, Wautier J-C, Pidard D, Newman PJ: A single amino acid substitution flanking the fourth calcium binding domain of α_{IIb} prevents maturation of the $\alpha_{IIb}\beta_{IIIa}$ integrin complex. J Biol Chem 269:4450, 1994

206. Wilcox DA, Gill J, Newman PJ: Glanzmann thrombasthenia resulting from a single amino acid substitution flanking the fibrinogen γ-chain dodecapeptide binding domain on GPIIb, abstracted. Blood, suppl. 1. 82:210a, 1993

207. Li L, Bray PF: Homologous recombination among three intragene Alu sequences causes an inversion-deletion resulting in the hereditary bleeding disorder Glanzmann thrombasthenia. Am J Hum Genet 53:140, 1993

208. Bray PF, Shuman MA: Identification of an abnormal gene for the GPIIIa subunit of the platelet fibrinogen receptor resulting in Glanzmann's thrombasthenia. Blood 75:881, 1990

209. Simsek S, Heyboer H, Bruijne-Admiraael LG et al: Glanzmann's thrombasthenia caused by homozygosity for a splice defect that leads to deletion of the first coding exon of the glycoprotein IIIa mRNA. Blood 81:2044, 1993

210. Jin Y, Dietz HC, Bray PF: A mutation in the GPIIIa gene results in a mRNA splicing abnormality and suggests maintenance of reading frame is a deliberate process. Blood, abstracted. suppl. 1. 82:210a, 1993

211. Chen F, Coller BS, French DL: Homozygous mutation of platelet glycoprotein IIIa (β₃) Cys374-Tyr in a Chinese patient with Glanzmann thrombasthenia, Blood, abstracted. suppl. 1. 82:163a, 1993

212. Chen Y, Djaffar I, Pidard D et al: Ser-752-Pro mutation in the cytoplasmic domain of integrin β₃ subunit and defective activation of platelet integrin $\alpha_{IIb}\beta_3$ (glycoprotein IIb-IIIa) in a variant of Glanzmann thrombasthenia. Proc Natl Acad Sci USA 89:10169, 1992

213. Loftus JC, O'Toole TE, Plow EF et al: A β3 integrin mutation abolishes ligand binding and alters divalent cation-dependent conformation. Science 249:915, 1990

214. Lanza F, Stierle A, Fournier D et al: A new variant of Glanzmann's thrombasthenia (Strasbourgl). J Clin Invest 89:1995, 1992

215. Bajt ML, Ginsberg MH, Frelinger AL III et al: A spontaneous mutation of integrin $\alpha_{IIb}\beta_3$ (platelet glycoprotein IIb-IIIa) helps define a ligand binding site. J Biol Chem 267:3789, 1992

216. D'Souza SE, Ginsberg MH, Burke TA et al: Localization of an Arg-Gly-Asp recognition site within an integrin adhesion receptor. Science 242:91, 1988

217. Charo IF, Nannizzi L, Phillips DR et al: Inhibition of fibrinogen binding to GPIIb-IIIa by a GP IIIa peptide. J Biol Chem 266:1415, 1991

218. Nurden AT, Rosa JP, Fournier D et al: A variant of Glanzmann's thrombasthenia with abnormal glycoprotein IIb-IIIa complexes in the platelet membrane. J Clin Invest 79:962, 1987

219. Fournier DJ, Kabal A, Castaldi PA, Berndt MC: A variant of Glanzmann's thrombasthenia characterized by abnormal glycoprotein IIb/IIIa complex formation. Thromb Haemost 62:977, 1989

220. Legrand C, Dubernard V, Nurden AT: Studies on the mechanism of expression of secreted fibrinogen on the surface of activated human platelets. Blood 73:1226, 1989

221. Escolar G, Diaz Ricart M et al: A variant of Glanzmann's thrombasthenia which fails to express a GPIIb-IIIa related epitope that is recognized by a specific monoclonal antibody (C17). Br J Haematol 81:545, 1992

222. Tanoue K, Hasegawa S, Yamaguchi A et al: A new variant of thrombasthenia with abnormally glycosylated GP IIb/IIIa. Thromb Res 47:323, 1987

223. Jung SM, Yoshida N, Aoki N et al: Thrombasthenia with an abnormal platelet membrane glycoprotein IIb of different molecular weight. Blood 71:915, 1988

224. Hardisty R, Pidard D, Cox A et al: A defect of platelet aggregation associated with an abnormal distribution of glycoprotein IIb-IIIa complexes within the platelet: the cause of a lifelong bleeding disorder. Blood 80:696, 1992

225. Fujisawa K, Tani P, McMillan R: Platelet-associated antibody to glycoprotein IIb/IIIa from chronic immune thrombocytopenic purpura patients often binds to divalent cation-dependent antigens. Blood 81:1284, 1993

226. Berchtold P, Wenger M: Autoantibodies against platelet glycoproteins in autoimmune thrombocytopenic purpura: their clinical significance and response to treatment. Blood 81:1246, 1993

227. Niessner H, Clemetson KL, Panzer S et al: Acquired thrombasthenia due to GPIIb/IIIa-specific platelet autoantibodies. Blood 68:571, 1986

228. Kubota T, Tanoue K, Murohashi I et al: Autoantibody against platelet glycoprotein IIb/IIIa in a patient with non-Hodgkin's lymphoma. Thromb Res 53:379, 1989

229. Meyer M, Kirchmaier CM, Schirmer A et al: Acquired disorder of platelet function associated with autoantibodies against membrane glycoprotein IIb-IIIa complex—1. Glycoprotein analysis. Thromb Haemost 65:491, 1991

230. DiMinno G, Coraggio F, Cerbone AM et al: A myeloma paraprotein with specificity for platelet glycoprotein IIIa in a patient with a fatal leeding disorder. J Clin Invest 77:157, 1986

231. DiMinno G, Cerbone AM, Mattioli PL et al: Functionally thrombasthenic state in normal platelets following the administration of ticlopidine. J Clin Invest 75:328, 1985

232. Weiss HJ, Rogers J: Fibrinogen and platelets in the primary arrest of bleeding. N Engl J Med 285:369, 1971

233. Bierling P, Fromont P, Elbez A et al: Early immunization against platelet glycoprotein IIIa in a newborn Glanzmann type I patient. Vox Sang 55:109, 1988

234. Ito K, Yoshida H, Hatoyama H et al: Antibody removal therapy used successfully at delivery of a pregnant patient with Glanzmann's thrombasthenia and multiple anti-platelet antibodies. Vox Sang 61:40, 1991

235. Mannucci PM: Desmopressin: a non-transfusional form of treatment for congenital and acquired bleeding disorders. Blood 72:1449, 1988

236. Belluci S, Devergie A, Gluckman E et al: Complete correction of Glanzmann's thrombasthenia by allogenic bone-marrow transplantation. Br J Haematol 59:635, 1985

237. Stenberg PE, Bainton DF: Storage organelles in platelets and megakaryocytes. p. 257. In Phillips DR, Shuman MA (eds): Biochemistry of Platelets. Academic Press, San Diego, 1986

238. Weiss HJ: Congenital disorders of platelet function. Semin Hematol 17:228, 1980

239. Nieuwenhuis HK, Akkerman JW, Sixma JJ: Patients with a prolonged bleeding time and normal aggregation tests may have storage pool deficiency: studies on one hundred six patients. Blood 70:620, 1987

240. Harrison P, Savidge GF, Cramer EM: The origin and physiological relevance of α-granule adhesive proteins. Br J Haematol 74:125, 1990

241. Holt JC, Niewiarowski S: Biochemistry of α granule proteins. Semin Hematol 22:151, 1985

242. Sporn LA, Chavin SI, Marder VJ, Wagner DD: Biosynthesis of von Willebrand protein by human megakaryocytes. J Clin Invest 76:1102, 1985

243. Gewirtz AM, Keefer M, Doshi K et al: Biology of human megakaryocyte factor V. Blood 67:1639, 1986

244. Cramer EM, Savidge GF, Vainchenker W et al: Alpha-granule pool of glycoprotein IIb-IIIa in normal and pathologic platelets and megakaryocytes. Blood 75:1220, 1990

245. Stenberg PE, McEver RP, Shuman MA et al: A platelet alpha-granule membrane protein (GMP-140) is expressed on the plasma membrane after activation. J Cell Biol 101:880, 1985

246. Berman CL, Yeo EL, Wencel-Drake JD et al: A platelet alpha granule membrane protein that is associated with the plasma membrane after activation. J Clin Invest 78:130, 1986

247. Breton-Gorius J, Clezardin P, Guichard J et al: Localization of platelet osteonectin at the internal face of the α-granule membranes in platelets and megakaryocytes. Blood 79:936, 1992

248. Bevilacqua MP, Nelson RM: Selectins. J Clin Invest 91:379, 1993

249. White JG: Ultrastructural studies of the gray platelet syndrome. Am J Pathol 95:445, 1979

250. Cramer EM, Vainchenker W, Vinci G et al: Gray platelet syndrome: immuno-electron microscopic localization of fibrinogen and von Willebrand factor in platelets and megakaryocytes. Blood 66:1309, 1985

251. Rosa JP, George JN, Bainton DF et al: Gray platelet syndrome. Demonstration of alpha granule membranes that can fuse with the cell surface. J Clin Invest 80:1138, 1987

252. Levy-Toledano S, Caen JP, Breton-Gorius J et al: Gray platelet syndrome: α-granule deficiency. Its influence on platelet function. J Lab Clin Med 98:831, 1981

253. Gebrane-Younes J, Cramer EM, Orcel L, Caen JP: Gray platelet syndrome. Dissociation between abnormal sorting in megakaryocyte α-granules and

normal sorting in Weibel-Palade bodies of endothelial cells. J Clin Invest 92:3023, 1993

254. Gootenberg JE, Buchanan GR, Holtkamp CA, Casey CS: Severe hemorrhage in a patient with gray platelet syndrome. J Pediatr 109:1017, 1986

255. Srivastava PC, Powling MJ, Nokes TJ et al: Grey platelet syndrome: studies on platelet alpha-granules, lysosomes and defective response to thrombin. Br J Haematol 65:441, 1987

256. Rendu F, Marche P, Hovig T et al: Abnormal phosphoinositide metabolism and protein phosphorylation in platelets from a patient with the grey platelet syndrome. Br J Haematol 67:199, 1987

257. Berndt MC, Castaldi PA, Gordon S et al: Morphological and biochemical confirmation of gray platelet syndrome in two siblings. Aust NZ J Med 13: 387, 1983

258. Pfueller SL, David R: Platelet-associated immunoglobulins G,A, and M are secreted during platelet activation: normal levels but defective secretion in grey platelet syndrome. Br J Haematol 68:235, 1988

259. Jackson CW, Hutson NK, Steward SA et al: Platelets of the Wistar Furth rat have reduced levels of alpha-granule proteins. An animal model resembling gray platelet syndrome. J Clin Invest 87:1985, 1991

260. Pfueller SL, Howard MA, White JG et al: Shortening of bleeding time by 1-deamino-8-arginine vasopressin (DDAVP) in the absence of platelet von Willebrand factor in gray platelet syndrome. Thromb Haemost 58:1060, 1987

261. Weiss HJ, Lages B, Vicic W et al: Heterogeneous abnormalities of platelet dense granule ultrastructure in 20 patients with congenital storage pool deficiency. Br J Haematol 83:282, 1993

262. Gerrard JM, Lint D, Sims PJ et al: Identification of a platelet dense granule membrane protein that is deficient in a patient with the Hermansky-Pudlak syndrome. Blood 77:101, 1991

263. Israels SJ, Gerrard JM, Jacques YV et al: Platelet dense granule membranes contain both granulophysin and P-selectin (GMP-140). Blood 80:143, 1992

264. Charo IF, Feinman RD, Detweiler TC: Interrelations of platelet aggregation and secretion. J Clin Invest 60:866, 1977

265. Weiss HJ, Lages B: The response of platelets to epinephrine in storage pool deficiency—evidence pertaining to the role of adenosine diphosphate in mediating primary and secondary aggregation. Blood 72:1717, 1988

266. Lages B, Dangelmaier CA, Holmsen H, Weiss HJ: Specific correction of impaired acid hydrolase secretion in storage pool-deficient platelets by adenosine diphosphate. J Clin Invest 81:1865, 1988

267. Depinho RA, Kaplan KL: The Hermansky-Pudlak syndrome. Report of three cases and review of pathophysiology and management considerations. Medicine 64:192, 1985

268. Buchanan GR, Handin RI: Platelet function in the Chediak-Higashi syndrome. Blood 47:941, 1976

269. Novak EK, Hui S-W, Swank RT: Platelet storage pool deficiency in mouse pigment mutations associated with seven distinct genetic loci. Blood 63: 536, 1984

270. Tschopp TB, Zucker MB: Hereditary defect in platelet function in rats. Blood 40:217, 1972

271. Menard M, Meyers KM: Storage pool deficiency in cattle with the Chediak-Higashi syndrome results from an absence of dense granule precursors in their megakaryocytes. Blood 72:1726, 1988

272. Cowles BE, Meyers KM, Wardrop KJ et al: Prolonged bleeding time of Chediak-Higashi cats corrected by platelet transfusion. Thromb Haemost 67:708, 1992

273. Meyers KM, Holmsen H, Seachord CL et al: Characterization of platelets from normal mink and mink with the Chediak-Higashi syndrome. Am J Hematol 7:137, 1979

274. Sjaastad OV, Blom AK, Stormorken H, Nes N: Adenine nucleotides, serotonin, and aggregation properties of platelets of blue foxes (Alopex lagopus) with the Chediak-Higashi syndrome. Am J Med Genet 35:373, 1990

275. Holmsen H, Weiss HJ: Secretable storage pools in platelets. Annu Rev Med 30:119, 1979

276. Pareti FI, Day HJ, Mills DCB: Nucleotide and serotonin metabolism in platelets with defective secondary aggregation. Blood 44:789, 1974

277. Grottum KA, Hovig T, Holmsen H et al: Wiskott-Aldrich syndrome: qualitative platelet defects and short platelet survival. Br J Haematol 17:373, 1969

278. Day HJ, Holmsen H: Platelet adenine nucleotide "storage pool deficiency" in thrombocytopenic absent radii syndrome. JAMA 221:1053, 1972

279. Onel D, Ulutin SB, Ulutin ON: Platelet defect in a case of Ehlers-Danlos syndrome. Acta Haematol 50:238, 1973

280. Hathaway WE, Solomons C, Ott JE: Platelet function and pyrophosphates in osteogenesis imperfecta. Blood 39:500, 1972

281. Barak Y, Nir E: Chediak-Higashi syndrome. Am J Pediatr Hematol Oncol 9: 42, 1987

282. Shalev A, Michaud G, Israels SJ et al: Quantification of a novel dense granule

283. protein (granulophysin) in platelets of patients with dense granule storage pool deficiency. Blood 80:1231, 1992

283. Weiss HJ, Witte LD, Kaplan KL et al: Heterogeneity in storage pool deficiency: studies on granule-bound substances in 18 patients including variants deficient in α granules, platelet factor 4, β-thromboglobulin, and platelet-derived growth factor. Blood 54:1296, 1979

284. Lages B, Shattil SJ, Bainton DF, Weiss HJ: Decreased content and surface expression of alpha-granule membrane protein GMP-140 in one of two types of platelet alpha delta storage pool deficiency. J Clin Invest 87:919, 1991

285. Weiss HJ, Lages B: Studies of thromboxane B2, platelet factor 4, and fibrinopeptide A in bleeding-time blood of patients deficient in von Willebrand factor, platelet glycoproteins Ib and IIb-IIIa, and storage granules. Blood 82: 481, 1993

286. Weiss HJ, Lages B: Platelet malondialdehyde production and aggregation responses induced by arachidonate, prostaglandin-G2, collagen, and epinephrine in 12 patients with storage pool deficiency. Blood 58:27, 1981

287. Lages B, Weiss HJ: Biphasic aggregation responses to ADP and epinephrine in some storage pool deficient platelets: relationship to the role of endogenous ADP in platelet aggregation and secretion. Thromb Haemost 43:147, 1980

288. Ingerman CM, Smith JB, Shapiro S et al: Hereditary abnormality of platelet aggregation attributable to nucleotide storage pool deficiency. Blood 52: 332, 1978

289. Weiss HJ, Tschopp TB, Rogers J, Brand H: Studies of platelet 5-hydroxytryptamine (serotonin) in storage pool disease and albinism. J Clin Invest 54: 421, 1974

290. Weiss HJ, Chervenick PA, Zalusky R, Factor A: A familial defect in platelet function associated with impaired release of adenosine diphosphate. N Engl J Med 281:1262, 1969

291. Novak EK, Sweet HO, Prochazka M et al: Cocoa: a new mouse model for platelet storage pool deficiency. Br J Haematol 69:371, 1988

292. Swank RT, Reddington M, Howlett O, Novak EK: Platelet storage pool deficiency associated with inherited abnormalities of the inner ear in the mouse pigment mutants muted and mocha. Blood 78:2036, 1991

293. Swank RT, Sweet HO, Davisson MT et al: Sandy: a new mouse model for platelet storage pool deficiency. Genet Res 58:51, 1991

294. Swank RT, Jiang SY, Reddington M et al: Inherited abnormalities in platelet organelles and platelet formation and associated altered expression of low molecular weight guanosine triphosphate-binding proteins in the mouse pigment mutant gunmetal. Blood 81:2626, 1993

295. White RA, Peters LL, Adkison LR et al: The murine pallid mutation is a platelet storage pool disease associated with the protein 4.2 (pallidin) gene. Nat Genet 2:80, 1992

296. Gerritsen SW, Akkerman JW, Sixma JJ: Correction of the bleeding time in patients with storage pool deficiency by infusion of cryoprecipitate. Br J Haematol 40:153, 1978

297. Kobrinsky NL, Gerrard JM, Watson CM et al: Shortening of bleeding time by 1-deamino-8-arginine vasopressin in various bleeding disorders. Lancet 1:1145, 1984

298. Nieuwenhuis HK, Sixma JJ: 1-Desamino-8-D-arginine vasopressin (desmopressin) shortens the bleeding time in storage pool deficiency. Ann Intern Med 108:65, 1988

299. Mannucci PM: Desmopressin (DDAVP) for treatment of disorders of hemostasis. Prog Hemost Thromb 8:19, 1986

300. Sonnenberg A, Modderman PW, Hogervorst F: Laminin receptor on platelets is the integrin VLA-6. Nature 336:487, 1988

301. Watson AJ, Whelton A: Therapeutic manipulations in uremic bleeding. Clin Pharmacol 25:315, 1985

302. Smith TJ, Gill JC, Ambruso DR, Hathaway WE: Hyponatremia and seizures in young children given DDAVP. Am J Hematol 31:199, 1989

303. Brynes JJ, Larcada A, Moake JL: Thrombosis following desmopressin for uremic bleeding. Am J Hematol 28:63, 1988

304. Bond L, Bevan D: Myocardial infarction in a patient with hemophilia treated with DDAVP. N Engl J Med 318:121, 1988

305. Albert SG, Salvato-Lechner V, Joist JH: Venous thromboembolism and transient thrombocytopenia in a patient with diabetes insipidus treated with desmopressin acetate. Thromb Res 50:695, 1988

306. Mielke CH Jr, Levine PH, Zucker S: Preoperative prednisone therapy in platelet function disorders. Thromb Res 21:655, 1981

307. Thong KL, Mant MJ, Grace MG: Lack of effect of prednisone administration on bleeding time and platelet function of normal subjects. Br J Haematol 38:373, 1978

308. Sahud MA, Aggeler PM: Platelet dysfunction-differentiation of a newly recognized primary type from that produced by aspirin. N Engl J Med 280:453, 1969

309. Czapek EE, Deykin D, Salzman E et al: Intermediate syndrome of platelet dysfunction. Blood 52:103, 1978

310. Stenberg PE, Shuman MA, Levine SP, Bainton DF: Redistribution of alpha-granules and their contents in thrombin-stimulated platelets. J Cell Biol 98: 748, 1984

311. White JG, Krumwiede M: Further studies of the secretory pathway in thrombin-stimulated human platelets. Blood 69:1196, 1987

312. Brass LF, Manning DR, Shattil SJ: GTP-binding proteins and platelet activation. Prog Hemost Thromb 10:127, 1990

313. Golden A, Nemeth SP, Brugge JS: Blood platelets express high levels of the pp60c-src-specific tyrosine kinase activity. Proc Natl Acad Sci USA 83:852, 1986

314. Shattil SJ, Brugge JS: Protein tyrosine phosphorylation and the adhesive functions of platelets. Curr Opin Cell Biol 3:869, 1991

315. Taniguchi T, Kitagawa H, Yasue S et al: Protein-tyrosine kinase p72syk is activated by thrombin and is negatively regulated through Ca^{2+} mobilization in platelets. J Biol Chem 268:2277, 1993

316. Wilson DB, Neufeld EJ, Majerus PW: Phosphoinositide interconversion in thrombin-stimulated human platelets. J Biol Chem 260:1046, 1985

317. Brass LF, Joseph SK: A role for inositol triphosphate in intracellular Ca^{2+} mobilization and granule secretion in platelets. J Biol Chem 260:15172, 1985

318. Ferrell JE Jr, Martin GS: Platelet tyrosine-specific protein phosphorylation is regulated by thrombin. Mol Cell Biol 8:3603, 1988

319. Nakamura S, Yamamura H: Thrombin and collagen induce rapid phosphorylation of a common set of cellular proteins on tyrosine in human platelets. J Biol Chem 264:7089, 1989

320. Ferrell JE Jr, Martin GS: Thrombin stimulates the activities of multiple previously unidentified protein kinases in platelets. J Biol Chem 264:20723, 1989

321. Rao AK, Koke K, Willis J et al: Platelet secretion defect associated with impaired liberation of arachidonic acid and normal myosin light chain phosphorylation. Blood 64:914, 1984

322. Fuse I, Mito M, Hattori A et al: Defective signal transduction induced by thromboxane A_2 in a patient with a mild bleeding disorder: impaired phospholipase C activation despite normal phospholipase A_2 activation. Blood 81:994, 1993

323. Malmsten C, Hamberg M, Svensson J, Samuelsson B: Physiological role of endoperoxide in human platelets: hemostatic defect due to platelet cyclo-oxygenase deficiency. Proc Natl Acad Sci USA 72:1446, 1975

324. Lagarde M, Byron PA, Vargaftig BB, Dechavanne M: Impairment of platelet thromboxane A2 generation and of the platelet release reaction in two patients with congenital deficiency of platelet cyclo-oxygenase. Br J Haematol 38:251, 1978

325. Nyman D, Eriksson AW, Lehmann W, Blomback M: Inherited defective platelet aggregation with arachidonate as the main expression of a defective metabolism of arachidonic acid. Thromb Res 14:739, 1979

326. Pareti FI, Mannucci PM, D'Angelo A et al: Congenital deficiency of thromboxane and prostacyclin. Lancet 1:898, 1980

327. Horellou MH, Lecompte T, Lecrubier C et al: Familial and constitutional bleeding disorder due to platelet cyclo-oxygenase deficiency. Am J Hematol 14:1, 1983

328. Ehara H, Yoshimoto T, Yamamoto S, Hattori A: Enzymological and immunological studies on a clinical case of platelet cyclooxygenase abnormality. Biochim Biophys Acta 960:35, 1988

329. Mestel F, Oetliker O, Beck E et al: Severe bleeding associated with defective thromboxane synthetase. Lancet 1:157, 1980

330. Defreyn G, Machin SJ, Carreras LO et al: Familial bleeding tendency with partial platelet thromboxane synthetase deficiency: reorientation of cyclic endoperoxide metabolism. Br J Haematol 49:29, 1981

331. Wu KK, Le Breton GC, Tai H-H, Chen Y-C: Abnormal platelet response to thromboxane A2. J Clin Invest 67:1801, 1981

332. Lages B, Malmsten C, Weiss HJ, Samuelsson B: Impaired platelet response to thromboxane-A2 and defective calcium mobilization in a patient with a bleeding disorder. Blood 57:545, 1981

333. Machin SJ, Keenan JP, McVerry BA: Defective platelet aggregation to the calcium ionophore A23187 in a patient with a lifelong bleeding disorder. J Clin Pathol 36:1140, 1983

334. Hardisty RM, Machin SJ, Nokes TJC et al: A new congenital defect of platelet secretion: impaired responsiveness of the platelets to cytoplasmic free calcium. Br J Haematol 53:543, 1983

335. Rao AK, Kowalska MA, Disa J: Impaired cytoplasmic ionized calcium mobilization in inherited platelet secretion defects. Blood 74:664, 1989

336. Holmsen H, Walsh PN, Koike K et al: Familial bleeding disorder associated with deficiencies in platelet signal processing and glycoproteins. Br J Haematol 67:335, 1987

337. Lages B, Weiss HJ: Impairment of phosphotidylinositol metabolism in a patient with a bleeding disorder associated with defects of initial platelet responses. Thromb Haemost 59:175, 1988

338. Cattaneo M, Lecchi A, Randi AM et al: Identification of a new congenital defect of platelet function characterized by severe impairment of platelet responses to adenosine diphosphate. Blood 80:2787, 1993

339. Scrutton MC, Clare KA, Hutton RA, Bruckdorfer KR: Depressed responsiveness to adrenaline in platelets from apparently normal human donors: a familial trait. Br J Haematol 49:303, 1981

340. Tamponi G, Pannocchia A, Arduino C et al: Congenital deficiency of alpha-2-adrenoceptors on human platelets: description of two cases. Thromb Haemost 58:1012, 1987

341. Stormorken H, Gogstad G, Solum NO: A new bleeding disorder: lack of platelet aggregatory response to adrenalin and lack of secondary aggregation to ADP and platelet activating factor (PAF). Thromb Res 29:391, 1982

342. Pelczar-Wissner CJ, McDonald EG, Sussman II: Absence of platelet activating factor (PAF) mediated platelet aggregation: a new platelet defect. Am J Hematol 16:419, 1984

343. Lages B, Weiss HJ: Heterogeneous defects of platelet secretion and responses to weak agonists in patients with bleeding disorders. Br J Haematol 68:53, 1988

344. Koike K, Rao AK, Holmsen H, Mueller PS: Platelet secretion defect in patients with the attention deficit disorder and easy bruising. Blood 63:427, 1984

345. Rosing J, van Rijn JLML, Bevers EM et al: The role of activated human platelets in prothrombin and factor X activation. Blood 65:319, 1985

346. Zwaal RF, Comfurius P, Bevers EM: Platelet procoagulant activity and microvesicle formation. Its putative role in hemostasis and thrombosis. Biochim Biophys Acta 1180:1, 1992

347. Weiss HJ, Vicic WJ, Lages BA, Rogers J: Isolated deficiency of platelet procoagulant activity. Am J Med 67:206, 1979

348. Miletich JP, Kane WH, Hofmann SL et al: Deficiency of factor X_a-factor V_a binding sites on the platelets of a patient with a bleeding disorder. Blood 54:1015, 1979

349. Ahmad SS, Rawala Sheikh R, Ashby B, Walsh PN: Platelet receptor-mediated factor X activation by factor IXa. High-affinity factor IXa receptors induced by factor VIII are deficient on platelets in Scott syndrome. J Clin Invest 84: 824, 1989

350. Rosing J, Bevers EM, Comfurius P et al: Impaired factor X and prothrombin activation associated with decreased phospholipid exposure in platelets from a patient with a bleeding disorder. Blood 65:1557, 1985

351. Sims PJ, Wiedmer T, Esmon CT et al: Assembly of the platelet prothrombinase complex is linked to vesiculation of the platelet plasma membrane. Studies in Scott syndrome: an isolated defect in platelet procoagulant activity. J Biol Chem 264:17049, 1989

352. Bevers EM, Wiedmer T, Comfurius P et al: Defective Ca(2+)-induced microvesiculation and deficient expression of procoagulant activity in erythrocytes from a patient with a bleeding disorder: a study of the red blood cells of Scott syndrome. Blood 79:380, 1992

Acquired Disorders of Platelet Function

130

James N. George and Sanford J. Shattil

INTRODUCTION

The acquired disorders of platelet function are among the most common of all hematologic abnormalities, an observation supported by the predictable effect on platelet function caused by the ubiquitous drug, aspirin. This chapter discusses the clinical disorders associated with acquired defects in platelet function (Table 130-1). A major goal of this discussion is to attempt to provide the reader with a balanced view of the clinical significance of each particular acquired platelet defect. This task may not be possible in all cases. An illustration of the real difficulty in predicting the risk of hemorrhage is the clinical experience with Glanzmann thrombasthenia, a congenital platelet disease that is well defined by a long bleeding time and absent platelet aggregation—abnormalities similar to but typically more severe than those found in many acquired disorders. Among thrombasthenic patients who have equally severe abnormalities of platelet function the range of bleeding symptoms is great, and some patients experience no excessive bleeding throughout their lives. In most patients, severe hemorrhagic episodes are sporadic and unpredictable.[1] Therefore, since acquired platelet function defects are generally milder than Glanzmann thrombasthenia, it should be expected that bleeding in patients with acquired defects will be even less predictable and will often occur only when there are additional hemostatic defects. The preservation of normal hemostasis in spite of diminished platelet function is consistent with the observation that spontaneous bleeding does not usually occur in thrombocytopenic patients until the platelet count is <10,000/ml, <5% of the normal value.[2]

Part of the problem in the clinical assessment of these disorders is the difficulty in interpreting the laboratory measures of platelet function by which they are defined: platelet aggregation and the bleeding time. These diagnostic procedures are discussed more fully elsewhere, but their interpretation requires emphasis here. There are several reasons why it cannot be assumed that abnormal in vitro platelet aggregation or a prolonged bleeding time predict an increased risk for bleeding. First, it is difficult to express aggregation studies in quantitative terms, accurately and no definition of a normal range of values is universally accepted. Second, aggregation studies can be inconsistent and "abnormal" in normal subjects who have ingested no medication[3] and may vary with the age of the subject.[4] Third, aspirin ingestion is widespread in our society, and this drug causes abnormal patterns of aggregation (see below). Fourth, the secondary wave of aggregation following ADP stimulation occurs in citrate-anticoagulated platelet-rich plasma but not in the presence of physiologic concentrations of calcium, suggesting that this "normal" aggregation pattern occurs in vitro but that it may not occur in vivo. Even with these limitations, platelet aggregation studies can be useful in the diagnostic evaluation of selected patients, but the ability of abnormal results to predict an increased risk of bleeding is unknown. Finally, although the bleeding time is an important aid in the diagnosis of selected congenital disorders,[5] its value in predicting a risk of hemorrhage is unproved.[6]

In spite of the difficulty in assessing individual risks, acquired platelet function disorders do have a clear effect on hemostasis and thrombosis in large studies. Again the case of aspirin is pertinent, as recent data demonstrate that a small but sustained dose of aspirin (325 mg every other day) may cause a reduction in the risk for myocardial infarction in a selected study group but also may cause an increased risk for hemorrhage.[7]

DRUGS THAT AFFECT PLATELET FUNCTION

A vast array of drugs are known to affect platelet function (Table 130-2). Some of the agents listed in Table 130-2 are used specifically for their antithrombotic activity, with diminished platelet function being the therapeutic goal. These agents are also discussed in Chapter 124. For the others, the occurrence of abnormal platelet function is an unwanted side effect. For all of these drugs, their effect on platelet function is defined by an abnormality of platelet aggregation or the bleeding time, but whether they contribute to a risk of excessive bleeding is definitively established only for aspirin.

Aspirin

Aspirin has become a common household drug since its introduction nearly 100 years ago, and estimates of its current use in the United States are staggering: 10–20 thousand tons annually, which is equivalent to almost one tablet for every person every day.[8] A survey performed at the American Heart Association in 1992 reported that 57% of attendees thought aspirin should be used by everyone to protect against heart attack.[9] With the subsequent publicity on studies demonstrating that aspirin diminishes the risk of common disorders such as cardiovascular disease[7,10,11] and pre-eclampsia,[12] the use of aspirin will certainly increase.

Definition of the Aspirin-Induced Platelet Defect

Aspirin was first noticed to impair platelet function in 1967,[13] and the mechanism was found to be the acetylation and irreversible inhibition of platelet cyclo-oxygenase.[14–16] For platelets, which have minimal protein synthetic capacity, a single small dose of aspirin (40–100 mg)[17–19] or as little as 10 mg taken daily for 1 week,[20] can totally inhibit thromboxane production and therefore impair the function of a cohort of platelets for its entire circulating life span of about 10 days. These observations are consistent with data suggesting a therapeutic antithrombotic effect of aspirin at doses as low as 30 mg/day.[21,22] Although the effect of aspirin on platelet cyclo-oxygenase function is clear, it may not be the only mechanism by which aspirin interferes with hemostasis.[23–25] Aspirin depresses thrombin formation in clotting blood, possibly by acetylating prothrombin,[26] and the acetylation of fibrinogen after therapeutic doses of aspirin significantly interferes with fibrin formation and allows accelerated fibrinolysis.[25] Aspirin at therapeutic doses

Table 130-1. Principal Causes of Acquired Disorders of Platelet Function

Drugs that affect platelet function
    Nonsteroidal anti-inflammatory drugs
    Ticlopidine
    β-Lactam antibiotics
    Other drugs (see Table 130-2)
    Foods and food additives
Systemic conditions associated with abnormal platelet function
    Chronic renal disease
    Cardiopulmonary bypass surgery
    Antiplatelet antibodies
Hematologic diseases associated with abnormal platelet function
    Chronic myeloproliferative disorders
    Leukemias and myelodysplastic syndromes
    Dysproteinemias

does not significantly diminish the function of the vitamin K-dependent coagulation factors and factor V.[27]

Aspirin also acetylates cyclo-oxygenase in endothelial cells, blocking synthesis of the final product of endothelial cell eicosanoid metabolism, prostacyclin, which is a strong inhibitor of platelet function. However, the endothelial enzyme is less sensitive than platelet cyclo-oxygenase to low doses of aspirin and, in contrast to platelets, endothelial cells can recover cyclo-oxygenase activity by synthesizing new enzyme.[28] Therefore a consideration for therapeutic trials with aspirin has been to use a low dose, minimizing the inhibition of endothelial cell prostacyclin synthesis, which could have a prothrombotic effect. A significant portion of aspirin's effect on platelets occurs in the portal circulation[29]; one-half of an oral dose is deacetylated in the liver to form inactive salicylic acid. This provides an additional therapeutic advantage by allowing small oral doses of aspirin to react more effectively with circulating platelets than with endothelial cells in the systemic circulation.

Aspirin and Platelet Aggregation

A predictable abnormality after exposure of platelets to aspirin either in vivo or in vitro is impaired aggregation with epinephrine, ADP, arachidonic acid, and low concentrations of collagen and thrombin.[13] These abnormalities are a direct result of inhibition of cyclo-oxygenase, with the resulting deficient synthesis of the final product of platelet arachidonic acid metabolism, thromboxane A_2.[14–16,30] Thromboxane A_2 diffuses out of the platelet, binds to specific platelet membrane receptors, and reinforces aggregation by promoting α-granule and dense granule secretion. With cyclo-oxygenase inhibition, only a primary, reversible wave of platelet aggregation without platelet secretion occurs following stimulation by epinephrine and low concentrations of ADP, thrombin, and collagen. The aspirin-induced abnormality of platelet aggregation is so characteristic that abnormal platelet aggregation patterns of any etiology are often termed aspirin-like. Stronger agonists (high concentrations of thrombin and collagen) do not require thromboxane A_2 synthesis to cause platelet secretion and irreversible aggregation. The occurrence of a complete platelet response in the presence of total inhibition of the enzyme cyclo-oxygenase demonstrates the presence of multiple pathways of platelet activation, and this may explain why normal subjects almost always have normal hemostasis while taking aspirin.

Aspirin and the Bleeding Time

Aspirin also prolongs the bleeding time, but in individual subjects this is less consistent than the platelet aggregation abnormality. Initial studies demonstrated that 2 hours after two to three aspirin tablets (650–975 mg), the mean template bleeding time of a group of normal subjects was significantly increased.[31] Prolongation of the bleeding time can be demonstrated for ≤4 days after a single dose of aspirin,[32] until normal platelet turnover results in the appearance of new platelets with normal function.[33] However, aspirin actually prolongs the bleeding time to a value greater than the normal range in only about one-half of normal subjects.[31] It is assumed, but it has not been clearly demonstrated, that individual subjects demonstrate a consistent bleeding time response to aspirin on repeated challenges.[32] Smaller single doses of aspirin (150–160 mg) that consistently cause abnormal platelet aggregation do not cause a prolonged bleeding time[24]; however daily ingestion of 30 mg of aspirin (but not 10 mg) does cause an increased bleeding time.[20]

The bleeding time has a reputation for being the most accurate test of platelet function, because it is performed directly on the patient and because it correlates with the platelet count in selected patients.[5] However, its limitations need to be recognized.[6] For example, to demonstrate an effect of aspirin on the template bleeding time, certain technical details must be followed. If the bleeding time is performed with a vertical rather than the traditional transverse skin incision, and without the usual venostasis, there is no prolongation after aspirin treatment, despite the characteristic changes in platelet aggregation and secretion.[32] An older bleeding time technique, the Duke earlobe puncture, is insensitive to aspirin treatment.[31] It is usually assumed that the skin bleeding time can be used to assess the risk of bleeding from other organs. However, in one study of patients on aspirin for rheumatic disease undergoing gastric endoscopic biopsy, this assumption was shown not to be true.[34] These data emphasize that the bleeding time cannot be blindly accepted as an accurate representation of systemic hemostasis.[6]

The most dramatic demonstrations of the aspirin's effect on the bleeding time have been in patients with severe hemophilia.[35,36] The bleeding time is already slightly prolonged in some patients with severe hemophilia A.[37] However, following the administration of two or three aspirin tablets, sustained hemorrhage from the bleeding time incision was observed in 5 to 11 patients with severe hemophilia A, and this ultimately required an infusion of plasma or factor VIII to arrest the bleeding.[35] Patients with mild hemophilia appeared to have less risk from aspirin, as none of 16 patients prolonged their bleeding time greater than the normal control group.[35] Also small doses of aspirin cause a greater than normal prolongation of the bleeding time in patients with chronic renal failure[24] and have been associated with reports of major bleeding.[38] The combination of ethanol and aspirin has a synergistic effect on increasing the bleeding time in normal subjects,[39] an observation that may have clinical significance in some subjects.[40]

Aspirin and Gastrointestinal Bleeding

In contrast to its antithrombotic effect, which appears not to be dose related above small threshold doses,[19,41] aspirin-induced gastrointestinal mucosal toxicity is dose related.[42,43] The mechanism of mucosal injury appears to be separate from the effect on hemostasis.[44] The risk of gastrointestinal bleeding with aspirin, from both the upper and lower gastrointestinal tracts and from both discrete ulceration and from more diffuse mucosal damage,[45] is increased 1.5–2.0-fold,[43] even with low doses of aspirin (100 mg/day).[46]

Clinical Significance of the Aspirin-Induced Defect in Platelet Function

The clinical significance of aspirin on hemostasis was demonstrated by the administration of a low dose of aspirin (325 mg every other day) or a placebo to 22,071 physicians over 5 years[7]

Table 130-2. Drugs that Inhibit Platelet Function[a]

Nonsteroidal anti-inflammatory drugs
- Aspirin[b]
- Sulfinpyrazone (Anturane)[b]
- Indomethacine (Indocin)
- Ibuprofen (Advil, Motrin, Nuprin, Rufen)
- Sulindac (Clinoril)
- Naproxen (Naprosyn)
- Phenylbutazone (Butazolidin)
- Meclofenamic acid (Meclomen)
- Mefanamic acid (Ponstel)
- Diflunisal (Dolobid)
- Piroxican (Feldene)
- Tolmetin (Tolectin)
- Zompirac (Zomax)[c]

β-Lactam antibiotics
- Penicillin G
  - Penicillin G
  - Carbenacillin (Geopen)
  - Ticarcillin (Ticar, Timentin)
  - Methicillin (Staphcillin)
  - Ampicillin (Polycillin, Omnipen)
  - Nafcillin (Nafcil, Unipen)
  - Piperacillin (Pipracil)
  - Azlocillin (Axlin)
  - Mezlocillin (Mezlin)
  - Apalcillin
  - Sulbenicillin
  - Temocillin
- Cephalosporins
  - Cephalothin (Keflin, Seffin)
  - Moxalactam (Moxam)
  - Cefoxitin (Mefoxin)
  - Cefotaxime (Claforan)
  - Cefazolin (Ancef, Kefzol)

Other drugs
- Antibiotics
  - Nitrofurantoin (Furadantin, Macrodantin)
- Drugs that increase platelet cAMP concentration
  - Prostacyclin
  - Iloprost
  - Dipyridamole (Persantin)[b]
- Anticoagulant
  - Heparin
- Fibrinolytic agents
- Plasma expanders
  - Dextrans
  - Hydroxyethyl starch (hetastarch)
- Cardiovascular drugs
  - Nitroglycerin
  - Isosorbide dinitrate (Isordil, Diltrate)
  - Propranolol (Inderal)
  - Nitroprusside (Nitropress)
  - Nifedipine (Procardia)

- Verapamil (Calan, Isoptin)
- Diltiazem (Cardizem)
- Quinidine

Psychotropic drugs
- Tricyclic antidepressants
  - Imiprimine (Tofranil)
  - Amitriptyline
  - Nortryptaline (Pamelor)
- Phenothiazines
  - Chlorpromazine (Thorazine)
  - Promethazine (Phenergan)
  - Trifluoperazine (Stelazine)

Anesthetics
- Local
  - Dibucaine (Lidocaine)
  - Tetracaine (Carbocaine)
  - Metycaine
  - Cyclaine
  - Butacaine
  - Nepercaine
  - Procaine
  - Cocaine
  - Plaquenil
- General
  - Halothane (Fluothane)
- Narcotic
  - Heroin

Oncologic drugs
- Mithramycin
- Daunorubicin
- BCNU

Miscellaneous drugs
- Ticlopidine
- Clofibrate (Atromid-S)
- Ketanserin
- Antihistamines
  - Diphenhydramine (Benadryl, Allerdryl)
  - Chlorpheniramine (Donatussin, Probahist)
  - Mepyramine
- Radiographic contrast agenst
  - Renografin-76
  - Renovist II
  - Conray-60

Foods and food additives
- ω-3 Fatty acids (eicosapentanoic acid)
- Ethanol
- Chinese black tree fungus
- Onion extract
- Ajoene (garlic component)
- Cumin
- Turmeric
- Clove

[a] Of these drugs, only aspirin has been demonstrated to cause a significant increase in bleeding (Table 130-3). The other drugs are described as affecting platelet aggregation or the bleeding time, and case reports have suggested an association with increased bleeding. Brand names for these agents are given in parentheses when they may be more familiar.
[b] Used as a therapeutic antithrombotic agent.
[c] Withdrawn from the US market in 1983.

(Table 130-3). Aspirin-treated subjects had a 44% decrease in risk of myocardial infarction. Aspirin treatment was also associated with a small but significant increased risk of serious hemorrhage. In the aspirin group, 2,979 subjects and in the placebo group, 2,248 subjects reported problems such as easy bruising, hematemesis, melena, and epistaxis (relative risk 1.32; $P < 0.00001$); 48 subjects in the aspirin group compared with 28 in the placebo group required a blood transfusion during this 5-year period ($P = 0.02$). Therefore, in spite of the difficulty in assessing the effect of aspirin on the hemostatic function of individual normal subjects, the clinical significance of aspirin-induced impairment of hemostasis is certain. Aspirin may cause more bleeding symptoms in patients with other hemostatic defects. The risk of bleeding is increased if aspirin is given simultaneously with warfarin, although the occurrence of major hemorrhagic events may not be increased.[47] These

Table 130-3. Effect of Aspirin on the Risk of Bleeding in Normal Subjects[a]

	Aspirin	Placebo	Relative Risk	P Value
No. of subjects	11,037	11,034	—	—
No. with hemorrhagic complications	2,979	2,248	1.32	<0.00001
Easy bruising	1,587	1,027	1.55	<0.0001
Epistaxis	862	640	1.35	<0.0001
Melena	364	246	1.48	<0.00001
Hematemesis	38	28	1.36	0.22
Nonspecific gastrointestinal bleeding[b]	440	422	1.04	0.55
Other bleeding[c]	724	596	1.21	0.0004
Number of requiring blood transfusion	48	28	1.71	<0.02

[a] These data are adapted from the Physicians' Health Study Research Group,[7] and they represent the only definitive documentation of a hemorrhagic risk from drug-induced platelet dysfunction. The subjects were healthy male physicians, treated with one aspirin tablet (325 mg) every other day or a placebo, and followed for an average of 60.2 months.

[b] No further defined.

[c] Hemorrhagic complications described as "other bleeding": 29% were related to shaving or brushing the teeth (32% in the aspirin group and 27% in the placebo group), and 72% were hematuria (70% in the aspirin group and 75% in the placebo group).

studies used high-intensity regimens of 3.0–4.5[47]; it is possible (but not yet proved) that aspirin may not accentuate the bleeding risk with less intense warfarin therapy. Also aspirin may increase the risk of spontaneous hemorrhage when it is given during treatment with recombinant tissue plasminogen activator.[48,49]

The hemostatic risks of aspirin treatment may be similar to the congenital disorder of platelet function, Glanzmann thrombasthenia, in which the hemorrhagic complications are greater when there is an additional cause for bleeding, such as during childbirth.[1] In a small group of patients, aspirin ingestion within 5 days of delivery was associated with an increased occurrence of both maternal vaginal blood loss and systemic bleeding in the infants.[50] Aspirin is known to cross the placenta,[51] and the risk of neonatal bleeding after maternal aspirin ingestion appears to be greater in premature infants weighing <1,500 g.[52]

Several studies have addressed the risk of postoperative hemorrhage in patients taking aspirin. The results, as may be expected with a very mild hemostatic defect, are not consistent. One study gave a single dose of aspirin to 23 patients the evening prior to elective coronary bypass graft surgery and found that there was no difference in bleeding (measured as the amount of chest tube drainage and red cell transfusions required) in these patients compared with 26 control patients who had specifically avoided aspirin and related drugs. By contrast, a retrospective study of 100 patients undergoing elective coronary artery bypass surgery found that 13 patients who had taken aspirin preoperatively (dose and duration not stated) had significantly more bleeding (measured as the volume of mediastinal blood loss and the duration of chest tube drainage) compared with 64 patients who had taken no drugs.[53] In this study, 3 patients required re-exploration for significant postoperative hemorrhage (1 patient in the aspirin group, 1 in the control group, and 1 of 6 patients who had taken Coumadin before surgery), and all were found to have a surgically correctable lesion. Other reports have also noted an increased blood loss during cardiopulmonary bypass surgery following aspirin treatment[54] and an increased rate of reoperation for bleeding, transfusion requirement, and duration of hospitalization.[55]

In two studies of 224 patients undergoing elective total hip replacement by a single surgeon aspirin treatment (1.2–3.6 g/day) was begun the day before surgery and continued for 7 days.[56,57] The blood loss was 20% greater in the treated group in one study, but this was considered clinically insignificant and required no additional care.[57] In the other study, there was no difference in blood loss, although the aspirin group had more wound hematomas (3 in 44 patients versus 1 in 51 control patients).[56] A study of 200 patients undergoing general or gynecologic surgery also suggested that there was greater operative

blood loss in patients who had taken aspirin.[58] The surgeon and the anesthesiologist observed "greater than expected bleeding" in 12 of 55 patients who had taken aspirin and had abnormal platelet aggregation studies, compared with 7 to 97 patients who had not taken aspirin and had normal aggregation studies. The other 48 patients in this study either claimed they had not taken aspirin but were found to have abnormal platelet aggregation—a frequent occurrence in many studies due to habitual and forgotten aspirin use (33 patients)—or had taken aspirin but their platelet aggregation was normal (15 patients). Of these 48 patients, 8 were thought to have excessive bleeding at surgery. Although the results were interpreted as demonstrating increased operative bleeding following aspirin treatment, it is important to note that "greater than expected bleeding" sometimes occurred in the control patients. This observation is inevitable in all subjective evaluations of bleeding, either surgical or medical. The observer always expects—hopes for—the normal bleeding response to be minimal, but the range of "normal bleeding" is great, and patients with more bleeding are often viewed with concern. It may be concluded from the sum of these reports that aspirin has a small, inconsistent, but significant effect on surgical bleeding. Minimally invasive trauma, such as epidural anesthesia at the time of obstetric delivery, is not associated with increased bleeding in patients on daily small doses of aspirin (60 mg).[59]

These data on aspirin present the clinical paradigm for acquired disorders of platelet function: (1) their occurrence is common; (2) the defect is usually mild; (3) individuals vary in their sensitivity to aspirin; (4) platelet aggregation and bleeding time are subject to technical vagaries; (5) the risk of increased bleeding in the individual subject who is otherwise normal is minimal and unpredictable; and (6) nevertheless, a definite risk for increased bleeding with aspirin can be demonstrated when large groups of normal subjects are analyzed or when individuals are studied who have concomitant pathologic (e.g., hemophilia) or physiologic (e.g., childbirth) conditions that can predispose to hemorrhage.

Other Nonsteroidal Anti-Inflammatory Drugs

In addition to aspirin, many other drugs used for their anti-inflammatory and analgesic properties can also cause decreased platelet function[66,67] (Table 130-2). Like aspirin, their mechanism of action appears to be the inhibition of the activity of platelet cyclo-oxygenase. In contrast to aspirin, each of these agents has only a temporary effect on cyclo-oxygenase function, causing enzyme inhibition only as long as the active drug is present in the circulation. Therefore, among these agents

MANAGEMENT OF PATIENTS TAKING ASPIRIN

The therapeutic recommendations for management of a patient on aspirin are straightforward. In a patient with a clear therapeutic indication for aspirin, whether it be a headache or unstable angina,[60] and no apparent increased risk of bleeding, aspirin is one of our safest drugs. In patients who already have greatly increased hemorrhagic risks, such as severe hemophilia, aspirin must be avoided.[35,36] When a hemostatically normal patient who is taking aspirin requires an invasive procedure, aspirin should be discontinued for $\geq$5 days.[50] This period is sufficient for about one-half of the circulating platelets to be replaced by platelets from megakaryocytes that were not exposed to aspirin[33]; one-half of the normal number of platelets (e.g., approximately 100,000/mm^3) is sufficient for normal hemostasis during any surgical procedure.[61] However, since aspirin use is so common[8] and since the drug is present in hundreds of pharmaceutical products,[62] it may be feasible to discontinue aspirin and wait 5 days for a procedure in most patients. Then only careful observation is required. Significant excessive bleeding due to aspirin will be a rare occurrence, and if serious bleeding does occur during an operative procedure, it is likely due to a surgically correctible lesion. If severe hemorrhage due to deficient platelet function is suspected, either DDAVP[63] or a platelet transfusion would be promptly effective, but this will be indicated only very rarely. Perhaps the recommendations for surgery in a patient who has taken aspirin should parallel the recommendations for surgery in patients receiving prophylactic subcutaneous heparin.[64,65] With both aspirin and the conventional fixed doses of subcutaneous heparin (5,000 U twice daily), the risk of increased bleeding during and after surgery is significant in large studies but is a negligible risk in any individual patient. Therefore, except for those patients in whom the nature of the surgical procedure requires the absolute minimum risk of excessive bleeding—as in some plastic surgical, neurosurgical, or ophthalmologic procedures—the increased risk of bleeding with aspirin does not appear to be a reason to delay necessary surgery. The use of "prophylactic" platelet transfusions in this clinical setting is to be discouraged.

only drugs such as piroxicam, which has a plasma half-life of >2 days, affects platelets for more than a few hours.[67] As with aspirin, the most sensitive indication of impaired platelet function is the inhibition of in vitro aggregation and secretion. These agents prolong the bleeding time minimally and transiently[66,68] or not at all, consistent with the bleeding time being a less sensitive measure of the aspirin-induced defect.[20]

Clinical reports are consistent with the observations on platelet function and suggest that these drugs cause less risk of increased bleeding than aspirin. As with aspirin, they may increase the bleeding time in patients with severe hemophilia,[37,68,69] although in two studies therapeutic doses of ibuprofen had no effect on the bleeding time in 19 to 20 patients with hemophilia.[68] Therefore, the clinical approach to patients taking any drug that can inhibit platelet cyclo-oxygenase should be similar, although the hemostatic risk with drugs other than aspirin usually disappears a few hours after the drug is stopped. The additional risk of bleeding with surgery should be negligible, but a prudent course would be to discontinue these drugs the day before a procedure. Analgesics such

as acetaminophen and sodium or choline salicylate do not inhibit platelet function and have no adverse effect on hemostasis.[36,68,70,71]

Ticlopidine

Ticlopidine is used to reduce the risk of thrombotic strokes in patients who have cerebrovascular disease and who are intolerant to aspirin, and it is being studied for its effect in preventing myocardial infarction.[72-74] The degree of prolongation of the bleeding time is equivalent to aspirin.[75] Ticlopidine impairs fibrinogen binding to GPIIb/IIIa and inhibits platelet aggregation to many agonists, particularly ADP.[74,76] The major site of action appears to be on the pathway providing stimulus-response coupling between the ADP receptor and fibrinogen binding.[74,76] The effects of ticlopidine on platelet function appear within 24–48 hours after ingestion, are maximal in 4–6 days, and continue for 4–10 days after the drug has been discontinued.[74] Ticlopidine may be associated with a small increased risk of bruising and epistaxis,[77] but the major potential complications are neutropenia, aplastic anemia, and thrombocytopenia.[73,74,78,79] It is recommended that ticlopidine be discontinued $\geq$10 days before elective surgical procedures.

β-Lactam Antibiotics

Antibiotics are the other major category of therapeutic agents, along with the nonsteroidal anti-inflammatory drugs, that affect platelet function[80-99] (Table 130-2). Like nonsteroidal anti-inflammatory drugs, the use of antibiotics is extremely common. It has been estimated that one-third of hospitalized patients receive antimicrobial therapy.[100] The antibiotics that affect platelet function all share a common β-lactam ring structure, a characteristic of the penicillins and cephalosporins. Some of the antibiotics listed in Table 130-2 have been shown to have a predictable dose- and duration-related effect on the bleeding time.[89,90] Because the effect on the bleeding time is seen only in patients who are receiving large parenteral doses of antibiotics, this is a problem only for hospitalized patients. Also the effect of these drugs on platelets may be greater in chronically ill patients with low serum albumin levels, who have less albumin binding of the antibiotic in the plasma.[101] In a study of 74 hospitalized patients with a consistently prolonged bleeding time, the likely cause was penicillin in 39 patients (30 patients were receiving penicillin G [>15,000,000 U/day] and 9 were receiving ampicillin [6–8 gm/day]) and aspirin or related drugs in 7 patients.[102] The frequency of clinically significant hemorrhage is not predicted by a prolonged bleeding time, the causal relationship to antibiotic treatment is unproved, and fortunately its occurrence is rare.[91]

The structural properties that cause some, but not all, of the penicillins and cephalosporins to affect platelet function are unknown. The diversity of side chain structure alters the antibacterial and pharmacologic properties of the penicillins and cephalosporins and may also determine their effect on platelet function. It is postulated that the antibiotic associates with the platelet plasma membrane by a lipophilic mechanism, causing a perturbation that blocks multiple receptor-agonist interactions or stimulus-response coupling.[103-109] Another plasma membrane function inhibited by penicillin in vivo is the influx of calcium in response to platelet stimulation by thrombin or arachidonate.[110] The characteristic clinical observation is the occurrence of a prolonged bleeding time and abnormal platelet aggregation after several days of high-dose parenteral therapy.[89,90] These abnormalities do not subside until several days after the antibiotic is discontinued.

Although the penicillins can cause a prolonged bleeding time in a predictable, dose-dependent manner, their association with a significant hemostatic defect is much less clear.[80,81,83, 88,90,91,93–97] In fact, it appears that the frequency of clinically significant hemorrhage due solely to the effect of antibiotics on platelet function is rare, and the bleeding time is not helpful in predicting who will bleed.[91] Certainly many patients who need to receive high doses of these antibiotics have risk factors for hemorrhage, such as thrombocytopenia, sepsis, malignancy, and renal failure. Typical case reports of antibiotic-related hemorrhage, such as those with carbenicillin and nafcillin,[94,96] occur in such complicated patients. In these cases, the antibiotic was assumed to have contributed to the bleeding because the diagnostic bleeding times were markedly abnormal. An alternative explanation is that the bleeding time is not related to a risk for hemorrhage and that the antibiotics were innocent.[6] For each report implicating an antibiotic as a cause of hemorrhage, many more patients receive the same antibiotics in large doses without bleeding complications.[91] In conclusion, antibiotic-induced platelet dysfunction appears to have little clinical significance in most patients, and the potential effect on platelet function should not be considered in the decision to use any antibiotic. In the difficult case in which antibiotic-induced platelet dysfunction cannot be excluded as a contributory cause of bleeding, only the passage of time allows a clear diagnosis, since the antiplatelet effect disappears within several days of discontinuation of the drug.

An exception to this conclusion may be moxalactam. The frequency of clinically significant hemorrhagic complications with moxolactam appears to be greater than with other antibiotics.[91,97] Its effect on the bleeding time and platelet aggregation are no different from other antibiotics, so it probably has no more profound effect on platelet function.[90] However, unlike most other β-lactam antibiotics, moxalactam contains a methylthiotetrazole-leaving group that has been implicated in the inhibition of synthesis of vitamin K-dependent proteins.[111] Therefore moxalactam-induced bleeding may be due to the combination of deficiencies of coagulation factors II, VII, IX, and X and impaired platelet function.

Other Drugs

Antibiotic

Nitrofurantoin, an antibiotic structurally unrelated to the β-lactam antibiotics, may cause a mild prolongation of the bleeding time and impair platelet aggregation when blood levels of the drug are >20 μM.[112] Nitrofurantoin is not known to cause clinical bleeding.

Drugs that Increase Platelet cAMP Concentration

Elevation of the platelet concentration of cAMP by any mechanism inhibits platelet function.[113] Prostacyclin and its analogue increase cAMP synthesis by stimulation of adenyl cyclase, and they have been studied as antithrombotic substitutes for heparin in cardiopulmonary bypass surgery and hemodialysis.[114–117] In spite of the potent inhibition of platelet aggregation by prostacyclin in vitro, the effects on the bleeding time are minimal and inconsistent.[114–118] Dipyridamole increases cAMP concentration by inhibition of the cAMP phosphodiesterase.[119] This drug has been used extensively as an antithrombotic agent, in spite of its approval by the US Food and Drug Administration solely as an adjunctive therapy with Coumadin in the treatment of patients with artificial heart valves. A recent review concluded that dipyridamole has no efficacy as an antithrombotic drug.[119] There are no data to suggest that dipyridamole causes increased bleeding.

Anticoagulant

Although heparin is best known for its anticoagulant effect and its adverse effect in causing thrombocytopenia (see Chs. 121 and 128), it has the potential to affect platelet function. Heparin can bind to the platelet surface,[120] cause platelet aggregation and secretion,[121,122] and impair von Willebrand factor-dependent platelet function.[123] Heparin can also cause a prolonged bleeding time.[124,125] Whether these phenomena have relevance to the bleeding complications of heparin is unknown. The prolonged bleeding time is probably due to heparin's inhibition of thrombin generation, analogous to the slight but significantly increased bleeding time in patients with hemophilia.[37]

Fibrinolytic Agents

Bleeding during therapy with plasminogen activators is predominantly due to the effects of hypofibrinogenemia and increased fibrin(ogen) degradation products on fibrin clot formation, usually combined with a structural lesion in the blood vessel wall (see Ch. 122). Recent data also suggest that pharmacologic doses of streptokinase, urokinase, and tissue plasminogen activator may impair platelet function.[126] Several mechanisms may be involved. First, very high levels of fibrin(ogen) degradation products coupled with very low levels of fibrinogen may impair platelet aggregation. Second, plasminogen can bind to the platelet surface, where it is converted to the proteolytic enzyme plasmin by plasminogen activator.[27] On the platelet surface, plasmin can degrade both GPIb (thereby impairing the interaction of the platelet with von Willebrand factor[128]) and fibrinogen (thereby dispersing platelet aggregates[129]). Third, plasmin can inhibit platelet aggregation by blocking the release of arachidonic acid from platelet membranes, thereby limiting thromboxane production.[130] The clinical significance of these observations is unknown, but recent observations suggest that infusions of rt-PA can potentiate the risk of aspirin-associated bleeding.[48,49]

Plasma Expanders

Dextrans are partially hydrolyzed branched polysaccharides of glucose. The two preparations in clinical use have average molecular sizes of 70,000–75,000 (often termed dextran 70) and 40,000 (termed dextran 40, or low-molecular-weight dextran). Both preparations are effective plasma expanders and both can affect platelet function,[131,132] although there are some data to suggest that the high-molecular-weight molecules have a greater effect on hemostasis.[131] An infusion of 1 L of 6% dextran solution over 1 hour prolonged the bleeding time in about one-half of 163 normal subjects, with some bleeding times prolonged to >30 minutes.[131] Dextran infusion also impairs platelet aggregation and platelet procoagulant activity[133] and can cause a modest reduction in plasma von Willebrand factor concentration.[134] However, dextran has no effect on platelet function when added directly to platelet-rich plasma in vitro.[133] Because of these effects on platelet function, dextran has been used extensively as an antithrombotic agent,[135,136] and its efficacy in preventing fatal postoperative pulmonary emboli appears to be equivalent to that of subcutaneous heparin.[135] This therapeutic effect is achieved without any increased risk of bleeding.[136] Therefore, dextran infusions represent yet another example of an agent that can alter platelet function and prolong the bleeding time without an apparent increased risk of hemorrhage. Whether patients who are also receiving another antithrombotic agent, such as aspirin or heparin, or who have a hemostatic defect, would have a greater risk for hemorrhage is suggested but uncertain.[137] Hydroxyethyl starch, known as hetastarch, is a synthetic glucose polymer with an average molecular weight of 450,000 (range 10,000–1,000,000) that is also used for plasma expansion. Like dextran, it may prolong the bleeding time, particularly if administered in doses of >20 ml/kg of a 6% solution, and may predispose to bleeding if administered simultaneously with heparin or used in a patient with a pre-existant hemostatic defect.[132]

Cardiovascular Drugs

Administration of nitroglycerin,[138,139] isosorbide dinitrate,[140] propranolol,[141] and nitroprusside[142] can decrease platelet aggregation and secretion, although the effects are minimal and inconsistent in some studies.[143] Some of the observed effects may also be mediated by desensitization of platelets by increased plasma concentrations of epinephrine.[144] There are also numerous reports on the effect on platelets by drugs used clinically for their ability to inhibit the influx of Ca^{2+} across the membranes of excitable cells, a heterogeneous group known as organic calcium channel blockers: nifedipine, verapamil, and diltiazem.[145-148] These studies have demonstrated inhibition of platelet aggregation in vitro using high concentrations (micromolar) of the drug with washed platelets.[145] This effect is seen primarily with epinephrine as the agonist, and it does not appear to be related to inhibition of Ca^{2+} flux. The proposed mechanisms of action include inhibition of epinephrine binding to α_2-adrenergic receptors, inhibition of the platelet response to thromboxane A_2, and inhibition of serotonin-induced aggregation.[146-148] In therapeutic doses, the calcium channel blockers do not prolong the bleeding time. Quinidine, an antiarrhythmic drug, can act as an antagonist at platelet α_2-adrenergic receptors when used at high concentrations.[149] In a single report, a patient taking quinidine (800 mg) and aspirin (650 mg) daily developed melena and generalized petechiae with a normal platelet count and a bleeding time of >35 minutes.[150] Subsequent studies on two normal volunteers showed that quinidine caused a mild increase in the bleeding time that was apparently potentiated by aspirin.

Psychotropic Agents

Platelets from patients taking tricyclic antidepressent drugs (imiprimine, amitryptyline, nortryptaline) or phenothazines (chlorpromazine, promethazine, trifluoroperazine) may have impaired in vitro aggregation and secretion responses to ADP, epinephrine, and collagen, but this effect is not associated with an increased risk of bleeding.

Anesthetics

Both local and general anesthetics may impair in vitro platelet aggregation.[151] Halothane may cause a slight prolongation of the bleeding time, but it has no adverse effect on surgical hemostasis.[152,153] Cocaine may increase platelet responsiveness to ADP.[154]

Heroin

A study of 10 patients admitted to a methadone program who denied intake of any other drugs for the previous 2 weeks, demonstrated a long bleeding time in 2 and abnormal platelet aggregation in 8.[155] None of these patients had any evidence of a clinically significant hemostatic defect, and the cause of the abnormalities is unclear.

Oncologic Drugs

Administration of mithramycin to a total dose of 6–21 mg has been associated with decreased platelet aggregation, an increased bleeding time, and mucocutaneous bleeding.[156] Daunorubicin and BCNU can each inhibit platelet aggregation

and secretion when added to platelet-rich plasma, but there has been no suggestion of clinically significant bleeding caused by defective platelet function.[157-159]

Miscellaneous Drugs

Clofibrate, a drug that can lower the plasma concentration of lipoproteins, diminishes platelet responsiveness to ADP, collagen, and epinephrine when given to patients with type II hyperbetalipoproteinemia and can diminish the responsiveness of normal platelets to ADP and epinephrine in vitro.[160] Ketanserin, which has been studied for its potential to prevent atherosclerotic complications, causes decreased platelet aggregation in response to serotonin.[161,162] Antihistamines[163] and some radiographic contrast agents[164,165] can also impair platelet aggregation. The mechanism of action of these agents is not known.

Foods and Food Additives

In our nutrition-conscious society, the effect of certain food components on platelet function is an increasingly important issue. A diet rich in fish and other marine oils, which contain a high concentration of ω-3 fatty acids (eicosapentaeoic acid [EPA], C20:5ω-3; and docosahexaenoic acid [DCHA], C22:6ω-3) may decrease the development of atherosclerosis and the occurrence of myocardial infarction.[166] One proposed mechanism of this effect is inhibition of the platelet's role in the pathogenesis of atherosclerosis.[167] Subjects ingesting a diet rich in marine oils or supplemented with ω-3 fatty acids have a slight prolongation of the bleeding time. These lipids act by reducing the platelet content of arachidonic acid and by competing with arachidonic acid for cyclo-oxygenase, thereby reducing thromboxane production.[167] Whether these subjects have any increased risk of clinically significant bleeding is unknown.

Ethanol is a commonly imbibed substance, which, as noted above, has a synergistic effect with aspirin to prolong the bleeding time.[39] Ethanol can itself significantly impair platelet function in vitro,[168] and a blood level as low as 0.05% can impair platelet adhesion to vessel subendothelium in an in vitro perfusion system.[169]

Other food components or additives may affect platelet function and have been suspected of increasing the risk of minor bleeding. Easy bruising noted after eating Chinese food has been attributed to an effect on platelets by a black tree fungus.[170] A component of onion extract can inhibit platelet arachidonic acid metabolism.[171] Ajoene, a component of garlic, is an inhibitor of fibrinogen binding to platelets and platelet aggregation.[172] Extracts from frequently consumed spices (cumin, turmeric, and clove) can decrease platelet thromboxane production and inhibit platelet aggregation.[173]

It can be concluded that platelets are sensitive to an enormous variety of therapeutic and dietary compounds. The inhibition of platelet aggregation is a common observation in patients receiving a wide variety of agents; prolongation of the bleeding time is less common. However, an increased risk of clinically significant bleeding has been demonstrated only for aspirin[7] (Table 130-3). Reports of increased bleeding with all other agents must be viewed with caution. Despite this qualification, it would be prudent for the clinician to have a thorough understanding of the antiplatelet effects of drugs prescribed, and always to consider the potential impact of drug-induced platelet dysfunction, particularly in patients with coexistent hemostatic defects.

SYSTEMIC DISORDERS THAT AFFECT PLATELET FUNCTION

Chronic Renal Failure

Clinical Manifestations

The clinical significance of bleeding in chronic renal failure is difficult to assess. The recognition of severe hemorrhage as a distinct complication of renal failure is generally attributed to Reisman's[174] description in 1907 of two patients with Bright disease who had severe and generalized bleeding. Reisman proposed that the etiology was "a toxin analogous to the hemorrhagins of snake venom." However, there could have been multiple etiologies for the observed bleeding problems in both of Reisman's patients.[174] Others observed a "tendency to hemorrhage" in patients with chronic glomerulonephritis in the predialysis era, and the descriptions of epistaxis and menometrorrhagia[175] are similar to the symptoms of patients with a primary platelet abnormality. Chronic nephritis was also noted to be one of the common causes of cerebral hemorrhage in young people.[175] However, before dialysis, death occurred primarily from hyperkalemia and pulmonary edema.[176] After dialysis became an established treatment, the major causes of death became infection and the underlying cause of the renal failure, such as trauma and poisoning. Hemorrhage caused 6 of 100 deaths in one series, but additional factors could have contributed in each patient.[176] Others noted that management with dialysis, allowing better nutrition and improved general health, appeared to diminish the occurrence of hemorrhagic symptoms.[177] The current prognosis for patients with end-stage renal disease is excellent. Patients who are <46 years old have a 97% 5-year survival with no medical complications; for patients <61 years old, the 5-year survival is 84%.[178] Bleeding problems were not mentioned in this discussion,[178] nor was bleeding considered in general reviews during the past 25 years on the clinical course and management of patients with chronic renal failure.[179]

A more objective indication of the rarity of a significant bleeding diathesis in patients with renal failure is the extensive experience with percutaneous renal biopsy. A study of 1,000 consecutive percutaneous renal biopsies at the Mayo Clinic reported that 69 patients had hematuria, of whom 50 cleared within 2 days and 2 required blood transfusions.[180] Fourteen patients had clinically detectable perirenal hematomas, and two required surgical exploration and evacuation. A bleeding time was performed in 707 of these patients before biopsy; it was abnormal in 24 (3%), and one of these patients had a perirenal hematoma. The other 13 patients with perirenal hematoma had had a normal bleeding time. Hypertension was a more significant factor than the bleeding time in predicting the occurrence of complications.[180] Another study of 183 consecutive renal biopsies reported three hemorrhagic complications that required surgical intervention, and all were the result of needle lacerations of the kidney or spleen.[181] In a discussion of 5,120 renal biopsies from 15 institutions, no fatalities occurred, and the severe bleeding complications appeared to be related to anomalous vessels, heparin anticoagulation, or the presence of amyloid in the kidney.[182] The incidence of small perirenal hematomas following percutaneous renal biopsy, as diagnosed by computed tomography, is high (85%[183]), but this may not be unexpected for the puncture of an organ that receives 20% of the cardiac output. The reports with other invasive procedures in patients with chronic renal disease are few, but they suggest that bleeding complications following abdominal surgery, liver and bone marrow biopsies, and tooth extractions may be rare.[184]

By contrast, gastrointestinal hemorrhage is a common complication and frequent cause of death in patients with acute renal failure,[185,186] and patients with chronic renal failure account for a significant proportion of those requiring endoscopy for upper gastrointestinal bleeding.[186] Experimental data suggest that chronic uremia causes increased susceptibility of gastric mucosa to acid injury.[187] Over 90% of patients with renal failure and gastrointestinal bleeding have an anatomic diagnosis at endoscopy: angiodysplasia is most common, with "peptic" lesions (gastric or duodenal ulcer, erosive esophagitis, gastritis, or duodenitis) also being very common.[186] Rectal ulcers

can also be a cause of sudden, massive lower gastrointestinal hemorrhage.[188]

These observations suggest that serious, spontaneous hemorrhage is very uncommon in patients with chronic renal failure. However, the many individual case reports of serious, spontaneous hemorrhage support the existence of a hemostatic defect in at least some uremic patients. Patients have been reported with subdural hematoma,[189] subarachnoid hemorrhage,[190] hemorrhagic pericardial effusion,[191] hemorrhagic pleural effusion,[192] subcapsular liver hematoma,[193] retroperitoneal hematoma,[194] mediastinal hemorrhage,[195] and bleeding into the anterior chamber of the eye.[196] In these patients, the heparin therapy used for hemodialysis could have been a factor in their bleeding because the nature of the bleeding, primarily visceral hematomas, is more consistent with a heparin-induced coagulopathy than with the typical mucocutaneous bleeding of a platelet function disorder.

The primary hemostatic abnormality in uremia is thought to be a defect in platelet function.[184,197–201] These discussions of bleeding in uremia often focused on the laboratory phenomena of abnormal platelet aggregation or a prolonged bleeding time, rather than actual hemorrhagic episodes in patients. Like the drug-induced disorders of platelet function discussed above, abnormal platelet function in uremia is far more common than clinically significant bleeding. Furthermore, laboratory evaluation of platelet function may not be a good predictor for the risk of hemorrhage.

Tests of Hemostasis and Platelet Function in Uremia

Platelet aggregation studies are frequently abnormal in uremic patients, and the occurrence of the abnormality does not appear to correlate with the severity of the renal failure or the occurrence of bleeding.[200] The bleeding time is characteristically prolonged in uremia and does appear to correlate with the severity of the renal failure.[199,200,202] The bleeding time has also been reported to correlate with the occurrence of clinically significant bleeding in uremic patients,[184,199,200,203,204] but a recent analysis of these data suggests that the correlation may not be clinically significant.[6]

The severity of anemia also correlates with the severity of real failure,[202,205] and it is now clear that anemia itself is an independent cause of a prolonged bleeding time.[203,206–211] The relationship of the hematocrit to the bleeding time was first made by Duke in 1910, who found that the bleeding time in thrombocytopenic patients was corrected by transfusion of fresh whole blood, but when thrombocytopenia recurred the bleeding time was less abnormal in the presence of a higher hematocrit. Bleeding times can be prolonged with severe anemia due to vitamin B_{12} or iron deficiency, and are corrected when the anemia is corrected with transfusions of washed red cells.[206] Therefore, it should be expected that severely anemic patients with chronic renal failure will have a long bleeding time. The relationship of the bleeding time to hematocrit in these patients has been confirmed by the correction of the bleeding time with transfusion of washed red cells[207] and by treatment with recombinant human erythropoietin.[209,210] There was a suggestion in these reports that bleeding symptoms were also improved with the correction of the anemia.[207,209] A similar dependence of platelet function on the hematocrit has been demonstrated in studies of platelet adhesion to deendothelialized rabbit vessels using perfusion of whole blood from uremic patients: platelet adhesion was decreased in the patients, but corrected when the blood was supplemented with red cells.[204] In other experiments, it has been shown that the presence of red cells displaces the less dense platelets to the periphery of the column of circulating blood, thereby increasing the interaction of platelet with the vessel wall.[212] Since a prolonged bleeding time, rather than clinical bleeding, has been the focus for concern and discussion in many studies of the hemostatic defect in uremia, it is likely that this issue will receive less emphasis as patients with chronic renal failure are routinely treated with erythropoietin.

In contrast to the studies of platelet function performed to understand the possible increased risk of bleeding in patients with chronic renal failure, coagulation and fibrinolytic activities have been investigated to understand the increased risk of thrombotic complications—a major cause of mortality. Although the data are inconsistent, with some suggesting diminished fibrinolytic activity[213] and some consistent with accelerated fibrinolysis,[214] markers of activated coagulation are commonly present and suggest the presence of a prothrombotic state.[214,215] The extent of these changes may be related to differences among hemodialysis membranes.[216]

Pathogenesis of Abnormal Platelet Function in Uremia

Even though the anemia of renal failure appears to be the major cause of the prolonged bleeding time, there is other evidence for abnormal platelet function. Platelet aggregation abnormalities persist when the hematocrit is normalized by red cell transfusion[203] or erythropoietin treatment.[210] Washed uremic platelets suspended in normal plasma do not adhere normally to deendothelialized rabbit vessels at a high shear rate, and normal platelets suspended in uremic plasma acquire an adhesion defect,[204] which may be related to an abnormality of the interaction of von Willebrand factor with GPIIb/IIIa.[217] This has led to the suggestion that there may be an abnormality of von Willebrand factor in uremia, but measurement of von Willebrand factor antigen and activity (measured as ristocetin cofactor activity) demonstrates that the values are normal or elevated.[201] Other studies have found that von Willebrand factor function is diminished relative to the amount of immunologic von Willebrand factor present, consistent with an observation that the proportion of the more hemostatically effective larger multimers is decreased.[218,219] However, these observations have not always been confirmed, and no abnormalities of the interaction of von Willebrand factor with its constitutive platelet membrane receptor, GPIb/IX, have been reported.[204,218,219]

Platelets from uremic patients frequently exhibit reduced fibrinogen binding, aggregation, and secretion in response to a wide variety of agonists. This abnormality may be retained by the platelets after their separation from uremic plasma, and in some experiments uremic plasma has induced these defects in normal platelets.[220,221] Uremic platelets may also also exhibit a reduction in several of the biochemical responses necessary for aggregation and secretion, including the rise in cytoplasmic free calcium levels,[222] release of arachidonic acid from membrane phospholipids,[220] conversion of arachidonic acid to thromboxane A_2,[223–225] and dense-granule and α-granule secretion.[226,227] In addition, a decrease in the dense-granule content of ADP and serotonin[228] and an increase in cAMP[229] have been demonstrated. However, others have noted increased mobilization of internal calcium stores in platelets from patients with chronic renal failure.[230]

The pathogenesis of the diverse platelet function defects in uremia remains undefined. They may be caused by both dialyzable and nondialyzable substances present in uremic plasma. For example, platelet aggregation can be inhibited by dialyzable substances, such as guanidinosuccinic acid or phenolic acids, and by poorly characterized substances of intermediate molecular sizes at concentrations found in uremic plasma.[231,232] The reduced aggregation responses may improve after the uremia is corrected by dialysis.[197,233] Venous and arterial segments from uremic patients produce more of the platelet inhibitor prostacyclin than normal vessels, and this abnormality is not corrected by dialysis.[226] In rats, uremic plasma can be shown to stimulate excessive prostacyclin production by endothelial cells.[234] Endothelial cells from uremic patients also generate more nitric oxide, possibly related to higher plasma levels of the nitric oxide precursor L-arginine, and nitric oxide may be responsible for the higher platelet concentrations of cGMP and deficient platelet function.[235–237] Furthermore, the response of platelets from patients on hemodialysis to nitric oxide may be impaired.[236] Some substances found in high concentrations in uremic plasma, such as urea and parathyrin, appear to have no role in inhibiting platelet function,[184,197,238] although ingestion of large amounts of urea by normal subjects causes abnormal platelet aggregation.[199]

Procoagulant activity describes an important ability of platelets to provide a catalytic membrane surface for accelerating the generation of thrombin. Congenital deficiency of platelet procoagulant activity is not associated with an abnormality of aggregation or the bleeding time but may be associated with increased bleeding.[239] Based on crude tests, the serum prothrombin time, and "platelet factor 3" assay, this property of platelets is consistently diminished in patients with uremia.[184,198,221] Since optimal procoagulant activity requires platelet activation, decreased procoagulant activity in uremia may reflect the abnormalities of activation described above.

Platelets from uremic patients may be unusually sensitive to medicines that decrease platelet function. Aspirin has been reported to be more effective in prolonging the bleeding time in uremic patients than in control subjects, and this effect may occur by mechanisms other than the irreversible inhibition of cyclo-oxygenase function.[24,240] Similarly, β-lactam antibiotics that prolong the bleeding time may have a greater effect in uremic patients and may increase the occurrence of bleeding, particularly if the renal clearance of the antibiotic is reduced.[241]

Mild thrombocytopenia has been reported in chronic renal failure,[231] probably due to a combination of diminished marrow production and diminished platelet survival.[242] Also mean platelet volume may be diminished in uremic patients, resulting in a decreased total platelet mass (estimated from platelet count × platelet volume), which in turn may contribute to the increased bleeding time.[243] However, a platelet count <100,000/mm^3 should alert the physician to the possibility of thrombocytopenia due to a systemic disease, such as multiple myeloma, systemic vasculitis, hemolytic uremic syndrome, eclampsia, renal allograft rejection, or an adverse reaction to a medicine such as heparin.

Cardiopulmonary Bypass Surgery

Clinical Manifestations and Laboratory Evaluation

Although cardiopulmonary bypass is accompanied by decreased plasma levels of coagulation factors and increased fibrinolytic activity, abnormal platelet function is a prominent observation is these patients. A fall in the platelet count and platelet dysfunction are seen in most patients undergoing bypass surgery with either a bubble or membrane oxygenator.[264–267] A prolonged bleeding time—longer than expected for the degree of thormbocytopenia—decreased platelet aggregation, decreased platelet agglutination in response to ristocetin, and a decreased concentration of α- and/or dense-granule contents are typically found in patients following bypass surgery.[264,267–269] In spite of these abnormalities, excessive bleeding is uncommon, occurring in only about 5% of patients. Bleeding, usually presenting as excessive chest tube blood loss (defined as >100 ml/hr), is due to a surgical cause in more than one-half of cases, while platelet function abnormalities account for most of the remainder.[270,271]

MANAGEMENT OF PATIENTS WITH CHRONIC RENAL FAILURE AND ABNORMAL PLATELET FUNCTION STUDIES

The first principle of management for patients with chronic renal failure and abnormal platelet assays is to determine whether an increased risk of clinically significant bleeding is present. This must be determined by a careful history and examination (see Ch. 103). Since the presence of abnormal platelet aggregation and a prolonged bleeding time are common in uremic patients and they do not predict an increased risk of hemorrhage, they are not an indication for transfusion or therapeutic intervention. If a patient with abnormal platelet function and a long bleeding time requires an invasive procedure (e.g., a kidney biopsy, lung biopsy, or laparotomy) and there is no history to suggest an increased risk of bleeding, there is probably less risk in doing the procedure without specific treatment to correct the platelet defect than to delay and attempt to normalize a laboratory value.[180–182,184] If bleeding does complicate a procedure, a surgical complication is the most likely etiology and the initial management is no different than in patients without renal failure. If a patient with chronic renal failure presents with a hemorrhagic episode, the cause of bleeding should be evaluated without assuming that uremia is the etiology. Several treatment modalities may improve the bleeding time, and anecdotal observations suggest that they may also improve hemostasis. However, these modalities have not been uniformly effective, and prospective studies have not been performed. Therefore therapy for bleeding in a patient with chronic renal failure should involve consideration of the severity of bleeding, the anticipated severity of the hemostatic risk from surgery or trauma, and the risks of the therapy.

Dialysis with correction of the renal failure is often, but not always, effective in correcting the abnormal platelet function and the long bleeding time in uremia, diminishing the risk of clinical bleeding.[184,197,227,233,244,245] For example, intensive dialysis decreases the occurrence of acute gastrointestinal bleeding, a major cause of morbidity and mortality in acute renal failure, probably by decreasing the ulcerative intestinal complication.[185] Peritoneal dialysis and hemodialysis are equally effective.[197,244,245]

Infusion of DDAVP (desmopressin) avoids the risk of blood-born infection and has been used in the management of bleeding in uremia. DDAVP has less pressor effect than natural vasopressin, and side effects are uncommon.[63] However, reported complications of DDAVP therapy include facial flushing, mild tachycardia, water retention, hyponatremia severe enough to cause seizures,[246–248] arterial thrombosis,[249] and memory loss.[250] DDAVP stimulates the release of von Willebrand factor from endothelial cells, and this may be the reason for its therapeutic effect in uremia, although other mechanisms may be involved.[251,252] DDAVP, administered intravenously or subcutaneously in a dose of 0.3 μg/kg over 15–30 minutes, shortens the bleeding time in 50–75% of uremic patients.[253–256] This correction occurs within 30–60 minutes and lasts for about 4 hours, correlating with an increase in the plasma concentration of von Willebrand factor and an increase in the proportion of the higher-molecular-weight multimers of von Willebrand factor.[255,257,258] There are reports of the effectiveness of DDAVP in preventing bleeding at surgery in uremic patients,[254] but no controlled trial has been performed, and the occurrence of excessive bleeding with surgery in uremic patients who have not received specific treatment may be negligible.[180–182,184,208]

An increase of the hematocrit, either by red cell transfusion or by treatment with recombinant human erythropoietin, is associated with a correction of the bleeding time and a suggestion of diminished clinical bleeding.[203,207,208] It seems unusual to suggest red cell transfusions as a therapeutic measure for correction of abnormal hemostasis, but if hemorrhage occurs and red cell replacement is required, transfusion up to a hematocrit ≥30% may provide some improvement in hemostasis. However, the inevitable risk of infection associated with transfusion of blood products outweighs the potential benefit unless red cell replacement is required. Similarly, the use of cyroprecipitate infusions, which have been reported to shorten the bleeding time in some studies[39,257] but not others.[259] may have greater risk than benefit for patients with chronic renal failure.

Conjugated estrogens have also been reported to shorten prolonged bleeding times in uremic patients.[260–262] Given intravenously in a dose of 0.6 mg/kg/day for 5 days, the effects may be seen after the first dose and may persist for 2 weeks. One report suggests that oral conjugated estrogens are effective at a dose of 50 mg/day, but this regimen has not been prospectively studied.[263] The mechanism of this effect and its clinical relevance are unknown.

Pathogenesis of the Platelet Disorder

The platelet defect caused by cardiopulmonary bypass is most likely due to the effects of platelet activation and fragmentation within the extracorporeal circulation. The severity of the platelet abnormalities correlates with the duration of the bypass procedure.[264,272] Following uncomplicated surgery, platelet function returns to normal within 1 hour,[264] although a much longer time may be required in some patients,[267] and the platelet count typically does not return to normal for several days. Thrombocytopenia is caused by hemodilution, by accumulation of platelets within the bypass circuit, and to a lesser extent by sequestrations of damaged platelets in the liver.[273] Platelet dysfunction following bypass may be due to reversible adhesion and aggregation of platelets to fibrinogen absorbed from plasma onto the bypass circuit material,[274,275] mechanical trauma and shear stress,[276] cardiotomy suction,[277] trace concentrations of circulating thrombin and ADP,[278,279] complement activation,[280] hypothermia,[281] blood conservation devices,[282] bypass priming solutions,[283,284] and—with bubble oxygenators—exposure of platelets to the blood-air interface.[285] Cardiopulmonary bypass also consistently causes the appearance of platelet fragments, or membrane "microparticles," evidence that the platelet surface membrane is subjected to severe mechanical stress during the procedure.[272] Surface membrane alterations may play a significant role in platelet dysfunction.[286–288] Other data suggest that the hemostatic abnormality is not intrinsic to platelets, but rather primarily due to reduced formation of the platelet agonist thrombin during heparin administration.[289]

Management

Whether to perform a bleeding time preoperatively in patients without a bleeding history, hoping to identify those patients more likely to have excessive postoperative bleeding, is controversial.[290–292] However in cardiac surgery, as well as in other major surgery,[293] the bleeding time should not be relied on as a good predictor of postoperative hemorrhage.[6] In fact, if a careful history is taken, few laboratory assays are helpful in the preoperative evaluation.[294] Prophylactic platelet transfusions are not routinely indicated for cardiopulmonary bypass surgery.[294] However, patients who have a prolonged bleeding time and excessive blood loss in the postoperative period usually will respond to platelet transfusions.[264]

Postoperative blood loss may be diminished by the use of desamino-D-arginine-vasopressin (DDAVP) after cessation of bypass,[296–298] but most clinical trials have not demonstrated a beneficial effect for this drug.[299–302] In these studies, a benefit of DDAVP seemed more apparent in patients undergoing more complex cardiac surgical procedures.[303] Potential risks of DDAVP include hyponatremia,[247,248] hypotension,[301] and thrombosis,[304] although an increased risk for postoperative thrombosis has not been observed in recent clinical trials.[303,305]

Attempts have been made to prevent platelet activation during bypass surgery in both humans and experimental animals by infusion of prostaglandin E_1 or prostacyclin. By increasing the platelet concentration of cAMP and reducing platelet responsiveness, these agents partially prevent the occurrence of thrombocytopenia and platelet function abnormalities.[115,116] However, the hypotensive properties of these agents limit their usefulness. Aprotinin (Trasylol), a peptide serine protease inhibitor, has been studied for its potential to protect platelets from activation by thrombin, plasmin, and other proteases generated during cardiopulmonary bypass.[270,306–309] Allergic reactions preclude its use in patients who have previously been treated with aprotinin. Currently aprotinin is not approved for use in the United States, and further studies will be required to define its risks and potential benefits clearly.[310,311]

Antiplatelet Antibodies

Immunoglobulin molecules can bind to the platelet surface in several pathologic conditions, including idiopathic thrombocytopenic purpura (ITP), systemic lupus erythematosus (SLE), and platelet alloimmunization.[312,313] The common pathologic result of antibody binding, with or without complement binding, is accelerated platelet destruction and thrombocytopenia.[314] In most cases, the surviving platelets appear to function normally; indeed, bleeding times in ITP may be shorter than expected for the degree of thrombocytopenia.[5] On the other hand, some individuals with circulating antiplatelet antibodies appear to have impaired platelet function, although the frequency of this problem, compared with the occurrence of thrombocytopenia, must be very uncommon. Immune thrombocytopenia is a common disease; significantly impaired hemostasis caused primarily by antibody-mediated platelet dysfunction has been demonstrated in only a few reports.

Clinical Manifestations and Laboratory Evaluation

In some patients with ITP or SLE, platelet dysfunction may be suspected because mucocutaneous bleeding symptoms occur at a platelet count that is usually sufficient for normal hemostasis ($>50,000/mm^3$), and the bleeding time may be longer than expected for the degree of thrombocytopenia.[315–318] The clinical spectrum of autoimmune platelet dysfunction may include some patients (predominantly young women) with mild purpura, often described as easy bruising,

and a normal platelet count.[319] It has been suggested that these patients have accelerated platelet destruction but a normal platelet count due to compensatory increased thrombopoiesis.[319]

Patients with antiplatelet antibodies may exhibit defective platelet function in vitro, even if they do not manifest a prolonged bleeding time or clinical symptoms of excessive bleeding—a situation like that described above for the effects of aspirin ingestion and renal disease. For example, in two studies, 13 of 19 patients with ITP demonstrated impaired platelet aggregation to ADP, epinephrine, or collagen.[315,320] In two other studies, 22 of 35 patients with SLE were found to have decreased platelet aggregation in response to these agonists.[321,322] These platelet function abnormalities appeared to be antibody mediated because IgG purified from the plasma or eluted from the platelets of some of the patients inhibited the aggregation of normal platelets.

Several aspects of platelet function may be impaired by antiplatelet antibodies. The most frequently observed abnormality is absence of platelet aggregation in response to low concentrations of collagen and absence of the second wave of irreversible aggregation in response to ADP or epinephrine. This pattern is identical to the abnormalities caused by aspirin. In ITP and SLE, the abnormal aggregation may be related to a decreased platelet content of dense- and α-granule contents.[316,317,323] In one report, platelets in ITP also exhibited an activation defect manifested by diminished conversion of arachidonic acid to thromboxane A_2.[318] In addition, experiments using an ex vivo perfusion system indicated that some antiplatelet antibodies may inhibit the adhesion of platelets to subendothelial matrix.[324]

Pathogenesis

How autoantibodies on alloantibodies may impair platelet function is unknown. Antibody binding to specific platelet membrane proteins[325–331] or glycosphingolipids[332] could affect the participation of these membrane components in stimulus-response coupling. For example, antibodies against β_2-microglobulin from the sera of patients with SLE or rheumatoid arthritis inhibit ADP-induced platelet aggregation, although the normal function of β_2-microglobulin on the surface of platelets is unknown.[333] Some HLA antibodies inhibit the uptake of serotonin by platelets.[334] Anti-PI^{A1} alloantibodies bind to GPIIIa, and some inhibit aggregation by interfering with fibrinogen binding to the GPIIb/IIIa complex.[335] Autoantibodies in two patients with clinical syndromes similar to ITP bound to GPIIb/IIIa and caused a functional platelet disorder indistinguishable from Glanzmann thrombasthenia.[336–340] Isoantibodies from several patients with Glanzmann thrombasthenia have had this same effect on normal platelets in vitro.[341,342] One patient has been reported who developed an IgG autoantibody reacting with platelet membrane GPIb and GPV, producing a platelet function disorder indistinguishable from Bernard-Soulier syndrome.[343] A similar patient has also been described.[344]

Some antiplatelet antibodies can induce aggregation and secretion. In fact, the ability of ITP sera to induce platelet secretion of serotonin formed the basis of an early test for antiplatelet antibodies.[345] In vitro, antibodies may activate platelets through the binding of IgG-immune complexes to platelet Fc receptors[346]; the deposition onto the cell of sublytic quantities of C5b-9, the membrane attack complex of the complement system[347,348]; and the binding of the Fab portion of an antibody to a specific membrane antigen.[328,333] If bound antibody were to cause platelet secretion in vivo and the platelets continued to circulate, they might be expected to be refractory to platelet agonists and deficient in secretory granule contents. While such activation of circulating platelets is an attractive hypothesis for the the "acquired storage pool deficiency" seen occasionally in ITP or SLE, alternative mechanisms need to be considered. For example, some antibodies may affect the uptake of substances into platelet granules, either during megakaryocytopoiesis[349] or in the circulation.[350]

Management

Antibody-mediated platelet dysfunction is a syndrome of only investigative interest and not of clinical importance, except when an acquired platelet disorder was responsible for bleeding symptoms.[336,337,339,343,344]

Miscellaneous Disorders

In addition to an autoimmune etiology, acquired thrombasthenia can also occur due to an abnormality of chromosome 17, at the site of the genes for the platelet membrane GPIIb and GPIIIa.[351] Patients with the adult respiratory distress syndrome often have thrombocytopenia. In some instances, those platelets remaining in the circulation appear to have undergone extensive secretion, as evidenced by the presence of the α-granule membrane protein P-selectin and secreted thrombospondin on the platelet surface.[272] This may be caused by extensive damage of pulmonary vessels. Patients with disseminated intravascular coagulation (DIC) may have reduced platelet aggregation associated with a deficiency of secretory granule contents, a phenomenon termed acquired storage pool disease or, more graphically, exhausted platelets,[352] resulting from platelet stimulation by thrombin or other agonists. It has also been suggested that the elevated fibrin(ogen) degradation products and low fibrinogen levels that occur in DIC may inhibit platelet function. Although purified fibrin(ogen) degradation products can impair platelet aggregation in vitro, this requires high concentrations that are unlikely to occur in vivo. Furthermore, hypofibrinogenemia would contribute to a defect in platelet aggregation only in extreme cases (plasma fibrinogen <10 mg/dl) because concentrations above that are sufficient to saturate platelet membrane fibrinogen receptors.[353] Chronic liver disease and hepatic cirrhosis of various etiologies have been reported to cause a prolonged bleeding time and other platelet function abnormalities.[354–356] However, studies demonstrating that the bleeding time and platelet aggregation abnormalities correlated with the degree of thrombocytopenia suggest that no specific platelet function defect exists in liver disease.[351] Bartter syndrome, a disorder of primary renal potassium wasting and hypokalemic alkalosis, has been reported to be associated with a prolonged bleeding time and decreased platelet aggregation and secretion in response to ADP and epinephrine.[358] There are isolated reports of a slight prolongation of the bleeding time and/or platelet aggregation defects in a number of other clinical conditions: nonthrombocytopenic purpura with eosinophilia,[359,360] atopic asthma and hay fever,[361] acute respiratory failure,[362] and Wilms tumor.[363] The clinical significance of these observations is unknown.

HEMATOLOGIC DISORDERS THAT AFFECT PLATELET FUNCTION

Chronic Myeloproliferative Disorders

Bleeding and thrombosis represent significant causes of morbidity and mortality in the chronic myeloproliferative disorders, which include essential thrombocythemia, polycythemia rubra vera, myelofibrosis with myeloid metaplasia, and chronic myeloid leukemia. Abnormal platelet function has been postulated as a contributing cause for these complications. Thrombocytosis is present by definition in thrombocythemia and may

also occur in each of the other disorders. Bleeding occurs in about one-third of patients with myeloproliferative disorders and contributes to mortality in about 10% of patients. Thrombosis also occurs in about one-third of patients, contributing to mortality in 15–40%.[364] Most symptomatic patients experience either bleeding or thrombosis; however, some will develop both complications. Bleeding is usually mucocutaneous in nature, suggesting a platelet defect. Both arterial and venous thromboses can occur, and they may involve unusual locations, such as the hepatic, portal, and mesenteric circulations.[364–366] Patients with thrombocythemia can develop ischemia of the fingers and toes due to digital artery thrombosis, microvascular occlusion in the coronary circulation, and transient neurologic symptoms due to cerebrovascular occlusion.[367–370] Despite these potentially serious problems, it is difficult to predict the risk of bleeding or thrombosis in asymptomatic patients. For example, a retrospective study of 38 untreated patients with various myeloproliferative disorders followed for an average of 6.5 years found that vaso-occlusive symptoms were no more frequent than in an age-matched control group. Bleeding, primarily gastrointestinal, occurred in 11 patients and was more likely in patients >59 years of age.[371]

Pathogenesis of the Bleeding and Thrombosis

A number of intrinsic platelet function defects have been reported, but their clinical significance is uncertain. The bleeding time is prolonged in only a few patients, and significant bleeding complications can occur in patients with a normal bleeding time.[372] Elevation of the platelet count per se correlates poorly with the risk of hemorrhage or thrombosis.[364,373–375] A clear risk factor for excessive bleeding, particularly after surgery, is the increased whole blood viscosity in patients with uncontrolled polycythemia vera and a high hematocrit.[376,377]

Platelets in these disorders may be larger or smaller than normal, abnormally shaped, and have a decreased number of secretory granules.[378] Platelet survival may be decreased in essential thrombocythemia.[379] The most common platelet abnormality is decreased aggregation and secretion in response to epinephrine (60% of patients), ADP (40%), and collagen (35%).[364,380] These abnormalities are not due merely to the high platelet count, since patients with reactive thrombocytosis have functionally normal platelets.[381] In what may appear to be a paradox, some patients may demonstrate spontaneous in vitro platelet aggregation in platelet-rich plasma.[364] The significance of this is unknown because it is also occasionally seen in normal individuals. Decreased platelet aggregation or secretion, and decreased procoagulant activity, may be caused by (1) decreased agonist-induced release of arachidonic acid from membrane phospholipids,[382] (2) decreased conversion of arachidonic acid to prostaglandin endoperoxides or lipoxygenase products,[383] (3) decreased platelet responsiveness to thromboxane A_2,[384] (4) decreased dense-granule or α-granule contents,[382,385–387] or (5) decreased α_2-adrenergic receptors.[388,389] Specific platelet membrane abnormalities have also been reported, including a deficiency of GPIb and GPIX, causing an acquired form of the Bernard-Soulier syndrome[390]; a deficiency of receptors for prostaglandin D_2[391]; an increased number of receptors for the Fc portion of IgG[392]; and a relative increase in the concentration of GPIV compared with GPIb.[393,394] Myeloproliferative disorders are thought to be clonal in origin, and therefore the platelet abnormalities may develop from a clone of abnormal megakaryocytes. An acquired form of von Willebrand disease has also been reported in these patients.[387,395–397]

It is important to emphasize several features about the platelet function defects reported in myeloproliferative disorders. First, none has consistently predicted a risk of bleeding or thrombosis. Second, none are unique to a particular myeloproliferative disorder. Third, their relative frequency has varied widely in different reported series. Therefore, the clinical significance of the described abnormalities of platelet function in myeloproliferative disorders is unknown.

Management

The most effective preventive treatment is to maintain the hematocrit at <45% in patients with polycythemia vera.[398] Decreasing the platelet count with alkylating agents (busulfan or hydroxyurea) or with plateletpheresis is of less certain benefit. Anecdotal data exist on clinical improvement associated with lowering of the platelet count,[364,365,369,370,399,400] but a lack of symptoms associated with untreated extreme thrombocytosis of long duration has also been documented.[373,401] Knowing the potential leukemogenic risks of alkylating agents, asymptomatic patients should probably not be treated with such drugs to decrease their platelet count, especially if they are young, except for specific indications of serious thrombotic or hemorrhagic complications, or both.[401] Aspirin may be effective therapy for acute digital ischemia, but it should not be used in asymptomatic patients to diminish the risk of thrombosis because it can increase the risk of hemorrhagic complications.[364] Anegrilide is a new drug that decreases the platelet count by inhibiting platelet production[402]; it may become a useful agent to control thrombocytosis in certain patients with myeloproliferative disorders.[403]

Leukemias and Myelodysplastic Syndromes

Bleeding in these disorders is most always due to thrombocytopenia, although abnormalities of platelet function have been described. In acute myeloid leukemia and its variants, platelets may be larger than normal, abnormally shaped, and have a marked variation in the number of granules. There may be decreased aggregation and secretion in response to ADP, epinephrine, or collagen, as well as decreased platelet procoagulant activity.[404,405] Identical abnormalities can be seen in the myelodysplastic syndromes, although the platelets may be less uniformly affected, perhaps due to the presence of normal platelets mixed with those produced by the neoplastic clone.[386,404] Abnormal platelet function and acquired von Willebrand disease have been reported in hairy cell leukemia.[406–409]

Dysproteinemias

Clinical Manifestations

Platelet dysfunction is observed in approximately one-third of patients with IgA myeloma or Waldenström's macroglobulinemia, 5% of patients with IgG myeloma, and occasionally in patients with benign monoclonal gammopathy.[410–412] However, thrombocytopenia is much more likely to be a major cause of bleeding. Additional hemostatic problems in these patients can be due to the hyperviscosity syndrome,[412] a heparin-like coagulation inhibitor,[413,414] or to complications of amyloidosis (i.e., acquired factor X deficiency[415,416] or fibrinolysis[417,418]). A diagnostic problem in patients with myeloma can be the interpretation of laboratory assays of coagulation when the paraprotein interferes with fibrin polymerization and the function of other coagulation proteins.[410–412] Patients may have markedly abnormal laboratory tests (for example, the thrombin time) with no evidence of clinical bleeding.[410] Also the bleeding time may be prolonged in patients with dysproteinemias in the absence of clinical bleeding.

Pathogenesis

Abnormalities of platelet function correlate with the concentration of the plasma paraprotein.[412] Myeloma proteins can inhibit all platelet functions: aggregation, secretion, procoagu-

lant activity, and clot retraction, and normal platelets can acquire these defects when incubated with the purified monoclonal immunoglobulin.[411,412,419] In some cases, specific interactions of the monoclonal protein have been described. One IgA myeloma protein inhibited the ability of a suspension of aortic connective tissue to aggregate normal platelets.[420] The bleeding time and bleeding symptoms of the patient from whom this paraprotein was isolated were corrected when the IgA myeloma protein was removed by plasmapheresis. In another patient, an IgGκ myeloma protein bound specifically to platelet membrane GPIIIa.[421] Both the intact IgG and its F(ab')$_2$ fragment inhibited binding of fibrinogen to activated platelets, thus inducing a defect comparable to thrombasthenia. This patient also had bleeding reminiscent of classical Glanzmann thrombasthenia[1] and died of hemorrhage from a gastic ulcer.[421] There are a number of reports of acquired von Willebrand disease in patients with myeloma, benign monoclonal gammopathy, or chronic lymphocytic leukemia.[422–426] In some the plasma concentration of von Willebrand factor was decreased, and in others the larger multimers were deficient. The myeloma protein may interact with von Willebrand factor and accelerate its clearance from plasma, or may interfere with its binding to platelet GPIb. Another hypothesis is that the plasma concentration of von Willebrand factor may be decreased by adsorption of the protein onto the tumor cells.[409,427] In fact, in one patient, plasma cells were purported to express GPIb/IX and to bind von Willebrand factor.[428]

Management

A high plasma concentration of myeloma protein can cause severe hemorrhagic symptoms, in part due to hyperviscosity and in part to platelet dysfunction. Under these conditions, bleeding should be regarded as a medical emergency and treatment initiated by means of plasmapheresis to reduce the concentration of the myeloma protein.[412,422,429,430] The goal of therapy is the cessation of bleeding. Chemotherapy for the underlying plasma cell neoplasm should be begun to effect more long-lasting reduction of the paraprotein. DDAVP infusion, with or without plasmapheresis, may be transiently effective in patients with acquired von Willebrand disease.[422,423,425,431]

REFERENCES

1. George JN, Caen JP, Nurden AT: Glanzmann's thrombasthenia: the spectrum of clinical disease. Blood 75:1383, 1990
2. Slichter SL, Harker LA: Thrombocytopenia: mechanisms and management of defects in platelet production. Clin Haematol 7:523, 1978
3. O'Brien JR: Variability in the aggregation of human platelets by adrenaline. Nature 202:1188, 1964
4. Vilen L, Jacobsson S, Wadenvik H, Kutti J: ADP-induced platelet agregation as a function of age in healthy humans. Thromb Haemost 61:490, 1989
5. Harker LA, Slichter SJ: The bleeding time as a screening test for evaluation of platelet function. N Engl J Med 287:155, 1972
6. Rodgers RPC, Levin J: A critical reappraisal of the bleeding time. Semin Thromb Hemost 16:1, 1990
7. Steering Committee of the Physicians' Health Study Research Group: Final report of the aspirin component of the ongoing physicians' health study. N Engl J Med 321:129, 1989
8. Flower RJ, Moncada S, Vane JR: Analgesic-antipyretics and anti-inflammatory agents. p. 674. In Gilman AG, Goodman LS, Rall TW, Murad F (eds): Goodman and Gilman's The Pharmacological Basis of Therapeutics. 7th Ed. Macmillan, New York, 1985
9. Editorial: Aspirin and heart attack. Am Heart News 65:7, 1992
10. Willard JE, Lange RA, Hillis LD: The use of aspirin in ischemic heart disease. N Engl J Med 327:175, 1992
11. Fuster V, Dyken ML, Vokonas PS, Hennekens C: Aspirin as a therapeutic agent in cardiovascular disease. Circulation 87:659, 1993
12. Cunningham FG, Gant NF: Prevention of preeclampsiava reality? N Engl J Med 321:606, 1989
13. Weiss HJ, Aledort LM: Impaired platelet-connective tissue reaction in man after aspirin ingestion. Lancet 2:495, 1967

14. Smith JB, Willis AL: Aspirin selectively inhibits prostaglandin production in human platelets. Nature 231:235, 1971

15. Roth GJ, Siok CJ: Acetylation of the NH_2-terminal serine of prostaglandin synthetase by aspirin. J Biol Chem 253:3782, 1978

16. Burch JW, Stanford N, Majerus PW: Inhibition of platelet prostaglandin synthetase by oral aspirin. J Clin Invest 61:314, 1978

17. Patrignani P, Filabozzi P, Patrono C: Selective cumulative inhibition of platelet thromboxane production by low-dose aspirin in healthy subjects. J Clin Invest 69:1366, 1982

18. Tohgi H, Konno S, Tamura K et al: Effects of low-to-high doses of aspirin on platelet aggregability and metabolites of thromboxane A_2 and prostacyclin. Stroke 23:1400, 1992

19. Kearon C, Hirsh J: Optimal dose for starting and maintaining low-dose aspirin. Arch Intern Med 153:700, 1993

20. Kallmann R, Nieuwenhuis HK, de Groot PG et al: Effects of low doses of aspirin, 10 mg and 30 mg daily, on bleeding time, thromboxane production and 6-keto-PGF1a excretion in healthy subjects. Thromb Res 45:355, 1987

21. The Dutch TIA Trial Study Group: A comparison of two doses of aspirin (30 mg vs. 283 mg a day) in patients after a transient ischemic attack or minor ischemic stroke. N Engl J Med 325:1261, 1991

22. Hoffman W, Förster W: Two year Cottbus Reinfarction Study with 30 mg aspirin per day. Prostaglandins Leukot Essent Fatty Acids 44:159, 1991

23. Hanson SR, Harker LA, Bjornsson TD: Effects of platelet-modifying drugs on arterial thromboembolism in baboons. Aspirin potentiates the antithrombotic actions of dipyridamole and sulfinpyrazone by mechanism(s) independent of platelet cyclooxygenase inhibition. J Clin Invest 75:1591, 1985

24. Gaspari F, Vigano G, Orisio S et al: Aspirin prolongs bleeding time in uremia by a mechanism distinct from platelet cyclooxygenase inhibition. J Clin Invest 79:1788, 1987

25. Bjornsson TD, Schneider DE, Berger H Jr: Aspirin acetylates fibrinogen and enhances fibrinolysis. Fibrinolytic effect is independent of changes in plasminogen activator levels. J Pharm Exp Ther 250:154, 1989

26. Szczeklik A, Krzanowski M, Gora P, Radwan J: Antiplatelet drugs and generation of thrombin in clotting blood. Blood 80:2006, 1992

27. Cattaneo M, D'Angelo A, Canciani MT et al: Effect of oral aspirin on plasma levels of vitamin K-dependent clotting factors—studies in healthy volunteers. Thromb Haemost 59:540, 1988

28. Clarke RJ, Mayo G, Price P, FitzGerald GA: Suppression of thromboxane A2 but not systemic prostacyclin by controlled-release aspirin. N Engl J Med 325:1137, 1991

29. Pedersen AK, FitzGerald GA: Dose-related kinetics of aspirin. Presystemic acetylation of platelet cyclooxygenase. N Engl J Med 311:1206, 1984

30. FitzGerald GA, Oates JA, Hawiger J et al: Endogenous biosynthesis of prostacyclin and thromboxane and platelet function during chronic administration of aspirin in man. J Clin Invest 71:676, 1983

31. Mielke CH Jr: Influence of aspirin on platelets and the bleeding time. Am J Med, suppl. 6A. 74:72, 1982

32. Mielke CH Jr: Aspirin prolongation of the template bleeding time: influence of venostasis and direction of incision. Blood 60:1139, 1982

33. Catalano PM, Smith JB, Murphy S: Platelet recovery from aspirin inhibition in vivo: differing patterns under various assay conditions. Blood 57:99, 1981

34. O'Laughlin JC, Hoftiezer JW, Mahoney JP, Ivey KJ: Does aspirin prolong bleeding from gastric biopsies in man? Gastrointest Endosc 27:1, 1981

35. Kaneshiro MM, Mielke CH Jr, Kasper CK, Rapaport SI: Bleeding time after aspirin in disorders of intrinsic clotting. N Engl J Med 281:1039, 1969

36. Kasper CK, Rapaport SI: Bleeding times and platelet aggregation after analgesics in hemophilia. Ann Intern Med 77:189, 1972

37. Eyster ME, Gordon RA, Ballard JO: The bleeding time is longer than normal in hemophilia. Blood 58:719, 1981

38. Vigano G, Remuzzi G: Low-dose aspirin and bleeding in uremia. Am J Hematol 42:235, 1993

39. Deykin D, Janson P, McMahon L: Ethanol potentiation of aspirin-induced prolongation of the bleeding time. N Engl J Med 6:852, 1982

40. Kageler WV, Moake JL, Garcia CA: Spontaneous hyphema associated with ingestion of aspirin and ethanol. Am H Ophth 82:631, 1976

41. Hirsh J, Salzman EW, Harker LA et al: Aspirin and other platelet active drugs. Relationship among dose, effectiveness, and side effects. Chest, suppl. 85: 12S, 1989

42. Hawthorne AB, Mahida YR, Cole AT, Hawkey CJ: Aspirin-induced gastric mucosal damage: prevention by enteric-coating and relation to prostaglandin synthesis. Br J Clin Pharmacol 32:77, 1991

43. Roderick PJ, Wilkes HC, Meade TW: The gastrointestinal toxicity of aspirin: an overview of randomised controlled trials. Br J Clin Pharmacol 35:219, 1993

44. Hawkey CJ, Hawthorne AB, Hudson N et al: Separation of the impairment

of haemostasis by aspirin from mucosal injury in the human stomach. Clin Sci 81:565, 1991

45. Lanas A, Sekar MC, Hirschowitz BI: Objective evidence of aspirin use in both ulcer and nonulcer upper and lower gastrointestinal bleeding. Gastroenterology 103:862, 1992

46. Leivonen M, Sipponen P, Kivilaakso E: Gastric changes in coronary-operated patients with low-dose aspirin. Scand J Gastroenterol 27:912, 1992

47. Turpie AGG, Gent M, Laupacis A et al: A comparison of aspirin with placebo in patients treated with warfarin after heart-valve replacement. N Engl J Med 329:524, 1993

48. Gimple LW, Gold HK, Leinbach RC et al: Bleeding time measurement predicts spontaneous bleeding during thrombolysis with recombinant tissue-type plasminogen activator (rt-PA). J Am Coll Cardiol, suppl. A. 11:231A, 1988

49. Vaughan DE, Declerck PJ, De Mol M, Collen D: Recombinant plasminogen activator inhibitor-1 reverses the bleeding tendency associated with combined administration of tissue-type plasminogen activator and aspirin in rabbits. J Clin Invest 84:586, 1989

50. Stuart MJ, Gross SJ, Elrad H, Graeber JE: Effects of acetylsalicylic-acid ingestion on maternal and neonatal hemostasis. N Engl J Med 307:909, 1982

51. Jacobson RL, Brewer A, Eis A et al: Transfer of aspirin across the perfused human placental cotyledon. Am J Obstet Gynecol 165:939, 1991

52. Rumack CM, Guggenheim MA, Rumack BH et al: Neonatal intracranial hemorrhage and maternal use of aspirin. Obstet Gynecol, suppl. 58:52S, 1981

53. Torosian M, Micelson EL, Morganroth J, MacVaugh H: Aspirin and Coumadin-related bleeding after coronary artery bypass graft surgery. Ann Intern Med 89:325, 1978

54. Bick RF: Alterations of hemostasis associated with cardiopulmonary bypass. Semin Thromb Hemost 3:59, 1976

55. Bashein G, Nessly ML, Rice AL et al: Preoperative aspirin therapy and reoperation for bleeding after coronary artery bypass surgery. Arch Intern Med 151:89, 1991

56. Harris WH, Salzman EW, Athanasoulis CA et al: Aspirin prophylaxis of venous thromboembolism after total hip replacement. N Engl J Med 297:1246, 1977

57. Amrein PC, Ellman L, Harris WH: Aspirin-induced prolongation of the bleeding time and perioperative blood loss. JAMA 245:1825, 1981

58. Kitchen L, Erichson RB, Sideropoulos H: Effect of drug-induced platelet dysfunction on surgical bleeding. Am J Surg 143:215, 1982

59. De Swiet M, Redman CWG: Aspirin, extradural anaesthesia and the MRC Collaborative Low-Dose Aspirin Study in Pregnancy (CLASP). Br J Anaesth 69:109, 1992

60. Theroux P, Ouimet H, McCans J et al: Aspirin, heparin, or both to treat acute unstable angina. N Engl J Med 319:1105, 1988

61. Counts RB, Haisch C, Simon TL et al: Hemostasis in massively transfused trauma patients. Ann Surg 190:91, 1979

62. Leist ER, Banwell JG: Products containing aspirin. N Engl J Med 291:710, 1974

63. Mannucci PM: Desmopressin: a nontransfusional form of treatment for congenital and acquired bleeding disorders. Blood 72:1449, 1988

64. Salzman EW, Hirsh J: Prevention of venous thromboembolism. p. 1252. In Colman RW, Hirsh J, Marder VJ, Salzman EW (eds): Hemostasis and Thrombosis. Basic Principles and Clinical Practice. 2nd Ed. JB Lippincott, Philadelphia, 1987

65. Collins R, Scrimgeour A, Yusuf S, Peto R: Reduction in fatal pulmonary embolism and venous thrombosis by perioperative administration of subcutaneous heparin. Overview of results of randomized trials in general, orthopedic, and urologic surgery. N Engl J Med 318:1162, 1988

66. Simon LS, Mills JA: Non-steroidal anti-inflammatory drugs. N Engl J Med 302:1179, 1980

67. McQueen EG, Facoory B: Non-steroidal anti-inflammatory drugs and platelet function. NZ Med J 99:358, 1986

68. Thomas P, Hepburn B, Kim HC, Saidi P: Nonsteroidal anti-inflammatory drugs in the treatment of hemophilic arthropathy. Am J Hematol 12:131, 1982

69. Ragni MV, Miller BJ, Whalen R, Ptachcinski R: Bleeding tendency, platelet function, and pharmacokinetics of ibuprofen and zidovudine in HIV(+) hemophilic men. Am J Hematol 40:176, 1992

70. Mielke CH Jr, Heiden D, Britten AF: Hemostasis, antipyretics, and mild analgesics: acetoaminophen vs aspirin. JAMA 235:613, 1976

71. Sutor AH, Bowie EJW, Owen CA Jr: Effect of aspirin, sodium salicylate, and acetaminophen on bleeding. Mayo Clin Proc 46:178, 1971

72. Hass WK, Easton JD, Adams HP Jr et al: A randomized trial comparing ticlopidine hydrochloride with aspirin for the prevention of stroke in high-risk patients. N Engl J Med 321:501, 1989

73. Gent M, Blakely JA, Easton JD et al: The Canadian American Ticlopidine Study (CATS) in thromboembolic stroke. Lancet 1:1215, 1989

74. McTavish D, Faulds D, Goa KL: Ticlopidine: an updated review of its pharmacology and therapeutic use in platelet-dependent disorders. Drugs 40:238, 1990

75. DeCaterina R, Sicari R, Bernini W et al: Benefit/risk profile of combined antiplatelet therapy with ticlopidine and aspirin. Thromb Haemost 65:504, 1991

76. Hardisty RM, Powling MJ, Nokes TJC: The action of ticlopidine on human platelets. Studies on aggregation, secretion, calcium mobilization and membrane glycoproteins. Thromb Haemost 64:150, 1990

77. DiMinno G, Cerbone AM, Mattioli PL et al: Functionally thrombasthenic state in normal platelets following the administration of ticlopidine. J Clin Invest 75:328, 1985

78. Mataiz R, Ojeda E, Perez MDC, Jiminez S: Ticlopidine and severe aplastic anemia. Br J Haematol 80:125, 1992

79. Garnier G, Taillan B, Pesce A et al: Ticlopidine and severe aplastic anemia. Br J Haematol 81:459, 1992

80. Lurie A, Ogilvie M, Townsend R et al: Carbenicillin-induced coagulopathy. Lancet 1:1114, 1970

81. McClure PD, Casserly JG, Monsier C, Crozier D: Carbenicillin-induced bleeding disorder. Lancet 2:307, 1970

82. Ikeda Y, Kichuchi M, Matsuda S et al: Inhibition of platelet function by sulbenicillin and its metabolite. Antimicrob Agents Chemother 5:881, 1978

83. Leading Article: Antimicrobials and haemostasis. Lancet 1:510, 1983

84. Brown CH III, Natelson EA, Bradshaw MW et al: Studies of the effects of ticarcillin on blood coagulation and platelet function. Antimicrob Agents Chemother 7:652, 1975

85. Gentry LO, Jemsek JG, Natelson EA: Effects of sodium piperacillin on platelet function in normal volunteers. Antimicrob Agents Chemother 19:532, 1981

86. Dukmans BAC, van der Meer JWM, Bockhout-Mussert MJ et al: Prolonged bleeding time during azlocillin therapy. J Antimicrob Chemother 6:554, 1980

87. Natelson EA, Brown CH III, Bradshaw MW et al: Influence of cephalosporin antibiotics on blood coagulation and platelet function. Antimicrob Agents Chemother 9:91, 1976

88. Lerner PI, Lubin A: Coagulopathy with cefazolin in uremia. N Engl J Med 290:1324, 1974

89. Brown CH III, Natelson EA, Bradshaw MW: The hemostatic defect produced by carbenicillin. N Engl J Med 291:265, 1974

90. Sattler FR, Weitekamp MR, Ballard JO: Potential for bleeding with the new beta-lactam antibiotics. Ann Intern Med 105:924, 1986

91. Brown RB, Klar J, Lemeshow S: Enhanced bleeding with cefoxitin or moxolactam: statistical analysis within a defined population. Arch Intern Med 146:2159, 1986

92. Pillgram-Larsen J, Wisloff F, Jorgensen JJ: Effect of high-dose ampicillin and cloxacillin on bleeding time and bleeding in open-heart surgery. Scand J Thorac Cardiovasc Surg 19:45, 1985

93. Fass RJ, Copelan EA, Brandt ML et al: Platelet-mediated bleeding caused by broad-spectrum penicillins. J Infect Dis 155:1242, 1987

94. Harburchak DR, Head DR, Everett ED: Postoperative hemorrhage associated with carbenicillin administration. Report of two cases and review of the literature. Am J Surg 134:630, 1977

95. Andrassy KE, Ritz B, Hasper M: Penicillin-induced coagulation disorder. Lancet 2:1039, 1976

96. Alexander DP, Russo ME, Fohrman DE, Rothstein G: Nafcillin-induced platelet dysfunction and bleeding. Antimicrob Agents Chemother 23:59, 1983

97. Weitekamp MR, Aber RC: Prolonged bleeding times and bleeding diathesis associated with moxolactam administration. JAMA 249:69, 1983

98. Bang NU, Tessler SS, Heidenreich RO: Effects of moxalactam on blood coagulation and platelet function. Rev Infect Dis, suppl. 4:S546, 1982

99. Kaplan SL, Courtney JT, Kenal KA: Effect of Haemophilus influenzae infection and moxalactam on platelet function in children. Antimicrob Agents Chemother 31:467, 1987

100. Dunagan WC, Woodward RS, Medoff G et al: Antimicrobial misuse in patients with positive blood cultures. Am J Med 87:253, 1989

101. Sloand EM, Pierce P, Klein HG: Effect of albumin concentration on inhibition of platelet aggregation by beta lactam antibiotics, abstracted. Blood 741989

102. Wisloff F, Godal HC: Prolonged bleeding time with adequate platelet count in hospital patients. Scand J Haematol 27:45, 1981

103. Henry D, Audet P, Shattil SJ: Relationships between the structure of penicillins and their anti-platelet activity, abstracted. Blood 54:243a, 1979

104. Fletcher C, Pearson C, Choi SC: In vitro comparison of antiplatelet effects of beta-lactam penicillins. J Lab Clin Med 108:217, 1986

105. Cazenave JP, Packham MA, Guccione MA, Mustard JF: Effects of penicillin G on platelet aggregation, release, and adhesion to collagen. Proc Soc Exp Biol Med 142:159, 1973

106. Shattil SJ, Bennett JS, McDonaugh M, Turnbull J: Carbenicillin and penicillin G inhibit platelet function in vitro by impairing the interaction of agonists with the platelet surface. J Clin Invest 65:329, 1980

107. Pastakia KB, Terle D, Producz KN: Penicillin-induced dysfunction of platelet membrane glycoproteins. J Lab Clin Med 121:546, 1993

108. Johnson GJ: Platelets, penicillin, and purpura: what does it all mean? J Lab Clin Med 121:531, 1993

109. Burroughs SF, Johnson GJ: β-Lactam antibiotic-induced platelet dysfunction: evidence for irreversible inhibition of platelet activation in vitro and in vivo after prolonged exposure to penicillin. Blood 75:1473, 1990

110. Burroughs SF, Johnson GJ: Beta-lactam antibiotics alter calcium transport across platelet membranes, abstracted. Blood 741989

111. Lipsky JJ: Antibiotic-associated hypoprothrombinaemia. J Antimicrob Chemother 21:281, 1988

112. Rossi EC, Levin NW: Inhibition of primary ADP-induced platelet aggregation in normal subjects after the administration of nitrofurantoin (Furadantin). J Clin Invest 52:2457, 1973

113. Hawiger J, Steer ML, Salzman EW: Intracellular regulatory processes in platelets. p. 710. In Colman RW, Hirsh J, Marder VJ, Salzman EW (eds): Hemostasis and Thrombosis. Basic Principles and Clinical Practice. 2nd Ed. JB Lippincott, Philadelphia, 1987

114. Huddleston CB, Wareing TH, Clanton JA, Bender HW Jr: Amelioration of the deleterious effects of platelets activated during cardiopulmonary bypass: comparison of a thromboxane synthetase inhibitor and a prostacyclin analogue. J Thorac Cardiovasc Surg 89:190, 1985

115. Walker ID, Davidson JF, Faichney A: A double-blind study of prostacyclin in cardiopulmonary bypass surgery. Br J Haematol 49:415, 1981

116. Malpass TW, Amory DW, Harker LA: The effect of prostacyclin infusion on platelet hemostatic function in patients undergoing cardiopulmonary bypass. J Thorac Cardiovasc Surg 87:550, 1984

117. Zusman RM, Rubin RH, Cato AE et al: Hemodialysis using prostacyclin instead of heparin as the sole antithrombotic agent. N Engl J Med 304:934, 1981

118. Fisher CA, Kappa JR, Sinha AK et al: Comparison of equimolar concentrations of iloprost, prostacyclin, and prostaglandin E1 on human platelet function. J Lab Clin Med 109:184, 1987

119. FitzGerald GA: Dipyridamole. N Engl J Med 316:1247, 1987

120. Horne MKIII, Chao ES: Heparin binding to resting and activated platelets. Blood 74:238, 1989

121. Zucker MB: Heparin and platelet function. Fed Proc 36:47, 1977

122. Salzman EW, Rosenberg RD, Smith MH et al: Effect of heparin and heparin fractions on platelet aggregation. J Clin Invest 65:64, 1980

123. Sobel M, McNeill PM, Carlson PL: Heparin inhibition of von Willebrand factor-dependent platelet function in vitro and in vivo. J Clin Invest 87:1787, 1991

124. Heiden D, Mielke CH Jr, Rodvien R: Impairment by heparin of primary haemostasis and platelet [^{14}C]5-hydroxytryptamine release. Br J Haematol 36:427, 1977

125. Fernandez F, N'guyen P, van Ryn J: Hemorrhagic doses of heparin and other glycosaminoglycans induce a platelet defect. Thromb Res 43:491, 1986

126. Coller BS: Platelets and thrombolytic therapy. N Engl J Med 322:33, 1990

127. Miles LA, Ginsberg MA, White JG, Plow EF: Plasminogen interacts with human platelets through two distinct mechanisms. J Clin Invest 77:2001, 1986

128. Adelman B, Michaelson AD, Loscalzo J: Plasmin effect on platelet glycoprotein Ib-von Willebrand factor interactions. Blood 65:32, 1985

129. Loscalzo J, Vaughan DE: Tissue plasminogen activator promotes platelet disaggregation in plasma. J Clin Invest 79:1749, 1987

130. Schafer AI, Adelman B: Plasmin inhibition of platelet function and of arachidonic acid metabolism. J Clin Invest 75:456, 1985

131. Langdell RD, Adelson E, Furth FW, Crosby WH: Dextran and prolonged bleeding time. Results of a sixty-gram, one-liter infusion given to 163 normal human subjects. JAMA 166:346, 1958

132. Mishler JMIV: Synthetic plasma volume expanders—their pharmacology, safety, and clinical efficacy. Clin Haematol 13:75, 1984

133. Weiss HJ: The effect of clinical dextran on platelet aggregation, adhesion, and ADP release in man: in vivo and in vitro studies. J Lab Clin Med 69:37, 1967

134. Aberg M, Hedner U, Bergentz SE: Effect of dextran 70 on factor VIII and platelet function in von Willebrand's disease. Thromb Res 12:629, 1978

135. Gruber UF, Duckert F, Fridrich R et al: Prevention of postoperative thromboembolism by dextran 40, low doses of heparin, or xantinol nicotinate. Br Med J 280:69, 1980

136. Kelton JG, Hirsh J: Bleeding associated with antithrombotic therapy. Semin Hematol 17:259, 1980

137. Kortilla K, Lauritsalo K, Sarmo A: Suitability of plasma expanders in patients

receiving low-dose heparin for prevention of venous thrombosis after surgery. Acta Anesthesiol Scand 27:104, 1983

138. Karlberg K-E, Ahlner J, Henriksson P et al: Effects of nitroglycerin on platelet aggregation beyond the effects of acetylsalicyclic acid in healthy subjects. Am J Cardiol 71:361, 1993

139. Chirkov YY, Naujalis JI, Sage RE, Horowitz JD: Antiplatelet effects of nitroglycerin in healthy subjects and in patients with stable angina pectoris. J Cardiovasc Pharmacol 21:384, 1993

140. De Caterina R, Giannessi D, Bernini W, Mazzone A: Organic nitrates: direct antiplatelet effects and synergism with prostacyclin. Thromb Haemost 59:207, 1988

141. Leon R, Tiarks CY, Pechet L: Some observations on the in vivo effect of propranolol on platelet aggregation and release. Am J Hematol 5:117, 1978

142. Saxon A, Kattlove H: Platelet inhibition by nitroprusside, a smooth muscle inhibitor. Blood 47:957, 1976

143. Pamphilon DH, Boon RJ, Prentice AG, Rozkovec A: Lack of significant effect of therapeutic propranolol on measurable platelet function in healthy subjects. J Clin Pathol 42:793, 1989

144. Wallen NH, Larsson PT, Bröijersen A et al: Effects of an oral dose of isosorbide dinitrate on platelet function and fibrinolysis in healthy volunteers. Br J Clin Pharmacol 35:143, 1993

145. Ring ME, Corrigan JJ Jr, Fenster PE: Effects of oral diltiazem on platelet function: alone and in combination with "low dose" aspirin. Thromb Res 44:391, 1986

146. Barnathan E, Addonzio VP, Shattil SJ: Interaction of verapamil with human platelet alpha-adrenergic receptors. Am J Physiol 242:H19, 1982

147. Johnson GJ, Leis LA, Francis GS: Disparate effects of the calcium-channel blockers, nifedipine and verapamil, on alpha$_2$-adrenergic receptors and thromboxane A$_2$-induced aggregation of human platelets. Circulation 73:847, 1986

148. Glusa E, Bevan J, Heptinstall S: Verapamil is a potent inhibitor of 5-HT-induced platelet aggregation. Thromb Res 55:239, 1989

149. Motulsky HJ, Maisel AS, Snavely MD, Insel PA: Quinidine is a competitive antagonist at alpha-1 and alpha-2-adrenergic receptors. Circ Res 55:376, 1984

150. Lawson D, Mehta J, Mehta P et al: Cumulative effects of quinidine and aspirin on bleeding time and platelet alpha-2-adrenoreceptors: potential of bleeding diathesis in patients receiving this combination. J Lab Clin Med 108:581, 1986

151. Ueda I: The effects of volatile general anesthetics on adenosine diphosphate-induced platelet aggregation. Anesthesiology 34:306, 1971

152. Dalsgaard-Nielsen J, Risbo A, Simmelkjaer P, Gormsen J: Impaired platelet aggregation and increased bleeding time during general anesthesia with halothane. Br J Anaesth 53:1039, 1981

153. Fyman PN, Triner L, Schranz H et al: Effect of volatile anesthetics and nitrous oxide-fentanyl anesthesia on the bleeding time. Br J Anaesth 56:1197, 1984

154. Rezkalla SH, Mazza JJ, Kloner RA et al: Effects of cocaine on human platelets in healthy subjects. Am J Cardiol 72:243, 1993

155. Puszkin E, Gutfreund D, Aledort LM: Hemostatic abnormalities in heroin addicts. Transfusion 12:9, 1972

156. Ahr DJ, Scialla SJ, Kimball DB Jr: Acquired platelet dysfunction following mithramycin therapy. Cancer 41:448, 1978

157. Pogliani EM, Fantasia R, Lambertenghi-Delliers G, Cofrancesco E: Daunorubicin and platelet function. Thromb Haemost 45:38, 1981

158. McKenna R, Ahmad T, Ts'ao CH, Frischer H: Glutathione reductase deficiency and platelet dysfunction induced by 1,3-bis(2-chloroethyl)-1-nitrosourea. J Lab Clin Med 102:102, 1983

159. Karolak L, Chandra A, Khan W et al: High-dose chemotherapy-induced platelet defect: inhibition of platelet signal transduction pathways. Mol Pharmacol 43:37, 1993

160. Carvalho ACA, Colman RW, Lees RS: Clofibrate reversal of platelet hypersensitivity in hyperbetalipoproteinemia. Circulation 50:570, 1974

161. PACK Trial Group: Platelet function during long-term treatment with ketanserin of claudicating patients with peripheral atherosclerosis. A multi-center, double-blind, placebo-controlled trial. Thromb Res 55:13, 1989

162. Coffman JD, Clement DL, Creager MA et al: International study of ketanserin in Raynaud's phenomenon. Am J Med 87:264, 1989

163. Thomson C, Forbes CD, Prentice CRM: A comparison of the effects of antihistamines on platelet function. Thromb Diath Haemorrh 30:547, 1973

164. Parvez Z, Moncada R, Fareed J, Messmore HL: Antiplatelet action of intravascular contrast media. Invest Radiol 19:208, 1984

165. Rao AK, Rao VM, Willis J et al: Inhibition of platelet function by contrast media: Iopamidol and Hexabrix are less inhibitory than Conray-60. Radiology 156:311, 1985

166. Kromhout D, Bosschieter EB, de Lezenne Coulander C: The inverse relation between fish consumption and 20-year mortality from coronary heart disease. N Engl J Med 312:1205, 1985

167. Leaf A, Weber PC: Cardiovascular effects of ω-3 fatty acids. N Engl J Med 318:549, 1988

168. Haut MJ, Cowan DH: The effect of ethanol on hemostatic properties of human blood platelets. Am J Med 56:22, 1974

169. Lawrence JB, Bodenheimer SL, Kramer WS, Zekert SL: Clinically relevant concentrations of ethanol inhibit platelet adherence on human arterial subendothelium and collagen-induced platelet aggregation, abstracted. Blood 74:402, 1989

170. Hammerschmidt DE: Szechwan purpura. N Engl J Med 302:1191, 1980

171. Srivastava KC: Onion exerts antiaggregatory effects by altering arachidonic acid metabolism in platelets. Prostaglandin Leukot Med 24:43, 1986

172. Apitz-Castro R, Badimon JJ, Badimon L: Effect of ajoene, the major antiplatelet compound from garlic, on platelet thrombus formation. Thromb Res 68:145, 1992

173. Srivastava KC: Extracts from two frequently consumed spices—cumin (Cuminum cyminum) and turmeric (Curcuma longa)—inhibit platelet aggregation and alter eicosanoid biosynthesis in human blood platelets. Prostaglandins Leukotr Essent Fatty Acids 37:57, 1989

174. Reisman D: Hemorrhages in the course of Bright's disease, with especial reference to the occurrence of a hemorrhagic diathesis of nephritic origin. Am J Med Sci 134:709, 1907

175. Ball WG, Evans G: Diseases of the Kidney. 1st Ed. p. 250. P Blakiston's Sons, Philadelphia, 1932

176. Maher JF, Schreiner GE: Cause of death in acute renal failure. Arch Intern Med 110:493, 1962

177. Hamberger J, Richet G, Crosnier J et al: Nephrology. 1st Ed. p. 347. WB Saunders, Philadelphia, 1968

178. Hakim RM, Lazarus JM: Medical aspects of hemodialysis. p. 1791. In Brenner BM, Rector FC Jr (eds): The Kidney. 3rd Ed. WB Saunders, Philadelphia, 1986

179. Morrison G, Geheb MA, Earley LE: Chronic renal failure. p. 1901. In Seldin DN, Giebisch G (eds): The Kidney: Physiology and Pathophysiology. 1st Ed. Raven Press, New York, 1985

180. Diaz-Buxo JA, Donadio JV Jr: Complications of percutaneous renal biopsy: an analysis of 1000 consecutive biopsies. Clin Nephrol 4:223, 1975

181. Schreiner GF: The nephrotic syndrome. p. 335. In Strauss MB, Welt LG (eds): Diseases of the Kidney. 1st Ed. Little, Brown, Boston, 1963

182. Ciba Foundation Symposium: Renal Biopsy. p. 371. Little, Brown, Boston, 1961

183. Rosenbaum R, Hoffstein PE, Stanley RJ, Klahr S: Use of computerized tomography to diagnose complications of percutaneous renal biopsy. Kidney Int 14:87, 1978

184. Hutton RA, O'Shea MJ: Haemostatic mechanism in uraemia. J Clin Pathol 21:406, 1968

185. Kleinknecht D, Jungers P, Chanard J et al: Uremic and non-uremic complications in acute renal failure: evaluation of early and frequent dialysis on prognosis. Kidney Int 1:190, 1972

186. Zuckerman GR, Cornette GL, Clouse RE, Harter HR: Upper gastrointestinal bleeding in patients with chronic renal failure. Ann Intern Med 102:588, 1985

187. Quintero E, Kaunitz J, Nishizaki Y et al: Uremia increases gastric mucosal permeability and acid back-diffusion injury in the rat. Gastroenterology 103:1762, 1992

188. Goldberg M, Hoffman GC, Wombolt DG: Massive hemorrhage from rectal ulcers in chronic renal failure. Ann Intern Med 100:397, 1984

189. Zarowny DP, Rose I: Acute subdural hematoma during maintenance hemodialysis. Can Med Assoc J 103:634, 1970

190. Pedigo GW, Nolan DE: Subarachnoid hemorrhage complicating hemorrhagic nephritis. Ohio State Med J 43:743, 1947

191. Alfrey AC, Goss JE, Ogden DA et al: Uremic hemopericardium. Am J Med 45:391, 1968

192. Galen MA, Steinberg SM, Lowrie EG et al: Hemorrhagic pleural effusion in patients undergoing chronic hemodialysis. Ann Intern Med 82:359, 1975

193. Borra S, Kleinfeld M: Subcapsular liver hematomas in a patient on chronic hemodialysis. Ann Intern Med 93:574, 1980

194. Brautbar N, Menz CL, Winston MA, Shonberg JH: Retroperitoneal bleeding in hemodialysis patients: a cause for morbidity and mortality. JAMA 1978:1530, 239

195. Ellison RT III, Corrao WM, Fox MJ, Braman SS: Spontaneous mediastinal hemorrhage in patients on chronic hemodialysis. Ann Intern Med 95:704, 1981

196. Slusher MM, Hamilton RW: Spontaneous hyphema during hemodialysis. N Engl J Med 293:561, 1975

197. Stewart JH, Castaldi PA: Uraemic bleeding: a reversible platelet defect corrected by dialysis. Q J Med 36:409, 1967

198. Rabiner SF, Hrodek O: Platelet factor 3 in normal subjects and patients with renal failure. J Clin Invest 47:901, 1968
199. Eknoyan G, Wacksman SJ, Glueck HI, Will JJ: Platelet function in renal failure. N Engl J Med 280:677, 1969
200. Steiner RW, Coggins C, Carvalho ACA: Bleeding time in uremia: a useful test to assess clinical bleeding. Am J Hematol 7:107, 1979
201. Deykin D: Uremic bleeding. Kidney Int 24:698, 1983
202. Gordge MP, Faint RW, Rylance PB, Neild GH: Platelet function and the bleeding time in progressive renal failure. Thromb Haemost 60:83, 1988
203. Fernandez F, Goudable C, Sie P et al: Low hematocrit and prolonged bleeding time in uraemic patients: effect of red cell transfusions. Br J Haematol 59:139, 1985
204. Castillo R, Lozano T, Escolar G et al: Defective platelet adhesion on vessel subendothelium in uremic patients. Blood 68:337, 1986
205. Adamson JW, Eschbach JW, Finch CA: The kidney and erythropoiesis. Am J Med 44:725, 1968
206. Hellem AJ, Borchgrevink CF, Ames SB: The role of red cells in haemostasis: the relation between haematocrit, bleeding time and platelet adhesiveness. Br J Haematol 7:42, 1961
207. Livio M, Gotti E, Marchesi D et al: Uraemic bleeding: role of anaemia and beneficial effect of red cell transfusions. Lancet 2:1013, 1982
208. Gotti E, Mecca G, Valentino C et al: Renal biopsy in patients with acute renal failure and prolonged bleeding time. Lancet 2:978, 1984
209. Moia M, Vizzotto L, Cattanea M et al: Improvement in the haemostatic defect of uraemia after treatment with recombinant human erythropoietin. Lancet 2:1227, 1987
210. van Geet C, Hauglustaine D, Vanrusselt M, Vermylen J: Haemostatic effects of recombinant human erythropoietin in chronic haemodialysis patients. Thromb Haemost 61:117, 1989
211. Small M, Lowe GDO, Cameron E, Forbes CD: Contribution of the hematocrit to the bleeding time. Haemostasis 13:379, 1983
212. Turrito VT, Weiss HJ: Red blood cells: their dual role in thrombus formation. Science 207:541, 1980
213. Doherty CC: Gastrointestinal bleeding in dialysis patients. Nephron 63:132, 1993
214. Nakamura Y, Chida Y, Tomura S: Enhanced coagulation-fibrinolysis in patients on regular hemodialysis treatment. Nephron 58:201, 1991
215. Sagripanti A, Cupisti A, Baicchi U et al: Plasma parameters of the prothrombotic state in chronic uremia. Nephron 63:273, 1993
216. Verbeelen D, Jochmans K, Herman AG et al: Evaluation of platelets and hemostasis during hemodialysis with six different membranes. Nephron 59:567, 1991
217. Escolar G, Cases A, Bastida E et al: Uremic platelets have a functional defect affecting the interaction of von Willebrand factor with glycoprotein IIb-IIIa. Blood 76:1336, 1990
218. Turney JH, Woods HF, Fewell MR, Weston MJ: Factor VIII complex in uraemia and effects of haemodialysis. Br Med J 282:1653, 1981
219. Gralnick HR, McKeown I, Williams S et al: Plasma and platelet von Willebrand factor in uremia. Blood 70:374a, 1987
220. DiMinno G, Cerbone A, Usberti M et al: Platelet dysfunction in uremia. II. Correction by arachidonic acid of the impaired exposure of fibrinogen receptors by adenosine diphosphate or collagen. J Lab Clin Med 108:246, 1986
221. Horowitz HI, Cohen BD, Martinez P, Papayoanou MF: Defective ADP-induced platelet factor 3 activation in uremia. Blood 30:331, 1967
222. Ware JA, Clark BA, Smith M, Salzman EW: Abnormalities of cytoplasmic calcium in platelets from patients with uremia. Blood 73:172, 1989
223. Remuzzi G, Benigni A, Dodesini P et al: Reduced platelet thromboxane formation in uremia. Evidence for a functional cyclooxygenase defect. J Clin Invest 71:762, 1983
224. Winter M, Frampton G, Bennett A et al: Synthesis of thromboxane B2 in uraemia and the effects of dialysis. Thromb Res 30:265, 1983
225. Bloom A, Greaves M, Preston FE, Brown CB: Evidence against a platelet cyclooxygenase defect in uraemic subjects on chronic dialysis. Br J Haematol 62:143, 1986
226. Kyrle PA, Stockenhuber F, Brenner B et al: Evidence for an increased generation of prostacyclin in the microvasculature and an impairment of the platelet alpha-granule release in chronic renal failure. Thromb Haemost 60:205, 1988
227. DiMinno G, Martinez J, McKean M et al: Platelet dysfunction in uremia. Multifaceted defect partially corrected by dialysis. Am J Med 79:552, 1985
228. Eknoyan G, Brown CH III: Biochemical abnormalities of platelets in renal failure. Evidence for decreased platelet serotonin, adenosine diphosphate, and Mg-dependent adenosine triphosphatase. Am J Nephrol 1:17, 1981
229. Vlachoyannis J, Schoeppe W: Adenylate cyclase activity and cAMP content of human platelets in uraemia. Eur J Clin Invest 12:379, 1982
230. Tokumoto A, Uemasu J, Kawasaki H: Increased internal calcium mobilization in platelets of patients with chronic renal failure. Horm Metab Res 24:588, 1992
231. Rabiner SF: Uremic bleeding. Prog Hemost Thromb 1:233, 1972
232. Bazilinski N, Shaykh M, Dunea G et al: Inhibition of platelet function by uremic middle molecules. Nephron 40:423, 1985
233. Remuzzi G, Livio M, Marchiaro et al: Bleeding in renal failure: altered platelet function in chronic uremia only partially corrected by haemodialysis. Nephron 22:347, 1978
234. Remuzzi G, Livio M, Cavenaghi AE et al: Unbalanced prostaglandin synthesis and plasma factors in uraemic bleeding: a hypothesis. Thromb Res 13:531, 1978
235. Remuzzi G, Perico N, Zoja C et al: Role of endothelium-derived nitric oxide in the bleeding tendency of uremia. J Clin Invest 86:1768, 1990
236. Gordge MP, Neild GH: Platelets from patients on haemodialysis show impaired responses to nitric oxide. Clin Sci 83:313, 1992
237. Noris M, Benigni A, Boccardo P et al: Enhanced nitric oxide synthesis in uremia: implications for platelet dysfunction and dialysis hypotension. Kidney Int 44:445, 1993
238. Docci D, Turci F, Delvecchio C et al: Lack of evidence for the role of secondary hyperparathyroidism in the pathogenesis of uremic thrombocytopathy. Nephron 43:28, 1986
239. Weiss HJ, Vicic WJ, Lages BA, Rogers J: Isolated deficiency of platelet procoagulant activity. Am J Med 67:206, 1979
240. Livio M, Vigano G, Benigni A et al: Moderate doses of aspirin and risk of bleeding in renal failure. Lancet 2:414, 1986
241. Andrassy K, Ritz E: Uremia as a cause of bleeding. Am J Nephrol 5:313, 1985
242. George CRP, Slichter SJ, Quadracci LJ et al: A kinetic evaluation of hemostasis in renal disease. N Engl J Med 291:1111, 1974
243. Michalak E, Walkowiak B, Paradowski M, Cierniewski CS: The decreased circulating platelet mass and its relation to bleeding time in chronic renal failure. Thromb Haemost 65:11, 1991
244. Lindsay RM, Friesen M, Koens F et al: Platelet function in patients on long-term peritoneal dialysis. Clin Nephrol 6:335, 1976
245. Nenci GG, Berrettini M, Agnelli G et al: Effect of peritoneal dialysis, hemodialysis, and kidney transplantation on blood platelet function. Nephron 23:287, 1979
246. Shepherd LL, Hutchinson RJ, Worden EK: Hyponatremia and seizures after intravenous administration of desmopressin acetate for surgical hemostasis. J Pediatr 114:470, 1989
247. Weinstein RE, Bona RD, Altman AJ et al: Severe hyponatremia after repeated intravenous administration of desmopressin. Am J Hematol 32:258, 1989
248. Hamed M, Mitchell H, Chow DJ: Hyponatremic convulsion associated with desmopressin and imiprimine treatment. Br Med J 306:1169, 1993
249. Editorial: Desmopressin and arterial thrombosis. Lancet 1:938, 1989
250. Beckwith BE, Till RE, Reno CR, Poland RE: Dose-dependent effects of DDAVP on memory in healthy young adult males: a preliminary study. Peptides 11:473, 1990
251. Escolar G, Cases A, Monteagudo J et al: Uremic plasma after infusion of desmopressin (DDAVP) improves the interaction of normal platelets with vessel subendothelium. J Lab Clin Med 114:36, 1989
252. Soslau G, Schwartz AB, Putatunda B et al: Desmopressin-induced improvement in bleeding times in chronic renal failure patients correlates with platelet serotonin uptake and ATP release. Am J Med Sci 300:372, 1990
253. Livio M, Benigni A, Remuzzi G: Coagulation abnormalities in uremia. Semin Nephrol 5:82, 1985
254. Mannucci PM, Remuzzi G, Pusineri F et al: Deamino-8-D-arginine vasopressin shortens the bleeding time in uremia. N Engl J Med 308:8, 1983
255. Mannucci PM: Desmopressin (DDAVP) for treatment of disorders of hemostasis. Prog Hemost Thromb 8:19, 1986
256. Vigano G, Mannucci PM, Lattuada A et al: Subcutaneous desmopressin (DDAVP) shortens the bleeding time in uremia. Am J Hematol 31:32, 1989
257. Juhl A: DDAVP, cryoprecipitate, and highly "purified" factor VIII concentrate in uremia. Nephron 43:305, 1986
258. Ruggeri ZM, Mannucci PM, Lombardi R et al: Multimeric composition of factor VIII/von Willebrand factor following administration of DDAVP: implications for pathophysiology and therapy of von Willebrand's disease subtypes. Blood 59:1272, 1982
259. Triulzi DJ, Blumber N: Variability in response to cryoprecipitate treatment for hemostatic defects in uremia. Yale J Biol Med 63:1, 1990
260. Liu YK, Kosfeld RE, Marcum SG: Treatment of uremic bleeding with conjugated estrogen. Lancet 2:887, 1984
261. Vigano G, Marchesi E, Remuzzi G, Mecca G: Conjugated estrogens (CE) to reduce bleeding in uremics. Thromb Haemost 58:81, 1987
262. Livio M, Mannucci PM, Vigano G et al: Conjugated estrogens for the management of bleeding associated with renal failure. N Engl J Med 315:731, 1986
263. Shemin D, Elnour M, Amarantes B et al: Oral estrogens decrease bleeding

time and improve clinical bleeding in patients with renal failure. Am J Med 89:436, 1990

264. Harker LA, Malpass TW, Branson HE et al: Mechanism of abnormal bleeding in patients undergoing cardiopulmonary bypass: acquired transient platelet dysfunction associated with selective alpha-granule release. Blood 56:824, 1980

265. Bachmann F, McKenna R, Cole ER, Najafi H: The hemostatic mechanism after open heart surgery. I. Studies on plasma coagulation factors and fibrinolysis in 512 patients after extracorporeal circulation. J Thorac Cardiovasc Surg 70:76, 1975

266. Bick RF: Hemostasis defects associated with cardiac surgery, prosthetic devices, and other extracorporeal circuits. Semin Thromb Hemost 11:249, 1985

267. Holloway DS, Summaria L, Sandesara J et al: Decreased platelet number and function and increased fibrinolysis contribute to postoperative bleeding in cardiopulmonary bypass patients. Thromb Haemost 59:62, 1988

268. Pumphrey CW, Dawes J: Platelet alpha granule depletion: findings in patients with prosthetic heart valves and following cardiopulmonary bypass surgery. Thromb Res 30:257, 1983

269. Mammen EF, Koets MH, Washington BC et al: Hemostasis changes during cardiopulmonary bypass. Semin Thromb Hemost 11:281, 1985

270. Woodman RC, Harker LA: Bleeding complications associated with cardiopulmonary bypass. Blood 76:1680, 1990

271. Khuri SF, Wolfe JA, Josa M et al: Hematologic changes during and after cardiopulmonary bypass and their relationship to the bleeding time and nonsurgical blood loss. J Thorac Cardiovasc Surg 104:94, 1992

272. George JN, Pickett EB, Saucerman S et al: Platelet surface glycoproteins. Studies on resting and activated platelets and platelet membrane microparticles in normal subjects, and observations in patients during adult respiratory distress syndrome and cardiac surgery. J Clin Invest 78:340, 1986

273. Hope AF, Heyns duPA, Lotter MG et al: Kinetics and sites of sequestration of indium 111-labeled human platelets during cardiopulmonary bypass. J Thorac Cardiovasc Surg 81:880, 1981

274. Lindon JN, McManama, Kushner L et al: Does the conformation of adsorbed fibrinogen dictate platelet interactions with artificial surfaces? Blood 68:355, 1986

275. Gluszko P, Rucinski B, Musial J, et al: Fibrinogen receptors in platelet adhesion to surfaces of excorporeal circuits. Am J Physiol 252:H615, 1987

276. Brown CHIII, Lemuth RF, Hellums JD et al: Response of human platelets to shear stress. Trans Am Soc Artif Organs 21:35, 1975

277. deJong JCF, ten Duis HJ, Sibinga TS, Wildevuur CRH: Hematologic aspects of cardiotomy suction in cardiac operations. J Thorac Cardiovasc Surg 79:227, 1980

278. Davies GC, Sobel M, Salzman EW: Elevated plasma fibrinopeptide A and thromboxane A2 during cardiopulmonary bypass surgery. Circulation 61:808, 1980

279. Teufelsbauer H, Proidl S, Havel M, Vukovich T: Early activation of hemostasis during cardiopulmonary bypass: evidence for thrombin mediated hyperfibrinolysis. Thromb Haemost 68:250, 1992

280. Chenoweth DE, Cooper SW, Hugli TE et al: Complement activation during cardiopulmonary bypass. N Engl J Med 304:497, 1981

281. Boldt J, Knothe C, Zickmann B et al: Platelet function in cardiac surgery: influence of temperature and aprotinin. Ann Thorac Surg 55:652, 1993

282. Boldt J, Zickmann B, Czeke A et al: Blood conservation techniques and platelet function in cardiac surgery. Anesthesiology 75:426, 1991

283. Boldt J, Zickmann B, Ballesteros MBM et al: Influence of five different priming solutions on platelet function in patients undergoing cardiac surgery. Anesth Analg 74:219, 1992

284. Boldt J, Knothe C, Zickmann B et al: Influence of different intravascular volume therapies on platelet function in patients undergoing cardiopulmonary bypass. Anesth Analg 76:1185, 1993

285. van den Dungen JJAM, Karliczek GF, Branken U et al: Clinical study of blood trauma during perfusion with membrane and bubble oxygenators. J Thorac Cardiovasc Surg 83:108, 1982

286. Rinder CS, Bohnert J, Rinder HM et al: Platelet activation and aggregation during cardiopulmonary bypass. Anesthesiology 75:388, 1991

287. Rinder CS, Mathew JP, Rinder HM et al: Modulation of platelet surface adhesion receptors during cardiopulmonary bypass. Anesthesiology 75:563, 1991

288. Metzelaar MJ, Korteweg J, Sixma JJ, Nieuwenhuis HK: Comparison of platelet membrane markers for the detection of platelet activation in vitro and during platelet storage and cardiopulmonary bypass surgery. J Lab Clin Med 121:579, 1993

289. Kestin AS, Valeri CR, Khuri SF et al: The platelet function defect of cardiopulmonary bypass. Blood 82:107, 1993

290. Burns ER, Billett HH, Frater RWM et al: The preoperative bleeding time as a predictor of postoperative hemorrhage after cardiopulmonary bypass. J Thorac Cardiovasc Surg 92:310, 1986

291. Ferraris VA, Berry W, Lough F: Routine template bleeding time determinations before cardiac procedures. J Thorac Cardiovasc Surg 93:474, 1987

292. Ratnatunga CP, Rees GM, Kovacs IB: Preoperative hemostatic activity and excessive bleeding after cardiopulmonary bypass. Ann Thorac Surg 52:250, 1991

293. Barber A, Green D, Galluzzo T, Ts'ao CH: The bleeding time as a preoperative screening test. Am J Med 78:761, 1985

294. Rapaport SI: Preoperative hemostatic evaluation: which tests, if any? Blood 61:229, 1983

295. Simon TL, Akl BF, Murphy W: Controlled trial of routine administration of platelet concentrates in cardiopulmonary bypass surgery. Ann Thorac Surg 37:359, 1984

296. Czer LSC, Bateman TM, Gray RJ et al: Treatment of severe platelet dysfunction and hemorrhage after cardiopulmonary bypass: reduction in blood product usage with desmopressin. J Am Coll Cardiol 9:1139, 1987

297. Salzman EW, Weinstein MJ, Weintraub RM et al: Treatment with desmopressin acetate to reduce blood loss after cardiac surgery. A double-blind randomized trial. N Engl J Med 314:1402, 1986

298. Gratz I, Koehler J, Olsen D et al: The effect of desmopressin acetate on postoperative hemorrhage in patients receiving aspirin therapy before coronary artery bypass operations. J Thorac Cardiovasc Surg 104:1417, 1992

299. Rocha E, Llorens R, Paramo JA: Does desmopressin acetate reduce blood loss after surgery in patients on cardiopulmonary bypass? Circulation 77:1319, 1988

300. Hackmann T, Gascoyne RD, Naiman SC et al: A trial of desmopressin (1-desamino-8-D-arginine vasopressin) to reduce blood loss in uncomplicated cardiac surgery. N Engl J Med 321:1437, 1989

301. Frankville DD, Harper GB, Lake CL, Johns RA: Hemodynamic consequences of desmopressin administration after cardiopulmonary bypass. Anesthesiology 74:988, 1991

302. De Prost D, Barbier-Boehm G, Hazebroucq J et al: Desmopressin has no beneficial effect on excessive postoperative bleeding or blood product requirements associated with cardiopulmonary bypass. Thromb Haemost 68:106, 1992

303. Salzman EW, Weinstein MJ, Reilly D, Ware JA: Adventures in hemostasis: desmopressin in cardiac surgery. Arch Surg 128:212, 1993

304. Mannucci PM, Lusher JM: Desmopressin and thrombosis. Lancet 2:675, 1989

305. Flordal PA, Ljungström K-G, Fehrm A: Desmopressin and postoperative thromboembolism. Thromb Res 68:429, 1992

306. Van Oeveren W, Harder MP, Roozendaal KJ et al: Aprotinin protects platelets against the initial effect of cardiopulmonary bypass. J Thorac Cardiovasc Surg 99:788, 1990

307. Lavee J, Raviv Z, Smolinsky A et al: Platelet protection by low-dose aprotinin in cardiopulmonary bypass: electron microscopic study. Ann Thorac Surg 55:114, 1993

308. Nagaoka H, Innami R, Murayama F: Effects of aprotinin on prostaglandin metabolism and platelet function in open heart surgery. J Cardiovasc Surg 32:31, 1991

309. Bidstrup BP, Underwood SR, Sapsford RN, Streets EM: Effect of aprotinin (Trasylol) on aorta-coronary bypass graft patency. J Thorac Cardiovasc Surg 105:147, 1993

310. Hardy JF, Desroches J: Natural and synthetic antifibrinolytics in cardiac surgery. Can J Anesth 39:353, 1992

311. Horrow JC, Ellison N: Effective hemostasis during cardiac surgery. Can J Anesth 39:309, 1992

312. George JN: The origin and significance of platelet IgG. p. 305. In Kunicki TJ, George JN (eds): Platelet Immunobiology. Molecular and Clinical Aspects. JB Lippincott, Philadelphia, 1989

313. George JN: Platelet IgG: measurement, interpretation, and clinical significance. Prog Hemost Thromb 10:97, 1991

314. Aster RH: The immunologic thrombocytopenias. p. 387. In Kunicki TJ, George JN (eds): Platelet Immunobiology. Molecular and Clinical Aspects. JB Lippincott, Philadelphia, 1989

315. Clancy R, Jenkins E, Firkin B: Qualitative platelet abnormalities in idiopathic thrombocytopenic purpura. N Engl J Med 286:622, 1972

316. Zahavi J, Marder VJ: Acquired "storage pool disease" of platelets associated with circulating antiplatelet antibodies. Am J Med 56:883, 1974

317. Weiss HJ, Rosove MH, Lages BA, Kaplan KL: Acquired storage pool deficiency with increased platelet-associated IgG. Am J Med 69:711, 1980

318. Stuart MJ, Kelton JG, Allen JB: Abnormal platelet function and arachidonate metabolism in chronic idiopathic thrombocytopenic purpura. Blood 58:326, 1981

319. Lackner H, Karpatkin S: On the "easy bruising" syndrome with normal platelet count: a study of 75 patients. Ann Intern Med 83:190, 1975

320. Heyns AD, Fraser J, Retief FP: Platelet aggregation in chronic idiopathic thrombocytopenic purpura. J Clin Pathol 31:1239, 1978

321. Regan MG, Lackner H, Karpatkin S: Platelet function and coagulation profile in lupus erythematosus. Am J Med 81:462, 1974

322. Dorsch CA, Meyerhoff J: Mechanisms of abnormal platelet aggregation in systemic lupus erythematosus. Arthritis Rheum 25:966, 1982

323. Meyerhoff J, Dorsch CA: Decreased platelet serotonin levels in systemic lupus erythematosus. Arthritis Rheum 24:1495, 1981

324. Nieuwenhuis HK, Zwaginga JJ, Sixma JJ: Analysis of patients with a prolonged bleeding time. Thromb Haemost 58:527, 1987

325. Devine DV, Rosse WF: Identification of platelet proteins that bind alloantibodies and autoantibodies. Blood 64:1240, 1984

326. Woods VL Jr, Oh EH, Mason D, McMillan R: Autoantibodies against the platelet glycoprotein IIb-IIIa complex in patients with chronic ITP. Blood 63:368, 1984

327. Szatkowski NS, Kunicki TJ, Aster RH: Identification of glycoprotein Ib as a target for autoantibody in idiopathic (autoimmune) thrombocytopenic purpura. Blood 67:310, 1986

328. Sugiyama T, Okuma M, Ushikubi F et al: A novel platelet aggregating factor found in a patient with defective collagen-induced platelet aggregation and autoimmune thrombocytopenia. Blood 69:1712, 1987

329. Tomiyama Y, Kurata Y, Mizutani H et al: Platelet glycoprotein IIb as a target antigen in two patients with chronic idiopathic thrombocytopenic purpura. Br J Haematol 66:535, 1987

330. McMillan R, Tani P, Millard F et al: Platelet-associated and plasma anti-glycoprotein autoantibodies in chronic ITP. Blood 70:1040, 1987

331. Beardsley DS: Platelet autoantigens. p. 121. In Kunicki TJ, George JN (eds): Platelet Immunobiology. Molecular and Clinical Aspects. JB Lippincott, Philadelphia, 1989

332. Koerner TAW, Weinfeld HM, Bullard LSB, Williams LCJ: Antibodies against platelet glycosphingolipids: detection in serum by quantitative HPTLC-autoradiography and association with autoimmune and alloimmune processes. Blood 74:274, 1989

333. Falus A, Merety K, Bagdy D et al: Beta-2-microglobulin-specific autoantibodies cause platelet aggregation and interfere with ADP-induced aggregation. Clin Exp Immunol 47:103, 1982

334. Mueller-Eckhardt C, Monch H: The effect of platelet specific alloantibodies on the aggregation of human thrombocytes induced by ADP and collagen. Thromb Diath Haemorrh 25:379, 1971

335. van Leeuwen EF, Leeksma OC, van Mourik JA et al: Effect of the binding of anti-Zwa antibodies on platelet function. Vox Sang 47:280, 1984

336. Niessner H, Clemetson KJ, Panzer S et al: Acquired thrombasthenia due to GP IIb-IIIa-specific autoantibodies. Blood 68:571 1986

337. Kubota T, Tanoue K, Murohashi I et al: Autoantibody against platelet glycoprotein IIb-IIIa in a patient with non-Hodgkin's lymphoma. Thromb Res 53:379, 1989

338. Meyer M, Kirchmaier CM, Schirmer A et al: Acquired disorder of platelet function associated with autoantibodies against membrane glycoprotein IIb-IIIa complex-1. Glycoprotein analysis. Thromb Haemost 65:491, 1991

339. Balduini CL, Grignani G, Sinigaglia F: Severe platelet dysfunction in a patient with autoantibodies against membrane glycoproteins IIb-IIIa. Haemost 7:98, 1987

340. Balduini CL, Bertolino G, Noris P et al: Defect of platelet aggregation and adhesion induced by autoantibodies against platelet glycoprotein IIIa. Thromb Haemost 68:208, 1992

341. Levy-Toledano S, Tobelem G, Legrand C et al: Acquired IgG antibody occurring in a thrombasthenia patient: its effect on human platelet function. Blood 51:1965, 1978

342. Coller BS, Peerschke EIB, Seligsohn U et al: Studies on the binding of an alloimmune and two murine monoclonal antibodies to the platelet glycoprotein IIb-IIIa complex receptor. J Lab Clin Med 107:384, 1986

343. Devine DV, Currie MS, Rosse WF, Greenberg CS: Pseudo-Bernard-Soulier syndrome: thrombocytopenia caused by autoantibody to platelet glycoprotein Ib. Blood 70:428, 1987

344. Stricker RB, Wong D, Saks SR et al: Acquired Bernard-Soulier syndrome. J Clin Invest 76:1274, 1985

345. Hirschman RJ, Shulman NR: The use of platelet serotonin release as a sensitive method for detecting anti-platelet antibodies and a plasma anti-platelet factor in patients with idiopathic thrombocytopenic purpura. Br J Haematol 24:793, 1973

346. Rosenfeld SI, Anderson CL: Fc receptors of human platelets. p. 337. In Kunicki TJ, George JN (eds): Platelet Immunobiology. Molecular and Clinical Aspects. JB Lippincott, Philadelphia, 1989

347. Weidmer T, Ando B, Sims PJ: Complement C5b-9-stimulated platelet secretion is associated with a calcium-initiated activation of cellular protein kinases. J Biol Chem 262:13674, 1987

348. Sims PJ: Interaction of human platelets with the complement system. p 354. In Kunicki TJ, George JN (eds): Platelet Immunobiology. Molecular and Clinical Aspects. JB Lippincott, Philadelphia, 1989

349. Handagama PJ, Shuman MA, Bainton DF: Incorporation of intravenously injected albumin, immunoglobulin G, and fibrinogen in guinea pig megakaryocyte granules. J Clin Invest 84:73, 1989

350. Harrison P, Wilbourn BR, Debili N et al: Uptake of plasma fibrinogen into the alpha granules of human megakaryocytes and platelets. J Clin Invest 84:1320, 1989

351. Chen Y, Li J, Wu Q et al: Acquired platelet glycoprotein IIb-IIIa deficiency (Glanzmann thrombasthenia) in acute promyelocytic leukemia. 1993 (submitted)

352. Pareti FI, Capitanio A, Mannucci PM et al: Acquired dysfunction due to circulation of "exhausted" platelets. Am J Med 69:235, 1980

353. Bennett JS, Vilaire G: Exposure of platelet fibrinogen receptors by ADP and epinephrine. J Clin Invest 64:1393, 1979

354. Ingeberg S, Jacobsen P, Fischer E, Bentsen KD: Platelet aggregation and release of ATP in patients with hepatic cirrhosis. Scand J Gastroenterol 20:285, 1985

355. Hillbom M, Muuronen A, Neiman J: Liver disease and platelet function in alcoholics. Br Med J 295:581, 1987

356. Ordinas A, Maragall S, Castillo R, Nurden AT: A glycoprotein I defect in the platelets of three patients with severe cirrhosis of the liver. Thromb Res 13:297, 1978

357. Stein SF, Harker LA: Kinetic and functional studies of platelets, fibrinogen, and plasminogen in patients with hepatic cirrhosis. J Lab Clin Med 99:217, 1982

358. Stoff JS, Stemerman M, Steer M et al: A defect in platelet aggregation in Bartter's syndrome. Am J Med 68:171, 1980

359. Kueh YK: The syndrome of nonthrombocytopenic purpura with eosinophilia: an acquired platelet dysfunction. N Engl J Med 306:365, 1982

360. Muthiah MM, Mitchell TR, Thorn CT: Acquired platelet dysfunction with eosinophilia. Br Med J 289:1044, 1984

361. Szczeklik A, Milner PC, Birch J et al: Prolonged bleeding time, reduced aggregation, altered PAF-ether sensitivity and increased platelet mass are a trait of asthma and hay fever. Thromb Haemost 56:283, 1986

362. Carvalho ACA, Quinn DA, DeMarinis SM et al: Platelet function in acute respiratory failure. Am J Hematol 25:377, 1987

363. Bracey AW, Wu AHB, Aceves J et al: Platelet dysfunction associated with Wilms' tumor and hyaluronic acid. Am J Hematol 24:247, 1987

364. Schafer AI: Bleeding and thrombosis in the myeloproliferative disorders. Blood 64:1, 1984

365. Murphy S: Thrombocytosis and thrombocythaemia. Clin Haematol 12:89, 1983

366. Mitchell MC, Boitnott JK, Kaufman S et al: Budd-Chiari syndrome: etiology, diagnosis, and management. Medicine 61:199, 1982

367. Singh AK, Wetherly-Mein G: Microvascular occlusive lesions in primary thrombocythemia. Br J Haematol 36:553, 1977

368. Jabaily J, Iland H, Laszlo J et al: Neurologic manifestations of essential thrombocythemia. Ann Intern Med 99:513, 1983

369. Hussein S, Schwartz JM, Friedman SA, Chua SN: Arterial thrombosis in essential thrombocythemia. Am Heart J 96:31, 1978

370. Preston FE, Martin JF, Stewart RM, Davies-Jones GAB: Thrombocytosis, circulating platelet aggregates, and neurological dysfunction. Br Med J 2:1561, 1979

371. Kessler CM, Klein HG, Havlik RJ: Uncontrolled thrombocytosis in chronic myeloproliferative disorders. Br J Haematol 50:157, 1982

372. Murphy S, Davis JL, Walsh PN, Gardner FH: Template bleeding time and clinical hemorrhage in myeloproliferative disease. Arch Intern Med 138:1251, 1978

373. Hoagland HC, Silverstein MN: Primary thrombocythemia in the young patient. Mayo Clin Proc 53:578, 1978

374. Mitus AJ, Barbui T, Shulman LN et al: Hemostatic complications in young patients with essential thrombocythemia. Am J Med 88:371, 1990

375. McIntyre KJ, Hoagland HC, Silverstein MN, Petitt RM: Essential thrombocythemia in young adults. Mayo Clin Proc 66:149, 1991

376. Wasserman LR, Gilbert H: Complications of polycythemia vera. Semin Hematol 3:199, 1966

377. Murphy S: Polycythemia vera. Dis Mon 38:165, 1992

378. Maldonado JE, Pintado T, Pierre RV: Dysplastic platelets and circulating megakaryocytes in chronic myeloproliferative diseases. I. The platelets. Ultrastructure and peroxidase reaction. Blood 43:797, 1974

379. Bautista AP, Buckler PW, Towler HMA et al: Measurement of platelet lifespan in normal subjects and patients with myeloproliferative disease with indium oxine labelled platelets. Br J Haematol 58:679, 1984

380. Yamamoto K, Sekiguchi E, Takatani O: Abnormalities of epinephrine-in-

duced platelet aggregation and adenine nucleotides in myeloproliferative disorders. Thromb Haemost 52:292, 1984

381. Ginsberg AD: Platelet function in patients with high platelet counts. Ann Intern Med 82:506, 1975

382. Pareti FI, Gugliotti L, Mannucci PM et al: Biochemical and metabolic aspects of platelet dysfunction in chronic myeloproliferative disorders. Thromb Haemost 47:84, 1982

383. Schafer AI: Deficiency of platelet lipoxygenase activity in myeloproliferative disorders. N Engl J Med 306:381, 1982

384. Ushikubi F, Okuma M, Kanaji K et al: Hemorrhagic thrombocytopathy with platelet thromboxane A2 receptor abnormality: defective signal transduction with normal binding activity. Thromb Haemost 57:158, 1987

385. Malpass TW, Savage B, Hanson SR et al: Correlation between prolonged bleeding time and depletion of platelet dense granule ADP in patients with myelodysplastic and myeloproliferative disorders. J Lab Clin Med 103:894, 1984

386. Meschengieser S, Blanco A, Maugeri N et al: Platelet function and intraplatelet von Willebrand factor antigen and fibrinogen in myelodysplastic syndromes. Thromb Res 46:601, 1987

387. Mohri H: Acquired von Willebrand disease and storage pool disease in chronic myelocytic leukemia. Am J Hematol 22:391, 1986

388. Kaywin P, McDonough M, Insel PA, Shattil SJ: Platelet function in essential thrombocythemia: decreased epinephrine responsiveness associated with a deficiency of platelet alpha-adrenergic receptors. N Engl J Med 299:505, 1978

389. Swart SS, Pearson D, Wood JK, Barnett DB: Functional significance of the platelet alpha2-adrenoreceptor: studies in patients with myeloproliferative disorders. Thromb Res 33:531, 1984

390. Berndt MC, Kabral A, Grimsley P et al: An acquired Bernard-Soulier-like platelet defect associated with juvenile myelodysplastic syndrome. Br J Haematol 68:97, 1988

391. Cooper B, Schafer AI, Puchalsky D, Handin RI: Platelet resistance to prostaglandin D2 in patients with myeloproliferative disorders. Blood 52:618, 1978

392. Moore A, Nachman RL: Platelet Fc receptor: increased expression in myeloproliferative disease. J Clin Invest 67:1064, 1981

393. Bolin RB, Okumura T, Jamieson GA: Changes in distribution of platelet membrane glycoproteins in patients with myeloproliferative disorders. Am J Hematol 3:63, 1977

394. Eche N, Sie P, Caranobe C et al: Platelets in myeloproliferative disorders. III. Glycoprotein profile in relation to platelet function and platelet density. Scand J Haematol 26:123, 1981

395. Mohri H, Ohkubo T: Acquired von Willebrand's syndrome due to an inhibitor of IgG specific for von Willebrand's factor in polycythemia rubra vera. Acta Haematol 78:258, 1987

396. Budde U, Schaefer G, Mueller N et al: Acquired von Willebrand's disease in the myeloproliferative syndrome. Blood 64:981, 1984

397. Duran-Suarez JR, Pico M, Zuazu J et al: Acquired von Willebrand's disease caused by chronic grnaulocytic leukemia. Br J Haematol 48:173, 1981

398. Kaplan ME, Mack K, Goldberg JD: Long-term management of polycythemia vera with hydroxyurea: a progress report. Semin Hematol 23:167, 1986

399. Murphy S, Iland H, Resenthal D, Laszlo J: Essential thrombocythemia: an interim report from the polycythemia vera study group. Semin Hematol 23:177, 1986

400. Greenberg BR, Watson-Williams EJ: Successful control of life-threatening thrombocytosis with a blood processor. Transfusion 15:620, 1975

401. McIntyre KJ, Hoagland HC: Essential thrombocythemia in young persons, abstracted. Blood 741989

402. Silverstein MN, Pettit RM, Solberg LA: Anagrelide: a new drug for treating thrombocytosis. N Engl J Med 318:1292, 1988

403. Anagrelide Study Group: Anagrelide, a therapy for thrombocythemic states: experience in 577 patients. Am J Med 92:69, 1992

404. Sultan Y, Caen JP: Platelet dysfunction in preleukemic states and in various types of leukemia. Ann NY Acad Sci 201:300, 1972

405. Cowan DH, Graham RR Jr, Baunack D: The platelet defect in leukemia: plate-

let ultrastructure, adenine nucleotide metabolism, and the release reaction. J Clin Invest 56:188, 1975

406. Westbrook CA, Golde DW: Clinical problems in hairy cell leukemia: diagnosis and management. Semin Oncol 11:514, 1984

407. Sweet DL, Golomb HL: Correction of platelet defect after splenectomy in hairy cell leukemia. JAMA 241:1684, 1979

408. Rosove MH, Naeim F, Harwig S, Zighelboim J: Severe platelet dysfunction in hairy cell leukemia with improvement after splenectomy. Blood 55:903, 1980

409. Roussi JH, Houbouyan LL, Alterescu R et al: Acquired von Willebrand's syndrome associated with hairy cell leukemia. Br J Haematol 46:503, 1980

410. Lackner H, Hunt V, Zucker MB, Pearson J: Abnormal fibrin ultrastructure, polymerization, and clot retraction in multiple myeloma. Br J Haematol 18:625, 1970

411. Lackner H: Hemostatic abnormalities associated with dysproteinemias. Semin Hematol 10:125, 1973

412. Perkins HA, MacKenzie MR, Fudenberg HH: Hemostatic defects in dysproteinemias. Blood 35:695, 1970

413. Palmer RN, Rick ME, Rick PD et al: Circulating heparan sulfate anticoagulant in a patient with a fatal bleeding disorder. N Engl J Med 310:1696, 1984

414. Chapman GS, George CB, Danley DL: Heparin-like anticoagulant associated with plasma cell myeloma. Am J Clin Pathol 83:764, 1985

415. Furie B, Greene E, Furie BC: Syndrome of acquired factor X deficiency and systemic amyloidosis. N Engl J Med 297:81, 1977

416. McPherson RA, Onstad JW, Ugoretz RJ et al: Coagulopathy in amyloidosis: combined deficiency of factors IX and X. Am J Hematol 3:225, 1977

417. Liebman H, Chinowsky M, Valdin J et al: Increased fibrinolysis and amyloidosis. Arch Intern Med 143:678, 1983

418. Meyer K, Williams EC: Fibrinolysis and acquired alpha-2 plasmin inhibitor deficiency in amyloidosis. Am J Med 79:394, 1985

419. Kasturi J, Saraya AK: Platelet functions in dysproteinemia. Acta Haematol 59:104, 1978

420. Vigliano EM, Horowitz HI: Bleeding syndrome in a patient with IgA myeloma: interaction of protein and connective tissue. Blood 29:823, 1967

421. DiMinno G, Coraggio F, Cerbone AM et al: A myeloma paraprotein with specificity for platelet glycoprotein IIIa in a patient with a fatal bleeding disorder. J Clin Invest 77:157, 1986

422. Mohri H, Noguchi T, Kodama F et al: Acquired von Willebrand disease due to inhibitor of human myeloma protein specific for von Willebrand factor. Am J Clin Pathol 87:663, 1987

423. Takahashi H, Nagayama R, Tanabe Y et al: DDAVP in acquired von Willebrand syndrome associated with multiple myeloma. Am J Hematol 22:421, 1986

424. Mannucci PM, Lombardi R, Bader R et al: Studies of the pathophysiology of acquired von Willebrand's disease in seven patients with lymphoproliferative disorders or benign monoclonal gammopathies. Blood 64:614, 1984

425. Bovill EG, Ershler WB, Golden EA et al: A human myeloma-produced myeloma protein directed against the active subpopulation of von Willebrand factor. Am J Clin Pathol 85:115, 1986

426. Castaman G, Tosetto A, Rodeghiero F: Effectiveness of high-dose intravenous immunoglobulin in a case of acquired von Willebrand syndrome with chronic melena not responsive to desmopressin and factor VIII concentrate. Am J Hematol 41:132, 1992

427. Scott JP, Montgomery RR, Tubergen DG, Hays T: Acquired von Willebrand's disease in association with Wilms' tumor: regression following treatment. Blood 48:665, 1981

428. Scrobohaci ML, Daniel MT, Levy Y et al: Expression of GPIb on plasma cells in a patient with monoclonal IgG and acquired von Willebrand disease. Br J Haematol 84:471, 1993

429. Wallace MR, Simon SR, Ershler WB, Burns SL: Hemorrhagic diathesis in multiple myeloma. Acta Haematol 72:340, 1984

430. Hyman BT, Westrick MA: Multiple myeloma with polyneuropathy and coagulopathy. Arch Intern Med 146:993, 1986

431. Silberstein LE, Abraham J, Shattil SJ: The efficacy of intensive plasma exchange in acquired von Willebrand's disease. Transfusion 27:234, 1987

Human Blood Group Antigens and Antibodies

131

Part 1
Carbohydrate Determinants

Steven L. Spitalnik

INTRODUCTION

Biochemical studies demonstrated that many important blood group antigens are complex carbohydrates. These are grouped together in this section, as there are some similarities in their biosynthesis, in the human immune response to these antigens, in the serologic methods for detecting antibodies specific for these antigens, and in the outcome in vivo after transfusion of incompatible blood.

The biosynthetic pathways used in forming antigens in the ABH, Lewis, P, and I blood group systems are interrelated. These oligosaccharide antigens may exist free in solution. In addition, they may be covalently attached to lipid molecules (ceramide) to form glycosphingolipids, or to polypeptides to form mucins, integral membrane glycoproteins, or soluble glycoproteins. The glycosidic linkages (i.e., the bonds between monosaccharides) are specifically catalyzed by glycosyltransferases. Some glycosyltransferases, found in all individuals, form framework structures. Other glycosyltransferases are allelically inherited and specify the synthesis of variable structures. Because of their variable inheritance and expression, the latter may form blood group antigens. As described below, antigens in the ABH, Lewis, P, and I blood group systems are synthesized on common precursor framework molecules. Competition between genetically inherited blood group-specific glycosyltransferases results in a rich mixture of antigenic molecules. In addition, a single oligosaccharide may contain several different blood group specificities. The absence of particular blood group antigens in certain individuals may result in specific antibody production after antigenic stimulation.

The immune response to carbohydrate antigens, particularly when presented as repetitive epitopes, is usually thymus independent. In this case, multivalent antigens directly stimulate B cells to synthesize antibodies without the aid of helper T cells. Thymus-independent immune responses classically result in the production of IgM antibodies, and most antibodies to carbohydrate blood group antigens are, in fact, IgM. Surprisingly, individuals lacking a carbohydrate blood group antigen on their red cells often have "naturally occurring" IgM antibodies to that particular antigen in their serum. The current understanding of this phenomenon is not that these antibodies spontaneously arise without prior antigenic stimulation, but that cross-reacting antigens present in the environment, such as on gut bacteria, stimulate specific IgM production. By contrast, high-titer IgG antibodies to carbohydrate antigens can be found in certain individuals. The latter may be stimulated by a thymus-dependent form of these oligosaccharides, perhaps as individual epitopes on glycoproteins, in which T-cell help leads to an isotype switch from IgM to IgG production. A clear understanding of this phenomenon is not yet available.

Since carbohydrate-specific blood group antibodies are predominantly IgM, these pentameric molecules directly agglutinate antigen-positive human red cells without the aid of an antiglobulin reagent. These antibodies, for unclear reasons, often cause more significant agglutination in vitro at temperatures <37°C. Since most IgM molecules directly fix complement, these antibodies can cause immediate intravascular hemolysis after transfusion of incompatible, antigen-positive red cells. In unusual cases, high-titer IgG carbohydrate-specific antibodies coat red cells and lead to extravascular hemolysis after incompatible transfusion. Alternatively, they may cross the placenta resulting in hemolytic disease of the newborn.

ABH, SECRETOR, AND LEWIS SYSTEMS

ABH Antigens

At the turn of the century, Karl Landsteiner discovered the ABO blood group system, which is the most important one with respect to blood transfusion and renal transplantation. He was fortunate to discover the first human alloantigens, using a conceptually simple experiment (Table 131-1). Each individual was found either to lack or to have one or both of the two antigens, A and B, on the red cells. In addition, the serum of each subject contained "naturally occurring" directly agglutinating antibodies that recognized the antigens absent from their own red cells. This experiment can be explained in modern terms as follows: cross-reacting carbohydrate structures on environmental agents stimulate the thymus-independent production of IgM anti-A and/or anti-B in individuals not tolerant to these antigens. The IgM antibodies then directly agglutinate the appropriate antigen-positive red cells, preferentially at room temperature. There are interesting variations in the frequencies of these blood types in different human populations[1,2] (Table 131-2).

Although the ABH antigens (the H antigen is the relevant carbohydrate structure present on group O red cells) are typically described as blood group antigens because of their presence on red cells, they are also found on other tissues, and may be more appropriately termed histo-blood group antigens.[3] In blood they exist in both a cellular form on platelets and a soluble form as blood group active glycosphingolipids coupled to plasma lipoproteins. They exist as membrane antigens on such diverse cells as vascular endothelial cells and intestinal, cervical, urothelial, and mammary epithelial cells. Soluble forms are also found in various secretions and excretions, such as saliva, milk, urine, and feces. In some tissues, their appearance is developmentally regulated. Despite their wide distribution, genetic inheritance, developmental regulation, and importance in transfusion and transplantation, their normal physiologic function, if any, remains a mystery.

To appreciate the structure and antigenicity of ABH antigens and their relationship to other blood group systems fully, it is necessary to understand the underlying biochemistry.

Early studies indicated that anti-A, anti-B, and anti-H specifically recognize epitopes composed of the terminal trisaccharides or disaccharides illustrated in Figure 131-1. From these

Table 131-1. ABO Blood Group Antigens and Antibodies

Blood Group	Red Blood Cell Antigens		Serum Antibodies	
	A	B	Anti-A	Anti-B
A	+	−	−	+
B	−	+	+	−
AB	+	+	−	−
O	−	−	+	+

Table 131-2. Frequencies of ABO Groups in Selected Populations

Population[a] (No. Tested)	Various Phenotypes (%)					
	O	A_1	A_2	B	A_1B	A_2B
South American Indians (539)	100	0	0	0	0	0
Vietnamese (220)	45	21	0	29	4	0
Australian aborigines (126)	44	55	0	0	0	0
Germans (100,000)	43	33	9	11	3	1
Bengalese (241)	22	22	2	38	15	1
Lapps (324)	18	36	19	15	6	6

[a] Figures are for selected populations and do not necessarily apply to the racial group as a whole.
(Data from Mourant et al.[1] and Walker.[2])

H: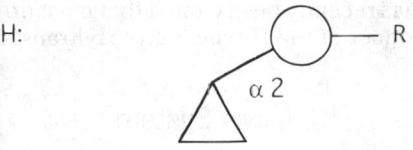

A: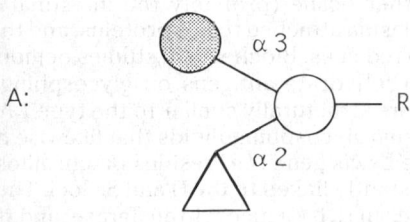

B: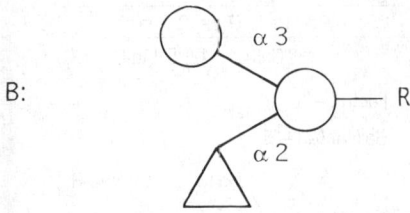

Fig. 131-1. Biochemical structures of the immunodominant oligosaccharides of the A, B, and H antigens. Open circle, D-galactose; closed circle, D-N-acetylgalactosamine; open triangle, L-fucose. Disaccharide linkages are from C-1 of the nonreducing terminal monosaccharide to the indicated carbon of the reducing terminal disaccharide; for example, α2 represents the α1−2 linkage.

results it is possible to conclude that the A, B, and H antigens are not directly encoded by the corresponding genes, but rather the genes code for particular glycosyltransferases, commonly called the A, B, and H transferases, or, equivalently, the A, B, and H enzymes. The H enzyme is a fucosyltransferase that specifically adds fucose in an (α1−2) linkage to a terminal galactose. The A or B enzymes then add N-acetylgalactosamine or galactose, respectively, in an (α1−3) linkage to the same terminal galactose. However, the substrate for the A or B enzymes is a terminal H antigen sequence; these enzymes do not transfer the appropriate sugar to galactose in the absence of (α1−2)-linked fucose. Similarly, the H enzyme does not function if this galactose is substituted with a different sugar. Thus, the biosynthetic pathway is as follows:

$$\text{Gal-R} \xrightarrow{\;1\;} \text{H} \xrightarrow{\;2\;} \text{A or B}$$

where reaction 1 is catalyzed by the H enzyme and reaction 2 by the A or B enzyme.

The finding that the A and B genes code for glycosyltransferases explains some results obtained from classic genetic analysis of family pedigrees. In particular, the A and B genes are inherited in a strict mendelian fashion and are dominant compared to O, but the A and B genes are co-dominant with each other. That is, an individual with the genotype AO (or BO) is phenotypically A (or B), an individual of genotype AB is also phenotypically AB, and an individual of genotype OO is phenotypically group O. Since the A and B enzymes both use the H antigen as substrate, even the presence of only approximately 50% of these enzymes in an AO (or BO) heterozygote is sufficient to convert the red cells to the corresponding A (or B) phenotype. Similarly, if both the A and B enzymes are present, they each convert approximately 50% of the available H antigen substrate, yielding red cells expressing both antigens A and B.

Recent studies have begun to elucidate the biology of the ABH system at the level of the gene. The genes encoding the A and B enzymes are located on chromosome 9. They encode membrane-bound glycosyltransferases containing 354 amino acids (Fig. 131-2). Interestingly, these two enzymes exhibit a great degree of mutual homology and, at the amino acid level, differ at only four residues.[4] Their substrate specificity is primarily determined by the two adjacent residues near the C terminus of the protein, amino acids 266 and 268[5] (Fig. 131-2). The allele corresponding to blood group O contains a single nucleotide deletion near the N terminus of the protein, leading to a shift in reading frame and a prematurely terminated translation product lacking enzymatic activity[4] (Fig. 131-2). Not only do these findings confirm and extend the results obtained from carbohydrate biochemistry and enzymology, but they also suggest new ways of blood typing using molecular biology techniques.[6]

Secretor Gene

The ABH antigens are found not only on red cells but also in secretions, particularly saliva and plasma. The ability to secrete ABH is genetically inherited: approximately 80% of whites are secretors and 20% are nonsecretors. This trait is inherited as a single locus gene in simple mendelian fashion. The secretor gene (*Se*) is dominant; nonsecretor (*se*) is recessive. The terminal carbohydrate sequences of the ABH antigens in saliva and plasma are identical to those on red cells. However, the backbone or framework carbohydrate structures are different. ABH antigens on glycosphingolipids and glycoproteins synthesized by red cell precursors are primarily coupled to framework type 2 chains (Gal(β1−4)GlcNAc-R); the same antigens on plasma

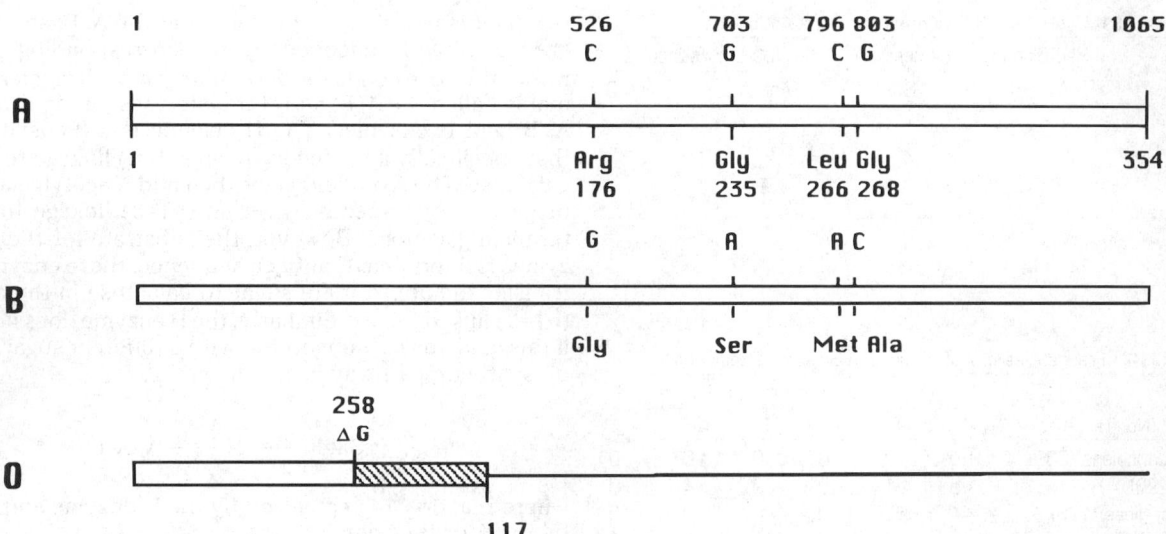

Fig. 131-2. cDNA structures of the A and B glycosyltransferases. Each of the A and B transferases encodes a 354-amino acid protein and differs at the four amino acid residues indicated.[4,5] The corresponding cDNA from group O individuals contains a single nucleotide deletion, resulting in a frameshift, premature termination of the translated polypeptide, and no enzymatic activity.[4]

glycosphingolipids and salivary mucins are coupled to type 1 chains (Gal(β1–3)GlcNAc-R) (Table 131-3). Since ABH blood group-active glycosphingolipids on plasma lipoproteins are also passively transferred onto red cells, red cells of secretors have ABH antigens on both type 1 and type 2 precursor chains, but red cells of nonsecretors only have ABH antigens on type 2 chains.

Initially, the *H* gene was thought to be a structural gene coding for the H enzyme and the secretor locus coded for a regulatory gene that permitted expression of the *H* gene in the appropriate tissues. This hypothesis suggested that a single H enzyme transferred fucose residues onto either type 1 or type 2 precursor chains. In this model, the H enzyme is always expressed in red cell precursors, but its expression in secretory tissues (e.g., salivary epithelium) comes under the control of the secretor locus. However, this does not explain all the available information, and recent biochemical, immunologic, and genetic studies demonstrate that an alternative model is correct.[7,8] The latter hypothesizes that there are two different H transferases: one that adds fucose to type 1 chains (H type 1 enzyme) and one that acts on type 2 chains (H type 2 enzyme). Therefore, the H type 1 enzyme is the structural protein coded for by the secretor gene and is expressed in secretory tissues. At least one copy of this gene (*Se*) is found in approximately 80% of the population and leads to the expression of ABH antigens in secretions. By contrast, the traditional H locus is a structural gene for the H type 2 enzyme. This gene (*H*) is active

in virtually all individuals (see below) and leads to the formation of ABH antigens on red cells and other tissues. These two enzymes are encoded by genes at two closely linked loci on chromosome 19. A human cDNA encoding an (α1–2) fucosyltransferase has recently been cloned that most probably represents the product of the H type 2 glycosyltransferase gene.[9]

Lewis System

The two Lewis blood group antigens Le^a (Lewis *a*) and Le^b (Lewis *b*) were discovered in the 1940s (Fig. 131-3). Virtually all individuals fall into one of three different Lewis types: Le(a+b−), Le(a−b+), and Le(a−b−) (Table 131-4). These molecules are not intrinsic red cell antigens; they are synthesized in another tissue (probably the intestinal epithelium), circulate in plasma attached to lipoproteins, and then passively transfer onto red cells. Biochemical studies demonstrated that these are carbohydrate antigens on glycosphingolipids (Fig. 131-3). They are structurally similar to the type 1 ABH antigens found on plasma glycosphingolipids that likewise transfer onto red cells. The Lewis gene (*Le*) resides on chromosome 19 and its locus is distantly linked to the H and Se loci. The gene codes for an enzyme, an (α1–4) fucosyltransferase, and thus behaves in a dominant fashion. A human cDNA derived from the *Le* gene has recently been cloned.[10] Approximately 95% of whites and 75% of blacks have at least one *Le* allele. The transfer of fucose

Table 131-3. Biochemical Structures of ABH Antigens

Blood Group	Secretions (Type 1 Chain)	Red Cells (Type 2 Chain)
H	Gal(β1–3)GlcNAc-R / Fuc(α1–2)	Gal(β1–4)GlcNAc-R / Fuc(α1–2)
A	GalNAc(α1–3) \ Gal(β1–3)GlcNAc-R / Fuc(α1–2)	GalNAc(α1–3) \ Gal(β1–4)GlcNAc-R / Fuc(α1–2)
B	Gal(α1–3) \ Gal(β1–3)GlcNAc-R / Fuc(α1–2)	Gal(α1–3) \ Gal(β1–4)GlcNAc-R / Fuc(α1–2)

Table 131-4. The Lewis Blood Group System

	Red Cell Antigens		Serum Antibodies	
Blood Group	Le^a	Le^b	Anti-Le^a	Anti-Le^b
Le(a+b−)	+	−	—	Very rarely
Le(a−b+)	−	+	Very rarely	—
Le(a−b−)	−	−	Occasionally	Occasionally

Table 131-5. Interactions of the ABH, Lewis, and Secretor Systems

Genes	A LeSe	A Lese	A leSe	A lese
Red cell antigens	A type 1	—	A type 1	—
	A type 2	A type 2	A type 2	A type 2
	Le^b (type 1)	Le^a (type 1)	—	—
	ALe^b (type 1)	—	—	—
Salivary blood	A type 1	Le^a (type 1)	A type 1	—
group antigens	Le^b (type 1)	—	—	—
	ALe^b (type 1)	—	—	—

to a type 1 precursor by the Lewis enzyme results in the formation of the Le^a antigen; the addition of (α1–4) linked fucose to the H type 1 structure leads to the formation of the Le^b antigen. Thus, the latter is formed through the cooperation of two glycosyltransferases encoded by two genes, one gene from the Lewis system (*Le* on chromosome 19) and one from the ABH system (*Se* or, equivalently, H type 1 at a different, unlinked locus on chromosome 19). The biosynthetic pathways demonstrating the connections of the ABH, Secretor, and Lewis systems (encoded by genes at three distinct loci on two chromosomes, 9 and 19) are illustrated in Figure 131-4. Interestingly, cooperation of the *Le, Se,* and *A* (or *B*) genes leads to the formation of a minor antigen, ALe^b (or BLe^b), recognized by both anti-A (or -B) and anti-Le^b antibodies. Since the H type 1 enzyme converts virtually all type 1 precursor into H type 1, whether or not the Lewis enzyme is present, Lewis-positive secretors have virtually no Le^a antigen and their red cells type as Le(a−b+). By contrast, Lewis-positive nonsecretors have Le(a+b−) red cells. This is summarized in Table 131-5.

Antigenic Variants of the ABH System

The ABH system has several unusual but instructive antigenic variants. The most striking is the Bombay phenotype (O$_h$). The red cells of these individuals type as group O, and they are nonsecretors of ABH antigens. However, they do not express H antigens on their red cells and their serum contains high-titer hemolytic anti-H antibodies that lyse red cells of any ABO group, except those from another individual of the Bombay phenotype. Based on the premise that the H gene codes for the H type 2 glycosyltransferase, then the allelic h gene codes for a nonfunctional enzyme. In addition, since individuals of the Bombay phenotype are nonsecretors (i.e., they lack a functional H type 1 transferase), their genotype is *hh sese.* Interestingly, some of these individuals do express active A and/or B enzymes, but the A (or B) antigen is not detected because the appropriate substrate for these enzymes is not synthesized. Nonetheless, the functional *A* or *B* genes can be transmitted to the next generation, yielding the apparently paradoxical pedigree O × O → A (or B). On rare occasions, individuals are identified with ABH deficient red cells but with ABH antigens in their secretions; this is referred to as the para-Bombay phenotype.[7] Again, in terms of the model described above, these individuals have the *hh Sese* or *hh SeSe* genotype. They are able to synthesize functional H type 1 glycosyltransferase, but not H type 2 transferase. These variations are summarized in Table 131-6. In the future, the use of molecular biology techniques to clone and sequence the genes at *H* and *Se* loci should lead to a clear understanding of the causes of the Bombay and para-Bombay phenotypes.[9]

Subgroups of A

Some relatively common variations in the ABH system relate to the "strength" of the A antigen on group A cells. Several subgroups of A that have weak expression of the A antigen have been identified. The red cells of most group A individuals

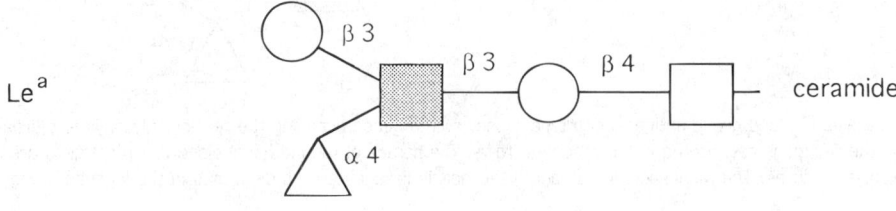

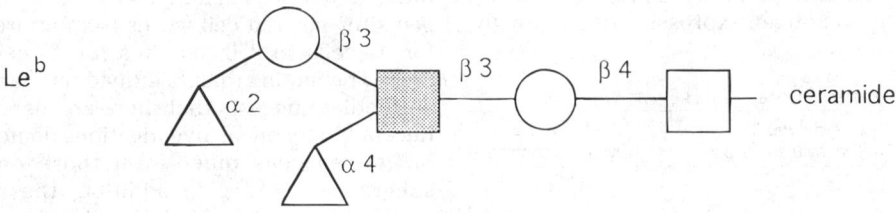

Fig. 131-3. Structure of Lewis-active glycosphingolipids. Open circle, D-galactose; open triangle, L-fucose; open square, D-glucose; closed square, D-*N*-acetylglucosamine. Linkages are as described in the legend of Figure 131-1.

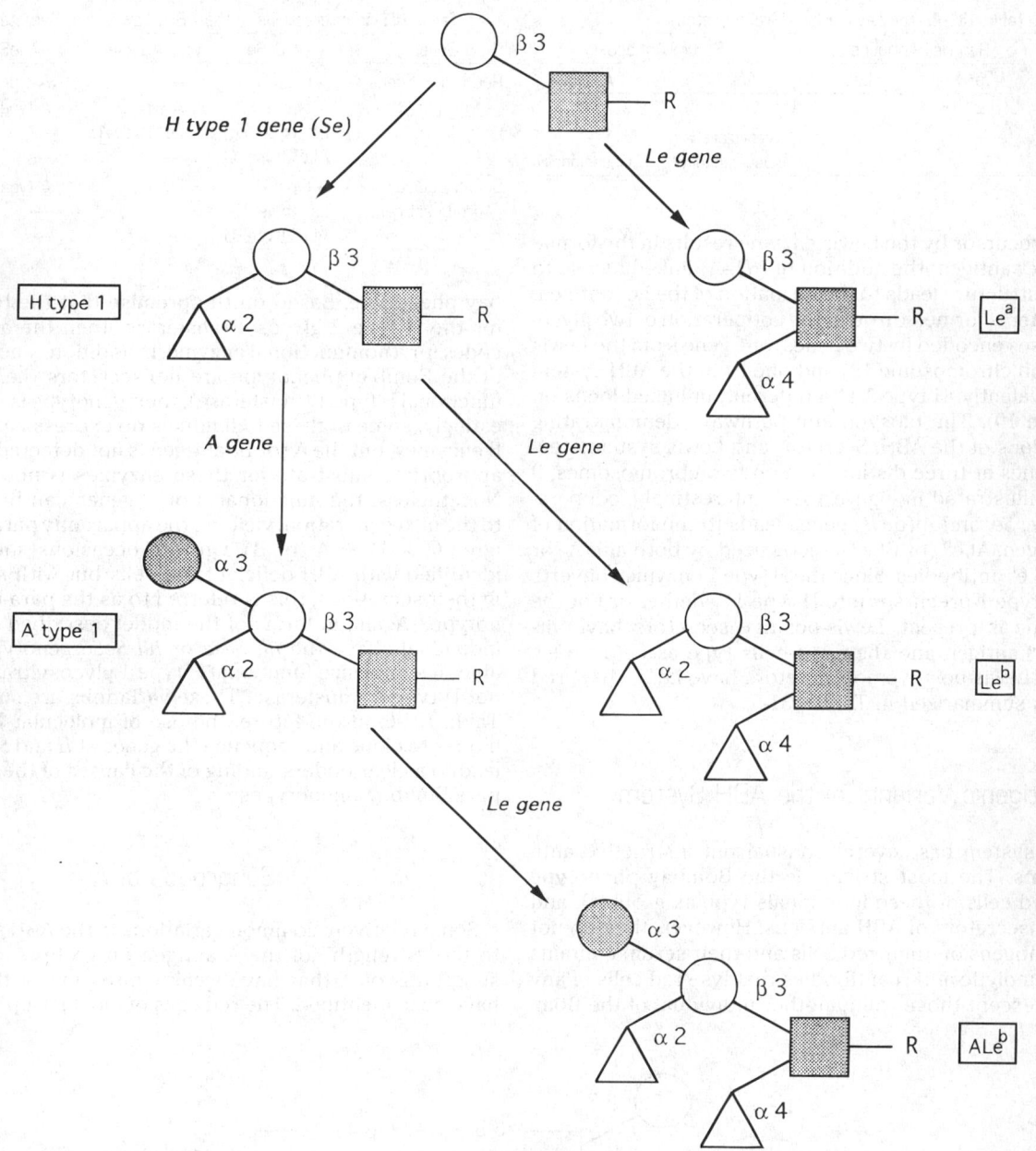

Fig. 131-4. Biosynthesis of blood group antigens with type 1 chains. The genes encoding the relevant glycosyltransferases are denoted in bold italics and the reactions catalyzed are indicated by arrows. The names of the individual blood group antigens are shown in boxes next to the relevant structures. The monosaccharides and disaccharide linkages are as described in the legends of Figures 131-1 and 131-3.

(80% of whites) type as A_1 (Table 131-2) and correspond to the results originally described by Landsteiner. Most of the remaining group A individuals have weaker expression and are denoted A_2. Other rarer subgroups of A (i.e., A_3, A_x, A_m, A_{el}) have progressively weaker A antigen expression. Interestingly,

many of these people produce an antibody, anti-A_1, which does not agglutinate their own red cells but does agglutinate A_1 red cells. This phenomenon is explained by quantitative and qualitative differences in antigen expression. The number of A antigen sites per red cell varies from approximately 800,000 sites for A_1 cells to 250,000 sites for A_2 cells to 700 sites for A_m cells. The finding that A_2 individuals can synthesize A_1-specific antibodies suggests that there are also qualitative differences. Recent biochemical investigations demonstrate that A antigens on A_1 red cells differ from those on cells of the various subgroups of A.[3,11] In addition, the molecular biologic approach has identified polymorphisms in allelic A glycosyltransferase cDNA sequences in individuals with red cells expressing weak A activity.[12,13] These polymorphisms may result in weak-

Table 131-6. Genetic Inheritance of H Enzymes

	H Type 1 Glycosyltransferase	H Type 2 Glycosyltransferase
Normal secretor	+	+
Normal nonsecretor	−	+
Bombay phenotype	−	−
Para-Bombay phenotype	+	−

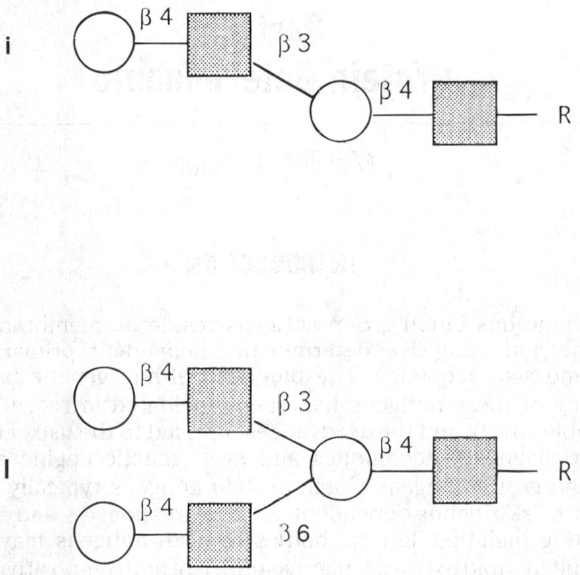

Fig. 131-5. Ii blood group antigens. The monosaccharides and disaccharide linkages are as described in the legends of Figures 131-1 and 131-3.

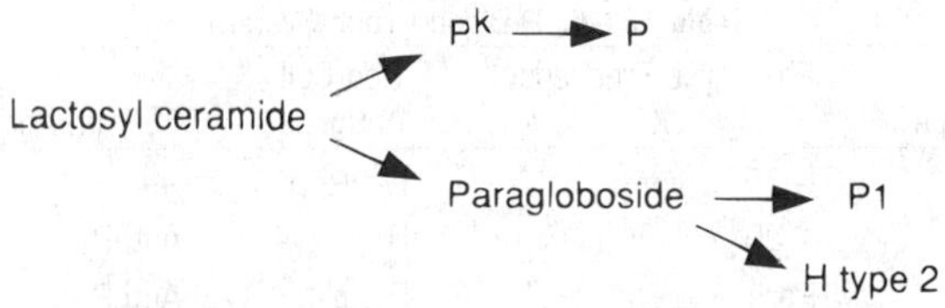

Fig. 131-6. Biosynthetic pathway of antigens in the P blood group system.

ened or variant enzyme activity in the encoded glycosyltransferases.[12]

I SYSTEM

The I blood group system has been intensively studied but is not well understood. The I antigens are oligosaccharides that form the type 2 chain precursors for ABH antigens (Fig. 131-5). The best available evidence indicates that the difference between I and i antigens relates to branching of the oligosaccharide chain; anti-i antibodies recognize an unbranched oligosaccharide chain, and anti-I antibodies recognize a similar chain that is also branched. Fetal and cord red cells contain mostly i antigen with small amounts of I; adult red cells demonstrate the opposite pattern. This suggests that the glycosyltransferase necessary for synthesis of the branched structure, a (β1–6) N-acetylglucosaminyltransferase, is developmentally regulated. The availability of the cloned cDNA encoding this enzyme will now allow this hypothesis to be tested.[14] Rare adults have red cells that type as i; presumably their red cell precursors lack this glycosyltransferase. Antibodies specific for the I antigens are clinically relevant in the setting of cold type autoimmune hemolytic anemia. The sera of these patients typically contain high titers of a monoclonal antibody, usually with anti-I specificity. In patients demonstrating hemolysis in vivo, the antibodies bind to red cells at or near 37°C in vitro and have the ability to fix complement. Surprisingly, almost all normal individuals have low titers of presumably polyclonal anti-I. These autoantibodies have a low thermal amplitude, agglutinating red cells only at room temperature or below, and do not cause accelerated red cell destruction in vivo. Patients with particular infectious diseases such as infectious mononucleosis and mycoplasma pneumonia often develop cold agglutinins, typically with anti-i and anti-I specificity, respectively. In unusual cases, this may result in immune-mediated hemolytic anemia. At present, no satisfactory explanation that describes, at a molecular level, the differences between cold agglutinins that cause hemolysis in vivo, and those that do not, is available.

P BLOOD GROUP SYSTEM

The P blood group system consists of three glycosphingolipid antigens: pk, P, and P_1 (Fig. 131-6 and Table 131-7). These carbohydrate chains are structurally and biosynthetically re-

lated.[15] Each has a common precursor, Gal(β1–4)Glc-ceramide; the pk antigen is the biosynthetic precursor of the P antigen; both pk and P_1 share a common disaccharide structure, Gal(α1–4)Gal(β1–4)-R, at the nonreducing end of the glycosphingolipid. Five different red cell phenotypes in which various combinations of these three antigens are present have been described (Table 131-8). The P_1 and P_2 phenotypes are common and account for almost all of the population. The serum of some P_2 individuals contains anti-P_1 antibodies. These antibodies are usually IgM low-titer cold agglutinins and are rarely of clinical significance. By contrast, the rare individuals with the p_1k, p_2k, and p phenotypes have naturally occurring high-titer IgM antibodies with specificity either for the P antigen (anti-P) or for all the antigens in the P blood group system (anti-P_1Ppk, or, equivalently, anti-Tj[a]). These antibodies are clinically relevant in that they can cause severe hemolytic transfusion reactions. An unusual syndrome of recurrent spontaneous abortions has also been associated with these antibodies, presumably due to the presence of pk- and P-active glycosphingolipids on trophoblastic tissue. In addition, the syndrome of paroxysmal cold hemoglobinuria, originally associated with syphilis, is caused by Donath-Landsteiner antibodies. The latter are complement-fixing IgG antibodies with anti-P specificity that cause immune-mediated hemolysis in vivo. Finally, recent studies have shown that the P blood group antigen is the receptor for B19 parvovirus on erythropoietic precursors.[16] This virus causes both transient aplastic crises in patients with underlying hemolysis and anemia in immunocompromised patients.

POLYAGGLUTINATION AND T AND Tn ANTIGENS

The major glycoproteins on red cell membranes, glycophorins A, B, and C, each carry 15, 11, and 12 O-linked oligosaccharides per molecule, respectively. These oligosaccharides are disialylated tetrasaccharides with the structure shown in Figure 131-7. In certain individuals, cryptic carbohydrate antigens are exposed by removing sialic acid residues from the mature tetrasaccharide (T activation) revealing the T antigen. In other individuals, cryptic antigens are exposed by preventing enzymatic attachment of (β1–3) linked galactose (Tn activation) resulting in expression of the Tn antigen.[17] Interestingly, the T and Tn structures are also tumor associated antigens.[18]

Red cells expressing the T or Tn antigens are "polyagglutinable" because they are agglutinated by IgM antibodies present in all adult sera. These "naturally occurring" anti-T and anti-Tn antibodies presumably arise after exposure of individuals to cross-reacting structures present on bacteria.

The T antigen is transiently exposed on red cells in vivo by

Table 131-7. Biochemistry of the P Blood Group System

pk	Gal(α1–4)Gal(β1–4)Glc-ceramide
P	GalNAc(β1–3)Gal(α1–4)Gal(β1–4)Glc-ceramide
P_1	Gal(α1–4)Gal(β1–4)GlcNAc(β1–3)Gal(β1–4)Glc-ceramide

Table 131-8. P Blood Group System

Phenotype	Phenotype Frequency (%)	Red Cell Antigens	Serum Antibodies
P_1	~ 75	P_1, P, p^k	—
P_2	~ 25	P, p^k	Anti-P_1
p_1^k	Rare	P_1, p^k	Anti-P
p_2^k	Rare	p^k	Anti-P, anti-P_1
p	Rare	—	Anti-P_1Ppk (anti-Tj^a)

the action of microbial neuraminidases (sialidases), typically in individuals with a bacterial infection caused by organisms such as Escherichia coli. However, T activation has also been reported to occur in normal individuals. Although this phenomenon causes serologic problems in Blood Banks, it rarely, if ever, causes hemolysis in vivo.

The Tn phenotype is an acquired condition of unknown etiology that may be transient, but is usually persistent. It is a clonal disorder resulting from diminished (β1–3) galactosyltransferase activity arising in hematopoietic stem cells.[19] Thus, the Tn antigen is not only expressed on red cells, but it is also found on platelets and granulocytes. In most affected individuals, two populations of red cells are found: one normal and one polyagglutinable. Although this disorder may occur in healthy individuals, patients may present with immune-mediated hemolytic anemia, thrombocytopenia, or granulocytopenia or may subsequently develop acute leukemia.[20,21]

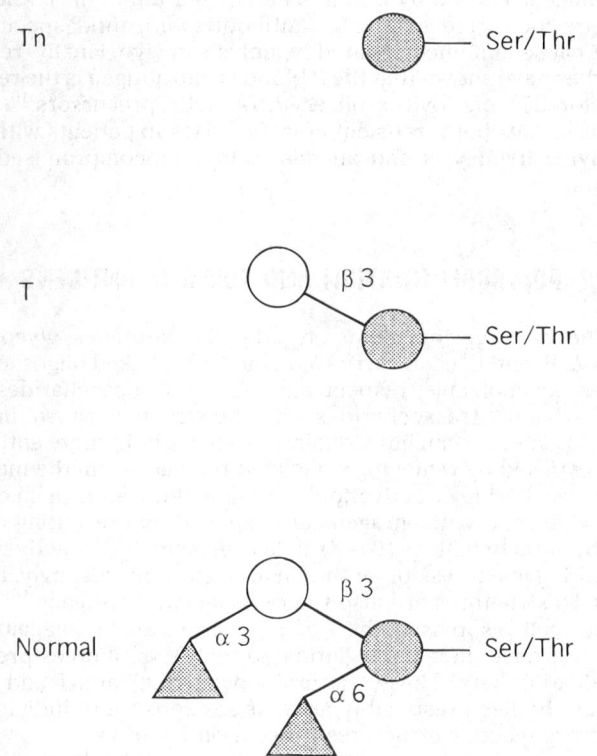

Fig. 131-7. Biochemical structures of O-linked oligosaccharides on glycophorins of normal red cells and of T- and Tn-activated polyagglutinable red cells. Oligosaccharides with the NeuAc(α2–6)GalNAc(α1–O)Ser/Thr structure are also found on Tn-activated red cells.[16] Closed triangle, N-acetylneuraminic acid (sialic acid). Disaccharide linkages involve C_2 on sialic acid. The other monosaccharides and disaccharide linkages are as described in the legends of figures 131-1 and 131-3.

Part 2
Protein Determinants

Marilyn J. Telen

INTRODUCTION

Numerous blood group antigens reside on membrane proteins and comprise determinants dependent primarily on amino acid sequence. The biochemical and genetic basis of many of these antigens has been elucidated in recent years (Table 131-9), and these advances have led to the use of molecular diagnostic techniques and even genetic engineering of blood group antigens. Some protein antigens typically stimulate brisk thymus-dependent immune responses, and the resulting high-titer IgG antibodies to such antigens may often result in rapid extravascular clearance of antigen-positive cells. These IgG antibodies may also cross the placenta, resulting in hemolytic disease of the newborn. For unknown reasons, other antigens, however, only rarely stimulate antibody production.

Rh BLOOD GROUP

The Rh blood group antigens are clinically the most important protein antigens. They are the most frequent targets of alloantibodies produced by transfusion recipients as well as

Table 131-9. Blood Group Antigens that Reside on Identified Erythrocyte Membrane Proteins

Blood Group System	Symbols for System and Major Antigens	Molecular Characterization, Other Nomenclature
Rh	Rh: D,E/e,C/c	30–32-kd Integral protein, highly fatty acid acylated
MN	M/N	Glycophorin A, sialoglycoprotein α
SsU	S/s,U	Glycophorin B, sialoglycoprotein δ
Kell	K/k, Js^a/Js^b, Kp^a/Kp^b, etc.	93-kd Protein of zinc-binding neutral endopeptidase family
Kidd	Jk^a/Jk^b	Poorly characterized
Duffy	Fy^a/Fy^b	35–46-kd Glycoprotein of the chemokine receptor family
Lutheran	Lu^a/Lu^b	78- and 85-kd Glycoprotein
Gerbich	Ge:2,3	Glycophorins C and D, sialoglycoproteins β and γ
Cromer	Cr^a, Tc^a, Dr^a, etc.	Decay accelerating factor (CD55)
Landsteiner-Weiner	LW^a/LW^b	37–47 kd-Glycoprotein
Cartwright	Yt^a/Yt^b	Acetylcholinesterase
Dombrock	Hy, Gy^a, Do^a/Do^b	46–57-kd Phosphatidylinositol-anchored glycoprotein
Indian	In^a/In^b	Hyaluronan receptor, CD44
Knops/McCoy	Kn^a, McC^a	Complement receptor type 1, CR1, CD35
Diego	Di^a/Di^b	Band 3, anion transport protein
Chido/Rodgers	Ch^a, Rg^a	C4 complement component
Colton	Co^a/Co^b	CHIP 28-kd Water channel protein
Scianna	Sc:1,2	60-kd Glycoprotein
JMH	JMH	76-kd Phosphatidylinositol-linked glycoprotein

by mothers alloimmunized to fetal antigens. The Rh antigen proteins are also frequent targets of autoantibodies responsible for idiopathic and drug-induced hemolytic anemias. Antibodies to Rh antigens are usually IgG and rarely fix complement. Nevertheless, they may induce rapid extravascular clearance of antibody-sensitized cells.

The Rh blood group comprises >40 individual antigens, of which 5 are routinely identified: D, C, c, E, and e. These 5 reside on three proteins, which are themselves the products of two extremely closely linked genes. The first Rh antigen to be defined was the Rh_o, or D, antigen. This antigen may be expressed or absent, giving rise to the so-called Rh-positive (D-positive) and Rh-negative (D-negative) phenotypes, respectively. No antigen antithetical to D has ever been identified. However, the other four antigens comprise two antithetical pairs: C and c, and E and e. Because of the tight linkage between the D and C/c/E/e loci, however, these five antigens are inherited en bloc. Certain genotypes are more common than others, although gene frequencies vary from one population to another (Table 131-10).[22]

LABORATORY METHODS FOR DETECTING BLOOD GROUP ANTIGENS AND ANTIBODIES

Manual methods based on agglutination of red blood cells are still the most common serologic assays performed in Blood Banks. Automated assays based on agglutination, and manual or automated solid-phase assays adherence assays not based on agglutination, are used in large blood centers or in research environments.

The serologic behavior of red blood cell antibodies primarily relates to their immunoglobulin isotype. Thus, most antibodies to carbohydrate antigens, such as those in the ABO, Lewis II, and P blood group systems, are naturally occurring and are of the IgM isotype. These multivalent antibodies optimally bind to red blood cells at temperatures below 37°C and directly agglutinate these cells suspended in saline. By contrast, antibodies occurring following immunization to protein antigens, such as those in the Rh, Kell, and Duffy blood group systems, are of the IgG isotype. These bivalent antibodies optimally bind to red blood cells at 37°C and will bind to, but not directly agglutinate, red cells suspended in saline. The addition of an antiglobulin reagent (i.e., rabbit anti-human IgG) is required to induce agglutination.

Antigen Typing of Human Red Blood Cells

Commercially available human polyclonal and mouse monoclonal IgM anti-A and anti-B antibodies are used to determine the ABO type of patient and donor red blood cells. These antibodies will directly agglutinate red blood cells at room temperature. To confirm a patient's ABO type, the presence of the corresponding serum isoagglutinins is also determined by incubating the serum at room temperature with commercially available group A and group B red blood cells. In both cases, hemagglutination is macroscopically visible, and an antiglobulin reagent is not required.

Patient and donor red blood cells are also routinely tested for the presence of the D antigen in the Rh system. A commonly used anti-D reagent is a chemically reduced IgG antibody that directly agglutinates D-positive red blood cells suspended in saline at room temperature.

Identification of Serum Alloantibodies or Autoantibodies Directed Against Red Blood Cells

Most alloantibodies found in patient sera are of the IgG isotype and therefore do not directly agglutinate antigen-positive red blood cells. Thus, the most common assay used to detect these antibodies is the indirect antiglobulin test, formerly known as the indirect Coombs test. In this assay, patient serum is incubated at 37°C with commercially available reagent red blood cells of known antigen type. Following incubation, unbound antibodies are removed from the red blood cells by washing with saline, and an antiglobulin reagent containing either rabbit anti-human IgG or a mixture of rabbit anti-human IgG and anti-human complement is added. If the red cells are agglutinated, this indicates the presence of an alloantibody or an autoantibody, or both. The distinction between alloantibody and autoantibody and the determination of the specificity of the alloantibody are determined by performing this assay with a panel of 10 different reagent red blood cells varying in antigen phenotype. Agglutination of all panel cells suggests the presence of an autoantibody; differential reactivity suggests the presence of an alloantibody to a specific red blood cell antigen.

The indirect antiglobulin test is also used to cross-match donor blood for transfusion into patients. In this case, patient serum is tested against red blood cells from a donor with a compatible ABO and D antigen type. A positive reaction indicates the probable presence of an alloantibody in the recipient directed against a donor red blood cell antigen. The specificity of this alloantibody can be determined by the approach outline above.

Detection of Red Blood Cells Coated In Vivo with Immunoglobulin and Complement

The direct antiglobulin test, formerly known as the direct Coombs test, detects the presence of antibody or complement (or both) on the surface of red blood cells. This technique is used in the analysis of delayed hemolytic transfusion reactions and in the evaluation of patients with suspected autoimmune hemolytic anemia. In this assay, unagglutinated patient red blood cells are obtained from EDTA anticoagulated blood, washed with saline, and then incubated with a commercially available antiglobulin reagent containing either rabbit anti-human IgG or a mixture of rabbit anti-human IgG and anti-human complement. The test is positive if agglutination is seen after the addition of the antiglobulin reagent. Antiglobulin reagents containing anti-IgM or anti-IgA are available in specialized centers to detect coating of red blood cells in vivo by antibodies of these isotypes.

(Continues)

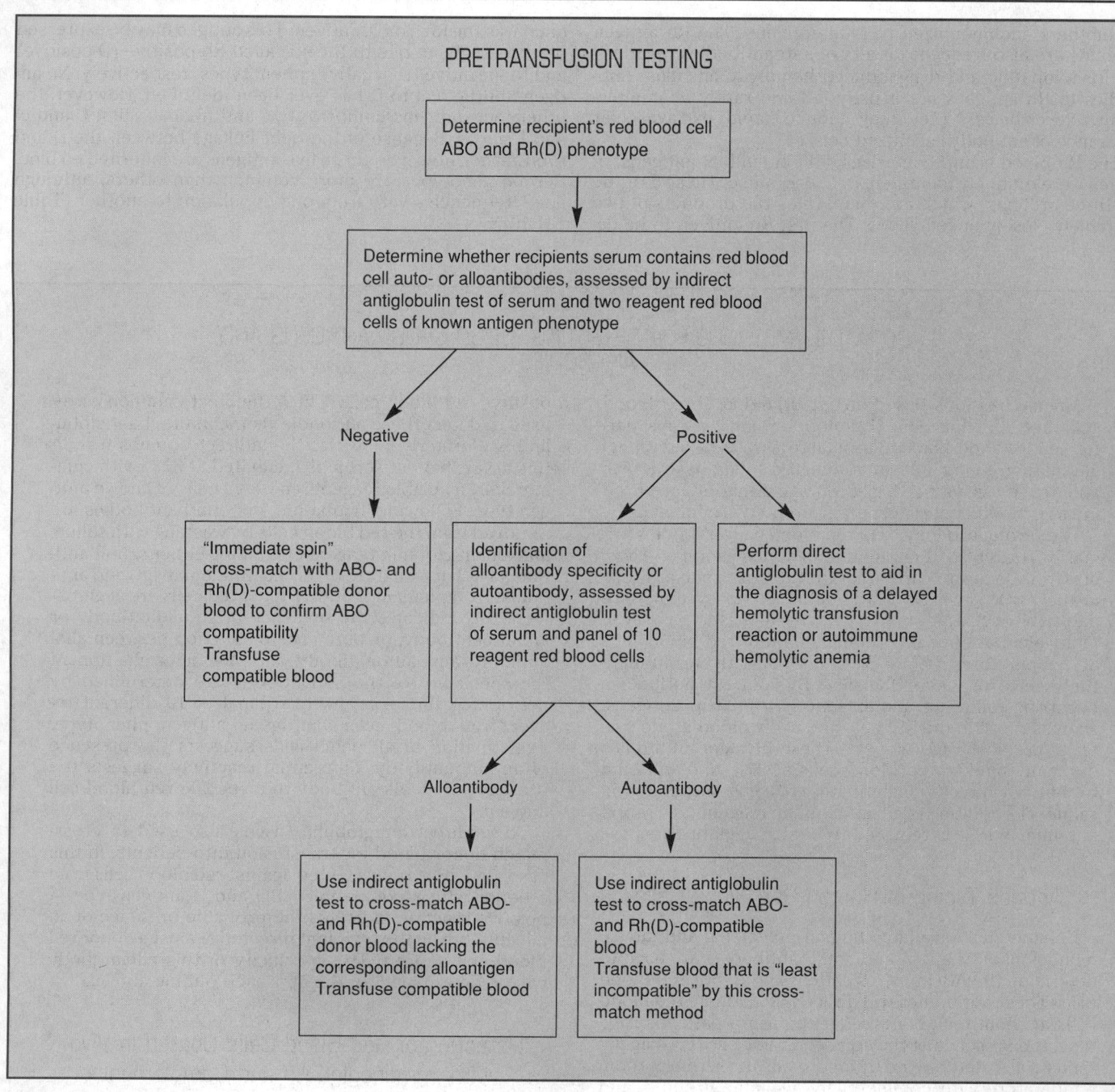

PRETRANSFUSION TESTING

Determine recipient's red blood cell ABO and Rh(D) phenotype

Determine whether recipients serum contains red blood cell auto- or alloantibodies, assessed by indirect antiglobulin test of serum and two reagent red blood cells of known antigen phenotype

Negative

Positive

"Immediate spin" cross-match with ABO- and Rh(D)-compatible donor blood to confirm ABO compatibility
Transfuse compatible blood

Identification of alloantibody specificity or autoantibody, assessed by indirect antiglobulin test of serum and panel of 10 reagent red blood cells

Perform direct antiglobulin test to aid in the diagnosis of a delayed hemolytic transfusion reaction or autoimmune hemolytic anemia

Alloantibody

Autoantibody

Use indirect antiglobulin test to cross-match ABO- and Rh(D)-compatible donor blood lacking the corresponding alloantigen
Transfuse compatible blood

Use indirect antiglobulin test to cross-match ABO- and Rh(D)-compatible blood
Transfuse blood that is "least incompatible" by this cross-match method

Table 131-10. Frequencies of Rh Gene Complexes in Different Populations

Gene Complex	Frequency	
	White Population	Black Population
DCe	0.40	0.17
dce	0.39	0.26
DcE	0.14	0.11
Dce	0.04	0.44
dCe	0.02	0.02
dcE	0.01	<0.001
DCE	<0.001	<0.001
dCE	<0.001	<0.001

The Rh blood group system also encompasses a large number of antigens that represent epitopes determined by rare Rh protein polymorphisms or epitopes common to most Rh proteins but recognized immunologically by those rare persons who are deficient in Rh proteins or whose cells carry only abnormal Rh protein molecules. These are the low- and high-frequency antigens of the Rh system. In addition, some Rh antigens exist when certain antigens are encoded in cis. The most common example is the f antigen, produced when the c and e antigens are encoded in cis. For example, f is expressed by the genotype *CDE/ce,* but not by the genotype *CDe/cDE,* even though both lead to expression of both the c and e antigens. Numerous other "cis" antigens have also been identified.

The null phenotype in the Rh blood group system has been

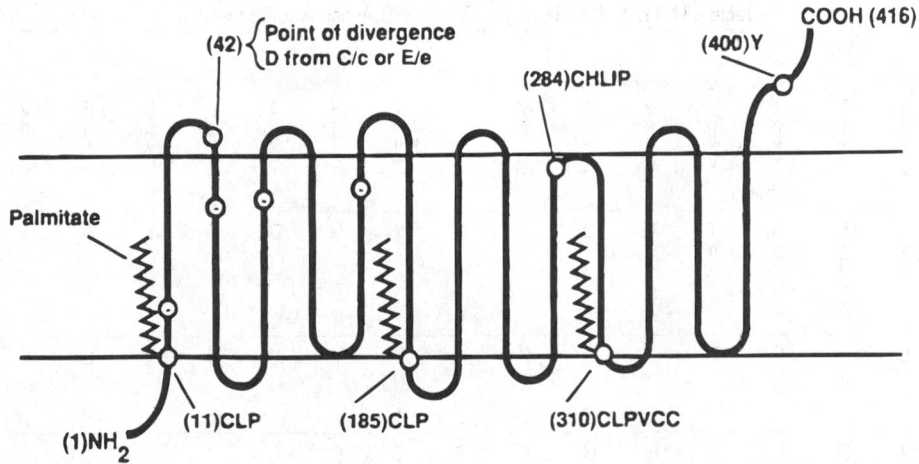

Fig. 131-8. Schematic representation of an Rh polypeptide corresponding to an E/e cDNA transcript. Analysis of predicted hydrophilic and hydrophobic domains generates a protein model that has 13 membrane spanning domains, a cytoplasmic N terminus, and an extracellular C terminus. Three cysteines located adjacent to the inner membrane leaflet cytoplasmic surface are likely to be sites for reversible fatty acid acylation. Some membrane spanning domains contain negatively charged amino acids (as indicated). The D polypeptide cDNA is compatible with a similar predicted structure and membrane orientation. (From Agre and Cartron,[57] with permission.)

extensively studied. Rh$_{null}$ erythrocytes express no Rh antigens. Most interestingly, these cells also exhibit a wide range of abnormalities,[23–25] including stomatocytosis, reduced cation and water content, increased ATPase activity, abnormal membrane phospholipid distribution, reduced membrane stability, and shortened survival in vivo. Thus, individuals with this phenotype have a mild-to-moderate chronic hemolytic anemia.

Biochemistry

Several proteins bearing Rh antigens have been identified and characterized[26,27] (Figure 131-8). Some investigators have used immunoaffinity purification methods, while others have used physicochemical methods.[28] Ultimately, these efforts resulted in isolation of 28,000–33,000-kd membrane proteins, all with common N-terminal sequences and a high degree of homology over the remaining protein domains. These proteins are highly hydrophobic and lack any detectable glycosylation, a highly unusual trait for membrane proteins. The Rh proteins make up a large portion of the fatty acid acylated proteins of the plasma membrane[29] and may also interact with the cytoskeleton.[30,31] Fatty acid acylation appears to be the result of a continuous "on and off" process of constant exchange of free palmitate for palmitate esterified onto cysteine residues within the portion of the molecule residing near the cytoplasmic border of the inner membrane leaflet.

Despite the marked abnormalities demonstrated by Rh$_{null}$ erythrocytes, in which Rh peptides are not expressed, no function has yet been attributed to these proteins. The multiple membrane spanning domains of the Rh peptides are reminiscent of transport proteins, but no transport function has been successfully demonstrated for Rh peptides. When Rh proteins are deficient, abnormalities in the expression of other membrane proteins are also detected. These include reduced or absent expression of the U antigen, known to be at least partly dependent on expression of glycophorin B. Expression of another glycoprotein, CD47 (see below), is also markedly reduced in Rh$_{null}$ cells. Some human and murine monoclonal antibodies coprecipitate several membrane proteins, including the Rh peptides and either CD47 and/or another glycoprotein, Rh50. This and additional evidence has led to the belief that the Rh

peptides exist in the membrane as part of a multiprotein complex that may include the Rh peptides, the Rh50 protein, CD47, and glycophorin B. Serologic evidence suggests that expression of the Rh and Duffy proteins may also be related.

Genetics

Two closely linked genes on chromosome 1 encode the proteins bearing the D, C/c, and E/e antigens.[32–34] One encodes the D protein; in persons with the Rh-negative (D-negative) phenotype, this gene is missing, so that Southern blots of genomic DNA show absence of a set of bands corresponding to a single Rh gene.[34] The other gene encodes either E or e, along with either C or c. Analysis of cDNAs shows that the E or e antigen is borne by a protein comprising all 10 exons of this gene, while the C or c antigen is presented by a protein formed without the use of exons 4, 5, and possibly 6. The difference between the coding regions of the D and E/e cDNAs consist of scattered nucleotide differences encoding only a relatively small number of amino acid differences. Both the D and E/e proteins have similar overall structure, including approximately 30% hydrophobic amino acid residues and 13 predicted transmembrane domains (Fig. 131-9). The C/c protein is slightly smaller, due to splicing out of some internal exons. The difference between the E and e proteins depends on a single amino acid polymorphism in one of the extracellular domains. The difference between the C and c proteins consists of four amino acid substitutions.

The cDNAs of two additional Rh-associated proteins have been cloned. The Rh-related glycoprotein Rh50 is encoded by chromosome 6 and its cDNA bears partial sequence homology to the Rh cDNAs encoded by chromosome 1.[35] In addition, the predicted structure of the protein is analogous to the D and C/c/E/e proteins. However, the Rh50 protein is glycosylated, unlike the Rh proteins.

The second Rh-related protein, which is widely expressed by human tissues, has been described by a number of names. Identification on leukocytes via monoclonal antibodies has led to its designation as CD47,[36] while its association with integrins in certain tissues has led to its description as an integrin-associated protein.[37] Unlike the Rh50 protein, CD47 bears no significant homology to the Rh polypeptides.

Table 131-11. Comparison of GPA and GPB Amino Acid Sequences[a]

M/N

GPA 1	(L)S	S	T	T	(E)G	V	A	M	H	T	S	T	S	S	S	V	T	K	S	Y
GPB 1	L	S	T	T	E	V	A	M	H	T	S	T	S	S	S	V	T	K	S	Y

GPA 21	I	S	S	Q	T	N	D	T	H	K	R	D	T	Y	A	A	T	P	R	A
GPG 21	I	S	S	Q	T	N	.	.	.	.	.	.	.	.	.	.	.	.	.	.

GPA 41	H	E	V	S	E	I	S	R	V	T	V	Y	P	P	E	E	E	T	G	E
GPG	.	.	.	.	.	.	.	.	.	.	.	.	.	.	.	.	.	.	G	E

GPA 61	R	V	Q	L	A	H	H	F	S	E	P	E			I	T	L	I	I
GPB 29	M/T	G	Q	L	V	H	R	F	T	V	P	A	P	V	V	I	I	L	I	I

S/s

GPA 78	F	G	V	M	A	G	V	I	G	T	I	L	L	I	S	Y	G	I	R	R
GPB 49	L	C	V	M	A	G	I	I	G	T	I	L	L	I	S	Y	S	I	R	R

GPA 98	L	I	K	K	S	P	S	D	V	K	P	L	P	S	P	D	T	D	V	P
GPB 69	L	I	K	A																

GPA 118	L	S	S	V	E	I	E	N	P	E	T	S	D	Q

[a]GPA and GPB genes are identical in the N-terminal domain (encoded by exon 2 of each gene). (Identity is indicated by vertical arrows between the two amino acid sequences.) However, the region corresponding to GPA exon 3 is a pseudoexon in the GPB gene due to mutation at one of the intron-exon junctions, preventing usage of the exon. Thus, a large midportion of GPA has no homologue in GPB. In the extracellular domain nearest to the membrane, as well as in the intramembranous domain, the two proteins are again highly homologous. However, GPA has a cytoplasmic tail that is lacking from GPB. The locations of the polymorphisms responsible for the M/N and S/s antigens on GPA and GPB, respectively, are indicated.

LW Antigens

The LW antigen, named for two pioneers in blood group antigens, Landsteiner and Weiner, is more strongly expressed by D+ than D− red cells. Indeed, LW is the true Rh antigen originally identified by these investigators using heterologous antisera to rhesus monkey red cells. Since its original identification, LW has been subdivided into LW[a] and LW[b]. Both antigens are borne by 37–47-kd glycoproteins encoded by a gene on chromosome 19.[38] Expression of these antigens is also abolished in the Rh$_{null}$ phenotype. However, the full relationship between the LW antigens and the Rh system remains to be determined.

MNSs BLOOD GROUP ANTIGENS

The M, N, and S/s antigens reside on two highly related integral membrane glycoproteins most often called glycophorin A (GPA) and glycophorin B (GPB).[39] GPA is one of the two most abundant erythrocyte integral membrane proteins, each of which exists as about 1×10^6 copies per cell. GPB is somewhat less abundant (0.8–3 $\times 10^5$ copies per cell). Together they account for 95% of the PAS-staining material in the red cell membrane and bear the great majority of the sialic acid residues that confer a negative surface charge to erythrocytes.

Antibodies to the M and N determinants of GPA may be immune or naturally occurring and may be allo- or autoimmune. These antibodies are rarely of clinical significance in transfusion, hemolytic disease of the newborn, and autoimmune he-

molysis. Antibodies to the S and s antigens, however, are most often IgG alloimmune antibodies that are capable of stimulating immune clearance of transfused or fetal red cells.

Biochemistry and Genetics

The glycophorins are highly homologous proteins whose genes lie close to each other on chromosome 4, apparently due to gene duplication.[40] GPB is smaller than GPA, because the region of the GPB gene corresponding to exon 3 of GPA is not used due to mutation of the intron-exon junction in the GBP gene. In addition, the cytoplasmic portion of the molecule is truncated (Table 131-11).

GPA bears an M or N antigen at its N terminus, depending on whether the N terminus comprises Ser-Ser-Thr-Thr-Gly··· or Leu-Ser-Thr-Thr-Glu···, respectively.[39] However, human anti-M and anti-N, which are usually IgM antibodies, often depend both on primary amino acid structure as well as appropriate glycosylation of the second, third and fourth amino acids (-Ser-Thr-Thr-).

GPB's N-terminal structure is homologous to that of the N variant of GPA through residue 26. At amino acid 29, GPB is polymorphic; the existence of a methionine corresponds to expression of the S antigen, while a threonine at this site gives rise to the s antigen.[39]

Null and Variant Phenotypes

Red cells may be totally deficient in either GPA or GPB, or both, without apparent shortening of red cell half-life or functional abnormalities. Lack of GPA or GPB, or both, are denoted as the En(a−), S−s−U−, and M^kM^k phenotypes, respectively.

The GPA and GPB genes also account for a large number of genetic variants, often associated with unique antigens. The variant phenotypes created by these genetic events have been designated Miltenberger phenotypes. These phenotypes arise from a number of different genetic events. Some represent simple point mutations. Others appear to arise from formation of variant GPA/B-type genes via unequal crossing over,[41,42] a phenomenon apparently dependent on the existence in close proximity to one another of the highly homologous GPA and GPB genes, along with a third homologous gene, denoted glycophorin E; thus, some molecules may consist of the N terminal portion of GPA, along with the C-terminal portion of GPB, or vice versa. Other variant glycophorin genes appear to result from gene-conversion events that result in genes that have small internal segments that correspond to the homologous gene.

Antibodies to the En^a and U antigens made by En(a−), U−, and M^kM^k individuals are almost always capable of markedly accelerating clearance of antigen-positive cells. Likewise, antibodies made to antigens carried by variant glycophorin molecules are frequently capable of causing hemolytic transfusion reactions and hemolytic disease of the newborn.

GERBICH ANTIGENS

Although antibodies to the Gerbich antigens are rarely encountered, their mention is appropriate, as they reside on two molecules that also bear the name glycophorins. Glycophorins C and D (GPC/D) are membrane glycoproteins that arise from a single gene by the use of alternate translation start sites.[43,44] Unlike GPA and GPB, to which they are unrelated, GPC/D are physiologically important membrane proteins that interact with the peripheral membrane protein band 4.1 to mediate attachment of the cytoskeleton to the membrane.[45] Complete lack of these glycoproteins, a phenotype designated Leach, results in absence of the Gerbich blood group antigens as well as a rare form of hereditary elliptocytosis.[46,47]

KELL BLOOD GROUP ANTIGENS

The Kell blood group system is extremely important from the point of view of transfusion medicine, as antibodies to the K antigen are among the alloantibodies most often identified. Antibodies to K, as well as to other Kell system antigens (Table 131-12), are in general IgG antibodies that are capable of rapidly clearing antigen-positive cells. The Kell blood group system includes three sets of well-defined antithetical antigens that have been mapped to chromosome 7.

Null and Variant Kell Phenotypes

Although most Kell system-related immune problems are caused by antibodies to antigens that belong to one of the three antithetical antigen pairs listed in Table 131-12, the unusual

Table 131-12. Commonly Identified Kell System Antigens

Symbol and Original Name	ISBT Alphanumeric Symbol	Frequency
K (Kell)	K1	Low
k (Cellano)	K2	High
Kp^a (Penney)	K3	Low
Kp^b (Rautenberg)	K4	High
Js^a (Sutter)	K6	Low
Js^b (Matthews)	K7	High

Abbreviation: ISBT, International Society of Blood Transfusion.

Kell phenotypes are quite interesting from a number of points of view. Rare individuals have been found who fail to express all Kell antigens, apparently due to inheritance of two nonfunctional (amorphic) Kell alleles. This phenotype, designated K_o, is associated with no morphologic or physiologic red cell abnormalities. However, another phenotype, associated with weakened Kell antigens, presents with acanthocytosis and mild chronic hemolytic anemia. This latter phenotype is associated with absence of the Kx antigen, and is often designated the McLeod phenotype. The Kx antigen is encoded at a locus on the X chromosome located near the loci for X-linked chronic granulomatous disease and Duchenne muscular dystrophy.[48]

Biochemistry and Genetics

The protein carrying the Kell antigens has been purified and its cDNA isolated and cloned.[49] This protein belongs to the family of zinc-binding neutral endopeptidases and is highly homologous to CD10 (CALLA, common acute lymphocytic leukemia antigen). The Kell protein comprises 732 amino acids, organized with one membrane-spanning domain, so that the C terminus is extracellular and the N terminus is in the cytoplasm.

Immunoprecipitation studies using antibodies to various Kell system antigens consistently isolate a protein of approximately 93,000 daltons. It thus appears that most or all Kell system antigens reside on a single protein, and that the various antithetical antigen pairs represent polymorphic epitopes on a single protein. However, these studies also demonstrated a second protein, of about 34,000 daltons, that appeared to be coprecipitated with the Kell protein. A similar 34,000-dalton protein is also precipitated by anti-Kx, and thus it is thought to be the *Kx* gene product.[50] The serologic characteristics of the K_o and McLeod phenotypes are thought to result from failure of the normal interaction of the Kell and Kx proteins.

KIDD BLOOD GROUP SYSTEM

The Kidd antigens are clinically important antigens, although their biochemistry and genetics remains poorly understood. Antibodies to these antigens are relatively common alloimmune antibodies that often fix complement. This property, as well as that antibodies to Kidd antigens often wane to undetectable levels after primary or secondary exposure, makes these antibodies frequent causes of delayed hemolytic transfusion reactions.

The two common alleles in this system—*Jk^a* and *Jk^b*—occur at about the same frequency in the white population. A rare allele that apparently encodes no Kidd protein is denoted *Jk*. Individuals homozygous for this amorphic allele express no Kidd antigens and may, after exposure to normal red cells, make anti-Jk3, an antibody that reacts with all cells that express Jk antigens. The Jk(a−b−) phenotype is of added interest because it can be shown to have a defect in urea transport; unlike normal red cells, Jk(a−b−) red cells will not lyse in 2M urea.[51,52]

DUFFY BLOOD GROUP ANTIGENS

The Duffy (Fy) antigens—Fy^a and Fy^b—occur with nearly similar frequencies in the white population, while approximately two-thirds of American and 90% of West African blacks are Fy(a−b−). Antibodies to Fy antigens are relatively common, most often IgG and immune in nature. Anti-Fy^a is slightly more common that anti-Fy^b. The Fy antigens appear to reside on a protein of 35,000–46,000 daltons that has recently been shown to be part of the chemokine receptor family of proteins.[53] The Duffy antigens have been investigated with intense interest because of their relationship to malarial resistance. *Plasmodium vivax,* a cause of human malaria, and *Plasmodium knowlesi,* a causative agent of malaria in monkeys, cannot invade Fy(a−b−) red cells, although *Plasmodium falciparum*—the malarial parasite causing the most serious human morbidity and mortality—can both attach to and invade Fy(a−b−) red cells.

LUTHERAN ANTIGENS AND RELATED PROTEIN ANTIGENS

The Lutheran blood group system is another system that comprises a large number of individual antigens, of which eight comprise four antithetical pairs. Only Lu^a and Lu^b, however, are frequently identified. Lu^b is expressed by >99% of individuals, while Lu^a is expressed by about 8%. In general, antibodies to Lutheran antigens are IgG in nature, although IgA and IgM antibodies have been reported; most are not effective in causing accelerated clearance of antigen-positive red cells. Lutheran antigens appear to reside on related proteins of 78,000 and 85,000 daltons[54]; little else is known about these proteins, other than that they are encoded by a gene on chromosome 19 at a locus linked to that of the secretor (*Se*) gene.

The Lutheran blood group system is of especial interest, however, because of the unusual genetic regulation of expression of Lutheran antigens. Although some Lu(a−b−) persons have inherited two amorphic (nonfunctional) Lutheran alleles, most examples of the Lu(a−b−) phenotype are due to inheritance of a single, dominant *In(Lu)* gene. This gene causes markedly reduced expression of Lutheran antigens, so that routine typing results in identification of a Lu(a−b−) phenotype. However, more sensitive techniques demonstrate expression of very small amounts of apparently normal Lutheran protein and antigens by these cells. In addition, the *In(Lu)* gene also suppresses expression of unrelated proteins, including the CD44 hyaluronan receptor,[55] a protein that carries another blood group, In.[56] In addition, *In(Lu)* may affect expression of other antigens, including the Knops and AnWj antigens.

A third type of Lu(a−b−) phenotype has also been identified. Like the *In(Lu)* phenotype, Lutheran antigens are suppressed but not totally absent. Other molecules, such as CD44, are not suppressed. Finally, this phenotype is inherited in an X-linked recessive manner, whereas the *In(Lu)* phenotype is inherited as an autosomal dominant trait.

OTHER BLOOD GROUP SYSTEMS

A large number of blood group systems and individual unrelated blood group antigens have been identified. However, a complete review of all these is beyond the scope of this chapter. The reader should keep in mind that some proteins bearing blood group antigens are functionally important, and that some—but by no means all—polymorphisms or deficiencies of such proteins may be accompanied by physiologically significant changes in red cell morphology, function, or survival. Antibodies to blood group antigens will continue to serve as obstacles to transfusion, as well as tools for investigating the surface structure of the erythrocyte.

REFERENCES

1. Mourant AE, Kopec AC, Domaniewska-Sobczak K: The Distribution of Human Blood Groups and Other Polymorphisms. 2nd Ed. Oxford University Press, London, 1976, p. 215
2. Walker RH (ed): Technical Manual. 10th Ed. American Association of Blood Banks, Arlington, VA, 1990, p. 178
3. Clausen H, Hakomori S-I: ABH and related histo-blood group antigens; immu-nochemical differences in carrier isotypes and their distribution. Vox Sang 56:1, 1989
4. Yamamoto F-I, Clausen H, White T et al: Molecular genetic basis of the histo-blood group ABO system. Nature 345:229, 1990
5. Yamamoto F-I, Hakomori S-I: Sugar-nucleotide donor specificity of histo-blood group A and B transferases is based on amino acid substitutions. J Biol Chem 265:19257, 1990
6. Ugozzoli L, Wallace RB: Application of an allele-specific polymerase chain reaction to the direct determination of ABO blood group genotypes. Genomics 12:670, 1992
7. Oriol R, Le Pendu J, Mollicone R: Genetics of ABO, H, Lewis, X and related antigens. Vox Sang 51:161, 1986
8. Sarnesto A, Kohlin T, Hindsgaul O et al: Purification of the secretor-type beta-galactoside alpha 1-2-fucosyltransferase from human serum. J Biol Chem 267:2737, 1992
9. Larsen RD, Ernst LK, Nair RP et al: Molecular cloning, sequence, and expression of a human GDP-L-fucose: beta-D-galactoside 1-alpha-L-fucosyltransferase cDNA that can form the H blood group antigen. Proc Natl Acad Sci USA 87:6674, 1990
10. Kukowska-Latallo JF, Larsen RD, Nair RP et al: A cloned human cDNA determines expression of a mouse stage-specific embryonic antigen and the Lewis blood group alpha(1,3/1,4)fucosyltransferase. Genes Dev 4:1288, 1990
11. Clausen H, Levery SB, Nudelman E et al: Further characterization of Type 2 and Type 3 chain blood group A glycosphingolipids from human erythrocyte membranes. Biochemistry 25:7075, 1986
12. Yamamoto F-I, McNeill PD, Hakomori S-I: Human histo-blood group A^2 transferase coded by A^2 allele, one of the A subtypes, is characterized by a single base deletion in the coding sequence, which results in an additional domain at the carboxyl terminal. Biochem Biophys Res Commun 187:366, 1992
13. Yamamoto F-I, McNeill PD, Yamamoto M et al: Molecular analysis of the ABO blood group system. 1. Weak subgroups: A^3 and B^3 alleles. Vox Sang 64:116, 1993
14. Bierhuizen MF, Mattei MG, Fukuda M: Expression of the developmental I antigen by a cloned human cDNA encoding a member of a beta-1,6-N-acetyl-glucosaminyltransferase gene family. Genes Dev 7:168, 1993
15. Bailly P, Piller F, Gillard B et al: Biosynthesis of the blood group P^k and P$_1$ antigens by human kidney microsomes. Carbohydr Res 228:277, 1992
16. Brown KE, Anderson SM, Young NS: Erythrocyte P antigen: cellular receptor for B19 parvovirus. Science 262:114, 1993
17. Blumenfeld OO, Lalezari P, Khorshidi M et al: O-linked oligosaccharides of glycophorins A and B in erythrocytes of two individuals with the Tn polyag-glutinability syndrome. Blood 80:2388, 1992
18. Springer GF: T and Tn, general carcinoma autoantigens. Science 224:1198, 1974
19. Cartron JP, Andreu G, Cartron J et al: Demonstration of T-transferase deficiency in Tn-polyagglutinable blood samples. Eur J Biochem 92:111, 1978
20. Dausset J, Moullec J, Bernard J: Acquired hemolytic anemia with polyagglutinability or red blood cells due to a new factor present in normal human serum (anti-Tn). Blood 14:1079, 1959
21. Ness PM, Garratty G, Morel PA et al: Tn polyagglutination preceding acute leukemia. Blood 54:30, 1979
22. Walker RH (ed): Technical Manual. 10th Ed. American Association of Blood Banks, Arlington, VA, 1990, p. 201
23. Sturgeon P: Hematological observations on the anemia associated with blood type Rh$_{null}$. Blood 36:310, 1970
24. Lauf PK, Joiner CH: Increased potassium transport and ouabain binding in human Rh null red blood cells. Blood 48:457, 1976
25. Kuypers F, van Linde-Sibenius-Trip M, Roelofsen B et al: Rh$_{null}$ human erythrocytes have an abnormal membrane phospholipid organization. Biochem J 221:931, 1984
26. Moore S, Woodrow CF, McClelland DBL: Isolation of membrane components associated with human red cell antigens (Rh)(D), (C), (E) and Fy(a). Nature 285:529, 1982
27. Gahmberg CG: Molecular characterization of the human red cell Rh$_0$(D) antigen. EMBO J 2:223, 1982
28. Agre P, Saboori AM, Asimos A, Smith BL: Purification and partial characterization of the Mr 30,000 integral membrane protein associated with the erythrocyte Rh(D) antigen. J Biol Chem 262:17497, 1987
29. de Vetten MP, Agre P: The Rh polypeptide is a major fatty-acid acylated erythrocyte membrane protein. J Biol Chem 263:18193, 1988
30. Ridgwell K, Tanner MJA, Anstee DJ: The Rhesus (D) polypeptide is linked to the human erythrocyte cytoskeleton. FEBS Lett 174:7, 1984
31. Gahmberg CG, Karhi KK. Association of Rho(D) polypeptides with the membrane skeleton in Rh$_0$(D)-positive human red cells. J Immunol 133:334, 1984
32. Cherif-Zahar B, Bloy C, Le Van Kim C et al: Molecular cloning and protein

structure of a human blood group Rh polypeptide. Proc Natl Acad Sci USA 87:6243, 1990

33. Avent ND, Ridgwell K, Tanner MJA, Anstee DJ. cDNA cloning of a 30 kDa erythrocyte membrane protein associated with Rh (Rhesus)-blood-group-antigen expression. Biochem J 271:821, 1990

34. Colin Y, Cherif-Zahar B, Le Van Kim C et al: Genetic basis of the RhD-positive and RhD-negative blood group polymorphism as determined by Southern analysis. Blood 78:2747, 1991

35. Ridgwell K, Spurr NK, Laguda B et al: Isolation of cDNA clones for a 50 kDa glycoprotein of the human erythrocyte membrane associated with Rh (rhesus)-blood-group antigen expression. Biochem J 287:223, 1992

36. Avent ND, Judson PA, Parsons SF et al: Monoclonal antibodies that recognize different membrane proteins that are deficient in Rh-null human erythrocytes. Biochem J 251:499, 1988

37. Rosales C, Gresham HD, Brown EJ: Expression of the 50-kDa integrin-associated protein on myeloid cells and erythrocytes. J Immunol 149:2759, 1992

38. Mallinson G, Martin PG, Anstee DJ et al: Identification and partial characterization of the human erythrocyte membrane component(s) which express the antigens of the LW blood group system. Biochem J 234:649, 1986

39. Chasis JA, Mohandas N: Red blood cell glycophorins. Blood 80:1869, 1992

40. Cartron J-P, Colin Y, Kudo S, Fukuda M: Molecular genetics of human erythrocyte sialoglycoproteins, glycophorins A, B, C, and D. p. 299. In Harris JR (ed): Blood Cell Biochemistry. Vol. 1: Erythroid cells. Plenum, London, 1990

41. Vignal A, Rahuel C, El Maliki B et al: Molecular analysis of glycophorin A and B gene structure and expression in homozygous Miltenberger class V (Mi.V) human erythrocytes. Eur J Biochem 184:337, 1989

42. Huang C-H, Blumenfeld OO: Molecular genetics of human erythrocyte MiIII and MiVI glycophorins: use of a pseudoexon in construction of two delta-alpha-delta hybrid genes resulting in antigenic diversification. J Biol Chem 266:7248, 1991

43. Colin Y, Le Van Kim C, Tsapis A et al: Human erythrocyte glycophorin C: gene structure and rearrangement in genetic variants. J Biol Chem 264:3773, 1989

44. El Maliki B, Blanchard D, Dahr W et al: Structural homology between glycophorins C and D of human erythrocytes. Eur J Biochem 183:639, 1989

45. Reid ME, Chasis JA, Mohandas N: Identification of a functional role for human erythrocyte sialoglycoproteins beta and gamma. Blood 69:1068, 1987

46. Daniels GL, Shaw M-A, Judson PA et al: A family demonstrating inheritance of the Leach phenotype: a Gerbich-negative phenotype associated with elliptocytosis. Vox Sang 50:117, 1986

47. Telen MJ, Le Van Kim M, Chung A et al: Molecular basis for elliptocytosis associated with glycophorin C and D deficiency in the Leach phenotype. Blood 78:1603, 1991

48. Frey D, Maechler M, Seger R et al: Gene deletion in a patient with chronic granulomatous disease and McLeod syndrome: fine mapping of the Xk gene locus. Blood 71:252, 1988

49. Lee S, Zambas ED, Marsh LW, Redman CM: Molecular cloning and primary structure of Kell blood group protein. Proc Natl Acad Sci USA 88:6353, 1991

50. Redman CM, Marsh WL, Scarborough A et al: Biochemical studies on McLeod phenotype red cells and isolation of the Kx antigen. Br J Haematol 68:131, 1988

51. Heaton DC, McLoughlin K: Jk(a−b−) red blood cells resist urea lysis. Transfusion 22:70, 1982

52. Frohlich O, Macey RI, Edwards-Moulds J et al: Urea transport deficiency in Jk(a−b−) erythrocytes. Am J Physiol 260:C778, 1991

53. Horuk R, Chitnis CE, Darbonne WC et al: A receptor for the malarial parasite *Plasmodium vivax*: the erythrocyte chemokine receptor. Science 261:1182, 1993

54. Parsons SF, Mallinson G, Judson PA et al: Evidence that the Lu[b] blood group antigen is located on red cell membrane glycoproteins of 85 and 78 kD. Transfusion 27:61, 1987

55. Telen MJ, Eisenbarth GS, Haynes BF: Human erythrocyte antigens. Regulation of a novel red cell surface antigen by the inhibitor Lutheran *In(Lu)* gene. J Clin Invest 71:1978, 1983

56. Spring FA, Dalchau R, Daniels GL et al: The In[a] and In[b] blood group antigens are located on a glycoprotein of 80,000 MW (the CDw44 glycoprotein) whose expression is influenced by the *In(Lu)* gene. Transfusion 64:37, 1988

57. Agre P, Cartron JP: Molecular biology of the Rh antigens: a review. Blood 78:555, 1991

Human Platelet Antigens

132

Thomas J. Kunicki

INTRODUCTION

A brief overview of the molecular biology of selected platelet membrane constituents is presented before an in-depth review of the antigens associated with them, so that the molecular basis of platelet antigenicity may be better understood. This overview focuses on those membrane constituents that are the most frequent antigenic targets of the human immune response to platelets, namely the integrins $\alpha_{IIb}\beta_3$ and $\alpha_2\beta_1$, the glycoprotein (GP)Ib/IX complex, and selected glycolipids.

Platelet Membrane Glycoproteins

Our understanding of platelet immunogenicity has closely paralleled progress in the identification and characterization of platelet glycoproteins during the past 10 years. The apparent molecular weight and subunit composition of platelet glycoproteins relevant to this chapter are summarized in Table 132-1.

Table 132-1. Selected Platelet Membrane Glycoproteins

Glycoprotein	Approximate Molecular Weight		
	Intact Molecule	Large Subunit	Small Subunit
Ib	170	143	22
α_5	150	134	27
α_{IIb}	136.5	114	22.5
α_v	160	135	25
α_2	155/170[a]		
β_1	130/145[a]		
β_3	95/115[a]		
IIIb (IV)	95		
V	80		
IX	20		

[a] Nonreduced/reduced.

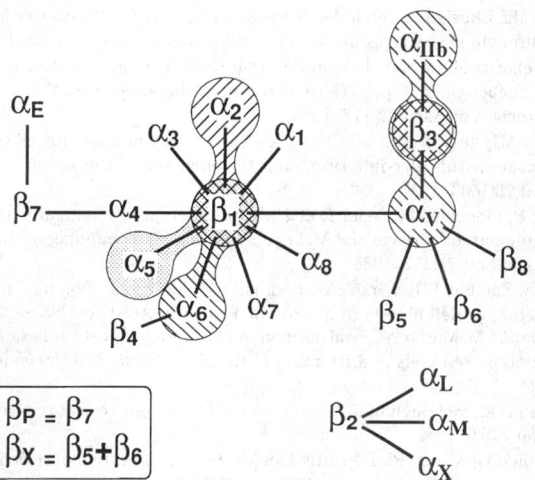

$$\beta_P = \beta_7$$
$$\beta_X = \beta_5 + \beta_6$$

Fig. 132-1. The integrin receptor family. Integrin α- and β-subunits are paired to form functional receptors, as indicated by solid connecting lines. Those integrins that exist on human platelets are highlighted and include $\alpha_2\beta_1$, $\alpha_5\beta_1$, $\alpha_6\beta_1$, $\alpha_v\beta_3$, and $\alpha_{IIb}\beta_3$.

Two membrane receptors that figure prominently in the antigenic profile of platelets, $\alpha_{IIb}\beta_3$ and $\alpha_2\beta_1$, are members of a large family of ubiquitous adhesion receptors known as the integrins.[1] Each integrin is a noncovalently associated heterodimer formed by a combination of α- and β-subunits (Fig. 132-1). Initial attempts to distinguish subgroups of the integrin family based on utilization of one of at least eight β-subunits have been thwarted by the finding that certain α-subunits (e.g., α_v, α_4, or α_6) can form functional complexes with several β-subunits. β_3 (Fig. 132-2), first cloned and sequenced from endothelial cell cDNA,[2] is a component of at least two receptors—$\alpha_{IIb}\beta_3$ and the vitronectin receptor $\alpha_v\beta_3$—and has been found to be expressed by a number of cell types, including platelets, endothelial cells, activated monocytes, and fibroblasts. However, α_{IIb} (Fig. 132-3) is a megakaryocyte-specific integrin subunit that has thus far been found only on platelets, megakaryocytes, or human erythroleukemic cell lines with a megakaryocytic phenotype.[3]

On platelets, $\alpha_{IIb}\beta_3$ functions as an activation-dependent receptor that recognizes at least two adhesive peptide motifs: the tripeptide-binding site Arg-Gly-Asp (RGD) found on numerous adhesive proteins and the C-terminal decapeptide sequence of the fibrinogen γ-chain[4,5] (Table 132-2). $\alpha_{IIb}\beta_3$ is considered the primary mediator of fibrinogen-dependent platelet cohesion (aggregation) and thus plays a pivotal role in platelet function. In addition, $\alpha_{IIb}\beta_3$ is involved in platelet clot retraction, although its role in this process is not precisely known. Glanzmann thrombasthenia (GT) is an inherited disorder of platelet function characterized by an inability of platelets to bind fibrinogen and to undergo agonist-induced aggregation.[6] The molecular defect in this disease is specific but heterogeneous and involves either a quantitative or a qualitative abnormality of $\alpha_{IIb}\beta_3$. The $\alpha_{IIb}\beta_3$ heterodimer complex is depicted schematically in Figure 132-4.

The platelet integrin $\alpha_2\beta_1$ functions as a receptor for various collagen types, including I and III[7,8] (Table 132-2). Unlike α_{IIb}, the α_2 subunit is a single-chain molecule[9] that contains an additional 129-amino acid segment known as the I domain (Fig. 132-5). Inherited platelet deficiencies of the α_2 subunit have been

Table 132-2. Functional Properties of Selected Platelet Membrane Glycoprotein Complexes

GP Complex	Receptor Function (Adhesive Protein Ligand)
IbIX	vWF
$\alpha_{IIb}\beta_3$	Collagen
	Fibrinogen
	Fibronectin
	Vitronectin
	vWF
$\alpha_2\beta_1$	Collagen
$\alpha_5\beta_1$	Fibronectin
$\alpha_6\beta_1$	Laminin
IIIb (IV; CD36)	Collagen
	Thrombospondin

Abbreviations: vWF, von Willebrand factor.

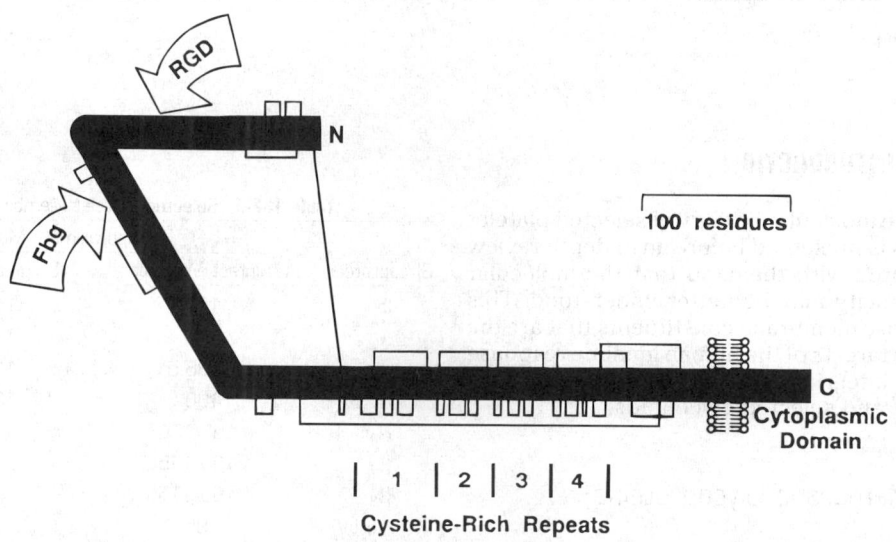

Fig. 132-2. Schematic diagram of the β_3 subunit. The β_3 subunit is a single-chain (thick solid line) transmembrane molecule. Twenty-eight intrachain disulfide bonds (thin lines) are present, at least one of which is thought to bring the N-terminal domain (N) proximal to the cysteine-rich domain consisting of at least four cystine-rich repeats at the C-terminal (C) third of the molecule. Regions of β_3 considered to bind to the RGD peptide motif and an unidentified segment of the fibrinogen (Fbg) molecule are indicated.

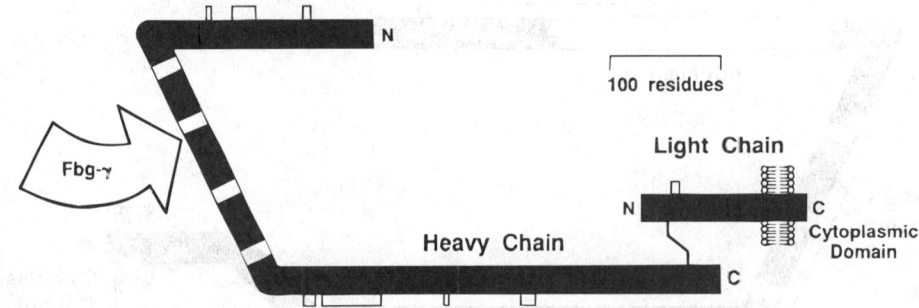

Fig. 132-3. Schematic diagram of the α_{IIb} subunit. α_{IIb} is composed to two chains (solid, thick lines) linked by a single interchain disulfide bond. The heavy chain contains seven intrachain disulfides (thin lines), four consensus calcium-binding repeats (open bars) and a recognition site for the C-terminal decapeptide sequence of the fibrinogen γ-chain (Fbg-γ). The light chain is a transmembrane molecule with a single intrachain disulfide.

described; these patients exhibit chronic mucocutaneous bleeding and prolonged bleeding times.[10,11] The expression of $\alpha_2\beta_1$ on platelets also differs markedly between normal subjects, as a result of an undefined but heritable polymorphism(s) in the α_2 subunit.[12] Moreover, the activity of $\alpha_2\beta_1$ on platelets of female subjects has been found to cycle in synchrony with plasma levels of estradiol,[13] suggesting that this integrin may be transcriptionally regulated by estrogen. The regulation of $\alpha_2\beta_1$ expression by these factors would certainly modulate the antigenicity of this membrane receptor. It is also possible that these or similar factors influence expression of other platelet

integrins, including $\alpha_{IIb}\beta_3$, but the extent to which that occurs remains to be determined. Two other integrins, the fibronectin receptor $\alpha_5\beta_1$[14] and the laminin receptor $\alpha_6\beta_1$,[15] are expressed by platelets, but neither has been shown to contribute significantly to platelet immunogenicity.

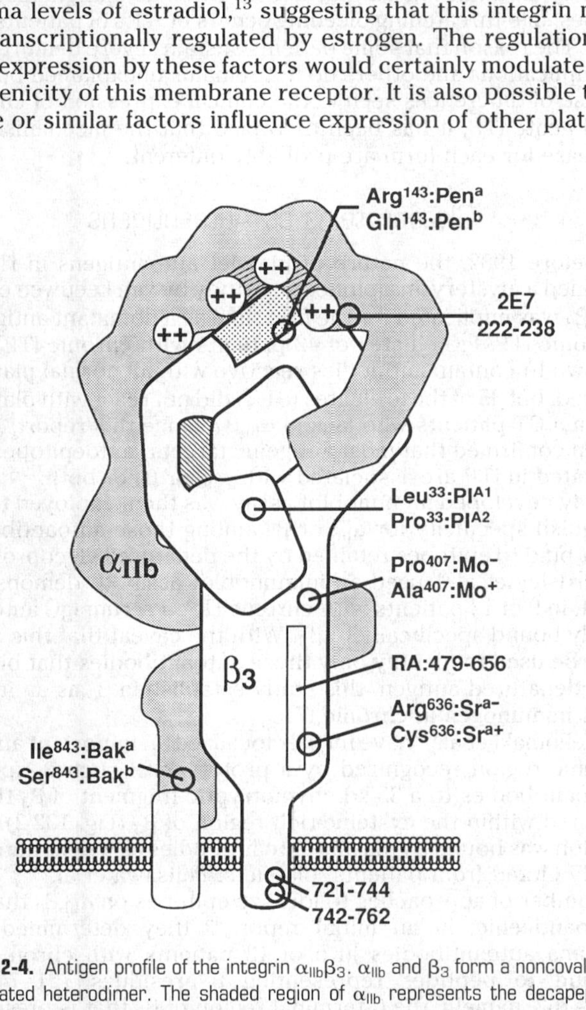

The pattern of membrane glycoproteins existing as noncovalent functional complexes is repeated in the case of the nonintegrin adhesion receptor GPIb/IX[16,17] (Fig. 132-6). GPIb/IX is the receptor for von Willebrand factor (Table 132-2), which is thought to be a primary mediator of platelet adhesion to the vessel wall under conditions of flow and high shear stress. Bernard-Soulier syndrome (BSS) is an inherited disorder of platelet function characterized by defective platelet adhesion to subendothelium and a quantitative or qualitative defect in GPIb/IX.

Platelet Glycolipids

Preliminary indications are that platelet glycolipids may represent significant autoantigens on the platelet surface. Although less is known about platelet glycolipid structure and immunogenicity, compared with the platelet glycoproteins, important contributions have recently been made to this area.[18] Glycolipids represent 3.2% of the total platelet lipid content, consisting of both acidic and neutral glycolipids. The predominant glycolipid on human platelets is lactosylceramide, representing 64% of neutral glycolipids. Other neutral glycolipids include trihexosylceramide, glycosylceramide, and globoside. The principal fatty acids associated with these neutral glycolipids are behenic acid (22:0), arachiditic acid (20:0), and lignoceric acid (24:0). Ganglioside I (identified as hematoside or GM3) represents 92% of the acidic glycolipids; ganglioside II represents 5% of the platelet acidic glycolipid composition. Recently, Koerner et al.[19] purified 13 platelet glycosphingolipid components and showed that two uncharacterized platelet glycosphingolipids may represent platelet-specific autoantigens.

ISOANTIGENS

Isoantibodies are produced against an epitope expressed by all normal individuals that is not polymorphic. In the area of human platelet immunology, a classic example of isoimmunization can and does occur when a patient with an inherited deficiency of a membrane glycoprotein has been subjected to multiple platelet transfusions in order to correct a bleeding diathesis. GT and BSS are such inherited disorders, wherein the individual either lacks or expresses an altered form of $\alpha_{IIb}\beta_3$ (GT) or GPIb/IX (BSS), respectively. Isoantibodies developed by transfused patients do not distinguish any of the allelic

Fig. 132-4. Antigen profile of the integrin $\alpha_{IIb}\beta_3$. α_{IIb} and β_3 form a noncovalently associated heterodimer. The shaded region of α_{IIb} represents the decapeptide recognition site. On β_3, the stippled region represents the RGD recognition site; the shaded region, an alternative fibrinogen recognition site. Divalent cations (positively charged spheres) are required for both complex integrity and ligand binding. The locations of the polymorphisms that give rise to alloantigens Pl^A, Pen, Bak, Mo, and Sr^a are indicated. Autoantigens have been localized to two sequences on the cytoplasmic tail of β_3, to a portion of the cysteine-rich domain bound by the RA prototype, and to a discrete sequence on α_{IIb} (2E7).

Figure labels:
Arg[143]:Pen[a]
Gln[143]:Pen[b]
2E7 222-238
Leu[33]:Pl[A1]
Pro[33]:Pl[A2]
Pro[407]:Mo[-]
Ala[407]:Mo[+]
RA:479-656
Arg[636]:Sr[a-]
Cys[636]:Sr[a+]
Ile[843]:Bak[a]
Ser[843]:Bak[b]
721-744
742-762
α_{IIb}
β_3

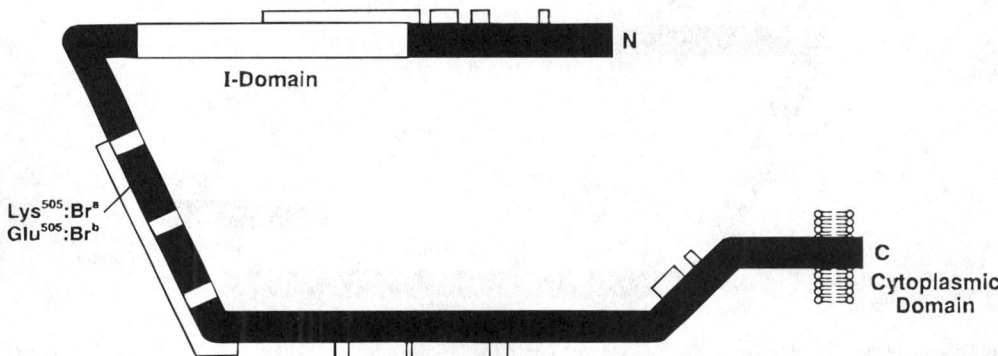

Fig. 132-5. The α_2 subunit. α_2 belongs to the subgroup of α-subunits that are single-chain molecules with an additional I-domain (large open bar) sequence. Three putative calcium-binding repeats are indicated (small open bars), as is the site of the alloantigenic Br polymorphism. Ten intrachain disulfides are depicted by thin lines.

forms of the glycoproteins (e.g., Bak or Pl^A alloantigens on $\alpha_{IIb}\beta_3$) but react with the platelets or all normal persons tested. Since the propositus does not express the platelet glycoprotein that carries the epitope in question, these antibodies do not bind to the patient's own platelets. Several cases have been documented wherein GT patients have produced antibodies specific for α_{IIb}, β_3, or the $\alpha_{IIb}\beta_3$ complex.[20–24] Since BSS is less frequently encountered than GT, it follows that isoantibodies produced in conjunction with this syndrome are also less frequently encountered. In the only clear-cut case of such an iso-antibody,[25] the isolated IgG impaired both normal platelet adhesion to subendothelial elements and in vitro aggregation in response to ristocetin and bovine factor VIII.

AUTOANTIGENS

Autoimmune (or idiopathic) thrombocytopenia (AITP or ITP) is the most frequently encountered form of immune thrombocytopenia.[26,27] This disorder can be classified as acute or

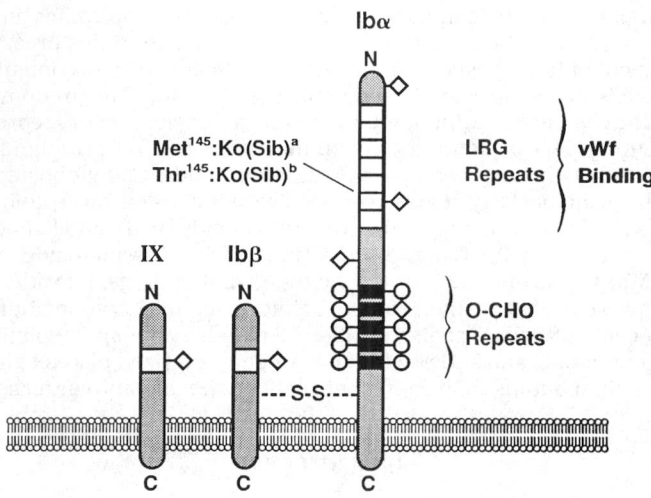

Fig. 132-6. GPIb/IX. GPIb is composed of a heavy chain (Ibα) and light chain (Ibβ) linked by a disulfide bond. The GPIb molecule is noncovalently associated with GPIX. All three polypeptides span the membrane, are glycosylated (open diamonds or circles), and contain repetitive sequences known as leucine-rich glycoprotein (LRG) repeats. In the case of Ibα, von Willebrand factor (vWF) binds at the N-terminal region of the molecule; five additional O-glycosylated repeats generate a carbohydrate-rich C region. The position of the Ibα polymorphism that gives rise to the Ko (Sib) alloantigen system is indicated.

chronic on the basis of the duration of the thrombocytopenia, the chronic form persisting >6–12 months (see Ch. 125). The acute, self-limiting form occurs predominantly in children, often following a viral illness or immunization, and affects males and females with equal frequency. The chronic form is mainly an adult illness that affects twice as many females as males. Life-threatening bleeding occurs in ≤1% of patients with ITP. The reason that some patients sustain severe hemorrhagic complications and others do not remains unexplained but, because of differences seen in the clinical expression of chronic and acute ITP, it has been theorized that the mechanisms of disease for each form are probably different.

Glycoproteins as Autoantigens

Before 1982, the nature of platelet autoantigens in ITP remained a mystery. In a pioneering study by van Leeuwen et al.[28] $\alpha_{IIb}\beta_3$ was implicated for the first time as a dominant antigen in chronic ITP. IgG eluates of 42 patients with chronic ITP were shown to contain antibodies reactive with all normal platelets tested, but 35 of these eluates (91%) did not react with platelets from a GT patients who lacked $\alpha_{IIb}\beta_3$. Since this report, it has been confirmed that most antigenic targets (autoepitopes) implicated in ITP are associated with α_{IIb} or β_3 or both.[29–35] The newly developed immunoblot assay was then employed to distinguish specificity for α_{IIb} or β_3 among those autoantibodies that bind to epitopes retained by the denatured glycoproteins. Beardsley et al.[30] used an immunoblot assay to demonstrate that, in 9 of 13 patients with chronic ITP, a serum IgG autoantibody bound specifically to β_3. With the caveat that this assay can be used to identify only those autoantibodies that bind to the denatured antigen, this study established β_3 as an important immunogen in chronic ITP.

Kekomaki et al.[35] have further localized an important autoantigenic region recognized by a prototype of such β_3-specific autoantibodies to a 33-kd chymotryptic fragment of β_3 that is located within the cysteine-rich region of β_3 (Fig. 132-2). This region was bound by plasma autoantibodies as well as autoantibody eluted from patients' platelets. Fujisawa et al.[36–38] used a number of approaches to localize epitopes on $\alpha_{IIb}\beta_3$ that are autoantigenic. In an initial report,[36] they determined that plasma autoantibodies in 5 of 13 patients with chronic ITP bound to peptides representing β_3 residues 721–744 or 742–762, namely, the C-terminal region of β_3 that is presumed to be located in the cytoplasm of the platelet. Subsequently,[37] these investigators observed that autoantibodies eluted from the platelets of additional ITP patients bind to other areas of β_3 within the extracellular portion of the molecule (perhaps to the 33-kd region defined by Kekomaki et al.[35]). Lastly, they determined that certain platelet-associated autoantibodies bind preferentially to cation-dependent conformational antigens on the $\alpha_{IIb}\beta_3$ complex.[38]

Autoantibodies reactive with α_{IIb} were identified in two patients with chronic ITP[33,34] in one of these patients, the antibody was subsequently shown to react with a chymotryptic 65-kd C-terminal fragment of the α_{IIb} heavy chain[34] (Fig. 132-3). EDTA-dependent autoantibodies represent a special category that are adsorbed by autologous platelets when whole blood is drawn in EDTA.[39] In one such case of EDTA-dependent "pseudothrombocytopenia," an IgM antibody was shown to bind to α_{IIb} by immunoblot assay and crossed immunoelectrophoresis.[40] One recent and particularly intriguing case of cyclic thrombocytopenia of apparent autoimmune origin was also found to be associated with an autoantibody to $\alpha_{IIb}\beta_3$.[41] As a final note, it should be remembered that, although most autoantibodies apparently induce thrombocytopenia, some can induce platelet dysfunction without an increase in platelet clearance (see Ch. 130). Two cases of "acquired thrombasthenia" due to autoantibodies against $\alpha_{IIb}\beta_3$ have been reported.[42,43] Indeed, one is led to speculate, not unreasonably, that the proportion of the two types of autoantibody—one leading to platelet clearance and one blocking platelet function—may be a very important factor controlling the unpredictable clinical severity of ITP.

$\alpha_{IIb}\beta_3$ is not the only integrin implicated as the antigen target for human autoantibodies. Serum IgG autoantibodies specific for GPIa (integrin subunit α_2) were identified in a unique case of autoimmune platelet dysfunction following myasthenia gravis.[44] This autoantibody inhibited aggregation of normal platelets induced by collagen or wheat germ agglutinin. This is the first case wherein autoantibodies to GPIa were associated with a chronic hemorrhagic disorder, and this study actually provides strong indirect support for a role of the platelet integrin $\alpha_2\beta_1$ in hemostasis in vivo.

Autoantibodies to GPIb/IX are the second most frequently encountered autoantibodies in adult chronic ITP.[45] In some cases in which autoantibody to GPIb/IX was detected, the clinical presentation proved particularly severe and refractory to therapy.[46] One case of pseudo-BSS (dysfunction of GPIb/IX) was reported to be caused by an autoantibody to GPIb.[47]

It had been hoped that the antigenic targets in acute and chronic forms of ITP might be different so that antigen identity might one day be used as an early indicator of clinical outcome. Early comparisons between antigens in acute and chronic ITP raised hopes that this would be the case. In one study, four children with acute varicella-associated thrombocytopenia were found to have autoantibodies reactive with a thrombin-sensitive 85-kd glycoprotein fitting the description of GPV.[48] A possible association of GPV with acute ITP was also proposed by a second study in which six of seven patients were observed to have antibody of this specificity.[49] Subsequent studies have shed more light on the similarities between autoantibody specificity in chronic versus acute ITP, particularly in children.[50,51] In the report of Berchtold et al.,[50] serum IgG autoantibodies specific for $\alpha_{IIb}\beta_3$ were detected, by immunobead assay, in 14 of 24 (58.3%) children with chronic ITP. By the same method, autoantibodies to $\alpha_{IIb}\beta_3$ were detected in 4 of 15 (26.7%) children with acute ITP. Additional findings were as follows: none of the patients had IgG antibodies specific for GPIb/IX; the level of IgG autoantibody to $\alpha_{IIb}\beta_3$ was about fourfold higher, on average, in chronic ITP; in chronic ITP, there was no correlation between serum IgG autoantibody level and platelet count. These results in chronic childhood ITP were essentially identical to previous findings in adults, where 56% of patients had autoantibody to $\alpha_{IIb}\beta_3$.[31] Along the same lines, Winiarski,[51] using an immunoblot assay, found that sera from 13 of 21 children with acute ITP had IgG or IgM antibodies that bound to

platelet proteins. Of these 13 sera; 5 bound to β_3; 1 to α_{IIb}; 4 to GPIb, 1 to an unidentified 250-kd protein; and 12 to smaller protein antigens ranging in size from 25 to 52 kd. Comparing these last two reports, one finds conspicuous differences in the latter report: the somewhat higher frequency of antibodies reactive with $\alpha_{IIb}\beta_3$ (67%) and the finding of antibodies against GPIb. This can be attributed to differences in the methods used to detect antibodies but may also reflect that Winiarski[51] measured both IgG and IgM, while Berchtold et al.[50] screened only for IgG.

Despite this retrospective evidence, a distinction between antigen specificity and an acute versus chronic course in ITP may yet be found in the early stages of the autoimmune response. Clearly, prospective studies aimed at answering this question are still warranted.

How large is the autoepitope repertoire on a given glycoprotein antigen? This important question needs to be addressed, because the answer will have an impact on the feasibility of developing therapeutic and diagnostic measures based on epitope specificity. Since the autoantibodies that react with a given epitope are likely to share idiotypes, two approaches can be used, analyzing either the epitope repertoire or the idiotype repertoire, or both. Two studies have addressed the extent of the autoantigen repertoire on $\alpha_{IIb}\beta_3$ by analyzing the competitive binding between human autoantibodies and murine monoclonal antibodies.[52,53] In the earlier report,[52] the binding of one murine monoclonal antibody, 3B2, was found to show decreased reactivity with platelets from 16 ITP patients, presumably because the platelet-associated autoantibodies bound to sites at or close by the 3B2 epitope. This finding would argue for homogeneity of autoepitopes on $\alpha_{IIb}\beta_3$. In the latter study,[53] the ability of four murine monoclonal antibodies specific for $\alpha_{IIb}\beta_3$ to block autoantibody binding to heterologous platelets was analyzed. IgG fractions from six different ITP patients were found to react with apparently different epitopes on $\alpha_{IIb}\beta_3$. On the basis of the limited number of studies in which this approach was used and the conflicting results to date, insufficient data are available with which to judge the size of the autoepitope repertoire on $\alpha_{IIb}\beta_3$. Additional analyses aimed at epitope localization will be necessary, and perhaps novel approaches will expedite this task. One such novel approach is the development of human monoclonal autoantibodies specific for $\alpha_{IIb}\beta_3$ and other platelet glycoproteins.

Human monoclonal antibodies are a promising new tool used in the search for glycoprotein epitopes that are autoimmunogenic in humans. The first human monoclonal antibody against a platelet glycoprotein was developed by Nugent et al.,[54] derived from an ITP individual producing an antibody against β_3. This human monoclonal antibody detects a neoantigen associated with β_3 that is expressed only on stored or thrombin-activated platelets. A number of human monoclonal autoantibodies specific for the heavy chain of GPIb were generated from the lymphocytes of an ITP patient with serum autoantibody specific for GPIb.[55] The heavy chain variable region genes of four of these antibodies have been sequenced and found to be markedly homologous to human immunoglobulin germline heavy chain variable region genes.[55] Most recently, another human monoclonal autoantibody was produced that is specific for the heavy chain of α_{IIb}.[56] The epitope recognized by this antibody has been identified as a contiguous amino acid sequence with residues 231–238 with an immunodominant tryptophan residue at position 235[57] (Fig. 132-3). This is the first identification of the precise epitope on α_{IIb} or β_3 recognized by a human antibody.

From the foregoing analysis, it is clear that further studies are required to determine the extent to which the production of human autoantibodies to platelet glycoproteins is clonally restricted. Given a selected number of idiotypes related to autoimmunity to $\alpha_{IIb}\beta_3$, one could potentially use the anti-idiotype to modulate immunization to $\alpha_{IIb}\beta_3$. Along these lines, it has been reported that intravenous immunoglobulin, which is routinely used to reverse acute thrombocytopenia in ITP, may contain anti-Id directed to idiotypes of autoantibody but not alloantibodies that recognize $\alpha_{IIb}\beta_3$.[58] Recently, Nugent et al.[46] defined a DM idiotype that is characteristic of human autoantibodies specific for the GPIb heavy chain. The latter study clearly suggests that the repertoire of idiotypes expressed by human autoantibodies specific for membrane glycoproteins, such as those of the human platelet, will be narrowly defined and, thus, amenable to study.

Platelet Protein Autoantigens in ITP Secondary to Other Immune Disorders

Autoimmune thrombocytopenia secondary to another autoimmune disorder, such as systemic lupus erythematosus (SLE) (e.g., SLE-ITP) or primary biliary cirrhosis, are conditions in which the platelet autoantigens are largely different from those implicated in primary ITP. The immunoblot assay has been the principal method used to identify platelet protein antigens in SLE-ITP. By means of this approach, IgG autoantibodies have been detected that react with protein antigens with apparent molecular weights of 65, 80, 108, and 120.[59–61] Howe and Lynch[59] were the first to detect antibodies to both the 80- and 120-kd antigens in 10 of 10 patients with SLE. This antigen-binding pattern was not observed in sera from 20 normal individuals and infrequently in 20 patients with ITP.

We have determined that the 120- and 80-kd antigens frequently detected by immunoblot assay with sera from thrombocytopenic patients are intact and fragmented vinculin, respectively.[62] In contrast to the report by Howe and Lynch,[59] we find antibodies reactive with vinculin in 67% of patients with primary ITP or secondary immune thrombocytopenia and in 40% of normal subjects. The finding of antivinculin antibodies in the sera of normal individuals by immunoblot assay had previously been made by Pfueller et al.[63] More recently, Reid et al.[64] confirmed the presence of immunoglobulin reactivity against vinculin or talin in the sera of normal subjects. In our studies, however, the levels of these antibodies in sera of patients with active autoimmune thrombocytopenia were at least two orders of magnitude higher than found in sera of normal individuals.[62]

Additional studies of another of these protein antigens, the 65-kd protein, have determined that it is a membrane-associated internal protein with a pI of 4.7–5.2, which is not recognized by polyclonal rabbit antisera specific for vimentin, a previously identified antigen target of SLE autoantibodies that has similar electrophoretic characteristics.[65]

Autoantibodies reactive with $\alpha_{IIb}\beta_3$ were detected in a patient who unexpectedly developed thrombocytopenia after a 4-year history of primary biliary cirrhosis.[66] Additional platelet-reactive antibodies were found that bound to the 70-kd mitochondrial antigen M2, considered a primary antigenic target in about 95% of cases of primary biliary cirrhosis. On the basis of these findings, the intriguing hypothesis was put forward that $\alpha_{IIb}\beta_3$ and the 70-kd mitochondrial antigen bear cross-reactive epitopes. Indeed, two short sequences were found to be homologous when human β_3 and human M2 antigens were compared, but neither corresponds to the reported immunodominant epitope of the M2 protein.[67] Unfortunately, cross-adsorption studies were not performed, and it has not been established that both antigens are bound by the same population of autoantibodies. The putative immunologic association between the two proteins was not strengthened by the fact that sera from 10 other patients with primary biliary cirrhosis did not contain antibodies reactive with platelet antigens, and sera from an undisclosed number of patients with ITP known

Table 132-3. Glycolipid Antigens of Platelets

Cardiolipin
Lactosylceramide
Glycosphingolipids
Acidic (sulfatides/gangliosides, monogalactosyl sulfatide [16/6 idiotype])
Neutral (globotriosylceramide, globotetraosylceramide)

to contain antibodies to $\alpha_{IIb}\beta_3$ did not contain antibodies that bind to the M2 protein.

Caution is also advised in the exclusive use of immunoblot assays to detect less dominant protein antigens as targets for autoantibodies. Reid et al.[68] have very convincingly pointed out that control normal sera often generate antigen profiles very similar to those considered characteristic of autoimmune disease; 85% of normal sera were found to contain IgG that bound to protein bands at 90–95 kd. Less often, positive bands at 100–110 kd, 80–85 kd, 60–75 kd, and 50–60 kd were also seen with normal sera. This study emphasizes the need for a rigorous distinction of quantitative variations in the patterns produced by normal sera before attributing positive reactions to the presence of true disease-associated autoantibodies. Naturally, this distinction is one of association. The argument is clearly being made that true disease-associated pathogenic autoantibodies will be associated with clinically definable autoimmune disease and will not be present in apparently normal individuals. One could also make the argument that autoantibodies identical to those characteristic of patients with bona fide clinical autoimmune disease might well exist in the sera of normal individuals and remain nonpathologic, as long as their effector functions are actively controlled.

Glycolipids as Antigens

A number of reports have implicated cardiolipin, lactosylceramide and other glycosphingolipids (GSLs) as autoantigenic targets[19,69–74] (Table 132-3). van Vliet et al.[72] analyzed the binding of serum IgG/IgM antibodies from 30 ITP patients to platelet GSLs separated by high-performance thin-layer chromatography. Acidic GSLs, namely sulfatides and gangliosides, were identified as the major targets of serum autoantibodies. Of the 30 sera, 13 (5 with anticardiolipin antibodies) had antibodies that bound to sulfatides, while 4 sera showed antibody binding to gangliosides. Koerner et al.[19] employed a more efficient phase-partition separation of acidic GSL from neutral GSL and were able to demonstrate that serum antibodies specific for neutral GSL were more characteristic of ITP. Two classes of GSL autoantigens were defined: those associated with general autoimmunity and detected in the sera of patients with either SLE or ITP, and those peculiar to platelet-specific autoimmunity and detected only in the sera of ITP patients. Two GSL forms belong to the platelet-specific group, but they are present at minute levels, and further characterization awaits large-scale purification. One-half (6 of 12) of patients with ITP had serum IgG or IgM antibodies that bound these platelet-specific GSLs. Sera from none of 10 patients with nonimmune thrombocytopenia, none of 10 patients with SLE, and only 1 of 18 normal subjects gave positive reactions with the platelet-specific GSL group. The general GSL antigen group includes globotriaosylceramide, globotetraosylceramide, and a third unidentified neutral GSL. Antigens in the general group were bound by IgG or IgM antibodies in the sera of 10 of 10 patients with SLE, 8 of 12 patients with ITP, and none of 10 patients with nonimmune thrombocytopenia or 18 control subjects. These findings provide compelling support for a role of neutral GSL as antigenic targets in ITP.

Autoantibodies that cross-react with single-stranded or double-stranded DNA, cardiolipin, and platelet-surface antigens are among the serologic findings in patients with active SLE. Monoclonal IgM anti-DNA autoantibodies have been produced from hybridomas prepared from lymphocytes of SLE patients and shown to react with platelet acidic glycolipids.[75,76] Several antibodies of this type express a dominant 16/6 idiotype[77]; the complete amino acid sequences of the heavy and light chain variable regions of one prototype HF2-1/17 were determined by Lampman et al.[78] The heavy chain is characterized by a V_HIII subgroup framework and is nearly identical to the product of the VH26 germline gene. The framework of the light chain is typical of the $V_κI$ subgroup and is homologous to other immunoglobulins of known primary structure, including WEA, GAL, HAU, HK101, and DEE.[78] These findings indicate that the 16/6 idiotype is derived with little or no modification from germline genes. In an effort to define the molecular basis for the polyreactivity of antibodies bearing the 16/6 idiotype, Lampman et al.[78] generated a molecular model of the combining site of the prototype antibody HF2-1/17. Arg 24 and Arg 30 within CDR1 of the light chain are the only positively charged residues in any of the CDR of the heavy or light chains. These residues are exposed in the hypothetical model and would consequently be available for contact with negatively charged phosphate groups of DNA or sulfate groups of platelet glycolipid antigens. A correlation between the DNA-binding properties of 16/6 idiotype antibodies and the presence of light chain Arg 24 and Arg 30 is strengthened by the finding that the light chains of each of the DNA-binding antibodies 1/17, 16/6, 18/2, 21/28, WEA, and GAL have arginine residues at both positions. The platelet autoantigen bound by the cross-reactive antibodies bearing the 16/6 idiotype has very recently been identified as monogalactosylsulfatides.[79]

HIV-Associated ITP

Immune thrombocytopenia associated with human immunodeficiency virus (HIV) infection occurs predominantly among three groups of individuals, patients with hemophilia who previously were exposed to contaminated concentrates of factor VIII,[80] narcotic addicts[81] and homosexuals.[82] Clinically, HIV-associated ITP is indistinguishable from classic primary ITP, although there is some indication that the immune mechanisms involved in the etiology of ITP among narcotics addicts and homosexuals may be different from those operative in classic primary ITP and HIV-infected hemophilic patients.[26,81–83] Hemophilic patients and classic ITP patients exhibit notable similarities that distinguish them from the other two disorders; that is, one sees an inverse relationship between platelet count and platelet-bound IgG, anti-platelet IgG can be eluted from patients' platelets, and one does not see a significant increase in circulating immune complexes. Compared with patients with classic ITP, all three groups of HIV-associated patients with immune thrombocytopenia present with significantly higher levels of platelet-bound IgG and complement components C3 and C4.[81,82,84,85]

While an initial report showed that the antigens involved in HIV-associated ITP might be unique,[86] subsequent studies have not substantiated this finding. Using an immunoblot assay, Stricker et al.[86] found antibodies in the sera of 29 of 30 patients with HIV-related ITP that bound to a 25-kd platelet protein. They concluded that antibodies specific for HIV antigen(s) cross-react with this unidentified platelet protein. This protein antigen was not further characterized, and the presence of antibody reactive with this protein did not correlate with the presence of thrombocytopenia in these patients. The prevalence of this antibody specificity in HIV-associated ITP has not been established since this initial report. By contrast, Klaasen et al.[87] found that autoantibodies both in sera and eluted from the platelets of 16 patients with acquired immunodeficiency syndrome (AIDS) have specificities largely the same as those seen in primary chronic ITP, most specific for antigens on $α_{IIb}β_3$.

Bettaieb et al.[88] analyzed antiplatelet antibodies in the sera and on the platelets of 68 HIV-infected, but AIDS-free, patients with ITP. Serum IgG specific for platelet antigens was detected in 72% of these patients. These IgG antibodies did not bind to surface antigens but reacted with intracytoplasmic constituents. Platelet-bound antibodies were detected in 75% of patients and isolated in ether eluates. In 44% of cases, the eluted antibodies were found to bind to normal, but not to thrombasthenic, platelets. By immunoprecipitation, the specificity of autoantibodies in six eluates was determined. In two cases, $α_{IIb}$ was the target; in one case, $β_3$. In three other cases, reactivity with an unidentified 150-kd protein was observed. This study confirms the generalization that autoantibody specificity in HIV-ITP is not different from that reported for classic primary ITP.

Anticardiolipin antibodies (ACAs) are frequently detected in the sera of HIV-infected patients,[89] and a role for ACAs in the etiology of the ITP that often accompanies HIV infection has been postulated. This association is based largely on reports that ACAs are prevalent in sera of patients with chronic ITP,[70] a correlation is observed between ACAs and thrombocytopenia in SLE,[69] and human hybridomas established from peripheral blood lymphocytes of patients with SLE produce monoclonal antibodies that bind both to cardiolipin and human platelets.[75,76,90] Conflicting evidence also exists in the literature. For example, Klaassen et al.[87] noted the important discrepancy that, although ACAs were detected in the sera of every patient with AIDS they analyzed, ACAs were never present in eluates prepared from the platelets of the same patients.

Indeed, while several laboratories argue that thrombocytopenia in HIV-infected persons is a direct result of platelet-specific autoantibodies,[86,87,91,92] it has also been proposed that it results from deposition on platelets of immune complexes.[84,93] This conclusion is based on the findings that (1) the amount of platelet-associated immunoglobulin in HIV-infected persons with ITP is much higher than that observed in cases of classic primary ITP[84]; (2) the amount of platelet-bound complement is increased in the case of HIV-infected patients with ITP[84]; and (3) in eluates of platelets from HIV-infected patients with ITP, not only anti-HIV antibodies but also anti-anti-HIV antibodies (anti-idiotypic antibodies) can be detected.[93] Although the level of such complexes was not measured in HIV-infected persons without thrombocytopenia as a control, Karpatkin et al.[93] argued that immune complexes composed of anti-HIV (idiotype) bound by anti-idiotypic antibodies are the cause of Fc receptor-mediated thrombocytopenia in HIV-infected persons. This conclusion is not supported by the study conducted by Klaassen et al.,[87] wherein only weak reactivity against HIV antigens was observed in eluates of patient platelets and equivalent weak reactivity was observed in all HIV-infected patients regardless of the presence or degree of thrombocytopenia. Clearly, the relative contribution of autoantibodies specific for GSLs, phospholipids, or glycoproteins to the pathology of ITP warrants further investigation.

DRUG-DEPENDENT IMMUNE THROMBOCYTOPENIA: A UNIQUE FORM OF AUTOIMMUNITY

Quinine/Quinidine Purpura

Although drug-induced thrombocytopenia (DITP) may be a complication of therapy employing a variety of drugs, it is most frequently seen in the Untied States with the administration of quinine and quinidine.[94] It has been proposed that the following criteria be met before an individual can be considered to have DITP: (1) the patient is not thrombocytopenic before administration of the drug; (2) thrombocytopenia follows drug ingestion and begins to reverse shortly after cessation of drug; (3) thrombocytopenia does not recur after cessation of drug treatment; and (4) all other causes of thrombocytopenia are ruled out.[95]

The precise mechanism for platelet clearance is not certain. However, cumulative evidence favors a mechanism whereby the drug induces the expression of a neoantigen on the platelet surface[96-101] that is recognized by circulating antibodies only in the presence of the drug. The observation that platelets from BSS patients (lacking in GPIb/IX, and GPV) failed to lyse in the presence of drug-dependent antibody (ddAb), specific drug, and complement, was the first indication that a specific platelet antigen is recognized by ddAb.[101] This finding led other laboratories to confirm that purified GPIb/IX would compete for drug plus ddAb and was therefore likely to contain the antigenic epitope in question. Evidence of direct binding of ddAb to GPIb/IX was first provided by Chong et al.,[99] and Berndt et al.[98] established that the complex of both GPIb and GPIX is likely required for maximum antigen expression. Whereas epitope(s) on GPIb/IX are almost certainly a major antigen in DITP,[101-104] $\alpha_{IIb}\beta_3$, in soluble form, has been shown to react with certain ddAb.[105] Continued study of the drug-dependent autoimmune phenomena and their relationship to platelets is warranted, with particular attention to a comparison of the clinical significance of drug-dependent autoantibodies that bind to either GPIb/IX or $\alpha_{IIb}\beta_3$.

In order to understand the mechanism whereby drugs such as quinine or quinidine induce neoantigen formation, one must first consider the direct effects of these drugs on platelet membrane components, a subject that has not received enough attention by those interested in DITP. Deykin and Hellerstein[106] were probably the first to show that quinidine inhibits in vitro platelet aggregation induced by ADP, collagen, or epinephrine. Lawson et al.[107] demonstrated that quinidine administration will induce the prolongation of the bleeding time without thrombocytopenia. Connellan et al.[108] recently extended these findings and showed that quinine, both ex vivo and in vitro, will inhibit platelet aggregation induced by weak agonists such as ADP or epinephrine. Aggregation by strong agonists (e.g., collagen, thrombin, or arachidonate) was inhibited only in vitro. The combination of ddAb and quinine inhibited the binding of two monoclonal antibodies, HuPlml (specific for β_3) and FMC25 (specific for GPIX). By contrast, the binding of another antibody AN51 (specific for GPIb) was enhanced. The studies clearly point to a general platelet dysfunction that can be attributed to exposure to these drugs. That this dysfunction should be the result of perturbations of specific membrane glycoprotein receptors is not surprising. Nor should it be surprising that one effect of such perturbations might be the development of neoantigens or the exposure of cryptic antigens.

Chong et al.[109] used a panel of murine monoconal antibodies in competitive binding assays to map the domains on GPIb/IX bound by ddAbs from 12 patients with DITP. The combined data showed that one quinine-ddAb binds to an epitope on the N-terminal portion of the GPIb heavy chain, and five other quinine-ddAbs recognize a complex-specific epitope proximal to the membrane-associated region GPIb/IX. Each of six quinidine-ddAbs contained two specificities, one for the same GPIb/IX complex epitope described above, the other for GPIX alone. Additional observations were that ddAbs reactive with GPIb/IX are more predominant (12 of 12 patients) than those that bind $\alpha_{IIb}\beta_3$ (3 of 12 patients) and ddAbs specific for GPIb/IX are present in titers 8- to 32-fold higher than the corresponding antibodies that bind to $\alpha_{IIb}\beta_3$ in the same patient samples. In each case, those antibodies that bound to GPIb/IX were distinct from those that recognized $\alpha_{IIb}\beta_3$.

Regions of $\alpha_{IIb}\beta_3$ that bind to ddAb have also been further localized by Visentin et al.[110] Of 13 patient sera containing qui-

nine- or quinidine-ddAb, 10 were reactive with both GPIb/IX and $\alpha_{IIb}\beta_3$, two reacted with GPIb/IX alone and one reacted with $\alpha_{IIb}\beta_3$ alone. Again, in those sera in which both specificities were identified, the anti-GPIb/IX antibodies were distinct from those that bound to $\alpha_{IIb}\beta_3$. Seven sera containing anti-$\alpha_{IIb}\beta_3$ antibodies were further characterized. Three bound only to the $\alpha_{IIb}\beta_3$ complex, one bound to α_{IIb} alone, and three bound to β_3 alone. Those that recognized β_3 alone were found to bind to epitopes on the major 61-kd chymotryptic fragment of β_3 that are resistant to deglycosylation with endo-H.

Heparin-Associated Thrombocytopenia

Heparin-associated immune thrombocytopenia (HAT) represents a unique form of platelet clearance, and the detailed mechanism of platelet destruction remains to be elucidated. Unlike quinine- or quinidine-dependent antibodies, the actual binding of heparin-dependent antibodies (HDA) to the platelet surface appears to be of very low affinity, and has been difficult to demonstrate, having been accomplished only by Lynch and Howe.[111] HDA also differ from other forms of ddAbs in that they are activating, causing not only thrombocytopenia, but heparin-dependent platelet aggregation, thromboxane synthesis, and granule release that can be quantitated by preloading platelets with [^{14}C]serotonin. The consequences of HAT therefore are multiplied by often serious thrombotic complications. Approximately 30% of these patients die, with an additional 20% developing vascular occlusions that result in gangrene and subsequent amputation.[112]

Two mechanisms by which HDA interact with platelets have been proposed. The first is similar to the case for quinine- and quinidine-dependent antibodies, in which the Fab region of the antibody binds to neoantigens formed on the platelet surface as a result of the interaction of heparin with an undefined membrane component. The second is that heparin forms an immune complex with HDA in the plasma that subsequently binds to the platelet surface via the Fc region of the molecule. Recent evidence would suggest that the latter of these two scenarios is most certainly the case. Kelton et al.[113] showed that the platelet-release reaction induced by HDA could be blocked by pretreating platelets with human or goat IgG Fc fragments. Adelman et al.[114] showed that the Fab region of HDA alone are not sufficient to cause platelet activation. Similar studies were performed by Chong et al.,[115] who showed that purified rabbit IgG and its Fc, but not Fab, fragments markedly inhibited platelet aggregation induced by HDA. Further evidence of Fc receptor involvement in HAT has been provided by a number of laboratories that employed the monoclonal anti-Fc receptor antibody, IV.3, to block platelet activation by HDA, further supporting the notion that HAT is an Fc receptor-mediated event that involves both the Fab (for heparin binding) and Fc (for Fc receptor binding) regions of a heparin/IgG immune complex to achieve platelet activation and destruction.[113,116] Finally, although monoclonal antibodies to GPIb/IX can interfere with HDA binding to the platelet surface,[114] this is most probably due to stearic hindrance caused by the close proximity of the Fc receptor to GPIb/IX, as two different laboratories have convincingly demonstrated that HDA bind normally to Bernard-Soulier platelets, which lack expression of surface GPIb/IX/V.[113,116]

ALLOANTIGENS

Two clinically significant syndromes are the direct result of sensitization to platelet-specific alloantigens: neonatal alloimmune thrombocytopenia (NATP) and post-transfusion purpura

Table 132-4. Platelet-Specific Alloantigen Systems

Name	System	Allele	Phenotype Frequency (%) Western	Oriental	Glycoprotein Association
HPA-1a	P1ᴬ(Zw)	1(a)	98	>99	β₃
1b		2(b)	27		
				4	
HPA-2a	Ko(Sib)	b	99	NT	Iᵦ (H chain)
2b		a	15	25	
HPA-3a	Bak(Lek)	a	88	79	αᵢᵢᵦ (H chain)
3b		b	64	NT	
HPA-4a	Pen(Yuk)	a(b)	>99	>99	β₃
4b		b(a)	0.2		
				1.7	
HPA-5a	Br	b	99	NT	α₂
5b		a	21	NT	
	P1ᵀ	?	>98	NT	V
	Mo		<99	NT	β₃
	Serᵃ		NT	NT	β₃
	GOV	a	81	NT	
		b	74	NT	

Abbreviation: NT, not tested.

(PTP). Table 132-4 lists the established alloantigens: P1ᴬ (Zw),[117,118] Bak (Lek),[119–123] Pen (Yuk),[124,125] Ko (Sib),[126,127] P1ᵀ,[128] Br (Hc),[129,130] Srᵃ,[131] Mo,[132] Gov,[133] and Nak.[134] These were the original names of these alloantigens, although a uniform nomenclature has been proposed.[135]

Neonatal Alloimmune Thrombocytopenia and Post-transfusion Purpura

NATP is caused by maternal sensitization to paternal alloantigens on fetal platelets (Table 132-5). It is intriguing that only a fraction of those mothers negative for the platelet antigen in question deliver infants affected with NATP. The frequency of P1ᴬ¹-negative mothers in the general western population is 2%, while estimates put the incidence of NATP at ≤0.5%. A key to understanding this discrepancy lies in the finding by Reznikoff-Etievant et al.[136,137] that the frequency of HLA-DR3 in mothers delivering infants with NATP is 80–90%, while the frequency of HLA-DR3 in the general population is only about 22%. Further analyses have indicated that the propensity to develop such antibodies is associated with the DRw52a allele at the DR3 locus.[138] Thus, the risk among HLA-DR3-positive P1ᴬ¹-negative women to be immunized by P1ᴬ¹-positive fetal platelets is increased.

In a recent large study of 349 cases of clinically suspected NATP,[139] 78% of serologically confirmed cases were due to anti-P1ᴬ¹ and 19%, to anti-Brᵃ. All other specificities accounted for ≤5% of cases. The association of NATP with other alloantigens, such as Bakᵃ, Bakᵇ, P1ᴬ², and Koᵃ, is rare.[119,140–142] By contrast, in the Japanese population, anti-P1ᴬ¹ has never been shown to be involved in cases of NATP, and antibodies specific for Yukᵃ play a dominant clinical role.[143]

Table 132-5. Neonatal Alloimmune Thrombocytopenia

Incidence: 1 per 3,000 in a retrospective study, 1 per 2,200 births in one prospective study

Maternal antibodies produced against paternal antigens on fetal platelets

Similar to erythroblastosis fetalis, except that 50% of cases occur during first pregnancy

Most frequently implicated antigen is P1ᴬ¹ (United States/Europe)

High-risk association with HLA-DRw52a (DR3 locus)

Table 132-6. Post-transfusion Purpura

Nearly all reported patients have been females previously sensitized by pregnancy or transfusion (≤5% were males)

Thrombocytopenia usually occurs 1 week after transfusion

P1ᴬ¹-negative individuals account for most (>60%) cases

High-risk association with HLA-DR3

Enigmatically, the recipient's antigen-negative platelets are destroyed by autologous antibody

PTP follows 7–10 days after an immunogenic blood (platelet) transfusion (Table 132-6). It most often affects previously non-transfused multiparous women. As with NATP, there is an increased risk of the development of PTP among HLA-DR3-positive individuals.[136,144]

The precise mechanism by which the recipient's antigen-negative platelets are also cleared from the circulation in PTP is not fully understood. Proposed mechanisms include the following: (1) during the first phase of PTP, the recipient develops antibodies that recognize "framework" determinants (conserved protein structures surrounding the specific polymorphic sites), and these react with each of the allelic forms of the antigen; (2) recipient antibodies form immune complexes with soluble antigens from donor platelets, and these interact with autologous platelets via an Fc receptor-dependent mechanism; and (3) soluble antigen from the transfused product is adsorbed onto recipient platelets, rendering them passively positive for the antigen in question. Platelet membrane microparticles are known to be a constituent of fresh frozen plasma and platelet concentrates.[145] The αᵢᵢᵦβ₃ complex could conceivably become adsorbed onto neighboring platelets via this process. At this time, evidence to support or refute any one of the proposed mechanisms for the pathology of PTP is not conclusive. See Chapter 125 for further discussion of NATP and PTP. P1ᴬ¹-negative platelets have been reported to become P1ᴬ¹ positive when incubated with plasma from P1ᴬ¹-positive individuals.[146–148] Although this passive form of transfer of soluble antigen has been proposed as a mechanism of clearance of the recipient platelets in PTP, Ehmann et al.[149] contend that this is an in vitro artifact. These investigators provide evidence in patients with post-transfusion purpura for the presence of immune complexes composed of donor antigen and recipient antibody. We have found that centrifugation, even at forces exceeding 10,000g, fails to remove antigen-positive material (residual platelets and/or fragments) from plasma preparations. However, the clearance of antigen-positive material is reliably accomplished by the passage of such plasma through a 0.45-μm filter (Warejka D, Aster RH, Kunicki TJ, unpublished observations). These findings support the Ehmann contention that antigen transfer using nonfiltered plasmas is an in vitro artifact.

IMMUNOCHEMISTRY OF PLATELET ALLOANTIGENS

β₃ Alloantigens

Alloantigens are phenotypically definable differences in a single protein often created by inherited polymorphisms of amino acid residues and can be detected by antibodies from individuals of the same species. The human P1ᴬ alloantigen system is a diallelic system on β₃ associated with a Leu 33/Pro 33 β₃ polymorphism thought to be enclosed within a small 13-amino acid loop formed by the pairing of Cys 26 with Cys 38 (Fig. 132-2).[150–154] A long-range disulfide bond linking Cys 5 and Cys 435 creates a large loop[155] that brings the N-terminal region of β₃, including the small Cys 26-Cys 38 loop, proximal to the cysteine-rich region of the middle of β₃. Lacking the precise three-dimensional structure of β₃, it is not yet possible to explain why synthetic peptides that mimic the P1ᴬ epitope sequences are not antigenic.[156] Murine monoclonal antibodies raised against linear peptides containing the Leu 33 or Pro 33 polymorphisms will bind to the corresponding synthetic peptides or to denatured and reduced β_3 of the appropriate phenotype but fail to bind to native β_3.[157] The structural basis for the alloantigen phenotype remains to be precisely determined. Direct binding analysis with murine monoclonal antibodies has determined that about 40,000–50,000 $\alpha_{IIb}\beta_3$ complexes are available on the surface of nonactivated platelets.[158–160] Thus, each molecule of GPβ_3 has a single Pl^A epitope, and all GPβ_3 molecules appear to express one or the other of the two alleles.

Anti-Pl^{A1} antibodies inhibit clot retraction and platelet aggregation; in the latter case, presumably because they block the binding of fibrinogen.[161,162] Ryu et al.[163] have also reported that there is a dose-dependent stimulation versus inhibition of fibrinogen binding induced by anti-Pl^{A1}. A similar effect has been attributed to other platelet inhibitors, particularly the disintegrins, RGD peptides, and certain snake venoms.[164]

Another diallelic human alloantigen system known as Pen (or Yuk) is found on β_3 and is associated with an Arg 143/Gln 143 polymorphism.[162,165–168] Given the proximity of the Pen polymorphism to the RGD-binding domain (residues 109–171) of β_3, it is not surprising that anti-Pen^a antibodies completely inhibit aggregation of Pen$^{a/a}$ homozygous platelets.[162]

Two novel alloantigens, Sr^a and Mo, have recently been localized to β_3.[131,132] The alloantigen Sr^a is classified as a private alloantigen, since it appears to be inherited within a single family or family group, but not expressed by the general population. The unique feature of the Sr^a polymorphism is that it is associated with an Arg 636/Cys 636 substitution, resulting in an additional unpaired cysteine residue.[131] Since its initial characterization, it has been accepted that all cysteine residues in β_3 are involved in disulfide bridges. Despite the addition of this new sulfhydryl group, the Sr^a-positive β_3 subunit still associates with α_{IIb} and contributes to an expressed $\alpha_{IIb}\beta_3$ complex without apparent impairment of function. The alloantigen Mo results from a C → G substitution at base pair 1,267 of β_3, resulting in replacement of Pro 407 by Ala 407.[132] Mo is a very low-frequency alloantigen that has been detected in only 1 of 450 random donors outside of the initial family of the propositus.

Other cells that express β_3, as the β-subunit of the vitronectin receptor, including endothelial cells, fibroblasts, and smooth muscle cells, also express Pl^A and Pen epitopes.[169–172] This could contribute to the complexity of the clinical symptoms in alloimmune-mediated thrombocytopenia. Little is known about the involvement of tissues other than platelets in these conditions.

α_{IIb} Alloantigens

The Bak system is associated with an Ile 843/Ser 843 polymorphism of α_{IIb}[123] (Fig. 132-3). In addition, Take et al.[173] reported that the binding of certain anti-Bak^a antisera to α_{IIb} is decreased after desialation of α_{IIb}, raising the possibility that glycosylation of α_{IIb} may contribute to or influence the expression of the Bak epitopes. Anti-Bak alloantibodies do not bind to the precursor form of the α_{IIb} molecule, pro-α_{IIb}.[153] Thus, O-glycosylation at the polymorphic Ser 843 may influence specificity or accessibility of anti-Bak alloantibodies.

No report has appeared concerning the effect of antibodies specific for Bak(Lek) antigens on fibrinogen binding, platelet aggregation, or clot retraction. Since the α_{IIb} molecule is expressed only on platelets, megakaryocytes, or cells with a megakaryocyte lineage, the Bak(Lek) epitopes are not found on other cells types, as noted above.

α_2 Alloantigens

The Br^a (Hc^a) platelet-specific alloantigen system is located on the integrin subunit α_2[129,130] (Fig. 132-5). The detection of this system was facilitated by the recent development of a highly sensitive murine monoclonal antibody-based monoclonal antibody immobilization of platelet antigen assay.[32] Like the preceding alloantigenic systems, the Br^a system is diallelic. Roughly 2,000 copies of α_2 are present on the surface of normal platelets, and each α_2 molecule expresses a single Br epitope.[129] α_2 is distributed on a wide variety of cells, but nothing is known about the distribution of the Br (Hc) antigens.

GPIb/IX Alloantigens

Two reported polymorphisms of the Ib/IX/V complex, termed Ko and Sib, have been localized to the GPIbα subunit. The Ko^a/Ko^b antigens comprise a diallelic system,[174,175] and Kuijpers et al.[176] have found that anti-Ko antibodies bind to the N-terminal elastase-sensitive fragment of the GPIbα chain, where a Thr/Met polymorphism at residue 145 is associated with Ko^a/Ko^b phenotype (Fig. 132-6). Molecular variants of GPIbα at residue 145 have also been independently reported by Ware et al.[177] The molecular basis of the Sib polymorphism is less well understood. First reported by Saji et al.,[178] the Sib system has recently been found to be associated with a molecular-weight polymorphism of GPIb[179] formed by allelic variation in the number of 13-amino acid repeat structures present within the macroglycopeptide region of the GPIbα chain.[177,180] Somewhat puzzling is the recent co-classification of the Sib antigen system with the Ko system as the HPA-2 platelet antigen system.[135] It is not clear how the two systems are related, however, since the 13-amino acid repeats in GPIb associated with Sib are >200 residues from the Thr 145/Met 145 polymorphism associated with Ko. One possible explanation for this apparent discrepancy is that one of these polymorphisms has been evolutionarily superimposed on the other, resulting in a co-inheritance as a common haplotype.

Alloantigens on Other Platelet Membrane Glycoproteins

Pl^T, a recently described platelet alloantigen, has been implicated in a single case of NATP. Beardsley et al.[128] localized this antigen to GPV by immunoblot assay. In platelets tested from 50 normal donors, all were found to contain this allele.

Kelton et al.[133] described another alloantigen system carried by a novel platelet protein with an apparent molecular weight of 150/175 (nonreduced/reduced). Alloantibodies defining each of two alleles (Gov^a/Gov^b) were detected in two patients who had received multiple platelet transfusions. The phenotypic frequencies in the Canadian population are for Gov^a, 81%; and for Gov^b, 74%.

Ikeda et al.[134] defined another platelet antigen, Nak^a, that was implicated in a thrombocytopenic patient with refractoriness to HLA-matched platelet transfusions. Tomiyama et al.[181] later showed that anti-Nak^a antibodies reacted specifically with GPIV (CD36), an 88-kd membrane glycoprotein believed to be involved in the interaction of platelets with collagen[182] or thrombospondin.[183] Interestingly, Nak^a-negative platelets fail to synthesize biochemically or immunochemically detectable amounts of GPIV,[184] even though their platelets contain mRNA transcripts for this glycoprotein.[185] Interestingly, these GPIV-negative individuals had no platelet functional defects and no hematologic disorders, suggesting that the putative functions of GPIV can be compensated for by other platelet membrane components in its absence. Since anti-Nak^a antibodies do not recognize a molecular variant of the GPIV molecule, Nak^a is more properly classified as an iso-, rather than an allo-, antigen.

REFERENCES

1. Hynes RO: Integrins: versatility, modulation, and signaling in cell adhesion. Cell 69:11, 1992
2. Fitzgerald LA, Steiner B, Rall SC Jr et al: Protein sequence of endothelial glycoprotein IIIa derived from a cDNA clone. Identity with platelet glycoprotein IIIa and similarity to "integrin." J Biol Chem 262:3936, 1987
3. Poncz M, Eisman R, Heidenreich R et al: Structure of the platelet membrane glycoprotein IIb. Homology to the alpha subuntis of the vitronectin and fibronectin membrane receptors. J Biol Chem 262:8476, 1987
4. D'Souza S, Ginsberg MH, Burke TA et al: Localization of an Arg-Gly-ASP recognition site within an integrin adhesion recepter. Science 242:91, 1988
5. D'Souza SE, Ginsberg MH, Burke TA et al: The ligand binding site of the platelet integrin receptor GPIIb-IIIa is proximal to the second calcium binding domain of its α subunit. J Biol Chem 265:3440, 1990
6. George JN, Caen JP, Nurden AT: Glanzmann thrombasthenia: the spectrum of clinical disease. Blood 75:1383, 1990
7. Santoro SA: Identification of a 160,000 dalton platelet membrane protein that mediates the initial divalent cation-dependent adhesion of platelets to collagen. Cell 46:913, 1986
8. Kunicki TJ, Nugent DJ, Staats S et al: The human fibroblast class II extracellular matrix receptor mediates platelet adhesion to collagen and is identical to the platelet glycoprotein Ia-IIa complex. J Biol Chem 263:4516, 1988
9. Takada Y, Hemler ME: The primary structure of the VLA-2/collagen receptor alpha 2 subunit (platelet GPIa): homology to other integrins and the presence of a possible collagen-binding domain. J Cell Biol 109:397, 1989
10. Nieuwenhuis HK, Akkerman JWN, Houdijk WPM et al: Human blood platelets showing no response to collagen fail to express surface glycoprotein Ia. Nature 318:470, 1985
11. Kehrel B, Balleisen L, Kokott R et al: Deficiency of intact thrombospondin and membrane glycoprotein Ia in platelets with defective collagen-induced aggregation and spontaneous loss of disorder. Blood 71:1074, 1988
12. Kunicki TJ, Orchekowski R, Annis D et al: Variability of integrin $\alpha_2\beta_1$ activity on human platelets. Blood 82:2693, 1993
13. Tarantino M, Kunicki T, Nugent D: Identification of the estrogen receptor in human megakaryocytes. Arterioscler Thromb 1994 (in press)
14. Piotrowicz RS, Orchekowski RP, Nugent DJ et al: Glycoprotein Ic-IIa functions as an activation-independent fibronectin receptor on human platelets. J Cell Biol 106:1359, 1988
15. Sonnenberg A, Modderman PW, Hogervorst F: Laminin receptor on platelets is the integrin VLA-6. Nature 336:487, 1988
16. Lopez JA, Chung DW, Fujikawa K et al: Cloning of the alpha chain of human platelet glycoprotein Ib: a transmembrane protein with homology to leucine-rich alpha-2-glycoprotein. Proc Natl Acad Sci USA 84:5615, 1987
17. Titani K, Takio K, Handa M, Ruggeri ZM: Amino acid sequence of the von Willebrand factor-binding domain of platelet membrane glycoprotein Ib. Proc Natl Acad Sci USA 84:5610, 1987
18. Schick PK: Platelet glycolipids. p. 31. In Kunicki TJ, George JN (eds): Platelet Immunobiology: Molecular and Clinical Aspects. JB Lippincott, Philadelphia, 1989
19. Koerner TAW, Weinfeld HM, Bullard LSB, Williams LCJ: Antibodies against platelet glycosphingolipids: detection in serum by quantitative HPTLC-autoradiography and association with autoimmune and alloimmune processes. Blood 73:273, 1989
20. Degos L, Dautigny A, Brouet JC et al: A molecular defect in thrombasthenic platelets. J Clin Invest 56:236, 1974
21. Coller BS, Peerschke EI, Seligsohn U et al: Studies on the binding of an alloimmune and two murine monoclonal antibodies to the platelet glycoprotein IIb-IIIa receptor. J Lab Clin Med 107:384, 1986
22. Kunicki TJ, Furihata K, Bull B, Nugent D: The immunogenicity of platelet membrane glycoproteins. Transfus Med Rev 1:21, 1987
23. Nurden AT, Jallu V, Hourdille P et al: Evidence for multiple antibodies in the sera of two patients with immune thrombocytopenia of different origins. Thromb Haemost 62:565, 1989
24. Bierling P, Fromont P, Elbez A et al: Early immunization against platelet glycoprotein IIIa in a newborn Glanzmann type I patient. Vox Sang 55:109, 1988
25. Tobelem G, Levy-Toledano S, Bredoux et al: New approach to determination of specific functions of platelet membrane sites. Nature 263:427, 1975
26. Karpatkin S: Autoimmune thrombocytopenia purpura. Semin Hematol 22:260, 1985
27. Beardsley DS: Platelet autoantigens. p. 121. In Kunicki TJ, George JN (eds): Platelet Immunobiology: Molecular and Clinical Aspects. JB Lippincott, Philadelphia, 1989
28. van Leeuwen EF, van der Ven JTM, Engelfriet CP, von dem Borne AEGK: Specificity of autoantibodies in autoimmune thrombocytopenia. Blood 59:23, 1982
29. Woods VL, Oh EH, Mason D, McMillan R: Autoantibodies against the platelet glycoprotein IIb/IIIa complex in patients with chronic ITP. Blood 63:368, 1984
30. Beardsley D, Spiegel J, Jacobs M et al: Platelet membrane glycoprotein IIIa contains target antigens that bind antiplatelet antibodies in immune thrombocytopenias. J Clin Invest 73:1701, 1984
31. McMillan R, Tani P, Millard F, Woods VL: Platelet-associated and plasma anti-glycoprotein autoantibodies in chronic ITP. Blood 70:1040, 1987
32. Kiefel V, Santoso S, Weisheit M, Mueller-Eckhardt C: Monoclonal antibody-specific immobilization of platelet antigens (MAIPA): a new tool for the identification of platelet-reactive antibodies. Blood 70:1732, 1987
33. Tomiyama Y, Kurata Y, Mizutani H et al: Platelet glycoprotein IIb as a target antigen in two patients with chronic idiopathic thrombocytopenic purpura. Br J Haematol 66:535, 1987
34. Tomiyama Y, Kurata Y, Shibata Y et al: Immunochemical characterization of an autoantigen on platelet glycoprotein IIb in chronic ITP: comparison with the Bakª alloantigen. Br J Haematol 71:76, 1989
35. Kekomaki R, Dawson B, McFarland J et al: Localization of human platelet autoantigens to the cysteine-rich region of glycoprotein IIIa. J Clin Invest 88:847, 1991
36. Fujisawa K, O'Toole TE, Tani P et al: Autoantibodies to the presumptive cytoplasmic domain of platelet glycoprotein IIIa in patients with chronic immune thrombocytopenic purpura. Blood 77:2207, 1991
37. Fujisawa K, Tani P, O'Toole TE et al: Different specificities of platelet-associated and plasma autoantibodies to platelet GPIIb-IIIa in patients with chronic ITP. Blood 79:1441, 1992
38. Fujisawa K, Tani P, McMillan R: Platelet-associated antibody to glycoprotein IIb/IIIa from chronic immune thrombocytopenic purpura patients often binds to divalent cation-dependent antigens. Blood 81:1284, 1993
39. Von dem Borne AEGK, van der Lelie H, Vos JJE et al: Antibodies against cryptantigens of platelets. p. 33. In Decary F, Rock G (eds): Platelet Serology. Research Progress and Clinical Implications. S Karger, Basel, 1986
40. van Vliet H, Kappers-Klunne M, Abels J: Pseudothrombocytopenia: a cold antibody against platelet glycoprotein GPIIb. Br J Haematol 62:501, 1986
41. Menitove J, Pereira J, Hoffman R et al: Cyclic thrombocytopenia of apparent autoimmune etiology. Blood 73:1561, 1989
42. Niessner H, Clemetson KJ, Panzer S et al: Acquired thrombasthenia due to GPIIb/IIIa-specific autoantibodies. Blood 68:571, 1986
43. Balduini C, Grignani G, Sinigaglia F et al: Severe platelet dysfunction in a patient with autoantibodies against membrane glycoproteins IIb/IIIa. Haemostasis 7:98, 1987
44. Deckmyn H, Chew SL, Vermylen J: Lack of platelet response to collagen associated with an autoantibody against glycoprotein Ia: A novel cause of acquired qualitative platelet dysfunction. Thromb Haemost 64:74, 1990
45. Szatkowski NS, Kunicki TJ, Aster RH: Identification of glycoprotein Ib as a target for autoantibody in idiopathic (autoimmune) thrombocytopenic purpura. Blood 67:310, 1986
46. Nugent DJ: Human monoclonal antibodies in the characterization of platelet antigens. p. 273. In Kunicki TJ, George JN (eds): Platelet Immunobiology: Molecular and Clinical Aspects. JB Lippincott, Philadelphia, 1989
47. Devine DV, Curie MS, Rosse WF, Greenberg CS: Pseudo-Bernard-Soulier syndrome: thrombocytopenia caused by autoantibody to platelet glycoprotein Ib. Blood 70:428, 1987
48. Beardsley DJS, Ho J, Beyer EC: Varicella-associated thrombocytopenia: antibodies against an 85-KDa thrombin sensitive protein (?GPV), abstracted. Blood, suppl. 1. 66:1030, 1985
49. Stricker RB, Koerper MA, Bussel J, Shuman MA: Target platelet antigens in childhood immune thrombocytopenic purpura, abstracted. Blood, suppl. 1. 68:118a, 1986
50. Berchtold P, Tani P, McMillan R, Blanchette VS: Autoantibodies against platelet membrane glycoproteins in children with acute and chronic ITP. Blood, suppl. 1. 73:261a, 1988
51. Winiarski J: IgG and IgM antibodies to platelet membrane glycoprotein antigens in acute childhood idiopathic thrombocytopenic purpura. Br J Haematol 73:88, 1989
52. Varon D, Karpatkin S: A monoclonal anti-platelet antibody with decreased reactivity for autoimmune thrombocytopenic platelets. Proc Natl Acad Sci USA 80:6992, 1983
53. Tsubakio T, Tani P, Woods VL, McMillan R: Autoantibodies against platelet GPIIb/IIIa in chronic ITP react with different epitopes. Br J Haematol 67:345, 1987
54. Nugent DJ, Kunicki TJ, Berglund C, Bernstein ID: A human monoclonal autoantibody recognizes a neoantigen on glycoprotein IIIa expressed on stored and activated platelets. Blood 70:16, 1987
55. Hiraiwa A, Nugent DJ, Milner ECB: Sequence analysis of monoclonal antibod-

ies derived from a patient with idiopathic thrombocytopenic purpura. J Autoimmun 8:107, 1990

56. Kunicki TJ, Furihata K, Kekomaki R et al: A human monoclonal autoantibody specific human platelet glycoprotein IIb (integrin α_{IIb}) heavy chain. Hum Antibodies Hybridomas 1:83, 1990

57. Kunicki TJ, Plow EF, Kekomaki R, Nugent DJ: Human monoclonal autoantibody 2E7 is specific for a peptide sequence of platelet glycoprotein IIb. Localization of the epitope to IIb$_{231-238}$ with an immunodominant Trp$_{235}$. J Autoimmun 4:415, 1991

58. Berchtold P, Dale G, Tani P, McMillan R: Inhibition of autoantibody binding to platelet glycoprotein (GP) IIb/IIIa by anti-idiotypic antibodies (anti-Id) in intravenous immunoglobulin (IvIgG). Blood, suppl. 1. 73:261a, 1988

59. Howe SE, Lynch DM: Platelet antibody binding in systemic lupus erytematosus. J Rheumatol 14:482, 1987

60. Kaplan C, Champeix P, Blanchard D et al: Platelet antibodies in systemic lupus erythematosus. Br J Haematol 67:89, 1987

61. Jouhikainen T, Kekomaki R, Leirisalo-Repo M et al: Platelet antibodies detected by immunoblotting in systemic lupus erythematosus: association with the lupus anticoagulant, thrombosis and thrombocytopenia, abstracted. Thromb Haemost 62:373, 1989

62. Tomiyama Y, Kekomaki R, McFarland J et al: Anti-vinculin antibodies in sera of patients with immune thrombocytopenia and normal subjects. Blood 79:161, 1992

63. Pfueller SL, Logan D, Tran TT et al: Naturally occurring IgG antibodies to intracellular and cytoskeletal components of human platelets. Clin Exp Immunol 79:367, 1990

64. Reid DM, Jones CE, Luo C-Y et al: Immunoglobulins from normal sera bind platelet vinculin and talin and their proteolytic fragments. Blood 81:745, 1993

65. Kekomaki R, Jouhikainen J, Kunicki T: Characterization of a 65 kDa platelet antigen frequently presenting as an immunogen in thrombocytopenic patients, abstracted. Blood, suppl. 1. 73:34a, 1989

66. Panzer S, Penner E, Nelson PJ et al: Identification of the platelet glycoprotein IIb/IIIa complex as a target antigen in primary biliary cirrhosis-associated autoimmune thrombocytopenia. J Autoimmun 3:473, 1990

67. Van de Water J, Gershwin ME, Leung P et al: Autoepitope of the 74-kD mitochondrial autoantigen of primary biliary cirrhosis corresponds to the functional site of dihydrolipoamide acetyltransferase. J Exp Med 167:1791, 1988

68. Reid DM, Jones CE, Vostal JG et al: Western blot identification of platelet proteins that bind normal serum immunoglobulins. Characteristics of a 95-Kd reactive protein. Blood 75:2194, 1990

69. Harris EN, Asherson RA, Gharavi AE et al: Thrombocytopenia in SLE and related autoimmune disorders: association with anticardiolipin antibody. Br J Haematol 59:227, 1985

70. Harris EN, Gharavi AE, Hegde U et al: Anticardiolipin antibodies in autoimmune thrombocytopenia. Br J Haematol 59:231, 1985

71. Kaise S, Yasuda T, Kasukawa et al: Antiglycolipid antibodies in normal and pathologic human sera and synovial fluids. Vox Sang 49:292, 1985

72. Van Vliet HHDM, Kappers-Klunne MC, van der Hel JWB, Abels J: Antibodies against glycosphingolipids in sera of patients with idiopathic thrombocytopenic purpura. Br J Haematol 67:103, 1987

73. dePosba NK, Pfueller SL: Characterization of platelet components to which antiplatelet IgG antibodies bind in idiopathic thrombocytopenic purpura, abstracted. Clin Exp Pharmacol Physiol 9:532, 1982

74. Weinfeld HM, Williams LCJ, Koerner TAW: Detection and frequency of platelet antibodies with glycolipid specificity, abstracted. Transfusion 26:583, 1986

75. Shoenfeld YS, Hsu-Lin SC, Gabriels JE et al: Production of autoantibodies by human-human hybridomas. J Clin Invest 170:205, 1982

76. Asano T, Furie BC, Furie B: Glycolipid is the platelet autoantigen of platelet-binding monoclonal lupus autoantibodies produced by human hybridomas. Clin Res 34:654, 1986

77. Atkinson PM, Lampman GW, Furie BC et al: Homology of the NH$_2$-terminal amino acid sequences of the heavy and light chains of human monoclonal lupus autoantibodies containing the dominant 16/6 idiotype. J Clin Invest 74:1138, 1985

78. Lampman GW, Furie B, Schwartz RS et al: Amino acid sequence of a platelet-binding human anti-DNA monoclonal autoantibody. Blood 73:262, 1989

79. Murakami H, Lam Z, Furie BC et al: Sulfated glycolipids are the platelet autoantigens for human platelet-binding monoclonal anti-DNA autoantibodies. J Biol Chem 266:15414, 1991

80. Ratnoff OD, Menitove JE, Aster RH et al: Coincident classic hemophilia and "idiopathic" thrombocytopenic purpura in patients under treatment with concentrates of anti-hemophilic factor (factor VIII). N Engl J Med 308:439, 1983

81. Savona S, Nardi MA, Lennette ET et al: Thrombocytopenic purpura in narcotic addicts. Ann Intern Med 102:737, 1985

82. Morris L, Distenfeld A, Amorosi E et al: Autoimmune thrombocytopenic purpura in homosexual men. Ann Intern Med 96:714, 1982

83. Karpatkin S, Nardi MA: Immunologic thrombocytopenic purpura in human immunodeficiency virus-seropositive patients with hemophilia. Comparison with patients with classic autoimmune thrombocytopenic purpura, homosexuals with thrombocytopenia, and narcotic addicts with thrombocytopenia. J Lab Clin Med 111:441, 1988

84. Walsh CM, Nardi MA, Karpatkin S: On the mechanism of thrombocytopenic purpura in sexually active homosexual men. N Engl J Med 311:635, 1984

85. Walsh C, Krigel R, Lennette ET et al: Thrombocytopenia in homosexual patients. Prognosis, response to therapy, and prevalence of antibody to the retrovirus assocaited with the acquired immunodeficiency syndrome. Ann Intern Med 103:542, 1985

86. Stricker RB, Abrams DI, Corash L et al: Target antigens in homosexual men with immune thrombocytopenia. N Engl J Med 313:1374, 1985

87. Klaassen RJL, van der Lelie J, Vlekke ABJ et al: The serology and immunochemistry of HIV-induced platelet-bound immunoglobulin. Blut 59:75, 1989

88. Bettaieb A, Oksenhendler E, Fromont P et al: Immunochemical analysis of platelet autoantibodies in HIV-related thrombocytopenic purpura: a study of 68 patients. Br J Haematol 73:241, 1989

89. Canoso RT, Zon LI, Groopman JE: Anticardiolipin antibodies associated with HTLV-III-infection. Br J Haematol 65:495, 1987

90. Rauch J, Qiang-Hua Meng, Tannenbaum H: Lupus anticoagulant and antiplatelet properties of human hybridoma antibodies. J Immunol 139:2598, 1987

91. van der Lelie J, Lang JMA, Vos JJE et al: Autoimmunity against peripheral blood cells in human immunodeficiency virus (HIV) infection. Br J Haematol 67:109, 1987

92. Murphy MF, Metcalfe P, Waters AH et al: Incidence and mechanism of neutropenia and thrombocytopenia in patients with human immunodeficiency virus infection. Br J Haematol 66:337, 1987

93. Karpatkin S, Nardi M, Lennette ET et al: Anti-human immunodeficiency virus type 1 antibody complexes on platelets of seropositive thrombocytopenic homosexuals and narcotic addicts. Proc Natl Acad Sci USA 85:9763, 1988

94. Shulman NR: Immunoreactions involving platelets. I. A steric and kinetic model for formation of a complex from a human antibody, quinidine as a haptene, and platelets; and for fixation of complement by the complex. J Exp Med 107:665, 1958.

95. Hackett T, Kelton JG, Powers P: Drug induced platelet destruction. Semin Thromb Hemost 8:116, 1982

96. Van Leeuwen EF, Engelfriet CP, von dem Borne AEGK: Studies on quinine and quinidine-dependent antibodies against platelets and their reaction with platelets in the Bernard-Soulier syndrome. Br J Haematol 51:551, 1982

97. Pfueller SL, Kerlero de Posbo N, Bilston RA: Platelets deficient in glycoprotein I have normal Fc receptor expression. Br J Haematol 56:607, 1984

98. Berndt MC, Chong BH, Bull HA et al: Molecular characterization of quinine/quinidine drug-dependent antibody platelet interaction using monoclonal antibodies. Blood 66:1292, 1985

99. Chong BH, Berndt MC, Koutts J et al: Quinidine-induced thrombocytopenia and leukopenia; demonstration and characterization of distinct antiplatelet and antileukocyte antibodies. Blood 62:1218, 1983

100. Christie DJ, Mullen PC, Aster RH: Fab-mediated binding of drug-dependent antibodies to platelets in quiidine- and quinine-induced thrombocytopenia. J Clin Invest 74:310, 1985

101. Kunicki TJ, Aster RH: Absence of the platelet receptor for drug dependent antibodies in the Bernard-Soulier syndrome. J Clin Invest 62:716, 1979

102. Kunicki TJ, Russell N, Nurden AT et al: Further studies of the human platelet receptor for quinine- and quinidine-dependent antibodies. J Immunol 126:398, 1981

103. Christie DJ, Aster RH: Drug-antibody-platelet interaction in quinine and quinidine-induced thrombocytopenia. J Clin Invest 70:989, 1982

104. George JN, Reimmann TA, Moake JL et al: Bernard-Soulier disease. A study of four patients and their parents. Br J Haematol 48:459, 1981

105. Christie DJ, Mullen PC, Aster RH: Quinine- and quinidine platelet antibodies can react with GPIIb/IIIa. Br J Haematol 67:213, 1987

106. Deykin D, Hellerstein LJ: The assessment of drug-dependent and isoimmune antiplatelet antibodies by the use of platelet aggregometry. J Clin Invest 51:3142, 1972

107. Lawson D, Mehta J, Mehta P et al: Cumulative effects of quinidine and aspirin on bleeding time and platelet α_2-adenoreceptors: potential mechanism of bleeding diathesis in patients receiving this combination. J Lab Clin Med 108:581, 1986

108. Connellan JM, Deacon S, Thurlow PJ: Changes in platelet function and reac-

tivity induced by quinine in relation to quinine (drug) induced immune thrombocytopenia. Thromb Res 61:501, 1991

109. Chong BH, Du X, Berndt MC et al: Characterization of the binding domains on platelet glycoproteins Ib-IX and IIb-IIIa complexes for the quinine/quinidine-dependent antibodies. Blood 77:2190, 1991

110. Visentin GP, Newman PJ, Aster RH: Characteristics of quinine- and quinidine-induced antibodies specific for platelet glycoproteins IIb and IIIa. Blood 77:2668, 1991

111. Lynch DM, Howe SE: Heparin-associated thrombocytopenia: antibody binding specificity to platelet antigens. Blood 66:1176, 1985

112. Berndt MC, Chong BH, Andrews RK: Biochemistry of drug-dependent platelet autoantigens. p. 132. In Kunicki TJ, George JN (eds): Platelet Immunobiology. JB Lippincott, Philadelphia, 1989

113. Kelton JG, Sheridan D, Santos A et al: Heparin-induced thrombocytopenia: laboratory studies. Blood 72:925, 1988

114. Adelman B, Sobel M, Fujimura YY et al: Heparin-associated thrombocytopenia: observations on the mechanism of platelet aggregation. J Lab Clin Med 113:204, 1989

115. Chong BH, Castaldi PA, Berndt MC: Heparin-induced thrombocytopenia: effects of rabbit IgG, and its Fab and Fc fragments on antibody-heparin-platelet interaction. Thromb Res 55:291, 1989

116. Chong BH, Fawaz I, Chesterman CN et al: Heparin-induced thrombocytopenia: mechanism of interaction of the heparin-dependent antibody with platelets. Br J Haematol 73:235, 1989

117. Van Loghem J, Dorfmeijer H, van der Hart M: Serological and genetical studies on a platelet antigen (Zw). Vox Sang 4:161, 1959

118. Shulman NR, Marder V, Hiller M, Collier E: Platelet and leukocyte isoantigens and their antibodies: serologic, physiologic and clinical studies. Prog Hematol 4:222, 1964

119. von dem Borne A, von Riesz E, Verheugt F et al: Bak^a, a new platelet-specific antigen involved in neonatal alloimmune thrombocytopenia. Vox Sang 39:113, 1980

120. Boizard B, Wautier J-L: Lek^a, a new platelet antigen absent in Glanzmann's thrombasthenia. Vox Sang 46:47, 1984

121. Kieffer N, Boizard B, Didry D et al: Immunochemical characterization of the platelet-specific alloantigen Lek^a. A comparable study with the P1^{A1} alloantigen. Blood 64:1212, 1984

122. von dem Borne A, van der Plas-van Dalen CM: Bak^a and Lek^a are identical antigens. Br J Haematol 62:404, 1986

123. Lyman S, Aster RH, Visentin GP et al: Polymorphism of human platelet membrane glycoprotein IIa associated with the Bak^a/Bak^b alloantigen system. Blood 75:2343, 1990

124. Friedman JM, Aster RH: Neonatal alloimmune thrombocytopenic purpura and congenital porencephaly in two siblings associated with a "new" maternal antiplatelet antibody. Blood 65:1412, 1985

125. Shibata Y, Miyaji T, Ichikawa Y, Matsuda I: A new platelet antigen system Yuk^a/Yuk^b. Vox Sang 51:334, 1986

126. van der Weerdt C: The platelet agglutination test. p. 161. In Histocompatibility Testing. Vol. II. Munksgaard, Copenhagen, 1965

127. Saji H, Maruya E, Fujii H et al: New platelet antigen, Sib^a, involved in platelet transfusion refractoriness in a Japanese man. Vox Sang 56:283, 1989

128. Beardsley DS, Ho JS, Moulton T: P1^T: a new platelet specific antigen on glycoprotein V, abstracted. Blood, suppl. 1. 70:347a, 1987

129. Kiefel V, Santoso S, Katzmann B et al: The Br^a/Br^b alloantigen system on human platelets. Blood 73:2219, 1989

130. Woods VL, Pischel KD, Avery ED et al: Antigenic polymorphism of human very late activation protein-2 (platelet glycoprotein Ia-IIa). J Clin Invest 83:9, 1989

131. Santoso S, Newman P, Kalb R et al: An unpaired cysteine residue is involved in epitope formation but has no influence on platelet GPIIIa expression and function, abstracted. Blood, suppl. 1. 80:128a, 1992

132. Kuijpers RWAM, Simsek S, Faber NM et al: Single point mutation in human glycoprotein IIIa is associated with a new platelet-specific alloantigen (Mo) involved in neonatal alloimmune thrombocytopenia. Blood 81:70, 1993

133. Kelton JG, Smith JW, Horsewood P et al: Gov$^{a/b}$ alloantigen system on human platelets. Blood 75:2172, 1990

134. Ikeda H. Mitani T, Ohnuma M et al: A new platelet-specific antigen, Nak^a, involved in the refractoriness of HLA-matched platelet transfusion. Vox Sang 57:213, 1989

135. von dem Borne AEGKr: Nomenclature of platelet antigen systems. Br J Haematol 74:239, 1990

136. Reznikoff-Etievant MF, Dangu C, Lobet R: HLA-B8 antigen and anti-P1^{A1} alloimmunization. Tissue Antigens 18:66, 1981

137. Reznikoff-Etievant MF, Muller JY, Julien F et al: An immune response gene linked to MHC in man. Tissue Antigens 22:312, 1983

138. Valentin N, Vergracht A, Bignon JD et al: HLA-DRw52a is involved in alloimmunization against PL-A1 antigen. Hum Immunol 27:73, 1990

139. Mueller-Eckhardt C, Kiefel V, Grubert A et al: 348 cases of suspected neonatal alloimmune thrombocytopena. Lancet 1:363, 1989

140. McGrath K, Minchinton R, Cunningham I et al: Platelet anti-Bak^b antibody associated with neonatal alloimmune thrombocytopenia. Vox Sang 57:182, 1989

141. Mueller-Eckhardt C, Becker T, Weisheit M et al: Neonatal alloimmune thrombocytopenia due to fetomaternal Zw^b incompatibility. Vox Sang 50:94, 1986

142. Grenet P, Dausset J, Dugas M et al: Purpura thrombopénique neonatal avec isoimmunisation foeto-maternelle anti-Ko^a. Arch Fr Pediatr 22:1165, 1965

143. Shibata Y, Matsuda I, Miyaji T et al: Yuk^a, a new platelet antigen involved in two cases of neonatal alloimmune thrombocytopenia. Vox Sang 50:177, 1986

144. Mueller-Eckhardt C: HLA-B8 antigen and anti-P1^{A1} allo-immunization. Tissue Antigens 19:154, 1982

145. George JN, Pickett EB, Heinz R: Platelet membrane microparticles in blood bank fresh frozen plasma and cryoprecipitate. Blood 68:307, 1987

146. Warejcka D, Janson M, Aster RH: The P1^{A1} antigen, but not HLA antigens, can be acquired by platelets from plasma, abstracted. Blood, suppl. 1. 66:109a, 1985

147. Kickler TS, Ness PM, Herman JH, Bell WR: Studies on the pathophysiology of posttransfusion purpura. Blood 68:347, 1986

148. Dancis A, Ehmann C, Ferzinger R et al: Studies on the mechanism of P1^{A1} post-transfusion purpura (PTP), abstracted. Blood, suppl. 1. 68:106a, 1986

149. Ehmann EC, Dancis A, Ferzinger R et al: Post-transfuson purpura: evidence that conversion of P1A-1 negative platelets to the P1A-1 positive phenotype is an in vitro artifact, abstracted. Blood, suppl. 1. 70:339a, 1987

150. Kunicki TJ, Aster RH: Isolation and immunologic characterization of the human platelet alloantigen, P1A1. Mol Immunol 16:353, 1979

151. Newman PJ, Derbes RS, Aster RH: The human platelet alloantigens, PLA1 and PLA2, are associated with a leucine33/proline33 amino acid polymorphism and are distinguishable by DNA typing. J Clin Invest 83:1778, 1989

152. Bowditch RD, Tani PH, Halloran CE et al: Localization of a P1^{A1} epitope to the amino terminal 66 residues of platelet glycoprotein IIIa. Blood 79:559, 1992

153. Goldberger A, Kolodziej M, Poncz M et al: Effect of single amino acid substitutions on the formation of the P1A and Bak alloantigenic epitopes. Blood 78:681, 1991

154. Calvete JJ, Henschen A, Gonzalez-Rodriguez J: Assignment of disulphide bonds in human platelet GPIIIa. A disulphide pattern for the beta-subunits of the integrin family. Biochem J 274:63, 1991

155. Beer J, Coller BS: Evidence that platelet glycoprotein IIIa has a large disulfide-bonded loop that is susceptible to proteolytic cleavage. J Biol Chem 264:17564, 1989

156. Flug F, Espinola R, Liu L-X et al: A 13-mer peptide straddling the leucine^{33}/proline^{33} polymorphism in glycoprotein IIIa does not define the PLA$_1$ epitope. Blood 77:1964, 1991

157. Ryckewaert J-J, Schweizer B, Chapel A et al: Production of anti-P1^A monoclonal antibodies. J Lab Clin Med 19:52, 1992

158. McEver RP, Bennett EM, Martin MN: Identification of two structurally and functionally distinct sites on human platelet membrane glycoprotein IIb-IIIa using monoclonal antibodies. J Biol Chem 258:5269, 1983

159. Pidard D, Montgomery RR, Bennett JS, Kunicki TJ: Interaction of AP2, a monoclonal antibody specific for the human platelet glycoprotein IIb-IIIa complex, with intact platelets. J Biol Chem 258:12582, 1983

160. Newman PJ, Allen RW, Kahn RA, Kunicki TJ: Quantitation of membrane glycoprotein IIIa on intact human platelets using the monoclonal antibody, AP3. Blood 65:227, 1985

161. van Leeuwen E, Leeksma O, van Mourik J et al: Effect of the binding of anti-Zw^a antibodies on platelet function. Vox Sang 47:280, 1984

162. Furihata K, Nugent DJ, Bissonette A et al: On the association of the platelet-specific alloantigen, Pen^a, with glycoprotein IIIa. Evidence for heterogeneity of glycoprotein IIIa. J Clin Invest 80:1624, 1987

163. Ryu T, Davis JM, Schwartz KA: Dose-dependent platelet stimulation and inhibition induced by anti-P1A1 IgG. J Lab Clin Med 116:91, 1990

164. Du X, PLow EF, Frelinger AL et al: Ligands "activate" integrin $\alpha_{IIb}\beta_3$ (platelet GPIIb-IIIa). Cell 65:409, 1991

165. Santoso S, Shibata Y, Kiefel V et al: Identification of Yuk(b) alloantigen on platelet glycoprotein IIIa, abstracted. Thromb Haemostas 58:197, 1987

166. Shibata Y, Mori H: A new platelet-specific alloantigen system, Yuk^a/Yuk^b, is located on platelet membrane glycoprotein IIIa. Proc Jpn Acad 63:36, 1987

167. Wang L, Juji T, Shibata Y et al: Sequence variation of human platelet membrane glycoprotein IIIa associated with the Yuk^a/Yuk^b alloantigen system. Proc Jpn Acad 67:102, 1991

168. Wang R, Furihata K, McFarland JG et al: An amino acid polymorphism within the RGD binding domain of platelet membrane glycoprotein IIIa is responsible for the formation of the Pen^a/Pen^b alloantigen system. J Clin Invest 90: 2038, 1992

169. Newman PJ, Kawai Y, Montgomery RR et al: Synthesis by cultured human umbilical vein endothelial cells of two proteins structurally and immunologically related to platelet membrane glycoproteins IIb and IIIa. J Cell Biol 103: 81, 1986

170. Giltay JC, Leeksma OC, von dem Borne AEGK et al: Alloantigenic composition of the endothelial vitronectin receptor. Blood 72:230, 1988

171. Kawai Y, Montgomery RR, Furihata K et al: Expression of platelet alloantigens on human endothelial cells and HEL cells, abstracted. Thromb Haemost 58:4, 1987

172. Giltay JC, Brinkman H-JM, von dem Borne AEGK et al: Expression of the alloantigen Zw^a (or P1^{A1}) on human vascular smooth muscle cells and foreskin fibroblasts: a study on normal individuals and a patient with Glanzmann's thrombasthenia. Blood 74:965, 1989

173. Take H, Tomiyama, Y, Shibata Y et al: Demonstration of the heterogeneity of epitopes of the platelet-specific alloantigen, Baka. Br J Haematol 76:395, 1990

174. van der Weerdt CM, van de Wiel-Dorfmeyer H, Engelfriet CP et al: A new platelet antigen. p. 379. In Proceedings of the Eighth Congress of the European Society of Haematology. S Karger, Basel, 1961

175. Dausset J, Berg P: Un nouvel exemple d'anticorps antiplaquettaire Ko. Vox Sang 8:341, 1963

176. Kuijpers R, Faber NM, Cuypers H TM et al: The N-terminal globular domain of human platelet glycoprotein Ibα has a methionine^{145}/threonine^{145} amino-acid polymorphism, which is associated with the HPA-2 (Ko) alloantigens. J Clin Invest 89:381, 1992

177. Ware J, Russell S, Ruggeri ZM: Genetic basis for the molecular polymorphisms of platelet glycoprotein Ibα. Thromb Haemost 65:347a, 1991

178. Saji H, Maruya E, Fujii H et al: New platelet antigen, Sib^a, involved in platelet transfusion refractoriness in a Japanese man. Vox Sang 56:283, 1989

179. Ishida F, Saji H, Maruya E et al: Human platelet-specific antigen Sib^a is associated with a structural polymorphism of glycoprotein Ibα. Thromb Haemost 65:417a, 1991

180. Lopez JA, Ludwig EH: Molecular basis of platelet glycoprotein Ib polymorphism. Clin Res 39:327a, 1991

181. Tomiyama Y, Take H, Ikeda H: Identification of the platelet-specific alloantigen, Nak^a, on platelet membrane glycoprotein IV. Blood 75:684, 1990

182. Tandon NN, Kralisz U, Jamieson GA: Identification of GPIV (CD36) as a primary receptor for platelet-collagen adhesion. J Biol Chem 264:7576, 1989

183. Asch AS, Barnwell J, Silverstein RL, Nachman RL: Isolation of the thrombospondin membrane receptor. J Clin Invest 79:1054, 1987

184. Yamamoto N, Ikeda H, Tandon NN: A platelet membrane glycoprotein (GP) deficiency in healthy blood donors: Nak^{a-} platelets lack detectable GPIV (CD36). Blood 76:1698, 1990

185. Lipsky RH, Sobieski DA, Tandon NN et al: Detection of GPIV (CD36) mRNA in Nak^{a-} platelets. Thromb Haemost 65:456, 1991

Leukocyte Antigens and Antibodies

133

Parviz Lalezari

INTRODUCTION

The development of antileukocyte antibodies after blood transfusion was first reported by Doan in 1926.[1] Later, the presence of leukoagglutinins was described in association with agranulocytosis.[2,3] The demonstration of leukocyte antibodies in sera of multiparous women[4,5] subsequently led to the discovery of the HLA antigens. Concurrent with this event, neonatal neutropenia due to fetal/maternal incompatibility was described,[6] and investigation of the involved antibodies demonstrated the existence of several alloantigens that were expressed only on neutrophils.[7-9] Further studies of these antigens established their polymorphism and their role in autoimmune neutropenia,[10-13] as well as in febrile and pulmonary transfusion reactions.[14-16] More recently, neutrophil-specific antigens have been implicated in quinine-induced neutropenia,[17] and in some neutropenias following bone marrow transplantation.[18]

With the advent of monoclonal antibodies, additional neutrophil surface markers[19] were identified, some with important clinical implications.[20,21] Attempts are now being made to clarify possible relationships between neutrophil alloantigens and the markers defined by monoclonal antibodies and to determine their chemical structures and regulating genes.

This section provides a general classification for leukocyte antigens, emphasizing neutrophil alloantigens and their related clinical disorders.

NEUTROPHIL ANTIGEN CLASSIFICATION

The classification in Table 133-1 is based on various properties of neutrophil antigens, including their distribution patterns, serology, ontogeny, relationships with maturation, and function. Neutrophil antigens are divided into two major subgroups: antigens identified by alloantibodies and those defined by monoclonal antibodies. The alloantigens are divided into those expressed only on neutrophils, those shared by neutrophils and other blood cells, and those with wide tissue distribution. The antigens recognized by monoclonal antibodies are classified according to their known functional properties.

Neutrophil Antigens Defined by Alloantibodies

Neutrophil-Specific Antigens (N Series)

The letter N used in the nomenclature of neutrophil-specific antigens indicates their restriction to neutrophilic leukocytes; genetic loci and individual alleles are identified alphabetically and numerically, respectively. The allelomorphs, gene frequen-

Table 133-1. Neutrophil Antigens[a]

Antigens identified by alloantibodies
  Neutrophil-specific antigens (N)
    NA, NB, NC, ND, NE, HGA-3, LAN
  Antigens shared with other hematopoietic cells
    Granulocyte antigens (G)
    Granulocyte/monocyte antigens (GM): HGA-1
    Granulocyte/monocyte/lymphocyte/platelets (GMLP): Mart, Ond
  Antigens with wide tissue distribution
    HLA, group 5
    Defined by cold-reactive antibodies: I, i
Antigens defined by monoclonal antibodies (associated with functional structures)
  Fc receptors
    FcγR1, FcγRII, FcγRIII-1, FcαR
  β_2 Integrins
    LFA-1, CR_3, P150,95
  Other receptors for complement and chemotactic agents

[a] NA and LAN are located on FcγRIII-1, Ond on LFA-1, and Mart on CR3 molecules.

cies, and the known clinical implications of these antigens are described in Table 133-2.

Antigens NA,[7] NB,[8] and NC[22] were identified during the study of neonatal neutropenia, and ND1[23] and NE1[24] were associated with autoimmune neutropenia.

In the NA system, TO1, an antigen identical to NA1, has been subjected to extensive genetic analysis,[25] and the existence of a third member has been suggested.[10,26] An association has been found between NA2 and NC1.[11,26,27] NB2[28] is reported to be identical with 9[a], an antigen described in 1965.[29] HGA-3,[30] detected by fluorochromasia, has at least five alleles. Unfortunately, limited availability of antisera has prohibited further investigation of these antigens.

A common property of neutrophil-specific alloantigens is their absence from myeloid precursors and their concurrent development on differentiating cells. These features suggest a relationship between neutrophil-specific antigens and the cell functions that depend on and require cell maturity. The association found between NA and low-affinity Fc receptors for IgG[31] is consistent with this assumption. The low-affinity receptor for IgG (FcγRIII), as defined by monoclonal antibodies (CD16), is expressed on neutrophils, natural killer cells, large granular lymphocytes, T_s lymphocytes, and monocytes. The FcγRIII receptor has two distinct types regulated by two separate genes: FcγR111-1, exclusively expressed on neutrophils, is attached

Table 133-2. Frequencies and Clinical Significance of Neutrophil-Specific Antigens

Locus	Alleles	Frequency Phenotype (%)	Genotype	Clinical Significance
NA	NA1	46	0.367	Alloimmune neutropenia, autoimmunic neutropenia, febrile
	NA2	88	0.633	Pulmonary transfusion reaction
NB	NB1	97	0.827	Alloimmune neutropenia, febrile transfusion reaction
	NB2	32	0.173	Alloimmune neutropenia
NC	NC1	91	0.72	Alloimmune neutropenia
ND	ND1	98.5	0.88	Autoimmune neutropenia
NE	NE1	23	0.12	Autoimmune neutropenia
HGA-3	1–5			Not determined
Mart		90.1		Not determined
Ond		>90		Not determined

to the outer leaflet of the cell membrane bilayer by a glycosyl-phosphatidylinositol (GPI)—anchoring mechanism.[32] By contrast, FcγR111-2, expressed on various mononuclear cells, is a transmembrane glycoprotein. NA antigens represent polymorphisms of FcγRIII-1 on neutrophils; LAN, another neutrophil-specific antigen, is located on this receptor as well.[33] No polymorphism has been described for FcγR111-2. Several cases of alloimmune neonatal neutropenia have been described in which the maternal neutrophils did not react with either anti-NA1 or anti-NA2 antibodies.[34–37] Since neutrophils from these individuals do not react with monoclonal anti-FcγR111, they are considered to be NA[null]. Fromont et al.[37] found four NA[null] individuals among 3,377 randomly tested French donors. Clark et al.[38] reported on a patient with systemic lupus erythematosus whose neutrophils failed to react with anti-CD16. The possibility was not excluded that the two abnormalities were unrelated and merely coincidental. The absence of an NA gene does not seem to lead to clinically discernible neutrophil dysfunction. In this laboratory, several members of a family were identified to be NA[null], and all have remained in perfect health during 17 years of observation. CD16 antigen has been found in the soluble form in plasma, presumably originating from neutrophils.[39] Plasma CD16 level is considered to be of prognostic value in human immunodeficiency virus infection.[40] The GPI-anchoring mechanism is defective in paroxysmal nocturnal hemoglobinuria.[41] Consequently, the NA antigens are poorly expressed on neutrophils from these patients. NB and group 5 antigens are also poorly expressed on paroxysmal nocturnal hemoglobinuria neutrophils and are therefore likely to be attached to the cell membrane by a GPI-anchoring mechanism. NA and NB antigens have relative molecular weights of 46[39] and 56–62[42,43] respectively.

The neutrophil-specific antigens, defined by human antibodies, are not detected on nonprimate neutrophils. In primates, NA2 and NB1 (and 5[b]) are expressed on chimpanzee neutrophils and NB1 is detected in baboons.[11]

Antigens Shared by Neutrophils and Other Hematopoietic Cells

Granulocyte Antigens

The granulocyte (G) antigens,[44,45] presumably expressed on neutrophils and other granulocytes, have been identified by standard granulocytotoxicity assays.

Granulocyte/Monocyte Antigens

HGA-1[30] is an example of a granulocyte/monocyte (GM) antigen, expressed on both granulocytes and monocytes. The corresponding antibodies are found in the sera of recipients of bone marrow or kidney transplantation and have been thought to be involved in allograft rejection.

Granulocyte/Monocyte/Lymphocyte/Platelet Antigens

Two antigens with high frequencies, designated Mart[46] and Ond,[47] have been found on granulocytes, monocytes, lymphocytes, and platelets (GMLP); these antigens have been determined to be associated with the α-chains αM and αL of β-integrin, respectively.[47]

Antigens with Wide Tissue Distribution

ABH

Early reports on the expression of ABH antigens on human neutrophils have not been confirmed.[48–51] ABO incompatibility does not alter the in vivo survival of ^{111}In-labeled granulocytes or their ability to localize at the sites of infection.[52] Failure to

Table 133-3. Fc Receptors on Human Cells

Types	Ligand	Affinity	Molecular Weight ($\times 10^3$)	Site/Cell $\times 10^3$	Monoclonal Antibodies	Expression
FcγRI	Monomeric IgG	High	72	20	32.2, 10.1	Monocyte, PMN[a]
FcγRII	Complexed IgG	Low	40	PMN: 31	CD$_w$32[b]	Myeloid, monocyte, platelet, B cells, some T cells, some endothelial and epithelial cells
				Monocyte: 36		
				B: 38		
				Platelt: 1.2		
FcγRIII	Complexed IgG	Low	50–80	PMN: 100–200	CD16[a]	PMN, monocytes, LGL, NK, T cells
FcαR	IgA		50–70			PMN

Abbreviations: PMN, polymorphonuclear neutrophil; NK, natural killer; LGL, large granular lymphocytes.
[a] Inducible by interferon-γ.
[b] IV.3, CIKM5.
[c] 3G8, B73.1, Gran CLB-1, VEP-13, NKP-13, 80H3, and Leu-11.

demonstrate the ABH antigens on neutrophils does not exclude the possibility that some are acquired through adsorption from plasma.

HLA Antigens

A general feature of HLA antigens, in contrast to neutrophil-specific antigens, is their reduction or loss concurrent with cell maturation and differentiation. In general, HLA antigens, particularly class II, cannot be detected on the cells that do not proliferate. Accordingly, class II molecules are not demonstrable on neutrophils either by absorption[53] or by the use of monoclonal antibodies.[54] Class I antigens are detected on neutrophils but at a level much lower than that found on lymphocytes.[55] This low density may be the reason for the reported failure of anti-HLA antibodies to cause in vitro granulocytotoxicity.[56]

Group 5

Antigens 5[a] and 5[b], the two alleles known in group 5, have gene frequencies of 0.181 and 0.819, respectively.[57] These antigens have demonstrated a wide distribution, expressed on all blood and solid tissue cells except erythrocytes.[58] Antibodies to 5[b] have been involved in febrile[58] and pulmonary transfusion reactions.[59]

Leukocyte Antigens Defined by Cold-Reactive Antibodies

Anti-I and anti-i antibodies cause reversible "cold agglutination" of neutrophils similar to red cell hemagglutination; the presence of I and i antigens has been confirmed by antibody absorption and elution methods.[60] These antigens also have been demonstrated on lymphocytes by cytotoxicity assays. Cold-reactive antigens, other than I and i, have been described on leukocytes: sera of 25% normal donors contain a low titer neutrophil cold agglutinin,[60] and a high-titer cold leukoagglutinin is reported in the serum of a severely neutropenic patient.[61] Similar cold-reactive antibodies, detected by cytotoxicity assay, have been reported.[62] The antigens related to these cold-reactive antibodies appear to be expressed on neutrophils and other granulocytes.

Antigens Identified by Monoclonal Antibodies

The screening of monoclonal antihuman neutrophil antibodies has led to the identification of several antigens associated with various neutrophil functions. These include antigens associated with Fc receptors[63,64] and the adhesive protein receptors,[21,47,65] integrins composed of a common β-chains and varying α-chains. The current information on Fc receptors is summarized in Table 133-3; integrins are described in detail in other chapters. Monoclonal antibodies reacting with NA1,[41] NA2,[66] and NB1[45] alloantigens have also been described.

METHODS FOR DETECTION OF NEUTROPHIL ANTIGEN/ANTIBODY REACTIONS

The agglutination technique is the method of choice for detection of antibodies against the N series and group 5.[67] These antibodies are not usually cytotoxic. Unlike hemagglutination, antibody-induced neutrophil agglutination is not a passive reaction mediated by formation of "immunologic bridges." Rather, neutrophil agglutination is a time- and temperature-dependent active process that requires viable cells. Neutrophils become "activated" by the effects of antibodies, form pseudopods, and move toward each other until aggregates are formed.[11] At physiologic temperatures, therefore, leukoagglutination can be considered a test of neutrophil function. The immunofluorescence (IF) assays,[14] including flow cytometry,[67] are also suitable methods. NB2 (9[a]) and 5[b], however, do not react in the IF tests, indicating the need for the use of multiple techniques for neutrophil antibody screening. Also, it should be recognized that the direct IF test, employed for detection of neutrophil-bound IgG, may produce misleading results. This fact became apparent when we detected positive IF tests on neutrophils of patients who had received colony-stimulating factor-granulocyte (CSF-G).[68] Subsequent studies in this and other laboratories[69,70] revealed that CSF-G treatment induces expression on neutrophils of high-affinity receptor for IgG (FcγR1, CD64), which is absent from normal neutrophils. FcγR1 nonspecifically binds serum IgG, which is then detected on neutrophils by a direct IF reaction. Thus, for proper interpretation of a positive direct IF reaction, it would be necessary to demonstrate that the neutrophils being tested do not express FcγR1. For monoclonal antibodies, flow cytometry remains the method of choice. Other methods used for detection of leukocyte antibodies, including radiolabeling and avidin/biotin immunoassays, enzyme-linked immunosorbent assay, and various complement-binding and cytotoxic assays, are reviewed elsewhere.[71]

CLINICAL DISORDERS RELATED TO NEUTROPHIL ANTIGENS AND ANTIBODIES

The clinical disorders discussed in this section are immunologically induced neutropenias and pulmonary and febrile transfusion reactions.

Immunologically Induced Neutropenias

The balance between the rates of cell production and destruction determines the level at which various blood cells are maintained. Leukocytes are composed of heterogeneous cell types, each with a distinct proliferative property and life span and independent antigenic structures and functions. Accordingly, the production/destruction imbalance can occur for each leukocyte population independently, and each can present a distinct clinical entity. For these reasons, the terms leukopenia, granulocytopenia, and neutropenia should not be used interchangeably.[72] Leukopenia should define conditions in which all the granulocytes, monocytes, and lymphocytes are affected; granulocytopenia should refer to a reduction in the number of granulocytes; and neutropenia should indicate selective paucity of neutrophils. Such discrimination applies readily to immune neutropenias of infancy in which only neutrophils are affected. In adults, however, these disorders appear to be more complex.

Immunologically Induced Neutropenias During Infancy

Four etiologic types of immunologically induced neutropenias are recognized during infancy: alloimmune neonatal neutropenia (ANN), transient neutropenia secondary to maternal autoimmune neutropenia, autoimmune neutropenia of infancy (AINI), and autoimmune neutropenia associated with hemolytic anemia and/or thrombocytopenia.

Alloimmune Neonatal Neutropenia

ANN[6,9,73] is a disorder analogous to erythroblastosis, caused by transplacental transfer of maternal neutrophil-specific alloantibodies into fetal circulation.

Etiology and Pathophysiology. ANN frequently occurs in the first pregnancy, without a history of maternal blood transfusion. Assuming immunogenicity of the fetal neutrophils,[74] it is likely that maternal alloimmunization is initiated after the first trimester of pregnancy, at the time the hematopoietic cells are developed. The incidence of pregnancy-induced neutrophil alloimmunization has been estimated to be 0.1–0.2%,[75,76] in contrast to 20% for the HLA antigens. The difference has been attributed to the multiplicity of the sources of stimuli for the HLA.[11] ABH and other red cell incompatibilities are irrelevant. By contrast, HLA compatibility may even facilitate an immune response to tissue-specific antigens.

The target for antineutrophil antibodies in the fetus is a small mass confined to mature neutrophils. This results in selective destruction of the mature cells but sparing of the immature myeloid cells as well as the monocytes and eosinophils, which proliferate in the bone marrow. These effects are distinct from those anticipated for the HLA-type antibodies. Anti-HLA antibodies must overcome the placental barrier where some of the cells express the HLA antigens. Antibodies that cross this barrier are likely to be neutralized by the soluble HLA molecules in circulation and by the antigens present on the surfaces of various tissue cells. This reduces efficacy of anti-HLA antibodies against individual cell types to the extent that an adverse effect can occur only if the antibody concentration is overwhelming.

Infants affected by ANN are, as a rule, neutropenic at birth. In several cases, however, neutropenia did not occur at birth but was recognized after a delay of 1–3 days. The immaturity of the macrophages and other mechanisms involved in neutrophil destruction may be one explanation for this delay.

Among various neutrophil specificities, NA1 is involved in 34%, NB1 in 13%, and NA2 in 12% of ANN. In one-third of the cases other specificities, not as yet defined, have been involved, and in 4% no antibodies are detected.[73] A heretofore unexplained high incidence of spontaneous abortion, stillbirth, prematurity, and twin pregnancy has been reported in the affected families.[73]

Pathogenesis. Complement-dependent cell lysis analogous to intravascular hemolysis does not seem to occur, because most antineutrophil antibodies found in association with ANN do not fix complement. Phagocytosis of the opsonized neutrophils by macrophages has been shown in vitro and in the bone marrow of some of the patients affected with AINI.[77] Antibody-dependent neutrophil agglutination may also prove to be a factor. Neutrophil aggregates, produced by activated C5[78] or by phorbol myristate acetate[79] experimentally, become trapped in the lung capillaries. Entrapment of the circulating neutrophils may similarly occur in the splenic sinusoids and liver capillaries, thereby reducing the number of circulating neutrophils.

Clinical Presentation and Laboratory Evaluation. ANN in newborn infants is often asymptomatic. The absence of neutrophils is discovered only if a routine blood examination is performed at birth. In symptomatic cases, fever and respiratory, urinary, or skin infections develop within 1 or 2 weeks. These complications are, in general, self-limited and without sequelae. The bacteria involved are mostly staphylococci, β-hemolytic streptococcus, and *Escherichia coli*. Neutropenia may last from 2 weeks to 6 months. In a total of 95 affected cases studied in this laboratory, we have recorded only four deaths due to sepsis, all occurring before the disease was recognized.

Diagnosis of neutropenia requires examination of blood smears. The total leukocyte count is usually normal and would be misleading unless differentials are determined manually. The blood smear reveals paucity or complete absence of the mature neutrophils, often with absolute monocytosis and eosinophilia. Band forms or more immature myeloid cells may also be seen. The presence of monocytosis should be verified by an experienced morphologist, since monocytes may be reported as "atypical lymphocytes." Red blood cells and platelets are normal unless the patient has an associated neonatal thrombocytopenia. This association has been reported. In a retrospective study of sera from 33 affected families, 10 contained both antineutrophil and antiplatelet antibodies. The bone marrow shows myeloid cell hyperplasia with a characteristic left shift often described as "maturation arrest" at either myelocyte, metamyelocyte, or band stage. Occasionally, the segmented neutrophils are found in the marrow in near-normal numbers.

Once neutropenia is recognized, the alloimmune nature of the disorder must be established by demonstrating neutrophil-specific alloantibodies in the maternal sera. A systematic investigation should include examination of the blood samples from the infant and both parents. Neutrophil specificity of the antibodies should be established by absorption of the maternal serum with paternal platelets to remove non-neutrophilic antibodies, and the parental neutrophils should be typed to facilitate determination of the specificity involved.

Transient Congenital Neutropenia

Mothers with autoimmune neutropenia may give birth to infants who develop transient neutropenia.[80] I have observed this disorder in two families. In one case, the mother had a persistent total leukocyte count of 1,300–3,500/mm^3, mild Crohn disease, and a palpable spleen. The fourth child of this mother was a premature infant who, at birth, had a leukocyte count of 4,500/mm^3 with 21% neutrophils and 4% bands. On day 5, the neutrophil count was only 1%. The severe neutropenia lasted 6 weeks, followed by a complete recovery. Four years later, this mother gave birth to her fifth child, who also developed a transient but severe neutropenia, lasting 2 weeks. The agglutination and IF test results in the mother and her infants were negative. In the second family, the mother had been neutropenic (leukocyte count of 1,200–3,000/mm^3 with 13–26% neutrophils) and was told she had a slightly enlarged spleen. Three years later, she gave birth to her first infant, who was found on the second day to have an absolute neutrophil count of 500. Neutrophils returned to normal within 4 months. The following year, a second child was born to the family and was initially reported to have a normal neutrophils. Repeat evaluation after 1 week, however, determined the infant to be neutropenic. The recovery this time occurred within 4 weeks. The autoimmune nature of the mother's neutropenia was established by positive serologic tests.

Autoimmune Neutropenia of Infancy

Chronic benign neutropenia of infancy and early childhood[81] and chronic granulocytopenia in childhood[82] have long been recognized. The autoimmune nature of this disorder was established when autoantibodies with specificity for neutrophils were demonstrated.[10] AINI is the most common form of chronic neutropenia in infants.[13] Severe neutropenia is usually recognized when the child is 5–7 months old. Diagnosis of neutropenia is made either by a routine blood test or during evaluation of an infection. The chronicity becomes apparent when the blood tests, repeated after recovery from infection, remain abnormal. The clinical course of AINI is relatively mild, with occasional stomatitis, otitis, diarrhea, and respiratory infection. The incidence of these complications diminishes as the child grows older. Occasionally, chronic otitis results in hearing loss, and persistent gingivitis in older children leads to tooth loss. Neutropenia is self-limited, and complete recovery within 1–6 years is the rule. Recurrence of the autoimmunity has not thus far been observed in the long-term follow-up of these patients. The etiology and the reason for the spontaneous loss of the autoantibodies have not been clarified.

Autoimmune Neutropenias Associated with Hemolytic Anemia and Thrombocytopenia

Autoimmune neutropenia may occur in combination with autoimmune hemolytic anemia and thrombocytopenia during the perinatal period. In these cases, the clinical course is often severe.

Management of Immune Neutropenias in Infancy. Immune neutropenias in infancy are usually self-limited and are compatible with normal growth and development. The affected infants, however, should receive protective mouth and skin care and avoid exposure to potential sources of infection. Hospitalization and vigorous antibiotic therapy are required only for severe infections. Intravenous administration of large doses of γ-globulin has been shown to reverse the neutropenia in AINI.[83] This treatment is necessary only in cases complicated by refractory infections. In ANN, demonstration of neutrophil antibodies in the maternal sera implies the likelihood that infants born in future pregnancies will be affected. Possible prevention of this occurrence by intravenous administration of γ-globulin during the last trimester of pregnancy, as recommended in alloimmune neonatal thrombocytopenia,[84] is not warranted because of the benign nature of the disorder. Mothers with neutrophil alloantibodies should be warned about the possibility of febrile reactions if they receive blood transfusions in the future. They should also be advised that transfusion of their blood, or even their packed red blood cells, into normal recipients may cause a severe and potentially fatal pulmonary transfusion reaction.

Differential Diagnosis of Neutropenias in Infants. The prognosis of neutropenias in infancy varies according to etiology. Therefore, once neutropenia is diagnosed, efforts should be made to determine the cause. Immunologically induced neutropenias, with the exception of those associated with hemolytic anemia and thrombocytopenia, have a benign course, whereas the nonimmune congenital forms last for life and may become complicated by repeated life-threatening infections. In ANN, alloantibodies are demonstrated in the maternal sera. In AINI, documentation of a normal neutrophil count before the apparent onset of the disease is most valuable. Diagnosis of AINI is established by demonstrating antibodies in the affected children rather than in the maternal sera. Positive diagnosis of the transient congenital form is made by documenting an autoimmune neutropenia in the mother. Differential diagnosis should include disorders of neutrophil production, stem cell abnormalities (see Ch. 18), and neutropenias associated with infection.

Neutropenia Associated with Infection

The relative neutrophil reserve (the total number of neutrophils, bands, and metamyelocytes) in the bone marrow in newborn infants is small compared with adults. The bone marrow reserve in newborn rats has been estimated to be $2 \pm 0.1 \times 10^6/kg$ as compared to $4.5 \pm 0.2 \times 10^6/kg$ in adult rats.[85] Moreover, newborn rats, unlike adults, cannot increase the rate of their stem cell proliferation in response to bacterial inoculation, presumably because their myeloid cells are already maximally stimulated. Similar limitations may be contributing to the development of neutropenia in association with viral and bacterial infections in infants. In such cases, other etiologies should be suspected if neutropenia persists after the acute inflammation has subsided.

Primary Autoimmune Neutropenias in Adolescence and Adults

The hematologic profile is that of the absence or reduction in the number of neutrophils, often with preservation of other granulocytes and lymphocytes. Monocytosis is commonly present. The bone marrow typically reveals an absence of the mature cells with increased number of precursors. Clinically, manifestations vary from mild to severe forms. Patients may develop mucocutaneous infections, but overwhelming sepsis is rare. Splenomegaly is not a consistent finding in this disorder. Serologic diagnosis is made by demonstrating neutrophil antibodies as described for infants. In some cases, the antibody may have specificity for the known antigens,[11] similar to those described in AINI. In rare instances, neutropenia may be caused by cold-reactive antibodies.

Secondary Immune Neutropenias in Adults

Autoimmune neutropenias may be associated with systemic lupus erythematosus, rheumatoid arthritis, Sjögren syndrome, Graves disease, and lymphoproliferative disorders (e.g., T cell, hairy cell leukemia). A combination with hemolytic anemia and/or thrombocytopenia, in a characteristic sequence, has been designated alternating autoimmune hemocytopenia.[72] In this form, the disease is multiphasic, initially being limited to only one cell population. Remissions occur, with or without treatment, only to relapse but involving another cell type. Alternation between neutropenia, thrombocytopenia, and hemolytic anemia continues until a pancytopenia often resistant to treatment prevails. Neutropenia may also occur in infectious mononucleosis or *Mycoplasma* pneumonia. In these cases, cold-reactive antibodies have been considered to be a contributory factor.

Febrile Transfusion Reactions

The association between leukoagglutinins and febrile transfusion reaction has long been established. Anti-HLA, 5[b,] and antibodies against neutrophil-specific antigens have been implicated. Since these antibodies do not occur naturally, the patients are alloimmunized either by previous transfusions or by pregnancies. The reaction has been defined by Brittingham and Chaplin[86] in three phases. Immediate reaction may occur within 5 minutes and is manifested by palpitation, cough, flush, and tachycardia. The second phase is silent and may last for 1 hour. The third phase starts with chills, headache, fever, irritability, and occasionally nausea and vomiting. These symptoms usually subside spontaneously within a few hours and require only symptomatic treatment. Future reactions usually can be prevented by use of leukocyte-depleted blood.

Pulmonary Transfusion Reaction

Volume overload, transmission of infectious agents, and hemolytic, febrile, and allergic reactions are familiar hazards of blood transfusion. A less appreciated but serious complication is a noncardiogenic pulmonary edema, attributed to the presence of leukocyte antibodies in the donors' plasma. This complication was first reported by Barnard[87] in 1951. In 1957, Brittingham[88] observed a severe febrile reaction that was associated with cyanosis, dyspnea, hypotension, and radiographic evidence of bilateral pulmonary infiltrates after 50 ml of whole blood had been infused into a normal recipient. The blood was from a multitransfused donor and contained leukoagglutinins. Many cases with similar symptoms in which the reactions were attributed to leukocyte antibodies in the donors' or in the recipients' plasmas were subsequently reported.[89] Additional cases were reported after granulocyte transfusion.[90]

Pathogenesis of the lung injury in this complication is not fully understood. Three phases are suggested. In the initial phase, the recipient's neutrophils are activated by direct effects of the antibodies or by complement activation and release of C5a. In the second phase, the activated neutrophils adhere to the pulmonary capillary bed. In the third phase, disintegration of neutrophils and release of their proteolytic enzymes and/or generation of free radicals lead to breakdown of the capillary wall and accumulation of fluid in the alveolar space.

Pulmonary transfusion reaction is clinically manifested by an acute respiratory distress syndrome that develops after or during administration of blood or blood products. It is usually manifested by an abrupt onset of chills, fever, tachycardia, cough, and severe dyspnea, often leading to cyanosis, hypotension, and occasionally death. In patients under anesthesia or in debilitated persons, the onset may be more insidious and frequently the diagnosis is made when a chest radiograph is obtained to clarify the cause of the patients' respiratory symptoms. The radiologic appearance of bilateral pulmonary infiltrates, without cardiomegaly or pulmonary vascular congestion, in a patient who had normal lungs before transfusion strongly suggests this diagnosis. In most cases, the lung infiltrates disappear within a few days, and recovery is complete. The antibodies implicated in these reactions have included those against 4^a,[91] HLA,[92] NA1, NA2,[15] 5^b,[59] and NB1.[16] The incidence of transfusion-associated lung injury is estimated to be 1 in 5,000 units of blood transfused, or 0.16% in transfused patients.[89] Despite this high incidence, to date only 66 cases have been reported in the literature. Among these and five additional examples observed in our laboratory, eight deaths have been recorded, indicating an 11% mortality rate. Differential diagnoses include sepsis, volume overload, aspiration pneumonia, hypersensitivity reaction, shock, uremia, neurogenic pulmonary edema, narcotic or salicylate overdose, hypoxia, inhalation of toxic gases, trauma, and pancreatitis.

Therapy for this complication is supportive. Prevention by routine screening of blood donors for neutrophil antibodies would not be cost effective but may be necessary at least for multiparous female donors. The use of packed cells may reduce the severity but would not eliminate the reaction (see also Ch. 141).

Future Directions

Because of the diversities of the neutrophil surface structures, many new neutrophil-specific antigens are expected to be defined in the future. Development of new techniques for detection of leukocyte antigen/antibody reactions should facilitate characterization of these antigens. The more difficult challenges are in the areas of pathophysiology and autoimmunity. Leukocyte differentials vary in autoimmune disorders affecting leukocytes. In the autoimmune neutropenias, involvement of neutrophil-specific antigens is a plausible explanation for selective destruction of neutrophils, and the commonly associated monocytosis and eosinophilia may reflect the bone marrow response to compensatory increased levels of growth factors. Neutrophil specificity, however, does not explain the changes observed in the lymphocyte counts in many cases of leukopenias, particularly in adults and adolescents. It is likely that in these cases, targets of autoimmunity are antigens with wider cell distribution, such as leukocyte adhesion molecules. Determination of specificities of autoantibodies in autoimmune neutropenia has practical and therapeutic implications. The chemical structure and regulating genes for various neutrophil surface antigens are likely to be defined by application of modern techniques of molecular biology. Large quantities of these antigens can then be produced by genetic engineering and bound covalently to absorbing filters. Such filters may provide a means for selective removal of the auto- and alloantibodies, temporarily reducing damage to the target cells.

In the management of autoimmune diseases, steroids and immunosuppressive agents are commonly used to the limit of compromising the patient's defense mechanism. Benefit from these therapeutic procedures in patients in whom neutrophils are already compromised is not clear. The use of intravenous γ-globulin is helpful, mostly in cases affecting children. The mechanism by which intravenous IgG modifies the immune-mediated cell destruction must be clarified if this therapy is to be optimally exploited. It is likely that not all substructural components of the IgG molecule are necessary. A promising new approach to the treatment of autoimmune neutropenia is the administration of CSF-G. Treatment with low doses of CSF-G has led to elevated neutrophil counts and complete elimination of clinical symptoms in several patients (Lalezari P, unpublished data). In these patients, treatment with CSF-G is believed to convert the "uncompensated" disorder to a "compensated" form, analogous to compensated autoimmune hemolytic anemia in which the patient maintains a normal blood count. High doses of CSF-G in these patients has been found to cause thrombocytopenia, a complication that can be corrected by reducing the dose of the growth factor.

The ultimate control of autoimmune neutropenia requires the clarification and correction of the underlying irregularities of the immune system. Moreover, an understanding of the mechanism of cell destruction, including the indications for splenectomy (which occasionally is recommended), is necessary in order to develop more logical therapeutic strategies.

ACKNOWLEDGMENT

This work was supported by the Jimmy Pollock Research Foundation.

REFERENCES

1. Doan CA: The recognition of a biologic differentiation in the white blood cells with a specific reference to blood transfusion. JAMA 86:1593, 1926
2. Dausset J, Nenna A: Presence d'une leuco-agglutinine dans le serum d'un cas d'agranulocytose chronique. C R Soc Biol 146:1539, 1952

3. Moeschlin S, Wagner K: Agranulocytosis due to the occurrence of leukocyte agglutinins (pyramidon and cold agglutinins). Acta Haematol 8:29, 1952

4. Payne R, Folfs MR: Fetomaternal leukocyte incompatibility. J Clin Invest 37:1756, 1958

5. van Rood JJ, van Leeuwen A, Ernisse JG: Leukocyte antibodies in sera of pregnant women. Vox Sang 4:427, 1959

6. Lalezari P, Nussbaum M, Gelman S, Spaet TH: Neonatal neutropenia due to maternal isoimmunization. Blood 15:236, 1960

7. Lalezari P, Bernard JE: An isologous antigen-antibody reaction with human neutrophils related to neonatal neutropenia. J Clin Invest 45:1741, 1966

8. Lalezari P, Murphy GB, Allen FH: NB1, a new neutrophil antigen involved in the pathogenesis of neonatal neutropenia. J Clin Invest 50:1108, 1971

9. Lalezari P, Radel E: Neutrophil-specific antigens: immunology and clinical significance. Semin Hematol 11:281, 1974

10. Lalezari P, Jiang AF, Yegen L, Santorineou M: Chronic autoimmune neutropenia due to anti-NA2 antibody. N Engl J Med 293:744, 1975

11. Lalezari P: Neutrophil antigens: immunology and clinical implications. p. 209. In Greenwalt TJ, Jamieson GA (eds): The Granulocyte: Function and Clinical Utilization: Progress in Clinical and Biological Research. Alan R Liss, New York, 1977

12. McCullough J, Clay ME, Priest JR et al: A comparison of methods for detecting leukocyte antibodies in autoimmune neutropenia. Transfusion 21:483, 1981

13. Lalezari P, Khorshidi M, Petrosova M: Autoimmune neutropenia of infancy. J Pediatr 109:764, 1986

14. Verheugt FWA, von dem Borne AEGK, Decary S, Engelfriet CP: The detection of granulocyte alloantibodies with an indirect immunofluorescence test. Br J Haematol 36:533, 1977

15. Yomtovian R, Kline W, Press C et al: Severe pulmonary hypersensitivity associated with passive transfusion of a neutrophil-specific antibody. Lancet 1:244, 1984

16. van Buren N, Stonek D, Clay M et al: Transfusion related lung injury caused by a NB2 granulocyte-specific antibody, abstracted. Transfusion 28:27S, 1988

17. Stroncek DF, Shankar RA, Herr GP: Quinine-dependent antibodies to neutrophils react with a 60-Kd glycoprotein on which neutrophil-specific antigen NB1 is located and an 85-Kd glycosylphosphatidylinositol-linked N-glycosylated plasma membrane glycoprotein. Blood 81:2758, 1993

18. Stroncek DF, Shapiro R, Philipovich A et al: Prolonged neutropenia following marrow transplant due to antibodies to neutrophil-specific antigen NB1. Transfusion 33:158, 1993

19. McMichael AJ: Leukocyte Typing. Vol. III: White Cell Differentiation Antigens. Oxford University Press, Oxford, 1987

20. Crowley CA, Curnutte JT, Rosin RE et al: An inherited abnormality of neutrophil adhesion. Its genetic transmission and its association with a missing protein. N Engl J Med 302:1163, 1980

21. Ross GD: Clinical and laboratory features of patients with an inherited deficiency of neutrophil membrane complement receptor type 3 (CR3) and the related membrane antigens LFA-1. J Clin Immunol 6:107, 150, 1986

22. Lalezari P, Thalenfeld B, Weinstein WJ: The third neutrophil antigen. p. 319. In Terasaki PI (ed): Histocompatibility Testing, 1970. Williams & Wilkins, Baltimore, 1970

23. Verheugt FWA, von dem Borne AEG Kr, van Noord-Bokhorst JC: NDI, a new neutrophil granulocyte antigen. Vox Sang 35:13, 1978

24. Claas FHJ, Langerak J, Sabre LJM, van Roor JJ: NE1, a new neutrophil specific antigen. Tissue Antigens 13:129, 1979

25. Ceppellini R, Curtoni ES, Mattiuz PL et al: Genetics of leukocyte antigens: a family study of segregation and linkage. p. 149. In Curtoni ES, Mattiuz PL, Tosi RM (eds): Histocompatibility Testing, 1967. Munksgaard, Copenhagen, 1967

26. McCullough J, Clay M, Press C, Kline W: Granulocyte Serology, A Clinical and Laboratory Guide. American Society of Clinical Pathologists, Chicago, 1989

27. Schacter B, Kadushin J, Hsieh K: Neutrophil antigens: population and family studies in Caucasians and blacks. Hum Immunol 1:280, 1980

28. Lalezari P, Petrosova M, Jiang AF: NB2, an allele of NB1 neutrophil specific antigen: relationship to 9a. Transfusion 22:433, 1982

29. van Rood JJ, van Leeuwen A, Schippers AMJ. Leukocyte groups, the normal lymphocyte transfer test and homograft sensitivity. p. 37. In Amos DB, van Rood JJ (eds): Histocompatibility Testing, 1965. Munksgaard, Copenhagen, 1965

30. Thompson JS, Overlin VL, Herbick JM et al: New granulocyte antigens demonstrated by microgranulocytotoxicity assay. J Clin Invest 65:1431, 1980

31. Werner G, von dem Borne AEGK, Bos MJE et al: Localization of the human NA1 alloantigen on neutrophil-Fc receptors. p. 109. In Reinherz EL, Haynes BF, Nadler LM, Berstein ID (eds): Leukocyte Typing. Vol. II: Human Myeloid and Hematopoietic Cells. Springer-Verlag, New York, 1985

32. Selveraj P, Rosse WF, Silber R, Springer TA: The major Fc receptor in blood has a phosphatidylinositol anchor and is deficient in paroxysmal nocturnal hemoglobinuria. Nature 333:565, 1988

33. Metcalfe P, Waters AH: Location of the granulocyte-specific antigen LAN on FcγRIII. Transfus Med 2:283, 1992

34. Huizinga WJ, Kuijpers WAM, Kleijer M et al: Maternal genomic neutrophil FcRIII deficiency leading to neonatal isoimmune neutropenia. Blood 76:1927, 1990

35. Stroncek DF, Skubitz KM, Plachta LB et al: Alloimmune neonatal neutropenia due to an antibody to the neutrophil Fc-gamma-receptor III with maternal deficiency at CD16 antigen. Blood 77:1572, 1991

36. Cartron J, Celton JL, Gane P et al: Iso-immune neonatal neutropenia due to an anti-FCRIII-1 (CD16) antibody. Eur J Pediatr 151:438, 1992

37. Fromont P, Bettaieb A, Skouri H et al: Frequency of the PMN-FcRIII deficiency in the French population and its involvement in the development of neonatal alloimmune neutropenia. Blood 79:2131, 1992

38. Clark MR, Liu L, Clarkson SB et al: An abnormality of the gene that encodes neutrophil Fc receptor III in a patient with systemic lupus erythematosus. J Clin Invest 86:341, 1990

39. Huizinga TWJ, Haas MD, Kleijer M et al: Soluble Fcγ receptor III in human plasma originates from release by neutrophils. J Clin Invest 86:416, 1990

40. Khayat D, Soubrane C, Andrieu JM et al: Changes of soluble CD16 levels in serum of HIV-infected patients: correlation with clinical and biologic prognostic factors. J Infect Dis 161:430, 1990

41. Huizinga TWJ, Shoot E, van der Jost G et al: PI-linked receptor FcRIII is released on stimulation of neutrophils. Nature 333:667, 1988

42. Stroncek DF, Skubitz KM, McCullough J: Biochemical characterization of neutrophil-specific antigen NB1. Blood 75:744, 1990

43. Goldschmedine R, van Dalen CM, Faber N et al: Further characterization of the NB1 antigen as a variably expressed 56–62 kD GPI-linked glycoprotein of plasma membranes and specific granules of neutrophils. Br J Haematol 81:336, 1992

44. Drew SI, Bergh O, McClelland J et al: Antigenic specificities detected on papainized human granulocytes by microgranulocytotoxicity. Transplant Proc 9:639, 1977

45. Korinkova P, Vorlicek J, Majsky A: A study of granulocyte cytotoxins and detection of granulocyte allospecific antigens. Transfusion 22:379, 1982

46. Kline WE, Press C, Clay M et al: Three sera defining a new granulocyte-monocyte-T-lymphocyte antigen. Vox Sang 50:181, 1986

47. van der Schoot CE, Daams M, Huiskes E et al: Antigenic polymorphism of the leu-CAM family recognized by human leukocyte alloantisera. Br J Haematol (in press)

48. Karhi KK, Andersson LC, Vuopio P, Gahmberg CG: Expression of blood group A antigens in human bone marrow. Blood 57:147, 1981

49. Lalezari P: Biological roles of tissue-specific and systemic alloantigens. p. 55. In McCullough J, Sandler SG (eds): Blood Cell Antigens and Bone Marrow Transplantation Advances in Immunobiology: Progress in Clinical and Biological Research. Alan R Liss, New York, 1984

50. Kelton JG, Bebenek G: Granulocytes do not have surface ABO antigens. Transfusion 25:567, 1985

51. Dunstan RA, Simpson MB, Borowitz M: Absence of ABH antigens on neutrophils. Br J Haematol 60:651, 1985

52. McCullough J, Clay M, Press C, Kline W: Granulocyte Serology, A Clinical Laboratory Guide. American Society for Clinical Pathology, Chicago, 1988

53. Thompson JS, Severson CD: Granulocyte antigens. p. 151. In Bell CA (ed): A Seminar on Antigens on Blood Cells and Body Fluid. American Association of Blood Banks, Washington, DC, 1980

54. Dunstan RA, Simpson MB, Sanfilippo FP: Absence of specific HLA-DR antigens on human platelets and neutrophils. Blood 64:85a, 1984

55. Thompson JS: Antileukocyte capillary agglutinating antibody in pre- and post-transplantation sera. p. 868. In Rose NR, Friedman H (eds): Manual of Clinical Immunology. American Society of Microbiology, Washington, DC, 1976

56. Blaschke J, Goeken NE, Thompson JS et al: Acquired agranulocytosis with granulocyte specific cytotoxic autoantibody. Am J Med 66:862, 1979

57. van Leeuwen A, Eernise JG, van Rood JJ: A new leukocyte group with two alleles: leukocyte group five. Vox Sang 9:431, 1964

58. Lalezari P, Bernard GE: Identification of a specific leukocyte antigen, another presumed example of 5b. Transfusion 5:135, 1965

59. Nordhagen R, Conradi M, Dromtorp SM: Pulmonary reaction associated with transfusion of plasma containing anti-5b. Vox Sang 51:102, 1986

60. Lalezari P, Murphy GB: Cold reacting leukocyte agglutinins and their significance. p. 421. In Curtoni ES, Mattinuz PL, Tosi RM (eds): Histocompatibility Testing, 1967. Williams & Wilkins, Baltimore, 1967

61. Markenson AL, Lalezari P, Markenson JA: In Proceedings of the Eighteenth Congress of the American Society of Hematology, Dallas. Grune & Stratton, Orlando, FL, 1975

62. Drew SI, Terasaki PI: Autoimmune cytotoxic granulocyte antibodies in normal persons and various diseases. Blood 52:941, 1978

63. Fleit HB, Wright SD, Unkeless JC: Human neutrophil Fc receptor distribution and structure. Proc Natl Acad Sci USA 79:3275, 1982

64. Hogg N: The structure and function of Fc receptors. Immunol Today 9:185, 1988

65. Hemler ME: Adhesive protein receptors on hematopoietic cells. Immunol Today 9:109, 1988

66. Huizinga TWJ, Kleijer M, Roos D, von dem Borne AEGK: Leucocyte Typing. Vol. IV. Oxford University Press, New York, 1990

67. Lalezari P, Khorshidi M: Detection of neutrophil and platelet antibodies: agglutination, immunofluorescence and flow cytometry. p. 149. In Greenwalt TJ (ed): Methods in Hematology. Blood Transfusion. Churchill Livingstone, Edinburgh, 1988

68. Lalezari P, Khorshidi M, Warshaw T et al: Treatment of an adult case of Job's syndrome with recombinant granulocyte colony stimulating factor. Blood 78:4a, 1991

69. Repp R, Valerius TH, Sendler A et al: Neutrophils express the high affinity receptor for IgG (FcRI, CD64) after in vivo application of recombinant human granulocyte colony-stimulating factor. Blood 78:885, 1991

70. Kerst JM, Van de Winkel JGJ, Evans AH et al: G-CSF induces hFcgammaRI (CD64 antigen) positive neutrophils via an effect on myeloid precursor cells. Blood 81:1457, 1993

71. McCullough J, Clay M, Press C, Kline W: Leukocyte Serology, a Clinical and Laboratory Guide. American Society of Clinical Pathologists, Chicago, 1988

72. Lalezari P: Autoimmune Neutropenia. p. 523. In Rose NR, Mackay IR (eds): The Autoimmune Diseases. Academic Press, San Diego, 1985

73. Lalezari P: Alloimmune neonatal neutropenia. p. 443. In Engelfriet CP, Von Dem Borne AEGK (eds): Alloimmune and Autoimmune Cytopenias. Baillieres Clinical Immunology and Allergy. Bailliere Tindall, London, 1987

74. Madyastha PR, Glassman AB, Levine DH: Incidence of neutrophil antigens on human cord neutrophils. Am J Reprod Immunol 6:124, 1984

75. Clay M, Kline W, McCullough J: Serological examination of postpartum sera for the presence of neutrophil-specific antibodies. Transfusion 21:616, 1981

76. Levine DH, Madyastha P, Wade R, Levkoff AH: Neonatal isoimmune neutropenia. Pediatr Res 15:296a, 1981

77. Boxer LA, Stossel TP: Effects of anti-human neutrophil antibodies in vitro. J Clin Invest 53:1534, 1974

78. Craddock PR, Fehr J, Brigham KL: Complement and leukocyte-mediated pulmonary dysfunction in hemodialysis. N Engl J Med 296:769, 1977

79. O'Flaherty JT, Cousart S, Lineberger AS: Phorbol myristate acetate. Am J Pathol 101:79, 1980

80. Stefanini M, Mele RH, Skimer D: Transitory congenital neutropenia: a new syndrome, a report of two cases. Am J Med 25:749, 1958

81. Stahlie TD: Chronic benign neutropenia in infancy and early childhood. Report of a case and review of literature. J Pediatr 48:710, 1956

82. Zuelzer WW, Bajoghli M: Chronic granulocytopenia in childhood. Blood 23:359, 1964

83. Bussel JB, Lalezari P, Hilgartner M: Reversal of neutropenia with intravenous gammaglobulin in autoimmune neutropenia of infancy. Blood 62:398, 1983

84. Bussel JB, Berkowitz RL, McFarland JG: Antenatal treatment of neonatal alloimmune thrombocytopenia. N Engl J Med 319:1374, 1988

85. Christensen RD, Rothstein G, Hill HR, Anstall HB: Why do septic neonates develop profound neutropenia? Transfusion 22:434, 1982

86. Brittingham TE, Chaplin H: Febrile transfusion reactions caused by sensitivity to donor leukocytes and platelets. JAMA 16:819, 1957

87. Barnard RD: Indiscriminate transfusion: a critique of case reports illustrating hypersensitivity reactions. NY State J Med 51:2399, 1951

88. Brittingham TE: Immunologic studies on leukocytes. Vox Sang 2:242, 1957

89. Popovsky MA, Moore SB: Diagnostic and pathogenetic considerations in transfusion related acute lung injury. Transfusion 25:573, 1985

90. Karp DD, Ervin TJ, Tuttle S: Pulmonary complications during granulocyte transfusion: incidence and clinical features. Vox Sang 42:57, 1982

91. Andrews AT, Zmijewski CM, Bowman HS, Reihart JK: Transfusion reaction with pulmonary infiltration associated with HL-A specific leukocyte antibodies. Am J Clin Pathol 66:483, 1976

92. Carilli AD, Ramanamurty MV, Chang YS: Noncardiac pulmonary edema following blood transfusion. Chest 74:310, 1978

Principles of Red Blood Cell Transfusion

134

Paul M. Ness and Kate Rothko

INTRODUCTION

Approximately 12 million units of blood was transfused in the United States in 1992. This is striking, considering that the era of blood transfusion began less than a century ago, with the discovery of the ABO system by Landsteiner.[1] Actually, it was not until about four decades later, with the description of the Rh system by Levine, Stetson, Landsteiner, Wiener, and Peters[2-4] and, perhaps even more critically, with the introduction of a safe and effective anticoagulant-preservative solution suggested by Loutit and Mollison,[5] that the clinical practice of transfusion as we know it began. Another important landmark at about the same time was the development of the antiglobulin test by Coombs,[6] which permitted the detection of antibodies in recipient plasma that did not produce direct agglutination in the test tube but might be capable of causing in vivo red cell destruction.

After these initial breakthroughs, the next several decades of development in transfusion practice focused on improvements in the preservation of red cells and on expansion of our knowledge of red cell antigens and their clinical significance. However, it was not until the mid-1960s, with the introduction of plastic blood packs by Walter and Murphy,[7] that a new phase, the era of component therapy, began. This innovation, combined with the ability to store blood for extended periods, again revolutionized transfusion practice.

The next two decades saw major advances in transplantation and open heart surgery and in therapy for many malignancies, supported by the ready availability of blood component support. During this period, although some adverse effects of transfusion, such as transmission of hepatitis, were well established, the new found benefits of transfusion seemed to outweigh any risks.

Since the recognition in late 1982 that the human immunodeficiency virus is transmissible by blood transfusion, the risks of transfusion are weighed more heavily against the benefits. Donor blood is subjected to an ever-growing battery of tests to detect potentially transmissible infectious agents, and the era in which ABO compatibility was the major hurdle seems eons away.

RED BLOOD CELL PRESERVATION AND STORAGE

The first key to storage of blood for later transfusion is a stable, minimally toxic anticoagulant with preservative properties. During the early 1900s, it was recognized[8-10] that citrate met these criteria. Although slightly more toxic than heparin, if given rapidly and in large amounts, citrate has preservative action that heparin lacks. Citrate has the added advantage of not causing systemic anticoagulation in the recipient.

The other essential for long-term storage is a mechanism to maintain cell viability and function. Fresh transfused red cells have a good survival rate in the recipient's circulation, having a destruction rate approximately equal to that of the recipient's own cells: 1%/day.[11] The arbitrary standard used for stored red cells requires 70% to remain in the circulation for 24 hours.

Adenosine Triphosphate Levels

ATP levels appear to be a major determinant of red cell viability.[12-14] The drop in cellular ATP levels, during storage has been correlated with change from disc to sphere configuration, increased cell rigidity, and loss of membrane lipid leading to decreased critical hemolytic volume.[15] For this reason, most efforts to extend the period of red cell storage have focused on ways to maintain intracellular ATP levels. First, dextrose was introduced into the citrate solution (citrate phosphate dextrose [CPD]: 21 days), to which adenine was added (CPDA-1: 35 days). Most recently, two additive solutions containing additional dextrose and adenine (Nutricell or AS-3) or dextrose and adenine plus mannitol (Adsol or AS-1) have been licensed, extending the maximum storage time to 42 days (Table 134-1). Unfortunately, it is clear that ATP is not the sole determinant of red blood cell viability.[16] It appears that when intracellular ATP is maintained at >1.5 μmol/g hemoglobin (Hb), other factors also predict viability. Since these factors remain undefined, no in vitro test is available to predict in vivo survival rate of stored red cells.

2,3-Diphosphoglycerate Levels

Stored red cells must also maintain their capacity to deliver oxygen. It was not until 1967 that the central role of 2,3-diphosphoglycerate (2,3-DPG) in releasing oxygen from oxyhemoglobin was recognized.[17,18] Interestingly, it had already been observed that the oxygen dissociation curve of stored red cells was shifted to the left.[19] Attention was then focused on ways to maintain high levels of 2,3-DPG in stored cells. The first anti-

coagulant introduced on a large scale, acid citrate dextrose, was ineffective because of its low initial pH, so that the new CPD, with its higher initial pH and slower fall in pH, was superior. CPDA-1, Adsol, and Nutricell have not further improved 2,3-DPG maintenance. Although 2,3-DPG depletion of stored red cells is known to decrease their oxygen delivery, the clinical significance of these findings is unclear. 2,3-DPG levels of stored cells are rapidly regenerated in vivo, rising to ≥50% of normal within several hours and to normal within 24 hours.[20] Although a patient with normal cardiac status should be able to compensate by increasing cardiac output to maintain normal oxygen delivery until 2,3-DPG levels are regenerated, an improvement in 2,3-DPG preservation in stored red cells is still desirable. New additive systems containing ascorbate, ascorbate-2-phosphate, or other materials that maintain pH and 2,3-DPG levels are under study but have not yet been licensed for clinical use.[21,22]

By-products of Red Cell Storage with Potential Adverse Effects

Infusion of large volumes of blood with citrate anticoagulant over a short period may cause plasma citrate levels to reach the toxic range. The primary concern is cardiovascular effects of hypocalcemia caused by chelation of calcium by citrate. The risk of citrate toxicity is exacerbated in the setting of liver dysfunction or liver immaturity, so that the situations of greatest risk appear to be exchange transfusion of premature infants and massive transfusion. Despite these theoretical considerations, there is little documented evidence of clinical citrate toxicity, and the problem can usually be prevented by slower infusion.[23] If large amounts of blood have to be infused over a very short period, administration of calcium gluconate can be considered, but whether the benefits justify the risk is controversial.[24]

Another issue with prolonged storage is the question of excess potassium in the red cell supernatant that could cause cardiac problems. At a storage temperature of 4°C the red cell sodium-potassium pump is essentially nonfunctional and intra- and extracellular levels gradually equilibrate. In addition, the hemolysis that occurs during the storage period results in increased potassium in the supernatant. However, because the total volume of plasma in red cell concentrates is low (approximately 70 ml), the total potassium burden is only about 5.5 mEq at product expiration. Practically speaking, the potassium load is rarely a clinical problem except in the setting of pre-existing hyperkalemia and renal failure. In this situation, fresher units of red cells or washed red cells may be used.

Microaggregates consisting of platelets, leukocytes, and fibrin form during blood storage. Although several studies have shown that pulmonary dysfunction after massive transfusion may be significantly diminished by the use of a microaggregate filter of pore size 20–40 μm,[25,26] other studies have not confirmed microaggregates as the cause of hypoxia.[27,28] Since microaggregate filters have been found to slow the infusion rate, their use is not uniformly recommended in cases of trauma. Some authorities suggest their application in cardiopulmonary bypass and when more than 5 U of blood is to be given.[29]

Since their introduction in the 1960s, plastic blood bags used for storing red cells have been made from polyvinylchloride containing the plasticizer di(2-ethyl)phthalate (DEHP), which confers pliability. Nevertheless, questions have been raised for many years about the safety of DEHP, which is known to be lipophilic, to leach from the bag, and to be present at levels of 50–70 mg/L in stored red cells.[30] Numerous studies in animal models have addressed the toxicity of the substance and are summarized in a comprehensive review.[31] The DEHP effects found in animals range from a shock lung-like picture, to loss

Table 134-1. Biochemical Changes in Stored Red Cells

Variable	Fresh	CPDA-1 35 Days	Adsol 35 Days
In vivo survival (at 24 hours)(%)	100	71.0	88.0
pH	7.5	6.7	6.7
ATP (% initial)	100	45.0	76.0
2,3-DPG (% initial)	100	<10.0	<10.0
Plasma K$^+$ (mEq/L)	5.1	78.5	49.0

(Data from Fenwal Laboratories,[95] Zuck et al.,[96] and Moore et al.[97])

of fertility, to hepatocarcinogenicity, to teratogenicity. While none of these adverse effects has been documented in humans, the question of potential toxicity has obviously been raised, initiating a search for alternative materials.[32] The situation is complicated by DEHP having been shown to have a significant stabilizing effect on the red blood cell membrane, and red cells stored in various containers lacking DEHP have shown unacceptable recovery at the end of the storage period. The decreased recovery has been shown to be due to increased hemolysis and increased osmotic fragility.[33] Recently, however, Baxter-Fenwal has introduced a new plastic, PL 2209™, a polyvinylchloride plasticized with butyryl-n-trihexyl-citrate (BTHC) in place of DEHP. BTHC undergoes less leaching from the bag than does DEHP and has passed numerous safety tests. In addition, the 24-hour post-transfusion recovery of red cells held in these bags to the end of the permitted storage period is excellent (83%), and hemolysis is minimal.[34]

RED BLOOD CELL COMPONENTS

Modern transfusion medicine assumes that it is preferable to give the patient the specific portion of the blood required rather than whole blood: red cells for oxygen-carrying capacity, plasma for coagulation proteins, and platelets for microvascular bleeding. The component therapy approach allows for optimal use of a limited community resource (Table 134-2). Methods for extended storage of red cells do not result in optimal preservation of other blood elements.

Today the clinician wishing to increase the patient's oxygen-carrying capacity is more likely to be using a red cell concentrate than whole blood, although there may still be situations in which whole blood, if available, is appropriate. Several modifications can be made to red cell products to render them leukocyte or plasma depleted that have particular clinical applications. Red cells can also be frozen for long-term storage.

Whole Blood

A unit of whole blood is collected in CPDA-1 anticoagulant, giving it a shelf life of 35 days and a volume of approximately 510 ml (450 ml blood plus 63 ml CPDA-1). Within 24 hours of collection, the platelets in the unit,[35] as well as the granulocytes, are dysfunctional and several plasma coagulation factors have fallen to suboptimal levels.[36]

Whole blood has the single advantage of correcting simultaneous deficits in oxygen-carrying capacity and blood volume. Therefore, whole blood is indicated in the management of trauma or in surgical cases involving extensive blood loss. In this setting, whole blood has two distinct advantages: (1) it provides colloid osmotic pressure and some coagulation factors not supplied by crystalloid solutions, and (2) it does not expose the recipient to red cells and plasma from different donors.

However, the goal of using whole blood for all cases of concomitant red cell and volume deficit is a very difficult one to achieve in practice. Not only is it difficult to balance the overall community need for production of other blood components, but it may be difficult for the hospital to predict inventory needs. Most cases requiring massive transfusion involve either trauma victims or emergency cardiovascular surgeries. Although various studies of this issue maintain that 20–50% of red cell transfusions should be met with whole blood,[37–39] some trauma centers manage patients exclusively with red cell concentrates.[40]

In the absence of whole blood, the simultaneous need for volume and oxygen-carrying capacity can be met by combining red cell concentrates with one of several volume expanders. If blood loss is mild to moderate, volume can generally be replaced with crystalloid (e.g., normal saline), which has the combined advantage of sterility and economy. In the setting of massive transfusion, there may be a need to replace intravascular proteins. Colloid solutions (albumin and plasma protein fraction) are expensive but are preferred to plasma because they carry no risk of disease transmission. In fact, plasma is rarely indicated, even in the setting of massive transfusion, unless there is a well-documented coagulopathy, as in the setting of liver failure.[41,42] In addition, in some cases of trauma and cardiovascular surgery platelet transfusion may be indicated to combat microvascular bleeding from dilutional thrombocytopenia or bypass-associated platelet dysfunction. The transfusion of an average adult dose of platelets usually supplies the equivalent of several units of relatively fresh plasma, so that there is no reason for further donor exposure by the administration of frozen plasma.

Whole blood <5 days old is indicated for exchange transfusion in infants to provide the proper hematocrit and coagulation factors while limiting donor exposure. For elective surgery commonly associated with massive transfusion, particularly liver transplantation, in which large amounts of plasma are transfused, whole blood would certainly be advantageous if it could be made available.

Red Cell Concentrates

Red cell concentrates are obtained from whole blood after removal of most of the plasma for the production of frozen plasma, or platelets, or both. At most blood centers, the red cells are then mixed with 100 ml of an additive nutrient solution that extends the storage period to 42 days[43] and results in flow properties similar to those of whole blood.[44] Alternatively, red cells can be produced from CPDA-1 anticoagulated blood and stored for 35 days.

Red cell concentrates are the product of choice for the correction of an isolated defect of oxygen-carrying capacity, as in chronic anemia. These concentrates have a particular advantage over whole blood in patients with cardiovascular compromise who might be unable to deal with the volume of whole blood.

Another setting in which packed cells, rather than whole

Table 134-2. Red Cell Components: Characteristics and Indications

Component	Characteristics	Indications
Whole blood	High volume; good flow	Combined red cell/ volume deficit (massive hemmorrhage; exchange transfusion)
Red blood cells	Lower volume Higher hematocrit Good flow in AS-1	Red cell deficit
Leukocyte-reduced red blood cells	85–90% leukccyte depletion <10⁶ leukocytes	Prevention of febrile reactions ?Prevention of alloimmunization
Washed red cells	Plasma depletion Leukocyte depletion Must use within 24 hr	Prevention of severe allergic reactions Prevention of anaphylaxis in IgA deficiency
Frozen red cells	Long-term storage Plasma and leukocyte depletion Must use within 24 hr of thawing	Rare donor unit storage Autologous storage for postponed surgery

blood, must be used is emergency transfusion of patients of unknown ABO type. Concentrated type O red cells are transfused after the plasma containing isohemagglutinins is removed to prevent potential hemolysis of the recipient's red cells.

Leukocyte-Poor Red Cells

Leukocyte-poor red cells (LPRCs) can be prepared by a variety of methods, resulting in differing degrees of white cell removal. The minimum requirement is a leukocyte number in the final component of $<5 \times 10^8$.[45] Earlier techniques involved the centrifugation or washing with saline, whereby the buffy coat was repeatedly removed. A more modern technique, known as the "spin-cool-filter" method, requires use of 1 week-old red cells, which are centrifuged and then cooled for 4 hours to enhance microaggregate formation before passage through a microaggregate filter.[46,47] Leukocyte depletion is reported to be 85% and red cell recovery 90%. The method is economical and feasible to perform on a large scale. Most recently, in-line leukocyte removal filters that eliminate 98% of leukocyte contamination while depleting $<10\%$ of the red cells have been introduced.[48]

The major indication for the use of LPRCs has been the prevention of the nonhemolytic febrile transfusion reaction, which is the most common adverse effect of transfusion, particularly in multiply transfused patients or multiparous females.[49] It is clear that these reactions are mediated by antibodies directed against leukocyte antigens,[50] but whether lymphocyte HLA antigens or granulocyte-specific antigens are the major targets has remained a subject of controversy.[51] Depletion of leukocytes has been shown to prevent, or at least ameliorate, such reactions in some patients.[52,53]

Another indication for LPRCs is the prevention of alloimmunization to HLA antigens that can adversely affect post-transfusion platelet increments, for example, in cancer patients undergoing chemotherapy.[54,55] This approach will only be effective if platelets for transfusion can also be white cell depleted. With the recent introduction of in-line filters for both red cells and platelets, this may be an achievable goal. However, there is little consensus on the degree of leukocyte depletion necessary to diminish significantly or eliminate alloimmunization.[56,57] According to AABB Standards,[45] the total leukocyte number must be $<5 \times 10^6$. Ultraviolet irradiation has also been shown to prevent alloimmunization in experimental settings[58,59] and may offer another practical approach to this problem. These issues are being addressed in a multicenter clinical trial sponsored by the National Institutes of Health.

Washed Red Cells

Red cells are washed, using isotonic saline solutions, by either automated or manual techniques. Automated techniques are more efficient, but there is always some degree of red cell loss with each wash cycle. Because the washing is performed in an open system, the resulting product must be transfused within 24 hours.

The primary aim of washing is to remove plasma proteins, although some leukocytes and platelets are removed simultaneously. The major indication for washed red cells is the prevention of severe allergic transfusion reactions, thought to be mediated by recipient antibodies (most likely IgE) to donor plasma proteins. Washing is recommended when reactions are recurrent and severe, even in the face of antihistamine administration. In IgA-deficient patients who have preformed antibody to IgA, IgA-containing plasma can actually cause anaphylaxis[60] (see Ch. 141). Multiple cell washes may be required to remove the contaminating plasma protein.[61,62]

Another setting in which washed cells may be indicated is paroxysmal nocturnal hemoglobinuria.[63] However, one study has suggested that these patients do not require washed cells.[64] In theory, washing removes complement components that could cause lysis of the patient's complement-sensitive red cells.

Frozen Red Cells

Red cells can be frozen using glycerol as a cryoprotective agent and stored in liquid nitrogen or mechanical freezers. The required concentration of glycerol depends on the rate and the temperature of freezing.[65-67] The freezing process destroys other blood constituents, except for a small percentage of immunocompetent lymphocytes.[68] Red cells are prepared for transfusion by thawing and washing away the glycerol using a series of progressively less hypertonic saline solutions, allowing glycerol to diffuse gradually from the cells to prevent hemolysis. The cells are resuspended in isotonic saline containing glucose. The extensive washing removes approximately 99.9% of the plasma,[69] as well as cellular debris.

Red cells can be stored in the frozen state for 10 years by regulation[45] and for considerably longer periods with good viability.[70] After thawing and washing, storage is limited to 24 hours because of the open system. The 24-hour post-transfusion survival rate has been shown to be about 85-90%.[67]

Frozen cells have been shown to maintain prefreezing ATP and 2,3-DPG levels. The standard is to freeze within 6 days of collection while these factors are still high. When it is necessary to freeze older units, rejuvenation with a solution containing pyruvate, glucose, phosphate, and adenine has provided excellent results.[71]

The major indication for frozen red cells is the maintenance of a collection of rare donor units for transfusion of patients with unusual red cell phenotypes who have developed alloantibodies. Sometimes patients with such rare phenotypes can make autologous donations that can be frozen for later use. Cells from autologous donors can be frozen if more units are required than can be collected in the 42-day liquid storage period or if surgery is postponed. One other legitimate use for frozen red cells deserves mention. In patients with severe aplastic anemia awaiting bone marrow transplantation in whom transfusion cannot be avoided, frozen cells have been shown to have the least adverse effect on subsequent graft survival.[72,73]

Because of the high cost and cumbersome nature of freeze-thaw procedures, other uses of frozen red cells are somewhat difficult to justify. Occasionally, frozen red cells are effective in preventing severe febrile transfusion reactions when LPRCs in conjunction with medications have failed.

APPROPRIATE TRANSFUSION PRACTICE IN VARIOUS CLINICAL SETTINGS

Response to red cell transfusion varies from patient to patient. In the absence of increased red cell destruction or sequestration, 1 U of red cells can be expected to increase the Hb level by 1 g/dl or the hematocrit by approximately 3%. This rise is usually not measurable until about 24 hours after transfusion, when the plasma volume has had time to return to normal. On the basis of a half-life of about 57.7 days for donor red cells, Mollison et al[11] calculated that an average size adult requires 24 ml red cells/day to maintain a given hematocrit, assuming no red cell production. Petz and Tomasulo[74] estimated this requirement to be 2 U of red cells every 2 weeks.

Several factors can adversely affect the survival of transfused red cells. Hemolysis caused by either immune red cell damage or mechanical trauma shortens the survival of transfused cells much as it does the survival of the patient's own cells. Hypersplenism can lead to initial sequestration as well as increased destruction of red cells. Continued blood loss is another obvious cause of suboptimal response to transfusion. It should also be emphasized that transfusion has been shown to suppress erythropoiesis, so that the net result of transfusion may be less than expected.[75]

Chronic Anemia

As a rule, signs and symptoms attributable to anemia are unlikely to develop at a hemoglobin level of >7–8 g/dl.[74] When the anemia is of gradual onset, the body's compensatory mechanisms for maintaining oxygen delivery to the tissues come into play. Cardiac output is increased and intracellular 2,3-DPG is increased; thus, oxygen unloads at a lower oxygen saturation of Hb. When chronic anemia is due to red cell destruction, the healthy bone marrow can respond by increasing production by up to sixfold.

Red cell transfusion is always symptomatic and supportive rather than definitive therapy for anemia. Transfusion should be used only when there is no definitive treatment for the underlying cause, or when the severity of the anemia and the clinical manifestations in the patient make it impossible to wait for the effects of the treatment to be realized.

Generalizations about whether or when to transfuse red cells—and how many—are difficult to make and are usually inappropriate. The clinical impact of anemia varies, depending on its pathogenesis, rate of onset, presence or absence of accompanying hypovolemia, and, most importantly, the individual patient. The Hb level at which a given individual experiences the signs and symptoms of anemia relates, in part, to underlying health status, cardiorespiratory reserve, and activity level.

Perioperative Period

Many generalizations have been made about appropriate transfusion management of acute blood loss, often with very little hard data to support the arguments. One rule of thumb is that blood losses of ≤10% of total blood volume require no replacement therapy at all, losses of ≤20% can be replaced exclusively with crystalloid solutions, while losses of >25% generally require red cell transfusion to restore oxygen-carrying capacity, along with crystalloid and sometimes colloid solutions to restore intravascular volume and maintain perfusion. For years the figure of 10 g/dl of Hb has been used as the gold standard for the red cell transfusion trigger during the perioperative period.[76]

In the acquired immunodeficiency syndrome era, however, this approach is no longer justified. Each case must be evaluated individually on the basis of clinical signs and symptoms, rather than on the basis of laboratory values. If the cardiovascular system is healthy and the degree of hypoperfusion is not significant, good tissue oxygenation can be maintained at much lower Hb levels. A recent National Institutes of Health consensus conference suggested that many surgical patients do not require transfusion unless the Hb level falls to <7 g/dl.[76] Recent re-examination of these issues has laid to rest the long-held belief that these lower Hb levels interfere with wound healing[77] or automatically make general anesthesia a risk.[78]

Given that red blood cell transfusion should be tailored to individual needs, the question logically arises, is there any readily available, objective measurement that can be used to determine how low the Hb level can safely be allowed to fall before red cell transfusion is initiated? Several recent studies of acute, normovolemic anemia in rats,[79] dogs,[80] and baboons[81,82] have focused on the whole body oxygen extraction ratio (ER) as an indicator of when to transfuse. These studies make the seemingly valid assumption that the heart is the major organ at risk. With progressive hemodilution, healthy animals with normal coronary trees were able to maintain normal levels of oxygen consumption through a moderate increase in cardiac output, an increase in coronary blood flow, and a linear increase in the ER up to a ratio of 50%. As the hematocrit fell to <10%, however, oxygen consumption began to fall off, and the animals were no longer able to increase the ER enough to compensate for the low oxygen blood tension. An ER of 50% was found to represent the critical point at which the myocardium converted from aerobic to anaerobic metabolism, reflected in net lactate production. At this point, metabolic acidosis set in, resulting in hemodynamic instability. Most recently, experimenters compared the response to acute normovolemic anemia in healthy dogs to the response in dogs with a critical coronary stenosis and found that both groups converted to anaerobic metabolism and went into congestive heart failure at an ER of >50%, but that an ER of >50% occurred at a Hct of 17.0% in the dogs with critical stenosis compared to a Hct of 8.6% in the healthy group.[83] On the basis of these studies, it seems reasonable to extrapolate to humans and to suggest that the ER, which is a variable readily obtainable from standard hemodynamic monitoring devices, can used to help assess transfusion need and that an ER of 50% can be used as a red cell transfusion trigger, since it appears to be a valid indicator of marginal myocardial oxygen reserve in both normal persons and individuals with coronary artery disease.

Red Cell Transfusion in Neonates

In full-term infants, red cell transfusion is rarely indicated unless acute blood loss has occurred at birth or an intrauterine situation has led to prenatal anemia. In severe hemolytic disease of the newborn, red cell transfusion may be essential even in the full-term infant. The two triggers for transfusion are (1) rapidly rising, unconjugated bilirubin that is inadequately responding to phototherapy techniques and that may lead to kernicterus and permanent central nervous system damage; or (2) congestive heart failure secondary to severe anemia. In either case, exchange transfusion is most often the preferred approach because it clears the bilirubin and the offending antibody from the circulation, while removing antibody-coated red cells before lysis. A two-blood-volume exchange is commonly performed by using a fresh unit of blood concentrated to a final hematocrit of about 50%.[84]

Premature infants exhibit several additional indications for transfusion. As a result of the inability of the immature liver to conjugate bilirubin, unconjugated bilirubin levels may rise to dangerous levels shortly after birth and exchange transfusion may be essential. In the intensive care setting, the premature infant is subjected to frequent blood sampling, and iatrogenic anemia may necessitate transfusion. The clinical signs and symptoms that trigger transfusion in these infants are somewhat unique. Congestive heart failure, recurrent apnea, and severe respiratory distress are clearly ameliorated by raising the hematocrit.[85] Failure to thrive as an indication for transfusion is somewhat more controversial. One study[86] showed a significant improvement in weight gain after transfusion, but this has not been corroborated by others.[87]

Newborn physiology is unique in several other ways that may have an impact on transfusion therapy. The newborn does not handle metabolites in a mature fashion. Renal immaturity may lead to problems in clearing potassium or acid from stored red cells, and the immature liver may not catabolize citrate efficiently. These problems are accentuated and protracted in the premature infant. To handle the potassium load, fresh or washed red cells may be used. The citrate problem is best handled by use of slow infusion rates.[23] The use of bicarbonate or calcium replacement to counteract the acid load or calcium-chelating effects of citrate is controversial.[24] Finally, the use of red cells stored in the newer preservative solutions (Adsol, Nutricell) is rejected by some authorities because of the potential risk of renal damage and renal stones due to adenine metabolites.[88,89]

The humoral and cellular immune systems of the neonate are also immature; again,this problem is accentuated in the premature infant. This has two implications for transfusion therapy. There is a small but real risk of transfusion-induced graft-versus-host disease in premature infants receiving red cell transfusions[90] and in the fetus undergoing intrauterine transfusion.[91] The irradiation of red cells is performed in these two settings. Another risk of transfusion in low birth weight (<1,500 g) premature infants is the development of clinical cytomegalovirus (CMV) infection in infants of CMV-seronegative mothers.[92] CMV-seronegative blood is now routinely used in these neonates. However, it appears that leukodepletion by freezing or filtration methods may offer an alternative to CMV screening.[93,94]

REFERENCES

1. Landsteiner K: Über Agglutinationserscheinungen normalen menschlichen Blutes. Wien Klin Wochenschr 14:1132, 1901
2. Levine P, Stetson RE: An unusual case of intragroup agglutination. JAMA 113:126, 1939
3. Landsteiner K, Wiener AS: An agglutinable factor in human blood recognized by immune sera for Rhesus blood. Proc Soc Exp Biol NY 43:223, 1940
4. Wiener AS, Peters HR: Hemolytic reactions following transfusions of blood of the homologous group, with three cases in which the same agglutinogen was responsible. Ann Intern Med 13:2306, 1940
5. Loutit JF, Mollison PL: Advantages of a disodium-citrate-glucose mixture as a blood preservative. Br Med J 2:744, 1943
6. Coombs RRA, Mourant AE, Race RR: A new test for the detection of weak and "incomplete" Rh agglutinins. Br J Exp Pathol 26:255, 1945
7. Walter CW, Murphy WP: A closed gravity technique for the preservation of whole blood in ACD solution utilizing plastic equipment. Surg Gynecol Obstet 94:687, 1952
8. Hustin A: Principe d'une nouvelle méthode de transfusion muqueuse. J Med Brux 12:436, 1914
9. Rous P, Turner JR: The preservation of living red blood cells in vitro. J Exp Med 23:219, 1916
10. Lewisohn R: Blood transfusion by the citrate method. Surg Gynecol Obstet 21:37, 1915
11. Mollison PL, Engelfreit CP, Contreras M: Blood transfusion. p. 97. In Mollison PL (ed): Blood Transfusion in Clinical Medicine. 8th Ed. Mosby-Year Book, St. Louis, MO, 1987
12. Rapoport S: Dimensional, osmotic and clinical changes of erythrocytes in stored blood. I: blood preserved in sodium citrate, neutral and acid citrate-glucose (ACD) mixtures. J Clin Invest 26:591, 1947
13. Gabrio BW, Hennessey M, Thomasson J, Finch CA: Erythrocyte preservation. IV: the in vitro reversibility of the storage lesion. J Biol Chem 215:357, 1955
14. Nakao KT, Wade T, Kamiyama M: A direct relationship between adenosine triphosphate level and in vivo viability of erythrocytes. Nature 194:877, 1962
15. Haradin AR, Weed RI, Reed CF: Changes in physical properties of stored erythrocytes: relationship to survival in vivo. Transfusion 9:229, 1969
16. Dern RJ, Brewer GJ, Wiorkowski JJ: Studies on the preservation of human blood. II: the relationship of erythrocyte adenosine triphosphate levels and other in vitro measures to red cell storageability. J Lab Clin Med 69:968, 1967
17. Chanutin A, Curnish RR: Effect of organic and inorganic phosphates on oxygen equilibrium of human erythrocytes. Arch Biochem Biophys 121:96, 1967
18. Benesch R, Benesch RE: The influence of organic phosphates on the oxygenation of hemoglobin. Fed Proc 26:673, 1967
19. Valtis DJ, Kennedy AC: Defective gas-transport function of stored red blood cells. Lancet 2:119, 1954
20. Beutler E, Wood L: The in vivo regeneration of red cell 2,3-diphosphoglyceric acid (DPG) after transfusion of stored blood. J Lab Clin Med 74:300, 1969
21. Moore GL, Ledford ME: Development of an optimized additive solution containing ascorbate-2-phosphate for the preservation of red cells with retention of 2,3-diphosphoglycerate. Transfusion 25:319, 1985
22. Dawson RB, Fagan DS, Meyer DR: Dihydroxyacetone, pyruvate, and phosphate effects on 2,3-DPG and ATP in citrate phosphate dextrose adenine blood preservation. Transfusion 24:237, 1984
23. Veall N, Mollison PL: The rate of red cell exchange in replacement transfusions. Lancet 2:792, 1950
24. Howland WS, Bellville JW, Zucker MB: Massive blood transfusion. V: failure to demonstrate citrate intoxication. Surg Gynecol Obstet 105:529, 1957
25. McNamara JJ, Molot MD, Stremple JF: Screen filtration pressure in combat casualties. Ann Surg 172:334, 1970
26. Reul GT, Beall AC, Greenberg SD: Protection of pulmonary microvasculature by fine screen blood filtration. Chest 66:4, 1974
27. Tobey RE, Kopriva CJ, Homer LD: Pulmonary gas exchange following hemorrhagic and massive transfusion in the baboon. Ann Surg 179:316, 1974
28. Bredenberg CE: International forum: does a relationship exist between massive blood transfusion and the adult respiratory distress syndrome? Vox Sang 32:311, 1977
29. Solis RT, Walker BD: International forum: does a relationship exist between massive blood transfusion and the adult respiratory distress syndrome? Vox Sang 32:319, 1977
30. Jaeger RJ, Rubin RJ: Contamination of blood stored in plastic packs. Lancet 2:151, 1970
31. Rubin RJ, Ness PM: What price progress? An update on vinyl plastic blood bags. Transfusion 29:358, 1989
32. Carmen R: The selection of plastic materials for blood bags. Transf Med Rev 7:1, 1993
33. Horowitz B, Stryker MH, Waldman AA et al: Stabilization of red blood cells by the plasticizer, diethylhexylphthalate. Vox Sang 48:150, 1985
34. Hogman CF, Eriksson L, Ericson A, Reppucci AJ: Storage of saline-adenine-glucose-mannitol-suspended red cells in a new plastic container: polyvinyl-chloride plasticized with butyryl-n-trihexyl-citrate. Transfusion 31:26, 1991
35. Baldini M, Costea N, Dameschek W: The viability of stored human platelets. Blood 16:1969, 1960
36. Rapaport SI, Ames SB, Mikkelsen S: The level of antihemophilic globulin and proaccelerin in fresh and bank blood. Am J Clin Pathol 31:297, 1959
37. Chaplin H: Packed red cells. Current concepts. N Engl J Med 281:364, 1969
38. Schmidt PJ: Red cells for transfusion. N Engl J Med 299:1411, 1978
39. Schmidt PJ: Whole blood transfusion. Transfusion 24:368, 1984
40. Sohmer PR, Dawson RB: Transfusion therapy in trauma: a review of the principles and techniques used in the MIEMS program. Am Surg 45:109, 1979
41. Braunstein AH, Oberman HA: Transfusion of plasma components. Transfusion 24:281, 1984
42. National Institute of Health Consensus Conference: Fresh frozen plasma: indications and rules. Transfus Med Rev 1:201, 1987
43. Valeri CR, Pivacek LE, Ouellet R, Gray A: A comparison of methods of determining the 100% survival of preserved red cells. Transfusion 24:109, 1984
44. Pineda AD, Viggiano NR, Clare D, Bukowski B: Flow rate of AS-1 preserved red cells and whole blood—a comparison. Transfusion 25:449, 1985
45. Widman FK (ed): Standards for Blood Banks and Transfusion Services, American Association of Blood Banks, Bethesda, MD, 1993
46. Wenz B, Gurtlinger KF, O'Toole AM, Dugan EP: Preparations of granulocyte-poor red blood cells by microaggregate filtration: a simplified method to minimize febrile transfusion reactions. Vox Sang 39:282, 1980
47. Parravcini A, Rebulla P, Apuzzo J et al: The preparation of leukocyte-poor red cells for transfusion by a simple cost-effective technique. Transfusion 24:508, 1984
48. Domen RE, Williams L: Use of the Sepacell filter for preparing white-cell depleted red cells. Transfusion 28:506, 1988
49. Payne R: Leukocyte agglutinins in human sera. Arch Intern Med 99:587, 1957
50. Payne R: The association of febrile transfusion reactions with leuko-agglutinins. Vox Sang 2:233, 1957
51. Heinrich D, Muller-Eckhardt C, Steir W: The specificity of leukocyte and platelet alloantibodies in sera of patients with non-hemolytic transfusion reactions: absorption and elution studies. Vox Sang 25:442, 1973
52. Brittingham TE, Chaplin H: Febrile transfusion reaction caused by sensitivity to donor leukocytes and platelets. JAMA 165:819, 1957
53. Menitove JE, McElligott, Aster RH: Febrile transfusion reactions: what blood component should be given next? Vox Sang 42:318, 1982
54. Schiffer CA, Lichtenfeld JL, Wiernik PH et al: Antibody response in patients with acute non-lymphocytic leukemia. Cancer 37:2177, 1976
55. Tejada F, Bias WB, Santos GW, Zieve PD: Immunologic response of patients with acute leukemia to platelet transfusions. Blood 42:405, 1973
56. Murphy MF, Metcalfe P, Thomas H et al: Use of leukocyte-poor blood components and HLA matched-platelet donor to prevent HLA alloimmunization. Br J Haematol 62:529, 1986
57. Myllylä E, Ruutu T, Kekomak R et al: Prevention of HLA-alloimmunization by using leukocyte-free blood components. Abs IXX Congress of the International Society of Blood Transfusion, London, 1988

58. Kahn RA, Duffy BF, Rodey GG: Ultraviolet irradiation of platelet concentrates abrogates lymphocyte activation without affecting platelet function in vitro. Transfusion 25:547, 1985

59. Slichter SJ, Deeg HJ, Kennedy MS: Prevention of alloimmunization in dogs with systemic cyclosporine and by UV-irradiation or cyclosporine-loading of donor platelets. Blood 69:414, 1987

60. Vyas GN, Holmdahl L, Perkins HA, Fudenberg HH: Serologic specificity of human anti-IgA and its significance in transfusion. Blood 34:573, 1969

61. Staveley L, Jakway J, Schoeppner S et al: Quantitation of IgA in blood components and plasma derivatives. Transfusion 24:421, 1984

62. Yap PL, Pryde EAD, McClelland DBL: IgA content of frozen-thawed washed red blood cells and blood products measured by radioimmunoassay. Transfusion 22:36, 1982

63. Dacie JV: Transfusion of saline-washed red cells in nocturnal hemoglobinuria. Clin Sci 7:65, 1948

64. Hartmann RC, Kolhouse JF: Viewpoints in the management of PNH. Ser Haematol 5:42, 1972

65. Rowe AW, Exster E, Kellner A: Liquid nitrogen preservation of red blood cells for transfusion. A low glycerol-rapid freeze procedure. Cryobiology J 1:193, 1968

66. Meryman HT, Hornblower M: A method for freezing and washing red blood cells using high glycerol concentration. Transfusion 12:145, 1972

67. Valeri CR: Factors influencing the 24 hour post-transfusion survival and oxygen transport function of previously frozen red cells preserved with 40% W/V glycerol and frozen at $-80°$. Transfusion 14:1, 1974

68. Kurtz SR, Van Deinse WH, Valeri CR: Immunocompetence of residual lymphocytes at various stages of red cell cryopreservation with 40% W/V glycerol in an ionic medium at $-80°C$. Transfusion 18:441, 1978

69. Contreras TJ, Valeri CR: A comparison of methods to wash liquid-stored red blood cells and red blood cells frozen with high or low concentrations of glycerol. Transfusion 16:339, 1976

70. Meryman HT: The cryopreservation of blood cells for clinical use. Prog Hematol 9:193, 1979

71. Valeri CR, Zaroulis CG: Rejuvenation and freezing of outdated stored human red cells. N Engl J Med 287:1307, 1972

72. Storb R: Marrow transplantation in thirty "untransfused" patients with severe aplastic anemia. Ann Intern Med 92:30, 1980

73. Storb R, Weiden PL: Transfusion in transplantation with emphasis on bone marrow transplantation. p. 578. In Petz LD, Swisher SN (eds): Clinical Practice of Blood Transfusion. Churchill Livingstone, New York, 1982

74. Petz LD, Tomasulo PA: Red blood cell transfusion. p. 1. In Kolins J, McCarthy LJ (eds): Contemporary Transfusion Practice. American Association of Blood Banks, Arlington, VA, 1987

75. Pace N, Lozner EL, Consolazio WV et al: The increase in hypoxia tolerance of normal men accompanying the polycythemia induced by transfusion of erythrocytes. Am J Physiol 148:152, 1947

76. NIH Consensus Conference: Perioperative red blood cell transfusion. JAMA 260:2700, 1988

77. Hunt TK: Perioperative anemia and wound healing. p. 37. In NIH Consensus Development Conference on Perioperative Red Cell Transfusion, Program and Abstracts, Bethesda, MD, 1988

78. Stehling L: Surgery without transfusion: the anesthesiologist's viewpoint. p. 45. In NIH Consensus Conference on Perioperative Red Cell Transfusion. National Institutes of Health Consensus Development Conference, Bethesda, MD, 1988

79. Adams RP, Dielman LA, Cain SA: A critical value for oxygen transport in the rat. J Appl Physiol 53:660, 1982

80. Cain SM: Oxygen delivery and uptake in dogs during anemic and hypoxic hypoxia. J Appl Physiol 42:228, 1977

81. Wilkerson DK, Rosen AL, Gould SA et al: Oxygen extraction ratio: a valid indicator of myocardial metabolism in anemia. J Surg Res 42:629, 1987

82. Wilkerson DK, Rosen AL, Sehgal LR et al: Limits of cardiac compensation in anemic baboons. Surgery 103:665, 1988

83. Levy PS, Chavez RP, Crystal GJ et al: Oxygen extraction ratio: a valid indicator of transfusion need in limited coronary vascular reserve? J Trauma 32:769, 1992

84. Widman FK: Technical Manual. 9th Ed. American Association of Blood Banks, Arlington, VA, 1985

85. Strauss RG: Current issues in neonatal transfusions. Vox Sang 51:1, 1986

86. Stockman JA, Clark DA: Weight gain: a response to transfusion in selected preterm infants. Am J Dis Child 138:828, 1984

87. Blank JP, Sheagren TG, Vajaria J et al: The role of RBC transfusion in the premature neonate. Am J Dis Child 138:831, 1984

88. Peck CC, Bailey FJ, Morre GL, Zuck TF: Urinary supersaturation by 2,8-dihydroxyadenine (DOA). Transfusion 15:518, 1975

89. Kreuger AO: Exchange transfusion with ACD adenine blood: a follow-up study. Transfusion 13:69, 1973

90. Seemayer TA, Bolande RP: Thymic involution mimicking thymic dysplasia. A consequence of transfusion induced graft-versus-host disease in a premature infant. Arch Pathol Lab Med 104:141, 1980

91. Parkman M, Mosier D, Umansky I et al: Graft-versus-host disease after intra-uterine and exchange transfusions for hemolytic disease of the newborn. N Engl J Med 290:359, 1974

92. Tegtmeier GE: Transfusion-transmitted cytomegalovirus infections: significance and control. Vox Sang, suppl. 1:22, 1986

93. Lang DJ, Ebert PA, Rodgers BM et al: Reduction of postperfusion cytomegalovirus-infections following the use of leukocyte depleted blood. Transfusion 17:391, 1977

94. Brady M, Anderson D, Milam J et al: Prevention of posttransfusion cytomegalovirus infection in neonates by the use of frozen-washed red blood cells. Clin Res 30:895A, 1982

95. Fenwal Laboratories

96. Zuck TF, Bensinger TA, Peck CC et al: The in vivo survival of red cells stored in modified CPD with adenine: report of a multi-institutional cooperative effort. Transfusion 17:374, 1977

97. Moore GL, Peck CC, Sohmer RR, Zuck TF: Some properties of blood stored in anticoagulant CPDA-I solution: a brief summary. Transfusion 21:135, 1981

Principles of Platelet Transfusion Therapy

135

Sherrill J. Slichter

INTRODUCTION

As early as 1910, Duke[1] reported the efficacy of transfusing platelets into patients with bleeding disorders. However, not until the advent of plastic bags for blood collection in the 1960s did it become feasible to centrifuge the blood easily to produce platelet concentrates. The subsequent development of methods to improve the preparation and storage of platelet concentrates has had a major impact on the use of this product. Several studies have subsequently demonstrated the efficacy of platelet therapy in controlling bleeding in leukemic patients. Specifically, in 57 autopsied patients, bleeding was the proximate cause of death in 65% of the 30 patients who were not treated with platelet transfusions and in only 15% of the 27 patients given platelet transfusions.[2] In a prospective controlled study, 18 patients with acute leukemia and platelet counts of $<30 \times 10^9$/L were randomized to receive either platelets or platelet-poor plasma.[3] Eight of 9 in the plasma-treated group bled, compared with only 4 of 12 in the platelet-treated group. Thus, these early studies clearly demonstrated the efficacy of platelet therapy to control thrombocytopenic bleeding.

Currently, platelet transfusions (random donor platelet concentrates and single donor apheresis platelets) are being administered at an ever-increasing rate compared with red blood cell (RBC) products. For example, transfusions of platelet concentrates have increased from 2,857,000 in 1980 to 4,855,000 in 1987; similarly, apheresis platelets transfusions rose from 56,000 to 262,000.[4] Furthermore, the fraction of platelets transfused as apheresis platelets has increased from 11% to 23%. This 191% increase in total platelet use during this time compares with a 15% increase in red cell products (packed RBCs and whole blood).

Undoubtedly many reasons exist for this accelerated platelet use. Advances in patient care have contributed to the increased need for platelets; for example, more aggressive chemotherapy programs have produced more prolonged and more severe thrombocytopenia in cancer patients. In addition, sophisticated open heart surgery procedures frequently result in dilutional as well as consumptive thrombocytopenias.

A substantial number of platelet transfusions are given for inappropriate reasons, either to patients who are not at risk of platelet-related bleeding, or repeatedly to patients who demonstrate no post-transfusion platelet increments. Platelet transfusions that do not increase the platelet count are unlikely to benefit the patient. Thus, additional efforts to define the indications for platelet transfusions better and to improve both the quality and the compatibility of the transfused platelets are clearly needed. Unfortunately, many physicians consider platelet transfusions a relatively innocuous form of therapy, and they are often prescribed with little thought to appropriate indications. Inappropriate platelet transfusions are not only an unnecessary expense for the patient and third-party payers in a time of escalating medical costs, but also a costly burden on the community that has to supply the donors. In addition, inappropriate platelet transfusions represent unnecessary infectious and immunologic risks to the patient. Chronically thrombocytopenic patients (usually with a malignant disorder) who are prophylactically transfused represent the largest transfusion group.[5] If the platelet transfusion therapy of these patients could be reduced, it would have a substantial impact on platelet inventory requirements, cost/benefit ratios, and transfusion-related risks to the patient.

NORMAL PLATELET HEMOSTASIS IN THROMBOCYTOPENIC PATIENTS

Platelet hemostasis requires combined adequacy of number and function of the circulating platelets. Abnormalities in either of these two parameters may be associated with bleeding. If a decrease in both platelet number and function occurs, the bleeding risk is substantially increased.

To determine whether transfused platelets have produced the expected result, the recovery, survival, and function of autologous platelets in thrombocytopenic patients must be characterized as a performance standard; detailed autologous platelet recovery and survival measurements have been performed in thrombocytopenic patients.[6] In 27 patients with stable, untreated thrombocytopenia secondary to bone marrow failure who had platelet counts ranging from 12 to 70 $\times$ 10[9]/L, radiochromium-labeled autologous platelet survival measurements demonstrated a direct relationship between platelet

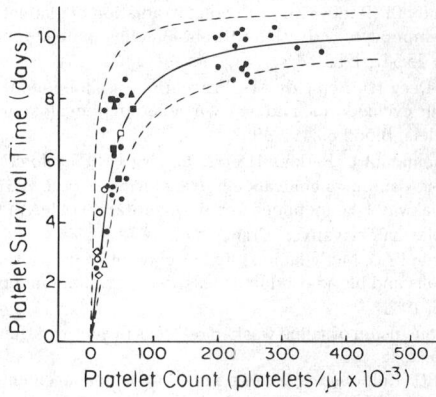

Fig. 135-1. Relationship between platelet count and survival of autologous or homologous platelets. The relationship between platelet count and survival of autologous (closed symbols) and donor (open symbols) ^{51}Cr platelets in normal and thrombocytopenic subjects with no evidence of hypersplenism (circles). Complications include splenectomy (squares), splenomegaly (triangles), and prior transfusions (diamonds). The data are well correlated (solid line) under the assumption of a finite platelet life span of 10½ days and a fixed rate of platelet destruction averaging 4,700 platelets/mm³/day. The data are bounded by the region shown between the dashed lines. (From Hanson and Slichter,[6] with permission.)

count and platelet survival (Fig. 135–1). Platelet life span was only modestly reduced in patients who had counts in the range of 50–100 $\times$ 10[9]/L (7.0 $\pm$ 1.5 days versus 9.6 $\pm$ 0.6 days in normal controls; $P <0.01$) but was markedly reduced when the platelet count fell to $<50 \times 10^9$/L (5.1 $\pm$ 1.9 days; $P <0.001$). The recovery of autologous platelets was normal when the platelet count was $>50 \times 10^9$/L (74 $\pm$ 15%) but was reduced in patients with low counts (50 $\pm$ 20%; $P <0.01$). The survival of homologous platelets in these thrombocytopenic patients was equivalent to their autologous survival; it thus correlated directly with the post-transfusion platelet count. By contrast, the recovery of donor platelets in severely thrombocytopenic patients was 60 $\pm$ 15% and was equivalent to the control values determined in 16 normal individuals (66 $\pm$ 8%; $P >0.20$). Furthermore, analysis of these data indicated that platelets are removed from circulation by two mechanisms: a fixed number of platelets are removed daily, presumably in an endothelial supportive function, and the remainder are lost through senescent mechanisms. This fixed daily random loss of platelets from the circulation accounts for the progressive decrease in platelet survival at low platelet counts. This fixed fraction represents only 18% of the daily platelet loss at normal platelet counts and, therefore, has little impact on platelet survival. However, at lower platelet counts a progressively larger fraction of the circulating platelets is involved in this process, with a direct effect on measured platelet survival.

The usual in vitro technique of measuring platelet function involves adding a variety of platelet-aggregating agents to platelets as they are stirred in an aggregometer. Changes in light transmission, as the stirred platelets agglutinate in response to the aggregating agents, are recorded as a measure of platelet function. However, aggregation studies generally require a platelet concentration of $\geq100 \times 10^9$/L for accurate measurements. Although the preparation of platelet-rich plasma from whole blood for aggregation studies increases the platelet concentration about twofold, it is still a technique that cannot be used for severely thrombocytopenic patients. Therefore, most investigators have relied on bleeding time measurements as an in vivo measure of platelet function. The relationship between bleeding time and platelet count was determined in 70 individuals with marrow failure and platelet counts of $<150 \times 10^9$/L.[7] As long as the platelet count remained at levels $>100 \times 10^9$/L, the bleeding time was within the normal range of 4.5 $\pm$ 1.5

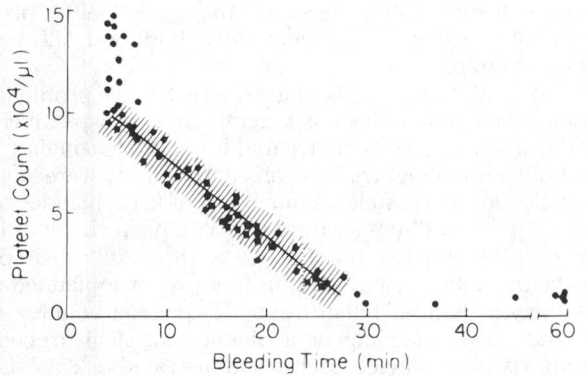

Fig. 135-2. Relationship between bleeding time and platelet count (see text). From Harker and Slichter,[7] with permission.)

minutes. However, in patients with platelet counts between 10 and 100 × 10^9/L, a direct, inverse relationship between bleeding time and platelet count existed that could be predicted by the equation:

$$\text{Bleeding time (minutes)} = 30.5 - \frac{\text{platelet count} \times 10^9/\text{L}}{3.85}$$

At platelet counts of <10 × 10^9/L, the bleeding time is >30 minutes (Fig. 135-2). Similar observations were obtained when platelet transfusions were given to thrombocytopenic patients. This measure permits the bleeding time to be used as a method of documenting whether any transfused platelets demonstrate the expected relationship between platelet count and bleeding time or whether they are dysfunctional (bleeding time disproportionately prolonged for the platelet count) or hyperfunctional (bleeding time disproportionately reduced for the platelet count).

INDICATIONS FOR PLATELET TRANSFUSIONS

Thrombocytopenia

Both the response to platelet transfusions and the indications may vary based on the mechanism of the thrombocytopenia, which has four major causes: (1) decreased platelet production, (2) splenomegaly, (3) increased platelet destruction, and (4) dilutional thrombocytopenia caused by large volume replacement with nonplatelet-containing fluids.

Decreased Platelet Production

Platelet transfusions are often provided prophylactically at low platelet counts to prevent bleeding, or, alternatively, are given at higher platelet counts in the presence of significant bleeding manifestations. In the latter situation, the platelets are frequently dysfunctional because of medications or disease-related platelet abnormalities; alternatively, the vascular system may have been disrupted, requiring higher platelet counts in order to maintain hemostasis.

To determine when platelet transfusions are needed, it is important to understand how platelets are involved in maintaining normal hemostasis. Platelets are postulated to maintain hemostasis by plugging gaps in the endothelium of blood vessels. In rabbits with severe thrombocytopenia, electron microscopy studies demonstrated thinning of the endothelial cells, with gaps between the cells.[8] Others have proposed that endothelial cells retract and expand intermittently, leaving uncovered gaps on the subendothelial basement membrane. Thus, there may be a continuous requirement for platelets to be pres-

ent to prevent extravasation of RBCs through these gaps. Animal studies have shown a clear correlation between the degree of thrombocytopenia and the amount of spontaneous hemorrhage into the lymphatic system.[9] If indeed platelets maintain hemostasis by plugging gaps in the endothelium, the question becomes how many platelets are required to perform this vital function. As previously discussed,[6] a small fixed fraction of about 7.1 × 10^9 platelets/L/day are removed randomly, presumably to provide for the endothelial supportive function suggested by the animal studies.[8,9] Thus, these data would suggest that, if the average blood volume is assumed to be about 5 L, then approximately 5 times 7.1 × 10^9, or 3.6 × 10^{10}, platelets/day would be needed to maintain hemostasis. However, as only about two-thirds of the transfused platelets circulate—the remaining one-third are pooled in a normal-sized spleen[10]—the actual number of platelets required may be 4.8 × 10^{10}, which can be met by transfusing 1 platelet concentrate/day that should contain ≥5.5 × 10^{10} platelets (by Food and Drug Administration guidelines). However, in addition to these physiologic platelet requirements, many clinically ill thrombocytopenic patients also demonstrate platelet consumption secondary to sepsis, malignancy, and other conditions.[11] Thus, >1 platelet concentrate/day may be required to meet both physiologic and pathogenic platelet requirements and provide for some margin of safety. Based on these calculations, transfusing relatively large amounts of platelets each day as pools of random donor platelets or an apheresis transfusion may not be the best method of meeting platelet hemostatic requirements. However, the use of small doses of platelets given daily has never been tested.

Reductions in platelet transfusion therapy can be made through changes in indications (triggers or decision points) used to initiate therapy. Unfortunately, the guidelines for prophylactic transfusions (and even the need for such a policy, rather than providing platelet transfusions only when bleeding occurs) remain controversial.[12–14] Most clinicians use the level of the patient's count as an indicator for transfusing platelets rather than transfusing some fixed number of platelets per day. Although a 20 × 10^9/L platelet count has often been used as an indication for prophylactic platelet transfusions in chronically thrombocytopenic patients with decreased platelet production (a policy reaffirmed by a Consensus Conference Statement[15]), little direct evidence substantiates this practice.

For example, in one of the earliest studies, published in 1962,[16] the authors could not determine a threshold platelet level to prevent bleeding. Serious bleeding, such as grossly visible hemorrhage (hematuria, melena, and hematemesis), was most often present (10–30% of the days) at platelet counts <5 × 10^9/L in children with acute leukemia. Patients whose platelet counts were at any level between 5 and 100 × 10^9/L had little difference in serious bleeding episodes (between 8% and 4%, respectively). Of the 92 patients analyzed, 16 died of intracerebral bleeding. One-half of these bleeding patients had chronic myeloid leukemia in blast crisis, and autopsy revealed leukostasis and leukemic nodules. In this group, platelet levels were relatively high at the time of hemorrhage (median 10 × 10^9/L), and only one patient had a platelet count <5 × 10^9/L. By contrast, in patients without blastic crisis, only one of the eight patients had a platelet count >5 × 10^9/L at the time of the intracerebral bleed, and that count was <10 × 10^9/L. Thus, in this study, intracerebral bleeding was commonly related to high white blood cell (WBC) counts and leukostasis. In patients without this complication, intracerebral bleeding was usually found only in patients with platelet counts <5 × 10^9/L. It is of note that significant bleeding did not occur at higher platelet counts, even though many of these children may have been on aspirin because of fever. It was not demonstrated until later that aspirin causes significant platelet dysfunction and should not be given to thrombocytopenic patients.

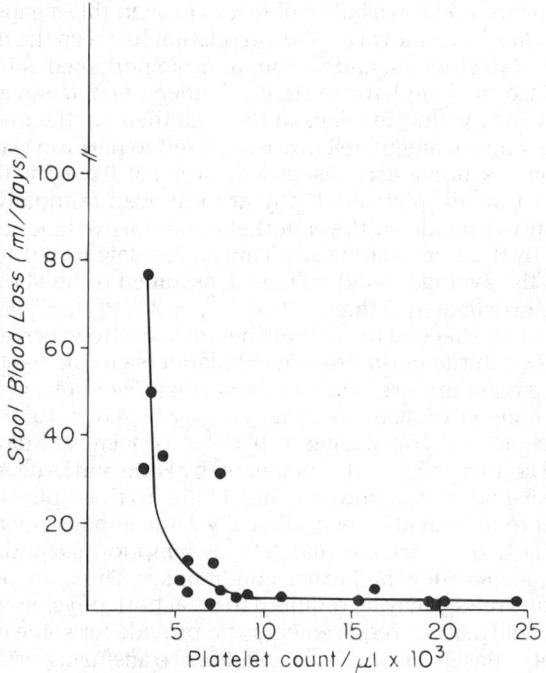

Fig. 135-3. Stool blood loss as a measure of thrombocytopenic bleeding. When stool blood loss (expressed as milliliters of blood/day) was determined in 20 aplastic thrombocytopenic patients (closed circles), blood loss was <5 ml/day at platelet counts >10,000/mm³. At platelet counts between 5,000 and 10,000/mm³, blood loss averaged 9 ± 7 ml/day. At levels <5,000/mm³, blood loss averaged 9 ± 7 ml/day. At levels <5,000/mm³, blood loss was markedly elevated, at 50 ± 20 ml/day. (From Slichter and Harker,[17] with permission.)

Additional evidence for the occurrence of spontaneous bleeding only at very low platelet counts comes from observations of radiochromium-labeled stool blood loss measurements in 20 patients with aplastic thrombocytopenia. In these patients, stool blood loss was <5 ml/day (within the normal range) at platelet counts >10 × 10⁹/L. At platelet counts between 5 and 10 × 10⁹/L, blood loss averaged 9 ± 7 ml/day. At levels <5 × 10⁹/L, blood loss was markedly elevated, at 50 ± 20 ml[17] (Fig. 135–3).

In another study in which the relationship between bleeding manifestations and platelet count was assessed, serious bleeding (gross bleeding from the gastrointestinal or genitourinary tracts) occurred in 26% of the leukemic children with platelet counts between 0 and 10 × 10⁹/L, in 10% of the patients with platelet counts between 10 and 20 × 10⁹/L, and in 4–5% of the patients with platelet counts between 20 and 40 × 10⁹/L.[18] Minor bleeding into skin or mucous membranes, microscopic hematuria, guaiac-positive stools, and epistaxis were found in approximately 50% of the persons with platelet counts between 0 and 40 × 10⁹/L, but no correlation was found between bleeding and platelet count in these patients.

In a retrospective study, bleeding manifestations were evaluated in leukemic patients with platelet counts of <10 × 10⁹/L compared with platelet counts between 10 and 20 × 10⁹/L. A clear increase in bleeding risk existed for patients with platelet counts of <10 × 10⁹/L; at higher platelet counts, the risk of severe bleeding (gastrointestinal, or genitourinary, or intracerebral) was only 3%.[19] In general, for all types of bleeding (major or minor), the bleeding risk was increased for leukemic versus chemotherapy-induced thrombocytopenia, for patients with falling rather than stable or rising platelet counts, and for febrile versus afebrile patients. This study also indicated that the bleeding risk was greater in patients <18 years of age and in those with acute lymphocytic leukemia (ALL) versus acute

myeloid leukemia (AML), suggesting that guidelines for platelet therapy might differ for patients with childhood ALL versus adults with AML.

The safety and practicality of a more restrictive prophylactic platelet transfusion policy has recently been prospectively assessed in 102 patients being treated for acute leukemia.[20] The indications for platelet transfusions in this study were any one of the following: (1) platelet count <5 × 10⁹/L; (2) platelet count of 6–10 × 10⁹/L and temperature of >38°C or fresh minor hemorrhages; (3) platelet count of 11–20 × 10⁹/L and other coagulation factor deficiencies, heparin therapy, or a planned marrow biopsy or lumbar puncture; or (4) platelet count >20 × 10⁹/L and major bleeding or a planned surgical procedure. Bleeding risk by platelet count demonstrated a 2.5% risk of major bleeding with a platelet count of <5 × 10⁹/L and <1% risk at a platelet count of 6–10 × 10⁹/L. There was no measurable risk of major bleeding at higher platelet counts. The correlation coefficient between platelet counts of <20 × 10⁹/L and bleeding was $r = 0.963$ (P <0.01). Three hemorrhagic deaths occurred in this study, one a patient with a platelet count of 1 × 10⁹/L who was alloimmunized and did not have a compatible donor, and two other patients on low doses of heparin with platelet counts of 35 × 10⁹/L and 55 × 10⁹/L at the time of death, suggesting an increased bleeding risk with further compromises to the overall hemostatic system. Thus, the overall mortality with this platelet transfusion program was very low.

However, the authors of this study made additional assumptions about factors other than the platelet count that they assumed would affect the bleeding risk, such as fever, fresh minor hemorrhages, and associated plasma coagulation factor deficiencies. If any of these factors were present, then the patient was transfused at a higher platelet count. Since the study was not designed simply to randomize patients to be prophylactically transfused at a given platelet count, it cannot be determined from the data whether any of these other factors had an effect or whether just transfusing all patients with platelet counts of <5 × 10⁹/L would have produced the same results. In addition, 78% of the platelets given to patients in this study were transfused within 6 hours of collection. Thus, these results may not be applicable to routine transfusion practice, in which platelets may be stored for ≤5 days before transfusion. Data that are presented later suggest that the quality of long-term stored platelets may be inferior to fresh platelets, which may indicate that patients transfused with older platelets may not be as hemostatically protected as those receiving fresher platelets.

In summary, in all the studies in which bleeding risk was evaluated in patients with platelet counts <5 × 10⁹/L, a clear increase in bleeding manifestations was seen. In studies in which patients were segregated into those with platelet counts of <10 × 10⁹/L versus >10 × 10⁹/L, a greater bleeding risk was seen in patients with counts of <10 × 10⁹/L. Whether these results mainly reflected bleeding in patients with platelet counts of <5 × 10⁹/L, rather than 5–10 × 10⁹/L, was not determined. As our ability to count low numbers of platelets accurately and to reduce high WBC counts rapidly with chemotherapy has markedly improved, it should be easy to justify reducing the prophylactic platelet transfusion level from the current 20 × 10⁹/L to at least 10 × 10⁹/L, if not 5 × 10⁹/L.[21]

However, lowering the prophylactic platelet transfusion level is acceptable only if it can be demonstrated that, when bleeding manifestations occur at higher-than-expected levels, a platelet transfusion given as therapy to control bleeding will be successful. Only two studies have attempted to address the question of prophylactic versus therapeutic platelet transfusions in a prospective controlled fashion. In both studies prophylactic platelet transfusions were given to one group of leukemic patients when their platelet counts were <20 × 10⁹/L; the second group of leukemic patients received therapeutic

INDICATIONS FOR PLATELET TRANSFUSIONS IN THROMBOCYTOPENIA

Patients with production-related thrombocytopenia and platelet counts $<5 \times 10^9/L$ should be given prophylactic platelet transfusions to prevent the risk of substantial bleeding. At platelet counts between 5 and $10 \times 10^9/L$, clinical judgment should be used to assess the severity of bleeding and the need for platelet therapy. When a patient has significant bleeding at a platelet count $>10 \times 10^9/L$, either platelet dysfunction is usually present (as evidenced by a longer-than-expected bleeding time for the platelet count), or else the vascular system has been disrupted. A direct approach should be made to eliminate the platelet dysfunction, which is often drug-related, or to repair the vascular system; platelets should be given only to control significant bleeding until the underlying problem can be eliminated.

platelet transfusions only for bleeding that involved more than skin and mucous membranes or epistaxis.[22,23] There were no differences in RBC transfusion requirements or hemorrhagic deaths when comparing the two groups of patients; these data suggest that therapeutic transfusions given only for active bleeding are effective in controlling bleeding and that prophylactic platelet transfusions are not necessary. In addition, patients in the prophylactic arm received two to three times as many platelet transfusions as those in the therapeutic arm, substantially increasing the costs of the platelet therapy, with no added benefits.

Hypersplenism

Normally, approximately one-third of the platelets produced by the bone marrow are pooled in the spleen, accounting for the normal platelet recovery value of $66 \pm 8\%$.[10] However, if the spleen becomes enlarged, more platelets are pooled in the spleen, and thrombocytopenia may ensue. Nonetheless, it is unusual for hypersplenism alone to cause a platelet count of $<40-50 \times 10^9/L$ (these levels should not require platelet support). Even though the patient may have a large spleen, a platelet count of $<40 \times 10^9/L$ should provoke a search for an additional cause of thrombocytopenia. Hypersplenism per se is usually not an indication for platelet transfusions; its contribution to the thrombocytopenia is only of concern if a hypersplenic patient develops an additional cause of a low platelet count, and platelet transfusions are required. In this situation, there will also be increased pooling of donor as well as autologous platelets, requiring a higher dose of platelets to achieve the desired increment. However, platelet survival is not reduced by the hypersplenism, so transfusion frequency does not have to be increased.

Increased Platelet Destruction

In disorders of increased platelet destruction, the frequency of transfusions may have to be substantially increased to compensate for reduced platelet survival. In certain situations, platelet survival may be so compromised that it is difficult to maintain at adequate platelet level.

Consumptive Thrombocytopenia

Two basic types of platelet consumption exist. The first represents an exaggeration of the physiologic hemostatic response, in which not only platelets but other coagulation factors are removed from circulation at an accelerated rate. This type of consumption occurs in a wide variety of patients: those with venous thrombosis, tissue trauma (accidental or surgically related), widespread malignancy, obstetric complications, and bacteremia.[11] Furthermore, when two or more of these events occur in the same patient, the effects are often additive. For example, one of the first indications of bacteremia in patients with acute leukemia may be an unusually rapid fall in the platelet count, often accompanied by markedly decreased responses to transfused platelets. Management of patients who are consuming platelets calls for therapy directed at the underlying disease process that is causing the consumptive state. For many of these patients, platelet transfusions are required only until the disease process is resolved. These situations may be associated not only with reduced platelet survivals, necessitating frequent transfusions, but also with very poor platelet increments, making transfusion support extremely difficult.

The second consumptive process is characterized by selective platelet destruction and appears to reflect platelet thrombus formation on abnormal surfaces in the arterial system, including prosthetic devices (artificial heart valves, prosthetic aortic grafts, plastic arteriovenous cannula) and conditions such as arterial thrombosis, thrombotic thrombocytopenic purpura, hemolytic uremic syndrome, and other disorders associated with vasculitis.[11] These processes can often be managed by providing platelet function inhibitors or other forms of therapy. However, if platelet transfusions are required, lower survival rates can be anticipated.

Immunologic Conditions

Neonatal Alloimmune Thrombocytopenia. Neonatal alloimmune thrombocytopenia (NAIT) occurs when nonshared paternal antigens expressed on the platelets of the fetus result in the formation of maternal alloantibodies that cross the placenta.[24] If the mother has had one thrombocytopenic newborn, then intravenous immunoglobulin can be administered prophylactically to prevent NAIT.[25] Unfortunately, approximately 30–60% of the time, this disorder occurs during the course of the first pregnancy,[26] unlike maternal-fetal Rh incompatibility, which usually requires an initial pregnancy to produce sensitization.

If a thrombocytopenic infant is delivered, compatible platelets can be obtained from the mother. However, because her plasma contains the offending antibody, these platelets should be washed before transfusion to prevent further administration of the maternal alloantibody.[27] If the mother has a prior history of an infant with NAIT, maternal platelets can be harvested before delivery to have available as needed. Often only one platelet transfusion is required, but as the half-life disappearance time for an immunoglobulin antibody is approximately 30 days, some infants may require additional platelet support until the maternal alloantibody falls to low levels.

In addition, in about 10% of cases, intracranial bleeding in utero may occur.[28] As the recurrence rate of NAIT in subsequent pregnancies is almost 90% and hemorrhagic manifestations are often more severe,[24] intrauterine transfusions of compatible platelets should be considered in repeat pregnancies, particularly if the first pregnancy resulted in a severely effected infant.[29-32]

Post-Transfusion Purpura. In post-transfusion purpura, approximately 5–10 days after a blood product transfusion that contains an incompatible platelet antigen, an amnestic recall of and antibody occurs in a previously transfused or pregnant individual.[33] In the process of recalling this alloantibody, autologous platelets of the transfused recipient are also destroyed.

The mechanism whereby this destruction of autologous platelets occurs in the process of recalling an alloantibody is not well understood.[34] However, when the identity of the platelet-specific alloantibody has been determined and compatible platelets administered, there has been no increase in the circulating platelet count in 60% of the cases.[35]

Individuals with post-transfusion purpura seem to be hyperimmune responders. They form not only platelet-specific but also HLA as well as red cell alloantibodies.[36] Therefore, either the transfused platelets may have been destroyed because of HLA incompatibility between donor and recipient, or, alternatively, a platelet autoantibody may develop in these patients that may destroy their own as well as homologous platelets.[37] Some evidence shows that an antibody that cross-reacts with autologous platelets forms as part of the immune response to foreign antigens in these patients. Indeed, in some of these patients, platelet counts are increased by autoimmune thrombocytopenic purpura (AITP) therapy such as steroids, intravenous immunoglobulin, or plasma exchange.[36,38,39]

Autoimmune Thrombocytopenic Purpura. Although it has now been demonstrated that a major mechanism of thrombocytopenia in AITP is ineffective platelet production (as demonstrated by autologous platelet survivals that are relatively normal for the patient's degree of thrombocytopenia), homologous platelets in the presence of the patient's autoantibody demonstrate a markedly reduced platelet life span.[40] This finding suggests that those autologous platelets that are released from the marrow and do circulate in AITP are relatively antibody resistant, as opposed to the heterogeneous population of donor platelets, some of which may be highly sensitive to the patient's antibody. Since a variety of therapies are now available that rapidly increase the autologous platelet count in patients with AITP, the only indication for platelet transfusions in this disorder is evidence of central nervous system or other life-threatening bleeding. Even surgical procedures such as splenectomy do not require platelet transfusions in these patients; the platelet count can usually be increased preoperatively into a relatively normal range with either steroids or intravenous immunoglobulin. In addition, some patients may have a shorter-than-expected bleeding time for the platelet count, demonstrating that young, hyperfunctional platelets are in circulation, further reducing the need for platelet therapy.[7] However, if platelet transfusions are deemed to be necessary for splenectomy, they should not be given until the splenic pedicle has been clamped to prevent the transfused platelets from immediately being sequestered in the organ that is to be removed.

Drug-Induced Thrombocytopenias. Drug-related thrombocytopenias may be related to either decreased platelet production or increased platelet removal. Bone marrow examination may be helpful in distinguishing the two potential mechanisms. If an immunologic mechanism is identified, patients are usually refractory to transfusion therapy.[41]

Dilutional Thrombocytopenia

Mathematical models have been formulated to predict the disappearance rate of a substance confined to the intravascular volume when blood is periodically removed and replaced with a fluid not containing that substance.[42] An exchange transfusion of 1 blood volume will reduce the concentration of any substance by approximately two-thirds. The next equivalent exchange will reduce the remaining one-third by two-thirds, and so on. During massive blood loss and replacement with 4°C stored blood (which contains no viable platelets), exchange of 1 blood volume (about 11 U of blood in a man weighing 75 kg)

will decrease the platelet count from its normal value of 250 ± 40 × 10^9/L to approximately 80 × 10^9/L. It may require ≥100 × 10^9 platelets/L to maintain hemostasis with a nonintact vascular system (as would likely be the situation in a massively bleeding patient); even a 1-volume exchange may thus increase the bleeding risk. Other factors besides dilution that might contribute to an even lower than calculated postexchange platelet count are (1) a lower-than-normal pre-exchange platelet count and (2) any complicating condition causing accelerated platelet destruction. For example, if massive bleeding occurs during the course of a major operative procedure such as open heart surgery or with severe traumatic injuries, then accelerated platelet consumption, due to the tissue injury, may result in a lower-than-expected postexchange platelet count. Furthermore, if the tissue injury might be expected to release tissue thromboplastic directly into the circulation, as may occur with head trauma, thrombocytopenia is likely to be severe.[43]

Increased platelet mobilization from the splenic storage pool may mitigate the low platelet count that might be expected from dilution or consumption. In young soldiers transfused for combat injuries, the postexchange platelet count was higher than predicted, particularly in those given >20 U of blood.[44] This finding suggests that, in a basically healthy population, platelet mobilization from the spleen and perhaps premature release of marrow platelets may prevent platelet counts from falling to predicted levels.

Platelet Dysfunction

The most common causes of platelet dysfunction in thrombocytopenic patients are those related to drugs (aspirin or other anti-inflammatory drugs as well as semisynthetic penicillins)[45–47] or to specific disorders such as uremia,[48] hyperfibrinolysis secondary to disseminated intravascular coagulation,[49] or other aspects of the patient's underlying disease process. For example, dysfunctional platelets are often found in patients with leukemia,[50] myeloproliferative disorders,[51] or fever/infection.[52] Aspirin or other anti-inflammatory drugs should be avoided in any thrombocytopenic patient. However, it has been documented that a platelet transfusion given to a patient who has aspirin-induced platelet dysfunction will improve the bleeding time as long as the transfused platelets constitute ≥10% of the circulating platelet number.[53] This observation may be particularly important for patients undergoing emergency open heart surgery, who may be receiving aspirin as antithrombotic therapy. It has been documented that such patients have a larger RBC transfusion requirement than patients not on aspirin; thus, the aspirin-treated patients may benefit from platelet transfusions.[54]

The ability of platelet transfusions to correct the platelet dysfunction associated with other drugs or diseases has not been well documented. However, it is probably reasonable to give platelet transfusions if bleeding is severe. Their efficacy can be documented by performing pre- and post-transfusion bleeding times as well as by monitoring RBC transfusion requirements.

It is unlikely that platelet dysfunction will substantially contribute to any bleeding problem in patients with platelet counts of >50 × 10^9/L if the vascular system is intact. Even with a disrupted vascular system, 100 × 10^9 platelets/L are usually sufficient to form a hemostatic platelet plug. However, in one clinical situation—after open heart surgery—some patients have been documented to have significant bleeding even in the presence of platelet counts >100 × 10^9/L. The bleeding time becomes infinite in patients undergoing cardiopulmonary bypass, but this dysfunction rapidly corrects itself in most patients during the postoperative period.[55] However, in 10 patients who were documented to have significant blood loss in he immediate postsurgical period, the bleeding time did not correct, and these patients benefited from platelet transfusions. In animal studies, prolongation of the bleeding time during cardiopulmonary bypass could be produced either by inducing hypothermia or by just performing a bypass procedure.[56] Interestingly, aprotinin given during cardiopulmonary bypass may substantially reduce the platelet dysfunction associated with cardiopulmonary bypass procedures, resulting in significant reductions in RBC transfusion requirements.[57-60] The mechanism whereby aprotinin improves platelet function has been postulated to be either preservation of membrane integrity with maintenance of membrane receptor function,[61] or, alternatively, prevention of platelet dysfunction induced by fibrinolysis.[58] Although platelet quality was improved by aprotinin, postoperative decreases in platelet counts were similar in the treated and control groups.[57-60] If aprotinin consistently improves platelet function even though platelet counts are not protected, this should result in the need for fewer platelet transfusions.

The congenital disorders of platelet dysfunction (i.e., von Willebrand disease, Glanzmann thrombasthenia, Bernard-Soulier syndrome, hereditary storage pool deficiencies) are usually not associated with thrombocytopenia. Therefore, even though the patients' bleeding times may be >30 minutes, the likelihood of hemorrhage is small as long as the vascular system remains intact. The lifelong nature of these defects mandates against prophylactic platelet transfusion. This conservative approach prevents needless alloimmunization and thereby maintains the capacity for effective platelet support to control bleeding during surgical or traumatic events.

EXPECTED RESPONSE TO PLATELET TRANSFUSIONS AND DOSE CONSIDERATIONS

The measurements required to determine the efficacy of transfused platelets are (1) platelet increment, (2) platelet survival, (3) platelet function, and (4) clinical evaluation of hemostasis.

Platelet Increment

The increment is usually determined by subtracting the pretransfusion platelet count from the count measured 1 hour after the transfusion; however, a similar result can be obtained using the 10-minute post-transfusion platelet count instead of the 1-hour count.[62] Normally, about 60 ± 15% of the transfused platelets circulate in thrombocytopenic patients,[6] calculated by the following formula:

$$\text{Platelet recovery (\%)} = \left[\frac{\begin{array}{c}(\text{platelet increment}) \\ \times (\text{patient's weight in kg}) \\ \times (\text{blood volume estimated at 75 ml/kg})\end{array}}{\begin{array}{c}(\text{platelet count of infused product}) \times \\ (\text{volume of product in ml})\end{array}} \right] \times 100$$

Any noncirculating platelets are pooled in the spleen. Thus, in asplenic individuals, the post-transfusion platelet recovery approaches 100%; in hypersplenism the recovery is reduced proportionally to the size of the spleen.[10]

As an alternative measure of initial platelet response, a corrected count increment (CCI) can be calculated:

$$\text{CCI} = \frac{(\text{platelet increment}) \times (\text{body surface area in m}^2)}{\text{number of platelets transfused} \times 10^{11}}$$

A CCI of 30×10^9/L represents 100% recovery, and a CCI corresponding to a 60% recovery would be 18×10^9/L.[63]

Each platelet concentrate is expected to contain a minimum of 5.5×10^9 platelets/U. Thus, a single platelet concentrate should increase the peripheral platelet count in a 75-kg recipient by approximately 6×10^9/L; however, if the average platelet yield is higher, at 7.0×10^{10} (a reasonable expectation for most blood centers to achieve), the increment will be about 8×10^9/L. These estimates assume normal splenic pooling. Therefore, the usual pooled transfusion dose of 4–6 U of platelet concentrates should be adequate to control bleeding in most patients.

Survival

Although normal autologous platelet survivals average 9.6 ± 0.6 days, there exists a direct relationship between platelet count and survival at platelet counts $<100 \times 10^9$/L. The survival of transfused platelets in thrombocytopenic patients can be determined by following daily platelet counts, and this determines transfusion frequency. However, in addition to the fixed platelet/vessel wall loss and platelet senescence (as determinants of platelet life span), numerous clinical events may also adversely affect the survival of transfused platelets (e.g., any condition associated with disseminated intravascular coagulation [bacteremia, metastatic malignancies, leukemia, obstetric catastrophes],[11,64] viral infections,[65,66] increased platelet utilization associated with wound healing,[67] amphotericin therapy,[65,66] fever,[68] and, undoubtedly, other factors that have not yet been identified).

Function

Further documentation of the efficacy of transfused platelets is demonstrated by measuring the bleeding time and correlating it with the platelet count (Fig. 135–2). Evidence of post-transfusion platelet dysfunction implies either some extrinsic factor (usually the patient's medications or disease processes) that alters the function of the transfused platelets, or, alternatively, defective transfused platelets. The latter finding usually suggests either poor platelet collection techniques, inadequate platelet storage procedures, or aspirin use by the platelet donor within the preceding several days. Surprisingly, aspirin-impaired donor platelets show progressive improvement in function with time after a transfusion. Usually only 4–9 hours is required to achieve their expected function.[69] The reversibility of the platelet dysfunction means that whole blood donors who are taking aspirin can be used as a source of platelet concentrates. Adequate recipient hemostasis is ensued by giving pooled platelet concentrates; by chance, at least one-half the donors will not be taking aspirin, and these nonaspirinized platelets will substantially reduce the initial impact of any dysfunctional aspirin-affected platelets. However, if aspheresis platelets are to be used and the transfusion is being given for active bleeding rather than prophylaxis, then platelets from a nonaspirinized donor, if possible, should be used.

Hemostasis

The most important parameter reflecting the efficacy of a platelet transfusion is cessation of bleeding. Hemostasis can be evaluated directly by clinical observations and indirectly by reduction in RBC transfusion requirements.

PLATELET PRODUCTS AVAILABLE FOR TRANSFUSION

Platelet concentrates are either prepared from routinely donated units of whole blood, or, alternatively, platelets are obtained by apheresis procedures. To reduce the need for platelet transfusions, platelet products that have been appropriately prepared and stored must be available for transfusion. It is important to optimize the yield of platelets in the product while ensuring that neither the preparation nor the storage procedure has compromised the viability or the function (or both) of the platelets.

Random Donor Platelet Concentrates

The yield of platelets in a platelet concentrate varies with the time and force of centrifugation used to prepare the platelet-rich plasma (PRP) from whole blood and subsequently to sediment platelets from the PRP. It is possible to harvest 85–90% of the whole blood platelets consistently into a platelet concentrate.[70] Federal guidelines require $\geq 5.5 \times 10^{10}$ platelets/concentrate, and optimum techniques should produce an average yield of $\geq 7.0 \times 10^{10}$.

PLATELET TRANSFUSION PROGRAM OF THE AUTHOR

First, any medications given to a thrombocytopenic patient should be evaluated for their likelihood to cause drug-related thrombocytopenia or induce platelet dysfunction. Any nonessential medications, or those considered to be potentially associated with thrombocytopenia or platelet dysfunction, should be discontinued.

Any patient who has a decrease in platelet number or function associated with substantial bleeding either from operative incisions or occurring spontaneously from the gastrointestinal or genitourinary tract or the central nervous system is a candidate for platelet transfusions. For prophylactic platelet therapy, patients with production-related thrombocytopenia should receive platelet therapy if their count is $<5 \times 10^9$/L.

Since only about one-half of chronically thrombocytopenic patients develop alloimmunization (it is not possible to predict which patients will develop this problem) and since it is not clear that the currently available techniques will consistently prevent platelet alloimmunization, the initial therapy for patients expected to be chronically thrombocytopenic remains pooled random donor platelet concentrates in a dose of 4–6 U/transfusion episode.

When an individual becomes platelet refractory (as demonstrated by a failure to increase the circulating platelet count by $\geq 5 \times 10^9$ platelets/L on two sequential occasions after the transfusion of 4–6-U pools of random donor platelet concentrates), the following algorithm can be used to identify mechanisms of refractoriness and their appropriate management. This algorithm proceeds from the simplest potential approaches to improving platelet transfusion responses to those that require either more sophisticated laboratory tests to establish a diagnosis or the provision of platelets from specially selected donors, or both.

As ABO compatibility between donor and recipient may be a major cause not only of the development of alloimmunization but also of poor platelet responses in platelet-refractory patients, ABO-compatible products should be provided to any platelet-refractory patients—if they are not already receiving this product.

If ABO-compatible platelets do not improve the transfusion response, fresh platelets should be provided. As some patients demonstrate a poorer response to stored platelets than to fresh platelets, this may be a simple method of obtaining better platelet increments. It is not clear how fresh the platelets need to be in any given patient to obtain a benefit. However, the freshest platelets available—preferably, <24 hours old—should be given as the "test" transfusion to document whether this is helpful. It can then be determined for each individual patient how long the platelets can be stored

while maintaining the desired improvement in platelet increments.

If providing ABO-compatible or fresh platelets is not successful, the presumption is that the patient is alloimmunized. To test by both platelet and lymphocytotoxic antibody tests with panel platelets and lymphocytes, respectively, a serum sample should be obtained from the patient to determine whether antibodies can be detected using either type of assay.

If any of the antibody tests are positive, compatible platelet donors can be selected by any one of several techniques, as outlined in the text, (i.e., (1) determine antibody specificity by means of lymphocyte or platelet panel reactivity and avoid antigen-incompatible donors; (2) select HLA or platelet antigen-compatible donors from within the family or from antigen-typed community donor apheresis panels; or (3) perform platelet crossmatch tests with family or community platelet donors).

In the event that a compatible donor cannot be identified by any of these techniques, then a trial of intravenous IgG can be considered if the patient is considered to be at risk of a fatal hemorrhage. After this treatment, the most compatible donors should be selected, since, even with intravenous IgG, an improved response may only be observed with compatible donors. If compatible donors are successful, then less compatible donors can be tested to see whether the intravenous IgG produces a benefit from any platelet donor.

Alternatively, if the antibody tests are negative, adverse clinical factors or drugs may be compromising transfusion responses. As discussed in the text, a variety of clinical factors and drugs may affect post-transfusion platelet increments or survivals. These situations should be corrected as much as possible, but often the adverse factors cannot be identified or corrected. Frequent doses (every 4–8 hours) of small amounts of pooled random donor platelet concentrates (4 U) may be effective in providing some hemostasis. In addition, it should be remembered that these adverse events may also compromise the response to an otherwise compatible donor in patients who do have evidence of alloantibodies.

For patients who become platelet refractory and who have not responded to ABO-compatible or fresh platelets, weekly antibody samples should be obtained for testing as long as they continue to require platelet support. For antibody-positive patients, antibodies may be lost over time, allowing them to, again, respond to the less expensive random donor platelet therapy. In addition, periodic testing of initially antibody-negative patients permits the indentification of those patients who develop antibodies over time and who might then benefit from antigen-compatible donors.

(Continues)

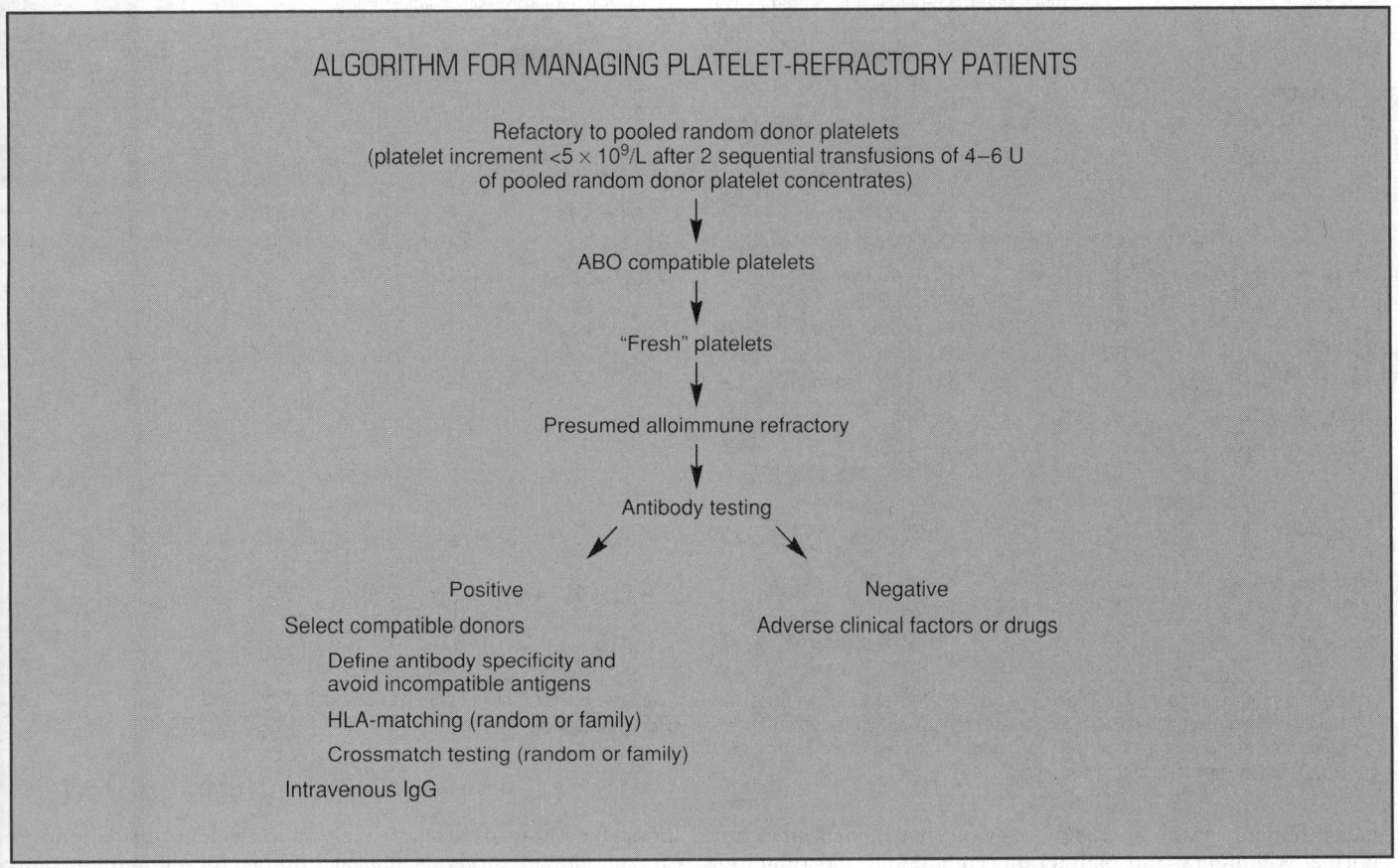

ALGORITHM FOR MANAGING PLATELET-REFRACTORY PATIENTS

Refactory to pooled random donor platelets
(platelet increment $<5 \times 10^9$/L after 2 sequential transfusions of 4–6 U
of pooled random donor platelet concentrates)

↓

ABO compatible platelets

↓

"Fresh" platelets

↓

Presumed alloimmune refractory

↓

Antibody testing

↙   ↘

Positive   Negative

Select compatible donors   Adverse clinical factors or drugs

Define antibody specificity and
avoid incompatible antigens

HLA-matching (random or family)

Crossmatch testing (random or family)

Intravenous IgG

Another factor that may need to be considered in preparing platelet concentrates is the number of contaminating white cells. This variable has not been systematically addressed, but high WBC counts in the platelet concentrate appear to contribute to a pH fall during storage, leading to loss of platelet viability.[71,72] In addition, these contaminating white cells may also contribute to platelet alloimmunization.[73–78] Prolonged centrifugation of the whole blood at low g forces to prepare the PRP gives the greatest reduction in white cell contamination of platelet concentrates.[79]

A substantial amount of work has been done to determine the variables that must be controlled in order to provide platelets with normal recovery, survival, and function after storage. Unfortunately, a "storage lesion" remains, in spite of major advances in our understanding storage conditions that must be maintained to ensure a quality product.[80] Specifically, excessive g forces used in the centrifugation of the PRP to concentrate the platelets will reduce poststorage platelet viability; an anticoagulant solution with a relatively high initial pH of ≥ 7 is required to maintain pH levels of ≥ 6 throughout the storage interval (pH values of <6 are associated with unacceptable decreases in platelet viability); the storage bag must have a large enough surface area and sufficient gas permeability to permit oxygen intake and carbon dioxide loss during storage; the temperature must be maintained at 22°C; and an appropriate type of constant, gentle agitation is required throughout the storage interval. In spite of all these recent advances in platelet concentrate storage techniques, normal volunteer autologous radiolabeled platelet viability studies performed after 5 days of storage demonstrate platelet recoveries in the range of only 38 ± 7% to 48 ± 6% and survivals of 5.1 ± 1.4 days to 6.3 ± 1.3 days, compared with fresh recoveries of 59 ± 4% and survivals of 8.1 ± 0.2 days.[81–85]

Some investigators have also performed stored platelet concentrate transfusion studies in thrombocytopenic patients[85–90] (Table 135-1). In general, these data indicate that, no matter how long the platelets are stored, 1-hour post-transfusion platelet increments are consistently less than expected, and platelet survivals are only about 3 days. As platelet survivals are decreased in proportion to the platelet count in thrombocytopenic patients, estimated survivals of 3 days are probably within the anticipated range for severely thrombocytopenic patients requiring platelet transfusions.[6]

Some studies have suggested that clinically unstable patients show good responses only to fresh platelets, while clinically stable patients respond equally well to either fresh or stored platelets.[89,91] However, other investigators who studied only clinically stable patients still demonstrated poorer responses to stored compared with fresh platelets.[86,88,90] Thus, these data raise the question of whether thrombocytopenic patients in general, or at least some subsets of these patients, are being adequately supported by stored platelets.

Apheresis Platelets

Plateletpheresis procedures are well established and have a long history of efficacy for collecting large numbers of viable and functional platelets without affecting donor safety.[92,93] In addition, within the past 3–4 years, the apheresis collection bags have been prepared from the same plastic materials that have facilitated 5-day storage of platelet concentrates prepared from whole blood donations. The platelet apheresis storage studies performed to date suggest that the quality of stored apheresis platelets is similar to that of stored platelet concentrates based on in vitro pre- and poststorage platelet function

Table 135-1. Transfusion of Stored Platelet Concentrates into Thrombocytopenic Patients

Investigators	Recipients (N)	Storage Time (days)	Bag	Corrected Platelet Count Increment ($\times 10^3/mm^3$)[a]		Platelet Recovery (%)	
				1-Hour	18–48 Hours	1-Hour	18–48 Hours
Snyder et al.[85]	13	5	PL 1240 (Fenwall)	13.6 ± 10.4		59 ± 40[b]	
	8	5	PL 1240 (Fenwall)	15.6 ± 12.2		74 ± 52[b]	47 ± 38[b]
Hogge et al.[86]	16	Fresh	CL 3861 (Cutter)	20.1 ± 8.4 ⎱	10.8 ± 4.4 ⎱		
	16	3	CL 3861 (Cutter)	12.2 ± 8.1 ⎰ P = 0.02	7.5 ± 5.6 ⎰ P < 0.0001	61[c]	
	16	7	CLX (Cutter)	10.0 ± 7.2	7.0 ± 5.5	50[c]	
Schiffer et al.[87d]	135	1	PL 1240 (Fenwall)	15.5 ± 6.3	10.9 ± 5.3		
	81	2	PL 1240 (Fenwall)	16.1 ± 5.9	10.5 ± 5.5		
	53	3	PL 1240 (Fenwall)	13.6 ± 5.5	10.0 ± 5.2		
	60	4	PL 1240 (Fenwall)	13.0 ± 5.0	8.5 ± 4.4		
	33	5	PL 1240 (Fenwal)	13.2 ± 6.0	8.9 ± 5.0		
Lazarus et al.[88]	15	<1	Fenwal	9.5 (5.0–18.0)			
	15	1–2	Fenwal	7.2 (5.4–14.5) ⎱ P = 0.01		76[c]	
	15	2–3	Fenwal	1.0 (0.0–4.8)		11[c]	
Peter-Salonen et al.[89]	51	Fresh	Biotest, FRG	9.5 ± 7.0 ⎱ P = 0.014	4.7 ± 2.8 ⎱ P = 0.004		
	20	1–4	Biotest, FRG	5.6 ± 4.9 ⎰	2.4 ± 2.8 ⎰	68[c]	
Duguid et al.[90]	52	1	PL 1240 (Fenwall)	12.3 ± 0.7 ⎱ P = 0.08	8.6 ± 0.7 ⎱ P = 0.001		
	7	5	PL 1240 (Fenwall)	5.7 ± 1.4 ⎰	2.9 ± 1.0 ⎰		

[a] Corrected platelet count increment = absolute platelet increment $\times$ body surface area (m^2)/number of platelets transfused $\times 10^{11}$).
[b] Calculated from actual number of platelets transfused and adjusted for blood volume and splenic pooling.
[c] Calculated as percentage of observed/expected based on concurrent fresh transfusions.
[d] Data from nonsplenectomized patients.

measurements, radiolabeled platelet survival measurements in normal volunteers, and platelet increments and bleeding time measurements in thrombocytopenic patients.[94–102]

One additional concern with the transfusion of stored platelet concentrates is the possibility of bacterial contamination during the collection or processing of the platelets or the collection of platelets from a bacteremic donor with subsequent bacterial overgrowth during room temperature platelet storage.[103] The major cause of bacterial contamination is inadequate sterilization of the venipuncture site. Good donor quality control procedures and the use of a sterile docking device to facilitate pooling of platelet concentrates prior to transfusion should prevent most instances of inadvertent bacterial contamination.

Although chills and fever following a platelet transfusion are usually caused by a reaction to contaminating white cells (suggesting the use of leukocyte-poor platelets and/or premedication with antihistamines or steroids to reduce these side effects), the question of bacterial contamination of the platelet product should always be considered, particularly if an associated drop in blood pressures occurs.[104,105] Highly contaminated platelet products can often be detected by Gram staining the residual platelet product, and recipient blood and platelet product cultures can be used to identify the organism.

In summary, the evidence suggests that the optimum methods of maintaining the viability and function of platelets during storage have not yet been identified. For some patients, storing platelets for a relatively short period (24–48 hours) may improve their transfusion responses; this may be worth trying in refractory patients before presuming they are alloimmunized and changing their therapy from random donor platelets to HLA-matched apheresis donor platelets.

PREVENTION OF PLATELET ALLOIMMUNIZATION

Alloimmune platelet destruction was recognized as a consequence of repeated platelet transfusions as early as the 1950s. Three of four chronically transfused patients with marrow hy-

poplasia showed progressively poorer increments and reduced platelet survivals, classic findings for alloimmune platelet destruction.[106] Yankee and co-workers[63] demonstrated that matching for HLA antigens between donor and recipient would provide compatible platelet support for most patients alloimmunized to random donor platelets. However, the complexity of the HLA system makes donor selection difficult, and for some patients compatible donors are not found even when the donor pool is expanded by using HLA cross-reactive specificities. Furthermore, 18–39% of alloimmunized patients do not respond even to fully HLA-matched platelets[107–113] (Table 135–2). Although such nonresponsive patients may have complicating clinical factors that cause rapid platelet consumption, others undoubtedly destroy their transfused platelets because of incompatible platelet-specific antigens.

Clearly, there are abundant reasons to develop strategies to at least delay, if not prevent, platelet alloimmunization. As it requires 10–14 days to develop a primary immune response, patients who need only one or two platelet transfusions for an acute event (such as cardiopulmonary bypass surgery) are not candidates for programs designed to prevent platelet alloimmunization. Rather, the patients with an anticipated prolonged period of marrow failure (requiring chronic platelet support) should be considered for transfusion programs designed to prevent platelet alloimmunization. Most of these patients

Table 135-2. Failure Rate of HLA-A-Matched Platelets

Investigators	No. Refractory/No. Tested	%
Brand et al.[107]	12/31	39
Duquesnoy et al.[108]	5/47	12
Gmur et al.[109]	1/18	6
Kickler et al.[110]	10/45	22
Lohrman et al.[111]	2/11	18
Slichter[112]	2/11	18
Tosato et al.[113]	9/49	18
	41/212	19

either have idiopathic marrow failure, or they are cancer patients who have chemotherapy- or radiotherapy-induced marrow suppression.

In order to evaluate the data on the success of programs designed to prevent platelet alloimmunization, criteria for alloimmunization must be established. Alloimmune platelet refractoriness is present when there is a significant reduction in platelet recovery or survival, or both, in association with alloantibodies. Although this definition appears straightforward, it is often difficult to determine mechanisms of platelet refractoriness in any given patient, for two reasons: (1) many additional factors may be associated with poor platelet recoveries and survivals besides alloimmunization (e.g., fever, infection, drugs, splenomegaly, and so forth)[64-66]; and (2) the simple presence of antibodies does not mean that these antibodies are causing the patient's poor response to transfused platelets. To conclusively demonstrate that alloimmunization is the cause of platelet refractoriness, antigen-compatible platelets must provide consistently better responses than random donor platelets. However, even if a compatible platelet transfusion does not improve a patient's response to platelets, the patient may still be alloimmune refractory, but additional clinical or product factors must be present that are impairing the response to any transfused platelets.

Criteria

Abnormal Platelet Responses

Guidelines of <30% recovery at 1 hour or a survival of <2 days can be used as indicators of an abnormal response. These values correspond to less than one-half the expected recovery measurement, and the survival is shorter than that seen in thrombocytopenic patients.[6]

By the CCI criterion, an unsuccessful transfusion is a CCI of <7.5 or <10.0 × 10⁹/L (depending on the investigator) within 1 hour of a transfusion, and <4.5 or <7.5 × 10⁹/L at 18–24 hours.[63,107,114-116] A CCI of 7.5–10 × 10⁹/L is equivalent to a 25–30% recovery, and a CCI of 4.5–7.5 × 10⁹/L equals 15–25% recovery. Thus, the two reported criteria for determining abnormal platelet responses, based on either platelet recovery or CCI measurements, are roughly equivalent.

On a practical level, the number of platelets transfused is often not counted, and, therefore, it is not possible to calculate a platelet recovery or CCI. In these circumstances, an increment of <5 × 10⁹ platelets/L after two sequential transfusions of 6 U of platelet concentrates is sufficiently abnormal to identify patients who are in need of further evaluation for the identification of causes and the management of their platelet refractoriness.

Detection of Platelet Alloantibodies

As HLA antigens are the major immunogens present on the surface of platelets, lymphocytotoxic antibodies to HLA antigens expressed on lymphocytes are often used as a marker of platelet alloimmunization. However, major improvements have been seen in direct platelet antibody testing using a variety of techniques, and this approach has several advantages.[117] Some HLA antigens may not be as well expressed on platelets as on lymphocytes.[118-121] Thus, detecting a strong lymphocytotoxic antibody against HLA antigens on lymphocytes may not necessarily correlate with platelet transfusion outcomes. In addition, there is increasing interest in the role of platelet-specific, non-HLA antigens in alloimmune platelet refractoriness.[117] These types of antibodies can only be detected by direct platelet antibody assays.

As another guide to the significance of any alloantibodies detected, several studies have demonstrated that the higher the frequency of antibody reactivity with panel lymphocytes or platelets, the more likely is the patient to demonstrate poor responses to pooled random donor platelet transfusions.[62,114,122] Thus, the more panreactive the antibody, the more likely is any platelet unresponsiveness due to alloimmunization.

In summary, neither laboratory (antibody positivity) nor clinical (markedly reduced platelet increment or survival, or both) criteria are sufficiently sensitive or specific, respectively, to establish definitively that platelet alloimmunization is the cause of a poor response to transfused platelets (i.e., platelet refractoriness). However, they represent the best measures available and have been used either alone or in combination to determine rates of platelet alloimmunization.

The incidence of platelet alloimmunization in chronically transfused thrombocytopenic patients ranges between 8% and 100%, with the average being 69%.[123] The variability in reported immunization rates is likely related to differences in the blood products transfused, the administration schedules used, the immunocompetence of the transfused recipient, and/or the criteria for platelet alloimmunization. Several strategies have been applied to the prevention of platelet alloimmunization, which can generally be categorized as follows: (1) immunosuppress the transfused recipient, (2) reduce the exposure to donor antigens, (3) provide leukocyte-poor blood products, or (4) inactive or remove antigen-presenting cells from the transfused blood products. Although these techniques aimed at prevention of platelet alloimmunization have associated expenses that are greater than providing pooled random donor platelet transfusions, they may be less expensive than the costs of providing antigen-compatible platelet donors, if the patient becomes alloimmunized.

Methods

Immunosuppression of the Platelet Transfusion Recipient

Patients with malignant disorders have a much lower rate of immunization to platelet transfusions than do patients with aplastic anemia. In one study, only 20 of 65 (31%) transfused patients with AML developed alloantibodies, compared with 7 of 8 (88%) patients with aplastic anemia.[124] The difference is likely due to the potentially immunosuppressive chemotherapy given to leukemia patients while they are being transfused. In addition, the high-dose steroids received by patients with ALL compared with patients with AML may produce a lower incidence of alloimmunization (i.e., 18% for ALL versus 44% for AML patients [$P <0.0002$]).[125] However, in another study, immunization frequency was the same—38% in AML and 35% in ALL.[126] In neither study were the doses of the chemotherapeutic agents used detailed, and clear differences in immunization rates may exist, depending on the patients' chemotherapy.[124,126] Overall, in a series of studies, 380 of 944 (40%) patients with malignant disorders receiving chemotherapy developed alloantibodies.[124,125,127-131]

In a dog platelet transfusion model, none of the nine recipients given Cyclosporin A therapy became refractory to platelets from a single random donor dog—even after eight weekly transfusions. Furthermore, six of nine recipients (67%) remained responsive to an additional eight weekly transfusions after the cyclosporine was stopped.[132] In six of seven baboons (86%) given either prednisone, antithymocyte globulin, or a combination of these two agents, platelet refractoriness did not occur after repeated weekly platelet transfusions from a single random donor baboon.[133]

In summary, it is unlikely that specific immunosuppressive therapy given to prevent platelet alloimmunization—as was done in the animal transfusion experiments—would ever be accepted for patients because of the increased infectious disease and tumor recurrence risks that might result from such therapy. However, it is quite likely that patients with malignancy who are receiving chemotherapy have a reduced rate of immunization because of the immunosuppressive effect of some of these treatments. Furthermore, it is also possible that some of the other methods that have been used to prevent platelet alloimmunization, such as modifying the transfused blood products, are in part successful because the transfused patients are at least partially immunoincompetent because of their disease or its treatment.

Reduce Exposure To Donor Antigens

Limit the Number of Transfusions

A fundamental hypothesis has been that limiting the number of platelet transfusions reduces the incidence of platelet alloimmunization.[123] Although some studies have suggested that there is a dose-response relationship between the number of transfusions given and the incidence of alloimmunization, other investigations have demonstrated that only a few transfusions may result in immunization. A likely confounding variable in these studies is the failure to control for the effects of time on immunization rates. Usually 2–3 weeks is required for primary immunization, and, whether the patient receives few or many transfusions during this time, the final outcome is often alloimmunization.

Limit the Number of Donors

Three prospective randomized trials have attempted to determine the relative benefits of providing single random donor apheresis platelets compared with pooled random donor platelet transfusions to prevent platelet alloimmunization[134–136] (Table 135-3). Only one of these studies showed a significant decrease in rates of platelet refractoriness and lymphocytotoxic antibody formation, even though the number of donor exposures for the patients who received pooled random donor platelets was ≥10 times that of the patients receiving single-donor random apheresis platelets.[136]

As only a subset of chronically transfused patients with malignant disorders become alloimmunized, the question becomes whether it is worthwhile to provide all chronically thrombocytopenic patients with the more expensive single-donor apheresis transfusions when only a fraction of the patients need protection and, at best, alloimmunization is likely to be only delayed rather than prevented.[123]

Select Compatible Donors

ABO Compatibility. A and B antigens are expressed on the surface of platelets.[137] To determine the effect of ABO mismatching on platelet alloimmunization, 40 leukemic patients undergoing induction chemotherapy were randomly assigned to receive two sets of paired transfusions of ABO-compatible or -incompatible pooled random donor platelet transfusions.[138] Although no difference in platelet recoveries was seen with the first set of transfusions, the CCI for the second ABO-compatible transfusion averaged 14.9×10^9/L, compared with 9.5×10^9/L for the ABO-incompatible transfusion ($P < 0.0007$); survivals were similar. Eleven patients had serial isohemagglutination titers for anti-A and anti-B antibodies performed; in the six patients with consistently poor results to ABO-incompatible platelets, the relevant anti-A or anti-B titers were either elevated at baseline or became elevated after the incompatible transfusions (isohemagglutination titers were 256–1,024). By contrast, only one of the five patients with consistently good responses to ABO-incompatible platelets had elevated titers.

In another study of 26 patients undergoing treatment for acute leukemia or autografting for relapsed Hodgkin disease who were randomly assigned to receive either ABO-compatible or ABO-incompatible platelets, platelet refractoriness was significantly lower in the group receiving ABO-compatible platelets—not only because patients did not increase their anti-A or anti-B isohemagglutinin titers but also because the ABO-compatible recipients had a much lower incidence of lymphocytotoxic and platelet-specific alloantibodies.[139] Nine of the 13 patients (69%) who were given ABO-mismatched platelet transfusions became platelet-refractory, compared with only 1 of 13 patients (8%) who received ABO-compatible platelets ($P < 0.0014$) (Fig. 135-4). The repeated administration of ABO-mismatched platelets produced a significant rise in anti-AB titers in 7 of 13 patients (54%) that were generally correlated with poor platelet increments. In addition, 5 of 13 recipients (38%) of the ABO-mismatched platelets developed lymphocytotoxic antibodies, and 4 of 13 (31%) developed platelet-specific alloantibodies, compared with only 1 of 13 (8%) and 1 of 13 (8%), respectively, of the recipients of ABO-compatible platelets. The close temporal association between the development of HLA and platelet-specific alloantibodies and rises in anti-A/B titers suggests that, in the process of responding to the ABO-incompatible antigens, recognition of other antigen incompatibilities also occurred. Data from these two studies suggest that provi-

Table 135-3. Transfusion of Single Random Donor Apheresis Platelets Versus Pooled Random Donor Platelet Concentrates[a]

| | Pooled Random Donor Platelet Concentrates | | | | | | | Single Random Donor Apheresis Platelets | | | | | | |
| | | Transfusion Events[b] (no.) | | Platelet Refractory | | Alloantibodies | | | Transfusion Events (no.) | | Platelet Refractory | | Alloantibodies | |
Investigators	Patients (N)	Platelet	RBC	N	%	N	%	Patients (N)	Platelet	RBC	N	%	N	%
Sintnicolaas et al.[134] (1981)	17	2.4 (1–75) NS	8 (3–20)	NI		2 NS	12	17	1.7 (1–75)	5 (2–19)	NI		1	6
Kakaiya et al.[135] (1981)	7	8 ± 6 NS	NI	NI		2 NS	29	9	10 ± 9	NI	NI		5	56
Gmur et al.[136] (1983)	27	5.5 ± 3.0 NS	10.7 ± 5.5	14	52 $P < 0.005$	15	56 $P < 0.002$	27	6.0 ± 3.0	12.8 ± 6.0	4	15	4	15

Abbreviations: NI, no information; NS, not significant.

[a] Significance values compare the results of transfusions with pooled random donor platelet concentrates to single random donor apheresis platelets.

[b] Average transfusions per patient (range), or ± SD. In studies by Sintnicolaas et al. and Kakaiya et al., each pooled random donor transfusion consisted of 10 platelet concentrates; in Gmur et al.'s study, 5–10 platelet concentrates/transfusion were given. In Sintnicolaas et al.'s study, all RBCs were buffy-coat-poor; in Gmur et al.'s study, the RBCs were made leukocyte-poor by filtration.

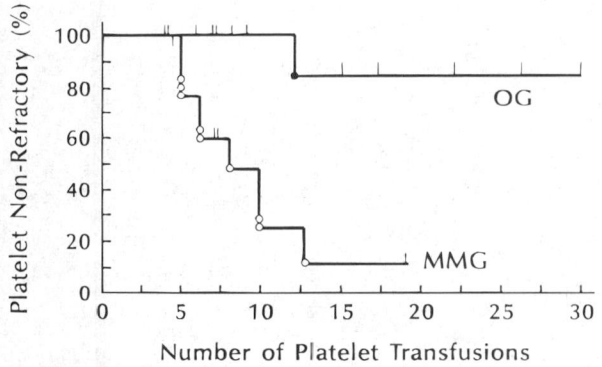

Fig. 135-4. Estimated survival curves of refractoriness by number of platelet transfusions. Ordinate: probability (percent) of not becoming refractory. Log rank statistic = 10.3 (P = 0.00114). (From Carr et al.,[139] with permission.)

sion of ABO-compatible platelets may be a simple method of reducing the incidence of alloimmune platelet refractoriness.

HLA Compatibility. As HLA antigens are the predominant immunogens expressed on the surface of platelets and the major cause of refractoriness to ABO-compatible platelets, in two transfusion trials the benefits of HLA compared with random single-donor apheresis platelet transfusions were evaluated.[74,140] In one trial, 18 cancer patients receiving chemotherapy for a variety of malignant disorders received only HLA-matched platelets, and another 15 patients received single-donor platelets mismatched for one or more HLA antigens.[140] No significant difference was seen between total number of platelet transfusions per patient (median 3 versus 5, respectively; P = 0.076), number of platelet transfusions per thrombocytopenic episode (median 3.0 versus 3.5, respectively; P = 0.28), or days between transfusions (median 2 versus 2, respectively; P >0.40). Only one study patient developed antiplatelet antibodies.

In the other study, 30 patients with newly diagnosed acute leukemia were given red cells and platelet apheresis transfusions that were both made leukocyte-poor prior to transfusion.[74] Nineteen patients received single random donor apheresis transfusions, and 11 patients received apheresis transfusions compatible for at least three of the four HLA-A and -B locus antigens. The single random donor apheresis group received a mean of 33 U of RBCs and 19 random apheresis transfusions, compared with 23 U of RBCs and 9 HLA-matched apheresis transfusions. Three of the 19 recipients (16%) who were given random single-donor apheresis platelets developed lymphocytotoxic antibodies, and 1 of 19 (5%) became platelet-refractory, compared with 0 of 11 and 0 of 11, respectively, for the recipients of the HLA-selected transfusions. No significant differences were seen in platelet refractoriness or antibody development between the groups. Thus, in neither of these two studies was there evidence that provision of HLA-matched apheresis platelets provided an additional benefit over that achieved with single random donor apheresis transfusions, possibly because thrombocytopenic patients not only receive platelets but also red cell transfusions. Since the red cell transfusions were obtained from non-HLA-selected donors, this may have been enough of a challenge to the recipient's immune system that any expected benefits from HLA matching of platelet donor and recipient were obscured—even if the RBC products were made leukocyte-poor by filtration in an attempt to prevent platelet alloimmunization from the contaminating WBCs.[74]

Modification of the Transfused Platelets and RBCs to Reduce their Immunogenicity

For some of the investigations to be discussed, only the transfused platelets were modified and evaluated. However, it should be remembered that chronically thrombocytopenic patients require both RBC and platelet transfusions, and transfusion studies modifying both products will be needed to determine the efficacy of any of these methods in preventing platelet alloimmunization.

Leukocyte Reduction

It has been well documented that alloantigen recognition requires the expression of both class I and class II HLA antigens on the surface of the transfused cells.[141,142] As platelets, in contrast to WBCs, express only class I but not class II HLA antigens and RBCs do not express HLA antigens, the question of whether leukocyte-poor blood components will prevent platelet alloimmunization has been investigated. Early animal studies in both rats[141] and mice[143] demonstrated that leukocyte-depleted platelets were not associated with alloantibody development.

In humans, administration of $<5 \times 10^6$ leukocytes did not result in lymphocytotoxic antibody formation following a limited number of injections.[144,145] Although centrifugation techniques have been used to produce leukocyte-poor blood products, in the last several years a number of highly efficient leukocyte reduction filters have been developed. A review of the literature between 1980 and 1990 provides data on the residual leukocyte levels in RBC and platelet products using these filters.[146] In fact, the efficacy of some of these filters is so good that newer techniques are required to count accurately the very low number of white cells remaining in the filtered products.[147]

To date, six prospective randomized clinical trials in 299 patients have evaluated the efficacy of leukocyte-poor RBCs and platelets in preventing platelet alloimmunization[73–78] (Table 135-4). Substantial variability existed in patient selection, methods of leukocyte reduction, and end-point criteria. Not unexpectedly, differences were also seen in the leukocyte concentration of the control blood products and the leukocyte-poor blood products, as well as in the results of these transfusion trials (Table 135-4). Four of the six studies showed a significant reduction in the development of lymphocytotoxic antibodies in patients given leukocyte-poor products; however, in the three studies that tested for platelet-specific alloantibodies, no difference was found between the control and leukocyte-poor arms. The incidence of clinical refractoriness to transfused platelets was reduced by leukocyte-poor blood products in only three of the six trials.

Two recent editorials have suggested caution in interpreting the data from these leukocyte-poor transfusion trials because of the small numbers of patients in the studies and conflicting data on the levels of leukocytes that either produce or prevent platelet alloimmunization or platelet refractoriness, or both.[148,149] Furthermore, in another recent study, although the 27% incidence of antibody formation in 71 previously pregnant women was the same as the 19% found in 264 non-presensitized patients (all patients were receiving leukocyte-poor RBCs and platelet products), the rate of platelet refractoriness was significantly higher in the previously pregnant women—15 of 71 (21%) compared with 16 of 264 (6%) in the non-presensitized patients (P <0.001).[150] This finding suggests that the subgroup of patients with prior antigenic exposure through pregnancy, or probably by transfusions as well—although the latter patients were excluded from the trial—may not benefit clinically from filtration procedures.

One technical issue that has been raised in the performance of these trials is the timing of the leukocyte reduction. One

Table 135-4. Leukocyte-Poor Transfusion Trials—Results

Investigators	Patients (N)	Control[a] Platelets (WBC × 10^6)	Control[a] RBC[b] (WBC × 10^6)	Leukocyte-Poor[a] Platelets (WBC × 10^6)	Leukocyte-Poor[a] RBC[b] (WBC × 10^6)	Antibody Positive (%) Lymphocytotoxic Control	Antibody Positive (%) Lymphocytotoxic Leukocyte-Poor	Antibody Positive (%) Platelet Control	Antibody Positive (%) Platelet Leukocyte-Poor	Clinically Platelet Refractory (%) Control	Clinically Platelet Refractory (%) Leukocyte-Poor
Schiffer et al.[73] (1983)	56	65	Frozen,[b] washed	12	Frozen,[b] washed	42 ($P = 0.07$)	20	NT	NT	19 (NS)	16
Murphy et al.[74] (1986)	50	5,380[c]	NI	90–220[c]	≤8	48 ($P < 0.02$)	16	10 (NS)	11	23 (NS)	5
Sniecinski et al.[75] (1988)	40	530	3,900	6	50	50 ($P < 0.01$)	15	35 (NS)	15	50 ($P < 0.01$)	15
Andreu et al.[76] (1988)	69	477–678	2,300	47–151	61	31 ($P < 0.05$)	12	NT	NT	47 ($P < 0.05$)	21
Oksanen et al.[77] (1991)	31	800	1,000	0.2	0.1	26 (NS)	13	33 (NS)	31	26 (NS)	13
van Marwijk Kooy et al.[78] (1991)	53	35[d]	5[d]	<5	<5	42 ($P < 0.004$)	7	NT	NT	46 ($P < 0.005$)	11

Abbreviations: NI, no information; NT, not tested; NS, no significant difference between control and leukocyte-poor data.
[a] Leukocyte data are reported as average number or range of residual WBCs per transfusion event for platelets or per unit of RBCs transfused.
[b] Frozen washed red cells have no identifiable intact white cells.
[c] Single random donor apheresis transfusions were given rather than the pooled random donor transfusions used in all other studies, except for the study of Andreu et al., in which one of four trial sites used single random donor apheresis transfusions.
[d] Control platelets leukocyte-reduced by centrifugation and RBCs made leukocyte-poor by filtration.

investigator suggested that an intact white cell is required for induction of an immune response[141] while another found that WBC fragments were immunogenic.[151] As WBCs break down during storage and no information is available on whether the leukocyte reduction filters will remove these fragments, it may be important to filter the blood products shortly after collection to prevent the transfusion of potentially immunogenic fragments. The question of the immunogenicity of WBC fragments has been evaluated in a rabbit transfusion model.[151,152] In one study, 24 control rabbits received eight weekly fresh whole blood transfusions prepared from a single donor of a different strain.[152] At the end of 8 weeks, platelets from the donor rabbit were radiolabeled and given to the recipient of the whole blood transfusions. Donor platelet survivals averaged 18.5 hours compared with autologous platelet survivals of 41.9–75.1 hours. The platelet refractory rate (defined as a donor platelet survival of <42 hours) was 96% in these recipients. By contrast, immediate leukocyte depletion and storage of the whole blood for 1 week prior to transfusion resulted in mean donor platelet survivals of 54.7 hours and a refractory rate of 33%. However, if the blood was stored for 1 week and then leukocyte depleted and transfused, after eight weekly transfusions of the poststorage leukocyte-depleted whole blood, donor platelet survivals were only 31.0 hours, and 67% of the recipients were platelet refractory ($P < 0.05$ for both end points, compared with prestorage leukocyte-depleted transfusions). During the week of storage, the WBC count in the unfiltered blood decreased by approximately 20%. In the other study, rabbits received RBCs made leukocyte-poor immediately after collection or after 3 days of storage, or they received frozen/thawed deglycolized RBCs.[151] None of the recipients of the immediately filtered blood developed lymphocytotoxic antibodies, while all the recipients of the other blood products became immunized.

Ultraviolet Irradiation

Instead of removing white cells from the transfused blood products (with the inherent problems of complete and effective removal), another approach would be to alter the transfusions to eliminate their immunogenicity. In that regard, an important observation demonstrated that ultraviolet (UV) irradiation renders lymphocytes unable either to stimulate or respond in mixed lymphocyte culture (MLC), even though HLA antigens are still expressed on the surface of the UV-irradiated lymphocytes.[153] It has been known for some time that γ-irradiation prevents lymphocytes from responding in MLC, but γ-irradiated cells are still able to act as stimulating cells in MLC. Several explanations were postulated for the failure of UV radiation-treated lymphocytes to stimulate in MLC: (1) other unrecognized antigens on the cell surface important for MLC reactivity are altered by UV radiation, (2) lymphocytes release mediators for the MLC reaction that are inhibited by UV radiation, or (3) the motility of UV-irradiated cells is impaired, preventing appropriate cell-to-cell interaction—a function known to be required for MLC reactivity. Since this initial publication, all these potential mechanisms for failure of UV-irradiated cells to stimulate in MLC have been evaluated, and more than one of these mechanisms may be involved in producing the UV radiation effect.[154]

In a dog transfusion model, 11 of 12 recipients (92%) of UV-irradiated donor platelets did not become platelet-refractory after eight weekly single random donor transfusions ($P < 0.01$); compared with unmodified controls, only 3 of 21 (14%) were not refractory.[132] In addition, when unmodified platelet transfusions were continued from the same random donor, tolerance to the unmodified platelets was observed in 8 of 11 (73%) of the nonrefractory recipient dogs. To determine whether the tolerance induced was specific to the platelets of only the treated donor, the eight nonrefractory recipients were also given unmodified transfusions from at least two other random donor dogs (called secondary donors). A high degree of nonspecific tolerance to platelets from other donors had been induced in these transfused animals: 10 of 23 (43%) secondary donors transfusions were tolerated by the dogs who had previously received UV-irradiated platelets.

These encouraging results in the dog model have led to several recent attempts to evaluate the effects of UV irradiation on human platelets. The in vivo viability and function of human platelets remains intact after the platelets have been UV irradiated in special plastic bags that permit adequate UV penetrance.[155–157] Furthermore, platelets could be UV-B irradiated and then stored with no adverse effects on poststorage platelet viability.

A large multi-institutional trial sponsored by the National Heart, Lung, and Blood Institute has recently been initiated in the United States to explore the relative merits of leukocyte reduction and UV-B irradiation in the prevention of platelet alloimmunization.[158] Certainly either of these two approaches—which require only a manipulation of the product prior to transfusion to prevent platelet alloimmunization—is preferable to the other approaches discussed previously, which would involve either some type of immunosuppression of the recipient or donor selection.

MANAGEMENT OF PLATELET REFRACTORINESS

The major problem in planning the management of platelet-refractory patients is the multiplicity of factors that may be adversely affecting the transfused platelets. The most helpful method of initially categorizing patients (useful for both diagnostic and therapeutic purposes) is to perform platelet or lymphocytotoxic antibody screening assays, or both. This allows patients to be classified as either nonimmune or alloimmune platelet-refractory. However, classification of a patient as alloimmune, based on positive antibody tests between the patient's serum and donor platelets/lymphocytes, does not exclude the possibility that concurrent nonimmune causes of platelet refractoriness may also exist; such causes may compromise response, even to platelets from compatible donors.

Nonimmune Platelet Refractoriness

If the platelet or lymphocytotoxic antibody screening assays (or both) are negative, the patient is presumed to have nonimmune causes of platelet refractoriness.

Stored Platelets

On a practical level, the easiest test in platelet-refractory patients, and one that may produce a high yield of improved responses, is to give fresh platelets. Of 108 patients who were refractory to pooled random donor platelets and had no evidence of antibodies, only 3 (3%) did not show improved platelet responses when they were given single random donor apheresis platelets that had been stored for ≤36 hours.[159] If fresh platelet transfusions are not successful in improving platelet responses, then other potential causes of platelet refractoriness should be considered.

Splenomegaly

To compensate for the platelet pooling associated with hypersplenism,[10] the number of units of platelets transfused will need to be increased to achieve the desired platelet increment. However, as platelet survival is not affected by the size of the spleen, transfusion frequency will not have to be modified.

Fever

Undoubtedly, it is not the fever per se that reduces the platelet increment,[68] but the factors that cause the fever. Thus, antipyretics are unlikely to be associated with improved platelet increments, although clinical studies to test this approach have not been reported. It is more likely that the underlying problem producing the fever will have to be resolved before platelet increments will improve.

Disseminated Intravascular Coagulation

Prompt and aggressive treatment of the underlying disease state producing the disseminated intravascular coagulation, in order to eliminate hemostatic factor consumption, is the most important step in the management of these patients. Until the underlying pathologic state responds to treatment, hemostatic factor replacement therapy, as indicated by the results of platelet counts, coagulation tests, and bleeding manifestations, should be provided.[160] Both the amount and frequency of platelet therapy may need to be increased in order to maintain adequate hemostasis.

Alloimmune Platelet Refractoriness

Obviously, the best method of managing platelet alloimmunization is to prevent its occurrence. However, if this is not successful, selection of antigen-compatible donors will be needed. Alternatively, intravenous IgG may provide transient platelet increments in some patients if antigen-compatible platelets are not available.

Selection of Compatible Donors for Alloimmunized Patients

Determination of Antibody Specificity Using Lymphocyte Panels

Significant information can sometimes be gained by testing patients' sera for antibody reactivity with antigen-selected lymphocyte panels. If HLA antibody specificity is determined, HLA-typed donors can be selected to avoid the offending antigen. Avoiding a limited number of incompatible antigens rather than matching for antigens will greatly expand the available donor pool for some patients. However, this approach is likely to be successful only with antibodies of limited specificity. Unfortunately, many patients become broadly alloimmunized, reducing the effectiveness of antiserum analysis.[123]

Antigen Matching

ABO. Several large platelet transfusion studies have established the transfusion relevance of donor-recipient ABO antigen compatibility. The effects of ABO compatibility on transfusion responses were documented in 91 platelet-refractory patients who received 389 HLA-selected apheresis platelet transfusions.[161] For the ABO-compatible platelets, recoveries averaged $73 \pm 4\%$ at 1 hour, compared with $55 \pm 5\%$ for ABO-mismatched transfusions ($P <0.01$); at 24 hours post-transfusion, recoveries were $37 \pm 3\%$ versus $29 \pm 4\%$, respectively ($P <0.05$). In a second, similar study of 51 platelet-refractory patients given 316 HLA-selected donor apheresis transfusions, ABO-compatible platelet transfusions gave average CCIs of 10 $\times$ 10^9/L, compared with 5.9 $\times$ 10^9/L for ABO-incompatible platelets ($P <0.01$).[162] However, there was no effect of ABO incompatibility on platelet survivals.

HLA. Although HLA-matched donors may give compatible transfusion responses in patients who have become refractory to random donor platelets, the complexity of the HLA system often makes it difficult to find HLA-matched donors.[63,163] Therefore, the effectiveness of platelets mismatched for cross-reactive HLA antigens has been evaluated.[164] A total of 421 single donor apheresis transfusions were administered to 59 alloimmunized platelet-refractory patients. Partially matched single-donor platelets were effective when the mismatch at one or two loci involved cross-reactive groups only. However, approximately 30% of even the best matched donors did not provide acceptable post-transfusion platelet increments. Possible immunologic explanations for these incompatible transfusion results are the presence of platelet-specific antibodies or antibodies against cross-reactive HLA antigens.

Platelet-Specific Antibodies. Evidence that platelet-specific antibodies may produce platelet refractoriness comes from transfusion studies using HLA fully matched family or unrelated donors. Seven studies reported a failure rate of HLA-A-matched platelets from either family members or unrelated donors of 6–39%, with an average of 19% (41 of 212) (Table 135-2). Unfortunately, there are not enough platelet-specific antisera available to type community donor platelet apheresis panels for these antigens. Therefore, the most likely source of platelet-specific antigen-compatible donors may be within the patient's family. Family member compatibility can be determined either by platelet antigen typing, by platelet cross-match testing, or by platelet transfusion trials.

Platelet Cross-match Testing

The platelet antibody tests that have been adapted for platelet cross-match testing have relatively good sensitivity and specificity. Many investigators are successfully predicting ≥70% of the transfusion outcomes using these assays.[64,165–169] Cross-matching can be performed either with random donor platelet concentrates followed by pooling of the compatible units to constitute a transfusion dose, or with single random or HLA-selected apheresis platelets.

However, patients selected for these platelet cross-matching studies have often been restricted to those who are not clinically ill at the time of the transfusion. Although this approach permits a more reliable evaluation of the platelet cross-match assays, it does not reflect the actual situation, in which compatible platelet support must be available for all patients regardless of their clinical status. In addition, detailed information on the clinical condition of most patients is not usually available to the laboratory performing the cross-match tests. Therefore, platelet cross-match testing in the routine clinical situation is likely to be less reliable than has been suggested by these carefully controlled clinical trials. The major problem with the platelet antibody tests is a relatively high incidence of false-negative cross-match tests results, that is, a poor platelet increment with a negative cross-match test. The question then becomes whether the assay is sensitive enough to pick up all relevant antibodies, or, alternatively, whether the patient has a clinical condition that results in an inappropriate transfusion increment. Only additional studies will permit documentation of the true relevance of platelet cross-match testing to select compatible donors for all alloimmunized patients who require platelet support.

Reversal of Platelet Alloimmunization

Even using the best available methods of preventing platelet alloimmunization, some patients will still become immunized. In addition, those individuals with prior antigenic exposures through pregnancy or transfusions that were not modified to reduce their immunogenicity may become alloimmunized in spite of any preventative measures. For some of these alloimmunized patients, compatible platelet donors will not be identified using either antigen-matched donors or platelet cross-match testing. For these patients, it is important to determine whether techniques are available to reverse, temporarily or permanently, an already established immune response.

Spontaneous Antibody Loss

It has been well documented that many patients will lose their antibodies over time, often in spite of continued platelet and RBC transfusions; thus, active approaches to alloimmune reversal will not be required for these individuals. Overall, in six studies, antibody loss was documented in 144 of 340 patients (42%).[124,125,127,128,130,131] In one study, none of 7 aplastic patients versus 10 of 20 (50%) leukemic patients lost their antibodies, suggesting that there may be an influence of chemotherapy on antibody loss.[124] In addition, although some variability in the data exist, approximately equal numbers of patients lose antibodies over time whether they are continuing to receive transfusions or not. Some evidence also exists showing that individuals who have not been previously exposed to incompatible antigens by prior pregnancies or transfusions tend to lose their current transfusion-induced antibodies more frequently. Five of 10 patients (50%) who had prior antigen exposure lost their antibodies, compared with 25 of 27 (93%) who had no prior antigenic exposure.[130] In another study, the types of prior antigen exposure also affected antibody loss.[131] If the patient had a history of both prior pregnancies and transfusions, only one of five (20%) lost their antibodies while antibodies resolved in all nine (100%) with a history of only one type of exposure (i.e., either prior transfusions or pregnancies).

It is of great practical importance that once antibodies disappear, patients may regain their responsiveness to random donor platelet transfusions. For example, of 34 patients who lost their antibodies, all had good initial responses to reinstitution of random donor platelet transfusions, and 21 of 34 (62%) never again became platelet-refractory even with multiple additional transfusions.[125] These data clearly suggest that a prudent strategy is to measure antibodies serially over time in platelet-refractory patients, with the goal of returning those patients who lose their antibodies to random donor platelet therapy.

Administration of Intravenous IgG

The effectiveness of intravenous IgG in managing patients with alloimmune platelet destruction is unclear. Studies have shown improved platelet responses in some treated patients,[170–173] while other patients have shown no response.[174–176] In the only randomized controlled trial in which platelets from the same donor were given both before and after intravenous IgG, a significant increase in platelet counts occurred in the treated group compared with the untreated group at 1 hour post-transfusion (8,413 versus 1,050 $\times$ 10^9/L CCI, respectively [$P < 0.007$]).[171] Although platelet increments were improved, platelet survival was increased in only one of the treated patients. Considering the high cost of intravenous IgG and the very transient improvement this therapy was not considered cost-effective. At present, intravenous IgG should be given only to patients who are refractory to all forms of platelet therapy and who have clinically significant bleeding.

Management of the Persistently Refractory Patient

For those patients who are consuming platelets from any available donor, or, alternatively, who have drug-related antibodies or both multispecific HLA antibodies and platelet-specific alloantibodies (making the selection of compatible donors virtually impossible), the question of how they should be supported remains. The primary question is whether transfusions that do not increase the platelet count provide any hemostatic benefit. A definitive study on this question has never been performed, but the clinical observations of many physicians would suggest that some hemostatic benefit does result from platelet transfusions that do not increase the platelet count. In these situations, it may be advisable to give small numbers of platelet concentrates on a frequent basis (e.g., four platelet concentrates every 6–8 hours), rather than a single large daily infusion. For patients who actually show a decrease in platelet count with transfusions, it may be better not to transfuse. In addition, there is some evidence that medications such as aminocaproic acid,[177,178] estrogens,[179] and/or desmopressin[180] may improve hemostasis in chronically thrombocytopenic patients who are refractory to platelet transfusions.

REFERENCES

1. Duke WW: The relation of blood platelets to hemorrhagic disease: description of a method for determining the bleeding time and coagulation time and report of three cases of hemorrhagic disease relieved by transfusion. JAMA 55:1185, 1910
2. Han T, Stutzman L, Cohen E, Kim U: Effect of platelet transfusion on hemorrhage in patients with acute leukemia. Cancer 19:1937. 1966
3. Higby DJ, Cohen E, Holland JF, Sinks L: The prophylactic treatment of thrombocytopenic leukemic patients with platelets: a double blind study. Transfusion 14:440, 1974
4. Surgenor DM, Wallace EL, Hao SH, Chapman RH: Collection and transfusion of blood in the United States, 1982–1988. N Engl J Med 322:1646, 1990
5. McCullough J, Steeper TA, Connelly DP et al: Platelet utilization in a university hospital. JAMA 259:2414, 1988
6. Hanson SR, Slichter SJ: Platelet kinetics in patients with bone marrow hypoplasia: evidence for a fixed platelet requirement. Blood 66:1105, 1985
7. Harker LA, Slichter SJ: The bleeding time as a screening test for evaluating platelet function. N Engl J Med 287:155, 1972
8. Kitchens CS, Weiss L: Ultrastructural changes of endothelium associated with thrombocytopenia. Blood 46:567, 1975
9. Aursnes I: Blood platelet production and red cell leakage to lymph during thrombocytopenia. Scand J Haematol 13:184, 1974
10. Harker LA: The role of the spleen in thrombokinetics. J Lab Clin Med 77:247, 1971
11. Harker LA, Slichter SJ: Platelet and fibrinogen consumption in man. N Engl J Med 297:999, 1972
12. Schiffer CA: Prophylactic platelet transfusion, editorial. Transfusion 32:295, 1992
13. Patten E: Controversies in transfusion medicine. Prophylactic platelet transfusion revisited after 25 years: con. Transfusion 32:381, 1992
14. Baer MR, Bloomfield CD: Controversies in transfusion medicine. Prophylactic platelet transfusion therapy: pro. Transfusion 32:381, 1992
15. Consensus Conference: National Institutes of Health Consensus Development Conference On Platelet Transfusion Therapy. JAMA 257:1777, 1987
16. Gaydos LA, Freireich EJ, Mantel N: The quantitative relation between platelet count and hemorrhage in patients with acute leukemia. N Engl J Med 266:905, 1962
17. Slichter SJ, Harker LA: Thrombocytopenia: mechanisms and management of defects in platelet production. Clin Haematol 7:523, 1978
18. Roy AJ, Jaffe N, Djerassi I: Prophylactic platelet transfusions in children with acute leukemia: a dose response study. Transfusion 13:283, 1973
19. Aderka D, Praff G, Santo M, Weinberger A: Bleeding due to thrombocytopenia in acute leukemias and reevaluation of the prophylactic platelet transfusion policy. Am J Med Sci 291:147, 1986
20. Gmur J, Burger J, Schanz U et al: Safety of a stringent prophylactic platelet transfusion policy for patients with acute leukemia. Lancet 338:1223, 1991
21. Beutler E: Platelet transfusions: the 20,000/μl trigger. Blood 81:1411, 1993
22. Solomon J, Bokefkamp T, Fahey JL et al: Platelet prophylaxis in acute non-lymphocytic leukemia. Lancet 1:267, 1978
23. Murphy S, Litwin S, Koch P et al: The indications for platelet transfusion in children with acute leukemia. Am J Hematol 12:347, 1982
24. Pearson HA, Schulman NR, Marder VJ, Cone TE Jr: Isoimmune neonatal thrombocytopenic purpura: clinical and therapeutic considerations. Blood 23:154, 1964
25. Bussel JB, Berkowitz RL, McFarland JG et al: Antenatal treatment of neonatal alloimmune thrombocytopenia. N Engl J Med 319:1374, 1988

26. Kakaiya RM, Cable RG, Pisciotto P et al: Clinical and serological findings in alloimmune neonatal thrombocytopenia. Conn Med 50:220, 1986

27. Adner MM, Fisch GR, Starobin SG, Aster RH: Use of "compatible" platelet transfusions in treatment of congenital isoimmune thrombocytopenic purpura. N Engl J Med 280:244, 1969

28. Reznikoff-Etievant MF: Management of alloimmune neonatal and antenatal thrombocytopenia. Vox Sang 55:193, 1988

29. Muller JY: Alloimmune thrombocytopenia in the newborn. Curr Stud Hematol Blood Transfus 55:94, 1988

30. Blanchette VS, Peters MA, Pegg-Feige K: Alloimmune thrombocytopenia. Platelet serology. Curr Stud Hematol Blood Transfus 52:87, 1986

31. Kaplan C: Prenatal treatment in neonatal alloimmune thrombocytopenia. Platelet immunology. Curr Stud Hematol Blood Transfus 55:142, 1988

32. Murphy MF, Pullon HWH, Metcalfe P et al: Management of fetal alloimmune thrombocytopenia by weekly in utero platelet transfusion. Vox Sang 58:45, 1990

33. Mueller-Eckhardt C, Lechner K, Heinrich D et al: Post-transfusion thrombocytopenic purpura: immunological and clinical studies in two cases and review of the literature. Blut 40:249, 1980

34. Kickler TS, Ness PM, Herman JH, Bell WR: Studies on the pathophysiology of posttransfusion purpura. Blood 68:347, 1986

35. Lippman SM, Lizak GE, Foung SKH, Grumet FC: The efficacy of PL^{A1}-negative platelet transfusion therapy in posttransfusion purpura. West J Med 148:86, 1988

36. Slichter SJ: Post-transfusion purpura: response to steroids and association with red blood cell and lymphocytotoxic antibodies. Br J Haematol 50:599, 1982

37. Morrison FS, Mollison PL: Post transfusion purpura. N Engl J Med 275:243, 1966

38. Mueller-Eckhardt C, Kuenzlen E, Thilo-Koenner D, Pralle H: High dose intravenous immunoglobulin for post-transfusion purpura. N Engl J Med 308:287, 1983

39. Cimo PL, Aster RH: Post-transfusion purpura. Successful treatment by exchange transfusion. N Engl J Med 6:290, 1972

40. Ballem PJ, Segal GM, Stratton JR et al: Mechanisms of thrombocytopenia in chronic autoimmune thrombocytopenic purpura. Evidence of both impaired platelet production and increased platelet clearance. J Clin Invest 80:33, 1987

41. Hackett T, Kelton JG, Powers P: Drug-induced platelet destruction. Semin Thromb Hemost 8:116, 1982

42. Marsaglia G, Thomas ED: Mathematical consideration of cross-circulation in exchange transfusion. Transfusion 11:216, 1971

43. Slichter SJ: Identification and management of defects in platelet hemostasis in massively transfused patients. p. 225. In Collins JA, Murawski K, Shafer AW (eds): Massive Transfusion in Surgery and Trauma. Alan R Liss, New York, 1982

44. Miller RD, Robins TO, Tong MJ, Barton SL: Coagulation defects associated with massive blood transfusion. Ann Surg 174:794, 1971

45. Brown CH, Bradshaw MW, Natelson EA et al: Effect on platelet function following the administration of penicillin compounds. Blood 47:949, 1976

46. Brown CH, Natelson EA, Bradshaw MW et al: The hemostatic defect produced by carbenicillin. N Engl J Med 291:265, 1974

47. Weiss HJ, Aledort LM, Kochwa S: The effect of salicylates on the hemostatic properties of platelets in man. J Clin Invest 47:2169, 1968

48. Remuzzi G, Marchesi D, Livio M et al: Altered platelet function and vascular prostaglandin-generation in patients with renal failure and prolonged bleeding time. Thromb Res 13:1007, 1978

49. McKay DG: Disseminated Intravascular Coagulation. Harper & Row, New York, 1965

50. Van Der Weyden MB, Clancy RL, Howard MA, Firkin BG: Qualitative platelet defects with reduced life-span in acute leukemia. Aust NZ J Med 4:339, 1972

51. Cardamon JM, Edson R, McArthur J, Jacob H: Abnormalities of platelet function in the myeloproliferative disorders. JAMA 221:270, 1972

52. Freeman G, Buckley ES: Serum polysaccharide and fever in thrombocytopenic bleeding in leukemia. Blood 9:586, 1954

53. Cerskus AL, Ali M, Davies BJ, McDonald JWD: Possible significance of small numbers of functional platelets in a population of aspirin-treated platelets in vitro and in vivo. Thromb Res 18:389, 1980

54. Torosian M, Michelson EL, Morganroth J, MacVaugh H: Aspirin- and Coumadin-related bleeding after coronary artery bypass graft surgery. Ann Intern Med 89:325, 1978

55. Harker LA, Malpass TW, Branson HE et al: Mechanisms of abnormal bleeding in patients undergoing cardio-pulmonary bypass: acquired transient platelet dysfunction associated with selected alpha granule release. Blood 56:824, 1980

56. Malpass TW, Hanson SR, Savage B et al: Prevention of acquired transient defect in platelet plug formation by infused prostacyclin. Blood 57:736, 1981

57. Bidstrup BP, Royston D, Sapsford RN et al: Reduction in blood loss and blood use after cardiopulmonary bypass with high dose aprotinin. J Thorac Cardiovasc Surg 97:364, 1989

58. Blauhut B, Gross C, Necek S et al: Effects of high-dose aprotinin on blood loss, platelet function, fibrinolysis, complement, and renal function after cardiopulmonary bypass. J Thorac Cardiovasc Surg 101:958, 1991

59. Dietrich W, Spannagl M, Jochum M et al: Influence of high-dose aprotinin treatment on blood loss and coagulation patterns in patients undergoing myocardial revascularization. Anesthesiology 73:1119, 1990

60. Lavee J, Savion N, Smolinsky A et al: Platelet protection by aprotinin in cardiopulmonary bypass: electron microscopic study. Ann Thorac Surg 53:477, 1992

61. van Oeveren W, Eijsman L, Roozendaal KJ, Wildevuur CRH: On the mechanism of platelet preservation during cardiopulmonary bypass by aprotinin. Lancet 1:644, 1988

62. O'Connell B, Lee EJ, Schiffer CA: The value of 10-minute posttransfusion platelet counts. Transfusion 28:66, 1988

63. Yankee RA, Grumet FC, Rogentine GN: Platelet transfusion therapy: the selection of compatible platelet donors for refractory patients by lymphocyte HLA typing. N Engl J Med 281:1208, 1969

64. McFarland JG, Anderson AJ, Slichter SJ: Factors influencing the response to HLA-selected apheresis platelets in patients refractory to random platelet concentrates. Br J Haematol 73:380, 1989

65. Bishop JF, McGrath K, Wolf MM et al: Clinical factors influencing the efficacy of pooled platelet transfusions. Blood 71:383, 1988

66. Bishop JF, Matthews JP, McGrath K et al: Factors influencing 20-hour increments after platelet transfusion. Transfusion 31:392, 1991

67. Slichter SJ, Funk DD, Leandoer LE, Harker LA: Kinetic evaluation of hemostasis during surgery and wound healing. Br J Haematol 27:115, 1974

68. Yam P, Petz LD, Scott EP, Santos S: Platelet crossmatch tests using radiolabeled staphylococcal protein A or peroxidase antiperoxidase in alloimmunized patients. Br J Haematol 57:337, 1984

69. Slichter SJ, Harker LA: Separation and storage of platelet concentrates. II. Storage variables influencing platelet viability and function. Br J Haematol 34:403, 1976

70. Slichter SJ, Harker LA: Preparation and storage of platelet concentrates. I. Factors influencing the harvest of viable platelets from whole blood. Br J Haematol 34:393, 1976

71. Gottschall TL, Johnston VL, Rzad L et al: Importance of white blood cells in platelet storage. Vox Sang 47:101, 1984

72. Moroff G, Friedman A, Robkin-Kline L: Factors influencing changes in pH during storage of platelet concentrates at 20–24°C. Vox Sang 42:33, 1982

73. Schiffer CA, Dutcher JP, Aisner J et al: A randomized trial of leukocyte-depleted platelet transfusions to modify alloimmunization in patients with leukemia. Blood 62:815, 1983

74. Murphy MF, Metcalfe P, Thomas H et al: Use of leukocyte-poor blood components in HLA-matched-platelet donors to prevent HLA alloimmunization. Br J Haematol 62:529, 1986

75. Sniecinski I, O'Donnell MR, Nowicki B, Hill LR: Prevention of refractoriness and HLA-alloimmunization using filtered blood products. Blood 71:1402, 1988

76. Andreu G, Dewailly J, Leberre C et al: Prevention of HLA immunization with leukocyte-poor packed red cells and platelet concentrates obtained by filtration. Blood 72:964, 1988

77. Oksanen K, Kekomaki R, Ruutu T et al: Prevention of alloimmunization in patients with acute leukemia by use of white cell-reduced blood components—a randomized trial. Transfusion 41:588, 1991

78. van Marwijk Kooy M, van Prooijen HC, Moes M et al: Use of leukocyte-depleted platelet concentrates for the prevention of refractoriness and primary HLA alloimmunization: a prospective, randomized trial. Blood 77:201, 1991

79. Slichter SJ: Optimum platelet concentrate preparation and storage. p. 1. In Garratty G (ed): Current Concepts in Transfusion Therapy. American Association of Blood Banks, Arlington, VA, 1985

80. Chernoff A, Snyder EL: The cellular and molecular basis of the platelet storage lesion: a symposium summary. Transfusion 32:386, 1992

81. Rock G, Sherring VA, Tittley P: Five-day storage of platelet concentrates. Transfusion 24:147, 1984

82. Murphy S, Holme S, Nelson E, Carmen R: Paired comparison of the in vivo and in vitro results of storage of platelet concentrates in two containers. Transfusion 24:31, 1984

83. Simon TL, Nelson EJ, Murphy S: Extension of platelet concentrate storage to 7 days in second-generation bags. Transfusion 27:6, 1987

84. Holme S, Heaton A, Momoda G: Evaluation of a new, more oxygen-permeable, polyvinylchloride container. Transfusion 29:159, 1989

85. Snyder EL, Ezekowitz M, Aster R et al: Extended storage of platelets in a new plastic container. II. In vivo response to infusion of platelets stored for 5 days. Transfusion 25:209, 1985

86. Hogge DE, Thompson BW, Schiffer CA: Platelet storage for 7 days in second-generation blood bags. Transfusion 26:131, 1986

87. Schiffer CA, Lee EJ, Ness PM, Reilly J: Clinical evaluation of platelet concentrates stored for one to five days. Blood 67:1591, 1986

88. Lazarus HM, Herzig RH, Warm SE, Fishman DJ: Transfusion experience with platelet concentrates stored for 24 to 72 hours at 22°C. Transfusion 22:39, 1982

89. Peter-Salonen K, Bucher U, Nydegger UE: Comparison of posttransfusion recoveries achieved with either fresh or stored platelet concentrates. Blut 54:207, 1987

90. Duguid JKM, Carr R, Jenkins JA et al: Clinical evaluation of the effects of storage time and irradiation on transfused platelets. Vox Sang 60:151, 1991

91. Norol F, Kuentz M, Haloun C et al: Relative effect of clinical factors on the efficacy of fresh and stored platelet transfusions, abstracted. Rev Paul Med 110:06, 1992

92. Slichter SJ: Efficacy of platelets collected by semicontinuous flow centrifugation (Haemonetics model 30). Br J Haematol 38:131, 1978

93. Puig LI, Mazzara R, Gelabert A, Castillo R: Plateletpheresis: a comparative study of six different protocols. J Clin Apheresis 3:129, 1986

94. Ross DG, Holme S, Heaton WAL: In vitro and in vivo comparison of platelet concentrates collected by automated versus manual apheresis. Vox Sang 57:25, 1989

95. Read EJ, Goetzman H, Moroff G et al: Pair-controlled comparison of apheresis and manually collected platelets stored for 5 days, abstracted. Transfusion, suppl. 29:8S, 1989

96. Shanwell A, Gulliksson H, Berg BK et al: Evaluation of platelets prepared by apheresis and stored for 5 days. In vitro and in vivo studies. Transfusion 29:783, 1989

97. Rock G, Tittley P, McCombie N: 5-day storage of single-donor platelets obtained using a blood cell separator. Transfusion 29:288, 1989

98. Rock G, Senack E, Tittley P: 5-day storage of platelets collected on a blood cell separator. Transfusion 29:626, 1989

99. Simon TL, Sierra ER, Ferdinando B, Moore R: Collection of platelets with a new cell separator and their storage in a citrate-plasticized container. Transfusion 31:335, 1991

100. Buchholz DH, Porten JH, Grode G et al: Extended storage of single-donor platelet concentrates collected by a blood cell separator. Transfusion 25:557, 1985

101. Kenney DM, Peterson JJ, Smith JW: Extended storage of single-donor apheresis platelets in CLX blood bags: effects of storage on platelet morphology, viability, and in vitro function. Vox Sang 54:24, 1988

102. Anderson NAB, Pamphilon DH, Tandy NJ et al: Comparison of platelet-rich plasma collection using the Haemonetics PCS and Baxter Autopheresis C. Vox Sang 60:155, 1991

103. Goldman M, Blajchman MA: Blood product-associated bacterial sepsis. Transfus Med Rev 5:73, 1991

104. Mintz PD: Febrile reactions to platelet transfusions. Am J Clin Pathol 95:609, 1991

105. Wenz B, Ciavarella B, Freundlich L: Effect of prestorage white cell reduction on bacterial growth in platelet concentrates. Transfusion 33:520, 1993

106. Stefanini M, Dameshek W, Adelson E: Platelets. VII. Shortened "platelet survival time" and development of platelet agglutinins following multiple platelet transfusions. Proc Soc Exp Biol Med 80:230, 1952

107. Brand A, van Leeuwen A, Eernisse JG, van Rood JJ: Platelet transfusion therapy. Optimal donor selection with a combination of lymphocytotoxicity and platelet fluorescence tests. Blood 51:781, 1978

108. Duquesnoy RJ, Filip DJ, Rodey GE et al: Successful transfusion of platelets "mismatched" for HLA antigens to alloimmunized thrombocytopenic patients. Am J Hematol 2:219, 1977

109. Gmur J, von Felten A, Frick P: Platelet support in polysensitized patients: role of HLA specificities and crossmatch testing for donor selection. Blood 51:903, 1978

110. Kickler TS, Braine H, Ness PM: The predictive value of crossmatching platelet transfusions for alloimmunized patients. Transfusion 25:385, 1985

111. Lohrmann HP, Bull MI, Decter JA et al: Platelet transfusions from HLA compatible unrelated donors to alloimmunized patients. Ann Intern Med 80:9, 1974

112. Slichter SJ: Selection of compatible platelet donors. p. 83. In Schiffer CA (ed): Platelet Physiology And Transfusion. American Association of Blood Banks, Washington, DC 1978

113. Tosato G, Appelbaum FR, Deisseroth AB: HLA-matched platelet transfusion therapy of severe aplastic anemia. Blood 52:846, 1978

114. Hogge DE, Dutcher P, Aisner J, Schiffer CA: Lymphocytotoxic antibody is a predictor of response to random-donor platelet transfusion. Am J Hematol 14:363, 1983

115. Kakaiya RM, Gudino MD, Miller MV et al: Four crossmatch methods to select platelet donors. Transfusion 24:35, 1984

116. Daly PA, Schiffer CA, Aisner J, Wiernik PH: Platelet transfusion therapy. One-hour-post-transfusion increments are valuable in predicting the need for HLA-matched preparations. JAMA 243:435, 1980

117. von dem Borne AEGK, Ouwehand WH, Kuijpers RWAM: Theoretic and practical aspects of platelet crossmatching. Transfus Med Rev 4:265, 1990

118. Leibert M, Aster RH: Expression of HLA-B12 on platelets, on lymphocytes, and in serum: a quantitative study. Tissue Antigens 9:199, 1977

119. Schiffer CA, O'Connell B, Lee EJ: Platelet transfusion therapy for alloimmunized patients: selective mismatching for HLA-B12, an antigen with variable expression on platelets. Blood 74:1172, 1989

120. Aster RH, Szatkowski N, Liebert M, Duquesnoy RJ: Expression of HLA-B12, HLA-B8, Bw4, and w6 on platelets. Transplant Proc 9:4, 1977

121. Szatkowski NS, Aster RH: HLA antigens of platelets. IV. Influence of "private" HLA-B locus specificities on the expression of Bw4 and Bw6 on human platelets. Tissue Antigens 15:361, 1980.

122. Pegels JG, Bruynes ECE, Engelfriet CP, von dem Borne AEGK: Serological studies in patients on platelet- and granulocyte-substitution therapy. Br J Haematol 52:59, 1982.

123. Slichter SJ: Prevention of platelet alloimmunization. p. 83. In Murawski K (ed): Transfusion Medicine: Recent Technological Advances. Alan R Liss, New York, 1985

124. Holohan W, Terasaki PI, Diesseroth AB: Suppression of transfusion-related alloimmunization in intensively treated cancer patients. Blood 58:122, 1981

125. Lee EJ, Schiffer CA: Serial measurement of lymphocytotoxic antibody and response to nonmatched platelet transfusions in alloimmunized patients. Blood 70:1727, 1987

126. Ford JM, Brown LM, Cullen MH et al: Combined granulocyte and platelet transfusions. Development of alloimmunization as reflected by decreasing cell recovery values. Transfusion 22:498, 1982.

127. Pamphilon DH, Farrell DH, Donaldson C et al: Development of lymphocytotoxic and platelet reactive antibodies: a prospective study in patients with acute leukemia. Vox Sang 57:177, 1989

128. Tejada F, Bias WB, Santos GW, Zieve PD: Immunologic response of patients with acute leukemia to platelet transfusions. Blood 42:405, 1973

129. Howard JE, Perkins HA: The natural history of alloimmunization to platelets. Transfusion 18:496, 1978

130. Murphy MF, Metcalfe P, Ord J et al: Disappearance of HLA and platelet-specific antibodies in acute leukaemia patients alloimmunized by multiple transfusions. Br J Haematol 67:255, 1987

131. McGrath K, Wolf M, Bishop J et al: Transient platelet and HLA antibody formation in multitransfused patients with malignancy. Br J Haematol 68:345, 1988

132. Slichter SJ, Deeg JH, Kennedy MS: Prevention of platelet alloimmunization in dogs with systemic cyclosporine and by UV-irradiation or cyclosporine-loading of donor platelets. Blood 69:414, 1987

133. Slichter SJ, Weiden PL, Kane PJ, Storb RF: Approaches to preventing or reversing platelet alloimmunization using animal models. Transfusion 28:103, 1988

134. Sintnicolaas K, Sizoo W, Haije WG et al: Delayed alloimmunization by random single donor platelet transfusions. Lancet 1:750, 1981

135. Kakaiya RM, Hezzey AJ, Bove JR et al: Alloimmunization following apheresis platelets vs. pooled platelet concentrate transfusion—a prospective randomized study, abstracted. Transfusion 21:600, 1981

136. Gmur J, von Felten A, Osterwalder B et al: Delayed alloimmunization using random single donor platelet transfusions: a prospective study in thrombocytopenic patients with acute leukemia. Blood 62:473, 1983

137. Dunstan RA, Simpson MB, Rosse WF: Origin of ABH antigens on human platelets. Blood 65:615, 1985

138. Lee EJ, Schiffer CA: ABO compatibility can influence the results of platelet transfusion. Results of a randomized trial. Transfusion 29:384, 1989

139. Carr R, Hutton JL, Jenkins JA et al: Transfusion of ABO-mismatched platelets leads to early platelet refractoriness. Br J Haematol 75:408, 1990

140. Messerschmidt G, Makuch R, Appelbaum F et al: A prospective randomized trial of HLA-matched versus mismatched single-donor platelet transfusions in cancer patients. Cancer 62:795, 1988

141. Welsh J, Burgos H, Batchelor JR: The immune response to allogeneic rat platelets; Ag-B antigens in matrix form lacking Ia. Immunology 7:267, 1977

142. Batchelor JR, Welsh KI, Burgos H: Transplantation antigens per se are poor immunogens within a species. Nature, 273:54, 1978

143. Claas FHJ, Smeenk RJT, Schmidt R et al: Alloimmunization against the MHC antigens after platelet transfusions is due to contaminating leukocytes in the platelet suspension. Exp Hematol 9:84, 1981

144. Fisher M, Chapman JR, Ting A, Morris PJ: Alloimmunization to HLA antigens following transfusion with leukocyte-poor and purified platelet suspensions. Vox Sang 49:331, 1985

145. Petranyi GG, Padanyi A, Horuzsko A et al: Mixed lymphocyte culture—evidence that pre-transplant transfusion with platelets induces FcR and blocking antibody production similar to that induced by leukocyte transfusion. Transplantation 45:823, 1988

146. Chambers LA, Garcia LW: White blood cell content of transfusion components. Lab Med 22:857, 1991

147. Friedman LI, Stromberg RR: White cell counting in red cells and platelets: how few can we count?, editorial Transfusion 30:387, 1990

148. Schiffer CA: Prevention of platelet alloimmunization, editorial. Blood 77:1, 1991

149. Snyder EL: Clinical use of white cell-poor blood components. Transfusion 29:568, 1989

150. Brand A, Claas FHJ, Voogt PJ et al: Alloimmunization after leukocyte-depleted multiple random donor platelet transfusions. Vox Sang 54:160, 1988

151. Englefriet CP, van Loghem JJ: HL-A in connection with blood transfusion. Haematologia 8:267, 1974

152. Blajchman MA: The effect of leukodepletion on allogeneic donor platelet survival and refractoriness in an animal model. Semin Hematol 28:14, 1991

153. Lindahl-Kiessling K, Safwenberg J: Inability of UV-irradiated lymphocytes to stimulate allogeneic cells in mixed lymphocyte culture. Int Arch Allergy 41:670, 1971

154. Slichter SJ: UV irradiation: effects on the immune system and on platelet function, viability, and alloimmunization. p. 205. In Sibinga CTS, Kater L (eds): Advances in Haemapheresis, Proceedings of the Third International Congress of the World Apheresis Association. Kluwer Academic Publishers, Dordrecht, The Netherlands, 1991

155. Pamphilon DH, Potter M, Cutts M et al: Platelet concentrates irradiated with ultraviolet light retain satisfactory in vitro storage characteristics and in vivo survival. Br J Haematol 75:240, 1990

156. Andreu G, Boccaccio C, Lecrubier C et al: Ultraviolet irradiation of platelet concentrates: feasibility in transfusion practice. Transfusion 30:401, 1990

157. Buchholz DH, Miripol J, Aster RH et al: Ultraviolet irradiation of platelets to prevent recipient alloimmunization, abstract. Transfusion 28:26S, 1988

158. Nemo GJ, McCurdy PR: Prevention of platelet alloimmunization, editorial. Transfusion 31:584, 1991

159. Skodlar J, Bolgiano D, Teramura G, Slichter SJ: Distinguishing between mechanisms of platelet refractoriness: abnormal post-storage platelet viability vs. Immune destruction, abstracted. Blood, suppl. 1. 80:260a, 1992

160. Feinstein DI: Treatment of disseminated intravascular coagulation. Semin Thromb Hemost 14:351, 1988

161. Duquesnoy RJ, Anderson AJ, Tomasulo PA, Aster RH: ABO compatibility and platelet transfusions of alloimmunized thrombocytopenic patients. Blood 54:595, 1979

162. Heal JM, Blumberg N, Masel D: An evaluation of crossmatching, HLA, and ABO matching for platelet transfusions to refractory patients. Blood 70:23, 1987

163. Yankee RA, Graff KS, Dowling R et al: Selection of unrelated compatible platelet donors by lymphocyte HL-A matching. N Engl J Med 288:760, 1973

164. Duquesnoy RJ, Filip DJ, Rodey GE et al: Successful transfusion of platelets "mismatched" for HLA antigens to alloimmunized thrombocytopenic patients. Am J Hematol 2:19, 1977

165. Kickler TS, Nedd PM, Braine HG: Platelet crossmatching. A direct approach to the selection of platelet transfusions for the alloimmunized thrombocytopenic patient. Am J Clin Pathol 90:69, 1988

166. Rachel JM, Summers TC, Sinor LT, Plapp FV: Use of a solid phase red blood cell adherence method for pretransfusion platelet compatibility testing. Am J Clin Pathol 90:63, 1988

167. Freedman J, Hooi C, Garvey MB: Prospective platelet crossmatching for selection of compatible random donors. Br J Haematol 56:9, 1984

168. Freedman J, Garvey MB, Salomon de Friedberg Z et al: Random donor platelet crossmatching: comparison of four platelet antibody detection methods. Am J Hematol 28:1, 1988

169. O'Connell BA, Schiffer CA: Donor selection for alloimmunized patients by platelet crossmatching of random-donor platelet concentrates. Transfusion 30:314, 1990

170. Kekomaki R, Elfenbein G, Gardner R et al: Improved response of patients refractory to random-donor platelet transfusions by intravenous gamma globulin. Am J Med 76:199, 1984

171. Kickler T, Braine HG, Piantadosi S et al: A randomized, placebo-controlled trial of intravenous gammaglobulin in alloimmunized thrombocytopenic patients. Blood 75:313, 1990

172. Zeigler ZR, Shadduck RK, Rosenfeld CS et al: High-dose intravenous gamma globulin improves responses to single-donor platelets in patients refractory to platelet transfusion. Blood 70:1433, 1987

173. Ziegler ZR, Shadduck RK, Rosenfeld CS et al: Intravenous gamma globulin decreases platelet-associated IgG and improves transfusion responses in platelet refractory states. Am J Hematol 38:15, 1991

174. Knupp C, Chamberlain JK, Raab SO: High-dose intravenous gamma globulin in alloimmunized platelet transfusion recipients, letter. Blood 65:776, 1985

175. Lee EJ, Norris D, Schiffer CA: Intravenous immune globulin for patients alloimmunized to random donor platelet transfusion. Transfusion 27:245, 1987

176. Schiffer CA, Hogge DE, Aisner J et al: High-dose intravenous gammaglobulin in alloimmunized platelet transfusion recipients. Blood 64:937, 1984

177. Gardner FH, Helmer RE: Aminocaproic acid: use in control of hemorrhage in patients with amegakaryocytic thrombocytopenia. JAMA 243:35, 1980

178. Bartholomew JR, Salgia R, Bell WR: Control of bleeding in patients with immune and nonimmune thrombocytopenia with aminocaproic acid. Arch Intern Med 149:1959, 1989

179. Livio M, Mannucci PM, Vigano G et al: Conjugated estrogens for the management of bleeding associated with renal failure. N Engl J Med 315:731, 1986

180. Mannucci PM: Desmopressin: a nontransfusional form of treatment for congenital and acquired bleeding disorders. Blood 72:1449, 1988

Principles of White Blood Cell Transfusion

136

Ronald G. Strauss

INTRODUCTION

Current technology permits collection of highly enriched fractions of several types of blood leukocytes from healthy donors and from patients for further processing, study, or transfusion. Because neutrophils are donated routinely and issued as a standard blood product (granulocyte concentrate), this chapter focuses on an analysis of the use of granulocyte transfusions (GTX) as an adjunct to antimicrobial drugs in the treatment of progressive infections. Serious and repeated bacterial and fungal infections are an undeniable consequence of both severe neutropenia ($<0.5 \times 10^9$ neutrophils/L blood) and disorders of abnormal neutrophil function. GTX have proven efficacy as treatment for infections in certain clinical settings, both in animals and in humans.[1] Despite considerable data supporting the transfusion of granulocyte concentrates in these settings, the use of GTX has diminished strikingly. Although this can be explained, in part, by the development of alternative therapies such as recombinant myeloid growth factors, many physicians hold strong negative opinions about the value of GTX. This excessively negative attitude seems to be based on antiquated information, and it is reasonable to reassess the role of GTX in the light of modern technology and current standards of practice.

THERAPEUTIC GRANULOCYTE TRANSFUSIONS IN NEUTROPENIC PATIENTS

Thirty papers[2] reporting the use of GTX plus antimicrobial drugs to treat bacterial and fungal infections in severely neutropenic patients (usually $<0.5 \times 10^9$/L blood) were analyzed for this report. Data from all 30 studies were combined; Table 136-1 displays the number of patients treated with GTX for specific types of infections. Patients are listed according to the index infection that prompted GTX; additional infections recognized during therapy or at postmortem examination are not tabulated. All patients with septicemia are listed in the septicemia section even if they did not exhibit another infection such as pneumonia or abscess. All patients who received therapeutic GTX for a designated type of infection are accounted for in the column labeled "Treated." Treated patients, whose actual course and mortality could be clearly documented, are again listed in the "Evaluable" column. GTX are considered successful in patients who could be evaluated, if so stated.

Many of these reports are uncontrolled studies that consist of small numbers of patients with a diversity of underlying diseases, types of infections, antimicrobial management, and both quantity and quality of GTX. Because of these complex issues, most reports are of limited value, and it is useful to analyze critically the seven controlled studies in more detail.[3–9] In these seven studies, the response of infected neutropenic patients to treatment with GTX plus antibiotics (study group) was compared to that of comparable patients given antibiotics alone and evaluated concurrently (control group). The design, size, and results of these seven studies are presented in Tables 136-2 and 136-3. Three of the seven reported a significant overall benefit for GTX.[6–8] In two additional studies,[3,5] overall success was not demonstrated for all patients given GTX, but certain subgroups of patients were found to benefit significantly. In the first controlled study,[3] many patients received an inadequate dose of GTX by current standards. Thus, overall success was not demonstrated. However, 100% of patients who received GTX on at least four occasions and 80% of those receiving at least three, survived, as compared to only 30% survival among controls. In the other study that found partial benefit,

Table 136-2. Results of Seven Controlled Studies Evaluating Therapeutic Granulocyte Transfusions in Neutropenic Patients

Investigators	Success	Study Group		Control Group	
		N	Survival (%)	N	Survival (%)
Higby et al.[7]	Yes	17	76	19	26
Vogler et al.[8]	Yes	17	59	13	15
Herzig et al.[6]	Yes	13	75	14	36
Alavi et al.[3]	Partial	12	82	19	62
Graw et al.[5]	Partial	39	46	37	30
Winston et al.[9]	No	48	63	47	72
Fortuny et al.[4]	No	17	78	22	80

no advantage for GTX could be demonstrated when all patients were analyzed. However, when the subgroup of patients with persistent bone marrow failure were analyzed separately, 75% of those receiving GTX responded favorably, compared with only 20% of controls. Thus, some measure of success for GTX was evident in five of the seven controlled studies. However, this was counterbalanced by four studies that were negative in some respect, with two totally negative[4,9] and two partially negative.[3,5]

An explanation of these inconsistent results is evident on critical analysis of the adequacy of GTX support (Table 136-3). Patients in the three successful trials received relatively high doses of neutrophils; the usual dose was $\geq 1.7 \times 10^{10}$/day.[6–8] Moreover, donors were selected on the basis of both erythrocyte and leukocyte compatibility. By contrast, the four negative controlled studies can be legitimately criticized in light of current technology. Of major importance, data for three[3–5] of the four negative studies were collected before 1977, and both the quality and quantity of granulocytes transfused at that time were clearly inferior to those available today. Two of the four negative studies used granulocytes collected by filtration leukapheresis for at least some patients.[3,5] The functions of these cells are now known to be defective, and the neutrophils collected by this technique are no longer transfused. Although three of the four negative studies used neutrophils collected by centrifugation leukapheresis,[4,5,9] the dose was extremely low (0.41–0.56 × 10^{10} per concentrate). This daily dose is approximately one-fourth the number that could be given currently, and it is not surprising that GTX were unsuccessful, when given in such a grossly inadequate fashion. As another factor, investigators in two of the four negative studies[3,9] made no provisions for the possibility of leukocyte alloimmunization and selected donors solely on the basis of erythrocyte compatibility. Finally, control subjects responded reasonably well to antibiotics alone in three of the four negative studies,[4,5,9] suggesting that some patients have no apparent need for additional therapeutic modalities.

The most frequent infection for which GTX are considered is bacterial sepsis; many patients transfused with neutrophil concentrates for septicemia have been reported (Table 136-1). Most neutropenic patients with bacterial sepsis who experience bone marrow recovery during the early days of infections will respond to antibiotics alone.[1,2] Most patients with newly diagnosed acute leukemia who experience successful induction chemotherapy fit into this category; these patients generally will not require GTX. By contrast, septic patients with persistent severe neutropenia due to continuing bone marrow failure may benefit when GTX is added to antibiotic therapy.[1] Examples are patients in the later stages of leukemia undergoing investigational chemotherapy or recipients of bone marrow grafts in whom marrow recovery may be delayed for >2–3 weeks. Regarding other types of systemic infection (fungemia) and the other infections listed in Table 136-1, information published to date is insufficient to determine definitively whether therapeutic GTX offer benefits over those antibiotics alone. However, on the basis of studies in animals and occasional

Table 136-1. Episodes of Infection from 30 Reports of Neutropenic Patients Treated with Therapeutic Granulocyte Transfusions

Type of Infection	Treated	Evaluable	Successful
Total septicemias	436	248	147/248 = 59%
Gram-negative	238	172	103/172 = 60%
Gram-positive	44	18	16/18 = 89%
Polymicrobial	16	16	8/16 = 50%
Fungal	6	3	—
Organism unspecified	132	39	18/39 = 46%
Total pneumonias	130	45	23/45 = 51%
Bacterial	5	—	
Fungal	10	9	1/9 = 11%
Organism unspecified	115	11	7/11 = 64%
Total localized infections	143	47	39/47 = 83%
Fever of unknown cause	184	85	65/85 = 75%

(From Strauss,[2] with permission.)

Table 136-3. Design of Seven Controlled Studies Evaluating Therapeutic Granulocyte Transfusions in Neutropenic Patients

Investigators	Randomized	Collection Method	Characteristics of Neutrophil Concentrates			
			Dose ($\times 10^{10}$)	Schedule	HLA[a]	WBC[a]
Higby et al.[7]	Yes	Filtration	2.2	Daily	No	Yes
Vogler et al.[8]	Yes	Centrifugation	2.7	Daily	Yes	Yes
Herzig et al.[6]	Yes	Filtration	1.7	Daily	No	Yes
		Centrifugation	0.4	Daily	No	Yes
Alavi et al.[3]	Yes	Filtration	5.9	Daily	No	No
Graw et al.[5]	No	Filtration	2.0	Daily	No	Yes
		Centrifugation	0.6	Daily	No	Yes
Winston et al.[9]	Yes	Centrifugation	0.5	Daily	No	No
Fortuny et al.[4]	No	Centrifugation	0.4	Daily	No	Yes

[a] Donors selected to compatible with recipient either by HLA typing (A and B loci matched, at least in part) or by leukocyte cross-matching.

reports in humans, therapeutic GTX might be considered treatment for fungal infections—particularly those accompanied by fungemia. Recently, a retrospective study reported lack of benefit for GTX in fungal infections occurring in bone marrow transplant patients.[9a] Of 87 patients reviewed, 50 received GTX without apparent benefit. This study must be interpreted very cautiously because it contains several methodologic limitations: (1) patients were not randomized; (2) types of infections varied between patients given GTX or not; (3) the dose of neutrophils given was known for only 15% of GTX administered; and (4) no attempt was made to select donors on the basis of leukocyte compatibility.

To determine the optimal role for therapeutic GTX, individual physicians should survey the outcome of bacterial and fungal sepsis in their own neutropenic patients. If infections in these patients respond promptly to antibiotics alone and survival approaches 100%, GTX are unnecessary and should not be used, as the benefits would not outweigh the potential risks. However, if significant numbers of infected neutropenic patients fail to respond to antibiotics alone, the addition of GTX should be considered along with other modifications of therapy (e.g., selection of different antibiotics, closer monitoring of antibiotic blood levels, intravenous γ-globulin therapy, recombinant myeloid growth factors, interferon).

Once the decision to use therapeutic GTX has been made, it must be given effectively. A daily infusion of approximately $2-3 \times 10^{10}$ neutrophils ($\geq 1 \times 10^{10}$) should be given to patients with severe persistent neutropenia ($<0.5 \times 10^9$/L) who have infections (usually gram-negative sepsis) who have failed to respond to a reasonable course (approximately 48 hours) of combination antibiotics. GTX is continued until the infection has resolved or until the blood neutrophil count has risen to $>0.5 \times 10^9$/L. It seems logical that patients with evidence of alloimmunization (platelet refractoriness, antileukocyte antibodies, repeated febrile transfusion reactions, or post-transfusion pulmonary infiltrates) should receive GTX from donors selected to be as leukocyte compatible as possible by HLA matching and/or leukocyte cross-matching. However, it has not been clearly shown that these attempts to improve compatibility, in fact, increase success of GTX in alloimmunized patients.

THERAPEUTIC GRANULOCYTE TRANSFUSIONS IN SPECIAL CIRCUMSTANCES

Most patients with congenital disorders of qualitative neutrophil dysfunction have adequate numbers of blood neutrophils, but they are susceptible to serious infections because their neutrophils fail to perform one or more of the tasks required to kill pathogenic microorganisms. Patients with severe forms of neutrophil dysfunction are relatively rare, and no definitive studies have been reported to establish the efficacy of therapeutic GTX in their management. Thus, firm recommendations about the use of GTX to treat infections in patients with

severe neutrophil dysfunction cannot be made. However, a few patients with chronic granulomatous disease complicated by progressive life-threatening fungal infections have been reported to benefit.[10–18] Because of the possibility of alloimmunization and concern over transfusion-transmitted infections, therapeutic GTX is recommended only for progressive infections that cannot be controlled with antimicrobial drugs. Prophylactic GTX is impractical and is unlikely to be effective.

Neonates (infants within the first month of life) are another group of patients who may suffer life-threatening bacterial infections caused, at least in part, by neutrophil dysfunction and neutropenia.[19,20] Neutropenia must be viewed differently in neonates than in older patients, in whom GTX are usually considered only when the blood neutrophil count falls to $<0.5 \times 10^9$/L. By contrast, absolute blood neutrophil counts as high as 3.0×10^9/L might prompt consideration for GTX in neonates.[19,20] The blood neutrophil count varies greatly during the first few days of life, and a transient neutrophilia normally occurs, with absolute neutrophil counts of $10-25 \times 10^9$/L commonly seen in healthy neonates. Although not completely specific, sepsis should be suspected in any sick neonate with an absolute neutrophil count of $<3.0 \times 10^9$/L during the first week of life. The mechanism of neutropenia cannot always be identified, but in some infants a marked decrease in the neutrophil storage pool of the bone marrow can be demonstrated. These forms (metamyelocytes and segmented neutrophils) account for 26–65% of all nucleated cells in normal bone marrow. Some neonates with sepsis during the first days of life and with absolute blood neutrophil counts of $<3.0 \times 10^9$/L will exhibit diminished marrow storage pool ($<10\%$ of nucleated marrow cells). Several

AUTHOR'S APPROACH TO THERAPY FOR NEONATAL SEPSIS

For an infant <1 month of age, who has fulminant sepsis with a relative neutropenia in the blood of $<3 \times 10^9$/L at the first week of life or $<1 \times 10^9$/L after the first week of life the following treatment is provided:

Appropriate antibiotic therapy
1 g/kg intravenous immunoglobulin[a]
1×10^9/kg neutrophils collected by automated leukapheresis

The above treatment is continued daily until the relative neutropenia is corrected.

[a] The efficacy of immunoglobulin is debatable, but it may serve two purposes: (1) it may increase low plasma γ-globulin levels of premature infants, and (2) it may provide a therapeutic effect during the 4–8-hour delay needed to obtain quality neutrophils through leukapheresis.

Table 136-4. Five Controlled Trials (Six Reports) of Neonatal Granulocyte Transfusions

Investigators	Randomized	Infants Transfused	Survival (%)	Infants Not Transfused	Survival (%)
Laurenti et al.[22]	No	20	90[a]	18	28
Christensen et al.[21]	Yes	7	100[a]	9	11
	No[b]	—	—	10	100
Cairo et al.[23]	Yes	13	100[a]	10	60
Cairo et al.[24]	Yes[c]	21	95[a]	14	64
Baley et al.[25]	Yes	12	58	13	69
Wheeler et al.[26]	Yes	4	50	5	40
	No[b]	—	—	11	91

[a] Transfused infants survival significantly better than nontransfused.
[b] Additional nontransfused infants who were not randomized because all had adequate marrow storage pools.
[c] Expanded version of study reported earlier by Baley et al.[25]

investigators have reported the use of GTX to treat neonatal sepsis.[20] Six reports were of controlled studies[21–26]; four of the six reports[21–24] demonstrated a significant benefit of GTX (Table 136-4). However, these studies can easily be criticized because of small size, faulty design, and heterogeneity of both patients and quality of granulocyte concentrates transfused. Thus, the use of GTX as treatment of neonatal sepsis remains controversial.[20]

ALTERNATIVE OR ADDITIVE MEASURES TO THERAPEUTIC GRANULOCYTE TRANSFUSIONS

Many patients with severe neutropenia, particularly those experiencing chemotherapy or bone marrow transplantation, exhibit a variety of abnormalities in body defense mechanisms. Moreover, infections that occur in these patients do not always respond to GTX. Consequently, a number of alternative therapies have been evaluated—two that appear to hold promise are the use of recombinant myeloid growth factors and intravenous immunoglobulin (IVIg).

Recombinant myeloid growth factors (colony-stimulating factors, e.g., colony-stimulating factor-granulocyte and 1-granulocyte/macrophage [CSF-G and CSF-GM]) are glycoprotein cytokines that enhance the production, differentiation, and function of myeloid cells.[27–29] Both CSF-G and CSF-GM have been used successfully to accelerate bone marrow recovery following chemotherapy, and the development of infections and need for prolonged hospitalization have been diminished.[27] In contrast to the success in preventing neutropenic infections, the role of CSF-G and CSF-GM in the treatment of established infections is more controversial—particularly following dose-intensified regimens for the treatment of acute myeloid leukemia.[27] Currently, it seems reasonable to consider adding GTX to the treatment of patients with severe bacterial or fungal infections that are progressing despite the use of appropriate antibiotics plus recombinant myeloid growth factors.

The use of IVIg, either to prevent or to treat neonatal sepsis, has appeal because this therapy may correct abnormalities of both humoral immunity and neutrophil function. In several studies of experimental infections in animals, IVIg proved beneficial by increasing opsonic activity and by improving neutrophil kinetics. Although the precise role for IVIg in the treatment of human infants is incompletely defined, this therapy has been given with promising effects both in the prevention and treatment of infections.[30,31] However, caution is warranted before

IVIg is broadly applied in the treatment of neonatal sepsis. At high doses, IVIg has been demonstrated to impair body defense mechanisms and to increase susceptibility to fatal infections. Because of the ease with which IVIg can be prescribed, its apparent benefits to multiple body defense systems and, finally, its safety in terms of failing to transmit donor infectious diseases, IVIg has great appeal. However, the genuine benefits and risks of IVIg must be carefully examined before it can be considered as a replacement for GTX in the treatment of fulminant sepsis in neutropenic neonates.

PROPHYLACTIC GRANULOCYTE TRANSFUSIONS IN NEUTROPENIC PATIENTS

Prophylactic GTX are considered by nearly all investigators to be of marginal value. In 12 reports,[32–43] the benefits were few, while the risks and expenses were substantial. However, partial success was demonstrated when certain subgroups of patients were examined separately. Some measure of success was found in 7 of 12 studies; the remaining 5 studies failed to show a benefit for prophylactic GTX.[39–43] In none of these five studies were large numbers of neutrophils obtained from matched donors and transfused daily. Thus, in a situation analogous to that for the negative therapeutic GTX trials, the failure of prophylactic GTX might be explained, at least in part, by inadequate transfusions.

The main concern raised by prophylactic GTX has been that of transfusion-related risks, a concern heightened because of the limited benefits of prophylactic GTX. In the therapeutic setting, the benefits of GTX are more apparent, making the risks more acceptable. Leukocyte alloimmunization poses a risk of special importance for GTX therapy. Although reports are controversial, it seems likely that most patients receiving multiple GTX from random donors will develop antileukocyte antibodies. Antileukocyte antibodies have been reported to mediate transfusion reactions, to have an adverse effect on post-transfusion increments of blood polymorphonuclear neutrophil counts, to alter the circulating kinetics of infused polymorphonuclear neutrophils, and to decrease the antimicrobial effects of GTX.[44–47] Many of the other risks of GTX have been greatly diminished by current practices, such as γ-irradiation to prevent graft-versus-host disease and the use of cytomegalovirus-negative units to eliminate cytomegalovirus transmission.

Thus, prophylactic GTX cannot be recommended for the treatment of neutropenic patients (except on an investigational basis), as the benefits are few and the risks and costs are substantial. Unfortunately, definitive studies using modern blood bank technology (e.g., high doses of neutrophils, donors selected by leukocyte matching) have not been reported. As is true for all blood products, prophylactic GTX should be given only after the likelihood of benefit has been demonstrated to outweigh the risks.

PREPARATION AND STORAGE OF NEUTROPHIL CONCENTRATES

To ensure adequate numbers and quality of neutrophils, granulocyte concentrates must be prepared by automated leukapheresis using an erythrocyte sedimenting agent such as hydroxyethyl starch.[48] In addition, donors should be stimulated with adrenal corticosteroids (e.g., prednisone) a few hours before collection.[49] Granulocyte concentrates should be transfused as soon as possible after collection because neutrophil functions begin to deteriorate almost immediately.[50,51] Some delay between collection and transfusion is inevitable, and granulocyte concentrates are usually stored briefly at 22°C, with little or no agitation. Lane et al.[51] have published a number of reports about the properties of neutrophils collected for transfusion, and aberrations of nearly every function become evident within 24–72 hours. It is highly desirable to transfuse granulocyte concentrates within 6 hours of collection; they should not be given if >24 hours old. In the future, GTX may be obtained from donors stimulated with granulocyte colony stimulating factor.[52]

ACKNOWLEDGMENT

Ronald G. Strauss is a recipient of Research Career Development award K04 HD00255 and Transfusion Medicine Academic award K07 HL01426 from the National Institutes of Health.

REFERENCES

1. Strauss RG: Granulocyte transfusions: uses, abuses and indications. p. 65. In Kolins J, McCarthy LJ (eds): Contemporary Transfusion Practice. American Association of Blood Banks, Arlington, VA, 1987
2. Strauss RG: Granulocyte transfusions. p. 287. In Rossi EC, Simon TL, Moss GS (eds): Principles of Transfusion Medicine. Williams & Wilkins, Baltimore, MD, 1991
3. Alavi JB, Root RK, Djerassi I et al: A randomized clinical trial of granulocyte transfusions for infection in acute leukemia. N Engl J Med 296:706, 1977
4. Fortuny IE, Bloomfield CD, Hadlock DC et al: Granulocyte transfusion: a controlled study in patients with acute non-lymphocytic leukemia. Transfusion 15:548, 1975
5. Graw RG Jr, Herzig G, Perry S, Henderson IS: Normal granulocyte transfusion therapy. N Engl J Med 287:367, 1972
6. Herzig RH, Herzig GP, Graw RG Jr et al: Successful granulocyte transfusion therapy for gram-negative septicemia. N Engl J Med 396:702, 1977
7. Higby DJ, Yates JW, Henderson ES, Holland JF: Filtration leukapheresis for granulocytic transfusion therapy. N Engl J Med 292:761, 1975
8. Vogler WR, Winton EF: A controlled study of the efficacy of granulocyte transfusions in patients with neutropenia. Am J Med 63:548, 1977
9. Winston DJ, Ho WG, Gale RP: Therapeutic granulocyte transfusions for documented infections: a controlled trial in 95 infectious granulocytopenic episodes. Ann Intern Med 97:509, 1982
9a. Bhatia S, McCullough JJ, Perry EH et al: Granulocyte transfusions: efficacy in fungal infections in neutropenic patients following bone marrow transplantation. Transfusion 34:226, 1994
10. Maybee DA, Milan AP, Ruymann FB: Granulocyte transfusion therapy in children. South Med J 70:320, 1977
11. Yomtovian R, Abramson J, Quie P, McCullough J: Granulocyte transfusion therapy in chronic granulomatous disease; report of a patient and review of the literature. Transfusion 21:739, 1981
12. Raubitschek AA, Levin AS, Stites DP et al: Normal granulocyte infusion therapy for aspergillosis in chronic granulomatous disease. Pediatrics 51:230, 1973
13. Chusid MJ, Tomasulo PA: Survival of transfused normal granulocytes in a patient with chronic granulomatous disease. Pediatrics 61:556, 1978
14. Pedersen FK, Johansen KS, Rosenkrist J et al: Refractory pneumocystis carinii infection in chronic granulomatous disease: successful treatment with granulocytes. Pediatrics 64:935, 1979
15. Buescher ES, Gallin JI: Leukocyte transfusion in chronic granulomatous disease; persistence of transfused leukocytes in sputum. N Engl J Med 307:800, 1982
16. Brzica SM, Rhodes KH, Rineda AA, Taswell HF: Chronic granulomatous disease and the McLeod phenotype; successful treatment of infection with granulocyte transfusion resulting in subsequent hemolytic transfusion reaction. Mayo Clin Proc 52:153, 1977
17. Bujak JS, Kwon-chung KJ, Chusid MJ: Osteomyelitis and pneumonia in a boy with chronic granuomatous disease of childhood caused by a mutant strain of aspergillus nidulans. Am J Clin Pathol 61:361, 1974
18. Haddad HL, Beatty DW, Dowdle EB: Chronic granulomatous disease of childhood. S Afr Med J 50:2068, 1976
19. Strauss RG: Granulopoiesis and neutrophil function in the neonate. p. 88. In Stockman JA, Pochedly C (eds): Developmental and Neonatal Hematology. Raven Press, New York, 1988
20. Strauss RG: Current status of granulocyte transfusions to treat neonatal sepsis. J Clin Apheresis 5:25, 1989
21. Christensen RD, Rothstein G, Anstall HB, Bybee B: Granulocyte transfusions in neonates with bacterial infection, neutropenia, and depletion of mature marrow neutrophils. Pediatrics 70:1, 1982
22. Laurenti F, Ferro R, Isacchi G et al: Polymorphonuclear leukocyte transfusion for the treatment for sepsis in the newborn infant. J Pediatr 98:118, 1981
23. Cairo MS, Rucker R, Bennetts GA et al: Improved survival of newborns receiving leukocyte transfusions for sepsis. Pediatrics 74:887, 1984
24. Cairo MS, Worcester C, Rucker R et al: Role of circulating complement and polymorphonuclear leukocyte transfusion in treatment and outcome in critically ill neonates with sepsis. J Pediatr 110:935, 1987
25. Baley JE, Stork EK, Warkentin PI, Shurin SB: Buffy coat transfusions in neutropenic neonates with presumed sepsis: a prospective, randomized trial. Pediatrics 80:712, 1987
26. Wheeler JC, Chauvenet AR, Johnson CA et al: Buffy coat transfusions in neonates with sepsis and neutrophil storage pool depletion. Pediatrics 79:422, 1987
27. Gabrilove J: The development of granulocyte colony-stimulating factor in its various clinical applications. Blood 80:1382, 1992
28. Gasson JC: Molecular physiology of granulocyte-macrophage colony-stimulating factor. Blood 77:1131, 1991
29. Greenberg PL: Treatment of myelodysplastic syndromes with hemopoietic growth factors. Semin Onco 19:106, 1992
30. Schreiber JR, Berger M: Intravenous immune globulin therapy for sepsis in premature neonates. J Pediatr 121:401, 1992
31. Fischer GW, Weisman LE, Hemming VG: Directed immune globulin for the prevention or treatment of neonatal group B streptococcal infections: a review. Clin Immunol Immunopathol 62:S92, 1992
32. Mannoni P, Rodet M, Vernant JP et al: Efficiency of prophylactic granulocyte transfusions in preventing infections in acute leukaemia. Blood Transfus Immunohaematol 22:503, 1979
33. Gomez-Villagran JL, Torres-Gomez A, Gomez-Garcia P et al: A controlled trial of prophylactic granulocyte transfusions during induction chemotherapy for acute nonlymphoblastic leukemia. Cancer 54:734, 1984
34. Clift RA, Sanders JE, Thomas ED et al: Granulocyte transfusions for the prevention of infection in patients receiving bone-marrow transplants. N Engl J Med 298:1052, 1978
35. Strauss RG, Connett JE, Gale RP et al: A controlled trial of prophylactic granulocyte transfusions during initial induction chemotherapy for acute myelogenous leukemia. N Engl J Med 305:597, 1981
36. Hester JP, McCredie KB, Freireich EJ: Advances in supportive care: blood component transfusions. p. 93. In Care of the Child with Cancer. American Cancer Society, Atlanta, 1979
37. Buckner CD, Clift RA, Thomas ED et al: Early infections complications in allogenic marrow transplant recipients with acute leukemia: effects of prophylactic measures. Infection 11:243, 1983
38. Curtis, JE, Hasselback R, Bergsagel DE: Leukocyte transfusions for the prophylaxis and treatment of infections associated with granulo-cytopenia. Can Med Assoc J 117:341, 1977
39. Schiffer CA, Aisner J, Daly PA et al: Alloimmunization following prophylactic granulocyte transfusion. Blood 54:766, 1979
40. Sutton DMC, Shumak KH, Baker MA: Prophylactic granulocyte transfusions in acute leukemia. Plasma Ther Transfus Technol 3:45, 1982
41. Ford JM, Cullen MH, Roberts MM et al: Prophylactic granulocyte transfusions: results of a randomized controlled trial in patients with acute myelogenous leukemia. Transfusion 22:311, 1982
42. Cooper MR: Personal communication update of earlier study, Cooper MR, Heise E, Richards F et al (1975): A prospective study of histocompatible leukocyte and platelet transfusions during chemotherapeutic induction of acute myeloblastic leukemia. p. 436. In Goldman JM, Lowenthal RM (eds): Leukocytes: Separation, Collection and Transfusion. Academic Press, San Diego, 1981
43. Winston DJ, Ho WG, Young LS, Gale RP: Prophylactic granulocyte transfusions during human bone marrow transplantation. Am J Med 68:893, 1982
44. Goldstein IM, Eyre JH, Terasaki PI et al: Leukocyte transfusions: role of leukocyte alloantibodies in determining transfusion response. Transfusion 11:19, 1971
45. McCullough JJ, Weiblen BJ, Clay ME, Forstrom L: Effect of leukocyte antibodies on the fate, in vivo, of Indium-111-labelled granulocytes. Blood 58:164, 1981
46. Dutcher JP, Schiffer CA, Johnston GS et al: Alloimmunization prevents the migration of transfused [111]Indium-labeled granulocytes to sites of infection. Blood 62:354, 1983
47. Dahlke MB, Keashen M, Alavi JB et al: Granulocyte transfusions and outcome of alloimmunized patients with gram-negative sepsis. Transfusion 22:347, 1982
48. Strauss RG, Rohert PA, Randels MJ, Winegarden D: Granulocyte collection. J Clin Apheresis 6:241, 1991
49. Strauss RG, Hester JP, Vogler WR et al: A multi-center trial to document the efficacy and safety of a rapidly excreted analogue of hydroxyethyl starch for leukapheresis; with a note on steroid stimulation. Transfusion 26:258, 1986
50. Strauss RG: Function of granulocytes collected for transfusion. p. 9. In Vogler WR (ed): Cytapheresis and Plasma Exchange: Clinical Indications. Alan R Liss, New York, 1982
51. Lane TA, Lamkin GE: Adherence to fresh and stored granulocytes to endothelial cells, effect of storage temperature. Transfusion 28:237, 1988
52. Bensinger WI, Price TH, Dale DC et al: The effects of daily recombinant human granulocyte colony stimulating factor administration on normal granulocyte donors undergoing leukapheresis. Blood 81:1883, 1993

Transfusion of Plasma Derivatives: Fresh Frozen Plasma, Cryoprecipitate, Albumin, and Immunoglobulins

137

Christopher D. Hillyer and Eugene M. Berkman

INTRODUCTION

The use of plasma and plasma derivatives has risen dramatically over the past two decades. While plasma and its derivatives represent a valuable resource, these blood products can transmit infectious diseases and therefore should be used appropriately. The value of plasma and plasma derivatives has led to a decline in the use and availability of whole blood. Furthermore, it is most cost effective to fractionate whole blood into plasma and packed red blood cells at collection. Plasma may then undergo further fractionation (Cohn fractionation), which was described in the 1940s and exploits the use of ethanol and protein precipitation in the cold.[1] This chapter discusses the features and uses of fresh frozen plasma (FFP), cryoprecipitate, albumin, intravenous immunoglobulin (IVIg), intramuscular immunoglobulins, and Alpha$_1$-Proteinase Inhibitor (Human) Prolastin. The use of FFP, cryoprecipitate, and specific coagulation factor concentrates in the treatment of congenital clotting factor deficiencies is discussed in Chapter 139.

FRESH FROZEN PLASMA

Plasma is the fluid compartment of blood, consisting of 90% water, 7% protein and colloids, and 2–3% nutrients, crystalloids, hormones, and vitamins. The protein fraction contains the soluble clotting factors, the constituents for which transfusion of FFP is most often required.

Plasma frozen at $\leq -18°C$ within 6 hours of donation is labeled fresh frozen plasma. This product may be stored ≤1 year before use, at which time it is thawed over 20–30 minutes. The activities of the labile coagulation factors (V and VIII) decrease after thawing but remain adequate for ≥24 hours. Plasma that is not immediately frozen as FFP becomes either liquid plasma (stored at 1–6°C) or source plasma (stored at $\leq -18°C$). These latter products are used for the preparation of plasma derivatives: albumin, clotting factor concentrates, and immunoglobulin preparations.

Indications

The indications for FFP administration are listed in Table 137-1, as are the conditions for which FFP transfusions are not indicated. Audits of transfusion practices have consistently demonstrated that FFP use is inappropriately high.[2,3] Specifically, FFP should not be used (1) to reconstitute "whole blood" by co-administration with red blood cells, (2) as a volume expander or (3) as a source of nutrients. Appropriate uses are described in detail below.

Liver Disease and Transplantation

Patients with severe liver disease may have low levels of the vitamin K-dependent clotting factors (II, VII, IX, and X) (see Ch. 147). These patients develop a prolonged prothrombin time (PT) and partial thromboplastin time (PTT). In addition, the thrombin time may be prolonged and fibrin-split products may be elevated. The plasma fibrinogen level is elevated in early liver disease but decreases in the later stages. Hemorrhage, most often secondary to an anatomic lesion, may be complicated by the coagulopathy represented by these abnormalities.

FFP infusion is indicated during severe bleeding if the coagulation test results are abnormal. In the absence of anatomic lesions, bleeding is not usually seen until the PT is >16–18 seconds or the PTT is >55–60 seconds. FFP is not recommended prophylactically prior to a surgical challenge or liver biopsy, unless these values are exceeded.[4] In fact, the PT and PTT are poor predictors of surgical bleeding, and mild abnormalities in these coagulation tests may be impossible to correct, even with infusion of large quantities of FFP.[5] Thus, in patients with liver disease and no clinical bleeding, infusion of FFP, regardless of test results, is wasteful.[6] Unfortunately, patients with liver disease still represent a significant propor-

Table 137-1. Administration of Fresh Frozen Plasma

Indicated
- Multiple coagulation factor deficiency
  - Liver disease
  - Massive transfusion
- Disseminated intravascular coagulation
- Rapid reversal of warfarin effect
- Thrombotic thrombocytopenia purpura (hemolytic uremic syndrome)
- Congenital coagulation defects (see Ch. 139)
- C1-esterase inhibitor deficiency (life-threatening edema)
- Fluid replacement during plasma exchange for hemolytic uremic syndrome/ thrombotic thrombocytopenic purpura or Refsum disease

Not indicated
- Immunodeficiency
- Burns
- Reconstitution of "packed" red blood cells
- Volume expansion
- Source of nutrients

tion of those for whom FFP is ordered.[7,8] Large volumes of FFP are required, however, during liver transplantation complicated by severe liver disease preoperatively, lack of clotting factor synthesis during the anhepatic stage, massive red blood cell transfusion, and disseminated intravascular coagulation (DIC).[9,10]

Massive Transfusion

The administration of FFP to patients receiving large quantities of red blood cells (>1 blood volume within 24 hours) is often recommended because of a dilutional coagulopathy arising from blood replacement with packed red blood cells and crystalloid solutions, both of which lack coagulation factors. Studies addressing the use of FFP transfusion in massive transfusion have yielded confusing and conflicting results.[11,12] Dilutional thrombocytopenia may also complicate the coagulopathy in these patients.[13,14]

In general, FFP transfusions are of little value in nonbleeding patients who have received <6–10 U of red blood cells. In some patients, however, shock associated with DIC and dilutional coagulopathy may occur necessitating FFP.[15] While several studies have demonstrated the ineffectiveness of routine FFP infusions in patients receiving >10 U of red blood cells within 24 hours, many physicians still opt to transfuse FFP in the face of continued bleeding of unknown cause. Predetermined formulations (e.g., 1 U of FFP for every 5 U of red blood cells transfused) are attractive but result in excessive transfusion.[16] It is far more effective to use FFP to replace depleted clotting factors documented by abnormal laboratory tests.[17]

Disseminated Intravascular Coagulation

DIC may be secondary to sepsis, liver disease, hypotension, surgery with poor perfusion, trauma, obstetric complications, leukemia (usually promyelocytic) or underlying malignancy (see Ch. 116). Successful treatment of the underlying cause is paramount. Patients with DIC and bleeding should be given FFP in amounts sufficient to correct the abnormalities of the coagulation tests. The use of heparin in DIC is discussed in Chapter 116. In patients with severe liver disease, bleeding, and laboratory abnormalities consistent with DIC, FFP infusions in any amount often fail to correct the PT and PTT.[18]

Rapid Reversal of Warfarin Effect

Warfarin changes the state of carboxylation of the vitamin K-dependent clotting factors (II, VII, IX, and X) in the liver (see Ch. 120). Thus, patients anticoagulated with warfarin have functional deficiencies of these factors. After discontinuation of the warfarin, these deficiencies correct within 48 hours if diet and vitamin K absorption are normal. Vitamin K administration permits correction within 12–18 hours.[19] In bleeding patients anticoagulated with warfarin, patients requiring emergency surgery, or patients with serious trauma, the deficient clotting factors can be immediately provided by FFP transfusion and the PT normalized. In patients not experiencing bleeding but with significantly prolonged PT, the potential danger of significant hemorrhage is often overemphasized and must be weighed against the risks of FFP infusion. FFP is overused in this situation.

Thrombotic Thrombocytopenic Purpura and Hemolytic Uremic Syndrome

In some patients with thrombotic thrombocytopenic purpura (TTP) or hemolytic uremic syndrome (HUS), FFP infusions alone have induced clinical remission.[20–22] The mechanism by which FFP works is unknown but may be due to high-molecular-weight von Willebrand factor (vWF) multimers. Most patients, however, should undergo plasmapheresis, with FFP used as the replacement fluid (see Ch. 127). Some authorities have suggested the use of cryo-poor plasma (cryosupernatant) for refractory patients.[23] This is not a licensed product, nor has it been prospectively compared with other transfusion therapies in controlled trials.

Antithrombin III Deficiency

FFP has been used as a source of antithrombin III (AT III) in congenitally deficient patients. Purified AT III concentrates are now available and have replaced FFP for this indication[24] (see Ch. 119).

Plasma Exchange

Plasma is used as the replacement fluid during plasma exchange in patients with TTP/HUS and Refsum disease. FFP infusion and plasma exchange with FFP have also been espoused in the treatment of meningococcal sepsis, although this requires confirmation.[25]

Dosage

One unit of FFP contains 200–280 ml. On average, there are 0.7 to 1 U/ml of activity of each coagulation factor per milliliter of FFP and 1–2 mg/ml fibrinogen. The appropriate dose of FFP may be estimated from the plasma volume, the desired increment of factor activity, and the expected half-life of the factor being replaced. Alternatively, FFP dosage may be estimated as 8–10 ml/kg.[26] The frequency of administration depends on the response to infusion, the half-life of the factor being replaced, and the patient's clinical response. Laboratory confirmation of efficacy is suggested. The practice of ordering FFP by numbers of units should be replaced by ordering the number of milliliters to be infused.

Compatibility and Side Effects

FFP has been screened for unexpected red blood cell antibodies and should be ABO type compatible. Tests for serologic compatibility are not performed before administration. The $Rh_o(D)$ type is matched in only some parts of the United States, as immunization to $Rh_o(D)$ antigen has rarely been reported because of transfusion of $Rh_o(D)$-positive plasma to $Rh_o(D)$-negative patients.[27] Plasma from multiparous women should not be used. Hemolytic reactions due to infusion of an undetected antibody directed toward recipient red blood cell antigens have been reported, but these cases are extremely rare.[28] Alloimmunization to red blood cell antigens may occur with FFP transfusion but is also rare.[29]

Fever, chills, and allergic reactions may occur and are treated symptomatically. Occasionally, severe allergic reactions with pulmonary symptoms or noncardiogenic pulmonary edema are seen. These cases are thought to be due to antibodies present in donor plasma that react with recipient leukocytes. These severe reactions are usually transient; in rare cases, they are prolonged and can result in death. Anaphylactic reactions may occur after infusion of plasma (containing IgA) into patients with IgA deficiency and antibodies to IgA.[30] These reactions are exceedingly rare, but a national registry of IgA-deficient donors does exist and thus it is possible to obtain IgA-deficient plasma for patients who exhibit this complication. Transmission of infectious disease by FFP has been significantly reduced but not yet completely eliminated, although FFP is not thought to transmit the cell-associated cytomegalovirus (CMV).[31]

CRYOPRECIPITATE

Cryoprecipitate is the precipitate formed when FFP is thawed at 4°C. The precipitate is then refrozen in 10–15 ml of plasma and stored at ≤ -18°C for a period of 1 year. Cryoprecipitate contains 80–100 U of factor VIII, 100–250 mg of fibrinogen, and 50–60 mg of fibronectin, as well as 40–70% of the vWF originally in the plasma. Anti-A and anti-B antibodies may also be present.

For clinical purposes, cryoprecipitate should be considered the blood product most rich in factor VIII, vWF, and fibrinogen. Cryoprecipitate is used predominately to treat bleeding in fibrinogen deficiency states, occasionally in vWF deficiency, and only rarely in factor VIII deficiency. Congenital deficiencies of these factors are discussed in Chapters 108, 111, and 113.

Indications

The indications for the administration of cryoprecipitate are listed in Table 137-2, as well as, a list of conditions in which cryoprecipitate transfusions are not indicated. Specific indications and inappropriate uses are discussed in detail below.

Fibrinogen Deficiency

Fibrinogen deficiency is the primary indication for cryoprecipitate transfusion and may be in the form of congenital afibrinogenemia (rare) or dysfibrinogenemia due to severe liver disease and DIC.[32] These patients often have concomitant decreases in clotting factor levels and require the co-administration of FFP as above. It is important in these complicated cases to obtain fibrinogen measurements. A fibrinogen level <100 mg/dl will cause prolongation of both the PT and PTT despite adequate clotting factor replacement. Very low levels of fibrinogen occur during liver transplantation for which transfusion support with cryoprecipitate is vital.[9]

von Willebrand Disease

vWF, required for platelet binding to ruptured vascular endothelium, is low or dysfunctional in vWD. Desamino-D-arginine vasopressin (DDAVP) remains the treatment of choice, although severe bleeding may require cryoprecipitate. Recent advances in clotting factor concentrates and viral inactivation methods may make the use of "wet" cryoprecipitate obsolete.[33]

Fibrin Glue

An adhesive made of fibrin precipitated by the addition of bovine thrombin to cryoprecipitate has been used in some surgical procedures, including liver and ear procedures, and in burn patients.[34–40] This is not a licensed product, and its use has not been well studied, but its use is increasing. In some instances (i.e., ear surgery) autologous fibrin glue can be supplied. Anaphylaxis secondary to the bovine thrombin has been reported.[41] In addition, life-threatening hemorrhage may be

Table 137-2. Administration of Cryoprecipitate

Indicated
    Some patients with hemophilia A or von Willebrand disease[33]
    Fibrinogen deficiency
    Dysfibrinogenemia[32]
    Fibrin glue[34–40]
    Renal stone removal[26]
Not indicated
    Uremic bleeding
    Sepsis (postoperative)

caused by the formation of clotting factor inhibitors that cross-react to epitopes on bovine and human coagulant proteins.[42–44]

Fibronectin

Fibronectin, in cryoprecipitate or purified from plasma, has been used in surgical and trauma patients to promote wound healing.[45] No clear indication has been found, and further study is required to prove efficacy and safety.

Uremic Bleeding

Abnormal bleeding is a common complication of uremia. In 1980, a single study led to the widespread but temporary use of cryoprecipitate as treatment for uremic bleeding.[46] No data currently support this use.[47] Still, the literature continues to recognize cryoprecipitate as a therapeutic option.[48] Cryoprecipitate should not be used in the routine management of uremic bleeding.

Dosage

The dosage of cryoprecipitate is calculated on the basis of the amount of fibrinogen present in 1 U of cryoprecipitate, the plasma volume, and the desired increment. The difficulty in determining the correct dosage is due primarily to variability in the fibrinogen content of cryoprecipitate, secondary to variable storage volume and pooling methods used. The goal of therapy should be to maintain the measured fibrinogen at >100 ml/dl. This can usually be accomplished by transfusion of 2–4 U/10 kg if the fibrinogen content of the concentrate is low and by 1–2 U/10 kg if the fibrinogen content is high.

Compatibility and Side Effects

Since cryoprecipitate can contain anti-A and/or anti-B antibody, infused units should be ABO compatible. The risks of fevers, chills, allergic reactions, and infectious disease transmission are similar to those associated with FFP.

ALBUMIN

Albumin, a very important plasma protein, contributes primarily to the maintenance of plasma colloid oncotic pressure. It is clinically available in three forms: a 5% solution in saline, a 25% solution in distilled water, and as purified protein fraction, which is 5% total protein (88% albumin, 12% globulins). These products are heat-treated and unable to transmit viruses. The high cost, periodic shortages, and lack of efficacy in some clinical situations has led to increased scrutiny over the appropriate use of this important plasma derivative.[49] In many clinical situations, the use of albumin remains controversial and is the subject of continued debate. Some favor the use of crystalloid solutions over albumin, while others insist on the use of albumin. We believe that albumin is extensively overused. Thus, in Table 137-3, under Authors' Recommendations, we have listed our preferences for indications, possible indications, and investigational indications for albumin administration, as well as situations in which we believe albumin administration is not indicated; under Common Usages, we have listed clinical situations in which albumin is used.

Indications

A decrease in measured plasma albumin is found in many situations and often is not a clinical concern. Mild edema due to hypoalbuminemia does not require albumin therapy. However,

Table 137-3. Administration of Albumin

Authors' Recommendations

Indicated
Following large volume paracentesis[69]
Nephrotic syndrome resistant to potent diuretics[70]
Volume/fluid replacement in plasmapheresis[115]

Possibly indicated
Adult respiratory distress syndrome
Cardiopulmonary bypass pump priming[56–59]
Fluid resuscitation in shock/sepsis/burns[51–55,65]
Neonatal kernicterus
To improve enteral feeding intolerance[116,117]

Not indicated
Correction of measured hypoalbuminemia or hypoproteinemia[51]
Nutritional deficiency, total parenteral nutrition[118,119]
Pre-eclampsia[120]
Red blood cell suspension
Simple volume expansion (surgery, burns)[61,62]
Wound healing

Investigational
Cadaveric renal transplantation[121]
Cerebral ischemia[122,123]
Stroke[124]

Common Usages
Serum albumin <2.0 g/dl
Nephrotic syndrome, proteinuria and hypoalbuminemia
Labile pulmonary, cardiovascular status
Cardiopulmonary bypass, pump priming
Extensive burns
Plasma exchange
Hypotension
Liver disease, hypoalbuminemia, diuresis
Protein losing enteropathy, hypoalbuminemia
Resuscitation
Intraoperative fluid requirement >5–6 L in adults
Premature infant undergoing major surgery

---

inadequate synthesis, as seen in several liver disease and severe malnutrition, and excessive loss, as seen in nephrotic syndrome and protein-losing enteropathy, can lead to significant hypoalbuminemia with intravascular volume depletion, anasarca, ascites, and pleural effusions. Historically, albumin had been advocated for nutritional support, to correct measured hypoalbuminemia, as volume replacement, and in the care of burned and critically ill patients. Recent studies support the use of albumin in only a few situations, which include nephrotic syndrome resistant to potent diuretic therapy and following large volume paracentesis.[50] These indications and the appropriate and inappropriate uses of albumin are described in detail below.

Intravascular Volume Expansion

Albumin provides most (80%) plasma colloid oncotic pressure. Infused albumin will provide colloid oncotic pressure, however, 50% of the infused protein is lost to the extravascular fluid compartment within 4 hours. Crystalloid may also provide volume expansion and is more quickly redistributed into total body fluids. Many studies have compared albumin with crystalloids for volume expansion[51–55] during and/or after thoracic/abdominal surgery or trauma with no improvement in outcome for patients treated with albumin. Studies in cardiac surgery patients in whom albumin was used in cardiopulmonary bypass also showed no clinical differences as compared with controls.[56–59] Studies investigating intensive care unit patients failed to show beneficial outcome to those whose colloid oncotic pressure was maintained with albumin.[60–62] An apparent benefit of albumin followed by diuretic therapy may be found

in postoperative patients with intrapulmonary shunting, although the studies have been criticized.[63,64] One prospective trial of colloid and crystalloid solutions has been accomplished in burn patients[65] and, while showing a difference in cardiac index in the albumin group, failed to show a significant difference in outcome. Thus, albumin therapy cannot be recommended for simple volume expansion or for the maintenance of albumin levels or colloid oncotic pressure.

Cirrhosis

The use of albumin in cirrhotic patients dates back to before 1950. In this setting, albumin is recommended for temporary improvement in hyponatremia[66] or to prevent complications, including volume shifts and hyponatremia, associated with paracentesis.[67–69] One study demonstrated that both hyponatremia and renal insufficiency were increased in the saline versus the albumin-treated group after large-volume paracentesis, which were associated with decreased patient survival.[69]

Nephrotic Syndrome

Albumin has been used to increase colloid oncotic pressure with the intention of increasing diuresis. This use is limited to those patients in whom diuretic therapy is poorly tolerated or ineffective[70] or in those with massive ascites or anasarca.[71]

Dosage

The volume and speed of administration should be determined by the patient's volume status, condition, and response to the product. Albumin 5% is oncotically equal to normal human plasma. Albumin 25% provides less infusion volume for the equivalent amount of albumin.

Compatibility and Side Effects

Albumin is a widely used plasma derivative, and adverse reactions are rare. Still, allergic reactions, including urticaria, may be encountered. Volume overload may occur with excessive doses and a decrease in ionized calcium is at least a theoretical possibility. Albumin is an excellent growth medium for bacteria, and bacterial contamination can lead to febrile, and more serious, reactions. Albumin lots are tested for contaminants and pyrogens before being shipped. Transmission of infectious diseases is no longer a concern.

Hypotension with PPF infusion has been reported and was secondary to prekallikrein activator in lots manufactured during the 1970s. This, too, is no longer a concern.

INTRAVENOUS IMMUNOGLOBULIN

IVIg is prepared by fractionation of large pools of human plasma. Numerous preparations are available in the United States and throughout the world. Each preparation is slightly different and has theoretical advantages and disadvantages and specific licensed indications. Ideally, IVIg should contain each IgG subclass; retain Fc receptor activity; have a normal half-life; demonstrate virus neutralization, opsonization, and intracellular killing; and have antibacterial capsular polysaccharide antibody. Furthermore, vasoactive impurities should be absent, and no transmissible infectious agents should be present.[72]

Table 137-4. Administration of Intravenous Immunoglobulins

Indicated (licensed)
    Primary immunodeficiency syndromes
        Common variable immunodeficiency[86]
        X-linked agammaglobulinemia
        Sever combined immunodeficiency
        Ataxia-telangiectasia
        Wiskott-Aldrich syndrome
        IgG subclass deficiency[77,78]
    Chronic lymphocytic leukemia[79,80]
    Mucocutaneous lymph node syndrome[93,94]
    Idiopathic thrombocytopenic purpura[81–92,125]
Investigational
    Acquired von Willebrand disease[126]
    Amyotrophic lateral sclerosis[127]
    Autoimmune hemolytic anemia[128 129]
    Burn patients[130–133]
    Chronic inflammatory demyelinating polyneuropathy[133,134]
    Factor VIII inhibitors[135]
    Graft-versus-host disease[136]
    Guillain-Barré syndrome[137]
    Human immunodeficiency virus infection[138,139]
    Immune mediated aplastic anemia[87]
    Immune neutropenia[140]
    Inflammatory bowel disease[141]
    Multiple myeloma[141]
    Myasthenia gravis[143]
    Neonatal and premature infants[144,145]
    Prevention of nosocomial postoperative infections[146,147]
    Prophylaxis in transplant recipients against cytomegalovirus infection[148–151]
    Rheumatoid arthritis[152]
    Systemic lupus erythematosus[153]
    Thrombocytopenia refractory to platelet transfusion[154–157]
    Vasculitis[158]

Indications

Indications for the administration of IVIg are listed in Table 137-4, as well as a list of conditions for which IVIg administration is being investigated.

Primary Immunodeficiency Syndromes

Primary congenital immunodeficiency syndromes have been treated with intramuscular immunoglobulin for the past 30 years. The use of intramuscular immunoglobulin has certain disadvantages. In patients with small muscle mass, it may be difficult to give adequate amounts to achieve desired serum concentrations. Pain at the injection site is also a problem. Absorption of the immunoglobulin is delayed and maximum blood levels are not achieved for several days. IVIg has been developed to overcome these disadvantages and the prophylactic use of IVIg in these patients has gained acceptance.[73–75] Primary immunodeficiency patients treated with IVIg have less fever, fewer infectious episodes, and improved survival rate.[76] IVIg use in IgG subclass deficiencies is also beneficial.[77,78]

Chronic Lymphocytic Leukemia

Chronic lymphocytic leukemia (CLL) may be associated with hypogammaglobulinemia and complications of repeated bacterial infections (see Ch. 83). IVIg decreases the incidence of bacterial infection and serious complications in patients with CLL and secondary immunodeficiency and has become accepted prophylactic therapy.[79,80] Viral and fungal infections are not prevented.

Idiopathic Thrombocytopenic Purpura

The use of IVIg represents a major advance in the treatment of both acute and chronic idiopathic thrombocytopenic purpura (ITP) (see Ch. 125). IVIg will significantly raise the platelet count within 5 days in both adults with chronic ITP and children with acute ITP.[81–84] The mechanism of action of IVIg in ITP is unknown, but most believe that Fc receptor blockade decreases the removal of antibody-coated platelets.[85] Other proposed mechanisms include suppressed antiplatelet antibody synthesis, increased antiviral immunity, and inhibition by anti-idiotypic antibodies.[86] In general, most patients respond initially to IVIg, with platelet increments that occur within 1–2 days and continue for >5–10 days. Sustained responses are uncommon, although maintenance therapy may be of some value.[87] IVIg may be effective even after previous therapy with corticosteroids or splenectomy.[88] A recent comparison of IVIg versus oral corticosteroids in acute ITP in children showed IVIg to be superior.[89] IVIg given in conjunction with corticosteroids may be even more effective.[83,90]

IVIg is therefore indicated in patients when rapid elevation of platelet count is required, especially in those who are bleeding or require urgent surgery, including splenectomy. It is also indicated in patients who are at high risk of intracranial hemorrhage and in those for whom corticosteroids are contraindicated.[91] IVIg has been used to treat ITP during pregnancy.[92] Although corticosteroids and splenectomy remain the cornerstone of treatment in adults, IVIg is being used more frequently. In children, many centers are using IVIg routinely.[90]

Mucocutaneous Lymph Node Syndrome

The mucocutaneous lymph node syndrome (Kawasaki disease) has been treated with aspirin or aspirin combined with IVIg in randomized prospective trials. A serious complication seen in the disease, coronary artery aneurysm, was significantly reduced in the IVIg-treated group.[93] Other studies have confirmed these findings.[94]

Investigational Uses

A variety of diseases are listed in Table 137-4 for which IVIg has been used but for which IVIg is not licensed for use in the United States. Prospective well-designed studies are needed to determine in which of these diseases the treatment is clearly effective. The use of IVIg in CMV prevention in bone marrow and solid organ transplant patients, and for the prevention of infections in critically ill patients, appears promising.

Dosage

Patients with primary immunodeficiency syndromes and IgG levels of <200 mg% are candidates for immunoglobulin replacement. Most patients require 100–200 mg/kg IV every 3–4 weeks to achieve adequate IgG levels (usually >800 mg%) and protection against infection. Initially, frequent determinations of IgG levels allow the treating physician to individualize the dose and schedule. These are affected by the recovery and half-life of the infused product as well as the redistribution and catabolism of IVIg, which vary from product to product and patient to patient. Doses can be given more frequently or increased to 400 mg/kg if the clinical response or level of circulating IgG is not adequate. Patients with ITP are usually treated with 400 mg/kg/day for 5 days or 1,000 mg/kg/day for 2 days (see Ch. 125). Repeat single doses (400 mg/kg) have been used intermittently in some patients (particularly children) to maintain platelet counts of >50,000/mm³. Kawasaki disease has also been treated with 400 mg/kg/day for 3–5 days, but the optimal dose and schedule have not been determined.

Compatibility and Side Effects

It is recommended that IVIg infusions be started slowly and that the patients be closely monitored. If the initial rate (0.5 ml/kg/hr) is well tolerated, the rate can be increased gradually but not more than eightfold. Fever, headache, nausea, vomiting, fatigue, backache, leg cramps, urticaria, flushing, elevation of blood pressure, and thrombophlebitis may be seen. IgA-deficient patients may have IgG anti-IgA antibodies, which can cause anaphylactic reactions.[95] This complication is rare and may be avoided by using products with lower concentration of IgA.[96] Chills, nausea, flushing, chest tightness, and wheezing have been ascribed to serum sickness or aggregated IgG. The presence of aggregated IgG has been largely resolved by the addition of maltose as a stabilizing agent in the diluent.[97] Rarely, IVIg may produce hemolysis secondary to infusion of IgG anti-A and/or anti-B red blood cell antibodies present in the preparation.[98] Infectious disease transmission, although present several years ago, is no longer a concern due to newer products rendered free of infectious agents by improved methods of viral inactivation or elimination.[99,100] It is necessary to remember that IVIg may contain antibodies that could interfere with serologic evaluations, including red blood cell compatibility testing.[101]

HYPERIMMUNE AND INTRAMUSCULAR IMMUNOGLOBULINS

Hyperimmune immunoglobulins are prepared from large pools of plasma known to contain elevated antibody titers against specific infectious agents. The intramuscular and hyperimmune immunoglobulins are listed in Table 137-5.

Antithymocyte globulin (ATG) is a purified concentrated γ-globulin made from hyperimmune serum of horses immunized with human T lymphocytes. ATG is used in renal transplant patients as an adjunct therapy in the treatment of graft rejection.[102,103] It is also used in patients with aplastic anemia who are not candidates for bone marrow transplantation[104,105] (see Ch. 22).

CMV immunoglobulin is indicated in all kidney transplant recipients who are seronegative for CMV who receive a kidney from a seropositive donor,[106] and is being evaluated in bone marrow transplant patients with CMV-induced pneumonia.[107]

Hepatitis B immunoglobulin is used to provide passive immunity to hepatitis B virus because of needle-stick exposure to HbSAg positive blood or sexual contact with HbSAg-positive people.[108]

Table 137-5. Available Hyperimmune and Intramuscular Immunoglobulins

Antithymocyte globulin
Cytomegalovirus immunoglobulin[a]
γ-Globulin
Hepatitis β-immunoglobulin
Rabies immunoglobulin
Rh$_o$(D) immunoglobulin
Tetanus immunoglobulin
Vaccinia immunoglobulin[b]
Varicella-zoster immunoglobulin[c]
Western equine encephalitis immunoglobulin[b]

[a] Available on treatment IND, American Red Cross Blood Services Northeast Region, Dedham, MA.
[b] Available on treatment IND, United States Centers for Disease Control, Atlanta, GA.
[c] Available from Massachusetts Department of Public Health, Jamaica Plain, MA.

Intramuscular immunoglobulin may be used as replacement therapy in primary immunodeficiency syndromes. The trend, however, is toward the use of IVIg. Intramuscular immunoglobulin is also used to provide passive immunity to hepatitis A infection in exposed individuals and as pre-exposure prophylaxis in individuals traveling to an endemic area.

Rabies immunoglobulin is used to provide passive immunity to individuals exposed to the disease. It should be given in conjunction with active immunization.

Rh immunoglobulin is used when fetal Rh$_o$(D)-positive red blood cells may have entered the maternal circulation of an Rh$_o$(D)-negative mother. This means that Rh$_o$(D) immunoglobulin is given to Rh$_o$(D)-negative mothers after abortion or amniocentesis as well as before delivery and again postpartum if the child is proved Rh$_o$(D) positive.[109–111] The mechanism by which anti-Rh$_o$(D) antibody is prevented is not known but may involve antibody feedback with T-cell suppression of the B-cell clones responsible for the formation of anti-Rh antibody.

Rh immunoglobulin can also be given to prevent immunization in Rh$_o$(D)-negative individuals given Rh$_o$(D)-positive components such as platelets. Transfusion of Rh$_o$(D)-positive red blood cells to Rh$_o$(D)-negative recipients is occasionally necessary and prevention of immunization require much larger doses and is not possible unless *intravenous* Rh immunoglobulin is made available by the manufacturers. Rh immunoglobulin has also been used to treat ITP[112] and is discussed in Chapter 125.

Tetanus immunoglobulin is indicated in patients who are injured who have no reliable history of prior immunization. If the history of immunization is >10 years old, a booster injection of tetanus toxoid is the preferred treatment.

Varicella-zoster immunoglobulin is used to provide passive immunization in exposed immunodeficient patients. Immunodeficient states include patients with primary or acquired immunodeficiency syndromes and neoplastic diseases, those treated with steroids or other immunosuppressive drugs, and those receiving organ or bone marrow transplants.

Western equine encephalitis immunoglobulin and *vaccinia immunoglobulin* are available from the Centers for Disease Control. The route of dosage administration and side effects of the hyperimmune and intramuscular immunoglobulin preparations can be ascertained from information on the product inserts.

ALPHA$_1$-PROTEINASE INHIBITOR (HUMAN) PROLASTIN

Alpha$_1$-Proteinase Inhibitor (Human) Prolastin (α_1-antitrypsin) is used to treat patients with congenital α_1-antitrypsin deficiency.[113,114] This product is prepared from pooled human plasma and has been heat treated in solution for 10 hours at 60°C. Viral inactivation is probably achieved but total effectiveness of the method has not yet been demonstrated with this product. Mild adverse reactions have been reported rarely and include fever, light-headedness, dizziness, mild leukocytosis, and dilutional anemia. Dosage can be obtained from the package insert.

REFERENCES

1. Cohn EJ, Oncley JL, Strong LE et al: Chemical, clinical and immunological studies on the products of human plasma fractionation. I: the characterization of the protein fractions in human plants. J Clin Invest 23:417, 1944
2. National Institute of Health Consensus Conference: Fresh frozen plasma: indications and risks. JAMA 253:551, 1985
3. Braunstein AH, Oberman HA: Transfusion of plasma components. Transfusion 24:281, 1984
4. Gazzard BG, Henderson JM, Williams R: The use of fresh frozen plasma or a concentrate of factor IX as replacement therapy before liver biopsy. Gut 16:621, 1975

5. Spector I, Corn M, Ticktin HE: Effect of plasma transfusion on the prothrombin time and clotting factors in liver disease. N Engl J Med 275:1032, 1966

6. McVay PA, Toy PT: Lack of increased bleeding after paracentesis and thoracentesis in patients with mild coagulation abnormalities. Transfusion 31:164, 1991

7. Oberman HA: Uses and abuses of fresh frozen plasma. p. 109. In Garratty G (ed): Current Concepts in Transfusion Therapy. American Association of Blood Banks, Arlington, VA, 1985

8. Blumberg N, Laczin J, McMican A et al: A critical survey of fresh-frozen plasma use. Transfusion 26:511, 1986

9. Nusbacher J: Blood transfusion support in liver transplantation. Transfusion 5:207, 1991

10. Motschman TI, Taswell HF, Brecher ME et al: Intraoperative blood loss and patient and graft survival in orthotopic liver transplantation: their relationship to clinical and laboratory data. Mayo Clin Proc 64:346, 1989

11. Mannucci PM, Federici AB, Sirchia G: Hemostasis testing during massive blood replacement. Vox Sang 42:113, 1982

12. Harke H, Rahman S: Haemostatic disorders in massive transfusion. Bibli Haematol 46:179, 1980

13. Reed RL, Clavarella D, Heimbach DM et al: Prophylactic platelet administration during massive transfusion. Ann Surg 203:40, 1986

14. Lomanto C, Howland WS: A re-evaluation of massive blood replacement. Clin Anesth 9:33, 1972

15. Hewson JR, Neame PB, Kumar N et al: Coagulopathy related to dilution and hypotension during massive transfusion. Crit Care Med 13:387, 1985

16. Counts RB, Haisch C, Simon TL et al: Hemostasis in massively transfused trauma patients. Ann Surg 190:91, 1979

17. Kruskall MS, Mintz PD, Bergin JJ et al: Transfusion therapy in emergency medicine. Ann Emerg Med 17:327, 1988

18. Colman RW, Robboy SJ, Minna JD: Disseminated intravascular coagulation: a reappraisal. Annu Rev Med 30:359, 1979

19. Shearer MJ, Barkhan P: Vitamin K1 and therapy of massive warfarin overdose. Lancet 1:266, 1979

20. Breckenridge RL, Solberg LA, Pineda AA et al: Treatment of thrombocytopenic purpura with plasma exchange, antiplatelet agents, corticosteroid and plasma infusion: Mayo Clinic experience. J Clin Apheresis 1:6, 1982

21. Byrnes JJ, Moake JL: Thrombotic thrombocytopenic purpura and the haemolytic-uraemic syndrome: evolving concepts of pathogenesis and therapy. Clin Haematol 15:413, 1986

22. Blitzer JB, Granfortuna JM, Gottlieb AJ et al: Thrombotic thrombocytopenic purpura: treatment with plasmapheresis. Am J Hematol 24:329, 1987

23. Byrnes JJ, Moake JL, Klug P et al: Effectiveness of the cryosupernatant fraction of plasma in the treatment of refractory thrombotic thrombocytopenic purpura. Am J Hematol 34:169, 1990

24. Vinazzer H: Clinical use of anti-thrombin III concentrates. Vox Sang 53:193, 1987

25. van Deuren M, Santman FW, van Dalen R et al: Plasma and whole blood exchange in meningococcal sepsis. Clin Infect Dis 15:424, 1992

26. Snyder EL (ed): Blood Transfusion Therapy, A Physician's Handbook. American Association of Blood Banks, Arlington, VA, 1983

27. McBride JA, O'Hoski P, Blajchman MA et al: Rhesus alloimmunization following intensive plasmapheresis. Transfusion 18:626, 1978

28. Abbott D, Hussain S: Intravascular coagulation due to inter-donor incompatibility. Can Med Assoc J 103:752, 1970

29. Ching EP, Poon M, Neurath D et al: Red blood cell alloimmunization complicating plasma transfusion. Am J Clin Pathol 96:201, 1991

30. Pineda AA, Taswell HF: Transfusion reactions associated with anti-IgA antibodies: report of four cases and review of the literature. Transfusion 15:10, 1975

31. Bowden R, Sayers M: The risk of transmitting cytomegalovirus infection by fresh frozen plasma. Transfusion 30:762, 1990

32. Francis JL, Armstrong DJ: Acquired dysfibrinogenemia in liver disease. J Clin Pathol 35:667, 1982

33. Rodeghiero F, Castaman G, Meyer D et al: Replacement therapy with virus inactivated plasma concentrates in von Willebrand disease. Vox Sang 62:193, 1992

34. Brennan M: Fibrin glue. Blood 5:240, 1991

35. Boeckx W, Vandevoort M, Blondeel P et al: Fibrin glue reduces seroma formation in the rat after mastectomy. Burns 175:450, 1992

36. Fischer CP, Sonda LP, Dionko AC: Further experience with cryoprecipitate coagulum in renal calculus surgery: a review of 60 cases. J Urol 126:432, 1981

37. Silberstein LE, Williams IJ, Hughlett MA et al: An autologous fibrinogen-based adhesive for use in otologic surgery. Transfusion 28:319, 1988

38. Spotnitz WD, Dalton MS, Baker JW, Nolan SP: Successful use of fibrin glue during 2 years of surgery at a university medical center. Am Surg 55:166, 1989

39. Kram HB, Ocampo HP, Yamaguchi MP et al: Fibrin glue in renal and ureteral trauma. Urology 33:2151, 1989

40. Kram HB, Nathan RC, Stafford FJ et al: Fibrin glue achieves hemostasis in patients with coagulation disorders. Arch Surg 124:385, 1989

41. Berguer R, Staerkel RL, Moore EE et al: Warning: fatal reaction to the use of fibrin glue in deep hepatic wounds. Case reports. J Trauma 31:408, 1991

42. Rapaport SI, Zivelin A, Minow RA et al: Clinical significance of antibodies to bovine and human thrombine and factor V after surgical use of bovine thrombin. Am J Clin Pathol 97:84, 1992

43. Ortel TL, Quinn-Allen MA, Charles LA et al: Characterization of an acquired inhibitor to coagulation factor V: antibody binding to the second C-type domain of factor V inhibits the binding of factor V to phosphatidylserine and neutralizes procoagulant activity. J Clin Invest 90:2340, 1992

44. Berruyer M, Amiral J, Ffrench P et al: Immunization by bovine thrombin used with fibrin glue during cardiovascular operations. J Thorac Cardiovasc Surg 105:892, 1993

45. Powell FS, Doran JE: Current status of fibronectin in transfusion medicine: focus on clinical studies. Vox Sang 60:193, 1991

46. Janson PA, Jubelirer SJ, Weinstein MJ, Deykin D: Treatment of the bleeding tendency in uremia with cryoprecipitate. N Engl J Med 303:1318, 1980

47. Triulzi DJ, Blumberg N: Variability in response to cryoprecipitate treatment for hemostatic defects in uremia. Yale J Biol Med 63:1, 1990

48. Mannucci PM: Desmorpressin: a nontransfusional form of treatment for congenital and acquired bleeding disorders. Blood 72:1449, 1988

49. Subcommittee of the Victorian Drug Usage Advisory Committee: Human albumin solutions: consensus statements for use in selected clinical situations. Med J Aust 157:340, 1992

50. Erstad BL, Gales BJ, Rappaport WD: The use of albumin in clinical practice. Arch Intern Med 51:901, 1991

51. Lucas CE, Ledgerwood AM, Higgins RF, Weaver DW: Impaired pulmonary function after albumin resuscitation from shock. J Trauma 20:446, 1980

52. Lowe RJ, Moss GS, Jilek J, Levine HD: Crystalloid vs colloid in the etiology of pulmonary failure after trauma: a randomized trial in man. Surgery 81:676, 1977

53. Moss GS, Lowe RJ, Jilek J, Levine HD: Colloid or crystalloid in the resuscitation of hemorrhagic shock: a controlled clinical trial. Surgery 89:434, 1981

54. Zetterstrom H: Albumin treatment following major surgery. II: effects on postoperative lung function and circulatory adaptation. Acta Anesthesiol Scand 25:133, 1981

55. Virgilio RW, Rice CL, Smith DE et al: Crystalloid vs. Colloid resuscitation: is one better? Surgery 85:129, 1979

56. Hallowell P, Bland JHL, Dalton BC et al: The effect of hemodilution with albumin or Ringer's lactate on water balance and blood use in open-heart surgery. Ann Thorac Surg 25:22, 1979

57. Ohqvist G, Settergren G, Bergstrom K, Lundberg S: Plasma colloid osmotic pressure during open-heart surgery using noncolloid or colloid priming solution in the extracorporeal circuit. Scand J Thorac Cardiovasc Surg 15:251, 1981

58. Marelli D, Samson R, Edgell D et al: Does the addition of albumin to the prime solution in cardiopulmonary bypass affect clinical outcome? J Thorac Cardiovasc Surg 98:751, 1989

59. Bodenhamer RM, Johnson RG, Randolph JD et al: The effect of adding mannitol or albumin to a crystalloid cardioplegic solution: a prospective, randomized clinical study. Ann Thorac Surg 40:374, 1985

60. Grundmann R, Heistermann S: Postoperative albumin infusion therapy based on colloid osmotic pressure. Arch Surg 120:911, 1985

61. Grootendorst AF, van Wilgenburg MGM, de Laat PHJM, van der Hoven B: Albumin abuse in intensive care medicine. Intensive Care Med 14:554, 1988

62. Zadrobilek E, Hackl W, Sporn P, Steinbereithner K: Effect of large volume replacement with balanced electrolyte solutions on extravascular lung water in surgical patients with sepsis syndrome. Intensive Care Med 15:505, 1989

63. Skillman JJ, Parikh BM, Tanenbaum BJ: Pulmonary arteriovenous admixture: improvement with albumin and diuresis. Am J Surg 119:440, 1970

64. Vinocur B, Artz JS, Sampliner JE, Perse EJ: The effect of albumin and diuretics on the alveolar-arterial oxygen gradient in patients with pulmonary insufficiency. Chest 68:429, 1975

65. Demling RH: Fluid replacement in burned patients. Surg Clin North Am 67:15, 1987

66. McCormick PA, Mistry P, Kaye G et al: Intravenous albumin infusion is an effective therapy for hyponatremia in cirrhotic patients with ascites. Gut 31:204, 1990

67. Gines P, Arroyo V, Quintero E et al: Comparison of paracentesis and di-

uretics in the treatment of cirrhotics with tense ascites. Gastroenterology 93:234, 1987

68. Gines P, Tito L, Arroyo V et al: Randomized comparative study of therapeutic paracentesis with and without intravenous albumin in cirrhosis. Gastroenterology 94:1493, 1988

69. Tito L, Gines P, Arroyo V et al: Total paracentesis associated with intravenous albumin management of patients with cirrhosis and ascites. Gastroenterology 98:146, 1990

70. Davison AM, Lambie AT, Verth AH, Cash JD: Salt-poor human albumin in management of nephrotic syndrome. Br Med J 1:481, 1974

71. Weiss RA, Schoeneman M, Greifer I: Treatment of severe nephrotic edema with albumin and furosemide. NY State J Med 84:384, 1984

72. Seligmann M, Cunningham-Rundles C, Hanson LA et al: Appropriate uses of human immunoglobulin in clinical practice: IUIS WHO Notice 1983. Clin Exp Immunol 52:417, 1983

73. Cunningham-Rundles C, Siegal FP, Smithwick EM et al: Efficacy of intravenous immunoglobulin in primary humoral immunodeficiency disease. Ann Intern Med 101:435, 1984

74. Nolte MT, Pirofsky B, Gerritz GA et al: Intravenous immunoglobulin therapy for antibody deficiency. Clin Exp Immunol 36:237, 1979

75. Pirofsky B: Intravenous immune globulin therapy in hypogammaglobulinemia. Am J Med 76:53, 1984

76. Hauser GJ, Spirer Z: Point: gamma globulin therapy for children with recurrent respiratory infections. Pediatr Infect Dis 5:393, 1986

77. Page R, Friday G, Stillwagon P et al: Asthma and selective immunoglobulin subclass deficiency: improvement of asthma after immunoglobulin replacement therapy. J Pediatr 112:127, 1988

78. Silk H, Geha RS: Asthma, recurrent infections and IgG2 deficiency. Ann Allergy 60:98, 1988

79. Besa EC: Use of intravenous immunoglobulin in chronic lymphocytic leukemia. Am J Med 76:209, 1984

80. Cooperative Group for the Study of Immunoglobulin in chronic lymphocytic Leukemia: intravenous immunoglobulin for the prevention of infection in chronic lymphocytic leukemia: a randomized, controlled clinical trial. N Engl J Med 319:902, 1988

81. Bussell JB, Kimberly RP, Inman RD et al: Intravenous gammaglobulin treatment of chronic idiopathic thrombocytopenic purpura. Blood 62:480, 1983

82. Blanchette VS: Review of ITP in children and the therapeutic role of IV IgG. p. 33. In Imbach P (ed): Idiopathic Thrombocytopenic Purpura—Proceedings of a Workshop. Pharma Libri, Morristown, NJ, 1987

83. Hara T, Miyazaki S, Yoshida N, Goya N: High doses of gammaglobulin and methylprednisolone therapy for idiopathic thrombocytopenic purpura in children. Eur J Pediatr 144:240, 1985

84. Imbach P, Barnadun S, d'Apuzzo V et al: High-dose intravenous gammaglobulin for idiopathic thrombocytopenic purpura in childhood. Lancet 1:228, 1981

85. Fehr J, Hofmann V, Kappeler U: Transient reversal of thrombocytopenia in idiopathic thrombocytopenic purpura by high-dose intravenous gamma globulin. N Engl J Med 306:1254, 1982

86. Berkman SA, Lee ML, Gale RP: Clinical uses of intravenous immunoglobulins. Semin Hematol 25:140, 1988

87. Bussel JB, Pham LC, Aledort L, Nachman R: Maintenance treatment of adults with chronic refractory immune thrombocytopenic purpura using repeated intravenous infusions of gammaglobulin. Blood 72:121, 1988

88. Imholz B, Imbach P, Baumgartner C et al: Intravenous immunoglobulin (i.v. IgG) for previously treated acute or for chronic idiopathic thrombocytopenic purpura (ITP) in childhood: a prospective multicenter study. Blut 56:63, 1988

89. Imbach P, Wagner HP, Berchtold W et al: Intravenous immunoglobulin versus oral corticosteroids in acute immune thrombocytopenic purpura in childhood. Lancet 2:464, 1985

90. Bussel JB: Intravenous gammaglobulin therapy for immune cytopenias. Antibody Ther 1:1, 1988

91. Woerner SJ, Abildgaard CF, French BN: Intracranial hemorrhage in children with idiopathic thrombocytopenia purpura. Pediatrics 67:453, 1981

92. Carloss HW, McMillan R, Crosby WH: Management of pregnancy in women with thrombocytopenic purpura. JAMA 244:2756, 1980

93. Furusho K, Kamiya T, Nakano H et al: High-dose intravenous gammaglobulin for Kawasaki disease. Lancet 2:1055, 1984

94. Newburger JW, Takahashi M, Burns JC et al: The treatment of Kawasaki syndrome with intravenous gamma globulin. N Engl J Med 315:341, 1986

95. Wadsworth C, Hanson LA: IgA in commercial gamma globulin preparations. Scand J Immunol 5:15, 1976

96. Apfelzweig R, Piszkiewicz D, Hooper JA: Immunoglobulin A concentrations in commercial immune globulins. J Clin Immunol 7:46, 1987

97. Ochs HD, Buckley RH, Pirofsky B et al: Safety and patient acceptability of intravenous immunoglobulin in 10% maltose. Lancet 2:1158, 1980

98. Copelan EA, Strohm PL, Kennedy MS, Tutschka PJ: Hemolysis following intravenous immunoglobulin therapy. Transfusion 26:410, 1986

99. Bossell J: Safety of therapeutic immune globulin preparations with respect to transmission of human T-lymphotropic virus type III/lymphadenopathy-associated virus infection. MMWR 35:231, 1986

100. Tedder RS, Uttley A, Cheingsong-Popov R: Safety of immunoglobulin containing anti-HTLV-III. Lancet 1:815, 1985

101. Lichtiger B, Rogge K: Spurious serologic test results in patients receiving infusions of intravenous immune gammaglobulin. Arch Pathol Lab Med 115:467, 1991

102. Arndt R, Hammerer P, Huland E et al: Treatment of acute cellular rejection in renal transplantation patients on cyclosporin with anti-thymocyte globulin. Urol Int 43:139, 1983

103. Norman DJ, Barry JM, Bennett WM et al: The use of OKT3 in cadaveric renal transplantation for rejection that is unresponsive to conventional anti-rejection therapy. Am J Kidney Dis 11:90, 1988

104. Marsh JC, Gordon-Smith EC: The role of antilymphocyte globulin in the treatment of chronic acquired bone marrow failure. Blood Rev 2:141, 1988

105. Hunter RF, Huang AT: Antithymocyte globulin: a realistic approach to therapy for severe aplastic anemia. South Med J 79:1121, 1986

106. Snydman DR, Werner BG, Heinze-Lacey B et al: Use of cytomegalovirus immune globulin to prevent cytomegalovirus disease in renal transplant recipients. N Engl J Med 317:1049, 1987

107. Reed EC, Bowden RA, Dandliker PS: Treatment of cytomegalovirus pneumonia with ganciclovir and intravenous cytomegalovirus immunoglobulin in patients with bone marrow transplants. Ann Intern Med 109:783, 1988

108. Practices Advisory Committee: Recommendations for protection against viral hepatitis. MMWR 34:313, 1985

109. Bowman JM: Suppression of Rh isoimmunization: a review. Obstet Gynecol 52:385, 1978

110. Bowman JM, Chown B, Lewis M, Pollock JM: Rh immunization during pregnancy: antenatal prophylaxis. Can Med Assoc J 118:623, 1978

111. Keith L, Bozorgl N: Small dose anti-Rh therapy after first trimester abortion. Int J Gynaecol Obstet 15:235, 1977

112. Baglin TP, Smith MP, Boughton BJ: Rapid and complete response of immune thrombocytopenic purpura to a single injection of rhesus anti-D immunoglobulin. Lancet 1:1329, 1986

113. Larsson C: Natural history and life expectancy in severe alpha$_1$-antitrypsin deficiency, Pi Z. J Intern Med 204:345, 1978

114. Gadek JE, Klein HG, Holland PV et al: Replacement therapy of alpha$_1$-antitrypsin deficiency: reversal of protease-antiprotease imbalance within the alveolar structures of PiZ subjects. J Clin Invest 68:1158, 1981

115. French Cooperative Group on plasma Exchange in Guillain-Barre Syndrome: Efficiency of plasma exchange in Guillain-Barre syndrome: role of replacement fluids. Ann Neurol 22:753, 1987

116. Brinson RR, Kolts BE: Hypoalbuminemia as an indicator of diarrheal incidence in critically ill patients. Crit Care Med 15:506, 1987

117. Ford EG, Jennings M, Andrassy RJ: Serum albumin (oncotic pressure) correlates with enteral feeding tolerance in the pediatric surgical patient. J Pediatr Surg 22:597, 1987

118. Brown RO, Bradley JE, Bekemeyer WB, Luther RW: Effect of albumin supplementation during parenteral nutrition on hospital mortality. Crit Care 16:1177, 1988

119. Foley EF, Borlase BC, Dzik WH et al: Albumin supplementation in the critically ill. Arch Surg 125:739, 1990

120. Stratta P, Canavese C, Dogliani M et al: Repeated albumin infusions do not lower blood pressure in preeclampsia. Clin Nephrol 36:234, 1991

121. Dawidson IJ, Sandor ZF, Coorpender L et al: Intraoperative albumin administration affects the outcome of cadaver renal transplantation. Transplantation 53:774, 1992

122. Awad AI, Carter LP, Spetzler RF et al: Clinical venospasm after subarachnoid hemorrhage: response to hypervolemic hemodilution and arterial hypertension. Stroke 18:365, 1987

123. Yamakami I, Isobe K, Yamaura A: Effects of intravascular volume expansion on cerebral blood flow in patients with ruptured cerebral aneurysms. Neurosurgery 21:303, 1987

124. Goslinga H, Eijzenbach V, Heuvelmans JH et al: Custom-tailored hemodilution with albumin and crystalloids in acute ischemic stroke. Stroke 23:181, 1992

125. Rarick MU, Montgomery T, Groshen S et al: Intravenous immunoglobulin in the treatment of human immunodeficiency virus-related thrombocytopenia. Am J Hematol 38:261, 1991

126. Macik BG, Gabriel DA, White GC et al: The use of high dose intravenous

gamma globulin in acquired von Willebrand syndrome. Arch Pathol Lab Med 112:143, 1988

127. Savery F, Hang LM: Immunodeficiency associated with motor neuron disease treated with intravenous immunoglobulin. Clin Ther 8:700, 1986

128. Besa EC: Rapid transient reversal of anemia and long-term effects of maintenance intravenous immunoglobulin for autoimmune hemolytic anemia in patients with lymphoproliferative disorders. Am J Med 84:691, 1988

129. MacIntyre EA, Linch DC, Macey MG, Newland AC: Successful response to intravenous immunoglobulin in autoimmune haemolytic anaemia. Br J Haematol 60:387, 1985

130. Munster AM: Infections in burns. p. 339. In Morell A, Nydegger UE (eds): Clinical Uses of Intravenous Immunoglobulins. Academic Press, San Diego, 1986

131. Jones RJ, Roe EA, Gupta JL: Controlled trial of Pseudomonas immunoglobulin and vaccine in burn patients. Lancet 2:1263, 1980

132. Shirani KZ, Vaughan GM, McManas AT et al: Replacement therapy with modified immunoglobulin G in burn patients: preliminary kinetic studies. Am J Med 76:175, 1984

133. Faed JM, Day B, Pollock M et al: High-dose intravenous human immunoglobulin in chronic inflammatory demyelinating polyneuropathy. Neurology 39:422, 1989

134. Vermeulen M, van der Meche FG, Speelman JD et al: Plasma and gammaglobulin infusion in chronic inflammatory polyneuropathy. J Neurol Sci 70:317, 1985

135. Gianella-Borradori A, Hirt A, Luthy A et al: Haemophilia due to factor VIII, inhibitors in a patient suffering from an autoimmune disease treatment with intravenous immunoglobulin: a case report. Blut 48:403, 1984

136. Sullivan KM: Immunoglobulin therapy in bone marrow transplantation. Am J Med 83:37, 1987

137. van der Meche FG, Kleijwcg RP, Meulstee J: Intravenous gammaglobulin (IVGG) versus plasmapheresis trial in patients with acute Guillain-Barre syndrome (GBS). Clin Neurol Neurosurg 89:62, 1987

138. Yap PL, Williams PE: Immunoglobulin preparation for HIV-infected patients. Vox Sang 55:65, 1988

139. Beard J, Savidge CF: High-dose intravenous immunoglobulin and splenectomy for the treatment of HIV-related immune thrombocytopenia in patients with severe haemophilia. Br J Haematol 68:303, 1988

140. Bussel JB, Hilgartner MW: The use and mechanism of action of intravenous immunoglobulin in the treatment of immune haematologic disease. Br J Haematol 56:1, 1984

141. Levine DS, Fischer SH, Christie DL et al: Intravenous immunoglobulin therapy for active, extensive, and medically refractory idiopathic ulcerative or Crohn's colitis. Am J Gastroenterol 87:91, 1992

142. Schedel I: Application of immunoglobulin preparations in multiple myeloma.

p. 123. In Morell A, Nydegger VE (eds): Clinical Use of Intravenous Immunoglobulins. Academic Press, San Diego, 1986

143. Arsura EL, Bick A, Brunner NG et al: High dose immunoglobulin in the treatment of myasthenia gravis. Arch Intern Med 146:1365, 1986

144. Fischer GW, Weisman LB, Hemming VG et al: Intravenous immunoglobulin in neonatal group B streptococcal disease. Am J Med 76:117, 1984

145. Chirico G, Rondini G, Plebani A et al: Intravenous gammaglobulin therapy for prophylaxis of infection in high-risk neonates. J Pediatr 110:437, 1987

146. The Intravenous Immunoglobulin Collaborative Study Group: Prophylactic intravenous administration of standard immune globulin as compared with core-lipopolysaccharide immune globulin in patients at high risk of postsurgical infection. N Engl J Med 327:234, 1992

147. Baker CJ, Melish ME, Hall RT et al: Intravenous immune globulin for the prevention of nosocomial infection in low-birth-weight neonates. N Engl J Med 327:213, 1992

148. Winston DJ, Pollard RB, Ho WG et al: Cytomegalovirus immune plasma in bone marrow transplantation recipients. Ann Intern Med 97:11, 1982

149. Condie RM, O'Reilly RJ: Prevention of cytomegalovirus infection by prophylaxis with an intravenous, hyperimmune, native, unmodified cytomegalovirus globulin. Am J Med 76:134, 1984

150. Winston DJ, Ho WG, Lin CH et al: Intravenous immunoglobulin for modification of cytomegalovirus infections associated with bone marrow transplantation. Am J Med 76:128, 1984

151. Filipovich AH, Peltier MH, Bechtel MK et al: Circulating cytomegalovirus (CMV) neutralizing activity in bone marrow transplant recipients: comparison of passive immunity in a randomized study of four intravenous IgG products administered to CMV-seronegative patients. Blood 80:2656, 1992

152. Combe B, Cosso B, Clot J et al: Human placenta-eluted gammaglobulins in immunomodulating treatment of rheumatoid arthritis. Am J Med 78:920, 1985

153. Pahwa RN: New and controversial uses of intravenous gamma-globulin. Pediatr Infect Dis J 7:S34, 1988

154. Kekomaki R, Elfenbein G, Gardner R et al: Improved response of patients refractory to random-donor platelet transfusions by intravenous gamma globulin. Am J Med 76:199, 1984

155. Schiffer CA, Hogge DE, Aisner J et al: High-dose intravenous gammaglobulin in alloimmunized platelet transfusion recipients. Blood 64:937, 1984

156. Becton, DL, Kinney TR, Chaffee S et al: High dose intravenous immunoglobulin for severe platelet alloimmunization. Pediatrics 74:1120, 1984

157. Kickler T, Braine HG, Piantadosi S et al: A randomized, placebo-controlled trial of intravenous gammaglobulin in alloimmunized thrombocytopenic patients. Blood 75:313, 1990

158. Tuso P, Moudgil A, Hay J et al: Treatment of antineutrophil cytoplasmic autoantibody-positive systemic vasculitis and glomerulonephritis with pooled intravenous gammaglobulin. Am J Kidney Dis 5:504, 1992

Preparation of Plasma-Derived and Recombinant Human Plasma Proteins 138

William N. Drohan and Craigenne A. Williams

INTRODUCTION

The development of large-scale methods for the preparation of human plasma proteins began >50 years ago. In 1940, after the outbreak of World War II, a meeting was called to discuss the urgent request of the United States Armed Forces for

300,000 U of human whole blood or plasma for transfusion, which at that time seemed an impossibly large amount.[1,2] Dr. Edwin J. Cohn of the Harvard Medical School was approached to determine whether animal plasma could be made safe for human use. Cohn drew together a task force of investigators and developed a method for the fractionation of bovine plasma based on differential precipitation of various plasma proteins achieved by appropriate combinations of ethanol concentration, pH, low temperature, ionic strength, and protein concentration. Within a short time, highly purified preparations of bovine serum albumin were available for clinical trials. Although there were no immediate reactions, the frequency of severe delayed reactions made it obvious that these preparations were unsuitable for clinical use. Meanwhile, Cohn had arranged with the American Red Cross to provide his laboratory with a supply of human plasma, and the ethanol method was quickly adapted for human plasma fractionation. While albumin was the only product distributed during the war, the remaining plasma fractions were carefully preserved, and other preparations, including fibrinogen and immunoglobulins, were soon developed.

Since World War II, major improvements have occurred in the preparation of human plasma proteins. The ethanol process has been supplemented by more selective purification techniques. A variety of methods have been developed for inactivation or removal of viruses that might be present in the starting materials, which may be pooled from the plasma of thousands of human donors.[3] During the past decade, advances in recombinant DNA technology have allowed recombinant human plasma proteins to be produced in tissue culture systems. This chapter describes current methods and future directions for the preparation of plasma-derived and recombinant human plasma proteins for clinical use.

FRESH FROZEN PLASMA

Plasma that has been frozen solid within 6 hours after phlebotomy and stored at $\leq 18°C$ meets the criteria for labeling as fresh frozen plasma (FFP).[4] Clinical indications for the administration of FFP are described in Chapter 137. At the present time, the viral safety of FFP depends entirely on donor selection and blood screening techniques. However, a method has recently been developed for the treatment of plasma with a solvent/detergent mixture to inactivate any lipid-enveloped viruses that might be present. The coagulation factor content of solvent/detergent-treated plasma has been found to be comparable to that of untreated FFP, but the safety and efficacy of solvent detergent-treated plasma will need to be determined in appropriate clinical trials.[5]

ALBUMIN AND PLASMA PROTEIN FRACTION

Albumin is still one of the major products of human plasma fractionation. During the 50 years since the initial use of human serum albumin in treating the casualties at Pearl Harbor, tons of albumin have been isolated and millions of units have been infused.[6] Cohn's method 6 is the basis for most of the large-scale production of albumin today.[7] Most manufacturers use cryoprecipitation as the first step in order to obtain the factor VIII/von Willebrand factor (vWF) complex, which can then be further purified by a variety of techniques. Factor IX complex and antithrombin III (AT III) may be separated from the cryosupernatant before it is processed by the ethanol method to obtain immunoglobulins and albumin. Albumin, having the highest solubility and the lowest isoelectric point of all the major plasma proteins, remains in solution as the ethanol concentration is raised in stages from 0% to 40%, with an overall decrease in pH from neutrality to 5.8 and a temperature adjustment to $-5°C$. It is only when the pH is adjusted to 4.8, in the presence of 40% ethanol at $-5°C$, that the bulk of the albumin is finally precipitated in fraction V.[6,8] After the removal of ethanol and salts, sodium acetyltryptophanate and sodium caprylate are added as stabilizers, and the albumin is filtered and

bottled. The vials are then held for 10 hours at $60°C$ to inactivate any remaining blood-borne viruses.

Three albumin products are manufactured in the United States: Albumin (human) 25%, Albumin (human) 5%, and plasma protein fraction (PPF). To be designated Albumin, $>96\%$ of the protein content must be albumin. PPF is an albumin product of lower purity, obtained by coprecipitating fraction IV-4 with fraction V.[9] The total protein in PPF must be $\geq 83\%$ albumin, with $\leq 17\%$ globulins, and $\leq 1\%$ γ-globulin. PPF is more economical to produce than albumin,[10] but the rapid infusion of PPF has been associated with hypotensive episodes.[11,12] Clinical indications for the use of Albumin and PPF are described in Chapter 137.

IMMUNOGLOBULINS

Immuno- and Hyperimmunoglobulins

Since the early 1950s, immunoglobulins have been prepared from the fraction II + III precipitate obtained by Cohn's method 6.[7] The precipitate is extracted to solubilize lipoproteins before IgA, IgM, and other plasma proteins are removed by an additional precipitation step.[13] The pH, ethanol concentration, and ionic strength at this step have a significant effect on the purity, recovery, and viral safety of these products.[14] Variations of this scheme continue to be used worldwide.[15] Immunoglobulin is prepared from the plasma of unselected normal donors, while hyperimmunoglobulins are prepared from the plasma of donors with high antibody titers against specific antigens (e.g., $Rh_0(D)$, hepatitis B, rabies, and tetanus). These donors may be identified during convalescent periods after infection or transfusion, or they may be specifically immunized to produce the desired antibodies. Immunoglobulin products currently available in the United States are described in Chapter 137.

These immunoglobulin concentrates are usually administered by the intramuscular route. The volumes injected are limited by the capacity of the muscle mass. Even moderate volumes may cause considerable discomfort at the injection site. The bioavailability may be diminished because of degradation by tissue proteases, and maximum blood levels may be reached only after delays of 2–7 days.[16] Attempts to overcome these problems by using the intravenous route caused serious clinical reactions, attributed to complement-activating aggregates in these products.[17] The removal of aggregates by centrifugation reduced the frequency of adverse reactions, but aggregates have reappeared during storage.

Intravenous Immunoglobulins

Intravenous immunoglobulin (IVIg) products have been developed using a variety of methods to remove or inactivate any anticomplementary aggregates. Processing and formulation techniques have been improved, and conditions have been identified to permit these products to be stored in liquid states.[18] In 1990, at the Consensus Development Conference on Intravenous Immunoglobulin, the Consensus Panel commented on the low incidence of adverse reactions to IVIg therapy and stressed that transmission of hepatitis B and human immunodeficiency virus-1 infection had not been reported following administration of products licensed in the United States at that time.[19] However, the potential for the transmission of hepatitis C virus cannot be disregarded, and most manufacturers have incorporated viral inactivation or removal steps in the production of IVIg.[20]

The development of IVIg has permitted the administration of much higher doses, with a subsequent expansion in immuno-

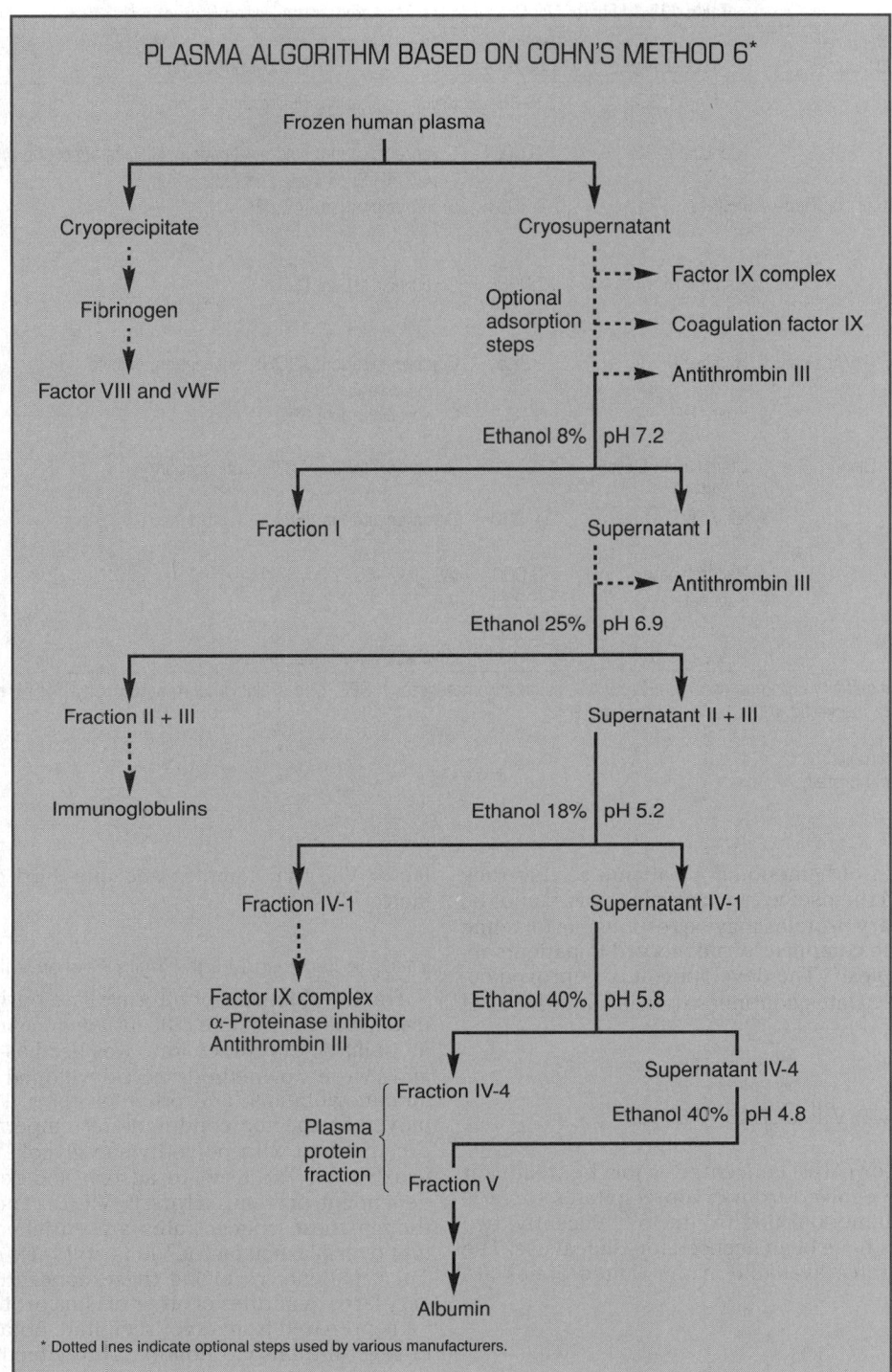

PLASMA ALGORITHM BASED ON COHN'S METHOD 6*

* Dotted lines indicate optional steps used by various manufacturers.

globulin therapy. In addition to providing passive immune protection, IVIg has been found to modulate the immune response to autoimmune diseases such as idiopathic thrombocytopenic purpura. Clinical indications for the use of IVIg are described in Chapter 137. It has been suggested that the clinical demand for this plasma derivative will become the driving factor in plasma fractionation by 1994.[21,22]

COAGULATION FACTOR CONCENTRATES

The distinction between hemophilia A and B was unknown when it was first shown that the transfusion of whole blood could be used to curtail bleeding in patients with hemophilia.[23]

By 1940, bleeding episodes were treated routinely with plasma. However, large amounts of plasma were needed, and this method of therapy could not provide normal levels of coagulation factors without producing hypervolemia.[24] The development of coagulation factor concentrates has resulted in dramatic increases in the life expectancy and the quality of life of patients with hemophilia.

The major issues in the preparation and use of coagulation factor concentrates are viral safety and purity. With the exception of cryoprecipitate, all these concentrates are now subjected to some form of treatment for the inactivation or removal of viruses that might be present in the starting materials. The purity may be important for both immediate and long-term safety. The use of low-purity factor VIII concentrates may affect

Table 138-1. Factor VIII Concentrates Marketed in the United States[a]

Antihemophilic Factor	Manufacturer/ Distributor	Product Name	Specific Activity[b]	Purification Methods	Virus Inactivation/ Removal Methods
Human	Alpha	Profilate OSD	2–10	Cryoprecipitation, PEG precipitation	Solvent/detergent: TNBP/polysorbate 80
	Armour	Monoclate-P	>3,000[c]	Cryoprecipitation, cold purification, Al(OH)$_3$ adsorption, IAC, AH-Sepharose chromatography	Pasteurization at 60°C for 10 hr
	Baxter/American Red Cross	AHF-M	~2,000[c]	Cryoprecipitation, IAC, IEC	Solvent/detergent: TNBP/Triton X-100; IAC, IEC
	Baxter	Hemofil M	~2,000[c]	Cryoprecipitation, IAC, IEC	Solvent/detergent: TNBP/Triton X-100; IAC, IEC
	Behringwerke/Armour	Humate-P	2–5	Cryoprecipitation, Al(OH)$_3$ adsorption, glycine precipitation	Pasteurization at 60°C for 10 hr
	Miles	Koāte-HP	9–22	Cryoprecipitation, SEC	Solvent/detergent: TNBP/polysorbate 80
	New York Blood Center	Coagulation factor VIII-SD	~1	Cryoprecipitation, Al(OH)$_3$ adsorption	Solvent/detergent: TNBP/sodium cholate
		MelATE	20–200	Cryoprecipitation, IEC	Solvent/detergent: TNBP/polysorbate 80
Recombinant	Baxter	Recombinate	>3,000[c]	IAC, IEC, IEC	Purification steps
	Miles	Kogenate	>3,000[c]	IAC, SEC, IEC	Inactivation/purification steps
Porcine	Porton	Hyate-C	>15[d]	Polyelectrolyte fractionation	Unknown

Abbreviations: IAC, immunoaffinity chromatography; IEC, ion exchange chromatography; SEC, size exclusion chromatography; TNBP, tri-n-butyl phosphate.
[a] These concentrates were marketed in the United States in 1993.
[b] Factor VIII U/mg protein.
[c] Prior to addition of human albumin.
[d] Porcine factor VIII μm/mg protein.

the immune responses of hemophilia A patients so that they are less able to defend themselves against infections,[25] and the presence of unnecessary proteins may be responsible for some of the thromboembolic complications observed in patients receiving factor IX complex.[26] The development of improved coagulation factor concentrates continues to be a major focus of research.[27]

Factor VIII Concentrates

Antihemophilic factor (AHF) concentrates for the treatment of hemophilia A have evolved from cryoprecipitates to very-high-purity immunoaffinity-purified products.[28] Recently, two recombinant products have been licensed for clinical use. The various AHF concentrates available in the United States are shown in Table 138-1.

Cryoprecipitate

In 1959, Pool and Robinson[29] reported that when frozen plasma is slowly thawed, a residual cryoprecipitate contains most of the factor VIII activity from the original plasma. By 1965, single-donor cryoprecipitate with factor VIII concentrations 5–20 times that of plasma became widely available for use in the treatment of hemophilia A.[30] While single-donor cryoprecipitate now has only limited clinical use, cryoprecipitation has become an established procedure for the preparation of plasma fractions containing high concentrations of the factor VIII/vWF complex, fibrinogen, fibronectin, and factor XIII.[31] Cryoprecipitation results from the formation of regions of high concentrations of proteins and salts during the freezing of plasma. Under these conditions, some of the higher molecular weight plasma proteins undergo a phase transition. The cryoprecipitate formed may contain approximately one-half of the

factor VIII/vWF complex and one-third of the fibrinogen and factor XIII.[32]

Intermediate- and High-Purity Factor VIII Concentrates

The development of intermediate-purity factor VIII concentrates was the next significant advance in the treatment of hemophilia A. Cryoprecipitate was used as the starting material, and a variety of methods were developed to remove fibrinogen, immunoglobulins, and other proteins. Fibrinogen can be removed at specific conditions of temperature and pH[33] or by precipitation with polyethylene glycol,[34] while aluminum hydroxide may be used to adsorb and remove the vitamin K-dependent protein factors II, VII, IX, and X.[34] However, even though these concentrates are enriched approximately 400-fold over plasma, factor VIII is still >1% of the total protein.[35] Thus, patients receiving these concentrates are exposed to very large quantities of other plasma proteins. In addition, each lot is prepared from cryoprecipitate obtained from the plasma of several thousand donors. Until effective methods were developed for viral inactivation, patients receiving these concentrates were exposed to all blood-borne viruses in the donor population. It is not surprising that frequently treated patients uniformly became infected with hepatitis B[36] and hepatitis C.[37]

Intermediate-purity factor VIII concentrates were the mainstay of hemophilia A treatment until the development of high-purity concentrates in the late 1980s. Various ion-exchange and gel filtration techniques have been added to the precipitation methods so that concentrates have specific activities of 10–50 U/mg of protein, in contrast to <10 U/mg for intermediate-purity factor VIII and <1 U/mg for cryoprecipitate.[22,25,38] However, even though these concentrates are highly purified in comparison with the intermediate-purity concentrates, high-molecular-weight proteins that tend to fractionate with factor VIII remain in these preparations. The major contaminants continue to be fibrinogen, fibronectin, and vWF.[39]

Factor VIII Concentrates Purified by Immunoaffinity Chromatography

The next major advance in the preparation of factor VIII concentrates was the use of murine monoclonal antibodies to factor VIII or to vWF for the immunoaffinity purification of factor VIII. Two different procedures are used in this approach. Both start with low-purity factor VIII concentrates partially purified by conventional means. In one procedure, the factor VIII concentrate is pasteurized in aqueous solution for viral inactivation, and a monoclonal anti-vWF is used to bind the factor VIII/vWF complex. After washing the column to remove other proteins and possible residual viral contaminants, factor VIII is separated from vWF by a high-ionic-strength calcium chloride solution, leaving the vWF bound to the immobilized antibody.[40] The factor VIII is further purified using an aminohexyl/agarose column to remove any remaining impurities, including any murine IgG that might have been leached from the column. After elution from the aminohexyl/agarose column, the product is approximately 99% pure. Human albumin is added as a stabilizer.[41]

The other procedure employs a monoclonal antibody to factor VIII itself. After treating a low-purity factor VIII concentrate with a solvent/detergent mixture, the factor VIII is bound directly to the column. The column is washed using buffers that remove other proteins, including vWF, and the factor VIII is eluted with 40% ethylene glycol. After further purification by ion exchange chromatography to remove any murine IgG and other impurities, this product is also stabilized by the addition of human albumin.[42]

Recombinant Factor VIII Concentrates

One of the remarkable accomplishments of molecular biologists during the past decade has been the elucidation of the structure of factor VIII, as well as its molecular cloning and the successful production of recombinant human factor VIII. Almost simultaneously, two groups cloned the entire factor VIII gene, the largest gene cloned at that time, and isolated a cDNA encoding the structural regions of the factor VIII molecule.[43–46]

Because post-translational processing is essential to factor VIII, both groups have expressed the factor VIII molecule in mammalian cells. Both groups manufactured sufficient quantities of recombinant factor VIII to allow extensive in vitro characterization and clinical evaluation.[47,48] The production of recombinant factor VIII by one group was initially achieved by expression of the protein in a Chinese hamster ovary tissue culture cell line. It was then recognized that co-expression of vWF cDNA in the same cells resulted in an increased secretion of factor VIII into the culture medium.[48] The recombinant factor VIII is purified by immunoaffinity and ion-exchange chromatography, so that the final product contains minimal vWF and only trace quantities of mouse immunoglobulin, hamster protein, and cellular DNA. The product is essentially pure prior to the addition of human albumin to stabilize the recombinant factor VIII. This factor has been shown to be similar to plasma-derived factor VIII in its peptide and carbohydrate composition.[49]

The other process for recombinant factor VIII manufacture uses baby hamster kidney cells; the product is also immunoaffinity purified and it contains minimal amounts of mouse IgG, hamster protein, and cellular DNA.[50] The electrophoretic pattern of the recombinant factor VIII in sodium dodecyl sulfate polyacrylamide gels is the same as that of purified plasma-derived factor VIII.[47,51–53] In vitro analysis has established that recombinant factor VIII can not be distinguished from plasma-derived factor VIII in functional clotting assays or in its response to thrombin and other proteases.[47,50–52,54]

On the basis of clinical studies, two recombinant factor VIII preparations have been licensed for the treatment of hemophilia A.[53,55,56] The synthesis of large quantities of safe material may permit the prophylactic treatment of hemophilic patients so that joint and soft tissue bleeds can be prevented.

Factor IX Concentrates

Two types of factor IX concentrates are available today: factor IX complex, which contains significant amounts of the other vitamin K-dependent proteins, including factors II, VII, and X; and coagulation factor IX, a generic name for preparations that are substantially free of these other proteins. The factor IX concentrates available in the United States are shown in Table 138-2.

Factor IX Complex Concentrates

The vitamin K-dependent clotting factors, because of their similar structures, tend to co-purify by most of the methods used to isolate them from plasma. Thus, the initial preparations containing factor IX for treatment of hemophilia B were in fact complex mixtures of the vitamin K-dependent proteins. Because the protein in highest concentration in these materials is prothrombin, they have also been identified as prothrombin

Table 138-2. Factor IX Concentrates and Other Related Products Marketed in the United States[a]

Product Type	Manufacturer/ Distributor	Product Name	Specific Activity[b]	Purification Methods	Virus Inactivation/ Removal Methods
Factor IX complex	Alpha	Profilnine heat-treated	4–5	IEC	Heat treatment in n-heptane suspension at 60°C for 20 hr
	Baxter	Proplex T	NA	Tricalcium phosphate adsorption	Dry heat treatment at 60°C for 144 hr
	Immuno	Bebulin VH	NA	NA	Vapor heating[c]
	Miles	Konÿne 80	~1	IEC	Dry heat treatment at 80°C for 72 hr
Coagulation factor IX (human)	Alpha	AlphaNine SD	≥50	IEC, barium citrate adsorption, dual AC steps	Solvent/detergent: TNBP/polysorbate 80; IEC, dual AC steps
	Armour	Mononine	≥150	IEC, IAC, AH-Sepharose chromatography	Sodium thiocyanate; IAC, ultrafiltration
Anti-inhibitor coagulant complex	Baxter	Autoplex T	NA	NA	Dry heat treatment at 60°C for 144 hr
	Immuno	FEIBA VH	NA	NA	Vapor heating[c]

Abbreviations: NA, not available; AC, affinity chromatography; IAC, immunoaffinity chromatography; IEC, ion exchange chromatography; TNBP, tri-n-butyl phosphate.
[a] These concentrates were marketed in the United States in 1993.
[b] Factor IX U/mg protein.
[c] At 60°C for 10 hr at 190 ± 25 mbar, then at 80°C for 1 hr at 375 ± 35 mbar.

complex concentrates. However, factor IX complex is the generic name in the United States.

The first factor IX-rich concentrate used for the treatment of hemophilia B was developed in France >30 years ago.[57] It was produced by the adsorption of the plasma vitamin K-dependent clotting factors with tricalcium phosphate and was successfully used to treat hemophilia B for a number of years. However, the original production process had a number of disadvantages, including the need to collect the plasma specially in EDTA, a step that prevented factor VIII preparation from the plasma, and it was eventually discontinued.[58] However, this method led to the development of several other processes based on tricalcium phosphate adsorption in ways that did not interfere with the purification of other products.[59] Factor IX complex produced by these methods contains approximately equal amounts of factors II, VII, IX, and X activity units.

The next major development in the production of prothrombin complex concentrates was the introduction of ion exchange chromatography using DEAE-cellulose or DEAE-Sephadex.[60] This represented one of the first major uses of chromatography in plasma fractionation. As shown in the box, the vitamin K-dependent clotting factors can be removed from the cryosupernatant of plasma by adsorption onto DEAE-cellulose or DEAE-Sephadex and the plasma can then be further fractionated by Cohn's method for the production of immunoglobulin and albumin. The eluate from the DEAE resin may be further purified by additional precipitation or adsorption steps.[61,62] Such processes give 100-fold or more purification of factors II, IX, and X. Factor VII does not bind to DEAE under the conditions used, however, and is present at only very low concentrations in concentrates prepared in this way.

Coagulation Factor IX

With the widespread use of factor IX complex, it became apparent that thromboembolic episodes were a serious complication of their infusion, especially when used in large quantities for extended periods, such as for surgical procedures or in patients with liver disease.[63] As discussed in Chapter 139, the cause of the thrombogenicity has not been rigorously defined; it is thought to be due to the presence of activated clotting factors,[64] and possibly contaminating phospholipids.[65] It has also been suggested that these complications may be the result of zymogen overload, that is, the administration of large and unnecessary quantities of factors II and X in the factor IX complex preparations.[66,67] These factors persist in the circulation (half-lives of about 4 days and 30–50 hours, respectively, compared with about 20 hours for factor IX), so that they accumulate after repeated infusions of the complex, upsetting the normal balance and leading to a hypercoaguable state.[68]

On the basis of this hypothesis, methods have been developed for the preparation of second-generation factor IX concentrates that are essentially free of the other vitamin K-dependent clotting factors. These have been designated coagulation factor IX concentrates. Coagulation factor IX concentrates are manufactured from factor IX complex by one or more additional steps, either chromatography on sulfated dextran,[67] a second DEAE column and a heparin-Sepharose column,[69] or barium citrate adsorption followed by an affinity column.[70] All these methods also include a viral inactivation step. These preparations have been shown to be nonthrombogenic when compared with factor IX complex in animal models[67,69–72] and also in clinical studies.[70,73–77] Coagulation factor IX concentrates have also been prepared by immunoaffinity chromatography using monoclonal antibodies to factor IX.[78,79] Clinical studies with one of these preparations has shown it to be effective in stopping bleeding episodes. The evidence for absence of thrombogenicity includes measurement of prothrombin fragment F_{1+2} levels as a marker for activation of the clotting system, as well as clinical observations.[80]

Other Coagulation Factor Concentrates

As described in Chapter 139, one of the major complications in the treatment of hemophilic patients is the development of inhibitors, antibodies directed against factors VIII or IX. While low-titer inhibitors can be saturated by administering large amounts of factor VIII or factor IX, this may not be feasible when the inhibitor level is >5–10 Bethesda U/ml plasma.[81] It is known that some antibodies to factor VIII inactivate porcine factor VIII less readily than the human protein.[82] A porcine factor VIII concentrate has been developed to take advantage of this difference and has been quite effective in the treatment of patients with inhibitor antibodies to factor VIII.[82–85] The critical factor for repeated use of porcine factor VIII, anamnesis with development of high-titer inhibitor levels against porcine factor VIII, is seen in approximately one-third of patients.[84]

In that case, one method of treatment for hemophilia A inhibitor patients is to administer either factor IX complex or a specially activated factor IX complex termed anti-inhibitor coagulant complex to "bypass" factor VIII.[86,87] These concentrates are effective in 50–60% of the cases, but thromboembolic complications have occurred in some patients treated in this way. The "bypass" rationale has led to the use of activated factor VII for treatment of both hemophilia A and B patients with inhibitors.[88] Highly purified plasma-derived factor VIIa has been infused in two hemophiliacs with antibodies to factor VIII.[89] The bleeding episodes appeared to respond, encouraging the belief that factor VIIa has an effective factor VIII bypassing activity. Subsequently, the cDNA for factor VII was cloned in 1986, and a mammalian expression system was used to produce the protein.[90] Factor VII produced in these cells possesses full biologic activity, and the biochemical characterization of the recombinant protein demonstrated complete modification of the γ-carboxyglutamic acid residues. Activation to factor VIIa occurs spontaneously during purification. Clinical trials with the recombinant product are now under way, and preliminary results are encouraging in that a number of factor VIII inhibitor patients have been successfully treated. As it is impossible to purify enough factor VIIa from plasma to prepare a useful therapeutic concentrate for widespread patient use, the recombinant molecule provides an opportunity to evaluate the potential of this approach.[88,91] A recombinant factor VIIa preparation is now in clinical trials.[92] Should it be shown to be effective, recombinant factor VIIa may replace anti-inhibitor coagulant complex in the treatment of hemophilic patients with inhibitors to factor VIII or factor IX.

Patients with von Willebrand disease (vWD) have been treated with plasma, with cryoprecipitate, and with factor VIII concentrates that contain variable amounts of vWF. It is known that lyophilized factor VIII concentrates are usually deficient in the higher molecular weight multimeric forms of vWF. As early as 1984, Nilsson et al.[93] recognized that intermediate-purity and high-purity concentrates of factor VIII lacking these multimers did not correct the vWD hemostatic defect. This observation was confirmed in 1988, when it was shown that nine high-purity concentrates lacking the largest vWF multimers also failed to correct the vWD defect.[94] While not a good in vitro predictor of hemostatic response, ristocetin cofactor activity is usually less than expected from the amount of vWF protein in factor VIII concentrates. By contrast, cryoprecipitate has a population of vWF multimers similar to that of normal plasma, and the ratio of ristocetin cofactor activity to vWF antigen is close to 1.[95–99] Numerous studies have verified that the infusion of cryoprecipitate temporarily corrects the vWD hemostatic defect, and consequently it would be the treatment of choice for vWF if it could be sterilized to avoid transmission of blood-borne viruses.

Mannucci et al.[100] compared the effectiveness of four lyophilized virus-inactivated concentrates for their ability to establish factor VIII and vWF plasma levels and to correct bleeding time in patients with severe vWD. The concentrates examined were an intermediate-purity, pasteurized factor VIII/vWF concentrate; an intermediate-purity, dry-heated factor VIII/vWF concentrate; a solvent/detergent-treated vWF concentrate, containing little factor VIII; and a high-purity solvent/detergent-treated factor VIII/vWF concentrate. Although the pasteurized factor VIII/vWF concentrate transiently corrected the bleeding times in most patients, partially or completely, none of the four concentrates consistently normalized it.

FIBRIN SEALANTS

Fibrin sealants, or fibrin glues, are topical hemostatic agents that have been used in a variety of surgical situations for their hemostatic and adhesive properties.[101–105] The preparations consist of two components that are mixed together immediately prior to use. The first component is derived from human plasma and contains fibrinogen, factor XIII, fibronectin, and small amounts of other plasma proteins, while the second component is a thrombin solution derived from either bovine or human plasma. The preparation of the fibrinogen component is particularly critical, because the fibrinogen quality and concentration are the primary determinants of the tensile strength of the clot. Depending on the manufacturer, the fibrinogen may be isolated directly from plasma by an ethanol precipitation step[106] or from cryoprecipitate as a by-product of the preparation of factor VIII.[107]

Although preparations of fibrin sealant have been available in Europe since the mid-1970s, the U.S. Food and Drug Administration revoked all licenses for the manufacture of fibrinogen concentrates in 1978. These high-molecular-weight protein preparations, obtained from pooled plasma, had hepatitis virus contamination.[108] Although the several fibrinogen preparations are now treated for viral inactivation, none has yet been approved for use in the United States.[29,106,107]

Fibrin sealant has been advocated by many surgeons as the material that best approaches the ideal operative sealant.[104] It appears to have no tissue toxicity, forms a firm seal within seconds, is completely readsorbed within days or weeks following application, and may promote local tissue growth and repair.[101,103,104] In the absence of licensed products, a variety of methods have been used to prepare fibrin sealant for use in the treatment of individual patients.[105] However, the methods are somewhat cumbersome, and the concentration of fibrinogen in these preparations is highly variable.[102] The use of a standardized manufactured product should increase the likelihood of uniform performance in the surgical field.[104]

PLASMA PROTEINASE INHIBITORS

The proteinase inhibitors that are present in human plasma play critical roles in the regulation of the proteolytic cascades of the coagulation, fibrinolytic, complement, and kinin systems. Most of these inhibitors have similar amino acid and structural properties and are members of a superfamily of proteins designated serpins, (serine proteinase inhibitors).[109] Hereditary deficiencies of α_1-antitrypsin, AT III, and C1 esterase inhibitor can cause specific disease states, and inhibitor concentrates have

been developed. The plasma proteinase inhibitor concentrates available in the United States are shown in Table 138-3.

α_1-Proteinase Inhibitor

α_1-Proteinase inhibitor (API) was the first of the serpins to be isolated and characterized.[110] Although the protein was originally named for its antitrypsin activity, its primary physiologic function appears to be the inhibition of neutrophil elastase. Patients with hereditary deficiencies of this inhibitor develop pulmonary emphysema and liver disease.

API therapy is indicated for chronic treatment of individuals with hereditary deficiency who have clinical evidence of panacinar emphysema. Weekly intravenous infusions are recommended in order to maintain an adequate level of functional API in the epithelial lining of the lower respiratory tract.[111] However, intravenous administration is an inefficient therapy; it has been estimated that only 2% of the infused API is present in the lung. A recent clinical study suggests that it may be possible to deliver API to the lung by aerosol. If confirmed in larger trials, aerosol therapy could replace intravenous administration because of its lower cost and greater convenience.[112]

An API concentrate prepared from human plasma is licensed for use in the United States. The product is prepared from Cohn fraction IV-1 by fractional precipitation with polyethylene glycol followed by ion exchange chromatography on DEAE-Sepharose. The API is pasteurized by heating in solution for 10 hours at 60°C to ensure viral inactivation.[113,114]

A recombinant API concentrate has also been prepared.[115] Unlike plasma-derived API, recombinant API made in *Escherichia coli* is not glycosylated. This means that aerosol therapy would be the only method of administering recombinant API, since the nonglycosylated recombinant protein is rapidly excreted in the urine after intravenous administration.[116] However, using recombinant DNA techniques, it may be possible to modify the API molecule so as to give it advantageous new properties, such as resistance to oxidation and a broader antiprotease inhibitory spectrum.[112]

Antithrombin III

AT III, as the major physiologic inhibitor of thrombin and factor Xa, plays a critical role in the regulation of hemostasis. Heterozygous hereditary deficiency of AT III has been linked to an increased tendency toward thrombosis.[117] Acquired deficiencies have also been reported in women on oral contraceptives and as a consequence of pregnancy, surgery, cirrhosis, and hepatic malignancies.

The affinity of heparin for AT III, essential for the pharmacologic effect of the drug, can also be employed as a means of purifying AT III. Use of immobilized heparin as an affinity adsorbent for AT III[118] is the key step in large-scale preparation of AT III concentrates for clinical use.[119] As shown in the box, AT III may be isolated from cryosupernant,[120] from Cohn fraction I supernatant,[107,121] or from Cohn fraction IV-1.[122] While heparin-based adsorbents are not specific for AT III, other plasma proteins are bound less tightly and may be washed off with medium-ionic-strength buffers prior to the elution of AT III with a high-ionic-strength buffer. Although these eluates may contain small amounts of other proteins, an additional purification step makes possible concentrates that contain >95% AT III.[119] All the AT III concentrates now being manufactured are pasteurized by heating in solution for 10 hours at 60°C to inactivate blood-borne viruses. Clinical studies by a number of investigators have shown that these AT III concentrates are effective in the prophylaxis or treatment of thromboembolic disorders in patients with hereditary AT III deficiency.[123,124] However, the

Table 138-3. Plasma Proteinase Inhibitor Concentrates Marketed in the United States[a]

Product Type	Manufacturer/ Distributor	Product Name	Specific Activity	Purification Methods	Virus Inactivation/ Removal Methods
α_1-Proteinase inhibitor (human)	Miles	Prolastin	≥ 0.35[b]	Ethanol fractionation, PEG precipitation, IEC	Pasteurization at 60°C for 10 hr
Antithrombin III (human)	Kabi/Baxter	ATnativ	NA	AC, IEC	Pasteurization at 60°C for 10 hr
	Miles	Thrombate III	~8[c]	Ethanol fractionation, dual AC steps	Pasteurization at 60°C for 10 hr

Abbreviations: AC, affinity chromatography; IEC, ion exchange chromatography; NA, not available.
[a] These concentrates were marketed in the United States in 1993.
[b] Milligrams functional α_1-PI/mg protein.
[c] AT III U/mg protein.

benefit of AT III therapy in acquired deficiencies is as yet uncertain, and careful clinical trials are needed.

C1 Esterase Inhibitor

C1 esterase inhibitor (C$\bar{\text{I}}$-INH) plays an important role in the regulation of the complement system cascade. In 1963, it was established that a deficiency of C$\bar{\text{I}}$-INH is the underlying biochemical defect in hereditary angioedema, an autosomal-dominant disease that is characterized by episodic swelling of the subcutaneous tissues and the mucosa of the gastrointestinal and respiratory tracts.[125] The swelling can lead to acute airway obstruction, a major cause of mortality among patients with this disease.[126] FFP has been used in replacement therapy for the treatment of acute attacks as well as for short-term prophylaxis prior to surgery, but the volume of plasma needed and the time required for thawing and infusion are drawbacks to this approach.[127]

C$\bar{\text{I}}$-INH concentrates are not yet licensed in the United States, although preparations have been available in Europe for several years.[107,128–131] C$\bar{\text{I}}$-INH concentrates have been used there for short-term and long-term prophylaxis, as well as for treatment of acute episodes of hereditary angioedema. The products are treated for viral inactivation and are supplied as freeze-dried concentrates that can be stored in a refrigerator.

FUTURE DIRECTIONS

During the previous several years almost all plasma proteins licensed for human use have been cloned and expressed in a biologically active form in animal cells.[132] However, since most of these proteins include a complex post-translational modification, few have been produced at commercially viable levels in animal cells. A notable exception to this observation is the recent licensure of two recombinant human factor VIII preparations.[49,54] Recombinant human factor VIII, while synthesized in mammalian cells at relatively low levels, appears to be very similar in structure and function to factor VIII isolated from human plasma. More importantly, after worldwide evaluation of recombinant factor VIII in clinical trials, the in vivo recovery and half-life were seen to be similar to that reported for the plasma-derived material.[53,133] After comprehensive clinical evaluation recombinant factor VIII was deemed to be safe[134] and effective in preventing and treating hemorrhagic episodes in hemophilia A patients.[55,135]

It is not yet evident which recombinant plasma protein will be next to be licensed in the United States. Although factors IX and VII have been cloned and the encoded recombinant proteins produced in animal cells for many years, neither protein is licensed in the United States. It appears that overproduction of vitamin K-dependent proteins in tissue culture systems generates protein that is not properly modified and consequently is biologically inactive.[136] In general, as the expression level of these proteins increases in mammalian tissue culture systems, the specific activity of the protein decreases, suggesting that one or more of the post-translational modifications is limiting during overexpression.[137] Other plasma proteins such as fibrinogen and albumin have been cloned and expressed by a variety of laboratories, but remain untested in clinical trials. The reasons for this include the inability to produce these proteins in adequate quantities or in the inappropriate post-translational modification of the recombinant protein.[138,139]

Transgenic Animal Production of Human Plasma Proteins

Advances in molecular biology and embryology have led to the production of plasma proteins in the milk of genetically engineered farm animals.[140] This technology has overcome at least one of the apparent shortcomings of tissue culture production systems. Farm animals (goats, pigs, and sheep) can produce large quantities of human proteins whose genes have been genetically engineered to be expressed in mammary epithelial cells and subsequently secreted into the animals' milk (1–10 g/L), while animal tissue culture systems routinely produce substantially less protein ($\leq 10–100$ mg/L).[141] In addition, transgenic animals appear to be able to perform most of the post-translational modifications required for protein activity, even when the protein is being made at relatively high levels of production.[141] The production of biologically active human protein C at >1 g/L and API at >6 g/L has been reported.[142] Although neither of these proteins is yet being evaluated in clinical trials, the production of human plasma proteins in transgenic animals is an attractive alternative to their isolation from human plasma or production in tissue culture systems. Proteins produced in transgenic animals should be free of human viruses, less expensive to produce, and available in unlimited quantities.

Gene Therapy

Of course, the most satisfying solution to human gene deficiencies would be the replacement of the functional gene in the affected individual so the consequence of the gene abnormality goes unnoticed. To this end, numerous investigators have attempted to insert a functional gene encoding a plasma protein into animals, with the hope of demonstrating the permanent expression of the encoded protein in the animals' plasma. A number of issues must be addressed before this approach can be applied to human disease. An appropriate cell type must be identified that can permanently express the recombinant protein in a biologically active form in the host. Expression levels of the protein must be optimized and controlled, and the long-term effect of gene expression on the animal needs to be better understood. These and other difficult questions must be answered before gene therapy can become a reality in the treatment of human disease.

REFERENCES

1. Janeway CA: Human serum albumin: historical review. p. 3. In Sgouris JT, René A (eds): Proceedings of the Workshop on Albumin. US Government Printing Office, Washington, DC, 1976
2. Palmer JW: The evolution of large-scale human plasma fractionation in the United States. p. 255. In Sgouris JT, René A (eds): Proceedings of the Workshop on Albumin. US Government Printing Office, Washington, DC, 1976
3. Suomela H: Inactivation of viruses in blood and plasma products. Transfus Med Rev 7:42, 1993
4. Consensus Conference: Fresh-frozen plasma: indications and risks. JAMA 253:551, 1985
5. Horowitz B, Bonomo R, Prince AM et al: Solvent/detergent-treated plasma: a virus-inactivated substitute for fresh frozen plasma. Blood 79:826, 1992
6. Finlayson JS: Albumin products. Semin Thromb Hemost 6:85, 1980
7. Cohn EJ, Strong LE, Hughes WL Jr et al: Preparation and properties of serum and plasma proteins. IV. A system for the separation into fractions of the proteins and lipoprotein components of biological tissues and fluids. J Am Chem Soc 68:459, 1946
8. More JE, Harvey MJ: Purification technologies for human plasma albumin. p. 261. In Harris JR (ed): Blood Separation and Plasma Fractionation. Wiley-Liss, New York, 1991
9. Hink JH Jr, Hidalgo J, Seeberg VP, Johnson FF: Preparation and properties of a heat-treated human plasma protein fraction. Vox Sang 2:174, 1957
10. Ng PK, Fournel MA, Lundblad JL: Plasma protein fraction: product improvement studies. Transfusion 21:682, 1981
11. Bland JHL, Laver MB, Lowenstein E: Vasodilator effect of commercial 5% plasma protein fraction solutions. JAMA 224:1721, 1973
12. Alving BM, Hojima Y, Pisano JJ et al: Hypotension associated with prekallikrein activator (Hageman-factor fragments) in plasma protein fraction. N Engl J Med 299:66, 1978
13. Oncley JL, Melin M, Richert A et al: The separation of the antibodies, isoagglutinins, prothrombin, plasminogen and β_1-lipoprotein into subfractions of human plasma. J Am Chem Soc 71:541, 1949
14. Rousell RH, McCue JP: Antibody purification from plasma. p. 307. In Harris J (ed): Blood Separation and Plasma Fractionation. Wiley-Liss, New York, 1991
15. Stryker MH, Bertolini MJ, Hao Y: Blood fractionation: proteins. p. 275. In Mizrahi A, Van Wezel AL (eds): Advances in Biotechnological Processes 4. Wiley-Liss, New York, 1985
16. Nydegger UE: Immunoglobulins in clinical medicine. p. 383. In Rossi EC, Simon TL, Moss GL (eds): Principles of Transfusion Medicine. Williams & Wilkins, Baltimore, 1991
17. Barandun S, Kistler P, Jeunet F, Isliker H: Intravenous administration of human γ-globulin. Vox Sang 7:157, 1962
18. Drohan WN, Hoyer LH: Preparation of plasma products. In Anderson KC, Ness PM (eds): Scientific Basis of Transfusion Medicine. WB Saunders, Philadelphia, 1993
19. NIH Consensus Conference: Intravenous immunoglobulin: prevention and treatment of disease. JAMA 264:3189, 1990
20. Hämäläinen E, Suomela H, Ukkonen P: Virus inactivation during intravenous immunoglobulin purification. Vox Sang 63:6, 1992
21. Stagnaro TP: Impact of new technology on plasma industry marketplace. PLASMApheresis 3:206, 1989
22. Brodniewicz-Proba T: Human plasma fractionation and the impact of new technologies on the use and quality of plasma-derived products. Blood Rev 5:245, 1991
23. Lane S: Haemorrhagic diathesis. Successful transfusion of blood. Lancet 1:185, 1840
24. Roberts HR: Highly purified factor VIII concentrates. p. 167. In Kasper CK (ed): Recent Advances in Hemophilia Care. Alan R Liss, New York, 1990
25. Smith JK: Trends in the production and use of coagulation factor concentrates. p. 93. In Smit Sibinga CT, Das PC, Mannucci PM (eds): Coagulation and Blood Transfusion. Kluwer Academic Publishers, Dordrecht, The Netherlands, 1990
26. Smith KJ: Factor IX concentrates: the new products and their properties. Transfus Med Rev 6:124, 1992
27. Clark DB, Drohan WN, Miekka SI, Katz AJ: Strategy for purification of coagulation factor concentrates. Ann Clin Lab Sci 19:196, 1989
28. Kasper CK, Lusher JM, Transfusion Practices Committee: Recent evolution of clotting factor concentrates for hemophilia A and B. Transfusion 33:422, 1993
29. Pool JG, Robinson J: Observations on plasma banking and transfusion procedures for haemophilic patients using a quantitative assay for antihaemophilic globulin (AHG). Br J Haematol 5:24, 1959
30. Pool JG, Shannon AE: Production of high-potency concentrates of antihaemophilic globulin in a closed bag system. N Engl J Med 273:1443, 1965
31. Farrugia A, Grasso S, Douglas S et al: Modulation of fibrinogen content in cryoprecipitate by temperature manipulation during plasma processing. Transfusion 32:755, 1992
32. Feldman P, Winkelman L: Preparation of special plasma products. In Harris JR (ed): Blood Separation and Plasma Fractionation. Wiley-Liss, New York, 1991
33. Smith JK, Evans DR, Stone V, Snape TJ: A factor VIII concentrate of intermediate purity and higher potency. Transfusion 19:299, 1979
34. Newman J, Johnson AJ, Karpatkin MH, Puszkin S: Methods for the production of clinically effective intermediate- and high-purity factor-VIII concentrates. Br J Haematol 21:1, 1971
35. Weinstein RE: Immunoaffinity purification of factor VIII. Ann Clin Lab Sci 19:84, 1989
36. Gerety RJ, Eyster ME, Tabor E et al: Hepatitis B virus, hepatitis A virus, and persistently elevated aminotransferases in hemophiliacs. J Med Virol 6:111, 1980
37. Kim HC, Saidi P, Ackley AM et al: Prevalence of type B and non-A, non-B hepatitis in hemophilia: relationship to chronic liver disease. Gastroenterology 79:1159, 1980
38. Bloom AL: Progress in the clinical management of haemophilia. Thromb Haemost 66:166, 1991
39. Gomperts ED, de Biasi R, De Vreker R: The impact of clotting factor concentrates on the immune system in individuals with hemophilia. Tranfus Med Rev 6:44, 1992
40. Tuddenham EGD, Trabold NC, Collins JA, Hoyer LW: The properties of factor VIII coagulant activity prepared by immunoadsorbent chromatography. J Lab Clin Med 93:40, 1979
41. Zimmerman TS: Purification of factor VIII by monoclonal antibody affinity chromatography. Semin Hematol, suppl. 1. 25:25, 1988
42. Griffith MJ: Biochemical characterization of method M AHF process developed to reduce the risk of hepatitis transmission. p. 69. In Roberts HH (ed): Proceedings of the Symposium on Biotechnology and the Promise of Pure Factor VIII. Baxter Healthcare Publications, Brussels, Belgium, 1988
43. Gitschier J, Wood WI, Goralka TM et al: Characterization of the human factor VIII gene. Nature 312:326, 1984
44. Wood WI, Capon DJ, Simonsen CC et al: Expression of active human factor VIII from recombinant DNA clones. Nature 312:330, 1984
45. Vehar GA, Keyt B, Eaton D et al: Structure of human factor VIII. Nature 312:337, 1984
46. Toole JJ, Knopf JL, Wozney JM et al: Molecular cloning of a cDNA encoding human antihaemophilic factor. Nature 312:342, 1984
47. Eaton DL, Hass PE, Riddle L et al: Characterization of recombinant human factor VIII. J Biol Chem 262:3285, 1987
48. Kaufman RJ, Wasley LC, Dorner AJ: Synthesis, processing and secretion of recombinant human factor VIII expressed in mammalian cells. J Biol Chem 263:6352, 1988
49. Gomperts E, Lundblad R, Adamson R: The manufacturing process of recombinant factor VIII, Recombinate. Transfus Med Rev 6:247. 1991
50. Klein U: Production and characterization of recombinant factor VIII. Semin Hematol 28:17, 1991
51. Giles AR, Tinlin S, Hoogendoorn H et al: In vivo characterization of recombinant factor VIII on a canine model of hemophilia A (factor VIII deficiency) Blood 72:335, 1988
52. Fournel MA: Preclinical and in vitro studies of recombinant factor VIII. Semin Hematol 28:22, 1991
53. Schwartz RS: Clinical trials of factor VIII produced by recombinant technology. p. 229. In Hoyer LW, Drohan WN (eds): Recombinant Technology in Hemostasis and Thrombosis. Plenum Press, New York, 1991
54. Boedeker BGD: The manufacturing of the recombinant factor VIII, Kogenate. Transfus Med Rev 6:256, 1992
55. White GC II, McMillan CW, Gomperts ED et al: Clinical trials of recombinant factor VIII. p. 235. In Hoyer LW, Drohan WN (eds): Recombinant Technology in Hemostasis and Thrombosis. Plenum Press, New York, 1991
56. Mannucci PM, Gringeri A, Cattaneo M: Use of recombinant factor VIII in the management of hemophilia. p. 46. In Albertini A, Lenfant CL, Mannucci PM, Sixma JJ (eds): Biotechnology of Plasma Proteins. Karger, Basel, 1991
57. Didisheim P, Loeb J, Blatrix C, Soulier JP: Preparation of a human plasma fraction rich in pro-thrombin, proconvertin, Stuart factor, and PTC and a study of is activity and toxicity in rabbits and man. J Lab Clin Med 53:322, 1959
58. Soulier JP: The history of PPSB. Vox Sang 46:58, 1984
59. White GC, Lundblad RL, Kingdon HS: Prothrombin complex concentrates: preparation, properties, and clinical uses. Curr Top Hematol 2:203, 1979
60. Heysteck J, Brummelhuis HGJ, Krijnen HW: Contributions to the optimal use of human blood. II. The large-scale preparation of prothrombin complex.

A comparison between two methods using the anion exchangers DEAE-cellulose DE 52 and DEAE-Sephadex A-50. Vox Sang 25:113, 1973

61. Bidwell E, Dike GW, Snape TJ: Therapeutic materials. p. 275. In Biggs R (ed): Human Blood Coagulation, Haemostasis and Thrombosis. 2nd Ed. Blackwell Scientific Publications, Oxford, 1976

62. Aronson DL: Factor IX concentrates. p. 78. In Sandberg HE (ed): Proceedings of the International Workshop on Technology for Protein Separation and Improvement of Blood Plasma Fractionation. US Government Printing Office, Washington, DC, 1978

63. Kasper CK: Thromboembolic complications. Thromb Diath Haemorrh 33: 640, 1975

64. Hultin MB: Activated clotting factors in factor IX concentrates. Blood 54: 1028, 1979

65. Giles AR, Nesheim ME, Hoogendorn H et al: The coagulant-active phospholipid content is a major determinant of in vivo thrombogenicity of prothrombin complex (factor IX) concentrates in rabbits. Blood 59:401, 1982

66. Magner A, Aronson DL: Toxicity of factor IX concentrates in mice. Dev Biol Stand 44:185, 1979

67. Menache D, Behre HE, Orthner CL et al: Coagulation factor IX concentrate: method of preparation and assessment of potential in vivo thrombogenicity in animal models. Blood 64:1220, 1984

68. Murano G: Commercial preparations of vitamin-K dependent factors and their use in therapy. p. 131. In Seegers WH, Walz DA (eds): Prothrombin and Other Vitamin K Proteins, Vol. II. CRC Press, Boca Raton, FL 1986

69. Burnouf T, Michalski C, Goudemand M et al: Properties of a highly purified human plasma factor IX:c therapeutic concentrate prepared by conventional chromatography. Vox Sang 57:225, 1989

70. Herring S, Abramson S, Kasper C et al: A highly purified factor IX concentrate. XVIII International Congress, World Federation of Hemophilia, Madrid, 1988

71. Clark DB, Menache D, Gee DM et al: Coagulation factor IX for replacement therapy in hemophilia B patients. p. 315. In Stoltz JF, Rivat C (eds): Biotechnology of Plasma Proteins. Colloque INSERM, 175, Paris, 1989

72. Macgregor IR, Ferguson JM, McLaughlin LF et al: Comparison of high purity factor IX concentrates and a prothrombin complex concentrate in a canine model of thrombogenicity. Thromb Haemost 66:609, 1991

73. Menache D: Coagulation factor IX concentrate: properties and clinical evaluation. Thromb Haemost 54:282, 1985

74. Novak P, Kasper C, Goldsmith J, Gomperts E: Clinical studies using a highly purified factor IX concentrate. Thromb Haemost 62:182, 1989

75. Bardin JM, Sultan Y: Factor IX concentrate versus prothrombin complex concentrate for the treatment of hemophilia B during surgery. Transfusion 30:441, 1990

76. Novak P, Bauer K, Blatt P et al: Clinical studies using a coagulation factor IX concentrate. XIX International Congress, World Federation of Hemophilia, Washington, DC, 1990

77. Menache D, Clark DB, Miekka SI et al: Coagulation factor IX (human). p. 301. In Lusher JM, Kessler CM (eds): Hemophilia and von Willebrand's Disease in the 1990's. Elsevier, Amsterdam, 1991

78. Tharakan J, Strickland D, Burgess W et al: Development of an immunoaffinity process for factor IX purification. Vox Sang 58:21, 1990

79. Hrinda ME, Huang C, Tarr GC et al: Preclinical studies of a monoclonal antibody-purified factor IX, Mononine™. Semin Hematol, suppl. 6. 28:6, 1991

80. Kim HC, Matts L, Eisele J et al: Monoclonal antibody-purified factor IX—comparative thrombogenicity to prothrombin complex concentrate. Semin Hematol 28:15, 1991

81. Kasper CK, Aledort LM, Counts RB et al: A more uniform measurement of factor VIII inhibitors. Thromb Diath Haemorrh 34:869, 1975

82. Kernoff PBA, Thomas ND, Lilley PA et al: Clinical experience with polyelectrolyte-fractionated porcine factor VIII concentrate in the treatment of hemophiliacs with antibodies to factor VIII. Blood 63:31, 1984

83. Hultin MB, Hennessey J: The use of polyelectrolyte-fractionated porcine factor VIII in the treatment of a spontaneously acquired inhibitor to factor VIII. Thromb Res 55:51, 1989

84. Brettler DB, Forsberg AD, Levine PH et al: The use of porcine factor VIII concentrate (Hyate:C) in the treatment of patients with inhibitor antibodies to factor VIII: a multicenter US experience. Arch Intern Med 149:1381, 1989

85. Kernoff PBA: The clinical use of porcine factor VIII. p. 47. In Kasper CK (ed): Recent Advances in Hemophilia Care. Alan R Liss, New York, 1990

86. Fekete L, Holst S, Peetoom F et al: Auto factor IX concentrate: a new therapeutic approach to treatment of hemophilia A patients with inhibitors. The XIV International Congress of Hematology, 1972

87. Lusher JM, Blatt PM, Penner JA et al: Autoplex versus proplex: a controlled double-blind study of effectiveness in acute hemarthroses in hemophiliacs with inhibitors to factor VIII. Blood 62:1135, 1983

88. Hedner U: Experiences with recombinant factor VIIa in hemophiliacs in recombinant technology. p. 223. In Hoyer LH, Drohan WN (eds): Hemostasis and Thrombosis. Plenum Press, New York, 1991

89. Hedner U, Kisiel W: Use of human FVIIa in the treatment of two haemophilia A patients with high titre inhibitors. J Clin Invest 71:1836, 1983

90. Hagen FS, Gray CL, O'Hara P et al: Characterization of a cDNA coding for human factor VII. Proc Natl Acad Sci USA 83:2412, 1986

91. Hedner U, Glazer S, Pingel K et al: Successful use of recombinant factor VIIa in patient with severe haemophilia A during synovectomy. Lancet 2:1193, 1988

92. Meulien P, Tuddenham EGD: Genetically engineered and affinity purified plasma proteins. Baillieres Clin Haematol 3:451, 1990

93. Nilsson IM, Borge L, Gunnarsson M, Kristoffersson AC: Factor VIII related activities in concentrates. Scand J Hematol, suppl. 41. 33:157, 1984

94. Berntorp E, Nilsson IM: Biochemical and in vivo properties of commercial virus-inactivated factor VIII concentrates. Eur J Haematol 40:205, 1988

95. Weinstein M, Deykin D: Comparison of factor VIII-related von Willebrand factor proteins prepared from human cryoprecipitate and factor VIII concentrates. Blood 53:1095, 1979

96. Barrowcliffe TW, Kemball-Cook G, Morris G et al: Factor VIII-related activities in therapeutic concentrates. J Lab Clin Med 97:429, 1981

97. Hill FGH, Enayat MS: Multimeric analysis of eight lyophilized factor VIII concentrates. Br J Haematol 60:201, 1985

98. Fricke AF, Yu MW: Characterization of von Willebrand factor in factor VIII concentrates. Am J Hematol 31:41, 1989

99. Lawrie AS, Harrison P, Armstrong AL et al: Comparison of the in vitro characteristics of von Willebrand factor in British and commercial factor VIII concentrates. Br J Haematol 73:100, 1989

100. Mannucci PM, Tenconi PM, Castaman G, Rodeghiero F: Comparison of four virus-inactivated plasma concentrates for treatment of severe von Willebrand disease: a cross-over randomized trial. Blood 79:3130, 1992

101. Matras H: Fibrin seal: the state of the art. J Oral Maxillofac Surg 43:605, 1985

102. Thompson DF, Letassy NA, Thompson GD: Fibrin glue: a review of its preparation, efficacy, and adverse effects as a topical hemostat. Drug Intell Clin Pharm 22:946, 1988

103. Toti F, Follea G, Delannee C et al: Biological glues: present status and further prospects. p. 81. In Stoltz JF, Rivat C (eds): Biotechnology of Plasma Proteins: Fractionation and Applications. Inserm, Paris, 1989

104. Gibble JW, Ness PM: Fibrin glue: the perfect operative sealant? Transfusion 30:741, 1990

105. Brennan M: Fibrin glue. Blood Rev 5:240, 1991

106. Burnouf-Radosevich M, Burnouf T, Huart JJ: Biochemical and physical properties of a solvent-detergent-treated fibrin glue. Vox Sang 58:77, 1990

107. Fuhge P, Gratz P, Geiger H: Modern methods for the manufacture of coagulation factor concentrates. Transfus Sci 11:23S, 1990

108. Bove JR: Fibrinogen: is the benefit worth the risk? Transfusion 18:129, 1978

109. Carrell R, Travis J: α_1-Antitrypsin and the serpins: variation and countervariation. Trends Biochem Sci 10:20, 1985

110. Schultze HE, Heide K, Haupt H: Alpha$_1$-antitrypsin aus Humanserum. Klin Wochenschr 40:427, 1962

111. Hubbard RC, Crystal RG: Alpha-1-antitrypsin augmentation therapy for alpha-1-antitrypsin deficiency. Am J Med 84:52, 1988

112. Hubbard RC, Crystal RG: Strategies for aerosol therapy of α_1-antitrypsin deficiency by the aerosol route. Lung, suppl.:565, 1990

113. Hein RH, Van Beveren SM, Shearer MA, et al: Production of alpha$_1$-proteinase inhibitor (human). Eur Respir J, suppl. 9. 3:16s, 1990

114. Coan MH, Dobkin MB, Brockway WJ, Mitra G: Characterization and virus safety of alpha$_1$-proteinase inhibitor. Eur Respir J, suppl. 9. 3:35s, 1990

115. Hubbard RC, McElvaney NG, Sellers SE et al: Recombinant DNA-produced α_1-antitrypsin administered by aerosol augments lower respiratory tract antineutrophil elastase defenses in individuals with α_1-antitrypsin deficiency. J Clin Invest 84:1349, 1989

116. Courtney M, Jallat A, Tessier L-H et al: Synthesis in E. coli of alpha 1-antitrypsin variants with potential in the therapy of emphysema and thrombosis. Nature 313:149, 1985

117. Bock SC: Antithrombin III, genetics, structure and function in recombinant technology. p. 25. In Hoyer LW, Drohan WN (eds): Recombinant Technology in Hemostasis and Thrombosis. Plenum Press, New York, 1991

118. Miller-Andersson M, Borg H, Andersson LO: Purification of antithrombin III by affinity chromatography. Thromb Res 5:439, 1974

119. Nunez H, Drohan WN: Purification of antithrombin III (human). Semin Hematol 28:24, 1991

120. Wickerhauser M, Williams C, Mercer J: Development of large scale fractionation methods. VII. Preparation of antithrombin III concentrate. Vox Sang 36: 281, 1979

121. Eketorp R, Engman L, Johansson L et al: A large-scale purification method for antithrombin III (applied to the Cohn fractionation procedure). p. 321.

In Sandberg HE (ed): Proceedings of the International Workshop on Technology for Protein Separation and Improvement of Blood Plasma Fractionation. US Government Printing Office, Washington, DC, 1978

122. Hoffman DL: Purification and large-scale preparation of antithrombin III. Am J Med, suppl. 3B. 87:23S, 1989

123. Menache D: Replacement therapy in patients with hereditary antithrombin III deficiency. Semin Hematol 28:31, 1991

124. Hathaway WE: Clinical aspects of antithrombin III deficiency. Semin Hematol 28:19, 1991

125. Donaldson VH, Evans RR: A biochemical abnormality in hereditary angioneurotic edema: absence of serum inhibitor of C1-esterase. Am J Med 35: 37, 1963

126. Atkinson JP: Diagnosis and management of hereditary angioedema (HAE). Ann Allergy 42:348, 1979

127. van Aken WG: Preparation of plasma derivatives. p. 323. In Rossi EC, Simon TL, Moss GL (eds): Principles of Transfusion Medicine. Williams & Wilkins, Baltimore, 1991

128. Bergamaschini L, Cicardi M, Tucci A et al: C1 INH concentrate in the therapy of hereditary angioedema. Allergy 38:81, 1983

129. Logan RA, Greaves MW: Hereditary angio-oedema: treatment with C1 esterase inhibitor concentrate. J R Soc Med 77:1046, 1984

130. Bork K, Günther W: Long-term prophylaxis with C1-inhibitor (C1 INH) concentrate in patients with recurrent angioedema caused by hereditary and acquired C1-inhibitor deficiency. J Allergy Clin Immunol 83:677, 1989

131. Laxenaire MC, Audibert G, Janot C: Use of purified C_1 esterase inhibitor in patients with hereditary angioedema. Anesthesiology 72:956, 1990

132. Drohan WN, Hoyer LH: Plasma protein products. p. 381. In Anderson KC,

Ness PM (eds): Scientific Basis of Transfusion Medicine. WB Saunders, Philadelphia, 1993

133. Harrison JFM, Bloom AL, Abildgaard CF: The pharmacokinetics of recombinant factor VIII. Semin Hematol 28:29, 1991

134. Kasper CK: Comments on adverse reactions with recombinant factor VIII. Semin Hematol 28:43, 1991

135. Arkin S, Rose E, Forster A, Aledort LM: Clinical efficacy of recombinant factor VIII. Semin Hematol 28:47, 1991

136. Limentani SA, Roth DA, Furie BC, Furie B: Recombinant blood clotting proteins for hemophilia therapy. Semin Thromb Hemost 19:62, 1993

137. Kaufman RJ, Wasley LC, Furie BC et al: Expression, purification, and characterization of recombinant carboxylated factor IX synthesized in Chinese hamster ovary cells. J Biol Chem 261:9622, 1986

138. Saunders LW, Schmidt BJ, Mallona RL et al: Secretion of human serum albumin from *Bacillus subtilis*. J Bacteriol 169:2917, 1987

139. Latta M, Kanpp M, Sarmientos P et al: Synthesis and purification of mature human serum albumin from *E. coli*. Bio/Technology 5:1309, 1987

140. Paleyanda R, Young J, Velander W, Drohan W: The expression of therapeutic proteins in transgenic animals. p. 197. In Hoyer LW, Drohan WN (eds): Recombinant Technology in Hemostasis and Thrombosis. Plenum Press, New York, 1991

141. Wright G, Carver A, Cottom D et al: High level expression of active human alpha-1-antitrypsin in the milk of transgenic sheep. Bio/Technology 9:830, 1991

142. Velander WH, Johnson JL, Page RL et al: High-level expression of a heterologous protein in the milk of transgenic swine using the cDNA encoding human protein C. Proc Natl Acad Sci USA 89:12003, 1992

Transfusion Principles for Congenital Coagulation Disorders

139

Joan Cox Gill

INTRODUCTION

Rapid advances in knowledge over the past several decades have led to an increased understanding of both hemorrhagic and thrombophilic plasma deficiency states and to the development of sophisticated therapeutic products to replace many of the deficient proteins. This chapter outlines the general principles of replacement transfusion therapy for clotting factor and other plasma protein deficiencies and provides recommendations for the use of transfusion and pharmacologic products for these disorders.

GENERAL PRINCIPLES OF PLASMA PROTEIN TRANSFUSION THERAPY

Of major importance in the consideration of therapeutic options for a particular patient is the establishment of an accurate diagnosis and determination of the severity of the patient's coagulopathy. Because hemostasis testing is often technically difficult and time-consuming, the clinician who relies on an inexperienced laboratory will have great difficulty in the treatment of a patient when the proper diagnosis is masked by laboratory artifact. Therefore, a high-quality and experienced coagulation laboratory should be used.

Once an accurate diagnosis has been established and the severity of the plasma protein deficiency has been determined, replacement therapy and other therapeutic maneuvers can be planned to restore balance to the hemostatic system. For a rational approach, one must first know the hemostatic level that must be achieved to treat a particular clinical manifestation.[1] For example, it has been established that patients with hemophilia A require 30–40% of normal factor VIII levels to control joint hemorrhages[2]; however, for major surgery, a 100% correction is desirable.[3] Hemostatic levels have been established for most of the coagulation factors and are summarized in Table 139-1.

Second, the in vivo volume of distribution of the plasma pro-

Table 139-1. Characteristics of Coagulation Factors Important for Transfusion Therapy

Factor	Factor Source (Concentration)	Minimal Hemostatic Level[a] (U/dl)	Desired Initial Level for Major Surgery (U/dl)	Increase in Plasma Level with Dose of 1 U/kg (U/dl)	Biologic Half-Life	Initial Dose[e]
Fibrinogen (I)	Cryoprecipitate (200–300 mg/bag)	75–150 mg/dL	150 mg/dL	—[b]	4–5 days	2–3 bags/15 kg daily
Prothrombin (II)	Fresh frozen plasma[c] PCC[d]	15–40	40	1.0	3 days	12–20 ml/kg 40 U/kg
V	Fresh frozen plasma	10–25	30	1.5	12–36 hr	15–20 ml/kg
VII	Fresh frozen plasma PCC[d]	5–10	25	1.0	4–6 hr	10–20 ml/kg 20–50 U/kg
VIII[f]	Cryoprecipitate (100 U/bag) Factor VIII concentrate (preferred)	30–50	100	2.0	12–15 hr	50 U/kg
IX[f]	Factor IX concentrate (preferred)	20–50	80	1.0	18–30 hr	80 U/kg
X	Fresh frozen plasma PCC[d]	10–20	25	1.0	1.5–2.5 days	15–20 ml/kg 25 U/kg
XI	Fresh frozen plasma	10–30	30	2.0	1–3 days	15–20 ml/kg
XIII	Fresh frozen plasma Cryoprecipitate (50–100 U/bag)	1–5	5	1–3	3–10 days	10 ml/kg 1 bag/20 kg
von Willebrand factor	Humate P	30–50	80	2.0	12–15 hr	40 U/kg

[a] The lower value is the minimal hemostatic level required for treatment of minor bleeding and the higher value is the maintenance nadir level required for treatment of major bleeds and surgery.

[b] 10–20 ml/kg fresh frozen plasma or 1 donor U (bag)/5 kg cryoprecipitate will raise the plasma fibrinogen level 50–100 mg/dl.

[c] One ml of plasma containing approximately 1 U factor activity.

[d] Prothrombin complex concentrate; factor VII content variable; see text of this chapter and Chapters 106, 108, 110, 111, and 138 for further details.

[e] For severe deficiency for surgery.

[f] See Table 139-2.

tein must be considered. The volume of distribution differs for each protein because of varying molecular size, interaction with other plasma proteins, and interaction with cellular elements of blood as well as the endothelial cell. The dose needed to raise the plasma level a desired amount has been determined by recovery and half-life studies for the various coagulation factor proteins and is included in Table 139-1. For example, it is known that infusion of 1 U factor VIII/kg body weight will result in a 2% (2 U/dl) rise in plasma factor VIII. Thus, a 70-kg man with severe hemophilia A (<1 U/dl factor VIII) would require 20 U/kg or 1,400 U factor VIII to achieve a 40% (U/dl) factor VIII level, the effective hemostatic level known to achieve hemostasis for a significant hemarthrosis.

Third, knowledge of the half-life of the infused protein is necessary if the plasma level of the coagulation factor must be maintained over time as is necessary in perioperative management. For example, in the postoperative treatment of hemophilia A, since factor VIII has a 12-hour half-life, in order to maintain a plasma factor VIII level >40–50% (U/dl), a 50% (25 U/kg) correction every 12 hours must be administered. The biologic half-lives of the coagulation factors are listed in Table 139-1.

Finally, the concentration of the coagulation factor in the product must be known in order to calculate the amount of product to be administered. Fresh frozen plasma, because of its content of approximately 1 IU/ml of each of the coagulation factors, can theoretically be used to treat any plasma protein deficiency, but frequently the dose needed to attain a particular in vivo hemostatic level would result in circulatory volume overload. Therefore, the coagulation factor concentrates, because of their convenience and now increased safety over most

plasma and cryoprecipitate products, have become the preferred method of treatment for most disorders; the amount contained in each vial is printed on the label. In cases of life-threatening bleeding or major surgery, or if the patient is not responding clinically as expected, daily laboratory monitoring of factor levels is advisable. A detailed description of the preparation and properties of products containing coagulation factor proteins is found in Chapter 138.

THERAPY FOR PROCOAGULANT DEFICIENCIES

Hemophilia A

Once the diagnosis of hemophilia A (factor VIII deficiency) has been established, the clinician may choose from a variety of therapeutic alternatives to treat bleeding manifestations or to prepare the patient for surgery, tooth extractions, or other invasive procedures. The desired concentration of plasma factor VIII (hemostatic level) to be achieved depends on the type and location of the bleed or planned procedure. Two dose classifications are generally accepted. For tooth extractions, routine joint and muscle hemorrhages, and lacerations one should attain a plasma factor VIII level of 30–40% (U/dl) (Table 139-2). By contrast, more aggressive replacement therapy (80–100% [U/dl] plasma factor VIII) should be instituted for patients undergoing major surgery or with limb- or life-threatening bleeding episodes such as central nervous system bleeding, hemorrhage around the neck or retroperitoneum, and compartment syndromes from muscle or subcutaneous

Table 139-2. Treatment of Specific Hemorrhages in Hemophilia

Type of Bleed	Hemophilia A	Hemophilia B
Hemarthrosis[a]	20 U/kg factor VIII concentrate[b]; 15 U/kg if treated early; repeat dose the following day if severe bleed	30 U/kg factor IX concentrate[c]; 20 U/kg if treated early
Muscle or significant subcutaneous hematoma	20 U/kg factor VIII concentrate; may need q48h treatment until well controlled	30 U/kg factor IX concentrate[c]; may need q2–3d treatment until well controlled
Mouth, deciduous tooth, or tooth extraction	20 U/kg factor VIII concentrate; antifibrinolytic therapy; remove loose deciduous tooth	30 U/kg factor IX concentrate[c]; antifibrinolytic therapy[d]; remove loose deciduous tooth
Epistaxis	Pressure for 15–20 minutes; pack with vaseline gauze; antifibrinolytic therapy; 20 U/kg factor VIII concentrate if above fails	Pressure for 15–20 minutes; pack with vaseline gauze; antifibrinolytic therapy; 30 U/kg factor IX concentrate if above fails (4 hours after antifibrinolytic dose)
Major surgery, life-threatening hemorrhage (e.g., central nervous system, gastrointestinal, airway)	50 U/kg factor VIII concentrate, then 25 U/kg q12h or continuous infusion to maintain factor VIII >50 U/dl for 5–7 days and then >30 U/dl for 5–7 days	80 U/kg factor IX concentrate[c], then 20–40 U/kg q12–24h to maintain factor IX >40 U/dl for 5–7 days and then >30 U/dl for 5–7 days[c]
Ileopsoas hemorrhage	50 U/kg factor VIII concentrate, then 25 U/kg q12h until asymptomatic, then 20 U q48h for total 10–14 days[e]	80 U/kg factor IX concentrate,[c] then 20–40 U/kg q12–24h to maintain factor IX >40 U/dl until asymptomatic, then 30 U q48h for total 10–14 days[c][e]
Hematuria	Bed rest; 1.5 × maintenance fluids; if not controlled in 1–2 days, 20 U/kg factor VIII concentrate; if not controlled, prednisone if HIV negative	Bed rest; 1.5 × maintenance fluids; if not controlled in 1–2 days, 30 U/kg factor IX concentrate; if not controlled, prednisone if HIV negative

[a] For hip hemarthrosis, orthopedic evaluation for possible aspiration is advisable.

[b] For mild or moderate hemophilia, DDAVP, 0.3 μg/kg should be used instead of factor VIII concentrate if patient is known to respond with a hemostatic level of factor VIII; if repeated doses are given, monitor factor VIII levels for tachyphylaxis.

[c] If repeated doses of factor IX concentrate are given, highly purified coagulation factor IX concentrate should be used.

[d] Do not give antifibrinolytic therapy until 4–6 hours following a dose of prothrombin complex factor IX concentrate.

[e] Repeat radiologic assessment should be performed prior to discontinuation of therapy.

hemorrhage. Calculation of the dose required to achieve a desired hemostatic level is based on the following formula[4]:

$$\begin{aligned}\text{Dose of factor VIII (IU)} &= \% \text{ (U/dl) desired rise} \\ &\quad \text{plasma factor VIII} \times \text{body weight (kg)} \times 0.5\end{aligned}$$

Thus, for treatment of a hemarthrosis in a 70-kg man with severe hemophilia A, the dose would be 40 (U/dl) × 70 (kg) × 0.5 = 1,400 IU factor VIII.

For patients undergoing major surgery or with serious hemorrhage, the plasma factor VIII level should initially be corrected to 100% (U/dl) immediately prior to the procedure, if for surgery, and then maintained at >40–50% (U/dl) for 5–7 days and then at >20–30% (U/dl) for an additional 5–7 days (Table 139-2). This can be accomplished by infusion of intermittent doses of factor VIII based on the half-life of 12 hours, for example, by administration of 25 U/kg (50% [U/dl] correction) every 12 hours. Alternatively, a 50% (U/dl) level can be maintained by continuous infusion of 2 IU factor VIII/kg/hr (0.4 IU/kg/hr/% [U/dl] desired factor VIII level).[5] It is advisable to administer a 50% (U/dl) correction of factor VIII concentrate immediately following major surgery in order to compensate for the loss of factor VIII by increased consumption and blood loss during the surgical procedure. For surgical procedures and limb- and life-threatening hemorrhages, a factor VIII assay should be monitored at least daily. Central nervous system bleeding requires a full 2 weeks of therapy, and patients are at increased risk of recurrence for approximately 6 months after an episode. Iliopsoas and other retroperitoneal hemorrhage must be treated aggressively with maintenance of a 50% (U/dl) plasma factor VIII level until symptoms have abated; it is then possible to taper the factor VIII therapy to every other day for a total of 10–14 days.

For treatment of more routine bleeding, such as hemarthro-

sis, usually only a single dose of clotting factor replacement (plasma factor VIII level 30–40% [U/dl]) is required. However, with severe joint bleeds or in the case of many muscle bleeds, additional infusions of factor VIII must be given. Generally, administration of a 40% correction every other day for 7–10 days, or until a muscle hemorrhage or large subcutaneous hematoma has nearly resolved, is adequate. For tooth extractions, mouth lacerations, or recurrent epistaxis, it is often helpful to use antifibrinolytic therapy as an adjunct (Table 139-2).

Therapy Products

Recombinant Factor VIII Concentrates

The factor VIII gene has been cloned, sequenced, and successfully transfected into mammalian cell cultures to produce recombinant factor VIII.[6,7] Two recombinant factor VIII products have recently been licensed (Recombinate and Kogenate). Clinical trials have documented that the half-life, recovery, and efficacy of recombinant factor VIII is indistinguishable from plasma-derived factor VIII.[8,9] The clear advantage to use of recombinant factor VIII is safety from human viral contamination, making these products preferable to plasma-derived concentrates in most cases if cost is not an issue. Speculation that the incidence of inhibitor development may be increased in previously untreated patients awaits larger studies with longer follow-up.[10,11]

Plasma-Derived Factor VIII Concentrates

At present, several commercial plasma-derived factor VIII concentrates are available. Concentrates of intermediate purity are produced from large pools of plasma by combinations of cryoprecipitation and precipitation with glycine, polyethylene glycol, or ethanol.[12] These products contain, on the average, 2–5 antihemophilic factor (AHF) (factor VIII) U/mg protein.

More recently, products of high purity have been developed. These products, also derived from large pools of human plasma, are produced by immunopurification of cryoprecipitate on monoclonal antibody columns utilizing mouse monoclonal antibodies to factor VIII[13] or von Willebrand factor (vWF).[14] Extraneous proteins are washed from the column, the factor VIII is eluted, albumin is added as a stabilizer (resulting in 2–15 AHF U/mg protein), and the final product is lyophilized. Products produced by gel filtration chromatography are also considered to be of high purity and contain approximately 9–22 AHF U/mg protein, similar to the monoclonal antibody-purified factor VIII concentrates after albumin has been added during the formulation. The diversity of foreign antigens contaminating the products is higher, however, since the specific activity is 35–60 AHF U/mg protein prior to the addition of albumin, whereas the monoclonal antibody immunopurification results in 1,500–2,500 AHF U/mg protein prior to the addition of albumin.

With improved purity of plasma-derived products, the frequency of complications due to exposure to extraneous plasma proteins has greatly diminished. Complications such as allergic reactions, isohemagglutinin-induced hemolytic anemia, immune complex-mediated hematuria, and granulocyte antibody-induced acute lung injury are rarely seen. Use of monoclonal antibody immunopurified concentrates appears to stabilize CD4 counts in human immunodeficiency virus-(HIV)-infected hemophilic patients.[15,16]

All plasma protein concentrates now undergo a viral attenuation process in addition to purification. Dry heating in the lyophilized state from 60°C to 68°C for 30–72 hours, initially developed to eliminate hepatitis from concentrates, was soon shown to be ineffective for this purpose: hepatitis C developed in most treated patients[17]; however, it was fairly effective in reduction of HIV transmission, although a few cases were reported. With the development of improved viral attenuation methods, all dry-heated factor VIII concentrates of intermediate purity were removed from the market. Newer virus attenuation methods include heating in the "wet" state (pasteurization), solvent/detergent treatment with a variety of agents, vapor heating, superdry heat (80°C for 72 hours), and affinity chromatography plus dry heat or solvent/detergent treatment; these methods have been successful in eliminating HIV seroconversions and possibly hepatitis C.[18] The exceptions have included the transmission of hepatitis C in products heated in n-heptane and probable transmission of hepatitis A in products treated with a particular solvent/detergent method.[19] Parvovirus can be transmitted by all current virus-inactivated human plasma-derived concentrates.[20] The risk of hepatitis B transmission can be further diminished by scrupulous immunization at the time of diagnosis of all patients, including infants, with one of the currently approved hepatitis B vaccines.[21] If clotting factor replacement therapy is needed at the time of diagnosis, hepatitis B immunoglobulin with the first dose of vaccine may provide passive protection until vaccine-induced antibodies are formed. Family members of chronic carriers of hepatitis B antigen and those involved in the preparation and administration of clotting factor concentrates should be immunized as well.

Factor VIII concentrates are formulated in vials that may be stored either refrigerated or, for short periods, at room temperature. These commercial products are packaged in vials with the number of units of activity of the coagulation factor printed on the label, and most packages also contain diluent and needles necessary for reconstitution and administration of the product; thus, they are very convenient for outpatient use and home care.

Cryoprecipitate

The first widely used concentrated factor VIII preparation, cryoprecipitate, was prepared by Judith Graham Poole in 1965.[22] Since that time technical advances have improved the yield of factor VIII in cryoprecipitate, and the preparations now generally contain approximately 100 IU factor VIII/bag. Thus, the patient with hemophilia A would require exposure to 2–16 donor U (bags) for treatment of a single routine hemorrhage, in comparison with the 10,000–20,000 donor exposures associated with exposure to a single lot of commercial concentrate. Prior to the development of effective viral attenuation of commercial lyophilized factor VIII concentrates, cryoprecipitate was safer from transfusion-transmitted viral disease because of the reduced number of donor exposures. However, with the exception of carefully screened, small-donor-pool cryoprecipitate, viral attenuated concentrates are now preferred because cryoprecipitate cannot easily be viral attenuated.[15]

Desmopressin

Desmopressin (1-desamino-8-D-arginine vasopressin [DDAVP]), a synthetic vasopressin analogue, increases factor VIII and vWF levels, allowing for successful treatment of dental and surgical patients with mild and moderate hemophilia A and von Willebrand disease with DDAVP alone.[23,24] DDAVP is now considered the treatment of choice in those patients with mild and moderate hemophilia A who respond to the drug. It is not efficacious in the treatment of severe hemophilia A or severe type III von Willebrand disease (vWD) or in patients with any form of hemophilia B.

The individual response to DDAVP is variable[25]; in hemophilia A the range of responses have been reported to be 2–25-fold over baseline factor VIII levels. Thus, it is recommended that patients undergo a trial dose with laboratory measurement of the factor VIII (or vWF) response prior to the use of DDAVP for treatment of bleeding episodes and prophylaxis for dental and other surgical procedures. A single individual usually responds to a similar degree with repeated doses[26]; thus, the plasma level of factor VIII attained following a trial dose of DDAVP can be used to predict responses for the design of future therapy. For example, a patient with mild hemophilia A who achieves a 40% factor VIII level following DDAVP stimulation should be treated with DDAVP for routine hemarthroses, tooth extractions, and so forth, but DDAVP would not be sufficient for treatment of limb- or life-threatening hemorrhages or preparation for major surgery, situations in which a 100% factor VIII level is indicated.

In this country, DDAVP is presently available only in an intravenous form, but clinical trials to evaluate a concentrated intranasal form are ongoing.[27] The dilute intranasal preparation for diabetes insipidus is not effective for treatment of hemophilia and vWD. The recommended dose is 0.3 µg/kg body weight[23,25]; the calculated dose is diluted in 25–50-ml normal saline and given as an intravenous infusion over 20–30 minutes. Since the maximal rise in factor VIII occurs at 30–60 minutes, it is advisable to time the infusion as close to the surgical procedure as possible.

Tachyphylaxis may occur with repeated doses of DDAVP and varies from patient to patient.[28] Therefore, if repeated dosing is contemplated, factor VIII levels should be monitored and exogenous factor VIII given as needed. In general, if 2–4 days have elapsed between doses, a response similar to baseline can be expected.

Side effects are usually minimal and include facial flushing, headache, or mild increases in pulse rate or blood pressure that resolve when the infusion is slowed or discontinued. Rare cases of seizures associated with hyponatremia have been reported.[29] Fluids should be restricted to maintenance for ≥24 hours when DDAVP is administered, and serum sodium should be monitored in the patient treated with repeated doses; hyponatremia generally responds to fluid restriction. Thrombosis has occurred rarely[30]; thus, the drug should be used with caution in patients with an increased risk of thrombosis.

Antifibrinolytic Therapy

Antifibrinolytic therapy is a useful adjunctive therapy, particularly for treatment of injuries involving the oral and nasal mucous membranes. It is not effective in obtaining initial hemostasis, but it prevents clot lysis once hemostasis has been achieved by clotting factor replacement or local measures. For example, in the treatment of dental extractions, usually a single dose of clotting factor replacement prior to the procedure is sufficient for hemostasis, and maintenance with an antifibrinolytic agent can be substituted for maintenance clotting factor replacement.[31,32] Tranexamic acid has recently been shown to be effective when used as a mouthwash, as well.[33] Antifibrinolytic agents have not shown any efficacy in the treatment of hemarthroses and are contraindicated in the presence of hematuria. Patients treated with prothrombin complex concentrates should not be given antifibrinolytic drugs simultaneously with an infusion (it is advisable to wait ≥4–6 hours), because of the increased risk of thrombotic complications.

Two antifibrinolytic agents are presently available in the United States, ε-aminocaprioc acid (EACA; Amicar) and tranexamic acid (Cyclokapron). EACA is formulated in both an oral tablet and oral elixir form. The tablet is a very large 500-mg size, and with the usual adult dose of 5 g (10 capsules), even adults prefer the elixir. The oral dose of EACA is 100 mg/kg (maximum 10 g) initial dose followed by 50 mg/kg/dose (maximum 5 g) every 6 hours. The second agent, tranexamic acid, is also available in 500-mg capsules, but they are smaller and the lower recommended oral dose (25 mg/kg/dose every 6–8 hours) is more tolerable. Both are available in intravenous forms but the dosing schedules are different.

Hemophilia B

The clinical manifestations of hemophilia B (factor IX deficiency) are quite similar to hemophilia A. Therefore, the approach to management of hemorrhages with products containing factor IX is analogous to that using factor VIII in hemophilia A. Recovery of factor IX in plasma following an infusion is approximately one-half that of factor VIII (1% [U/dl] rise following 1 U/kg) and therefore, twice as much product must be given to achieve a desired plasma level (Table 139-1). However, the minimal hemostatic level is lower than that of factor VIII and the biologic half-life of factor IX is longer (18–24 hours).[34]

Two generally accepted dose classifications are used for hemophilia B as well (Table 139-2). Routine bleeds such as hemarthrosis and muscle hemorrhage require 20–30% (U/dl) plasma factor IX levels; with major surgery and life-threatening hemorrhage, an 80% (U/dl) factor IX level should be achieved initially and factor IX levels maintained at >30–45% (U/dl) for 5–7 days and then >15–20% (U/dl) for another 5–7 days. Calculation of the dose required to achieve a desired rise in plasma factor IX is as follows:

Dose of factor IX (IU)
= % (U/dl) desired rise × body weight (kg)

Thus, for treatment of hemarthrosis in a 70-kg man with severe hemophilia B, the dose would be 30% (U/dl) × 70 kg = 2,100 IU factor IX. For maintenance therapy for major bleeds, doses are smaller because of the longer biologic half-life of factor IX. For major hemorrhage, factor IX levels should be monitored.

Therapy Products

Prothrombin Complex Concentrates

Fractionation procedures developed to produce factor IX concentrates for the treatment of hemophilia B utilize barium sulfate precipitation and column chromatography with a variety of adsorbents.[35,36] Because the physical and chemical properties of the vitamin K–dependent clotting factors are highly similar, factors II and X, as well as varying amounts of factor VII and the physiologic anticoagulant protein C, are co-purified with factor IX. Although this similarity has been used for treatment of other vitamin K–dependent coagulation factor deficiencies, the presence of these factors in an "activated" form is thought to be the cause of rare but life-threatening thrombotic complications, including deep venous thrombosis, pulmonary emboli, myocardial infarctions, and disseminated intravascular coagulation.[37,38] The risk appears to be increased in patients receiving high or multiple doses of concentrate or concurrent antifibrinolytic therapy or in those with significant liver disease and impaired ability to clear activated clotting factors from the circulation. Therefore, the recommendation was made to add 100 U heparin/500 U factor IX concentrate to the vials after the product is reconstituted when using these products in high doses or when more than a single infusion is anticipated.[39] However, nonthrombogenic highly purified factor IX concentrates for treatment of hemophilia B have recently been licensed and should be used when more than a single dose of factor IX is anticipated.[40] Currently available prothrombin complex concentrates undergo dry heating at high temperatures (80°C) or vapor heating to inactivate viruses; no HIV seroconversions have been noted, and hepatitis C transmission may also be eliminated.[18]

Coagulation Factor IX Concentrates

Coagulation factor IX concentrates, the most recent advance for treatment of hemophilia B, are highly purified plasma-derived products that are nonthrombogenic.[41] It is strongly recommended that they be used, instead of prothrombin complex concentrates when treating with high or repeated doses of factor IX for major surgery or life-threatening hemorrhages, in patients with impaired ability to clear activated coagulation factors such as those with hepatocellular disease or infants, those with crush injuries or massive muscle hemarthroses, or those with a history of thrombosis. The two currently available products are virus inactivated by solvent/detergent treatment (AlphaNine) in one and ultrafiltration plus thiocyanate treatment (MonoNine) in the other.

Fresh Frozen Plasma

Until the recent availability of pure, safe factor IX concentrates, fresh frozen plasma was used, particularly in young children and mild and moderate hemophilia B patients in whom infrequent use and smaller doses did not result in untoward numbers of donor exposures; however, the highly purified, viral attenuated concentrates are now preferred for treatment of hemophilia B. If fresh frozen plasma is used for the treatment of coagulation deficiencies for which there is no safe, effective concentrate, consideration should be given to use of small pools of well-screened volunteer donors in order to limit the possibility of HIV or hepatitis transmission. A viral attenuated solvent/detergent fresh frozen plasma is currently undergoing clinical trials. If parental heterozygous carriers are considered for directed donations, clotting factor levels should be evaluated before donation of plasma for affected children. Maternal plasma should be avoided because it is more likely to be implicated in the rare complication of transfusion-related acute lung injury, mediated by granulocyte antibodies.[42] Fresh frozen plasma should be ABO type-compatible to avoid the complication of isohemagglutinin-induced hemolytic anemia. Fresh frozen plasma should be administered immediately after thawing.[43] Patients with intact cardiovascular systems can safely tolerate a dose of 15–20 ml/kg.

Hemophilia with Inhibitors

Of patients with severe hemophilia A, 15–25% develop a circulating inhibitor (antibody) to factor VIII, and thus treatment with factor VIII concentrates becomes extremely difficult or impossible. Development of an inhibitor should be suspected in a patient who does not respond to coagulation factor replacement therapy in the expected manner. Clinically, inhibitor patients can be divided into two general categories: those who develop higher titers of antibody with exposure to factor VIII (high responders) and those who maintain a low-titer inhibitor in spite of repeated doses of factor VIII (low responders).[44] Treatment recommendations differ for the two groups.

Low-Responder Factor VIII Inhibitors

Patients whose inhibitor titers, measured by the standard method of Kasper et al.,[45] do not rise >10 Bethesda Units in spite of exposure to factor VIII, are considered low responders. Most of these individuals can continue to be treated with factor VIII concentrate, but in higher doses. For serious limb- or life-threatening bleeding, current recommendations include a bolus infusion of 100 U/kg of factor VIII initially, followed by 20 U/kg/hr. Factor VIII assays should be obtained 1 hour after the bolus infusion has been given and then at least daily so that the dose may be adjusted depending on the factor VIII level.

Joint and muscle hemorrhages and other more minor hemorrhages can usually be successfully managed with bolus infusions of factor VIII; the exact dose should be determined in each patient based on a factor VIII recovery study following an infusion of factor VIII. Adjunctive therapy with antifibrinolytic agents is effective in the management of dental extraction and nasal and mucous membrane injury, as discussed above for noninhibitor patients.

High-Responder Factor VIII Inhibitors

Numerous therapies and combinations of therapies have been devised for treatment of the high-responder inhibitor patient; to date, none of these is as uniformly successful as factor VIII replacement in the noninhibitor patient.

Prothrombin Complex Concentrates

Prothrombin complex concentrates are often used to treat routine joint and muscle hemorrhages in inhibitor patients. A multicenter study conducted in the late 1970s showed that the two prothrombin complex concentrates then available promoted hemostasis in 50% of bleeding episodes at a dose of 75 factor IX U/kg in comparison with a 25% placebo effect with albumin.[46] The addition of heat treatment to the manufacturing process has not altered the response rate.[47] Most physicians initially manage hemarthroses and other routine bleeds in these hemophilia patients with prothrombin complex concentrates. The treatment dose for joint and muscle bleeds has varied from 50 to 100 U/kg, with most physicians presently administering 75 U/kg/dose in this setting. If no response occurs after 2–3 infusions given 12 hours apart, it is unlikely that additional infusions will achieve hemostasis and instead will only increase the risk of thrombotic complications.

Activated Prothrombin Complex Concentrates

Currently two activated prothrombin complex concentrates (APCC) are commercially available, Autoplex and FEIBA, that have been purposefully "activated" during fractionation, resulting in increased amounts of activated factor VII, factor X, and perhaps thrombin; these products are intended for use in patients with circulating inhibitors. Two double-blind controlled trials comparing the efficacy of APCC with standard prothrombin complex concentrates showed a small but significant advantage of FEIBA (64% efficacy) over a standard prothrombin complex concentrate (52% efficacy) in one trial[48] and no additional benefit of Autoplex over Proplex (standard prothrombin complex concentrate) in the second trial.[49] The introduction of viral attenuation of these products has had no apparent effect on their hemostatic efficacy or safety in noncontrolled studies.[50] Although the high cost of the APCCs and their unproved efficacy over standard prothrombin complex concentrates has led most investigators to discourage their use for routine management of inhibitor patients, anecdotal reports of their utility in the management of serious bleeding episodes have led to the recommendation of their use as an initial therapy in serious hemorrhages when other available therapy would not be expected to be efficacious (e.g., patients with inhibitor titers >50 Bethesda units). The dose usually recommended is 75 U/kg. This can be repeated within 6–12 hours, but more than three consecutive doses and simultaneous use of antifibrinolytic therapy should be avoided, if possible. If not, the patient should be monitored for the possibility of disseminated intravascular coagulation and myocardial infarction, which has been reported with the use of APCCs as well as the standard prothrombin complex concentrates.[51]

Recombinant Factor VIIa

Recently a recombinant factor VIIa (activated factor VII) concentrate has been reported to achieve hemostasis in surgical and life-threatening hemorrhage in high-responder inhibitor patients who have failed conventional therapy.[52] It is postulated to interact with tissue factor expressed on endothelial cells at the site of vascular injury and to activate factor X, thus bypassing the inhibited factor VIII cofactor step in factor X activation.[53] This promising product is currently undergoing clinical trials and is available only for investigational or compassionate use.

Porcine Factor VIII Concentrates

Most investigators prefer to use a factor VIII-containing product for limb- or life-threatening bleeding if it is at all feasible to achieve a hemostatic level. Human factor VIII concentrate in high doses (see recommendations above for low-responder inhibitors) can be tried if the inhibitor titer is <10 Bethesda units or can be lowered to ≤10 with plasma exchange or immunoadsorbant columns, but this is a temporary solution, since a rapid anamnestic response usually limits the ability to maintain a hemostatic level for >1–3 days in high-responder inhibitors.[54] A porcine factor VIII concentrate, highly purified by polyelectrolyte ion exchange chromatography, is particularly useful for treatment of hemorrhages in patients with an inhibitor titer <50 Bethesda units.[55] Occasionally, it has been efficacious in patients with higher titer inhibitors who have antibodies that are less cross-reactive with porcine factor VIII. It is preferable to high-dose human factor VIII because of the lower risk of anamnesis.[56] In those patients who do not have anamnesis, the product can be considered for routine bleeding as well. The recommended starting dose is 100–150 U/kg, with measurement of plasma factor VIII levels to guide continued therapy. It is advisable to determine periodically the antiporcine factor VIII antibody titer in high-responder inhibitor patients to be prepared when a life-threatening hemorrhage occurs.

Other Therapy

In the 1970s, the first attempts were made to induce immune tolerance to factor VIII in inhibitor patients by infusions of twice daily high doses of factor VIII (100–150 U/kg) plus APCC over prolonged periods (months to years).[57] This very expen-

Table 139-3. Therapeutic Alternatives for vWD

Type of vWD	DDAVP	vWF or Factor VIII Concentrate	Platelets
I	Preferred treatment if DDAVP results in therapeutic level in trial	If DDAVP is not effective or if higher levels are required	Not indicated
IIA	Not usually effective; may cause improvement for 1–2 hr	Preferred treatment	Not indicated
IIB	May cause further decrease in platelet count	Preferred treatment	If thrombocytopenia remains severe after vWF replacement; not usually effective alone
Platelet-type vWD	May cause further decrease in platelet count	May cause further decrease in platelet count	Preferred treatment
Untyped vWD	Use with caution; follow platelet count and vWF levels	Preferred treatment in untyped patient with vWD	Not usually required unless patient has platelet-type vWD

sive and demanding treatment, although successful in 15 who completed the Bonn Protocol, led others to modify the regimen by eliminating the APCC and reducing the amount and frequency of factor VIII infusions with some success.[58] Other modifications reported to have varying success rates have included the use of intravenous γ-globulin, immunosuppressive therapy, removal of antibody by extracorporeal immunoadsorption on Staph Protein A columns, and combinations of those modalities.[59] Induction of immune tolerance in four of five patients on home-based therapy with porcine factor VIII was also recently reported.[60]

Factor IX Inhibitors

In patients with hemophilia B and factor IX inhibitors, treatment with prothrombin complex concentrates for routine hemorrhages or APCCs for more serious bleeding at the dose recommended for factor VIII inhibitor patients has been successful. If recombinant factor VIIa is proved to be efficacious for factor VIII inhibitor patients, it should theoretically also be successful in this group.

von Willebrand Disease

Treatment of vWD depends on the type of vWF defect and on the patient's individual response to DDAVP. Either quantitative or qualitative vWF defects may be present. Transfusion products appropriate for each type are summarized in Table 139-3.

The most common quantitative defect, a functional molecule present in decreased amounts (hypoproteinemia), is termed type I vWD[61]; most vWD patients (approximately 90%) are type I, and most of these respond to administration of DDAVP with a three- to fivefold increase in plasma vWF.[23–26,28] A single dose of DDAVP is generally sufficient for minor bleeding and tooth extractions. For oral bleeding and tooth extractions, antifibrinolytic therapy is also recommended, as discussed for hemophilia. It is advisable to perform a DDAVP trial to determine the individual response before its use for major surgical procedures; in general, if the vWF activity (ristocetin cofactor) rises to ≥100% (U/dl), the patient can be treated with DDAVP alone. For major surgery, doses given every 12–24 hours for 2–3 days postoperatively are usually sufficient to maintain hemostatic levels of vWF ≥40–50 U/dl (%); vWF:Ristocetin cofactor levels should be measured daily and exogenous vWF (Humate-P or vWF concentrate) administered if tachyphylaxis occurs. In patients in whom factor VIII:C levels are also low, factor VIII:C should be monitored and maintained at a hemostatic level as recommended for hemophilia A with either DDAVP or factor VIII concentrate as needed.

Patients with qualitative vWF defects (type II)[62] can be subgrouped into those with absent high-molecular-weight multimers on the basis of failure of multimerization or increased proteolysis of vWF (type IIA), or those with a loss of high-molec-

ular-weight multimers from plasma on the basis of an increased affinity of vWF for the platelet surface due either to a vWF defect (type IIB)[63] or to a platelet glycoprotein Ib defect (platelet-type vWD).[64] Some patients with type IIA vWD have a transient response to DDAVP, and minor bleeding may be treated with DDAVP. However, for major bleeds and surgery, replacement therapy with factor VIII concentrate containing normal vWF multimers (Humate-P) (see Ch. 138) is usually required. Type IIB patients and those with platelet-type vWD may have thrombocytopenia that is exacerbated by the administration of DDAVP; therefore, DDAVP is generally considered to be contraindicated in this group. Replacement therapy with Humate-P or vWF concentrate is required for treatment of type IIB vWD; platelets may need to be given if thrombocytopenia is severe, but normal vWF should be given first. For patients with platelet-type vWD, platelet transfusion is indicated for treatment of hemorrhages; rarely, vWF replacement is also needed.

Patients with severe type III vWD lack detectable vWF; factor VIII:C is also low (3–5%) because vWF serves as a stabilizer for factor VIII in the circulation. DDAVP is ineffective in this group because vWF stores are also absent. Therefore, vWF and factor VIII must be replaced for treatment of hemorrhages. Since vWF has a 12-hour half-life in the circulation, management of bleeding episodes with vWF replacement is similar to that described above for factor VIII replacement for hemophilia A. Humate-P is currently the only licensed factor VIII concentrate in the United States that contains normal vWF. A vWF concentrate is currently in clinical trials.

Other Inherited Procoagulant Deficiencies

Factors II, VII, and X

Transfusion therapy for these very rare vitamin K-dependent procoagulant deficiencies should be approached through analysis of minimal hemostatic levels, as well as recovery and half-life of the transfused protein (Table 139-1). As with other clotting factor deficiencies, the use of fresh frozen plasma may be limited by volume constraints but is usually quite efficacious at a dose of 10–20 ml/kg because of the low minimal hemostatic levels of these procoagulants. If higher plasma levels of the vitamin K-dependent clotting factors are needed, one can either use plasma exchange procedures or begin the use of prothrombin complex concentrate. The content of the various vitamin K-dependent procoagulants in each prothrombin complex concentrate is variable[65,66]; the specific concentration of the required clotting factor in a concentrate can often be obtained from the manufacturer. Precautions regarding adverse effects are outlined above for plasma and prothrombin complex concentrates. A factor VII concentrate is in development. Vitamin K administration has no role in the treatment of these inherited coagulopathies.

Fibrinogen and Factors V, XI, and XIII

Although most patients with fibrinogen deficiencies are asymptomatic, the afibrinogenemic and some of the dysfibrinogenemic patients may occasionally have hemorrhage that requires replacement therapy. Fibrinogen can be replaced with either fresh frozen plasma (10–20 ml/kg) or cryoprecipitate (1 donor U/5 kg) to raise the fibrinogen level to 50–100 mg/dl.[67,68] Because of its long half-life, repeated infusions need only be given every 4–5 days if prolonged correction of the deficiency is required.

Factor V deficiency, also called parahemophilia, is rarely associated with bleeding severe enough to require replacement therapy. When required, the only available product is fresh frozen plasma; preferably the product should be <1 month old. Hemostatic level is approximately 25%, and the half-life of the transfused protein is 36 hours; thus, the condition is highly amenable to treatment with fresh frozen plasma.[69,70]

Factor XI deficiency, also known as hemophilia C, is variably associated with symptoms, even in those with moderate or severe deficiencies. Therefore, treatment should be reserved for bleeding episodes or for surgery in those who are known to be symptomatic. Fresh frozen plasma (10–20 ml/kg body weight), will result in a rise of 25–50% of factor XI, which is an adequate dose for hemostasis even for severe bleeding episodes and surgery[71]; plasma exchange may also be useful.[72] Cryoprecipitate supernatant and one of the prothrombin complex concentrates (Konyne) contain factor XI and have been used in the extraordinary circumstance in which prolonged high-dose therapy is needed.[73] A factor XI concentrate is available in Europe.

Congenital factor XIII deficiency is an extremely rare deficiency characterized by bleeding with injuries and delayed healing. The very low hemostatic level (2–3%) and long half-life (6 days) permit most bleeding to be treated with fresh frozen plasma.[74] Alternatively, cryoprecipitate may be used[75]; a factor XIII concentrate is available in Europe.[76]

The contact factors, factor XII (Hageman factor), prekallekrein (Fletcher factor), and high-molecular-weight kininogen (Fitzgerald factor), are not associated with bleeding manifestations and require no transfusion therapy.

THERAPY FOR INHERITED ANTICOAGULANT DEFICIENCIES

Inherited deficiencies of the naturally occurring anticoagulants are associated with an increased risk of thrombosis, both arterial and venous. The most widely recognized is antithrombin III deficiency, but deficiencies of other physiologic anticoagulants, such as the vitamin K-dependent factors protein C and protein S, as well as the fibrinolytic protein plasminogen, have also been implicated in thrombophilic disorders.[77] The general approach for management of the heterozygous states is similar. Specific treatment is not instituted until the first thrombotic episode occurs because many heterozygotes never develop a thrombotic complication. At that point, after treatment of the acute thrombosis with standard therapy, lifelong anticoagulation with coumarin is usually recommended after the first thrombotic episode. In some cases, replacement therapy is warranted.

Antithrombin III Deficiency

Antithrombin III deficiency, a fairly rare heterozygous deficiency, has been well described as associated with venous thrombosis and pulmonary emboli.[77] Because heparin's anticoagulant activity to inactive thrombin and factor Xa is effected through induction of a conformational change in antithrombin III, patients with antithrombin III deficiency often manifest heparin resistance when attempts are made to treat their thrombotic episodes. If significant heparin resistance is encountered, treatment with antithrombin III may be indicated. Antithrombin III may be replaced by infusion of a pasteurized antithrombin

III concentrate licensed for prophylaxis of deep vein thrombosis and treatment of thrombosis in patients with inherited antithrombin III deficiency.[78] The transfused protein has a recovery of 1.4% (U/dl)/U/kg of antithrombin III administered and a biologic half-life of 3.8 days.

Protein C Deficiency

Heterozygous protein C deficiency has been variably associated with thrombotic tendencies.[79] Therefore, the incidental discovery of protein C deficiency is not an indication for lifelong anticoagulation. However, if thrombotic complications occur after treatment of the acute thrombotic event, long-term anticoagulation with coumarin is indicated. It is important that the patient be adequately heparinized during the initial administration of coumarin because protein C is a vitamin K-dependent protein with a very short half-life (4–6 hours); a more thrombophilic state is induced until the level of the procoagulants is also lowered and may be the cause of coumarin-induced skin necrosis.[80]

Homozygous protein C deficiency is an extremely rare disorder; affected infants have nearly all presented in the newborn period with purpura fulminans and disseminated intravascular coagulation.[81] Infants presenting with these symptoms should have assays obtained for protein C and then be treated immediately with fresh frozen plasma (9–12 ml/kg every 12 hours has been shown to control symptoms) or, if available, the vapor-heated protein C concentrate currently in clinical trials.[82] Replacement therapy should be continued until all lesions are healed. Once lesions have healed most patients can be maintained on coumarin with occasional replacement therapy if symptoms recur.

Other Inherited Anticoagulant Deficiencies

Protein S, another vitamin K-dependent plasma anticoagulant, functions as a cofactor in protein C inactivation of factors Va and VIIIa. Heterozygous deficiency of free protein S has been described in families with an increased incidence of thrombotic episodes.[83] Currently no replacement product for protein S deficiency is available, and patients should be placed on lifelong anticoagulation after treatment of the initial thrombotic episode. Coumarin-induced skin necrosis has also been reported in association with heterozygous protein S deficiency.[84]

Other inherited deficiencies associated with hypercoagulability include dysfibrinogenemias (abnormal plasmin-binding site), plasminogen deficiencies, and tissue plasminogen activator release defects.[85] No replacement products are currently available for treatment, and therapy depends on anticoagulation.

REFERENCES

1. Rizza CR: Coagulation factor therapy. Clin Haematol 5:113, 1976
2. Allain JP: Principles of *in vivo* recovery and survival studies. Scand J Haematol suppl 40:161, 1984
3. Kasper CK, Boylen AL, Ewing NP et al: Hematologic management of hemophilia A for surgery. JAMA 253:1279, 1985
4. Abildgaard CF, Simone JV, Corrigan JJ et al: Treatment of hemophilia with glycine-precipitated factor VIII. N Engl J Med 275:471, 1966
5. Hathaway WE, Christian MJ, Clarke SL et al: Comparison of continuous and intermittent factor VIII concentrate therapy in hemophilia A. Am J Hematol 17:85, 1984
6. Gitschier J, Wood WI, Goralka TM et al: Characterization of the human factor VIII gene. Nature 312:326, 1984
7. Wood WI, Capon DJ, Simonsen CC et al: Expression of active human factor VIII from recombinant DNA clones. Nature 312:330, 1984
8. White GC, McMillan CW, Kingdon HS et al: Use of recombinant antihemophilic

factor in the treatment of two patients with classic hemophilia. N Engl J Med 320:166, 1989

9. Schwartz RS, Abildgaard CF, Aledort LM et al: Human recombinant DNA-derived antihemophilic factor (factor VIII) in the treatment of hemophilia A. N Engl J Med 323:1800, 1990

10. Lusher JM, Arkin S, Abildgaard CF et al: Recombinant factor VIII for the treatment of previously untreated patients with hemophilia A. N Engl J Med 328: 453, 1993

11. Ehrenforth S, Kreuz W, Scharrer I et al: Incidence of development of factor VIII and factor IX inhibitors in haemophiliacs. Lancet 339:594, 1992

12. Webster WP, Roberts HR, Thelin GM et al: Clinical use of a new glycine-precipitated antihemophilic fraction. Am J Med Sci 250:643, 1965

13. Piszkiewicz D, Sun CS, Tondreau SC et al: Inactivation and removal of human immunodeficiency virus in monoclonal purified antihemophilic factor (human) (Hemofil M). Thromb Res 55:627, 1989

14. Brettler DB, Forsberg AD, Levine PH et al: Factor VIII concentrate purified from plasma using monoclonal antibodies: human studies. Blood 73:1859, 1989

15. Brettler DB, Levine PH: Factor concentrates for treatment of hemophilia: which one to choose? Blood 73:2067, 1989

16. de Biasi R, Rocino A, Miraglia E et al: The impact of a very high purity factor VIII concentrate on the immune system of human immunodeficiency virus-infected hemophiliacs. Blood 78:1919, 1991

17. Columbo M, Mannucci PM, Carnelli V et al: Transmission of non-A, non-B hepatitis by heat-treated factor VIII concentrate. Lancet 2:1, 1985

18. Fricke WA, Lamb MA: Viral safety of clotting factor concentrates. Semin Haemost Thromb 19:54, 1993

19. Vermylen J, Briet E: Factor VIII preparations: need for prospective pharmaco-vigilance. Lancet 342:693, 1993

20. Azzi A, Ciappi S, Zakvrzewska K et al: Human parvovirus B19 infection in hemophiliacs first infused with two high purity, virally attenuated factor VIII concentrates. Am J Hematol 39:228, 1992

21. Health and Public Policy Committee, American College of Physicians: Hepatitis B vaccine. Ann Intern Med 100:149, 1984

22. Pool JG, Shannon AE: Production of high-potency concentrates of antihemophilic globulin in closed-bag system. N Engl J Med 273:1443, 1965

23. Mannucci PM, Canciani MT, Rota L et al: Response of factor VIII/von Willebrand factor to DDAVP in healthy subjects and patients with haemophilia A and von Willebrand's disease. Br J Haematol 47:283, 1981

24. de la Fuente B, Kasper CK, Rickles FR et al: Response of patients with mild and moderate hemophilia A and von Willebrand's disease to treatment with desmopressin. Ann Intern Med 103:6, 1985

25. Warrier AI, Lusher JM: DDAVP: A useful alternative to blood components in moderate hemophilia A and von Willebrand disease. J Pediatr 102:228, 1983

26. Rodeghiero F, Castaman G, Bona ED et al: Consistency of responses to repeated DDAVP infusions in patients with von Willebrand's disease and hemophilia A. Blood 74:1997, 1989

27. Nilsson IM, Mikaelsson M, Vilharot H: The effect of intranasal DDAVP on coagulation and fibrinolytic activity in normal persons. Scand J Haematol 29: 70, 1982

28. Mannucci PM: Desmopressin: a nontransfusional form of treatment for congenital and acquired bleeding disorders. Blood 75:1449, 1988

29. Smith TJ, Gill JC, Hathaway WE et al: Hyponatremia and seizures in young children given DDAVP. Am J Hematol 31:191, 1989

30. Mannucci PM, Lusher JM: Desmopressin and thrombosis. Lancet 2:675, 1989

31. Walsh PN, Rizza CR, Matthews J et al: Epsilon-aminocaproic acid therapy for dental extractions in haemophilia and Christmas disease: a double-blind controlled trial. Br J Haematol 20:463, 1971

32. Forbes CD, Barr RD, Reid G et al: Tranexamic acid in control of haemorrhage after dental extraction in haemophilia and Christmas disease. BMJ 2:311, 1972

33. Sindet-Pedersen S, Ramstrom G, Bernvil S et al: Hemostatic effect of tranexamic acid mouthwash in anticoagulant-treated patients undergoing oral surgery. N Engl J Med 320:840, 1989

34. Smith KJ, Thompson AR: Labeled factor IX kinetics in patients with hemophilia-B. Blood 58:625, 1981

35. Hoag MS, Johnson FF, Robinson JA et al: Treatment of hemophilia B with a new clotting-factor concentrate. N Engl J Med 280:581, 1969

36. Gunay U, Choi HS, Maurer HS et al: Commercial preparations of prothrombin complex. Am J Dis Child 126:775, 1973

37. Kasper CK: Postoperative thromboses in hemophilia B. N Engl J Med 289: 160, 1973

38. Campbell EW, Neff S, Bowdler AJ: Therapy with factor IX concentrate resulting in DIC and thromboembolic phenomena. Transfusion 18:94, 1978

39. Gobel U, Voss H, Petrich C: Use of heparin in combination with factor-VII-rich prothrombin complex concentrate. Lancet 1:279, 1975

40. Kim HC, McMillan CW, White CC et al: Clinical experience of a new monoclonal antibody purified factor IX: half-life, recovery, and safety in patients with hemophilia B. Semin Hematol 27:30, 1990

41. Mannucci PM, Bauer KA, Gringeri A et al: No activation of the common pathway of the coagulation cascade after a highly purified factor IX concentrate. Br J Haematol 79:606, 1991

42. Popovsky MA, Moore SB: Diagnostic and pathogenetic considerations in transfusion-related acute lung injury. Transfusion 25:573, 1985

43. Urbaniak SJ, Cash JD: Blood replacement therapy. Br Med Bull 33:273, 1977

44. Lusher JM: Management of patients with factor VIII inhibitors. Transfusion Med Rev 1:123, 1987

45. Kasper CK, Aledort LM, Counts RB et al: A more uniform measurement of factor VIII inhibitors. Thromb Diath Haemarth 34:869, 1985

46. Lusher JM, Shapiro SS, Palascak JE et al: Efficacy of prothrombin-complex concentrates in hemophiliacs with antibodies to factor VIII. N Engl J Med 303:421, 1980

47. Schwartz RS, Ewing NP, Gorenc TJ et al: Comparative efficacy of nonheated and heat-treated factor IX complex concentrate in treatment of hemophiliacs with inhibitors. Am J Hematol 30:22, 1989

48. Sjamsoedin LJM, Heijnen L, Mauser-Bunzschuten EP et al: The effect of activated prothrombin-complex concentrate (FEIBA) on joint and muscle bleeding in patients with hemophilia A and antibodies to factor VIII. N Engl J Med 305:717, 1981

49. Kurczynski EM, Penner JA: Activated prothrombin concentrate for patients with factor VIII inhibitors. N Engl J Med 291:164, 1974

50. Hilgartner M, Aledort L, Gill JC et al: Efficacy and safety of vapor-heated anti-inhibitor coagulant complex in hemophilia patients. Transfusion 30:626, 1990

51. Chavin SI, Siegel DM, Rocco TA et al: Acute myocardial infarction during treatment with an activated prothrombin complex concentrate in a patient with factor VIII deficiency and a factor VIII inhibitor. Am J Med 85:245, 1988

52. Hedner U, Glazer S, Pingel K et al: Successful use of recombinant factor VIIa in patients with severe haemophilia A during synovectomy. Lancet 2:1193, 1988

53. Rao LVM, Rapaport SI: Factor VIIa-catalyzed activation of factor X independent of tissue factor: its possible significance for control of hemophilic bleeding by infused factor VIIa. Blood 75:1069, 1990

54. Bloom AL: Factor VIII inhibitors revisited. Br J Haematol 49:319, 1981

55. Brettler DB, Forsberg AD, Levine PH et al: The use of procine factor VIII concentrate (Hyate:C) in the treatment of patients with inhibitor antibodies to factor VIII. Arch Intern Med 149:1381, 1989

56. Verroust F, Allain JP: Immune response induced by porcine factor VIII in severe hemophiliacs with antibody to factor VIII. Thromb Haemost 48:238, 1982

57. Brackmann HH, Gormsen J: Massive factor VIII infusion in haemophiliac with factor VIII, high responder. Lancet 2:933, 1977

58. Ewing NP, Sanders NL, Dietrich SL et al: Induction of immune tolerance to factor VIII in hemophiliacs with inhibitors. JAMA 259:65, 1988

59. Nilsson IM, Berntorp E, Zetterval O et al: Induction of immune tolerance in patients with hemophilia and antibodies to factor VIII by combined treatment with intravenous IgG, cyclophosphamide, and factor VIII. N Engl J Med 318: 947, 1988

60. Hay CRM, Laurian Y, Verroust F et al: Induction of immune tolerance in patients with hemophilia A and inhibitors treated with porcine VIIIC by home therapy. Blood 76:882, 1990

61. Ruggeri ZM, Zimmerman TS: The classification of variant von Willebrand's disease subtypes by analysis of functional characteristics and multimeric conposition of factor VIII/von Willebrand factor. Ann NY Acad Sci 370:205, 1981

62. Ruggeri ZM, Zimmerman TS: Variant von Willebrand's disease. Characterization of two subtypes by analysis of multimeric composition of factor VIII/von Willebrand factor in plasma and platelets. J Clin Invest 64:1318, 1980

63. Ruggeri ZM, Pareti FI, Mannucci PM et al: Heightened interaction between platelets and factor VIII/von Willebrand factor in a new subtype of von Willebrand's disease. N Engl J Med 32:1047, 1980

64. Miller JL, Kupinski JM, Castella A et al: von Willebrand factor binds to platelets and induces aggregation in platelet-type but not type IIB von Willebrand disease. J Clin Invest 72:1532, 1983

65. Breen F, Tullis J: Prothrombin concentrates in treatment of Christmas disease and allied disorders. JAMA 208:1848, 1969

66. Kohler M, Hellstern P, Pindur G et al: Factor VII half-life after transfusion of a steam-treated prothrombin complex concentrate in a patient with homozygous factor VII deficiency. Vox Sang 56:200, 1989

67. Hattersley PG, Dimick ML: Cryoprecipitates in treatment of congenital fibrinogen deficiency. Transfusion 9:261, 1969

68. McLeod B, McKenna R, Sassetti RJ: Treatment of von Willebrand's disease

and hypofibrinogenemia with single donor cyoprecipitate from plasma exchange donation. Am J Hemotol 32:112, 1989

69. National Institutes of Health Consensus Conference: Fresh-frozen plasma. Plasma 253:551, 1985

70. Melliger EJ, Duckert F: Major surgery in a subject with factor V deficiency: cholecystectomy in a parahaemophilic woman and review of the literature. Thromb Diath Haemorrh 25:438, 1971

71. Rosenthal RL, Sloan E: PTA levels and coagulation studies after plasma infusions in PTA deficient patients. J Lab Clin Med 66:709, 1965

72. Novakova IRO, van Ginneken CAM, Verbruggen HW et al: Factor XI kinetics after plasma exchange in severe factor XI deficiency. Haemostasis 16:51, 1986

73. Bick RL, Adams T, Radack K et al: Surgical hemostasis with a factor XI-containing concentrate. JAMA 229:163, 1974

74. Losowsky MS, Miloszewski KJA: Annotation: factor XIII. Br J Haematol 37:1, 1977

75. Amris CJ, Hilden M: Treatment of factor XIII deficiency with cryoprecipitate: Thromb Diath Haemorrh 20:528, 1968

76. Daly HM, Haddon ME: Clinical experience with a pasteurised human plasma concentrate in factor XIII deficiency. Thromb Haemost 59:171, 1988

77. Moake JL: Hypercoagulable states. Adv Intern Med 35:235, 1990

78. Schwartz RS, Bauer KA, Rosenberg RD et al: Clinical experience with antithrombin III concentrate in treatment of congenital and acquired deficiency of antithrombin. Am J Med 87:3B, 1989

79. Griffin JH, Zimmerman EB, Evatt B et al: Deficiency of protein C in congenital thrombotic disease. J Clin Invest 68:1370, 1981

80. Vigano-D'Angelo S, Comp PC, Esmon CT et al: Relationship between protein C antigen and anticoagulant activity during oral anticoagulation and in selected disease stages. J Clin Invest 77:416, 1986

81. Sills RH, Marlar RA, Montgomery RR et al: Severe homozygous protein C deficiency. J Pediatr 150:409, 1984

82. Marlar RA, Montgomery RR, Broekmans AW et al: Report on the diagnosis and treatment of homozygous proten C deficiency. Thromb Haemost 61:529, 1989

83. Comp PC, Esmon CT: Recurrent venous thromboembolism in patients with a partial deficiency of protein S. N Engl J Med 331:1525, 1984

84. Friedman KD, Marlar RA, Gill JC et al: Warfarin-induced skin necrosis in a patient with protein S deficiency. Blood 68:333a, 1986

85. Rosenberg RD: The biochemistry and pathophysiology of the prethrombotic state. Annu Rev Med 38:493, 1987

Hemapheresis and Cellular Therapy

140

Harvey G. Klein

INTRODUCTION

Bloodletting is an ancient therapy, fashionable, albeit unproved, well into the nineteenth century. About the time that scientific skepticism began to temper the widespread use of therapeutic phlebotomy, a new technique for blood removal, apheresis, appeared in the research laboratory.[1] The term *apheresis,* derived from a Greek verb meaning "to take away or withdraw," was coined to describe removal of one component of blood with return of the remaining components to the donor. Like phlebotomy, apheresis was used first to treat patients but later became more important for collecting blood components for transfusion. In the United States, >6 million units of platelets are collected by plateletpheresis and >10 million plasmapheresis procedures are performed annually. Physicians still perform an estimated 50,000 therapeutic apheresis procedures each year for a wide variety of indications.

PRINCIPLES OF APHERESIS

The principal objective of apheresis is efficient removal of some circulating blood component, either cells (cytapheresis) or some plasma solute (plasmapheresis). For most disorders, the treatment goal is to deplete the circulating cell or substance directly responsible for the disease process. Apheresis can also mobilize cells and plasma components from tissue depots. For example, peripheral lymphocytes may be mobilized from the spleen and lymph nodes of some patients with chronic lymphocytic leukemia and low-density lipoproteins can be re-

moved from tissue stores in patients with familial hyperlipoproteinemia. Apheresis may have other, less obvious effects. Lymphocyte depletion may modify immune responsiveness in some disease states, possibly by disturbing the control mechanisms of cellular immune regulation. Plasmapheresis enhances splenic clearance of immune complexes in certain autoimmune disorders.[2] When therapeutic effect is judged by clinical improvement rather than by efficiency of solute removal, apheresis is more often a helpful adjunct than a form of first-line therapy.

Several mathematical models formulated for different clinical conditions describe the kinetics of apheresis.[3-5] Removal of most blood components follows a logarithmic curve (Fig. 140-1). This model assumes that the component removed is neither synthesized nor degraded substantially during the procedure, remains within the intravascular compartment, and mixes instantaneously and completely with any plasma replacement solution. When the goal of plasmapheresis is to supply a deficient substance, for example plasma factors in the treatment of thrombotic thrombocytopenic purpura, replacement follows logarithmic kinetics similar to those developed for solute removal. From Figure 140-1 it is evident that removal of 1.5–2 volumes will reduce an intravascular substance by about 60% and that processing larger volumes results in little additional gain.

Specific cell removal with centrifugal automated cell separators depends on the number of cells available, the volume of blood processed, the efficiency of the particular instrument, and the separation characteristics of the different cells. Most commercially available instruments remove platelets and lym-

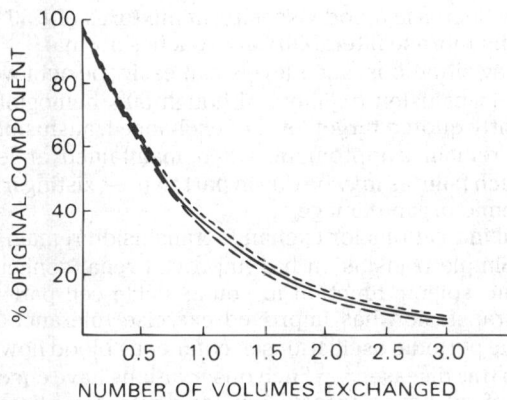

Fig. 140-1. Relationship between volumes removed by apheresis and percentage of the target component remaining. The relationship is valid for blood volumes during red cell exchange or for plasma volumes during plasmapheresis if the target solute remains primarily within the intravascular compartment. Solid line, continuous exchange; large dashes, discontinuous exchange with initial removal; small dashes, discontinuous exchange with initial infusion.

phocytes extremely efficiently. Granulocytes and monocytes cannot be cleanly separated from other cells by standard centrifugal apheresis equipment (Fig. 140-2). Optimal harvesting of these cells requires special techniques such as stimulating the donor with corticosteroids or cytokines and adding sedimenting agents to enhance cell separation.

TECHNOLOGY AND TECHNIQUES

The plasmapheresis technique that originated in the animal laboratory required manual resuspension of red cells and posed a substantial risk of microbial contamination of the com-

ponents being reinfused.[1] With the introduction of sterile, disposable, interconnected plastic blood bags, plasmapheresis became relatively safe and easy. However, manual apheresis proved too inefficient and labor intensive for collecting large component volumes and raised concerns that the separated units of red blood cells might be reinfused accidentally into the wrong donor or patient. The introduction of automated on-line blood cell separators solved these problems.[6,7]

Automated apheresis instruments use microprocessor technology to draw and anticoagulate blood, separate components either by centrifugation or by filtration, collect the desired component, and recombine the remaining components for return to the patient.[8] The equipment puts disposable plastic software in the blood path and uses anticoagulants containing citrate or combinations of citrate and heparin that do not result in clinical anticoagulation of the patient. Most instruments function well at blood flow rates of 30–80 ml/min and can operate from peripheral venous access or from a variety of multilumen central venous catheters.

Since the ideal method for treating disorders mediated by abnormal plasma components is to remove the offending substance selectively, a variety of on-line filtration and column adsorption techniques have been introduced or proposed. Ligands bound to a column matrix may be relatively nonspecific chemical sorbents such as charcoal or heparin, or specific ligands such as monoclonal antibodies and recombinant protein antigens. The two most successful clinical columns use staphylococcal protein A and dextran sulfate cellulose. Staphylococcal protein A has high affinity for the Fc portion of IgG1, 2, and 4, and for immune complexes containing these IgG subtypes. The dextran sulfate cellulose columns selectively remove low-density lipoproteins and have proved effective in managing patients with homozygous hyperlipoproteinemia (Fig. 140-3).

A procedure related to hemapheresis, although not strictly a removal technique, has been termed photopheresis.[9] Photopheresis is an automated extracorporeal photochemotherapy treatment that involves oral administration of a light-sensitizing agent, 8-methoxypsoralen followed by leukapheresis and ex vivo ultraviolet A irradiation of leukocytes. The treated cells are reinfused. Photopheresis has induced remissions in patients with Sézary syndrome and is being investigated as a

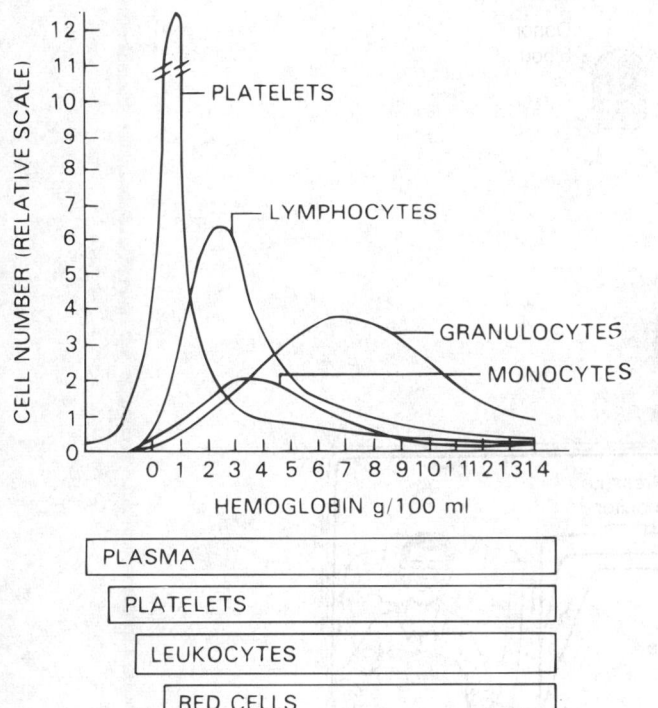

Fig. 140-2. Schematic distribution of cells at the collection port of a centrifugal cell separator. The number and percentage of each cell type collected can be varied by adjusting the site of collection along the interface or by changing centrifugal force, blood flow rate, or rate of cell removal.

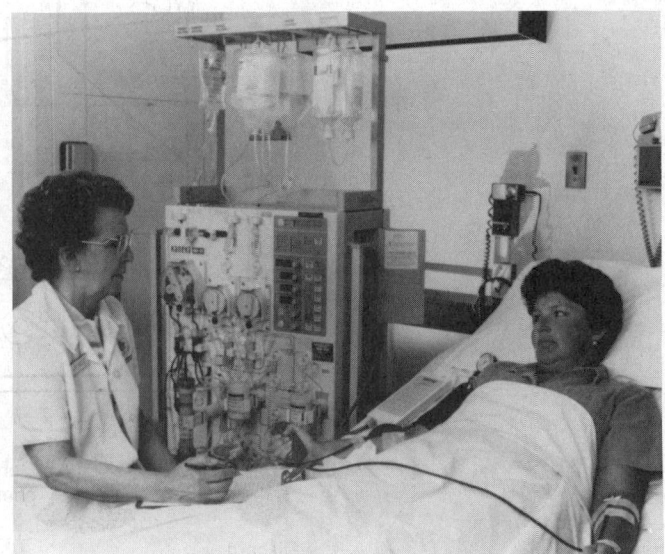

Fig. 140-3. Two-stage therapeutic plasmapheresis. Plasma is separated from cells by filtration, then passed through parallel adsorption columns to remove low-density lipoproteins from a patient with homozygous familial hyperlipoproteinemia.

Table 140-1. Common Indications for Therapeutic
Cytapheresis

Red cell exchange
    Sickle cell disease
        Acute complications
        Prophylaxis for recurrent stroke
        Frequent severe pain crises
    Malaria with hyperparasitemia
Leukapheresis
    Leukemia with hyperleukocytosis syndrome
    Rheumatoid arthritis
    Peripheral blood progenitor cell collection
Plateletpheresis
    Symptomatic thrombocythemia

treatment for scleroderma and organ graft rejection. The mechanism of action of photopheresis is unknown.

THERAPEUTIC CYTAPHERESIS

Common indications for therapeutic cell removal are listed in Table 140-1. Red cell exchange (erythrocytapheresis) is used most often to manage complications of sickle cell disease. When such exchanges are indicated, mechanical cell separators offer the advantages of speed and ease. Automated procedures can be performed with all centrifugal instruments (Fig. 140-4). The rationale behind exchange transfusion involves improving tissue oxygenation and preventing microvascular sickling by diluting the patient's abnormal red cells, simultaneously correcting anemia and favorably altering whole blood viscosity and rheology. No clinical data support a single optimal level of hemoglobin A; however, as few as 30% of transfused cells markedly decrease blood viscosity; at mixtures of ≥50%, resistance to membrane filterability approaches normal.[10,11] In nonemergency situations, such levels can easily be achieved with a simple transfusion regimen. Although 50% hemoglobin A is a frequently quoted target level of exchange transfusion, some patients remain symptomatic when maintained at levels of ≥80%. Such failures may be due in part to pre-existing irreversible ischemic organ damage.

Clinical indications for exchange transfusion remain controversial. Simple transfusion has improved renal concentrating ability and splenic function in young sickle cell patients; exchange transfusion has improved exercise tolerance and reversed the periodic oscillations in cutaneous blood flow associated with this disease.[12-15] Such observations have encouraged the use of exchange transfusion for acute complications of sickle cell disease such as acute chest syndrome, priapism, retinal artery occlusion, and intrahepatic cholestasis. Exchange transfusion for sickle cell patients has also been used for prophylaxis during pregnancy, before surgery, or for patients who have suffered a stroke.[16] However a multicenter randomized trial of transfusion during pregnancy has reported that transfusion sufficient to reduce the incidence of painful crises did not reduce other maternal morbidity or perinatal mortality, suggesting that effects of transfusion on the pathophysiology of sickle cell disease may be more complex than originally believed.[17]

Exchange transfusion, although relatively safe and convenient, carries all the complications of red cell transfusion. Patients are exposed to a large number of donors and are at substantial risk of contracting hepatitis and other blood-borne infections. As many as one-third of all patients develop alloantibodies, and life-threatening delayed hemolytic transfusion reactions have been reported.[18,19] Despite the removal of cells during exchange, patients remain in positive iron balance, al-

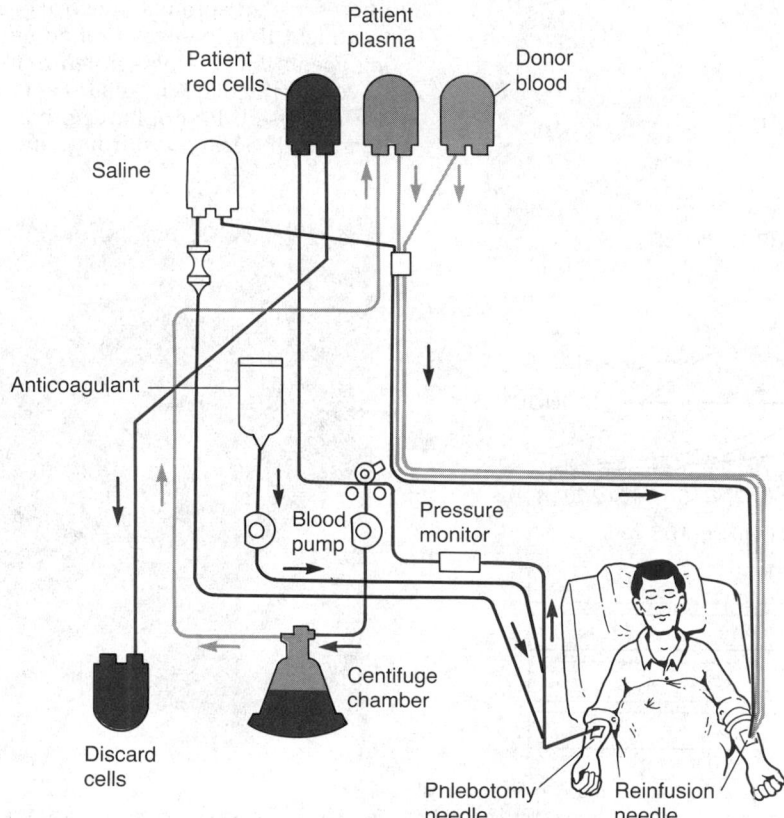

Fig. 140-4. Schematic of an automated red cell exchange transfusion using a two-arm procedure.

hough iron accumulation is slow and chelation is rarely required to prevent transfusional hemosiderosis.

Other indications for red cell exchange are rare. The procedure has been used for patients with overwhelming red cell parasitic infections, such as severe and complicated malaria and babesiosis.[20,21] In these situations, red cell exchange decreases the concentration of circulating parasites and may help sustain life until conventional therapy and natural immunity take effect. Automated red cell removal with volume replacement, isovolemic hemodilution, can be performed rapidly and safely in polycythemic subjects.[22] This maneuver should be reserved for polycythemic patients with an urgent clinical indication to lower the hematocrit, for example, evolving thrombotic stroke, for which standard single-unit manual phlebotomy might be inadvisably slow.

Therapeutic leukapheresis has been used most successfully to help manage patients with acute or chronic leukemia and extremely high white blood cell (WBC) numbers, so-called hyperleukocytic leukemias.[23,24] When the fractional volume of leukocytes (leukocrit) exceeds 20%, blood viscosity increases and leukocytes can interfere with pulmonary and cerebral blood flow and compete with tissue for oxygen in the microcirculation.[25] A single leukapheresis procedure generally reduces the WBC count by 20–50%. Ordinarily, leukapheresis is indicated when the blast count is >100,000/mm^3 or when rapidly rising blast counts are >50,000/mm^3 (leukocrit >10%), especially when evidence of central nervous system or pulmonary symptoms appears.[26] Although repeated leukapheresis has adequately reduced the WBC count in a series of patients with chronic myeloid leukemia (CML), median patient survival rate was not significantly different from that of similar patients treated with conventional chemotherapy.[27] Chronic leukapheresis can provide acceptable control of the peripheral WBC count in clinical situations such as pregnancy, when cytotoxic agents may best be avoided, but cytoreduction alone does not appear to alter the course of CML.

Cytoreduction for managing other leukemic processes has limited value. Some studies of patients with chronic lymphocytic leukemia suggested short-term clinical benefit, but long-term support of patients when disease is refractory to chemotherapy does not appear to prolong life.[28] Transient responses to leukapheresis used alone or in combination with low-dose chemotherapy have been reported in a variety of lymphoproliferative disorders. However, most patients relapse quickly and do not respond to further leukapheresis therapy.[29–32]

Lymphocyte depletion has been used therapeutically to modify patient immune responsiveness. Removal of large numbers of lymphocytes over a period of a few weeks can suppress peripheral lymphocyte counts in rheumatoid arthritis patients for ≤1 year and alter skin-test reactivity and lymphocyte mitogen responsiveness to a variety of stimulants.[33] Selected patients experience a modest but significant reduction in disease activity; however, the subset of patients who may derive substantial benefit from this therapy is difficult to identify.[34,35] Lymphocyte removal by apheresis has also been used to treat patients with multiple sclerosis, to enhance allograft survival, and to reverse graft rejection, but evidence of clinical efficacy in these situations is sparse.

Therapeutic plateletpheresis is generally reserved for patients with myeloproliferative disorders and hemorrhage or thrombosis associated with an increase in circulating platelets. Since thrombocytosis from other causes, such as iron deficiency or splenectomy, rarely causes such problems, other factors, such as a clone of functionally abnormal cells, may cause the symptoms attributed to elevated platelets in myeloproliferative disorders. Many centers consider using plateletpheresis when the patient's peripheral platelet count is >10^6/mm^3, although no consistent relationship between the level of platelet elevation and the occurrence of symptoms has been found.[36,37]

Unfortunately, no generally accepted assay of platelet dysfunction predicts which patients are at risk.

When therapeutic plateletpheresis is indicated, generally in symptomatic patients, a single procedure can lower the platelet count by 30–50%. Attempts to maintain thrombocythemic patients at normal platelet counts by cytapheresis alone have not been successful, so that more practical long-term therapy, such as chemotherapy, should be instituted concurrently with the cytapheresis program. Since most patients with thrombocytosis, even those with myeloproliferative disorders, do not develop symptoms, prophylactic plateletpheresis seems unwarranted, regardless of the platelet count.[38]

THERAPEUTIC PLASMAPHERESIS

Growth of therapeutic plasmapheresis during the past 50 years owes more to the development of new technology than to new insight into the pathophysiology of the diseases under treatment. Technical developments continue to outpace clinical applications. The prevailing developmental strategy has been to complement plasmapheresis with more specific procedures to remove pathologic plasma constituents. An impressive array of immunologic and physicochemical techniques, including cascade filtration, adsorption, immunoadsorption, cryoprecipitation, and photoinactivation, have been added to the plasmapheresis system for laboratory research and early clinical studies.[39]

Common clinical indications for therapeutic plasmapheresis are outlined in Table 140-2. Comprehensive reviews describing the rationale for using plasmapheresis in a wide variety of disease states can be found elsewhere.[40] Some of the least controversial indications for plasmapheresis are supported by small series of uncontrolled cases that rely on some objective clinical or laboratory measurement of patient improvement. This is the case for the hyperviscosity syndrome resulting from paraproteinemia and for cold agglutinin disease, cryoglobulinemia, and poisoning with albumin-bound toxins.[41–45] Evidence that both cutaneous and vascular lesions regress in familial hypercholesterolemia as low-density lipoprotein levels are controlled by plasmapheresis has encouraged the use of several related procedures in patients with homozygous disease and in poorly controlled heterozygous patients. By extension, plasmapheresis is used in patients with other inherited metabolic disorders such as Refsum disease.[46–48] The frequency of exchange depends primarily on total body burden, rate of synthesis, and plasma concentration of the solute to be removed (Fig. 140-5).

Plasmapheresis appears to have at least a temporary adjunctive role in managing some disorders characterized by circulat-

Table 140-2. Common Indications for Therapeutic Plasmapheresis

Paraproteinemia with hyperviscosity syndrome
Cold agglutinin disease
Cryoglobulinemia
Drug overdose and poisoning
Familial hypercholesterolemia
Refsum disease
Coagulation factor inhibitors
Immune thrombocytopenic purpura
Myasthenia gravis
Post-transfusion purpura
Goodpasture syndrome
Pemphigus vulgaris
Chronic demyelinating polyneuropathy
Guillain-Barré syndrome
Thrombotic thrombocytopenic purpura

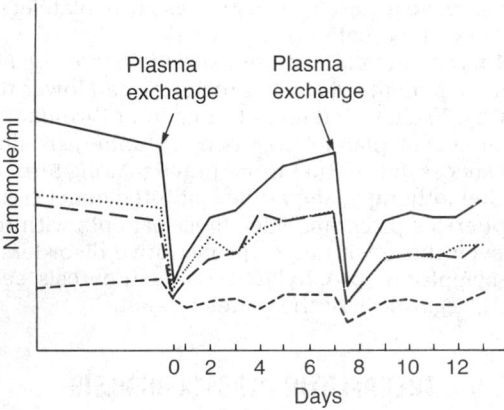

Fig. 140-5. Plasma exchange to remove plasma neutral glycolipids in a patient with Fabry disease. The plasma lipid recovery curve appears to be biphasic, reflecting initial re-equilibration from tissue stores and subsequent new synthesis of that glycolipid. Solid line, cerebrosides; dotted line, dihexosylceramides; large dashes, trihexosylceramides; small dashes, globosides.

ing autoantibodies. Early success was reported in patients with Goodpasture syndrome, a disorder characterized by specific pathogenic autoantibody directed against the renal glomerular and pulmonary alveolar basement membrane. Plasmapheresis has enjoyed similar success in a variety of disorders associated with specific autoantibodies, including myasthenia gravis, pemphigus, and Eaton-Lambert syndrome. In other autoimmune disorders, such as immune thrombocytopenic purpura and immune inhibitors to coagulation proteins, plasmapheresis may be helpful during a catastrophic event, but benefit in chronic disorders is less well established.[49-55] Controlled clinical trials of plasmapheresis have demonstrated efficacy in at least two of the polyradiculoneuropathies.[56,57] Although therapeutic plasma exchange has been used in a variety of other "immune" disorders, such as systemic lupus erythematosus and rheumatoid vasculitis, such use remains unproved and should be reserved for circumstances where a vital organ or life itself is endangered.

Controversy surrounds the practice of combining cytotoxic drug therapy with plasmapheresis to prevent rapid resynthesis of antibody, so-called antibody rebound. Although the rebound phenomenon is well established in animal models, investigational studies in healthy volunteers suggest that antibody rebound is not common. Controlled trials of plasmapheresis therapy in lupus nephritis and polymyositis have been criticized for not including a plasmapheresis-with-immunosuppression arm. Since many uncontrolled treatment protocols stipulate simultaneous use of immunosuppressive drugs and plasmapheresis, an apparent favorable outcome may result from the independent effects of the different treatments or some synergistic effect, or from neither.

The success of therapeutic apheresis procedures seldom depends on the composition of the replacement solution that is used. The single exception seems to be thrombotic thrombocytopenic purpura. Numerous reports support the use of fresh frozen plasma or cryoprecipitate-poor plasma as a specific therapeutic replacement fluid, possibly to replace a labile inhibitor of platelet aggregation.[58,59] Since <500-ml volume is removed during most cell collections and depletions, no replacement beyond the anticoagulant and saline priming solution is required. With therapeutic plasmapheresis, the primary function of the replacement solution is to maintain intravascular volume, but additional features deemed desirable include restoration of important plasma proteins, maintenance of colloid osmotic pressure, maintenance of electrolyte balance, and preservation of trace elements lost during a prolonged course

of plasmapheresis procedures. In moderately well-nourished subjects, homeostatic mechanisms normally obviate the need for precise plasma replacement. Other patients should receive solutions prepared specifically to meet their individual requirements. Routine supplementation with calcium, potassium, or immunoglobulins is unnecessary.

Automated apheresis is a minimal risk procedure for normal healthy donors. The current generation of blood cell separators is remarkably reliable and equipped with sensitive detection and alarm systems to alert the operator to potential problems. Nevertheless, ≥59 deaths have been associated with therapeutic procedures, an estimated mortality of 3 in 10,000 procedures. However most deaths are related to cardiac and respiratory causes in patients critically ill prior to apheresis.[60] If citrate-induced hypocalcemia, vasovagal reactions, clotting of fistulas and catheters, and urticaria are included, about 10% of procedures have medical complications. The frequency of adverse reactions is influenced primarily by the experience of the operator and the nature of the patient population under treatment. The most severe allergic complications occur when plasma is used as the replacement solution, and this risk increases with the number of procedures.[61] A decade of experience has confirmed the safety of these procedures when carried out in appropriate clinical circumstances by experienced operators under close medical supervision.

CELLULAR THERAPY

Blood cell separators developed for hemapheresis are used increasingly for novel forms of cellular therapy. In the cell-processing laboratory, separation techniques have been developed for removing T lymphocytes from allogeneic bone marrow, for purging tumor cells, and for selecting progenitor cells from autologous bone marrow harvests.[62] Hematopoietic progenitor cells can be collected from peripheral blood and cryopreserved. Such progenitors have been used to reconstitute bone marrow in patients who receive ablative chemotherapy.[63,64] Lymphocyte concentrates prepared from leukocyte collections have been used as immunotherapy for solid tumors and leukemia. Preliminary studies promise a role for both circulating hematopoietic progenitor cells and for lymphocytes in the therapy of immunosuppressed patients and in gene therapy.

Peripheral Blood Stem Cells

Pluripotential hematopoietic progenitor cells, most likely including primordial hematopoietic stem cells capable of reconstituting the bone marrow and the immune system, have long been known to circulate in the peripheral blood.[65] Substantial numbers of peripheral blood ("progenitor") stem cells (PBSCs), as measured by colony-forming assays, can be identified in plateletpheresis collections from normal donors. Recently, large volume hemapheresis collection protocols have been developed to recruit into the peripheral circulation sufficient numbers of PBSCs for marrow repopulation.[66,67] PBSC infusions have been used both for complete marrow replacement and for bone marrow rescue after high-dose chemotherapy. PBSC collections have several potential advantages compared to bone marrow harvests: (1) eliminates risk associated with anesthesia, (2) permits performance of peripheral collection despite tumor involvement of the marrow or previous pelvic irradiation, (3) theoretically reduces the risk of tumor cell contamination, and (4) permits collection as often as necessary. One disadvantage of PBSC collection is the large number of contaminating T lymphocytes in the collection. A secondary processing technique may be necessary to decrease the risk of graft-versus-host disease when PBSC are used for allogeneic transplantation.

Ordinarily, PBSCs circulate in small numbers. Efforts to define optimal collection conditions have been hindered by the lack of a standardized assay. The number of circulating PBSCs increases severalfold during the recovery phase following chemotherapy and may be further enhanced by administering recombinant hematopoietic growth factors. The optimal combination of cytokines and sequence of administration has not yet been established. Although definition of a therapeutic dose remains controversial, most centers recommend a minimum of 6×10^8/kg mononuclear cells or 5×10^5/kg colony-forming unit-granulocyte/macrophage by clonogenic assay. Assays that use the CD34 antigen as a marker of early progenitors may more accurately reflect true stem cell content of the component. Techniques are being developed to select and concentrate these cells from leukapheresis collections with monoclonal antibodies. The method of PBSC recruitment may alter the heterogeneity of cells at different stages of differentiation. Infusion of committed progenitor cells has been shown to decrease the period of myelosuppression that follows intensive chemotherapy, but such changes may adversely affect the permanence of the graft.

Several problems complicate the widespread use of PBSCs. Venous access requires large-bore multilumen catheters, and these appear particularly susceptible to clotting, especially when patients receive recombinant cytokine stimulation. PBSCs are stored frozen in liquid nitrogen with the cryoprotectant, dimethylsulfoxide. Cryopreservation is expensive and rapid infusion of dimethylsulfoxide causes bradycardia, hypertension, fever, nausea, and vomiting. The best times to begin and repeat PBSC collection are difficult to predict, and the quality of the component is difficult to assess in vitro. Finally, while PBSC shortens the period of post-transplant aplasia following intensive chemotherapy and irradiation, when used solely as an adjunct to marrow transplantation, decreased mortality has yet to be demonstrated in this setting.

Adoptive Immunotherapy

Advancements in cellular immunology and cell culture technology, the availability of recombinant human cytokines, and the ability to collect large numbers of lymphocytes have resulted in the development of adoptive immunotherapy, the passive transfer of immunologically active cells. The most extensive clinical studies have been performed with autologous lymphocytes, collected by hemapheresis or separated from resected tumors, and expanded ex vivo 100–1,000-fold.[68,69] Peripheral blood lymphocytes, cultured in high concentrations of the lymphokine interleukin-2, generate clones of cells capable of lysing fresh tumor cells in short-term cytotoxicity assays. The effector cells, termed lymphokine-activated killer (LAK) cells, consist of a heterogeneous population of cells, primarily natural killer cells and T cells, that mediate tumor regression in animal models, have produced objective responses in patients with advanced renal cell carcinoma, melanoma, colorectal cancer, and non-Hodgkin lymphoma. The effects appear to be dose dependent and non-MHC restricted and require the simultaneous administration of high-dose systemic interleukin-2. The postulated mechanism of action involves lymphocyte trafficking to the site of tumor followed by local expansion and cytokine release under the influence of interleukin-2. The cellular mechanisms of tumor targeting, recognition, binding, and lysis have not been identified. Lymphocytes separated from resected tumors, termed tumor-infiltrating lymphocytes (TIL) can be similarly expanded, to $\leq 10^{12}$ cells, and infused. TIL are reportedly 50–100 times more potent than are LAK cells.[70] Un-like LAK cells, TIL often recognize specific tumor antigens, and their action is MHC restricted.

While adoptive immunotherapy has been used primarily in the treatment of solid tumors, cellular immunotherapy has also been investigated for the treatment of acquired immunodeficiency syndrome and for relapsed CML after allogeneic bone marrow transplantation. Initial studies in acquired immunodeficiency syndrome involved adoptive transfer of syngeneic peripheral blood lymphocytes and bone marrow; treatment resulted in short-term immune reconstitution but no antiviral benefit.[71] Subsequent studies with cells expanded 15–24-fold in culture have resulted in increased circulating CD4 cell numbers sustained for ≤ 6 weeks. Infusion of donor leukocytes in CML patients who relapsed after bone marrow transplantation resulted in cytogenetic remission after inducing graft-versus-host disease, suggesting a role for infusional cellular graft-versus-leukemia therapy.[72] While all these clinical studies are encouraging, effective and practical adoptive immunotherapy awaits additional basic understanding of the underlying cellular immunology.

Cellular Gene Therapy

Cells collected by hemapheresis have been used in the first therapeutic gene transfer protocol.[73] Two children with severe combined immunodeficiency as a result of an inherited deficiency of adenosine deaminase (ADA), received autologous T cells that had been expanded ex vivo and corrected by the insertion of a normal ADA gene. Monthly collections and reinfusions of gene-corrected cells have resulted in increased levels of ADA in both children and in improved immune function and clinical status. In these cases, lymphocytes have functioned as a temporary biologic drug-delivery system. Permanent correction of the genetic defect might be effected by inserting the ADA gene into hematopoietic stem cells. Hematopoietic stem cell gene insertion with retroviral vectors has been accomplished in murine and primate models, but the numbers of gene-marked cells are small and gene expression is poor. Recently retrovirus-mediated gene transfer into CD34-enriched human PBSC has been reported.[74] The ability to collect large numbers of leukocytes and PBSCs and to expand and manipulate their growth and differentiation in vitro makes these cells logical candidates for cellular gene therapy. Leukocytes are potential vehicles for replacing defective or deficient genes in a variety of inherited disorders and for delivery of new genes, for example, in the immunotherapy of cancer. The ability to insert and express genes in hematopoietic stem cells would create the opportunity to correct a variety of genetic and acquired disorders.

REFERENCES

1. Abel JJ, Rowntree LG, Turner BB: Plasma removal with return of corpuscles (plasmaphaeresis). J Pharmacol Exp Ther 5:625, 1914
2. Lockwood SM, Worlledge S, Nicholas A et al: Reversal of impaired splenic function in patients with nephritis or vasculitis by plasma exchange. N Engl J Med 300:524, 1979
3. Weiner AS, Wexler IB: The use of heparin when performing exchange blood transfusions in newborn infants. J Lab Clin Med 31:1016, 1946
4. Collins JA: Problems associated with the massive transfusion of stored blood. Surgery 75:274, 1974
5. McCullough J, Chopek M: Therapeutic plasma exchange. Lab Med 12:745, 1981
6. Tullis JL, Surgenor DM, Tinch RJ et al: New principle of closed system centrifugation. Science 124:792, 1956
7. Freireich EJ, Judson G, Levin RH: Separation and collection of leukocytes. Cancer Res 25:1516, 1965
8. Hester JP, Kellogg RM, Mulzet AP et al: Principles of blood separation and component extraction in a disposable continuous-flow single-stage channel. Blood 54:254, 1978

9. Koh HK: Extracorporeal photopheresis. p. 87. In Sacher RA, Brubaker DB, Kasprisin DO, McCarthy LJ (eds): Cellular and Humoral Immunotherapy and Apheresis. American Association of Blood Banks, Arlington, VA, 1991

10. Anderson R, Cassell M, Mullinax GL et al: Effect of normal cells on viscosity of sickle-cell blood: in vitro studies and report of six years experience with a prophylactic program of "partial exchange transfusion." Arch Intern Med 111:286, 1963

11. Lessin LS, Kurantsin-Mills J, Klug PP et al: Determination of rheologically optimal mixtures of AA and SS erythrocytes for transfusion. Prog Clin Biol Res 20:123, 1978

12. Keitel HG, Thompson D, Itano HA: Hyposthenuria in sickle cell anemia: a reversible renal defect. J Clin Invest 35:998, 1956

13. Pearson HA, Cornelius EA, Schwartz AD et al: Transfusion-reversible functional asplenia in young children with sickle-cell anemia. N Engl J Med 283:334, 1970

14. Miller DM, Winslow RM, Klein HG et al: Improved exercise performance after exchange transfusion in subjects with sickle cell anemia. Blood 56:1127, 1980

15. Rodgers GP, Schechter AN, Noguchi CT et al: Periodic microcirculatory flow in patients with sickle cell disease. N Engl J Med 311:1534, 1984

16. Klein HG: Transfusion support of hemoglobinopathies. p. 198. In Cash J (ed): Progress in Transfusion Medicine. Vol. 3. Churchill Livingstone, Edinburgh, 1987

17. Koshy M, Burd L, Wallace D et al: Prophylactic red-cell transfusions in pregnant patients with sickle cell disease. N Engl J Med 319:1447, 1988

18. Coles SM, Klein HG, Holland PV: Alloimmunization in two multitransfused patient populations. Transfusion 21:462, 1981

19. Diamond WJ, Brown FL, Bitterman P et al: Delayed hemolytic transfusion reactions presenting as sickle cell crisis. Ann Intern Med 93:231, 1980

20. Miller KD, Greenberg AE, Campbell CC: Treatment of severe malaria in the United States with a continuous infusion of quinidine gluconate and exchange transfusion. N Engl J Med 321:65, 1989

21. Jacoby JA, Hunt JV, Kosinski KS et al: Treatment of transfusion-transmitted babesiosis by exchange transfusion. N Engl J Med 303:1098, 1980

22. Winslow RM, Monge CC, Brown EG et al: The effect of hemodilution on O_2 transport in high altitude polycythemia. J Appl Physiol 59:1495, 1985

23. Freireich EJ, Thomas LB, Frei E III et al: A distinctive type of intracerebral hemorrhage associated with "blastic crisis" in patients with leukemia. Cancer 13:146, 1960

24. Lester TJ, Johnson JW, Cuttner J: Pulmonary leukostasis as the single worst prognostic factor in patients with acute myelocytic leukemia and hyperleukocytosis. Am J Med 79:43, 1985

25. Lichtman MA, Rowe JM: Hyperleukocytic leukemias: rheological, clinical, and therapeutic considerations. Blood 60:279, 1982

26. Cuttner J, Holland JF, Norton L et al: Therapeutic leukapheresis in acute myelocytic leukemia. Med Pediatr Oncol 11:76, 1983

27. Hester JP, McCredie KB, Freireich EJ: Response to chronic leukapheresis procedures and survival of chronic myelogenous leukemia patients. Transfusion 22:305, 1982

28. Lowenthal RM, Buskard NA, Goldman JM et al: Intensive leukapheresis as an initial therapy for chronic granulocytic leukemia. Blood 46:835, 1975

29. Goldfinger D, Capostagno V, Lowe C et al: Use of long-term leukapheresis in the treatment of chronic lymphocytic leukemia. Transfusion 20:450, 1980

30. Cooper IA, Ding JC, Adams PB: Intensive leukapheresis in the management of cytopenias in patients with chronic lymphocytic leukemia (CLL) and lymphocytic lymphoma. Am J Hematol 6:387, 1979

31. Fay JW, Moore JO, Logue GL et al: Leukopheresis therapy of leukemic reticuloendotheliosis (hairy cell leukemia). Blood 54:747, 1979

32. Golomb HM, Kraut EH, Oviatt DL et al: Absence of prolonged benefit of initial leukapheresis therapy for hairy cell leukemia. Am J Hematol 14:49, 1983

33. Wright DG, Karsh J, Fauci AS et al: Lymphocyte depletion and immunosuppression with repeated leukapheresis by continuous flow centrifugation. Blood 58:451, 1981

34. Karsh J, Klippel JH, Plotz PH et al: Lymphapheresis in rheumatoid arthritis: a randomized trial. Arthritis Rheum 24:867, 1981

35. Wallace DJ, Goldfinger D, Lowe C et al: A double-blind controlled study of lymphoplasmapheresis versus sham apheresis in rheumatoid arthritis. N Engl J Med 306:1406, 1982

36. Chievitz E, Thiede T: Complications and causes of death in polycythemia vera. Acta Med Scand 172:51, 1962

37. Dawson AA, Ogston D: The influence of the platelet count on the incidence of thrombotic and hemorrhagic complications in polycythemia vera. Postgrad Med J 46:76, 1970

38. Kessler CM, Klein HG, Havlik RJ: Uncontrolled thrombocythemia in myeloproliferative disorders. Br J Haematol 50:157, 1982

39. Klein HG: Plasma exchange in the future: innovations and new indications.

p. 557. In Rossi EC, Simon TL, Moss GS (eds): Principles of Transfusion Medicine. Williams & Wilkins, Baltimore, 1991

40. Strauss RG, Ciavarella D, Gilcher R et al: Clinical applications of therapeutic apheresis: report of the Clinical Applications Committee. J Clin Apheresis 8:4, 1993

41. Solomon A, Fahey JL: Plasmapheresis therapy in macroglobulinemia. Ann Intern Med 58:799, 1963

42. Taft EG, Propp RP, Sullivan SA: Plasma exchange for cold agglutinin hemolytic anemia. Transfusion 17:173, 1977

43. Silberstein LE, Berkman EM: Plasma exchange in autoimmune hemolytic anemia. J Clin Apheresis 1:238, 1983

44. Geltner D, Kohn RW, Gorevic PD et al: The effect of combination chemotherapy (steroids, immunosuppressives and plasmapheresis) on 5 mixed cryoglobulinemia patients with renal, neurologic and vascular involvement. Arthritis Rheum 24:1121, 1981

45. Miller J, Sanders E, Webb D: Plasmapheresis for paraquat poisoning. Lancet 1:875, 1978

46. King ME, Breslow JL, Lees RS: Plasma-exchange therapy of homozygous familial hypercholesterolemia. N Engl J Med 302:1457, 1979

47. Leitman SF, Smith JW, Gregg RE: Homozygous familial hypercholesterolemia: selective removal of low density lipoproteins by secondary membrane filtration. Transfusion 29:341, 1989

48. Gibberd FB, Billimoria JD, Page NGR, Retsas S: Heredopathia atactica polyneuritiformis (Refsum's disease) treated by diet and plasma-exchange. Lancet 1:575, 1979

49. Pintado T, Taswell HF, Bowie EJW: Treatment of life-threatening hemorrhage due to acquired factor VIII inhibitor. Blood 46:535, 1975

50. Nilsson I, Jonsson S, Sundquist S et al: A procedure for removing high titer antibodies by extracorporeal protein-A-sepharose adsorption in hemophilia substitution therapy and surgery in a patient with hemophilia B antibodies. Blood 58:38, 1981

51. Marder VJ, Nusbacher J, Anderson FW: One-year follow-up of plasma exchange therapy in 14 patients with idiopathic thrombocytopenic purpura. Transfusion 21:291, 1981

52. Kornfeld P, Ambinder EP, Mittag T et al: Plasmapheresis in generalized refractory myasthenia gravis. Arch Neurol 38:478, 1972

53. Cimo PL, Aster RH: Post-transfusion purpura: successful treatment by exchange transfusion. N Engl J Med 287:290, 1972

54. Johnson JP, Whitman W, Briggs WA et al: Plasmapheresis and immunosuppressive agents in antibasement membrane antibody-induced Goodpasture's syndrome. Am J Med 64:354, 1978

55. Roujeau JC, Kalis B, Lauret P et al: Plasma exchange in corticosteroid-resistant pemphigus. Br J Dermatol 106:103, 1982

56. Dyck PJ, Daube J, O'Brien P et al: Plasma exchange in chronic inflammatory demyelinating polyradiculoneuropathy. N Engl J Med 314:461, 1986

57. Guillain-Barré Study Group: Plasmapheresis and acute Guillain-Barré syndrome. Neurology 35:1096, 1985

58. Rock GA, Shumak KH, Buskard NA et al: Comparison of plasma exchange and plasma infusion in the treatment of thrombotic thrombocytopenic purpura. N Engl J Med 325:393, 1991

59. Bell WR, Braine HG, Ness PM, Kickler TS: Improved survival in thrombotic thrombocytopenic purpura-hemolytic uremic syndrome. N Engl J Med 325:398, 1991

60. Huestis DW: Complications of therapeutic apheresis. p. 179. In Valbonesi M, Pineda AA, Biggs JC (eds): Therapeutic Hemapheresis. Wichtig Editore, Milan, 1986

61. Sutton DMC, Nair RC, Rock G, and the Canadian Apheresis Study Group: Complications of plasma exchange. Transfusion 29:124, 1989

62. Lasky LC: The role of the laboratory in marrow manipulation. Arch Pathol Lab Med 115:293, 1991

63. Korbling M, Dorken B, Ho AD et al: Autologous transplantation of blood-derived hemopoietic stem cells after myeloablative therapy in a patient with Burkitt's lymphoma. Blood 67:529, 1986

64. Kessinger A, Armitage JO, Landmark JD et al: Autologous peripheral hematopoietic stem cell transplantation restores hematopoietic function following marrow ablative therapy. Blood 71:723, 1988

65. Storb R, Graham TC, Epstein RB et al: Demonstration of hemopoietic stem cells in the peripheral blood of baboons by cross circulation. Blood 50:537, 1977

66. Hillyer CD, Lackey DA, Hart KK et al: CD34+ progenitors and colony-forming units-granulocyte macrophage are recruited during large-volume leukapheresis and concentrated by counterflow centrifugl elutriation. Transfusion 33:316, 1993

67. Peters WP, Drago SS, Teppenberg M, Vredenburgh JJ: Collection, cryopreservation and use of peripheral blood progenitor cells primed with colony-stimulating growth factors. p. 51. In Sacher RA, AuBuchon JP (eds): Marrow Trans-

plantation: Practical and Technical Aspects of Stem Cell Reconstitution. American Association of Blood Banks, Bethesda, MD, 1992

68. Klein HG, Leitman SF: Adoptive immunotherapy in the treatment of malignant disease. Transfusion 29:170, 1989

69. Rosenberg SA: The immunotherapy and gene therapy of cancer. J Clin Oncol 10:180, 1992

70. Rosenberg SA, Spiess P, Lafreniere R: A new approach to the adoptive immunotherapy of cancer with tumor infiltrating lymphocytes. Science 233:1318, 1986

71. Lane HC, Zunich KM, Wilson W et al: Syngeneic bone marrow transplantation

and adoptive transfer of peripheral blood lymphocytes combined with zidovudine in human immunodeficiency virus infection. Ann Intern Med 113:512, 1990

72. Bar BMAM, Schattenberg A, Mensink EJBM et al: Donor leukocyte infusions for chronic myeloid leukemia relapsed after allogeneic bone marrow transplantation. J Clin Oncol 11:513, 1993

73. The ADA human gene therapy clinical protocol. Hum Gene Ther 1:441, 1990

74. Cassel A, Cottler-Fox M, Doren S, Dunbar C: Retroviral-mediated gene transfer into CD34-enriched human peripheral blood stem cells. Exp Hematol 21:585, 1993

Transfusion Reactions

141

Edward L. Snyder

INTRODUCTION

A transfusion reaction can be defined as any untoward reaction that occurs as a consequence of infusion of blood or one of its components. Reactions are considered to be *acute* when they occur during transfusion or within several hours after the transfusion has been terminated (Table 141-1). Reactions can also be classified as *delayed*. Delayed hemolytic transfusion reactions, for example, usually occur days after the transfusion. Other types of delayed reactions occur long after the blood has been infused—months or even years—as in the case of some transfusion-transmitted diseases. This chapter reviews various types of transfusion reactions.

HEMOLYTIC TRANSFUSION REACTIONS

Hemolytic transfusion reactions are caused by the immune-mediated lysis of transfused red cells. Immune-mediated hemolysis can be conveniently divided into four categories: by time of reaction (into acute or delayed) and by site of hemolysis (into intravascular or extravascular). Thus, the four types are

acute intravascular, acute extravascular, delayed intravascular, and delayed extravascular reactions (Table 141-2).

Acute Intravascular Hemolytic Transfusion Reactions

Acute reactions occur when incompatible red cells are transfused into a patient who already possesses the corresponding antibody and a reaction occurs within minutes. Because of naturally occurring ABO antibodies, infusion of ABO-incompatible blood is the most likely cause of a clinically significant acute intravascular hemolytic transfusion reaction.[1] Such a reaction could occur, for example, after transfusion of A red cells into an O recipient who has significant amounts of circulating anti-A. Although the titer and avidity of the antibody affect the extent of the hemolytic reaction, the clinical severity of an ABO-incompatible blood transfusion is greatly influenced by the degree of complement activation. In an ABO-incompatible transfusion reaction, fixation of the C5b-9 complex occurs with release of C3a and C5a (anaphylatoxins 1 and 2, respectively). These low-molecular-weight peptides produce bronchospasm, mast cell degranulation, hypotension (C3a), and pulmonary dysfunction (C5a); the latter is secondary to migration of granulocytes to the pulmonary capillary bed, resulting in $\dot{V}/\dot{Q}$ abnormalities.[2] Fixation of the C5b-9 complement membrane attack complex produces pores in the red cell membrane, and the resultant osmotic lysis produces hemoglobinuria and hemoglobine-

Table 141-1. Differential Diagnosis of Acute Transfusion Reactions

Reaction Type	Presenting Signs and Symptoms
Acute intravascular hemolytic	Fever, chills, dyspnea, hypotension, tachycardia, flushing, vomiting, back pain, hemoglobinuria, hemoglobinemia, shock
Acute extravascular hemolytic	Fever, indirect hyperbilirubinemia, post-transfusion hematocrit increment lower than expected
Febrile reaction	Fever, chills
Allergic (mild)	Urticaria, pruritus, rash
Anaphylactic	Dyspnea, bronchospasm, hypotension, tachycardia, shock
Hypervolemic	Dyspnea, tachycardia, hypertension, headache, jugular venous distension
Septic	Fever, chills, hypotension, tachycardia, vomiting, shock

Table 141-2. Hemolytic Transfusion Reactions: Serologic Presentation

Type	Antibody Detectable Initially	Primary Antibody Type	Degree of Complement Binding	Example
Acute intravascular	Yes	IgM	Full (C1–9)	ABO system
Acute extravascular	Yes	IgG	None/partial	Rh system
Delayed intravascular	No	IgG	Full (C1–9)	Kidd system
Delayed extravascular	No	IgG	None/partial	Duffy system

(Adapted from American Association of Blood Banks,[133] with permission.)

mia.[2,3] Indeed, the sine qua non of an acute intravascular hemolytic transfusion reaction is the presence of both red plasma and red urine. It is critically important to distinguish, as quickly as possible, hemoglobinuria and hemoglobinemia secondary to an acute hemolytic transfusion reaction from similar signs due to other causes. Such confusion can arise from a variety of reasons. Hemoglobinuria can be confused with hematuria from bladder hemorrhage, or myoglobinuria. Hemoglobinemia due to non-immune-mediated lysis can occur secondary to mechanical hemolysis from an improperly collected blood sample. The direct antiglobulin test (DAT) usually becomes positive in an immune hemolytic reaction; preparation of an antibody eluate is necessary to identify the offending antibody. An antibody elution is the removal of antibody from the red cell by various physical or chemical techniques with concentration of the antibody in the eluting solution, which is usually albumin/saline. This antibody-containing solution, the eluate, is then treated as a serum sample and used to identify the offending blood group antibody. The time lost in making a clinical diagnosis can turn a mild treatable reaction into one that is life-threatening. Indeed, a full-blown acute intravascular hemolytic transfusion reaction is a true medical emergency. Antibody-coated red cell stroma produced during an immune hemolytic transfusion reaction induces renal vasoconstriction, resulting in acute tubular necrosis.[2,4] The C3a and C4a generated may cause hypotension and tachycardia and may produce shock. Clinical symptoms include shortness of breath, chest pain, dizziness, and nausea. Patients often report a sense of impending doom. C3a can also cause bronchospasm, and C5a generation causes further pulmonary dysfunction. Many patients, curiously even anephric patients, often complain of lower back pain.[5] This is believed to be due to ischemic muscle pain or vasospasm, rather than to kidney pain from developing renal failure.

It is now appreciated that in addition to complement components, another class of biologic response modifiers, cytokines and interleukins (ILs) also play a role in the clinical symptom complex associated with acute intravascular hemolytic transfusion reactions. For example IL-1β, IL-6, and tumor necrosis factor-α (TNF-α) have pyrogenic activity; IL-8 is a neutrophil chemotactic and activating factor. These four cytokines have been generated in in vitro models of intravascular hemolysis and IgG-mediated red cell incompatibility.[6–9]

Therapy

Initial therapy consists of immediately stopping the transfusion, maintaining a patent intravenous line, supporting the patient's cardiorespiratory system, and ensuring a brisk diuresis. Increasing renal blood flow is the best way to prevent acute oliguric renal failure. The usual therapeutic maneuver used to induce a diuresis is infusion of 0.9% NaCl or some other suitable crystalloid solution. Crystalloid should be given to maintain a urine output of 100 ml/hr for about 24 hours. Diuretics, such as furosemide, can also be used and are preferred by some to infusion of mannitol to increase intravascular volume.[10,11] Mannitol, if chosen, must be used with caution; if acute tubular necrosis (ATN) occurs before mannitol infusion, pulmonary edema due to the acute increase in intravascular volume secondary to fluid expansion may occur. Similarly, excessive crystalloid infusion should be prevented in patients with borderline congestive heart failure. Renal damage must be minimized, however, and increasing renal blood flow helps to prevent anuric renal failure. Creatinine and BUN should be closely monitored; dialysis may be necessary for therapy of acute renal failure. As difficult as ATN therapy is, it is easier to treat a patient in the diuretic phase than in the oliguric phase of ATN. Support of blood pressure and respiration may require the use of vasopressors, bronchodilators, and, when necessary, intu-

---

APPROACH TO WORKUP OF AN ACUTE INTRAVASCULAR HEMOLYTIC TRANSFUSION REACTION

If an acute transfusion reaction occurs:

1. *Stop blood component infusion immediately*
2. Maintain intravenous access with a suitable crystalloid or colloid solution
3. Maintain blood pressure, heart rate
4. Maintain an adequate airway
5. Give a diuretic or institute a fluid diuresis, or both
6. Obtain blood/urine for transfusion reaction workup
   Blood bank workup of suspected transfusion reaction:
   Check paperwork to ensure correct blood component was transfused to the right patient
   Observe plasma for hemoglobinemia
   Perform direct antiglobulin test
   Repeat compatibility testing (cross-match)
   Repeat other serologic testing as needed (ABO, Rh)
   Analyze urine for hemoglobinuria

If intravascular hemolytic reaction confirmed:

7. Monitor renal status (BUN, creatinine)
8. Monitor coagulation status (prothrombin time, partial thromboplastin time, fibrinogen)
9. Monitor for signs of hemolysis (LDH, bilirubin, haptoglobin)
10. If sepsis is suspected, culture as appropriate

---

bation. Disseminated intravascular coagulation (DIC) can occur in severe cases, and heparin may be indicated if a significant coagulopathy is evident. Heparin, however, is rarely needed in mild cases. The prothrombin time, partial thromboplastin time, and fibrinogen level should be closely monitored.

Laboratory Evaluation

Laboratory findings include hemoglobinuria, hemoglobinemia, and a haptoglobin level that is low to 0 mg/dl. During the hemolytic episode, the bilirubin usually increases only to 2–3 mg/dl if the patient has normal liver function. Elevations of bilirubin to 20–30 mg/dl are not seen in otherwise normal patients even with florid hemolysis. Very elevated bilirubin levels are only seen in patients with concurrent hepatocellular disease such as viral hepatitis or hepatic carcinoma. Due to the lysis of red cells, levels of lactate dehydrogenase (LDH) may rise markedly. If the patient shows no signs of vasomotor instability and if hemostatic and renal function are unchanged 24 hours after the incompatible transfusion, the episode can be considered to be over, with serious sequelae unlikely. Although ABO-incompatible blood transfusions are the most common cause of an acute intravascular hemolytic transfusion reaction, other complement-fixing antigen-antibody systems, such as the Jk^a (Kidd) or Fy^a (Duffy) blood group systems, can also produce these reactions.[12]

Acute Extravascular Hemolytic Transfusion Reaction

In an extravascular hemolytic transfusion reaction, complement either is not fixed at all or it may be fixed only to C3b. In either situation, because of the nature of the antigen-antibody eaction, complement activation with fixation of the C5b-9 complex does not occur. The presence of IgG on the red cell or ixation of complement to C3b, or both, results in an extravascular reaction, since the antibody-coated cells are cleared by either the IgG receptors in the spleen or the C3b receptors in the liver, but red cell lysis does not occur in the intravascular space. Largely as a result of the lack of generation C3a or C5a, an extravascular hemolytic transfusion reaction does not usually present as a clinical emergency. It is characterized, as are all immune hemolytic transfusion reactions, by development of a positive DAT due to recipient red cell alloantibody binding to the circulating donor red cells. Moreover, an increase in indirect bilirubin, an increase in LDH, a decline in hematocrit, and an increase in colorless urine urobilinogen occurs; hemoglobinuria and hemoglobinemia, however, are rarely present. The patient typically remains clinically stable, and renal failure, shock, and hemostatic abnormalities such as DIC are rarely seen unless the amount of incompatible blood infused is excessive. However, patients often have a low-grade fever, some of which may be attributable to the generation of IL-1 or other pyrogenic cytokines.

The diagnostic test of choice is, again, a DAT with an eluate. The eluate is performed to identify the antibody coating the red cells.[12] It must be remembered that the positive DAT result is due to the patient's antibody coating the donor red cells. This is not autoantibody, and the patient's own red cells are not involved in the reaction. Usually an acute extravascular hemolytic transfusion reaction requires no therapy, and the patient characteristically recovers in a few days as the offending donor red cells are cleared from the circulation. The pathogenic alloantibody can often be identified in the patient's serum. These acute transfusion reactions may occur either if the patient's pre-existing alloantibody was missed by the blood bank during the antibody screening process, or, more often, if the unit of blood was mislabeled or was hung in error on the wrong patient by the house or nursing staff.[1]

Delayed Hemolytic Reactions

The pathogenesis of a delayed intravascular transfusion reaction is similar to that described for acute intravascular hemolytic reactions. However, in the delayed type, the patient develops the antigen-antibody reaction some time (5–10 days) after the transfusion. The process thus occurs more slowly and is less likely to present as a clinical emergency. Hemoglobinuria and hemoglobinemia can occur but often are less profound and pronounced than are seen with an acute intravascular reaction. This is likely due to the continual and gradual removal of antibody-coated red cells as the antibody titer rises, as well as to more gradual generation of C3a and C5a. The same serologic diagnostic and treatment concepts used for an acute intravascular hemolytic reaction apply here. However, the need for acute intervention is much less likely. Initiating a diuresis and monitoring renal and hemostatic function may be sufficient.

Delayed extravascular hemolytic transfusion reactions occur as well. Such antigen-antibody reactions often involve the Rh system. The clinical presentation is similar to that of an acute extravascular reaction in that the patient often has no acute clinical symptoms but may present with a fever, a falling hematocrit, and the development of a new DAT. Serologic evaluation of a transfusion reaction in a patient who had a positive pretransfusion antiglobulin test result, caused by autoantibody or medication, may be confusing. Such a workup requires an expert serologist to detect the new alloantibody in the patient's serum and make a diagnosis of a hemolytic transfusion reaction.

FEBRILE NONHEMOLYTIC TRANSFUSION REACTIONS

A febrile nonhemolytic transfusion reaction (FNHTR) is suspected when a temperature rise of $\geq 1°C$ occurs during or after transfusion when no other cause can be found. In addition to fever, an FNHTR is often accompanied by shaking chills. These reactions are due to cytotoxic or agglutinating antibodies in the patient's plasma reacting against antigens present on transfused donor lymphocytes, granulocytes, or platelets.[13–16] The antibodies often have HLA specificity, although they also may be neutrophil- or platelet-specific.[17,18] Conversely, the donor plasma can also contain antibody that can react with the corresponding cellular antigens in the recipient's blood.[19] The cause of the fever relates to antibody-leukocyte or antibody-platelet interactions. The febrile reaction is mediated largely by the release of cytokines such as IL-1β, IL-6, and TNF-α from macrophages, monocytes, granulocytes, or lymphocytes.[20] IL-1 (endogenous pyrogen), via prostaglandin E_2 synthesis, probably stimulates the thermoregulatory center of the hypothalamus to produce fever. Other mediators such as macrophage inflammatory proteins (MIP-1) may also participate in the febrile response, but this reaction is not mediated through prostaglandin synthesis.[21]

The cytokines could be derived from three possible sources in the transfusion setting. The first is synthesis by recipient leukocytes in response to transfusion. The second is production by donor leukocytes after infusion into the recipient. The third mechanism is generation by donor leukocytes in vitro during storage prior to transfusion.[22] Red cells and units of platelet concentrates have sufficient potential sources of cytokines in the ample number (10^7–10^8) of mononuclear leukocytes capable of cytokine synthesis. Studies have shown that generation of cytokines does indeed occur in units of blood during storage and that such generation is directly proportional to the leukocyte count of the unit, as well as the duration of storage.[23–25] Use of third-generation leukocyte reduction filters can lower the incidence of febrile reactions. Judging from reports of persistent febrile reactions despite use of these 3–4 $\log_{10}$ leukocyte reduction filters, such filtration needs to occur before storage and before the donor leukocytes begin to generate these proinflammatory cytokines in the blood storage bag. These cytokines are not removed by bedside blood filters and enter the circulation.[26]

The frequency of febrile reactions has been estimated to be 0.5%/U transfused.[27,28] Reactions are most commonly seen in recipients who have been exposed to multiple white cell or platelet antigens, such as oncology patients or multiparous women. The oncology patients are at risk as a result of frequent transfusions and multiparous women are at risk from multiple exposures during childbirth. Both of these groups of patients can form multiple HLA, granulocyte, or platelet-specific antibodies that will react with white cells or platelets on subsequent exposure. Antigen-antibody reactions are capable of stimulating cellular activation with resultant complement fixation, cytokine (IL) generation, and activation of other biologic response modifiers.[29,30]

Clinical Manifestations

Clinically, an FNHTR is characterized by fever and chills occurring shortly after the transfusion has begun.[31] The patient may have nausea and vomiting. Various factors, including rate of infusion of the blood and leukocyte content of the transfused blood (antigen load), may have an effect on the severity of the clinical presentation of the febrile reaction. Febrile reactions also can occur several hours after the transfusion has ended.[14] Although an FNHTR often starts with the patient's complaint of feeling uneasy or "chilly," symptoms often progress from a slight tremor to true rigors. The chills or rigors are a manifestation of heat-conserving cutaneous vasoconstriction and result in muscular heat production.[32] These thermogenic responses, coupled with any effects due to release of IL-1β or other cytokines, may cause the patient's temperature to rise several degrees above pretransfusion levels. Although these reactions are rarely dangerous, the severity often increases as the rate and dose of the infusion increases. Mild reactions are generally more uncomfortable and frightening than life-threatening. FNHTRs are usually self-limited, with fever persisting for ≤8–10 hours. Elderly patients with a tenuous cardiovascular status and critically ill patients may develop respiratory complications, hypotension, or shock. Young adults, however, are less likely to become seriously ill even with development of a high fever. As in any transfusion reaction, the onset of fever and chills requires that the transfusion be stopped, the intravenous line kept open with normal saline or a suitable crystalloid, and appropriate samples sent to the blood bank. The patient should be reassured, as anxiety may be extreme.

Laboratory Evaluation

The workup of a febrile reaction must be undertaken promptly. Fever may also be the first sign of an acute hemolytic reaction or infusion of a unit of red cells or platelets contaminated with bacteria. The workup consists of ruling out a hemolytic reaction by reconfirming the ABO type of the patient and the donor unit, re-cross-matching to confirm patient-donor compatibility, evaluating the results of the pre- and post-transfusion DATs, evaluating the serum for hemolysis, and rechecking accuracy of paperwork.[33–35] The post-transfusion DAT should yield negative findings, as an FNHTR does not involve red cell alloantibody. As laboratory testing is being completed, the workup should extend beyond the blood bank to include bedside patient evaluation. As fever and chills also may be caused by drugs or by diseases associated with infection or inflammation, these factors should also be evaluated. Blood cultures of both the patient and the blood product, to rule out infusion of a contaminated unit of blood, is becoming more common at many medical centers. The difficulty lies in knowing when to order blood cultures. Not only are blood cultures expensive, but there is a 3% incidence of positive cultures due to contamination during collection (see the section Bacterial Contamination). Most routine hospital blood banks do not have the expertise or reagents needed to identify specific HLA, platelet, or granulocyte antibodies. Accordingly, the diagnosis of a febrile hemolytic transfusion reaction is usually made without isolating an identifiable antibody. The FNHTR is often a diagnosis of exclusion arrived at after ruling out a hemolytic reaction, a septic transfusion, or other possible causes of fever.

Fever usually responds to antipyretics, including aspirin and acetaminophen. For thrombocytopenic adult patients, acetaminophen (325–650 mg PO) is the antipyretic of choice. Thrombocytopenic patients should avoid aspirin, as this will further compromise platelet function because of its inhibitory effect on platelet cyclo-oxygenase, an enzyme involved in the release reaction. Nonthrombocytopenic patients may receive aspirin if its use is not contraindicated for other medical reasons. Many house officers routinely order diphenhydramine for treatment of febrile reactions. This therapy, however, should be reserved for pretreatment of possible allergic reactions. Unless the patient has a history of allergic reactions or shows signs of an allergic component to an FNHTR, such as flushing, hives, or pruritis, there is no benefit from the use of antihistamines for febrile reactions. In addition, antihistamines may produce drowsiness in some patients.

For patients with no history of febrile reactions, routine premedication is unnecessary. Adult patients with severe reactions despite premedication may require more intensive pharmacotherapy, including hydrocortisone sodium succinate (100 mg IV) given immediately before transfusion. Patients with severe shaking chills can be treated with meperidine intramuscularly or subcutaneously. Meperidine can stop shaking chills almost immediately.[36] Febrile reactions after granulocyte transfusions and, less frequently, after platelet transfusions can be so severe that hypotension and cardiovascular collapse can occur.

Prevention of febrile reactions when pharmacologic therapy fails relies on the use of leukocyte-depleted blood components. Several leukocyte depletion techniques are available. Centrifugation can remove approximately 70% of the leukocytes in 1 U of blood, and cell washing or use of frozen deglycerolized red cells can remove ≤95% of contaminating white cells. Older microaggregate blood filters can reduce leukocyte content by approximately 1–2 logs (90–93%).[37–43] Third-generation leukocyte depletion red cell filters are also useful for preventing febrile reactions.[44–46] They can remove ≤4 logs (99.99%) of white cells, often lowering the level of white cells in 1 U of blood from 10^9 to 10^5. They also may be useful for preventing or delaying the onset of HLA alloimmunization.[47,48] Leukocyte-depletion platelet filters are also available.[49–55] Use of leukocyte-depleted blood components is currently controversial.[56,57] Data show that a patient who has had one febrile transfusion reaction has a 1:8 chance of having another one.[28] Thus, although they clearly are indicated for people with multiple and recurrent febrile reactions, many physicians question whether leukocyte-depleted blood products should be used indiscriminately for all patients.[56,57] Individuals with a history of recurrent severe febrile reactions should have notations made in their blood bank record to ensure continued future use of leukocyte-depleted components.

ALLERGIC TRANSFUSION REACTIONS

Allergic transfusion reactions are believed to be most commonly due to infusion of plasma proteins.[58] The allergic manifestations produced vary; they include skin erythema with mild associated urticaria and pruritus; a confluent rash, which is intensely pruritic; extensive urticaria; severe vasomotor instability; bronchospasm; and anaphylaxis. It is important to note that a patient who develops hives and a mild allergic reaction during a blood transfusion does not progress to a more severe anaphylactic reaction after infusion of additional blood from the same unit. Thus, the severity of allergic transfusion reactions is not necessarily dose related.

The exact nature of the antibodies involved in the various types of allergic reactions is unclear. The mild allergic reactions are usually IgG mediated, but IgE may also be involved; anaphylactic reactions are most often IgG mediated.[5] Allergic transfusion reactions are quite common, occurring in approximately 1% of all transfusions.[59,60] Most of these reactions start with the patient's complaining of pruritus followed by the development of hives. At this point, the transfusion should be stopped and the patient given 25–50 mg of diphenhydramine, if there are no medical contraindications and if the patient had not been already maximally premedicated. After a short interval the transfusion can be continued *but only if* the rash decreases and/or the hives disappear and the patient feels well and shows no signs of fever, chills, or vasomotor instability. For mild allergic transfusion reactions not associated with any cardiorespiratory problems, such as bronchospasm, dyspnea, hypotension, or tachycardia, it is acceptable to continue the transfusion after the reaction has subsided, as it is not likely to recur. The risk of transfusion-transmitted disease posed by infusion of another unit of blood is greater than the risk posed by continuing a transfusion that has produced mild urticaria.

This is not true, however, if the patient shows signs of systemic toxicity from the transfusion, such as hypotension, bronchospasm, or tachycardia.

The treatment of mild allergic reactions involves the use of diphenhydramine. Reactions are rarely serious and often do not recur with subsequent transfusions. The pathogenesis is thought to be recipient antibody directed against donor plasma proteins. Most blood banks, however, are not able to identify the etiologic antibody; identification usually requires research laboratory techniques. Accordingly, the diagnosis of an allergic transfusion reaction is a diagnosis of exclusion. Washed red cells can be used to prevent reactions.[37,38] Leukocyte depletion or microaggregate filters are of no value since the plasma protein passes through the filter. Most patients who have one allergic reaction should continue to receive routine bank blood. Washed cells should not be provided until a second reaction has occurred and generally should be provided only for patients with severe or recurrent reactions. The occurrence of one or two hives or mild pruritus after transfusion is not an indication for use of washed cells. Anaphylactic reactions, however, can be life-threatening and may require intubation and pressor agents. Washed cells for patients experiencing these reactions are appropriate. Although it is convenient to characterize a transfusion reaction as purely febrile or allergic, in reality the two symptoms are often mixed, and the reaction is designated according to the predominant clinical sign.

OTHER ADVERSE EFFECTS OF TRANSFUSION

Microaggregate Debris and Adult Respiratory Distress Syndrome

Much has been published regarding the use of microaggregate filters for preventing adult respiratory distress syndrome (ARDS) after massive transfusion.[56,57,61-65] Microaggregate debris consists of dead platelets, granulocytes, and fibrin strands that form in blood during storage.[66-68] It has been hypothesized that infusion of blood containing microaggregate debris through standard 170-μm-pore filters results in the passage of these 20-120-μm-size microaggregates into the pulmonary vasculature, producing occlusion of the pulmonary capillaries and pulmonary failure. Published studies have shown, however, that microaggregate filters are not required and do not appear to influence the onset of ARDS.[69,70] This syndrome is most likely, and most often, attributable to concurrent hypotension and sepsis, rather than to infusion of microaggregate debris per se. Microaggregate filters may be of value during cardiopulmonary bypass surgery, when the microaggregate debris can enter the arterial circulation directly. It is likely that improvements in surgical techniques, post-trauma medical care, perfusion technology, and especially treatment of shock and sepsis have contributed more to the decreased incidence of postperfusion ARDS than has use of microaggregate filters.[71]

Leukocyte Reduction

Multiple reasons are emerging to perform leukocyte reduction of units of blood and components. Standards of the American Association of Blood Banks recommend that to prevent febrile reactions levels of leukocytes should be $<5 \times 10^8$ and for other purposes $<5 \times 10^6$.[72] The "other" indications for leukocyte reduction range from those for which some data exist (such as to decrease the incidence of HLA-alloimmunization[47,48]) to other areas with fewer data (such as to decrease the incidence of tumor recurrence[73]). As more data are published, the indications for use of leukocyte reduction filters will become clearer. For now, a conservative approach to their use for well-established indications would seem most prudent.

Bacterial Contamination

Bacterial contamination of stored blood can pose grave risks to the recipient. Bacteria can enter the blood bag during venipuncture as a result of inadequate skin preparation or during component preparation.[74] Some bacteria grow best at room temperature; other (psychrophilic) organisms grow optimally at refrigerated blood bank (1°–6°C) temperatures. Gram-negative bacteria, including *Pseudomonas, Yersinia, Enterocolitica,* and *Flavobacterium,* are organisms commonly associated with a contaminated unit of refrigerated blood.[75,76] Platelet concentrates, stored at room temperature, are also known to be subject to bacterial contamination; several reports have described fatal septic transfusion reactions due to platelets containing *Salmonella* or *Staphylococcus.*[77-79] Units of blood that are contaminated need not be obviously discolored, malodorous, or clotted; by simple visual inspection it is usually impossible to determine whether a unit is contaminated.

Individuals who receive a unit of contaminated blood may develop fever, rigors, skin flushing, abdominal cramps, myalgias, DIC, renal failure, cardiovascular collapse, and cardiac arrest. Clinically the patient presents in warm shock. These reactions may be immediate or there may be a delay of several hours before the symptom complex becomes apparent. Reaction to infusion of a unit of contaminated blood is distinguishable from FNHTR by the former's more severe clinical presentation and is distinguishable from intravascular hemolytic transfusion reaction by the absence of the latter's characteristic hemoglobinuria and hemoglobinemia. Reactions following transfusion of infected units of blood are often attributable to endotoxin produced by gram-negative bacteria. The presence of bacteria alone, however, can also cause many of these symptoms. Additionally, evidence is accumulating that the symptom complex is attributable, in part, to cytokines and ILs generated in the contaminated, stored blood in vitro. These biologic response modifiers could produce severe reactions in vivo after transfusion.[23-25,80]

If, during transfusion, a patient who appeared well suddenly develops rigors and shock, infusion of an infected component should be considered. If, on further evaluation, this diagnosis is still considered likely, the patient should be treated immediately, since delay significantly contributes to the chance of a fatal outcome. The need to support blood pressure, pulse, respiration, and renal blood flow should be remembered. Blood infusion should be stopped the moment any transfusion reaction is suspected and appropriate samples sent to the blood bank for a DAT and other studies. Cultures of the untransfused blood remaining in the blood bag should be sent, as they may be diagnostic. Broad-spectrum antibiotics should be started immediately if infusion of contaminated blood is suspected and continued until the culture results are reported. These reactions are rare, but when they occur they can be fatal. Use of recombinant IL or cytokine inhibitors is still too experimental to be useful clinically.

Circulatory Overload

Hypervolemia

Hypervolemia is a form of transfusion reaction that should be considered in patients who, during a blood infusion, develop sudden severe headache, dyspnea, tachycardia, tachypnea, congestive heart failure, or other signs of fluid overload. Unless the patient is actively hemorrhaging, blood should never be infused rapidly, as the acute expansion of the patient's intravascular volume may exceed the capacity of the cardiovascular system to compensate.[81] Rapidly transfusing a patient who is anemic but who is euvolemic and not actively bleeding produces no benefit and may cause harm. This caveat applies to transfusion of any blood component. Patients with compromised cardiopulmonary status may not tolerate acute blood volume expansion and may develop right- or left-sided heart failure. This is especially true for infants and the elderly. If symptoms occur, the transfusion should be stopped and some form of volume reduction, either diuretics or phlebotomy, instituted. If a concern exists that the patient may not tolerate infusion of a full unit of blood or component within the 4-hour period allotted for infusion of blood components, the blood bank can divide the product into smaller portions, which can be transfused in aliquots. As a general guide, infusions in adults should occur at a rate that is not >2–4 ml/kg/hr. The rate should be lowered to 1 ml/kg/hr for patients at risk of fluid overload. Diuretics may be given to patients with compromised cardiopulmonary status before transfusion. The initial stages of transfusion-induced hypervolemia may be difficult to distinguish from hemolytic transfusion reactions as well as from febrile or allergic reactions. The absence of hemoglobinuria and hemoglobinemia or absence of a positive post-transfusion DAT result should serve to distinguish this group from the set of reactions due to immune hemolysis, and the absence of fever, chills, or urticaria from the febrile or allergic types of reactions.

Transfusion-Related Acute Lung Injury

Noncardiogenic Pulmonary Edema

On rare occasions individuals being transfused with red cells or platelets develop pulmonary edema without an elevation in cardiac pressure.[82–86] Several reports of this type of transfusion-related acute lung injury suggest that these cases may be more common than expected. The chest radiograph reveals a pulmonary edema pattern, and there is respiratory insufficiency but without development of elevated left-side cardiac pressure. Copious amounts of pulmonary edema fluid are produced, as is characteristic of hypervolemia; however, the noncardiogenic reaction usually follows infusion of volumes of blood too small to produce fluid overload. The patient may also develop fever, chills, cyanosis, or hypotension. The postulated pathologic mechanism includes a reaction between donor-derived antibodies to HLA or neutrophil antigens and recipient leukocytes; complement activation also may occur when leukoagglutinins present in the recipient react with leukocytes contained in the infused donor blood, with aggregation of white cells.[87,88] As a result, the activated leukocytes generate adhesive molecules on their surface—CD11/CD18. These proteins permit the leukocytes to attach to the cell membrane of the pulmonary endothelial cells and by diapedesis enter the interstitial space between the pulmonary capillaries and the alveolar epithelium. Once they are in the interstitial space, the neutrophils degranulate and release destructive enzymes, which produce a capillary leak, resulting in fluid filling the alveolar air sacs. Thus, pulmonary leukostasis with pulmonary edema occurs as a result of microvascular occlusion and capillary leakage.[89,90] Complement-activated granulocytes also produce oxygen radicals that damage pulmonary endothelial cells, resulting in an increase in pulmonary vascular permeability and further passage of fluid into aveolar spaces. Since this diagnosis usually requires that cardiac monitoring (Swan-Ganz) catheters be in place, it is difficult to make outside the operating room or intensive care unit. When a patient shows signs of noncardiogenic pulmonary edema, the infusion should be stopped, as with all other reactions. These HLA/neutrophil antigen-antibody reactions may be idiosyncratic and often do not recur. To remove leukocyte antigens from units of red cells or platelets, leukocyte reduction filters may be useful; washed red cells are useful for that component as well. Multiparous women who are blood donors and blood donors who have been multiply transfused should not be used as plasma donors, as their serum may contain high titers of leukoagglutinating antibodies.[91]

Hypothermia

Hypothermia can occur with rapid infusion of large quantities of refrigerated (1–6°C) blood.[92–94] Data have shown that rapid infusion of blood (1 U every 5 minutes) may lower the temperature of the sinoatrial node to <30°C, at which point ventricular fibrillation may occur.[95] Most transfusions need not be given this rapidly. Thus, for routine transfusion, blood does not have to be warmed. Indeed, overwarming blood can cause thermal injury and produce hemolysis, DIC, or shock. Furthermore, a delay in infusing blood due to the extra time required for warming could impede resuscitation. Thus, routine warming of blood for trauma patients is not recommended. If blood is to be warmed, only an electric blood warmer should be used. The temperature must be monitored and kept at <38°C.[96] Heating blood under running hot tap water or heating in a microwave device is unacceptable; microwave devices produce hot spots that can cause hemolysis.[97,98]

Electrolyte Toxicity

Citrate, a component of the preservative solution used in blood storage, functions as an anticoagulant by chelating calcium and interfering with the coagulation cascade. Rapid transfusion of citrated blood can thus be associated with a drop in ionized calcium levels.[99–101] Citrate-containing blood products, however, are routinely infused without any problem, as the citrate is rapidly metabolized to bicarbonate. In patients with normal liver function, citrate infusion is thus highly unlikely to produce reactions. Mild citrate toxicity can be seen, however, in individuals undergoing cytapheresis when large volumes of citrated plasma are reinfused.[102]

The effects of hypocalcemia range from mild circumoral paresthesias to frank tetany. However, severe citrate toxicity even with massive transfusion is very rare. More commonly the reaction is mild and self-limiting and can be treated by merely slowing the rate of reinfusion.[103] If prolonged Q-T intervals or signs of tetany are seen, calcium can be administered. It is important to bear in mind that infusion of calcium is itself often associated with the development of ventricular arrhythmias and cardiac arrest.[104] Calcium should not be infused routinely, even after large-volume blood transfusions. *Under no circumstances should calcium be added to a unit of blood as it would recalcify the unit and cause clots to form in the bag.* Hypomagnesemia, presumably due to chelation of magnesium by citrate, has also been reported. Actual clinical complications of transfusion-induced hypomagnesemia, however, have not been well documented.[105] Hyperkalemia due to infusion of stored blood is a rare occurrence. Although hyperkalemia is often thought to be a problem in massive transfusion, in reality development of hypokalemia is of greater concern. With storage, leakage of potassium from red cells to the extracellular fluid occurs. However, following infusion into a recipient, the red cells reverse this biochemical storage lesion and intracellular potassium levels are restored. Furthermore, as the citrate is metabolized to bicarbonate the blood becomes alkalotic, contributing to hypokalemia.[106–108] In massive transfusion this may not uncommonly result in the need for administration of potassium. Extracellular potassium increases in a blood bag at the rate of about 1 mEq/day during the first few weeks of storage. If this presents a concern for neonates or patients with renal failure, fresher blood can be requested. Ammonia toxicity was previously thought to be a problem with stored blood but rarely is a problem today.[109]

Plasticizers

Plasticizers are chemicals used to make the rigid polyvinyl chloride plastic used in blood bags more malleable. The traditional plasticizer is di-2-ethylhexylphthalate (DEHP).[110] There has been some question as to whether DEHP is carcinogenic and whether its breakdown product, monoethylhexylphthalate, may produce problems due to production of peroxisomes, which may be destructive to vital organs.[111–114] This plasticizer is being replaced with a citrate-based plasticizer, and new generation blood bags are commercially available.[115,116] Ironically, DEHP plasticizers may actually serve a useful function in that they appear to stabilize the red cell membrane and also may have a beneficial effect on platelet morphology.[117–119]

Graft-Versus-Host Disease

Graft-versus-host disease (GVHD) occurs when immunologically competent lymphocytes are introduced into an immunoincompetent host who is unable to destroy the donor lymphocytes. The immunocompetent donor lymphocytes engraft, recognize the host as foreign, and then attack host tissues. GVHD occurs after allogeneic bone marrow transplantation and (less often) after transfusion of nonirradiated cellular blood components, especially when the blood donor and recipient share some HLA antigens.[120] There is an increased danger from post-transfusion GVHD, in part because of the frequent failure of physicians to recognize and treat the reaction promptly. Another major factor, however, is the propensity of the donor's lymphocytes to produce recipient bone marrow aplasia. In post-bone marrow transplant GVHD, the bone marrow is of donor origin and bone marrow aplasia does not occur. In post-transfusion GVHD, however, the bone marrow is of foreign (host) origin and the donor's lymphocytes attack it, thus producing aplasia.

Post-transfusion GVHD is fatal in 90% of cases, primarily because of aplasia of the recipient's bone marrow. Reports have shown that haploidentical directed donor units of blood may produce fatal post-transfusion GVHD even in immunocompetent recipients.[121,122] The use of irradiated blood (≥2,500 cGy) is now recommended in clinical situations in which post-transfusion GVHD is considered likely, such as when patients receive blood transfusions from their relatives. Leukocyte reduction filters should not be used as prophylaxis against GVHD, as the exact number of leukocytes needed to produce the disease is not known with certainty. Case reports of fatal GVHD in patients who received leukocyte reduced, but not irradiated blood have been published.[123] Recent articles have addressed this subject in depth.[124–127] Radiation of red cells produces a membrane defect, however, which causes a slow leakage of potassium and hemoglobin.[128] Accordingly, the Food and Drug Administration has ruled that irradiated units of red cells shall have an outdate not to exceed 28 days from the time of irradiation.

Hemosiderosis

One milliliter of red cells contains 1 mg iron. A unit of blood with 250 ml of red cells thus contains approximately 250 mg iron, and 4 U of blood contain 1 g iron, roughly the amount stored in the bone marrow. Males and nonmenstruating women lose only about 1 mg iron/day. Continued use of transfusion

---

GENERAL GUIDELINES FOR USE OF IRRADIATED BLOOD COMPONENTS

Absolute indications
    Bone marrow transplant recipients
    Congential immunodeficiency syndrome patients
Relative indications
    Infants receiving intrauterine/exchange transfusion for hemolytic disease of the newborn
    Premature infants
    Patients with hematologic malignancies
    Patients receiving intensive chemo/radiotherapy for solid tumors
    Directed donor units from family relatives
    Immunosuppressed patients receiving organ transplants
No definite indications
    Patients with the acquired immunodeficiency syndrome

(Adapted from American Association of Blood Banks,[133] with permission.)

---

therapy in individuals with an extravascular type of hemolytic anemia, such as those with thalassemia or sickle cell anemia, in which iron is not lost from the body but is recycled, can thus result in the accumulation of excessive tissue stores of iron. Over long periods, the iron that is stored in parenchymal cells results in death of the cell and eventual organ failure.[129] Despite early signs of promise, transfusion of reticulocyte-rich blood (neocytes) has not been found to be of value for decreasing the transfusion requirement in patients with chronic hemolytic anemias.[130] While young red cells have a longer half-life and should decrease the transfusion requirement, neocytes are not widely accepted as clinically useful. Iron chelation therapy such as that with deferoxamine is now widely used and actually may be able to maintain patients with chronic hemolytic anemias in negative iron balance.[131] Oral iron chelators are under development.

Air Emboli

With replacement of evacuated glass bottles by plastic blood bags, the risk of air embolism from phlebotomy or transfusion has virtually disappeared from transfusion practice. Air, however, may still be pumped into patients by the roller pumps contained in various transfusion devices.[132] Most devices contain in-line air sensors. However, any operators using this equipment must be well trained and remain alert to the potential risk of air embolization at all times while the patient is being treated. Patients who receive air intravenously experience acute cardiopulmonary insufficiency. The air tends to lodge in the right ventricle, preventing blood from entering the pulmonary circulation. Acute cyanosis, pain, cough, shock, and arrhythmia may occur, and death may result unless immediate action is taken. The patient should be placed head down on the left side. This will usually displace the air bubble from the pulmonary valve.

REFERENCES

1. Honig CL, Bove JR: Transfusion-associated fatalities: a review of Bureau of Biologics reports 1976–1978. Transfusion 20:653, 1980
2. Frank MM: Complement in the pathophysiology of human disease. N Engl J Med 316:1525, 1987

3. Williams LW, Burks AW, Steele RW: Complement: function and clinical relevance. Ann Allergy 60:293, 1988

4. Schmidt PJ, Holland PV: Pathogenesis of the acute renal failure associated with incompatible transfusion. Lancet 2:1169, 1967

5. Mollison PL, Engelfriet CP, Contreras M (eds): Blood Transfusion in Clinical Medicine. 8th Ed. Blackwell Scientific Publications, London, 1987, p. 601

6. Davenport RD, Strieter RM, Standiford TJ, Kunkel SL: Interleukin-8 production in red blood cell incompatibility. Blood 76:2439, 1990

7. Davenport RD, Burdick M, Moore SA, Kunkel SL: Cytokine production in IgG-mediated red cell incompatibility. Transfusion 33:19, 1993

8. Davenport RD, Strieter RM, Kunkel SL: Red cell ABO incompatibility and production of tumour necrosis factor-alpha. Br J Haematol 78:540, 1991

9. Blajchman MA: Cytokines in transfusion medicine. Transfusion 33:1, 1993

10. Barry KG, Crosby WH: The prevention and treatment of renal failure following transfusion reactions. Transfusion 3:34, 1963

11. Goldfinger D: Acute hemolytic transfusion reactions—a fresh look at pathogenesis and considerations regarding therapy. Transfusion 17:85, 1977

12. Issitt PD: Applied Blood Group Serology. 3rd Ed. Montgomery Press, Miami, 1985

13. Brittingham TE, Chaplin H Jr: Febrile transfusion reactions caused by sensitivity to donor leukocytes and platelets. JAMA 165:819, 1957

14. Payne R: The association of febrile transfusion reactions with leukoagglutinins. Vox Sang 2:233, 1957

15. Perkins HA, Payne R, Ferguson J, Wood M: Nonhemolytic febrile transfusion reactions. Vox Sang 11:578, 1966

16. Decary F, Ferner P, Giavedoni L et al: An investigation of nonhemolytic transfusion reactions. Vox Sang 46:277, 1984

17. Heinrich D, Mueller-Eckhardt C, Stier W: The specificity of leukocyte and platelet alloantibodies in sera of patients with nonhemolytic transfusion reactions. Vox Sang 25:442, 1973

18. de Rie MA, van der Plas-van Dalen CM, Engelfriet CP, von dem Borne AEGK: The serology of febrile transfusion reactions. Vox Sang 49:126, 1985

19. Popovsky MA, Moore SB: Diagnostic and pathogenetic considerations in transfusion-related acute lung injury. Transfusion 25:573, 1985

20. Dinarello CA, Cannon JG, Wolff SM: New concepts on the pathogenesis of fever. Rev Infect Dis 10:168, 1988

21. Davatelis G, Wolpe SD, Sherry B et al: Macrophage inflammatory protein-1, a prostaglandin independent endogenous pyrogen. Science 243:1066, 1989

22. Stack G, Snyder EL: Cytokine generation in stored platelet concentrates. Transfusion 34:20, 1994

23. Stack G, Cole S, Campbell et al: Interleukin-8 generation in bacterially contaminated platelet concentrates, abstracted (S190). Transfusion 33:50S, 1993

24. Stack G, Baril L, Napychank P, Snyder EL: Cytokine generation in stored units of red blood cells. Transfusion 1994 (in press)

25. Cole S, Stack E: Macrophage inflammatory protein-1-α generation in stored platelets. Blood, Suppl. 1. 82:398a, 1993

26. Mangano MM, Chamber LA, Kruskall MS: Limited efficiency of leukopoor platelets for prevention of febrile transfusion reactions. Am J Clin Pathol 95:733, 1991

27. Walker RH: Special report: transfusion risks. Am J Clin Pathol 88:374, 1987

28. Menitove JE, McElligott MC, Aster RH: Febrile transfusion reaction: what blood component should be given next? Vox Sang 42:318, 1982

29. Muylle L, Joos M, Wouters E et al: Increased tumor necrosis factor-α (TNF-α), interleukin-1, and interleukin-6 (IL-6) levels in plasma of stored platelet concentrate: relationship between TNF-α and IL-6 levels and febrile transfusion reactions. Transfusion 33:195, 1993

30. Hoffman M: Antibody-coated erythrocytes induce secretion of tumor necrosis factor by human monocytes: a mechanism for the production of fever by incompatible transfusions. Vox Sang 60:184, 1991

31. Rush B, Lee NLY: Clinical presentation of nonhemolytic transfusion reactions. Anaesth Intensive Care 8:125, 1980

32. Braunwald E, Isselbacher KJ, Petersdorf RG et al (eds): Principles of Internal Medicine. 11th Ed. McGraw-Hill, New York, 1987

33. Walker R (ed): Technical Manual. 10th Ed. American Association of Blood Banks, Arlington, VA, 1989

34. McCord RG, Myhre BA: A method for rapid and thorough work-up of febrile and allergic transfusion reactions. Lab Med 9:39, 1978

35. Myhre BA, Van Antwerp R: Diagnosis of unexpected reactions to transfusion. Lab Med 14:153, 1983

36. Burks LC, Aisner J, Fortner CL, Wiernik PH: Meperidine for the treatment of shaking chills and fever. Arch Intern Med 140:483, 1980

37. Goldfinger D, Lowe C: Prevention of adverse reactions to blood transfusion by the administration of saline-washed red blood cells. Transfusion 21:277, 1981

38. Meryman HT, Hornblower M: The preparation of red cells depleted of leukocytes: review and evaluation. Transfusion 26:101, 1986

39. Hughes A, Mijovic V, Brozovic B, Davies TD: Leukocyte-depleted blood: a comparison of cell-washing techniques. Vox Sang 42:145, 1982

40. Meryman MT, Bross J, Lebovitz R: The preparation of leukocyte-poor red blood cells: a comparative study. Transfusion 20:285, 1980

41. Schned AR, Silver H: The use of microaggregate filtration in the prevention of febrile transfusion reactions. Transfusion 21:675, 1981

42. Wenz B: Microaggregate blood filtration and the febrile transfusion reaction. Transfusion 23:95, 1983

43. Parravicini A, Rebulla P, Apuzzo J et al: The preparation of leukocyte-poor red cells for transfusion by a simple cost-effective technique. Transfusion 24:508, 1984

44. Sirchia G, Rebulla P, Parravicini A et al: Leukocyte depletion of red cell units at the bedside by transfusion through a new filter. Transfusion 27:402, 1987

45. Domen RE, Williams L: Use of the Sepacell filter for preparing white cell depleted red cells. Transfusion 28:506, 1988

46. Shannon JA, Sepulveda PS, Holland PV: Comparison of two preparation techniques for white cell-poor red cells. Transfusion 28:507, 1988

47. Sniecinski I, O'Donnell MR, Nowicki B, Hill LR: Prevention of refractoriness and HLA-alloimmunization using filtered blood products. Blood 71:1402, 1988

48. Andreu G, Dewailly J, Leberre C et al: Prevention fo HLA immunization with leukocyte-poor packed red cells and platelet concentrates obtained by filtration. Blood 72:964, 1988

49. Sirchia G, Parravicini A, Rebulla P et al: Preparation of leukocyte-free platelets for transfusion by filtration through cotton wool. Vox Sang 44:115, 1983

50. Brubaker DB, Romine CM: The in vitro evaluation of two filters (Erypur and Imugard IG 500) for white cell-poor platelet concentrates. Transfusion 28:383, 1988

51. Rydberg L, Ulfvin A, Stigendal L: White cell depletion of platelet concentrates using different filters. Transfusion 6:604, 1988

52. Koerner K, Kubanek B: Comparison of three different methods used in the preparation of leukocyte-poor platelet concentrates. Vox Sang 53:26, 1987

53. Miyamoto M, Sasakawa S, Ishikawa Y et al: Leukocyte-poor platelet concentrates at the bedside by filtration through Sepacell-PL. Vox Sang 57:164, 1989

54. Kickler TS, Bell W, Ness PM et al: Depletion of white cells from platelet concentrates with a new adsorption filter. Transfusion 29:411, 1989

55. Snyder EL, DePalma L, Napychank P: Use of polyester filters for the preparation of leukocyte-poor platelet concentrates. Vox Sang 54:21, 1988

56. Snyder EL: Clinical use of white cell-poor blood components. Transfusion 29:68, 1989

57. Snyder EL, Bookbinder M: Role of microaggregate blood filtration in clinical medicine. Transfusion 23:460, 1983

58. Lichtenstein LM: Allergy and the immune system. Sci Am 269:116, 1993

59. Ahrons S, Kissmeyer-Nielsen F: Serological investigation of 1,358 transfusion reactions in 74,000 transfusions. Dan Med Bull 15:259, 1968

60. Kevy SV, Schmidt PJ, McGinniss MH, Workman WG: Febrile, nonhemolytic transfusion reactions and the limited role of leukoagglutinins in their etiology. Transfusion 2:7, 1966

61. Mosely RV, Doty DB: Death associated with multiple pulmonary emboli soon after battle injury. Ann Surg 171:336, 1970

62. McNamara JJ, Molot MD, Stremple JF: Screen filtration pressure in combat casualties. Ann Surg 172:334, 1970

63. Simmons RL, Heisterkamp CA III, Collins JA et al: Respiratory insufficiency in combat casualties. IV. Hypoxemia during convalescence. Ann Surg 170:53, 1962

64. Bredenberg CE: Does a relationship exist between massive blood transfusions and the adult respiratory distress syndrome? If so, what are the best preventive measures? Vox Sang 32:311, 1977

65. Collins JA, James PM, Bredenberg CE et al: The relationship between transfusion and hypoxemia in combat casualties. Ann Surg 188:513, 1978

66. Suehiro A, Leinberger H, McNamara JJ: Counting microaggregate particles in blood. Transfusion 18:281, 1978

67. Swank RL: Alteration of blood on storage: measurement of adhesiveness of "aging" platelets and leukocytes and their removal by filtration. N Engl J Med 265:728, 1961

68. McNamara JJ, Anderson BS, Hayashi T: Stored blood platelets and microaggregate formation. Surg Gynecol Obstet 147:507, 1978

69. Snyder EL, Underwood PS, Spivack M et al: An in vivo evaluation of microaggregate blood filtration during total hip replacement. Ann Surg 190:75, 1979

70. Snyder EL, Hezzey A, Barash PG, Palermo G: Microaggregate blood filtration in patients with compromised pulmonary function. Transfusion 22:21, 1982

71. Swank DW, Moore SB: Roles of the neutrophil and other mediators in adult respiratory distress syndrome. Mayo Clin Proc 64:1118, 1989

72. Widmann FW (ed): Standards for Blood Banks and Transfusion Services. 15th Ed. American Association of Blood Banks, Bethesda, MD, 1993, p. 10, B4.240.

73. Blajchman MA, Bardossy L, Carmen R et al: Allogeneic blood transfusion-induced enhancement of tumor growth: two animal models showing amelioration by leukodepletion and passive transfer using spleen cells. Blood 81: 1880, 1993

74. Anderson KC, Lew MA, Gorgone BC et al: Transfusion-related sepsis after prolonged platelet storage. Am J Med 81:405, 1986

75. Scott J, Boulton FE, Govan JRW et al: A fatal transfusion reaction associated with blood contaminated with *Pseudomonas fluorescens.* Vox Sang 54:201, 1988

76. Brown SE, White SE: *Yersinia enterocolitica* and transfusion-induced septicemia. Anesth Analg 67:415, 1988

77. Braine HG, Kickler TS, Charache P et al: Bacterial sepsis secondary to platelet transfusion: an adverse effect of extended storage at room temperature. Transfusion 26:391, 1986

78. Heal JM, Jones ME, Forey J et al: Fatal *Salmonella* septicemia after platelet transfusion. Transfusion 27:2, 1987

79. Arnow PM, Weiss LM, Weil D, Rosen NR: *Escherichia coli* sepsis from contaminated platelet transfusion. Arch Intern Med 146:321, 1986

80. Bone RC: The pathogenesis of sepsis. Ann Intern Med 115:457, 1991

81. Mariott HL, Kekwick A: Volume and rate in blood transfusion for the relief of anemia. BMJ 1:1043, 1940

82. DeWolf AM, Van Den Berg BW, Hoffman HJ, Van Zundert AA: Pulmonary dysfunction during one-lung ventilation caused by HLA-specific antibodies against leukocytes. Anesth Analg 66:463, 1987

83. Latson TW, Kickler TS, Baumgartner WA: Pulmonary hypertension and noncardiogenic pulmonary edema following cardiopulmonary bypass associated with an antigranulocyte antibody. Anesthesiology 64:106, 1986

84. Ebert JP, Grimes B, Niemann KMW: Respiratory failure secondary to homologous blood transfusion. Anesthesiology 65:104, 1985

85. Popovsky MA, Abel MD, Moore SB: Transfusion-related acute lung injury associated with passive transfer of antileukocyte antibodies. Am Rev Respir Dis 128:185, 1983

86. Dubois M, Lotze MT, Diamond WJ et al: Pulmonary shunting during leukoagglutin-induced noncardiac pulmonary edema. JAMA 244:2186, 1980.

87. Ward HN, Lipscomb TS, Cawley LP: Pulmonary hypersensitivity reaction after blood transfusion. Arch Intern Med 122:362, 1968

88. Wolf CFW, Canale VC: Fatal pulmonary hypersensitivity reaction to HL-A incompatible blood transfusion: report of a case and review of the literature. Transfusion 16:135, 1976

89. Jacob HS, Craddock PR, Hammerschmidt DE, Moldow CF: Complement-induced granulocyte aggregation. N Engl J Med 302:789, 1980

90. Hammerschmidt DE, Jacob HS: Adverse pulmonary reactions to transfusion. Adv Intern Med 27:511, 1982

91. Yomtovian R, Kline W, Press C et al: Severe pulmonary hypersensitivity associated with passive transfusion of a neutrophil specific antibody. Lancet 1:244, 1984

92. Boyan CP: Cold or warmed blood for massive transfusions. Ann Surg 160:282, 1964

93. Collins JA: Problems associated with massive transfusion of stored blood. Surgery 75:274, 1974

94. Boyan CP, Howland WS: Cardiac arrest and temperature of bank blood. JAMA 183:58, 1963

95. Boyan CP, Howland WS: Blood temperature: a critical factor in massive transfusion. Anesthesiology 22:559, 1961

96. Holland PV: Standards for Blood Banks and Transfusion Services. 13th Ed. American Association of Blood Banks, Arlington, VA, 1989

97. Staples PJ, Griner PF: Extracorporeal hemolysis of blood in a microwave blood warmer. N Engl J Med 285:317, 1971

98. Linko K, Hynynen K: Erythrocyte damage caused by the Haemotherm microwave blood warmer. Acta Anaesth Scand 23:320, 1979

99. Denlinger JK, Nahrwold ML, Gibbs PS: Hypocalcemia during rapid blood transfusion in an anaesthetized man. Br J Anaesth 48:995, 1976

100. Dzik WH, Kirkley SA: Citrate toxicity during massive blood transfusion. Transfus Med Rev 2:76, 1988

101. Marquez J, Martin D, Virji MA et al: Cardiovascular depression secondary to ionic hypocalcemia during hepatic transplantation in humans. Anesthesiology 65:457, 1986

102. Watson DK, Penny AF, Marshall RW, Robinson EAE: Citrate induced hypocalcemia during cell separation. Br J Haematol 44:503, 1980

103. Hester JP, McCullough J, Mishler JM, Szymanski IO: Dosage regimens for citrate anticoagulants. J Clin Apheresis 1:149, 1983

104. Wolf PL, McCarthy LJ, Hafleight B: Extreme hypercalcemia following blood transfusion combined with intravenous calcium. Vox Sang 19:544, 1970

105. McLellan BA, Reid SR, Lane PL: Massive blood transfusion causing hypomagnesemia. Crit Care Med 12:146, 1984

106. Blanchette VS, Gray E, Hardie MJ et al: Hyperkalemia after neonatal exchange transfusion: risk eliminated by washing red cell concentrates. J Pediatr 105:321, 1984

107. Carmichael D, Hosty T, Kastl D, Beckman D: Hypokalemia and massive transfusion. South Med J 77:315, 1984

108. Driscoll DF, Bistrian BR, Jenkins RL et al: Development of metabolic alkalosis after massive transfusion during orthopedic liver transplantation. Crit Care Med 15:905, 1987

109. Spear PW, Sass M, Cincotti JJ: Ammonia levels in transfused blood. J Lab Clin Med 48:702, 1956

110. Myhre BA: Toxicological quandary of the use of bis (2-diethylhexyl) phthalate (DEHP) as a plasticizer for blood bags. Ann Clin Lab Sci 18:131, 1988

111. Rock G, Secours VE, Franklin CA et al: The accumulation of mono-2-ethylhexylphthalate (MEHP) during storage of whole blood and plasma. Transfusion 18:553, 1978

112. Kluwe WM, Haseman JK, Huff JE: The carcinogencity of di(2-ethylhexyl) phthalate (DEHP) in perspective. J Toxicol Environ Health 12:159, 1983

113. Barry YA, Labow RS, Rock G, Keon WJ: Cardiotoxic effects of the plasticizer metabolite, mono(2-ethylhexyl) phthalate (MEHP), on human myocardium. Blood 72:1438, 1988

114. Rubin RJ, Ness PM: What price progress? An update on vinyl plastic blood bags. Transfusion 29:358, 1989

115. Snyder EL, Hedberg SL, Napychank PA et al: Stability of red cell antigens and plasma coagulation factors stored in a non-diethylhexyl phthalate-plasticized container. Transfusion 33:515, 1993

116. Snyder EL, Aster RH, Heaton A et al: Five day storage of platelets in a non-diethylhexyl phthalate-plasticized container. Transfusion 32:736, 1992

117. Rock G, Tocchi M, Ganz PR, Tackaberry ES: Incorporation of plasticizer into red cells during storage. Transfusion 24:493, 1984

118. Labow RS, Tocchi M, Rock G: Platelet storage: effects of leachable materials on morphology and function. Transfusion 26:351, 1986

119. Waldman A: Effects of plasticizers on red blood cells and platelets during storage. Plasma Ther Transfus Technol 9:317, 1988

120. Holland PV: Prevention of transfusion-associated graft-vs-host disease. Arch Pathol Lab Med 113:285, 1989

121. Otsuka S, Kunieda K, Hirose M et al: Fatal erythroderma (suspected graft-versus-host disease) after cholecystectomy. Transfusion 29:544, 1989

122. Thaler M, Shamiss A, Orgad S et al: The role of blood from HLA homozygous donors in fatal transfusion-associated graft-vrsus-host disease after open-heart surgery. N Engl J Med 321:25, 1989

123. Akahoshi M, Takanashi M, Masuda M et al: A case of transfusion-associated graft-versus-host disease not prevented by white-cell reduction filters. Transfusion 32:169, 1992

124. Dzik WH, Jones KS: The effects of gamma irradiation versus white cell reduction in the mixed lymphocyte reaction. Transfusion 33:493, 1993

125. Moroff G, Luban NLC: Prevention of transfusion-associated graft-versus-host disease. Transfusion 32:102, 1992

126. Shivdasani RA, Anderson KC: Transfusion-associated graft-versus-host disease: scratching the surface. Transfusion 33:696, 1993

127. Petz LD, Calhoun L, Yam P et al: Transfusion-associated graft-versus-host disease in immunocompetent patients: report of a fatal case associated with transfusion of blood from a second-degree relative and a survey of predisposing factors. Transfusion 33:742, 1993

128. Rivet C, Baxter A, Rock G: Potassium levels in irradiated blood, letter. Transfusion 29:185, 1989

129. Marcus CS, Huehns ER: Transfusional iron overload. Clin Lab Haematol 7:195, 1985

130. Propper RD, Button LN, Nathan DG: New approach to the transfusion management of thalassemia. Blood 55:1, 1980

131. Miller DR, Giardina PV: Congenital hemolytic anemias. p. 583. In Petz LD, Swisher SN (eds): Clinical Practice of Transfusion Medicine. 2nd Ed. Churchill Livingstone, New York, 1989

132. Schmidt PJ, Kevy SV: Air embolism. N Engl J Med 258:424, 1958

133. American Association of Blood Banks: Blood Transfusion Therapy: An Audiovisual Program. American Association of Blood Banks, Arlington, VA, 1991

Transfusion-Transmitted Diseases

142

Jay E. Menitove

INTRODUCTION

Volunteer blood donors undergo screening and testing procedures to impede the transmission by transfusion of hepatitis viruses, retroviruses, cytomegalovirus (CMV), spirochetes, parasites, and bacteria. These measures are highly effective but do not eliminate all transmission risk (Table 142-1).

HEPATITIS

Hepatitis A

The viremic phase of hepatitis A, a DNA virus, is limited to a few weeks before and after the onset of clinical symptoms. A carrier state does not exist, although recurrence or relapse of hepatitis A virus (HAV) may occur within 3 months of onset. Post-transfusion hepatitis A is a result of donation during the brief asymptomatic (7–28-day) interval before the onset of illness. In general, the recipients develop clinical symptoms 22–31 days after transfusion. Secondary and tertiary transmission occurs from the transfusion-associated index patient to others.

Since HAV is nonenveloped, it is not inactivated by the solvent/detergent treatment used to reduce the risk of transfusion-transmitted infection by factor VIII and coagulation factor IX concentrates. Hepatitis A outbreaks occurred in hemophilic patients in Italy, Germany, and Ireland who received solvent/detergent-treated products, but hepatitis A was not reported in patients in other countries who infused similarly treated products.[1-3]

Hepatitis B

Hepatitis B is a double-stranded, circular DNA virus comprising a surface antigen (HBsAg) surrounded by a central core that has its own antigenic component (HBcAg).[4] Of those infected with hepatitis B, 6–10% become asymptomatic carriers and are at risk of chronic liver dysfunction and hepatoma.[5,6]

Post-transfusion hepatitis B has a 6-week to 6-month incubation period. Approximately 67% of patients who receive 1 U of HBsAg-positive blood develop hepatitis, and 20–50% become icteric.[7] In studies conducted during the late 1970s hepatitis B accounted for approximately 10% of post-transfusion hepatitis cases. Currently, the incidence is estimated as 1 in 50,000/recipient or 1 in 200,000/U.[8] The risk relates to infection by hepatitis

Table 142-1. Transfusion-Transmitted Disease Risk

Hepatitis B	~1/200,000
Hepatitis C	~1/5,000
Human T-Lymphotropic virus	1/50,000
Human immunodeficiency virus-1	~1/225,000
Human immunodeficiency virus-2	Very rare
Transfusion-associated sepsis	Rare
Cytomegalovirus	Variable

B carriers who have no serologic markers of infection (i.e., assays for HBsAg and anti-HBcAg are negative, the alanine aminotransferase [ALT] level is within the acceptable range, but hepatitis B virus [HBV] DNA is detectable with amplification techniques using the polymerase chain reaction [PCR]).[9]

Hepatitis C

The term, non-A, non-B hepatitis was introduced in the mid-1970s to characterize a viral-like illness with hepatic dysfunction that was not caused by hepatitis A, hepatitis B, cytomegalovirus, or Epstein-Barr virus.[10] It is now called hepatitis C.

The etiologic agent of most hepatitis C cases was identified through molecular biology techniques in 1988.[11] The virus was not cultured, visualized, or isolated. Instead, nucleic acids were extracted from a plasma pool prepared from a chimpanzee infected with hepatitis through transfusion from another chimpanzee that previously received nonvirally inactivated factor VIII concentrates. Using reverse transcriptase, cDNA was isolated and inserted into λ gt 11 vectors. The cDNA was expressed in *Escherichia coli* and screened with serum from a patient infected with the putative agent, presumably containing antibodies against the agent. Eventually, a 126-base pair, single-stranded RNA clone, 5-1-1, was isolated. The sequence was expanded to encompass a 363-amino acid polypeptide, c100-3, fused with human superoxide dismutase gene and expressed in recombinant yeast cultures.

At least three hepatitis C viral groups exist, with varying degrees of sequence homology. Some types may be associated with more severe liver disease.[12] The genomic structure indicates that hepatitis C virus (HCV) is similar to the flaviviruses and pestiviruses. Enzyme immunoassays (EIAs) developed on the basis of the c100-3 clone and licensed in the United States in May, 1990, are considered first-generation HCV assays.

Initial studies using the c100-3-based assay detected HCV antibodies in 15 of 15 patients with well-characterized chronic transfusion-associated hepatitis C followed at the National Institutes of Health.[13] Anti-HCV (anti-c100-3) seroconversion occurs 10–78 weeks post-transfusion and 4–78 weeks after the onset of hepatitis. Anti-HCV antibodies were present in 44–85% of patients with post-transfusion hepatitis C in the United States, Italy, Japan, the Netherlands, Spain, and Germany and in 64–98% of hemophilic patients. Approximately 90% of recipients of HCV-infected blood seroconvert to anti-HCV.[14-17]

Multiple-antigen or second-generation anti-HCV EIAs were licensed in the United States in March, 1992. These tests contained additional epitopes derived from the core or nucleocapsid part of the genome (c22-3) and the NS-3 nonstructural region (c33c), in addition to c100-3. During development of second-generation assays, the c33c and c100-3 clones were combined into a c200 expression product. The second generation tests detect approximately 20% more patients with acute post-transfusion hepatitis and are positive 30–90 days earlier than first-generation assays.[18,19]

In chimpanzee studies, second-generation assays detected anti-HCV, 13.8 weeks after infection or approximately 5 weeks earlier than first-generation assays and persisted longer than antibodies against c100-3.[20] Antibodies against c22-3 present in second-generation assays are retained in HCV-infected hemophilic patients who lose antibodies against c100-3.[21] Among patients with community-acquired hepatitis C, loss of antibodies against second-generation assays occurred in 2 of 85 patients. Antibody titers were below detectable limits in 10 of 81 according to first-generation assays.[22]

Third-generation EIAs, under development, contain epitopes for the NS-5 region. First-generation assays contain amino acids from 12% of the HCV genome, second-generation assays have epitopes from 26% of the genome, and third-generation assays expand the potential determinants to 60% of the genome. Third-generation assays provide an increase in sensitivity over second-generation assays.

In practice, positive second-generation anti-HCV EIA screening test results are subjected to supplemental testing using strip immunoassays or other solid-phase assays for detecting antibodies against recombinant HCV antigens corresponding to 5-1-1, c100-3, c33c, and c22-3. A specimen is considered reactive in these assays if reactivity to two or more gene products is demonstrated.[23] Evidence that supplemental assays are helpful in resolving nonspecific reactions is shown by detection of HCV RNA using nested PCR assays with primers from the conserved 5′ untranslated region of the HCV genome or other regions.[24] PCR assays provide the most sensitive method of documenting HCV infection; HCV RNA is found in serum within 1–2 weeks after infection.[20,25]

Clinical Manifestations

Approximately one-half of those infected with HCV have symptoms consisting of fatigue, anorexia, nausea and/or vomiting, abdominal pain, and weight loss. One-quarter become icteric. Most cases occur 49–56 days after transfusion, but considerable variation exists. The acute illness persists for ≤10 weeks. Chronic hepatitis develops in approximately two-thirds of patients, approximately 10% of these patients develop cir-

rhosis, and one- to two-thirds have chronic active hepatitis.[22,26] Persons at high risk of HCV infection include recipients of blood transfusion, injection-drug users, occupational or household contacts of patients with HCV, or persons with low socioeconomic status. Chronic active hepatitis may be more frequent if HCV is acquired through blood transfusion. ALT levels vary in persons with HCV and do not predict histologic severity; normal ALT levels occur in patients with persistent evidence of HCV infection.[22]

Despite the high incidence of histologic and biochemical evidence of chronic hepatitis, long-term follow-up studies indicate the clinical outcome is less dire. In a case-control study involving patients enrolled in transfusion-associated hepatitis trials between 1967 and 1980, no difference in mortality was observed between patients with post-transfusion hepatitis and those who received transfusions but did not have hepatitis an average of 18 years after transfusion (Fig. 142-1). The statistically significant increase in death related to liver disease noted in this study in patients with post-transfusion hepatitis (3.3% versus 1–2% of those without hepatitis) probably reflects an adverse impact of alcoholism in HCV-infected patients.[27] Another study analyzed prospectively monitored patients who contracted post-transfusion hepatitis between 1972 and 1980.[28] The minimum time between acute hepatitis C and clinical evidence of liver failure was 6 years. After 16 years, demonstrable liver failure was present in 18% of patients with post-transfusion hepatitis.

The possibility of hepatitis C transmission through sexual contact is an important issue for donors and for HCV-seropositive patients. Available data indicate that transmission occurs infrequently, possibly because of low titers of HCV in serum and nondetectable levels in secretions.[29,30]

Occurrence of vertical transmission between mother and fetus is controversial. Reported cases may reflect confusion arising from passive antibody transfer to the fetus, an increased risk of HCV infectivity when the mothers are co-infected with HIV and HCV, and the reliability of HCV RNA detection by PCR testing.[31]

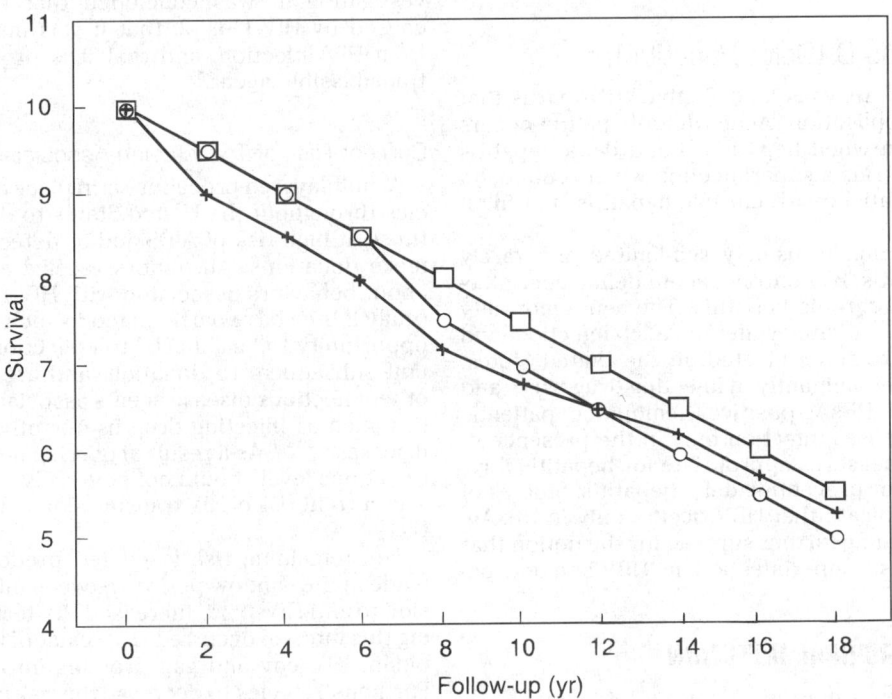

Fig. 142-1. Overall mortality of patients enrolled in five separate studies of transfusion-associated hepatitis between 1967 and 1980 as of December, 1991. All the patients received transfusions. Patients with hepatitis C had elevated ALT levels between 2 and 24 weeks after transfusion. Subjects in each of the two control groups had repeatably normal ALT values. (From Seeff et al.,[27] with permission.)

Severe aplastic anemia is a reported complication of hepatitis. However, HCV is not present before onset of illness, and hepatitis A and B are not implicated in the etiology. A non-A, non-B, non-C virus is postulated as a potential agent.[32,33]

An increased incidence of hepatocellular carcinoma has been reported in HCV-infected persons, but a direct causative relationship between the two entities has not been proved. Hepatitis C infection leads to cirrhosis, and this condition may increase the risk of primary liver cancer.[34]

Prevention of Transfusion-Transmitted Hepatitis C

The Transfusion-Transmitted Virus (TTV) Study[35,36] and an evaluation of patients undergoing open heart surgery at the National Institutes of Health (NIH) Clinical Center[37,38] provided data showing that donors with elevated ALT levels or anti-HBcAg antibodies (or both) were at risk for post-transfusion hepatitis C. If the donor ALT levels were elevated, there was a three- to fivefold increased chance that the recipient would develop post-transfusion hepatitis (TTV Study: 37.5% versus 7.1% incidence of post-transfusion hepatitis; NIH Study: 28.8% versus 9.1%). The risk was two- to three-fold higher for recipients of anti-HBcAg-positive blood (TTV Study: 18.7% versus 7.2%; NIH Study: 11.9% versus 4.2%). These studies and a subsequent report from Germany partly led to the adoption of these surrogate, or nonspecific, tests to reduce the incidence of post-transfusion hepatitis in 1986 and 1987.[39] The efficacy of surrogate testing was demonstrated by retrospectively testing post-transfusion blood samples collected between 1985 and 1991 for anti-HCV. ALT and anti-HBcAg testing decreased the incidence of post-transfusion hepatitis from 3.84%/patient and 0.45%/U to 1.54/patient and 0.19%/U.[40]

Currently, donor blood is tested for anti-HCV and the surrogate markers, ALT and anti-HBcAg. Second-generation screening tests detect 82–91%[41] of post-transfusion hepatitis C. Implementation of first-generation tests prevented 1.6–2 HCV infections/1,000 U transfused,[16,40] and second-generation tests reduced this further by 1/1,000 U transfused.[19] The current estimate of HCV transmission risk is approximately 1/3,300–5,000/U transfused.[8]

Hepatitis D (Delta Hepatitis)

Hepatitis delta virus (HDV) is a "defective" RNA virus that requires HBV for its replication. Acute delta hepatitis occurs either as a co-infection when hepatitis B and delta hepatitis occur simultaneously or as a superinfection when acute delta hepatitis occurs in a patient with chronic hepatitis B or in an HBsAg carrier.[4]

Acute delta co-infection is usually self-limited and rarely leads to chronic hepatitis. By contrast, acute delta superinfection is associated with chronic hepatitis. The acute mortality rate is 1–10% among patients suffering a co-infection and 5–20% in those who are superinfected. In the United States, the disease is found predominantly in injecting drug users and approximately 20% of HBsAg-positive hemophilic patients. Since delta hepatitis causes infection only in the presence of active HBV infection, measures appropriate for hepatitis B reduction are indicated for preventing delta hepatitis. Studies of hemophilia patients indicate that HDV occurs only in HBsAg-positive patients, providing further support for the notion that HDV is unable to cause superinfection in HBV-immune patients.[14]

RETROVIRAL INFECTION

Human Immunodeficiency Virus-1 Infection

The human immunodeficiency virus-1 (HIV-1) is the etiologic agent of the acquired immunodeficiency syndrome (AIDS). By September 30, 1993, 340,000 AIDS cases had been reported in the United States; approximately 6,300 (2%) are transfusion related, and almost 3,200 (1%) occurred in patients treated with coagulation factor concentrates. Sixty-eight percent of patients with severe hemophilia A and 46% of those with severe hemophilia B are HIV seropositive.[42]

Transfusion-associated AIDS associated with voluntarily donated whole blood was reported in December, 1982,[43] 4 months after a report of three cases of *Pneumocystis carinii* pneumonia in patients with hemophilia.[44] Changes were made in screening blood donors in early 1983 to defer donations by persons at high risk of AIDS. HIV antibody testing was introduced in March, 1985. In a retrospective review, the number of transfusion-associated AIDS cases by year of transfusion was found to have increased each year between 1978 and 1984. The incidence dropped precipitously in 1985, and current estimates suggest that ≤20 infectious units enter the blood supply annually[45] (Fig. 142-2).

The trend in clinically diagnosed transfusion-associated AIDS cases is influenced by the age of the patient. In children <5 years of age and adults >65 years, the interval between infection and progression to AIDS is shorter than in other age groups.[45] As a result, new transfusion-associated AIDS cases in adults but not in children are expected to occur over the next several years despite the paucity of recent transmission by transfusion.

A series of in vitro experiments indicates that peripheral blood mononuclear cells from patients with HIV-1, exposed to allogeneic mononuclear cells, underwent activation of HIV-1 expression followed by dissemination to uninfected cells.[46] Although in vivo studies have not been reported, these preliminary findings suggest that there is a potential benefit in using leukocyte-depleted blood and components for HIV-infected patients requiring transfusion.

Initial reports of an AIDS-like illness occurring in patients with no serologic evidence of HIV infection, <300 CD4$^+$ T lymphocytes/mm^3, and no underlying immunologic disorder were accompanied by suggestions that an unidentified pathogen was transmitted by blood transfusion. After extensive investigation, it was concluded that the syndrome was not caused by HIV-1 or -2, that it was immunologically different from HIV infection, and that it is probably not caused by a transmissible agent.[47]

Current Risk of Transfusion-Associated HIV Infection

A multilayered procedure is in place at blood collection agencies throughout the United States to defer blood donation by those at high risk of AIDS and to detect infected persons who make donations. All donors receive educational information about behaviors associated with HIV infection risk, are asked orally if they have participated in such activities, are given the opportunity to "call-back" to collection agencies to remove a unit subsequent to donation, and are tested for HIV-1/2 and other infectious disease agents associated with AIDS risk activities such as injecting drug use or other sexually transmitted diseases.[8,48–50] As a result of overlap between these layers, failure at one level should not adversely affect transfusion safety. The current risk of HIV transmission is approximately 1/225,000 U.

The remaining risk is related predominantly to donations made in the window period between infection and seroconversion to anti-HIV-1.[51,52] Increased HIV test sensitivity by shortening this interval occurred as a result of incorporation of recombinant HIV env and gag proteins into test kit configuration. Further strategies to decrease the risk include improved donor screening techniques and possibly the use of computer-generated donor history questioning.[53]

The HIV p24 antigen is detected briefly prior to development of anti-HIV, but none of >1,100,000 volunteer blood donors

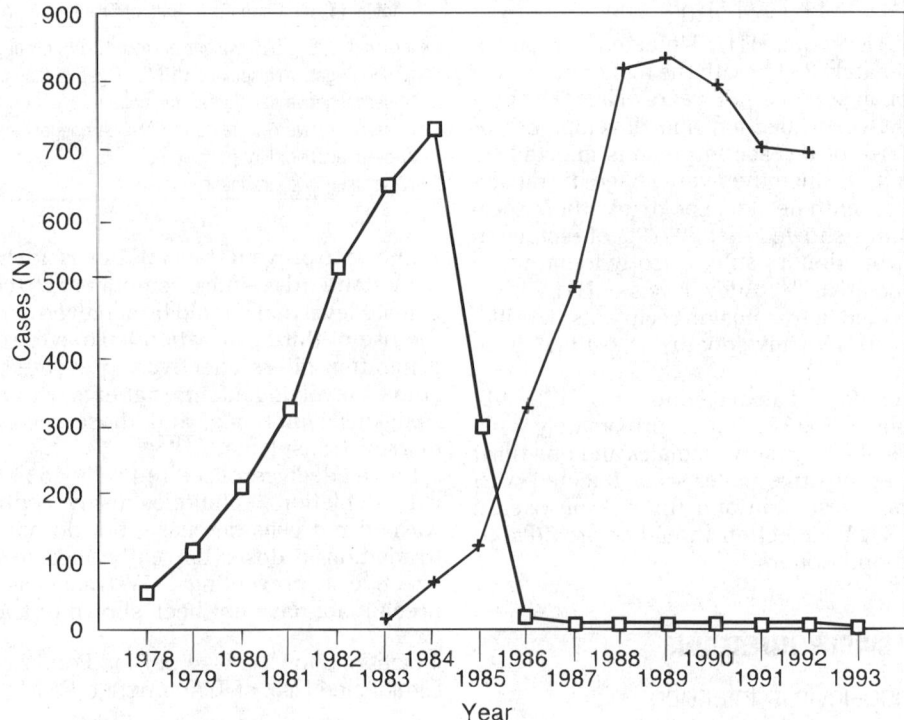

Fig. 142-2. Transfusion-associated AIDS cases in patients with a single year of transfusion according to the year of transfusion and the number of cases occurring in patients with known, unknown or multiple years of transfusion analyzed by year of diagnosis. (From Selik et al.,[45] with permission.)

were found to be HIV antigen positive and antibody negative in Bavaria, Austria, and the United States.[54,55] HIV antigen testing is not recommended for screening blood donors in the United States. PCR-based assays are under development, but probably will be more helpful as confirmatory and investigational tools than as diagnostic screening tests.[9]

Human Immunodeficiency Virus-2 Infection

A second human immunodeficiency retrovirus, HIV-2, reported in 1985, was shown subsequently to have 42% nucleotide homology with HIV-1 and 75% similarity to simian immunodeficiency virus.[56,57] A relatively high prevalence of HIV-2 infection is found in West Africa and in former Portuguese colonies in southern Africa. As of April, 1992, 32 cases of HIV-2 had been reported in the United States. Since the route of transmission is similar to that of HIV-1, there was concern about transmission through blood transfusion. The Food and Drug Administration (FDA) mandated testing of blood donors in June, 1992.

HIV-2 causes AIDS, but the clinical course may be significantly longer than that of HIV-1.[57] Carriers of the virus are detected by HIV-2 EIA tests or HIV-1/HIV-2 combination kits. The latter is preferred for testing blood donors since separate tests for HIV-1 and HIV-2 are not needed. The use of recombinant DNA-derived HIV-1 core and envelope amino acid sequences and HIV-2 envelope antigens has increased test sensitivity for the detection of HIV-1- and HIV-2-infected donors. Before implementation of the combination assays, HIV-1 tests were cross-reactive with approximately 60% of HIV-2 antibodies.[56] On the basis of this assumption, the estimated prevalence of HIV-2-infected blood donors was approximately 2–6 in 10,000,000 at the time HIV-2 testing was required by the FDA.

Human T-Lymphotropic Virus-I and -II

The human T-lymphotropic virus-I (HTLV-I) is a transforming retrovirus that integrates into genomic DNA. The virus is associated with two distinct diseases: adult T-cell leukemia (ATL),

and HTLV-I myelopathy, previously known as tropical spastic paraparesis.[58,59] The two conditions, with rare exception, occur in different patients. Recently, a new entity, HTLV-I-associated arthropathy, has been described. Cases of uveitis and infectious dermatitis in pediatric patients have also been linked with HTLV-I.[59]

HTLV-II is detected, in part, by testing for HTLV-I and is prevalent among injecting drug users, some Native American populations, and approximately one-half of HTLV-I-positive blood donors.[58–61] It is unclear whether HTLV-II is linked to a specific disease entity. However, HTLV-II-infected patients have been reported with neurologic disorders similar to HTLV-I myelopathy, mycosis fungoides, and large granular lymphocyte leukemia. The role of HTLV-II in the pathogenesis of these conditions is under investigation.[62–64]

Transmission by Transfusion

HTLV-I, a highly cell-associated virus, is transmitted by transfusion of cellular components, with seroconversion occurring in 14–63% of recipients.[58,61] Lack of seroconversion in cryoprecipitate, plasma, or coagulation factor concentrate recipients, other than those presumably infected by cellular components, is interpreted as evidence that HTLV-I is not transmitted by these products.

HTLV-II is also transmitted by transfusion. The detection of HTLV-II-infected donors is carried out by HTLV-I/II EIA screening tests, although some HTLV-II transmissions may be missed. The risk of HTLV-II transmission by transfusion may be lower than that of HTLV-I.[61,65] HTLV-I testing was implemented in the winter of 1988/89 in the United States. Approximately 0.016% of U.S. blood donors have antibodies against HTLV I/II.[58,66] Since the sensitivity of tests licensed in November, 1988 has been questioned, recombinant HTLV-I p21 envelope protein was added to the viral lysate-based assays.[58] In the absence of this modification, the risk of HTLV-I/II infection by transfusion is approximately 1/50,000 U transfused.[8]

Risk of Disease as a Result of HTLV-I/II Infection

The lifetime risk of ATL among HTLV-I-infected persons is estimated to be approximately 2–4%, with the higher incidence associated with infection in persons <20 years of age. The prolonged latent period between infection and development of ATL suggests that the risk of disease in persons infected by blood transfusion is limited, since the average age of transfusion recipients is in the seventh decade. Lookback studies performed in the United States showed that 30–39% of recipients of untested donations from donors subsequently found to be seropositive were seropositive.[61,67] A few cases of HTLV-I myelopathy have been detected in transfusion recipients. The lifetime risk of developing HTLV-I myelopathy is estimated as 0.25%.[59]

Interviews with household and sexual contacts of HTLV I/II-seropositive blood donors found that approximately one-quarter of male partners of seropositive females and one-third of female partners of seropositive males were infected with HTLV-I or HTLV-II. This information and the risk of disease development following HTLV-I infection should be provided to HTLV I/II-seropositive blood donors.[66]

HERPESVIRUS INFECTIONS

Cytomegalovirus Infection

CMV is a large, enveloped, double-stranded DNA human herpesvirus that is associated with latent infection and reactivation. The presence of antibody denotes previous exposure but not resolution of the infection or immunity to reactivation or possibly reinfection. In a recent study only 8% of CMV-seropositive donors were found to have CMV DNA using a PCR assay.[68] These data are consistent with previous reports of CMV transmission by transfusion of 0.9–17% if some CMV-seropositive blood is transfused, and estimates that 0.14–12% of blood donors are latently infected.[69–71] In patients with systemic infection, CMV is found principally in polymorphonuclear leukocytes but is present also in lymphocytes and monocytes.

In general, most immunocompetent patients exposed to CMV become infected but only rarely have symptoms. By contrast, immunocompromised patients or transplant recipients are at risk of fever, arthralgias, enteritis, hepatitis, thrombocytopenia, leukopenia, encephalitis, interstitial pneumonia, and delayed engraftment of allogenic bone marrow.[72,73] Low-birthweight neonates and fetuses in utero have a higher likelihood of severe morbidity and mortality from primary CMV infection. The incubation period is ≤12 weeks.

Methods for Reducing Transfusion-Transmitted CMV Infection

Blood components from donors who are anti-CMV negative should not transmit CMV to transfusion recipients. The efficacy of seronegative blood in preventing CMV transmission is supported by studies in infants of seronegative mothers and seronegative recipients of seronegative bone marrow or renal transplants. Approximately 50% of blood donors are CMV seropositive, but the prevalence varies according to age, sex, geographic region, and socioeconomic status. The highest rates occur in females, older persons, those in the southern part of the United States, and those individuals with lower socioeconomic status. Serologic screening is used primarily for identifying donors at reduced risk of transmitting the virus.[69,71] However, additional techniques are needed to meet the demand for platelet transfusion.

Since leukocytes represent the site of latent CMV infection, leukocyte reduction has been studied as an alternative to CMV-seronegative components. The degree of leukocyte reduction

Table 142-2. Patients at Risk of Transfusion-Associated CMV Disease

Infants <1,200 g birthweight born to CMV-seronegative mothers
CMV-seronegative recipients of CMV-negative allogeneic bone marrow transplants
CMV-seronegative candidates for bone marrow or solid organ transplantation
CMV-seronegative recipients of CMV-seronegative solid organ allografts
CMV-seronegative, HIV-positive patients
CMV-seronegative pregnant women

required to prevent transmission is not known. However, blood bank standards require components to contain $<5 \times 10^6$ leukocytes, a level that should be achieved >95% of the time through the use of third-generation leukocyte reduction filters. Third-generation filters effectively prevented CMV transmission in studies involving infants, patients with acute leukemia or non-Hodgkins lymphoma, and those receiving autologous bone marrow transplants.[72,74–77]

Frozen deglycerolized red cells do not transmit CMV; leukocyte depletion techniques using centrifugation and saline-washed red cells decrease, but do not eliminate, the risk. γ-Irradiation in doses currently used to irradiate blood is not effective in preventing CMV transmission. Plasma and cryoprecipitiate have not been shown to transmit CMV.[69,71]

Indications for the Use of Blood and Components with Diminished Risk of Transmitting CMV

Immunocompetent Patients

Since primary CMV infection during pregnancy poses a risk of intrauterine transmission and adverse outcome in the fetus, components with diminished risk of transmitting CMV should be considered for seronegative pregnant women or pregnant women of unknown status requiring transfusion therapy and for intrauterine transfusions[78] (Table 142-2). Otherwise, screened units are not provided for immunocompetent patients.

Neonates of Less Than 1,200 Birthweight Born to CMV-Seronegative Mothers

Two studies published in the early 1980s found that approximately 30% of low-birthweight infants born to CMV-seronegative mothers and transfused with unscreened blood developed CMV infection, with a mortality rate of approximately 40%.[79,80] Subsequent studies have not reproduced the high morbidity and mortality rates, although precise reasons for the disparate findings have not been identified. American Association of Blood Bank Standards suggest using CMV-screened blood and cellular components with a reduced risk of CMV transmission for neonates <1,200 g at birth where transfusion-associated CMV disease is a problem, when either the recipient or the mother is CMV seronegative, or that information is unknown.

The exclusive use of CMV-seronegative blood components for low-birthweight infants whose serostatus is either positive or unknown has been questioned because some infants born to seropositive mothers develop symptomatic CMV infection when passively transferred maternal antibody titers decline.[81] However, some neonatologists request CMV-seronegative cellular components for all low-birthweight neonates in this patient population despite lack of data to support his approach. Others use CMV-negative blood for all neonates undergoing extracorporeal membrane oxygenation or for children with congenital immunodeficiency disorders. A recommendation to use CMV risk-reduced blood in these patients is controversial.

Seronegative Solid-Organ Transplant Recipients and Candidates

CMV-seronegative candidates for solid-organ transplant should receive CMV-screened blood components to prevent primary infection. Approximately 20–30% of seronegative individuals who receive cadaveric renal transplants from a sero-negative donor develop primary CMV infection, presumably as a result of blood transfusion.[69,71] The remainder developing CMV are infected by the graft. Serum creatinine levels in infected patients are higher than in noninfected persons. Additionally, patient survival is decreased in patients with primary CMV infection who received antilymphocyte globulin. CMV-screened blood reduces the risk of CMV infection in seronegative recipients of cadaveric grafts from CMV antibody-negative donors.

The CMV serostatus of the organ donor is more significant than blood transfusion as a source of CMV infection in cardiac transplantation.[69,71] Seronegative cardiac transplant recipients who receive hearts from CMV-seronegative donors should receive CMV-negative blood components since allograft rejection and atherosclerosis are accelerated in CMV-infected patients.

Serious morbidity has been associated with CMV infection in patients undergoing liver transplantation. The CMV status of the donor organ represents the major risk to seronegative recipients; infection risk is reported as 24-fold higher for seronegative recipients who receive seropositive rather than seronegative organs.[82] It is possible that immunosuppressive effects of transfusion increase the severity of CMV infection in patients receiving multiple transfusions at the time of transplant. Difficulties in supplying the large quantities of blood components required during hepatic transplantation surgery often preclude the ability to supply CMV-screened components. However, third-generation leukocyte depletion filters should be considered when avoidance of CMV infection is necessary.

Bone Marrow Transplantation

Seronegative bone marrow transplant patients who receive bone marrow from a seronegative donor are at risk of acquiring CMV infection through transfusion and should receive blood and components with a reduced risk of CMV transmission.[69,71,72,77]

Components with a reduced risk of CMV transmission are also recommended for seronegative patients who are potential candidates for allogenic bone marrow transplantation. Recommendations for seronegative recipients of autologous marrow transplantation are less clear. The risk of CMV infection is lower in this group than in patients receiving allogeneic marrow transplants, but CMV pneumonia occurs. The risk may be reduced by providing components with reduced CMV transmission risk.[73] It appears that CMV-seronegative components, although desirable, are less critical for patients receiving autologous transplants.

Granulocyte Transfusions

Granulocyte transfusions from CMV-seropositive donors represent a significant source of CMV transmission and should be avoided when granulocyte transfusions are given to CMV-seronegative or unknown serostatus recipients.[69,71]

Acquired Immunodeficiency Syndrome

CMV-seronegative patients with AIDS (e.g., children born to HIV-infected mothers and hemophilic patients) are at risk of CMV-associated morbidity. CMV-screened blood components should be considered for this group.[69,71]

Patients Undergoing Splenectomy

Symptomatic CMV infections have occurred in patients undergoing splenectomy following traumatic injury. Since there are only a few reports of this complication, the use of CMV-screened components for this group of patients is controversial.[69,71]

Epstein-Barr Virus Infection

Epstein-Barr virus (EBV), another human herpesvirus, is rarely transmitted by transfusion because 90% of the adult population has evidence of previous exposure and immunity is substantial in seropositive individuals; susceptible recipients usually receive >1 U of blood and are likely to have passive infusion of EBV neutralizing antibodies; and viability of B lymphocytes (the cells harboring EBV) declines during blood storage.[83] EBV has been transmitted through transfusion when only a single unit from a donor who was incubating an acute infection was involved or when the recipient had a T-cell deficiency that permitted transfused B lymphocytes to survive longer than passively transferred protective antibody. The postperfusion syndrome that occurs following open-heart surgery is usually linked to CMV, not EBV infection.

PARVOVIRUS INFECTION

Parvovirus B19, a single-stranded DNA virus, is the etiologic agent of fifth disease. Acute infection with parvovirus B19 in a few patients with congenital hemolytic disorders or those with immunodeficiencies is associated with transient aplastic crises. Since 50% of the adult population has been previously exposed to the virus, and only a few cases of hypoplastic anemia have been reported, the significance of transfusion-transmitted parvovirus infection is unclear. Factor VIII concentrates subjected to viral inactivation techniques by pasteurization or solvent/detergent treatment have infected susceptible individuals.[84]

SPIROCHETE INFECTIONS

Syphilis

Syphilis is caused by *Treponema palladium*. Transfusion-associated cases occur very infrequently because the viability of *T. palladium* in blood stored at 4°C is only 48–120 hours, donors are screened by Venereal Disease Research Laboratory or rapid plasmin reagin testing, many patients receiving platelet transfusions also receive antibiotic therapy, and the viability of *T. palladium* is decreased in components stored under more aerobic conditions (e.g., platelets). Serologic testing for syphilis, once questioned, is now regarded as valid to guard against syphilis transmission by components stored for a few days and as a surrogate marker of those at high risk of sexually transmitted diseases, including HIV.[85,86] Interestingly, the benefit of syphilis testing to detect heterosexually infected HIV carriers who present for blood donation was questioned by data collected by Centers for Disease Control investigators.[87] The average incubation period for post-transfusion-associated syphilis is 9–10 weeks, but varies from 4 to 18 weeks.

Lyme Borreliosis

Lyme disease or Lyme borreliosis is caused by a spirochete, *Borrelia burgdorferi*. Most infections with *B. burgdorferi* occur following *Ixodes scapularis* and *I. pacificus* tick bites.[88] All patients in whom the spirochete was recovered from blood cultures were symptomatic at the time the cultures were taken. It is expected that spirochetemic donors would be symptomatic and, therefore, not be accepted for donation. In experimental studies, spirochetes remain viable in red cells and platelet concentrates stored under standard conditions throughout the shelf life of these components and remain viable in fresh frozen plasma stored at −18°C for 45 days. Nonetheless, cases of transfusion-associated Lyme disease have not been reported. Serologic testing results are inconsistent.[89]

Health care workers have been advised to be alert for the diagnosis of Lyme borreliosis and to determine whether such patients have previously been a blood donor or transfusion recipient.

PARASITIC INFECTIONS

Malaria

Between 1972 and 1988, 45 cases of transfusion-associated malaria were reported in the United States. *Plasmodium malariae* was implicated in 38% of the cases, *P. falciparum* in 29%, *P. vivax* in 24%, and *P. ovale* in 9%. Of the 45 patients, 3 died as a result of the malaria infection, 2 with *P. falciparum* and 1 with *P. malariae*.[90] Most of the donors were born in countries in which malaria is prevalent. The incubation period following transfusion is approximately 20 days (range 7–50 days). Platelet concentrates may transmit malaria, but they probably carry a smaller risk than do red cell products because relatively few erythrocytes are contained in them. Plasma components do not transmit malaria.

Prevention of transfusion-transmitted malaria is predicated on deferring donation by those with identifiable risk of malaria or a diagnosis of malaria. Travelers to endemic regions and those residing in these areas are deferred for 1 year after returning to nonendemic areas, provided they do not have symptoms suggestive of malaria. If they emigrated from a country considered endemic for malaria the deferral is 3 years. Serologic tests, including enzyme-linked immunosorbent assay and immunofluorescent assays, have been used to identify donors implicated in transfusion-associated cases, but donor deferral is a more efficient mechanism for screening blood donors.

Babesiosis

Babesiosis, caused by *Babesia microtia* and *B. equi,* is an infection of red cells that is transmitted by the *I. scapularies* and possibly *I. pacificus* ticks.[88] It causes a malaria-like illness that is generally mild but may be associated with hemolysis and renal failure; on occasion, it is fatal. Immunocompromised, asplenic, and elderly patients appear to be at highest risk of morbidity. At least seven transfusion-associated cases have been reported, including recipients of platelet, red cell, and frozen-thawed red cell transfusions.[91,92] The reported incubation period varies from 17 days to 8 weeks. Current blood bank recommendations for decreasing potential transmission by transfusion include indefinitely deferring donors who give a history of babesiosis, encouraging health care providers to be alert to making the diagnosis of babesiosis, and notifying blood collection and transfusion services of potential cases of transfusion-transmitted *B. microtia* infection.

Chagas Disease

Chagas disease (American Trypanosomiasis) is caused by the protozoan parasite *Trypanosoma cruzi,* an organism that is endemic in Mexico and Central and South America. Triatomine bugs (kissing bugs) spread infection to humans, and low levels of parasitemia persist throughout life. Severe myocarditis develops in a small percentage of patients with acute symptoms. Chronic Chagas disease occurs in 10–30% of infected persons

and is manifest by dilated cardiomyopathy and dysrhythmias, megaesophagus, or megacolon.[93,94]

Only a few cases of transfusion-transmitted Chagas disease have been reported in the United States. The risk of transmission is estimated as 13–23% per infected unit of blood. The incidence of transfusion-associated Chagas disease may increase as a result of extensive migration of Central and South Americans to the United States; as many as 50,000–100,000 immigrants with *T. cruzi* infection may be in the United States.[94] Adequate screening tests are currently unavailable. It may be more appropriate to exclude donors by questioning about risks of *T. cruzi* infection such as prolonged residence in endemic areas under conditions leading to exposure to insect vectors, or by obtaining a history of transfusion or previous exposure to *T. cruzi*.[95]

Toxoplasmosis

Toxoplasmosis is caused by the intracellular protozoan parasite *Toxoplasma gondii*. It persists in white blood cells throughout the shelf life of blood. Transfusion-transmitted cases have occurred in immunosuppressed patients receiving leukocyte concentrates.[96]

Leishmaniasis

More than 500,000 U.S. military personnel were stationed in the Persian Gulf region during 1990–1991. By November, 1991 approximately 24 cases of infection caused by *Leishmania tropica* had been reported, including 7 patients with visceral organ involvement. Although only five reported cases of leishmaniasis are known to be associated with blood transfusion and all were caused by *L. donovani,* the potential risk of transfusion-transmitted leishmaniasis led to deferral from blood donation of all returning military personnel through December 31, 1992. No cases of *L. tropica* attributed to transfusions were reported.[97]

BACTERIAL INFECTION

Septic complications associated with transfusion of red cells, whole blood, platelets, and cryoprecipitate have been reported. Between 1986 and 1991, of 182 transfusion-related fatalities reported to the FDA, 29 (16%) were caused by bacterial contamination.[98] Organisms isolated included *Pseudomonas, Yersinia, Enterobacter, Staphylococcus aureus* and *epidermidis, Clostridium, Klebsiella, Salmonella,* and *Proteus.*[99]

Recipients develop fever, chills, vomiting, tachycardia, and hypotension during transfusion or several hours later. Reactions occurring immediately are attributed to endotoxin rather than bacterial load. A 25% mortality rate is reported.[100] In general, bacteria contaminate the blood or components as a result of asymptomatic bacteremia and multiply during storage. Occasional contamination occurs because of inadequate skin sterilization at the site of venipuncture during collection.

Recognition of transfusion-related sepsis is imperative so that the transfusion may be discontinued and antibacterial therapy instituted immediately. The diagnosis must be suspected and treated on clinical grounds since Gram stains are not always informative; no organisms were seen with high-speed centrifugation and gram stain when 10^5/ml organisms are present. Organisms are seen 50% of the time when preparations containing 10^8/ml organisms are spun at high speed and Gram stained.[101]

CREUTZFELDT-JAKOB DISEASE

Creutzfeldt-Jakob disease (CJD) is a central nervous system disorder with a prolonged latent period associated with other scrapie-like or prion diseases. Some affected patients received growth hormone prepared from extracts or human pituitary glands from persons with unsuspected CJD, and other cadaver-derived materials, including corneas and dura mater grafts. Since some recipients of human pituitary-derived growth hormone may harbor the CJD agent and may be at risk of transmitting it through transfusion, donors are deferred if they received human growth hormone extracted from pituitary glands. It is unclear whether CJD has been transmitted by blood transfusion.[102]

REFERENCES

1. Forbes A, Williams R: Changing epidemiology and clinical aspects of hepatitis A. Br Med Bull 46:303, 1990
2. Mannucci PM: Outbreak of hepatitis A among Italian patients with hemophilia. Lancet 339:819, 1992
3. Shouval D, Gerlich WH, Temperly IJ et al: Clotting factors and hepatitis A. Lancet 340:1465, 1992
4. Foster GR, MRCP, Carman WF et al: Replication of hepatitis B and delta viruses: appearance of viral mutants. Semin Liver Dis 11:121, 1991
5. Centers for Disease Control: Recommendations for preventing transmission of human immunodeficiency virus and hepatitis B virus to patients during exposure-prone invasive procedures. MMWR 40:1, 1991
6. Zuckerman AJ: Viral hepatitis. Transfus Med 3:7, 1993
7. Alter HJ, Holland PV, Purcell RH et al: Posttransfusion hepatitis after exclusion of commercial and hepatitis-B antigen-positive donors. Ann Intern Med 77:691, 1972
8. Dodd RY: The risk of transfusion transmitted infection. N Engl J Med 327:419, 1992
9. Barbara JAJ, Garson JA: Polymerase chain reaction and transfusion microbiology. Vox Sang 64:73, 1993
10. Alter HJ, Holland PV, Morrow AG et al: Clinical and serological analysis of transfusion-associated hepatitis. Lancet 2:838, 1975
11. Choo QL, Kuo G, Weiner AJ et al: Isolation of a cDNA clone derived from a blood-borne non-A non-B viral hepatitis genome. Science 244:359, 1989
12. McOmish F, Chan SW, Dow BC et al: Detection of three types of hepatitis C virus in blood donors: investigation of type-specific differences in serologic reactivity and rate of alanine aminotransferase abnormalities. Transfusion 33:7, 1993
13. Alter HJ, Purcell RH, Shh JW et al: Detection of antibody to hepatitis C virus in prospectively followed transfusion recipients with acute and chronic non-A, non-B hepatitis. N Engl J Med 321:1494, 1989
14. Troisi CL, Hollinger BF, Hoots WK et al: A multicenter study of viral hepatitis in a United States hemophilic population. Blood 81:412, 1993
15. Skaug K, Li H, Jonassen TO et al: Hepatitis C virus (HCV) RNA among anti-HCV-positive blood donors and their recipients. Vox Sang 64:215, 1993
16. Aoki SK, Holland PV, Fernando LP et al: Evidence of hepatitis in patients receiving transfusions of blood components containing antibody to hepatitis C. Blood 82:1000, 1993
17. Estevan JI, Gonzalez A, Hernandez JM et al: Evaluation of antibodies to hepatitis C virus in a study of transfusion associated hepatitis. N Engl J Med 323:1107, 1990
18. Alter J: New kit on the block: evaluation of second-generation assays for detection of antibody to the hepatitis C virus. Hepatology 15:350, 1992
19. Kleinman S, Alter H, Busch M et al: Increased detection of hepatitis C virus (HCV)-infected blood donors by a multiple-antigen HCV enzyme immunoassay. Transfusion 32:805, 1992
20. Farci P, London WT, Wong DC et al: The natural history of infection with hepatitis C virus (HCV) in chimpanzees: comparison of serologic responses measured with first- and second-generation assays and relationship to HCV viremia. J Infect Dis 165:1006, 1992
21. Ragni MV, Ndimbie OK, Rice EO et al: The presence of hepatitis C virus (HCV) antibody to human immunodeficiency virus-positive hemophilic men undergoing HCV "seroconversion." Blood 82:1010, 1993
22. Alter MJ, Margolis HS, Krawczynski K et al: The natural history of community-acquired hepatitis C in the United States. N Engl J Med 327:1899, 1992
23. Busch MP, Tobler L, Quan S et al: A pattern of 5-1-1 and c100-3 only on hepatitis C virus (HCV) recombinant immunoblot assay does not reflect HCV infection in blood donors. Transfusion 33:84, 1993
24. Zaaijer HL, Cuypers HTM, Reesink HW et al: Reliability of polymerase chain reaction for detection of hepatitis C virus. Lancet 341:722, 1993
25. Farci P, Alter HJ, Wong D et al: A long-term study of hepatitis C virus replication in non-A, non-B hepatitis. N Engl J Med 325:98, 1991
26. Esteban JI, Lopez Talavera JC, Genesca J et al: High rate of infectivity and liver disease in blood donors with antibodies to hepatitis C virus. Ann Intern Med 115:443, 1991
27. Seeff LB, Buskell-Bales Z, Wright EC et al: Long-term mortality after transfusion-associated non-A, non-B hepatitis. N Engl J Med 327:1906, 1992
28. Koretz RL, Abbey H, Coleman E, Gitnick G: Non-A, non-B post-transfusion hepatitis. Ann Intern Med 119:110, 1993
29. Bresters D, Mauser-Bunschoten EP, Reesink HW et al: Sexual transmission of hepatitis C virus. Lancet 342:210, 1993
30. Brackmann SA, Gerritzen A, Oldenburg J et al: Search for intrafamilial transmission of hepatitis C virus in hemophilia patients. Blood 81:1077, 1993
31. Reinus JF, Leikin EL, Alter HJ et al: Failure to detect vertical transmission of hepatitis C. Ann Intern Med 117:881, 1992
32. Pol S, Driss F, Devergie A et al: Is hepatitis C virus involved in hepatitis-associated aplastic anemia? Ann Intern Med 113:435, 1990
33. Hibbs JR, Frickhofen N, Rosenfeld SJ et al: Aplastic anemia and viral hepatitis non-A, non-B, non-C? JAMA 267:2051, 1992
34. Simonetti RG, Camma C, Fiorello F et al: Hepatitis C virus infection as a risk factor for hepatocellular carcinoma in patients with cirrhosis. Ann Intern Med 116:97, 1992
35. Aach RD, Szmuness W, Mosley JW et al: Serum alanine aminotransferase of donors in relation to the risk of non-A, non-B hepatitis in recipients. The transfusion-transmitted viruses study. N Engl J Med 304:989, 1981
36. Stevens CE, Aach RD, Hollinger FB et al: Hepatitis B virus antibody in blood donors and the occurrence of non-A, non-B hepatitis recipients. An analysis of the transfusion-transmitted viruses study. Ann Intern Med 101:733, 1984
37. Alter HJ, Purcell RH, Holland PV et al: Donor transaminase and recipient hepatitis. Impact on blood transfusion services. JAMA 246:630, 1981
38. Koziol DE, Holland PV, Alling DW et al: Antibody to hepatitis B core antigen as a paradoxical marker for non-A, non-B hepatitis agents in donated blood. Ann Intern Med 104:488, 1986
39. Sugg U, Schenzle D, Hess G: Antibodies to hepatitis B core antigen in blood donors screened for alanine aminotransferase level and hepatitis non-A, non-B in recipients. Transfusion 28:386, 1988
40. Donahue JG, Munoz A, Ness PM et al: The declining risk of post-transfusion hepatitis C virus infection. N Engl J Med 327:369, 1992
41. Aach RD, Stevens CE, Hollinger FB et al: Hepatitis C virus infection in post-transfusion hepatitis. N Engl J Med 325:1325, 1991
42. Fricke W, Augustyniak L, Lawrence D et al: Human immunodeficiency virus infection due to clotting factor concentrates: results of the Seroconversion Surveillance Project. Transfusion 32:707, 1992
43. Centers for Disease Control: Possible transfusion associated acquired immunodeficiency syndrome (AIDS)—California. MMWR 31:652, 1982
44. Centers for Disease Control: *Pneumocystis carinii* pneumonia among persons with hemophilia A. MMWR 31:365, 1982
45. Selik R, Ward J, Buehler J: Trends in transfusion-associated acquired immunodeficiency syndrome in the United States, 1982–1991. Transfusion 33:890, 1993
46. Busch MP, Lee HT, Heitman J: Allogeneic leukocytes but not therapeutic blood elements induce reactivation and dissemination of latent human immunodeficiency virus type I infection: implications for transfusion support of infected patients. Blood 80:2128, 1992
47. Fauci AS: CD4+ T-lymphocytopenia without HIV infection—no lights, no camera, just facts. N Engl J Med 328:429, 1993
48. Silvergleid AJ, Leparc GF, Schmidt PJ: Impact of explicit questions about high-risk activities on donor attitudes and donor deferral patterns. Transfusion 29:362, 1989
49. Leitman SF, Klein HG, Melpolder JJ et al: Clinical implications of positive tests for antibodies to human immunodeficiency virus type I in asymptomatic blood donors. N Engl J Med 321:917, 1989
50. Menitove JE: Current risk of transfusion-associated human immunodeficiency virus infection. Arch Pathol Lab Med 114:330, 1990
51. Ward JW, Homberg SD, James RA et al: Transfusion of human immunodeficiency virus (HIV) by blood transfusion screened as negative for HIV antibody. N Engl J Med 318:473, 1988
52. Ping W, Miller B, Gallana J: Early detection of IGM antibodies to HIV-I by recombinant antigen enzyme immunoassay. W.C. 3184. VIIth International AIDS Conference, Florence, Italy, 1991
53. Locke SE, Kuwaloff HB, Hoff RG et al: Screening blood donors by computer interview. JAMA 268:1301, 1992
54. Alter HJ, Epstein JS, Swenson SG et al: Prevalence of human immunodeficiency virus type I p24 antigen in U.S. blood donors—an assessment of the efficacy of testing in donor screening. N Engl J Med 323:1312, 1990
55. Busch MP, Taylor PE, Lenes BA: Screening of selected male blood donors

for p24 antigen of human immunodeficiency virus type I. N Engl J Med 323: 1308, 1990

56. O'Brien TR, George JR, Holberg SD: Human immunodeficiency virus type 2 infection in the United States. JAMA 267:2775, 1992

57. Markovitz DM: Infection with the human immunodeficiency virus type 2. Ann Intern Med 118:211, 1993

58. Centers for Disease Control and Prevention, the U.S.P.H.S. Working Group: Guidelines for counseling persons infected with human T-lymphotropic virus type I (HTLV-I) and type II (HTLV-II). Ann Intern Med 118:448, 1993

59. Hollsberg P, Hafler DA: Pathogenesis of disease induced by human lymphotropic virus type I infection. N Engl J Med 328:1173, 1993

60. Khabbaz RF, Onorato IM, Cannon RO et al: Seroprevalence of HTLV-I and HTLV-II among intravenous drug users and persons in clinics for sexually transmitted diseases. N Engl J Med 326:375, 1992

61. Kleinman S, Swanson P, Allain JP et al: Transfusion transmission of human T-lymphotropic virus types I and II: serologic and polymerase chain reaction results in recipients identified through look-back investigations. Transfusion 31:14, 1993

62. Hjelle B, Appenzeller O, Mills R et al: Chronic neurodegenerative disease associated with HTLV-II infection. Lancet 339:645, 1992

63. Zucker-Franklin D, Hooper WC, Evatt BL: Human lymphotropic retroviruses associated with mycosis fungoides: evidence that human T-cell lymphotropic virus type II (HTLV-II) as well as HTLV-I may play a role in the disease. Blood 80:1537, 1992

64. Loughran TP Jr, Coyle T, Sherman MP et al: Detection of human T-cell leukemia/lymphoma virus, type II, in a patient with large granular lymphocyte leukemia. Blood 80:1116, 1992

65. Hjelle B, Wilson C, Cyrus S et al: Human T-cell leukemia virus type II infection frequently goes undetected in contemporary US blood donors. Blood 81: 1641, 1993

66. Sullivan MT, Williams AE, Fang CT et al: Human T-lymphotropic virus (HTLV) types I and II infection in sexual contacts and family members of blood donors who are seropositive for HTLV type I or II. Transfusion 33: 585, 1993

67. Herr V, Ambruso D, Fairfax M et al: Transfusion-associated transmission of human T-lymphotropic virus types I and II: experience of a regional blood center. Transfusion 33:208, 1993

68. Smith KL, Kulski JK, Cobain T, Duston RA: Detection of cytomegalovirus in blood donors by the polymerase chain reaction. Transfusion 33:497, 1993

69. Hillyer CD, Snydman DR, Berkman EM: The risk of cytomegalovirus infection in solid organ and bone marrow transplant recipients: transfusion of blood products. Transfusion 30:659, 1990

70. Lamberson HV, Dock NL: Prevention of transfusion-transmitted cytomegalovirus infection. Transfusion 32:196, 1992

71. Sayers MH, Anderson KC, Goodnough LT et al: Reducing the risk for transfusion-transmitted cytomegalovirus infection. Ann Intern Med 116:55, 1992

72. Verdonck LF, de Gast GC, Van Heugten HG: Cytomegalovirus infection causes delayed platelet recovery after bone marrow transplantation. Blood 78:844, 1991

73. Reusser P, Fisher LD, Buckner CD et al: Cytomegalovirus infection after autologous bone marrow transplantation: occurrence of cytomegalovirus disease and effect on engraftment. Blood 75:1888, 1990

74. Gilbert GL, Hayes K, Hudson IL et al: Prevention of transfusion-acquired cytomegalovirus infection in infants by blood filtration to remove leucocytes. Lancet 2:1228, 1989

75. Eisenfeld L, Silver H, McLaughlin J et al: Prevention of transfusion-associated cytomegalovirus infection in neonatal patients by the removal of white cells from blood. Transfusion 32:205, 1992

76. De Graan-Hentzen YCE, Gratama JW, Mudde GC et al: Prevention of primary cytomegalovirus infection in patients with hematologic malignancies by intensive white cell depletion of blood products. Transfusion 29:757, 1989

77. Bowden RA, Slichter SJ, Sayers MH et al: Use of leukocyte-depleted platelets and cytomegalovirus-seronegative red blood cells for prevention of primary cytomegalovirus infection after marrow transplant. Blood 78:246, 1991

78. Fowler KB, Stagno S, Pass RF et al: The outcome of congenital cytomegalovirus infection in relation to maternal antibody status. N Engl J Med 326:663, 1992

79. Yeager AS, Grumet FC, Hafleigh EB et al: Prevention of transfusion-acquired cytomegalovirus infection in newborn infants. J Pediatr 98:281, 1981

80. Adler SP, Chandrika T, Lawrence L, Baggett J: Cytomegalovirus infections in neonates acquired by blood transfusions. Pediatr Infect Dis 2:114, 1983

81. Yeager AS, Palumbo PE, Malachowski N et al: Sequelae of maternally derived cytomegalovirus infections in premature infants. J Pediatr 102:918, 1983

82. Manez R, Kusne S, Martin M et al: The impact of blood transfusion on the occurrence of pneumonitis in primary cytomegalovirus infection after liver transplantation. Transfusion 33:594, 1993

83. Klein G: Epstein-Barr virus-carrying cells in Hodgkin's disease. Blood 80: 299, 1992

84. Zakrzewska K, Azzi A, Patou G et al: Human parvovirus B19 in clotting factor concentrates: B19 DNA detection by the nested polymerase chain reaction. Br J Haematol 81:407, 1993

85. de Schryver A, Meheus A: Syphilis and blood transfusion: a global perspective. Transfusion 30:844, 1990

86. Seidl S: Syphilis screening in the 1990's. Transfusion 30:773, 1990

87. Petersen LR, Doll LS, White CR et al: Heterosexually acquired human immunodeficiency virus infection and the United States blood supply: considerations for screening of potential blood donors. Transfusion 33:552, 1993

88. Spach D, Liles WC, Campbell GL et al: Tick-borne diseases in the United States. N Engl J Med 329:936, 1993

89. Bakken LL, Case KL, Callister SM et al: Performance of 45 laboratories participating in a proficiency testing program for lyme disease serology. JAMA 268:891, 1992

90. Nahlen BL, Lobel HO, Cannon SE, Campbell CC: Reassessment of blood donor selection criteria for United States travelers to malarious areas. Transfusion 31:798, 1991

91. Guerrero IC, Weniger BC, Shultz MG: Transfusion malaria in the United States, 1972–1981. Ann Intern Med 99:221, 1983

92. Mintz ED, Anderson JF, Cable RG, Hadler JR: Transfusion-transmitted babesiosis: a case report from a new endemic area. Transfusion 31;365, 1991

93. Wendel S, Gonzaga AL: Chagas' disease and blood transfusion a new world problem? Vox Sang 64:1, 1993

94. Kirchhoff LV: American trypanosomiasis (Chagas' disease)—a tropical disease now in the United States. N Engl J Med 329:639, 1993

95. Appleman MD, Shulman IA, Saxena S, Kirchhoff LV: Use of a questionnaire to identify potential blood donors at risk for infection with *Trypanosoma cruzi*. Transfusion 33:61, 1993

96. Nelson JC, Kauffmann DJH, Ciavarella D, Senisi WJ: Acquired toxoplasmic retinochoroiditis after platelet transfusions. Ann Ophthalmol 21:253, 1989

97. Magill AJ, Grogl M, Gasser RA Jr et al: Visceral infection caused by *Leishmania tropica* in veterans of operation Desert Storm. N Engl J Med 328:1383, 1993

98. Hoppe PA: Interim measures for detection of bacterially contaminated red cell components. Transfusion 32:199, 1992

99. Tipple MA, Bland LA, Murphy JJ et al: Sepsis associated with transfusion of red cells contaminated with yersinia enterocolitica. Transfusion 30:207, 1990

100. Goldman M, Blajchman MA: Blood product-associated bacterial sepsis. Transfus Med Rev V:73, 1991

101. Barrett BB, Andersen JW, Anderson KC: Strategies for the avoidance of bacterial contamination of blood components. Transfusion 33:228, 1993

102. Klein R, Dumble LJ: Transmission of Creutzfeldt-Jakob disease by blood transfusion. Lancet 341:768, 1993

Autologous Blood Transfusion

143

Margot S. Kruskall

INTRODUCTION

Although the concept of collecting, saving, and transfusing autologous blood has existed for >100 years, practical applications for these techniques appeared limited until recently. With the emergence of the human immunodeficiency virus and its facility for highly efficient transmission via blood has come an increased interest in using the patient's own blood for transfusion.

ADVANTAGES OF AUTOLOGOUS BLOOD TRANSFUSION

The substitution of autologous blood components for those collected from other (allogeneic) donors eliminates transfusion-transmitted diseases such as hepatitis and acquired immunodeficiency syndrome. Immunologic complications related to the transfusion of foreign cells, including hemolysis and febrile reactions to white cells, are also prevented. Other advantages, while possible, are less clearly established. For example, erythropoiesis may be sufficiently stimulated in the repeatedly bled autologous donor to hasten recovery from postoperative anemia.[1] Intraoperatively salvaged red cells are spared the acquired membrane defects ("storage lesion") and 2,3-diphosphoglycerate deficiency of refrigerated allogeneic cells.[2] Some investigators believe that allogeneic blood transfusions may contribute to immunosuppression in the recipient,[3] and therefore to an increased risk of cancer spread[4]; autologous blood should not. However, a recent randomized trial of autologous versus allogeneic blood transfusion in colon cancer was unable to detect any differences in prognosis, thereby disputing the contribution to immunosuppression by allogeneic blood.[5] An important drawback to these techniques is their increased expense, in contrast to the technically and administratively simpler allogeneic transfusions they replace.[6] Other potential problems, such as the risks of blood donation in patients with cardiac disorders[7] or complications from reinfusion of red cells damaged during their salvage from the surgical field,[8,9] are of unknown significance.

METHODS OF COLLECTION

Three approaches are popular and sometimes used in combination in an individual patient: autologous blood donations in advance of an anticipated blood loss during surgery, salvage of intra- and postoperatively shed blood, and intraoperative acute hemodilution.

Autologous Blood Donations

Preoperative

The typical volunteer allogeneic blood donor is allowed to give 1 unit of blood (450 ml ±10%) no more than once every 8 weeks, in order to prevent such complications as iron deficiency. However, provided that bone marrow erythropoiesis can be stimulated, and satisfactory iron supplies maintained, blood can be collected as frequently as once a week from an autologous donor.[10] Although the shelf life of refrigerated red blood cells is limited to 42 days, storage for ≤10 years is possible at ≤ −65°C, using glycerol as a cryopreservative.

From a cardiovascular standpoint, phlebotomy is well tolerated by a variety of seemingly high-risk donors, including the elderly,[11,12] children,[13] pregnant women,[14,15] and patients with coronary artery disease.[1,16] By contrast, anemia frequently develops during the donation interval and limits the number of autologous units that can be collected. In addition to marginal iron stores, erythropoietin levels often do not increase during the donation interval, probably because the hematocrit of most donors is not allowed to fall to <30%.[17] Recent research suggests that this situation may be improved by the administration to autologous donors of the recombinant growth hormone erythropoietin.[18] Many variables affect the response to this drug in blood donors, and are under active study, including the route of administration (intravenous versus subcutaneous), baseline iron stores, and the method of iron supplementation (oral versus parenteral).[19] The expense of recombinant growth hormone erythropoietin therapy has limited its application to situations in which autologous blood donation might otherwise be difficult or impossible, such as in the already anemic patient.[20]

Patients planning to undergo an elective orthopaedic surgical procedure make ideal autologous donors (Table 143-1): these patients typically require blood transfusions either during surgery or during the first few postoperative days, and most have sufficient time before the operative date to make multiple donations.[21,22] Autologous blood has also been collected from patients undergoing elective open heart surgery and other vascular bypass grafts.[1,12] The reduction or elimination of allogeneic blood use by these patients is testimony to the value of

Table 143-1. Common Indications for Autologous Blood Techniques

Surgical/Obstetric Procedures	Preoperative Donations	Perioperative Salvage
Intra-abdominal vascular procedures	Yes	Yes
Open heart surgery	Yes	Yes
Total hip replacement	Yes	Yes[a]
Total knee replacement	Yes	Yes[b]
Scoliosis repairs	Yes	Yes
Radical prostatectomy	Yes	Yes[c]
Placenta previa	Yes	No[d]
Multiple gestations	Yes	No[d]

[a] The need for postoperative salvage has not been conclusively established.

[b] Intraoperative salvage is unnecessary when a tourniquet technique is used; postoperative salvage may be of value when procedure is performed without cement.

[c] The risk of cancer spread after transfusion of intraoperatively salvaged blood has not been established.

[d] The safety of blood containing amniotic fluid has not been conclusively established.

(Adapted from Kruskall,[97] with permission.)

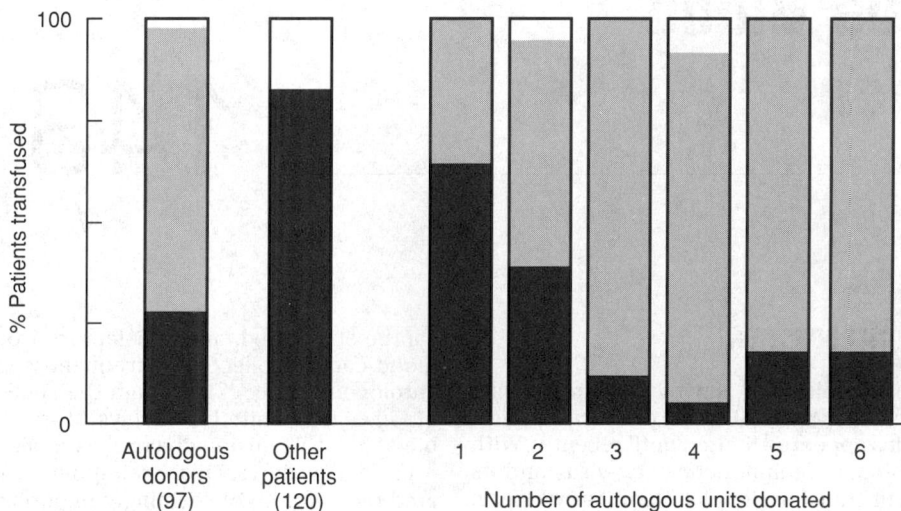

Fig. 143-1. Proportion of patients undergoing first-time elective coronary artery bypass surgery who required transfusion. **(Left)** Autologous donors versus other patients. **(Right)** Autologous donors according to the number of units of autologous blood donated. White bars, no transfusion; gray bars, autologous blood transfusions only; red bars, allogeneic blood transfusions. (From Owings et al.,[1] with permission.)

autologous collections in such operations (Fig. 143-1). The use of preoperatively donated autologous blood has also been reported for a variety of other surgical procedures, including radical prostatectomy; hysterectomies and other gynecologic procedures; colorectal, biliary, and gastric surgery; and neurosurgery.[12,23,24] With their growing popularity, autologous donations have also been used unnecessarily, particularly in plastic surgery procedures, in which allogeneic blood transfusions are rarely necessary.[25]

Other Uses

Autologous blood has been collected from women during pregnancy for use during childbirth, but this approach is controversial. A number of recent clinical studies of blood donations during pregnancy have found no complications for either the mother or the fetus.[14,15] Nevertheless, the transfusion rate at delivery is quite low, at <2.5% in many institutions,[26] and most autologous donations are unused. The use of autologous donations may best be directed toward patients with multiple gestations or placenta previa, in which the likelihood of transfusion may exceed 25%.[27]

Long-term (frozen) storage of autologous red cells in the absence of a planned transfusion episode is largely ineffective and expensive. Medical emergencies requiring transfusion are of an unpredictable but low incidence, and the likelihood is not very great that sufficient blood could be donated and stored and that such blood could be sent where it was needed and prepared in a timely fashion (i.e., thawed and washed free of its glycerol cryoprotectant).

Other autologous components have applications in surgery. Although autologous plasma is easily separated and stored, there is little need for this component in elective surgery.[28] However, autologous "fibrin glue" can be prepared using the cryoprecipitated portion of the plasma mixed immediately before use with thrombin. This tissue adhesive has been used for a variety of purposes in surgical procedures, including the control of bleeding in cardiovascular and thoracic surgery,[29] adhesion in middle ear surgery,[30] closure of the dura in neurosurgery,[31] adhesion of skin grafts,[32] and closure of gastrointestinal fistulas.[33] Fibrin glue has been also used in pancreatic and hepatic resection and trauma,[34,35] although episodes of severe hypotension have been reported, possibly related to allergic reactions to systemically absorbed bovine thrombin.[36] Another rare complication, the development of life-threatening bleeding in association with acquired factor inhibitors, is caused by immunization to small amounts of bovine factor V in the thrombin; these antibodies recognize cross-reactive epitopes on human factor V.[37–39]

Autologous platelet-rich plasma has been prepared at the start of open heart surgery, before bypass, using apheresis equipment, for return to the patient following heparin reversal.[40] Both thrombocytopenia and an acquired platelet defect, due to activation and α-granule release, occur when blood passes through the membrane oxygenator during cardiopulmonary bypass.[41] The theoretical advantage of transfusing autologous platelet-rich plasma should be an improvement in hemostasis and a reduction in transfusion requirements. Initial studies provided enthusiastic confirmation.[40,42–44] More recent prospective, blind studies have been unable to demonstrate a reduction in blood use after either primary or repeat open heart surgery.[45,46] Furthermore, the harvesting of platelet-rich plasma has been followed by intraoperative heparin resistance, possibly due to the release of platelet factor 3 and other procoagulants from platelets damaged during collection.[47] Further studies of this autologous component are needed before its utility can be advocated.

Intraoperative Blood Salvage

Interest in salvaging blood shed at surgery has been stimulated by the introduction of automated instruments for autologous blood salvage over the past 30 years. The first model suctioned blood from the surgical field into a reservoir, from which it could be rapidly reinfused to the patient.[8] Unfortunately, a design flaw allowed the reinfusion pump to continue to operate even when the reservoir was empty, and several deaths from air embolism were reported.[48] This situation has since been improved by the appearance of other high-speed models with safer air detectors. Techniques for washing blood to remove excess surgical irrigant fluids and other contaminants appeared at around the same time.[49]

Systems for blood collection without further washing are usually modifications of disposable suction devices (Table 143-2). Blood is collected under low vacuum pressure into a plastic bag seated within a hard outer cannister. An anticoagulant such as citrate can be added. As soon as the bag is full, or within 4 hours of the start of collection (to prevent bacterial

Table 143-2. Autologous Blood Salvage Systems[a]

			Characteristics of Collected Blood				
System	Hardware	Software	Hematocrit	Free Hemoglobin	Platelet Count	Coagulation Factors	Fibrin Degradation Products
Collection without washing	Rigid plastic cannister	Plastic bag	Low (25%)	Very high (200 mg%)	Low (100,000/mm³)	Low (35–75%)	High (300 mg%)
Collection followed by washing	Integral or separate blood cell processor	Disposable plastic bowl and tubing	High (60%)	Low (<50 mg%)	Very low (10,000/mm³)	Absent (0%)	Absent (0%)

[a] Typical results of laboratory tests are shown. Transfusion of large volumes of salvaged blood results in similar alterations in these tests in the recipient. (Data from Noon[2] and Silva et al.[98])

overgrowth), the contents of the bag are reinfused into the patient by gravity without any further processing, except passage through a standard blood filter.

Alternatively, the contents in the bag can be washed to remove free hemoglobin, surgical irrigant solutions, and other debris. Although this step is theoretically attractive and increasingly popular, its necessity before reinfusion of shed blood has not been established.[50,51] Instruments that include both a reservoir for collecting salvaged blood and a centrifugal washer have been developed. Large aliquots (≥500 ml) can be fully washed in as little as 3 minutes. As a result of this speed, autologous blood salvage has become practical in situations in which blood loss may be extremely rapid, such as trauma or liver transplantation.

The hematocrit of unwashed blood is typically low because of dilution from irrigating surgical fluids and some degree of mechanical hemolysis.[52] Free hemoglobin levels are sometimes >1,000 mg% in unwashed blood, and hemoglobinemia and hemoglobinuria may occur after the transfusion, but renal sequelae are surprisingly low.[51,53] Despite this evidence of red cell injury, the survival rate of ^{51}Cr-labeled salvaged cells is normal in most patients studied.[54,55]

Transfusion of salvaged blood has resulted in coagulation abnormalities in animals and humans, including hypofibrinogenemia, prolonged prothrombin time and partial thromboplastin time, elevated fibrin degradation products, and thrombocytopenia.[9,56] Some authors originally interpreted these results as evidence of disseminated intravascular coagulation, possibly incited by phospholipids and other material released from damaged red cells and platelets. A more likely alternative is that the laboratory data reflect the characteristics of the salvaged blood itself, which, after exposure to serosal surfaces, becomes deficient in coagulation factors and platelets and, in the case of unwashed blood, has high levels of fibrin degradation products[57] (Table 143-2). In those few cases in which the progression of coagulation abnormalities over time has pointed to disseminated intravascular coagulation, rather than simple hemodilution,[8,58] the patient's underlying condition (shock due to massive hemorrhage) appears to have been the cause. A relationship between postoperative coagulopathies and salvaged autologous blood remains tenuous.

Fat, fibrin, bone fragments, and microaggregates often contaminate salvaged autologous blood. However, infusion of unwashed blood has not been proved harmful in either animals or humans, possibly because most particulate material is removed by routine blood filters.[59,60] Other contaminants, such as heparin, topical antibiotics, hemostatic agents, and biologic substances such as tissue enzymes, can be removed, but not necessarily completely, by washing.[61,62] Complete removal of bacteria is also not possible, even when the salvaged blood is washed with antibiotics.[63] Thus, collection of blood from a contaminated site, (e.g., with intestinal contents) is probably contraindicated, although some investigators have argued

that, if no other blood is available, such transfusions may be lifesaving.[64,65] Tumor cells have also been found in blood salvaged during cancer operations; their malignant potential after salvage and transfusion is unknown, and many consider cancer another contraindication.[66,67]

Approximately one-half the blood lost during surgery can be salvaged; the rest is usually irretrievably absorbed in drapes and sponges or damaged during collection.[55] The use of salvaged autologous blood has been associated with a 50% reduction in allogeneic blood use in orthopaedic procedures such as spinal surgery[68] and hip replacement[69,70] and is also effective in such vascular surgical procedures as aortic reconstruction.[71] In cardiac surgery, the largest volume of blood that can be processed for return to the patient comes from the membrane oxygenator.[72,73] Although the blood is technically not "shed," in that it is still in the extracorporeal circuit, the processing is helpful in concentrating the red cells and removing cardioplegic solutions. Autologous blood salvage has also proved useful in large volume blood loss such as that occurring in liver transplantation, in which the volume salvaged averaged 25 U in one study,[74,75] and in trauma.[76] Blood has also been salvaged from the hemoperitoneum associated with ectopic pregnancy,[77] during radical prostatectomy,[78] and during splenectomy.[79] Autologous salvage has been a useful adjunct in the treatment of some Jehovah's Witnesses, whose literal acceptance of the Bible includes abstention from routine allogeneic blood transfusions.[80]

Both the cannister systems and red cell processors used to collect intraoperative autologous blood can also be employed to collect postoperative blood drainage, such as that from the mediastinum after open heart surgery,[81] from the knee or hip after orthopaedic procedures,[82] or from the peritoneal cavity after hepatic injury.[83] Because blood salvaged from a serosal cavity has little residual fibrinogen and platelets, clotting is not a problem, and the addition of anticoagulants is usually unnecessary.[84] Although the volume of postoperative drainage is often substantial in orthopaedic surgery,[85,86] red cells may represent only a small portion; thus, one study reported a mean of only 55 ± 29 ml of red cells in drains following hip surgery.[87] Arthroplasty procedures performed without cement are associated with larger perioperative blood losses, and postoperative red cell salvage may be more effective in such cases.[88]

Hemodilution

The collection of autologous blood during surgery for later reinfusion at the end of the procedure was first suggested in open heart operations, in which it was hoped that a supply of platelets undamaged by exposure to the membrane oxygenator might reduce the incidence of coagulopathies.[89] Hemodilution itself reduces red cell loss: a patient with a hematocrit of 45% and a 2-L blood loss during surgery loses roughly 900 ml of red cells but with a hematocrit of 20% from hemodilution loses only 400 ml of red cells. Proponents claim that the induced anemia may even be beneficial to the patient, in that oxygen delivery at a hematocrit of 30% is enhanced by an increased cardiac output resulting from the decreased blood viscosity.[90]

Reductions in allogeneic blood needs have been reported after marked intraoperative hemodilution (after the hematocrit is lowered by 50%).[91] More modest hemodilution (e.g., removal of 2 U of blood at the beginning of open heart surgery) is also beneficial, according to some workers[92,93] but not others.[94,95] Furthermore, one group has provided evidence that hemodilution may jeopardize patients at risk of ischemic myocardial injury.[96] More research is needed to establish the safety and ideal protocols for this form of blood conservation.

FUTURE DIRECTIONS

Even if human immunodeficiency virus and hepatitis could be completely eliminated from blood components, the risk of other transfusion-transmissible diseases (both known and undiscovered) is ample reason for the continued use of autologous blood protocols, wherever feasible. Recombinant erythropoietin is likely to play an increasingly important role in facilitating autologous blood donation, as are improvements in blood salvage devices that make their use easier and less costly.

REFERENCES

1. Owings DV, Kruskall MS, Thurer RL, Donovan LM: Autologous blood donations prior to elective cardiac surgery: safety and effect on subsequent blood use. JAMA 262:1963, 1989
2. Noon GP: Intraoperative autotransfusion. Surgery 84:719, 1978
3. Blumberg N, Heal J: Transfusions and recipient immune function. Arch Pathol Lab Med 113:246, 1989
4. Blumberg N, Heal J, Chuang C et al: Further evidence supporting a cause and effect relationship between blood transfusions and earlier cancer recurrence. Ann Surg 207:410, 1988
5. Busch OR, Hop WC, van Papendrecht MAH et al: Blood transfusion and prognosis in colorectal cancer. N Engl J Med 328:1372, 1993
6. Birkmeyer JD, Goodnough LT, Aubuchon JP et al: The cost-effectiveness of preoperative autologous blood donation in total hip and knee replacement. Transfusion 33:544, 1993
7. Spiess BD, Sassetti RJ, McCarthy RJ et al: Autologous blood donation: hemodynamics in a high-risk patient population. Transfusion 32:17, 1992
8. Duncan SE, Klebanoff G, Rogers W: A clinical experience with intraoperative autotransfusion. Ann Surg 180:296, 1974
9. Stillman RM, Wrezlewicz WW, Stanczewski BS et al: The haematological hazards of autotransfusion. Br J Surg 63:651, 1976
10. Coleman DH, Stevens AR Jr, Dodge HT, Finch CA: Rate of blood regeneration after blood loss. Arch Intern Med 92:341, 1953
11. Greenwalt TJ: Autologous and aged blood donors. JAMA 257:1220, 1987
12. Kruskall MS, Glazer EE, Leonard SS et al: Utilization and effectiveness of a hospital autologous preoperative blood donor program. Transfusion 26:335, 1986
13. Silvergleid AJ: Safety and effectiveness of predeposit autologous transfusions in preteen and adolescent children. JAMA 257:3403, 1987
14. Kruskall MS, Leonard S, Klapholz H: Autologous blood donation during pregnancy: analysis of safety and blood utilization. Obstet Gynecol 70:938, 1987
15. McVay PA, Hoag RW, Hoag MS, Toy PT: Safety and use of autologous blood donation during the third trimester of pregnancy. Am J Obstet Gynecol 160:1479, 1989
16. Goldfinger D, Capon S, Czer L et al: Safety and efficacy of preoperative donation of blood for autologous use by patients with end-stage heart or lung disease who are awaiting organ transplantation. Transfusion 33:336, 1993
17. Kickler TS, Spivak JL: Effect of repeated whole blood donations on serum immunoreactive erythropoietin levels in autologous donors. JAMA 260:65, 1988
18. Goodnough LT, Rudnick S, Price TH et al: Increased preoperative collection of autologous blood with recombinant human erythropoietin: a controlled trial. N Engl J Med 321:1163, 1989
19. Brugnara C, Chambers LA, Malynn E et al: Red blood cell regeneration in-

20. Mercuriali F, Zanella A, Barosi G et al: Use of erythropoietin to increase the volume of autologous blood donated by orthopedic patients. Transfusion 33:55, 1993
21. Haugen RK, Hill GE: A large-scale autologous blood program in a community hospital: a contribution to the community's blood supply. JAMA 257:1211, 1987
22. Woolson ST, Pottorff G: Use of preoperatively deposited autologous blood for total knee replacement. Orthopedics 16:137, 1993
23. Toy PTCY, Menozzi D, Strauss RG et al: Efficacy of preoperative donation of blood for autologous use in radical prostatectomy. Transfusion 33:721, 1993
24. Toy PTCY, Strauss RG, Stehling LC et al: Predeposited autologous blood for elective surgery. N Engl J Med 316:517, 1987
25. Kruskall MS: Autologous blood transfusions and plastic surgery, editorial. Plast Recontr Surg 84:662, 1989
26. Kamani AA, McMorland GH, Wadsworth LD: Utilization of red blood cell transfusion in an obstetric setting. Am J Obstet Gynecol 159:1177, 1988
27. Klapholz H: Blood transfusion in contemporary obstetric practice. Obstet Gynecol 75:940, 1990
28. Consensus conference: Fresh-frozen plasma: indications and risks. JAMA 253:551, 1985
29. Matthew TL, Spotnitz WD, Kron IL et al: Four years' experience with fibrin sealant in thoracic and cardiovascular surgery. Ann Thorac Surg 50:40, 1990
30. Silberstein LE, Williams LJ, Hughlett MA et al: An autologous fibrinogen-based adhesive for use in otologic surgery. Transfusion 28:319, 1988
31. Stechison MT: Rapid polymerizing fibrin flue from autologous or single-donor blood: preparation and indications. J Neurosurg 76:626, 1993
32. Dahlstrom KK, Weis-Fogh US, Medgyesi S et al: The use of autologous fibrin adhesive in skin transplantation. Plast Reconstr Surg 89:968, 1992
33. Abel ME, Chui YS, Russell TR, Volpe PA: Autologous fibrin glue in the treatment of rectovaginal and complex fistulas. Dis Colon Rectum 36:447, 1993
34. Kram HB, Clark SR, Ocampo HP et al: Fibrin glue sealing of pancreatic injuries, resections, and anastomoses. Am J Surg 161:479, 1991
35. Dulchavsky SA, Geller ER, Maurer J et al: Autologous fibrin gel: bactericidal properties in contaminated hepatic injury. J Trauma 31:991, 1991
36. Berguer R, Staerkel RL, Moore EE et al: Warning: fatal reaction to the use of fibrin glue in deep hepatic wounds. Case reports. J Trauma 31:408, 1991
37. Rapaport SI, Zivelin A, Minow RA et al: Clinical significance of antibodies to bovine and human thrombin and factor V after surgical use of bovine thrombin. Am J Clin Pathol 97:84, 1992
38. Ortel TL, Quinn-Allen MA, Charles LA et al: Characterization of an acquired inhibitor to coagulation factor V: antibody binding to the second C-type domain of factor V inhibits the binding of factor V to phosphatidylserine and neutralizes procoagulant activity. J Clin Invest 90:2340, 1992
39. Berruyer M, Amiral J, Ffrench P et al: Immunization by bovine thrombin used with fibrin glue during cardiovascular operations. J Thorac Cardiovasc Surg 105:892, 1993
40. Giordano GF, Rivers SL, Chung GK et al: Autologous platelet-rich plasma in cardiac surgery: effect on intraoperative and postoperative transfusion requirements. Ann Thorac Surg 46:416, 1988
41. Harker LA, Malpass TW, Branson HE et al: Mechanism of abnormal bleeding in patients undergoing cardiopulmonary bypass: acquired transient platelet dysfunction associated with selective alpha-granule release. Blood 56:824, 1980
42. Boldt J, von Bormann B, Kling D et al: Preoperative plasmapheresis in patients undergoing cardiac surgery procedures. Anesthesiology 72:282, 1990
43. Davies GG, Wells DG, Mabee TM et al: Platelet-leukocyte plasmapheresis attenuates the deleterious effects of cardiopulmonary bypass. Ann Thorac Surg 53:274, 1992
44. DelRossi AJ, Cernaianu AC, Vertrees RA et al: Platelet-rich plasma reduces postoperative blood loss after cardiopulmonary bypass. J Thorac Cardiovasc Surg 100:281, 1990
45. Tobe CE, Vocelka C, Sepulvada R et al: Infusion of autologous platelet rich plasma does not reduce blood loss and product use after coronary artery bypass. J Thorac Cardiovasc Surg 105:1007, 1993
46. Ereth MH, Oliver WC, Beynen FMK et al: Autologous platelet-rich plasma does not reduce transfusion of homologous blood products in patients undergoing repeat valvular surgery. Anesthesiology 79:540, 1993
47. Wickey GS, Keifer JC, Larach DR et al: Heparin resistance after intraoperative platelet-rich plasma harvesting. J Thorac Cardiovasc Surg 103:1172, 1992
48. Deysine M: Intraoperative autotransfusion and air embolism, letter. Surgery 81:729, 1977
49. Wilson JD, Utz DC, Taswell HF: Autotransfusion during transurethal resection of the prostate: technique and preliminary clinical evaluation. Mayo Clin Proc 44:374, 1969

50. Ouriel K, Shortell CK, Green RM, DeWeese JA: Intraoperative autotransfusion in aortic surgery. J Vasc Surg 18:16, 1993
51. Long GW, Glover JL, Bendick PJ et al: Cell washing versus immediate reinfusion of intraoperatively shed blood during abdominal aortic aneurysm repair. Am J Surg 166:97, 1993
52. Aaron RK, Beazley RM, Riggle GC: Hematologic integrity after intraoperative allotransfusion: comparison with bank blood. Arch Surg 108:831, 1974
53. Brener BJ, Raines JK, Darling RC: Intraoperative autotransfusion in abdominal aortic resections. Arch Surg 107:78, 1973
54. Ansell J, Parrilla N, King M et al: Survival of autotransfused red blood cells recovered from the surgical field during cardiovascular operations. J Thorac Cardiovasc Surg 84:387, 1982
55. O'Hara PJ, Hertzer NR, Santilli PH, Beven EG: Intraoperative autotransfusion during abdominal aortic reconstruction. Am J Surg 145:215, 1983
56. Moore EE, Dunn EL, Breslich DJ, Galloway WB: Platelet abnormalities associated with massive autotransfusion. J Trauma 20:1052, 1980
57. Griffith LD, Billman GF, Daily PO, Lane TA: Apparent coagulopathy caused by infusion of shed mediastinal blood and its prevention by washing of the infusate. Ann Thorac Surg 47:400, 1989
58. Klebanoff G: Early clinical experience with a disposable unit for the intraoperative salvage and reinfusion of blood loss (intraoperative autotransfusion). Am J Surg 120:718, 1970
59. Dorang LA, Klebanoff G, Kemmerer WT: Autotransfusion in long-segment spinal fusion: an experimental model to demonstrate the efficacy of salvaging blood contaminated with bone fragments and marrow. Am J Surg 123:686, 1972
60. Bennett SH, Geelhoed GW, Terrill RE, Hoye RC: Pulmonary effects of autotransfused blood: a comparison of fresh autologous and stored blood with blood retrieved from the pleural cavity in an insitu lung perfusion mode. Am J Surg 125:696, 1973
61. Umlas J, O'Neill TP: Heparin removal in an autotransfusor device. Transfusion 21:70, 1981
62. Paravicini D, Thys J, Hein H: Use of neomycin-bacitracin irrigating solution with intraoperative autotransfusions during orthopedic operations. Arzneimittleforschung 33:997, 1983
63. Rumisek JD, Weddle RL: Autotransfusion in penetrating abdominal trauma. p. 105. In Hauer JM, Thurer RL, Dawson RB (eds): Autotransfusion. Elsevier/North-Holland, New York, 1981
64. Timberlake GA, McSwain NE: Autotransfusion of blood contaminated by enteric contents: a potentially life-saving measure in the massively hemorrhaging trauma patient? J Trauma 28:855, 1988
65. Ozmen V, McSwain NE Jr, Nichols RL et al: Autotransfusion of potentially culture-positive blood (CPB) in abdominal trauma: preliminary data from a prospective study. J Trauma 32:36, 1992
66. Yaw PB, Sentany M, Link WJ et al: Tumor cells carried through autotransfusion: contraindication to intraoperative blood recovery? JAMA 231:490, 1975
67. Lane TA: The effect of storage on the metastatic potential of tumor cells collected in autologous blood: an animal model. Transfusion 29:418, 1989
68. Lennon RL, Hosking MP, Gray JR et al: The effects of intraoperative blood salvage and induced hypotension on transfusion requirements during spinal surgical procedures. Mayo Clin Proc 62:1090, 1987
69. Bovill DF, Moulton CW, Jackson WST et al: The efficacy of intraoperative autotransfusion in major orthopedic surgery: a regression analysis. Orthopedics 9:1403, 1986
70. Kruger LM, Colbert JM: Intraoperative autologous transfusion in children undergoing spinal surgery. J Pediatr Orthop 5:330, 1985
71. Hallett JW Jr, Popovsky M, Ilstrup D: Minimizing blood transfusions during abdominal aortic surgery: recent advances in rapid autotransfusion. J Vasc Surg 5:601, 1987
72. Keeling MM, Gray LA, Brink MA et al: Intraoperative autotransfusion: experience in 725 consecutive cases. Ann Surg 197:536, 1983
73. McCarthy PM, Popovsky MA, Schaff HV et al: Effect of blood conservation efforts in cardiac operations at the Mayo Clinic. Mayo Clin Proc 63:225, 1988
74. Dzik WH, Jenkins R: Use of intraoperative blood salvage during orthotopic liver transplantation. Arch Surg 120:946, 1985
75. Williamson KR, Taswell HF, Rettke SR, Krom RAF: Intraoperative autologous transfusion: its role in orthotopic liver transplantation. Mayo Clin Proc 64:340, 1989
76. Reul GJ Jr, Solis RT, Greenberg SD et al: Experience with autotransfusion in the surgical management of trauma. Surgery 76:546, 1974
77. Merrill BS, Mitts DL, Rogers W, Weinberg PC: Autotransfusion: intraoperative use in ruptured ectopic pregnancy. J Reprod Med 24:14, 1980
78. Klimberg I, Sirois R, Wajsman Z, Baker J: Intraoperative autotransfusion in urologic oncology. Arch Surg 121:1326, 1986
79. Witte CL, Esser MJ, Rappaport WD: Updating the management of salvageable splenic injury. Ann Surg 215:261, 1992
80. Spence RK, Alexander JB, DelRossi AJ et al: Transfusion guidelines for cardiovascular surgery: lessons learned from operations in Jehovah's Witnesses. J Vasc Surg 16:825, 1992
81. Johnson RG, Rosenkrantz KR, Preston RA et al: The efficacy of postoperative autotransfusion in patients undergoing cardiac operations. Ann Thorac Surg 36:173, 1983
82. Semkiw LB, Schurman DJ, Goodman SB, Woolson ST: Postoperative blood salvage using the Cell Saver after total joint arthroplasty. J Bone Joint Surg 71A:823, 1989
83. Reiner DS, Tortolani AJ: Postoperative peritoneal blood salvage with autotransfusion after hepatic trauma. Surg Gynecol Obstet 173:501, 1991
84. Glover JL, Broadie TA: Intraoperative autotransfusion. World J Surg 11:60, 1987
85. Gannon DM, Lombardi AV, Mallory TH et al: An evaluation of the efficacy of postoperative blood salvage after total joint arthroplasty. J Arthroplasty 1:109, 1991
86. Majkowski RS, Currie IC, Newman JH: Postoperative collection and reinfusion of autologous blood in total knee arthroplasty. Ann R Coll Surg Engl 73:381, 1991
87. Umlas J, Foster R, Dalal S et al: Postoperative red cell loss following hip or knee surgery compared to total blood loss: the case against postoperative salvage. Transfusion 34:402, 1994
88. Martin JW, Whiteside LA, Milliano MT, Reedy ME: Postoperative blood retrieval and transfusion in cementless total knee arthroplasty. J Arthroplasty 7:205, 1992
89. Cooley DA, Beall AC Jr, Grondin P: Open-heart operations with disposable oxygenators, 5 per cent dextrose prime, and normothermia. Surgery 52:713, 1962
90. Messmer K: Hemodilution. Surg Clin North Am 55:659, 1975
91. Milam JD, Austin SF, Nihill MR et al: Use of sufficient hemodilution to prevent coagulopathies following surgical correction of cyanotic heart disease. J Thorac Cardiovasc Surg 89:623, 1985
92. Hallowell P, Bland JHL, Buckley MJ, Lowenstein E: Transfusion of fresh autologous blood in open-heart surgery. J Thorac Cardiovasc Surg 64:941, 1972
93. Ness PM, Bourke DL, Walsh PC: A randomized trial of perioperative hemodilution versus transfusion of preoperatively deposited autologous blood in elective surgery. Transfusion 32:226, 1992
94. Pliam MB, McGoon DC, Tarhan S: Failure of transfusion of autologous whole blood to reduce banked-blood requirements in open-heart surgical patients. J Thorac Cardiovasc Surg 70:338, 1975
95. Sherman MM, Dobnik DB, Dennis RC, Berger RL: Autologous blood transfusion during cardiopulmonary bypass. Chest 70:592, 1976
96. Weisel RD, Charlesworth DC, Mickleborough LL et al: Limitations of blood conservation. J Thorac Cardiovasc Surg 88:26, 1984
97. Kruskall MS: On measuring the success of an autologous blood donation program, editorial. Transfusion 31:481, 1991
98. Silva R, Moore EE, Bar-Or D et al: The risk:benefit ratio of autotransfusion—comparison to banked blood in a canine model. J Trauma 24:557, 1984

Pharmacologic Alternatives to Blood Transfusion

144

Lawrence T. Goodnough

INTRODUCTION

Renewed emphasis has been placed on alternatives to blood transfusion. The changing environment of transfusion medicine includes increased awareness on the part of patients and physicians about issues of blood safety, blood conservation, and informed consent (Table 144-1) before elective blood transfusion is undertaken.[1] For example, more conservative transfusion policy of physicians toward surgical patients has been noted with regard to the "transfusion trigger"[2] in patients undergoing elective orthopaedic[3] and urologic[4] surgery who choose to predeposit autologous blood. Similarly, the use of blood and blood components has been reduced in programs using surgical blood conservation methods; an example is coronary artery bypass graft surgery, in which a combination of interventions, such as preoperative autologous blood donation, acute hemodilution, use of nonhemic pump prime solutions, intra- and postoperative autologous blood salvage and reinfusion, and, most importantly, acceptance of postoperative normovolemic anemia, was reported to reduce blood transfusions markedly.[5] In addition to these blood conservation approaches, a growing list (Table 144-2) of pharmacologic agents shows promise in further reducing, or perhaps eliminating, allogeneic blood transfusion, particularly when used in combination with other blood conservation interventions. This chapter reviews developments in this area. Other potential interventions to reduce or eliminate allogeneic blood transfusion, including the use of blood substitutes, are reviewed in Chapters 143 and 146.

THERAPY TO STIMULATE ERYTHROPOIESIS

The history of the development of recombinant human erythropoietin (rHuEPO), from its identification as the hormone responsible for regulating erythropoiesis[6] to the purification of human urinary EPO,[7] and subsequently to cloning, expression, and characterization as a recombinant product[8-10] has taken place within the relatively brief span of only 32 years (1953–1985).

EPO is a glycoprotein produced by the kidney in a feedback control system in which the kidney responds to hypoxia or hyperoxia to enhance or reduce the production of the circulating hormone.[11] The relationship between red blood cell mass and EPO level is arithmetic/logarithmic.[12] Normal plasma levels of EPO in nonanemic patients are within 12–32 μ/ml. As illustrated in Figure 144-1, EPO levels can be demonstrated to increase exponentially with progressive anemia, so that at a hematocrit level of <20%, production of EPO increases ≥100-fold.[13,14] The biology of EPO and its mechanism of action, along with results of clinical trials of rHuEPO therapy in anemic patients, have recently been reviewed.[11,15,16]

Anemia in Medical Patients

The purification of EPO[7] led to the development of an easy and accurate radioimmunoassay.[17] As would be expected, levels of EPO were subsequently found to be low in anemic patients with chronic renal disease.[11] The anemia of chronic renal disease was subsequently demonstrated to respond to rHuEPO therapy.[18-20] On the basis of these studies, its use in this setting was approved for anemic (hematocrit ≤30%) patients with elevated serum creatinine levels (>1.8 mg/dl). The response to rHuEPO therapy was shown to be accompanied by reduced blood transfusion needs[19,20] and an enhanced sense of well-being.[21,22] In patients with chronic renal failure, rHuEPO therapy has been associated with the development or exacerbation of pre-existing hypertension.[20,22,23] In addition, an increased incidence of shunt thrombosis has been reported in renal dialysis patients treated with rHuEPO.[22] The dose of rHuEPO approved in renal failure patients is 50–100 U/kg body weight given intravenously or subcutaneously three times weekly, with a dose reduction once the patient's hematocrit reaches 0.30–0.34. However, <45% of dialysis patients have been recorded to achieve hematocrits of >30% when treated with rHuEPO for ≥6 months.[24] If efficacy of rHuEPO therapy in dialysis patients is defined as elimination of the need for blood transfusion,[25] recommendations of lower doses for rHuEPO than approved initially, such as an average initial starting dose of 34 U/kg three times weekly,[26] may be reasonable.[11] Whether lower target hemoglobin levels will be associated with an improved quality of life seen with target levels of 95–130 g/L hemoglobin,[21,22] however, remains to be determined.

rHuEPO therapy has also been demonstrated to be effective in raising hematocrit levels in predialysis patients with chronic

Table 144-1. Medical Elements of Informed Consent for Elective Blood Transfusion

Risks of allogeneic blood
Benefits of blood (or risks of anemia)
Alternatives to allogeneic blood
  No transfusion (alteration of the "transfusion trigger" hematocrit, pharmacologic therapy, refusal of blood on religious grounds)
  Designated trasnfusion (blood from a donor known to the transfusion recipient)
  Autologous transfusion
Opportunity to ask questions
Documented consent

Table 144-2. Pharmacologic Alternatives to Blood Transfusion

Blood replacement
  Recombinant human erythropoietin
Blood loss
  Aprotinin
  Desamino-D-arginine vasopressin
  Tranexamic acid
  Fibrin glue
Blood substitute
  Hemoglobin solutions
  Perfluorochemicals

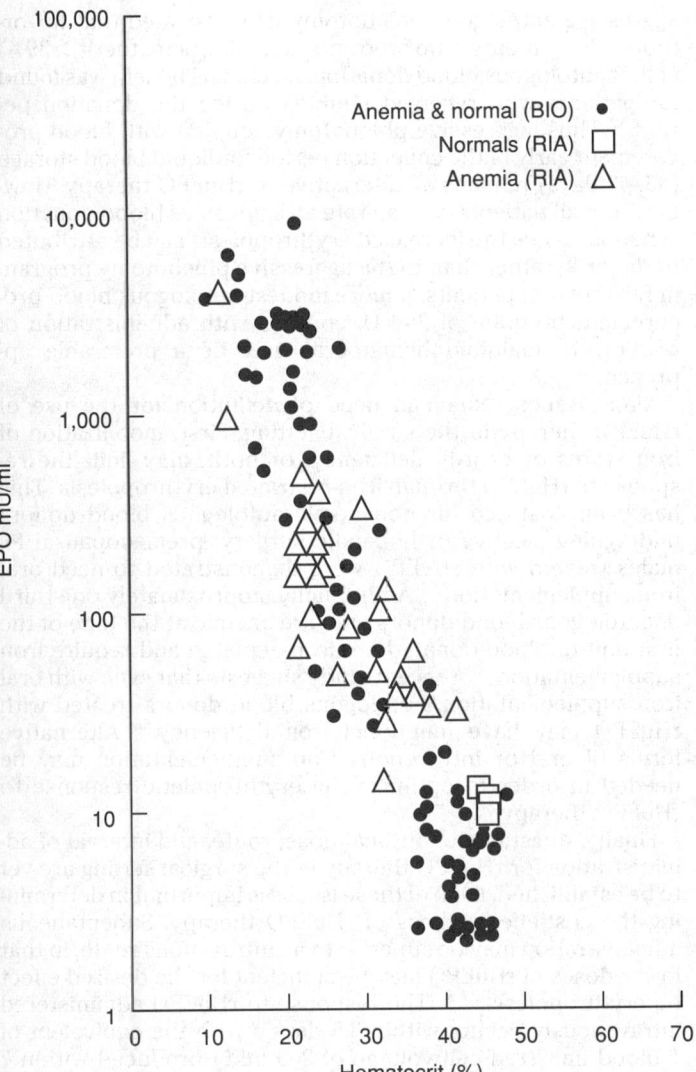

Fig. 144-1. EPO titers measured by bioassay and radioimmunoassay and reported in milliunits per milliliter of plasma from normal volunteers and from patients with anemias not complicated by renal or chronic disease. Red circles, bioassay measurement of patients with anemia and normal individuals; squares, radioimmunoassay of normal individuals; triangles, radioimmunoassay of anemic patients.) (From Erslev and Caro,[13] with permission.)

renal disease.[23,26] However, these patients are usually not transfusion dependent, and subjective improvement or increase in exercise capacity has been more difficult to demonstrate.[26] In this setting, and in patients undergoing chronic ambulatory peritoneal dialysis, rHuEPO is administered subcutaneously, since intravenous access is inconvenient. Nevertheless, the pharmacokinetics of subcutaneously administered rHuEPO would be more advantageous than the intravenous route, since slow release from subcutaneous depots results in a longer circulating half-life than the 6–8 hours of intravenous rHuEPO, providing lower but more sustained plasma levels of EPO.[27]

A second currently approved indication for rHuEPO therapy is the treatment of zidovudine (AZT)-induced anemia in patients who are serologically positive for human immunodeficiency virus (HIV). Anemia with hemoglobin levels of <7.5 g/dl were reported in 24% of acquired immunodeficiency syndrome (AIDS) patients undergoing a clinical trial of AZT therapy, compared with only 4% of placebo recipients. This observation led to randomized, placebo-controlled trials of rHuEPO therapy in

patients with AIDS treated with AZT.[28] Reductions in the number of units of red cells transfused and the number of patients transfused per month were observed in patients with endogenous EPO levels of <500 U/L at baseline, but not in those whose levels were ≥500 U/L at the beginning of the study.

Decreased EPO response to anemia has also been reported in patients with cancer, indicating that EPO deficiency contributes to the development of this anemia of chronic disease.[29] A randomized placebo-controlled trial of rHuEPO therapy at 100–150 U/kg SC three times weekly over 3 months was conducted in 413 cancer patients treated with or without cisplatinum-containing chemotherapy regimens, as well as in untreated cancer patients.[30] On the basis of the results of this clinical trial, EPO therapy has been approved for treatment of anemia related to cancer chemotherapy, particularly for patients whose serum EPO level is <200 μ/mL. Another potential setting for rHuEPO therapy in malignancy is bone marrow transplantation. The endogenous EPO response to anemia has been shown to be inadequate during the post-transplant period.[31] A subsequent study, however, showed that these patients receive only 42 (5.8%) of total allogeneic blood component exposures by red blood cell transfusion when pharmacologic doses of rHuEPO might be of benefit, indicating the need for interventions to reduce platelet donor exposure as well.[32]

Similar studies of the relationship between hemoglobin and serum immunoreactive EPO have been conducted in the anemia of rheumatoid arthritis.[33,34] A subsequent randomized placebo-controlled trial of rHuEPO therapy (50–150 U/kg IV three times weekly over 32 weeks), showed that all 11 patients receiving rHuEPO attained a normal hematocrit,[35] demonstrating that rHuEPO therapy may be clinically useful in those whose magnitude of anemia would require red cell transfusion. The anemia in chronic disorders due to other inflammatory conditions, such as cirrhosis, has been similarly demonstrated to respond to rHuEPO therapy before elective surgery.[36]

Serum EPO levels in 46 patients with myelodysplastic syndromes suggest that although an overall relationship between the degree of anemia and circulating EPO can be demonstrated in some patients, the EPO response does not match the degree of anemia.[12,37] However, in a randomized placebo-controlled trial, only 4 (24%) of 17 patients responded to rHuEPO doses of 1,200–1,600 U/kg IV given twice weekly.[38] While this study indicated that rHuEPO could be administered safely in very high doses to patients with myelodysplastic syndromes, and that a few of these patients responded with increased erythropoiesis, those most in need of a response failed to show much benefit.

A number of studies have examined the relationship between EPO and the anemia of prematurity. Taken together, these studies suggest that the erythropoietic response to anemia in infants with the anemia of prematurity is limited by inadequate EPO production, rather than by inadequate erythroid marrow potential.[39] Recent clinical trials of rHuEPO in this setting found that while a lower dose of rHuEPO (100 U/kg twice weekly) did not affect the hematocrit levels or transfusion requirements in rHuEPO-treated premature infants compared with placebo controls,[40] substantially higher doses of rHuEPO have been reported to be effective in reducing transfusion requirements.[41] While higher exogenous doses of rHuEPO to achieve logarithmic, rather than arithmetic, increases of EPO in plasma may be of benefit, the economic costs of rHuEPO are likely to restrict trials with very high doses in adult patients.[42]

EPO responses in patients with sickle cell anemia have also been found to be blunted, with marked increases in serum EPO occurring only with hemoglobin levels of <90 g/L.[43] A study in five patients with sickle cell disease treated with escalating doses of rHuEPO (1,200–3,000 U/kg/wk) failed to demonstrate an effect on the percentage of hemoglobin F-containing reticulocytes. Other subsequent studies of higher escalating doses of rHuEPO (≤9,000 U/kg/wk) supplemented with oral iron sulfate, along with less myelosuppressive doses of hydroxyurea, reported increases in the number of reticulocytes containing fetal hemoglobin and in the percentage of fetal hemoglobin as compared with hydroxyurea therapy alone.[44] The small number of patients reported to date precludes any analysis of clinical benefit with this therapeutic approach.

Anemia in Surgical Patients

Interest in rHuEPO therapy as a surgical blood conservation intervention, as in blood conservation in medical anemias, has been similarly stimulated by recent emphasis on issues of blood safety, blood inventory, and alternatives to allogeneic blood transfusion. Published guidelines have recommended that if elective surgical patients require transfusion, autologous blood is the preferred therapy.[25] Despite autologous blood donation, however, 15–20% of elective orthopaedic patients[46] and urologic patients[4] receive allogeneic blood transfusions. Studies of endogenous EPO levels in autologous blood donors suggested that treatment of autologous blood donors with rHuEPO would diminish or prevent the development of anemia in these patients and would also increase the volume of autologous blood that could be collected before surgery.[47–49] A recent clinical trial in anemic (hematocrit ≤0.40%) orthopaedic patients asked to predonate ≥4 autologous units reported that rHuEPO therapy reduced subsequent allogeneic blood needs compared with placebo controls.[50] However, this effect was seen only with supplemental intravenous iron administration. In another clinical trial, analysis of preoperative red blood cell production, taking into account both in vivo and ex vivo (stored) red blood cell volumes, indicated that patients who underwent aggressive autologous blood phlebotomy (procurement of 6 U beginning 25–35 days before surgery) had a significant (27%) expansion of red blood cell volume preoperatively, along with accelerated erythropoiesis at surgery.[51] As illustrated in Figure 144-2, the red cell volume expansion (47%) in the patients treated with rHuEPO was significantly greater, generating the equivalent of nearly 5 blood units preoperatively compared to 3 blood units for the control group. The major difference in red blood cell expansion between the placebo and EPO groups occurred early in the collection period; by the time of surgery, the endogenous EPO effect in the placebo patients diminished the differences between groups. These results were achieved with an aggressive phlebotomy program involving the attempted removal of 2 U/wk of blood. A recent clinical trial using aggressive autologous phlebotomy demonstrated that for orthopaedic patients who were not anemic (hematocrit >39%) at first autologous blood donation, no clinical benefit was found for patients who received rHuEPO during the donation period.[52] Thus, aggressive phlebotomy coupled with blood procurement early in the collection period for liquid blood storage (35–42 days) remains an alternative to rHuEPO therapy. However, not all patients can tolerate an aggressive blood donation schedule. Since the increased erythropoiesis can be attributed to the drug rather than to the aggressive phlebotomy program in EPO-treated patients, a more modest autologous blood procurement program of 3–4 U, coupled with administration of rHuEPO to maintain hematocrit, may be a preferable approach.[53]

Many issues remain in need of definition for the use of rHuEPO therapy in the surgical setting. First, mobilization of iron stores or of iron deficiency, or both, may limit the response to rHuEPO through iron-restricted erythropoiesis. This has been analyzed for nonanemic autologous blood donors undergoing elective orthopaedic surgery; premenopausal females treated with rHuEPO were demonstrated to need oral iron supplementation.[54] Additionally, approximately one-third of autologous blood donors who are anemic at the time of the first unit of blood donated are iron-depleted and require iron supplementation.[55] A recent study suggests that even with oral iron supplementation, autologous blood donors treated with rHuEPO may have functional iron deficiency.[56] Alternative forms of oral or intravenous iron supplementation may be needed in order to optimize the erythropoietic response to rHuEPO therapy.[50]

Finally, questions of optimal dose, route, and interval of administration for rHuEPO therapy in the surgical setting are yet to be established. Each of these issues is important in determining the cost-effectiveness of rHuEPO therapy. Subcutaneous administration may be superior to an intravenous route, in that lower doses of rHuEPO may be sufficient for the desired effect on erythropoiesis.[27,57] The response to rHuEPO administered intravenously occurs within 3.5 days[49] with the equivalent of 1 blood unit (red cell volume of 200 ml[58]) produced within 7 days.[51] The rHuEPO dosage (600 U/kg given twice over 1 week) for a 70-kg patient to achieve this effect would total 84,000 U; at current costs of $0.01/U,[42] rHuEPO therapy to produce the equivalent of 1 blood unit can be estimated to cost $840, compared to a mean cost of $119 (range 60–233) for procurement of 1 autologous blood unit.[59] Alternative routes of iron administration may significantly improve the cost/benefit ratio of

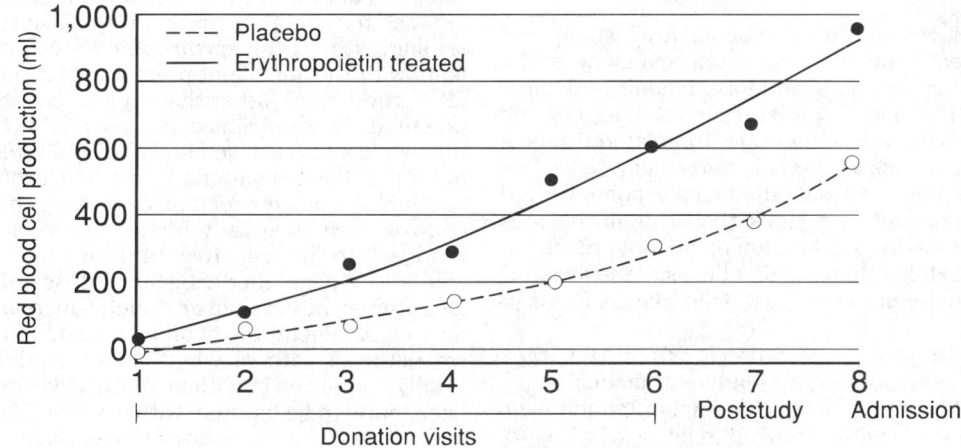

Fig. 144-2. Red blood cell (RBC) production during autologous blood donation, in 23 placebo (open circles) and 21 EPO (closed circles) -treated patients. Data points represent calculated RBC production from donation visits 1–6, poststudy visit, and hospital admission. (From Goodnough et al.,[51] with permission.)

rHuEPO therapy. Recent estimates of the high cost-effectiveness of preoperative autologous blood donation[60,61] emphasize that blood conservation interventions, including pharmacologic agents, must be held accountable for their costs as well as their benefits.

Side Effects

The prevalence of serious adverse concomitant events in patients treated with rHuEPO should be monitored carefully and compared to untreated control groups. The prevalence of hypertension reported in an initial trial in dialysis patients[19] and in subsequent placebo-controlled trials in patients with chronic renal insufficiency[21,23] suggests that the interrelationship of hematocrit level, blood viscosity, and peripheral vascular resistance is important in this setting.[62] A recent study suggested that renal dialysis patients with a family of hypertension have an increased likelihood of developing hypertension with rHuEPO therapy.[63] Two studies of orthopaedic surgical patients without renal insufficiency who underwent aggressive autologous blood phlebotomy, with or without rHuEPO therapy, reported thromboembolic events in 2 (1 placebo, 1 rHuEPO treated) of 47 patients[49] and 2 (1 placebo, 1 rHuEPO treated) of 116 patients;[52] the overall prevalence of 4 (2.4%) of 163 patients compares favorably to the prevalence of such events reported in patients undergoing orthopaedic joint replacement surgery.[64] Clinical trials in progress will provide additional information on the prevalence of possible adverse events in patients undergoing rHuEPO therapy.

Current Guidelines

The use of rHuEPO in patients with medical anemia should be limited to those who do not have correctable anemias (e.g., iron, folate, or vitamin B_{12} deficiency) and who are candidates for blood transfusion because of symptoms or signs that are related to the degree of anemia. Additionally, data from clinical trials should provide clear evidence that correction of anemia is accompanied either by avoidance of blood transfusion or by improved quality of life. Current guidelines for use of rHuEPO on the basis of published results are summarized in Table 144-3.[16]

The use of rHuEPO in patients with surgical anemia should similarly be restricted to clinical settings in which avoidance of blood transfusion has been demonstrated. Therapy should

Table 144-3. Guidelines for Recombinant Human Erythropoietin Therapy

I. Currently approved indications
   A. Anemia[a] in chronic renal failure (creatinine ≥1.8 mg%)
   B. Anemia with HIV infection undergoing treatment with AZT (EPO level <500 U/L)
   C. Anemia in cancer patients undergoing therapy (EPO level <200 U/L)

II. Indications under investigation
   A. Anemia of chronic disease (e.g., rheumatoid arthritis)
   B. Autologous blood donation
   C. Surgical blood loss
   D. Bone marrow transplantation
   E. Anemia of prematurity
   F. Myelodysplastic syndromes
   G. Sickle cell anemia

III. Current contraindications
   A. Patients in whom therapy will result in polycythemia
   B. Patients with uncontrolled hypertension

[a] Anemia is defined as a reduced patient red cell volume, for which a blood transfusion is anticipated or needed.
(Adapted from Goodnough et al.,[16] with permission.)

be linked to ongoing blood losses to avoid potential complications related to polycythemia and hyperviscosity. Ideally, the use of this agent to correct preoperative anemia should be coupled with autologous blood procurement not only for these safety concerns, but to enhance the effectiveness of this therapy in reducing perisurgical allogeneic blood transfusions. Until clinical trials that use allogeneic blood exposure as outcome are completed, the role of rHuEPO therapy in surgical anemia remains investigational.

The identification of an increasingly complex network of stimulatory and inhibitory molecules that regulate normal hematopoiesis, such as stem cell growth factor, holds great promise for the development of other growth factors that stimulate in vivo and ex vivo hematopoiesis.[65] These can be anticipated to have significant effects in transfusion medicine, particularly in areas of solid tumor chemotherapy, bone marrow transplantation, and treatment of the leukemias. Clinical trials in this rapidly moving field are planned or in progress. No clinical effect of rHuEPO therapy on platelet production in human trials has been seen.[28,29,49,52] Other hematopoietic growth factors, such as colony-stimulating factor-granulocyte/macrophage, colony-stimulating factor-megakaryocyte, and interleukin-3, are known to stimulate platelet precursor expansion.[66] Most recently, several groups have successfully identified, purified, and cloned the platelet-regulatory factor thrombopoietin.[67] Eventually, hematopoietic growth factors may be used in combination in clinical circumstances such as allogeneic and autologous bone marrow transplantation in order to achieve significant reductions in requirements for red blood cell and platelet transfusion support, as well as reduction of morbidity and mortality due to complications of infections.

THERAPY TO REDUCE BLOOD LOSSES

Desamino-D-arginine vasopressin (DDAVP) is a synthetic analogue of antidiuretic hormone (vasopressin) that has no clinically significant vasomotor effects. This drug has been shown to increase plasma levels of factor VIII and the high-molecular-weight forms of von Willebrand factor.[68] Thus, DDAVP can be used to treat patients with mild hemophilia, patients with von Willebrand disease, and some patients with circulating anticoagulants for factor VIII.[69,70] When DDAVP is given as a dose of 0.3 µg/kg body weight IV, factor VIII activity increases three-to fivefold. In patients with von Willebrand disease, the bleeding time is shortened or even normalized. Because of the antidiuretic effect, excessive free water administration should be avoided. DDAVP has also been shown to reduce operative blood loss and blood transfusion requirements in patients without clotting factor deficiencies who undergo complex cardiac surgery with ex vivo corporeal circulation,[71] but not first-time coronary artery bypass graft surgery.[72] In addition, DDAVP has been described to reduce operative blood loss in patients with normal platelet function who undergo Harrington rod spinal fusion surgery.[73] Finally, DDAVP has been shown to improve or correct the prolonged bleeding times in patients with acquired platelet defects, such as in uremia,[74] cirrhosis,[75] and aspirin ingestion.[76] The potential role of DDAVP in these clinical settings is discussed further in Chapters 106, 113, and 129.

Other agents that affect platelet function have been studied and show considerable promise. Significant reductions in perioperative blood loss have been associated with the administration of aprotinin (an inhibitor of human trypsin), plasmin, and kallikrein. In low concentrations, aprotinin inhibits plasmin and therefore fibrinolysis.[77] At intermediate concentrations, aprotinin inhibits platelet aggregation and activation, possibly through an effect on platelet von Willebrand factor, thrombin, and fibrinogen receptors.[78,79] Aprotinin has been shown to reduce postoperative bleeding after open heart surgery in adults and to decrease the need for transfusion.[77,80] The use of this agent in pediatric surgical patients in association with other blood conservation interventions also shows promise.[81] A related antifibrinolytic agent, tranexamic acid, was shown in a recent report to decrease blood loss and transfusion requirements in cardiac surgical patients when compared with placebo and desmopressin-treated patients.[82] Prostenol (prostacyclin, prostaglandin I_2) was reported to have a platelet-sparing effect during cardiopulmonary bypass,[83] presumably by inhibition of platelet aggregation[84]; however, another study failed to confirm any platelet-sparing effect of prostacyclin during cardiopulmonary bypass.[85] The antiplatelet agent dipyridamole has also been reported to reduce platelet activation and depletion during bypass surgery. In a prospective randomized trial of oral and intravenous dipyridamole compared with placebo, significant reductions in postoperative blood loss and transfusion requirements were reported.[86]

Fibrin glue is a blood derivative rather than a pharmacologic agent, but its rapidly increasing use as an intervention in surgical hemostasis and blood conservation deserves mention. This preparation is derived from a source of fibrinogen and factor XIII (fibrin-stabilizing factor), in which a solution of fibrinogen is mixed with a solution of bovine thrombin and applied to a surgical field.[87] It is important to note that preparations derived from cryoprecipitate or single donor plasma[87,88] representing additional allogeneic blood donor exposure. Alternatively, the source of fibrinogen and factor XIII can be derived from ≥40 ml of the patient's autologous blood[89] or prepared from an autologous plasma unit. Potential clinical applications of this intervention include patients undergoing thoracic surgery[90] as well as otologic surgery.[91] A review of the potential use of this product has recently been published.[92]

The use of allogeneic cryoprecipitate as a fibrinogen source for fibrin glue carries a risk. Patients should be made aware of the potential complications as well as the potential benefits of its use. To date there has been one case report of anaphylactic reaction after a total of only 8 ml of fibrin glue administration and one case of HIV transmission.[93,94] The use of autologous donation as a source of fibrinogen would be the safest and therefore preferable approach. A solvent detergent-treated fibrin glue preparation is currently under evaluation and appears promising; however, this is still under investigation.[95] A recent report of nine cardiac surgery patients who presented with acquired bovine thrombin-induced factor V deficiency, each of whom had been previously exposed to bovine thrombin,[96] is a cause of concern over the potential toxicities associated with the use of both allogeneic and autologous fibrin glue. Issues of informed consent for administration of this blood product and criteria for use need to be addressed by transfusion medicine services.

REFERENCES

1. Goodnough LT, Shuck J: Blood transfusion in elective surgery: review of risks, options and informed consent. Am J Surg 159:602, 1990
2. Friedman BA, Burns TL, Schork MA: An analysis of blood transfusion of surgical patients by sex: a quest for the transfusion trigger. Transfusion 20:179, 1980
3. Wasman J, Goodnough LT: Autologous blood donatioin for elective surgery: effect on physician transfusion behavior. JAMA 258:3135, 1987
4. Goodnough LT, Riddell J, Kursh E, Resnick MI: Utilization and efficacy of autologous blood predeposit in radical prostatectomy with lymphadenectomy: implications for blood conservation and physician education programs. Urology 40:201, 1992
5. Cosgrove DM, Coop FP, Lytle BW et al: Determinants of blood utilization during myocardial revascularization. Ann Thorac Surg 40:380, 1985
6. Erslev A: Humoral regulation of red cell production. Blood 8:349, 1953
7. Miyake T, Kung CK, Goodwasser E: Purification of human erythropoietin. J Biol Chem 252:5558, 1977
8. Lee-Huang S: Cloning and expression of human erythropoietin cDNA in *Escherichia coli.* Proc Natl Acad Sci USA 81:2708, 1984
9. Egrie JC, Strickland TW, Lane J et al: Characterization and biologic effects of recombinant human erythropoietin. Immunobiology 172:213, 1986
10. Lin FK, Suggs S, Liln CH et al: Cloning and expression of the human erythropoietin gene. Proc Natl Acad Sci USA 82:7580, 1985
11. Erslev AJ: Erythropoietin. N Engl J Med 324:1339, 1991
12. Gaines Das RE, Milne A Rowley M et al: Serum immunoreactive erythropoietin in patients with idiopathic aplastic and Fanconi's anemia. Br J Haematol 82:601, 1992
13. Erslev AJ, Caro J: Physiology and molecular biology of erythropoietin. Med Oncol Tumor Pharmacother 2:154, 1986
14. Adamson JW: The erythropoietin/hematocrit relationship in normal and polycythemic: implications of marrow regulation. Blood 32:597, 1968
15. Krantz SB. Erythropoietin. Blood 77:419, 1991
16. Goodnough LT, Anderson KC, Kurtz S et al: Indications and guidelines for the use of hematopoietic growth factors. Transfusion 33:944, 1993
17. Sherwood JB, Goldwasser E: A radioimmunoassay for erythropoietin. Blood 54:885, 1979
18. Winnearls CG, Oliver DO, Pippard MJ et al: Effects of human erythropoietin derived from recombinant DNA on the anemia of patients maintained by chronic haemodialysis. Lancet 2:1175, 1986
19. Eschbach JW, Egrie JC, Downing MR et al: Correction of the anemia of end-stage renal disease with recombinant human erythropoietin. N Engl J Med 316:3, 1987
20. Eschbach JB, Abdulhadi MH, Browne JK et al: Recombinant human erythropoietin in anemic patients with end stage renal disease. Ann Intern Med 111:992, 1989
21. Evans RW, Rader B, Manninen DL, Cooperative Multicenter EPO Clinical Trial Group: The quality of life of haemodialysis recipients treated with recombinant human erythropoietin. JAMA 263:825, 1990
22. Canadian Erythropoietin Study Group: Association between recombinant human erythropoietin and quality of life and exercise capacity of patients receiving haemodialysis. Br Med J 300:573, 1990
23. Eschbach JB, Kelley MR, Haley NR et al: Treatment of the anemia of progressive renal failure with recombinant human erythropoietin. N Engl J Med 32:158, 1989
24. Sisk JE, Gianfrancesco FD, Coster JM: Recombinant erythropoietin and medicare payment. JAMA 266:247, 1991
25. American College of Physicians: Practice strategies for elective red blood cell transfusion. Ann Intern Med 116:403, 1992
26. Lim VS, DeGowin RL, Zavala D et al: Recombinant human erythropoietin treatment in pre-dialysis patients. Ann Intern Med 110:108, 1989
27. McMahon FG, Vargas R, Ryan M et al: Pharmacokinetics and effects of recombinant human erythropoietin after intravenous and subcutaneous injections in healthy volunteers. Blood 76:1718, 1990
28. Henry DH, Beall GN, Benson CA et al: Recombinant human erythropoietin in the treatment of anemia associated with human immunodeficiency virus (HIV) infection and zidovudine therapy. Ann Intern Med 117:739, 1992
29. Miller CB, Jones RJ, Piantadosi S et al: Decreased erythropoietin response in patients with the anemia of cancer. N Engl J Med 322:1689, 1990
30. Abels RI, Larholt KM, Krantz KD, Bryant EC: Recombinant human erythropoietin for the treatment of the anemia of cancer. p. 121. In Murphy MJ Jr (ed): Blood Cell Growth Factors: Their Present and Future Use in Hematology and Oncology. Alpha Medical Press, Dayton, OH, 1991
31. Miller CB, Jones RJ, Burns WH et al: Impaired erythropoietin response after bone marrow transplantation. Exp Hematol 18:700A, 1990
32. Lazarus HM, Goodnough LT, Goldwasser E et al: Serum erythropoietin levels and blood component therapy after autologous bone marrow transplantation: implications for erythropoietin therapy in this setting. Bone Marrow Transplant 63:90, 1992
33. Baer AN, Dessypris EN, Goldwasser E, Krantz SB: Blunted erythropoietin response to anemia in rheumatoid arthritis. Br J Haematol 66:559, 1987
34. Hochberg MC, Arnold CM, Hogans BB, Spivak JL: Serum immunoreactive erythropoietin in rheumatoid arthritis: impaired response to anemia. Arthritis Rheum 31:1318, 1988
35. Pincus T, Olsen NJ, Russell J et al: Multicenter study of recombinant human erythropoietin in correction of anemia in rheumatoid arthritis. Am J Med 89:161, 1990
36. Thompson FL, Powers JS, Graber SE, Krantz SB: Use of recombinant human erythropoietin to enhance autologous blood donation in a patient with multiple red cell allo-antibodies and the anemia of chronic disease. Am J Med 90:398, 1991
37. Jacobs A, Janowska-Wieczorek A, Caro J et al: Circulating erythropoietin in patients with myelodysplastic syndromes. Br J Haematol 73:36, 1989
38. Stein RS, Abels RI, Krantz SB: Pharmacologic doses of recombinant human erythropoietin in the treatment of myelodysplastic syndromes. Blood 78:1658, 1991

39. Mentzer WC, Shannon KM, Phibbs RH: Recombinant human erythropoietin in patients with the anemia of prematurity. p. 374. In Erslev AJ (ed): Erythropoietin. Johns Hopkins University Press, Baltimore, 1991

40. Shannon KS, Mentzer WC, Abels RI et al: Enhancement of erythropoiesis by recombinant human erythropoietin in low birth weight infants: a pilot study. J Pediatr 120:586, 1992

41. Carnielli V, Montini G, Da Riol R et al: Effect of high doses of human recombinant erythropoietin on the need for blood transfusions in preterm infants. J Pediatr 121:98, 1992

42. Doolittle RF: Biotechnology—the enormous cost of success. N Engl J Med 324:1360, 1991

43. Sherwood JB, Goldwasser E, Chilcote R et al: Sickle cell anemia patients have low erythropoietin level for their degree of anemia. Blood 67:46, 1986

44. Rodgers GP, Dover GJ, Uyesaka N et al: Augmentation by erythropoietin of the fetal-hemoglobin response to hydroxyurea in sickle cell disease. N Engl J Med 328:73, 1993

45. Goodnough LT, Shaffron D, Marcus RE: Impact of preoperative autologous blood donation in elective orthopaedic surgery. Vox Sang 59:65, 1990

46. Goodnough LT, Verbrugge D, Vizmeg K, Riddell J: Identification of elective orthopaedic surgical patients transfused with blood volume in excess of blood needs: the "transfusion trigger" revisited. Transfusion 32:648, 1992

47. Kickler TS, Spivak JL: Effect of repeated whole blood donations on serum immunoreactive erythropoietin levels in autologous donors. JAMA 260:65, 1988

48. Goodnough LT, Brittenham G: Limitations of the erythropoietic response to serial phlebotomy: implications for autologous blood donor programs. J Lab Clin Med 115:28, 1990

49. Goodnough LT, Rudnick S, Price TH et al: Increased collection of autologous blood preoperatively with recombinant human erythropoietin therapy. N Engl J Med 321:1163, 1989

50. Mercuriali F, Zanella A, Barosi G et al: Use of erythropoietin to increase the volume of autologous blood donated by orthopaedic patients. Transfusion 33:55, 1993

51. Goodnough LT, Price TH, Rudnick S: Preoperative red blood cell production in patients undergoing aggressive autologous blood phlebotomy with and without erythropoietin therapy. Transfusion 32:441, 1992

52. Goodnough LT, Price TH, EPO Study Group: A phase III trial of recombinant human erythropoietin therapy in non-anemic orthopaedic patients subjected to aggressive autologous blood phlebotomy: dose, response, toxicity, and efficacy. Clin Res 41:199a, 1993

53. Watanabe Y, Fuse K, Konishi T et al: Autologous blood transfusion with recombinant human erythropoietin in heart operations. Ann Thorac Surg 51:767, 1991

54. Goodnough LT, Price TH, Rudnick S: Iron-restricted erythropoiesis as a limitation to autologous blood donation in the erythropoietin-stimulated bone marrow. J Lab Clin Med 188:289, 1991

55. Goodnough LT, Vizmeg K, Riddell J, Soegiarso W: Prevalence of anemia in autologous blood donors prior to elective orthopaedic surgery: implications for blood conservation programs. Vox Sang 63:96, 1992

56. Brugnara C, Chambers LA, Malynn E et al: Red blood cell regeneration induced by subcutaneous recombinant erythropoietin: iron-deficient erythropoiesis in iron-replete subjects. Blood 81:956, 1993

57. Hughes RT, Cotes PM, Oliver DO et al: Correction of the anemia of chronic renal failure with erythropoietin: pharmacokinetic studies in patients on haemodialysis and CAPD. Contrib Nephrol 76:122, 1989

58. Goodnough LT, Bravo J, Hsueh Y et al: Red blood cell volume in autologous and homologous blood units: implications for risk/benefit assessment for autologous blood "crossover" and directed blood transfusion. Transfusion 29:821, 1989

59. Goodnough LT, Soegiarso RW, Birkmeyer JD, Welch HG: The economic impact of inappropriate blood transfusions in coronary artery bypass graft surgery. Am J Med 94:1, 1993

60. Birkmeyer JD, Aubuchon JP, Littenberg B et al: Cost-effectiveness of preoperative autologous blood donation in coronary artery bypass grafting. Ann Thorac Surg 57:161, 1994

61. Birkmeyer JD, Goodnough LT, Aubuchon JP et al: The cost-effectiveness of preoperative autologous blood donation in total hip and knee replacement. Transfusion 33:544, 1993

62. Raine AEG: Hypertension, blood viscosity and cardiovascular morbidity in renal failure: implications for erythropoietin therapy. Lancet 1:97, 1988

63. Ishimitsu T, Tsukada H, Ogawa Y et al: Genetic predisposition to hypertension facilitates blood pressure elevation in hemodialysis patients treated with erythropoietin. Am J Med 94:401, 1993

64. Harris WH, Sledge CB: Total hip and total knee replacement. N Engl J Med 323:725, 1990

65. Shiohara M, Koike K, Nahahata T: Synergism of interferon-δ and stem cell factor on the development of murine hematopoietic progenitors in serum-free culture. Blood 81:1435, 1993

66. Hoffman R: Thrombopoiesis. In Hematopoietic Growth Factors, Twentieth Annual Scientific Sessions of the American Red Cross, Bethesda, MD, May 10–11, 1989

67. Metcalf D: Thrombopoietin—at last. Nature 369:519, 1994

68. Sakariassen KS, Cattaneo M, Van Denberg A et al: DDAVP enhances platelet adherence and platelet aggregate growth on human artery subendothelium. Blood 64:229, 1984

69. Mannucci PM, Canciani MT, Rota L et al: Response of factor VIII von Willebrand factor to DDAVP in healthy subjects and patients with hemophilia A and von Willebrand's disease. Br J Haematol 47:283, 1981

70. Naorose-Abidi SM, Bond LR, Chitolie A, Bevan DH: Desmopressin therapy in patients with acquired factor VIII inhibitors. Lancet 1:366, 1988

71. Salzman EW, Weinstein MJ, Weintraub RM et al: Treatment with desmopressin acetate to reduce blood loss after cardiac surgery: a double-blind randomized trial. N Engl J Med 314:1402, 1986

72. Hackman T, Gasconne RD, Naiman SC et al: A trial of desmopressin to reduce blood loss in uncomplicated cardiac surgery. N Engl J Med 321:1437, 1989

73. Kobrinsky NL, Letts M, Gatel LR et al: DDAVP (desmopressin) decreases operative blood loss in patients having Harrington rod spinal fusion surgery. Ann Intern Med 107:446, 1987

74. Mannuccio PM, Remuzzi G, Pusineri F et al: Deamino-8-D-arginine vasopressin shortens the bleeding time in uremia. N Engl J Med 308:8, 1983

75. Burrhoughs AK, Matthews K, Qadiri M et al: Desmopressin and bleeding time in patients with cirrhosis. Br Med J 291:1377, 1985

76. Kobrinsky NL, Gerrard JM, Watson CM et al: Shortening of bleeding time by deamino-D-arginine vasopressin in various bleeding disorders. Lancet 1:1145, 1984

77. Royston D, Taylor KM, Bidstrup BD, Sapsford RN: Effect of aprotinin on need for blood transfusion after repeat open-heart surgery. Lancet 2:1289, 1987

78. Fritz H, Wunderer G: Biochemistry and applications of aprotinin, the kallikrein inhibitor from bovine organs. Arzneimi ellforschung 33:479, 1983

79. Ruggiero M, Lapetina EG: Protease and cyclooxygenase inhibitors synergistically prevent activation of human platelets. Proc Natl Acad Sci USA 83:3456, 1986

80. Alajmo F, Calamai G, Perna AM et al: High-dose aprotinin: hemostatic effects in open heart operations. Ann Thorac Surg 48:536, 1989

81. Kawaguchi A, Bergeland J, Subramanian S: Total bloodless open heart surgery in the pediatric age group. Circulation, suppl. 70:30, 1984

82. Horrow JC, Van Riper OF, Strong MD et al: The hemostatic effects of tranexamic acid and desmopressin during cardiac surgery. Circulation 84:1, 1991

83. Fish KJ, Sarnquist FH, Van Steennis C et al: A prospective randomized study of the effects of prostacyclin on platelets and blood loss during coronary bypass operations. J Thorac Cardiovasc Surg 91:436, 1986

84. Szczeklik A, Gryglewski RJ, Nizankowski R, Musial J: Pulmonary and antiplatelet effects on intravenous and inhaled prostacyclin in man. Prostaglandins 16:654, 1978

85. Disesa VJ, Huval W, Lelcuck S et al: Disadvantages of prostacyclin infusion during cardiopulmonary bypass. A double-blind study of 50 patients having coronary revascularization. Ann Thorac Surg 38:514, 1984

86. Teoh KH, Christakis GT, Weisel RD et al: Dipyridamole preserved platelets and reduced blood loss after cardiopulmonary bypass. J Thorac Cardiovasc Surg 96:332, 1988

87. Baker JW, Spotnitz WD, Nolan SP: A technique for spray application of fibrin glue during cardiac operations. Ann Thorac Surg 43:564, 1987

88. Dresdale A, Bowman FO, Malm JR et al: Hemastatic effectiveness of fibrin glue derived from single-donor fresh frozen plasma. Ann Thorac Surg 40:385, 1985

89. Silberstein LE, Williams LJ, Hughlett MA et al: An autologous fibrinogen-based adhesive for use in otologic surgery. Transfusion 28:319, 1988

90. Jessen C, Sharma P: Use of fibrin glue in thoracic surgery. Ann Thorac Surg 39:521, 1985

91. Moretz WH Jr, Shea JJ Jr, Emmett JR, Shea JJ III: A simple autologous fibrinogen glue for otologic surgery. Otolaryngol Head Neck Surg 95:122, 1986

92. Gibble JW, Ness P: Fibrin glue: the perfect operative sealant? Transfusion 30:741, 1990

93. Milde LN: An anaphylactic reaction to fibrin glue. Anesth Analg 69:684, 1989

94. Wilson SM, Pell P, Donegan EA: HIV-1 transmission following the use of cryoprecipitated fibrinogen as gel/adhesive, abstracted. Transfusion 31:51S, 1991

95. Burnouf-Radosevich M, Burnouf T, Huart JJ: Biochemical and physical properties of a solvent-detergent-treated fibrin glue. Vox Sang 58:77, 1990

96. Cmolik BL, Spero JA, Magovern GJ, Clark RE: Redo cardiac surgery: late bleeding complications from topical thrombin-induced Factor V deficiency. J Thorac Cardiovasc Surg 105:222, 1993

Transfusion Medicine in Hematopoietic Stem Cell and Solid Organ Transplantation

145

Kenneth C. Anderson and Walter H. Dzik

BONE MARROW TRANSPLANTATION

Introduction

Bone marrow transplantation (BMT) is currently being used to treat a broad spectrum of malignant and nonmalignant diseases. Refinements in testing for HLA compatibility, coupled with new approaches both to prevent and to treat graft-versus-host disease (GVHD), have resulted in widespread use of allogeneic BMT.[1] Only 40% of patients have HLA-matched related donors; however, allogeneic BMT, using either related donors other than HLA-identical siblings or unrelated HLA-matched donors has demonstrated promising preliminary results.[2] Moreover, autologous BMT is being used increasingly, with or without purging of marrow tumor cells, in the treatment of both hematologic cancers and solid tumors.[3] This chapter focuses specifically on the following aspects: donor typing and recruitment; ABO compatibility in allogeneic BMT; avoidance of transfusion-related alloimmunization, GVHD, and infection in patients undergoing BMT; bone marrow processing and cryopreservation; documentation of engraftment; immune cytopenia post-BMT; and the use of peripheral blood stem cells (PBSCs) and recombinant growth factors to hasten engraftment and lessen toxicity of high-dose ablative treatments. Transfusion medicine expertise is central and essential in all these aspects of hematopoietic stem cell transplantation, both in current practice and in furthering research efforts.[4]

Donor Typing and Recruitment

In some cases, the blood component laboratory may play a role in the typing of potential donors for allogeneic BMT. Donors are matched for HLA class I and II antigens. Classically, HLA compatibility testing is done serologically (class I) and using mixed-lymphocyte culture (class II); however, molecular technology is currently available for typing both class I and II HLA antigens and will likely come into routine use in the future.[5] The incidence of GVHD and graft rejection is equivalent when relatives who are either completely matched or mismatched by 1 antigen are used as marrow donors, but the incidence of either GVHD or rejection rises markedly with increasing degrees of HLA disparity between donor and recipient. Once a related donor is identified, prior transfusion of the blood components to the potential transplant recipient should be avoided, to prevent sensitization to HLA antigens and related problems with marrow engraftment. After allogeneic BMT, the marrow donor can then be recruited specifically to provide HLA-matched platelets to the marrow recipient.

Only 30–40% of patients requiring allogeneic BMT have histocompatible related donors. In this setting, unrelated but histocompatible donors have been employed, markedly expanding the number of patients eligible for allogeneic BMT. Preliminary findings (i.e., in patients with chronic myeloid leukemia in first remission[2]) suggest that such patients receiving allografts from HLA-matched unrelated donors have results similar to those receiving marrow from HLA-matched related donors. To facilitate the search for unrelated HLA-matched marrow donors, registries have been established.[6–8] The National Marrow Donor Program,[9,10] for example, was established in 1986 and has a computerized registry of >750,000 potential unrelated marrow donors HLA typed for A and B antigens, some of whom are already DR typed as well. Many blood banks, given their established expertise in recruitment of both blood and apheresis platelet donors, now also play an integral role in the recruitment and evaluation of donors for the National Marrow Donor Program.

Blood Component Support

The blood component laboratory plays a critical role in BMT by providing appropriate red blood cell (RBC), platelet, and blood component support both before and after BMT. The criteria for transfusion of blood components to patients undergoing BMT are not different from those used more generally, but the magnitude of support required is great. Moreover, transfusion strategy to avoid alloimmunization, cytomegalovirus (CMV) infection, and transfusion-associated (TA) GVHD may be necessary. Finally, as in other settings, the blood bank should not only determine which products are required but should also review ongoing transfusion practice.

Several donor and patient factors can influence hematologic engraftment, immune reconstitution, and the blood product support required after BMT.[11] In all marrow recipients, engraftment may be compromised by disease or by treatment-related effects on the marrow microenvironment, or by both factors. Reconstitution after allogeneic BMT may be relatively enhanced, since the donor marrow is healthy; however, engraftment may be adversely affected by regimens employed in the recipient either to prevent or to treat GVHD. Moreover, in some patients, in vitro T-cell depletion of donor marrow, which can effectively abrogate GVHD, has resulted in failure to engraft and in graft rejection. Autologous marrow may be intrinsically compromised due to the patient's underlying disease and cytotoxic therapy received before marrow harvesting, due to in vitro techniques used for removal of tumor cells or to cryopreservation. In syngeneic BMT, donor marrow is histocompatible and healthy and is neither manipulated nor cryopreserved. However, the underlying disease and previous treatment of the recipient may, as is true in other types of BMT, compromise the marrow microenvironment, thereby adversely affecting engraftment.

BMT is followed by a period of pancytopenia lasting ≥2–4 weeks in patients requiring multiple RBC and platelet transfusions.[4,12–14] For example, patients with aplastic anemia undergoing allogeneic BMT received a median of 9 (1–82) and 44 (6–468) U of RBCs and platelets, respectively, primarily during the first 4 weeks postgraft.[13] Clinical parameters may correlate with transfusion needs. In BMT patients with acute myeloid leukemia in first remission, for example, such factors as method of prophylaxis against GVHD, the development of acute GVHD, method of prophylaxis against infection, and donor/recipient ABO compatibility influenced the magnitude of transfusion support required.[15] In particular, patients with grade 3–4 acute GVHD required more blood product support than did those with grade 1–2 acute GVHD: a median of 217 U of platelets and 27.5 U of RBCs in the former group, compared to 91 U of platelets and 14 U of RBCs in the latter patients.

Although complications related to GVHD and infection are fewer in autologous than in allogeneic BMT recipients, the magnitude of transfusion support is nonetheless significant in recipients of autografts as well. In a study of patients with non-T-cell acute lymphocytic leukemia who underwent either monoclonal antibody (mAb)-purged autologous BMT or allogeneic BMT, autologous marrow recipients engrafted more quickly, had shorter hospital stays, and had fewer early deaths, suggesting that they may have less transfusion requirements than do allogeneic BMT recipients.[16] However, the time to hematologic engraftment and transfusion needs for patients undergoing either autologous or allogeneic BMT or autologous PBSC transplantation for hematologic cancers and solid tumors at our institute are similar, regardless of the source of stem cells or underlying disease.[4] The blood component laboratory must therefore be an integral part of the planning for and daily management of the BMT service, in order to meet these demands in a timely fashion.

Importance of ABO Compatibility in Allogeneic BMT

ABO incompatibility between marrow donor and recipient may be either major, with isohemagglutinin in the recipient directed against donor RBC antigens; or minor, with isohemagglutinin in the donor directed against recipient RBC antigens. Major ABO incompatibility has an attendant potential risk of severe hemolytic reactions, graft rejection, or delayed engraftment in the setting of high-titer hemolytic isohemagglutinin in the marrow recipient.[4,14] Attempts to overcome major ABO incompatibility have included depletion of RBCs from the bone marrow graft prior to BMT[17,18] and/or the removal of isohemagglutinin from the recipient by large-volume plasma exchanges or immunoadsorption.[19] In addition, some investigators have supplemented these techniques with pre-BMT transfusions of donor type blood or purified A or B substance to adsorb recipient isohemagglutinins completely.[20,21] Although studies suggest that major ABO-incompatible HLA-matched transplants have resulted in no increase in patient mortality, incidence of rejection, delayed engraftment, or GVHD compared with ABO-compatible controls,[22–24] some reports suggest that RBC engraftment can be delayed in this setting.[4,14,18] Current practice in major ABO-incompatible HLA-matched BMT is to deplete RBCs from all marrow before BMT, but to use methods for depletion of recipient isohemagglutinin only when it is present in high titer and may result in delayed erythropoiesis and hemolysis after BMT.

Potential adverse outcomes of minor ABO incompatibility between marrow donor and recipient include rapid immune hemolysis at infusion of donor marrow due to passive transfer of isohemagglutinin in the marrow plasma, or delayed immune hemolysis caused by anti-RBC antibodies produced by the donor marrow.[4,14] Minor ABO incompatibility does not have an effect on graft rejection, the incidence or severity of GVHD, or patient survival.[22,23] Although exchange transfusion of the recipient before BMT using red cells of the donor's blood group has been employed to prevent hemolysis caused by passive transfer of isohemagglutinin in the marrow product, this is rarely a clinically significant problem and can more easily be avoided by removing plasma from the marrow before infusion. Minor ABO incompatibility can result in adverse reactions due to the production of anti-A and/or anti-B antibodies by donor marrow lymphocytes early (1–3 weeks) post-transplant, particularly in patients on cyclosporine therapy or in those receiving T-cell-depleted allografts.[25–27] This may be particularly severe and associated with reactive hemolysis in the setting of minor ABO-incompatible HLA-matched BMT, using unrelated donors.[28] The rapidity of engraftment and early related production of isohemagglutinins is somewhat surprising, given the delay in humoral reconstitution noted after BMT.[11] Current practice involves transfusion of either group O or donor group RBCs to dilute the recipient RBCs and to monitor patients closely for evidence of hemolysis; in rare cases, exchange transfusion has been required due to very rapid engraftment of donor lymphocytes, production of anti-RBC antibodies, and related hemolysis.

Alloimmunization

Patients undergoing BMT require large numbers of cellular blood product transfusions, often before, and always after, BMT. Since some studies suggest that sensitization to HLA antigens has increased with number of transfusions and related donor exposures,[29] it might be expected that patients eligible to undergo BMT would be at high risk of the development of alloimmunization. The adverse effect of such HLA sensitization on marrow engraftment is most evident in the setting of aplastic anemia. An analysis of 625 patients with aplastic anemia who received allografts from HLA-identical donors demonstrated either no or transient engraftment in 68 (11%) patients.[30] Of a variety of clinical parameters analyzed, post-BMT treatment with cyclosporine and avoidance of pre-BMT blood transfusions were associated with improved survival.

Although graft failure associated with histocompatibility differences between donor and recipients is often attributed to rejection by host T lymphocytes, persistent host antibodies specific for donor antigen may also mediate graft failure, whether by antibody-dependent cell-mediated cytotoxicity or by complement-mediated cytotoxicity. Specifically, host anti-HLA class I antibodies have been associated with graft failure and death, and host anti-ABO antibodies have persisted for ≤18 months post-BMT and resulted in erythroid hypoplasia.[31] Therefore, the need for transfusions should be critically evaluated in patients eligible for subsequent allogeneic marrow grafting. Although the use of family members as blood donors pre-BMT has been reported not to be harmful in patients with malignancy,[32] transfusions from the potential marrow donor should be avoided due to the risk of sensitization of the patient both to HLA and non-HLA antigens.

Patients are also at high risk of becoming alloimmunized post-BMT. A retrospective analysis of patients with severe aplastic anemia who underwent allogeneic BMT documented the development of refractoriness to transfusion of random donor platelets in 34% of patients; indeed, the number of platelets transfused (if ≥40 U) as well as lymphocytotoxic antibodies correlated with refractoriness.[33] Finally, Galel and colleagues[34] also documented alloimmunization in 31% of transplant patients, with a similar incidence in recipients of autologous (34%) and allogeneic (27%) recipients. One-half of the alloimmunization in each group was demonstrated pre-BMT. Galel's group identified patients with Hodgkin disease and women with children to be at particular risk of the development of alloimmunization. Most importantly, these investigators concluded that BMT does not prevent the development of alloimmunization in either autologous or allogeneic BMT recipients. It is therefore important to test for anti-HLA antibodies whenever transplant recipients become refractory to random donor platelet transfusion, since the response to random donor platelet transfusion is poor in the sensitized host, and HLA-matched, family member, or cross-match-compatible platelets may be useful in this setting.[35–39]

It would appear that patients undergoing BMT would be an appropriate group in which to employ strategies to avoid alloimmunization (i.e., use of single-donor platelets[40,41] or HLA-matched platelets,[42] or ultraviolet [UV] irradiation[43,44] or leukocyte depletion[45–48] of platelets for transfusion). Leukocyte depletion of platelets for transfusion can be achieved by filtration, centrifugation, or apheresis technology and results in $<10^6$ residual leukocytes in platelets and a delay or avoidance of alloimmunization in transfusion recipients. The only potential adverse effect of depleting leukocytes from blood products would be the removal of a purported graft-versus-leukemia effect,[49] but whether white blood cells within transfused cellular blood components mediate such an effect remains controversial.[50] One should therefore consider the use of measures to avoid alloimmunization (i.e., transfusion of exclusively leukocyte-poor blood components) to patients who are eligible to undergo BMT.

Cytomegalovirus Infection

Cellular blood components transfused from CMV-seropositive donors to CMV-seronegative transplant recipients and neonates can cause CMV seroconversion and infection.[51] In allogeneic BMT, it has long been known that the serologic status of the patient pre-BMT is the most important predictor of CMV infection post-BMT and that transfusions from CMV-seropositive donors to CMV-seronegative recipients can cause CMV seroconversion and infection.[52] In an early study of prophylactic granulocytes in recipients of allogeneic BMT, for example, lack of infection was documented only in the setting of seronegative recipients who received granulocytes from seronegative donors.[53] Transfusion with seronegative blood products appears to lessen CMV infection after allogeneic BMT when both donor and patient are seronegative, but not when either are seropositive[54]; in some studies, treatment of patients with immunoglobulin has been efficacious in this setting and may also reduce CMV sequelae in seropositive recipients.[55] The use of both immunoglobulin and CMV-seronegative blood products appears to confer no additional benefit. CMV antigen can be detected in peripheral blood leukocytes after allogenic transplantation, but whether antigenemia is more sensitive than rapid culture methods to focus antiviral prophylaxis in BMT patients remains to be determined.[56] CMV infection, strongly associated with acute GVHD,[57] may become less frequent in all patients undergoing allogeneic BMT due to the development of effective prophylaxis for GVHD. In addition, acyclovir therapy can lessen the incidence of CMV infection and related morbidity, thereby improving the survival of seropositive allogeneic BMT recipients.[58] Finally, reports document successful therapy for CMV pneumonia that has developed after BMT with ganciclovir and either intravenous immunoglobulin or CMV immunoglobulin.[59,60] On the basis of these and other studies, it has been standard practice to reserve the exclusive use of CMV-seronegative blood components for allogeneic BMT when both donor and recipient are seronegative.

CMV infection in autologous BMT recipients is less common, perhaps related to the rarity of GVHD in autologous BMT recipients. Indeed, equivalent numbers of autologous and allogeneic BMT recipients either seroconvert to or excrete CMV, but clinical sequelae develop only in allogeneic BMT recipients who have GVHD.[61] Therefore, methods for CMV prophylaxis, such as immunoglobulin, seronegative blood products, or post-transplant acyclovir therapy, have not been used in autologous BMT recipients. It has been noted, however, that pretransplant CMV serology is also predictive of CMV infection after autologous BMT[62] and that engraftment may be delayed after autologous BMT in patients with CMV infection. Moreover, recent analysis of 159 autologous BMT recipients, all of whom received CMV unscreened blood products, documented a probability of CMV infection of 22.5% in CMV-seronegative patients and 61.1% in CMV-seropositive recipients.[63] In this series, CMV pneumonia developed in 11 patients at a median of 100 days post-BMT and was fatal in 9 cases. Although an area of active study, the standard of practice is not to use CMV-seronegative blood products in the setting of autologous BMT.

The traditional CMV-seronegative cellular blood products have been frozen deglycerolized RBCs and platelets harvested from CMV-seronegative donors and should be used in appropriate BMT patients. However, filtration of RBCs has been shown to decrease transfusion-acquired CMV infection in infants[64]; moreover, filtered blood components have also been shown to decrease CMV seroconversion in patients undergoing treatment for acute leukemia.[65,66] Preliminary data from Seattle suggest that provision of filtered RBCs and platelet transfusions from unscreened donors to CMV-seronegative patients undergoing autologous BMT may prevent seroconversion or infection in the recipient.[67] In addition, De Witte and colleagues[68] recently showed that leukocyte depletion of blood products by centrifugation coupled with acyclovir prophylaxis may also prevent primary CMV infection in CMV-seronegative allogeneic BMT recipients. Although further confirmation in larger studies is needed before it can be attempted more generally, the ability to use filtered blood products as CMV-seronegative would markedly expand the donor pool, and hence the supply of noninfectious components.

Transfusion-Associated Graft-Versus-Host Disease

All patients undergoing BMT are at risk of the development of TA-GVHD after receiving cellular blood products. The most commonly reported manifestations are skin rash, abnormal liver function tests, and severe pancytopenia. The degree of pancytopenia has generally been profound, perhaps related to the HLA disparity evident between donor and recipient in TA-GVHD. By contrast, GVHD occurs after allogeneic BMT when marrow and donor have been chosen by virtue of histocompatibility. TA-GVHD results in an overall 84% mortality rate after a median of 21 days (range 8–1,050 days).[69]

TA-GVHD is effectively prevented by γ-irradiation of the blood product prior to transfusion. Moreover, if any transfusions are given to the patient during autologous marrow harvest, they must also be irradiated. A survey of blood component irradiation practices in the United States found that 88% and 81.4% of allogeneic and autologous BMT recipients, respectively, received irradiated cellular components.[70] Although it is reassuring that the overwhelming majority of patients do receive irradiated components, it is disturbing that not all patients receive them. A recent documentation of several cases of fatal TA-GVHD in recipients of autologous BMT[71] further suggests that irradiation of cellular components transfused to BMT recipients is not yet uniform practice. Moreover, doses of radiation used to treat cellular blood components before transfusion are also not uniform, varying from 15 to 35 Gy.[70] Recent studies suggest that irradiation at 15–20 Gy can reduce mitogen-responsive lymphocytes by 5–6 logs, compared with unirradiated controls,[72] and it has recently been recommended that all cellular products be irradiated with ≥25 Gy to avoid TA-GVHD.

A potential alternative method to prevent TA-GVHD would be to deplete lymphocytes from blood products before transfusion. It has been demonstrated in murine systems, as well as in humans, that T lymphocytes mediate GVHD and that the incidence and severity of GVHD after allogeneic BMT can be reduced if T cells are eliminated from the donor marrow prior to grafting by a variety of techniques.[73,74] While techniques are available for the preparation of leukocyte-poor red cells and platelets containing 10^6 lymphocytes, the precise number and type of T cells required to mediate TA-GVHD remain undefined. It remains unproven as to whether leukocyte depletion from blood components would decrease the risk of TA-GVHD, and indeed cases of GVHD after transfusion of leukocyte-poor components have been reported.[75] A canine model has been used to demonstrate that UV rather than γ-irradiation of transfused leukocytes can abrogate TA-GVHD in recipient animals.[76] However, future studies are needed to determine whether UV light can avoid TA-GVHD in transfusion recipients without leading to adverse effects on in vitro function or in vivo recovery of UV-treated red cells or platelets. Finally, immunocompetent patients who share an HLA haplotype with HLA homozygous blood donors also appear to be at risk of TA-GVHD.[77,78] Homozygosity for HLA types is more likely to occur among first-degree family members (e.g., parents, children, and siblings). Moreover, the risk of transfusion of blood from HLA-homozygous donors to unrelated HLA-heterozygous patients is 1 in 874 in Japan and may be as high as 1 in 7,174 in the United States, suggesting that γ-irradiation may be of more widespread use.[79]

Leukocyte-Depleted Products

Potential adverse consequences of residual white blood cells within platelet products include febrile nonhemolytic transfusion reactions (FNHTRs), alloimmunization, transmission of infection, GVHD, and immunomodulation.[80] Current filtration and apheresis technologies can yield leukocyte-poor cellular components, red cells and platelets containing $<10^6$ residual leukocytes.[45–48] It would appear that transfusion of such components can abrogate alloimmunization and avoid CMV transmission. FNHTRs are associated with antibodies to HLA and other leukocyte antigens and can sometimes be avoided, even in patients with a history of prior FNHTRs, by removal of leukocytes before transfusion[48]; however, studies to date have not examined the value of transfusing exclusively leukocyte-poor blood products, as described above to avoid alloimmunization and CMV infection, and thereby FNHTRs. Studies in animals have demonstrated that transfusion of 10^7 leukocytes/kg recipient weight are necessary to mediate TA-GVHD, suggesting that leukocyte depletion before transfusion may be useful to avoid TA-GVHD.[69] In humans, however, the precise number and type of T cells that mediate TA-GVHD are not defined; the potential value of blood product leukocyte depletion to avoid TA-GVHD is also unknown. Finally, it is clear that transfusion recipients may already be immunocompromised as a result of their underlying illness or its treatment, or both, and would be at additional risk from the effects of additional transfusion-associated immunosuppression. However, the effects of this complication of transfusion (i.e., increased risk of postoperative infections and cancer recurrence)[81] and its mechanism of action are also undefined. Therefore, avoidance of FNHTRs, TA-GVHD, and immunomodulation remains a potential but unproven benefit of providing exclusively leukocyte-poor cellular blood components.

In summary, it would appear that transfusion of exclusively leukocyte-poor cellular blood components has proven efficacy in abrogating alloimmunization in patients at risk. It also seems very likely that the exclusive use of leukocyte-poor blood components can avoid transfusion-related CMV infection; ongoing studies should confirm initial encouraging reports. It seems likely that BMT recipients should receive only leukocyte-poor blood components.[82] Obviously, the cost-effectiveness of transfusing leukocyte-poor components would improve if their use could achieve more than one of these desirable outcomes.

Bone Marrow Processing

As the use of BMT has increased as a treatment strategy, the blood component laboratory has become increasingly involved in marrow processing. However, bone marrow is not a licensed blood component, and no federal regulations concerning its collection, transportation, processing, storage, or transfusion are available. It was recently suggested that bone marrow processing laboratories adopt the laboratory standards already in existence for blood banks (e.g., regulations concerning storage, freezing, transfusion), thereby treating marrow as any other blood component[83]; such standards have recently been developed.[84]

Bone marrow processing may consist of several steps: concentration and washing; sedimentation with hydroxyethyl starch, Ficoll-Hypaque, or Percoll; purging and washing; cryopreservation and storage; and thawing and transfusion. The goal of marrow processing is depletion of RBCs, plasma, and fat, with minimal loss of progenitor cells. Processing was originally done manually by simple centrifugation; however, cell separators are used for the preferential concentration of progenitor cells with increased elimination of other hematopoietic cells. A variety of automated procedures have now been published for marrow processing, using various cell separators; engraftment has been documented after transfusion of such marrow.[85–88] As is true in the preparation of other blood components, it is also critical to develop techniques to avoid bacterial contamination during the collection and processing of bone marrow.[89]

Marrow processing may also include depletion (purging) of tumor cells from autologous marrow before grafting. The various methods of purging are based on physical properties, sensitivity to chemotherapy, and/or expression of cell-surface antigens.[90] Each of these has its own set of optimal conditions, some well defined and others under investigation. It may be postulated that malignancies that either arise from the marrow (i.e., leukemias, myelomas) or that are histologically evident within the marrow (i.e., relapsed lymphomas) will require purging; however, the need for purging in any setting remains undefined. Purging of tumor cells from autologous marrow is being evaluated: (1) to allow patients with overt tumor involvement to undergo autologous BMT, and (2) to deplete subclinical residual malignant cells when tumor is not evident on cytopathologic examination. In particular, three lines of evidence suggest that $≤10^8$ tumor cells may be in marrow when histopathologic examination is normal: (1) the ability to derive tumor cell lines from marrows that appear to be pathologically normal[91]; (2) the observed time to relapse and known tumor-doubling times in patients with hematologic cancers, which suggest that tumor cells were present when not pathologically evident; and (3) the use of more sensitive techniques, such as gene rearrangement or polymerase chain reaction (PCR) technology,[92] which can confirm the presence of a single malignant cell within 10^6 marrow cells.

The conditions for pharmacologic purging of autologous

marrow tumor cells on a cell separator (i.e., marrow RBC and drug concentration) have been established.[93,94] Moreover, when using cell separator technology for mAb-based purging of autologous marrow tumor cells, a 4–5 $\log_{10}$ depletion can be achieved using only 50% of the mAb and complement with in 50% of the time required for manual techniques.[93] Purging of tumor cells from autologous grafts prior to BMT has permitted the use of this approach in patients with ≤20% histopathologic involvement with tumor.[95] PCR has recently demonstrated that immunologic purging using anti-B cell mAbs and complement lysis could successfully remove PCR-detectable lymphoma cells from autografts in only one-half of patients[96]; importantly, those patients who were reinfused with autologous marrow containing residual lymphoma cells detectable by PCR had an increased incidence of relapse.[92] Sharp and co-workers[97] recently used a culture technique sensitive for detecting occult lymphoma cells in marrow to analyze histologically normal marrow harvested from patients with lymphoma who were candidates for high-dose therapy and autologous BMT; detection of lymphoma cells in marrow was found to be an adverse prognostic factor, independent of other clinical features. Finally, Gorin and colleagues[98] recently examined 263 patients with standard-risk acute myeloid leukemia in first complete remission who underwent autografting after total body irradiation; a higher leukemia-free survival rate and a lower relapse rate in recipients of mafosfamide-purged marrows than in recipients of non purged marrows were noted. To date, however, no study has proved the need for purging.

In allogeneic BMT, purging has been used to deplete T cells in donor marrow before grafting to prevent GVHD.[73,90] Although the incidence of GVHD has thereby been decreased, concomitant increases in graft failure, rejection, and relapse rates have lessened enthusiasm for this approach to abrogate GVHD. After processing and/or purging of either autologous or allogeneic marrow, quality control measures should include assessment of viability, sterility, and number of stem cells present, using currently available blood stem cell assays. Although there is no standardized assay for the pluripotential hematopoietic stem cell, some investigators have found a relationship between colony-forming unit-granulocyte/macrophage (CFU-GM) and engraftment.[99]

Autologous marrow depleted of erythrocytes, granulocytes, and plasma is usually frozen in 10% dimethylsulfoxide (DMSO) in a rate-controlled freezer, set to cool at a constant 1°C/min, and then stored until infusion in either liquid or vapor phase of liquid nitrogen.[100] Alternatively, recovery of CFU-GM from unfractionated bone marrow stored in vapor phase liquid nitrogen has been reported to be higher in 5% DMSO and 6% hydroxyethyl starch than that from marrow stored in 10% DMSO alone.[101] Moreover, marrows frozen by simple immersion in a −80°C freezer, without controlled rate freezing, and stored at this temperature have resulted in satisfactory engraftment after autotransplantation. Quality control measures in both cryopreservation and thawing again must ensure both sterility and viability of stem cells.

The RBCs separated from donated marrow can be transfused to the marrow donor (either the patient undergoing autologous BMT or the allogeneic marrow donor) after the marrow harvest.[102,103] Thus, homologous transfusions can be avoided.

Documentation of Engraftment

Use of BMT in the treatment of patients with hematologic malignancies is based on the assumption that the high doses of chemotherapy eradicate the malignant clone but also result in permanent ablation of host hematopoiesis and lymphopoiesis. Ablation of the recipient's marrow eliminates cells that could cause rejection of the donor bone marrow and also provides space for engraftment of donor cells. Free of competition, allogeneic marrow can then replace normal recipient marrow and re-establish normal hematologic and immune function.

Although the transplant preparative regimens are thought to be ablative, several previous reports have demonstrated the recovery of recipient hematopoiesis after BMT.[104,105] These surviving recipient cells can either be normal hematopoietic host cells or tumor cells. When neoplastic cells are identified post-BMT, they often, but not invariably, result in clinical relapse.[106] When these cells are normal recipient hematopoietic cells, they can either reject the donor bone marrow cells[107] or become tolerant to donor cells and contribute to the establishment of mixed hematopoietic chimerism.[108] The phenomenon of graft rejection has been studied extensively both in experimental animal models and in clinical transplants, but the phenomenon of coexisting donor and recipient cells has only recently been recognized.

Several techniques have been used to evaluate mixed chimerism after allogeneic BMT. Cytogenetic analysis has frequently been used to differentiate between donor and recipient cells in patients with sex-mismatched donors; when donor and recipient are sex matched, characteristic polymorphic regions or satellites can be used to distinguish the donor or recipient origin of the dividing cells.[109] Donor and recipient RBCs have been distinguished by analysis of surface antigens and enzymatic content.[110,111] This is only possible if donor and recipient differ in a given red cell antigen, and transfusion with red cells bearing this antigen is avoided. More recently, DNA analysis using Y-chromosome probes[112] or probes for highly polymorphic regions on other chromosomes have been used to evaluate chimerism.[113,114] These DNA restriction fragment length polymorphisms are used more often because they allow distinction and quantitation of donor and recipient cells in almost all BMT patients and also because they can identify the origin of nondividing cells. In an analysis at our institution, mixed chimerism after transplant was found by restriction fragment length polymorphism analysis in 53% of patients, by cytogenetic analysis in 21% of patients, and by RBC phenotyping in 44% of patients.[115]

Immune-Mediated Cytopenias

Hemolysis can be avoided in the setting of ABO incompatibility between donor and recipient of allogeneic BMT as described above. Autoimmune hemolytic anemia has also rarely been reported after allogeneic BMT.[116] After bone marrow grafting, severe unexplained thrombocytopenia and granulocytopenia may also complicate the post-graft recovery of the patient.[117] Antibodies to platelets and granulocytes of donor origin have been demonstrated in recipients of both allogeneic and autologous bone marrow grafts. In the case of autografts, such antibodies are by definition autoantibodies, and similar antibodies after allografting may also have an autoimmune origin. It is likely that this is the result of transient immune system imbalance, common to both allografts and autografts, in the early post-graft period. The extent to which these antibodies affect the peripheral counts probably depends on the ability of the grafted marrow to compensate for the rate of antibody-mediated cell destruction. Many patients have responded to conventional therapy, including steroids, splenectomy, and intravenous immunoglobulin.

Role of Recombinant Hematopoietic Growth Factors

The hematopoietic growth factors are glycoprotein hormones that regulate the proliferation and differentiation of hematopoietic progenitor cells and function of mature blood cells. Erythropoietin (EPO), a glycoprotein produced in response to hypoxia in the kidney, induces RBC production by stimulating the mitotic activity of erythroid progenitor cells—burst-forming unit-erythroid (BFU-E) and colony-forming unit-erythroid (CFU-E) and early erythroid precursor cells—in the bone marrow. Recombinant human (rHu) EPO is already of proven efficacy in the treatment of the anemia of chronic renal failure[118] and of acquired immunodeficiency syndrome treated with zidovudine.[119] It may also be useful to treat the anemia of cancer, since endogenous EPO levels may be inappropriately low.[120-122] Specifically, levels of endogenous EPO have been reported to be inappropriately low for the degree of anemia in patients after both autologous and allogeneic BMT.[122,123] Supplemental rHuEPO may therefore also be useful to hasten RBC engraftment and to decrease RBC transfusion requirements.[122-124]

Recombinant human colony-stimulating factor-granulocyte/macrophage (rHuCSF-GM) may also be useful post-BMT. It has been shown to accelerate hematopoietic recovery in primates undergoing autologous BMT.[125] Administration of rHuCSF-GM after autologous BMT in humans led to accelerated total leukocyte and granulocyte recovery and reduced morbidity and mortality compared to historical controls.[126,127] However, a temporary reduction of granulocytes occurred with discontinuation of the growth factor, emphasizing the need to determine whether engraftment is not only enhanced, but also sustained, by growth factor stimulation. Due to a randomized trial demonstrating that rHuCSF-GM hastens myeloid recovery and shortens hospital stay,[128] it has now been approved to accelerate myeloid recovery in patients with non-Hodgkin lymphoma, acute lymphocytic leukemia, and Hodgkin disease undergoing autologous bone marrow transplantation. A study of the effect of rHuCSF-GM on hematopoietic recovery in patients who underwent autologous BMT demonstrated enhanced engraftment only in patients who received adequate CFU-GM in the marrow grafts.[129] Finally, it has recently been demonstrated that rHuCSF-GM can be used effectively to treat patients with graft failure after BMT[130] and appears not to exacerbate GVHD when used early after allogeneic BMT.[131]

Peripheral Blood Stem Cell Autotransplantation

Hematopoietic stem cells can be collected from the peripheral blood of laboratory animals by cytapheresis and successfully reconstitute myelopoiesis following marrow lethal treatment.[132] In humans, autologous PBSCs have been collected from patients during the chronic phase of chronic myeloid leukemia and have subsequently been infused after the patient has received high-dose therapy for accelerated or blastic phase disease.[133] These cells engraft, as evidenced by return to the chronic phase. Other investigators have also used reinfusion of PBSCs to achieve hematopoietic reconstitution after high-dose chemotherapy and total body irradiation.[134,135] The potential advantages of PBSCs are several: leukapheresis is an outpatient procedure similar to platelet donation and avoids the need for hospitalization, general anesthesia, and bone marrow harvest; adequate numbers of stem cells can be collected from patients with hemipelvectomies, tumor involving the pelvic bones, or after pelvic irradiation; and it may be possible to harvest adequate numbers of PBSCs from patients with tumor-involved marrow. In multiple myeloma, for example, studies have demonstrated that the relative number of malignant stem cells is markedly reduced in peripheral blood relative to bone marrow, suggesting a potential benefit for PBSC grafting.[136] It should be noted, however, that even patients with solid tumors may have tumor cells contaminating PBSC collections.[137]

There are two concerns of PBSC transplantation: the need for multiple collections to obtain adequate numbers of stem cells, and the question of whether PBSCs provide long-term engraftment of all lineages. The number of collection procedures can be decreased if leukapheresis is done when increased numbers of hematopoietic progenitor cells are mobilized into the peripheral blood by administration of recombinant growth factors[138,139] or with the use of growth factors at recovery from high-dose chemotherapy.[140-143] The precise subpopulations of progenitor cells mobilized by chemotherapy or growth factor and the potential depletion of stem cells related to the repeated use of restorative growth factor regimens are currently being defined.[144,145]

The CD34 antigen is expressed by 1–4% of human and baboon marrow cells, including virtually all hemotopoietic progenitors detectable by in vitro assays. These CD34+ cells are capable of reconstituting hematopoiesis in both baboons and humans.[146,147] Siena and colleagues[140] demonstrated that CD34+ cells in the peripheral blood can be increased fivefold by rHu-CSF-GM after high-dose cyclophosphamide and that these cells possess qualitatively normal hematopoietic colony growth and high cloning efficiency compared with bone marrow CD34+ cells. Moreover, CD34+ cells isolated from bone marrow or umbilical cord blood from healthy donors can be induced to proliferate rapidly in vitro with differentiation to multiple myeloid lineages, while certain subsets maintain expression of CD34.[148,149] Additional purification of CD34+HLA-DR-CD15- rhodamine 123 dull cells yields a fraction of human bone marrow highly enriched for human primitive hematopoietic progenitor cells, which can be expanded in vitro by stimulation with c-kit ligand and a synthetic interleukin-3 (IL-3)/CSF-GM fusion protein.[150] Further studies will define optimal conditions for expansion of these CD34+ progenitor cells for transplantation.

Preliminary data suggest that umbilical cord and placental blood from an HLA-identical sibling is a rich source of hematopoietic progenitor cells and may produce stable donor-derived lymphohematopoietic engraftment.[151,152] Placental blood also has a potential use in unrelated BMT, because of the predominance of stem cells coupled with the lack of mature T lymphocytes that could mediate GVHD.[153] Finally, as described for PBSCs, positive selection of CD34+ human umbilical cord blood hematopoietic progenitors has demonstrated that they have high proliferative and replating potential,[154] suggesting their use in transplantation.

Summary

The provision of appropriate blood component support has been critical for the development of curative treatment programs (i.e., aggressive combination chemotherapy in childhood leukemias). The blood component laboratory will continue to play a central broadening role in the treatment of cancer, specifically in the harvesting, processing, and transfusion of hematopoietic stem cells from marrow and peripheral blood sources to restore hematologic and immune function after high-dose ablative therapy. The use of recombinant growth factors appears both to facilitate the harvesting of hematopoietic stem cells from peripheral blood and to hasten engraftment after transplantation. Innovative treatment strategies, including intensive myeloablative therapies, may now be used for a broad spectrum of patients with presently incurable cancers. Transfusion medicine expertise will be essential to ensure that appropriate blood components are provided before and after hematopoietic stem cell transplantation, to collect hematopoietic stem cells, and to avoid immune and infectious complications in patients so treated.

SOLID ORGAN TRANSPLANTATION

Introduction

The tremendous growth in solid organ transplantation has resulted in part from improved antirejection therapy. In addition to prednisone and azathioprine, the use of cyclosporine, FK506, and OKT3, either singly or in combination, has greatly improved graft survival.[155] Cyclosporine and FK506 are not cytotoxic agents and thus lack marrow toxicity. These drugs block transcription of IL-2 by interfering with Ca^{2+}-activated transcription factors.[156] Release of other T-cell cytokines, such as interferon-γ is also down-regulated. The overall effect is directed primarily at suppression of T-cell activation. Because corticosteroids prevent the release of IL-1 from accessory cells, the combination of cyclosporine or FK506 with prednisone has been highly successful. Newer agents, such as Rapamycin, RS61443, and deoxyspergualin, are under investigation.[157]

Renal Transplantation

Pretransplant Blood Transfusions

Following the initial investigations by Opelz et al[158] numerous studies documented that pretransplant blood transfusions promoted prolonged renal allograft survival.[159] As a result, deliberate use of random donor transfusions before cadaver donor renal transplantation and donor-specific transfusions before living-related donor transplants became widespread.[160] A proportion of such patients became HLA alloimmunized, however, and the resulting HLA incompatibility—detected during pretransplant cross-matching—eliminated them as candidates for transplantation. The introduction of cyclosporine in the 1980s led to improved overall graft survival and the beneficial effect of pretransplant transfusions became more difficult to document.[161,162] As a result, most transplant centers abandoned programs of immunologic conditioning by deliberate transfusion in favor of avoiding HLA sensitization through the use of EPO and leukocyte-reduced blood components.[163] The role of pretransplant transfusions before kidney transplantation remains controversial.[164,165]

Despite decades of investigation the exact mechanism of the beneficial effect of pretransplant transfusions remains uncertain. Three basic mechanisms have been proposed: (1) pretransplant transfusions may select for patients who are immunologic "nonresponders" because patients developing HLA antibodies would be restricted from access to transplant by pretransplant HLA cross-matching; (2) transfusions may serve to "prime" the recipient immune system, which is then stimulated to undergo a rapid secondary antigraft immune response at transplant (the rapid clonal expansion of the secondary immune response is then eliminated by immunosuppressive drugs given after surgery[166]); and (3) recipient exposure to residual allogeneic leukocytes in blood components may exert an immunosuppressive effect. Numerous immunomodulatory effects of transfusion have been investigated, including the development of anti-idiotypes,[167,168] production of antigen-specific suppressor T cells,[169] elimination of alloreactive cytotoxic T cells,[170] and changes in natural killer cell function. Recently, it has been suggested that residual allogeneic leukocytes may transiently engraft in the recipient and induce anergy through transient microchimerism.[171]

Antigen Matching and Compatibility

ABO Compatibility

ABO compatibility between donor antigens and recipient antibodies is critical for successful renal transplantation. ABH antigens are richly expressed on vascular endothelial cells[172] and renal cells[173] and are excreted in the urine.[174] As a result, ABO-incompatible grafts are at high risk of rejection and transplantation against ABO barriers is contraindicated.[175,176] Because group O recipients are restricted to group O donors, several experimental protocols have investigated preoperative preparation to permit the use of group A_2 donors for group O recipients.[177,178] Other experimental protocols have been used to attempt ABO-incompatible renal grafting.[179] Transplantation of nonmatched but compatible grafts (e.g., group O donor for a group A recipient) is commonly done. However, passenger lymphocytes that accompany the graft may continue to secrete ABO antibodies during the early postoperative period. Therefore, recipients of ABO-compatible, but mismatched, allografts may experience hemolysis secondary to ABO alloantibodies of graft (lymphocyte) origin (see the section Orthotopic Liver Transplantation, ABO Compatibility).

HLA Compatibility

The importance of serologic HLA compatibility between donor antigens and recipient antibodies is well established in renal transplantation. Recipients who express warm-reactive antibodies to HLA class I antigens of the donor generally reject in a pattern termed hyperacute rejection[180] characterized by complement activation, intravascular coagulation, organ ischemia, and necrosis that may occur within minutes of establishing blood flow to the graft.[181] A variety of techniques are used for HLA cross-matching, which methods have the highest predictive value is controversial.[182] ASHI Standards require that the cross-match techniques have increased sensitivity compared with the basic microlymphocytotoxicity test.

The recognition that HLA-serologic incompatibility predicts hyperacute rejection and that HLA antibodies are often transient has led to the practice of monthly HLA antibody screening of serum from potential kidney graft recipients. Identified antibody specificities are recorded and the corresponding antigens avoided when allocating suitable kidney grafts. Identification of antibodies to public specificities may be more clinically meaningful than specificities to private antigens.[183] Previously collected serum with HLA reactivity is no longer required to be cross-match compatible with the donor lymphocytes at transplant; successful renal transplantation has been performed in patients who were compatible with the donor using the current serum but incompatible when using previously collected serum.[184]

HLA Matching

Evidence that greater degrees of HLA matching between donor and recipient result in longer graft survival has led to efforts to allocate cadaver organs based on the degree of matching in addition to the results of pretransplant HLA compatibility.[185,186] First-time transplants from HLA-identical sibling donors have a 10-year actuarial survival rate of 68% compared with 43% from HLA-identical parental donors and 26% from HLA-identical cadaver donors.[187] The poorer graft survival rate for recipients of matched cadaver donors may reflect the influence of histocompatibility mismatches not recognized by current HLA typing techniques or incorrect HLA antigen assignments using traditional serologic typing methods.[188] The application of molecular biologic techniques has revealed an unexpected extraordinary complexity to HLA antigen assignments.[189,190] As many as 25% of samples may be incorrectly typed by serologic techniques as compared with DNA typing.[191] As current serologic methods are replaced by more accurate HLA DNA typing, it is expected that the improved graft survival using matched donor/recipient pairs, which has already been documented, will continue to advance.[186,188,192] Allocation by HLA matching may be of particular value for those patients awaiting transplant who are highly sensitized.[193,194]

In addition to ABO and HLA, other antigen systems may play a role in renal allograft survival. Evidence for a contribution by the Lewis blood group system,[195,196] by a poorly characterized vascular endothelial cell antigen system,[197-199] and by other non-HLA organ kidney-specific antigens[200] has been reported.

Orthotopic Liver Transplantation

Orthotopic liver transplantation (OLT) entails the removal of the patient's liver and placement of the donor organ in the same anatomic location. OLT has become an established therapy for end-stage life-threatening hepatic failure.[201,202] Successful OLT requires a close working relationship between the surgical team and blood services because the operation sometimes requires spectacular quantities of blood support. Better patient selection, improved surgical technique, use of venovenous bypass while the inferior vena cava is being clamped, argon/laser directed electrocoagulation, and better preservative solutions used for storing the donor liver ex vivo have all contributed to decreased transfusion requirements during surgery.[203]

Causes of Extreme Bleeding

Intraoperative transfusion requirements cannot be predicted solely on the basis of preoperative coagulation screening.[204] Rather, the presence of severe portal hypertension, previous right upper quadrant surgery, vascular abnormalities of the portal vein or hepatic artery, poor left ventricular function, poor nutritional state, or comorbid diseases are the most important predictors of massive transfusion and decreased survival rate.

OLT requires a difficult right upper quadrant dissection of the recipient hepatic bed that can be complicated by severe portal hypertension and multiple friable collateral blood vessels. Removal of the recipient liver requires clamping and cutting the portal vein, the hepatic artery and the inferior vena cava above and below the liver. The period after the recipient hepatectomy and before re-establishing blood flow to the new graft is referred to as the anhepatic phase of surgery. During the anhepatic phase, venous blood draining the bowel and lower extremities is usually diverted through a nonanticoagulated venovenous extracorporeal bypass circuit to an axillary vein. During the anastomoses of donor and recipient vessels, rapid surgical blood loss may occur.

Patients who require OLT usually have multiple hemostatic abnormalities associated with acute or chronic liver failure. Decreased coagulation factors, splenomegaly with thrombocytopenia, dysfibrinogenemia, and chronic fibrinolysis may all be present in varying combinations. In addition, some patients develop a profound intraoperative fibrinolysis.[205,206] Tissue plasminogen activator (t-PA), presumably released from recipient blood vessels or from the vessels of the allograft in response to shock, acidosis, pharmacologic pressors, ischemia, or preservation injury, circulates in high concentration. Normally cleared by the liver, t-PA released during and immediately after the anhepatic phase of surgery is not cleared from the bloodstream. As a result, t-PA activity can reach 10–100 times normal, and a pathologic systemic lytic state ensues. A sudden decrease in all coagulation factors occurs with particularly marked declines in fibrinogen and factor VIII.[207] Less severe cases may not demonstrate systemic lysis but may lyse fibrin clot at sites of previous hemostasis. As the liver allograft begins to function, t-PA is rapidly cleared and fibrinolysis decreases. Administration of antifibrinolytic agents such as ∈-aminocaproic acid[208] or aprotinin[209] can significantly improve hemostasis and may prevent exsanguination in some patients.

A properly functioning graft is essential to the success of OLT. Grafts damaged during the demise of the donor, during harvesting or ex vivo preservation, or during implantation are associated with both severe hypotension and coagulopathy. Hypotension results from a pronounced decline in total systemic vascular resistance and is often refractory to aggressive pharmacologic pressor support. The ensuing shock exacerbates the derangement in hemostasis. With the introduction of better graft-preserving solutions, such as that developed at the University of Wisconsin (UW solution), the incidence of severe graft ischemia and massive blood requirements has decreased.[210] Postoperatively, there may be transient diminished production of those coagulant and anticoagulant proteins that require high synthetic rates.[211]

Transfusion Support

A rapid transfusion device designed to deliver large volumes of blood components in a rapid fashion is essential for OLT. These devices consist of a sterile holding reservoir, high-capacity blood filter, roller pump, in-line blood warmer, and air-detection device. Blood is directed through large-bore tubing and infused under pump pressure through very large-bore catheters placed in the antecubital or central veins. Intraoperative blood recovery devices are a useful adjunct to blood support during OLT, particularly in cases requiring massive transfusion.[212,213] Blood suctioned from the operative field is anticoagulated with citrate and collected in a sterile holding reservoir. The shed blood is then centrifuged, the supernatant discarded, and the residual packed red cells washed with saline. The saline-suspended packed red cells may then be pumped to the rapid transfusion device for immediate reinfusion.

Careful but aggressive component therapy guided by the clinical course and the results of intraoperative coagulation monitoring is essential for successful OLT. Serial intraoperative hematocrit and coagulation monitoring using a limited number of tests with rapid turnaround time provides valuable information for rational blood component support. Some OLT centers monitor coagulation using the thromboelastogram, a device that measures whole blood coagulation by impedance to an oscillating cylinder.[214] Other programs use traditional measurements such as the prothrombin time, fibrinogen, and platelet count. Either method of monitoring is valuable, provided that testing is done serially, that results are reported rapidly, that changes are correlated in the operating room with the clinical picture, and that abnormalities are interpreted by someone experienced in the coagulopathy of OLT.

Red cell support for patients with multiple red cell alloantibodies can present a special challenge to blood services supporting OLT.[215] Preoperative plasmapheresis can be used to remove clinically significant, low-titer, high-frequency alloantibodies. Patients with medium titer clinically significant alloantibodies can sometimes be managed initially with antigen-negative red cells and then switched to antigen-positive cells, should massive blood support be required. Antigen-negative units are then reinstituted at the end of surgery to prevent postoperative hemolysis. Patients with high-titer alloantibodies may require special planning and cooperation among blood suppliers to provide a sufficient quantity of antigen-negative blood. Rh-negative women of childbearing age without anti-D are initially supported with a reasonable number of D-negative units and then switched to D-positive cells should more units be needed.[216]

The use of fresh frozen plasma (FFP), platelet concentrates, and cryoprecipitate is guided by the clinical course and by the results of intraoperative monitoring.[217,218] Although care must be given to prevent dilutional coagulopathy, it is not necessary to mix equal ratios of red cells and FFP or platelet concentrates. Reasonable goals of component therapy in the absence of fibrinolytic or other complications include a prothrombin time of $<1.3 \times$ normal, a platelet count of $>50,000–100,000/mm^3$, and a fibrinogen level of >100 mg/dl. Antifibrinolytic agents are indicated during or shortly after the anhepatic phase of surgery in those patients who demonstrate a systemic lytic state. A loading dose and continuous infusion or simply multiple boluses of 2.5–5 g of ϵ-aminocaproic acid has been used with success. Local hemostasis provided by meticulous and advanced surgical skill is critical to the overall transfusion support of OLT.

Complications of Massive Transfusion

Patients undergoing massive transfusion during OLT are susceptible to all the major complications of massive blood transfusion, including hypothermia, dilutional coagulopathy, electrolyte imbalances, pulmonary dysfunction, and transfusion-transmitted infections. However, OLT patients are uniquely at risk of life-threatening hypocalcemia as a result of citrate toxicity.[219] Since the liver is the main organ for citrate metabolism in the Krebs cycle and since OLT patients can receive very rapid infusions of large volumes of blood components such as FFP that are rich in Na_3-citrate, the quantity of citrate infused per kilogram body weight per minute can quickly exceed the rate of citrate removal.[220] Citrate toxicity is more pronounced if concomitant renal failure is present because the kidney is the major organ of citrate excretion. The principal effects of citrate toxicity are cardiovascular. An initial blunted response of cardiac output to left ventricular volume loading is followed by hypotension resulting from decreased left ventricular performance and decreased systemic vascular resistance. If misinterpreted as hypotension due to hypovolemia, a more rapid transfusion of citrate-rich blood components worsen cardiac output. Citrate toxicity is aggravated by hypothermia and hyperkalemia. Because widened $Q\text{-}T_c$ intervals on the electrocardiogram have low specificity and poor predictive value, intraoperative monitoring of the ionized calcium level is very important. With severe hypocalcemia and hypomagnesemia, bizarre electrocardiographic disturbances and fatal arrhythmias can develop.

Antigen Matching and Compatibility

ABO Compatibility

Under normal circumstances, the donor liver must be ABO compatible with recipient antibodies. Transplantation of ABO incompatible livers has occurred by error or under urgent circumstances and has had limited success.[221,222] However, survival of emergency ABO-incompatible grafts was 30% compared with 76% in emergency ABO compatible grafts.[223] ABO-incompatible hepatic grafts undergo immunologic attack in a manner consistent with hyperacute rejection.[223,224] Transfusion support for ABO-incompatible grafts is not standardized, but the use of RBCs and FFP compatible with both donor and recipient would seem desirable. ABO-nonmatched but compatible donors (e.g., group O donor for group A recipient) is common in OLT, but nonmatched compatible grafts may have decreased survival rates compared with matched grafts. Approximately 30% of patients transplanted with compatible but nonmatched livers suffer postoperative hemolysis of recipient red cells due to ABO antibodies produced by passenger lymphocytes of donor origin.[225] This complication has been reported after all major solid organ transplants, including liver,[225] kidney,[226,227] lung,[228] heart-lung,[229] spleen,[230] and pancreas.[231] It is most common after liver transplantation, probably by virtue of the greater number of passenger lymphocytes that accompany this large organ. Hemolysis develops approximately 1 week after surgery and is generally detected by the development of a positive direct antiglobulin test (DAT) with ABO alloantibodies recovered in the eluate. Although the direct antiglobulin test may only be weakly reactive, rather brisk hemolysis typical of complement fixing ABO antibodies can occur

with a rapid fall in hematocrit and dramatic rise in bilirubin. Acute renal failure from hemolysis was reported in one patient.[232] Treatment is based on transfusion of red cells compatible with antibodies produced by both the recipient and the graft. Red cell exchange is usually not required. Care must be taken in routine postoperative compatibility testing for these patients. A group A_2 recipient whose group O hepatic graft is producing warm-reactive IgG anti-A_1 can have an acute hemolytic transfusion reaction to a group A_1 donor unit transfused postoperatively despite a negative antibody screen, negative DAT, and compatible immediate-spin pretransfusion crossmatch.

HLA Testing

HLA testing for OLT has not reached the clinical importance found in renal transplantation. Donor livers are not allocated on the basis of the degree of donor/recipient HLA antigen matching and incompatible HLA cross-matches do not preclude use of the graft. Three interesting observations regarding HLA testing and OLT have emerged. First, evidence suggests that recipient HLA antibody may contribute to graft rejection in some circumstances.[233–235] Second, recipients with demonstrable HLA antibodies reacting with donor antigens in a pretransplant serum sample often no longer react with those antigens post-transplant, suggesting that HLA antibodies are "absorbed" from the recipient's serum by the incompatible graft.[236,237] As a result, patients have had successful kidney transplants using donor organs that were originally HLA incompatible but that became compatible 48 hours after liver transplantation from the same donor. Third, data from Pittsburgh suggest that donor/recipient liver transplant pairs who match at HLA class I loci have a diminished graft survival rate compared with mismatched donor/recipient pairs.[238] This seemingly paradoxical finding may result from the MHC-restricted cellular immune attack against viral antigens expressed on the graft.[239]

Cardiac Transplantation and Other Solid Organ Transplantations

Advances in the detection of rejection via the use of endomyocardial biopsies coupled with the general improvement in immunosuppressive regimens have gradually improved results for cardiac transplantation.[240] As with the case of kidney and liver allografts, donor hearts are ABO compatible with the antibodies of the recipient. ABH antigens have been detected on the cardiovascular endothelium, but not on cardiac myocytes.[241] The importance of pretransplant HLA serologic compatibility is less established. If the recipient is not broadly HLA alloimmunized, transplantation is done without preoperative HLA cross-matching. For sensitized patients, a pretransplant cross-match is generally performed.[157,240] Cardiac allografts are not allocated on the basis of HLA matching, and the importance of HLA matching in cardiac graft survival remains controversial.

During the postoperative period, the development of accelerated coronary atherosclerosis (coronary occlusive disease) occurs in approximately 40% of patients by 3 years. This serious complication is believed to be a manifestation of allograft rejection and may correlate with post-transplant HLA sensitization.[242] Among 107 patients who received cardiac allografts at Columbia University in New York, actuarial survival was 90% among those who did not form HLA antibodies in response to transplantation versus 38% among those who did.[243] These results were not confirmed however in a report from a different transplant center.[244]

Heart-lung, single lung, pancreas, and small bowel transplants all present unique problems and special demands for effective transfusion support.[157] Information on the relative importance of HLA matching and compatibility is not as highly developed for these systems as for kidney transplants. In addition, transplantation of these organs does not generally require the intensive blood component support seen in liver transplantation. Nevertheless, careful patient selection, compatibility of dominant antigen systems such as ABO, and effective surgical support with blood components that will neither jeopardize graft survival nor transmit viruses dangerous to immunocompromised recipients remain common themes of transfusion medicine in organ transplantation.

Transfusion-Transmitted CMV Infection

Although transfusion-transmitted CMV can be an important source of postoperative morbidity for recipients of solid organ allografts, the mortality from CMV infection is considerably lower after solid organ transplantation than after BMT. When either the donor or the recipient is CMV-positive, the use of CMV-negative blood should be considered investigational. Most transplant centers provide either leukocyte-reduced blood components or blood from CMV-seronegative donors for the transfusion support of CMV-negative recipients of CMV-negative renal or heart allografts. CMV-negative blood is generally not used for liver transplantation because of the large number of blood components required. For CMV-negative renal transplant recipients the use of CMV hyperimmunoglobulin has provided protective passive immunity. In a randomized trial among 59 CMV-seronegative recipients of seropositive kidneys, the incidence of virologically confirmed CMV syndromes was reduced from 60% in control subjects to 21% in patients receiving globulin.[245] CMV immunoglobulin may also have benefit in prophylaxis against primary infection during liver transplantation.[246] Because CMV globulin may not be cost-effective therapy,[247] antiviral agents such as ganciclovir may be preferred to reduce morbidity from CMV after solid organ transplantation.[248,249]

REFERENCES

1. Ferrara JLM, Deeg HJ: Graft-versus-host disease. N Engl J Med 324:667, 1991
2. Kernan NA, Bartsch G, Ash RC et al: Analysis of 462 transplantations from unrelated donors facilitated by the National Marrow Donor Program. N Engl J Med 328:593, 1993
3. Cheson BD, Lacerna L, Leyland-Jones B: Autologous bone marrow transplantation. Ann Intern Med 110:51, 1989
4. Anderson KC: The role of the blood bank in hematopoietic stem cell transplantation. Transfusion 32:272, 1992
5. Bidwell JL, Bidwell EA, Klouda PT et al: DNA-RFLP typing in the selection of related bone marrow donors, letter. Bone Marrow Transplant 1:413, 1987
6. McCullough J: Bone marrow transplantation from unrelated volunteer donors: summary of a conference on scientific, ethical, legal, financial, and other practical issues. Transfusion 22:78, 1982
7. McCullough J, Rogers G, Dahl R et al: Development and operation of a program to obtain volunteer bone marrow donors unrelated to the patient. Transfusion 26:315, 1986
8. McEligott MC, Menitove JE, Aster RH: Recruitment of unrelated persons as bone marrow donors: a preliminary experience. Transfusion 26:309, 1986
9. McCullough J, Hansen J, Perkins HA et al: Establishment of National Marrow Donor Registry. p. 641. In Gale RP, Champlin RE (eds): Bone Marrow Transplantation: Current Controversies. Alan R Liss, New York, 1989
10. Stroncek DF, Holland PV, Bartch G et al: Experiences of the first 493 unrelated marrow donors in the National Marrow Donor Program. Blood 81:1940, 1993
11. Lum LG: The kinetics of immune reconstitution after human marrow transplantation. Blood 69:369, 1987
12. Brand A, Class HJ, Falkenburg JHF et al: Blood component therapy in bone marrow transplantation. Semin Hematol 21:141, 1984
13. Wulff JC, Santner TJ, Storb R et al: Transfusion requirements after HLA identical marrow transplantation in 82 patients with aplastic anemia. Vox Sang 44:366, 1983
14. Petz LD: Immunohematologic problems associated with bone marrow transplantation. Transfus Med Rev 1:85, 1987

15. Bensinger W, Peterson FB, Banaji M et al: Engraftment and transfusion requirements after allogeneic marrow transplantation for patients with acute non-lymphocytic leukemia in first complete remission. Bone Marrow Transplant 4:409, 1989
16. Kersey JH, Weisdorf D, Nesbit ME et al: Comparison of autologous and allogeneic bone marrow transplantation for treatment of high-risk refractory acute lymphoblastic leukemia. N Engl J Med 317:461, 1987
17. Braine HG, Sensenbrenner L, Wright SK et al: Bone marrow transplantation with major ABO blood group incompatibility using erythrocyte depletion of marrow prior to infusion. Blood 60:420, 1982
18. Blacklock HA, Gilmore MJ, Prentice HG et al: ABO-incompatible bone marrow transplantation: removal of red blood cells from donor marrow avoiding recipient antibody depletion. Lancet 2:1061, 1982
19. Bensinger WI, Buckner CD, Thomas ED et al: ABO-incompatible marrow transplants. Transplantation 33:427, 1982
20. Bleyer WA, Blaese RM, Bujak JS et al: Long term remission from acute myelogenous leukemia after bone marrow transplantation and recovery from acute graft-versus-host reaction and prolonged immunocompetence. Blood 45:171, 1975
21. Gorgone BC, Ritz J, Anderson KC: In vivo neutralization of isohemagglutinin (IH) prior to HLA matched ABO incompatible bone marrow transplantation. Blood 66:267a, 1985
22. Buckner CD, Clift RA, Sanders JE et al: ABO-incompatible marrow transplants. Transplantation 26:233, 1978
23. Lasky LC, Warkentin PI, Kersey JH et al: Hemotherapy in patients undergoing blood group incompatible bone marrow transplantation. Transfusion 23:277, 1983
24. Marmont AM, Domasio EE, Bacigalupo A et al: A to O bone marrow transplantation in severe aplastic anemia: dynamics of blood group conversion and demonstration of early dyserythropoiesis in the engrafted marrow. Br J Haematol 36:511, 1978
25. Rowley S, Braine H: Probable hemolysis following minor and incompatible marrow transplantation (IMT). Blood, suppl. 60:171a, 1982
26. Hows J, Beddow K, Gordon-Smith E et al: Donor-derived red blood cell antibodies and immune hemolysis after allogeneic bone marrow transplantation. Blood 67:177, 1986
27. Hazelhurst GR, Brenner MK, Wimperis JZ et al: Hemolysis after T-cell depleted bone marrow transplantation involving minor ABO incompatibility. Scand J Haematol 37:1, 1986
28. Gajewski JL, Petz LD, Calhoun L et al: Immune mediated hemolysis followed by massive reactive hemolysis associated with minor ABO incompatible bone marrow transplants from unrelated donors. Blood, suppl. 76:158a, 1990
29. Bensinger WI, Hadlock J, Slichter SJ: Identification of alloimmunized patients: use of radiolabeled allogeneic platelet kinetic measurements and platelet antibody tests. Blood 77:2372, 1991
30. Champlin RE, Horowitz MM, van Bekkum DW et al: Graft failure following bone marrow transplantation for severe aplastic anemia: risk factors and treatment results. Blood 73:606, 1989
31. Barge AJ, Johnson G, Witherspoon R, Torok-Storb B: Antibody-mediated marrow failure after allogeneic bone marrow transplantation. Blood 74:1477, 1989
32. Ho WG, Champlin RE, Winston DJ et al: Bone marrow transplantation in patients with leukemia previously transfused with blood products from family members. Br J Haematol 67:67, 1987
33. Klingemann HG, Self S, Banaji M et al: Refractoriness to random donor platelet transfusions in patients with aplastic anemia: a multivariate analysis of data from 264 cases. Br J Haematol 66:115, 1987
34. Galel S, Vayntrub T, Grumet FC: HLA alloimmunization in bone marrow transplant patients. p. S787. In the Proceedings of the Joint Congress of ISBT and AABB, 1990
35. Yankee RA, Grumet FC, Rogentine GN: Platelet transfusion therapy: the selection of compatible donors for refractory patients by lymphocyte HLA-typing. N Engl J Med 281:1208, 1969
36. Yankee RA, Graffs KS, Dowling R et al: Selection of unrelated compatible platelet donors by lymphocyte HL-A matching. N Engl J Med 288:760, 1973
37. Lohrmann HP, Bull MI, Decter JA et al: Platelet transfusions from HL-A compatible unrelated donors to alloimmunized patients. Ann Intern Med 80:9, 1974
38. Kickler TS, Braine H, Ness PM: The predictive value of crossmatching platelet transfusion for alloimmunized patients. Transfusion 25:385, 1985
39. Moroff G, Garraty G, Heal JM et al: Selection of platelets for refractory patients by HLA matching and prospective crossmatching. Transfusion 32:633, 1992
40. Gmur J, von Felton A, Osterwalder B et al: Delayed alloimmunization using

random single donor platelet transfusions: a prospective study in thrombocytopenic patients with acute leukemia. Blood 2:473, 1983

41. Sintnicolaas K, Vriesendorp HM, Sizoo W et al: Delayed alloimmunization by random single donor platelet transfusions. A randomized study to compare single donor and multiple donor platelet transfusions in cancer patients with severe thrombocytopenia. Lancet 1:750, 1981

42. Murphy MF, Metcalf P, Thomas H et al: Use of leukocyte-poor blood components and HLA-matched platelet donors to prevent HLA alloimmunization. Br J Haematol 62:529, 1986

43. Sherman L, Menitove J, Kagen LR et al: Ultraviolet-B irradiation of platelets: a preliminary trial of efficacy. Transfusion 32:402, 1992

44. Andreu G, Boccaccio C, Lecrubier C et al: Ultraviolet irradiation of platelet concentrates: feasibility in transfusion practice. Transfusion 30:401, 1990

45. Van Marwijk Kooy M, van Prooijen HC, Moes M et al: Use of leukocyte-depleted platelet concentrates for the prevention of refractoriness and primary HLA alloimmunization: a prospective, randomized trial. Blood 77:201, 1991

46. Saarinen UM, Kekomaki R, Siimes MA et al: Effective prophylaxis against platelet refractoriness in multitransfused patients by use of leukocyte-free components. Blood 75:512, 1990

47. Schiffer CA: Prevention of alloimmunization against platelets. Blood 77:1, 1991

48. Anderson KC, Gorgone BC, Wahlers E et al: Preparation and utilization of leukocyte poor apheresis platelets. Transfus Sci 12:163, 1991

49. Tucker J, Murphy MF, Gregory W et al: Removal of graft-versus-leukemia effect by the use of leukocyte-poor blood components in patients with acute myeloblastic leukemia, letter. Br J Haematol 69:118, 1988

50. Lopez J, Fernandez-Villalta MJ, Gomez-Reino F, Fernandez-Ramada JM: Absence of graft-versus-leukemia effect of standard hemotherapy in patients with acute myeloblastic leukemia, letter. Transfusion 30:191, 1990

51. Sayers MH, Anderson KC, Goodnough LT et al: Reducing the risk for transfusion-transmitted cytomegalovirus infection. Ann Intern Med 116:55, 1992

52. Rubie H, Attal M, Campardou AM et al: Risk factors for cytomegalovirus infection in BMT recipients transfused exclusively with seronegative blood products. Bone Marrow Transplant 11:209, 1993

53. Hersman J, Meyers JD, Thomas ED et al: The effect of granulocyte transfusions upon the incidence of cytomegalovirus infection after allogeneic marrow transplantation. Ann Intern Med 96:149, 1982

54. Bowden RA, Sayers M, Fluornoy N et al: Cytomegalovirus immune globulin and seronegative blood products to prevent primary cytomegalovirus infection after marrow transplantation. N Engl J Med 314:1006, 1986

55. Winston DJ, Ho WG, Lin CH et al: Intravenous immune globulin for prevention of cytomegalovirus infection and interstitial pneumonia after bone marrow transplantation. Ann Intern Med 106:12, 1987

56. Filipovich AH, Peltier MH, Bechtel MK et al: Circulating cytomegalovirus (CMV) neutralizing activity in bone marrow transplant recipients: comparison of passive immunity in a randomized study of four intravenous IgG products administered to CMV-seronegative patients. Blood 80:2656, 1992

57. Miller W, Flynn P, McCullough J et al: Cytomegalovirus infection after bone marrow transplantation: an association with acute graft-versus-host disease. Blood 67:1162, 1986

58. Meyers JD, Reed EC, Shepp DH et al: Acyclovir for prevention of cytomegalovirus infection and disease after allogeneic marrow transplantation. N Engl J Med 318:70, 1988

59. Reed EC, Bowden RA, Dindliker PS et al: Treatment of cytomegalovirus pneumonia with ganciclovir and intravenous cytomegalovirus immunoglobulin in patients with bone marrow transplants. Ann Intern Med 109:783, 1988

60. Emmanuel D, Cunningham I, Jules-Elysse K et al: Cytomegalovirus pneumonia after bone marrow transplantation successfully treated with the combination of ganciclovir and high-dose intravenous immune globulin. Ann Intern Med 109:777, 1988

61. Wingard JR, Chen DYH, Burns WH et al: Cytomegalovirus infection after autologous bone marrow transplantation with comparison to infection after allogeneic bone marrow transplantation. Blood 71:1432, 1988

62. Reusser P, Fisher LD, Buckner CD et al: Cytomegalovirus infection after autologous bone marrow transplantation: occurrence of cytomegalovirus disease and effect on engraftment. Blood 75:1988, 1990

63. Verdonck LF, van der Linden JA, Bast BJEG et al: Influence of cytomegalovirus infection on the recovery of humoral immunity after autologous bone marrow transplantation. Exp Hematol 15:864, 1987

64. Gilbert GL, Hayes K, Hudson IL et al: Prevention of transfusion-acquired cytomegalovirus infection in infants by blood filtration to remove leukocytes. Lancet 1:1228, 1989

65. Murphy MF, Grint PCA, Hardiman AE et al: Use of leukocyte-poor blood components to prevent primary cytomegalovirus (CMV) infections in patients with acute leukaemia. Br J Haematol 70:253, 1988

66. De Graan-Hentzen YCE, Gratama JW, Mudde GC et al: Prevention of primary cytomegalovirus infection in patients with hematologic malignancies by intensive white cell depletion of blood products. Transfusion 29:757, 1989

67. Bowden RA, Slichter SJ, Sayers MH et al: The use of leukocyte-depleted platelets and cytomegalovirus seronegative red cells for prevention of primary cytomegalovirus infection after marrow transplant. Blood 78:246, 1991

68. De Witte T, Schattenberg A, Van Djik BA et al: Prevention of primary cytomegalovirus infection after allogeneic bone marrow transplantation by using leukocyte-poor random donor blood products from cytomegalovirus unscreened blood bank donors. Transplantation 50:964, 1990

69. Anderson KC, Weinstein HJ: Transfusion-associated graft versus host disease. N Engl J Med 323:315, 1990

70. Anderson KC, Goodnough LT, Pisciotto P et al: Variation in blood component irradiation practice: implications for prevention of transfusion associated graft versus host disease. Blood 73:2096, 1991

71. Postmus PE, Mulder NH, Elema JD: Graft versus host disease after transfusions of non-irradiated blood cells in patients having received autologous marrow. Eur J Cancer Clin Oncol 24:839, 1988

72. Drobyski W, Thibodeau S, Truitt RL et al: Third party mediated graft rejection and graft-versus-host disease after T cell depleted bone marrow transplantation, as demonstrated by hypervariable DNA probes and HLA-DR polymorphism. Blood 74:2285, 1989

73. Anderson KC, Nadler LM, Takvorian T et al: Monoclonal antibodies: their use in bone marrow transplantation. p. 137. In Brown E (ed): Progress in Hematology. Grune & Stratton, Orlando, FL, 1987

74. Sprent J, Von Boehmer H, Nabholz M: Association of immunity and tolerance to host H-2 determinants in irradiated F1 hybrid mice reconstituted with bone marrow cells from one parental strain. J Exp Med 142:321, 1975

75. Akahoshi M, Takanashi M, Masuda M et al: A case of transfusion-associated graft-versus-host disease not prevented by white cell-reduction filters. Transfusion 32:169, 1992

76. Deeg HJ, Graham TC, Gerhard Miller L et al: Prevention of transfusion-induced graft-versus-host disease in dogs by ultraviolet irradiation. Blood 74:2592, 1989

77. Shivdasani RA, Haluska FG, Dock NL et al: Brief report: graft-versus-host disease associated with transfusion of blood from unrelated HLA-homozygous donors. N Engl J Med 328:766, 1993

78. Thaler M, Shamiss A, Orgad S et al: The role of the blood from HLA-homozygous donors in fatal transfusion-associated graft-versus-host disease after open heart surgery. N Engl J Med 321:25, 1989

79. Ohto H, Yasuda H, Noguchi M, Abe K: Risk of transfusion-associated graft-versus-host disease as a result of directed donations from relatives. Transfusion 32:691, 1992

80. Lane TA, Anderson KC, Goodnough LT et al: Leukocyte reduction in blood component therapy. Ann Intern Med 117:151, 1992

81. Blumberg N, Heal JM: Transfusion and host defense against cancer recurrence and infection. Transfusion 29:236, 1989

82. Anderson KC: Current trends: evolving concepts in transfusion medicine: who should receive leukodepleted blood components? Transfus Sci 13:107, 1992

83. Rowley SD, Davis JM: Standards for bone marrow processing laboratories. Transfusion 30:571, 1990

84. Widmann FK (ed): Standards for Blood Banks and Transfusion Services. American Association of Blood Banks, Bethesda, MD, 1993, p.45.

85. Faradji A, Andreu G, Pillier-Loriette C et al: Separation of mononuclear bone marrow cells using the COBE 2997 blood cell separator. Vox Sang 55:133, 1988

86. English D, Lamberson R, Graves V et al: Semiautomated processing of bone marrow grafts for transplantation. Transfusion 29:12, 1989

87. Areman EM, Cullis H, Spitzer T, Sacher RA: Automated processing of human bone marrow can result in a population of mononuclear cells capable of achieving engraftment following transplantation. Transfusion 31:724, 1991

88. Saarinen UM, Lahteenoja KM, Juvonen E: Bone marrow fractionation by the Haemonetics system: reduction of red cell mass before marrow freezing, with special reference to pediatric marrow volumes. Vox Sang 63:16, 1992

89. Rowley SD, Davis J, Dick J et al: Bacterial contamination of bone marrow grafts intended for autologous and allogeneic bone marrow transplantation. Transfusion 28:109, 1988

90. Anderson KC: Malignant cell purging: monoclonal antibodies. In Lasky (ed): Stem Cell and Marrow Processing for Transplantation: Review and Update. American Association of Blood Banks, Rockville, MD, (in press)

91. Benjamin D, Magrath IT, Douglas EC, Corash LM: Derivation of lymphoma cell lines from microscopically normal bone marrow in patients with undif-

ferentiated lymphomas: evidence of occult bone marrow involvement. Blood 61:1017, 1983

92. Gribben JG, Freedman AS, Neuberg D et al: Immunologic purging of marrow assessed by PCR before autologous bone marrow transplantation for B cell lymphoma. N Engl J Med 325:1525, 1991

93. Leach MF, Howell AL, Ball ED et al: Automated elimination of leukemic cells using antibody and complement, abstracted. Transfusion 27:526, 1987

94. Rowley SD, Jones RJ, Piantadosi S: Efficacy of ex vivo purging for autologous bone marrow transplantation in the treatment of acute nonlymphoblastic leukemia. Blood 74:501, 1989

95. Freedman AS, Takvorian T, Anderson KC et al: Autologous bone marrow transplantation in B-cell non-Hodgkin's lymphoma: very low treatment-related mortality in 100 patients in sensitive relapse. J Clin Oncol 8:784, 1990

96. Gribben JG, Saporito L, Barber M et al: Bone marrows of non-Hodgkin's lymphoma patients with a bcl-2 translocation can be purged of polymerase chain reaction-detectable lymphoma cells using monoclonal antibodies and immunomagnetic bead depletion. Blood 80:1083, 1992

97. Sharp JG, Joshi SS, Armitage JO et al: Significance of detection of occult non-Hodgkin's lymphoma in histologically uninvolved bone marrow by a culture technique. Blood 79:1074, 1992

98. Gorin NC, Aegerter P, Auvert B et al: Autologous bone marrow transplantation for acute myelocytic leukemia in first remission: a European survey of the role of marrow purging. Blood 75:1606, 1990

99. Rowley SD, Zuehlsdorf M, Braine HG et al: CFU-GM content of bone marrow graft correlates with time to hematologic reconstitution following autologous bone marrow transplantation with 4-hydroperoxycyclophosphamide-purged bone marrow. Blood 70:271, 1987

100. Rowley SD, Byrne DV: Low-temperature storage of bone marrow in nitrogen vapor-phase refrigerators: decreased temperature gradients with an aluminum racking system. Transfusion 32:750, 1992

101. Stiff PJ, Koester AR, Weidner MK et al: Autologous bone marrow transplantation using unfractionated cells cryopreserved in dimethylsulfoxide and hydroxyethyl starch without controlled-rate freezing. Blood 70:974, 1987

102. Sonneveld P, deLeeuw CA, Schipperus M et al: Transfusion of red cells after autologous bone marrow harvest in patients with acute leukemia and malignant lymphoma. Transfusion 30:310, 1990

103. Ciobanu N, Weinberg V, Sparano JA et al: Experience with autologous bone marrow harvesting and transfusion of marrow-derived red cells. Transfusion 32:231, 1992

104. Thomas ED, Storb R, Giblett ER et al: Recovery from aplastic anemia following attempted marrow transplantation. Exp Hematol 4:97, 1975

105. Sparkes MC, Crist ML, Sparkes RS et al: Gene markers in human bone marrow transplantation. Vox Sang 33:202, 1977

106. Zaccaria A, Rosti G, Testoni N et al: Chromosone studies in patients with Philadelphia chromosome-positive chronic myeloid leukemia submitted to bone marrow transplantation. Results of a European cooperative study. Cancer Genet Cytogenet 26:5, 1987

107. Bosserman LD, Murray C, Takvorian T et al: Mechanism of graft failure in HLA-matched and HLA-mismatched bone marrow transplant recipients. Bone Marrow Transplant 4:239, 1989

108. Walker H, Singer CRJ, Patterson J et al: The significance of host haematopoietic cells detected by cytogenetic analysis of bone marrow from recipients of bone marrow transplants. Br J Haematol 62:385, 1986

109. Khokhar MT, Lawler S, Powles RL, Millar BL: Cytogenetic studies using Q-band polymorphisms in patients with AML receiving marrow from like-sex donors. Hum Genet 76:176, 1987

110. Schattenberg A, DeWitte T, Salden M et al: Mixed hematopoietic chimerism after allogeneic transplantation with lymphocyte-depleted bone marrow is not associated with a higher incidence of relapse. Blood 73:1367, 1989

111. Grahovac B, Labar B, Stavljenic A: Phenotyping of phosphoglucomutase (PGM1) isoenzymes—a method for the follow-up of chimerism after bone marrow transplantation. Enzyme 40:37, 1988

112. Morisaki H, Morisaki T, Nakahori Y et al: Genotypic analysis using a Y-chromosome-specific probe following bone marrow transplantation. Am J Hematol 27:30, 1988

113. Knowlton RG, Brown VA, Braman JC et al: Use of highly polymorphic DNA probes for genotypic analysis following bone marrow transplantation. Blood 68:378, 1986

114. Blazar BR, Orr HT, Arthur DC et al: Restriction fragment length polymorphisms as markers of engraftment in allogeneic marrow transplantation. Blood 66:1436, 1985

115. Roy DC, Tantravahi R, Murray C et al: Natural history of mixed chimerism after bone marrow transplantation with CD6-depleted allogeneic marrow: a stable equilibrium. Blood 75:296, 1990

116. Klumpp T, Caligiuri MA, Rabinowe SA et al: Autoimmune pancytopenia fol-

lowing allogeneic bone marrow transplantation. Bone Marrow Transplant 6:445, 1990

117. Minchinton RM, Waters AH, Malpas JS et al: Platelet and granulocyte-specific antibodies after allogeneic and autologous bone marrow grafts. Vox Sang 46:125, 1984

118. Eschbach JW, Kelly MR, Halley NR et al: Treatment of the anemia of progressive renal failure with recombinant human erythropoietin. N Engl J Med 321:158, 1989

119. Fischl M, Galpin JE, Levine JD et al: Recombinant human erythropoietin for patients with AIDS treated with zidovudine. N Engl J Med 322:1488, 1990

120. Ludwig H, Fritz E, Kotzmann H et al: Erythropoietin treatment of anemia associated with multiple myeloma. N Engl J Med 322:1693, 1990

121. Miller CB, Jones RJ, Piantadosi S et al: Decreased erythropoietin response in patients with the anemia of cancer. N Engl J Med 322:1689, 1990

122. Schapira L, Antin JH, Ransil BJ et al: Serum erythropoietin levels in patients receiving intensive chemotherapy and radiotherapy. Blood 76:2354, 1990

123. Beguin Y, Clemons GK, Oris R, Fillet G: Circulating erythropoietin levels after bone marrow transplantation: inappropriate response to anemia in allogeneic transplants. Blood 77:868, 1991

124. Ayash L, Elias A, Demetri G et al: Recombinant human erythropoietin (EPO) in anemia associated with autologous bone marrow transplantation (ABMT), abstracted. Blood, suppl. 1. 76:131a, 1990

125. Nienhius AW, Donahue RE, Karlsson S et al: Recombinant human granulocyte-macrophage colony stimulating factor (GM-CSF) shortens the period of neutropenia after autologous marrow transplantation in a primate model. J Clin Invest 80:573, 1987

126. Brandt SJ, Peters WP, Atwater SK et al: Effects of recombinant human granulocyte-macrophage colony-stimulating factor on hematopoietic reconstitution after high-dose chemotherapy and autologous bone marrow transplantation. N Engl J Med 318:869, 1988

127. Nemunaitis J, Singer JW, Buckner CD et al: Use of recombinant human granulocyte-macrophage colony-stimulating factor in autologous marrow transplantation for lymphoid malignancies. Blood 72:834, 1988

128. Nemunaitis J, Rabinowe SN, Singer JW et al: Recombinant granulocyte-macrophage colony-stimulating factor after autologous bone marrow transplantation for lymphoid cancer. N Engl J Med 324:1773, 1991

129. Blazar BR, Kersey JH, McGlave PB et al: In vivo administration of recombinant human granulocyte-macrophage colony-stimulating factor in acute lymphoblastic leukemia patients receiving purged autografts. Blood 73:849, 1989

130. Nemunaitis J, Singer JW, Buckner CD et al: Use of recombinant human granulocyte-macrophage colony-stimulating factor in graft failure after bone marrow transplantation. Blood 76:245, 1990

131. Nemunaitis J, Buckner CD, Appelbaum FR et al: Phase I/II trial of recombinant human granulocyte-macrophage colony-stimulating factor following allogeneic bone marrow transplantation. Blood 77:2065, 1991

132. Sarpel SC, Axel Z, Harvath L et al: The collection, preservation and function of peripheral blood hematopoietic cells in dogs. Exp Hematol 7:113, 1979

133. Goldman JR, Catovsky D, Galton DAG: Reversal of blast cell crisis in CGL by transfusion of stored autologous buffy-coat cells. Lancet 1:437, 1978

134. Kessinger A, Armitage JO, Landmark JD et al: Autologous peripheral hematopoietic stem cell transplantation restores hematopoietic function following marrow ablative therapy. Blood 71:723, 1988

135. Lasky LC: Hematopoietic reconstitution using progenitors recovered from blood. Transfusion 29:552, 1989

136. Griepp PR, Ahmann G, Katzman JA et al: Peripheral blood as a source of stem cells in myeloma, abstracted. Blood, suppl. 72:243a, 1988

137. Moss TJ, Sanders DG, Lasky LC, Bostrom B: Contamination of peripheral blood stem cell harvests by circulating neuroblastoma cells. Blood 76:1879, 1990

138. Molineux G, Pojda Z, Hampson N et al: Transplantation potential of peripheral blood stem cells induced by granulocyte colony-stimulating factor. Blood 76:2153, 1990

139. Peters WP, Rosner G, Ross M et al: Comparative effects of granulocyte-macrophage colony-stimulating factor (GM-CSF) and granulocyte colony-stimulating factor (G-CSF) on priming peripheral blood progenitor cells for use with autologous bone marrow after high-dose chemotherapy. Blood 81:1709, 1993

140. Siena S, Bregni M, Brando B et al: Circulation of CD34$^+$ hematopoietic stem cells in the peripheral blood of high-dose cyclophosphamide-treated patients: enhancement by intravenous recombinant human granulocyte-macrophage colony-stimulating factor. Blood 74:1905, 1989

141. Elias AD, Ayash L, Anderson KC et al: Mobilization of peripheral blood progenitor cells by chemotherapy and granulocyte-macrophage colony-stimulating factor for hematologic support after high-dose intensification for breast cancer. Blood 79:3036, 1992

142. Brugger W, Bross K, Frisch J et al: Mobilization of peripheral blood progenitor cells by sequential administration of interleukin-3 and granulocyte-macrophage colony-stimulating factor following polychemotherapy with etoposide, ifosfamide, and cisplatin. Blood 79:1193, 1992

143. Shea TC, Mason JR, Storniolo AM et al: Sequential cycles of high-dose carboplatin administered with recombinant human granulocyte-macrophage colony-stimulating factor and repeated infusions of autologous peripheral-blood progenitor cells: a novel and effective method for delivering multiple courses of dose-intensive therapy. J Clin Oncol 10:464, 1992

144. Neben S, Marcus K, Mauch P: Mobilization of hematopoietic stem and progenitor cell subpopulations from the marrow to the blood of mice following cyclophosphamide and/or granulocyte colony-stimulating factor. Blood 81:1960, 1993

145. Hornung RL, Longo DL: Hematopoietic stem cell depletion by restorative growth factor regimens during repeated high-dose cyclophosphamide therapy. Blood 80:77, 1992

146. Andrews RG, Bryant EM, Bartelmez SH et al: CD34$^+$ marrow cells, devoid of T and B lymphocytes, reconstitute stable lymphopoiesis and myelopoiesis in lethally irradiated allogeneic baboons. Blood 80:1693, 1992

147. Berenson RJ, Bensinger WI, Hill RS et al: Engraftment after infusion of CD34$^+$ marrow cells in patients with breast cancer or neuroblastoma. Blood 77:1717, 1991

148. Egeland T, Steen R, Quarsten H et al: Myeloid differentiation of purified CD34$^+$ cells after stimulation with recombinant human granulocyte-monocyte colony-stimulating factor (CSF), granulocyte-CSF, monocyte-CSF, and interleukin-3. Blood 78:3192, 1991

149. Haylock DN, To LB, Dowse TL et al: Ex vivo expansion and maturation of peripheral blood CD34$^+$ cells into the myeloid lineage. Blood 80:1405, 1992

150. Srour EF, Brandt JE, Briddell RA et al: Long-term generation and expansion of human primitive hematopoietic progenitor cells in vitro. Blood 81:661, 1993

151. Gluckman E, Broxmeyer HE, Auerbach AD et al: Hematopoietic reconstitution in a patient with Fanconi's anemia by means of umbilical-cord blood from an HLA-identical sibling. N Engl J Med 321:1174, 1989

152. Wagner JE, Broxmeyer HE, Byrd RL et al: Transplantation of umbilical cord blood after myeloablative therapy: analysis of engraftment. Blood 79:1874, 1992

153. Rubinstein P, Rosenfield RE, Adamson JW, Stevens CE: Stored placental blood for unrelated bone marrow reconstitution. Blood 81:1679, 1993

154. Lu L, Xiao M, Shen R-N et al: Enrichment, characterization, and responsiveness of single primitive CD34^{+++} human umbilical cord blood hematopoietic progenitors with high proliferative and replating potential. Blood 81:41, 1993

155. Flye MW: Immunosuppressive therapy. p. 155. In Flye MW (ed): Principles of Organ Transplantation. WB Saunders, Philadelphia, 1989

156. Sigal NH, Dumont FJ: Cyclosporin A, FK-506, and rapamycin: pharmacologic probes of lymphocyte signal transduction. Annu Rev Immunol 10:519, 1992

157. Keown PA: Annual review of transplantation. p. 205. In Terasaki PI, Cecka JM (eds): Clinical Transplants. UCLA Tissue Typing Laboratory, Los Angeles, 1991

158. Opelz G, Sengar DPS, Mickey MR et al: Effect of blood transfusion on subsequent kidney transplants. Transplant Proc 4:253, 1973

159. Terasaki PI (ed): Blood Transfusion and Transplantation. Grune & Stratton, Orlando, FL, 1982, p. 1

160. Rodney GE: Blood transfusions and their influence on renal allograft survival. Prog Hematol 14:99, 1986

161. Opelz G: Improved kidney graft survival in nontransfused recipients. Transplant Proc 19:149, 1987

162. Lundgren G, Albrechtsen D, Flatmark A et al: HLA-matching and pretransplant blood transfusions in cadaveric renal transplantation—a changing picture with cyclosporine. Lancet 2:66, 1986

163. Deierhol MH, Barger BO, Hudson SL et al: The effect of erythropoietin and blood transfusions on highly sensitized patients on a single cadaver renal allograft waiting list. Transplantation 53:363, 1992

164. Kerman RH, Van Buren CT, Lewis RM et al: Successful transplantation of 100 untransfused cyclosporine-treated primary recipients of cadaveric renal allografts. Transplantation 45:37, 1988

165. Cecka JM, Cicciarelli J, Mickey MR et al: Blood transfusions and HLA matching—an either/or situation in cadaveric renal transplantation. Transplantation 45:81, 1988

166. Terasaki PI: The beneficial transfusion effect on kidney graft survival attributed to clonal deletion. Transplantation 37:119, 1984

167. Reed E, Hardy M, Benvenisty A et al: Effect of antiidiotypic antibodies to HLA on graft survival in renal-allograft recipients. N Engl J Med 316:1450, 1987

168. Barkley SC, Sakai RB, Ettenger RN et al: Determination of antiidiotypic antibodies to anti-HLA IgG following blood transfusion. Transplantation 44:30, 1987

169. Reinsmoen NL, Kaufman D, Matas A et al: A new in vitro approach to determine acquired tolerance in long-term kidney allograft recipients. Transplantation 50:783, 1990

170. Grailer AP, Sollinger HW, Kawamura T et al: Donor-specific cytotoxic T lymphocyte hyporesponsiveness following renal transplantation in patients pretreated with donor-specific transfusions. Transplantation 51:320, 1991

171. Starzl TE, Demetris AJ, Murase N et al: Cell migration, chimerism, and graft acceptance. Lancet 339:1579, 1992

172. Szulman AE: The histological distribution of blood group substances A and B in man. J Exp Med 111:785, 1960

173. Bariety J, Oriol R, Hinglais N et al: Distribution of blood group antigen A in normal and pathologic human kidneys. Kidney Int 17:820, 1980

174. Oriol R, Cartron JP, Cartron J et al: Biosynthesis of ABH and Lewis antigens in normal and transplanted kidneys. Transplantation 29:184, 1980

175. Starzl TE, Marchioro TC, Holmes JH et al: Renal homografts in patients with major donor-recipient blood group incompatibilities. Surgery 55:195, 1964

176. Willbrant R, Tung KSK, Deodar SD et al: ABO blood group incompatibility in human renal transplantation. Am J Clin Pathol 51:15, 1969

177. Nelson PW, Helling TS, Pierce GE et al: Successful transplantation of blood group A$_2$ kidneys into non-A recipients. Transplantation 45:316, 1988

178. Rydberg L, Breimer ME, Brynger H et al: ABO-incompatible kidney transplantation (A$_2$ to O). Transplantation 49:954, 1990

179. Alexandre GPJ, Squifflet JP, DeBruyere M et al: Present experience in a series of 26 ABO-incompatible living donor renal allografts. Transplant Proc 19:4538, 1987

180. Kissmeyer-Nielson F, Olsen S, Peterson VP et al: Hyperacute rejection of kidney allografts associated with pre-existing humoral antibodies against donor cells. Lancet 2:662, 1966

181. Sibley RK, Snover DC: The use and interpretation of biopsies in the management of the post-transplant patient. p. 396. In Cerilli GJ (ed): Organ Transplantation and Replacement. JB Lippincott, Philadelphia, 1988

182. Scornik JC, Brunson ME, Howard RJ et al: Alloimmunization, memory, and the interpretation of crossmatch results for renal transplantation. Transplantation 54:389, 1992

183. Duquesnoy RJ, White LT, Fierst JW et al: Multiscreen serum analysis of highly sensitized renal dialysis patients for antibodies toward public and private class I HLA determinants. Transplantation 50:427, 1990

184. Matas AJ, Tellis VA, Quinn TA et al: Successful transplantation of highly sensitized patients without regard to HLA matching. Transplantation 45:338, 1988

185. Thorogood J, Persijn GG, Schreuder GMTH et al: The effect of HLA matching of kidney graft survival in separate posttransplantation intervals. Transplantation 50:146, 1990

186. Takemoto S, Cecka JM, Gjertson DW et al: Six-antigen-matched transplants. Transplantation 55:1005, 1993

187. Takiff H, Cook DJ, Himaya NS et al: Dominant effect of histocompatibility on ten-year transplant survival. Transplantation 45:410, 1988

188. Opelz G, Mytilineos J, Scherer S et al: Survival of DNA HLA-DR typed and matched cadaver kidney transplants. Lancet 338:461, 1991

189. Bodmer JG, Marsh SGE, Albert ED et al: Nomenclature for factors of the HLA system, 1991. Tissue Antigens 39:161, 1992

190. Spies T, Blanck G, Bresnahan M et al: A new cluster of genes within the human major histocompatibility complex. Science 243:214, 1989

191. Mytilineos J, Scherer S, Dunckley H et al: DNA HLA-DR typing results of 4000 kidney transplants. Transplantation 55:778, 1993

192. Opelz G, Mytilineos J, Scherer S et al: Analysis of HLA-DR matching in DNA-typed cadaver kidney transplants. Transplantation 55:782, 1993

193. Takiff H, Iwaki Y, Cecka M et al: The benefit and underutilization of sharing kidneys for better histocompatibility. Transplantation 47:102, 1989

194. Opelz G: Collaborative transplant study kidney exchange trial for highly sensitized recipients. p. 61. In Terasaki PI, Cecka JM (eds): Clinical Transplants. UCLA Tissue Typing Laboratory, Los Angeles, 1992

195. Wick MR, Moore SB: The role of the Lewis antigen system in renal transplantation and allograft rejection. Mayo Clin Proc 59:423, 1984

196. Gratama JWC, Hendriks GFJ, Persijn GG et al: The interaction between the Lewis blood group system and HLA-matching in renal transplantation. Transplantation 45:926, 1988

197. Cerilli J, Clarke J, Abrams A et al: Overview: significance of vascular endothelial cell antigen. Transplant Proc 19:4468, 1987

198. Joyce S, Flye MW, Mohanakumar T: Characterization of kidney cell-specific, non-major histocompatibility complex alloantigen using antibodies eluted from rejected human renal allografts. Transplantation 46:362, 1988

199. Cerilli J, Clarke J, Doolin T et al: The significance of a donor-specific vessel crossmatch in renal transplantation. Transplantation 46:359, 1988

00. Joyce S, Mathew JM, Flye MW et al: A polymorphic human kidney-specific non-MHC alloantigen. Transplantation 53:1119, 1992
01. Calne R (ed): Liver Transplantation: The Cambridge/King's College Experience. 2nd Ed. Grune & Stratton, London, 1987
02. Winter P, Kang YG: Hepatic Transplantation: Anesthetic and Perioperative Management. Praeger Scientific, New York, 1986
03. Lewis JH, Bontempo FA, Cornell F et al: Blood use in liver transplantation. Transfusion 27:222, 1987
04. Bontempo FA, Lewis JH, Van Thiel DH et al: The relation of preoperative coagulation findings to diagnosis, blood usage, and survival in adult liver transplantation. Transplantation 39:532, 1985
05. Dzik WH, Arkin CF, Jenkins RL et al: Fibrinolysis during liver transplantation in humans: role of tissue-type plasminogen activator. Blood 71:1090, 1988
06. Porte RJ, Bontempo FA, Knot EAR et al: Systemic effects of tissue plasminogen activator-associated fibrinolysis and its relation to thrombin generation in orthotopic liver transplantation. Transplantation 47:978, 1989
07. Lewis JH, Bontempo FA, Awad SA et al: Liver transplantation: intraoperative changes in coagulation factors in 100 first transplants. Hepatology 9:710, 1989
08. Kang Y, Lewis JH, Navalgund A et al: Epsilon-aminocaproic acid for treatment of fibrinolysis during liver transplantation. Anesthesiology 66:766, 1987
09. Himmelreich G, Muser M, Neuhaus P et al: Different aprotinin applications influencing hemostatic changes in orthotopic liver transplantation. Transplantation 53:132, 1992
10. Blankensteijn JD, Terpstra OT: Liver preservation: the past and the future. Hepatology 13:1235, 1991
11. Velasco F, Villalba R, Fernandez M et al: Diminished anticoagulant and fibrinolytic activity following liver transplantation. Transplantation 53:1256, 1992
12. Dzik WH, Jenkins RL: Use of intraoperative blood salvage during orthotopic liver transplantation. Arch Surg 120:946, 1985
13. Williamson KR, Taswell HF, Rettke SR et al: Intraoperative autologous transfusion: its role in orthotopic liver transplantation. Mayo Clin Proc 64:340, 1989
14. Kang YG, Martin DJ, Marquez J et al: Intraoperative changes in blood coagulation and thrombelastographic monitoring in liver transplantation. Anesth Analg 64:888, 1985
15. Ramsey G, Cornell FW, Hahn LF et al: Red cell antibody problems in 1000 liver transplants. Transfusion 27:552, 1987
16. Motschman TL, Taswell HF, Brecher ME: Blood bank support of a liver transplantation program. Mayo Clin Proc 64:103, 1989
17. Dzik WH: Blood component therapy during liver transplantation in adults. p. 1. In Gambino SR (ed): Check Sample—Immunohematology. American Society of Clinical Pathologists, Chicago, 1988
18. Kang YG, Gelman S: Liver transplantation. p. 139. In Gelman S (ed): Anesthesia and Organ Transplantation. WB Saunders, Philadelphia, 1987
19. Marquez JM Jr: Citrate intoxication during hepatic transplantation. p. 110. In Winter PM, Kang YG (eds): Transplantation: Anesthetic and Perioperative Management. Praeger Scientific, New York, 1986
20. Dzik WH, Kirkley S: Citrate toxicity during massive blood transfusion. Transfus Med Rev 2:76, 1988
21. Gordon RD, Shunzaburo I, Ewquivel CO et al: Liver transplantation across ABO blood groups. Surgery 100:342, 1986
22. Bismuth H, Samuel D, Gugenheim J et al: Emergency liver transplantation for fulminant hepatitis. Ann Intern Med 107:337, 1987
23. Gugenheim J, Samuel D, Reynes M et al: Liver transplantation across ABO blood group barriers. Lancet 336:519, 1990
24. Demetris AJ, Jaffe R, Tzakis A et al: Antibody-mediated rejection of human orthotopic liver allografts: a study of liver transplantation across ABO blood group barriers. Am J Pathol 132:489, 1988
25. Ramsey G, Nusbacher J, Starzl TE et al: Isohemagglutinins of graft origin after ABO-unmatched liver transplantation. N Engl J Med 311:1167, 1984
26. Ahmed KY, Nunn G, Brazier DM et al: Hemolytic anemia resulting from autoantibodies produced by the donor's lymphocytes after renal transplantation. Transplantation 43:163, 1987
227. Mangal AK, Growe GH, Sinclair M et al: Acquired hemolytic anemia due to "auto" anti-A or "auto" anti-B induced by group O homograft in renal transplant recipients. Transfusion 24:201, 1984
228. Beck ML, Haines RF, Oberman HA: Unexpected serologic findings following lung homotransplantation, abstracted. p. 98. In the Proceedings of the Second Annual Meeting of the American Association of Blood Banks. American Association of Blood Banks, Chicago, 1971
229. Hunt BJ, Yacoub M, Amin S et al: Induction of red blood cell destruction by graft-derived antibodies after minor ABO-mismatched heart and lung transplantation. Transplantation 46:246, 1988
230. Salamon DJ, Ramsey G, Nusbacher J et al: Anti-A production by a group O spleen transplanted to a group A recipient. Vox Sang 48:309, 1985
231. Swanson J, Sastomoinen R, Steeper T et al: Production of anti-A and B by donor lymphocytes following transplantation of group O organs to ABO incompatible patients receiving cyclosporin A. Transfusion 24:431, 1984
232. Dzik WH, Jenkins RL: Renal failure from ABO hemolysis due to anti-A of graft origin following liver transplantation. Transfusion 27:550, 1987
233. Ratner LE, Phelan D, Brunt EM et al: Probable antibody-mediated failure of two sequential ABO-compatible hepatic allografts in a single recipient. Transplantation 55:814, 1993
234. Karuppan S, Ericzon BG, Moller E: Relevance of a positive crossmatch in liver transplantation. Transplant Int 4:18, 1991
235. Takaya S, Bronsther O, Iwaki Y et al: The adverse impact on liver transplantation of using positive cytotoxic crossmatch donors. Transplantation 53:400, 1992
236. Fung J, Makowka L, Tzakis A et al: Combined liver-kidney transplantation: analysis of patients with preformed lymphocytotoxic antibodies. Transplant Proc 20:88, 1988
237. Gonwa TA, Nery JR, Husberg BS et al: Simultaneous liver and renal transplantation in man. Transplantation 46:690, 1988
238. Markus BH, Duquesnoy RJ, Gordon RD et al: Histocompatibility and liver transplant outcome: does HLA exert a dualistic effect? Transplantation 46:372, 1988
239. Manez R, White LT, Linden P et al: The influence of HLA matching on cytomegalovirus hepatitis and chronic rejection after liver transplantation. Transplantation 55:1067, 1993
240. Baldwin JC, Wolfgang TC, Shumway NE et al: Cardiac transplantation. p. 385. In Flye MW (ed): Principles of Organ Transplantation. WB Saunders, Philadelphia, 1989
241. Thorpe SJ, Hunt B, Yacoub M: Expression of ABH blood group antigens in human heart tissue and its relevance to cardiac transplantation. Transplantation 51:1290, 1991
242. Salomon RN, Hughes CCW, Schoen FJ et al: Human coronary transplant-associated arteriosclerosis: evidence for a chronic immune reaction to activated graft endothelial cells. Am J Pathol 138:791, 1991
243. Suciu-Foca N, Reed E, Marboe C et al: The role of anti-HLA antibodies in heart transplantation. Transplantation 51:716, 1991
244. Smith JD, Danskine AJ, Rose ML et al: Specificity of lymphocytotoxic antibodies formed after cardiac transplantation and correlation with rejection episodes. Transplantation 53:1358, 1992
245. Snydman DR, Werner BG, Heinze-Lacey B et al: Use of cytomegalovirus immune globulin to prevent cytomegalovirus disease in renal-transplant recipients. N Engl J Med 317:1049, 1987
246. Stratta RJ, Shaefer MS, Cushing KA et al: Successful prophylaxis of cytomegalovirus disease after primary CMV exposure in liver transplant recipients. Transplantation 51:90, 1991
247. Tsevat J, Snydman DR, Pauker SG et al: Which renal transplant patients should receive cytomegalovirus immune globulin? Transplantation 52:259, 1991
248. Harbison MA, DeGirolami PC, Jenkins RL et al: Ganciclovir therapy of severe cytomegalovirus infections in solid-organ transplant recipients. Transplantation 46:82, 1988
249. Paya CV, Hermans PE, Smith TF et al: Efficacy of ganciclovir in liver and kidney transplant recipients with severe cytomegalovirus infection. Transplantation 46:229, 1988

Red Cell Substitutes

146

Robert M. Winslow

INTRODUCTION

Red cell substitutes are designed to replace red blood cells for transfusion. These substitutes would carry out the primary function of red cells: transport of oxygen to tissues. The goal of developing a red cell substitute has been elusive: for centuries, an alternative to allogeneic blood for transfusion has been sought by scientists, the military, and by industry. Early attempts included the use of milk, wine, gum, and red cell hemolysates. In the modern era (since about 1965), three general types of products have been under development: modified hemoglobin solutions, perfluorocarbon emulsions, and lipid vesicle-encapsulated hemoglobin. None is as yet approved for clinical use.

The current driving force for the development of red cell substitutes is the perceived danger of transfusion of allogenic blood (Table 146-1). In fact, blood is safer now than it ever has been. However, the aggregate risks listed in Table 146-1 are frightening to many patients, their families, and their doctors as well, and the demand for a safe and efficacious alternative is increasing. Beyond the risks listed in Table 146-1, it should be emphasized that in regions of the world where the frequency of human immunodeficiency virus infection is high, development of these solutions would be particularly important.

Because of the risks of allogenic blood transfusion, and because of the large markets that could be generated for red cell substitutes, considerable efforts are now being expended by industry and academia to develop safe products. It is likely that red cell substitutes will find their way into clinical practice within the next decade.

PRINCIPLES

Several major issues must be addressed in order to develop a successful red cell substitute.

1. *Oxygen transport:* Must a red cell substitute transport oxygen in the same way as red cells do? Oxygen affinity and cooperatively of cell-free or encapsulated hemoglobin may be very different from that of red cells. Perfluorocarbons carry oxygen physically dissolved, rather than chemically bound, and therefore the dissociation curve is linear. Whether these factors are important, physiologically or clinically, is not yet known.
2. *Plasma retention:* The normal red cell life span is about 120 days. However, the plasma half-life of cell-free hemoglobin may be only 12 hours and that of encapsulated hemoglobin

and perfluorocarbon emulsions 24–48 hours. Are these times clinically useful? If the effect of a red cell substitute is so short that a transfusion with allogeneic blood is only delayed, not eliminated, then the usefulness of the product becomes questionable.
3. *Efficacy:* It will be necessary to demonstrate efficacy for any red cell substitute to be used clinically. At present, it is taken as a matter of faith that a solution carrying oxygen will be more useful than one with no oxygen, if it is without side effects. However, conclusive demonstrations will be necessary because no red cell substitutes currently being developed are without side effects. For example, if a particular substitute increases systemic pressure and vascular resistance (as many hemoglobin-based solutions do), this property could counteract any increase in oxygen transported.
4. *Toxicity:* No candidate product developed to date is without toxicity. Cell-free hemoglobin has vasoconstrictor properties that could limit its use in shock and trauma. Lipid vesicles and perfluorocarbon emulsions stimulate macrophages to elaborate cytokines that can produce diverse effects, including fever and flu-like symptoms.
5. *Commercial viability:* To be successful, a red cell substitute must be competitive with allogeneic red blood cells in effect, toxicity, and cost. The cost of providing human red cells for transfusion is now very low.[1] The technology required for the production of red cell substitutes is complex, and likely to be expensive.

CLINICAL APPLICATIONS

Products

Hemoglobin-Based Products

The red cell substitute products that have gained the most attention are based on hemoglobin, an extraordinarily complex molecule consisting of four polypeptide chains, each one made up of about 140 amino acids. Normally packaged in the red cell, free in solution it is fragile: it tends to oxidize, is unstable and toxic, and is excreted by the kidneys as the subunits fall apart. Over the years, the strategy for making a hemoglobin-based red cell substitute has been based on cross-linking hemoglobin to correct these problems.[2]

Hemoglobin has the desirable properties of a high capacity to bind oxygen and to release it cooperatively; this makes it attractive for use as a red cell substitute. However, hemoglobin, free in solution, has several unique properties: (1) its oxygen affinity is high because outside of the red cell the normal allosteric effectors, 2,3-diphosphoglycerate (2,3-DPG) and ATP, for example, are not present; (2) its effectiveness as an oxygen carrier is limited because it dissociates into half-molecules ($\alpha\beta$ dimers) (haptoglobin is rapidly saturated, and excess dimers are quickly removed from the circulation by the kidney after filtration in the glomerulus); (3) once filtered, a high concentration of protein in the renal tubules can cause tubular obstruction and consequent renal failure; (4) cell-free hemoglobin binds nitric oxide, an endothelium-derived relaxing factor, to produce vasoconstriction; (5) outside the red cell, hemoglobin exerts an oncotic pressure similar to that of albumin; thus, if large amounts are to be administered to a patient, shifts of

Table 146-1. Risks of Transfusion of Allogeneic Blood in the United States

Event	Risk
HIV	1/225,000
Hepatitis	1/3,300
HTLV I/II	1/50,000
Fever, chills	1/100
Hemolytic transfusion reaction	1/6,000
Fatal hemolytic transfusion reaction	1/100,000

(Data from Klein[1] and Winslow.[2])

Table 146-2. Classes of Hemoglobin Modification

Class	Examples
Amino-terminal modification	Carbamylation
	Carboxymethylation
	Pyridoxylation
	Acetaldehyde
Lysine (EF6(82)β modification	Mono-(3,5-dibromosalicyl) fumarate
Valine NA1(1)β-lysine EF6(82)ββ-cross-link	2-Nor-2-formylpyridoxal 5'-phosphate (NFPLP) (Bis-PL)P$_4$
Lysine G6(99)α$_1$-lysine G6(99)α$_2$-cross-link	Bis-(3,5-dibromosalicyl) fumarate (DBBF)
Three-point	Trimesoyl tris(methyl phosphate)
2,3-DPG analogue	Pyridoxal 5'-phosphate
	Bezafibrate, Clofibrate
Surface, multisite	Glutaraldehyde
	Ring-opened dials
	Diimidate esters
Conjugated hemoglobin	Dextran-aldehyde
	Polyethylene glycol
	Polyoxyethylene

(Modified from Winslow,[2] with permission.)

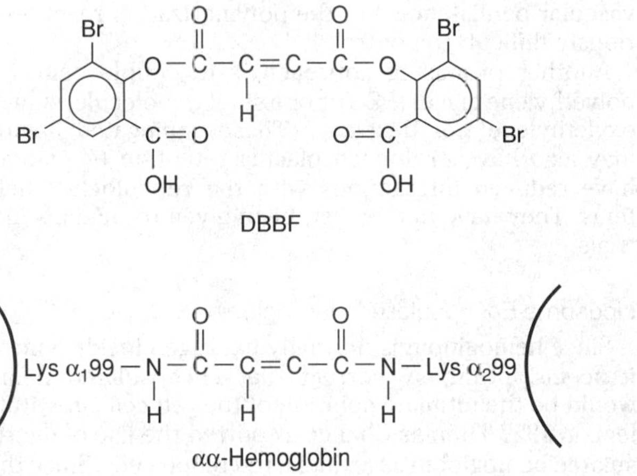

Fig. 146-1. The reaction of DBBF with hemoglobin. (From Winslow,[2] with permission.)

fluid between the interstitial and intravascular spaces would be expected; and (6) iron, when released from hemoglobin, can promote the formation of toxic oxygen radicals.

Thus, to be an effective oxygen carrier in the cell-free state, hemoglobin must be chemically modified to avoid these problems. Whether all these must be solved completely for a product to be useful is a matter of intense current debate.

All the reactions currently considered useful in the production of hemoglobin-based red substitutes use chemical modification at one or more sites on the surface of the protein (Table 146-2). Differences in the reactions are determined by the dimensions and reactivity of the cross-linking reagents. Since the function of hemoglobin in binding and releasing oxygen is intricately connected to the transition between T and R conformations (see Ch. 35), it is not surprising that the P$_{50}$ and yield are highly variable. Even small differences among structures of the reagents can yield products with quite different properties. In addition, the conditions of the reaction are very important, not only in regard to the state of ligation (i.e., oxygen saturation) but also in regard to the presence of agents or molecules that block or compete for certain reactive sites.

A further complication of these reactions is that many nonhemoglobin proteins, co-purified with hemoglobin, contain reactive groups and may also be modified to produce new, potentially toxic, contaminants. It is understandable that it has been difficult to produce a "pure" modified hemoglobin for toxicity studies when most processes start with relatively crude "stroma-free" hemoglobin.[3]

An example of a cross-linked hemoglobin currently being commercialized is a product studied intensively by the U.S. Army and a number of academic laboratories. Cross-linking of hemoglobin isolated from outdated human blood is carried out with bis-(3,5-dibromosalicyl)fumarate (DBBF)[4] (Table 146-2). The reaction results in a four-carbon covalent link between adjacent α-chains at position 99 (Lys α$_1$99-Lys α$_2$99) (Fig. 146-1). This covalently cross-linked hemoglobin cannot break down into subunits in the circulation and, therefore, cannot be excreted as filtered globin chains.

The production process is complex. Stroma-free hemoglobin is separated from red cell membranes, deoxygenated to achieve the proper molecular conformation for cross-linking, and the 2,3-DPG pocket is blocked reversibly with an allosteric effector. It is then cross-linked, heated to pasteurize it and also to remove unreacted hemoglobin, and passed through a series

of cross-flow filters. It is finally sterilized by filtration through a 0.2-μm filter.

The product has many favorable properties (Table 146-3). Oxygen-dissociation curves show a P$_{50}$ under physiologic conditions of 28 mmHg. The degree of cooperativity (the slope of the dissociation curve) is quite similar to that of blood (2.62 for blood, 2.31 for cross-linked hemoglobin) and the Bohr[5] and carbon dioxide[6] effects are nearly intact.

Theoretically, this product should have in vivo oxygen transport properties quite similar to those of whole blood. The intravascular persistence is markedly extended in the rat: uncross-linked hemoglobin has a half-life of about 1.2 hours and cross-linked hemoglobin one of 4.3 hours. In the rabbit, the persistence is longer, ≤16 hours for cross-linked hemoglobin, for monkey about 14 hours, and for pig about 7 hours.[7] There is no doubt that cell-free hemoglobin transports oxygen: many studies in the literature have demonstrated the ability of hemoglobin solutions to resuscitate animals in lethal hemorrhagic shock.[2]

Other hemoglobin-based products are also being developed. For example, a product very similar to the αα-cross-linked hemoglobin described above has been produced as a recombinant protein in *Escherichia coli*.[8] Starting material for hemoglobin modification can also be produced in transgenic animals. Hemoglobin also can be polymerized using a number of polyfunctional reagents (Table 146-2) to yield molecules with markedly increased molecular weights. One example is human hemoglobin reacted first with pyridoxal-5' phosphate and then polymerized with glutaraldehyde.[9] This product has the advantages of a reduced colloidal osmotic pressure and longer intra-

Table 146-3. Properties of a Single Batch of Cross-Linked Hemoglobin

Property	Measurement/Value
Formulation	Ringer's acetate
Volume	16.1 L
Hemoglobin concentration	9.8 g/dl
P$_{50}$, 37°C	29 mmHg
Hill's parameter (n)	2.31
Inorganic phosphate	<1 μg/ml
pH	7.4
Sterility	Pass
Pyrogen test	Negative
Endotoxin	<0.1 EU/ml

(From Winslow,[26] with permission.)

vascular persistence, but the polymerization reaction is notoriously difficult to control.[10,11]

Another promising approach is to couple hemoglobin to polyethylene glycol (PEG)[12] or a similar molecule, such as polyoxylethylene[13] or dextran.[14] These conjugated hemoglobins may also have prolonged plasma retention times and might have reduced interactions with the reticuloendothelial systems. They have not, as yet, been given to humans in clinical trials.

Liposome-Encapsulated Hemoglobin

Since hemoglobin is normally packaged inside a membrane, it seems intuitively correct that encapsulated hemoglobin would be the ultimate solution of the red cell substitute problem. In 1957 Thomas Chang[15] reported the use of microencapsulated hemoglobin as artificial red blood cells. Since that time, dramatic results have been reported in the complete exchange transfusion of laboratory animals,[16,17] but progress toward development of an artificial red cell for human use has been slow because of problems of reticuloendothelial and other macrophage stimulation.[18] Other problems include maintaining sterility and large-scale production.

In the 30 years that have followed Chang's initial descriptions of encapsulated hemoglobin, much work with lipid vesicles (liposomes) has been carried out. Liposomes have served as models for understanding natural cell membranes. They also have been used investigationally as vehicles for gene transfer, as targeted carriers, for pharmacologic agents, and even as lubricants for degenerated joint surfaces. They have also found applications in the cosmetic, vaccine, and paint industries.[19]

The most extensively studied liposomes used to encapsulate hemoglobin are composed of phospholipid in combination with cholesterol and other lipids that confer flexibility and stability, such as ganglioside GM_1 or cholesterol.[20] When injected into animals, such liposomes are rapidly coated with IgG, albumin, and other opsonins.[21] Newer formulations include the use of surface components like PEG or dextran, which can stabilize the liposomes in the circulation.[22]

The limitations to the development of liposome-encapsulated hemoglobin as a red cell substitute are difficulties in stabilizing the final product and the massive scale-up that would be required to produce a commercial product. The size of most liposome particles is approximately $0.2-1.0$ μm, too large to be filter sterilized. Also, neither the liposome nor its hemoglobin contents can withstand pasteurization temperature. Two approaches to the solution of these problems involve non-phospholipic liposomes[23] and those made from polymerizable phospholipids.[24]

Perfluorocarbon-Based Products

A recent resurgence has occurred in the development of perfluorocarbons for two reasons. First, Fluosol-DA 20% (Fluosol, Green Cross Corporation, Osaka, Japan) was approved for marketing by the Food and Drug Administration (FDA) for use in coronary angioplasty in 1990. Second, new perfluorocarbon emulsions now being developed by industry carry much more oxygen than previous products.[25] Still, there is a fundamental difference between fluorocarbon- and hemoglobin-based red cell substitutes: oxygen is transported by perfluorocarbons as dissolved gas, whereas hemoglobin carries oxygen chemically bound to the protein itself (Fig. 146-2). The oxygen dissociation curve for hemoglobin is sigmoid, while oxygen dissociation from perfluorocarbons is linear. The lower curve in Figure 146-2 is for Fluosol, and the upper one is for an emulsion of perfluorooctylbromide (Perflubron) and egg-yolk phospholipid (Oxygen HT, Alliance Pharmaceutical Corporation, San Diego, CA), which contains about five times more fluorocarbon, and therefore, five times more dissolved oxygen.

Initially, it would appear that it is better to have a sigmoid oxygen dissociation curve because (1) it is natural and (2) maximum oxygen carriage in blood is achieved at an alveolar PO_2 of about 100 mmHg, whereas only about 20% of the perfluorocarbon carries oxygen at the same PO_2. In order to carry as much oxygen in this fluorocarbon as 7 g/dl hemoglobin, an arterial PO_2 of about 280 mmHg is needed. Therefore, it seems that the utility of fluorocarbon red cell substitutes will depend on a high inspired PO_2. However, in many elective surgical procedures, arterial PO_2 well above 300 mmHg is quite achievable.

In practice, a margin of safety could be achieved with relatively low doses of perfluorocarbon emulsions, which could have a significant impact; increased tolerance to a reduced hematocrit would further reduce the "transfusion trigger." In a theoretical analysis of transfusion, mixed venous PO_2 is nearly constant from a hematocrit of 25–45% because as oxygen is added in the form of transfused red cells, cardiac output decreases.[26] If the hematocrit is kept low but oxygen is added in the form of perfluorocarbon, a significant increase in mixed venous PO_2 occurs because the cardiac output remains high. Cell-free hemoglobin solutions would not offer this advantage if their use does not result in an increased cardiac output.

Safety

Demonstration of safety of red cell substitutes is a critical issue, because the risks of transfusion of allogeneic blood are well known. A substitute should be as least as safe as red cells in order to be used, unless a decisive therapeutic advantage can be demonstrated.

In a review of almost a century of clinical trials with red cell substitutes, reported side effects involved renal dysfunction, systemic symptoms (fever, chills, nausea, headache, flushing, vomiting), allergic reactions, tachycardia, bradycardia, hypertension, rigors, low back pain, chest pain, abdominal pain, decreased platelets, and increased partial thromboplastin time.[2] Many of these effects could be explained by the depletion of nitric oxide, in the case of hemoglobin-based products, or by stimulation of macrophages, in the case of liposomes or perfluorocarbon emulsions. Many are smooth muscle effects and some involve macrophages and platelets. Recent clinical trials with hemoglobin-based products have not been extensively reported in the literature. However, it is clear that preclinical animal studies have not been completely successful in predicting human reactions to the products.[27]

Cell-free hemoglobin is widely distributed in the tissues after administration. Studies of the distribution of cross-linked hemoglobin in the intact animal show that significant amounts of hemoglobin are retained in the kidney, spleen, liver, adrenal gland, lung, heart, brain, and muscle well after any hemoglobin is detected in the plasma.[28-30] Thus, cell-free hemoglobin is distributed in almost every tissue of the body, and therefore we might expect toxic effects that could be quite unpredictable or unknown. Extensive histologic studies have been carried out in animals after exchange transfusion and have been summarized.[2]

Perhaps the effect of cell-free hemoglobin of most concern is its known ability to cause vasoconstriction. This vasoconstriction is thought to be mediated by the reaction of hemoglobin with nitric oxide, an endothelium-derived relaxing factor.[31] Nitric oxide is synthesized from arginine in endothelial cells (as well as in other cells) by an enzyme, nitric oxide synthase, that produces nitric oxide and citrulline. It binds to a heme group in guanyl cyclase that activates cGMP. Nitric oxide diffuses extremely rapidly out of endothelial cells into the interstitium, and into smooth muscle cells, where it binds to a heme group in guanyl cyclase, activating cGMP and moving calcium from the unbound to bound state. The result is smooth muscle relaxation.

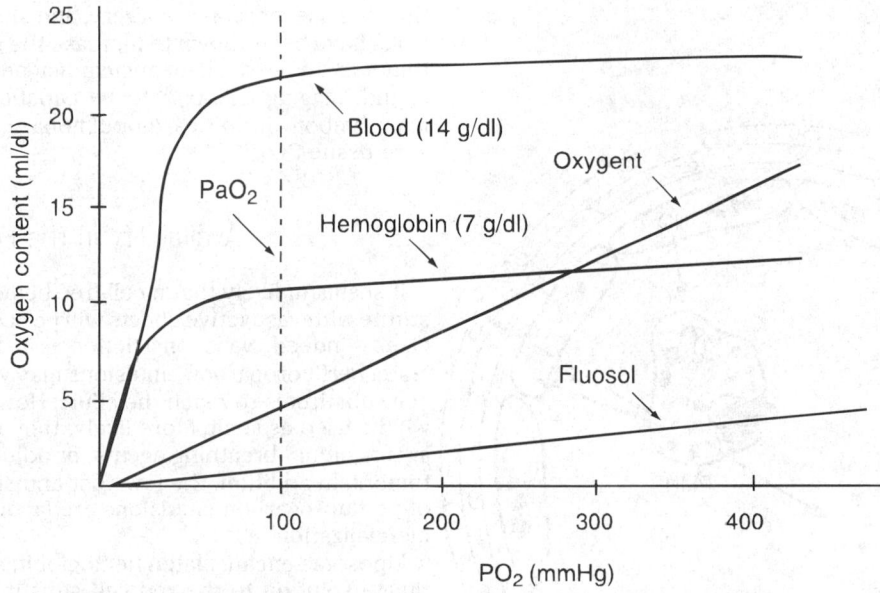

Fig. 146-2. *Comparison of the oxygen capacity of isooncotic blood (14 g/dl), cell-free hemoglobin (7 g/dl), Fluosol, and Oxygent HT. Note that the cooperativity of hemoglobin leads to nearly complete saturation at arterial oxygen partial pressure of 100 mmHg. At 280 mmHg, Oxygent HT carries approximately the same amount of oxygen as blood with a hemoglobin concentration of 7 g/dl. At PO$_2$ levels >280 mmHg, the perfluorocarbon emulsion can continue to take up more oxygen while the hemoglobin cannot. (From Winslow,[26] with permission.)*

It has been known for many years that hemoglobin binds nitric oxide very tightly, more tightly, in fact, than it binds oxygen, whether hemoglobin is in the red cell or free in solution.[32] The reaction is virtually irreversible. After synthesis of nitric oxide in endothelial cells, it diffuses into the smooth muscle cells, causing relaxation (Fig. 146-3). It also diffuses into the lumen of the vessel, where it stimulates platelets and polymorphonuclear leukocytes. Nitric oxide also diffuses into tissue, where it can stimulate macrophages and, since it is also a free radical, can kill bacteria. Whether this interaction of hemoglobin with nitric oxide will limit clinical usefulness of hemoglobin-based red cell substitutes remains to be determined.

Perfluorocarbon emulsions have the most extensive history of use in humans. Fluosol is approved by the FDA for use in coronary angioplasty and therefore has been given to many human subjects. In addition, similar formulations have been used on the battlefield in China and Afghanistan, although data are generally not available. Perfluorocarbon emulsions have also been tested in humans as imaging agents.

The principle toxicity of perfluorocarbon emulsions appears to be in their stimulation of macrophages.[33,34] This can result in pulmonary hypertension and elaboration of thromboxane in swine and could lead to nonspecific symptoms such as fever, chills, and flu-like symptoms in humans.[35]

Biocompatibility studies with liposome-encapsulated hemoglobin have been generally favorable[17] but such products tend to be removed from the circulation by the phagocytic cells in the reticuloendothelial system.[36] This leads to significant enlargement of the liver and spleen. The direction of current research is to attempt to prolong the intravascular persistence to minimize this problem.

Efficacy

It seems intuitively obvious that a plasma expander that carries oxygen would be superior to one that does not, and that experimental proof of this concept would be relatively straightforward. However, the problem of efficacy can be appreciated by considering the difficulties in showing efficacy for red cell transfusion. The problem is a lack of clear end points: no single

measures of oxygen transport are accurate and easily obtainable. It might be possible to show improved clinical outcome after transfusion of red cells to patients with extremely low hematocrits, but the bulk of allogeneic blood is given intraoperatively in response to blood loss, not severe anemia.

Most demonstrations of efficacy have been either by exchange transfusions with test material, or resuscitation from shock.[21] However, exchange transfusion is not a situation encountered clinically, and shock resuscitation is particularly complex: the most urgent requirement is for volume replacement. Clinical trials involving trauma patients are particularly difficult to design because of the problems of controls and informed consent. Future clinical trials will most likely be aimed at, for example, reduced use of allogeneic blood, rather than at specific oxygen transport parameters, which may be controversial, at best. For example, one trial with Fluosol during surgery showed that its use did not reduce the need for allogeneic blood transfusions in the postoperative period.[37]

Clinical Trials

A number of hemoglobin preparations are now in phase I clinical trials (safety), and the greatest fear is that the known vasoactivity of the solutions could lead to hypertension or underperfusion of ischemic tissue. Perfluorocarbon emulsions also have been tested in humans, but no data are available in the peer-reviewed literature. No liposome-based product has yet been approved for use in human trials.

Early trials with various cell-free hemoglobin solutions were reviewed and showed an array of side effects that affect every organ of the body.[2] However, most of these are mild or reversible, and only 1 death in >211 patients was reported; this patient was terminally ill and would likely have died even without administration of hemoglobin.[38]

IMPLICATIONS/FUTURE APPLICATIONS
Potential Clinical Applications

The need for red cell substitutes to replace all use of allogeneic blood is both unnecessary and naive. The red cell substitute candidates now being developed will probably be used

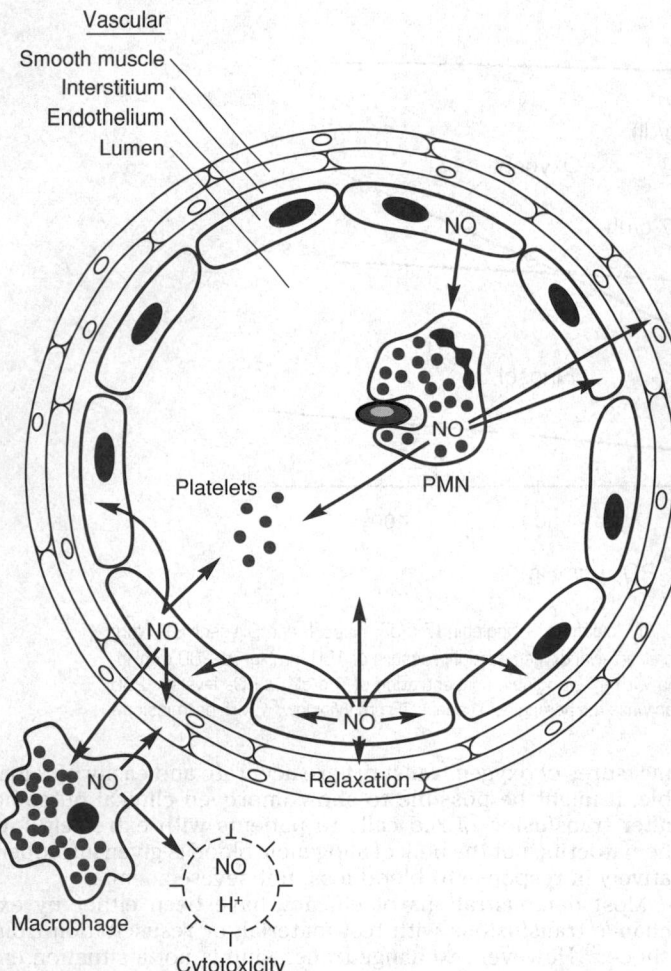

Vascular
Smooth muscle
Interstitium
Endothelium
Lumen

NO

NO

PMN

Platelets

NO

NO

Relaxation

NO

Macrophage

NO
H⁺

Cytotoxicity

Fig. 146-3. Schematic illustration of the scope of the transcellular signaling that is possible when nitric oxide is synthesized and released from the vascular endothelium, circulating neutrophils, and tissue macrophages. Nitric oxide triggers diverse but complementary cellular responses by stimulating different cells within a local environment. (From Winslow,[26] with permission.)

initially in surgical hemodilution to provide a margin of safety and perhaps to reduce the need for the 2 or 3 U of blood used in most surgeries.

Many clinical applications in addition to hemodilution for the products now being developed will be targeted by industry (Table 146-4). Applications for perfluorocarbon emulsions other than as red cell substitutes could be even more important

Table 146-4. Potential Clinical Applications for Red Cell Substitutes

Trauma
Hemodilution (elective surgery)
Red cell incompatibility
Ischemic disease (e.g., percutaneous transluminal coronary angiography, stroke)
Extracorporeal circulation
Cell culture media
Hematopoietic stimulation
High-blood-use surgery
Cardioplegia
Tumor therapy
Chronic anemia
Organ transplantation
Sickle cell anemia
Research

than the use in trauma, surgery, and shock. For example, emulsions have been shown to increase the radiosensitivity of solid tumors,[39] to be excellent nuclear magnetic resonance and ultrasound imaging agents,[40] to be capable of removing gaseous microemboli during cardiopulmonary bypass,[41] and to measure tissue PO_2.[42]

Availability in the Future

It seems unlikely that a cell-free hemoglobin as red cell substitute with vasoactive effects will be accepted broadly by clinicians—indeed, vasoconstriction is a hallmark of the shock state. Perfluorocarbon emulsions may very well be the first red cell substitutes to reach the clinic. However, it is unlikely they will be used as such. More likely, they will find use as imaging agents, liquid-breathing agents, or adjuncts to radiotherapy of tumors. In addition, the low cost and simplicity of production of perfluorocarbon emulsions are favorable qualities for commercialization.

Liposome-encapsulated hemoglobin may very well be the ultimate solution to the red cell substitute problem. However, to be successful, an inexpensive and simple process will need to be developed, and any problems of reticuloendothelial system blockade and engorgement of organs such as liver and spleen will have to be thoroughly studied and understood.

The present commercial climate is such that few, if any, of these products will be used in scientific studies that can be reviewed in the peer-reviewed literature until they are approved for use by the FDA. This unfortunate situation has retarded development in the past and is likely to do so in the future.[27]

REFERENCES

1. Klein HK: Role of blood substitutes in transfusion medicine. Biomater Artif Cells Immobil Biotechnol 1994 (in press)
2. Winslow RM: Hemoglobin-Based Red Cell Substitutes. Johns Hopkins University Press, Baltimore, 1992
3. Christensen SM, Medina F, Winslow RM et al: Preparation of human hemoglobin Ao for possible use as a blood substitute. J Biochem Biophys Methods 17:143, 1988
4. Walder JA, Chatterjee R, Arnone A: Electrostatic effects within the central cavity of the hemoglobin tetramer, abstracted (2228). Fed Proc 41:651, 1982
5. Vandegriff KD, Medina F, Marini MA, Winslow RM: Equilibrium oxygen binding to human hemoglobin cross-linked between the α chains by bis(3,5-dibromosalicyl) fumarate. J Biol Chem 264:17824, 1989
6. Vandegriff KD, Benazzi L, Ripamonti M et al: Carbon dioxide binding to human hemoglobin cross-linked between the α chains. J Biol Chem 266:2697, 1991
7. Hess JR, Fadare SO, Tolentino LSL et al: The intravascular persistence of crosslinked human hemoglobin. p. 351. In Brewer G (ed): The Red Cell: Seventh Ann Arbor Conference. Alan R Liss, New York, 1989
8. Hoffman SJ, Looker DL, Roehrich JM et al: Expression of fully functional tetrameric human hemoglobin in *Escherichia coli*. Proc Natl Acad Sci USA 87:8521, 1990
9. Gould SA, Sehgal LR, Sehgal HL, Moss GS: Artificial blood: current status of hemoglobin solutions. Crit Care Clin 8:293, 1992
10. Marini MA, Moore GL, Fishman RM et al: A critical examination of the reaction of pyridoxal 5-phosphate with human hemoglobin Ao. Biopolymers 28:2071, 1989
11. Marini MA, Moore GL, Fishman RM et al: Reexamination of the polymerization of pyridoxylated hemoglobin with glutaraldehyde. Biopolymers 29:871, 1990
12. Nho K, Glower D, Bredehoeft S et al: PEG-bovine hemoglobin: safety in a canine dehydrated hypovolemic-hemorrhagic shock model. Biomater Artif Cells Immobil Biotechnol 20:511, 1992
13. Malchesky PS, Takahashi T, Iwasaki K et al: Conjugated human hemoglobin as a physiological oxygen carrier—pyridoxalated hemoglobin polyoxyethylene conjugate (PHP). Int J Artif Organs 13:442, 1990
14. Wong JTF: Righshifted dextran-hemoglobin as blood substitute. Biomater Artif Cells Artif Organs 16:237, 1988
15. Chang TMS: Red blood cell substitutes: microencapsulated hemoglobin and cross-linked hemoglobin including pyridoxalated polyhemoglobin & conjugated hemoglobin. Biomater Artif Cells Artif Organs 16:11, 1988

16. Djordjevich L, Mayoral J, Ivankovich A: Synthetic erythrocytes: cardiorespiratory changes during exchange transfusions. Anesthesiology 63:A109, 1985

17. Hunt CA, Burnette RR, MacGregor RD: Synthesis and evaluation of a prototypal artificial red cell. Science 230:1165, 1985

18. Rabinovici R, Rudolph AS, Feuerstein G: Characterization of hemodynamic, hematologic, and biochemical responses to administration of liposome-encapsulated hemoglobin in the conscious, freely moving rat. Circ Shock 29:115, 1989

19. Bangham AD: Liposomes: realizing their promise. Hosp Pract [Off] 27:51, 1992

20. Farmer MC, Gaber BP: Liposome-encapsulated hemoglobin as an artificial oxygen-carrying system. Methods Enzymol 149:184, 1987

21. MacGregor RD, Hunt CA: Artificial red cells. A link between the membrane skeleton and RES detectability? Biomater Artif Cells Artif Organs 18:329, 1990

22. Allen TM, Hansen C, Martin F: Liposomes containing synthetic lipid derivatives of poly(ethylene glycol) show prolonged circulation half-times *in vivo*. Biochim Biophys Acta 1066:29, 1991

23. Wallach DFH, Philippot JR: New type of lipid vesicle: Novasomes™. p. 141. In Gregoriadis G (ed): Liposome Technology: Liposome Preparation and Related Techniques. CRC Press, Boca Raton, FL, 1993

24. Satoh T, Kobayashi K, Sekiguchi S, Tsuchida E: Characteristics of artificial red cells. Hemoglobin encapsulated in poly-lipid vesicles. ASAIO J 38:M580, 1992

25. Long C, Long DM, Riess J: Preparation and application of highly concentrated perfluoroctylbromide fluorocarbon emulsions. Biomater Artif Cells Artif Organs 16:441, 1988

26. Winslow RM: Red cell substitutes: current status, 1992. p. 151. In Nance SJ (ed): Blood Safety: Current Challenges. American Association of Blood Banks, Bethesda, MD, 1992

27. Naval Research Advisory Committee Report: Requirements for Delivery of "Artifical Blood" to the Military. U.S. Navy, Washington, D.C., 1992

28. Keipert PE, Verosky M, Triner L: Metabolism, distribution, and excretion of HbXL: a nondissociating interdimerically crosslinked hemoglobin with exceptional oxygen offloading capability. Biomater Artif Cells Artif Organs 16:643, 1988

29. Keipert PE, Gomez CL, Gonzales A et al: Organ distribution and long-term excretion of diaspirin crosslinked hemoglobin after major exchange transfusion. Biomater Artif Cells Immobil Biotechnol 1994

30. Hsia JC, Song DL, Er SS et al: Pharmacokinetic studies in the rat on o-raffinose polymerized human hemoglobin. Biomater Artif Cells Immobil Biotechnol 20:587, 1992

31. Palmer RMJ, Ferrige A, Moncada S: Nitric oxide release accounts for the biological activity of endothelium-derived relaxing factor. Nature 327:524, 1987

32. Gibson QH: The kinetics of reactions between haemoglobin and gases. p. 1. In Butler JAV, Katz B (eds): Progress in Biophysics and Biophysical Chemistry. Pergamon Press, New York, 1959

33. Ingram DA, Forman MB, Murray JJ: Phagocytic activation of human neutrophils by the detergent component of Fluosol. Am J Pathol 140:1081, 1992

34. Bucala R, Kawakami M, Cerami A: Cytotoxicity of a perfluorocarbon blood substitute to macrophages *in vitro*. Science 220:965, 1983

35. Flaim SF, Hazard DR, Hogan J, Peters RM: Characterization and mechanism of side-effects of Imagent BP (highly concentrated fluorocarbon emulsion) in swine. Invest Radiol, suppl. 1. 26:S122-4, 1991

36. Beach MC, Morley J, Spiryda L, Weinstock SB: Effects of liposome encapsulated hemoglobin on the reticuloendothelial system. Biomater Artif Cells Immobil Biotechnol 20:771, 1992

37. Gould SA, Rosen AL, Sehgal LR et al: Fluosol-DA as a red-cell substitute in acute anemia. N Engl J Med 314:1653, 1986

38. Amberson WR, Jennings JJ, Rhodes CM: Clinical experience with hemoglobin-saline solutions. J App. Physiol 1:469, 1949

39. Teicher BA, Herman TS, Menon K: Enhancement of fractionated radiation therapy by an experimental concentrated perflubron emulsion (Oxygent) in the Lewis lung carcinoma. Biomater Artif Cells Immobil Biotechnol 20:899, 1992

40. Mattrey RF: Perfluorooctylbromide: a new contrast agent for CT, sonography, and MR imaging. AJR 152:247, 1988

41. Blauth C, Smith P, Newman S et al: Retinal microembolism and neuropsychological deficit following clinical cardiopulmonary bypass: comparison of a membrane and a bubble oxygenator. A preliminary communication. Eur J Cardiothorac Surg 3:135, 1989

42. Mason RP, Shukla H, Antich PP: Oxygent: a novel probe of tissue oxygen tension. Biomater Artif Cells Immobil Biotechnol 20:929, 1992

CONSULTATIVE HEMATOLOGY

Part IX

Hematologic Complications of Liver Disease and Alcoholism

147

Ralph Zalusky and Bruce Furie

INTRODUCTION

Liver disease and its major handmaiden, alcohol abuse, have profound effects on hemostasis and hematopoiesis. Liver disease, regardless of etiology, can be associated with abnormal bleeding due to anatomic derangements and impairment of hepatic synthetic and clearance functions. Abnormal lipid metabolism can cause red cell structural defects. Alcohol and its metabolites have direct effects on hematopoiesis, behaving as a toxin and impairing nutritional physiology. Although a few well-described hematologic syndromes have been described, in most instances multiple and complex derangements are present simultaneously in the same patient, challenging the diagnostic and therapeutic skills of the hematologist.

EFFECTS OF LIVER DISEASE ON HEMOSTASIS

Abnormal hemostasis is a common complication of liver disease, and a determination of its underlying pathogenesis is essential for rational management. Mechanisms resulting in these defects include (1) diminished hepatic synthesis of coagulation factors V, VII, IX, X, and XI, prothrombin, and fibrinogen (reflected in prolongation of the prothrombin time [PT] and partial thromboplastin time [PTT]), (2) dietary vitamin K deficiency due to inadequate intake or malabsorption (based on intrahepatic or extrahepatic cholestasis or intestinal malabsorption), (3) dysfibrinogenemia, (4) enhanced fibrinolysis, due to decreased synthesis of α_2-plasmin inhibitor, (5) disseminated intravascular coagulation (DIC), and (6) thrombocytopenia due to hypersplenism.

Abnormalities of Protein Synthesis

With the exception of factor VIII,[1] the liver is the site of synthesis of the blood coagulation proteins and related regulatory proteins.[2–4] Parenchymal diseases of the liver, including cirrhosis, hepatitis, and infiltrative disorders can impair synthesis, leading to a deficiency of plasma proteins involved in hemostasis.[5–8] Often, these abnormalities may be subclinical. Measurement of specific coagulation factors may be reduced but not attended by clinical bleeding or prolongation of the PT or PTT. In inflammatory liver disorders, the plasma levels of some coagulation proteins, such as factor VIII and fibrinogen, may increase as an acute-phase reaction.[6,9,10] When the PT and PTT are prolonged, however, more extensive hepatic dysfunction is present and is associated with a poor prognosis. Hypofibrinogenemia, with plasma fibrinogen levels <100 mg/dl, is an especially grave sign.[11]

Acquired Defects of Vitamin K-Dependent Carboxylation

The vitamin K-dependent blood coagulation proteins, including prothrombin and factors II, VII, IX, and X, are synthesized in the liver. These proteins undergo a unique post-translational processing step whereby glutamic acid residues in the N-terminal region of these proteins are converted to γ-carboxyglutamic acid residues by a vitamin K-dependent carboxylase.[12–16] In some liver disorders, such as cirrhosis and hepatitis, an acquired deficiency of this carboxylation step may occur. Although generally mild, it may lead to the circulation of des-γ-carboxylated proteins in the blood (Fig. 147-1). Although biologically inactive and synthesized at the expense of biologically active forms, their levels are sufficiently low that they do not contribute significantly, if at all, to coagulation abnormalities associated with liver disease. They can, however, serve as useful markers of this acquired vitamin K-dependent carboxylation defect. Des-γ-carboxy (abnormal) prothrombin, normally absent from plasma, circulates at detectable levels in >90% of patients with hepatoma[18–20] (Fig. 147-2). The tumor itself is responsible for the production of this protein since surgical removal or reduction in tumor mass with chemotherapy is associated with reduction or elimination of the abnormal prothrombin. Unlike the situation in vitamin K deficiency, levels of both the abnormal and normal prothrombin may be high simultaneously in patients with hepatoma. Therefore, this defect is not associated pathophysiologically with bleeding that may complicate management in primary hepatocellular carcinoma. Together with measurement of serum levels of α-fetoprotein, abnormal prothrombin is able to identify >84% of patients with hepatomas.

Vitamin K Deficiency

Nutritional deficiencies are common in alcoholism and alcoholic liver disease. However, with a daily minimal requirement of 100–200 μg,[21] inadequate intake does not lead to clinically significant vitamin K deficiency even with substandard diets. Since vitamin K is a fat-soluble vitamin, defects related to absorption can occur. This is especially so when impairment of bile acid metabolism occurs in primary biliary cirrhosis,[22] intrahepatic or extrahepatic cholestasis,[23] and during therapy with bile acid binders (e.g., cholestyramine).[24] In addition, since vitamin K is synthesized by intestinal bacteria, the use of oral antibiotics may result in frank deficiency.[25]

Dysfibrinogenemias

A defective functional form of fibrinogen has been described in some patients with liver disease, including cirrhosis and hepatocellular carcinoma.[26,27] The defect in the molecule appears to be a post-translational event resulting in excess sialic acid residues following glycosylation in the hepatocyte.[26,28] The action of thrombin on this abnormal fibrinogen appears to result in the formation of defective fibrin monomers with impaired ability to polymerize.[29,30] Both the thrombin time and

MANAGEMENT OF THE HEMOSTATIC DEFECTS IN PATIENTS WITH LIVER DISEASE

Evaluation and management of defective hemostasis in patients with liver disease should include a careful history and physical examination, appropriate laboratory testing to establish etiology, and institution of corrective therapy when required. Laboratory abnormalities in the absence of clinically significant bleeding may require only careful monitoring, whereas overt bleeding or preparation for invasive or surgical procedures requires replacement therapy.

Prolongation of the PT and PTT usually indicates plasma clotting factor deficiency, ether as a result of impaired hepatic synthesis or secondary to vitamin K deficiency. When combined with diminished levels of factor V, factor XI, or fibrinogen, which are not vitamin K dependent, then liver dysfunction is apparent. Some of these abnormalities may be complicated by the presence of inhibitory activity in the plasma such as fibrin degradation products (FDP). In addition, a low fibrinogen level can result from increased fibrinolysis/fibrinogenolysis, DIC, or structurally abnormal fibrinogen. Measurement of the thrombin time shows a prolongation under all these conditions. Evidence for increased fibrinolytic activity is obtained by finding elevated FDP or the D dimer. Distinction between plasma clotting factor deficiency and plasma inhibitory activity is obtained by determining whether the PT and PTT can be corrected in a 1:1 mix of normal plasma and patient plasma. Reduction of the platelet count commonly accompanies the coagulation factor disturbances and is attributable to hypersplenism, recent alcohol abuse, and, if especially severe, DIC.

If the PT is prolonged >3 seconds, and if the patient is not actively bleeding, a trial of vitamin K can be given when the laboratory findings are consistent with plasma clotting factor deficiency. A dose of 10 mg/day SC for 3 successive days is sufficient to correct the abnormality in those few patients in whom malabsorption of the vitamin is present.

More characteristically, hepatic dysfunction is the underlying mechanism, and replacement therapy is warranted in patients who are actively bleeding or who are to undergo invasive diagnostic or therapeutic procedures. Fresh frozen plasma (FFP) remains the mainstay of replacement therapy. Its major drawback is the large volume that may be required in patients with unstable cardiovascular conditions. Although small-volume replacement factor IX concentrates, which are rich in vitamin K-dependent factors, have occasionally been used, their administration has been associated with thromboembolic problems or DIC. The amount of FFP infused will vary with the clinical status of the patient and the frequency of administration dictated by the plasma half-life of the clotting factors. The desired initial infusion is 25–30% of the plasma volume (approximately 1,200–1,500 ml in a 70-kg adult), to achieve at least partial correction of the hemostatic defect. With continued active bleeding, one-half the initial dose may be required as often as every 6 hours, considering that the half-life of several clotting factors varies from 5 to 8 hours. In the presence of ascites, in which the volume of distribution is increased, or in the presence of fibrinolysis or DIC, an increased dose of FFP will be required as determined by serial measurement of the PT and PTT. Red cell transfusions will also be required in the actively bleeding patient to maintain adequate hemoglobin levels and a normotensive state. In very advanced liver disease, hypofibrinogenemia may be severe (i.e., <100 mg/dl), and cryoprecipitate can be transfused at the rate of 1 U/3 kg body weight. Each bag contains about 300 mg of fibrinogen and, because one-half the transfused fibrinogen is metabolized within 3 or 4 days, a daily transfusion of 1 U/15 kg body weight can maintain the fibrinogen concentration at adequate levels. Many of these patients may have some degree of thrombocytopenia, but when the platelet count is <20,000/mm^3 and bleeding is active, platelet transfusions should be considered. Determining the platelet count 1 hour after transfusion provides a useful guide to the adequacy of retention. In the presence of splenomegaly, this may be minimal due to platelet pooling in the spleen. When a qualitative platelet dysfunction is suspected, desmopressin may be tried at a dose of 0.3 µg/kg IV.

Establishing a diagnosis of DIC in bleeding patients with liver disease is especially challenging. Prolongation of the PT, PTT, and thrombin time, low fibrinogen levels, elevated FDP, and thrombocytopenia may have multiple pathophysiologic mechanisms. Since factor VIII coagulant activity is often elevated in liver disease and reduced in DIC, its measurement helps to distinguish these disorders. A diagnosis of DIC is more likely to be associated with precipitating factors such as sepsis, shock, or peritoneovenous shunts. The use of heparin in these situations has always been controversial, especially in the presence of active bleeding, so reliance must be placed on replacement therapy with FFP, cryoprecipitate, and platelets. In the setting of liver diseases and DIC, a role for antithrombin III concentrates or antifibrinolytic agents has not been established.

---

the reptilase time are usually prolonged, while the fibrinogen level measured immunochemically remains normal.

Increased Fibrinolysis/Fibrinogenolysis

Several types of pathophysiologic derangements can lead to factor deficiencies through increased factor consumption. Depressed synthesis of the major plasma inhibitor of plasmin, α_2-plasmin inhibitor, which is produced by the liver, results in enhanced fibrinolytic activity of the blood.[31,32] This plasma protease inhibitor forms a complex with and inactivates plasmin.[33] Impaired synthesis correlates with the severity of the liver disease, and pathologic fibrinolysis is manifested by decreased fibrinogen levels, increased fibrin degradation products, and accelerated euglobulin lysis time.[34,35]

Tissue plasminogen activator (t-PA) levels and its plasma inhibitors have been studied in patients with liver cirrhosis. Abnormal fibrinolysis, as measured by the dilute whole blood clot lysis time, correlated with a disproportionate reduction in t-PA-inhibitor activity, even when t-PA and its inhibitor were increased.[36] Attempts to inhibit fibrinolysis through the use of

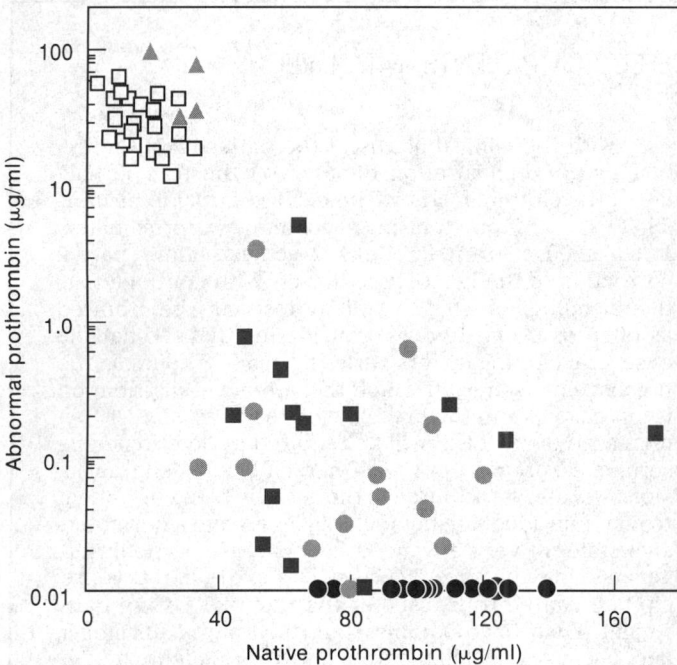

Fig. 147-1. Plasma levels of abnormal (des-γ-carboxy) prothrombin in liver disease. The abnormal prothrombin level is displayed on the y axis on a logarithmic scale. The fully carboxylated native prothrombin is shown on a linear scale on the x axis. Severe vitamin K deficiency, pink triangle; warfarin therapy, white square; acute hepatitis, gray circle; cirrhosis, red square; normal, black circle. (From Blanchard et al.,[17] with permission.)

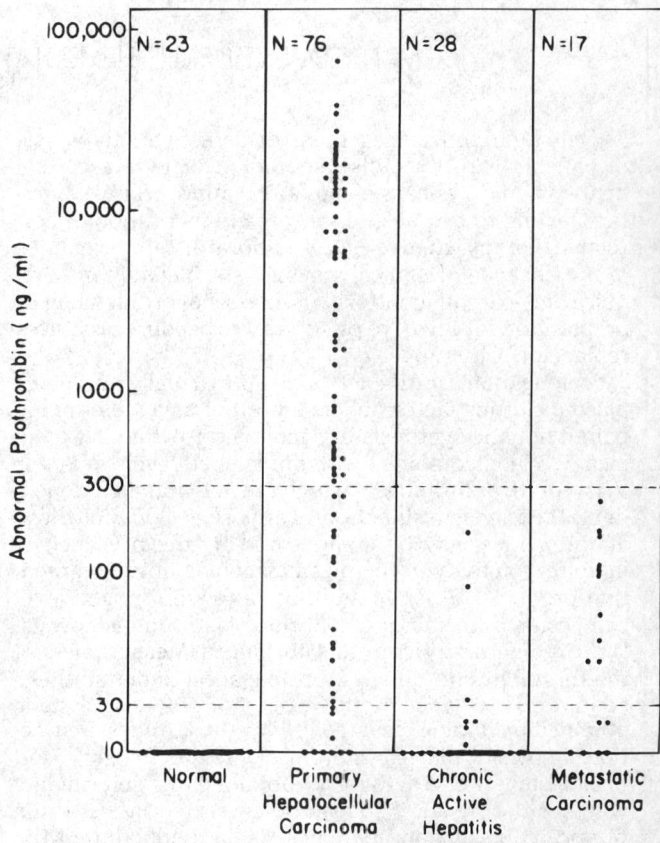

Fig. 147-2. Plasma levels of abnormal (des-γ-carboxy) prothrombin in primary hepatocellular carcinoma. Comparison in patients with primary hepatocellular carcinoma, chronic active hepatitis, and metastatic carcinoma. The abnormal prothrombin level is displayed on the y axis on a logarithmic scale. (From Liebman et al.,[18] with permission.)

antifibrinolytic agents have not been uniformly successful[37] and in the presence of possible DIC are contraindicated.[5]

Disseminated Intravascular Coagulation

A clear role for DIC in the pathogenesis of bleeding in liver disease is complicated by other causes of factor and platelet depletion, the cardinal signs of this disorder. Thus, decreased levels of clotting factors, as enumerated above, and thrombocytopenia secondary to hypersplenism make it difficult to assess the contribution of DIC in an individual case.[38] In some patients with cirrhosis, accelerated catabolism of fibrinogen, prothrombin, and plasminogen has been described that is improved by administration of heparin.[37–40] Accelerated catabolism of fibrinogen occurs in acute liver necrosis, biliary tract obstruction, cholangitis, and liver contusion.[41–43] Entry of endotoxin into the circulation from the gastrointestinal tract in patients with portal hypertension has been suggested as another mechanism inducing DIC, as has impaired reticuloendothelial function, especially in alcohol-induced liver disease.[44]

Although the pathogenesis of DIC in cirrhosis is often puzzling, DIC is frequent in patients who have had surgical peritoneovenous shunts (LeVeen and Denver shunts) placed between ascitic fluid and the venous circulation.[45–48] The cells suspended in ascitic fluid may induce coagulation.[48,49] Collagen-like protein may induce platelet aggregation[50] or activate factor XII.[5] A concomitant drop in fibrinogen level and platelet count occurs, and occasionally a disproportionate fall in the former has suggested a primary role for activation of fibrinolysis.[51] Clinically significant bleeding requires interruption of the shunt. Therapy with heparin has not been helpful, and although a role for antiplatelet agents, aspirin, and dipyridamole, has been suggested,[50] they may add to the bleeding tendency in these patients.

Reduced levels of antithrombin III in chronic liver disease

may contribute to the development of DIC and reflect impaired hepatic synthesis.[52] Correction of the antithrombin III deficiency by transfusion increases the survival of fibrinogen.[52] Low levels of heparin cofactor II have been reported in a few patients who may have undergone DIC.[53]

Platelets

Thrombocytopenia is commonly observed in patients with chronic liver disease and is ascribed to portal hypertension with its accompanying congestive splenomegaly.[54] This results in a shift in the platelets from the circulation to the enlarged spleen and may not affect platelet survival.[55] The reduction in the effective circulation is seldom in itself sufficient to induce a bleeding diathesis, but may contribute by additive effects to the other coagulation factor disturbances.

EFFECTS OF LIVER DISEASE ON HEMATOPOIESIS

Chronic liver disease causing cirrhosis leads to portal hypertension and congestive splenomegaly. The former can then lead to excessive blood loss from variceal and other types of upper gastrointestinal bleeding, while the latter represents a major cause of hypersplenism. When blood loss continues on a chronic basis, iron deficiency can supervene. Thrombocytopenia, leukopenia, and anemia, or any combination thereof, may result from excessive trapping by the enlarged, congested spleen. In addition, the anemia of chronic disease, as seen in other disorders of inflammation, infection, or malignancy, further complicates the hematologic presentation in these patients. Altered lipid metabolism may lead to structural changes in the red cell membrane, occasionally causing unusual hemolytic syndromes.

Hypersplenism

Splenomegaly is a common finding in patients with chronic liver disease and portal hypertension. The degree of reduction in the blood counts is a reflection of both splenic size and the capacity of the bone marrow to compensate for this reduction. Anemia results from (1) red cell pooling in the enlarged spleen, (2) decreased red cell survival, and (3) increased plasma volume.[56–58] Neutropenia has been attributed both to increased pooling and decreased survival.[56,59] Thrombocytopenia is primarily the result of increased platelet pooling.[55] Because of the moderate degree of these cytopenias and the operative risks in these patients, splenectomy is rarely indicated. Shunting procedures, both splenorenal and portocaval, have been shown to have variable results on the hematologic manifestations.[60–62]

Effects of Liver Disease on Erythrocyte Membranes

Structural abnormalities causing red cell shape changes are common in liver disease. Target cells are frequently seen in the peripheral blood smear and result from increased surface area due to excess membrane cholesterol and phospholipid transferred from lipoproteins in the plasma.[63] These cells have a normal survival and resist osmotic lysis.[63]

Spur cells are a grave finding in some patients with advanced liver disease. This shape transformation can occur in normal red blood cells incubated with plasma from affected patients.[64] Although membrane cholesterol is increased, total phospholipids are normal, and the cells show decreased resistance to osmotic lysis.[65] Splenic modeling of these cells contributes to their reduced survival, and hemolysis is usually moderate to severe.[66] Although splenectomy may improve the anemia, patients with this acquired disorder are rarely surgical candidates.

A unique feature of patients with chronic liver disease is the presence of "thin macrocytes" in the peripheral smear, unrelated to vitamin B_{12} or folic acid deficiency.[67] Red cell diameter is increased, but the mean corpuscular volume (MCV) remains normal. Unlike target cells and spur cells, thin macrocytes do not become normal when transfused into normal subjects, nor are normal cells transformed into thin macrocytes when transfused into patients with liver disease.[67,68] Red cell survival does not appear to be affected.

Anemia Associated with Viral Hepatitis

Viral hepatitis may be associated with mild anemia secondary to bone marrow suppression and shortened red cell survival.[69,70] Since hepatic clearance of oxidizing metabolites may be impaired in patients with viral hepatitis, depression of reduced glutathione occurs.[71] This is of special concern for patients with glucose-6-phosphate dehydrogenase deficiency.[72,73]

Aplastic anemia (see Ch. 21) is a potential consequence of viral hepatitis; one study has estimated an incidence of 0.1–0.2%.[74] The average age is 18 years, with a male preponderance.[75] Hepatitis C is a more common cause of hepatitis-associated aplastic anemia.[76] Aplasia usually develops within 2 months of this hepatitis and without bone marrow transplantation has a high mortality rate.

HEMATOLOGIC EFFECTS OF ALCOHOL ABUSE

Metabolism of Ethanol

Hepatocyte cytosol contains alcohol dehydrogenase, which constitutes the major pathway for the catalytic conversion of ethanol to acetaldehyde.[77] In this reaction, hydrogen is transferred from the substrate to the cofactor, nicotinamide adenine dinucleotide (NAD), and then to its reduced form, NADH, producing acetaldehyde. This oxidation step results in an excess of reducing capacity of the cell, and the shift in redox potential alters the lactate pyruvate ratio.[78,79] The acetaldehyde produced is then converted in the mitochondria to acetate, which is catalyzed by acetaldehyde dehydrogenase, generating further NADH, a major factor in the toxicity of ethanol.[77] Increased lactic acid contributes to acidosis, and decreased uric acid excretion by the kidney leads to hyperuricemia. Gluconeogenesis is impaired and triglyceride accumulation favored. Impaired oxidation of fatty acids, resulting from reduced availability of NAD in the citric acid cycle, leads to the accumulation of esterified fatty acids. Further deposition of triglyceride and phospholipids occurs as a result of activation of the second pathway for ethanol metabolism, the cytochrome P-450-dependent microsomal ethanol-oxidizing system located in the endoplasmic reticulum. In the presence of oxygen and NAD phosphate (NADPH) as cofactor, acetaldehyde accumulates. With heavy ethanol intake, ≤20% of the substrate is metabolized through this pathway.[77,80] The lipid accumulation in the hepatocyte is further enhanced by the direct toxic effect of acetaldehyde. Mitochondrial function is altered, as is the impairment of microtubule formation. This effect of acetaldehyde on protein synthesis interferes with the transport of lipoprotein from the liver, thus participating in the formation of the fatty liver. Engorgement of the hepatocyte by an increased protein load when accompanied by necrosis and polymorphonuclear inflammation characterizes alcoholic hepatitis. Although this manifestation is not necessarily a precursor to the development of cirrhosis, it is frequently a prelude.[77]

The hematologic sequelae of alcoholism are the consequences of those alterations secondary to portal hypertension and hypersplenism, lipid abnormalities reflected in membrane structural defects, disturbed synthesis of the coagulation factors, and the direct toxic effects of alcohol and acetaldehyde.

DIRECT EFFECTS OF ETHANOL ON HEMATOPOIESIS

Bone Marrow

Excessive alcohol consumption affects the bone marrow in several ways. These include vacuolization of hematopoietic precursors, megaloblastic changes in the absence of folate deficiency, sideroblastic changes, hypocellularity, and increased numbers of plasma cells.[81–87] Since a characteristic pattern of bone marrow injury is not diagnostic of alcoholism, some or all of these features may not necessarily coexist. Since the progeny of bone marrow precursors may lack certain synthetic capacities, it is likely that some of the described abnormalities of the peripheral blood cells may have been inflicted at the bone marrow level.[88]

Vacuolization of proerythroblasts occurs with high frequency in heavy imbibers (1–2 pints of 80-proof whiskey daily). Vacuoles can be seen within 1 week of such intake and quickly disappear within a few days of abstinence.[82] They appear to result from surface invagination of the cell membrane, leading to endocytosis and subsequent vacuole formation.[89] Cytoplasmic localization in the proerythroblast is characteristic, although occasional nuclear vacuoles can be seen. Promyelocytes share the injury to a lesser extent, as do other precursor cells. In vitro studies with normal bone marrow incubated in the presence of alcohol reproduce these findings.[89] Chemical identification of the inclusions has not been achieved. Similar morphologic changes had been described in association with chloramphenicol use, and in other clinical disorders.[90]

Marrow hypocellularity has been observed in occasional patients with excessive alcohol intake and was attributed to the toxic effect of ethanol or its metabolites because of the absence of other factors.[85,91] Further evidence of a toxic effect of alcohol on the bone marrow has come from in vitro studies of this agent on in vitro colony formation.[92–94] Depressed burst-forming unit-erythroid and colony-forming unit (CFU)-erythroid have been observed,[92] whereas higher ethanol concentrations impair CFU-granulocyte/macrophage and CFU-macrophage.[93,94] The pluripotential stem cell escapes this injury, which may account for the common in vivo observation that these toxic effects are reversible on cessation of alcohol abuse.[92,95]

Sideroblastic changes are commonly present in erythroid precursors of alcoholic patients.[96–98] Structural studies show accumulation of siderotic granules in the mitochondria, which surround the nucleus and give the characteristic ringed appearance on Prussian blue stains of the marrow. Generally, these morphologic findings are more readily appreciated in the more mature erythroid cells. Defective iron utilization for hemoglobin synthesis underlies this process, producing a dimorphic anemia that generally reverses within days to 2 weeks of alcohol withdrawal.[99] In most instances, this is not the sole cause of the anemia but may occur in up to one-third of alcoholic patients, usually in association with folate deficiency and acute blood loss.[96,98] Earlier studies suggested that the defect resulted from ethanol impairment of the conversion of pyridoxine to pyridoxal phosphate, which is catalyzed by pyridoxine kinase.[99] Pyridoxal phosphate, the cofactor for aminolevulinic acid synthase, although measurably low in the serum of chronic alcoholics, does not necessarily correlate with the finding of ringed sideroblasts.[97,100,101] In addition, decreased kinase activity has not clearly been demonstrated to account for low pyridoxal phosphate levels, although the latter has been shown to undergo enhanced degradation in the presence of acetaldehyde.[101–103] Since a direct role for vitamin B_6 deficiency has not been clearly shown in these alcoholic patients, an inhibitory role of ethanol on heme biosynthetic pathways (see Ch. 35) may be more likely. Overall heme production is reduced in the presence of ethanol, as is globin synthesis.[104,105]

Macrocytosis

Macrocytic red cells are a common finding in alcoholism.[106] When present in the absence of folate deficiency or reticulocytosis, a diagnosis of alcohol abuse can be considered.[107,108] The MCV is generally in the 100–110 fl range, the cells are round and not ovalocytic, and, together with the finding of an elevated γ-glutamyl transpeptidase in the serum, can be of diagnostic import. Mechanisms underlying this alteration have not been clarified. In a significant number of heavy drinkers, an increased value for red cell distribution width obtained from automated cell counters has also been described,[109] but others have not substantiated the value of this determination.[107] Unlike the readily reversible cell injury described for alcohol-mediated toxicity, this form of red cell change remains for ≤2–4 months of abstinence.

Folate and Vitamin B_{12} Metabolism

When megaloblastic anemia is found in the alcoholic patient, it is almost always secondary to folate deficiency; the hematologic manifestations of macrovalocytosis, hypersegmentation of polymorphonuclear leukocytes, leukopenia, and thrombocytopenia are indistinguishable from other causes of folate deficiency (see Ch. 41). Although liver disease is common in this group of patients, the vitamin deficiency primarily arises as a result of poor dietary intake and the effect of ethanol on folate metabolism.[87,110,111] Other causes of nonalcoholic cirrhosis are uncommonly associated with folate deficiency, nor is it seen in well-nourished drinkers. Secondary effects on folate homeostasis may occur as a result of poor retention by the cirrhotic liver and increased urinary loss.[112,113]

Evidence for a direct effect of ethanol on folate metabolism has come from several studies, both human and animal, in which alcohol and dietary intake were carefully controlled. In folate-deficient humans, megaloblastic changes can be seen within a few days when ethanol is added, but such changes take longer to develop when it is not.[87] Furthermore, giving folate supplements prevents these morphologic changes. Characteristically, hematosuppression, including white cell and platelet counts, reverts to normal within 1–2 weeks of a hospital diet.[98] The explanation for these observations has not been fully clarified. Among the suggested mechanisms have been (1) impairment of jejunal absorption,[114] (2) block in the delivery of N-5-methylfolate from the liver to the circulation,[110] (3) interruption of a putative enterohepatic circulation,[111,115] and (4) increased urinary excretion of folate.[112,113] In animal models, conflicting data have emerged on the effect of ethanol on hepatic polyglutamate folate synthesis and retention. Both increased synthesis and decreased formation have been described.[110,116] Furthermore, the clearance of methyltetrahydrofolic acid is normal in alcoholic patients, and its uptake is stimulated by ethanol in hepatocytes in vitro.[117,118] Extraneous factors such as gastrointestinal blood loss, hypersplenism, hemolysis, and infection further confound the interpretation of folate balance in these patients.

Clinically significant vitamin B_{12} deficiency rarely occurs in the alcoholic patient. This is rather surprising since impairment of absorption could occur secondarily to the frequently seen gastritis (parietal cell injury), pancreatitis (interference with pancreatic enzyme release of vitamin B_{12} from GR binders), or ileal malabsorption (vitamin B_{12} uptake) in these patients.[119,120] Whether as a result of liver injury or abnormal transcoalbumin binding, serum levels of the vitamin are frequently elevated. Even when low serum levels have been observed, concomitant folate deficiency may have been causal, since serum vitamin B_{12} levels reverted to normal within a few days of adequate folate intake.[121]

Iron Metabolism

Iron deficiency is commonly seen in alcoholic patients, usually as a result of gastrointestinal bleeding. However, because of the frequent association with folic acid deficiency, the usual laboratory parameters (MCV, serum iron, and transferrin saturation) may be normal or even increased.[82,87] Serum ferritin levels may be unreliable because of coexisting liver disease or complicating inflammatory disorders.[122] Simple chronic anemia, with low serum iron and low serum iron-binding capacity, will be found in those patients with infection or malignancy. Bone marrow iron stores are probably the most reliable means of ruling out iron deficiency in this complicated setting when folate deficiency has been ruled out.

Alcohol abuse may increase the body iron burden. This can result from excessive ingestion of iron-containing spirits (e.g., red wine) or increased iron absorption.[123,124] There has been some confusion between idiopathic hemochromatosis and alcoholic cirrhosis with increased stainable iron in the liver. Patients with alcoholic cirrhosis can be divided into two groups: (1) those patients who have a mild-to-moderate increase in stainable iron, but relatively normal body iron stores, and (2) those patients with gross iron deposition and increased total body iron stores of the magnitude seen in idiopathic hemochromatosis (15–50 g iron stores). Based on studies of HLA antigens, the first group shows no evidence of the genetic disease and the liver iron concentration is usually less than twice the upper limits of normal.[125] The second group appears to have idiopathic hemochromatosis in addition to alcoholism.[126] Additionally, in alcoholic patients the synthesis of desialated transferrin may lead to preferential hepatic uptake of iron.[127,128]

Red Cell Survival

A direct effect of alcohol on red cell survival once cells leave the bone marrow has not been demonstrated.[63] However, alcohol is the most common etiologic factor in acute and chronic liver disease that may be associated with hemolysis. A mild hemolytic state is relatively common in cirrhosis, reducing red cell survival to 50% of normal.[129] In the Zieve syndrome, alcohol-induced fatty liver is associated with hypertriglyceridemia, hemolysis, and jaundice.[130] Hemolysis is usually transient, and its pathophysiology appears to be unrelated to the hypertriglyceridemia.[63] A similar transient hemolytic state showing red cell stomatocytosis has been described.[131] Rarer still has been the hemolytic anemia associated with severe hypophosphatemia.[132] In many of these alcoholic patients, additional features such as bleeding, alcohol withdrawal, folate repletion, and hypersplenism make interpretation of the reticulocyte count difficult.

Platelet Production and Function

Thrombocytopenia is a well-recognized consequence of excessive ethanol intake.[82,84,87] With abstinence, the platelet count begins to rise within a few days, return to normal by 1 week, and may reach supranormal levels (rebound thrombocytosis) within 1–3 weeks. It should be emphasized that ethanol (or its metabolites) is the etiologic agent, and thrombocytopenia may be present in the absence of complicating liver disease, hypersplenism, nutritional deficiency, or DIC. The major toxic effect appears to be mediated at the bone marrow level, although there is some evidence for decreased platelet survival.[133] Megakaryocytes in the bone marrow are usually adequate in number[134,135] but may be reduced.[87,94,136] CFU-megakaryocyte grown in the presence of ethanol show diminished numbers in vitro.[93]

Not only does alcohol affect platelet production, but immoderate drinking can lead to several abnormalities of platelet function. Impaired platelet aggregation,[137–139] decreased thromboxane A_2 release,[137] and prolongation of the bleeding time, even in the absence of thrombocytopenia, have been observed.[133,140] Effects on storage pool ADP and platelet cAMP have also been described.[133,141] The degree to which impaired platelet function contributes to abnormal bleeding in alcoholic patients is not clear. Whether the decreased risk of cardiovascular disease, but an increased risk of cerebrovascular accidents, observed in these patients can be attributed to platelet function defects requires further study.[142,143]

Granulocyte Production and Function

The effect of ethanol consumption on granulocyte production is less clear than its effect on red cells and platelets. Neutropenia is more commonly a result of hypersplenism or folate deficiency.[144] Even though alcohol injury to bone marrow can produce vacuolization of myeloid precursors, the white cell count and marrow granulocyte reserve remain normal.[82,145] In vitro incubation of bone marrow with high levels of alcohol can inhibit granulocyte colony formation.[95] In occasional patients, the combination of heavy alcohol intake in combination with severe bacterial infections has been associated with marked neutropenia and bone marrow myeloid arrest at the myelocyte stage.[146]

The effect of alcohol on granulocyte function has long been suggested by the poor delivery of neutrophils to sites of acute infection. Movement into skin abrasions is decreased and has been attributed to defective adherence.[145,147] Although chemotaxis is reduced, phagocytosis and intracellular bacterial killing are not affected.[147–149]

Immune Function

Decreased numbers of circulating lymphocytes have been described in alcoholic subjects.[144] Active drinkers fail to develop expected, increased antibody titer responses to immune challenge and delayed hypersensitivity responses to new antigens.[144] In animal studies, ethanol ingestion decreases natural killer cell activity and delayed hypersensitivity responses.[150] Although the mechanisms underlying impaired cellular and humoral immune functions in alcoholic subjects have not been fully clarified, epidemiologic data support the association.

REFERENCES

1. Wion KL, Kelly D, Summerfield JA et al: Distribution of factor VII mRNA and antigen in human liver and other tissues. Nature 317:726, 1985
2. Mann FD, Shonyo ES, Mann FC: Effect of removal of the liver on blood coagulation. Am J Physiol 164:111, 1951
3. Pool J, Robinson J: In vitro synthesis of coagulation factors by rat liver slices. Am J Physiol 196:423, 1959
4. Olson JP, Miller LL, Troup SB: Synthesis of clotting factors by the isolated perfused rat liver. J Clin Invest 45:690, 1966
5. Ratnoff OD: Hemostatic defects in liver and biliary tract disease and disorders of vitamin K metabolism. p. 459. In Ratnoff OD, Forbes CD (eds): Disorders of Hemostasis. WB Saunders, Philadelphia, 1991
6. Rapaport SI, Ames SB, Mikkelsen S, Goodman JR: Plasma clotting factors in chronic hepatocellular disease. N Engl J Med 263:278, 1960
7. Donaldson GWK, Davies SH, Darg A, Richmond J: Coagulation factors in chronic liver disease. J Clin Pathol 22:199, 1969
8. Lechner K, Nisser H, Tahler E: Coagulation abnormalities in liver disease. Semin Thromb Hemost 4:40, 1977
9. Cederblad G, Korsan-Bengtsen K, Olson R: Observations of increased levels of blood coagulation factors and other plasma proteins in cholestatic liver disease. Scand J Gastroenterol 11:391, 1976
10. Maisonneuve P, Sultan Y: Modifications of factor VII complex properties in patients with liver disease. J Clin Pathol 30:221, 1977
11. Dymock IW, Tucher JS, Woolf IL et al: Coagulation studies as a prognostic index in acute liver failure. Br J Haematol 29:385, 1975
12. Furie B, Furie BC: The molecular basis of blood coagulation. Cell 53:505, 1988
13. Suttie JW: Vitamin K-dependent carboxylation. CRC Crit Rev Biochem 8:191, 1980
14. Nelsestuen GL, Zykowicz TH, Howard JB: The mode of action of vitamin K: identification of γ-carboxyglutamic acid as a component of prothrombin. J Biol Chem 249:6342, 1974
15. Stenflo J, Fernlund P, Egan W, Roepstorff P: Vitamin K-dependent modifications of glutamic acid residues in prothrombin. Proc Natl Acad Sci USA 71:2730, 1974
16. Esmon CT, Sadowski JA, Suttie JW: A new carboxylation reaction. The vitamin K-dependent incorporation of $H^{14}CO_3^-$ into prothrombin. J Biol Chem 250:4744, 1975
17. Blanchard RA, Furie BC, Jorgenson MJ et al: Acquired vitamin K-dependent carboxylation deficiency in liver disease. N Engl J Med 305:242, 1981
18. Liebman HA, Furie BC, Tong MJ et al: Des-γ-carboxy (abnormal) prothrombin as a serum marker of primary hepatocellular carcinoma. N Engl J Med 310:1427, 1984

19. Fujiyama S, Morishita T, Hashiguichi O, Sato T: Plasma abnormal prothrombin (des-γ-carboxy prothrombin) as a marker of hepatocellular carcinoma. Cancer 61:1621, 1988

20. Fujiyama S, Morishita T, Sagara K et al: Clinical evaluation of plasma abnormal prothrombin (PIVKA-II) in patients wtih hepatocellular carcinoma. Hepatogastroenterology 33:201, 1986

21. Frick PG, Riedler G, Brogli H: Dose response and minimal daily requirement for vitamin K in man. J Appl Physiol 23:387, 1967

22. Kaplan MM, Elta GH, Furie B et al: Fat soluble vitamin nutriture in primary biliary cirrhosis. Gastroenterology 95:787, 1988

23. Mombelli G, Monotti R, Haeberli A et al: Relationship between fibrinopeptide A and fibrinogen/fibrin fragment E in thromboembolism, DIC and various non-thromboembolic diseases. Thromb Haemost 58:758, 1987

24. vanDeWater L, Carr JM, Aronson D et al: Analysis of elevated fibrin(ogen) degradation product levels in patients with liver disease. Blood 67:1468, 1986

25. Sherlock S, Alpert L: Bleeding in surgery in relation to liver disease. Proc R Soc Med 58:257, 1965

26. Gralnick HR, Givelber H, Abrams E: Dysfibrinogenemia associated with hepatoma. Increased carbohydrate content of the fibrinogen molecule. N Engl J Med 299:221, 1978

27. Palascak J, Martinez J: Dysfibrinogenemia associated with liver disease. J Clin Invest 60:89, 1977

28. Martinez J, Palascak JE, Kwasniak D: Abnormal sialic acid content of the dysfibrinogenemia associated with liver disease. J Clin Invest 61:535, 1978

29. Green G, Thomson JM, Dymock IW, Poller L: Abnormal fibrin polymerization in liver disease. Br J Haematol 34:425, 1970

30. Martinez J, Keane PM, Gilman PB, Palascak JE: The abnormal carbohydrate composition of the dysfibrinogenemia associated with liver disease. Ann NY Acad Sci 408:388, 1983

31. Fletcher AP, Biederman O, Moore D et al: Abnormal plasminogen-plasmin system activity (fibrinolysis) in patients with hepatic cirrhosis. Its cause and consequences. J Clin Invest 43:681, 1964

32. Pises P, Bick R: Hyperfibrinolysis in cirrhosis. Am J Gastroenterol 60:280, 1973

33. Collen D: On the regulation and control of fibrinolysis. Thromb Haemost 43:77, 1980

34. Aoki N, Yamanaka T: The α₂-plasmin inhibitor levels in liver disease. Clin Chim Acta 84:99, 1978

35. Knot EAR, Drijfhout HR, ten Cate JW et al: α₂-Plasmin inhibitor metabolism in patients with liver cirrhosis. J Lab Clin Med 105:353, 1985

36. Hersch SL, Kunelis T, Francis RB Jr: The pathogenesis of accelerated fibrinolysis in liver cirrhosis: a critical role for tissue plasminogen activator inhibitor. Blood 69:1315, 1987

37. Tytgat GN, Collen D, Verstraete M: Metabolism of fibrinogen in cirrhosis of the liver. J Clin Invest 50:1690, 1971

38. Straub PW: Diffuse intravascular coagulation in liver disease. Semin Thromb Hemost 4:29, 1977

39. Stein SF, Harker LA: Kinetic and functional studies of platelets, fibrinogen and plasminogen in patients with hepatic cirrhosis. J Lab Clin Med 99:217, 1982

40. Coleman M, Finlayson N, Bettigole et al: Fibrinogen survival in cirrhosis: improvement by low dose heparin. Ann Intern Med 83:79, 1975

41. Singh R, Singh MM, Hazra DK et al: A study of disseminated intravascular coagulopathy in hepatic coma complicating acute viral hepatitis. Angiology 34:470, 1983

42. Rake MO, Flute PT, Panell G et al: Intravascular coagulation in acute hepatic necrosis. Lancet 1:533, 1970

43. Wardle EN: Fibrinogen in liver disease. Arch Surg 109:741, 1974

44. Lahnborg G, Friman L, Berghem L: Reticuloendothelial function in patients with alcoholic liver cirrhosis. Scand J Gastroenterol 16:481, 1981

45. Harmon DC, Demirjian Z, Ellman L et al: Disseminated intravascular coagulation with the peritoneovenous shunt. Ann Intern Med 90:774, 1979

46. Rubinstein D, McInnes I, Dudley F: Morbidity and mortality after peritoneovenous shunt surgery for refractory ascites. Gut 26:1070, 1985

47. Stein SF, Fulenwider JT, Ansley JD et al: Accelerated fibrinogen and platelet destruction after peritoneovenous shunting. Arch Intern Med 141:1149, 1981

48. Phillips LL, Rodger JB: Procoagulant activity of ascitic fluid in hepatic cirrhosis in vivo and in vitro. Surgery 86:714, 1979

49. Lerner RG, Nelson JC, Corines P et al: Disseminated intravascular coagulation: complication of peritoneovenous shunts. JAMA 240:2064, 1978

50. Salem HH, Dudley FJ, Merrett A et al: Coagulopathy of peritoneovenous shunts: studies on the pathogenic role of ascitic fluid collagen and value of antiplatelet therapy. Gut 24:412, 1983

51. LeVeen HH: The LeVeen shunt. Annu Rev Med 36:453, 1985

52. Schipper HG, ten Cate JW: Antithrombin III transfusion in patients with hepatic cirrhosis. Br J Haematol 52:25, 1982

53. Tollefson DM, Pestka CA: Heparin cofactor II activity in patients with disseminated intravascular coagulation and hepatic failure. Blood 66:769, 1985

54. Aster RH: Pooling of platelets in the spleen: role in the pathogenesis of "hypersplenic" thrombocytopenia. J Clin Invest 45:645, 1966

55. Harker LA: Kinetics of thrombopoiesis. J Clin Invest 47:458, 1968

56. Jacob HS: Hypersplenism: mechanisms and management. Br J Haematol 27:1, 1974

57. Hess CE, Ayers CR, Sandusky WR et al: Mechanism of dilutional anemia in massive splenomegaly. Blood 47:629, 1976

58. Lieberman FL, Reynolds TB: Plasma volume in cirrhosis of the liver. J Clin Invest 46:1297, 1967

59. Brubaker LH, Johnson CA: Correlation of splenomegaly and abnormal neutrophil pooling (margination). J Lab Clin Med 92:508, 1978

60. Ferrara J, Ellison C, Martin EW et al: Correction of hypersplenism following distal splenorenal shunt. Surgery 86:570, 1979

61. Morris PW, Patton TB, Balint JA et al: Portal hypertension, congestive splenomegaly and portacaval shunt. Gastroenterology 42:555, 1962

62. Mutchnick MG, Lerner E, Conn HO: Effect of portacaval anastomosis on hypersplenism. Dig Dis Sci 25:929, 1980

63. Cooper RA: Hemolytic syndromes and red cell membrane abnormalities in liver disease. Semin Hematol 17:103, 1980

64. Cooper RA: Anemia with spur cells: a red cell defect acquired in serum and modified in the circulation. J Clin Invest 48:1820, 1969

65. Cooper RA, Diloy-Puray M, Lando P et al: An analysis of lipoproteins, bile acids and red cell membranes associated with target cells and spur cells in patients with liver disease. J Clin Invest 51:3182, 1972

66. Cooper RA, Kimball DB, Durocher JR: Role of the spleen in membrane conditioning and hemolysis of spur cells in liver disease. N Engl J Med 290:1279, 1974

67. Bingham J: The macrocytosis of hepatic disease. I. Thin macrocytosis. Blood 14:694, 1958

68. Werre JM, Helleman PW, Verloop MC et al: Causes of macroplania of erythrocytes in diseases of the liver and biliary tract with special reference to leptocytosis. Br J Haematol 19:223, 1970

69. Conrad ME, Schwartz FD, Young AA: Infectious hepatitis—a generalized disease. A study of renal, gastrointestinal and hematologic abnormalities. Am J Med 37:789, 1964

70. Raffensperger EC: Acute acquired hemolytic anemia in association with acute viral hepatitis. Ann Intern Med 65:1210, 1966

71. Pitcher CS, Williams R: Reduced red cell survival in jaundice and its relation to abnormal glutathione metabolism. Clin Sci 24:239, 1963

72. Salen G, Goldstein F, Hauran F et al: Acute hemolytic anemia complicating viral hepatitis in patients with glucose-6-phosphate dehydrogenase deficiency. Ann Intern Med 65:1210, 1966

73. Chan TK, Todd D: Haemolysis complicating viral hepatitis in patients with glucose-6-phosphate dehydrogenase deficiency. BMJ 1:131, 1975

74. Bottiger LE, Westerholm B: Aplastic anemia—III. Aplastic anemia and infectious hepatitis. J Intern Med 192:323, 1972

75. Young N, Mortimer P: Viruses and bone marrow failure. Blood 63:729, 1984

76. Zeldis JB, Dienstag JL, Gale RP: Aplastic anemia and non-A, non-B hepatitis. Am J Med 74:64, 1983

77. Lieber CS: Metabolism and metabolic effects of alcohol. Med Clin North Am 68:3, 1984

78. Domshke S, Domshke W, Lieber CS: Hepatic redox state: attenuation of the acute effects of ethanol induced by chronic ethanol consumption. Life Sci 15:1327, 1974

79. Veech RL, Guyan R, Veloso D: The time-course of the effects of ethanol on the redox and phosphorylation states of rat liver. Biochem J 127:387, 1972

80. Lieber CS, Savolainen M: Ethanol and lipids. Alcohol Clin Exp Res 8:409, 1984

81. McCurdy PR, Pierce LE, Rath CE: Abnormal bone marrow morphology in acute alcoholism. N Engl J Med 266:505, 1962

82. Lindenbaum J, Lieber CS: Hematologic effects of alcohol in man in the absence of nutritional deficiency. N Engl J Med 281:333, 1969

83. Chanarin I: Hemopoiesis and alcohol. Med Clin North Am 68:179, 1982

84. Colman N, Herbert V: Hematologic complications of alcoholism. Semin Hematol 17:164, 1980

85. Ballard HS: Alcohol-associated pancytopenia with hypocellular bone marrow. Am J Clin Pathol 73:830, 1980

86. Casagrande G, Michot F: Alcohol-induced bone marrow damage: status before and after a 4-week period of abstinence from alcohol with or without disulfiram. A randomized bone marrow study in alcohol-dependent individuals. Blut 59:231, 1989

87. Sullivan LW, Herbert V: Suppression of hematopoiesis by ethanol. J Clin Invest 43:2048, 1964
88. Goldstein DB, Chin JH: Interactions of ethanol with biological membranes. Fed Proc 40:2073, 1981
89. Yeung KY, Klug PP, Lessin LS: Alcohol-induced vacuolization in bone marrow cells: ultrastructure and mechanism of formation. Blood Cells 13:487, 1988
90. Saidi P, Wallerstein RP, Aggeler PM: Effect of chloramphenicol on erythropoiesis. J Lab Clin Med 57:249, 1961
91. Norgard MJ, Carpenter JT, Conrad ME: Bone marrow necrosis and degeneration. Arch Intern Med 139:905, 1970
92. Meagher RC, Sieber F, Spivak JL: Suppression of hematopoietic-progenitor-cell proliferation by ethanol and acetaldehyde. N Engl J Med 307:845, 1982
93. Clark DA, Krantz SB: Effects of ethanol on cultured human megakaryocyte progenitors. Exp Hematol 14:951, 1986
94. Gewirtz AM, Hoffman R: Transitory hypomegakaryocytic thrombocytopenia: aetiological association with ethanol abuse and implications regarding regulation of human megakaryocytopoiesis. Br J Haematol 62:333, 1986
95. Tisman G, Herbert V: In vitro myelosuppression and immunosuppression by ethanol. J Clin Invest 52:1410, 1973
96. Eichner ER, Hillman RS: The evolution of anemia in alcoholic patients. Am J Med 50:218, 1971
97. Pierce HI, McGuffin RG, Hillman RS: Clinical studies in alcoholic sideroblastosis. Arch Intern Med 136:283, 1975
98. Savage D, Lindenbaum J: Anemia in alcoholics. Medicine 65:322, 1986
99. Hines JD, Cowan DH: Studies on the pathogenesis of alcohol-induced sideroblastic bone marrow abnormalities. N Engl J Med 283:441, 1970
100. Parker TH, Marshall JP, Roberts RK et al: Effect of acute alcohol ingestion on plasma pyridoxal 5'-phosphate. Am J Clin Nutr 32:1246, 1979
101. Lumeng L, Li TK: Vitamin B_6 metabolism in chronic alcohol abuse: pyridoxal phosphate levels in plasma and the effects of acetaldehyde on pyridoxal phosphate synthesis and degradation in human erythrocytes. J Clin Invest 53:693, 1974
102. Solomon LR, Hillman RS: Vitamin B_6 metabolism in anemic and alcoholic man. Br J Haematol 41:343, 1979
103. Lumeng L: The role of acetaldehyde in mediating the deleterious effect of ethanol on pyxridoxal 5'-phosphate metabolism. J Clin Invest 62:286, 1978
104. Ali MAM, Brain MC: Ethanol inhibition of haemoglobin synthesis: in vitro evidence for a haem correctable defect in normal subjects and in alcoholics. Br J Haematol 28:311, 1974
105. Freedman ML, Cohen HS, Rosman J et al: Ethanol inhibition of reticulocyte protein synthesis: the role of haem. Br J Haematol 30:351, 1975
106. Wu A, Chanarin I, Levi AJ: Macrocytosis of chronic alcoholism. Lancet 1:829, 1974
107. Unger KW, Johnson D: Red blood cell MCV: a potential indicator of alcohol usage in a working population. Am J Med Sci 267:281, 1974
108. Seppa K, Laippala P, Saarni M: Macrocytosis as a consequence of alcohol abuse among patients in general practice. Alcohol Clin Exp Res 15:871, 1991
109. Seppa K, Sillanaukee P, Koivula T: Abnormalities of hematologic parameters in heavy drinkers and alcoholics. Alcohol Clin Exp Res 16:117, 1992
110. Lindenbaum J: Folate and vitamin B_{12} deficiencies in alcoholism. Semin Hematol 17:119, 1980
111. Hillman RS, Steinberg SE: The effects of alcohol on folate metabolism. Annu Rev Med 33:345, 1982
112. Russell RM, Rosenberg IH, Wilson PD et al: Increased urinary excretion and prolonged turnover time of folic acid during ethanol ingestion. Am J Clin Nutr 38:64, 1983
113. McMartin KE, Collins TD, Shiao CQ et al: Study of dose-dependence and urinary folate excretion produced by ethanol in humans and rats. Alcohol Clin Exp Res 10:419, 1986
114. Halsted CH, Robles EA, Mezey E: Intestinal malabsorption in folate-deficient alcoholics. Gastroenterology 64:526, 1973
115. Steinberg SE, Campbell CL, Hillman RS: Kinetics of the normal folate enterohepatic cycle. J Clin Invest 64:83, 1979
116. Wilkinson JA, Shane B: Folate metabolism in the ethanol-fed rat. J Nutr 112:604, 1982
117. Lane F, Godd P, McGuffin R et al: Folic acid metabolism in normal, folate deficient and alcoholic man. Br J Haematol 34:489, 1976
118. Horne DW, Briggs WT, Wagner C: Studies on the transport mechanism of 5 methyltetrahydrofolic acid in freshly isolated hepatocytes: effect of ethanol. Arch Biochem Biophys 19:557, 1979
119. Allen RH, Seetharam B, Allen NC et al: Correction of cobalamin malabsorption in pancreatic insufficiency with a cobalamin analogue that binds with high affinity to R protein but not to intrinsic factor: in vivo evidence that a failure to partially degarde R protein is responsible for cobalamin malabsorption in pancreatic insufficiency. J Clin Invest 62:1628, 1978
120. Rubin E, Rybak BJ, Lindenbaum J et al: Ultrastructural changes in the small intestine induced by ethanol. Gastroenterology 63:801, 1972
121. Johnson S, Swaminathan SP, Baker SJ: Changes in serum vitamin B_{12} levels in patients with megaloblastic anemia treated with folic acid. J Clin Pathol 15:274, 1962
122. Lipschitz DA, Cook JD, Finch CA: A clinical evaluation of serum ferritin as an index of iron stores. N Engl J Med 290:1213, 1974
123. Charlton RW, Jacobs P, Seftel H et al: Effect of alcohol on iron absorption. BMJ 2:1427, 1964
124. Weintraub LR, Conrad ME, Crosby WH: Regulation of intestinal iron absorption by the rate of erythropoiesis. Br J Haematol 11:432, 1965
125. Simon M, Bourel M, Genetet B et al: Idiopathic hemochromatosis and iron overload in alcoholic liver disease: differentiation by HLA phenotype. Gastroenterology 73:655, 1977
126. Halliday JW, Powell LW: Iron overload. Semin Hematol 19:42, 1982
127. Beguin Y, Bergmaschi G, Huebers H et al: The behavior of asialotransferrin in the rat. Am J Hematol 29:204, 1988
128. Storey EL, Anderson GJ, Mack U et al: Desialylated transferrin as a serological marker of excessive alcohol ingestion. Lancet 1:1292, 1987
129. Jandl JH: The anemia of liver disease: observations on its mechanism. J Clin Invest 34:390, 1955
130. Zieve L: Jaundice hyperlipemia and hemolytic anemia: a heretofore unrecognized syndrome associated with alcoholic fatty liver and cirrhosis. Ann Intern Med 48:471, 1958
131. Douglass CC, Twomey JJ: Transient stomatocytosis with hemolysis: a previously unrecognized complication of alcoholism. Ann Intern Med 72:159, 1970
132. Territo MC, Tanaka KR: Hypophosphatemia in chronic alcoholism. Arch Intern Med 134:445, 1974
133. Cowan DH: Effect of alcoholism on hemostasis. Semin Hematol 17:137, 1980
134. Lindenbaum J, Hargrove RL: Thrombocytopenia in alcoholics. Ann Intern Med 68:526, 1968
135. Levine RF, Spivak JL, Maegher RC et al: Effect of ethanol on thrombopoiesis. Br J Haematol 62:345, 1986
136. Fink R, Hutton RA: Changes in the blood platelets of alcoholics during withdrawal. J Clin Pathol 36:337, 1983
137. Mikhailidis DP, Jenkins WJ, Barradas MA et al: Platelet function defects in chronic alcoholism. BMJ 293:715, 1986
138. Mikhailidis DP, Barradas MA, Epemolu O et al: Ethanol ingestion inhibits human whole blood platelet impedance aggregation. Am J Clin Pathol 88:342, 1987
139. Rand ML, Neiman J, Jakower DM et al: Effects of alcohol withdrawal on response of platelets from alcoholics—a study using platelet-rich plasma from blood anticoagulated with D-phenylalanyl-L-prolyl-L-arginyl chloromethyl ketone (FPRCH2C1). Thromb Hemost 63:178, 1990
140. Deykin D, Janson P, McMahon L: Ethanol potentiation of aspirin-induced prolongation of the bleeding time. N Engl J Med 306:852, 1982
141. DePetrillo PB, Swift RM: Ethanol exposure results in a transient decreased in human platelet cAMP levels: evidence for a protein kinase C mediated process. Alcoholism 16:290, 1992
142. Stampfer MJ, Colditz GA, Willett WC et al: A prospective study of moderate alcohol consumption and the risk of coronary disease and stroke in women. N Engl J Med 319:267, 1988
143. Gill JS, Vezulka AV, Shipkey MJ et al: Stroke and alcohol consumption. N Engl J Med 315:1041, 1986
144. Liu YK: Effects of alcohol on granulocytes and lymphocytes. Semin Hematol 17:130, 1980
145. Gluckman SJ, MacGregor RR: Effect of acute alcohol intoxication on granulocyte mobilization and kinetics. Blood 52:551, 1978
146. McFarland E, Libre EP: Abnormal leucocyte response in alcoholism. Ann Intern Med 59:865, 1963
147. Brayton RG, Stokes PE, Schwartz MS et al: Effect of alcohol and various diseases on leukocyte mobilization, phagocytosis, and intracellular bacterial killing. N Engl J Med 282:123, 1970
148. Spagnuolo PJ, MacGregor RR: Acute ethanol effect on chemotaxis and other components of host defense. J Lab Clin Med 86:24, 1975
149. Gluckman SJ, Dvorak VC, MacGregor RR: Host defenses during prolonged alcohol consumption in a controlled environment. Arch Intern Med 137:1539, 1977
150. Meadows GG, Blank SE, Duncan DD: Influence of ethanol consumption on natural killer cell activity in mice. Alcohol Clin Exp Res 13:476, 1989

Hematologic Complications of Renal Disease

148

Nicholas Dainiak

INTRODUCTION

Chronic renal insufficiency is characterized by an elevation in serum urea nitrogen and creatinine concentrations with or without reduced urine output. It leads ultimately to functional disorders involving virtually every organ system in the body, including the fluid and electrolyte, endocrine and metabolic, neuromuscular, cardiovascular, pulmonary, dermatologic, gastrointestinal, hematologic, and immunologic systems. Disturbances of the hematopoietic system range from cytopenias and hypocomplementemia to disorders of hemostasis. These disturbances may lead to the development of splenomegaly and hypersplenism and to increased susceptibility to infection. In turn, these sequelae may worsen cytopenias and bleeding. Unfortunately, most of the hematologic and immunologic disturbances present in chronic renal insufficiency progress or develop even after an optimal program of dialysis and related therapy has been initiated.[1]

PATHOPHYSIOLOGY OF RENAL DYSFUNCTION

The classic evolution of renal failure to terminal uremia and azotemia was first described by Bright[2] in 1936. Although the full clinical spectrum of abnormalities in uremia is rarely seen today because of therapeutic intervention, pallor and anemia persist as hallmarks of severe renal insufficiency. Patients with a blood urea nitrogen concentration of >100 mg/dl rarely have a hematocrit value >30%.[3] Attempts to explain this relationship have changed in concert with evolving concepts concerning the pathogenesis of uremia.[4] Although excretory failure leading to retention of nitrogenous waste products is pathogenetically more closely related to acute neurobehavioral abnormalities, failure of renal biosynthetic processes and hormonal regulation has been recognized as related to chronic organ abnormalities. Renal biosynthetic failure encompasses not only impaired secretion of metabolites (including serine, leucine, and arginine) by the kidney but also impaired production of renal hormones.[5] Among the renal hormones are erythropoietin (EPO), renin, 1,25-dihydroxycholecalciferol-vitamin D_3, and prostaglandins. Defective production or release of these hormones leads to a wide spectrum of organ dysfunction, including anemia, hypertension, disturbed calcium metabolism, altered renal blood flow, and impaired sodium and water excretion.[6-8] Recently, the concept that defective hormonal feedback systems may lead to uremia has been advanced.[9,10] Since the diseased kidney maintains sodium balance in spite of a loss of functioning nephrons, circulating inhibitors of sodium transport may be present. Although little is known about the chemical identity of such inhibitors (or uremic "toxins"), considerable evidence indicates that sodium transport is inhibited and sodium/potassium/ATPase levels are decreased.[11-14] Such abnormal regulators appear to be distinct from low molecular mass "toxins," which include >70 nitrogenous compounds, and also distinct from oligopeptides and polypeptides (i.e., "middle molecules" ranging in molecular mass from 300 to 2,000 daltons), which may be retained as a consequence of impaired renal excretory function.[5] In addition, endocrine "toxins," including parathyrin and natriuretic hormone, may be present in increased quantities in response to reduced renal mass. As a result of the ubiquitous actions of these substances, many features of uremia may be explained by disruption of normal hormonal feedback systems.[15,16]

ETIOLOGY AND PATHOGENESIS OF HEMATOLOGIC AND IMMUNOLOGIC DISTURBANCES

Abnormalities in renal excretory function, renal biosynthetic processes, or hormonal regulation may be responsible for the hematologic sequelae of renal failure. Except for defective production of the hematopoietic hormone EPO, evidence that a direct relationship exists between a specific abnormality in renal function and a hematologic complication remains circumstantial.

Hypoproliferative Anemia

Anemia characteristically accompanies the uremic syndrome. It is virtually always present in acute forms of renal failure associated with interstitial nephritis, tubular necrosis, and glomerulonephritis,[17] and it is often the presenting symptom of chronic renal insufficiency as well.[3] Over 90% of patients receiving chronic dialysis therapy have anemia, and in 25% of these individuals, anemia is severe enough (hematocrit <25%) to require repeated blood transfusions.[18] Although the etiology of renal failure correlates poorly with degree of anemia, patients with polycystic disease are less anemic than those with other renal disorders on a per-milligram serum creatinine basis. This may in part be related to induction of EPO synthesis or release in response to local renal hypoxia that develops as a consequence of pressure exerted by space-occupying cysts. By contrast, renal failure associated with other disorders may be complicated by a greater degree of anemia than anticipated. For example, blood loss and iron deficiency invariably complicate renal failure due to Goodpasture syndrome and Henoch-Schönlein purpura. Likewise, hemolysis may be more severe in patients with renal insufficiency associated with connective tissue disease (such as systemic lupus erythematosus), and production of EPO by kidneys that have been damaged by radiation may be inordinately depressed.[19-21]

A low red blood cell mass in uremia is most often the result of diminished red cell production. The principal cause of this defect is a decrease in renal EPO production relative to the degree of anemia that is present. Although low, normal, and high levels of plasma EPO have been measured by radioimmunoassay and bioassay,[22-27] they are inappropriately low when adjusted for degree of anemia[23-30] (Fig. 148-1). Furthermore, a positive correlation is present between serum EPO level and hematocrit, and between hematocrit and creatinine clearance in patients with a relatively mild degree of renal failure (i.e., creatinine clearance of 2–40 ml/min[28]). Anephric patients have the lowest EPO levels, a finding that complements the observa-

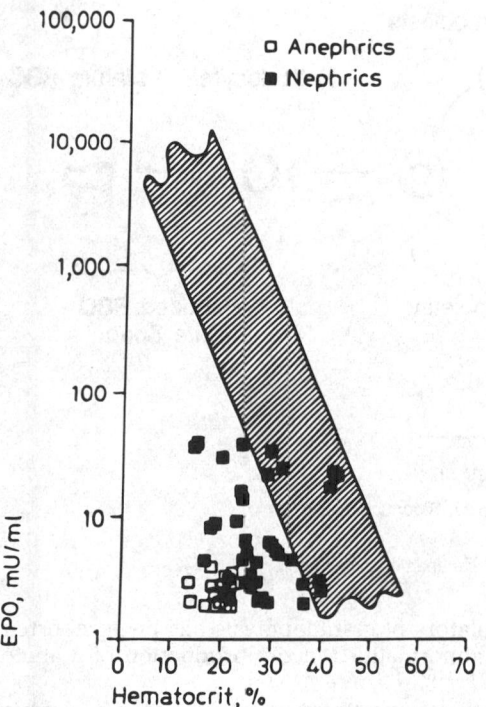

Fig. 148-1. Levels of EPO versus hematocrit in uremic patients with or without intact kidneys. Shaded area represents predicted values. (From Caro et al.,[6] with permission.)

tion that erythropoiesis is severely impaired (but not abolished) in patients who have undergone bilateral nephrectomy.[28-31] As shown in Figure 148-1, anephric individuals have extremely low but nevertheless detectable plasma EPO. The source of this extrarenal EPO is unknown but may be macrophages in the bone marrow or spleen,[31] Kupffer cells in the liver,[33-36] or possibly cellular components of submandibular glands.[37,38] In addition to EPO, plasma from anephric individuals may also contain an insulin growth factor-like activity that supports the growth of mature erythroid progenitor cells.[39]

Although the presence of a circulating erythropoietic factor was postulated at the turn of the century,[40] was confirmed to exist in 1953,[41] and was demonstrated to be of renal origin in 1957,[42] remarkably little is known about its cellular site of production. The renal cellular origin of the hormone has been ascribed to glomerular,[43-47] mesangial,[48,49] cortical,[50-53] tubular,[54] medullary,[55,56] and juxtaglomerular[57,58] cells at one time or another. Recently, the EPO gene has been used as a probe to detect EPO mRNA accumulation under hypoxic conditions.[59,60] Results of this experimental approach suggest that tubular[61] or peritubular[62] cells produce EPO in response to hypoxia. Nevertheless, because the healthy kidney contains no detectable stores of EPO,[63] insight concerning cellular or subcellular mechanisms leading to defective production in renal failure has not been forthcoming.

Even less is known about the forces that drive EPO production and release. Clinical observations in patients with patent ductus arteriosus and erythrocyte overproduction suggested that an oxygen sensor for hypoxia is located below the diaphragm.[64,65] Although the sensing mechanism for hypoxia is believed to reside in the kidneys, virtually no information concerning its cellular localization is available. It has been suggested that the regulatory feedback mechanism for EPO production remains intact in patients with mild renal insufficiency but that the entire system operates at a reduced level.[29,30] This may result in a suboptimal EPO response to hypoxia. Such a mechanism may be the antithesis of an abnormally high "set

point" for EPO production, which has been suggested to be responsible for EPO-dependent erythrocytosis.[65]

In addition to relative EPO deficiency, other processes may contribute to hypoproliferative anemia in renal disease (Fig. 148-2). Uremic "toxins" that impair proliferation of erythroid progenitor cells and erythroid precursors in the bone marrow have been described. These include serum inhibitors of erythroblast maturation and heme synthesis,[67-69] as well as inhibitors directed at progenitor cells. The latter toxins have been identified in in vitro marrow culture systems as spermine,[70] parathyrin,[71] ribonuclease,[72] and various serum lipoproteins. However, the physiologic relevance of these in vitro observations is not established. Uremic serum has been found to inhibit colony-forming unit-granulocyte/macrophage (CFU-GM) proliferation as well as megakaryocyte cell line growth[73]; spermine has been found to inhibit CFU-GM proliferation.[74] These observations are discordant with in vivo findings that both the white blood cell count and platelet count are characteristically normal in renal insufficiency. Furthermore, uremic serum contains normal levels of polyamines.[75] Likewise, serum lipoproteins from healthy (nonanemic) individuals have been found to suppress hematopoietic progenitor cell proliferation.[76] Finally, the concentration of ribonuclease required for in vitro inhibition of erythroid progenitor cell growth exceeds levels found in uremic serum.[72] On the other hand, the pathogenesis of hypoproliferative anemia may be more complex than a mere hormone (i.e., EPO) deficiency state.[77]

Hemolytic Anemia

A diminished red cell mass may result not only from impaired red cell production but also from decreased red cell life span (Fig. 148-2). Reductions in red cell survival rates to approximately one-half normal have been measured in patients with advanced renal failure.[78-81] This defect has been shown to be extracorpuscular and may be due to retention of uremic solutes that function as abnormal metabolites or to mechanical factors in the environment of the red cell as it travels through abnormal vasculature. Cross-transfusion studies indicate that uremic red cells survive normally in normal recipients, whereas the life span of normal red cells is shortened when transfused into uremic patients.[82,83] Moreover, red cell life span occasionally normalizes after intensification of dialysis[84] or change to continuous ambulatory peritoneal dialysis,[85] thereby suggesting that metabolic factors are involved.

In contrast to its environment, the red cell appears to be generally normal in renal failure. Laboratory evidence for appropriately increased activities (for age) of many red cell enzymes and ATP[14,86,87] supports this concept. An appropriately elevated 2,3-diphosphoglycerate level and depressed hemoglobin affinity for oxygen suggest that the red cell carries and releases oxygen in a normal fashion. Nevertheless, slightly decreased transketolase and superoxide dismutase levels[88,89] as well as depressed Na$^+$/K$^+$-ATPase[90] have been reported; these findings may be physiologically important when the red cell membrane is exposed to oxidant drugs or compounds.[91] Therefore, therapy generating factors that stress the red cell antioxidant system may result in accelerated hemolysis (see below). In the absence of such stress, only a small minority of uremic patients have underlying anemia principally due to diminished red cell survival.

Erythrocytosis

In some patients with impaired renal function the red cell mass is elevated rather than depressed. Isolated erythrocytosis has been described in association with a variety of renal

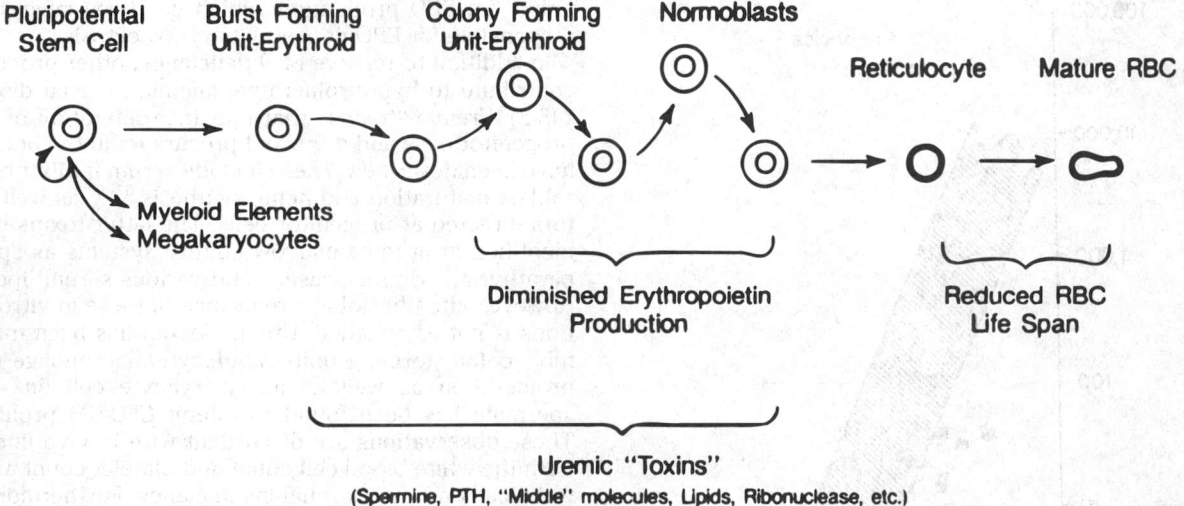

Fig. 148-2. Levels of defects in the production and life span of the red cell.

disorders, including hypernephroma, cystic renal disease, ureteral obstruction, and renal artery stenosis.[90-92] In addition, it may complicate the clinical course of 10–20% of patients receiving renal transplantation.[93,94] Erythrocytosis may be the harbinger of acute or chronic allograft rejection[95,96] and transplant renal artery stenosis.[92,97,98] In many patients, it is accompanied by excessive EPO production.[95,97,98-102] Even moderate levels of erythrocytosis can be associated with elevated serum EPO levels.[103-105] The etiology of increased EPO levels is unclear, but may be related to impaired renal blood flow, resulting in local hypoxia and stimulation of the renal oxygen sensor.[93,94] Selective catheterization of veins of native and transplanted kidneys has demonstrated elevated EPO levels in blood exiting from native (diseased) kidney or kidney remnants.[94,106] Whether such EPO production is autonomous or subject to feedback regulation (but at an elevated EPO "set point") is unknown.[94] Alternatively, hepatic EPO production may be stimulated by unknown mechanisms, or EPO production may be induced by administration of androgenic steroids.[107-109] It appears that administration of exogenous EPO at the time of renal transplantation does not predispose to development of posttransplant erythrocytosis, although follow-up has been for only 15 months.[110]

Since erythrocytosis may occur in patients lacking native kidneys and since confounding variables such as androgenic steroid administration, smoking, hepatic insufficiency, diabetes mellitus, cardiac dysfunction, and pulmonary disease often complicate renal failure, the etiology of EPO-dependent erythrocytosis in the renal transplant recipient may be multifactorial.[95] Moreover, because uremic serum from patients with renal failure contains factors that are recognized by anti-EPO antibody (i.e., share antigenic determinants with EPO) but that are free of biologic activity and are smaller in molecular mass than native EPO, the relationship between elevated EPO levels and erythrocytosis requires further characterization.[111]

Leukocyte Dysfunction

Renal failure is accompanied by a high incidence of infection that often leads to death.[112,113] Multiple defects in the complex network of immunoregulation have been described, although a clear explanation for infection has been elusive. Granulopoiesis is appropriately stimulated, provided that cytotoxic immunotherapy is not being used. Megaloblastic morphologic changes are only rarely seen and when present are usually unexplained.[114] Conflicting evidence for stimulatory and inhibitory regulators of granulopoiesis has been reported, suggesting that abnormalities in the production of granulocytes are unusual.[115,116]

By contrast, granulocyte pool sizes may be prominently disturbed in uremia, particularly during hemodialysis. Mild neutrophilia is commonly seen, a finding that may be related to alterations in the distribution of granulocyte pools.[114,117,118] A low mobilizable marrow pool of granulocytes has been found in uremic patients after hydrocortisone injection.[119] Presumably, marrow granulocyte reserves have already been called on, leading to diminished pool sizes that are assessed by steroid release tests. On the other hand, marrow release appears to be normal in response to complement, as assessed by the C3e-responsive pool.[120] More marked changes occur in granulocytes during hemodialysis. Severe transient neutropenia occurs within 2 hours after dialysis is begun, a finding that initially appeared to be due to sequestration of granulocytes in the dialysis apparatus.[121] Further study of this phenomenon, however, disclosed that administration of autologous plasma that had been incubated with dialyzer cellophane resulted in complement-mediated leukostasis in pulmonary vessels.[122,123] Precisely how complement activation alters granulocyte adhesiveness and whether this mechanism fully explains hypoxemia during hemodialysis remain unknown.

Mild functional abnormalities of granulocytes have also been observed in uremia. Impaired granulocyte migration into a Rebuck skin window,[124] abnormal chemotactic activity in the presence of autologous uremic plasma or serum,[125] and uremic "factors" capable of inhibiting chemotaxis[126] have all been described. Some of these defects are reversible with successful renal transplantation.[127]

In contrast to mild disturbances of granulocytes, significant lymphopenia and lymphocyte dysfunction have been described in uremia. Absolute lymphopenia occurs in patients with renal failure with or without hemodialytic therapy.[115-120] Lymphopoietic hypoplasia and thymic hypoplasia have been described in neonates of women with renal insufficiency as well.[5] Whereas T cells are depressed in number, B-cell lymphopenia is more prominent.[128-130] In addition, a variety of immunologic abnormalities have been found in nephrotic syndrome (Table 148-1). These include hypocomplementemia, defective opsonization, impaired immunoglobulin production, abnormal humoral function (assessed by presence of soluble factors that inhibit lymphocyte proliferation and factors that inhibit monocyte migration), and impaired cellular immunity.

Although serum immunoglobulin A, G, and M levels have

Table 148-1. Immunologic Disturbances in Nephrotic Syndrome

Immune Response	Disturbance	Reference
Opsonization	Low factor B, D serum levels	131, 132
	Impaired neutrophil chemotaxis/ chemiluminescence	133
	Impaired reticuloendothelial cell function	134
Immunoglobulin production	Low serum immunoglobulin levels	135, 136
	Diminished immunoglobulin systhesis in vitro	138
	Decreased immunoglobulin reactivity	139, 140
Humoral immunity	Serum inhibition of lymphyocyte proliferation	141, 142
	Serum toxicity to lymphoctyes	143
	Production of soluble inhibitors, including monocyte migration inhibitory factor, immune response suppressor	144, 145, 146
Cellular immunity	Impaired lymphocyte blastogenesis	147
	Reduced delayed hypersensitivity reactions	148, 149
	Suppression of antibody-dependent cell-mediated cytotoxicity	150, 151
	Impaired transfer of tuberculin sensitivity	152, 153
	Cutaneous anergy	154, 155

been reported to be diminished,[135,136] some researchers have found normal values in uremic patients.[128,137] On the other hand, striking defects in cellular immunity have been observed consistently, both in vitro (Table 148-1) and in vivo. Reduced delayed hypersensitivity reactions to common antigens such as mumps, *Trichophyton,* and *Candida* are well described.[149,156,157] Extended survival of skin allotransplants[158–160] and prolonged cardiac transplant survival[161] occur as well. In addition, alterations in the immune surveillance system may be related to the high incidence of malignancy known to occur in uremic patients.[151,162] Both natural killer cell activity and antibody-dependent cell-mediated cytotoxicity are inhibited by uremic serum, an observation that may be important in host defense against malignancy.[120,150,151]

Abnormalities of Hemostasis

Abnormal hemostasis, with a proclivity for bruising and bleeding, is commonly seen in chronic renal disease. Although qualitative and quantitative disturbances of the platelets, clotting cascade proteins, and blood vessels are known to occur in uremia, the pathogenesis of these defects remains obscure. One potentially important factor may be retention of low-molecular-weight toxins. Guanidinosuccinic acid and phenolic acid are known to reduce platelet factor III availability and to inhibit ADP-induced platelet aggregation.[163,164] By contrast, prostaglandins that have a tonic vasodilating effect in chronic renal disease[165,166] activate platelets and induce coagulation, particularly within glomerular capillary loops.[167] Dialyzer membrane composition and flow design may also play a role in activating platelets of hemodialyzed patients.[168]

In addition, it is possible that the clotting abnormalities, particularly those involving the platelet, develop as a consequence of fluctuations in the hematocrit value. According to this hypothesis, platelet adhesion to the subendothelium increases progressively as the hematocrit rises.[169] As red cells flow through vessels at relatively high shear rates, platelets diffuse radially, increasing the chances of platelet collision with the vessel wall, thereby favoring thrombus formation.[170] Disproportionate increases in hematocrit value and whole blood viscosity may be further aggravated by the therapeutic use of

diuretics. An inverse correlation exists between bleeding time and hematocrit, and red cell transfusion improves several clotting parameters, including platelet retention on glass beads, prothrombin consumption, serum thromboxane B_2 production, and intraplatelet cAMP levels.[171,172]

Alterations in clotting factor levels occur in uremia as well. Decreased blood levels of factors IX, XI, and XII have been reported and are believed to result from increased urinary losses of these relatively low-molecular-weight proteins.[168] Blood levels of other clotting factors (factors II, V, VII, VIII, X, and XIII) are often increased.[173–176] Because the latter changes correlate with degree of hypoalbuminemia, it is possible that they develop secondary to increased hepatic synthesis.[177] Nevertheless, no direct relationship has been established between clotting factor levels and development of the thrombotic diatheses (such as renal vein thrombosis) that are known to complicate renal insufficiency.[178]

An abnormality of the von Willebrand factor (vWF) has also been identified in uremia, a finding that may bear directly on the role of platelets in primary hemostasis. Ristocetin cofactor activity is lower than normal in chronic renal failure patients, and elevated vWF antigen levels are detected.[179] These findings are supported by the observation that in uremia, the vWF activity is consistently lower than its antigen level and that hemorrhagic tendency is corrected by infusion of either cryoprecipitate[180] or the synthetic derivation of the antidiuretic hormone 1-desamino-8-D-arginine vasopressin (DDAVP).[181] These findings correlate with shortening of an abnormal bleeding time, suggesting that abnormalities in the factor VIII/vWF antigen level and functional activity lead to a prolonged bleeding time.

Disturbances of coagulation are also common in pre-eclampsia and eclampsia.[182,183] Intravascular hemolysis and coagulation abnormalities are no more severe in women who develop acute renal failure than in those who do not.[184] It is unknown whether the deposition of thrombi and development of renal cortical necrosis occur as the primary event or as a secondary event in obstetric acute renal failure.[185]

CLINICAL MANIFESTATIONS AND LABORATORY EVALUATION

Signs and symptoms of uremia, including hypertension, metabolic acidosis, fluid overload, and disturbances of the gastrointestinal, cardiovascular, and nervous systems, are usually the major clinical manifestations of renal insufficiency. In addition, pallor, fatigue, and high-output cardiac failure due to anemia and bleeding and/or intravascular coagulation may become major clinical problems that demand appropriate therapy.

Anemia

Normocytic, normochromic anemia with a corrected reticulocyte count of approximately 1% (i.e., "normal" reticulocyte index in the face of anemia) are characteristically present. Morphologically, the red blood cells frequently show the characteristic even scalloping of echinocytes or burr cells.[186] The clinical significance of this morphologic change is uncertain since the presence or absence of echinocytes does not correlate with severity of hemolysis and because even normal red blood cells reversibly transform into echinocytes in vitro.[187] Occasionally, asymmetrically distributed, large spicules appear on the surface of uremic red blood cells (acanthocytes), or gross red blood cell deformities and fragmentation (schistocytes) appear. In contrast to echinocyte formation, their presence is a manifestation of a pathologic process involving the microcirculation that has occurred in vivo. When severe, these changes are the hallmark of the hemolytic uremic syndrome (see below).

In the absence of a complicating nutritional deficiency or drug-related hemolytic process, the bone marrow aspirate appears normal. Mild granulocyte hyperplasia may be observed, and erythroid precursors are normal in appearance and maturation.[188] Occasionally marrow fibrosis (i.e., osteitis fibrosa) is apparent on bone biopsy. Here, decreased marrow space is available for erythropoiesis, regardless of circulating EPO levels. Osteitis fibrosa, a complication of secondary hyperparathyroidism and renal insufficiency, may play a pathogenic role in the production of anemia since the amount of marrow fibrosis correlates well with correction of anemia that follows parathyroidectomy.[189,190] The extent of fibrosis also correlates with response to EPO treatment[191] (see below). The relationship of elevated parathyrin levels to in vivo suppression of erythropoiesis[71] or to reduction in red cell survival[192] is unknown. As osteitis fibrosa progresses, alkaline phosphatase levels rise, and ultimately myelofibrosis accompanied by extramedullary hematopoiesis and hepatosplenomegaly develop.

Frequently, iron deficiency associated with blood loss or folic acid deficiency complicates renal anemia (Table 148-2). Gastrointestinal tract blood loss (believed to be due to platelet dysfunction) or iatrogenic blood loss (via phlebotomy, dialyzer, or fistula) may lead to depletion of iron stores and erythroid hyperplasia. Blood losses may average as much as

Table 148-2. Correctable Causes of Anemia of Renal Failure

Mechanism	Etiology	Reference
Blood loss, iron deficiency	Iatrogenic loss	193
	Dialyzer loss	194
	Shunt or fistula loss	195, 196
	Gastrointestinal loss	197
	Urinary loss of transferrin	198
Folate deficiency	Increased demand	78–81, 199
	Restricted oral intake	200, 201
	Dialyzer loss	200
	Drug-inhibition of absorption or metabolism	202, 203
Accelerated hemolysis		
Dialysis-associated toxicity	Toxicity due to exposure to copper, chloramine, formaldehyde, or nitrates	211–214
	Overheating of erythrocytes	215
	Mechanical erythrocyte fragmentation	216
	Dehydration/overhydration of erythrocytes	217
Drug-associated	High oxidative potential agents: thiol-containing drugs, phenylhydrazine-like drugs	91, 207, 218
	Immunohemolytic agents: α-methyldopa, penicillin, quinidine, etc.	
Microangiopathic	Malignant hypertension Vasculitis	219
Red cell phosphate depletion	Excessive antacid intake	220
Hypersplenism	Red cell sequestration/work hypertrophy	221–223
	Chronic hepatitis	221
	Transfusion-induced hemosiderosis	222
	Marrow fibrosis	224
	Silicone toxicity	225

1 L/mo in patients receiving chronic hemodialysis.[193–197] By contrast, patients dialyzed peritoneally do not develop iron deficiency without gastrointestinal blood loss. Rarely, iron deficiency may develop in association with urinary loss of transferrin.[198]

Several factors contribute to development of clinically apparent folic acid deficiency. Since red cell survival is decreased, demand for folate is higher than normal.[78–81,199] This demand may not be met when patients are advised to restrict protein intake, although the need for supplemental folic acid is not clearly established.[200–201] Nevertheless, folate is removed during dialysis.[200] In addition, absorption and metabolism of dietary folate may be suppressed by many of the drugs used in treating uremic patients, including diphenylhydantoin, barbiturates, cholestyramine, dietary amino acids, oral contraceptives, and inhibitors of dihydrofolate reductase (such as methotrexate and pyrimethamine).[202] Megaloblastic maturation and dyshematopoiesis are characteristically present in marrow aspirates of uremic patients with folate deficiency.

Red blood cells from uremic patients with renal insufficiency are hypersensitive to oxidant challenge.[91,204] Most enzymes of the oxidant defense system have been shown to be normal or slightly below normal in activity,[205–208] rendering cells hypersensitive to hydrogen peroxide-induced hemolysis.[209] Cross-incubation studies suggest that increased oxidant sensitivity is due to uremic plasma factors since normal red cells can be made hypersensitive to ascorbate-generated oxidants by incubation in uremic plasma.[210] The production of oxidants such as chloramine during dialysis leads to brisk hemolysis (Table 148-2). Other dialysis-associated alterations in uremic red cells, such as overheating, mechanical fragmentation, and dehydration/overhydration, may also lead to accelerated hemolysis. Drugs having a high oxidative potential may also induce hemolysis and worsen anemia. Furthermore, since malignant hypertension and vasculitis are frequently observed, uremic patients are prone to develop microangiopathic hemolysis.[219] Finally, hypophosphatemia associated with excessive use of phosphate-binding antacids (i.e., aluminum gels) may lead to several red cell abnormalities, including depletion of ATP stores, impaired glycolysis, reduced red cell deformability, and, ultimately, hemolysis.[220]

Although many uremic patients develop hypersplenism as a complication of their underlying disease or its therapy (Table 148-2), a small percentage actively sequester and destroy red cells in the spleen.[221] The latter patients have a red cell survival rate one-fourth of normal, demonstrate increased uptake of radioactive chromium-labeled red cells, and have a beneficial response to splenectomy. However, most patients with mild splenomegaly do not actively sequester red cells in the spleen, suggesting that they will have a poor response to splenectomy.[226]

Recently, aluminum toxicity has been recognized in dialysis patients. High levels of aluminum develop as a consequence of long-term use of aluminum-containing antacids that facilitate phosphate binding or of aluminum-containing dialysates. The precise level at which aluminum becomes toxic is debatable and is in part determined by exclusion of other known causes of organ dysfunction.[227,228] An early manifestation of aluminum toxicity is microcytosis.[229,230] Later, hypochromic anemia, dialysis encephalopathy, vitamin D-resistant osteomalacia, and muscle weakness develop.[230,231] The mechanism responsible for development of microcytic anemia may involve suppression of enzymes involved in heme synthesis.[232] Alternatively, aluminum may interfere with iron uptake by the red cell since it is similar to iron with respect to trivalency and avid binding to transferrin.[233] Aluminum-induced anemia can be reversed by use of a dialysate containing deionized water[234] or by chelation with desferrioxamine, or both.[235]

Bleeding and Abnormal Coagulation Tests

Clinical bleeding in uremia presents most often as purpura, menorrhagia, or occult or frank gastrointestinal blood loss. Bleeding occurs in up to one-half of all patients with chronic renal insufficiency.[236] Characteristically, the platelets are quantitatively normal, although dialysis-associated thrombocytopenia with clinical bleeding may occur.[168,173] Platelet dysfunction characterized by abnormalities in bleeding time, platelet aggregation and adhesiveness, prostacyclin production, and factor VIII/vWF complex activity is well documented.[163–168,236,237] Dialysis has been reported to improve abnormalities in many of these tests and to ameliorate bleeding by an unknown mechanism(s).[238]

Hemolytic Uremic Syndrome

Occasionally brisk hemolysis and thrombocytopenia occur in the setting of acute renal failure. This clinical picture has emerged as a distinct syndrome, the hemolytic uremic syndrome. It is relatively common in infants and children who develop sudden anemia, renal failure, central nervous system dysfunction, and gastrointestinal bleeding. This syndrome often follows a prodrome of infectious symptoms involving the digestive or respiratory tracts, or both. Although the inciting agent may be viruses, bacteria, drugs, or pregnancy, little is known of the pathogenetic mechanisms involved.

The peripheral blood smear classically shows fragmented red cells and thrombocytopenia. These may result from mechanical trauma as cellular elements traverse renal arteriolar and glomerular vessels whose endothelial lining is injured. The reticulocyte index is invariably elevated, and signs of overt hemolysis, including indirect hyperbilirubinemia, elevated blood lactate dehydrogenase, and low or undetectable haptoglobin level, are evident. Consistent with hemolysis, EPO levels are elevated even though uremia is present.[239] Prognosis is related to degree of renal insufficiency and to extent of central nervous system involvement. The latter sequelae may be permanent. Hematologic alterations are completely reversible in surviving patients and do not recur. Therapy is supportive in nature and includes dialysis and blood component replacement. The role of heparin is controversial; other forms of therapy, such as steroids, immunosuppressive agents, and antimetabolites, have not produced clear-cut benefit.

THERAPY AND PROGNOSIS

The management of anemia in acute and chronic renal insufficiency consists of nutritional replacement, including repletion of low iron stores, conservative blood component transfusion

---

APPROACH TO THE EVALUATION OF WORSENING ANEMIA IN RENAL FAILURE

Hematologists are frequently asked to evaluate worsening anemia in patients with chronic renal insufficiency. A logical approach to the diagnostic workup of such patients is outlined here. Baseline laboratory information includes examination of the blood smear and calculation of the reticulocyte index (corrected for level of hematocrit). Individuals with hypoproliferative red cell production indices may have nutritional deficiency or an abnormal process involving the bone marrow (i.e., dyshematopoiesis, myelofibrosis, or an unrelated disorder such as myelophthisis). When microcytosis is present, a serum ferritin level measurement usually confirms the diagnosis of iron deficiency. If inflammation is present, a marrow aspiration to assess tissue iron stores may be required. Alternatively, microcytic anemia can also be observed in patients with aluminum toxicity. Because aluminum is ubiquitous (being particularly concentrated in glassware), aluminum measurements may be erroneous because of contamination of plasma samples by collecting and transport material.[273] Recently, a red cell aluminum assay whose measurements are not altered by aluminum contamination of blood samples has been developed.[274] Alternatively, aluminum excretion after deferoxamine administration can be measured[273] and aluminum concentrations in the bone can be quantitated[275] to establish the diagnosis of aluminum toxicity.

The diagnosis of macrocytic, hypoproliferative anemia should be approached by measurement of serum and red cell folate and vitamin B_{12} levels. If results are normal or equivocal, a bone marrow aspiration may be required to establish the diagnosis of nutritional deficiency or another marrow disorder. Furthermore, liver function tests must be obtained since macrocytic anemia may be associated with liver disease even in the absence of folate deficiency, and particularly because uremic patients are at risk of developing hepatic dysfunction. The presence of hyperproliferative anemia characterized by an elevated reticulocyte index necessitates a hemolytic workup. Careful examination of the blood smear for spherocytes and schistocytes is necessary when chemical evidence of hemolysis is present. The spectrum of microangiopathic changes on the blood smear, thrombocytopenia, and renal insufficiency should raise the possibility of hemolytic uremic syndrome. Alternatively, microangiopathic changes can be seen with underlying vasculitis, malignant hypertension, or connective tissue disorders that may be responsible for both renal disease and hemolysis. Sudden development of accelerated hemolysis accompanied by spherocytes should raise the possibilities of immune hemolysis, dialysis-associated hemolysis (i.e., that associated with copper, chloramine, formaldehyde, nitrate, or zinc toxicity) or drug-related hemolysis (either drugs with high oxidative potential or those known to induce antibody-medicated hemolysis; Table 148-2). Excessive use of phosphate-binding antacids may cause a similar hemolytic picture.

Assessment of hyperproliferative anemia in the absence of chemical evidence for intravascular hemolysis should raise the possibilities of brisk erythropoietic response to blood loss and red cell sequestration in an enlarged spleen. If splenomegaly is present, one should measure uptake of ^{51}Cr-tagged red cells over the spleen. Increased uptake occurs with splenic sequestration, suggesting several possible etiologies and indicating splenectomy as a potential therapeutic option. Alternatively, splenomegaly may develop as a consequence of hepatic disease and portal hypertension. In the absence of splenomegaly, a careful search should be made for blood loss (via the gastrointestinal tract, into the retroperitoneum, or via dialysis). An ultrasound examination to evaluate for a retroperitoneal collection of blood and multiple stool guaiac tests to evaluate for gastrointestinal loss may yield the appropriate diagnosis.

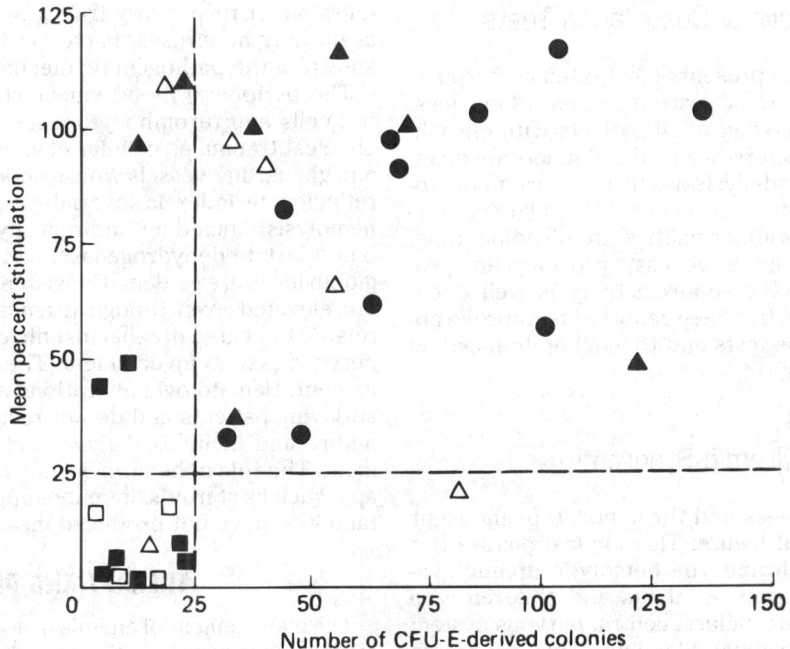

Fig. 148-3. Correlation of erythroid colony formation with androgen responsiveness (stimulation) in androgen-treated patients studied retrospectively (closed symbols) or prospectively (open symbols). Each clinical responder (triangles), clinical nonresponder (squares), and hematologically normal donor (circles) is identified as a single observation. The formation of <25 colonies together with <25% androgen-induced stimulation identifies clinical nonresponders to the drug. (From Kalmanti et al.,[251] with permission.)

therapy, and an optimal program of dialysis and related therapy aimed at correcting uremia or reversing its effects. Recently, specific therapies for anemia and bleeding complications have been employed.

Correction of Anemia

Hemodialysis may ameliorate symptoms of anemia, but rarely does anemia fully resolve.[240] Although EPO levels appear to be unchanged after dialysis, suggesting that removal of uremic inhibitors of stem cells or EPO action may be clinically important, it is unknown whether amelioration of anemia is due to improved renal function or removal of uremic "toxins." When the clinical spectrum of tachypnea, tachycardia, and other symptoms of high-output cardiac failure develop in association with tissue hypoxia disproportionate to the degree of azotemia, blood component therapy is required. Because transfusion of whole blood may place patients at risk of development of pulmonary edema, infusion of packed red blood cells is usually recommended. When laboratory parameters for folic acid deficiency are evident, oral supplementation should be given. Routine folate administration, however, may be unnecessary.[201] Iron deficiency is easily correctable when documented in uremic patients. Because intestinal absorption of iron is normal in renal failure, oral supplementation of elemental iron (65 mg) twice daily with meals is recommended.[203,241] Occasionally parenteral iron administration may be necessary in individuals whose total rate of iron losses (Table 148-2) exceeds the daily iron absorption rate.

Androgens effectively increase the red cell mass in one-half of patients undergoing dialysis.[108] Their efficacy in treating the anemia of primary bone marrow failure is debatable,[242,243] but their utility in treating anemia of end-stage renal disease is well established[244–247] even though the hematocrit usually remains at <36% and rarely achieves normal levels. Symptomatic individuals with a hematocrit of <25% are good candidates for androgen therapy, keeping in mind potential toxicities that include masculinzation, acne, fluid retention, and hepatotoxicity (i.e., cholestasis, peliosis hepatitis, and hepatic adenomas). Parenteral administration of androgens may be more effective than administration by other routes.[248] Agents belonging to several classes (testosterone esters, 17 α-alkylated compounds, and nonsteroids) are commonly used.[108] It has been suggested that androgens having an angular configuration (5-β-epimers) stimulate stem cell proliferation to a greater degree than those whose configuration is planar (5-α-epimers), which

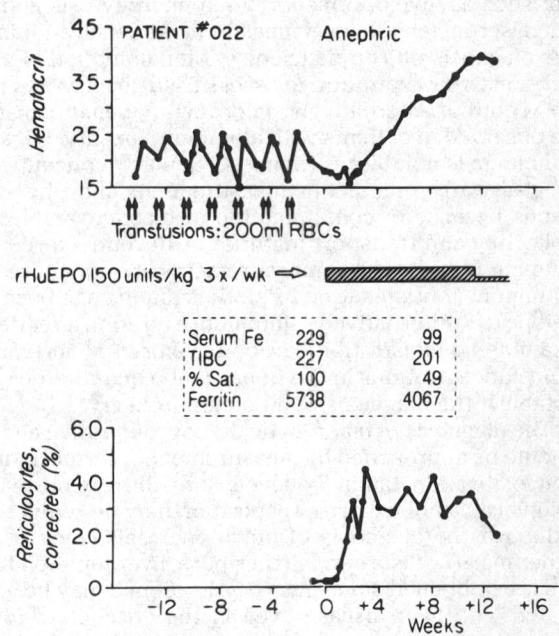

Fig. 148-4. Effect of recombinant human EPO on transfusion requirement, hematocrit, reticulocyte index, and serum iron parameters in a patient with renal insufficiency. (From Eschbach et al.,[254] with permission.)

may act primarily by enhancing EPO production.[108] Nandrolone decanoate (Deca-Durabolin) and fluoxymesterone are popular choices for both nephrectomized and non-nephrectomized individuals.[249,250] Patients are unlikely to respond to androgens if, after 6–9 months of therapy at different dosages, a favorable clinical outcome has not been achieved.[108] Since androgens of one class may be effective, whereas drugs of another class may be ineffective, a method to select appropriate androgen therapy may be helpful. An in vitro marrow culture assay has been found to predict which individuals will respond to androgens of a specific class.[251] It appears that an adequate number of erythroid progenitor cells must be present and normal sensitivity to androgens of a specific class must be retained to achieve a favorable clinical response (Fig. 148-3).

Perhaps in no other way has the therapy of renal anemia been more affected than by the introduction of human EPO to clinical medicine. By analogy with other hormone deficiency states, it is predictable that a hormone will be effective when administered to individuals who either lack the capacity to generate a sufficient hormone level in response to a physiologic stimulus or produce a hormone fragment that is biologically inactive. In view of the central role played by EPO in erythropoiesis, the finding that EPO corrects the anemia of end-stage renal disease in humans[252–256] and small animals[257] is not surprising. Typically, recombinant human EPO administration results in a dose-related, sequential increase in the reticulocyte count and hematocrit accompanied by complete loss of a transfusion requirement (Fig. 148-4). Increases in red cell transferrin uptake accompany this erythropoietic effect.[254] Both intravenous and subcutaneous routes of administration are effective in raising the hematocrit of healthy volunteers.[258] Improvement in ane-

mia after EPO administration is accompanied by loss of fatigue, amelioration of Raynaud's phenomenon,[255] shortening of bleeding time and improved platelet adhesion to subendothelium,[259] improved sexual function,[257] improved brain function, and psychological sense of well-being.[260,261]

Side effects of EPO rarely require discontinuation of therapy. Most patients develop a mild sensation of aching in the long bones during administration of the drug. Approximately one-third of patients develop diastolic hypertension, an effect that is not explained by hypervolemia since blood pressure elevation occurs in spite of intensive efforts to prevent hypervolemia by maintaining patients at their "dry weight."[255] It has been suggested that hemodialysis patients with a positive family history of hypertension are particularly susceptible to EPO-induced hypertension, whereas age, sex, gender, etiology of renal dysfunction, and duration of hemodialysis therapy have no predisposing effect.[262] A perplexing observation is that cardiac output, cardiac index, and left ventricular ejection fraction are increased after therapy, contrary to what would be expected with the correction of anemia. Sporadic cases of thrombotic episodes with clotting of fistulae and elevated predialysis creatinine, potassium, and phosphate levels, as well as thrombocytosis have also been reported but may not be the result of EPO administration per se. Interestingly, correction of erythropoiesis to "normal" levels by EPO therapy may uncover iron deficiency and aluminum toxicity. Finally, in theory, it is unclear whether raising the hematocrit worsens or improves renal function.[260] Since an increased red cell mass is invariably accompanied by a proportional decrease in plasma volume, changes in dialysis requirements are anticipated. Recently, it has been suggested that high-flux dialysis of EPO recipients

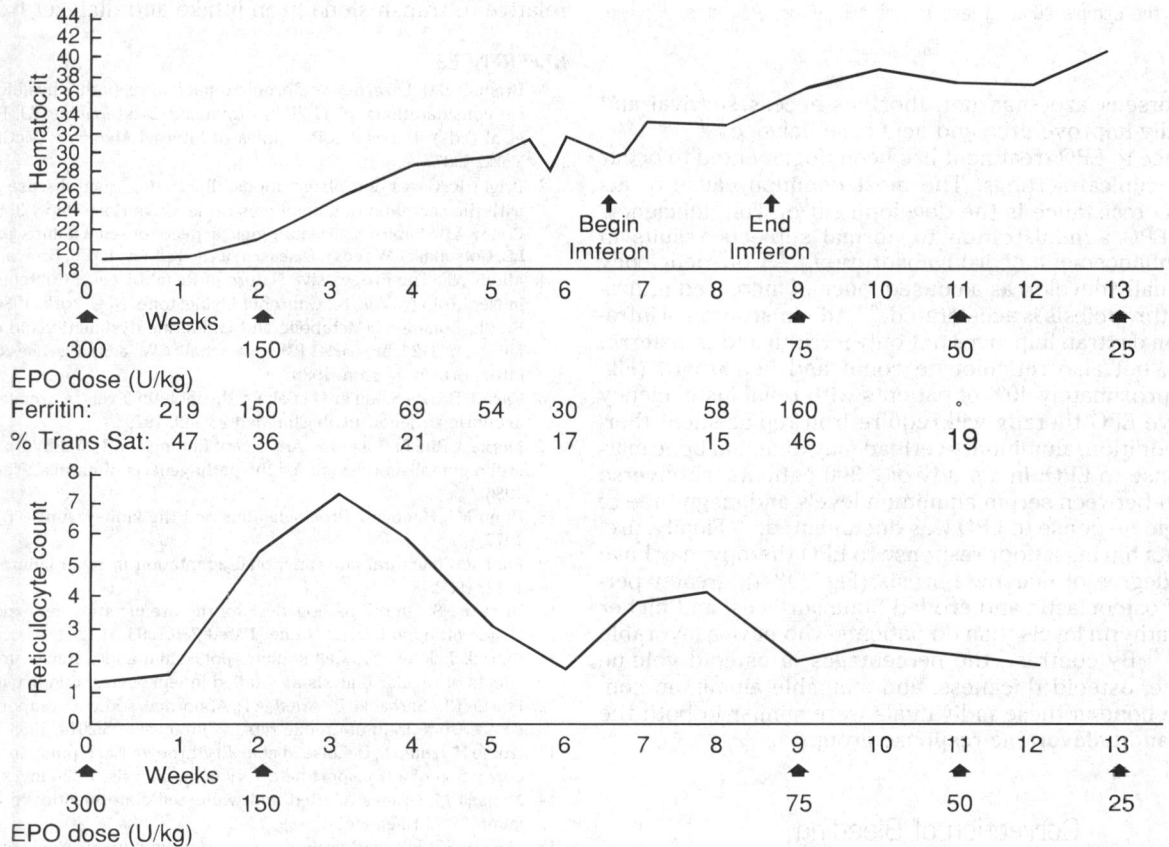

Fig. 148-5. Effect of iron dextran (Imferon) administration on iron deficiency state (as measured by ferritin level and percentage of transferrin saturation), and hematologic response to treatment with recombinant human EPO (as measured as by hematocrit and reticulocyte count). (From Nissenson et al.,[265] with permission).

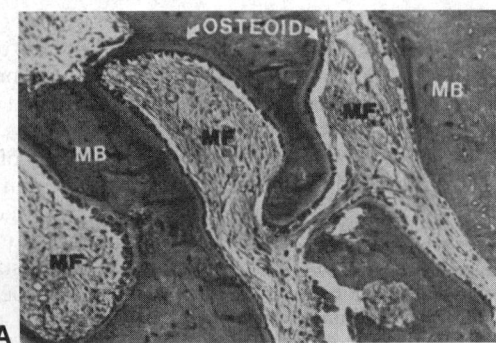

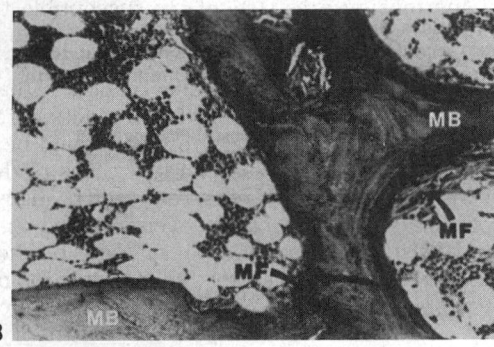

Fig. 148-6. Photomicrographs of cancellous bone tissue from iliac crest biopsies stained with toluidine blue. **(A)** Extensive marrow fibrosis (MF) in a specimen from a patient with severe hyperparathyroidism. Mineralized bone (MB) appears as solid dark areas. **(B)** Mild paraosseous marrow fibrosis in a specimen from a patient with less severe hyperparathyroidism. Note that whereas the marrow space is completely obliterated in the sample showing extensive MF, it is readily detectable in the sample showing less severe MF. (From Rao et al.,[191] with permission).

neither worsens azotemia nor shortens access survival and may actually improve urea and acid-base balance.[261]

Resistance to EPO treatment has been documented to occur in several clinical settings. The most common cause of acquired EPO resistance is the development of iron deficiency. Although EPO administration to normal subjects results in striking enhancement of iron absorption,[263] iron deficiency may eventually develop as a consequence of increased utilization as erythropoiesis is accelerated.[264] Administration of intravenous iron dextran improves not only ferritin and transferrin saturation, but also reticulocyte count and hematocrit (Fig. 148-5). Approximately 40% of patients with renal insufficiency who receive EPO therapy will require iron replacement therapy.[265] In addition, aluminum overload may diminish bone marrow response to EPO. In a study of >300 patients, an inverse correlation between serum aluminum levels and magnitude of hematologic response to EPO was documented.[266] Finally, uremic patients having a poor response to EPO therapy may have a greater degree of marrow fibrosis (Fig. 148-6), greater percentage of osteoclastic and eroded bone surfaces, and higher serum parathyrin levels than do patients who have a favorable response.[191] By contrast, the percentages of osteoid volume and surface, osteoid thickness, and stainable aluminum content of the bone in these individuals were similar in both the favorable and unfavorable response groups.

Correction of Bleeding

Cryoprecipitate shortens the bleeding time in patients with uremia.[174] More importantly, major surgical or invasive procedures have been undertaken without clinical bleeding in pa-

tients treated by cryoprecipitate infusion. Minor increases in plasma concentrations of factor VIII-vWF properties, factor VIII-related antigen, and ristocetin cofactor are also observed after cryoprecipitate therapy.[180] In addition, DDAVP has been administered in a double-blind, controlled study of patients with prolonged bleeding times.[181] DDAVP infusion caused a shortening of the bleeding time and the appearance of larger factor VIII-vWF multimers in the circulation than were present in pretreatment plasma. These results suggest that coagulation abnormalities may be abrogated by therapy directed at correction of abnormalities of the factor VIII molecule.[171] Conjugated estrogens have also been used successfully to shorten the prolonged bleeding time and correct the hemostatic defect of uremia.[267-268]

Transfusional Hemosiderosis

Iron overload due to iron administration in the form of blood transfusion or parenteral iron supplementation frequently complicates end-stage renal failure. Serum ferritin levels >300 mg/ml may be anticipated when iron intake exceeds daily losses over a protracted period. Since hemodialyzed patients with transfusional iron overload may develop widespread organ dysfunction, including glucose intolerance, impaired cardiac ventricular function, reduced pituitary reserves, and noncardiac myopathy, care must be taken not to administer parenteral iron without careful assessment of iron stores.[269] Because gastrointestional absorption is diminished in iron-overloaded uremic patients, oral iron may be administered safely, unless the patient is genetically predisposed to hemochromatosis.[270] Desferrioxamine may be used to remove iron stores from dialysis patients who are iron overloaded.[271,272] When using chelators, it is important to calculate the interval of treatment relative to transfusional iron intake and dialyzer iron loss.

REFERENCES

1. Brenner BM, Lazarus JM: Chronic renal failure: pathophysiologic and clinical considerations. p. 1155. In Braunuald E, Issebacher KJ, Petersdorf RG et al (eds): Harrison's Principles of Internal Medicine. McGraw-Hill, New York, 1987
2. Bright R: Cases and observations, illustrating renal disease accompanied with the secretion of albuminous urine. Guys Hosp Rep 1:338, 1986
3. Erslev AJ, Shapiro SS: Hematologic aspects of renal failure, p. 227. In Early LE, Gotschalk CW (eds): Diseases of the Kidney. Little, Brown, Boston, 1979
4. Mitch WE: The Progressive Nature of Renal Disease. Contemporary Issues in Nephrology. Vol. 14. Churchill Livingstone, New York, 1986
5. Ritz E, Bommer J: Metabolic and endocrine dysfunctions in chronic renal failure. p. 3127. In Schrier RW, Gottschalk CW (eds): Diseases of the Kidney. Little, Brown, Boston, 1988
6. Caro J, Brown S, Miller O et al: Erythropoietin levels in uremic, nephric and anephric patients. J Lab Clin Med 93:449, 1979
7. Merke J, Ritz E, Boland R: Are recent findings on 1,25-dihydroxycholecalciferol metabolism relevant for the pathogenesis of uremia? Nephron 42:277, 1986
8. Dunn MJ, Hood VL: Prostaglandins and the kidney. Am J Physiol 233:169, 1977
9. Platt R: Structural and functional adaptation in renal failure. Br Med J 1: 1313, 1952
10. Bricker NS: On the pathogenesis of the uremic state: an exposition of the "trade off hypothesis." N Engl J Med 286:1093, 1972
11. Patrick J, Jones NF: Cell sodium, potassium and water in uremia and the effects of regular dialysis as studied in leukocytes. Clin Sci 46:583, 1974
12. Fraser CL, Sarnacki P, Arieff AT: Abnormal sodium tranport in synaptosomes from brain of uremic rats. J Clin Invest 75:2014, 1985
13. Izumo H, Izumo S, DeLuise M et al: Erythrocyte Na, K pump in uremia. Acute correction of a transport defect by hemodialysis. J Clin Invest 74:581, 1984
14. Mansell M, Grimes AJ: Red and white cell abnormalities in chronic renal failure. Br J Haematol 42:169, 1979
15. Massry SG: Is parathyroid hormone a uremic toxin? Nephron 19:125, 1977
16. Hayslett JP: Functional adaptation to reduction in renal mass. Physiol Rev 59:137, 1979
17. Eschbach JW, Adamson JW: Anemia in renal disease. p. 3019. In Schrier RW, Gottschalk CW (eds): Diseases of the Kidney. Little, Brown, Boston, 1988

18. Nissenson AR, Nimer SD, Wolcott DL: Recombinant human erythropoietin and renal anemia: molecular biology, clinical efficacy and neurons system effects. Ann Intern Med 114:402, 1991

19. Frenkle EP, Douglas CC, McCall MS: Hypoerythropoietinemia and anemia. Arch Intern Med 125:1050, 1970

20. Cameron JS: Henoch-Schönlein purpura. p. 6. In Massry SG, Glassock RJ (eds): Textbook of Nephrology. Williams & Wilkins, Baltimore, 1983

21. Glassrock RJ, Cohen AH, Adler SG, Ward HJ et al: Secondary glomerular lesions. p. 1014. In Brenner BM, Rector FC Jr (eds): The Kidney. 3d Ed. WB Saunders, Philadelphia, 1986

22. Davies S, Glynnejo E, Bisson et al: Plasma erythropoietin assay in patients with chronic renal failure. J Clin Pathol 28:875, 1975

23. Radtke HW, Erbes PM, Fassbinder W et al: The variable role of erythropoietin deficiency in the pathogenesis of dialysis anemia. Proc Eur Dial Transplant Assoc 14:177, 1977

24. Lertora JJL, Dargon PA, Rege AB et al: Studies on a radioimmunoassay for erythropoietin. J Lab Clin Med 86:140, 1975

25. Sherwood JB, Goldwasser E: A radioimmunoassay for erythropoietin. Blood 54:885, 1979

26. McGonigle RJS, Wallin JD, Shadduck RR et al: Erythropoietin deficiency and inhibition of erythropoiesis in renal insufficiency. Kidney Int 25:437, 1984

27. Fisher JW, Modder BH, Foley JE et al: Role of erythropoietin and inhibitors of erythropoiesis in the anemia of renal insufficiency. p. 551. In Fisher JW (ed): Kidney Hormones. Vol. 2. Academic Press, San Diego, 1977

28. Erslev AJ: Anemia of chronic renal failure. p. 417. In Williams WJ, Beutler E, Erslev AJ, Lichtman MA (eds): Hematology. McGraw-Hill, New York, 1983

29. Radtke HW, Claassner A, Erbes PM et al: Serum erythropoietin concentrations in chronic renal failure: relationship to degree of anemia and excretory renal function. Blood 54:877, 1979

30. Pavlovic-Kentera V, Clemons GK, Dkukanovic L et al: Erythropoietin and anemia in chronic renal failure. Exp Hematol 15:785, 1987

31. Nathan DG, Schupack E, Stohlman F Jr et al: Erythropoietin in anephric man. J Clin Invest 43:2158, 1964

32. Rich IN, Heit W, Kubanek B: Extrarenal erythropoietin production by macrophages. Blood 60:1007, 1982

33. Fried W, Anagnostou A: Extrarenal erythropoietin production. p. 231. In Fisher JW (ed): Kidney Hormones. Vol. 2. Academic Press, San Diego, 1977

34. Peschle C, Marone G, Genovese A et al: Increased erythropoietin production in anephric rats with hyperplasia of the reticuloendothelial system induced by colloidal carbon or zymosan. Blood 47:325, 1976

35. Peschle C, Marone G, Arturo G et al: Hepatic erythropoietin enhanced production in anephric rats with hyperplasia of Kupffer cells. Br J Haematol 32:105, 1976

36. Paul P, Rothman SA, McMahon JT et al: Erythropoietin secretion by isolated rat Kupffer cells. Exp Hematol 12:825, 1984

37. Zangheri EO, Lopez OI, Honorato LO et al: The role of the submandibular glands in erythropoietin production in mice. Exp Hematol 5:237, 1977

38. Clemons GK, DeManincor D, Fitzsimmons SL et al: Immunoreactive erythropoietin studies in hypoxic rats and the role of the salivary glands. Exp Hematol 15:18, 1987

39. Brox AG, Congote LF, Fafard J et al: Indentification and characterization of our 8-kd peptide stimulating late erythropoiesis. Exp Hematol 17:769, 1989

40. Carnot P, Deflandre C: Sur l'activité hematopoietique de serum au cours de la régénération du sang. CR Acad Sci (Paris) 143:384, 1906

41. Erslev AJ, Lavietes PH, van Wagenen G: Erythropoietic stimulation induced by "anemic serum." Proc Soc Exp Biol 83:548, 1953

42. Jacobson LO, Goldwasser E, Fried W et al: The role of the kidney in erythropoiesis. Nature 179:633, 1957

43. Fisher JW, Taylor G, Porteous DD: Localization of erythropoietin in glomeruli of sheep kidney by fluorescent antibody technique. Nature 205:611, 1965

44. Frankel EP, Suke W, Baum J: Some observations on the localization of erythropoietin. Ann NY Acad Sci 149:292, 1968

45. Busuttil RW, Roh BL, Fisher JW: The cytological localization of erythropoietin in the human kidney using the fluorescent antibody technique. Proc Soc Exp Biol Med 137:327, 1971

46. Burlington H, Cronkite EP, Reincke U et al: Erythropoietin production in cultures of goat renal glomeruli. Proc Natl Acad Sci USA 69:3547, 1972

47. Jelkman W, Kurtz A, Bauer C: Extraction of erythropoietin from isolated renal glomeruli of hypoxic rats. Exp Hematol 11:581, 1983

48. McCully KS, Rinehimer LA, Gillies CG et al: Erythrocytosis, glomerulomegaly, mesangial, hyperplasia, sialyl and arteriosclerosis induced in rats by nickel subsulfide. Virchows Arch 394:207, 1982

49. Kurtz A, Jelkmann W, Sinowatz F et al: Renal mesangial cell cultures as a model for study of erythropoietin production. Proc Natl Acad Sci USA 80:4008, 1983

50. Penington DG: Erythropoietin in tissues: features of the erythropoietin-producing system. p. 201. In Williams P (ed): Hormones and the Kidney. Academic Press, San Diego, 1963

51. Zanjani ED, Cooper GW, Gordon AS et al: The renal erythropoietic factor (REF). Distribution in mammalian kidneys. Proc Soc Exp Biol Med 126:540, 1967

52. Ozawa S: Erythropoietin from the kidney cells cultured in vitro. Keio J Med 16:193, 1967

53. Fried W, Barone-Varelas J, Barone T et al: Extraction of erythropoietin from kidneys. Exp Hematol 8:41, 1980

54. Caro J, Erslev AJ: Biologic and immunologic erythropoietin in extracts from hypoxic whole rat kidneys and in their glomerular and tubular fractions. J Lab Clin Med 103:922, 1984

55. Chowdhurry RR, Datta AG: Studies on the in vitro formation of erythropoietin in sheep kidney medulla and the effect of cobalt theron. Biochem Biophys Res Commun 52:1329, 1973

56. Reissman KR, Namura T, Gunn RW et al: Erythropoietic response to anemia or erythropoietin injection in uremic rats with or without functioning renal tissue. Blood 16:1411, 1960

57. Jepson J, McGarry EE: Polycythemia and increased erythropoietin production in a patient with hypertrophy of the juxtaglomerular apparatus. Blood 32:370, 1968

58. Hartroft PM, Bischoff MB, Bucci TJ: Effects of chronic exposure to high altitude on the juxtaglomerular complex and adrenal cortex of dogs, rabbits and rats. Fed Proc 28:1234, 1969

59. Lin FK, Suggs S, Lin CH et al: Cloning and expression of the human erythropoietin gene. Proc Natl Acad Sci USA, 82:7580, 1985

60. Bondurant MC, Koury MJ: Anemia induces accumulation of erythropoietin mRNA in the kidney and liver. Mol Cell Biol 6:2731, 1986

61. Schuster SJ, Wilson JH, Erslev AJ et al: Physiologic regulation and tissue localization of renal erythropoietin messenger RNA. Blood 70:316, 1987

62. LaCombe C, DaSilva J-L, Bruneval P et al: Identification of tissues and cells producing erythropoietin in the anemic mouse. Contrib Nephrol 66:17, 1988

63. Sherwood JB, Goldwasser E: Extraction of erythropoietin from normal kidneys. Endocrinology 103:866, 1978

64. Stohlman F Jr, Rath CE, Rose JC: Evidence for a humoral regulation of erythropoiesis. Blood 9:721, 1954

65. Schmid R, Gilbertson AS: Fundamental observations on the production of compensatory polycythemia in a case of patent ductus arteriosus with reversed blood flow. Blood 10:247, 1955

66. Dainiak N, Hoffman E, Lebowitz AI et al: Erythropoietin-dependent primary pure erythropoiesis. Blood 53:1076, 1979

67. Wallner SF, Ward HP, Vautrin R et al: The anemia of chronic renal failure. In vitro response of bone marrow to erythropoietin. Proc Soc Exp Biol Med 149:939, 1971

68. Wallner SF, Vautrin R: The anemia of chronic renal failure: studies of the effect of organic solvent extraction of serum. J Lab Clin Med 92:363, 1978

69. Urabe A, Chiba S, Kosaka K et al: Response of uremic bone marrow cells to erythropoietin in vitro. Scand J Haematol 17:335, 1976

70. Radtke HW, Rege AB, LaMouche MB et al: Identification of spermine as an inhibitor of erythropoiesis in patients with chronic renal failure. J Clin Invest 67:1623, 1981

71. Meytes D, Bogin A, Dukes P et al: Effect of parathyroid hormone on erythropoiesis. J Clin Invest 67:1263, 1981

72. Freedman M, Saunders E, Cattran D et al: Ribonuclease inhibition of erythropoiesis in anemia of uremia. Am J Kidney Dis 2:530, 1983

73. Delwiche F, Segal GM, Eschbach JW et al: Erythropoietin inhibitors in chronic renal failure: studies of clinical correlations and in vitro specificity. Kidney Int 29:641, 1984

74. Caro J, Hickey J, Erslev AJ: Is spermine the uremic inhibitor? Clin Res 31:309A, 1983

75. Spragg BP, Bentley DP, Coles GA: Anemia of chronic renal failure. Polyamines are not increased in uraemic serum. Nephron 38:65, 1984

76. Dainiak N, Warren HB, Kreczko S et al: Acetylated lipoproteins impair erythroid growth factor release from endothelial cells. J Clin Invest 81:834, 1988

77. Caro J, Erslev AJ: Uremic inhibitors of erythropoiesis. Semin Nephrol 5:128, 1985

78. Eschbach JW, Korn D, Finch CA: ^{14}C cyanate as a tag for red cell survival in normal and uremic man. J Lab Clin Med 89:823, 1977

79. Shaw AB: Haemolysis in chronic renal failure. Br Med J 2:213, 1967

80. Stewart JH: Haemolytic anemia in acute and chronic renal failure. Q J Med 36:85, 1967

81. Hocken AG: Haemolysis in chronic renal failure. Nephron 32:28, 1982

82. Joske RA, McCallister JM, Prankerd TAJ: Isotope investigations of red cell production and destruction in chronic renal disease. Clin Sci 15:511, 1956

83. Desferges JF, Dawson JP: The anemia of renal failure. Arch Intern Med 101:326, 1958

84. Berry ER, Rambach WA, Alt HL et al: Effect of peritoneal dialysis on erythro-

kinetics and ferrokinetics of azotemic anemias. Trans Am Soc Artif Intern Organs 10:415, 1965

85. Summerfield GP, Gyde OHB, Forbes AMW et al: Hemoglobin concentration and serum erythropoietin in renal dialysis and transplant patients. Acta Haematol 30:389, 1963

86. Wallas CH: Metabolic studies on the erythrocytes from patients with chronic renal disease or hemodialysis. Br J Haematol 27:145, 1974

87. Chauhan DP, Gupta PH, Nampoothiri MRN et al: Determination of erythrocyte superoxide dismutase, catalase, glucose-6-phosphatase dehydrogenase, reduced glutathione, and malonyldialdehyde in uremia. Clin Chim Acta 123:153, 1982

88. Lonergan ET, Semar M, Sterzel RB et al: Erythrocyte transketolase activity in dialyzed patients. A reversible metabolic lesion of uremia. N Engl J Med 284:1399, 1971

89. Vanella A, Geremia E, Pintura R et al: Superoxide dismutase activity and reduced glutathione content in erythrocytes of uremic patients on chronic dialysis. Acta Haematol 70:312, 1983

90. Francavila A, Albano O, Mastrangelel R et al: Erythrocyte membrane ATPase in patients with acute or chronic renal disease. Clin Chim Acta 37:298, 1972

91. Yawata Y, Howe R, Jacob HS: Abnormal red cell metabolism causing hemodialysis. Ann Intern Med 79:362, 1973

92. Luke RG, Kennedy AC, Stirling WB: Renal artery stenosis, hypertension and polycythemia. Br Med J 5428:164, 1965

93. Wickre CG, Norman DJ, Bennison A et al: Post-renal transplant erythrocytosis: a review of 53 patients. Kidney Int 23:731, 1983

94. Thevenod F, Radtke HW, Grutzmacher P et al: Deficient feed-back regulation of erythropoiesis in kidney transplant patients with polycythemia. Kidney Int 24:227, 1983

95. Westerman MP, Kenkins JL, Dekker A et al: Significance of erythrocytosis and increased erythropoietin secretion after renal transplantation Lancet 2:755, 1967

96. Wales JD, Evans DB: Erythemia in renal transplantation. Br Med J 2:80, 1969

97. Hammond D, Winnicks S: Paraneoplastic erythrocytosis and ectopic erythropoietins. Ann NY Acad Sci 230:219, 1974

98. Thorling EB: Paraneoplastic erythrocytosis and inappropriate erythropoietin production. Scand J Haematol, suppl. 17. 9:25, 1972

99. Schramek A, Adler O, Hashmonai M et al: Hypertensive crisis, erythrocytosis and uremia due to renal artery stenosis of kidney transplants. Lancet 1:70, 1975

100. Bacon BR, Rothman SA, Ricanti ES et al: Renal artery stenosis with erythrocytosis after renal transplantation. Arch Intern Med 140:1206, 1980

101. Jepson JH, DeLeeuw NKM, Gault MH et al: Characteristics of erythrocytosis following human renal hemotransplantation. Transplant Proc 3:353, 1971

102. Nellans R, Otis P, Martin DC: Polycythemia following renal transplantation. Urology 6:158, 1975

103. Wikstrom B, Goch J, Danielson BG, et al: Serum erythropoietin in renal transplant patients. Transplant Proc 21:2043, 1989

104. Sun CH, Ward HJ, Wellington WL, et al: Serum erythropoietin levels after renal transplantation. N Engl J Med 321:151, 1989

105. Shih L-Y, Leu M-L: Erythropoiesis in patients with renal failure on hemodialysis: study of underlying mechanism by in vitro erythroid culture assay. Exp Hematol 21:1239, 1993

106. Dagher FJ, Ramos E, Erslev AJ et al: Are the native kidneys responsible for erythrocytosis in renal allografts? Transplantation 28:496, 1979

107. Meyrier A, Simon P, Boffa G et al: Uremia and the liver: the liver and erythrocytosis in chronic renal failure. Nephron 29:3, 1981

108. Dainiak N: The role of androgens in the treatment of anemia of chronic renal failure. Semin Nephrol 5:147, 1985

109. Fried W: The liver as a source of extrarenal erythropoietin production. Blood 40:671, 1972

110. Kessler M, Legrand E, Mertes M et al: Treatment of chronic renal failure-anemia by recombinant erythropoietin and polycythemia following kidney transplantation. Nephron 62:370, 1992

111. Goldwasser E: The action of erythropoietin as the inducer of erythroid differentiation. p. 77. In Cronkite EP, Dainiak N, McCaffrey R et al (eds): Hematopoietic Stem Cell Physiology. Alan R Liss, New York, 1985

112. Montgomerie JZ, Kulmanson GM, Guze LB: Renal failure and infection. Medicine 47:1, 1968

113. Siddiqui JY, Fitzae L, Lawton R: Causes of death in patients receiving long-term hemodialysis. JAMA 139:1255, 1979

114. Jensson O: Observations on the blood picture of acute uraemia. Br J Haematol 4:422, 1958

115. Foster RS, Mirand EA: Bone marrow colony-stimulating factor following ureteral ligation in germ-free mice. Proc Soc Exp Biol Med 133:1223, 1970

116. Vincent PC, Sutherland R, Morris TCM et al: Inhibitor of in vitro granulopoiesis in plasma of patients with renal failure. Lancet 2:864, 1978

117. Gallen IR, Limarzi LR: Blood and bone marrow studies in renal disease. Am J Clin Pathol 20:3, 1950

118. Riis P, Stuugaard G: The peripheral blood leukocytes in chronic renal insufficiency. Dan Med Bull 6:85, 1959

119. Perescenschi G, Zakouth V, Spirer Z et al: Leukocyte mobilization by epinephrine and hydrocortisone in patients with chronic renal failure. Experentia 33:1529, 1977

120. Hammerschmidt DE, Goldberg R, Raij L et al: Leukocyte abnormalities in renal failure and hemodialysis. Serum Nephrol 5:91, 1985

121. Kaplow LS, Goffinet JA: Profound neutropenia during the early phase of hemodialysis. JAMA 203:1135, 1968

122. Craddock PR, Fehr J, Brigham KL et al: Complement and leukocyte-mediated pulmonary dysfunction in hemodialysis. N Engl J Med 296:769, 1977

123. Craddock PR, Fehr J, Dalmasso AP et al: Hemodialysis leukopenia: pulmonary vascular leukostasis resulting from complement activation by dialyzer cellophane membrane. J Clin Invest 59:879, 1977

124. Perille PE, Nolan JP, Finch SC: Studies of the resistance to infection in diabetes mellitus: local exudative cellular response. J Lab Clin Med 59:1008, 1962

125. Clark RA, Hamory BH, Ford GH et al: Chemotaxis in acute renal failure. J Infect Dis 126:460, 1972

126. Siriwatrananonta P, Sinsakul V, Stern K et al: Defective chemotaxis in uremia. J Lab Clin Med 92:402, 1978

127. Greene WH, Ray CR, Mauer SM et al: The effect of hemodialysis on neutrophil chemotactic responsiveness. J Lab Clin Med 88:971, 1976

128. Hosking CA, Atkings RC, Scott DF et al: Immune and phagocytic functions in patients on maintenance dialysis and post-transplantation. Clin Nephrol 6:501, 1976

129. Raska K, Raskova J, Shea SM et al: T cell subsets and cellular immunity in end-stage renal disease. Am J Med 75:734, 1983

130. Hoy WE, Cestero RVM, Freeman RBL: Deficiency of T and B lymphocytes in uremic subjects and partial improvement with maintenance hemodialysis. Nephron 20:182, 1978

131. McLean RH, Forsgren A, Bjorksten B et al: Decreased serum factor B concentration associated with decreased opsonization of *Escherichia coli* in the idiopathic nephrotic syndrome. Pediatr Res 11:910, 1977

132. Ballow M, Kennedy TL, Gaudio KM et al: Serum hemolytic factor D values in children with steroid-responsive idiopathic nephrotic syndrome. J Pediatr 100:192, 1982

133. Anderson DC, York TL, Rose G et al: Assessment of serum factor B, serum opsonins, granulocyte chemotaxis and infection in nephrotic syndrome of children. J Infect Dis 140:1, 1979

134. Davin JC, Foidart JB, Mahieu PR: Fc receptor function in minimal change nephrotic syndrome of childhood. Clin Nephrol 20:280, 1983

135. Brouhard BH, Goldblum RM, Bunce H III et al: Immunoglobulin synthesis and urinary IgG excretion in the idiopathic nephrotic syndrome of children. Int J Nephrol 2:163, 1983

136. Giangiacomo J, Cleary TG, Cole BR et al: Serum immunoglobulins in the nephrotic syndrome. A possible cause of minimal change nephrotic syndrome. N Engl J Med 293:8, 1975

137. McIntosh J, Hansen P, Ziegler J et al: Defective immune and phagocytic functions in uremia and renal transplantation. Int Arch Allergy Appl Immunol 51:544, 1976

138. Heslan JM, Lautie JP, Intrator L et al: Impaired IgG synthesis in patients with the nephrotic syndrome. Clin Nephrol 18:144, 1982

139. Lange K, Ahmed U, Seligson G et al: Depression of endostreptosin, streptolysin O and streptozyme antibodies in patients with idiopathic nephrosis with and without nephrotic syndrome. Clin Nephrol 15:279, 1981

140. Spika JS, Halsey NA, Fish AJ et al: Serum antibody response to pneumococcal vaccine in children with nephrotic syndrome. Pediatrics 69:219, 1982

141. Lenarsky C, Jordan SC, Ladisch S: Plasma inhibition of lymphocyte proliferation in nephrotic syndrome: correlation with hyperlipidemia. J Clin Immunol 2:276, 1982

142. Moorthy AV, Zimmerman SW, Burkholder PM: Inhibition of lymphocyte blastogenesis by plasma of patients with minimal-change nephrotic syndrome. Lancet 1:1160, 1976

143. Ooi BS, Orlina AR, Masaitis L: Lymphocytotoxins in primary renal disease. Lancet 2:1160, 1976

144. Mallick NP, Williams RJ, McFarlane H, et al: Cell-mediated immunity in nephrotic syndrome. Lancet 1:507, 1972

145. Schnaper HW, Aune TM: Identification of the lymphokine soluble immune response suppressor in urine of nephrotic children. J Clin Invest 76:341, 1985

146. Lagrue G, Xheneumont S, Branellec A et al: A vascular permeability factor elaborated from lymphocytes. I: demonstration in patients with nephrotic syndrome. Biomedicine 23:37, 1975

147. Minchin MA, Turner KJ, Bower GD: Lymphocyte blastogenesis in nephrotic syndrome. Clin Exp Immunol 42:241, 1980

148. Fodor P, Saitua MT, Rodriguez E et al: T-cell dysfunction in minimal-change nephrotic syndrome of childhood. Am J Dis Child 136:713, 1982

149. Matsumoto K, Osakabe K, Harada M et al: Impaired cell-mediated immunity in lipid nephrosis. Nephron 29:190, 1981

150. Badger AM, Benward DB, Idelson BA et al: Depressed spontaneous cellular cytotoxicity associated with normal or enhanced antibody-dependent cellular cytotoxicity in patients on chronic haemodialysis. Clin Exp Immunol 45:568, 1981

151. Lang I, Taraba I, Hering A et al: Effect of haemodialysis on the antibody-dependent and spontaneous cell-mediated cytotoxicity of patients with chronic renal failure. Immunology 5:55, 1982

152. Rutsky EA, Rostand SG: Mycobacteriosis in patients with chronic renal failure. Arch Intern Med 140:57, 1980

153. Andrew OT, Schoenfeld PY, Hopewell PC et al: Tuberculosis in patients with end-stage renal disease. Am J Med 68:59, 1980

154. Huber H, Pastner D, Dittrich P et al: In vitro reactivity of human lymphocytes in uremia—a comparison with the impairment of delayed hypersensitivity. Clin Exp Immunol 5:75, 1969

155. Sengar DPS, Rashid A, Harris JE: In vitro cellular immunity and in vivo delayed hypersensitivity in uremic patients maintained on hemodialysis. Int Arch Allergy 47:829, 1974

156. Kirkpatrick CH, Wilson WEC, Talmage DW: Immunologic studies in human organ transplantation. I: observation and characterization of suppressed cutaneous reactivity in uremia. J Exp Med 119:727, 1964

157. Wilson WEC, Kirkpatrick CH, Talmage DW: Suppression of immunologic responsiveness in uremic patients. Ann Intern Med 62:1, 1965

158. Couch NP, Murray JE, Dammin GJ et al: The fate of the skin homograft in the chronically uremic patient. Surg Forum 7:626, 1956

159. Dammin GJ, Couch NP, Murray JE: Prolonged survival of skin homografts in uremic patients. Ann NY Acad Sci 64:967, 1957

160. Shackman R, Castro JE: Prelusive skin grafts in live-donor kidney transplantation. Lancet 2:521, 1975

161. Souhami RL, Smith J, Bradfield JWB: The effect of uremia on organ graft survival in the rat. Br J Exp Pathol 54:183, 1973

162. Matas AJ, Simmons RL, Kellstrand CM et al: Increased incidence of malignancy during chronic renal failure. Lancet 1:883, 1975

163. Horowitz HI, Stein IM, Cohen BD et al: Further studies on the platelet inhibitory effect of guanidinosuccinic acid and its role in uremic bleeding. Am J Med 49:336, 1970

164. Rabiner SF, Molinas F: The role of phenol and phenolic acid on the thrombocytopathy and defective platelet aggregation of patients with renal failure. Am J Med 49:346, 1970

165. Kimberly RP, Gill JR, Bowden RE et al: Elevated urinary prostaglandins and the effects of aspirin on renal function in lupus erythematosus. Ann Intern Med 89:336, 1978

166. Nath KA, Chmielewski D, Hostetter TH: Regulatory role of prostaglandins in the remnant glomerulus. Am J Physiol 252:F829, 1987

167. Purkeson ML, Joist JH, Yates J et al: Inhibition of thromboxane synthesis ameliorates the progressive kidney disease of rats with subtotal renal ablation. Proc Natl Acad Sci USA 82:193, 1985

168. Schmitt GW, Moake JL, Rudy CK et al: Alteration in hemostatic parameters during hemodialysis with dialyzers of different membrane compositional and flow design. Am J Med 83:411, 1987

169. Turitto VT, Baumgartner HR: Platelet interaction with subendothelium in flowing rabbit blood: effects of blood shear rate. Microvasc Res 17:38, 1979

170. Turitto VT, Weiss HJ: Red blood cells: their dual role in thrombus formation. Science 207:541, 1980

171. Livio M, Benigni A, Remuzzi G: Coagulation abnormalities in uremia. Semin Nephrol 5:82, 1985

172. Livio M, Marchesi D, Remuzzi G et al: Uraemic bleeding: role of anemia and beneficial effect of red cell transfusions. Lancet 2:1013, 1982

173. Lynch RE, Bosl RH, Steifel AJ et al: Dialysis thrombocytopenia: parallel plate vs hollow fiber dialyzer. Trans Am Soc Artif Intern Organs 24:704, 1978

174. Vaziri ND, Ngo J-CT, Ibsen KH et al: Deficiency and urinary loss of factor XII in nephrotic syndrome. Nephron 32:342, 1982

175. Thomson C, Forbes CD, Prentice CR et al: Changes in blood coagulation and fibrinolysis in the nephrotic syndrome. Q J Med 43:399, 1974

176. Kendall AG: Nephrotic syndrome: a hypercoagulable state. Arch Intern Med 127:1021, 1971

177. Kanfer A, Kleinknecht D, Broyer M et al: Coagulation studies in 45 cases of nephrotic syndrome without uremia. Thromb Diathes Haemorrh 24:5622, 1970

178. Wagoner RD, Stanson AW, Holley KE: Renal vein thrombosis in idiopathic membranous glomerulopathy and nephrotic syndrome: incidence and significance. Kidney Int 23:368, 1983

179. Kazatchkine M, Sultan Y, Caen JP et al: Bleeding in renal failure: a possible cause. Br Med J 2:216, 1976

180. Janson PA, Jubelirer SJ, Weinstein M et al: Treatment of the bleeding tendency in uremia with cryoprecipitate. N Engl J Med 303:318, 1980

181. Mannucci PM, Remuzzi G, Pusineri F et al: Deamino-8-D-arginine vasopressin shortens the bleeding time in uremia. N Engl J Med 308:8, 1983

182. Howie PW, Prentice CR, McNicol GP: Coagulation, fibrinolysis and placental function in pre-eclampsia, essential hypertension and placental insufficiency. Br J Obstet Gynaecol 78:952, 1971

183. Pollack VE: The role of intravascular coagulation in toxemia of pregnancy. In McIntosh RM, Guggenheim SJ, Schrier RW (eds): Kidney Disease: Hematologic and Vascular Problems. Wiley, New York, 1977

184. Grunfeld JP, Ganeval D, Bournerias F: Acute renal failure in pregnancy. Kidney Int 18:179, 1980

185. Sheehan HL, Lynch JB: Pathology of Toxemia of Pregnancy. Williams & Wilkins, Baltimore, 1973

186. Schwartz SO, Motto SA: The diagnostic significance of "burr" red blood cells. Am J Med Sci 218:563, 1949

187. Williams WJ: Examination of the blood. p. 9. In Williams WJ, Beutler E, Erslev AJ, Lichtman MA (eds): Hematology. 3rd Ed. McGraw-Hill, New York, 1983

188. Callen JR, Limarzi LR: Blood and bone marrow studies in renal disease. Am J Clin Pathol 2:3, 1950

189. Zingraff J, Drueket T, Marie P et al: Anemia and secondary hyperparathyroidism. Arch Intern Med 138:1650, 1978

190. Barbour GL: Effect of parathyroidectomy on anemia in chronic renal failure. Arch Intern Med 139:889, 1979

191. Rao DS, Shih M-S, Mohini R: Effect of serum parathyroid hormone and bone marrow fibrosis on the response to erythropoietin in uremia. N Engl J Med 328:171, 1993

192. Bogin E, Massry SG, Levi J et al: Effects of parathyroid hormone on osmotic fragility of human erythrocytes. J Clin Invest 69:1017, 1982

193. Logue JP, Lange Rd, Moore CV: Characterization of the anemia associated with chronic insufficiency. Am J Med 24:4, 1958

194. Eschbach JW, Cook JD, Scribner BH et al: Iron balance in hemodialysis patients. Ann Intern Med 87:710, 1977

195. Holken AG, Marwah PK: Iatrogenic contribution to anemia of renal failure. Lancet 1:164, 1971

196. Longnecker RE, Goffinet JA, Hendler ED: Blood loss during maintenance hemodialysis. Trans Am Soc Artif Intern Organs 20:135, 1974

197. Linton AL, Clark WF, Driedger AA et al: Correctable factors contributing to the anemia of dialysis patients. Nephron 19:95, 1977

198. Rifkind D, Kravetz HM, Knight V et al: Urinary excretion of iron-binding protein in the nephrotic syndrome. N Engl J Med 265:115, 1961

199. Paine CJ, Hargrove MD, Jr, Eichner ER: Folic acid binding protein and folate balance in uremia. Arch Intern Med 136:756, 1979

200. Hampers CL, Streiff R, Nathan DG et al: Megaloblastic hematopoiesis in uremia and in patients on long-term hemodialysis. N Engl J Med 276:551, 1961

201. Swainson SP, Winney RJ: Do dialysis patients need extra folate? Lancet 1:239, 1983

202. Weir DG, Scott JM: Interrelationships of folate and cobalamins. p. 121. In Lindenbaum J (ed): Contemporary Issues in Clinical Nutrition: Nutrition in Hematology. Churchill Livingstone, New York, 1983

203. Hutchins L, Lipschitz D: Iron and folate metabolism in renal failure. Semin Nephrol 5:142, 1985

204. Yawata Y, Hacob HS: Abnormal red cell metabolism in patients with chronic uremia: nature of the defect and its persistance despite adequate hemodialysis. Blood 45:231, 1975

205. Le Leeuw NKM, Shapiro L, Lowenstein L: Drug-induced hemolytic anemia. Ann Intern Med 58:592, 1963

206. Melissinos KG, Vlassopoulous K, Drivas G et al: The catalase activity of erythrocytes in chronic renal failure. Clin Chim Acta 66:267, 1976

207. Rosenmund A, Binswanger U, Straub PW: Oxidative injury to erythrocytes, cell rigidity, and splenic hemolysis in hemodialyzed uremic patients. Ann Intern Med 82:460, 1975

208. Giardini O, Taccone-Gallucci M, Lubrano R et al: Evidence of red blood cell membrane lipid peroxidation in haemodialysis patients. Nephron 35:235, 1984

209. Albright RK, White RP: Red blood cell susceptibility to hydrogen peroxide (H_2O_2) lysis in chronic hemodialysis patients. Clin Exp Dial Apheresis 6:223, 1982

210. Eaton JW, Leida MN: Hemolysis in chronic renal failure. Semin Nephrol 5:133, 1985

211. Manzler AD, Schreiner AW: Copper-induced acute hemolytic anemia: a new complication of hemodialysis. Ann Intern Med 73:409, 1970

212. Higgins MR, Grace M, Ulan RA et al: Anemia in hemodialysis patients. Arch Intern Med 137:172, 1977

213. Carlson DJ, Shaprio FL; Methemoglobinemia from well water nitrates: a complication of heme dialysis. Ann Intern Med 73:757, 1970

214. Punk, Yeung CK, Chan TK: Acute intravascular hemolysis due to accidental formation intoxication during hemodialysis. Clin Nephrol 21:188, 1984

215. Berkes SL, Kahn SI, Chazan JA et al: Prolonged hemolysis from overheated dialysate. Ann Intern Med 83:363, 1975

216. Francos GC, Burke JF Jr, Besarb A et al: An unsuspected cause of acute hemolysis during hemodialysis. Trans Am Artif Intern Organs 29:140, 1983

217. Said R, Quintanilla A, Levin H et al: Acute hemolysis due to profound hypo-osmolality. A complication of hemodialysis. J Dial 1:447, 1977

218. Eaton JW, Kolpin CF, Swofford HS et al: Chlorinated urban water: a cause of dialysis-induced hemolytic anemia. Science 181:463, 1973

219. Anagnostou A, Kurtzman NA: The anemia of chronic renal failure. Semin Nephrol 5:115, 1985

220. Jacob HS, Amsden T: Acute hemolytic anemia with rigid red cells in hypophosphatemia. N Engl J Med 285:1446, 1971

221. Bischel MD, Neimea RS, Berne TV et al: Hypersplenism in the uremic hemodialysis patient. Nephron 9:146, 1972

222. Hartley LCJ, Mortan TO, Innis MD et al: Splenectomy for anemia in patients on hemodialysis. Lancet 2:1343, 1971

223. Neiman RS, Bischel MD, Lukes RJ: Hypersplenism in the uremic hemodialyzed patient. Am J Clin Pathol 60:602, 1973

224. Weinberg SG, Lubin A, Wiener S et al: Myelofibrosis and renal osteodystrophy. Am J Med 63:755, 1977

225. Bommer J, Ritz E, Woldherr R: Silicone-induced splenomegaly. N Engl J Med 305:1077, 1981

226. Clark KGA: Splenectomy for anemia of chronic renal failure. Lancet 1:325, 1972

227. Sherrard DJ: The role of aluminum in renal osteodystrophy. Mayo Clin Proc 68:510, 1993

228. Romanski SA, McCarthy JT, Kluge K, et al: Detection of subtle aluminum-related renal osteodystrophy. Mayo Clin Proc 68:419, 1993

229. Elliot HL, Dryburgh F, Fell GS et al: Aluminum toxicity during regular haemodialysis. Br J Med 1:1101, 1978

230. Short AI, Winney RJ, Robson JS: Reversible microcytic hypochromic anaemia in dialysis patients due to aluminum intoxication. Proc Eur Dial Transplant Assoc 17:226, 1980

231. Parkinson IS, Ward MK, Kerr DN: Dialysis encephalitis, bone disease and anaemia. The aluminum intoxication syndrome during regular hemodialysis. J Clin Pathol 34:1285, 1981

232. Huber CT, Frieden E: The inhibition of ferroxidase by trivalent and other metal ions. J Biol Chem 245:3979, 1970

233. Cochran M, Cochran M, Coates JH et al: Direct spectrophotometric determination of the two site binding of aluminum to transferrin. Life Sci 40:2337, 1987

234. Ohare JA, Murnoghan DJ: Reversal of aluminum-induced hemodialysis anemia by a low-aluminum dialysate. N Engl J Med 306:654, 1982

235. Dombroski J, Kluin K, Burnatowska-Hledin M et al: Microcytic anemia and aluminum toxicity, abstracted. Kidney Int 27:128, 1985

236. Rabiner SF: Uremic bleeding. p. 223. In Spaet TH (ed): Progress in Hemostasis and Thrombosis. Grune & Stratton, Orlando, FL, 1972

237. Castaldi PA, Rozenberg MC, Stewart JH: The bleeding disorder of uremia: a qualitative platelet defect. Lancet 2:66, 1966

238. Rabiner SF, Drake RF: Platelet function as an indicator of adequate dialysis. Kidney Int, suppl. 2. 17:S144, 1975

239. Miller RP, Denny WF: Hemolytic anemia during acute renal failure: observations on plasma erythropoietin levels. South Med J 61:2, 1968

240. Radtke HW, Frei U, Erbes PM et al: Improving anemia by hemodialysis: effect on serum erythropoietin. Kidney Int 17:382, 1980

241. Milman N: Iron absorption in patients with chronic uraemia. Scand J Haematol 29:5, 1982

242. Camitta BM, Thomas ED, Nathan DG et al: A prospective study of androgens and bone marrow transplantation for treatment of severe aplastic anemia. Blood 53:504, 1979

243. Gardner FH: Introduction. p. 1. In Najean Y (ed): Medullary Aplasia. Masson, New York, 1980

244. DeGowin RL, Lavender AR, Forland M et al: Erythropoiesis and erythropoietin in patients with chronic renal failure treated with hemodialysis and testosterone. Ann Intern Med 72:913, 1970

245. Fried W, Johansson O, Lang C et al: The hematologic effect of androgens in uremic patients. Ann Intern Med 79:823, 1973

246. Eschbach JW, Adamson JW: Improvement in the anemia of chronic renal failure with fluoxymesterone. Ann Intern Med 78:527, 1973

247. Hendler ED, Goffinet JA, Ross S et al: Controlled study of androgen therapy in anemia of patients on maintenance hemodialysis. N Engl J Med 291:1046, 1974

248. Neff MS, Goldberg J, Slifkin RF et al: A comparison of androgens for anemia in patients on hemodialysis. N Engl J Med 304:871, 1981

249. Williams JS, Stein JH, Ferris TF: Nandrolone decanoate therapy for patients receiving hemodialysis. A controlled study. Arch Intern Med 134:289, 1974

250. Acchiardo SR, Black WD: Fluoxymesterone therapy in anemia of patients on maintenance hemodialysis: comparison between patients with kidneys and anephric patients. J Dial, suppl. 4. 1:357, 1977

251. Kalmanti M, Dainiak N, Martino J et al: Correlations of clinical and in vitro erythropoietic responses to androgens in renal failure. Kidney Int 22:383, 1982

252. Winearls CG, Oliver D, Pippard MJ et al: Effect of human erythropoietin derived from recombinant DNA on the anemia of patients maintained by chronic hemodialysis. Lancet 2:1175, 1986

253. Zin B, Drueke T, Zinpratt J et al: Erythropoietin treatment in anemic patients on hemodialysis. Lancet 2:1329, 1986

254. Eschbach JW, Egrie JC, Downing MR et al: Correction of the anemia of end stage renal disease with recombinant human erythropoietin. N Engl J Med 316:73, 1987

255. Bommer J, Alexiou C, Muller-Buhl E et al: Recombinant human erythropoietin therapy in hemodialitis patients: dose determination and clinical experience. Nephrol Dial Transplant 2:238, 1987

256. Erslev A: Erythropoietin coming of age. N Engl J Med 316:101, 1987

257. Anagnostou A, Barone J, Kedo A et al: Effect of erythropoietin therapy on the red cell volume of uremic and nonuremic rats. Br J Haematol 37:85, 1977

258. McMahon FG, Vargas R, Ryan M et al: Pharmacokinetics and effects of recombinant human erythropoietin following intravenous and subcutaneous injections in healthy volunteers. (in press)

259. Moia M, Mannucci PM, Vizzotto L et al: Improvement in the hemostatic defect of uraemia after treatment with recombinant human erythropoietin. Lancet 2:1227, 1987

260. Eschbach JW, Adamson JW: Modern aspects of the pathophysiology of renal anemia, discussion. Contrib Nephrol 66:63, 1988

261. Stivelman J, Vanwyck D, Kirlin L et al: Use of recombinant erythropoietin (R-HuEPO) with high-flux dialysis (HFD) does not worsen azotemia or shorten access survival, abstracted. Kidney Int 33:239, 1988

262. Ishimitsu T, Tsukada H, Ogawa Y, et al: Genetic predisposition to hypertension facilitates blood pressure elevation in hemodialysis patients treated with erythropoietin. Am J Med 94:401, 1993

263. Skikne BS, Cook JD: Effect of enhanced erythropoiesis on iron absorption. J Lab Clin Med 120:746, 1992

264. Brugnara C, Chambers LA, Malynn E, et al: Red blood cell regeneration induced by subcutaneous recombinant erythropoietin: iron-deficient erythropoiesis in iron-replete subjects. Blood 81:956, 1993

265. Nissenson AR, Nimer SD, Wolcott DL: Recombinant human erythropoietin and renal anemia: molecule biology, clinical efficacy, and nervous system effects. Ann Intern Med 114:402, 1991

266. Grutzmacher P, Ehmer B, Messinger D, et al: Effect of aluminum overload on the bone marrow response to recombinant human erythropoietin. p. 315. In Baldamus CA, Scigalla P, Wieczorek L, Koch KM (eds): Erythropoietin: From Molecular Structure to Clinical Application. Karger, Basel, 1989

267. Liu YK, Kosfield RE, Marcum SG: Treatment of uraemic bleeding with erythroid oestrogen. Lancet 2:887, 1984

268. Livio M, Mannucci PM, Vigano G et al: Conjugated estrogens for the management of bleeding associated with renal failure. N Engl J Med 315:731, 1986

269. Schaefer AI, Cheron RG, Dluhy R et al: Clinical consequences of acquired transfusional iron overload in adults. N Engl J Med 304:319, 1981

270. Eschbach JW, Cook JD, Finch CA: Iron absorption in chronic renal disease. Clin Sci 38:191, 1970

271. Falk RJ, Mattern WD, Lamanna RW et al: Iron removal during continuous ambulatory peritoneal dialysis using desferrioxamine. Kidney Int 24:110, 1983

272. Hilfenhaus M, Koch K-M, Bechstein PB et al: Therapy and monitoring of hypersiderosis in chronic renal insufficiency. Contrib Nephrol 38:167, 1984

273. Adan L, Hainline BW, Zackson D: The importance of accurate and precise aluminum levels. N Engl J Med 313:1609, 1985

274. Abreo K, Brown ST, Sella ML et al: Application of an erythrocyte aluminum assay in the diagnosis of aluminum-associated microcytic anemia in patients undergoing dialysis and response to deferoxamine therapy. J Lab Clin Med 13:50, 1984

275. Maloney NA, Oh SM, Alfrey AC et al: Histologic quantitation of aluminum in iliac bone from patients with renal failure. J Lab Clin Med 99:206, 1982

Hematologic Aspects of Pregnancy

149

Thomas P. Duffy

INTRODUCTION

Pregnancy constitutes a major challenge for the hematologic and hemostatic resources of a woman's body and requires a dual focus on the mother and fetus in order to recognize and treat any complications in this arena. As pregnancy progresses, a hypercoagulable state develops in anticipation of the hemorrhagic insult that accompanies placental separation.[1,2] The expectant mother is thus doubly jeopardized by an increased risk of thromboembolism and the many hemorrhagic complications of the pregnant state. In addition, therapies chosen to manage a maternal problem must be modulated according to their potential for damage to the fetus.[3] Any antecedent hematologic lesion will obviously further complicate and be complicated by a pregnancy. The hematologic problems of pregnancy are therefore the shared responsibility of the obstetrician, pediatrician, and the hematologist as their varied expertise and knowledge are integrated for the benefit of the mother and child.

ANEMIA

The physiologic expansion of the expectant mother's blood volume consists of an increase in plasma volume (40–60%), which is approximately twice the simultaneous expansion in the red blood cell (RBC) mass (20–50%); this "hydremia" of pregnancy results in a fall in hematocrit to the 30–32% range, requiring a revision downward (to 10 g%) of the lower limits of a normal hemoglobin during pregnancy[4] (Table 149-1). The expanded blood pool of the mother compensates for the increased metabolic and perfusion needs of the fetal-placental unit and serves as a reservoir to compensate for blood loss at delivery of the infant.

Anemia occurring during pregnancy is most frequently a reticulocytopenic, hyporegenerative anemia attributable to deficiencies of iron or folate, or both. In order to provide iron for fetal hemoglobin synthesis and to anticipate the losses due to bleeding, approximately 1,000 mg of additional iron is needed during the course of pregnancy. This amount is greater than the normal 500-mg iron storage pool present in most women, and an iron-deficient state with low ferritin levels frequently occurs in the mother.[5,6] However delivery of iron to the placenta continues, with a rerouting of the normal vector of iron transport to the heavy concentration of transferrin receptors on the placental trophoblastic membranes.[7] This major demand on the iron stores overwhelms most women's marginal storehouses of iron. Iron supplementation (300 mg ferrous sulfate/day) is administered to pregnant women in anticipation of this drain on their limited stores.[8]

Folate deficiency may also complicate pregnancy because of a similar escalation in the need for this essential cofactor in nucleic acid synthesis during pregnancy.[9] The total body stores of this vitamin are small and short-lived. Nausea and vomiting during pregnancy may significantly impair its intake. Pure folate deficiency results in a macrocytic anemia or even pancytopenia, but the expected elevation of RBC mean corpus-cular volume may be masked during pregnancy by the contribution of concomitant iron deficiency.[10] This combined deficiency may produce normocytic indices, although review of the peripheral smear often reveals a dimorphic population of RBCs and the hypersegmentation of polymorphonuclear neutrocytes that indicates megaloblastic hematopoiesis. RBC sizing index curves may uncover the two distinct cell populations that characterize combined iron-folate deficiency. Most prenatal vitamins contain folate in addition to iron, so proper prenatal care of expectant mothers should obviate these problems.[11,12] There is little concern that folate will mask vitamin B_{12} deficiency, since women with this deficiency are usually older or infertile, or both.

A few other causes of reticulocytopenic anemia are directly related to pregnancy. Several cases of aplastic anemia complicating pregnancy have been described; the outcome is usually determined by the severity of the marrow lesion and the threat of leukopenia-associated infection.[13,14] Although some consider this a chance association, the resolution of the aplasia after delivery or abortion and the documented recurrence of aplasia in subsequent pregnancies makes a causal, perhaps immunologic, mechanism likely. The severity of the aplasia and the ability to support the patient help to determine the decision regarding continuation or termination of the pregnancy. Pure red cell aplasia has also been associated temporally with pregnancy.[15] Congenital aplastic anemia or Fanconi anemia may paradoxically not be manifest until the childbearing age. Instances of successful childbirth have occurred in such patients with meticulous hematologic support.[16]

LEUKOCYTOSIS

An elevated white blood cell (WBC) count with a differential revealing a rare myelocyte or metamyelocyte can occur in pregnancy.[17] Döhle bodies may also be present; this may lead to confusion in assessing the possibility of intercurrent infection. Since the count returns to normal after-delivery, it is likely that the WBC elevation is secondary to the steroid or cytokine alterations that accompany pregnancy.

Differentiation of a leukemoid reaction from leukemia should not present any unique difficulties when this question arises during pregnancy. Flow analysis and chromosomal studies help resolve any confusion in the rare pregnant patient with leukemia. When leukemia or other hematologic malignancies complicate pregnancy, management is influenced by the stage of pregnancy at which diagnosis is made, the clinical effects of the disease, and the anticipated toxic effects of chemotherapy or radiotherapy (or both) on the mother and child.[18] Since the most active stage of organogenesis is the first trimester, recommendations regarding the continuation of pregnancy would differ greatly in this setting from those of a woman with leukemia or lymphoma at a later stage of pregnancy. There are several reports of successful, uncomplicated births after chemotherapy for leukemia and lymphoma,[19,20] but the most common outcomes are abortion and fetal loss. When chronic leukemias occur during pregnancy, leukapheresis may serve as a delaying device until delivery is possible.[21]

Table 149-1. Plasma Volume, Red Cell Volume, Total Blood Volume, and Hematocrit in Pregnancy

| | Nonpregnant | Weeks of Pregnancy | | |
		20	30	40
Plasma volume (ml)	2,600	3,150	3,750	3,850
Red cell mass (ml)	1,400	1,450	1,550	1,650
Total blood volume (ml)	4,000	4,600	5,300	5,500
Body hematocrit (%)	35.0	32.0	29.0	30.0
Venous hematocrit (%)	39.8	36.4	33.0	34.1

(From Hytten,[4] with permission.)

THROMBOCYTOPENIA

Although some of the data conflict, ample evidence shows that the platelet count does not deviate from normal limits during an uncomplicated pregnancy.[22] Thrombocytopenia (<150,000/L) in the expectant mother requires consideration of the usual causes of a lowered platelet count as well as diatheses unique to pregnancy. Most authors would restrict these concerns to women with platelet counts of <100,000/L; a platelet count of 100,000–150,000/L, newly discovered during an otherwise uncomplicated pregnancy, is not thought to pose any threat to the fetus.[23] This so-called gestational thrombocytopenia is not considered an indication for fetal blood sampling or therapeutic intervention, although the cause of the thrombocytopenia should be investigated and identified if possible.[24] Finding and eliminating the cause have special significance since thrombocytopenia can threaten both the mother and the fetus. Thrombocytopenia in the fetus has important implications for determining the method of delivery and defining the postnatal needs of the infant. The situation is even more complicated in those patients with qualitative platelet abnormalities such as the Bernard-Soulier syndrome and Glanzmann thrombosthenia; these patients require platelet support during delivery, even if the numbers of platelets are normal, to compensate for their lack of effective platelet function.[25]

IMMUNE THROMBOCYTOPENIC PURPURA

Immune thrombocytopenic purpura (ITP) has a pronounced incidence in young adult women. The immunologic alterations of pregnancy may create the same sensitization, and thus, it is not surprising that ITP may complicate the course of pregnancy. The same diagnostic criteria are used as for standard ITP.[26] Platelet-associated IgG is frequently detectable in ITP, but this sensitive assay is relatively nonspecific. Demonstrable serum antiplatelet antibodies are more specific for this diagnosis and are usually directed against platelet glycoproteins GPIIb/IIIa or GPIb/9.[27]

Therapy for ITP during pregnancy is basically the same as during the nonpregnant state. Steroids, starting at 1 mg/kg of prednisone and titering according to the platelet response, are initiated for platelet counts <50,000/L; some clinicians reserve steroid use for thrombocytopenic patients with prolonged bleeding times (>20 minutes) or with demonstrated bleeding.[28] If the patient is steroid refractory or if there are contraindications to their use, intravenous immunoglobulins are now administered as a first line of intervention.[29] Since the platelet-elevating effect of the latter is relatively short-lived (3 weeks), it may be necessary to punctuate the regimen with weekly to biweekly immunoglobulin infusions. With the availability of these two modalities, it is usually possible to avoid splenectomy, an operation that carries the risk of fetal loss. If splenectomy is required, the first portion of the second trimester is probably the optimal time for this intervention.

The fetus is also a candidate for development of thrombocytopenia because of transplacental passage of antiplatelet IgG in ITP. Either fetal scalp vein sampling during labor[30] or umbilical vein sampling before labor[31] is used for diagnosis and to determine the method of delivery of the affected fetus; a fetal platelet count of >50,000/L is considered adequate for vaginal delivery. Initial enthusiasm for using the presence or absence of maternal serum antiplatelet antibodies as a means for anticipating thrombocytopenia in the fetus has waned.[32] There is still support for the administration of steroids to ITP mothers in the 3 weeks before delivery for their effect on the platelet count of the fetus[33]; however, there is controversy as to the transplacental passage of steroids and their postulated positive effects upon the fetal platelet count.[34,35]

PRE-ECLAMPSIA AND ECLAMPSIA

The specific pathophysiologic mechanisms that cause eclampsia are not known. Abnormal platelet-endothelium interactions, with excessive platelet consumption, are thought to be major components of this hypertensive disorder.[36,37] There is also support for a more minor contribution from disseminated intravascular coagulation (DIC) in eclampsia,[38] since low antithrombin III levels[39] and elevated dimers of fibrin split products[40] are observed. The platelet decrement usually outdistances any evidence for fibrinogen consumption in eclampsia. The marked imbalance in the thromboxane/prostacyclin placental levels in eclamptic patients has been suggested as a causal factor in the development of this process. The sevenfold thromboxane excess contributes to both increased platelet consumption and vasoconstriction.[41] Successful prophylaxis against eclampsia with daily ingestion of acetylsalicylic acid in several studies also supports a causal role of platelets and arachidonic metabolites.[42,43] Plasma endothelin levels are also elevated, suggesting some causal role for this potent vasoconstrictor as well.[44]

When thrombocytopenia is discovered in a patient with classic evidence for pre-eclampsia (>30-mmHg rise in systolic or >15-mmHg rise in diastolic pressures from baseline, proteinuria >0.3 g/L/24 hr, and edema) or eclampsia (seizures/coma), the cause of the thrombocytopenia is easy to identify. Thrombocytopenia develops in ≤50% of patients with pre-eclampsia. However, thrombocytopenia may also accompany hepatic forms of toxemia, in which the more classic signs of pre-eclampsia are absent.[45] Acute fatty liver of pregnancy is one of these variants. Clinical attention is drawn to and focused on the hepatic abnormalities. Liver biopsy specimens of eclamptic patients demonstrate the same fatty changes with the fat content of the liver paralleling the degree of thrombocytopenia.[46]

The hematologic alterations in pregnancy sometimes extend to encompass a clinical entity that includes a hemolytic anemia.[47] The so-called HELLP syndrome (*h*emolysis, *e*levated *l*iver enzymes, and *low p*latelets) may or may not be associated with increased blood pressure, edema, or proteinuria.[48] Most patients with the HELLP syndrome present with malaise and right upper quadrant or epigastric pain, often diverting the physician's attention from the recognition of a "toxemic" state.

THROMBOTIC THROMBOCYTOPENIC PURPURA

Several cases of thrombotic thrombocytopenic purpura (TTP) during pregnancy have been reported in the literature, but the appearance of a TTP-like picture during the third trimester of pregnancy may actually be toxemia masquerading as TTP.[50] The pentad of TTP (fever, hemolytic anemia, thrombocytopenia, renal and central nervous system disease) may all be present in toxemia except for fever. The management of a patient with this constellation during the last trimester of pregnancy is delivery of the infant and not the complex interventions used to treat classic TTP. When TTP appears earlier in pregnancy, steroids and plasma infusions[51] with and without plasmapheresis have been successfully employed; uterine evacuation has also been used with successful reversal of the picture.[52]

DISSEMINATED INTRAVASCULAR COAGULATION

The most frequent causes of bleeding in obstetric patients are the many pathologic precipitants of DIC. These have their origin in the entrance of the products of conception into the systemic circulation.[53] "Slow" DIC is now infrequently a problem because its cause, fetal death in utero, is easily recognized by ultrasound and can be corrected by induction of delivery with blood component support to correct any coagulation abnormalities; delivery of the dead fetus removes the source of the DIC, which is thought to be the tissue thromboplastin released from the decomposing fetus.[54]

A rapid and frequently fatal form of DIC accompanies clostridial sepsis; this unfortunate aftermath of illegal abortions is also characterized by severe intravascular hemolysis, attributable to the direct bacterial by-product attack of lecithinase on the lipid component of the RBC membrane.[55] "Fast" DIC also accompanies abruptio placentae[56] and amniotic fluid embolism.[57] The major complication of the former is hemorrhage, whereas the latter is usually complicated by cardiopulmonary collapse in addition to hemorrhage. Treatment of DIC associated with abruptio placentae consists of stabilization of the clotting disorder with the necessary blood component support, followed by delivery of the infant. The epidemic of cocaine addiction has seen an increased incidence of abruptio placentae in which cocaine is thought to play a causal role. Amniotic fluid embolism is usually fatal (85% mortality), primarily as a result of cardiovascular collapse. This life-threatening entity occurs most frequently during a difficult delivery in a multiparous woman. Hypoxemia, shock, and hemorrhage in this setting should suggest the diagnosis, and aggressive cardiopulmonary support, blood component administration, and steroids have been recommended for its management.

"Fast" and "slow" DIC represent the most dramatic occurrences of DIC during pregnancy. However, evidence for DIC also exists in patients who have hypertonic saline- and urea-induced abortions.[58] This complication is usually fleeting and disappears shortly after the fetus is delivered. No therapeutic intervention is usually necessary. Heparin therapy is not indicated in this situation or in the other forms of DIC complicating pregnancy. Successful heparin treatment of DIC associated with a single fetal death in a twin pregnancy has been reported[59]; this may have implications for management of a multiple pregnancy now that selective destruction of some of the fetuses is performed.

PREGNANCY AND THROMBOSIS

Pregnancy constitutes a hypercoagulable state with a progressive increase in the concentration of clotting factors and a decrease in the body's fibrinolytic capacity. A specific plasminogen activator inhibitor is produced by the placenta.[60] This situation, when coupled with stasis due to obstruction of venous return by an enlarging uterus, explains the dramatically increased incidence of venous thrombosis that occurs during pregnancy and the puerperium.[61] Thrombosis of the pelvic and lower extremity vessels is common. Diagnosis and treatment are influenced by their potential for damage to the fetus.

No form of anticoagulation is without significant risk during pregnancy.[62] A firm diagnosis of thrombosis or embolism, or both, must be made before initiating any therapy. This may entail using the gold standard of venography, with shielding of the uterus, to document the thrombosis if impedance plethysmography is not available. The risk of the radiographic procedure is thought to be offset by the greater certainty that venography allows in dictating the need for anticoagulation.[63] The same is true for ventilation/perfusion scans or pulmonary angiography as a means of diagnosing pulmonary embolism in the same population.

The maternal and fetal morbity and mortality due to anticoagulation make family planning counseling essential for an individual who requires chronic anticoagulation.[66] Patients with artificial prosthetic valves require continuation of anticoagulation throughout pregnancy and must recognize that only one-third of pregnancies in which Coumadin is administered during the first trimester result in normal liveborn infants.[67,68] Heparin administration is not clearly superior, although the risk of abnormalities in liveborn infants is less. Heparin does not cross the placenta and is not associated with any specific embryopathy. Heparin, however, leads to bone demineralization in the mother and in about 10% of patients results in thrombocytopenia.[69] Since both agents pose serious risks during pregnancy, most clinicians use them sequentially to dampen the risk of one and capitalize on the convenience of the other. Heparin is used during the first trimester, with a subsequent switch to oral Coumadin; close to the end of pregnancy, heparin (10,000 U bid) is used and then stopped as described above at the time of delivery. Heparin or Coumadin can be reintroduced postpartum because neither drug is a threat to nursing infants.

Thrombolytic agents are contraindicated in pregnancy because of their risk of severe hemorrhage.

Because of the high incidence of recurrent thrombotic events with subsequent pregnancies, expectant mothers with a previous history of deep venous thrombosis or pulmonary embolism have usually been prophylactically anticoagulated. This practice is no longer universal. Anticoagulation is sometimes withheld as prophylaxis; dextran is administered at and around the time of delivery, and heparin is initiated in the postpartum period; a small series has demonstrated the safety and utility of this alternative management.[70]

PREGNANCY AND THE HEMOGLOBINOPATHIES

The vogue for prophylactic exchange transfusions in sickle cell anemia has waned and has given way to watchful anticipation of the patient's course by the hematologist and obstetrician together.[71] Many series have demonstrated a high risk of stillbirths, abortions, and fetal growth retardation as the outcome of nontransfused sickle cell pregnancies, but the contribution of poor prenatal care in this socioeconomically deprived group may have been the critical factor in these fetal losses. With good antenatal care and recognition of any backdrop of organ dysfunction, the usual patient with hemoglobin SS disease tolerates pregnancy without major morbidity for mother or child. Transfusions are reserved for any acceleration of the sickling disorder, worsening of anemia (hemoglobin <6 g%), or obstetric complications.[72] In light of the severe hemolytic component of this disease, folic acid must be adequately supplemented to guarantee that a hyporegenerative megaloblastic crisis does not occur. Iron therapy may also be needed, since these young women frequently have meager iron stores even in the setting of hemolytic anemia.

Management of the patient with sickle cell disorder during the delivery period remains controversial. Some would exchange transfuse such individuals if general anesthesia is required for delivery; the potential for an anesthetic accident with hypoxemia is the basis for this recommendation. Epidural anesthesia lessens this risk, but hypotension secondary to venous pooling may occur even with this modality; attention to fluid expansion, use of pressure leg wraps, and unweighting uterine compression of the vena cava by positioning the patient on the left lateral side lessen this risk.

The same concerns apply to individuals with other interacting hemoglobins (SC, S thal, and others) that participate in the sickling phenomenon. Sickle trait should pose no threat to pregnancy except for the need to recognize and treat properly the higher incidence of kidney infections. The probable contribution of infection to precipitation of premature labor makes such infections a more significant threat during pregnancy.

Thalassemia major is not a frequent problem for the obstetrician because such patients often suffer with failure of pubertal growth and delayed sexual development. Hypogonadotropic hypogonadism due to hemosiderin deposition in the hypothalamus makes these patients anovulatory and afertile.[73] However, there have been reports of 14 pregnancies in this patient population, with five fetal losses. Cardiac iron disease may be present and may lead to heart failure during pregnancy; close attention to maintaining the hemoglobin at a level of 10 g/dl is important. Thalassemia intermedia and minor are not characterized by any special problems during pregnancy; ferritin levels in these groups may be adequate to permit dispensation from the need for iron supplementation during pregnancy.[74]

COAGULOPATHIES DURING PREGNANCY

The most common coagulopathy creating problems during pregnancy and delivery is von Willebrand disease (vWD).[75] Recommendations regarding the management of vWD must take into consideration the spectrum of severity of the different subtypes of vWD and the relatively sparse experience in managing some of the more recently defined subtypes. Fortunately, in most of these patients, an increase in factor VIII coagulant and factor VIII antigen accompanying pregnancy frequently permits delivery without undue risk of bleeding. There remains the delayed risk of bleeding after delivery in these individuals because of the rapid return of coagulant levels to a nonpregnant deficient state. In such patients, the bleeding time is an important parameter to monitor and correct with desmopressin or concentrate as necessary.

Some individuals with vWD, especially those with the type III variant, have persisting very low to absent von Willebrand factor (vWF) levels throughout pregnancy and demonstrate a poor response to desmopressin infusions. Factor VIII concentrates that contain vWF should be administered to these patients if a cesarean section is performed; support should continue for 5–7 days after the delivery. The previous recommendation, that all such patients with severe vWD undergo cesarean section to protect the fetus, should be modified now that prenatal sampling of fetal blood allows identification of infants with the disorder.

The type IIB subtype presents an additional layer of complexity since a progressive diminution in platelet count accompanies the pregnancy-associated increased synthesis of this variant form of vWF.[76] The appearance of thrombocytopenia during pregnancy is, in fact, grounds for considering this diagnosis, wherein the interaction of the abnormal vWF and platelets results in thrombocytopenia.[77] Because of this interaction, administration of desmopressin to such patients has been prohibited, although there remains some question as to the appropriateness of this admonition. Patients with type IIB vWD have had normal vaginal deliveries without excessive bleeding even in the presence of significant thrombocytopenia. Factor VIII concentrate that contains vWF can successfully prevent bleeding in this condition when needed.

The remainder of the inherited coagulopathies are not a major threat unless the coagulant levels are <25% of normal.[78] Fresh frozen plasma infusions during and 4–5 days after delivery are the universal solution to these deficiencies, with monitoring of coagulant levels to gauge the adequacy of the replacement therapy. Factor XIII deficiency presents a special problem during pregnancy because of its association with spontaneous recurrent abortions and marked uterine bleeding; regular plasma infusions during pregnancy have sustained a normal pregnancy in the presence of factor XIII deficiency.[79]

LUPUS ANTICOAGULANT AND PREGNANCY: ANTIPHOSPHOLIPID SYNDROME

The lupus anticoagulant (LA), an immunoglobulin of the IgG or IgM subclass prolongs phospholipid-dependent coagulation tests by interfering with the essential phospholipid skeleton of the coagulation cascade.[80] A positive test result for syphilis, a so-called biologic false-positive test, and anticardiolipin antibodies (both tests having phospholipids as their target antigens) are frequent accompaniments of the LA. Individuals possessing such antibodies often develop thrombocytopenia and thromboses involving both the arterial and venous circuits[81]; the antibodies may be a factor implicated in creating the thromboses, since plasma from LA patients inhibit vessel wall generation of prostacyclin, a vasodilator and powerful inhibitor of platelet aggregation. The procoagulant role of LA plasma may not be restricted to prostacyclin inhibition, since other investigators have demonstrated defective thrombomodulin activation of protein C in the presence of LA plasma.[82] Whatever the role of the phospholipid antibody in the process, the LA is

THERAPY FOR LUPUS ANTICOAGULANT

Optimal treatment of the pregnant patient with the LA remains to be determined. Use of prednisone (30–40 mg/day) and acetylsalicylic acid (80 mg/day) has reversed the previous near-total loss of such pregnancies and has permitted approximately 70% to be salvaged. This therapy is not without complications since the incidence of steroid side effects and supervention of eclampsia in these treated patients is high. Therapeutic intervention with heparin has also permitted successful pregnancies. Doppler ultrasound monitoring of placental blood flow has been suggested as a means of charting the pathologic effects of the antibody on the vascular bed and helping define the need for infant delivery.[87] The complex clinical scenarios in these patients and the gaps in our knowledge regarding the pathophysiology of the disease make necessary a close collaboration among obstetricians, hematologists, and pediatricians in their care.

paradoxically a marker for an increased risk of thrombotic episodes, including strokes.

Nowhere is this thrombotic tendency more threatening than in the association of the LA with first-trimester abortions and fetal deaths in the second and third trimesters.[83] The lesion in many of these women is a thrombotic process involving the decidual and placental vessels; the absence of such findings in other LA patients forces the conclusion that the pathogenetic mechanisms of the antiphospholipid antibodies must still be clarified. Since the fetal loss syndrome is well identified in mothers with anticardiolipin antibodies who lack LA, the phospholipid target of the antibody appears to have the most significance.

Any mother with systemic lupus erythematosus (SLE) or a history of fetal loss should be screened for antiphospholipid antibodies; the LA is not restricted to women with SLE, and there is no relationship of the antibody to the activity of the disease or even to anti-DNA activity. The activated partial thromboplastin time[84] or the more sensitive Russell's viper venom time[85] is a good screen for the presence of the LA; a low-titer positive serologic test result for syphilis is sometimes the clue that LA is complicating a pregnancy. Because the anticardiolipin antibody is only loosely associated with LA in SLE patients, separate testing for this antibody should also be performed since it may be an earlier and more important predictor of fetal distress.[86]

HYPERCOAGULABLE STATES AND PREGNANCY

Primary or essential thrombocythemia in a pregnant woman may lead to the development of multiple placental infarcts, fetal loss, or fetal growth retardation.[88,89] A combination of dipyridamole and aspirin has been administered with a successful outcome in such pregnancies; plateletpheresis has been performed immediately before delivery with effective lowering of the platelet counts. Monitoring of thrombocythemic pregnancies with Doppler ultrasound studies of placental blood flow has been recommended as a means of gauging the need for platelet reduction by pheresis earlier in the pregnancy.

Pregnancy complicated by polycythemia vera has been infrequently reported; the perinatal outcome has been poor, with significant fetal loss.[90] Attention must be paid to maintenance of a hematocrit in the 40% range with phlebotomy used to maintain that level. Because of the frequent association of thrombocythemia with erythrocytosis in polycythemia vera, some clinicians recommend the use of low-dose heparin during and after delivery, although this approach is not without controversy. There is usually a rapid rebound in the hematocrit after delivery, requiring special vigilance to prevent threatening erythrocytosis at that time. Interferon-α has been used successfully to control disease activity in myeloproliferative disorders during pregnancy without damage to the fetus; this agent may permit a smoother control of the blood counts, but experience with its use during pregnancy is still limited.[91]

Protein C deficiency dramatically increases the risk of deep venous thromboses (DVT) during pregnancy[92,93]; there is a 25% incidence of DVT in pregnancy and the puerperium in patients with this autosomal dominant inherited disorder. Therapy recommended for management of protein C deficiency is ambulatory full-dose subcutaneous heparin.

Antithrombin III deficiency is the most common inherited procoagulant state. Thrombotic events may occur during pregnancy or after delivery in 70% of such cases.[94,95] Management of these patients has included heparin (20,000 U SC bid) during the first 4–4.5 months and Coumadin in the remainder of pregnancy to the 36th or 37th week; heparin is then reintroduced and withdrawn before delivery, at which time a single infusion of antithrombin III (3,500 U) has been given. Heparin is again restarted in the postdelivery period until Coumadin is introduced.

Approximately 50 cases of pregnancy in women with paroxysmal nocturnal hemoglobinuria have been reported[96]; these pregnancies have been complicated by venous thromboses involving the lower extremities and the hepatic and cerebral vasculatures. Anticoagulation with low-dose heparin is recommended for these patients if they are confined to bed during the pregnancy. This disease may also witness worsening of marrow aplasia during pregnancy and an increased number and severity of hemolytic crises. Transfusions with washed RBCs to maintain the hemoglobin at 10 g% is suggested, with particular attention toward preventing hemolytic crises after delivery. The fetus in such pregnancies needs monitoring for neonatal isoimmune hemolysis because of the risk of maternal sensitization after transfusions.

REFERENCES

1. Crowley JP: Coagulopathy and bleeding in the parturient patient. Rhode Island Med J 72:135, 1989
2. Todd M, Thompson JH Jr, Bowie EJ et al: Changes in blood coagulation during pregnancy. Mayo Clinic Proc 40:370, 1975
3. Hall J, Pauli R, Wilson K: Maternal and fetal sequelae of anticoagulation during pregnancy. Am J Med 68:122, 1980
4. Hytten F: Blood volume changes in normal pregnancy. Clin Haematol 14:601, 1985
5. Foulkes J, Goldie DJ: The use of ferritin to assess the need for iron supplements in pregnancy. J Obst Gynecol 3:11, 1982
6. Romslo I, Haram K, Sagen V, Augensen K: Iron requirement in normal pregnancy as assessed by serum ferritin, serum transferrin saturation and erythrocyte protoporphyrin determinations. Br J Obstet Gynecol 90:101, 1988
7. Okuyama T, Tawada T, Furuya H, Villee CA: The role of transferrin and ferritin in the fetal-maternal-placental unit. Am J Obstet Gynecol 152:344, 1985
8. Bentley DP: Iron metabolism and anemia in pregnancy. Clin Haematol 14:613, 1985
9. Chanarin I: Folate and cobalamin. Clin Hematol 14:629, 1985
10. Solano FX Jr, Couricell RB: Folate deficiency presenting as pancytopenia in pregnancy. Am J Obstet Gynecol 154:1117, 1986
11. Horn E: Iron and folate supplements during pregnancy: supplementing everyone treats those at risk and is cost effective. Br Med J 297:1325, 1988
12. McGrath K: Treatment of anaemia caused by iron, vitamin B$_{12}$ or folate deficiency. Med J Aust 151:693, 1989
13. Aitchison RG, Marsh JC, Hows JM et al: Pregnancy associated aplastic anemia: a report of 5 cases and review of current management. Br J Haematol 73:541, 1989

14. Pajor A, Kelemen E, Szakacs Z et al: Pregnancy in idiopathic aplastic anemia. Eur J Obstet Gynecol Reprod Biol 42:590, 1991

15. Banavali SD, Parikh PM, Charak BS et al: Corticosteroid-responsive pure red cell aplasia in rheumatoid arthritis and its association with pregnancy. Am J Hematol 31:58, 1989

16. Alter BP, Frissora CL, Halperin DS et al: Fanconi's anaemia and pregnancy. Br J Haematol 77:410, 1991

17. Kuvin SF, Brecker G: Differential neutrophil counts in pregnancy. N Engl J Med 266:877, 1962

18. Caligiuri M, Mayer R: Pregnancy and leukemia. Semin Oncol 16:388, 1989

19. Doll DC, Ringenberg QS, Yarbro JW: Antineoplastic agents and pregnancy. Semin Oncol 16:337, 1989

20. Ward F, Weiss R: Lymphoma and pregnancy. Semin Oncol 16:397, 1989

21. Fitzgerald D, Rowe JM, Heal J: Leukapheresis for control of chronic myelogenous leukemia during pregnancy. Am J Hematol 22:213, 1986

22. Romero R, Duffy TP: Platelet disorders in pregnancy. Clin Perinatol 7:327, 1980

23. Burrows RF, Kelton JG: Incidentally detected thrombocytopenia in healthy mothers and their infants. N Engl J Med 319:142, 1988

24. Copplestone JA: Asymptomatic thrombocytopenia developing during pregnancy (gestational thrombocytopenia)—clinical study. Q J Med 8:593, 1992

25. Peng TC, Kickler TS, Bell WR et al: Obstetric complications in a patient with Bernard-Soulier syndrome. Am J Obstet Gynecol 165:425, 1991

26. McCrae K, Samuels P, Schreiber A: Pregnancy-associated thrombocytopenia. Pathogenesis and management. Blood 80:2697, 1992

27. Kunicki T, Newman P: The molecular immunology of human platelet proteins. Blood 80:1386, 1992

28. Cook RL, Miller RC, Katz VL et al: Immune thrombocytopenic purpura in pregnancy: a reappraisal of management. Obstet Gynecol 78:578, 1991

29. Bussel JB, Hilgartner MW: Intravenous immunoglobulin therapy of idiopathic thrombocytopenic purpura. Hematol Oncol Clin North Am 1:465, 1987

30. Christiaens GG, Helmerhorst FM: Validity of intrapartum diagnosis of fetal thrombocytopenia. Am J Obstet Gynecol 157:864, 1987

31. Moise KJ Jr, Carpenter RJ Jr, Cotton DB et al: Percutaneous umbilical cord blood sampling in the evaluation of fetal platelet counts in pregnant patients with autoimmune thrombocytopenia purpura. Obstet Gynecol 72:346, 1988

32. Samuels P, Bussel JB, Braitman LE et al: Estimation of the risk of thrombocytopenia in the offspring of pregnant women with presumed immune thrombocytopenia. N Engl J Med 323:229, 1990

33. Karpatkin M, Porges RF, Karpatkin S: Platelet counts in infants of women with autoimmune thrombocytopenia: effect of steroid administration to the mother. N Engl J Med 305:936, 1981

34. Christiaeus GC, Nienwenhuis HK, von Dem Borne AE et al: Idiopathic thrombocytopenic purpura in pregnancy: a randomized trial on the effect of antenatal low dose corticosteroids on neonatal platelet count. Br J Obstet Gynecol 97:893, 1990

35. Strother SV, Wagner AM: Prednisone in pregnant women with idiopathic thrombocytopenic purpura, letter. N Engl J Med 319:178, 1988

36. Burrows RF, Hunter DJ, Andrew M et al: A prospective study investigating the mechanism of thrombocytopenia in preeclampsia. Obstet Gynecol 70:334, 1987

37. Redman CW: Platelets and the beginning of preeclampsia. N Engl J Med 323:478, 1990

38. Leduc L, Wheeler JM, Kirshon B et al: Coagulation profile in severe preeclampsia. Obstet Gynecol 79:14, 1992

39. Weiner CP: The mechanism of reduced antithrombin III activity in women with preeclampsia. Obstet Gynecol 72:847, 1988

40. Gaffney PJ, Creighton LJ, Callus M: Monoclonal antibodies to crosslinked fibrin degradation products. II. Evaluation in a variety of clinical conditions. Br J Haematol 68:91, 1988

41. Walsh S: Preeclampsia: an imbalance in placental prostacyclin and thromboxane production. Am J Obstet Gynecol 152:335, 1985

42. Wallenburg HC, Dekker GA, Makovitz JW et al: Low dose aspirin prevents pregnancy-induced hypertension and pre-eclampsia in angiotensin-sensitive primigravida. Lancet 1:1, 1986

43. Sureau C: Prevention of perinatal consequences of pre-eclampsia with low-dose aspirin; results of the epreda trial. Eur J Obstet Gynecol Reprod Biol 41:71, 1991

44. Schiff E, Ben-Baruch G, Peleg E et al: Immunoreactive circulating endothelin-1 in normal and hypertensive pregnancies. Am J Obstet Gynecol 166:624, 1992

45. Riely CA, Latham PS, Romero R, Duffy TP: Acute fatty liver of pregnancy—a reassessment based on observations in nine patients. Ann Intern Med 106:703, 1987

46. Minakami H, Oka N, Sato T et al: Preeclampsia: a microvesicular fat disease of the liver? Am J Obstet Gynecol 159:1043, 1988

47. Schrocksnadel H, Sitte B, Stekel-Berger G et al: Hemolysis in hypertensive disorders of pregnancy. Gynecol Obstet Invest 34:211, 1992

48. Baca L, Gibbons R: The HELLP syndrome: a serious complication of pregnancy with hemolysis, elevated levels of liver enzymes, and low platelet count. Am J Med 85:590, 1988

49. Mimouni F, Miodovinik M: How often does maternal preeclampsia-eclampsia create thrombocytopenia in the fetus?, letter. Obstet Gynecol 70:811, 1987

50. Schwartz M, Brenner W: The obfuscation of eclampsia by thrombotic thrombocytopenia purpura. Am J Obst Gynecol 131:18, 1978

51. Upshaw JD Jr, Reidy TJ, Groshart K: Thrombotic thrombocytopenic purpura in pregnancy: response to plasma manipulations. South Med J 78:677, 1985

52. Natelson EA, White D: Recurrent thrombotic thrombocytopenic purpura in early pregnancy: effect of uterine evacuation. Obstet Gynecol 66:545, 1985

53. Weiner CP: The obstetric patient and disseminated intravascular coagulation. Clin Perinatol 13:705, 1986

54. Romero R, Copel JA, Hobbins JC: Intrauterine fetal demise and hemostatic failure: the fetal death syndrome. Clin Obstet Gynecol 28:24, 1985

55. Pritchard J, Whalley PJ: Abortion complicated by *Clostridium perfringens* infection. Am J Obstet Gynecol 111:484, 1971

56. Lowe TW, Cunningham FG: Placental abruption. Clin Obstet Gynecol 33:406, 1990

57. Sprung J, Cheng EY, Patel S et al: Understanding and management of amniotic fluid embolism. J Clin Anesth 4:235, 1992

58. Brown FD, Davidson EC, Phillips F et al: Coagulation changes after hypertonic saline infusion for late abortions. Obstet Gynecol 39:538, 1972

59. Romero R, Duffy TP, Berkowitz R et al: Prolongation of a preterm pregnancy complicated by death of a single twin in utero and disseminated intravascular coagulation: effects of treatment with heparin. N Engl J Med 310:772, 1984

60. Lecander I, Astedt B: Isolation of a new specific plasminogen activator inhibitor from pregnancy plasma. Br J Haematol 62:221, 1986

61. Rutherford SE, Phelan JP: Thromboembolic disease in pregnancy. Clin Perinatol 13:719, 1986

62. Ginsberg JS, Hirsh J: Anticoagulants during pregnancy. Annu Rev Med 40:79, 1989

63. Ginsberg JS, Hirsh J, Rainbow A, Coates G: Risks to the fetus of radiologic procedures used in the diagnosis of maternal thromboembolic disease. Thromb Haemost 61:189, 1989

64. Letsky E, de Swiet M: Thromboembolism in pregnancy and its management. Br J Haematol 57:543, 1984

65. Hux CH, Wapner RJ, Chayen B et al: Use of the Greenfield filter for thromboembolic disease in pregnancy. Am J Obstet Gynecol 155:734, 1986

66. Ginsberg JS, Hirsh J, Turner D et al: Risks to the fetus of anticoagulant therapy during pregnancy. Thromb Haemost 61:197, 1989

67. McColgin SW, Martin JN Jr, Morrison JC: Pregnant women with prosthetic heart valves. Clin Obstet Gynecol 32:76, 1989

68. Sareli P, England MJ, Berk M et al: Maternal and fetal sequelae of anticoagulation during pregnancy in patients with mechanical heart valve prostheses. Am J Cardiol 63:1462, 1989

69. Calhoun BC, Hesser JW: Heparin-associated antibody with pregnancy: discussion of two cases. Am J Obstet Gynecol 156:964, 1987

70. Lao TT, de Swiet M, Letsky et al: Prophylaxis of thromboembolism in pregnancy: an alternative. Br J Obstet Gynaecol 92:202, 1985

71. Wayne A, Kevy S, Nathan D: Transfusion in sickle cell disease. Blood 81:1109, 1993

72. Koshy M, Burd L, Wallace D et al: Prophylactic red-cell transfusions in pregnant patients with sickle cell disease. A randomized cooperative study. N Engl J Med 319:1447, 1988

73. Mordel N, Birkenfeld A, Goldfarb AN et al: Successful full-term pregnancy in homozygous beta-thalassemia major. Obstet Gynecol 73:837, 1989

74. VanderWeyden MB, Fong H, Hallam, LI et al: Red cell ferritin and iron overload in heterozygous beta-thalassemia. Am J Hematol 30:201, 1989

75. Chediak JR, Alban GM, Maxey B: von Willebrand's disease and pregnancy: management during delivery and outcome of offspring. Am J Obstet Gynecol 155:618, 1986

76. Rick ME, Williams SB, Sacher RA et al: Thrombocytopenia associated with pregnancy in a patient with type II B von Willebrand's disease. Blood 69:786, 1987

77. Giles AR, Hoogendoorn H, Benford K: Type II B von Willebrand's disease presenting as thrombocytopenia during pregnancy. Br J Haematol 67:349, 1987

78. Greer IA, Lowe GD, Walker JJ et al: Hemorrhagic problems in obstetrics and gynecology in patients with congenital coagulopathies. Br J Obstet Gynecol 98:909, 1991

79. Boda Z, Pfliegler G, Muszbek L et al: Congenital factor XIII deficiency with multiple benign breast tumors and successful pregnancy with substitute therapy. Haemostasis 19:348, 1989

80. Feinstein D: Lupus anticoagulant, thrombosis and fetal loss. N Engl J Med 313:1348, 1985

81. Averbuch M, Koifman B, Levo Y: Lupus anticoagulant, thrombosis and thrombocytopenia in systemic lupus erythematosus. Am J Med Sci 293:2, 1987

82. Carion R, Tobelem G, Soria C et al: Inhibitor of protein C activation by endothelial cells in the presence of lupus anticoagulant, letter. N Engl J Med 314: 1193, 1986

83. Lockslin MD, Druzin MC, Goei S et al: Antibody to cardiolipin as a predictor of fetal distress or death in pregnant patients with systemic lupus erythematosus. N Engl J Med 313:152, 1985

84. Petri M, Rheinschmidt M, Whiting-OKeefe P et al: The frequency of lupus anticoagulant in systemic lupus erythematosus. A study of sixty consecutive patients by activated partial thromboplastin time, Russell viper venom time, and anticardiolipin antibody level. Ann Intern Med 106:524, 1987

85. Thiagarajan P, Pengo V, Shapiro SS: The use of the dilute Russell viper venom time for the diagnosis of lupus anticoagulants. Blood 68:869, 1986

86. Branca DW, Scott JR, Kochenour NK et al: Obstetric complications associated with the lupus anticoagulant. N Engl J Med 313:1322, 1985

87. Trudinger BJ, Stewart G, Cook C et al: Monitoring lupus anticoagulant positive pregnancies with umbilical artery flow velocity waveforms. Obstet Gynecol 72:215, 1988

88. Jones EC, Mosesson MW, Thomason JL, Jackson TC: Essential thrombocythemia in pregnancy. Obstet Gynecol 71:501, 1988

89. Mercer B, Drouin J, Jolly E, D'Anjou G: Primary thrombocythemia in pregnancy: a report of two cases. Am J Obstet Gynecol 159:127, 1988

90. Ferguson JE II, Ueland K, Aronson W: Polycythemia rubra vera and pregnancy. Obstet Gynecol 62:16S, 1983

91. Baer MR, Ozer H, Foon KA: Interferon-alpha therapy during pregnancy in chronic myelogenous leukemia and hairy cell leukemia. Br J Haematol 81: 167, 1992

92. Morrison AE, Walker IO, Black WP: Protein C deficiency presenting as deep venous thrombosis in pregnancy. Case report. Br J Obstet Gynaecol 95:1077, 1988

93. Vogel J, de Moerloose PA, Bounameaux H: Protein C deficiency and pregnancy: a case report. Obstet Gynecol 73:455, 1989

94. De Stefano V, Leone G, De Carolis S et al: Management of pregnancy in women with anti-thrombin III congenital defect: report of four cases. Thromb Haemost 59:193, 1988

95. Winter JH, Fenech A, Ridler W et al: Familial antithrombin III deficiency. Q J Med 204:373, 1982

96. Solal-Celigney P, Tertian G, Fernandez H et al: Pregnancy and paroxysmal nocturnal hemoglobinuria. Arch Intern Med 148:593, 1988

Hematologic Problems in the Surgical Patient: Bleeding and Thrombosis

150

Charles W. Francis

INTRODUCTION

Surgery represents a dual challenge to the hemostatic system. First, bleeding must be rapidly stopped at the operative site, and also unwanted thrombosis must be prevented. Hemostatic failure can result in a variety of bleeding complications that are well known to the surgeon. They may be mild, with an increased transfusion requirement or excessive oozing at the operative site, or more severe, resulting in blood loss with shock in the postoperative period, internal hematomas that compromise organ function, or occasionally death from uncontrolled hemorrhage. On the other hand, thrombotic complications occur frequently in the postoperative period. They are related to hemostatic changes resulting from surgery, including local damage to vessels, venous stasis, and alterations in the fibrinolytic and coagulation systems. The prevention and treatment of thrombosis in surgical patients requires difficult choices and administration of drugs that interfere with hemostasis in the perioperative period when the risk of bleeding is high. Surgeons are well aware of the hemostatic requirements of operative procedures and manage routine cases and many cases with hemostatic problems without assistance. However, consultation is often requested for complex or difficult problems, including preoperative evaluation of hemostasis in patients with known hemostatic defects, treatment of unexpected intra- or postoperative bleeding, prophylaxis of deep vein thrombosis (DVT) in high-risk patients, and treatment of thrombosis in the postoperative period.

PREOPERATIVE EVALUATION OF HEMOSTATIC RISK

Preoperative evaluation of hemostasis occurs at two levels. First is the routine evaluation needed in all patients before surgery to identify those with potential abnormalities of hemostasis. An adequate history is the most effective screening modality for adults and may be based on a questionnaire[1] (see Ch. 103), while the need for routine laboratory testing is controversial. Recommendations that it is not useful[2] point to retrospective studies[3-5] indicating that it rarely detects unexpected bleeding disorders and often requires further workup to evaluate false-positive abnormalities. This has also been emphasized in a recent review indicating that the bleeding time used as a screening test is not predictive of abnormal surgical bleeding.[6] Screening programs that recommend laboratory testing point to the asymptomatic nature of some hemostatic abnormalities that may cause surgical bleeding and the occasional failure to obtain a detailed history.[1,7,8] A prospective study of preoperative screening in children before tonsillectomy found both history and laboratory screening to have high specificity but a low positive predictive value for perioperative bleeding.[8] Given

Table 150-1. Risk of Bleeding with Surgical Procedures

Risk	Type of Surgery	Examples
Low	Nonvital organs involved, exposed surgical site, limited dissection	Lymph node biopsy, dental extraction
Moderate	Vital organs involved, deep or extensive dissection	Laparotomy, thoracotomy, mastectomy
High	Bleeding likely to compromise surgical result, bleeding complications frequent	Neurosurgery, ophthalmic surgery, plastic surgery, cardiopulmonary bypass, prostatic surgery, surgery to stop bleeding

the variety of potential hemostatic defects, no simple screening system will identify all patients at increased of bleeding. The level of hemostatic risk for the proposed surgery (Table 150-1) forms the basis for an approach to preoperative evaluation (Table 150-2). A hemostatic history should be obtained in all patients, and in patients with negative histories having low-risk surgery, no laboratory tests are required. For moderate- to high-risk surgery additional screening would include an activated partial thromboplastin time (PTT) and an assessment of platelet count either by examination of a peripheral blood smear or by automated counting.

In practice, a hematologist is rarely consulted for routine screening since surgeons have adopted approaches based on their training and local practice patterns. Rather, consultation is sought because of a history suggesting a bleeding disorder or an abnormal test that is found on initial screening. The approach of the consultant cannot be one of "screening" since the judgment of the referring physician that a bleeding disorder may be present indicates a greatly increased probability of finding an abnormality. If a referral is obtained as a result of an abnormal screening test result, this finding must be pursued and the abnormality fully explained. However, for all referrals the history is of central importance and must include a thorough review of any bleeding episodes, including hospital records and results of prior hemostatic testing, as well as careful attention to the family history. The physical examination should focus on evidence of bleeding and on identifying systemic disorders such as hepatic or renal disease. If the history of bleeding is negative or minimal, appropriate laboratory testing would include a prothrombin time (PT) and PTT and a biochemical profile to evaluate hepatic and renal function. A CBC and examination of the peripheral blood smear are useful to identify a myeloproliferative disorder or thrombocytopenia. If the history is suggestive of a hemostatic abnormality, a full evaluation is indicated and specific testing beyond the screening procedures is usually required, since von Willebrand dis-

Table 150-2. Preoperative Hemostatic Evaluation

Routine Screening	
Surgical Risk	Approach
Low	History only
Moderate or high	History, PTT, platelet count
Consultation	
History	Approach
Negative or minimal for bleeding	PT, PTT, platelet count, biochemical profile, CBC and differential, review of peripheral blood smear
Suggestive of bleeding disorder	Add to above as indicated, consider bleeding time, ristocetin cofactor, von Willebrand antigen, factor VIII, factor IX, factor XI, factor XIII assays

ease, mild factor VIII, factor IX, and factor XI deficiencies, factor XIII deficiency, platelet function defects, and abnormalities of the fibrinolytic system are not identified by routine screening tests.

MANAGEMENT OF PATIENTS WITH HEMOSTATIC ABNORMALITIES

Patients with known hemostatic abnormalities are often referred in anticipation of surgery for assessment of bleeding risk and recommendations regarding perioperative management. Generally, surgery in the presence of a hemostatic defect is associated with increased operative risk, and this should be adequately discussed with both patient and surgeon. Even when the diagnosis is clearly established and adequate replacement therapy is available, the operative risk is increased by the possibility of bleeding. Several general considerations affect evaluation of risk and planning management. First, the risk of bleeding with the specific contemplated surgery must be evaluated (Table 150-1). The support of hemostasis for an extensive procedure such as pneumonectomy will be much more difficult than that for a lymph node biopsy. Second, both the need for surgery and its urgency must be carefully considered. Greater risks are more warranted for correction of a life-threatening condition such as bowel perforation than for elective cosmetic surgery. Finally, the nature and severity of the hemostatic abnormality and the ability to correct it during the operative period are of fundamental importance. Consideration must also be given to the duration of replacement that will be required with appreciation of potential bleeding associated with events in the postoperative period such as removal of sutures and deep drains and the need for physical therapy, especially after orthopaedic surgery.

The following sections discuss perioperative management of some of the more common acquired coagulation abnormalities; therapy for congenital factor deficiencies and von Willebrand disease is discussed elsewhere in this text.

Thrombocytopenia

Thrombocytopenia is one of the most common acquired hemostatic abnormalities in hospitalized patients, and the availability of platelet transfusion has made consideration of both emergency and elective surgery reasonable even in severely thrombocytopenic patients. The bleeding time is one measure of primary hemostasis and is used by many clinicians as a guide to assessing the bleeding risk associated with thrombocytopenia. The relationship between bleeding time and the severity of thrombocytopenia is clear, with prolongation beyond normal with a count of $<100,000/mm^3$ and very long bleeding times with platelet counts of $<20,000/mm^3$.[9,10] Spontaneous bleeding occurs with increased frequency at platelet counts of $<20,000/mm^3$ and is common at platelet counts of $<5,000/mm^3$.[10,11] Differences in platelet function must also be considered in evaluating the risk of thrombocytopenic bleeding since large platelets that may be seen in idiopathic thrombocytopenic purpura (ITP) are more effective than normal, whereas dysfunctional platelets seen in myeloproliferative disease and uremia, and after administration of drugs that affect platelet function, will be less effective. Other critical considerations include clinical conditions that reduce platelet recovery or life span after transfusion, including splenomegaly, fever, infection, active bleeding, and the presence of auto- or alloantibodies.

In preparation for elective surgery, therapy for the disorder causing the thrombocytopenia is the most satisfactory approach. For example, steroid or intravenous γ-globulin therapy for ITP may increase the platelet count so that transfusion is ot needed, and surgery in patients with leukemia should be scheduled, if possible, after achievement of hematologic remission. The platelet count required for safe performance of surgery is controversial. A recent National Institutes of Health Consensus Development Conference recommended transfusion at a platelet count of <50,000/mm³ [12]; others suggest transfusion at platelet counts of <80,000/mm³ for general surgery and <100,000/mm³ for cardiopulmonary bypass.[13] A reasonable approach involves considering the bleeding risks associated with surgical intervention (Table 150-1) in deciding both the necessary platelet count to be achieved and the duration of required platelet support after surgery. For low-risk surgery, a single transfusion to increase the platelet count >50,000/mm³ followed by close observation may suffice. Transfusion to keep the platelet count >75,000/mm³ for moderate-risk surgery and >100,000/mm³ for high-risk surgery is appropriate. The duration of platelet support required has not been carefully studied, but for moderate- or high-risk surgery platelets may be needed for ≤1 week, and the platelet count should be monitored closely, with the expectation that platelet survival will be shortened by infection, fever, or bleeding. A special case is splenectomy for patients with ITP when the primary site of platelet destruction is being removed. Platelet transfusion in anticipation of splenectomy is not effective because of the short platelet survival, but transfusion after the splenic artery has been clamped may prove effective.

Liver Disease

The hemostatic abnormality of liver disease is complex and is due to a number of factors, including decreased synthesis of enzymes and inhibitors of the coagulation and fibrinolytic systems, synthesis of abnormal fibrinogen, decreased clearance of activated factors, abnormal platelet function, and thrombocytopenia[14,15] (see Ch. 147). The severity of the hemostatic abnormality parallels the overall severity of the liver disease, which also represents the greatest determinant of surgical risk. Patients with severe decompensated liver disease and markedly abnormal coagulation tests are at great risk of bleeding, and surgery should be avoided except as a lifesaving measure. In evaluating hemostasis in patients with less severe disease, the PT provides a good measure of decreased synthesis of coagulation factors. In addition, platelet count and bleeding time are needed to identify thrombocytopenia or abnormal platelet function; a fibrinogen assay, a test for fibrinogen/fibrin degradation products (FDP), and the euglobulin clot lysis time are useful in evaluating disseminated intravascular coagulation (DIC) or accelerated fibrinolysis.

In patients with mild disease and a PT prolongation of <3 seconds, serious surgical bleeding is unlikely in the absence of other hemostatic abnormalities, and prophylactic intervention is not necessary for low- or moderate-risk surgery. For high-risk surgery or greater degrees of hemostatic abnormality, transfusion of fresh frozen plasma is the most useful approach for correcting the coagulation abnormality. The volume of plasma needed is guided by the correction of the PT, and the success of this approach is limited by the volume required in patients with low levels of coagulation factors. Plasma exchange may be of value in extreme circumstances. Administration of platelets should be considered for thrombocytopenia, although recovery will be decreased in the presence of splenomegaly. Administration of desmopressin acetate (DDAVP) is useful in correcting abnormal platelet function in some cases.[16] Prothrombin complex concentrates provide vitamin K-dependent factors in a smaller volume than plasma and have been used successfully before liver biopsy or surgery[17,18] but cannot be generally recommended because of the occasional occurrence of severe thrombotic complications[19,20] due to the pres-

ence of activated factors in available preparations. Vitamin K deficiency is a correctable abnormality in patients with associated bile duct obstruction or those taking broad-spectrum antibiotics, and parenteral administration of vitamin K (10 mg) will usually shorten the PT if vitamin K deficiency is a contributory factor (see Ch. 114). Insertion of peritoneovenous shunts is frequently associated with development of a consumption coagulopathy[21,22] due to entry into the circulation of procoagulants from ascitic fluid. Treatment with antithrombin III (AT III) replacement has not been successful,[23] but administration of heparin has led to decreased consumption of fibrinogen and platelets in this condition.[24]

Platelet Dysfunction

Patients with platelet dysfunction represent a large group in whom preoperative consultation is sought, usually because of finding a prolonged bleeding time with a normal platelet count (see Ch. 130). The etiology may be obvious in cases of renal or liver disease or myeloproliferative syndromes, but may also require evaluation for storage pool disease or platelet activation defects. The most frequent cause of platelet dysfunction is administration of drugs such as aspirin. A careful drug history is therefore essential.

Drugs that interfere with platelet function should be discontinued before surgery and avoided in the perioperative period if possible. Treatment of the underlying disease is the most effective approach in many acquired disorders of platelet function such as renal disease (see the section Renal Disease) or myeloproliferative syndromes. Platelet transfusion is an effective treatment for intrinsic platelet dysfunction, but the dose required to achieve hemostasis is difficult to predict and depends in part on the severity of the underlying platelet abnormality. Recently, DDAVP has been shown to shorten the bleeding time effectively in some patients with platelet dysfunction due to either congenital or acquired abnormalities.[16,25–29] As described in more detail in Chapter 130, the bleeding time has not been shown to be useful as a predictor of bleeding in qualitative platelet disorders. However, it can be used to assess the efficacy of therapeutic modalities such as DDAVP.

Renal Disease

Patients with renal disease may experience platelet dysfunction accompanied by increased bleeding times and abnormal in vitro platelet function studies.[30–32] The approach to therapy is given in Chapter 130.

Antiplatelet, Anticoagulant, and Fibrinolytic Therapy

The most frequent hemostatic abnormalities encountered in patients before surgery occur in those receiving antiplatelet, anticoagulant, or fibrinolytic drugs. Patients taking aspirin as antiplatelet therapy or for its anti-inflammatory or analgesic effects represent the largest such group. Some studies have shown a mild increase in surgical bleeding in patients taking aspirin,[33–35] although this has not been confirmed in other studies.[36,37] For elective surgery it is prudent to discontinue aspirin approximately 1 week before the operation, although in the absence of other hemostatic abnormalities, recent or current aspirin use should not represent a contraindication to surgery and requires no prophylactic therapy. The effect of aspirin may, however, seriously potentiate the bleeding tendency in the presence of other hemostatic abnormalities such as thrombocytopenia, uremia, or congenital factor deficien-

Table 150-3. Surgery on Patients Taking Anticoagulants

	Bleeding Risk	Elective Surgery	Emergency Surgery
Warfarin	Low	Adjust dose to INR <2.5	Discontinue warfarin
	Moderate	Adjust dose to INR <2.5	Discontinue warfarin; FFP to reduce INR to <2.5
	High	Discontinue and allow PT to normalize Substitute heparin if needed and hold heparin in perioperative period	Discontinue warfarin; FFP-vitamin K to normalize PT
Heparin	Low or moderate	Discontinue high dose and give low-dose SQ heparin	Discontinue high-dose and give low-dose SQ heparin
	High	Discontinue 6–12 hr before surgery[a]	Discontinue; give protamine sulfate if needed

[a] 12–24 hr for LMWH.

cies, and in such patients may contribute significantly to postoperative bleeding.

Subcutaneous heparin in low doses such as 5,000 U bid is recommended as prophylaxis for postoperative venous thromboembolic disease in some patient groups (see the section Prophylaxis of Deep Vein Thrombosis and Chs. 121 and 123). Its use results in minimal prolongation of the PTT[38] with a slight increased frequency of wound hematomas.[39,40] Higher doses of heparin given as treatment for thrombosis cause increased surgical bleeding, but the management of such patients is not difficult because the half-life of heparin is <2 hours[41,42] (Table 150-3). Consequently, the heparin can be withheld 6–12 hours before anticipated surgery, and the PTT should return to control levels. If more rapid neutralization is required for emergency surgery, heparin can be neutralized by protamine sulfate in a dose of 1 mg IV for every 100 U of heparin expected to be in the circulation. In patients requiring therapy for thrombosis, heparin should be interrupted for the minimum time consistent with obtaining good surgical hemostasis. In these patients, low-dose subcutaneous heparin can be administered in the immediate preoperative period and continued until therapeutic heparin in higher doses can be restarted between the third and seventh postoperative days, depending on the type of surgery and the clinical course. Low molecular weight heparin (LMWH) has greater bioavailability after subcutaneous administration and a longer half-life.[43] Consequently, it should be discontinued 12–24 hours before surgery.

Perioperative management of patients taking warfarin is more difficult because of the longer duration of its anticoagulant effect (Table 150-3) (see Ch. 120). The risk of thrombosis or embolism during interruption of anticoagulant therapy must be balanced against the benefit of surgery, and this may be difficult in patients with recent venous thromboembolic disease, intracardiac thrombosis, or prosthetic heart valves. For elective surgery with low-to-moderate bleeding risk (Table 150-1), a reasonable approach is to reduce the dose preoperatively to achieve an International Normalized Ratio (INR) of <2.5,[44–46] at which level surgery can be safely performed. For high-risk patients, this degree of anticoagulation is unacceptable; warfarin should be withheld long enough before surgery to allow the PT to correct, and the patient should be switched to heparin, given either subcutaneously or intravenously, if continued antithrombotic therapy is needed. Heparin can then be withheld 6–12 hours before surgery, allowing the PTT to return to

normal, and anticoagulation reinstituted postoperatively with heparin. Finally, the patient should be switched back to oral anticoagulants for long-term care. For emergency surgery in patients at moderate or high risk of bleeding, rapid reversal of the anticoagulant effect is required, and this can be achieved with vitamin K or fresh frozen plasma, or both. Fresh frozen plasma contains all vitamin K-dependent coagulation factors reliably and rapidly corrects the PT, and is the preferred approach in patients needing immediate correction. Its value is limited by the volume that must be administered, although 2 U of fresh frozen plasma usually corrects a therapeutic PT to within a level safe for surgery. Another limitation is that the half-life of factor VII is short, only about 7 hours, so that the PT should be monitored and additional fresh frozen plasma administered as needed. Parenteral administration of vitamin K (10–20 mg) also reverses the effect of warfarin with a delay of 6–12 hours, although its use is complicated by the relative resistance to warfarin effect after its administration, so that reinstituting oral anticoagulation can be difficult. Administration of vitamin K in a low dose (0.5–1.0 mg IV) is also effective in reversing the anticoagulant effect and does not result in warfarin resistance.[47] Administration of both fresh frozen plasma and vitamin K is prudent in patients needing emergency surgery with high risk of bleeding. If the volume of plasma needed to correct the PT is too large, then prothrombin complex concentrates can be substituted.

Fibrinolytic therapy results in pronounced hemostatic abnormalities including decreases in plasma plasminogen, α_2-plasmin inhibitor, fibrinogen, factor VIII, and factor V, and increases in FDP and abnormalities in platelet function.[48,49] In combination with the capacity of fibrinolytic therapy to lyse needed hemostatic plugs, these abnormalities contribute to the bleeding complications seen with fibrinolytic therapy and make surgery hazardous.[50] Elective surgery should be postponed after fibrinolytic therapy until the hemostatic abnormalities are corrected. However, the need for emergency surgery is not uncommon, particularly with the increased use of fibrinolytic therapy for acute myocardial infarction and the occasional need for revascularization procedures soon after its administration. There are several reports[51–55] of successful coronary artery bypass graft surgery immediately after fibrinolytic therapy, although bleeding was excessive and increased transfusion requirements were observed.

The two issues that must be considered in a patient receiving fibrinolytic therapy who requires emergency surgery are the presence of plasminogen activator in the circulation and its effects on the hemostatic system. The effect of circulating plasminogen activator can be inhibited by administration of ε-aminocaproic acid (EACA), usually given in a loading dose of 6 g, administered either orally or intravenously, followed by a dose of 1 g/hr. This will have the unwanted effect of inhibiting physiologic fibrinolysis and potentially increasing the chance of developing a thrombosis, a potentially serious problem in a patient with recent myocardial infarction. However, the half-life of fibrinolytic agents is short, varying from 6 minutes for tissue plasminogen activator (t-PA)[56] to 23 minutes for streptokinase and 16 minutes for urokinase,[48] although in the case of t-PA, a low level of fibrinolytic activity can be identified for longer periods.[57] Because of the short half-life of fibrinolytic agents, administration of EACA should be required only if surgery is needed within 1–2 hours after discontinuing the fibrinolytic agent.

When surgery is delayed for longer periods, one must correct the hypocoagulable state resulting from fibrinolytic degradation of coagulation proteins. Cryoprecipitate, which is rich in fibrinogen, von Willebrand factor, and factor VIII, is the first approach to replacement in this situation. Ten bags can be given initially, along with 2 U of fresh frozen plasma to help replete factor V. Monitoring improvement of coagulation abnormalities can be difficult in the emergency setting, although the thrombin time is a useful guide to fibrinogen replacement. If operative bleeding occurs despite administration of cryoprecipitate and fresh frozen plasma, EACA should be given, and platelet transfusion considered to correct potential platelet dysfunction.[58,59]

INTRAOPERATIVE AND POSTOPERATIVE BLEEDING

Excessive bleeding during or after surgery represents a significant and potentially life-threatening complication that requires immediate evaluation and a rapid approach to diagnosis and institution of treatment. The first consideration is to determine whether the bleeding is related to a hemostatic defect or to a local lesion that requires surgery (Table 150-4). Failure to ligate bleeding vessels at the operative site is the most frequent cause of postoperative bleeding and results in excessive blood loss limited to the site of surgery that may be very rapid if a larger vessel is involved. Very rapid bleeding confined only to the operative site is usually due to a surgical problem. Evidence of bleeding at sites outside the operative field favors a contribution from hemostatic failure, and the patient should be examined for signs of petechiae or purpura, or oozing from venipuncture sites or indwelling catheters; the urine, stool, and nasogastric aspirate should be examined for blood if available. Laboratory tests are an essential part of the evaluation, and screening tests are nearly always ordered before consultation is requested. In addition to the PT, PTT, and platelet count, it may be useful to obtain a bleeding time to evaluate platelet function if the platelet count is normal. A fibrinogen level, a test for FDP, and euglobulin lysis time are needed to search for evidence of DIC or fibrinolysis, and a thrombin clotting time and reptilase time can identify a heparin effect (see Ch. 104). The peripheral blood smear should be reviewed to examine platelet size and number and to identify possible red cell fragmentation that may occur in DIC. When evaluating hemostatic tests, one must consider changes that normally occur in response to surgery, including a decrease in AT III concentration immediately postoperatively,[60,61] the dilutional thrombocytopenia that occurs after transfusion of more than one blood volume of banked blood,[62,63] and the increase in platelet count, fibrinogen, FDP, von Willebrand factor, and factor VIII that occurs in the first postoperative week.[64,65]

If hemostatic failure is thought to contribute to bleeding, the potential causes should be quickly considered (Table 150-4). A pre-existing hemostatic abnormality may have been undetected before surgery, and the family history and patient's past medical history should be reviewed. Results of preoperative coagulation tests should be checked and interpreted, realizing

Table 150-4. Approach to Intra- or Postoperative Bleeding

1. Decide whether the bleeding is due to a local cause or to hemostatic failure
   Local: single site of bleeding, rapid rate, minimal or no abnormalities of coagulation tests
   Hemostatic failure: multiple sites of bleeding, unusual bleeding pattern, abnormal coagulation tests

2. Causes of perioperative hemostatic failure
   Pre-existing hemostatic abnormality, DIC, primary fibrinolysis; also consider contribution of dilutional thrombocytopenia and drug effects
   Special cases: cardiopulmonary bypass, platelet dysfunction, prostatic surgery, local fibrinolysis

3. Diagnosis of hemostatic failure
   Review preoperative coagulation tests and operative record; interview family members; obtain PT, PTT, thrombin clotting time, platelet count, peripheral blood smear; consider reptilase time, fibrinogen, FDP, euglobulin lysis time, bleeding time

that mild deficiencies of factor VIII, factor IX, factor XI, and factor XIII may be present without prolongation of the PTT and that platelet functional abnormalities will not be identified without a bleeding time. Fibrinolytic abnormalities, including deficiency of α_2-plasmin inhibitor[66,67] and of plasminogen activator inhibitor-1,[68,69] can cause postoperative bleeding and are not identified by screening coagulation tests. Consumption coagulopathy, possibly due to a mismatched blood transfusion, a period of profound hypotension, fat embolism, or amniotic fluid embolization may be a cause of the hemostatic defect.

Massive transfusion is often discussed as a cause of intraoperative coagulopathy but rarely causes bleeding by itself. Transfusion of more than 1 vol of banked blood predictably decreases the platelet count, but the microvascular bleeding occasionally seen in patients receiving massive transfusion cannot be directly related to the thrombocytopenia.[62,63] Therefore, routine platelet transfusion in the absence of unusual bleeding has not been recommended even during massive transfusion.[62,63] However, in the presence of other hemostatic abnormalities such as drugs affecting platelet function, the dilutional thrombocytopenia may be a significant contributing factor to the development of bleeding, particularly if suggestive of a hemostatic defect. In the presence of excessive operative bleeding, aggressive platelet transfusion to a platelet count $<100,000/mm^3$ is indicated. Excessive urinary bleeding after prostatectomy can be caused by local fibrinolysis related to high concentrations of urokinase; therapy with EACA is often beneficial,[70,71] but care must be taken to avoid treatment of patients with upper urinary tract bleeding, in whom fibrinolytic inhibition can result in ureteral obstruction.

Patients with excessive bleeding after cardiopulmonary bypass require special consideration[72] (see Ch. 130). The platelet count, hematocrit, and levels of coagulation and fibrinolytic factors are reduced to approximately 50% of baseline after starting bypass as a result of hemodilution.[73,74] These levels are maintained throughout the bypass, with the exception of factor V, which shows further reduction to $<20\%$. The large doses of heparin given during bypass to prevent clotting are neutralized by protamine sulfate at termination. The bypass procedure results in significant platelet dysfunction reflected by release of the α-granule constituents, platelet factor IV, and β-thromboglobulin, abnormal in vitro aggregation tests, and a prolonged bleeding time that usually corrects within 1 hour postoperatively.[73,75] Several hemostatic abnormalities may contribute to postoperative bleeding after cardiopulmonary bypass. Inadequate neutralization of heparin by protamine sulfate may result in prolonged PTT and thrombin time with a normal reptilase time and can be corrected by administration of additional protamine sulfate. The most significant contributor to post-bypass hemostatic failure is persistently abnormal platelet function that can be detected by an excessively prolonged bleeding time with a normal platelet count. This platelet abnormality can be treated with platelet transfusions.[73] The appearance of the heparin effect several hours after adequate protamine sulfate neutralization, termed "heparin rebound," has been suggested as a cause of post-bypass bleeding[76] but is rare. Excessive fibrinolysis and DIC have also been reported[77] but are uncommon and should be well documented prior to instituting therapy with heparin or EACA.

DDAVP has been administered to patients undergoing surgery with cardiopulmonary bypass because of the frequent development of abnormal platelet function and the ability of DDAVP to improve hemostasis in a variety of conditions with abnormal platelet function. Salzman and colleagues[78] conducted a double-blind prospective randomized trial in 70 patients undergoing cardiopulmonary bypass. Patients receiving DDAVP at the conclusion of bypass had reduced operative and early postoperative blood loss compared with those receiving placebo. Reduced blood loss was related to an increase in plasma von Willebrand factor concentration.[79] In another study, patients with a prolonged bleeding time and excessive bleeding after bypass received standard treatment with or without administration of DDAVP, and those who received DDAVP had a lower transfusion requirement.[80] However, another trial reported no decrease in blood transfusion or blood loss after cardiopulmonary bypass in patients receiving DDAVP.[81–83] Preoperative administration of DDAVP decreased the bleeding time and reduced blood loss in a prospective randomized trial in patients having surgery for scoliosis.[84] These studies suggest that routine use of DDAVP in "high-risk" surgery associated with excessive blood loss or evidence of platelet dysfunction, or both, can result in significant reduction in transfusion requirements. Further studies are required to determine whether this treatment also decreases the incidence of clinically significant bleeding complications.

PROPHYLAXIS OF DEEP VEIN THROMBOSIS

The clinical consequences of postoperative venous thromboembolic disease include DVT with sequelae of venous valvular damage and postphlebitic syndrome as well as pulmonary embolism, which may be fatal (see Ch. 123). Accurate epidemiologic information regarding postoperative venous thrombosis has relied on the development of sensitive detection methods because venous thrombosis is frequently asymptomatic. The most widely used diagnostic technique has been the radioactive fibrinogen uptake test (RFUT), which depends on the ability of a forming clot to incorporate radiolabeled fibrinogen that can then be detected by external counting. As defined by RFUT, the risk of developing venous thrombosis varies in different surgical groups, but in patients >40 years of age undergoing general abdominal or thoracic surgery, the incidence is approximately 20–30%.[40,85] Thrombi begin forming during or soon after surgery, initially in the calf veins.[86] Most clots are asymptomatic, and many spontaneously regress, although in the absence of treatment, 20% extend into veins proximal to the knee,[87] where most pulmonary emboli originate.[88] In patients at moderate risk (Table 150-5) the incidence of proximal vein thrombosis is between 2% and 10% and fatal pulmonary embolism between 0.1% and 0.7%.[85]

Strategies for management are based on the frequency of thromboembolic disease in different surgical groups, expected clinical outcomes, and cost effectiveness. The simplest approach relies on treatment of clinically diagnosed disease but is unacceptable in moderate- or high-risk groups because postoperative DVT is frequently asymptomatic, and the initial presentation of pulmonary embolism may be sudden death. A second potential strategy is monitoring with noninvasive tests such as RFUT or plethysmography. This approach would be both expensive and cumbersome and also raises difficult problems in management of false-positive results. The most effective approach is primary prophylaxis in moderate- or high-risk patients using anticoagulants or methods to reduce venous stasis.

Anesthesia, operative pain, bed rest, and lack of leg muscle activity reduce venous blood flow, which predisposes the patient to the development of thrombosis. Simple measures to counteract venous stasis that are applicable to nearly all patients include leg and foot exercises while in bed and early ambulation. The use of elastic stockings is of little documented benefit, but graduated compression stockings that exert greater pressure at the ankles and less pressure proximally may be of some value in low- or moderate-risk patients.[89,90] External pneumatic compression employs active leg compression with inflatable boots that rhythmically compress calf or both calf and thigh sequentially. Such compression increases venous blood flow[91,92] and also raises blood fibrinolytic activity[93]; both effects may contribute to its efficacy. The absence of side effects makes it an attractive prophylactic modality, particularly in patients at increased bleeding risk. External pneumatic compression has been shown to be effective in patients after general abdominal surgery,[91,94,95] urologic,[96] neurologic,[97,98] and gynecologic surgery (including that for malignancy[99]), and knee replacement.[100]

The greatest experience with anticoagulant prophylaxis of postoperative venous thromboembolic disease has been with low doses of heparin, based on the rationale that lower concentrations are needed to prevent than to treat venous thrombosis. Heparin administered in a dose of 5,000 U subcutaneously results in a peak plasma level of 0.05–0.15 U/ml approximately 2 hours after injection[101,102] with a slight but detectable increase in the PTT.[38] Administration of this dose every 8–12 hours beginning 2 hours before surgery results in a risk reduction of 67% as determined by meta-analysis of >70 controlled studies.[40] A single large trial[39] demonstrated a significant reduction in both total pulmonary embolism and fatal pulmonary embolism in patients >40 years of age undergoing major surgery who received low-dose heparin prophylaxis compared with control patients. Although this study has been criticized,[103,104] an analysis of the published experience suggests a 47% reduction in risk from postoperative pulmonary embolism with the use of low-dose heparin.[40] Side effects of this regimen include bruising at injection sites that can be minimized by proper technique and a 2% increase in wound hematomas.[39,40] The generally accepted effectiveness and safety have led to recommendations[105] that low-dose heparin be used in most moderate-risk surgical patients. However, surveys indicate that only a few surgeons use low-dose heparin prophylaxis because of the perceived infrequency of clinically significant thromboembolic complications and fear of bleeding.[106–109]

There have been several approaches to improve the effectiveness of low-dose heparin, including the addition of ergot, a venoconstricting agent, to decrease venous capacitance.[110,111] This has not met with wide acceptance because of the occasional occurrence of vasospastic side effects and the limited evidence of the superiority of the combination compared with low-dose heparin alone. Some studies have suggested that adjusting the heparin dosage based on PTT may increase its effectiveness and extend the usefulness of heparin prophylaxis to high-risk patients.[112,113] Postoperatively, the plasma concentration of AT III declines, and this observation led to consideration that heparin prophylaxis could be improved by supplementation with AT III. This was tested in two prospective, randomized trials following total hip[114] and knee[115] replacement, demon-

Table 150-5. Prophylaxis for Deep Vein Thrombosis in Surgical Patients

Risk	Patients	Recommendation
Low	Age <40, surgery <30 min, no additional risk factors	Early ambulation, leg exercises
Moderate	Age >40, abdominal or thoracic surgery >30 min	Heparin 5,000 U SQ q12h beginning 2 hr preoperatively
	Neurosurgery	External pneumatic compression
High	Hip fracture	LMWH, warfarin[a]
	Hip replacement	LMWH, warfarin,[a] adjusted-dose heparin
	Knee replacement	LMWH, warfarin,[a] external pneumatic compression
	Open prostatectomy	External pneumatic compression
	Gynecologic malignancy	External pneumatic compression

[a] Given in low-dose regimen.

strating that the combination of AT III and heparin was safe and more effective than a standard regimen of dextran. Also, the risk of developing DVT was related to the postoperative decline in AT III.

Heparin preparations with a restricted low molecular-weight range (LMWH) have relatively greater activity in promoting the inactivation of factor Xa by AT III than in promoting inactivation of thrombin.[116] They were developed as therapeutic agents based on this property and on the results of animal studies[117,118] suggesting that they could have greater antithrombotic effectiveness with a reduced risk of bleeding complications. Several LMWH preparations have demonstrated effectiveness in preventing venous thrombosis after general surgery.[43] In comparison with standard heparin, LMWH has greater bioavailability, particularly after subcutaneous injection. This property, in addition to a longer plasma half-life, allows for once daily injection, rather than two or three times daily for unfractionated heparin. Data are conflicting regarding the relative effectiveness of LMWH in comparison with unfractionated heparin in prevention of venous thrombosis. A meta-analysis of a large number of clinical trials suggests that LMWH may be slightly more effective after general surgery.[119]

The protection afforded by low-dose heparin is insufficient in some surgical patients with a particularly high risk of developing venous thrombosis, including those undergoing open prostatectomy and surgery for gynecologic malignancies and especially following certain orthopaedic procedures. For example, after hip fracture, total hip replacement, or total knee replacement, the risk of venous thrombosis without prophylaxis is 40–70%, with the frequent development of proximal leg vein clots and an incidence of pulmonary embolism of 5–10% and fatal pulmonary embolism of 1–5%.[12,120] Several alternative prophylactic modalities have been tested in these high-risk patients. Dextran has been shown to be effective after total hip replacement or fracture[121,122] but is not widely used because of the need for intravenous administration and the precipitation of congestive heart failure, especially in older individuals, who frequently require such procedures. External pneumatic compression has been shown to be effective in a limited number of studies after total knee replacement,[100] prostatectomy,[96] and gynecologic surgery for malignancy.[99] It is more effective than no prophylaxis after total hip replacement[123,124] but is less effective than warfarin in preventing proximal vein thrombosis.[125] Although the usual low-dose heparin regimen has not been sufficiently effective in high-risk patients, some evidence suggests that subcutaneous heparin given in a dose that would increase the PTT to the upper normal range may be more efficacious.[112] LMWH is more effective than no prophylaxis after total hip replacement and has been compared directly with unfractionated heparin in several studies with conflicting results.[43] A meta-analysis of available studies indicates that LMWH is clearly superior to unfractionated heparin after hip replacement.[119] Adequate clinical studies comparing LMWH with warfarin in this patient group are not available.

Oral anticoagulants have been shown to be consistently effective in preventing venous thrombosis in high-risk patients. In a classic study, Sevitt and Gallagher[126] demonstrated a reduction in both clinical and autopsy evidence of pulmonary embolism and DVT with coumarin prophylaxis compared with a control group. Although the effectiveness of warfarin has been amply confirmed in subsequent studies, concern over bleeding complications has limited its general acceptance. However, recent studies have demonstrated that a lower intensity of anticoagulation is effective without increasing the bleeding risk. Hull and colleagues[127] demonstrated that less intense oral anticoagulation was equally effective in preventing recurrent DVT and resulted in fewer bleeding complications. Paiement et al.[128] have reported a low incidence of venous thrombosis and bleeding complications following elective surgery with

the use of warfarin, keeping the PT to <15 seconds. Francis and colleagues[129] have suggested a two-step approach in which a low dose of warfarin is begun 7–10 days before surgery to increase the PT at the time of operation to 1.1–1.3 times control (INR 1.4–2.0). The dose is then increased postoperatively to increase the PT further to 1.5 times control (INR 2.5). In a prospective randomized study, this regimen decreased the rate of venous thrombosis compared with a dextran control group and was associated with a low bleeding risk. A similar approach was effective in patients following general surgery.[130] The two-step method has the advantage of providing individual dose adjustment before surgery, thereby preventing the problems of over- and underdosage; it also provides some protection at the time of surgery, with an increased effect in the first postoperative week.

Recommendations for prophylaxis are given in Table 150-5; patients are classified by three risk groups. For patients at low risk, early ambulation and leg exercises are recommended. If low-risk patients have additional factors predisposing to thrombosis, such as congestive heart failure, history of venous thromboembolic disease, severe obesity, AT III, protein C or protein S deficiency, or a procedure requiring prolonged bed rest, then low-dose heparin is indicated. Patients >40 years old having general abdominal or thoracic surgery lasting >30 minutes represent a moderate-risk group, and the use of low-dose heparin (5,000 U bid) beginning 2 hours before surgery and continuing until the patient is fully ambulatory, is recommended. Patients in whom any increased risk of bleeding (e.g., after neurosurgery) is unacceptable are exceptions; external pneumatic compression is the best alternative. Following hip fracture, hip replacement, or knee replacement, warfarin can be given in a low-dose regimen to minimize bleeding complications. Alternatives to warfarin in hip fracture, hip replacement, and knee replacement are LMWH or adjusted-dose heparin, the latter particularly in hip replacement. External pneumatic compression is recommended after surgery for gynecologic malignancy or open prostatectomy.

THERAPY FOR THROMBOSIS

The principles of treatment of thrombotic disease following surgery do not differ from those in other settings except there must be a careful consideration of the risk of bleeding related to the surgical procedure (see Ch. 123). This often results in a difficult clinical decision, balancing the risks of worsening of the thrombotic disease due to suboptimal anticoagulant therapy against the risk of bleeding with more intensive anticoagulation. Consideration of the risks associated with surgical bleeding in the postoperative period (Table 150-1) is important in making these decisions. For patients at highest risk, such as those who have had intracranial or ophthalmologic surgery, anticoagulant therapy may not be appropriate until 10 or more days after surgery, and fibrinolytic therapy should be delayed for even a longer time. By contrast, after minor external procedures patients at low risk for bleeding can be treated aggressively with anticoagulants 1–2 days after surgery with close observation of the surgical site. Patients at moderate bleeding risk represent a difficult group because of the potentially serious results of internal bleeding in the thoracic cavity, abdomen, or retroperitoneum. This concern must be tempered by the report of successful abdominal or thoracic surgery[131,132] or orthopaedic surgery[128,129] in patients receiving oral anticoagulation having PTs corresponding to an INR of 2.0–2.5.

Heparin is preferred for treatment of thrombosis in the postoperative period because of its shorter half-life and ease of dose adjustment. Each case must be individually considered, but experience would suggest that heparin may be given in the early postoperative period by continuous infusion to keep the

PTT in the range of 1.5 times control, with close observation for evidence of bleeding. For fibrinolytic therapy, the risks of bleeding are higher because of the potential for dissolution of fibrin in hemostatic plugs at the surgical site. Most recommendations suggest that fibrinolytic therapy be given no sooner than 7–10 days following surgery.[133,134] This is appropriate in treatment of venous thromboembolic disease for which heparin anticoagulation is an acceptable alternative treatment. However, there is clear evidence that thrombolytic therapy reduced morbidity and mortality from acute myocardial infarction. This must be carefully considered in the risk/benefit analysis in treating patients who develop myocardial infarction in the postoperative period.

REFERENCES

1. Rapaport SI: Preoperative hemostatic evaluation: which tests, if any? Blood 61:229, 1983
2. Suchman AL, Griner PF: Diagnostic uses of the activated partial thromboplastin time and prothrombin time. Ann Intern Med 104:810, 1986
3. Robbins JA, Rose SD: Partial thromboplastin time as a screening test. Ann Intern Med 90:796, 1979
4. Eisenberg JM, Clarke JR, Sussman SA: Prothrombin and partial thromboplastin times as preoperative screening tests. Arch Surg 117:48, 1982
5. Kaplan EB, Sheiner LB, Boeckmann AJ et al: The usefulness of preoperative laboratory screening. JAMA 253:3576, 1985
6. Lind SE: The bleeding time does not predict surgical bleeding. Blood 77:2547, 1991
7. Bowie EJW, Owen CA Jr: The significance of abnormal preoperative hemostatic tests. Prog Hemost Thromb 5:179, 1980
8. Burk CD, Miller L, Handler SD, Cohen AR: Preoperative history and coagulation screening in children undergoing tonsillectomy. Pediatrics 89:691, 1992
9. Harker LA, Slichter SJ: The bleeding time as a screening test for evaluation of platelet function. N Engl J Med 287:155, 1972
10. Slichter SJ, Harker LA: Thrombocytopenia: mechanisms and management of defects in platelet production. Clin Haematol 7:523, 1978
11. Gaydos LA, Freireich EJ, Mantel N: The quantitative relation between platelet count and hemorrhage in patients with acute leukemia. N Engl J Med 266:905, 1962
12. Consensus Development Conference: Platelet transfusion therapy. JAMA 257:1777, 1987
13. McCullough J, Steeper TA, Connelly DP et al: Platelet utilization in a university hospital. JAMA 259:2414, 1988
14. Lechner K, Neissner H, Thaler E: Coagulation abnormalities in liver disease. Semin Thromb Hemost 4:40, 1977
15. Kelly DA, Tuddenham EGD: Haemostatic problems in liver disease. Progress report. Gut 27:339, 1986
16. Mannucci PM, Vicente V, Vianello L et al: Controlled trial of desmopressin in liver cirrhosis and other conditions associated with a prolonged bleeding time. Blood 67:1148, 1986
17. Sandler G, Rath CE, Ruder A: Prothrombin complex concentrates in acquired hypoprothrombinemia. Ann Intern Med 70:485, 1973
18. Mannucci PM, Franchi F, Dioguardi N: Correction of abnormal coagulation in chronic liver disease by combined use of fresh-frozen plasma and prothrombin complex concentrates. Lancet 2:542, 1976
19. Blatt PM, Lundblatt RL, Kingdon HS, Roberts HK: Thrombogenic materials in prothrombin complex concentrates. Ann Intern Med 81:766, 1972
20. Marassi A, DiCarlo V, Manzullo V, Mannucci PM: Thromboembolism following a prothrombin complex concentrate and major surgery in severe liver disease. Thromb Haemost 39:787, 1978
21. Ragni MV, Lewis JH, Spero JA: Ascites-induced LeVeen shunt coagulopathy. Ann Surg 198:91, 1983
22. LeVeen HH: The LeVeen shunt. Annu Rev Med 36:453, 1985
23. Buller HR, tenCate JW: Antithrombin III infusion in patients undergoing peritoneovenous shunt operation: failure in the prevention of disseminated intra-vascular coagulation. Thromb Haemost 49:128, 1983
24. Stein SF, Harker LA: Kinetic and functional studies of platelets, fibrinogen, and plasminogen in patients with hepatic cirrhosis. J Lab Clin Med 99:217, 1982
25. Richardson DW, Robinson AG: Desmopressin. Ann Intern Med 103:228, 1985
26. Mannucci PM: Desmopressin: a nontransfusional form of treatment for congenital and acquired bleeding disorders. Blood 72:1449, 1988
27. Nieuwenhuis HK, Sixma JJ: 1-Desamino-8-D-arginine vasopressin (desmopressin) shortens the bleeding time in storage pool deficiency. Ann Intern Med 108:68, 1988
28. DiMichele DM, Hathaway WE: Use of DDAVP in inherited and acquired platelet dysfunction. Am J Hematol 33:39, 1990
29. Bichet DG, Razi M, Lonergan M et al: Hemodynamic and coagulation responses to 1-desamino-8-D-arginine vasopressin in patients with congenital nephrogenic diabetes insipidus. N Engl J Med 318:881, 1988
30. DiMinno G, Martinez J, McKean M-L et al: Platelet dysfunction in uremia: multifaceted defect partially corrected by dialysis. Am J Med 79:552, 1985
31. Remuzzi G: Bleeding in renal failure. Lancet 1:1205, 1988
32. Castillo R, Lozano T, Escolar G et al: Defective platelet adhesion on vessel subendothelium in uremic patients. Blood 68:337, 1986
33. Rubin RN: Aspirin and postsurgery bleeding. Ann Intern Med 89:1006, 1978
34. Torosian M, Michelson EL, Morganroth J, MacVaugh H, III: Aspirin- and Coumadin-related bleeding after coronary-artery bypass graft surgery. Ann Intern Med 89:325, 1978
35. Goldman S, Copeland J, Moritz T et al: Improvement in early saphenous vein graft patency after coronary artery bypass surgery with antiplatelet therapy: results of a Veterans Administration cooperative study. Circulation 77:1324, 1988
36. Amrein PC, Ellman L, Harris WH: Aspirin-induced prolongation of bleeding time and perioperative blood loss. JAMA 245:1825, 1981
37. Ferraris VA, Swanson E: Aspirin usage and perioperative blood loss in patients undergoing unexpected operations. Surg Gynecol Obstet 156:439, 1983
38. Gallus AS, Hirsh J, Tuttle RJ et al: Small subcutaneous doses of heparin in prevention of venous thrombosis. N Engl J Med 288:545, 1973
39. International Multicentre Trial: Prevention of fatal postoperative pulmonary embolism by low doses of heparin. Lancet 2:45, 1975
40. Collins R, Scrimgeour A, Yusuf S, Peto R: Reduction in fatal pulmonary embolism and venous thrombosis by perioperative administration of subcutaneous heparin. N Engl J Med 318:1162, 1988
41. Simon TL, Hyers TM, Gaston JP, Harker LA: Heparin pharmacokinetics: increased requirements in pulmonary embolism. Br J Haematol 39:111, 1978
42. Hirsh J: Heparin. N Engl J Med 324:1565, 1991
43. Hirsh J, Levine MN: Low molecular weight heparin. Blood 779:1, 1992
44. International Committee on Thrombosis and Haemostasis/International Committee for Standardization in Hematology: Report of the expert panel on oral anticoagulant control. Thromb Haemost 42:1073, 1979
45. Loeliger EA, Lewis SM: Progress in laboratory control of oral anticoagulants. Lancet 2:318, 1982
46. Hirsh J, Poller L, Deykin D et al: Optimal therapeutic range for oral anticoagulants. Chest 95:5S, 1989
47. Shetty HGM, Backhouse G, Bentley DP. Routledge PA: Effective reversal of warfarin-induced excessive anticoagulation with low dose vitamin K₁. Thromb Haemost 67:13, 1992
48. Marder VJ, Sherry S: Thrombolytic therapy: current status. N Engl J Med 318:1512, 1988
49. Coller BS: Platelets and thrombolytic therapy. N Engl J Med 322:33, 1990
50. Sane DC, Califf RM, Topol EJ et al: Bleeding during thrombolytic therapy for acute myocardial infarction: mechanisms and management. Ann Intern Med 111:1010, 1989
51. Skinner JR, Phillips SJ, Zeff RH, Kongtahworn C: Immediate coronary bypass following failed streptokinase infusion in evolving myocardial infarction. J Thorac Cardiovasc Surg 87:567, 1984
52. Kay P, Ahmad A, Floten S, Starr A: Emergency coronary artery bypass surgery after intracoronary thrombolysis for evolving myocardial infarction. Br Heart J 53:260, 1985
53. Anderson JL, Battistessa SA, Clayton PD et al: Coronary bypass surgery early after thrombolytic therapy for acute myocardial infarction. Ann Thorac Surg 41:176, 1986
54. Mantia AM, Lolley DM, Stullken EH Jr et al: Coronary artery bypass grafting within 24 hours after intracoronary streptokinase thrombolysis. J Cardiothorac Anesth 1:392, 1987
55. Lee KF, Mandell J, Rankin JS et al: Immediate versus delayed coronary grafting after streptokinase treatment. J Thorac Cardiovasc Surg 95:216, 1988
56. Loscalzo J, Braunwald E: Tissue plasminogen activator. N Engl J Med 319:925, 1988
57. Eisenberg PR, Sherman LA, Tiefenbrunn AJ et al: Sustained fibrinolysis after administration of t-PA despite its short half-life in the circulation. Thromb Haemost 57:35, 1987
58. Adelman B, Michelson AD, Loscalzo J et al: Plasmin effect on platelet glycoprotein 1B—von Willebrand factor interactions. Blood 65:32, 1985
59. Schafer AI, Adelman B: Plasmin inhibition of platelet function and of arachidonic acid metabolism. J Clin Invest 75:455, 1985
60. Jorgensen KA, Stoffersen E, Sorensen PJ et al: Alterations in plasma antithrombin III following total hip replacement and elective cholecystectomy. Scand J Haematol 24:101, 1980

61. Seyler AE, Seaber AV, Dombrose FA, Urbaniak JR: Coagulation changes in elective surgery and trauma. Ann Surg 193:210, 1981

62. Counts RB, Haisch C, Simon TL et al: Hemostasis in massively transfused trauma patients. Ann Surg 190:91, 1979

63. Reed RL II, Ciavarella D, Heimbach DM et al: Prophylactic platelet administration during massive transfusion: a prospective, randomized, double-blind clinical study. Ann Surg 203:40, 1986

64. Egan EL, Bowie EJW, Kazmier FJ et al: Effect of surgical operations on certain tests used to diagnose intravascular coagulation and fibrinolysis. Mayo Clin Proc 49:658, 1974

65. Slichter SJ, Funk DD, Leandoer LE, Harker LA: Kinetic evaluation of haemostasis during surgery and wound healing. Br J Haematol 27:115, 1974

66. Koie E, Kamiya T, Ogata K, Takamatsu J: α_2-Plasmin-inhibitor deficiency (Miyasato disease). Lancet 2:1334, 1978

67. Saito H: α_2-Plasmin inhibitor and its deficiency states. J Lab Clin Med 112:671, 1988

68. Schleef RR, Higgins DL, Pillemer E, Levitt LJ: Bleeding diathesis due to decreased functional activity of type 1 plasminogen activator inhibitor. J Clin Invest 83:1747, 1989

69. Fay WP, Shapiro AD, Shih JL et al: Brief report: complete deficiency of plasminogen-activator inhibitor type 1 due to a frame-shift mutation. N Engl J Med 327:1729, 1992

70. Sack E, Spaet TH, Gentile RL et al: Reduction of postprostatectomy bleeding by epsilon-aminocaproic acid. N Engl J Med 266:541, 1962

71. Vinnicombe J, Shuttleworth KED: Aminocaproic acid in the control of haemorrhage after prostatectomy: a controlled trial. Lancet 1:230, 1966

72. Woodman RC, Harker LA: Bleeding complications associated with cardiopulmonary bypass. Blood 76:1680, 1990

73. Harker LA, Malpass TW, Branson HE et al: Mechanism of abnormal bleeding in patients undergoing cardiopulmonary bypass: acquired transient platelet dysfunction associated with selective α-granule release. Blood 56:824, 1980

74. Mammen EF, Koets MH, Washington BC et al: Hemostasis changes during cardiopulmonary bypass surgery. Semin Thromb Hemos 11:281, 1985

75. Zilla P, Fasol R, Groscurth P et al: Blood platelets in cardiopulmonary bypass operations. Recovery occurs after initial stimulation, rather than continual activation. J Thorac Cardiovasc Surg 97:379, 1989

76. Ellison N, Beatty CP, Blake DR et al: Heparin rebound: studies in patients and volunteers. J Thorac Cardiovasc Surg 67:723, 1974

77. Bick RL: Hemostasis defects associated with cardiac surgery, prosthetic devices, and other extracorporeal circuits. Semin Thromb Hemost 11:249, 1985

78. Salzman EW, Weinstein MJ, Weintraub RM et al: Treatment with desmopressin acetate to reduce blood loss after cardiac surgery: a double-blind randomized trial. N Engl J Med 314:1402, 1986

79. Weinstein M, Ware AJ, Troll J, Salzman E: Changes in von Willebrand factor during cardiac surgery: effect of desmopressin acetate. Blood 71:1648, 1988

80. Czer LSC, Bateman TM, Gray RJ et al: Treatment of severe platelet dysfunction and hemorrhage after cardiopulmonary bypass: reduction in blood product usage with desmopressin. J Am Coll Cardiol 9:1139, 1987

81. Rocha E, Llorens R, Paramo JA et al: Does desmopressin acetate reduce blood loss after surgery in patients on cardiopulmonary bypass? Circulation 77:1319, 1988

82. Hackmann T, Gascoyne RD, Naiman SC et al: A trial of desmopressin (1-desamino-8-D-arginine vasopressin) to reduce blood loss in uncomplicated cardiac surgery. N Engl J Med 321:1437, 1989

83. de Prost D, Barbier-Boehm G, Hazebroucq J et al: Desmopressin has no beneficial effect on excessive postoperative bleeding or blood product requirements associated with cardiopulmonary bypass. Thromb Haemost 68:106, 1992

84. Kobrinsky NL, Letts RP, Patel RL et al: DDAVP shortens the bleeding time and decreases blood loss in hemostatically normal subjects undergoing spinal fusion surgery. Ann Intern Med 107:446, 1987

85. Clagett GP, Anderson FA Jr, Levine MN et al: Prevention of venous thromboembolism. Chest 102:391S, 1992

86. Maynard MJ, Sculco TP, Ghelman B: Progression and regression of deep vein thrombosis after total knee arthroplasty. Clin Orthop Rel Res 273:125, 1991

87. Kakkar VV, Flanc C, Howe CT, Clarke MB: Natural history of postoperative deep-vein thrombosis. Lancet 2:230, 1969

88. Moser KM, LeMoine JR: Is embolic risk conditioned by location of deep venous thrombosis? Ann Intern Med 94:439, 1981

89. Scurr JH, Ibrahim SZ, Faber RG, LeQuesne LP: The effect of graduated compression stockings in the prevention of deep vein thrombosis. Br J Surg 64:371, 1977

90. Fasting H, Andersen K, Nielsen HK et al: Prevention of postoperative deep venous thrombosis: low-dose heparin versus graded pressure stockings. Acta Chir Scand 151:245, 1985

91. Nicolaides AN, Fernandes FJ, Pollock AV: Intermittent sequential pneumatic compression of the legs in the prevention of venous stasis and postoperative deep venous thrombosis. Surgery 87:69, 1980

92. Mühe E: Intermittent sequential high-pressure compression of the leg: a new method of preventing deep vein thrombosis. Am J Surg 147:781, 1984

93. Allenby F, Pflug JJ, Boardman L, Calnan JS: Effects of external pneumatic intermittent compression on fibrinolysis in man. Lancet 2:1412, 1973

94. Hills NH, Pflug JJ, Jeyasingh K et al: Prevention of deep vein thrombosis by intermittent pneumatic compression of calf. Br Med J 1:131, 1972

95. Clark WB, MacGregor AB, Prescott RJ et al: Pneumatic compression of the calf and postoperative deep-vein thrombosis. Lancet 2:5, 1974

96. Coe NP, Collins REC, Klein LA et al: Prevention of deep vein thrombosis in urological patients: a controlled, randomized trial of low-dose heparin and external pneumatic compression boots. Surgery 83:230, 1978

97. Skillman JJ, Collins REC, Coe NP et al: Prevention of deep vein thrombosis in neurosurgical patients: a controlled, randomized trial of external pneumatic compression boots. Surgery 83:354, 1978

98. Turpie AGG, Delmore T, Hirsch J et al: Prevention of venous thrombosis by intermittent sequential calf compression in patients with intracranial disease. Thromb Res 15:611, 1979

99. Clarke-Pearson DL, Synan IS, Hinshaw WM et al: Prevention of postoperative venous thromboembolism by external pneumatic calf compression in patients with gynecologic malignancy. Obstet Gynecol 63:92, 1984

100. Hull R, Delmore TJ, Hirsh J et al: Effectiveness of intermittent pulsatile elastic stockings for the prevention of calf and thigh vein thrombosis in patients undergoing elective knee surgery. Thromb Res 16:37, 1979

101. Kakkar VV, Spindler J, Flute PT et al: Efficacy of low doses of heparin in prevention of deep-vein thrombosis after major surgery. Lancet 2:101, 1972

102. Brozovic M, Stirling Y, Abbosh J: Plasma heparin levels after low dose subcutaneous heparin in patients undergoing hip replacement. Br J Haematol 31:461, 1975

103. Gruber UF, Duckert F, Fridrich R et al: Prevention of postoperative thromboembolism by dextran 40, low doses of heparin, or xantinol nicotinate. Lancet 1:207, 1977

104. International Multicentre Trial Co-ordinating Centre: Prevention of fatal postoperative pulmonary embolism by low doses of heparin: reappraisal of results of International Multicentre Trial. Lancet 1:567, 1977

105. Prevention of venous thrombosis and pulmonary embolism. National Institutes of Health Consensus Development Conference Statement 6:2, 1986

106. Simon TL, Stengle JM: Antithrombotic practice in orthopedic surgery: results of a survey. Clin Orthop 102:181, 1974

107. Conti S, Daschbach M: Venous thromboembolism prophylaxis: a survey of its use in the United States. Arch Surg 117:1036, 1982

108. Morris GK: Prevention of venous thromboembolism: a survey of methods used by orthopaedic and general surgeons. Lancet 2:572, 1980

109. Anderson FA Jr, Wheeler HB, Goldberg RJ et al: Physician practices in the prevention of venous thromboembolism. Ann Intern Med 115:591, 1991

110. Multicenter Trial Committee: Dihydroergotamine-heparin prophylaxis of postoperative deep vein thrombosis. JAMA 251:2960, 1984

111. Gent M, Roberts RS: A meta-analysis of the studies of dihydroergotamine plus heparin in the prophylaxis of deep vein thrombosis. Chest 89:396S, 1986

112. Leyvraz PF, Richard J, Bachmann F et al: Adjusted versus fixed-dose subcutaneous heparin in the prevention of deep-vein thrombosis after total hip replacement. N Engl J Med 309:954, 1983

113. Green D, Lee MY, Ito VY et al: Fixed- vs adjusted-dose heparin in the prophylaxis of thromboembolism in spinal cord injury. JAMA 260:1255, 1988

114. Francis CW, Pellegrini VD Jr, Marder VJ et al: Prevention of venous thrombosis after total hip arthroplasty. Antithrombin III and low dose heparin compared with dextran 40. J Bone Joint Surg 71A:327, 1989

115. Francis CW, Pellegrini VD Jr, Stulberg BN et al: Prevention of venous thrombosis following total knee arthroplasty: comparison of antithrombin III plus low dose heparin to dextran. J Bone Joint Surg 72A:976, 1990

116. Holmer E, Jurachi K, Söderström G: The molecular-weight dependence of the rate-enhancing effect of heparin on the inhibition of thrombin, factor Xa, factor IXa, factor XIa, factor XIIa and kallikrein by antithrombin. Biochem J 193:395, 1981

117. Carter CJ, Kelton JH, Hirsh J et al: The relationship between the hemorrhagic and antithrombotic properties of low molecular weight heparin in rabbits. Blood 59:1239, 1982

118. Holmer E, Matsson C, Nilsson S: Anticoagulant and antithrombotic effects of heparin and low molecular weight heparin fragments in rabbits. Thromb Res 25:475, 1982

119. Nurmohamed MT, Rosendaal RF, Büller HR et al: Low-molecular weight hep-

arin versus standard heparin in general and orthopaedic surgery: a meta-analysis. Lancet 340:152, 1992

120. Hull RD, Raskob GE: Prophylaxis of venous thromboembolic disease following hip and knee surgery. J Bone Joint Surg 68-A:146, 1986

121. Evarts CM, Feil EJ: Prevention of thromboembolic disease after elective surgery of the hip. J Bone Joint Surg 53-A:1271, 1971

122. Harris WH, Salzman EW, Athanasoulis C et al: Comparison of warfarin, low-molecular weight dextran, aspirin, and subcutaneous heparin in prevention of venous thromboembolism following total hip replacement. J Bone Joint Surg 56-A:1552, 1974

123. Gallus A, Raman K, Darby T: Venous thrombosis after elective hip replacement—the influence of preventive intermittent calf compression and of surgical technique. Br J Surg 70:17, 1983

124. Hull RD, Raskob GE, Gent M et al: Effectiveness of intermittent pneumatic leg compression for preventing deep vein thrombosis after total hip replacement. JAMA 263:2313, 1990

125. Francis CW, Pellegrini VD Jr, Marder VJ et al: Comparison of warfarin and external pneumatic compression in prevention of venous thrombosis after total hip replacement. JAMA 267:2911, 1992

126. Sevitt S, Gallagher NG: Prevention of venous thrombosis and pulmonary embolism in injured patients. Lancet 2:981, 1959

127. Hull R, Hirsh J, Jay R: Different intensities of oral anticoagulant therapy i the treatment of proximal-vein thrombosis. N Engl J Med 307:1676, 1982

128. Paiement G, Weissinger SJ, Waltman AC, Harris WH: Low-dose warfarin ve sus external pneumatic compression for prophylaxis against venous throm boembolism following total hip replacement. J Arthroplasty 2:23, 1987

129. Francis CW, Marder VJ, Evarts CM, Yaukoolbodi S: Two-step warfarin the apy: prevention of postoperative venous thrombosis without excessiv bleeding. JAMA 249:374, 1983

130. Taberner DA, Poller L, Burslem RW, Jones JB: Oral anticoagulants controlle by the British comparative thromboplastin versus low-dose heparin in pro phylaxis of deep vein thrombosis. Br Med J 1:272, 1978

131. Müllertz S, Storm O: Anticoagulant therapy with dicumarol maintained du ing major surgery. Circulation 10:213, 1954

132. Rustad H, Myhre E: Surgery during anticoagulant treatment: the risk of in creased bleeding in patients on oral anticoagulant treatment. Acta Me Scand 173:115, 1963

133. Bell WR, Meek AG: Guidelines for the use of thrombolytic agents. N Engl Med 301:1266, 1979

134. Marder VJ: The use of thrombolytic agents: choice of patient, drug adminis tration, laboratory monitoring. Ann Intern Med 90:802, 1979

Hematologic Manifestations of Childhood Illness

151

A. Kim Ritchey and Karen A. Zaboy

INTRODUCTION

The hematologic response to systemic illness in children is similar to that in adults. However, a number of disorders occur more frequently in children, and some are unique to the pediatric population. In addition, interpretation of the hematologic response is predicated on knowledge of the normal developmental changes that occur within the hematopoietic system throughout childhood (Table 151-1). This chapter focuses on the hematologic manifestations of common or unique systemic diseases that occur in the neonate, child, or adolescent. Illnesses that often require hematologic consultation are emphasized. Systemic diseases that produce hematologic abnormalities similar in adults and children are discussed in other chapters. For a comprehensive review of the subject, the reader is referred to a published textbook.[1]

INFECTIOUS DISEASE

Infection, especially viral infection, is the most common problem encountered by the pediatrician. Although most infections do not produce significant hematologic sequelae, all classes of microorganisms have been implicated in the pathogenesis of hematologic abnormalities that range from mild and clinically irrelevant to severe and life-threatening. In this section, changes seen in red cells, white cells, platelets, or the coagulation system that are either routinely encountered or associated with a specific infection, or that have a potentially serious clinical impact are discussed.

Red Cells

The anemia of chronic inflammation/infection in children is similar to that seen in adults in terms of both clinical and hematologic findings and pathogenesis. However, anemia with acute infections occurs more commonly in children than in adults.

Anemia of Acute Infections

A mild-to-moderate anemia of uncertain etiology may occur in the setting of both acute viral infection or more serious bacterial infections. In a study of children with mild viral or bacterial infections in the outpatient setting, anemia was documented in 5% of children 4–12 years, 17% of children 0.5–4 years, and 33% of infants 6–11 months of age.[2] In 14 of 15 young children, the anemia resolved within 3–4 weeks. However, multiple mild infections may predispose the infant to develop a more chronic, mild anemia or "low normal" hemoglobin, which may be due to iron deficiency, thus warranting a trial of iron.[3] In children hospitalized with moderately severe inflammatory processes, the incidence of mild anemia (hemoglobin 10.1–11.0 g/dl) is as high as 78%.[4] Specific acute bacterial infections associated with a high incidence of anemia (44–74%) include bone and joint infection,[5] typhoid fever,[6] brucellosis,[7] and invasive *Haemophilus influenzae* type b infections.

The anemia associated with *H. influenzae* type b meningitis has been the most thoroughly studied of the anemias of acute infection. Most children with *H. influenzae* meningitis have mild anemia on admission with hemoglobin in the 9–11 g/dl range,

Table 151-1. Normal Hematologic Values in Childhood

	Red Cells						White Cells		Neutro-phils (%)	Lympho-cytes (%)	Coagulation			
	Hb (g/dl)		Hct (%)		MCV (fl)		Total				PT (sec)[a]		PTT (sec)[a]	
Age	Mean	(Range)	Mean	(Range)	Mean	(Range)	Mean	(Range)	Mean	Mean	Mean	(Range)	Mean	(Range)
Birth (term)	18.5	(14.5–22.5)	56	(45–69)	108	(95–121)	18.1	(9.0–30.0)	61	31	16	(13–20)	55	(45–65)
2 mo	11.2	(9.4–14.0)	35	(28–42)	96	(77–115)								
6 mo–2 yr	12.5	(11.0–14.0)	37	(33–41)	77	(70–84)	11.3	(6.0–17.5)	32	61				
2–6 yr	12.5	(11.5–13.5)	37	(34–40)	81	(75–87)	8.5	(5.0–15.5)	42	50				
6–12 yr	13.5	(11.5–15.5)	40	(35–45)	86	(77–95)	8.1	(4.5–13.5)	53	39				
12–18 yr							7.8	(4.5–13.5)	57	35				
Male	14.5	(13.0–16.0)	43	(37–49)	88	(78–98)								
Female	14.0	(12.0–16.0)	41	(36–46)	90	(78–102)								

Abbreviations: Hb, hemoglobin; Hct, hematocrit; MCV, mean corpuscular volume.

[a] The normal range for the PT and PTT varies between laboratories. The time at which normal adult values are attained is 1 week for the PT and 2–9 months for the PTT. The platelet count is within the adult range from birth.

(Data from Dallman and Rudolph[232] and Nathan and Oski.[233])

and up to 90% become anemic during the course of the illness.[8–12] This is in contrast to meningitis secondary to *Streptococcus pneumoniae* or *Neisseria meningitidis*, in which anemia is uncommon. The pathophysiology of the anemia of *H. influenzae* disease appears to be multifactorial. Shurin et al.[13] have shown that *H. influenzae* type b capsular polysaccharide, polyribosyl ribitol phosphate, binds to erythrocytes and in the presence of antibody and complement can result in intravascular and extravascular hemolysis. They further hypothesize that polyribosyl ribitol phosphate alone may induce more rapid clearance of red cells, perhaps on the basis of decreased red cell deformability.[11] In addition, hypoferremia may limit bone marrow response to hemolysis.[10]

Acute Hemolytic Anemia

Acute hemolysis has been observed with infections from all classes of microorganisms but is relatively uncommon.[14,15] The anemia may be mild to severe and occurs in two clinical settings: (1) the child who presents predominantly with symptoms and signs of infection and is found to have anemia, and (2) the child who presents with the manifestations of autoimmune hemolytic anemia.

The mechanism of hemolysis in patients presenting with an infectious disorder depends on the infecting organism, but in most cases hemolysis is extravascular. Reported mechanisms include the following:

1. Release of hemolysins (*Clostridium perfringens* sepsis)
2. Invasion of the red cell (malaria)
3. Alteration of red cell surface
   a. By direct adherence by the organism (*Bartonella*)
   b. By alterations of antigenic phenotype by neuraminidase (influenza)
   c. By cold agglutinin (mycoplasma, *Listeria*, Epstein-Barr virus [EBV])
   d. By absorption of capsular polysaccharide (*H. influenzae*)
4. Mechanical mechanisms (microangiopathy associated with disseminated intravascular coagulation [DIC] or hemolytic-uremic syndrome)
5. Oxidative damage in individuals with congenital enzyme deficiencies (hepatitis and glucose-6-phosphate dehydrogenase [G6PD] deficiency,[16] *Campylobacter jejuni* in the neonate).[17]

Autoimmune hemolytic anemia in children is usually transient, is not associated with underlying systemic disease, and has a low mortality rate.[18,19] Children frequently have a history of concurrent or recently resolved infection, especially viral upper respiratory infection. In the typical acute, transient situations, 59–68% of children have such a history, whereas 0–20% of those with the less common chronic course have a history of infection.

Aplastic Crisis

Temporary arrest of red cell production has been observed in children with infections,[20] but anemia is uncommon because of the long red cell life span. However, in two situations severe anemia has been linked to infection and cessation of erythropoiesis: (1) B19 parvovirus infection in patients with an underlying hemolytic anemia, and (2) transient erythroblastopenia of childhood.

The B19 parvovirus has been a known pathogen in animals for years, but has only recently been linked to human disease.[21] It is the etiologic agent of fifth disease (erythema infectiosum), a mild illness with a characteristic "slapped cheek" facial erythema and a generalized reticular rash. In normal children this infection is not associated with hematologic abnormalities, although in normal volunteers infected with B19 parvovirus a mild, transient, and clinically irrelevant drop in the hemoglobin and reticulocyte count was observed.[22] However, in children with sickle cell disease, spherocytosis, and other hemolytic anemias, B19 parvovirus infection can produce a severe anemia associated with peripheral reticulocytopenia and marrow erythroblastopenia: the "aplastic crisis." Recovery within 1–2 weeks is the rule, but transfusion may be necessary. B19 parvovirus infection has also been associated with prolonged anemia and reticulocytopenia in children with acute lymphocytic leukemia (ALL) in remission,[23,24] immunodeficiency,[25,26] and autoimmune hemolytic anemia[27]; it can also be an initial manifestation of human immunodeficiency virus (HIV) infection.[28]

Transient erythroblastopenia of childhood (TEC) is a syndrome characterized by temporary arrest of red cell production with moderate-to-severe anemia in previously normal infants and toddlers. Although no specific infectious agent has been linked to TEC, the frequency of a history of infection within 1–3 months, the seasonal clustering, and the similarity to childhood idiopathic thrombocytic purpura (ITP) all suggest a possible viral etiology. B19 parvovirus has not been associated with TEC.

White Cells

Children, as a rule, have the expected leukocyte response to infection. It should be remembered that infants and young children normally have a lymphocyte predominance (Table

151-1), and any leukocyte response to infection must be judged on the basis of age-related normal values.

The predictive value of the peripheral white blood cell (WBC) and differential counts in suspected bacterial infections has been extensively evaluated in infants and children.[29] Todd[30] has shown in hospitalized children that a neutrophil count >10,000/mm^3 or bands >500/mm^3 are associated with an 80% chance of bacterial infection. Febrile children between the ages of 3 and 48 months are at increased risk of bacteremia, especially with *S. pneumoniae*. McCarthy et al.[31] demonstrated a threefold increase in risk of bacteremia in febrile (>40°C) children <2 years old who had a WBC count of ≥15,000/mm^3. In this setting, the WBC count was a more sensitive indicator of the presence of pneumonia or bacteremia than was the absolute neutrophil or band count.

Exceptions to the anticipated leukocyte response to infection are recognized that may serve as a clue to the diagnosis. In typhoid fever and brucellosis, leukopenia and neutropenia are prominent early in the illness. Shigellosis is associated with a variable leukocyte count, but it is often normal, with a greater percentage of bands than neutrophils. Illnesses associated with lymphocytosis include pertussis (whooping cough), infectious lymphocytosis, infectious mononucleosis, and other viral infections. Neutropenia can be seen in bacterial sepsis from meningococcus, pneumococcus, staphylococcus, and other bacteria, and is associated with a poor prognosis. Black children normally have lower WBC and neutrophil counts than do white children; they also have less of a leukocytosis and neutrophilic response to serious infection.[32]

Neutropenia

The most common cause of neutropenia (neutrophil count <1,500/mm^3) in childhood is viral infection. A number of specific viruses have been associated with neutropenia, including hepatitis, roseola, rubella, mumps, adenovirus, coxsackievirus A21, EBV, and influenza.[33] However, the most common clinical setting is the incidental discovery of neutropenia in the child with a nonspecific viral syndrome. Usually the neutropenia in this situation continues for <30 days and is rarely associated with infectious complications.[34] Neutropenia has also been associated with a number of bacterial, rickettsial, and fungal infections.[35]

Eosinophilia

The most common cause of eosinophilia worldwide is parasitic infection. In the United States, visceral larva migrans is the most common cause of exaggerated eosinophilia (WBC 30,000–100,000/mm^3 with 50–90% mature eosinophils) in children.[36,37] Mild-to-moderate eosinophilia (≥400/mm^3) is most often seen in allergic children, but is also characteristic of *Chlamydia* pneumonitis in infants.

Platelets/Coagulation

Thrombocytosis

Thrombocytosis (>500,000/mm^3) is an acute-phase reaction to infection, but it has been infrequently identified in children in the past.[38] The incidence of thrombocytosis is particularly high in patients with *H. influenzae* type b meningitis, with 45% of patients having a platelet count of >500,000/mm^3 at some time during the course of the disease, and counts as high as 1.2 million have been reported.[39] Inflammatory cytokines such as interleukin-1 may play an etiologic role in the reactive thrombocytosis of infection.[40] Thrombocytosis may be more common in simple acute infections than previously recognized. Heath and Pearson[41] documented a 13% incidence of thrombo-

cytosis in ambulatory patients; children with an increased platelet count were more likely to have a diagnosis of infection. All children with platelets >700,000/mm^3 had a presumptive diagnosis of infection. There were no apparent sequelae to the thrombocytosis. Antiplatelet therapy is usually not indicated. While the most common cause of thrombocytosis in children is infection,[42] the differential diagnosis of an elevated platelet count is extensive[43] and rarely includes underlying childhood malignancy.[44]

Thrombocytopenia

Thrombocytopenia can be seen in patients suffering from infections with all types of organisms. Common viral agents include varicella, EBV, rubella, mumps, measles (wild or vaccine strains), and cytomegalovirus (CMV). The primary mechanism of the thrombocytopenia is immune destruction, although a direct viral effect on the platelet or megakaryocyte has been demonstrated. Since childhood ITP is believed to be secondary to infection in most instances, the definitions of "thrombocytopenia with infection" and "childhood ITP" tend to merge. Children with thrombocytopenia from infection (regardless of the title) usually have a transient course, although chronic thrombocytopenia from specific viral infections (e.g., varicella) have been documented.[45]

Thrombocytopenia is associated with bacterial sepsis. The low platelet count may be an isolated finding or may be associated with DIC. Corrigan[46] documented a 61% incidence of thrombocytopenia in 45 children with sepsis. The degree of thrombocytopenia was mild to moderate (64% had >50,000/mm^3 platelets) but ranged as low as 8,000/mm^3. DIC was not evident in 39% of those with low platelet counts. Thrombocytopenia in the setting of bacterial sepsis is probably mediated by an immune mechanism with elevated platelet-associated IgG.[47]

Petechial bleeding without thrombocytopenia can be found in both bacterial and viral disease, especially with the meningococcus and streptococcus organisms and the echoviruses. The mechanism for the petechial rash in these infections is either a vasculitis or platelet dysfunction.

Disseminated Intravascular Coagulation/Purpura Fulminans

DIC is uncommon after childhood infections and if present is usually accompanied by shock and mortality rate of ≥50%. The most common organisms producing DIC are bacterial, especially the gram-negative bacteria (meningococcus, *H. influenzae*, *Aerobacter*, and others) but also gram-positive organisms (*Staphylococcus aureus*, group B streptococcus, and *S. pneumoniae*—particularly in the asplenic host). DIC is also associated with disseminated viral (varicella, measles, rubella), rickettsial (Rocky Mountain spotted fever), fungal, mycoplasma, and parasitic infections.

Purpura fulminans is a rare syndrome, seen in extremely ill children with DIC. Purpura fulminans is characterized by the rapid progression of ecchymotic skin lesions, especially of the extremities, that may progress to gangrene and ultimately result in amputation.[48] This syndrome has been described as a postinfectious purpura; scarlet fever, upper respiratory tract infection, and varicella are the most common preceding illnesses, with a latent period of 0–90 days following infection.[49] A similar clinical picture can be seen in children with DIC and acute bacterial sepsis, especially meningococcemia. Treatment of purpura fulminans consists of antibiotics for suspected bacterial infection, volume replacement for shock, and heparin. Although there is controversy regarding the routine use of heparin in DIC, its use in purpura fulminans has been associated with an improved outcome, especially when started early in the course of the disease and continued for 2–3 weeks. To improve the efficacy of heparin, it is reasonable to infuse fresh frozen plasma (or antithrombin III [AT III] concentrates when available)[50] if the AT III level is low. Furthermore, fresh frozen plasma would replace proteins C and S, which have been shown to be low in children with infectious purpura.[51-53] Other treatments, such as regional sympathetic blockade, topical nitroglycerin, and tissue plasminogen activator have been employed to improve regional blood flow to the affected part.[54-56] The mortality of postinfectious purpura fulminans has declined from 90% in the past to 18%,[49] although patients with acute bacterial sepsis with purpura fulminans continue to have a high mortality rate.

Coagulation Inhibitors

Acquired inhibitors of coagulation in children with infection are uncommon, transient, and usually mild,[57,58] but may be associated with severe bleeding.[59] They are usually detected after a viral illness, during penicillin therapy,[60] or incidentally. Both specific inhibitors of coagulation factors (especially factors VIII and IX) and lupus anticoagulants have been demonstrated, with significant bleeding found only in those with specific factor inhibitors. Treatment of symptomatic patients with prednisone has been associated with improvement in bleeding manifestations. Complete resolution without recurrence is the most common course.

Pancytopenia

Pancytopenia in a child should alert the clinician to disorders such as leukemia, aplastic anemia, or disseminated neuroblastoma. Infectious causes of pancytopenia are uncommon, and disseminated disease is most often present. Organisms implicated in patients with pancytopenia include *Mycobacterium tuberculosis,* atypical mycobacteria, *Histoplasma capsulatum, Salmonella typhi, Mucor* spp., *Brucella* spp., and *Fusobacterium necrophorum.*[35,61] Recently *Erlichia canis,* a tick-borne rickettsia, has been identified as a cause of pancytopenia in a child.[62] Virus-associated or reactive hemophagocytic syndrome is an additional, although rare, cause of pancytopenia.[63]

Human Immunodeficiency Virus Infection in Children/Adolescents

HIV infection is more common in adults but is now recognized as a leading cause of immunodeficiency in infants and children. Acquisition of HIV in the majority of infected children (most of whom are <2 years old) is by vertical transmission from an infected mother to her infant. In children with acquired immunodeficiency syndrome (AIDS) who are <13 years old, 80% have a parent with AIDS or AIDS-related complex (ARC), 13% have a history of blood transfusion, and 5% have hemophilia or another coagulation disorder.[64] Other "adult" routes of infection (homosexuality, intravenous needle use) are possible, especially in the adolescent and the sexually abused child.

The definition of AIDS in childhood differs from that for adults in two ways.[65] Multiple, serious bacterial infections and lymphocytic interstitial pneumonitis/pulmonary lymphoid hyperplasia are accepted as indicative of AIDS among children but not adults. Because of the possibility of passively acquired maternal antibody in children <15 months, the diagnosis of HIV infection is difficult, and laboratory criteria are more stringent.

Most children with AIDS present with oral thrush, chronic interstitial pneumonitis, hepatosplenomegaly, lymphadenopathy, or failure to thrive. Other clinical characteristics distinguishing pediatric HIV infection include a shorter incubation period, more pronounced hypergammaglobulinemia, more serious bacterial and CMV disease, and the rare occurrence of Kaposi sarcoma or other malignancies. However, as in adults, the spectrum of disease manifestations is broad; all organ systems may be affected, with progressive immune and clinical deterioration.

The hematologic manifestations of AIDS in children are similar to those in adults (see Ch. 155) and depend on the state of the HIV infection and the presence of coexistent disease.[66,67] Anemia is by far the most common finding (>90%). Severe anemia (hematocrit <25%) correlates with development of an opportunistic infection and death within 7 months.[68] Leukopenia and neutropenia are commonly seen in HIV-infected children (47% and 41%, respectively) with severe neutropenia associated with opportunistic infections. Immune neutropenia, as well as circulating anticoagulants, has been described.[69,70] Lymphopenia is progressive but less prominent in children than adults, until late in the course. Thrombocytopenia is present in 13–30% of pediatric patients with AIDS, and can be associated with clinically significant, and even fatal, hemorrhage. In most instances, the mechanism of the thrombocytopenia is immune destruction, with a high percentage of patients having antiplatelet antibodies or immune complexes.[71] Amegakaryocytic thrombocytopenia has also been reported.[72] Variable therapeutic responses to both corticosteroids and intravenous IgG have been demonstrated, and some children will have spontaneous remissions.[71,73] The evaluation and treatment of hematologic abnormalities in HIV-infected children have been reviewed by Hilgartner.[74] Consensus guidelines for the diagnosis and overall management of children with HIV infection have also been published.[75]

Isolated thrombocytopenia as a presenting manifestation of HIV infection has been reported in a number of children, usually infants.[76,77] No associated clinical stigmata of AIDS or ARC have been found, and patients have been responsive to standard treatment (intravenous IgG or prednisone), often with sustained remissions. In a few patients with prolonged follow-up, no further manifestations of HIV infection were seen. Although it has been suggested that HIV testing may be indicated in all children with ITP, it seems most reasonable to check the HIV status of those with risk factors for AIDS, and those outside the typical age group for ITP, especially infants.[77]

COLLAGEN VASCULAR DISEASE/ACUTE VASCULITIS

Juvenile Rheumatoid Arthritis

Juvenile rheumatoid arthritis (JRA) includes a group of disorders with a varied clinical presentation, course, and outcome.[78] Systemic JRA, which occurs in 30% of patients, is a multisystem disease characterized by fever, rash, polyarticular (often destructive) arthritis, hepatosplenomegaly, and lymphadenopathy. These patients commonly demonstrate hematologic abnormalities that are proportional to disease activity. In the polyarticular presentation, more than four joints are involved, but the systemic findings are absent. This group, which makes up 25% of patients, may also exhibit hematologic findings. Pauciarticular JRA is characterized by involvement of fewer than four joints and is rarely associated with hematologic abnormalities.

The incidence of anemia is 50–60% in patients with systemic or polyarticular JRA and 10% in pauciarticular arthritis. The anemia usually correlates with disease activity, worsening during acute flare-ups, but there is no relationship to the duration of illness.[79] The red blood cells may be normochromic, normocytic or microcytic, or hypochromic. The reticulocyte count is usually low.[80,81] Iron studies often show low serum iron, increased free erythrocyte protoporphyrin, low-normal or elevated total iron binding capacity, and normal or low serum ferritin. Serum erythropoietin levels are usually mildly elevated (but not as high as in iron deficiency).[82] The bone marrow does not show erythroid hyperplasia in response to the anemia and has diminished (but not absent) iron stores.[83] The etiology of the anemia may be anemia of chronic disease or iron deficiency anemia, or both. It is difficult to differentiate the two, as the laboratory findings in anemia of chronic disease may overshadow those of iron deficiency.[81]

True iron deficiency may be more prevalent than expected, because patients often have impaired intestinal absorption of iron and chronic blood loss due to aspirin-induced gastritis. A clinical trial of iron may be indicated in children with a low hemoglobin or mean corpuscular volume for their age even when associated with normal ferritin.[80] Less common causes of anemia are erythroid aplasia,[84] suppression of erythropoiesis by circulating inhibitors,[85] hemolysis, and a macrocytic anemia probably related to increased folate clearance and low plasma and red cell folate levels.[86,87]

In systemic JRA, leukocytosis with mean WBC counts $\leq 30,000/mm^3$ and neutrophilia with a left shift occur in 90% of patients, especially those with active disease. Leukocytosis is less common in polyarticular arthritis and is usually absent in pauciarticular disease.[88–90] Leukocytosis is so prevalent in systemic JRA that the presence of neutropenia should alert the clinician to question the diagnosis and ensure that other possibilities such as systemic lupus erythematosus (SLE) and ALL are not overlooked.[91,92] Acute leukemia in children may present with fever, joint pain, hepatosplenomegaly, and isolated cytopenias. Since about 4% of children with acute leukemia are misdiagnosed as having JRA,[93] it is important to perform a bone marrow aspirate to rule out leukemia in any patient thought to have systemic JRA before corticosteroid therapy is instituted.

Nonetheless, neutropenia has been reported in several patients with JRA.[94,95] Other causes of neutropenia are bone marrow suppression due to therapy with gold or nonsteroidal anti-inflammatory drugs[96] and, in adults, Felty syndrome—the triad of rheumatoid arthritis, splenomegaly, and neutropenia.[97] Studies of neutrophil function have demonstrated mild defects in chemotaxis and phagocytosis.[98,99] About 50% of patients with systemic JRA have >5% eosinophils on the peripheral smear.[100] Basophilia[101] and plasmacytoid lymphocytes[102] have also been reported. Studies of cellular immunity are conflicting, demonstrating normal or increased T- and B-lymphocyte number, increased immunoglobulin synthesis and secretion, and either impaired or normal delayed hypersensitivity and lymphoproliferative response to mitogens.[103–106] Monocyte dysfunction with decreased Fc receptor expression, decreased nitroblue tetrazolium activity, and decreased complement-mediated phagocytosis has been described.[107,108]

The platelet count is elevated in 50% of patients with systemic JRA.[88] Thrombocytopenia may result from bone marrow suppression by gold therapy,[96,109] rare consumptive coagulopathy,[110] or platelet trapping in Felty syndrome.[79] Since thrombocytopenia is uncommon in JRA, an unexplained low platelet count should lead one to consider alternative diagnoses, such as SLE or ALL.[111] On the other hand, isolated thrombocytopenia may be the only presenting sign in a child who later develops JRA or another collagen vascular disease. Therefore, one should consider JRA and SLE in the differential diagnosis of ITP in a girl who is >9 years. Appropriate screening tests for autoantibodies (e.g., antinuclear antibody, direct Coombs test) should be performed at diagnosis and periodically if new symptoms develop.[112,113]

A consumptive coagulopathy may occur in children with systemic JRA after hepatic damage from aspirin or gold therapy, or during disease flare-ups treated with nonsteroidal anti-inflammatory drugs when serum albumin is low. These patients are often very ill and may require corticosteroid therapy as well as platelet and coagulation factor replacement to control the coagulopathy.[110,114] The incidence of coagulation abnormalities in nonbleeding patients with systemic JRA is controversial. One study demonstrated prolonged prothrombin time (PT) and partial thromboplastin time (PTT), as well as elevated fibrinogen, factor VIII, and fibrinopeptide A levels in $\leq 50\%$ of these patients.[115] Other reports have not confirmed such findings.[114] Antibodies against factor VIII[116] and the lupus anticoagulant[117] are occasionally seen in these children.

Kawasaki Disease

Kawasaki disease is an acute multisystem disorder characterized by abrupt onset of fever unresponsive to antibiotics; bilateral conjunctival infection; reddening of the lips, tongue, or oral mucosa; reddening, induration, or peeling of the hands or feet; polymorphous truncal rash; and cervical lymphadenopathy. This disorder occurs most commonly in children <2 years old and has many features of a severe vasculitis. The most serious complication is the development of coronary artery aneurysms, which occur in 20% of children and are responsible for the 3% mortality rate associated with coronary artery thrombosis or rupture.[118–120]

Children with Kawasaki disease may have a mild normochromic, normocytic anemia with reticulocytopenia.[121] Leukocytosis is almost universal, with mean neutrophil counts of 21,000/mm³. Ninety-five percent of patients have neutrophilia with a left shift persisting for ≤ 3 weeks.[122] The role of activated neutrophils and monocytes in aneurysm development is unclear, since both impaired and enhanced phagocyte function have been described.[123,124] Studies of cellular immunity show normal total T-cell numbers but decreased suppressor T cells, causing relatively elevated T-helper-cell levels during the first 4 weeks of disease.[125] The change in T-cell subsets plus B-lymphocyte stimulation may contribute to the exaggerated production of all major immunoglobulin classes during the first 8 weeks of the disease.[126] Circulating immune complexes and high C3 (but not C4) levels are found during weeks 1–3. Impressive thrombocytosis occurs in 85% of patients by the second week, peaking during the third.[120] Platelet counts of ≤ 2 million are not uncommon, and the mean platelet count is 700,000/mm³.[122,127] However, 2% of patients may have thrombocytopenia caused by a consumptive coagulopathy.[128] Platelets demonstrate hyperaggregation on exposure to ADP, epinephrine, and collagen in vitro. These abnormalities may persist for as long as 9 months after diagnosis.[129,130] During the first month, levels of factor VIII, fibrinogen, thromboxane B_2, and thromboglobulin are increased. AT III and fibrinolytic activity are decreased. The PT, PTT, and thrombin time are usually normal.[131,132]

Prevention and treatment of existing coronary aneurysms are the primary therapeutic goal. Aspirin suppresses platelet aggregation[129] but does not affect aneurysm formation. Combining aspirin with high-dose intravenous γ-globulin infusions reduces aneurysm formation, decreases fever, and normalizes laboratory signs of inflammation.[133–135] Corticosteroid therapy increases aneurysm formation and should be avoided.[136] The treatment of Kawasaki syndrome has recently been reviewed.[137]

Henoch-Schönlein Purpura

Henoch-Schönlein purpura (HSP) is a systemic vasculitis characterized by unique purpuric skin lesions, transient arthralgias or arthritis (especially affecting the knees and ankles), olicky abdominal pain, and nephritis.[138] Recognition of HSP is important not so much for its hematologic abnormalities (which are rare) as for the unusual nonthrombocytopenic purpuric lesions that are frequently confused with the hemorrhagic rash of ITP.

HSP occurs most commonly in children 3–7 years old, often 1–3 weeks after an upper respiratory illness. The presenting complaint in 50% of children is a characteristic rash, which may begin as urticaria. As these eruptions fade, they are replaced by brownish red maculopapular lesions and petechiae. The petechiae coalesce, forming areas of raised or "palpable" purpura on the buttocks, legs, and extensor surfaces of the arms with a symmetric distribution. The rash may fade and recur for months, especially with increased activity. Children <3 years of age often have painful soft tissue swellings of the scalp and face (especially periorbital areas) and dorsum of hands and feet.[138]

Sixty-seven percent of patients experience colicky abdominal pain, often associated with vomiting, hematemesis, or melena, from submucosal hemorrhage and edema of the small bowel wall. With severe edema, the bowel wall may become a leading point for intussception.[138,139]

Renal involvement occurs in 50% of patients, especially boys and older children. Hematuria, either microscopic or gross, may occur with proteinuria during the first 3 weeks of the illness. With progressive involvement, hypertension, impaired renal function, and, finally, renal failure in 15% of children may occur, with an associated mortality rate of 3%.[138,140]

Anemia occasionally develops as a result of gastrointestinal tract blood loss or decreased red cell production caused by renal failure. The leukocyte count is normal. Despite the impressive purpura, the platelet count is normal or increased, with normal platelet function.[138,141] Coagulation factor levels are usually normal, although transient decreases in factor XIII activity[142,143] and vitamin K deficiency from severe vasculitis-induced intestinal malabsorption[144] have been reported. Bleeding in the gastrointestinal tract, the lungs, or (rarely) the central nervous system is due to a necrotizing vasculitis and not a hemostatic defect.[139,141]

HSP may be a systemic form of IgA nephropathy.[145] Both disorders have identical renal biopsy findings and are characterized by mesangial proliferation, occasional focal sclerosis, and crescent formation.[146,147] Immune complexes of IgA with complement, IgG, or IgM have been found circulating in the serum[148,149] and deposited in blood vessel walls of the kidney and in intestinal and skin lesions.[150] The mechanism of production, accumulation, and deposition of IgA immune complexes in the blood vessel is unclear.[151]

Treatment is mainly supportive, although corticosteroids have been used to provide symptomatic relief with severe joint or abdominal complaints.[152] They do not alter skin or renal involvement. The prognosis is good for full recovery except for the children with renal failure.

CARDIOPULMONARY DISEASE

Congenital Heart Disease

Congenital heart disease occurs in about 1% of live births.[153] Structural heart malformation usually follows predictable patterns, so six defects account for 70% of all cardiac disorders: ventricular septal defect, atrial septal defect, tetralogy of Fallot, patent ductus arteriosus, pulmonary stenosis, and aortic stenosis. Children with cardiac abnormalities may be acyanotic or cyanotic, depending on the underlying lesion. Hematologic abnormalities occur most often in children with cyanotic congenital heart disease (CCHD).

Polycythemia, an increased red cell mass for age, is the bone marrow response to chronic hypoxemia in patients with CCHD. The decreased arterial oxygen saturation stimulates erythropoietin production, which in turn increases erythropoiesis. The resultant increased red cell mass increases the oxygen-carrying capacity of the blood, resulting in improved tissue oxygenation.[154] With adequate compensation, erythropoietin levels fall to normal, while higher red cell production is maintained.[155] A second compensatory mechanism is an increase in 2,3-diphosphoglycerate levels in the red cell when the arterial oxygen tension is <70 mmHg. The higher 2,3-diphosphoglycerate levels cause a right shift of the oxyhemoglobin curve, resulting in greater oxygen release to the tissues.

Polycythemia in the cyanotic child is beneficial up to a point. Because the relationship between the hematocrit and blood viscosity is a hyperbolic curve, minor increases in the hematocrit above 70% cause marked increases in blood viscosity.[156] This higher viscosity results in impaired blood flow through the smaller vessels, with less tissue oxygen delivery. This impairment is magnified in severe polycythemia (hematocrit >75%) such that headache, irritability, dyspnea, and even pulmonary, renal, or central nervous system thrombi may occur.[157] To prevent these complications, the hematocrit should be maintained around 60% through the use of therapeutic erythropheresis. Small aliquots of the patient's blood are slowly removed and replaced by equal volumes of plasma or 5% albumin.[158] Care should be taken to remove blood slowly, as vascular collapse, cyanosis, stroke, and seizures have been reported with too rapid an exchange.[159]

Infants with CCHD are at risk of developing iron deficiency anemia. This may result from the combination of poor iron stores at birth (especially in premature infants), increased iron needed for enhanced erythropoiesis, poor iron intake due to poor feeding, and ongoing iron losses as a consequence of phlebotomy or erythropheresis. These children may exhibit symptoms of iron deficiency (irritability, anorexia, poor weight gain) or worsening cyanosis. The hemoglobin may be normal or high for age, but inappropriately low for the degree of hypoxemia. Hypochromic and microcytic red cells are better indices of iron deficiency in this setting.[160,161] Polycythemic children with iron deficiency anemia are at increased risk of cerebral vascular thrombosis because of the poor deformability of the iron-deficient red cell, which further increases blood viscosity.[162–164] To prevent this complication and to allow for maximal tissue oxygenation, all infants with CCHD should be fed iron-rich infant formula and receive iron replacement therapy as needed.[165]

Routine screening of patients with congenital heart disease has demonstrated coagulation abnormalities in 20–59% of children with acyanotic defects and in 40–50% of those with CCHD[166] (Table 151-2). Only 11% of children with CCHD have any clinical evidence of bleeding preoperatively.[167] However, children with underlying hemostatic defects have a greater frequency and severity of postoperative bleeding.[166,168] Presurgical testing should include at least the platelet count, bleeding time, PT, and PTT. Fibrinogen, fibrin split products, thrombin time, platelet function, and clot lysis time should be assessed with any history of bleeding or any abnormality revealed on the screening tests. Children with polycythemia have contracted plasma volumes. Therefore, when collecting blood samples, extra care should be taken to ensure the proper 1:9 ratio of 3.8% sodium citrate to blood, to prevent artificial abnormalities of coagulation tests.

The etiology of the coagulation abnormalities in CCHD is unclear. Earlier reports suggesting a role for consumptive coagulopathy have not been confirmed.[156,169,170] Protein C levels in 8 of 29 term infants with CCHD were significantly lower than controls, with no evidence of familial deficiency. Of these, 2 had thrombotic complications and 4 had consumptive coagulo-

Table 151-2. Coagulation Abnormalities in Congenital Heart Disease

	Acyanotic (%)	Cyanotic (%)
Prolonged bleeding time	11	28
Prolonged PT		20
Prolonged PTT		19
Thrombocytopenia	12–40	0–36
Abnormal platelet aggregation	14	38–70
Increased fibrinolysis	12	0–10
Abnormal clot retraction	10	
Low fibrinogen	16	12
Increased fibrin split products		Occasionally
Decreased factors II, V, VII, VIII, IX, X, XI, XII		Occasionally
Decreased protein C		25%[171]
Decreased large multimers of von Willebrand factor		100[a]

[a] Twelve patients studied; true prevalence unknown.[177]
(Adapted from Lascari,[1] with permission.)

pathy.[171] Platelets have shortened survival times (even with normal counts), and normal to increased numbers of megakaryocytes in the bone marrow are reported.[172] This increased platelet destruction does not appear to be due to DIC. Both the platelet and coagulation abnormalities are directly proportional to the degree of hypoxemia and polycythemia.[168,170] For example, children with oxygen saturation >60% have mean platelet counts of 315,000/mm^3, whereas those with saturation <60% have a mean of 185,000/mm^3.[172] The mild platelet and coagulation abnormalities are usually improved or corrected after surgical repair of the heart defect.[166,173] With bleeding, or if surgery is not possible, the coagulopathy may be improved by correction of polycythemia to a hematocrit of 60% by using slow plasma exchange transfusion.[158,174–176]

Cystic Fibrosis

Cystic fibrosis (CF) is a multisystem disorder of exocrine gland dysfunction characterized by chronic pulmonary disease, pancreatic exocrine insufficiency, hepatic dysfunction, abnormal reproductive organ function, and intestinal obstruction associated with abnormally high sweat electrolyte levels.[178] It is an autosomal recessive disease with an incidence of 1 in 2,000 live births.

Most children with CF are chronically hypoxic, yet they do not have the expected augmented erythroid response. In a study of 42 children with CF, Vichinsky et al[179] showed that none had polycythemia and 30% (especially the boys and the older children) had a normochromic, normocytic, or hypochromic, microcytic anemia with reticulocytopenia. Compared with children with CCHD, there was no appropriate increase in red cell 2,3-DPG levels, no right shift of oxyhemoglobin curve, and either a low or a normal erythropoietin level. In vitro assays showed normal erythroid progenitor cell numbers and no serum inhibitor of erythropoiesis. Of the 25 children studied, ≤ 66% had abnormalities consistent with iron deficiency, and all responded to oral or parenteral iron therapy. It appears that the etiology of anemia in CF is multifactorial. A blunted erythropoietic response to hypoxia plus iron deficiency secondary to iron malabsorption or poor dietary iron intake (or both) may all be partially responsible for the development of anemia. If iron deficiency persists despite adequate oral supplementation, one should consider the possibility of ongoing

blood loss or iron malabsorption that may necessitate the use of parenteral iron replacement.

Studies of neutrophil function in children with CF give conflicting results. Some reports indicate impaired chemotaxis, chemiluminescence, granule release, and superoxide production[180–182]; others have demonstrated factors in patient sputum that actually enhance neutrophil and monocyte responses to stimulants.[183–185] Although these sputum factors may improve neutrophil killing ability, they may also worsen neutrophil-mediated lung damage. Evaluation of immune function has revealed impaired lymphoproliferative responses to *Pseudomonas* and other gram-negative bacterial antigens, defective opsonization, increased levels of circulating immune complexes, and decreased numbers of T-helper cells in 30% of patients.[186] The contribution of these findings to frequent pulmonary infection is still under investigation.

Children with CF usually do not experience clinically significant bleeding due to impaired hemostasis, despite the risk of liver disease and vitamin K deficiency from malabsorption in this patient population. Routine coagulation tests usually yield normal results with an occasional prolonged PTT reported. A study by Corrigan et al.[187] revealed that 60% of 24 patients had a more subtle deficiency of prothrombin activity thought to be due to vitamin K deficiency. Another 11% had decreased prothrombin antigen levels, suggesting impaired liver production. Measurement of prothrombin coagulant activity may be used to assess efficacy of vitamin K replacement.

ANOREXIA NERVOSA

Anorexia nervosa is a psychiatric disorder occurring in about 1 in 800 adolescent girls; it is characterized by an inability to maintain a minimal normal body weight, intense fear of being fat, body image distortion, and amenorrhea. The profound weight loss is accompanied by hypothermia, hypotension, edema, lanugo, and metabolic changes and has a mortality rate of 5–18%.[188]

A mild, normochromic, normocytic anemia with reticulocytopenia occurs in 30% of patients.[189] Acanthocytes or spur cells have been reported and may be due to low serum β-lipoprotein levels. The causes of the anemia are most likely decreased red cell production and a relative increase in plasma volume. A few patients have had a slightly decreased red cell survival. Despite low serum iron and decreased marrow iron stores in 80% of patients, iron deficiency anemia is uncommon, except during recovery, when iron supplementation is necessary. Serum vitamin B$_{12}$ and folate are usually normal.[190]

Fifty percent of patients have leukopenia with an absolute decrease in numbers of neutrophils, lymphocytes, and monocytes.[189,191] The neutropenia may be quite severe, yet an increased incidence of infection does not occur. Studies of neutrophil compartments have shown normal bone marrow reserves despite marrow hypoplasia and a normal to slightly decreased size of the marginated pool, suggesting an ability to respond to infection.[190,191] Impaired neutrophil chemotaxis, intracellular killing of staphylococcus, and decreased complement levels have been demonstrated in patients. These are associated with occasional skin abscess formation.[189] Lymphocytes may have impaired proliferative response to mitogens or poor or absent delayed hypersensitivity, or the number of circulating T cells may be decreased.[192]

Patients with anorexia nervosa have no apparent bleeding diathesis. The platelet count is normal to slightly decreased,[189,193] and in vitro platelet aggregation to epinephrine, ADP, and collagen is exaggerated.[194,195] Coagulation defects are ıncommon except for vitamin K deficiency reported in buımia.[196]

The bone marrow in anorexia nervosa becomes hypoplastic, with loss of fat stores and replacement by a gelatinous acid mucopolysaccharide ground substance.[197] Focal or extensive necrosis may be present.[198] Bone marrow histiocytes are relatively increased in number and have prominent blue-green granules.[190] With nutritional treatment, bone marrow hypoplasia reverses, the gelatinous material disappears, and the hematologic abnormalities, including the neutrophil defects and low complement levels, resolve in 8 weeks.[189,190]

HEMATOLOGIC ASPECTS OF POISONING

Poisoning is an important problem in children.[199–201] It has been estimated that approximately 6 million children, most <5 years old, ingest toxins each year. The effects of toxins on the blood are diverse, usually nonspecific, and in most situations are overshadowed by the nonhematologic manifestations of the exposure.[202] However, with certain toxins, bleeding, anemia, or change in the appearance of the blood may be an important component of the clinical sequelae of an acute exposure.

The abnormalities of hemostasis after poisoning are numerous, and the mechanisms vary. Bleeding may be the only manifestation of warfarin toxicity secondary to an overdose of the drug or ingestion of a rodenticide containing warfarin. Any hepatotoxic substance (e.g., iron or acetaminophen) may lead to decreased synthesis of clotting factors and a resultant coagulopathy. Bleeding in these circumstances is delayed for ≥24 hours, although there appears to be an early coagulopathy in iron poisoning that may be due to a direct effect on clotting protein function and not hepatotoxicity.[203] DIC has been seen after ingestion of mushrooms of the *Amanita* genus[204] or a bite from the brown recluse spider *(Loxosceles reclusa)*.[205] Poisonous snake bites can result in coagulation abnormalities characterized by hypofibrinogenemia with or without thrombocytopenia or a DIC-like syndrome.[202]

Acute hemolytic anemia may be the presenting manifestation of exposure to drugs and toxins in children with G6PD deficiency or hemoglobin Zürich[206,207] or (rarely) in normal children.[208] Severe hemolytic anemia has been seen after the bite of the brown recluse spider[205,209] and after a wasp sting.[210]

Exposure to certain toxins may result in characteristic color changes of the blood, which in turn may be reflected clinically in abnormal skin color. The child with methemoglobinemia (see below) presents with a "slate gray" cyanosis unresponsive to 100% oxygen administration. On exposure to air, the blood retains a distinct brown color. Patients with toxic exposure to carbon monoxide or cyanide have increased levels of carboxyhemoglobin or cyanohemoglobin, respectively, resulting in a "cherry-red" color of the blood and skin, but only with relatively high concentrations of the offending hemoglobin.

Infants (≤4 months of age) are at particular risk of developing methemoglobinemia because of a reduced amount (about 60% of normal) of cytochrome b_5 reductase present in neonatal red cells. Nursery epidemics of methemoglobinemia have been reported in normal newborns exposed to disinfectants or aniline dyes used to mark diapers.[211] Infants fed formulas made with well water containing a high concentration of nitrates have developed methemoglobinemia. Although the list of oxidants reported to cause methemoglobinemia is long,[212] methemoglobinemia is uncommonly seen in infants and children. Nonetheless, a recent report of methemoglobinemia after metoclopramide overdose in an infant emphasizes the need to be alert to this complication.[213]

Lead Poisoning

Lead poisoning in children has been a serious public health problem for decades. However, the most serious toxicities of lead (e.g., encephalopathy) commonly seen in the past are rarely encountered today, primarily because of measures instituted to decrease lead exposure (no-lead paint, no-lead gasoline) and the screening programs in high-risk areas. Nonetheless, lead toxicity remains a problem, especially in large metropolitan areas, where an estimated 2,380,600 children have levels >15 μg/dl.[214] Of these children, 5.2% have levels >20 μg/dl, and 1.4% have levels >25 μg/dl. There is recent concern that long-term neurobehavioral, cognitive, and developmental effects can be seen at lower levels of lead (>15 μg/dl) than were previously thought harmful.[215]

The primary hematologic effect of lead is interference at multiple points along the heme synthetic pathway.[216] The two most important effects are inhibition of δ-aminolevulinic acid dehydratase[217] and ferrochelatase,[218] resulting in the accumulation of heme intermediates such as protoporphyrin. A shortened red cell survival accompanies lead poisoning and is probably due to decreased activity of pyrimidine 5′-nucleotidase (also resulting in basophilic stippling of the red cell) and possibly inhibition of G6PD and the pentose shunt.[219]

The anemia of lead poisoning has classically been described as a hypochromic, microcytic anemia, as might be expected from the effects of lead on heme synthesis. Although anemia has been said to be a common finding in lead intoxication, in reality anemia is uncommon unless the lead poisoning is severe, or associated iron deficiency is present.

The association between lead poisoning and iron deficiency in children is strong. Both tend to occur in the same population of predominantly lower socioeconomic status children. Experimentally, iron deficiency has been shown to increase lead absorption, retention in tissues, and toxicity.[220] Lead may impede iron absorption and metabolism, thus leading to a vicious cycle of increasing lead toxicity and worsening iron deficiency. In a study of children with lead poisoning (blood lead levels of ≥30 μg/dl), 86% were found to have iron deficiency, and 100% of those with more severe lead poisoning (Centers for Disease Control [CDC] risk classification III)[221] were iron deficient.[222]

There have now been a number of reports of children with lead toxicity documenting the infrequent occurrence of anemia without concomitant iron deficiency. Cohen et al.[223] found anemia in 12% and microcytosis in 21% of iron-sufficient children with severe lead poisoning (CDC classes III and IV). The combination of anemia plus microcytosis, however, was found in only 1 of the 58 children. In less severely affected children (CDC classes I–III) Yip et al.[222] found a 30% incidence of anemia, but of those with either mild or no iron deficiency, only 6% were anemic. Clark et al.,[224] using multiple linear regression analysis, found transferrin saturation to be the most important predictor of mean corpuscular volume, hemoglobin, and zinc protoporphyin levels in children with lead poisoning. Two important points emerge from the foregoing information: (1) children with significant lead poisoning may have neither anemia nor microcytosis, and (2) children with documented lead poisoning should be screened for underlying iron deficiency. The immediate treatment and long-term management of lead poisoning are beyond the scope of this chapter.[225]

SPLENOMEGALY

Splenomegaly is a problem frequently encountered by both the pediatrician and the pediatric hematologist. Although the spleen is rarely a site of primary disease, it may reflect systemic involvement with a variety of disorders. The spleen is the largest collection of lymphoid tissue in the body. It demonstrates a unique association between the bloodstream and the reticuloendothelial compartment.[226] Splenomegaly may result when there is antigenic stimulation of the lymphoid system (e.g., infection), obstruction of blood flow within or distal to the spleen (e.g., portal vein obstruction), exaggeration of one of the normal functions of the spleen due to an underlying abnormality (e.g., hemolytic anemia, splenic sequestration), or infiltration of the spleen by a foreign cell (e.g., leukemia, storage diseases).

The spleen tip is normally palpable in preterm infants; ≤30% of full-term neonates have a palpable spleen.[227] A spleen can be felt in ≤5–10% of normal children, but most of these are in the infant/toddler age group. As a general rule, a spleen easily palpable below the costal margin in any child >3–4 years of age must be considered abnormal until proven otherwise. That some palpable spleens may indeed be normal is attested to by the often-quoted study of McIntyre and Ebaugh,[228] reporting that 3% of healthy college freshmen have palpable spleens, of which about one-third persist. "Pretenders" of splenomegaly include the left lobe of the liver, a left upper quadrant tumor such as Wilms tumor or neuroblastoma, the "wandering spleen,"[229] and the proptotic spleen (seen in children with depressed diaphragms from obstructive pulmonary disease, such as asthma or bronchiolitis).

A list of causes of splenomegaly in children is presented in Table 151-3.[230] The most common cause of acute splenomegaly in children, especially young children, is a viral infection. Splenic enlargement in this setting is mild to moderate and usually transient. When history and physical examination suggest a viral etiology, a CBC with differential count, platelet count, and reticulocyte count should be performed to rule out unsuspected leukemia or hemolytic anemia, and to determine whether an atypical lymphocytosis is present. The child should be rechecked in approximately 4 weeks (or sooner if symptoms persist). If splenomegaly persists beyond 4–6 weeks, the splenic enlargement may be considered chronic.

When evaluating the child with chronic splenomegaly, one must consider all the possibilities noted in Table 151-3. However, clues from the history and physical examination may suggest a specific etiology and direct an approach tailored to the diagnostic laboratory evaluation. If, on the other hand, no cause is apparent for the enlarged spleen, a number of "screening" laboratory tests should be performed, including a CBC with differential count, platelet count, and reticulocyte count; evaluation of the peripheral smear; sedimentation rate; liver function tests; antibody titers to EBV, CMV, and toxoplasmosis; antinuclear antibody; and ultrasonic evaluation of the liver, spleen, and portal system (the latter with Doppler flow technique). Further evaluation, including bone marrow examination, may be necessary if the screening tests do not reveal the cause of the splenic enlargement.

Symptoms from splenic enlargement are uncommon, although massive splenomegaly may cause abdominal discomfort and early satiety. If the spleen is sufficiently large, destruction and sequestration of one or more of the formed elements of the blood may be increased. This phenomenon, termed *hypersplenism,* is associated with a mild to moderate degree of cytopenia and infrequent symptoms.

Management of splenomegaly is usually related to treatment of the underlying disease, when such treatment exists. Splenectomy may be indicated in selected conditions, but the potential benefits from splenectomy must be weighed against the risk of postsplenectomy sepsis, a rapidly progressive bacteremia, most commonly due to *S. pneumoniae,* with a mortality rate of approximately 50%.[231] The risk of postsplenectomy sepsis depends on the age of the patient and the nature of the underlying disorder. Patients <3 years old, and those with a compromised immune or reticuloendothelial system, are most susceptible. When elective splenectomy is indicated, it is advisable to (1) postpone surgery until the patient is ≥5–6 years of age, (2) administer pneumococcal vaccine ≥1–2 weeks before splenectomy, (3) use prophylactic penicillin for ≥2–4 years, and (4) manage significant febrile illnesses as possible postsplenectomy sepsis at all times.

Table 151-3. Splenomegaly in Children

Disorders of the blood
    Hemolytic anemia: congenital/acquired
    Thalassemia
    Sickle cell disease
    Leukemia
    Osteopetrosis
    Myelofibrosis/myeloid metaplasia
Infections: acute and chronic
    Viral
        Congenital (TORCH)
        Mononucleosis (EBV, CMV)
        Virus associated hemophagocytic syndrome
        Human immunodeficiency virus
    Bacteria
        Sepsis/abscess
        Brucellosis
        Salmonella
        Tularemia
        Tuberculosis
        Subacute bacterial endocarditis
        Syphilis
        Lyme disease
    Fungal
        Histoplasmosis (disseminated)
    Rickettsial
        Rocky Mountain spotted fever
        Cat scratch disease
    Parasitic
        Toxoplasmosis
        Malaria
        Leishmaniasis (kala-azar)
        Schistosomiasis
        Echinococcosis
Hepatic/portal system disorder
    Acute/chronic active hepatitis
    Cirrhosis/hepatic fibrosis/biliary atresia
    Portal or splenic venous obstruction (Banti syndrome)
Connective tissue disease
    Juvenile rheumatoid arthritis
    Systemic lupus erythematosus
Neoplasms/cysts
    Lymphomas (Hodgkin and non-Hodgkin)
    Hemangiomas/lymphangiomas
    Hamartomas
    Congenital or acquired (post-traumatic) cysts
Storage diseases/inborn errors of metabolism
    Lipidoses: Gaucher disease, Niemann-Pick disease, etc.
    Mucopolysaccharidoses
    Defects in carbohydrate metabolism: galactosemia, fructose intolerance
    Sea blue histiocyte syndrome
Miscellaneous
    Histiocytoses
        Reactive
        Langerhans cell
        Malignant
    Sarcoidosis
    Congestive heart failure

REFERENCES

1. Lascari AD: Hematologic Manifestations of Childhood Diseases. Thieme-Stratton, New York, 1984
2. Jansson LT, Kling S, Dallman PR: Anemia in children with acute infection seen in primary care pediatric outpatient clinic. Pediatr Infect Dis 5:424, 1986
3. Reeves JD, Yip R, Kiley VA et al: Iron deficiency in infants: the influence of mild antecedent infection. J Pediatr 105:874, 1984
4. Abshire TC, Reeves JD: Anemia of acute inflammation in children. J Pediatr 103:868, 1983
5. Odio C, Buchanan GR: Anemia in children with acute bacterial infection. Clin Res 31:901A, 1983
6. Chow CB, Leung NK: Anemia with typhoid fever (letter). Pediatr Infect Dis 5:495, 1986
7. Crosby E, Llosa L, MiroQuesada M et al: Hematologic changes in brucellosis. J Infect Dis 150:419, 1984
8. Schiavone DJ, Rublo S: Anemia associated with *Haemophilus influenzae* meningitis. Lancet 2:696, 1953
9. Kaplan KM, Oski FA: Anemia with *Haemophilus influenzae* meningitis. Pediatrics 65:1101, 1980
10. O'Brien RT, Santos JI, Glasgow L et al: Pathophysiologic basis for anemia associated with *Haemophilus influenzae* meningitis: preliminary observations. J Pediatr 98:928, 1981
11. Sills RH, Caserta MT, Landaw SA: Decreased erythrocyte deformability in the anemia of bacterial meningitis. J Pediatr 101:395, 1982
12. Buchanan GR: The mild anemia of acute infection. Pediatr Infect Dis 4:225, 1985
13. Shurin SB, Anderson P, Zollinger J et al: Pathophysiology of hemolysis in infections with *Hemophilus influenzae* type b. J Clin Invest 77:1340, 1986
14. Dacie JV: The auto-immune hameolytic anemias. p. 525. In: The Haemolytic Anemias. Congenital and Acquired. J&A Churchill, London, 1962
15. Dacie JV: Secondary or symptomatic haemolytic anemia. p. 908. In: The Haemolytic Anemias. Congenital and Acquired. J&A Churchill, London, 1967
16. Kattanis CA, Tjortjatou F: The hemolytic process of viral hepatitis in children with normal or deficient glucose-G-phosphate dehydrogenase activity. J Pediatr 77:422, 1970
17. Smith MA, Shah NR, Lobel JS et al: Methemoglobinemia and hemolytic anemia associated with *Campylobacter jejuni* enteritis. Am J Pediatr Hematol Oncol 10:35, 1988
18. Habibi B, Homberg JC, Schaisan G et al: Autoimmune hemolytic anemia in children. Am J Med 56:61, 1974
19. Buchanan GR, Boxer LA, Nathan DG: The acute and transient nature of idiopathic immune hemolytic anemia in childhood. J Pediatr 88:780, 1976
20. Gasser C: Aplasia of erythropoiesis. Acute and chronic erythroblastopenias or pure (red cell) aplastic anaemias in childhood. Pediatr Clin North Am 4:445, 1957
21. Young N: Hematologic and hematopoietic consequences of B19 parvovirus infection. Semin Hematol 25:159, 1988
22. Anderson MJ, Higgins PG, Davies LR et al: Experimental parvovirus infection in humans. J Infect Dis 152:257, 1985
23. Van Horn DK, Mortimer PP, Young NS et al: Human parvovirus associated red cell aplasia in the absence of underlying hemolytic anemia. Am J Pediatr Hematol Oncol 8:235, 1986
24. Carstensen H, Ornvold K, Cohen BJ: Human parvovirus B19 infection associated with prolonged erythroblastopenia in a leukemic child. Pediatr Infect Dis J 8:56, 1989
25. Kurtzman G, Ozawa K, Cohen B et al: Bone marrow failure due to chronic B19 parvovirus infection. N Engl J Med 317:287, 1987
26. Kurtzman G, Frickhofen N, Kimball J et al: Pure red-cell aplasia of 10 years' duration due to persistent parvovirus B19 infection and its cure with immunoglobulin therapy. N Engl J Med 321:519, 1989
27. Smith MA, Shah NS, Lobel JS: Parvovirus B19 infection associated with reticulocytopenia and chronic autoimmune hemolytic anemia. Am J Pediatr Hematol Oncol 11:167, 1989
28. Griffin TC, Squires JC, Timmons CF, Buchanan GR: Chronic human parvovirus B19-induced erythroid hypoplasia as the initial manifestation of human immunodeficiency virus infection. J Pediatr 118:899, 1991
29. Weitzman M: Diagnostic utility of white blood cell and differential cell counts. Am J Dis Child 129:1183, 1975
30. Todd JK: Childhood infections. Diagnostic value of peripheral white blood cell and differential cell counts. Am J Dis Child 127:810, 1974
31. McCarthy PL, Jekel JF, Dolan TF: Temperature greater than or equal to 40C in children less than 24 months of age. A prospective study. Pediatrics 59:663, 1977
32. Sadowitz PD, Oski FA: Differences in polymorphonuclear cell counts between healthy white and black infants: response to meningitis. Pediatrics 72:405, 1983
33. Buranski B, Young N: Hematologic consequences of viral infections. Hematol Oncol Clin North Am 1:167, 1987
34. Alario AJ, O'Shea JS: Risk of infectious complications in well-appearing children with transient neutropenia. Am J Dis Child 143:973, 1989
35. Strausbaugh LJ: Hematologic manifestations of bacterial and fungal infections. Hematol Oncol Clin North Am 1:185, 1987
36. Lukens JN: Eosinophilia in children. Pediatr Clin North Am 19:969, 1972
37. Shantz PM, Glickman LT: Current conception in parasitology. Toxocaral visceral larva migrans. N Engl J Med 298:436, 1978
38. Addegio JE, Mentzer WC, Dallman PR: Thrombocytosis in infants and children. J Pediatr 85:805, 1974
39. Thomas GA, O'Brien RT: Thrombocytosis in children with *Hemophilus influenzae* meningitis. Clin Pediatr 25:610, 1986
40. Kelpi T, Anttila M, Kallio MJT, Peltola H: Thrombocytosis and thrombocytopenia in childhood bacterial meningitis. Pediatr Infect Dis J 11:456, 1992
41. Heath HW, Pearson HA: Thrombocytosis in pediatric outpatients. J Pediatr 114:805, 1989
42. Chan KW, Kaikov Y, Wadsworth LD: Thrombocytosis in childhood. Pediatrics 84:1064, 1989
43. Nathan DG, Oski FA (eds): Platelet abnormalities in infancy and childhood. p. 1587. In Hematology of Infancy and Childhood. 4th Ed. WB Saunders, Philadelphia, 1993
44. Blatt J, Penchansky L, Horn M: Thrombocytosis as a presenting feature of acute lymphoblastic leukemia in childhood. Am J Hematol 31:46, 1989
45. Ware R, Kurtzberg J, Friedman HS et al: Chronic immune-mediated thrombocytopenia after varicella infection. J Pediatr 112:742, 1988
46. Corrigan JJ: Thrombocytopenia: a laboratory sign of septicemia in infants and children. J Pediatr 85:219, 1974
47. Kelton JG, Neame PB, Gauldie J et al: Elevated platelet-associated IgG in the thrombocytopenia of septicemia. N Engl J Med 300:760, 1979
48. Francis RB: Acquired purpura fulminans. Semin Thromb Hemost 16:310, 1990
49. Spicer TE, Rau JM: Purpura fulminans. Am J Med 61:566, 1976
50. Hanada T, Abe T, Takita H: Antithrombin III concentrates for treatment of disseminated intravascular coagulation in children. Am J Pediatr Hematol Oncol 7:3, 1985
51. Powars DR, Rogers ZR, Patch MJ et al: Purpura fulminans in meningococcemia: association with acquired deficiencies of proteins C and S. N Engl J Med 317:571, 1987
52. Madden RM, Gill JC, Marlar RA: Protein C and protein S levels in two patients with acquired purpura fulminans. Br J Haematol 75:112, 1990
53. Leclerc F, Hazelzet J, Jude B et al: Protein C and S deficiency in severe infectious purpura of children: a collaborative study of 40 cases. Intensive Care Med 18:202, 1992
54. Anderson CT, Berde CB, Sethna NF, Pribas JJ: Meningococcal purpura fulminans: treatment of vascular insufficiency in a two year old child with lumbar epidural sympathetic blockade. Anesthesiology 71:463, 1989
55. Irazuzta J, McManus ML: Use of topically applied nitroglycerin in the treatment of purpura fulminans. J Pediatr 117:993, 1990
56. Keeley SR, Matthews NT, Brust M: Tissue plasminogen activator for gangrene in fulminant meningococi anemia. Lancet 2:1359, 1991
57. Brodeur GM, O'Neill PJ, Wilimas JA: Acquired inhibitors of coagulation in nonhemophiliac children. J Pediatr 96:439, 1980
58. Currimbhoy Z: Transitory anticoagulants in healthy children. Am J Pediatr Hematol Oncol 6:210, 1984
59. Ryan HR, Arkel Y, Walters TR et al: Acquired symptomatic inhibitors of plasma clotting factors in nonhemophilic children. Am J Pediatr Hematol Oncol 8:144, 1986
60. Orris DJ, Lewis JH, Spero JA et al: Blocking coagulation inhibitors in children taking penicillin. J Pediatr 97:426, 1980
61. Epstein M, Pearson ADJ, Hudson SJ et al: Necrobacillosis with pancytopenia. Arch Dis Child 67:958, 1992
62. Doran TI, Parmley RT, Logas PC et al: Infection with *Erlichia canis* in a child. J Pediatr 114:809, 1989
63. McClain K, Gehrz R, Grierson H et al: Virus-associated histiocytic proliferations in children. Am J Pediatr Hematol Oncol 10:196, 1988
64. Falloon J, Eddy J, Wiener L et al: Human immunodeficiency virus infection in children. J Pediatr 114:1, 1989

65. Revision of the CDC surveillance case definition for acquired immunodeficiency syndrome. MMWR, suppl. 36:35, 1987
66. Ryan B, Connor E, Minnefor A et al: Human immunodeficiency virus (HIV) infection in children. Hematol Oncol Clin North Am 1:381, 1987
67. Zon LI, Groopman JE: Hematologic manifestations of the human immune deficiency virus (HIV). Semin Hematol 25:208, 1988
68. Ellaurie M, Burns ER, Rubenstein A: Hematologic manifestations in pediatric HIV infection: severe anemia as a prognostic factor. Am J Pediatr Hematol Oncol 12:449, 1990
69. McCance-Katz EF, Hoecker JC, Vitalo NB: Severe neutropenia associated with anti-neutrophil antibody in a patient with acquired immunodeficiency syndrome-related complex. Pediatr Infect Dis J 6:417, 1987
70. Burns ER, Krieger B-Z, Bernstein L et al: Acquired circulating anticoagulants in children with acquired immunodeficiency syndrome. Pediatrics 82:763, 1988
71. Ellaurie M, Burns ER, Bernstein LJ et al: Thrombocytopenia and human immunodeficiency virus in children. Pediatrics 82:905, 1988
72. Weinblatt ME, Scimeca PG, James-Herry AG et al: Thrombocytopenia in an infant with AIDS. Am J Dis Child 141:15, 1987
73. Bussel JB, Haimi JS: Isolated thrombocytopenia in patients infected with HIV: treatment with intravenous gamma-globulin. Am J Hematol 28:79, 1988
74. Hilgartner M: Guidelines for the care of children and adolescents with HIV infection. Hematologic manifestations in HIV-infected children. J Pediatr 119:S47, 1991
75. Working Group on Antiretroviral Therapy: National Pediatric HIV Resource Center: antiretroviral therapy and medical management of the human immunodeficiency virus-infected child. Pediatr Infect Dis J 12:513, 1993
76. Saulsbury FT, Boyle RJ, Wykoff RF et al: Thrombocytopenia as the presenting manifestation of human T-lymphotropic virus type III infection in infants. J Pediatr 109:301, 1986
77. Kurtzberg J, Friedman HS, Kinney TR et al: Management of human immunodeficiency virus-associated thrombocytopenia with intravenous gamma globulin. Am J Pediatr Hematol Oncol 9:299, 1987
78. Behrman RE, Vaughan VC III (eds): Rheumatic diseases of childhood. p. 515. In: Nelson Textbook of Pediatrics. 13th Ed. WB Saunders, Philadelphia, 1987
79. Mowat AG: Connective tissue diseases. Clin Haematol 1:573, 1972
80. Koerper M, Stempel D, Dallman P: Anemia in patients with juvenile rheumatoid arthritis. J Pediatr 92:930, 1978
81. Harvey A, Peppard M, Ansell B: Microcytic anemia in juvenile chronic arthritis. Scand J Rheumatol 16:53, 1987
82. Ward H, Gordon B, Pickett J: Serum levels of erythropoietin in rheumatoid arthritis. J Lab Clin Med 74:93, 1969
83. Cavill I, Bentley D: Erythropoiesis in the anaemia of rheumatoid arthritis. Br J Haemotol 50:583, 1982
84. Rubin R, Walker B, Ballas S et al: Erythroid aplasia in juvenile rheumatoid arthritis. Am J Dis Child 132:760, 1978
85. Dainiak N, Hardin J, Floyd V et al: Humoral suppression of erythropoiesis in systemic lupus erythematosus (SLE) and rheumatoid arthritis. Am J Med 69:537, 1980
86. Omer A, Mowat AG: Nature of anemia in rheumatoid arthritis. IX: Folate metabolism in patients with rheumatoid arthritis. Ann Rheum Dis 27:414, 1968
87. Alter H, Zvaifler N, Rath C: Interrelationship of rheumatoid arthritis, folic acid, and aspirin. Blood 38:405, 1971
88. Calabro J, Staley H, Burnstein I et al: Laboratory findings in juvenile rheumatoid arthritis. Arthritis Rheum 20:268, 1977
89. Calabro J, Holgerson W, Sonpal G et al: Juvenile rheumatoid arthritis: a general review and report of 100 patients observed for 15 years. Semin Arthritis Rheum 5:257, 1976
90. Griffen P, Tachdjian M, Green W: Pauciarticular arthritis in children. JAMA 184:23, 1963
91. Sills E: Errors in diagnosis of juvenile rheumatoid arthritis. Johns Hopkins Med J 133:88, 1973
92. Ostrov BE, Goldsmith DP, Athreya BH: Differentiation of systemic juvenile rheumatoid arthritis from acute leukemia near the onset of disease. J Pediatr 122:595, 1993
93. Schaller J: Arthritis as a presenting manifestation of malignancy in children. J Pediatr 81:793, 1972
94. Scopelitis E, Perez M, Biundo J: Leukopenia in Still's disease. JAMA 252:2450, 1984
95. Scopelitis E, Perez M, Biundo J: Letters to the editor. JAMA 253:2194, 1985
96. Thompson D, Pegelow C, Singsen B et al: Neutropenia associated with chryso therapy for juvenile rheumatoid arthritis. J Pediatr 93:871, 1978
97. Felty A: Chronic arthritis in the adult associated with splenomegaly and leukopenia. Bull Johns Hopkins Hosp 35:16, 1924
98. Mowat A, Baum J: Chemotaxis of polymorphonuclear leukocytes from patients with rheumatoid arthritis. J Clin Invest 50:2541, 1971
99. Turner R, Schumacker H, Myers A et al: Phagocytic function of polymorphonuclear leukocytes in rheumatic diseases. J Clin Invest 52:1632, 1973
100. Sylvester R, Pinals R: Eosinophilia in rheumatoid arthritis. Ann Allergy 28:565, 1970
101. Athreya B, Moser G, Raghaven T: Increased circulating basophils in juvenile rheumatoid arthritis. Am J Dis Child 129:935, 1975
102. Delborre F, LeGo A, Kahan A: Hyperbasophilic immunoblasts in circulating blood in chronic inflammatory rheumatic and collagen diseases. Ann Rheum Dis 34:422, 1975
103. Tsokos G, Mauridis A, Ingherami G et al: Cellular immunity in patients with systemic juvenile rheumatoid arthritis. Clin Immunol Immunopathol 42:86, 1987
104. Alarcon-Requelme M, Vasquez-Mellado J, Gomez-Cordillo M et al: Immunoregulatory defect in juvenile rheumatoid arthritis: comparison between patients with the systemic or polyarticular forms. J Rheumatol 15:1547, 1988
105. Silverman ED, Somma C, Khan MM et al: Abnormal T-cell suppressor cell function in juvenile rheumatoid arthritis. Arthritis Rheum 33:205, 1990
106. DeBendetti F, Marconi M, Ravelli A et al: Multiple inhibitors of mitogen-induced proliferation of normal lymphocytes in juvenile chronic arthritis sera. Clin Exp Rheumatol 8:505, 1990
107. Marek-Szydlowski T, Uracz W, Ruggiero I et al: Juvenile rheumatoid arthritis: monocyte dysfunction in selected patients. Clin Pediatr 27:551, 1988
108. Hurst N, Nuki G: Evidence for defect of complement-mediated phagocytosis by monocytes from patients with rheumatoid arthritis and cutaneous vasculitis. Br Med J 282:2081, 1982
109. Coblyn J, Weinblatt M, Holdsworth D et al: Gold-induced thrombocytopenia: a clinical and immunogenetic study of twenty-three patients. Ann Intern Med 95:178, 1981
110. Silverman E, Miller J, Bernstein B et al: Consumption coagulopathy associated with systemic juvenile rheumatoid arthritis. J Pediatr 103:872, 1983
111. Sherry D, Kredich D: Transient thrombocytopenia in systemic onset juvenile rheumatoid arthritis. Pediatrics 76:600, 1985
112. Miller B, Beardsley D: Autoimmune pancytopenia of childhood associated with multisystem disease manifestations. J Pediatr 103:877, 1983
113. McClure P: Idiopathic thrombocytopenic purpura in children: diagnosis and management. Pediatrics 55:68, 1975
114. Mukamel M, Bernstein B, Brik R et al: Prevalence of coagulation abnormalities in juvenile rheumatoid arthritis. J Rheumatol 14:1147, 1987
115. Scott J, Gerber P, Maryjowski M et al: Evidence for intravascular coagulation in systemic onset, but not polyarticular juvenile rheumatoid arthritis. Arthritis Rheum 28:256, 1985
116. Green D, Schuelte P, Wallace W: Factor VIII antibodies in rheumatoid arthritis: effect of cyclophosphamide. Arch Intern Med 140:1232, 1980
117. Schleider M, Nachman R, Jaffle E et al: A clinical study of the lupus anticoagulant. Blood 48:499, 1976
118. Hicks R, Melish M: Kawasaki's disease. Pediatr Clin North Am 33:1151, 1986
119. Melish M: Kawasaki's syndrome: a 1986 perspective. Rheum Dis Clin Am 13:7, 1987
120. Monens D, Anderson L, Hurwitz E: National surveillance of Kawasaki's disease. Pediatrics 65:21, 1980
121. Yanagihara R, Todd J: Acute febrile mucocutaneous lymph node syndrome. Am J Dis Child 134:603, 1980
122. Melish M, Hicks R, Larson E: Mucocutaneous lymph node syndrome in the United States. Am J Dis Child 130:599, 1976
123. Ono S, Onimaru T, Kawakami K et al: Impaired granulocyte chemotaxis and increased circulating immune complexes in Kawasaki's disease. J Pediatr 106:567, 1985
124. Kuratsuji T, Takagi K, Tsunawaki S: Etiologic role of phagocytes in Kawasaki disease. Acta Paediatr Jpn 33:778, 1991
125. Abe J, Katzin BL, Meissner C et al: Characterization of T-cell repertoire changes in acute Kawasaki's disease. J Exp Med 177:791, 1993
126. Kawamori J, Miyake T, Yoshidu T: B-cell function in Kawasaki disease and the effect of high dose gammaglobulin therapy. Acta Paediatr Jpn 31:537, 1989
127. Centers for Disease Control: Kawasaki's disease—United States. MMWR 27:9, 1978
128. Hara T, Mizuno Y, Akida H: Thrombocytopenia: a complication of Kawasaki's disease. Eur J Pediatr 147:51, 1988
129. Yamada K, Fukumoto T, Shinkai A et al: The platelet functions in acute febrile mucocutaneous lymph node syndrome: a trial for prevention of thrombosis by antiplatelet agents. Acta Haematol Jpn 41:113, 1978

130. Levin M, Holland P, Nokes T et al: Platelet immune complex interaction in pathogenesis of Kawasaki's disease and childhood polyarteritis. Br Med J 290:1456, 1985

131. Burns J, Glode M, Clarke I et al: Coagulopathy and platelet activation in Kawasaki syndrome: identification of patients at high risk for development of coronary artery aneurysms. J Pediatr 105:206, 1984

132. Hidaka T, Nakano M, Ueta T et al: Increased synthesis of thromboxane A_2 by platelets from patients with Kawasaki's disease. J Pediatr 102:94, 1983

133. Furusho K, Nakano H, Shinomuja K et al: High-dose intravenous gammaglobulin for Kawasaki's disease. Lancet 2:1055, 1984

134. Newburger J, Takahashi M, Burns J et al: Treatment of Kawasaki syndrome with intravenous gammaglobulin. N Engl J Med 315:341, 1986

135. Rowley A, Shulman S: What is the status of intravenous gammaglobulin for Kawasaki syndrome in the United States and Canada? Pediatr Infect Dis J 7:463, 1988

136. Kato H: Kawasaki's disease: effect of treatment on coronary artery involvement. Pediatrics 63:175, 1979

137. Rowley AH, Shulman ST: Current therapy for acute Kawasaki syndrome. J Pediatr 118:987, 1991

138. Allen D, Diamond L, Howell D: Anaphylactoid purpura in children (Schönlein-Henoch syndrome): review with a follow-up of the renal complications. Am J Dis Child 99:833, 1960

139. Clark J, Fitzgerald J: Hemorrhagic complications of Henoch-Schönlein syndrome. J Pediatr Gastroenterol Nutr 4:311, 1985

140. Meadow R: Schönlein-Henoch syndrome. Arch Dis Child 54:822, 1979

141. Byrn J, Fitzgerald J, Northway J et al: Unusual manifestations of Henoch-Schönlein syndrome. Am J Dis Child 130:1335, 1976

142. Henriksson P, Hedner U, Nelsson I: Factor XIII (fibrin stabilizing factor) in Henoch-Schönlein purpura. Acta Pediatr Scand 66:273, 1977

143. Dalen B, Travade P, Labbe A et al: Diagnostic and prognostic value of fibrin stabilizing factor in Schönlein-Henoch syndrome. Arch Dis Child 58:12, 1983

144. McNairy SL, Milins J, Phyliky R et al: Vitamin K-responsive coagulopathy in Henoch-Schönlein purpura. Mayo Clin Proc 52:746, 1977

145. Waldo F: Is Henoch-Schönlein purpura the systemic form of IgA nephropathy? Am J Kidney Dis 12:373, 1988

146. Urizor R, Michael A, Herdman R et al: Anaphylactoid purpura. II: Immunofluorescent and electron microscopic studies of the glomerular lesions. Lab Invest 119:437, 1969

147. Heaton J, Turner D: Localization of glomerular deposits in Henoch-Schönlein purpura. Histopathology 1:93, 1977

148. Levinsky R, Barrott T: IgA immune complexes in Henoch-Schönlein purpura. Lancet 2:1100, 1979

149. Kauffmann R, Herrmann W, Meyer C: Circulating IgA-immune complexes in Henoch-Schönlein purpura: a longitudinal study of their relationship to disease activity and vascular deposition of IgA. Am J Med 69:859, 1980

150. Giangiacomo J, Tsai C: Dermal and glomerular deposition of IgA in anaphylactoid purpura. Am J Dis Child 131:981, 1977

151. Saulsbury F: Role of IgA rheumatoid factor in the formation of IgA-containing immune complexes in Henoch-Schönlein purpura. J Clin Lab Immunol 23:123, 1987

152. Rosenblum N: Steroid effects on the course of abdominal pain in children with Henoch-Schönlein purpura. Pediatrics 79:1018, 1987

153. Bayne E: Etiology, diagnosis, and management of congenital cardiac disorders. Compr Ther 14:31, 1988

154. Gidding S, Stockman J: Erythropoietin in cyanotic heart disease. Am Heart J 116:128, 1988

155. Haja P, Cotes P, Till J et al: Is oxygen supply the only regulator of erythropoietin levels? Acta Pediatr Scand 76:907, 1987

156. Maurer H: Hematologic effects of cardiac disease. Pediatr Clin North Am 19:1083, 1972

157. Strong WB: Complications of polycythemia in patients who have cyanotic congenital heart disease. Pediatr Rev 13:379, 1992

158. Komp D, Carpenter M, Nolan S et al: Preoperative phlebotomy in children with cyanotic heart disease (letter to the editor). J Pediatr 84:313, 1974

159. Rosenthal A, Nathan D, Marty A et al: Acute hemodynamic effects of red cell volume reduction in polycythemia of cyanotic congenital heart disease. Circulation 42:297, 1970

160. Gidding S, Stockman J: Effect of iron deficiency on tissue oxygen delivery in cyanotic congenital heart disease. Am J Cardiol 61:605, 1988

161. Gedding S, Bessel M, Liao Y: Determinant of hemoglobin concentration in cyanotic heart disease. Pediatr Cardiol 11:121, 1990

162. Cottrill C, Kaplan S: Cerebral vascular accidents in cyanotic congenital heart disease. Am J Dis Child 125:484, 1973

163. Linderkamp O, Klose H, Betke K et al: Increased blood viscosity in patients with cyanotic congenital heart disease and iron deficiency. J Pediatr 95:567, 1979

164. West D, Scheel J, Stoverk et al: Iron deficiency in children with cyanotic congenital heart disease. J Pediatr 117:266, 1990

165. Gidding S, Rosenthal A: Iron supplementation in cyanotic congential heart disease. Clin Pediatr 27:261, 1988

166. Kontras S, Sirak H, Newton W: Hematologic abnormalities in children with congenital heart disease. JAMA 195:611, 1966

167. Maurer H, McCue C, Caul J et al: Impairment in platelet aggregation in congenital heart disease. Blood 40:207, 1972

168. Ekert H, Gilchrist G, Stanton R et al: Hemostasis in cyanotic congenital heart disease. J Pediatr 76:221, 1970

169. Waldman J, Czapek E, Paul M et al: Shortened platelet survival in cyanotic heart disease. J Pediatr 87:77, 1975

170. Wedemeyer A, Edson J, Krivit W: Coagulation in cyanotic congenital heart disease. Am J Dis Child 124:656, 1972

171. Macdonald PD, Gibson BE, Braunlie J et al: Protein C activity in severely ill newborns with congenital heart disease. J Perinat Med 20:421, 1992

172. Gross I, Keefer V, Liebman J et al: The platelet in cyanotic congenital heart disease. Pediatrics 42:651, 1968

173. Ekert H, Sheers M: Preoperative and postoperative platelet function in cyanotic congenital heart disease. J Thorac Cardiovasc Surg 67:184, 1974

174. Kontras S, Bodenbender J, Craenen J et al: Hyperviscosity in congenital heart disease. J Pediatr 76:214, 1970

175. Maurer H, McCue C, Robertson L et al: Correction of platelet dysfunction and bleeding in cyanotic congenital heart disease by simple red cell volume reduction. Am J Cardiol 35:831, 1975

176. Von Kaulla K, Paton B, Rosenkrantz J et al: Preoperative correction of coagulation in tetralogy of Fallot. Arch Surg 94:107, 1967

177. Gill J, Wilson A, Endres-Brooks J et al: Loss of largest von Willebrand factor multimers from the plasma of patients with congenital cardiac defects. Blood 67:758, 1986

178. Behrman RE, Vaughan VC III (eds): Cystic fibrosis. p. 926. In: Nelson Textbook of Pediatrics. 13th Ed. WB Saunders, Philadelphia, 1987

179. Vichinsky E, Pennathur-Das R, Nickerson B et al: Inadequate erythroid response to hypoxia in cystic fibrosis. J Pediatr 105:15, 1984

180. Kemp T, Schram-Doumont A, Van Geffel R et al: Alteration on the N-formyl-methionyl-leucyl-phenylalanine-induced response in cystic fibrosis neutrophils. Pediatr Res 20:520, 1986

181. Lawrence RH, Sorrelli TC: Decreased polymorphonuclear leukocyte chemotactic response to leukotriene B_4 in cystic fibrosis. Clin Exp Immunol 89:321, 1992

182. Graff I, Schran Doumount A, Szpirer C: Defective protein kinase C-mediated actions in cystic fibrosis neutrophils. Cell Signal 3:259, 1991

183. Kharazmi A, Rechnitzer C, Schiotz P et al: Priming of neutrophils for enhanced oxidative burst by sputum from cystic fibrosis patients with *Pseudomonas aeruginosa* infection. Eur J Clin Invest 17:256, 1987

184. Regilmann W, Lundi N, Porter P: Increased monocyte chemiluminescence in cystic fibrosis patients and in their parents. Pediatr Res 20:619, 1986

185. Roberts RL, Stiehm R: Increased phagocytic cell chemiluminescence in patients with cystic fibrosis. Am J Dis Child 143:944, 1989

186. Krutsen A, Slavin R, Roodman S et al: Decreased T-helper cell function in patients with cystic fibrosis. Int Arch Allergy Appl Immunol 85:208, 1988

187. Corrigan J, Taussig L, Beckerman R et al: Factor II (prothrombin) coagulant activity and immunoreactive protein: detection of vitamin K deficiency and liver disease in patients with cystic fibrosis. J Pediatr 99:254, 1981

188. Anorexia Nervosa (307.10). In: Diagnostic and Statistical Manual of Mental Disorders. 3rd Ed. American Psychiatric Association, Washington, 1987

189. Kay J, Strickler RB: Hematologic and immunologic abnormalities in anorexia nervosa. South Med J 76:1008, 1983

190. Mant MJ, Faragher BS: The haematology of anorexia nervosa. Br J Haematol 23:727, 1972

191. Bowers TK, Eckert E: Leukopenia in anorexia nervosa: lack of increased risk of infection. Arch Intern Med 138:1520, 1978

192. Cason J, Ainley CC, Wolstencroft RA et al: Cell-mediated immunity in anorexia nervosa. Clin Exp Immunol 64:370, 1986

193. Amrun PC, Friedman R, Kosinski K et al: Hematologic changes in anorexia nervosa. JAMA 241:2190, 1979

194. Luck P, Mikhailidis DP, Dashwood R et al: Platelet hyperaggregability and increased adrenocepter density in anorexia nervosa. J Clin Endocrinol Metab 57:911, 1983

195. Mikhailidis DP, Barradas MA, DeSouza V et al: Adrenaline-induced hyperaggregability of platelets and enhanced thromboxane release in anorexia nervosa. Prostaglandins Leukotr Med 24:27, 1986

196. Nuya K, Kitagaiva T, Fujishita M: Bulemia nervosa complicated by deficiency of vitamin K-dependent coagulation factors. JAMA 250:792, 1983

197. Pearson H: Marrow hypoplasia in anorexia nervosa. J Pediatr 71:211, 1967
198. Smith R, Spivak JL: Marrow cell necrosis in anorexia nervosa and involuntary starvation. Br J Haematol 60:525, 1985
199. Dickerman JD, Lucey JF (eds): Smith's The Critically Ill Child: Diagnosis and Medical Management. 3rd Ed. WB Saunders, Philadelphia, 1985, p. 78
200. Arena JM: Poisoning. Toxicology. Symptoms. Treatment. 5th Ed. Charles C Thomas, Springfield, IL, 1986
201. Behrman RE, Vaughan VC III (eds): Poisonings from food, drugs, chemicals, pollutants, and venomous bites; mammalian bites. p. 1491. In: Nelson Textbook of Pediatrics. 13th Ed. WB Saunders, Philadelphia, 1987
202. Sauter D, Goldfrank L: Hematologic aspects of toxicology. Hematol Oncol Clin North Am 1:335, 1987
203. Tenenbein M, Israels SJ: Early coagulopathy in severe iron poisoning. J Pediatr 113:695, 1988
204. Sanz P, Reig R, Borrias L et al: Disseminated intravascular coagulation and mesenteric venous thrombosis in fatal *Amanita* poisoning. Hum Toxicol 7: 199, 1988
205. Wasserman GS, Anderson PL: Loxoscelism and necrotic arachnidism. J Toxicol 21:451, 1984
206. Beutler E: Drug-induced hemolytic anemia. Pharmacol Rev 21:73, 1969
207. Kattamis CS, Kyriazakou M, Chaidas S: Favism: clinical and biochemical data. J Med Genet 6:34, 1969
208. Wong KY, Boose GM, Issitt MS: Erythromycin-induced hemolytic anemia. J Pediatr 98:647, 1981
209. Ginsburg CM, Weinberg AG: Hemolytic anemia and multiorgan failure associated with localized cutaneous lesion. J Pediatr 112:496, 1988
210. Monzon C, Miles J: Hemolytic anemia following a wasp sting. J Pediatr 96: 1039, 1980
211. Scott EP, Prince GE, Rotondo C: Dye poisoning in infancy. J Pediatr 28:713, 1946
212. Curry S: Methemoglobinemia. Ann Emerg Med 11:214, 1982
213. Kearns GL, Fiser DH: Metoclopramide-induced methemoglobinemia. Pediatrics 82:364, 1988
214. Childhood lead poisoning—United States: report to the Congress by the Agency for Toxic Substances and Disease Registry. MMWR 37:481, 1988
215. Needleman HL, Schell A, Bellinger D et al: The longterm effects of exposure to low doses of lead in childhood. An 11 year follow-up report. N Engl J Med 322:83, 1990
216. Piomelli S: Lead poisoning. p. 472. In Nathan DG, Oski FA (eds): Hematology of Infancy and Childhood. 4th Ed. WB Saunders, Philadelphia, 1993

217. deBruin A, Hoolboom H: Early signs of lead-exposure. A comparative study of laboratory tests. Br J Ind Med 24:203, 1967
218. Gibson SM, Goldberg A: Defects in haeme synthesis in mammalian tissues in experimental lead poisoning and experimental porphyria. Clin Sci 38:63, 1970
219. Lachant NA, Tomoda A, Tanaka KR: Inhibition of the pentose phosphate shunt by lead: a potential mechanism for hemolysis in lead poisoning. Blood 63:518, 1984
220. Six KM, Goyer RA: The influence of iron deficiency on tissue content and toxicity of ingested lead in rats. J Lab Clin Med 79:128, 1972
221. United States Public Health Service Statement: Preventing Lead Poisoning in Young Children. Centers for Disease Control, Atlanta, 1978
222. Yip R, Norris TN, Anderson AS: Iron status of children with elevated blood lead concentrations. J Pediatr 98:922, 1981
223. Cohen AR, Trotzky MS, Pincus D: Reassessment of the microcytic anemia of lead poisoning. Pediatrics 67:904, 1981
224. Clark M, Royal J, Seeler R: Interaction of iron deficiency and lead and the hemotologic findings in children with severe lead poisoning. Pediatrics 81: 247, 1988
225. Mofensan HC, Caraccio TR, Gruef JW: Chronic lead poisoning in children. p. 757. In Burg FD, Ingelfinger JR, Wald ER (eds): Current Pediatric Therapy. WB Saunders, Philadelphia, 1993
226. Baehner RC, Miller DR. The spleen and disorders of the monocyte-macrophage (reticuloendothelial) system. p. 722. In Miller DR, Bachner RL, McMillan CW (eds): Blood Diseases of Infancy and Childhood. CV Mosby, St. Louis, 1984
227. Munolini F, Merlob P, Ashkenazi S et al: Palpable spleens in newborn term infants. Clin Pediatr 24:197, 1985
228. McIntyre CR, Ebaugh FG Jr: Palpable spleens in college freshmen. Ann Intern Med 66:301, 1967
229. Vermylen C, Lebecque P, Claus D et al: The wandering spleen. Eur J Pediatr 140:112, 1983
230. Oclan LF, Tubergen DG: Splenomegaly in children. Identifying the cause. Postgrad Med 64:191, 1979
231. Singer DB: Postsplenectomy sepsis. p. 285. In Rosenberg HS, Bolander RP (eds): Perspectives in Pediatric Pathology. Year Book Medical Publishers, Chicago, 1973
232. Dallman PR, Rudolph AM (eds): Pediatrics. 17th Ed. Appleton-Century-Crofts, East Norwalk, CT, 1982
233. Nathan DG, Oski FA (eds): Hematology of Infancy and Childhood. 3rd Ed. WB Saunders, Philadelphia, 1987, p. 1679.

Hematologic Problems in Patients with Cancer and Chronic Inflammatory Disorders

152

Irwin M. Weinstein and Barry E. Rosenbloom

HEMATOLOGIC PROBLEMS IN PATIENTS WITH CANCER

In patients with malignancy, hematologic abnormalities are encountered with considerable frequency.[1-8] These abnormalities result directly from the malignancy or as a consequence of treatment.

Red Blood Cells

Anemia

Anemia is the most common hematologic abnormality seen in association with cancer, occurring in approximately 50% of patients during the course of their illness.[1,2] Review of the red

Table 152-1. Causes of Anemia in Cancer

Anemia of chronic disease
Tumor invasion
Pure red cell aplasia
Anemia due to blood loss
    Acute hemorrhage
    Iron deficiency (chronic blood loss)
Treatment-related anemia
Anemia due to nutritional causes
Hemolytic anemias
    Immunohemolytic anemia
    Microangiopathic hemolytic anemia
    Drug-associated hemolytic anemia
    Hemophagocytic syndrome

blood cell indices, reticulocyte count, peripheral smear, iron studies, hemolytic studies, and bone marrow examination usually delineate the etiology (Table 152-1).

Anemia of Chronic Disease

Anemia of chronic disease (ACD) is the most common type seen with nonhematologic malignancies.[9-11] It can manifest early in the course of disease in association with cancer, and the severity of anemia can parallel the extent of the underlying cancer. Although bone marrow involvement may be present, it is not required to cause this type of anemia. The etiology of ACD is unclear.

Treatment has until recently been limited to treatment of the underlying disease or blood transfusions. However, regular administration of human erythropoietin (EPO) can ameliorate the ACD associated with cancer.[12-17]

Tumor Invasion of the Marrow

Marrow invasion by solid tumors can be seen most frequently with small cell lung cancer, breast cancer, prostate cancer, and lymphoma. Anemia occurs as a direct result of replacement of the marrow with tumor. Peripheral smears may show a leukoerythroblastic pattern; with severe involvement, pancytopenia can occur. Extensive bone marrow fibrosis can accompany marrow invasion, further exaserbating the peripheral blood abnormalities. Treatment of the underlying malignancy, blood transfusions, and more recently EPO administration have been beneficial.[15]

Pure Red Cell Aplasia

Although rare, pure red cell aplasia has been reported with neoplasms other than thymoma, including lymphoid tumors, non-small cell lung cancer, breast cancer, and gastric cancer. The bone marrow typically shows a marked reduction of erythroid precursors, and plasma EPO levels are markedly increased. In approximately one-half the cases, an autoantibodiy directed against red blood cell progenitors can be observed.[18,19] In T-cell chronic lymphocytic leukemia, T-lymphocyte suppression of erythropoiesis has been described, and this may be operative in patients with other types of malignancies.[20,21] Treatment of pure red cell aplasia in patients with thymoma by thymectomy is successful in one-third of cases. Resection of the malignancy in patients with other types of tumors is also successful. However, most such patients need immunosuppressive therapy, including corticosteroids, high-dose immunoglobulin, antithymocyte globulin, danazol, and cytotoxic agents. Blood transfusion support is invariably required.

Anemia Due to Blood Loss

Iron deficiency is frequently the initial manifestation of patients with gastrointestinal malignancies. Renal carcinoma and bladder carcinoma may lead to blood loss through hematuria. Postgastrectomy patients may re-bleed at sites of marginal ulcerations, and achlorhydria can impair iron absorption. The clinical distinction between iron deficiency and ACD may be difficult. Serum iron and transferrin levels can be low in both, but serum ferritin levels <10 mg/L are almost always due to iron deficiency. The presence of blood in the stools or urine is presumptive evidence for iron deficiency. Bone marrow iron stores are markedly reduced or absent.

Appropriate diagnostic studies to determine the site of blood loss should be the initial step. Treatment with oral iron preparations or parenteral iron dextran administration can improve the anemia. However, the hemoglobin level may not return to normal because, concomitantly, ACD may be present.

Therapy-Related Anemia

Treatment of solid tumors with cytotoxic agents usually leads to bone marrow depression, which can result in anemia. Although granulocytopenia and thrombocytopenia induced by such treatments reverse within 4–7 days after their onset, the anemia may be chronic and persist throughout the course of treatment secondary to depressed erythropoiesis. Macrocytic red cell indices and megaloblastic dysplasia of the bone marrow are frequently seen.[22] Blood transfusions may be needed, and EPO administration may benefit some patients.[23]

Nutritional Causes of Anemia

Folic acid deficiency due to poor dietary intake can be seen as a result of anorexia associated with cancer. In addition, postgastrectomy patients with achlorhydria will develop vitamin B_{12} malabsorption, although anemia may take 3–5 years to develop.[24] Malnutrition per se can lead to ACD.

Hemolytic Anemias Associated with Cancer

Immunohemolytic Anemia. Autoimmune hemolytic anemia is principally associated with lymphoid malignancies. Approximately 45% of patients with angioimmunoblastic lymphadenopathy will develop this type of hemolysis, and 20–25% of patients with chronic lymphocytic leukemia will develop autoimmune hemolysis during the course of their illness.[25,26] Additionally, patients with non-Hodgkin lymphoma can develop typical autoimmune hemolytic anemia.[27] With solid tumors, this is less frequent but is well documented with squamous carcinomas of the lung and cervix, adenocarcinomas of the breast, lung, ovaries, stomach, and colon, as well as others (Table 152-2). Most patients exhibit the warm antibody pattern with a positive direct antiglobulin test (Coombs test). However, cold agglutinins can be seen with non-Hodgkin lymphoma. When treatment directed at the underlying illness is successful, hemolysis can be ameliorated. However, more often other measures, including corticosteroids, cytotoxic agents, high-dose intravenous immunoglobulins, and splenectomy, are necessary.

Microangiopathic Hemolytic Anemia. Mechanical intravascular destruction of red blood cells is relatively common with metastatic adenocarcinomas, especially those that secrete mucin.[28-30] Gastric cancer is the most frequently associated malignancy. The clinical laboratory findings associated with hemolysis are present, and, in addition, the peripheral smear will show schistocytes, helmet cells, and sometimes thrombocytopenia. In severe cases, nucleated red cells are seen in the periperal blood along with hemoglobinemia, hemoglobinuria,

Table 152-2. Immunohemolytic Anemias
Associated with Malignancy

Warm-reactive antibody type
  Hodgkin disease
  Non-Hodgkin lymphoma
  Chronic lymphocytic leukemia
  Multiple myeloma
  Wäldenstrom disease
  Angioimmunoblastic lymphadenopathy
  Ovarian teratoma
  Thymoma
  Enteric adenocarcinoma
  Breast cancer
  Kaposi sarcoma
  Seminoma
  Renal cell carcinoma
Cold-reactive antibody type
  As above plus
    Chronic granulocytic leukemia
    Carcinoid tumor
    Adrenocorticocarcinoma

(Data from Doll and Weiss.[1])

and hemosiderinuria. The etiology appears, in part, to be due to low-grade disseminated intravascular coagulation (DIC) occurring in response to tumor products in the circulation that activate coagulation. Tumor products can also cause enhanced circulating platelet aggregates, which may also cause mechanical red blood cell destruction.[31,32] Treatment is directed at the underlying tumor, but is usually incomplete because of the advanced state of the neoplasms associated with this complication.

Drug-Associated Hemolysis. Mitomycin C has been associated with a syndrome of microangiopathic hemolytic anemia of a severe nature, with thrombocytopenia and renal insufficiency mimicking de novo hemolytic uremic syndrome.[33–35] Many of these patients have circulating immune complexes, and therefore an interaction of the drug with the tumor or some tumor product has been postulated as the etiology of the hemolysis. Another hypothesis is that Mitomycin C is toxic to the renal endothelium, activating clotting with resultant deposition of fibrin thrombi in the renal microvasculature. This would explain the finding of fibrin deposition in small vessels seen on renal biopsy. However, proliferative glomerular changes are also seen that are compatible with immune complex deposition. Another mechanism is that the formed immune complexes bind platelets, IgG, and complement along with tumor-associated antigens such as carcinoembryonic antigen. This type of hemolytic uremic syndrome is usually refractory to treatment, with an almost invariably fatal course. However, recent reports suggest that plasma exchange, immunoperfusion, and azothioprine may benefit some patients, especially when circulating immune complexes are etiologic.[36] A similar clinical picture has been reported with the bleomycin/cisplatinum-related Raynaud syndrome.[37,38]

Some chemotherapeutic agents have caused a warm antibody type of hemolytic anemia. This has been reported with cisplatinum, tenoposide, melphalan, and methotrexate. The mechanism appears similar to that seen with high-dose penicillin-associated hemolytic anemia.[39] Discontinuation of the drug usually leads to resolution of this hemolysis.

In patients with glucose-6-phosphate dehydrogenase deficiency, administration of doxorubicin can cause an oxidant stress, producing a hemolytic anemia.[40] Discontinuation of this drug leads to resolution.

Hemophagocytic Syndrome. The hemophagocytic syndrome has rarely been reported with gastric cancer, lymphoma, and acute leukemia.[41] This syndrome is characterized by pancytopenia, fever, lymphadenopathy, and splenomegaly. The bone marrow resembles a histiocytosis with hemophagocytosis by benign-appearing macrophages. This syndrome is unresponsive to treatment and is usually fatal within a few weeks.

Polycythemia

True erythrocytosis has been reported with certain neoplasms, including renal cell carcinoma, hepatocellular carcinoma, and cerebellar hemagioblastoma.[42–44] This phenomenon has been noted in approximately 1–3% of patients with renal cell carcinoma, and in many of these cases elevated serum EPO levels are found. Although tumor cells from these patients do contain immunoreactive EPO, erythrocytosis in patients with Wilms tumor is due to pressure-induced hypoxia of the adjacent normal renal parenchyma.[45,46] Removal of the kidney in patients with renal cell carcinoma has frequently led to reversion of the red cell mass to normal, and recurrence of the polycythemia has occurred when metastatic disease develops.

The association of secondary polycythemia and hepatocellular carcinoma may be due to the production of extrarenal EPO.[47,48] However, this mechanism has not been convincingly proved. Other mechanisms such as diminished metabolism of androgenic-like substances have been postulated.[49,50] Regardless of the etiology, if the tumor can be completely excised, reversal of this abnormality can ensue.

White Blood Cells

Leukocytosis

Mild-to-moderate leukocytosis can be seen with malignancies such as bronchogenic carcinoma, gastric carcinoma, and renal cell carcinoma. When the tumors are widespread and necrotic, a typical neutrophilic leukemoid reaction can be seen, with white counts of 50,000/mm^3 or more.[51] Counts as high as 200,000/mm^3 have been reported. The distinction between a leukemoid reaction and leukemia is sometimes confusing, but in the leukemoid reaction, immaturity is typically absent and the leukocyte alkaline phosphate score is high. The cause of this phenomenon may be tumor-elaborated colony-stimulating factors (CSF).[52,53] No specific therapy is warranted for this problem.

Leukopenia and Neutropenia

Leukopenia can be seen in association with marrow invasion due to malignancy and the associated leukoerythroblastic blood picture. More typically, leukopenia is a result of bone marrow depression due to chemotherapy. This is usually reversible within 4–7 days of onset. More rarely, prolonged leukopenia may be seen after a chemotherapeutic course with antileukemic therapy. The use of growth factors, including CSF-granulocyte (G) CSF-granulocyte/macrophage (GM), has led to an earlier recovery for these patients.[54] The use of these growth factors has become increasingly routine in treating infected neutropenic patients.[55] Furthermore, these agents are being increasingly used with high-dose chemotherapy regimens to ameliorate or prevent severe neutropenia.[56–58]

Neutropenia is frequently associated with the Tγ-cell lymphoproliferative syndrome.[59] In this disorder, T-suppressor cells appear to inhibit granulopoiesis directly. This syndrome has responded to corticosteroids, cyclophosphamide, and CSF-G (authors' personal observations).

Platelets

Thrombocytosis

Thrombocytosis associated with malignancy probably represents a reactive response to the presence of malignancy and is seen with frequency in patients with cancer,[60,61] with or without bone marrow hypercellularity and increased megakaryocytes. Whether thrombocytosis per se in part causes the hypercoaguable state seen in association with cancer is unclear. No specific treatment for this abnormality is available.

Thrombocytopenia

Modest thrombocytopenia is frequent after treatment of solid tumors with cytotoxic agents.[62] Severe life-threatening thrombocytopenia can occur in such patients, especially if they have had prior radiotherapy or incomplete recovery from prior bone marrow depressive treatment. The bleeding risk may be enhanced by concurrent infection as a result of treatment-induced granulocytopenia. In addition, the risk of gastrointestinal hemorrhage may be enhanced by breaks in mucosal integrity due to chemotherapy. Recovery from most chemotherapy occurs within 1 week after onset. However, some agents such as mitomycin C or the nitrosoureas may cause prolonged thrombocytopenia. Bone marrow invasion can also lead to thrombocytopenia, and bleomycin damage of pulmonary endothelium may lead to platelet destruction.[63]

Treatment for thrombocytopenia due to chemotherapeutic agents should follow the same guidelines established for leukemic patients. Although most patients have a spontaneous recovery of their platelets after chemotherapy, in those who have any bleeding or whose platelet counts fall too low, platelet transfusions may be necessary.

Autoimmune thrombocytopenia is most commonly seen in association with lymphoid malignancies, but also can be seen with lung cancer, breast cancer, and testicular carcinoma.[64,65] Treatment with corticosteroids, cytotoxic agents, high-dose intravenous γ-globulin, and splenectomy may be necessary if treatment of the underlying neoplasm does not improve this condition.

Coagulation Abnormalities

Cancer-Related Thrombosis

Patients with cancer have a greater tendency to thrombosis as a result of a number of causal mechanisms. This hypercoaguable state has been characteristic of patients with various malignancies. In addition to cancer patients being debilitated and possibly requiring prolonged bed rest, tumors can compress or invade blood vessels, leading to stasis, and the normal hemostatic mechanisms may become disrupted.[66–69] Also, release of tumor products into the circulation may be thrombogenic.

It has been demonstrated that many of the procoagulants are increased in patients with cancer. Fibrinogen and factors V, VII, VIII, IX, and XI have been found to be elevated.[70,71] When DIC is present, antithrombin III, protein C, and protein S can be consumed, leading to an increased tendency to thrombosis.[72] Neoplastic cells themselves can initiate the clotting cascade by releasing tissue factor, which complexes with factor VIIa in the blood to activate factor X.[73] Tissue factors have been described with lung, kidney, colon, and breast cancer. The migratory thrombotic syndrome known as Trousseau syndrome may be caused by this latter mechanism.[74,75] This clinical syndrome has sometimes been called chronic DIC when a thrombotic tendency dominates the syndrome instead of a bleeding tendency.[76]

Mucinous adenocarcinomas of the lung, gastrointestinal tract, and ovary are associated with a high risk of thrombosis. In addition, systemic trypsin from pancreatic carcinoma can activate the clotting cascade.[77]

Other mechanisms may be active, including monocytic production of procoagulant substances.[78–81] The substances expressed include tissue factor, factor X activators, and prothrombinase complex. The lupus inhibitor and anticardiolipins are seen with some malignancies. They increase the thrombotic risk, although the actual mechanism is unknown. Increased platelet aggregation is seen in patients with cancer, which may add to the risk of thrombosis.[82,83]

Treatment of cancer-related thrombosis starts with minimizing the conditions associated with thrombosis, such as prolonged bed rest and lower extremity edema. Although successful treatment of the underlying tumor can benefit these patients, many of these tumors are resistant to therapy and therefore anticoagulation should be considered. Some can be treated with warfarin, but heparin may be useful because it potentiates the anticoagulant activity of tissue-factor pathway inhibitor, which neutralizes factor VIIa-tissue factor coagulant activity.[76] In addition, warfarin lowers protein C levels and may add to the thrombotic tendency. Anticoagulation in cancer patients can be fraught with difficulties, including heparin resistance and a greater bleeding risk.[84,85] The use of thrombolytic agents is discouraged because the bleeding risk in cancer patients is high.[86]

Nonbacterial Thrombotic Endocarditis

Nonbacterial thrombotic endocarditis is a paraneoplastic thrombotic syndrome associated with predominantly neurologic complications and (less frequently) systemic embolization.[87,88] Such patients can present with embolic strokes manifested by focal or generalized neurologic findings (or both). Cardiac findings are minimal, and fever is absent. Emboli to other sites such as the spleen, kidneys, gastrointestinal tract, and coronary arteries are detected at autopsy but are rarely clinically manifest. Additional findings at autopsy include fibrin-platelet vegetations on the mitral and aortic valves. Tumors most commonly associated with this complication include non-small cell lung cancer, prostate cancer, and pancreatic cancer. Anticoagulants are of no benefit in this condition.

Cancer-Related Bleeding

DIC is a frequent cause of cancer-related bleeding. Although it is most frequently seen with prostate cancer, it has been reported with cancers of the gastrointestinal tract, ovary, and lung, as well as melanoma. Many of these patients bleed, usually mildly; bleeding can become massive after manipulating the tumor, as in prostate cancer surgery. Infections may exacerbate a compensated DIC and lead to bleeding. The treatment of DIC associated with cancer can be challenging. Treating the underlying disease is frequently inadequate. Judicious use of heparin may benefit some patients.[89]

Certain chemotherapeutic agents have been associated with hemostatic defects. L-Asparaginase can lead to the production of a functionally impaired fibrinogen, which may cause bleeding.[90] Mithramycin can cause platelet dysfunction and increased fibrinolysis, leading to an enhanced bleeding risk.[91] Suramin, which is used for refractory prostate cancer, has been associated with clinical bleeding.[92] Actinomycin D can antagonize vitamin K, and the anthracyclines have been reported to cause primary fibrinogenolysis. These effects will reverse with discontinuation of the agents.

HEMATOLOGIC PROBLEMS IN PATIENTS WITH CHRONIC INFLAMMATORY DISORDERS

Rheumatic Diseases

Inflammatory rheumatic disorders are commonly associated with hematologic abnormalities, especially anemia. The anemia of rheumatoid arthritis (RA) has been a classic model for studying ACD. Anemia and other hematopoietic dysfunctions also occur frequently in systemic lupus erythematosus (SLE). Other inflammatory states associated to a lesser degree with hematopoietic disorders include mixed connective tissue disease, polymyalgia rheumatica, dermatomyositis, scleroderma, and Sjögren syndrome.

Anemia of Rheumatic Disorders

Anemia of Chronic Disease

Anemia, usually ACD, is the most common hematologic abnormality found in rheumatic disorders.[93] The exact pathogenesis of ACD still remains a matter of debate. In 1966, Cartwright[10] postulated three basic abnormalities: impaired marrow response, possibly due to diminished production of EPO; impaired release of iron from the reticuloendothelial system; and a mild decrease in red cell survival. More recently, several studies have clarified the relationship of EPO to the anemia of RA.[94–97] The EPO level is inversely correlated with the hemoglobin level. Although EPO levels rise in response to the anemia of RA, the rise is less than that found in patients with the same degree of anemia who have other illnesses. However, the blunted EPO effect is not the primary cause of the anemia of RA since the EPO levels are still greater than normal.[98,99] Recent investigations have studied the failure of the bone marrow to respond to higher levels of EPO in chronic inflammatory disorders, particularly RA. Several cytokines involved in the inflammatory response are elevated in chronic inflammatory diseases.[100,101] These include tumor necrosis factor-α (TNF-α), interleukin (IL)-1, IL-6, interferon-α and -γ, and the pteridine neopterin, which is a marker of immune activation. IL-6, which has been shown to be increased in RA patients, produces anemia in animals and correlates with the other more common markers of inflammation such as the sedimentation rate. However, it is not clear in humans whether IL-6 is important in the pathogenesis of the anemia of RA or is merely a marker of RA activity.[102,103] Cytokines may be involved in the impaired EPO response to anemia in rheumatic disorders. IL-1 and TNF-α have been shown to inhibit EPO production from a hepatoma cell line. This effect may occur at the level of EPO mRNA.[104,105]

The pathogenesis of the disturbances of iron metabolism in rheumatoid disorders (decreased serum iron and iron binding capacity, normal or increased tissue iron) has been extensively studied. Early studies demonstrating a block in the release of reticuloendothelial iron utilizing ^{59}Fe-labeled iron have not been confirmed when smaller doses of radiolabeled iron were used.[106–110] These more recent studies also suggest that the disturbances of iron metabolism may be secondary to decreased erythropoiesis. The role of cytokines in the erythropoiesis of inflammatory disorders shows their involvement in the impairment of iron metabolism. Recombinant TNF induces anemia and hypoferremia in animals.[111,112] IL-I increases ferritin production, and this additional ferritin may trap iron, making it unavailable for red cell production.[113]

Treatment options for the ACD associated with rheumatic disorders have increased since the availability of EPO. Pharmacologic doses of EPO often ameliorate the anemia in RA patients.[114–117] EPO can also correct cytokine-induced inhibition of erythropoiesis in animals.[118,119] EPO does not correct the anemia of chronic renal disease in humans or in anemic rats in the presence of concomitant iron deficiency.[120,121]

CONSIDERATIONS REGARDING THE USE OF EPO IN INFLAMMATORY DISORDERS

1. Pretreatment EPO level is not predictive of an optimal response.
2. Therapeutic dosage usually needs to be larger than that used in patients with renal failure.
3. It is prudent to delay therapy until the effects of treatment of the underlying disorder are evaluated.
4. Coexisting iron deficiency will blunt the response of EPO, and iron deficiency can develop during EPO treatment.
5. In most circumstances an EPO trial should be avoided in mild anemia (i.e., hematocrit > 30 vol%).
6. An adequate response to EPO is an increase of the hematocrit ≥6 vol% in 6–8 weeks of therapy or relief of symptoms of anemia, or both.
7. A maintenance dose must be determined for each responder. A useful hint is to start by decreasing the dose by one-third.
8. Chronic administration of EPO is not justifiable for trivial improvement in the hematocrit or in the absence of an overall clinical improvement.

Iron-Deficiency Anemia

Iron-deficiency anemia may coexist with ACD in rheumatoid disorders. If the serum ferritin level is <10 ng/L, the diagnosis of coexisting iron deficiency is established. When levels of ferritin are this low, gastrointestinal blood loss, particularly in patients on nonsteroidal anti-inflammatory drugs,[122] is suggested. When the serum ferritin level is between 40 and 50 ng/L in patients with rheumatic disorders,[123,124] it is worthwhile to search for a source of iron loss and to begin oral iron therapy. If no response to the oral iron therapy occurs, it is recommended that a bone marrow study be done to exclude iron deficiency firmly and to see whether any unexpected reasons for the anemia are present.

Hemolytic Anemia

Acquired hemolytic anemia, usually secondary to immune mechanisms, is frequently associated with rheumatic disorders, particularly SLE. The anemia may vary from mild to severe and is typically characterized by the presence of spherocytes on the peripheral blood film. Autoimmune hemolytic anemia associated with autoimmune thrombocytopenia is occasionally seen in SLE (Evan syndrome).

Therapy of autoimmune hemolytic anemia depends on the severity of the red cell destruction. Some patients have a compensated hemolytic state and need no therapy. More often, the anemia is severe enough that treatment should be instituted with corticosteroids. Large doses are usually required (prednisone 60–100 mg/day PO). Beneficial responses occur in most patients, especially those with SLE.[125] Patients with severe anemia who have not responded to corticosteroids or in whom a large maintenance dose is required should be managed by splenectomy. However, poor-risk patients with SLE or other rheumatic syndromes may be treated first on immunosuppressive drugs, danazol, plasmapheresis, or high-dose intravenous γ-globulin. Reported results with these therapeutic modalities are contradictory.[126–131]

Acquired Pure Red Cell Aplasia

Pure red cell aplasia is an uncommon immunologic disorder that has been reported in association with both RA and SLE. Pure red cell aplasia should not be mistaken for ACD. Distinctive features are moderate-to-severe anemia, marked reticulo-cytopenia, and the findings in the bone marrow of severe hypoplasia of the red cell series and normal production of the other marrow cell lines.

Spontaneous remission occurs in about 10–15% of these patients. The management of this condition requires withdrawal of all medications. If there is no response to withdrawal nor any spontaneous remission occurring within a few weeks, corticosteroids, cytotoxic agents, antithymocyte globulin, danazol, cyclosporine, plasmapheresis, high-dose γ-globulin, and splenectomy may be considered.[132–139] Because EPO levels are very high, EPO therapy is not helpful. About two-thirds of patients in need of treatment will respond to one or more of the other modalities.

Neutropenia

With the exception of patients with SLE, neutropenia is seen infrequently in the inflammatory arthritides. In SLE, a neutropenia has been reported to occur in about one-half of patients.[140] The neutropenia in this setting is usually not severe and is not often associated with an infectious complication. Therefore, initiation of therapy is usually not indicated. Indeed, the neutropenia may worsen with cytotoxic therapy, even though the neutropenia is thought to be due to immune destruction of mature neutrophils or marrow progenitors.[141] Occasionally the neutropenia of SLE is secondary to hypersplenism.

Felty syndrome is an uncommon but important hematologic abnormality that occurs in 1% of patients with RA, developing about 15 years after the onset of the disease and usually when the arthritis is not active.[142] The characteristic triad of Felty syndrome is RA, splenomegaly, and neutropenia. The syndrome is also associated with recurrent infections, leg ulceration, rheumatoid nodules, and lymph node enlargement. The neutropenia is usually severe, ranging between 500 and 2,500/mm[3]. The mechanism of the neutropenia has been attributed to antineutrophil antibodies, increased occurrence of immune complexes, inhibition of neutrophil production mediated by T cells, altered neutrophil distribution, reduced neutrophil function, and hypersplenism.[143–145] Elevated levels of neutrophil-bound IgG and serum IgG neutrophil-binding activity are found in about one-half of RA patients with Felty syndrome.[146]

Appropriate therapy for Felty syndrome is often difficult. If infections have been infrequent and mild in nature, no intervention is needed. Repeated and serious infections or chronic leg ulceration usually require treatment. In addition to the administration of appropriate antibiotics, other therapies are usually tried with mixed results. These include cytotoxic agents, corticosteroids, methotrexate, cyclosporine, penicillamine, plasmapheresis, gold salts, and splenic radiation. The role of splenectomy remains a matter of controversy. For decades, it has been known that splenectomy normalizes the neutrophil count in about one-half of RA patients. Prior to the modern antibiotic era, mortality following splenectomy was high. It still continues to be an increased risk, and postoperative morbidity is common. In addition, the relapse rate is about a 20% with recurrence of neutropenia associated with infection and leg ulceration. Splenectomy may be more effective in patients who have high levels of serum granulocyte-binding IgG.[147] With the recent availability of leukocyte growth factors, reports are encouraging and suggest that CSF-GM may ameliorate the neutropenia of Felty syndrome.[148–153] It would appear that growth factors are useful therapy in seriously ill RA patients with Felty syndrome, but further and better controlled studies are needed. CSF-GM therapy has resulted in a flare-up of previously inactive arthritis due to the release of IL-6.[154]

Certain similarities are apparent among Felty syndrome, the T-γ lymphoproliferative disorder, and hairy cell leukemia. Both hairy cell leukemia and the Tγ lymphoproliferative disorder are malignancies that have a known association with RA.[155] Patients with hairy cell leukemia may present with complaints of arthralgias or arthritis.[156] Table 152-3 summarizes some clinical and laboratory findings of these three syndromes.

Coagulation Disturbances
Thrombocytopenia

Thrombocytopenia, usually autoimmune in type, frequently occurs in the rheumatoid disorders, especially in patients with SLE.[157] It has also been reported in dermatomyoisitis, scleroderma, and mixed connective tissue disease. Thrombocytopenia is rare in RA, and its presence should alert the consultant to the possibility of a drug-related etiology or an unrelated primary bone marrow disorder. The therapy of autoimmune thrombocytopenic purpura in SLE is similar to that used in the management of idiopathic thrombocytopenic purpura, except that some evidence shows that splenectomy is less likely to be effective in SLE patients.[158] Patients with SLE who fail corticosteroid therapy should be considered for alternative therapies other than splenectomy. These include cyclophosphamide, azothiaprine, vincristine, danazol, or high-dose

Table 152-3. Differential Diagnosis of Syndromes Associated with Rheumatoid Arthritis

	Peripheral Blood	Bone Marrow	Spleen Size	Lymph Node Size	Tartaric Acid Phosphatase Activity	Renal Abnormalities	Cell Markers
Felty syndrome	Absolute neutropenia Cytopenias No characteristic cell	Normal Hypercellular Hypocellular	Splenomegaly prominent	Enlargement common	Negative	Usually absent	Normal or variable abnormalities
T-γ lymphoproliferative disorder	Lymphocytosis Cytopenias (neutropenia) Characteristic large granular lymphocyte	Lymphocytic infiltration	Splenomegaly present, not prominent	Enlargement rare	Rarely positive	Commonly present	Suppressor cytotoxic T cells CD2+, CD3+, CD8+, CD16+
Hairy cell leukemia	Cytopenias Characteristic hairy cell	Dry aspirate Hairy cells on biopsy	Splenomegaly present, not prominent	Enlargement rare	Positive Nearly pathognomonic	Usually absent	B-cell origin CD11+, CD19+, CD20+, CD22+

intravenous γ-globulin. The prognostic significance of autoimmune thrombocytopenia in SLE patients has been a matter of dispute. The platelet count is probably not a prognostic indicator in SLE.[159]

While thrombotic thrombocytopenic purpura is associated with SLE, the relationship appears to be an example of distinct clinical entities occurring together in an immunologically compromised host, rather than a causal association. In patients with SLE who have neurologic symptoms along with thrombocytopenia, thrombotic thrombocytopenic purpura should be considered. Aggressive plasmapheresis is the treatment of choice and is usually effective.[160,161]

Thrombocytosis

Thrombocytosis occurs in about one-half of patients with RA. The increased platelet count is an acute-phase reactant correlating positively with the sedimentation rate and the clinical activity of the disease.[162] This reactive thrombocytosis is almost never in excess of 1 million/mm^3. Usually, the increased platelet count is 400,000–700,000/mm^3. The reactive thrombocytosis in these patients is only rarely associated with abnormal bleeding or clotting.

The Lupus Inhibitor

An elevated partial thromboplastin time (PTT) is frequently found in patients with rheumatoid disorders, especially SLE. Typically, these patients have no history of bleeding nor any familial bleeding tendency. Most often, this elevation of the PTT is due to the presence of a lupus anticoagulant. Although the first reported case was of a hemorrhagic disorder,[163] this syndrome is generally not associated with bleeding but with an increase of both venous and arterial thrombotic events. In pregnancy, the lupus inhibitor is associated with increased spontaneous abortions, presumably secondary to placental infarctions. The correlation between the lupus inhibitor and an elevated anticardiolipin antibody titer is strong. Anticardiolipin antibody titers are found in about 40% of patients with SLE and 30% of patients with RA. Hughes[164] has described an "antiphospholipid antibody syndrome" in which these elevated antibodies are associated with thrombosis, recurrent fetal loss, and thrombocytopenia. The diagnosis of a lupus inhibitor is easily established.

Since the important clinical association is between the lupus inhibitor and thrombotic events, a program to prevent recurrent thrombosis is essential. Most patients do not have a history of thrombotic events even when their cardiolipin antibody level is quite high. Such patients should not be placed on an oral anticoagulant. However, if there is a history of thrombosis, warfarin should be administered. If thrombosis occurs in patients on warfarin, aspirin or immunosuppressive agents may be tried, although their effectiveness in this setting is not well defined. The management of pregnant patients with the lupus inhibitor is the subject of debate. The literature suggests that both aspirin and corticosteroids are useful.[165,166] However, these agents may be dangerous in pregnancy.

Hematologic Malignancies

An increased incidence of lymphoproliferative disorders has been reported in patients with many of the rheumatoid disorders but most frequently with Sjögren syndrome. The incidence of eventual lymphoma in Sjögren syndrome is >40 times that expected in the general population. The incidence of leukemia and myeloma is two to eight times expected.[167] The association of hairy cell leukemia and the γ lymphoproliferative disorder with RA has been discussed above.

Infectious Diseases

The hematologic consequences of viral, bacterial, and fungal infections are extremely common and protean in nature. A complete review of this relationship is beyond the scope of this discussion, which is restricted to hematologic manifestations of infectious diseases that might typically result in a hematologic consultation. Human immunodeficiency virus infection and hematologic disturbances are discussed elsewhere (see Ch. 155).

Viral Infections

Neutropenia

Contrary to common perception, although neutropenia is frequently seen in viral infections, mild leukocytosis, both granulocytic and lymphocytic, is probably more frequent, particularly early in the course of the viral illness.[168] Certain viral illnesses are particularly prone to be associated with neutropenia. They include influenza, hepatitis, rubella, rubeola, adenovirus, coxsackie virus A21, dengue, and mumps. The specific cause(s) for neutropenia is still not well defined.[169] The neutropenia of common viral infections is almost never profound and is generally self-limiting. A hematology consultation is often requested when there is a severe neutropenia ($\leq$1,500/mm^3) that has persisted for >1 or 2 weeks. This situation should be investigated further, including a bone marrow study to rule out a primary bone marrow disorder.

Lymphocytosis

Lymphocytosis occurs frequently in viral disorders. A childhood illness, acute infectious lymphocytosis, often occurs in outbreaks and is usually caused by the coxsackie virus.[170,171]

Atypical lymphocytosis is characteristically seen in infectious mononucleosis as a result of an Epstein-Barr virus (EBV) infection. The primary cell target of EBV is B lymphocytes. The response of activated suppressor CDA$^+$ T cells to the attack on B lymphocytes results in the characteristic large lymphocytes seen in this disorder. Atypical lymphocytosis may also be found in cytomegaloviral disease, hepatitis, mumps, varicella, rubeola, rubella, herpes simplex, herpes zoster, influenza, and roseola infantum. The appearance of infectious mononucleosis-like illness in an older adult may raise a concern about a lymphocytic leukemia, usually of the acute variety. In this uncommon setting, lymphocyte phenotyping and bone marrow evaluation will quickly resolve the concern. Some patients maintain the clinical and serologic manifestations of infectious mononucleosis for some period following the acute infection.[172] This sequela is rare but may especially be seen in families with a genetic disposition to disorders such as the X-linked lymphoproliferative syndrome.[173]

Thrombocytopenia

Mild-to-moderate thrombocytopenia is frequently seen in patients with measles, dengue, varicella, rubella, rubeola, mumps, EBV disease, and cytomegaloviral disease. Thrombocytopenia is rare in hepatitis B and in herpes simplex virus. Important bleeding events are rare in this viral-associated thrombocytopenia. Idiopathic thrombocytopenic purpura is known to occur in the aftermath of a viremia in children. Usually this complication is self-limited, but at times the thrombocytopenia is severe and prolonged, and intervention is necessary. In children, corticosteroid therapy is usually successful, and splenectomy is only rarely needed. DIC has occurred during the course of viral infections, especially rubella, rubeola, varicella, vaccinia, and variola. This is often a frightening complication unexpectedly accompanying a seemingly common childhood viral infection, but it is rarely fatal.[174] Hemorrhagic complications may also be alarming in other viral infections such as those caused by the arbovirus, the arenavirus, and the enterovirus. In these settings, fatal reactions have occurred and are attributed to DIC-like mechanisms.[175]

Virus-Related Bone Marrow Failure

EBV and other viral infections have been reported to cause the hemophagocytic syndrome. This peculiar disorder is characterized by fever, hepatosplenomegaly, lymph node enlargement, rashes, and pancytopenia. Bone marrow study reveals hemophagocytosis and histocytic hyperplasia. It may be a self-limiting process, but death can occur.[176] A fatal outcome is frequent when this illness occurs in patients with malignancies.

Hematologic abnormalities have been associated with uncomplicated hepatitis, including leukopenia, thrombocytopenia, anemia with macrocytosis, and atypical lymphocytosis. Fatal aplastic anemia is a rare occurrence (0.22%) in patients with infectious hepatitis.[177] Conversely, patients with aplastic anemia may have an antecedent history of abnormal liver function tests, suggesting a subclinical hepatitis. Most cases of aplastic anemia, especially the fatal ones, occur within 6 months of the onset of the hepatitis and often when the illness is improving. Bone marrow transplantation after high-dose chemotherapy is effective in 70–80% of these patients.[178] Transient aplastic crises due to infection with the parvovirus B19 has been described in patients with sickle cell disease and hereditary spherocytosis. In hematologically healthy children, parvovirus B19 causes fifth disease. In adults, this virus causes arthralgias. Parvovirus B19 has been described as the causal agent for pure red cell anemia and transient aplastic anemia in immunodeficient patients.[179] The myriad of hematologic manifestations of human immunodeficiency virus positivity and the acquired immunodeficiency syndrome are discussed elsewhere (see Ch. 155).

Bacterial and Fungal Infections

Neutrophilia

Neutrophilia is the hallmark of bacterial infection. Children have higher white counts in response to these infections than do adults. Neutrophil counts of 12,000–15,00/mm^3 are usual in moderate and localized infections. Systemic infections are commonly associated with neutrophil counts of 15,000–25,000/mm^3, and in severe pyogenic infections neutrophil counts may reach 50,000–75,000/mm^3. Neutrophilic leukemoid reactions (>50,000/mm^3) in adults can be confused with chronic myeloid leukemia. The presence of known infection and the finding of an elevated leukocyte alkaline phosphatase generally excludes chronic myeloid leukemia. Usual causes of leukemoid reactions include metastatic disease of the bone marrow, Hodgkin disease, and carcinoma of the stomach, breast, liver, and lung. When evaluating patients with neutrophilia of uncertain origin, a review of the morphologic changes in the peripheral blood film may be helpful. Infection as the etiology of the neutrophilia should be considered when findings such as toxic granulation, cytoplasmic vacuolization, Döhle bodies, and the Pelger-Huët anomaly are found. However, these morphologic changes are more commonly seen when infection is obvious. They are also found in a diverse variety of noninfectious states, including myeloproliferative disorders, burns, pregnancy, and drug reactions.[180] Most fungal infections do not produce neutrophilia.

Neutropenia

Neutropenia is unusual in patients with bacterial infections. However, it is found with some frequency in patients who have salmonellosis, brucellosis, pertussis, rickettsial infections, disseminated tuberculosis, and disseminated histoplasmosis, as well as in the presence of overwhelming infection. Neutropenia in overwhelming infection as an indication of exhaustion of the bone marrow neutrophil reserve and is generally considered a poor prognostic sign. Usually the neutropenia associated with bacterial infections is modest and not clinically important. Severe neutropenia in patients with bacterial infection is more likely to occur in the elderly, in alcoholics and other drug abusers, and in patients who are myelosuppressed. The therapeutic value of CSF-G and CSF-GM for the amelioration of severe neutropenia in these settings is under investigation. Most fungal infections do not produce neutropenia.

Lymphocytosis

Lymphocytosis >400/mm^3 is seen most often in pertussis. In this infection the lymphocytosis is usually 15,000–25,000/mm,^{3} but occasionally it may rise to 150,000/mm^3. Other bacterial infections commonly associated with lymphocytosis are rickettsial illnesses, tuberculosis, syphilis, and burcellosis. Lymphocytosis is often seen as part of a neutrophilic leukemoid reaction. A lymphocytic leukemoid reaction has rarely been seen in patients with tuberculosis.

Lymphocytopenia

Lymphocyte counts <1,000/mm^3 are common in many acute infections, particularly when marked neutrophilia is present. Tuberculosis, brucellosis, and disseminated histoplasmosis infections frequently cause lymphocytopenia. Lymphocytopenia in elderly patients with a bacterial infection is a poor prognostic sign.[181]

Monocytosis

A low-grade monocytosis of >800/mm^3 often accompanies the recovery phase of acute infections. Of patients with disseminated tuberculosis and patients with subacute bacterial endocarditis, 15–20% have a monocytosis.[182,183] Persistant monocytosis following recovery from an infectious disorder suggests the possibility of an underlying primary marrow disorder and should be investigated.

Eosinophilia

Eosinophilia >350/mm^3 is rare in patients with bacterial or fungal diseases. Exceptions are bronchopulmonary aspergillosis, coccidiomycosis, and chlamydia pneumonitis of infancy. Fungal infections with eosinophilia appear to be related to immune responses, particularly high serum concentrations of IgE. The most common causes of infection-induced eosinophilia are parasites in the gastrointestinal tract. Occasionally eosinophilia from parasitic infections can be quite high and can mimic that degree of eosinophilia seen in the hypereosinophilic syndrome.

Thrombocytosis

Thrombocytosis (500,000–700,000/mm^3) is fairly common in some chronic bacterial infections, including tuberculosis, subacute bacterial endocarditis, and osteomyelitis. However, thrombotic events accompanying this degree of platelet elevation are quite rare.

Thrombocytopenia

Any acute bacterial or fungus infection causing bacteremia or fungemia can cause thrombocytopenia. Several mechanisms are responsible for this development, but increased consumption is probably the most common. Tuberculosis, histoplasmosis, and rickettsial diseases may be associated with thrombocytopenia in the absence of bloodstream infection. The finding of thrombocytopenia in bacterial and fungal infections usually raises the specter of DIC. In the absence of this complication, severe bleeding from thrombocytopenia in acute bacterial and fungus infections is rare. However, severe infections are the most common cause of DIC, particularly in those caused by gram-negative bacilli. Fungal infections are only rarely associated with DIC. The prognosis of infection-induced DIC is relatively good because of the likelihood of control of the infection with appropriate antibiotic therapy. Platelet transfusions are valuable while the infectious etiology is being treated. Extreme forms of DIC, such as that seen with purpura fulminans, may prove fatal.[184]

Anemia

A significant anemia is uncommon in acute bacterial and fungal infections. An exception is the complication of a hemolytic anemia seen with a *Clostridium welchii* or *Bartonella bacilliformis* infections. The anemia of chronic bacterial infection is usually the result of ACD.

REFERENCES

1. Doll DC, Weiss R: Neoplasia and the erythron. J Clin Oncol 3:429, 1985
2. Zucker S: Anemia in cancer. Cancer Invest 3:249, 1985
3. Dutcher JP: Hematologic abnormalities in patients with nonhematologic malignancies. Hematol Oncol Clin North Am 1:281, 1987
4. Schwartzberg LS, Holbert JM: Hemorrhagic and thrombotic abnormalities of cancer. Crit Care Clin 4:107, 1988
5. Bunn P, Ridgway EC: Paraneoplastic syndromes. p. 1986. In DeVita VT, Hellman S, Rosenberg SA (eds): Cancer Principles and Practice of Oncology. JB Lippincott, Philadelphia, 1989
6. Schafer AI: The hypercoagulable states. Ann Intern Med 102:814, 1985
7. Auger MJ, MacKie MJ: Hemostasis in malignant disease. J R Coll Physicians Lond 22:74, 1988
8. Laszlo J: Hematologic effects of cancer. p. 1275. In Holland JF, Frei E (eds): Cancer Medicine. Lea & Febiger, Philadelphia 1982
9. Bentley DP: Anemia and chronic disease. Clin Haematol 11:465, 1982
10. Cartwright GE: The anemia of chronic disorders. Semin Hematol 3:351, 1966
11. Cartwright GE, Lee GR: The anemia of chronic disorders. Br J Haematol 21:147, 1971
12. Miller CB, Jones RJ, Piantadosi S et al: Decreased erythropoietin response in patients with the anemia of cancer. N Engl J Med 322:1689, 1990
13. Henry DH, Rudnick SA, Bryant E et al: Preliminary reports of two double blind placebo controlled studies using recombinant erythropoietin (rHu EPO) in the anemia associated with cancer, abstracted. Blood, suppl. 1. 74: 6a, 1989
14. Ludwig H, Fritz E, Kotzmann H et al: Erythropoietin treatment for chronic anemia of malignancy, abstracted. Blood, suppl. 1. 74:16a, 1989
15. Oster W, Herrmann F, Gamm H et al: Erythropoietin (EPO) for the treatment of anemia of malignancy associated with neoplastic bone marrow infiltration. J Clin Oncol 8:956, 1990
16. Nelson RA, Guilfoyle MC, Abels RI et al: Long-term treatment of anemic cancer patients with recombinant human erythropoietin, abstracted. Blood, suppl. 1. 80:537a, 1992
17. Means RT, Krantz SB: Progress in understanding the pathogenesis of anemia of chronic disease. Blood 80:1639, 1992
18. Krantz SB: Pure red cell aplasia. N Engl J Med 241:345, 1974
19. Jepson JH, Lowenstein L: Inhibition of erythropoiesis by a factor present in the plasma of patients with erythroblastopenia. Blood 27:425, 1966
20. Akard LP, Brandt J, Lu L et al: Chronic T-cell lymphoproliferative disorder and pure red cell aplasia. Am J Med 83:1069, 1987
21. Shlonoya S, Amaro M, Imamura Y et al: Suppressor T-cell chronic lymphocytic leukemia associated with pure red cell aplasia. Scand J Haematol 33: 231, 1984
22. Doll DC, Weiss RB: Chemotherapeutic agents and the erythron. Cancer Treat Rev 10:185, 1983
23. Henry D, Keller A, Kugler J et al: Treatment of anemia in cancer patients on cisplatin chemotherapy with recombinant human erythropoietin, abstracted. Proc Am Soc Clin Oncol 9:182, 1990
24. Hines JD, Hoffbrand AV, Mollin DL: The hematologic complications following partial gastrectomy. A study of 292 patients. Am J Med 43:555, 1967
25. Petz LD: Autoimmune hemolytic anemia. Hum Pathol 141:251, 1983
26. Pirofsky B: Clinical aspects of autoimmune hemolytic anemia. Semin Hematol 13:251, 1976
27. Jones SE: Autoimmune disorders and malignant lymphoma. Cancer 31:1092 1973
28. Murgo AJ: Thrombotic microangiopathy in the cancer patient including those induced by chemotherapy. Semin Hematol 24:161, 1987
29. Anyman KH, Skarin T, Mayor RJ et al: Microangiopathic hemolytic anemia and cancer: a review. Medicine 58:377, 1979
30. Lohrman HP, Adam W, Heymer B et al: Microangiopathic hemolytic anemia in metastatic carcinoma: a report of eight cases. Ann Intern Med 79:368, 1973
31. Gasic GJ, Gasic TB, Galanti N et al: Platelet-tumor cell interactions in mice. The role of platelets in the spread of malignant disease. Int J Cancer 11: 704, 1973
32. Zacharski LR, Memoli VA, Rousseau SM: Coagulation cancer interaction in situ in renal cell carcinoma. Blood 68:394, 1986
33. Kressel BR, Ryan KP, Duong AF et al: Microangiopathic hemolytic anemia, thrombocytopenia and renal failure in patients treated for adenocarcinoma. Cancer 48:1738, 1981
34. Lesesne JB, Rothschild N, Erikson B et al: Cancer-associated hemolytic-uremic syndrome: analysis of 85 cases from a national registry. J Clin Oncol 7:791, 1989
35. Cantrell JE, Phillips TM, Schein PS: Carcinoma-associated hemolytic-uremic: a complication of mitomycin-C chemotherapy. J Clin Oncol 3:723, 1985
36. Korec S, Schein PS, Smith FP et al: Treatment of cancer associated hemolytic syndrome with a staphylococcal protein A immunoperfusion. J Clin Oncol 4:219, 1986
37. Vogelzang NJ, Bosl GJ, Johnson K, Kennedy BJ: Raynaud's phenomenon: a common toxicity after combination chemotherapy for testicular cancer. Ann Intern Med 95:288, 1981
38. Doll DC, Weiss RB: Hemolytic anemia associated with antineoplastic agents. Cancer Treat Rep 69:777, 1985
39. Getaz EP, Beckley S, Fitzpatrick J, Dozier A: Cisplatin-induced hemolysis. N Engl J Med 302:334, 1980
40. Doll DC: Oxidative hemolysis after administration of doxorubicin. Br Med J 287:180, 1983
41. Reiner AP, Spivak JL: Hemophagocytic histiocytosis—a report of 23 new patients and a review of the literature. Medicine 67:369, 1988
42. Hammond D, Winnick S: Paraneoplastic erythrocytosis and ectopic erythropoietin. Ann NY Acad Sci 230:219, 1974
43. Sytkowski AJ, Richie WR, Bicknell KA: New human renal carcinoma cell line established from a patient with erythrocytosis. Cancer Res 43:1415, 1983
44. Tsu SC, Hua ASP: Erythrocytosis in hepatocellular carcinoma: a compensatory phenomena. Br J Haematol 28:497, 1974
45. Thurman WG, Grabstajd H, Lieberman PH: Elevation of erythropoietin levels in association with Wilms' tumor. Arch Intern Med 117:280, 1966
46. Kenny GM, Murad EA, Stanbitz WJ et al: Erythropoietin levels in Wilms' tumor patients. J Urol 104:758, 1970
47. Gordon AS, Zanjani ED, Zalusky R: A possible mechanism for erythrocytosis associated with hepatocellular carcinoma in man. Blood 35:151, 1970
48. Fried W: The liver as a source of renal erythropoietin production. Blood 40:671, 1972
49. Kan YW, McFadzean AJS, Todd D, Tso SC: Further observations on polycythemia in hepatocellular carcinoma. Blood 18:592, 1961
50. Lehman AJ, Erslev AJ, Myerson RM: Erythrocytosis associated with hepatocellular carcinoma. Am J Med 35:439, 1963
51. Robinson WA: Granulocytosis in neoplasia. Ann NY Acad Sci 230:212, 1974
52. Clark SC, Kamen R: The human hematopoietic colony stimulating factors. Science 236:1229, 1987
53. Sato N, Shigetaka A, Ueyama Y et al: Granulocytosis and colony-stimulating activity produced by human squamous cell carcinoma. Cancer 43:605, 1979
54. Morstyn G, Campbell L, Lieschke G et al: Treatment of chemotherapy-induced neutropenia by subcutaneously administered granulocyte colony-stimulating factor with optimization of dose of therapy. J Clin Oncol 7:1554, 1989
55. Crawford J, Ozer H, Stoller R et al: Reduction by granulocyte colony-stimulating factor and neutropenia induced by chemotherapy in patients with small-cell lung cancer. N Engl J Med 325:164, 1991
56. Brouchud MH, Howell A, Crowther D et al: The use of granulocyte colony-stimulating factor to increase the intensity of treatment with doxorubicin in patients with advanced breast and ovarian cancer. Br J Cancer 60:121, 1989
57. Sheridan WP, Morstyn G, Wolf M et al: Granulocyte colony-stimulating factor and neutrophil recovery after high-dose chemotherapy and autologous bone marrow transplantation. Lancet 2:891, 1989
58. Taylor KM, Jagannath S, Spitzer G et al: Recombinant human granulocyte colony-stimulating factor hastens granulocyte recovery after high-dose chemotherapy and autologous bone marrow transplantation in Hodgkin's disease. J Clin Oncol 7:1791, 1989

59. Aisenberg AC, Wilkes BM, Harris N et al: Chronic T-cell lymphocytosis with neutropenia: report of a case with monoclonal antibody. Blood 58:818, 1981
60. Levin J, Conley CL: Thrombocytosis associated with malignant disease. Arch Intern Med 114:497, 1964
61. Silvis SE, Turklas N, Duscherholman A: Thrombocytosis in patients with lung cancer. JAMA 211:1852, 1970
62. Livingston RB, Carter SK: Single Agents in Cancer Chemotherapy. IFI/Plenum, New York, 1970
63. Hilgard H, Hossfeld DK: Transient bleomycin-induced thrombocytopenia: a clinical study. Eur J Cancer 14:1261, 1978
64. Kaden BR, Rosse WF, Hauch TW: Immune thrombocytopenia in lymphoproliferative diseases. Blood 53:545, 1979
65. Kim HD, Boggs DR: A syndrome resembling idiopathic thrombocytopenic purpura in ten patients with diverse forms of cancer. Am J Med 67:371, 1979
66. Hedderich GS, O'Connor RJ, Reid EC et al: Caval tumor thrombus complicating renal cell carcinoma: a surgical challenge. Surgery 102:614, 1987
67. Pritchett TR, Lieskowsky G, Skinner DG: Extension of renal cell carcinoma into the vena cava: clinical review and surgical approach. J Urol 135:460, 1986
68. Sharifi R, Ray P, Schade SG et al: Inferior vena cava thrombosis. Unusual presentation of testicular tumor. Urology 32:146, 1988
69. Fujisaki M, Kurihara E, Kikuchi K et al: Hepatocellular carcinoma with tumor thrombus extending into the right atrium: report of a successful resection with the use of cardiopulmonary bypass. Surgery 109:214, 1991
70. Miller SP, Sanchez-Avalos J, Stefanski T: Coagulation disorders in cancer. I. Clinical and laboratory studies. Cancer 20:1452, 1967
71. Schafer AI: The hypercoagulable states. Ann Intern Med 102:814, 1985
72. Nand S, Gross Fisher S, Salgia R et al: Hemostatic abnormalities in untreated cancer: incidence and correlation with thrombotic and hemorrhagic complications. J Clin Oncol 5:1998, 1987
73. Gralnick HR, Abrell BA: Studies of the procoagulant and fibrinolytic activity of promyelocytes in acute promyelocytic leukemia. Br J Haematol 24:89, 1973
74. Rickles FR, Edwards RL: Activation of blood coagulation in cancer: Trousseau's syndrome revisited. Blood 62:14, 1983
75. Callander N, Rapaport, SI: Trousseau's syndrome. West J Med 158:364, 1993
76. Rapaport SI: Blood coagulation and its alterations in hemorrhagic and thrombotic disorders. West J Med 158:153, 1993
77. Gore I: Thrombosis and pancreatic cancer. Am J Pathol 29:1093, 1953
78. Bevilacqua MP, Poper JS, Wheeler ME et al: Interleukin 1 acts on cultured human vascular endothelium to increase the adhesion of polymorphonuclear leukocytes, monocytes, and related leukocyte cell lines. J Clin Invest 76:2003, 1985
79. Greczy CL: Induction of macrophage procoagulant by products of activated lymphocytes. Haemaostasis 14:400, 1984
80. Morgan D, Edwards RL, Rickles FR: Monocyte procoagulant activity as a peripheral marker of clotting activation in cancer patients. Haemostasis 18:55, 1988
81. Dean RT, Leoni P, Rossi BC: Regulation of procoagulant factors in mononuclear phagocytes. Haemostasis 14:412, 1984
82. Grignani G, Jamieson GA: Platelets in tumor metastases: generation of adenosine diphosphate by tumor cells is specific but unrelated to metastatic potential. Blood 71:844, 1988
83. Honn KV, Busse WD, Sloane BF: Prostacyclin and thromboxanes. Implications for their role in tumor cell metastases. Biochem Pharmacol 32:1, 1983
84. Bick RL: Alterations of hemostasis in malignancy. p. 262. In Disorders of Hemostasis and Thrombosis: Principles of Clinical Practice. Thieme, New York, 1985
85. Slickter SJ, Harker LA: Hemostasis in malignancy. Ann NY Acad Sci 230:252, 1974
86. Gray W, Bell W: Fibrinolytic agents in the treatment of thrombotic disorders. Semin Oncol 17:228, 1990
87. Rosen P, Armstrong D: Nonbacterial thrombotic endocarditis in patients with malignant diseases. Am J Med 54:23, 1973
88. Studdy P, Wiloughby JMT: Non-bacterial thrombotic endocarditis in early cancer. Br J Med 1:752, 1976
89. Rosen PJ: Bleeding problems in the cancer patient. Hematol Oncol Clin North Am 6:1315, 1992
90. Gralnick HR, Henderson E: Hypofibrinogenemia and coagulation factor deficiencies with L-asparaginase treatment. Cancer 27:131, 1970
91. Monto RW, Talley RW, Coldwell MJ et al: Observations on the mechanism of hemorrhagic toxicity in mithramycin (NSC-24559) therapy. Cancer Res 29:697, 1969
92. Stein CA, Larocca RV, Thomas R et al: Suramin: an anticancer drug with a unique mechanism of action. J Clin Oncol 7:499, 1989
93. Schilling, RF: Anemia of chronic disease: a misnomer. Ann Intern Med 115:572, 1991
94. Erslev AJ, Caro J, Miller O, Silver R: Plasma erythropoietin in health and disease. Ann Lab Clin Sci 10:250, 1980
95. Birgegard G, Hallgren R, Caro J: Serum erythropoietin in rheumatoid arthritis and other inflammatory arthritides: relationship to anaemia and the effect of anti-inflammatory treatment. Br J Haematol 65:479, 1987
96. Ward HP, Gordon B, Pickett JC: Serum levels of erythropoietin in rheumatoid arthritis. J Lab Clin Med 74:93, 1969
97. Pavlovic-Kentera V, Ruvidic R, Milenkovic P, Marinkovic D: Erythropoietin in patients with anemia in rheumatoid arthritis. Scand J Haematol 23:141, 1979
98. Baer, AN, Dessypris EN, Goldwasser E, Krantz SB: Blunted erythropoietin response to anaemia in rheumatoid arthritis. Br J Haematol 66:559, 1987
99. Hochberg MC, Arnold CM, Hogans BB, Spivak JL: Serum immunoreactive erythropoietin in rheumatoid arthritis: impaired response to anemia. Arthritis Rheum 31:1318, 1988
100. Maury CPJ: Anaemia in rheumatoid arthritis: role of cytokines. Scand J Rheumatol 18:3, 1989
101. Fuchs D, Hausen A, Reibnegger G et al: Immune activation and the anaemia associated with chronic inflammatory disorders. Eur J Haematol 46:65, 1991
102. Houssiau FA, Devogelaer J-P, Van Damme J et al: Interleukin-6 in synovial fluid and serum of patients with rheumatoid arthritis and other inflammatory arthritides. Arthritis Rheum 31:784, 1988
103. Vreugdenhil G, Lowenberg B, van Ejik HG, Swaak AJG: Anaemia of chronic disease in rheumatoid arthritis: raised serum interleukin-6 (IL-6) levels and the effects of IL-6 and anti-IL-6 on in vitro erythropoiesis. Rheumatol Int 10:127, 1990
104. Faquin WC, Schneider TJ, Goldberg MA: Effect of inflammatory cytokines on hypoxia-induced erythropoietin production. Blood 79:1987, 1992
105. Jelkman W, Pagel H, Wolff M, Fandrey J: Monokines inhibiting erythropoietin production in human hepatoma cultures and in isolated perfused rat kidneys. Life Sci 50:31, 1991
106. Bennett RM, Holt PJL, Lewis SM: Role of the reticuloendothelial system in the anaemia of rheumatoid arthritis: a study using the ^{59}Fe-labelled dextran model. Ann Rheum Dis 33:147, 1974
107. Haurani FI, Burke WM, Martnez EJ: Effective reutilization of iron in the anemia of inflammation. J Lab Clin Med 65:560, 1965
108. Konijn AM, Hershko C: Ferritin synthesis and inflammation. I. Pathogenesis of impaired iron release. Br J Haematol 37:7, 1977
109. Williams RA, Samson D, Tikerpac J et al: In vitro studies of ineffective erythropoiesis in rheumatoid arthritis. Ann Rheum Dis 41:502, 1982
110. Zarrabi MH, Lysik R, DiStefano J, Zucker S: The anaemia of chronic disorders: studies of iron reutilization in the anaemia of experimental malignancy and chronic inflammation. Br J Haematol 35:647, 1977
111. Moldawer LL, Marano MA, Wei He et al: Cachectin/tumor necrosis factor alters red blood cell kinetics and induces anemia in vivo. FASEB J 3:1637, 1989
112. Alvarez-Hernandez X, Liceaga J, McKay IC, Brock JH: Induction of hypoferremia and modulation of macrophage iron metabolism by tumor necrosis factor. Lab Invest 61:319, 1989
113. Rogers J, Durmowicz G, Kasschau K et al: A motif within the 5' non-coding regions of acute phase mRNAs mediates ferritin translation by IL-1β and may contribute to the anemia of chronic disease, abstracted. Blood, suppl. 1. 78:367a, 1991
114. Means RT, Olsen NJ, Krantz SB et al: Treatment of the anemia of rheumatoid arthritis with recombinant human erythropoietin: clinical and in vitro studies. Arthritis Rheum 32:638, 1989
115. Pincus T, Olsen NJ, Russell, IJ et al: Multicenter study of recombinant human erythropoietin in correction of anemia in rheumatoid arthritis. Am J Med 89:161, 1990
116. Tauchi T, Ohyashiki JH, Fujieda H et al: Suppressed erythropoietin response to anemia and the efficacy of recombinant erythropoietin in the anemia of rheumatoid arthritis. J Rheumatol 17:885, 1990
117. Biregegard G, Gudbjronsson B, Hallgren R, Wide L: Anemia of chronic inflammatory arthritides: treatment with recombinant erythropoietin. Contrib Nephrol 88:295, 1991
118. Johnson CS, Keckler CS, Topper MI et al: In vivo hematopoietic effects of recombinant interleulin-1α in mice: stimulation of granulocytic, monocytic, megakaryocytic, and early erythroid progenitors, suppression of late erythroid progenitors, and reversal of erythroid suppression with erythropoietin. Blood 73:678, 1989
119. Johnson CS, Cook CA, Furmanski P: In vivo suppression of erythropoiesis by tumor necrosis factor-α: reversal with exogenous erythropoietin (EPO). Exp Hematol 18:109, 1990
120. Eschbach JW, Egrie JC, Downing MR et al: Correction of the anemia of end-stage renal disease with recombinant erythropoietin: results of a combined phase I and II clinical trial. N Engl J Med 316:73, 1987

121. Masunga H, Murakami A, Goto M, Ueda M: Effects of erythropoietin injection on the anemic rats with different serum erythropoietin titer. Jpn J Vet Sci 19:1, 1986

122. Graham DY, Agarwal NM, Roth SH: Prevention of NSAID-induced gastric ulcer with misoprostol: multicentre, double-blind, placebo-controlled trial. Lancet 2:1277, 1988

123. Bentley DP, Williams P: Serum ferritin concentrations as an index of storage iron in rheumatoid arthritis. J Clin Pathol 27:786, 1974

124. Hansen TM, Hansen NE, Birgens HS et al: Serum ferritin and the assessment of iron deficiency in rheumatoid arthritis. Scand J Rheumatol 12:353, 1983

125. Dacie JV: Autoimmune hemolytic anemia. Arch Intern Med 135:1293, 1975

126. Shumak KH, Rock GA: Therapeutic plasma exchange. N Engl J Med 310:762, 1984

127. Council Report: Current status of therapeutic plasmapheresis and related techniques. JAMA 253:819, 1985

128. Ahn YS, Harrington WJ, Byrnes JJ et al: Treatment of autoimmune hemolytic anemia with vinca-loaded platelets. JAMA 249:2189, 1983

129. Leickly FE, Buckley RH: Successful treatment of autoimmune hemolytic anemia in common variable immunodeficiency with high-dose intravenous gamma globulin. Am J Med 82:159, 1987

130. Salama A, Mahn I, Neuzner J et al: IgG therapy in autoimune haemolytic anaemia of warm type. Blut 48:391, 1984

131. Ahn YS, Harrington WJ, Mylvaganam R et al: Danazol therapy for autoimmune hemolytic anemia. Ann Intern Med 102:298, 1985

132. Dessypris EN: Pure Red Cell Aplasia. Johns Hopkins University Press, Baltimore, 1988

133. Clark DA, Dessypris EN, Krantz SB: Studies on pure red cell aplasia. XI. Results of immunosuppressive treatment of 37 patients. Blood 63:227, 1984

134. Marmont A, Peschle C, Sanguinetti M, Condorelli M: Pure red cell aplasia: response of three patients to cyclophosphamide and/or antilymphocyte globulin (ALG) and demonstration of two types of serum IgG inhibitors to erythropoiesis. Blood 45:247, 1975

135. Zaentz SD, Krantz SB, Brown EB: Studies on pure red cell aplasia. VIII. Maintenance therapy with immunosuppressive drugs. Br J Haematol 32:47, 1976

136. Totterman TH, Bengtsson M: Treatment of pure red cell aplasia with cyclosporin: suppression of activated T supressor/cytotoxic and NK-like cells in marrow and blood correlates with haematological response. Eur J Haematol 41:204, 1988

137. Lippman SM, Durie BGM, Garewal HS et al: Efficacy of danazol in pure red cell aplasia. Am J Hematol 23:373, 1986

138. Khelif A, Van HV, Tremis JP et al: Remission of acquired pure red cell aplasia following plasma exchanges. Scand J Haematol 34:13, 1985

139. McGuire WA, Yang HH, Bruno E et al: Treatment of antibody-mediated pure red cell aplasia with high-dose intravenous gamma globulin therapy. N Engl J Med 317:1004, 1987

140. Budman DR, Steinberg AD: Hematologic aspects of systemic lupus erythematosus. Ann Intern Med 86:220, 1977

141. Bagby GC, Gaborrel JD: Neutropenia in three patients with rheumatic disorders: suppression of granulopoiesis by cortisol-sensitive thymus dependent lymphocytes. J Clin Invest 64:72, 1979

142. Bishop CR: The neutropenia of Felty's syndrome. Am J Hematol 2:203, 1977

143. Abdou NI: Heterogeneity of bone marrow directed immune mechanisms in the pathogenesis of neutropenia of Felty's syndrome. Arthritis Rheum 26:947, 1983

144. Bagby GC, Lawrence HJ, Neerhout RC: T-lymphocyte mediated granulopoietic failure: in vitro identification of prednisone-responsive patients. N Engl J Med 309:1073, 1983

145. Abdou NI, NaPombejara C, Balentine L et al: Suppressor cell-mediated neutropenia in Felty's syndrome. J Clin Invest 61:738, 1978

146. Starkebaum JW, Singer WP, Arrend WP: Humoral and cellular immune mechanisms of neutropenia in patients with Felty's syndrome. Clin Exp Immunol 39:307, 1980

147. Blumfelder TM, Logue GL, Shimm DS: Felty's syndrome: effects of splenectomy upon granulocyte count and granulocyte associated IgG. Ann Intern Med 94:623, 1981

148. Gari-Bai AR, Rochlitz C, Riewald M et al: Treatment of neutropenia in Felty's syndrome with granulocyte-macrophage colony-stimulating factor—hematological response accompanied by pulmonary complications with lethal outcome. Ann Hematol 65:232, 1992

149. Watanabe F, Satoh M: Improvement of pancytopenia and articular findings by splenectomy in a patient with Felty's syndrome. Ryumachi 32:347, 1992

150. Kaiser U, Klausmann M, Kolb G et al: Felty's syndrome: favorable response to granulocyte-macrophage colony-stimulating factor in the acute phase. Acta Haematol 87:190, 1992

151. Ito T, Miyairi Y, Kuwabara T et al: Granulocyte-colony stimulating factor corrects granulocytopenia in Felty's syndrome. Am J Hematol 40:318, 1992

152. Joseph G, Neustadt DH, Hamm J et al: GM-CSF in the treatment of Felty syndrome. Am J Hematol 37:55, 1991

153. Lubbe AS, Schwella N, Riess H, Huhn D: Improvement of pneumonia and arthritis in Felty's syndrome by treatment with granulocyte-macrophage colony-stimulating factor (GM-CSF). Blut 61:379, 1990

154. Hazenberg BP, Van Leeuwen MA, Van Rijswijk MH et al: Correction of granulocytopenia in Felty's syndrome by granulocyte-macrophage colony-stimulating factor. Simultaneous induction of interleukin-6 release and flare-up of the arthritis. Blood 74:2769, 1989

155. Loughran TP, Starkebaum G: Large granular lymphocytic leukemia. Medicine 66:397, 1987

156. Sattar MA, Cawley ID: Arthritis associated with hairy cell leukaemia. Case report. Ann Rheum Dis 41:289, 1982

157. Karpatkin S, Garg SK, Siskind GW: Autoimmune thrombocytopenic purpura and the compensated thrombocytolyic state. Am J Med 51:1, 1971

158. Hall S, McCormick JL, Greipp PR et al: Splenctomy does not cure the thrombocytopenia of systemic lupus erythematosus. Ann Intern Med 102:325, 1985

159. Miller MH, Urowitz MB, Galdman DD: The significance of thrombocytopenia in systemic lupus erythematosus. Arthritis Rheum 26:1181, 1983

160. Stricker RB, Davis JA, Gershow J et al: Thrombotic thrombocytopenic purpura complicating systemic lupus erythematosus. Case report and literature review from the plasmapheresis era. J Rheumatol 19:1469, 1992

161. Hess DC, Sethi K, Awad E: Thrombotic thrombocytopenic purpura in systemic lupus erythematosus and antiphospholipid antibodies: effective treatment with plasma exchange and immunosuppression. J Rheumatol 19:1474, 1992

162. Smith AF, Castor CW: Connective tissue activation: platelet abnormalities in patients with rheumatoid arthritis. J Rheumatol 5:177, 1978

163. Conley CL, Hartman RC: A hemorrhagic disorder caused by circulating anticoagulant in patients with disseminated lupus erythematosus. J Clin Invest 31:621, 1952

164. Hughes GRV: Thrombosis, abortion, cerebral disease, and the lupus anticoagulant. Br Med J 287:1088, 1983

165. Branch DW, Scott JR, Kochenour NK et al: Obstetric complications associated with the lupus anticoagulant. N Engl J Med 313:1322, 1985

166. Lubbe WF, Butler WS, Palmer SJ et al: Fetal survival after prednisone suppression of maternal lupus-anticoagulant. Lancet 1:1361, 1983

167. Richert-Boe, KE: Hematologic complications of rheumatic disease. Hematol Oncol Clin North Am 1:301, 1987

168. Douglas Rg, Alfoed RH, Cate TR et al: The leukocyte response during viral respiratory illness in man. Ann Intern Med 64:521, 1965

169. Zoumbos N, Raefsky E, Young NS: Lymphokines and hematopoiesis. Prog Hematol 16:201, 1985

170. Horowitz MS, Moore GH: Acute infectious lymphocytosis: an epidemiologic study of an outbreak. N Engl J Med 279:399, 1968

171. Saulsbury FT: B cell proliferation in acute infectious lymphocytosis. Pediatr Infect Dis 6:1127, 1987

172. Straus SE, Tosato G, Armstrong G et al: Persisting illness and fatigue in adults with evidence of Epstein-Barr virus infection. Ann Intern Med 102:7, 1985

173. Purtilo DT, Sakamoto K, Barnabei V et al: Epstein-Barr virus-induced diseases in boys with the linked lymphoproliferative syndrome (XLP). Am J Med 73:49, 1982

174. Baker WF: Clinical aspects of disseminated intravascular coagulation: a clinicians' point of view. Semin Thromb Hemost 15:1, 1989

175. Halfon N, Spector SA: Fatal echovirus type 11 infection. Am J Dis Child 135:1017, 1981

176. Wilson ER, Malluh A, Stagno S et al: Fatal Epstein-Barr virus-associated hemophagocytic syndrome. J Pediatr 98:260, 1981

177. Bottinger LE, Westerholm B: Aplastic anaemia I: Incidence and aetiology. Acta Med Scand 192:315, 1972

178. Storb R, Doney, KC, Thomas, ED et al: Marrow transplantation with or without donor buffy coat cells for 65 transfused aplastic anemic patients. Blood 59:236, 1982

179. Kurtzman G, Frickhofen N, Kimball J et al: Pure red cell aplasia of 10 years duration due to persistent parvovirus B19 infection and its care with immunoglobulin therapy. N Engl J Med 321:519, 1989

180. Mandell GL, Douglas RG, Bennett JE (eds): Principles and Practice of Infectious Diseases. 4th Ed. Churchill Livingstone, New York, 1994

181. Proust J, Rosenzweig P, Debouzy C et al: Lymphopenia induced by acute bacterial infections in the elderly: a sign of age-related immune dysfunction of major prognostic significance. Gerontology 31:178, 1985

182. Glasser RM, Walker RI, Herion JC: The significance of hematologic abnormalities in patients with tuberculosis. Arch Intern Med 125:691, 1970

183. Wintrobe MM, Lee GR, Boggs DR et al (eds): Clinical Hematology. Lea & Febiger, Philadelphia, 1981

184. Spicer TE, Rau JM: Purpura fulminans. Am J Med 61:566, 1976

Hematologic Manifestations of Endocrine Disorders

153

Jane F. Desforges

INTRODUCTION

The physiologic environment provides the determining factors that control hematopoiesis. When that environment is disrupted by an endocrinologic disorder, it may be reflected in abnormalities of the bone marrow or peripheral blood. Growth factors that can be demonstrated to have specific targets in the hematopoietic population of cells are now well defined and their receptors identified. However, other factors secreted by cells of the endocrine system may affect hematopoiesis in more subtle ways.

Hormones secreted by endocrine glands may exert effects on hematopoiesis directly on the progenitor cell, or indirectly, by regulating production of another growth factor. It is not clear that any of the hormones are vital to hematopoiesis, but evidence is abundant, in vivo and ex vivo, that deficiencies may affect marrow function. Deficiency states are more likely to be associated with hematologic abnormalities than hyperfunctioning glands, but abnormalities may be seen in either case. Those endocrine glands most commonly associated with hematologic changes are the thyroid, pituitary, adrenal, and testes.

Hormones differ in their site of action from the traditional hematologic growth factors. For the latter, the receptors are on the cell membrane, and the signal is then transmitted via a series of steps to the nucleus. By contrast, thyroid hormone and steroids do not require a membrane receptor, but passively enter the cell, and are bound to their specific receptors in the nucleus. Presumably, it is from this vantage point that they exert some control over hematopoiesis.

ENDOCRINOPATHIES AND HEMATOPOIESIS

Anemia is the most common hematologic manifestation of an endocrine disorder and usually reflects an endocrine deficiency state. It is not a predictable finding in these states but, in general, is more likely to be seen as the deficiency becomes more profound. Moreover, it is seldom of a degree to cause signs or symptoms per se, and is therefore usually found in routine testing, sometimes providing the first clue to the presence of an endocrinopathy.

Thyroid Disease

The basic hematologic disturbance in hypothyroidism is a productive deficit leading to moderate normochromic, normocytic, or slightly macrocytic anemia (Table 153-1). Since the plasma volume may be decreased, the anemia may not be recognized.[1] Just as the onset of the endocrinologic disease itself is subtle and slow, specific symptoms or signs may not be present that one could attribute to the anemia. It is not predictable, either in degree or in relation to other manifestations of thyroid failure. In fact, when the diagnosis of hypothyroidism is made, patients have hematocrit within normal limits.

The mechanism of erythropoietic suppression in hypothy-

EVALUATION OF THE PATIENT WITH NONDESCRIPT ANEMIA

Every hematologist is consulted regarding the puzzling patient who has unexplained anemia with no other specific findings. Hints of the cause may be provided by the history (e.g., exposure to tuberculosis) or on physical examination (e.g., a changing cardiac murmur). In some, the underlying cause may be demonstrated in a routine laboratory test, such as an elevated creatinine revealing previously unrecognized uremia. A proportion of such patients, however, may have normocytic, normochromic anemia secondary to an endocrine disorder, and one should approach these puzzling cases with minimal testing to assess the broad possibilities.

If the patient has a moderate degree of anemia, a boring smear with all cells appearing normal, reticulocytes present but not appropriately increased to compensate for the anemia, normal white cell and platelet count, normal erythrocyte sedimentation rate, and no adenopathy or splenomegaly, the patient is unlikely to have a primary hematologic disease. The search should be for an internal environmental factor that is suppressing the erythropoietic response. Imaging studies are not indicated, and a marrow aspirate will not help; instead, the potential for EPO response should be explored. Normal concentration of serum creatinine is adequate to rule out deficiency of receptors to stimulate production of that growth factor. At the same time, evaluation of the endocrine status should be carried out with attention to thyroid, pituitary, adrenal, and, if male, gonadal function. Deficiency of any of these glands may cause anemia due to decreased erythropoiesis. In most patients, a careful history and physical examination will reveal which hormonal deficiency is most likely. the thyroid probably being the most common offender, and a few specific tests will confirm the diagnosis. Treatment of the anemia involves not only replacing the deficient hormone, but also determining the underlying problem, be it simply a primary deficiency of a single gland or lack of appropriate stimulus secondary to disease in the pituitary or hypothalamus.

roidism is not clear. However, that the thyroid hormone receptor in the nucleus associates with a triiodothyronine receptor auxiliary protein to bind to DNA in regulating development processes suggests that it may play a regulatory role in normoblast proliferation and maturation.[2-6] Moreover, ex vivo studies have demonstrated an effect of thyroid hormone in stimulating hemoglobin synthesis and erythropoiesis.[7-9] Thyroid hormone may also play a regulatory role in production of erythropoietin (EPO),[10] and triiodothyronine has been shown to augment release of burst-promoting activity from blood and bone marrow mononuclear cells.[11] EPO secretion may be stimulated by sym-

Table 153-1. Hematologic Manifestations of Thyroid Disease

Abnormality	Comment
Hypothyroid	
Red cells	
Normocytic/macrocytic anemia	Decreased EPO production; erythroid hypoplasia
Microcytic anemia	Iron deficiency usually due to menorrhagia
Macrocytic anemia	Megaloblastic; pernicious anemia, rarely folic acid deficiency
Platelets and coagulation	
Decreased platelet function	
Nonspecific changes	Bleeding tendency occasionally
Decreased adhesiveness	No definite bleeding tendency
Thrombocytopenia	Autoimmune; occurs in Hashimoto thyroiditis
Factor VIII decreased	Related to down-regulation of catechol receptors (?)
Factors VII, IX, X decreased	No clinical problems; may reflect general suppression of protein synthesis
Hyperthyroid	
Red cells	
Microcytic	Not iron deficient
Erythrocytosis, mild degree	Increased EPO; increased erythropoiesis
Platelets and coagulation	
Thrombocytopenia	Autoimmune
Easy bruising	Associated with platelet antibodies
Factor VIII increased	Related to up-regulation of catechol receptors (?)

pathetic discharge of adrenergic receptors, although it is primarily regulated by oxygen, and the stimulus of thyroxine for EPO production may be the increased metabolic rate producing relative hypoxia. In hypothyroidism, an analogous physiologic adjustment to the lower metabolic rate may occur, with a decrease in EPO production.[1,12] Treatment of the underlying deficiency will result in gradual improvement to normal values as other clinical evidence of hypothyroidism disappears.

In some patients, the anemia may be microcytic. This condition is seen in women who develop menorrhagia secondary to the hypothyroid state, and thereby iron deficiency, which is then superimposed on the anemia directly related to hypothyroidism. Treatment with iron in such an instance will produce normochromic, normocytic red cells but will give a suboptimal response, unless the hormone deficiency is also treated.

Pernicious anemia occurs in patients with hypothyroidism approximately 10% of the time. It is also found in thyroiditis and, to a lesser degree, in hyperthyroidism. Presumably, it has in common with these diseases a pathogenetic relationship of autoimmunity.[13] Occasionally megaloblastic anemia precedes the development of myxedema. When the two occur in parallel, the latter may not be immediately recognized unless care is taken in a careful clinical evaluation of the patient. On rare occasions folic acid deficiency has also been seen in patients with hypothyroidism, and there is some suggestion that malabsorption can be a factor. However, the mechanism of folic acid deficiency is not clear.[14] Patients with hypothyroidism and associated megaloblastic anemia should therefore also be considered a challenge in differential diagnosis, and in view of the hazards of treating cobalamin deficiency with folic acid, the latter drug should not be given until cobalamin deficiency is ruled out or appropriately treated.

The relationship between thyroxine's effect on metabolism and erythropoiesis is not clear. Although the stimulus it provides for expression of catechol receptors[15] and for increased

metabolic rate might be expected to affect demand for hemoglobin, the erythropoietic response in hyperthyroidism is limited. Some evidence shows increased erythropoiesis in this state, but the hemoglobin and hematocrit are not above normal limits. A mild erythrocytosis may be obscured, however, by the increased plasma volume.[16] One finding in thyrotoxicosis that is not well explained is the presence of microcytosis without evidence of iron deficiency. An associated finding in these patients is evaluation of hemoglobin A_2, although not to the degree seen in β-thalassemia.[17] Shortened red cell survival has also been reported to occur in hyperthyroidism.[1] These abnormalities are reversed with treatment of the endocrine disorder. By contrast, macrocytic anemia can also be seen in hyperthyroidism, reflecting the autoimmune complication of pernicious anemia that may occur in this disease.[18]

Other hematologic abnormalities may complicate diseases of the thyroid. Hashimoto thyroiditis, an autoimmune disease, is often associated with other manifestations of autoimmunity. A significant number of these patients, as well as patients with Graves disease, have easy bruising associated with antiplatelet antibodies, and a proportion of these have thrombocytopenia.[19-21] In hypothyroidism, platelet adhesiveness has been reported to be decreased and is responsive to thyroid replacement therapy.[22] Factors VIII, VII, IX, and X have been reported to be low in hypothyroidism, while euglobulin lysis time has been reported to be increased or decreased, and fibrinolytic activity is said to be increased.[23-25] By contrast, in thyrotoxicosis, euglobulin lysis time is increased with decreased fibrinolytic activity, and factor VIII is occasionally elevated. These changes are not associated with overt clinical manifestations and revert to normal with hormone replacement.

In rare situations disease in the thyroid may be confused with primary hematologic disease. This can occur when lymphoma involves the thyroid and may be the presenting finding in that disease. This differential diagnosis may also be a problem when following patients with lymphoma who have been treated. In patients who have received radiotherapy in a field that includes the thyroid, thyroiditis may occur and may manifest as a positive gallium scan over the organ, confusing the interpretation of a follow-up evaluation of the patient.

Pituitary Disorders

The major hematologic effects of pituitary deficiency are the result of this gland's role in affecting function of other endocrine glands. Thus, the patient may present with anemia as a complication of secondary hypothyroidism, hypogonadism, or adrenal insufficiency. Evidence is equivocal that growth hormone itself plays a role in regulation of erythropoiesis. After hypophysectomy both anemia and leukopenia may occur, and some in vitro evidence shows that granulocytic colony growth may be enhanced by growth hormone through a pathway involving insulin-like growth factor/somatomedin C.[26] Moreover, mice deficient in acidophilic anterior pituitary cells have pancytopenia, which responds to recombinant human growth hormone.[27]

Two hormones, activin and inhibin, which are produced by several tissues and affect the pituitary, also affect hematopoiesis ex vivo, although their physiologic role in regulation of hematopoiesis is uncertain. Activin enhances human erythroid colony formation and inhibin suppresses this activity.[28] Similarly, activin enhances release of follicle-stimulating hormone from the pituitary and inhibin suppresses this action. Activin has also been shown to suppress the response of colony-forming unit-granulocyte/macrophage (CFU-GM) to interleukin-3.[29] These hormones appear to play a role in both development and reproduction[30]; how important they are in regulating hematopoiesis is not clear.

IATROGENIC ENDOCRINE DISORDERS

In practice, the hematologist may induce a number of endocrinologic abnormalities, and careful follow-up of patients includes an assessment of these problems.

First, in the treatment of Hodgkin disease, mantle irradiation may suppress thyroid function. The incidence of this complication has been fairly high, with the performance of lymphangiograms contributing to the risk. Hypothyroidism usually occurs within 5 years of treatment. As is usually the case with diminished thyroid function, recognition depends on careful history and physical examination. In this setting, anemia can be a special challenge because of the potential for other hematologic problems. A second problem related to the thyroid is the development of nodules, which can occur at any time throughout the life of the patient.

Second, alkylating agents or radiotherapy may result in endocrinologic complications. Hypogonadism and sterilization, a predictable result in males with such therapy as MOPP (mechlorethamine, vincristine [Oncovin], procarbazine, prednisone) or total nodal irradiation, may also occur in females receiving similar chemotherapy. In general older women are more susceptible, but attention should be paid to ovarian function during and after such treatment. Early menopause has been found in long-term survivors of childhood Hodgkin disease.

Some complications of chemotherapy may be transient. An example is the possible induction of diabetes insipidus with administration of vincristine.[44] Since most chemotherapy is given in the clinic and at home, patients must be involved in monitoring urinary output as well as intake when receiving this drug. Fortunately the stimulus to release antidiuretic hormone rarely achieves enough effect to have clinical significance, and the syndrome is reversible with cessation of the drug.

Hormones themselves may induce incidental hematologic side effects. In patients with idiopathic thrombocytopenia purpura receiving steroids, unexplained leukocytosis with neutrophilia usually reflects the effect of the hormone on granulocyte release. When using androgens for the treatment of myeloid metaplasia, one may see not only the desired effect of an increased hematocrit, but the undesirable effect of a larger spleen, reflecting the hormone's stimulatory effect on erythropoietic colonies, and to a lesser extent on myelopoiesis.

Gonadal Dysfunction

Androgens have long been recognized as stimulants of erythropoiesis and until the advent of recombinant EPO were the most effective agents available for therapeutic trial in management of anemias that occur in myelofibrosis with myeloid metaplasia, hypoplastic marrow, or renal failure. In the era before hematologic growth factors were available, they were used in therapeutic trials to stimulate hematopoiesis, and some evidence showed that they could enhance recovery after suppression of marrow with chemotherapy.[31–33] That androgens play a role in the physiologic increase in hematocrit that occurs in males with puberty is assumed. The agents active in regulating erythropoiesis are probably metabolic products of testosterone rather than the hormone itself.[34] The 5-β metabolites upregulate erythrocyte progenitors,[35,36] and the 5-α metabolites appear to stimulate EPO production.[37,38] Moreover, different metabolites may affect progenitors at different stages.[39]

Table 153-2. Hematologic Manifestations of Adrenal Disease

Abnormality	Comment
Adrenal insufficiency	
Red cells	
Normocytic anemia	Decreased erythropoiesis; may be masked by decreased plasma volume
Macrocytic anemia	Pernicious anemia; associated with other autoimmune diseases
Cushing syndrome	
Red cells	
Erythrocytosis	Mild, with increased plasma volume
White cells	
Neutrophilia	Increased mobilization; increased production
Eosinopenia	
Lymphopenia	Redistribution
Platelets and coagulation	
Bruisability	No measurable abnormality

While hematologists may be more familiar with androgens as pharmacologic agents, their physiologic role in hematopoiesis is apparent in the anemia associated with hypogonadism. This is one of the endocrinologic syndromes that may be subtle and that may manifest primarily as a mild or moderate anemia. In such an instance, however, history and physical examination usually provide adequate clues, and the patient will have an appropriate hematologic response to hormone replacement therapy. The burden still remains on the physician to determine the mechanism. The cause is often related to pituitary deficiency rather than primary gonadal failure, and the situation demands a careful search for intracranial lesions, as well as for impaired function of other endocrine glands that could be secondary to pituitary deficiency.

In females, hypogonadism is not associated with specific hematologic abnormalities, but the administration of estrogens may produce some hematologic changes. Persons taking birth control pills may have increased total iron binding capacity with lowered serum iron concentration, mimicking pregnancy. An increase in platelet count and adhesiveness, and in concentration of factors II, VII, IX, and X, with a decrease in antithrombin III may also occur.[40] Whether these changes account for an increased thrombotic tendency in women who are at risk because of smoking is not clear. The leukemoid reaction occasionally seen in pregnancy has not been attributed to a specific hormone, and its rarity makes a physiologic role of estrogens unlikely. Estradiol has, however, been found to augment myelomonocytic colony formation, and an increase in circulating monocytes has been demonstrated during the time of ovulation in the menstrual cycle.[41] Some experiments in animals have suggested that estrogen metabolites may play an indirect role in inhibiting hematopoiesis,[42,43] but there evidence for this in humans is small, and it is unlikely that they play any part in the development of aplastic anemia, which occurs as an extremely rare but recognized complication of pregnancy.

Adrenal Disorders

Corticosteroids may be the most commonly used medications in hematologic practice. While their use is usually attributed to their potential effects on immunoregulation, the adrenal steroids play a role in hematopoietic regulation as well (Table 153-2). Just as deficiency of thyroid hormone or testosterone may result in suppression of erythropoiesis, Addison disease also results in anemia secondary to a productive deficit. The degree may be masked by the associated decrease in plasma volume, giving a falsely high hematocrit. Glucocorti-

THERAPY FOR ENDOCRINE-RELATED HEMATOLOGIC DISORDERS

Anemia is the main hematologic target for treatment in endocrine disorders. It is the most common hematologic manifestation of endocrine insufficiency and reflects a productive deficit in erythropoietic function. This is seldom, if ever, apparent as a hypoplastic marrow, but is evident in the inappropriately low reticulocyte response to anemia. While the white cells may have some changes in differential such as the eosinophilia seen in adrenal insufficiency or the lymphopenia of Cushing syndrome, the changes are not reflected in clinical disease.

Treatment of the anemia cannot be considered separately from treatment of the disease. Since anemia develops in these endocrine disorders because of impairment of hormonal adjustment of red cell output, the mechanism of which is poorly understood, hormonal replacement alone is adequate therapy to increase erythroid output to normal levels. In follow-up of these patients, one cannot evaluate symptomatic relief of the anemia, since the patient is at the same time responding to treatment of the endocrine insufficiency. Moreover, the anemia is not of a degree to generate a brisk reticulocyte response, nor is the amount of hormone necessarily the dose that would produce immediate maximal response of erythropoiesis. Therefore, it is not advantageous to check a reticulocyte response after 1 week of therapy, since the climb in hematocrit is slow and steady, and reassessment in 4–8 weeks should find the values within the normal range.

If the response is not complete, other causes of anemia must be reconsidered, and in treating a single hormone deficiency, the first possibility to consider is multiple hormone deficiencies, secondary to a lesion in the pituitary or hypothalamus. Besides the appropriate measurements of trophic hormones, a search should be made with indicated imaging studies to evaluate the possibility of tumor, infection, or vascular problems involving this area of the brain. Treatment is determined by the findings but includes replacement of all of the relevant hormones that have been secondarily affected. Complete replacement is necessary for complete response.

Besides the anemia directly attributable to a state of hormone deficiency, there are associated hematologic disorders that may require specific treatment. Autoimmune disorders are a complication of diseases of the thyroid and more rarely of diseases of the other endocrine glands. Both idiopathic thrombocytopenic purpura and acquired hemolytic anemia occur in this setting and must be treated independently of the endocrinopathy. They are treated with prednisone, intravenous IgG, and, when indicated, other immunosuppressive drugs as well as splenectomy. Pernicious anemia, another autoimmune disease, requires vitamin B_{12} replacement and responds appropriately. As in pernicious anemia unassociated with endocrine disease, the patient should be continued on parenteral therapy indefinitely. A complete response of the anemia in these autoimmune diseases depends on the maintenance of adequate hormone replacement in the patient.

Studies of hemostasis in hypothyroidism may reveal some minor changes in platelet function and in clotting factors. These require no treatment, since they are seldom associated with any clinical problems. The values revert to normal after hormone replacement.

The one setting in which anemia occurs with excessive hormone is hyperparathyroidism. In these patients, hematologic response occurs following parathyroidectomy and appears to be related to an increased output of EPO. Whether these patients would respond to recombinant EPO has not been reported, but it appears that in those patients who are uremic with secondary hyperparathyroidism, EPO will elicit a response.

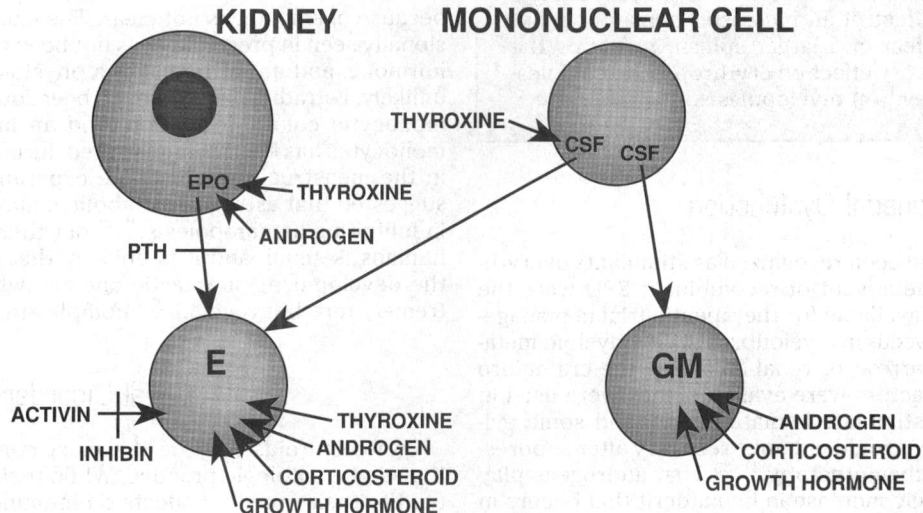

Fig. 153-1. Possible sites of hormones on hematopoiesis. Indirect stimulatory effects are noted by arrows directed toward production of growth factors, erythropoietin (EPO) and colony-stimulating factor (CSF), in the appropriate cells. Direct stimulatory effects of hormones are noted by arrows projecting across the cell membrane of erythroid (E) and granulocytic/monocytic precursors (GM). Production of EPO and CSF is noted by arrows to cell membrane of these precursors, where their receptors receive the signal. Suppression is noted by perpendicular lines intersecting arrows. PTH, parathyrin.

coids also play a role in the distribution of neutrophils by stimulating release from marrow to blood, and in adrenal insufficiency, associated white cell changes may occur with the development of mild neutropenia along with eosinophilia. These steroids also affect lymphocyte traffic, causing lymphopenia, and patients with adrenal insufficiency may have a relative lymphocytosis.[45] Study of the effects of hydrocortisone on progenitor cell growth has also demonstrated stimulation of growth of CFU-GM.[46] Thus, this hormone may participate in regulating production as well as delivery of granulocytes. In mice, adrenalectomy appears to result in relocation of the stem cells to the circulating blood and spleen, suggesting that adrenal steroids may play a physiologic role in migration of these cells as well.[47]

Addison disease may occasionally present as part of a polyglandular autoimmune syndrome, in which a macrocytic anemia may be seen. In this setting multiple mechanisms can account for the hematologic changes. One must consider the possibilities already mentioned in terms of hematologic manifestations of hypothyroidism, hypopituitarism, and pernicious anemia.

Cushing syndrome may also be associated with hematologic changes. Although patients with this disease may have an increase in red cell mass, more commonly they simply have facial plethora. In the peripheral blood, they often have lymphopenia and eosinopenia in response to the increased glucocorticoids.[45] The presence of an excess of steroids also leads to easy bruisability without a measurable hemostatic abnormality.

Vitamin D and the Parathyroid Glands

Vitamin D plays a broad role in development and may affect cell growth in many tissues. This is also evident in the hematopoietic system. Patients with rickets due to vitamin D deficiency may have anemia with a hypocellular marrow and are subject to increased frequency of infection, perhaps related to impairment of phagocytosis. These abnormalities are corrected by vitamin D_3.[48] 1,25-Dihydroxyvitamin D_3 has been shown to inhibit proliferation and to stimulate differentiation in several culture systems, and appears to direct myeloid cells toward macrophage differentiation.[48] It may affect colony growth by modulating the production of CSF-GM in human T cells.[49] No clinical hematologic syndromes are induced by hypervitaminosis D, but vitamin D_3 has been used as a potential differentiation agent in some settings of hematoproliferative disease, with as yet uncertain results. Diverse biologic activities are governed by this compound, suggesting its involvement in regulation of a number of genes.[50] How important its function is in physiologic hematopoiesis is not clear.

Anemia is a known but not predictable complication of primary hyperparathyroidism. It has been reported in 3–29% of patients.[51,52] The anemia is normochromic and normocytic and is corrected by successful parathyroidectomy. It tends to be of a mild degree and is not associated with other abnormal hematologic findings. It does not appear to be a myelophthisic process. While myelofibrosis may be seen in these patients, it does not correlate with the anemia, and evidence does not show a leukoerythroblastic picture. In some series, the anemia appeared to correlate with the degree of hyperparathyroidism,[53,54] but in others it did not.[52] Some observations of colony formation suggest that parathyrin may directly inhibit erythropoiesis.[55]

Secondary hyperparathyroidism may also be associated with anemia, but it is more difficult to evaluate because of the underlying renal failure. However, it does appear to occur by a mechanism separate from that of the anemia of uremia. Following parathyroidectomy, serum EPO levels increase, a reticu-

locytosis occurs, and the anemia responds.[56] Thus, the anemia appears to be related to suppression of EPO production beyond that explained by the renal failure itself.

SUMMARY

Most of the endocrine glands have some regulatory effect on the rate of red cell production (Fig. 153-1). They may act as a fine adjustment to the system, without being a necessary requirement, and the hematopoietic response may reflect the broader physiologic response that goes on in many tissues when the hormonal environment changes. The minor changes seen in white cells, platelets, and clotting factors have little clinical relevance but occasionally offer an aid in diagnosis.

REFERENCES

1. Das KC, Mukherjee M, Sarker TJ et al: Erythropoiesis and erythropoietin in hypo- and hyperthyroidism. J Clin Endocrinol Metab 40:211, 1975
2. Chatterjee VK, Tata JR: Thyroid hormone receptors and their role in development. Cancer Surv 14:147, 1992
3. Lazar MA: Steroid and thyroid hormone receptors. Endocrinol Metab Clin North Am 20:681, 1991
4. Thomson KL, Santon JB, Shephard LB et al: A nuclear protein is required for thyroid hormone receptor binding to an inhibitory half-site in the epidermal growth factor receptor promoter. Mol Endocrinol 6:627, 1992
5. Darling DS, Beebe JS, Burnside J et al: 3,5,3′-Triiodothyronine (T_3) receptor auxiliary protein (TRAP) binds DNA and forms heterodimers with the T_3 receptor. Mol Endocrinol 5:73, 1991
6. Hudson LG, Santon JB, Glass CK, Gill GN: Ligand-activated thyroid hormone and retinoic acid receptors inhibit growth factor receptor promoter expression. Cell 62:1165, 1990
7. Malgor LA, Blanc CC, Klainer E et al: Direct effects of thyroid hormone on bone marrow erythroid cells in rats. Blood 45:671, 1975
8. Golde DW, Bersch N, Chopra IJ et al: Thyroid hormones stimulate erythropoiesis in vitro. Br J Haematol 37:173, 1977
9. Dainiak N, Hoffman R, Maffei LA et al: Potentiation of human erythropoiesis in vitro by thyroid hormone. Nature 272:260, 1978
10. Peschle C, Zanjani ED, Gidari AS et al: Mechanisms of thyroxine action on erythropoiesis. Endocrinology 89:609, 1971
11. Dainiak N, Sutter D, Kreczko S: L-triiodothyronine augments erythropoietic growth factor release from peripheral blood and bone marrow leukocytes. Blood 68:1289, 1986
12. Ganong WF: Neuroendocrinology. p. 75. In Greenspan FS (ed): Basic and Clinical Endocrinology. Appleton & Lange, E. Norwalk, CT, 1991, p. 75
13. Irvine WJ, Davies SH, Delamore JW et al: Immunologic relationship between pernicious anemia and thyroid disease. Br Med J 2:454, 1962
14. Vassilopoulou R, Sellin JH: The gastrointestinal tract and liver in hypothy-

roidism. p. 1017. In Braverman LE, Utiger RD (eds): Werner and Ingbar's The Thyroid. 6th Ed. JB Lippincott, Philadelphia, 1991

15. Greenspan FS, Rapoport B: Thyroid gland, p. 205. In Greenspan FS (ed): Basic and Clinical Endocrinology. 3rd Ed. Appleton & Lange, E. Norwalk, CT, 1991

16. Ansell JE: The blood in thyrotoxicosis. p. 785. In Braverman LE, Utiger RD (eds): Werner and Ingbar's The Thyroid. 6th Ed. JB Lippincott, Philadelphia, 1991

17. Kuhn JM, Riew M, Rochete J et al: Influence of thyroid status on hemoglobin A$_2$ expression. J Clin Endocrinol Metab 57:344, 1983

18. Carmel R, Spencer CA: Clinical and subclinical thyroid disorders associated with pernicious anemia. Arch Intern Med 142:1465, 1982

19. Hymes K, Blum M, Lackner H et al: Easy bruising, thrombocytopenia and elevated platelet immunoglobulin G in Graves' disease and Hashimoto's thyroiditis. Ann Intern Med 94:27, 1981

20. Branehog I, Olsson KS, Weinfield A et al: Association of hyperthyroidism with idiopathic thrombocytopenic purpura and hemolytic anemia. Acta Med Scand 205:125, 1979

21. Ansell JE: The blood in hypothyroidism. p. 1022. In Braverman LE, Utiger RD, (eds): Werner and Ingbar's The Thyroid. 6th Ed. JB Lippincott, Philadelphia, 1991

22. Edson JR, Fecher DR, Doe RP: Low platelet adhesiveness and other hemostatic abnormalities in hypothyroidism. Ann Intern Med 82:342, 1975

23. Farid NR, Griffiths BL, Collins JR et al: Blood coagulation and fibrinolysis in thyroid disease. Thromb Haemost 35:415, 1976

24. Rennie JAN, Bewsher PD, Murchison LE, Ogston D: Coagulation and fibrinolysis in thyroid disease. Acta Haematol 59:171, 1978

25. Simone JV, Abilgaard CF, Schulman I: Blood coagulation in thyroid dysfunction. N Engl J Med 273:1057, 1965

26. Merchov S, Tartasky I, Hochberg Z: Enhancement of human granulopoiesis in vitro by biosynthetic insulin-like growth factor 1/somatomedin C and human growth hormone. J Clin Invest 81:791, 1988

27. Murphy WJ, Durum SK, Anver MR, Longo DL: Immunologic and hematologic effects of neuroendocrine hormones. J Immunol 148:3799, 1992

28. Broxmeyer HE, Lu L, Cooper S et al: Selective and indirect modulation of human multipotential and erythroid hematopoietic progenitor cell proliferation by recombinant human activin and inhibin. Proc Natl Acad Sci USA 85:9052, 1988

29. Mizuguchi T, Kosaka M, Saito S: Activin A suppresses proliferation of interleukin-3-responsive granulocyte-macrophage colony-forming progenitors and stimulates proliferation and differentiation of interleukin-3-responsive erythroid burst-forming progenitors in peripheral blood. Blood 81:2891, 1993

30. Krummen LA, Woodruff TK, DeGuzman G et al: Identification and characterization of binding proteins for inhibin and activin in human serum and follicular fluids. Endocrinology 132:431, 1993

31. Udupa KB, Reissman KR: Acceleration of granulopoietic recovery by androgenic steroids in mice made neutropenic by cytotoxic drugs. Cancer Res 34:2517, 1974

32. Ambrus JL, Mirand EA: Effect of autologous bone marrow transplantation and an anabolic steroid on erythropoietin production and hemopoietic recovery after whole body irradiation and treatment with alkylating agents. J Med 4:65, 1973

33. Gallicchio G, Chen MG, Watts TD: Regeneration of murine megakaryoctopoiesis and the hematopoietic inductive microenvironment after sublethal whole body irradiation by treatment with anabolic steroid. Acta Haematol 73:80, 1985

34. Mooradian AD, Morley JE, Korenmen SG: Biological actions of androgens. Endocrinol Rev 8:1, 1987

35. Singer JW, Samuels AI, Adamson JW: Steroids and hematopoiesis. I: The effects of steroids on in vivo erythroid colony growth: structure/activity relationships. J Cell Physiol 88:127, 1976

36. Modder B, Foley JE, Fisher JW: The in vitro and in vivo effects of testosterone on erythroid colony forming cells (CFU-E). J Pharmacol Exp Ther 207:1004, 1978

37. Dainiak N: The role of androgens in the treatment of anemia of chronic renal failure. Semin Nephrol 5:147, 1985

38. Shahidi N: Androgens and erythropoiesis. N Engl J Med 289:72, 1973

39. Singer JW, Adamson JW: Steroids and hematopoiesis. II. The effect of steroids on in vitro erythroid colony growth: evidence for different target cells for different classes of steroids. J Cell Physiol 88:135, 1976

40. Weindling H, Henry JB: Laboratory tests altered by "the pill." JAMA 229:1762, 1974

41. Maoz H, Kaiser N, Halimi M et al: The effect of estradiol on human myelomonocytic cells. 1. Enhancement of colony formation. J Reprod Immunol 7:325, 1985

42. Crandall TL, Joyce RA, Boggs DR: Estrogens and hematopoiesis: characterization and studies on the mechanism of neutropenia. J Lab Clin Med 95:857, 1980

43. Sherrill A, Gorham J: Bone marrow hypoplasia associated with estrus in ferrets. Lab Anim Sci 35:280, 1985

44. Robertson GL, Bhoopalam N, Zelkowitz IJ: Vincristine neurotoxicity and abnormal secretion of antidiuretic hormone. Arch Intern Med 132:717, 1973

45. Orth DN, Kovaks WJ, Debold CR: The adrenal cortex. p. 517. In Wilson JD, Foster DW (eds): Williams' Textbook of Endocrinology. 8th Ed. WB Saunders, Philadelphia, 1992

46. Barr RD, Koekebakker H, Milner RA: Hydrocortisone—a possible physiological regulator of human granulopoiesis. Scand J Haematol 31:31, 1985

47. Khaitov RM, Petrov RV, Moroz BB, Bezin GI: The factors controlling stem cell migration. I. Migration of hemopoietic stem cells in adrenalectomized mice. Blood 46:73, 1975

48. Reichel H, Koeffler P, Norman AW: The role of the vitamin D endocrine system in health and disease. N Engl J Med 320:980, 1989

49. Tobler A, Gasson J, Reichel H et al: Granulocyte-macrophage colony-stimulating factor. Sensitive and receptor-mediated regulation by 1,25-dihydroxyvitamin D$_3$ in normal human peripheral blood lymphocytes. J Clin Invest 79:1700, 1987

50. Minghetti PP, Norman AW: 1,25(OH)$_2$-Vitamin D$_3$ receptors: gene regulation and genetic circuitry. FASEB J 2:3043, 1988

51. Abarca J, Trigonis C, Hamberger B, Granberg PO: Anaemia in primary hyperparathyroidism—fantasy or reality. Ann Chir Gynaecol 74:74, 1985

52. Bernheim J, Rathaus V, Rathaus M, Bernheim J: L'anemie de l'hyperparathyroidie primitive. Nephrologie 7:28, 1986

53. Mallette L-E: Hyporegenerative anemia in primary hyperparathyroidism. South Med J 70:1199, 1977

54. Boxer M, Ellman L, Geller R, Wang CA: Anemia in primary hyperparathyroidism. Arch Intern Med 137:588, 1977

55. Meytes D, Bogin A, Dukes P et al: Effect of parathyroid hormone on erythropoiesis. J Clin Invest 67:1263, 1981

56. Urena P, Eckardt KU, Sarfati E et al: Serum erythropoietin and erythropoiesis in primary and secondary hyperparathyroidism: effect of parathyroidectomy. Nephron 59:384, 1991

57. Bichet DG, Razi M, Lonergan M: Haemodynamic and coagulation responses to 1-desamino[8-D-arginine] vasopressin in patients with congenital nephrogenic diabetes insipidus. N Engl J Med 318:881, 1988

58. Eadington DW: Hypoglycaemia and metabolic acidosis in a patient with acute leukaemia. Scott Med J 33:309, 1988

59. Schmid C, Beham A, Seewann HL: Extramedullary hematopoiesis in the thyroid gland due to agnogenic myeloid metaplasia is reported. Histopathology 15:423, 1989

60. Balducci L, Chapman SW, Little DD, Hardy CL: Paraneoplastic eosinophilia. Report of a case with in vitro studies of hemopoiesis. Cancer 64:2250, 1989

61. Swelstad JA, Scanlon EF, Murphy ED et al: Thyroid disease following irradiation for benign conditions. Arch Surg 112:380, 1977

62. Scholefield JH, Quayle AR, Harris SC, Talbot CH: Primary lymphoma of the thyroid, the association with Hashimoto's thyroiditis. Eur J Surg Oncol 18:89, 92

63. Edson JR, Fecher DR, Doe RP: Low platelet adhesiveness and other hemostatic abnormalities in hypothyroidism. Ann Intern Med 82:342, 1975

64. Dalton RG, Dewar MS, Sowidge GF et al: Hypothyroidism as a cause of von Willebrand's disease. Lancet 1:1007, 1987

Hematologic Manifestations of Infectious Disease

154

David S. Rosenthal

INTRODUCTION

The hematologist is all too aware of the many catastrophic infections that affect the patient with hematologic-oncologic diseases. From the fungal lung infections of the acute leukemia patient to the salmonella osteomyelitis of the sickle cell individual, the infectious disease consultant is of tremendous support in the overall management of hematologic diseases. Just as important is the role of the blood specialist in assisting the clinician to manage the many and various types of hematologic manifestations of infections. Some infectious diseases may cause a number of different and occasionally opposite blood dyscrasias. For example, tuberculosis, depending on its degree of severity, can present as pancytopenia with myelophthisis in one individual but can mimic acute or chronic myeloid leukemia (AML, CML) in another. Infection with aspergilli can cause disseminated intravascular coagulation (DIC) in one instance and thrombosis in another. A wide range of abnormalities and effects on primitive and adult hematopoietic cells occurs with bacteria, viruses, fungi, and protozoa and serves as the basis for this chapter.[1] Discussions of the human immunodeficiency virus (HIV) and the acquired immunodeficiency syndrome (AIDS) (see Ch. 155) and infectious mononucleosis (see Ch. 58) appear elsewhere.

ANEMIA

Anemia that results from infection can be categorized by the same pathophysiologic mechanisms that apply to anemias in general: blood loss, decreased production, and increased destruction (Table 154-1). Anemia secondary to gastrointestinal blood loss can occur in patients with hookworm infestation and bowel involvement with shigella or typhoid. *Campylobacter pyloridis* has been implicated in gastric and duodenal ulcer dis-

ease and may cause upper gastrointestinal hemorrhage,[2] while blood loss can be significant from hematuria due to bacterial cystitis or hemoptysis due to large cavitary pulmonary disease from tuberculosis or aspergillosis. Blood loss anemia, usually of an acute nature in these disorders, will be associated with iron-deficiency anemia as well if it is chronic.

Most infections can cause some degree of marrow suppression or decreased production. In an acute or self-limited illness, the effect on blood counts may be imperceptible. If the illness is prolonged, the blood count changes will be more striking. Infection-induced myelosuppression can involve red cells alone or all three hematopoietic cell lines, thus resulting in (1) aplastic or hypoplastic anemia, or (2) the anemia of acute and chronic infection.

Aplastic Anemia

Aplastic anemia is extremely uncommon but can result directly or indirectly from an infectious agent. Hepatitis, usually hepatitis C, has been shown to carry a significant risk for aplasia.[3,4] Approximately 0.1–0.2% of all cases of hepatitis can develop pancytopenia, while 5% of aplastic anemia cases have a recent history of hepatitis. The incidence is unrelated to the severity of the infection, and the prognosis is grave. The marrow suppression generally occurs during the convalescent phase, and the mechanism is not clear. Certain viruses like hepatitis B are known to be trophic for hematopoietic cells.[5] The ability to transplant compatible marrow cells into affected patients suggests that the virus does not cause damage to the marrow microenvironment.[6]

Other viral illnesses such as HIV, infectious mononucleosis, and B19 parvovirus are also associated with aplastic anemia. Although anemia associated with parvovirus usually occurs in individuals with other underlying hematologic conditions such as hemolytic anemias, cases in previously normal individuals have been reported.[7] Replacement of the marrow by granulomas of tuberculosis and histoplasmosis, marrow necrosis caused by overwhelming gram-negative and gram-positive infections, mucor, dengue fever, rubella, brucella, or *Salmonella typhi* may result in pancytopenia and marrow failure.[8–10] In these latter instances, possible mechanisms for pancytopenia include (1) a direct toxic effect causing marrow necrosis, (2) myelophthisis due to replacement with granulomas, (3) histiocytic hemophagocytosis, or (4) nutritional deficiencies as seen in anorexia nervosa. Experimental studies with B19 parvovirus suggest an inhibitory effect of the organism.[7] Addition of infected sera to human marrow culture systems caused significant inhibition of erythropoiesis as measured by colony-forming unit-erythroid and burst-forming unit-erythroid. Indirectly, infectious organisms can interfere with hematopoiesis by activating macrophages or lymphocytes to release inhibitory mediators.[11] Whatever the mechanism of infection-related marrow failure, the incidence is greater in patients previously compromised by poor nutrition, alcohol abuse, or previous exposure to chemotherapy.

Pancytopenia may also result from persistence of congestive

Table 154-1. Pathophysiology of Anemia

Blood loss
  Gastrointestinal (hookworm)
  Genitourinary (schistosomiasis)
  Pulmonary (tuberculosis)

Decreased production
  Aplasia
  Anemia of chronic disease
  Anemia of acute infection

Increased destruction
  Intraerythrocyte parasitization
  Immunohemolytic conditions
    Autoimmune
    "Innocent bystander"
    Polyagglutination
  Enzyme deficiency (G6PD)
  Pathologic changes
    Hemolytic uremic syndrome
    DIC
    Hypersplenism

Table 154-2. Anemia of Chronic Disease

Laboratory findings
  Normochromic normocytic or microcytic hypochromic
  Decreased reticulocyte count
  Decreased serum iron
  Decreased serum transferrin
  Slight-to-moderate decrease in iron saturation
  Slight-to-moderate decrease in sideroblasts
  Normal to increased iron stores
Disorders
  Endocarditis (bacterial or fungal)
  Meningitis
  Emphysema
  Cavitary pulmonary disease
  Abscess
  Chronic peritonitis
  Chronic osteomyelitis
  Chronic infectious arthritis
Agents
  Tuberculosis
  Leprosy
  Typhoid
  Tularemia
  Brucellosis
  Lyme disease

splenomegaly related to malaria, infectious mononucleosis, toxoplasmosis, hepatitis, salmonellosis, tularemia, syphilis, subacute bacterial endocarditis, tuberculosis, or schistosomiasis.

Anemia of Chronic Disease

Anemia of chronic disease (ACD) (Table 154-2) is probably the most common blood dyscrasia seen as a result of infection.[12-15] The degree of anemia tends to correlate with the intensity of the fever or the degree of inflammation. The anemia may be normocytic, normochromic or microcytic, hypochromic and is characterized by decreased reticulocytes, low serum iron, low serum transferrin, and slight-to-moderate decrease in percent saturation and marrow sideroblasts but a normal-to-increased amount of body iron stores. The commonest infectious diseases are bacterial or fungal endocarditis, meningitis, empyema, cavitary pulmonary disease, abscess (especially intra-abdominal), chronic peritonitis, chronic osteomyelitis, and chronic infectious arthritis (Table 154-2). In addition, any chronic infection such as tuberculosis, leprosy, typhoid, tularemia, brucellosis, or Lyme disease can be associated with ACD.

The mechanism proposed for this anemia was initially put forth by Cartwright and Lee.[12] The reticuloendothelial system becomes activated by the chronic infection, resulting in a block in the normal iron transfer. The result is that iron released by senescent red cells is picked up by stimulated macrophages and blocked from release to marrow erythropoietic precursors. Thus, marrow stores of iron (in macrophages) are sufficient but sideroblasts are reduced to absent. Another theory relates to the effect of various cytokines whose activity is enhanced by the infection.[13] Interleukin-1 (IL-1) and tumor necrosis factor-α are two such proteins.[17] Bacteria and fungi, as well as certain endotoxins and other infectious agent by-products, are enhancers of IL-1 production and release. Among other biologic properties, IL-1 activates neutrophils to release lactoferrin and inhibits liver cells from synthesizing transferrin, thus resulting in decreased serum iron.[18] The IL-1-induced hypoferremia is thought to be a homeostatic mechanism to decrease

the virulence of infection. Infusing iron into experimental animals increases the severity of infection, while reducing the iron level by chelation decreases the virulence.[16,19] A similar mechanism involves the role of TNF in ACD. As one author commented "the anemia of chronic infection may be the 'cost' paid by the host to deprive microbial invaders of this essential nutrient."[1]

Anemia of Acute Infection

The anemia of acute infection has been described in children admitted for *Haemophilus influenzae* meningitis.[20] Although this infection is more commonly associated with hemolysis, the reticulocyte count has been reported to be low in some cases, implying marrow suppression. The anemia is usually mild and rebounds without hematinics when the infection is resolved. Other acute infections in the pediatric age group such as osteomyelitis, arthritis, and pneumonia can also cause a picture not too dissimilar to ACD.

Hemolytic Anemia

Hemolytic anemia, the rapid destruction of red cells, can occur due to infections from many of the same mechanisms classically described for hemolysis in general, such as immune mechanisms, underlying red cell defects, or increased susceptibility to phagocytosis by macrophages in the spleen.[1,21] Table 154-3 categorizes the infection-induced hemolysis into those associated with normal red cells, those associated with an underlying red cell defect such as an enzyme deficiency, and those related to pathologic changes secondary to the infection. These anemias can be clinically quite dramatic as well as demanding and exciting for the laboratory involved in their evaluation.

Parasitic and Bacterial Infection

Intraerythrocyte parasitization and red cell destruction occurs with malaria and babesiosis as well as with *Bartonella bacilliformis*. In these disorders, the red cells are either directly

Table 154-3. Categories of Infection-Related Hemolytic Anemias

Intraerythrocyte parasitization
  Malaria
  Babesiosis
  Bartonellosis
  Clostridia perfringens
Immunohemolytic conditions
  Autoimmune states
    Cold hemagglutinin disease
      Mycoplasma
      EBV
    Donath-landsteiner antibodies (paroxysmal cold hemoglobinuria)
      Secondary and congenital syphilis
      Measles
      Measles vaccination
  "Innocent bystander"
    Haemophilus influenzae
  Polyagglutination
    Enteric bacteria
Oxidative effect on enzyme-deficient red cells
  G6PD deficiency
Pathologic changes
  Hemolytic uremic syndrome
  Endocarditis
  Hypersplenism
  DIC

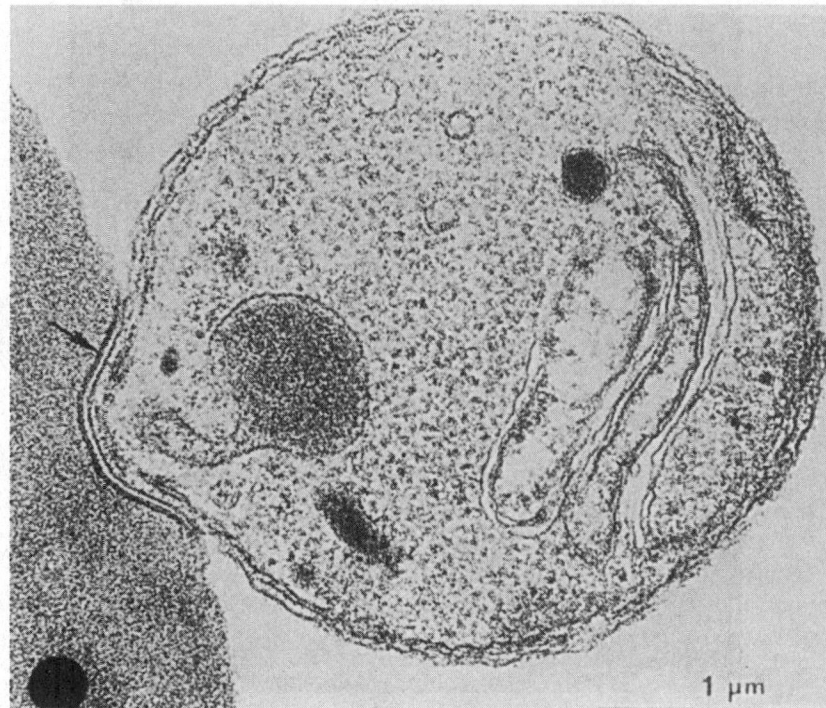

Fig. 154-1. Interaction of *Plasmodium falciparum* with a red cell. The parasite creates a depression in the membrane, which becomes thickened at the site of invagination. (From Aikawa and Miller,[86] with permission.)

lysed, deformed, and/or removed by the spleen directly or through immune mechanisms. Malaria-infected tissues release millions of merozoites into the circulation that adhere to erythrocytes through specific red cell surface antigens.[22] *Plasmodium falciparum* merozoites adhere to red cell glycophorin and then invade the membrane, creating entry for the parasite. The cytoskeleton structure opens up to allow passage and then reforms itself after the organism has entered the cytoplasm. Some red cells are lysed immediately by the resulting parasitization, while others, containing the characteristic Wright-Giemsa appearance (Fig. 154-1) and shapes, feed on hemoglobin and produce various proteins. These malaria by-products can protrude through the membrane and cause the cell to adhere to vascular endothelium or to other red cells, or to both. IgG is attracted to these abnormal proteins and sets up the cell for immune destruction by the splenic reticuloendothelial system. With continued splenic hemolysis, the spleen enlarges, causing increased red cell destruction by trapping and removing partially damaged or deformed erythrocytes. The most serious hemolytic complication is blackwater fever. In rare instances of *P. falciparum* infection, an overwhelming and acute intravascular hemolysis occurs due to a direct autoimmune reaction associated with a positive Coombs test.

Babesiosis-induced hemolysis is similar to malaria. The disease occurs along the coast of New England, is caused by *Bacillus microti,* and is transmitted from infected deer mice by the tick from the *Ixodes* species. The parasite invades the red cell directly by a complement-mediated mechanism. The symptoms range from a generalized malaise to a hectic fever and hemolytic anemia.[23] Infection in splenectomized patients can lead to catastrophic intravascular hemolysis and acute renal failure.[24]

Bartonellosis (Oroya fever) is transmitted by a sandfly, not uncommon in Peru.[25] Within 2–3 weeks of the bite, fever, chills, and hemolysis occurs. The hemolysis is quite dramatic and severe. The organism attaches to the surface of the red cell and may or may not invade the membrane (Fig. 154-2). If untreated, the patient can die from the event.

Although it is well known that bacteria produce hemolytic toxins (microbiology culture systems), rarely is there a direct effect in humans. An exception occurs in *Clostridium perfringens* infection, which can cause severe hemolysis through an α-toxin, a lecithinase, which reacts with red cell membrane lipoproteins to release lysolecithin, a red cell lysing agent.[26,27] The resultant intravascular hemolysis can be quite sudden and dramatic. Suspicion of this infection is raised after septic abortion, biliary tract disease, or traumatic wound infection, or in malignancy. A patient with CML developed a hemolytic crisis secondary to clostridia sepsis. She was able to survive for almost 5 hours with a hematocrit of 0% on the oxygen-carrying capacity of free hemoglobin.[28]

Many other bacterial infections, when severe in nature, have been associated with hemolysis.[29] Rapidly falling hematocrits, increased reticulocytes without evidence of bleeding, have been reported with septicemia and endocarditis due to gram-negative or -positive organisms. Intravascular hemolysis has been cited secondary to cholera, while hemoglobinuria has been seen with miliary tuberculosis and some spirochetal infections such as those caused by borrelia. The mechanism for these types of hemolysis is unclear, but evidence points to a direct effect of the infectious agent or its by-product.

Immunohemolytic Conditions

A large number of infection-related hemolytic anemias can be due to an immunohemolytic condition. The immunohemolytic conditions can be divided into three categories: (1) autoimmune, (2) antigen/antibody complexes or "innocent bystander" reactions, and (3) polyagglutination.[21] An infectious agent or its by-product can stimulate antibody production with an affinity for a red cell surface-specific protein and cause an autoimmune hemolytic anemia (AHA). The inciting agent need not be present. The resultant hemolysis can be either intravascular secondary to IgM or "cold" antibodies or extravascular secondary to the IgG antibodies, which are usually of the "warm" type and are directed against one of the Rh antigens.

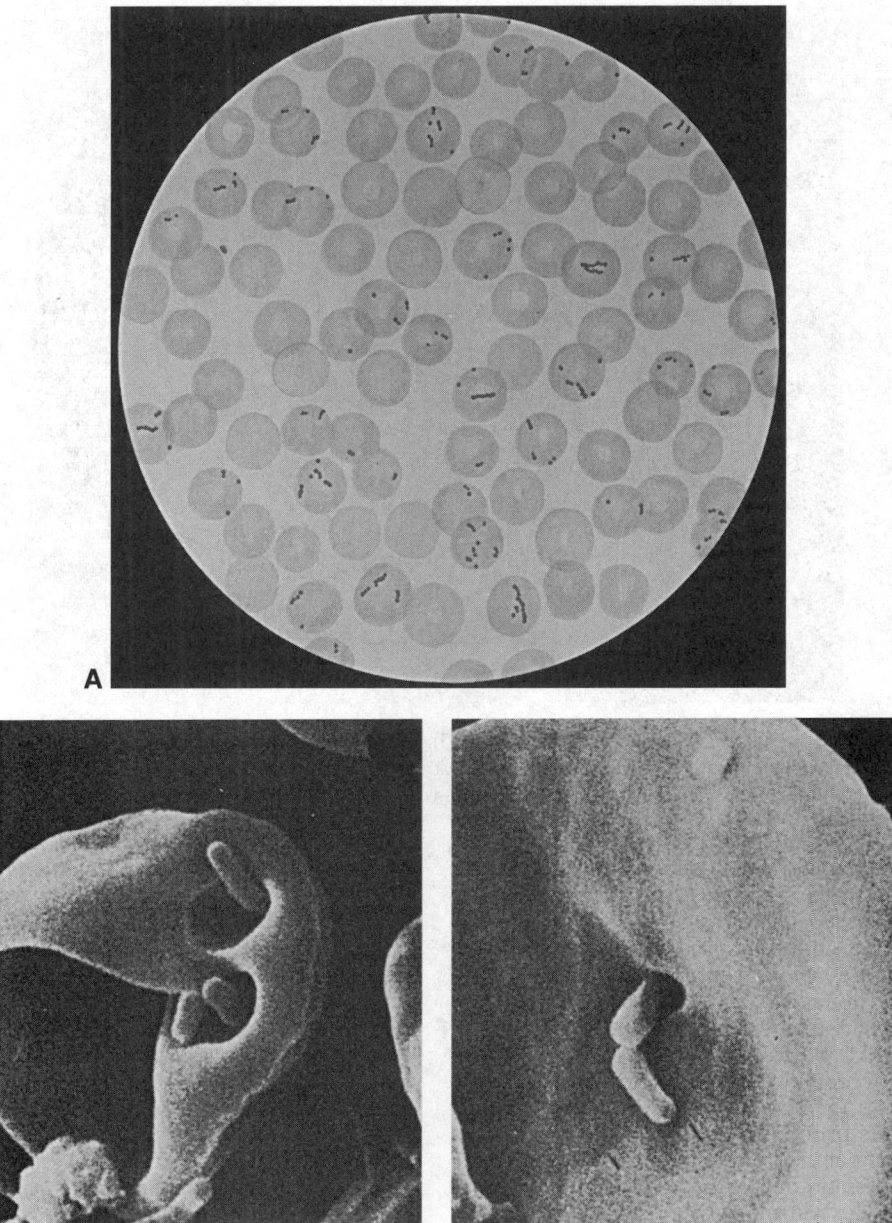

Fig. 154-2. (A) Wright-stained blood smear from Oroya fever *(Bartonella bacilliformis)*. The parasites are pleomorphic, stain bright red, are usually spherical, and can form small chains (× 1,100). (From Bogemann and Rastetter,[87] with permission.) **(B)** Scanning electron microscopy showing bartonella burrowing into and penetrating the membranes of red cells during hemolytic septicemia. (From Benson et al.,[88] with permission.)

Most of the infection-induced AHAs are of the "cold" antibody type and are referred to as cold hemagglutinin disease (CHAD). Two of the commonest infections causing CHAD are *Mycoplasma pneumoniae* and Epstein-Barr virus (EBV) of infectious mononucleosis.[30–32] Both infectious agents are associated with IgM antibodies to the I,i red cell antigens; mycoplasma with anti-I and infectious mononucleosis with anti-i antibodies. These cold agglutinin antibodies bind to the red cell at low temperatures, fix complement, and cause hemolysis. The incidence of CHAD with *M. pneumoniae* and EBV infections is low but is aggravated by low external temperatures. Other organisms such as mumps, cytomegalovirus, and legionella have also been known to produce CHAD.[33,34]

In secondary and congenital syphilis, an AHA can result from the production of Donath-Ladsteiner antibodies. Even though these proteins are of the IgG class and react against the P anti-gen of red cells, they do so at cold temperatures, and the resultant clinical picture has been labeled paroxysmal cold hemoglobinuria.[35] In affected patients this can be a chronic illness and can require patients to live in warm climates. Paroxysmal cold hemoglobinuria can also occur as an acute illness following varicella, infectious mononucleosis, mumps, measles, MMR (measles, mumps, rubella) vaccination, and mycoplasma infections.[36] During the convalescent stage of these infections or when the patient is exposed to low environmental temperatures, the individual suddenly develops pallor, jaundice, hemoglobinuria, and splenomegaly.

The "innocent bystander" mechanism for AHA is caused by the complex of the antigen with the antibody nonspecifically, in proximity to the red cell. An infectious agent or antibiotic medication, or both, can cause an antibody formation. The resultant antigen/antibody complex in the bloodstream can nonspecifically attach to the red cell and lead to hemolysis, the red cell being the "innocent bystander." *H. influenzae* type b meningitis in children can cause this type of hemolysis.[37] It is cause for suspicion that the capsular antigen of the bacteria and its resultant antibody are simultaneously present in the bloodstream of children with this infection.[38] The protein complex binds in some way to red cells, fixes complement, and causes intravascular hemolysis. Drugs that have been implicated in the "innocent bystander" type of hemolysis include antibiotics such as quinine, quinidine, sulfonamide, P-aminosalicylic acid (PAS), and sulfanilic acid derivatives.

The third mechanism for AHA has been termed polyagglutination.[21] Antigens, normally hidden or masked from contact with the red cell membrane called Thomson-Friedenreich cryptoantigens or T antigens, may become exposed by infectious agent enzyme digestion and make the red cell membrane more susceptible to normal plasma antibodies.[39] For example, neuraminidase, produced by enteric bacteria, can break down red cell surface glycoproteins, unmask the T antigen and expose the red cell to natural blood IgM antibodies, resulting in cell agglutination or polyagglutination and eventual hemolysis.[40]

AHA can be detected by the sudden clinical picture and by a positive antiglobulin or Coombs test. The direct Coombs test will detect red cells with antibody coating the red cell membrane. The indirect Coombs test will demonstrate the presence of circulating antibody in the plasma.

Hemolysis Due to Infection in G6PD-Deficient Patients

Normal red cells cope with the oxidative stresses of infections and drugs with the help of reducing enzymes.[41] Four enzymes keep the red cell membrane and hemoglobin in the reduced state. Once oxidized, the membrane becomes rigid and susceptible to extravascular hemolysis within the spleen (Fig. 154-3). Oxidized hemoglobin or methemoglobin form inclusions within the cell (Heinz bodies) that cling to the surface of the membrane and further initiate extravascular hemolysis. The Heinz body/membrane interface is subject to splenic macrophage stimulation that causes the red cell to look as if a piece had been removed, a "bite cell." Of the four enzymes involved, glucose 6-phosphate dehydrogenase (G6PD) is most frequently deficient in various populations. Several common genetic variants such as G6PD^{A-}, G6PD^{Mediterranean}, and G6PD^{Canton} are associated with decreased enzyme activity. Historically, a higher incidence of infection-related hemolysis had

Table 154-4. Causes of Hemolysis in Infected G6PD-Deficient Patients

Infectious agents	Medications
Salmonella	Antimalarials
Escherichia coli	Primaquine
β-Hemolytic streptococci	Paraquine
Rickettsia	Pentaquine
Viral hepatitis	Sulfonamides
Influenza A	Sulfones
	Nitrofurans
	Analgesics

been noted in blacks versus whites in the United States, which led to the hypothesis that infection causes hemolysis in G6PD-deficient patients.[42,43] Infection-activated neutrophils produce superoxide, which converts hemoglobin to methemoglobin. In the absence of the enzyme, methemoglobin interacts with hydrogen peroxide, Heinz bodies are formed, the red cell membrane becomes rigid, and hemolysis results.[44–46]

G6PD-deficient patients may not have had any prior clinically evident hemolysis when they first present. Affected patients have sudden hemolysis, scleral icterus, and increased reticulocytes, with or without splenomegaly. The blood film may initially show "bite cells" along with polychromatophilia. Heinz body preparations may be positive if performed during the acute hemolytic episode. G6PD enzyme assays can be falsely normal during the hemolytic period, since enzyme activity is highest in young red cells, in some variants high enough to give a normal result. The cyanide-ascorbate test detects the red cells' ability to prevent hemoglobin oxidation by ascorbate and can be sensitive enough to detect as few as 10–15% of deficient cells on a slide.[47]

The most frequent infectious organisms associated with hemoglobin oxidation are listed in Table 154-4 and include salmonella, *Escherichia coli,* β-streptococci, various rickettsiae, and viral hepatitis organisms. In addition, the influenza A virus has been shown to have a direct lytic effect in vitro on G6PD-deficient cells.[48] Many antibiotics and medications used in managing infections are direct oxidants and cause hemolysis in enzyme-deficient patients during convalescence. Table 154-4 lists the more common agents implicated clinically.

Pathologic Changes

The final group of infection-induced hemolytic diseases can be categorized by tissue damage or hypertrophy. Pathologic changes in tissues created directly or indirectly by the infecting organism is the mechanism of hemolysis, as in the hemolytic uremic syndrome, DIC, bacteria endocarditis, or hypersplenism. The hemolytic uremic syndrome primarily affects young adults, children, and infants and follows a nonspecific infection.[49] For example, after an upper respiratory infection or bout of gastroenteritis, the youngster suddenly develops hemolysis, thrombocytopenia, and renal failure. Pathologic changes noted in the renal glomeruli are consistent with a thrombotic microangiopathy. The blood film is characteristic of a traumatic or microangiopathic hemolytic anemia, with fragmented cells, burr cells, helmet cells, and schistocytes. Whatever the inciting agent, endothelial injury occurs and leads to platelet aggregation, microthrombi formation, and the mechanical destruction of platelets and red cells. A direct toxic effect on the hematopoietic cells may occur as well. DIC and thrombotic thrombocytopenic purpura are in the differential diagnosis. Usually no organism can be identified, but documented relationships have been reported with *E. coli* (verotoxin-producing strains), shigella, and *S. pneumoniae.*[50] The *E. coli* verotoxin is known to cause vascular injury, while shigella infections may involve an endotoxin effect and streptococcus infections may be me-

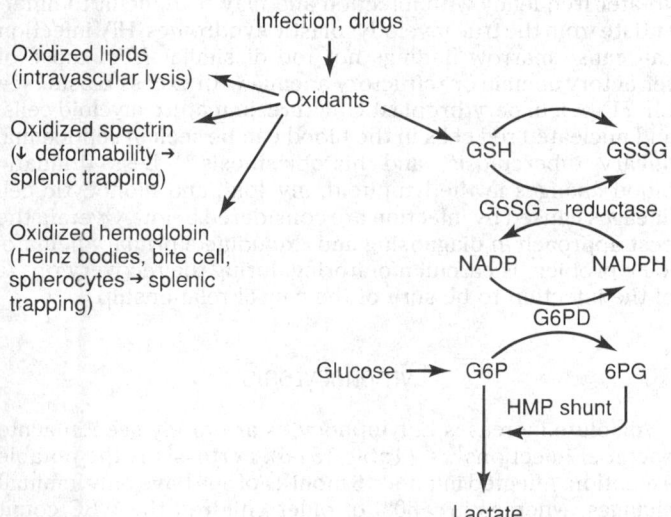

Fig. 154-3. Pathophysiology of infection-induced hemolysis in G6PD-deficient patients. (From Beck and Tepper,[89] with permission.)

diated by the neuraminidase effect on cells through the organism's ability to unmask the T antigens[51] (see above).

Traumatic valvular hemolysis, a result of high blood flow through abnormal mitral and aortic valves, can occasionally be seen with rheumatic heart disease and in infective endocarditis due to organisms such as *Candida albicans*.[52] Hypersplenism and DIC, further causes of increased red cell destruction, are considered elsewhere in this chapter.

WHITE BLOOD CELL DISORDERS

Leukocyte disorders vary considerably from infection to infection and from individual to individual. A bacterial infection may cause a neutrophilia in one instance and a neutropenia in another. In addition to the absolute changes in numbers of lymphoid and myeloid cells, morphologic, immunologic, and functional alteration can result from infection.

Leukocytosis

The leukemoid blood picture is of great alarm to the clinician. It is most frequently caused by infection[53,54] (Table 154-5). Although the definition varies, the basis for the entity is (1) no evidence of leukemia, (2) a white blood cell (WBC) count $>50 \times 10^9$/L, and/or (3) the presence of immature cells. With some infections, the added complication of anemia and thrombocytopenia can create a difficult differential diagnostic problem, solved only by a marrow examination or cell marker studies.

Infections can mimic myeloid or lymphoid leukemia, acute or chronic. CML is probably the most common differential diagnosis with infection. A high WBC count with little or no immaturity can be seen with infections accompanying other disorders such as malignancy, inflammatory arthritis, or glomerulonephritis. More difficult to differentiate is the exaggerated response to disseminated tuberculosis, with WBC counts as high as 200×10^9/L accompanied by a moderate left shift in the differential.[55–57] Similar blood pictures have been seen with staphylococcal septicemia and pneumonia, meningitis secondary to *H. influenzae* and *Neisseria meningitidis*, pneumococcal

Table 154-5. Differential Diagnosis of Leukemoid Reaction Conditions

CML
> Infection with underlying disorders
> Meningitis *(Haemophillis influenzae, Nelsseria meningitidis)*
> Staphylococcus sepsis
> Pneumococcal endocarditis
> Diphtheria
> Bubonic plague
> Tuberculosis
> Salmonellosis

AML
> Tuberculosis
> Pseudoleukemia (rebound from neutropenia)

CLL
> Pertussis
> Varicella
> Viral exanthems

ALL
> Tuberculosis
> Infectious mononucleosis

Acute monocytic leukemia
> Tuberculosis

Myelodysplasia
> HIV
> Other viruses

Table 154-6. Infections that Cause Lymphocytosis

Acute infection	Chronic infection
Pertussis	Tuberculosis
Acute infectious lymphocytosis	Brucellosis
Infectious mononucleosis	Syphilis
Infectious hepatitis	Congenital
Toxoplasmosis	Secondary
Cytomegalovirus	Rickettsia

endocarditis, salmonella, diphtheria, and bubonic plague.[58] In the event of an elevated WBC count without a source of infection, it may be necessary to order a leukocyte alkaline phosphatase and in some instances obtain a marrow for cytogenetics.

An AML picture has also been described with tuberculosis either in its disseminated form or when the organism invades lymphoid tissue and the spleen.[56,59] Discussion continues about the presence of Auer rods in tuberculosis and the coexistence of AML and tuberculosis.[58] A pseudoleukemic blood picture is not uncommon as a rebound phenomenon in antibiotic-induced agranulocytosis and after marrow suppression from severe bacterial and protozoan infections. This scenario may be extremely difficult to diagnose on the spot and requires careful follow-up observations after appropriate therapy.

Chronic lymphocytic (CLL) and acute lymphocytic (ALL) leukemias are less frequently confused with infections. In the preantibiotic era, potentially fatal cases of pertussis were reported to have WBC counts as high as 200×10^9/L.[60] Similarly, chickenpox and the viral exanthems may be associated with extremely high adult lymphocyte counts. The age of the patient, associated symptoms, clinical absence of adenopathy, and splenomegaly will often suffice in diagnosis. Rarely will it be necessary to perform a bone marrow aspirate or analyze for lymphocyte clonality. Disseminated tuberculosis has also been reported to give high WBC counts, with immature lymphoid cells resembling lymphoblasts and ALL.[57,61] The blood findings of infectious mononucleosis (see Ch. 58) often instill the greatest fear of a diagnosis of ALL in young adults. The clinical picture, the "atypically atypical" lymphocytes (i.e., nonuniform population of lymphocytes), in addition to abnormal liver function tests, serologic findings, and a normal marrow, will exclude ALL.

Disseminated tuberculosis may also mimic acute monocytic leukemia.[62] The recovery phase of many other infections may occasionally give rise to a high WBC count with monocytosis. Myelodysplastic blood smears and marrows are being seen in greater frequency with infection and may be difficult to differentiate from the true myelodysplastic syndromes. HIV infection can cause marrow findings not too dissimilar from those of refractory anemia or refractory anemia with excess blasts (see Ch. 71). A leukoerythroblastic picture, immature myeloid cells, and nucleated red cells in the blood can be seen in septicemia, miliary tuberculosis, and histoplasmosis.[63] Less dramatic blood changes in the lymphoid, myeloid, and monocytic cell lineages caused by infection are considered below. Overall, the best approach in diagnosing and excluding a primary hematologic problem is careful monitoring during the recovery phase of the infection to be sure of the causal relationship.

Lymphocytosis

Absolute increases in lymphocytes are rarely seen in acute bacterial infections[15,64] (Table 154-6). Pertussis is the notable exception. Affected infants <6 months of age have only minimal changes, whereas in >50% of older children the WBC count can rise to $15–20 \times 10^9$/L during the first 2 weeks of illness, and rarely to the leukemoid range discussed above. *Bordetella pertussis* toxin, known as pertussigen or lymphocytosis-promoting factor, has been shown to increase lymphocytes in experimental animals.[65] It is suspected that pertussigen blocks the normal migration of lymphocytes out of the bloodstream and into the tissues. The cells are normal B and T cells.

Rickettsial infections such as scrub typhus, tuberculosis, syphilis, and brucellosis can also cause an absolute lymphocytosis. Acute infectious lymphocytosis varies from a very mild nonspecific illness to a more acute disorder characterized by fever, diarrhea, upper respiratory symptoms, central nervous system involvement, and dramatic absolute lymphocyte counts of 30 to as high as 100×10^9/L. Although no definite etiologic agent is known, an adenovirus and coxsackievirus A with incubation periods of 12–21 days have been implicated.

Lymphocytopenia

Lymphocyte counts $<1 \times 10^9$/L are quite common in acute infections, malaria, HIV infection, and a number of chronic infections such as tuberculosis, histoplasmosis, and brucellosis.[66] The decreased lymphocyte count (often in association with neutrophilia) probably results from elevated plasma cortisol levels. The degree of lymphocytopenia seems to correlate with the severity of the infection.

Morphologic and immunologic lymphoid changes may occur with disease. Atypical lymphoid cells characterized by an abnormal nuclear/cytoplasmic ratio with resultant increased cytoplasm are not uncommon in infectious mononucleosis, infectious hepatitis, and some chronic infections. Changes in the numbers of B and T cells and in the ratio of T-cell subsets are hallmark findings in HIV infection (see Ch. 155) but have also been shown to occur in other viral infections and in bacterial and fungal disease.[67,68] For example, in acute bacterial infections, T cells of all types can decline in number early in infection, while B cells rise. Prolonged T-cell lymphopenia in the face of active infection is more frequent in aging patients and is considered a poor prognostic finding. In leprosy and tuberculosis, T-cell subset ratios may change, and decreased cellular immunity has been associated with a decrease in T-helper cells an an increase in T suppressors.[69]

Neutrophilia

Leukocytosis with neutrophilia and a left shift commonly accompanies bacterial infections. Most bacteria produce a 12–14 $\times 10^9$/L WBC count, while systemic infections will be as high as 15–30 $\times 10^9$/L, and massive infections such as the leukemoid type $\geq$50 $\times 10^9$/L.[65] Neutrophilia is most common with suppurative infections such as an abscess, empyema, or meningitis and is usually associated with bacteria like staphylococcus and streptococcus. Over two-thirds of infection-related neutrophilia cases are secondary to bacteria.[1,70] The lack of an increased count directs the clinician to a problem with the host or to the type of infectious agent. Most healthy individuals respond with some degree of neutrophilia. Patients with alcohol-related problems may have a limited or no increase in WBC count, like the malnourished patient and a high percentage of the elderly population. Infections with chlamydia, fungi, mycoplasma, and rickettsiae may have little effect on the WBC count. The neutrophilic response results from increased release from the marginal pool secondary to endogenous catecholamines and increased levels of IL-1.[71] Animal research has demonstrated an almost immediately accelerated egress of neutrophils from the storage pools into the blood after bacterial innoculation.[72]

Table 154-7. Infections that Cause Neutropenia

Bacterial	Rickettsial
Salmonella infection	Rickettsial pox
Tularemia	Rocky Mountain spotted fever
Brucellosis	Protozoan
Viral	Malaria
Measles	Kala-azar
Chickenpox	Relapsing Fever
Rubella	Massive
Influenza	Miliary tuberculosis
Infectious hepatitis	
Yellow fever	
Sandfly fever	
HIV	
Colorado tick fever	
Dengue fever	

Neutropenia

Neutropenia defined as absolute counts $<1.5 \times 10^9$/L, can occur paradoxically in almost any bacterial infection and more likely in patients with compromised marrows due to chemotherapy, nutritional deficiency, or chronic debilitation. Certain viral, rickettsial, and protozoal infections may be associated with low counts, while it would be unusual to find neutropenia in fungal infections[1] (Table 154-7). Were neutropenia to occur during the second week or recovery phase of the infection, it might be difficult to distinguish between a drug and an infection-induced etiology. Medications such as analgesics, sulfonamides, and other microbials can be implicated.

Bacterial infections such as typhoid, paratyphoid, and tularemia may cause an initial rise in neutrophils and then a fall during the bacteremic phase of the disease.[73] Low counts are typical of many viral infections. Infectious hepatitis, HIV infection, yellow fever, influenza, measles, Colorado tick fever, and many others characteristically present with neutropenia. Well-documented cases of neutropenia have been shown to be caused by experimentally induced sandfly fever[74] (Fig. 154-4) and infectious hepatitis (Fig. 154-5). Almost 90% of patients with sandfly fever have a neutropenia during the course of their disease.

The cause of infection-related neutropenia is either due to a direct toxic effect or to increased utilization. With sepsis, neutrophils are mobilized, and the circulating pool acutely decreases before the accelerated marrow egress can compensate. Many individuals will overshoot, with a marrow rebound, producing a pseudoleukemia or leukemoid picture. There is some speculation that neutropenia is a result of an inhibition of growth factors, a decrease in colony-stimulating factors, or lysis of WBCs through activation of the complement system.[11]

Neutrophil Morphologic Abnormalities

Some infected patients may show no change in the number of myeloid cells but instead either a shift to the left, with increased bands and metamyelocytes, or morphologic changes such as toxic granulations, cytoplasmic vacuolization, or the formation of Döhle bodies. With massive bacterial infection, organisms can rarely be seen within the neutrophil cytoplasm, and nuclear changes can result, such as the Pelger-Huët anomaly. In patients with frequent infections, especially children, one should be alerted to the possibility of an inherited or acquired functional neutrophil abnormality. These are consid-

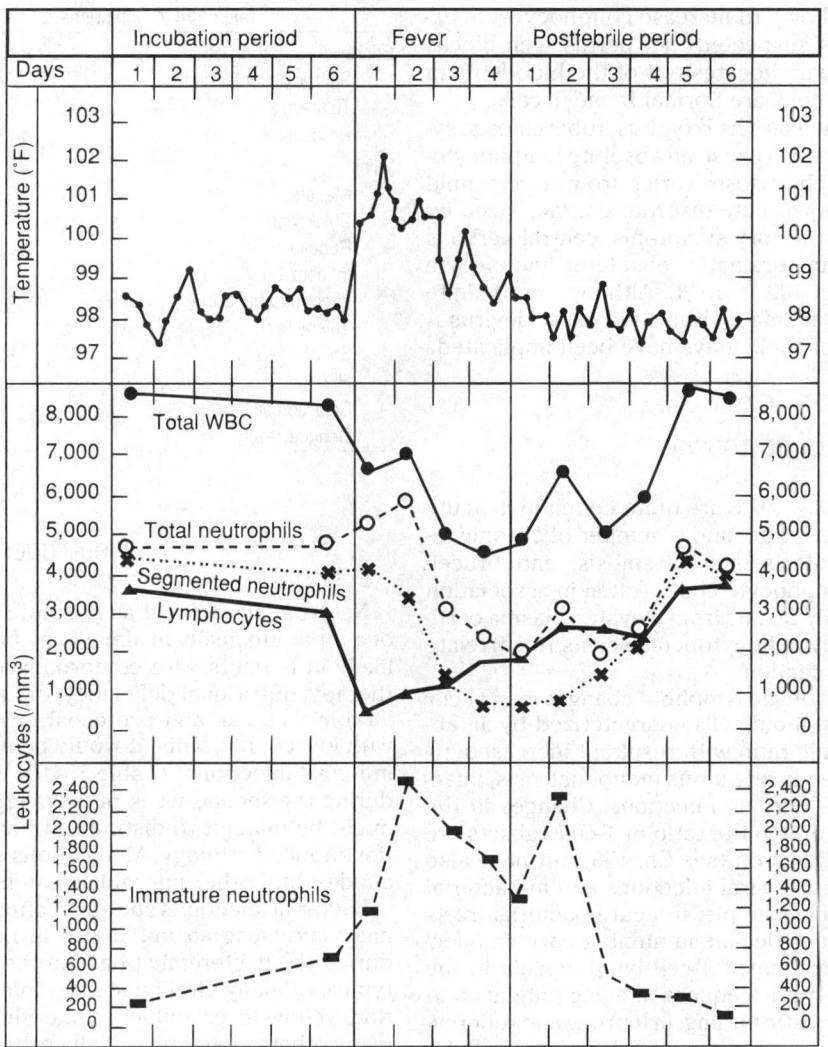

Fig. 154-4. Changes in white blood cell, neutrophil, and lymphocyte counts in experimentally induced sandfly *(Phlebotomus)* fever. (From Sabin and Paul,[74] with permission.)

ered elsewhere and include problems in phagocytosis, motility, chemotaxis and adherence, and bactericidal activity.

Monocytosis

Monocytosis, defined as WBC counts $>0.95 \times 10^9$/L, may be seen with a subacute or chronic infection such as tuberculosis, subacute bacterial endocarditis, syphilis, and brucellosis as well as with many rickettsial and protozoan infections such as malaria, typhus, trypanosomiasis, and kala-azar.[15] Monocytosis may also develop transiently during the recovery phase of any infection. In tuberculosis, the monocytosis may reflect a high rate of turnover and new tubercle formation. The monocyte/lymphocyte ratio (M/L) may be a useful measure of the activity of the tuberculosis infection.[75] With activity, the M/L increases due to an absolute increase in monocytes, and the ratio may exceed 1, the normal being 0.3. A ratio greater than 1 has been associated with active exudates and a poor overall prognosis.[76] The healing phase is characterized by an increase in lymphocytes, a decrease in monocytes, and a return to the normal M/L ratio.

Cells resembling histiocytes or macrophages may accompany monocytes in chronic infections, and the monocytes may become vacuolated. A bedside diagnosis for subacute bacterial endocarditis consisted of obtaining a blood smear from the ear lobe and demonstrating abundant macrophage-like cells.[77]

Eosinophilia

Eosinophilia, defined as a WBC count $>0.25 \times 10^9$/L, is frequent in parasitic infections that invade tissues, such as trichiniasis and echinococcal disease, and rare in bacterial and fungal infections.[78] With involvement by schistosomiasis, filiariasis, gnathostomia, the liver fluke *Clonorchis sinensis,* and *Capillaria hepatica,* eosinophilia is frequently observed. Intestinal parasites are less likely to stimulate eosinophils if tissue invasion does not occur. In patients with bronchopulmonary aspergillosis, coccidioidomycosis, and chlamydia pneumonitis of infancy, absolute eosinophil counts may range from 0.5 to 1.0×10^9/L, with rare elevations to as high as 44×10^9/L. A mild eosinophilia has also been seen in the early phases of scarlet fever.

Eosinopenia

Eosinopenia correlates with the severity of various infections. The absence of eosinophils in infection is the sign of a bad prognosis. The mechanism for eosinopenia is probably not

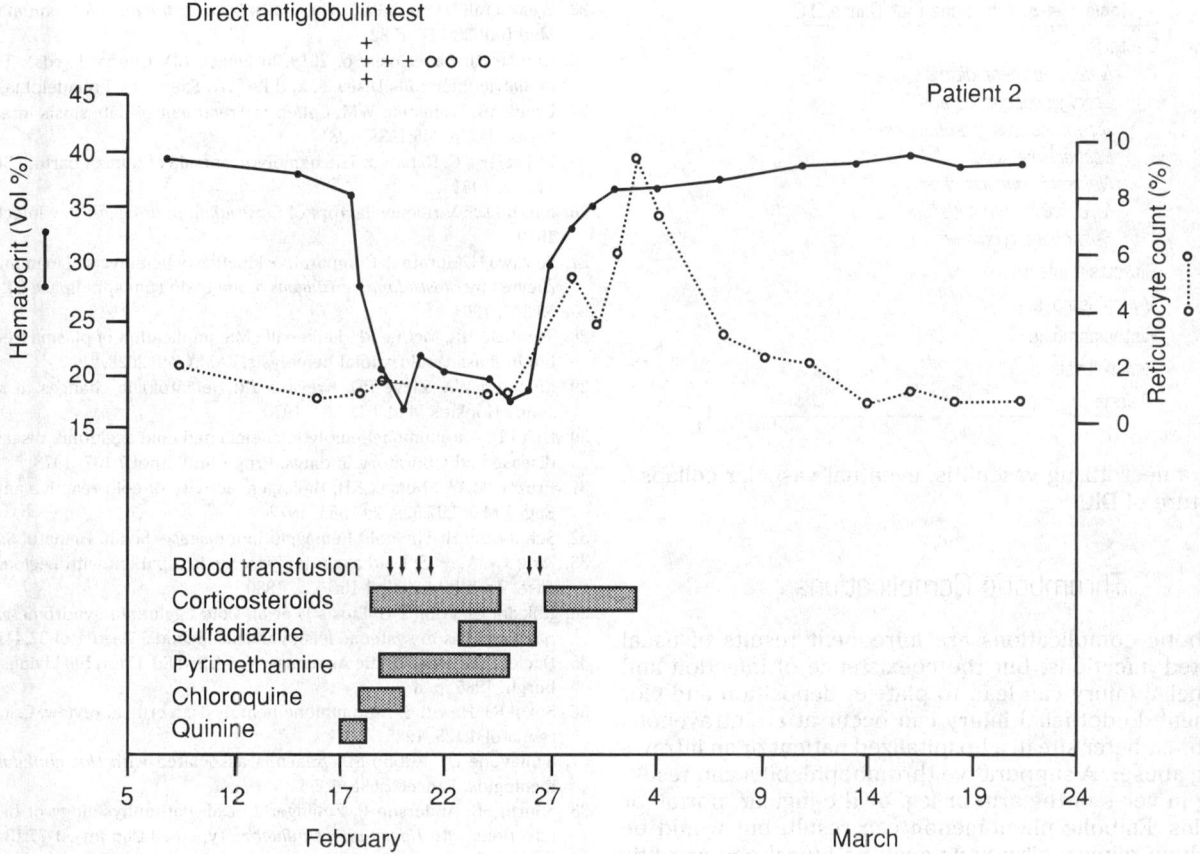

Fig. 154-5. Changes in white blood cell, neutrophil, and leukocyte counts in experimentally induced infectious hepatitis. (From Havens and Marck,[90] with permission.)

corticosteroid related but due to other chemotactic factors such as C5a, which causes intravascular cell destruction, tissue margination, and/or intravascular margination.[79] Cytokine inhibition may also play a role in decreasing marrow production and release. Basophils are rarely affected by infection and in general are not part of the leukemoid blood picture. Basophilia should alert the clinician to a chronic myeloproliferative disorder.

PLATELET AND CLOTTING DISORDERS

Thrombocytopenia

Thrombocytopenia is a frequent complication of septicemia due to any bacterium, virus, or fungus.[1,80,81] Of patients with bacteremia, >65% have thrombocytopenia to some degree, while 33% will have a more significant drop to levels of <50 × 10^9/L. Despite the high incidence of abnormal counts, the thrombocytopenia is rarely associated with clinical bleeding unless simultaneous evidence of DIC is present. Occasionally a severe infection with bloodstream involvement (e.g., peritonitis, pneumonia, and abscess) can cause a drop in count.

The mechanism of thrombocytopenia without DIC may be due to (1) decreased production, (2) increased platelet utilization, (3) binding of platelets to exposed and infected subendothelial tissue, and/or (4) an immune phenomenon. Infection-induced immune thrombocytopenia may be IgG mediated and caused by gram-positive and -negative septicemias or the development of platelet aggregates and subsequent lysis by complement or infection-related immune complexes.

Thrombocytosis

Thrombocytosis, frequently as high as 500–700 × 10^9/L, is seen in chronic infections such as tuberculosis, osteomyelitis, and subacute bacterial endocarditis, as well as in the recovery period of a variety of fungal and bacterial infections.[82,83] Despite reactive platelet counts as high as 900–1,000 × 10^9/L, the incidence of thrombosis is rare and reportable, and no anticoagulation is necessary. The mechanism of reactive thrombocytosis is poorly understood. Some patients have impaired splenic function, raising the possibility of a hyposplenic state with resultant increased platelets, Howell-Jolly bodies, and target cells.

DIC and Vascular Purpura

Up to 65% of all cases of DIC occur secondary to infections.[84] Serious infections often lead to the development of rapid and massive activation of the coagulation system. DIC can be caused by tissue necrosis, endothelial surface damage, and blood stagnation, all potential complications of an infectious disease. In Rocky Mountain spotted fever, for example, endothelial damage is the pathogenetic mechanism. Many causative agents are implicated; bacterial, viral, parasitic, and fungal (Table 154-8). Most impressive clinically are purpura fulminans and the Waterhouse-Friderichsen syndrome. The latter condition refers to the triad in meningococcemia of vascular collapse, mucosal and cutaneous hemorrhage, and bleeding into the adrenal gland. In addition to the direct effect of the infecting agent, bacterial products and toxins such as meningococcal endotoxin can cause endothelial destruction.[86] These endotox-

Table 154-8. Infections that Cause DIC

Bacteria
  Neisseria meningitidis
  Staphylococcus aureus
  Streptococcus pneumoniae
  Escherichia coli
  Neisseria gonorrhoeae
  Mycobacterium tuberculosis
  Salmonella typhimurium
Rickettsia infection
Mycoplasmosis
Histoplasmosis
Aspergillosis
Malaria

ins cause a necrotizing vasculitis, eventual vascular collapse, and a picture of DIC.

Thrombotic Complications

Thrombotic complications are infrequent results of usual and isolated infections, but the coexistence of infection and an endothelial injury can lead to platelet deposition and clot development. Endothelial injury can occur at an intravenous long line or catheter site in a hospitalized patient or an intravenous drug abuser. A suppurative thrombophlebitis can result, occurring in veins of the arm or leg, or the jugular, portal, or pelvic veins. Embolic phenomenon can result, but would be more likely in clinical situations such as fungal endocarditis with aspergillosis.

REFERENCES

1. Strausbaugh LJ: Hematologic manifestations of bacterial and fungal infections. Hematol Oncol Clin North Am 1:185, 1987
2. Marshall BJ: *Campylobacter pyloridis* and gastritis. J Infect Dis 153:650, 1986
3. Levy RN: Fatal aplastic anemia after hepatitis. N Engl J Med 273:1118, 1965
4. Zeldis JB: Aplastic anemia and non-A, non-B hepatitis. Am J Med 74:64, 1983
5. Foon KA: Immunologic defects in young male patients with hepatitis-associated aplastic anemia. Ann Intern Med 100:657, 1984
6. Witherspoon RP: Marrow transplantation in hepatitis-associated aplastic anemia. Am J Hematol 17:269, 1984
7. Young N: Hematologic and hematopoietic consequences of B19 parvovirus infection. Semin Hematol 25:159, 1988
8. Brown CH III: Bone marrow necrosis. A study of seventy cases. Johns Hopkins Med J 131:189, 1972
9. Caraveo J, Trowbridge AA, Amarel BW et al: Bone marrow necrosis associated with a mucor infection. Am J Med 52:679, 1972
10. Katzen H, Spagnolo SV: Bone marrow necrosis from miliary tuberculosis. JAMA 244:2438, 1980
11. Bagby GC, Gilbert DN: Suppression of granulopoiesis by T-lymphocytes in two patients with disseminated mycobacterial infection. Ann Intern Med 94:478, 1981
12. Cartwright GE, Lee GR: The anaemia of chronic disorders. Br J Haematol 21:147, 1971
13. Lee GR: The anemia of chronic disease. Semin Hematol 20:61, 1983
14. Samson D: The anaemia of chronic disorders. Postgrad Med 59:543, 1943
15. Murdoch JM, Smith CC: Infection. Clin Haematol 1:619, 1972
16. Bullen JJ: The significance of iron in infection. Rev Infect Dis 3:1127, 1981
17. Le J, Vilcek J: Tumor necrosis factor and interleukin I: cytokines with multiple overlapping biological activities. Lab Invest 56:234, 1987
18. Klempner MS, Dinarello CA, Gallin JJ: Human leukocyte pyrogen induces release of specific granule contents from human neutrophils. J Clin Invest 61:1330, 1978
19. Weinberg ED: Iron withholding: a defense against infection and neoplasia. Physiol Rev 64:65, 1984
20. Buchanan GR: The mild anemia of acute infection. Pediatr Infect Dis 4:225, 1985
21. Berkowitz FE: Hemolysis and infection. Categories and mechanisms. Rev Infect Dis 13:1151, 1991
22. Weatherall DJ, Abdalla S: The anaemia of *Plasmodium falciparum* malaria. Br Med Bull 38:147, 1982
23. Krause PJ: Babesiosis. p. 2019. In Feigen RD, Cherry J (eds): Textbook of Pediatric Infectious Disease. 2nd Ed. WB Saunders, Philadelphia, 1987
24. Bredt AB, Weinstein WM, Cohen S: Treatment of babesiosis in asplenic patients. JAMA 245:1938, 1981
25. Reynafarje C, Ramos J: The hemolytic anemia of human bartonellosis. Blood 17:562, 1961
26. Smith LDS: Virulence factors of *Clostridium perfringens*. Rev Infect Dis 1:254, 1979
27. Ikezawa H, Murata R: Comparative kinetics of hemolysis of mammalian erythrocytes by *Clostridium perfringens* alpha-toxin (phospholipase C). J Biochem 55:217, 1964
28. Terebelo HR, McCue RL, Lenneville MS: Implication of plasma free hemoglobin in massive clostridial hemolysis. JAMA 248:2028, 1982
29. Emerson WA, Zieve PD, Krevans JR: Hematologic changes in septicemia. Johns Hopkins Med J 122:69, 1970
30. Issit PD: Autoimmunehemolytic anemia nad cold agglutinin disease. Clinical disease and laboratory findings. Prog Clin Pathol 7:137, 1978
31. Pruzanski W, Shumak KH: Biological activity of cold reactive antibodies. N Engl J Med 297:538, 297:583, 1977
32. Schubothe H: The cold hemagglutinin disease. Semin Hematol 3:27, 1966
33. King JW, May JS: Cold agglutinin release in a patient with Legionnaire's disease. Arch Intern Med 10:1537, 1980
34. Kokkini G, Vrionis G, Liosis G et al: Cold agglutinin syndrome and haemophagocytosis in systemic leishmaniasis. Scand J Haematol 32:441, 1984
35. Dacie J: The Haemolytic Anaemias. Vol. I. 3rd Ed. Churchill Livingstone, Edinburgh, 1985, p. 4
36. Sokol RJ, Hewitt S: Autoimmune hemolysis: a critical review. Crit Rev Oncol Hematol 4:125, 1985
37. Schiavone DJ, Rubbo SD: Anaemia associated with *Haemophilus influenza* meningitis. Lancet 2:696, 1953
38. Shurin SB, Anderson P, Zollinger J et al: Pathophysiology of hemolysis in infections with *Haemophilus influenza* type b. J Clin Invest 77:1340, 1986
39. Lenz G, Goes U, Baron D et al: Red blood cell T-activation and hemolysis in surgical intensive care patients with severe infection. Blut 54:89, 1987
40. Obeid D, Bird GWG, Wingham J: Prolonged erythrocyte T-polyagglutination in two children with bowel disorders. J Clin Pathol 30:953, 1977
41. Gordon-Smith EC: Drug-induced oxidative hemolysis. Clin Haematol 9:557, 1980
42. Mengel CE, Metz E, Yancey WS: Anemia during acute infections. Role of glucose-6-phosphate dehydrogenase deficiency in negroes. Arch Intern Med 119:287, 1967
43. Shannon K, Buchanan GR: Severe hemolytic anemia in black children with glucose-6-phosphate dehydrogenase deficiency. Pediatrics 70:364, 1982
44. Baehner RL, Nathan DG, Castle WB: Oxidant injury of Caucasian glucose-6-phosphate dehydrogenase-deficient red blood cells by phagocytosing leukocytes during infection. J Clin Invest 50:2466, 1971
45. Weiss SJ: The role of superoxide in the destruction of erythrocyte targets by human neutrophils. J Biol Chem 257:2947, 1982
46. Claster S, Chiu DT-Y, Quintanilha A et al: Neutrophils mediate lipid peroxidation in human red cells. Blood 64:1079, 1984
47. Jacob HS, Jandl JH: A simple visual screening test for G-6-PD deficiency employing ascorbate and cyanide. N Engl J Med 274:1162, 1966
48. Lukens JN: Glucose-6-phosphate dehydrogenase deficiency and related deficiencies involving the pentose phosphate pathway and glutathione metabolism. p. 1006. In Lea GR, Bithell TC, Foerster J et al (eds): Wintrobe's Clinical Hematology. 9th Ed. Lea & Febiger, Philadelphia, 1993
49. Kaplan BS, Proesmans W: The hemolytic uremic syndrome of childhood and its variants. Semin Hematol 24:148, 1987
50. Cleary TG: Cytotoxin-producing *Escherichia coli* and the hemolytic uremic syndrome. Pediatr Clin North Am 35:485, 1988
51. Novak RW, Martin CR: Hemolytic-uremic syndrome and T-cryptantigen exposure by neuraminidase-producing pneumococci: an emerging problem? Pediatr Pathol 1:409, 1983
52. Krishnaswami S, Cherian G, John S: Red cell hemolysis in rheumatic valvular disease and following prosthetic and heterograft valve replacement surgery: a study of 40 cases and review of the literature. Indian J Med Res 63:130, 1975
53. Hill JM, Duncan CN: Leukemoid reactions. Am J Med Sci 201:847, 1941
54. Hilts SV, Shaw CC: Leukemoid blood reactions. N Engl J Med 249:434, 1953
55. Coley WB, Ewing J: Acute lymphocytic tuberculosis with purpura hemorrhagica. Proc NY Pathol Soc 10:1945, 1911
56. Twomey JJ, Leavell BS: Leukemoid reactions to tuberculosis. Arch Intern Med 116:21, 1965

57. Hughes JT, Johnstone RM, Scott AC, Stewart PD: Leukemoid reactions in disseminated tuberculosis. J Clin Pathol 12:307, 1959

58. Krumbhaar EB: Leukemoid blood pictures in various clinical conditions. Am J Med Sci 172:519, 1926

59. Leibowitz S: Tuberculous sepsis with a myeloblastic blood picture. Arch Pathol Lab Med 25:365, 1938

60. Albert J, Jongco AP: Leucemoid blood as a malignant sign in pertussis. J Philippine Med Assoc 21:63, 1941

61. Gardner FH, Mettier SR: Lymphocytic leukemoid reaction of the blood associated with miliary tuberculosis. Blood 4:767, 1949

62. Gibson A: Monocytic leukaemoid reaction associated with tuberculosis and a mediastinal teratoma. J Pathol 58:469, 1946

63. Burkett LL, Cox ML, Fields ML: Leukoerythroblastosis in the adult. Am J Clin Pathol 44:494, 1965

64. Chanarin I, Harrisingh D, Tidmarsh E et al: Significance of lymphocytosis in adults. Lancet 2:897, 1984

65. Mandell GL, Douglas RG, Bennett JE: Principles and Practice of Infectious Diseases. 4th Ed. Churchill Livingstone, New York, 1985

66. Zacharski LR, Linman JW: Lymphocytopenia: its causes and siginficance. Mayo Clin Proc 46:168, 1971

67. Williams RC, Koster FT, Kilpatrick KA: Alterations in lymphocyte cell surface markers during various human infections. Am J Med 75:807, 1983

68. Niklasson PM, Williams RC Jr: Studies of peripheral blood T- and B-lymphocytes in acute infections. Infect Immun 9:1, 1974

69. Blumberg RS, Schooley RT: Lymphocytes. III: lymphocyte markers and infectious diseases. Semin Hematol 22:81, 1985

70. Emerson WA, Zieve PD, Krevens JR: Hematologic changes in septicemia. Johns Hopkins Med J 126:69, 1969

71. Dinarellop CA: Interleukin I. Rev Infect Dis 6:51, 1984

72. Christensen RD, Hill HR, Rothstein G: Granulocytic stem cell (CFUc) proliferation in experimental group B streptococcal sepsis. Pediatr Res 17:278, 1983

73. Austin JH, Leopold SS: An extraordinary polymorphonuclear leukopenia in typhoid fever. JAMA 66:1084, 1916

74. Sabin AB, Paul JR: Phlebotomus fever. JAMA 125:603, 1944

75. Schmitt E, Meuret G, Stix L: Monocyte recruitment in tuberculosis and sarcoidosis. Br J Haematol 35:11, 1977

76. Blackfan KD, Diamond LK: The monocyte in active tuberculosis. Am J Dis Child 37:233, 1929

77. Hill RW, Bayrd ED: Phagocytic reticuloendothelial cells in subacute bacterial endocarditis with negative cultures. Ann Intern Med 52:310, 1960

78. Weller PF: Eosinophilia. J Allergy Clin Immunol 73:1, 1984

79. Bass DA, Gonwa TA, Szejda P et al: Eosinopenia of acute infection: production of eosinopenia by chemotactic factors of acute inflammation. J Clin Invest 65:1265, 1980

80. Cohen P, Gardner FH: Thrombocytopenia as a laboratory sign and complication of gram negative bacteremic infection. Arch Intern Med 117:113, 1966

81. Bithell TC: Miscellaneous form of thrombocytopenia. p. 1363. In Lee GR, Bithell TC, Foerster J et al (eds): Wintrobe's Clinical Hematology. 9th Ed. Lea & Febiger, Philadelphia, 1993

82. Murphy S: Thrombocytosis and thrombocythemia. Clin Hematol 12:89, 1983

83. Iland H, Laszlo J: Thrombocytosis. Med Grand Rounds 3:225, 1984

84. McKay DG: Disseminated Intravascular Coagulation. Harper & Row, New York, 1964

85. McGarth JM, Stewart GJ: The effects of endotoxin on vascular endothelium. J Exp Med 129:883, 1969

86. Aikawa M, Miller LH: Malaria and the red cell. Ciba Found Symp 94:45, 1983

87. Bogemann H, Rastetter J: Atlas of Clinical Hematology. 4th Ed. Springer-Verlag, Berlin, 1989, p. 293

88. Benson LA, Car S, McLaughlin G, Ihler GM: Entry of *Bartonella bacilliformis* into erythrocytes. Infect Immun 54:347, 1986

89. Beck WS, Tepper RI: Hemolytic anemia. p. 287. In Beck WS (ed): Metabolic Disorders in Hematology. Vol. 4. 5th Ed. MIT Press, Cambridge, 1991

90. Havens WP, Marck E: The leukocyte response of patients with experimentally induced infectious hepatitis. Am J Med Sci 212:129, 1946

Hematologic Manifestations of AIDS

155

James A. Hoxie

INTRODUCTION

The acquired immunodeficiency syndrome (AIDS) is caused by infection with the human immunodeficiency virus (HIV). This retrovirus produces a slow but usually progressive deterioration in the host immune system that in its most advanced stage is complicated by particular opportunistic infections, neurologic disorders, and neoplasms. Hematologic abnormalities occur in most individuals during the course of this infection, reflecting alterations in the host immune system as well as complications of secondary infections, malignancies, and therapy. Evidence has also implicated a direct role for HIV infection itself on some hematopoietic precursor cells and other cells in the bone marrow. This chapter presents a general overview of the basic epidemiologic, virologic, and immunologic aspects of HIV infection, followed by a more specific discussion of its hematologic complications.

DEFINITION AND EPIDEMIOLOGY

A diagnosis of AIDS is established when HIV infection is complicated by particular opportunistic infections, neoplasms, or neurologic disorders. The current definition of AIDS includes a number of clinical complications[1] (Table 155-1). In addition, this surveillance case definition has recently been expanded to include individuals with laboratory evidence of severe immunodeficiency, as manifested by a reduction in the number of $CD4^+$ T lymphocytes to $<200/mm^3$ or in the $CD4^+$ T-lymphocyte percentage of total lymphocytes to <14.[1] It is clear, however, that AIDS is simply an advanced stage in a spectrum of clinical complications that occur following HIV infection.

An earlier classification system defined a symptomatic state of HIV infection as AIDS-related complex (ARC), characterized most commonly by persisting generalized lymphadenopathy with or without a number of nonspecific complaints, including arthralgias, fatigue, intermittent diarrhea, or chronic sinus-

Table 155-1. Centers for Disease Control Classification of Clinical Categories for HIV Infection

Category A: Acute HIV infection, asymptomatic infection, persisting generalized lymphadenopathy

Category B: Symptomatic HIV infection (excluding conditions in category C) complicated by conditions attributable to compromised cellular immunity (i.e., idiopathic thrombocytopenic purpura, thrush, listerosis, peripheral neuropathy)

Category C: AIDS (any one of the following laboratory or clinical criteria)
  Laboratory criteria
    $CD4^+$ T-cell number $<200/mm^2$
    $CD4^+$ % of lymphocytes <14
  Clinical criteria
    Opportunistic infections
      Candidiasis of bronchi, trachea, lungs, or esophagus
      Coccidioidomycosis, disseminated or extrapulmonary
      Cryptococcosis, extrapulmonary
      Cryptosporidiosis, chronic intestinal
      Cytomegalovirus (other than liver, spleen, or nodes)
      Herpes simplex (chronic ulcers, bronchitis, esophagitis)
      Histoplasmosis, disseminated or extrapulmonary
      Isosporiasis (chronic intestinal)
      Mycobacterium avium complex or *kansasii,* disseminated or extrapulmonary
      Mycobacterium tuberculosis, pulmonary or extrapulmonary
      Mycobacterium, other species (disseminated or extrapulmonary)
      Pneumocystis carinii pneumonia
      Pneumonia, recurrent
      Salmonella septicemia
      Toxoplasmosis of brain
    Neoplasms
      Cervical cancer, invasive
      Kaposi sarcoma
      Lymphoma (non-Hodgkin)
    Central nervous system
      Encephalopathy, HIV-related
      Progressive multifocal leukoencephalopathy
    Wasting syndrome due to HIV

(Modified from Centers for Disease Control.[1])

itis.[2,3] Although in the current revised definition, many of these individuals would now be defined as having AIDS if their CD4 cell number were $<200/mm^3$, the term ARC has been extensively incorporated into many clinical studies and is used periodically here.

The epidemic of AIDS and HIV infection continues to be an international health crisis with, as of mid-1993, a cumulative total of approximately 13 million adults and 1 million children infected worldwide.[4] In addition to the increasing incidence of HIV infection in North America, Central Europe, and sub-Sahara Africa, recent surveys have shown a dramatic rise in the incidence of HIV infection in Latin America, the Middle East, and, particularly, southeast Asia.[4] In the United States, approximately 300,000 adults and 5,000 children ≤13 years of age had developed AIDS as of July, 1993, and current estimates for the prevalence of HIV infection in the United States range between 1 and 2 million individuals.[5] As the epidemic in the United States enters its second decade, changes in the distribution of cases have been noted, with an increase in the proportion of individuals who have become infected through heterosexual contact, particularly adolescents and black and Hispanic women in urban areas.[6]

Although HIV has been cultured from a variety of body fluids, including blood, semen, saliva, urine, and tears,[7] infection occurs almost exclusively by sexual contact (homosexual and heterosexual), by parenteral inoculation of infected blood or blood products, and perinatally from mother to infant.[7,8] In unusual circumstances, infection has also occurred as a result of skin or mucous membrane contact (or both) with blood from an infected individual,[9] although this mode of transmission appears to be exceedingly uncommon.[10–13] Overall, the incidence of seroconversion to HIV following occupational exposure via needle stick has been estimated to be approximately 0.3%.[14] Studies evaluating the incidence of HIV infection in nonsexual household contacts of patients with AIDS have clearly shown that transmission does not occur through casual contact.[7,15]

Two major groups of retroviruses have been associated with AIDS. HIV-1 is the cause of the AIDS epidemic in Europe, Central Africa, Asia, and the Americas, while a closely related but molecularly distinct virus, HIV-2, has been isolated from AIDS patients originating from West Africa, where this virus has been shown to be endemic.[16,17] Prospective epidemiologic studies have indicated that HIV-2 may be less pathogenic in vivo than HIV-1 with respect to the development of immunologic abnormalities and disease.[18] However, in view of the long time interval between infection and the development of AIDS, which for HIV-1 may average 10-years or more,[19–24] longer periods of follow-up will clearly be needed before the true pathologic potential of HIV-2 is known. Several different isolates of HIV-related simian immunodeficiency viruses (SIVs) have been obtained from a number of non-human primate species in Africa.[25] Recent molecular studies of healthy humans in West Africa have identified variants of HIV-2 that are closely related to some SIVs, suggesting a zoogenic origin, at least for HIV-2.[26]

PATHOGENESIS OF HIV INFECTION IN VITRO AND IN VIVO

In Vitro Pathogenesis

The genetic organization of HIV-1 (Fig. 155-1) is remarkably complex compared with other retroviruses and encodes at least nine genes.[27] Like other retroviruses, HIV-1 contains *gag, pol,* and *env* genes that encode viral core proteins, enzymes (reverse transcriptase, integrase, and a viral protease), and envelope glycoproteins, respectively. In addition, a number of other viral proteins have been identified, including tat and rev, which play critical roles in regulating the transcription and processing of viral mRNAs[27]; nef, which may exert a negative effect on viral production[28,29] and may modulate CD4 expression in infected cells[30,31]; and vif, which enhances the infectivity of cell-free virions in vitro.[32,33] The *vpr* gene[34,35] and *vpu* gene of HIV-1,[36,37] as well as the *vpx* gene of HIV-2 and some SIVs,[38–40] encode proteins whose functions are as yet unknown.

The structure of the HIV virion and the viral life cycle at the cellular level are shown in Figures 155-2 and 155-3. The mature virus particle contains two coding strands of RNA and reverse transcriptase molecules packaged in a core by the gag proteins p24, p17, p9, and p7. This core is surrounded by an icosahedral sphere containing a lipid membrane and the viral envelope glycoproteins that consist of oligomers of an external molecule of 120 kd (gp120) and a 41-kd transmembrane molecule (gp41).[22,27] gp120 binds with high affinity to the CD4 molecule expressed on the surface of a number of cells that play essential roles in the function of the immune system.[41] These cells include a subset of T lymphocytes, monocytes, follicular dendritic cells, and Langerhans cells, all of which have been shown to be infectable by HIV.[22,42–51] As described in a later section, CD4 has also been demonstrated on human megakaryocytes and likely mediates infection of this hematopoietic cell type by HIV.[52–54] The function of CD4 on nonlymphoid cells, including megakaryocytes, remains an interesting but unresolved question. Binding of the envelope to CD4 is required for attachment of the virion to the cell surface and determines, at least in part, the range of cells that are susceptible to infection.[22,27] In addition, other molecules may facilitate viral binding, including cellular adhesion molecules,[55,56] complement receptors,[57] and Fc receptors.[58,59] CD4-independent mechanisms of viral entry

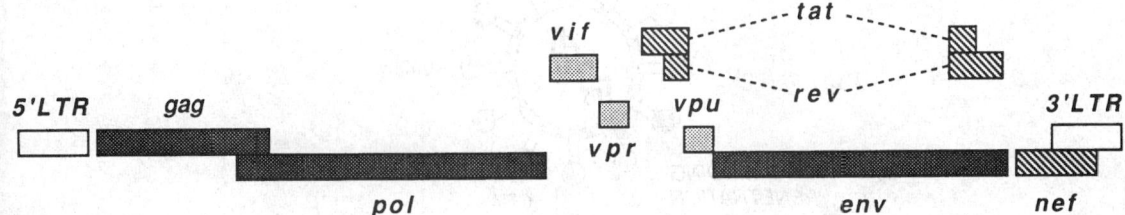

Fig. 155-1. Genetic organization of HIV-1. The nine genes of HIV-1 are shown. Structural proteins of the virion and enzymes required for replication are encoded by *gag*, *pol*, and *env* (darkly shaded regions); regulatory proteins (cross-hatched areas) are encoded by *tat* and *rev*, arising from doubly spliced messages, and *nef*. The *vif*, *vpr*, and *vpu* genes are dispensable for viral replication, and their function is unclear. Two identical long terminal repeats (LTRs) are present at the 5' and 3' end of the genome and contain sequences critical for viral transcription and activation by cellular and viral factors.

have also been demonstrated in vitro in a number of non-lymphoid cells,[60–63] and for some glial-derived and colon carcinoma cell lines, the glycolipid galactosyl ceramide has been shown to mediate infection in a CD4-independent manner.[64,65] The relevance of these findings for viral entry to the pathogenesis of HIV in vivo remains to be determined.

Following adsorption of the virion to the cell surface, HIV penetrates the cellular plasma membrane and is uncoated in the cytosol. Viral RNA is reverse transcribed to single- and then double-stranded DNA by the viral reverse transcriptase enzyme and translocated to the nucleus, where it circularizes and integrates at random positions in host chromosomes. Transcription of this provirus leads to the production of genomic RNA as well as viral proteins; following an obligatory processing step in which the gag and pol precursor proteins are cleaved by the viral protease, the virion is assembled at the inner surface of the plasma membrane, buds outward from the infected cell, and is released as an infectious particle. A number of factors have been shown to up-regulate virus production markedly, including cellular activation,[66–71] trans-acting factors of other viruses,[71–76] cytokines,[77–81] and ultraviolet light.[82] These cofactors, along with the balance of viral regulatory gene products tat and rev, could have relevance in vivo in determining the extent of virus production in an infected individual.[27,83]

In Vivo Pathogenesis

The mechanism by which HIV infection produces immunodeficiency in vivo remains under intense investigation and likely reflects a complex interplay of viral and host factors. The evolution from asymptomatic HIV infection to full-blown AIDS probably involves a gradual increase in a systemic viral load that leads to a progressive and irreversible depression of cellular immunity. Central to the immune abnormalities in AIDS are both quantitative[22,24] and qualitative[22,24,84,85] abnormalities in CD4+ lymphocytes. Proposed mechanisms for the depletion of these cells are listed in Table 155-2 and include both direct effects of viral infection on mature and progenitor CD4 cells, as well as the destruction by cellular or humoral mechanisms of uninfected CD4 cells that display adsorbed or processed viral antigens on their surface.[22,24,86,87] Recent studies have shown that the attachment of gp120 to CD4 on the surface of T lymphocytes can lead to programmed cell death or apoptosis when these cells are subsequently stimulated through their antigen receptor or when CD4 is cross-linked by anti-gp120 antibodies.[88–90] Moreover, recent animal models have indicated that CD4+ cell depletion may also result from defective maturation of CD4+ T cells in the thymus.[91,92] In addition, immune defects are present prior to a severe depletion in CD4

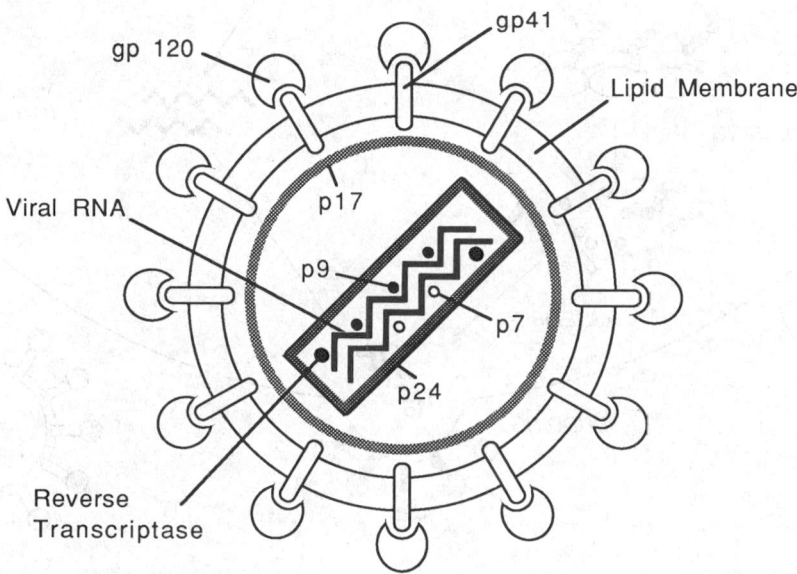

Fig. 155-2. Structure of the HIV virion. Two coding strands of genomic RNA are packaged in a nucleoid core with the p7, p9, and p24 proteins and reverse transcriptase. The core is surrounded by the p17 matrix protein lining the inner surface of the envelope. The envelope consists of a lipid bilayer derived from the infected cell and glycoprotein spikes that consist of the outer gp120 molecule, which contains the binding site for the CD4 molecule, and gp41, which serves both to anchor the glycoprotein complex to the envelope and to mediate fusion of the viral membrane with the cell membrane during viral penetration.

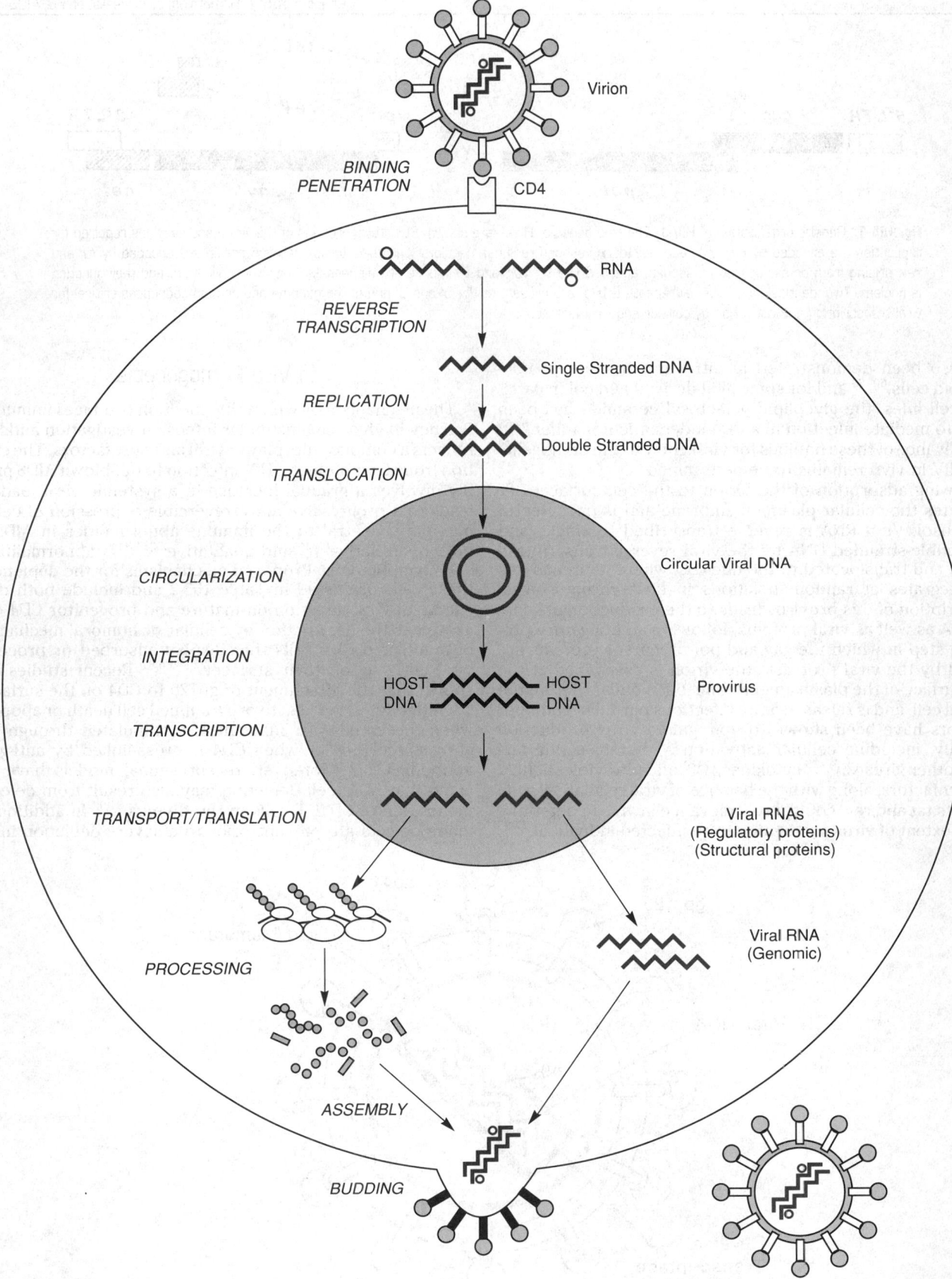

Fig. 155-3. HIV life cycle. Binding of the virion to the cell surface is mediated by a specific interaction of the GP120 envelope glycoprotein with the cellular CD4 molecule. Penetration occurs as the viral membrane fuses with the cellular membrane in a process that requires the gp41 envelop molecule. The viral capsid is uncoated, and viral genomic RNA is reverse transcribed and duplicated by the viral reverse transcriptase to produce a double-stranded copy of viral DNA. The DNA duplex is translocated to the nucleus, where it circularizes and integrates into host chromosomes. Following appropriate activating signals, the provirus is transcribed by a cellular RNA polymerase and transported to the cytoplasm. Proteins are translated and processed through biochemical steps that, depending on the protein, involve glycosylation (envelope), cleavage (envelope, gag, pol), myristoylation (p17), and phosphorylation (rev, nef). Packaging of genomic RNA with viral proteins occurs as envelope glycoproteins are inserted into the cell membrane, and a new virion subsequently buds.

Table 155-2. Possible Mechanisms for Depletion of CD4 Lymphocytes During HIV Infection

Direct killing of CD4 cells by HIV

Syncytia formation between infected and uninfected cells

Cytotoxic humoral or cellular immune responses to gp120 adsorbed on uninfected CD4 cells

Induction of programmed cell death (apoptosis) by the interaction of gp120 with CD4 molecule

Defective maturation of CD4 cells in the thymus

Infection and killing of lymphoid stem cells or supporting cells required for stem cell proliferation or differentiation, or both

Antilymphocyte antibodies

---

lymphocytes and may reflect an imbalance of particular T-lymphocyte subsets resulting from a selective effect of HIV on memory as opposed to naive T cells.[93,94] Alternatively, an initial dysregulation in immunity may result from a depletion of CD4 cells involved in helping cellular immunity (T_{H1} cells), in contrast to those involved in promoting humoral immunity (T_{H2} cells).[95,96] True autoimmune mechanisms have also been suggested by the demonstration of antilymphocyte antibodies in HIV-infected patients with clinical evidence of immunodeficiency.[97–100] In addition to the role of CD4[+] lymphocyte depletion in the pathogenesis of AIDS, it is clear that monocytes and macrophages are targets for HIV infection and probably represent a major reservoir for virus production in vivo.[42,43,101,102] In view of the central role of the monocyte in processing and presenting antigens to T and B lymphocytes and in its ability to migrate to the central nervous system, it is likely that infection of this cell type by HIV plays a significant role in the development of both immunologic and neurologic disease in infected individuals.[22,103]

As indicated by the current surveillance definition of AIDS (Table 155-1), neurologic abnormalities in both the central and peripheral nervous systems, as well as the development of Kaposi sarcoma and B-cell lymphomas, are common clinical manifestations of AIDS.[1] In the central nervous system, glial and other reticuloendothelial cells,[47,103–105] and possibly endothelial cells,[106] have been shown to be productively infected by HIV, raising the possibility that dementia and other neurologic defects could arise from the direct effects of viral infection, inflammatory responses, or the elaboration of toxic cytokines by infected cells.[103,107] Kaposi sarcoma is a proliferative disorder of endothelial cells that occurs predominantly in homosexual and bisexual men with HIV infection.[108,109] Although the endothelial cells of Kaposi sarcoma lesions are not themselves infected by HIV, recent findings have suggested that factors promoting angiogenesis are produced by HIV-infected cells and may stimulate endothelial cell proliferation.[109–112] Consequently, Kaposi sarcoma, while reflecting a dysregulation of cell growth, may not represent a true neoplasm. Moreover, the long recognized association of Kaposi sarcoma in AIDS with homosexual and bisexual males provides strong epidemiologic evidence that cofactors or, alternatively, other transmissible agents may be involved in its pathogenesis besides HIV infection.[113]

A dramatic rise in the incidence of B-cell lymphomas has been reported in patients with HIV infection[114–125]; in contrast to Kaposi sarcoma, this complication has been observed in all patient groups, including hemophiliacs and children.[120,122–124,126–128] The malignant B cells from these lymphomas are not infected by HIV[123,129,130] and are likely derived from a clonal outgrowth of polyclonal populations of proliferating B cells present in patients with HIV infection.[123,131–134] Possible mechanisms for the B-cell stimulation observed in these individuals include a dysregulation in CD4 helper function,[95,96]

the direct mitogenic effects of Epstein-Barr virus (EBV) infection,[123,135,136] cytomegalovirus (CMV),[137] or HIV antigens.[138] Approximately 30–70% of lymphomas have been found to contain EBV DNA, strongly implicating this virus in at least some of these neoplasms.[123,126,130,136,139,140] Hodgkin disease has also been reported with increased frequency in HIV-infected patients,[114,141–146] although the reason for this association is unclear. In at least a subset of non-AIDS, HIV-infected patients with Hodgkin disease, Reed-Sternberg cells were shown to contain integrated copies of the EBV genome[143,147] or to express EBV RNA,[140] raising the possibility that the reactivation of EBV seen in patients with HIV infection[148] may be implicated in the development of AIDS-associated Hodgkin disease. Although less common than B-cell lymphomas, peripheral as well as cutaneous T-cell lymphomas have also been reported in patients with HIV infection.[115,149–153] A more complete discussion of AIDS-associated lymphomas is presented in Chapter 86.

A number of phases of HIV infection have been recognized, including an acute viral syndrome, an asymptomatic stage, a variety of symptomatic conditions in which generalized lymphadenopathy is common, and full-blown AIDS[1] (Table 155-1). Patients with the acute viral syndrome typically present 2–6 weeks after exposure with fever, malaise, myalgias, maculopapular rash, diarrhea, lymphadenopathy, or aseptic meningitis.[154–160] Laboratory findings include lymphocytosis with atypical plasmacytoid lymphocytes, a negative heterophil count, and mild thrombocytopenia.[154–157] In one recent series of 23 patients with symptomatic primary HIV-1 infection, thrombocytopenia was the most frequent hematologic finding, observed in 17 patients (74%), and leukopenia without lymphocytosis was reported in approximately 50%.[161] It is important in the diagnosis of acute HIV infection that individuals may be serologically negative during the viral prodrome but typically develop anti-HIV antibodies 1–2 months after the onset of this illness. Circulating viral p24 antigen in the absence of anti-HIV antibody may be detectable during this acute phase.[155,161] Probably most HIV-infected individuals in the United States are asymptomatic, and exhibit serologic evidence of infection by enzyme-linked immunosorbent assay, Western blot, or immunofluorescence assays.[5] That asymptomatic but seropositive patients are persistently infected with HIV has been clearly established by epidemiologic studies,[162,163] positive viral cultures,[164,165] and the presence of viral DNA and RNA in peripheral blood mononuclear cells and plasma, respectively, detected by the polymerase chain reaction.[166–168] Recent studies evaluating lymph nodes of HIV-infected patients have shown that even in this asymptomatic period there is an abundance of replicating virus in these tissues, indicating that while these individuals may be clinically well, contrary to earlier views, HIV is clearly not latent during this period.[166,169] This prolonged period of clinical latency may be complicated by persistent generalized lymphadenopathy with or without a number of nonspecific complaints, including arthralgias, fatigue, intermittent diarrhea, and chronic sinusitis.[1–3] As noted previously, prospective studies of homosexual men and hemophiliacs infected with HIV indicate that the median duration between HIV infection and the onset of full-blown AIDS is ≥10 years.[20–24,170] In HIV-infected patients a low CD4 lymphocyte number (<200/mm^3), an elevated level of β_2-microglobulin, and a persistence of the viral p24 antigen in serum are each associated with an increased risk of opportunistic infections.[171–176] The clinical course of HIV infection is summarized in Figure 155-4, which emphasizes that clinical progression over time is associated with a progressive and irreversible loss of CD4 lymphocytes as well as a gradual increase in a systemic viral load, particularly in peripheral blood.

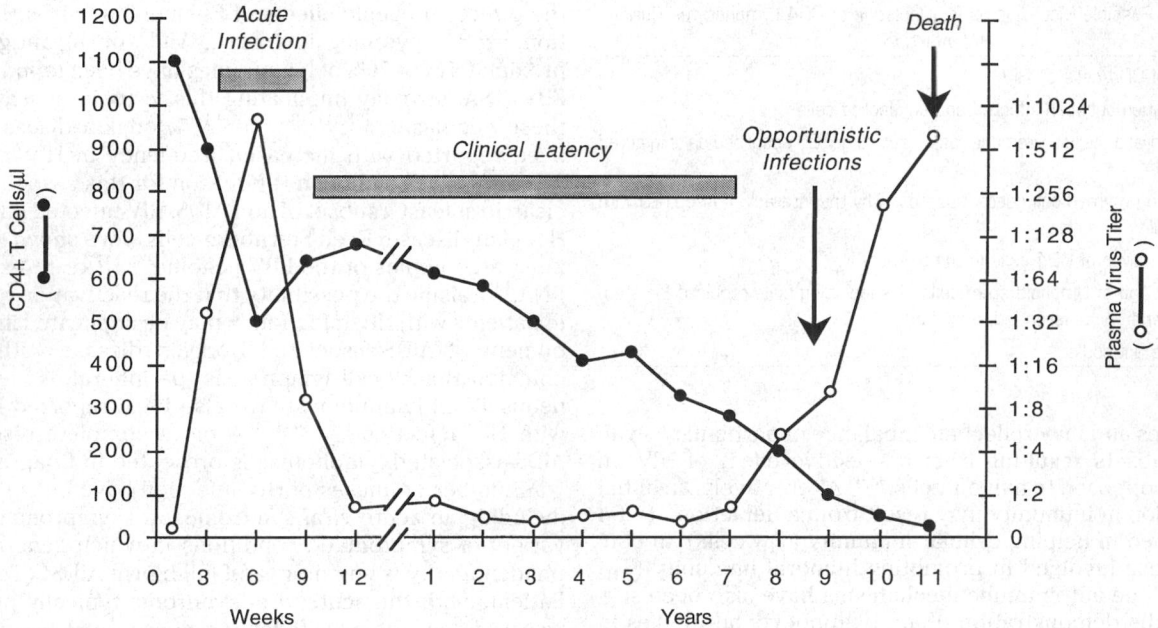

Fig. 155-4. Natural history of HIV infection in an infected individual. A typical course of HIV infection is shown. During primary infection there is active viral replication with viremia and widespread dissemination of virus to lymph organs, during which time a sharp decline in the number of CD4+ lymphocytes occurs. This is followed by a prolonged period of clinical latency, characterized by a slow but progressive decline in CD4+ lymphocytes. When the CD4+ cell number falls <200/mm³ the clinical course is generally complicated by opportunistic infections. A quantitative increase in viremia occurs during this time, reflecting increased viral replication, an increasing viral load, and/or redistribution of virus from damaged lymph organs. (Modified from Pantaleo et al.,[22] with permission.)

HEMATOLOGIC ABNORMALITIES IN PATIENTS WITH HIV INFECTION

It is clear that hematologic abnormalities in infected individuals may arise from a number of causes, including (1) direct infection by HIV of bone marrow cells or other supporting cells required for hematopoiesis; (2) dysregulation of the host immune system, leading to destruction or inhibition of hematopoietic cells; and (3) secondary complications of either opportunistic infections, malignancies, and/or therapy for these disorders. Not surprisingly, the principle hematologic problems encountered in patients with HIV infection include cytopenias of red cells, neutrophils, lymphocytes, and platelets, as well as a variety of polyclonal and oligoclonal gammopathies. Several general reviews of the hematologic complications in AIDS have been published.[177–182]

Abnormalities in Hematopoietic Cells

Anemia and Red Blood Cell Abnormalities

Anemia occurs in most HIV-infected patients at some point in the natural history of their disease,[181,183,184] and both the incidence and degree of anemia have been shown to correlate with the severity of the clinical syndrome.[181] When HIV infection is complicated by opportunistic infections, anemia is seen in 70–95% of patients with mean hemoglobin and hematocrit levels of 9.7–11.7 g/dl and 36%, respectively.[181,185] However, even in asymptomatic patients with HIV infection or those with minimal symptoms, a mild but significant reduction in hematocrit has been reported in 15–20% of patients.[2,3,181] Anemia and granulocytopenia tend to occur concurrently, with one series showing that 68% of patients with hematocrits of <40 were also neutropenic, with white blood cell (WBC) counts <1.4 × 10³/μl, while 88% of patients with neutropenia were also anemic.[181]

Anemia in patients with HIV infection who are not undergoing antiretroviral therapy with zidovudine is typically normochromic normocytic, although a mild degree of anisocytosis and poikilocytosis is common.[186–190] Macrocytosis occurs in most patients treated with zidovudine,[191,192] and in the experience of some urban hospitals, zidovudine therapy has become the most common cause of macrocytosis.[193] Schistocytes are prominent in the setting of thrombotic thrombocytopenic purpura (TTP), which may complicate HIV infection.[194–199]

Depressed or ineffective erythropoiesis in patients with AIDS is suggested by a low or inappropriately "normal" reticulocyte count; in HIV-infected patients, the reticulocyte count cannot be used as a reliable indicator of either hemolysis or bleeding.[178,183,184,190,200] Moreover, the finding on bone marrow examination of normal to increased numbers of erythroid precursor cells[181,183,185,201] along with a variable degree of dyserythropoiesis[181,189,201–203] has indicated that ineffective erythropoiesis may be a major factor in the anemia of AIDS.[177,202–204] A syndrome resembling paroxysmal nocturnal hemoglobinuria was described in a patient presenting with intravascular hemolytic anemia, markedly dysplastic erythroid hyperplasia on bone marrow examination, and abnormal acid hemolysis and sucrose-lysis tests.[205] Megaloblastic changes in erythroid precursors are uncommonly seen[189,206] but have been described during therapy with trimethoprim sulfamethoxazole, dapsone, and zidovudine.[189,191,192,202–204,207] Several reports have noted profound erythroid hypoplasia as well as pure red cell aplasia in the setting of *Mycobacterium avium* complex infection[185–187,189,208]; one study demonstrated a selective suppression of erythroid progenitors due to the presence of soluble factors in serum, possibly produced by macrophages.[208] A low hematocrit (<25%) has been shown to be a highly significant negative predictor for survival in patients with *M. avium* complex infection.[209] Pure red cell aplasia has also been reported in HIV-infected patients receiving zidovudine[210] and without any associated cause.[211] In both adults and children infected with HIV, a severe depression of erythropoiesis may occur due to chronic parvovirus B19 infection, in which the presence of giant pronormoblasts in bone marrow may be diagnostic.[212–215]

Serum erythropoietin (EPO) levels in patients with HIV-associated anemia may be increased[192,216] or reduced[217]; one series found reduced serum levels in 22 of 29 AIDS patients.[217] Although for untreated patients there is an inverse correlation between hematocrit and serum EPO levels, the EPO response to anemia is inappropriately low compared with patients who have iron deficiency anemia or bleeding.[216,218,219] Similar findings have been described in patients with the anemia of chronic disease.[220] Interestingly, for some patients treated with zidovudine, serum EPO levels may increase dramatically in response to anemia, suggesting a restoration of the EPO response.[216,219] Early clinical trials evaluating the role of recombinant EPO in the treatment of anemia in patients receiving zidovudine have found that patients with low pretreatment serum EPO levels (≤500 IU/L) are more likely to respond to EPO therapy, as shown by an improvement in hematocrit and a decreased transfusion requirement.[217,221]

Iron stores in anemic patients with HIV infection are typically adequate or increased; and iron indices are similar to those seen in chronic disease states and show low serum iron and transferrin and elevated serum ferritin.[187,206,222,223] In one report, the level of serum ferritin was found to correlate with the severity of the clinical status showing a mean value of 961 μg/dl in patients with AIDS compared with 318 μg/dl in patients with ARC.[224] Bone marrow iron is usually adequate or increased in reticuloendothelial cells,[181,183,189] although in one study, reduced or absent bone marrow iron was found in 16 of 32 patients with AIDS.[186] Ringed sideroblasts, while uncommon, have been described in ≤5% of AIDS patients in some series.[181,185,189,203]

Reduced serum vitamin B$_{12}$ levels are seen in 7–20% of patients with AIDS,[225–228] although this typically occurs in the absence of neutrophilic hypersegmentation, red blood cell (RBC) macrocytosis, or megaloblastic changes on bone marrow aspirate.[226–228] A slightly higher prevalence of vitamin B$_{12}$ deficiency (20%) has been observed in HIV-infected patients referred for neurologic evaluation, particularly for peripheral neuropathy.[229] When present, a low plasma vitamin B$_{12}$ level in HIV-infected patients does not appear to be due to a reduction in the vitamin B$_{12}$-binding proteins transcobalamin or haptocorrin.[230] Moreover, malabsorption of vitamin B$_{12}$ with an abnormal Schilling test has been found in AIDS patients both with[226,231] and without[225,227,229] chronic diarrhea syndromes, suggesting that a true negative balance of vitamin B$_{12}$ may exist in some patients. Correction of the Schilling test by intrinsic factor in these patients has been variable.[228,229] In one study, patients with an abnormal Shilling test were noted to have chronic inflammatory changes on colonic and duodenal biopsy, as well as evidence by in situ hybridization of HIV-infected mononuclear cells within the lamina propria.[227] These findings have suggested that HIV infection within the gut mucosa could contribute directly to vitamin B$_{12}$ malabsorption. Nonetheless, normal Schilling tests in patients with low serum vitamin B$_{12}$ levels have also been reported.[226,229] Although patients with reduced serum vitamin B$_{12}$ levels are more likely to be anemic, the absence of megaloblastic changes and the lack of a hematologic response to vitamin B$_{12}$ therapy have indicated that in most patients this reduction is not clinically significant.[178,226,228] However, using a reduction in serum holotranscobalamin II levels as a more sensitive indicator of negative vitamin B$_{12}$ balance, reduced levels were reported in approximately one-half of patients with AIDS[232] and have raised the possibility that subclinical vitamin B$_{12}$ deficiency may be more significant than previously recognized. Clinically, reduced serum vitamin B$_{12}$ levels may increase the hematologic toxicity associated with zidovudine therapy,[191] consistent with the findings of one in vitro study.[233] Alterations in folate metab-

olism have also been reported in AIDS patients with reduced intestinal absorption of folate,[234] as well as increased serum and RBC folate levels[235,236] even in the absence of reduced serum vitamin B$_{12}$ levels.[236] The underlying mechanism and clinical significance of these findings are unknown.

Positive direct antiglobulin tests have been reported in 20–43% of hospitalized AIDS patients or patients undergoing transfusion therapy[177,188,222,237,238] and in 8% of asymptomatic individuals.[239] These reactions are usually weak, involve either IgG or complement, or both, and are likely due, at least in part, to the deposition of immune complexes on RBCs similar to that seen in non-AIDS patients with hypergammaglobulinemia.[237] Nonetheless, sensitive assays have documented the presence of true anti-RBC antibodies with anti-i and anti-U specificity in 64% and 32% of AIDS patients, respectively,[238] as well as anti-PI and anti-LEB antibodies in some patients.[177,238] Anti-i antibodies are known to occur during acute EBV infection, and it is possible that the increased frequency of this antibody in patients with HIV infection results from active EBV or possibly CMV infection.[238] Although uncommon, severe autoimmune hemolytic anemia has been reported, with responses observed to steroids, intravenous γ-globulin, splenectomy, and zidovudine.[214,240–243] The relative reticulocytopenia frequently observed in patients with HIV infection may mask the diagnosis of autoimmune hemolytic anemia.[242]

Leukopenia and White Blood Cell Abnormalities

Leukopenia is common in HIV-infected individuals and, similar to anemia, occurs with a frequency that generally correlates with the severity of the clinical syndrome. Between 57% and 85% of patients with AIDS[177,183,187] and between 10% and 21% of patients with ARC[177,185,244] are leukopenic while 5% of asymptomatic seropositive patients present with leukopenia.[181,185] In one series only 12% of patients with AIDS were found to have WBC counts >7,000/mm^3.[183] Leukopenia typically involves both lymphocytes and granulocytes, although monocytopenia has also been reported in 8–75% of patients with AIDS.[180,185,189] In patients with advanced immunodeficiency, all lymphocyte subsets are decreased. However, as noted previously, a reduction in the absolute number of CD4$^+$ T cells occurs as one of the earliest immunologic abnormalities of HIV infection, and the number of these cells declines progressively over time[22] (Fig. 155-4). A low number of CD4$^+$ lymphocytes is one of the most important prognostic indicators for the risk of developing opportunistic infections.[172–175]

A number of morphologic abnormalities have been described in peripheral blood and bone marrow WBCs of patients with HIV infection. Particularly in the setting of granulocytopenia, neutrophils may show nuclear hyposegmentation with an apparent left shift, along with the presence of monolobed or Pelger-Huët forms[189,190,222] (Fig. 155-5A). In addition, other dysplastic changes of neutrophils have been described, including increased size, prominent granulation, and increased peroxidase activity.[177,189,190,222,245] Nonspecific morphologic findings include large vacuolated monocytes and atypical lymphocytes, particularly in patients who are lymphopenic.[189,200,222] Although myelodysplastic changes are common and likely do not represent a preleukemic syndrome,[178,190] rare cases of acute myeloid leukemia evolving from a pre-existing myelodysplastic state have been reported in HIV-infected individuals.[202,246–249]

Granulocytopenia is a common complication of several drugs used in the therapy for AIDS-related infections, including trimethoprim sulfamethoxozole and pentamidine for *Pneumocystis carinii* pneumonia, pyrimethamine sulfadiazine for central nervous system toxoplasmosis, flucytosine for cryptococcal or other fungal infections, and ganciclovir for CMV infection.[250] Between 19% and 28% of patients receiving tri-

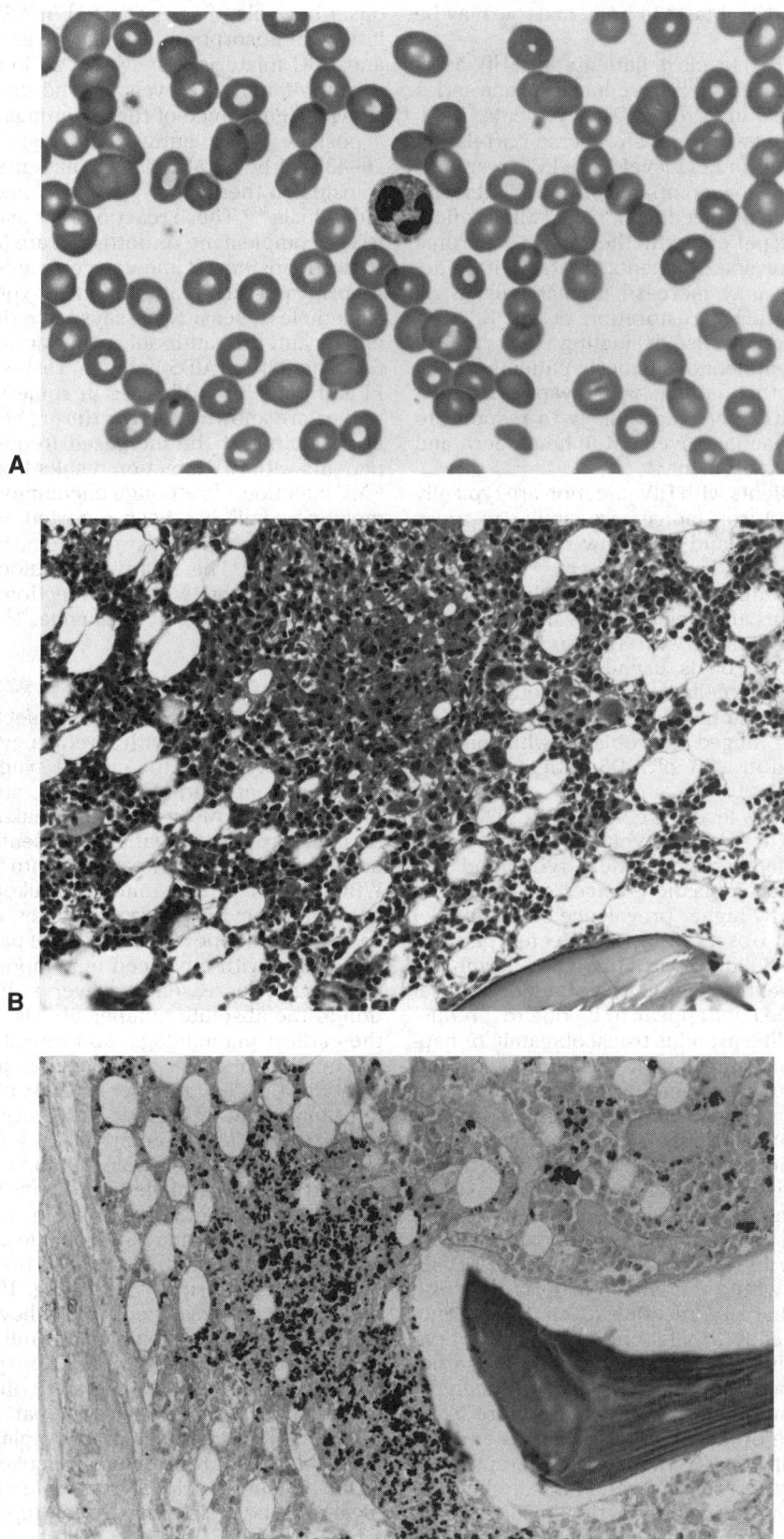

Fig. 155-5. Peripheral blood and bone marrow morphologic abnormalities in AIDS. **(A)** Pelger-Huët cell and macrocytes in a patient with AIDS-related complex undergoing therapy with zidovudine. The mean corpuscular volume on this blood sample was 118 μm^3. **(B)** "Loose granuloma" formation from a bone marrow biopsy in patient with disseminated *Mycobacterium avium* complex infection involving bone marrow. Acid-fast stains of this specimen showed numerous organisms within the granuloma. **(C)** Grocott stain showing cryptococcal involvement of bone marrow. Organisms in this panel are darkly stained. *(Figure continues.)*

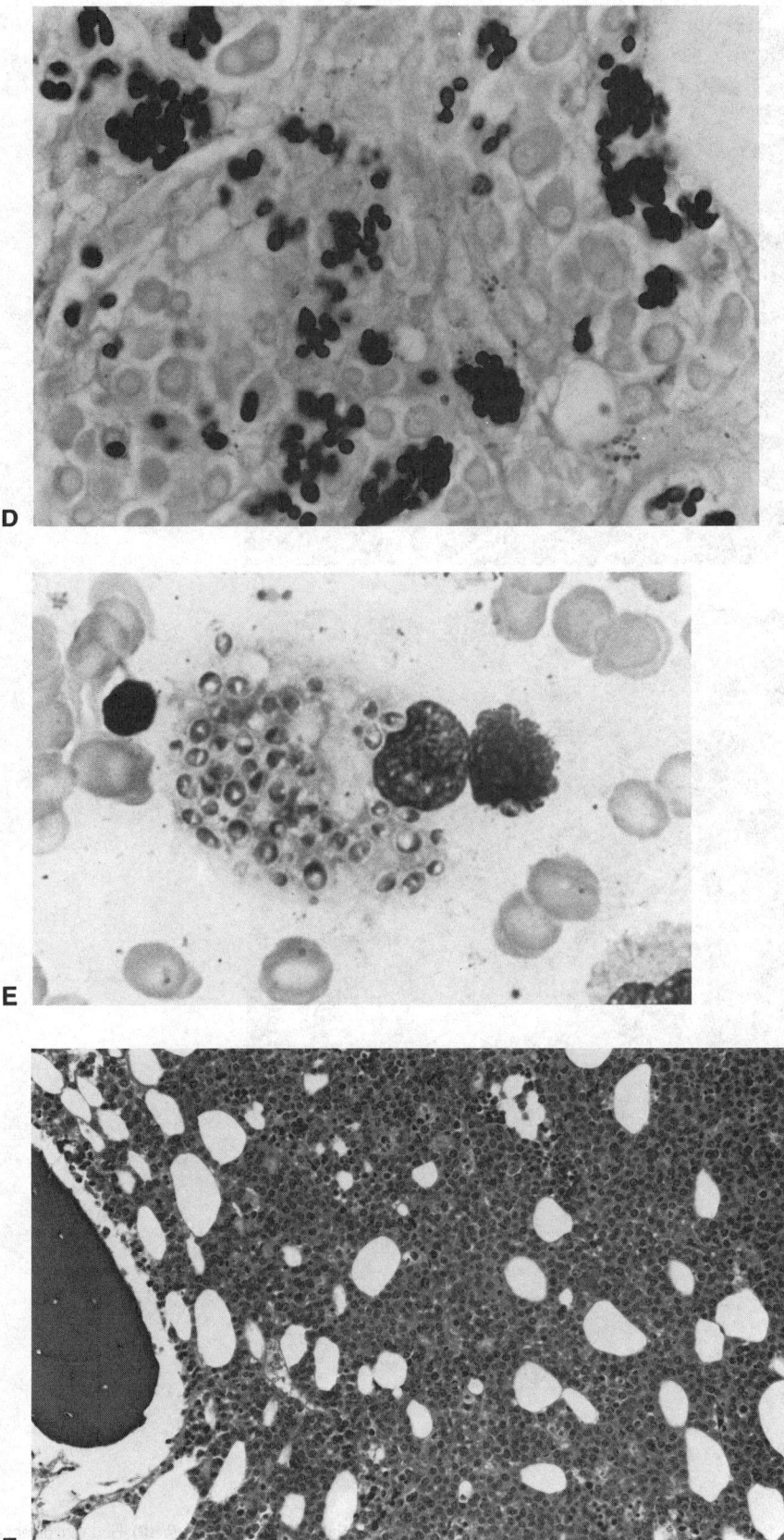

Fig. 155-5 *(Continued).* **(D)** High magnification of this specimen shows numerous budding yeast forms. **(E)** Histoplasma within a macrophage seen on Wright-Giemsa stain of a bone marrow aspirate. **(F)** Non-Hodgkin lymphoma involvement of marrow (diffuse non-Burkitt type), showing a hypercellular marrow completely replaced by malignant cells. *(Figure continues.)*

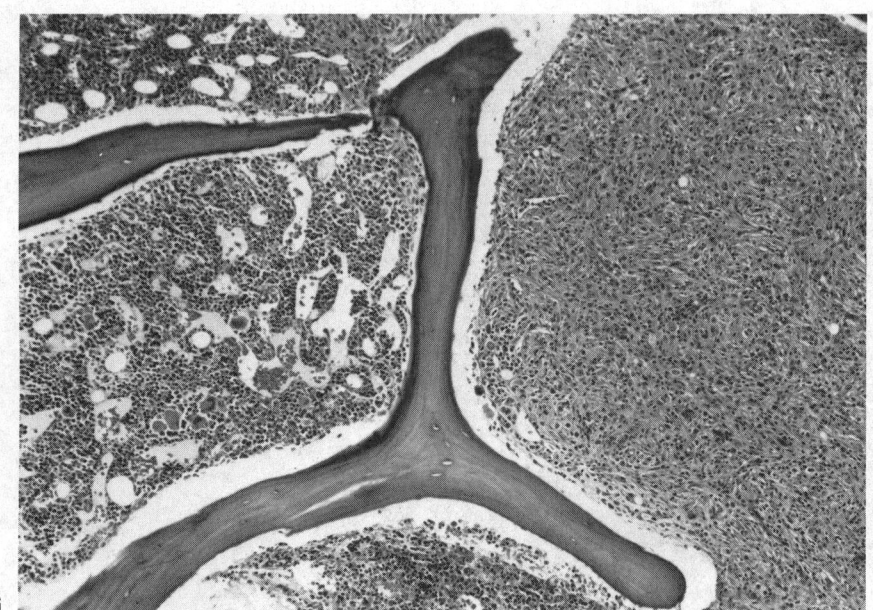

G

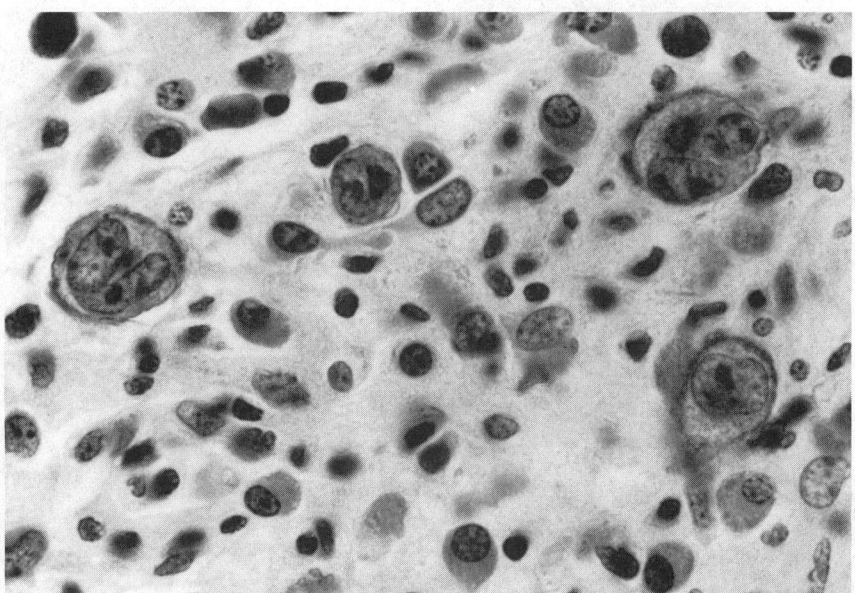

H

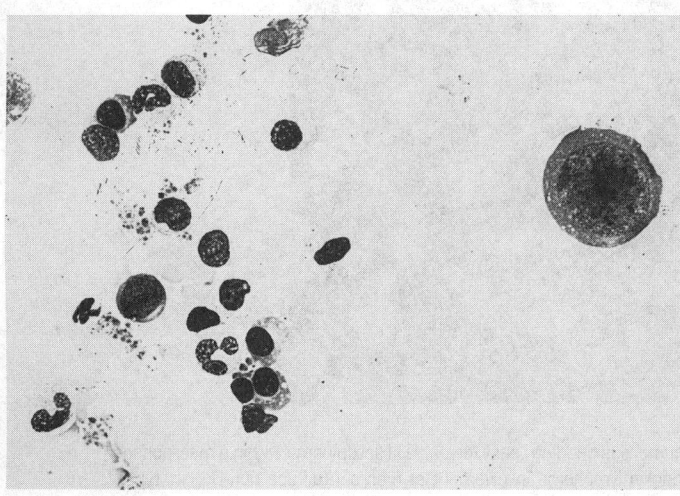

I

Fig. 155-5 *(Continued).* **(G)** Hodgkin disease involving marrow, showing normal cellularity (left) and a pleomorphic desmoplastic reactive process (right). **(H)** High-magnification view of this specimen shows numerous Reed-Sternberg cells. **(I)** Giant pronormoblast in parvovirus B19 infection. *(Figure continues).*

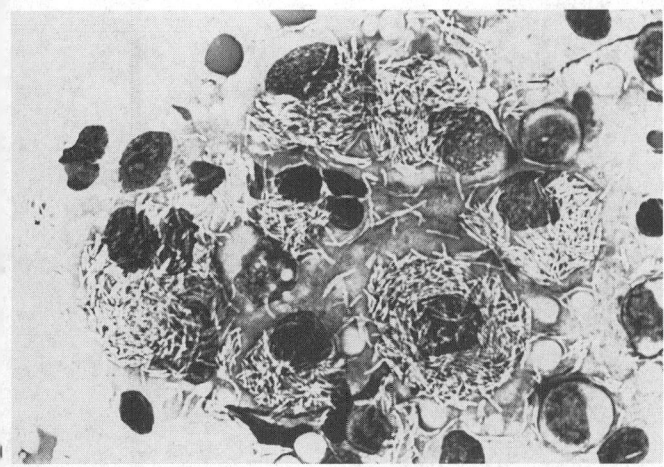

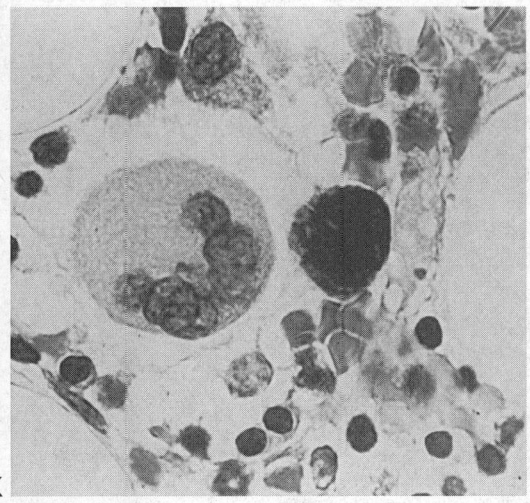

ig. 155-5 *(Continued).* **(J)** Pseudo-Gaucher cell resulting from bone marrow hisiocytes engorged with *Mycobacterium avium* complex organisms. **(K)** Condensed obulated nucleus of a dysplastic megakaryocyte from a patient is shown adjacent o a normal megakaryocyte. (Figs. I–K from Bauer et al.,[316] with permission.)

methoprim sulfamethoxozole for *P. carinii* pneumonia develop neutropenia,[251–254] usually in the setting of fever, rash, and elevated liver transaminases.[253,254] Dose-dependent neutropenia in patients receiving zidovudine has been reported in 8–16% of patients during long-term therapy[191,255] but may also occur in an apparently idiosyncratic manner with profound bone marrow hypoplasia[256] and agranulocytosis.[257]

Although the mechanism of granulocytopenia in AIDS remains under intense investigation, the role of HIV infection in bone marrow function has remained controversial. Bone marrow biopsies in patients with AIDS and symptomatic HIV infection are either normocellular or hypercellular in 60–100%[181,183,185,187,189,190,201,206,222,258] and are frequently associated with dysplastic changes,[185,190,201] suggesting that ineffective myelopoiesis may be occurring. In vitro cultures of bone marrow from HIV-infected patients for colony-forming unit-granulocyte/macrophage (CFU-GM) and burst-forming unit-erythroid (BFU-E) or of CD34+ progenitor cells have been reported to be either normal[259–261] or reduced.[262–267] Infection of cultured bone marrow cells by HIV-1 has been demonstrated in vitro, and in some[265,268–270] but not all studies,[259] has been reported to inhibit colony formation. However, directly evaluating CD34+ cells or CFUs from patients with AIDS for HIV DNA by the highly sensitive polymerase chain reaction technique has, in several studies, failed to show a significant degree of infection.[259,260,264,265,271] A single study using in situ hybridization of bone marrow

from patients did report HIV genomes in a high proportion of patients, detectable in immature myeloid cells, histiocytes, endothelial cells, and nucleated RBCs.[204] Nonetheless, the predominant view emerging from most studies is that (with the exception of the megakaryocyte) few hematopoietic progenitor cells are directly infected by HIV.

A number of indirect mechanisms of HIV-mediated suppression of hematopoiesis have also been suggested. Suppressive effects of the viral envelope gp120 on hematopoietic colony formation have been observed in vitro in some,[270,272] but not all, studies.[259] In addition, earlier studies have implicated suppression of myelopoiesis by T lymphocytes,[252] anti-gp120 antibodies,[261] and a glycoprotein produced by cultured bone marrow cells.[263] It is also possible that HIV infection of CD4 lymphocytes or monocytes, or both, may induce the production of endogenous lymphokines and other growth factors that either positively or negatively regulate myelopoiesis.[273] Recently the viral gene product tat has been shown to suppress cultured bone marrow cells by inducing macrophages to produce transforming growth factor, a potent inhibitor of hematopoiesis.[274] A possible autoimmune mechanism for the destruction of peripheral blood granulocytes has also been suggested by the presence of antineutrophil immunoglobulins in as high as 67% of patients with AIDS and ARC.[100,275–277] One interesting study raised the possibility that bone marrow stromal fibroblasts may be infectable by HIV, implying that hematopoiesis could be affected through viral-induced alterations in the bone marrow microenvironment.[179] Nonetheless, whatever the mechanism of AIDS-associated leukopenia, a dramatic rise in peripheral blood neutrophils is typically seen in AIDS patients following therapy with recombinant colony-stimulating factor-granulocyte/macrophage (CSF-GM)[278] (see Fig. 155-8) or CSF-G,[279] clearly indicating that competent myeloid stem cells with the capacity for differentiation are present, even in patients with advanced immunodeficiency.

Thrombocytopenia

Thrombocytopenia is a frequently reported complication of HIV infection,[281] and has been described in a variety of patient populations, including homosexual men,[282–285] heterosexuals,[286] intravenous drug users,[287] hemophiliacs,[288,289] and children.[290–292] Depending on the patient population analyzed, thrombocytopenia, defined as a platelet count <100,000/mm^3 has been reported in 3–8% of seropositive individuals[188,285,293–296] and in 30–45% of patients with fully developed AIDS.[177,294] In some studies an inverse correlation was found between the platelet count and the CD4+ lymphocyte number.[293,295] However, it is important to recognize that isolated and occasionally severe thrombocytopenia may occur even in asymptomatic individuals as the presenting manifestation of HIV infection. Thrombocytopenia has also been reported during acute HIV infection as part of the acute viral syndrome described earlier.[157,161,297]

The degree of HIV-related thrombocytopenia is generally mild to moderate, with mean counts ranging from 43,000 to 57,000/mm^3.[283,287] However, a severe reduction to levels <10,000/mm^3 has also been described.[283,284,286,287] Roughly one-third of patients with thrombocytopenia present with a history of easy bruising, petechiae, or bleeding,[284,298] although in most, significant spontaneous clinical bleeding usually does not occur.[177,280,299] Not surprisingly, life-threatening hemorrhagic complications primarily due to central nervous system bleeding may occur in HIV-infected hemophiliacs, particularly with platelet counts <50,000/mm^3.[300] Unlike classic idiopathic thrombocytopenic purpura (ITP), HIV-related thrombocytopenia is frequently accompanied by other hematologic abnormalities, usually neutropenia with or without anemia (60% of cases).[177,178] However, particularly in asymptomatic seropositive patients, it generally occurs as an isolated hematologic abnormality.[181,284] The presence or absence of thrombocytopenia in seropositive individuals does not appear to be a prognostic indicator for the development of AIDS.[283,288] Interestingly, in as many as 11–50% of patients, thrombocytopenia may regress spontaneously without therapy.[177,283,284,288,295]

The mechanism of thrombocytopenia in HIV infection appears to involve both increased platelet destruction and ineffective platelet production. In one recent study, the survival of ^{111}In-labeled autologous platelets was found to be significantly reduced compared with normal controls in both untreated and zidovudine-treated patients with HIV-related thrombocytopenia.[301] Platelet survival was also decreased in HIV-infected patients without thrombocytopenia, although to a lesser extent.[301] While there continues to be some controversy concerning the extent to which platelet clearance is mediated by the spleen,[301,302] the high response rate of HIV-related thrombocytopenia to splenectomy suggests that the spleen is probably a major site of platelet sequestration or destruction, or both.[283,284,303–309] The observed decrease in platelet survival is most likely immunologically mediated. In HIV-related thrombocytopenia, there is a marked increase in platelet-associated immunoglobulin and complement and in circulating immune complexes to levels two to four times higher than that seen in classic ITP.[286,288,310] An analysis of circulating as well as platelet-associated immune complexes has shown anti-idiotypic antibodies directed against antibodies to the HIV-1 envelope glycoprotein gp120.[311] In at least some individuals, a true autoimmune process has been suggested by the detection of antiplatelet activity in IgG eluted from platelets,[275,287,288,310,312] including one study suggesting that at least some patients may exhibit antibodies to platelet glycoproteins GPIIb/IIIa,[313] similar to that seen in classic ITP, although this has been somewhat controversial.[312] Interestingly, one report demonstrated that antibodies eluted from patient platelets could recognize both platelet GPIIIa as well as HIV envelope glycoproteins, suggesting that cross-reactive epitopes between viral envelope and platelet glycoproteins could potentially mediate a true autoimmune destruction of platelets in some patients.[314]

Although megakaryocytes are typically increased in HIV-related thrombocytopenia, a kinetic analysis has shown a significant reduction in platelet production.[301] Megakaryocytes are characteristically dysplastic,[190,201,315,316] and circulating platelets have been shown to exhibit an inappropriately low mean platelet volume, similar to that seen in myelosuppressive disorders.[317] A number of studies have strongly suggested that this dysplasia may be related to direct infection of the megakaryocyte by HIV.[318] Megakaryocytes have been shown to express CD4 on the cell surface and to be able to bind HIV.[52,53] Megakaryocytic cell lines are susceptible in vitro to infection by particular isolates of HIV,[53,319] and one report indicated that this infection could be markedly enhanced by tumor necrosis factor-α,[320] similar to the effects of this cytokine on T-cell and monocytic cell lines.[78,81,321,322] Finally, studies of megakaryocytes directly from HIV-infected patients have shown viral RNA by in situ hybridization (Fig. 155-6) and viral proteins by immunofluorescence microscopy, strongly suggesting that these cells are infected in vivo.[323,324] Interestingly, in one study HIV transcripts were not detected in megakaryocyte colonies, suggesting that megakaryocytes may not be susceptible to infection until they are more differentiated or that infected megakaryocytes may be unable to proliferate or differentiate in vitro.[324] A recent study has described an isolate of HIV-1 that was selectively cytopathic for megakaryocytic cell lines, indicating that viral factors could be involved in determining the extent to which megakaryocyte dysfunction and thrombocytopenia occur in infected patients.[325] Thus, unlike other hematopoietic precursors, there is mounting evidence that HIV directly infects megakaryocytes, contributes to ineffective thrombopoiesis,

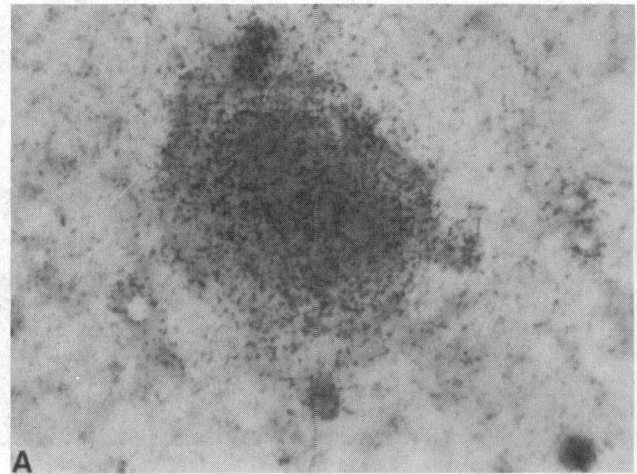

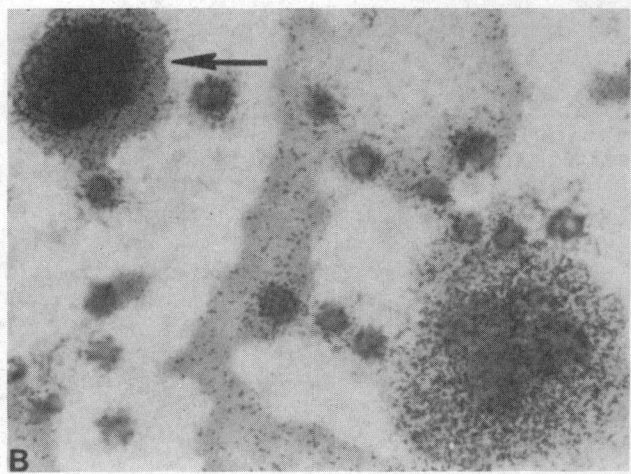

Fig. 155-6. (A & B) Megakaryocyte infection by HIV. In situ hybridization with a ^{35}S-labeled HIV-specific probe in a bone marrow biopsy from an HIV-seropositive patient. In both figures, numerous grains are apparent, indicating the presence of HIV RNA within the megakaryocyte cytoplasm. In Fig. B, a dysplastic megakaryocyte largely denuded of cytoplasm is shown (arrow) that also is reactive with the HIV probe. (From Zucker-Franklin and Cao,[323] with permission.)

and, coupled with antiviral immune responses, leads to thrombocytopenia in a subpopulation of patients.

Abnormalities in Coagulation

Antiphospholipid antibodies detectable as lupus anticoagulants or anticardiolipin antibodies (ACAs) have been identified in 22–82% of patients with HIV infection, including homosexual men, intravenous drug users, and hemophiliacs.[326–330] Interestingly, despite the association in non-HIV-infected patients among lupus anticoagulants, ACA, and a false-positive Venereal Disease Research Laboratory (VDRL) test, the VDRL test in HIV-infected patients without a history of syphilis is usually nonreactive, probably reflecting differences in specificity of the antiphospholipid antibodies in patients with and without HIV infection.[327]

Patients with a lupus anticoagulant typically present in the absence of a bleeding history with a prolonged activated partial thromboplastin time (PTT)[177,178] that does not correct after mixing with normal plasma and incubation at 37°C.[177,326] A prolongation in the tissue thromboplastin time is also usually seen.[326,327] The Russell's viper venom clotting time, which mea-

...ures clot formation by the direct activation of factor X, is the most specific indicator of a lupus anticoagulant.[177,326,327] In HIV-infected patients, lupus anticoagulants are typically IgMs[327] and can be partially adsorbed with phospholipids obtained from commercially available lipid extracts or platelet membranes.[177,326] In one recent study of HIV-infected patients with prolonged PTTs, lupus anticoagulants were described that were not detectable by a mixing test. However, a functional inhibitory activity was demonstrated by a prolonged Russell's viper venom clotting time or by correction of the PTT with increasing concentrations of exogenous phospholipid.[331] Lupus inhibitors were initially described in 20–73% of patients with AIDS[178,326,327,332] and in as many as 43% of asymptomatic seropositive patients[333,334]; in a more recent series, however, lupus inhibitors were considerably less frequent, particularly in nonhospitalized patients, in whom they were not observed in 142 HIV-infected patients.[330]

ACAs that may or may not have activity as lupus inhibitors are detectable by enzyme-linked immunosorbant assays; in HIV-infected patients they are usually IgG immunoglobulins.[328,349] In one study a higher frequency of ACAs in patients with AIDS compared with asymptomatic patients (84% versus 50%, respectively) was found,[328] although another study of hemophiliacs found no difference in the frequency of ACAs among hemophiliacs with or without AIDS.[334] In a more recent study, ACAs were detectable in 30% of hospitalized and 8% of nonhospitalized seropositive patients.[330] No correlation has been found between the presence of ACAs and the presence or absence of thrombocytopenia,[335] the CD4 cell number,[334] or the risk of progression to AIDS.[334] Despite the association of a positive ACA titer with antinuclear antibodies in >90% of patients with lupus, antinuclear antibodies have rarely been reported in patients with AIDS,[328] although one study did note low-titer antinuclear antibodies in 19 of 151 patients with AIDS or ARC.[336]

The presence of a lupus inhibitor or ACAs does not predispose to clinical bleeding and, in the absence of thrombocytopenia or an elevated prothrombin time, is not a contraindication to an invasive procedure.[177,178,326,327] However, depending on the specificity of the antiphospholipid antibody, other coagulation defects may be present, including a reduced level of factor VII, resulting in a prolongation in the prothrombin time[367] and abnormal platelet aggregation studies associated with an abnormal bleeding time.[327] Consequently, the decision to perform invasive procedures on an HIV-infected patient in whom a lupus anticoagulant is identified should be individualized and requires a careful bleeding history. In addition, the presence of a lupus inhibitor in hemophiliacs may complicate factor replacement therapy: the resulting prolongation of the PTT may be misinterpreted as a factor VIII inhibitor and may interfere with monitoring for factor VIII replacement therapy.[177] In contrast to patients without HIV infection, in whom the presence of a lupus inhibitor is associated with thrombotic events and fetal loss,[338–340] a lupus inhibitor is rarely associated with thrombosis in patients with HIV infection.[326,327]

The mechanism for the high frequency of antiphospholipid antibodies in HIV-infected patients is unclear but presumably involves the generation of phospholipids from either endogenous or exogenous sources. Destruction of immune or hematopoietic cells directly or indirectly by HIV could induce membrane damage and the liberation of phospholipids as immunogens. Alternatively, secondary infections could provide exogenous phospholipids or further contribute to the release of endogenous phospholipids from damages tissues. The combined results of two studies noted a frequency of lupus anticoagulants or ACAs in 39 of 50 AIDS patients with *P. carinii* pneumonia and in only 1 of 34 AIDS patients with other opportunistic infections, suggesting an association between *P. carinii* and antiphospholipid antibodies.[332,341] Moreover, in both studies, patients were described who developed these antibodies

with the onset of the pneumonia and who subsequently lost the antibody with successful therapy of the infection. However, another study found no correlation between the presence of an opportunistic infection and a lupus inhibitor.[177] The high frequency of ACAs even in asymptomatic individuals,[333] however, as described above, indicates that other factors aside from *P. carinii* infection are likely involved.

Several recent reports have described a remarkably high frequency of acquired protein S deficiency in HIV-infected patients, with a reduction noted in 17–73% of seropositive patients.[342–345] This deficiency reflects a true reduction in both free and total protein S levels, with no alteration found in the level of C4b-binding protein, which binds 60–70% of circulating protein S.[342,343] One study did note a correlation of reduced protein S levels with a diagnosis of AIDS and a low CD4 cell number,[344] while another study found an association with an increasing duration of HIV infection and elevated levels of ACAs.[343] The mechanism of protein S deficiency in these patients is unclear and could involve decreased synthesis or abnormalities in endothelial cell function. Protein S is synthesized in liver and endothelial cells, and the presence of normal levels of other hepatic coagulation factors in patients studied does suggest that endothelial cell dysfunction could be involved.[343,344] Increased levels of antigenic von Willebrand factor have been described in seropositive patients, possibly reflecting abnormal endothelial cell function.[343,345] Importantly, of 159 patients studied in three published reports, 8 had thromboembolic complications and reduced protein S levels.[342–344] Thus, in contrast to the presence of a lupus anticoagulant, it is possible that protein S deficiency may predispose to thrombosis in HIV-infected patients in certain settings. Further studies will clearly be needed to address this point.

Gammopathies

Polyclonal hypergammaglobulinemia was among the first of the immunologic abnormalities described in AIDS and is seen in both asymptomatic and symptomatic seropositive patients.[131,346–350] Elevated levels of IgG, IgA, and IgM are present in spite of depressed in vitro B-cell proliferative responses to mitogens.[131,132] Interestingly, in 3–18% of HIV-infected patients, monoclonal or oligoclonal immunoglobulin bands can be demonstrated by serum protein electrophoresis or immunofixation.[351–358] This high frequency of monoclonal gammapathy in patients with a mean age of 35 is in marked contrast to a frequency of 0.09% for age-matched controls.[352,359] Paraproteins can be either IgG or IgM and usually occur in the absence of a depression of other immunoglobulins and without Bence Jones proteinuria.[351,352] In one study, an analysis of paraproteins in seven HIV-infected patients demonstrated that five had a polyclonal response to HIV antigens, suggesting an exaggerated humoral immune response to particular viral components.[357]

Clinically, hypergammaglobulinemia may contribute to rouleaux formation of RBCs on a peripheral blood smear,[185,222] the generation of circulating of immune complexes,[310,360,361] and the formation of a number of abnormal antibodies reactive with platelets,[275,287,294,312] RBCs,[177,237,238] lymphocytes,[97–100] granulocytes,[275,276,294] and phospholipids.[326–328,330] Remarkable cases of a hyperviscosity syndrome secondary to diffuse polyclonal hypergammaglobulinemia have also been described in AIDS patients presenting with visual blurring, characteristic changes on fundoscopic examination, and epistaxis with a documented elevation in serum viscosity.[362,363] Hyperviscosity syndromes have also been reported in HIV-infected children during the administration of intravenous γ-globulin.[364] Although uncommon, both multiple myeloma and isolated plasmacytomas have been described in HIV-infected patients,[204,365–367] including one case of myeloma in which the paraprotein was directed against the HIV p24 gag gene product.[367] Amyloidosis with AA-type fibrils has been reported in a single patient with AIDS who presented with nephrotic syndrome and demonstrated characteristic green birefringence after Congo red staining of kidney, liver, spleen, and bone marrow.[369] Paradoxically, HIV-infected hemophiliacs with a history of acquired inhibitors to factor VIII frequently lose this activity during the course of their HIV infection and may benefit from the reintroduction of factor VIII as part of their management.[370]

The mechanism of hypergammaglobulinemia in HIV-infected individuals appears to involve polyclonal activation of B cells in vivo, possibly through mechanisms independent of help normally provided by T lymphocytes. although B cells obtained from patients are poorly responsive to mitogens in vitro, Lane and co-workers[131] demonstrated that cultured B cells from patients with HIV infection secrete immunoglobulin spontaneously, suggesting that circulating B cells in these patients were "preactivated" in vivo and, paradoxically, refractory to further stimulation in vitro. B cells from normal donors can be directly activated without T-cell help by EBV infection[135] as well as CMV[137] and HIV antigens,[138] and it is possible that one or more of these factors could be responsible for the apparent activation of B cells in HIV-infected patients. As noted previously, paraproteins in these patients may have anti-HIV activity,[357,368,371] indicating that one component of the hypergammaglobulinemia may be an appropriate albeit exaggerated response to particular HIV antigens. Alternatively, as noted earlier, immune dysregulation may result from an imbalance of CD4 lymphocyte subsets that help either cellular or humoral immune responses, resulting in sustained polyclonal B-cell activation.[95,96] The profound stimulation of B cells present even in asymptomatic individuals with HIV infection is closely linked to the development of generalized lymphadenopathy[350] and likely plays a role in the pathogenesis of B-cell lymphomas observed in these patients,[68,115-118] discussed further in Chapter 86. Although the risk of developing B-cell lymphomas is greatest in patients with a severe depletion of CD4$^+$ lymphocytes ($<50/mm^3$),[372] unlike opportunistic infections, lymphomas may also occur in the absence of clinically significant immunodeficiency.[114,115,146]

Thrombotic Thrombocytopenic Purpura

TTP is an uncommon but well-described complication of HIV infection.[194-199,373] Although reported in patients with fully developed AIDS, TTP has been described as the initial manifestation of HIV infection in previously asymptomatic individuals.[195,196,199] TTP has also been described in two patients 10 and 32 months after a diagnosis of HIV-related ITP.[374] Clinically, patients present with the typical TTP syndrome of fulminant microangiopathic hemolytic anemia and thrombocytopenia; a variable proportion of individuals exhibits fever, elevated creatinine, and neurologic abnormalities.[199,375] A single case with a more protracted course of TTP has also been described.[376] Schistocytes and an elevated lactate dehydrogenase (LDH) are present, although the reticulocyte count may be less than expected for the degree of anemia, depending on the degree of bone marrow compromise by the underlying HIV infection. Neurologic abnormalities have included mental status changes, seizures, transient focal neurologic defects, and coma.[194-196,199] Examinations of tissues from autopsy specimens, as well as lymph node and gingival biopsies, have documented characteristic histologic changes of fibrin deposition in the microvasculature.[194-196,377] Responses to therapy in HIV-associated TTP are similar to that seen for the classic syndrome, with 50–85% of patients responding to regimens that included plasmapheresis with or without fresh frozen plasma infusions, antiplatelet agents, corticosteroids or vincris-

tine.[194-199] One case report of a patient with relapsing TTP suggested a response to zidovudine therapy.[378]

The mechanism for HIV-associated TTP and its relationship to HIV infection itself is unclear. As with TTP in the absence of HIV infection, the pathogenesis of this disorder may involve primary endothelial cell damage[379-382] and/or platelet agglutination as a result of a platelet-agglutinating agent[383] or the lack of a circulating inhibitor to platelet agglutination.[384] The hemolytic uremic syndrome has also been reported in HIV-infected patients presenting with renal failure and microangiopathic hemolytic anemia.[385,386] Interestingly, TTP has also been reported in a patient infected with a different human retrovirus, human T-cell lymphotropic virus (HTLV-I),[387] which is closely associated with adult T-cell leukemia and a demyelinating neurologic disorder termed HTLV-associated myelopathy.[388,389]

Porphyria Cutanea Tarda

Several recent reports have described acquired porphyria cutanea tarda (PCT) in HIV-seropositive patients.[390-395] Acquired PCT is a disorder of heme synthesis characterized by a reduction in uroporphyrin decarboxylase activity in liver cells with an elevation in heme precursors in plasma, primarily uroporphyrinogen; such precursors are oxidized and excreted in the urine as uroporphyrin, causing an increased urinary uroporphyrin/coproporphyrin ratio (see Ch. 39). As in non-HIV-associated PCT, patients present with manifestations of delayed-type photosensitivity—increased skin fragility, vesicles, bullae, hyperpigmentation, and hypertrichosis, particularly on the face and dorsum of the hands.[390] However, in contrast to classic PCT, polycythemia and sclerodermoid changes are uncommon.[390] Hepatic dysfunction appears to be a common cofactor, since most patients have abnormal liver function tests, serologic evidence of viral hepatitis, or a history of excessive alcohol consumption.[390,391,394,395] Therapeutic measures directed at avoiding sun exposure and removing precipitating agents (ethanol, estrogens, barbiturates) are generally successful, although additional measures, including phlebotomy, antimalarials,[390,392] and, in one case, therapy with zidovudine[392] may also be beneficial.

Diffuse Infiltrative CD8 Lymphocytosis Syndrome

A remarkable syndrome characterized clinically by bilateral parotid gland enlargement, xerostomia, and xeropthalmia has been described in HIV-infected patients.[396,397] Biopsies of minor salivary or parotid glands have shown diffuse infiltration by benign CD8$^+$ lymphocytes. Extraglandular infiltration by CD8$^+$ cells is also common; 10 of 17 patients exhibited lymphocytic interstitial pneumonitis, and smaller numbers of patients had infiltration of gastric mucosa, kidney, thymus, and liver.[396] Peripheral blood typically shows normal total WBC counts with a CD8$^+$ T-cell lymphocytosis of approximately 50% and an elevated total CD8 count. CD4$^+$ T cells in these patients are mildly to moderately depressed, indicating that this syndrome usually occurs in patients with minimal immune deficits. In contrast to patients with Sjögren syndrome, serologic markers of rheumatologic disorders (rheumatoid factor, antinuclear antibodies, anti-Ro/SS-A, anti-La/SS-B) are negative, and HLA typing shows an association with HLA-DR5. Complete responses in individual patients have been observed following treatment with zidovudine or chlorambucil.[396] However, the numbers of treated patients are too small to permit general therapeutic recommendations. Phenotypic analysis of peripheral and infiltrating CD8$^+$ lymphocytes, the detection of HIV antigens in salivary tissue, and the association of this syndrome with HLA-DR5 suggest that this disorder results from a genetically determined nd exuberent polyclonal cellular immune response to HIV it-elf, possibly correlated with an abnormal tissue expression f adhesion molecules.[397]

MORPHOLOGY OF HEMATOPOIETIC CELLS IN HIV INFECTION

Peripheral Smear

Cytopenias of all peripheral blood cells have been observed n patients with HIV infection (Table 155-3). With the exception f thrombocytopenia, which can occur in asymptomatic indi-viduals with relatively mild immune deficiency, anemia and leu-xopenia are both more frequent and more severe in patients vith advanced immunodeficiency.[177,181] Peripheral red blood :ells in patients with anemia are typically normochromic and iormocytic and exhibit a varying degree of anisocytosis and poikilocytosis.[185,188-190,202] The perturbation in RBC size and shape is reflected in an increased red cell distribution width.[178,245] Macrocytosis is rarely seen.[185] However, in pa-tients receiving therapy with zidovudine, macrocytosis is pres-ent in most patients, occasionally with mean corpuscular vol-umes ≥ 120[191-193] (Fig. 155-5A). Rouleaux formation of RBCs may also be seen and likely reflects the presence of concomi-tant hypergammaglobulinemia.[185,189,202] As noted above, schistocytes and nucleated RBCs are present in patients with HIV-associated TTP.[194-196,199]

Peripheral blood neutrophils are typically left shifted[183,185,222] and may exhibit a number of morphologic ab-normalities, including enlarged size, hyposegmentation, and Pelger-Huët anomalies[185,190,245] (Fig. 155-5A). In one study of peripheral blood smears from AIDS patients, atypical neutro-phils were described that were larger than normal, had irregu-lar nuclei and abundant cytoplasm, and showed striking in-creases in peroxidase activity.[245] Atypical plasmacytoid lymphocytes are occasionally seen in asymptomatic individu-als but are particularly common in lymphopenic patients with AIDS[185,189,202,222] and during acute HIV infection.[154,155,157,398] Large atypical monocytes have also been described with prom-inent vacuolization and fine nuclear chromatin.[185,189,200,222]

Bone Marrow Histology

Bone marrow examinations in HIV-infected patients are usu-ally performed to evaluate peripheral cytopenias or when sys-temic infections or malignancies are suspected. Thus, with the exception of patients presenting with isolated thrombocyto-penia, most data available on bone marrow histology in pa-tients with HIV infection are from individuals with advanced immunodeficiency. It is clear, however, that in this population, abnormalities are frequently seen in all marrow cellular ele-ments, as well as in the marrow matrix itself (Table 155-3). With the possible exception of particular types of dysplastic changes in megakaryocytes,[315,316] there appear to be no dis-tinctive features of bone marrow histology in patients with HIV infection or AIDS.[177,178]

Marrow cellularity is typically normocellular to hypercellular even in the setting of peripheral cytopenias, although 5–25% of AIDS patients in some series have exhibited hypocellular marrows.[181,183,186,187,201,202,204,206,222,258] In general, the periph-eral blood counts do not correlate with the overall degree of marrow cellularity, and patients with granulocytopenia and anemia are more likely to have normocellular or hypercellular than hypocellular marrows.[181] The myeloid/erythroid ratio is usually in the range of 2–7:1, reflecting the combined effects of myeloid hyperplasia seen even in patients with peripheral granulocytopenia, and erythroid hypoplasia.[178,183,190,201,204,399] A higher degree of erythroid hypoplasia, described in more recent series, likely reflects the increased use of zidovudine, which can suppress erythropoiesis.[202]

A remarkable degree of dysplasia has been noted in the mor-phology of myeloid, erythroid, and platelet precursors. Mye-loid maturation is in general left-shifted,[181,183,201,222] and one series noted a relative maturation arrest at the metamyelocyte stage.[185] A number of myelodysplastic changes in the myeloid lineage have been described, including the presence of abnor-mal myeloblasts with high nuclear/cytoplasmic ratios and ab-normal folded or cleaved nuclei,[190] as well as large myelocytes, metamyelocytes, and bands with megaloblastic-appearing nu-clei.[185,190,201,203] In contrast to the megaloblastic changes of myeloid cells seen in vitamin B_{12} deficiency, granulocytes in patients with AIDS are often hyposegmented rather than hyper-segmented.[185,190,245]

Dyserythropoiesis, although initially reported less often than myelodysplasia, has been increasingly recognized.[202-204] Ab-normalities have included erythroblasts with lobulated, binu-cleated, and fragmented nuclei as well as basophilic stippling in more mature RBCs.[185,190,201] In one series, all patients with dysplastic changes were found to be anemic and exhibited marked anisocytosis and poikilocytosis on peripheral

Table 155-3. Morphologic and Histologic Abnormalities of Peripheral Blood and Bone Marrow in Patients with ARC and AIDS

Peripheral blood
  Red cells
    Normochromic normocytic anemia
    Anisocytosis and poikilocytosis
    Rouleaux
    Schistocytes
    Reticulocytopenia
    Basophilic stippling
    Macrocytosis (during zidovudine therapy)
  Neutrophils
    Enlarged
    Left shifted
    Hyposegmented with Pelger-Huët forms
  Other
    Plasmacytoid lymphocytes
    Large vacuolated monocytes
Bone marrow
  Cytologic features
    Myelocytic/erythrocytic ratio 2–5:1
    Hypercellular, normocellular or hypocellular
    Erythroid dysplasia
    Erythroid hypoplasia (*M. avium* complex infection, zidovudine)
    Myeloid dysplasia
      Left shifted, hyposegmented, maturation arrest at metamyelocyte stage
    Megakaryocytes
      Adequate to increased
      Dysplastic (hypersegmented, micromegakaryocytes, denuded nuclei)
    Plasmacytosis
    Lymphoid aggregates/infiltrates
    Histiocytes
    "Loose granulomas" (aggregates of plasma cells, lymphocytes, histiocytes)
    Erythrophagocytosis
    Increased eosinophils
    Iron adequate to increased (reticuloendothelial cell distribution)
  Marrow matrix
    Increased reticulin
    Necrosis
    Serous atrophy

(Data from Zon and Groopman[177] and Perkocha and Rodgers.[178])

smear.[181] Frank megaloblastic changes in erythroid precursors have been reported but appear to be less common than megaloblastic features of myeloid cells.[190] However, erythroid megaloblastic changes have been described and are probably more common in patients receiving folate antagonists or zidovudine.[189,191,192,202–204,207] Erythroid hypoplasia that may be severe has been reported in some patients with AIDS or ARC,[206] in patients receiving zidovudine,[192,202,210,256] and in the setting of systemic *M. avium* complex infection.[180,185,189,208,209] Pure red cell aplasia or severe hypoplasia secondary to persistent parvovirus B19 infection have also been described in immunocompromised patients with[212,214,215,400–403] and without[400,404–406] HIV infection. Remarkable responses have been observed with intravenous γ-globulin therapy resulting from the administration of neutralizing antibodies.[212,215,400,401,404] Chronic parvovirus B19 infection should be suspected if characteristic vacuolated giant pronormoblasts are seen on marrow aspirates or biopsies[212,214,215,403,404,407] (Fig. 155-5I), but such infection may warrant consideration in any patient in whom a profound depression in erythropoiesis occurs out of proportion to other marrow elements.

Megakaryocytic dysplasia has become increasingly recognized in patients with fully developed AIDS as well as in those with isolated thrombocytopenia.[204,275,316] Dysplastic changes that have been described include micromegakaryocytes with denuded nuclei and megakaryocytes with hyposegmented or fragmented nuclei[190,201,203,204,315,316,308] (Fig. 155-5K). Ultrastructure analysis of megakaryocytes from AIDS patients with thrombocytopenia has demonstrated marked ballooning or blebbing of the peripheral zone, a finding not encountered in megakaryocytes from individuals with non-HIV ITP.[315] In addition, abnormal clustering of megakaryocytes on bone marrow biopsy sections similar to that seen in myeloproliferative syndromes has also been described.[190] As noted previously, dysplastic changes observed in megakaryocytes (Fig. 155-6), the detection of HIV RNA in megakaryocytes from infected patients, and the clinical response of 50–68% of patients with HIV-related thrombocytopenia to zidovudine are all consistent with the view that the megakaryocyte itself is a target for HIV infection in vivo.[323,324]

Although several of the dysplastic changes noted in HIV-infected patients resemble those seen in preleukemia syndromes, myeloid leukemia in AIDS, although reported, is very uncommon.[202,246–249] Thus, it appears that the significance and the etiology of dysplasia in patients with HIV infection is different from that described for patients without HIV infection who present with peripheral cytopenias and marrow dysplasia.[178,190] As noted previously, it is possible that direct infection of marrow precursors by HIV may contribute to these defects, although this issue remains controversial.[259–261,265,268–270,323,409]

Lymphoid aggregates are common and have been reported in 10–50% of patients with AIDS and ARC.[181,183,186–188,190,201–204,206,222,258] Lymphoid aggregates may be either small, well circumscribed, and composed of small round lymphocytes or large, poorly defined, and mixed with histiocytes.[189,203] Infiltrating lymphocytes have also been described that are atypical or cleaved and located in paratrabecular areas.[201,206,399] However, when paratrabecular localization of lymphocytes is seen, it is important to rule out the possibility of a non-Hodgkin lymphoma, since lymphomas in AIDS patients involve bone marrow in ≤50% of cases.[114,115] The bone marrow has also been described as the initial or only site of involvement for both non-Hodgkin and Hodgkin lymphomas, which can complicate HIV infection[122,410,411] (Fig. 155-5F).

Plasmacytosis is also extremely common in bone marrow and has been seen in 31–85% of patients.[181,183,186,202–204,258] In individual patients, plasma cells may represent as much as 40% of bone marrow cells in the absence of a neoplastic disorder.[202]

The morphology of plasma cells has varied from normal to moderately dysplastic with large bi- or trinucleated cells. Russell bodies with multiple globules have also been described.[20] Although myeloma has clearly been reported in AIDS, it is important to recognize that patients may present with monoclonal spikes on serum protein electrophoresis and marrow plasmacytosis with plasma cell aggregates and atypical forms but without a clonal proliferation of plasma cells.[412] Thus, in the absence of lytic bone lesions or other clinical evidence of a plasma cell neoplasm, a diagnosis of myeloma should be made with caution.

Additional cellular abnormalities of bone marrow include increased numbers of histiocytes, noncaseating granulomas, and "loose granulomas" consisting of aggregated histiocytes, lymphocytes, and plasma cells[186,187,190,201,202,204,206,222] (Fig. 155-5B). Pseudo-Gaucher cells have also been described from a patient with *M. avium* complex infection in which large foamy histiocytes seen on Wright-Giemsa stain were shown to contain numerous mycobacterial organisms by periodic acid-Schiff and Ziehl-Neelsen stains.[413] An additional case of this morphologic manifestation of *M. avium* complex infection is shown in Figure 155-5J. Histiocytic phagocytosis of erythroid cells and occasionally granulocytes and platelets has been described[189,200,222,414] but is a nonspecific finding that may also occur in a variety of viral, fungal, and bacterial infections. Severe hemophagocytic syndromes have been reported in HIV-infected patients presenting with pancytopenia.[415,416] Although peripheral blood eosinophilia is rarely seen,[185,245] marrow eosinophilia is common and has been reported in 9–61% of patients with AIDS.[181,201,202,206,222,399]

In most series, bone marrow iron stores are adequate to increased[181,187,189,190,203,206] in reticuloendothelial cells, indicating a defect in iron utilization similar to that seen in other chronic disease states.[220] Sideroblasts with or without ringed forms have been described but are uncommon.[181,185,187,203]

Abnormalities in the bone marrow matrix are frequently seen and include increased reticulin or fibrosis,[181,185,187,190,201–204,206,222] serous atrophy or "gelatinous transformation,"[186,201,202,204,206,222,258] and bone marrow necrosis.[222,258] The increase in marrow reticulin may be focal or diffuse and may be increased in areas of granuloma formation[187,206] or lymphoid aggregates.[206] In most patients in some series, bone marrow aspiration is either difficult or, not uncommonly, dry,[185,187,189,222] probably as a result of one or more of these abnormalities. While atypical proliferation of endothelial cells has been noted on histologic sections of marrow,[206] Kaposi sarcoma involving bone marrow is rarely seen.[203,417,418]

Bone marrow histology or culture may be particularly useful for documenting opportunistic infection and should be performed in HIV-infected patients with undiagnosed fevers or constitutional symptoms.[419,420] In one series of 47 patients with AIDS in whom a bone marrow aspiration or biopsy was performed to evaluate unexplained fever, pathogens were detected in 20 patients (42.5%).[419] Although it has been argued in the diagnosis of mycobacterial infection that blood cultures have a sensitivity comparable to that of bone marrow cultures in diagnosing disseminated infection,[421] bone marrow examination with special histologic staining can certainly provide a more rapid method of diagnosis for both opportunistic mycobacterial and fungal infections.[422] Infectious agents reported to involve the bone marrow in patients with AIDS are listed in Table 155-4 and include *M. avium* complex,[185–187,189,419,420,422,423] *M. tuberculosis*,[419,422] *M. xenopi* and *kansasii*,[421] histoplasma,[186,258,422] (Fig. 155-5E), cryptococcus[258,419,422,424] (Fig. 155-5C & D), toxoplasma,[187] CMV,[201,203] leishmania,[180] disseminated cat scratch disease,[425] and *P. carinii*.[426–429] Marrow granuloma in patients with mycobacterial infection may be either loosely formed or absent, despite the presence of abundant

Table 155-4. Infections Involving the Bone Marrow in Patients with AIDS

	References
Mycobacterium avium complex	185–187,189,419,420,422,423
Mycobacterium tuberculosis	419,422
Mycobacterium xenopi and kansasii	422
Histoplasma	186,258,422
Cryptococcus	258,419,422,424
Toxoplasma	187
Cytomegalovirus	201,203
Leishmania	180
Pneumocystis carinii	426–429
Disseminated cat scratch disease	425
Parvovirus B19	212,214,215,400–403

organisms on acid-fast stains[183,186,419] (Fig. 155-5B). Parvovirus B19 infection should be suspected in the setting of profound erythroid hypoplasia if giant pronormoblasts are present[212,214,215,400–403] (Fig. 155-5I).

Extralymphatic presentation of non-Hodgkin lymphomas occurs in ≤90% of patients with HIV infection and has been reported to involve the bone marrow in 50% of cases. As noted previously, the bone marrow may be the presenting site of lymphoma.[114,115,117] The lymphomas are typically high-grade Burkitt or non-Burkitt lymphomas (Fig. 155-5F), although more well-differentiated types have also been described.[114,115,117,203] Lymphomas should be suspected in the clinical setting of constitutional symptoms, an elevated LDH, and the presence of teardrop or nucleated RBCs on peripheral blood smear. Hodgkin disease, also noted with increased frequency in HIV-infected patients is, in comparison to patients without HIV infection, more likely to involve extralymphatic sites including the bone marrow[115,117,146,203,411,430] (Fig. 155-5G & H). A more complete discussion of HIV-related lymphomas is presented in Chapter 86.

HEMATOLOGIC COMPLICATIONS AND EFFICACY OF ANTIRETROVIRAL THERAPY

Zidovudine

Zidovudine or 3′-azido-2′,3′-dideoxythymidine (AZT) is the first antiretroviral drug shown to improve the survival of patients with AIDS.[431–433] This thymidine analogue contains an azido group in place of the 3′ hydroxyl group of the nucleoside sugar moiety. Zidovudine is phosphorylated by cellular kinases; after incorporation into an elongating strand of viral DNA by reverse transcriptase, AZT-triphosphate prevents subsequent 5′ to 3′ phosphodiester linkages from forming, resulting in premature termination of the viral DNA chain.[431,432,434] An increased sensitivity of reverse transcriptase to zidovudine compared with cellular DNA polymerases is thought to confer greater activity of this drug on viral than on cellular DNA synthesis.[431,434,435] The antiviral effects of zidovudine depend on its phosphorylation by cellular kinases.[434] In addition to its activity as a chain terminator, AZT-monophosphate competitively inhibits thymidine kinase, resulting in a reduced level of intracellular thymidine-5′-triphosphate and an inhibition of DNA synthesis.[431,432]

In the first double-blind placebo-controlled trial of zidovudine in patients with AIDS complicated by *P. carinii* pneumonia, a remarkable decrease in the incidence of opportunistic infections and an improvement in survival was noted in patients receiving zidovudine 200 mg every 4 hours,[217] a dose two to three times that currently recommended.[432,436] After 9 months of therapy, 1 of 145 patients receiving zidovudine had died,

compared with 19 of 137 patients receiving placebo. Hematologic toxicity in this group of patients with severe immune dysfunction was considerable: 34% of zidovudine-treated patients developed anemia with hemoglobin values <7.5 g/dl, and 21% required blood transfusions.[191,217] In addition, 16% of the zidovudine-treated patients developed neutropenia, with WBC counts <500/mm^3. Other toxicities related to zidovudine therapy included fever, rash, headache, fatigue, increased nail pigmentation, abnormal liver function tests, myositis, and, less commonly, seizures, encephalopathy, or the Stevens-Johnson syndrome.[432] In addition to the improved survival seen in patients with advanced immunodeficiency treated with zidovudine, other reports in adults[437,438] and children[439] have provided encouraging indications that in at least some patients, AIDS-related neurologic deficits and even dementia may respond to therapy.

More recent studies have addressed the issue of whether a clinical benefit can be achieved by the use of zidovudine in asymptomatic seropositive individuals.[440–443] Although two studies of patients with <500 and <400 CD4$^+$ cells found an approximately two- to threefold reduction in the rate of progression to AIDS,[440,441] two other studies found no survival advantage for patients who received early zidovudine therapy.[442,443] Given that the median interval between HIV infection and the development of AIDS has been estimated to be approximately ≥10 years,[22–24] it is clear that studies of asymptomatic seropositive individuals will require an extensive period of follow-up before data on survival are conclusive. However, given the emerging evidence for active retroviral replication throughout the asymptomatic period[166,169] and a gradual increase over time in the viral burden in an infected host,[166,444] it is likely that antiviral therapies early in the course of infection will have a significant impact on the natural history of infection.

Hematologic toxicities associated with zidovudine are in general dose related and are more likely to develop in patients with pre-existing neutropenia and anemia, low serum vitamin B$_{12}$ levels, and CD4 cell numbers <100/mm^3.[191,445] However, severe pancytopenia occurring within 4–6 weeks of starting zidovudine has also been reported as an apparent idiosyncratic reaction and may persist for several months after discontinuation of therapy.[256] Patients on chronic zidovudine therapy typically develop macrocytic RBC indices, although generally without hypersegmentation of neutrophils.[191,446] Unlike thrombocytopenia, HIV-related anemia and neutropenia usually do not respond to zidovudine therapy. As noted previously, bone marrow examinations of patients receiving zidovudine have demonstrated a number of abnormalities in the erythroid lineage including erythroid hypoplasia, aplasia, or maturation arrest.[192] Interestingly, among patients who develop severe pancytopenia and marrow hypoplasia as an early complication of zidovudine therapy, macrocytosis is not seen.[256] Zidovudine is metabolized primarily by glucuronidation in the liver, and drugs that are also glucuronidated, particularly probenecid,[432,447] may prolong the half-life of zidovudine and potentiate its toxicity. It is also probable that the effects of myelosuppressive drugs such as chemotherapeutic agents will be worsened by concomitant therapy with zidovudine.

The hematologic toxicity of zidovudine is likely related to inhibition of cellular DNA polymerases as well as a depletion of intracellular thymidine pools.[431,432,448] Studies on the effects of zidovudine on bone marrow progenitor cells have demonstrated a time and dose dependent inhibition of marrow erythroid and granulocyte/macrophage precursors, with the BFU-E exhibiting five- to eightfold more sensitivity to zidovudine than colony-forming unit-erythroid (CFU-E), CFU-GM, and colony-forming unit-granulocyte/erythrocyte/macrophage/megakaryocyte (CFU-GEMM).[448] The concurrent administration of recombinant EPO or myeloid CSFs (CSF-GM or CSF-G) can ameliorate the anemia and leukopenia that may complicate zidovudine therapy.[221,279,449-451]

Dideoxyinosine, Dideoxycytidine, and Non-Nucleoside Analogue Reverse Transcriptase Inhibitors

A number of other nucleoside analogues that have potent inhibitory effects on HIV replication in vitro are undergoing clinical evaluation.[432,433] Two agents recently approved for clinical use, 2′,3′-dideoxyinosine (DDI) and 2′,3′-dideoxycytidine (DDC), have shown clinical activity, including a transient improvement in immunologic parameters and a reduction in serum p24 antigen levels.[452-457] In contrast to zidovudine, hematologic toxicity with DDI and DDC has been relatively mild, with thrombocytopenia and leukopenia described for DDC only at high doses.[444,455] In one retrospective study of patients receiving DDI, a significant improvement in hemoglobin level, granulocyte number, and platelet count was observed and found to persist for ≤1 year following therapy.[458] Macrocytosis has not been observed with either DDC or DDI.[455,457] However, for both DDI and DDC nonhematologic toxicities are common and often dose limiting; they include peripheral neuropathy (for DDI and DDC) and gastrointestinal toxicity (for DDI), particularly acute pancreatitis.[445,455-458]

A number of non-nucleoside reverse transcriptase inhibitors with distinct mechanisms of action have also been identified and are undergoing clinical trials.[433,459-463] However, for both nucleoside analogue and non-nucleoside-based reverse transcriptase inhibitors, drug-resistant strains of HIV emerge due to the selection of viral mutants with specific amino acid changes in the reverse transcriptase molecule.[433,463,464] Studies to circumvent this problem by using different reverse transcriptase inhibitors in combination or sequentially are in progress and may provide a more rational approach to the use of pharmacologic agents to inhibit HIV replication in vivo.[432,433,465-467] In addition, the combination of a reverse transcriptase inhibitor with interferons may also provide synergistic antiviral effects, although clinical trials using zidovudine with interferon-α have demonstrated significant leukopenia as a dose-limiting toxicity.[468-470]

THERAPY FOR HEMATOLOGIC COMPLICATIONS OF HIV INFECTION

The evaluation and treatment of cytopenias in patients with HIV infection must take into account a number of possible contributing factors, including (1) the effects of drugs used to treat the underlying retroviral infection or complicating opportunistic infections; (2) direct marrow involvement by infectious pathogens or neoplasms, particularly lymphomas; (3) generalized suppressive effects of chronic disease states on myelo- and erythropoiesis; (4) possible nutritional deficiencies; (5) immune-mediated destruction of mature or immature hematopoietic cells; and (6) direct effects of the underlying HIV infection itself on bone marrow stem cells (Table 155-5). Consequently, the approach to the treatment of cytopenias in patients with HIV infection requires a careful consideration of multiple iatrogenic, infectious, neoplastic, and immune etiologies, many of which are potentially reversible. As described further below, the development of hematopoietic growth factors for both anemia and neutropenia has added considerably to the therapeutic options available for these patients.[471-473]

Table 155-5. General Approach to the Differential Diagnosis of Cytopenias in Patients with HIV Infection

Hematologic toxicity of drugs
  Antiretroviral therapy (i.e., zidovudine, interferon)
  Antibiotics (i.e., trimethoprim sulfamethoxazole, dapsone, pentamidine, ganciclovir, flucytosine)
Direct marrow involvement by infections (i.e., *Mycobacterium avium* complex, parvovirus B19)
Marrow involvement by malignancies (i.e., non-Hodgkin and Hodgkin lymphomas)
Autoimmune destruction of hematopoietic cells
Nutritional deficiencies (vitamin B_{12}, folate)
Generalized myelosuppressive effects of chronic disease states
Direct effects of HIV infection of marrow stem cells (i.e., megakaryocytes)
Miscellaneous (i.e., blood loss, TTP, DIC)

Anemia

As in any patient with a low hematocrit, the diagnostic evaluation of anemia in a patient with HIV infection requires a careful consideration of factors that contribute to decreased or ineffective red cell production, increased peripheral destruction, and blood loss. In addition to direct effects of HIV or chronic disease states, or both, on hematopoietic precursors, other important etiologies include marrow involvement by lymphomas and opportunistic infections, particularly *M. avium* complex or fungal pathogens. Pure red cell aplasia secondary to persisting parvovirus B19 infection has been well described in HIV-infected patients and typically responds to intravenous γ-globulin therapy.[212,214,215,400-402] Available evidence does not indicate that decreased iron, vitamin B_{12}, or folate levels contribute to the chronic anemia that is typically seen in HIV-infected patients, although consideration of these potentially reversible etiologies is always warranted.[178] Immune hemolytic anemia, although reported, is similarly rare,[240,242,243,431,474] despite the frequency of positive anti-RBC immunoglobulin tests[177,237,238]; when present, it has been reported to respond to corticosteroids, splenectomy, and, in a single case, zidovudine.[242,243,475] Microangiopathic hemolytic anemia secondary to TTP, although uncommon, may be fulminant, and in the limited number of reported cases, has responded to regimens that included plasmapheresis with or without antiplatelet agents and plasma infusion.[194-197,199]

Potentially reversible drug etiologies of anemia include zidovudine, trimethoprim sulfamethoxazole, dapsone, and, in the setting of antimycobacterial therapy, isoniazid. Reversible megaloblastic panhypoplasia has been reported secondary to trimethoprim and dapsone therapy for *P. carinii* pneumonia, and folinic acid has been recommended, particularly with suspected vitamin B_{12} deficiency, to ameliorate the hematopoietic toxicity of these and other folate antagonists.[207] Although patients receiving dapsone frequently exhibit manifestations of low-grade hemolysis with an increase in LDH, severe hemolysis may also occur, particularly in the setting of glucose-6-phosphate dehydrogenase deficiency.[475,476]

As noted previously, therapy with zidovudine is frequently complicated by anemia and occurs more commonly in patients with advanced immunodeficiency and low serum vitamin B_{12} levels.[191] Although the anemia secondary to zidovudine therapy is generally dose related and typically responds to dose reduction, apparently idiosyncratic reactions have been reported that may cause profound and prolonged marrow hypoplasia even after zidovudine is discontinued.[256] The long-term administration of zidovudine to some patients may require transfusion support, although in some patients this may be ameliorated by the use of recombinant EPO.[221,449,450]

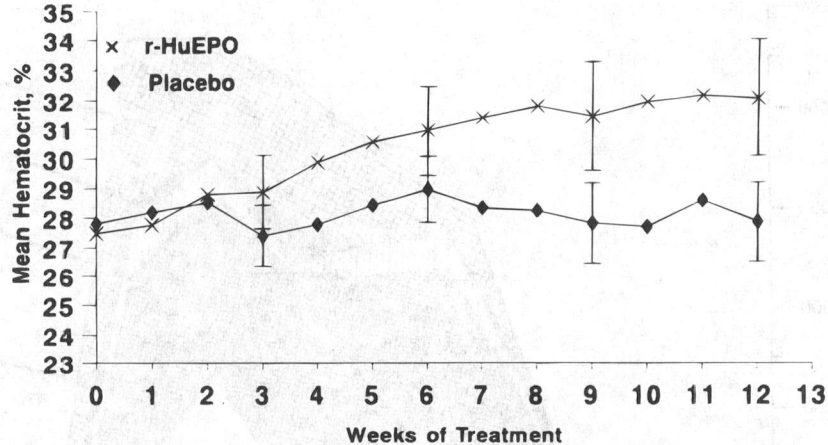

Fig. 155-7. Response to recombinant erythropoietin in patients on zidovudine therapy. Mean hematocrit concentrations are shown for zidovudine-treated patients with endogenous EPO levels of ≤500 mU/ml who were treated with either recombinant human EPO (rHuEPO) or placebo. rHuEPO dose in the treated group was 100–200 U/kg IV or SC three times per week. Bars represent 95% confidence intervals. No benefit was seen in patients with endogenous EPO levels >500 mU/ml. (From Henry et al.,[221] with permission.)

Several clinical trials have evaluated the effects of recombinant human EPO in treating anemia in HIV-infected patients receiving zidovudine.[221,449,450] Two placebo-controlled trials using EPO doses of 100–200 U/kg IV or SC three times per week demonstrated an improved hematocrit and a decreased transfusion requirement in patients whose levels of endogenous EPO were <500 IU/L (Fig. 155-7). No benefit was seen in patients with pretreatment EPO levels >500 IU/L, who comprised approximately one-third of the zidovudine-treated patients.[221,449] A similar clinical benefit was also seen in zidovudine-treated patients who received EPO in combination with recombinant CSF-G.[450] Although fewer data are available on the use of recombinant EPO for anemia in HIV-infected patients not receiving zidovudine, one placebo-controlled study with small numbers of patients did demonstrate a trend toward increased hemoglobin and decreased transfusion requirement in the treated group, although this was not statistically significant.[477] Nonetheless, the available data indicate that a subpopulation of HIV-infected patients, particularly those on zidovudine with a low endogenous EPO level (<500 IU/L), will benefit from EPO therapy. Although studies in AIDS patients did not demonstrate significant side effects from EPO therapy, toxicities are well described in other patient groups and include rash, fatigue, and headache, as well as more severe cerebrovascular and cardiovascular complications, including stroke, seizure, hypertension, and myocardial infarction.[478,479] Finally, an additional study has demonstrated that CSF-G in the absence of EPO treatment may also increase RBC production and the number of circulating BFU-E, raising the possibility that additional therapeutic approaches using combinations of hematopoietic growth factors may be useful in the treatment of HIV-associated anemia.[480]

Neutropenia

A number of drugs or infectious and neoplastic complications of AIDS can produce leukopenia, although reversible iatrogenic or secondary etiologies are often not found. Common drugs associated with neutropenia include zidovudine (for HIV infection), interferons (for HIV infection or Kaposi sarcoma, or both), folate antagonists (especially trimethoprim sulfamethoxazole for *P. carinii* pneumonia or sulfadiazine for toxoplasmosis infections), ganciclovir (for CMV infection), and chemotherapeutic agents (for lymphomas or Kaposi sarcoma).[250,251,253,254,445,470,481] However, even when drugs can be implicated as the cause of neutropenia, management decisions are frequently complicated by risks associated with discontinuing or reducing the dose of drugs that are required for medical complications of AIDS.

The early observation that AIDS-related neutropenia could respond dramatically to therapy with CSF-GM provided a rationale for using hematopoietic growth factors in a number of clinical settings in which neutropenia is common. Groopman and co-workers[278] initially described responses in 16 of 16 AIDS patients who were treated with intravenous recombinant CSF-GM. A remarkably rapid and dose-dependent increase in peripheral blood neutrophils, monocytes, and eosinophils was observed (Fig. 155-8). Increased marrow cellularity was seen even in patients who had hypocellular marrows prior to therapy. Toxicities were mild and included fever, myalgias, headache, and flushing. Similar responses of granulocytes have been described for patients treated with CSF-G.[279] Although responses to intravenous CSF-GM and CSF-G were transient, subsequent studies have demonstrated that long-term subcutaneous therapy with these growth factors can produce a sustained increase in granulocyte counts from weeks to months without an apparent depletion in marrow stem cell activity.[450,451,482] This effect has been observed in a variety of clinical settings in which neutropenia is common, including (1) patients receiving zidovudine either with[468,469] or without[279,450,451,482] interferon, (2) patients with CMV infection receiving ganciclovir,[483] and (3) patients with HIV-related lymphomas receiving chemotherapy.[484] In general, the addition of CSFs improved the ability of patients to tolerate myelosuppressive therapy; in one study of patients with non-Hodgkin lymphoma, CSF-GM therapy reduced the number of febrile episodes and days of hospitalization.[484] However, although these early results are encouraging, future studies will be needed to determine the cost-effectiveness and ultimate impact of hematopoietic growth factors on quality of life and survival.

Although some in vitro studies have shown that CSF-GM but not CSF-G could stimulate replication of particular HIV isolates,[78] with one exception,[451] clinical trials to date have not demonstrated laboratory evidence of a sustained enhancement of viral replication in vivo.[468,469,482,484,485] However, this potentially important issue will need to be readdressed as more quantitative and sensitive assays for HIV replication are used to monitor patients receiving these growth factors.[166] Interestingly, CSF-GM has been shown to augment markedly the antiretroviral effects of zidovudine in vitro, apparently by increasing intracellular levels of the biologically active triphosphate

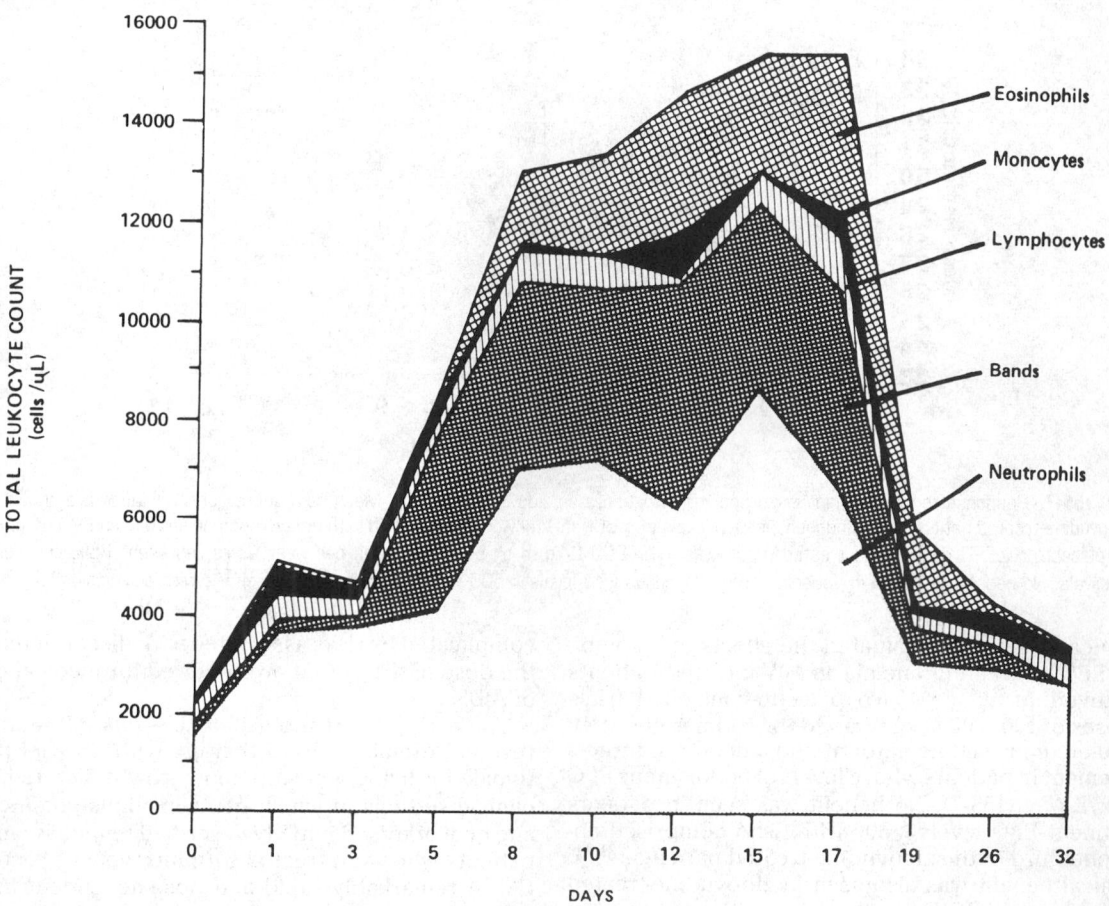

Fig. 155-8. Response to recombinant CSF-GM in an AIDS patient with neutropenia. Total leukocyte counts and differentials are shown for an AIDS patient treated with intravenous recombinant CSF-GM (1.0 × 10⁴ U/kg/day) from days 1 through 17. (From Groopman et al.,[278] with permission.)

form.[486,487] In addition, several reports have described functional defects in neutrophils from patients with HIV infection (depending on the assay used), although no consensus exists as to the specific defects involved.[488–492] In two studies, neutrophil function was observed to be enhanced following CSF-GM therapy.[492,493] Neutrophils from patients treated with CSF-GM have also exhibited enhanced killing of HIV-infected target cells in the presence of antibodies to the HIV envelope glycoprotein.[79] Thus, myeloid growth factors may have a number of therapeutic roles both in promoting antiviral effects and in augmenting host immunity. However, the significance of these findings in terms of clinical benefit to patients will require carefully controlled trials.

Thrombocytopenia

As noted previously, studies on the mechanism of thrombocytopenia in HIV-infected patients have demonstrated decreased platelet survival[301] and the presence of circulating and platelet-associated immune complexes,[288,310,360,361] as well as the presence of true antiplatelet antibodies in some patients.[275,287,288,294,310,312] A number of medical approaches that have been successfully used to treat classic ITP have also been used in HIV-related thrombocytopenia with varying degrees of success; they include corticosteroids,[283,285,298,494] intravenous γ-globulin,[495–499] and danazol.[298] Although responses are seen in as many as 60–85% of patients receiving prednisone, usually in 4-week courses of 1 mg/kg/day followed by rapid taper, these responses are sustained in only 10–20% of patients.[283,285,298,494]

However, the long-term or repetitive use of an immunosuppressive agent in the setting of HIV infection is a major concern. Intravenous γ-globulin may produce a rapid improvement in the platelet count, as seen in classic ITP, in approximately 90% of patients, and it represents the treatment of choice in the setting of a medical emergency or as a supportive measure for an invasive procedure.[495,496,499] Responses typically last for several days or weeks but, as with corticosteroids, are usually transient, although infrequently, long-term remissions have been described.[495] Therapy with anti-Rh(D) immunoglobulin[500–502] or dapsone[503] has been an effective temporizing measure, presumably as a result of reticuloendothelial modulation from IgG-coated or hemolyzed RBCs, respectively. Vincristine has also been reported to improve the platelet count in small numbers of AIDS patients with thrombocytopenia.[285,504] In a more investigational approach, long-term correction of the platelet count was observed in a single AIDS patient following treatment with an anti-CD16 monoclonal antibody, reactive with the low-affinity Fcγ receptor, again indicating that therapeutic measures to induce reticuloendothelial blockade may improve platelet survival.[505]

In contrast to the typically transient improvement following medical management of HIV-related ITP, splenectomy has been highly effective in producing a sustained increase in platelet counts in approximately 90% of patients.[283,284,303–309] Improvement has been seen even in patients who are refractory to steroids and γ-globulin before splenectomy and those with severe thrombocytopenia with platelet counts <10,000/mm³.[283,304,305,307] Although in most reported series there has been no increase in the morbidity of splenectomy in HIVıfected patients,[304,305,307,308] the use of this procedure, while ffective, clearly must be individualized. In one small series of ıatients with hemophilia, in which relatively mild thrombocy-ıopenia can lead to life-threatening hemorrhagic complica-ıons,[300] complete and lasting responses were seen following plenectomy in four of four patients studied.[506] Most reported eries have shown that splenectomy does not accelerate the linical progression to AIDS.[283,298,307,309] As a possible alterna-ıve to splenectomy, a single report also showed responses to ow-dose splenic irradiation in three of three patients who ailed to respond to zidovudine or γ-globulin.[507]

Several reports have shown responses to zidovudine in ap-ıroximately 50% of patients with HIV-related thrombocyto-ıenia.[281,508–513] In one blinded placebo-controlled trial of 10 ıatients with platelet counts of 20,000–100,000/mm^3 (mean ـ3,000/mm^3), zidovudine therapy (250 mg q6h) resulted in a ınean increase of 53,000/mm^3 in all patients during 8 weeks of reatment, while no patients receiving placebo showed im-ırovement.[509] Relapses occurred in three of five patients on liscontinuation of drug. In spite of concern that the well-docu-nented myelosuppressive effects of zidovudine could present risks for thrombocytopenic patients, thrombocytopenia, in :ontrast to neutropenia and anemia, is a rare complication of zidovudine.[191,217] However, a mild decrease in the platelet :ount has been noted in patients on long-term zidovudine ther-apy (>36 weeks), particularly in those who develop anemia.[510] The mechanism for the beneficial effects of zidovudine on HIV-related thrombocytopenia is unclear, but in view of the evi-dence for HIV infection of megakaryocytes, it is likely that the antiviral activity of this agent acts to promote more effective thrombopoiesis. One kinetic analysis of platelet production demonstrated a significant improvement following zidovudine treatment.[300] Successful therapy of HIV-related thrombocyto-penia has also been described for another anti-retroviral drug, DDI, in both children[513a] and adults.[513b] One large series of patients receiving long-term DDI therapy showed a general im-provement in hemoglobin, granulocyte, and platelet counts.[458] Interestingly, in one report, a beneficial effect on HIV-related thrombocytopenia was seen for zidovudine but not DDI.[513c] Clearly, more information will be needed to determine if DDI and other anti-retroviral agents besides zidovudine can be used to treat HIV-related thrombocytopenia. Interferon-α has been reported to produce an increase in the platelet count in thrombocytopenic patients with HIV infection,[514–516] although it is unclear if this benefit is mediated by its antiviral, cytotoxic, or immunosuppressive effects.[280]

FUTURE DIRECTIONS

The pandemic of AIDS and HIV infection will continue well into the next decade and is certain to pose major health care problems throughout the world. Although recent studies with an SIV model have shown that animals can be successfully vaccinated with an attenuated virus,[517] the prospect for an ef-fective human vaccine for HIV in the near future is remote.[518] Moreover, no current approaches can kill or eliminate HIV from an infected host, and all HIV-infected individuals will likely re-main infected for life. However, while the hope for cure is dim, there is considerable optimism that HIV infection will be con-trollable and that the complications resulting from progressive immune and hematopoietic dysfunction will be preventable and treatable. Dideoxynucleoside analogues that inhibit re-verse transcriptase have provided the first encouraging clinical data that viral replication in vivo can be retarded and that the natural history of HIV infection can be altered. Although cur-rent studies have shown either equivocal or modest effects on survival,[441–443] it is likely that early therapy with reverse transcriptase inhibitors will be beneficial, particularly when

combinations of drugs are employed in strategies to deal with the emerging problem of HIV drug resistance.[464] The develop-ment of highly sensitive quantitative assays for viral replication in vivo will add considerably to the ability to monitor the ef-fects of antiviral protocols.[166] In addition, aside from reverse transcriptase inhibitors, other antiviral agents that target dif-ferent stages in the viral life cycle may provide novel and syner-gistic approaches to therapy.[432,433] Of particular interest are viral protease inhibitors that, unlike reverse transcriptase in-hibitors, have the ability to interfere with viral production in cells already infected by HIV.[519,520] The viral regulatory pro-teins tat and rev, which are essential for viral replication, are ideal targets for novel antiviral agents or the production of hematopoietic cells genetically engineered to be resistant to HIV infection.[433,521–524] Finally, specific viral genes can be tar-geted using highly innovative molecular approaches, including antisense oligonucleotides, ribozymes, and the delivery of trans-dominant mutant proteins[521,524–527] that may represent future directions for antiviral therapy.

As with antimicrobial and antineoplastic chemotherapy, it is likely that strategies for controlling HIV infection will arise from combinations of effective agents each targeted at different parts of the viral life cycle.[433,528] In addition, with a better un-derstanding of the mechanisms that underlie HIV-induced dis-ease, it is probable that novel supportive modalities such as recombinant CSF-GM or CSF-G, EPO, and other growth factors will gain increasing importance in conjunction with antiviral agents for stabilizing or restoring hematopoietic and immuno-logic function in infected patients. Clearly, hematologic compli-cations of HIV infection will remain an active area for basic research and a challenge to clinicians for many years.

ACKNOWLEDGMENTS

The author gratefully acknowledges Drs. Kevin Salhany and David Hicks for technical assistance in preparing photomicro-graphs and Drs. Hugh Bonner, Neal Merapol, and Dennis Corn-feld for providing the patient specimens photographed in Fig-ure 155-5.

REFERENCES

1. Centers for Disease Control: 1993 Revised classification system for HIV in-fection and expanded surveillance case definition for AIDS among adoles-cents and adults. MMWR 41(RR-17):1, 1993
2. Abrams DI: Lymphadenopathy related to the acquired immunodeficiency syndrome in homosexual men. Med Clin North Am 70:693, 1986
3. Metroka CE, Cunningham-Rundles S, Pollack MS et al: Generalized lymphad-enopathy in homosexual men. Ann Intern Med 99:585, 1983
4. Merson MH: Slowing the spread of HIV: agenda for the 1990s. Science 260: 1266, 1993
5. Centers for Disease Control: Projections of the number of persons diag-nosed with AIDS and the number of immunosuppressed HIV-infected per-sons—United States, 1992–1994. MMWR 41 (RR-18):1, 1992
6. Centers for Disease Control: Update: acquired immunodeficiency syn-drome—United States, 1992. MMWR 42:547, 1993
7. Friedland GH, Klein RJ: Transmission of the human immunodeficiency virus. N Engl J Med 317:1125, 1989
8. Ryder RW, Hassig SE: The epidemiology of perinatal transmission of HIV. AIDS, suppl. 1. 2:S83, 1988
9. Centers for Disease Control: Update: human immunodeficiency virus infec-tions in health care workers exposed to blood of infected patients. MMWR 36:286, 1987
10. McEvoy M, Porter K, Mortimer P et al: Prospective study of clinical, labora-tory, and ancillary staff with accidental exposures to blood or body fluids from patients infected with HIV. BMJ 294:1595, 1987
11. Klein RS, Phelan JA, Freeman K et al: Low occupational risk of human immu-nodeficiency virus infection among dental professionals. N Engl J Med 318: 86, 1988
12. Centers for Disease Control: Update: acquired immunodeficiency syndrome and human immunodeficiency virus infection among health care workers. MMWR 37:229, 1988

13. Marcus R, CDC Cooperative Needlestick Surveillance Group: Surveillance of health care workers exposed to blood from patients infected with the human immunodeficiency virus. N Engl J Med 319:1118, 1988

14. Henderson DK, Fahey BJ, Willy M et al: Risk for occupational transmission of human immunodeficiency virus type 1 (HIV-1) associated with clinical exposures. A prospective evaluation. Ann Intern Med 113:729, 1990

15. Friedland GH, Saltzman BR, Rodgers MF et al: Lack of transmission of HTLV-III/LAV infection to household contacts of patients with AIDS or AIDS-related complex with oral candidiasis. N Engl J Med 314:344, 1986

16. Clavel F, Guetard D, Brun-Vezinet F et al: Isolation of a new human retrovirus from West African patients with AIDS. Science 233:343, 1986

17. Clavel F, Mansinho K, Chamaret S et al: Human immunodeficiency virus type 2 infection associated with AIDS in West Africa. N Engl J Med 316:1180, 1987

18. Marlink RG, Ricard D, M'Boup S et al: Clinical, hematologic, and immunologic cross-sectional evaluation of individuals exposed to human immunodeficiency virus type-2 (HIV-2). AIDS Res Hum Retroviruses 4:137, 1988

19. Medley GF, Anderson RM, Cox DR, Billard L: Incubation period of AIDS in patients infected via blood transfusion. Nature 328:719, 1987

20. Bacchetti P, Moss AR: Incubation period of AIDS in San Francisco. Nature 338:251, 1989

21. Goedert JJ, Kessler CM, Aledort LM et al: A prospective study of human immunodeficiency virus type 1 infection and the development of AIDS in subjects with hemophilia. N Engl J Med 321:1141, 1989

22. Pantaleo G, Graziosi C, Fauci AS: New concepts in the immunopathogenesis of human immunodeficiency virus infection. N Engl J Med 328:327, 1993

23. Sabin C, Phillips A, Elford J et al: The progression of HIV disease in a haemophilic cohort followed for 12 years. Br J Haematol 83:330, 1993

24. Weiss RA: How does HIV cause AIDS? Science 260:1273, 1993

25. Desrosiers RC: The simian immunodeficiency viruses. Annu Rev Immunol 8:557, 1990

26. Gao F, Yue L, White AT et al: Human infection by genetically diverse SIVsm-related HIV-2 in west Africa. Nature 358:495, 1992

27. Greene WC: the molecular biology of human immunodeficiency virus type 1 infection. N Engl J Med 324:308, 1991

28. Luciw PA, Cheng-Mayer C, Levy JA: Mutational analysis of the human immunodeficiency virus (HIV): the orf-B region down regulates virus replication. Proc Natl Acad Sci USA 84:1434, 1987

29. Ahmad N, Venkatesan S: Nef protein of HIV-1 is a transcriptional repressor of HIV-1 LTR. Science 241:1481, 1988

30. Garcia JV, Miller AD: Serine phosphorylation independent downregulation of cell-surface CD4 by Nef. Nature 350:508, 1991

31. Benson RE, Sanfridson A, Ottinger JS et al: Downregulation of cell-surface CD4 expression by simian immunodeficiency virus Nef prevents viral super infection. J Exp Med 177:1561, 1993

32. Fisher AG, Ensoli B, Ivanoff L et al: The sor gene of HIV-1 is required for efficient virus transmission in vitro. Science 237:888, 1987

33. Strebel K, Daugherty D, Clouse K et al: The HIV-1 'A' (sor) gene product is essential for virus infectivity. Nature 328:728, 1987

34. Wong-Staal F, Chanda PKI, Ghrayeb J: Human immunodeficiency virus: the eighth gene. AIDS Res Hum Retroviruses 3:33, 1987

35. Dedera D, Hu W, Heyden NV, Ratner L: Viral protein R of human immunodeficiency virus types 1 and 2 is dispensable for replication and cytopathogenicity in lymphoid cells. J Virol 63:3205, 1989

36. Strebel K, Klimkait T, Martin MA: A novel gene of HIV-1, vpu, and its 16-kilodalton product. Science 241:1221, 1988

37. Cohen EA, Terwilliger EF, Sodroski JG, Haseltine WA: Identification of a protein encoded by the vpu gene of HIV-1. Nature 334:532, 1988

38. Henderson LE, Sowder RC, Copeland TD et al: Isolation and characteristics of a novel protein (x-orf product) from SIV and HIV-2. Science 241:199, 1988

39. Yu XF, Ito S, Essex M, Lee TH: A naturally immunogenic virion-associated protein specific for HIV-2 and SIV. Nature 335:262, 1988

40. Kappes JC, Morrow CD, Lee SW et al: Identification of a novel retroviral gene unique to human immunodeficiency virus type 2 and simian immunodeficiency virus SIVmac. J Virol 62:3501, 1988

41. Sattentau QJ, Weiss RA: the CD4 antigen, physiological ligand and HIV receptor. Cell 52:631, 1988

42. Gartner S, Markovits P, Markovitz DM et al: The role of mononuclear phagocytes in HTLV-III/LAV infection. Science 233:215, 1986

43. Gendelman HE, Orenstein JM, Baca LM et al: The macrophage in the persistence and pathogenesis of HIV infection. AIDS 3:475, 1989

44. Tschachler E, Groh V, Popovic M et al: Epidermal Langerhans cells—a target for HTLV-III/LAV infection. J Invest Dermatol 88:233, 1987

45. Rappersberger K, Gartner S, Schenk P et al: Langerhans' cells are an actual site of HIV-1 replication. Intervirol 29:185, 1988

46. Tenner-Racz K, Racz P, Dietrich M, Kern P: Altered follicular dendritic cells and virus-like particles in AIDS and AIDS-related lymphadenopathy. Lancet 1:105, 1985

47. Gabuzda DH, Ho DD, de la Monte SM et al: Immunohistochemical identification of HTLV-III antigen in brains of patients with AIDS. Ann Neurol 20:28 1986

48. Giannetti A, Zambruno G, Cimarelli A et al: Direct detection of HIV-1 RNA in epidermal Langerhans cells of HIV-infected patients. J Acquir Immun Defic Syndr 6:329, 1993

49. Langhoff E, Terwilliger EF, Bos HJ et al: Replication of human immunodeficiency virus type 1 in primary dendritic cell cultures. Proc Natl Acad Sci USA 88:7998, 1991

50. Spiegel H, Herbst G, Niedobitek G et al: Follicular dendritic cells are a major reservoir for human immunodeficiency virus type I in lymphoid tissue facilitating infection of CD4+ T-helper cells. Am J Pathol 140:15, 1992

51. Parmentier HK, van Wichen D, Sie-Go DM et al: HIV-1 infection and virus production in follicular dendritic cells in lymph nodes. A case report, with analysis of isolated follicular dendritic cells. Am J Pathol 137:247, 1990

52. Basch RS, Kouri YH, Karpatkin S: Expression of CD4 by human megakaryocytes. Proc Natl Acad Sci USA 87:8085, 1990

53. Kouri YH, Borkowsky W, Nardi M et al: Human megakaryocytes have a CD molecule capable of binding human immunodeficiency virus-1. Blood 81 2664, 1993

54. Gewirtz AM, Boghosian-Sell L, Catani L et al: Expression of Fc gamma RI and CD4 receptors by normal human megakaryocytes. Exp Hematol 20:512 1992

55. Hildreth JEK, Orentas RJ: Involvement of a leukocyte adhesion receptor (LFA-1) in HIV-induced syncytium formation. Science 244:1075, 1989

56. Pantaleo G, Butini L, Graziosi C et al: Human immunodeficiency virus (HIV infection in CD4+ T lymphocytes genetically deficient in LFA-1: LFA-1 is required for HIV-mediated cell fusion but not for viral transmission. J Exp Med 173:511, 1991

57. Montefiori DC, Stewart K, Ahearn JM et al: Complement-mediated binding of naturally glycosylated and glycosylation-modified human immunodeficiency virus type 1 to human CR2 (CD21). J Virol 67:2699, 1993

58. McKeating JA, Griffiths PD, Weiss RA: HIV susceptibility conferred to human fibroblasts by cytomegalovirus-induced Fc receptor. Nature 343:659, 1990

59. Homsy J, Meyer M, Tateno M et al: The Fc and not CD4 receptor mediates antibody enhancement of HIV infection in human cells. Science 244:1357 1989

60. Cao Y, Friedman-Kein AE, Huang Y et al: CD4-independent, productive human immunodeficiency virus type 1 infection of hepatoma cell lines in vitro. J Virol 64:2553, 1990

61. Bachelerie F, Alcami J, Hazan U et al: Constitutive expression of human immunodeficiency virus (HIV) nef protein in human astrocytes does not influence basal or induced HIV long terminal repeat activity. J Virol 64:3059, 1990

62. Ikeuchi K, Kim S, Byrn RA et al: Infection of nonlymphoid cells by human immunodeficiency virus type 1 or type 2. J Virol 64:4226, 1990

63. Li XL, Moudgil T, Vinters HV, Ho DD: CD4-independent, productive infection of a neuronal cell line by human immunodeficiency virus type 1. J Virol 64:1383, 1990

64. Harouse JM, Bhat S, Spitalnik SL et al: Inhibition of entry of HIV-1 in neural cell lines by antibodies against galactosyl ceramide. Science 253:320, 1991

65. Yahi N, Baghdiguian S, Moreau H, Fantini J: Galactosyl ceramide (or a closely related molecule) is the receptor for human immunodeficiency virus type 1 on human colon epithelial HT29 cells. J Virol 66:4848, 1992

66. Cullen BR, Greene WC: Regulatory pathways governing HIV-1 replication. Cell 58:423, 1989

67. Shaw JP, Utz PJ, Durand DB et al: Identification of a putative regulator of early T cell activation genes. Science 241:202, 1988

68. Jones KA, Kadonaga JT, Luciw PA, Tijan R: Activation of AIDS retrovirus promoter by the cellular transcription factor Spl. Science 232:755, 1986

69. Nabel G, Baltimore D: An inducible transcription factor activates expression of human immunodeficiency virus in T cells. Nature 326:711, 1987

70. Garcia JA, Wu FK, Mitsuyasu R, Gaynor RB: Interactions of cellular proteins involved in the transcriptional regulation of the human immunodeficiency virus. EMBO J 6:3761, 1987

71. Siekevitz M, Josephs SF, Dukovich M et al: Activation of the HIV-1 LTR by T cell mitogens and the trans-activator protein of HTLV-1. Science 238:1575, 1987

72. Mosca JD, Bednarik DP, Raj NBK et al: Activation of human immunodeficiency virus by herpes virus infection: identification of a region within the long terminal repeat that responds to a trans-acting factor encoded by herpes simplex virus 1. Proc Natl Acad Sci USA 84:7408, 1987

73. Gendelman HE, Phelps W, Feigenbau L et al: Transactivation of the human immunodeficiency virus long terminal repeat sequence by DNA viruses. Proc Natl Acad Sci USA 83:9759, 1986

74. Kenney A, Kamine J, Markovitz D et al: An Epstein-Barr virus immediate-early gene product trans-activates gene expression from the human immu-

nodeficiency virus long terminal repeat. Proc Natl Acad Sci USA 85:1652, 1988

75. Rando RF, Pellett PE, Luciw PA et al: Transactivation of human immunodeficiency virus by herpes viruses. Oncogene 1:13, 1987

76. Davis M, Kenney SC, Kamine J et al: Immediate-early gene region of human cytomegalovirus trans-activates the promoter of human immunodeficiency virus. Proc Natl Acad Sci USA 84:8642, 1987

77. Folks TM, Justement J, Kinter A et al: Cytokine-induced expression of HIV-1 in a chronically infected promonocyte cell line. Science 238:800, 1987

78. Koyanagi Y, O'Brien WA, Zhao JQ et al: Cytokines alter production of HIV-1 from primary mononuclear phagocytes. Science 241:1673, 1988

79. Baldwin GC, Fuller ND, Roberts RL et al: Granulocyte- and granulocyte-macrophage colony-stimulating factors enhance neutrophil cytotoxicity toward HIV-infected cells. Blood 74:1673, 1989

80. Poli G, Bressler P, Kinter A et al: Interleukin-6 induces human immunodeficiency virus expression in infected monocytic cells alone and in synergy with tumor necrosis factor alpha by transcriptional and post-transcriptional mechanisms. J Exp Med 172:151, 1990

81. Poli G, Kinter A, Justement JS et al: Tumor necrosis factor alpha functions in an autocrine manner in the induction of human immunodeficiency virus expression. Proc Natl Acad Sci USA 87:782, 1990

82. Valerie K, Delers A, Bruck C et al: Activation of human immunodeficiency virus type-1 by DNA damage in human cells. Nature 333:78, 1988

83. Pomerantz RJ, Trono D, Feinberg MB, Baltimore D: Cells nonproductively infected with HIV-1 exhibit an aberrant pattern of viral RNA expression: a molecular model for latency. Cell 61:1271, 1990

84. Lane HC, Depper JM, Greene WC et al: Qualitative analysis of immune function in patients with acquired immunodeficiency syndrome. N Engl J Med 313:79, 1984

85. Gurley RJ, Ikeuchi K, Byrn RA et al: CD4+ lymphocyte function with early human immunodeficiency virus infection. Proc Natl Acad Sci USA 86:1993, 1989

86. Siliciano RF, Lawton T, Knall C et al: Analysis of host-virus interactions in AIDS with anti-gp120 T cell clones: effect of HIV sequence variation and a mechanism for CD4+ cell depletion. Cell 54:561, 1988

87. Lyerly HK, Matthews TJ, Langlois AJ et al: Human T-cell lymphotropic virus IIIB glycoprotein (gp120) to CD4 determinants on normal lymphocytes and expressed by infected cells serves as target for immune attack. Proc Natl Acad Sci USA 84:4601, 1987

88. Terai C, Kornbluth RS, Pauza CD et al: Apoptosis as a mechanism of cell death in cultured T lymphoblasts acutely infected with HIV-1. J Clin Invest 87:1710, 1991

89. Groux H, Torpier G, Monte D et al: Activation-induced death by apoptosis in CD4+ T cells from human immunodeficiency virus-infected asymptomatic individuals. J Exp Med 175:331, 1992

90. Banda NK, Bernier J, Kurahara DK et al: Crosslinking CD4 by human immunodeficiency virus gp120 primes T cells for activation-induced apoptosis. J Exp Med 176:1099, 1992

91. Bonyhadik ML, Rabink L, Salimi S et al: HIV induces thymus depletion in vivo. Nature 363:728, 1993

92. Aldrovandi GM, Feuer G, Gao L et al: The SCID-hu mouse as a model for HIV-1 infection. Nature 363:732, 1993.

93. van Noesel CJM, Gruters RA, Terpstra FG et al: Functional and phenotypic evidence for a selective loss of memory T cells in asymptomatic human immunodeficiency virus-infected men. J Clin Invest 86:293, 1990

94. Schnittman SM, Lane HC, Greenhouse J et al: Preferential infection of CD4+ memory T cells by human immunodeficiency virus type 1: evidence for a role in the selective T-cell functional defects observed in infected individuals. Proc Natl Acad Sci USA 87:6058, 1990

95. Clerici M, Shearer GM: A TH1 → TH2 switch is a critical step in the etiology of HIV infection. Immunol Today 14:107, 1993

96. Clerici M, Hakim FT, Venzon DJ et al: Changes in interleukin-2 and interleukin-4 production in asymptomatic, human immunodeficiency virus-seropositive individuals. J Clin Invest 91:759, 1993

97. Stricker RB, McHugh TM, Moody DJ et al: An AIDS-related cytotoxic autoantibody reacts with a specific antigen on stimulated CD4+ T cells. Nature 327:710, 1987

98. Kirprov DD, Anderson RE, Morand PR et al: Antilymphocyte antibodies and seropositivity of retroviruses in groups at high risk for AIDS. N Engl J Med 312:1517, 1985

99. Dorsett B, Cronin W, Chuma V, Ioachim HL: Antilymphocyte antibodies in patients with the acquired immune deficiency syndrome. Am J Med 78:621, 1985

100. Williams RC, Masur H, Spira TJ: Lymphocyte-reactive antibodies in acquired immunodeficiency syndrome. J Clin Immunol 4:118, 1984

101. Embretson J, Zupancic M, Ribas JL et al: Massive covert infection of helper T lymphocytes and macrophages by HIV during the incubation period of AIDS. Nature 362:359, 1993

102. Gendelman HE, Orenstein JM, Martin MA: Efficient isolation and propagation of human immunodeficiency virus on recombinant colony stimulating factor 1-treated monocytes. J Exp Med 167:1428, 1988

103. Price RW, Brew B, Sidtis J et al: The brain in AIDS: central nervous system HIV-1 infection and AIDS-dementia complex. Science 239:586, 1988

104. Koenig S, Gendelman HE, Orenstein JM et al: Detection of AIDS virus in macrophages in brain tissue from AIDS patients with encephalopathy. Science 233:1089, 1986

105. Gartner S, Markovits P, Markovitz DM et al: Virus iolation and identification of HTLV-III/LAV producing cells in brain tissue from a patient with AIDS. JAMA 256:2365, 1986

106. Wiley CA, Schrier RD, Nelson JA et al: Cellular localization of human immunodeficiency virus infection within the brains of acquired immunodeficiency syndrome patients. Proc Natl Acad Sci USA 83:7089, 1986

107. Geleziunas R, Schipper HM. Wainberg MA: Pathogenesis and therapy of HIV-1 infection of the central nervous system. AIDS 6:1411, 1992

108. Groopman JE: Biology and therapy of epidemic Kaposi's sarcoma. Cancer 59:633, 1987

109. Ensoli B, Barillari G, Gallo RC: Pathogenesis of AIDS-associated Kaposi's sarcoma. Hematol Oncol Clin North Am 5:281, 1991

110. Ensoli B, Nakamura S, Salahuddin SZ et al: AIDS-Kaposi's sarcoma-derived cells express cytokines with autocrine and paracrine growth factors. Science 243:223, 1989

111. Nair BC, DeVico AL, Nakamura S et al: Identification of major growth factor for AIDS-Kaposi's sarcoma cells as oncostatin M. Science 255:1430, 1992

112. Miles SA, Martinez-Maza O, Rezai A et al: Oncostatin M as a potent mutagen for AIDS-Kaposi's sarcoma-derived cells. Science 255:1432, 1992

113. Beral V, Peterman TA, Berkelman RL, Jaffe HW: Kaposi's sarcoma among persons with AIDS: a sexually transmitted infection? Lancet 335:123, 1990

114. Ziegler JL, Beckstead JA, Volberding PA et al: Non-Hodgkin's lymphoma in 90 homosexual men. N Engl J Med 311:565, 1984

115. Knowles DM, Chamaluk GA, Subar M et al: Lymphoid neoplasia associated with the acquired immunodeficiency syndrome (AIDS). Ann Intern Med 108:744, 1988

116. Levine AM: Non-Hodgkin's lymphoma and other malignancies in the acquired immune deficiency syndrome. Semin Oncol 14:34, 1987

117. Lowenthal DA, Straus DJ, Campbell SW et al: AIDS-related lymphoid neoplasia: the Memorial Hospital Experience. Cancer 61:2325, 1988

118. Ergerter DA, Beckstead JH: Malignant lymphomas in the acquired immunodeficiency syndrome. Additional evidence for a B-cell origin. Arch Pathol Lab Med 112:602, 1988

119. Gail MH, Pluda JM, Rabkin CS et al: Projections of the incidence of non-Hodgkin's lymphoma related to acquired immunodeficiency syndrome. J Natl Cancer Inst 83:662, 1991

120. Pluda JM, Yarchoan R, Jaffe ES et al: Development of non-Hodgkin lymphoma in a cohort of patients with severe human immunodeficiency virus (HIV) infection on long-term antiretroviral therapy. Ann Intern Med 113:276, 1990

121. Beral V, Peterman T, Berkelman R, Jaffe H: AIDS-associated non-Hodgkin lymphoma. Lancet 337:805, 1991

122. Ioachim HL, Dorsett B, Cronin W et al: Acquired immunodeficiency syndrome-associated lymphomas: clinical, pathologic immunologic, and viral characteristics of 111 cases. Hum Pathol 22:659, 1991

123. Karp JE, Broder S: Acquired immunodeficiency syndrome and non-Hodgkin's lymphomas. Cancer Res 51:4743, 1991

124. Levine AM: Acquired immunodeficiency syndrome-related lymphoma. Blood 80:8, 1992

125. Centers for Disease Control: Opportunistic non-Hodgkin's lymphomas among severely immunocompromised HIV-infected patients surviving for prolonged periods on antiretroviral therapy—United States. MMWR 40:591, 1991

126. Ragni MV, Belle SH, Jaffe RA et al: Acquired immunodeficiency syndrome-associated non-Hodgkin's lymphomas and other malignancies in patients with hemophilia. Blood 81:1889, 1993

127. Goldstein J, Dickson DW, Rubenstein A et al: Primary central nervous system lymphoma in a pediatric patient with acquired immune deficiency syndrome. Treatment with radiation therapy. Cancer 66:2503, 1990

128. Esptein LG, DiCarlo FJ Jr, Joshi VV et al: Primary lymphoma of the central nervous system in children with acquired immunodeficiency syndrome. Pediatrics 82:355, 1988

129. Groopman JE, Sullivan JL, Mulder C et al: Pathogenesis of B cell lymphoma in a patient with AIDS. Blood 67:612, 1986

130. Shiramizu B, McGrath MS: Molecular pathogenesis of AIDS-associated non-Hodgkin's lymphoma. Hematol Oncol Clin North Am 5:323, 1991

131. Lane HC, Masur H, Edgar LC et al: Abnormalities of B-cell activation and immunoregulation in patients with the acquired immunodeficiency syndrome. N Engl J Med 309:453, 1989

132. Pahwa SG, Quilop MTJ, Lange M et al: Defective B-lymphocyte function in homosexual men in relation to the acquired immunodeficiency syndrome. Ann Intern Med 101:757, 1984

133. Barriga F, Whang-Peng J, Lee E et al: Development of a second clonally discrete Burkitt's lymphoma in a human immunodeficiency virus-positive homosexual patient. Blood 72:792, 1988

134. McGrath MS, Shiramizu B, Meekder TC et al: AIDS-associated polyclonal lymphoma: identification of a new HIV-associated disease process. J Acquir Immune Defic Syndr 4:408, 1991

135. Bird AG, Britton S, Ernberg I, Nilsson K: Characteristics of Epstein-Barr virus activation of human B lymphocytes. J Exp Med 154:832, 1981

136. Shibata D, Weiss LM, Hernandez AM et al: Epstein-Barr virus associated non-Hodgkin's lymphoma in patients infected with the human immunodeficiency virus. Blood 81:2102, 1993

137. Hutt-Fletcher LM, Balachandran N, Elkins MH: B cell activation by cytomegalovirus. J Exp Med 158:2171, 1983

138. Schnittman SM, Lane HC, Higgins SE et al: Direct polyclonal activation of human B lymphocytes by the acquired immune deficiency syndrome virus. Science 233:1084, 1986

139. Levine AM, Shibata D, Sullivan-Halley J et al: Epidemiological and biological study of acquired immunodeficiency syndrome-related lymphoma in the country of Los Angeles: preliminary results. Cancer Res 52:5482s, 1992

140. Hamilton-Dutoit SJ, Raphail M, Audouin J et al: In situ demonstration of Epstein-Barr virus small RNAs (EBER 1) in acquired immunodeficiency syndrome-related lymphomas: correlation with tumor morphology and primary site. Blood 82:619, 1993

141. Gold JE, Altarac D, Ree HJ et al: HIV-associated Hodgkin disease: a clinical study of 18 cases and review of the literature. Am J Hematol 36:93, 1991

142. Pelstring RJ, Zellmer RB, Sulak LE et al: Hodgkin's disease in association with human immunodeficiency virus infection. Cancer 67:1865, 1991

143. Uccini S, Monardo F, Stoppacciaro A et al: High frequency of Epstein-Barr virus genome detection in Hodgkin's disease of HIV-positive patients. Int J Cancer 46:581, 1990

144. Ames ED, Conjalka MS, Goldberg AF et al: Hodgkin's disease and AIDS. Hematol Oncol Clin North Am 5:343, 1991

145. Hessol NA, Katz MH, Liu JY et al: Increased incidence of Hodgkin's disease in homosexual men with HIV infection. Ann Intern Med 117:309, 1992

146. Italian Cooperative Group for AIDS-Related Tumors: Malignant lymphomas in patients with or at risk for AIDS in Italy. J Natl Cancer Inst 80:855, 1988

147. Weiss LM, Movahed LA, Warnke RA, Sklar J: Detection of Epstein-Barr viral genomes in Reed-Sternberg cells of Hodgkin's disease. N Engl J Med 320:502, 1989

148. Birx DL, Redfield RR, Tosato G: Defective regulation of Epstein-Barr virus infection in patients with acquired immunodeficiency syndrome (AIDS) or AIDS-related disorders. N Engl J Med 314:847, 1986

149. Presant CA, Gala K, Wiseman C et al: Human immunodeficiency virus-associated T-cell lymphoblastic lymphoma in AIDS. Cancer 60:1459, 1987

150. Nasr SA, Byrnes RK, Garrison CP, Chan WC: Peripheral T-cell lymphoma in a patient with acquired immunodeficiency syndrome. Cancer 61:947, 1988

151. Lust JA, Banks PM, Hooper WC et al: T-cell non-Hodgkin's lymphoma in human immunodeficiency virus-1-infected individuals. Am J Hematol 31:181, 1989

152. Crane GA, Variakojis D, Rosen ST et al: Cutaneous T-cell lymphoma in patients with human immunodeficiency virus infection. Arch Dermatol 127:989, 1991

153. Nahass GT, Kraffert CA, Penneys NS: Cutaneous T-cell lymphoma associated with the acquired immunodeficiency syndrome. Arch Dermatol 127:1020, 1991

154. Goldman R, Lang W, Lyman D: Acute AIDS viral infection. Am J Med 81:1122, 1986

155. Kessler HA, Blaauw B, Spear J et al: Diagnosis of human immunodeficiency virus infection in seronegative homosexuals presenting with an acute viral syndrome. JAMA 258:1196, 1987

156. Ho DD, Sarngadharan MG, Resnick L et al: Primary human T-lymphotropic virus type III infection. Ann Intern Med 103:880, 1985

157. Cooper DA, Gold J, Maclean P et al: Acute AIDS retrovirus infection. Definition of a clinical illness associated with seroconversion. Lancet 1:537, 1985

158. Ho DD, Rota TR, Schooley RT et al: Isolation of HTLV-III from cerebrospinal fluid and neural tissues of patients with neurological syndromes related to the acquired immunodeficiency syndrome. N Engl J Med 313:1493, 1985

159. Carne CA, Smith A, Elkington SG et al: Acute encephalopathy coincident with seroconversion for anti-HTLV-III. Lancet 2:1206, 1985

160. Hollander H, Stringari S: Human immunodeficiency virus-associated meningitis: clinical course and correlations. Am J Med 83:813, 1987

161. Klinoch-de Loës S, de Saussure P. Saurat J-H et al: Symptomatic primary infection due to human immunodeficiency virus type 1: review of 31 cases. Clin Infect Dis 17:59, 1993

162. Feorino PM, Jaffe HW, Palmer E et al: Transfusion-associated acquired immunodeficiency syndrome: evidence for persistent infection in blood donors. N Engl J Med 312:1293, 1985

163. Laurence J, Brun-Vezinet F, Schutzer SE et al: Lymphadenopathy-associated viral antibody in AIDS. Immune correlations and definition of a carrier state. N Engl J Med 311:1269, 1984

164. Åsjö B, Albert J, Karlsson A et al: Replication properties of human immunodeficiency virus from patients with varying severity of HIV infection. Lancet 2:660, 1986

165. Cheng-Mayer C, Seto D, Tateno M, Levy JA: Biological features of HIV-1 that correlate with virulence in the host. Science 240:80, 1988

166. Piatak M Jr, Saag MS, Yang LC et al: High levels of HIV-1 in plasma during all stages of infection determined by competitive PCR. Science 259:1749, 1993

167. Schnittman SM, Psallidopoulos MC, Lane HC et al: The reservoir for HIV in the peripheral blood of HIV-infected individuals is a T cell that maintains expression of the CD4 molecule. Science 245:305, 1989

168. Ou C-Y, Kwok S, Mitchell SW et al: DNA amplification for direct detection of HIV-1 in DNA of peripheral blood mononuclear cells. Science 239:295, 1988

169. Pantaleo G, Graziosi C, Demarest JF et al: HIV infection is active and progressive in lymphoid tissue during the clinically latent stage of disease. Nature 362:355, 1993

170. Jason J, Lui K-J, Ragni MV et al: Risk of developing AIDS in HIV-infected cohorts of hemophiliac and homosexual men. JAMA 261:725, 1989

171. Eyster ME, Ballard JO, Gail MH et al: Predictive markers for the acquired immunodeficiency syndrome (AIDS) in hemophiliacs: persistence of p24 antigen and low T4 cell count. Ann Intern Med 110:963, 1989

172. Polk BF, Fox R, Brookmeyer R et al: Predictors of the acquired immunodeficiency syndrome developing in a cohort of seropositive homosexual men. N Engl J Med 316:61, 1987

173. Moss AR, Bacchetti P, Osmond D et al: Seropositivity for HIV and the development of AIDS or AIDS related condition: three year follow up of the San Francisco General Hospital Cohort. BMJ 296:745, 1988

174. Masur H, Ognibene FP, Yarchoan R et al: CD4 counts as predictors of opportunistic pneumonias in human immunodeficiency virus (HIV) infection. Ann Intern Med 111:223, 1989

175. Burcham J, Marmor M, Dubin N et al: CD4% is the best predictor of development of AIDS in a cohort of HIV-infected homosexual men. AIDS 5:365, 1991

176. Anderson RE, Lang W, Shiboski S et al: Use of β_2-microglobulin level and CD4 lymphocyte count to predict development of acquired immunodeficiency syndrome in persons with human immunodeficiency virus infection. Arch Intern Med 150:73, 1990

177. Zon LI, Groopman JE: Hematologic manifestations of the human immune deficiency virus (HIV). Semin Hematol 25:208, 1988

178. Perkocha LA, Rodgers GM: Hematologic aspects of human immunodeficiency virus infection: laboratory and clinical considerations. Am J Hematol 29:94, 1988

179. Scadden DT, Zeira M, Woon A et al: Human immunodeficiency virus infection of human bone marrow stromal fibroblasts. Blood 76:317, 1990

180. Costello C: Haematological abnormalities in human immunodeficiency virus (HIV) disease. J Clin Pathol 41:711, 1988

181. Zon LI, Arkin C, Groopman JE: Haematologic manifestations of human immune deficiency virus (HIV). Br J Haematol 66:251, 1987

182. Aboulafia DM, Mitsuyasu RT: Hematologic abnormalities in AIDS. Hematol Oncol Clin North Am 5:195, 1991

183. Frontiera M, Myers AM: Peripheral blood and bone marrow abnormalities in the acquired immunodeficiency syndrome. West J Med 147:157, 1987

184. Doukas MA: Human immunodeficiency virus associated anemia. Med Clin North Am 76:699, 1992

185. Mir N, Costello C, Luckit J, Lindley R: HIV-disease and bone marrow changes: a study of 60 cases. Eur J Haematol 42:339, 1989

186. Osborne BM, Guarda LA, Butler JJ: Bone marrow biopsies in patients with the acquired immunodeficiency syndrome. Hum Pathol 15:1048, 1984

187. Costella A, Croxson TS, Mildvan D et al: The bone marrow in AIDS. A histologic, hematological and microbiologic study. Am J Clin Pathol 84:425, 1985

188. Abrams DI, Chinn EK, Lewis BJ et al: Hematologic manifestations in homosexual men with Kaposi's sarcoma. Am J Clin Pathol 81:13, 1984

189. Treacy M, Lai L, Costello C, Clark A: Peripheral blood and bone marrow abnormalities in patients with HIV related disease. Br J Haematol 65:289, 1987

190. Schneider DR, Picker LJ: Myelodysplasia in the acquired immune deficiency syndrome. Am J Clin Pathol 84:144, 1985

191. Richman DD, Fischl MA, Grieco MH et al: The toxicity of azidothymidine (AZT) in the treatment of patients with AIDS and AIDS-related complex. N Engl J Med 317:192, 1987

192. Walker RE, Parker RI, Kovacs JA et al: Anemia and erythropoiesis in patients with the acquired immunodeficiency syndrome (AIDS) and Kaposi's sarcoma, treated with zidovudine. Ann Intern Med 108:372, 1988

193. Snower DP, Weil SC: Changing etiology of macrocytosis. Hematopathology 99:57, 1993

194. Leaf AN, Laubenstein LJ, Raphael B et al: Thrombotic thrombocytopenic purpura associated with human immunodeficiency virus type I (HIV-1) infection. Ann Intern Med 109:194, 1988

195. Nair JMG, Bellevue R, Bertoni M, Dosik H: Thrombotic thrombocytopenic purpura in patients with the acquired immunodeficiency syndrome (AIDS)-related complex. Ann Intern Med 109:209, 1988

196. Meisenberg BR, Robinson WL, Mosley CA et al: Thrombotic thrombocytopenic purpura in human immunodeficiency HIV-seropositive males. Am J Hematol 27:212, 1988

197. Henry K, Flynn T: Association of thrombotic thrombocytopenic purpura (TTP) and human immunodeficiency virus (HIV) infection. Am J Hematol 29:182, 1988

198. Jokela J, Flynn T, Henry K: Thrombotic thrombocytopenic purpura in a human immunodeficiency virus (HIV)-positive homosexual man. Am J Hematol 25:341, 1987

199. Rarick MU, Espina B, Mocharnuk R et al: Thrombotic thrombocytopenic purpura in patients with human immunodeficiency virus infection: a report of three cases and review of the literature. Am J Hematol 40:103, 1992

200. Spivak JL, Selonick SE, Quinn TC: Acquired immune deficiency syndrome and pancytopenia. JAMA 250:3084, 1983

201. Delacretaz F, Perey L, Schmidt P-M et al: Histopathology of bone marrow in human immunodeficiency virus infection. Virchows Arch A Pathol Anat Histopathol 411:543, 1987

202. Harris CE, Biggs JC, Concannon AJ, Dodds AJ: Peripheral blood and bone marrow findings in patients with acquired immune deficiency syndrome. Pathology 22:206, 1990

203. Karcher DS, Frost AR: The bone marrow in human immunodeficiency virus (HIV)-related disease. Am J Clin Pathol 95:63, 1991

204. Sun NCJ, Shapshak P, Lachant NA et al: Bone marrow examination in patients with AIDS and AIDS-related complex (ARC). Am J Clin Pathol 92:589, 1989

205. Baumann MA, Pacheco J, Paul CC et al: Paroxysmal nocturnal hemoglobinuria associated with the acquired immunodeficiency syndrome. Arch Intern Med 148:212, 1988

206. Shenoy CM, Lin JH: Bone marrow findings in acquired immunodeficiency syndrome (AIDS). Am J Med Sci 292:372, 1986

207. McKinsey DS, Durfee D, Kurtin PJ: Megaloblastic pancytopenia associated with dapsone and trimethoprim treatment of Pneumocystis carinii pneumonia in the acquired immunodeficiency syndrome. Arch Intern Med 149:965, 1989

208. Gascon P, Sathe SS, Rameshwar P: Impaired erythropoiesis in the acquired immunodeficiency syndrome with disseminated Mycobacterium avium complex. Am J Med 94:41, 1993

209. Sathe SS, Gascone P, Lo W et al: Severe anemia is an important negative predictor for survival with disseminated Mycobacterium avium-complex in acquired immunodeficiency syndrome. Am Rev Respir Dis 142:1306, 1990

210. Cohen H, Williams I, Matthey F et al: Reversible zidovudine-induced pure red-cell aplasia. AIDS 3:177, 1989

211. Parmentier L, Boucary D, Salmon D: Pure red cell aplasia in an HIV-infected patient. AIDS 6:234, 1992

212. Frickhofen N, Abkowitz JL, Safford M et al: Persistent B19 parvovirus infection in patients infected with human immunodeficiency virus type 1 (HIV-1): a treatable cause of anemia in AIDS. Ann Intern Med 113:926, 1990

213. Nigro G, Gattinara GC, Mattia S et al: Parvovirus-B19-related pancytopenia in children with HIV infection. Lancet 340:115, 1992

214. Mitsuyasu RT, Lambertus M, Goetz MB: Transfusion-dependent anemia in a patient with AIDS. Clin Infect Dis 15:533, 1992

215. Griffin TC, Squires JE, Timmons CF, Buchanan GR: Chronic human parvovirus B19-induced erythroid hypoplasia as the initial manifestation of human immunodeficiency virus infection. J Pediatr 118:899, 1991

216. Rarick MU, Loureiro C, Groshen S et al: Serum erythropoietin titers in patients with human immunodeficiency virus (HIV) infection and anemia. J Acquir Immune Defic Syndr 4:593, 1991

217. Fischl MA, Richman DD, Grieco MH: The efficacy of azidothymidine (AZT) in the treatment of patients with AIDS and AIDS-related complex: a double blind, placebo-controlled trial. N Engl J Med 317:185, 1987

218. Camacho J, Poveda F, Zamorano AF et al: Serum erythropoietin levels in anaemic patients with advanced human immunodeficiency virus infection. Br J Haematol 82:608, 1992

219. Spivak JL, Barnes DC, Fuchs E, Quinn TC: Serum immunoreactive erythropoietin in HIV-infected patients. JAMA 261:3104, 1989

220. Lee GR: The anemia of chronic disease. Semin Hematol 20:61, 1983

221. Henry DH, Beal GN, Benson CA et al: Recombinant human erythropoietin in the treatment of anemia associated with human immunodeficiency virus (HIV) infection and zidovudine therapy. Ann Intern Med 117:739, 1992

222. Spivak JL, Bender BS: Hematologic abnormalities in the acquired immunodeficiency syndrome. Am J Med 77:224, 1984

223. Gupta S, Imam A, Licorish K: Serum ferritin in acquired immune deficiency syndrome. J Clin Lab Immunol 20:11, 1986

224. Blumberg BS, Hann H-WL, Mildvan D et al: Iron and iron binding proteins in persistent generalized lymphadenopathy and AIDS. Lancet 1:347, 1984

225. Herbert V: B$_{12}$ deficiency in AIDS JAMA 260:2837, 1988

226. Burkes RL, Cohen H, Krailo M et al: Low serum cobalamin levels occur frequently in the acquired immune deficiency syndrome and related disorders. Eur J Haematol 38:141, 1987

227. Harriman GR, Smith PD, Horne McK et al: Vitamin B$_{12}$ malabsorption in patients with acquired immunodeficiency syndrome. Arch Intern Med 149:2039, 1989

228. Remacha AF, Riera A, Cadafalch J, Gimferrer E: Vitamin B-12 abnormalities in HIV-infected patients. Eur J Haematol 47:60, 1991

229. Kieburtz KD, Giant DW, Schiffer RB, Vakil N: Abnormal vitamin B12 metabolism in human immunodeficiency virus infection. Arch Neurol 48:312, 1991

230. Hansen M, Gimsing P, Ingeberg S et al: Cobalamin binding proteins in patients with HIV infection. Eur J Haematol 48:228, 1992

231. Modigliani R, Bories C, LeCharpentier Y et al: Diarrhoea and malabsorption in acquired immune deficiency syndrome: a study of four cases with special emphasis on opportunistic protozoan infections. Gut 26:179, 1985

232. Herbert V, Fong W, Gulle V, Stopler T: Low holotranscobalamin II is the earliest serum marker for subnormal vitamin B12 (cobalamin) absorption in patients with AIDS. Am J Hematol 34:132, 1990

233. Herzlich BC, Ranginwala M, Nawabi I, Herbert V: Synergy of inhibition of DNA synthesis in human bone marrow by azidothymidine plus deficiency of folate and/or vitamin B12. Am J Hematol 33:177, 1990

234. Revell P, O'Doherty MJ, Tang A, Savidge GF: Folic acid absorption in patients infected with the human immunodeficiency virus. J Intern Med 230:227, 1991

235. Beach RS, Mantero Atienza E: Altered folate metabolism in early HIV infection. JAMA 259:519, 1988

236. Beach RS, Mantero-Atienza E: Altered folate metabolism in early HIV infection. JAMA 259:3128, 1988

237. Toy PTCY, Reid ME, Burns M: Positive direct antiglobulin test associated with hyperglobulinemia in acquired immunodeficiency syndrome (AIDS). Am J Hematol 19:145, 1985

238. McGinnis MH, Macher AM, Rook AH, Alter HJ: Red cell autoantibodies in patients with acquired immune deficiency syndrome. Transfusion 26:405, 1986

239. Lepennec P-Y, LeFrere J-J, Rouzaud A-M, Rouger P: Red cell autoantibodies in asymptomatic HIV-infected subjects. Transfusion 29:465, 1989

240. Rapoport AP, Rowe JM, McMican A: Life threatening autoimmune hemolytic anemia in a patient with the acquired immune deficiency syndrome. Transfusion 28:190, 1988

241. Puppo F, Torresin A, Lotti G: Autoimmune hemolytic anemia and human immunodeficiency virus (HIV) infection. Ann Intern Med 109:250, 1988

242. Telen MJ, Roberts KB, Bartlett JA: HIV-associated autoimmune hemolytic anemia: report of a case and review of the literature. J Acquir Immune Defic Syndr 3:933, 1990

243. Tongol JM, Gounder MP, Butala A, Rabinowitz M: HIV-related autoimmune hemolytic anemia: good response to zidovudine. J Acquir Immune Defic Syndr 4:1163, 1991

244. Carne CA, Weller IVD, Loveday C, Adler MW: From persistent generalized lymphadenopathy to AIDS: who will progress? BMJ 294:868, 1987

245. D'Onofrio G, Mancini S, Tamburrini E et al: Giant neutrophils with increased peroxidase activity—another evidence of dysgranulopoiesis in AIDS. Am J Clin Pathol 87:584, 1987

246. Napoli VM, Stein SF, Spira TJ, Raskin D: Myelodysplasia progressing to acute myeloblastic leukemia in an HTLV-III virus positive homosexual man with AIDS-related complex. Am J Clin Pathol 86:788, 1986

247. Willumsen L, Ellegaard J, Pedersen B: HIV infection in acute myeloblastic leukemia: a similar case. Am J Clin Pathol 88:536, 1987

248. Rivers JK, Laubenstein LJ, Postel AH: Acute monocytic leukaemia in a HIV-seropositive man. Clin Exp Dermatol 17:203, 1992

249. Peters BS, Matthews J, Gompels M et al: Acute myeloblastic leukemia in AIDS. AIDS 4:367, 1990

250. Glatt AE, Chirgwin K, Landesman SH: Current concepts: treatments of infections associated with human immunodeficiency virus. N Engl J Med 318: 1439, 1988

251. Gordin FM, Simon GL, Wofsy CB, Mills JM: Adverse reactions to trimethoprim-sulfamethoxazole in patients with the acquired immunodeficiency syndrome. Ann Intern Med 100:495, 1984

252. Mitsuyasa R, Groopman J, Volberding P: Cutaneous reaction to trimethoprim-sulfamethoxazole in patients with AIDS and Kaposi's sarcoma. N Engl J Med 308:1535, 1989

253. Wharton JM, Coleman DL, Wofsy CB et al: Trimethoprim-sulfamethoxazole or pentamidine for *Pneumocystis carinii* pneumonia in the acquired immunodeficiency syndrome: a prospective randomized trial. Ann Intern Med 105: 37, 1986

254. Jaffe HS, Abrams DI, Ammann AJ et al: Complications of cotrimoxazole in treatment of AIDS-associated *Pneumocystis carinii* pneumonia in homosexual men. Lancet 2:1109, 1983

255. Creagh-Kirk T, Doi P, Andrews E et al: Survival experience among patients with AIDS receiving zidovudine. Follow-up of patients in a compassionate plea program. JAMA 25:3009, 1988

256. Gill PS, Rarick M, Byrnes RK et al: Azidothymidine associated with bone marrow failure in the acquired immunodeficiency syndrome (AIDS). Ann Intern Med 107:502, 1987

257. Goldsmith JC, Irvine W: Reversible agranulocytosis related to azidothymidine. Am J Hematol 30:263, 1989

258. Namiki TS, Boone DC, Meyer PR: A comparison of bone marrow findings in patients with acquired immunodeficiency syndrome (AIDS) and AIDS related conditions. Hematol Oncol 5:99, 1987

259. Molina J-M, Scadden DT, Sakaguchi M et al: Lack of evidence for infection of or effect on growth of hematopoietic progenitor cells after in vivo or in vitro exposure to human immunodeficiency virus. Blood 76:2476, 1990

260. Kaczmarski RS, Davison F, Blair E et al: Detection of HIV in haemopoietic progenitors. Br J Haematol 82:764, 1992

261. Donahue RE, Johnson MM, Zon LI et al: Suppression of in vitro haematopoiesis following human immunodeficiency virus infection. Nature 326:200, 1987

262. Stella CC, Ganser A, Hoelzer D: Defective in vitro growth of the hemopoietic progenitor cells in the acquired immunodeficiency syndrome. J Clin Invest 80:286, 1987

263. Leiderman IZ, Greenberg ML, Adelsberg BR, Siegal FP: A glycoprotein inhibitor of in vitro granulopoiesis associated with AIDS. Blood 70:1267, 1987

264. Louache F, Henri A, Bettaieb A et al: Role of human immunodeficiency virus replication in defective in vitro growth of hematopoietic progenitors. Blood 80:2991, 1992

265. Zauli G, Re MC, Visani G et al: Evidence for a human immunodeficiency virus type 1-mediated suppression of uninfected hematopoietic (CD34+) cells in AIDS patients. J Infect Dis 166:710, 1992

266. Geissler RG, Kleiner OK, Mentzel U et al: Decreased haematopoietic colony growth in long-term bone marrow cultures of HIV-positive patients. Res Virol 144:69, 1993

267. Ganser A, Ottmann OG, von Briesen H et al: Changes in the haematopoietic progenitor cell compartment in the acquired immunodeficiency syndrome. Res Virol 141:185, 1990

268. Folks TM, Kessler SW, Orenstein JM et al: Infection and replication of HIV-1 in purified progenitor cells of normal human bone marrow. Science 242: 919, 1988

269. Steinberg HN, Crumpacker CS, Chatis PA: In vitro suppression of normal human bone marrow progenitor cells by human immunodeficiency virus. J Virol 65:1765, 1991

270. Zauli G, Re MC, Furlini G et al: Evidence for an HIV-1 mediated suppression of in vitro growth of enriched (CD34+) hematopoietic progenitors. J Acquir Immune Defic Syndr 4:1251, 1991

271. von Laer D, Hufert FT, Fenner TE et al: CD34+ hematopoietic progenitor cells are not a major reservoir of the human immunodeficiency virus. Blood 76:1281, 1990

272. Zauli G, Re MC, Visani G et al: Inhibitory effect of HIV-1 envelope glycoproteins gp120 and gp160 on the in vitro growth of enriched (CD34+) hematopoietic progenitor cells. Arch Virol 122:271, 1992

273. Murray HW, Rubin BY, Masur H, Roberts RB: Impaired production of lymphokines and immune (gamma) interferon in the acquired immunodeficiency syndrome. N Engl J Med 310:883, 1984

274. Zauli G, Davis BR, Re MC et al: tat protein stimulates production of transforming growth factor-b1 by marrow macrophages: a potential mechanism for human immunodeficiency virus-1-induced hematopoietic suppression. Blood 80:3036, 1992

275. van der Lelie J, Lange JMA, Vos JJE et al: Autoimmunity against blood cells in human immunodeficiency virus (HIV) infection. Br J Haematol 67:109, 1987

276. Murphy MF, Metcalfe P, Waters AH: Immune neutropenia in homosexual men. Lancet 1:217, 1985

277. Kaplan C, Morinet F, Cartron J: Virus-induced autoimmune thrombocytopenia an neutropenia. Semin Hematol 29:34, 1992

278. Groopman JE, Mitsuyasu RT, DeLeo MJ et al: Effect of recombinant human granulocyte-macrophage colony-stimulating factor on myelopoiesis in the acquired immunodeficiency syndrome. N Engl J Med 317:593, 1987

279. Kimura S, Matsuda J, Ikematsu S et al: Efficacy of recombinant human granulocyte colony-stimulating factor on neutropenia in patients with AIDS. AIDS 4:1251, 1990

280. Ratner L: Human immunodeficiency virus-associated autoimmune thrombocytopenic purpura: a review. Am J Med 86:194, 1989

281. Walsh CM, Karpatkin S: Thrombocytopenia and human immunodeficiency virus-1 infection. Semin Oncol 17:367, 1990

282. Morris L, Distenfeld A, Amorosi E, Karpatkin S: Autoimmune thrombocytopenic purpura in homosexual men. Ann Intern Med 96:714, 1982

283. Walsh C, Krigel R, Lennette E, Karpatkin S: Thrombocytopenia in homosexual patients: prognosis, response to therapy, and prevalence of antibody to the retrovirus asociated with the acquired immunodeficiency syndrome. Ann Intern Med 103:542, 1985

284. Goldsweig HG, Grossman R, William D: Thrombocytopenia in homosexual men. Am J Hematol 21:243, 1986

285. Abrams DI, Kiprov DD, Goedert JJ et al: Antibodies to human T-lymphotrophic virus type III and development of the acquired immunodeficiency syndrome in homosexual men presenting with immune thrombocytopenia. Ann Intern Med 104:47, 1986

286. Karpatkin S, Nardi MA, Hymes KB: Immunologic thrombocytopenic purpura after heterosexual transmission of human immunodeficiency virus (HIV). Ann Intern Med 109:190, 1988

287. Savona S, Nardi M, Lennette E, Karpatkin S: Thrombocytopenic purpura in narcotics addicts. Ann Intern Med 102:737, 1985

288. Karpatkin S: Immunologic thrombocytopenic purpura in HIV-seropositive homosexuals, narcotic addicts and hemophiliacs. Semin Hematol 25:219, 1988

289. Ratnoff OD, Menitove JE, Aster RH, Lederman MM: Coincident classic hemophilia and "idiopathic" thrombocytopenic purpura in patients under treatment with concentrates of antihemophilic factor (factor VIII). N Engl J Med 308:439, 1982

290. Saulsbury FT, Boyle RJ, Wykoff RF, Howard RH: Thrombocytopenia as the presenting manifestation of human T-lymphotropic virus type III infection in infants. J Pediatr 109:30–34, 1986

291. Labrune P, Blanche S, Catherine N et al: Human immunodeficiency virus-associated thrombocytopenia in infants. Acta Paediatr Scand 78:811, 1989

292. Rigaud M, Leibovitz E, Quee CS et al: Thrombocytopenia in children infected with human immunodeficiency virus: long-term follow-up and therapeutic considerations. J Acquir Immune Defic Syndr 5:450, 1992

293. Kaslow RA, Phair JP, Friedman HB et al: Infection with the human immunodeficiency virus: clinical manifestations and their relationship to immune deficiency. A report of the Multicenter AIDS Cohort Study. Ann Intern Med 107: 474, 1987

294. Murphy MF, Metcalfe P, Waters AH et al: Incidence and mechanism of neutropenia and thrombocytopenia in patients with human immunodeficiency virus infection. Br J Haematol 66:337, 1987

295. Peltier J-Y, Lambin P, Doinel C et al: Frequency and prognostic importance of thrombocytopenia in symptom-free HIV-infected individuals: a 5-year prospective study. AIDS 5:381, 1991

296. Mientjes GHC, van Amerijden EJC, Mulder JW et al: Prevalence of thrombocytopenia in HIV-infected and non-HIV infected drug users and homosexual men. Br J Haematol 82:615, 1992

297. Lima J, Ribera A, Garcia-Bragado F et al: Antiplatelet antibodies in primary infection by human immunodeficiency virus. Ann Intern Med 106:333, 1987

298. Oskenhendler E, Bierling P, Farcet JP et al: Response to therapy in 37 patients with HIV-related thrombocytopenic purpura. Br J Haematol 66:491, 1987

299. Finazzi G, Mannucci PM, Lazzarin A et al: Low incidence of bleeding from HIV-related thrombocytopenia in drug addicts and hemophiliacs: implications for therapeutic strategies. Eur J Haematol 45:82, 1990

300. Ragni MV, Bontempo FA, Myers DJ et al: Hemorrhagic sequelae of immune thrombocytopenic purpura in human immunodeficiency virus-infected hemophiliacs. Blood 75:1267, 1990

301. Ballem PJ, Belzberg A, Devine DV et al: Kinetic studies of the mechanism of the thrombocytopenia in patients with human immunodeficiency virus infection. N Engl J Med 327:1779, 1992

302. Bel-Ali Z, Dufour V, Najean Y: Platelet kinetics in human immunodeficiency virus induced thrombocytopenia. Am J Hematol 26:299, 1987

303. Schneider PA, Abrams DI, Rayner AA, Hahn DC: Immunodeficiency-associ-

ated thrombocytopenic purpura (IDTP): response to splenectomy. Arch Surg 122:1175, 1987

304. Ferguson CM: Splenectomy for immune thrombocytopenia related to human immunodeficiency virus. Surg Gynecol Obstet 167:300, 1988

305. Ravikumar TS, Allen JD, Bothe A, Steele G: Splenectomy. The treatment of choice for human immunodeficiency virus-related immune thrombocytopenia? Arch Surg 124:625, 1989

306. Costello C, Treacy M, Lai L: Treatment of immune thrombocytopenia in homosexual men. Scand J Haematol 36:507, 1986

307. Alonso M, Gossot D, Bourstyn E et al: Splenectomy in human immunodeficiency virus-related thrombocytopenia. Br J Surg 80:330, 1993

308. Tyler DS, Shaunak S, Bartlett JA, Inglehard JD: HIV-1-associated thrombocytopenia. Ann Surg 211:211, 1990

309. Oskenhendler E, Bierling P, Chevret S et al: Splenectomy is safe and effective in human immunodeficiency virus-related immune thrombocytopenia. Blood 82:29, 1993

310. Walsh CM, Nardi MA, Karpatkin S: On the mechanism of thrombocytopenic purpura in sexually active homosexual men. N Engl J Med 311:635, 1984

311. Karpatkin S, Nardi M: Autoimmune anti-HIV-1gp120 antibody with antiidiotype-like activity in sera and immune complexes of HIV-1-related immunologic thrombocytopenia. J Clin Invest 89:356, 1992

312. Magnac C, de Saint Martin J, Pidard D et al: Platelet antibodies in serum of patients with human immunodeficiency virus (HIV) infection. AIDS Res Hum Retroviruses 6:1443, 1990

313. Bettaieb A, Oskenhendler E, Fromont P et al: Immunochemical analysis of platelet autoantibodies in HIV-related thrombocytopenic purpura: a study of 68 patients. Br J Haematol 73:241, 1989

314. Bettaieb A, Fromont P, Louache F et al: Presence of cross-reactive antibody between human immunodeficiency virus (HIV) and platelet glycoproteins in HIV-related immune thrombocytopenic purpura. Blood 80:162, 1992

315. Zucker-Franklin D, Termin CS, Cooper MC: Structural changes in megakaryocytes of patients infected with the human immunodeficiency virus (HIV-1). Am J Pathol 134:1295, 1989

316. Bauer S, Khan A, Klein A, Starasoler L: Naked megakaryocyte nuclei as an indicator of human immunodeficiency virus infection. Arch Pathol Lab Med 116:1025, 1992

317. Koenig C, Sidhu GS, Schoentag RA: The platelet volume-number relationship in patients infected with the human immunodeficiency virus. Am J Clin Pathol 96:500, 1991

318. Nieuwenhuis HK, Sixma JJ: Thrombocytopenia and the neglected megakaryocyte. N Engl J Med 327:1812, 1992

319. Sakaguchi M, Sato T, Groopman JE: Human immunodeficiency virus infection of megakaryocytic cells. Blood 77:481, 1991

320. Monté D, Groux H, Raharinivo B et al: Productive human immunodeficiency virus-1 infection of megakaryocytic cells is enhanced by tumor necrosis factor alpha. Blood 79:2670, 1992

321. Rosenberg ZF, Fauci AS: Immunopathogenic mechanisms of HIV infection: cytokine induction of HIV expression. Immunol Today 11:176, 1990

322. Folks TM, Clouse KA, Justement JS: TNF induces expression of HIV in a chronically infected T-cell clone. Proc Natl Acad Sci USA 86:2365, 1989

323. Zucker-Franklin D, Cao Y: Megakaryocytes of human immunodeficiency virus-infected individuals express viral RNA. Proc Natl Acad Sci USA 5599:5595, 1989

324. Louache F, Bettaieb A, Henri A et al: Infection of megakaryocytes by human immunodeficiency virus in seropositive patients with immune thrombocytopenic purpura. Blood 78:1697, 1991

325. Kunzi MS, Groopman JE: Identification of a novel human immunodeficiency virus strain cytopathic to megakaryocytic cells. Blood 81:3336, 1993

326. Bloom EJ, Abrams DI, Rodgers G: Lupus anticoagulant in the acquired immunodeficiency syndrome. JAMA 256:491, 1986

327. Cohen AJ, Philips TM, Kessler CM: Circulating coagulation inhibitors in the acquired immunodeficiency syndrome. Ann Intern Med 104:175, 1986

328. Canoso RT, Zon LI, Groopman JE: Anticardiolipin antibodies associated with HTLV-III infection. Br J Haematol 65:495, 1987

329. Cohen H, Mackie IJ, Anagnostopoulos N et al: Lupus anticoagulant anticardiolipin antibodies, and human immunodeficiency virus in haemophilia. J Clin Pathol 42:629, 1989

330. Capel P, Janssens A, Clumeck N et al: Anticardiolipin antibodies (ACA) are most often not associated with lupus-like anticoagulant (LLAC) in human immunodeficiency virus (HIV) infection. Am J Hematol 37:234, 1991

331. Clyne LP, Yen Y, Kriz NS, Breitenstein MG: The lupus anticoagulant. High incidence of "negative" mixing studies in a human immunodeficiency virus-positive population. Arch Pathol Lab Med 117:595, 1993

332. Gold JE, Haubenstock A, Zalusky R: Lupus anticoagulants and AIDS. N Engl J Med 314:1252, 1986

333. LeFrere J-J, Gozin D, Modai J, Vittecoq D: Circulating anticoagulant in the acquired immunodeficiency syndrome. Ann Intern Med 107:429, 1987

334. Panzer S, Stain C, Hartl H et al: Anticardiolipin antibodies are elevated in HIV-1 infected haemophiliacs but do not predict for disease progression. Thromb Haemost 61:81, 1989

335. Intrator L, Oksenhendler E, Desforges L, Bierling P: Anticardiolipin antibodies in HIV infected patients with or without thrombocytopenic purpura. Br J Haematol 68:269, 1988

336. Kopelman RG, Zolla-Pazner S: Association of human immunodeficiency virus infection and autoimmune phenomena. Am J Med 84:82, 1988

337. Ndimbie OK, Raman BKS, Saeed SM: Lupus anticoagulant associated with specific inhibition of factor VII in a patient with AIDS. Am J Clin Pathol 91:491, 1989

338. Mueh JR, Kerbst KP, Rappaport SI: Thombosis in patients with lupus anticoagulant. Ann Intern Med 92:156, 1980

339. Carreras LO, Vermylen JB: 'Lupus' anticoagulant and thrombosis: possible inhibition of prostacyclin formation. Thromb Haemost 48:38, 1982

340. Lubbe WF, Butler WS, Palmer SJ, Liggins GC: Lupus anticoagulant in pregnancy. Br J Obstet Gynaecol 91:357, 1984

341. DiPrima MA, Sorice M, Vullo V et al: Anticardiolipin antibody in the acquired immunodeficiency syndrome: a marker of Pneumocystis carinii infection? J Infect 18:100, 1989

342. Lafeuillade A, Alssi MC, Poizot-Martin I et al: Protein S deficiency and HIV infection. N Engl J Med 1220, 1991

343. Stahl CP, Wideman CS, Spira TJ et al: Protein S deficiency in men with long-term human immunodeficiency virus infection. Blood 81:1801, 1993

344. Bissuel F, Berruyer M, Causse X et al: Acquired protein S deficiency: correlation with advanced disease in HIV-1-infected patients. J Acquir Immune Defic Syndr 5:484, 1992

345. Lafeuillade A, Alessi MD, Poizot-Martin I et al: Endothelial cell dysfunction in HIV infection. J Acquir Immune Defic Syndr 5:127, 1992

346. Masur H, Michelis MA, Greene JB et al: An outbreak of community acquired Pneumocystis carinii pneumonia. N Engl J Med 305:1431, 1981

347. Siegal FP, Lopez C, Hammer GS et al: Severe acquired immunodeficiency in male homosexuals, manifested by chronic perianal ulcerative herpes simplex lesions. N Engl J Med 305:1439, 1981

348. Friedman-Kien AE, Laubenstein LJ, Rubenstein P et al: Disseminated Kaposi's sarcoma in homosexual men. Ann Intern Med 96:693, 1982

349. Stahl RE, Friedman-Kien A, Dubin R et al: Immunologic abnormalities in homosexual men. Relationship to Kaposi's sarcoma. Am J Med 73:171, 1982

350. Jacobson DL, McCutchan JA, Spechko PL et al: The evolution of lymphadenopathy and hypergammaglobulinemia are evidence of early and sustained polyclonal B lymphocyte activation during human immunodeficiency virus infection. J Infect Dis 163:240, 1991

351. Crapper RM, Deam DR, Mackay IR: Paraproteins in homosexual men with HIV infection. Lack of association with abnormal clinical or immunologic findings. Am J Clin Pathol 88:348, 1987

352. LeFrere J-J, Fine J-M, Lambin P et al: Monoclonal gammopathies in asymptomatic HIV-seropositive patients. Clin Chem 33:1697, 1987

353. Kouns DM, Marty AM, Sharpe RW: Oligoclonal bands in serum protein electrophoretograms of individuals with human immunodeficiency virus antibodies. JAMA 256:2343, 1986

354. Papadopoulos NM, Lane HC, Costello R et al: Oligoclonal immunoglobulins in patients with the acquired immunodeficiency syndrome. Clin Immunol Immunopathol 35:43, 1985

355. Heriot K, Hallquist AE, Tomar RH: Paraproteinemia in patients with acquired immunodeficiency syndrome (AIDS) or lymphadenopathy syndrome (LAS). Clin Chem 31:1224, 1985

356. Sala PG, Mazzolini S, Tonutti E, Bramezza M: Monoclonal immunoglobulins in HTLV-III-positive sera. Clin Chem 32:574, 1986

357. Ng VL, Chen KH, Hwang KM et al: The clinical significance of human immunodeficiency virus type 1-associated paraproteins. Blood 74:2471, 1989

358. Rapoport P, Cart-Tanneur E, Fischer AM et al: Monoclonal immunoglobulins in haemophiliac patients with HIV infection. Thromb Haemost 65:636, 1991

359. Fine JM, Lambin P, Leroux P: Frequency of monoclonal gammopathy (M components) in 13,400 sera from blood donors. Vox Sang 23:336, 1972

360. Yu J-R, Lennette ET, Karpatkin S: Anti-F(ab')2 antibodies in thrombocytopenic patients at risk for acquired immunodeficiency syndrome. J Clin Invest 77:1756, 1986

361. Karpatkin S, Nardi M, Lennette ET et al: Anti-human immunodeficiency virus type I antibody complexes on platelets of seropositive thrombocytopenic homosexuals and narcotic addicts. Proc Natl Acad Sci USA 85:9763, 1988

362. Martin CM, Matlow AG, Chew E et al: Hyperviscosity syndrome in a patient with acquired immunodeficiency syndrome. Arch Intern Med 149:1435, 1989

363. Beverley P, Houston S, Latif AS: HIV infection associated with the plasma hyperviscosity syndrome: a report of two fatal cases. AIDS 4:1302, 1990

364. Hague RA, Eden OB, Yap PL et al: Hyperviscosity in HIV infected children—a potential hazard during intravenous immunoglobulin therapy. Blut 61:66, 1990

365. Israel AM, Koziner B, Straus DJ: Plasmacytoma and the acquired immunodeficiency syndrome. Ann Intern Med 99:635, 1983

366. Thomas MAB, Isbister JP, Ibels LS et al: IgA kappa multiple myeloma and lymphadenopathy syndrome associated with AIDS virus infection. Aust N Z J Med 16:402, 1986

367. Shokunbi WA, Okpala IE, Shokunbi MT et al: Multiple myeloma co-existing with HIV-1 infection in a 65-year-old Nigerian man. AIDS 5:115, 1991

368. Konrad RJ, Kricka LJ, Goodman DBP et al: Myeloma-associated paraprotein directed against the HIV-1 p24 antigen in an HIV-1 seropositive patient. N Engl J Med 328:1817, 1993

369. Cozzi PJ, Abu-Jawdeh GM et al: Amyloidosis in association with human immunodeficiency virus infection. Clin Infect Dis 14:189, 1991

370. Bray GL, Kroner BL, Arkin S et al: Loss of high-responder inhibitors in patients with severe hemophilia A and human immunodeficiency virus type 1 infection: a report from the multi-center hemophilia cohort study. Am J Hematol 42:375, 1993

371. Ng VL, Hwang KM, Reyes GR et al: High titer anti-HIV antibody reactivity associated with a paraprotein spike in a homosexual male with AIDS related complex. Blood 71:1397, 1988

372. Pluda JM, Venzon DJ, Tosato G et al: Parameters affecting the development of non-Hodgkin's lymphoma in patients with severe human immunodeficiency virus infection receiving antiretroviral therapy. J Clin Oncol 6:1099, 1993

373. Botti AC, Hyde P, DiPillo F: Thrombotic thrombocytopenic purpura in a patient who subsequently developed the acquired immunodeficiency syndrome (AIDS). Ann Intern Med 109:242, 1988

374. Routy J-P, Beaulieu R, Monte M et al: Immunologic thrombocytopenia followed by thrombotic thrombocytopenic purpura in two HIV-1 patients. Am J Hematol 38:327, 1991

375. Thompson CE, Damon LE, Ries CA, Linker CA: Thrombotic microangiopathies in the 1980s: clinical features, response to treatment, and the impact of the human immunodeficiency virus epidemic. Blood 80:1890, 1992

376. Veenstra J, van der Lelie J, Mulder JW, Reiss P: Low-grade thrombotic thrombocytopenic purpura associated with HIV-1 infection. Br J Haematol 83:346, 1993

377. Charesse C, Michelet C, LeTulzo Y et al: Thrombotic thrombocytopenic purpura with the acquired immunodeficiency syndrome: a pathologically documented case report. Am J Kidney Dis 17:80, 1991

378. Salem G, Terebelo H, Raman S: Human immunodeficiency virus associated with thrombotic thrombocytopenic purpura. Successful treatment with zidovudine. South Med J 84:483, 1991

379. Kwann HC, Pierre RV, Potter EV, Gallo GF: The nature of vascular lesions in thrombotic thrombocytopenic purpura. Blood 28:986, 1966

380. Lian EC: Pathogenesis of thrombotic thrombocytopenic purpura. Semin Hematol 24:82, 1987

381. Moake JL, Rudy CK, Troll JH et al: Unusually large plasma factor VIII: von Willebrand factor multimers in chronic relapsing thrombotic thrombocytopenic purpura. N Engl J Med 307:1432, 1982

382. Sporn LA, Marder VJ, Wagner DD: von Willebrand factor released from Wiebel-Palade bodies binds more avidly to extracellular matrix than that secreted constitutively. Blood 69:1531, 1987

383. Kelton JG, Moore J, Santos A, Sheridan D: Detection of a platelet-agglutinating factor in thrombotic thrombocytopenic purpura. Ann Intern Med 101:589, 1984

384. Lian EC, Harkness DR, Byrnes JJ et al: The presence of a platelet aggregating factor in the plasma of patients with thrombotic thrombocytopenic purpura and its inhibition by normal plasma. Blood 53:333, 1979

385. Boccia RV, Gelman EP, Baker CC et al: A hemolytic-uremic syndrome with the acquired immunodeficiency syndrome. Ann Intern Med 101:716, 1984

386. Esforzado N, Poch E, Almirall J et al: Hemolytic uremic syndrome associated with HIV infection. AIDS 5:1041, 1991

387. Dixon AC, Kwock DW, Nakamura JM et al: Thrombotic thrombocytopenic purpura and human T-lymphotropic virus, type 1 (HTLV-I). Ann Intern Med 110:93, 1989

388. Höllsberg P, Hafler DA: Pathogenesis of diseases induced by human lymphotropic virus type I infection. N Engl J Med 328:1173, 1993

389. Palker TJ: Human T-cell lymphotropic viruses: review and prospects for antiviral therapy. Antiviral Chem Chemother 3:127, 1992

390. Cohen PR: Porphyria cutanea tarda in human immunodeficiency virus-seropositive men: case report and literature review. J Acquir Immune Defic Syndr 4:1112, 1991

391. Scannell KA: Porphyria cutanea tarda and acquired immunodeficiency syndrome: case reports and literature review. Arch Dermatol 126:1658, 1990

392. Conlan MG, Hoots WK: Porphyria cutanea tarda in association with human immunodeficiency virus infection in a hemophiliac. J Am Acad Dermatol 26:857, 1992

393. Lafeuillade A, Dhiver C, Martin I et al: Porphyria cutanea tarda associate with HIV infection. AIDS 4:924, 1990

394. deSalamanca RE, Sanchez-Perez J, Diaz-Mora F et al: Porphyria cutane tarda associated with HIV infection: are those conditions pathogenetical related or merely coincidental? AIDS 4:926, 1990

395. Boisseau A-M, Couzigou P, Forestier J-F et al: Porphyria cutanea tarda associated with human immunodeficiency virus infection. Dermatologica 18: 155, 1991

396. Itescu S, Dalton J, Zhang H-Z, Winchester R: Tissue infiltration in a CD lymphocytosis syndrome associated with human immunodeficiency virus 1 infection has the phenotypic appearance of an antigenically driven response. J Clin Invest 91:2216, 1993

397. Itescu S, Brancato LJ, Buxbaum J et al: A diffuse infiltrative CD8 lymphocytosis syndrome in human immunodeficiency virus (HIV) infection: a host immune response associated with HLA-DR5. Ann Intern Med 112:3, 1990

398. Buchanan JG, Goldwater PN, Somerfield SD, Tobias MI: Mononucleosis-like syndrome associated with acute AIDS retrovirus infection. N Z Med J 9: 405, 1986

399. Geller SA, Muller R, Greenberg ML, Siegal FP: Acquired immunodeficienc syndrome. Distinctive features of bone marrow biopsies. Arch Pathol Lab Med 109:138, 1985

400. Kurtzman GJ, Cohen BJ, Field AM et al: The immune response to B19 parvovirus and an antibody defect in persistent viral infection. J Clin Invest 84 1114, 1989

401. Mitchell SA, Welch JM, Weston-Smith S et al: Parvovirus infection and anaemia in a patient with AIDS: case report. Genitourin Med 66:95, 1990

402. Bowman CA, Cohen BJ, Norfolk DR, Lacey CJN: Red cell aplasia associated with human parvovirus B19 and HIV infection: failure to respond clinically to intravenous immunoglobulin. AIDS 4:1038, 1990

403. DeMayolo JA, Temple JD: Pure red cell aplasia due to parvovirus B19 infection in a man with HIV infection. South Med J 83:1480, 1990

404. Kurtzman G, Frickhofer N, Kimball J et al: Pure red-cell aplasia of 10 years duration due to persistent parvovirus B19 infection and its cure with immunoglobulin therapy. N Engl J Med 321:519, 1989

405. Kurtzman GJ, Ozawa K, Cohen B et al: Chronic bone marrow failure due to persistent B19 parvovirus infection. N Engl J Med 317:287, 1987

406. Kurtzman G, Cohen B, Meyers P et al: Persistent B19 parvovirus infection as a cause of severe chronic anemia in children with acute lymphoblastic leukemia. Lancet 2:1159, 1988

407. Young N: Hematologic and hematopoietic consequences of B19 parvovirus infection. Semin Hematol 25:159, 1988

408. Hromas RA, Murray JL: Bone marrow in the acquired immunodeficiency syndrome. Ann Intern Med 101:877, 1984

409. Folks TM: Human immunodeficiency virus in bone marrow: still more questions than answers. Blood 77:1625, 1991

410. DiCarlo EF, Amberson JB, Metroka CE et al: Malignant lymphoma and the acquired immunodeficiency syndrome. Evaluation of 30 cases using a working formulation. Arch Pathol Lab Med 110:1012, 1986

411. Karcher DS: Clinically unsuspected Hodgkin disease presenting initially in the bone marrow of patients infected with the human immunodeficiency virus. Cancer 71:1235, 1993

412. Turbat-Herrera EA, Hancock C, Cabello-Inchausti B, Herrera GA: Plasma cell hyperplasia and monoclonal paraproteinemia in human immunodeficiency virus-infected patients. Arch Pathol Lab Med 117:497, 1993

413. Solis OG, Belmonte AH, Ramaswamy G, Tchertkoff V: Pseudogaucher cells in mycobacterium avium complex infections in acquired immune deficiency syndrome (AIDS). Am J Clin Pathol 85:233, 1986

414. Bello JL, Burgaleta C, Magallon M et al: Hematological abnormalities in hemophilic patients with human immunodeficiency virus infection. Am J Hematol 33:230, 1990

415. Lortholary A, Raffi F, Aubertin P, Barrier JH: HIV-associated haemophagocytic syndrome. Lancet 336:1128, 1990

416. Sasadeusz J, Buchanan M, Speed B: Reactive haemophagocytic syndrome in human immunodeficiency virus infection. J Infect 20:65, 1990

417. Little BJ, Spivak JL, Quinn TC, Mann RB: Case report: Kaposi's sarcoma with bone marrow involvement: occurrence in a patient with the acquired immunodeficiency syndrome. Am J Med Sci 292:44, 1986

418. Ahluwalia C, Bernstein-Singer M, Beckstead J, Brynes RK: Kaposi's sarcoma in the bone marrow of a patient with AIDS. Am J Clin Pathol 95:561, 1990

419. Bishburg E, Eng RHK, Smith SM, Kapila R: Yield of bone marrow culture in the diagnosis of infectious diseases in patients with acquired immunodeficiency syndrome. J Clin Microbiol 24:312, 1986

420. Horsburgh CR, Mason HG, Farhi DC, Iseman ND: Disseminated infection with mycobacterium avium-complex. A report of 13 cases and a review of the literature. Medicine 64:36, 1985

421. Northfelt DW, Mayer A, Kaplan LD et al: The usefulness of diagnostic bone marrow examination in patients with human immunodeficiency virus (HIV) infection. J Acquir Immune Defic Syndr 4:659, 1991

22. Nichols L, Florentine B, Lewis W et al: Bone marrow examination for the diagnosis of mycobacterial and fungal infections in the acquired immunodeficiency syndrome. Arch Pathol Lab Med 115:1125, 1991

23. Poropatich CO, Labriola AM, Tuazon CU: Acid-fast smear and culture of respiratory secretions, bone marrow, and stools as predictors of disseminated mycobacterium avium complex infection. J Clin Microbiol 25:929, 1987

24. Wong KF, Ma SK, Chan JKC, Lam KW: Acquired immunodeficiency syndrome presenting as marrow cryptococcosis. Am J Hematol 42:392, 1993

25. Milam MW, Balerdi MJ, Toney JF et al: Epithelioid angiomatosis secondary to disseminated cat scratch disease involving the bone marrow and skin in a patient with acquired immune deficiency syndrome: a case report. Am J Med 88:180, 1990

26. Heyman MR, Rasmussen P: *Pneumocystis carinii* involvement of the bone marrow in acquired immunodeficiency syndrome. Am J Clin Pathol 87:780, 1987

27. Rossi J-F, Dubois A, Bengler C et al: *Pneumocystis carinii* in bone marrow. Ann Intern Med 102:868, 1985

28. Raviglione MC, Garner GR, Mullen MP: *Pneumocystis carinii* in bone marrow. Ann Intern Med 109:253, 1988

29. Rossi J-F, Eledjam J-J, Delage A et al: *Pneumocystis carinii* infection of bone marrow in patients with malignant lymphoma and acquired immunodeficiency syndrome. Arch Intern Med 150:450, 1990

30. Unger PD, Stauchen JA: Hodgkin's disease in AIDS complex patients. Cancer 58:821, 1986

31. Yarchoan R, Mitsuya H, Myers CE, Broder S: Clinical pharmacology of 3'-dideoxythymidine (zidovudine) and related dideoxynucleosides. N Engl J Med 321:726, 1989

32. Yarchoan R, Pluda JM, Perno C-F et al: Anti-retroviral therapy of human immunodeficiency virus infection: current strategies and challenges for the future. Blood 78:859, 1991

33. Hirsch MS, D'Aquila RT: Therapy for human immunodeficiency virus infection. N Engl J Med 328:1686, 1983

34. Furman PA, Fyfe JA, St Clair MH et al: Phosphorylation of 3'-azido-3'-deoxythymidine and selective interaction with human immunodeficiency virus reverse transcriptase. Proc Natl Acad Sci USA 83:8333, 1986

35. Waqar MA, Evans MJ, Manly KF et al: Effects of 2',3'-dideoxynucleosides on mammalian cells and viruses. J Cell Physiol 121:402, 1984

36. Fischl MA, Parker CB, Pettinelli C et al: A randomized controlled trial of a reduced daily dose of zidovudine in patients with the acquired immunodeficiency syndrome. N Engl J Med 323:1009, 1990

37. Schmitt FA, Bigley JW, McKinnis R et al: Neuropsychological outcome of zidovudine (AZT) treatment of patients with AIDS and AIDS-related complex. N Engl J Med 319:1573, 1988

38. Yarchoan R, Berg G, Brouwers P et al: Response of human immunodeficiency-virus associated neurological disease to 3'-azido-3'-deoxythymidine. Lancet 1:132, 1987

39. Pizzo PA, Eddy J, Falloon J et al: Effect of continuous intravenous infusion of zidovudine (AZT) in children with symptomatic HIV infection. N Engl J Med 319:889, 1988

40. Volberding PA, Lagakos SW, Koch MA et al: Zidovudine in asymptomatic human immunodeficiency virus infection. A controlled trial in persons with fewer than 500 CD4-positive cells per cubic millimeter. N Engl J Med 322:941, 1990

41. Cooper DA, Gatell JM, Kroon S et al: Zidovudine in persons with asymptomatic HIV infection and CD4+ cell counts greater than 400 per cubic millimeter. N Engl J Med 329:297, 1993

42. Hamilton JD, Hartigan PM, Simberkoff MS et al: A controlled trial of early versus late treatment with zidovudine in symptomatic human immunodeficiency virus infection. Results of the Veterans Affairs Cooperative Study. N Engl J Med 326:437, 1992

43. Aboulker JP, Swart AM: Preliminary analysis of the Concorde trial. Lancet 341:889, 1993

44. Schnittman SM, Greenhouse JJ, Psallidopoulos MC et al: Increasing viral burden in CD4+ T cells from patients with human immunodeficiency virus (HIV) infection reflects rapidly progressive immunosuppression and clinical disease. Ann Intern Med 113:438, 1993

45. Pluda JM, Mitsuya H, Yarchoan R: Hematologic effects of AIDS therapies. Hematol Oncol Clin North Am 5:229, 1991

46. Yarchoan R, Klecker RW, Weinhold KJ et al: Administration of 3'-azido-3'deoxythymidine, an inhibitor of HTLV-III/LAV replication to patients with AIDS or AIDS-related complex. Lancet 1:575, 1986

47. Kornhauser DM, Petty BG, Hendrix CW et al: Probenecid and zidovudine metabolism. Lancet 2:473, 1989

48. Dainiak N, Worthington M, Riordan MA et al: 3'-azido-3'-deoxythymidine (AZT) inhibits proliferation in vitro of human haematopoietic progenitor cells. Br J Haematol 69:299, 1988

49. Fischl M, Galpine JE, Levine JD et al: Recombinant human erythropoietin for patients with AIDS treated with zidovudine. N Engl J Med 322:1488, 1990

450. Miles SA, Mitsuyasu RT, Moreno J et al: Combined therapy with recombinant granulocyte colony-stimulating factor and erythropoietin decreases hematologic toxicity from zidovudine. Blood 77:2109, 1991

451. Pluda JM, Yarchoan R, Smith PD et al: Subcutaneous recombinant granulocyte-macrophage colony-stimulating factor used as a single agent and in an alternating regimen with azidothymidine in leukopenic patients with severe human immunodeficiency virus infection. Blood 76:463, 1990

452. Butler KM, Husson RN, Balis FM et al: Dideoxyinosine in children with symptomatic human immunodeficiency virus infection. N Engl J Med 324:137, 1991

453. Kahn JO, Lagakos SW, Richman DD et al: A controlled trial comparing continued zidovudine with didanosine in human immunodeficiency virus infection. N Engl J Med 327:581, 1992

454. Merigan TC, Skowron G, Bozzette S et al: Circulating p24 antigen levels and responses to dideoxycytidine in human immunodeficiency virus (HIV) infections: a phase I and II study. Ann Intern Med 110:189, 1989

455. Yarchoan R, Perno CF, Thomas RV et al: Phase I studies of 2',3'-dideoxycytidine in severe human immunodeficiency virus infection as a single agent and alternating with zidovudine (AZT). Lancet 1:76, 1988

456. Yarchoan R, Mitsuya H, Thomas RV et al: In vivo activity against HIV and favorable toxicity profile of 2',3'-dideoxyinosine. Science 245:412, 1989

457. Lambert JS, Seidlin M, Reichman RC et al: 2',3'-Dideoxyinosine (ddI) in patients with the acquired immunodeficiency syndrome or AIDS-related complex. A phase I trial. N Engl J Med 322:1333, 1990

458. Schacter LP, Rozencweig M, Beltangady M et al: Effects of therapy with didanosine on hematologic parameters in patients with advanced human immunodeficiency virus disease. Blood 80:2969, 1992

459. Grob PM, Wu JC, Cohen KA et al: Nonnucleoside inhibitors of HIV-1 reverse transcriptase: nevirapine as a prototype drug. AIDS Res Hum Retroviruses 8:145, 1992

460. Romero DL, Busso M, Tan C-K et al: Nonnucleoside reverse transcriptase inhibitors that potently and specifically block human immunodeficiency virus type 1 replication. Proc Natl Acad Sci USA 88:806, 1991

461. Pauwels R, Andries K, Desmyter J et al: Potent and selective inhibition of HIV-1 replication in vitro by a novel series of TIBO derivatives. Nature 343:470, 1990

462. Merluzzi MJ, Hargrave KD, Labadia M et al: Inhibition of HIV-1 replication by a nonnucleoside reverse transcriptase inhibitor. Science 250:1411, 1990

463. Nunberg JH, Schleif WA, Boots EJ et al: Viral resistance to human immunodeficiency virus type 1-specific pyridinone reverse transcriptase inhibitors. J Virol 65:4887, 1991

464. Richman DD: HIV drug resistance. AIDS Res Hum Retroviruses 8:1065, 1992

465. Merigan TC: Treatment of AIDS with combinations of antiretroviral agents. Am J Med, suppl. 4A. 90:8S, 1991

466. Meng TC, Fischl MA, Boota AM et al: Combination therapy with zidovudine and dideoxycytidine in patients with advanced human immunodeficiency virus infection. Ann Intern Med 116:13, 1992

467. Fauci A: Combination therapy for HIV infection: getting closer. Ann Intern Med 116:85, 1992

468. Krown SE, Paredes J, Bundow D et al: Interferon-α, zidovudine, and granulocyte-macrophage colony-stimulating factor: a phase I AIDS clinical trials group study in patients with Kaposi's sarcoma associated with AIDS. J Clin Oncol 10:1344, 1992

469. Scadden DT, Bering HA, Levine JD et al: Granulocyte-macrophage colony-stimulating factor mitigates the neutropenia of combined interferon alfa and zidovudine treatment of acquired immune deficiency syndrome-associated Kaposi's sarcoma. J Clin Oncol 9:802, 1991

470. Mitsuyasu RT: Use of recombinant interferons and hematopoietic growth factors in patients infected with human immunodeficiency virus. Rev Infect Dis 13:979, 1991

471. Scadden DT: The clinical applications of colony-stimulating factors in acquired immunodeficiency syndrome. Semin Hematol 29:33, 1992

472. Miles SA, Golde DW, Mitsuyasu RT: The use of hematopoietic hormones in HIV infection and AIDS-related malignancies. Hematol Oncol Clin North Am 5:267, 1991

473. Groopman JE, Feder D: Hematopoietic growth factors in AIDS. Semin Oncol 19:408, 1992

474. Gaffuri L, Repetto L, Rossi E et al: Haemolitic anaemia with positive cryoglobulin test in a HIV positive man. Eur J Cancer 27:304, 1991

475. Blum RN, Miller LA, Gaggini LC, Cohn DL: Comparative trial of dapsone versus trimethoprim/sulfamethoxazole for primary prophylaxis of *Pneumocystis carinii* pneumonia. J Acquir Immune Defic Syndr 5:341, 1991

476. Kemper CA, Tucker RM, Lang OS et al: Low-dose dapsone prophylaxis of *Pneumocystis carinii* pneumonia in AIDS and AIDS-related complex. AIDS 4:1145, 1990

477. Henry DH, Jemsek JG, Levin AS et al: Recombinant human erythropoietin and the treatment of anemia in patients with AIDS or advanced ARC not receiving ZDV. J Acquir Immune Defic Syndr 5:847, 1992

478. Eschbach JW, Egrie JC, Downing MR: Correction of the anemia of end-stage renal disease with recombinant human erythropoietin. N Engl J Med 316:73, 1987

479. Casati S, Passerini P, Campise MR et al: Benefits and risks of protracted treatment with human recombinant erythropoietin in patients having haemodialysis. BMJ 295:1017, 1987

480. Miles SA, Mitsuyasu RT, Lee K et al: Recombinant human granulocyte colony-stimulating factor increases circulating burst forming unit-erythron and red blood cell production in patients with severe human immunodeficiency virus infection. Blood 75:2137, 1990

481. Merigan TC: Treatment of cytomegalovirus infection in the AIDS patient. Transplant Proc, 3 suppl. 3. 23:122, 1991

482. Levine JD, Allan JD, Tessitore JH et al: Recombinant human granulocyte-macrophage colony-stimulating factor ameliorates zidovudine-induced neutropenia in patients with acquired immunodeficiency syndrome (AIDS)/AIDS-related complex. Blood 78:3148, 1991

483. Grossberg HS, Bonnem EM, Buhles WC: GM-CSF with ganciclovir for the treatment of CMV retinitis in AIDS. N Engl J Med 320:1560, 1989

484. Kaplan LD, Kahn JO, Crowe S et al: Clinical and virologic effects of recombinant human granulocyte-macrophage colony-stimulating factor in patients receiving chemotherapy for human immunodeficiency virus-associated non-Hodgkin's lymphoma: results of a randomized trial. J Clin Oncol 9:929, 1991

485. Israel RJ, Levine JD: Granulocyte-macrophage colony-stimulating factor and azidothymidine in patients with acquired immunodeficiency syndrome. Blood 77:2085, 1991

486. Perno C-F, Yarchoan R, Cooney DA et al: Replication of human immunodeficiency virus in monocytes. Granulocyte macrophage colony-stimulating factor (GM-CSF) potentiates viral production yet enhances the antiviral effect mediated by 3'-azido-2'3'-deoxythymidine (AZT) and other dideoxynucleoside congeners of thymidine. J Exp Med 169:933, 1989

487. Perno C-F, Cooney DA, Gao W-Y et al: Effects of bone marrow stimulatory cytokines on human immunodeficiency virus replication and the antiviral activity of dideoxynucleosides in cultures of monocytes/macrophages. Blood 80:995, 1992

488. Nielsen H, Kharazmi A, Faber V: Blood monocyte and neutrophil functions in the acquired immunodeficiency syndrome. Scand J Immunol 24:291, 1986

489. Ellis M, Gupta S, Galant S et al: Impaired neutrophil function in patients with AIDS or AIDS-related complex: a comprehensive evaluation. J Infect Dis 158:1268, 1988

490. Murphy PM, Lane HC, Fauci AS, Gallin JI: Impairment of neutrophil bactericidal capacity in patients with AIDS. J Infect Dis 158:627, 1988

491. Lazzarin A, Uberti Foppa C, Galli M et al: Impairment of polymorphonuclear leucocyte function in patients with acquired immunodeficiency syndrome and with lymphadenopathy syndrome. Clin Exp Immunol 65:105, 1986

492. Roilides E, Mertins S, Eddy J et al: Impairment of neutrophil chemotactic and bactericidal function in children infected with human immunodeficiency virus type 1 and partial reversal after in vitro exposure to granulocyte-macrophage colony-stimulating factor. J Pediatr 117:531, 1990

493. Baldwin GC, Gasson JC, Quan SG et al: Granulocyte-macrophage colony-stimulating factor enhances neutrophil function in acquired immunodeficiency syndrome patients. Proc Natl Acad Sci USA 85:2763, 1988

494. Rosenfelt FP, Rosenbloom BE, Weinstein IM: Immune thrombocytopenia in homosexual men. Ann Intern Med 104:583, 1986

495. Bussel JB, Haimi JS: Isolated thrombocytopenia in patients infected with HIV: treatment with intravenous gammaglobulin. Am J Hematol 28:79, 1988

496. Pollak AN, Janinis J, Green D: Successful intravenous immune globulin therapy for human immunodeficiency virus-associated thrombocytopenia. Arch Intern Med 148:695, 1988

497. Tertian G, Risler N, Lebras P et al: Intravenous gammaglobulin treatment for thrombocytopenic purpura in patients with human immunodeficiency virus (HIV) infection. Eur J Haematol 39:180, 1987

498. Beard J, Savidge GF: High-dose intravenous immunoglobulin and splenectomy for treatment of HIV-related immune thrombocytopenia in patients with severe haemophilia. Br J Haematol 68:303, 1988

499. Rarick MU, Montgomery T, Groshen S et al: Intravenous immunoglobulin in the treatment of human immunodeficiency virus-related thrombocytopenia. Am J Hematol 38:261, 1991

500. Biniek R, Malessa R, Brockmeyer NH, Luboldt W: Anti-Rh(D) immunoglobulin for AIDS-related thrombocytopenia. Lancet 2:627, 1986

501. Cattaneo M, Gringeri A, Capitanio AM et al: Anti-D immunoglobulins for treatment of HIV-related immune thrombocytopenic purpura. Blood 73:357, 1989

502. Oskenhendler E, Bierling P, Brossard Y et al: Anti RH immunoglobulin therapy for human immunodeficiency virus-related immune thrombocytopenic purpura. Blood 71:1499, 1988

503. Durand JM, Lefévre P, Hovette et al: Dapsone for thrombocytopenic purpura related to human immunodeficiency virus infection. Am J Med 90:675, 199

504. Mintzer DM, Real FX, Jovino L, Krown SE: Treatment of Kaposi's sarcoma and thrombocytopenia with vincristine in patients with the acquired immunodeficiency syndrome. Ann Intern Med 102:200, 1985

505. Soubrane C, Tourani JM, Andrieu JM et al: Biologic response to anti-CD1 monoclonal antibody therapy in a human immunodeficiency virus-related immune thrombocytopenic purpura patient. Blood 81:15, 1993

506. Leissinger CA, Andes WA: Role of splenectomy in the management of hemophilic patients with human immunodeficiency virus-associated immunopathic thrombocytopenic purpura. Am J Hematol 40:207, 1992

507. Needleman SW, Sorace J, Poussin-Rosillo H: Low-dose splenic irradiation in the treatment of autoimmune thrombocytopenia in HIV-infected patients. Ann Intern Med 116:310, 1992

508. Gottlieb MS, Wolfe PR, Chafey S: Case report: response of AIDS-related thrombocytopenia to intravenous oral azidothymidine (3'-azido-3'-deoxy thymidine). AIDS Res Hum Retroviruses 3:109, 1987

509. The Swiss Group for Clinical Studies on the Acquired Immunodeficiency Syndrome (AIDS): Zidovudine for the treatment of thrombocytopenia associated with human immunodeficiency virus (HIV). A prospective study. Ann Intern Med 109:718, 1988

510. Flegg PJ, Jones ME, MacCallum LR et al: The effect of zidovudine on platelet count. BMJ 298:1074, 1989

511. Hymes KB, Greene JB, Karpatkin S: The effect of azidothymidine on HIV-related thrombocytopenia. N Engl J Med 318:516, 1988

512. Pottage JC, Benson CA, Spear JB et al: Treatment of human immunodeficiency virus-related thrombocytopenia with zidovudine. JAMA 260:3045, 1988

513. Rarick MU, Espina B, Montgomery T et al: The long-term use of zidovudine in patients with severe immune-mediated thrombocytopenia secondary to infection with HIV. AIDS 5:1357, 1991

513a. Butler KM, Husson RN, Balis FM et al: Dideoxyinosine in children with symptomatic human immunodeficiency virus infection. N Engl J Med 324:137, 1991

513b. Piketty C, Gilquin J, Kazatchkine MD: Successful treatment of HIV-related thrombocytopenia with didanosine (ddI). J Acquir Immune Defic Syndr 7:521, 1994

513c. Pechere M, Samii K, Hirschel B: HIV-related thrombocytopenia. N Engl J Med 328:1785, 1993

514. Ellis ME, Neal KR, Leen CLS, Newland AC: Alfa-2a recombinant interferon in HIV-associated thrombocytopenia. BMJ 295:1519, 1987

515. Lever AML, Brook MG, Yap I, Thomas HC: Treatment of thrombocytopenia with alfa interferon. BMJ 295:1519, 1987

516. Murphy KP, Stein MD, D'Amico RP: Correction of HIV-associated thrombocytopenia with low doses of interferon alfa. South Med J 85:557, 1992

517. Daniel MD, Kirchhoff F, Czajak SC et al: Protective effects of a live attenuated SIV vaccine with a deletion in the nef gene. Science 258:1938, 1992

518. Haynes BF: Scientific and social issues of human immunodeficiency virus vaccine development. Science 260:1279, 1993

519. Meek TD, Lambert DM, Dreyer GM et al: Inhibition of HIV-1 protease in infected T-lymphocytes by synthetic peptide analogues. Nature 343:90, 1990

520. Lambert DM, Petteway SR Jr, McDanal CE et al: Human immunodeficiency virus type 1 protease inhibitors irreversibly block infectivity of purified virions from chronically infected cells. Antimicrob Agents Chemother 36:982, 1992

521. Malim MH, Bohnlein S, Hauber J, Cullen BR: Functional dissection of the HIV-1 rev trans-activator-derivation of a trans-dominant repressor of rev function. Cell 58:205, 1989

522. Green M, Ishino M, Loewenstein PM: Mutational analysis of HIV-1 tat minimal domain peptides: identification of trans-dominant mutants that suppress HIV-1-driven gene expression. Cell 58:215, 1989

523. Hsu MC, Schutt AD, Holly M et al: Inhibition of HIV replication in acute and chronic infections in vitro by a tat antagonist. Science 254:1799, 1991

524. Malim MH, Freimuth WW, Liu J et al: Stable expression of transdominant rev protein in human T cells inhibits human immunodeficiency virus replication. J Exp Med 176:1197, 1992

525. Rossi JJ, Elkins D, Zaia JA, Sullivan S: Ribozymes as anti-HIV-1 therapeutic agents: principles, applications, and problems. AIDS Res Hum Retroviruses 8:183, 1992

526. Heidenreich O, Eckstein F: Hammerhead ribozyme-mediated cleavage of the long terminal repeat RNA of human immunodeficiency virus type 1. J Biol Chem 267:1904, 1992

527. Rhodes A, James W: Inhibition of heterologous strains of HIV by antisense RNA. AIDS 5:145, 1991

528. Johnston JI, Hoth DF: Present status and future prospects for HIV therapies. Science 260:1286, 1993

SPECIAL TESTS AND PROCEDURES IN HEMATOLOGY

Part X

Preparation and Interpretation of Peripheral Blood Smears

156

Jean A. Shafer

INTRODUCTION

Examination of the well-prepared and well-stained blood smear is one of the most efficient and important initial laboratory tests in the evaluation of a patient with an abnormal blood count. In addition, in some instances, despite a normal blood count, the blood smear morphology reveals important diagnostic or therapy-related information. This chapter discusses proper blood smear preparation and staining as well as many diagnostic clues that can be provided by careful examination of a properly stained specimen.

BLOOD SMEAR PREPARATION

The push or wedge type of smear continues to be the most prevalent technique and the easiest to master.

Place a small to medium (approximately 2-μm diameter) drop of capillary, needle-drop, or well-mixed ethylenediamine tetra acetic acid (EDTA) anticoagulated blood in the center of a 1″ by 3″ clean glass slide, about 1/2″ in from the end of a clear slide or 1/3″ from the frosted area of a frosted end slide (Fig. 156-1A). The slide should be on a flat surface and held fixed by one or two fingers of one hand (Fig. 156-1C).

Hold spreader slide between the thumb and middle finger of the other hand with the index finger at the top center to provide slight weight and stability. The spreader slide should have a polished end and be slightly narrower than the slide on which the blood smear is made (Fig. 156-1B).

Completely back the spreader slide into the blood drop, which will run along the rear edge to the side edges of the spreader slide (Fig. 156-1C).

Hold the spreader slide at a 30-degree angle for best distribution. A higher angle produces a thick smear; a lesser angle produces a thin smear.

When the blood reaches the side edges, quickly move the spreader slide to the opposite end with an even motion.

Speed of the spread affects the distribution. Rapid motion produces a thick smear; slow motion produces a thin, uneven spread.

Anemic blood should be spread with a faster motion or a greater spreader/slide angle. Polycythemia and newborns' blood should be spread more slowly or with a smaller spreader/slide angle. Adding a drop of 22% bovine albumin to a drop of blood with an elevated hematocrit dilutes the blood and reduces cell distortion.

APPEARANCE OF PROPER PUSH-WEDGE BLOOD SMEAR

The push-wedge blood smear should have the following appearance:

The smear should cover approximately two-thirds the length of the slide (minimum of 1″).

It should be narrower than the slide with smooth margins so cells at side edges may be examined.

The spread should be smooth with gradual transition from thick to thin areas, terminating in a straight feathered end (tail area).

The smear should be free of holes, scratches, ridges, grease, and dirt contaminants.

Its color should be reddish brown to orangish brown.

STAINING THE BLOOD SMEAR

Wright stain, one of the Romanowsky-type stains, commonly is used for the routine examination of blood and bone marrow smears in the United States and Canada. Variations are Leishmann, Jenner, and May-Grünwald. Giemsa frequently is added to one of these stain solutions or employed separately as a counterstain. Methylene blue and eosin are the prime constituents of each stain. Basic cellular elements (i.e., hemoglobin and some cytoplasmic granules) react with the acidic dye eosin and stain variations of orange-red. Acidic cellular elements (i.e., cytoplasmic RNA and nuclear DNA) react with the basic dye, methylene blue, and stain variation of blue. Structures, such as neutrophil-specific granules, are neutral and show little color; other organelles are blended shades of color such as purple. Stain solutions can be purchased ready for use.

Most laboratories use an automatic staining instrument for blood and bone marrow smears. The Ames Hema-Tek slide stainer, the most popular, utilizes a platen tray to move the slide, face down, through flushes of stain, stain plus buffer, and washes. Other methodology automatically transfers a dish of slides in and out of dishes of stain, stain buffer, and wash solutions. The traditional and still widely used manual technique employs the staining rack.

Staining-Rack Procedure

Place a completely dry, properly prepared blood slide on a level staining rack, smear side up.

Flood slide with Wright stain until completely covered. Leave it on for 3 minutes.

Add almost the same amount of dilute phosphate buffer (pH 6.4 to 6.8), mix by gently blowing on the fluids, and allow to stain for 5 to 6 minutes.

Flush off the stain solution completely with fresh distilled water; do not overwash.

Remove slide from rack, clean residue off back with moist gauze, stand on end and allow to air-dry.

Staining quality is important for proper evaluation of the cells. Red cells should be orange-gray; platelets light blue with distinct red-purple granules; white cells should show a sharp demarcation between nucleus and cytoplasm. The eosinophil's large bright orange granules are an excellent indicator of the quality of the stain. Smears with overly orange-red and light

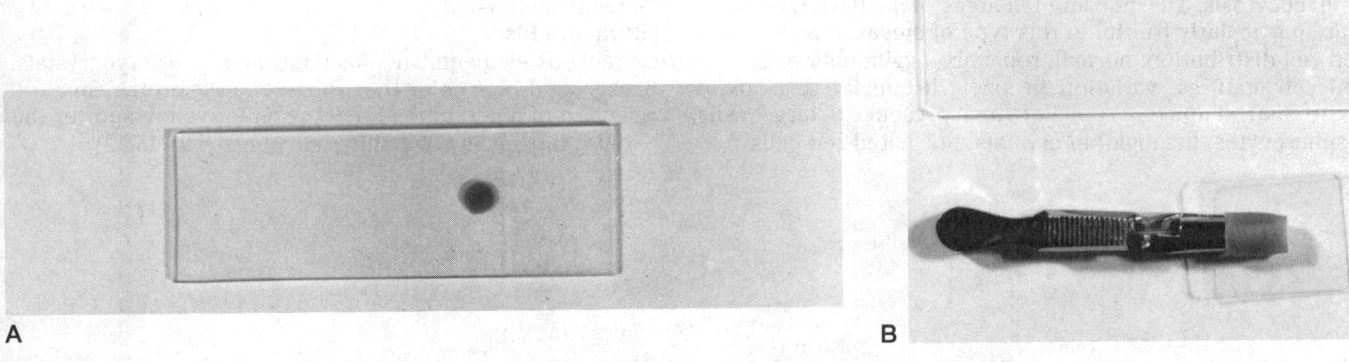

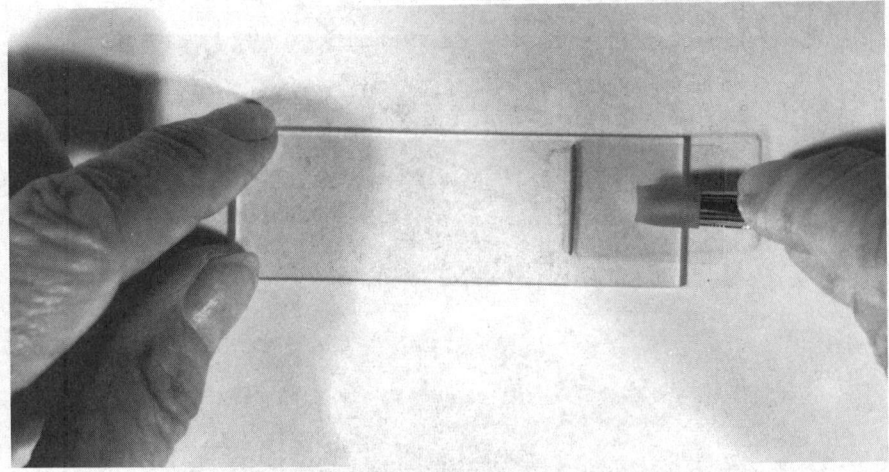

Fig. 156-1. **(A)** Microslide with proper size drop of blood. **(B)** "Spreader" slides: microslide with chipped-off corners and polished ends; "special pusher" consisting of a 20 × 26-mm hemocytometer cover glass held by a straight artery clamp with rubber tubing enclosing the prongs. **(C)** Position of finger and angle of spreader slide at beginning of smear preparation.

blue colors result from too much buffer, a low pH buffer, short staining time, excessive washing, or use of tap water or old stain. Green or brown-red cells, invisible platelets, light cytoplasm, or nuclei in white cells result from too little buffer, high pH buffer, inadequate wash time, use of tap water, very short drying time, thick smear, or old smear.

EXAMINATION OF THE BLOOD SMEAR

Each smear examiner should develop a systematic approach to ensure that all features are reviewed and to prevent abnormalities from being missed. This format should include the following:

Review of smear with low power.
Review of a minimum of 100 leukocytes with high-power, noting immaturity, abnormalities in nucleus or cytoplasm, variance from normal number of any cell if a differential is not performed.
Review of red cells for size, hemoglobin content, shape changes, polychromatophilia, inclusions.
Review of platelets for number estimate and morphology.
Correlation with results of other hematologic laboratory values (white blood cell count, platelet count, reticulocyte count, indices).

LOW-POWER EXAMINATION

Evaluation of a blood smear should commence with a review of the body, side, and tail areas of the push-wedge smear with low-power objective, preferably 20 or 25×. Features to examine include the following:

Staining quality of the smear.
Leukocyte distribution, which will affect differential cell count accuracy.
Body of smear for uniform distribution of various types of cells.
Tail and side edges of push-wedge type smear for an increase in the total number of cells and for a disproportionate increase in the number of neutrophils and monocytes. If there are more than three times as many cells at the edges as at the center, the smear is inadequate for a leukocyte differential count.
Clumping of leukocytes.
Leukocyte number estimate. Depending on magnification and size of field, a formula can be computed to check the white cell count. With the low- (20 or 25×) power lens, count the number of leukocytes in 10 proper fields on a blood smear. Calculate the average number of leukocytes per field. Divide the instrument counted total white cell count for that sample by this average number. Repeat this process for about 25 different blood smears from various individuals. The most consistent quotient number should represent each white cell in similar fields on other smears. If, for example, the quotient for most patients is 200, it becomes the multiplier for the average number of white cells per field, for estimating the leukocyte count using the same lens.
Type of nucleated cells.
Increase or decrease in normal leukocytes.
Smudge cell increase.
Immature or abnormal cells. Low-power examination can be very helpful in finding rare nucleated red cells, immature

leukocytes, blast cells, plasma cells, tumor cells, and erythro-phagocytosis. The side and tail areas of push-wedge smears are particularly fruitful in this type of smear.

Red cell distribution: normal, rouleaux, agglutination.

Red cell features: variation in size, chromicity (e.g., hypo-chromia), shape (e.g., poikilocytes), presence of target cells, spherocytes, hemoglobin crystals, nucleated red cells.

Platelet clumps and uneven distribution of platelets.

Platelet satellitism.

Fibrin strands.

Extraneous elements such as microfilariae or cryocrystals.

Background blue color that suggests a dysproteinemia.

Selection of a good area for representative high-power (50 o 100× oil) review of cellular elements (Fig. 156-2).

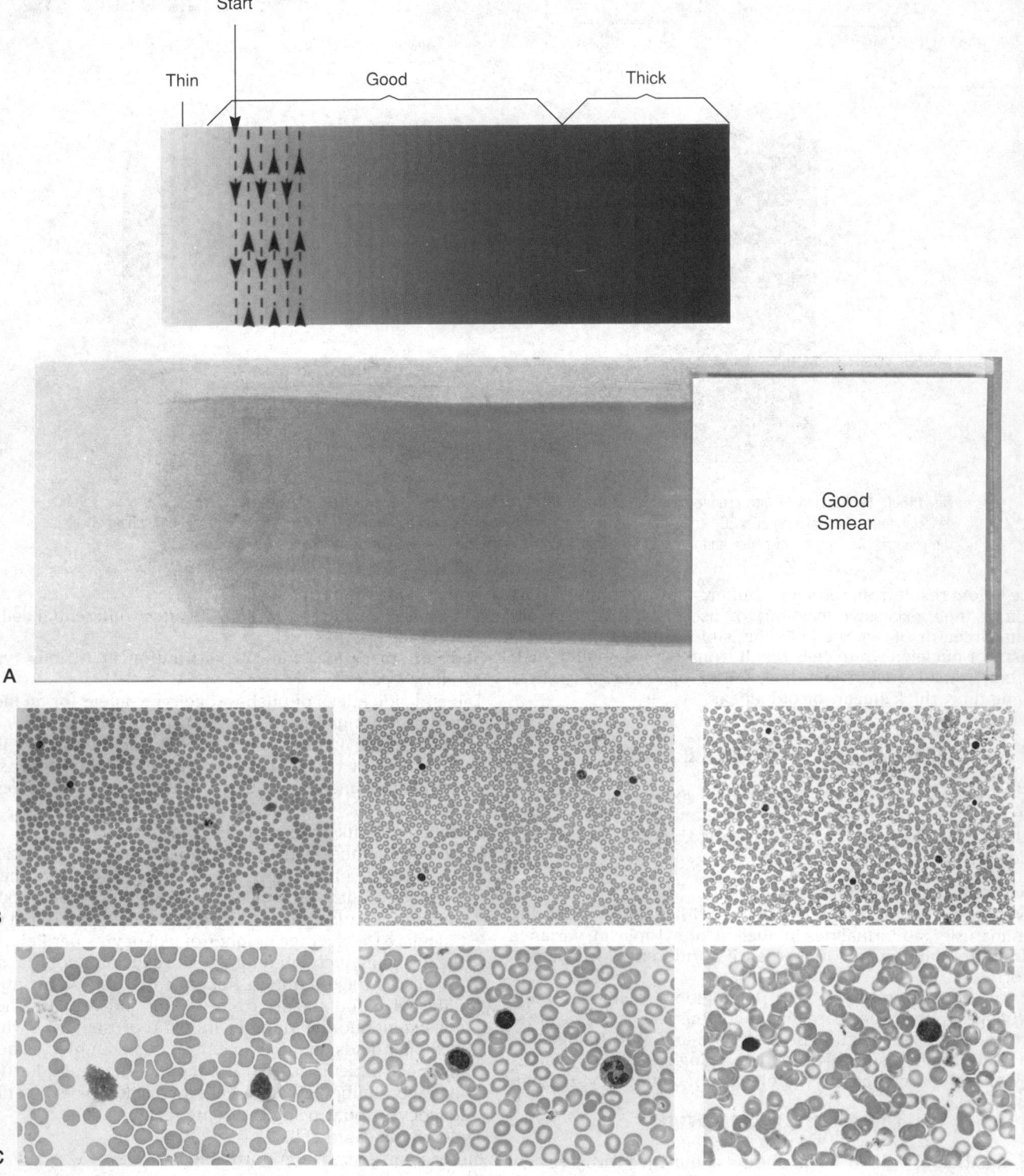

Fig. 156-2. (A) Gross appearance of well-prepared and stained blood smear. **(B)** Low- (20×) power field of thin, proper, and thick areas of a blood smear. **(C)** Oil (100×) immersion power field of thin, proper, and thick areas of a blood smear.

HIGH-POWER EXAMINATION

After selection of a proper field, the examiner should switch to higher power for evaluation of the following:

Leukocyte differential count and individual morphology.
Platelet number estimate and morphology. Some laboratories have calculated a factor to estimate the platelet count using methodology similar to that described for a leukocyte factor. This varies according to the brand of microscope, total magnification, size of field, and type of smear preparation. The product of this factor, which is usually between 10,000 and 20,000, multiplied by the average number of platelets/oil field gives a rough total platelet count estimate.
Red cell morphology.
Cellular artifacts.

MICROSCOPE OBJECTIVES

Traditionally, microscopes in the hematology laboratory were equipped with 10, 40, and 100× oil objectives. Since the automatic particle counters replaced the hemocytometer counting procedures, the need for the 10× objective has been greatly reduced. The 20 or 25× objective has become a useful replacement. Although the high dry 40–45× objective is still popular, it has been replaced or supplemented by the 40, 50, or 63× oil-immersion objective. Use of an oil-immersion medium objective allows one to switch easily to the 100× oil objective without oil contamination of the former when one returns to it.

VARIOUS AREAS ON PUSH-WEDGE SMEAR

A proper area for high-power examination should comprise ≥25% of the smear (Fig. 156-2). On the push-wedge smear it is found just behind the tail end. The straight tail end provides a larger area than the bullet-shaped one in addition to having a more reliable distribution of leukocytes.[1] Red cells, which barely touch or slightly overlap, demonstrate a definite center pallor. Figure 156-2 illustrates this area on a wedge smear with gross, 20×, and oil-immersion observation.

An area too thin for proper evaluation shows flattened red cells that lack a central pallor, mocking spherocytes and thus termed spheroid. Red cells may have an irregular squared-off shape and smudge leukocytes may be frequent. On a well-made push-wedge smear, this area is adjacent to and at the tail area. Figure 156-2 illustrates such an area with gross, 20×, and oil-immersion observation. Too thin smears will have many fields showing above artifacts and may be inadequate for evaluation.

Toward the point of origin on a push-wedge smear there is a more dense distribution of the cells, the thick area, which should comprise <50% of the smear (Fig. 156-2). It is characterized by rouleaux or a stacking appearance of red cells that is normal in thick areas. As a result of this crowding, individual red cell and leukocyte morphology is not assessible. During preparation much plasma is deposited in this area, causing it to dry more slowly than the other areas. Leukocytes tend to shrink during prolonged drying and to stain more densely.[2] Consequently, it may be difficult to distinguish the type of mononuclear cells or identify neutrophils that stain darkly and show poor nuclear-cytoplasmic demarcation. Excessive plasma may cause the "drying" or "moisture" artifact in red cells in this area. Despite its faults, a thick area may be fruitful when looking for red cell hemoglobin C and S-C crystals, coarse basophilic stippling, even nucleated red cells, or other "rare" invaders such as microfilariae.

Review of the tail, or feathered end of a push-wedge smear, can provide valuable information, since larger cells and clumps of cells tend to be carried to this area during smear preparation. Among the cells likely to be found in the region are immature leukocytes, nucleated red cells, megakaryocyte nuclei, platelet clumps, mitotic forms, tumor cells, macrophages, microfilariae, and monocytes and neutrophils containing red cells, bacteria, and parasites. Smudge cells and partly disintegrated cells are increased in this area, so one must be cautious in interpretation.

The side edges of the push-wedge smear are also fruitful in the search for abnormal and immature cells, especially nucleated red cells, reactive lymphocytes, young neutrophils, blasts, and Sézary and other lymphoma cells. Cells found in the tail area also are more likely to be found at the side edges than in the body of the smear.

LEUKOCYTE DIFFERENTIAL COUNT

Differentiation or classification of the percentage of the various types of white cells present on the blood smear has been termed the *leukocyte differential count*. Generally, 100 consecutive leukocytes are counted and classified, but for validity, this number should be greater, especially with elevated white cell counts containing a heterogeneous population of cells. Various pathways have been advocated, but the one most followed is shown in Figure 156-2. On the push-wedge smear, select an area just behind the tail end where the red cells are barely touching. Using a high-power oil objective, crisscross the smear from side to side, including two to four side edge fields, gradually moving toward the thicker end of the smear. Since there is an increased tendency for the larger cells, especially monocytes, to accumulate at the side edge, including several fields should provide a more representative differential count. If there are a disproportionate (three times) number of large cells at the side and/or tail area compared with the body of the film, the differential count should not be performed on that smear.

The most commonly encountered cells are segmented and band neutrophils, lymphocytes, monocytes, eosinophils, and basophils. Some laboratories group segmented and band neutrophils together or separate small lymphocytes and reactive (atypical) lymphocytes. All identifiable white cells should be included in the count. Smudge cells (>25/100 white blood cells), nucleated red cells, and megakaryocyte nuclear fragments are counted outside the leukocyte differential and reported as the number noted per 100 identifiable white cells.

The Normal Leukocyte Differential for Adults	
56 ± 10	Mature neutrophils
5 ± 3	Band neutrophils
3 ± 2	Eosinophils
<1	Basophils
30 ± 10	Lymphocytes
6 ± 4	Monocytes
<0.1	Plasma cell

Traditionally, the leukocyte differential count has been one of the principal tests performed in the hematology laboratory. In addition to providing data as to the percentage of each type of leukocyte present on the blood smear, performance of the differential reassures the physician that someone has reviewed the smear for any cellular abnormalities. In 1974, automatic differential instruments became available; they have replaced a significant number of manual differentials in many laboratories. Studies[3,4] have questioned the value of the leukocyte differential itself, in the clinical evaluation of the patient. Some laboratories are relying completely on one of the flow cytometry systems with smear preparation and review only when there are abnormalities in the quantitative data (counts, indices, histograms, automated differential). Others are performing a screen review of the smear to accompany the automated differential. Because of cost restrictions, some laboratories are providing the screen scan with a differential performed only when leukocyte histogram abnormalities are noted. A *screening scan* is a low- (20 or 40×) power review of the blood smear for red cell morphology and distribution, platelet number and morphology, and impression of the percentage of the types of leukocytes present. When an abnormal or immature cell is observed, examination of that cell with higher power is indicated. Depending on laboratory policy, any increases in cell type either is reported as such or mandates a differential cell count. A brief oil-immersion examination can check for red cell inclusions, polychromatophilia, and platelet morphology. Generally 200–300 leukocytes can be examined, correctly identified mentally, and approximate percentages reported in <3 minutes by an experienced observer.

NORMAL LEUKOCYTES AND PLATELETS

Normal leukocytes and platelets have the following characteristics:

Neutrophil, mature (segmented or polymorphonuclear)
  Medium size (10–15 μm diameter) with two to five unequal nuclear lobes connected by a filament
  Purple chromatin coarsely clumped with a few open areas randomly distributed
  Pinkish tan or light lilac cytoplasm; specific neutrophil granules too tiny to be visible; may contain a few red-purple residual primary granules
Neutrophil, band
  Similar to mature except for nuclear shape, which is a non-segmented continuous band of chromatin that may contain more open areas than the later segmented form
Eosinophil
  Similar to the mature or band neutrophil except for a two-lobed nucleus and presence of numerous bright orange spherical cytoplasmic granules
Basophil
  Similar to the mature neutrophil except for a round or indented light red-purple staining nucleus and presence of large purple-black granules that may obscure the nucleus
Lymphocyte
  Small to large (8–14 μm) in size and mononuclear with a high nuclear/cytoplasmic (N/C) ratio
  Nucleus: round, oval, or slightly indented with semidensely blocked red-purple chromatin; the larger the cell, the less dense the nucleus; nucleolus occasionally visible, especially in larger cells and in thin areas
  Cytoplasm: pale or medium blue, translucent, and may contain several azurophilic (red-purple) granules; larger lymphocytes have a smaller N/C ratio than small ones
Plasma cell
  10–15 μm diameter with a round or oval shape and low N/C ratio
  Nucleus: usually eccentrically located with semicoarsely blocked chromatin similar to lymphocyte
  Cytoplasm: medium to deep blue with a prominent perinuclear clear area
Monocyte
  Medium to large (12–20 μm), mononuclear, with a medium N/C ratio
  Nucleus: usually convoluted or horseshoe-shaped, containing evenly distributed chromatin that is pale and delicate staining
  Cytoplasm: usually abundant, dull gray-blue; a few coarse red-purple or tiny dust-like granules may be present

Table 156-1. Reactive or Toxic Changes in Leukocytes

	Nucleus	Cytoplasm
Neutrophil	Dense chromatin	Small to medium size dark granules (toxic)
	Hypersegmentation	1–3 μm size light blue or gray inclusion (Döhle body)
		Vacuoles
Monocyte	Dense chromatin	Irregular outline with obvious pseudopods
	Increased lobulation	Increased vacuolization
Lymphocyte	Convoluted shape	Irregular outline
	Immature chromatin (pink-red)	Increased amount
		Peripheral basophilia
	Nucleoli	Vacuolization
		Azurophilic granules

Platelets
  2–3 μm diameter cytoplasmic fragments with red-purple granules and no nucleus
  Clumps frequent on capillary or needle drop smears
  Megathrombocytes, which represent prematurely released platelets; 3–6 μm diameter, usually round, containing multiple red-purple granules that are more darkly stained on a direct capillary or needle drop specimen

Tables 156-1 and 156-2 describe the reactive, toxic, and pathologic changes found in leukocytes in a peripheral blood smear.

MORPHOLOGY OF ERYTHROCYTES

The predominant red blood cell (RBC) is approximately 7–8 μm in diameter (normocytic), about the same size as the nucleus of a small, mature lymphocyte. A few RBCs, representing the recently released cells, are slighter larger (macrocytic). As RBCs age they lose membrane and become smaller (microcytic). The normal blood smear demonstrates a few microcytic and macrocytic RBCs. Variation in cell size is termed *anisocytosis.*

The hemoglobinized area comprises about two-thirds of the diameter in the normochromic cell. An increase in the pale center suggests reduced hemoglobin content (hypochromia)

Table 156-2. Pathologic Changes in Leukocytes

Increased size

Increased or reduced N/C ratio

Nuclear changes
  Shape: convolutions, clefts, folds in lymphocytes and monocytes; hypersegmentation in neutrophils in megaloblastic states and as a result of chemotherapy
  Chromatin: dense pattern in neutrophils and eosinophils
  Size: increased for size of cell
  Numerous, large, prominent, or bizarre nucleoli in immature cells
  Distinct nucleolar membrane in lymphoma cells

Cytoplasmic changes
  Hypo- or agranular neutrophils, eosinophils, basophils
  Hybrid granulation: mixture of eosinophilic and basophilic
  Bizarre granulation: large azurophilic
  Inclusion bodies: Auer rods, spheroid bodies in blasts, crystals in lymphocytes
  Vacuolization
  Fragmentation

Table 156-3. Red Cell Morphology Terminology

Greek Term	Other Terms	Appearance	
Discocyte	Normocyte	Normal round RBC (biconcave with SEM)	
Elliptocyte	Elliptocyte, ovalocyte	Elongated with parallel sides or egg-shaped	
Megalocyte	Oval macrocyte	Large and egg-shaped	
Spherocyte	Spherocyte	Round with little or no central pallor	
Stomatocyte	Stomatocyte	Slit-like central pale area (unicave with SEM)	
Codocyte	Target cell	Hemoglobin color in center and periphery; bullseye	
Keratocyte	Helmet or bitten cell	One or more pointed projections (horns) on cell of near-normal size	
Dacrocyte	Teardrop	Pulled out, hand mirror or pear shape	
Schistocyte	Fragment	Small cell with at least one irregular edge	
Drepanocyte	Sickle cell	Crescent-shaped with dense center	
Echinocyte	Crenated or spiculated cell	Numerous regular scalloped projections evenly distributed	
Acanthocyte	Burr, spur, or spiculated cell or pyknocyte	A few irregular spiny projections unevenly distributed on membrane of a cell with reduced volume	

Abbreviation: SEM, scanning electron microscopy.

but is best judged by the automated instrument indices, unless normochromic cells are present for comparison.

Poikilocytes or abnormally shaped erythrocytes frequently are diagnostic clues in anemia. In order to achieve a universal and standardized terminology, Greek names are applied to these poikilocyte changes[6] (Table 156-3 and Plate 156-1).

Inclusions in red cells are always abnormal and should be noted. Table 156-4 lists and Plate 156-2 illustrates the more common ones.

Polychromatophilic red cells have a gray-pink color due to the mixture of remnant RNA and incomplete hemoglobinization. These large cells recently released from the marrow show numerous individual or a network (reticulum) of blue granules when vitally stained with New Methylene Blue reticulocyte stain. Younger forms (stress, shift, or marrow reticulocytes) show a gray-blue coloration and are not normally found in the blood (Plate 156-3).

In the thick areas of the smear red cells tend to form chains or rouleaux, whereas they are separate in the thin areas. Rouleaux formation in the thin and proper areas suggests a protein abnormality. Amorphous clumping of red cells suggests a cold antibody disorder and may cause a falsely high mean corpuscular volume and low RBC count (Plate 156-4).

MORPHOLOGIC ARTIFACTS

Anticoagulated Samples

Most blood smears are made from EDTA anticoagulated blood that may be several hours old. Standing at room temperature enhances cellular morphologic changes, which are especially pronounced in reactive and pathologic cells. Refrigeration retards but does not eliminate these alterations. Some of the more common changes are the following:

RBCs are spiculated or crenated.

Spherocytes, especially if RBCs are abnormal.

Platelets become rounded, swell, and lose granules. Clumping occasionally occurs. Platelet satellitism, the adhesion of platelet fragments to a mature neutrophil, is rare. Clumping and platelet satellitism may cause falsely low platelet counts.

Neutrophils die and display a pyknotic nucleus with 2–10 separate lobes. Numerous small granules help distinguish them from nucleated red cells. Cytoplasm may show increased peripheral raggedness or become vacuolated or even bluish after long standing. Toxic neutrophils may lose their toxic

Table 156-4. Red Cell Inclusions

Name	Nature	Significance	Description	Appearance
Coarse basophilic stippling	Residual RNA	Abnormal marrow Erythropoiesis	Small to medium purple granules diffusely distributed in RBC	
Fine basophilic stippling	Residual RNA	Premature release of young RBC, similar to polychromatophilia or reticulocyte	Fine purple granules diffusely distributed in RBC	
Howell-Jolly body	DNA (chromosome remnant)	Ineffective or absent spleen; erythroblast nuclear abnormality	One or two medium to large round purple granules in RBC	
Siderotic granules (Pappenheimer bodies)	Nonhemoglobin iron	Ineffective or absent spleen; erythroblast nuclear and/or cytoplasmic abnormality with increased marrow iron stores	Cluster of small purple granules in localized area of RBC or 1–2 medium or large size granule	
Malaria parasite	Parasite	Malaria	Ring form with 1 or 2 purple chromatin dots and light blue cytoplasm, gamete forms sometimes present	
Babesia parasite	Parasite	Babesiosis	Small, ring-shaped with filmy blue cytoplasm and one or more purple chromatin granules or a tetrad of tiny dot-like dark staining granules	
Erythroblast (nucleated RBC)	Normal marrow cell	Abnormal in blood other than newborn	8–12 μm cell with gray or orange cytoplasm and dense nucleus	
Megaloblast	Abnormal marrow cell	Abnormal marrow erythropoiesis (pernicious anemia, folate deficiency, chemotherapy)	10–20 μm cell with gray or orange cytoplasm and dense or semidense nucleus	

granulation and Döhle bodies and develop cytoplasmic vacuolization.

Clumping of white cells is rare.

Lymphocytes very rarely show a dense nucleus after standing several hours.

Reactive lymphocytes may display a contorted (cloverleaf) nucleus, increased vacuolization (swiss cheese appearance), or expanded cytoplasm with poor color.

Lymphoma cells and leukemic blasts, especially lymphoblasts, may display a contorted nucleus.

Monocytes may show one or numerous cytoplasmic vacuoles of variable size immediately after anticoagulation. Nuclear convolution may increase with standing.

"Reactive" monocytes may show excess vacuolization and peripheral cytoplasmic fragmentation.

Other Artifacts

Basophil granules are water soluble and may wash out during staining. The resultant cell may resemble a lymphocyte. Excessive humidity may cause red cells to concentrate their hemoglobin in the periphery with a prominent pale center. The sharp demarcation rim identifies this as artifact (torocyte) rather than true hypochromia. Slow drying in a humid environment also may cause a spiculated or crenated appearance.

BUFFY COAT

In leukopenic patients, especially if immature or abnormal cells are suspected, an examination of a concentrate of the nucleated cells can be very helpful and time saving. One milliliter of well-mixed EDTA anticoagulated blood is placed in one or two Wintrobe hematocrit tubes and centrifuged for 6 minutes at 1,500–1,800 rpm or three-fourths of the maximum speed. With a capillary pipette, remove and discard most of the plasma, leaving an amount equal to the light-appearing layer above the packed red cells. Remove the remaining plasma, the buffy coat, and the very top of the mature red cell layer and express onto a clean glass slide. Mix and make several push smears. Air dry and stain as for the usual blood smear.

An accurate leukocyte differential cannot be obtained on the buffy coat preparation, nor can red cell morphology be evaluated, nor platelets quantified. However, the nucleated cells should be representative of the general population of cells in that sample of blood, so a description of the findings may be very important. In instances of leukopenia or even a normal white blood cell count, a few minutes of careful examination of a well-prepared buffy coat preparation permits one to review many times the number of cells seen in routine examination of a direct blood smear, and abnormalities are more likely to be discovered.

Indications for a blood buffy coat preparation are the following:

Pancytopenia for the presence of immature or abnormal cells

Treated leukemia: for the presence of blasts and early return of granulocytes

Leukoerythroblastic blood: for the presence of nucleated RBCs and immature myeloid cells

Macrocytic anemia: for the presence of megaloblastic nucleated RBCs and hypersegmented neutrophils

Multiple myeloma: for the presence of plasma cells

Tumor cells circulating in blood

Parasite infections such as histoplasmosis

A smear of the top of the red cell layer in the Wintrobe hematocrit is helpful when looking for the malaria and babesia parasites.

From the above discussion it should be clear that the proper preparation and examination of a peripheral blood smear can be very helpful in the diagnosis and follow-up of many hematologic, infectious, inflammatory, metabolic, and immunologic disorders.

REFERENCES

1. Stiene-Martin EA: Causes for poor leukocyte distribution in manual spreader-slide blood film. Am J Med Technol 46:624, 1980
2. Cuadra M: The spreading of leukocytes released from their liquid environment. Blut 37:95, 1978
3. Dutcher TF: Leukocyte differentials: are they worth the effort? Clin Lab Med 4:1, 1984
4. Rick EC, Crowson TW, Connelly DP: Effectiveness of differential leukocyte count in case finding in the ambulatory case setting. JAMA 249:633, 1983
5. Shapiro MF, Hatch RL, Greenfield S: Cost containment and labor-intensive tests: the case of the leukocyte differential count. JAMA 232:231, 1984
6. Bessis M: Blood Smears Reinterpreted. Becker G (trans) Singer International, New York, 1977

Bone Marrow Aspiration 157

Harvey J. Cohen and Daniel H. Ryan

INTRODUCTION

After the blood itself, the bone marrow is the largest and most widely distributed organ in the body. Our bone marrow contains about 1 trillion cells and releases approximately 200 billion red blood cells (RBCs), 100 billion white blood cells (WBCs), and 400 billion platelets each day.[1]

For centuries, the marrow was considered a source of warmth and energy. Before its discovery as a blood-forming organ, it was believed to be the source of bone nutrition. It was not until the work of Neumann[2] and Bizzozero[3,4] that a relationship between the blood and bone marrow was established. In 1868, Neumann[2] noted that bone marrow was an important organ for blood formation and was involved in de novo formation of red blood cells. Bizzozero[3,4] independently concluded that non-nucleated cells form from bone marrow nucleated cells and that WBCs are also made in the bone marrow. Neumann[5] continued to investigate bone marrow and was the first to identify leukemia as a disease of the marrow. He also coined the term *myelogenous leukemia.*[6] Neumann[7] was also the first to recognize that at birth, all bones containing marrow contain red marrow. As the individual ages, the peripheral marrow becomes more fatty and develops into yellow marrow.

Bone marrow is the last site of hematopoiesis during the prenatal period. In humans, bone marrow hematopoiesis becomes apparent at approximately 20 weeks' gestation.[8] However, some observers have found evidence for bone marrow activity as early as 12–15 weeks' gestation.[9] Under normal conditions, at the time of birth almost all hematopoiesis occurs in the bone marrow. Extramedullary hematopoiesis is sometimes observed in stressed situations, such as severe hemolytic anemia.

BONE MARROW ANATOMY

The marrow exists as a richly cellular and highly vascular tissue. It consists of two components: the hematopoietic cell compartment and a highly organized stromal component that appears to support the proliferation of these hematopoietic cells. Whereas the hematopoietic cells are transient in the marrow, the stroma remains and serves as a backbone on which the hematopoietic cells grow and differentiate. Within the hematopoietic areas of the bone marrow, hematopoiesis appears to be highly compartmentalized. Erythropoiesis takes place in distinct anatomic units surrounding a central macrophage (an erythroid island).[10] Granulopoiesis appears to take place in somewhat less appreciable morphologic foci and is often associated with a reticular cell.[11,12] Megakaryopoiesis occurs adjacent to the sinus endothelium, with cytoplasmic processes of the megakaryocytes appearing to penetrate the endothelial wall.[13,14] Both the hematopoietic cells and the stromal cells of the bone marrow are separated from the blood by a large-caliber, relatively thin-walled, vascular wall. The mature cells of the bone marrow migrate through these vessel walls, probably as a transendothelial process; the exiting cells appear to make pores within the endothelial cells.[15]

At birth all bone cavities are completely filled with hematopoietic cells and hence appear red, but with advancing age the hematopoietic elements are gradually replaced by adipose tissue. By adolescence, hematopoietic marrow is found only in the cavities of the centrally located bones, such as the sternum, ribs, vertebrae, clavicles, scapulae, skull, pelvis, and proximal ends of the femurs and humeri. A slow reduction in the red marrow mass then continues throughout life. This phenomenon has age-related implications for deciding where bone marrow aspirations and biopsies might be performed. Thus, for the tibia and femur, approximately one-half of the hematopoietic cells are replaced by fatty material after the first decade of life, whereas for the vertebral column and iliac crest, one-half of the bone marrow remains hematopoietic for ≤60 years of life.

HISTORICAL PERSPECTIVE ON BONE MARROW EXAMINATIONS

The first bone marrow biopsy (performed in an infant with leishmaniasis) was reported in 1905 by Pianese.[16,17] He also trephined the tibia and femur, aspirating the marrow with a needle attached to a syringe in 1909.[18] In 1923, Seyfarth[19] used a surgical trephine for obtaining marrow from the ribs and the sternum. Because trephination resulted in excessive bleeding and infection, it was not generally well accepted. In 1927, Airinkin[20] eliminated the trephine complications by using a short lumbar needle to puncture the menubrium and sternum. He obtained marrow aspiration by placing a syringe on the needle hub. In 1945, Vandenberghe and Blitstein[21] were the first to use the iliac crest to obtain bone marrow, and Heidenreich and Heidenreich[22] obtained marrow from the spinous processes. In 1952, Bierman[23] used the posterior iliac crest as the site for bone marrow aspiration, claiming it to be a safe site.

ASPIRATION AND BIOPSY

Criteria

Bone marrow aspiration and biopsy are now well-accepted procedures for evaluating both the cellularity of the marrow and the nature of the cells present. Before deciding whether, or what kind of, bone marrow examination is necessary, it is important to obtain a clinical history and to determine what question is being asked. Although in most instances both aspiration and biopsy are necessary to evaluate the clinical situation fully, sometimes aspiration alone will give the information required. In the evaluation of a patient who is thought to have immune thrombocytopenia, an appropriately handled bone marrow aspiration allows the hematologist to determine whether the thrombocytopenia is associated with increased numbers of megakaryocytes. The hematologist is sometimes asked to perform a bone marrow to determine whether a pediatric patient has a constitutional chromosomal abnormality. Such consultations frequently occur in the neonatal intensive care unit. A bone marrow aspiration is adequate and often gives results on potential chromosomal abnormalities within 1–2 days. The only other instance in which a aspiration alone is indicated is in the follow-up of patients with leukemia or neuroblastoma, when the only question being asked is: Are these patients still in remission? Otherwise bone marrow biopsy along with aspiration is the norm; it is especially helpful in assessing the cellularity of the bone marrow (for example, in patients with cytopenias) and in searching for evidence of infiltration associated with either malignancies or storage diseases. Bone marrow cytologic examination may also be obtained by an incisional biopsy. This is usually performed by the surgeon at a staging laparotomy for Hodgkin disease.

Even though bone marrow obtained by aspiration may yield excellent particles for the preparation of smears and sections, it is still important to study histologic sections of bone marrow obtained by biopsy. Stromal reactions in the bone marrow, granulomas, metastatic involvement, and vascular lesions can be best appreciated when a biopsy is examined cytologically. Occasionally the site at which the bone marrow aspiration and biopsy are performed is determined by a prior examination of the patient. For example, when looking for metastatic cancer or multiple myeloma, it is of value (if possible) to aspirate a tender area or an area showing radiologic evidence of potential infiltration.

The only contraindication to bone marrow biopsy and aspiration is the presence of hemophilia or other related disorders. (Thrombocytopenia, no matter how severe, is not a contraindication.) Complications are possible, and fatalities, although rare, have been reported, especially with sternal aspirations and biopsies. Rarely, a bone marrow needle may break, and an attempt to extract the distal segment with a hemostat should be made. If it is unsuccessful, a surgeon should be consulted. Hemorrhage from bone marrow aspiration can occur at any site, especially in the thrombocytopenic individual. This can usually be prevented by applying a pressure bandage at the site. Other rare complications include pulmonary emboli following sternal aspiration and infected bone marrow aspiration sites, especially in immunocompromised patients.

Although the sternum is the traditional site for bone marrow aspiration (but not for biopsy), our preferred site for both aspiration and biopsy in the adult as well as the child and infant is the posterior iliac crest and spine. In many premature infants and some full-term infants, however, the iliac bone has not completely ossified, and an alternative bone such as the anterior tibia should be utilized. Because of both ease and safety, to attempt to use the iliac bone initially is still worthwhile, even in neonates.

Aspiration of the posterior iliac bone marrow is usually quite cellular, even in the elderly. However, if an individual has had total nodal radiotherapy for Hodgkin disease, this bone may be permanently altered. In obese patients, a long needle is required for posterior iliac crest aspiration.

Procedure

The patient should be assured that the study is safe and that although some pain will occur, analgesic agents will be used and pain will terminate at the end of the procedure. For the overly anxious patient, a tranquilizer can be helpful. In children, especially those with procedure phobias, the use of lorazapam under carefully controlled conditions has been very beneficial. This drug produces both relaxation and an antegrade amnesia that many children prefer.

Adults, and some older or heavier children, are asked to lie on one side after removing their clothing. In young or thin patients, it may be easier to perform the aspiration with the patient lying prone or with a pillow under the abdomen and pelvis. Since this procedure is performed without the patient seeing it, it is important to tell the patient what will be, and is being, done. The iliac crest and spine are felt with the fingers, and a small mark is made in the appropriate area with the fingernail. After double gloving, the area is swabbed with an antiseptic solution, and then the outer pair of gloves is removed. Lidocaine, or some other anesthetic agent, is then injected where the mark was made. We use an air gun to give the initial anesthetic agent and follow it with a needle long enough to anesthetize the periosteum directly. It is worthwhile to allow 1–2 minutes for the anesthetic to produce a maximum effect.

The kinds of needles used for aspiration are numerous. We prefer a needle with a stylet fixed by a Luer-Lok or some other locking device. It is important to use a sharp needle, one long enough to penetrate the bone easily. To be sure the needle is entering correctly, the second and third fingers on the hand not being used to insert the needle should be placed on the iliac crest or spine and the needle inserted between them. The needle and stylet are pushed into the bone with a slight rotary motion. When it is felt that the needle is firmly in place, the stylet is removed and a 10- or 20-ml plastic syringe is attached. The patient is then told that an unpleasant sensation may ensue, and the plunger of the syringe is pulled back vigorously with no more than 0.5 ml of bone marrow and blood aspirated. The smaller the volume, the less the contamination with peripheral blood. The sample is then given to an assistant, who prepares it as described below. If additional samples are needed, another syringe may then be placed on the needle. When the procedure is completed, the stylet is reinserted, the needle removed, and pressure applied to the area.

If a biopsy is performed, a small incision with a #11 scalpel blade is made before insertion of the biopsy needle and stylet. A different site should be chosen for the biopsy, if it is performed after the aspiration. After insertion of the biopsy needle into the bone, the stylet is removed. The needle is then advanced between 1 and 2 cm, depending on the size of the patient. This is performed with very little rotation of the needle. After advancing the needle, the hub is rotated a few times in one direction and then a few times in the other direction. The needle is advanced a small additional amount to break the attachment, and the rotations are repeated. The thumb is then placed on the hub of the needle, and the needle is extracted, with slight lateral movements accompanying the removal. The bone marrow biopsy is then placed on a slide, where imprints are made before processing for cytologic investigations.

MORPHOLOGIC PREPARATIONS OF BONE MARROW

A complete diagnostic evaluation of a bone marrow sample may involve any or all of the following techniques: morphologic examination of stained smears, cytochemistry, culture for microorganisms, histologic examination of stained sections, immunocytochemistry, cell marker analysis by flow cytometry, cell culture assays, cytogenetics, and molecular biologic studies of gene rearrangements or translocations. It is important that the sample be prepared in a fashion that allows the maximal use of as many of these techniques as is necessary to answer the clinical question.

Several morphologic preparations can be made from the bone marrow sample obtained by aspiration or biopsy.[24] Each has its advantages and limitations, as listed in Table 157-1. The sample considered to have the best morphology and most representative distribution of cell types is the direct smear, since its preparation involves the least manipulation of the sample, and no anticoagulant is present. This is the preparation that should preferably be used for a bone marrow differential count. In some patients, the marrow is too hypocellular to allow an

Table 157-1. Morphologic Preparations Made from the Bone Marrow Sample

Preparation	Major Purpose	Limitations
Direct smear	Relative percentage of marrow elements; best morphology	Too few cells to evaluate in some hypocellular marrows
Particle	Marrow cellularity	Parts of smear (near particles) may be too thick for best morphology
Concentrate	Concentrates nucleated cells, especially megakaryocytes and tumor clumps	Relative proportions of cells may be distorted; morphologic changes due to EDTA
Mixed layer	Enriched for macrophages; evaluation of iron stores	Similar to particle
Biopsy imprint	Tumor cells; useful in case of a "dry tap"	Similar to particle

adequate number of cells to be examined on the direct smear. Here the bone marrow concentrate (essentially a buffy coat preparation) is useful since the leukocytes are enriched relative to RBCs. Megakaryocytes and tumor cell clumps are also enriched, particularly at the feathered and side edges of the smear. However, since the buffy coat layer is not sharply demarcated and merges imperceptibly with the red cell layer, there is some variability in the degree of enrichment of nucleated cell types of differing densities. Often, erythroid precursors are significantly enriched relative to granulocyte precursors. Furthermore, the exposure to an anticoagulant such as EDTA, required during the preparation of the buffy coat, may result in artifactual nuclear clefting and cytoplasmic vacuolation, particularly of abnormal cells.[25]

The bone marrow particle preparation is useful for estimating overall cellularity, since large spicules are concentrated in this specimen. However, the morphology is often not as good as in the direct smear, since portions of the smear near the particles may be relatively thick. Macrophages are frequently enriched in the particles found in the mixed layer and are useful in evaluating iron stores. The bone marrow biopsy imprint is helpful in detecting metastatic tumor in patients in whom the aspirate is uninformative, and in allowing immediate morphologic examination of the marrow when a "dry tap" occurs (found in about 4% of marrow aspirations.[26] Examination of the biopsy imprint is useful in view of the high incidence of pathologic changes (93%) with a "dry tap."[26] Considerable evidence shows that metastatic malignancy, lymphoma, or multiple myeloma are missed more frequently on the aspirate than the biopsy.[27-29] However, the sensitivity of bone marrow aspirate for detection of metastatic tumor depends on the thoroughness of examination of all smear preparations. A recent study in which the presence of tumor cells on each aspirate smear was examined separately has shown that tumor cell clumps are found in only one of eight smears in 5% of patients with positive aspirates.[30]

Bone Marrow Smears at the Bedside

In addition to the syringes and needles required for the actual aspiration, it is important to have the following materials ready for the preparation of the sample:

Glass slides, coverslips
Gauze
Forceps
Sample collection tube with EDTA (liquid EDTA for best morphology)
Heparinized tubes with culture medium for special studies
Pusher device (forceps with hemacytometer cover glass)

The glass slides should be placed in a convenient location before the procedure so that no time is lost in the preparation of the direct smears. The technical considerations that apply to blood smears (see Ch. 156) are also important for bone marrow smears. About 0.25 ml of marrow is placed on a glass slide and the remainder immediately added to the EDTA-anticoagulated sample collection tube and mixed well. The marrow placed on the glass slide is examined to determine whether bone marrow has been obtained, as indicated by the presence of "spicules," which appear as fatty droplets, granules, or small chunks of bone. These concentrate at the feathered edge when a smear of the bone marrow is made.

Nine bone marrow direct smears are made from the pool of marrow by placing a tiny drop on a clean glass slide and making a smear in the same fashion as a blood smear. Alternatively, the pusher may be dipped directly into the pool of marrow and the smear then rapidly pushed out on a fresh glass slide.

This step should be done quickly, as the marrow sample is not anticoagulated. Four bone marrow direct-particle coverslips are made by placing a small drop of the spicule-containing marrow pool on a coverslip or the end of a glass slide, placing another coverslip/slide on top, allowing the marrow to spread, and quickly pulling apart. It is very important to get spicules on this preparation so that the cellularity of the particles can be assessed. In addition, two direct "squash" particle slides are made by draining the marrow pool on a gauze (leaving behind the particles), placing a slide on top, and slowly pulling apart.

When a biopsy is performed, the bone is pushed out onto the slide. Several touch preparations (usually five) are made without damaging the bone (by lightly touching the bone on different sites on the slide). The bone is placed into 10% formalin for fixation and histologic sectioning. Several blood smears should also be prepared.

Bone Marrow Concentrate

The EDTA tube containing marrow is mixed and pipetted into Wintrobe tubes as would be done for a buffy coat. The Wintrobe tube is spun at 1,500g for 10 minutes. The layers of the Wintrobe tube are shown in Figure 157-1, with approximate normal ranges for the nucleated cell, containing layers (the plasma and red cell layers are variable and reflect the amount of blood aspirated with the marrow).

The fat layer is discarded. The mixed layer is placed on a slide to make a "squash" particle preparation, as described above. A drop of plasma is placed on a Parafilm watchglass. The myeloid/erythroid layer is removed (if this layer is small, the top of the RBC layer is taken also) and mixed with an equal amount of plasma. Several (10–15) push smears of this concentrated bone marrow sample are made in the usual fashion. Smears containing any particles that are seen in the concentrated sample can also be made.

It is important to retain several unstained smears from each preparation for special stains. Unstained slides are labeled before storage at room temperature on the side opposite the smear with an identifying number using a marker. When special stains are performed, the slides should be marked on the edge

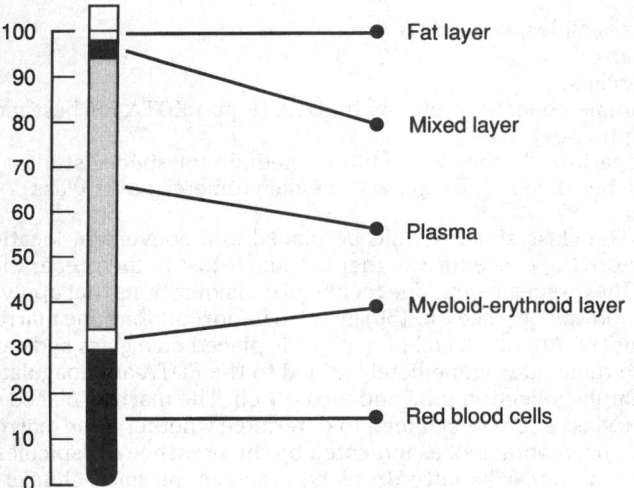

Fig. 157-1. Layers of the Wintrobe tube: the fatty layer is on top and is yellow or milky in color (1–2 %); the mixed layer is second, and is not always present. It contains particles with a high content of fat cells (<1%). The plasma layer is next, followed by the myeloid/erythroid layer. This layer appears as a buffy coat and contains nucleated cells not associated with fat cells (3–8%). At the bottom of the tube are the RBCs (i.e., the hematocrit of the marrow sample).

with a diamond-point pencil to prevent sample mixup. The completed bone marrow slide folder should contain Wright-Giemsa-stained smears of blood, direct marrow smear, marrow particle, marrow concentrate, and marrow biopsy imprint, as well as unstained smears of the mixed layer. Marked iron accumulation in macrophages can be seen on the unstained mixed layer smear as a golden-brown pigment.

Sample for Special Studies

At the time of bone marrow aspiration, it is important to consider whether cell marker studies, cell culture assays, cytogenetic analyses, or molecular biologic assays are likely to be required for clinical diagnosis. Fortunately, the initial sample preparation at the bedside is similar for most special studies, so that an extra sample may be obtained to be used if later morphologic examination suggests the need for additional testing of the bone marrow aspirate.

The general rule is to obtain a viable, sterile, anticoagulated marrow specimen sufficient for the required assays. It is essential to determine the sample preparation and storage requirements of the individual laboratory performing each test, since assay procedures may vary. The most commonly used procedures are outlined below.

Sample for Cell Marker Studies

Before the marrow aspiration, sterile glass sample collection tubes containing RPMI 1640 tissue culture medium, 100 u/ml penicillin, 100 mg/ml streptomycin, 10 u/ml of preservative-free heparin (or 0.15% EDTA), and 10% fetal bovine serum are prepared under sterile conditions and stored at 4°C. Alternatively, sterile EDTA or heparinized sample collection tubes may be used to collect the bone marrow specimen. The standard storage protocol when precise quantitation of cell populations is required (for instance, CD4+ T-cell enumeration in blood) is to store samples at room temperature for ≤24 hours prior to staining. This is also recommended for bone marrow phenotyping. Some evidence shows that cellular phenotypes are generally stable if cells are maintained in sterile tissue culture medium at room temperature for ≤3 days.[31] Since precise quantitation is seldom critical for diagnosis and classification of leukemic cells, this may be an option if samples need to be shipped to another laboratory for analysis, or if further marker studies are needed after the initial panel is run. Either EDTA or heparin is suitable for cell marker analysis, but EDTA may be preferable due to the possible interference of heparin with some molecular studies, as discussed below. EDTA has also become the standard anticoagulant for CD4+ T-cell phenotyping in peripheral blood. If the aspirate is inadequate and phenotypic data are critical, mechanical or collagenase disaggregation of the biopsy preparation may permit cell marker analysis.[32,33]

Long-term storage of interesting or complex samples is often desired to permit later testing with additional antibodies or specialized molecular biology techniques. The best way to accomplish this is to freeze aliquots of the marrow sample for storage in liquid nitrogen. The standard technique of freezing cells in DMSO using a controlled-rate (1°C/min) liquid nitrogen freezer, followed by rapid rewarming from liquid nitrogen storage, has been shown to preserve lymphocyte markers.[34] If a controlled-rate freezer is not available, a modification of the two-step method published by McGann and Farrant[35,36] can be used. Ficoll/Hypaque-separated cells (10^7/ml in RPMI 1640, 10% fetal bovine serum, and 5% DMSO) are held in 1-ml vials at −30°C for 5 minutes (in methanol cooled with dry ice) and then quickly plunged into liquid nitrogen. Cells are thawed by rapid rewarming at 40°C and gradual addition, over 5 minutes, of 5 volumes of tissue culture medium with 10% fetal bovine serum before centrifugation to remove the DMSO. Cell viability should be determined after thawing, as this may be variable, especially if the sample contains many myeloid cells.

Sample for Cytogenetic and Cell Culture Studies

In order to maintain cells in an optimal condition for assays requiring cell proliferation, it is advisable to store marrow at room temperature in a tube containing tissue culture medium with anticoagulant, as described above. The shorter the storage period the better, although overnight storage in general does not significantly affect the validity of cytogenetic results. The considerations for bone marrow colony assays are similar to those for cytogenetic studies. However, it is necessary to test proposed storage conditions to be sure they will yield valid results with the specific assay being performed.

Sample for Molecular Analysis

Examples of molecular assays include detection of clinically relevant gene translocations (for instance, *bcl-2*, *bcr/abl*, *PML/RARa*) or clonal rearrangements (immunoglobulin gene or T-cell antigen receptor). The most commonly used assay end points are Southern blotting and polymerase chain reaction (PCR). The preparation and storage of marrow cells for these tests is similar to cell marker studies, although sample requirements must be checked with the specific laboratory before obtaining the marrow sample. Interestingly, heparin may interfere with digestion of occasional samples using certain restriction endonucleases, particularly *Eco*RI and *Hind*III.[37] The major requirement for assays of DNA structure is that the cells remain viable until they can be lysed in the presence of nuclease inhibitors and proteases. Excessive cell death during storage may result in the fragmentation of nucleic acids by intracytoplasmic nucleases. This is particularly relevant for those assays that use PCR to detect a chimeric mRNA arising from a hybrid translocated gene. Since mRNA is easily degraded and may have a short half-life even in viable cells, sample requirements for such assays must be carefully evaluated.

REFERENCES

1. Tavassoli M, Yoffey JM: Bone Marrow: Structure and Function. Alan R Liss, New York, 1983, p. 1
2. Neumann E: Über die Bedentung des Knochenmarkes für die Blutbildung. Zentralbl Med Wissensch 6:689, 1868
3. Bizzozero G: Sulla funzione ematopoetica del midollo delle ossa. Zentralbl Med Wissensch 6:885, 1868
4. Bizzozero G: Sulla funzione ematopoetica del midollo delle ossa. Seconda communicazione preventiva. Zentralbl Med Wissensch 10:149, 1869
5. Neumann E: Ein Fall von Leukamie mit Erkrankung des Knochenmarkes. Arch Heilk 10:1, 1870
6. Neumann E: Ueber myelogene Leukamie. Berl Klin Wochenschr 15:69, 1878
7. Neumann E: Das Gesetz der Verbreitung des gelben und roten Markes in den Extremitatenknochen. Zentralbl Med Wissensch 20:321, 1882
8. Knoll W, Pingel E: Der Erythropoese beim menschlichen Embryo. Acta Haematol 2:369, 1949
9. Yoffey JM, Thomas DB: The development of bone marrow in the human fetus. J Anat 98:463, 1964
10. Shaklai M, Tavassoli M: Cellular relationship in the rat bone marrow studied by freeze fracture and lanthanum impregnation thin-sectioning electron microscopy. J Ultrastruct Res 69:343, 1979
11. LaPushin RW, Trentin JJ: Identification of distinctive stromal elements in erythroid and neutrophil granuloid spleen colonies. Exp Hematol 5:505, 1971
12. Westen H, Bainton DF: Association of alkaline phosphatase-positive reticulum cells in bone marrow with granulocytic precursors. J Exp Med 150:919, 1979
13. Tavassoli M: Fusion-fission reorganization of membrane. A developing membrane model for thrombocytogenesis in megakaryocytes. Blood Cells 5:89, 1979
14. Tavassoli M, Aoki M: Migration of entire megakaryocytes through the marrow blood barrier. Br J Haematol 48:25, 1979
15. Tavassoli M, Crosby WH: Fate of the nucleus of the marrow erythroblast. Science 179:912, 1973
16. Schleicher EM: Bone Marrow Morphology and Mechanics of Biopsy. Charles C Thomas, Springfield, IL, 1973, p. 60
17. Pianese G: Sull'anemia splenia infantile: anemia infantum a *Leishmania*. Gas Int Med Chir 8:265, 1905
18. Pianese G: Caratteri clinici e reperti ematologici e istopathologici onde si differenzia l'anaemia infantum a *Leishmania* (Pianese) da l'anaemia infantum pseudoleucemia (Jaksch). Atti R Acc Med Chir Napoli 63:155, 1909
19. Seyfarth C: Die Sternumtrepanation, eine einfache Methode zur diagnostischen Entnahme von Knochenmark bei Lebenden. Dtsch Med Wochenschr 49:180, 1923
20. Airinkin MI: Concerning methods of bone marrow research during the life of patients with diseases of the blood-producing organs [Translation from Russian]. Vestn Khir 10:57. 1927
21. Vandenberghe L, Blitstein I: Advantages du prélevement de la moelle osseuse par punction de la crête iliaque. Presse Med 53:419, 1945
22. Heidenreich AJ, Heidenreich GL: La biopsia de la medula osea por puncion de las apofisis espinosas de las vertebras lumbares. Prensa Med Argent 23: 2818, 1936
23. Bierman HR: Bone marrow aspiration: the posterior iliac crest, an additional safe site. Calif Med 77:138, 1952
24. Byrnes RK, McKenna RW, Sundberg RD: Bone marrow aspiration and trephine biopsy. Am J Clin Pathol 70:753, 1978
25. Shafer JA: Artifactual alterations in phagocytes in the blood smear. Am J Med Technol 48:507, 1982
26. Humphries JE: Dry tap bone marrow aspiration: Clinical significance. Am J Hematol 35:247, 1990
27. James LP, Stass SA, Schumacher HR: Value of imprint preparation of bone marrow biopsies in hematologic diagnosis. Cancer 46:173, 1980
28. Juneja SK, Wolf MM, Cooper IA: Value of bilateral bone marrow biopsy specimens in non-Hodgkin's lymphoma. J Clin Pathol 43:630, 1990
29. Terpstra WE, Lokhorst HM, Blomjous F et al: Comparison of plasma cell infiltration in bone marrow biopsies and aspirates in patients with multiple myeloma. Br J Haematol 82:46, 1992
30. Atac B, Lawrence C, Goldberg SN: Metastatic tumor: the complementary role of the marrow aspirate and biopsy. Am J Med Sci 302:211, 1991
31. Muirhead KA, Wallace PK, Schmitt TC et al: Methodological considerations for implementation of lymphocyte subset analysis in a clinical laboratory. Ann NY Acad Sci 486:113, 1986
32. Maung ZT, Bown NP, Hamilton PJ: Collagenase digestion of bone marrow trephine biopsy specimens: an important adjunct to haematological diagnosis when marrow aspiration fails. J Clin Pathol 46:576, 1993
33. Pihan GA, Woda BA: Immunophenotypic analysis of cells isolated from bone marrow biopsies in patients with failed bone marrow aspiration ('dry tap'). Am J Clin Pathol 93:545, 1990
34. Glassman AB, Christopher JB: Effect of cryopreservation on lymphocyte markers evaluated by monoclonal antibodies. Transfusion 24:538, 1984
35. McGann LE, Farrant J: Survival of tissue culture cells frozen by a two-step procedure to −196°C. I. Holding temperature and time. Cryobiology 13:261, 1976
36. McGann LE, Farrant J: Survival of tissue culture cells frozen by a two-step procedure to −196°C. II. Warming rate and concentration of dimethyl sulfoxide. Cryobiology 13:269, 1976
37. Todd DM, Buccini FJ: Apparent heparin interference with restriction enzyme digestion of genomic DNA. Clin Chem 39:362, 1993

Examination and Interpretation of Bone Marrow Biopsies and Aspirate Smears

158

Patrick J. Buckley

INTRODUCTION

Bone marrow aspiration and biopsy are fundamentally important procedures in hematology. Evaluation of the histology and cellular morphology of the marrow, marrow culture for infectious pathogens, tissue culture assay of progenitors, and assessment of marrow iron stores together form indispensible aspects of the workup for almost every disorder of blood cells. In this chapter, I emphasize the hematopathologist's approach to examination of the morphology and histology of bone marrow specimens.

BONE MARROW BIOPSY AND ASPIRATION

Bone marrow biopsy and aspiration each provide valuable and unique information. Neither alone contributes all of the information needed to assess the status of the marrow. Considered together, they provide a complete hematologic evaluation. Therefore, both procedures should be performed, whenever feasible, as part of the marrow examination. To a first approximation, biopsies provide *histologic* information, whereas aspirates provide *cytologic* information.

An additional type of specimen, the clot section, may be obtained by the marrow aspiration technique. In some institutions, aspirate smears are prepared quickly from marrow that has not been anticoagulated. The remaining marrow clots. This clot should be placed in the same fixative as the biopsy for processing into tissue sections. Rather large, intact particles of marrow in these sections often provided valuable additional morphologic information.

In the following sections, the principles of bone marrow biopsy and aspirate examination and interpretation are discussed. Because these sections are not intended to be an encyclopedia of the manifestations of diseases in the bone marrow, principles are stressed and the morphologic features of selected marrow abnormalities are presented.

EXAMINATION AND INTERPRETATION

For reasons outlined previously, both biopsies and aspirate smears should be examined in each case. It is helpful to have a recent blood smear available as well. Ideally, the examinations are performed by the same person. However, the smears and biopsies are often interpreted by different individuals, perhaps because of a lack of expertise or because the two types of specimens are processed in different locations, with an overnight delay in preparation of the biopsy sections. In any case, the interpretations should be coordinated to prevent confusion, to ensure proper patient management, and to prevent seemingly discrepant reports. The differences are often easily explained in terms of the unique information provided by each type of specimen.

The importance of considering the patient's clinical and laboratory information cannot be overemphasized. Thus, the bone marrow is examined in the full context of the patient's disease manifestations, for a more informative interpretation. In addition, comparing previous bone marrow biopsies and aspirate smears from each patient with current specimens is quite helpful to the pathologist or hematologist in understanding the course of various diseases. Such comparisons may also allow advance warning of impending change in disease behavior.

The microscope is an absolute necessity for the examination of hematologic materials. It must be well maintained, adjusted correctly, and kept clean.

Bone Marrow Biopsy

Adequacy of the Biopsy

The first decision is whether the biopsy is adequate for the clinical question(s) being asked. No set rule exists on how much marrow is enough, since the amount differs depending on the clinical situation. For example, a 0.5-cm-long core of marrow may be insufficient to exclude metastatic carcinoma but may be entirely adequate to determine whether megakaryocytes are present or to evaluate iron stores. In the first case, the patient is not being well served if the small marrow biopsy is interpreted as "negative" rather than "insufficient for diagnosis." Thus, the biopsy examiner must assess adequacy.

Technical Aspects

Bone marrow biopsies must be fixed, gently decalcified, dehydrated, embedded in paraffin wax, sectioned on a microtome, mounted on glass slides, and stained with hematoxylin (a nuclear stain) and eosin (a cytoplasmic stain). Most variability occurs with fixation and cutting of sections. Fixation is a process that cross-links or coagulates proteins, preventing their deterioration. The net result is preservation of tissue architecture and cell morphology. Common fixatives are 10% neutral buffered formalin and those that are mercury based, such as Zenker's fluid and B5.[1,2] The latter is particularly well suited to morphologic preservation of bone marrow and results in excellent cytologic detail.

Good histologic sections are of equal importance. They must be 3–5 μm thick to provide cytologic detail. Cutting sections to this thickness is difficult and requires skill, time, and patience on the part of the histotechnologist. Sections of bone marrow biopsies that are > 3–5 μm thick are difficult to interpret, and new sections should be obtained.

BONE MARROW BIOPSY AND BONE MARROW ASPIRATE SMEARS

A *bone marrow biopsy* provides particularly useful information about the following:

1. *Cellularity:* The relatively large areas of intact fat and hematopoietic tissue provide a reasonably accurate estimation of total cellularity; this is especially helpful in hypoplastic states such as those encountered after chemotherapy, in aplastic anemia, and in some myelodysplasic syndromes.
2. *Architecture:* Bone marrow architecture is intact in properly obtained and processed biopsies. The location and relationships among granulocytic, erythrocytic, and megakaryocytic precursors, for example, are important in distinguishing regenerating marrow from recurrent or persistent leukemia; the abnormal location of immature granulocytic precursors can be a clue to some preleukemic states. Moreover, the architectural preservation in biopsies routinely allows rapid and reasonably acurate estimates of the myelocytic/erythrocytic (M/E) ratio.
3. *Assessment of marrow involvement by malignant lymphoma and Hodgkin disease:* The cytologic differences between certain common lymphomas and "reactive" lymphoid aggregates can be very subtle; the paratrabecular location of these lymphomas (along the bony trabeculae) in biopsies is a helpful discriminating feature. Hodgkin disease in the marrow is invariably accompanied by a fibrotic reaction, preventing its aspiration; thus, biopsy is essentially the only way to evaluate Hodgkin disease in the marrow.
4. *Evaluation of marrow involvement by metastatic neoplasms:* Most metastatic carcinomas and other types of metastatic neoplasms, such as Hodgkin disease, elicit a fibrotic reaction in the bone marrow and usually can only be detected by marrow biopsy.
5. *Detection of certain myeloproliferative disorders:* These disorders, often catalogued under the term *myelofibrosis,* are characterized by an increase in reticulin, a precursor of mature collagen, which often prevents adequate aspiration.
6. *Diagnosis of diseases eliciting a granulomatous response:* Granulomas are difficult to aspirate; they may also disturb the marrow architecture in a subtle way that is appreciated only in biopsy sections; furthermore, the granulomas have structural features that are disrupted by aspiration and smear preparation.
7. *Evaluation of bone morphology:* The morphology of the bone in a marrow biopsy can give clues to hematologic disorders such as plasma cell myeloma (increased osteoclastic and osteoblastic activity), to metabolic diseases (hyperparathyroidism, osteoporosis), and to primary bone disease (Paget disease).

Aspirate smears are especially useful for the following:

1. *Evaluation of cytoplasmic and nuclear morphology:* The technique of smear preparation flattens marrow cells, spreading out the nucleus and especially the cytoplasm; the cytoplasmic accentuation aids in the assessment of (1) granularity (e.g., detection of Auer rods in acute leukemias and abnormal granules in myelodysplastic syndromes); (2) phagocytosis by monocytes and macrophages (useful in hemophagocytic syndromes); and (3) presence of ringed sideroblasts (using an iron stain). Evaluation of nuclear morphology and chromatin staining patterns is aided by the smear technique and helps in the analysis of the nuclear changes associated with dyserythropoiesis and dysmyelopoiesis. Finally, the combination of good nuclear and cytoplasmic morphology in aspirate smears allows precise assessment of maturation of the various cell lines and of such abnormalities as megaloblastosis.
2. *Cytochemical analysis:* The fixation and processing of bone marrow biopsies cause denaturation of most nuclear and cytoplasmic enzymes; thus, air-dried aspirate smears are required for such cytochemical analyses as leukocyte alkaline phosphatase, myeloperoxidase, nonspecific esterase, and the nuclear enzyme terminal deoxynucleotidyl transferase, which are necessary for the classification of acute leukemias.
3. *Assessment of iron stores:* The processing of bone marrow biopsies may result in the loss of some stainable iron; although there is good correlation between the amounts of detectable iron in biopsies and smears, iron staining of the latter is a more sensitive indicator of storage iron; also, as noted above, ringed sideroblasts are much more easily detected on aspirate smears.
4. *Analysis of cell surface antigens by flow cytometry:* Cell suspensions obtained by bone marrow aspiration may be analyzed by flow cytometry using antibodies to myelocytic and lymphocytic antigens. These antigens are, for the most part, destroyed during the processing of bone marrow biopsies.

Examination at Low Magnification

A routine that divides the complex process into manageable steps is helpful. First, examine the biopsy that the lowest magnification objective (usually ×4, but preferably ×2). Answer the following questions:

Is the biopsy of sufficient size to assess the clinical problem?
Is there any artifact (e.g., biopsy artifacts such as crushed tissue or hemorrhage into the marrow) that will impede interpretation?
Is there any significant alteration of the marrow architecture, such as solid areas, indicating possible metastatic tumor or lymphoma?

Second, search the specimen for the following features: (1) cellularity, (2) myelocytic/erythrocytic ratio, (3) maturation, (4) megakaryocytes, (5) lymphocytes, (6) plasma cells, (7) macrophages, (8) bone, (9) iron, and (10) reticulin.

Cellularity

Bone marrow is composed of hematopoietic cells, stromal elements (including blood vessels and sinusoids), and fat. Cellularity is the ratio of hematopoietic cells and stromal elements to fat, expressed as a percentage. It is most easily assessed by using a low (×4–10) objective. This method of estimating marrow cellularity has been found to be quite accurate. Cellularity may be variable, differing from one part of the biopsy to another. It is usually possible to give an overall estimate in such cases. If the variation is extreme, give the range and an estimated total cellularity. Older people (>60 years) sometimes have an accumulation of subcortical fat (just below the heavy, outer shell of bone of the iliac crest). If the biopsy needle is angled improperly (i.e., parallel to the cortex), this fat may occupy a large portion of the biopsy and cause an inaccurately low estimate of total cellularity. The presence of cortical bone along the side of the biopsy specimen, rather than at the end of the core, signals this problem.

Cellularity is age dependent. In infants and young children, 90% cellular marrows are common. Healthy young adults may average 60–70%, and individuals >60 years of age average about 50% cellularity.

Myelocytic/Erythrocytic Ratio

The M/E ratio is most easily assessed by using the ×10–20 microscope objectives. The intact marrow architecture in bone marrow biopsies allows a reasonably accurate estimate of the M/E ratio (Plate 158-1). Erythrocytic precursors tend to aggregate in clusters that are scattered relatively evenly throughout the marrow. They are easily recognized in marrow sections by the presence of many normoblasts with very round nuclei that stain evenly and darkly. They have relatively little cytoplasm. The granulocytic elements are mostly situated between the clusters of red cell precursors. The presence of mature neutrophils with their lobulated nuclei makes them easily distinguishable from the erythrocytic precursors. A crude analogy for the relationship between the M and the E is clusters of dark, round pebbles evenly distributed on a somewhat dirty sand beach. In most instances in which cellularity is not below normal, as the M/E ratio increases (i.e., increased M) the clusters of red cell precursors are farther apart; decreased M/E ratio (i.e., increased E) is usually evidenced by closer proximity (and sometimes larger size) of the red cell precursor clusters.

The normal M/E ratio varies between 2:1 and about 4:1. Once the visual relationship between the clusters of red cell precursors and the granulocytic elements for a "normal" M/E ratio is firmly in ones mind's "eye," it is generally easy to estimate the actual ratio. As a rough guide, for an M/E ratio of 3:1, the clusters of erythrocyte precursors are separated from each other by a distance equal to approximately two to three fat spaces (the latter tend to be of rather uniform size).

Maturation

The maturational status of granulocytic, erythrocytic, and megakaryocytic elements is determined most easily by a combination of ×20 and ×40 microscopic objectives. In the normal marrow, immature myelocytic precursors are concentrated in relatively large numbers along the bony trabeculae (Plate 158-2) and are present as scattered clusters in the areas between the trabeculae of bone. Normal granulocytic maturation is considered to be present when about 75% of the myelocytic elements are mature polymorphonuclear leukocytes with distinct nuclear lobulations. The immature precursors are scattered among these cells and form only very small clusters of three to five cells. They are easily recognized (Plate 158-3) by their size (about two times the size of a red blood cell), round or oval nuclei with lightly stained chromatin, nucleoli (myeloblasts and promyelocytes), and pink, granular cytoplasm (promyelocytes, myelocytes).

A left shift in maturation is characterized by a decrease in mature granulocytes, an increase in the number and size of the clusters of immature precursors, and an increase in the number of immature granulocytic precursors along the trabeculae of bone. The term left shift implies that at least some normal maturation is present; it may be characterized as mild, moderate, or prominent. It is very important to indicate when a left shift in maturation is not accompanied by some normal mature cells (i.e., maturation arrest). This is an ominous sign, usually

associated with impending acute leukemia. Many immature myelocytic precursors are located around the trabeculae of bone and in small clusters between the trabeculae. Sometimes larger than normal clusters of immature granulocytes are identified in the latter area. This phenomenon, termed abnormal localization of immature precursors, has been associated with myeloproliferative disorders and myelodysplasic syndromes.[2] By itself, this finding is somewhat "soft," but it is worth noting, especially if a reason exists to suspect one of the above disorders.

Erythrocytic maturation is usually normal when about 75% of the cells in the clusters of red cell precursors are normoblasts. In a normocellular marrow, a left shift in erythrocytic maturation is detected by an increase in the number of immature red cells precursors within the erythrocytic clusters. These precursors have relatively distinct morphologic features: they are about three times the size of a red cell and have round nuclei with very delicate lightly stained chromatin, tiny nucleoli, a distinct sharply demarcated nuclear membrane (as if drawn with a sharp pencil), and blue-gray cytoplasm (Plate 158-4). Megaloblastic maturation (usually related to vitamin B_{12} or folate deficiency) is more easily appreciated in aspirate smears. In biopsies, mild-to-moderate degrees of megaloblastic maturation usually manifest as a decreased M/E ratio (i.e., an increased number of red cell precursors) and a left shift in maturation. Florid cases may exhibit such an extreme left shift that they may resemble acute leukemia (Plate 158-5).

Megakaryocytes are scattered singly and rather uniformly throughout normal marrow. They are the largest cells in the marrow (approximately six times the diameter of a red blood cell). The mature forms have abundant light pink cytoplasm and multilobulated folded nuclei (Plate 158-6). Immature megakaryocytes are smaller (one-third to two-thirds normal size), with relatively less cytoplasm, fewer nuclear lobes, and more darkly staining chromatin (Plate 158-7). The smallest (so-called micromegakaryocytes) may have only a single round, dark nucleus. Immature megakaryocytes are most often seen in platelet-consumption states (e.g., idiopathic thrombocytopenic purpura [ITP] and thrombotic thrombocytopenic purpura [TTP]), in which there is a compensatory increase in megakaryocyte production by the marrow.

Megakaryocytes

Megakaryocyte maturation has been considered above. These cells are normally distributed singly throughout the marrow. Number and distribution are most easily determined with the medium-power (×10–20) microscope objectives. An increase in number is obvious when three or four times the normal number is seen. Less pronounced increases are more difficult to assess, particularly because a baseline marrow examination is not available for most patients. A rough guide to the "normal" number of megakaryocytes is about three to five on average high-power (×40) microscopic field. More than this number (averaged) indicates an increase. This information is particularly relevant to conditions such as those described previously (ITP, TTP) and to certain myeloproliferative disorders, including essential thrombocythemia.

Megakaryocyte distribution may also be informative (e.g., pronounced clustering is generally an abnormal finding associated with myeloproliferative disorders). Furthermore, megakaryocytes in these disorders may be morphologically abnormal (Plate 158-8): the nuclear/cytoplasmic ratio may be increased; nuclei frequently have bizarre shapes with angulated contours and are very darkly stained (hyperchromatic). These morphologic features are often associated with pronounced variation in size, from micromegakaryocytes to giant forms.

Lymphocytes

Small lymphocytes are scattered among the other hematopoietic elements in normal marrows in no discernible pattern. They constitute about 5% of the total cellularity in adults but are more numerous in the marrows of infants and young children. Lymphocytes may be difficult to recognize when very few are seen, and they are often confused with normoblasts in marrow sections. Careful examination using the ×20 or ×40 objective shows that lymphocytes are slightly smaller, have little cytoplasm, and, rather than the round, uniformly dark nucleus of the normoblast, have slightly irregular nuclear outlines and clumped chromatin.

Aggregates of lymphocytes are present in 10–15% of the marrow biopsies from patients >40 years old. These benign lymphoid aggregates are apparently unrelated to any detectable disease process (Plate 158-9). Aggregates of lymphoid tissue in bone marrow may indicate autoimmune disease, in particular rheumatoid arthritis. The number and size may be quite large, and they may be confused with the aggregates of certain kinds of malignant lymphoma. The cytologic features of the cells in these lymphoid aggregates may also be difficult to differentiate from those seen in some lymphomas. Although certain special techniques may be helpful in this decision (see the section Malignant Lymphoma), a good clinical history is imperative.

Plasma Cells

Like lymphocytes, plasma cells are scattered randomly throughout normal marrows and comprise <5% of the total cellularity. The cytologic features of plasma cells in marrow biopsies are quite characteristic: a size that is about 2.5 times the diameter of a red cell; an oval, eccentric nucleus with a chromatin pattern that resembles the face of a clock; a perinuclear clear zone (representing a well-developed Golgi apparatus); and an abundance of bluish pink cytoplasm (Plate 158-10). Plasma cells are sometimes seen lying along the course of blood vessels in marrow biopsies, a phenomenon that can result in a rather large local concentration of plasma cells. It is, however, seldom encountered as a sole manifestation of plasma cell dyscrasias.

The number of plasma cells is increased during immune responses, so that patients with infectious or autoimmune diseases often have a greater than normal number in the marrow. They tend to be distributed randomly, do not form sheets or large aggregates, and are morphologically normal. Furthermore, the proportion of the total cellularity accounted for by plasma cells rarely exceeds 20% in non-neoplastic conditions and is usually far lower.

Macrophages

Macrophages, sometimes called histiocytes or tissue macrophages, are ubiquitous tissue constituents. They are particularly numerous in tissues with rapid cell turnover and are present in normal bone marrow. Their size is variable but typically they are about three times the diameter of a red cell. Macrophages have a large amount of pale pink cytoplasm that may contain phagocytized debris and a small, round, usually eccentric nucleus. The nuclear features are rather "bland" in most instances (Plate 158-11). However, when macrophages are newly activated by, for example, a phagocytic stimulus, their nuclei may be larger and have a distinct nucleolus. They are most easily assessed at medium (×20) to high (×40) magnification.

The number of macrophages in a normal marrow is difficult to determine because these cells are hard to see. They tend to blend into the background because their cytoplasm may be very pale; phagocytized debris may obscure the cytoplasm. In marrows with increased iron stores, macrophages are more easily seen, since they contain hemosiderin or storage iron, in the form of refractile, brown, variably sized clumps of material in their cytoplasm. *If macrophages are readily apparent in marrow biopsies, their number is increased, and the cause of the increase should be sought.* Clinically important causes of this phenomenon, for example, are the hemophagocytic syndromes, which may be familial (seen in young infants) or related to infections (e.g., virus-induced hemophagocytic syndrome). The bone marrow, liver, and spleen are filled with actively phagocytic macrophages. The familial form is frequently lethal. The infection-related syndrome must be recognized as such so that proper supportive care may be provided.

Bone

A bone marrow biopsy contains some bone. This part of the biopsy is frequently neglected. A typical biopsy from the iliac crest (the most common biopsy site) contains a variable amount of cartilage and some thick, heavy bone at one end, derived from the cortex; the cortex is often covered by a layer of pink, collagenous tissue that represents periosteum. Thinner, elongated spicules or trabeculae of medullary bone (within the marrow cavity) are also present, interspersed with hematopoietic and stromal tissue as well as fat.

The surfaces of the bony trabeculae are lined by osteoblasts, hardly recognizable as such in adults because they are elongated and flattened against the bone (visible only as spindle-shaped cells with long, thin nuclei), as befits their relatively inactive state. Although bone remodeling is an ongoing process, it is much slower in adults than in children. Thus osteoblasts are inconspicuous. The same is true of osteoclasts. In fact, it is uncommon to see even a single osteoclast in an adult bone marrow biopsy.

The opposite is true in growing children and early adolescents. The bony trabeculae are lined by plump osteoblasts with round nuclei, relatively abundant bright pink cytoplasm, and prominent perinuclear clear zones (Golgi zones). Osteoclasts are also easily found. They are located near the bone or in reabsorption lacunae near the surface of the bone, are five to six times the diameter of a red cell, and have multiple small, round nuclei.

The presence of osteoblastic and osteoclastic activity (i.e., increased bone remodeling) in a biopsy from an adult may be a manifestation of a metabolic disease (hyperparathyroidism) or renal dysfunction; furthermore, in the absence of the above conditions, these findings indicate the possibility of certain neoplastic diseases associated with osteoclast activation and hypercalcemia, such as multiple myeloma and certain T-cell lymphomas/leukemias that are related to infection by human T-cell leukemia virus I.

Examination of the bone may provide some clues to other diseases. For example, thinning of the bony trabeculae may indicate the osteoporosis or bone loss seen in postmenopausal women. Excessively thick trabeculae with prominent disordered "cement" lines are signs of Paget disease of bone (Plate 158-12). Normal bone stains uniformly pink and has evenly spaced parallel "cement" lines, representing successive waves of previous bone deposition (Plate 158-2). In Paget disease, bone deposition is increased (thicker bones) and disordered (unevenly spaced, nonparallel "cement" lines).

Iron

Iron is present in storage form (hemosiderin) in the cytoplasm of macrophages (Plate 158-13). Iron stores are most easily evaluated by using medium ($\times 20$) and high-power ($\times 40$) objectives. Only bright blue particles (using the Prussian blue stain for iron) located within the cytoplasm of macrophages are considered. Iron stores may be quantitated as follows: present (nearly every microscopic field ($\times 40$) has an iron-positive cell), increased (more than two iron-positive cells for each $\times 40$ field), decreased (less than one iron-positive cell, on the average, for each $\times 40$ field), and absent.

Stainable iron stores vary with age: children up to the age of about 14 years do not have detectable stainable iron in their marrow, presumably because of a homeostasis that balances gastrointestinal iron absorption with metabolic use in these growing children. Iron-deficiency anemia is probably the most common cause of decreased or absent iron stores. Abnormally large amounts of marrow storage iron arise from a number of causes, including those that result in increased systemic iron, such as numerous blood transfusions or altered iron use, for example, after chemotherapy and in myeloproliferative and myelodysplastic syndromes.

Reticulin

Reticulin is an early form of collagen synthesized by marrow stromal fibroblasts.[4] It is detected by a special staining technique that results in the deposition of silver on the delicate reticulin fibers, causing them to appear as a fine interlacing meshwork of thin black filaments. A larger concentration of reticulin is normally present around marrow blood vessels. Increased reticulin in the bone marrow is, with few exceptions (e.g., within some "benign" lymphoid aggregates and around granulomas), an ominous warning sign, usually indicative of a primary hematopoietic or metastatic neoplasm. Presumably, the neoplastic cells produce growth factors that stimulate reticulin synthesis by normal marrow fibroblasts. (One of these may be platelet-derived growth factor synthesized by neoplastic megakaryocytes in some leukemias and myeloproliferative disorders.)

Since a true increase in marrow reticulin is highly significant, careful evaluation of reticulin stains is mandatory. The somewhat difficult staining technique, which may produce variable results, can complicate the evaluation. Thus, comparison with a control marrow stained at the same time is mandatory. Since obtaining normal marrow controls is difficult, a "non-neoplastic" bone marrow may have to suffice. Typically, abnormal reticulin appears as an increase in the number and thickness of fibers (Plate 158-14). The thickness may be quite striking, and the fibers often have an uneven texture and irregular surfaces.

INCREASED RETICULIN

Reticulin is an early form of collagen synthesized by marrow fibroblasts. Increased reticulin in the bone marrow is, with few exceptions, an ominous warning sign, and usually indicates a primary hematopoietic or metastatic neoplasm.

Reticulin increase in bone marrow is a reversible phenomenon. After chemotherapy, it frequently decreases to normal (e.g., in leukemias that exhibited abnormal amounts of reticulin before treatment). Some patients with so-called myelofibrosis related to myeloprofilerative disorders have what appears to be permanent ("mature") collagen in their marrows revealed by standard staining procedures. The reticulin is markedly elevated as well, yet when a stain for "mature" collagen is applied to such marrows (trichrome), the result is frequently negative. The implication is that perhaps even long-standing myelofibrosis may be, to some degree, reversible if the underlying cause can be successfully treated.

Morphologic Features of Selected Abnormalities

Infection

Granulomatous inflammation induced by such agents as fungi and acid-fast bacteria and the granulomas of sarcoidosis are often detectable in bone marrow biopsies. Granulomas are most easily assessed at relatively low magnification (about $\times 10$) because they cause a distortion of the marrow architecture: focal expansions of the hematopoietic tissue between the fat cells that appear as small nodules, which stain pinker than the surrounding cells because of the abundant cytoplasm of the macrophages that make up the granulomas (Plate 158-15). Some granulomas, such as those in patients with sarcoidosis, may be discrete, tightly woven collections of macrophages, sometimes containing multinucleated forms, that are easily detected. More frequently the granulomas associated with other infections are loose aggregates of macrophages, sometimes very small and relatively indistinct, causing a quite subtle distortion of the marrow architecture. Furthermore, only one or two may be present in sections of the marrow biopsy. Thus, careful examination of each of the multiple sections typically cut from the biopsy specimen is mandatory. Any apparent abnormality detected at low magnification can then be observed at higher power ($\times 20-40$) to check for the presence of macrophage aggregates. The presence of granulomas in a biopsy mandates that stains for acid-fast bacteria and fungi be performed. Even if the marrow has been cultured, the presence of these relatively slow-growing organisms may be detected before cultures are positive, allowing the institution of appropriate therapy.

Viral inclusions are sometimes detectable in bone marrow cells. The characteristic cytopathic effects of cytomegalovirus (i.e., giant cells with huge, red-staining nucleoli surrounded by a clear halo) have been observed in marrow biopsies, particularly in immunosuppressed patients. Of the latter group, patients with the acquired immunodeficiency syndrome (AIDS) are especially prone to viral infections as well as to infection by acid-fast bacteria. These patients sometimes do not mount a normal granulomatous response, and the presence of such an infection may be especially subtle. Any suspicion of AIDS, often suggested only by the history, provides sufficient reason to obtain stains for acid-fast organisms and fungi.

Metastatic Neoplasms

As noted in the Introduction, metastatic neoplasms, especially carcinomas, often elicit an intense increase in reticulin or even actual fibrosis and are usually detectable only by biopsy. The reaction to the tumor deposits and the typically cohesive property of the malignant cells (i.e., carcinoma and sarcoma cells tend to stick together in tight groups; this is unusual for lymphoid or hematopoietic cells) cause enough distortion of the marrow to be recognizable at low ($\times 4-10$) magnification (Plate 158-16).

Closer inspection of the metastatic tumor deposits often gives clues to their origin (i.e., gland formation by adenocarcioma, spindle-shaped cells of certain sarcomas, and so forth). . stain for mucin is easily performed and may help to identify ertain adenocarcinomas. The detection of cytoplasmic and ell membrane antigens on metastatic cells in marrow biopsies ay be quite useful in the identification of the cell type and in ome instances even the primary site. Many of these antigens re preserved in routinely fixed and processed biopsies and re detected with the appropriate monoclonal or polyclonal ntibodies by using indicator systems such as the peroxidase or alkaline phosphatase techniques (Plate 158-17). Examples re cytokeratins (present in epithelial cells and carcinomas), prostate-specific acid phosphatase, and leukocyte common antigen (present only on hematopoietic and lymphoid cells).

Multiple Myeloma

In a previous section the morphology and distribution of nonneoplastic plasma cells in bone marrow biopsies were outlined. The diagnosis of plasma cell neoplasms, specifically plasma cell (multiple) myeloma, is facilitated in bone marrow biopsies. n addition to the simple increase in number of plasma cells found in most cases, the presence of sheets and large aggregates of plasma cells and the architectural distortion caused by them are features seldom, if ever, encountered in conditions that cause reactive plasmacytosis. Furthermore, since plasma cell myeloma is frequently a focal disease, these findings strongly suggest the diagnosis even when the number of plasma cells is not higher than is typical for reactive conditions (as a rough guide, >20%).

The cytologic features of the plasma cells in plasma cell myeloma may also indicate neoplasia, but these features are quite variable. The cells often closely resemble mature plasma cells. Careful examination at high magnification ($\times 40$) usually reveals the presence of cells with distinct nucleoli that often stain pink to bright red (Plate 158-18). Such cells are rarely seen in non-neoplastic conditions. The stage of maturation of the cells in various cases of plasma cell myeloma can resemble the less mature precursors of plasma cells: the cells may be larger, with increased nuclear size and less pronounced nuclear eccentricity, more prominent nucleoli, and less evident paranuclear clear zones (Golgi regions). In some cases, they have no recognizable plasma cell features and resemble the transformed B lymphocytes (immunoblasts) that are the precursors of plasma cells. In these latter cases, the clinical features (e.g., multiple lytic bone lesions, serum paraprotein) help to classify the neoplasm.

Utilization of antibodies to immunoglobulin heavy and light chains and immunodetection methods such as the immunoperoxidase technique can confirm the diagnosis of malignancy by showing that the cells are monoclonal (i.e., produce only a single immunoglobulin light chain). Such techniques can be performed with routinely processed biopsies because the plasma cells usually produce such large amounts of cytoplasmic immunoglobulin that some of it is preserved (Plate 158-19).

Malignant Lymphoma

Bone marrow biopsy examination is quite useful in the detection of marrow involvement by lymphoma. As a general rule, lymphoma in the marrow is present as "nodules" or large aggregates that are visible at low magnification ($\times 2–4$). They push aside the normal marrow, often replace the local marrow fat, and, even at low magnification, have recognizably different staining qualities from the surrounding marrow. Another architectural feature of some lymphomas in the bone marrow, especially the common "low-grade" lymphomas of follicular center cell origin, is a propensity to form aggregations along the bony trabeculae (Plate 158-20). This property is unusual in the so-

LYMPHOMA IN THE MARROW

Aggressive lymphomas, such as large cell lymphomas, often contain a minor component of small cleaved lymphocytes, which may circulate to the marrow. Since the presence of large cell lymphoma in the marrow is an ominous prognostic sign, it is important to specify in such cases exactly which cells are present.

called benign lymphoid aggregates that may be seen in the marrows of patients >40 years old (Plate 158-9).

The cytologic features of lymphomas in bone marrow biopsies tend to resemble those seen in lymph nodes. For this reason, it is quite helpful to review a previous lymph node biopsy when assessing a bone marrow biopsy for the presence of lymphoma. A detailed description of the morphologic features of the numerous types of lymphomas has been provided by Jaffe.[5]

Several aspects of lymphoma diagnosis in bone marrow biopsies must be considered. First, "benign" lymphoid aggregates, mentioned previously, resemble certain low- and intermediate grade-lymphomas so closely that it may be difficult to be certain of the correct diagnosis. This is problematic, either when the initial diagnosis of lymphoma is based on the marrow biopsy, or when serial biopsies are used to follow the effects of treatment. The lymphomas in question are the common follicular center cell-derived lymphomas, including the follicular small cleaved cell, follicular mixed small cleaved and large cell, and diffuse small cleaved cell types, as well as the somewhat heterogeneous group of diffuse mixed small and large cell lymphomas (National Cancer Institute Working Formulation[6]). These lymphomas have either a predominance or large proportion of small, irregular (cleaved) lymphocytes, the component that presumably circulates and involves bone marrow. Because these cells so closely resemble those that constitute "benign" lymphoid aggregates, minimal involvement of the marrow by lymphoma or residual lymphoma after treatment may be difficult to diagnose with certainty. My experience is that the presence of small cleaved cells in the marrow of patients with large cell lymphomas does not imply the dismal prognosis associated with large cells in the marrow. This phenomenon has been reported by others.[7]

Another important point is that the follicular pattern of growth of some low-grade lymphomas is not usually recapitulated in the bone marrow. Since this growth pattern is associated with a more indolent clinical course, the primary diagnosis of such lymphomas by bone marrow biopsy does not provide this important information. Also, the presence of small cleaved cells in the marrow, even when the amount and paratrabecular pattern strongly suggest lymphoma, does not indicate whether the patient has a mixed lymphoma (small and large cells) or even whether the cells in the marrow are a minor component of a large cell lymphoma elsewhere.

In certain circumstances a bone marrow biopsy reveals extensive involvement by lymphoid tissue. Such marrows are usually not aspirable. Furthermore, lymph nodes may not be accessible for biopsy. Cell-surface antigen studies may be helpful in such cases to define the lymphoproliferative disorder better. Since most of these antigens are destroyed by routine fixation and processing, an alternative is to perform a repeat biopsy of the marrow, to freeze the fresh non-decalcified biopsy, and to cut sections with a cryostat. Some shattering of the biopsy occurs, but large enough fragments are usually produced to allow the frozen-section immunoperoxidase technique to be performed using a panel of antibodies to selected lymphocyte antigens. This technique has been described by

Wood and Warnke[8] and has been successfully used by our diagnostic service.

Bone Marrow Aspiration

Adequacy of the Aspirate and Technical Aspects

Aspirate smears should be examined at low magnification (×4) to determine the adequacy of the specimen. At least a few marrow particles should be present in most cases, and several slides should be screened to find them. If the smears show large amounts of mature, non-nucleated red cells interspersed by few nucleated cells, peripheral blood rather than marrow may have been obtained. Such specimens are not adequate for marrow examination. The marrow should be well spread so that the cells on at least a portion of each slide can be examined in detail. Small clusters, especially of erythrocytic precursors, are seen, even on well-prepared smears. The cells within marrow particles cannot usually be seen clearly because of high cell density; however, the cells thin out at the edges of the particles in technically good smears, and this is a good place to examine the cellular composition of the particles (Plate 158-21).

The number of damaged cells and "naked nuclei" should be assessed. These cells are not suitable for cytologic evaluation. The smearing process always causes some cell damage, particularly to the cytoplasm. Mechanical shearing away of the cytoplasm results in the "naked nucleus" phenomenon. If a large number of such damaged cells is present, the cause(s) should be sought. Too vigorous smear preparation may render some of the specimens technically inadequate, especially in highly cellular marrows. On the other hand, because neoplastic cells, such as those in acute and certain chronic leukemias, are very delicate, it is difficult to prevent damage to them. Added care in smear preparation is necessary when such conditions are suspected.

Finally, the adequacy of staining must be determined. Too dark a stain obscures cytologic detail, especially of nuclear features. If the stain is not dark enough, certain morphologic aspects may be overlooked. An example is cytoplasmic granules. Several smears may have to be examined or additional smears stained to obtain adequate specimens.

Examination of Bone Marrow Aspirate Smears

The following sections outline the procedure for the examination and interpretation of aspirate smears. Numerous excellent publications address the morphology of normal hematopoietic cells in marrow aspirates in great detail. The focus here is on examination of aspirates and the more important sorts of deviations from normal that may be encountered in the clinical setting. For reasons similar to those discussed above in the section Bone Marrow Biopsy, using an established routine for examining aspirate smears is essential. At each step the use of a particular microscopic objective facilitates gathering of certain types of information. Developing the ability to appreciate certain aspects of a bone marrow aspirate smear before examining it with the oil immersion object is important.

Examination at Low Magnification

Scan the aspirate smear at low magnification (×2–4) for the presence of marrow particles, an estimate of cellularity, and the number of megakaryocytes (see the section Megakaryocytes). At slightly increased magnification (×10) scan for technical adequacy and for clumps of nonhematopoietic cells that may signal the presence of a metastatic neoplasm. Occasionally small "benign" lymphoid aggregates or, more rarely, clumps of lymphoma cells may be recognized during a low-magnification scan.

Cellularity

Cellularity should be described in broad categories: hypercellular, normocellular, and hypocellular. Hypercellularity is generally characterized by a large number of marrow particles with broad, gradually thinned-out borders created by the smearing process (Plate 158-21). By contrast, hypocellular marrows have fewer than the normal number of particles, and these may be smaller than usual, often with thin borders. In extreme cases, such as hypoplastic ("aplastic") anemia and after chemotherapy, the aspiration process itself collapses the cell-poor particles, making more detailed analysis difficult. Sometimes a "hypocellular" marrow is the result of mechanical problems such as misplacement of the aspiration needle. Furthermore, paucicellular aspirates may result from extremely cellular marrows ("packed" marrows) or from marrows that are replaced by either a metastatic neoplasm or a lymphocytic/hematopoietic malignancy that stimulates increased reticulin formation. A biopsy is necessary for proper evaluation in such cases.

Myelocytic/Erythrocytic Ratio

The M/E ratio may be determined by using either a ×40 (high dry) or oil immersion (×50–100) objective, depending on preference. Two methods may be used: actual differential counts of granulocytic and erythrocytic precursors in several different fields, or estimates of the proportions of these cells in a number of fields. The former is quite tedious, and different fields (100–200 cells/field) on several smears should be evaluated. Such counts are necessary because of the intrinsic variability of the M/E ratio in these preparations, especially due to the inclusion of clusters of erythrocytic and granulocytic elements in some fields, which may bias the ratio considerably. The second method, estimation of the M/E ratio, is subject to the same field-to-field variability noted above. However, the variability is mitigated to some degree because the technique is more rapid and a larger number of areas can be examined. One microscopic field, using the oil immersion (×100) objective, contains approximately 100 cells in areas where the cells are not quite touching one another. In such fields, the M/E ratio can be estimated rather easily and the results of 8–10 random fields averaged.

Maturation

Evaluation of maturation includes two broad aspects: overall completeness of cellular maturation and cytologic detail of the maturation of the various types of cells in the marrow. The former is most easily evaluated at intermediate (×20) to high (×40) magnification and should be done before oil is placed on the slide. As described in the section Bone Marrow Biopsy, granulocytic and erythrocytic maturation is generally thought to be complete when >75% of the cells are mature granulocytes (polymorphonuclear leukocytes and eosinophils) and normoblasts, respectively. This is generally rather easy to determine, but a number of different areas on each slide and several slides should be examined to prevent misinterpretation due to local variations. An increased number of immature precursors (left shift in maturation), at the expense of more mature elements, should be noted and correlated with the clinical information. Some causes are bleeding, infection, myeloproliferative disorders, and myelodysplastic syndromes. An important aspect of the evaluation of overall maturation is to record the presence of maturation arrest (i.e., the paucity or complete absence of the more mature elements of a cell line). This is usually an ominous finding, often associated with incipient acute leukemia.

Cytology

The detailed cytologic examination of the components of the various hematopoietic cell lines is typically performed by the oil immersion objective. I find, however, that a scan of the aspirate smear using the ×40 (high dry) objective is an efficient way to gain a general picture of cellular morphology and to identify cell types that need closer scrutiny.

Myelocytic/Monocytic Series. Begin the cytologic evaluation by determining the approximate sizes of the various elements of the myelocytic series (including monocytes and precursors). Abnormally large cells, particularly metamyelocytes and the band forms of neutrophils, may be seen in the megaloblastic anemias and in some preleukemic states (megaloblastoid change). The following are the approximate sizes of myelocytic precursors, using the diameter of the mature erythrocyte as the internal standard of measurement: myeloblast, ×2.5–3; promyelocyte, ×3.5–4; myelocyte, ×3–3.5; metamyelocyte, ×3–3.5; band, ×2.5–3; neutrophil, basophil, eosinophil, ×2–2.5; and monocyte, ×3–4.

Next examine the cytoplasm for the quality and quantity of granules. Auer rods are sometimes present in acute myeloblastic leukemias (M1 and M2 of the French-American-British classification), and bundles of these structures may be seen in acute promyelocytic leukemias (M3). Hypogranular mature elements of this series may be a finding in myeloproliferative and myelodysplastic (preleukemic) disorders. In some cases of the latter, careful examination can sometimes reveal the presence of eosinophilic and basophilic granules within the cytoplasm of the same cell. Increased granularity can be a feature in infections, myeloproliferative disorders, and acute promyelocytic leukemia (M3).

Finally, evaluate the cells for nuclear abnormalities, particularly of shape and lobation. Incomplete segmentation of the nuclei of mature neutrophils is a hallmark of the Pelger-Huët anomaly, in which the nuclei are shaped like peanuts; more importantly, similar nuclear morphology (pseudo-Pelger-Huët change) may indicate some preleukemic states. Hypersegmented neutrophils (more than five lobes) are associated with the megaloblastic anemias. Complex, folded nuclear contours in early granulocytic precursors constitute another important abnormality because they are seldom present except in acute leukemias.

Erythrocytic Series. Erythroblasts are approximately three to four times the size of a mature red cell. The various stages of normoblastic differentiation usually vary from twice the size of a mature red cell for the earlier precursors to about the same size for the later elements. Larger than normal erythrocytic precursors are found in the megaloblastic anemias, in myelodysplastic syndromes, and in erythroleukemia (M6). Cytoplasmic alterations in erythrocytic precursors include coarse, basophilic granule-like stippling and vacuolization. The former usually indicate abnormal iron metabolism and may be associated with hemoglobinopathies, sideroblastic anemias, erythroleukemia (M6), and megaloblastic anemias. Cytoplasmic vacuoles may be seen in such conditions as myelodysplasia, erythroleukemia, and alcohol intoxication. A note of caution about cytoplasmic vacuoles: these and nuclear vacuoles may be formed artifactually during the preparation of aspirate smears. If significant nuclear vacuolization is also present, it usually indicates that the cytoplasmic changes are artifactual.

A variety of nuclear variations can occur in erythrocytic precursors. Most of them (exceptions noted) may be seen in the megaloblastic anemias, myelodysplastic syndromes, and erythroleukemias (M6). These include bi- or multinucleated precursors, sometimes with nuclei at dissimilar stages of maturation (Plate 158-22); multiple nuclear lobulations; folded nuclei (M6); giant nuclei (M6); nuclear fragmentation; and accelerated pyknosis (condensation of chromatin). Since many of these changes have more than one cause, clinical correlation is highly important.

A hallmark of both vitamin B_{12} or folate deficiency and the abnormal metabolism encountered in some preleukemic states is dyschrony of nuclear and cytoplasmic maturation (megaloblastic or megaloblastoid change). This is characterized by cytoplasm that exhibits varying degrees of hemoglobin formation (indicated by a range of color changes from gray-blue to various shades of red) with nuclei that are less mature than normal for the degree of hemoglobinization (i.e., they show a retarded degree of chromatin condensation, resulting in a more lightly staining and more diffuse chromatin pattern) (Plate 158-23).

Megakaryocytes

Normal mature megakaryocytes are approximately 6–10 times the diameter of a red cell. The nucleus is extensively and smoothly lobulated, and the cytoplasm is reddish blue with a few scattered, tiny red granules.

When megakaryocyte turnover is high, such as in accelerated platelet consumption (ITP, TTP) and myeloproliferative disorders, megakaryocytes may be small, with attenuated cytoplasm and small, round, dark, hypolobated nuclei (so-called micromegakaryocytes). In other words, there is a bias in maturation toward smaller, immature forms that have not yet undergone extensive nuclear division. At the opposite extreme, giant megakaryocytes may be encountered in myeloproliferative disorders. These may have distinctly abnormal nuclear morphology: hyperchromatic (very dark staining) with angulated (rather than smooth) contours.

Megakaryocytes may sometimes be confused with osteoclasts, particularly in marrows from children and in conditions of increased bone turnover such as hyperparathyroidism. The latter cells are truly multinucleated rather than multilobulated, with distinct, small round nuclei. Furthermore, the cytoplasm is pink and agranular.

Finally, a phenomenon often encountered in the examination of normal megakaryocytes is the presence of neutrophils and other hematopoietic elements within the cytoplasm of megakaryocytes (Plate 158-24). This process, which is unexplained, is called *emperipolesis*. It is not phagocytosis in the strict sense, since the engulfed cells are not in true phagolysosomes, nor are they destroyed.

Lymphocytes

Normal lymphocytes are about the size of a mature erythrocyte in aspirate smears; have slightly oval, darkly staining nuclei with indistinct nucleoli and a thin rim of blue cytoplasm; and constitute <5% of the total cellularity. During an immunologic response, transformed lymphocytes may be found in the marrow. These are larger, have more cytoplasm, and may exhibit prominent nucleoli. Such cells may resemble quite closely those of some large cell lymphomas, and clinical correlation is required for proper interpretation. In general, however, the number of such reactive lymphocytes is usually small and is accompanied by a population of normal small lymphocytes and, often, plasma cells, indicating a maturation sequence not found with most lymphomas. Small aggregates of lymphocytes, normally present in the marrows of some individuals >40 years of age, may be aspirated.

The appearance of sheets of small lymphocytes on an aspirate smear may suggest a diagnosis of lymphoma. Careful examination of the cells for the cytologic features of normal lymphocytes and the presence of such sheets on only a few of the smears prepared from the aspirate support an interpretation of benign lymphoid aggregate. Comparison with the bone marrow biopsy may be very helpful. The lymphocytic malignancies that most frequently involve the bone marrow are the low-grade lymphomas of follicular center cell origin, chronic lymphocytic leukemia (CLL), and acute lymphocytic leukemia (ALL). Each has cytologic features in aspirate smears that help to distinguish it from normal lymphocytes.

The low-grade lymphomas that derive from the germinal centers of lymph node follicles frequently involve the bone marrow, often in a spotty distribution. The characteristic cell is the small, cleaved follicular center cell: a lymphocyte that is slightly larger than a normal small lymphocyte, has little cytoplasm, and has folded (cleaved), somewhat twisted nuclear contours. This feature has given rise to the term *buttock cell* to describe the deep nuclear groove sometimes seen in this type of lymphoma cell. The abnormal nuclear contours may be difficult to appreciate in many of the cells, and their detection requires careful examination of well-smeared and -stained cells.

The cytology of CLL cells, although similar to that of normal lymphocytes, has some distinctive features. Although of comparable size, CLL cells have distinctly round nuclei and very clumped chromatin, with lighter-staining areas between the chromatin clumps. These cells seem to be somewhat more fragile than normal cells, and a typical finding on aspirate smears from patients with CLL is numerous damaged "smudge" cells. ALL cells vary from the same size to somewhat larger than a normal small lymphocyte and may exhibit more size heterogeneity than is typical of normal lymphocytes. The key distinguishing features are a fine, uniform staining pattern of nuclear chromatin and nuclear convolutions. The former results in a much lighter-staining nucleus. The latter is variable (i.e., not present in all cells) and can best be described as smooth, undulating folds of the nuclear membrane.

Plasma Cells

Plasma cells in normal marrows make up <5% of the total cellularity. Their cytologic features are characteristic in that they are about two times the diameter of a mature erythrocyte, and they have an eccentric nucleus with clumped, somewhat peripherally arranged chromatin resembling the face of a clock, as well as intensely blue cytoplasm and a perinuclear clear (Golgi) zone (Plate 158-25). Their number is increased in infections and other conditions eliciting an immune response but is virtually never >20% of the cellularity. Plasma cell dyscrasias, particularly plasma cell myeloma, usually cause an increased number of plasma cells in the marrow, aggregates of these cells in aspirate smears, and sometimes distinct cytologic changes. The most frequent change is a prominent nucleolus, a feature seldom found in reactive plasmacytoses (Plate 158-26). Other findings include larger than normal size, increased nuclear/ cytoplasmic ratio, and central nuclei. In some cases of plasma cell myeloma (as noted in the section Bone Marrow Biopsy) the cells may resemble the precursors of plasma cells, exhibiting the cytologic features of immunoblasts (transformed lymphocytes), with plasmacytoid features. In such cases the clinical history may be important in helping to make the diagnosis of plasma cell myeloma.

Macrophages

Macrophages are typically large cells, about three to five times the diameter of a red cell (Plate 158-27). They have a small, eccentric nucleus (approximately one red cell diameter) and voluminous gray-blue cytoplasm that often contains phagocytosed debris or hemosiderin (storage iron), or both. Macrophages make up <1% of the cells in the marrow and are usually concentrated in the marrow particles. An increase in number of these cells is uncommon; one example occurs after chemotherapy, in which macrophages play a clean-up role.

The so-called hemophagocytic syndromes are clinically important situations involving increased numbers of macrophages. Some of these syndromes are hereditary, others are infection induced, and both types are characterized by large increases in actively phagocytic macrophages in the liver, spleen, and bone marrow. These are often difficult to detect in marrow biopsies without a high index of suspicion. Such phagocytic macrophages are easier to see in aspirate smears. In fact, if macrophages are easily detected in the smears, their number is almost certainly increased, and clinical correlation should be obtained.

REFERENCES

1. Luna L (ed): Manual of Histologic Staining Methods of the Armed Forces Institute of Pathology. 3rd Ed. McGraw-Hill, New York, 1968
2. Troyer H (ed): Principles and Techniques of Histochemistry. Little, Brown, Boston, 1980
3. Tricot G, DeWolf-Peters C, Hendrickx B, Verwilghen RL: Bone marrow histology in myelodysplasic syndromes. I. Histological findings in myelodysplastic syndromes and comparison with bone marrow smears. Br J Haematol 57:423, 1984
4. Hay ED (ed): Cell Biology of Extra-Cellular Matrix. Plenum, New York, 1982, p. 3
5. Jaffe ES (ed): Surgical Pathology of the Lymph Nodes and Related Organs. Vol. 16. Major Problems in Pathology. WB Saunders, Philadelphia, 1985
6. The Non-Hodgkin's Lymphomas Pathologic Classification Project: National Cancer Institute sponsored study of classifications of non-Hodgkin's lymphomas: summary and description of a working formulation for clinical usage. Cancer 49:2112, 1982
7. Robertson LE, Redman JR, Bulter JJ et al: Discordant bone marrow involvement in diffuse large-cell lymphoma: a distinct clinical-pathologic entity associated with a continuous risk of relapse. J Clin Oncol 9:236, 1991
8. Wood G, Warnke R: The immunologic phenotyping of bone marrow biopsies and aspirates: frozen section techniques. Blood 59:913, 1982

Automated Analysis of Blood Cells

159

Daniel H. Ryan

INTRODUCTION

Automated blood cell analysis and manual morphologic examination of the blood smear each possess significant advantages and disadvantages. It is unlikely that either approach will totally supplant the other. Without the speed and walk-away capabilities of modern automated instruments, clinical laboratories would be unable to handle a large volume of samples efficiently. Automated instruments also provide superior accuracy and precision in quantitative blood cell measurements. By contrast, the complexity and remarkable variation of the formed blood elements should be recognized as a formidable challenge for any automated instrument, present or future. Therefore, some samples analyzed on an automated blood cell counter will require manual examination of the blood smear for definitive diagnosis of morphologic abnormalities. Even as powerful a technique as flow cytometry is useless unless correlated with the morphology of the cells being analyzed.

AUTOMATED ANALYSIS TECHNIQUES

Packed cell volume: The oldest method of quantitative measurement of blood cells is the measurement of packed volume of formed elements of the blood after centrifugation. A clinical instrument provides a rapid estimate of hematocrit, leukocyte, and platelet count using an inserted float to expand the buffy coat region of blood stained with a fluorescent nuclear dye. This approach has been used for screening applications[1] and to detect microfilaria[2] and malaria,[2] but may not possess sufficient precision for following hematologic disorders.[3]

Image analysis: Computerized image analysis has been extensively utilized in the past for routine blood smear analysis, but it is hampered by slow throughput requirement for smear preparation and the need to perform the cell counts on a separate instrument.[4] This approach has largely been superseded by blood counters that analyze cells in flow.

Impedance particle counting (the Coulter principle): Cells can be counted and their size measured by measuring change in electrical resistance as cells in solution flow through a narrow aperture across which a DC current is maintained.[5] The magnitude of the voltage change is directly proportional to particle size for objects of similar shape, but is affected by the relative deformability of particles as they pass through the aperture.[6] Red cells are easily deformable as they pass through the aperture[7]; platelets and leukocytes have intermediate "shape factors." Therefore it is critical to calibrate instruments according to the cell type being analyzed.

Light scatter: A focused light beam striking a cell will be scattered in all directions. The amount of light scattered at a relatively low angle from the incident light path is primarily dependent on cell size. The amount of light scattered at wide angle is primarily affected by structural complexity within the cell (granules, nuclear shape). Simultaneous measurement of light scattered at different angles allows certain leukocyte types to be distinguished, although there is some overlap. For this reason, an unanticipated excess of any one cell type (for instance, incompletely lysed red cells in a leukocyte analysis) may invalidate the quantitative results.

Light absorption: Absorption of incident light by cells as a result of accumulation of a cytochemical dye for detection of peroxidase activity is used by some instruments in conjunction with light scatter measurements to identify the five major leukocyte populations.[8] This method is generally less sensitive than fluorescence labeling but has been used for immunophenotyping with alkaline-phosphatase conjugated antibodies.[9]

Conductivity: A relatively new technique in clinical instruments is measurement of conductivity of cells to high-frequency alternating current to identify granulocytes.

Fluorescence: Measurement of the emission of fluorescent light is sensitive and broadly applicable to analysis of multiple cellular characteristics, such as immunophenotype (using labeled antibodies), DNA content, RNA content, and other cellular characteristics.

Blood analyzers increasingly combine analytical principles, such as light scatter and fluorescence (flow cytometers), impedance, conductivity, and light scatter (Coulter STKS), progressively blurring distinctions between flow cytometers and automated cell counters. Newer instruments, including flow cytometers, will automate sample identification, preparation, aspiration, analysis, identification of problematic results, and quality control. These instruments represent significant clinical advances but require an increasing degree of interpretive sophistication on the part of the laboratory technologist.

INTERPRETATION OF AUTOMATED BLOOD CELL ANALYSIS

In a typical automated blood cell counter, a portion of the aspirated sample is lysed for hemoglobin and leukocyte analysis. A separate aliquot is diluted without lysis for red cell and platelet analysis. Some parameters are calculated from the primary data, including hematocrit (= red blood cell [RBC] count × mean corpuscular volume [MCV]), mean corpuscular hemoglobin concentration (MCHC) (= hemoglobin/hematocrit), mean corpuscular hemoglobin (MCH) (= hemoglobin/RBC count), and red cell distribution width (RDW) or platelet distribution width (PDW) (= estimate of variance in the red cell or platelet volume distribution).

Hemoglobin and Hematocrit

All hemoglobins in the lysed aliquot, including oxy-, carboxy-, carbonmonoxy-, and methemoglobin, are converted by potassium ferricyanide to cyanmethemoglobin, which has a broad and easily measured absorbance peak at 540 nm.[10] The hemoglobin is preferable to the hematocrit, since it is directly measured and is not subject to some of the infrequent artifacts that affect the hematocrit measurement. Lipemia may falsely elevate the hemoglobin measurement, but this artifact is usually detectable by examination of the sample and comparison of the hemoglobin and (independently calculated) hematocrit. Hematocrit measured as packed cell volume (spun hematocrit) is slightly higher than the automated hematocrit, due to the inclusion of trapped plasma in the packed red cell column.[11] The amount of this trapped plasma, typically about 2–3% of the packed red cell volume,[11] varies depending on red cell morphology and technical factors, and may be as high as 6% in microcytic anemias.[12] Although blood counters are typically calibrated to yield a hematocrit equivalent to the packed cell volume for normal blood, the spun hematocrit is likely to be higher than the automated hematocrit in patients with hypochromic or poorly deformable (i.e., sickled) red cells, due to increased plasma trapping.

Erythrocyte Count and Indices

The MCV is directly calculated as the average red cell volume determined by impedance or light scatter, while the other indices are calculated as described above. The MCV is the most clinically useful red cell index.[13,14] Although the MCV has been widely used to direct the workup of hypoproductive anemias, its diagnostic sensitivity in both iron-deficiency anemia and megaloblastic anemia has been questioned.[15,16] The MCH closely parallels the MCV and provides little additional diagnostic information.[14] The MCHC is more frequently reduced in iron-deficiency anemia than other causes of microcytosis,[17] but the drop in MCHC occurs relatively late,[18] and the diagnostic utility of the parameter is poor.[19] An elevated MCHC is classically associated with hereditary spherocytosis or autoimmune hemolytic anemia, but this finding is not always present. The dynamic range of the MCHC measurement is limited by the tendency of certain cells with truly high MCHCs, such as spherocytes or sickled cells, to deform less in the aperture, overestimating the MCV and consequently reducing the measured MCHC. Numerous discriminant functions based on red cell indices have been proposed to differentiate iron deficiency from thalassemia trait, but they cannot substitute for definitive tests in diagnosing individual patients.[17]

The MCV and red cell count are subject to several artifacts. The most common of these is autoreactive red cell antibodies active at room temperature, which aggregate red cells in the instrument, lowering the red cell count while increasing the MCV.[20] Typically, the red cell count is lowered to a greater degree than the MCV is increased (since large aggregates are not counted), causing a falsely elevated MCHC. Warming or prediluting the sample usually reverses this effect, which may occur in healthy subjects. Artifactually low MCV measurements due to osmotic effects have been infrequently reported in extreme hyperglycemia.[21]

Red Cell Distribution Width

The RDW is a quantitative estimation of anisocytosis, and is typically computed as the coefficient of variation of red cell size distribution. Anemic disorders can be classified on the basis of RDW.[22] In particular, the RDW is more frequently elevated in iron-deficiency anemia than in thalassemia or anemia of chronic disease.[22,23] However, the overlap among these patient groups is significant, even when only clear-cut presentations are considered,[17] complicating interpretation of the results in individual patients.[24] This parameter may be useful in screening high-prevalence populations or in conjunction with other more specific tests, such as serum ferritin.[25] The RDW is used in the clinical laboratory as an indicator of anisocytosis to select samples from the automated blood counter for morphologic red cell analysis.

Reticulocyte Count

Standard method: In the standard manual reticulocyte count, new methylene blue is used to stain residual RNA and aggregate the RNA to make it easily visible. Flow cytometers are sufficiently sensitive to detect fluorescence from RNA binding dyes in single cells. Dedicated clinical flow instruments capable of staining and analyzing reticulocytes in whole blood are now available.[26] Leukocytes and large platelets or platelet aggregates must be carefully excluded by light scatter measurements, as these cells will contain variable amounts of RNA. A major advantage of automated reticulocyte counting is improved precision,[27] especially in the low-normal range, in which manual methods are imprecise due to the small number of reticulocytes counted.[28] The reference range by manual and automated methods is similar.[29] Recovery after bone marrow transplantation may be detectable slightly earlier by the automated reticulocyte count as compared with standard reticulocyte, platelet, or neutrophil counts.[30,31]

Reticulocyte maturity index: Immature or "shift" reticulocytes with increased RNA can be recognized by increased staining with precipitating RNA dyes[32] or as polychromatophilic cells on a blood smear.[33] Increased RNA content by flow cytometry may be an indicator of reticulocyte immaturity. Increased reticulocyte RNA content is an early sign of erythroid recovery following bone marrow transplantation.[31,34] Standardization of staining procedures, data analysis,[35] and quality control[36,37] are important, since the reticulocyte RNA content is a continuous variable without clearly separated positive and negative populations. (This is also a problem with manual reticulocyte counting.[38])

Platelet Count

Counting of platelets in whole blood has traditionally been difficult because of their small size, wide size range, tendency to aggregate, and potential overlap with more numerous red cells or debris.[39] Current instruments deal with these problems by mathematical analysis of the platelet volume distribution to ensure that it represents the log-normal distribution (skewed to the higher volumes) expected in both normal and diseased subjects. If the volume distribution does not conform to this shape, the presence of cell fragments or microcytic red cells is suspected, and manual techniques must be used. Like the MCV and RDW, mean platelet volume (MPV) and PDW are calculated from the platelet volume distribution.

Even with automated instruments, the platelet count is measured less precisely than the other components of the blood count (expected analytic variability of about 22%).[40] Variability tends to be higher in the markedly thrombocytopenic range, in which there may be the greatest need to measure small changes in platelet number accurately. The lower limit of linearity in these instruments is 5–20,000/mm^3, below which the platelet count must be performed manually, with further loss of precision. Therefore, care should be exercised in clinical interpretation of small changes in reported platelet counts in thrombocytopenic patients.

The most important cause of falsely low platelet count is inadequate anticoagulation (indicated by small clots or fibrin strands visible on smear). Some individuals possess autoreactive antibodies that recognize platelet surface epitopes, which are exposed under divalent cation-free conditions (i.e., EDTA or citrate-anticoagulated blood).[41] The resulting platelet clumps show up as an abnormal peak in the leukocyte volume histogram (the aggregated platelets are incompletely lysed by detergent) and can also be observed in the feathered edge of the smear. Platelet adequacy can be estimated from a heparinized sample or fingerstick smear (both of which typically show ome platelet clumping due to incomplete inhibition of platelet ctivation). Falsely high platelet counts can be caused by cytolasmic fragments of degenerated leukocytes, microcytic red ells, cryoglobulins, or debris. In all these instances, the platet volume distribution would demonstrate a significant deviaon from the expected log-normal relationship and would be agged as abnormal.

Platelet Analysis

MPV: The MPV is inversely correlated with platelet count,[42] nd must therefore be interpreted in conjunction with the latelet count using a nomogram of reference ranges.[43] An elerated MPV is associated with destructive thrombocytopenia,[44] nd decreased MPV with hypoproliferative thrombocytoenia.[43] Increased MPV may be due to stimulation of megakarypoiesis,[45] rather than simply decreased platelet age.[44,46] MPV nay be a risk factor for recurrent myocardial infarction[47] and estenosis after coronary angioplasty.[48] Interpretation of MPV

is complicated by the continuously changing MPV observed in patients recovering from destructive thrombocytopenia[44] and the instability of MPV in EDTA anticoagulated blood.[49,50] The clinical significance of the PDW is unclear.

"Reticulated" platelets: The RNA content of platelets can be quantitated by flow cytometry using the RNA-binding dye thiazole orange. Due to their small size, platelets must be carefully distinguished from cellular fragments and debris using light scatter parameters or platelet-specific markers.[51] An increased percentage, but not absolute number, of "reticulated" or RNA-containing platelets is observed in destructive thrombocytopenia,[52–54] suggesting that young platelets are also subject to destruction.[52–54] A subset of patients with clinically defined idiopathic thrombocytopenic purpura do not show increased RNA-containing platelets[53]; it is not known whether these patients represent a subgroup complicated by deficient thrombopoiesis.[55] By contrast, patients with hypoproliferative thrombocytopenia have a normal percentage, but a markedly decreased absolute number, of RNA-containing platelets.[52]

Platelet function: Decreased surface expression of platelet

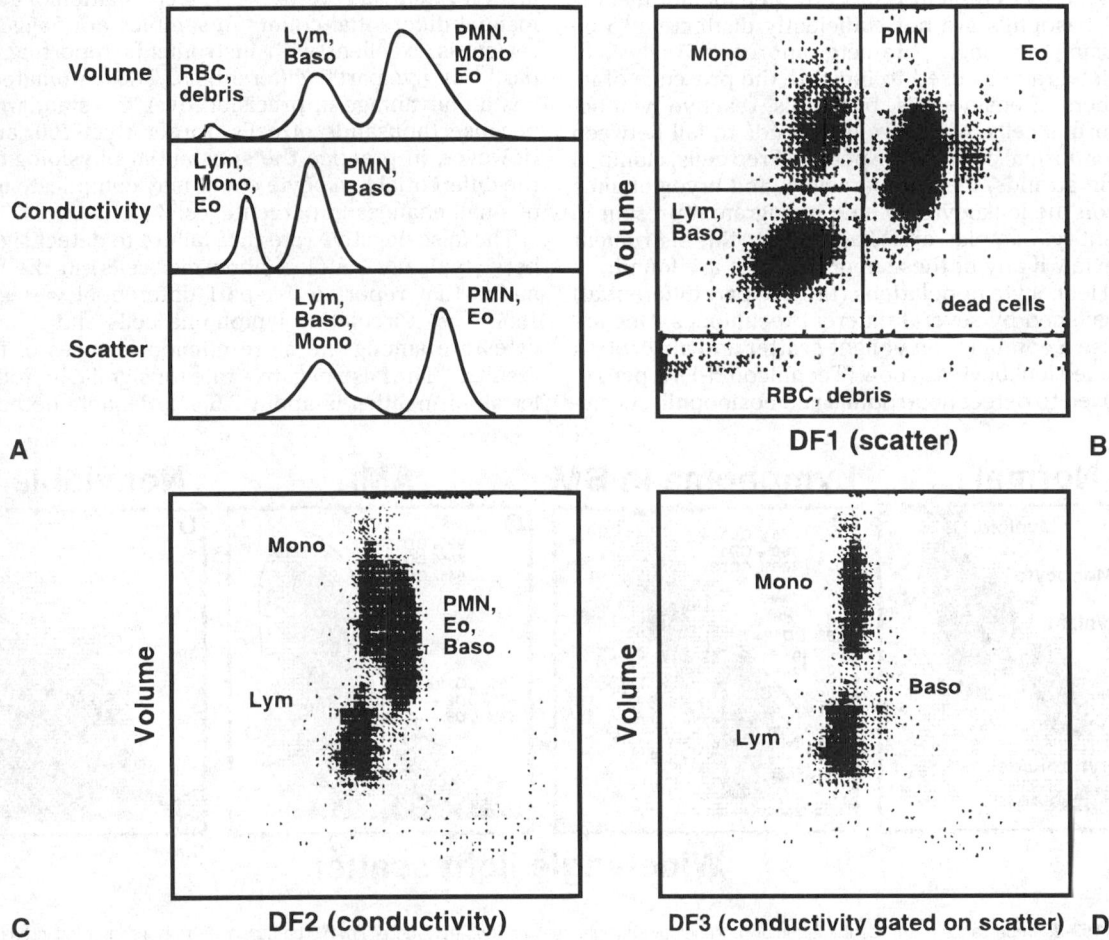

Fig. 159-1. Automated five-part leukocyte differential. **(A)** Simultaneously measured volume, electrical conductivity, and light scatter in lysed whole blood analyzed by the Coulter STKS automated blood counter. As shown, each parameter distinguishes different groups of leukocytes, allowing numerical estimation of the five major leukocyte subgroups by comparing data from each measurement. Abnormal cells lie in between these normal populations. **(B)** Two-parameter histogram of discriminant function (DF)1 (derived from scatter data) versus volume, showing the cell populations identified. Basophils are indistinguishable from lymphocytes on the basis of scatter and volume alone. **(C)** Two-parameter histogram of DF2 (derived from conductivity data) versus volume). Basophils have higher conductivity than lymphocytes, but are not separable from other granulocytes. **(D)** Two-parameter histogram of DF3 (conductivity, gated on scatter to eliminate cells with high light scatter) versus volume. Basophils can now be seen as a separate population, since they have lower light scatter than other granulocytes, but higher conductivity than lymphocytes or monocytes. Lym, lymphocyte; Baso, basophil; PMN, polymorphonuclear neutrophil; Mono, monocyte; Eo, eosinophil.

surface integrin adhesion molecules in congenital platelet function disorders has been detected by flow cytometry.[56] Surface expression of certain adhesion molecules, such as P-selectin, is induced by platelet activation and can be detected by flow cytometry.[57] The clinical significance of such measurements in cardiovascular disease and thrombosis remains to be established.

Platelet-associated IgG: Flow cytometric detection of platelet-associated immunoglobulin[58] has some advantages (no requirement for platelet isolation, sample volume, ability to identify subpopulations) as well as disadvantages (poorer sensitivity and quantitation) in comparison with standard immunoassay methods.[51]

Leukocyte Count and Differential

Three major normal leukocyte populations (lymphocytes, monocytes, and neutrophils—the three-part differential), can be distinguished by electrical impedance volume measurement of leukocytes in which the cytoplasmic contents have been partially removed by detergent lysis of the cell membrane. Eosinophils and basophils are not sufficiently distinctive to be enumerated using this single-parameter approach. Analysis of the volume histograms is used to indicate the presence of increased numbers of eosinophils, basophils, reactive lymphocytes, or abnormal cells, whose volume tends to fall between the three major normal cell types. Nucleated red cells, clumped platelets, fibrin strands, malaria parasites, and cryoglobulins will show up on the leukocyte volume histogram if present in sufficient quantity. Samples are "flagged" by the instrument for manual review if any of these abnormalities are found.

Five normal leukocyte populations (the five-part differential) can be distinguished by several different techniques. One approach is to use a combination of light scatter and absorption to identify stained leukocytes in flow (Technicon H-1). A peroxidase stain is used to detect neutrophils and eosinophils. Eosin-

ophils have very high peroxidase staining but relatively lo[w] forward light scatter, because their large granules scatter mo[st] of the incident light at high angles rather than low angles. Bas[o]phils are identified by resistance to lysis using a different dete[r]gent. Leukemic cells are typically large but lack peroxidas[e] positivity ("large unstained cells"). This approach has the a[d]vantage of using a more biologically relevant end point for le[u]kocyte identification, but may require more maintenance an[d] is somewhat slower in operation.[59]

A commonly used instrument (Coulter STKS) identifies th[e] five major blood leukocyte types by electrical impedance, ligh[t] scatter, and electrical conductivity, as shown in Figure 159-[1.] Other approaches to the five-part leukocyte differential includ[e] differential resistance to lysis of eosinophils and basophils [in] specific detergents at different temperatures (Sysmex E-5000[)] or patterns of light scatter determined by measurements a[t] four different angles, using a polarized light source (Cell-Dy[n] 3000).

A significant proportion of samples submitted for automate[d] blood count and differential (about 10–40% depending on pa[-] tient population and instrument type) are flagged by the instru[-] ment for manual review.[60,61] The correlation of automated an[d] manual differential counts in samples not flagged for manua[l] review is excellent with instruments reporting either three[-] part[62] or five-part[63] differentials. The automated differentia[l] has an advantage in precision over the standard differentia[l] because thousands of cells, rather than 100, are counted.[6] However, in practice the substantial physiologic variation i[n] the differential leukocyte count may complicate interpretatio[n] of small changes in percentages.[65]

The false-negative rate (i.e., failure to detect significant num[-] bers [typically ≥5%] of abnormal cells) in the newer instru[-] ments that report a five-part differential varies from 1% t[o] 15%.[60,66,67] Circulating lymphoma cells and reactive lympho[-] cytes are among the more common causes of false-negative results.[60] The false-negative rate for significant red cell or plate[-] let abnormalities is about 2.5%.[68] Reliable detection of infre[-]

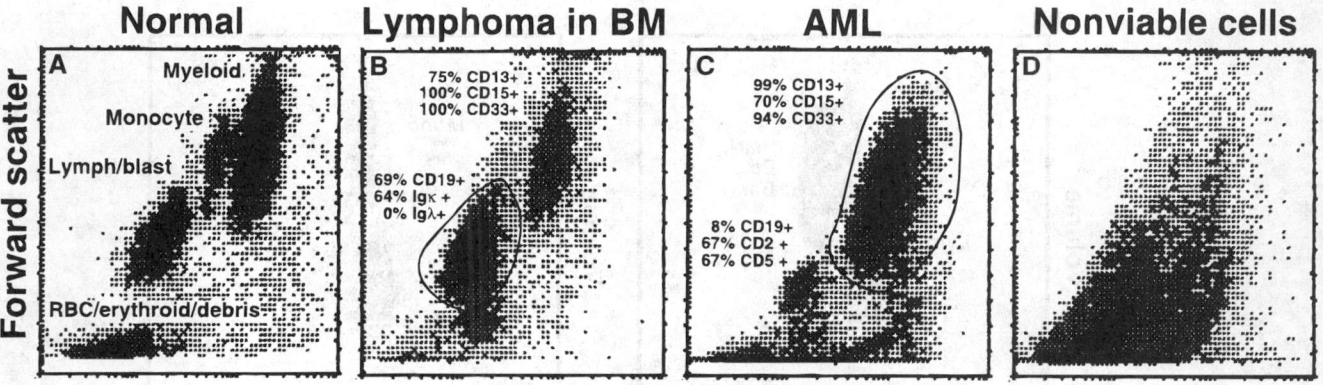

Fig. 159-2. Importance of cell identification by morphology and light scatter. Two-parameter flow cytometry histograms displaying intensity of wide-angle versus forward light scatter. Cells are plotted on the histogram according to their light scatter intensity; density of the dot pattern indicates numbers of cells. **(A)** Scatter histogram of whole blood after erythrocyte lysis. Bone marrow scatter histograms are similar in appearance. The location of major blood and bone marrow cells is indicated. **(B)** Scatter histogram of light density bone marrow cells involved with B-cell lymphoma. The phenotype of the two major populations of cells evident by light scatter is indicated. The monoclonal B cells are contained in the circled region, while cells in the upper region express myeloid-associated markers and represent normal myeloid elements that were abundant in the marrow smear. **(C)** Scatter histogram of light density cells from bone marrow of a patient with AML. In this case, the lower "lymphoid" region contained normal lymphocytes (67% T cells and 8% B cells), while the upper circled region (90% of total cells) was positive for myeloid-associated markers. Since the bone marrow smear contained >90% abnormal leukemic cells, these results indicated that the leukemia was of myeloid origin. Note that the percentage of cells positive for myeloid markers in the myeloid light scatter region was similar in Figs. b and c, and correlation with morphology was absolutely essential for proper interpretation. **(D)** Scatter histogram of light density cells from bone marrow containing a high proportion of dead cells. Note the absence of a defined population with light scatter characteristics similar to lymphoid or myeloid cells.

uent abnormal cells is a problem for both automated counters and conventional microscopy. The best approach is to use all available clinical and laboratory information to identify patients in whom careful morphologic examination of the blood smear for a specific abnormality is of diagnostic relevance.[69] The data generated by automated blood counters can be used to direct attention to those blood films most likely to contain diagnostic information.[70]

The blood count[71] and leukocyte differential count[72] are considered by many observers to be overused as screening tests relative to their diagnostic utility. Given the current ordering patterns for these tests, automated differential counters offer a rapid and cost-effective means of screening blood for significant quantitative and qualitative leukocyte abnormalities, but definitive characterization of any cell population flagged by these instruments as atypical still requires visual examination of the blood smear by a trained observer.

CELL MARKER ANALYSIS BY FLOW CYTOMETRY

Principles of Flow Cytometry

Flow cytometers use the general principles of automated cell analysis mentioned above, particularly light scatter, but are especially designed for sensitive and quantitative fluorescence measurements of single cells. A very brief overview of technical aspects of flow cytometry is presented here. Excellent reviews and textbooks covering this subject in detail are available.[73]

Cell preparation and staining: For accurate surface labeling, cells must be viable and contamination with irrelevant cells or debris kept to a minimum. Staining and analysis of neoplastic cells is typically performed after density gradient centrifugation to remove RBCs in mature neutrophils. Improper specimen processing resulting in cell death is a common cause of decreased or nonspecific labeling. The requirement of flow cytometers for single cell suspensions can be problematic in solid tissue samples, which must be mechanically or enzymatically disaggregated, sometimes resulting in loss of the cells of interest and a false-negative result. Cells are typically stained using directly conjugated monoclonal antibodies.

Recognition of cells by light scatter: The flow cytometer senses particles passing through the light beam by detection of scattered light. The major subpopulations of hematopoietic cells can be recognized (albeit with some overlap) by analysis of light scatter (Fig. 159-2A). Because monocytes and myeloid cells may nonspecifically bind antibodies, it is critical to select the proper cell population for analysis. Accurate fluorescence data is absolutely dependent on correct recognition of the location of the cells of interest using light scatter (Fig. 159-2B & C). Understanding expected light scattering patterns is critical: lymphoid malignancies and undifferentiated acute myeloid leukemia (AML) are similar to normal lymphoid cells, while differentiated myeloid/monocytic leukemias have high forward or wide-angle scatter[74]; dead cells show decreased light scatter (Fig. 159-2D).

Fluorescence measurement: The fluorescence emitted by each cell as it passes through the light beam is optically focused and amplified. Discrimination of two to three colors of fluorescence emission is accomplished by optical filters placed in front of separate light detectors. The combination of intense incident light and sensitive photomultiplier tubes makes the flow cytometer well suited for fluorescence measurements of individual cells.

Principles of Cell Marker Analysis

Flow cytometry is broadly applicable beyond the field of hematology.[73] The most common applications in hematology are detection of differentiation- or maturation-related cellular pro-

Table 159-1. Lineage Association of Diagnostically Useful Hematopoietic Markers[a]

Marker	Lineage Association
B cell	
Immunoglobulin	B
CD22	B
CD20	B
CD21	B
CD19	B, AMoL
T cell	
CD3/TCR	T
CD2	T, NK
CD5	T, B subset
CD4	T, Mo, eos, Mk
CD7	T, myeloid progenitor
CD1	Thymocyte, Langerhans
Progenitors	
CD34	All progenitors
TdT	Lymphoid progenitors
CD10	Pre-B, activated B, PMN
Myeloid/monocyte	
MPO	My, Mo
CD33	My, Mo
CD13	My, Mo
CD14	Mo
CD15	My, Mo
CD11c	My, Mo
Megakaryocyte	
plt. perox.	Mk
CD41a	Mk, endothelium
CD61	Mk, endothelium
Erythroid	
Glycophorin	Erythroid
Spectrin	Erythroid
NK/cytotoxic T	
CD56	NK, plasma cell
CD16	NK, PMN
CD57	Cytotoxic T

Abbreviations: B, B cell; T, T cell; AMoL, acute monocytic leukemia; NK, natural killer cell; Mo, monocyte; TdT, terminal deoxynucleotidyl transferase; MPO, myeloperoxidase; My, myeloid cell; Mk, megakaryocyte; eos, eosinophil; PMN, polymorphonuclear neutrophil; TCR, T-cell receptor; plt. perox., platelet peroxidase.

[a] Commonly used markers are grouped according to their major lineage association. The more specific markers are at the top of the list in each lineage category.

teins using labeled monoclonal antibodies, or DNA content using DNA binding dyes. Numerous cellular proteins have been recognized using monoclonal antibodies (CDs).[75] Some clinically useful lineage-associated markers are listed in Table 159-1, and the pattern of expression of selected markers in the major hematopoietic lineages is shown in Figure 159-3.

The clinical relevance of immunophenotyping is based on the assumptions that the phenotype of the abnormal cell is an interpretable pattern and not a random collection of markers and that the phenotype of a cell reflects important biologic characteristics (i.e., clinical aggressiveness, drug sensitivity). In view of their markedly altered genotype and clinical behavior, it is remarkable that leukemic cells usually phenotypically resemble some normal stage of differentiation. However, the biologic role of most cell markers is incompletely understood. Therefore, these markers are likely to be only surrogates for the actual proteins that determine response to chemotherapy and clinical aggressiveness.

Lineage specificity of markers: Although terms such as myeloid marker are convenient and commonly used, the functional

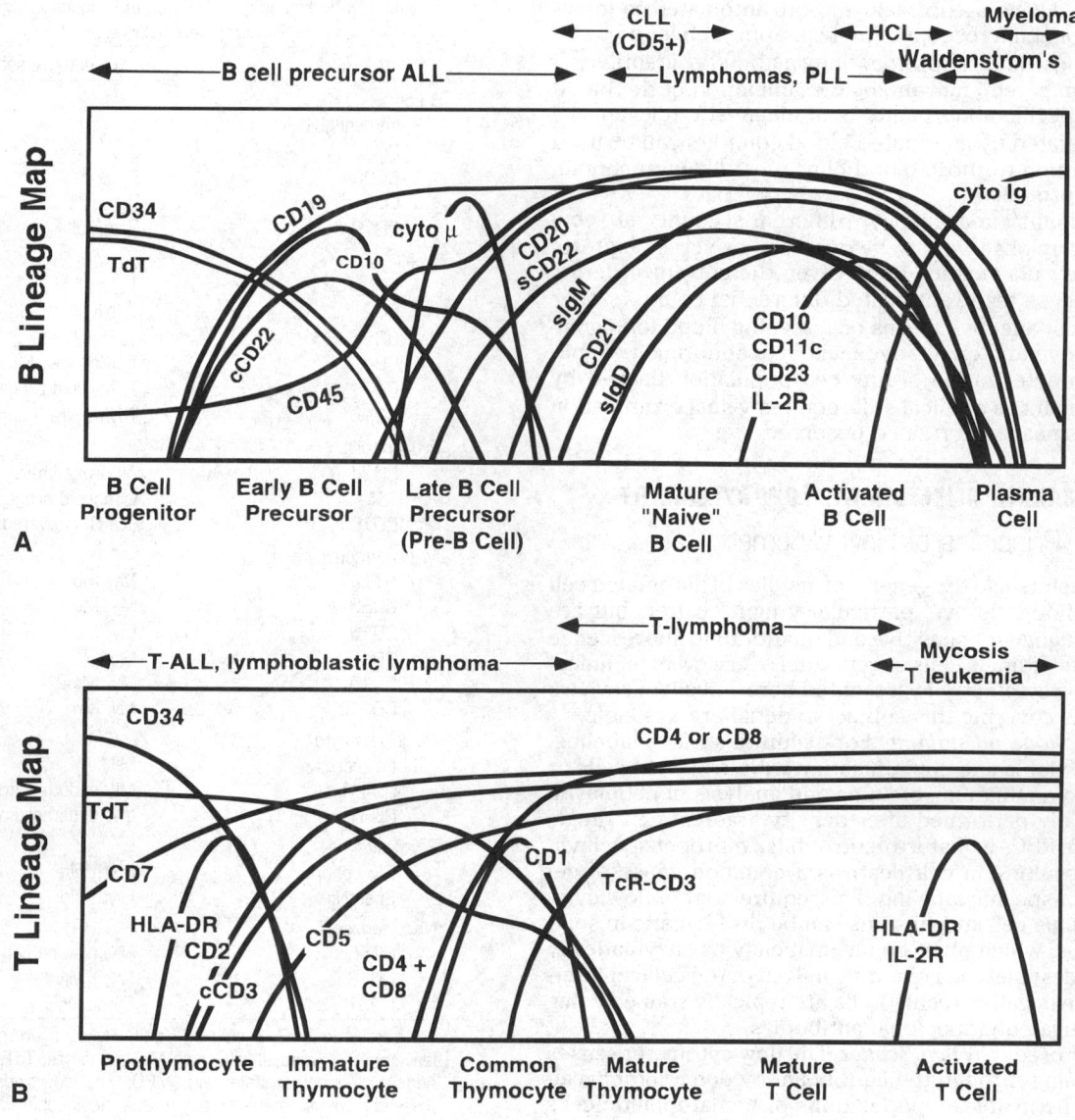

Fig. 159-3. Differentiation-based expression of cell markers (lineage maps). Expression of clinically useful surface markers during differentiation in the **(A)** B-cell, **(B)** T-cell. *(Figure continues.)*

role of any surface protein is seldom restricted to cells of a given lineage. For instance, the neutral endopeptidase CD10, initially identified as a marker of immature B cells, is expressed by other cell types, including neutrophils and renal tubular epithelium. Although neoplastic cells do tend to resemble normal cells in a particular lineage at a particular stage of differentiation, on close examination neoplastic cells often display an "incorrect" phenotype when compared with any known normal cell. This can take the form of "asynchronous" (lineage-correct markers appearing in the wrong order) or "mixed lineage" (markers associated with different lineages appearing in one cell) differentiation. It should be recognized that "aberrant" marker expression may also reflect leukemic expansion of a rare normal population that is difficult to detect by standard techniques.[76]

Interpretation of marker studies: In general, the diagnostic or prognostic value of any single marker is limited due to the lack of absolute specificity of any marker, and the complex biologic abnormalities involved in neoplastic transformation. The diagnostic importance of recognizing characteristic combinations of surface markers in lymphoid malignancies is illustrated in

Figure 159-4. Flow cytometry analysis of neoplasms requires pattern recognition; it has been stated that "flow cytometric diagnosis is more analogous to reading a bone marrow aspirate than determining a serum sodium level."[77] The recognition of populations of cells with distinctive immunophenotype and correlation of these populations with morphologically relevant cells is the key skill of flow cytometric interpretation. The major steps in cell marker analysis and interpretation by flow cytometry are summarized in Table 159-2. A recent study has emphasized the importance of pattern recognition over numerical analysis in diagnosis of hematologic neoplasia.[78] The importance of visual analysis of histograms for recognizing abnormal expression density or co-expression of markers is often obscured by the standard practice of reporting percentage of positive cells for each marker, which may be misleading when a weakly staining population of neoplastic cells is present[79,80] (Fig. 159-5). Immunohistochemical staining of tissue sections is complementary to flow cytometry because of the additional morphologic information that can only be gained from the tissue section. However, many surface markers, in particular surface immunoglobulin, are not consistently detectable after fixation.

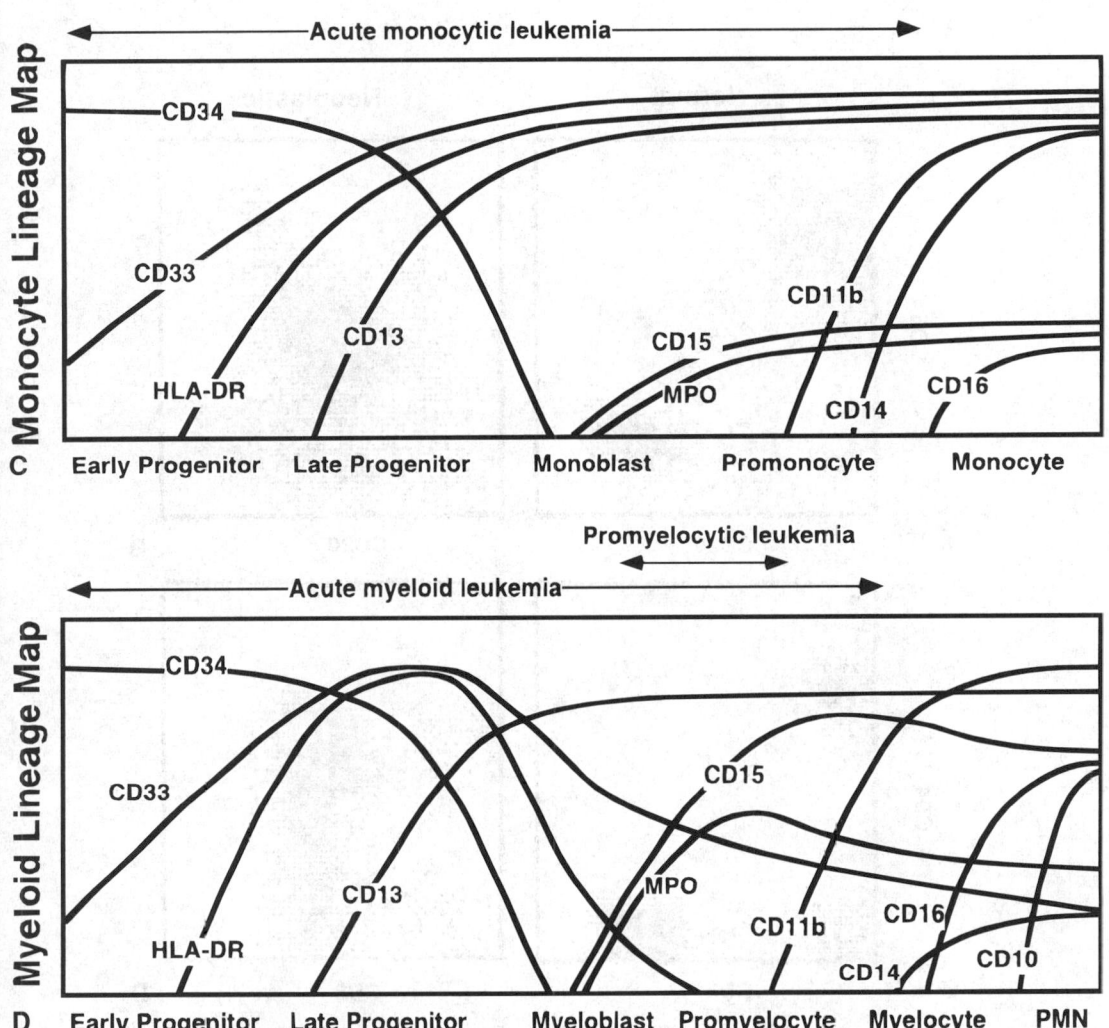

Fig. 159-3 *(Continued).* **(C)** myeloid, and **(D)** monocytic lineages.[129,130] A general idea of the variation of expression intensity of a specific marker is indicated by the height of the line corresponding to each marker. CD5 is expressed on a subset of normal B cells and on B-CLL. The phenotype of activated B cells and corresponding lymphomas is complex and varied. While most normal pre-B cells are TdT⁻, pre-B ALL is TdT⁺, an example of asynchronous differentiation. Asynchronous differentiation is also seen in myeloid leukemias: they often express late markers such as CD11b and CD15 along with the earlier markers CD34 and HLA-DR. HCL, hairy cell leukemia; PLL, prolymphocytic leukemia; cyto, cytoplasmic; Ig, immunoglobulin; TdT, terminal deoxynucleotidyl transferase; MPO, myeloperoxidase.

Demonstration of monoclonality: Monoclonal origin can be detected in immunoglobulin expressing B-cell malignancies by light chain restriction (i.e., a population expressing only κ or λ light chain).[81] There is no comparable phenotypic marker for monoclonality in T cells. Light chain analysis is more sensitive in identifying B-cell lymphoma than the percentage of total B cells, with a κ/λ ratio of >3:1 or <1:2 strongly suggesting a monoclonal population.[82] Quantitatively restricted expression of surface immunoglobulin by monoclonal B cells has been used to detect small monoclonal B-cell populations undetectable by analysis of the κ/λ ratio.[83] Nonspecific binding should be excluded by simultaneous staining with anti-κ- and anti-λ-antibodies or combining the anti-light chain antibody with a B-cell marker[84] (Fig. 159-6).

Cell Marker Analysis in Acute Leukemia

Classification of Acute Leukemia: Because of phenotypic overlap between leukemic and normal progenitors and the lack of leukemia-specific markers, immunophenotyping is generally more useful in classifying a recognizable leukemia than in diag-

nosing leukemia when it is not morphologically evident. Immunophenotyping allows reproducible lineage assignment of some leukemias that would otherwise be difficult to classify, particularly in differentiating lymphoid from immature myeloid leukemias.[85] Cytoplasmic markers (peroxidase, cCD22,[86] cCD3,[87] cCD13[88]) may be more specific indicators than are surface markers of lineage commitment in acute leukemia.[86] There is significant immunophenotypic overlap among the different French-American-British categories,[89] but some associations have been noted: CD14 expression in M4/M5[90]; aberrant expression of CD2 in M3[91] and M4eo, lack of HLA-DR in M3,[92] and CD19 expression in M2.[93] Phenotypic changes are generally not sufficiently characteristic to allow diagnosis of myelodysplastic syndromes or to differentiate the various subgroups of myelodysplastic syndrome.

Aberrant phenotypes: Detection of mixed lineage differentiation (i.e., myeloid markers in an otherwise clear-cut acute lymphocytic leukemia [ALL] or vice-versa) has been associated with poor prognosis,[94,95] but the prognostic significance of these phenotypes is treatment dependent and may not always be demonstrable.[96] Certain cytogenetically defined leukemias with poor prognostic outcomes [i.e., t(4;11), t(9;22)] are espe-

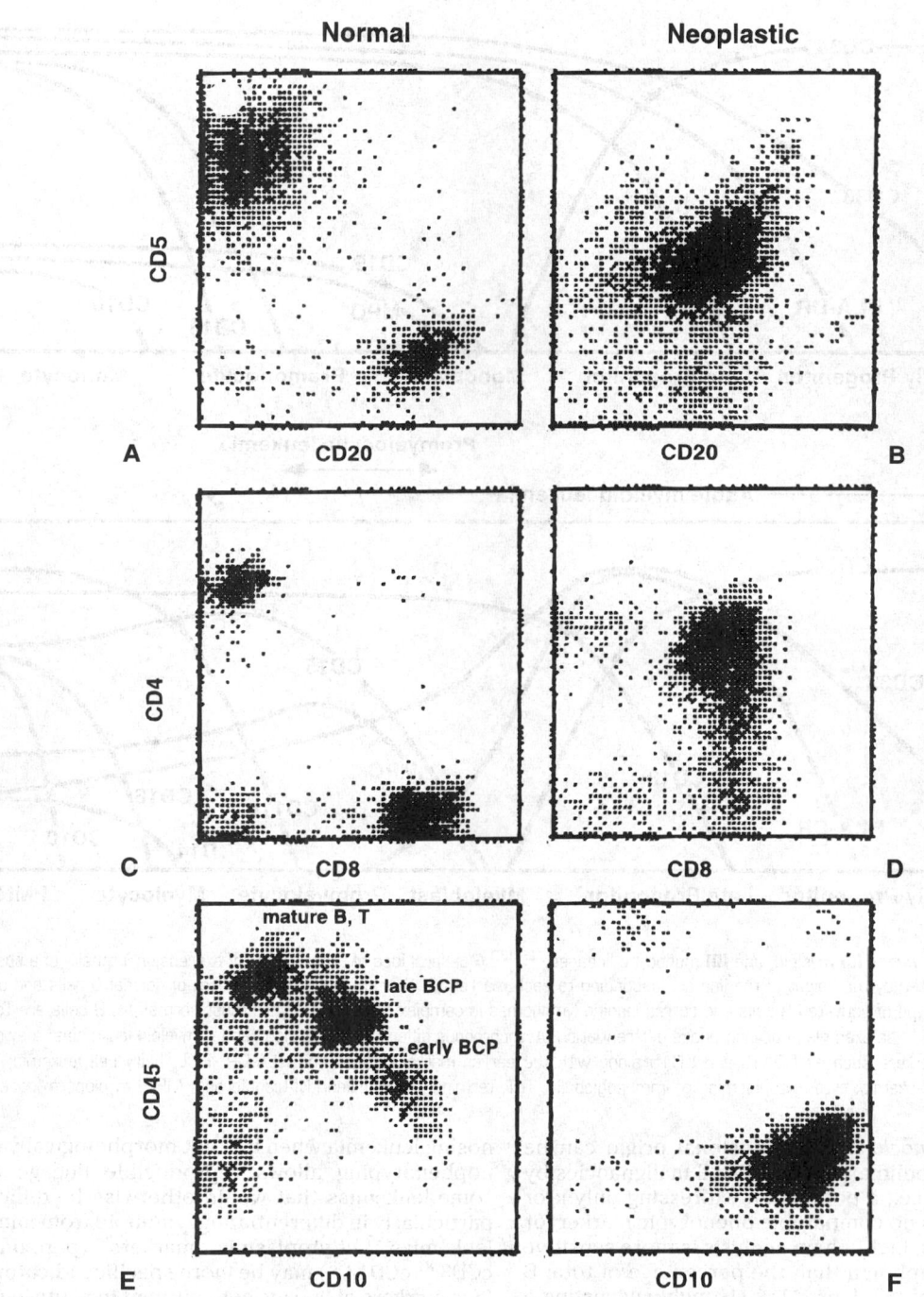

Fig. 159-4. Diagnostic importance of multiparameter analysis. **(A)** Fluorescence histogram of CD8 versus CD4 in normal blood mononuclear cells. Note virtually exclusive expression of the two markers on different subsets (T suppresser/cytotoxic and T helper/inducer). **(B)** Fluorescence histogram of CD8 versus CD4 in T-cell lymphoblastic lymphoma, showing co-expression of CD4 and CD8, a common thymocyte phenotype that is typical of T-ALL and T-cell lymphoblastic lymphoma. **(C)** Fluorescence histogram of CD20 versus CD5 in normal lymph node. Only a small number of CD20$^+$/CD5$^+$ cells are typically observed in normal tissues. **(D)** Fluorescence histogram of CD20 versus CD5 in B-cell CLL. The characteristic co-expression of CD5 by the malignant B cells is clearly demonstrated by two-color analysis. Note that expression of both CD20 and CD5 is quantitatively lower in the malignant cells than the normal B (CD20$^+$) or T (CD5$^+$) cells. **(E)** Fluorescence histogram of CD10 versus CD45 in remission bone marrow after chemotherapy. Although 60% of the lymphoid cells are CD10$^+$, they show a sequence of loss of CD10 correlated with increasing CD45 expression characteristic of normal B-cell maturation, as indicated in the histogram. **(F)** Fluorescence histogram of CD10 versus CD45 in B-cell precursor ALL. Note the high CD10 expression, CD45 negativity, and lack of evidence of progressive maturation of the cells.

Table 159-2. Practical Considerations in Hematopoietic Immunophenotyping

Morphologically identify cells of interest

Formulate the clinical question

Select appropriate antibody panel

Identify light scatter population likely to contain cells of interest

Verify identity of light scatter populations with lineage markers

Identify phenotypic pattern of cells of interest

Compare composite phenotype with expected lineage patterns
  Diagnostic: ≥2 lineage-specific markers + appropriate negative markers
  Probable: 1 lineage-specific marker + appropriate negative markers
  Aberrant expression if single inappropriate lineage marker is present
  Mixed lineage differentiation likely if ≥2 inappropriate markers are present

Identify differentiation stage within lineage

Restain with additional markers if lineage assignment is ambiguous

cially prone to multilineage differentiation. Co-expression of mixed lineage markers should be confirmed by two-color analysis or a 20% numerical overlap in cells positive for each marker.[78] Recent efforts to standardize the diagnosis of mixed lineage leukemia reserve this category for those acute leukemias (about 10%) that display at least two specific markers of two or more lineages.[96,97]

Residual disease: Aberrant marker expression may also be useful in detection of residual disease.[98,99] At present, the ability of flow cytometry-based immunophenotyping to detect residual acute leukemia is limited by the substantial overlap between normal and leukemic cells. Recently, detailed dual-color studies have shown that 85% of AML cells express at least one unusual marker combination that is rare (<0.1%) in normal marrow. Persistence of these residual cells can be identified by flow cytometry and may be prognostically important.[100]

Prognostic significance of phenotype: B-cell precursor ALL has a better prognosis than pre-B-, T-, or mature B-cell ALL. Improvements in treatment tend to narrow these prognostic differences, provided therapy is tailored to the phenotype.[101] Increasingly, specific phenotypes are associated with molecular

abnormalities: pre-B ALL [t(1;19), E2A/PBX-1[102]], B-ALL (*myc* translocation), CD34$^+$ AML (chromosome 5 or 7 abnormalities[103,104]), and mixed lineage leukemia [t(4;11), ALL-1/AF-4[105]]. Other prognostic categories may be recognizable by phenotypic studies. For instance, expression of CD34 is a favorable prognostic feature in B-precursor ALL,[106] but is unfavorable in T-ALL[107] and AML,[90,104] while expression of the multidrug resistance transport protein MDR in acute leukemia may be unfavorable.[108]

Cell Marker Analysis in Lymphoproliferative Disorders

B-cell neoplasms: B-cell chronic lymphoproliferative disorders are identified by B-cell-associated markers and expression of monotypic surface immunoglobulin. Infrequently, follicular lymphomas (similar to some normal germinal center cells in reactive hyperplasia) may lack detectable surface immunoglobulin.[109] Generally, lymphoproliferative disorders cannot be classified on the basis of phenotype alone.[110] A distinctive CD20$^+$/CD11c$^+$ phenotype is characteristic of hairy cell leukemia,[111] but may also be found in some patients with B-CLL or other lymphoproliferative disorders.[112] Interestingly, both normal[113] and neoplastic[114] plasma cells co-express several myeloid-associated markers. The CD20$^+$/CD5$^+$ phenotype, which is found in about 90% of B-cell chronic lymphocytic leukemia (CLL),[115] most instances of well-differentiated or intermediate[116] lymphoma, and a minority of other lymphoproliferative disorders,[117] also identifies a subset of normal B cells that may be involved in autoimmunity. Monoclonal light chain expression and an expanded CD20$^+$/CD5$^+$ population may permit diagnosis of early CLL in patients with relative lymphocytosis but normal absolute lymphocyte counts.[118] Diagnosis of Hodgkin lymphoma by flow cytometry is seldom practical due to the infrequency of the abnormal cells.

T-cell neoplasms: Immunophenotypic diagnosis of T-cell lymphoproliferative disorders is more difficult, since these cells usually express markers found normally in mature T cells. However, on careful analysis, most of both mature and immature T-cell lymphomas show either loss of an expected T-cell marker (typically CD7 or CD5), loss or co-expression of CD4 and CD8, or expression of CD1, suggesting aberrant or asynchronous differentiation.[119] Due to the phenotypically complex mixture of cells that make up the normal T-cell population, detection of small malignant T-cell populations (e.g., 2% Sézary cells) on this basis is generally not feasible. Most patients with large granular cell lymphoproliferative disease display a characteristic cytotoxic T-cell phenotype (CD3$^+$/CD57$^+$/CD56$^\pm$/CD16$^-$), while a minority display a phenotype of true natural killer cells (CD3$^-$/CD57$^\pm$/CD56$^+$/CD16$^+$).[120] Only the former type can be identified by T-cell antigen receptor gene rearrangement.

Prognostic significance: Subtle phenotypic differences occur within specific lymphoproliferative disorders and have been reported in some patients to provide prognostic information. For instance, high fluorescence intensity of surface IgM and expression of CD23 in B-cell CLL are associated with poorer prognosis.[121] The prognostic significance of immunophenotype in lymphoma is controversial.[122,123]

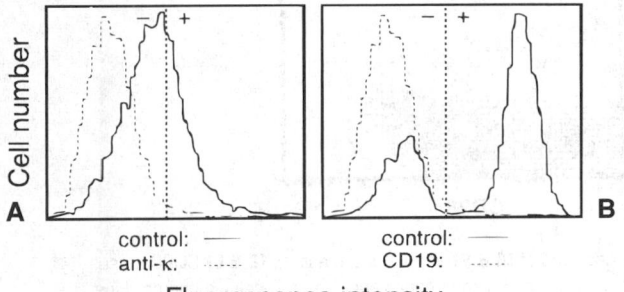

Fig. 159-5. Problems in interpretation of numerical cell marker results. Single-parameter histogram of fluorescence intensity versus cell number in blood cells from a patient with B-cell CLL. Each peak represents a population of cells; position on the x-axis corresponds to fluorescence intensity on a log scale. **(A)** Fluorescence of cells stained with either control (dashed line) or anti-κ antibody (solid line). Dashed vertical line represents cut-off point for positive cells, as determined by fluorescence of cells stained with control antibody (which places the cut-off so that only 1–2% of cells in the control would be considered positive). **(B)** Fluorescence of cells stained with either control (dashed line) or anti-CD19 antibody (solid line). Note that by standard convention, only 30% of the cells would be considered to be surface κ-positive, even though the histogram clearly indicate a shift (albeit small) in fluorescence intensity of the majority of cells when stained with anti-κ antibody. This is confirmed by staining of 70% of cells with the B-cell CD19 markers.

Other Flow Cytometry Applications in Hematology

DNA content: Staining of fixed cells with dyes that bind stoichiometrically to DNA permits direct analysis of DNA content in individual cells. Flow cytometry can detect a gain or loss of 5–20% (depending on instrument precision and a percentage of aneuploid cells) in DNA content of G_0/G_1 cells. B-precursor

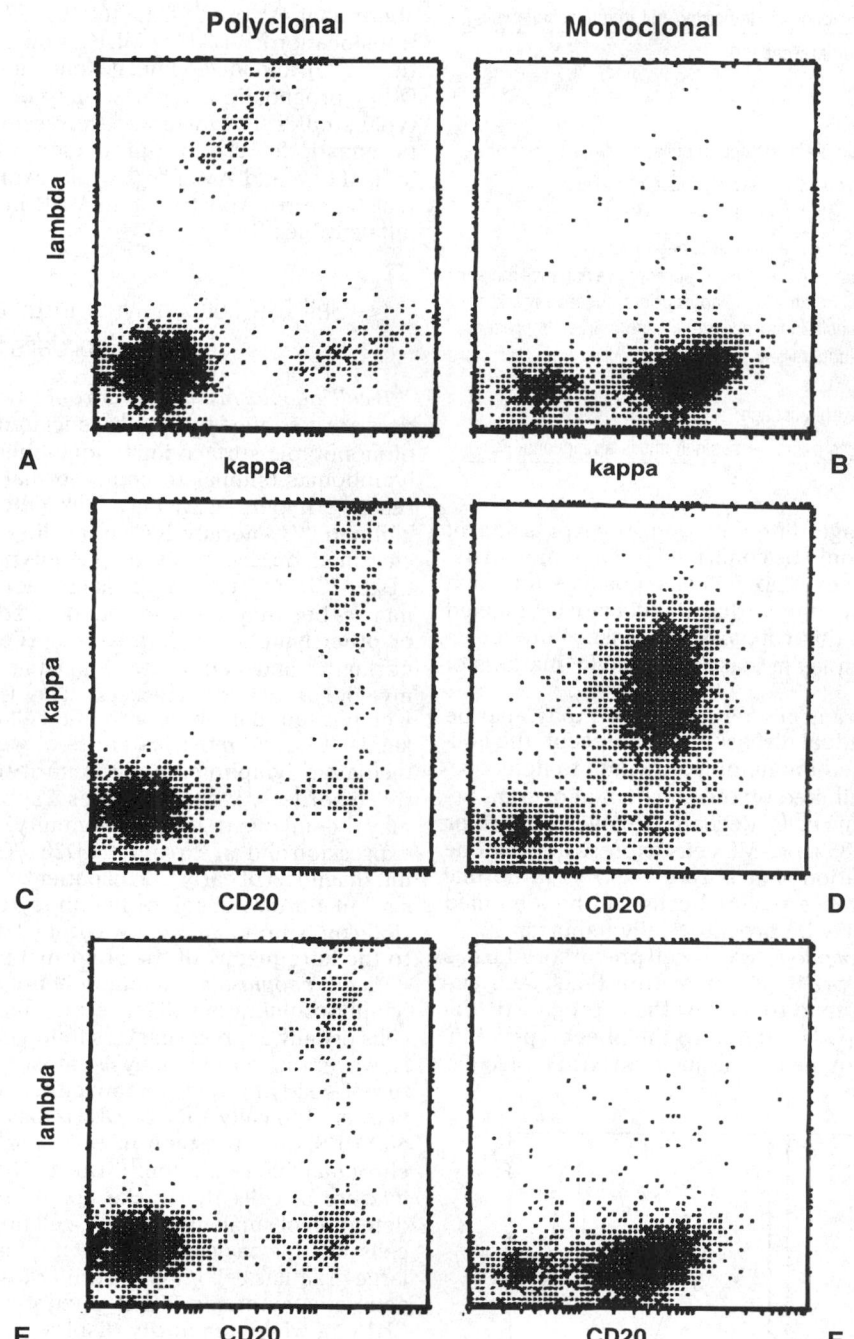

Fig. 159-6. Detection of monoclonality by flow cytometry. Fluorescence histograms of **(A & B)** anti-κ versus anti-λ, **(C & D)** CD20 versus anti-κ, and **(E & F)** CD20 versus anti-λ in a reactive lymph node (Figs. A, C, & E), or a lymph node replaced by B-cell lymphoma (Figs. B, D, & F). Note the separate κ$^+$/λ$^-$ (15%) and κ$^-$/λ$^+$ (12%) populations in the benign reactive node (Fig. A), each of which is identified as a true B-cell population by co-expression of CD20 (Figs. C & E). Note the κ$^+$/λ$^-$ (81%) population without a corresponding κ$^-$/λ$^+$ (<1%) population in B-cell lymphoma, consistent with a B-cell monoclonal proliferation.

ALL patients with a DNA index (DNA content relative to normal cells) of >1.16 have significantly better relapse-free survival regardless of age or white cell count than those with a DNA index of ≤1.16.[124] DNA content is of limited diagnostic value in chronic lymphoproliferative disorders and myeloid leukemia. Cells in the S phase of cell cycle can be recognized by DNA content between G_0/G_1 and G_2. Estimation of the percentage of S phase cells by DNA content analysis in lymphomas is correlated with morphologic risk categories, and may provide additional prognostic information.[125] Reproducible estimation of

percentage of S phase cells presents considerably more technical challenges than measurement of DNA content, due to the greater complexity in modeling the S phase to account for variability in G_0/G_1 and G_2 peaks, as well as the presence of nuclear fragments and debris.[126]

Paroxysmal nocturnal hemoglobinuria: Deficiency of phosphatidylinositol-anchored surface molecules (e.g., CD48, CD55, CD59, CD14) in hematopoietic cells in paroxysmal nocturnal hemoglobinuria can be detected by immunophenotyping.[127]

Leukocyte adhesion deficiency: A congenital defect in produc-on of the common β_2 chain of the leukocyte integrin adhesion molecule family causes defective migration of neutrophils and an increased susceptibility to recurrent infections and is detectable by loss of either the α- (CD11a, CD11b, CD11c) or the -chain (CD18) of the leukocyte integrin molecule.[128]

REFERENCES

1. Solomon HM, Rau JJ: Quantitative buffy coat analysis. A hematologic screen applicable to the selection of apheresis donors. Am J Clin Pathol 84:490, 1985
2. Long GW, Rickman LS, Cross JH: Rapid diagnosis of *Brugia malayi* and *Wuchereria bancrofti* filariasis by an acridine orange/microhematocrit tube technique. J Parasitol 76:278, 1990
3. Lindhardt PT, Kjaersgaard E, Plesner T: Quantitative buffy coat analysis in haematological patients compared to standard laboratory methods. Scand J Clin Lab Invest 50:657, 1990
4. Wilding P, Leboy EL: Use of pattern recognition technology for determination of the human differential leukocyte count. Blood Cells 11:187, 1985
5. Coulter WH: High speed automatic blood cell counter and cell size analyzer. Proc Natl Elect Conf 12:1034, 1956
6. Segel GB, Cokelet GR, Lichtman MA: The measurement of lymphocyte volume: importance of reference particle deformability and counting solution tonicity. Blood 57:894, 1981
7. Bator JM, Groves MR, Price BJ et al: Erythrocyte deformability and size measured in a multiparameter system that includes impedance sizing. Cytometry 5:34, 1984
8. Mansberg HP, Saunders AM, Groner W: The Hemalog D white cell differential system. J Histochem Cytochem 22:711, 1974
9. Kim YR, Paseltiner L, Kling G et al: Subtyping lymphocytes in peripheral blood by direct immunoalkaline phosphatase labeling and light scatter/absorption flow cytometric analysis. Am J Clin Pathol 97:331, 1992
10. Recommendations for reference method for haemoglobinometry in human blood (ICSH standard 1986) and specifications for international haemiglobincyanide reference preparation. 3rd Ed. Clin Lab Haematol 9:73, 1987
11. England JM, Walford DM, Waters DAW: Re-assessment of the reliability of the hematocrit. Br J Haematol 23:247, 1972
12. England JM: Blood cell sizing. p. 109. In Koepke JA (ed): Practical Laboratory Hematology. Churchill Livingstone, New York, 1991
13. Hillman RS: After sixty years: the MCV is still alive and well, editorial; comment. J Gen Intern Med 5:264, 1990
14. Rund D, Filon D, Strauss N et al: Mean corpuscular volume of heterozygotes for beta-thalassemia correlates with the severity of mutations. Blood 79:238, 1992
15. Seward SJ, Safran C, Marton KI et al: Does the mean corpuscular volume help physicians evaluate hospitalized patients with anemia? J Gen Intern Med 5:187, 1990
16. Carmel R: Pernicious anemia. The expected findings of very low serum cobalamin levels, anemia, and macrocytosis are often lacking. Arch Intern Med 148:1712, 1988
17. Bentley SA, Ayscue LH, Watson JM et al: The clinical utility of discriminant functions for the differential diagnosis of microcytic anemias. Blood Cells 15:575, 1989
18. Conrad ME, Crosby WH: The natural history of iron deficiency induced by phlebotomy. Blood 20:173, 1962
19. Mahu JL, Leclercq C, Suquet JP: Usefulness of red cell distribution width in association with biological parameters in an epidemiological survey of iron deficiency in children. Int J Epidemiol 19:646, 1990
20. Bessman JD, Banks D: Spurious macrocytosis: a common clue to erythrocytic cold agglutinins. Am J Clin Pathol 74:797, 1980
21. Holt JT, DeWandler MJ, Arvan DA: Spurious elevation of the electronically determined mean corpuscular volume and hematocrit caused by hyperglycemia. Am J Clin Pathol 77:561, 1982
22. Bessman JD, Gilmer PR, Gardner FH: Improved classification of anemias by MCV and RDW. Am J Clin Pathol 80:322, 1983
23. Lin CK, Lin JS, Chen SY et al: Comparison of hemoglobin and red blood cell distribution width in the differential diagnosis of microcytic anemia. Arch Pathol Lab Med 116:1030, 1992
24. Flynn MM, Reppun TS, Bhagavan NV: Limitations of red cell distribution width (RDW) in evaluation of microcytosis. Am J Clin Pathol 85:445, 1986
25. van Zeben D, Bieger R, van Wermeskerken R et al: Evaluation of microcytosis using serum ferritin and red blood cell distribution width. Eur J Haematol 44:106, 1990
26. Kojima K, Niri M, Setoguchi K et al: An automated optoelectronic reticulocyte counter. Am J Clin Pathol 92:57, 1989

27. Metzger DK, Charache S: Flow cytometric reticulocyte counting with thioflavin T in a clinical hematology laboratory. Arch Pathol Lab Med 111:540, 1987
28. Savage RA, Skoog DP, Rabinovitch A: Analytic inaccuracy and imprecision in reticulocyte counting: a preliminary report from the College of American Pathologists Reticulocyte Project. Blood Cells 11:97, 1985
29. Nobes PR, Carter AB: Reticulocyte counting using flow cytometry. J Clin Pathol 43:675, 1990
30. Lazarus HM, Chahine A, Lacerna K et al: Kinetics of erythrogenesis after bone marrow transplantation. Am J Clin Pathol 97:574, 1992
31. Davies SV, Cavill I, Bentley N et al: Evaluation of erythropoiesis after bone marrow transplantation: quantitative reticulocyte counting. Br J Haematol 81:12, 1992
32. Heilmeyer L, Westhäuser: Reifunsstadien an überlebenden Reticulocyten in vitro und ihre Bedeutung für die Schätzung der täglichen Hamoglobinproduktion in vivo. Z Kinder Med 121:361, 1932
33. Crouch JY, Kaplow LS: Relationship of reticulocyte age to polychromasia, shift cells, and shift reticulocytes. Arch Pathol Lab Med 109:325, 1985
34. Davis BH, Bigelow N, Ball ED et al: Utility of flow cytometric reticulocyte quantification as a predictor of engraftment in autologous bone marrow transplantation. Am J Hematol 32:81, 1989
35. Davis BH, DiCorato M, Bigelow NC et al: Proposal for the standardization of flow cytometric reticulocyte maturity index (RMI) measurements. Cytometry 14:318, 1992
36. van Hove L, Goossens W, van Duppen V et al: Reticulocyte count using thiazole orange. A flow cytometry method. Clin Lab Haematol 12:287, 1990
37. Davis BH, Bigelow NC: Flow cytometric reticulocyte analysis and the reticulocyte maturity index. Ann NY Acad Sci 677:281, 1993
38. Gilmer PR, Koepke JA: The reticulocyte: an approach to definition. Am J Clin Pathol 66:262, 1976
39. Haynes JL: High-resolution particle analysis—its application to platelet counting and suggestions for further application in blood cell analysis. Blood Cells 6:201, 1980
40. Klee GG: Performance goals for internal quality control of multichannel haematology analysers. Clin Lab Haematol 1:65, 1990
41. Pegels JG, Bruynes ECE, Engelfreit CP et al: Pseudothrombocytopenia: an immunological study on platelet antibodies dependent on ethylene diamine tetra-acetate. Blood 59:152, 1982
42. Bessman JD, Williams LF, Gilmer PR: Mean platelet volume. The inverse relation of platelet size and count in normal subjects and an artifact of other particles. Am J Clin Pathol 76:289, 1981
43. Bessman JD, Gilmer PR, Gardner FH: Use of mean platelet volume improves detection of platelet disorders. Blood Cells 11:127, 1985
44. Levin J, Bessman JD: The inverse relation between platelet volume and platelet number. Abnormalities in hematologic disease and evidence that platelet size does not correlate with platelet age. J Lab Clin Med 101:295, 1983
45. Bessman JD: The relation of megakaryocyte ploidy to platelet volume. Am J Hematol 16:161, 1984
46. Thompson CB, Love DG, Quinn PG et al: Platelet size does not correlate with platelet age. Blood 62:487, 1983
47. Martin JF, Bath PM, Burr ML: Influence of platelet size on outcome after myocardial infarction. Lancet 338:1409, 1991
48. Smyth DW, Martin JF, Michalis L et al: Influence of platelet size before coronary angioplasty on subsequent restenosis. Eur J Clin Invest 23:361, 1993
49. Reardon DM, Hutchinson D, Preston FE et al: The routine measurement of platelet volume: a comparison of aperture-impedance and flow cytometric systems. Clin Lab Haematol 7:251, 1985
50. Lippi U, Cappelletti P, Schinella M et al: Mean platelet volumes: facts or artifacts? Am J Clin Pathol 84:111, 1985
51. Ault KA: Flow cytometric analysis of platelets. p. 389. In Bauer KD, Duque RE, Shankey TV (eds): Clinical Flow Cytometry. Williams & Wilkins, Baltimore, 1993
52. Kienast J, Schmitz G: Flow cytometric analysis of thiazole orange uptake by platelets: a diagnostic aid in the evaluation of thrombocytopenic disorders. Blood 75:116, 1990
53. Rinder HM, Munz UJ, Ault KA et al: Reticulated platelets in the evaluation of thrombopoietic disorders. Arch Pathol Lab Med 117:606, 1993
54. Ault KA, Rinder HM, Mitchell J et al: The significance of platelets with increased RNA content (reticulated platelets). A measure of the rate of thrombopoiesis. Am J Clin Pathol 98:637, 1992
55. Ballem PJ, Segal GM, Stratton JR et al: Mechanisms of thrombocytopenia in chronic autoimmune thrombocytopenic purpura: evidence of both impaired platelet production and increased platelet clearance. J Clin Invest 80:33, 1987
56. Marti GE, Magruder L, Schuette WE et al: Flow cytometric analysis of platelet surface antigens. Cytometry 9:448, 1988

57. Shattil SJ, Cunningham M, Hoxie JA: Detection of activated platelets in whole blood using activation dependent monoclonal antibodies and flow cytometry. Blood 70:307, 1987

58. Lazarchick J, Hall SA: Platelet associated IgG assay using flow cytometric analysis. J Immunol Methods 87:257, 1986

59. Warner BA, Reardon DM, Marshall DP: Automated haematology analysers: a four-way comparison. Med Lab Sci 47:285, 1990

60. Cornbleet PJ, Myrick D, Levy R: Evaluation of the Coulter STKS five-part differential. Am J Clin Pathol 99:72, 1993

61. Duncan KL, Gottfried EL: Utility of the three-part leukocyte differential count. Am J Clin Pathol 88:308, 1987

62. Pierre RV, Payne BA, Lee WK et al: Comparison of four leukocyte differential methods with the National Committee for Clinical Laboratory Standards (NCCLS) reference method. Am J Clin Pathol 87:201, 1987

63. Robertson EP, Lai HW, Wei DC: An evaluation of leucocyte analysis on the Coulter STKS. Clin Lab Haematol 14:53, 1992

64. Breakell ES, Marchand A, Marcus R et al: Comparison of performance for leukocyte differential counting of the Technicon H6000 system with a manual reference method using the NCCLS standard. Blood Cells 11:257, 1985

65. Saunders AM: Sources of physiological variation in differential leukocyte counting. Blood Cells 11:31, 1985

66. Warner BA, Reardon DM: A field evaluation of the Coulter STKS. Am J Clin Pathol 95:207, 1991

67. Zaccaria A, Celso B, Raspadori D et al: Comparative evaluation of differential leukocyte counts by Coulter VCS cytometer and direct microscopic observation. Haematologica 75:412, 1990

68. Vinatier I, Lorriaux C, Capiod JC et al: Evaluation of the erythrocyte and platelet morphological analysis given by the hematology analyzer Coulter STKS. Nouv Rev Fr Hematol 34:205, 1992

69. Morse EE, Nashed A, Spilove L: Automated differential leukocyte counts. Ann Clin Lab Sci 19:155, 1989

70. Koepke JA, Dotson MA, Shifman MA et al: A flagging system for multichannel hematology analyzers. Blood Cells 11:113, 1985

71. Ruttimann S, Clemencon D, Dubach UC: Usefulness of complete blood counts as a case-finding tool in medical outpatients. Ann Intern Med 116:44, 1992

72. Shapiro MF, Hatch RL, Greenfield S: Cost containment for labor-intensive tests. The case of the leukocyte differential count. JAMA 252:231, 1984

73. Bauer KD, Duque RE, Shankey TV: Clinical Flow Cytometry: Williams & Wilkins, Baltimore, 1993

74. Terstappen LW, Konemann S, Safford M et al: Flow cytometric characterization of acute myeloid leukemia. Part 1. Significance of light scattering properties. Leukemia 5:315, 1991

75. Knapp W, Dörken B, Rieber EP et al: Leucocyte Typing IV: White Cell Differentiation Antigens. Oxford University Press, Oxford, 1987

76. Hurwitz CA, Gore SD, Stone KD et al: Flow cytometric detection of rare normal human marrow cells with immunophenotypes characteristic of acute lymphoblastic leukemia cells. Leukemia 6:233, 1992

77. Smith BR: Qualitative versus quantitative immunophenotyping. Ann NY Acad Sci 677:152, 1993

78. van't Veer MB, Kluin-Nelemans JC, van der Schoot CE et al: Quality assessment of immunological marker analysis and the immunological diagnosis in leukaemia and lymphoma: a multi-center study. Br J Haematol 80:458, 1992

79. Braylan RC, Benson NA, Iturraspe J: Analysis of lymphomas by flow cytometry. Current and emerging strategies. Ann NY Acad Sci 677:364, 1993

80. Braylan RC: Acute leukemias. p. 206. In Bauer KD, Duque RE, Shankey TV (eds): Clinical Flow Cytometry. Williams & Wilkins, Baltimore, 1993

81. Levy R, Warnke R, Dorfman RF et al: The monoclonality of human B-cell lymphomas. J Exp Med 145:1014, 1977

82. Geary WA, Frierson HF, Innes DJ et al: Quantitative criteria for clonality in the diagnosis of B-cell non-Hodgkin's lymphoma by flow cytometry. Mod Pathol 6:155, 1993

83. Ault KA: Detection of small numbers of monoclonal B lymphocytes in the blood of patients with lymphoma. N Engl J Med 300:1401, 1979

84. Letwin BW, Wallace PK, Muirhead KA et al: An improved clonal excess assay using flow cytometry and B-cell gating. Blood 75:1178, 1990

85. Bowman GP, Neame PB, Soambonsrup P: The contribution of cytochemistry and immunophenotyping to the reproducibility of the FAB classification in acute leukemia. Blood 68:900, 1986

86. Janossy G, Coustan-Smith E, Campana D: The reliability of cytoplasmic CD3 and CD22 antigen expression in the immunodiagnosis of acute leukemia: a study of 500 cases. Leukemia 3:170, 1989

87. Campana D, Thomson JS, Amlot P et al: The cytoplasmic expression of CD3 antigen in normal and malignant cells of the T lymphoid lineage. J Immunol 138:648, 1987

88. Pombo de Oliveira MS, Matutes E, Rani S et al: Early expression of MC (CD13) in the cytoplasm of blast cells from acute myeloid leukemia. Ac Haematol 80:61, 1988

89. Kuerbitz SJ, Civin CI, Krischer JP et al: Expression of myeloid-associate and lymphoid-associated cell-surface antigens in acute myeloid leukem of childhood: a Pediatric Oncology Group study. J Clin Oncol 10:1419, 199

90. Solary E, Casasnovas RO, Campos L et al: Surface markers in adult acu myeloblastic leukemia: correlation of CD19+, CD34+ and CD14+ DR—phenotypes with shorter survival. Groupe d'Etude Immunologique de Leucemies (GEIL). Leukemia 6:393, 1992

91. Reading CL, Estey EH, Huh YO et al: Expression of unusual immunophen type combinations in acute myelogenous leukemia. Blood 81:3083, 1993

92. Griffin JD, Mayer RJ, Weinstein HJ et al: Surface marker analysis of acut myeloblastic leukemia: identification of differentiation-associated phen types. Blood 62:557, 1983

93. Kita K, Nakase K, Miwa H et al: Phenotypic characteristics of acute myel cytic leukemia associated with the t(8;21)(q22;q22) chromosomal abno mality: frequent expression of immature B-cell antigen CD19 together wit stem cell antigen CD34. Blood 80:470, 1992

94. Cantu-Rajnoldi A, Putti C, Saitta M et al: Co-expression of myeloid antigen in childhood acute lymphoblastic leukaemia: relationship with the stage o differentiation and clinical significance. Br J Haematol 79:40, 1991

95. Urbano-Ispizua A, Matutes E, Villamor N et al: The value of detecting surfac and cytoplasmic antigens in acute myeloid leukaemia. Br J Haematol 81 178, 1992

96. Pui C-H, Raimondi SC, Head DR et al: Characterization of childhood acute leukemia with multiple myeloid and lymphoid markers at diagnosis and relapse. Blood 78:1327, 1991

97. Buccheri V, Matutes E, Dyer MJ et al: Lineage commitment in biphenotypic acute leukemia. Leukemia 7:919, 1993

98. Reading CL, Estey EH, Huh YO et al: Expression of unusual immunopheno type combinations in acute myelogenous leukemia. Blood 81:3083, 1993

99. Coustan-Smith E, Behm FG, Hurwit CA et al: N-CAM (CD56) expression by CD34+ malignant myeloblasts with implications for minimal residual disease detection in acute myeloid leukemia. Leukemia 7:853, 1993

100. Reading CL, Estey EH, Huh YO et al: Expression of unusual immunopheno type combinations in acute myelogenous leukemia. Blood 81:3083, 1993

101. Crist W, Shuster J, Look T et al: Current results of studies of immunopheno type-, age- and leukocyte-based therapy for children with acute lymphoblastic leukemia. The Pediatric Oncology Group. Leukemia 2:162, 1992

102. Crist WM, Carroll AJ, Shuster JJ et al: Poor prognosis of children with pre-B acute lymphoblastic leukemia is associated with the t(1;19)q23;p13): A Pediatric Oncology Group study. Blood 76:117, 1990

103. Borowitz MJ, Gockerman JP, Moore JO et al: Clinicopathologic and cytogenic features of CD34 (My 10)-positive acute nonlymphocytic leukemia. Am J Clin Pathol 91:265, 1989

104. Geller RB, Zahurak M, Hurwitz CA et al: Prognostic importance of immunophenotyping in adults with acute myelocytic leukaemia: the significance of the stem-cell glycoprotein CD34 (My10). Br J Haematol 76:340, 1990

105. Hayashi Y, Pui C-H, Behm FG et al: 14q32 translocations are associated with mixed-lineage expression in childhood acute leukemia. Blood 76:150, 1990

106. Borowitz MJ, Shuster JJ, Civin CI et al: Prognostic significance of CD34 expression in childhood B-precursor acute lymphocytic leukemia: a Pediatric Oncology Group study. J Clin Oncol 8:1389, 1990

107. Pui CH, Hancock ML, Head DR et al: Clinical significance of CD34 expression in childhood acute lymphoblastic leukemia. Blood 82:889, 1993

108. Marie JP, Zittou R, Sikic BI: Multidrug resistance (mdr1) gene expression in adult acute leukemias: correlations with treatment outcome and in vitro drug sensitivity. Blood 78:586, 1991

109. Picker LJ, Weiss LM, Medeiros LJ et al: Immunophenotypic criteria for the diagnosis of non-Hodgkin's lymphoma. Am J Pathol 128:181, 1987

110. Schwonzen M, Pohl C, Steinmetz T et al: Immunophenotyping of low-grade B-cell lymphoma in blood and bone marrow: poor correlation between immunophenotype and cytological/histological classification. Br J Haematol 83:232, 1993

111. Schwarting R, Stein H, Wang CY: The monoclonal antibodies S-HCL (Leu-14) and S-HCL 3 (Leu-M5) allow the diagnosis of hairy cell leukemia. Blood 69:1011, 1985

112. Oertel J, Kastner M, Bai AR et al: Analysis of chronic lymphoid leukaemias according to FAB. Leuk Res 16:919, 1992

113. Terstappen LWMM, Johnsen S, Segers-Nolten IMJ et al: Identification and characterization of plasma cells in normal human bone marrow by high-resolution flow cytometry. Blood 76:1739, 1990

114. Grogan TM, Durie BG, Spier CM et al: Myelomonocytic antigen positive multiple myeloma. Blood 73:763, 1989

115. Geisler CH, Larsen JK, Hansen NE et al: Prognostic importance of flow cyto-

metric immunophenotyping of 540 consecutive patients with B-cell chronic lymphocytic leukemia. Blood 78:1795, 1991

16. Strickler JG, Medeiros LJ, Copenhauer CM et al: Intermediate lymphocytic lymphoma: an immunophenotypic study with comparison to small lymphocytic lymphoma and diffuse small cleaved cell lymphoma. Hum Pathol 19: 550, 1988

17. Burns BF, Warnke RA, Doggett RS et al: Expression of a T cell antigen (Leu 1) by B cell lymphomas. Am J Pathol 113:165, 1983

18. Batata A, Shen B: Chronic lymphocytic leukemia with low lymphocyte count. Cancer 71:2732, 1993

19. Hastrup N, Ralfkiaer E, Pallesen G: Aberrant phenotypes in peripheral T cell lymphomas. J Clin Pathol 42:398, 1989

20. Chan WC, Link S, Mawle A et al: Heterogeneity of large granular lymphocyte proliferations: delineation of two major subtypes. Blood 68:1142, 1986

21. Geisler CH, Larsen JK, Hansen NE et al: Prognostic importance of flow cytometric immunophenotyping of 540 consecutive patients with B-cell chronic lymphocytic leukemia. Blood 78:1795, 1991

22. Armitage JO, Vose JM, Linder J et al: Clinical significance of immunophenotype in diffuse aggressive non-Hodgkin's lymphoma. J Clin Oncol 7:1783, 1989

23. Lippman SM, Miller TP, Spier CM et al: The prognostic significance of the

immunophenotype in diffuse large cell lymphoma: a comparative study of the T cell and B cell phenotype. Blood 72:436, 1988

124. Trueworthy R, Shuster J, Look T et al: Ploidy of lymphoblasts is the strongest predictor of treatment outcome in B-progenitor cell acute lymphoblastic leukemia of childhood: a Pediatric Oncology Group study. J Clin Oncol 10: 606, 1992

125. Christensson B, Lindemalm C, Johansson B et al: Flow cytometric DNA analysis: a prognostic tool in non-Hodgkin's lymphoma. Leuk Res 13:307, 1989

126. Rabinovitch PS. Practical considerations for DNA content and cell cycle analysis. p. 117. In Bauer KD, Duque RE, Shankey TV (eds): Clinical Flow Cytometry. Williams & Wilkins, Baltimore, 1993

127. Schubert J, Alvarado M, Uciechowski P et al: Diagnosis of paroxysmal nocturnal haemoglobinuria using immunophenotyping of peripheral blood cells. Br J Haematol 79:487, 1991

128. Arnaout MA, Spits H, Terhorst C et al: Deficiency of a leukocyte surface glycoprotein (LFA-1) in two patients with Mo1 deficiency: effects of cell activation on Mo-1/LFA-1 surface expression in normal and deficient leukocytes. J Clin Invest 74:1291, 1984

129. Civin CI: Human monomyeloid cell membrane antigens. Exp Hematol 18: 461, 1990

130. Terstappen LWMM, Safford M, Loken MR: Flow cytometric analysis of human bone marrow. III. Neutrophil maturation. Leukemia 4:657, 1990

Estimation of the Bleeding Time

160

Jan J. Sixma

INTRODUCTION

Primary hemostasis is a complex process in which many different mechanisms are involved. The overall efficacy of this process cannot be determined by any in vitro test. Direct measurement of the bleeding from a small skin wound is still the best overall test that is presently available. The bleeding time is defined as the time between initiation of a standardized skin wound and complete hemostasis at the wound.

The first bleeding time test was introduced by Duke[1] in 1910, when he made a small cut in an earlobe and observed prolonged bleeding in thrombocytopenia. Important progress was made by Ivy et al.,[2] who used standardized venous pressure of 40 mmHg and selected the skin of the volar side of the forearm, because thickness is more reproducible at that site. Later modification entailed the use of a surgical blade instead of a lancet[3] and the use of a template.[4]

In the present overview, the histology of the bleeding time wound and the variables that help to determine the length of the bleeding time are discussed. The value of the bleeding time for the diagnosis of various bleeding disorders is briefly reviewed and the optimal test procedure described.

HISTOLOGY

The skin consists of two layers: the epidermis and the dermis beneath it. The epidermis consists of various layers of squamous epithelial cells, the thickness varying with the localiza-

tion. Forearm skin thickness varies relatively little between individuals (60 ± 20 μm, mean ± 1 SD) and is equal in men and women.[5] There is a gradual increase in thickness with age. The dermis can be divided into a papillary layer just below the epidermis and a deeper reticular layer. The papillary layer sends finger-like projections, or papillae, into the epidermis. The dermal vasculature consists of a superficial papillary plexus linked to a deeper reticular plexus. Arcades of capillaries loop upward from the superficial plexus into the papillae.

When a bleeding time is performed, the depth of the vessels transected depends on the depth of the wound. With the template bleeding time and its variations, in which the knife protrudes at most 1 mm, the vessels transected are the arterioles and venules of the superficial papillary plexus.[6]

The wound has a V shape and is first filled with red blood cells. Fibrin fibrils form quickly along the edges of the wound and are already visible before platelet plugs occlude the severed vessels. No or only a few platelet aggregates are seen in a normal wound.[6] At later time points, the fibrin fibers grow in number and thickness and begin to bridge the wound, but this is usually seen after bleeding from the wound has stopped. The actual hemostasis is brought about by hemostatic plugs that occlude arterioles and venules. These hemostatic plugs have the shape of capsules, but in many instances an extension into the vessel is observed. This extension often consists of platelets that are loosely aggregated and not degranulated, indicating that it is formed by the recent accumulation of platelets. The platelet plug consists at first of loosely packed and nondegranulated platelets, but degranulation occurs within a few minutes, and a tight three-dimensional mosaic of intertwined platelets is formed.[6,7] Studies in hemophilia A show that this degranulation and interdigitation are due to the action of thrombin. Primary hemostatic plugs in hemophilia A are loosely packed and larger than normal. They are often disrupted because of their fragility, resulting in blood flow through the channel that is formed. They subsequently grow to become occlusive again by new deposition of platelets. Channels containing red blood cells are therefore often observed in the plugs of hemophilia A patients but not in the plugs of normal individuals.[8] Fibrin is seen at the edge of the plug but not in the primary plug. Platelets near the edge change in shape to become large lytic balloons with holes in their plasma membrane and loss of the intracellular contents.

The primary hemostatic plug undergoes a fibrinous transformation by which it changes from a platelet plug into a fibrin mass. During this process, platelets change into empty rounded balloon-shaped vesicles, and the space between them is filled with fibrin fibers that thicken with time. This process starts at the periphery of the hemostatic plug and moves slowly to the more central areas. The process is accompanied by a pronounced infiltration of leukocytes around the vessels and into the hemostatic plugs. The fibrinous transformation process occurs in the first 2 hours after a wound has been made.[6] The characteristic abnormalities in hemophilia occur in this phase of hemostasis.[8] The lytic changes in the platelets do occur, but the lysed platelets are not stabilized by a fibrin network, leading to an extremely fragile hemostatic plug.

STANDARDIZATION OF TEST VARIABLES

The bleeding time test value obtained depend on a large number of variables that should be controlled as strictly as possible to obtain optimal results.

Experience of the Operator

The experience of the operator is of major importance for the standardization of the bleeding time. Only after >60 assays have been performed are good duplicates obtained. This was true for the Ivy bleeding time and is also true for the automated devices.[9]

Temperature of the Skin

Cold prolongs the bleeding time.[10–12] Care should therefore be taken to standardize the skin temperature. The bleeding time varies little between skin temperatures of 25° and 33°C. Prolongation is seen at temperatures <16°C. Prolongation is also seen at temperatures >43.5°C, and old wounds may start to rebleed at this temperature.

Venous Pressure

A continuous venous pressure of 40 mmHg increases the sensitivity and reproducibility of the bleeding time.[2] The effect of aspirin on the bleeding time is not observed when there is no increase in venous pressure.[13] Higher venous pressure (80 mmHg) has been used to make the bleeding time suitable for demonstration of increased platelet reactivity in patients who have suffered a myocardial infarction. These patients had a shorter bleeding time.[14] However, the test is very stressful and its predictive value is doubtful.

Length and Number of Incisions

Increasing the length of the freehand incision has bee shown to increase the sensitivity of the technique,[3] but simila sensitivity was found for 3- and 9-mm incisions with an auto mated device. For the Ivy bleeding time, three punctures wer performed and the mean value of these used.[15] For the Simplat technique two incisions with a length of 5 mm are made. Th two values are usually similar, and perhaps a single valu would suffice. However, some investigators prefer the greate certainty of a duplicate assay.[16]

Direction of the Incision

The incision for the template bleeding time can be eithe horizontal or vertical (i.e., perpendicular to the elbow crease) The vertical direction is more often preferred, probably be cause it produces less scarring.[17] On the other hand, the hori zontal direction gives longer times (a mean of 5 minutes, 3 seconds versus 4 minutes, 21 seconds), and the test is some what more sensitive for detecting the effects of aspirin.[13,18]

Depth of the Incision

The introduction of a template has done much to standardize the depth of the wound. A histologic study showed that wounds with a depth of 0.4 mm were made with a template device and a knife protruding 1 mm through the template.[7] Deeper wounds are probably made by spring-loaded devices such as the Simplate II, as can be deduced by the longer bleeding times found (the knife may also protrude a little more: 1.2 mm instead of 1 mm).[14] An important factor determining the depth of the wound is the amount of pressure with which the device is applied to the skin. Skin is pliable, and increased local pressure produces deeper wounds. The Simplate device has some disadvantage in this respect because it has a relatively narrow convex bottom plate with which it rests on the skin, and it may therefore indent the skin more easily. Part of the experience needed to obtain reproducible results may reside in the control of this variable.

Normal Values

The upper limit of the original template bleeding time was 5.5 minutes, but longer times have been quoted, depending on the device used.[14] The upper limits of the bleeding times obtained with the Simplate II device are usually not >8.5 minutes,[19] but the values vary with geographic location[20] and other unknown factors, and each laboratory should establish its own upper limits. The skin becomes less elastic with age, and a significant but slight shortening of the bleeding time has been observed with increasing age.[21] A peculiar type of subcutaneous bleeding is sometimes seen in puncture wounds in the elderly, and this may stop the blood flow from the wound, giving artificially low values. There is a dispute about the effect of gender on the bleeding time. Some authors have found longer values in women,[16,22] but others could not confirm this finding.[21,23] The bleeding time becomes longer during pregnancy, probably because of the lower hematocrit and platelet number. The higher von Willebrand factor (vWF) level does not compensate for this.[24] There is dispute as to whether the bleeding time in normals is related to blood group. Normals with blood group O have lower vWF levels, and one group found longer bleeding times,[25] whereas two other groups could not confirm this finding.[26,27] A weak but statistically significant correlation between the bleeding time in normals and platelet

TEST PROCEDURE

1. Inform the patient of possible scarring. Do not perform a template bleeding time if there is a tendency toward keloid formation.
2. Avoid extreme temperatures in the room.
3. Seat the subject with the arm slightly flexed; place the forearm on a steady support with the volar side exposed. Neither arm is preferred over the other.
4. Select the area on the volar side of the forearm approximately 5 cm below the elbow crease.
5. Clean the skin gently with alcohol and allow it to dry. If a lot of hair is present shave the area.
6. Place a sphygmomanometer cuff (width 12–14 cm) around the upper arm and inflate the cuff to a pressure of 40 mmHg. Take care that the pressure is maintained during the entire procedure.
7. Wait 30 seconds before making the incisions.
8. Place the template device firmly on the arm, without pressing too hard. Make one or two horizontal incisions. Remove the template and start the stopwatches.
9. Blot the outflowing blood at 30-second intervals with filter paper (Whatman no. 1 or equivalent). Do not touch the wound.
10. Stop the stopwatch when the filter paper no longer turns red. Note whether a wound starts to bleed again.
11. Remove the cuff and apply a butterfly bandage across the wound to minimize scar formation.
12. The value obtained with a single wound or mean value of two wounds is the bleeding time.

vWF has been reported.[27] Determining the bleeding time in preterm infants requires special consideration. The wounds inflicted by current devices are too large and too deep to be appropriate in these babies. Good results have been obtained using a template with a length of 5 mm and a knife protrusion of 0.5 mm.[14] Stab wounds of the thumb have also been used in newborns and have been shown to be reproducible. A template-type device is available for this purpose (Autolet, Owen Mumford, Oxford, UK).[28] An additional important consideration for neonates is the use of a standardized venous pressure. It was found that a pressure of 40 mmHg is too high for preterm infants: 20 mmHg was recommended for a birthweight <1,000 g; 25 mmHg for birthweights between 1,000 and 2,000 g; and 30 mmHg for infants with a birthweight >2,000 g. Recently, a spring-loaded templated device, Simplate Paediatric, has been marketed with a retractable blade making a single incision 3 mm long. The blade protrudes 0.5 mm from the device.[29]

WHICH METHOD TO USE

The first method, described by Duke,[1] consisted of a deep puncture in the earlobe. This method cannot be recommended because it is not reliable; it can be very difficult to obtain adequate hemostasis in patients who have prolonged bleeding times. The choice at present is between the standardized Ivy bleeding time using a puncture, or one of the commercial devices employing a template to make a standardized incision. The template bleeding times are at present more popular, and the Simplate II device (General Diagnostics, Organon Teknika, Turnhout, Belgium) is frequently used.[17] The Simplate II-R has recently been introduced and gives similar results; it has a retractable blade to avoid accidental cuts and transmission of blood-borne viruses.[29] Preference is generally given to the template techniques, because they may be more sensitive. An advantage of the commercial devices is that they are disposable and safe to use. A disadvantage is that they are in general much more expensive, in both cost and operator time. Recent data have indicated that the Ivy technique may not differ much in sensitivity and specificity for aspirin-induced changes, when it is rigorously standardized, and when the upper limits of a normal population have been defined precisely.[15,30] In these studies the Ivy test was performed by making three puncture wounds with a blade depth of 2.5 mm and a width of 1.5 mm. Similar specificity and sensitivity were found for aspirin-induced changes with the Ivy technique performed in this way and the Simplate technique performed with either a vertical or a horizontal incision. The Ivy technique was preferred by the patients because it caused less scarring. The horizontal Simplate II caused the most scarring. The Ivy was also preferred because it takes less time to perform. The horizontal Simplate II takes the longest time to perform. The question remains as to whether these data can be extrapolated to other disorders. Our own unpublished data indicate that the Simplate II is more sensitive than the Ivy for patients with the uremic defect in platelet function (see below).

CLINICAL DISORDERS

Vascular Disorders

Petechiae, purpura, and easy bruising are regular features of vascular diseases (see Ch. 103) such as allergic vasculitis, Henoch-Schönlein purpura, and scurvy. Superficial subcutaneous bleeding is also observed in Cushing syndrome and is often seen in patients on cortisone treatment. Notwithstanding these features of a vascular bleeding disorder, the bleeding time is most often not prolonged, and major bleeding is not observed in these patients. Prolonged bleeding times have been found in connective tissue disorders, such as the Ehlers-Danlos syndrome, and in some patients with osteogenesis imperfecta.[31]

von Willebrand Disease

Von Willebrand disease (see Chs. 104 and 113) is characterized by quantitative or qualitative abnormalities of vWF.[32] vWF is necessary for platelet adhesion at high shear rates,[33] and it plays a role in platelet-platelet interaction.[34] It also serves as a carrier molecule for factor VIII and protects it against proteolytic degradation.[35,36] For the in vitro assessment of the ability of vWF to support platelet adhesion, the ristocetin cofactor assay is used. This test shows a reasonable correlation with the support of adhesion by vWF, but discrepant results are sometimes found.[37] Recent studies have indicated that the bleeding time is dependent not only on the quantity or quality (or both) of the vWF present in plasma, but also on platelet vWF.[38–40]

Thrombocytopenia

A good inverse correlation was found between the template bleeding time and a platelet count between 10,000 and 100,000/mm^3. At levels >100,000/mm^3, the bleeding time remained constant; at <10,000/mm^3, a bleeding time of >30 minutes was observed.[41] These findings have been confirmed, although the correlation was not completely linear and the values were in general more widely scattered.[42,43] Caution is therefore needed in the interpretation of the correlation between the bleeding time and the platelet count. As a general guideline for the length of the bleeding time in thrombocytopenia, the following equation may be used:

$$\text{Bleeding time (in minutes)} = 30 - \frac{\text{platelet count/mm}^3}{4{,}000}$$

A disproportionate prolongation may indicate an accompanying functional disorder of the platelet. Disproportionate shortening is caused by the presence of young functionally active platelets, such as those that may be present in immune thrombocytopenic purpura.[41]

Platelet Function Disorders

Platelet function disorders (see Chs. 129 and 130) cause prolongation of the bleeding time at least as frequently as von Willebrand disease. Abnormalities in the contribution of blood platelets to the coagulant system, such as abnormal phospholipid exposure[44] and abnormal platelet factor V,[45] are not reflected in a prolongation of the bleeding time.

Coagulation Factor Abnormalities

Prolongation of the bleeding time is found in patients with severe factor V and factor VII deficiencies. From the histologic observations of the hemostatic plug it has become clear that thrombin formation via the extrinsic pathway is involved in making the hemostatic plug impermeable, but abnormalities are only observed in severe deficiencies. This is also true in hemophilia A and B. About one-half of the patients with hemophilia A showed a relatively mild prolongation of the bleeding time,[46,47] although the hemostatic plug formation in hemophilia A and B is abnormal.[8] As has been mentioned, the central abnormality causing bleeding resides in the abnormal fibrin formation during the fibrinous transformation of the plug, and this is not reflected in the bleeding time. Prolongation of the bleeding time is observed in afibrinogenemia. Fibrinogen is the main adhesive protein required for platelet aggregation.[48] Levels of fibrinogen >25 mg/dl are sufficient for normal hemostasis.[49]

Uremia

Many patients with uremia (see Ch. 130) have a prolonged bleeding time,[50] partly due to the presence of anemia in these patients; at least partial correction can be obtained by transfusion of red cells or by erythropoietin treatment.[51] The abnormality is also caused by the presence of toxins in uremic plasma, which inhibit adhesion and aggregation in flow.[52] A pronounced discrepancy exists between the bleeding time values as measured with the Ivy method when compared with the Simplate II device in uremia. The Ivy values are often normal in patients on chronic hemodialysis, whereas the Simplate II values are prolonged (H. K. Nieuwenhuis, personal observation).

Other Disorders

Prolongation of the bleeding time has been found in severe anemia.[53] It is possible, though, that subthreshold platelet abnormalities are present in the occasional anemic patients with very long bleeding times. Long bleeding times have been observed in some patients with multiple myeloma and Waldenström disease. This prolongation is attributed to the interference with platelet function by abnormal monoclonal immunoglobulins.[54]

Short Bleeding Times

Short bleeding times have been observed in patients with atherosclerotic vessel disease during myocardial infarction[55] and in those who have survived a myocardial infarction.[57–] The difference is even more pronounced when a higher venous pressure of 80 mmHg is used.[14] Shortened bleeding times have also been reported in patients with diabetes mellitus and in those with hyperlipoproteinemia,[60] but not in patients with unstable angina.[55]

EFFECTS OF DRUGS

Prolongation of the Bleeding Time

Many drugs may affect the bleeding time.[61] The most prominent among them are the nonsteroidal anti-inflammatory agents, aspirin in particular,[4,62] and antibiotics such as penicillin and various cephalothins.[63,64] The effects of these drugs are most pronounced in patients with a pre-existing bleeding disorder. Dipyridamole, a weak platelet function inhibitor, may prolong the bleeding time in uremia and when high doses of the drug are used.[65] Another drug that gives a pronounced prolongation of the bleeding time is ticlopidine, an effective platelet function inhibitor with an unknown mechanism of action.[66–68] Anticoagulants, heparin and coumarin, usually have no effect on the bleeding time at normal therapeutic levels, but a prolonged bleeding time is observed when patients have received too high a dose of heparin, or when very low doses of factor VII are caused by overdosage of coumarin.[69] Heparin or oral anticoagulants cause a further prolongation of the bleeding time in patients in whom the bleeding time is already prolonged by platelet function inhibitors.[70,71]

Shortening of a Prolonged Bleeding Time

Antifibrinolytic agents such as ε-aminocaproic acid or tranexamic acid have been shown to diminish bleeding in menorrhagia or in hemophilic patients after dental extraction.[72–74] These drugs are also used in patients with a prolonged bleeding time due to thrombocytopenia or a platelet function disorder or in von Willebrand disease, but there is currently no proof that such therapy has any effect.

The use of corticosteroids to prevent bleeding is disputed. A large dose of corticosteroids has been shown to shorten the bleeding time in normal and thrombocytopenic rabbits,[75] but consistent data are not present for the use of corticosteroids in humans. Correction of the bleeding time has been observed in several patients with "aspirin-like" platelet function disorders.[76] Administration of prednisone (80 mg) had no effect on the bleeding time before and after administration of aspirin to normal individuals,[77] and corticosteroids were also shown to be ineffective in von Willebrand disease and Glanzmann thrombasthenia.[41] 1-Desamino-8-D-arginine vasopressin (DDAVP) (0.3 μg/kg body weight IV infused over 20–30 minutes) has been shown to increase factor VIII and vWF levels in normal individuals, in those having mild hemophilia A, and in many patients with von Willebrand disease. In the latter group a temporary shortening of the bleeding time was also observed.[78,79] More recently, shortening of a prolonged bleeding time with DDAVP has also been observed in uremia,[80] liver disease,[81] and various platelet function disorders, such as defects in prostaglandin metabolism, and in many cases of storage pool deficiency.[82,83] No effect was seen in Glanzmann thrombasthenia.[82] The effect in storage pool deficiency is unpredictable, and a test administration is therefore justified. A hemostatic effect of DDAVP administration has also been shown in normal children undergo-

PREDICTIVE VALUE AND IMPORTANCE OF THE BLEEDING TIME

The bleeding time[68] is used to (1) diagnose hereditary bleeding disorders, (2) find an explanation for previous bleeding, (3) determine a cause for ongoing bleeding, (4) to screen patients for invasive procedures, (5) evaluate the quality of vWF concentrates and stored blood platelets, and (6) follow the effect of platelet function inhibitors.

The bleeding time is not a good predictor of the chance of bleeding (see Ch. 130). Studies in uremic patients have shown no correlation between subcapsular kidney bleeding after renal biopsy and bleeding time.[89] In extensive review of the literature showed no evidence that the bleeding time in a general population has any predictive value at all.[90] This is important because the bleeding time is still generally used as a preoperative screening test, and this practice should be abandoned. A much better procedure is to obtain a good history of previous bleeding and to determine bleeding times only in patients with a positive history as part of a preoperative diagnostic workup of hemostasis.

The recent disenchantment with the bleeding time as a predictive test occasionally leads to the belief that the bleeding time is useless altogether. We believe this is incorrect. The bleeding time is still a useful component of the workup of a patient suspected of having a bleeding disorder. It is perhaps less useful in determining the cause of ongoing bleeding, and critical studies should be performed to determine its role in that situation. The role of the bleeding time as an intermediary end point in the study of hemostatic agents and platelet function inhibitors is less self evident than it seems at first glance. A vWF concentrate that corrects the prolonged bleeding time in von Willebrand disease is more likely to prevent bleeding than a concentrate that does not, and the same is true for stored platelet concentrates in thrombocytopenia. There is no hard proof for this contention, however. The situation is more complicated in the case of prolongation of the bleeding time by platelet function inhibitors. Although in general drugs that prolong the bleeding time may cause increased bleeding, it is becoming evident that the length of the bleeding time in this instance is not a good predictor for the risk of bleeding: drugs with different mechanisms of actions may lead to similar prolongations of the bleeding time but may carry different bleeding risks.

ing spinal surgery for scoliosis.[84] The reason for this beneficial action of DDAVP is not explained. The vWF level in normal blood may be suboptimal, and an increase in this level may lead to a shortening of the bleeding time, but the action of DDAVP may be more complex. A synergistic shortening of the bleeding time was found with a combination of DDAVP and ethamsylate, a drug that inhibits prostacyclin formation and that has no effect on the bleeding time on its own.[85]

Another measure that has been shown to cause a shortening of the bleeding time in patients with uremia and in many with storage pool deficiency is the administration of cryoprecipitate.[86,87] At present, cryoprecipitate preparations are treated to eradicate the human immunodeficiency virus; such treatment may make cryoprecipitates less effective. Pasteurization of high-purity factor VIII concentrates may eradicate the human immunodeficiency virus and keep vWF functionally intact.[88]

REFERENCES

1. Duke W: The relation of blood platelets to hemorrhagic disease: description of a method for determining the bleeding time and coagulation time and report of three cases of hemorrhagic disease relieved by transfusion. JAMA 55:1185, 1910
2. Ivy AC, Shapiro PF, Melnick P: The bleeding tendency in jaundice. Surg Gynecol Obstet 60:781, 1935
3. Borchgrevink CF, Waaler BA: The secondary bleeding time: a new method for the differentation of hemorrhagic diseases. J Intern Med 162:361, 1958
4. Mielke CH Jr, Kaneshiro MM, Maher IA et al: The standardized normal Ivy bleeding time and its prolongation by aspirin. Blood 34:204, 1969
5. Ivy AC, Nelson D, Bucher G: The standardization of certain factors in the cutaneous "venostasis" bleeding time technique. J Lab Clin Med 26:1812, 1941
6. Wester J, Sixma JJ, Geuze JJ, Heynen H: Morphology of the haemostatic plug in human skin wounds: transformation of the plug. Lab Invest 41:182, 1979
7. Wester J, Sixma JJ, Geuze JJ, van der Veen J: Morphology of the early hemostasis in human skin wounds: influence of acetyl salicylic acid. Lab Invest 39:298, 1978
8. Sixma JJ, van den Berg A: The haemostatic plug in haemophilia A: a morphological study of haemostatic plug formation in bleeding time skin wounds of patients with severe haemophilia A. Br J Haematol 58:741, 1984
9. Brown CH, Natelson EA, Bradshaw MV et al: Study of the effects of ticarcillin on blood coagulation and platelet function. Antimicrob Agents Chemother 7:652, 1975
10. König L: Versuche über Blutstillung. Klin Wochenschr 1:2376, 1922
11. Quick AJ: The Duke bleeding time. Am J Clin Pathol 47:459, 1967
12. Sutor AH, Bowie EJW, Owen CAJ: Effect of temperature on haemostasis: a cold tolerance test. Blut 22:27, 1970
13. Mielke CH: Aspirin prolongation of the template bleeding time: influence of venostasis and direction of incision. Blood 60:1139, 1982
14. Babson SR, Babson AL: Development and evaluation of a disposable device for performing simultaneous duplicate bleeding time determinations. Am J Clin Pathol 70:406, 1978
15. Koster TMS, Caekebeke-Peerlinck KMJ, Briet E: A randomized and blinded comparison of the sensitivity and the reproducibility of the Ivy and Simplate II bleeding time techniques. Am J Clin Pathol 92:315, 1989
16. Mielke CH: Measurement of the bleeding time. Thromb Haemost 52:210, 1984
17. Poller L, Thomson JM, Tomenson JA: The bleeding time: current practice in the UK. Clin Lab Haematol 6:369, 1984
18. Buchanan GR, Holtkamp BS: A comparative study of variables affecting the bleeding time using two disposable devices. Am J Clin Pathol 91:45, 1989
19. Thorngren M: Bleeding times in southern Sweden, letter. Lancet 1:450, 1982
20. Nieuwenhuis HK, Sixma JJ: Bleeding time measurements. p. 26. In Harker LA, Zimmerman TS (eds): Measurements of Platelet Function. Methods in Hematology. Churchill Livingstone, Edinburgh, 1983
21. Macpherson CR, Jacobs P: Bleeding time decreases with age. Arch Pathol Lab Med 111:328, 1987
22. Parkin JD, Smith IL: Sex and bleeding time. Thromb Haemost 3:731, 1985
23. Nieuwenhuis HK, Akkerman JWN, Sixma JJ: Patients with a prolonged bleeding time and normal aggregation tests may have storage pool deficiency: studies on one hundred six patients. Blood 70:620, 1987
24. Ivankovic M, Pereira J, Germain A et al: Pregnancy and the bleeding time. Thromb Haemost 68:375, 1992
25. Caekebeke-Peerlinck KMJ, Koster T, Briët E: Bleeding time, blood groups and von Willebrand Factor. Br J Haematol 73:217, 1987
26. Wahlberg TB, Blombäck M, Magnusson D: Influence of sex, blood group, secretor character, smoking habits, acetyl salicylic acid, oral contraceptives, fasting and general health state on blood coagulation variables in randomly selected young adults. Haemostasis 14:312, 1984
27. Rodeghiero F, Castaman G, Ruggeri M, Tosetto A: The bleeding time in normal subjects is mainly determined by platelet von Willebrand factor and is independent from blood group. Thromb Res 65:605, 1992
28. Rennie JM, Gibson T, Cooke RWI: Micromethod for bleeding time in the newborn. Arch Dis Child 60:51, 1985
29. Lethagen S, Kling S: New bleeding time devices with retractable blades evaluated in children, healthy volunteers and patients with prolonged bleeding time. Thromb Haemost 70:595, 1993
30. Srámek R, Srámek A, Koster T et al: A randomized and blinded comparison of three bleeding time techniques: the Ivy method, and the Simplate II method in two directions. Thromb Haemost 67:514, 1992
31. Hindriks GA, de Boer HC, Nieuwenhuis HK et al: Adhesion of blood platelets to the extracellular matrix of cultured cells in which collagen synthesis is impaired or induced. Thromb Haemost 58:206, 1987
32. Ruggeri ZM, Zimmerman TS: Von Willebrand factor and von Willebrand disease. Blood 70:895, 1987

33. Weiss HT, Turitto VT, Baumgartner HR: Effect of shear rate on platelet interaction in von Willebrand's disease and Bernard-Soulier syndrome. J Lab Clin Med 92:750, 1978

34. Turitto VT, Weiss HJ, Baumgartner HR: Platelet interaction with rabbit subendothelium in von Willebrand's disease: altered thrombus formation distinct from platelet adhesion. J Clin Invest 74:1730, 1984

35. Weiss HJ, Sussman II, Hoyer LW: Stabilization of factor VIII in plasma by the von Willebrand factor: studies on posttransfusion and dissociated factor VIII and in patients with von Willebrand's disease. J Clin Invest 60:390, 1977

36. Koedam JA, Meijers JCM, Sixma JJ, Bouma BN: Inactivation of factor VIII by activated protein C. Cofactor activity of protein S and protective effect of von Willebrand factor. J Clin Invest 82:1236, 1988

37. Sixma JJ, Sakariassen KS, Beeser-Visser NH et al: Adhesion of platelets to human artery subendothelium: effect of factor VIII-von Willebrand factor of various multimeric composition. Blood 63:128, 1984

38. Gralnick HR, Rick ME, McKeown LP et al: Platelet von Willebrand factor: an important determinant of the bleeding time in type I von Willebrand's disease. Blood 68:58, 1986

39. Fressinaud E, Baruch D, Rothschild C et al: Platelet von Willebrand factor: evidence for its involvement in platelet adhesion to collagen. Blood 70:1214, 1987

40. D'Alessio PA, Zwaginga JJ, de Boer HC et al: Platelet adhesion to collagen in subtypes of type I von Willebrand's disease is dependent on platelet von Willebrand factor. Thromb Haemost 64:227, 1990

41. Caen JP, Castaldi PA, Leclerc JC: Congenital bleeding disorders with long bleeding time and normal platelet count. I: Glanzmann's thrombasthenia (report of fifteen patients). Am J Med 41:4, 1966

42. Heiden D, Mielke CH Jr, Rodvien R: Impairment by heparin of primary haemostasis and platelet [^{14}C]5-hydroxytryptamine release. Br J Haematol 36:427, 1977

43. Kahn RA, Meryman HT: Storage of platelet concentrates. Transfusion 16:13, 1976

44. Weiss HJ, Vicic WJ, Lages BA, Rogers J: Isolated deficiency of platelet procoagulant activity. Am J Med 67:206, 1979

45. Tracy PB, Giles AR, Mann KG et al: Factor V Quebec: a bleeding diathesis associated with a qualitative platelet factor V deficiency. J Clin Invest 74:1221, 1984

46. Buchanan GR, Holtkamp CA: Prolonged bleeding time in children and young adults with hemophilia. Pediatrics 66:951, 1980

47. Eyster ME, Gordon RA, Ballard JO: The bleeding time is longer than normal in haemophilia. Blood 58:719, 1981

48. Bennet JS, Hoxie JA, Leitman SF et al: Inhibition of fibrinogen binding to stimulated human platelets by a monoclonal antibody. Proc Natl Acad Sci USA 80:2417, 1983

49. Caen J, Inceman S: Considérations sur l'allongement du temps de saignement dans l'afibrinogenémie congénitale. Nouv Rev Fr Hematol 3:614, 1963

50. Steiner RW, Coggins C, Carvalho ACA: Bleeding time in uremia: a useful test to assess clinical bleeding. Am J Hematol 7:107, 1979

51. Moia M, Vizzotto L, Cattaneo M et al: Improvement in the haemostatic defect of uraemia after treatment with recombinant erythropoietin. Lancet 2:1227, 1987

52. Zwaginga JJ, IJsseldijk MJW, Beeser-Visser N et al: High von Willebrand factor concentration compensates a relative adhesion defect in uremic blood. Blood 75:1498, 1990

53. Hellem AJ, Borchgrevink CF, Ames SB: The role of red cells in haemostasis: the relation between haematocrit, bleeding time and platelet adhesiveness. Br J Haematol 7:42, 1961

54. Kasturi J, Saraya AK: Platelet function in dysproteinaemia. Acta Haematol 59:104, 1978

55. Kristensen SD, Bath PMW, Martin JF: Differences in bleeding time, aspirin sensitivity and adrenaline between acute myocardial infarction and unstable angina. Cardiovasc Res 24:19, 1990

56. Bath PMW, Kristensen SD, Martin JF, Milner PC: Bleeding time and diagnosis of acute myocardial infarction. Haemostasis 21:181, 1991

57. Milner PC, Martin JF: Shortened bleeding time in acute myocardial infarction and its relation to platelet mass. BMJ 290:1767, 1985

58. O'Brien JR, Etherington MD, Jamieson S et al: Blood changes in atherosclerosis and long after myocardial infarction and venous thrombosis. Thromb Diath Haemorrh 34:483, 1975

59. O'Brien JR, Jamieson S, Etherington M et al: Stressed template bleeding time and other platelet function tests in myocardial infarction. Lancet 1:694, 1973

60. Joist JH, Balser K, Schoenfeld G: Increased in vivo platelet function in type II and type IV hyperbetalipoproteinemia. Thromb Res 15:95, 1979

61. Quick AJ: Salicylates and bleeding: the aspirin tolerance test. Am J Med S 252:265, 1966

62. Bick RL: Platelet function defects: a clinical review. Semin Thromb Hemo 18:167, 1992

63. Brown CH, Bradshaw MW, Natelson EA et al: Defective platelet function following the administration of penicillin compounds. Blood 47:949, 1976

64. McClure PD, Casserly JG, Monsier C, Crozier D: Carbenicillin-induced bleeding disorder. Lancet 2:1307, 1970

65. Weston MJ, Rubin MH, Langly PG et al: Effects of sulphinpyrazone and dipyridamole on capillary bleeding time in man. Thromb Res 10:833, 1977

66. David JL, Monfort F, Herion F, Raskinet P: Compared effect of three dose levels of ticlopidine on platelet function in normal subjects. Thromb Res 1 35, 1979

67. O'Brien JR, Etherington MD, Shuttleworth RD: Ticlopidine—an antiplatelet drug: effects in human volunteers. Thromb Res 14:245, 1978

68. Lind SE: The bleeding time does not predict surgical bleeding. Blood 77:254 1991

69. Hjort PF, Borchgrevink CF, Iversen OH, Stormorken H: The effect of heparin on the bleeding time. Thromb Diath Haemorrh 4:389, 1960

70. De Boer A, Kroon M, Van Vliet A et al: Pronounced effects of the combination of a new thromboxane antagonist (GR32191) and heparin on bleeding time in man. Thromb Haemost 86:24, 1992

71. Bang CJ, Riedel B, Talstad I, Berstad A: Interaction between heparin and acetylsalicylic acid on gastric mucosal and skin bleeding in humans. Scan J Gastroenterol 27:489, 1992

72. Nilsson L, Rybo G: Treatment of menorrhagia with an antifibrinolytic agent, tranexamic acid (AMCA). Acta Obstet Gynecol Scand 46:572, 1967

73. Vermijlen J, Verhaegen-Declercq ML, Verstraete M, Fierens F: A double blind study of the effect of tranexamic acid in essential menorrhagia. Thromb Diath Haemorrh 20:583, 1968

74. Callender ST, Warner GT, Cope E: Treatment of menorrhagia with tranexamic acid: a double-blind trial. BMJ 4:214, 1979

75. Blajchman MA, Senyi AF, Hirsch J et al: Shortening of the bleeding time in rabbits by hydrocortisone caused by inhibition of prostacyclin generation by the vessel wall. J Clin Invest 63:1026, 1979

76. Mielke CH Jr, Levine PH, Zucker S: Preoperative prednisone therapy in platelet function disorders. Thromb Res 21:655, 1981

77. Thong KL, Mant MJ, Grace MG: Lack of effect of prednisone administration on bleeding time and platelet function of normal subjects. Br J Haematol 38:373, 1978

78. Mannucci PM, Canciani MT, Rota L, Donovan BS: Response of factor VIII/von Willebrand factor to DDAVP in healthy subjects and patients with haemophilia A and von Willebrand's disease. Br J Haematol 47:283, 1981

79. Sakariassen KS, Cattaneo M, van den Berg A et al: DDAVP enhances platelet adherence and platelet aggregate growth on human artery subendothelium. Blood 64:229, 1984

80. Mannucci PM, Remuzzi G, Pusineri F et al: Desamino-8-D-arginine vasopressin shortens the bleeding time in uremia. N Engl J Med 308:8, 1983

81. Mannucci PM, Vicente V, Vianello L et al: Controlled trial of desmopressin in liver cirrhosis and other conditions associated with a prolonged bleeding time. Blood 4:1148, 1986

82. Nieuwenhuis HK, Sixma JJ: 1-Desamino-8-D-arginine vasopressin (desmopressin) shortens the bleeding time in storage pool deficiency. Ann Intern Med 108:65, 1988

83. Kobrinsky NL, Israels ED, Gerrard JM et al: Shortening of bleeding time by 1-desamino-8-arginine in various bleeding disorders. Lancet 1:145, 1984

84. Kobrinsky NL, Letts M, Patel LR et al: 1-Desamino-8-D-arginine vasopressin (desmopressin) decreases operative blood loss in patients having Harrington rod spinal fusion surgery. Ann Intern Med 107:446, 1987

85. Kobrinsky NL, Israels ED, Bickis MG: Synergistic shortening of the bleeding time by desmopressin and ethamsylate in patients with various constitutional bleeding disorders. Am J Pediatr Hematol Oncol 13:437, 1991

86. Janson PA, Jubelirer SJ, Weinstein MJ, Deykin D: Treatment of the bleeding tendency in uremia with cryoprecipitate. N Engl J Med 303:1318, 1980

87. Gerritsen SW, Akkerman JWN, Sixma JJ: Correction of the bleeding time in patients with storage pool deficiency by infusion of cryoprecipitate. Br J Haematol 40:153, 1978

88. Berntorp E, Nilsson IM: Use of a high-purity factor VIII concentrate (Hemate P) in von Willebrand's disease. Vox Sang 56:212, 1989

89. Gotti E, Mecca G, Valentino C et al: Renal biopsy in patients with acute renal failure and prolonged bleeding time: a preliminary report. Am J Kidney Dis 6:397, 1985

90. Rogers RPC, Levin J: A critical reappraisal of the bleeding time. Semin Thromb Hemost 16:1, 1990

Laboratory Detection of Hemoglobinopathies and thalassemias

161

Martin H. Steinberg and Junius G. Adams III

INTRODUCTION

Hemoglobin electrophoresis has been the most widely used technique for the identification of hemoglobinopathies and thalassemias. Isoelectric focusing (IEF) and high-performance liquid chromatography (HPLC) have also been employed extensively for hemoglobinopathy detection. These methods can provide preliminary and sometimes definitive diagnosis of disorders of hemoglobin structure or synthesis. The hemoglobinopathies have been reviewed in detail along with methods for their detection.[1-4] No single laboratory test alone is adequate for the detection of all hemoglobinopathies and thalassemias in both adults and neonates. The various techniques in current use and their pitfalls are discussed below. Blood counts and erythrocyte indices can modulate the interpretation of the results of hemoglobin electrophoresis and are briefly reviewed first.

MEASUREMENT OF HEMATOLOGIC PARAMETERS

Hematologic indices play an extremely important role in the differential diagnosis of hemoglobinopathies and the thalassemia syndromes. The measurement of mean corpuscular volume (MCV) and other red cell indices, by electronic cell counting, are particularly useful in this regard.[5,6] In thalassemia, microcytosis (MCV <80 fl) is usually present. However, in sickling hemoglobinopathies without associated thalassemia or iron deficiency, the erythrocytes are usually normocytic.[7] The Hb E syndromes, and the Hb C disorders to a lesser extent, are also associated with a decreased MCV. A normal value for the MCV generally excludes the possibility of Hb E or β-thalassemia trait. The red cell distribution width (RDW) can be used to differentiate thalassemia carriers from people with iron deficiency. In iron deficiency the RDW is high; in most other conditions it is normal. However, abnormal erythrocyte indices are nonspecific and can arise from a number of conditions, such as iron deficiency, α-thalassemia, and other uncommon hematologic entities. In addition, microcytosis is not present in all instances of thalassemia and can be masked by concurrent megaloblastic erythropoiesis.[8]

HEMOGLOBIN ELECTROPHORESIS

Of the many methods available to characterize and quantitate hemoglobin, electrophoresis remains the most useful for practical clinical application.

Hemoglobin Electrophoresis at Alkaline pH

Hemoglobin is negatively charged at alkaline pH and it migrates anodically (toward the positive pole) from its point of application in an electrical field. Some variant hemoglobins have different charges than normal hemoglobin at alkaline pH. For example, Hb S has two more positive charges than Hb A per hemoglobin tetramer. Hb C has four more positive charges, and Hb J has two less positive charges. Thus, Hb S migrates more slowly than Hb A toward the anode, Hb C migrates more slowly than Hb S, and Hb J migrates more rapidly than Hb A, since a protein's migration in an electrical field is in part determined by its charge.

Hemoglobin electrophoresis utilizes various solid support media, and cellulose acetate membranes are now the material of choice. They are inexpensive, can be prepared quickly and easily, provide sharp resolution of hemoglobin bands, allow measurement of the relative quantities of the major hemoglobin bands by densitometry, and furnish a permanent record after the membranes are fixed and cleared.[9-12]

However, when applied to newborn screening, Hb A and Hb S are poorly resolved on cellulose acetate at alkaline pH from Hb F, which makes up about 80% of the newborn hemolysate. It is therefore imperative that in newborns some other method, such as citrate agar gel electrophoresis, be used in conjunction with cellulose acetate. Cellulose acetate electrophoresis of some common hemoglobin variants is shown in Figure 161-1 (top), and more complex patterns are diagrammatically depicted in Figure 161-2.

Citrate Agar Gel Electrophoresis

To identify abnormal hemoglobins more definitively it is often useful to examine their electrophoretic mobility using more than one support medium, buffer, and pH. Electrophoresis on agar gels with citrate buffer at pH 6.1 causes most hemoglobins to move cathodically (i.e., to the negative pole) from the point of origin and with different relative mobilities than those seen with cellulose acetate electrophoresis at alkaline pH.[13-15] Citrate agar electrophoresis is capable of resolving some variants that do not separate from Hb A, S, or C by cellulose acetate electrophoresis and should be employed in conjunction with cellulose acetate electrophoresis to resolve confusion in the identification of many common variants. It is especially useful for detecting hemoglobinopathies in the newborn owing to the distinct separation of Hb F from Hb A and the major common variants. The migration patterns of some common hemoglobin variants on citrate agar gels at pH 6.1 are shown in Figures 161-1 (middle) and 161-2. Hb D and G, which co-migrate with Hb S on cellulose acetate, migrate with Hb A on citrate agar. Citrate agar gel electrophoresis is extremely helpful for differentiating between Hb E, Hb C, and Hb O-Arab, which all co-migrate on alkaline electrophoresis (Fig. 161-2). Thus, although citrate agar gel electrophoresis is one of the oldest screening tools, it remains one of the few methods that unambiguously distinguishes Hb S and Hb C from other common variants, and it is an important adjunct to cellulose acetate electrophoresis.

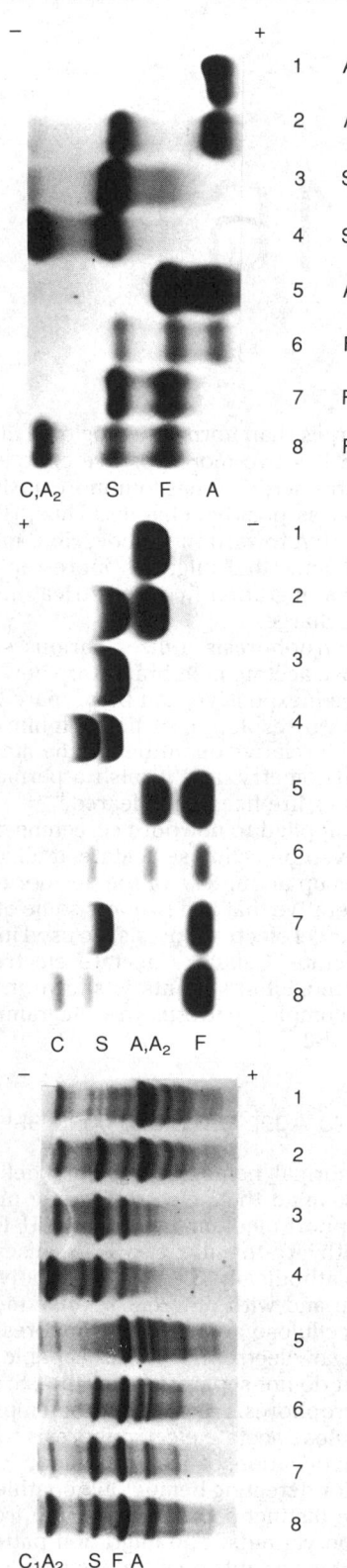

Fig. 161-1. (Top) Cellulose acetate electrophoresis (TRIS, EDTA, borate buffe pH 8.6) of some common hemoglobinopathies. Migration is from cathode to anod The samples are (1) Hb AA (adult, normal); (2) Hb AS (adult, sickle cell trait (3) Hb SS (adult, sickle cell anemia); (4) Hb SC (adult, Hb SC disease); (5) H FA (newborn, normal); (6) Hb FAS (newborn, sickle cell trait); (7) Hb FS (newborn sickle cell anemia); and (8) Hb FSC (newborn, Hb SC disease). When high concer trations of Hb A and Hb F are present, the resolution is poor. Hb A$_2$ is a ver faint band and does not show up well in all samples. **(Middle)** Citrate agar g electrophoresis, pH 6.1. The samples are arranged as in the top panel. Note th excellent resolution of Hb F from all other hemoglobin types. The migrations c Hb C and to a lesser extent Hb S depend somewhat on their concentrations Thus, there are differences in the mobilities in samples 4 and 8. Controls o appropriate concentrations eliminate any confusion in this regard. **(Bottom)** IEI using pH 5–9 ampholines in polyacrylamide gel. The samples are arranged as i the top panel. Note that Hb F is more clearly resolved from Hb A and Hb S that on cellulose acetate. The high resolving power of this technique leads to th resolution of several minor hemoglobin bands that are not seen by other methods These bands represent glycosylated and acetylated hemoglobins as well as variou methemoglobin hybrids. (Electrophoretograms courtesy of Robert L. Barlow).

sharp, distinct bands at their isoelectric points. As can be seen in Figure 161-1 (bottom), many hemoglobin variants that are resolved poorly by cellulose acetate electrophoresis are clearly differentiated by this technique. Although more costly than cellulose acetate electrophoresis, the resolving power of this technique has made it the method of choice for initial screening in many laboratories, especially for neonatal screening. However, considerable skill is required to interpret IEF gels, as many extraneous minor hemoglobin bands are often present and only qualitative information is obtained.

High-Performance Liquid Chromatography

Hemoglobins can also be separated on the basis of charge by HPLC[19,20] (Fig. 161-5). The advantages of this technique are (1) the resolution of various hemoglobins, including Hb F, is excellent; (2) the procedure is usually automated by an interface to a microcomputer, which can produce a reliable interpretation of the chromatogram; and (3) the various hemoglobin fractions are quantified by this method. This technique is used as the primary screening procedure in some newborn screening programs. Its limitation is that it cannot always resolve Hb S or Hb C from other variants with the same charge. Also, the equipment is expensive to purchase and maintain, and greater technical skills are required with some systems.

Practical Approach to Interpretation of Hemoglobin Electrophoresis

Electrophoresis, IEF, and HPLC of hemoglobin are usually performed for a limited number of clinical indications: (1) neonatal or population screening; (2) evaluation of anemia, erythrocytosis, syndromes suggestive of a sickling disorder, or microcytosis; or (3) quantitation of the percentage of normal and abnormal hemoglobin components in order to monitor chronic transfusion programs and for diagnostic purposes. With the exception of chronic transfusion monitoring and neonatal screening, repeating the electrophoresis once a diagnosis has been established is rarely indicated because the vast majority of patients will have a stable distribution of normal and abnormal hemoglobins after the neonatal period.

The major clinical questions to be resolved when ordering a hemoglobin electrophoresis are (1) Is an abnormal variant present? (2) What is (are) the abnormal variant(s)? (3) How abundant is (are) the variant(s)? (4) Is (are) the variant hemoglobin(s) relevant to the clinical picture that prompted the electrophoresis in the first place? Most electrophoreses will

Isoelectric Focusing

The limited sensitivity of cellulose acetate electrophoresis often necessitates use of supplementary procedures in newborn screening. Isoelectric focusing is capable of overcoming this limited sensitivity by its superior resolution of hemoglobin fractions.[16–18] IEF utilizes a pH gradient in a polyacrylamide gel. The electric field "focuses" the hemoglobin fractions into

CELLULOSE ACETATE (pH 8.6)   **CITRATE AGAR GEL (pH 6.1)**

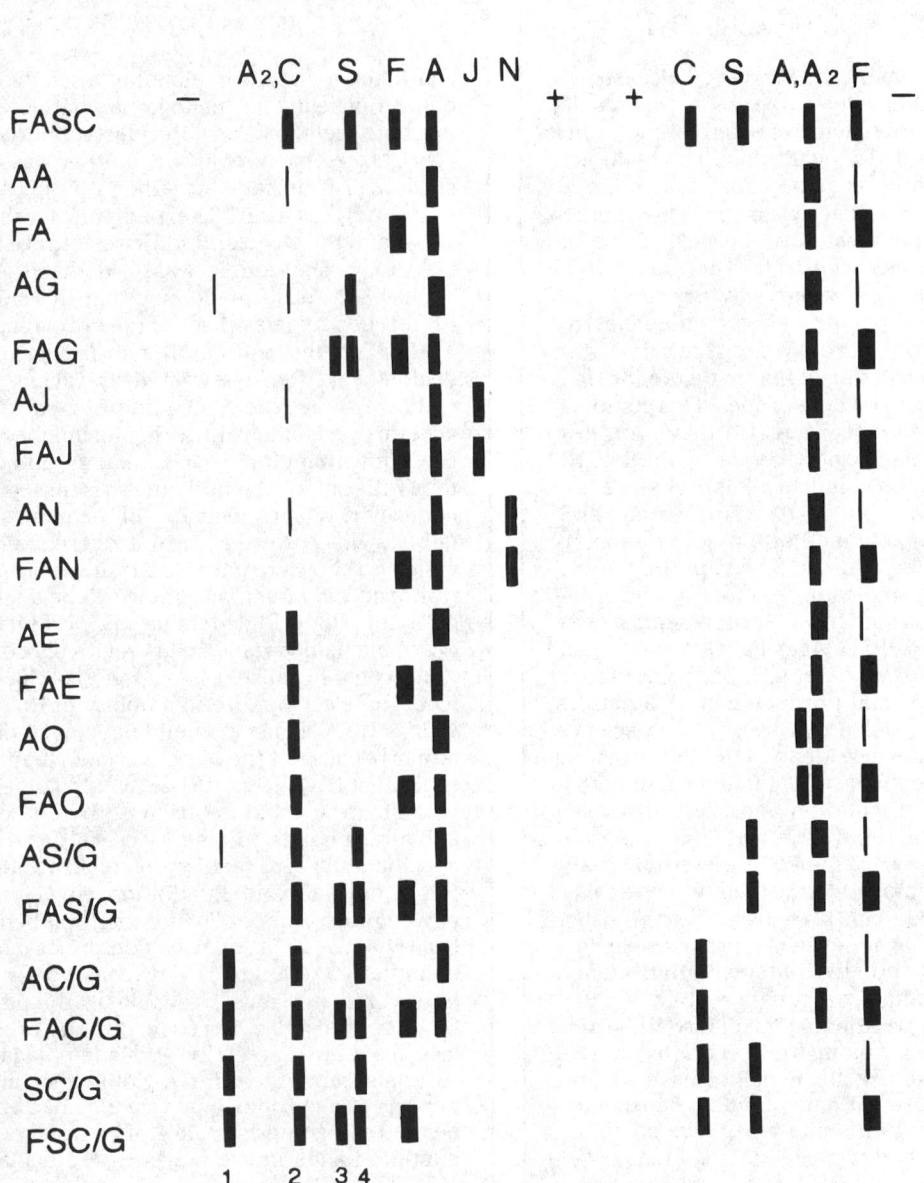

Fig. 161-2. Diagrammatic representation of some common electrophoretic patterns on cellulose acetate (pH 8.6) and citrate agar gel (pH 6.1). The electrophoretic mobilities of the common variants are listed above the electrophoretograms. The numbers beneath the cellulose acetate electrophoretic patterns indicate the positions of hybrid hemoglobins formed with Hb G-Philadelphia (an α-globin mutant). Position 1 can be occupied by $\alpha_2{}^G\delta_2$ (e.g., see Hb AG) or by this hybrid and $\alpha_2{}^G\beta_2{}^C$ (e.g., see Hb AC/G). Position 2 can be occupied by $\alpha_2{}^G\beta_2{}^S$ (e.g., see Hb AS/G) or by this hybrid and Hb C (e.g., Hb see SC/G). Position 3 is occupied by $\alpha^G{}_2\gamma_2$ (e.g., see Hb FA/G). Position 4 can be occupied by Hb G (e.g., see Hb AG) or by Hb S and Hb G (e.g., see Hb AS/G).

be ordered to evaluate the possibility of a sickle cell syndrome, a thalassemia syndrome, or the presence of common hemoglobin variants such as Hbs E, D, C, O, and G, which often accompany these conditions.

The use of hemoglobin electrophoresis to detect an unstable hemoglobin as a cause of an unexplained hemolytic anemia, a hemoglobin with altered oxygen affinity as the cause of erythrocytosis or cyanosis, or the presence of methemoglobinemia must be approached with a proper appreciation of the actual value of electrophoresis in these special situations. Hemoglobin electrophoresis is usually reliable only for confirmation and further characterization of variants causing these clinical syndromes. Functional tests to establish the presence of an abnormal hemoglobin that is likely to be relevant to these clinical syndromes should be the primary diagnostic maneuver. A

heat or isopropanol stability test and a search for Heinz bodies are obtained when evaluating the possibility of hemolysis from unstable hemoglobins. The oxygen half-saturation pressure (P_{50}) should be measured when a variant with high- or low-affinity hemoglobin oxygen affinity is suspected. Spectrophotometric analysis for methemoglobin first detects this oxidized form of hemoglobin. As discussed in Chapters 37 and 44, one should also search for characteristic clinical and hematologic features of these syndromes. Many variants that are unstable or have altered oxygen affinity are silent elecrophoretically, so normal electrophoresis will not rule these out. Electrophoresis will be informative only if it reveals an abnormal band; the mobility of the abnormal band in various electrophoretic systems may also provide clues as to the likely identity of the hemoglobin.

A VARIANT MIMICKING HEMOGLOBIN S

A 24-year-old black woman with sickle cell disease was referred for further testing because of conflicting results of hemoglobin studies that were reported in one of her children who had attended a health fair. The child was told that she had only normal hemoglobin, but she knew from recent studies in her science class that if her mother had sickle cell anemia she must have the sickle cell trait. An older sibling had sickle cell trait. The mother had symptoms of sickle cell disease and was anemic.

The predigree and the results of hemoglobin electrophoresis in the reference laboratory are shown in Figure 161-3. The mother (I 2) is a mixed heterozygote for Hb S and the β-globin variant, Hb D-Los Angeles. This combination results in sickle cell disease, as Hb D-Los Angeles, present in 0.1–0.4% of blacks, polymerizes with Hb S. Hb D-Los Angeles is also found in Indian Sikhs. Cellulose acetate electrophoresis does not resolve Hb D from Hb S. Therefore, if this is the sole method of electrophoresis used, the single major band of Hb S seen in the mother will be misinterpreted as indicating homozygosity for the sickle hemoglobin gene when in fact it represents a composite of both Hb S and Hb D. Agar gel electrophoresis at pH 6.1 causes Hb D to migrate with Hb A, permitting its distinction from Hb S and producing in I 2 a pattern that appears to be like sickle cell trait. At the science fair, hemoglobin screening was done by solubility testing only. This method is incapable of detecting variants that do not contain the Hb S mutation and is an ill-advised screening test, hence the report that this child was "normal." When her blood was examined by electrophoresis, (II 2) the pattern on cellulose acetate membranes at alkaline pH resembled sickle cell trait, as was seen in her brother (II 1). However, agar gel electrophoresis showed only an Hb A band that actually contains both Hb A and Hb D. The child is thus heterozygous for Hb D.

There are several Hb D variants and all have the same electrophoretic behavior. Among these variants, only Hb D-Los Angeles causes severe sickle cell disease when it coexists with Hb S. These variants should be suspected when sickle cell trait patterns show negative solubility tests. Hb D trait is innocuous.

A VARIANT MIMICKING HEMOGLOBIN D

A black couple was planning a family and sought genetic counseling for hemoglobinopathies. After performing both cellulose acetate electrophoresis and citrate agar gel electrophoresis, the mother was diagnosed with sickle cell trait and the father was diagnosed with Hb D-Los Angeles trait. The pedigree is shown in Figure 161-4, and the electrophoretic results are included in Figure 161-2. The couple was told that there was a 25% chance with each pregnancy that the child would have Hb S/D-Los Angeles disease (see previous box).

After lengthy and emotional discussions, the couple decided that the risk was worth taking. When the first child was born, the electrophoretic pattern on cellulose acetate at alkaline pH was confusing, because Hb A was present with multiple variant bands, and was not consistent with any of the outcomes discussed by the genetic counselor. When specimens of the child's blood and the father's blood were sent to a reference laboratory, the child was shown to have Hb S trait with Hb G-Philadelphia trait, and the father was shown to be a simple heterozygote for Hb G-Philadelphia. Hb G-Philadelphia is an α-globin chain variant that is relatively common in black Americans. Because it is an α-globin chain variant, it affects the electrophoretic mobility of Hb A_2 and Hb F as well as Hb A. Thus, it should have been picked up in the father because of the minor variant Hb A_2 band cathodic to normal Hb A_2 (Fig. 161-2, AG). In some instances, the variant Hb A_2 band is obscured by one of the carbonic anhydrase bands and is missed. In these cases, a heme-specific stain will readily demonstrate the presence of this abnormal band. In addition, Hb G-Philadelphia usually comprises about 20% of the total hemolysate, while Hb D-Los Angeles usually comprises about 40%. The quantitative differences between the two hemoglobins, however, is not always reliable, as the percentage of Hb D-Los Angeles may be reduced in the presence of α-thalassemia. Conversely, Hb G-Philadelphia is usually linked to a deletion of the other α-globin gene in cis, and when in trans to a chromosome that also has an α-globin gene deleted can comprise ≤45% of the total hemolysate. The multiple bands in the newborn are explained in Figure 161-2 (FAS/G).

The distinction between Hb G-Philadelphia and Hb D-Los Angeles is not a trivial one. Unlike Hb D-Los Angeles, Hb G-Philadelphia does not participate in the polymerization of Hb S. Thus, the newborn in this case would not have any clinical manifestations associated with her variant hemoglobins, and it would be impossible for these parents to have a child with a clinically significant hemoglobinopathy. With proper interpretation of the electrophoretic patterns, the parents in this case would not have been subjected to unnecessary concern and anguish.

Although there are >800 known mutants of hemoglobin, the bulk of abnormal electrophoresis results will arise from a handful of variants like Hbs S, C, D, E, G-Philadelphia, and Lepore. This reflects that sickling syndromes, thalassemias, and a few other hemoglobinopathies account for >99% of the abnormal hemoglobins encountered. Most remaining variants occur rarely and sporadically among human populations, and the bulk of them are clinically silent.[3]

Interpreting electrophoresis results is not always straightforward because several common variants have identical charge differences and co-migrate (Figs. 161-1 and 161-2). For example, on cellulose acetate electrophoresis, Hb D co-migrates with Hb S, and Hb E, C, and A_2 have identical mobilities. Hb C and A_2 are well separated, however, on citrate agar, where Hb A_2 travels with Hb A. Both Hb D and E co-migrate with Hb A on citrate agar electrophoresis. By using both techniques of separation it is possible to distinguish among these variants.

The fractional percentage of each hemoglobin is an important factor in abnormal hemoglobin identification and in the diagnosis of certain types of thalassemia. For example, Hb A_2 rarely accounts for >6% and is never >12% of the total hemo-

globin. A band in the position of Hb A_2 on cellulose acetate that comprises 25–50% of the total hemoglobin is probably Hb C or E. Hb Lepore co-migrates with Hb S on cellulose acetate but is never >10–15% of the total hemoglobin; Hb S, by contrast, is rarely <25–30% of the total hemoglobin.

For most common hemoglobinopathies, hemoglobin electrophoresis results can usually be interpreted by considering: (1) the number of abnormally migrating bands seen, and their electrophoretic mobility relative to Hb A; (2) the amount of each

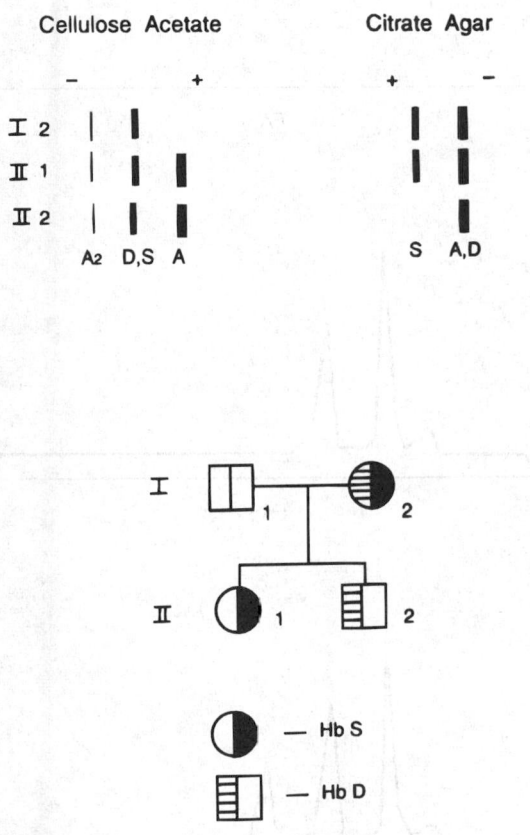

Fig. 161-3. Electrophoretic results and pedigree of a family with the β-globin variants Hb D-Los Angeles and Hb S.

hemoglobin found, expressed as percentage of the total; and (3) placing this information into the clinical context of the case by considering the patient's age, hematologic parameters, and red cell morphology.

The normal electrophoretogram of an adult will have three bands on cellulose acetate electrophoresis: Hb A $(\alpha_2\beta_2)$, constituting 95% of the total; Hb A$_2$ $(\alpha_2\delta_2)$, constituting 2–3% of the total; and Hb F $(\alpha_2\gamma_2)$, barely visible, if seen at all, and accounting for 0.5–1% of the total. These components should be employed as a frame of reference when evaluating abnormalities; one should focus not simply on the abnormal bands but also on the deviations of the overall pattern from the normal. For example, are the Hb A$_2$ and Hb F bands present at the appropriate positions but in altered amounts? Are any normal bands missing from their usual positions?

Specific globin gene mutations will have very different im-

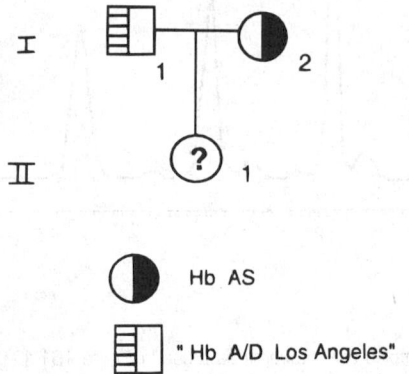

Fig. 161-4. Pedigree of a family with Hb S and Hb G-Philadelphia.

pacts on the pattern of electrophoretic variants. The hemoglobin profile of a patient represents the complex interaction of products of several globin genes: two α-loci, one β-locus, two γ-loci, and one δ-locus. The following principles should be kept in mind when reviewing electrophoresis results:

1. *Mutations affecting the β-globin locus will tend to change only one band on the electrophoretogram, and this will usually be a major band, in terms of the quantity of hemoglobin.* This is because there is only one copy of the β-globin gene per haploid cell and that β-globin is a constituent of only Hb A. Two β-globin genes are expressed in the diploid adult erythroid cell, and this accounts for ≥95% of the total non-α-globin chains. On the basis of gene dosage and this level of output, one would expect, as a first approximation, heterozygosity for a β-globin variant to yield a single new band that would account for about one-half of the total hemoglobin. As a corollary, Hb A levels are reduced by about one-half. The actual quantity of normal and abnormal hemoglobins may deviate somewhat from 50% for complex reasons.

2. *By contrast, α-globin variants should give rise to altered Hb A, A$_2$, and F bands because each of these hemoglobins contains α-globin.* There are four functioning α-globin genes in the diploid erythroid cell. Therefore, a mutation of one α-globin gene might then be expected to create variants constituting 25% of the total Hb A, 25% of the total Hb A$_2$, and 25% of the Hb F. This approximation is reasonable in practice, but is not precise, because the two α-globin alleles are not equally expressed. Moreover, the frequent occurrence of α-globin variants in areas of the world where α-thalassemia is extremely common often results in complex linkages of structural variants to thalassemic alleles, a feature that complicates predictions of the quantity of hemoglobin types based on gene dosage alone. Importantly, α-globin variants usually, but not always, amount to ≤25% of the total hemoglobin and tend to give rise to multiple new hemoglobin bands.

3. *γ-Globin variants will alter a single major hemoglobin band during fetal and neonatal life but, after the first year of life, will alter only the faint Hb F band and are rarely detected.*

4. *Mutants of the δ-globin gene will alter only the Hb A$_2$ band and are never clinically significant.* However, an elevation of the amounts of normal Hb A$_2$ indicates the probable presence of β-thalassemia trait.

The actual amounts of different hemoglobin types that accumulate in vivo depend on the output from individual globin genes, on the stability of the globin and hemoglobin products, and on the post-translational assembly of αβ dimers. From a practical point of view, this is most relevant to sickle cell disease.

The more positively charged the β-variant, the lower its affinity for α-chains. This usually has little impact on the steady-state accumulation of hemoglobin tetramers because a slight excess of α-chains is always available to bind non-α-chains. However, mild forms of α-thalassemia are extraordinarily common in the same populations in which sickle cell anemia and other β-chain variants are often found. Thus, individuals heterozygous for β-chain variants who also carry α-thalassemia genes exhibit altered ratios of the individual hemoglobin components. The positively charged β^S-globin chain binds α-chain less well than does β^A-chain. Since α-thalassemia limits the number of α-chains available to bind the β^A- and β^S-chains, normal β^A- and abnormal β^S-chains compete for the limited α-globin pool. More Hb A than Hb S forms because of the higher affinity of β^A-chain for α-chain. Therefore, a typical Hb A/Hb S ratio in individuals with sickle cell trait and α-thalassemia is 70:30 compared with 60:40 in uncomplicated sickle cell trait.[21] By contrast, Hb S is slightly *less* positively charged than Hb C. In patients inheriting both β^S- and β^C-genes (Hb SC disease),

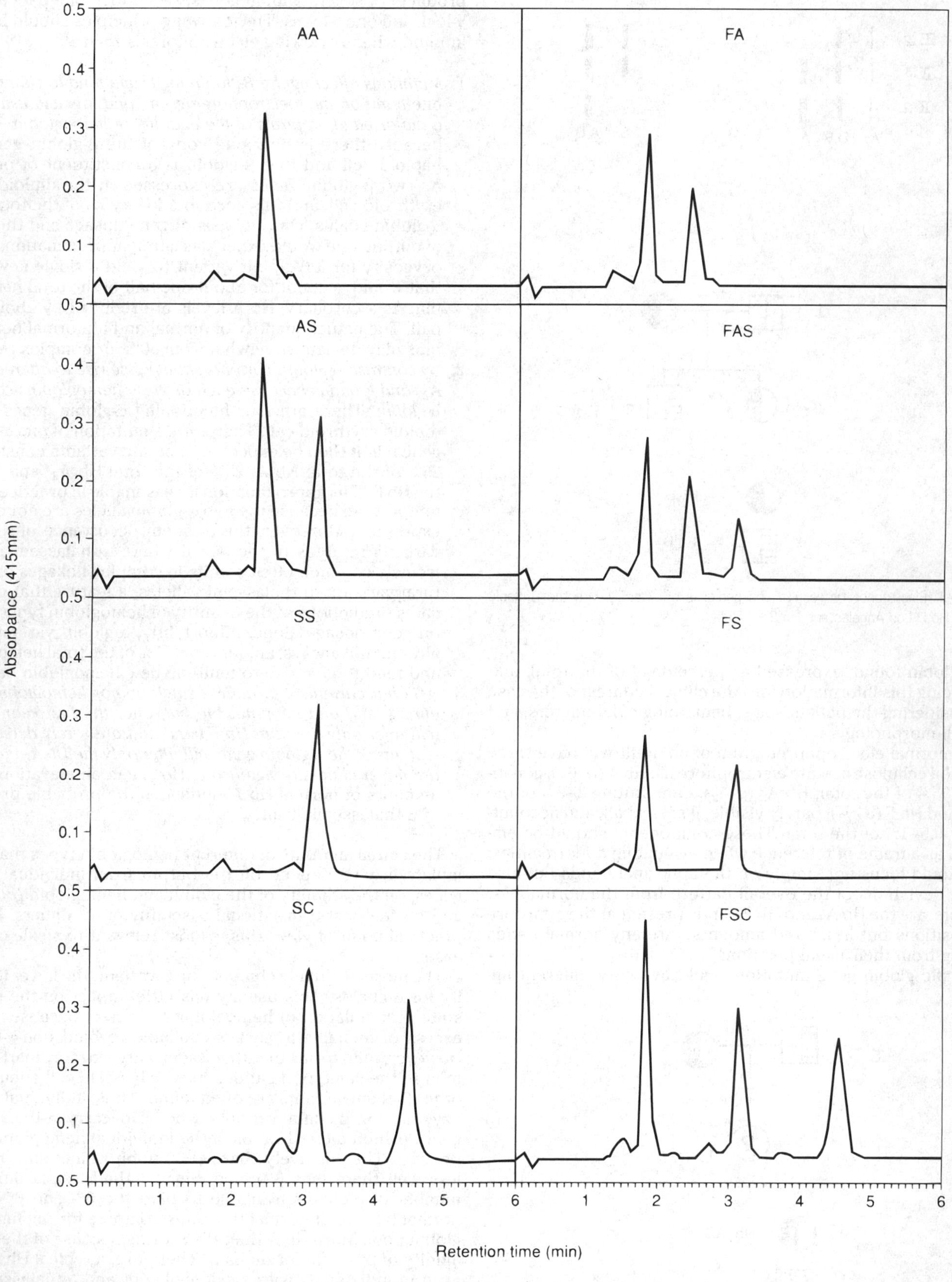

Fig. 161-5. HPLC on a CS-300 cation exchange column (Brownlee Labs). The samples are the same as those in Figure 161-1.

he Hb S/Hb C ratio is approximately 55:45, reflecting a very lose degree of charge distribution.

Heterozygosity for both Hb S and β^+-thalassemia causes igher amounts of Hb S than Hb A because the output of the -thalassemia locus is usually reduced to <30% of normal. Typ-:al Hb S/Hb A ratios in Hb S-β^+-thalassemia are 70:30–90:10.[22]

Hb E is a very common variant in southeast Asians and is aefficiently expressed (see Ch. 42). It rarely constitutes -25–30% of the total hemoglobin. Since it is highly positively harged, its percentage drops dramatically to 10–15% in pa-ients who also inherit α-thalassemia. Hb C and Hb O, by con-rast, usually accumulate in amounts close to those of Hb A. individuals with Hb E will have a thalassemic phenotype (mi-rocytosis) and a lower percentage of the abnormal hemoglo-oin, which provides strong evidence for the diagnosis.

Hb Lepore is moderately common among southern Europe-ans. As noted in Chapter 42, Hb Lepore arises from fusion of he δ- and β-genes, eliminating the normal β- and δ-globin loci rom that chromosome and replacing them with a poorly ex-oressed thalassemic $\delta\beta$ gene. Therefore, heterozygous Hb Lep-ore should be suspected if the electrophoresis shows a hemo-globin band that migrates like Hb S but comprises only 5–10% of the hemolysate. Homozygotes for Hb Lepore have no Hb A. The cells of these patients should also be profoundly mi-crocytic, like those of patients with classic forms of β-thalas-semia.

By employing the above-stated principles, interpretation of the most common types of hemoglobinopathies should be pos-sible. To recapitulate: α-globin variants affect multiple bands and are usually <25% of total hemoglobin in heterozygotes; β-globin variants affect one band and form about 50% of total hemoglobin; γ- and δ-globin variants affect only the minor Hb F and A_2 bands in adult life; the fractional percent of the variant can be as informative as its point of migration in the electropho-resis system.

ADDITIONAL METHODS FOR CHARACTERIZING HEMOGLOBINS

Sickle Solubility Test

Sickle hemoglobin has unique properties that allow its chem-ical detection. It is insoluble and precipitates in high-molarity phosphate buffer at neutral pH when reduced with sodium di-thionite. This observation forms the basis for the sickle solubil-ity tests.[23–25] A reliable solubility test should be an adjunct to the electrophoretic identification of Hb S in adults, since it is quite specific for this hemoglobin and will help distinguish it from other variants that may electrophoretically mimic Hb S. The sickle solubility test has no role as a primary screening test or as the sole means of detecting Hb S. It identifies only the presence of Hb S and not its quantity and so cannot distinguish among sickle cell trait, sickle cell anemia, and Hb S-β-thalas-semia, nor can it detect other nonsickling variants. The solubil-ity test is not applicable in neonates who have a large amount of Hb F. This test is useful in identification of the rare variants with two amino acid substitutions, one of which is the sickle mutation (Hb C-Harlem, C-Ziguinchor, S-Antilles, S-Travis, S-Providence, and S-Oman). Solubility tests sometimes give false-positive results, but with reliable reagents this problem is very rare.

Globin Chain Electrophoresis

The hemoglobin tetramer is readily separated from its heme groups and dissociated into its component globin chains by treatment with urea and 2-mercaptoethanol. The globin sub-

units can then be separated according to their relative charges by cellulose acetate electrophoresis, which is usually carried out under alkaline (pH 8.9) and acid (pH 6.0) conditions.[26–28] By measuring the relative mobilities of the hemoglobins on cellulose acetate and agar gels and of the globin chains at alka-line and acid pH, many hemoglobin variants may be identified without the necessity for further structural analysis.[28,29] These methods are technically demanding and require special inter-pretation. They are thus rarely available in the clinical labora-tory.

Quantitation of Hemoglobin and Globin Chain Fractions

Measuring the fractional percentages of the hemoglobin components that are separated by cellulose acetate electro-phoresis is useful. For example, quantitation of Hb S and Hb A levels helps to distinguish Hb S-β^+-thalassemia from sickle cell trait; the proportion of Hb S in sickle cell trait is often reduced in the presence of α-thalassemia; the quantitation of Hb A_2 in adults is important because it is so often elevated in β-thalas-semia carriers.[21,30]

A number of reliable procedures for hemoglobin quantitation are available. These include elution from cellulose acetate strips and spectrophotometric analysis of the eluted fraction, densitometry of stained and cleared cellulose acetate strips, chromatography on "minicolumns," and HPLC.[5,31] The elution method is highly reliable for measuring Hb A_2 and variant he-moglobin levels in adults. Because Hb F migrates between Hb A and Hb S, this method is not used for newborn samples. Densitometry is unreliable for measuring Hb A_2 and Hb F.[32,33] The "minicolumn" method is reliable but has been largely sup-planted by HPLC, which is probably the method of choice for quantitation of the major hemoglobins in the newborn.[18]

The quantitation of Hb F is extremely important in the diag-nosis of the thalassemias, sickle cell disease, the Hb E syn-dromes, and the hereditary persistence of Hb F syndromes in adults. Most human hemoglobins rapidly denature at alkaline pH and can then be precipitated with ammonium sulfate. Hb F, however, is not denatured and remains soluble under these conditions. The alkali resistance of Hb F provides a rapid and reasonably simple technique for quantifying Hb F in human blood samples.[34–38] Fetal hemoglobin can also be quantified by HPLC and radial immunodiffusion.[37,38] The analysis of the distribution of Hb F in the red cells is useful in distinguishing among various forms of $\delta\beta$-thalassemia and hereditary persis-tence of Hb F (HPFH). The $^A\gamma$- and $^G\gamma$-globin chains of Hb F can be separated and quantified either by HPLC or by Triton-acid-urea gel electrophoresis; the procedure is useful in differentiat-ing some of the forms of HPFH.[39,40] Hb F-specific antibodies can measure the number of "F cells" as well as the amount of Hb F/F cell[41] (see Ch. 42).

Hemoglobin Functional Studies

Some variant hemoglobins are characterized by abnormal functional properties. Variants with abnormal oxygen affinity may be recognized by abnormal oxygen dissociation curves or determination of the P_{50}. Several automatic methods of obtain-ing oxyhemoglobin dissociation curves have been de-scribed.[42–44] Most unstable hemoglobins have been found to precipitate more readily than Hb A when exposed to heat (50°C) or when incubated at 37°C in a buffer containing isopro-pyl alcohol.[45,46] The Hb M variants can be identified by their spectral changes.[47]

PRIMARY EVALUATION OF HEMOGLOBINOPATHIES

Initial Laboratory Determinations
    Measurement of hemoglobin concentration
    Measurement of mean corpuscular volume and RDW
    Hemoglobin separation by cellulose acetate electrophoresis (pH 8.6), IEF, or HPLC
Procedure and Evaluation
    Hemoglobin concentration measurement
        If a normal value is obtained, proceed with other studies as clinically indicated
        If a decreased value is obtained, complete the studies and refer the patient for hematologic evaluation
        If an abnormally high value is obtained, measure hemoglobin oxygen affinity and complete other studies as clinically indicated
    Measurement of the mean corpuscular volume
        If a normal value is obtained, proceed with the other studies
        If a decreased value is obtained, quantify Hb A_2 and Hb F and determine the iron and iron-binding capacity or serum ferritin level.
            If the findings indicate β-thalassemia, refer for appropriate family studies and counseling
            If the findings indicate iron deficiency, refer for medical evaluation and treatment
            If normal values are obtained, refer the patient for family studies and for specialized laboratory determinations for the detection of α-thalassemia or other abnormalities and then refer the patient for counseling or treatment.
    Hemoglobin separation study
        If a normal pattern is seen and the other determinations are normal, notify the patient that all results appear normal
        If the hemoglobin separation study shows SS, SA, SC, or CC, do confirmatory testing and then refer the patient for hematologic evaluation, family studies, counseling, and long-term care
        If an AS pattern is obtained, confirm by citrate agar gel electrophoresis (pH 6.1), and perform sickle solubility test
            If sickle cell trait is confirmed, refer patient with counseling
            If sickle cell trait is not confirmed, refer to reference laboratory to determine the hemoglobin abnormality and refer the individual for counseling
        If an AC or AE pattern is obtained, perform the sickle solubility test
            If a negative result is obtained, perform citrate agar gel electrophoresis (pH 6.1) to confirm Hb E or Hb C trait, and refer the patient for counseling
            If a positive result is obtained, refer to reference laboratory to determine the hemoglobin abnormality and refer the patient to counseling
        If another pattern is obtained, refer to reference laboratory to determine the hemoglobin abnormality and then refer the patient for counseling

(Adapted from Honig and Adams,[1] with permission.)

NEWBORN SCREENING FOR HEMOGLOBINOPATHIES

Hemoglobin separation by cellulose acetate electrophoresis (pH 8.6), IEF, HPLC
If a normal result (FA) is obtained, notify the patients that the results appear normal; if clinically or hematologically indicated, the analysis should be repeated at 6 months
If the study shows an FS or FSC pattern, confirm by citrate agar gel electrophoresis (pH 6.1) and refer the patient for hematologic evaluation, family studies, parental counseling, long-term care, and prophylactic penicillin therapy; perform confirmatory studies as outlined in the adult protocol at 6 months of age
If the study shows an FSA, FCA, FE, or FC pattern, confirm by citrate agar gel electrophoresis (pH 6.1) and refer the patient for hematologic evaluation, family studies, parental counseling, and long-term care; perform confirmatory studies as outlined in the adult protocol at 6 months of age
If the study shows an FAS, FAC, or FAE pattern, perform citrate agar gel electrophoresis (pH 6.1)
    If the results indicate sickle cell trait, Hb C trait, Hb E trait, or Hb O-Arab trait, the parents should be referred for counseling
    If the results indicate the presence of another variant, obtain another sample at 6 months of age and refer to reference laboratory
If other patterns are detected, obtain another sample at 6 months of age and refer to reference laboratory

Hemoglobin Structural Studies

In some instances a variant hemoglobin will be found that cannot be identified by any of the above techniques. In these instances detailed structural analysis of the variant may be required; it is most easily accomplished by DNA-based methods.[48,49] These methods provide the DNA sequence encoding the variant.

LABORATORY PROTOCOL

Although all the procedures discussed above are useful at times, most clinical laboratories will have access to only a limited number. To provide basic hemoglobin diagnostic studies, a typical clinical hematology facility should be able to perform the following techniques: (1) cellulose acetate electrophoresis at alkaline pH, (2) citrate agar electrophoresis at pH 6.1, (3) sickle solubility testing, (4) electronic cell counting for the determination of hematologic indices, (5) accurate determination of Hb A_2 and Hb F levels, (6) testing of blood for abnormal hemoglobin-oxygen affinity, and (7) heat or isopropyl alcohol stability of the hemolysate. Access to a major reference laboratory should be established. Newborn screening laboratories have successfully used cellulose acetate electrophoresis coupled with citrate agar gel electrophoresis, isoelectric focusing, or HPLC.

REFERENCES

1. Honig GR, Adams JG: Human Hemoglobin Genetics. Springer-Verlag, Vienna, 1986
2. Bunn HF, Forget BG: Hemoglobin: Molecular, Genetic, and Clinical Aspects. WB Saunders, Philadelphia, 1986

3. International Hemoglobin Information Center: IHIC variants list. Hemoglobin 176:89, 1993

4. Adams JG III, Baine R, Eckman J et al: In Steinberg MH (ed): Newborn Screening for Hemoglobinopathies: Program Development and Laboratory Methods. National Institutes of Health, Washington, DC, 1991

5. Steinberg MH, Adams JG III: Laboratory diagnosis of sickling hemoglobinopathies. South Med J 71:413, 1978

6. Lubin BH, Witkowska HE, Kleman K: Laboratory diagnosis of hemoglobinopathies. Clin Biochem 24:363, 1991

7. West MS, Wethers D, Smith J et al: Laboratory profile of sickle cell disease: a cross-sectional analysis. J Clin Epidemiol 45:893, 1992

8. Green R, Kuhl W, Jacobson R et al: Masking of macrocytosis by α-thalassemia in blacks with pernicious anemia. N Engl J Med 307:1322, 1982

9. Graham JL, Grunbaum BW: A rapid method for microelectrophoresis and quantitation of hemoglobins on cellulose acetate. Am J Clin Pathol 39:567, 1963

10. Bartlett RC: Rapid cellulose acetate electrophoresis. II. Qualitative and quantitative hemoglobin fractionation. Clin Chem 9:325, 1963

11. Briere RO, Golias T, Batsakis JG: Rapid qualitative and quantitative hemoglobin fractionation: cellulose acetate electrophoresis. Am J Clin Pathol 14:695, 1965

12. Schmidt RM, Holland S: Standardization in abnormal hemoglobin detection. An evaluation of hemoglobin electrophoresis kits. Clin Chem 20:501, 1964

13. Robinson AR, Robson M, Harrison AP et al: A new technique for differentiation of hemoglobin. J Lab Clin Med 50:745, 1957

14. Marder VJ, Conley CL: Electrophoresis of hemoglobins on agar gels: frequency of hemoglobin D in a Negro population. Johns Hopkins Med J 105: 77, 1959

15. Winter WP, Yodh J: Interaction of human hemoglobin and its variants with agar. Science 221:175, 1983

16. Drysdale JW, Rhigetti P, Bunn HF: The separation of human and animal hemoglobins by isoelectric focusing in polyacrylamide gel. Biochim Biophys Acta 229:42, 1971

17. Basset P, Beuzard Y, Garel MC et al: Isoelectric focusing of human hemoglobin: its application to screening, to the characterization of 70 variants, and to the study of modified fractions of normal hemoglobins. Blood 51:971, 1978

18. Galacteros F, Kleman K, Caburi-Martin J et al: Cord blood screening for hemoglobinopathies by thin layer isoelectric focusing. Blood 56:1068, 1980

19. Wilson JB, Headlee ME, Huisman THJ: A new high performance liquid chromatographic procedure for the separation and quantiation of various hemoglobins in adults and newborn babies. J Lab Clin Med 10:174, 1983

20. Kutlar F, Kutlar A, Nuguid E et al: Usefulness of HPLC methodology for the characterization of combinations of the common β chain variants Hbs S, C, and O-Arab, and the α chain variant Hb G-Philadelphia. Hemoglobin 17:55, 1993

21. Steinberg MH: The interactions of α-thalassemia with hemoglobinopathies. Hematol Oncol Clin North Am 5:453, 1991

22. Divoky V, Baysal E, Schiliro G et al: A mild type of Hb S-β⁺-thalassemia [-92(C → T)] in a Sicilian family. Am J Hematol 42:225, 1993

23. Schmidt RM, Wilson SM: Standardization in detection of abnormal hemoglobins. I. Solubility tests for hemoglobin S. JAMA 225:1225, 1973

24. Itano HA: Solubilities of naturally occurring mixtures of human hemoglobin. Arch Biochem Biophys 47:148, 1953

25. Greenberg MS, Harvey HA, Morgan C: A simple and inexpensive screening test for sickle hemoglobin. N Engl J Med 286:1143, 1972

26. Ueda S, Schneider RG: Rapid identification of polypeptide chains of hemoglobin by cellulose acetate electrophoresis of hemolysates. Blood 34:230, 1969

27. Schneider RG: Differentiation of electrophoretically similar hemoglobins—such as S, D, G, and P; or A₂, C, E, and O—by electrophoresis of the globin chains. Clin Chem 20:1111, 1974

28. Schneider RG, Barwick RC: Measuring relative electrophoretic mobilities of mutant hemoglobins and globin chains. Hemoglobin 2:417, 1978

29. Schneider RG, Hightower B, Hosty TS et al: Abnormal hemoglobins in a quarter million people. Blood 48:629, 1976

30. Steinberg MH, Adams JG III: Hemoglobin HbA₂: origin, evolution, and aftermath. Blood 78:2165, 1991

31. Huisman THJ, Schroeder WA, Brodie AN et al: Microchromatography of hemoglobins. III. A simplified method for the determination of hemoglobin A₂. J Lab Clin Med 86:700, 1975

32. Schmidt RM, Rucknagel DL. Necheles TF: Comparison of methodologies for thalassmia screening by Hb A₂ quantitation. J Lab Clin Med 86:700, 1975

33. Schmidt RM, Brosious EM, Holland S: Quantitation of fetal hemoglobin by densitometry. J Lab Clin Med 84:740, 1975

34. Singer K, Chernoff AI, Singer L: Studies of abnormal hemoglobins. I. Their demonstration in sickle cell anemia and other hematologic disorders by means of alkali denaturation. Blood 6:413, 1951

35. Betke K, Marti HR, Schlicht I: Estimation of small percentages of foetal haemoglobin. Nature 184:1877, 1959

36. Pembrey ME, McWade P, Weatherall DJ: Reliable routine measurement of small amounts of foetal haemoglobin by alkali denaturation. J Clin Pathol 25: 738, 1972

37. Shelton JB, Shelton JR, Schroeder WA: Separation of globin chains on a large pore C4 column. J Liquid Chromatogr 1:1969, 1984

38. Chudwin DS, Rucknagel DL: Immunological quantification of hemoglobins F and A₂. Clin Chim Acta 50:413, 1974

39. Rovera G, Magarian C, Borun TW: Resolution of hemoglobin subunits by electrophoresis in acid urea polyacrylamide gels containing Triton X-100. Anal Biochem 85:506, 1978

40. Alter BP, Goff SC, Efremov G et al: Globin chain electrophoresis: a new approach to the determination of the ᴳγ/ᴬγ ratio in fetal hemoglobin and to studies of globin synthesis. Br J Haematol 44:527, 1980

41. Dover GJ, Boyer SH: Quantitation of hemoglobins within individual red cells: asynchronous biosynthesis of fetal and adult hemoglobin during erythroid maturation in normal subjects. Blood 56:1082, 1980

42. Duvellroy MA, Buckles RG, Rosenkeimer S et al: An oxygen dissociation analyzer. J Appl Physiol 28:229, 1970

43. Rossi-Benardi L, Lazzana M, Samaja M et al: Continuous determination of the oxygen dissociation curve for whole blood. Clin Chem 21:1747, 1975

44. Imai K, Yoshioka Y, Tyuma I et al: Studies on the function of abnormal hemoglobin. I. An improved method for automatic measurement of the oxygen equilibrium curve of hemoglobin. Biochim Biophys Acta 200:189, 1970

45. Dacie JV, Grimes AJ, Meisler A et al: Hereditary Heinz body anaemia. Br J Haematol 10:388, 1964

46. Carrell RW, Kay R: A simple method for the detection of unstable haemoglobins. Br J Haematol 23:615, 1972

47. Tonz O: The Congenital Methemoglobinemias. Karger. Basel, 1968

48. Jones RT: Recent developments in structural analysis. Tex Rep Biol Med 40: 157, 1981

49. Kazazian HH Jr, Boehm CD: Molecular basis and prenatal diagnosis of β-thalassemia. Blood 72:1107, 1988

Antenatal Diagnosis of Hematologic Disorders

162

Kim Kramer and Harvey J. Cohen

INTRODUCTION

The past three decades have taken the concept of antenatal diagnosis from a blind needle uterine insertion for acquisition of amniotic cells to a refined real-time ultrasound-guided transcervical swab for villous sampling. Once able to perform only karyotyping within ≥4 weeks, recent advances have resulted in the ability to detect single gene defects within 24 hours. What once necessitated 50 ml of amniotic fluid in the 20th week of gestation now routinely requires as little as 20 mg from chorionic villus sampling, at as early as 6 weeks of gestation.[1] Indeed, in the 1990s the ability exists to detect DNA base pair alterations in one blastomere from an extracorporeal embryo.

With this explosive surge in methods to detect molecular defects earlier, more quickly, and more effectively, comes the desire to make possible earlier, safer, and more effective interventional and therapeutic techniques. The practice of antenatal diagnosis once served for elective termination of those fetuses affected by a known genetic disorder, it is now possible to provide in utero treatments that conceivably could alter the natural history of many genetic disorders. This concept holds particular relevance for the hematologist, who is involved with an entire array of clinical conditions that can be detected and treated in the antenatal period.

METHODS OF ANTENATAL DIAGNOSIS

Amniocentesis

The concept of obtaining amniotic fluid cells shed from fetal skin, lung, and gastrointestinal tract for diagnostic purpose had its origin in 1930 in the setting of amniography.[2] This procedure involved the transabdominal, intrauterine injection of strontium iodide, frequent withdrawals of amniotic fluid to dilute the solution, and the subsequent imaging of abdominal plain films by conventional radiography. Visualization of fetal soft spots and localization of the placenta was thereby possible. It was not until the 1950s, however, that amniocentesis was introduced as a method of diagnosing and managing erythroblastosis fetalis.[3–5] By knowing the normal chemical composition of amniotic fluid, an assessment of by-products of heme metabolism led to the diagnosis of Rh immunization.[4] In the same decade, Fuchs and Riis[6,7] used desquamated fetal cells in the amniotic fluid for sex chromatin analysis. The field of fetal cytogenetic studies further advanced when Steele and Breg[8] cultured amniotic fluid cells in sufficient quantity to be karyotyped. Although early attempts at culture were difficult, and were associated with poor culture survival and low viability, this led to the first diagnosis of Down syndrome in utero by Valenti in 1968.[9] In the same year, Nadler[10] reported the first antenatal detection of the hereditary disorders galactosemia and mucopolysaccharidosis. By 1970, an estimated 10,000 procedures had been performed in high-risk pregnancies, with a fetal morbidity and mortality of <1%.[11]

Although routine amniocentesis is performed at 16–20 weeks' gestation, the clinical and laboratory experience with procedures at 11–15 weeks has been encouraging.[12–15] In the outpatient setting, the procedure is performed after a thorough ultrasound examination of the fetus, placenta, and uterus. With a 22-gauge spinal needle, approximately 1 ml/wk of gestation is withdrawn either transabdominally or transvaginally.[12] Successful fluid acquisition approaches 99.8%, and the fluid can be used for cytogenetic and biochemical studies.[12] Recent improvements in methods to enhance cell growth can result in prenatal diagnoses as early as 5 days.[16] The procedure boasts an extremely high diagnostic reliability, with an estimate of 1 miskaryotype per 5,000 procedures and a culture failure rate <1%.[17] A procedure-related fetal loss rate is approximately 0.5%.[18] Complications are rare but may include amniotic fluid leakage, severe cramping, fetal trauma, blood-stained amniotic fluid, and infection.[19–21] Concern over the possibility of positional deformities and pulmonary hypoplasia due to removal of amniotic fluid early in gestation has been expressed, although no conclusive evidence exists for such an association.[22]

Chorionic Villus Sampling

Although fetal chorionic villi were successfully sampled using a transvaginal hysteroscope as early as 1968,[23] chromosome analysis from chorionic villus sampling (CVS) in the first trimester became possible in the early 1980s. Since that time, CVS has emerged as a means of making prenatal diagnosis earlier, more quickly, and as reliably as amniocentesis. The number of CVS procedures performed thus far is >80,000 worldwide.[24] The test is commonly performed under ultrasound guidance between 9 and 12 weeks' gestation; it involves the aspiration of 20–30 mg of villi from the placenta via a transabdominal, or more conventionally, transcervical approach.[25] Analysis of maternal outcomes in women randomly assigned to undergo either transabdominal or transcervical villus sampling indicates the same yield of tissue suitable for diagnosis and no difference in risk.[25,26] A shift towards transabdominal CVS occurs with increasing gestational age as the placenta becomes more bulky and moves away from the cervix.[27] Both a "direct" method of analyzing metaphases present in the villi to yield a rapid karyotype analysis, and a conventional culture of slowly dividing cells from the mesenchymal cores, are performed. CVS provides large amounts of metabolically active material and DNA for enzyme and gene probe diagnosis of genetic defects.[28,29] Whereas standard blot techniques require ≤1 week to detect a specific molecular mutation, application of the polymerase chain reaction (PCR) has shortened the time to a few hours (see Ch. 164). Early concerns over both the safety and accuracy of CVS led to randomized trials between first-trimester CVS and second-trimester amniocentesis.[25,30–32] It is generally held that CVS permits earlier detection of a genetic defect. This must be weighed against a slightly poorer performance with respect to fetal loss rate and diagnostic accuracy.[25,30–34] Few other potential and avoidable complications appear to exist with CVS. Maternal contamination is a potential pitfall that can be avoided with experience in the dissection and preparation of the samples for assay.[33] Likewise, fetal hemor-

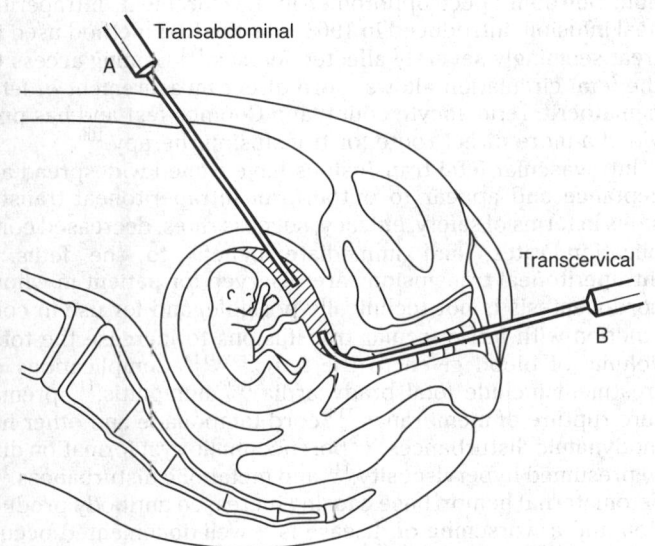

Fig. 162-1. Chorionic villus sampling depicting the transabdominal (A) and transcervical approach (B).

rhagic lesions after CVS can occur, likely secondary to inexperience and overtraumatization of the placental bed.[34,35] The controversial link between CVS and limb and oromandibular malformations continues to exist.[36-41] This seemingly rare but apparent causal association is greatest in CVS obtained <9 weeks' gestation.[29] Appropriate timing of the procedure can avoid this potential complication. CVS is likely to remain the optimum procedure used to diagnose 100 fetal metabolic disorders, and >260 single gene defect disorders currently assessed (Fig. 162-1).

Fetal Blood Sampling

Whereas amniocentesis and CVS both allow rapid early cytogenetic diagnosis of fetal disorders, direct access to the fetal circulation has become indispensable for both diagnosis and treatment of many fetal disorders. In utero blood sampling via fetoscopy was first introduced in 1973; a fiberoptic endoscope is passed transabdominally into the amniotic cavity.[42] Fetal blood may then be sampled by passage of a needle through the fetoscope into the umbilical vessels. Although it is a reliable method of obtaining pure fetal blood, procedure-related fetal deaths approach 2–5%.[43] Placental aspiration is another method for accessing fetal blood, but the technique is associated with a high rate of contamination of maternal blood or amniotic fluid, or both, making it unreliable for determining most hematologic disorders.[44,45] As of 1983, percutaneous umbilical blood sampling, also called cordocentesis, has become the safest and most reliable means of accessing the fetal circulation.[46] It is much less invasive than fetoscopy. It is generally performed from 15 weeks' gestation until the last trimester of pregnancy but has been used to make prenatal diagnoses as early as 12 weeks' gestation.[47] Under direct high-resolution ultrasound guidance, a spinal needle is inserted transabdominally through the uterus and into the umbilical vessel. Approximately 1–3 ml of blood are aspirated, and the purity of the sample is assessed to exclude maternal blood/amniotic fluid contamination.[44] Difficulty in obtaining the sample occurs if fetal movements are frequent and strong enough to dislodge the needle, if the placenta is placed posteriorly, if the umbilical cord is small or if oligohydramnios and maternal obesity are present; both of the latter result in poor ultrasound visualization.[48] Serious complications are unusual, with clinically insig-

nificant bleeding from the umbilical puncture site being the most common. Fetal bradycardia, which occurs in about 10% of procedures, is generally transient.[49] Other complications such as irregular uterine contractions, chorioamnionitis, cord hematoma, and premature rupture of membranes are rare.[44] The procedure-related fetal loss rate is approximately 1%.[49,50]

When cordocentesis is technically impossible, hepatic vein sampling and cardiac puncture have been used for fetal blood sampling.[51] With cardiocentesis, the rate of transient bradycardia (9%) compares with that found in cardiocentesis, but hemopericardium is a serious complication, leading to a fetal loss rate ≤6.5%.[51]

Cordocentesis remains the most desirable way of accessing the fetal circulation. In addition to its role in the diagnosis and management of hematologic conditions, it has been used for rapid karyotyping,[44,49,52,53] diagnosing congenital infections such as rubella and toxoplasmosis,[44,49,54-56] assessing fetal blood pH and acid-base status,[44,57] assessment of intrauterine growth retardation,[44,57-59] and fetal pharmacologic therapy.

RED BLOOD CELL DISORDERS

Hemoglobinopathies

The hemoglobinopathies are the most commonly inherited recessive diseases in humans, with an estimated 240 million heterozygotes worldwide and 200,000 homozygotes or compound heterozygotes born each year.[60] The global nature of these conditions, coupled with the desire for their prevention and prediction, has propelled research into the molecular biology of the hemoglobinopathies. Application to antenatal assessment has progressed at a comparable rate, leading to the International Registry for Prenatal Monitoring of Hereditary Anemias, a documentation of the thousands of patients examined to date.[61] The combination of heterozygote screening, counseling, and prenatal testing has dramatically reduced the number of affected infants born in many countries throughout the world.[60,62-65]

Sickle Cell Anemia

An 8% incidence of the homozygous sickle cell trait is found in American blacks,[66] for a prevalence of 1 in 573 newborns.[67] Approximately 60,000 persons are affected by the disease in the United States.[68] Hollenberg et al.[69] first predicted that the detection of sickle cell hemoglobin in utero could identify affected fetuses. In 1972, Kan and associates[68] detected sickle cell trait in a 15-week-old fetus by incubating umbilical cord blood with radioactive leucine followed by separation of the globin chains using carboxymethyl cellulose chromatography (CMC). Other methods for globin chain analysis have been devised, including electrophoresis on polyacrylamide gels containing urea, acetic acid, and Triton X-100,[70] as well as hemoglobin immunofluorescence.[71] High-pressure liquid chromatography (HPLC) by ion exchange has recently been shown to correlate highly with CMC and can separate globin chains to provide an answer within 15 minutes.[72] Isoelectric focusing is an alternative method for analysis of hemoglobin tetramers, instead of globin chain synthesis, in pure fetal blood samples.[73,74] Maternal blood contamination is a potential source of error in any of the above methods, skewing globin chain percentages.[75]

Southern blot analysis was first used in the antenatal diagnosis of sickle cell disease at the DNA level. As polymorphism of the DNA sequence adjacent to the β-globin gene was established, the normal Hb A fragment was differentiated from the

Hb S allele of a different length.[76] Several altered restriction endonuclease sites have been found using the enzymes *Hpa*I, *Dde*I, *Mst*II, *Cvn*I, and *Oxa*NI.[77–82] PCR techniques allow for restriction digestion and direct visualization of DNA fragments more rapidly and without the need for radioisotopes.[83–85] Direct assays that detect the Hb S mutation in enzymatically amplified fetal DNA are possible with allele-specific oligonucleotide probes.[86,87] Using allele-specific oligonucleotide primers conjugated to fluorescein, the sickle cell base alteration may also be detected by the color complementation methods described by Chehab and Kan.[88,89]

Thalassemias

In contrast to the structural variant of Hb S, the thalassemias are characterized by decreased production of α- or β-globin chain synthesis. Screening programs and elective reproduction cessation were the initial methods of preventing the birth of an affected child. More precise methods were devised with the use of second-trimester fetal blood sampling and evaluation of globin chain synthesis. Since a rise in the β/γ ratio occurs normally throughout gestation, CMC was used to calculate the β/γ synthetic ratio.[90] A quantitative decrease in β-chain production was highly suggestive of the homozygous state.[90] Diagnostic errors were known to occur in those patients with high β-producing B⁺-thalassemia major and low β-producing B-thalassemia.[61,90] CMC was gradually replaced by HPLC,[91] isoelectric focusing,[92,93] and electrophoresis on polyacrylamide gels or cellulose acetate membranes.[94] Other mutant β-globin chain variants such as Hb E, Hb Lepore, Hb C, and Hb O-Arab are also detectable by CMC using fetal blood.[61]

As the molecular defects in the β-globin gene producing β-thalassemia were characterized, the use of restriction enzymes, gene mapping, and oligonucleotide probes specific for point mutations of interest has become more common in antenatal diagnosis.[60,95–98] PCR has also been used in the β-globin gene using oligonucleotide restriction and dot blot analysis.[98–101]

Detecting α-thalassemia by testing for the gene deletion causing decreased α-chain production was made possible in 1976 by Kan and associates.[102] A quantitated reduced amount of fibroblast DNA hybridization could indicate α-thalassemia trait, Hb H disease, or α-thalassemia fetal hydrops syndrome.[102,103] Such hybridization techniques can be used to detect Hb Lepore and other rare forms of β-thalassemia caused by gene deletions.[95,104–105] Lack of amplified globin gene DNA is a more recent test for thalassemia.[106]

Although rarer alleles are expected to be identified in the future, it is estimated that the 54 known alleles account for 99% of β-thalassemia gene defects in the world.[96] The combination of PCR and specific restriction enzymes or probes is the most commonly used method of antenatal assessment today and continues to revolutionize programs aimed at disease prevention.

Rh Disease

In the 1950s, severe hemolytic disease due to red blood cell alloimmunization accounted for >1,000 deaths/yr.[107] Since the introduction of anti-D immunoglobulin prophylaxis in the 1970s, a dramatic decrease to 34 deaths/yr has occurred.[108] Nevertheless, maternal Rh sensitization and fetal hemolytic disease due to other blood group antibodies remain significant problems that may lead to anasarca, fetal cardiac failure, and death.[109] Diagnostic and therapeutic advances were made in the late 1950s by Liley[110] and associates whereby an indirect index of fetal red cell destruction was estimated by amniotic

fluid bilirubin spectrophotometric measurement. Intraperitoneal infusion, introduced in 1963, was the first method used to treat seemingly severely affected fetuses.[111] Gaining access to the fetal circulation allows more direct measurement of fetal hematocrit, reticulocyte count, and Coombs test and has provided a more direct route for transfusion therapy.[109]

Intravascular fetal transfusions have gained widespread acceptance and appear to outperform intraperitoneal transfusions in terms of safety, efficacy, success rates, decreased complication rates, and immediate benefit to the fetus.[112] Intraperitoneal transfusions are reserved for patient in whom cordocentesis is not technically possible, and for use in conjunction with intravascular transfusions to increase the total volume of blood given to the fetus.[112–114] Complications of treatment include fetal bradycardia,[109] amnionitis,[114] premature rupture of membranes,[114] cord tamponade and other hemodynamic disturbances,[115] porencephalic cyst formation due to presumed hyperviscosity,[116] and metabolic disturbances.[117] Fetomaternal hemorrhage causing increased antibody production and a worsening of disease is a well-documented occurrence.[118,119] Despite the known risk, many centers quote a 90% survival rate for early severe hydrops, a once devastating prenatal disorder.[114]

Nonimmune hydrops fetalis may occur in a number of conditions, among which is the fetal aplastic anemia associated with parvovirus B19 infection. The gestational age with the greatest risk for fetal hydrops appears to be the second trimester.[120] Parvovirus B19 DNA has been obtained from fetal blood using PCR and parvovirus B19-specific primers; along with fetal ultrasound, the DNA has been used to diagnose fetuses at risk of severe disease because of maternal exposure to parvovirus B19. Reversal of parvovirus B19 hydrops has occurred with antenatal transfusion therapy.[121,122]

Enzymopathies

Inherited red blood cell enzyme defects may result in clinically undetectable altered red cell survival or function, intermittent hemolytic crises, or a state of chronic hemolytic anemia. The most common enzyme defects include glucose-6-phosphate dehydrogenase and pyruvate kinase deficiency. The diagnosis rests on demonstrating decreased activity of the enzyme in red blood cells. Lestas et al.[123,124] characterized the normal enzymatic activities of >12 glycolytic enzymes in fetal erythrocytes at 17–24 weeks of gestation and proposed that these reference values be used to assess those at risk of congenital deficiencies. Two other disorders in the heme synthetic pathway, acute intermittent porphyria and protoporphyria, can also be detected by assays of uroporphyrinogen I synthetase and heme synthetase, respectively.[125,126] Analysis at the molecular level would serve as a more reliable means in the antenatal diagnosis of these disorders.

Other Congenital Anemias

Two other rare fetal congenital anemias may be diagnosed in utero, Fanconi anemia and Diamond-Blackfan anemia.[127] Fetal blood counts and the number of circulating erythroid progenitor cells can be compared with normal values for gestational age.[128–130] Ultrasound demonstrating abnormalities of the radii or thumbs would support these diagnoses.[127] A more definitive test for Fanconi anemia is based on demonstrating hypersensitivity of chorionic villus samplings and amniocytes to clastogen-induced chromosomal breakage.[131–133]

WHITE BLOOD CELL DISORDERS

Severe inherited immunodeficiency states encompass a wide spectrum of disorders involving absent or abhorrent components of the lymphoid or phagocytic system. Although rare, many of these disorders are life-threatening. The issue of prenatal diagnosis arises in those families with a severely affected child. A prerequisite for antenatal diagnosis includes extensive phenotyping of the abnormality affecting an index sibling.

The relatively late development of the fetal immune system largely restricts confident antenatal diagnosis using fetal blood analysis during the second trimester of pregnancy. The most primitive lymphoid stem cell arises in the fetal liver by 7 weeks' gestation and is detectable in the developing thymus by 8–9 weeks.[134,135] Phenotypically mature T cells can be detected in the fetal circulation and peripheral lymphoid tissues by 12–13 weeks.[136–138] Synthesis of IgM, IgG, and IgA has been demonstrated by B cells at this stage.[137,139] Likewise, the synthesis of fetal liver complement components C2, C3, C4, C5, and C1q inhibitor takes place in the first trimester.[135] Insufficient numbers of neutrophils in the fetal circulation before 7 weeks' gestation restrict phenotypic phagocytic disorder identification until the second trimester.[140,141] Entertaining antenatal diagnosis of the congenital white blood cell disorders at an earlier stage is only recently possible with molecular techniques and a greater understanding of the genetic defects associated with these disorders.

Chronic Granulomatous Disease

Granulocyte oxidative metabolism in chronic granulomatous disease (CGD) has been evaluated by demonstrating the inability of affected neutrophils to reduce nitroblue tetrazolium (NBT) dye to blue formazan particles as well as absent superoxide anion production.[142–145] Prenatal diagnosis of CGD was first successfully performed by Newberger et al.[146] in 1979, who adapted the NBT test for use on blood samples obtained by placental vessel puncture visualized by fetoscopy. Unsuccessful attempts were made to perform NBT reduction on cultured amniotic fluid cells.[147] No consistent differences have been observed between normal cultured amniotic cells and those from CGD patients.[148,149] Matthay et al.[150] adapted the luminol-enhanced chemiluminescence method on pure fetal blood samples to exclude the diagnosis in one fetus at risk.

Analysis at the DNA level is now possible. Using the information of closely linked flanking markers to the CGD gene, Lindof et al.[151] performed the antenatal diagnosis of X-linked CGD on cultured amniotic fluid cells. In 1990, Nakamura et al.[152] demonstrated monoclonal antibody staining against cytochrome b_{558} villous macrophages to make the diagnosis of an unaffected fetus at 8 weeks' gestation. This was confirmed by NBT positivity in cord blood granulocytes at delivery.

When the gene mutation in a family is known, direct sequence analysis of amplified DNA can demonstrate a single base pair substitution. Using PCR-amplified DNA obtained by CVS, deBoer et al.[153] demonstrated a G-A substitution, the known genetic defect in question. The diagnosis was confirmed on phagocytic cells that failed to reduce NBT obtained by cardiocentesis at week 15.

It is likely that direct mutation analysis of PCR-amplified genomic DNA from CVS will be the method of choice for antenatal diagnosis of X-linked CGD.

Chédiak-Higashi Syndrome

Antenatal assessment of Chédiak-Higashi syndrome has relied on secondary manifestations of the disorder, including the identification of characteristic abnormally large granules present in neutrophils, eosinophils, basophils, lymphocytes, and fibroblasts.[154,155] The possibility of diagnosing this syndrome by examining fetal blood was suggested[135,140,156] and later performed in the feline model by Kahraman and Prieur[141] in 1989. Identification of peroxidase-positive granules in neutrophils from midgestation fetal blood samples led to the positive phenotypic identification of affected fetuses. This method has been employed in excluding and diagnosing affected human fetuses via cordocentesis.[155,157,158] More recently, such phenotypic expression in the feline model has been tested in cultured amniotic fluid cells[159] and in human chorionic villus samplings.[155] Until the molecular defect is further characterized, antenatal diagnosis will rely on the presence or absence of large acid phosphate-positive lysosomes in chorionic villus samplings, amniotic cells, or granulocytes obtained from fetal blood samplings.

Leukocyte Adhesion Deficiency

Leukocyte adhesion deficiency is a rare autosomal recessive disease caused by deficient leukocyte adhesion, which leads to severe and often fatal infections. Five distinct mutations of the gene encoding the common β-subunit CD18 shared by three leukocyte surface glycoproteins (Integrins) have been identified and mapped to chromosome 21.[160,161] Prenatal diagnosis has been reported twice. Weisman et al.[162] used cordocentesis at 22 weeks' gestation to demonstrate normal monoclonal antibody binding to the α-chain and β-chain of the Mol (CD18) complex: the affected sibling demonstrated <10% binding. Weening et al.[163] used the same technique to demonstrate normal fetal granulocyte expression at 20 weeks. Recent identification of distinct mutations on the leukocyte adhesion molecule gene on chromosome 21 suggests the potential of utilizing PCR-amplified CVS or amniocentesis in antenatal diagnosis. Genetic heterogeneity of the common β-unit, however, currently restricts antenatal diagnosis to the measurement of CD18 expression on fetal blood leukocytes.

Severe Combined Immunodeficiency Syndromes

The severe combined immunodeficiency (SCID) syndromes include a heterogeneous group of disorders. The inherited defect is largely X-linked, although several different autosomal recessive defects produce the SCID phenotype in 20% of cases.[164] About 20% of instances are associated with ADA and purine nucleoside phosphorylose deficiencies, resulting in a virtual absence or functional deficiency of T and B cells.[165,166] The high lethality of the disorder makes prenatal diagnosis and identification of the carrier states desirable. The goal has been complicated by the unknown molecular nature of the defect in 80% of patients and a negative family history in 75%; roughly 33% of instances represent the first manifestation of a new mutation.[164,167]

Antenatal diagnosis of SCID was once limited to the small percentage of infants with associated ADA deficiency.[168] The amount of ADA measured in chorionic villous biopsies has also been reported and has resulted in the potential for antenatal diagnosis in the first trimester.[169,170] Enzyme activity is similar to that in cultured amniotic fluid cells. Variation in the amount of residual ADA activity may represent genetic heterogeneity and has been recognized as a potential pitfall of this method.[168] The direct measurement of fetal red cell ADA and dATP has also been used to perform rapid prenatal diagnosis[171] but the most promising method is a result of the isolation of the ADA gene and cloning of the cDNA.[172,173] PCR-amplified DNA may permit direct detection of a known specific mutation. The value of fetal blood sampling in the antenatal diagnosis of other forms of SCID has been recognized by many investigators.[175–178] Monoclonal antibodies and flow cytometry have been used to determine leukocyte and lymphoid cell subsets. As reference ranges for fetal leukocyte subpopulations have been established such phenotypic analysis can be used to identify a fetus at risk.[179] T- and B-cell membrane HLA-DR and β_2-microglobulin can be detected by immunofluorescence.[180] A profound lymphopenia and an absence of T- and B-cell markers in pure fetal blood confirm the diagnosis of SCID.[180,181] A similar approach has been used in the antenatal diagnosis of the bare lymphocyte syndrome, a SCID variant in which T and B cells lack expression of HLA antigens.[182,183] Demonstrating HLA antigen expression on fetal blood lymphocytes using immunofluorescent monoclonal antibodies and flow cytometry has excluded the diagnosis in one infant at risk.[183]

Wiskott-Aldrich Syndrome

The X-linked recessively inherited Wiskott-Aldrich syndrome is characterized by eczematoid dermatitis, thrombocytopenia, and reduced cellular and humeral immunity. The absence of a defined lymphocyte population, or a constant immunologic abnormality, has made antenatal diagnosis difficult. Normal mean platelet volumes and platelet counts from fetal blood samples have been used to exclude the diagnosis,[184] but these measures are known to be unreliable in those individuals whose hematologic parameters alter after birth.[185] Kenney et al.[186] found that patients with Wiskott-Aldrich syndrome had qualitatively abnormal lymphocytes with short blunted microvilli under electron microscopy and used this morphologic marker to identify an affected fetus correctly. Recent progress has been made by indirect DNA analysis as early as 9 weeks' gestation.[187] The Wiskott-Aldrich syndrome gene has recently been mapped to the proximal arm of the X chromosome between Xp11.22 and 11.3.[188,189] Five DNA flanking markers are known and can be used in informative families.[190] Carrier status is also possible based on maternal X-chromosome inactivation patterns. All nucleated lineages of maternal blood cells appear to be affected, as demonstrated by non-random X inactivation in T cells, B cells, and monocytes in obligate heterozygotes.[191–193]

X-Linked Agammaglobulinemia

X-linked agammaglobulinemia is a congenital antibody deficiency disease caused by defective B-cell differentiation. In those families seeking genetic counseling, carrier status can be identified by assessing nonrandom X-chromosome inactivation patterns in the maternal B-cell population.[194–200] Because of the variability in the number of B cells in the midtrimester fetus, prenatal diagnosis using lymphocyte subpopulations is only helpful in excluding the disease if a normal number of cells are seen.[196]

The gene has recently been mapped to the region Xq21.3-Xq22.[197] Three flanking markers surrounding the locus are known and have been used to diagnose the disorder as early as 10 weeks' gestation in chorionic villus samplings.[198] Nonallelic genetic heterogeneity may complicate the diagnosis with the use of restriction fragment length polymorphisms, (RFLPs), although a method of calculating this risk has been developed.[199,200] It is now recommended that X-inactivation patterns be used to determine carrier status, that RFLPs be used for direct DNA analysis in fetuses at risk, and that confirmational immunologic studies be performed later in gestation.

Immunodeficiency With Ataxia-Telangiectasia

Ataxia-telangiectasia (AT) is an autosomal recessive disorder characterized by progressive cerebellar ataxia, oculocutaneous telangiectasia, immunodeficiency, increased incidence of malignancy, and a two- to threefold increased sensitivity to ionizing radiation.[201] Although the molecular defect of the disorder is unknown, defective DNA replication and repair appear to exist.[202] Recent evidence suggests that AT is associated with single gene defects of at least four different AT genes, ATA, ATC, ATD, and ATE.[203] The ATA gene has been localized to chromosome 11q22-23.[203] Lack of identification of the gene(s) responsible for this heterogeneous disorder makes a combined approach to the known abnormalities (cited above) a necessity in antenatal assessment. Cultured amniotic fluid cells have been used to demonstrate spontaneous chromosome breakage,[204] and the diagnosis has been excluded by demonstrating a normal response of amniocytes to x-ray stress.[205] This method of measuring the rate of DNA replication and inhibition in cultured villus samplings following exposure to ionizing radiation has been used to exclude AT in fetuses at risk.[205,206] The presence of a clastogenic factor (a low-molecular-weight protein in the serum of affected patients) has also been noted in the amniotic fluid of an affected fetus.[205] Until a better understanding of the molecular defects exists, the ability to monitor pregnancies at risk for this disease relies on the above methods.

Congenital C3 Deficiency

Congenital absence of C3 is an extremely rare disease resulting in failure of activation of the later components of the complement cascade. The clinical syndrome resembles that of X-linked agammaglobulinemia.[207] The disorder is inherited in an autosomal recessive manner, with heterozygotes having one-half the normal C3 levels. Since no placental transfer of C3 occurs, its detection in fetal serum as early as 8 weeks can exclude the homozygous condition.[208]

PLATELET DISORDERS

The antenatal diagnosis of platelet disorders is aimed at identifying and treating those infants at risk of hemorrhagic complications. Early detection can aid in determining those fetuses who would benefit from in utero treatment, delivery by cesarean section, or treatment in the immediate neonatal period.

Alloimmune Thrombocytopenia

Neonatal alloimmune thrombocytopenia (NAIT) is a potentially severe disease caused by fetal-maternal incompatibility for platelet-specific antigens, most commonly the PlA antigen system. An estimated 1 in 2,000 to 1 in 5,000 fetuses may be affected,[210] with a mortality rate as high as 13%.[211] One-half of all cases occur in a first-born child.[212] Although the risk of intracranial hemorrhage appears to be highest during delivery, 25–50% of such hemorrhages appear to occur earlier in gestation.[213,214]

Prenatal diagnosis is generally indicated in families in which an affected infant was born, since the risk of subsequent pregnancies being affected is as high as 97%.[215] Parental platelet phenotyping is first performed to determine pregnancies at risk. PlA1-negative women who are HLA-B8, -DR3 appear to be at greatest risk of having an affected infant.[216] As maternal anti-PlA1 antibody levels have not been useful in predicting the severity of fetal thrombocytopenia,[217,218] fetal blood sampling at 20–22 weeks' gestation is the most reliable method of assessing fetal platelet phenotype and platelet count.[219] Fetuses with platelet counts severely depressed early in gestation (i.e., by 20 weeks) appear to be at greatest risk of developing intracranial hemorrhage.[220] Early therapeutic interventions with in utero transfusions of PlA1-negative platelets together with frequent ultrasound examinations have been shown to increase the fetal platelet count and decrease the complication rate.[217,221–223] Fetal scalp vein platelet count estimations have been used at the time of delivery to determine which infants should be delivered by cesarean section. This procedure, however, is associated with a high frequency of falsely low fetal platelet counts in the setting of amniotic fluid contamination and does not address the percentage of neonates at risk of intracranial hemorrhage earlier in gestation.

Advances in the diagnosis of PlA1-associated NAIT using allele-specific oligonucleotide probes have been established by McFarland et al.[224] A single nucleic acid base substitution in the gene encoding glycoprotein (GP) IIIa of the PlA1 antigen differentiates it from PlA2 and accounts for the alloantigenic polymorphism in the PlA system.[225] This DNA-based platelet phenotyping has been used on fetal leukocytes and amniocytes and may also be applicable to CVS obtained earlier in pregnancy.[224] Its greatest advantage lies in the potential for earlier diagnosis with greater accuracy; and it also eliminates the problems and risks associated with platelet serologic typing from fetal blood samples.

Autoimmune Thrombocytopenia

Autoimmune thrombocytopenia in the neonate can occur by passive placental transfer of maternal IgG, resulting in the destruction of fetal platelets. For unclear reasons, the morbidity and mortality of fetal autoimmune thrombocytopenia is much lower than that associated with alloimmune thrombocytopenia.[227] Indeed, the nadir platelet count in an affected infant often occurs after delivery.[228] Given that idiopathic thrombocytopenic purpura (ITP) is a fairly common disease, both in childhood and in women of childbearing years, it is important to determine which fetuses may be at greatest risk of severe thrombocytopenia and thus would benefit from a cesarean section with postnatal observation. Little correlation exists between maternal and fetal platelet counts.[229] The observation that maternal platelet-associated IgG levels were predictive of neonatal thrombocytopenia has not been confirmed,[228,230,231] nor has the measurement of amniotic fluid or cord blood antibody levels.[232] Likewise, the platelet count of a previous baby is not a reliable predictor.[233] Fetal thrombocytopenia does appear to be more frequent when maternal thrombocytopenia is present at the time of delivery.[234] The only reliable way to establish the presence of fetal thrombocytopenia is by fetal blood sampling. Given the low risk of antenatal fetal morbidity, the benefit of an invasive procedure like cordocentesis has not been proven. Fetal blood sampling prior to delivery has been recommended by investigators.[235] Avoidance of fetal head trauma and delivery by cesarean section is generally reserved for pregnant patients with ITP and documented fetal platelet counts <50–70,000/mm^3.[228,229] Low doses of prednisone (10–15 mg/day) for the last 2–4 weeks of pregnancy have been shown to raise fetal platelet counts.[236]

It is important to note that many pregnant women have platelet counts in the range of 80–150,000/mm^3, especially in the second half of gestation.[237,238] This "benign thrombocytopenia of pregnancy," also called pseudo-ITP, poses no maternal or fetal risk and is not associated with neonatal thrombocytopenia. In the absence of an associated bleeding tendency, no specific antenatal or perinatal precautions need be taken. At times, this incidentally detected condition may be difficult to distinguish from chronic ITP.[228]

Glanzmann Thrombasthenia

Patients with Glanzmann thrombasthenia have normal circulating number and appearance of platelets but show failure to aggregate in response to any of the normal agonists, resulting in a variable hemorrhagic tendency. Absence or deficiency of GP IIb/IIIa, the fibrinogen receptor needed for normal platelet aggregation, causes the defect.[239,240] The GPIIb/IIIa complex is immunologically detectable as early as 19 weeks of gestation, allowing for radiolabeled anti-GPIIb/IIIa antibodies to be used in the assessment of fetuses at risk.[219,241] As the risk of fetal death due to postcordocentesis hemorrhage appears to be particularly high with this disorder, it is recommended that antenatal diagnosis be limited to those parents who have decided on terminating the pregnancy if the fetus is affected.[243] This risk may be removed by diagnosing the disorder at the gene level with CVS. Such use of gene markers would be limited because the Glanzmann phenotype corresponds to different genetic mutations, all resulting in a defect in GPIIb/IIIa synthesis and assembly.[244]

Bernard-Soulier Syndrome

Bernard-Soulier syndrome is a rare autosomal recessively inherited bleeding disorder characterized by mild thrombocytopenia, giant platelets, and absent ristocetin-induced von Willebrand factor (vWF) binding. The platelet membranes of affected individuals are known to have absent or deficient GPIb/IX and GPV.[245] Antenatal diagnosis of this disorder is theoretically possible by testing fetal cord blood samples at 18–22 weeks for membrane GPIb/IX content.[246,247] Affected women who have had multiple blood and platelet transfusions have an increased risk of fetal thrombocytopenia or immune hydrops fetalis.[248]

Other Inherited Platelet Disorders

Several other inherited platelet disorders have been detected in utero. Thrombocytopenia-absent radii syndrome is initially suspected by characteristic radiographic or ultrasonographic abnormalities and may be confirmed by cordocentesis documenting thrombocytopenia.[249–254] This syndrome is differentiated from amegakaryocytic thrombocytopenia, in which neonatal thrombocytopenia is followed by pancytopenia later in childhood. The disorder has been diagnosed in utero by detecting thrombocytopenia in an infant at risk.[255] Gray platelet syndrome, a rare platelet disorder caused by a defect in platelet α-granules, has been assessed antenatally by demonstrating the presence or absence of fetal platelet α-granules by electron microscopy.[243,244] Similarly, the demonstration of a normal platelet count and volume in the absence of abnormal spindle-shaped leukocyte inclusion bodies excluded the May-Hegglin anomaly in an infant at risk.[243]

COAGULOPATHIES

Components of the fetal hemostatic system begin to appear at approximately 10–11 weeks' gestation.[257] Reference values for an estimated 25 factors in the coagulation cascade have been obtained from fetal blood samples.[255,257–260] Important insights into the genetics of inherited coagulopathies enables prenatal diagnosis to be performed earlier and more accurately.

Von Willebrand Disease

One of the most commonly inherited bleeding disorders, von Willebrand disease (vWD), is a heterogeneous autosomally inherited disease caused by a qualitative or quantitative deficiency of vWF. More than 20 distinct clinical and laboratory subtypes of vWD have been described.[261] Variability of levels in the heterozygous state makes the phenotypic diagnosis by measurement of these levels difficult. vWF behaves like an acute-phase reactant and is often markedly elevated in the neonate.[262] Prenatal exclusion of severe vWD has been reported by many investigators using assays detecting factor VIII-related antigen and activity in fetal blood samples.[255,263–265] Conversely, finding little plasma factor VIII-related antigen and activity has supported the diagnosis of an affected infant.[258]

Advances in vWD molecular biology have already led to both prenatal diagnosis and rapid neonatal diagnosis of certain subtypes.[266–269] Knowing that the vWF gene on chromosome 12 contains a variable number of tandem repeats, Peake et al.[268] used PCR to amplify DNA from CVS at 10 weeks' gestation to identify a fetus with type III disease. The diagnosis was confirmed at 18 weeks by demonstrating undetectable levels of factor VIII, vWF:Ag, and ristocetin cofactor in fetal blood. Cord blood leukocyte DNA testing of this sequence has been reported, resulting in the rapid diagnosis of types I and IIb vWD in the neonatal period.[267,269]

Hemophilia

Deficiency or abnormality of human factor VIII or IX results in the inherited bleeding disorders hemophilia A or B, respectively. With an incidence of 1 in 5,000 males, the diseases are X-linked recessive. In the era prior to antenatal diagnosis, presumed carriers of severe hemophilia were advised not to conceive children.[270] With the technology offered by amniocentesis for prenatal sex determination, others practiced the termination of all male fetuses. Recognizing that measurements of fetal clotting factors may provide a method of detecting affected fetuses,[271] fetal blood sampling at 18–20 weeks offered known hemophilia carriers the chance of giving birth to a known unaffected son.[272–276] Since factor levels may vary widely with inflammation, stress, exercise, and pregnancy, ambiguous results at a fairly late stage of pregnancy were occasionally obtained.[277] Such fetal plasma assays have been surpassed by analysis at the DNA level.[278,279] Direct DNA analysis of the factor VIII and IX genes has identified a large number of point mutations, deletions, and insertions.[280–283] RFLPs have also been widely used in DNA analysis for those fetuses at risk.[278,284–296] RFLPs within or closely linked to the factor VIII gene can establish carrier status and give a rapid prenatal diagnosis by detecting a mutant factor VIII allele. In the United States and Italy, *Stl*4, *Bcl*I, and *Xba*I markers have been the most useful in diagnosing hemophilia A; *Stl*4 is informative 90% of the time.[279] The combined use of the enzymes *Taq*I, *Xmn*I, *Msp*I, *Bam*HI, *Sst*I, *Mnl*I, *Dde*I, and *Hha*I can ensure definitive diagnosis of hemophilia B in ≤90% of people of European descent.[283] Such technology is limited when mothers are not het-

erozygous for the mutant and marker gene, and when linkage disequilibrium exists.[297]

Other Factor Deficiencies

Congenital deficiencies of prothrombin[298,299] and factors V,[300] VII,[301] X,[302,303] XI,[304] XII,[305] and XIII[306] have all been described. Familial multiple factor deficiencies have also been characterized.[307] Prenatal diagnosis by conventional specific functional and antigenic assays on fetal blood samples had been performed.[308] Awareness of the diagnosis antenatally is important in providing parents with desired information, and in reducing the potential morbidity associated with vaginal delivery, scalp electrodes, vacuum extractions, forceps, and long labors.[308] Prompt use of factor concentrate given prior to delivery may benefit infants most at risk.

Hypercoagulable States

Severe thromboembolic disease may occur as a result of moderate-to-severe deficiency of the coagulation cascade inhibitory proteins S or C, or antithrombin III. Neonatal disseminated intravascular coagulation and purpura fulminans have been documented in infants within hours to days after birth, and in homozygous or compound heterozygous infants with protein S or C deficiency.[309–311]

Since protein S and C levels in newborns are 20–40% of normal adult levels,[312] detecting levels <1% in fetal blood samples may identify infants at greatest risk of purpura fulminans. Earlier and more reliable methods are now possible with molecular techniques. The gene for protein C has been localized to chromosome 2.[313] Family diagnosis in a pedigree of protein C deficiency was recently performed using a DNA polymorphism of the gene.[314] Several RFLP sites within or near the protein C gene have been discovered, implying the potential for prenatal diagnosis and improvement in carrier detection with such technology. Two protein S genes, PSα and PSβ, have been identified and localized near the centromere of chromosome 3,[315,316] with the PSα gene appearing to be responsible for protein S synthesis.[317] Further research is needed to reveal genetic alterations in affected individuals and the RFLPs that may be useful in prenatal diagnosis and carrier detection.

Deficiency of antithrombin III predisposes affected individuals to repeated thrombotic events. Inherited in an autosomal dominant pattern, homozygosity has been reported in children of consanguineous families.[318,319] Undetectable antithrombin III levels obtained by fetal blood sampling in the second trimester may detect infants severely affected. The diagnosis of the heterozygote forms is best deferred until later in the postnatal period.[320]

FUTURE DIRECTIONS

The future of antenatal assessment lies in the improvement both of methods of diagnosis and treatment of known hematologic abnormalities.

Every known invasive prenatal procedure carries the risk of fetal death. Several attempts have been made to detect fetal nucleated cells in the maternal circulation for the purpose of noninvasive diagnosis of selected inherited disorders.[321–326] Monoclonal antibodies directed at the syncytiotrophoblast antigen,[327] the HLA antigen,[328] and the transferrin receptor antigen OKT9 of fetal nucleated erythrocytes[324–326] have been used to detect these cells. PCR can then be used to detect fetal DNA sequences of interest, provided enough fetal blood is in the maternal circulation. The current high frequency of false-positive and -negative results, as well as the problems asso-

Table 162-1. Hematologic Disorders Diagnosed Antenatally

Disorder	Fetal Blood Sampling	DNA Analysis
Red blood cell disorders		
Sickle cell anemia	Globin chain analysis by carboxy methyl cellulose chromatography,[88] column chromatography electrophoresis,[70] hemoglobin immunofluorescence studies,[71] high-pressure liquid chromatography by ion exchange.[72] Isoelectric focusing[73,74]	Southern blot analysis[161] Restriction enzymes[77,82] Allele-specific probes[86,87] Color complementation method[88,89] or direct DNA fragments without the need for radioisotope[83–85] aided by PCR
β-Thalassemia	Globin chain analysis by methods described above[98,99] detecting β-chain production	Restriction enzymes, gene mapping, and oligonucleotide[95–98] and dot blot analysis Several RFLPs are available[98,99] Dot blot analysis aided by PCR[98–101]
α-Thalassemia	α-Globin chain analysis quantitated by fibroblast DNA hybridization[102,103,106]	Restriction enzymes[98] and RFLPs are available[134]
Other hemogloginopathies (HbE, HbC, HbD, HbO-Arab, Hb Lepore)	β-Globin chain analysis by carboxymethol cellulose or HPLC[61,98] and hybridization techniques[95,104,105]	
Rh disease	Spectrophotometric measurements of RBC destruction[110] may be replaced by accurate measurement of fetal hematocrit, reticulocyte count, and Coombs test[109,112]	PCR allows for RhD typing in amniotic cells without invading the maternal circulation
RBC Enzyme deficiencies	Fetal erythrocyte enzymatic activity may be measured as early as 17 weeks[123–120]	Gene probes are available for many RBC enzymopathies
Other congenital anemias Franconi anemia Diamond-Blackfan anemia	Erythroid progenitor cells can be measured[128–130] and compared with normal values for gestational age	Hypersensitivity of amniocytes and villous sampling to clastogen-induced chromosomal breakage support a diagnosis of Fanconi anemia[131–133]
White blood cell disorders		
Chronic granulomatous disease	Nitroblue tetrazolium dye test is available on cord blood[146] but is not reliable on cultured amniocytes;[147] luminol-enhanced chemiluminescence test and monoclonal antibodies against cytochrome b are also available[150,152]	Closely linked flanking markers in x-linked CGD are available[151] Direct gene sequencing on preamplified CVS data is possible[153]
Chediak-Higashi syndrome	Fetal neutrophils can be assessed for the characteristic abnormally large granules[141,155–159]	
Wiskott-Aldrich syndrome	Fetal blood mean platelet volume and platelet count may exclude the diagnosis,[184,185] and lymphocytes may demonstrate abnormal short blunted microvilli[186]	RFLPs are available in information families[190] Carrier detection is possible by skewed maternal X-chromosome inactivation patterns[191–193]
Leukocyte adhesion deficiency	Fetal granulocyte CD18 expression may be assessed,[163] and monoclonal antibody binding to the CD18 complex may be demonstrated[162]	
Severe combined immunodeficiency syndromes	Fetal RBC and dATP may be measured[171]; leukocyte and lymphoid T- and B-cell subsets may be analyzed, and HLA expression analyzed[175–178]	RFLPs are available in information families[174] PCR-amplified DNA may detect specific mutations at the ADA locus
X-linked agammaglobulinemia	Normal fetal lymphocyte subpopulations may exclude the diagnosis[196] but measurements of IgG or IgA levels are unreliable[201]	RFLPs are available[198]; carrier detection possible by skewed maternal X-chromosome inactivation patterns[195]
Ataxia-telangiectasia	Fetal blood cells and cultured amniocytes may demonstrate spontaneous and clastogen-induced chromosomal breakage[204–206]	
Congenital C3 deficiency	Measurement of C3 in fetal serum excludes the diagnosis[208]	
X-linked lymphoproliferative disorder		RFLPs are available in informative families[209]
Platelet disorders		
Alloimmune thrombocytopenia	Fetal platelet phenotype and platelet count can be assessed at 20 weeks[219]	Allele-specific oligonucleotide probe are available for the PLA system[224] and for the BAK phenotype[226]
Autoimmune thrombocytopenia	Fetal blood sampling establishes the degree of thrombocytopenia, as little correlation exists between maternal and fetal platelet counts[229] or the platelet count of a previous baby[233]	
Glanzmann thrombasthenia	Radiolabeled anti-GPIIb/IIIa antibodies as early as 19 weeks' gestation[219,241] and platelet aggregation studies from cord blood[242–244] can be diagnostic	The potential use of gene markers is limited by the different mutations, which all result in a defect in GPIIb/IIIa synthesis and assembly[244]
Bernard-Soulier syndrome	Fetal cord blood can be assessed for GPIb/1X content as early as 18 weeks' gestation[246,247]	

(Table continues)

Table 162-1. *(Continued)*

Disorder	Fetal Blood Sampling	DNA Analysis
Thrombocytopenia absent-radius syndrome	Fetal blood sampling documenting thrombocytopenia[249–254] and a characteristic ultrasonographic abnormality confirm the diagnosis	
Amegakaryocytic thrombocytopenia	Fetal blood demonstrating thrombocytopenia can confirm the diagnosis in infants at risk[255]	
Grey platelet syndrome	Electron microscopy can demonstrate the presence or absence of platelet α-granules in fetal blood samples[243,244]	
May-Hegglin anomaly	Demonstrating normal platelet counts and volume and the absence of leukocyte inclusion bodies can exclude the disease[243]	
Fechner syndrome	Fetal blood can be assessed for platlet size and leukocyte inclusion bodies[256]	
Hermansky-Pudlak syndrome	?Fetal blood may demonstrate abnormal platelet aggregation	
Coagulation disorders		
von Willebrand disease	Phenotypic diagnosis is difficult due to variability of VIII:Ag and vWF:Ag levels; immunodiametric assays detecting VIII:Ag can detect severe disease[255,262–265]	Identifying a known variable tandem repeat in PCR-amplified DNA from CVS has identified seven type III VWD[268]; RFLPs are available[268]; cord blood leukocyte DNA testing has been used to diagnose some infants in the neonatal period[267,269]
Hemophilia A	Clotting factor assays have been used to detect affected males,[271–276] although levels of factor VIII and IX may vary widely and yield ambiguous results[277]	Restriction enzymes can ensure diagnosis in 90% of cases of hemophilia A[279] and B[283], RFLPs have been widely used in fetal DNA.[278,284–296]; direct detection of point mutations, deletions, and insertions can be detected in fetal blood[278,279]
Hemophilia B		
Other factor deficiencies prothrombin[298,299] Factor V[300] Factor VII[301] Factor X[302,303] Factor XI[304] Factor XII[305] Factor XIII[306]	Conventional specific functional and antigenic assays have been performed on fetal blood sampling[308]	Cloning of any of the factor genes may permit antenatal diagnosis by direct DNA analysis
Hypofibrinogenemia		
Afibrinogenemia		
Thrombophilia Protein C deficiency Protein S deficiency Antithrombin III deficiency	Detecting levels <1% in fetal blood may identify infants most at risk of purpura fulminans, although diagnosis of the heterozygote forms is best deferred until the neonatal period[320]	Identification of RFLPs within or near the genes for protein S, protein C, and antithrombin III may allow for first-trimester diagnosis in fetuses at risk; family diagnosis in a pedigree of protein C deficiency has been performed by use of a DNA polymorphism in the gene[314]

ciated with maternal cell contamination, leaves the diagnostic value of this noninvasive procedure yet to be determined. The atraumatic retrieval of trophoblasts from the lower uterine cavity by a cotton wool swab from the cervix may be a more reliable alternative for fetal DNA analysis.[329]

Advances in the correction of selected hematologic disorders using in utero therapy continue to be made. The immaturity of the fetal immune system and the presence of marrow space make the fetus the ideal transplantation host, requiring neither extensive preconditioning regimens nor HLA-identical transfusions.[330–332] Hematopoietic stem cell transplantation, first demonstrated in mice,[333,334] sheep,[335,336] and non-human primates[335,337] led to several attempts in human fetuses.[332,338–343] The source of hematopoietic stem cells appears critical to engraftment, as isolated attempts to correct Rh immunization, metachromatic leukodystrophy, β-thalassemia major, SCID, and Chédiak-Higashi syndrome have been unsuccessful when using parental marrow donor cells.[332,340] Fetal liver cells, alone or with syngeneic fetal thymic cells and fetal skin cells, however, have shown engraftment following umbilical vein and intraperitoneal transfusions.[338,339,344] Full immunologic reconstitution of human fetuses with SCID has occurred following in utero stem cell transplantation.[331,339,345] Complete cure or significant improvements have been demonstrated in conditions associated with severe aplastic anemia, thalassemia, and inborn errors of metabolism.[331,339] In utero fetal stem cell transplantation offers the advantages of increased probability of engraftment and chimerism,[346] decreased risk of acute graft-versus-host disease,[332,347] and a more sterile environment.[347] Early gestational age improves the chance for full and rapid development of transplantated fetal stem cells. This exciting therapeutic modality has the potential to eliminate or ameliorate virtually all inherited hematologic disorders.[348]

Advances in gene transfer techniques may provide yet another avenue of treatment. When incorporated into a retroviral vector, foreign genes have been successfully incorporated into murine hematopoietic stem cells,[349,350] hepatocytes, skin cells, and endothelial cells.[351–353] In utero gene transfer and expression of neomycin-resistant genes in fetal sheep hematopoietic cells have been demonstrated.[354,355] We can expect direct gene targeting to fetal hepatocytes, as well as in utero genetically modified hematopoietic stem cell transplantation, to treat effectively a variety of the inherited hematologic disorders. The use of such technology may make prenatal diagnosis more palatable to individuals who would not consider termination of pregnancy (Table 162-1).

ETHICAL ISSUES IN ANTENATAL DIAGNOSES

The value of the dramatic advances in antenatal assessment can only be assessed by examining the personal, cultural, legal, religious, social, and economic factors. It has been argued that the foremost ethical justification for prenatal diagnosis lies in its potential to prevent the suffering of a future child, affected by a serious and untreatable genetic disorder, by selective abortion.[356] This in turn may prevent the inevitable suffering otherwise forced on a family and society. Such a premise would require clear distinctions as to what is a "serious and untreatable disorder." In a study of women's opinions on the use of prenatal diagnosis, strong positive attitudes toward diagnostic procedures were found, particularly if treatable abnormalities were detected.[357] In some instances, the availability of prenatal diagnosis has increased the birth rate, as in the Greek Cypriot population at risk of homozygous β-thalassemia; this group previously had a low birth rate, or terminated pregnancies without a diagnosis, because of the risk involved.[358] The >90% termination rate for fetuses with thalassemia major in Europe further emphasizes the cultural need for antenatal assessment.[359] For other diseases, however, prenatal diagnosis is not widely accepted, as is evident by its use in 4.1% of the estimated pregnancies at risk for sickle cell anemia in the United States in 1987.[360] The unpredictability of the severity of sickle cell anemia contributes to its infrequent antenatal assessment.

Many questions are raised regarding the purpose of prenatal diagnoses. A serious and controversial issue concerns assessment for fetal sex selection, a practice reportedly rare in industrialized countries but relatively common in developing countries.[361] Although unfounded fears of selective abortion for sex selection were raised with the development of amniocentesis, it is conceivable that this practice may be more common with the earlier assessment offered by CVS. Prenatal testing of the fetus conceived for the purpose of benefiting another sibling is another issue already reviewed by legal and ethical advisory committees.[356,362] In the instances of a family who sought prenatal diagnosis in order to bear a healthy child to serve as an HLA-identical bone marrow donor for their son affected by Wiskott-Aldrich syndrome, the

physicians involved concluded that prenatal testing should not be used to benefit a third party.[356] Here the concept of parental reproductive autonomy is a strong rebuttal. Prenatal diagnosis for the purpose of the prevention of late-onset genetic disorders is another issue arising with advanced antenatal technology. Our ability to detect offspring who have genes rendering them more susceptible to cancer, diabetes, heart disease, and depression further clouds the picture.

Although it is an arduous and yet to be perfected procedure, preimplantation genetic screening is now technically feasible. The genetic structure of the embryo formed by in vitro fertilization may be assessed, with uterine transfer of the genetically unaffected embryo following. Preconceptive testing of oocytes is yet another possibility, whereby biopsy of the first polar body permits knowledge of the DNA content remaining in the ovum.[363] Although strong ethical objections to such practices are raised, preimplantation genetic screening may appeal to those who are opposed to selective termination but who are at risk of a genetically affected offspring.

More universal acceptance of antenatal assessment can be expected with the development of intrauterine therapies, although procedures such as in utero fetal stem cell transplantation, fetal liver cell transplantation, and germline genetic therapy have posed ethical questions in and of themselves.[364-366] Selective termination is no longer the common conclusion in prenatal diagnosis. Genetic counseling has been shown to reduce anxiety and depression[367,368] and may serve to prepare a couple for parenting the child with special needs.[369] Immediate benefit may be offered to the pregnancy at hand, and anticipatory needs in the postnatal period may follow. Physicians have legal and ethical duties to inform parents of tests widely accepted in the medical community as standard prenatal care.[364] Although prenatal diagnosis involves many questions, the answers to which are openly debated, health care providers are obligated to help families make the most informed choices about reproduction, to allay parental anxiety where possible, to help manage pregnancies in the most optimum manner, and to care for the psychosocial needs of those involved.

REFERENCES

1. Evans MI, Johnson MP, Holzgrove W: Chorionic villus sampling. J Reprod Med 37:386, 1992
2. Menees T, Miller JP, Holly LE: Amniography: a preliminary report. AJR 24:363, 1930
3. Bevis DCA: Composition of liquor amnii in hemolytic disease of the newborn. J Obstet Gynecol Br Commun 60:244, 1953
4. Liley AW: Liquor amnii analysis in the management of pregnancy complicated by rhesus sensitization. Am J Obstet Gynecol 82:1359, 1961
5. Freda VJ: Rh problem in obstetrics and the new concept of its management using amniocentesis and spectrophotometric scanning of amniotic fluid. Am J Obstet Gynecol 92:341, 1965
6. Fuchs F, Riis P: Antenatal sex determination. Nature 177:330, 1956
7. Fuchs F, Riis P: Antenatal determination of foetal sex in prevention of hereditary diseases. Lancet 2:180, 1960
8. Steele MW, Breg WR: Chromosome analysis of human amniotic-fluid cells. Lancet 1:383, 1966
9. Valenti C, Schutta EJ, Kehay T: Prenatal diagnosis of Down's syndrome. Lancet 2:220, 1968
10. Nadler HL: Antenatal detection of heredity disorders. Pediatrics 42:912, 1968
11. Nadler HL, Gerbre AB: Role of amniocentesis in the intrauterine detection of genetic disorders. N Engl J Med 282:596, 1970
12. Henry GP, Miller WA: Early amniocentesis. J Reprod Med 37:396, 1992
13. Kennerknecht I, Baur-Aubele S, Grab D, Terinde R: First trimester amniocentesis between the 7th–13th weeks: evaluations of the earliest possible genetic defects. Prenat Diagn 12:595, 1992
14. Hanson FW, Tennaut F, Hune S, Brookhyser K: Early amniocentesis: outcome, risks and technical problems at <12.8 weeks. Am J Obstet Gynecol 166:1707, 1992
15. Jorgensen FS, Bang J, Lind AM et al: Genetic amniocentesis at 7–14 weeks of gestation. Prenat Diagn 12:227, 1992
16. Mathews T, Verma RS: Enhancement of amniotic fluid cell growth for genetic amniocentesis. Clin Genet 40:190, 1991
17. Thoulou JM: Amniocentesis vs. choroiocentesis (chorionic villus sampling) and cordocentesis (fetal blood sampling). Rev Fr Gynecol Obstet 85:101, 1990
18. Hogge WK: Prenatal diagnosis and treatment of genetic disorders. p. 138. In Merkatz IR, Thompson JE (eds): New Perspectives on Prenatal Care. Elsevier Science, 1990
19. Anandakumar C, Wong YC, Annapoorna V et al: Amniocentesis and its complications. Aust N Z J Obstet Gynecol 32:97, 1992
20. Ledbetter DJ, Hall DG: Traumatic arteriovenous fistula: a complication of amniocentesis. J Pediatr Surg 27:720, 1992
21. Naylor G, Roper JP, Willshaw HE: Ophthalmic complications of amniocentesis. Eye 4:845, 1990

22. Milner AD, Hoskyns EW, Hopkin JE: The efforts of mid-trimester amniocentesis on lung function in the neonatal period. Eur J Pediatr 151:458, 1992

23. Mohr J: Foetal genetic diagnosis: development of techniques for early sampling of foetal cells. Acta Pathol Microbiol Scand 73:73, 1968

24. Platt LD, Carlson DE: Prenatal diagnosis—when and how? N Engl J Med 327:636, 1992

25. Smidt-Jensen S, Philip J: Comparison of transabdominal and transcervical CVS and AC: sampling success and risk. Prenat Diagn II:529, 1991

26. Jackson LG, Zachary JM, Fowler SE et al: A randomized comparison of transcervical and transabdominal choriomic villus sampling. N Engl J Med 327:594, 1992

27. Hallak M, Johnson MP, Pryde PG et al: Chorionic villus sampling: transabdominal vs transcervical approach in more than 4,000 cases. Obstet Gynecol 80:349, 1992

28. Molecular analysis and chorionic vilus sampling (CVS): opportunities for rapid prenatal diagnosis in the military. Mil Med 156:678, 1991

29. Lilford RJ: The rise and fall of CVS. BMJ 303:936, 1991

30. Canadian Collaborative CVS-Amniocentesis Trial Group (1989): Multicentric trial comparing chorionic villus sampling and amniocentesis in prenatal diagnosis. Lancet 1:1, 1989

31. Rhoads GG, Jackson LG, Schlesselma SE et al: The safety and efficacy of CVS for early prenatal diagnosis of cytogenetic abnormalities. N Engl J Med 320:609, 1989

32. Medical Research Convert European Trial of Chorionic Villus Sampling. Lancet 337:1491, 1991

33. Desnick RJ, Schuette L, Golbus MS et al: First trimester biochemical and molecular diagnosis using chorionic villi: high accuracy in the US collaborative study, Prenat Diagn 12:357, 1992

34. Hurley PA, Rodeck CH: Fetal therapy. Curr Opin Obstet Gynecol 4:4, 1992

35. Quintero RA, Romero R, Mahoney MJ et al: Fetal hemorrhagic lesions after chorionic villus sampling. Lancet 339:193, 1992

36. Burton BK, Schulz CJ, Burd LI: Limb anomalies associated with chorionic villus samling. Obstet Gynecol 79:726, 1992

37. Firth HV, Boyd PA, Chamberlain P et al: Severe limb abnormalities after chorion villus sampling at 56–66 days gestation. Lancet 337:762, 1991

38. Dolk H, Bertrand F, Lechat MF: Chorionic villus sampling and limb abnormalities. Lancet 339:876, 1992

39. Froster VG: Limb reduction defects and chorionic villus sampling. Lancet 339:66, 1992

40. Boyd PA, Keeling JW, Selinger M et al: Limb reduction and chorion villus sampling. Prenat Diagn 10:437, 1990

41. Schloo R, Miny P, Holzgreve W et al: Distal limb deficiency following chorionic villus sampling? Am J Med Genet 42:404, 1992

42. Valenti C: Antenatal diagnosis of hemaglobinopathies: a prelim report. Am J Obstet Gynecol 115:851, 1973

43. Antsaklis A, Bang V, Benzie R et al: Special report. The status of fetoscopy and fetal tissue sampling. Prenat Diagn 4:79, 1984

44. Sacher RA, Falchnk SC: Percutaneous umbilical blood sampling. Clin Rev Clin Lab Sci 28:19, 1990

45. Kan YW, Valenti C, Carnazza V, et al: Fetal blood sampling in utero. Lancet 1:79, 1974

46. Daffos F, Capela-Pavlowsky M, Forestier F: A new procedure for fetal blood sampling in utero: preliminary report of 53 cases. Am J Obstet Gynecol 146:985, 1983

47. Trapani FD, Marino M, Dalcamo E et al: Prenatal diagnosis of hemoglobin disorders by cordocentesis at 12 weeks gestation. Prenat Diagn II:899, 1991

48. Boulet P, Deschamps F, Lefort G et al: Pure fetal blood samples obtained by cordocentesis: technical aspects of 322 cases. Prenat Diagn 10:93, 1990

49. Daffos F, Capella Pavlowsky, Forestier F: Fetal blood sampling during pregnancy with use of a needle guided by ultrasound. A study of 606 consecutive cases. Am J Obstet Gynecol 153:655, 1985

50. Nicolaides KH: Cordocentesis. Clin Obstet Gynecol 311:123, 1988

51. Antsaklis AL, Papantoniou NE, Mesogitis SA et al: Cardiocentesis: an alternative method of fetal blood sampling for the prenatal diagnosis of the hemoglobinopathies. Obstet Gynecol 79:630, 1992

52. Shah DM, Roussis P, Ulm J et al: Cordocentesis for rapid karyotyping. Am J Obstet Gynecol 162:1548, 1990

53. Boulet P, Courtier C, Lefort G et al: Fetal blood sampling for karyotype using echoguided puncture of the cord. Study of 103 pregnancies. J Gynecol Obstet Biol Reprod (Paris) 18:1007, 1989

54. Orlandi F, Damiani G, Jakil C et al: The risks of early cordocentesis. Prenat Diagn 10:425, 1990

55. Daffos F, Forestier F, Grangeot-Keros et al: Prenatal diagnosis of congenital rubella. Lancet 2:613, 1984

56. Morgan-Capner P, Rodeck CH, Nicolaides KH et al: Prenatal detection of rubella specific IgM in fetal sera. Prenat Diagn 5:21, 1985

57. Pardi G, Buscaglia M, Ferrazzi E et al: Cord sampling for the evaluation of oxygenation and acid-base balance in growth retarded human fetuses. Am J Obstet Gynecol 157:1221, 1987

58. Cox WL, Daffos F, Forestier F et al: Physiology and management of IUGR: biologic approach with fetal blood sampling. Am J Obstet Gynecol 159:36, 1988

59. Modaniou H, Smith E, Pane RH: Complications of fetal blood sampling during labor. Clin Pediatr 12:603, 1973

60. Modell B: Prevention of the haemoglobinopathies. Br Med Bull 39:386, 198

61. Alter BP: Advances in the prenatal diagnosis of hematologic diseases. Blood 64A:329, 1984

62. Alter BP: Prenatal diagnosis of haemoglobinopathies: a status report. Lancet 2:1152, 1981

63. Scriver CR, Bardanis M, Cartier L et al: β-Thalassemia disease prevention genetic medicine applied. Am J Hum Genet 36:1024, 1984

64. Tentori L, Marinucci M: Hemoglobinopathies and thalassemias in Italy and northern Africa. p. 299. In Bowman J (ed): Distribution and Evolution of Hemoglobin and Globin Loci. Elsevier, New York, 1983

65. Loukopoulos D: Prenatal diagnosis of thalassemia and of the hemoglobinopathies: a review. Hemaglobin 9:435, 1985

66. Eichner ER: Sickle cell trait: review of the literature. Am J Med 14:144, 1986

67. Vichinsky E, Hurst D, Earles A et al: Newborn screening for sickle cell disease: effect on mortality. Pediatrics 81:749, 1988

68. Kan YW, Dozy AM, Alter BP et al: Defection of the sickle gene in the human fetus. N Engl J Med 287:1, 1972

69. Hollenberg MD, Kaback MM, Kazazian HH Jr: Adult hemaglobin synthesis by reticulocytes from the human fetus at midtrimester. Science 174:698, 1971

70. Alter BP, Coupal E, Forget BF: Globin chain electrophoresis for prenatal diagnosis of beta thalassemia. Hemoglobin 5:357, 1981

71. Thorpe SJ, Huehns ER: A new approach for antenatal diagnosis of beta thalassemia: a double labelling immunofluorescence microscopy technique. Br J Haematol 53:103, 1983

72. Rouyer-Fessard P, Plazza F, Blouquit Y et al: Prenatal diagnosis of haemoglobinopathies by ion exchange HPLC of haemoglobins. Prenat Diagn 9:19, 1989

73. Dubart A, Goossens M, Beuzard Y et al: Prenatal diagnosis of hemoglobinopathies: comparison of the results obtained by isoelectric focusing of hemoglobins and by chromatography of radioactive globin chains. Blood 56:1091, 1980

74. Ferrari M, Crema A, Cantu-Rajnoldi A et al: Antenatal diagnosis of haemoglobinopathies by improved method of isoelectric focusing of haemoglobins. Br J Haematol 57:265, 1984

75. Chang H, Modell CB, Alter BP et al: Expression of the β-thalassemia gene in the first trimester fetus. Proc Natl Acad Sci USA 72:3633, 1975

76. Kan YW, Dozy AM: Polymorphism of DNA sequence adjacent to human β-globin structural gene: relationship to sickle mutation. Proc Natl Acad Sci USA 75:5631, 1978

77. Wilson JT, Milner PF, Summer ME et al: Use of restriction endonucleases to map the β-allele. Proc Natl Acad Sci USA 79:3628, 1982

78. Orkin SH, Kazazian HH Jr: The mutation and polymorphism of the human β-globin gene and its surrounding DNA. Annu Rev Genet 18:131, 1984

79. Chang JC, Kan YW: A sensitive new prenatal test for sickle cell anemia. N Engl J Med 307:30, 1982

80. Orkin SH, Little PFR, Kazazian HH Jr, Boehm CD: Improved detection of the sickle cell mutation of DNA analysis: application to prenatal diagnosis. N Engl J Med 307:32, 1982

81. Geever RF, Wilson LB, Nallaseth FS et al: Direct identification of sickle cell anemia by blot hybridization. Proc Natl Acad Sci USA 78:5081, 1981

82. Chehab FF, Doherty M, Cai S et al: Detection of sickle cell anaemia and thalassaemias. Nature 329:293, 1987

83. Posey YF, Shah D, Vlm JE et al: Prenatal diagnosis of sickle cell anemia. Am J Clin Pathol 92:347, 1989

84. Saiki RK, Scharf S, Faloona F et al: Enzymatic amplification of beta-globin genomic sequences and restriction site analysis for diagnosis of sickle cell anemia. Science 230:1350, 1985

85. Embury SH, Scharf SH, Saiki RK et al: Rapid prenatal diagnosis of sickle cell anemia by a new method of DNA analysis. N Engl J Med 316:656, 1987

86. Conner BJ, Reyes AA, Morin C et al: Detection of sickle cell β-S globin allele by hybridisation with synthetic oligonucleotides. Proc Natl Acad Sci USA 80:278, 1983

87. Cao A, Leoni GB, Sardu R, Piscaedd MC: Prenatal diagnosis of inherited hemoglobinopathies. Recent Prog Med 83:224, 1992

88. Chehab FF, Kan YW: Detection of specific DNA sequences by fluorescence amplification: a color complimentation assay. Proc Natl Acad Sci USA 86:9128, 1989

89. Chehab FF, Kan YW: Detection of sickle cell anaemia by mutation by colour DNA amplification. Lancet 1:15, 1990

90. Alter BP: Prenatal diagnosis of hemoglobinopathies and other hematologic diseases. J Pediatr 95:501, 1979

91. Congote LF: Rapid procedure for globin chain analysis in blood samples of normal and β-thalassemic fetuses. Blood 57:353, 1981

92. Valkonen KH, Gianazza E, Righetti PG: Human globin chain separation by isoelectric focusing in ultrathin polyacrylamide gels. Clin Chim Acta 107: 223, 1980

93. Manca M, Cossu G, Angioni G et al: Antenatal diagnosis of β-thalassemia by isoelectric focusing in immobilized pH gradients. Am J Hematol 22:285, 1986

94. Boccacci M, Massa A, Tentori L: Application of cellulose acetate electrophoresis to globin chain separation for antenatal diagnosis of β-thalassemias. Clin Chim Acta 116:137, 1981

95. Orkin SH, Alter BP, Atlay C et al: Application of endonuclease mapping to the analysis and prenatal diagnosis of thalassemias caused by globin gene deletion. N Engl J Med 299:166, 1978

96. Kazazian HH Jr, Boehm CD: Molecular basis and prenatal diagnosis of β-thalassemia. Blood 72:1107, 1988

97. Wallace RB, Schold M, Johnson MJ et al: Oligonucleotide directed mutagenesis of the human β-globin gene: a general method for producing specific point mutations in cloned DNA. Nucleic Acids Res 9:3647, 1981

98. Old JM, Ludlam CA: Antenatal diagnosis. Baillieres Clin Haematol 4:391, 1991

99. Kulozik AE, Lyons J, Kohne E et al: Ropia and non-radioactive prenatal diagnosis of β-thalassemia and sickle cell disease: application of the polymerase chain reaction (PCR). Br J Haematol 70:455, 1988

100. Faa V, Rosatelli MC, Sardu R et al: A simple electrophoretic procedure for fetal diagnosis of β-thalassaemia due to short deletions. Prenat Diagn 12: 903, 1992

101. Ristaldi MS, Pirastu M, Rosatelli C et al: Prenatal diagnosis of β-thalassaemia in Mediterranean populations by dot blot analysis with DNA amplification and allele specific digonucleotide probes. Prenat Diagn 9:629, 1989

102. Kan YW, Golbus MS, Dozy AM: Prenatal diagnosis of alpha-thalassemia. N Engl J Med 295:1165, 1976

103. Koenig HM, Vedvick TS, Golbus MS et al: Prenatal diagnosis of hemoglobin-H disease by molecular hybridization. Pediatr Res 11:459 (A), 1977

104. Orkin SH, Old J, Weatherall DJ, Nathan DG: Partial deletion of β-globin gene DNA in certain patients wtih β-thalassemia. Proc Natl Acad Sci USA 76:2400, 1979

105. Spiegelberg R, Aulehla-Scholz, Erlich H, Horst J: A β-thalassemia gene caused by a 290-base pair deletion: analysis by direct sequencing of enzymatically amplified DNA. Blood 73:1695, 1989

106. Chehab FF, Doherty M, Cai S et al: Detection of sickle cell anaemia and thalassaemia. Nature 329:293, 1987

107. Urbaniak SJ: Rh (D) haemolytic disease of the newborn: the changing scene. BMJ 291:4, 1985

108. Tovey LAD: Haemolytic disease of the newborn—the changing scene. Br J Obstet Gynaecol 93:960, 1986

109. Weiner CP, Williamson RA, Wenstrom KD et al: Management of fetal hemolytic disease by cordocentesis. I. Prediction of fetal anemia. Am J Obstet Gynecol 165:546, 1991

110. Liley AW. Liquor amnii analysis in the management of the pregnancy complicated by rhesus sensitization. Am J Obstet Gynecol 82:1359, 1961

111. Liley AW: Intrauterine transfusion of foetus in haemolytic disease. BMJ 2: 1107, 1963

112. Harman CR, Bowman JM, Manning FA, Menticoglou SM: Intrauterine transfusion-intraperitoneal versus intravascular approach: a case-control comparison. Am J Obstet Gynecol 162:1053, 1990

113. Nicolini U, Rodeck CH: A proposed scheme for planning intrauterine transfusion patients with severe Rh-immunization. J Obstet Gynecol 9:162, 1988

114. Rodeck CH, Letsky E: How the management of erythroblastosis fetalis has changed. Br J Obstet Gynaecol 96:759, 1989

115. Moise KJ, Mari G, Fisher DJ et al: Acute fetal hemodynamic alterations after intrauterine transfusion for treatment of severe red blood cell alloimmunization. Am J Obstet Gynecol 163:776, 1990

116. Dildy GA, Smith LG, Moise KJ et al: Porencephalic cyst: a complication of fetal intravascular transfusion. Am J Obstet Gynecol 165:76, 1991

117. Thorp JA, Plapp FV, Cohen GR et al: Hyperkalemia after irradiation of packed red blood cells: possible effects with intravascular fetal transfusion. Am J Obstet Gynecol 163:607, 1990

118. Bowell PJ, Selinger M, Ferguson J et al: Antenatal fetal blood sampling for alloimmunized pregnancies: effect upon maternal anti-D potency levels. Br J Obstet Gynaecol 95:759, 1988

119. Nicolini V, Kochenour NK, Greco P et al: Consequences of fetomaternal haemorrhage after intrauterine transfusion. BMJ 297:1379, 1988

120. Gloning K, Schramm TH, Brusis E et al: Successful intrauterine treatment of fetal hydrops caused by parvovirus B19 infection. Behring Inst Mitt 85: 79, 1990

121. Sahakian V, Weiner CP, Naides SJ et al: Intrauterine transfusion treatment of non-immune hydrops fetalis secondary to human parvovirus B19 infection. Am J Obstet Gynecol 164:1090, 1991

122. Peters MT, Nicolaides KH: Cordocentesis for the diagnosis and treatment of human fetal parvovirus infection. Obstet Gynecol 75:501, 1990

123. Lestas AN, Rodeck CH, White JM: Normal activities of glycolytic enzymes in fetal erythrocyes. Br J Haematol 50:439, 1982

124. Lestas AN, Bellingham AJ, Nicolaides KH: Red cell glycolytic intermediates in normal, anaemic and transfused human fetuses. Br J Haematol 73:387, 1989

125. Sassa S, Silish G, Levere RD, Kappas A: Studies in porphyria. IV. Expression of the gene defect of acute intermittent porphyria in cultured human skin fibroblasts and amniotic cells: prenatal diagnosis of the porphyric trait. J Exp Med 142:722, 1975

126. Bloomer JR, Bonkowsky HL, Ebert PS, Mahoney MJ: Inheritence in protoporphyria. Comparison of haem synthetase activity in skin fibroblasts with clinical features. Lancet 2:266, 1976

127. Alter BP, Nathan DG: Antenatal diagnosis of haematological disorders—"1978." Clin Haematol 7:195, 1978

128. Oski FA, Naiman JL: Hematologic problems in the Newborn. 3rd Ed. WB Saunders, Philadelphia, 1982, p. 4

129. Linch DC, Knott LJ, Rodeck CH, Huehns ER: Studies of circulating hematopoietic progenitor cells in human fetal blood. Blood 59:976, 1982

130. Forestier F: Biological characterization of prenatal samplings. Curr Stud Hematol Blood Transfus 55:130, 1988

131. Auerbach AD, Zhang M, Ghosh R et al: Clastogen-induced chromosomal breakage as a marker for first trimester prenatal diagnosis of Fanconi anemia. Hum Genet 73:86, 1986

132. Auerbach AD, Sagi M, Adler B: Fanconi anemia: prenatal diagnosis in 30 fetuses at risk. Pediatrics 76:794, 1985

133. Auerbach AD, Ghosh R, Pollio PC, Zhang M: Diepoxybutane (DEB) for prenatal and postnatal diagnosis of Fanconi anemia. p. 71. In Schroeder-Kurth TM, Auerbach AD, Obe G (eds): Fanconi Anemia: Clinical, Cytogenetic and Experimental Aspects. Springer-Verlag, Heidelberg, 1989

134. Boehm CD, Antonarakis SE, Phillips JA et al: Prenatal diagnosis using DNA polymorphisms: Report on 95 pregnancies at risk for sickle cell disease or β-thalassemia. N Engl J Med 308:1054, 1983

135. Linch DG: Prenatal diagnosis of immunodeficient disorders. Br Med Bull 39: 399, 1983

136. Hayward AR: The human fetus and newborn: development of the immune response. Birth Defects 19:289, 1983

137. Chandra RK, Matsumura T: Ontogenetic development of the immune system and effects of fetal growth retardation. J Perinat Med 71:279, 1979

138. Linch DC, Beverly PCL, Levinsky RJ, Rodeck CH: Phenotypic analysis of fetal blood leukocytes: potential for prenatal diagnosis of immunodeficiency disorders. Prenat Diagn 2:211, 1982

139. Gitlin D, Biasucci A: Development of the G, A, M, Cl esterase inhibitor, ceruloplasmin, transferrin, hemopexin, haptoglobin, fibrinogen, plasminogen, α_1-antitrypsin, B-lipoprotein, β_2-macroglobulin and prealbumin in the human conceptus. J Clin Invest 48:1433, 1969

140. Romero R, Hobbins JC, Mahoney MJ: Fetal blood sampling and fetoscopy. p. 571. In Milunsky A (ed): Genetic Disorders of the Fetus: Diagnosis, Prevention, Treatment. 2nd Ed. Plenum, New York, 1986

141. Kahraman MM, Prieur DJ: Chédiak Higashi syndrome: prenatal diagnosis by fetal blood examination in the feline model of the disease. Am J Med Genet 32:325, 1989

142. Baehner RL, Natran DG: Quantitative nitroblue terrazolium test in chronic granulomatous disease. N Engl J Med 278:971, 1968

143. Baehner RL, Boxer LA, Davis J: The biochemical basis of nitroblue tetrazolium reduction by normal human and chronic granulomatous disease polymorphonuclear leukocytes. Blood 48:309, 1976

144. Tatsuhito TO, Takahide M, Norihito V et al: Chemiluminescence of whole blood from various types of disease. Clin Immunol Immunopathol 29:333, 1983

145. Curnette JT, Whitten DM, Babior BM: Defective superoxide production by granulocytes from patients with chronic granulomatous disease. N Engl J Med 290:593, 1974

146. Newburger PE, Cohen HJ, Rothchild SB et al: Prenatal diagnosis of chronic granulomatous disease. N Engl J Med 300:178, 1979

147. Fikrig SM, Smithnick EM, Suniharalingam K, Good RA: Fibroblast nitroblue tetrazolium test and in-utero diagnosis of chronic granulomatous disease. Lancet 1:18, 1980

148. Seger R, Steinmann B: Prenatal diagnosis of chronic granulomatous disease: ureliability of fibroblast NBT. Lancet 1:1260, 1981

149. Borregaard N, Bang J, Berthelsen JG et al: Prenatal diagnosis of chronic granulomatous disease. Lancet 1:114, 1982

150. Matthay KK, Golbus MS, Wara DW, Mentzer WC: Prenatal diagnosis of chronic granulomatous disease. Am J Med Genet 17:731, 1984

151. Lindof M, Kere J, Ristola M et al: Prenatal diagnosis of X-linked chronic granulomatous disease using RFLP analysis. Genomics 1:87, 1987

152. Nakamura M, Imajoh-Ohmi S, Kanegasaki S et al: Prenatal diagnosis of cytochrome-deficient chronic granulomatous disease. Lancet 336:118, 1990

153. DeBoer M, Bolscher GJM, Sijmon RH et al: Prenatal diagnosis in a familiy with X-linked chronic granulomatous disease with the use of PCR. Prenat Diagn 12:773, 1992

154. Penner JD, Prieur DJ: A comparative study of the lesions in cultural fibroblast of humans and four species of mammals with Chédiak-Higashi syndrome. Am J Med Genet 28:445, 1987

155. Diukman R, Tanigawara S, Cowan MJ, Golbus MS: Prenatal diagnosis of Chédiak-Higashi syndrome. Prenat Diagn 12:877, 1992

156. Charrow J: Prenatal diagnosis and management of endocrine and metabolic disorders. Spe Topi Endocrinol Metab 7:31, 1985

157. Golbus MS, McGonigle KF, Goldberg JD et al: Fetal tissue sampling, the San Francisco experience with 190 pregnancies. West J Med 150:423, 1989

158. Fisher A, Durandy A, Griscelli C: Primary immunodeficiencies. p. 113. In Chaouat G (ed): The Immunology of the Fetus. CRC Press, Boca Raton, FL, 1990

159. Kahraman M, Prieur DJ: Chédiak-Higashi syndrome in the cat: prenatal diagnosis by evaluation of amniotic fluid cells. Am J Med Genet 36:321, 1990

160. Kishimoto TK, Hollander N, Roberts TM et al: Heterogeneous mutations in the B subunit common to the LFA-1, Mac-1 and p150, 95 glycoproteins causing leukocyte adhesion deficiency. Cell 50:193, 1987

161. Marlin SD, Morton CC, Anderson DC, Springer TA: LFA-1 immunodeficiency disease. Definition of the genetic defect and chromosomal mapping of and B subunits of the lymphocyte function-associated antigen (LFA-1) by complementation of hybrid cells. J Exp Med 164:855, 1986

162. Weisman SJ, Mahoney MJ, Anderson DC et al: Prenatal diagnosis for Mol (Cdw18) deficiency. Clin Res 35:435A, 1987

163. Weening RS, Brodius RGM, Wolf H, van der Schoot CE: Prenatal diagnostic procedure for leukocyte adhesion deficiency. Prenat Diagn 11:193, 1991

164. Puck J: Prenatal diagnosis and genetic analysis of X-linked immunodeficiency disorders. Pediatr Res 33:S29, 1993

165. Hirschhorn R: Genetic deficiencies of adenosine deaminase and purine nucleoside phosphorylase: overview, genetic heterogenity and therapy. Birth Defects 19:73, 1983

166. Meuwissen HJ, Pollara B, Pickering RJ: Combined immunodeficiency disease associated with adenosine deaminase deficiency. J Pediatr 86:169, 1975

167. Puck JM, Krauss CM, Puck SM et al: Prenatal test for X-linked sense combined immunodeficiency by analysis of maternal X-chromosome inactivation and linkage analysis. N Engl J Med 322:1063, 1990

168. Hirschhorn R, Beratis W, Rosen FS et al: Adenosine deaminase deficiency in a child diagnosed prenatally. Lancet 1:73, 1975

169. Aitken DA, Gilmore DH, Frew CA et al: Early prenatal investigation of a pregnancy at risk of adenosine deaminase deficiency using chorionic villi. J Med Genet 23:52, 1986

170. Dooley T, Fairbanks LD, Simmonds HA et al: First trimester diagnosis of adenosine deaminase deficiency. Prenat Diagn 7:561, 1987

171. Simmonds HA, Fairbanks LD, Webster DR: Rapid prenatal diagnosis of adenosine deaminase deficiency and other purine disorders using foetal blood. Biosci Rep 3:31, 1983

172. Wiginton DA, Kaplan DJ, States JC: Complete sequence and structure of the gene for human adenosine deaminase. Biochemistry 25:8234, 1986

173. Orkin SH, Daddona PE, Shewach DS: Molecular cloning of human adenosine deaminase gene sequences. J Biol Chem 258:1275, 1983

174. Tzall S, Ellenbogen A, Eng F, Hirshhorn R: Identification and characterization of nine RFLP's at the adenosine deaminase (ADA) locus. Am J Hum Genet 44:864, 1989

175. Levinsky RJ, Linch DC, Beverly PCL, Rodeck CH: Prenatal exclusion of severe combined immune deficiency. Arch Dis Child 57:958, 1982

176. Durandy A, Oury C, Griscelli C et al: Prenatal testing for inherited immune deficiencies by fetal blood sampling. Prenat Diagn 2:109, 1982

177. Durandy A, Dumez Y, Guy-Grand D et al: Prenatal diagnosis of severe combined immunodeficiency. J Pediatr 101:995, 1982

178. Blakemore K, Scioscia A, Grannum P et al: The value of fetal blood sampling in the prenatal diagnosis of severe combined immune deficiency syndrome. Am J Hum Genet, suppl. 41:A267, 1987

179. Linch DC, Rodeck CH, Simmonds HA, Levinsky RJ: Prenatal diagnosis for severe combined immune deficiency syndrome. Birth Defects 19:121, 1983

180. Durandy A, Griscelli C: Prenatal diagnosis of severe combined immune deficiency and X-linked agammaglobulinemia. Birth Defects 19:125, 1983

181. Hirschhorn R: Adenosine deaminase deficiency. Immunol Rev 2:175, 1990

182. Durandy A, Cerf-Bensussan N, Dumez Y, Griscelli C: Prenatal diagnosis of SCID with defective synthesis of HLA molecles. Prenat Diagn 7:27, 1989

183. Touraine JL, Raudrant D, Royo C et al: In-utero transplantation of stem cells in bare lymphocyte syndrome. Lancet 1:1382, 1989

184. Holmberg L, Gustavii B, Jonsson A: A prenatal study of fetal platelet coun and size with special application to a fetus at risk for Wiskott-Aldrich sy drome. J Pediatr 102:773, 1983

185. Lorenz P, Bollmann R, Hinkel GK, Machler M: False negative prenatal excl sion of Wiskott-Aldrich syndrome by measurement of fetal platelet coun and size. Prenat Diagn 11:819, 1991

186. Kenney D, Cairns L, Remold-O'Donnell E et al: Morphological abnormalitie in the lymphocytes of patients with Wiskott-Aldrich syndrome. Blood 68 1329, 1986

187. Schwartz M, Mibashan RS, Nicolaides KH et al: First trimester diagnosis o Wiskott-Aldrich syndrome by DNA markers. Lancet 2:1405, 1989

188. Kwan SP, Sandkuyl L, Blaese M et al: Genetic mapping of the Wiskott-Aldric syndrome with two highly linked polymorphic DNA markers. Genomics 3 39, 1988

189. de Saint Basile G, Fraser N, Craig L et al: Close linkage of hypervariabl markers DXS 255 to the disease locus of Wiskott-Aldrich syndrome. Lance 2:1319, 1989

190. Peacocke M, Siminovitch KA: Linkage of Wiskott-Aldrich syndrome wit polymorphic DNA sequences from the human X chromosome. Proc Nat Acad Sci USA 84:3430, 1987

191. Fearon ER, Kohn DB, Winkesteine JA et al: Carrier detection of the Wiskott Aldrich syndrome. Blood 72:1735, 1988

192. Greer WL, Kwong PC, Peacocke M et al: X chromosome inactivation in the Wiskott-Aldrich syndrome: a marker for detection of the carrier state and identification of cell lineages expressing the gene defect. Genomics 4:60 1989

193. Puck JM, Siminovitch KA, Poncz M et al: Atypical presentation of Wiskott-Aldrich syndrome: diagnosis in two unrelated males based on studies o maternal T cell X chromosome inactivation. Blood 75:2369, 1990

194. Conley ME, Brown P, Pickard AR: Expression of the gene defect in X-linked agammaglobulinemia. N Engl J Med 315:564, 1986

195. Fearon ER, Winkestein JA, Civin C et al: Carrier detection in X linked agam-maglobulinemia by analysis of X chromosome inactivation. N Engl J Med 316:427, 1987

196. Durandy A, Dumez Y, Griscelli C: Prenatal diagnosis of SCID: a five year experience. p. 323. In Vossen J, Griscelli C (eds): Progress in Immunodeficiency Research and Therapy II. Elsevier, Amsterdam, 1986

197. Kwan SP, Kunkel L, Bruns G et al: Mapping of the X-linked agammaglobulinemia locus by use of RFLP. J Clin Invest 77:649, 1986

198. Journet O, Durandy A, Doussau M et al: Carrier detection and prenatal diagnosis of X-linked agammaglobulinemia. Am J Med Genet 43:885, 1992

199. OH J, Mensink EJBM, Thompson A et al: Heterogeneity in the map distance between X-linked agammaglobulinemia and a map of 9 RFLP loci. Hum Genet 74:280, 1986

200. Lau YL, Levinksy RJ, Malcolm S et al: Genetic prediction of X-linked agamma-globulinemia. Am J Med Genet 31:437, 1988

201. Taalman ROFM, Jaspers NGJ, Scheres JMJC et al: Hypersensitivity in vitro to ionizing radiation in a new chromosome instability syndrome, the Nijmegen breakage syndrome. Mutat Res 112:23, 1983

202. Chan JYH, Becker FF, German J et al: Altered DNA ligase I activity in Bloom's syndrome cells. Nature 325:357, 1987

203. Gatti R: Ataxia-telangiectasia (group A): localization of ATA gene to chromosome 11q 22-23 and pathogenetic implication. Allergol Immunopathol 19: 42, 1991

204. Shaham M, Voss R, Becker Y et al: Prenatal diagnosis of ataxia-telangiecta-sia. J Pediatr 100:134, 1982

205. Jaspers NG, vanderKraan M, Linssen PCML et al: First trimester prenatal diagnosis of the Nijmegen breakage syndrome and ataxia-telangiectasia using an assay of radiosensitive DNA synthesis. Prenat Diagn 10:667, 1990

206. Lievena JC, Murer-Orlando M: Bloom syndrome and ataxia-telangiectasia. Semin Hematol 28:95, 1991

207. Alper CA, Colten HR, Gear JS et al: Homozygous human C3 deficiency: the role of C3 in antibody production, CI's induced vasopermeability and cobra venom-induced passive hemolysis. J Clin Invest 57:222, 1976

208. Kohler P: Maturation of the human complement system. J Clin Invest 52: 671, 1973

209. Davies KE, Mandel JL, Monaco AP et al: Report of the committee on the genetic constitution of the X chromosome, HGMII. Cell Genet 58:853, 1991

210. Blanchett VS, Peters MA, Pegg-Feige K: Alloimmune thrombocytopenia: review from a neonatal intensive care unit. Curr Stud Hematol Blood Transfus 52:87, 1986

211. Muller JY: Neonatal alloimmune thrombocytopenia. Baillieres Clin Immunol Allergy 1:427, 1987

212. Bussel JB, McFarland JG, Berkowitz RL: Antenatal management of fetal allo-immune and autoimmune thrombocytopenia. Trans Med Rev IV:149, 1990

213. Bussel JB, Kaplan C, McFarland J: Recommendations for the evaluation and

treatment of neonatal autoimmune and alloimmune thrombocytopenia. Thromb Haemost 65:631, 1991

14. Herman JH, Jumbelic MI, Ancoria RJ, Kicher TS: In utero cerebral hemorrhage in alloimmune thrombocytopenia. Am J Pediatr Hematol Oncol 8:12, 1986

15. Shulman NR, Jordan JV: Platelet immunology. p. 274. In Colman RW, Hirsh J, Marder VJ, Salzmann EW (eds): Haemostasis and Thrombosis: Basic Principles and Clinical Practice. JB Lippincott, Philadelphia, 1982

16. Muller JY, Reznikoff-Etievant MF, Patereau C, Julieu F: Thrombopenies neonatales par alloimmunization anti PLA1 et antigene DR 3. CR Acad Sci Paris 296:953, 1983

17. Kaplan C, Daffos F, Forestier F et al: Management of allothrombocytopenia: antenatal diagnosis and in utero transfusion of maternal platelets. Blood 72:340, 1988

18. Muller JY, Patereau C, Reznikoff-Etievant MF et al: Les thrombopenies neonatales alloimmunes. Rev Fr Transfus Immunohematol 28:625, 1985

19. Kaplan C, Patereau C, Reznikoff-Etievant MF et al: Antenatal PLA1 typing and detection of GP IIb-IIIa complex. Br J Haematol 60:586, 1984

220. Bussel JB, Berkowitz RL, McFarland JG et al: Antenatal treatment of neonatal alloimmune thrombocytopenia. N Engl J Med 319:1374, 1988

221. Murphy MF, Pullon HWH, Metcalfe P et al: Management of fetal alloimmune thrombocytopenia by weekly in utero platelet transfusions. Vox Sang 58:45, 1990

222. Daffos F, Forestier F, Muller JY et al: Prenatal treatment of alloimmune thrombocytopenia. Lancet 1:632, 1984

223. Nicolini V, Rodeck CH, Kochenour NK et al: In utero platelet transfusion for alloimmune thrombocytopenia. Lancet 1:506, 1988

224. McFarland JG, Aster RH, Bussel JB et al: Prenatal diagnosis of neonatal alloimmune thrombocytopenia using allele-specific oligonucleotide probes. Blood 78:2276, 1991

225. Newman PJ, Darbes RS, Aster RH: The human platelet allo-antigens PLA1 and PLA2 are associated with a leucine 33/proline 33 amino acid polymorphism in membrane glycoprotein IIIa, and are distinguishable by DNA typing. J Clin Invest 83:1728, 1989

226. Lyman S, Aster RH, Visentin GP et al: Polymorphism of human platelet membrane gycoprotein IIb associated with the Bak a/Bak b allo-antigen system. Blood 75:2343, 1990

227. Burrows RF, Kelton JG: Low fetal risks in pregnancies associated with immune thrombocytopenia. Am J Obstet Gynecol 163:1147, 1990

228. Tchernia G: Immune thrombocytopenia and pregnancy. Curr Stud Hematol Blood Transfus 55:81, 1988

229. Scott JR, Cruikshank DP, Kochenour NK et al: Fetal platelet counts in the obstetric management of immunologic thrombocytopenia. Am J Obstet Gynecol 136:495, 1980

230. Kitzmiller JL: Autoimmune disorders: maternal, fetal and neonatal risks. Clin Obstet Gynecol 21:385, 1978

231. Cines DB, Dusak B, Tomeski A et al: Immune thrombocytopenia and pregnancy. N Engl J Med 306:826, 1982

232. Scott JR, Rote NS, Cruikshank DP: Antiplatelet antibodies and platelet counts in pregnancies complicated by autoimmune thrombocytopenia. Am J Obstet Gynecol 145:932, 1983

233. Bussel JB: Management of infants of mothers with immune thrombocytopenia. J Pediatr 113:497, 1988

234. Territo M, Finkelstein J, Oh W et al: Management of autoimmune thrombocytopenia in pregnancy and in the neonate. Obstet Gynecol 41:579, 1973

235. Ayromloei J: A new approach to the management of immunologic thrombocytopenic purpura in pregnancy. Am J Obstet Gynecol 130:235, 1978

236. Karpatkin M, Porges R, Karpatkin S: Platelet counts in infants of women with autoimmune thrombocytopenia. N Engl J Med 305:936, 1981

237. Giles C, Inglis TCM: Thrombocytopenia and macrothrombocytosis in gestational hypertension. Br J Obstet Gynecol 163:1147, 1990

238. Burrows RF, Kelton JG: Incidentally detected thrombocytopenia in healthy mothers and their infants. N Engl J Med 319:142, 1988

239. Nurden AT, Caen JP: An abnormal platelet glycoprotein pattern in three cases of Glanzmann's thrombasthenia. Br J Haematol 28:253, 1974

240. Phillips DR, Agin PP: Platelet membrane defects in Glanzmann's thrombasthenia: evidence for decreased amounts of two major glycoproteins. J Clin Invest 60:535, 1977

241. Seligsohn V, Mibashan RS, Rodeck CS et al: Prenatal diagnosis of Glanzmann's thrombasthenia. Lancet 2:1419, 1985

242. Champeix P, Forestier F, Daffos F, Kaplan C: Prenatal diagnosis of a molecular variant of Glanzmann's thrombasthenia. Curr Stud Hematol Blood Transfus 55:180, 1988

243. Daffos F, Forestier F, Kaplan C et al: Prenatal diagnosis and management of bleeding disorders with fetal blood sampling. Am J Obstet Gynecol 158:939, 1988

244. Wautier JL, Gruel Y: Prenatal diagnosis of platelet disorders. Baillieres Clin Haematol 2:569, 1989

245. Beardsley DS: Platelet abnormalities of infancy and childhood. p. 1589. In Nathan DG, Oski FA (eds): Hematology of Infancy and Childhood. WB Saunders, Philadelphia, 1993

246. Peng TC, Kickler TS, Bell WR, Haller E: Obstetric complications in a patient with Bernard-Soulier syndrome. Am J Obstet Gynecol 165:425, 1991

247. Gruel Y, Boizard B, Daffos F et al: Determination of the platelet antigens and glycoproteins in the human fetus. Blood 68:488, 1986

248. Peaceman AM, Katz AR, Laville M: Bernard-Soulier syndrome complicating pregnancy: a case report. Obstet Gynecol 73:457, 1989

249. Omenn CS, Figley MM, Graham CB et al: Prospects for radiographic intrauterine diagnosis: the syndrome of thrombocytopenia with absent radii. N Engl J Med 288:777, 1973

250. Luthy DA, Hall JG, Graham CB: Prenatal diagnosis of thrombocytopenia with absent radii. Clin Genet 15:495, 1979

251. Shalev E, Weiner E, Feldman E et al: Micrognathia—prenatal ultrasonograpic diagnosis. Int J Gynaecol Obstet 21:343, 1983

252. Luthy DA, Mack L, Hirsch J et al: Prenatal ultrasound diagnosis of thrombocytopenia with absent radii. Am J Obstet Gynecol 141:350, 1981

253. Filkins K, Russo J, Bilinki I et al: Prenatal diagnosis of thrombocytopenia-absent radii syndrome using ultrasound and fetoscopy. Prenat Diagn 4:139, 1984

254. Donnenfeld AE, Wiseman B, Lari E, Weiner S: Prenatal diagnosis of thrombocytopenia absent radii syndrome by ultrasound and cordocentesis. Prenat Diagn 10:29, 1990

255. Mibashan RS, Millar DS: Fetal haemophilia and allied bleeding disorders. Br Med Bull 39:392, 1983

256. Greinacher A, Mueller-Eckhardt C: Hereditary types of thrombocytopenias with giant platelets and inclusion bodies in the leukocytes. Blut 60:53, 1990

257. Andrew M, Paes B, Johnston M: Development of the hemostatic system in the neonate and young infant. Am J Pediatr Hematol Oncol 12:95, 1990

258. Heikenheimo R: Coagulation studies with fetal blood. Biol Neonate 7:319, 1964

259. Holmberg L, Henriksson P, Ekelund H, Astedt B: Coagulation in the human fetus, comparison with term, newborn infants. J Pediatr 85:860, 1974

260. Forestier F, Daffos F, Galacteros F et al: Hematological values of 163 normal fetuses between 18 and 30 weeks of gestation. Pediatr Res 20:342, 1986

261. Ginsburg D: The von Willebrand's factor gene and genetics of von Willebrand's disease. Mayo Clin Proc 66:506, 1991

262. Andrew M, Paes B, Milner R et al: Development of the human coagulation system in the healthy premature infant. Blood 72:1651, 1988

263. Hoyer LW, Lindsten J, Blomback M et al: Prenatal evaluation of a fetus at risk for severe von Willebrand's disease. Lancet 2:191, 1979

264. Daffos F, Forestier F, Kaplan C, Cox W: Prenatal diagnosis and management of bleeding disorders with fetal blood sampling. Am J Obstet Gynecol 158:939, 1988

265. Rothschild C, Forestier F, Daffos F et al: Prenatal diagnosis in type IIA von Willebrand disease. Nouv Rev Fr Hematol 32:125, 1990

266. Inbal A, Kornbrot N, Zivelin A et al: The inheritance of type I and type III von Willebrand's disease in Israel: linkage analysis, carrier detection and prenatal diagnosis using three intragenic restriction fragment length polymorphisms. Blood Coagul Fibrinolysis 3:167, 1992

267. Ginsburg D, Handin RI, Bonthron DT et al: Human VWF: isolation of complementary DNA (cDNA) clones and chromosomal localization. Science 228:1401, 1985

268. Peake IR, Bowen D, Bignell P et al: Family studies and prenatal diagnosis in severe von Willebrand disease by PCR amplification of a variable number tandem repeat region of the von Willebrand factor gene. Blood 76:555, 1990

269. Mannhalter C, Kyrle PA, Brenner B, Lechner K: Rapid neonatal diagnosis of type IIB von Willebrand's disease using the PCR. Blood 77:2539, 1991

270. Tedgard V, Ljung R, McNeil T et al: How do carriers of hemophilia experience prenatal diagnosis? Acta Paediatr Scand 78:692, 1989

271. Nossel HL, Lanzkowsky P, Levy et al: A study of coagulation factor levels in women during labour and in the newborn infant. Thromb Diath Haemorrh 16:185, 1966

272. Firshein SI, Hoyer LW, Lazarchick J et al: Prenatal diagnosis of classic hemophilia. N Engl J Med 300:937, 1979

273. Mibashan RS, Rodeck CH, Thumpston JK et al: Plasma assay of fetal factors VIIIC and IX for prenatal diagnosis of haemophilia. Lancet 1:1309, 1979

274. Peake IR, Bloom AL, Giddings JC, Ludlam CA: An immunoradiometric assay for procoagulant factor VIII antigen. Results in haemophilia, von Willebrand's disease and fetal plasma and serum. Br J Haematol 42:269, 1979

275. Holmberg L, Gusdtavii B, Cordesius E: Prenatal diagnosis of Hemophilia B by an immunoradiometric assay of Factor IX. Blood 56:397, 1980

276. Forestier F, Daffos F, Sole Y, Rainaut M: Prenatal diagnosis of hemophilia by fetal blood sampling under ultrasound guidance. Haemostasis 16:346, 1986

277. Bloom AL: The biosynthesis of factor VIII. Clin Haematol 8:53, 1979

278. Brocker-Vriends AHJT, Briet E, Quadt R et al: Genotype assignment of hemophilia A by use of intragenic and extragenic restriction fragment length polymorphisms. Thromb Haemost 57:131, 1987

279. Oberle I, Camerino G, Heilig R et al: Genetic screening for hemophilia A (classic hemophilia) with a polymorphic DNA probe. N Engl J Med 312:682, 1985

280. Antonarakis SE, Youssoufian H, Kazazian HH Jr: Molecular genetics of hemophilia in man (factor VIII deficiency). Mol Biol Med 4:81, 1987

281. Kazazian HH Jr, Wong C, Youssoufian H et al: Haemophilia A resulting from de novo in insertion of L1 sequences represents a novel mechanism for mutation in man. Nature 332:164, 1988

282. White GC II, Shoemaker CE: Factor VIII gene and hemophilia A. Blood 73:1, 1989

283. Tsang TC, Bentley DR, Nilsson IM, Giannelli F: The use of DNA amplification for genetic counselling related diagnosis in haemophilia. Thromb Haemost 61:343, 1991

284. Brochev-Vriends AHJJ, Briet E, Kanhai HHH et al: First trimester prenatal diagnosis of haemophilia A. Two years' experience. Prenat Diagn 8:411, 1988

285. Pecorara M, Casavino L, Mori PG, Morfini M: Hemaophilia A: carrier detection and prenatal diagnosis by DNA analysis. Blood 70:531, 1987

286. Van de Water NS, Ockelford PA, Berry EW, Browett PJ: Hemophilia management: the application of DNA analysis for prenatal diagnosis. N Z Med J 104:443, 1991

287. Brocher-Vriends AHJT, Bakker E, Kanhai HHH et al: The contribution of DNA analysis to carrier detection and prenatal diagnosis of hemophilia A and B. Ann Hematol 64:2, 1992

288. Sampietro M, Camerino G, Romano M et al: Combined use of DNA probes in first trimester prenatal diagnosis of hemophilia A. Thromb Haemost 58:988, 1987

289. Yoshioka A, Naka H, Nishimma T et al: First trimester prenatal diagnosis of haemophilia A using a factor VIII gene probe. Jpn J Hum Genet 34:135, 1989

290. Chistolini A, Papacchini M, Mazzucconi MG et al: Carrier detection and prenatal diagnosis in haemophilia A and B. Haematologica 75:424, 1990

291. La Vergue JM, Laurian Y, Dudilleaux A et al: Carrier detection and prenatal diagnosis in 98 families of hemophilia A by linkage analysis and direct detection of mutations. Blood Coagul Fibrinolysis 2:293, 1991

292. Peake I: Carrier detection and prenatal diagnosis of hemophilia, present and future strategies. Res Clin Lab 20:177, 1990

293. Hay CW, Robertson KA, Yong 52 et al: Use of Bam HI polymorphism in the factor IX gene for the determination of haemophilia B carrier status. Blood 67:1508, 1986

294. Winship PR, Brownlee GG: Diagnosis of hemophilia B carriers using intragenic oligonucleotide probes. Lancet 2:218, 1986

295. Brocker-Vriends AHJT, Briet E, Quadt R et al: Carrier detection of haemophilia B by using an intragenic restriction fragment length polymorphism. Thromb Haemost 54:506, 1985

296. Tanimoto M, Kojima T, Ogata K et al: Extragenic factor IX gene RFLP is useful for detecting carriers of Japanese haemophilia B. Acta Haematol Jpn 52:774, 1989

297. Graham JB, Green PP, McGraw RA, Daws LM: Application of molecular genetics to prenatal diagnosis and carrier detection in the hemophilias: some limitations. Blood 66:759, 1985

298. Guillin MC, Bezeard A, Rabiet MJ, Elion J: Congenitally abnormal prothrombin and thrombin. Ann NY Acad Sci 485:56, 1986

299. Baude F, de Cataldo F, Josso F, Silvello L: Hereditary hypoprothmonbinaemia: the deficiency of factor II. Acta Haematol 47:243, 1972

300. WHO Scientific Group: Inherited blood clotting disorders. Tech Rep Ser WHO 1, 1972

301. Caldwell DC, Williamson RA, Goldsmith JC: Hereditary coagulopathies in pregnancy. Clin Obstet Gynecol 28:53, 1985

302. Watzke HH, Lechner K, Roberts HR et al: Molecular defect (Gla +14 − Lys) and its functional consequences in a hereditary factor X deficiency (factor X Vorarlberg). J Biol Chem 265:11982, 1990

303. Scambler PJ, Williamson R: The structural gene for human coagulation factor X is located on chromosome 13q34. Cytogenet Cell Genet 39:231, 1985

304. Bolton-Maggs PHB, Wan-Yin BY, McCraw AH et al: Inheritance and bleeding in factor XI deficiency. Br J Haematol 69:521, 1988

305. Ratnoff OD, Colopy JE: A familial hemorrhagic trait associated with a deficiency of a clot-promoting fraction of plasma. J Clin Invest 34:602, 1955

306. Dukert F: Documentation of the plasma factor XIII deficiency in man. Ann NY Acad Sci 202:190, 1972

307. Roberts HR, Lozier JN: Other clotting factor deficiencies. p. 1332. In Hoffman R, Benz EJ Jr, Shattil SJ. Hematology: Basic Principles and Practice. 1st Ed. Churchill Livingstone, New York, 1991

308. Daffos F, Forestier F, Kaplan C, Cox W: Prenatal diagnosis and management of bleeding disorders with fetal blood sampling. Am J Obstet Gynecol 158:939, 1988

309. Griffin JH, Evatt B, Zimmermann TS et al: Deficiency of protein C in congenital thrombolic disease. J Clin Invest 68:1370, 1981

310. Mahasandana C, Suvatte V, Marlar R et al: Neonatal purpura fulminans associated with homozygous protein S deficiency. Lancet 1:61, 1990

311. Marlar RA, Montgomery RR, Broekmans AW: Diagnosis and treatment of homozygous protein C deficiency. J Pediatr 114:5287, 1989

312. Polack B, Pouzol P, Amiral J, Kolodie L: Protein C level at birth. Thromb Haematol 52:188, 1984

313. Patracchini P, Aiello V, Pallazzi P et al: Sublocalization of human protein C gene in chromosome 2q13-q14. Hum Genet 81:191, 1989

314. Yamamoto K, Tanimoto M, Matsushita T et al: Genotype establishments for protein C deficiency by use of a DNA polymorphism in the gene. Blood 77:2633, 1991

315. Lundwall A, Dackowski W, Cohen E et al: Isolation and sequence of the cDNA for human protein S, a regulator of blood coagulation. Proc Natl Acad Sci USA 83:6716, 1986

316. Hoskins JA, Neuman K, Beckmann RJ, Long GL: Cloning and characterization of human liver cDNA encoding a protein S precursor. Proc Natl Acad Sci USA 84:349, 1987

317. Reitsma PH, Ploos van Amstel HK, Poort BR et al: Molecular basis of hereditary protein C and protein S deficiency. Curr Stud Hematol Blood Transfus 58:94, 1991

318. Fisher AM, Cornu P, Sternberg C et al: AT III Alger: a new homozygous AT II variant. Thromb Haemost 55:218, 1986

319. Boyer C, Wolf M, Vedrenne J et al: Homozygous variant of AT III: AT III Fontainebleau. Thromb Haemost 56:18, 1986

320. Andrew M, Paes B, Johnston M: Development of the hemostatic system in the neonate and young infant. Am J Pediatr Hematol Oncol 12:95, 1990

321. Aldinolfi M: On a noninvasive approach to prenatal diagnosis based on the detection of fetal nucleated cells in maternal blood samples. Prenat Diagn 11:799, 1991

322. Aldinolfi M: Fetal nucleated cells in the maternal circulation. In Brock DJ, Rodeck CH, Ferguson-Smith MA (eds): Prenatal Diagnosis Screening. Churchill Livingstone, Edinburgh, 1991

323. Aldinolfi M, Camporese C, Carr T: Gene amplification to detect fetal nucleated cell in pregnant women. Lancet 2:318, 1990

324. Bianchi DW, Flint AF, Pizziment MF et al: Isolation of fetal DNA from nucleated erythrocytes in maternal blood. Proc Natl Acad Sci USA 87:3279, 1990

325. Camaschella C, Alfarano A, Gottard E et al: Prenatal diagnosis of fetal hemoglobin Lepore-Boston disease on maternal peripheral blood. Blood 75:2102, 1990

326. Ganshirt-Ahlert D, Burschyk M, Garritsen HSP et al: Magnetic cell sorting and the transferrin receptor as potential means of prenatal diagnosis from maternal peripheral blood. Am J Obstet Gynecol 166:1350, 1992

327. Bruch JF, Metezean P, Garcia-Fonkechten N et al: Trophoblast like cells sorted from peripheral maternal blood using flow cytometry: a multi-parametric study involving transmission electron microscopy and fetal DNA amplification. Prenat Diagn 11:787, 1991

328. Covane AE, Mutton D, Van Dam M et al: Fetal lymphocytes and trophoblast cells in maternal circulation. p. 12. In Proceedings of the International Symposium on Early Diagnosis: Present and Future. Naples, 1984

329. Griffith-Jones MD, Miller D, Lilford RJ, Scott J: Detection of fetal DNA in trans-cervical swabs from first trimester pregnancies by gene amplification: a new route to prenatal diagnosis? Br J Obstet Gynecol 99:508, 1992

330. Touraine JL: Bone marrow and fetal liver transplantation in immunodeficiencies and inborn errors of metabolism: lack of significant restriction of T-cell function in long-term chimeras despite HLA-mismatch. Immunol Rev 71:103, 1983

331. Touraine JL, Raudrant D, Rebaud A et al: In utero transplantation of stem cells in humans: immunological aspects and clinical follow-up of patients. Bone Marrow Transplant 9:121, 1992

332. Diukman R, Golbus MS: In utero stem cell therapy. J Reprod Med 37:515, 1992

333. Sellers MJ, Poloni PE: Experimental chimerism in a genetic defect in the house mouse *Mus musculus*. Nature 212:80, 1966

334. Fleischman RA, Mintz B: Prevention of genetic anemias in mice by microinjection of normal hematopoietic stem cells into the fetal placenta. Proc Natl Acad Sci USA 76:5736, 1979

335. Zanjani ED, Mackintosh FR, Harrison MR: Hematopoietic chimerism, in sheep and nonhuman primates by in utero transplantation of fetal hematopoietic stem cells. Blood Cells 17:349, 1991

336. Crombleholme TM, Harrison MR, Zanjani ED: In utero transplantation of hematopoietic stem cells in sheep: the role of T cells in engraftment and graft-versus-host disease. J Pediatr Surg 25:885, 1990

37. Harrison MR, Stotnick RN, Crombleholme TM et al: In utero transplantation of fetal liver haemopoietic stem cells in monkeys. Lancet 2:1425, 1989

38. Touraine JL, Raudrant D, Royo C et al: In utero transplantation of stem cells in a patient with the bare lymphocyte syndrome. Lancet 1:1382, 1989

39. Touraine JL: The fetal liver as a source of stem cells for transplantation into fetuses in utero. Curr Top Microbiol Immunol 177:187, 1992

40. Linch DC, Rodeck CH, Nicolaides K et al: Attempted bone marrow transplantation in a 17 week fetus. Lancet 2:1953, 1986

41. Touraine JL, Raudrant D, Rebaud A et al: In utero stem cell transplantation in human fetuses. Exp Hematol 18:657, 1990

42. Slavin S, Naparstek E, Ziegler M et al: Intrauterine bone marrow transplantation for correction of genetic disorders in man. Exp Hematol 18:658, 1990

43. Touraine JL, Raudrant D, Vullo C et al: New developments in stem cell transplantation with special reference to the first in utero transplants in humans. Bone Marrow Transplant 7:92, 1991

44. Touraine JL, Roncarolo MG, Royo C, Touraine F: Fetal tissue transplantation, bone marrow transplantation and prospective gene therapy in severe immunodeficiencies and enzyme deficiencies. Thymus 10:75, 1987

45. Raudrant D, Touraine JL, Rebaud A: In utero transplantation of stem cells in humans: technical aspects and clinical experience during pregnancy. Bone Marrow Transplant 9:98, 1992

46. Flake AW, Harrison MR, Adzick S et al: Transplantation of fetal hematopoietic stem cells in utero: the creation of hematopoietic chimeras. Science 233:776, 1986

47. Touraine JL: Rationale and results of in utero transplants of stem cells in humans. Bone Marrow Transplant 9:121, 1992

48. Gluckman E: Fetal and neonatal hemopoietic stem cells: considerations in transplantation. Nouv Rev Fr Hematol 32:421, 1990

49. Constantini F, Chada K, Magram J: Correction of murine β-thalassemia by gene transfer into the germ line. Science 233:1192, 1986

50. Eglitis ME, Kantoff PW, Gilboa E, Anderson WF: Gene expression in mice after high efficiency retroviral-mediated gene transfer. Science 230:1395, 1985

51. Friedman T: Progress toward human gene therapy. Science 244:1275, 1989

52. Nabel EG, Plantz G, Boyce FM et al: Recombinant gene expression in vivo within endothelial cells of the arterial wall. Science 244:1342, 1989

353. Wilson JM, Birinyi LK, Salomon RN et al: Implantation of vascular grafts lined with genetically modified endothelial cells. Science 244:1344, 1989

354. Kantoff PW, Flake AW, Eglitis MA et al: In utero gene transfer and expression: a sheep transplantation model. Blood 73:1066, 1989

355. Ekhtarae D, Crombleholme T, Karson E et al: Retroviral vector-mediated transfer of the bacterial neomycin resistance gene into fetal and adult sheep and human hematopoietic progenitors in vitro. Blood 75:365, 1990

356. Clark RD, Fletcher J, Petersen G: Conceiving a fetus for bone marrow donation: an ethical problem in prenatal diagnosis. Prenat Diagn 9:329, 1989

357. Thymstra TJ, Bajema C, Beekhuis JR, Mantingh A: Women's opinions on the offer and use of prenatal diagnosis. Prenat Diagn 11:893, 1991

358. Modell BR, Ward HT, Fairweather VI: Effect of introducing antenatal diagnosis on reproductive behavior of families at risk for thalassemia major. BMJ 1:1347, 1980

359. Modell BP, Petron M: Review of control programs and future trends in the United Kingdom. p. 433. In Fucharoen S, Rowley PT, Paul NW (eds): Thalassemia: Pathology and Management. Alan R Liss, New York, 1988

360. Rowley PT: Prenatal diagnosis for sickle cell disease—a survey of the United States and Canada. Ann NY Acad Sci 565:48, 1989

361. Jeffery R, Jeffery P, Lyon A: Female infanticide and amniocentesis. Soc Sci Med 19:1207, 1984

362. Schaison GS: The child conceived to give life: the point of view of the hematologist. Bone Marrow Transplant 9:93, 1992

363. Satish J: Prenatal genetics in laboratory medicine: a cytogeneticist's perspective. Reprod Med 12:493, 1992

364. Robertson JA: Legal and ethical issues arising from the new genetics. J Reprod Med 37:521, 1992

365. Touraine JL: Transplantation of fetal haemopoietic and lymphopoietic cells in humans, with special reference to in utero transplantation. p. 155. In Edwards RG (ed): Fetal Tissue Transplants in Medicine. Cambridge University Press, Cambridge, 1992

366. Fine A: The ethics of fetal tissue transplants. Hastings Cent Rep 18:5, 1988

367. Antley RM: Variable in the outcome of genetic counseling. Soc Biol 23:108, 1976

368. Sorenson JR, Swazey JP, Scotch NA: Reproductive pasts, reproductive futures: genetic counseling and its effectiveness. Birth Defects 17:1, 1981

369. Rowley PT, Loader S, Sutera CJ, et al: Prenatal screening for hemoglobinopathies. I. A prospective regional trial. Am J Hum Genet 48:439, 1991

Electrophoretic and Immunochemical Analysis of Human Immunoglobulins

163

John P. Leddy

INTRODUCTION

Human immunoglobulins occur in five classes, based on amino acid sequence differences in the constant regions of their heavy polypeptide chains. A given immunoglobulin molecule may have either κ or λ light chains, a distinction determined by primary structural differences in the constant regions of the molecule. The various immunoglobulin heavy chain classes and subclasses (Table 163-1), termed isotypes, are encoded by immunoglobulin genes on chromosome 14. κ and λ light chain genes are encoded on chromosomes 2 and 22, respectively. Detailed information on immunoglobulin genes,

on B-cell development and activation, and on molecular structure and biologic functions of immunoglobulins is given in Chapter 8. The availability of heavy chain-specific antisera that identify γ-, μ-, α-, δ-, or ε-chains, and light chain-specific antisera that recognize κ- or λ-chains, is central to two of the principal methods for analysis of human immunoglobulins.[1] Of greatest utility in clinical diagnostic laboratories are polyclonal antisera, usually prepared in goats or rabbits. At this time, monoclonal antibodies have a more limited role because they precipitate poorly with the proteins to which they are directed, and their use therefore requires additional steps to immobilize the protein(s) of interest.

Table 163-1. Selected Properties of Immunoglobulins in Human Serum

Class (isotypes)	Heavy Chain Type	Light Chain Type	Molecular Weight	Normal Adult Serum Concentration[a]	Subclasses (%)	Normal Electrophoretic Mobility (range)	Half-Life (days)	Other Comments
IgG	γ	κ or λ	150,000	565–1,765 mg/dl[b]	IgG1 (62–70)[e] IgG2 (11–33) IgG3 (3–6) IgG4 (0.5–6)	From most cathodal portion of γ-globulin area to α_2-globulin region	23	Crosses placenta; neonatal levels approximate adult concentration; some IgG myelomas are euglobulins[f]
IgA	α	κ or λ	170,000 (monomer)	85–385 mg/dl[b]	IgA1 IgA2	From fast γ- to β_1-globulin area	6	In IgA myeloma a portion of paraprotein may form higher molecular weight polymers that differ from monomer in electrophoretic mobility
IgM	μ	κ or λ	900,000 (Pentamer)	45–250 mg/dl[b]	None recognized	From fast γ- to β_2-globulin area	5	In Waldenström macroglobulinemia significant IgM monomer may be present; IgM paraproteins often are euglobulins[f]
IgD	δ	κ or λ	185,000	0 to trace[c]	None recognized	Similar to IgM and IgA	2	Concentration in normal serum too low to be detected by zone electrophoresis, IEP, or IFE; rare myeloma; vary rare HCD
IgE	ϵ	κ or λ	200,000	10–200 IU/ml[d]	None recognized	Similar to IgM and IgA	2	Concentration in normal serum too low to be detected by zone electrophoresis, IEP, or IFE; very rare myeloma; elevated levels in allergic or parasitic diseases

Abbreviations: IEP, immunoelectrophoresis; IFE, immunofixation electrophoresis; HCD, heavy chain disease.
[a] See Table 163-2 for age-adjusted changes in concentrations of IgG, IgA, and IgM.
[b] By nephelometry.
[c] Undetectable in many normal individuals.
[d] By ELISA assay. Mayo Medical Laboratories (Rochester, MN), using a radioimmunoassay, lists a normal adult range of 20–367 U/ml.
[e] Approximate percentage of total IgG (data from Specialty Laboratories, Inc., Santa Monica, CA 90404).
[f] Euglobulins are insoluble in the low ionic strength buffers commonly employed in electrophoretic procedures, including IEP and IFE. This property often causes spontaneous precipitation at or near the origin and impedes analysis (see text).

Most pathologic immunoglobulin disorders involve IgG, IgA, and IgM, which are emphasized in this chapter. IgD and IgE occur in only trace amounts in normal sera (Table 163-1) and cannot be detected by the standard electrophoretic methods currently in use unless the concentration of these proteins is abnormally elevated, as in the rare IgD or IgE myelomas.

CONCEPTS OF MONOCLONAL AND POLYCLONAL IMMUNOGLOBULINS

One of the most striking features of the immunoglobulins synthesized by normal individuals is their heterogeneity, not only with respect to class, subclass, and light chain type, but also as reflected by an enormous diversity in antibody specificity. The latter property is related to amino acid differences in the variable regions of the heavy and light chains making up the immunoglobulin molecule. Each antibody with its unique primary structure arises from a unique B cell and its progeny (i.e., a clone). However, there are so many clones contributing to the immunoglobulin pool in normal serum that the immunoglobulin molecules produced by an individual clone cannot be detected within the collective background of immunoglobulins synthesized by all the other clones. Thus, the great heterogeneity of immunoglobulins in normal serum reflects their highly polyclonal origin.

All of the immunoglobulins synthesized by a clone of antibody-forming cells share identical amino acid sequences in both constant and variable regions and therefore are identical in class, subclass, and light chain type. Postsynthetic glycosylation of heavy chain constant regions varies among the immunoglobulin classes but is generally similar for immunoglobulin molecules formed by a given clone. It follows from these principles that the immunoglobulin proteins arising from a single clone typically have the same net electrical charge and therefore the same electrophoretic mobility. Such immunoglobulin proteins migrate electrophoretically as a very sharp, dense band. This is in contrast to the broader, polydisperse migration of normal serum immunoglobulins that reflect synthesis by a vast number of clones. At the molecular level, this electrophoretic (charge) heterogeneity of normal immunoglobulins is thought to be determined mainly by primary sequence differences in the immunoglobulin variable regions, but with some contributions from their class and subclass. Thus, antibodies with specificity for a given antigenic epitope may have a monoclonal origin and, if so, would be expected to exhibit a sharply restricted electrophoretic mobility. However, the quantity of immunoglobulin synthesized by each clone of antibody-forming cells is normally modulated in such a way that its immunoglobulin products do not "stand out from the pack" of immunoglobulins contributed by all the other clones. By contrast, in myeloma, Waldenström macroglobulinemia, some B-cell lymphomas, heavy chain diseases, or primary amyloidosis, a single clone of plasma cells or immunoglobulin-synthesizing B lymphocytes emerges from the general B-cell population, expands in an unregulated fashion, and synthesizes a homogeneous immunoglobulin product at a high enough rate to be detectable against the background of polyclonal immunoglobulins.

In this chapter, the historical term *paraprotein* is sometimes used to designate such a monoclonal immunoglobulin, even though the original concept that all monoclonal proteins represent intrinsically defective molecules, having no counterpart in the normal host, is no longer accepted. On the other hand, heavy chain disease, in which only portions of an immunoglobulin heavy chain are synthesized, and light chain disease (Bence Jones myeloma), in which qualitatively "normal" light chains are synthesized and secreted without heavy chains, do represent disordered synthesis beyond the abnormality of uncontrolled clonal expansion.

METHODS FOR CLINICAL EVALUATION OF HUMAN IMMUNOGLOBULINS

Current assessments of abnormalities of human immunoglobulins in serum, urine, or other body fluids utilize zone electrophoresis, immunoelectrophoresis (IEP), and immunofixation electrophoresis (IFE) for qualitative and semiquantitative analysis; nephelometry or radial immunodiffusion are used for quantitative assays. Other specialized procedures are employed for evaluation of anomalous proteins such as cryoglobulins.

Zone Electrophoresis

All electrophoretic methods separate proteins within a complex mixture by virtue of differences in their net electrochemical charges. Zone electrophoresis is a general term for procedures that subject proteins to an electrical field in or on a supporting matrix that permits subsequent fixation of the separated proteins and their detection by staining with protein-binding dyes. The supporting medium for historically the most familiar form of zone electrophoresis consists of strips of cellulose acetate. Agarose gels, supported on a clear plastic film sheet, are now widely used to produce a stained zone electrophoretic pattern and are replacing cellulose acetate as the standard medium because of their capacity to resolve serum into a greater number of discrete bands.[2] After fixation and drying, stained zone electrophoretic patterns (on cellulose acetate or dried agarose gels) can be scanned by a densitometer to produce a tracing in which each band in the stained pattern is "translated" into an inscribed peak whose height and width reflect the intensity and electrophoretic dispersity, respectively, of the band being scanned. When this is applied to serum separated on cellulose acetate, the traditional serum protein electrophoresis (SPEP) profile results (Fig. 163-1A). By determining the total protein concentration in the sample, each main peak (e.g., albumin, α_1- or α_2-globulins, β-globulin, or γ-globulin) can be assigned an approximate protein concentration (by mathematical integration). Similar analyses are performed with stained protein patterns obtained by zone electrophoresis in agarose. Such patterns are shown in the uppermost sections of

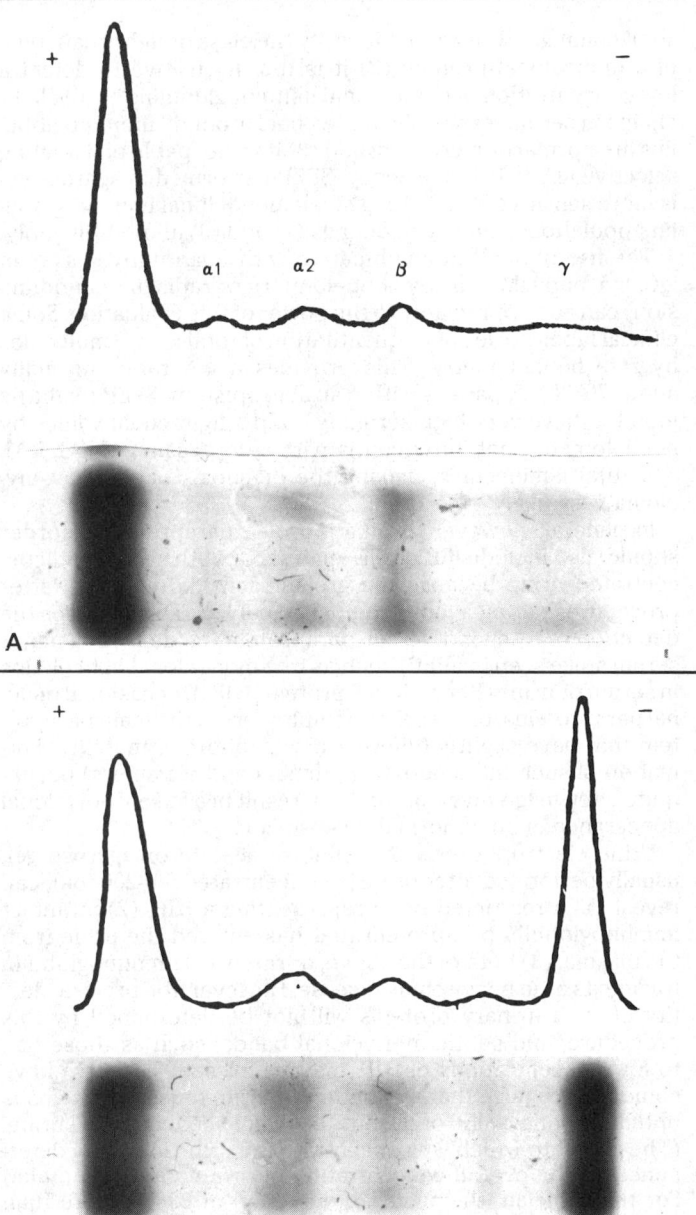

Fig. 163-1. Zone electrophoresis on cellulose acetate with densitometric scans. **(A)** Normal human serum. **(B)** Serum with large monoclonal spike in the mid γ-globulin area. Note that background of normal polyclonal γ-globulin on either side of the spike is severely diminished. Further evaluation by IEP revealed that the monoclonal spike was IgG-κ.

each of the immunofixation electrophoresis figures presented below.

It must be remembered that the classic γ-globulin peak does not encompass the full range of immunoglobulin mobilities. Some human immunoglobulins migrate as β-globulins and occasionally into the α_2-globulin area. By convention, an immunoglobulin population (with a negative net charge) that migrates more strongly toward the positive pole (anode) is said to have "fast" electrophoretic mobility, and immunoglobulin molecules found close to the cathode are said to be "slow."

SPEP performed on cellulose acetate has been widely employed for many years as a screening test for evaluation of serum immunoglobulins. This technique can establish the presence of moderate-to-large monoclonal spikes (Fig. 163-1B), polyclonal hypergammaglobulinemia, or generalized (pan-)hypogammaglobulinemia. By itself this method has significant shortcomings: (1) it cannot identify the class or light chain type of a monoclonal protein; (2) it is too insensitive to detect a low concentration of monoclonal immunoglobulins or free light chains in serum, especially if the "background" immunoglobulins are normal or increased; and (3) it is incapable of detecting selective IgA or IgM deficiency. SPEP performed in agarose gel is more sensitive in detecting small monoclonal immunoglobulin populations, but shortcomings (1) and (3) above still apply.

The use of SPEP in combination with quantitative assay of IgG, IgA, and IgM (e.g., by nephelometry or radial immunodiffusion) can add appreciably to the power of this evaluation. Some clinical laboratories offer quantitation of total κ- or λ-molecules by rate nephelometry. This provides a κ/λ ratio (normally about 70:30). A patient with a sizable spike by SPEP might be found to have very high serum IgA and λ light chain values by nephelometry, not infrequently with a depression of IgG, IgM, and total κ-molecules, making the diagnosis of an IgA λ-myeloma very likely.

In general, however, evaluation of a paraprotein disorder should also include IEP or IFE analysis of both serum and concentrated urine because the greater sensitivity of the latter procedures permit a more complete analysis. This includes the detection of a second, lesser paraprotein (aside from a major serum spike seen in SPEP) such as free monoclonal light chains in serum or urine (Bence Jones protein [BJP]), occasional biclonal paraproteins, or presence of multimers of the main paraprotein that have slightly different electrophoretic mobility. Formation of such multimers (e.g., dimers and tetramers) occurs quite often in IgA myeloma and can result in a falsely polyclonal appearance of an abnormal peak seen in SPEP.

Urine electrophoresis on cellulose acetate or agarose gel, usually performed after urine is concentrated 50–200-fold, can reveal (1) a restricted band representing a BJP, (2) an intact immunoglobulin paraprotein that has entered the urine from the plasma, (3) both of the above, or rarely (4) immunoglobulin fragments as in heavy chain disease. However, the precise identity of such urinary proteins will not be determined by this procedure, and subtle monoclonal bands, such as those due to low concentrations of BJP, may be missed. Thus, we have come to recognize that evaluation of urine for paraproteins is optimally done by IEP or IFE on 50–200-fold concentrated urine. (The extent to which we concentrate the urine is largely determined by the overall concentration of protein in the sample.) For the clinician, the accurate detection of BJP is more than academic, since the presence of BJP is associated with a greater risk of amyloidosis and renal disease ("myeloma kidney"). In some patients who eventually prove to have primary amyloidosis, a low concentration of monoclonal light chains in the urine may be a decisive clue. Thus, evaluation for a paraprotein disorder should always include appropriate studies of urine as well as serum. A 24-hour collection of urine is not necessary for this diagnostic study; the current, highly sensitive IEP or IFE analysis of concentrated urine requires only 100 ml of a random voiding. By contrast, serial quantitative assay of urinary light chains has been used in some centers for judging the efficacy of therapy; this type of assay does require a 24-hour collection.

Immunoelectrophoresis

IEP is a most versatile and broadly effective procedure for the detection of pathologic proteins in serum and urine.[1] In this method a thin (2–2.5 mm) layer of agar gel dissolved in 50 mM barbital buffer (pH 8.2) is formed on the surface of glass slides or on 85 × 100-mm clear, flexible plastic film sheets (Gel Bond). (Agar, rather than its purified constituent, agarose, is commonly used in IEP because its higher endosmotic [reverse] flow positions the immunoglobulins advantageously for analy-

sis.) The patient's serum or concentrated urine is placed in a small well punched into the agar, and a similar well on the same gel receives normal human serum as a control. The slides (or film sheets) are placed in the electrophoresis apparatus connected to the buffer wells by wicks, and then subjected to an electrical field at room temperature. After a predetermined period, or based on movement of a marker dye, the current is stopped, the agar-containing slides are removed from the electrophoresis apparatus, and narrow troughs are cut parallel to, and on either side of, the path of protein migration (Fig. 163-2). Each trough is filled with selected polyclonal antisera to human immunoglobulins, and the slides are kept in a moist environment overnight at room temperature. The antibodies then diffuse from the trough into the neutral agar, where they meet their corresponding antigens (i.e., human immunoglobulins or other serum proteins) that have migrated to various points in the agar during the electrophoretic phase of the procedure. When antigen and antibody meet, a smooth curvilinear arc of precipitation is formed (Fig. 163-2). This arc of precipitation demonstrates both the presence and the electrophoretic dispersion of the protein recognized by the antiserum. The intensity and position of the arc also provide a semiquantitative estimate of the concentration of that protein present in the patient's serum. Thus, IEP is a two-phase procedure: electrophoretic separation and immunoprecipitation. In common laboratory practice, the chief diagnostic interest concerns the immunoglobulins; accordingly, polyclonal anti-γ-, anti-α-, anti-μ-, anti-κ-, and anti-λ-antibodies are routinely employed to develop such precipitin arcs.

Figure 163-3 displays an IEP pattern of a serum with a large monoclonal IgG-κ spike (lower patterns in Fig. 163-3A&B). The key diagnostic feature is the localized bulge or bowing in both the IgG arc and the κ-arc. Note that these two arcs show bowing in precisely the same electrophoretic position (i.e., the abnormality in the IgG arc and in the κ-arc is attributable to the same molecule). The bulge or bowing in these IgG and κ-arcs result from an extremely high concentration of identical molecules that have the same net charge and migrate to one highly localized point during the electrophoretic separation; they then diffuse as a molecular cohort into the oncoming anti-γ- or anti-κ-antibodies from the troughs. The bowing or displacement of the IgG and κ-arcs toward the antibody source (lower patterns in Fig. 163-3A&B) actually result from the shift in the equilibrium point for antigen-antibody precipitation. Antigen excess (i.e., the high concentration of monoclonal IgG-κ) "drives" the region of optimal precipitation toward the antibody trough. By

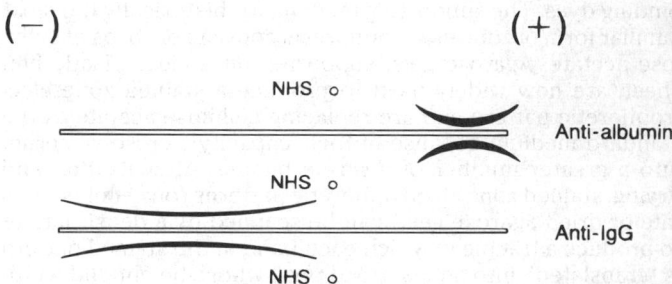

Fig. 163-2. Schematic diagram of IEP analysis of normal human serum (NHS) using each of two specific antisera. The serum was placed in each of the small wells and subjected to electrophoresis, resulting in migration of more negatively charged albumin to the anode and IgG toward the cathode. However, the distribution of albumin or IgG cannot be visualized until the long troughs in the gel are filled with specific antialbumin or anti-IgG and diffusion allowed to occur. Each antibody "finds" and precipitates with its corresponding protein antigen. These reactions produce curvilinear arcs of precipitation that identify the corresponding serum protein and delineate its electrophoretic distribution.

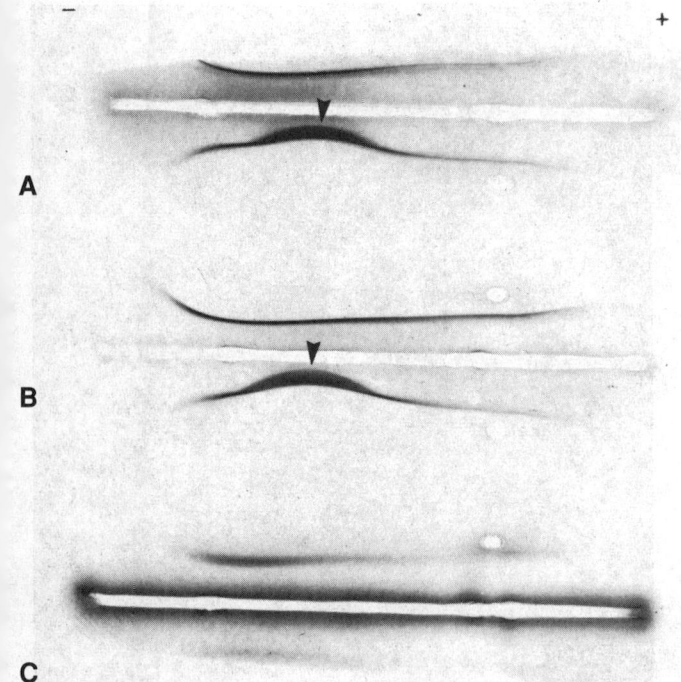

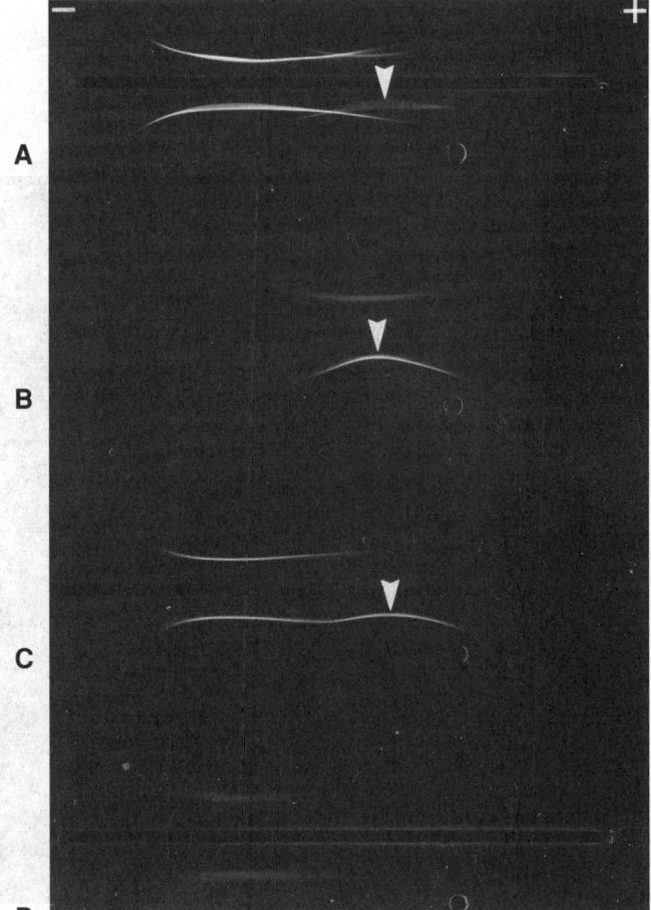

ig. 163-3. IEP analysis of a serum containing a large IgG-κ myeloma protein. or the initial electrophoretic separation in the agar gel, the upper small wells in ach pairing received normal serum and the lower wells received the patient's serum. At the conclusion of the electrophoretic separation, monospecific antisera o **(A)** human γ-chains (IgG-specific), **(B)** κ-chains, and **(C)** λ-chains were added .o the longitudinal troughs. For ease of illustration, results with antisera of other specificities are not shown. Arrowheads point to the abnormal bowing in the IgG and κ-arcs that indicates the presence of an IgG-κ monoclonal protein. This is a photograph of the stained, dried IEP pattern retained as a permanent record. Actual day-to-day readings are done on freshly developed, unstained "wet" gels visualized by indirect illumination (see Figs. 163-4, 163-5, and 163-7).

Fig. 163-4. IEP analysis of an IgA myeloma protein of moderate size. As in Figure 163-3, the upper wells in each pairing contained normal serum and the patient's serum was placed in the lower wells. The troughs contained antisera as follows: **(A)** Polyspecific antiserum to IgG, IgA, and IgM (the faint IgM arcs are not clearly seen in this photo); **(B)** antiserum to human α-chain (IgA-specific); **(C)** anti-κ-chains; and **(D)** anti-λ-chains. Localized bowing and thickening of the IgA arc (arrowheads) are apparent in both lane A and lane B, reflecting the presence of an IgA paraprotein. In lane C, the κ-curve is biphasic, with the more anodal portion mirroring the IgA paraprotein arc and the more cathodal portion reflecting the normal presence of κ-chains in the patient's polyclonal IgG population (compare the strong IgG curve in lane A). In lane D, λ-molecules in the patient's serum are polydisperse. This gel was photographed "wet."

contrast, the IgG and κ-precipitin arcs produced by normal serum are smooth, continuous curves without localized bowing or displacement (Fig. 163-3, upper patterns). Note that the polydisperse precipitin arc produced by anti-λ-antibody with this myeloma serum is significantly weaker than that obtained with normal serum (Fig. 163-3C). This indicates a depressed level of the polyclonal λ-immunoglobulin type in the serum containing the IgG-κ spike. Such reciprocal depression of normal (background) immunoglobulin concentrations is common in advanced myeloma.

The IEP pattern of an IgA-κ myeloma protein is shown in Figure 163-4. IgA paraproteins typically have a "fast" γ- or β-globulin mobility. This is also true of some IgM paraproteins, as well as the rarely encountered IgD or IgE paraproteins. However, some IgG paraproteins also migrate in this area. Figure 163-5A demonstrates a monoclonal protein with β-globulin mobility that proved to be IgG-λ. This patient had primary amyloidosis. Despite heavy generalized proteinuria, the same monoclonal IgG-λ protein was identified in the urine (Fig. 163-5B). Free λ light chains (BJP) were not detected.

The use of IEP to demonstrate λ-type BJP in concentrated urine is demonstrated in Figure 163-6. It should be borne in mind that 50- or 200-fold concentrated urine from healthy individuals often displays "free" *polyclonal* light chains (both κ-type and λ-type) by either IEP or IFE. Finally, Figure 163-7 illustrates an instance in which a myeloma *serum* contained two monoclonal populations, a more cathodally migrating IgG-λ paraprotein and slightly "faster" migrating type λ light chains without an associated heavy chain. The latter were present in the urine in even higher concentration as BJPs (not shown),

as would be expected for free light chains. BJPs often have a greater net negative charge (faster mobility) than the intact monoclonal immunoglobulin of the same patient.

IEP not only can establish the class and light chain type of an immunoglobulin population directly, but it also can provide critical evidence as to whether it is a monoclonal or polyclonal immunoglobulin and information on whether the "background" immunoglobulins are normal or depressed. In advanced myeloma, with a large monoclonal spike or with only BJP in the urine, it is common to observe depression of normal background immunoglobulin levels. When severe, this depression of normal polyclonal immunoglobulin may be associated with an increased risk of bacterial infection. Moreover, in the absence of a detectable serum paraprotein, hypogammaglobulinemia in an older patient may be an important clue to the presence of Bence Jones myeloma, in which case IEP or IFE of urine will provide decisive evidence.

The sensitivity of IEP is a major asset for the detection and isotyping of monoclonal proteins, yet there are situations in

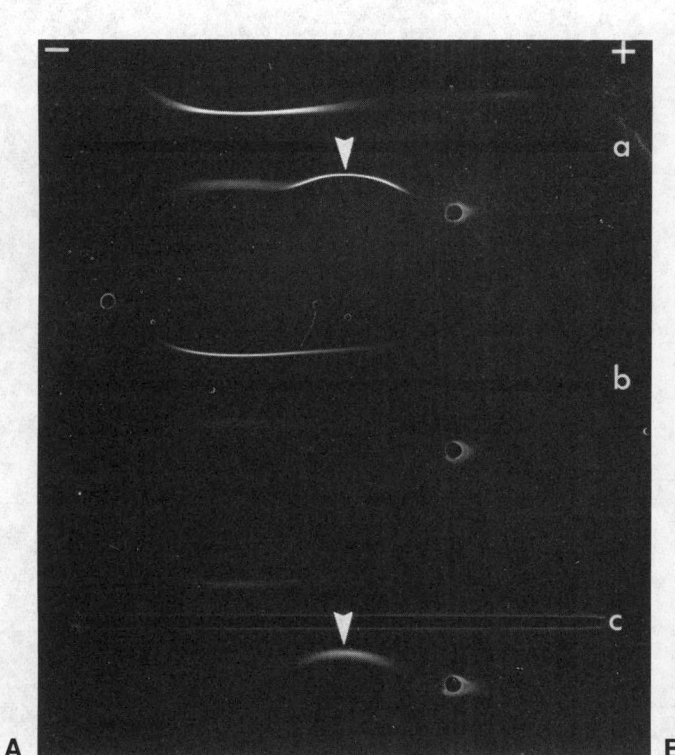

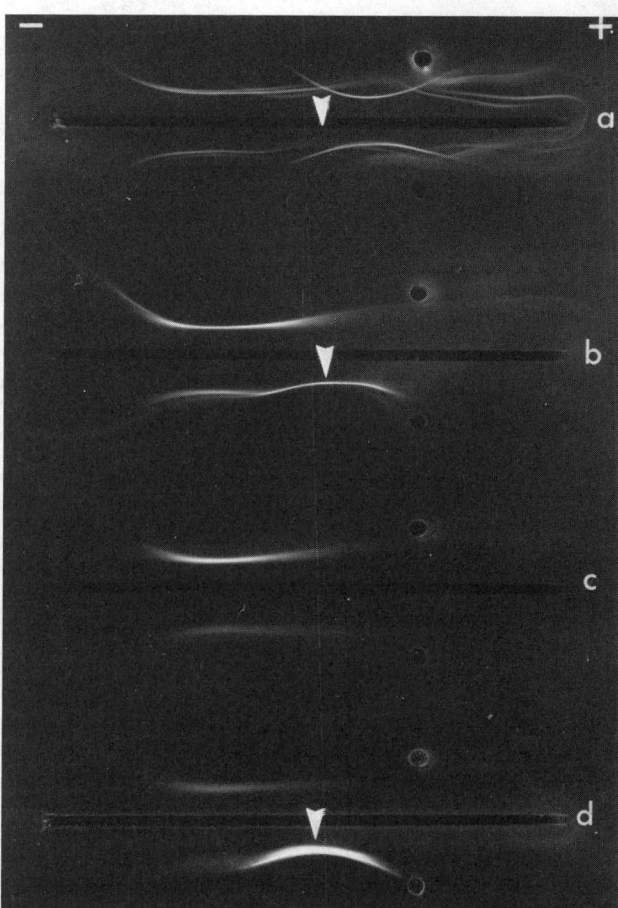

Fig. 163-5. (A) Immunoelectrophoresis of serum demonstrates an IgG-λ monoclonal protein with β-globulin mobility. Upper wells: normal serum. Lower wells: patient serum. Trough a, anti-IgG; trough b, anti-κ; trough c, anti-λ. **(B)** IEP of urine, which could only be concentrated 20-fold because of heavy nonselective proteinuria, revealed the same IgG-λ protein but no λ-BJP. Upper wells: normal serum. Lower wells: patient urine. Trough a, polyspecific antiserum to whole human serum; b, anti-IgG; c, anti-κ; d, anti-λ. Arrowheads mark the abnormal deflections in the relevant precipitin arcs. (Photograph of "wet" gel.)

which IEP yields an equivocal answer and then one must turn to the technique of IFE.

Immunofixation Electrophoresis

The more recently developed technique of IFE is even more sensitive than IEP in identifying monoclonal immunoglobulins or light chains at very low concentration in serum or urine[3]; it has emerged as a valuable supplementary technique to IEP or, in some laboratories, as the dominant immunospecific electrophoretic procedure. Two situations particularly warrant its use. In the presence of normal or increased background of polyclonal immunoglobulins standard IEP may fail to detect a very small monoclonal immunoglobulin. This occurs because the background immunoglobulins form unusually strong precipitin arcs within which it is difficult for a small quantity of paraprotein to produce a clear-cut deviation or bulge. Another problem sometimes encountered with IEP in this same setting is unsuccessful light chain typing of a monoclonal IgM protein because lower molecular weight and faster diffusing IgG and IgA molecules may preemptively bind the available anti-κ- or anti-λ-antibodies before the more slowly diffusing, high-molecular-weight IgM proteins can make contact. IFE is usually successful in these situations. IFE, however, is technically more demanding and labor-intensive than IEP. IFE has the advantage of being ready for interpretation on the same day as the electrophoretic run, and it requires less experience to interpret than IEP.

Like IEP, IFE employs a combination of zone electrophoresis and immunoprecipitation with a specific antisera. IFE begins with electrophoretic separation of suitably diluted serum or urine in 1% agarose gel (in 50 mM barbital buffer, pH 8.6). In our laboratory the agarose gel is applied to the surface of the same 85 × 100-mm Gel Bond clear plastic film sheets described in the discussion of IEP. The electrophoretic separation is performed on a cooling plate connected to a recirculating, temperature-controlled water bath at 5°–15°C (we favor 13°C). Immediately after the electrophoretic run, precut strips of cellulose acetate or lens paper, each soaked in a monospecific antiserum (e.g., anti-γ, anti-α, anti-μ, anti-κ, or anti-λ), are applied to the gel surface overlying individual electrophoretic lanes. The antibodies are allowed to diffuse (for approximately 10 minutes) from the strips into the gel, where they encounter and precipitate with their respective immunoglobulin antigens. The strips are removed and the agarose gel (on its plastic support) is then washed to remove all proteins that were not precipitated by a specific antibody. The final steps are drying the gel on the plastic sheet and staining with a protein dye such as Coomassie blue or amido black to reveal the bands of antibody-precipitated immunoglobulins. Figure 163-8 demonstrates an IFE pattern for normal serum, including both a Coomassie blue-stained agarose zone electrophoresis (upper segment) and the immunofixation patterns produced by each specific antiserum (see legend). All such patterns are polydisperse. Figures 163-9 and 163-10 depict sera with small monoclonal IgG or IgM bands, respectively, which were not clearly resolved by IEP.

Fig. 163-11 presents the serum IFE of a patient with IgD myeloma that had been classified at another hospital as Bence Jones myeloma because anti-IgD had not been tested. The patient has both an intact IgD-λ paraprotein and free type λ light chains. Similarly, IFE is even more sensitive than IEP in detecting very low concentrations of monoclonal light chains in concentrated urine.

Despite its superior sensitivity for detecting monoclonal immunoglobulins at low concentration, IFE does have some pitfalls. Optimal dilution of the serum or urine sample is essential. Too heavy a protein input can obscure monoclonal bands within the darkly staining background. Overdilution may result in loss of a potentially detectable monoclonal immunoglobulin. If the patient's serum concentrations of IgG, IgA, and IgM are known, that is helpful. One of the unique problems with IFE is that it is so sensitive that we are concerned about overdiagnosis of monoclonal proteins, with the potential to set in motion an expensive, anxiety-producing, and possibly unnecessary evaluation. For example, monoclonal gammopathies of undetermined significance[4] are detected by IFE with far greater frequency than by more traditional SPEP or IEP.[4] Clonally restricted light chains may also be detected in urine in the absence of other evidence for a plasma cell dyscrasia.[5,6] Moreover, using IFE, one or several faint but reproducible electrophoretically restricted bands are sometimes found in a strongly polyclonal hypergammaglobulinemic serum. Such oligoclonal bands are often undetectable by conventional SPEP or even by repeated careful IEP. This type of oligoclonal pattern in serum has been seen in acute and chronic infections, in rheumatologic diseases, in acquired immunodeficiency syndrome or asymptomatic human immunodeficiency virus infection, in chronic liver disease, in carcinoma, or in severe drug hypersensitivity.[7-10] These oligoclonal bands may be undetectable when the patient's serum is re-examined several months

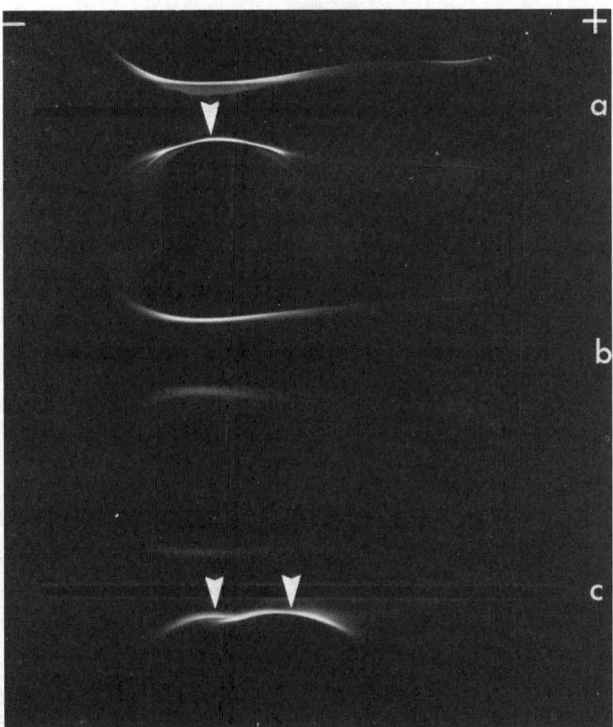

Fig. 163-7. IEP of a myeloma serum revealing evidence of two paraprotein populations. Upper wells: normal serum. Lower wells: patient serum. Trough a, anti-IgG; b, anti-κ; c, anti-λ. The more cathodal IgG-λ paraprotein caused an abnormal bowing of the IgG arc (a) and is also responsible for one of the double arcs seen with anti-λ-serum (c). The more anodal λ-arc represents free monoclonal λ-chains that have slightly "faster" mobility than the complete IgG-λ paraprotein.

later and thus may represent transient, accelerated immunoglobulin synthesis by vigorously expanded but nonmalignant clone(s) of antibody-forming cells stimulated by the acute illness or active flare. In other instances, such very weak monoclonal bands persist without change over time and should apparently be considered a variant form of monoclonal gammopathy of undetermined significance.

Overview of Electrophoretic Procedures

Some of the preceding discussion might leave the reader puzzled as to which electrophoretic procedure is best. In reply, it must be stated that the complete characterization of immunoglobulins often requires several different laboratory assays. A single method that will cover all situations does not exist.[1] A gradation, or hierarchy, of progressively more sensitive, and usually more expensive, methods has evolved. Some authors do not recommend the very sensitive IFE as an initial screening procedure; this view is not universally held, however.[11] We employ zone electrophoresis in agarose, IEP, and IFE in our laboratory. Increasingly, referring physicians, now aware of the greater sensitivity of IFE in detecting monoclonal immunoglobulins, are specifically requesting this procedure. As a result, a combination of SPEP in agarose and IFE is gradually becoming the norm of serum or urine evaluation.

This review has attempted to highlight the relative strengths and shortcomings of these diagnostic tools and thus diminish some of the mystery in their usage. Good communication between the clinician and diagnostic laboratory personnel should solve most problems.

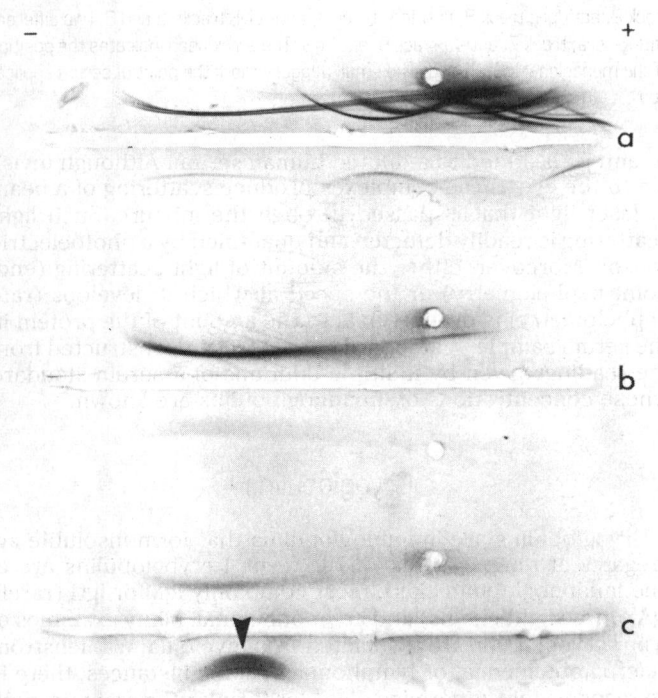

Fig. 163-6. IEP of 50-fold concentrated urine. Each of the upper wells contained normal serum; each lower well contained the concentrated urine of the patient. Trough a received polyspecific antiserum to whole human serum; trough b, anti-κ; trough c, anti-λ. Note the clear bowing or deviation of the precipitin arc formed by anti-λ but the smooth, polydisperse appearance of the arc formed by anti-κ. This urine sample contains λ-type BJP. (Photograph of dried, stained pattern.)

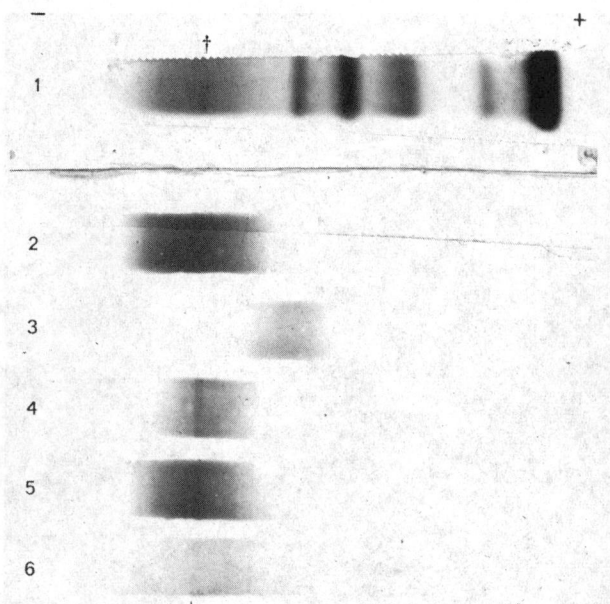

Fig. 163-8. IFE applied to normal serum. The upper pattern (track 1) represents zone electrophoresis in which Coomassie blue dye was applied to a strip cut from the plate after electrophoresis, without addition of antiserum. The major bands (from right to left) are albumin, α_1-antitrypsin, haptoglobin, transferrin, C3, and γ-globulin (with its normal polydisperse pattern). Below the zone electrophoresis strip, each horizontal track represents concurrently assayed immunoprecipitation (IFE) after overlay with antisera as follows: track 2, anti-IgG; track 3, anti-IgA; track 4, anti-IgM; track 5, anti-κ; track 6, anti-λ. The small daggers indicate the point of application of the serum sample; this process commonly leaves a narrow stripe that must not be confused with a monoclonal band.

Quantitative Assay of Immunoglobulins

Concentration ranges for immunoglobulins in adult human serum are included in Table 163-1; age-adjusted values are shown in Table 163-2. The technique of radial immunodiffusion was the dominant assay procedure for quantitative measurement of immunoglobulins for many years. In this technique, polyvalent antiserum specific for IgG, IgA, or IgM is incorporated into melted agarose, and the mixture is then allowed to gel on a glass or plastic slide, thus creating an anti-IgG slide, an anti-IgA slide, and an anti-IgM slide.[12] Multiple wells are punched into the gels. The wells are filled with serum from each patient to be assayed, but some wells receive serial dilutions of a standard serum or other preparation containing known concentrations of IgG, IgA, and IgM. From each well, the immunoglobulins diffuse into the surrounding antibody-impregnated agarose. Since excess antigen solubilizes antigen-antibody complexes, the point of equilibrium for maximum immunoprecipitation keeps moving outward as long as there is excess immunoglobulin antigen to solubilize the inner ring of precipitate. Ultimately, at about 24 hours, the system reaches equilibrium and each well shows a halo of surrounding precipitate. The diameter of the halo, measured accurately by special optical magnifiers, is proportional to the quantity of immunoglobulin in that serum. The diameter of the halo is converted to a milligram/deciliter concentration by constructing a standard curve relating halo diameter to several known concentrations of the respective immunoglobulin.

Nephelometry has recently emerged as the dominant technique for immunoglobulin quantitation in large laboratories since the procedure can be automated.[12] This method is possible because an extremely fine suspension of antigen-antibody complexes results when diluted antiserum (e.g., anti-γ, anti-α,

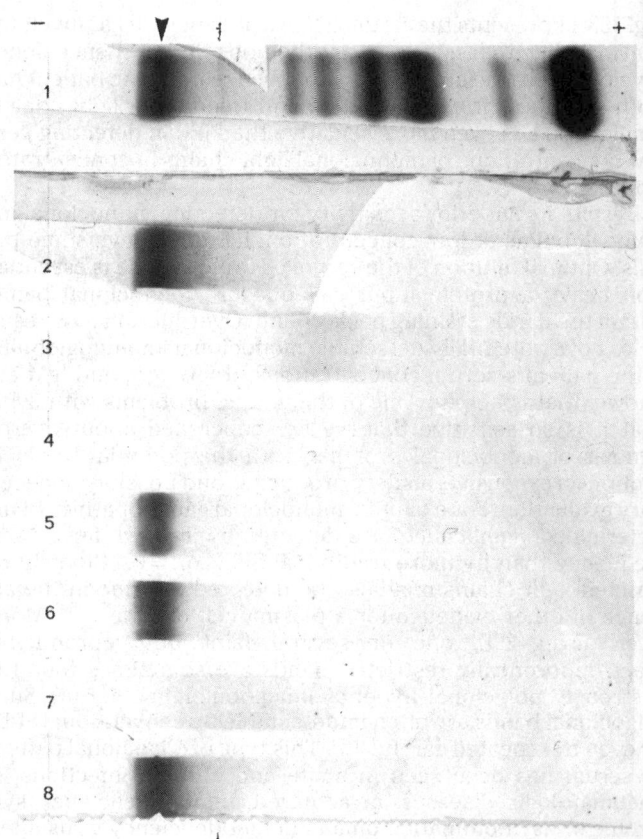

Fig. 163-9. IFE demonstrating a very small IgG-κ monoclonal protein. The upper segment is a stained zone electrophoresis of the patient's serum (no antibody was added). The other tracks, in descending order, were developed as follows: track 2, anti-IgG; track 3, anti-IgA; track 4, anti-IgM; tracks 5 and 6, two different anti-κ-sera; track 7, anti-λ; track 8, anti-IgG. The arrowhead indicates the position of the monoclonal IgG-κ band. The small daggers mark the point of serum application.

or anti-μ) is added to a diluted human serum. Although invisible to the eye, these complexes produce scattering of a beam of laser light that is passed through the mixture. Such light scattering is readily detected and quantified by a photoelectric sensor. Moreover, either the amount of light scattering (endpoint nephelometry) or the speed at which it develops (rate nephelometry) is proportional to the amount of the protein in the serum sample. A standard curve is again constructed from the readings given by multiple dilutions of a serum standard whose concentrations of immunoglobulins are known.

Cryoglobulins

Cryoglobulins are immunoglobulins that form insoluble aggregates at temperatures $<37°C$. Type I cryoglobulins are of one immunoglobulin class, most commonly IgM or IgG (rarely IgA or free light chains) and are monoclonal. Many examples of type I cryoglobulin are associated with myeloma, Waldenström macroglobulinemia, or lymphoma. In some instances, there is no recognizable underlying disorder (primary or essential type I cryoglobulinemia); such patients may, in time, develop an overt lymphoproliferative disease. The physical form of the type I cryoprecipitation may be amorphous, gelatinous, or crystalline.[13]

Types II and III cryoglobulins are termed mixed in that their formation involves the interaction of two or more classes of immunoglobulin. At least one of the immunoglobulin compo-

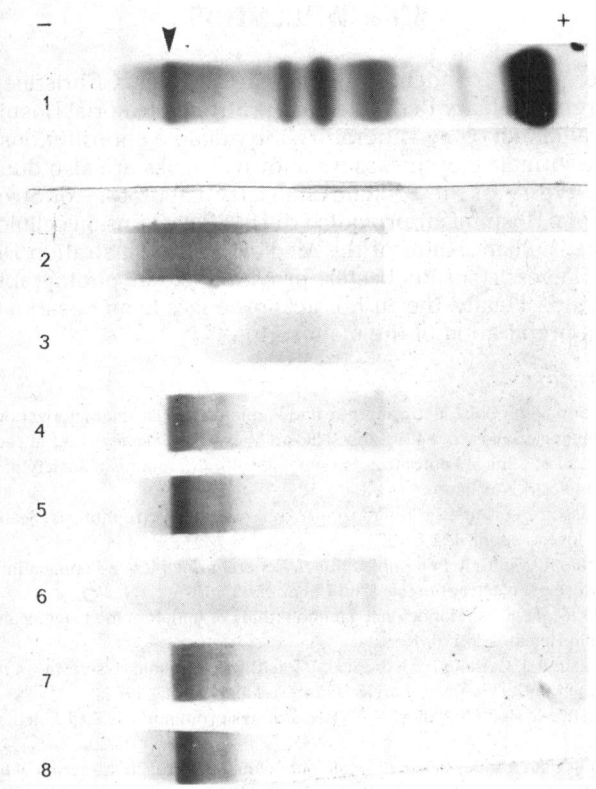

Fig. 163-10. IFE demonstrating a subtle IgM-κ monoclonal protein (arrowhead). Upper track: agarose zone electrophoresis. Other tracks, in descending order, were developed with anti-IgG (track 2), anti-IgA (track 3), anti-IgM (track 4), anti-κ (track 5), anti-λ (track 6), repeat anti-IgM (track 7), and repeat anti-κ (track 8).

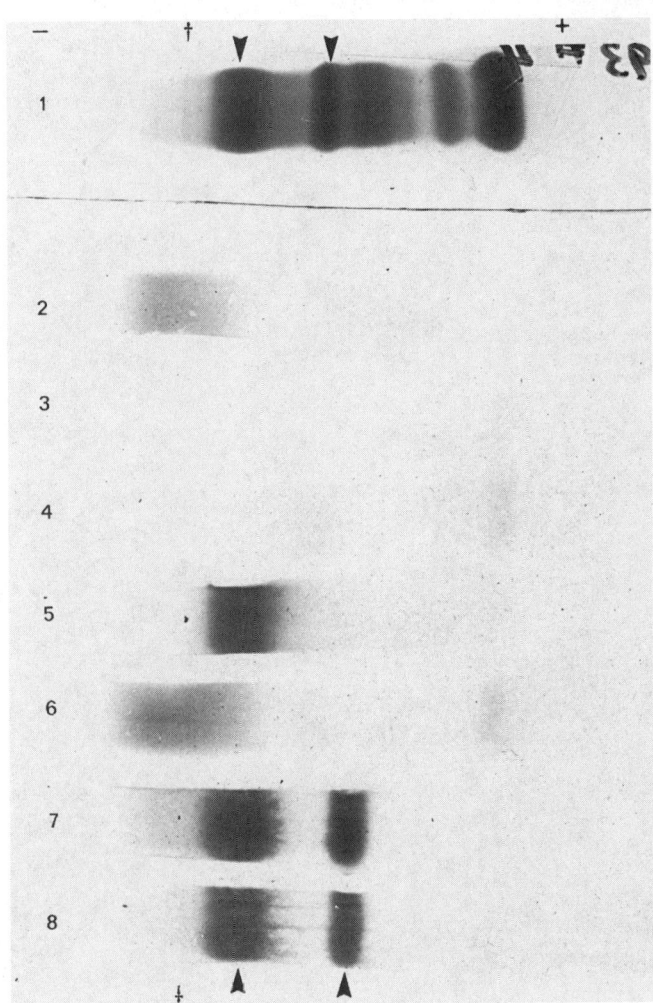

Fig. 163-11. IgD myeloma. Zone electrophoresis in agarose (track 1) revealed two abnormal, restricted bands (arrowheads). Concurrent IFE (tracks 2–8) was set up as follows: anti-IgG (lane 2), anti-IgA (lane 3), anti-IgM (lane 4), anti-IgD (lane 5), anti-κ (lane 6), anti-λ (lanes 7 and 8). The IFE results demonstrate that the more cathodal paraprotein is IgD-λ and the more anodal band contains free λ light chains.

nents is a cold-reactive anti-IgG (rheumatoid factor) that combines with the patient's polyclonal IgG (or any source of normal human IgG) to form a cryoprecipitate. This cryoprecipitate is a special type of immune complex possessing a definite capacity to activate and consume complement, both in vivo and in a test tube if cooling occurs. The anti-IgG antibody appears to be the critical component mediating cryoprecipitation. The essential immunochemical difference between types II and III cryoglobulinemia is that in type II the anti-IgG component is monoclonal, most commonly IgM-κ but in some cases it is IgG or IgA. In type III cryoglobulinemia the anti-IgG component is polyclonal; it may be polyclonal IgM alone or IgM in combination with IgG or IgA anti-IgG antibodies. Both type II and type III cryoglobulinemia, but particularly type II, have been associated with evidence of hepatitis C infection (i.e., detection of anti-hepatitis-C antibody or viral RNA in the serum or cryoprecipitate).[14] Distinguishing between type II and type III is important because patients with type II, but apparently not type III, cryoglobulinemia are at increased risk of concurrent or subsequently developing B-cell lymphoma. Many other instances of type II cryoglobulinemia in which an underlying disorder is not evident are termed essential or primary, but lymphomas have developed in a substantial proportion of such patients. Patients with type III cryoglobulinemia may have a collagen-vascular disease such as systemic lupus erythematosus or a systemic viral infection, but this disorder also occurs in an essential or primary form.

Blood drawn for cryoglobulin assay is ideally transported to the laboratory in a container of warm water, permitted to clot in a 37°C bath, and subjected to centrifugation in a warmed centrifuge. This 37°C serum is placed in the refrigerator in a graduated conical tube for 72–96 hours, to permit complete

precipitation. Many cryoglobulins, however, especially type I, precipitate far more rapidly. At the end of 72–96 hours, the tubes are spun and the packed precipitate volume (cryocrit) is measured in the same way as a hematocrit. Normal sera show no visible precipitate under these conditions.

If the test result is positive, the supernatant serum is removed, the cryoprecipitate is washed thoroughly in cold saline, and then redissolved in a small volume of warm 0.15 M NaCl for analysis of its immunoglobulin composition. For large cryoprecipitates, IEP is effective. Ouchterlony immunodiffusion is effective for analyzing type I cryoglobulins. For small cryoprecipitates and for distinction between type II and type III cryoglobulins, IFE has been highly effective in our laboratory (Fig. 163-12).

Table 163-2. Age-Adjusted Serum Immunoglobulin Levels (mg/dl)[a]

	IgG	IgA	IgM
Birth to 4 months	700–1,480	0–2.2	5–30
4–6 months	300–1,000	3–32	15–109
6 months–16 years	500–1,550	14–232	43–240

[a] Adult concentrations are shown in Table 163-1.

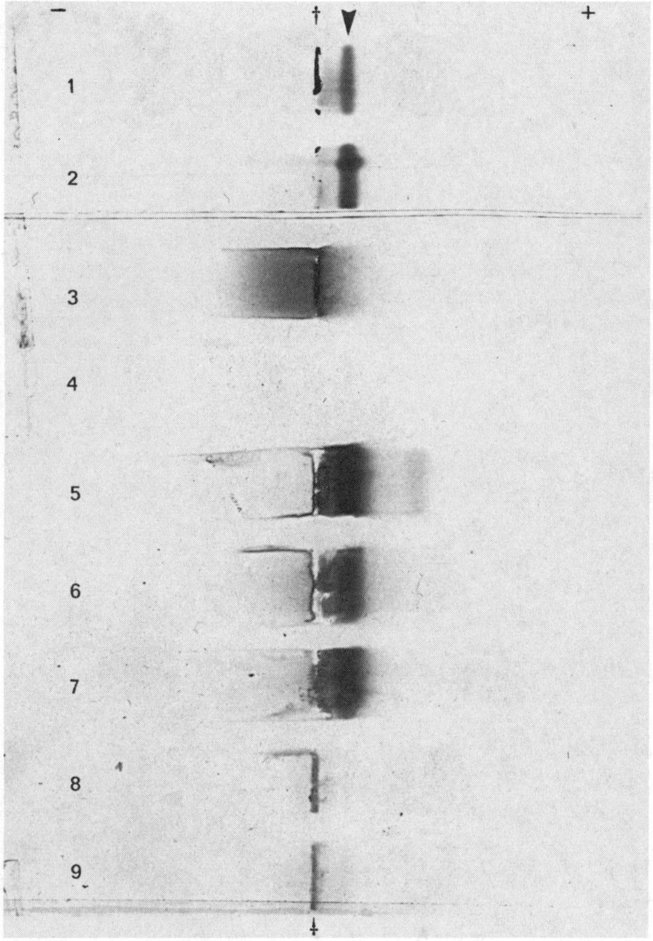

Fig. 163-12. IFE of an isolated, washed type II cryoglobulin. Upper two tracks: agarose zone electrophoresis of two concentrations of the redissolved cryoglobulin. Note the sharp monoclonal band (arrowhead) plus a very faint polyclonal background. IFE analysis revealed that the monoclonal band was IgM-κ (tracks 5–7) in association with polydisperse IgG (track 3). Anti-κ and anti-λ were each tested against two concentrations of the isolated cryoglobulin. Antisera were applied as follows: track 3, anti-IgG; track 4, anti-IgA; track 5, anti-IgM; tracks 6 and 7, anti-K; tracks 8 and 9, anti-λ.

ACKNOWLEDGMENTS

The author is indebted to Donna R. Graham, Christine C. Waldrop, and Mary Beth Chen of the Strong Memorial Hospital Clinical Immunology Laboratory for valuable contributions in the performance of the assays shown. Thanks are also due to Judith Sterry of the Protein Chemistry Laboratory of Strong Memorial Hospital for providing the SPEP patterns on cellulose acetate. William Smith of the Medical Photo/Illustration Division, University of Rochester, provided expert photographic assistance. Finally, the author acknowledges Lynn Kosarko for skillful preparation of the manuscript.

REFERENCES

1. Caron J, Penn GM: Electrophoretic and immunochemical characterization of immunoglobulins. p. 84. In Rose NR, de Macario EC, Fahey JL et al (eds): Manual of Clinical Laboratory Immunology. 4th Ed. American Society of Microbiology, Washington, DC, 1992
2. Jeppsson J-O, Laurell C-B, Franzen B: Agarose gel electrophoresis. Scand J Lab Invest, suppl. 124:7, 1972
3. Ritchie RF, Smith R: Immunofixation. I. General principles and application to agarose gel electrophoresis. Clin Chem 22:497, 1976
4. Kyle RA, Lust JA: Monoclonal gammopathies of undetermined significance. Semin Hematol 26:176, 1989
5. Cronstedt J, Carlong L, Ostberg H: Idiopathic light chain dyscrasia—a new distinct entity? Report of a case. J Intern Med 196:445, 1974
6. Kyle RA, Greipp PR: "Idiopathic" Bence Jones proteinuria. N Engl J Med 306:564, 1982
7. Keshgegian AA: Pevalence of small monoclonal proteins in the serum of hospitalized patients. Am J Clin Pathol 77:436, 1982
8. Kelly RH, Hardy TJ: Multiple clonally restricted immunoglobulins in human sera: disease associations. Int Arch Allergy Appl Immunol 69:56, 1982
9. Sinclair D, Galloway E, McKenzie S et al: Oligoclonal immunoglobulins in HIV infection. Clin Chem 35:1669, 1989
10. Del Carpio J, Espinosa LR, Lauater S, Osterland CK: Transient monoclonal proteins in drug hypersensitivity reactions. Am J Med 66:1051, 1979
11. Gerard SK, Chen KH, Khayam-Bashi H: Immunofixation compared with immunoelectrophoresis for the routine characterization of paraprotein disorders. Am J Clin Pathol 88:198, 1987
12. Check IJ, Piper M, Papadea C: Immunoglobulin quantitation. p. 71. In Rose NR, de Macario EC, Fahey JL et al (eds): Manual of Clinical Laboratory Immunology. 4th Ed. American Society of Microbiology, Washington, DC, 1992
13. Podell DN, Packman CH, Maniloff J, Abraham GN: Characterization of monoclonal IgG cryoglobulins: fine structural and morphological analysis. Blood 69:677, 1987
14. Abel G, Zhang Q-X, Agnello V: Hepatitis C virus infection in type II mixed cryoglobulinemia (review). Arthritis Rheum 36:1341, 1993

Use of Molecular Techniques in the Analysis of Hematologic Diseases

164

Nancy Berliner

INTRODUCTION

The dramatic advances in recombinant DNA technology in the last 20 years have yielded crucial insights into the processes involved in hematopoietic cell ontogeny. Equally impressive is the effect this technology has had on the diagnostic capabilities for defining, diagnosing, and predicting the natural history of hematologic diseases. The same techniques that have allowed the elucidation of the molecular mechanisms of hematologic abnormalities have provided powerful diagnostic

Table 164-1. Use of Molecular Techniques for Hematologic Diagnosis

Prenatal diagnosis
    Analysis of RFLPs linked to diseases of known genetic loci
    Direct oligonucleotide screening to detect single base changes defined as
        the basis of disease
    Use of PCR to amplify regions of DNA for further analysis for known or
        suspected molecular abnormalities within the gene of interest
Diagnosis of lymphoproliferative disease
    Defining clonality of poorly defined lymphoproliferative lesions lacking classic
        histology or lymphoid surface markers
    Determining extent of disease in patients with lymphoproliferative lesions
    Monitoring disease activity in patients undergoing treatment for lymphoproli-
        ferative disease
HLA typing for bone marrow transplantation
Analysis of cell origins in bone marrow transplantation patients
    Documentation of engraftment following marrow transplantation
    Identification of chimeric states and prediction of graft rejection
    Determination of cell implicated in relapse following bone marrow transplan-
        tation
Diagnosis of follow-up of diseases associated with known cytogenetic abnormalities
    Documenting aberrant translocations (i.e., Philadelphia chromosome-nega-
        tive CML)
    Detection of minimal residual disease by PCR across known chromosomal
        breakpoints

Abbreviations: RFLP, restriction fragment length polymorphism: PCR, polymerase chain reaction; CML, chronic myeloid leukemia.

tools, bringing our understanding of basic science into sharply relevant clinical focus. An exhaustive review of the application of these techniques is beyond the scope of this chapter; however, a brief summary of the areas outlined in Table 164-1 provides some insight into the current and evolving uses of DNA technology in clinical hematologic practice.

PRENATAL DIAGNOSIS

The interplay of basic science and clinical diagnostics is perhaps most dramatically reflected in the area of the hemoglobinopathies. The increasing precision with which the molecular lesions of thalassemia and sickle cell disease have been defined is paralleled by the increasing sensitivity and specificity of techniques for antenatal diagnosis of these disorders[1] (see Ch. 162). For the purposes of this discussion, the range of molecular techniques for antenatal diagnosis of sickle cell disease is described as a paradigm for these developing concepts.

With the exception of lymphocytes, as described below, the DNA content of all cells in a given individual is identical. Consequently, prenatal diagnosis by DNA analysis can be performed on DNA derived from any fetal tissue. The usual source of fetal DNA has been amniotic fluid cells. Obtaining adequate tissue for diagnosis requires 20–30 ml of amniotic fluid with growth of the cells in tissue culture prior to DNA isolation. Amniocentesis is performed at 16 weeks' gestation, and analysis may not be completed until 4 weeks later. Chorionic villus sampling has begun to supplant amniocentesis as a source of fetal tissue, because it can be performed at 8–12 weeks of gestation.[2,3] With the development of more sensitive methods of DNA diagnosis, notably the polymerase chain reaction (PCR), the cellular material necessary for genetic analysis has been reduced to a very few cells; consequently, it is likely that progressively less invasive procedures for obtaining fetal cells will evolve.

Analysis of Restriction Fragment Length Polymorphisms

Restriction fragment length polymorphisms (RFLPs) have been described in detail in Chapter 1. Briefly, RFLPs reflect DNA mutations that alter the recognition sites for restriction

endonucleases and persist as detectable polymorphisms on Southern blot analysis of genomic DNA.[4] These mutations are usually phenotypically silent, in that they usually lie within introns and do not affect the protein encoded by the gene locus in which they are found. The exception to this rule is discussed below.

RFLPs can be related to diseases caused by single gene defects in several ways (Fig. 164-1). A single base change causing a disease may itself give rise to an altered restriction site. Such a chance occurrence represents the exception to the usual rule that RFLPs arise from phenotypically silent mutations in intron regions; in this instance, finding the RFLP is diagnostic of the mutant allele. It allows the direct identification of both carriers and homozygous individuals with the disease and is not seen in any individual who does not carry the mutant allele. In such a situation, an individual can be diagnosed without knowing family inheritance patterns. With respect to the mutation in sickle cell anemia, the single A to T change at the DNA level that causes the conversion of glutamic acid to valine at position 6 of the β-chain can be detected directly using several restriction enzymes.[5–7]

In most instances, however, single base pair changes do not give rise to convenient restriction enzyme site alterations that allow direct detection of the mutation. Alternatively, RFLPs may arise within the gene of interest independently from the mutation that causes the disease. These reflect common mutations associated with, but not responsible for, the less frequent mutations that alter gene expression and cause disease. In these instances, the RFLP does not directly identify affected individuals in the general population but is diagnostic in a family known to carry a mutant gene in association with a given RFLP. The informativeness of such an RFLP depends on the origin of the disease-related mutation as a single event within a population at a time after the RFLP arose. Thus, it requires the selection for persistence of the original disease allele in the population rather than its continued renewal by new mutations. Both sickle cell disease and the thalassemias have been shown to have arisen in selected populations in association with such polymorphisms.[8–10] In stable populations, several such polymorphisms together have been used to define a "haplotype" with which a given disease is associated. This has been documented by Orkin and associates[11] for several specific β-thalassemia mutations.

Finally, an RFLP may not lie within the locus of the gene of interest at all, but may lie close enough to the gene that the two loci rarely, if ever, become separated by recombination. The diagnostic value of the RFLP then depends on statistical analysis of the proximity of the two genes. Diagnosis is based on the analysis of the RFLP patterns of a given affected family to ascertain whether the distribution of alleles allows identification of the RFLP associated with the disease within that individual pedigree. Although this kind of linkage analysis is the least direct application of RFLPs to disease diagnosis, it is the most generalizable to a wide range of diseases. Because the globin gene locus has been fully sequenced and the mutant alleles extensively analyzed, most diagnoses can be made by direct diagnosis using RFLP analysis based on either altered restriction sites at the site of mutation or haplotype analysis as described above. However, this more general application of RFLPs is the basis for gene mapping efforts that promise to allow diagnosis of diseases for which the mutations, and indeed the affected genes themselves, are yet to be identified.

The use of RFLPs for antenatal diagnosis was first undertaken for the diagnosis of hemoglobinopathies. The application of these techniques to the diagnosis of sickle cell disease is diagrammed in Figure 164-1. Similar techniques have been used in parallel fashion for the prenatal diagnosis of thalassemia. The earliest studies of sickle cell disease were based on a polymorphic site for the enzyme *Hpa*I, which was located 4 kb

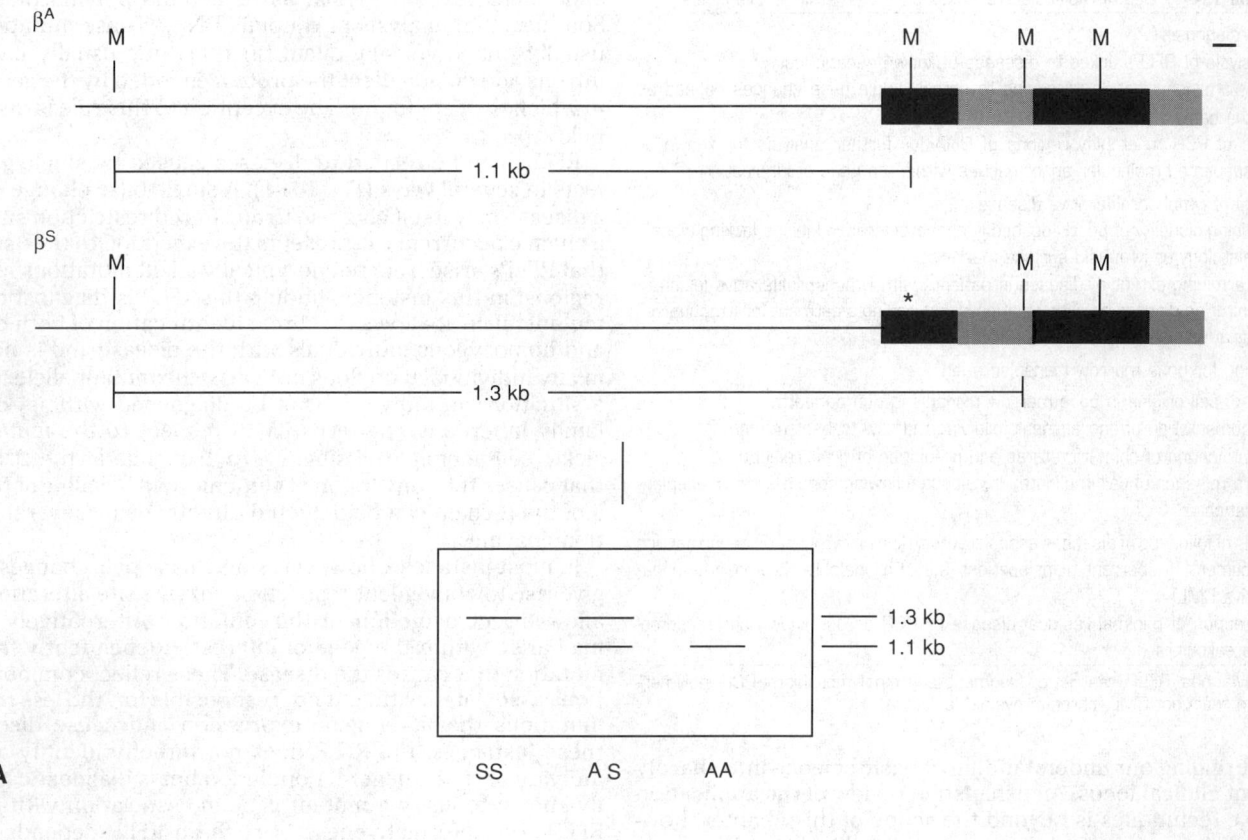

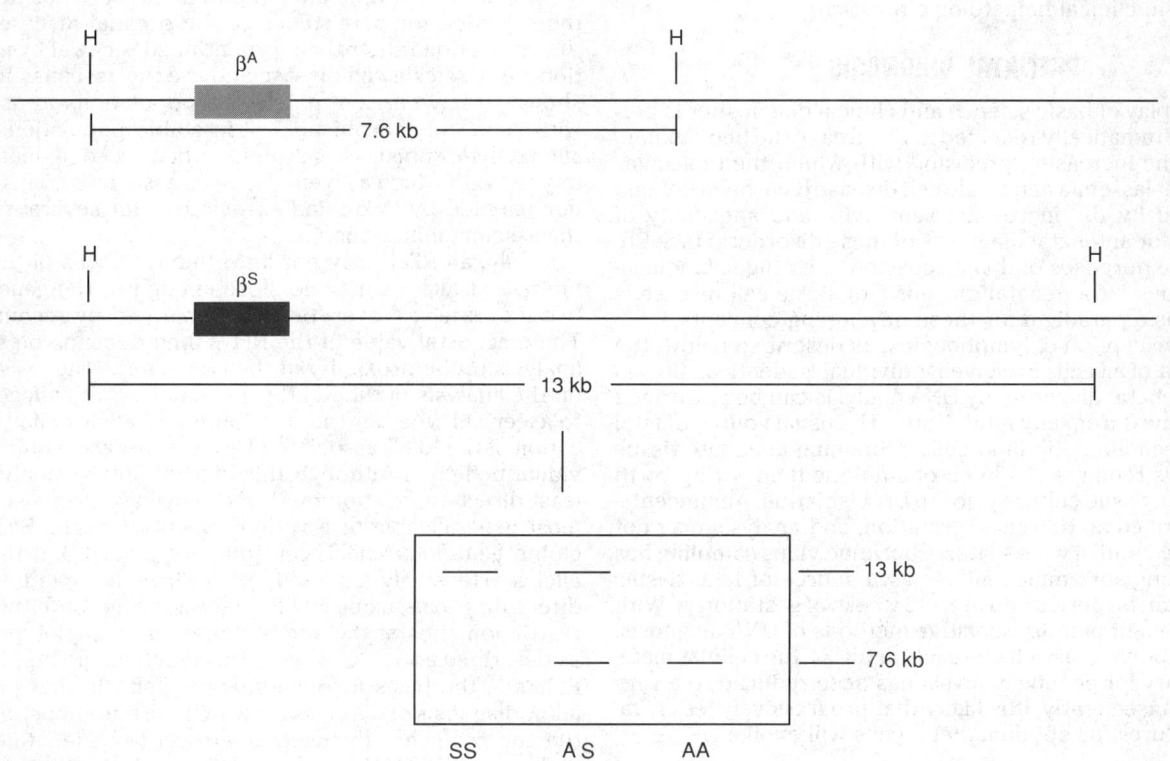

Fig. 164-1. Two different types of restriction fragment length polymorphisms used in the prenatal diagnosis of sickle cell disease. **(A)** The point mutation within the globin gene that gives rise to the sickle mutation alters the recognition site for the restriction endonuclease *Mst*II, giving rise to an altered restriction fragment when DNA containing the sickle gene is digested with that enzyme. **(B)** The sickle cell gene is associated with a DNA polymorphism in the 3′ flanking DNA of the globin gene. This polymorphism is clinically silent but can aid in the antenatal diagnosis of sickle cell disease. If carrier parents are heterozygous for the polymorphism in association with the sickle gene (AS in the Southern diagram), fetuses at risk can be identified by homozygous presence of the the same band (SS in diagram). M, *Mst*II; H, *Hpa*I; SS, sickle cell disease; AS, sickle trait; AA, normal.

wnstream of the β-globin gene.[3] Absence of the restriction e was seen in 87% of sickle genes in the population studied.[8] nsequently, if parents carrying the sickle gene were heterogous for the absent restriction site, affected fetuses could identified by homozygous absence of the same site (Fig. 164-). Subsequent techniques for diagnosing sickle cell disease ploited that sickle cell disease, unlike thalassemia, arises om a single defined mutation, namely a single A to T base bstitution. This allowed the identification of restriction enme sites that were altered by the mutation, as well as direct alysis of mutant alleles without family studies. Two enzymes at can be used to identify the sickle mutation have been iden- ied.[5–7] One of these, *Mst*II, results in an easily distinguishable attern diagnostic of the disease (Fig. 164-1A). This technique as also been used to diagnose other single-base mutations sulting in hemoglobins S, O-Arab, and others.[12,13] As previ- sly suggested, thalassemia is not readily amenable to this proach because of the heterogeneous lesions giving rise to e disease; however, certain predominant mutations within efined populations have been diagnosed in this manner.[14]

All of these studies are performed using Southern blotting chniques.[15] Genomic DNA from the fetus (and appropriate mily members as needed) is digested with a diagnostic re- riction enzyme, size fractionated by agarose gel electropho- sis, blotted on nitrocellulose, and hybridized to a radiola- led probe for the β-globin gene. Hybridization techniques re described in Chapter 1.

Direct Oligonucleotide Screening for Known Point Mutations

The full sequence of the β-globin gene is known, and the single base change responsible for the sickle mutation has been established. This knowledge allows more refined techniques for prenatal diagnosis of sickle cell disease, as well as for other hemoglobinopathies in which the responsible mutation is known at the level of the DNA sequence. Molecular hybridiza- tion techniques have been developed that can pinpoint single base changes in DNA sequence using short probes of 15–20 nucleotides. Under stringent washing conditions, hybridization between such a short probe and the DNA in question requires that the base pairing between the two be exact. Technology for the synthesis of such oligonucleotide probes now exists. Oligonucleotide sequences that are identical to either the na- tive or the mutant gene can be synthesized and the oligonucleo- tides radiolabeled and hybridized to DNA from the fetus at risk (Fig. 164-2). This DNA can be spotted directly onto nitrocellu- lose, since the hybridization does not require restriction en- zyme digestion of the DNA. The consequent rapidity of diagno- sis gives this technique its primary advantage over RFLP analysis by Southern blot hybridization. The method has been used successfully for prenatal diagnosis of both sickle cell dis- ease and thalassemias associated with known single base changes.[16–18]

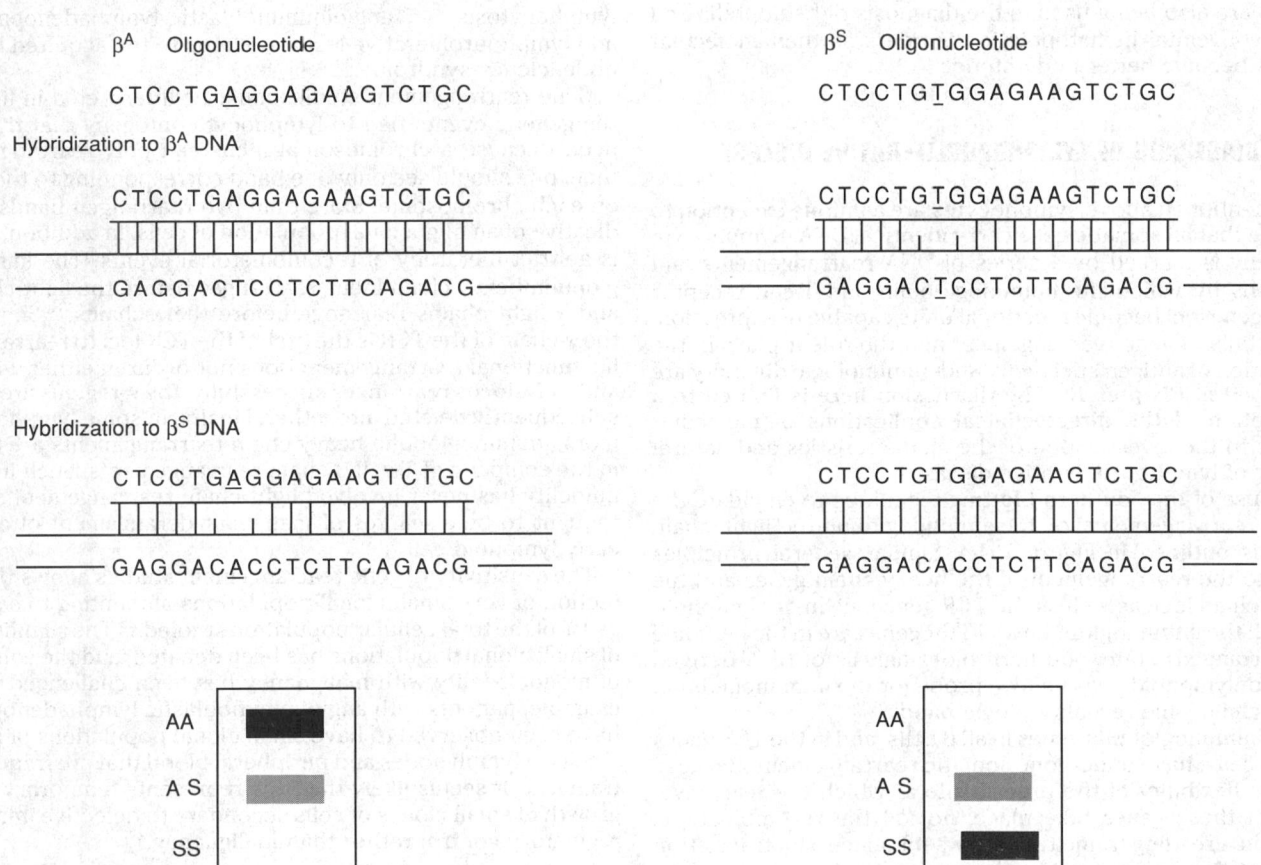

Fig. 164-2. Use of oligonucleotide probes to screen for sickle cell disease. Specific oligonucleotide probes that are homologous to the sequence of the β[A] and the β[S]-globin genes are synthesized. Because the oligonucleotides are only 19 nucleotides long, hybridization under appropriately stringent conditions will yield stable hybrids only if the DNA sequence is identical to the probe sequence. The single base change that gives rise to the sickle mutation is sufficient to destabilize the DNA-oligonucleotide duplex and allows the distinction of normal (AA), sickle trait (AS), and sickle cell disease (SS) DNA. After isolation, the DNA is blotted directly onto nitrocellulose without the necessity of restriction enzyme digestion and hybridized to the radiolabeled oligonucleotide probes. The blots are washed at high stringency and autoradiographed. Predicted results are as diagrammed in the lower panel.

Use of the Polymerase Chain Reaction in Prenatal Diagnosis

The development of PCR represents one of the most important technical advances in molecular diagnostics.[19] The technique is described elsewhere (see Ch. 1) and is summarized again in Figure 164-3. Using PCR, prenatal diagnosis is possible with as little as 1 μg of DNA. Diagnosis is performed by using oligonucleotides flanking the gene to amplify the DNA of interest from minute quantities of total cellular DNA. The amplified sequences can then be analyzed by any of the techniques described. The usual means of diagnosis is to hybridize the amplified DNA to oligonucleotide probes. This is currently the most rapid means of diagnosis of sickle cell disease[20,21] and thalassemias with known mutations.[22] These techniques can also be invaluable in the rapid analysis of unknown mutations.[22]

A fluorescence amplification technique has recently been developed that permits direct PCR analysis of DNA for known single base mutations. Oligonucleotide primers containing the normal and mutant sequence are synthesized, and the two primers are differentially labeled with red and green fluorescent tags. These primers are mixed with a common antisense primer, which is left unlabeled. PCR is then performed, and the reaction products are then directly analyzed in a fluorimeter for differential fluorescence.[23]

Although the primary focus of this discussion has been on the prenatal diagnosis of hemoglobinopathies, similar techniques are also being used in the diagnosis of hemophilia and other congenital hematopoietic disorders as their molecular origins become better understood.[24]

DIAGNOSIS OF LYMPHOPROLIFERATIVE DISEASE

As mentioned above, lymphocytes are a unique exception to the rule that all somatic cells carry identical DNA. Lymphocyte ontogeny is marked by a series of DNA rearrangements and deletions by which the immunoglobulin and T-cell receptor (TCR) gene loci become functional units capable of expression. The details of gene rearrangement and the role it plays in the generation of antigen specificity and immunologic diversity are described in Chapter 13. The discussion here is limited to a description of the direct clinical applications of molecular probes to the investigation of the characteristics and natural history of lymphoproliferative disease.

The use of the Southern blotting technique to elucidate the clonal rearrangements of the immunoglobulin κ light chain genes is outlined in Figure 164-4. Similar general principles apply to the rearrangement of the heavy chain genes and the λ light chain loci, as well as the TCR gene loci. In nonlymphoid cells, all the immunoglobulin and TCR genes are in the germline (unrearranged) state. Southern blot analysis of DNA derived from nonlymphoid cells using a probe for the immunoglobulin heavy chain gene reveals a single band.

The immunoglobulin genes in all β cells, and in the TCR genes in all T cells, have undergone somatic rearrangement. Because there is flexibility of the precise site at which the rearrangement of these genes take place, not all the recombinations maintain a reading frame that allows for successful translation of the mRNA into a functional protein. If a nonfunctional rearrangement takes place on one chromosome, a further rearrangement takes place on the homologous chromosome. Because of the large deletions that take place in the course of recombination, it is not possible for two rearrangements to take place on the same chromosome. Consequently, every lymphoid cell has either one or two rearranged heavy chain genes, and one or two rearranged light chain genes. If Southern blot analysis could be performed on a single cell, each lympho-

cyte would show either one or two rearranged bands. However, because the DNA from >10,000 cells is required to detect a single copy gene by Southern blot analysis, these bands will be undetectable in a polyclonal proliferation of lymphocytes. The only detectable band is the germline band contributed by the unrearranged heavy chain genes in the lymphocytes that have only rearranged one of the two heavy chain loci.

In a monoclonal proliferation of B cells, however, all the cells contain an identical pattern of heavy chain rearrangement. Southern blot analysis thus reveals one or two rearranged bands, corresponding to one or two rearranged heavy chain loci.

Defining Clonality of Lymphoproliferative Lesions

The process of malignant transformation "freezes" a tumor cell population at a given stage of differentiation and gives rise to a proliferation of cells manifesting an identical pattern of DNA rearrangement. Southern blot analysis consequently offers a sensitive means of establishing the clonality and lymphoid origin of cells showing somatic rearrangement of their immunoglobulin or TCR gene loci. Southern blot analysis of DNA from a range of tissues, including lymph nodes, pleural fluid, and peripheral blood, has been used to establish the diagnosis of lymphoma in lesions that lack either definitive histology or surface markers.[25] It has also been used to examine the clonality of poorly defined lymphoid lesions such as T-cell lymphocytosis,[26-28] angioimmunoblastic lymphadenopathy,[?] and lymphoproliferative lesions related to the acquired immunodeficiency syndrome.[30]

Gene rearrangement studies must be interpreted in light of the genetic events tied to lymphocyte ontogeny that they reflect. Because a chromosomal locus can only rearrange one time, one should see only one band corresponding to the DNA on each chromosome. More than two rearranged bands is indicative of an oligoclonal population of cells. In addition, there is a strict hierarchy of recombinatorial events. The immunoglobulin heavy chain locus rearranges before the light chains, and κ light chains rearrange before the λ-chains.[31] Similarly, the γ-chain of the TCR is the first of the TCR loci to rearrange.[3?] If a functional rearrangement does not occur in either κ-locus and the λ-locus rearranges successfully, the κ-regions are often subsequently deleted altogether. Finally, in some lymphoid tumors, immunoglobulin heavy chain rearrangements are found in the company of T-cell β-chain rearrangements. Such lineage infidelity has never involved light chain rearrangement and is thought to be a marker of malignant derangement of a very early lymphoid cell.

The sensitivity of gene rearrangement studies allows the detection of very small clonal populations amounting to as little as 1% of the total cellular population studied.[25] The significance of small clonal populations has been debated, and the equation of monoclonality with malignancy has been challenged.[32] For example, patients with angioimmunoblastic lymphadenopathy have been observed to have small clonal populations of B and T cells in lymph nodes and peripheral blood that are frequently transient. It seems likely that this represents temporary overgrowth of small clones of cells secondary to defective immunoregulatory control rather than malignancy.[29]

Determining Extent of Lymphoproliferative Disease

Immunoglobulin and TCR gene rearrangements have been used in the staging of patients with lymphoproliferative disease. Southern blot analysis using probes for these loci has been shown to be sensitive enough to detect clonal populations

Total genomic DNA as template

Denature

Anneal primers

Primer extension with TAQ polymerase

Denature, anneal primers, elongate

Repeat for total of thirty cycles

Products per original DNA molecule, where n=number of cycles

long-short hybrids=2n

short-short hybrids=2^n

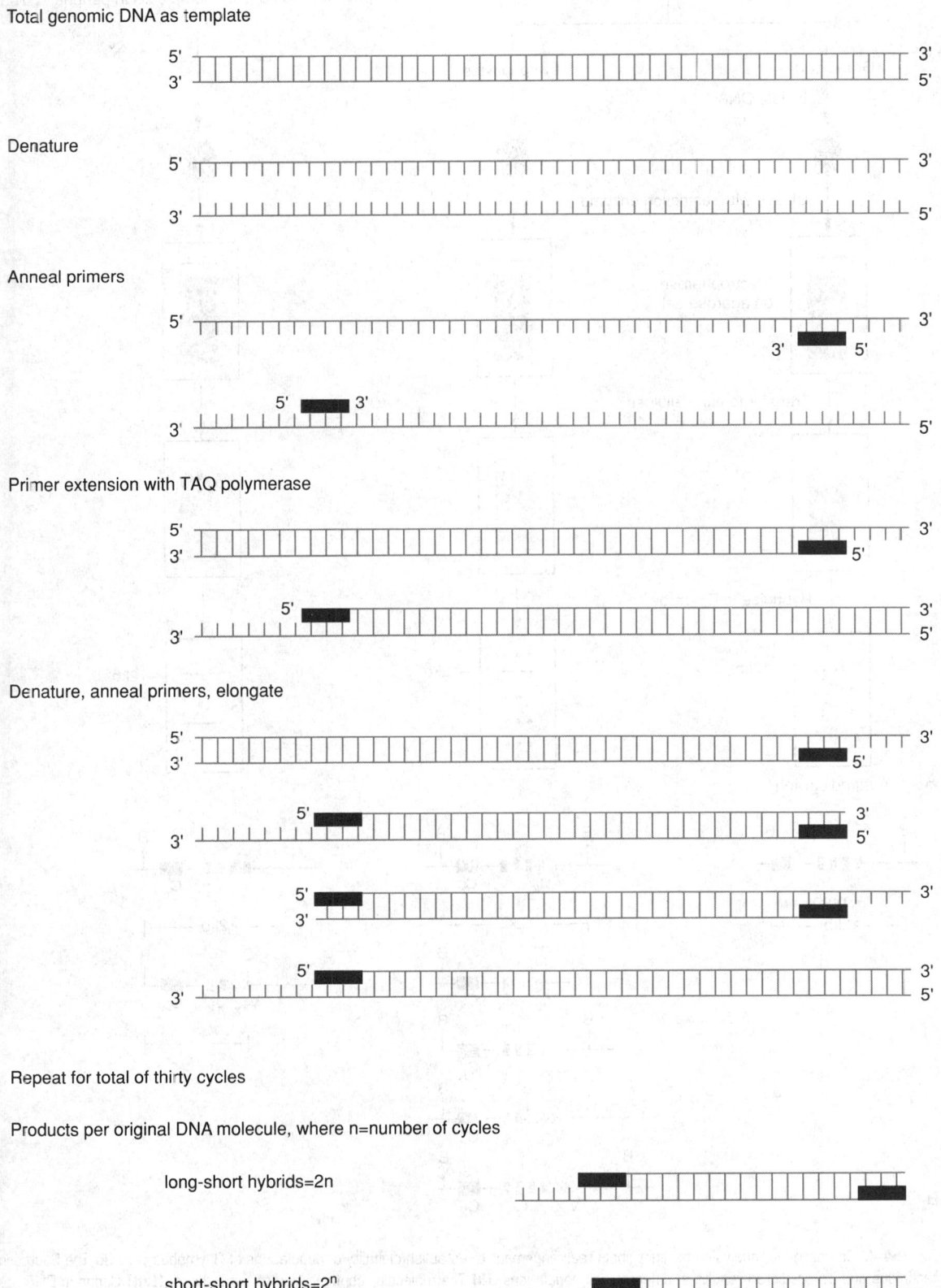

Fig. 164-3. Use of PCR to amplify a portion of DNA for analysis. One microgram of total genomic DNA is denatured at high temperature and annealed to oligonucleotide primers flanking the DNA of interest. By using the temperature-stable TAQ polymerase, the primers are extended to synthesize a copy of the DNA between the two primers. The temperature is then raised to denature the products, and the process is repeated for 30 cycles. The primary product of this reaction is a fragment of DNA bounded by the two oligonucleotide primers (short-short hybrids). By this means, a minute quantity of total DNA may be used to generate specific DNA in large quantity for analysis.

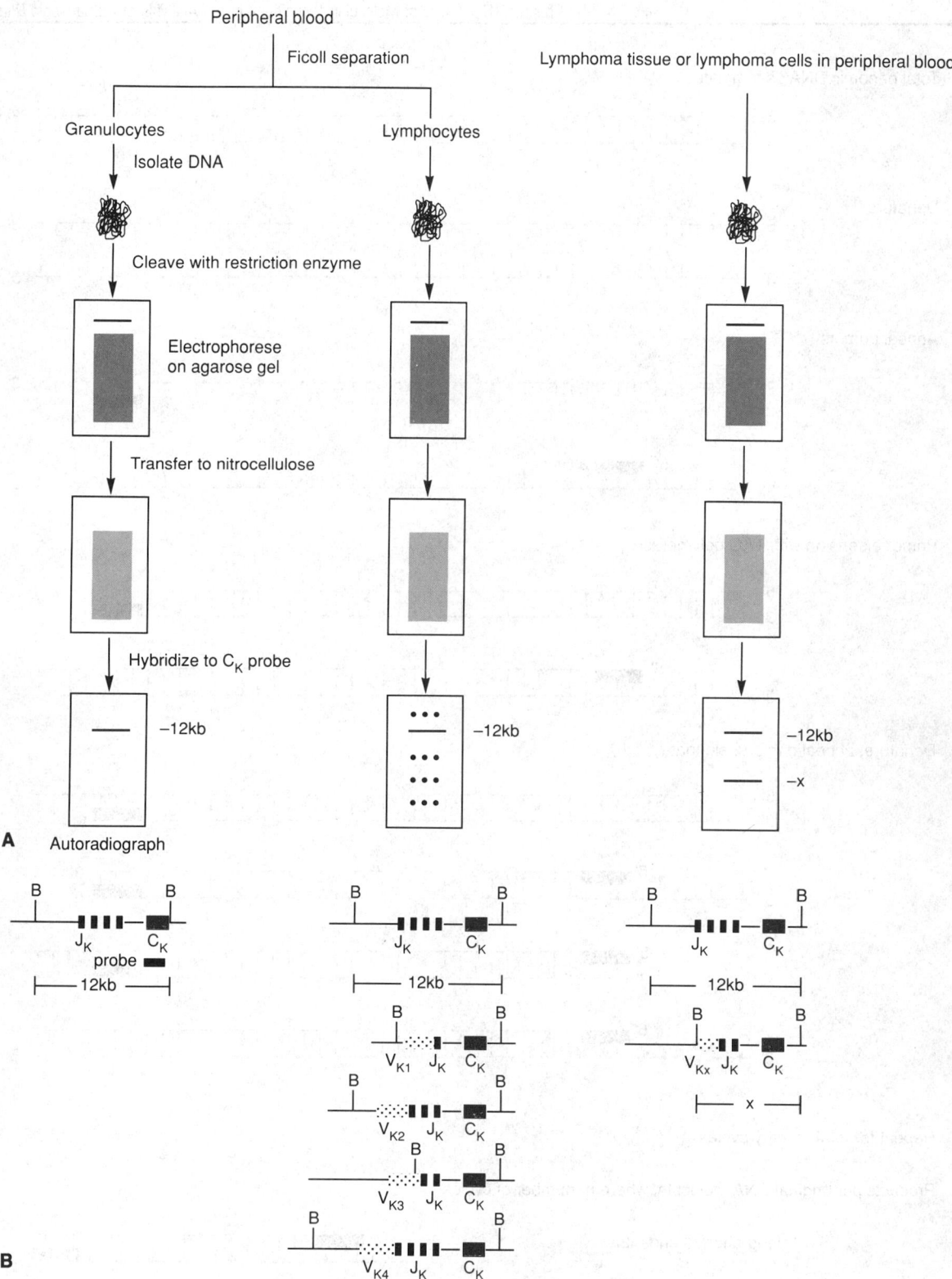

Fig. 164-4. Southern blot analysis of κ light chain rearrangement to establish clonality of populations of B lymphocytes. **(A)** The Southern technique and its predicted results in different cell populations. **(B)** The molecular configuration of the κ-locus. **(Left)** Genomic DNA, as represented in peripheral blood granulocytes is analyzed. As all of these cells retain their immunoglobulin genes in the germline configuration, a single band on Southern blot analysis corresponds to the germline κ-locus. **(Middle)** Polyclonal lymphocytes also show only a germline band on Southern analysis. However, as shown in Fig B, this does not show that the cells do not have rearrangement of the κ-locus. Instead, it demonstrates that there are insufficient cells of any one clone to be detectable as a discrete band on Southern analysis. Because a significant fraction of the cells will retain one κ-locus that is unrearranged, a germline band is detectable. (In normal peripheral lymphocytes, this band also partly reflects T cells, which do not rearrange their immunoglobulin gene loci). **(Right)** The Southern pattern produced by monoclonal tumor cells bearing a κ light chain. All the cells of the population will have an identical rearrangement of the κ-genes that will be apparent as a rearranged band on Southern blot analysis. The figure demonstrates the pattern of cells in which one κ-locus has rearranged. If both chromosomes are rearranged, then there will be two rearranged bands, and the germline band will no longer be present.

approximately 1% of the total cell population studied. This translates to detection of the DNA represented by 10^4 cells.[25,32] Consequently, it is a highly sensitive means of detecting peripheral blood or bone marrow involvement with lymphoma in patients with known lymphoproliferative disease in whom marrow involvement is insufficient for histologic diagnosis.

Gene rearrangement studies have also been used to validate the use of flow cytometry as a means of detecting peripheral blood involvement with B-cell lymphoma.[33] The κλ test allows cytofluorometric identification of small populations of clonal lymphocytes by detection of an imbalance in the normal distribution of surface immunofluorescent staining for κ and λ light chains. Peripheral blood mononuclear cells are labeled with fluorescent-tagged rabbit heteroantisera to κ and λ light chains and then analyzed in a flow cytometer. The success of the technique is based on the empirical observations that a given clone of B cells has a uniform expression of surface light chains, and that the histograms of κ and λ light chain distribution in normal polyclonal B cells are identical. The presence of a predominant clone distorts the histogram of the light chain expressed and causes the shift of one curve relative to the other. The difference between the curves may then be analyzed by computer.[34,35] The sensitivity of the flow cytometric technique allows detection of clonal populations in the 5–10% range. Gene rearrangement studies have confirmed that the finding of a positive κλ test result correlates with the finding of a circulating population of cells with the same DNA rearrangement as that found in the primary tumor.[32] Although Southern blot analysis is more sensitive than flow cytometry, it appears that the latter, simpler, technique is an extremely effective means of detecting minimal bone marrow involvement with lymphoma.

Monitoring Disease Activity in Treated Patients

The sensitivity of immunoglobulin and TCR gene rearrangement studies makes them an excellent method for detecting minimal residual involvement of the bone marrow in patients undergoing chemotherapy or bone marrow transplantation for the treatment of lymphoid malignancy. In a study of children treated with chemotherapy for acute lymphocytic leukemia (ALL), this technique allowed detection of an estimated 1 in 500–1,000 leukemic cells in remission marrows.[36,37] Subsequent studies have suggested that detection of any number of residual leukemic cells by this technique is highly predictive of relapse, although negative studies do not guarantee long-term remission.[37,38]

Use of Polymerase Chain Reaction Analysis of Immunoglobulin and T-Cell Receptor Loci in Lymphoproliferative Disease

Since PCR can potentially amplify the DNA of a single gene from a single cell to a detectable level, it can detect minimal involvement with cells carrying a characteristic gene rearrangement well below the limits of detectability by any other technique. However, PCR for diagnosis of lymphoproliferative disease is hampered because the sequence of rearranged immunoglobulin or TCR loci in a given lymphoma is specific to that patient's tumor and theoretically requires design of patient-specific primers to amplify tumor DNA. Modifications of the PCR technique have allowed for the design of primers that can monitor minimal residual disease by PCR. Two major techniques have been utilized. The first is to design two consensus primers, one to conserved sequences within the flanking DNA of the V region, and the other to a similarly conserved sequence

flanking the J region; these regions lie too far apart in unrearranged DNA to allow efficient PCR. Only rearranged immunoglobulin or TCR loci will allow amplification of a distinct fragment; clonal populations will yield an amplified species by this technique. PCR is then used to detect a characteristic "footprint" of the rearranged DNA within the tumor that can then be followed as a marker for residual disease.[39-41]

A more sensitive technique has been developed by which PCR fragments generated using consensus sequences are then subcloned and sequenced, with subsequent synthesis of patient-specific oligonucleotide probes, termed *allele-specific oligonucleotides*. PCR is then performed using one consensus primer and one allele-specific oligonucleotide; this has in fact resulted in the detection of malignant cells at the theoretical detection limits of PCR, namely 1 in 10^5–10^6 cells.[42]

Use of PCR of the immunoglobulin and TCR loci for detection of residual lymphoproliferative disease has proved highly predictive of relapse in patients with ALL.[43,44] However, absence of detectable diagnostic fragments by either Southern blot analysis or PCR has not been shown to guarantee ongoing remission. Some patients with previously normal results have been seen to develop positive PCR studies prior to relapse.[45]

It should be noted that the negative prognostic significance of detection of residual disease by these techniques contrasts with the results found for detection of residual *bcr-abl* transcripts following bone marrow transplantation for chronic myeloid leukemia (CML), as is discussed in greater detail below.

HLA TYPING FOR BONE MARROW TRANSPLANTATION

Molecular techniques are of growing importance in the analysis of potential donors for bone marrow transplantation. Serologic HLA testing identifies large groups of cross-reactive antigens. It has been found that genotypic incompatibility results in acute graft-versus-host disease, despite serologic identity.[46] When evaluating sibling donors, serologic testing and mixed lymphocyte culture (MLC) assays are usually adequate to confirm the haplotype identity of the donor and recipient. However, with the advent of unrelated donor transplantation, it has become increasingly important to guarantee genotypic identity by molecular techniques. In unrelated donor transplantation, MLC reactivity has been shown to be a very poor predictor of graft-versus-host-disease.[47] Many laboratories have abandoned MLC testing and are routinely using PCR amplification of DNA followed by hybridization to sequence-specific oligonucleotide probes to establish specific HLA-DR antigen typing.[48-50] Similar assays of HLA class I loci are also being developed and are anticipated to replace serologic testing in the future.[51]

ANALYSIS OF CELL ORIGINS IN BONE MARROW TRANSPLANT PATIENTS

RFLP analysis is a powerful technique for analyzing the engraftment of patients from their donors following bone marrow transplant. Southern blot analysis allows one to distinguish virtually any two individuals by the use of any of the growing panel of defined DNA polymorphisms.[52] Peripheral blood from the patient and the donor can be analyzed before transplantation to define polymorphic sites at which they differ. Alternatively, after transplantation, DNA from a nonhematopoietic tissue from the patient (i.e., skin) can be compared with DNA from the donor.

This approach has been used to document engraftment, graft failure, and graft loss. It has also been used to document hematopoietic chimerism in a patient with severe combined immunodeficiency, in whom the T cells were shown to be of donor origin and the B cells and granulocytes were shown to be of patient origin.[53,54] Similar studies can also be used to determine the cell implicated in the relapse of leukemia following transplantation.[55,56]

DIAGNOSIS AND FOLLOW-UP OF DISEASES ASSOCIATED WITH KNOWN CYTOGENETIC ABNORMALITIES

Several hematologic malignancies are associated with characteristic chromosomal translocations that mark the abnormal cell population. The Philadelphia chromosome in CML and the t(14;18) in follicular lymphoma are two examples of such translocations in which the genes involved in the chromosomal breakpoint have been defined. Southern blot analysis, using probes for the genes involved in the translocation event, permits the detection of a rearranged band in DNA from cells carrying the translation. In a manner similar to that used for the detection of small populations of lymphoma cells, this method can be used to detect small residual populations of malignant cells after treatment with chemotherapy or bone marrow transplantation.

The advent of PCR has rendered this methodology much more powerful. By means of probes for the *bcr-abl* translocation, this technique has been used to demonstrate residual CML cells in patients following chemotherapy and bone marrow transplantation.[57,58] Similarly, probes of the t(14;18) have been used to detect residual follicular lymphoma cells in patients apparently in remission in terms of histologic and conventional Southern blot analysis.[59] With respect to the t(14;18), detection of residual disease was highly predictive of relapse in one study.[60] However, in CML, *bcr-abl* transcripts were detectable by PCR in almost all patients within the first 6 months following bone marrow transplantation. This finding does not appear to be predictive of imminent cytogenetic or hematologic relapse and may support the hypothesis that the cure of CML depends on the graft-versus-leukemia effect, at least in some patients.[61] The long-term prognostic significance of repeated amplifiable *bcr-abl* transcripts in patients in remission remains to be determined. With this caveat in mind, PCR promises to be an extremely important tool for following the natural history and predicting the course of these diseases.

REFERENCES

1. Radin AI, Benz EJ Jr: Antenatal diagnosis of the hemoglobinopathies. Hematol Pathol 3:199, 1988
2. Williamson R, Eskdale J, Coleman DV et al: Direct gene analysis of chorionic villi: a possible technique for first-trimester antenatal diagnosis for haemoglobinopathies. Lancet 2:1125, 1981
3. Rodeck CH, Morsman JM: First-trimester chorion biopsy. Br Med Bull 39:338, 1983
4. Botstein D, White RL, Skolnick M et al: Construction of a genetic linkage map in man using restriction fragment length polymorphisms. Am J Hum Genet 32:314, 1980
5. Geever RF, Wilson LB, Nallaseth FS et al: Direct identification of sickle cell anemia by blot hybridization. Proc Natl Acad Sci USA 78:5081, 1981
6. Chang JC, Kan YW: A sensitive new prenatal test for sickle-cell anemia. N Engl J Med 307:30, 1982
7. Orkin SH, Little PFR, Kazazian HH et al: Improved detection of the sickle mutation by DNA analysis: application to prenatal diagnosis. N Engl J Med 307:32, 1982
8. Kan YW, Dozy AM: Polymorphism of DNA sequence adjacent to human β-globin structural gene: relationship to sickle mutation. Proc Natl Acad Sci USA 75:5631, 1978
9. Boehm CD, Antonarakis SE, Phillips JA et al: Prenatal diagnosis using DNA polymorphisms. N Engl J Med 308:1054, 1983
10. Kazazian JJ Jr, Phillips JA III, Boehm CD et al: Prenatal diagnosis of beta-thalassemia by amniocentesis: linkage analysis using multiple polymorphic restriction endonuclease sites. Blood 56:926, 1980
11. Orkin SH, Kazazian JJ, Antonarakis SE et al: Linkage of β-thalassaemia muta-

tions and β-globin gene polymorphisms with DNA polymorphisms in human β-globin gene cluster. Nature 296:627, 1982
12. Little PFR, Whitelaw E, Annison G et al: The detection and use of hemoglobin mutants in the direct analysis of human globin genes. Blood 55:1060, 198
13. Phillips JA III, Scott AF, Dazazian HH Jr: Prenatal diagnosis of hemoglobinopathies by restriction endonuclease analysis: pregnancies at risk for sickle-cell anemia and S-O (Arab) disease. Johns Hopkins Med J 145:57, 1979
14. Rowley PT, Benz EJ Jr, Nienhuis AW: Molecular genetics for the hematologist. Curr Hematol Oncol 4:1, 1986
15. Southern EM: Detection of specific sequences among DNA fragments separated by gel electrophoresis. J Mol Biol 98:503, 1975
16. Connor BJ, Reyes AA, Morin C et al: Detection of sickle cell β-S globin allele by hybridization with synthetic ologinucleotides. Proc Natl Acad Sci USA 80:278, 1983
17. Orkin SH, Markham AF, Kazazian HH Jr: Direct detection of the common Mediterranean β-thalassemia gene with synthetic DNA probes: an alternative approach for prenatal diagnosis. J Clin Invest 71:775, 1983
18. Piratsu M, Kan YW, Cao A et al: Prenatal diagnosis of β-thalassemia: detection of a single nucleotide mutation in DNA. N Engl J Med 309:284, 1983
19. Mullis K, Faloona F, Scharf S et al: Specific enzymatic amplification of DNA in vitro: the polymerase chain reaction. Cold Spring Harbor Symp Quant Biol LI:263, 1986
20. Saiki RK, Scharf S, Faloona F et al: Enzymatic amplification of β-globin genomic sequences and restriction site analysis for diagnosis of sickle-cell anemia. Science 230:1350, 1985
21. Embury SH, Scharf SH, Saiki RK et al: Rapid prenatal diagnosis of sickle cell anemia by a new method of DNA analysis. N Engl J Med 316:656, 1987
22. Wong C, Dowling CE, Saiki RK et al: Characterization of β-thalassemia mutations using direct genomic sequencing of amplified single copy DNA. Nature 330:384, 1987
23. Chebab FF, Kan YW: Detection of specific DNA sequences by fluorescence amplification: a color complementation assay. Proc Natl Acad Sci USA 86:9178, 1989
24. Kogan SC, Doherty M, Gitschier J: An improved method for prenatal diagnosis of genetic diseases by analysis of amplified DNA sequences: application to hemophilia A. N Engl J Med 317:985, 1987
25. Arnold A, Cossman J, Bakhshi A et al: Immunoglobulin-gene rearrangements as unique clonal markers in human lymphoid neoplasms. N Engl J Med 309:1593, 1983
26. Aisenberg A, Krontiris T, Mak T et al: Rearrangement of the gene for the β chain of the T-cell receptor in T-cell chronic lymphocytic leukemia and related disorders. N Engl J Med 313:529, 1985
27. Berliner N, Duby A, Linch D et al: T-cell receptor gene rearrangements define a monoclonal T-cell proliferation in patients with T-cell lymphocytosis and cytopenia. Blood 67:914, 1986
28. Bertness V, Kirsch I, Hollis G et al: T-cell receptor gene rearrangements as clinical markers of human T-cell lymphomas. N Engl J Med 313:534, 1985
29. Lipford EH, Smith HR, Pittaluga S et al: Clonality of angioimmunoblastic lymphadenopathy and implications for its evolution to malignant lymphoma. J Clin Invest 79:637, 1987
30. Pellici P-G, Knowles DM II, Arlin AZ et al: Multiple monoclonal B-cell expansions and c-*myc* oncogene rearrangements in acquired immune deficiency syndrome-related lymphoproliferative disorders: implications for lymphomagenesis. J Exp Med 164:2049, 1986
31. Korsmeyer SJ, Hieter PA, Ravetch JV et al: Developmental hierarchy of immunoglobulin gene rearrangements in human leukemic pre-B-cells. Proc Natl Acad Sci USA 78:7096, 1981
32. Minden MD, Mak TW: The structure of the T-cell antigen receptor genes in normal and malignant T-cells. Blood 68:327, 1986
33. Berliner N, Ault K, Martin P et al: Detection of clonal excess in lymphoproliferative disease by kappa/lambda analysis: correlation with immunoglobulin gene DNA rearrangement. Blood 67:80, 1986
34. Ault K: Detection of small numbers of monoclonal B lymphocytes in the blood of patients with lymphoma. N Engl J Med 300:1401, 1979
35. Weinberg DS, Pinkus GS, Ault KA: Cytofluorometric detection of B cell clonal excess: a new approach to the diagnosis of V cell lymphoma. Blood 63:1080, 1984
36. Zehnbauer BA, Pardoll DM, Burke PJ et al: Immunoglobulin gene rearrangements in remission bone marrow specimens from patients with acute lymphoblastic leukemia. Blood 67:835, 1986
37. Bregni M, Siena S, Neri A et al: Minimal residual disease in acute lymphoblastic leukemia detected by immune selection and gene rearrangement analysis. J Clin Oncol 7:338, 1989
38. Wright JJ, Poplack DT, Bakshi A et al: Gene rearrangements as markers of clonal variation and minimal residual disease in acute lymphoblastic leukemia. J Clin Oncol 5:735, 1987

Brisco MJ, Tan LW, Osborn AM, Morley AA: Development of a highly sensitive assay, based on the polymerase chain reaction, for rare B-lymphocyte clones in a polyclonal population. Br J Haematol 75:173, 1990

Trainor KJ, Brisco MJ, Wan JH et al: Gene rearrangement in B- and T-lymphoproliferative disease detected by the polymerase chain reaction. Blood 78:192, 1991

Deane M, Norton JD: Immunoglobulin gene 'fingerprinting': an approach to analysis of B lymphoid clonality in lymphoproliferative disorders. Br J Haematol 77:274, 1991

Billadeau D, Quam L, Thomas W et al: Detection and quantitation of malignant cells in the peripheral blood of multiple myeloma patients. Blood 80:1818, 1992

Zehnbauer BA, Pardoll DM, Burke PJ et al: Immunoglobulin gene rearrangements in remission bone marrow specimens from patients with acute lymphoblastic leukemia. Blood 67:835, 1986

Bregni M, Siena S, Neri A et al: Minimal residual disease in acute lymphoblastic leukemia detected by immune selection and gene rearrangement analysis. J Clin Oncol 7:338, 1989

Ito Y, Wasserman R, Galili N et al: Molecular residual disease status at the end of chemotherapy fails to predict subsequent relapse in children with B-lineage acute lymphoblastic leukemia. J Clin Oncol 11:546, 1993

Anasetti C, Beatty PG, Storb R et al: Effect of HLA incompatibility on graft-versus-host disease, relapse, and survival after bone marrow transplantation for patients with leukemia or lymphoma. Hum Immunol 29:79, 1990

Petersdorf EW, Smith AG, Mickelson EM et al: The role of HLA-DPB1 disparity in the development of acute graft-versus-host disease following unrelated donor morrow transplantation. Blood 81:1923, 1993

Erlich H, Bugawan T, Begovich AB et al: HLA-DR, DQ, and DP typing using PCR amplification and immobilized probes. Eur J Immunogen 18:33, 1991

Molkentin J, Gorski J, Baxter-Lowe L: Detection of 14 HLA-DQB1 alleles by oligotyping. Hum Immunol 31:114, 1991

Gyllensten U, Allen M: PCR-based HLA Class II typing. PCR Methods Applic 1:91, 1991

51. Fernandez-Vina MA, Falco M et al: DNA typing for HLA Class I alleles: I. Subsets of HLA-A2 and of -A28. Hum Immunol 33:163, 1992

52. Braman JC, Barker D, Schumm JW et al: Characterization of very highly polymorphic RFLP probes. 8th Human Gene Mapping Workshop. Cytogenet Cell Genet 40:739, 1985

53. Ginsberg D, Antin JH, Smith BR et al: Origin of cell populations after bone marrow transplantation: analysis using DNA sequence polymorphisms. J Clin Invest 75:596, 1985

54. Knowlton RG, Brown VA, Braman JC et al: Use of highly polymorphic DNA probes for genotypic analysis following bone marrow transplantation. Blood 68:378, 1986

55. Minden MD, Messner HA, Belch A: Origin of leukemic relapse after bone marrow transplantation detected by restriction fragment length polymorphism. J Clin Invest 75:91, 1985

56. Witherspoon RP, Schubach W, Neiman P et al: Donor cell leukemia developing six years after marrow grafting for acute leukemia. Blood 65:1172, 1985

57. Roth MS, Antin JH, Bingham EL et al: Detection of Philadelphia chromosome-positive cells by the polymerase chain reaction following bone marrow transplant for chronic myelogenous leukemia. Blood 74:882, 1989

58. Lange W, Snyder DS, Castro R et al: Detection by enzymatic amplification of bcr-abl mRNA in peripheral blood and bone marrow cells of patients with chronic myelogenous leukemia. Blood 73:1735, 1989

59. Lee MS, Chang KS, Cabanillas F: Detection of minimal residual cells carrying the t(14;18) by DNA sequence amplification. Science 237:175, 1987

60. Gribben JG, Saporito L, Barber M et al: Bone marrows of non-Hodgkin's lymphoma patients wth a bcl-2 translocation can be purged of polymerase chain reaction-detectable lymphoma cells using monoclonal antibodies and immunomagnetic bead depletion. Blood 80:1083, 1992

61. Lee M, Khouri I, Champlin R et al: Detection of minimal residual disease by polymerase chain reaction of bcr/abl transcripts in chronic myelogenous leukaemia following allogeneic bone marrow transplantation. Br J Hematol 82:708, 1992

ndex

ndogenous pyrogen. *See* IL-1.

ndomitosis, of megakaryocytes, 282–283

ndoperoxides, vasoconstrictive activity of, 1559

ndophthalmitis, *Candida*, management of, 1446

ndoplasmic reticulum (ER)
- in protein post-translational processing, 22–23
- in protein synthesis, 19, 20f
- in protein translocation, 21, 21f
- protein transport out of, vesicular, 23, 23f
- rough, 1516, 1518

ndoreduplication, 282–283

endothelial synthesis of, 1557

substances stimulating release of, 1559

vasodilation induced by, 1559

Endotoxemia, DIC caused by, 1762–1763

Endotoxin(s)
- in fibrinolysis inhibition, 1558
- in thrombomodulin regulation, 1557
- vascular purpura with, 2169–2170
- vessel wall damage with, 1830

Enteritis
- impaired vitamin K absorpt...

in nodular sclerosis Hodgkin disease, 765

normal blood smear, 2206

oxygen-dependent cytotoxicity in, 764

oxygen-independent cytotoxicity in, 764

PAF effects on, 266, 764

physical characteristics of, 188–189, 189f

plasma membrane activities of, 763–764

production of, 263–264, 265f

protein kinase C in, 765

Epinephrine
- adenylyl cyclase inhibition by, 1540
- cAMP inhibition by, 1539
- in platelet activation, 1537t, 1539–1540
- in platelet aggregation, 1529, 1529t, 1844

Epipodophyllin, AML due to, 1034

Epipodophyllotoxin(s), 922, 922t, 923t
- for AML, congenital, 1031
- AML due to, 996

Episome(s), in recombinant DNA technology, 13–15

Epistaxis
- bleeding history in, 1609t
- conditions associated with, 1608
- factor VII deficiency, 1695
- ...mophilia A, 1653
- ...rombin deficiency, 1692
- ...lebrand disease,

Epstein-Barr virus *(Continued)*
latent, 868
latent membrane protein (LMP-1 and LMP-2), 1346
molecular diagnostic techniques in, 873–874
neutropenia in, 870
non-Hodgkin lymphoma and, 1279
nuclear antigens (EBNA-2 through EBNA-5), 1346
pathogenesis of, 868–869, 869f
in pathogenesis of lymphoproliferative disease, 1204–1205, 1205t, 1345, 1345t
peripheral T-cell lymphoma and, 872
persistent, 870
post-transplant lymphoma and, 872
post-transplant lymphoproliferative syndrome and, 1392
primary, in congenital immunodeficiency syndrome, 1205
properties of, 1388
pure red cell aplasia in, 352
therapy and future directions in, 874
thrombopoiesis in, 871
transfusion-transmitted, 2059
transmission and persistence of, 867
virion infectivity in, 868
X-linked lymphoproliferative syndrome and, 1279
Epstein-Barr virus gene
BCRF-1 product, 1346
expression of, in AIDS-related lymphoma, 1346
ER. *See* Endoplasmic reticulum (ER).
*erb*A gene, 906
*erb*B gene, 902
Erythema multiforme, factor VIII inhibitors associated with, 1742
Erythroblast(s). *See also* Normoblast(s).
embryonic, characteristics of, 251
globin biosynthesis in, 465
internuclear bridging of, in congenital dyserythropoietic anemia type I, 383, 383f
suppression of, selective, 252
Erythroblastic anemia. *See* β-Thalassemia major.
Erythroblastic islet(s), of bone marrow, 195f, 197
Erythroblastic leukemia, cytogenetic analysis in, 883
Erythroblastopenia of childhood, transient (TEC), 2133
characteristics of, 350
congenital hypoplastic anemia vs., 354
Diamond-Blackfan anemia vs., 366, 366t, 480t, 481–482
immunoglobulin inhibitors in, 351
Erythroblastosis fetalis, treatment of, antibody feedback mechanisms in, 177

Erythrocyte(s). *See also* Red cell(s).
Erythrocyte mass, in polycythemia vera, 1130
Erythrocyte zinc protoporphyrin, for iron status, 506
Erythrocytopheresis. *See* Red cell transfusion, exchange.
Erythrocytosis, 484–491
in Bartter syndrome, 488
blood gas measurements in, 486
in chronic carbon monoxide intoxication, 487
in chronic mountain sickness, 486
in chronic pulmonary disease, 486–487
in cigarette smoking, 487
clinical manifestations of, 485
in cyanotic congenital heart disease, 487
differentiation of polycythemia vera from other causes of, 1133
EPO in
serum, 486
suppression of, 485
EPO receptor in, point mutations in, 247–248
etiology and pathogenesis of, 486–489, 2105–2106
evaluation and management of, 489
familial, 488
in glomerulonephritis, 488
in high oxygen-affinity hemoglobin, 487
in hypobaric hypoxia, 486
hypoxic, 486–487
in inappropriate EPO secretion, 487–488
in kidney transplantation, 488
laboratory evaluation of, 485–486
phlebotomy for, 489
physiologic causes of, 484
in polycythemia vera, 1122
in polycythemia vera rubra, 489
red cell mass determination in, 485–486
in renal artery stenosis, 487–488
in renal disease, 487–488
stress (spurious), in chronic carbon monoxide poisoning, 487
tumor-associated, 488
Erythroderma, 1336, 1337f, 1341
Erythrodermic disease, in systemic mastocytosis, 1406–1407
Erythrohepatic protoporphyria(s). *See* Protoporphyria(s), erythropoietic.
Erythroid ALA-synthase, iron-dependent translational regulation of, 500–501
Erythroid cell(s)
differentiation of, 80, 187, 193, 243f
adhesive interactions in, 186
c-*myb* in, 248
GATA factors in, 80, 183–184, 248

embryonic, phenotypic characteristics of, 249
ferritin in, 501
fetal
adult cells vs., 249, 251
antigenic profiles of, 251
EPO and, 249, 251
phenotypic characteristics of, 249
hematopoietic markers of, 2227t
heme synthesis in, iron for, 500
iron availability in, 501
iron uptake by, 500
maturation of, 245–247
EPO receptors in, 246
globin synthesis in, 245–246. *See also* Globin.
heme synthesis in, 245–246
red cell membrane changes in, 245. *See also* Red cell membrane.
transferrin receptors in, 246–247
transcription factors for, 80, 183–184
Erythroid iron turnover (EIT), 452f, 452–453, 453t
Erythroid precursor cell compartment (erythron), 245–247
Erythroid progenitor cell(s)
culture of, 243
in primary thrombocythemia, 1175
Erythroid progenitor cell compartment, 242–245
Erythroleukemia
acute, 1005–1006
Friend virus-induced, 985–986, 986f, 987f
Erythromelalgia
in polycythemia vera, 1128
in primary thrombocythemia, 1176–1177, 1180, 1181
Erythromycin, lymphadenopathy or atypical lymphoproliferation from, 1392t
Erythron, iron exchange in, 499–500
Erythropoiesis, 242–254
acute, accelerated differentiation and maturation in, 252
in bone marrow, 2209
cellular dynamics in, 251–252
CFS-GM in, 243
chronic, amplified late erythroid pool in, 252
commitment in, 242
cycle of, 468
depressed with HIV infection, 2176–2177
embryonic, 249
EPO in, 251–252, 484–485
in Epstein-Barr virus infection, 871
expansion of, fetal sites for, 252
fetal and postnatal, 249, 250f
growth factors influencing, 224f, 227
hematopoietic microenvironment for, 248–249
accessory cells in, 249
experimental models for, 248
extracellular matrix in, 249

stromal cells in, 248–249
hepatic, 249, 250f
IL-3 in, 243
ineffective, 187, 381
in congenital dyserythropoietic anemia, 382
interferon-γ, 243
iron deficient, 508
kinetics of, in vitro vs. in vivo 243
kit ligand in, 243
in megaloblastic anemia, 563
nurse cells in, 249
ontogeny of, 249–251, 250f
quantitative assessment of, 252
stress, 187
in β-thalassemia major, 591–592
therapy to stimulate, 2068–2071
transcriptional factors in, 248
transforming growth factor–β in, 243
in vivo imaging of, 454–455
Erythropoietic heme turnover, 456, 456t
Erythropoietic protoporphyria(s). *See* Protoporphyria(s), erythropoietic.
Erythropoietin (EPO), 247–248
after chemotherapy, 960–961
for AIDS or HIV infection, 960
for anemia, 2111–2112
of chronic disease, 2145, 2148
for anemia of prematurity, 961
for anemia of renal failure, 959–960
for autologous blood donation, 961
BFU-E effects of, 247
bioactivities of, 209t, 213
for bone marrow failure, 961
cellular processes stimulated by, 247–248
CFU-E effects of, 247
clinical applications of, 959–961, 982
in erythrocytosis, 2106
suppression of, 485
in erythroid differentiation, 80, 247
in erythroleukemias, Friend virus-induced, 985
in erythropoiesis, 251–252, 484–485
in feedback control, 2068
fetal erythroid cells and, 249, 251
hepatocellular production of, 484
in HIV-associated anemia, 2177
hypoxic response of, 484–485
impaired secretion of, 2104
for inflammatory disorders, 2148
for myelodysplastic syndrome, 1112, 1112t
myelodysplastic syndrome erythroid progenitor cell response to, 1101
plasma levels of in hypoproliferative anemia, 2104–2105
polycythemia related to, 2146
in polycythemia vera, 1122–1123, 1123t, 1124, 1125f

Bone marrow examination
in AML, 1000, 1016, 1035
in ALL, in adults, 1087
in agnogenic myeloid metaplasia, 1163, 1164f
in anemia of chronic disease, 475
in anemia, 472–473
1164–1165, 1165t
in anorexia nervosa, 472
in aplastic anemia, 339, 340f
in childhood lymphomas, 1302
in congenital dyserythropoiesis in CML, 1148
smears for, 2215
technical aspects of, 2214

Bone marrow transplantation, 2074
for ALL
in adults, 1095
in children, 1081
mismatched, 1093
allogeneic, 400–415
ABO compatibility in, 2075
for ALL, 402–403
in adults, 1092t
in children, 1092, 1092–1093
in advanced or refractory disease, 403
in first remission, 408
in children, 1080
for myelodysplastic syndrome, 404, 1109–1110
for myelodysplastic syndrome of childhood, 1188
for myeloid function disorders, 1186
for myeloproliferative disorders, 409
for non-Hodgkin lymphoma, 1187, 1188
407
for osteopetrosis, 410
for paroxysmal noc-

Cytomegaloviral pneumonia, 418–419. *See also* cytomegalovirus infection monia.
for congenital amegakaryocytic thrombocytopenia, 1874
noninfectious, 416t
late, 422–423
415–416
early-transplant associated,